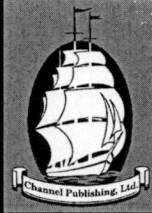

Errata #1
for
Channel Publishing's 2017 ICD-10-CM Code Books
2017 ICD-10-CM, The Educational Annotation of ICD-10-CM (All Versions)

Posting Date: October 10, 2016

Publication: 2017 ICD-10-CM, The Educational Annotation of ICD-10-CM (All Binding Versions)

Instructions: Make the Errata corrections below in your book, and keep this Errata page for your reference.

Coding Guidelines, pages: CG-11 and 721

Delete the lined-through words below:

9. **Chapter 9: Diseases of Circulatory System (I00-I99)**
   a. **Hypertension**
      1) **Hypertension with Heart Disease**
         Hypertension with heart conditions classified to I50.- or I51.4-I51.9, are assigned to, a code from category I11, Hypertensive heart disease, ~~when a causal relationship is stated (due to hypertension) or implied (hypertensive)~~.

Index to Diseases

Delete the lined-through 5th digits on the underlined codes as indicated. Although these 5th digit Index changes were included in the 2017 Official Addenda, the corresponding Tabular List codes were not added and therefore do not exist.

Abscess ... (p.6-7)
intra-abdominal ...
  postprocedural T81.4~~3~~
intra-muscular, postprocedural T81.4~~2~~
operative wound T81.4~~0~~
peritoneum, peritoneal ...
  postoperative T81.4~~3~~
postoperative (any site) T81.4~~0~~
stitch T81.4~~8~~
subcutaneous ...
  postprocedural T81.4~~1~~
subphrenic ...
  postoperative T81.4~~3~~
wound T81.4~~0~~

Cellulitis ... (p.61)
drainage site (following operation) T81.4~~8~~

Complication ... (p.80)
surgical procedure ...
  stitch abscess T81.4~~8~~
  wound infection T81.4~~0~~

Fever ... (p.166)
postoperative ...
  due to infection T81.4~~0~~

Infection ... (p.215, 217)
due to or resulting from
  surgery T81.4~~0~~
operation wound T81.4~~0~~
postoperative T81.4~~0~~
postoperative wound T81.4~~0~~
postprocedural T81.4~~0~~
  deep incisional surgical site T81.4~~2~~
  organ and space surgical site T81.4~~3~~
  sepsis T81.4~~9~~
  specified surgical site NEC T81.4~~8~~
  superficial incisional surgical site T81.4~~1~~

Sepsis ... (p.354-355)
localized ...
  in operation wound T81.4~~9~~
  postprocedural T81.4~~9~~

Stitch (p.367)
abscess T81.4~~8~~

D0904035

4750 Longley Lane, Suite 209 • Reno, NV 89502-5982 • (775) 825-0880 • Customer Service 1-800-248-2882 • FAX (775) 825-5633
WEB SITE: www.channelpublishing.com • E-MAIL: info@channelpublishing.com

2017 Annual
ICD-10-CM

The Educational Annotation of ICD-10-CM

DISEASES TABULAR LIST & INDEX

CRAIG D. PUCKETT

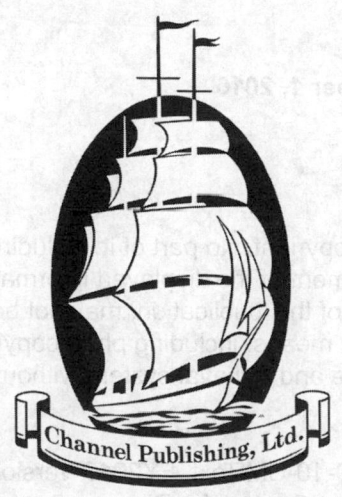

Channel Publishing, Ltd.

Complete Official ICD-10-CM Text, FY2017 Version
Effective October 1, 2016
as standardized by
U.S. DEPARTMENT OF HEALTH AND HUMAN SERVICES
CENTERS FOR DISEASE CONTROL AND PREVENTION
NATIONAL CENTER FOR HEALTH STATISTICS

ISBN: 978-1-933053-76-9

DISCLAIMER

Every effort has been made to ensure the accuracy and reliability of the information contained in this publication. However, complete accuracy cannot be guaranteed. The editor and publisher will not be held responsible or liable for any errors.

Corrections Identification and Reporting

In an effort to provide our customers with the best code books possible, Channel Publishing has added a "Channel Errata Page" for each of its ICD-10 code books on its web site: www.channelpublishing.com. These Channel Errata Pages will be updated whenever an error is identified. Check the appropriate web page periodically for any changes to your Channel Publishing ICD-10 code book.

In addition, if at any time you identify a potential error, please copy the page and fax/mail/e-mail it to: Channel Publishing, Ltd., Attn: ICD-10 Book Production Department, 4750 Longley Lane, Suite 110, Reno, NV 89502. FAX (775) 825-5633. E-mail: info@channelpublishing.com

ICD-10-CM, FY2017 Version, Effective October 1, 2016

This edition contains the Complete, Official ICD-10-CM Text, FY2017 Version as standardized by the U.S. Department of Health and Human Services, Centers for Disease Control and Prevention, National Center for Health Statistics.

Published by CHANNEL PUBLISHING, Ltd., Reno, Nevada

Produced by Craig Puckett, Editor; Susan Dely, Assistant Editor;
Jo Ann Jones, RHIA, CCS, Editorial Assistant; Charisse Puckett, Editorial Assistant;
Trey Puckett, Editorial Assistant

Printed in the United States of America

Additional sets may be ordered from Channel Publishing, Ltd., 4750 Longley Lane, Suite 110, Reno, Nevada 89502, 1-800-248-2882, www.channelpublishing.com

ISBN: 978-1-933053-76-9

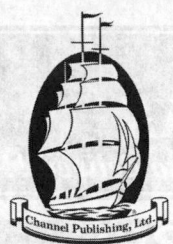

Channel Publishing, Ltd.

Publishers of

"THE EDUCATIONAL ANNOTATION OF ICD-10-CM & ICD-10-PCS"

August 2016

Dear ICD-10 Colleague:

First, I would like to personally thank each and every Channel Publishing customer who has purchased and enjoyed our ICD-9-CM and ICD-10 coding products and services over these past 30 years.

Thank you for purchasing Channel Publishing's *2017 Educational Annotation of ICD-10-CM* code book. I trust you will enjoy the design, layout, and all the new, coder-helpful features that we have created for you. I would also like to thank everyone who shared their ICD-10 comments and suggestions over the years from our "Preparing for ICD-10" seminars sixteen years ago, to those of you who called or wrote in, and those who stopped by our booth at AHIMA. We listened and made note of those comments and suggestions to bring you what we believe is an excellent ICD-10-CM code book, and at an incredibly low price.

In addition to this *2017 Educational Annotation of ICD-10-CM* code book, I'd like to remind you about all our ICD-10 products and services. Please visit our web site www.channelpublishing.com for details and sample content.

Once again, thank you for your purchase and I look forward to providing quality ICD-10 products and services to you in the years to come.

Sincerely,

Craig D. Puckett

Craig D. Puckett,
President, and Publisher

4750 Longley Lane, Suite 110 • Reno, NV 89502-5977 • (775) 825-0880 • Customer Service 1-800-248-2882 • FAX (775) 825-5633
WEB SITE: www.channelpublishing.com • E-MAIL: info@channelpublishing.com

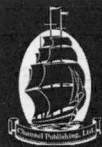
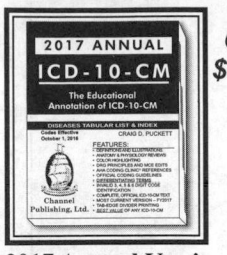
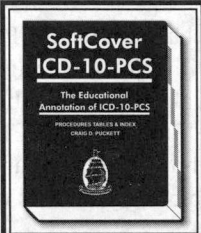
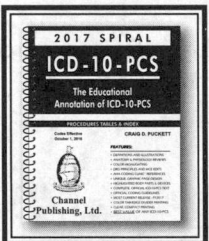

2016 FALL SALE ORDER FORM
Sale Prices Expire 12/31/16

1. CUSTOMER INFORMATION (Ship books to address below)

❑ Organization or ❑ Individual | ATTN: Name/Title/Dept. | Customer ID # | Order Date

Shipping Address (Street address required for FedEx delivery) | E-Mail Address

City | State | Zip | Telephone | Fax

2. ORDER INFORMATION

	Product — See Web Site for Complete Product Descriptions and Sample Pages	Quantity	Regular Price	Fall Sale Price	Total(s)
	2017 ICD-10-CM, The Educational Annotation of ICD-10-CM			Exp. 12/31/16	
C	Annual Version ICD-10-CM (Paperback) (ISBN: 9781933053-**76-9**)		$69⁹⁵ ea.	—	
O	Spiral Version ICD-10-CM (Spiral coil) (ISBN: 9781933053-**77-6**)		$74⁹⁵ ea.	—	
D	Spiral Version ICD-10-CM with Tabs (Spiral coil) (ISBN: 9781933053-**78-3**)		$89⁹⁵ ea.	—	
E	SoftCover Version ICD-10-CM (Vinyl cover, updateable) (ISBN: 9781933053-**79-0**)		$79⁹⁵ ea.	—	
	2017 Update ICD-10-CM (Full text replacement) (ISBN: 9781933053-**80-6**)		$55⁹⁵ ea.	—	
B	Tab Set for ICD-10-CM (SoftCover only, reusable) (ITEM: TABCM)		$17⁹⁵ ea.	—	
O	**2017 ICD-10-PCS, The Educational Annotation of ICD-10-PCS**				
O	Annual Version ICD-10-PCS (Paperback) (ISBN: 9781933053-**81-3**)		$59⁹⁵ ea.	—	
K	Spiral Version ICD-10-PCS (Spiral coil) (ISBN: 9781933053-**82-0**)		$64⁹⁵ ea.	—	
S	Spiral Version ICD-10-PCS with Tabs (Spiral coil) (ISBN: 9781933053-**83-7**)		$79⁹⁵ ea.	—	
	SoftCover Version ICD-10-PCS (Vinyl cover, updateable) (ISBN: 9781933053-**84-4**)		$69⁹⁵ ea.	—	
	2017 Update ICD-10-PCS (Full text replacement) (ISBN: 9781933053-**85-1**)		$48⁹⁵ ea.	—	
	Tab Set for ICD-10-PCS (SoftCover only, reusable) (ITEM: TABPCS)		$17⁹⁵ ea.	—	
	(Professional Version – Includes: PowerPoint Slides, Instructor's Manual, DVD set, Workbook & Code Book) (Individual Version – Includes: DVD set, Workbook & Code Book - CM-12 CEUs, PCS-20 CEUs)				
T	**Professional Version – Learning ICD-10-CM** (Step 1) (ITEM: SBCM-P)		~~$599⁹⁵~~ ea.	$559⁹⁵ ea.	
R	Additional Learning ICD-10-CM Workbook & Book Packages (ITEM: ACM16W)		$65⁹⁵ ea.		
A	**Professional Version – Learning ICD-10-PCS** (Step 1) (ITEM: SBPCS-P)		~~$699⁹⁵~~ ea.	$649⁹⁵ ea.	
I	Additional Learning ICD-10-PCS Workbook & Book Packages (ITEM: APCS16W)		$55⁹⁵ ea.		
N	**Individual Version – Learning ICD-10-CM** (Step 1) (12 CEUs) (ITEM: SBCM-I)		~~$299⁹⁵~~ ea.	$269⁹⁵ ea.	
I	**Individual Version – Learning ICD-10-PCS** (Step 1) (20 CEUs) (ITEM: SBPCS-I)		~~$399⁹⁵~~ ea.	$359⁹⁵ ea.	
N	**2016 Mastering ICD-10-CM Exercise Book** (Step 2) (ISBN: 9781933053-**88-2**)		$59⁹⁵ ea.		
G	**2016 Mastering ICD-10-PCS Exercise Book** (Step 2) (ISBN: 9781933053-**89-9**)		$59⁹⁵ ea.		
	2016 Mastering ICD-10-CM Guidelines Exercise Book (Step 3) (ISBN: 9781933053-**90-5**)		$59⁹⁵ ea.		
	2016 Mastering ICD-10-PCS Guidelines Exercise Book (Step 3) (ISBN: 9781933053-**91-2**)		$59⁹⁵ ea.		
	The Last Word on ICD-10 (Step 4) (ISBN: 9781933053-**61-5**)		$69⁹⁵ ea.		
O	**2017 Clinotes for ICD-10-CM** (ISBN: 9781933053-**87-5**)		~~$39⁹⁵~~ ea.	$29⁹⁵ ea.	
T	**2017 Expanded ICD-10-CM Table of Drugs & Chemicals** (ISBN: 9781933053-**86-8**)		~~$39⁹⁵~~ ea.	$29⁹⁵ ea.	
H	Acrylic Bookstand ❑ **One-piece** (ITEM: BSOP) ❑ **Two-piece** (ITEM: BSTP)		$34⁹⁵ ea.		
E	CPT® 2017 Standard Edition (ISBN: 978162202-**398-1**)		$94⁹⁵ ea.		
R	CPT® 2017 Professional Edition (ISBN: 978162202-**400-1**)		$119⁹⁵ ea.		

• OUTSIDE CONTINENTAL U.S.: Call for rates and shipping options. U.S. Dollars.
• EXPRESS SHIPPING: Call for delivery options and rates.

Fall Sale Prices Expire 12/31/16

Continental U.S. Shipping & Handling	
Less than $50	$7
$50-$99	$12
$100-$199	$19
$200-$299	$29
$300+	$39

Product Subtotal	
Shipping & Handling	
Nevada Res. Only Add Local Sales Tax	
Total Order Amount	

3. PAYMENT METHOD

❑ Purchase Order (Attach copy) ❑ Check Enclosed
❑ Credit Card: MC, VISA, DISC, AMEX (Charged date order received)

___ ___ ___ ___

___ / ___
Exp. Date | Sec. Code | Authorized Cardholder Signature

Billing Address (Street number or PO Box and Zip Code) ❑ Same as shipping

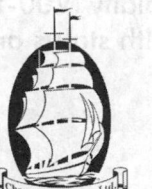

MAKE CHECKS PAYABLE AND MAIL TO:

Channel Publishing, Ltd.
4750 Longley Lane, Suite 110
Reno, NV 89502-5977
1-800-248-2882
(775) 825-0880
Fax (775) 825-5633
E-Mail: info@channelpublishing.com
Web Site: www.channelpublishing.com

THANK YOU FOR YOUR ORDER
FS99086-2

TABLE OF CONTENTS

Disease Index

Disease Tabular

ICD-10-CM PREFACE (FY 2017 Release)

Introduction

This FY 2017 update of the International Statistical Classification of Diseases and Related Health Problems, 10th revision, Clinical Modification (ICD-10-CM) is being published by the United States Government in recognition of its responsibility to promulgate this classification throughout the United States for morbidity coding. The International Statistical Classification of Diseases and Related Health Problems, 10th Revision (ICD-10), published by the World Health Organization (WHO), is the foundation of ICD-10-CM. ICD-10 continues to be the classification used in cause-of-death coding in the United States. The ICD-10-CM is comparable with the ICD-10. The WHO Collaborating Center for the Family of International Classifications in North America, housed at the Centers for Disease Control and Prevention's National Center for Health Statistics (NCHS), has responsibility for the implementation of ICD and other WHO-FIC classifications and serves as a liaison with the WHO, fulfilling international obligations for comparable classifications and the national health data needs of the United States.

Historical background

The historical background of ICD and ICD-10 can be found in the Introduction to the International Classification of Diseases and Related Health Problems (ICD-10), 2008, World Health Organization, Geneva, Switzerland.

Clinical modification

ICD-10-CM is the United States' clinical modification of the World Health Organization's ICD-10. The term "clinical" is used to emphasize the modification's intent: to serve as a useful tool in the area of classification of morbidity data for indexing of health records, medical care review, and ambulatory and other health care programs, as well as for basic health statistics. To describe the clinical picture of the patient the codes must be more precise than those needed only for statistical groupings and trend analysis.

Characteristics of ICD-10-CM

ICD-10-CM far exceeds its predecessors in the number of concepts and codes provided. The disease classification has been expanded to include health-related conditions and to provide greater specificity at the sixth and seventh character level. The sixth and seventh characters are not optional and are intended for use in recording the information documented in the clinical record.

ICD-10-CM extensions, interpretations, modifications, addenda, or errata other than those approved by the Centers for Disease Control and Prevention are not to be considered official and should not be utilized. Continuous maintenance of the ICD-10-CM is the responsibility of the aforementioned agencies. However, because the ICD-10-CM represents the best in contemporary thinking of clinicians, nosologists, epidemiologists, and statisticians from both public and private sectors, when future modifications are considered, advice will be sought from all stakeholders.

All official authorized addenda since the last update, October 1, 2015, have been included in this revision. For more information please see the complete official authorized addenda to ICD-10-CM, including the "ICD-10-CM Official Guidelines for Coding and Reporting," and a description of the ICD-10-CM updating and maintenance process.

The complete official authorized addenda to ICD-10-CM, including the "ICD-10-CM Official Guidelines for Coding and Reporting," can be accessed at the following website:

    http://www.cdc.gov/nchs/icd/icd10cm.htm#10update

A description of the ICD-10-CM updating and maintenance process can be found at the following website:

    http://www.cdc.gov/nchs/icd/icd9cm_maintenance.htm

INTRODUCTION TO ICD-10-CM (FY2017 Release)

The National Center for Health Statistics (NCHS), the Federal agency responsible for use of the International Statistical Classification of Diseases and Related Health Problems, 10th revision (ICD-10) in the United States, has developed a clinical modification of the classification for morbidity purposes. The ICD-10 is used to code and classify mortality data from death certificates, having replaced ICD-9 for this purpose as of January 1, 1999. ICD-10-CM is the replacement for ICD-9-CM, volumes 1 and 2.

The ICD-10 is copyrighted by the World Health Organization (WHO), which owns and publishes the classification. WHO has authorized the development of an adaptation of ICD-10 for use in the United States for U.S. government purposes. As agreed, all modifications to the ICD-10 must conform to WHO conventions for the ICD. ICD-10-CM was developed following a thorough evaluation by a Technical Advisory Panel and extensive additional consultation with physician groups, clinical coders, and others to assure clinical accuracy and utility.

The entire draft of the Tabular List of ICD-10-CM, and the preliminary crosswalk between ICD-9-CM and ICD-10-CM were made available on the NCHS website for public comment. The public comment period ran from December 1997 through February 1998. The American Hospital Association and the American Health Information Management Association conducted a field test for ICD-10-CM in the summer of 2003, with a subsequent report. All comments and suggestions from the open comment period and the field test were reviewed, and additional modifications to ICD-10-CM were made based on these comments and suggestions. Additionally, new concepts have been added to ICD-10-CM based on the established update process for ICD-9-CM (the ICD-9-CM Coordination and Maintenance Committee) and the World Health Organization's ICD-10 (the Update and Revision Committee). This represents ICD-9-CM modifications from 2003-2009 and ICD-10 modifications from 2002-2008.

The clinical modification represents a significant improvement over ICD-9-CM and ICD-10. Specific improvements include: the addition of information relevant to ambulatory and managed care encounters; expanded injury codes; the creation of combination diagnosis/symptom codes to reduce the number of codes needed to fully describe a condition; the addition of sixth and seventh characters; incorporation of common 4th and 5th digit subclassifications; laterality; and greater specificity in code assignment. The new structure will allow further expansion than was possible with ICD-9-CM.

On January 16, 2009 HHS published a Final Rule adopting ICD-10-CM (and ICD-10-PCS) to replace ICD-9-CM in HIPAA transactions, effective implementation date of October 1, 2013 (delayed two years to October 1, 2015).

ICD-10-CM Conventions (FY2017 Version)

The conventions for the ICD-10-CM are the general rules for use of the classification independent of the guidelines. These conventions are incorporated within the **Alphabetic Index** and **Tabular List** of the ICD-10-CM as instructional notes. The conventions and instructions of the classification take precedence over guidelines.

Organization of ICD-10-CM

The ICD-10-CM is divided into the Alphabetic Index, an alphabetical list of terms and their corresponding code, and the Tabular List, a chronological list of codes divided into chapters based on body system or condition.

Alphabetic Index

The Alphabetic Index consists of the following parts:
- Index of Diseases and Injury
- Table of Neoplasms
- Table of Drugs and Chemicals
- Index of External Causes of Injury

Tabular List

The Tabular List consists of the following chapters:
- Chapter 1 – Certain infectious and parasitic diseases (A00-B99)
- Chapter 2 – Neoplasms (C00-D49)
- Chapter 3 – Diseases of the blood and blood-forming organs and certain disorders involving the immune mechanism (D50-D89)
- Chapter 4 – Endocrine, nutritional and metabolic diseases (E00-E89)
- Chapter 5 – Mental, behavioral and neurodevelopmental disorders (F01-F99)
- Chapter 6 – Diseases of the nervous system (G00-G99)
- Chapter 7 – Diseases of the eye and adnexa (H00-H59)
- Chapter 8 – Diseases of the ear and mastoid process (H60-H95)
- Chapter 9 – Diseases of the circulatory system (I00-I99)
- Chapter 10 – Diseases of the respiratory system (J00-J99)
- Chapter 11 – Diseases of the digestive system (K00-K95)
- Chapter 12 – Diseases of the skin and subcutaneous tissue (L00-L99)
- Chapter 13 – Diseases of the musculoskeletal system and connective tissue (M00-M99)
- Chapter 14 – Diseases of the genitourinary system (N00-N99)
- Chapter 15 – Pregnancy, childbirth and the puerperium (O00-O99)
- Chapter 16 – Certain conditions originating in the perinatal period (P00-P96)
- Chapter 17 – Congenital malformations, deformations and chromosomal abnormalities (Q00-Q99)
- Chapter 18 – Symptoms, signs and abnormal clinical and laboratory findings, not elsewhere classified (R00-R99)
- Chapter 19 – Injury, poisoning and certain other consequences of external causes (S00-T88)
- Chapter 20 – External causes of morbidity (V00-Y99)
- Chapter 21 – Factors influencing health status and contact with health services (Z00-Z99)

Appendices

There are no appendices.

How to Use ICD-10-CM, General Coding Guidelines, and Chapter-Specific Coding Guidelines

See the 2017 ICD-10-CM Official Guidelines for Coding and Reporting following this Introduction.

Characteristics of ICD-10-CM

Format and Structure:

The ICD-10-CM Tabular List contains categories, subcategories and codes. Characters for categories, subcategories and codes may be either a letter or a number. All categories are 3 characters. A three-character category that has no further subdivision is equivalent to a code. Subcategories are either 4 or 5 characters. Codes may be 3, 4, 5, 6 or 7 characters. That is, each level of subdivision after a category is a subcategory. The final level of subdivision is a code. Codes that have applicable 7th characters are still referred to as codes, not subcategories. A code that has an applicable 7th character is considered invalid without the 7th character.

The ICD-10-CM uses an indented format for ease in reference.

Use of codes for reporting purposes

For reporting purposes only codes are permissible, not categories or subcategories, and any applicable 7th character is required.

Placeholder character

The ICD-10-CM utilizes a placeholder character "x". The "x" is used as a placeholder at certain codes to allow for future expansion. An example of this is at the poisoning, adverse effect and underdosing codes, categories T36-T50.

Where a placeholder "x" exists, the "x" must be used in order for the code to be considered a valid code.

7th Characters

Certain ICD-10-CM categories have applicable 7th characters. The applicable 7th character is required for all codes within the category, or as the notes in the Tabular List instruct. The 7th character must always be the 7th character in the data field. If a code that requires a 7th character is not 6 characters, a placeholder "x" must be used to fill in the empty characters.

Abbreviations

Alphabetic Index abbreviations

NEC "Not elsewhere classifiable"
This abbreviation in the Alphabetic Index represents "other specified." When a specific code is not available for a condition, the Alphabetic Index directs the coder to the "other specified" code in the Tabular List.

NOS "Not otherwise specified"
This abbreviation is the equivalent of unspecified.

Tabular List abbreviations

NEC "Not elsewhere classifiable"
This abbreviation in the Tabular List represents "other specified." When a specific code is not available for a condition the Tabular List includes an NEC entry under a code to identify the code as the "other specified" code.

NOS "Not otherwise specified"
This abbreviation is the equivalent of unspecified.

Punctuation

[ ] Brackets are used in the Tabular List to enclose synonyms, alternative wording or explanatory phrases. Brackets are used in the Alphabetic Index to identify manifestation codes.

( ) Parentheses are used in both the Alphabetic Index and Tabular List to enclose supplementary words that may be present or absent in the statement of a disease or procedure without affecting the code number to which it is assigned. The terms within the parentheses are referred to as nonessential modifiers.

: Colons are used in the Tabular List after an incomplete term which needs one or more of the modifiers following the colon to make it assignable to a given category.

Use of "and"

When the term "and" is used in a narrative statement it represents and/or.

Other and Unspecified codes

"Other" codes

Codes titled "other" or "other specified" are for use when the information in the medical record provides detail for which a specific code does not exist. Alphabetic Index entries with NEC in the line designate "other" codes in the Tabular List. These Alphabetic Index entries represent specific disease entities for which no specific code exists so the term is included within an "other" code.

"Unspecified" codes

Codes titled "unspecified" are for use when the information in the medical record is insufficient to assign a more specific code. For those categories for which an unspecified code is not provided, the "other specified" code may represent both other and unspecified.

Includes Notes

This note appears immediately under a three character code title to further define, or give examples of, the content of the category.

Inclusion terms

List of terms is included under some codes. These terms are the conditions for which that code is to be used. The terms may be synonyms of the code title, or, in the case of "other specified" codes, the terms are a list of the various conditions assigned to that code. The inclusion terms are not necessarily exhaustive. Additional terms found only in the Alphabetic Index may also be assigned to a code.

Excludes Notes

The ICD-10-CM has two types of excludes notes. Each type of note has a different definition for use but they are all similar in that they indicate that codes excluded from each other are independent of each other.

Excludes 1

A type 1 Excludes note is a pure excludes. It means "NOT CODED HERE!" An Excludes 1 note indicates that the code excluded should never be used at the same time as the code above the Excludes 1 note. An Excludes 1 is used when two conditions cannot occur together, such as a congenital form versus an acquired form of the same condition.

Excludes 2

A type 2 excludes note represents "Not included here". An Excludes 2 note indicates that the condition excluded is not part of the condition it is excluded from but a patient may have both conditions at the same time. When an Excludes 2 note appears under a code it is acceptable to use both the code and the excluded code together.

Etiology/manifestation convention ("code first", "use additional code" and "in diseases classified elsewhere" notes)

Certain conditions have both an underlying etiology and multiple body system manifestations due to the underlying etiology. For such conditions, the ICD-10-CM has a coding convention that requires the underlying condition be sequenced first followed by the manifestation. Wherever such a combination exists, there is a "use additional code" note at the etiology code, and a "code first" note at the manifestation code. These instructional notes indicate the proper sequencing order of the codes, etiology followed by manifestation.

In most cases the manifestation codes will have in the code title, "in diseases classified elsewhere." Codes with this title are a component of the etiology/manifestation convention. The code title indicates that it is a manifestation code. "In diseases classified elsewhere" codes are never permitted to be used as first-listed or principal diagnosis codes. They must be used in conjunction with an underlying condition code and they must be listed following the underlying condition. See category F02, Dementia in other diseases classified elsewhere, for an example of this convention.

There are manifestation codes that do not have "in diseases classified elsewhere" in the title. For such codes a "use additional code" note will still be present and the rules for sequencing apply.

In addition to the notes in the Tabular List, these conditions also have a specific Alphabetic Index entry structure. In the Alphabetic Index both conditions are listed together with the etiology code first followed by the manifestation codes in brackets. The code in brackets is always to be sequenced second.

An example of the etiology/manifestation convention is dementia in Parkinson's disease. In the Alphabetic Index, code G20 is listed first, followed by code F02.80 or F02.81 in brackets. Code G20 represents the underlying etiology, Parkinson's disease, and must be sequenced first, whereas codes F02.80 and F02.81 represent the manifestation of dementia in diseases classified elsewhere, with or without behavioral disturbance.

"Code first" and "Use additional code" notes are also used as sequencing rules in the classification for certain codes that are not part of an etiology/ manifestation combination.

"And"

The word "and" should be interpreted to mean either "and" or "or" when it appears in a title.

"With"

The word "with" should be interpreted to mean "associated with" or "due to" when it appears in a code title, the Alphabetic Index, or an instructional note in the Tabular List.

The word "with" in the Alphabetic Index is sequenced immediately following the main term, not in alphabetical order.

"See" and *"See Also"*

The *"see"* instruction following a main term in the Alphabetic Index indicates that another term should be referenced. It is necessary to go to the main term referenced with the *"see"* note to locate the correct code.

A *"see also"* instruction following a main term in the Alphabetic Index instructs that there is another main term that may also be referenced that may provide additional Alphabetic Index entries that may be useful. It is not necessary to follow the *"see also"* note when the original main term provides the necessary code.

"Code also note"

A "code also" note instructs that two codes may be required to fully describe a condition, but this note does not provide sequencing direction.

Default codes

A code listed next to a main term in the ICD-10-CM Alphabetic Index is referred to as a default code. The default code represents that condition that is most commonly associated with the main term, or is the unspecified code for the condition. If a condition is documented in a medical record (for example, appendicitis) without any additional information, such as acute or chronic, the default code should be assigned.

Syndromes

Follow the Alphabetic Index guidance when coding syndromes. In the absence of Alphabetic Index guidance, assign codes for the documented manifestations of the syndrome.

Typeface

Bold: Bold typeface is used for all codes and code titles in the Tabular List and for main terms in the Alphabetic Index.

Italics: Italicized typeface is used for all exclusion notes in the Tabular list and for *"see"* and *"see also"* instructions in the Alphabetic Index.

<u>Underscore</u>: See Channel Publishing Additional *Enhanced* Features.

DRG Pinciples and Medicare Code Editor Edits Key

DRG Principles

Identifies codes that are recognized and affected by the DRG Grouper.

CC – Identifies codes that are defined as a complication or comorbidity when used as a secondary diagnosis.

MCC – Identifies codes that are defined as a major complication or comorbidity when used as a secondary diagnosis.

[Not Allowed as PDX] – Identifies codes that are not allowed as a principal diagnosis for an acute care hospital admission.

[Questionable Admission] – Identifies some diagnoses that are usually not sufficient justification for admission to an acute care hospital.

[Unacceptable PDX] – Identifies codes that are considered unacceptable as a principal diagnosis for an acute care hospital admission.

[Wrong Procedure Performed] – Identifies codes that indicate that the wrong procedure was performed.

Medicare Code Editor Edits

Identifies codes that are edit-reviewed for age and sex-related discrepancies and principal diagnosis criteria.

[♂] – Identifies diagnoses allowed for males.

[♀] – Identifies diagnoses allowed for females.

[Age/0] – Identifies perinatal/newborn diagnoses for patient's age of 0 years only.

[Age/0-17] – Identifies pediatric diagnoses for patient's age range of 0-17 years inclusive.

[Age/12-55] – Identifies maternity diagnoses for patient's age of 12-55 years inclusive.

[Age/15-124] – Identifies adult diagnoses for patient's age of 15-124 years inclusive.

Channel Publishing Additional 2017 *Enhanced* Features

Definitions and Illustrations
Medical definitions of diseases written by a coder for coders. Anatomical illustrations with call outs of body parts.

Anatomy and Physiology Reviews
Anatomy and physiology reviews that help coders understand the anatomical structures and physiology of the various systems.

Color Highlighting
Color highlighting of key terms:
- Excludes 1 – Burgundy
- Excludes ❷ – Burgundy
- AHA Coding Clinic® Reference Notations – Burgundy
- Highlighted 7th Digit Subclassifications – Screened Burgundy
- Tab-Edge Printing – Screened Burgundy
- Index "continueds" – Burgundy
- Highlighted columns in Neoplasm Table – Screened Burgundy
- Highlighted columns in Drugs & Chemicals Table – Screened Burgundy

DRG Principles
Identifies codes that are recognized and affected by the DRG Grouper.

Medicare Code Editor Edits
Identifies codes that are edit-reviewed for age and sex-related discrepancies and principal diagnosis criteria.

AHA Coding Clinic® Reference Notations
Identifies AHA Coding Clinic® articles and Q&As (with descriptive title) that have relevant information for certain codes or code categories.

Highlighted Term <u>Differentiation</u>
Selected terms within code categories and code titles have been <u>underscored</u> to help coders more easily and accurately identify the correct code in the Tabular List.

Further use of dashes (-)
All code categories and codes requiring additional digits in the Tabular List have a dash (-) at the end of the last digit that helps coders be aware that additional characters are required for a complete code.

Further use of placeholder "x"
All codes requiring the coder to use the placeholder "x" to make a complete code have been placed in advance to help coders clearly identify when these "x" placeholders are required.

Excludes ❷:
All Excludes 2 listings have a graphic "❷" to help coders more clearly identify those unique excludes notations where a coder may code both conditions, if present.

Excludes 1 and Excludes ❷ key
The short descriptions of Excludes 1 and Excludes ❷ are listed on the bottom of each page throughout the Tabular List to help coders identify the difference between the two without referring back to the introduction.

Highlighted 7th digit subclassifications
Burgundy screen bars over the 7th digit subclassifications in the Tabular List help coders easily identify those code categories requiring a variable 7th digit.

Highlighted columns in the Neoplasm and Drugs & Chemical Tables
Burgundy screen bars over selected columns to help coders easily identify the appropriate column of codes.

Tab-Edge printing
Chapter-by-chapter, and section-by-section stair-stepped, tab-edge printing screen bars with code ranges for that page printed inside that helps coders locate the correct section quickly.

INTRODUCTION TO AHA CODING CLINIC® REFERENCE NOTATIONS

BACKGROUND

AHA Coding Clinic® is a registered trademark of the American Hospital Association. AHA Coding Clinic® Reference Notations is not a product of the American Hospital Association, and Channel Publishing, Ltd. is not affiliated with or endorsed by the American Hospital Association. The American Hospital coding website can be accessed at www.ahacentraloffice.org.

The AHA Coding Clinic® for ICD-10-CM/PCS is published quarterly by the American Hospital Association. The *Coding Clinic* is the official publication for *ICD-10-CM/PCS* coding guidelines and advice as designated by the four cooperating parties. The cooperating parties listed below have final approval of the coding advice provided in the *Coding Clinic*: American Hospital Association, American Health Information Management Association, Centers for Medicare and Medicaid Services, National Center for Health Statistics.

The *Coding Clinic* provides specific information and guidelines that are helpful for determining proper coding, and is used by CMS in reviewing claims. The goal of the *Coding Clinic* is to provide coding advice, official coding decisions, and news. It promotes accuracy and consistency in the use of ICD-10-CM/PCS. It offers coding guidelines and advice based on adherence to the statistical classification scheme of ICD-10-CM/PCS and the definitions specified in the Uniform Hospital Discharge Data Set (UHDDS).

INTRODUCTION

Channel Publishing has developed the AHA Coding Clinic® Reference Notations to help coders access the official coding advice found throughout all issues of the *Coding Clinic*. This information has been referenced in two ways: 1) direct code-by-code reference notations, 2) a categorical index of articles that are too broad in scope to be assigned to a particular code. Any comments regarding these reference notations should be directed to: *Coding Clinic* Reference Notations, c/o Channel Publishing, Ltd., 4750 Longley Lane, Suite 110, Reno, Nevada 89502.

GUIDANCE IN USE

Coders are encouraged to reference all relevant information contained in the *Coding Clinic* to promote the most accurate coding possible for their organization. It is important to understand the basic criteria for assigning the *Coding Clinic* Reference Notations. The basic criteria consists of: Assignment to codes with direct or indirect information concerning the proper use of each particular code, assignment to a code category when the information is relevant to all codes in that category, and assignment to codes where a coder might commonly attempt to use a code in error.

AHA CODING CLINIC® REFERENCE NOTATION INDEX

CODING CLINIC **INFORMATION**

AHA CODING CLINIC® REFERENCE NOTATION INDEX – *continued*

GUIDELINES

2017 OFFICIAL CODING GUIDELINES

IMPORTANT NOTE REGARDING THESE PRINTED GUIDELINES

These guidelines are effective for the 2017 Version of ICD-10-CM (guidelines posted August 8, 2016). A newer version may become available after this book has been printed. Coders should periodically check the National Center for Health Statistics (NCHS) web site for the most current version.

NCHS Web Site: www.cdc.gov/nchs/icd/icd10cm.htm

Channel Publishing, Ltd.

**2017 ICD-10-CM Official Guidelines for Coding and Reporting
FY 2017 (October 1, 2016 – September 30, 2017)**

Channel Publishing Changes Highlighting
The Channel Publishing highlighting is designed to show what has changed in the Official Coding Guidelines from the 2016 to 2017 version including text that has been deleted or replaced.
- **Additions and revisions are in burgundy-colored type**
- **Deletions are in burgundy-colored type with ~~strikethrough~~**
- **Items/text moved within the guidelines since the 2016 version are <u>underlined</u> in burgundy-colored type**
- **Revisions to headings are in burgundy-colored *italics* type**

The Centers for Medicare and Medicaid Services (CMS) and the National Center for Health Statistics (NCHS), two departments within the U.S. Federal Government's Department of Health and Human Services (DHHS) provide the following guidelines for coding and reporting using the International Classification of Diseases, 10th Revision, Clinical Modification (ICD-10-CM). These guidelines should be used as a companion document to the official version of the ICD-10-CM as published on the NCHS website. The ICD-10-CM is a morbidity classification published by the United States for classifying diagnoses and reason for visits in all health care settings. The ICD-10-CM is based on the ICD-10, the statistical classification of disease published by the World Health Organization (WHO).

These guidelines have been approved by the four organizations that make up the Cooperating Parties for the ICD-10-CM: the American Hospital Association (AHA), the American Health Information Management Association (AHIMA), CMS, and NCHS.

These guidelines are a set of rules that have been developed to accompany and complement the official conventions and instructions provided within the ICD-10-CM itself. The instructions and conventions of the classification take precedence over guidelines. These guidelines are based on the coding and sequencing instructions in the Tabular List and Alphabetic Index of ICD-10-CM, but provide additional instruction. Adherence to these guidelines when assigning ICD-10-CM diagnosis codes is required under the Health Insurance Portability and Accountability Act (HIPAA). The diagnosis codes (Tabular List and Alphabetic Index) have been adopted under HIPAA for all healthcare settings. A joint effort between the healthcare provider and the coder is essential to achieve complete and accurate documentation, code assignment, and reporting of diagnoses and procedures. These guidelines have been developed to assist both the healthcare provider and the coder in identifying those diagnoses and procedures that are to be reported. The importance of consistent, complete documentation in the medical record cannot be overemphasized. Without such documentation accurate coding cannot be achieved. The entire record should be reviewed to determine the specific reason for the encounter and the conditions treated.

The term encounter is used for all settings, including hospital admissions. In the context of these guidelines, the term provider is used throughout the guidelines to mean physician or any qualified health care practitioner who is legally accountable for establishing the patient's diagnosis. Only this set of guidelines, approved by the Cooperating Parties, is official.

The guidelines are organized into sections. Section I includes the structure and conventions of the classification and general guidelines that apply to the entire classification, and chapter-specific guidelines that correspond to the chapters as they are arranged in the classification. Section II includes guidelines for selection of principal diagnosis for non-outpatient settings. Section III includes guidelines for reporting additional diagnoses in non-outpatient settings. Section IV is for outpatient coding and reporting. It is necessary to review all sections of the guidelines to fully understand all of the rules and instructions needed to code properly.

TABLE OF CONTENTS

GUIDELINES

Section II.   Selection of Principal Diagnosis 26

Section III.   Reporting Additional Diagnoses 27

Section IV.   Diagnostic Coding and Reporting Guidelines for Outpatient Services ..27

Appendix I: Present on Admission Reporting Guidelines 29

SECTION I – CONVENTIONS
Section I. A. 1.

Section I. Conventions, general coding guidelines and chapter specific guidelines

The conventions, general guidelines and chapter-specific guidelines are applicable to all health care settings unless otherwise indicated. The conventions and instructions of the classification take precedence over guidelines.

A. Conventions for the ICD-10-CM

The conventions for the ICD-10-CM are the general rules for use of the classification independent of the guidelines. These conventions are incorporated within the Alphabetic Index and Tabular List of the ICD-10-CM as instructional notes.

1. The Alphabetic Index and Tabular List
The ICD-10-CM is divided into the Alphabetic Index, an alphabetical list of terms and their corresponding code, and the Tabular List, a structured list of codes divided into chapters based on body system or condition. The Alphabetic Index consists of the following parts: the Index of Diseases and Injury, the Index of External Causes of Injury, the Table of Neoplasms and the Table of Drugs and Chemicals.

See Section I.C2. General guidelines
See Section I.C.19. Adverse effects, poisoning, underdosing and toxic effects

2. Format and Structure
The ICD-10-CM Tabular List contains categories, subcategories and codes. Characters for categories, subcategories and codes may be either a letter or a number. All categories are 3 characters. A three-character category that has no further subdivision is equivalent to a code. Subcategories are either 4 or 5 characters. Codes may be 3, 4, 5, 6 or 7 characters. That is, each level of subdivision after a category is a subcategory. The final level of subdivision is a code. Codes that have applicable 7th characters are still referred to as codes, not subcategories. A code that has an applicable 7th character is considered invalid without the 7th character.

The ICD-10-CM uses an indented format for ease in reference.

3. Use of codes for reporting purposes
For reporting purposes only codes are permissible, not categories or subcategories, and any applicable 7th character is required.

4. Placeholder character
The ICD-10-CM utilizes a placeholder character "X". The "X" is used as a placeholder at certain codes to allow for future expansion. An example of this is at the poisoning, adverse effect and underdosing codes, categories T36-T50.

Where a placeholder exists, the X must be used in order for the code to be considered a valid code.

5. 7th Characters
Certain ICD-10-CM categories have applicable 7th characters. The applicable 7th character is required for all codes within the category, or as the notes in the Tabular List instruct. The 7th character must always be the 7th character in the data field. If a code that requires a 7th character is not 6 characters, a placeholder X must be used to fill in the empty characters.

6. Abbreviations

a. Alphabetic Index abbreviations
NEC "Not elsewhere classifiable"
This abbreviation in the Alphabetic Index represents "other specified". When a specific code is not available for a condition, the Alphabetic Index directs the coder to the "other specified" code in the Tabular List.

NOS "Not otherwise specified"
This abbreviation is the equivalent of unspecified.

b. Tabular List abbreviations
NEC "Not elsewhere classifiable"
This abbreviation in the Tabular List represents "other specified". When a specific code is not available for a condition, the Tabular List includes an NEC entry under a code to identify the code as the "other specified" code.

NOS "Not otherwise specified"
This abbreviation is the equivalent of unspecified.

7. Punctuation
[ ] Brackets are used in the Tabular List to enclose synonyms, alternative wording or explanatory phrases. Brackets are used in the Alphabetic Index to identify manifestation codes.

SECTION I – CONVENTIONS
Section I. A. 8.

( ) Parentheses are used in both the Alphabetic Index and Tabular List to enclose supplementary words that may be present or absent in the statement of a disease or procedure without affecting the code number to which it is assigned. The terms within the parentheses are referred to as nonessential modifiers. The nonessential modifiers in the Alphabetic Index to Diseases apply to subterms following a main term except when a nonessential modifier and a subentry are mutually exclusive, the subentry takes precedence. For example, in the ICD-10-CM Alphabetic Index under the main term Enteritis, "acute" is a nonessential modifier and "chronic" is a subentry. In this case, the nonessential modifier "acute" does not apply to the subentry "chronic".

: Colons are used in the Tabular List after an incomplete term which needs one or more of the modifiers following the colon to make it assignable to a given category.

8. Use of "and"
See Section I.A.14. Use of the term "And".

9. Other and Unspecified codes

a. "Other" codes
Codes titled "other" or "other specified" are for use when the information in the medical record provides detail for which a specific code does not exist. Alphabetic Index entries with NEC in the line designate "other" codes in the Tabular List. These Alphabetic Index entries represent specific disease entities for which no specific code exists so the term is included within an "other" code.

b. "Unspecified" codes
Codes titled "unspecified" are for use when the information in the medical record is insufficient to assign a more specific code. For those categories for which an unspecified code is not provided, the "other specified" code may represent both other and unspecified.

See Section I.B.18 Use of Sign/Symptom/Unspecified Codes.

10. Includes Notes
This note appears immediately under a three character code title to further define, or give examples of, the content of the category.

11. Inclusion terms
List of terms is included under some codes. These terms are the conditions for which that code is to be used. The terms may be synonyms of the code title, or, in the case of "other specified" codes, the terms are a list of the various conditions assigned to that code. The inclusion terms are not necessarily exhaustive. Additional terms found only in the Alphabetic Index may also be assigned to a code.

12. Excludes Notes
The ICD-10-CM has two types of excludes notes. Each type of note has a different definition for use but they are all similar in that they indicate that codes excluded from each other are independent of each other.

a. Excludes 1
A type 1 Excludes note is a pure excludes note. It means "NOT CODED HERE!" An Excludes1 note indicates that the code excluded should never be used at the same time as the code above the Excludes1 note. An Excludes1 is used when two conditions cannot occur together, such as a congenital form versus an acquired form of the same condition.

b. Excludes 2
A type 2 Excludes note represents "Not included here". An Excludes2 note indicates that the condition excluded is not part of the condition represented by the code, but a patient may have both conditions at the same time. When an Excludes2 note appears under a code, it is acceptable to use both the code and the excluded code together, when appropriate.

An exception to the Excludes1 definition is the circumstance when the two conditions are unrelated to each other. If it is not clear whether the two conditions involving an Excludes1 note are related or not, query the provider. For example, code F45.8, Other somatoform disorders, has an Excludes1 note for "sleep related teeth grinding (G47.63)," because "teeth grinding" is an inclusion term under F45.8. Only one of these two codes should be assigned for teeth grinding. However psychogenic dysmenorrhea is also an inclusion term under F45.8, and a patient could have both this condition and sleep related teeth grinding. In this case, the two conditions are clearly unrelated to each other, and so it would be appropriate to report F45.8 and G47.63 together.

13. Etiology/manifestation convention ("code first", "use additional code" and "in diseases classified elsewhere" notes)
Certain conditions have both an underlying etiology and multiple body system manifestations due to the underlying etiology. For such conditions, the ICD-10-CM has a coding convention that requires the underlying condition be sequenced first, if applicable, followed by the manifestation. Wherever such a combination exists, there is a "use additional code" note at the etiology code, and a "code first" note at the manifestation code. These instructional notes indicate the proper sequencing order of the codes, etiology followed by manifestation.

SECTION I – CONVENTIONS
Section I. A. 14.

In most cases the manifestation codes will have in the code title, "in diseases classified elsewhere." Codes with this title are a component of the etiology/ manifestation convention. The code title indicates that it is a manifestation code. "In diseases classified elsewhere" codes are never permitted to be used as first-listed or principal diagnosis codes. They must be used in conjunction with an underlying condition code and they must be listed following the underlying condition. See category F02, Dementia in other diseases classified elsewhere, for an example of this convention.

There are manifestation codes that do not have "in diseases classified elsewhere" in the title. For such codes, there is a "use additional code" note at the etiology code and a "code first" note at the manifestation code and the rules for sequencing apply.

In addition to the notes in the Tabular List, these conditions also have a specific Alphabetic Index entry structure. In the Alphabetic Index both conditions are listed together with the etiology code first followed by the manifestation codes in brackets. The code in brackets is always to be sequenced second.

An example of the etiology/manifestation convention is dementia in Parkinson's disease. In the Alphabetic Index, code G20 is listed first, followed by code F02.80 or F02.81 in brackets. Code G20 represents the underlying etiology, Parkinson's disease, and must be sequenced first, whereas codes F02.80 and F02.81 represent the manifestation of dementia in diseases classified elsewhere, with or without behavioral disturbance.

"Code first" and "Use additional code" notes are also used as sequencing rules in the classification for certain codes that are not part of an etiology/ manifestation combination.

See Section I.B.7. Multiple coding for a single condition.

14. "And"
The word "and" should be interpreted to mean either "and" or "or" when it appears in a title.

For example, cases of "tuberculosis of bones", "tuberculosis of joints" and "tuberculosis of bones and joints" are classified to subcategory A18.0, Tuberculosis of bones and joints.

15. "With"
The word "with" should be interpreted to mean "associated with" or "due to" when it appears in a code title, the Alphabetic Index, or an instructional note in the Tabular List. The classification presumes a causal relationship between the two conditions linked by these terms in the Alphabetic Index or Tabular List. These conditions should be coded as related even in the absence of provider documentation explicitly linking them, unless the documentation clearly states the conditions are unrelated. For conditions not specifically linked by these relational terms in the classification, provider documentation must link the conditions in order to code them as related.

The word "with" in the Alphabetic Index is sequenced immediately following the main term, not in alphabetical order.

16. "See" and "See Also"
The "see" instruction following a main term in the Alphabetic Index indicates that another term should be referenced. It is necessary to go to the main term referenced with the "see" note to locate the correct code.

A "see also" instruction following a main term in the Alphabetic Index instructs that there is another main term that may also be referenced that may provide additional Alphabetic Index entries that may be useful. It is not necessary to follow the "see also" note when the original main term provides the necessary code.

17. "Code also note"
A "code also" note instructs that two codes may be required to fully describe a condition, but this note does not provide sequencing direction.

18. Default codes
A code listed next to a main term in the ICD-10-CM Alphabetic Index is referred to as a default code. The default code represents that condition that is most commonly associated with the main term, or is the unspecified code for the condition. If a condition is documented in a medical record (for example, appendicitis) without any additional information, such as acute or chronic, the default code should be assigned.

19. Code assignment and Clinical Criteria
The assignment of a diagnosis code is based on the provider's diagnostic statement that the condition exists. The provider's statement that the patient has a particular condition is sufficient. Code assignment is not based on clinical criteria used by the provider to establish the diagnosis.

SECTION I – CONVENTIONS
Section I. B. 1.

B. General Coding Guidelines

1. Locating a code in the ICD-10-CM
To select a code in the classification that corresponds to a diagnosis or reason for visit documented in a medical record, first locate the term in the Alphabetic Index, and then verify the code in the Tabular List. Read and be guided by instructional notations that appear in both the Alphabetic Index and the Tabular List.

It is essential to use both the Alphabetic Index and Tabular List when locating and assigning a code. The Alphabetic Index does not always provide the full code. Selection of the full code, including laterality and any applicable 7th character can only be done in the Tabular List. A dash (-) at the end of an Alphabetic Index entry indicates that additional characters are required. Even if a dash is not included at the Alphabetic Index entry, it is necessary to refer to the Tabular List to verify that no 7th character is required.

2. Level of Detail in Coding
Diagnosis codes are to be used and reported at their highest number of characters available.

ICD-10-CM diagnosis codes are composed of codes with 3, 4, 5, 6 or 7 characters. Codes with three characters are included in ICD-10-CM as the heading of a category of codes that may be further subdivided by the use of fourth and/or fifth characters and/or sixth characters, which provide greater detail.

A three-character code is to be used only if it is not further subdivided. A code is invalid if it has not been coded to the full number of characters required for that code, including the 7th character, if applicable.

3. Code or codes from A00.0 through T88.9, Z00-Z99.8
The appropriate code or codes from A00.0 through T88.9, Z00-Z99.8 must be used to identify diagnoses, symptoms, conditions, problems, complaints or other reason(s) for the encounter/visit.

4. Signs and symptoms
Codes that describe symptoms and signs, as opposed to diagnoses, are acceptable for reporting purposes when a related definitive diagnosis has not been established (confirmed) by the provider. Chapter 18 of ICD-10-CM, Symptoms, Signs, and Abnormal Clinical and Laboratory Findings, Not Elsewhere Classified (codes R00.0 - R99) contains many, but not all codes for symptoms.

See Section I.B.18 Use of Sign/Symptom/Unspecified Codes.

5. Conditions that are an integral part of a disease process
Signs and symptoms that are associated routinely with a disease process should not be assigned as additional codes, unless otherwise instructed by the classification.

6. Conditions that are not an integral part of a disease process
Additional signs and symptoms that may not be associated routinely with a disease process should be coded when present.

7. Multiple coding for a single condition
In addition to the etiology/manifestation convention that requires two codes to fully describe a single condition that affects multiple body systems, there are other single conditions that also require more than one code. "Use additional code" notes are found in the Tabular List at codes that are not part of an etiology/manifestation pair where a secondary code is useful to fully describe a condition. The sequencing rule is the same as the etiology/manifestation pair, "use additional code" indicates that a secondary code should be added.

For example, for bacterial infections that are not included in chapter 1, a secondary code from category B95, Streptococcus, Staphylococcus, and Enterococcus, as the cause of diseases classified elsewhere, or B96, Other bacterial agents as the cause of diseases classified elsewhere, may be required to identify the bacterial organism causing the infection. A "use additional code" note will normally be found at the infectious disease code, indicating a need for the organism code to be added as a secondary code.

"Code first" notes are also under certain codes that are not specifically manifestation codes but may be due to an underlying cause. When there is a "code first" note and an underlying condition is present, the underlying condition should be sequenced first.

"Code, if applicable, any causal condition first" notes indicate that this code may be assigned as a principal diagnosis when the causal condition is unknown or not applicable. If a causal condition is known, then the code for that condition should be sequenced as the principal or first-listed diagnosis.

Multiple codes may be needed for sequela, complication codes and obstetric codes to more fully describe a condition. See the specific guidelines for these conditions for further instruction.

SECTION I – CONVENTIONS
Section I. B. 8.

8. Acute and Chronic Conditions

If the same condition is described as both acute (subacute) and chronic, and separate subentries exist in the Alphabetic Index at the same indentation level, code both and sequence the acute (subacute) code first.

9. Combination Code

A combination code is a single code used to classify:

> Two diagnoses, or
> A diagnosis with an associated secondary process (manifestation)
> A diagnosis with an associated complication

Combination codes are identified by referring to subterm entries in the Alphabetic Index and by reading the inclusion and exclusion notes in the Tabular List.

Assign only the combination code when that code fully identifies the diagnostic conditions involved or when the Alphabetic Index so directs. Multiple coding should not be used when the classification provides a combination code that clearly identifies all of the elements documented in the diagnosis. When the combination code lacks necessary specificity in describing the manifestation or complication, an additional code should be used as a secondary code.

10. Sequela (Late Effects)

A sequela is the residual effect (condition produced) after the acute phase of an illness or injury has terminated. There is no time limit on when a sequela code can be used. The residual may be apparent early, such as in cerebral infarction, or it may occur months or years later, such as that due to a previous injury. Examples of sequela include: scar formation resulting from a burn, deviated septum due to a nasal fracture, and infertility due to tubal occlusion from old tuberculosis. Coding of sequela generally requires two codes sequenced in the following order: The condition or nature of the sequela is sequenced first. The sequela code is sequenced second.

An exception to the above guidelines are those instances where the code for sequela is followed by a manifestation code identified in the Tabular List and title, or the sequela code has been expanded (at the fourth, fifth or sixth character levels) to include the manifestation(s). The code for the acute phase of an illness or injury that led to the sequela is never used with a code for the late effect.

See Section I.C.9. Sequelae of cerebrovascular disease.
See Section I.C.15. Sequelae of complication of pregnancy, childbirth and the puerperium.
See Section I.C.19. Application of 7th characters for Chapter 19.

11. Impending or Threatened Condition

Code any condition described at the time of discharge as "impending" or "threatened" as follows:

> If it did occur, code as confirmed diagnosis.
> If it did not occur, reference the Alphabetic Index to determine if the condition has a subentry term for "impending" or "threatened" and also reference main term entries for "Impending" and for "Threatened."
> If the subterms are listed, assign the given code.
> If the subterms are not listed, code the existing underlying condition(s) and not the condition described as impending or threatened.

12. Reporting Same Diagnosis Code More than Once

Each unique ICD-10-CM diagnosis code may be reported only once for an encounter. This applies to bilateral conditions when there are no distinct codes identifying laterality or two different conditions classified to the same ICD-10-CM diagnosis code.

13. Laterality

Some ICD-10-CM codes indicate laterality, specifying whether the condition occurs on the left, right or is bilateral. If no bilateral code is provided and the condition is bilateral, assign separate codes for both the left and right side. If the side is not identified in the medical record, assign the code for the unspecified side.

When a patient has a bilateral condition and each side is treated during separate encounters, assign the "bilateral" code (as the condition still exists on both sides), including for the encounter to treat the first side. For the second encounter for treatment after one side has previously been treated and the condition no longer exists on that side, assign the appropriate unilateral code for the side where the condition still exists (e.g., cataract surgery performed on each eye in separate encounters). The bilateral code would not be assigned for the subsequent encounter, as the patient no longer has the condition in the previously-treated site. If the treatment on the first side did not completely resolve the condition, then the bilateral code would still be appropriate.

SECTION I – CONVENTIONS
Section I. B. 14.

14. Documentation for BMI, *Depth of* Non-pressure ulcers, Pressure Ulcer Stages, *Coma Scale, and NIH Stroke Scale*

For the Body Mass Index (BMI), depth of non-pressure chronic ulcers, pressure ulcer stage, coma scale, and NIH stroke scale (NIHSS) codes, code assignment may be based on medical record documentation from clinicians who are not the patient's provider (i.e., physician or other qualified healthcare practitioner legally accountable for establishing the patient's diagnosis), since this information is typically documented by other clinicians involved in the care of the patient (e.g., a dietitian often documents the BMI, a nurse often documents the pressure ulcer stages, and an emergency medical technician often documents the coma scale). However, the associated diagnosis (such as overweight, obesity, acute stroke, or pressure ulcer) must be documented by the patient's provider. If there is conflicting medical record documentation, either from the same clinician or different clinicians, the patient's attending provider should be queried for clarification.

The BMI, coma scale, and NIHSS codes should only be reported as secondary diagnoses. ~~As with all other secondary diagnosis codes, the BMI codes should only be assigned when they meet the definition of a reportable additional diagnosis (see Section III, Reporting Additional Diagnoses).~~

15. Syndromes

Follow the Alphabetic Index guidance when coding syndromes. In the absence of Alphabetic Index guidance, assign codes for the documented manifestations of the syndrome. Additional codes for manifestations that are not an integral part of the disease process may also be assigned when the condition does not have a unique code.

16. Documentation of Complications of Care

Code assignment is based on the provider's documentaion of the relationship between the condition and the care or procedure, unless otherwise instructed by the classification. The guideline extends to any complications of care, regardless of the chapter the code is located in. It is important to note that not all conditions that occur during or following medical care or surgery are classified as complications. There must be a cause-and-effect relationship between the care provided and the condition, and an indication in the documentation that it is a complication. Query the provider for clarification, if the complication is not clearly documented.

17. Borderline diagnosis

If the provider documents a "borderline" diagnosis at the time of discharge, the diagnosis is coded as confirmed, unless the classification provides a specific entry (e.g., borderline diabetes). If a borderline condition has a specific index entry in ICD-10-CM, it should be coded as such. Since borderline conditions are not uncertain diagnoses, no distinction is made between the care setting (inpatient versus outpatient). Whenever the documentation is unclear regarding a borderline condition, coders are encouraged to query for clarification.

18. Use of Sign/Symptom/Unspecified Codes

Sign/symptom and "unspecified" codes have acceptable, even necessary, uses. While specific diagnosis codes should be reported when they are supported by the available medical record documentation and clinical knowledge of the patient's health condition, there are instances when signs/symptoms or unspecified codes are the best choices for accurately reflecting the healthcare encounter. Each healthcare encounter should be coded to the level of certainty known for that encounter.

If a definitive diagnosis has not been established by the end of the encounter, it is appropriate to report codes for sign(s) and/or symptoms(s) in lieu of a definitive diagnosis. When sufficient clinical information isn't known or available about a particular health condition to assign a more specific code, it is acceptable to report the appropriate "unspecified" code (e.g., a diagnosis of pneumonia has been determined, but not the specific type). Unspecified codes should be reported when they are the codes that most accurately reflects what is known about the patient's condition at the time of that particular encounter. It would be inappropriate to select a specific code that is not supported by the medical record documentation or conduct medically unnecessary diagnostic testing in order to determine a more specific code.

CHAPTER 1 – INFECTIOUS DISEASES
Section I. C. 1.

C. Chapter-Specific Coding Guidelines

In addition to general coding guidelines, there are guidelines for specific diagnoses and/or conditions in the classification. Unless otherwise indicated, these guidelines apply to all health care settings. Please refer to Section II for guidelines on the selection of principal diagnosis.

1. Chapter 1: Certain Infectious and Parasitic Diseases (A00-B99)

a. Human Immunodeficiency Virus (HIV) Infections

1) Code only confirmed cases

Code only confirmed cases of HIV infection/illness. This is an exception to the hospital inpatient guideline Section II, H.

In this context, "confirmation" does not require documentation of positive serology or culture for HIV; the provider's diagnostic statement that the patient is HIV positive, or has an HIV-related illness is sufficient.

2) Selection and sequencing of HIV codes

(a) Patient admitted for HIV-related condition

If a patient is admitted for an HIV-related condition, the principal diagnosis should be B20, Human immunodeficiency virus [HIV] disease followed by additional diagnosis codes for all reported HIV-related conditions.

(b) Patient with HIV disease admitted for unrelated condition

If a patient with HIV disease is admitted for an unrelated condition (such as a traumatic injury), the code for the unrelated condition (e.g., the nature of injury code) should be the principal diagnosis. Other diagnoses would be B20 followed by additional diagnosis codes for all reported HIV-related conditions.

(c) Whether the patient is newly diagnosed

Whether the patient is newly diagnosed or has had previous admissions/encounters for HIV conditions is irrelevant to the sequencing decision.

(d) Asymptomatic human immunodeficiency virus

Z21, Asymptomatic human immunodeficiency virus [HIV] infection status, is to be applied when the patient without any documentation of symptoms is listed as being "HIV positive," "known HIV," "HIV test positive," or similar terminology. Do not use this code if the term "AIDS" is used or if the patient is treated for any HIV-related illness or is described as having any condition(s) resulting from his/her HIV positive status; use B20 in these cases.

(e) Patients with inconclusive HIV serology

Patients with inconclusive HIV serology, but no definitive diagnosis or manifestations of the illness, may be assigned code R75, Inconclusive laboratory evidence of human immunodeficiency virus [HIV].

(f) Previously diagnosed HIV-related illness

Patients with any known prior diagnosis of an HIV-related illness should be coded to B20. Once a patient has developed an HIV-related illness, the patient should always be assigned code B20 on every subsequent admission/encounter. Patients previously diagnosed with any HIV illness (B20) should never be assigned to R75 or Z21, Asymptomatic human immunodeficiency virus [HIV] infection status.

(g) HIV Infection in Pregnancy, Childbirth and the Puerperium

During pregnancy, childbirth or the puerperium, a patient admitted (or presenting for a health care encounter) because of an HIV-related illness should receive a principal diagnosis code of O98.7-, Human immunodeficiency [HIV] disease complicating pregnancy, childbirth and the puerperium, followed by B20 and the code(s) for the HIV-related illness(es). Codes from Chapter 15 always take sequencing priority.

Patients with asymptomatic HIV infection status admitted (or presenting for a health care encounter) during pregnancy, childbirth, or the puerperium should receive codes of O98.7- and Z21.

(h) Encounters for testing for HIV

If a patient is being seen to determine his/her HIV status, use code Z11.4, Encounter for screening for human immunodeficiency virus [HIV]. Use additional codes for any associated high risk behavior.

If a patient with signs or symptoms is being seen for HIV testing, code the signs and symptoms. An additional counseling code Z71.7, Human immunodeficiency virus [HIV] counseling, may be used if counseling is provided during the encounter for the test.

When a patient returns to be informed of his/her HIV test results and the test result is negative, use code Z71.7, Human immunodeficiency virus [HIV] counseling.

If the results are positive, see previous guidelines and assign codes as appropriate.

CHAPTER 1 – INFECTIOUS DISEASES
Section I. C. 1. b.

b. Infectious agents as the cause of diseases classified to other chapters

Certain infections are classified in chapters other than Chapter 1 and no organism is identified as part of the infection code. In these instances, it is necessary to use an additional code from Chapter 1 to identify the organism. A code from category B95, Streptococcus, Staphylococcus, and Enterococcus as the cause of diseases classified to other chapters, B96, Other bacterial agents as the cause of diseases classified to other chapters, or B97, Viral agents as the cause of diseases classified to other chapters, is to be used as an additional code to identify the organism. An instructional note will be found at the infection code advising that an additional organism code is required.

c. Infections resistant to antibiotics

Many bacterial infections are resistant to current antibiotics. It is necessary to identify all infections documented as antibiotic resistant. Assign a code from category Z16, Resistance to antimicrobial drugs, following the infection code only if the infection code does not identify drug resistance.

d. Sepsis, Severe Sepsis, and Septic Shock

1) Coding of Sepsis and Severe Sepsis

(a) Sepsis

For a diagnosis of sepsis, assign the appropriate code for the underlying systemic infection. If the type of infection or causal organism is not further specified, assign code A41.9, Sepsis, unspecified organism.

A code from subcategory R65.2, Severe sepsis, should not be assigned unless severe sepsis or an associated acute organ dysfunction is documented.

(i) Negative or inconclusive blood cultures and sepsis

Negative or inconclusive blood cultures do not preclude a diagnosis of sepsis in patients with clinical evidence of the condition, however, the provider should be queried.

(ii) Urosepsis

The term urosepsis is a nonspecific term. It is not to be considered synonymous with sepsis. It has no default code in the Alphabetic Index. Should a provider use this term, he/she must be queried for clarification.

(iii) Sepsis with organ dysfunction

If a patient has sepsis and associated acute organ dysfunction or multiple organ dysfunction (MOD), follow the instructions for coding severe sepsis.

(iv) Acute organ dysfunction that is not clearly associated with the sepsis

If a patient has sepsis and an acute organ dysfunction, but the medical record documentation indicates that the acute organ dysfunction is related to a medical condition other than the sepsis, do not assign a code from subcategory R65.2, Severe sepsis. An acute organ dysfunction must be associated with the sepsis in order to assign the severe sepsis code. If the documentation is not clear as to whether an acute organ dysfunction is related to the sepsis or another medical condition, query the provider.

(b) Severe sepsis

The coding of severe sepsis requires a minimum of 2 codes: first a code for the underlying systemic infection, followed by a code from subcategory R65.2, Severe sepsis. If the causal organism is not documented, assign code A41.9, Sepsis, unspecified organism, for the infection. Additional code(s) for the associated acute organ dysfunction are also required.

Due to the complex nature of severe sepsis, some cases may require querying the provider prior to assignment of the codes.

2) Septic shock

(a) Septic shock

Septic shock generally refers to circulatory failure associated with severe sepsis, and therefore, it represents a type of acute organ dysfunction.

For cases of septic shock, the code for the systemic infection should be sequenced first, followed by code R65.21, Severe sepsis with septic shock or code T81.12, Postprocedural septic shock. Any additional codes for the other acute organ dysfunctions should also be assigned. As noted in the sequencing instructions in the Tabular List, the code for septic shock cannot be assigned as a principal diagnosis.

CHAPTER 1 – INFECTIOUS DISEASES
Section I. C. 1. d. 3)

3) Sequencing of severe sepsis

If severe sepsis is present on admission, and meets the definition of principal diagnosis, the underlying systemic infection should be assigned as principal diagnosis followed by the appropriate code from subcategory R65.2 as required by the sequencing rules in the Tabular List. A code from subcategory R65.2 can never be assigned as a principal diagnosis.

When severe sepsis develops during an encounter (it was not present on admission) the underlying systemic infection and the appropriate code from subcategory R65.2 should be assigned as secondary diagnoses.

Severe sepsis may be present on admission but the diagnosis may not be confirmed until sometime after admission. If the documentation is not clear whether severe sepsis was present on admission, the provider should be queried.

4) Sepsis and severe sepsis with a localized infection

If the reason for admission is both sepsis or severe sepsis and a localized infection, such as pneumonia or cellulitis, a code(s) for the underlying systemic infection should be assigned first and the code for the localized infection should be assigned as a secondary diagnosis. If the patient has severe sepsis, a code from subcategory R65.2 should also be assigned as a secondary diagnosis. If the patient is admitted with a localized infection, such as pneumonia, and sepsis/severe sepsis doesn't develop until after admission, the localized infection should be assigned first, followed by the appropriate sepsis/severe sepsis codes.

5) Sepsis due to a postprocedural infection

(a) Documentation of causal relationship

As with all postprocedural complications, code assignment is based on the provider's documentation of the relationship between the infection and the procedure.

(b) Sepsis due to a postprocedural infection

For such cases, the postprocedural infection code, such as, T80.2, Infections following infusion, transfusion, and therapeutic injection, T81.4, Infection following a procedure, T88.0, Infection following immunization, or O86.0, Infection of obstetric surgical wound, should be coded first, followed by the code for the specific infection. If the patient has severe sepsis the appropriate code from subcategory R65.2 should also be assigned with the additional code(s) for any acute organ dysfunction.

(c) Postprocedural infection and postprocedural septic shock

In cases where a postprocedural infection has occurred and has resulted in severe sepsis the code for the precipitating complication such as code T81.4, Infection following a procedure, or O86.0, Infection of obstetrical surgical wound should be coded first followed by code R65.20, Severe sepsis without septic shock and a code for the systemic infection. A code for the systemic infection should also be assigned.

If a postprocedural infection has resulted in postprocedural septic shock, the code for the precipitating complication such as T81.4, Infection following a procedure, or O86.0, Infection of obstetrical surgical wound should be coded first followed by code T81.12-, Postprocedural septic shock. A code for the systemic infection should also be assigned.

6) Sepsis and severe sepsis associated with a noninfectious process (condition)

In some cases a noninfectious process (condition), such as trauma, may lead to an infection which can result in sepsis or severe sepsis. If sepsis or severe sepsis is documented as associated with a noninfectious condition, such as a burn or serious injury, and this condition meets the definition for principal diagnosis, the code for the noninfectious condition should be sequenced first, followed by the code for the resulting infection. If severe sepsis, is present a code from subcategory R65.2 should also be assigned with any associated organ dysfunction(s) codes. It is not necessary to assign a code from subcategory R65.1, Systemic inflammatory response syndrome (SIRS) of non-infectious origin, for these cases.

If the infection meets the definition of principal diagnosis it should be sequenced before the non-infectious condition. When both the associated non-infectious condition and the infection meet the definition of principal diagnosis either may be assigned as principal diagnosis.

Only one code from category R65, Symptoms and signs specifically associated with systemic inflammation and infection, should be assigned. Therefore, when a non-infectious condition leads to an infection resulting in severe sepsis, assign the appropriate code from subcategory R65.2, Severe sepsis. Do not additionally assign a code from subcategory R65.1, Systemic inflammatory response syndrome (SIRS) of non-infectious origin.

See Section I.C.18. SIRS due to non-infectious process.

CHAPTER 1 – INFECTIOUS DISEASES
Section I. C. 1. d. 7)

7) Sepsis and septic shock complicating abortion, pregnancy, childbirth, and the puerperium

See Section I.C.15. Sepsis and septic shock complicating abortion, pregnancy, childbirth and the puerperium.

8) Newborn sepsis

See Section I.C.16.f. Bacterial sepsis of Newborn.

e. Methicillin Resistant *Staphylococcus aureus* (MRSA) Conditions

1) Selection and sequencing of MRSA codes

(a) Combination codes for MRSA infection

When a patient is diagnosed with an infection that is due to methicillin resistant *Staphylococcus aureus* (MRSA), and that infection that has a combination code that includes the causal organism (e.g., sepsis, pneumonia) assign the appropriate combination code for the condition (e.g., code A41.02, Sepsis due to methicillin resistant Staphylococcus aureus or code J15.212, Pneumonia due to methicillin resistant Staphylococcus aureus). Do not assign code B95.62, Methicillin resistant Staphylococcus aureus infection as the cause of the diseases classified elsewhere, as an additional code because the combination code includes the type of infection and the MRSA organism. Do not assign a code from subcategory Z16.11, Resistance to penicillins, as an additional diagnosis.

See Section C.1. for instructions on coding and sequencing of sepsis and severe sepsis.

(b) Other codes for MRSA infection

When there is documentation of a current infection (e.g., wound infection, stitch abscess, urinary tract infection) due to MRSA, and that infection does not have a combination code that includes the causal organism, assign the appropriate code to identify the condition along with code B95.62, Methicillin resistant Staphylococcus aureus infection as the cause of diseases classified elsewhere for the MRSA infection. Do not assign a code from subcategory Z16.11, Resistance to penicillins.

(c) Methicillin susceptible Staphylococcus aureus (MSSA) and MRSA colonization

The condition or state of being colonized or carrying MSSA or MRSA is called colonization or carriage, while an individual person is described as being colonized or being a carrier. Colonization means that MSSA and MSRA is present on or in the body without necessarily causing illness. A positive MRSA colonization test might be documented by the provider as "MRSA screen positive" or "MRSA nasal swab positive".

Assign code Z22.322, Carrier or suspected carrier of methicillin resistant Staphylococcus aureus, for patients documented as having MRSA colonization. Assign code Z22.321, Carrier or suspected carrier of methicillin susceptible Staphylococcus aureus, for patient documented as having MSSA colonization. Colonization is not necessarily indicative of a disease process or as the cause of a specific condition the patient may have unless documented as such by the provider.

(d) MRSA colonization and infection

If a patient is documented as having both MRSA colonization and infection during a hospital admission, code Z22.322, Carrier or suspected carrier of methicillin resistant Staphylococcus aureus, and a code for the MRSA infection may both be assigned.

f. Zika virus infections

1) Code only confirmed cases

Code only a confirmed diagnosis of Zika virus (A92.5, Zika virus disease) as documented by the provider. This is an exception to the hospital inpatient guideline Section II, H. In this context, "confirmation" does not require documentation of the type of test performed; the physician's diagnostic statement that the condition is confirmed is sufficient. This code should be assigned regardless of the stated mode of transmission.

If the provider documents "suspected", "possible" or "probable" Zika, do not assign code A92.5. Assign a code(s) explaining the reason for the encounter (such as fever, rash, or joint pain) or Z20.828, Contact with and (suspected) exposure to other viral communicable diseases.

CHAPTER 2 – NEOPLASMS
Section I. C. 2. a.

2. Chapter 2: Neoplasms (C00-D49)

<u>General guidelines</u>

Chapter 2 of the ICD-10-CM contains the codes for most benign and all malignant neoplasms. Certain benign neoplasms, such as prostatic adenomas, may be found in the specific body system chapters. To properly code a neoplasm it is necessary to determine from the record if the neoplasm is benign, in-situ, malignant, or of uncertain histologic behavior. If malignant, any secondary (metastatic) sites should also be determined.

Primary malignant neoplasms overlapping site boundaries

A primary malignant neoplasm that overlaps two or more contiguous (next to each other) sites should be classified to the subcategory/code .8 ('overlapping lesion'), unless the combination is specifically indexed elsewhere. For multiple neoplasms of the same site that are not contiguous such as tumors in different quadrants of the same breast, codes for each site should be assigned.

Malignant neoplasm of ectopic tissue

Malignant neoplasms of ectopic tissue are to be coded to the site of origin mentioned, e.g., ectopic pancreatic malignant neoplasms involving the stomach are coded to pancreas, unspecified (C25.9).

The neoplasm table in the Alphabetic Index should be referenced first. However, if the histological term is documented, that term should be referenced first, rather than going immediately to the Neoplasm Table, in order to determine which column in the Neoplasm Table is appropriate. For example, if the documentation indicates "adenoma," refer to the term in the Alphabetic Index to review the entries under this term and the instructional note to "see also neoplasm, by site, benign." The table provides the proper code based on the type of neoplasm and the site. It is important to select the proper column in the table that corresponds to the type of neoplasm. The Tabular List should then be referenced to verify that the correct code has been selected from the table and that a more specific site code does not exist.

See Section I.C.21. Factors influencing health status and contact with health services, Status, for information regarding Z15.0, codes for genetic susceptibility to cancer.

a. Treatment directed at the malignancy
If the treatment is directed at the malignancy, designate the malignancy as the principal diagnosis.

The only exception to this guideline is if a patient admission/encounter is solely for the administration of chemotherapy, immunotherapy or radiation therapy, assign the appropriate Z51.– code as the first-listed or principal diagnosis, and the diagnosis or problem for which the service is being performed as a secondary diagnosis.

b. Treatment of secondary site
When a patient is admitted because of a primary neoplasm with metastasis and treatment is directed toward the secondary site only, the secondary neoplasm is designated as the principal diagnosis even though the primary malignancy is still present.

c. Coding and sequencing of complications
Coding and sequencing of complications associated with the malignancies or with the therapy thereof are subject to the following guidelines:

1) Anemia associated with malignancy
When admission/encounter is for management of an anemia associated with the malignancy, and the treatment is only for anemia, the appropriate code for the malignancy is sequenced as the principal or first-listed diagnosis followed by the appropriate code for the anemia (such as code D63.0, Anemia in neoplastic disease).

2) Anemia associated with chemotherapy, immunotherapy and radiation therapy
When the admission/encounter is for management of an anemia associated with an adverse effect of the administration of chemotherapy or immunotherapy and the only treatment is for the anemia, the anemia code is sequenced first followed by the appropriate codes for the neoplasm and the adverse effect (T45.1X5, Adverse effect of antineoplastic and immunosuppressive drugs).

When the admission/encounter is for management of an anemia associated with an adverse effect of radiotherapy, the anemia code should be sequenced first, followed by the appropriate neoplasm code and code Y84.2, Radiological procedure and radiotherapy as the cause of abnormal reaction of the patient, or of later complication, without mention of misadventure at the time of the procedure.

3) Management of dehydration due to the malignancy
When the admission/encounter is for management of dehydration due to the malignancy and only the dehydration is being treated (intravenous rehydration), the dehydration is sequenced first, followed by the code(s) for the malignancy.

CHAPTER 2 – NEOPLASMS
Section I. C. 2. c. 4)

4) Treatment of a complication resulting from a surgical procedure
When the admission/encounter is for treatment of a complication resulting from a surgical procedure, designate the complication as the principal or first-listed diagnosis if treatment is directed at resolving the complication.

d. Primary malignancy previously excised
When a primary malignancy has been previously excised or eradicated from its site and there is no further treatment directed to that site and there is no evidence of any existing primary malignancy, a code from category Z85, Personal history of malignant neoplasm, should be used to indicate the former site of the malignancy. Any mention of extension, invasion, or metastasis to another site is coded as a secondary malignant neoplasm to that site. The secondary site may be the principal or first-listed with the Z85 code used as a secondary code.

e. Admissions/Encounters involving chemotherapy, immunotherapy and radiation therapy

1) Episode of care involves surgical removal of neoplasm
When an episode of care involves the surgical removal of a neoplasm, primary or secondary site, followed by adjunct chemotherapy or radiation treatment during the same episode of care, the code for the neoplasm should be assigned as principal or first-listed diagnosis.

2) Patient admission/encounter solely for administration of chemotherapy, immunotherapy and radiation therapy
If a patient admission/encounter is solely for the administration of chemotherapy, immunotherapy or radiation therapy assign code Z51.0, Encounter for antineoplastic radiation therapy, or Z51.11, Encounter for antineoplastic chemotherapy, or Z51.12, Encounter for antineoplastic immunotherapy as the first-listed or principal diagnosis. If a patient receives more than one of these therapies during the same admission more than one of these codes may be assigned, in any sequence.

The malignancy for which the therapy is being administered should be assigned as a secondary diagnosis.

3) Patient admitted for radiation therapy, chemotherapy or immunotherapy and develops complications
When a patient is admitted for the purpose of radiotherapy, immunotherapy or chemotherapy and develops complications such as uncontrolled nausea and vomiting or dehydration, the principal or first-listed diagnosis is Z51.0, Encounter for antineoplastic radiation therapy, or Z51.11, Encounter for antineoplastic chemotherapy, or Z51.12, Encounter for antineoplastic immunotherapy followed by any codes for the complications.

f. Admission/encounter to determine extent of malignancy
When the reason for admission/encounter is to determine the extent of the malignancy, or for a procedure such as paracentesis or thoracentesis, the primary malignancy or appropriate metastatic site is designated as the principal or first-listed diagnosis, even though chemotherapy or radiotherapy is administered.

g. Symptoms, signs, and abnormal findings listed in Chapter 18 associated with neoplasms
Symptoms, signs, and ill-defined conditions listed in Chapter 18 characteristic of, or associated with, an existing primary or secondary site malignancy cannot be used to replace the malignancy as principal or first-listed diagnosis, regardless of the number of admissions or encounters for treatment and care of the neoplasm.

See section I.C.21. Factors influencing health status and contact with health services, Encounter for prophylactic organ removal.

h. Admission/encounter for pain control/management
See Section I.C.6. for information on coding admission/encounter for pain control/management.

i. Malignancy in two or more noncontiguous sites
A patient may have more than one malignant tumor in the same organ. These tumors may represent different primaries or metastatic disease, depending on the site. Should the documentation be unclear, the provider should be queried as to the status of each tumor so that the correct codes can be assigned.

j. Disseminated malignant neoplasm, unspecified
Code C80.0, Disseminated malignant neoplasm, unspecified, is for use only in those cases where the patient has advanced metastatic disease and no known primary or secondary sites are specified. It should not be used in place of assigning codes for the primary site and all known secondary sites.

k. Malignant neoplasm without specification of site
Code C80.1, Malignant (primary) neoplasm, unspecified, equates to Cancer, unspecified. This code should only be used when no determination can be made as to the primary site of a malignancy. This code should rarely be used in the inpatient setting.

I. **Sequencing of neoplasm codes**

1) **Encounter for treatment of primary malignancy**
If the reason for the encounter is for treatment of a primary malignancy, assign the malignancy as the principal/first-listed diagnosis. The primary site is to be sequenced first, followed by any metastatic sites.

2) **Encounter for treatment of secondary malignancy**
When an encounter is for a primary malignancy with metastasis and treatment is directed toward the metastatic (secondary) site(s) only, the metastatic site(s) is designated as the principal/first-listed diagnosis. The primary malignancy is coded as an additional code.

3) **Malignant neoplasm in a pregnant patient**
When a pregnant woman has a malignant neoplasm, a code from subcategory O9A.1-, Malignant neoplasm complicating pregnancy, childbirth, and the puerperium, should be sequenced first, followed by the appropriate code from Chapter 2 to indicate the type of neoplasm.

4) **Encounter for complication associated with a neoplasm**
When an encounter is for management of a complication associated with a neoplasm, such as dehydration, and the treatment is only for the complication, the complication is coded first, followed by the appropriate code(s) for the neoplasm.
The exception to this guideline is anemia. When the admission/encounter is for management of an anemia associated with the malignancy, and the treatment is only for anemia, the appropriate code for the malignancy is sequenced as the principal or first-listed diagnosis followed by code D63.0, Anemia in neoplastic disease.

5) **Complication from surgical procedure for treatment of a neoplasm**
When an encounter is for treatment of a complication resulting from a surgical procedure performed for the treatment of the neoplasm, designate the complication as the principal/first-listed diagnosis. See guideline regarding the coding of a current malignancy versus personal history to determine if the code for the neoplasm should also be assigned.

6) **Pathologic fracture due to a neoplasm**
When an encounter is for a pathological fracture due to a neoplasm, and the focus of treatment is the fracture, a code from subcategory M84.5, Pathological fracture in neoplastic disease, should be sequenced first, followed by the code for the neoplasm.

If the focus of treatment is the neoplasm with an associated pathological fracture, the neoplasm code should be sequenced first, followed by a code from M84.5 for the pathological fracture.

m. **Current malignancy versus personal history of malignancy**
When a primary malignancy has been excised but further treatment, such as an additional surgery for the malignancy, radiation therapy or chemotherapy is directed to that site, the primary malignancy code should be used until treatment is completed.

When a primary malignancy has been previously excised or eradicated from its site, there is no further treatment (of the malignancy) directed to that site, and there is no evidence of any existing primary malignancy, a code from category Z85, Personal history of malignant neoplasm, should be used to indicate the former site of the malignancy.

See Section I.C.21. Factors influencing health status and contact with health services, History (of).

n. **Leukemia, Multiple Myeloma, and Malignant Plasma Cell Neoplasms in remission versus personal history**
The categories for leukemia, and category C90, Multiple myeloma and malignant plasma cell neoplasms, have codes indicating whether or not the leukemia has achieved remission. There are also codes Z85.6, Personal history of leukemia, and Z85.79, Personal history of other malignant neoplasms of lymphoid, hematopoietic and related tissues. If the documentation is unclear, as to whether the leukemia has achieved remission, the provider should be queried.

See Section I.C.21. Factors influencing health status and contact with health services, History (of).

o. **Aftercare following surgery for neoplasm**
See Section I.C.21. Factors influencing health status and contact with health services, Aftercare.

p. **Follow-up care for completed treatment of a malignancy**
See Section I.C.21. Factors influencing health status and contact with health services, Follow-up.

q. **Prophylactic organ removal for prevention of malignancy**
See Section I.C.21. Factors influencing health status and contact with health services, Prophylactic organ removal.

r. **Malignant neoplasm associated with transplanted organ**
A malignant neoplasm of a transplanted organ should be coded as a transplant complication. Assign first the appropriate code from category T86.-, Complications of transplanted organs and tissue, followed by code C80.2, Malignant neoplasm associated with transplanted organ. Use an additional code for the specific malignancy.

3. **Chapter 3: Disease of the Blood and Blood-forming Organs and Certain Disorders Involving the Immune Mechanism (D50-D89)**

Reserved for future guideline expansion

4. **Chapter 4: Endocrine, Nutritional, and Metabolic Diseases (E00-E89)**

a. **Diabetes mellitus**
The diabetes mellitus codes are combination codes that include the type of diabetes mellitus, the body system affected, and the complications affecting that body system. As many codes within a particular category as are necessary to describe all of the complications of the disease may be used. They should be sequenced based on the reason for a particular encounter. Assign as many codes from categories E08 – E13 as needed to identify all of the associated conditions that the patient has.

1) **Type of diabetes**
The age of a patient is not the sole determining factor, though most type 1 diabetics develop the condition before reaching puberty. For this reason type 1 diabetes mellitus is also referred to as juvenile diabetes.

2) **Type of diabetes mellitus not documented**
If the type of diabetes mellitus is not documented in the medical record the default is E11.-, Type 2 diabetes mellitus.

3) **Diabetes mellitus and the use of insulin *and oral hypoglycemics***
If the documentation in a medical record does not indicate the type of diabetes but does indicate that the patient uses insulin, code E11, Type 2 diabetes mellitus, should be assigned. Code Z79.4, Long-term (current) use of insulin, or Z79.84, Long term (current) use of oral hypoglycemic drugs, should also be assigned to indicate that the patient uses insulin or hypoglycemic drugs. Code Z79.4 should not be assigned if insulin is given temporarily to bring a type 2 patient's blood sugar under control during an encounter.

4) **Diabetes mellitus in pregnancy and gestational diabetes**
See Section I.C.15. Diabetes mellitus in pregnancy.
See Section I.C.15. Gestational (pregnancy induced) diabetes.

5) **Complications due to Insulin pump malfunction**

(a) **Underdose of insulin due to insulin pump failure**
An underdose of insulin due to an insulin pump failure should be assigned to a code from subcategory T85.6, Mechanical complication of other specified internal and external prosthetic devices, implants and grafts, that specifies the type of pump malfunction, as the principal or first-listed code, followed by code T38.3x6-, Underdosing of insulin and oral hypoglycemic [antidiabetic] drugs. Additional codes for the type of diabetes mellitus and any associated complications due to the underdosing should also be assigned.

(b) **Overdose of insulin due to insulin pump failure**
The principal or first-listed code for an encounter due to an insulin pump malfunction resulting in an overdose of insulin, should also be T85.6-, Mechanical complication of other specified internal and external prosthetic devices, implants and grafts, followed by code T38.3x1-, Poisoning by insulin and oral hypoglycemic [antidiabetic] drugs, accidental (unintentional).

CHAPTER 4 – ENDOCRINE & METABOLIC
Section I. C. 4. a. 6)

6) Secondary diabetes mellitus
Codes under categories E08, Diabetes mellitus due to underlying condition, and E09, Drug or chemical induced diabetes mellitus, and E13, Other specified diabetes mellitus, identify complications/manifestations associated with secondary diabetes mellitus. Secondary diabetes is always caused by another condition or event (e.g., cystic fibrosis, malignant neoplasm of pancreas, pancreatectomy, adverse effect of drug, or poisoning).

(a) Secondary diabetes mellitus and the use of insulin *or oral hypoglycemic drugs*
For patients who routinely use insulin or hypoglycemic drugs, code Z79.4, Long-term (current) use of insulin, or Z79.84, Long term (current) use of oral hypoglycemic drugs, should also be assigned. Code Z79.4 should not be assigned if insulin is given temporarily to bring a patient's blood sugar under control during an encounter.

(b) Assigning and sequencing secondary diabetes codes and its causes
The sequencing of the secondary diabetes codes in relationship to codes for the cause of the diabetes is based on the Tabular List instructions for categories E08, E09 and E13.

(i) Secondary diabetes mellitus due to pancreatectomy
For postpancreatectomy diabetes mellitus (lack of insulin due to the surgical removal of all or part of the pancreas), assign code E89.1, Postprocedural hypoinsulinemia. Assign a code from category E13 and a code from subcategory Z90.41-, Acquired absence of pancreas, as additional codes.

(ii) Secondary diabetes due to drugs
Secondary diabetes may be caused by an adverse effect of correctly administered medications, poisoning or sequela of poisoning.

See section I.C.19.e for coding of adverse effects and poisoning, and section I.C.20 for external cause code reporting.

---

5. Chapter 5: Mental and Behavioral Disorders (F01 – F99)

a. Pain disorders related to psychological factors
Assign code F45.41, for pain that is exclusively related to psychological disorders. As indicated by the Excludes1 note under category G89, a code from category G89 should not be assigned with code F45.41.

Code F45.42, Pain disorders with related psychological factors, should be used should be used with a code from category G89, Pain, not elsewhere classified, if there is documentation of a psychological component for a patient with acute or chronic pain.

See Section I.C.6. Pain.

b. Mental and behavioral disorders due to psychoactive substance use

1) In Remission
Selection of codes for "in remission" for categories F10-F19, Mental and behavioral disorders due to psychoactive substance use (categories F10-F19 with -.21) requires the provider's clinical judgment. The appropriate codes for "in remission" are assigned only on the basis of provider documentation (as defined in the Official Guidelines for Coding and Reporting).

2) Psychoactive Substance Use, Abuse And Dependence
When the provider documentation refers to use, abuse and dependence of the same substance (e.g. alcohol, opioid, cannabis, etc.), only one code should be assigned to identify the pattern of use based on the following hierarchy:
• If both use and abuse are documented, assign only the code for abuse
• If both abuse and dependence are documented, assign only the code for dependence
• If use, abuse and dependence are all documented, assign only the code for dependence
• If both use and dependence are documented, assign only the code for dependence

3) Psychoactive Substance Use
As with all other diagnoses, the codes for psychoactive substance use (F10.9-, F11.9-, F12.9-, F13.9-, F14.9-, F15.9-, F16.9-) should only be assigned based on provider documentation and when they meet the definition of a reportable diagnosis (see Section III, Reporting Additional Diagnoses). The codes are to be used only when the psychoactive substance use is associated with a mental or behavioral disorder, and such a relationship is documented by the provider.

CHAPTER 6 – NERVOUS SYSTEM
Section I. C. 6. a.

6. Chapter 6: Diseases of Nervous System and Sense Organs (G00-G99)

a. Dominant/nondominant side
Codes from category G81, Hemiplegia and hemiparesis, and subcategories, G83.1, Monoplegia of lower limb, G83.2, Monoplegia of upper limb, and G83.3, Monoplegia, unspecified, identify whether the dominant or nondominant side is affected. Should the affected side be documented, but not specified as dominant or nondominant, and the classification system does not indicate a default, code selection is as follows:
• For ambidextrous patients, the default should be dominant.
• If the left side is affected, the default is non-dominant.
• If the right side is affected, the default is dominant.

b. Pain - Category G89

1) General coding information
Codes in category G89, Pain, not elsewhere classified, may be used in conjunction with codes from other categories and chapters to provide more detail about acute or chronic pain and neoplasm-related pain, unless otherwise indicated below.

If the pain is not specified as acute or chronic, post-thoracotomy, postprocedural, or neoplasm-related, do not assign codes from category G89.

A code from category G89 should not be assigned if the underlying (definitive) diagnosis is known, unless the reason for the encounter is pain control/management and not management of the underlying condition.

When an admission or encounter is for a procedure aimed at treating the underlying condition (e.g., spinal fusion, kyphoplasty), a code for the underlying condition (e.g., vertebral fracture, spinal stenosis) should be assigned as the principal diagnosis. No code from category G89 should be assigned.

(a) Category G89 Codes as Principal or First-Listed Diagnosis
Category G89 codes are acceptable as principal diagnosis or the first-listed code:
• When pain control or pain management is the reason for the admission/encounter (e.g., a patient with displaced intervertebral disc, nerve impingement and severe back pain presents for injection of steroid into the spinal canal). The underlying cause of the pain should be reported as an additional diagnosis, if known.

• When a patient is admitted for the insertion of a neurostimulator for pain control, assign the appropriate pain code as the principal or first-listed diagnosis. When an admission or encounter is for a procedure aimed at treating the underlying condition and a neurostimulator is inserted for pain control during the same admission/encounter, a code for the underlying condition should be assigned as the principal diagnosis and the appropriate pain code should be assigned as a secondary diagnosis.

(b) Use of Category G89 Codes in Conjunction with Site Specific Pain Codes

(i) Assigning Category G89 and Site-Specific Pain Codes
Codes from category G89 may be used in conjunction with codes that identify the site of pain (including codes from chapter 18) if the category G89 code provides additional information. For example, if the code describes the site of the pain, but does not fully describe whether the pain is acute or chronic, then both codes should be assigned.

(ii) Sequencing of Category G89 Codes with Site-Specific Pain Codes
The sequencing of category G89 codes with site-specific pain codes (including chapter 18 codes), is dependent on the circumstances of the encounter/admission as follows:
• If the encounter is for pain control or pain management, assign the code from category G89 followed by the code identifying the specific site of pain (e.g., encounter for pain management for acute neck pain from trauma is assigned code G89.11, Acute pain due to trauma, followed by code M54.2, Cervicalgia, to identify the site of pain).

• If the encounter is for any other reason except pain control or pain management, and a related definitive diagnosis has not been established (confirmed) by the provider, assign the code for the specific site of pain first, followed by the appropriate code from category G89.

2) Pain due to devices, implants and grafts
See Section I.C.19. Pain due to medical devices.

CHAPTER 6 – NERVOUS SYSTEM
Section I. C. 6. b. 3)

3) Postoperative Pain

The provider's documentation should be used to guide the coding of postoperative pain, as well as *Section III. Reporting Additional Diagnoses and Section IV. Diagnostic Coding and Reporting in the Outpatient Setting.*

The default for post-thoracotomy and other postoperative pain not specified as acute or chronic is the code for the acute form.

Routine or expected postoperative pain immediately after surgery should not be coded.

(a) Postoperative pain not associated with specific postoperative complication

Postoperative pain not associated with a specific postoperative complication is assigned to the appropriate postoperative pain code in category G89.

(b) Postoperative pain associated with specific postoperative complication

Postoperative pain associated with a specific postoperative complication (such as painful wire sutures) is assigned to the appropriate code(s) found in Chapter 19, Injury, poisoning, and certain other consequences of external causes. If appropriate, use additional code(s) from category G89 to identify acute or chronic pain (G89.18 or G89.28).

4) Chronic pain

Chronic pain is classified to subcategory G89.2. There is no time frame defining when pain becomes chronic pain. The provider's documentation should be used to guide use of these codes.

5) Neoplasm Related Pain

Code G89.3 is assigned to pain documented as being related, associated or due to cancer, primary or secondary malignancy, or tumor. This code is assigned regardless of whether the pain is acute or chronic.

This code may be assigned as the principal or first-listed code when the stated reason for the admission/encounter is documented as pain control/pain management. The underlying neoplasm should be reported as an additional diagnosis.

When the reason for the admission/encounter is management of the neoplasm and the pain associated with the neoplasm is also documented, code G89.3 may be assigned as an additional diagnosis. It is not necessary to assign an additional code for the site of the pain.

See Section I.C.2 for instructions on the sequencing of neoplasms for all other stated reasons for the admission/encounter (except for pain control/pain management).

6) Chronic pain syndrome

Central pain syndrome (G89.0) and chronic pain syndrome (G89.4) are different than the term "chronic pain," and therefore codes should only be used when the provider has specifically documented this condition.

See Section I.C.5. Pain disorders related to psychological factors.

7. Chapter 7: Diseases of Eye and Adnexa (H00-H59)

a. Glaucoma

1) Assigning Glaucoma Codes

Assign as many codes from category H40, Glaucoma, as needed to identify the type of glaucoma, the affected eye, and the glaucoma stage.

2) Bilateral glaucoma with same type and stage

When a patient has bilateral glaucoma and both eyes are documented as being the same type and stage, and there is a code for bilateral glaucoma, report only the code for the type of glaucoma, bilateral, with the seventh character for the stage.

When a patient has bilateral glaucoma and both eyes are documented as being the same type and stage, and the classification does not provide a code for bilateral glaucoma (i.e. subcategories H40.10, H40.11 and H40.20) report only one code for the type of glaucoma with the appropriate seventh character for the stage.

3) Bilateral glaucoma stage with different types or stages

When a patient has bilateral glaucoma and each eye is documented as having a different type or stage, and the classification distinguishes laterality, assign the appropriate code for each eye rather than the code for bilateral glaucoma.

When a patient has bilateral glaucoma and each eye is documented as having a different type, and the classification does not distinguish laterality (i.e. subcategories H40.10, H40.11 and H40.20), assign one code for each type of glaucoma with the appropriate seventh character for the stage.

CHAPTER 7 – EYE AND ADNEXA
Section I. C. 7. a. 3)

When a patient has bilateral glaucoma and each eye is documented as having the same type, but different stage, and the classification does not distinguish laterality (i.e. subcategories H40.10, H40.11 and H40.20), assign a code for the type of glaucoma for each eye with the seventh character for the specific glaucoma stage documented for each eye.

4) Patient admitted with glaucoma and stage evolves during the admission

If a patient is admitted with glaucoma and the stage progresses during the admission, assign the code for highest stage documented.

5) Indeterminate stage glaucoma

Assignment of the seventh character "4" for "indeterminate stage" should be based on the clinical documentation. The seventh character "4" is used for glaucomas whose stage cannot be clinically determined. This seventh character should not be confused with the seventh character "0", unspecified, which should be assigned when there is no documentation regarding the stage of the glaucoma.

8. Chapter 8: Diseases of Ear and Mastoid Process (H60-H95)

Reserved for future guideline expansion

9. Chapter 9: Diseases of Circulatory System (I00-I99)

a. Hypertension

The classification presumes a causal relationship between hypertension and heart involvement and between hypertension and kidney involvement, as the two conditions are linked by the term "with" in the Alphabetic Index. These conditions should be coded as related even in the absence of provider documentation explicitly linking them, unless the documentation clearly states the conditions are unrelated.

For hypertension and conditions not specifically linked by relational terms such as "with," "associated with" or "due to" in the classification, provider documentaton must link the conditions in order to code them as related.

1) Hypertension with Heart Disease

Hypertension with heart conditions classified to I50.- or I51.4-I51.9, are assigned to, a code from category I11, Hypertensive heart disease, when a causal relationship is stated (due to hypertension) or implied (hypertensive). Use an additional code from category I50, Heart failure, to identify the type of heart failure in those patients with heart failure.

The same heart conditions (I50.-, I51.4-I51.9) with hypertension, ~~but without a stated causal relationship,~~ are coded separately if the provider has specifically documented a different cause. Sequence according to the circumstances of the admission/encounter.

2) Hypertensive Chronic Kidney Disease

Assign codes from category I12, Hypertensive chronic kidney disease, when both hypertension and a condition classifiable to category N18, Chronic kidney disease (CKD), are present. ~~Unlike hypertension with heart disease, ICD-10-CM presumes a cause-and-effect relationship and classifies chronic kidney disease with hypertension as hypertensive chronic kidney disease.~~ CKD should not be coded as hypertensive if the physician has specifically documented a different cause.

The appropriate code from category N18 should be used as a secondary code with a code from category I12 to identify the stage of chronic kidney disease.

See Section I.C.14. Chronic kidney disease.

If a patient has hypertensive chronic kidney disease and acute renal failure, an additional code for the acute renal failure is required.

3) Hypertensive Heart and Chronic Kidney Disease

Assign codes from combination category I13, Hypertensive heart and chronic kidney disease, when ~~both hypertensive kidney disease and hypertensive heart disease are stated in the diagnosis~~ there is hypertension with both heart and kidney involvement. ~~Assume a relationship between the hypertension and the chronic kidney disease, whether or not the condition is so designated.~~ If heart failure is present, assign an additional code from category I50 to identify the type of heart failure.

The appropriate code from category N18, Chronic kidney disease, should be used as a secondary code with a code from category I13 to identify the stage of chronic kidney disease.

See Section I.C.14. Chronic kidney disease.

CHAPTER 9 – CIRCULATORY SYSTEM
Section I. C. 9. a. 3)

The codes in category I13, Hypertensive heart and chronic kidney disease, are combination codes that include hypertension, heart disease and chronic kidney disease. The Includes note at I13 specifies that the conditions included at I11 and I12 are included together in I13. If a patient has hypertension, heart disease and chronic kidney disease then a code from I13 should be used, not individual codes for hypertension, heart disease and chronic kidney disease, or codes from I11 or I12.

For patients with both acute renal failure and chronic kidney disease, an additional code for acute renal failure is required.

4) Hypertensive Cerebrovascular Disease
For hypertensive cerebrovascular disease, first assign the appropriate code from categories I60-I69, followed by the appropriate hypertension code.

5) Hypertensive Retinopathy
Subcategory H35.0, Background retinopathy and retinal vascular changes, should be used with a code from category I10-I15, Hypertensive disease to include the systemic hypertension. The sequencing is based on the reason for the encounter.

6) Hypertension, Secondary
Secondary hypertension is due to an underlying condition. Two codes are required: one to identify the underlying etiology and one from category I15 to identify the hypertension. Sequencing of codes is determined by the reason for admission/encounter.

7) Hypertension, Transient
Assign code R03.0, Elevated blood pressure reading without diagnosis of hypertension, unless patient has an established diagnosis of hypertension. Assign code O13.-, Gestational [pregnancy-induced] hypertension without significant proteinuria, or O14.-, Pre-eclampsia, for transient hypertension of pregnancy.

8) Hypertension, Controlled
This diagnostic statement usually refers to an existing state of hypertension under control by therapy. Assign the appropriate code from categories I10-I15, Hypertensive diseases.

9) Hypertension, Uncontrolled
Uncontrolled hypertension may refer to untreated hypertension or hypertension not responding to current therapeutic regimen. In either case, assign the appropriate code from categories I10-I15, Hypertensive diseases.

10) Hypertensive Crisis
Assign a code from category I16, Hypertensive crisis, for documented hypertensive urgency, hypertensive emergency or unspecified hypertensive crisis. Code also any identified hypertensive disease (I10-I15). The sequencing is based on the reason for the encounter.

b. Atherosclerotic Coronary Artery Disease and Angina
ICD-10-CM has combination codes for atherosclerotic heart disease with angina pectoris. The subcategories for these codes are I25.11, Atherosclerotic heart disease of native coronary artery with angina pectoris and I25.7, Atherosclerosis of coronary artery bypass graft(s) and coronary artery of transplanted heart with angina pectoris.

When using one of these combination codes it is not necessary to use an additional code for angina pectoris. A causal relationship can be assumed in a patient with both atherosclerosis and angina pectoris, unless the documentation indicates the angina is due to something other than the atherosclerosis.

If a patient with coronary artery disease is admitted due to an acute myocardial infarction (AMI), the AMI should be sequenced before the coronary artery disease.

See Section I.C.9. Acute myocardial infarction (AMI).

c. Intraoperative and Postprocedural Cerebrovascular Accident
Medical record documentation should clearly specify the cause-and-effect relationship between the medical intervention and the cerebrovascular accident in order to assign a code for intraoperative or postprocedural cerebrovascular accident.

Proper code assignment depends on whether it was an infarction or hemorrhage and whether it occurred intraoperatively or postoperatively. If it was a cerebral hemorrhage, code assignment depends on the type of procedure performed.

CHAPTER 9 – CIRCULATORY SYSTEM
Section I. C. 9. d. 1)

d. Sequelae of Cerebrovascular Disease

1) Category I69, Sequelae of Cerebrovascular disease
Category I69 is used to indicate conditions classifiable to categories I60-I67 as the causes of sequela (neurologic deficits), themselves classified elsewhere. These "late effects" include neurologic deficits that persist after initial onset of conditions classifiable to categories I60-I67. The neurologic deficits caused by cerebrovascular disease may be present from the onset or may arise at any time after the onset of the condition classifiable to categories I60-I67.

Codes from category I69, Sequelae of cerebrovascular disease, that specify hemiplegia, hemiparesis and monoplegia identify whether the dominant or nondominant side is affected. Should the affected side be documented, but not specified as dominant or nondominant, and the classification system does not indicate a default, code selection is as follows:
- For ambidextrous patients, the default should be dominant.
- If the left side is affected, the default is nondominant.
- If the right side is affected, the default is dominant.

2) Codes from category I69 with codes from I60-I67
Codes from category I69 may be assigned on a health care record with codes from I60-I67, if the patient has a current cerebrovascular disease and deficits from an old cerebrovascular disease.

3) Codes from category I69 and Personal history of transient ischemic attack (TIA) and cerebral infarction (Z86.73)
Codes from category I69 should not be assigned if the patient does not have neurologic deficits.

See Section I.C.21.c.4. History (of) for use of personal history codes.

e. Acute myocardial infarction (AMI)

1) ST elevation myocardial infarction (STEMI) and non ST elevation myocardial infarction (NSTEMI)
The ICD-10-CM codes for acute myocardial infarction (AMI) identify the site, such as anterolateral wall or true posterior wall. Subcategories I21.0-I21.2 and code I21.3 are used for ST elevation myocardial infarction (STEMI). Code I21.4, Non-ST elevation (NSTEMI) myocardial infarction, is used for non ST elevation myocardial infarction (NSTEMI) and nontransmural MIs.

If NSTEMI evolves to STEMI, assign the STEMI code. If STEMI converts to NSTEMI due to thrombolytic therapy, it is still coded as STEMI.

For encounters occurring while the myocardial infarction is equal to, or less than, four weeks old, including transfers to another acute setting or a postacute setting, and ~~the patient requires continued care for~~ the myocardial infarction meets the definition for "other diagnoses" (see Section III, Reporting Additional Diagnoses), codes from category I21 may continue to be reported. For encounters after the 4 week time frame and the patient is still receiving care related to the myocardial infarction, the appropriate aftercare code should be assigned, rather than a code from category I21. For old or healed myocardial infarctions not requiring further care, code I25.2, Old myocardial infarction, may be assigned.

2) Acute myocardial infarction, unspecified
Code I21.3, ST elevation (STEMI) myocardial infarction of unspecified site, is the default for the unspecified acute myocardial infarction. If only STEMI or transmural MI without the site is documented, assign code I21.3.

3) AMI documented as nontransmural or subendocardial but site provided
If an AMI is documented as nontransmural or subendocardial, but the site is provided, it is still coded as a subendocardial AMI.

See Section I.C.21.3 for information on coding status post administration of tPA in a different facility within the last 24 hours.

4) Subsequent acute myocardial infarction
A code from category I22, Subsequent ST elevation (STEMI) and non ST elevation (NSTEMI) myocardial infarction, is to be used when a patient who has suffered an AMI has a new AMI within the 4 week time frame of the initial AMI. A code from category I22 must be used in conjunction with a code from category I21. The sequencing of the I22 and I21 codes depends on the circumstances of the encounter.

CHAPTER 10 – RESPIRATORY SYSTEM
Section I. C. 10. a.

10. Chapter 10: Diseases of the Respiratory System (J00-J99)

a. Chronic Obstructive Pulmonary Disease [COPD] and Asthma

1) Acute exacerbation of chronic obstructive bronchitis and asthma

The codes in categories J44 and J45 distinguish between uncomplicated cases and those in acute exacerbation. An acute exacerbation is a worsening or a decompensation of a chronic condition. An acute exacerbation is not equivalent to an infection superimposed on a chronic condition, though an exacerbation may be triggered by an infection.

b. Acute Respiratory Failure

1) Acute respiratory failure as principal diagnosis

A code from subcategory J96.0, Acute respiratory failure, or subcategory J96.2, Acute and chronic respiratory failure, may be assigned as a principal diagnosis when it is the condition established after study to be chiefly responsible for occasioning the admission to the hospital, and the selection is supported by the Alphabetic Index and Tabular List. However, chapter-specific coding guidelines (such as obstetrics, poisoning, HIV, newborn) that provide sequencing direction take precedence.

2) Acute respiratory failure as secondary diagnosis

Respiratory failure may be listed as a secondary diagnosis if it occurs after admission, or if it is present on admission, but does not meet the definition of principal diagnosis.

3) Sequencing of acute respiratory failure and another acute condition

When a patient is admitted with respiratory failure and another acute condition, (e.g., myocardial infarction, cerebrovascular accident, aspiration pneumonia), the principal diagnosis will not be the same in every situation. This applies whether the other acute condition is a respiratory or nonrespiratory condition. Selection of the principal diagnosis will be dependent on the circumstances of admission. If both the respiratory failure and the other acute condition are equally responsible for occasioning the admission to the hospital, and there are no chapter-specific sequencing rules, the guideline regarding two or more diagnoses that equally meet the definition for principal diagnosis *(Section II, C.)* may be applied in these situations.

If the documentation is not clear as to whether acute respiratory failure and another condition are equally responsible for occasioning the admission, query the provider for clarification.

c. Influenza due to certain identified influenza viruses

Code only confirmed cases of influenza due to certain identified influenza viruses (category J09), and due to other identified influenza virus (category J10). This is an exception to the hospital inpatient guideline Section II, H. (Uncertain Diagnosis).

In this context, "confirmation" does not require documentation of positive laboratory testing specific for avian or other novel influenza A or other identified influenza virus. However, coding should be based on the provider's diagnostic statement that the patient has avian influenza, or other novel influenza A, for category J09, or has another particular identified strain of influenza, such as H1N1 or H3N2, but not identified as novel or variant, for category J10.

If the provider records "suspected" or "possible" or "probable" avian influenza, or novel influenza, or other identified influenza, then the appropriate influenza code from category J11, Influenza due to unidentified influenza virus, should be assigned. A code from category J09, Influenza due to certain identified influenza viruses, should not be assigned nor should a code from category J10, Influenza due to other identified influenza virus.

d. Ventilator associated Pneumonia

1) Documentation of Ventilator associated Pneumonia

As with all procedural or postprocedural complications, code assignment is based on the provider's documentation of the relationship between the condition and the procedure.

Code J95.851, Ventilator associated pneumonia, should be assigned only when the provider has documented ventilator associated pneumonia (VAP). An additional code to identify the organism (e.g., Pseudomonas aeruginosa, code B96.5) should also be assigned. Do not assign an additional code from categories J12-J18 to identify the type of pneumonia.

Code J95.851 should not be assigned for cases where the patient has pneumonia and is on a mechanical ventilator and the provider has not specifically stated that the pneumonia is ventilator-associated pneumonia. If the documentation is unclear as to whether the patient has a pneumonia that is a complication attributable to the mechanical ventilator, query the provider.

CHAPTER 10 – RESPIRATORY SYSTEM
Section I. C. 11. d. 2)

2) Ventilator associated Pneumonia Develops after Admission

A patient may be admitted with one type of pneumonia (e.g., code J13, Pneumonia due to Streptococcus pneumonia) and subsequently develop VAP. In this instance, the principal diagnosis would be the appropriate code from categories J12-J18 for the pneumonia diagnosed at the time of admission. Code J95.851, Ventilator associated pneumonia, would be assigned as an additional diagnosis when the provider has also documented the presence of ventilator associated pneumonia.

11. Chapter 11: Diseases of the Digestive System (K00-K94)

Reserved for future guideline expansion

12. Chapter 12: Diseases of the Skin and Subcutaneous Tissue (L00-L99)

a. Pressure ulcer stage codes

1) Pressure ulcer stages

Codes from category L89, Pressure ulcer, ~~are combination codes that~~ identify the site of the pressure ulcer as well as the stage of the ulcer.

The ICD-10-CM classifies pressure ulcer stages based on severity, which is designated by stages 1-4, unspecified stage and unstageable.

Assign as many codes from category L89 as needed to identify all the pressure ulcers the patient has, if applicable.

2) Unstageable pressure ulcers

Assignment of the code for unstageable pressure ulcer (L89.--0) should be based on the clinical documentation. These codes are used for pressure ulcers whose stage cannot be clinically determined (e.g., the ulcer is covered by eschar or has been treated with a skin or muscle graft) and pressure ulcers that are documented as deep tissue injury but not documented as due to trauma. This code should not be confused with the codes for unspecified stage (L89.--9). When there is no documentation regarding the stage of the pressure ulcer, assign the appropriate code for unspecified stage (L89.--9).

3) Documented pressure ulcer stage

Assignment of the pressure ulcer stage code should be guided by clinical documentation of the stage or documentation of the terms found in the Alphabetic Index. For clinical terms describing the stage that are not found in the Alphabetic Index, and there is no documentation of the stage, the provider should be queried.

4) Patients admitted with pressure ulcers documented as healed

No code is assigned if the documentation states that the pressure ulcer is completely healed.

5) Patients admitted with pressure ulcers documented as healing

Pressure ulcers described as healing should be assigned the appropriate pressure ulcer stage code based on the documentation in the medical record. If the documentation does not provide information about the stage of the healing pressure ulcer, assign the appropriate code for unspecified stage.

If the documentation is unclear as to whether the patient has a current (new) pressure ulcer or if the patient is being treated for a healing pressure ulcer, query the provider.

For ulcers that were present on admission but healed at the time of discharge, assign the code for the site and stage of the pressure ulcer at the time of admission.

6) Patient admitted with pressure ulcer evolving into another stage during the admission

If a patient is admitted with a pressure ulcer at one stage and it progresses to a higher stage, ~~assign the code for the highest stage reported for that site~~ two separate codes should be assigned: one code for the site and stage of the ulcer on admission and a second code for the same ulcer site and the highest stage reported during the stay.

GUIDELINES

CHAPTER 13 – MUSCULOSKELETAL SYSTEM
Section I. C. 13. a.

13. Chapter 13: Diseases of the Musculoskeletal System and Connective Tissue (M00-M99)

a. Site and laterality

Most of the codes within Chapter 13 have site and laterality designations. The site represents the bone, joint or the muscle involved. For some conditions where more than one bone, joint or muscle is usually involved, such as osteoarthritis, there is a "multiple sites" code available. For categories where no multiple site code is provided and more than one bone, joint or muscle is involved, multiple codes should be used to indicate the different sites involved.

1) Bone versus joint

For certain conditions, the bone may be affected at the upper or lower end, (e.g., avascular necrosis of bone, M87, Osteoporosis, M80, M81). Though the portion of the bone affected may be at the joint, the site designation will be the bone, not the joint.

b. Acute traumatic versus chronic or recurrent musculoskeletal conditions

Many musculoskeletal conditions are a result of previous injury or trauma to a site, or are recurrent conditions. Bone, joint or muscle conditions that are the result of a healed injury are usually found in chapter 13. Recurrent bone, joint or muscle conditions are also usually found in chapter 13. Any current, acute injury should be coded to the appropriate injury code from chapter 19. Chronic or recurrent conditions should generally be coded with a code from chapter 13. If it is difficult to determine from the documentation in the record which code is best to describe a condition, query the provider.

c. Coding of Pathologic Fractures

7th character A is for use as long as the patient is receiving active treatment for the fracture. ~~Examples of active treatment are: surgical treatment, emergency department encounter, evaluation and continuing treatment by the same or a different physician.~~ While the patient may be seen by a new or different provider over the course of treatment for a pathological fracture, assignment of the 7th character is based on whether the patient is undergoing active treatment and not whether the provider is seeing the patient for the first time.

7th character D is to be used for encounters after the patient has completed active treatment. The other 7th characters, listed under each subcategory in the Tabular List, are to be used for subsequent encounters for routine care of fractures during the healing and recovery phase as well as treatment of problems associated with the healing, such as malunions, nonunions, and sequelae.

Care for complications of surgical treatment for fracture repairs during the healing or recovery phase should be coded with the appropriate complication codes.

See Section I.C.19. Coding of traumatic fractures.

d. Osteoporosis

Osteoporosis is a systemic condition, meaning that all bones of the musculoskeletal system are affected. Therefore, site is not a component of the codes under category M81, Osteoporosis without current pathological fracture. The site codes under category M80, Osteoporosis with current pathological fracture, identify the site of the fracture, not the osteoporosis.

1) Osteoporosis without pathological fracture

Category M81, Osteoporosis without current pathological fracture, is for use for patients with osteoporosis who do not currently have a pathologic fracture due to the osteoporosis, even if they have had a fracture in the past. For patients with a history of osteoporosis fractures, status code Z87.310, Personal history of (healed) osteoporosis fracture, should follow the code from M81.

2) Osteoporosis with current pathological fracture

Category M80, Osteoporosis with current pathological fracture, is for patients who have a current pathologic fracture at the time of an encounter. The codes under M80 identify the site of the fracture. A code from category M80, not a traumatic fracture code, should be used for any patient with known osteoporosis who suffers a fracture, even if the patient had a minor fall or trauma, if that fall or trauma would not usually break a normal, healthy bone.

CHAPTER 14 – GENITOURINARY SYSTEM
Section I. C. 14. a.

14. Chapter 14: Diseases of Genitourinary System (N00-N99)

a. Chronic kidney disease

1) Stages of chronic kidney disease (CKD)

The ICD-10-CM classifies CKD based on severity. The severity of CKD is designated by stages 1-5. Stage 2, code N18.2, equates to mild CKD; stage 3, code N18.3, equates to moderate CKD; and stage 4, code N18.4, equates to severe CKD. Code N18.6, End stage renal disease (ESRD), is assigned when the provider has documented end-stage-renal disease (ESRD).

If both a stage of CKD and ESRD are documented, assign code N18.6 only.

2) Chronic kidney disease and kidney transplant status

Patients who have undergone kidney transplant may still have some form of chronic kidney disease (CKD) because the kidney transplant may not fully restore kidney function. Therefore, the presence of CKD alone does not constitute a transplant complication. Assign the appropriate N18 code for the patient's stage of CKD and code Z94.0, Kidney transplant status. If a transplant complication such as failure or rejection or other transplant complication is documented, see section I.C.19.g for information on coding complications of a kidney transplant. If the documentation is unclear as to whether the patient has a complication of the transplant, query the provider.

3) Chronic kidney disease with other conditions

Patients with CKD may also suffer from other serious conditions, most commonly diabetes mellitus and hypertension. The sequencing of the CKD code in relationship to codes for other contributing conditions is based on the conventions in the Tabular List.

See I.C.9. Hypertensive chronic kidney disease.
See I.C.19. Chronic kidney disease and kidney transplant complications.

15. Chapter 15: Pregnancy, Childbirth, and the Puerperium (O00-O9A)

a. General Rules for Obstetric Cases

1) Codes from chapter 15 and sequencing priority

Obstetric cases require codes from chapter 15, codes in the range O00-O9A, Pregnancy, Childbirth, and the Puerperium. Chapter 15 codes have sequencing priority over codes from other chapters. Additional codes from other chapters may be used in conjunction with chapter 15 codes to further specify conditions. Should the provider document that the pregnancy is incidental to the encounter, then code Z33.1, Pregnant state, incidental, should be used in place of any chapter 15 codes. It is the provider's responsibility to state that the condition being treated is not affecting the pregnancy.

2) Chapter 15 codes used only on the maternal record

Chapter 15 codes are to be used only on the maternal record, never on the record of the newborn.

3) Final character for trimester

The majority of codes in Chapter 15 have a final character indicating the trimester of pregnancy. The timeframes for the trimesters are indicated at the beginning of the chapter. If trimester is not a component of a code it is because the condition always occurs in a specific trimester, or the concept of trimester of pregnancy is not applicable. Certain codes have characters for only certain trimesters because the condition does not occur in all trimesters, but it may occur in more than just one.

Assignment of the final character for trimester should be based on the provider's documentation of the trimester (or number of weeks) for the current admission/encounter. This applies to the assignment of trimester for pre-existing conditions as well as those that develop during or are due to the pregnancy. The provider's documentation of the number of weeks may be used to assign the appropriate code identifying the trimester.

Whenever delivery occurs during the current admission, and there is an "in childbirth" option for the obstetric complication being coded, the "in childbirth" code should be assigned.

4) Selection of trimester for inpatient admissions that encompass more than one trimesters

In instances when a patient is admitted to a hospital for complications of pregnancy during one trimester and remains in the hospital into a subsequent trimester, the trimester character for the antepartum complication code should be assigned on the basis of the trimester when the complication developed, not the trimester of the discharge. If the condition developed prior to the current admission/encounter or represents a pre-existing condition, the trimester character for the trimester at the time of the admission/encounter should be assigned.

[2017.CM] OFFICIAL CODING GUIDELINES – 2017 ICD-10-CM

GUIDELINES

CHAPTER 15 – PREGNANCY
Section I. C. 15. a. 5)

CHAPTER 15 – PREGNANCY
Section I. C. 15. d.

5) Unspecified trimester
Each category that includes codes for trimester has a code for "unspecified trimester." The "unspecified trimester" code should rarely be used, such as when the documentation in the record is insufficient to determine the trimester and it is not possible to obtain clarification.

6) 7th character for Fetus Identification
Where applicable, a 7th character is to be assigned for certain categories (O31, O32, O33.3 - O33.6, O35, O36, O40, O41, O60.1, O60.2, O64, and O69) to identify the fetus for which the complication code applies.

Assign 7th character "0":
• For single gestations
• When the documentation in the record is insufficient to determine the fetus affected and it is not possible to obtain clarification.
• When it is not possible to clinically determine which fetus is affected.

b. Selection of OB Principal or First-listed Diagnosis

1) Routine outpatient prenatal visits
For routine outpatient prenatal visits when no complications are present, a code from category Z34, Encounter for supervision of normal pregnancy, should be used as the first-listed diagnosis. These codes should not be used in conjunction with chapter 15 codes.

2) *Supervision of High-Risk Pregnancy*
Codes from category O09, Supervision of high-risk pregnancy, are intended for use only during the prenatal period. For complications during the labor or delivery episode as a result of a high-risk pregnancy, assign the applicable complication codes from Chapter 15. If there are no complications during the labor and delivery episode, assign code O80, Encounter for full-term uncomplicated delivery.

For routine prenatal outpatient visits for patients with high-risk pregnancies, a code from category O09, Supervision of high-risk pregnancy, should be used as the first-listed diagnosis. Secondary chapter 15 codes may be used in conjunction with these codes if appropriate.

3) Episodes when no delivery occurs
In episodes when no delivery occurs, the principal diagnosis should correspond to the principal complication of the pregnancy which necessitated the encounter. Should more than one complication exist, all of which are treated or monitored, any of the complications codes may be sequenced first.

4) When a delivery occurs
~~When a delivery occurs, the principal diagnosis should correspond to the main circumstances or complication of the delivery.~~ When an obstetric patient is admitted and delivers during that admission, the condition that prompted the admission should be sequenced as the principal diagnosis. If multiple conditions prompted the admission, sequence the one most related to the delivery as the principal diagnosis. A code for any complication of the delivery should be assigned as an additional diagnosis. In cases of cesarean delivery, ~~the selection of the principal diagnosis should be the condition established after study that was responsible for the patient's admission. If~~ if the patient was admitted with a condition that resulted in the performance of a cesarean procedure, that condition should be selected as the principal diagnosis. If the reason for the admission/~~encounter~~ was unrelated to the condition resulting in the cesarean delivery, the condition related to the reason for the admission/~~encounter~~ should be selected as the principal diagnosis.

5) Outcome of delivery
A code from category Z37, Outcome of delivery, should be included on every maternal record when a delivery has occurred. These codes are not to be used on subsequent records or on the newborn record.

c. Pre-existing conditions versus conditions due to the pregnancy
Certain categories in Chapter 15 distinguish between conditions of the mother that existed prior to pregnancy (pre-existing) and those that are a direct result of pregnancy. When assigning codes from Chapter 15, it is important to assess if a condition was pre-existing prior to pregnancy or developed during or due to the pregnancy in order to assign the correct code.

Categories that do not distinguish between pre-existing and pregnancy-related conditions may be used for either. It is acceptable to use codes specifically for the puerperium with codes complicating pregnancy and childbirth if a condition arises postpartum during the delivery encounter.

d. Pre-existing hypertension in pregnancy
Category O10, Pre-existing hypertension complicating pregnancy, childbirth and the puerperium, includes codes for hypertensive heart and hypertensive chronic kidney disease. When assigning one of the O10 codes that includes hypertensive heart disease or hypertensive chronic kidney disease, it is necessary to add a secondary code from the appropriate hypertension category to specify the type of heart failure or chronic kidney disease.

See Section I.C.9. Hypertension.

e. Fetal Conditions Affecting the Management of the Mother

1) Codes from categories O35 and O36
Codes from categories O35, Maternal care for known or suspected fetal abnormality and damage, and O36, Maternal care for other fetal problems, are assigned only when the fetal condition is actually responsible for modifying the management of the mother, i.e., by requiring diagnostic studies, additional observation, special care, or termination of pregnancy. The fact that the fetal condition exists does not justify assigning a code from this series to the mother's record.

2) In utero surgery
In cases when surgery is performed on the fetus, a diagnosis code from category O35, Maternal care for known or suspected fetal abnormality and damage, should be assigned identifying the fetal condition. Assign the appropriate procedure code for the procedure performed.

No code from Chapter 16, the perinatal codes, should be used on the mother's record to identify fetal conditions. Surgery performed in utero on a fetus is still to be coded as an obstetric encounter.

f. HIV Infection in Pregnancy, Childbirth and the Puerperium
During pregnancy, childbirth or the puerperium, a patient admitted because of an HIV-related illness should receive a principal diagnosis from subcategory O98.7-, Human immunodeficiency [HIV] disease complicating pregnancy, childbirth and the puerperium, followed by the code(s) for the HIV-related illness(es).

Patients with asymptomatic HIV infection status admitted during pregnancy, childbirth, or the puerperium should receive codes of O98.7- and Z21, Asymptomatic human immunodeficiency virus [HIV] infection status.

g. Diabetes mellitus in pregnancy
Diabetes mellitus is a significant complicating factor in pregnancy. Pregnant women who are diabetic should be assigned a code from category O24, Diabetes mellitus in pregnancy, childbirth, and the puerperium, first, followed by the appropriate diabetes code(s) (E08-E13) from Chapter 4.

h. Long-term use of insulin *and oral hypoglycemics*
Code Z79.4, Long-term (current) use of insulin, or code Z79.84, Long-term (current) use of oral hypoglycemic drugs, should also be assigned if the diabetes mellitus is being treated with insulin or oral medications. If the patient is treated with both oral medications and insulin, only the code for insulin-controlled should be assigned.

i. Gestational (pregnancy induced) diabetes
Gestational (pregnancy induced) diabetes can occur during the second and third trimester of pregnancy in women who were not diabetic prior to pregnancy. Gestational diabetes can cause complications in the pregnancy similar to those of pre-existing diabetes mellitus. It also puts the woman at greater risk of developing diabetes after the pregnancy. Codes for gestational diabetes are in subcategory O24.4, Gestational diabetes mellitus. No other code from category O24, Diabetes mellitus in pregnancy, childbirth, and the puerperium, should be used with a code from O24.4.

The codes under subcategory O24.4 include diet controlled, ~~and~~ insulin controlled, and controlled by oral hypoglycemic drugs. If a patient with gestational diabetes is treated with both diet and insulin, only the code for insulin-controlled is required. If a patient with gestational diabetes is treated with both diet and oral hypoglycemic medications, only the code for "controlled by oral hypoglycemic drugs" is required. Code Z79.4, Long-term (current) use of insulin or code Z79.84, Long-term (current) use of oral hypoglycemic drugs, should not be assigned with codes from subcategory O24.4.

An abnormal glucose tolerance in pregnancy is assigned a code from subcategory O99.81, Abnormal glucose complicating pregnancy, childbirth, and the puerperium.

j. Sepsis and septic shock complicating abortion, pregnancy, childbirth and the puerperium
When assigning a chapter 15 code for sepsis complicating abortion, pregnancy, childbirth, and the puerperium, a code for the specific type of infection should be assigned as an additional diagnosis. If severe sepsis is present, a code from subcategory R65.2, Severe sepsis, and code(s) for associated organ dysfunction(s) should also be assigned as additional diagnoses.

CHAPTER 15 – PREGNANCY
Section I. C. 15. k.

k. Puerperal sepsis
Code O85, Puerperal sepsis, should be assigned with a secondary code to identify the causal organism (e.g., for a bacterial infection, assign a code from category B95-B96, Bacterial infections in conditions classified elsewhere). A code from category A40, Streptococcal sepsis, or A41, Other sepsis, should not be used for puerperal sepsis. If applicable, use additional codes to identify severe sepsis (R65.2-) and any associated acute organ dysfunction.

l. Alcohol and tobacco use during pregnancy, childbirth and the puerperium

1) Alcohol use during pregnancy, childbirth and the puerperium
Codes under subcategory O99.31, Alcohol use complicating pregnancy, childbirth, and the puerperium, should be assigned for any pregnancy case when a mother uses alcohol during the pregnancy or postpartum. A secondary code from category F10, Alcohol related disorders, should also be assigned to identify manifestations of the alcohol use.

2) Tobacco use during pregnancy, childbirth and the puerperium
Codes under subcategory O99.33, Smoking (tobacco) complicating pregnancy, childbirth, and the puerperium, should be assigned for any pregnancy case when a mother uses any type of tobacco product during the pregnancy or postpartum. A secondary code from category F17, Nicotine dependence, Tobacco use, should also be assigned to identify the type of nicotine dependence.

m. Poisoning, toxic effects, adverse effects and underdosing in a pregnant patient
A code from subcategory O9A.2, Injury, poisoning and certain other consequences of external causes complicating pregnancy, childbirth, and the puerperium, should be sequenced first, followed by the appropriate injury, poisoning, toxic effect, adverse effect or underdosing code, and then the additional code(s) that specifies the condition caused by the poisoning, toxic effect, adverse effect or underdosing.

See Section I.C.19. Adverse effects, poisoning, underdosing and toxic effects.

n. Normal Delivery, Code O80

1) Encounter for full term uncomplicated delivery
Code O80 should be assigned when a woman is admitted for a full-term normal delivery and delivers a single, healthy infant without any complications antepartum, during the delivery, or postpartum during the delivery episode. Code O80 is always a principal diagnosis. It is not to be used if any other code from chapter 15 is needed to describe a current complication of the antenatal, delivery, or perinatal period. Additional codes from other chapters may be used with code O80 if they are not related to or are in any way complicating the pregnancy.

2) Uncomplicated delivery with resolved antepartum complication
Code O80 may be used if the patient had a complication at some point during the pregnancy, but the complication is not present at the time of the admission for delivery.

3) Outcome of delivery for O80
Z37.0, Single live birth, is the only outcome of delivery code appropriate for use with O80.

o. The Peripartum and Postpartum Periods

1) Peripartum and Postpartum periods
The postpartum period begins immediately after delivery and continues for six weeks following delivery. The peripartum period is defined as the last month of pregnancy to five months postpartum.

2) Peripartum and postpartum complication
A postpartum complication is any complication occurring within the six-week period.

3) Pregnancy-related complications after 6 week period
Chapter 15 codes may also be used to describe pregnancy-related complications after the peripartum or postpartum period if the provider documents that a condition is pregnancy related.

4) Admission for routine postpartum care following delivery outside hospital
When the mother delivers outside the hospital prior to admission and is admitted for routine postpartum care and no complications are noted, code Z39.0, Encounter for care and examination of mother immediately after delivery, should be assigned as the principal diagnosis.

5) Pregnancy associated cardiomyopathy
Pregnancy associated cardiomyopathy, code O90.3, is unique in that it may be diagnosed in the third trimester of pregnancy but may continue to progress months after delivery. For this reason, it is referred to as peripartum cardiomyopathy. Code O90.3 is only for use when the cardiomyopathy develops as a result of pregnancy in a woman who did not have pre-existing heart disease.

CHAPTER 15 – PREGNANCY
Section I. C. 16. p. 1)

p. Code O94, Sequelae of complication of pregnancy, childbirth, and the puerperium

1) Code O94
Code O94, Sequelae of complication of pregnancy, childbirth, and the puerperium, is for use in those cases when an initial complication of a pregnancy develops a sequelae requiring care or treatment at a future date.

2) After the initial postpartum period
This code may be used at any time after the initial postpartum period.

3) Sequencing of Code O94
This code, like all sequela codes, is to be sequenced following the code describing the sequelae of the complication.

q. Termination of Pregnancy and Spontaneous abortions

1) Abortion with Liveborn Fetus
When an attempted termination of pregnancy results in a liveborn fetus, assign code Z33.2, Encounter for elective termination of pregnancy and a code from category Z37, Outcome of Delivery.

2) Retained Products of Conception following an abortion
Subsequent encounters for retained products of conception following a spontaneous abortion or elective termination of pregnancy are assigned the appropriate code from category O03, Spontaneous abortion, or codes O07.4, Failed attempted termination of pregnancy without complication and Z33.2, Encounter for elective termination of pregnancy. This advice is appropriate even when the patient was discharged previously with a discharge diagnosis of complete abortion.

3) Complications leading to abortion
Codes from Chapter 15 may be used as additional codes to identify any documented complications of the pregnancy in conjunction with codes in categories in O07 and O08.

r. Abuse in a pregnant patient
For suspected or confirmed cases of abuse of a pregnant patient, a code(s) from subcategories O9A.3, Physical abuse complicating pregnancy, childbirth, and the puerperium, O9A.4, Sexual abuse complicating pregnancy, childbirth, and the puerperium, and O9A.5, Psychological abuse complicating pregnancy, childbirth, and the puerperium, should be sequenced first, followed by the appropriate codes (if applicable) to identify any associated current injury due to physical abuse, sexual abuse, and the perpetrator of abuse.

See Section I.C.19.f. Adult and child abuse, neglect and other maltreatment.

16. Chapter 16: Certain Conditions Originating in the Perinatal Period (P00-P96)

For coding and reporting purposes the perinatal period is defined as before birth through the 28th day following birth. The following guidelines are provided for reporting purposes

a. General Perinatal Rules

1) Use of Chapter 16 Codes
Codes in this chapter are <u>never</u> for use on the maternal record.

Codes from Chapter 15, the obstetric chapter, are never permitted on the newborn record. Chapter 16 codes may be used throughout the life of the patient if the condition is still present.

2) Principal Diagnosis for Birth Record
When coding the birth episode in a newborn record, assign a code from category Z38, Liveborn infants according to place of birth and type of delivery, as the principal diagnosis. A code from category Z38 is assigned only once, to a newborn at the time of birth. If a newborn is transferred to another institution, a code from category Z38 should not be used at the receiving hospital.

A code from category Z38 is used only on the newborn record, not on the mother's record.

3) Use of Codes from other Chapters with Codes from Chapter 16
Codes from other chapters may be used with codes from chapter 16 if the codes from the other chapters provide more specific detail. Codes for signs and symptoms may be assigned when a definitive diagnosis has not been established. If the reason for the encounter is a perinatal condition, the code from chapter 16 should be sequenced first.

4) **Use of Chapter 16 Codes after the Perinatal Period**
Should a condition originate in the perinatal period, and continue throughout the life of the patient, the perinatal code should continue to be used regardless of the patient's age.

5) **Birth process or community acquired conditions**
If a newborn has a condition that may be either due to the birth process or community acquired and the documentation does not indicate which it is, the default is due to the birth process and the code from Chapter 16 should be used. If the condition is community-acquired, a code from Chapter 16 should not be assigned.

6) **Code all clinically significant conditions**
All clinically significant conditions noted on routine newborn examination should be coded. A condition is clinically significant if it requires:
- clinical evaluation; or
- therapeutic treatment; or
- diagnostic procedures; or
- extended length of hospital stay; or
- increased nursing care and/or monitoring; or
- has implications for future health care needs

Note: The perinatal guidelines listed above are the same as the general coding guidelines for "additional diagnoses", except for the final point regarding implications for future health care needs. Codes should be assigned for conditions that have been specified by the provider as having implications for future health care needs.

b. **Observation and Evaluation of Newborns for Suspected Conditions not Found**
~~Reserved for future expansion~~

1) Assign a code from category Z05, Observation and evaluation of newborns and infants for suspected conditions ruled out, to identify those instances when a healthy newborn is evaluated for a suspected condition that is determined after study not to be present. Do not use a code from category Z05 when the patient has identified signs or symptoms of a suspected problem; in such cases code the sign or symptom.

2) A code from category Z05 may also be assigned as a principal or first-listed code for readmissions or encounters when the code from category Z38 code no longer applies. Codes from category Z05 are for use only for healthy newborns and infants for which no condition after study is found to be present.

3) **Z05 on a birth record**
A code from category Z05 is to be used as a secondary code after the code from category Z38, Liveborn infants according to place of birth and type of delivery.

c. **Coding Additional Perinatal Diagnoses**

1) **Assigning codes for conditions that require treatment**
Assign codes for conditions that require treatment or further investigation, prolong the length of stay, or require resource utilization.

2) **Codes for conditions specified as having implications for future health care needs**
Assign codes for conditions that have been specified by the provider as having implications for future health care needs.

Note: This guideline should not be used for adult patients.

d. **Prematurity and Fetal Growth Retardation**
Providers utilize different criteria in determining prematurity. A code for prematurity should not be assigned unless it is documented. Assignment of codes in categories P05, Disorders of newborn related to slow fetal growth and fetal malnutrition, and P07, Disorders of newborn related to short gestation and low birth weight, not elsewhere classified, should be based on the recorded birth weight and estimated gestational age. Codes from category P05 should not be assigned with codes from category P07.

When both birth weight and gestational age are available, two codes from category P07 should be assigned, with the code for birth weight sequenced before the code for gestational age.

e. **Low birth weight and immaturity status**
Codes from category P07, Disorders of newborn related to short gestation and low birth weight, not elsewhere classified, are for use for a child or adult who was premature or had a low birth weight as a newborn and this is affecting the patient's current health status.

See Section I.C.21. Factors influencing health status and contact with health services, Status.

f. **Bacterial Sepsis of Newborn**
Category P36, Bacterial sepsis of newborn, includes congenital sepsis. If a perinate is documented as having sepsis without documentation of congenital or community acquired, the default is congenital and a code from category P36 should be assigned. If the P36 code includes the causal organism, an additional code from category B95, Streptococcus, Staphylococcus, and Enterococcus as the cause of diseases classified elsewhere, or B96, Other bacterial agents as the cause of diseases classified elsewhere, should not be assigned. If the P36 code does not include the causal organism, assign an additional code from category B96. If applicable, use additional codes to identify severe sepsis (R65.2-) and any associated acute organ dysfunction.

g. **Stillbirth**
Code P95, Stillbirth, is only for use in institutions that maintain separate records for stillbirths. No other code should be used with P95. Code P95 should not be used on the mother's record.

17. **Chapter 17: Congenital Malformations, Deformations, and Chromosomal Abnormalities (Q00-Q99)**

Assign an appropriate code(s) from categories Q00-Q99, Congenital malformations, deformations, and chromosomal abnormalities when a malformation/deformation or chromosomal abnormality is documented. A malformation/deformation/or chromosomal abnormality may be the principal/first-listed diagnosis on a record or a secondary diagnosis.

When a malformation/deformation/or chromosomal abnormality does not have a unique code assignment, assign additional code(s) for any manifestations that may be present.

When the code assignment specifically identifies the malformation/deformation/or chromosomal abnormality, manifestations that are an inherent component of the anomaly should not be coded separately. Additional codes should be assigned for manifestations that are not an inherent component.

Codes from Chapter 17 may be used throughout the life of the patient. If a congenital malformation or deformity has been corrected, a personal history code should be used to identify the history of the malformation or deformity. Although present at birth, malformation/deformation/or chromosomal abnormality may not be identified until later in life. Whenever the condition is diagnosed by the physician, it is appropriate to assign a code from codes Q00-Q99.

For the birth admission, the appropriate code from category Z38, Liveborn infants, according to place of birth and type of delivery, should be sequenced as the principal diagnosis, followed by any congenital anomaly codes, Q00-Q99.

18. **Chapter 18: Symptoms, Signs, and Abnormal Clinical and Laboratory Findings, Not Elsewhere Classified (R00-R99)**

Chapter 18 includes symptoms, signs, abnormal results of clinical or other investigative procedures, and ill-defined conditions regarding which no diagnosis classifiable elsewhere is recorded. Signs and symptoms that point to a specific diagnosis have been assigned to a category in other chapters of the classification.

a. **Use of symptom codes**
Codes that describe symptoms and signs are acceptable for reporting purposes when a related definitive diagnosis has not been established (confirmed) by the provider.

b. **Use of a symptom code with a definitive diagnosis code**
Codes for signs and symptoms may be reported in addition to a related definitive diagnosis when the sign or symptom is not routinely associated with that diagnosis, such as the various signs and symptoms associated with complex syndromes. The definitive diagnosis code should be sequenced before the symptom code.

Signs or symptoms that are associated routinely with a disease process should not be assigned as additional codes, unless otherwise instructed by the classification.

c. **Combination codes that include symptoms**
ICD-10-CM contains a number of combination codes that identify both the definitive diagnosis and common symptoms of that diagnosis. When using one of these combination codes, an additional code should not be assigned for the symptom.

d. **Repeated falls**
Code R29.6, Repeated falls, is for use for encounters when a patient has recently fallen and the reason for the fall is being investigated.

Code Z91.81, History of falling, is for use when a patient has fallen in the past and is at risk for future falls. When appropriate, both codes R29.6 and Z91.81 may be assigned together.

GUIDELINES

CHAPTER 18 – SYMPTOMS & SIGNS
Section I. C. 18. e.

e. Coma scale

The coma scale codes (R40.2-) can be used in conjunction with traumatic brain injury codes, acute cerebrovascular disease or sequelae of cerebrovascular disease codes. These codes are primarily for use by trauma registries, but they may be used in any setting where this information is collected. The coma scale may also be used to assess the status of the central nervous system for other non-trauma conditions, such as monitoring patients in the intensive care unit regardless of medical condition. The coma scale codes should be sequenced after the diagnosis code(s).

These codes, one from each subcategory, are needed to complete the scale. The 7th character indicates when the scale was recorded. The 7th character should match for all three codes.

At a minimum, report the initial score documented on presentation at your facility. This may be a score from the emergency medicine technician (EMT) or in the emergency department. If desired, a facility may choose to capture multiple coma scale scores.

Assign code R40.24, Glascow coma scale, total score, when only the total score is documented in the medical record and not the individual score(s).

f. Functional quadriplegia

Functional quadriplegia (code R53.2) is the lack of ability to use one's limbs or to ambulate due to extreme debility. It is not associated with neurologic deficit or injury, and code R53.2 should not be used for cases of neurologic quadriplegia. It should only be assigned if functional quadriplegia is specifically documented in the medical record.

g. SIRS due to Non-Infectious Process

The systemic inflammatory response syndrome (SIRS) can develop as a result of certain non-infectious disease processes, such as trauma, malignant neoplasm, or pancreatitis. When SIRS is documented with a noninfectious condition, and no subsequent infection is documented, the code for the underlying condition, such as an injury, should be assigned, followed by code R65.10, Systemic inflammatory response syndrome (SIRS) of non-infectious origin without acute organ dysfunction, or code R65.11, Systemic inflammatory response syndrome (SIRS) of non-infectious origin with acute organ dysfunction. If an associated acute organ dysfunction is documented, the appropriate code(s) for the specific type of organ dysfunction(s) should be assigned in addition to code R65.11. If acute organ dysfunction is documented, but it cannot be determined if the acute organ dysfunction is associated with SIRS or due to another condition (e.g., directly due to the trauma), the provider should be queried.

h. Death NOS

Code R99, Ill-defined and unknown cause of mortality, is only for use in the very limited circumstance when a patient who has already died is brought into an emergency department or other healthcare facility and is pronounced dead upon arrival. It does not represent the discharge disposition of death.

i. NIHSS Stroke Scale

The NIH stroke scale (NIHSS) codes (R29.7- -) can be used in conjunction with acute stroke codes (I63) to identify the patient's neurological status and the severity of the stroke. The stroke scale codes should be sequenced after the acute stroke diagnosis code(s).

At a minimum, report the initial score documented. If desired, a facility may choose to capture multiple stroke scale scores.

See Section I.B.14. for information concerning the medical record documentation that may be used for assignment of the NIHSS codes.

19. Chapter 19: Injury, Poisoning, and Certain Other Consequences of External Causes (S00-T88)

a. Application of 7th Characters in Chapter 19

Most categories in chapter 19 have a 7th character requirement for each applicable code. Most categories in this chapter have three 7th character values (with the exception of fractures): A, initial encounter, D, subsequent encounter and S, sequela. Categories for traumatic fractures have additional 7th character values. While the patient may be seen by a new or different provider over the course of treatment for an injury, assignment of the 7th character is based on whether the patient is undergoing active treatment and not whether the provider is seeing the patient for the first time.

For complication codes, active treatment refers to treatment for the condition described by the code, even though it may be related to an earlier precipitating problem. For example, code T84.50xA, Infection and inflammatory reaction due to unspecified internal joint prosthesis, initial encounter, is used when active treatment is provided for the infection, even though the condition relates to the prosthetic device, implant or graft that was placed at a previous encounter.

CHAPTER 19 – INJURY & POISONING
Section I. C. 19. a.

7th character "A" initial encounter is used ~~while~~ for each encounter where the patient is receiving active treatment for the condition. ~~Examples of active treatment are: surgical treatment, emergency department encounter, and evaluation and continuing treatment by the same or a different physician.~~

7th character "D" subsequent encounter is used for encounters after the patient has ~~received~~ completed active treatment of the condition and is receiving routine care for the condition during the healing or recovery phase. ~~Examples of subsequent care are: cast change or removal, an x-ray to check healing status of fracture, removal of external or internal fixation device, medication adjustment, other aftercare and follow up visits following treatment of the injury or condition.~~

The aftercare Z codes should not be used for aftercare for conditions such as injuries or poisonings, where 7th characters are provided to identify subsequent care. For example, for aftercare of an injury, assign the acute injury code with the 7th character "D" (subsequent encounter).

7th character "S", sequela, is for use for complications or conditions that arise as a direct result of a condition, such as scar formation after a burn. The scars are sequelae of the burn. When using 7th character "S", it is necessary to use both the injury code that precipitated the sequela and the code for the sequela itself. The "S" is added only to the injury code, not the sequela code. The 7th character "S" identifies the injury responsible for the sequela. The specific type of sequela (e.g., scar) is sequenced first, followed by the injury code.

See Section I.B.10 Sequela (Late Effects).

b. Coding of Injuries

When coding injuries, assign separate codes for each injury unless a combination code is provided, in which case the combination code is assigned. Code T07, Unspecified multiple injuries should not be assigned in the inpatient setting unless information for a more specific code is not available. Traumatic injury codes (S00-T14.9) are not to be used for normal, healing surgical wounds or to identify complications of surgical wounds.

The code for the most serious injury, as determined by the provider and the focus of treatment, is sequenced first.

1) Superficial injuries

Superficial injuries such as abrasions or contusions are not coded when associated with more severe injuries of the same site.

2) Primary injury with damage to nerves/blood vessels

When a primary injury results in minor damage to peripheral nerves or blood vessels, the primary injury is sequenced first with additional code(s) for injuries to nerves and spinal cord (such as category S04), and/or injury to blood vessels (such as category S15). When the primary injury is to the blood vessels or nerves, that injury should be sequenced first.

c. Coding of Traumatic Fractures

The principles of multiple coding of injuries should be followed in coding fractures. Fractures of specified sites are coded individually by site in accordance with both the provisions within categories S02, S12, S22, S32, S42, S49, S52, S59, S62, S72, S79, S82, S89, S92 and the level of detail furnished by medical record content.

A fracture not indicated as open or closed should be coded to closed. A fracture not indicated whether displaced or not displaced should be coded to displaced.

More specific guidelines are as follows:

1) Initial vs. Subsequent Encounter for Fractures

Traumatic fractures are coded using the appropriate 7th character for initial encounter (A, B, C) ~~while~~ for each encounter where the patient is receiving active treatment for the fracture. ~~Examples of active treatment are: surgical treatment, emergency department encounter, and evaluation and continuing (ongoing) treatment by the same or different physician.~~ The appropriate 7th character for initial encounter should also be assigned for a patient who delayed seeking treatment for the fracture or nonunion.

Fractures are coded using the appropriate 7th character for subsequent care for encounters after the patient has completed active treatment of the fracture and is receiving routine care for the fracture during the healing or recovery phase. ~~Examples of fracture aftercare are: cast change or removal, an x-ray to check healing status of fracture, removal of external or internal fixation device, medication adjustment, and follow-up visits following fracture treatment.~~

Care for complications of surgical treatment for fracture repairs during the healing or recovery phase should be coded with the appropriate complication codes.

[2017.CM]   OFFICIAL CODING GUIDELINES – 2017 ICD-10-CM

CHAPTER 19 – INJURY & POISONING
Section I. C. 19. c. 1)

CHAPTER 19 – INJURY & POISONING
Section I. C. 19. d. 6)

GUIDELINES

Care of complications of fractures, such as malunion and nonunion, should be reported with the appropriate 7th character for subsequent care with nonunion (K, M, N,) or subsequent care with malunion (P, Q, R).

Malunion/nonunion: The appropriate 7th character for initial encounter should also be assigned for a patient who delayed seeking treatment for the fracture or nonunion.

The open fracture designations in the assignment of the 7th character for fractures of the forearm, femur and lower leg, including ankle are based on the Gustilo open fracture classification. When the Gustilo classification type is not specified for an open fracture, the 7th character for open fracture type I or II should be assigned (B, E, H, M, Q).

A code from category M80, not a traumatic fracture code, should be used for any patient with known osteoporosis who suffers a fracture, even if the patient had a minor fall or trauma, if that fall or trauma would not usually break a normal, healthy bone.

See Section I.C.13. Osteoporosis.

The aftercare Z codes should not be used for aftercare for traumatic fractures. For aftercare of a traumatic fracture, assign the acute fracture code with the appropriate 7th character.

2) **Multiple fractures sequencing**
Multiple fractures are sequenced in accordance with the severity of the fracture.

d. **Coding of Burns and Corrosions**
The ICD-10-CM makes a distinction between burns and corrosions. The burn codes are for thermal burns, except sunburns, that come from a heat source, such as a fire or hot appliance. The burn codes are also for burns resulting from electricity and radiation. Corrosions are burns due to chemicals. The guidelines are the same for burns and corrosions.

Current burns (T20-T25) are classified by depth, extent and by agent (X code). Burns are classified by depth as first degree (erythema), second degree (blistering), and third degree (full-thickness involvement). Burns of the eye and internal organs (T26-T28) are classified by site, but not by degree.

1) **Sequencing of burn and related condition codes**
Sequence first the code that reflects the highest degree of burn when more than one burn is present.

a. When the reason for the admission or encounter is for treatment of external multiple burns, sequence first the code that reflects the burn of the highest degree.

b. When a patient has both internal and external burns, the circumstances of admission govern the selection of the principal diagnosis or first-listed diagnosis.

c. When a patient is admitted for burn injuries and other related conditions such as smoke inhalation and/or respiratory failure, the circumstances of admission govern the selection of the principal or first-listed diagnosis.

2) **Burns of the same local site**
Classify burns of the same local site (three-character category level, T20-T28) but of different degrees to the subcategory identifying the highest degree recorded in the diagnosis.

3) **Non-healing burns**
Non-healing burns are coded as acute burns.

Necrosis of burned skin should be coded as a non-healed burn.

4) **Infected Burn**
For any documented infected burn site, use an additional code for the infection.

5) **Assign separate codes for each burn site**
When coding burns, assign separate codes for each burn site. Category T30, Burn and corrosion, body region unspecified is extremely vague and should rarely be used.

6) **Burns and Corrosions Classified According to Extent of Body Surface Involved**
Assign codes from category T31, Burns classified according to extent of body surface involved, or T32, Corrosions classified according to extent of body surface involved, when the site of the burn is not specified or when there is a need for additional data. It is advisable to use category T31 as additional coding when needed to provide data for evaluating burn mortality, such as that needed by burn units. It is also advisable to use category T31 as an additional code for reporting purposes when there is mention of a third-degree burn involving 20 percent or more of the body surface.

Categories T31 and T32 are based on the classic "rule of nines" in estimating body surface involved: head and neck are assigned nine percent, each arm nine percent, each leg 18 percent, the anterior trunk 18 percent, posterior trunk 18 percent, and genitalia one percent. Providers may change these percentage assignments where necessary to accommodate infants and children who have proportionately larger heads than adults, and patients who have large buttocks, thighs, or abdomen that involve burns.

7) **Encounters for treatment of sequela of burns**
Encounters for the treatment of the late effects of burns or corrosions (i.e., scars or joint contractures) should be coded with a burn or corrosion code with the 7th character "S" for sequela.

8) **Sequelae with a late effect code and current burn**
When appropriate, both a code for a current burn or corrosion with 7th character "A" or "D" and a burn or corrosion code with 7th character "S" may be assigned on the same record (when both a current burn and sequelae of an old burn exist). Burns and corrosions do not heal at the same rate and a current healing wound may still exist with sequela of a healed burn or corrosion.

See Section I.B.10 Sequela (Late Effects).

9) **Use of an external cause code with burns and corrosions**
An external cause code should be used with burns and corrosions to identify the source and intent of the burn, as well as the place where it occurred.

e. **Adverse Effects, Poisoning, Underdosing and Toxic Effects**
Codes in categories T36-T65 are combination codes that include the substance that was taken as well as the intent. No additional external cause code is required for poisonings, toxic effects, adverse effects and underdosing codes.

1) **Do not code directly from the Table of Drugs**
Do not code directly from the Table of Drugs and Chemicals. Always refer back to the Tabular List.

2) **Use as many codes as necessary to describe**
Use as many codes as necessary to describe completely all drugs, medicinal or biological substances.

3) **If the same code would describe the causative agent**
If the same code would describe the causative agent for more than one adverse reaction, poisoning, toxic effect or underdosing, assign the code only once.

4) **If two or more drugs, medicinal or biological substances**
If two or more drugs, medicinal or biological substances are reported, code each individually unless a combination code is listed in the Table of Drugs and Chemicals.

5) **The occurrence of drug toxicity is classified in ICD-10-CM as follows:**

(a) **Adverse Effect**
When coding an adverse effect of a drug that has been correctly prescribed and properly administered, assign the appropriate code for the nature of the adverse effect followed by the appropriate code for the adverse effect of the drug (T36-T50). The code for the drug should have a 5th or 6th character "5" (for example T36.0X5-). Examples of the nature of an adverse effect are tachycardia, delirium, gastrointestinal hemorrhaging, vomiting, hypokalemia, hepatitis, renal failure, or respiratory failure.

(b) **Poisoning**
When coding a poisoning or reaction to the improper use of a medication (e.g., overdose, wrong substance given or taken in error, wrong route of administration), first assign the appropriate code from categories T36-T50. The poisoning codes have an associated intent as their 5th or 6th character accidental, intentional self-harm, assault and undetermined. If the intent of the poisoning is unknown or unspecified, code the intent as accidental intent. The undetermined intent is only for use if the documentation in the record specifies that the intent cannot be determined. Use additional code(s) for all manifestations of poisonings.

If there is also a diagnosis of abuse or dependence of the substance, the abuse or dependence is assigned as an additional code.

Examples of poisoning include:

(i) Error was made in drug prescription
Errors made in drug prescription or in the administration of the drug by provider, nurse, patient, or other person.

(ii) **Overdose of a drug intentionally taken**
If an overdose of a drug was intentionally taken or administered and resulted in drug toxicity, it would be coded as a poisoning.

(iii) **Nonprescribed drug taken with correctly prescribed and properly administered drug**
If a nonprescribed drug or medicinal agent was taken in combination with a correctly prescribed and properly administered drug, any drug toxicity or other reaction resulting from the interaction of the two drugs would be classified as a poisoning.

(iv) **Interaction of drug(s) and alcohol**
When a reaction results from the interaction of a drug(s) and alcohol, this would be classified as poisoning.

See Section I.C.4. if poisoning is the result of insulin pump malfunctions.

(c) Underdosing
Underdosing refers to taking less of a medication than is prescribed by a provider or a manufacturer's instruction. For underdosing, assign the code from categories T36-T50 (fifth or sixth character "6").

Codes for underdosing should never be assigned as principal or first-listed codes. If a patient has a relapse or exacerbation of the medical condition for which the drug is prescribed because of the reduction in dose, then the medical condition itself should be coded.

Noncompliance (Z91.12-, Z91.13-) or complication of care (Y63.61, Y63.6-Y63.9) codes are to be used with an underdosing code to indicate intent, if known.

(d) Toxic Effects
When a harmful substance is ingested or comes in contact with a person, this is classified as a toxic effect. The toxic effect codes are in categories T51-T65.

Toxic effect codes have an associated intent: accidental, intentional self-harm, assault and undetermined.

f. Adult and child abuse, neglect and other maltreatment
Sequence first the appropriate code from categories T74.- (Adult and child abuse, neglect and other maltreatment, confirmed) or T76.- (Adult and child abuse, neglect and other maltreatment, suspected) for abuse, neglect and other maltreatment, followed by any accompanying mental health or injury code(s).

If the documentation in the medical record states abuse or neglect it is coded as confirmed (T74.-). It is coded as suspected if it is documented as suspected (T76.-).

For cases of confirmed abuse or neglect an external cause code from the assault section (X92-Y09) should be added to identify the cause of any physical injuries. A perpetrator code (Y07) should be added when the perpetrator of the abuse is known. For suspected cases of abuse or neglect, do not report external cause or perpetrator code.

If a suspected case of abuse, neglect or mistreatment is ruled out during an encounter code Z04.71, Encounter for examination and observation following alleged physical adult abuse, ruled out, or code Z04.72, Encounter for examination and observation following alleged physical child abuse, ruled out, should be used, not a code from T76.

If a suspected case of alleged rape or sexual abuse is ruled out during an encounter code Z04.41, Encounter for examination and observation following alleged ~~physical~~ adult rape ~~abuse, ruled out~~, or code Z04.42, Encounter for examination and observation following alleged child rape ~~or sexual abuse, ruled out~~, should be used, not a code from T76.

See Section I.C.15. Abuse in a pregnant patient.

g. Complications of care

1) General guidelines for complications of care

(a) Documentation of complications of care

See section I.B.16. for information on documentation of complications of care.

2) Pain due to medical devices
Pain associated with devices, implants or grafts left in a surgical site (for example painful hip prosthesis) is assigned to the appropriate code(s) found in Chapter 19, Injury, poisoning, and certain other consequences of external causes. Specific codes for pain due to medical devices are found in the T code section of the ICD-10-CM. Use additional code(s) from category G89 to identify acute or chronic pain due to presence of the device, implant or graft (G89.18 or G89.28).

3) Transplant complications

(a) Transplant complications other than kidney
Codes under category T86, Complications of transplanted organs and tissues, are for use for both complications and rejection of transplanted organs. A transplant complication code is only assigned if the complication affects the function of the transplanted organ. Two codes are required to fully describe a transplant complication: the appropriate code from category T86 and a secondary code that identifies the complication.

Pre-existing conditions or conditions that develop after the transplant are not coded as complications unless they affect the function of the transplanted organs.

See I.C.21. for transplant organ removal status.
See I.C.2. for malignant neoplasm associated with transplanted organ.

(b) Kidney transplant complications
Patients who have undergone kidney transplant may still have some form of chronic kidney disease (CKD) because the kidney transplant may not fully restore kidney function. Code T86.1- should be assigned for documented complications of a kidney transplant, such as transplant failure or rejection or other transplant complication. Code T86.1- should not be assigned for post kidney transplant patients who have chronic kidney (CKD) unless a transplant complication such as transplant failure or rejection is documented. If the documentation is unclear as to whether the patient has a complication of the transplant, query the provider.

Conditions that affect the function of the transplanted kidney, other than CKD, should be assigned a code from subcategory T86.1, Complications of transplanted organ, kidney, and a secondary code that identifies the complication.

For patients with CKD following a kidney transplant, but who do not have a complication such as failure or rejection, *see section I.C.14. Chronic kidney disease and kidney transplant status.*

4) Complication codes that include the external cause
As with certain other T codes, some of the complications of care codes have the external cause included in the code. The code includes the nature of the complication as well as the type of procedure that caused the complication. No external cause code indicating the type of procedure is necessary for these codes.

5) Complications of care codes within the body system chapters
Intraoperative and postprocedural complication codes are found within the body system chapters with codes specific to the organs and structures of that body system. These codes should be sequenced first, followed by a code(s) for the specific complication, if applicable.

20. Chapter 20: External Causes of Morbidity (V00-Y99)

The external causes of morbidity codes should never be sequenced as the first-listed or principal diagnosis.

External cause codes are intended to provide data for injury research and evaluation of injury prevention strategies. These codes capture how the injury or health condition happened (cause), the intent (unintentional or accidental; or intentional, such as suicide or assault), the place where the event occurred the activity of the patient at the time of the event, and the person's status (e.g., civilian, military).

There is no national requirement for mandatory ICD-10-CM external cause code reporting. Unless a provider is subject to a state-based external cause code reporting mandate or these codes are required by a particular payer, reporting of ICD-10-CM codes in Chapter 20, External Causes of Morbidity, is not required. In the absence of a mandatory reporting requirement, providers are encouraged to voluntarily report external cause codes, as they provide valuable data for injury research and evaluation of injury prevention strategies.

a. General External Cause Coding Guidelines

1) Used with any code in the range of A00.0-T88.9, Z00-Z99
An external cause code may be used with any code in the range of A00.0-T88.9, Z00-Z99, classification that is a health condition due to an external cause. Though they are most applicable to injuries, they are also valid for use with such things as infections or diseases due to an external source, and other health conditions, such as a heart attack that occurs during strenuous physical activity.

2) External cause code used for length of treatment
Assign the external cause code, with the appropriate 7th character (initial encounter, subsequent encounter or sequela) for each encounter for which the injury or condition is being treated.

Most categories in chapter 20 have a 7th character requirement for each applicable code. Most categories in this chapter have three 7th character values: A, initial encounter, D, subsequent encounter and S, sequela. While the patient may be seen by a new or different provider over the course of treatment for an injury or condition, assignment of the 7th character for external cause should match the 7th character of the code assigned for the associated injury or condition for the encounter.

3) Use the full range of external cause codes
Use the full range of external cause codes to completely describe the cause, the intent, the place of occurrence, and if applicable, the activity of the patient at the time of the event, and the patient's status, for all injuries, and other health conditions due to an external cause.

4) Assign as many external cause codes as necessary
Assign as many external cause codes as necessary to fully explain each cause. If only one external code can be recorded, assign the code most related to the principal diagnosis.

5) The selection of the appropriate external cause code
The selection of the appropriate external cause code is guided by the Alphabetic Index of External Causes and by Inclusion and Exclusion notes in the Tabular List.

6) External cause code can never be a principal diagnosis
An external cause code can never be a principal (first-listed) diagnosis.

7) Combination external cause codes
Certain of the external cause codes are combination codes that identify sequential events that result in an injury, such as a fall which results in striking against an object. The injury may be due to either event or both. The combination external cause code used should correspond to the sequence of events regardless of which caused the most serious injury.

8) No external cause code needed in certain circumstances
No external cause code from Chapter 20 is needed if the external cause and intent are included in a code from another chapter (e.g. T36.0x1- Poisoning by penicillins, accidental (unintentional)).

b. Place of Occurrence Guideline
Codes from category Y92, Place of occurrence of the external cause, are secondary codes for use after other external cause codes to identify the location of the patient at the time of injury or other condition.

Generally, a place of occurrence code is assigned only once, at the initial encounter for treatment. However, in the rare instance that a new injury occurs during hospitalization, an additional place of occurrence code may be assigned. No 7th characters are used for Y92.

Do not use place of occurrence code Y92.9 if the place is not stated or is not applicable.

c. Activity Code
Assign a code from category Y93, Activity code, to describe the activity of the patient at the time the injury or other health condition occurred.

An activity code is used only once, at the initial encounter for treatment. Only one code from Y93 should be recorded on a medical record.

The activity codes are not applicable to poisonings, adverse effects, misadventures or sequela.

Do not assign Y93.9, Unspecified activity, if the activity is not stated.

A code from category Y93 is appropriate for use with external cause and intent codes if identifying the activity provides additional information about the event.

d. Place of Occurrence, Activity, and Status Codes Used with other External Cause Code
When applicable, place of occurrence, activity, and external cause status codes are sequenced after the main external cause code(s). Regardless of the number of external cause codes assigned, there should be only one place of occurrence code, one activity code, and one external cause status code assigned to an encounter.

e. If the Reporting Format Limits the Number of External Cause Codes
If the reporting format limits the number of external cause codes that can be used in reporting clinical data, report the code for the cause/intent most related to the principal diagnosis. If the format permits capture of additional external cause codes, the cause/intent, including medical misadventures, of the additional events should be reported rather than the codes for place, activity, or external status.

f. Multiple External Cause Coding Guidelines
More than one external cause code is required to fully describe the external cause of an illness or injury. The assignment of external cause codes should be sequenced in the following priority:
If two or more events cause separate injuries, an external cause code should be assigned for each cause. The first-listed external cause code will be selected in the following order:

External codes for child and adult abuse take priority over all other external cause codes.
See Section I.C.19. Child and Adult abuse guidelines.

External cause codes for terrorism events take priority over all other external cause codes except child and adult abuse.

External cause codes for cataclysmic events take priority over all other external cause codes except child and adult abuse and terrorism.

External cause codes for transport accidents take priority over all other external cause codes except cataclysmic events, child and adult abuse and terrorism.

Activity and external cause status codes are assigned following all causal (intent) external cause codes.

The first-listed external cause code should correspond to the cause of the most serious diagnosis due to an assault, accident, or self-harm, following the order of hierarchy listed above.

g. Child and Adult Abuse Guideline
Adult and child abuse, neglect and maltreatment are classified as assault. Any of the assault codes may be used to indicate the external cause of any injury resulting from the confirmed abuse.

For confirmed cases of abuse, neglect and maltreatment, when the perpetrator is known, a code from Y07, Perpetrator of maltreatment and neglect, should accompany any other assault codes.

See Section I.C.19. Adult and child abuse, neglect and other maltreatment.

h. Unknown or Undetermined Intent Guideline
If the intent (accident, self-harm, assault) of the cause of an injury or other condition is unknown or unspecified, code the intent as accidental intent. All transport accident categories assume accidental intent.

1) Use of undetermined intent
External cause codes for events of undetermined intent are only for use if the documentation in the record specifies that the intent cannot be determined.

i. Sequelae (Late Effects) of External Cause Guidelines

1) Sequelae external cause codes
Sequela are reported using the external cause code with the 7th character "S" for sequela. These codes should be used with any report of a late effect or sequela resulting from a previous injury.

See Section I.B.10 Sequela (Late Effects).

2) Sequela external cause code with a related current injury
A sequela external cause code should never be used with a related current nature of injury code.

3) Use of sequela external cause codes for subsequent visits
Use a late effect external cause code for subsequent visits when a late effect of the initial injury is being treated. Do not use a late effect external cause code for subsequent visits for follow-up care (e.g., to assess healing, to receive rehabilitative therapy) of the injury when no late effect of the injury has been documented.

j. Terrorism Guidelines

1) Cause of injury identified by the Federal Government (FBI) as terrorism
When the cause of an injury is identified by the Federal Government (FBI) as terrorism, the first-listed external cause code should be a code from category Y38, Terrorism. The definition of terrorism employed by the FBI is found at the inclusion note at the beginning of category Y38. Use additional code for place of occurrence (Y92.-). More than one Y38 code may be assigned if the injury is the result of more than one mechanism of terrorism.

2) Cause of an injury is suspected to be the result of terrorism
When the cause of an injury is suspected to be the result of terrorism a code from category Y38 should not be assigned. Suspected cases should be classified as assault.

CHAPTER 20 – EXTERNAL CAUSES
Section I. C. 20. j. 3)

3) Code Y38.9, Terrorism, secondary effects
Assign code Y38.9, Terrorism, secondary effects, for conditions occurring subsequent to the terrorist event. This code should not be assigned for conditions that are due to the initial terrorist act.

It is acceptable to assign code Y38.9 with another code from Y38 if there is an injury due to the initial terrorist event and an injury that is a subsequent result of the terrorist event.

k.   External cause status
A code from category Y99, External cause status, should be assigned whenever any other external cause code is assigned for an encounter, including an Activity code, except for the events noted below. Assign a code from category Y99, External cause status, to indicate the work status of the person at the time the event occurred. The status code indicates whether the event occurred during military activity, whether a non-military person was at work, whether an individual including a student or volunteer was involved in a non-work activity at the time of the causal event.

A code from Y99, External cause status, should be assigned, when applicable, with other external cause codes, such as transport accidents and falls. The external cause status codes are not applicable to poisonings, adverse effects, misadventures or late effects.

Do not assign a code from category Y99 if no other external cause codes (cause, activity) are applicable for the encounter.

An external cause status code is used only once, at the initial encounter for treatment. Only one code from Y99 should be recorded on a medical record.

Do not assign code Y99.9, Unspecified external cause status, if the status is not stated.

21. Chapter 21: Factors Influencing Health Status and Contact with Health Services (Z00-Z99)

Note: The chapter specific guidelines provide additional information about the use of Z codes for specified encounters.

a.   Use of Z codes in any healthcare setting
Z codes are for use in any healthcare setting. Z codes may be used as either a first-listed (principal diagnosis code in the inpatient setting) or secondary code, depending on the circumstances of the encounter.
Certain Z codes may only be used as first-listed or principal diagnosis.

b.   Z Codes indicate a reason for an encounter
Z codes are not procedure codes. A corresponding procedure code must accompany a Z code to describe any procedure performed.

c. Categories of Z Codes

1)   Contact/Exposure
Category Z20 indicates contact with, and suspected exposure to, communicable diseases. These codes are for patients who do not show any sign or symptom of a disease but are suspected to have been exposed to it by close personal contact with an infected individual or are in an area where a disease is epidemic.

Category Z77, Other contact with and (suspected) exposures hazardous to health, indicates contact with and suspected exposures hazardous to health.

Contact/exposure codes may be used as a first-listed code to explain an encounter for testing, or, more commonly, as a secondary code to identify a potential risk.

2)   Inoculations and vaccinations
Code Z23 is for encounters for inoculations and vaccinations. It indicates that a patient is being seen to receive a prophylactic inoculation against a disease. Procedure codes are required to identify the actual administration of the injection and the type(s) of immunizations given. Code Z23 may be used as a secondary code if the inoculation is given as a routine part of preventive health care, such as a well-baby visit.

3)   Status
Status codes indicate that a patient is either a carrier of a disease or has the sequelae or residual of a past disease or condition. This includes such things as the presence of prosthetic or mechanical devices resulting from past treatment. A status code is informative, because the status may affect the course of treatment and its outcome. A status code is distinct from a history code. The history code indicates that the patient no longer has the condition.

CHAPTER 21 – FACTORS INFLUENCING HEALTH
Section I. C. 21. c. 3)

A status code should not be used with a diagnosis code from one of the body system chapters, if the diagnosis code includes the information provided by the status code. For example, code Z94.1, Heart transplant status, should not be used with a code from subcategory T86.2, Complications of heart transplant. The status code does not provide additional information. The complication code indicates that the patient is a heart transplant patient.

For encounters for weaning from a mechanical ventilator, assign a code from subcategory J96.1, Chronic respiratory failure, followed by code Z99.11, Dependence on respirator [ventilator] status.

The status Z codes/categories are:
Z14   Genetic carrier
          Genetic carrier status indicates that a person carries a gene, associated with a particular disease, which may be passed to offspring who may develop that disease. The person does not have the disease and is not at risk of developing the disease.

Z15   Genetic susceptibility to disease
          Genetic susceptibility indicates that a person has a gene that increases the risk of that person developing the disease.
          Codes from category Z15 should not be used as principal or first-listed codes. If the patient has the condition to which he/she is susceptible, and that condition is the reason for the encounter, the code for the current condition should be sequenced first. If the patient is being seen for follow-up after completed treatment for this condition, and the condition no longer exists, a follow-up code should be sequenced first, followed by the appropriate personal history and genetic susceptibility codes. If the purpose of the encounter is genetic counseling associated with procreative management, code Z31.5, Encounter for genetic counseling, should be assigned as the first-listed code, followed by a code from category Z15. Additional codes should be assigned for any applicable family or personal history.

Z16   Resistance to antimicrobial drugs
          This code indicates that a patient has a condition that is resistant to antimicrobial drug treatment. Sequence the infection code first.
Z17   Estrogen receptor status
Z18   Retained foreign body fragments
Z19   Hormone sensitivity malignancy status
Z21   Asymptomatic HIV infection status
          This code indicates that a patient has tested positive for HIV but has manifested no signs or symptoms of the disease.
Z22   Carrier of infectious disease
          Carrier status indicates that a person harbors the specific organisms of a disease without manifest symptoms and is capable of transmitting the infection.
Z28.3   Underimmunization status
Z33.1   Pregnant state, incidental
          This code is a secondary code only for use when the pregnancy is in no way complicating the reason for visit. Otherwise, a code from the obstetric chapter is required.
Z66   Do not resuscitate
          This code may be used when it is documented by the provider that a patient is on do not resuscitate status at any time during the stay.
Z67   Blood type
Z68   Body mass index (BMI)
          As with all other secondary diagnosis codes, the BMI codes should only be assigned when they meet the definition of a reportable diagnosis (see Section III, Reporting Additional Diagnoses).
Z74.01   Bed confinement status
Z76.82   Awaiting organ transplant status
Z78   Other specified health status
          Code Z78.1, Physical restraint status, may be used when it is documented by the provider that a patient has been put in restraints during the current encounter. Please note that this code should not be reported when it is documented by the provider that a patient is temporarily restrained during a procedure.
Z79   Long-term (current) drug therapy
          Codes from this category indicate a patient's continuous use of a prescribed drug (including such things as aspirin therapy) for the long-term treatment of a condition or for prophylactic use. It is not for use for patients who have addictions to drugs. This subcategory is not for use of medications for detoxification or maintenance programs to prevent withdrawal symptoms in patients with drug dependence (e.g., methadone maintenance for opiate dependence). Assign the appropriate code for the drug dependence instead.

CHAPTER 21 – FACTORS INFLUENCING HEALTH
Section I. C. 21. c. 3)

Assign a code from Z79 if the patient is receiving a medication for an extended period as a prophylactic measure (such as for the prevention of deep vein thrombosis) or as treatment of a chronic condition (such as arthritis) or a disease requiring a lengthy course of treatment (such as cancer). Do not assign a code from category Z79 for medication being administered for a brief period of time to treat an acute illness or injury (such as a course of antibiotics to treat acute bronchitis).

Z88   Allergy status to drugs, medicaments and biological substances
       Except: Z88.9, Allergy status to unspecified drugs, medicaments and biological substances status

Z89   Acquired absence of limb

Z90   Acquired absence of organs, not elsewhere classified

Z91.0-   Allergy status, other than to drugs and biological substances

Z92.82   Status post administration of tPA (rtPA) in a different facility within the last 24 hours prior to admission to a current facility.

Assign code Z92.82, Status post administration of tPA (rtPA) in a different facility within the last 24 hours prior to admission to current facility, as a secondary diagnosis when a patient is received by transfer into a facility and documentation indicates they were administered tissue plasminogen activator (tPA) within the last 24 hours prior to admission to the current facility.

This guideline applies even if the patient is still receiving the tPA at the time they are received into the current facility.

The appropriate code for the condition for which the tPA was administered (such as cerebrovascular disease or myocardial infarction) should be assigned first.

Code Z92.82 is only applicable to the receiving facility record and not to the transferring facility record.

Z93   Artificial opening status

Z94   Transplanted organ and tissue status

Z95   Presence of cardiac and vascular implants and grafts

Z96   Presence of other functional implants

Z97   Presence of other devices

Z98   Other postprocedural states

Assign code Z98.85, Transplanted organ removal status, to indicate that a transplanted organ has been previously removed. This code should not be assigned for the encounter in which the transplanted organ is removed. The complication necessitating removal of the transplant organ should be assigned for that encounter.

See section I.C19. for information on the coding of organ transplant complications.

Z99   Dependence on enabling machines and devices, not elsewhere classified
Note: Categories Z89-Z90 and Z93-Z99 are for use only if there are no complications or malfunctions of the organ or tissue replaced, the amputation site or the equipment on which the patient is dependent.

4) History (of)

There are two types of history Z codes, personal and family. Personal history codes explain a patient's past medical condition that no longer exists and is not receiving any treatment, but that has the potential for recurrence, and therefore may require continued monitoring.

Family history codes are for use when a patient has a family member(s) who has had a particular disease that causes the patient to be at higher risk of also contracting the disease.

Personal history codes may be used in conjunction with follow-up codes and family history codes may be used in conjunction with screening codes to explain the need for a test or procedure. History codes are also acceptable on any medical record regardless of the reason for visit. A history of an illness, even if no longer present, is important information that may alter the type of treatment ordered.

The history Z code categories are:

Z80   Family history of primary malignant neoplasm

Z81   Family history of mental and behavioral disorders

Z82   Family history of certain disabilities and chronic diseases (leading to disablement)

Z83   Family history of other specific disorders

Z84   Family history of other conditions

Z85   Personal history of malignant neoplasm

Z86   Personal history of certain other diseases

Z87   Personal history of other diseases and conditions

Z91.4-   Personal history of psychological trauma, not elsewhere classified

Z91.5   Personal history of self-harm

CHAPTER 21 – FACTORS INFLUENCING HEALTH
Section I. C. 21. c. 4)

Z91.8-   Other specified personal risk factors, not elsewhere classified
       Exception: Z91.83, Wandering in diseases classified elsewhere

Z92   Personal history of medical treatment
       Except: Z92.0, Personal history of contraception
       Except: Z92.82, Status post administration of tPA (rtPA) in a different facility within the last 24 hours prior to admission to a current facility

5) Screening

Screening is the testing for disease or disease precursors in seemingly well individuals so that early detection and treatment can be provided for those who test positive for the disease (e.g., screening mammogram).

The testing of a person to rule out or confirm a suspected diagnosis because the patient has some sign or symptom is a diagnostic examination, not a screening. In these cases, the sign or symptom is used to explain the reason for the test.

A screening code may be a first-listed code if the reason for the visit is specifically the screening exam. It may also be used as an additional code if the screening is done during an office visit for other health problems. A screening code is not necessary if the screening is inherent to a routine examination, such as a pap smear done during a routine pelvic examination.

Should a condition be discovered during the screening then the code for the condition may be assigned as an additional diagnosis.

The Z code indicates that a screening exam is planned. A procedure code is required to confirm that the screening was performed.

The screening Z codes/categories:

Z11   Encounter for screening for infectious and parasitic diseases

Z12   Encounter for screening for malignant neoplasms

Z13   Encounter for screening for other diseases and disorders
       Except: Z13.9, Encounter for screening, unspecified

Z36   Encounter for antenatal screening for mother

6) Observation

There are ~~two~~ three observation Z code categories. They are for use in very limited circumstances when a person is being observed for a suspected condition that is ruled out. The observation codes are not for use if an injury or illness or any signs or symptoms related to the suspected condition are present. In such cases the diagnosis/symptom code is used with the corresponding external cause code.

The observation codes are to be used as principal diagnosis only. The only exception to this is when the principal diagnosis is required to be a code from category Z38, Live-born infants according to place of birth and type of delivery. Then a code from category Z05, Encounter for observation and evaluation of newborn for suspected diseases and conditions ruled out, is sequenced after the Z38 code. Additional codes may be used in addition to the observation code but only if they are unrelated to the suspected condition being observed.

Codes from subcategory Z03.7, Encounter for suspected maternal and fetal conditions ruled out, may either be used as a first-listed or as an additional code assignment depending on the case. They are for use in very limited circumstances on a maternal record when an encounter is for a suspected maternal or fetal condition that is ruled out during that encounter (for example, a maternal or fetal condition may be suspected due to an abnormal test result). These codes should not be used when the condition is confirmed. In those cases, the confirmed condition should be coded. In addition, these codes are not for use if an illness or any signs or symptoms related to the suspected condition or problem are present. In such cases the diagnosis/symptom code is used.

Additional codes may be used in addition to the code from subcategory Z03.7, but only if they are unrelated to the suspected condition being evaluated.

Codes from subcategory Z03.7 may not be used for encounters for antenatal screening of mother. *See Section I.C.21. Screening.*

For encounters for suspected fetal condition that are inconclusive following testing and evaluation, assign the appropriate code from category O35, O36, O40 or O41.

The observation Z code categories:

Z03   Encounter for medical observation for suspected diseases and conditions ruled out

Z04   Encounter for examination and observation for other reasons
       Except: Z04.9, Encounter for examination and observation for unspecified reason

Z05   Encounter for observation and evaluation of newborn for suspected diseases and conditions ruled out

7) Aftercare

Aftercare visit codes cover situations when the initial treatment of a disease has been performed and the patient requires continued care during the healing or recovery phase, or for the long-term consequences of the disease. The aftercare Z code should not be used if treatment is directed at a current, acute disease. The diagnosis code is to be used in these cases. Exceptions to this rule are codes Z51.0, Encounter for antineoplastic radiation therapy, and codes from subcategory Z51.1, Encounter for antineoplastic chemotherapy and immunotherapy. These codes are to be first-listed, followed by the diagnosis code when a patient's encounter is solely to receive radiation therapy, chemotherapy, or immunotherapy for the treatment of a neoplasm. If the reason for the encounter is more than one type of antineoplastic therapy, code Z51.0 and a code from subcategory Z51.1 may be assigned together, in which case one of these codes would be reported as a secondary diagnosis.

The aftercare Z codes should also not be used for aftercare for injuries. For aftercare of an injury, assign the acute injury code with the appropriate 7th character (for subsequent encounter).

The aftercare codes are generally first-listed to explain the specific reason for the encounter. An aftercare code may be used as an additional code when some type of aftercare is provided in addition to the reason for admission and no diagnosis code is applicable. An example of this would be the closure of a colostomy during an encounter for treatment of another condition.

Aftercare codes should be used in conjunction with other aftercare codes or diagnosis codes to provide better detail on the specifics of an aftercare encounter visit, unless otherwise directed by the classification. Should a patient receive multiple types of antineoplastic therapy during the same encounter, code Z51.0, Encounter for antineoplastic radiation therapy, and codes from subcategory Z51.1, Encounter for antineoplastic chemotherapy and immunotherapy, may be used together on a record. The sequencing of multiple aftercare codes depends on the circumstances of the encounter.

Certain aftercare Z code categories need a secondary diagnosis code to describe the resolving condition or sequelae. For others, the condition is included in the code title.

Additional Z code aftercare category terms include fitting and adjustment, and attention to artificial openings.

Status Z codes may be used with aftercare Z codes to indicate the nature of the aftercare. For example code Z95.1, Presence of aortocoronary bypass graft, may be used with code Z48.812, Encounter for surgical aftercare following surgery on the circulatory system, to indicate the surgery for which the aftercare is being performed. A status code should not be used when the aftercare code indicates the type of status, such as using Z43.0, Encounter for attention to tracheostomy, with Z93.0, Tracheostomy status.

The aftercare Z category/codes:

Z42	Encounter for plastic and reconstructive surgery following medical procedure or healed injury
Z43	Encounter for attention to artificial openings
Z44	Encounter for fitting and adjustment of external prosthetic device
Z45	Encounter for adjustment and management of implanted device
Z46	Encounter for fitting and adjustment of other devices
Z47	Orthopedic aftercare
Z48	Encounter for other postprocedural aftercare
Z49	Encounter for care involving renal dialysis
Z51	Encounter for other aftercare and medical care

8) Follow-up

The follow-up codes are used to explain continuing surveillance following completed treatment of a disease, condition, or injury. They imply that the condition has been fully treated and no longer exists. They should not be confused with aftercare codes, or injury codes with a 7th character for subsequent encounter, that explain ongoing care of a healing condition or its sequelae. Follow-up codes may be used in conjunction with history codes to provide the full picture of the healed condition and its treatment. The follow-up code is sequenced first, followed by the history code.

A follow-up code may be used to explain multiple visits. Should a condition be found to have recurred on the follow-up visit, then the diagnosis code for the condition should be assigned in place of the follow-up code.

The follow-up Z code categories:

Z08	Encounter for follow-up examination after completed treatment for malignant neoplasm
Z09	Encounter for follow-up examination after completed treatment for conditions other than malignant neoplasm
Z39	Encounter for maternal postpartum care and examination

9) Donor

Codes in category Z52, Donors of organs and tissues, are used for living individuals who are donating blood or other body tissue. These codes are only for individuals donating for others, not for self-donations. They are not used to identify cadaveric donations.

10) Counseling

Counseling Z codes are used when a patient or family member receives assistance in the aftermath of an illness or injury, or when support is required in coping with family or social problems. They are not used in conjunction with a diagnosis code when the counseling component of care is considered integral to standard treatment.
The counseling Z codes/categories:

Z30.0-	Encounter for general counseling and advice on contraception
Z31.5	Encounter for genetic counseling
Z31.6-	Encounter for general counseling and advice on procreation
Z32.2	Encounter for childbirth instruction
Z32.3	Encounter for childcare instruction
Z69	Encounter for mental health services for victim and perpetrator of abuse
Z70	Counseling related to sexual attitude, behavior and orientation
Z71	Persons encountering health services for other counseling and medical advice, not elsewhere classified
Z76.81	Expectant mother prebirth pediatrician visit

11) Encounters for Obstetrical and Reproductive Services
See Section I.C.15. Pregnancy, Childbirth, and the Puerperium, for further instruction on the use of these codes.

Z codes for pregnancy are for use in those circumstances when none of the problems or complications included in the codes from the Obstetrics chapter exist (a routine prenatal visit or postpartum care). Codes in category Z34, Encounter for supervision of normal pregnancy, are always first-listed and are not to be used with any other code from the OB chapter.

Codes in category Z3A, Weeks of gestation, may be assigned to provide additional information about the pregnancy. Category Z3A codes should not be assigned for pregnancies with abortive outcomes (categories O00-O08), elective termination of pregnancy (code Z33.32), nor for postpartum conditions, as category Z3A is not applicable to these conditions. The date of the admission should be used to determine weeks of gestation for inpatient admissions that encompass more than one gestational week.

The outcome of delivery, category Z37, should be included on all maternal delivery records. It is always a secondary code. Codes in category Z37 should not be used on the newborn record.

Z codes for family planning (contraceptive) or procreative management and counseling should be included on an obstetric record either during the pregnancy or the postpartum stage, if applicable.

Z codes/categories for obstetrical and reproductive services:

Z30	Encounter for contraceptive management
Z31	Encounter for procreative management
Z32.2	Encounter for childbirth instruction
Z32.3	Encounter for childcare instruction
Z33	Pregnant state
Z34	Encounter for supervision of normal pregnancy
Z36	Encounter for antenatal screening of mother
Z3A	Weeks of gestation
Z37	Outcome of delivery
Z39	Encounter for maternal postpartum care and examination
Z76.81	Expectant mother prebirth pediatrician visit

12) Newborns and Infants
See Section I.C.16. Newborn (Perinatal) Guidelines, for further instruction on the use of these codes.

Newborn Z codes/categories:

Z76.1	Encounter for health supervision and care of foundling
Z00.1-	Encounter for routine child health examination
Z38	Liveborn infants according to place of birth and type of delivery

13) Routine and administrative examinations
The Z codes allow for the description of encounters for routine examinations, such as, a general check-up, or, examinations for administrative purposes, such as, a pre-employment physical. The codes are not to be used if the examination is for diagnosis of a suspected condition or for treatment purposes. In such cases the diagnosis code is used. During a routine exam, should a diagnosis or condition be discovered, it should be coded as an additional code. Pre-existing and chronic conditions and history codes may also be included as additional codes as long as the examination is for administrative purposes and not focused on any particular condition.

CHAPTER 21 – FACTORS INFLUENCING HEALTH
Section I. C. 21. c. 13)

Some of the codes for routine health examinations distinguish between "with" and "without" abnormal findings. Code assignment depends on the information that is known at the time the encounter is being coded. For example, if no abnormal findings were found during the examination, but the encounter is being coded before test results are back, it is acceptable to assign the code for "without abnormal findings." When assigning a code for "with abnormal findings," additional code(s) should be assigned to identify the specific abnormal finding(s).

Pre-operative examination and pre-procedural laboratory examination Z codes are for use only in those situations when a patient is being cleared for a procedure or surgery and no treatment is given.

The Z codes/categories for routine and administrative examinations:

Z00	Encounter for general examination without complaint, suspected or reported diagnosis
Z01	Encounter for other special examination without complaint, suspected or reported diagnosis
Z02	Encounter for administrative examination
	Except: Z02.9, Encounter for administrative examinations, unspecified
Z32.0-	Encounter for pregnancy test

14) Miscellaneous Z codes
The miscellaneous Z codes capture a number of other health care encounters that do not fall into one of the other categories. Certain of these codes identify the reason for the encounter; others are for use as additional codes that provide useful information on circumstances that may affect a patient's care and treatment.

Prophylactic Organ Removal
For encounters specifically for prophylactic removal of an organ (such as prophylactic removal of breasts due to a genetic susceptibility to cancer or a family history of cancer), the principal or first-listed code should be a code from category Z40, Encounter for prophylactic surgery, followed by the appropriate codes to identify the associated risk factor (such as genetic susceptibility or family history).

If the patient has a malignancy of one site and is having prophylactic removal at another site to prevent either a new primary malignancy or metastatic disease, a code for the malignancy should also be assigned in addition to a code from subcategory Z40.0, Encounter for prophylactic surgery for risk factors related to malignant neoplasms. A Z40.0 code should not be assigned if the patient is having organ removal for treatment of a malignancy, such as the removal of the testes for the treatment of prostate cancer.

Miscellaneous Z codes/categories:

Z28	Immunization not carried out
	Except: Z28.3, Underimmunization status
Z29	Encounter for other prophylactic measures
Z40	Encounter for prophylactic surgery
Z41	Encounter for procedures for purposes other than remedying health state
	Except: Z41.9, Encounter for procedure for purposes other than remedying health state, unspecified
Z53	Persons encountering health services for specific procedures and treatment, not carried out
Z55	Problems related to education and literacy
Z56	Problems related to employment and unemployment
Z57	Occupational exposure to risk factors
Z58	Problems related to physical environment
Z59	Problems related to housing and economic circumstances
Z60	Problems related to social environment
Z62	Problems related to upbringing
Z63	Other problems related to primary support group, including family circumstances
Z64	Problems related to certain psychosocial circumstances
Z65	Problems related to other psychosocial circumstances
Z72	Problems related to lifestyle
	Note: These codes should be assigned only when the documentation specifies that the patient has an associated problem
Z73	Problems related to life management difficulty
Z74	Problems related to care provider dependency
	Except: Z74.01, Bed confinement status
Z75	Problems related to medical facilities and other health care
Z76.0	Encounter for issue of repeat prescription
Z76.3	Healthy person accompanying sick person
Z76.4	Other boarder to healthcare facility
Z76.5	Malingerer [conscious simulation]
Z91.1-	Patient's noncompliance with medical treatment and regimen
Z91.83	Wandering in diseases classified elsewhere
Z91.89	Other specified personal risk factors, not elsewhere classified

CHAPTER 21 – FACTORS INFLUENCING HEALTH
Section I. C. 21. c. 15)

15) Nonspecific Z codes
Certain Z codes are so non-specific, or potentially redundant with other codes in the classification, that there can be little justification for their use in the inpatient setting. Their use in the outpatient setting should be limited to those instances when there is no further documentation to permit more precise coding. Otherwise, any sign or symptom or any other reason for visit that is captured in another code should be used.

Nonspecific Z codes/categories:

Z02.9	Encounter for administrative examinations, unspecified
Z04.9	Encounter for examination and observation for unspecified reason
Z13.9	Encounter for screening, unspecified
Z41.9	Encounter for procedure for purposes other than remedying health state, unspecified
Z52.9	Donor of unspecified organ or tissue
Z86.59	Personal history of other mental and behavioral disorders
Z88.9	Allergy status to unspecified drugs, medicaments and biological substances status
Z92.0	Personal history of contraception

16) Z Codes That May Only be Principal/First-Listed Diagnosis
The following Z codes/categories may only be reported as the principal/first-listed diagnosis, except when there are multiple encounters on the same day and the medical records for the encounters are combined:

Z00	Encounter for general examination without complaint, suspected or reported diagnosis Except: Z00.6
Z01	Encounter for other special examination without complaint, suspected or reported diagnosis
Z02	Encounter for administrative examination
Z03	Encounter for medical observation for suspected diseases and conditions ruled out
Z04	Encounter for examination and observation for other reasons
Z31.81	Encounter for male factor infertility in female patient
~~Z31.82~~	~~Encounter for Rh incompatibility status~~
Z31.83	Encounter for assisted reproductive fertility procedure cycle
Z31.84	Encounter for fertility preservation procedure
Z34	Encounter for supervision of normal pregnancy
Z39	Encounter for maternal postpartum care and examination
Z38	Liveborn infants according to place of birth and type of delivery
Z42	Encounter for plastic and reconstructive surgery following medical procedure or healed injury
Z51.0	Encounter for antineoplastic radiation therapy
Z51.1-	Encounter for antineoplastic chemotherapy and immunotherapy
Z52	Donors of organs and tissues
	Except: Z52.9, Donor of unspecified organ or tissue
Z76.1	Encounter for health supervision and care of foundling
Z76.2	Encounter for health supervision and care of other healthy infant and child
Z99.12	Encounter for respirator [ventilator] dependence during power failure

SECTION II – PRINCIPAL DIAGNOSIS
Section II.

Section II. Selection of Principal Diagnosis

The circumstances of inpatient admission always govern the selection of principal diagnosis. The principal diagnosis is defined in the Uniform Hospital Discharge Data Set (UHDDS) as "that condition established after study to be chiefly responsible for occasioning the admission of the patient to the hospital for care."

The UHDDS definitions are used by hospitals to report inpatient data elements in a standardized manner. These data elements and their definitions can be found in the July 31, 1985, Federal Register (Vol. 50, No, 147), pp. 31038-40.

Since that time the application of the UHDDS definitions has been expanded to include all non-outpatient settings (acute care, short term, long term care and psychiatric hospitals; home health agencies; rehab facilities; nursing homes, etc). The UHDDS definitions also apply to hospice services (all levels of care).

In determining principal diagnosis the coding conventions in the ICD-10-CM, the Tabular List and Alphabetic Index take precedence over these official coding guidelines. *(See Section I.A., Conventions for the ICD-10-CM)*

The importance of consistent, complete documentation in the medical record cannot be overemphasized. Without such documentation the application of all coding guidelines is a difficult, if not impossible, task.

A. Codes for symptoms, signs, and ill-defined conditions
Codes for symptoms, signs, and ill-defined conditions from Chapter 18 are not to be used as principal diagnosis when a related definitive diagnosis has been established.

B. Two or more interrelated conditions, each potentially meeting the definition for principal diagnosis.
When there are two or more interrelated conditions (such as diseases in the same ICD-10-CM chapter or manifestations characteristically associated with a certain disease) potentially meeting the definition of principal diagnosis, either condition may be sequenced first, unless the circumstances of the admission, the therapy provided, the Tabular List, or the Alphabetic Index indicate otherwise.

C. Two or more diagnoses that equally meet the definition for principal diagnosis
In the unusual instance when two or more diagnoses equally meet the criteria for principal diagnosis as determined by the circumstances of admission, diagnostic workup and/or therapy provided, and the Alphabetic Index, Tabular List, or another coding guidelines does not provide sequencing direction, any one of the diagnoses may be sequenced first.

D. Two or more comparative or contrasting conditions.
In those rare instances when two or more contrasting or comparative diagnoses are documented as "either/or" (or similar terminology), they are coded as if the diagnoses were confirmed and the diagnoses are sequenced according to the circumstances of the admission. If no further determination can be made as to which diagnosis should be principal, either diagnosis may be sequenced first.

E. A symptom(s) followed by contrasting/comparative diagnoses
Guideline has been deleted effective October 1, 2014

F. Original treatment plan not carried out
Sequence as the principal diagnosis the condition, which after study occasioned the admission to the hospital, even though treatment may not have been carried out due to unforeseen circumstances.

G. Complications of surgery and other medical care
When the admission is for treatment of a complication resulting from surgery or other medical care, the complication code is sequenced as the principal diagnosis. If the complication is classified to the T80-T88 series and the code lacks the necessary specificity in describing the complication, an additional code for the specific complication should be assigned.

H. Uncertain Diagnosis
If the diagnosis documented at the time of discharge is qualified as "probable", "suspected", "likely", "questionable", "possible", or "still to be ruled out", or other similar terms indicating uncertainty, code the condition as if it existed or was established. The bases for these guidelines are the diagnostic workup, arrangements for further workup or observation, and initial therapeutic approach that correspond most closely with the established diagnosis.

Note: This guideline is applicable only to inpatient admissions to short-term, acute, long-term care and psychiatric hospitals.

SECTION II – PRINCIPAL DIAGNOSIS
Section II. I.

I. Admission from Observation Unit

1. Admission Following Medical Observation
When a patient is admitted to an observation unit for a medical condition, which either worsens or does not improve, and is subsequently admitted as an inpatient of the same hospital for this same medical condition, the principal diagnosis would be the medical condition which led to the hospital admission.

2. Admission Following Post-Operative Observation
When a patient is admitted to an observation unit to monitor a condition (or complication) that develops following outpatient surgery, and then is subsequently admitted as an inpatient of the same hospital, hospitals should apply the Uniform Hospital Discharge Data Set (UHDDS) definition of principal diagnosis as "that condition established after study to be chiefly responsible for occasioning the admission of the patient to the hospital for care."

J. Admission from Outpatient Surgery
When a patient receives surgery in the hospital's outpatient surgery department and is subsequently admitted for continuing inpatient care at the same hospital, the following guidelines should be followed in selecting the principal diagnosis for the inpatient admission:
  • If the reason for the inpatient admission is a complication, assign the complication as the principal diagnosis.
  • If no complication, or other condition, is documented as the reason for the inpatient admission, assign the reason for the outpatient surgery as the principal diagnosis.
  • If the reason for the inpatient admission is another condition unrelated to the surgery, assign the unrelated condition as the principal diagnosis.

K. Admission/Encounters for Rehabilitation
When the purpose for the admission/encounter is rehabilitation, sequence first the code for the condition for which the service is being performed. For example, for an admission/encounter for rehabilitation right-sided dominant hemiplegia following a cerebrovascular infarction, report code I69.351, Hemiplegia and hemiparesis following cerebral infarction affecting right dominant side, as the first-listed or principal diagnosis.

If the condition for which the rehabilitation service is no longer present, report the appropriate aftercare code as the first-listed or principal diagnosis. For example, if a patient with severe degenerative osteoarthritis of the hip, underwent hip replacement and the current encounter/admission is for rehabilitation, report code Z47.1, Aftercare following joint replacement surgery, as the principal diagnosis.

See Section I.C.21.c.7, Factors influencing health status and contact with health services, Aftercare.

SECTION III – ADDITIONAL DIAGNOSES
Section III.

Section III. Reporting Additional Diagnoses

GENERAL RULES FOR OTHER (ADDITIONAL) DIAGNOSES

For reporting purposes the definition for "other diagnoses" is interpreted as additional conditions that affect patient care in terms of requiring:
    clinical evaluation; or
    therapeutic treatment; or
    diagnostic procedures; or
    extended length of hospital stay; or
    increased nursing care and/or monitoring.

The UHDDS item #11-b defines Other Diagnoses as "all conditions that coexist at the time of admission, that develop subsequently, or that affect the treatment received and/or the length of stay. Diagnoses that relate to an earlier episode which have no bearing on the current hospital stay are to be excluded." UHDDS definitions apply to inpatients in acute care, short-term, long term care and psychiatric hospital setting. The UHDDS definitions are used by acute care short-term hospitals to report inpatient data elements in a standardized manner. These data elements and their definitions can be found in the July 31, 1985, Federal Register (Vol. 50, No, 147), pp. 31038-40.

Since that time the application of the UHDDS definitions has been expanded to include all non-outpatient settings (acute care, short term, long term care and psychiatric hospitals; home health agencies; rehab facilities; nursing homes, etc). The UHDDS definitions also apply to hospice services (all levels of care).

The following guidelines are to be applied in designating "other diagnoses" when neither the Alphabetic Index nor the Tabular List in ICD-10-CM provide direction. The listing of the diagnoses in the patient record is the responsibility of the attending provider.

A. **Previous conditions**
If the provider has included a diagnosis in the final diagnostic statement, such as the discharge summary or the face sheet, it should ordinarily be coded. Some providers include in the diagnostic statement resolved conditions or diagnoses and status-post procedures from previous admission that have no bearing on the current stay. Such conditions are not to be reported and are coded only if required by hospital policy.

However, history codes (categories Z80-Z87) may be used as secondary codes if the historical condition or family history has an impact on current care or influences treatment.

B. **Abnormal findings**
Abnormal findings (laboratory, x-ray, pathologic, and other diagnostic results) are not coded and reported unless the provider indicates their clinical significance. If the findings are outside the normal range and the attending provider has ordered other tests to evaluate the condition or prescribed treatment, it is appropriate to ask the provider whether the abnormal finding should be added.

Please note: This differs from the coding practices in the outpatient setting for coding encounters for diagnostic tests that have been interpreted by a provider.

C. **Uncertain Diagnosis**
If the diagnosis documented at the time of discharge is qualified as "probable", "suspected", "likely", "questionable", "possible", or "still to be ruled out" or other similar terms indicating uncertainty, code the condition as if it existed or was established. The bases for these guidelines are the diagnostic workup, arrangements for further workup or observation, and initial therapeutic approach that correspond most closely with the established diagnosis.

Note: This guideline is applicable only to inpatient admissions to short-term, acute, long-term care and psychiatric hospitals.

SECTION IV – OUTPATIENT GUIDELINES
Section IV.

Section IV. Diagnostic Coding and Reporting Guidelines for Outpatient Services

These coding guidelines for outpatient diagnoses have been approved for use by hospitals/ providers in coding and reporting hospital-based outpatient services and provider-based office visits. Guidelines in Section I, Conventions, general coding guidelines and chapter-specific guidelines, should also be applied for outpatient services and office visits.

Information about the use of certain abbreviations, punctuation, symbols, and other conventions used in the ICD-10-CM Tabular List (code numbers and titles), can be found in Section IA of these guidelines, under "Conventions Used in the Tabular List." Section I.B. contains general guidelines that apply to the entire classification. Section I.C. contains chapter-specific guidelines that correspond to the chapters as they are arranged in the classification. Information about the correct sequence to use in finding a code is also described in Section I.

The terms encounter and visit are often used interchangeably in describing outpatient service contacts and, therefore, appear together in these guidelines without distinguishing one from the other.

Though the conventions and general guidelines apply to all settings, coding guidelines for outpatient and provider reporting of diagnoses will vary in a number of instances from those for inpatient diagnoses, recognizing that:

The Uniform Hospital Discharge Data Set (UHDDS) definition of principal diagnosis ~~applies only to inpatients in acute, short-term, long-term care and psychiatric hospitals~~ does not apply to hospital-based outpatient services and provider-based office visits.

Coding guidelines for inconclusive diagnoses (probable, suspected, rule out, etc.) were developed for inpatient reporting and do not apply to outpatients.

A. **Selection of first-listed condition**
In the outpatient setting, the term first-listed diagnosis is used in lieu of principal diagnosis.

In determining the first-listed diagnosis the coding conventions of ICD-10-CM, as well as the general and disease specific guidelines take precedence over the outpatient guidelines.

Diagnoses often are not established at the time of the initial encounter/visit. It may take two or more visits before the diagnosis is confirmed.

The most critical rule involves beginning the search for the correct code assignment through the Alphabetic Index. Never begin searching initially in the Tabular List as this will lead to coding errors.

1. **Outpatient Surgery**
When a patient presents for outpatient surgery (same day surgery), code the reason for the surgery as the first-listed diagnosis (reason for the encounter), even if the surgery is not performed due to a contraindication.

2. **Observation Stay**
When a patient is admitted for observation for a medical condition, assign a code for the medical condition as the first-listed diagnosis.

When a patient presents for outpatient surgery and develops complications requiring admission to observation, code the reason for the surgery as the first reported diagnosis (reason for the encounter), followed by codes for the complications as secondary diagnoses.

B. **Codes from A00.0 through T88.9, Z00-Z99**
The appropriate code(s) from A00.0 through T88.9, Z00-Z99 must be used to identify diagnoses, symptoms, conditions, problems, complaints, or other reason(s) for the encounter/visit.

C. **Accurate reporting of ICD-10-CM diagnosis codes**
For accurate reporting of ICD-10-CM diagnosis codes, the documentation should describe the patient's condition, using terminology which includes specific diagnoses as well as symptoms, problems, or reasons for the encounter. There are ICD-10-CM codes to describe all of these.

D. **Codes that describe symptoms and signs**
Codes that describe symptoms and signs, as opposed to diagnoses, are acceptable for reporting purposes when a diagnosis has not been established (confirmed) by the provider. Chapter 18 of ICD-10-CM, Symptoms, Signs, and Abnormal Clinical and Laboratory Findings Not Elsewhere Classified (codes R00-R99) contain many, but not all codes for symptoms.

E. **Encounters for circumstances other than a disease or injury**
ICD-10-CM provides codes to deal with encounters for circumstances other than a disease or injury. The Factors Influencing Health Status and Contact with Health Services codes (Z00-Z99) are provided to deal with occasions when circumstances other than a disease or injury are recorded as diagnosis or problems.

See Section I.C.21. Factors influencing health status and contact with health services.

SECTION IV – OUTPATIENT GUIDELINES
Section IV. F. 1.

F. Level of Detail in Coding

1. ICD-10-CM codes with 3, 4, 5, 6 or 7 characters
ICD-10-CM is composed of codes with 3, 4, 5, 6 or 7 characters. Codes with three characters are included in ICD-10-CM as the heading of a category of codes that may be further subdivided by the use of fourth, fifth, sixth or seventh characters to provide greater specificity.

2. Use of full number of characters required for a code
A three-character code is to be used only if it is not further subdivided. A code is invalid if it has not been coded to the full number of characters required for that code, including the 7th character, if applicable.

G. ICD-10-CM code for the diagnosis, condition, problem, or other reason for encounter/visit
List first the ICD-10-CM code for the diagnosis, condition, problem, or other reason for encounter/visit shown in the medical record to be chiefly responsible for the services provided. List additional codes that describe any coexisting conditions. In some cases the first-listed diagnosis may be a symptom when a diagnosis has not been established (confirmed) by the physician.

H. Uncertain diagnosis
Do not code diagnoses documented as "probable", "suspected," "questionable," "rule out," or "working diagnosis" or other similar terms indicating uncertainty. Rather, code the condition(s) to the highest degree of certainty for that encounter/visit, such as symptoms, signs, abnormal test results, or other reason for the visit.

Please note: This differs from the coding practices used by short-term, acute care, long-term care and psychiatric hospitals.

I. Chronic diseases
Chronic diseases treated on an ongoing basis may be coded and reported as many times as the patient receives treatment and care for the condition(s).

J. Code all documented conditions that coexist
Code all documented conditions that coexist at the time of the encounter/visit, and require or affect patient care treatment or management. Do not code conditions that were previously treated and no longer exist. However, history codes (categories Z80-Z87) may be used as secondary codes if the historical condition or family history has an impact on current care or influences treatment.

K. Patients receiving diagnostic services only
For patients receiving diagnostic services only during an encounter/visit, sequence first the diagnosis, condition, problem, or other reason for encounter/visit shown in the medical record to be chiefly responsible for the outpatient services provided during the encounter/visit. Codes for other diagnoses (e.g., chronic conditions) may be sequenced as additional diagnoses.

For encounters for routine laboratory/radiology testing in the absence of any signs, symptoms, or associated diagnosis, assign Z01.89, Encounter for other specified special examinations. If routine testing is performed during the same encounter as a test to evaluate a sign, symptom, or diagnosis, it is appropriate to assign both the Z code and the code describing the reason for the non-routine test.

For outpatient encounters for diagnostic tests that have been interpreted by a physician, and the final report is available at the time of coding, code any confirmed or definitive diagnosis(es) documented in the interpretation. Do not code related signs and symptoms as additional diagnoses.

Please note: This differs from the coding practice in the hospital inpatient setting regarding abnormal findings on test results.

L. Patients receiving therapeutic services only
For patients receiving therapeutic services only during an encounter/visit, sequence first the diagnosis, condition, problem, or other reason for encounter/visit shown in the medical record to be chiefly responsible for the outpatient services provided during the encounter/visit. Codes for other diagnoses (e.g., chronic conditions) may be sequenced as additional diagnoses.

The only exception to this rule is that when the primary reason for the admission/encounter is chemotherapy or radiation therapy, the appropriate Z code for the service is listed first, and the diagnosis or problem for which the service is being performed listed second.

M. Patients receiving preoperative evaluations only
For patients receiving preoperative evaluations only, sequence first a code from subcategory Z01.81, Encounter for pre-procedural examinations, to describe the pre-op consultations. Assign a code for the condition to describe the reason for the surgery as an additional diagnosis. Code also any findings related to the pre-op evaluation.

N. Ambulatory surgery
For ambulatory surgery, code the diagnosis for which the surgery was performed. If the postoperative diagnosis is known to be different from the preoperative diagnosis at the time the diagnosis is confirmed, select the postoperative diagnosis for coding, since it is the most definitive.

SECTION IV – OUTPATIENT GUIDELINES
Section IV. O.

O. Routine outpatient prenatal visits
See Section I.C.15. Routine outpatient prenatal visits.

P. Encounters for general medical examinations with abnormal findings
The subcategories for encounters for general medical examinations, Z00.0-, provide codes for with and without abnormal findings. Should a general medical examination result in an abnormal finding, the code for general medical examination with abnormal finding should be assigned as the first-listed diagnosis. An examination with abnormal findings refers to a condition/diagnosis that is newly identified or a change in severity of a chronic condition (such as uncontrolled hypertension, or an acute exacerbation of chronic obstructive pulmonary disease) during a routine physical examination. A secondary code for the abnormal finding should also be coded.

Q. Encounters for routine health screenings
See Section I.C.21. Factors influencing health status and contact with health services, Screening.

© 2016 Channel Publishing, Ltd.

Appendix I
Present on Admission Reporting Guidelines

Introduction

These guidelines are to be used as a supplement to the ICD-10-CM Official Guidelines for Coding and Reporting to facilitate the assignment of the Present on Admission (POA) indicator for each diagnosis and external cause of injury code reported on claim forms (UB-04 and 837 Institutional).

These guidelines are not intended to replace any guidelines in the main body of the ICD-10-CM Official Guidelines for Coding and Reporting. The POA guidelines are not intended to provide guidance on when a condition should be coded, but rather, how to apply the POA indicator to the final set of diagnosis codes that have been assigned in accordance with Sections I, II, and III of the official coding guidelines. Subsequent to the assignment of the ICD-10-CM codes, the POA indicator should then be assigned to those conditions that have been coded.

As stated in the Introduction to the ICD-10-CM Official Guidelines for Coding and Reporting, a joint effort between the healthcare provider and the coder is essential to achieve complete and accurate documentation, code assignment, and reporting of diagnoses and procedures. The importance of consistent, complete documentation in the medical record cannot be overemphasized. Medical record documentation from any provider involved in the care and treatment of the patient may be used to support the determination of whether a condition was present on admission or not. In the context of the official coding guidelines, the term "provider" means a physician or any qualified healthcare practitioner who is legally accountable for establishing the patient's diagnosis.

These guidelines are not a substitute for the provider's clinical judgment as to the determination of whether a condition was/was not present on admission. The provider should be queried regarding issues related to the linking of signs/symptoms, timing of test results, and the timing of findings.

Please see the CDC website for the detailed list of ICD-10-CM codes that do not require the use of a POA indicator (ftp://ftp.cdc.gov/pub/Health_Statistics/NCHS/Publications/ICD10CM/2017/). The conditions on this exempt list represent categories and/or codes for circumstances regarding the healthcare encounter or factors influencing health status that do not represent a current disease or injury or are always present on admission.

General Reporting Requirements

All claims involving inpatient admissions to general acute care hospitals or other facilities that are subject to a law or regulation mandating collection of present on admission information.

Present on admission is defined as present at the time the order for inpatient admission occurs — conditions that develop during an outpatient encounter, including emergency department, observation, or outpatient surgery, are considered as present on admission.

POA Indicator is assigned to principal and secondary diagnoses (as defined in Section II of the Official Guidelines for Coding and Reporting) and the external cause of injury codes.

Issues related to inconsistent, missing, conflicting or unclear documentation must still be resolved by the provider.

If a condition would not be coded and reported based on UHDDS definitions and current official coding guidelines, then the POA indicator would not be reported.

Reporting Options
Y - Yes
N - No
U - Unknown
W — Clinically undetermined
Unreported/Not used (or "1" for Medicare usage) — (Exempt from POA reporting)

Reporting Definitions
Y = present at the time of inpatient admission
N = not present at the time of inpatient admission
U = documentation is insufficient to determine if condition is present on admission
W = provider is unable to clinically determine whether condition was present on admission or not

Timeframe for POA Identification and Documentation

There is no required timeframe as to when a provider (per the definition of "provider" used in these guidelines) must identify or document a condition to be present on admission. In some clinical situations, it may not be possible for a provider to make a definitive diagnosis (or a condition may not be recognized or reported by the patient) for a period of time after admission. In some cases it may be several days before the provider arrives at a definitive diagnosis. This does not mean that the condition was not present on admission. Determination of whether the condition was present on admission or not will be based on the applicable POA guideline as identified in this document, or on the provider's best clinical judgment.

If at the time of code assignment the documentation is unclear as to whether a condition was present on admission or not, it is appropriate to query the provider for clarification.

Assigning the POA Indicator

Condition is on the "Exempt from Reporting" list
Leave the "present on admission" field blank if the condition is on the list of ICD-10-CM codes for which this field is not applicable. This is the only circumstance in which the field may be left blank.

POA Explicitly Documented
Assign Y for any condition the provider explicitly documents as being present on admission.

Assign N for any condition the provider explicitly documents as not present at the time of admission.

Conditions diagnosed prior to inpatient admission
Assign "Y" for conditions that were diagnosed prior to admission (example: hypertension, diabetes mellitus, asthma)

Conditions diagnosed during the admission but clearly present before admission
Assign "Y" for conditions diagnosed during the admission that were clearly present but not diagnosed until after admission occurred.

Diagnoses subsequently confirmed after admission are considered present on admission if at the time of admission they are documented as suspected, possible, rule out, differential diagnosis, or constitute an underlying cause of a symptom that is present at the time of admission.

Condition develops during outpatient encounter prior to inpatient admission
Assign Y for any condition that develops during an outpatient encounter prior to a written order for inpatient admission.

Documentation does not indicate whether condition was present on admission
Assign "U" when the medical record documentation is unclear as to whether the condition was present on admission. "U" should not be routinely assigned and used only in very limited circumstances. Coders are encouraged to query the providers when the documentation is unclear.

Documentation states that it cannot be determined whether the condition was or was not present on admission
Assign "W" when the medical record documentation indicates that it cannot be clinically determined whether or not the condition was present on admission.

Chronic condition with acute exacerbation during the admission
If a single code identifies both the chronic condition and the acute exacerbation, see POA guidelines pertaining to ~~combination~~ codes that contain multiple clinical concepts.

If a single code only identifies the chronic condition and not the acute exacerbation (e.g., acute exacerbation of chronic leukemia), assign "Y."

Conditions documented as possible, probable, suspected, or rule out at the time of discharge
If the final diagnosis contains a possible, probable, suspected, or rule out diagnosis, and this diagnosis was based on signs, symptoms or clinical findings suspected at the time of inpatient admission, assign "Y."

If the final diagnosis contains a possible, probable, suspected, or rule out diagnosis, and this diagnosis was based on signs, symptoms or clinical findings that were not present on admission, assign "N".

Conditions documented as impending or threatened at the time of discharge
If the final diagnosis contains an impending or threatened diagnosis, and this diagnosis is based on symptoms or clinical findings that were present on admission, assign "Y".

If the final diagnosis contains an impending or threatened diagnosis, and this diagnosis is based on symptoms or clinical findings that were not present on admission, assign "N".

Acute and Chronic Conditions
Assign "Y" for acute conditions that are present at time of admission and N for acute conditions that are not present at time of admission.

Assign "Y" for chronic conditions, even though the condition may not be diagnosed until after admission.

If a single code identifies both an acute and chronic condition, see the POA guidelines for ~~combination~~ codes that contain multiple clinical concepts.

GUIDELINES

Combination Codes That Contain Multiple Clinical Concepts

Assign "N" if ~~any part of the combination~~ at least one of the clinical concepts included in the code was not present on admission (e.g., COPD with acute exacerbation and the exacerbation was not present on admission; gastric ulcer that does not start bleeding until after admission; asthma patient develops status asthmaticus after admission).

Assign "Y" if all parts of the ~~combination~~ clinical concepts included in the code were present on admission (e.g., ~~patient with acute prostatitis admitted with hematuria~~ duodenal ulcer that perforates prior to admission).

If the final diagnosis includes comparative or contrasting diagnoses, and both were present, or suspected, at the time of admission, assign "Y".

For infection codes that include the causal organism, assign "Y" if the infection (or signs of the infection) ~~was~~ were present on admission, even though the culture results may not be known until after admission (e.g., patient is admitted with pneumonia and the provider documents Pseudomonas as the causal organism a few days later).

Same Diagnosis Code for Two or More Conditions

When the same ICD-10-CM diagnosis code applies to two or more conditions during the same encounter (e.g. two separate conditions classified to the same ICD-10-CM diagnosis code):

Assign "Y" if all conditions represented by the single ICD-10-CM code were present on admission (e.g. bilateral unspecified age-related cataracts).

Assign "N" if any of the conditions represented by the single ICD-10-CM code was not present on admission (e.g. traumatic secondary and recurrent hemorrhage and seroma is assigned to a single code T79.2, but only one of the conditions was present on admission).

Obstetrical conditions

Whether or not the patient delivers during the current hospitalization does not affect assignment of the POA indicator. The determining factor for POA assignment is whether the pregnancy complication or obstetrical condition described by the code was present at the time of admission or not.

If the pregnancy complication or obstetrical condition was present on admission (e.g., patient admitted in preterm labor), assign "Y".

If the pregnancy complication or obstetrical condition was not present on admission (e.g., 2nd degree laceration during delivery, postpartum hemorrhage that occurred during current hospitalization, fetal distress develops after admission), assign "N".
If the obstetrical code includes more than one diagnosis and any of the diagnoses identified by the code were not present on admission assign "N" (e.g., Category O11, Pre-existing hypertension with pre-eclampsia).

Perinatal conditions

Newborns are not considered to be admitted until after birth. Therefore, any condition present at birth or that developed in utero is considered present at admission and should be assigned "Y". This includes conditions that occur during delivery (e.g., injury during delivery, meconium aspiration, exposure to streptococcus B in the vaginal canal).

Congenital conditions and anomalies

Assign "Y" for congenital conditions and anomalies except for categories Q00-Q99, Congenital anomalies, which are on the exempt list. Congenital conditions are always considered present on admission.

External cause of injury codes

Assign "Y" for any external cause code representing an external cause of morbidity that occurred prior to inpatient admission (e.g., patient fell out of bed at home, patient fell out of bed in emergency room prior to admission).

Assign "N" for any external cause code representing an external cause of morbidity that occurred during inpatient hospitalization (e.g., patient fell out of hospital bed during hospital stay, patient experienced an adverse reaction to a medication administered after inpatient admission).

A

Aarskog's syndrome Q87.1
Abandonment — *see* Maltreatment
Abasia (-astasia) (hysterical) F44.4
Abderhalden-Kaufmann-Lignac
   syndrome (cystinosis) E72.04
Abdomen, abdominal — *see also* condition
  acute R10.0
  angina K55.1
  muscle deficiency syndrome Q79.4
Abdominalgia — *see* Pain, abdominal
Abduction contracture, hip or other joint
  — *see* Contraction, joint
Aberrant (congenital) — *see also* Malposition,
  congenital
  adrenal gland Q89.1
  artery (peripheral) Q27.8
    basilar NEC Q28.1
    cerebral Q28.3
    coronary Q24.5
    digestive system Q27.8
    eye Q15.8
    lower limb Q27.8
    precerebral Q28.1
    pulmonary Q25.79
    renal Q27.2
    retina Q14.1
    specified site NEC Q27.8
    subclavian Q27.8
    upper limb Q27.8
    vertebral Q28.1
  breast Q83.8
  endocrine gland NEC Q89.2
  hepatic duct Q44.5
  pancreas Q45.3
  parathyroid gland Q89.2
  pituitary gland Q89.2
  sebaceous glands, mucous membrane, mouth,
    congenital Q38.6
  spleen Q89.09
  subclavian artery Q27.8
  thymus (gland) Q89.2
  thyroid gland Q89.2
  vein (peripheral) NEC Q27.8
    cerebral Q28.3
    digestive system Q27.8
    lower limb Q27.8
    precerebral Q28.1
    specified site NEC Q27.8
    upper limb Q27.8
Aberration
  distantial — *see* Disturbance, visual
  mental F99
Abetalipoproteinemia E78.6
Abiotrophy R68.89
Ablatio, ablation
  retinae — *see* Detachment, retina
Ablepharia, ablepharon Q10.3
Abnormal, abnormality, abnormalities —
  see also Anomaly
  acid-base balance (mixed) E87.4
  albumin R77.0
  alphafetoprotein R77.2
  alveolar ridge K08.9
  anatomical relationship Q89.9
  apertures, congenital, diaphragm Q79.1
  auditory perception H93.29-
    diplacusis — *see* Diplacusis
    hyperacusis — *see* Hyperacusis
    recruitment — *see* Recruitment, auditory
    threshold shift — *see* Shift, auditory threshold
  autosomes Q99.9
    fragile site Q95.5
  basal metabolic rate R94.8
  biosynthesis, testicular androgen E29.1

Abnormal, abnormality, abnormalities
  (*see also* Anomaly) — *continued*
  bleeding time R79.1
  blood level (of)
    cobalt R79.0
    copper R79.0
    iron R79.0
    lithium R78.89
    magnesium R79.0
    mineral NEC R79.0
    zinc R79.0
  blood pressure
    elevated R03.0
    low reading (nonspecific) R03.1
  blood sugar R73.09
  blood-gas level R79.81
  bowel sounds R19.15
    absent R19.11
    hyperactive R19.12
  brain scan R94.02
  breathing R06.9
  caloric test R94.138
  cerebrospinal fluid R83.9
    cytology R83.6
    drug level R83.2
    enzyme level R83.0
    hormones R83.1
    immunology R83.4
    microbiology R83.5
    nonmedicinal level R83.3
    specified type NEC R83.8
  chemistry, blood R79.9
    C-reactive protein R79.82
    drugs — *see* Findings, abnormal, in blood
    gas level R79.81
    minerals R79.0
    pancytopenia D61.818
    PTT R79.1
    specified NEC R79.89
    toxins — *see* Findings, abnormal, in blood
  chest sounds (friction) (rales) R09.89
  chromosome, chromosomal Q99.9
    with more than three X chromosomes, female
      Q97.1
    analysis result R89.8
      bronchial washings R84.8
      cerebrospinal fluid R83.8
      cervix uteri NEC R87.89
      nasal secretions R84.8
      nipple discharge R89.8
      peritoneal fluid R85.89
      pleural fluid R84.8
      prostatic secretions R86.8
      saliva R85.89
      seminal fluid R86.8
      sputum R84.8
      synovial fluid R89.8
      throat scrapings R84.8
      vagina R87.89
      vulva R87.89
      wound secretions R89.8
    dicentric replacement Q93.2
    ring replacement Q93.2
    sex Q99.8
      female phenotype Q97.9
        specified NEC Q97.8
      male phenotype Q98.9
        specified NEC Q98.8
      structural male Q98.6
    specified NEC Q99.8
  clinical findings NEC R68.89
  coagulation D68.9
    newborn, transient P61.6
    profile R79.1
    time R79.1
  communication — *see* Fistula
  conjunctiva, vascular H11.41-
  coronary artery Q24.5

Abnormal, abnormality, abnormalities
  (*see also* Anomaly) — *continued*
  cortisol-binding globulin E27.8
  course, eustachian tube Q17.8
  creatinine clearance R94.4
  cytology
    anus R85.619
      atypical squamous cells cannot exclude
        high grade squamous intraepithelial
        lesion (ASC-H) R85.611
      atypical squamous cells of undetermined
        significance (ASC-US) R85.610
      cytologic evidence of malignancy R85.614
      high grade squamous intraepithelial lesion
        (HGSIL) R85.613
      human papillomavirus (HPV) DNA test
        high risk positive R85.81
        low risk positive R85.82
      inadequate smear R85.615
      low grade squamous intraepithelial lesion
        (LGSIL) R85.612
      satisfactory anal smear but lacking
        transformation zone R85.616
      specified NEC R85.618
      unsatisfactory smear R85.615
    female genital organs — *see* Abnormal,
      Papanicolaou (smear)
  dark adaptation curve H53.61
  dentofacial NEC — *see* Anomaly, dentofacial
  development, developmental Q89.9
    central nervous system Q07.9
  diagnostic imaging
    abdomen, abdominal region NEC R93.5
    biliary tract R93.2
    bladder R93.41
    breast R92.8
    central nervous system NEC R90.89
    cerebrovascular NEC R90.89
    coronary circulation R93.1
    digestive tract NEC R93.3
    gastrointestinal (tract) R93.3
    genitourinary organs R93.8
    head R93.0
    heart R93.1
    intrathoracic organ NEC R93.8
    kidney R93.42-
    limbs R93.6
    liver R93.2
    lung (field) R91.8
    musculoskeletal system NEC R93.7
    renal pelvis R93.41
    retroperitoneum R93.5
    site specified NEC R93.8
    skin and subcutaneous tissue R93.8
    skull R93.0
    ureter R93.41
    urinary organs specified NEC R93.49
  direction, teeth, fully erupted M26.30
  ear ossicles, acquired NEC H74.39-
    ankylosis — *see* Ankylosis, ear ossicles
    discontinuity — *see* Discontinuity, ossicles,
      ear
    partial loss — *see* Loss, ossicles, ear (partial)
  Ebstein Q22.5
  echocardiogram R93.1
  echoencephalogram R90.81
  echogram — *see* Abnormal, diagnostic
    imaging
  electro-oculogram [EOG] R94.110
  electrocardiogram [ECG] [EKG] R94.31
  electroencephalogram [EEG] R94.01
  electrolyte — *see* Imbalance, electrolyte
  electromyogram [EMG] R94.131
  electrophysiological intracardiac studies
    R94.39
  electroretinogram [ERG] R94.111
  erythrocytes
    congenital, with perinatal jaundice D58.9
  feces (color) (contents) (mucus) R19.5

Abnormal, abnormality, abnormalities
(*see also* Anomaly) — *continued*
finding — *see* Findings, abnormal, without
 diagnosis
fluid
  amniotic — *see* Abnormal, specimen,
   specified
  cerebrospinal — *see* Abnormal,
   cerebrospinal fluid
  peritoneal — *see* Abnormal, specimen,
   digestive organs
  pleural — *see* Abnormal, specimen,
   respiratory organs
  synovial — *see* Abnormal, specimen,
   specified
  thorax (bronchial washings) (pleural fluid) —
   see Abnormal, specimen, respiratory
   organs
  vaginal — *see* Abnormal, specimen, female
   genital organs
form
  teeth K00.2
  uterus — *see* Anomaly, uterus
function studies
  auditory R94.120
  bladder R94.8
  brain R94.09
  cardiovascular R94.30
  ear R94.128
  endocrine NEC R94.7
  eye NEC R94.118
  kidney R94.4
  liver R94.5
  nervous system
   central NEC R94.09
   peripheral NEC R94.138
  pancreas R94.8
  placenta R94.8
  pulmonary R94.2
  special senses NEC R94.128
  spleen R94.8
  thyroid R94.6
  vestibular R94.121
gait — *see* Gait
  hysterical F44.4
gastrin secretion E16.4
globulin R77.1
  cortisol-binding E27.8
  thyroid-binding E07.89
glomerular, minor (*see also* N00-N07 with
  fourth character .0) N05.0
glucagon secretion E16.3
glucose tolerance (test) (non-fasting) R73.09
gravitational (G) forces or states (effect of)
  T75.81
hair (color) (shaft) L67.9
  specified NEC L67.8
hard tissue formation in pulp (dental) K04.3
head movement R25.0
heart
  rate R00.9
   specified NEC R00.8
  shadow R93.1
  sounds NEC R01.2
hemoglobin (disease) (*see also* Disease,
  hemoglobin) D58.2
  trait — *see* Trait, hemoglobin, abnormal
histology NEC R89.7
immunological findings R89.4
  in serum R76.9
   specified NEC R76.8
increase in appetite R63.2
involuntary movement — *see* Abnormal,
  movement, involuntary
jaw closure M26.51
karyotype R89.8
kidney function test R94.4

Abnormal, abnormality, abnormalities
(*see also* Anomaly) — *continued*
knee jerk R29.2
leukocyte (cell) (differential) NEC D72.9
liver
loss of
  height R29.890
  weight R63.4
mammogram NEC R92.8
  calcification (calculus) R92.1
  microcalcification R92.0
Mantoux test R76.11
movement (disorder) — *see also* Disorder,
  movement
  head R25.0
  involuntary R25.9
   fasciculation R25.3
   of head R25.0
   spasm R25.2
   specified type NEC R25.8
   tremor R25.1
myoglobin (Aberdeen) (Annapolis) R89.7
neonatal screening P09
oculomotor study R94.113
palmar creases Q82.8
Papanicolaou (smear)
  anus R85.619
   atypical squamous cells cannot exclude
    high grade squamous intraepithelial
    lesion (ASC-H) R85.611
   atypical squamous cells of undetermined
    significance (ASC-US) R85.610
   cytologic evidence of malignancy R85.614
   high grade squamous intraepithelial lesion
    (HGSIL) R85.613
   human papillomavirus (HPV) DNA test
    high risk positive R85.81
    low risk postive R85.82
   inadequate smear R85.615
   low grade squamous intraepithelial lesion
    (LGSIL) R85.612
   satisfactory anal smear but lacking
    transformation zone R85.616
   specified NEC R85.618
   unsatisfactory smear R85.615
  bronchial washings R84.6
  cerebrospinal fluid R83.6
  cervix R87.619
   atypical squamous cells cannot exclude
    high grade squamous intraepithelial
    lesion (ASC-H) R87.611
   atypical squamous cells of undetermined
    significance (ASC-US) R87.610
   cytologic evidence of malignancy R87.614
   high grade squamous intraepithelial lesion
    (HGSIL) R87.613
   inadequate smear R87.615
   low grade squamous intraepithelial lesion
    (LGSIL) R87.612
   non-atypical endometrial cells R87.618
   satisfactory cervical smear but lacking
    transformation zone R87.616
   specified NEC R87.618
   thin preparaton R87.619
   unsatisfactory smear R87.615
  nasal secretions R84.6
  nipple discharge R89.6
  peritoneal fluid R85.69
  pleural fluid R84.6
  prostatic secretions R86.6
  saliva R85.69
  seminal fluid R86.6
  sites NEC R89.6
  sputum R84.6
  synovial fluid R89.6
  throat scrapings R84.6

Abnormal, abnormality, abnormalities
(*see also* Anomaly) — *continued*
Papanicolaou (smear) — *continued*
  vagina R87.629
   atypical squamous cells cannot exclude
    high grade squamous intraepithelial
    lesion (ASC-H) R87.621
   atypical squamous cells of undetermined
    significance (ASC-US) R87.620
   cytologic evidence of malignancy R87.624
   high grade squamous intraepithelial lesion
    (HGSIL) R87.623
   inadequate smear R87.625
   low grade squamous intraepithelial lesion
    (LGSIL) R87.622
   specified NEC R87.628
   thin preparation R87.629
   unsatisfactory smear R87.625
  vulva R87.69
  wound secretions R89.6
partial thromboplastin time (PTT) R79.1
pelvis (bony) — *see* Deformity, pelvis
percussion, chest (tympany) R09.89
periods (grossly) — *see* Menstruation
phonocardiogram R94.39
plantar reflex R29.2
plasma
  protein R77.9
   specified NEC R77.8
  viscosity R70.1
pleural (folds) Q34.0
posture R29.3
product of conception O02.9
  specified type NEC O02.89
prothrombin time (PT) R79.1
pulmonary
  artery, congenital Q25.79
  function, newborn P28.89
  test results R94.2
pulsations in neck R00.2
pupillary H21.56-
  function (reaction) (reflex) — *see* Anomaly,
   pupil, function
radiological examination — *see* Abnormal,
  diagnostic imaging
red blood cell(s) (morphology) (volume) R71.8
reflex — *see* Reflex
renal function test R94.4
response to nerve stimulation R94.130
retinal correspondence H53.31
retinal function study R94.111
rhythm, heart — *see also* Arrhythmia
saliva — *see* Abnormal, specimen, digestive
  organs
scan
  kidney R94.4
  liver R93.2
  thyroid R94.6
secretion
  gastrin E16.4
  glucagon E16.3
semen, seminal fluid — *see* Abnormal,
  specimen, male genital organs
serum level (of)
  acid phosphatase R74.8
  alkaline phosphatase R74.8
  amylase R74.8
  enzymes R74.9
   specified NEC R74.8
  lipase R74.8
  triacylglycerol lipase R74.8
shape
  gravid uterus — *see* Anomaly, uterus
sinus venosus Q21.1
size, tooth, teeth K00.2
spacing, tooth, teeth, fully erupted M26.30

DISEASE INDEX

Abnormal, abnormality, abnormalities
(*see also* Anomaly) — *continued*
specimen
  digestive organs (peritoneal fluid) (saliva)
    R85.9
    cytology R85.69
    drug level R85.2
    enzyme level R85.0
    histology R85.7
    hormones R85.1
    immunology R85.4
    microbiology R85.5
    nonmedicinal level R85.3
    specified type NEC R85.89
  female genital organs (secretions) (smears)
    R87.9
    cytology R87.69
      cervix R87.619
        human papillomavirus (HPV) DNA test
          high risk positive R87.810
          low risk positive R87.820
        inadequate (unsatisfactory) smear
          R87.615
        non-atypical endometrial cells
          R87.618
        specified NEC R87.618
      vagina R87.629
        human papillomavirus (HPV) DNA test
          high risk positive R87.811
          low risk positive R87.821
        inadequate (unsatisfactory) smear
          R87.625
      vulva R87.69
    drug level R87.2
    enzyme level R87.0
    histological R87.7
    hormones R87.1
    immunology R87.4
    microbiology R87.5
    nonmedicinal level R87.3
    specified type NEC R87.89
  male genital organs (prostatic secretions)
    (semen) R86.9
    cytology R86.6
    drug level R86.2
    enzyme level R86.0
    histological R86.7
    hormones R86.1
    immunology R86.4
    microbiology R86.5
    nonmedicinal level R86.3
    specified type NEC R86.8
  nipple discharge — *see* Abnormal,
    specimen, specified
  respiratory organs (bronchial washings)
    (nasal secretions) (pleural fluid) (sputum)
    R84.9
    cytology R84.6
    drug level R84.2
    enzyme level R84.0
    histology R84.7
    hormones R84.1
    immunology R84.4
    microbiology R84.5
    nonmedicinal level R84.3
    specified type NEC R84.8
  specified organ, system and tissue NOS
    R89.9
    cytology R89.6
    drug level R89.2
    enzyme level R89.0
    histology R89.7
    hormones R89.1
    immunology R89.4
    microbiology R89.5
    nonmedicinal level R89.3
    specified type NEC R89.8

Abnormal, abnormality, abnormalities
(*see also* Anomaly) — *continued*
specimen — *continued*
  synovial fluid — *see* Abnormal, specimen,
    specified
  thorax (bronchial washings) (pleural fluids)
    — *see* Abnormal, specimen, respiratory
    organs
  vagina (secretion) (smear) R87.629
  vulva (secretion) (smear) R87.69
  wound secretion — *see* Abnormal, specimen,
    specified
spermatozoa — *see* Abnormal, specimen,
  male genital organs
sputum (amount) (color) (odor) R09.3
stool (color) (contents) (mucus) R19.5
  bloody K92.1
  guaiac positive R19.5
synchondrosis Q78.8
thermography (*see also* Abnormal, diagnostic
  imaging) R93.8
thyroid-binding globulin E07.89
tooth, teeth (form) (size) K00.2
toxicology (findings) R78.9
transport protein E88.09
tumor marker NEC R97.8
ultrasound results — *see* Abnormal, diagnostic
  imaging
umbilical cord complicating delivery O69.9
urination NEC R39.198
urine (constituents) R82.90
  bile R82.2
  cytological examination R82.8
  drugs R82.5
  fat R82.0
  glucose R81
  heavy metals R82.6
  hemoglobin R82.3
  histological examination R82.8
  ketones R82.4
  microbiological examination (culture)
    R82.79
  myoglobin R82.1
  positive culture R82.79
  protein — *see* Proteinuria
  specified substance NEC R82.99
    chromoabnormality NEC R82.91
  substances nonmedical R82.6
uterine hemorrhage — *see* Hemorrhage, uterus
vectorcardiogram R94.39
visually evoked potential (VEP) R94.112
white blood cells D72.9
  specified NEC D72.89
X-ray examination — *see* Abnormal,
  diagnostic imaging
Abnormity (any organ or part) — *see* Anomaly
Abocclusion M26.29
  hemolytic disease (newborn) P55.1
  incompatibility reaction ABO — *see*
    Complication(s), transfusion,
    incompatibility reaction, ABO
Abolition, language R48.8
Aborter, habitual or recurrent — *see* Loss
  (of), pregnancy, recurrent
Abortion (complete) (spontaneous) O03.9
with
  retained products of conception — *see*
    Abortion, incomplete
attempted (elective) (failed) O07.4
  complicated by O07.30
    afibrinogenemia O07.1
    cardiac arrest O07.36
    chemical damage of pelvic organ(s)
      O07.34
    circulatory collapse O07.31
    cystitis O07.38
    defibrination syndrome O07.1
    electrolyte imbalance O07.33

Abortion (complete) (spontaneous) O03.9 —
  continued
attempted (elective) (failed) O07.4 —
  continued
  complicated by O07.30 — *continued*
    embolism (air) (amniotic fluid) (blood clot)
      (fat) (pulmonary) (septic) (soap)
      O07.2
    endometritis O07.0
    genital tract and pelvic infection O07.0
    hemolysis O07.1
    hemorrhage (delayed) (excessive) O07.1
    infection
      genital tract or pelvic O07.0
      urinary tract O07.38
    intravascular coagulation O07.1
    laceration of pelvic organ(s) O07.34
    metabolic disorder O07.33
    oliguria O07.32
    oophoritis O07.0
    parametritis O07.0
    pelvic peritonitis O07.0
    perforation of pelvic organ(s) O07.34
    renal failure or shutdown O07.32
    salpingitis or salpingo-oophoritis O07.0
    sepsis O07.37
    shock O07.31
    specified condition NEC O07.39
    tubular necrosis (renal) O07.32
    uremia O07.32
    urinary tract infection O07.38
    venous complication NEC O07.35
      embolism (air) (amniotic fluid) (blood
        clot) (fat) (pulmonary) (septic) (soap)
        O07.2
complicated (by) (following) O03.80
  afibrinogenemia O03.6
  cardiac arrest O03.86
  chemical damage of pelvic organ(s) O03.84
  circulatory collapse O03.81
  cystitis O03.88
  defibrination syndrome O03.6
  electrolyte imbalance O03.83
  embolism (air) (amniotic fluid) (blood clot)
    (fat) (pulmonary) (septic) (soap) O03.7
  endometritis O03.5
  genital tract and pelvic infection O03.5
  hemolysis O03.6
  hemorrhage (delayed) (excessive) O03.6
  infection
    genital tract or pelvic O03.5
    urinary tract O03.88
  intravascular coagulation O03.6
  laceration of pelvic organ(s) O03.84
  metabolic disorder O03.83
  oliguria O03.82
  oophoritis O03.5
  parametritis O03.5
  pelvic peritonitis O03.5
  perforation of pelvic organ(s) O03.84
  renal failure or shutdown O03.82
  salpingitis or salpingo-oophoritis O03.5
  sepsis O03.87
  shock O03.81
  specified condition NEC O03.89
  tubular necrosis (renal) O03.82
  uremia O03.82
  urinary tract infection O03.88
  venous complication NEC O03.85
    embolism (air) (amniotic fluid) (blood
      clot) (fat) (pulmonary) (septic) (soap)
      O03.7
failed — *see* Abortion, attempted
habitual or recurrent N96
  with current abortion — *see* categories O03-
    O06
  care in current pregnancy O26.2-
  without current pregnancy N96

Abortion (complete) (spontaneous) O03.9 — continued
  incomplete (spontaneous) O03.4
    complicated (by) (following) O03.30
      afibrinogenemia O03.1
      cardiac arrest O03.36
      chemical damage of pelvic organ(s) O03.34
      circulatory collapse O03.31
      cystitis O03.38
      defibrination syndrome O03.1
      electrolyte imbalance O03.33
      embolism (air) (amniotic fluid) (blood clot) (fat) (pulmonary) (septic) (soap) O03.2
      endometritis O03.0
      genital tract and pelvic infection O03.0
      hemolysis O03.1
      hemorrhage (delayed) (excessive) O03.1
      infection
        genital tract or pelvic O03.0
        urinary tract O03.38
      intravascular coagulation O03.1
      laceration of pelvic organ(s) O03.34
      metabolic disorder O03.33
      oliguria O03.32
      oophoritis O03.0
      parametritis O03.0
      pelvic peritonitis O03.0
      perforation of pelvic organ(s) O03.34
      renal failure or shutdown O03.32
      salpingitis or salpingo-oophoritis O03.0
      sepsis O03.37
      shock O03.31
      specified condition NEC O03.39
      tubular necrosis (renal) O03.32
      uremia O03.32
      urinary infection O03.38
      venous complication NEC O03.35
        embolism (air) (amniotic fluid) (blood clot) (fat) (pulmonary) (septic) (soap) O03.2
  induced (encounter for) Z33.2
    complicated by O04.80
      afibrinogenemia O04.6
      cardiac arrest O04.86
      chemical damage of pelvic organ(s) O04.84
      circulatory collapse O04.81
      cystitis O04.88
      defibrination syndrome O04.6
      electrolyte imbalance O04.83
      embolism (air) (amniotic fluid) (blood clot) (fat) (pulmonary) (septic) (soap) O04.7
      endometritis O04.5
      genital tract and pelvic infection O04.5
      hemolysis O04.6
      hemorrhage (delayed) (excessive) O04.6
      infection
        genital tract or pelvic O04.5
        urinary tract O04.88
      intravascular coagulation O04.6
      laceration of pelvic organ(s) O04.84
      metabolic disorder O04.83
      oliguria O04.82
      oophoritis O04.5
      parametritis O04.5
      pelvic peritonitis O04.5
      perforation of pelvic organ(s) O04.84
      renal failure or shutdown O04.82
      salpingitis or salpingo-oophoritis O04.5
      sepsis O04.87
      shock O04.81
      specified condition NEC O04.89
      tubular necrosis (renal) O04.82
      uremia O04.82
      urinary tract infection O04.88

Abortion (complete) (spontaneous) O03.9 — continued
  induced (encounter for) Z33.2 — continued
    complicated by O04.80 — continued
      venous complication NEC O04.85
        embolism (air) (amniotic fluid) (blood clot) (fat) (pulmonary) (septic) (soap) O04.7
  missed O02.1
  spontaneous — see Abortion (complete) (spontaneous)
    threatened O20.0
  threatened (spontaneous) O20.0
  tubal O00.10
    with intrauterine pregnancy O00.11
Abortus fever A23.1
Aboulomania F60.7
Abrami's disease D59.8
Abramov-Fiedler myocarditis (acute isolated myocarditis) I40.1
Abrasion T14.8
  abdomen, abdominal (wall) S30.811
  alveolar process S00.512
  ankle S90.51-
  antecubital space — see Abrasion, elbow
  anus S30.817
  arm (upper) S40.81-
  auditory canal — see Abrasion, ear
  auricle — see Abrasion, ear
  axilla — see Abrasion, arm
  back, lower S30.810
  breast S20.11-
  brow S00.81
  buttock S30.810
  calf — see Abrasion, leg
  canthus — see Abrasion, eyelid
  cheek S00.81
    internal S00.512
  chest wall — see Abrasion, thorax
  chin S00.81
  clitoris S30.814
  cornea S05.0-
  costal region — see Abrasion, thorax
  dental K03.1
  digit(s)
    foot — see Abrasion, toe
    hand — see Abrasion, finger
  ear S00.41-
  elbow S50.31-
  epididymis S30.813
  epigastric region S30.811
  epiglottis S10.11
  esophagus (thoracic) S27.818
    cervical S10.11
  eyebrow — see Abrasion, eyelid
  eyelid S00.21-
  face S00.81
  finger(s) S60.41-
    index S60.41-
    little S60.41-
    middle S60.41-
    ring S60.41-
  flank S30.811
  foot (except toe(s) alone) S90.81-
    toe — see Abrasion, toe
  forearm S50.81-
    elbow only — see Abrasion, elbow
  forehead S00.81
  genital organs, external
    female S30.816
    male S30.815
  groin S30.811
  gum S00.512
  hand S60.51-
  head S00.91
    ear — see Abrasion, ear
    eyelid — see Abrasion, eyelid
    lip S00.511
    nose S00.31

Abrasion — continued
  head S00.91 — continued
    oral cavity S00.512
    scalp S00.01
    specified site NEC S00.81
  heel — see Abrasion, foot
  hip S70.21-
  inguinal region S30.811
  interscapular region S20.419
  jaw S00.81
  knee S80.21-
  labium (majus) (minus) S30.814
  larynx S10.11
  leg (lower) S80.81-
    knee — see Abrasion, knee
    upper — see Abrasion, thigh
  lip S00.511
  lower back S30.810
  lumbar region S30.810
  malar region S00.81
  mammary — see Abrasion, breast
  mastoid region S00.81
  mouth S00.512
  nail
    finger — see Abrasion, finger
    toe — see Abrasion, toe
  nape S10.81
  nasal S00.31
  neck S10.91
    specified site NEC S10.81
    throat S10.11
  nose S00.31
  occipital region S00.01
  oral cavity S00.512
  orbital region — see Abrasion, eyelid
  palate S00.512
  palm — see Abrasion, hand
  parietal region S00.01
  pelvis S30.810
  penis S30.812
  perineum
    female S30.814
    male S30.810
  periocular area — see Abrasion, eyelid
  phalanges
    finger — see Abrasion, finger
    toe — see Abrasion, toe
  pharynx S10.11
  pinna — see Abrasion, ear
  popliteal space — see Abrasion, knee
  prepuce S30.812
  pubic region S30.810
  pudendum
    female S30.816
    male S30.815
  sacral region S30.810
  scalp S00.01
  scapular region — see Abrasion, shoulder
  scrotum S30.813
  shin — see Abrasion, leg
  shoulder S40.21-
  skin NEC T14.8
  sternal region S20.319
  submaxillary region S00.81
  submental region S00.81
  subungual
    finger(s) — see Abrasion, finger
    toe(s) — see Abrasion, toe
  supraclavicular fossa S10.81
  supraorbital S00.81
  temple S00.81
  temporal region S00.81
  testis S30.813
  thigh S70.31-
  thorax, thoracic (wall) S20.91
    back S20.41-
    front S20.31-
  throat S10.11
  thumb S60.31-

Abrasion — *continued*
  toe(s) (lesser) S90.416
    great S90.41-
  tongue S00.512
  tooth, teeth (dentifrice) (habitual) (hard tissues) (occupational) (ritual) (traditional) K03.1
  trachea S10.11
  tunica vaginalis S30.813
  tympanum, tympanic membrane — *see* Abrasion, ear
  uvula S00.512
  vagina S30.814
  vocal cords S10.11
  vulva S30.814
  wrist S60.81-

Abrism — *see* Poisoning, food, noxious, plant

Abruptio placentae O45.9-
  with
    afibrinogenemia O45.01-
    coagulation defect O45.00-
      specified NEC O45.09-
    disseminated intravascular coagulation O45.02-
    hypofibrinogenemia O45.01-
    specified NEC O45.8-

Abruption, placenta — *see* Abruptio placentae

Abscess (connective tissue) (embolic) (fistulous) (infective) (metastatic) (multiple) (pernicious) (pyogenic) (septic) L02.91
  with
    diverticular disease (intestine) K57.80
      with bleeding K57.81
      large intestine K57.20
        with
          bleeding K57.21
          small intestine K57.40
            with bleeding K57.41
      small intestine K57.00
        with
          bleeding K57.01
          large intestine K57.40
            with bleeding K57.41
    lymphangitis — *code by* site under Abscess
  abdomen, abdominal
    cavity K65.1
    wall L02.211
  abdominopelvic K65.1
  accessory sinus — *see* Sinusitis
  adrenal (capsule) (gland) E27.8
  alveolar K04.7
    with sinus K04.6
  ambic A06.4
    brain (and liver or lung abscess) A06.6
    genitourinary tract A06.82
    liver (without mention of brain or lung abscess) A06.4
    lung (and liver) (without mention of brain abscess) A06.5
    specified site NEC A06.89
    spleen A06.89
  anerobic A48.0
  ankle — *see* Abscess, lower limb
  anorectal K61.2
  antecubital space — *see* Abscess, upper limb
  antrum (chronic) (Highmore) — *see* Sinusitis, maxillary
  anus K61.0
  apical (tooth) K04.7
    with sinus (alveolar) K04.6
  appendix K35.3
  areola (acute) (chronic) (nonpuerperal) N61.1
    puerperal, postpartum or gestational — *see* Infection, nipple
  arm (any part) — *see* Abscess, upper limb
  artery (wall) I77.89
  atheromatous I77.2
  auricle, ear — *see* Abscess, ear, external

Abscess (connective tissue) (embolic) (fistulous) (infective) (metastatic) (multiple) (pernicious) (pyogenic) (septic) L02.91 — *continued*
  axilla (region) L02.41-
    lymph gland or node L04.2
  back (any part, except buttock) L02.212
  Bartholin's gland N75.1
    with
      abortion — *see* Abortion, by type complicated by, sepsis
      ectopic or molar pregnancy O08.0
      following ectopic or molar pregnancy O08.0
  Bezold's — *see* Mastoiditis, acute
  bilharziasis B65.1
  bladder (wall) — *see* Cystitis, specified type NEC
  bone (subperiosteal) — *see also* Osteomyelitis, specified type NEC
    accessory sinus (chronic) — *see* Sinusitis
    chronic or old — *see* Osteomyelitis, chronic
    jaw (lower) (upper) M27.2
    mastoid — *see* Mastoiditis, acute, subperiosteal
    petrous — *see* Petrositis
    spinal (tuberculous) A18.01
      nontuberculous — *see* Osteomyelitis, vertebra
  bowel K63.0
  brain (any part) (cystic) (otogenic) G06.0
    amebic (with abscess of any other site) A06.6
    gonococcal A54.82
    pheomycotic (chromomycotic) B43.1
    tuberculous A17.81
  breast (acute) (chronic) (nonpuerperal) N61.1
    newborn P39.0
    puerperal, postpartum, gestational — *see* Mastitis, obstetric, purulent
  broad ligament N73.2
    acute N73.0
    chronic N73.1
  Brodie's (localized) (chronic) M86.8x-
  bronchi J98.09
  buccal cavity K12.2
  bulbourethral gland N34.0
  bursa M71.00
    ankle M71.07-
    elbow M71.02-
    foot M71.07-
    hand M71.04-
    hip M71.05-
    knee M71.06-
    multiple sites M71.09
    pharyngeal J39.1
    shoulder M71.01-
    specified site NEC M71.08
    wrist M71.03-
  buttock L02.31
  canthus — *see* Blepharoconjunctivitis
  cartilage — *see* Disorder, cartilage, specified type NEC
  cecum K35.3
  cerebellum, cerebellar G06.0
    sequelae G09
  cerebral (embolic) G06.0
    sequelae G09
  cervical (meaning neck) L02.11
    lymph gland or node L04.0
  cervix (stump) (uteri) — *see* Cervicitis
  cheek (external) L02.01
    inner K12.2
  chest J86.9
    with fistula J86.0
    wall L02.213
  chin L02.01
  choroid — *see* Inflammation, chorioretinal
  circumtonsillar J36

Abscess (connective tissue) (embolic) (fistulous) (infective) (metastatic) (multiple) (pernicious) (pyogenic) (septic) L02.91 — *continued*
  cold (lung) (tuberculous) — *see also* Tuberculosis, abscess, lung
    articular — *see* Tuberculosis, joint
  colon (wall) K63.0
  colostomy K94.02
  conjunctiva — *see* Conjunctivitis, acute
  cornea H16.31-
  corpus
    cavernosum N48.21
    luteum — *see* Oophoritis
  Cowper's gland N34.0
  cranium G06.0
  cul-de-sac (Douglas') (posterior) — *see* Peritonitis, pelvic, female
  cutaneous — *see* Abscess, by site
  dental K04.7
    with sinus (alveolar) K04.6
  dentoalveolar K04.7
    with sinus K04.6
  diaphragm, diaphragmatic K65.1
  Douglas' cul-de-sac or pouch — *see* Peritonitis, pelvic, female
  Dubois A50.59
  ear (middle) — *see also* Otitis, media, suppurative
    acute — *see* Otitis, media, suppurative, acute
    external H60.0-
  entamebic — *see* Abscess, amebic
  enterostomy K94.12
  epididymis N45.4
  epidural G06.2
    brain G06.0
    spinal cord G06.1
  epiglottis J38.7
  epiploon, epiploic K65.1
  erysipelatous — *see* Erysipelas
  esophagus K20.8
  ethmoid (bone) (chronic) (sinus) J32.2
  external auditory canal — *see* Abscess, ear, external
  extradural G06.2
    brain G06.0
      sequelae G09
    spinal cord G06.1
  extraperitoneal K68.19
  eye — *see* Endophthalmitis, purulent
  eyelid H00.03-
  face (any part, except ear, eye and nose) L02.01
  fallopian tube — *see* Salpingitis
  fascia M72.8
  fauces J39.1
  fecal K63.0
  femoral (region) — *see* Abscess, lower limb
  filaria, filarial — *see* Infestation, filarial
  finger (any) — *see also* Abscess, hand
    nail — *see* Cellulitis, finger
  foot L02.61-
  forehead L02.01
  frontal sinus (chronic) J32.1
  gallbladder K81.0
  genital organ or tract
    female (external) N76.4
    male N49.9
      multiple sites N49.8
      specified NEC N49.8
  gestational mammary O91.11-
  gestational subareolar O91.11-
  gingival — *see* Peridontitis, aggressive, localized
  gland, glandular (lymph) (acute) — *see* Lymphadenitis, acute
  gluteal (region) L02.31
  gonorrheal — *see* Gonococcus
  groin L02.214

Abscess (connective tissue) (embolic) (fistulous) (infective) (metastatic) (multiple) (pernicious) (pyogenic) (septic) L02.91 — *continued*
gum — *see* Peridontitis, aggressive, localized
hand L02.51-
head NEC L02.811
    face (any part, except ear, eye and nose) L02.01
heart — *see* Carditis
heel — *see* Abscess, foot
helminthic — *see* Infestation, helminth
hepatic (cholangitic) (hematogenic) (lymphogenic) (pylephlebitic) K75.0
    amebic A06.4
hip (region) — *see* Abscess, lower limb
ileocecal K35.3
ileostomy (bud) K94.12
iliac (region) L02.214
    fossa K35.3
infraclavicular (fossa) — *see* Abscess, upper limb
inguinal (region) L02.214
    lymph gland or node L04.1
intestine, intestinal NEC K63.0
    rectal K61.1
intra-abdominal (*see also* Abscess, peritoneum) K65.1
    postprocedural T81.43
      retroperitoneal K68.11
intracranial G06.0
intramammary — *see* Abscess, breast
intra-muscular, postprocedural T81.42
intraorbital — *see* Abscess, orbit
intraperitoneal K65.1
intrasphincteric (anus) K61.4
intraspinal G06.1
intratonsillar J36
ischiorectal (fossa) K61.3
jaw (bone) (lower) (upper) M27.2
joint — *see* Arthritis, pyogenic or pyemic
    spine (tuberculous) A18.01
      nontuberculous — *see* Spondylopathy, infective
kidney N15.1
    with calculus N20.0
      with hydronephrosis N13.6
    puerperal (postpartum) O86.21
knee — *see also* Abscess, lower limb
    joint M00.9
labium (majus) (minus) N76.4
lacrimal
    caruncle — *see* Inflammation, lacrimal, passages, acute
    gland — *see* Dacryoadenitis
    passages (duct) (sac) — *see* Inflammation, lacrimal, passages, acute
lacunar N34.0
larynx J38.7
lateral (alveolar) K04.7
    with sinus K04.6
leg (any part) — *see* Abscess, lower limb
lens H27.8
lingual K14.0
    tonsil J36
lip K13.0
Littre's gland N34.0
liver (cholangitic) (hematogenic) (lymphogenic) (pylephlebitic) (pyogenic) K75.0
    amebic (due to Entamoeba histolytica) (dysenteric) (tropical) A06.4
      with
        brain abscess (and liver or lung abscess) A06.6
        lung abscess A06.5
loin (region) L02.211
lower limb L02.41-
lumbar (tuberculous) A18.01
    nontuberculous L02.212

Abscess (connective tissue) (embolic) (fistulous) (infective) (metastatic) (multiple) (pernicious) (pyogenic) (septic) L02.91 — *continued*
lung (miliary) (putrid) J85.2
    with pneumonia J85.1
      due to specified organism (*see* Pneumonia, in (due to))
    amebic (with liver abscess) A06.5
      with
        brain abscess A06.6
        pneumonia A06.5
lymph, lymphatic, gland or node (acute) — *see also* Lymphadenitis, acute
    mesentery I88.0
malar M27.2
mammary gland — *see* Abscess, breast
marginal, anus K61.0
mastoid — *see* Mastoiditis, acute
maxilla, maxillary M27.2
    molar (tooth) K04.7
      with sinus K04.6
    premolar K04.7
    sinus (chronic) J32.0
mediastinum J85.3
meibomian gland — *see* Hordeolum
meninges G06.2
mesentery, mesenteric K65.1
mesosalpinx — *see* Salpingitis
mons pubis L02.215
mouth (floor) K12.2
muscle — *see* Myositis, infective
myocardium I40.0
nabothian (follicle) — *see* Cervicitis
nasal J32.9
nasopharyngeal J39.1
navel L02.216
    newborn P38.9
      with mild hemorrhage P38.1
      without hemorrhage P38.9
neck (region) L02.11
    lymph gland or node L04.0
nephritic — *see* Abscess, kidney
nipple N61.1
    associated with
      lactation — *see* Pregnancy, complicated by
      pregnancy — *see* Pregnancy, complicated by
nose (external) (fossa) (septum) J34.0
    sinus (chronic) — *see* Sinusitis
omentum K65.1
operative wound T81.40
orbit, orbital — *see* Cellulitis, orbit
otogenic G06.0
ovary, ovarian (corpus luteum) — *see* Oophoritis
oviduct — *see* Oophoritis
palate (soft) K12.2
    hard M27.2
palmar (space) — *see* Abscess, hand
pancreas (duct) — *see* Pancreatitis, acute
parafrenal N48.21
parametric, parametrium N73.2
    acute N73.0
    chronic N73.1
paranephric N15.1
parapancreatic — *see* Pancreatitis, acute
parapharyngeal J39.0
pararectal K61.1
parasinus — *see* Sinusitis
parauterine (*see also* Disease, pelvis, inflammatory) N73.2
paravaginal — *see* Vaginitis
parietal region (scalp) L02.811
parodontal — *see* Peridontitis, aggressive, localized
parotid (duct) (gland) K11.3
    region K12.2
pectoral (region) L02.213

Abscess (connective tissue) (embolic) (fistulous) (infective) (metastatic) (multiple) (pernicious) (pyogenic) (septic) L02.91 — *continued*
pelvis, pelvic
    female — *see* Disease, pelvis, inflammatory
    male, peritoneal K65.1
penis N48.21
    gonococcal (accessory gland) (periurethral) A54.1
perianal K61.0
periapical K04.7
    with sinus (alveolar) K04.6
periappendicular K35.3
pericardial I30.1
pericecal K35.3
pericemental — *see* Peridontitis, aggressive, localized
pericholecystic — *see* Cholecystitis, acute
pericoronal — *see* Peridontitis, aggressive, localized
peridental — *see* Peridontitis, aggressive, localized
perimetric (*see also* Disease, pelvis, inflammatory) N73.2
perinephric, perinephritic — *see* Abscess, kidney
perineum, perineal (superficial) L02.215
    urethra N34.0
periodontal (parietal) — *see* Peridontitis, aggressive, localized
    apical K04.7
periosteum, periosteal — *see also* Osteomyelitis, specified type NEC
    with osteomyelitis — *see also* Osteomyelitis, specified type NEC
      acute — *see* Osteomyelitis, acute
      chronic — *see* Osteomyelitis, chronic
peripharyngeal J39.0
peripleuritic J86.9
    with fistula J86.0
periprostatic N41.2
perirectal K61.1
perirenal (tissue) — *see* Abscess, kidney
perisinuous (nose) — *see* Sinusitis
peritoneum, peritoneal (perforated) (ruptured) K65.1
    with appendicitis K35.3
    pelvic
      female — *see* Peritonitis, pelvic, female
      male K65.1
    postoperative T81.43
    puerperal, postpartum, childbirth O85
    tuberculous A18.31
peritonsillar J36
perityphlic K35.3
periureteral N28.89
periurethral N34.0
    gonococcal (accessory gland) (periurethral) A54.1
periuterine (*see also* Disease, pelvis, inflammatory) N73.2
perivesical — *see* Cystitis, specified type NEC
petrous bone — *see* Petrositis
phagedenic NOS L02.91
    chancroid A57
pharynx, pharyngeal (lateral) J39.1
pilonidal L05.01
pituitary (gland) E23.6
pleura J86.9
    with fistula J86.0
popliteal — *see* Abscess, lower limb
postcecal K35.3
postlaryngeal J38.7
postnasal J34.0
postoperative (any site) T81.40
    retroperitoneal K68.11
postpharyngeal J39.0
posttonsillar J36
post-typhoid A01.09

Abscess (connective tissue) (embolic) (fistulous) (infective) (metastatic) (multiple) (pernicious) (pyogenic) (septic) L02.91 — *continued*
pouch of Douglas — *see* Peritonitis, pelvic, female
premammary — *see* Abscess, breast
prepatellar — *see* Abscess, lower limb
prostate N41.2
  gonococcal (acute) (chronic) A54.22
psoas muscle K68.12
puerperal — *code by* site under Puerperal, abscess
pulmonary — *see* Abscess, lung
pulp, pulpal (dental) K04.01
  irreversible K04.02
  reversible K04.01
rectovaginal septum K63.0
rectovesical — *see* Cystitis, specified type NEC
rectum K61.1
renal — *see* Abscess, kidney
retina — *see* Inflammation, chorioretinal
retrobulbar — *see* Abscess, orbit
retrocecal K65.1
retrolaryngeal J38.7
retromammary — *see* Abscess, breast
retroperitoneal NEC K68.19
  postprocedural K68.11
retropharyngeal J39.0
retrouterine — *see* Peritonitis, pelvic, female
retrovesical — *see* Cystitis, specified type NEC
root, tooth K04.7
  with sinus (alveolar) K04.6
round ligament (*see also* Disease, pelvis, inflammatory) N73.2
rupture (spontaneous) NOS L02.91
sacrum (tuberculous) A18.01
  nontuberculous M46.28
salivary (duct) (gland) K11.3
scalp (any part) L02.811
scapular — *see* Osteomyelitis, specified type NEC
sclera — *see* Scleritis
scrofulous (tuberculous) A18.2
scrotum N49.2
seminal vesicle N49.0
septal, dental K04.7
  with sinus (alveolar) K04.6
serous — *see* Periostitis
shoulder (region) — *see* Abscess, upper limb
sigmoid K63.0
sinus (accessory) (chronic) (nasal) — *see also* Sinusitis
  intracranial venous (any) G06.0
Skene's duct or gland N34.0
skin — *see* Abscess, by site
specified site NEC L02.818
spermatic cord N49.1
sphenoidal (sinus) (chronic) J32.3
spinal cord (any part) (staphylococcal) G06.1
  tuberculous A17.81
spine (column) (tuberculous) A18.01
  epidural G06.1
  nontuberculous — *see* Osteomyelitis, vertebra
spleen D73.3
  amebic A06.89
stitch T81.48
subarachnoid G06.2
  brain G06.0
  spinal cord G06.1
subareolar — *see* Abscess, breast
subcecal K35.3
subcutaneous — *see also* Abscess, by site
  pheomycotic (chromomycotic) B43.2
  postprocedural T81.41
subdiaphragmatic K65.1

Abscess (connective tissue) (embolic) (fistulous) (infective) (metastatic) (multiple) (pernicious) (pyogenic) (septic) L02.91 — *continued*
subdural G06.2
  brain G06.0
  sequelae G09
  spinal cord G06.1
subgaleal L02.811
subhepatic K65.1
sublingual K12.2
  gland K11.3
submammary — *see* Abscess, breast
submandibular (region) (space) (triangle) K12.2
  gland K11.3
submaxillary (region) L02.01
  gland K11.3
submental L02.01
  gland K11.3
subperiosteal — *see* Osteomyelitis, specified type NEC
subphrenic K65.1
  postoperative T81.43
suburethral N34.0
sudoriparous L75.8
supraclavicular (fossa) — *see* Abscess, upper limb
suprapelvic, acute N73.0
suprarenal (capsule) (gland) E27.8
sweat gland L74.8
tear duct — *see* Inflammation, lacrimal, passages, acute
temple L02.01
temporal region L02.01
temporosphenoidal G06.0
tendon (sheath) M65.00
  ankle M65.07-
  foot M65.07-
  forearm M65.03-
  hand M65.04-
  lower leg M65.06-
  pelvic region M65.05-
  shoulder region M65.01-
  specified site NEC M65.08
  thigh M65.05-
  upper arm M65.02-
testis N45.4
thigh — *see* Abscess, lower limb
thorax J86.9
  with fistula J86.0
throat J39.1
thumb — *see also* Abscess, hand
  nail — *see* Cellulitis, finger
thymus (gland) E32.1
thyroid (gland) E06.0
toe (any) — *see also* Abscess, foot
  nail — *see* Cellulitis, toe
tongue (staphylococcal) K14.0
tonsil(s) (lingual) J36
tonsillopharyngeal J36
tooth, teeth (root) K04.7
  with sinus (alveolar) K04.6
  supporting structures NEC — *see* Peridontitis, aggressive, localized
trachea J39.8
trunk L02.219
  abdominal wall L02.211
  back L02.212
  chest wall L02.213
  groin L02.214
  perineum L02.215
  umbilicus L02.216
tubal — *see* Salpingitis
tuberculous — *see* Tuberculosis, abscess
tubo-ovarian — *see* Salpingo-oophoritis
tunica vaginalis N49.1
umbilicus L02.216

Abscess (connective tissue) (embolic) (fistulous) (infective) (metastatic) (multiple) (pernicious) (pyogenic) (septic) L02.91 — *continued*
upper
  limb L02.41-
  respiratory J39.8
urethral (gland) N34.0
urinary N34.0
uterus, uterine (wall) — *see also* Endometritis
  ligament (*see also* Disease, pelvis, inflammatory) N73.2
  neck — *see* Cervicitis
uvula K12.2
vagina (wall) — *see* Vaginitis
vaginorectal — *see* Vaginitis
vas deferens N49.1
vermiform appendix K35.3
vertebra (column) (tuberculous) A18.01
  nontuberculous — *see* Osteomyelitis, vertebra
vesical — *see* Cystitis, specified type NEC
vesico-uterine pouch — *see* Peritonitis, pelvic, female
vitreous (humor) — *see* Endophthalmitis, purulent
vocal cord J38.3
von Bezold's — *see* Mastoiditis, acute
vulva N76.4
vulvovaginal gland N75.1
web space — *see* Abscess, hand
wound T81.40
wrist — *see* Abscess, upper limb
Absence (of) (organ or part) (complete or partial)
adrenal (gland) (congenital) Q89.1
  acquired E89.6
albumin in blood E88.09
alimentary tract (congenital) Q45.8
  upper Q40.8
alveolar process (acquired) — *see* Anomaly, alveolar
ankle (acquired) Z89.44-
anus (congenital) Q42.3
  with fistula Q42.2
aorta (congenital) Q25.41
appendix, congenital Q42.8
arm (acquired) Z89.20-
  above elbow Z89.22-
    congenital (with hand present) — *see* Agenesis, arm, with hand present
    and hand — *see* Agenesis, forearm, and hand
  below elbow Z89.21-
    congenital (with hand present) — *see* Agenesis, arm, with hand present
    and hand — *see* Agenesis, forearm, and hand
  congenital — *see* Defect, reduction, upper limb
  shoulder (following explantation of shoulder joint prosthesis) (joint) (with or without presence of antibiotic-impregnated cement spacer) Z89.23-
    congenital (with hand present) — *see* Agenesis, arm, with hand present
artery (congenital) (peripheral) Q27.8
  brain Q28.3
  coronary Q24.5
  pulmonary Q25.79
  specified NEC Q27.8
  umbilical Q27.0
atrial septum (congenital) Q21.1
auditory canal (congenital) (external) Q16.1
auricle (ear), congenital Q16.0
bile, biliary duct, congenital Q44.5
bladder (acquired) Z90.6
  congenital Q64.5
bowel sounds R19.11

3

DISEASE INDEX

Absence (of) (organ or part) (complete or partial) — *continued*
brain Q00.0
  part of Q04.3
breast(s) (and nipple(s)) (acquired) Z90.1-
  congenital Q83.8
broad ligament Q50.6
bronchus (congenital) Q32.4
canaliculus lacrimalis, congenital Q10.4
cerebellum (vermis) Q04.3
cervix (acquired) (with uterus) Z90.710
  with remaining uterus Z90.712
  congenital Q51.5
chin, congenital Q18.8
cilia (congenital) Q10.3
  acquired — *see* Madarosis
clitoris (congenital) Q52.6
coccyx, congenital Q76.49
cold sense R20.8
congenital
  lumen — *see* Atresia
  organ or site NEC — *see* Agenesis
  septum — *see* Imperfect, closure
corpus callosum Q04.0
cricoid cartilage, congenital Q31.8
diaphragm (with hernia), congenital Q79.1
digestive organ(s) or tract, congenital Q45.8
  acquired NEC Z90.49
  upper Q40.8
ductus arteriosus Q28.8
duodenum (acquired) Z90.49
  congenital Q41.0
ear, congenital Q16.9
  acquired H93.8-
  auricle Q16.0
  external Q16.0
  inner Q16.5
  lobe, lobule Q17.8
  middle, except ossicles Q16.4
    ossicles Q16.3
  ossicles Q16.3
ejaculatory duct (congenital) Q55.4
endocrine gland (congenital) NEC Q89.2
  acquired E89.89
epididymis (congenital) Q55.4
  acquired Z90.79
epiglottis, congenital Q31.8
esophagus (congenital) Q39.8
  acquired (partial) Z90.49
eustachian tube (congenital) Q16.2
extremity (acquired) Z89.9
  congenital Q73.0
  knee (following explantation of knee joint prosthesis) (joint) (with or without presence of antibiotic-impregnated cement spacer) Z89.52-
  lower (above knee) Z89.619
    below knee Z89.51-
  upper — *see* Absence, arm
eye (acquired) Z90.01
  congenital Q11.1
  muscle (congenital) Q10.3
eyeball (acquired) Z90.01
eyelid (fold) (congenital) Q10.3
  acquired Z90.01
face, specified part NEC Q18.8
fallopian tube(s) (acquired) Z90.79
  congenital Q50.6
family member (causing problem in home) NEC (*see also* Disruption, family) Z63.32
femur, congenital — *see* Defect, reduction, lower limb, longitudinal, femur
fibrinogen (congenital) D68.2
  acquired D65
finger(s) (acquired) Z89.02-
  congenital — *see* Agenesis, hand
foot (acquired) Z89.43-
  congenital — *see* Agenesis, foot

Absence (of) (organ or part) (complete or partial) — *continued*
forearm (acquired) — *see* Absence, arm, below elbow
gallbladder (acquired) Z90.49
  congenital Q44.0
gamma globulin in blood D80.1
  hereditary D80.0
genital organs
  acquired (female) (male) Z90.79
  female, congenital Q52.8
    external Q52.71
    internal NEC Q52.8
  male, congenital Q55.8
genitourinary organs, congenital NEC
  female Q52.8
  male Q55.8
globe (acquired) Z90.01
  congenital Q11.1
glottis, congenital Q31.8
hand and wrist (acquired) Z89.11-
  congenital — *see* Agenesis, hand
head, part (acquired) NEC Z90.09
heat sense R20.8
hip (following explantation of hip joint prosthesis) (joint) (with or without presence of antibiotic-impregnated cement spacer) Z89.62-
hymen (congenital) Q52.4
ileum (acquired) Z90.49
  congenital Q41.2
immunoglobulin, isolated NEC D80.3
  IgA D80.2
  IgG D80.3
  IgM D80.4
incus (acquired) — *see* Loss, ossicles, ear
  congenital Q16.3
inner ear, congenital Q16.5
intestine (acquired) (small) Z90.49
  congenital Q41.9
    specified NEC Q41.8
  large Z90.49
    congenital Q42.9
      specified NEC Q42.8
iris, congenital Q13.1
jejunum (acquired) Z90.49
  congenital Q41.1
joint
  acquired
    hip (following explantation of hip joint prosthesis) (with or without presence of antibiotic-impregnated cement spacer) Z89.62-
    knee (following explantation of knee joint prosthesis) (with or without presence of antibiotic-impregnated cement spacer) Z89.52-
    shoulder (following explantation of shoulder joint prosthesis) (with or without presence of antibiotic-impregnated cement spacer) Z89.23-
  congenital NEC Q74.8
kidney(s) (acquired) Z90.5
  congenital Q60.2
    bilateral Q60.1
    unilateral Q60.0
knee (following explantation of knee joint prosthesis) (joint) (with or without presence of antibiotic-impregnated cement spacer) Z89.52-
labyrinth, membranous Q16.5
larynx (congenital) Q31.8
  acquired Z90.02
leg (acquired) (above knee) Z89.61-
  below knee (acquired) Z89.51-
  congenital — *see* Defect, reduction, lower limb
lens (acquired) — *see also* Aphakia
  congenital Q12.3
  post cataract extraction Z98.4-

Absence (of) (organ or part) (complete or partial) — *continued*
limb (acquired) — *see* Absence, extremity
lip Q38.6
liver (congenital) Q44.7
lung (fissure) (lobe) (bilateral) (unilateral) (congenital) Q33.3
  acquired (any part) Z90.2
menstruation — *see* Amenorrhea
muscle (congenital) (pectoral) Q79.8
  ocular Q10.3
neck, part Q18.8
neutrophil — *see* Agranulocytosis
nipple(s) (with breast(s)) (acquired) Z90.1-
  congenital Q83.2
nose (congenital) Q30.1
  acquired Z90.09
organ
  of Corti, congenital Q16.5
  or site, congenital NEC Q89.8
    acquired NEC Z90.89
osseous meatus (ear) Q16.4
ovary (acquired)
  bilateral Z90.722
  congenital
    bilateral Q50.02
    unilateral Q50.01
  unilateral Z90.721
oviduct (acquired)
  bilateral Z90.722
  congenital Q50.6
  unilateral Z90.721
pancreas (congenital) Q45.0
  acquired Z90.410
    complete Z90.410
    partial Z90.411
    total Z90.410
parathyroid gland (acquired) E89.2
  congenital Q89.2
patella, congenital Q74.1
penis (congenital) Q55.5
  acquired Z90.79
pericardium (congenital) Q24.8
pituitary gland (congenital) Q89.2
  acquired E89.3
prostate (acquired) Z90.79
  congenital Q55.4
pulmonary valve Q22.0
punctum lacrimale (congenital) Q10.4
radius, congenital — *see* Defect, reduction, upper limb, longitudinal, radius
rectum (congenital) Q42.1
  with fistula Q42.0
  acquired Z90.49
respiratory organ NOS Q34.9
rib (acquired) Z90.89
  congenital Q76.6
sacrum, congenital Q76.49
salivary gland(s), congenital Q38.4
scrotum, congenital Q55.29
seminal vesicles (congenital) Q55.4
  acquired Z90.79
septum
  atrial (congenital) Q21.1
  between aorta and pulmonary artery Q21.4
  ventricular (congenital) Q20.4
sex chromosome
  female phenotype Q97.8
  male phenotype Q98.8
skull bone (congenital) Q75.8
  with
    anencephaly Q00.0
    encephalocele — *see* Encephalocele
    hydrocephalus Q03.9
      with spina bifida — *see* Spina bifida, by site, with hydrocephalus
    microcephaly Q02
spermatic cord, congenital Q55.4
spine, congenital Q76.49

Absence (of) (organ or part) (complete or partial) — *continued*
- spleen (congenital) Q89.01
  - acquired Z90.81
- sternum, congenital Q76.7
- stomach (acquired) (partial) Z90.3
  - congenital Q40.2
- superior vena cava, congenital Q26.8
- teeth, tooth (congenital) K00.0
  - acquired (complete) K08.109
    - class I K08.101
    - class II K08.102
    - class III K08.103
    - class IV K08.104
    - due to
      - caries K08.139
        - class I K08.131
        - class II K08.132
        - class III K08.133
        - class IV K08.134
      - periodontal disease K08.129
        - class I K08.121
        - class II K08.122
        - class III K08.123
        - class IV K08.124
      - specified NEC K08.199
        - class I K08.191
        - class II K08.192
        - class III K08.193
        - class IV K08.194
      - trauma K08.119
        - class I K08.111
        - class II K08.112
        - class III K08.113
        - class IV K08.114
  - partial K08.409
    - class I K08.401
    - class II K08.402
    - class III K08.403
    - class IV K08.404
    - due to
      - caries K08.439
        - class I K08.431
        - class II K08.432
        - class III K08.433
        - class IV K08.434
      - periodontal disease K08.429
        - class I K08.421
        - class II K08.422
        - class III K08.423
        - class IV K08.424
      - specified NEC K08.499
        - class I K08.491
        - class II K08.492
        - class III K08.493
        - class IV K08.494
      - trauma K08.419
        - class I K08.411
        - class II K08.412
        - class III K08.413
        - class IV K08.414
- tendon (congenital) Q79.8
- testis (congenital) Q55.0
  - acquired Z90.79
- thumb (acquired) Z89.01-
  - congenital — *see* Agenesis, hand
- thymus gland Q89.2
- thyroid (gland) (acquired) E89.0
  - cartilage, congenital Q31.8
  - congenital E03.1
- toe(s) (acquired) Z89.42-
  - with foot — *see* Absence, foot and ankle
  - congenital — *see* Agenesis, foot
  - great Z89.41-
- tongue, congenital Q38.3
- trachea (cartilage), congenital Q32.1
- transverse aortic arch, congenital Q25.49
- tricuspid valve Q22.4
- umbilical artery, congenital Q27.0

Absence (of) (organ or part) (complete or partial) — *continued*
- upper arm and forearm with hand present, congenital — *see* Agenesis, arm, with hand present
- ureter (congenital) Q62.4
  - acquired Z90.6
- urethra, congenital Q64.5
- uterus (acquired) Z90.710
  - with cervix Z90.710
  - with remaining cervical stump Z90.711
  - congenital Q51.0
- uvula, congenital Q38.5
- vagina, congenital Q52.0
- vas deferens (congenital) Q55.4
  - acquired Z90.79
- vein (peripheral) congenital NEC Q27.8
  - cerebral Q28.3
  - digestive system Q27.8
  - great Q26.8
  - lower limb Q27.8
  - portal Q26.5
  - precerebral Q28.1
  - specified site NEC Q27.8
  - upper limb Q27.8
- vena cava (inferior) (superior), congenital Q26.8
- ventricular septum Q20.4
- vertebra, congenital Q76.49
- vulva, congenital Q52.71
- wrist (acquired) Z89.12-

Absorbent system disease I87.8

Absorption
- carbohydrate, disturbance K90.49
- chemical — *see* Table of Drugs and Chemcials
  - through placenta (newborn) P04.9
    - environmental substance P04.6
    - nutritional substance P04.5
    - obstetric anesthetic or analgesic drug P04.0
- drug NEC — *see* Table of Drugs and Chemicals
  - addictive
    - through placenta (newborn) P04.49
      - cocaine P04.41
  - medicinal
    - through placenta (newborn) P04.1
  - through placenta (newborn) P04.1
    - obstetric anesthetic or analgesic drug P04.0
- fat, disturbance K90.49
- pancreatic K90.3
- noxious substance — *see* Table of Drugs and Chemicals
- protein, disturbance K90.49
- starch, disturbance K90.49
- toxic substance — *see* Table of Drugs and Chemicals
- uremic — *see* Uremia

Abstinence symptoms, syndrome
- alcohol F10.239
  - with delirium F10.231
- cocaine F14.23
- neonatal P96.1
- nicotine — *see* Dependence, drug, nicotine, with, withdrawal
- opioid F11.93
  - with dependence F11.23
- psychoactive NEC F19.939
  - with
    - delirium F19.931
    - dependence F19.239
      - with
        - delirium F19.231
        - perceptual disturbance F19.232
      - uncomplicated F19.230
    - perceptual disturbance F19.932
  - uncomplicated F19.930

Abstinence symptoms, syndrome — *continued*
- sedative F13.939
  - with
    - delirium F13.931
    - dependence F13.239
      - with
        - delirium F13.231
        - perceptual disturbance F13.232
      - uncomplicated F13.230
    - perceptual disturbance F13.932
  - uncomplicated F13.930
- stimulant NEC F15.93
  - with dependence F15.23

Abulia R68.89

Abulomania F60.7

Abuse
- adult — *see* Maltreatment, adult
  - as reason for
    - couple seeking advice (including offender) Z63.0
- alcohol (non-dependent) F10.10
  - with
    - anxiety disorder F10.180
    - intoxication F10.129
      - with delirium F10.121
      - uncomplicated F10.120
    - mood disorder F10.14
    - other specified disorder F10.188
    - psychosis F10.159
      - delusions F10.150
      - hallucinations F10.151
    - sexual dysfunction F10.181
    - sleep disorder F10.182
    - unspecified disorder F10.19
  - counseling and surveillance Z71.41
- amphetamine (or related substance) — *see* Abuse, drug, stimulant NEC
- analgesics (non-prescribed) (over the counter) F55.8
- antacids F55.0
- antidepressants — *see* Abuse, drug, psychoactive NEC
- anxiolytic — *see* Abuse, drug, sedative
- barbiturates — *see* Abuse, drug, sedative
- caffeine — *see* Abuse, drug, stimulant NEC
- cannabis, cannabinoids — *see* Abuse, drug, cannabis
- child — *see* Maltreatment, child
- cocaine — *see* Abuse, drug, cocaine
- drug NEC (non-dependent) F19.10
  - with sleep disorder F19.182
  - amphetamine type — *see* Abuse, drug, stimulant NEC
  - analgesics (non-prescribed) (over the counter) F55.8
  - antacids F55.0
  - antidepressants — *see* Abuse, drug, psychoactive NEC
  - anxiolytics — *see* Abuse, drug, sedative
  - barbiturates — *see* Abuse, drug, sedative
  - caffeine — *see* Abuse, drug, stimulant NEC
  - cannabis F12.10
    - with
      - anxiety disorder F12.180
      - intoxication F12.129
        - with
          - delirium F12.121
          - perceptual disturbance F12.122
        - uncomplicated F12.120
      - other specified disorder F12.188
      - psychosis F12.159
        - delusions F12.150
        - hallucinations F12.151
      - unspecified disorder F12.19

Abuse — *continued*
  drug NEC (non-dependent) F19.10 —
    continued
    cocaine F14.10
      with
        anxiety disorder F14.180
        intoxication F14.129
          with
            delirium F14.121
            perceptual disturbance F14.122
          uncomplicated F14.120
        mood disorder F14.14
        other specified disorder F14.188
        psychosis F14.159
          delusions F14.150
          hallucinations F14.151
        sexual dysfunction F14.181
        sleep disorder F14.182
        unspecified disorder F14.19
    counseling and surveillance Z71.51
    hallucinogen F16.10
      with
        anxiety disorder F16.180
        flashbacks F16.183
        intoxication F16.129
          with
            delirium F16.121
            perceptual disturbance F16.122
          uncomplicated F16.120
        mood disorder F16.14
        other specified disorder F16.188
        perception disorder, persisting F16.183
        psychosis F16.159
          delusions F16.150
          hallucinations F16.151
        unspecified disorder F16.19
    hashish — *see* Abuse, drug, cannabis
    herbal or folk remedies F55.1
    hormones F55.3
    hypnotics — *see* Abuse, drug, sedative
    inhalant F18.10
      with
        anxiety disorder F18.180
        dementia, persisting F18.17
        intoxication F18.129
          with delirium F18.121
          uncomplicated F18.120
        mood disorder F18.14
        other specified disorder F18.188
        psychosis F18.159
          delusions F18.150
          hallucinations F18.151
        unspecified disorder F18.19
    laxatives F55.2
    LSD — *see* Abuse, drug, hallucinogen
    marihuana — *see* Abuse, drug, cannabis
    morphine type (opioids) — *see* Abuse, drug,
      opioid
    opioid F11.10
      with
        intoxication F11.129
          with
            delirium F11.121
            perceptual disturbance F11.122
          uncomplicated F11.120
        mood disorder F11.14
        other specified disorder F11.188
        psychosis F11.159
          delusions F11.150
          hallucinations F11.151
        sexual dysfunction F11.181
        sleep disorder F11.182
        unspecified disorder F11.19
    PCP (phencyclidine) (or related substance) —
      see Abuse, drug, hallucinogen

Abuse — *continued*
  drug NEC (non-dependent) F19.10 —
    continued
    psychoactive NEC F19.10
      with
        amnestic disorder F19.16
        anxiety disorder F19.180
        dementia F19.17
        intoxication F19.129
          with
            delirium F19.121
            perceptual disturbance F19.122
          uncomplicated F19.120
        mood disorder F19.14
        other specified disorder F19.188
        psychosis F19.159
          delusions F19.150
          hallucinations F19.151
        sexual dysfunction F19.181
        sleep disorder F19.182
        unspecified disorder F19.19
    sedative, hypnotic or anxiolytic F13.10
      with
        anxiety disorder F13.180
        intoxication F13.129
          with delirium F13.121
          uncomplicated F13.120
        mood disorder F13.14
        other specified disorder F13.188
        psychosis F13.159
          delusions F13.150
          hallucinations F13.151
        sexual dysfunction F13.181
        sleep disorder F13.182
        unspecified disorder F13.19
    solvent — *see* Abuse, drug, inhalant
    steroids F55.3
    stimulant NEC F15.10
      with
        anxiety disorder F15.180
        intoxication F15.129
          with
            delirium F15.121
            perceptual disturbance F15.122
          uncomplicated F15.120
        mood disorder F15.14
        other specified disorder F15.188
        psychosis F15.159
          delusions F15.150
          hallucinations F15.151
        sexual dysfunction F15.181
        sleep disorder F15.182
        unspecified disorder F15.19
    tranquilizers — *see* Abuse, drug, sedative
    vitamins F55.4
  hallucinogens — *see* Abuse, drug,
    hallucinogen
  hashish — *see* Abuse, drug, cannabis
  herbal or folk remedies F55.1
  hormones F55.3
  hypnotic — *see* Abuse, drug, sedative
  inhalant — *see* Abuse, drug, inhalant
  laxatives F55.2
  LSD — *see* Abuse, drug, hallucinogen
  marihuana — *see* Abuse, drug, cannabis
  morphine type (opioids) — *see* Abuse, drug,
    opioid
  non-psychoactive substance NEC F55.8
    antacids F55.0
    folk remedies F55.1
    herbal remedies F55.1
    hormones F55.3
    laxatives F55.2
    steroids F55.3
    vitamins F55.4
  opioids — *see* Abuse, drug, opioid
  PCP (phencyclidine) (or related substance) —
    see Abuse, drug, hallucinogen
  physical (adult) (child) — *see* Maltreatment

Abuse — *continued*
  psychoactive substance — *see* Abuse, drug,
    psychoactive NEC
  psychological (adult) (child) — *see*
    Maltreatment
  sedative — *see* Abuse, drug, sedative
  sexual — *see* Maltreatment
  solvent — *see* Abuse, drug, inhalant
  steroids F55.3
  vitamins F55.4
Acalculia R48.8
  developmental F81.2
Acanthamebiasis (with) B60.10
  conjunctiva B60.12
  keratoconjunctivitis B60.13
  meningoencephalitis B60.11
  other specified B60.19
Acanthocephaliasis B83.8
Acanthocheilonemiasis B74.4
Acanthocytosis E78.6
Acantholysis L11.9
Acanthosis (acquired) (nigricans) L83
  benign Q82.8
  congenital Q82.8
  seborrheic L82.1
    inflamed L82.0
  tongue K14.3
Acapnia E87.3
Acarbia E87.2
Acardia, acardius Q89.8
Acardiacus amorphus Q89.8
Acardiotrophia I51.4
Acariasis B88.0
  scabies B86
Acarodermatitis (urticarioides) B88.0
Acarophobia F40.218
Acatalasemia, acatalasia E80.3
Acathisia (drug induced) G25.71
Accelerated atrioventricular conduction
  I45.6
Accentuation of personality traits (type A)
  Z73.1
Accessory (congenital)
  adrenal gland Q89.1
  anus Q43.4
  appendix Q43.4
  atrioventricular conduction I45.6
  auditory ossicles Q16.3
  auricle (ear) Q17.0
  biliary duct or passage Q44.5
  bladder Q64.79
  blood vessels NEC Q27.9
    coronary Q24.5
  bone NEC Q79.8
  breast tissue, axilla Q83.1
  carpal bones Q74.0
  cecum Q43.4
  chromosome(s) NEC (nonsex) Q92.9
    with complex rearrangements NEC Q92.5
      seen only at prometaphase Q92.8
      13 — *see* Trisomy, 13
      18 — *see* Trisomy, 18
      21 — *see* Trisomy, 21
    partial Q92.9
    sex
      female phenotype Q97.8
  coronary artery Q24.5
  cusp(s), heart valve NEC Q24.8
    pulmonary Q22.3
  cystic duct Q44.5
  digit(s) Q69.9
  ear (auricle) (lobe) Q17.0
  endocrine gland NEC Q89.2
  eye muscle Q10.3
  eyelid Q10.3
  face bone(s) Q75.8
  fallopian tube (fimbria) (ostium) Q50.6
  finger(s) Q69.0
  foreskin N47.8

© 2016 Channel Publishing, Ltd.

DISEASE INDEX

Accessory (congenital) — *continued*
frontonasal process Q75.8
gallbladder Q44.1
genital organ(s)
female Q52.8
external Q52.79
internal NEC Q52.8
male Q55.8
genitourinary organs NEC Q89.8
female Q52.8
male Q55.8
hallux Q69.2
heart Q24.8
valve NEC Q24.8
pulmonary Q22.3
hepatic ducts Q44.5
hymen Q52.4
intestine (large) (small) Q43.4
kidney Q63.0
lacrimal canal Q10.6
leaflet, heart valve NEC Q24.8
ligament, broad Q50.6
liver Q44.7
duct Q44.5
lobule (ear) Q17.0
lung (lobe) Q33.1
muscle Q79.8
navicular of carpus Q74.0
nervous system, part NEC Q07.8
nipple Q83.3
nose Q30.8
organ or site not listed — *see* Anomaly, by site
ovary Q50.31
oviduct Q50.6
pancreas Q45.3
parathyroid gland Q89.2
parotid gland (and duct) Q38.4
pituitary gland Q89.2
preauricular appendage Q17.0
prepuce N47.8
renal arteries (multiple) Q27.2
rib Q76.6
cervical Q76.5
roots (teeth) K00.2
salivary gland Q38.4
sesamoid bones Q74.8
foot Q74.2
hand Q74.0
skin tags Q82.8
spleen Q89.09
sternum Q76.7
submaxillary gland Q38.4
tarsal bones Q74.2
teeth, tooth K00.1
tendon Q79.8
thumb Q69.1
thymus gland Q89.2
thyroid gland Q89.2
toes Q69.2
tongue Q38.3
tooth, teeth K00.1
tragus Q17.0
ureter Q62.5
urethra Q64.79
urinary organ or tract NEC Q64.8
uterus Q51.2
vagina Q52.10
valve, heart NEC Q24.8
pulmonary Q22.3
vertebra Q76.49
vocal cords Q31.8
vulva Q52.79
Accident
birth — *see* Birth, injury
cardiac — *see* Infarct, myocardium
cerebral I63.9

Accident — *continued*
cerebrovascular (embolic) (ischemic)
(thrombotic) I63.9
aborted I63.9
hemorrhagic — *see* Hemorrhage,
intracranial, intracerebral
old (without sequelae) Z86.73
with sequelae (of) — *see* Sequelae,
infarction, cerebral
coronary — *see* Infarct, myocardium
craniovascular I63.9
vascular, brain I63.9
Accidental — *see* condition
Accommodation (disorder) — *see also*
condition
hysterical paralysis of F44.89
insufficiency of H52.4
paresis — *see* Paresis, of accommodation
spasm — *see* Spasm, of accommodation
Accouchement — *see* Delivery
Accreta placenta O43.21-
Accretio cordis (nonrheumatic) I31.0
Accretions, tooth, teeth K03.6
Acculturation difficulty Z60.3
Accumulation secretion, prostate N42.89
**Acephalia, acephalism, acephalus,
acephaly** Q00.0
Acephalobrachia monster Q89.8
Acephalochirus monster Q89.8
Acephalogaster Q89.8
Acephalostomus monster Q89.8
Acephalothorax Q89.8
Acerophobia F40.298
Acetonemia R79.89
in Type 1 diabetes E10.10
with coma E10.11
Acetonuria R82.4
Achalasia (cardia) (esophagus) K22.0
congenital Q39.5
pylorus Q40.0
sphincteral NEC K59.8
Ache(s) — *see* Pain
Acheilia Q38.6
Achillobursitis — *see* Tendinitis, Achilles
Achillodynia — *see* Tendinitis, Achilles
Achlorhydria, achlorhydric (neurogenic)
K31.83
anemia D50.8
diarrhea K31.83
psychogenic F45.8
secondary to vagotomy K91.1
Achluophobia F40.228
Acholia K82.8
Acholuric jaundice (familial) (splenomegalic)
— *see also* Spherocytosis
acquired D59.8
Achondrogenesis Q77.0
Achondroplasia (osteosclerosis congenita)
Q77.4
Achroma, cutis L80
Achromat(ism), achromatopsia (acquired)
(congenital) H53.51
Achromia, congenital — *see* Albinism
Achromia parasitica B36.0
Achylia gastrica K31.89
psychogenic F45.8
Acid
burn — *see* Corrosion
deficiency
amide nicotinic E52
ascorbic E54
folic E53.8
nicotinic E52
pantothenic E53.8
intoxication E87.2
peptic disease K30
phosphatase deficiency E83.39
stomach K30
psychogenic F45.8

Acidemia E87.2
argininosuccinic E72.22
isovaleric E71.110
metabolic (newborn) P19.9
first noted before onset of labor P19.0
first noted during labor P19.1
noted at birth P19.2
methylmalonic E71.120
pipecolic E72.3
propionic E71.121
Acidity, gastric (high) K30
psychogenic F45.8
Acidocytopenia — *see* Agranulocytosis
Acidocytosis D72.1
Acidopenia — *see* Agranulocytosis
Acidosis (lactic) (respiratory) E87.2
in Type 1 diabetes E10.10
with coma E10.11
kidney, tubular N25.89
lactic E87.2
metabolic NEC E87.2
with respiratory acidosis E87.4
late, of newborn P74.0
mixed metabolic and respiratory, newborn
P84
newborn P84
renal (hyperchloremic) (tubular) N25.89
respiratory E87.2
complicated by
metabolic
acidosis E87.4
alkalosis E87.4
Aciduria
argininosuccinic E72.22
glutaric (type I) E72.3
type II E71.313
type III E71.5-
orotic (congenital) (hereditary) (pyrimidine
deficiency) E79.8
anemia D53.0
Acladiosis (skin) B36.0
Aclasis, diaphyseal Q78.6
Acleistocardia Q21.1
Aclusion — *see* Anomaly, dentofacial,
malocclusion
Acne L70.9
artificialis L70.8
atrophica L70.2
cachecticorum (Hebra) L70.8
conglobata L70.1
cystic L70.0
decalvans L66.2
excoriée (des jeunes filles) L70.5
frontalis L70.2
indurata L70.0
infantile L70.4
keloid L73.0
lupoid L70.2
necrotic, necrotica (miliaris) L70.2
neonatal L70.4
nodular L70.0
occupational L70.8
picker's L70.5
pustular L70.0
rodens L70.2
rosacea L71.9
specified NEC L70.8
tropica L70.3
varioliformis L70.2
vulgaris L70.0
Acnitis (primary) A18.4
Acosta's disease T70.29
Acoustic — *see* condition
Acousticophobia F40.298
Acquired — *see also* condition
immunodeficiency syndrome (AIDS) B20
Acrania Q00.0
Acroangiodermatitis I78.9
Acroasphyxia, chronic I73.89

Acrobystitis N47.7
Acrocephalopolysyndactyly Q87.0
Acrocephalosyndactyly Q87.0
Acrocephaly Q75.0
Acrochondrohyperplasia — see Syndrome, Marfan's
Acrocyanosis I73.8
  newborn P28.2
    meaning transient blue hands and feet — omit code
Acrodermatitis L30.8
  atrophicans (chronica) L90.4
  continua (Hallopeau) L40.2
  enteropathica (hereditary) E83.2
  Hallopeau's L40.2
  infantile papular L44.4
  perstans L40.2
  pustulosa continua L40.2
  recalcitrant pustular L40.2
Acrodynia — see Poisoning, mercury
Acromegaly, acromegalia E22.0
Acromelalgia I73.81
Acromicria, acromikria Q79.8
Acronyx L60.0
Acropachy, thyroid — see Thyrotoxicosis
Acroparesthesia (simple) (vasomotor) I73.89
Acropathy, thyroid — see Thyrotoxicosis
Acrophobia F40.241
Acroposthitis N47.7
Acroscleriasis, acroscleroderma, acrosclerosis — see Sclerosis, systemic
Acrosphacelus I96
Acrospiroma, eccrine — see Neoplasm, skin, benign
Acrostealgia — see Osteochondropathy
Acrotrophodynia — see Immersion
ACTH ectopic syndrome E24.3
Actinic — see condition
Actinobacillosis, actinobacillus A28.8
  mallei A24.0
  muris A25.1
Actinomyces israelii (infection) — see Actinomycosis
Actinomycetoma (foot) B47.1
Actinomycosis, actinomycotic A42.9
  with pneumonia A42.0
  abdominal A42.1
  cervicofacial A42.2
  cutaneous A42.89
  gastrointestinal A42.1
  pulmonary A42.0
  sepsis A42.7
  specified site NEC A42.89
Actinoneuritis G62.82
Action, heart
  disorder I49.9
  irregular I49.9
    psychogenic F45.8
Activated protein C resistance D68.51
Activation
  mast cell (disorder) (syndrome) D89.40
    idiopathic D89.42
    monoclonal D89.41
    secondary D89.43
    specified type NEC D89.49
Active — see condition
Acute — see also condition
  abdomen R10.0
  gallbladder — see Cholecystitis, acute
Acyanotic heart disease (congenital) Q24.9
Acystia Q64.5
Adair-Dighton syndrome (brittle bones and blue sclera, deafness) Q78.0
Adamantinoblastoma — see Ameloblastoma
Adamantinoma — see also Cyst, calcifying odontogenic
  long bones C40.90
    lower limb C40.2-
    upper limb C40.0-

Adamantinoma — see also Cyst, calcifying odontogenic — continued
  malignant C41.1
    jaw (bone) (lower) C41.1
      upper C41.0
    tibial C40.2-
Adamantoblastoma — see Ameloblastoma
Adams-Stokes(-Morgagni) disease or syndrome I45.9
Adaption reaction — see Disorder, adjustment
Addiction (see also Dependence) F19.20
  alcohol, alcoholic (ethyl) (methyl) (wood) (without remission) F10.20
    with remission F10.21
  drug — see Dependence, drug
  ethyl alcohol (without remission) F10.20
    with remission F10.21
  heroin — see Dependence, drug, opioid
  methyl alcohol (without remission) F10.20
    with remission F10.21
  methylated spirit (without remission) F10.20
    with remission F10.21
  morphine(-like substances) — see Dependence, drug, opioid
  nicotine — see Dependence, drug, nicotine
  opium and opioids — see Dependence, drug, opioid
  tobacco — see Dependence, drug, nicotine
Addison-Biermer anemia (pernicious) D51.0
Addisonian crisis E27.2
Addison's
  anemia (pernicious) D51.0
  disease (bronze) or syndrome E27.1
    tuberculous A18.7
  keloid L94.0
Addison-Schilder complex E71.528
Additional — see also Accessory
  chromosome(s) Q99.8
    21 — see Trisomy, 21
    sex — see Abnormal, chromosome, sex
Adduction contracture, hip or other joint — see Contraction, joint
Adenitis — see also Lymphadenitis
  acute, unspecified site L04.9
  axillary I88.9
    acute L04.2
    chronic or subacute I88.1
  Bartholin's gland N75.8
  bulbourethral gland — see Urethritis
  cervical I88.9
    acute L04.0
    chronic or subacute I88.1
  chancroid (Hemophilus ducreyi) A57
  chronic, unspecified site I88.1
  Cowper's gland — see Urethritis
  due to Pasteurella multocida (p. septica) A28.0
  epidemic, acute B27.09
  gangrenous L04.9
  gonorrheal NEC A54.89
  groin I88.9
    acute L04.1
    chronic or subacute I88.1
  infectious (acute) (epidemic) B27.09
  inguinal I88.9
    acute L04.1
    chronic or subacute I88.1
  lymph gland or node, except mesenteric I88.9
    acute — see Lymphadenitis, acute
    chronic or subacute I88.1
  mesenteric (acute) (chronic) (nonspecific) (subacute) I88.0
  parotid gland (suppurative) — see Sialoadenitis
  salivary gland (any) (suppurative) — see Sialoadenitis
  scrofulous (tuberculous) A18.2
  Skene's duct or gland — see Urethritis
  strumous, tuberculous A18.2

Adenitis (see also Lymphadenitis) — continued
  subacute, unspecified site I88.1
  sublingual gland (suppurative) — see Sialoadenitis
  submandibular gland (suppurative) — see Sialoadenitis
  submaxillary gland (suppurative) — see Sialoadenitis
  tuberculous — see Tuberculosis, lymph gland
  urethral gland — see Urethritis
  Wharton's duct (suppurative) — see Sialoadenitis
Adenoacanthoma — see Neoplasm, malignant, by site
Adenoameloblastoma — see Cyst, calcifying odontogenic
Adenocarcinoid (tumor) — see Neoplasm, malignant, by site
Adenocarcinoma — see also Neoplasm, malignant, by site
  acidophil
    specified site — see Neoplasm, malignant, by site
    unspecified site C75.1
  adrenal cortical C74.0-
  alveolar — see Neoplasm, lung, malignant
  apocrine
    breast — see Neoplasm, breast, malignant
    in situ
      breast D05.8-
      specified site NEC — see Neoplasm, skin, in situ
      unspecified site D04.9
    specified site NEC — see Neoplasm, skin, malignant
    unspecified site C44.99
  basal cell
    specified site — see Neoplasm, skin, malignant
    unspecified site C08.9
  basophil
    specified site — see Neoplasm, malignant, by site
    unspecified site C75.1
  bile duct type C22.1
    liver C22.1
    specified site NEC — see Neoplasm, malignant, by site
    unspecified site C22.1
  bronchiolar — see Neoplasm, lung, malignant
  bronchioloalveolar — see Neoplasm, lung, malignant
  ceruminous C44.29-
  cervix, in situ (see also Carcinoma, cervix uteri, in situ) D06.9
  chromophobe
    specified site — see Neoplasm, malignant, by site
    unspecified site C75.1
  diffuse type
    specified site — see Neoplasm, malignant, by site
    unspecified site C16.9
  duct
    infiltrating
      with Paget's disease — see Neoplasm, breast, malignant
      specified site — see Neoplasm, malignant, by site
      unspecified site (female) C50.91-
        male C50.92-
    specified site — see Neoplasm, malignant, by site
    unspecified site
      female C56.9
      male C61

Adenocarcinoma (see also Neoplasm, malignant, by site) — continued
eosinophil
  specified site — see Neoplasm, malignant, by site
  unspecified site C75.1
follicular
  with papillary C73
  moderately differentiated C73
  specified site — see Neoplasm, malignant, by site
  trabecular C73
  unspecified site C73
  well differentiated C73
Hurthle cell C73
in
  adenomatous
    polyposis coli C18.9
infiltrating duct
  with Paget's disease — see Neoplasm, breast, malignant
  specified site — see Neoplasm, by site, malignant
  unspecified site (female) C50.91-
    male C50.92-
inflammatory
  specified site — see Neoplasm, by site, malignant
  unspecified site (female) C50.91-
    male C50.92-
intestinal type
  specified site — see Neoplasm, by site, malignant
  unspecified site C16.9
intracystic papillary
intraductal
  breast D05.1-
  noninfiltrating
    breast D05.1-
    papillary
      with invasion
        specified site — see Neoplasm, by site, malignant
        unspecified site (female) C50.91-
          male C50.92-
      breast D05.1-
      specified site NEC — see Neoplasm, in situ, by site
      unspecified site D05.1-
    specified site NEC — see Neoplasm, in situ, by site
    unspecified site D05.1-
  papillary
    with invasion
      specified site — see Neoplasm, malignant, by site
      unspecified site (female) C50.91-
        male C50.92-
    breast D05.1-
    specified site — see Neoplasm, in situ, by site
    unspecified site D05.1-
  specified site NEC — see Neoplasm, in situ, by site
  unspecified site D05.1-
islet cell
  with exocrine, mixed
    specified site — see Neoplasm, malignant, by site
    unspecified site C25.9
  pancreas C25.4
  specified site NEC — see Neoplasm, malignant, by site
  unspecified site C25.4

Adenocarcinoma (see also Neoplasm, malignant, by site) — continued
lobular
  in situ
    breast D05.0-
    specified site NEC — see Neoplasm, in situ, by site
    unspecified site D05.0-
  specified site — see Neoplasm, malignant, by site
  unspecified site (female) C50.91-
    male C50.92-
mucoid — see also Neoplasm, malignant, by site
  cell
    specified site — see Neoplasm, malignant, by site
    unspecified site C75.1
nonencapsulated sclerosing C73
papillary
  with follicular C73
  follicular variant C73
  intraductal (noninfiltrating)
    with invasion
      specified site — see Neoplasm, malignant, by site
      unspecified site (female) C50.91-
        male C50.92-
    breast D05.1-
    specified site NEC — see Neoplasm, in situ, by site
    unspecified site D05.1-
  serous
    specified site — see Neoplasm, malignant, by site
    unspecified site C56.9
papillocystic
  specified site — see Neoplasm, malignant, by site
  unspecified site C56.9
pseudomucinous
  specified site — see Neoplasm, malignant, by site
  unspecified site C56.9
renal cell C64-
sebaceous — see Neoplasm, skin, malignant
serous — see also Neoplasm, malignant, by site
  papillary
    specified site — see Neoplasm, malignant, by site
    unspecified site C56.9
sweat gland — see Neoplasm, skin, malignant
water-clear cell C75.0
Adenocarcinoma-in-situ — see also Neoplasm, in situ, by site
breast D05.9-
Adenofibroma
clear cell — see Neoplasm, benign, by site
endometrioid D27.9
  borderline malignancy D39.10
  malignant C56-
mucinous
  specified site — see Neoplasm, benign, by site
  unspecified site D27.9
papillary
  specified site — see Neoplasm, benign, by site
  unspecified site D27.9
prostate — see Enlargement, enlarged, prostate
serous
  specified site — see Neoplasm, benign, by site
  unspecified site D27.9
specified site — see Neoplasm, benign, by site
unspecified site D27.9

Adenofibrosis
breast — see Fibroadenosis, breast
endometrioid N80.0
Adenoiditis (chronic) J35.02
with tonsillitis J35.03
acute J03.90
  recurrent J03.91
  specified organism NEC J03.80
    recurrent J03.81
  staphylococcal J03.80
    recurrent J03.81
  streptococcal J03.00
    recurrent J03.01
Adenoids — see condition
Adenolipoma — see Neoplasm, benign, by site
Adenolipomatosis, Launois-Bensaude E88.89
Adenolymphoma
specified site — see Neoplasm, benign, by site
unspecified site D11.9
Adenoma — see also Neoplasm, benign, by site
acidophil
  specified site — see Neoplasm, benign, by site
  unspecified site D35.2
acidophil-basophil, mixed
  specified site — see Neoplasm, benign, by site
  unspecified site D35.2
adrenal (cortical) D35.00
  clear cell D35.00
  compact cell D35.00
  glomerulosa cell D35.00
  heavily pigmented variant D35.00
  mixed cell D35.00
alpha-cell
  pancreas D13.7
  specified site NEC — see Neoplasm, benign, by site
  unspecified site D13.7
alveolar D14.30
apocrine
  breast D24-
  specified site NEC — see Neoplasm, skin, benign, by site
  unspecified site D23.9
basal cell D11.9
basophil
  specified site — see Neoplasm, benign, by site
  unspecified site D35.2
basophil-acidophil, mixed
  specified site — see Neoplasm, benign, by site
  unspecified site D35.2
beta-cell
  pancreas D13.7
  specified site NEC — see Neoplasm, benign, by site
  unspecified site D13.7
bile duct D13.4
  common D13.5
  extrahepatic D13.5
  intrahepatic D13.4
  specified site NEC — see Neoplasm, benign, by site
  unspecified site D13.4
black D35.00
bronchial D38.1
  cylindroid type — see Neoplasm, lung, malignant
ceruminous D23.2-
chief cell D35.1
chromophobe
  specified site — see Neoplasm, benign, by site
  unspecified site D35.2

DISEASE INDEX

Adenoma (see also Neoplasm, benign, by site) — continued
- colloid
  - specified site — see Neoplasm, benign, by site
  - unspecified site D34
- duct
- eccrine, papillary — see Neoplasm, skin, benign
- endocrine, multiple
  - single specified site — see Neoplasm, uncertain behavior, by site
  - two or more specified sites D44-
  - unspecified site D44.9
- endometrioid — see also Neoplasm, benign
  - borderline malignancy — see Neoplasm, uncertain behavior, by site
- eosinophil
  - specified site — see Neoplasm, benign, by site
  - unspecified site D35.2
- fetal
  - specified site — see Neoplasm, benign, by site
  - unspecified site D34
- follicular
  - specified site — see Neoplasm, benign, by site
  - unspecified site D34
- hepatocellular D13.4
- Hurthle cell D34
- islet cell
  - pancreas D13.7
  - specified site NEC — see Neoplasm, benign, by site
  - unspecified site D13.7
- liver cell D13.4
- macrofollicular
  - specified site — see Neoplasm, benign, by site
  - unspecified site D34
- malignant, malignum — see Neoplasm, malignant, by site
- microcystic
  - pancreas D13.6
  - specified site NEC — see Neoplasm, benign, by site
  - unspecified site D13.6
- microfollicular
  - specified site — see Neoplasm, benign, by site
  - unspecified site D34
- mucoid cell
  - specified site — see Neoplasm, benign, by site
  - unspecified site D35.2
- multiple endocrine
  - single specified site — see Neoplasm, uncertain behavior, by site
  - two or more specified sites D44-
  - unspecified site D44.9
- nipple D24-
- papillary — see also Neoplasm, benign, by site
  - eccrine — see Neoplasm, skin, benign, by site
- Pick's tubular
  - specified site — see Neoplasm, benign, by site
  - unspecified site
    - female D27.9
    - male D29.20
- pleomorphic
  - carcinoma in — see Neoplasm, salivary gland, malignant
  - specified site — see Neoplasm, malignant, by site
  - unspecified site C08.9

Adenoma (see also Neoplasm, benign, by site) — continued
- polypoid — see also Neoplasm, benign
  - adenocarcinoma in — see Neoplasm, malignant, by site
  - adenocarcinoma in situ — see Neoplasm, in situ, by site
- prostate — see Neoplasm, benign, prostate
- rete cell D29.20
- sebaceous — see Neoplasm, skin, benign
- Sertoli cell
  - specified site — see Neoplasm, benign, by site
  - unspecified site
    - female D27.9
    - male D29.20
- skin appendage — see Neoplasm, skin, benign
- sudoriferous gland — see Neoplasm, skin, benign
- sweat gland — see Neoplasm, skin, benign
- testicular
  - specified site — see Neoplasm, benign, by site
  - unspecified site
    - female D27.9
    - male D29.20
- tubular — see also Neoplasm, benign, by site
  - adenocarcinoma in — see Neoplasm, malignant, by site
  - adenocarcinoma in situ — see Neoplasm, in situ, by site
  - Pick's
    - specified site — see Neoplasm, benign, by site
    - unspecified site
      - female D27.9
      - male D29.20
- tubulovillous — see also Neoplasm, benign, by site
  - adenocarcinoma in — see Neoplasm, malignant, by site
  - adenocarcinoma in situ — see Neoplasm, in situ, by site
- villous — see Neoplasm, uncertain behavior, by site
  - adenocarcinoma in — see Neoplasm, malignant, by site
  - adenocarcinoma in situ — see Neoplasm, in situ, by site
- water-clear cell D35.1

Adenomatosis
- endocrine (multiple) E31.20
  - single specified site — see Neoplasm, uncertain behavior, by site
- erosive of nipple D24-
- pluriendocrine — see Adenomatosis, endocrine
- pulmonary D38.1
  - malignant — see Neoplasm, lung, malignant
- specified site — see Neoplasm, benign, by site
- unspecified site D12.6

Adenomatous
- goiter (nontoxic) E04.9
  - with hyperthyroidism — see Hyperthyroidism, with, goiter, nodular
  - toxic — see Hyperthyroidism, with, goiter, nodular

Adenomyoma — see also Neoplasm, benign, by site
- prostate — see Enlarged, prostate

Adenomyometritis N80.0
Adenomyosis N80.0
Adenopathy (lymph gland) R59.9
- generalized R59.1
- inguinal R59.0
- localized R59.0
- mediastinal R59.0
- mesentery R59.0
- syphilitic (secondary) A51.49

Adenopathy (lymph gland) R59.9 — continued
- tracheobronchial R59.0
  - tuberculous A15.4
    - primary (progressive) A15.7
  - tuberculous — see also Tuberculosis, lymph gland
    - tracheobronchial A15.4
    - primary (progressive) A15.7

Adenosalpingitis — see Salpingitis
Adenosarcoma — see Neoplasm, malignant, by site
Adenosclerosis I88.8
Adenosis (sclerosing) breast — see Fibroadenosis, breast
Adenovirus, as cause of disease classified elsewhere B97.0
Adentia (complete) (partial) — see Absence, teeth
Adherent — see also Adhesions
- labia (minora) N90.89
- pericardium (nonrheumatic) I31.0
  - rheumatic I09.2
- placenta (with hemorrhage) O72.0
  - without hemorrhage O73.0
- prepuce, newborn N47.0
- scar (skin) L90.5
- tendon in scar L90.5

Adhesions, adhesive (postinfective) K66.0
- with intestinal obstruction K56.5
- abdominal (wall) — see Adhesions, peritoneum
- appendix K38.8
- bile duct (common) (hepatic) K83.8
- bladder (sphincter) N32.89
- bowel — see Adhesions, peritoneum
- cardiac I31.0
  - rheumatic I09.2
- cecum — see Adhesions, peritoneum
- cervicovaginal N88.1
  - congenital Q52.8
  - postpartal O90.89
    - old N88.1
- cervix N88.1
- ciliary body NEC — see Adhesions, iris
- clitoris N90.89
- colon — see Adhesions, peritoneum
- common duct K83.8
- congenital — see also Anomaly, by site
  - fingers — see Syndactylism, complex, fingers
  - omental, anomalous Q43.3
  - peritoneal Q43.3
  - tongue (to gum or roof of mouth) Q38.3
- conjunctiva (acquired) H11.21-
  - congenital Q15.8
- cystic duct K82.8
- diaphragm — see Adhesions, peritoneum
- due to foreign body — see Foreign body
- duodenum — see Adhesions, peritoneum
- ear
  - middle H74.1-
- epididymis N50.89
- epidural — see Adhesions, meninges
- epiglottis J38.7
- eyelid H02.59
- female pelvis N73.6
- gallbladder K82.8
- globe H44.89
- heart I31.0
  - rheumatic I09.2
- ileocecal (coil) — see Adhesions, peritoneum
- ileum — see Adhesions, peritoneum
- intestine — see also Adhesions, peritoneum
  - with obstruction K56.5
- intra-abdominal — see Adhesions, peritoneum

DISEASE INDEX

Adhesions, adhesive (postinfective) K66.0 —
continued
　iris H21.50-
　　anterior H21.51-
　　goniosynechiae H21.52-
　　posterior H21.54-
　　to corneal graft T85.898
　joint — *see* Ankylosis
　　knee M23.8x
　　temporomandibular M26.61-
　labium (majus) (minus), congenital Q52.5
　liver — *see* Adhesions, peritoneum
　lung J98.4
　mediastinum J98.59
　meninges (cerebral) (spinal) G96.12
　　congenital Q07.8
　　tuberculous (cerebral) (spinal) A17.0
　mesenteric — *see* Adhesions, peritoneum
　nasal (septum) (to turbinates) J34.89
　ocular muscle — *see* Strabismus, mechanical
　omentum — *see* Adhesions, peritoneum
　ovary N73.6
　　congenital (to cecum, kidney or omentum)
　　　Q50.39
　paraovarian N73.6
　pelvic (peritoneal)
　　female N73.6
　　　postprocedural N99.4
　　male — *see* Adhesions, peritoneum
　　postpartal (old) N73.6
　　tuberculous A18.17
　penis to scrotum (congenital) Q55.8
　periappendiceal — *see also* Adhesions,
　　peritoneum
　pericardium (nonrheumatic) I31.0
　　focal I31.8
　　rheumatic I09.2
　　tuberculous A18.84
　pericholecystic K82.8
　perigastric — *see* Adhesions, peritoneum
　periovarian N73.6
　periprostatic N42.89
　perirectal — *see* Adhesions, peritoneum
　perirenal N28.89
　peritoneum, peritoneal (postinfective)
　　(postprocedural) K66.0
　　with obstruction (intestinal) K56.5
　　congenital Q43.3
　　pelvic, female N73.6
　　　postprocedural N99.4
　　postpartal, pelvic N73.6
　　to uterus N73.6
　peritubal N73.6
　periureteral N28.89
　periuterine N73.6
　perivesical N32.89
　perivesicular (seminal vesicle) N50.89
　pleura, pleuritic J94.8
　　tuberculous NEC A15.6
　pleuropericardial J94.8
　postoperative (gastrointestinal tract) K66.0
　　with obstruction K91.3
　　due to foreign body accidentally left in
　　　wound — *see* Foreign body, accidentally
　　　left during a procedure
　　pelvic peritoneal N99.4
　　urethra — *see* Stricture, urethra,
　　　postprocedural
　　vagina N99.2
　postpartal, old (vulva or perineum) N90.89
　preputial, prepuce N47.5
　pulmonary J98.4
　pylorus — *see* Adhesions, peritoneum
　sciatic nerve — *see* Lesion, nerve, sciatic
　seminal vesicle N50.89
　shoulder (joint) — *see* Capsulitis, adhesive
　sigmoid flexure — *see* Adhesions, peritoneum

Adhesions, adhesive (postinfective) K66.0 —
continued
　spermatic cord (acquired) N50.89
　　congenital Q55.4
　spinal canal G96.12
　stomach — *see* Adhesions, peritoneum
　subscapular — *see* Capsulitis, adhesive
　temporomandibular M26.61-
　tendinitis — *see also* Tenosynovitis, specified
　　type NEC
　　shoulder — *see* Capsulitis, adhesive
　testis N44.8
　tongue, congenital (to gum or roof of mouth)
　　Q38.3
　　acquired K14.8
　trachea J39.8
　tubo-ovarian N73.6
　tunica vaginalis N44.8
　uterus N73.6
　　internal N85.6
　　to abdominal wall N73.6
　vagina (chronic) N89.5
　　postoperative N99.2
　vitreomacular H43.82-
　vitreous H43.89
　vulva N90.89
Adiaspiromycosis B48.8
Adie(-Holmes) pupil or syndrome — *see*
　Anomaly, pupil, function, tonic pupil
Adiponecrosis neonatorum P83.8
Adiposis — *see also* Obesity
　cerebralis E23.6
　dolorosa E88.2
Adiposity — *see also* Obesity
　heart — *see* Degeneration, myocardial
　localized E65
Adiposogenital dystrophy E23.6
Adjustment
　disorder — *see* Disorder, adjustment
　implanted device — *see* Encounter (for),
　　adjustment (of)
　prosthesis, external — *see* Fitting
　reaction — *see* Disorder, adjustment
Administration of tPA (rtPA) in a
　different facility within the last 24
　hours prior to admission to current
　facility Z92.82
Admission (for) — *see also* Encounter (for)
　adjustment (of)
　　artificial
　　　arm Z44.00-
　　　　complete Z44.01-
　　　　partial Z44.02-
　　　eye Z44.2
　　　leg Z44.10-
　　　　complete Z44.11-
　　　　partial Z44.12-
　　brain neuropacemaker Z46.2
　　　implanted Z45.42
　　breast
　　　implant Z45.81
　　　prosthesis (external) Z44.3
　　colostomy belt Z46.89
　　contact lenses Z46.0
　　cystostomy device Z46.6
　　dental prosthesis Z46.3
　　device NEC
　　　abdominal Z46.89
　　　implanted Z45.89
　　　　cardiac Z45.09
　　　　　defibrillator (with synchronous
　　　　　　cardiace pacemaker) Z45.02
　　　　　pacemaker (cardiac resynchronization
　　　　　　therapy (CRT-P)) Z45.018
　　　　　　pulse generator Z45.010
　　　　　resynchronization therapy defibrillator
　　　　　　(CRT-D) Z45.02

Admission (for) (*see also* Encounter (for)) —
continued
　adjustment (of) — *continued*
　　device NEC — *continued*
　　　implanted Z45.89 — *continued*
　　　　hearing device Z45.328
　　　　　bone conduction Z45.320
　　　　　cochlear Z45.321
　　　　infusion pump Z45.1
　　　　nervous system Z45.49
　　　　　CSF drainage Z45.41
　　　　　hearing device — *see* Admission,
　　　　　　adjustment, device, implanted,
　　　　　　hearing device
　　　　　neuropacemaker Z45.42
　　　　　visual substitution Z45.31
　　　　specified NEC Z45.89
　　　　vascular access Z45.2
　　　　visual substitution Z45.31
　　　nervous system Z46.2
　　　　implanted — *see* Admission, adjustment,
　　　　　device, implanted, nervous system
　　　orthodontic Z46.4
　　　prosthetic Z44.9
　　　　arm — *see* Admission, adjustment,
　　　　　artificial, arm
　　　　breast Z44.3
　　　　dental Z46.3
　　　　eye Z44.2
　　　　leg — *see* Admission, adjustment,
　　　　　artificial, leg
　　　　specified type NEC Z44.8
　　substitution
　　　auditory Z46.2
　　　　implanted — *see* Admission,
　　　　　adjustment, device, implanted,
　　　　　hearing device
　　　nervous system Z46.2
　　　　implanted — *see* Admission,
　　　　　adjustment, device, implanted,
　　　　　nervous system
　　　visual Z46.2
　　　　implanted Z45.31
　　urinary Z46.6
　hearing aid Z46.1
　　implanted — *see* Admission, adjustment,
　　　device, implanted, hearing device
　ileostomy device Z46.89
　intestinal appliance or device NEC Z46.89
　neuropacemaker (brain) (peripheral nerve)
　　(spinal cord) Z46.2
　　implanted Z45.42
　orthodontic device Z46.4
　orthopedic (brace) (cast) (device) (shoes)
　　Z46.89
　pacemaker (cardiac resynchronization
　　therapy (CRT-P))
　　cardiac Z45.018
　　　pulse generator Z45.010
　　nervous system Z46.2
　　　implanted Z45.42
　portacath (port-a-cath) Z45.2
　prosthesis Z44.9
　　arm — *see* Admission, adjustment,
　　　artificial, arm
　　breast Z44.3
　　dental Z46.3
　　eye Z44.2
　　leg — *see* Admission, adjustment,
　　　artificial, leg
　　specified NEC Z44.8
　spectacles Z46.0
　aftercare (*see also* Aftercare) Z51.89
　postpartum
　　immediately after delivery Z39.0
　　routine follow-up Z39.2
　radiation therapy (antineoplastic) Z51.0

Admission (for) (*see also* Encounter (for)) — *continued*
- attention to artificial opening (of) Z43.9
  - artificial vagina Z43.7
  - colostomy Z43.3
  - cystostomy Z43.5
  - enterostomy Z43.4
  - gastrostomy Z43.1
  - ileostomy Z43.2
  - jejunostomy Z43.4
  - nephrostomy Z43.6
  - specified site NEC Z43.8
    - intestinal tract Z43.4
    - urinary tract Z43.6
  - tracheostomy Z43.0
  - ureterostomy Z43.6
  - urethrostomy Z43.6
- breast augmentation or reduction Z41.1
- breast reconstruction following mastectomy Z42.1
- change of
  - dressing (nonsurgical) Z48.00
  - neuropacemaker device (brain) (peripheral nerve) (spinal cord) Z46.2
    - implanted Z45.42
  - surgical dressing Z48.01
- circumcision, ritual or routine (in absence of diagnosis) Z41.2
- clinical research investigation (control) (normal comparison) (participant) Z00.6
- contraceptive management Z30.9
- cosmetic surgery NEC Z41.1
- counseling — *see also* Counseling
  - dietary Z71.3
  - gestational carrier Z31.7
  - HIV Z71.7
  - human immunodeficiency virus Z71.7
  - nonattending third party Z71.0
  - procreative management NEC Z31.69
- delivery, full-term, uncomplicated O80
  - cesarean, without indication O82
- desensitization to allergens Z51.6
- dietary surveillance and counseling Z71.3
- ear piercing Z41.3
- examination at health care facility (adult) (*see also* Examination) Z00.00
  - with abnormal findings Z00.01
  - clinical research investigation (control) (normal comparison) (participant) Z00.6
  - dental Z01.20
    - with abnormal findings Z01.21
  - donor (potential) Z00.5
  - ear Z01.10
    - with abnormal findings NEC Z01.118
  - eye Z01.00
    - with abnormal findings Z01.01
  - general, specified reason NEC Z00.8
  - hearing Z01.10
    - with abnormal findings NEC Z01.118
  - postpartum checkup Z39.2
  - psychiatric (general) Z00.8
    - requested by authority Z04.6
  - vision Z01.00
    - with abnormal findings Z01.01
- fitting (of)
  - artificial
    - arm — *see* Admission, adjustment, artificial, arm
    - eye Z44.2
    - leg — *see* Admission, adjustment, artificial, leg
  - brain neuropacemaker Z46.2
    - implanted Z45.42
  - breast prosthesis (external) Z44.3
  - colostomy belt Z46.89
  - contact lenses Z46.0
  - cystostomy device Z46.6
  - dental prosthesis Z46.3
  - dentures Z46.3

Admission (for) (*see also* Encounter (for)) — *continued*
- fitting (of) — *continued*
  - device NEC
    - abdominal Z46.89
    - nervous system Z46.2
      - implanted — *see* Admission, adjustment, device, implanted, nervous system
    - orthodontic Z46.4
    - prosthetic Z44.9
      - breast Z44.3
      - dental Z46.3
      - eye Z44.2
    - substitution
      - auditory Z46.2
        - implanted — *see* Admission, adjustment, device, implanted, hearing device
      - nervous system Z46.2
        - implanted — *see* Admission, adjustment, device, implanted, nervous system
      - visual Z46.2
        - implanted Z45.31
  - hearing aid Z46.1
  - ileostomy device Z46.89
  - intestinal appliance or device NEC Z46.89
  - neuropacemaker (brain) (peripheral nerve) (spinal cord) Z46.2
    - implanted Z45.42
  - orthodontic device Z46.4
  - orthopedic device (brace) (cast) (shoes) Z46.89
  - prosthesis Z44.9
    - arm — *see* Admission, adjustment, artificial, arm
    - breast Z44.3
    - dental Z46.3
    - eye Z44.2
    - leg — *see* Admission, adjustment, artificial, leg
    - specified type NEC Z44.8
  - spectacles Z46.0
- follow-up examination Z09
- intrauterine device management Z30.431
  - initial prescription Z30.014
- mental health evaluation Z00.8
  - requested by authority Z04.6
- observation — *see* Observation
- Papanicolaou smear, cervix Z12.4
  - for suspected malignant neoplasm Z12.4
- plastic and reconstructive surgery following medical procedure or healed injury NEC Z42.8
- plastic surgery, cosmetic NEC Z41.1
- postpartum observation
  - immediately after delivery Z39.0
  - routine follow-up Z39.2
- poststerilization (for restoration) Z31.0
  - aftercare Z31.42
- procreative management Z31.9
- prophylactic (measure) — *see also* Encounter, prophylactic measures
  - organ removal Z40.00
    - breast Z40.01
    - ovary Z40.02
    - specified organ NEC Z40.09
    - testes Z40.09
  - vaccination Z23
- psychiatric examination (general) Z00.8
  - requested by authority Z04.6
- radiation therapy (antineoplastic) Z51.0
- reconstructive surgery following medical procedure or healed injury NEC Z42.8
- removal of
  - cystostomy catheter Z43.5
  - drains Z48.03
  - dressing (nonsurgical) Z48.00
  - intrauterine contraceptive device Z30.432

Admission (for) (*see also* Encounter (for)) — *continued*
- removal of — *continued*
  - implantable subdermal contraceptive Z30.46
  - neuropacemaker (brain) (peripheral nerve) (spinal cord) Z46.2
    - implanted Z45.42
  - staples Z48.02
  - surgical dressing Z48.01
  - sutures Z48.02
  - ureteral stent Z46.6
- respirator [ventilator] use during power failure Z99.12
- restoration of organ continuity (poststerilization) Z31.0
  - aftercare Z31.42
- sensitivity test — *see also* Test, skin
  - allergy NEC Z01.82
  - Mantoux Z11.1
- tuboplasty following previous sterilization Z31.0
  - aftercare Z31.42
- vasoplasty following previous sterilization Z31.0
  - aftercare Z31.42
- vision examination Z01.00
  - with abnormal findings Z01.01
- waiting period for admission to other facility Z75.1

Adnexitis (suppurative) — *see* Salpingo-oophoritis

Adolescent X-linked adrenoleukodystrophy E71.521

Adrenal (gland) — *see* condition

Adrenalism, tuberculous A18.7

Adrenalitis, adrenitis E27.8
- autoimmune E27.1
- meningococcal, hemorrhagic A39.1

Adrenarche, premature E27.0

Adrenocortical syndrome — *see* Cushing's, syndrome

Adrenogenital syndrome E25.9
- acquired E25.8
- congenital E25.0
- salt loss E25.0

Adrenogenitalism, congenital E25.0

Adrenoleukodystrophy E71.529
- neonatal E71.511
- X-linked E71.529
  - Addison only phenotype E71.528
  - Addison-Schilder E71.528
  - adolescent E71.521
  - adrenomyeloneuropathy E71.522
  - childhood cerebral E71.520
  - other specified E71.528

Adrenomyeloneuropathy E71.522

Adventitious bursa — *see* Bursopathy, specified type NEC

Adverse effect — *see* Table of Drugs and Chemicals, categories T36-T50, with 6th character 5

Advice — *see* Counseling

Adynamia (episodica) (hereditary) (periodic) G72.3

Aeration lung imperfect, newborn — *see* Atelectasis

Aero-otitis media T70.0

Aerobullosis T70.3

Aerocele — *see* Embolism, air

Aerodermectasia
- subcutaneous (traumatic) T79.7

Aerodontalgia T70.29

Aeroembolism T70.3

Aerogenes capsulatus infection A48.0

Aerophagy, aerophagia (psychogenic) F45.8

Aerophobia F40.228

Aerosinusitis T70.1

Aerotitis T70.0

Affection — *see* Disease
Afibrinogenemia (*see also* Defect,
    coagulation) D68.8
  acquired D65
  congenital D68.2
  following ectopic or molar pregnancy O08.1
  in abortion — *see* Abortion, by type,
    complicated by, afibrinogenemia
  puerperal O72.3
African
  sleeping sickness B56.9
  tick fever A68.1
  trypanosomiasis B56.9
    gambian B56.0
    rhodesian B56.1
Aftercare (*see also* Care) Z51.89
  following surgery (for) (on)
    amputation Z47.81
    attention to
      drains Z48.03
      dressings (nonsurgical) Z48.00
        surgical Z48.01
      sutures Z48.02
    circulatory system Z48.812
    delayed (planned) wound closure Z48.1
    digestive system Z48.815
    explantation of joint prosthesis (staged
      procedure)
      hip Z47.32
      knee Z47.33
      shoulder Z47.31
    genitourinary system Z48.816
    joint replacement Z47.1
    neoplasm Z48.3
    nervous system Z48.811
    oral cavity Z48.814
    organ transplant
      bone marrow Z48.290
      heart Z48.21
      heart-lung Z48.280
      kidney Z48.22
      liver Z48.23
      lung Z48.24
      multiple organs NEC Z48.288
      specified NEC Z48.298
    orthopedic NEC Z47.89
    planned wound closure Z48.1
    removal of internal fixation device Z47.2
    respiratory system Z48.813
    scoliosis Z47.82
    sense organs Z48.810
    skin and subcutaneous tissue Z48.817
    specified body system
      circulatory Z48.812
      digestive Z48.815
      genitourinary Z48.816
      nervous Z48.811
      oral cavity Z48.814
      respiratory Z48.813
      sense organs Z48.810
      skin and subcutaneous tissue Z48.817
      teeth Z48.814
    specified NEC Z48.89
    spinal Z48.89
    teeth Z48.814
  fracture — *code to* fracture with seventh
    character D
  involving
    removal of
      drains Z48.03
      dressings (nonsurgical) Z48.00
      staples Z48.02
      surgical dressings Z48.01
      sutures Z48.02
  neuropacemaker (brain) (peripheral nerve)
    (spinal cord) Z46.2
    implanted Z45.42
  orthopedic NEC Z47.89

Aftercare (*see also* Care) Z51.89 — *continued*
  postprocedural — *see* Aftercare, following
    surgery
After-cataract — *see* Cataract, secondary
Agalactia (primary) O92.3
  elective, secondary or therapeutic O92.5
Agammaglobulinemia (acquired
  (secondary)) (nonfamilial) D80.1
  with
    immunoglobulin-bearing B-lymphocytes
      D80.1
    lymphopenia D81.9
  autosomal recessive (Swiss type) D80.0
  Bruton's X-linked D80.0
  common variable (CVAgamma) D80.1
  congenital sex-linked D80.0
  hereditary D80.0
  lymphopenic D81.9
  Swiss type (autosomal recessive) D80.0
  X-linked (with growth hormone deficiency)
    (Bruton) D80.0
Aganglionosis (bowel) (colon) Q43.1
Age (old) — *see* Senility
Agenesis
  adrenal (gland) Q89.1
  alimentary tract (complete) (partial) NEC
    Q45.8
    upper Q40.8
  anus, anal (canal) Q42.3
    with fistula Q42.2
  aorta Q25.41
  appendix Q42.8
  arm (complete) Q71.0-
    with hand present Q71.1-
  artery (peripheral) Q27.9
    brain Q28.3
    coronary Q24.5
    pulmonary Q25.79
    specified NEC Q27.8
    umbilical Q27.0
  auditory (canal) (external) Q16.1
  auricle (ear) Q16.0
  bile duct or passage Q44.5
  bladder Q64.5
  bone Q79.9
  brain Q00.0
    part of Q04.3
  breast (with nipple present) Q83.8
    with absent nipple Q83.0
  bronchus Q32.4
  canaliculus lacrimalis Q10.4
  carpus — *see* Agenesis, hand
  cartilage Q79.9
  cecum Q42.8
  cerebellum Q04.3
  cervix Q51.5
  chin Q18.8
  cilia Q10.3
  circulatory system, part NOS Q28.9
  clavicle Q74.0
  clitoris Q52.6
  coccyx Q76.49
  colon Q42.9
    specified NEC Q42.8
  corpus callosum Q04.0
  cricoid cartilage Q31.8
  diaphragm (with hernia) Q79.1
  digestive organ(s) or tract (complete) (partial)
    NEC Q45.8
    upper Q40.8
  ductus arteriosus Q28.8
  duodenum Q41.0
  ear Q16.9
    auricle Q16.0
    lobe Q17.8
  ejaculatory duct Q55.4
  endocrine (gland) NEC Q89.2
  epiglottis Q31.8

Agenesis — *continued*
  esophagus Q39.8
  eustachian tube Q16.2
  eye Q11.1
    adnexa Q15.8
  eyelid (fold) Q10.3
  face
    bones NEC Q75.8
    specified part NEC Q18.8
  fallopian tube Q50.6
  femur — *see* Defect, reduction, lower limb,
    longitudinal, femur
  fibula — *see* Defect, reduction, lower limb,
    longitudinal, fibula
  finger (complete) (partial) — *see* Agenesis,
    hand
  foot (and toes) (complete) (partial) Q72.3-
  forearm (with hand present) — *see* Agenesis,
    arm, with hand present
    and hand Q71.2-
  gallbladder Q44.0
  gastric Q40.2
  genitalia, genital (organ(s))
    female Q52.8
      external Q52.71
      internal NEC Q52.8
    male Q55.8
  glottis Q31.8
  hair Q84.0
  hand (and fingers) (complete) (partial) Q71.3-
  heart Q24.8
    valve NEC Q24.8
      pulmonary Q22.0
  hepatic Q44.7
  humerus — *see* Defect, reduction, upper limb
  hymen Q52.4
  ileum Q41.2
  incus Q16.3
  intestine (small) Q41.9
    large Q42.9
      specified NEC Q42.8
  iris (dilator fibers) Q13.1
  jaw M26.09
  jejunum Q41.1
  kidney(s) (partial) Q60.2
    bilateral Q60.1
    unilateral Q60.0
  labium (majus) (minus) Q52.71
  labyrinth, membranous Q16.5
  lacrimal apparatus Q10.4
  larynx Q31.8
  leg (complete) Q72.0-
    with foot present Q72.1-
    lower leg (with foot present) — *see* Agenesis,
      leg, with foot present
      and foot Q72.2-
  lens Q12.3
  limb (complete) Q73.0
    lower — *see* Agenesis, leg
    upper — *see* Agenesis, arm
  lip Q38.0
  liver Q44.7
  lung (fissure) (lobe) (bilateral) (unilateral)
    Q33.3
  mandible, maxilla M26.09
  metacarpus — *see* Agenesis, hand
  metatarsus — *see* Agenesis, foot
  muscle Q79.8
    eyelid Q10.3
    ocular Q15.8
  musculoskeletal system NEC Q79.8
  nail(s) Q84.3
  neck, part Q18.8
  nerve Q07.8
  nervous system, part NEC Q07.8
  nipple Q83.2
  nose Q30.1
  nuclear Q07.8

Agenesis — *continued*
  organ
    of Corti Q16.5
    or site not listed — *see* Anomaly, by site
  osseous meatus (ear) Q16.1
  ovary
    bilateral Q50.02
    unilateral Q50.01
  oviduct Q50.6
  pancreas Q45.0
  parathyroid (gland) Q89.2
  parotid gland(s) Q38.4
  patella Q74.1
  pelvic girdle (complete) (partial) Q74.2
  penis Q55.5
  pericardium Q24.8
  pituitary (gland) Q89.2
  prostate Q55.4
  punctum lacrimale Q10.4
  radioulnar — *see* Defect, reduction, upper limb
  radius — *see* Defect, reduction, upper limb,
      longitudinal, radius
  rectum Q42.1
    with fistula Q42.0
  renal Q60.2
    bilateral Q60.1
    unilateral Q60.0
  respiratory organ NEC Q34.8
  rib Q76.6
  roof of orbit Q75.8
  round ligament Q52.8
  sacrum Q76.49
  salivary gland Q38.4
  scapula Q74.0
  scrotum Q55.29
  seminal vesicles Q55.4
  septum
    atrial Q21.1
    between aorta and pulmonary artery Q21.4
    ventricular Q20.4
  shoulder girdle (complete) (partial) Q74.0
  skull (bone) Q75.8
    with
      anencephaly Q00.0
      encephalocele — *see* Encephalocele
      hydrocephalus Q03.9
        with spina bifida — *see* Spina bifida, by
            site, with hydrocephalus
      microcephaly Q02
  spermatic cord Q55.4
  spinal cord Q06.0
  spine Q76.49
  spleen Q89.01
  sternum Q76.7
  stomach Q40.2
  submaxillary gland(s) (congenital) Q38.4
  tarsus — *see* Agenesis, foot
  tendon Q79.8
  testicle Q55.0
  thymus (gland) Q89.2
  thyroid (gland) E03.1
    cartilage Q31.8
  tibia — *see* Defect, reduction, lower limb,
      longitudinal, tibia
  tibiofibular — *see* Defect, reduction, lower
      limb, specified type NEC
  toe (and foot) (complete) (partial) — *see*
      Agenesis, foot
  tongue Q38.3
  trachea (cartilage) Q32.1
  ulna — *see* Defect, reduction, upper limb,
      longitudinal, ulna
  upper limb — *see* Agenesis, arm
  ureter Q62.4
  urethra Q64.5
  urinary tract NEC Q64.8
  uterus Q51.0
  uvula Q38.5
  vagina Q52.0

Agenesis — *continued*
  vas deferens Q55.4
  vein(s) (peripheral) Q27.9
    brain Q28.3
    great NEC Q26.8
    portal Q26.5
  vena cava (inferior) (superior) Q26.8
  vermis of cerebellum Q04.3
  vertebra Q76.49
  vulva Q52.71
Ageusia R43.2
Agitated — *see* condition
Agitation R45.1
Aglossia (congenital) Q38.3
Aglossia-adactylia syndrome Q87.0
Aglycogenosis E74.00
Agnosia (body image) (other senses) (tactile)
    R48.1
  developmental F88
  verbal R48.1
    auditory R48.1
      developmental F80.2
    developmental F80.2
  visual (object) R48.3
Agoraphobia F40.00
  with panic disorder F40.01
  without panic disorder F40.02
Agrammatism R48.8
Agranulocytopenia — *see* Agranulocytosis
Agranulocytosis (chronic) (cyclical) (genetic)
    (infantile) (periodic) (pernicious) (*see also*
    Neutropenia) D70.9
  congenital D70.0
  cytoreductive cancer chemotherapy sequela
    D70.1
  drug-induced D70.2
    due to cytoreductive cancer chemotherapy
        D70.1
  due to infection D70.3
  secondary D70.4
    drug-induced D70.2
      due to cytoreductive cancer chemotherapy
          D70.1
Agraphia (absolute) R48.8
  with alexia R48.0
  developmental F81.81
Ague (dumb) — *see* Malaria
Agyria Q04.3
Ahumada-del Castillo syndrome E23.0
Aichomophobia F40.298
AIDS (related complex) B20
Ailment, heart — *see* Disease, heart
Ailurophobia F40.218
AIN — *see* Neoplasia, intraepithelial, anal
Ainhum (disease) L94.6
AIPHI (acute idiopathic pulmonary hemorrhage
    in infants (over 28 days old)) R04.81
Air
  anterior mediastinum J98.2
  compressed, disease T70.3
  conditioner lung or pneumonitis J67.7
  embolism (artery) (cerebral) (any site) T79.0
    with ectopic or molar pregnancy O08.2
    due to implanted device NEC — *see*
        Complications, by site and type,
        specified NEC
    following
      abortion — *see* Abortion by type,
          complicated by, embolism
      ectopic or molar pregnancy O08.2
    infusion, therapeutic injection or
        transfusion T80.0
    in pregnancy, childbirth or puerperium —
        see Embolism, obstetric
    traumatic T79.0
  hunger, psychogenic F45.8
  rarefied, effects of — *see* Effect, adverse, high
      altitude
  sickness T75.3

Airplane sickness T75.3
Akathisia (drug-induced) (treatment-induced)
    G25.71
  neuroleptic induced (acute) G25.71
Akinesia R29.898
Akinetic mutism R41.89
Akureyri's disease G93.3
Alactasia, congenital E73.0
Alagille's syndrome Q44.7
Alastrim B03
Albers-Schönberg syndrome Q78.2
Albert's syndrome — *see* Tendinitis, Achilles
Albinism, albino E70.30
  with hematologic abnormality E70.339
    Chédiak-Higashi syndrome E70.330
    Hermansky-Pudlak syndrome E70.331
    other specified E70.338
  I E70.320
  II E70.321
  ocular E70.319
    autosomal recessive E70.311
    other specified E70.318
    X-linked E70.310
  oculocutaneous E70.329
    other specified E70.328
    tyrosinase (ty) negative E70.320
    tyrosinase (ty) positive E70.321
  other specified E70.39
Albinismus E70.30
**Albright(-McCune)(-Sternberg)
    syndrome** Q78.1
Albuminous — *see* condition
Albuminuria, albuminuric (acute) (chronic)
    (subacute) (*see also* Proteinuria) R80.9
  complicating pregnancy — *see* Proteinuria,
      gestational
  with
    gestational hypertension — *see* Pre-
        eclampsia
    pre-existing hypertension — *see*
        Hypertension, complicating
        pregnancy, pre-existing, with, pre-
        eclampsia
  gestational — *see* Proteinuria, gestational
  with
    gestational hypertension — *see* Pre-
        eclampsia
    pre-existing hypertension — *see*
        Hypertension, complicating
        pregnancy, pre-existing, with, pre-
        eclampsia
  orthostatic R80.2
  postural R80.2
  pre-eclamptic — *see* Pre-eclampsia
  scarlatinal A38.8
Albuminurophobia F40.298
Alcaptonuria E70.29
Alcohol, alcoholic, alcohol-induced
  addiction (without remission) F10.20
    with remission F10.21
  amnestic disorder, persisting F10.96
    with dependence F10.26
  anxiety disorder F10.980
  bipolar and related disorder F10.94
  brain syndrome, chronic F10.97
    with dependence F10.27
  cardiopathy I42.6
  counseling and surveillance Z71.41
    family member Z71.42
  delirium (acute) (tremens) (withdrawal)
      F10.231
    with intoxication F10.921
    in
      abuse F10.121
      dependence F10.221
  dementia F10.97
    with dependence F10.27
  depressive disorder F10.94

Alcohol, alcoholic, alcohol-induced — *continued*
deterioration F10.97
   with dependence F10.27
hallucinosis (acute) F10.951
   in
      abuse F10.151
      dependence F10.251
insanity F10.959
intoxication (acute) (without dependence) F10.129
   with
      delirium F10.121
      dependence F10.229
         with delirium F10.221
         uncomplicated F10.220
      uncomplicated F10.120
jealousy F10.988
Korsakoff's, Korsakov's, Korsakow's F10.26
liver K70.9
   acute — *see* Disease, liver, alcoholic, hepatitis
major neurocognitive disorder, amnestic-confabulatory type F10.96
major neurocognitive disorder, nonamnestic-confabulatory type F10.97
mania (acute) (chronic) F10.959
mild neurocognitive disorder F10.988
paranoia, paranoid (type) psychosis F10.950
pellagra E52
poisoning, accidental (acute) NEC — *see* Table of Drugs and Chemicals, alcohol, poisoning
psychosis — *see* Psychosis, alcoholic
psychotic disorder F10.959
sexual dysfunction F10.981
sleep disorder F10.982
withdrawal (without convulsions) F10.239
   with delirium F10.231
Alcoholism (chronic) (without remission) F10.20
   with
      psychosis — *see* Psychosis, alcoholic
      remission F10.21
   Korsakov's F10.96
      with dependence F10.26
Alder (-Reilly) anomaly or syndrome (leukocyte granulation) D72.0
Aldosteronism E26.9
familial (type I) E26.02
glucocorticoid-remediable E26.02
primary (due to (bilateral) adrenal hyperplasia) E26.09
primary NEC E26.09
secondary E26.1
specified NEC E26.89
Aldosteronoma D44.10
Aldrich(-Wiskott) syndrome (eczema-thrombocytopenia) D82.0
Alektorophobia F40.218
Aleppo boil B55.1
Aleukemic — *see* condition
Aleukia
congenital D70.0
hemorrhagica D61.9
   congenital D61.09
splenica D73.1
Alexia R48.0
developmental F81.0
secondary to organic lesion R48.0
Algoneurodystrophy M89.00
ankle M89.07-
foot M89.07-
forearm M89.03-
hand M89.04-
lower leg M89.06-
multiple sites M89.0-
shoulder M89.01-
specified site NEC M89.08

Algoneurodystrophy M89.00 — *continued*
thigh M89.05-
upper arm M89.02-
Algophobia F40.298
Alienation, mental — *see* Psychosis
Alkalemia E87.3
Alkalosis E87.3
metabolic E87.3
   with respiratory acidosis E87.4
respiratory E87.3
Alkaptonuria E70.29
Allen-Masters syndrome N83.8
Allergy, allergic (reaction) (to) T78.40
air-borne substance NEC (rhinitis) J30.89
alveolitis (extrinsic) J67.9
   due to
      Aspergillus clavatus J67.4
      Cryptostroma corticale J67.6
      organisms (fungal, thermophilic actinomycete) growing in ventilation (air conditioning) systems J67.7
   specified type NEC J67.8
anaphylactic reaction or shock T78.2
angioneurotic edema T78.3
animal (dander) (epidermal) (hair) (rhinitis) J30.81
bee sting (anaphylactic shock) — *see* Toxicity, venom, arthropod, bee
biological — *see* Allergy, drug
colitis (*see also* Colitis, allergic) K52.2
dander (animal) (rhinitis) J30.81
dandruff (rhinitis) J30.81
dental restorative material (existing) K08.55
dermatitis — *see* Dermatitis, contact, allergic
diathesis — *see* History, allergy
drug, medicament & biological (any) (external) (internal) T78.40
   correct substance properly administered — *see* Table of Drugs and Chemicals, by drug, adverse effect
   wrong substance given or taken NEC (by accident) — *see* Table of Drugs and Chemicals, by drug, poisoning
due to pollen J30.1
dust (house) (stock) (rhinitis) J30.89
   with asthma — *see* Asthma, allergic extrinsic
eczema — *see* Dermatitis, contact, allergic
epidermal (animal) (rhinitis) J30.81
feathers (rhinitis) J30.89
food (any) (ingested) NEC T78.1
   anaphylactic shock — *see* Shock, anaphylactic, due to food
   dermatitis — *see* Dermatitis, due to, food
   dietary counseling and surveillance Z71.3
   in contact with skin L23.6
   rhinitis J30.5
   status (without reaction) Z91.018
      eggs Z91.012
      milk products Z91.011
      peanuts Z91.010
      seafood Z91.013
      specified NEC Z91.018
gastrointestinal — *see also* specific type of allergic reaction
   meaning colitis (*see also* Colitis, allergic) K52.29
   meaning gastroenteritis (*see also* Gastroenteritis, allergic) K52.29
   meaning other adverse food reaction not elsewhere classified T78.1
grain J30.1
grass (hay fever) (pollen) J30.1
   asthma — *see* Asthma, allergic extrinsic
hair (animal) (rhinitis) J30.81
history (of) — *see* History, allergy
horse serum — *see* Allergy, serum
inhalant (rhinitis) J30.89
   pollen J30.1
kapok (rhinitis) J30.89

Allergy, allergic (reaction) (to) T78.40 — *continued*
medicine — *see* Allergy, drug
milk protein (*see also* Allergy, food) Z91.011
   anaphylactic reaction T78.07
   dermatitis L27.2
   enterocolitis syndrome K52.21
   enteropathy K52.22
   gastroenteritis K52.29
   gastroesophageal reflux (*see also* Reaction, adverse, food) K21.9
      with esophagitis K21.0
   proctocolitis K52.82
nasal, seasonal due to pollen J30.1
pneumonia J82
pollen (any) (hay fever) J30.1
   asthma — *see* Asthma, allergic extrinsic
primrose J30.1
primula J30.1
proctocolitis K52.82
purpura D69.0
ragweed (hay fever) (pollen) J30.1
   asthma — *see* Asthma, allergic extrinsic
rose (pollen) J30.1
seasonal NEC J30.2
Senecio jacobae (pollen) J30.1
serum (*see also* Reaction, serum) T80.69
   anaphylactic shock T80.59
shock (anaphylactic) T78.2
   due to
      adverse effect of correct medicinal substance properly administered T88.6
      administration of blood and blood products T80.51
      immunization T80.52
      serum NEC T80.59
      vaccination T80.52
specific NEC T78.49
tree (any) (hay fever) (pollen) J30.1
   asthma — *see* Asthma, allergic extrinsic
upper respiratory J30.9
urticaria L50.0
vaccine — *see* Allergy, serum
wheat — *see* Allergy, food
Allescheriasis B48.2
Alligator skin disease Q80.9
Allocheiria, allochiria R20.8
Almeida's disease — *see* Paracoccidioidomycosis
Alopecia (hereditaria) (seborrheica) L65.9
androgenic L64.9
   drug-induced L64.0
   specified NEC L64.8
areata L63.9
   ophiasis L63.2
   specified NEC L63.8
   totalis L63.0
   universalis L63.1
cicatricial L66.9
   specified NEC L66.8
circumscripta L63.9
congenital, congenitalis Q84.0
due to cytotoxic drugs NEC L65.8
mucinosa L65.2
postinfective NEC L65.8
postpartum L65.0
premature L64.8
specific (syphilitic) A51.32
specified NEC L65.8
syphilitic (secondary) A51.32
totalis (capitis) L63.0
universalis (entire body) L63.1
X-ray L58.1
Alpers' disease G31.81
Alpine sickness T70.29
Alport syndrome Q87.81
ALTE (apparent life threatening event) in newborn and infant R68.13

Alteration (of), Altered
awareness
transient R40.4
unintended under general anesthesia, during procedure T88.53
mental status R41.82
pattern of family relationships affecting child Z62.898
sensation
following
cerebrovascular disease I69.998
cerebral infarction I69.398
intracerebral hemorrhage I69.198
nontraumatic intracranial hemorrhage NEC I69.298
specified disease NEC I69.898
subarachnoid hemorrhage I69.098
Alternating — see condition
Altitude, high (effects) — see Effect, adverse, high altitude
Aluminosis (of lung) J63.0
Alveolitis
allergic (extrinsic) — see Pneumonitis, hypersensitivity
due to
Aspergillus clavatus J67.4
Cryptostroma corticale J67.6
fibrosing (cryptogenic) (idiopathic) J84.112
jaw M27.3
sicca dolorosa M27.3
Alveolus, alveolar — see condition
Alymphocytosis D72.810
thymic (with immunodeficiency) D82.1
Alymphoplasia, thymic D82.1
Alzheimer's disease or sclerosis — see Disease, Alzheimer's
Amastia (with nipple present) Q83.8
with absent nipple Q83.0
Amathophobia F40.228
Amaurosis (acquired) (congenital) — see also Blindness
fugax G45.3
hysterical F44.6
Leber's congenital H35.50
uremic — see Uremia
Amaurotic idiocy (infantile) (juvenile) (late) E75.4
Amaxophobia F40.248
Ambiguous genitalia Q56.4
Amblyopia (congenital) (ex anopsia) (partial) (suppression) H53.00-
anisometropic — see Amblyopia, refractive
deprivation H53.01-
hysterical F44.6
nocturnal — see also Blindness, night
vitamin A deficiency E50.5
refractive H53.02-
strabismic H53.03-
suspect H53.04-
tobacco H53.8
toxic NEC H53.8
uremic — see Uremia
Ameba, amebic (histolytica) — see also Amebiasis
abscess (liver) A06.4
Amebiasis A06.9
with abscess — see Abscess, amebic
acute A06.0
chronic (intestine) A06.1
with abscess — see Abscess, amebic
cutaneous A06.7
cutis A06.7
cystitis A06.81
genitourinary tract NEC A06.82
hepatic — see Abscess, liver, amebic
intestine A06.0
nondysenteric colitis A06.2
skin A06.7
specified site NEC A06.89

Ameboma (of intestine) A06.3
Amelia Q73.0
lower limb — see Agenesis, leg
upper limb — see Agenesis, arm
Ameloblastoma — see also Cyst, calcifying odontogenic
long bones C40.9-
lower limb C40.2-
upper limb C40.0-
malignant C41.1
jaw (bone) (lower) C41.1
upper C41.0
tibial C40.2-
Amelogenesis imperfecta K00.5
nonhereditaria (segmentalis) K00.4
Amenorrhea N91.2
hyperhormonal E28.8
primary N91.0
secondary N91.1
Amentia — see Disability, intellectual
Meynert's (nonalcoholic) F04
American
leishmaniasis B55.2
mountain tick fever A93.2
Ametropia — see Disorder, refraction
AMH (asymptomatic microscopic hematuria) R31.21
Amianthosis J61
Amimia R48.8
Amino-acid disorder E72.9
anemia D53.0
Aminoacidopathy E72.9
Aminoaciduria E72.9
Amnesia R41.3
anterograde R41.1
auditory R48.8
dissociative F44.0
with dissociative fugue F44.1
hysterical F44.0
postictal in epilepsy — see Epilepsy
psychogenic F44.0
retrograde R41.2
transient global G45.4
Amnes(t)ic syndrome (post-traumatic) F04
induced by
alcohol F10.96
with dependence F10.26
psychoactive NEC F19.96
with
abuse F19.16
dependence F19.26
sedative F13.96
with dependence F13.26
Amnion, amniotic — see condition
Amnionitis — see Pregnancy, complicated by
Amok F68.8
Amoral traits F60.89
Amphetamine (or other stimulant) -induced
anxiety disorder F15.980
bipolar and related disorder F15.94
delirium F15.921
depressive disorder F15.94
obsessive-compulsive and related disorder F15.988
psychotic disorder F15.959
sexual dysfunction F15.981
sleep disorder F15.982
stimulant withdrawal F15.23
Ampulla
lower esophagus K22.8
phrenic K22.8
Amputation — see also Absence, by site, acquired
neuroma (postoperative) (traumatic) — see Complications, amputation stump, neuroma

Amputation (see also Absence, by site, acquired) — continued
stump (surgical)
abnormal, painful, or with complication (late) — see Complications, amputation stump
healed or old NOS Z89.9
traumatic (complete) (partial)
arm (upper) (complete) S48.91-
at
elbow S58.01-
partial S58.02-
shoulder joint (complete) S48.01-
partial S48.02-
between
elbow and wrist (complete) S58.11-
partial S58.12-
shoulder and elbow (complete) S48.11-
partial S48.12-
partial S48.92-
breast (complete) S28.21-
partial S28.22-
clitoris (complete) S38.211
partial S38.212
ear (complete) S08.11-
partial S08.12-
finger (complete) (metacarpophalangeal) S68.11-
index S68.11-
little S68.11-
middle S68.11-
partial S68.12-
index S68.12-
little S68.12-
middle S68.12-
ring S68.12-
ring S68.11-
thumb — see Amputation, traumatic, thumb
transphalangeal (complete) S68.61-
index S68.61-
little S68.61-
middle S68.61-
partial S68.62-
index S68.62-
little S68.62-
middle S68.62-
ring S68.62-
ring S68.61-
foot (complete) S98.91-
at ankle level S98.01-
partial S98.02-
midfoot S98.31-
partial S98.32-
partial S98.92-
forearm (complete) S58.91-
at elbow level (complete) S58.01-
partial S58.02-
between elbow and wrist (complete) S58.11-
partial S58.12-
partial S58.92-
genital organ(s) (external)
female (complete) S38.211
partial S38.212
male
penis (complete) S38.221
partial S38.222
scrotum (complete) S38.231
partial S38.232
testes (complete) S38.231
partial S38.232
hand (complete) (wrist level) S68.41-
finger(s) alone — see Amputation, traumatic, finger
partial S68.42-
thumb alone — see Amputation, traumatic, thumb
transmetacarpal (complete) S68.71-
partial S68.72-

DISEASE INDEX

Amputation (*see also* Absence, by site, acquired) — *continued*
  traumatic (complete) (partial) — *continued*
    head
      ear — *see* Amputation, traumatic, ear
      nose (partial) S08.812
        complete S08.811
        part S08.89
        scalp S08.0
    hip (and thigh) (complete) S78.91-
      at hip joint (complete) S78.01-
        partial S78.02-
      between hip and knee (complete) S78.11-
        partial S78.12-
      partial S78.92-
    labium (majus) (minus) (complete) S38.21-
      partial S38.21-
    leg (lower) S88.91-
      at knee level S88.01-
        partial S88.02-
      between knee and ankle S88.11-
        partial S88.12-
      partial S88.92-
    nose (partial) S08.812
      complete S08.811
    penis (complete) S38.221
      partial S38.222
    scrotum (complete) S38.231
      partial S38.232
    shoulder — *see* Amputation, traumatic, arm
      at shoulder joint — *see* Amputation, traumatic, arm, at shoulder joint
    testes (complete) S38.231
      partial S38.232
    thigh — *see* Amputation, traumatic, hip
    thorax, part of S28.1
      breast — *see* Amputation, traumatic, breast
    thumb (complete) (metacarpophalangeal) S68.01-
      partial S68.02-
      transphalangeal (complete) S68.51-
        partial S68.52-
    toe (lesser) S98.13-
      great S98.11-
        partial S98.12-
      more than one S98.21-
        partial S98.22-
      partial S98.14-
    vulva (complete) S38.211
      partial S38.212
Amputee (bilateral) (old) Z89.9
Amsterdam dwarfism Q87.1
Amusia R48.8
  developmental F80.89
Amyelencephalus, amyelencephaly Q00.0
Amyelia Q06.0
Amygdalitis — *see* Tonsillitis
Amygdalolith J35.8
Amyloid heart (disease) E85.4 *[I43]*
Amyloidosis (generalized) (primary) E85.9
  with lung involvement E85.4 *[J99]*
  familial E85.2
  genetic E85.2
  heart E85.4 *[I43]*
  hemodialysis-associated E85.3
  liver E85.4 *[K77]*
  localized E85.4
  neuropathic heredofamilial E85.1
  non-neuropathic heredofamilial E85.0
  organ limited E85.4
  Portuguese E85.1
  pulmonary E85.4 *[J99]*
  secondary systemic E85.3
  skin (lichen) (macular) E85.4 *[L99]*
  specified NEC E85.8
  subglottic E85.4 *[J99]*

Amylopectinosis (brancher enzyme deficiency) E74.03
Amylophagia — *see* Pica
Amyoplasia congenita Q79.8
Amyotonia M62.89
  congenita G70.2
Amyotrophia, amyotrophy, amyotrophic G71.8
  congenita Q79.8
  diabetic — *see* Diabetes, amyotrophy
  lateral sclerosis G12.21
  neuralgic G54.5
  spinal progressive G12.21
Anacidity, gastric K31.83
  psychogenic F45.8
Anaerosis of newborn P28.89
Analbuminemia E88.09
Analgesia — *see* Anesthesia
Analphalipoproteinemia E78.6
Anaphylactic
  purpura D69.0
  shock or reaction — *see* Shock, anaphylactic
Anaphylactoid shock or reaction — *see* Shock, anaphylactic
Anaphylactoid syndrome of pregnancy O88.01-
Anaphylaxis — *see* Shock, anaphylactic
Anaplasia cervix (*see also* Dysplasia, cervix) N87.9
Anaplasmosis, human A77.49
Anarthria R47.1
Anasarca R60.1
  cardiac — *see* Failure, heart, congestive
  lung J18.2
  newborn P83.2
  nutritional E43
  pulmonary J18.2
  renal N04.9
Anastomosis
  aneurysmal — *see* Aneurysm
  arteriovenous ruptured brain I60.8
  intestinal K63.89
    complicated NEC K91.89
      involving urinary tract N99.89
  retinal and choroidal vessels (congenital) Q14.8
Anatomical narrow angle H40.03-
Ancylostoma, ancylostomiasis (braziliense) (caninum) (ceylanicum) (duodenale) B76.0
  Necator americanus B76.1
Andersen's disease (glycogen storage) E74.09
Anderson-Fabry disease E75.21
Andes disease T70.29
Andrews' disease (bacterid) L08.89
Androblastoma
  benign
    specified site — *see* Neoplasm, benign, by site
    unspecified site
      female D27.9
      male D29.20
  malignant
    specified site — *see* Neoplasm, malignant, by site
    unspecified site
      female C56.9
      male C62.90
  specified site — *see* Neoplasm, uncertain behavior, by site
  tubular
    with lipid storage
      specified site — *see* Neoplasm, benign, by site
      unspecified site
        female D27.9
        male D29.20

Androblastoma — *continued*
  tubular — *continued*
    specified site — *see* Neoplasm, benign, by site
    unspecified site
      female D27.9
      male D29.20
  unspecified site
    female D39.10
    male D40.10
Androgen insensitivity syndrome (*see also* Syndrome, androgen insensitivity) E34.50
Androgen resistance syndrome (*see also* Syndrome, androgen insensitivity) E34.50
Android pelvis Q74.2
  with disproportion (fetopelvic) O33.3
    causing obstructed labor O65.3
Androphobia F40.290
Anectasis, pulmonary (newborn) — *see* Atelectasis
Anemia (essential) (general) (hemoglobin deficiency) (infantile) (primary) (profound) D64.9
  with (due to) (in)
    disorder of
      anaerobic glycolysis D55.2
      pentose phosphate pathway D55.1
    koilonychia D50.9
  achlorhydric D50.8
  achrestic D53.1
  Addison(-Biermer) (pernicious) D51.0
  agranulocytic — *see* Agranulocytosis
  amino-acid-deficiency D53.0
  aplastic D61.9
    congenital D61.09
    drug-induced D61.1
    due to
      drugs D61.1
      external agents NEC D61.2
      infection D61.2
      radiation D61.2
    idiopathic D61.3
    red cell (pure) D60.9
      chronic D60.0
      congenital D61.01
      specified type NEC D60.8
      transient D60.1
    specified type NEC D61.89
    toxic D61.2
  aregenerative
    congenital D61.09
  asiderotic D50.9
  atypical (primary) D64.9
  Baghdad spring D55.0
  Balantidium coli A07.0
  Biermer's (pernicious) D51.0
  blood loss (chronic) D50.0
    acute D62
  bothriocephalus B70.0 *[D63.8]*
  brickmaker's B76.9 *[D63.8]*
  cerebral I67.89
  childhood D58.9
  chlorotic D50.8
  chronic
    blood loss D50.0
    hemolytic D58.9
      idiopathic D59.9
    simple D53.9
  chronica congenita aregenerativa D61.09
  combined system disease NEC D51.0 *[G32.0]*
    due to dietary vitamin B12 deficiency D51.3 *[G32.0]*
  complicating pregnancy, childbirth or puerperium — *see* Pregnancy, complicated by (management affected by), anemia
  congenital P61.4
    aplastic D61.09
    due to isoimmunization NOS P55.9
    dyserythropoietic, dyshematopoietic D64.4

DISEASE INDEX

Anemia (essential) (general) (hemoglobin deficiency) (infantile) (primary) (profound) D64.9 — *continued*
congenital P61.4 — *continued*
  following fetal blood loss P61.3
  Heinz body D58.2
  hereditary hemolytic NOS D58.9
  pernicious D51.0
  spherocytic D58.0
Cooley's (erythroblastic) D56.1
cytogenic D51.0
deficiency D53.9
  2, 3 diphosphoglycurate mutase D55.2
  2, 3 PG D55.2
  6 phosphogluconate dehydrogenase D55.1
  6-PGD D55.1
  amino-acid D53.0
  combined B12 and folate D53.1
  enzyme D55.9
    drug-induced (hemolytic) D59.2
    glucose-6-phosphate dehydrogenase (G6PD) D55.0
    glycolytic D55.2
    nucleotide metabolism D55.3
    related to hexose monophosphate (HMP) shunt pathway NEC D55.1
    specified type NEC D55.8
  erythrocytic glutathione D55.1
  folate D52.9
    dietary D52.0
    drug-induced D52.1
  folic acid D52.9
    dietary D52.0
    drug-induced D52.1
  G SH D55.1
  G6PD D55.0
  GGS-R D55.1
  glucose-6-phosphate dehydrogenase D55.0
  glutathione reductase D55.1
  glyceraldehyde phosphate dehydrogenase D55.2
  hexokinase D55.2
  iron D50.9
    secondary to blood loss (chronic) D50.0
  nutritional D53.9
    with
      poor iron absorption D50.8
      specified deficiency NEC D53.8
  phosphofructo-aldolase D55.2
  phosphoglycerate kinase D55.2
  PK D55.2
  protein D53.0
  pyruvate kinase D55.2
  transcobalamin II D51.2
  triose-phosphate isomerase D55.2
  vitamin B12 NOS D51.9
    dietary D51.3
    due to
      intrinsic factor deficiency D51.0
      selective vitamin B12 malabsorption with proteinuria D51.1
    pernicious D51.0
    specified type NEC D51.8
Diamond-Blackfan (congenital hypoplastic) D61.01
dibothriocephalus B70.0 *[D63.8]*
dimorphic D53.1
diphasic D53.1
Diphyllobothrium (Dibothriocephalus) B70.0 *[D63.8]*
due to (in) (with)
  antineoplastic chemotherapy D64.81
  blood loss (chronic) D50.0
    acute D62
  chemotherapy, antineoplastic D64.81
  chronic disease classified elsewhere NEC D63.8
  chronic kidney disease D63.1

Anemia (essential) (general) (hemoglobin deficiency) (infantile) (primary) (profound) D64.9 — *continued*
due to (in) (with) — *continued*
  deficiency
    amino-acid D53.0
    copper D53.8
    folate (folic acid) D52.9
      dietary D52.0
      drug-induced D52.1
    molybdenum D53.8
    protein D53.0
    zinc D53.8
  dietary vitamin B12 deficiency D51.3
  disorder of
    glutathione metabolism D55.1
    nucleotide metabolism D55.3
  drug — *see* Anemia, by type — *see also* Table of Drugs and Chemicals
  end stage renal disease D63.1
  enzyme disorder D55.9
  fetal blood loss P61.3
  fish tapeworm (D.latum) infestation B70.0 *[D63.8]*
  hemorrhage (chronic) D50.0
    acute D62
  impaired absorption D50.9
  loss of blood (chronic) D50.0
    acute D62
  myxedema E03.9 *[D63.8]*
  Necator americanus B76.1 *[D63.8]*
  prematurity P61.2
  selective vitamin B12 malabsorption with proteinuria D51.1
  transcobalamin II deficiency D51.2
Dyke-Young type (secondary) (symptomatic) D59.1
dyserythropoietic (congenital) D64.4
dyshematopoietic (congenital) D64.4
Egyptian B76.9 *[D63.8]*
elliptocytosis — *see* Elliptocytosis
enzyme-deficiency, drug-induced D59.2
epidemic (*see also* Ancylostomiasis) B76.9 *[D63.8]*
erythroblastic
  familial D56.1
  newborn (*see also* Disease, hemolytic) P55.9
  of childhood D56.1
erythrocytic glutathione deficiency D55.1
erythropoietin-resistant anemia (EPO resistant anemia) D63.1
Faber's (achlorhydric anemia) D50.9
factitious (self-induced blood letting) D50.0
familial erythroblastic D56.1
Fanconi's (congenital pancytopenia) D61.09
favism D55.0
fish tapeworm (D. latum) infestation B70.0 *[D63.8]*
folate (folic acid) deficiency D52.9
glucose-6-phosphate dehydrogenase (G6PD) deficiency D55.0
glutathione-reductase deficiency D55.1
goat's milk D52.0
granulocytic — *see* Agranulocytosis
Heinz body, congenital D58.2
hemolytic D58.9
  acquired D59.9
    with hemoglobinuria NEC D59.6
    autoimmune NEC D59.1
    infectious D59.4
    specified type NEC D59.8
    toxic D59.4
  acute D59.9
    due to enzyme deficiency specified type NEC D55.8
    Lederer's D59.1
  autoimmune D59.1
    drug-induced D59.0

Anemia (essential) (general) (hemoglobin deficiency) (infantile) (primary) (profound) D64.9 — *continued*
hemolytic D58.9 — *continued*
  chronic D58.9
    idiopathic D59.9
  cold type (secondary) (symptomatic) D59.1
  congenital (spherocytic) — *see* Spherocytosis
  due to
    cardiac conditions D59.4
    drugs (nonautoimmune) D59.2
      autoimmune D59.0
    enzyme disorder D55.9
      drug-induced D59.2
    presence of shunt or other internal prosthetic device D59.4
  familial D58.9
  hereditary D58.9
    due to enzyme disorder D55.9
      specified type NEC D55.8
    specified type NEC D58.8
  idiopathic (chronic) D59.9
  mechanical D59.4
  microangiopathic D59.4
  nonautoimmune D59.4
    drug-induced D59.2
  nonspherocytic
    congenital or hereditary NEC D55.8
      glucose-6-phosphate dehydrogenase deficiency D55.0
      pyruvate kinase deficiency D55.2
    type
      I D55.1
      II D55.2
  type
    I D55.1
    II D55.2
  secondary D59.4
    autoimmune D59.1
  specified (hereditary) type NEC D58.8
  Stransky-Regala type (*see also* Hemoglobinopathy) D58.8
  symptomatic D59.4
    autoimmune D59.1
  toxic D59.4
  warm type (secondary) (symptomatic) D59.1
hemorrhagic (chronic) D50.0
  acute D62
Herrick's D57.1
hexokinase deficiency D55.2
hookworm B76.9 *[D63.8]*
hypochromic (idiopathic) (microcytic) (normoblastic) D50.9
  due to blood loss (chronic) D50.0
    acute D62
  familial sex-linked D64.0
  pyridoxine-responsive D64.3
  sideroblastic, sex-linked D64.0
hypoplasia, red blood cells D61.9
  congenital or familial D61.01
hypoplastic (idiopathic) D61.9
  congenital or familial (of childhood) D61.01
hypoproliferative (refractive) D61.9
idiopathic D64.9
  aplastic D61.3
  hemolytic, chronic D59.9
in (due to) (with)
  chronic kidney disease D63.1
  end stage renal disease D63.1
  failure, kidney (renal) D63.1
  neoplastic disease (*see also* Neoplasm) D63.0
intertropical (*see also* Ancylostomiasis) D63.8
iron deficiency D50.9
  secondary to blood loss (chronic) D50.0
    acute D62
  specified type NEC D50.8
Joseph-Diamond-Blackfan (congenital hypoplastic) D61.01

DISEASE INDEX

Anemia (essential) (general) (hemoglobin deficiency) (infantile) (primary) (profound) D64.9 — *continued*
Lederer's (hemolytic) D59.1
leukoerythroblastic D61.82
macrocytic D53.9
    nutritional D52.0
    tropical D52.8
malarial (*see also* Malaria) B54 [*D63.8*]
malignant (progressive) D51.0
malnutrition D53.9
marsh (*see also* Malaria) B54 [*D63.8*]
Mediterranean (with other hemoglobinopathy) D56.9
megaloblastic D53.1
    combined B12 and folate deficiency D53.1
    hereditary D51.1
    nutritional D52.0
    orotic aciduria D53.0
    refractory D53.1
    specified type NEC D53.1
megalocytic D53.1
microcytic (hypochromic) D50.9
    due to blood loss (chronic) D50.0
        acute D62
    familial D56.8
microdrepanocytosis D57.40
microelliptopoikilocytic (Rietti-Greppi-Micheli) D56.9
miner's B76.9 [*D63.8*]
myelodysplastic D46.9
myelofibrosis D75.81
myelogenous D64.89
myelopathic D64.89
myelophthisic D61.82
myeloproliferative D47.Z9
newborn P61.4
    due to
        ABO (antibodies, isoimmunization, maternal/fetal incompatibility) P55.1
        Rh (antibodies, isoimmunization, maternal/fetal incompatibility) P55.0
    following fetal blood loss P61.3
    posthemorrhagic (fetal) P61.3
nonspherocytic hemolytic — *see* Anemia, hemolytic, nonspherocytic
normocytic (infectional) D64.9
    due to blood loss (chronic) D50.0
        acute D62
    myelophthisic D61.82
nutritional (deficiency) D53.9
    with
        poor iron absorption D50.8
        specified deficiency NEC D53.8
    megaloblastic D52.0
of prematurity P61.2
orotaciduric (congenital) (hereditary) D53.0
osteosclerotic D64.89
ovalocytosis (hereditary) — *see* Elliptocytosis
paludal (*see also* Malaria) B54 [*D63.8*]
pernicious (congenital) (malignant) (progressive) D51.0
pleochromic D64.89
    of sprue D52.8
posthemorrhagic (chronic) D50.0
    acute D62
    newborn P61.3
postoperative (postprocedural)
    due to (acute) blood loss D62
        chronic blood loss D50.0
    specified NEC D64.9
postpartum O90.81
pressure D64.89
progressive D64.9
    malignant D51.0
    pernicious D51.0
protein-deficiency D53.0
pseudoleukemica infantum D64.89

Anemia (essential) (general) (hemoglobin deficiency) (infantile) (primary) (profound) D64.9 — *continued*
pure red cell D60.9
    congenital D61.01
pyridoxine-responsive D64.3
pyruvate kinase deficiency D55.2
refractory D46.4
    with
        excess of blasts D46.20
            1 (RAEB 1) D46.21
            2 (RAEB 2) D46.22
            in transformation (RAEB T) — *see* Leukemia, acute myeloblastic
        hemochromatosis D46.1
        sideroblasts (ring) (RARS) D46.1
    megaloblastic D53.1
    sideroblastic D46.1
    sideropenic D50.9
    without ring sideroblasts, so stated D46.0
    without sideroblasts without excess of blasts D46.0
Rietti-Greppi-Micheli D56.9
scorbutic D53.2
secondary to
    blood loss (chronic) D50.0
        acute D62
    hemorrhage (chronic) D50.0
        acute D62
semiplastic D61.89
sickle-cell — *see* Disease, sickle-cell
sideroblastic D64.3
    hereditary D64.0
    hypochromic, sex-linked D64.0
    pyridoxine-responsive NEC D64.3
    refractory D46.1
    secondary (due to)
        disease D64.1
        drugs and toxins D64.2
    specified type NEC D64.3
sideropenic (refractory) D50.9
    due to blood loss (chronic) D50.0
        acute D62
simple chronic D53.9
specified type NEC D64.89
spherocytic (hereditary) — *see* Spherocytosis
splenic D64.89
splenomegalic D64.89
stomatocytosis D58.8
syphilitic (acquired) (late) A52.79 [*D63.8*]
target cell D64.89
thalassemia D56.9
thrombocytopenic — *see* Thrombocytopenia
toxic D61.2
tropical B76.9 [*D63.8*]
    macrocytic D52.8
tuberculous A18.89 [*D63.8*]
vegan D51.3
vitamin
    B12 deficiency (dietary) pernicious D51.0
    B6-responsive D64.3
von Jaksch's D64.89
Witts' (achlorhydric anemia) D50.8
Anemophobia F40.228
Anencephalus, anencephaly Q00.0
Anergasia — *see* Psychosis, organic
Anesthesia, anesthetic R20.0
complication or reaction NEC (*see also* Complications, anesthesia) T88.59
    due to
        correct substance properly administered — *see* Table of Drugs and Chemicals, by drug, adverse effect
        overdose or wrong substance given — *see* Table of Drugs and Chemicals, by drug, poisoning
    unintended awareness under general anesthesia during procedure T88.53
        personal history of Z92.84

Anesthesia, anesthetic R20.0 — *continued*
cornea H18.81-
dissociative F44.6
functional (hysterical) F44.6
hyperesthetic, thalamic G89.0
hysterical F44.6
local skin lesion R20.0
sexual (psychogenic) F52.1
shock (due to) T88.2
skin R20.0
testicular N50.9
Anetoderma (maculosum) (of) L90.8
Jadassohn-Pellizzari L90.2
Schweniger-Buzzi L90.1
Aneurin deficiency E51.9
Aneurysm (anastomotic) (artery) (cirsoid) (diffuse) (false) (fusiform) (multiple) (saccular) I72.9
abdominal (aorta) I71.4
    ruptured I71.3
    syphilitic A52.01
aorta, aortic (nonsyphilitic) I71.9
    abdominal I71.4
        ruptured I71.3
    arch I71.2
        ruptured I71.1
    arteriosclerotic I71.9
        ruptured I71.8
    ascending I71.2
        ruptured I71.1
    congenital Q25.43
    descending I71.9
        abdominal I71.4
            ruptured I71.3
        ruptured I71.8
        thoracic I71.2
            ruptured I71.1
    root Q25.43
    ruptured I71.8
    sinus, congenital Q25.43
    syphilitic A52.01
    thoracic I71.2
        ruptured I71.1
    thoracoabdominal I71.6
        ruptured I71.5
    thorax, thoracic (arch) I71.2
        ruptured I71.1
    transverse I71.2
        ruptured I71.1
    valve (heart) (*see also* Endocarditis, aortic) I35.8
arteriosclerotic I72.9
    cerebral I67.1
        ruptured — *see* Hemorrhage, intracranial, subarachnoid
arteriovenous (congenital) — *see also* Malformation, arteriovenous
    acquired I77.0
        brain I67.1
        coronary I25.41
        pulmonary I28.0
    brain Q28.2
        ruptured I60.8
    peripheral — *see* Malformation, arteriovenous, peripheral
    precerebral vessels Q28.0
    specified site NEC — *see also* Malformation, arteriovenous
        acquired I77.0
basal — *see* Aneurysm, brain
basilar (trunk) I72.5
berry (congenital) (nonruptured) I67.1
    ruptured I60.7

Aneurysm (anastomotic) (artery) (cirsoid) (diffuse) (false) (fusiform) (multiple) (saccular) I72.9 — *continued*
- brain I67.1
  - arteriosclerotic I67.1
    - ruptured — *see* Hemorrhage, intracranial, subarachnoid
  - arteriovenous (congenital) (nonruptured) Q28.2
    - acquired I67.1
      - ruptured I60.8
    - ruptured I60.8
  - berry (congenital) (nonruptured) I67.1
    - ruptured (*see also* Hemorrhage, intracranial, subarachnoid) I60.7
  - congenital Q28.3
    - ruptured I60.7
  - meninges I67.1
    - ruptured I60.8
  - miliary (congenital) (nonruptured) I67.1
    - ruptured (*see also* Hemorrhage, intracranial, subarachnoid) I60.7
  - mycotic I33.0
  - ruptured — *see* Hemorrhage, intracranial, subarachnoid
  - syphilitic (hemorrhage) A52.05
- cardiac (false) (*see also* Aneurysm, heart) I25.3
- carotid artery (common) (external) I72.0
  - internal (intracranial) I67.1
    - extracranial portion I72.0
    - ruptured into brain I60.0-
  - syphilitic A52.09
    - intracranial A52.05
- cavernous sinus I67.1
  - arteriovenous (congenital) (nonruptured) Q28.3
    - ruptured I60.8
- celiac I72.8
- central nervous system, syphilitic A52.05
- cerebral — *see* Aneurysm, brain
- chest — *see* Aneurysm, thorax
- circle of Willis I67.1
  - congenital Q28.3
    - ruptured I60.6
  - ruptured I60.6
- common iliac artery I72.3
- congenital (peripheral) Q27.8
  - aorta (root) (sinus) Q25.43
  - brain Q28.3
    - ruptured I60.7
  - coronary Q24.5
  - digestive system Q27.8
  - lower limb Q27.8
  - pulmonary Q25.79
  - retina Q14.1
  - specified site NEC Q27.8
  - upper limb Q27.8
- conjunctiva — *see* Abnormality, conjunctiva, vascular
- conus arteriosus — *see* Aneurysm, heart
- coronary (arteriosclerotic) (artery) I25.41
  - arteriovenous, congenital Q24.5
  - congenital Q24.5
  - ruptured — *see* Infarct, myocardium
  - syphilitic A52.06
  - vein I25.89
- cylindroid (aorta) I71.9
  - ruptured I71.8
  - syphilitic A52.01
- ductus arteriosus Q25.0
- endocardial, infective (any valve) I33.0
- femoral (artery) (ruptured) I72.4
- gastroduodenal I72.8
- gastroepiploic I72.8
- heart (wall) (chronic or with a stated duration of over 4 weeks) I25.3
  - valve — *see* Endocarditis
- hepatic I72.8
- iliac (common) (artery) (ruptured) I72.3

Aneurysm (anastomotic) (artery) (cirsoid) (diffuse) (false) (fusiform) (multiple) (saccular) I72.9 — *continued*
- infective I72.9
  - endocardial (any valve) I33.0
- innominate (nonsyphilitic) I72.8
  - syphilitic A52.09
- interauricular septum — *see* Aneurysm, heart
- interventricular septum — *see* Aneurysm, heart
- intrathoracic (nonsyphilitic) I71.2
  - ruptured I71.1
  - syphilitic A52.01
- lower limb I72.4
- lung (pulmonary artery) I28.1
- mediastinal (nonsyphilitic) I72.8
  - syphilitic A52.09
- miliary (congenital) I67.1
  - ruptured — *see* Hemorrhage, intracerebral, subarachnoid, intracranial
- mitral (heart) (valve) I34.8
- mural — *see* Aneurysm, heart
- mycotic I72.9
  - endocardial (any valve) I33.0
  - ruptured, brain — *see* Hemorrhage, intracerebral, subarachnoid
- myocardium — *see* Aneurysm, heart
- neck I72.0
- pancreaticoduodenal I72.8
- patent ductus arteriosus Q25.0
- peripheral NEC I72.8
  - congenital Q27.8
    - digestive system Q27.8
    - lower limb Q27.8
    - specified site NEC Q27.8
    - upper limb Q27.8
- popliteal (artery) (ruptured) I72.4
- precerebral
  - congenital (nonruptured) Q28.1
  - specified site, NEC I72.5
- pulmonary I28.1
  - arteriovenous Q25.72
    - acquired I28.0
  - syphilitic A52.09
  - valve (heart) — *see* Endocarditis, pulmonary
- racemose (peripheral) I72.9
  - congenital — *see* Aneurysm, congenital
- radial I72.1
- Rasmussen NEC A15.0
- renal (artery) I72.2
- retina — *see also* Disorder, retina, microaneurysms
  - congenital Q14.1
  - diabetic — *see* Diabetes, microaneurysms, retinal
- sinus of Valsalva Q25.49
- specified NEC I72.8
- spinal (cord) I72.8
  - syphilitic (hemorrhage) A52.09
- splenic I72.8
- subclavian (artery) (ruptured) I72.8
  - syphilitic A52.09
- superior mesenteric I72.8
- syphilitic (aorta) A52.01
  - central nervous system A52.05
  - congenital (late) A50.54 *[I79.0]*
  - spine, spinal A52.09
- thoracoabdominal (aorta) I71.6
  - ruptured I71.5
  - syphilitic A52.01
- thorax, thoracic (aorta) (arch) (nonsyphilitic) I71.2
  - ruptured I71.1
  - syphilitic A52.01
- traumatic (complication) (early), specified site — *see* Injury, blood vessel
- tricuspid (heart) (valve) I07.8
- ulnar I72.1
- upper limb (ruptured) I72.1
- valve, valvular — *see* Endocarditis

Aneurysm (anastomotic) (artery) (cirsoid) (diffuse) (false) (fusiform) (multiple) (saccular) I72.9 — *continued*
- venous (*see also* Varix) I86.8
  - congenital Q27.8
    - digestive system Q27.8
    - lower limb Q27.8
    - specified site NEC Q27.8
    - upper limb Q27.8
- ventricle — *see* Aneurysm, heart
- vertebral artery I72.6
- visceral NEC I72.8

Angelman syndrome Q93.5

Anger R45.4

Angiectasis, angiectopia I99.8

Angiitis I77.6
- allergic granulomatous M30.1
- hypersensitivity M31.0
- necrotizing M31.9
  - specified NEC M31.8
- nervous system, granulomatous I67.7

Angina (attack) (cardiac) (chest) (heart) (pectoris) (syndrome) (vasomotor) I20.9
- with
  - atherosclerotic heart disease — *see* Arteriosclerosis, coronary (artery)
  - documented spasm I20.1
- abdominal K55.1
- accelerated — *see* Angina, unstable
- agranulocytic — *see* Agranulocytosis
- angiospastic — *see* Angina, with, documented spasm
- aphthous B08.5
- crescendo — *see* Angina, unstable
- croupous J05.0
- cruris I73.9
- de novo effort — *see* Angina, unstable
- diphtheritic, membranous A36.0
- equivalent I20.8
- exudative, chronic J37.0
- following acute myocardial infarction I23.7
- gangrenous diphtheritic A36.0
- intestinal K55.1
- Ludovici K12.2
- Ludwig's K12.2
- malignant diphtheritic A36.0
- membranous J05.0
  - diphtheritic A36.0
  - Vincent's A69.1
- mesenteric K55.1
- monocytic — *see* Mononucleosis, infectious
- of effort — *see* Angina, specified NEC
- phlegmonous J36
  - diphtheritic A36.0
- post-infarctional I23.7
- pre-infarctional — *see* Angina, unstable
- Prinzmetal — *see* Angina, with, documented spasm
- progressive — *see* Angina, unstable
- pseudomembranous A69.1
- pultaceous, diphtheritic A36.0
- spasm-induced — *see* Angina, with, documented spasm
- specified NEC I20.8
- stable I20.8
- stenocardia — *see* Angina, specified NEC
- stridulous, diphtheritic A36.2
- tonsil J36
- trachealis J05.0
- unstable I20.0
- variant — *see* Angina, with, documented spasm
- Vincent's A69.1
- worsening effort — *see* Angina, unstable

Angioblastoma — *see* Neoplasm, connective tissue, uncertain behavior

Angiocholecystitis — *see* Cholecystitis, acute

Angiocholitis (*see also* Cholecystitis, acute) K83.0

DISEASE INDEX

Angiodysgenesis spinalis G95.19
Angiodysplasia (cecum) (colon) K55.20
  with bleeding K55.21
  duodenum (and stomach) K31.819
    with bleeding K31.811
  stomach (and duodenum) K31.819
    with bleeding K31.811
Angioedema (allergic) (any site) (with urticaria) T78.3
  hereditary D84.1
Angioendothelioma — *see* Neoplasm, uncertain behavior, by site
  benign D18.00
    intra-abdominal D18.03
    intracranial D18.02
    skin D18.01
    specified site NEC D18.09
  bone — *see* Neoplasm, bone, malignant
  Ewing's — *see* Neoplasm, bone, malignant
Angioendotheliomatosis C85.8-
Angiofibroma — *see also* Neoplasm, benign, by site
  juvenile
    specified site — *see* Neoplasm, benign, by site
    unspecified site D10.6
Angiohemophilia (A) (B) D68.0
Angioid streaks (choroid) (macula) (retina) H35.33
Angiokeratoma — *see* Neoplasm, skin, benign
  corporis diffusum E75.21
Angioleiomyoma — *see* Neoplasm, connective tissue, benign
Angiolipoma — *see also* Lipoma
  infiltrating — *see* Lipoma
Angioma — *see also* Hemangioma, by site
  capillary I78.1
  hemorrhagicum hereditaria I78.0
  intra-abdominal D18.03
  intracranial D18.02
  malignant — *see* Neoplasm, connective tissue, malignant
  plexiform D18.00
    intra-abdominal D18.03
    intracranial D18.02
    skin D18.01
    specified site NEC D18.09
  senile I78.1
  serpiginosum L81.7
  skin D18.01
  specified site NEC D18.09
  spider I78.1
  stellate I78.1
  venous Q28.3
Angiomatosis Q82.8
  bacillary A79.89
  encephalotrigeminal Q85.8
  hemorrhagic familial I78.0
  hereditary familial I78.0
  liver K76.4
Angiomyolipoma — *see* Lipoma
Angiomyoliposarcoma — *see* Neoplasm, connective tissue, malignant
Angiomyoma — *see* Neoplasm, connective tissue, benign
Angiomyosarcoma — *see* Neoplasm, connective tissue, malignant
Angiomyxoma — *see* Neoplasm, connective tissue, uncertain behavior
Angioneurosis F45.8
Angioneurotic edema (allergic) (any site) (with urticaria) T78.3
  hereditary D84.1
Angiopathia, angiopathy I99.9
  cerebral I67.9
    amyloid E85.4 *[I68.0]*
  diabetic (peripheral) — *see* Diabetes, angiopathy

Angiopathia, angiopathy I99.9 — *continued*
  peripheral I73.9
    diabetic — *see* Diabetes, angiopathy
    specified type NEC I73.89
  retinae syphilitica A52.05
  retinalis (juvenilis)
    diabetic — *see* Diabetes, retinopathy
    proliferative — *see* Retinopathy, proliferative
Angiosarcoma — *see also* Neoplasm, connective tissue, malignant
  liver C22.3
Angiosclerosis — *see* Arteriosclerosis
Angiospasm (peripheral) (traumatic) (vessel) I73.9
  brachial plexus G54.0
  cerebral G45.9
  cervical plexus G54.2
  nerve
    arm — *see* Mononeuropathy, upper limb
      axillary G54.0
      median — *see* Lesion, nerve, median
      ulnar — *see* Lesion, nerve, ulnar
    axillary G54.0
    leg — *see* Mononeuropathy, lower limb
    median — *see* Lesion, nerve, median
    plantar — *see* Lesion, nerve, plantar
    ulnar — *see* Lesion, nerve, ulnar
Angiospastic disease or edema I73.9
Angiostrongyliasis
  due to
    Parastrongylus
      cantonensis B83.2
      costaricensis B81.3
  intestinal B81.3
Anguillulosis — *see* Strongyloidiasis
Angulation
  cecum — *see* Obstruction, intestine
  coccyx (acquired) (*see also* subcategory) M43.8
    congenital NEC Q76.49
  femur (acquired) — *see also* Deformity, limb, specified type NEC, thigh
    congenital Q74.2
  intestine (large) (small) — *see* Obstruction, intestine
  sacrum (acquired) (*see also* subcategory) M43.8
    congenital NEC Q76.49
  sigmoid (flexure) — *see* Obstruction, intestine
  spine — *see* Dorsopathy, deforming, specified NEC
  tibia (acquired) — *see also* Deformity, limb, specified type NEC, lower leg
    congenital Q74.2
  ureter N13.5
    with infection N13.6
  wrist (acquired) — *see also* Deformity, limb, specified type NEC, forearm
    congenital Q74.0
Angulus infectiosus (lips) K13.0
Anhedonia R45.84
  sexual F52.0
Anhidrosis L74.4
Anhydration E86.0
Anhydremia E86.0
Anidrosis L74.4
Aniridia (congenital) Q13.1
Anisakiasis (infection) (infestation) B81.0
Anisakis larvae infestation B81.0
Aniseikonia H52.32
Anisocoria (pupil) H57.02
  congenital Q13.2
Anisocytosis R71.8
Anisometropia (congenital) H52.31
Ankle — *see* condition
Ankyloblepharon (eyelid) (acquired) — *see also* Blepharophimosis
  filiforme (adnatum) (congenital) Q10.3
  total Q10.3

Ankyloglossia Q38.1
Ankylosis (fibrous) (osseous) (joint) M24.60
  ankle M24.67-
  arthrodesis status Z98.1
  cricoarytenoid (cartilage) (joint) (larynx) J38.7
  dental K03.5
  ear ossicles H74.31-
  elbow M24.62-
  foot M24.67-
  hand M24.64-
  hip M24.65-
  incostapedial joint (infectional) — *see* Ankylosis, ear ossicles
  jaw (temporomandibular) M26.61-
  knee M24.66-
  lumbosacral (joint) M43.27
  postoperative (status) Z98.1
  produced by surgical fusion, status Z98.1
  sacro-iliac (joint) M43.28
  shoulder M24.61-
  spine (joint) — *see also* Fusion, spine
    spondylitic — *see* Spondylitis, ankylosing
  surgical Z98.1
  temporomandibular M26.61-
  tooth, teeth (hard tissues) K03.5
  wrist M24.63-
Ankylostoma — *see* Ancylostoma
Ankylostomiasis — *see* Ancylostomiasis
Ankylurethria — *see* Stricture, urethra
Annular — *see also* condition
  detachment, cervix N88.8
  organ or site, congenital NEC — *see* Distortion
  pancreas (congenital) Q45.1
Anodontia (complete) (partial) (vera) K00.0
  acquired K08.10
Anomaly, anomalous (congenital) (unspecified type) Q89.9
  abdominal wall NEC Q79.59
  acoustic nerve Q07.8
  adrenal (gland) Q89.1
  Alder (-Reilly) (leukocyte granulation) D72.0
  alimentary tract Q45.9
    upper Q40.9
  alveolar M26.70
    hyperplasia M26.79
      mandibular M26.72
      maxillary M26.71
    hypoplasia M26.79
      mandibular M26.74
      maxillary M26.73
    ridge (process) M26.79
    specified NEC M26.79
  ankle (joint) Q74.2
  anus Q43.9
  aorta (arch) NEC Q25.40
    coarctation (preductal) (postductal) Q25.1
  aortic cusp or valve Q23.9
  appendix Q43.8
  apple peel syndrome Q41.1
  aqueduct of Sylvius Q03.0
    with spina bifida — *see* Spina bifida, with hydrocephalus
  arm Q74.0
  arteriovenous NEC
    coronary Q24.5
    gastrointestinal Q27.33
      acquired — *see* Angiodysplasia
  artery (peripheral) Q27.9
    basilar NEC Q28.1
    cerebral Q28.3
    coronary Q24.5
    digestive system Q27.8
    eye Q15.8
    great Q25.9
      specified NEC Q25.8
    lower limb Q27.8
    peripheral Q27.9
      specified NEC Q27.8
    pulmonary NEC Q25.79

Anomaly, anomalous (congenital) (unspecified type) Q89.9 — *continued*
- artery (peripheral) Q27.9 — *continued*
  - renal Q27.2
  - retina Q14.1
  - specified site NEC Q27.8
  - subclavian Q27.8
    - origin Q25.48
  - umbilical Q27.0
  - upper limb Q27.8
  - vertebral NEC Q28.1
- aryteno-epiglottic folds Q31.8
- atrial
  - bands or folds Q20.8
  - septa Q21.1
- atrioventricular
  - excitation I45.6
  - septum Q21.0
- auditory canal Q17.8
- auricle
  - ear Q17.8
    - causing impairment of hearing Q16.9
  - heart Q20.8
- Axenfeld's Q15.0
- back Q89.9
- band
  - atrial Q20.8
  - heart Q24.8
  - ventricular Q24.8
- Bartholin's duct Q38.4
- biliary duct or passage Q44.5
- bladder Q64.70
  - absence Q64.5
  - diverticulum Q64.6
  - exstrophy Q64.10
    - cloacal Q64.12
    - extroversion Q64.19
    - specified type NEC Q64.19
    - supravesical fissure Q64.11
  - neck obstruction Q64.31
  - specified type NEC Q64.79
- bone Q79.9
  - arm Q74.0
  - face Q75.9
  - leg Q74.2
  - pelvic girdle Q74.2
  - shoulder girdle Q74.0
  - skull Q75.9
    - with
      - anencephaly Q00.0
      - encephalocele — *see* Encephalocele
      - hydrocephalus Q03.9
        - with spina bifida — *see* Spina bifida, by site, with hydrocephalus
      - microcephaly Q02
- brain (multiple) Q04.9
  - vessel Q28.3
- breast Q83.9
- broad ligament Q50.6
- bronchus Q32.4
- bulbus cordis Q21.9
- bursa Q79.9
- canal of Nuck Q52.4
- canthus Q10.3
- capillary Q27.9
- cardiac Q24.9
  - chambers Q20.9
    - specified NEC Q20.8
  - septal closure Q21.9
    - specified NEC Q21.8
  - valve NEC Q24.8
    - pulmonary Q22.3
- cardiovascular system Q28.8
- carpus Q74.0
- caruncle, lacrimal Q10.6
- cascade stomach Q40.2
- cauda equina Q06.3
- cecum Q43.9

Anomaly, anomalous (congenital) (unspecified type) Q89.9 — *continued*
- cerebral Q04.9
  - vessels Q28.3
- cervix Q51.9
- Chédiak-Higashi(-Steinbrinck) (congenital gigantism of peroxidase granules) E70.330
- cheek Q18.9
- chest wall Q67.8
  - bones Q76.9
- chin Q18.9
- chordae tendineae Q24.8
- choroid Q14.3
  - plexus Q07.8
- chromosomes, chromosomal Q99.9
  - D(1) — *see* condition, chromosome 13
  - E(3) — *see* condition, chromosome 18
  - G — *see* condition, chromosome 21
  - sex
    - female phenotype Q97.8
    - gonadal dysgenesis (pure) Q99.1
    - Klinefelter's Q98.4
    - male phenotype Q98.9
    - Turner's Q96.9
  - specified NEC Q99.8
- cilia Q10.3
- circulatory system Q28.9
- clavicle Q74.0
- clitoris Q52.6
- coccyx Q76.49
- colon Q43.9
- common duct Q44.5
- communication
  - coronary artery Q24.5
  - left ventricle with right atrium Q21.0
- concha (ear) Q17.3
- connection
  - portal vein Q26.5
  - pulmonary venous Q26.4
    - partial Q26.3
    - total Q26.2
  - renal artery with kidney Q27.2
- cornea (shape) Q13.4
- coronary artery or vein Q24.5
- cranium — *see* Anomaly, skull
- cricoid cartilage Q31.8
- cystic duct Q44.5
- dental
  - alveolar — *see* Anomaly, alveolar
  - arch relationship M26.20
    - specified NEC M26.29
- dentofacial M26.9
  - alveolar — *see* Anomaly, alveolar
  - dental arch relationship M26.20
    - specified NEC M26.29
  - functional M26.50
    - specified NEC M26.59
  - jaw size M26.00
    - macrogenia M26.05
    - mandibular
      - hyperplasia M26.03
      - hypoplasia M26.04
    - maxillary
      - hyperplasia M26.01
      - hypoplasia M26.02
    - microgenia M26.06
    - specified type NEC M26.09
  - jaw-cranial base relationship M26.10
    - asymmetry M26.12
      - maxillary M26.11
    - specified type NEC M26.19
  - malocclusion M26.4
    - dental arch relationship NEC M26.29
    - jaw size — *see* Anomaly, dentofacial, jaw size
    - jaw-cranial base relationship — *see* Anomaly, dentofacial, jaw-cranial base relationship

Anomaly, anomalous (congenital) (unspecified type) Q89.9 — *continued*
- dentofacial M26.9 — *continued*
  - specified type NEC M26.89
  - temporomandibular joint M26.60-
    - adhesions M26.61-
    - ankylosis M26.61-
    - arthralgia M26.62-
    - articular disc M26.63-
    - specified type NEC M26.69
  - tooth position, fully erupted M26.30
    - specified NEC M26.39
- dermatoglyphic Q82.8
- diaphragm (apertures) NEC Q79.1
- digestive organ(s) or tract Q45.9
  - lower Q43.9
  - upper Q40.9
- distance, interarch (excessive) (inadequate) M26.25
- distribution, coronary artery Q24.5
- ductus
  - arteriosus Q25.0
  - botalli Q25.0
- duodenum Q43.9
- dura (brain) Q04.9
  - spinal cord Q06.9
- ear (external) Q17.9
  - causing impairment of hearing Q16.9
  - inner Q16.5
  - middle (causing impairment of hearing) Q16.4
    - ossicles Q16.3
- Ebstein's (heart) (tricuspid valve) Q22.5
- ectodermal Q82.9
- Eisenmenger's (ventricular septal defect) Q21.8
- ejaculatory duct Q55.4
- elbow Q74.0
- endocrine gland NEC Q89.2
- epididymis Q55.4
- epiglottis Q31.8
- esophagus Q39.9
- eustachian tube Q17.8
- eye Q15.9
  - anterior segment Q13.9
    - specified NEC Q13.89
  - posterior segment Q14.9
    - specified NEC Q14.8
  - ptosis (eyelid) Q10.0
  - specified NEC Q15.8
- eyebrow Q18.8
- eyelid Q10.3
  - ptosis Q10.0
- face Q18.9
  - bone(s) Q75.9
- fallopian tube Q50.6
- fascia Q79.9
- femur NEC Q74.2
- fibula NEC Q74.2
- finger Q74.0
- fixation, intestine Q43.3
- flexion (joint) NOS Q74.9
  - hip or thigh Q65.89
- foot NEC Q74.2
  - varus (congenital) Q66.3
- foramen
  - Botalli Q21.1
  - ovale Q21.1
- forearm Q74.0
- forehead Q75.8
- form, teeth K00.2
- fovea centralis Q14.1
- frontal bone — *see* Anomaly, skull
- gallbladder (position) (shape) (size) Q44.1
- Gartner's duct Q52.4
- gastrointestinal tract Q45.9

DISEASE INDEX

Anomaly, anomalous (congenital) (unspecified type) Q89.9 — *continued*
- genitalia, genital organ(s) or system
  - female Q52.9
    - external Q52.70
    - internal NOS Q52.9
  - male Q55.9
    - hydrocele P83.5
    - specified NEC Q55.8
- genitourinary NEC
  - female Q52.9
  - male Q55.9
- Gerbode Q21.0
- glottis Q31.8
- granulation or granulocyte, genetic (constitutional) (leukocyte) D72.0
- gum Q38.6
- gyri Q07.9
- hair Q84.2
- hand Q74.0
- hard tissue formation in pulp K04.3
- head — *see* Anomaly, skull
- heart Q24.9
  - auricle Q20.8
  - bands or folds Q24.8
  - fibroelastosis cordis I42.4
  - obstructive NEC Q22.6
  - patent ductus arteriosus (Botalli) Q25.0
  - septum Q21.9
    - auricular Q21.1
    - interatrial Q21.1
    - interventricular Q21.0
      - with pulmonary stenosis or atresia, dextraposition of aorta and hypertrophy of right ventricle Q21.3
    - specified NEC Q21.8
    - ventricular Q21.0
      - with pulmonary stenosis or atresia, dextraposition of aorta and hypertrophy of right ventricle Q21.3
  - tetralogy of Fallot Q21.3
  - valve NEC Q24.8
    - aortic
      - bicuspid valve Q23.1
      - insufficiency Q23.1
      - stenosis Q23.0
        - subaortic Q24.4
    - mitral
      - insufficiency Q23.3
      - stenosis Q23.2
    - pulmonary Q22.3
      - atresia Q22.0
      - insufficiency Q22.2
      - stenosis Q22.1
        - infundibular Q24.3
        - subvalvular Q24.3
    - tricuspid
      - atresia Q22.4
      - stenosis Q22.4
  - ventricle Q20.8
- heel NEC Q74.2
- Hegglin's D72.0
- hemianencephaly Q00.0
- hemicephaly Q00.0
- hemicrania Q00.0
- hepatic duct Q44.5
- hip NEC Q74.2
- hourglass stomach Q40.2
- humerus Q74.0
- hydatid of Morgagni
  - female Q50.5
  - male (epididymal) Q55.4
    - testicular Q55.29
- hymen Q52.4
- hypersegmentation of neutrophils, hereditary D72.0
- hypophyseal Q89.2
- ileocecal (coil) (valve) Q43.9
- ileum Q43.9

Anomaly, anomalous (congenital) (unspecified type) Q89.9 — *continued*
- ilium NEC Q74.2
- integument Q84.9
  - specified NEC Q84.8
- interarch distance (excessive) (inadequate) M26.25
- intervertebral cartilage or disc Q76.49
- intestine (large) (small) Q43.9
  - with anomalous adhesions, fixation or malrotation Q43.3
- iris Q13.2
- ischium NEC Q74.2
- jaw — *see* Anomaly, dentofacial
  - alveolar — *see* Anomaly, alveolar
- jaw-cranial base relationship — *see* Anomaly, dentofacial, jaw-cranial base relationship
- jejunum Q43.8
- joint Q74.9
  - specified NEC Q74.8
- Jordan's D72.0
- kidney(s) (calyx) (pelvis) Q63.9
  - artery Q27.2
  - specified NEC Q63.8
- Klippel-Feil (brevicollis) Q76.1
- knee Q74.1
- labium (majus) (minus) Q52.70
- labyrinth, membranous Q16.5
- lacrimal apparatus or duct Q10.6
- larynx, laryngeal (muscle) Q31.9
  - web(bed) Q31.0
- lens Q12.9
- leukocytes, genetic D72.0
  - granulation (constitutional) D72.0
- lid (fold) Q10.3
- ligament Q79.9
  - broad Q50.6
  - round Q52.8
- limb Q74.9
  - lower NEC Q74.2
    - reduction deformity — *see* Defect, reduction, lower limb
  - upper Q74.0
- lip Q38.0
- liver Q44.7
  - duct Q44.5
- lower limb NEC Q74.2
- lumbosacral (joint) (region) Q76.49
  - kyphosis — *see* Kyphosis, congenital
  - lordosis — *see* Lordosis, congenital
- lung (fissure) (lobe) Q33.9
- mandible — *see* Anomaly, dentofacial
- maxilla — *see* Anomaly, dentofacial
- May (-Hegglin) D72.0
- meatus urinarius NEC Q64.79
- meningeal bands or folds Q07.9
  - constriction of Q07.8
  - spinal Q06.9
- meninges Q07.9
  - cerebral Q04.8
  - spinal Q06.9
- meningocele Q05.9
- mesentery Q45.9
- metacarpus Q74.0
- metatarsus NEC Q74.2
- middle ear Q16.4
  - ossicles Q16.3
- mitral (leaflets) (valve) Q23.9
  - insufficiency Q23.3
  - specified NEC Q23.8
  - stenosis Q23.2
- mouth Q38.6
- Müllerian — *see also* Anomaly, by site
  - uterus NEC Q51.818
- multiple NEC Q89.7
- muscle Q79.9
  - eyelid Q10.3
- musculoskeletal system, except limbs Q79.9
- myocardium Q24.8

Anomaly, anomalous (congenital) (unspecified type) Q89.9 — *continued*
- nail Q84.6
- narrowness, eyelid Q10.3
- nasal sinus (wall) Q30.8
- neck (any part) Q18.9
- nerve Q07.9
  - acoustic Q07.8
  - optic Q07.8
- nervous system (central) Q07.9
- nipple Q83.9
- nose, nasal (bones) (cartilage) (septum) (sinus) Q30.9
  - specified NEC Q30.8
- ocular muscle Q15.8
- omphalomesenteric duct Q43.0
- opening, pulmonary veins Q26.4
- optic
  - disc Q14.2
  - nerve Q07.8
- opticociliary vessels Q13.2
- orbit (eye) Q10.7
- organ Q89.9
  - of Corti Q16.5
- origin
  - artery
    - innominate Q25.8
    - pulmonary Q25.79
    - renal Q27.2
    - subclavian Q25.48
- osseous meatus (ear) Q16.1
- ovary Q50.39
- oviduct Q50.6
- palate (hard) (soft) NEC Q38.5
- pancreas or pancreatic duct Q45.3
- papillary muscles Q24.8
- parathyroid gland Q89.2
- paraurethral ducts Q64.79
- parotid (gland) Q38.4
- patella Q74.1
- Pelger-Huët (hereditary hyposegmentation) D72.0
- pelvic girdle NEC Q74.2
- pelvis (bony) NEC Q74.2
  - rachitic E64.3
- penis (glans) Q55.69
- pericardium Q24.8
- peripheral vascular system Q27.9
- Peter's Q13.4
- pharynx Q38.8
- pigmentation L81.9
  - congenital Q82.8
- pituitary (gland) Q89.2
- pleural (folds) Q34.0
- portal vein Q26.5
  - connection Q26.5
- position, tooth, teeth, fully erupted M26.30
  - specified NEC M26.39
- precerebral vessel Q28.1
- prepuce Q55.69
- prostate Q55.4
- pulmonary Q33.9
  - artery NEC Q25.79
  - valve Q22.3
    - atresia Q22.0
    - insufficiency Q22.2
    - specified type NEC Q22.3
    - stenosis Q22.1
      - infundibular Q24.3
      - subvalvular Q24.3
  - venous connection Q26.4
    - partial Q26.3
    - total Q26.2
- pupil Q13.2
  - function H57.00
    - anisocoria H57.02
    - Argyll Robertson pupil H57.01
    - miosis H57.03
    - mydriasis H57.04

DISEASE INDEX

Anomaly, anomalous (congenital) (unspecified type) Q89.9 — *continued*
pupil Q13.2 — *continued*
  function H57.00 — *continued*
    specified type NEC H57.09
    tonic pupil H57.05-
pylorus Q40.3
radius Q74.0
rectum Q43.9
reduction (extremity) (limb)
  femur (longitudinal) — *see* Defect, reduction, lower limb, longitudinal, femur
  fibula (longitudinal) — *see* Defect, reduction, lower limb, longitudinal, fibula
  lower limb — *see* Defect, reduction, lower limb
  radius (longitudinal) — *see* Defect, reduction, upper limb, longitudinal, radius
  tibia (longitudinal) — *see* Defect, reduction, lower limb, longitudinal, tibia
  ulna (longitudinal) — *see* Defect, reduction, upper limb, longitudinal, ulna
  upper limb — *see* Defect, reduction, upper limb
refraction — *see* Disorder, refraction
renal Q63.9
  artery Q27.2
  pelvis Q63.9
    specified NEC Q63.8
respiratory system Q34.9
  specified NEC Q34.8
retina Q14.1
rib Q76.6
  cervical Q76.5
Rieger's Q13.81
rotation — *see* Malrotation
  hip or thigh Q65.89
round ligament Q52.8
sacroiliac (joint) NEC Q74.2
sacrum NEC Q76.49
  kyphosis — *see* Kyphosis, congenital
  lordosis — *see* Lordosis, congenital
saddle nose, syphilitic A50.57
salivary duct or gland Q38.4
scapula Q74.0
scrotum — *see* Malformation, testis and scrotum
sebaceous gland Q82.9
seminal vesicles Q55.4
sense organs NEC Q07.8
sex chromosomes NEC — *see also* Anomaly, chromosomes
  female phenotype Q97.8
  male phenotype Q98.9
shoulder (girdle) (joint) Q74.0
sigmoid (flexure) Q43.9
simian crease Q82.8
sinus of Valsalva Q25.49
skeleton generalized Q78.9
skin (appendage) Q82.9
skull Q75.9
  with
    anencephaly Q00.0
    encephalocele — *see* Encephalocele
    hydrocephalus Q03.9
      with spina bifida — *see* Spina bifida, by site, with hydrocephalus
    microcephaly Q02
specified organ or site NEC Q89.8
spermatic cord Q55.4
spine, spinal NEC Q76.49
  column NEC Q76.49
    kyphosis — *see* Kyphosis, congenital
    lordosis — *see* Lordosis, congenital
  cord Q06.9
  nerve root Q07.8
spleen Q89.09
  agenesis Q89.01
stenonian duct Q38.4
sternum NEC Q76.7

Anomaly, anomalous (congenital) (unspecified type) Q89.9 — *continued*
stomach Q40.3
submaxillary gland Q38.4
tarsus NEC Q74.2
tendon Q79.9
testis — *see* Malformation, testis and scrotum
thigh NEC Q74.2
thorax (wall) Q67.8
  bony Q76.9
throat Q38.8
thumb Q74.0
thymus gland Q89.2
thyroid (gland) Q89.2
  cartilage Q31.8
tibia NEC Q74.2
  saber A50.56
toe Q74.2
tongue Q38.3
tooth, teeth K00.9
  eruption K00.6
  position, fully erupted M26.30
  spacing, fully erupted M26.30
trachea (cartilage) Q32.1
tragus Q17.9
tricuspid (leaflet) (valve) Q22.9
  atresia or stenosis Q22.4
  Ebstein's Q22.5
Uhl's (hypoplasia of myocardium, right ventricle) Q24.8
ulna Q74.0
umbilical artery Q27.0
union
  cricoid cartilage and thyroid cartilage Q31.8
  thyroid cartilage and hyoid bone Q31.8
  trachea with larynx Q31.8
upper limb Q74.0
urachus Q64.4
ureter Q62.8
  obstructive NEC Q62.39
    cecoureterocele Q62.32
    orthotopic ureterocele Q62.31
urethra Q64.70
  absence Q64.5
  double Q64.74
  fistula to rectum Q64.73
  obstructive Q64.39
    stricture Q64.32
  prolapse Q64.71
  specified type NEC Q64.79
urinary tract Q64.9
uterus Q51.9
  with only one functioning horn Q51.4
uvula Q38.5
vagina Q52.4
valleculae Q31.8
valve (heart) NEC Q24.8
  coronary sinus Q24.5
  inferior vena cava Q24.8
  pulmonary Q22.3
  sinus coronario Q24.5
  venae cavae inferioris Q24.8
vas deferens Q55.4
vascular Q27.9
  brain Q28.3
  ring Q25.45
vein(s) (peripheral) Q27.9
  brain Q28.3
  cerebral Q28.3
  coronary Q24.5
  developmental Q28.3
  great Q26.9
    specified NEC Q26.8
vena cava (inferior) (superior) Q26.9
venous — *see* Anomaly, vein(s)
venous return Q26.8
ventricular
  bands or folds Q24.8
  septa Q21.0

Anomaly, anomalous (congenital) (unspecified type) Q89.9 — *continued*
vertebra Q76.49
  kyphosis — *see* Kyphosis, congenital
  lordosis — *see* Lordosis, congenital
vesicourethral orifice Q64.79
vessel(s) Q27.9
  optic papilla Q14.2
  precerebral Q28.1
vitelline duct Q43.0
vitreous body or humor Q14.0
vulva Q52.70
wrist (joint) Q74.0
Anomia R48.8
Anonychia (congenital) Q84.3
  acquired L60.8
Anophthalmos, anophthalmus (congenital) (globe) Q11.1
  acquired Z90.01
Anopia, anopsia H53.46-
  quadrant H53.46-
Anorchia, anorchism, anorchidism Q55.0
Anorexia R63.0
  hysterical F44.89
  nervosa F50.00
    atypical F50.9
    binge-eating type F50.2
      with purging F50.02
    restricting type F50.01
Anorgasmy, psychogenic (female) F52.31
  male F52.32
Anosmia R43.0
  hysterical F44.6
  postinfectional J39.8
Anosognosia R41.89
Anosteoplasia Q78.9
Anovulatory cycle N97.0
Anoxemia R09.02
  newborn P84
Anoxia (pathological) R09.02
  altitude T70.29
  cerebral G93.1
    complicating
      anesthesia (general) (local) or other sedation T88.59
      in labor and delivery O74.3
      in pregnancy O29.21-
      postpartum, puerperal O89.2
      delivery (cesarean) (instrumental) O75.4
    during a procedure G97.81
    newborn P84
    resulting from a procedure G97.82
  due to
    drowning T75.1
    high altitude T70.29
  heart — *see* Insufficiency, coronary
  intrauterine P84
  myocardial — *see* Insufficiency, coronary
  newborn P84
  spinal cord G95.11
  systemic (by suffocation) (low content in atmosphere) — *see* Asphyxia, traumatic
Anteflexion — *see* Anteversion
Antenatal
  care (normal pregnancy) Z34.90
  screening (encounter for) of mother Z36
Antepartum — *see* condition
Anterior — *see* condition
Antero-occlusion M26.220
Anteversion
  cervix — *see* Anteversion, uterus
  femur (neck), congenital Q65.89
  uterus, uterine (cervix) (postinfectional) (postpartal, old) N85.4
    congenital Q51.818
    in pregnancy or childbirth — *see* Pregnancy, complicated by
Anthophobia F40.228
Anthracosilicosis J60

Anthracosis (lung) (occupational) J60
  lingua K14.3
Anthrax A22.9
  with pneumonia A22.1
  cerebral A22.8
  colitis A22.2
  cutaneous A22.0
  gastrointestinal A22.2
  inhalation A22.1
  intestinal A22.2
  meningitis A22.8
  pulmonary A22.1
  respiratory A22.1
  sepsis A22.7
  specified manifestation NEC A22.8
Anthropoid pelvis Q74.2
  with disproportion (fetopelvic) O33.0
Anthropophobia F40.10
  generalized F40.11
Antibodies, maternal (blood group) — see
    Isoimmunization, affecting management of
    pregnancy
  anti-D — see Isoimmunization, affecting
    management of pregnancy, Rh
  newborn P55.0
Antibody
  anticardiolipin R76.0
    with
      hemorrhagic disorder D68.312
      hypercoagulable state D68.61
  antiphosphatidylglycerol R76.0
    with
      hemorrhagic disorder D68.312
      hypercoagulable state D68.61
  antiphosphatidylinositol R76.0
    with
      hemorrhagic disorder D68.312
      hypercoagulable state D68.61
  antiphosphatidylserine R76.0
    with
      hemorrhagic disorder D68.312
      hypercoagulable state D68.61
  antiphospholipid R76.0
    with
      hemorrhagic disorder D68.312
      hypercoagulable state D68.61
Anticardiolipin syndrome D68.61
Anticoagulant, circulating (intrinsic) (see also
    Disorder, hemorrhagic) D68.318
  drug-induced (extrinsic) (see also Disorder,
    hemorrhagic) D68.32
  iatrogenic D68.32
Antidiuretic hormone syndrome E22.2
Antimonial cholera — see Poisoning,
    antimony
Antiphospholipid
  antibody
    with hemorrhagic disorder D68.312
  syndrome D68.61
Antisocial personality F60.2
Antithrombinemia — see Circulating
    anticoagulants
Antithromboplastinemia D68.318
Antithromboplastinogenemia D68.318
Antitoxin complication or reaction — see
    Complications, vaccination
Antlophobia F40.228
Antritis J32.0
  maxilla J32.0
    acute J01.00
      recurrent J01.01
  stomach K29.60
    with bleeding K29.61
Antrum, antral — see condition

Anuria R34
  calculous (impacted) (recurrent) (see also
    Calculus, urinary) N20.9
  following
    abortion — see Abortion, by type,
      complicated by, renal failure
    ectopic or molar pregnancy O08.4
  newborn P96.0
  postprocedural N99.0
  postrenal N13.8
  traumatic (following crushing) T79.5
Anus, anal — see condition
Anusitis K62.89
Anxiety F41.9
  depression F41.8
  episodic paroxysmal F41.0
  generalized F41.1
  hysteria F41.8
  neurosis F41.1
  panic type F41.0
  reaction F41.1
  separation, abnormal (of childhood) F93.0
  specified NEC F41.8
  state F41.1
Aorta, aortic — see condition
Aortectasia — see Ectasia, aorta
  with aneurysm — see Aneurysm, aorta
Aortitis (nonsyphilitic) (calcific) I77.6
  arteriosclerotic I70.0
  Doehle-Heller A52.02
  luetic A52.02
  rheumatic — see Endocarditis, acute,
    rheumatic
  specific (syphilitic) A52.02
  syphilitic A52.02
    congenital A50.54 [I79.1]
Apathetic thyroid storm — see
    Thyrotoxicosis
Apathy R45.3
Apeirophobia F40.228
Apepsia K30
  psychogenic F45.8
Aperistalsis, esophagus K22.0
Apertognathia M26.29
Apert's syndrome Q87.0
Aphagia R13.0
  psychogenic F50.9
Aphakia (acquired) (postoperative) H27.0-
  congenital Q12.3
Aphasia (amnestic) (global) (nominal)
    (semantic) (syntactic) R47.01
  acquired, with epilepsy (Landau-Kleffner
    syndrome) — see Epilepsy, specified NEC
  auditory (developmental) F80.2
  developmental (receptive type) F80.2
    expressive type F80.1
    Wernicke's F80.2
  following
    cerebrovascular disease I69.920
      cerebral infarction I69.320
      intracerebral hemorrhage I69.120
      nontraumatic intracranial hemorrhage
        NEC I69.220
      specified disease NEC I69.820
      subarachnoid hemorrhage I69.020
  primary progressive G31.01 [F02.80]
    with behavioral disturbance G31.01
      [F02.81]
  progressive isolated G31.01 [F02.80]
    with behavioral disturbance G31.01
      [F02.81]
  sensory F80.2
  syphilis, tertiary A52.19
  Wernicke's (developmental) F80.2
Aphonia (organic) R49.1
  hysterical F44.4
  psychogenic F44.4

Aphthae, aphthous — see also condition
  Bednar's K12.0
  cachectic K14.0
  epizootic B08.8
  fever B08.8
  oral (recurrent) K12.0
  stomatitis (major) (minor) K12.0
  thrush B37.0
  ulcer (oral) (recurrent) K12.0
    genital organ(s) NEC
      female N76.6
      male N50.89
    larynx J38.7
Apical — see condition
Apiphobia F40.218
Aplasia — see also Agenesis
  abdominal muscle syndrome Q79.4
  alveolar process (acquired) — see Anomaly,
    alveolar
    congenital Q38.6
  aorta (congenital) Q25.41
  axialis extracorticalis (congenita) E75.29
  bone marrow (myeloid) D61.9
    congenital D61.01
  brain Q00.0
    part of Q04.3
  bronchus Q32.4
  cementum K00.4
  cerebellum Q04.3
  cervix (congenital) Q51.5
  congenital pure red cell D61.01
  corpus callosum Q04.0
  cutis congenita Q84.8
  erythrocyte congenital D61.01
  extracortical axial E75.29
  eye Q11.1
  fovea centralis (congenital) Q14.1
  gallbladder, congenital Q44.0
  iris Q13.1
  labyrinth, membranous Q16.5
  limb (congenital) Q73.8
    lower — see Defect, reduction, lower limb
    upper — see Agenesis, arm
  lung, congenital (bilateral) (unilateral) Q33.3
  pancreas Q45.0
  parathyroid-thymic D82.1
  Pelizaeus-Merzbacher E75.29
  penis Q55.5
  prostate Q55.4
  red cell (with thymoma) D60.9
    acquired D60.9
      due to drugs D60.9
    adult D60.9
    chronic D60.0
    congenital D61.01
    constitutional D61.01
    due to drugs D60.9
    hereditary D61.01
    of infants D61.01
    primary D61.01
    pure D61.01
      due to drugs D60.9
    specified type NEC D60.8
    transient D60.1
  round ligament Q52.8
  skin Q84.8
  spermatic cord Q55.4
  spleen Q89.01
  testicle Q55.0
  thymic, with immunodeficiency D82.1
  thyroid (congenital) (with myxedema) E03.1
  uterus Q51.0
  ventral horn cell Q06.1

Apnea, apneic (of) (spells) R06.81
  newborn NEC P28.4
    obstructive P28.4
    sleep (central) (obstructive) (primary) P28.3
  prematurity P28.4
  sleep G47.30
    central (primary) G47.31
      in conditions classified elsewhere G47.37
    obstructive (adult) (pediatric) G47.33
    primary central G47.31
    specified NEC G47.39
Apneumatosis, newborn P28.0
Apocrine metaplasia (breast) — see
  Dysplasia, mammary, specified type NEC
Apophysitis (bone) — see also
  Osteochondropathy
  calcaneus M92.8
  juvenile M92.9
Apoplectiform convulsions (cerebral
  ischemia) I67.82
Apoplexia, apoplexy, apoplectic
  adrenal A39.1
  heart (auricle) (ventricle) — see Infarct,
    myocardium
  heat T67.0
  hemorrhagic (stroke) — see Hemorrhage,
    intracranial
  meninges, hemorrhagic — see Hemorrhage,
    intracranial, subarachnoid
  uremic N18.9 [I68.8]
Appearance
  bizarre R46.1
  specified NEC R46.89
  very low level of personal hygiene R46.0
Appendage
  epididymal (organ of Morgagni) Q55.4
  intestine (epiploic) Q43.8
  preauricular Q17.0
  testicular (organ of Morgagni) Q55.29
Appendicitis (pneumococcal) (retrocecal) K37
  with
    perforation or rupture K35.2
    peritoneal abscess K35.3
    peritonitis K35.2
      generalized (with perforation or rupture)
        K35.2
      localized (with perforation or rupture)
        K35.3
  acute (catarrhal) (fulminating) (gangrenous)
    (obstructive) (retrocecal) (suppurative)
    K35.80
    with
      peritoneal abscess K35.3
      peritonitis K35.3
        generalized (with perforation or rupture)
          K35.2
        localized (with perforation or rupture)
          K35.3
    specified NEC K35.89
  amebic A06.89
  chronic (recurrent) K36
  exacerbation — see Appendicitis, acute
  gangrenous — see Appendicitis, acute
  healed (obliterative) K36
  interval K36
  neurogenic K36
  obstructive K36
  recurrent K36
  relapsing K36
  subacute (adhesive) K36
  subsiding K36
  suppurative — see Appendicitis, acute
  tuberculous A18.32
Appendicopathia oxyurica B80
Appendix, appendicular — see also
  condition
  epididymis Q55.4

Appendix, appendicular — see also
  condition — continued
  Morgagni
    female Q50.5
    male (epididymal) Q55.4
      testicular Q55.29
  testis Q55.29
Appetite
  depraved — see Pica
  excessive R63.2
  lack or loss (see also Anorexia) R63.0
    nonorganic origin F50.89
    psychogenic F50.89
  perverted (hysterical) — see Pica
Apple peel syndrome Q41.1
Apprehension state F41.1
Apprehensiveness, abnormal F41.9
Approximal wear K03.0
Apraxia (classic) (ideational) (ideokinetic)
  (ideomotor) (motor) (verbal) R48.2
  following
    cerebrovascular disease I69.990
      cerebral infarction I69.390
      intracerebral hemorrhage I69.190
      nontraumatic intracranial hemorrhage
        NEC I69.290
      specified disease NEC I69.890
      subarachnoid hemorrhage I69.090
  oculomotor, congenital H51.8
Aptyalism K11.7
Apudoma — see Neoplasm, uncertain
  behavior, by site
Aqueous misdirection H40.83-
Arabicum elephantiasis — see Infestation,
  filarial
Arachnitis — see Meningitis
Arachnodactyly — see Syndrome, Marfan's
Arachnoiditis (acute) (adhesive) (basal) (brain)
  (cerebrospinal) — see Meningitis
Arachnophobia F40.210
Arboencephalitis, Australian A83.4
Arborization block (heart) I45.5
ARC (AIDS-related complex) B20
Arches — see condition
Arcuate uterus Q51.810
Arcuatus uterus Q51.810
Arcus (cornea) senilis — see Degeneration,
  cornea, senile
Arc-welder's lung J63.4
Areflexia R29.2
Areola — see condition
Argentaffinoma — see also Neoplasm,
  uncertain behavior, by site
  malignant — see Neoplasm, malignant, by site
  syndrome E34.0
Argininemia E72.21
Arginosuccinic aciduria E72.22
**Argyll Robertson phenomenon, pupil or
  syndrome** (syphilitic) A52.19
  atypical H57.09
  nonsyphilitic H57.09
Argyria, argyriasis
  conjunctival H11.13-
  from drug or medicament — see Table of
    Drugs and Chemicals, by substance
Argyrosis, conjunctival H11.13-
Arhinencephaly Q04.1
Ariboflavinosis E53.0
Arm — see condition
**Arnold-Chiari disease, obstruction or
  syndrome** (type II) Q07.00
  with
    hydrocephalus Q07.02
      with spina bifida Q07.03
    spina bifida Q07.01
      with hydrocephalus Q07.03
  type III — see Encephalocele
  type IV Q04.8

**Aromatic amino-acid metabolism
  disorder** E70.9
  specified NEC E70.8
Arousals, confusional G47.51
Arrest, arrested
  cardiac I46.9
    complicating
      abortion — see Abortion, by type,
        complicated by, cardiac arrest
      anesthesia (general) (local) or other
        sedation — see Table of Drugs and
        Chemicals, by drug,
        in labor and delivery O74.2
        in pregnancy O29.11-
        postpartum, puerperal O89.1
      delivery (cesarean) (instrumental) O75.4
    due to
      cardiac condition I46.2
      specified condition NEC I46.8
    intraoperative I97.71-
    newborn P29.81
    postprocedural I97.12-
      obstetric procedure O75.4
  cardiorespiratory — see Arrest, cardiac
  circulatory — see Arrest, cardiac
  deep transverse O64.0
  development or growth
    bone — see Disorder, bone, development or
      growth
    child R62.50
    tracheal rings Q32.1
  epiphyseal
    complete
      femur M89.15-
      humerus M89.12-
      tibia M89.16-
      ulna M89.13-
    forearm M89.13-
      specified NEC M89.13-
      ulna — see Arrest, epiphyseal, by type,
        ulna
    lower leg M89.16-
      specified NEC M89.168
      tibia — see Arrest, epiphyseal, by type,
        tibia
    partial
      femur M89.15-
      humerus M89.12-
      tibia M89.16-
      ulna M89.13-
    specified NEC M89.18
  granulopoiesis — see Agranulocytosis
  growth plate — see Arrest, epiphyseal
  heart — see Arrest, cardiac
  legal, anxiety concerning Z65.3
  physeal — see Arrest, epiphyseal
  respiratory R09.2
    newborn P28.81
  sinus I45.5
  spermatogenesis (complete) — see
    Azoospermia
    incomplete — see Oligospermia
  transverse (deep) O64.0
Arrhenoblastoma
  benign
    specified site — see Neoplasm, benign, by
      site
    unspecified site
      female D27.9
      male D29.20
  malignant
    specified site — see Neoplasm, malignant,
      by site
    unspecified site
      female C56.9
      male C62.90
  specified site — see Neoplasm, uncertain
    behavior, by site

Arrhenoblastoma — *continued*
unspecified site
female D39.10
male D40.10
Arrhythmia (auricle) (cardiac) (juvenile)
(nodal) (reflex) (sinus) (supraventricular)
(transitory) (ventricle) I49.9
block I45.9
extrasystolic I49.49
newborn
bradycardia P29.12
occurring before birth P03.819
before onset of labor P03.810
during labor P03.811
tachycardia P29.11
psychogenic F45.8
specified NEC I49.8
vagal R55
ventricular re-entry I47.0
Arrillaga-Ayerza syndrome (pulmonary
sclerosis with pulmonary hypertension)
I27.0
Arsenical pigmentation L81.8
from drug or medicament — *see* Table of
Drugs and Chemicals
Arsenism — *see* Poisoning, arsenic
Arterial — *see* condition
Arteriofibrosis — *see* Arteriosclerosis
Arteriolar sclerosis — *see* Arteriosclerosis
Arteriolith — *see* Arteriosclerosis
Arteriolitis I77.6
necrotizing, kidney I77.5
renal — *see* Hypertension, kidney
Arteriolosclerosis — *see* Arteriosclerosis
Arterionephrosclerosis — *see* Hypertension,
kidney
Arteriopathy I77.9
Arteriosclerosis, arteriosclerotic (diffuse)
(obliterans) (of) (senile) (with calcification)
I70.90
aorta I70.0
arteries of extremities — *see* Arteriosclerosis,
extremities
brain I67.2
bypass graft
coronary — *see* Arteriosclerosis, coronary,
bypass graft
extremities — *see* Arteriosclerosis,
extremities, bypass graft
cardiac — *see* Disease, heart, ischemic,
atherosclerotic
cardiopathy — *see* Disease, heart, ischemic,
atherosclerotic
cardiorenal — *see* Hypertension, cardiorenal
cardiovascular — *see* Disease, heart, ischemic,
atherosclerotic
carotid (*see also* Occlusion, artery, carotid)
I65.2-
central nervous system I67.2
cerebral I67.2
cerebrovascular I67.2
coronary (artery) I25.10
bypass graft I25.810
with
angina pectoris I25.709
with documented spasm I25.701
specified type NEC I25.708
unstable I25.700
ischemic chest pain I25.709
autologous artery I25.810
with
angina pectoris I25.729
with documented spasm I25.721
specified type I25.728
unstable I25.720
ischemic chest pain I25.729

Arteriosclerosis, arteriosclerotic (diffuse)
(obliterans) (of) (senile) (with calcification)
I70.90 — *continued*
coronary (artery) I25.10 — *continued*
bypass graft I25.810 — *continued*
autologous vein I25.810
with
angina pectoris I25.719
with documented spasm I25.711
specified type I25.718
unstable I25.710
ischemic chest pain I25.719
nonautologous biological I25.810
with
angina pectoris I25.739
with documented spasm I25.731
specified type I25.738
unstable I25.730
ischemic chest pain I25.739
specified type NEC I25.810
with
angina pectoris I25.799
with documented spasm I25.791
specified type I25.798
unstable I25.790
ischemic chest pain I25.799
due to
calcified coronary lesion (severely) I25.84
lipid rich plaque I25.83
native vessel
with
angina pectoris I25.119
with documented spasm I25.111
specified type NEC I25.118
unstable I25.110
ischemic chest pain I25.119
transplanted heart I25.811
bypass graft I25.812
with
angina pectoris I25.769
with documented spasm I25.761
specified type I25.768
unstable I25.760
ischemic chest pain I25.769
native coronary artery I25.811
with
angina pectoris I25.759
with documented spasm I25.751
specified type I25.758
unstable I25.750
ischemic chest pain I25.759
extremities (native arteries) I70.209
bypass graft I70.309
autologous vein graft I70.409
leg I70.409
with
gangrene (and intermittent
claudication, rest pain and
ulcer) I70.469
intermittent claudication I70.419
rest pain (and intermittent
claudication) I70.429
bilateral I70.403
with
gangrene (and intermittent
claudication, rest pain and
ulcer) I70.463
intermittent claudication I70.413
rest pain (and intermittent
claudication) I70.423
specified type NEC I70.493

Arteriosclerosis, arteriosclerotic (diffuse)
(obliterans) (of) (senile) (with calcification)
I70.90 — *continued*
extremities (native arteries) I70.209 —
continued
bypass graft I70.309 — *continued*
autologous vein graft I70.409 —
continued
leg I70.409 — *continued*
left I70.402
with
gangrene (and intermittent
claudication, rest pain and
ulcer) I70.462
intermittent claudication I70.412
rest pain (and intermittent
claudication) I70.422
ulceration (and intermittent
claudication and rest pain)
I70.449
ankle I70.443
calf I70.442
foot site NEC I70.445
heel I70.444
lower leg NEC I70.448
midfoot I70.444
thigh I70.441
specified type NEC I70.492
right I70.401
with
gangrene (and intermittent
claudication, rest pain and
ulcer) I70.461
intermittent claudication I70.411
rest pain (and intermittent
claudication) I70.421
ulceration (and intermittent
claudication and rest pain)
I70.439
ankle I70.433
calf I70.432
foot site NEC I70.435
heel I70.434
lower leg NEC I70.438
midfoot I70.434
thigh I70.431
specified type NEC I70.491
specified type NEC I70.499
specified NEC I70.408
with
gangrene (and intermittent
claudication, rest pain and
ulcer) I70.468
intermittent claudication I70.418
rest pain (and intermittent
claudication) I70.428
ulceration (and intermittent
claudication and rest pain)
I70.45
specified type NEC I70.498
leg I70.309
with
gangrene (and intermittent
claudication, rest pain and ulcer)
I70.369
intermittent claudication I70.319
rest pain (and intermittent
claudication) I70.329
bilateral I70.303
with
gangrene (and intermittent
claudication, rest pain and
ulcer) I70.363
intermittent claudication I70.313
rest pain (and intermittent
claudication) I70.323
specified type NEC I70.393

Arteriosclerosis, arteriosclerotic (diffuse) (obliterans) (of) (senile) (with calcification) I70.90 — *continued*
  extremities (native arteries) I70.209 — *continued*
    bypass graft I70.309 — *continued*
      leg I70.309 — *continued*
        left I70.302
          with
            gangrene (and intermittent claudication, rest pain and ulcer) I70.362
            intermittent claudication I70.312
            rest pain (and intermittent claudication) I70.322
            ulceration (and intermittent claudication and rest pain) I70.349
              ankle I70.343
              calf I70.342
              foot site NEC I70.345
              heel I70.344
              lower leg NEC I70.348
              midfoot I70.344
              thigh I70.341
          specified type NEC I70.392
        right I70.301
          with
            gangrene (and intermittent claudication, rest pain and ulcer) I70.361
            intermittent claudication I70.311
            rest pain (and intermittent claudication) I70.321
            ulceration (and intermittent claudication and rest pain) I70.339
              ankle I70.333
              calf I70.332
              foot site NEC I70.335
              heel I70.334
              lower leg NEC I70.338
              midfoot I70.334
              thigh I70.331
          specified type NEC I70.391
        specified type NEC I70.399
      nonautologous biological graft I70.509
        leg I70.509
          with
            gangrene (and intermittent claudication, rest pain and ulcer) I70.569
            intermittent claudication I70.519
            rest pain (and intermittent claudication) I70.529
          bilateral I70.503
            with
              gangrene (and intermittent claudication, rest pain and ulcer) I70.563
              intermittent claudication I70.513
              rest pain (and intermittent claudication) I70.523
              specified type NEC I70.593
          left I70.502
           with
            gangrene (and intermittent claudication, rest pain and ulcer) I70.562
            intermittent claudication I70.512
            rest pain (and intermittent claudication) I70.522

Arteriosclerosis, arteriosclerotic (diffuse) (obliterans) (of) (senile) (with calcification) I70.90 — *continued*
  extremities (native arteries) I70.209 — *continued*
    bypass graft I70.309 — *continued*
      nonautologous biological graft I70.509 — *continued*
        leg I70.509 — *continued*
          left I70.502 — *continued*
           with — *continued*
            ulceration (and intermittent claudication and rest pain) I70.549
              ankle I70.543
              calf I70.542
              foot site NEC I70.545
              heel I70.544
              lower leg NEC I70.548
              midfoot I70.544
              thigh I70.541
          specified type NEC I70.592
        right I70.501
          with
            gangrene (and intermittent claudication, rest pain and ulcer) I70.561
            intermittent claudication I70.511
            rest pain (and intermittent claudication) I70.521
            ulceration (and intermittent claudication and rest pain) I70.539
              ankle I70.533
              calf I70.532
              foot site NEC I70.535
              heel I70.534
              lower leg NEC I70.538
              midfoot I70.534
              thigh I70.531
          specified type NEC I70.591
        specified type NEC I70.599
      specified NEC I70.508
        with
          gangrene (and intermittent claudication, rest pain and ulcer) I70.568
          intermittent claudication I70.518
          rest pain (and intermittent claudication) I70.528
          ulceration (and intermittent claudication and rest pain) I70.55
          specified type NEC I70.598
      nonbiological graft I70.609
        leg I70.609
          with
           gangrene (and intermittent claudication, rest pain and ulcer) I70.669
           intermittent claudication I70.619
           rest pain (and intermittent claudication) I70.629
          bilateral I70.603
           with
            gangrene (and intermittent claudication, rest pain and ulcer) I70.663
            intermittent claudication I70.613
            rest pain (and intermittent claudication) I70.623
            specified type NEC I70.693

Arteriosclerosis, arteriosclerotic (diffuse) (obliterans) (of) (senile) (with calcification) I70.90 — *continued*
  extremities (native arteries) I70.209 — *continued*
    bypass graft I70.309 — *continued*
      nonbiological graft I70.609 — *continued*
        leg I70.609 — *continued*
          left I70.602
           with
            gangrene (and intermittent claudication, rest pain and ulcer) I70.662
            intermittent claudication I70.612
            rest pain (and intermittent claudication) I70.622
            ulceration (and intermittent claudication and rest pain) I70.649
              ankle I70.643
              calf I70.642
              foot site NEC I70.645
              heel I70.644
              lower leg NEC I70.648
              midfoot I70.644
              thigh I70.641
          specified type NEC I70.692
        right I70.601
          with
            gangrene (and intermittent claudication, rest pain and ulcer) I70.661
            intermittent claudication I70.611
            rest pain (and intermittent claudication) I70.621
            ulceration (and intermittent claudication and rest pain) I70.639
              ankle I70.633
              calf I70.632
              foot site NEC I70.635
              heel I70.634
              lower leg NEC I70.638
              midfoot I70.634
              thigh I70.631
          specified type NEC I70.691
        specified type NEC I70.699
      specified NEC I70.608
        with
          gangrene (and intermittent claudication, rest pain and ulcer) I70.668
          intermittent claudication I70.618
          rest pain (and intermittent claudication) I70.628
          ulceration (and intermittent claudication and rest pain) I70.65
          specified type NEC I70.698
      specified graft NEC I70.709
        leg I70.709
          with
           gangrene (and intermittent claudication, rest pain and ulcer) I70.769
           intermittent claudication I70.719
           rest pain (and intermittent claudication) I70.729
          bilateral I70.703
           with
            gangrene (and intermittent claudication, rest pain and ulcer) I70.763
            intermittent claudication I70.713
            rest pain (and intermittent claudication) I70.723
            specified type NEC I70.793

Arteriosclerosis, arteriosclerotic (diffuse) (obliterans) (of) (senile) (with calcification) I70.90 — *continued*
  extremities (native arteries) I70.209 — *continued*
    bypass graft I70.309 — *continued*
      specified graft NEC I70.709 — *continued*
        leg I70.709 — *continued*
          left I70.702
            with
              gangrene (and intermittent claudication, rest pain and ulcer) I70.762
              intermittent claudication I70.712
              rest pain (and intermittent claudication) I70.722
              ulceration (and intermittent claudication and rest pain) I70.749
                ankle I70.743
                calf I70.742
                foot site NEC I70.745
                heel I70.744
                lower leg NEC I70.748
                midfoot I70.744
                thigh I70.741
            specified type NEC I70.792
          right I70.701
            with
              gangrene (and intermittent claudication, rest pain and ulcer) I70.761
              intermittent claudication I70.711
              rest pain (and intermittent claudication) I70.721
              ulceration (and intermittent claudication and rest pain) I70.739
                ankle I70.733
                calf I70.732
                foot site NEC I70.735
                heel I70.734
                lower leg NEC I70.738
                midfoot I70.734
                thigh I70.731
            specified type NEC I70.791
        specified type NEC I70.799
      specified NEC I70.708
        with
          gangrene (and intermittent claudication, rest pain and ulcer) I70.768
          intermittent claudication I70.718
          rest pain (and intermittent claudication) I70.728
          ulceration (and intermittent claudication and rest pain) I70.75
          specified type NEC I70.798
    specified NEC I70.308
      with
        gangrene (and intermittent claudication, rest pain and ulcer) I70.368
        intermittent claudication I70.318
        rest pain (and intermittent claudication) I70.328
        ulceration (and intermittent claudication and rest pain) I70.35
        specified type NEC I70.398
    leg I70.209
      with
        gangrene (and intermittent claudication, rest pain and ulcer) I70.269
        intermittent claudication I70.219
        rest pain (and intermittent claudication) I70.229

Arteriosclerosis, arteriosclerotic (diffuse) (obliterans) (of) (senile) (with calcification) I70.90 — *continued*
  extremities (native arteries) I70.209 — *continued*
    leg I70.209 — *continued*
      bilateral I70.203
        with
          gangrene (and intermittent claudication, rest pain and ulcer) I70.263
          intermittent claudication I70.213
          rest pain (and intermittent claudication) I70.223
          specified type NEC I70.293
      left I70.202
        with
          gangrene (and intermittent claudication, rest pain and ulcer) I70.262
          intermittent claudication I70.212
          rest pain (and intermittent claudication) I70.222
          ulceration (and intermittent claudication and rest pain) I70.249
            ankle I70.243
            calf I70.242
            foot site NEC I70.245
            heel I70.244
            lower leg NEC I70.248
            midfoot I70.244
            thigh I70.241
        specified type NEC I70.292
      right I70.201
        with
          gangrene (and intermittent claudication, rest pain and ulcer) I70.261
          intermittent claudication I70.211
          rest pain (and intermittent claudication) I70.221
          ulceration (and intermittent claudication and rest pain) I70.239
            ankle I70.233
            calf I70.232
            foot site NEC I70.235
            heel I70.234
            lower leg NEC I70.238
            midfoot I70.234
            thigh I70.231
        specified type NEC I70.291
    specified type NEC I70.299
    specified site NEC I70.208
      with
        gangrene (and intermittent claudication, rest pain and ulcer) I70.268
        intermittent claudication I70.218
        rest pain (and intermittent claudication) I70.228
        ulceration (and intermittent claudication and rest pain) I70.25
        specified type NEC I70.298
  generalized I70.91
  heart (disease) — *see* Arteriosclerosis, coronary (artery),
  kidney — *see* Hypertension, kidney
  medial — *see* Arteriosclerosis, extremities
  mesenteric (artery) K55.1
  myocarditis I51.4
  Mönckeberg's — *see* Arteriosclerosis, extremities
  peripheral (of extremities) — *see* Arteriosclerosis, extremities
  pulmonary (idiopathic) I27.0

Arteriosclerosis, arteriosclerotic (diffuse) (obliterans) (of) (senile) (with calcification) I70.90 — *continued*
  renal (arterioles) — *see also* Hypertension, kidney
    artery I70.1
  retina (vascular) I70.8 *[H35.0-]*
  specified artery NEC I70.8
  spinal (cord) G95.19
  vertebral (artery) I67.2
Arteriospasm I73.9
Arteriovenous — *see* condition
Arteritis I77.6
  allergic M31.0
  aorta (nonsyphilitic) I77.6
    syphilitic A52.02
  aortic arch M31.4
  brachiocephalic M31.4
  brain I67.7
    syphilitic A52.04
  cerebral I67.7
    in
      diseases classified elsewhere I68.2
      systemic lupus erythematosus M32.19
    listerial A32.89
    syphilitic A52.04
    tuberculous A18.89
  coronary (artery) I25.89
    rheumatic I01.8
      chronic I09.89
    syphilitic A52.06
  cranial (left) (right), giant cell M31.6
  deformans — *see* Arteriosclerosis
  giant cell NEC M31.6
    with polymyalgia rheumatica M31.5
  necrosing or necrotizing M31.9
    specified NEC M31.8
  nodosa M30.0
  obliterans — *see* Arteriosclerosis
  pulmonary I28.8
  rheumatic — *see* Fever, rheumatic
  senile — *see* Arteriosclerosis
  suppurative I77.2
  syphilitic (general) A52.09
    brain A52.04
    coronary A52.06
    spinal A52.09
  temporal, giant cell M31.6
  young female aortic arch syndrome M31.4
Artery, arterial — *see also* condition
  abscess I77.89
  single umbilical Q27.0
Arthralgia (allergic) — *see also* Pain, joint
  in caisson disease T70.3
  temporomandibular M26.62-
Arthritis, arthritic (acute) (chronic) (nonpyogenic) (subacute) M19.90
  allergic — *see* Arthritis, specified form NEC
  ankylosing (crippling) (spine) — *see also* Spondylitis, ankylosing
    sites other than spine — *see* Arthritis, specified form NEC
  atrophic — *see* Osteoarthritis
    spine — *see* Spondylitis, ankylosing
  back — *see* Spondylopathy, inflammatory
  blennorrhagic (gonococcal) A54.42
  Charcot's — *see* Arthropathy, neuropathic
    diabetic — *see* Diabetes, arthropathy, neuropathic
    syringomyelic G95.0
  chylous (filarial) (see also category M01) B74.9
  climacteric (any site) NEC — *see* Arthritis, specified form NEC
  crystal(-induced) — *see* Arthritis, in, crystals
  deformans — *see* Osteoarthritis
  degenerative — *see* Osteoarthritis

Arthritis, arthritic (acute) (chronic) (nonpyogenic) (subacute) M19.90 — *continued*
due to or associated with
  acromegaly E22.0
  brucellosis — *see* Brucellosis
  caisson disease T70.3
  diabetes — *see* Diabetes, arthropathy
  dracontiasis (*see also* category M01) B72
  enteritis NEC
    regional — *see* Enteritis, regional
  erysipelas (*see also* category M01) A46
  erythema
    epidemic A25.1
    nodosum L52
  filariasis NOS B74.9
  glanders A24.0
  helminthiasis (*see also* category M01) B83.9
  hemophilia D66 *[M36.2]*
  Henoch-(Schönlein) purpura D69.0 *[M36.4]*
  human parvovirus (*see also* category M01) B97.6
  infectious disease NEC — *see* category M01
  leprosy (*see also* category M01) (*see also* Leprosy) A30.9
  Lyme disease A69.23
  mycobacteria (*see also* category M01) A31.8
  parasitic disease NEC (*see also* category M01) B89
  paratyphoid fever (*see also* category M01) (*see also* Fever, paratyphoid) A01.4
  rat bite fever (*see also* category M01) A25.1
  regional enteritis — *see* Enteritis, regional
  respiratory disorder NOS J98.9
  serum sickness (*see also* Reaction, serum) T80.69
  syringomyelia G95.0
  typhoid fever A01.04
epidemic erythema A25.1
febrile — *see* Fever, rheumatic
gonococcal A54.42
gouty (acute) — *see* Gout
in (due to)
  acromegaly (*see also* subcategory M14.8-) E22.0
  amyloidosis (*see also* subcategory M14.8-) E85.4
  bacterial disease (*see also* category M01) A49.9
  Behçet's syndrome M35.2
  caisson disease (*see also* subcategory M14.8-) T70.3
  coliform bacilli (Escherichia coli) — *see* Arthritis, in, pyogenic organism NEC
  crystals M11.9
    dicalcium phosphate — *see* Arthritis, in, crystals, specified type NEC
    hydroxyapatite M11.0-
    pyrophosphate — *see* Arthritis, in, crystals, specified type NEC
    specified type NEC M11.80
      ankle M11.87-
      elbow M11.82-
      foot joint M11.87-
      hand joint M11.84-
      hip M11.85-
      knee M11.86-
      multiple sites M11.8-
      shoulder M11.81-
      vertebrae M11.88
      wrist M11.83-
  dermatoarthritis, lipoid E78.81
  dracontiasis (dracunculiasis) (*see also* category M01) B72
  endocrine disorder NEC (*see also* subcategory M14.8-) E34.9

Arthritis, arthritic (acute) (chronic) (nonpyogenic) (subacute) M19.90 — *continued*
in (due to) — *continued*
  enteritis, infectious NEC (*see also* category M01) A09
    specified organism NEC (*see also* category M01) A08.8
  erythema
    multiforme (*see also* subcategory M14.8-) L51.9
    nodosum (*see also* subcategory M14.8-) L52
  gout — *see* Gout
  helminthiasis NEC (*see also* category M01) B83.9
  hemochromatosis (*see also* subcategory M14.8-) E83.118
  hemoglobinopathy NEC D58.2 *[M36.3]*
  hemophilia NEC D66 *[M36.2]*
  Hemophilus influenzae M00.8- *[B96.3]*
  Henoch(-Schönlein) purpura D69.0 *[M36.4]*
  hyperparathyroidism NEC (*see also* subcategory M14.8-) E21.3
  hypersensitivity reaction NEC T78.49 *[M36.4]*
  hypogammaglobulinemia (*see also* subcategory M14.8-) D80.1
  hypothyroidism NEC (*see also* subcategory M14.8-) E03.9
  infection — *see* Arthritis, pyogenic or pyemic
    spine — *see* Spondylopathy, infective
  infectious disease NEC — *see* category M01
  leprosy (*see also* category M01) A30.9
  leukemia NEC C95.9- *[M36.1]*
  lipoid dermatoarthritis E78.81
  Lyme disease A69.23
  Mediterranean fever, familial (*see also* subcategory M14.8-) M04.1
  Meningococcus A39.83
  metabolic disorder NEC (*see also* subcategory M14.8-) E88.9
  multiple myelomatosis C90.0- [M36.1]
  mumps B26.85
  mycosis NEC (*see also* category M01) B49
  myelomatosis (multiple) C90.0- *[M36.1]*
  neurological disorder NEC G98.0
  ochronosis (*see also* subcategory M14.8-) E70.29
  O'nyong-nyong (*see also* category M01) A92.1
  parasitic disease NEC (*see also* category M01) B89
  paratyphoid fever (*see also* category M01) A01.4
  Pseudomonas — *see* Arthritis, pyogenic, bacterial NEC
  psoriasis L40.50
  pyogenic organism NEC — *see* Arthritis, pyogenic, bacterial NEC
  Reiter's disease — *see* Reiter's disease
  respiratory disorder NEC (*see also* subcategory M14.8-) J98.9
  reticulosis, malignant (*see also* subcategory M14.8-) C86.0
  rubella B06.82
  Salmonella (arizonae) (cholerae-suis) (enteritidis) (typhimurium) A02.23
  sarcoidosis D86.86
  specified bacteria NEC — *see* Arthritis, pyogenic, bacterial NEC
  sporotrichosis B42.82
  syringomyelia G95.0
  thalassemia NEC D56.9 *[M36.3]*
  tuberculosis — *see* Tuberculosis, arthritis
  typhoid fever A01.04
  urethritis, Reiter's — *see* Reiter's disease

Arthritis, arthritic (acute) (chronic) (nonpyogenic) (subacute) M19.90 — *continued*
in (due to) — *continued*
  viral disease NEC (*see also* category M01) B34.9
infectious or infective — *see also* Arthritis, pyogenic or pyemic
  spine — *see* Spondylopathy, infective
juvenile M08.90
  with systemic onset — *see* Still's disease
  ankle M08.97-
  elbow M08.92-
  foot joint M08.97-
  hand joint M08.94-
  hip M08.95-
  knee M08.96-
  multiple site M08.99
  pauciarticular M08.40
    ankle M08.47-
    elbow M08.42-
    foot joint M08.47-
    hand joint M08.44-
    hip M08.45-
    knee M08.46-
    shoulder M08.41-
    vertebrae M08.48
    wrist M08.43-
  psoriatic L40.54
  rheumatoid — *see* Arthritis, rheumatoid, juvenile
  shoulder M08.91-
  specified type NEC M08.80
    ankle M08.87-
    elbow M08.82-
    foot joint M08.87-
    hand joint M08.84-
    hip M08.85-
    knee M08.86-
    multiple site M08.89
    shoulder M08.81-
    specified joint NEC M08.88
    vertebrae M08.88
    wrist M08.83-
  wrist M08.93-
meaning osteoarthritis — *see* Osteoarthritis
meningococcal A39.83
menopausal (any site) NEC — *see* Arthritis, specified form NEC
mutilans (psoriatic) L40.52
mycotic NEC (*see also* category M01) B49
neuropathic (Charcot) — *see* Arthropathy, neuropathic
  diabetic — *see* Diabetes, arthropathy, neuropathic
  nonsyphilitic NEC G98.0
  syringomyelic G95.0
ochronotic (*see also* subcategory M14.8-) E70.29
palindromic (any site) — *see* Rheumatism, palindromic
pneumococcal M00.10
  ankle M00.17-
  elbow M00.12-
  foot joint — *see* Arthritis, pneumococcal, ankle
  hand joint M00.14-
  hip M00.15-
  knee M00.16-
  multiple site M00.19
  shoulder M00.11-
  vertebra M00.18
  wrist M00.13-
postdysenteric — *see* Arthropathy, postdysenteric
postmeningococcal A39.84
postrheumatic, chronic — *see* Arthropathy, postrheumatic, chronic

Arthritis, arthritic (acute) (chronic)
(nonpyogenic) (subacute) M19.90 —
continued
  primary progressive — see also Arthritis,
    specified form NEC
    spine — see Spondylitis, ankylosing
  psoriatic L40.50
  purulent (any site except spine) — see Arthritis,
    pyogenic or pyemic
    spine — see Spondylopathy, infective
  pyogenic or pyemic (any site except spine)
    M00.9
    bacterial NEC M00.80
      ankle M00.87-
      elbow M00.82-
      foot joint — see Arthritis, pyogenic,
        bacterial NEC, ankle
      hand joint M00.84-
      hip M00.85-
      knee M00.86-
      multiple site M00.89
      shoulder M00.81-
      vertebra M00.88
      wrist M00.83-
    pneumococcal — see Arthritis,
      pneumococcal
    spine — see Spondylopathy, infective
    staphylococcal — see Arthritis,
      staphylococcal
    streptococcal — see Arthritis, streptococcal
      NEC
    pneumococcal — see Arthritis,
      pneumococcal
  reactive — see Reiter's disease
  rheumatic — see also Arthritis, rheumatoid
    acute or subacute — see Fever, rheumatic
  rheumatoid M06.9
    with
      carditis — see Rheumatoid, carditis
      endocarditis — see Rheumatoid, carditis
      heart involvement NEC — see Rheumatoid,
        carditis
      lung involvement — see Rheumatoid, lung
      myocarditis — see Rheumatoid, carditis
      myopathy — see Rheumatoid, myopathy
      pericarditis — see Rheumatoid, carditis
      polyneuropathy — see Rheumatoid,
        polyneuropathy
      rheumatoid factor — see Arthritis,
        rheumatoid, seropositive
      splenoadenomegaly and leukopenia — see
        Felty's syndrome
      vasculitis — see Rheumatoid, vasculitis
      visceral involvement NEC —
        see Rheumatoid, arthritis, with
        involvement of organs NEC
    juvenile (with or without rheumatoid factor)
      M08.00
      ankle M08.07-
      elbow M08.02-
      foot joint M08.07-
      hand joint M08.04-
      hip M08.05-
      knee M08.06-
      multiple site M08.09
      shoulder M08.01-
      vertebra M08.08
      wrist M08.03-
    seronegative M06.00
      ankle M06.07-
      elbow M06.02-
      foot joint M06.07-
      hand joint M06.04-
      hip M06.05-
      knee M06.06-
      multiple site M06.09
      shoulder M06.01-
      vertebra M06.08

Arthritis, arthritic (acute) (chronic)
(nonpyogenic) (subacute) M19.90 —
continued
  rheumatoid M06.9 — continued
    seronegative M06.00 — continued
      wrist M06.03-
    seropositive M05.9
      specified NEC M05.80
        ankle M05.87-
        elbow M05.82-
        foot joint M05.87-
        hand joint M05.84-
        hip M05.85-
        knee M05.86-
        multiple sites M05.89
        shoulder M05.81-
        vertebra — see Spondylitis, ankylosing
        wrist M05.83-
      without organ involvement M05.70
        ankle M05.77-
        elbow M05.72-
        foot joint M05.77-
        hand joint M05.74-
        hip M05.75-
        knee M05.76-
        multiple sites M05.79
        shoulder M05.71-
        vertebra — see Spondylitis, ankylosing
        wrist M05.73-
    specified type NEC M06.80
      ankle M06.87-
      elbow M06.82-
      foot joint M06.87-
      hand joint M06.84-
      hip M06.85-
      knee M06.86-
      multiple site M06.89
      shoulder M06.81-
      vertebra M06.88
      wrist M06.83-
    spine — see Spondylitis, ankylosing
  rubella B06.82
  scorbutic (see also subcategory M14.8-) E54
  senile or senescent — see Osteoarthritis
  septic (any site except spine) — see Arthritis,
    pyogenic or pyemic
    spine — see Spondylopathy, infective
  serum (nontherapeutic) (therapeutic) — see
    Arthropathy, postimmunization
  specified form NEC M13.80
    ankle M13.87-
    elbow M13.82-
    foot joint M13.87-
    hand joint M13.84-
    hip M13.85-
    knee M13.86-
    multiple site M13.89
    shoulder M13.81-
    specified joint NEC M13.88
    wrist M13.83-
  spine — see also Spondylopathy, inflammatory
    infectious or infective NEC — see
      Spondylopathy, infective
    Marie-Strümpell — see Spondylitis,
      ankylosing
    pyogenic — see Spondylopathy, infective
    rheumatoid — see Spondylitis, ankylosing
    traumatic (old) — see Spondylopathy,
      traumatic
    tuberculous A18.01
  staphylococcal M00.00
    ankle M00.07-
    elbow M00.02-
    foot joint — see Arthritis, staphylococcal,
      ankle
    hand joint M00.04-
    hip M00.05-
    knee M00.06-

Arthritis, arthritic (acute) (chronic)
(nonpyogenic) (subacute) M19.90 —
continued
  staphylococcal M00.00 — continued
    multiple site M00.09
    shoulder M00.01-
    vertebra M00.08
    wrist M00.03-
  streptococcal NEC M00.20
    ankle M00.27-
    elbow M00.22-
    foot joint — see Arthritis, streptococcal, ankle
    hand joint M00.24-
    hip M00.25-
    knee M00.26-
    multiple site M00.29
    shoulder M00.21-
    vertebra M00.28
    wrist M00.23-
  suppurative — see Arthritis, pyogenic or
    pyemic
  syphilitic (late) A52.16
    congenital A50.55 [M12.80]
  syphilitica deformans (Charcot) A52.16
  temporomandibular M26.69
  toxic of menopause (any site) — see Arthritis,
    specified form NEC
  transient — see Arthropathy, specified form
    NEC
  traumatic (chronic) — see Arthropathy,
    traumatic
  tuberculous A18.02
    spine A18.01
  uratic — see Gout
  urethritica (Reiter's) — see Reiter's disease
  vertebral — see Spondylopathy, inflammatory
  villous (any site) — see Arthropathy, specified
    form NEC
Arthrocele — see Effusion, joint
Arthrodesis status Z98.1
Arthrodynia — see also Pain, joint
Arthrodysplasia Q74.9
Arthrofibrosis, joint — see Ankylosis
Arthrogryposis (congenital) Q68.8
  multiplex congenita Q74.3
Arthrokatadysis M24.7
Arthropathy (see also Arthritis) M12.9
  Charcot's — see Arthropathy, neuropathic
    diabetic — see Diabetes, arthropathy,
      neuropathic
    syringomyelic G95.0
  cricoarytenoid J38.7
  crystal(-induced) — see Arthritis, in, crystals
  diabetic NEC — see Diabetes, arthropathy
  distal interphalangeal, psoriatic L40.51
  enteropathic M07.60
    ankle M07.67-
    elbow M07.62-
    foot joint M07.67-
    hand joint M07.64-
    hip M07.65-
    knee M07.66-
    multiple site M07.69
    shoulder M07.61-
    vertebra M07.68
    wrist M07.63-
  following intestinal bypass M02.00
    ankle M02.07-
    elbow M02.02-
    foot joint M02.07-
    hand joint M02.04-
    hip M02.05-
    knee M02.06-
    multiple site M02.09
    shoulder M02.01-
    vertebra M02.08
    wrist M02.03-

Arthropathy (*see also* Arthritis) M12.9 — *continued*
 gouty — *see also* Gout
  in (due to)
   Lesch-Nyhan syndrome E79.1 *[M14.8-]*
   sickle-cell disorders D57- *[M14.8-]*
 hemophilic NEC D66 *[M36.2]*
  in (due to)
   hyperparathyroidism NEC E21.3 *[M14.8-]*
   metabolic disease NOS E88.9 *[M14.8-]*
 in (due to)
  acromegaly E22.0 *[M14.8-]*
  amyloidosis E85.4 *[M14.8-]*
  blood disorder NOS D75.9 *[M36.3]*
  diabetes — *see* Diabetes, arthropathy
  endocrine disease NOS E34.9 *[M14.8-]*
  erythema
   multiforme L51.9 *[M14.8-]*
   nodosum L52 *[M14.8-]*
  hemochromatosis E83.118 *[M14.8-]*
  hemoglobinopathy NEC D58.2 *[M36.3]*
  hemophilia NEC D66 *[M36.2]*
  Henoch-Schönlein purpura D69.0 *[M36.4]*
  hyperthyroidism E05.90 *[M14.8-]*
  hypothyroidism E03.9 *[M14.8-]*
  infective endocarditis I33.0 *[M12.80]*
  leukemia NEC C95.9- *[M36.1]*
  malignant histiocytosis C96.A *[M36.1]*
   (follows C96.6)
  metabolic disease NOS E88.9 *[M14.8-]*
  multiple myeloma C90.0- *[M36.1]*
  neoplastic disease NOS (*see also* Neoplasm) D49.9 *[M36.1]*
  nutritional deficiency (*see also* subcategory M14.8-) E63.9
  psoriasis NOS L40.50
  sarcoidosis D86.86
  syphilis (late) A52.77
   congenital A50.55 *[M12.80]*
  thyrotoxicosis (*see also* subcategory M14.8-) E05.90
  ulcerative colitis K51.90 *[M07.60]*
  viral hepatitis (postinfectious) NEC B19.9 *[M12.80]*
  Whipple's disease (*see also* subcategory M14.8-) K90.81
 Jaccoud — *see* Arthropathy, postrheumatic, chronic
 juvenile — *see* Arthritis, juvenile
  psoriatic L40.54
 mutilans (psoriatic) L40.52
 neuropathic (Charcot) M14.60
  ankle M14.67-
  diabetic — *see* Diabetes, arthropathy, neuropathic
  elbow M14.62-
  foot joint M14.67-
  hand joint M14.64-
  hip M14.65-
  knee M14.66-
  multiple site M14.69
  nonsyphilitic NEC G98.0
  shoulder M14.61-
  syringomyelic G95.0
  vertebra M14.68
  wrist M14.63-
 osteopulmonary — *see* Osteoarthropathy, hypertrophic, specified NEC
 postdysenteric M02.10
  ankle M02.17-
  elbow M02.12-
  foot joint M02.17-
  hand joint M02.14-
  hip M02.15-
  knee M02.16-
  multiple site M02.19
  shoulder M02.11-
  vertebra M02.18

Arthropathy (*see also* Arthritis) M12.9 — *continued*
 postdysenteric M02.10 — *continued*
  wrist M02.13-
 postimmunization M02.20
  ankle M02.27-
  elbow M02.22-
  foot joint M02.27-
  hand joint M02.24-
  hip M02.25-
  knee M02.26-
  multiple site M02.29
  shoulder M02.21-
  vertebra M02.28
  wrist M02.23-
 postinfectious NEC B99 *[M12.80]*
  in (due to)
   enteritis due to Yersinia enterocolitica A04.6 *[M12.80]*
   syphilis A52.77
   viral hepatitis NEC B19.9 *[M12.80]*
 postrheumatic, chronic (Jaccoud) M12.00
  ankle M12.07-
  elbow M12.02-
  foot joint M12.07-
  hand joint M12.04-
  hip M12.05-
  knee M12.06-
  multiple site M12.09
  shoulder M12.01-
  specified joint NEC M12.08
  vertebrae M12.08
  wrist M12.03-
 psoriatic NEC L40.59
  interphalangeal, distal L40.51
 reactive M02.9
  in (due to)
   infective endocarditis I33.0 *[M02.9]*
  specified type NEC M02.80
   ankle M02.87-
   elbow M02.82-
   foot joint M02.87-
   hand joint M02.84-
   hip M02.85-
   knee M02.86-
   multiple site M02.89
   shoulder M02.81-
   vertebra M02.88
   wrist M02.83-
 specified form NEC M12.80
  ankle M12.87-
  elbow M12.82-
  foot joint M12.87-
  hand joint M12.84-
  hip M12.85-
  knee M12.86-
  multiple site M12.89
  shoulder M12.81-
  specified joint NEC M12.88
  vertebrae M12.88
  wrist M12.83-
 syringomyelic G95.0
 tabes dorsalis A52.16
 tabetic A52.16
 transient — *see* Arthropathy, specified form NEC
 traumatic M12.50
  ankle M12.57-
  elbow M12.52-
  foot joint M12.57-
  hand joint M12.54-
  hip M12.55-
  knee M12.56-
  multiple site M12.59
  shoulder M12.51-
  specified joint NEC M12.58
  vertebrae M12.58
  wrist M12.53-

Arthropyosis — *see* Arthritis, pyogenic or pyemic
Arthrosis (deformans) (degenerative) (localized) (*see also* Osteoarthritis) M19.90
 spine — *see* Spondylosis
Arthus' phenomenon or reaction T78.41
 due to
  drug — *see* Table of Drugs and Chemicals, by drug
Articular — *see* condition
Articulation, reverse (teeth) M26.24
Artificial
 insemination complication — *see* Complications, artificial, fertilization
 opening status (functioning) (without complication) Z93.9
  anus (colostomy) Z93.3
  colostomy Z93.3
  cystostomy Z93.50
   appendico-vesicostomy Z93.52
   cutaneous Z93.51
   specified NEC Z93.59
  enterostomy Z93.4
  gastrostomy Z93.1
  ileostomy Z93.2
  intestinal tract NEC Z93.4
  jejunostomy Z93.4
  nephrostomy Z93.6
  specified site NEC Z93.8
  tracheostomy Z93.0
  ureterostomy Z93.6
  urethrostomy Z93.6
  urinary tract NEC Z93.6
  vagina Z93.8
 vagina status Z93.8
Arytenoid — *see* condition
Asbestosis (occupational) J61
Ascariasis B77.9
 with
  complications NEC B77.89
  intestinal complications B77.0
  pneumonia, pneumonitis B77.81
Ascaridosis, ascaridiasis — *see* Ascariasis
Ascaris (infection) (infestation) (lumbricoides) — *see* Ascariasis
Ascending — *see* condition
ASC-H (atypical squamous cells cannot exclude high grade squamous intraepithelial lesion on cytologic smear)
 anus R85.611
 cervix R87.611
 vagina R87.621
Aschoff's bodies — *see* Myocarditis, rheumatic
Ascites (abdominal) R18.8
 cardiac I50.9
 chylous (nonfilarial) I89.8
  filarial — *see* Infestation, filarial
 due to
  cirrhosis, alcoholic K70.31
  hepatitis
   alcoholic K70.11
   chronic active K71.51
  S. japonicum B65.2
 heart I50.9
 malignant R18.0
 pseudochylous R18.8
 syphilitic A52.74
 tuberculous A18.31
ASC-US (atypical squamous cells of undetermined significance on cytologic smear)
 anus R85.610
 cervix R87.610
 vagina R87.620
Aseptic — *see* condition
Asherman's syndrome N85.6
Asialia K11.7
Asiatic cholera — *see* Cholera

Asimultagnosia (simultanagnosia) R48.3

Askin's tumor — *see* Neoplasm, connective tissue, malignant

Asocial personality F60.2

Asomatognosia R41.4

Aspartylglucosaminuria E77.1

Asperger's disease or syndrome F84.5

Aspergilloma — *see* Aspergillosis

Aspergillosis (with pneumonia) B44.9
  bronchopulmonary, allergic B44.81
  disseminated B44.7
  generalized B44.7
  pulmonary NEC B44.1
    allergic B44.81
    invasive B44.0
  specified NEC B44.89
  tonsillar B44.2

Aspergillus (flavus) (fumigatus) (infection) (terreus) — *see* Aspergillosis

Aspermatogenesis — *see* Azoospermia

Aspermia (testis) — *see* Azoospermia

Asphyxia, asphyxiation (by) R09.01
  antenatal P84
  birth P84
  bunny bag — *see* Asphyxia, due to, mechanical threat to breathing, trapped in bed clothes
  crushing S28.0
  drowning T75.1
  gas, fumes, or vapor — *see* Table of Drugs and Chemicals
  inhalation — *see* Inhalation
  intrauterine P84
  local I73.00
    with gangrene I73.01
  mucus — *see also* Foreign body, respiratory tract, causing asphyxia
  newborn P84
  pathological R09.01
  postnatal P84
    mechanical — *see* Asphyxia, due to, mechanical threat to breathing
  prenatal P84
  reticularis R23.1
  strangulation — *see* Asphyxia, due to, mechanical threat to breathing
  submersion T75.1
  traumatic T71.9
    due to
      crushed chest S28.0
      foreign body (in) — *see* Foreign body, respiratory tract, causing asphyxia
      low oxygen content of ambient air T71.20
        due to
          being trapped in
            low oxygen environment T71.29
              in car trunk T71.221
                circumstances undetermined T71.224
                done with intent to harm by another person T71.223
                self T71.222
              in refrigerator T71.231
                circumstances undetermined T71.234
                done with intent to harm by another person T71.233
                self T71.232
            cave-in T71.21
      mechanical threat to breathing (accidental) T71.191
        circumstances undetermined T71.194
        done with intent to harm by another person T71.193
        self T71.192

Asphyxia, asphyxiation (by) R09.01 — *continued*
  traumatic T71.9 — *continued*
    due to — *continued*
      mechanical threat to breathing (accidental) T71.191 — *continued*
        hanging T71.161
          circumstances undetermined T71.164
          done with intent to harm by another person T71.163
          self T71.162
        plastic bag T71.121
          circumstances undetermined T71.124
          done with intent to harm by another person T71.123
          self T71.122
        smothering
          in furniture T71.151
            circumstances undetermined T71.154
            done with intent to harm by another person T71.153
            self T71.152
          under
            another person's body T71.141
              circumstances undetermined T71.144
              done with intent to harm T71.143
            pillow T71.111
              circumstances undetermined T71.114
              done with intent to harm by another person T71.113
              self T71.112
            trapped in bed clothes T71.131
              circumstances undetermined T71.134
              done with intent to harm by another person T71.133
              self T71.132
      vomiting, vomitus — *see* Foreign body, respiratory tract, causing asphyxia

Aspiration
  amniotic (clear) fluid (newborn) P24.10
    with
      pneumonia (pneumonitis) P24.11
      respiratory symptoms P24.11
  blood
    newborn (without respiratory symptoms) P24.20
      with
        pneumonia (pneumonitis) P24.21
        respiratory symptoms P24.21
      specified age NEC — *see* Foreign body, respiratory tract
  bronchitis J69.0
  food or foreign body (with asphyxiation) — *see* Asphyxia, food
  liquor (amnii) (newborn) P24.10
    with
      pneumonia (pneumonitis) P24.11
      respiratory symptoms P24.11
  meconium (newborn) (without respiratory symptoms) P24.00
    with
      pneumonitis (pneumonitis) P24.01
      respiratory symptoms P24.01
  milk (newborn) (without respiratory symptoms) P24.30
    with
      pneumonia (pneumonitis) P24.31
      respiratory symptoms P24.31
    specified age NEC — *see* Foreign body, respiratory tract
  mucus — *see also* Foreign body, by site, causing asphyxia
    newborn P24.10
      with
        pneumonia (pneumonitis) P24.11
        respiratory symptoms P24.11

Aspiration — *continued*
  neonatal P24.9
    specific NEC (without respiratory symptoms) P24.80
      with
        pneumonia (pneumonitis) P24.81
        respiratory symptoms P24.81
    newborn P24.9
      specific NEC (without respiratory symptoms) P24.80
        with
          pneumonia (pneumonitis) P24.81
          respiratory symptoms P24.81
    pneumonia J69.0
    pneumonitis J69.0
    syndrome of newborn — *see* Aspiration, by substance, with pneumonia
    vernix caseosa (newborn) P24.80
      with
        pneumonia (pneumonitis) P24.81
        respiratory symptoms P24.81
    vomitus — *see also* Foreign body, respiratory tract
      newborn (without respiratory symptoms) P24.30
        with
          pneumonia (pneumonitis) P24.31
          respiratory symptoms P24.31

Asplenia (congenital) Q89.01
  postsurgical Z90.81

Assam fever B55.0

Assault, sexual — *see* Maltreatment

Assmann's focus NEC A15.0

Astasia(-abasia) (hysterical) F44.4

Asteatosis cutis L85.3

Astereognosia, astereognosis R48.1

Asterixis R27.8
  in liver disease K71.3

Asteroid hyalitis — *see* Deposit, crystalline

Asthenia, asthenic R53.1
  cardiac (*see also* Failure, heart) I50.9
    psychogenic F45.8
  cardiovascular (*see also* Failure, heart) I50.9
    psychogenic F45.8
  heart (*see also* Failure, heart) I50.9
    psychogenic F45.8
  hysterical F44.4
  myocardial (*see also* Failure, heart) I50.9
    psychogenic F45.8
  nervous F48.8
  neurocirculatory F45.8
  neurotic F48.8
  psychogenic F48.8
  psychoneurotic F48.8
  psychophysiologic F48.8
  reaction (psychophysiologic) F48.8
  senile R54

Asthenopia — *see also* Discomfort, visual
  hysterical F44.6
  psychogenic F44.6

Asthenospermia — *see* Abnormal, specimen, male genital organs

Asthma, asthmatic (bronchial) (catarrh) (spasmodic) J45.909
  with
    chronic obstructive bronchitis J44.9
      with
        acute lower respiratory infection J44.0
        exacerbation (acute) J44.1
    chronic obstructive pulmonary disease J44.9
      with
        acute lower respiratory infection J44.0
        exacerbation (acute) J44.1
    exacerbation (acute) J45.901
  hay fever — *see* Asthma, allergic extrinsic
  rhinitis, allergic — *see* Asthma, allergic extrinsic
  status asthmaticus J45.902

Asthma, asthmatic (bronchial) (catarrh) (spasmodic) J45.909 — *continued*
  allergic extrinsic J45.909
    with
      exacerbation (acute) J45.901
      status asthmaticus J45.902
  atopic — *see* Asthma, allergic extrinsic
  cardiac — *see* Failure, ventricular, left
  cardiobronchial I50.1
  childhood J45.909
    with
      exacerbation (acute) J45.901
      status asthmaticus J45.902
  chronic obstructive J44.9
    with
      acute lower respiratory infection J44.0
      exacerbation (acute) J44.1
  collier's J60
  cough variant J45.991
  detergent J69.8
  due to
    detergent J69.8
    inhalation of fumes J68.3
  eosinophilic J82
  extrinsic, allergic — *see* Asthma, allergic extrinsic
  grinder's J62.8
  hay — *see* Asthma, allergic extrinsic
  heart I50.1
  idiosyncratic — *see* Asthma, nonallergic
  intermittent (mild) J45.20
    with
      exacerbation (acute) J45.21
      status asthmaticus J45.22
  intrinsic, nonallergic — *see* Asthma, nonallergic
  Kopp's E32.8
  late-onset J45.909
    with
      exacerbation (acute) J45.901
      status asthmaticus J45.902
  mild intermittent J45.20
    with
      exacerbation (acute) J45.21
      status asthmaticus J45.22
  mild persistent J45.30
    with
      exacerbation (acute) J45.31
      status asthmaticus J45.32
  Millar's (laryngismus stridulus) J38.5
  miner's J60
  mixed J45.909
    with
      exacerbation (acute) J45.901
      status asthmaticus J45.902
  moderate persistent J45.40
    with
      exacerbation (acute) J45.41
      status asthmaticus J45.42
  nervous — *see* Asthma, nonallergic
  nonallergic (intrinsic) J45.909
    with
      exacerbation (acute) J45.901
      status asthmaticus J45.902
  persistent
    mild J45.30
      with
        exacerbation (acute) J45.31
        status asthmaticus J45.32
    moderate J45.40
      with
        exacerbation (acute) J45.41
        status asthmaticus J45.42
    severe J45.50
      with
        exacerbation (acute) J45.51
        status asthmaticus J45.52
  platinum J45.998
  pneumoconiotic NEC J64

Asthma, asthmatic (bronchial) (catarrh) (spasmodic) J45.909 — *continued*
  potter's J62.8
  predominantly allergic J45.909
  psychogenic F54
  pulmonary eosinophilic J82
  red cedar J67.8
  Rostan's I50.1
  sandblaster's J62.8
  sequoiosis J67.8
  severe persistent J45.50
    with
      exacerbation (acute) J45.51
      status asthmaticus J45.52
  specified NEC J45.998
  stonemason's J62.8
  thymic E32.8
  tuberculous — *see* Tuberculosis, pulmonary
  Wichmann's (laryngismus stridulus) J38.5
  wood J67.8
Astigmatism (compound) (congenital) H52.20-
  irregular H52.21-
  regular H52.22-
Astraphobia F40.220
Astroblastoma
  specified site — *see* Neoplasm, malignant, by site
  unspecified site C71.9
Astrocytoma (cystic)
  anaplastic
    specified site — *see* Neoplasm, malignant, by site
    unspecified site C71.9
  fibrillary
    specified site — *see* Neoplasm, malignant, by site
    unspecified site C71.9
  fibrous
    specified site — *see* Neoplasm, malignant, by site
    unspecified site C71.9
  gemistocytic
    specified site — *see* Neoplasm, malignant, by site
    unspecified site C71.9
  juvenile
    specified site — *see* Neoplasm, malignant, by site
    unspecified site C71.9
  pilocytic
    specified site — *see* Neoplasm, malignant, by site
    unspecified site C71.9
  piloid
    specified site — *see* Neoplasm, malignant, by site
    unspecified site C71.9
  protoplasmic
    specified site — *see* Neoplasm, malignant, by site
    unspecified site C71.9
  specified site NEC — *see* Neoplasm, malignant, by site
  subependymal D43.2
    giant cell
      specified site — *see* Neoplasm, uncertain behavior, by site
      unspecified site D43.2
    specified site — *see* Neoplasm, uncertain behavior, by site
    unspecified site D43.2
  unspecified site C71.9
Astroglioma
  specified site — *see* Neoplasm, malignant, by site
  unspecified site C71.9
Asymbolia R48.8

Asymmetry — *see also* Distortion
  between native and reconstructed breast N65.1
  face Q67.0
  jaw (lower) — *see* Anomaly, dentofacial, jaw-cranial base relationship, asymmetry
Asynergia, asynergy R27.8
  ventricular I51.89
Asystole (heart) — *see* Arrest, cardiac
At risk
  for falling Z91.81
Ataxia, ataxy, ataxic R27.0
  acute R27.8
  brain (hereditary) G11.9
  cerebellar (hereditary) G11.9
    with defective DNA repair G11.3
    alcoholic G31.2
    early-onset G11.1
    in
      alcoholism G31.2
      myxedema E03.9 *[G13.2]*
      neoplastic disease (*see also* Neoplasm) D49.9 *[G32.81]*
      specified disease NEC G32.81
    late-onset (Marie's) G11.2
  cerebral (hereditary) G11.9
  congenital nonprogressive G11.0
  family, familial — *see* Ataxia, hereditary
  following
    cerebrovascular disease I69.993
      cerebral infarction I69.393
      intracerebral hemorrhage I69.193
      nontraumatic intracranial hemorrhage NEC I69.293
      specified disease NEC I69.893
      subarachnoid hemorrhage I69.093
  Friedreich's (heredofamilial) (cerebellar) (spinal) G11.1
  gait R26.0
    hysterical F44.4
  general R27.8
  gluten M35.9 *[G32.81]*
    with celiac disease K90.0 *[G32.81]*
  hereditary G11.9
    with neuropathy G60.2
    cerebellar — *see* Ataxia, cerebellar
    spastic G11.4
    specified NEC G11.8
    spinal (Friedreich's) G11.1
  heredofamilial — *see* Ataxia, hereditary
  Hunt's G11.1
  hysterical F44.4
  locomotor (progressive) (syphilitic) (partial) (spastic) A52.11
    diabetic — *see* Diabetes, ataxia
  Marie's (cerebellar) (heredofamilial) (late-onset) G11.2
  nonorganic origin F44.4
  nonprogressive, congenital G11.0
  psychogenic F44.4
  Roussy-Lévy G60.0
  Sanger-Brown's (hereditary) G11.2
  spastic hereditary G11.4
  spinal
    hereditary (Friedreich's) G11.1
    progressive (syphilitic) A52.11
  spinocerebellar, X-linked recessive G11.1
  telangiectasia (Louis-Bar) G11.3
Ataxia-telangiectasia (Louis-Bar) G11.3
Atelectasis (massive) (partial) (pressure) (pulmonary) J98.11
  newborn P28.10
    due to resorption P28.11
    partial P28.19
    primary P28.0
    secondary P28.19
  primary (newborn) P28.0
  tuberculous — *see* Tuberculosis, pulmonary
Atelocardia Q24.9

Atelomyelia Q06.1
Atheroembolism
of
extremities
lower I75.02-
upper I75.01-
kidney I75.81
specified NEC I75.89
Atheroma, atheromatous (*see also* Arteriosclerosis) I70.90
aorta, aortic I70.0
valve (*see also* Endocarditis, aortic) I35.8
aorto-iliac I70.0
artery — *see* Arteriosclerosis
basilar (artery) I67.2
carotid (artery) (common) (internal) I67.2
cerebral (arteries) I67.2
coronary (artery) I25.10
with angina pectoris — *see* Arteriosclerosis, coronary (artery),
degeneration — *see* Arteriosclerosis
heart, cardiac — *see* Disease, heart, ischemic, atherosclerotic
mitral (valve) I34.8
myocardium, myocardial — *see* Disease, heart, ischemic, atherosclerotic
pulmonary valve (heart) (*see also* Endocarditis, pulmonary) I37.8
tricuspid (heart) (valve) I36.8
valve, valvular — *see* Endocarditis
vertebral (artery) I67.2
Atheromatosis — *see* Arteriosclerosis
Atherosclerosis — *see also* Arteriosclerosis
coronary
artery I25.10
with angina pectoris — *see* Arteriosclerosis, coronary (artery)
due to
calcified coronary lesion (severely) I25.84
lipid rich plaque I25.83
transplanted heart I25.811
bypass graft I25.812
with angina pectoris — *see* Arteriosclerosis, coronary (artery)
native coronary artery I25.811
with angina pectoris — *see* Arteriosclerosis, coronary (artery)
Athetosis (acquired) R25.8
bilateral (congenital) G80.3
congenital (bilateral) (double) G80.3
double (congenital) G80.3
unilateral R25.8
Athlete's
foot B35.3
heart I51.7
Athrepsia E41
Athyrea (acquired) — *see also* Hypothyroidism
congenital E03.1
Atonia, atony, atonic
bladder (sphincter) (neurogenic) N31.2
capillary I78.8
cecum K59.8
psychogenic F45.8
colon — *see* Atony, intestine
congenital P94.2
esophagus K22.8
intestine K59.8
psychogenic F45.8
stomach K31.89
neurotic or psychogenic F45.8
uterus (during labor) O62.2
with hemorrhage (postpartum) O72.1
postpartum (with hemorrhage) O72.1
without hemorrhage O75.89
Atopy — *see* History, allergy
Atransferrinemia, congenital E88.09

Atresia, atretic
alimentary organ or tract NEC Q45.8
upper Q40.8
ani, anus, anal (canal) Q42.3
with fistula Q42.2
aorta (ring) Q25.29
aortic (orifice) (valve) Q23.0
arch Q25.21
congenital with hypoplasia of ascending aorta and defective development of left ventricle (with mitral stenosis) Q23.4
in hypoplastic left heart syndrome Q23.4
aqueduct of Sylvius Q03.0
with spina bifida — *see* Spina bifida, with hydrocephalus
artery NEC Q27.8
cerebral Q28.3
coronary Q24.5
digestive system Q27.8
eye Q15.8
lower limb Q27.8
pulmonary Q25.5
specified site NEC Q27.8
umbilical Q27.0
upper limb Q27.8
auditory canal (external) Q16.1
bile duct (common) (congenital) (hepatic) Q44.2
acquired — *see* Obstruction, bile duct
bladder (neck) Q64.39
obstruction Q64.31
bronchus Q32.4
cecum Q42.8
cervix (acquired) N88.2
congenital Q51.828
in pregnancy or childbirth — *see* Anomaly, cervix, in pregnancy or childbirth
causing obstructed labor O65.5
choana Q30.0
colon Q42.9
specified NEC Q42.8
common duct Q44.2
cricoid cartilage Q31.8
cystic duct Q44.2
acquired K82.8
with obstruction K82.0
digestive organs NEC Q45.8
duodenum Q41.0
ear canal Q16.1
ejaculatory duct Q55.4
epiglottis Q31.8
esophagus Q39.0
with tracheoesophageal fistula Q39.1
eustachian tube Q17.8
fallopian tube (congenital) Q50.6
acquired N97.1
follicular cyst N83.0-
foramen of
Luschka Q03.1
with spina bifida — *see* Spina bifida, with hydrocephalus
Magendie Q03.1
with spina bifida — *see* Spina bifida, with hydrocephalus
gallbladder Q44.1
genital organ
external
female Q52.79
male Q55.8
internal
female Q52.8
male Q55.8
glottis Q31.8
gullet Q39.0
with tracheoesophageal fistula Q39.1
heart valve NEC Q24.8
pulmonary Q22.0
tricuspid Q22.4

Atresia, atretic — *continued*
hymen Q52.3
acquired (postinfective) N89.6
ileum Q41.2
intestine (small) Q41.9
large Q42.9
specified NEC Q42.8
iris, filtration angle Q15.0
jejunum Q41.1
lacrimal apparatus Q10.4
larynx Q31.8
meatus urinarius Q64.33
mitral valve Q23.2
in hypoplastic left heart syndrome Q23.4
nares (anterior) (posterior) Q30.0
nasopharynx Q34.8
nose, nostril Q30.0
acquired J34.89
organ or site NEC Q89.8
osseous meatus (ear) Q16.1
oviduct (congenital) Q50.6
acquired N97.1
parotid duct Q38.4
acquired K11.8
pulmonary (artery) Q25.5
valve Q22.0
pulmonic Q22.0
pupil Q13.2
rectum Q42.1
with fistula Q42.0
salivary duct Q38.4
acquired K11.8
sublingual duct Q38.4
acquired K11.8
submandibular duct Q38.4
acquired K11.8
submaxillary duct Q38.4
acquired K11.8
thyroid cartilage Q31.8
trachea Q32.1
tricuspid valve Q22.4
ureter Q62.10
pelvic junction Q62.11
vesical orifice Q62.12
ureteropelvic junction Q62.11
ureterovesical orifice Q62.12
urethra (valvular) Q64.39
stricture Q64.32
urinary tract NEC Q64.8
uterus Q51.818
acquired N85.8
vagina (congenital) Q52.4
acquired (postinfectional) (senile) N89.5
vas deferens Q55.3
vascular NEC Q27.8
cerebral Q28.3
digestive system Q27.8
lower limb Q27.8
specified site NEC Q27.8
upper limb Q27.8
vein NEC Q27.8
digestive system Q27.8
great Q26.8
lower limb Q27.8
portal Q26.5
pulmonary Q26.3
specified site NEC Q27.8
upper limb Q27.8
vena cava (inferior) (superior) Q26.8
vesicourethral orifice Q64.31
vulva Q52.79
acquired N90.5
Atrichia, atrichosis — *see* Alopecia
At risk
for falling Z91.81
Atrophia — *see also* Atrophy
cutis senilis L90.8
due to radiation L57.8
gyrata of choroid and retina H31.23

DISEASE INDEX

Atrophia — *see also* Atrophy — *continued*
senilis R54
  dermatological L90.8
    due to radiation (nonionizing) (solar)
     L57.8
  unguium L60.3
  congenita Q84.6
Atrophie blanche (en plaque) (de Milian)
  L95.0
Atrophoderma, atrophodermia (of) L90.9
diffusum (idiopathic) L90.4
maculatum L90.8
  et striatum L90.8
    due to syphilis A52.79
    syphilitic A51.39
neuriticum L90.8
Pasini and Pierini L90.3
pigmentosum Q82.1
reticulatum symmetricum faciei L66.4
senile L90.8
  due to radiation (nonionizing) (solar) L57.8
vermiculata (cheeks) L66.4
Atrophy, atrophic (of)
adrenal (capsule) (gland) E27.49
  primary (autoimmune) E27.1
alveolar process or ridge (edentulous) K08.20
anal sphincter (disuse) N81.84
appendix K38.8
arteriosclerotic — *see* Arteriosclerosis
bile duct (common) (hepatic) K83.8
bladder N32.89
  neurogenic N31.8
blanche (en plaque) (of Milian) L95.0
bone (senile) NEC — *see also* Disorder, bone,
  specified type NEC
  due to
    tabes dorsalis (neurogenic) A52.11
brain (cortex) (progressive) G31.9
  frontotemporal circumscribed G31.01
    [F02.80]
    with behavioral disturbance G31.01
     [F02.81]
  senile NEC G31.1
breast N64.2
  obstetric — *see* Disorder, breast, specified
    type NEC
buccal cavity K13.79
cardiac — *see* Degeneration, myocardial
cartilage (infectional) (joint) — *see* Disorder,
  cartilage, specified NEC
cerebellar — *see* Atrophy, brain
cerebral — *see* Atrophy, brain
cervix (mucosa) (senile) (uteri) N88.8
  menopausal N95.8
Charcot-Marie-Tooth G60.0
choroid (central) (macular) (myopic) (retina)
  H31.10-
  diffuse secondary H31.12-
  gyrate H31.23
  senile H31.11-
ciliary body — *see* Atrophy, iris
conjunctiva (senile) H11.89
corpus cavernosum N48.89
cortical — *see* Atrophy, brain
cystic duct K82.8
Déjérine-Thomas G23.8
disuse NEC — *see* Atrophy, muscle
Duchenne-Aran G12.21
ear H93.8-
edentulous alveolar ridge K08.20
endometrium (senile) N85.8
  cervix N88.8
enteric K63.89
epididymis N50.89
eyeball — *see* Disorder, globe, degenerated
  condition, atrophy
eyelid (senile) — *see* Disorder, eyelid,
  degenerative
facial (skin) L90.9

Atrophy, atrophic (of) — *continued*
fallopian tube (senile) N83.32-
  with ovary N83.33-
fascioscapulohumeral (Landouzy-Déjérine)
  G71.0
fatty, thymus (gland) E32.8
gallbladder K82.8
gastric K29.40
  with bleeding K29.41
gastrointestinal K63.89
glandular I89.8
globe H44.52-
gum (*see also* Recession, gingival) K06.0
hair L67.8
heart (brown) — *see* Degeneration, myocardial
hemifacial Q67.4
  Romberg G51.8
infantile E41
  paralysis, acute — *see* Poliomyelitis,
    paralytic
intestine K63.89
iris (essential) (progressive) H21.26-
  specified NEC H21.29
kidney (senile) (terminal) (*see also* Sclerosis,
  renal) N26.1
  congenital or infantile Q60.5
    bilateral Q60.4
    unilateral Q60.3
  hydronephrotic — *see* Hydronephrosis
lacrimal gland (primary) H04.14-
  secondary H04.15-
Landouzy-Déjérine G71.0
laryngitis, infective J37.0
larynx J38.7
Leber's optic (hereditary) H47.22
lip K13.0
liver (yellow) K72.90
  with coma K72.91
  acute, subacute K72.00
    with coma K72.01
  chronic K72.10
    with coma K72.11
lung (senile) J98.4
macular (dermatological) L90.8
  syphilitic, skin A51.39
    striated A52.79
mandible (edentulous) K08.20
  minimal K08.21
  moderate K08.22
  severe K08.23
maxilla K08.20
  minimal K08.24
  moderate K08.25
  severe K08.26
muscle, muscular (diffuse) (general)
  (idiopathic) (primary) M62.50
  ankle M62.57-
  Duchenne-Aran G12.21
  foot M62.57-
  forearm M62.53-
  hand M62.54-
  infantile spinal G12.0
  lower leg M62.56-
  multiple sites M62.59
  myelopathic — *see* Atrophy, muscle, spinal
  myotonic G71.11
  neuritic G58.9
  neuropathic (peroneal) (progressive) G60.0
  pelvic (disuse) N81.84
  peroneal G60.0
  progressive (bulbar) G12.21
    adult G12.1
    infantile (spinal) G12.0
    spinal G12.9
     adult G12.1
     infantile G12.0
  pseudohypertrophic G71.0
  shoulder region M62.51-
  specified site NEC M62.58

Atrophy, atrophic (of) — *continued*
muscle, muscular (diffuse) (general)
  (idiopathic) (primary) M62.50 —
  continued
  spinal G12.9
    adult form G12.1
    Aran-Duchenne G12.21
    childhood form, type II G12.1
    distal G12.1
    hereditary NEC G12.1
    infantile, type I (Werdnig-Hoffmann)
     G12.0
    juvenile form, type III (Kugelberg-
     Welander) G12.1
    progressive G12.21
    scapuloperoneal form G12.1
    specified NEC G12.8
  syphilitic A52.78
  thigh M62.55-
  upper arm M62.52-
myocardium — *see* Degeneration, myocardial
myometrium (senile) N85.8
  cervix N88.8
myopathic NEC — *see* Atrophy, muscle
myotonia G71.11
nail L60.3
nasopharynx J31.1
nerve — *see also* Disorder, nerve
  abducens — *see* Strabismus, paralytic, sixth
    nerve
  accessory G52.8
  acoustic or auditory — *see* subcategory
    H93.3
  cranial G52.9
    eighth (auditory) — *see* subcategory
     H93.3
    eleventh (accessory) G52.8
    fifth (trigeminal) G50.8
    first (olfactory) G52.0
    fourth (trochlear) — *see* Strabismus,
     paralytic, fourth nerve
    second (optic) H47.20
    sixth (abducens) — *see* Strabismus,
     paralytic, sixth nerve
    tenth (pneumogastric) (vagus) G52.2
    third (oculomotor) — *see* Strabismus,
     paralytic, third nerve
    twelfth (hypoglossal) G52.3
  hypoglossal G52.3
  oculomotor — *see* Strabismus, paralytic,
    third nerve
  olfactory G52.0
  optic (papillomacular bundle)
    syphilitic (late) A52.15
    congenital A50.44
  pneumogastric G52.2
  trigeminal G50.8
  trochlear — *see* Strabismus, paralytic, fourth
    nerve
  vagus (pneumogastric) G52.2
neurogenic, bone, tabetic A52.11
nutritional E41
old age R54
olivopontocerebellar G23.8
optic (nerve) H47.20
  glaucomatous H47.23-
  hereditary H47.22
  primary H47.21-
  specified type NEC H47.29-
  syphilitic (late) A52.15
    congenital A50.44
orbit H05.31-
ovary (senile) N83.31-
  with fallopian tube N83.33-
oviduct (senile) — *see* Atrophy, fallopian tube
palsy, diffuse (progressive) G12.22
pancreas (duct) (senile) K86.89
parotid gland K11.0
pelvic muscle N81.84

Atrophy, atrophic (of) — continued
  penis N48.89
  pharynx J39.2
  pluriglandular E31.8
    autoimmune E31.0
  polyarthritis M15.9
  prostate N42.89
  pseudohypertrophic (muscle) G71.0
  renal (see also Sclerosis, renal) N26.1
  retina, retinal (postinfectional) H35.89
  rhinitis J31.0
  salivary gland K11.0
  scar L90.5
  sclerosis, lobar (of brain) G31.09 *[F02.80]*
    with behavioral disturbance G31.09
      [F02.81]
  scrotum N50.89
  seminal vesicle N50.89
  senile R54
    due to radiation (nonionizing) (solar) L57.8
  skin (patches) (spots) L90.9
    degenerative (senile) L90.8
    due to radiation (nonionizing) (solar) L57.8
    senile L90.8
  spermatic cord N50.89
  spinal (acute) (cord) G95.89
    muscular — see Atrophy, muscle, spinal
    paralysis G12.20
      acute — see Poliomyelitis, paralytic
      meaning progressive muscular atrophy
        G12.21
  spine (column) — see Spondylopathy, specified
    NEC
  spleen (senile) D73.0
  stomach K29.40
    with bleeding K29.41
  striate (skin) L90.6
    syphilitic A52.79
  subcutaneous L90.9
  sublingual gland K11.0
  submandibular gland K11.0
  submaxillary gland K11.0
  Sudeck's — see Algoneurodystrophy
  suprarenal (capsule) (gland) E27.49
    primary E27.1
  systemic affecting central nervous system
    in
      myxedema E03.9 *[G13.2]*
      neoplastic disease (see also Neoplasm)
        D49.9 *[G13.1]*
      specified disease NEC G13.8
  tarso-orbital fascia, congenital Q10.3
  testis N50.0
  thenar, partial — see Syndrome, carpal tunnel
  thymus (fatty) E32.8
  thyroid (gland) (acquired) E03.4
    with cretinism E03.1
    congenital (with myxedema) E03.1
  tongue (senile) K14.8
    papillae K14.4
  trachea J39.8
  tunica vaginalis N50.89
  turbinate J34.89
  tympanic membrane (nonflaccid) H73.82-
    flaccid H73.81-
  upper respiratory tract J39.8
  uterus, uterine (senile) N85.8
    cervix N88.8
    due to radiation (intended effect) N85.8
      adverse effect or misadventure N99.89
  vagina (senile) N95.2
  vas deferens N50.89
  vascular I99.8
  vertebra (senile) — see Spondylopathy,
    specified NEC
  vulva (senile) N90.5
  Werdnig-Hoffmann G12.0
  yellow — see Failure, hepatic

Attack, attacks
  with alteration of consciousness (with
    automatisms) — see Epilepsy, localization-
    related, symptomatic, with complex partial
    seizures
  Adams-Stokes I45.9
  akinetic — see Epilepsy, generalized, specified
    NEC
  angina — see Angina
  atonic — see Epilepsy, generalized, specified
    NEC
  benign shuddering G25.83
  cataleptic — see Catalepsy
  coronary — see Infarct, myocardium
  cyanotic, newborn P28.2
  drop NEC R55
  epileptic — see Epilepsy
  heart — see infarct, myocardium
  hysterical F44.9
  jacksonian — see Epilepsy, localization-
    related, symptomatic, with simple partial
    seizures
  myocardium, myocardial — see Infarct,
    myocardium
  myoclonic — see Epilepsy, generalized,
    specified NEC
  panic F41.0
  psychomotor — see Epilepsy, localization-
    related, symptomatic, with complex partial
    seizures
  salaam — see Epilepsy, spasms
  schizophreniform, brief F23
  shuddering, benign G25.83
  Stokes-Adams I45.9
  syncope R55
  transient ischemic (TIA) G45.9
    specified NEC G45.8
  unconsciousness R55
    hysterical F44.89
  vasomotor R55
  vasovagal (paroxysmal) (idiopathic) R55
  without alteration of consciousness — see
    Epilepsy, localization-related,
    symptomatic, with simple partial seizures

Attention (to)
  artificial
    opening (of) Z43.9
      digestive tract NEC Z43.4
        colon Z43.3
        ilium Z43.2
        stomach Z43.1
      specified NEC Z43.8
      trachea Z43.0
      urinary tract NEC Z43.6
        cystostomy Z43.5
        nephrostomy Z43.6
        ureterostomy Z43.6
        urethrostomy Z43.6
      vagina Z43.7
  colostomy Z43.3
  cystostomy Z43.5
  deficit disorder or syndrome F98.8
    with hyperactivity — see Disorder, attention-
      deficit hyperactivity
  gastrostomy Z43.1
  ileostomy Z43.2
  jejunostomy Z43.4
  nephrostomy Z43.6
  surgical dressings Z48.01
  sutures Z48.02
  tracheostomy Z43.0
  ureterostomy Z43.6
  urethrostomy Z43.6

Attrition
  gum (see also Recession, gingival) K06.0
  tooth, teeth (excessive) (hard tissues) K03.0

Atypical, atypism — see also condition
  cells (on cytolgocial smear) (endocervical)
    (endometrial) (glandular)
    cervix R87.619
    vagina R87.629
  cervical N87.9
  endometrium N85.9
    hyperplasia N85.00
  parenting situation Z62.9
Auditory — see condition
Aujeszky's disease B33.8
Aurantiasis, cutis E67.1
Auricle, auricular — see also condition
  cervical Q18.2
Auriculotemporal syndrome G50.8
Austin Flint murmur (aortic insufficiency)
  I35.1
Australian
  Q fever A78
  X disease A83.4
Autism, autistic (childhood) (infantile) F84.0
  atypical F84.9
  spectrum disorder F84.0
Autodigestion R68.89
Autoerythrocyte sensitization (syndrome)
  D69.2
Autographism L50.3
Autoimmune
  disease (systemic) M35.9
  inhibitors to clotting factors D68.311
  lymphoproliferative syndrome [ALPS] D89.82
  thyroiditis E06.3
Autointoxication R68.89
Automatism G93.89
  with temporal sclerosis G93.81
  epileptic — see Epilepsy, localization-related,
    symptomatic, with complex partial seizures
  paroxysmal, idiopathic — see Epilepsy,
    localization-related, symptomatic, with
    complex partial seizures
Autonomic, autonomous
  bladder (neurogenic) N31.2
  hysteria seizure F44.5
Autosensitivity, erythrocyte D69.2
Autosensitization, cutaneous L30.2
Autosome — see condition by chromosome
  involved
Autotopagnosia R48.1
Autotoxemia R68.89
Autumn — see condition
Avellis' syndrome G46.8
Aversion
  oral R63.3
    newborn P92-
    nonorganic origin F98.2
  sexual F52.1
Aviator's
  disease or sickness — see Effect, adverse, high
    altitude
  ear T70.0
Avitaminosis (multiple) (see also Deficiency,
  vitamin) E56.9
  B E53.9
    with
      beriberi E51.11
      pellagra E52
  B12 E53.8
  B2 E53.0
  B6 E53.1
  D E55.9
    with rickets E55.0
  G E53.0
  K E56.1
  nicotinic acid E52
AVNRT (atrioventricular nodal re-entrant
  tachycardia) I47.1
AVRT (atrioventricular nodal re-entrant
  tachycardia) I47.1

Avulsion (traumatic)
  blood vessel — *see* Injury, blood vessel
  bone — *see* Fracture, by site
  cartilage — *see also* Dislocation, by site
    symphyseal (inner), complicating delivery
      O71.6
  external site other than limb — *see* Wound,
    open, by site
  eye S05.7-
  head (intracranial)
    external site NEC S08.89
    scalp S08.0
  internal organ or site — *see* Injury, by site
  joint — *see also* Dislocation, by site
    capsule — *see* Sprain, by site
  kidney S37.06-
  ligament — *see* Sprain, by site
  limb — *see also* Amputation, traumatic, by site
    skin and subcutaneous tissue — *see* Wound,
      open, by site
  muscle — *see* Injury, muscle
  nerve (root) — *see* Injury, nerve
  scalp S08.0
  skin and subcutaneous tissue — *see* Wound,
    open, by site
  spleen S36.032
  symphyseal cartilage (inner), complicating
    delivery O71.6
  tendon — *see* Injury, muscle
  tooth S03.2
Awareness of heart beat R00.2
Axenfeld's
  anomaly or syndrome Q15.0
  degeneration (calcareous) Q13.4
Axilla, axillary — *see also* condition
  breast Q83.1
Axonotmesis — *see* Injury, nerve
Ayerza's disease or syndrome (pulmonary
  artery sclerosis with pulmonary
  hypertension) I27.0
Azoospermia (organic) N46.01
  due to
    drug therapy N46.021
    efferent duct obstruction N46.023
    infection N46.022
    radiation N46.024
    specified cause NEC N46.029
    systemic disease N46.025
Azotemia R79.89
  meaning uremia N19
Aztec ear Q17.3
Azygos
  continuation inferior vena cava Q26.8
  lobe (lung) Q33.1

B

Baastrup's disease — *see* Kissing spine
Babesiosis B60.0
Babington's disease (familial hemorrhagic
  telangiectasia) I78.0
Babinski's syndrome A52.79
Baby
  crying constantly R68.11
  floppy (syndrome) P94.2
Bacillary — *see* condition
Bacilluria R82.71
Bacillus — *see also* Infection, bacillus
  abortus infection A23.1
  anthracis infection A22.9
  coli infection (*see also* Escherichia coli) B96.20
  Flexner's A03.1
  mallei infection A24.0
  Shiga's A03.0
  suipestifer infection — *see* Infection, salmonella
Back — *see* condition
Backache (postural) M54.9
  sacroiliac M53.3
  specified NEC M54.89
Backflow — *see* Reflux
Backward reading (dyslexia) F81.0
Bacteremia R78.81
  with sepsis — *see* Sepsis
Bactericholia — *see* Cholecystitis, acute
Bacterid, bacteride (pustular) L40.3
Bacterium, bacteria, bacterial
  agent NEC, as cause of disease classified
    elsewhere B96.89
  in blood — *see* Bacteremia
  in urine — *see* Bacteriuria
Bacteriuria, bacteruria R82.71
  asymptomatic R82.71
Bacteroides
  fragilis, as cause of disease classified
    elsewhere B96.6
Bad
  heart — *see* Disease, heart
  trip
    due to drug abuse — *see* Abuse, drug,
      hallucinogen
    due to drug dependence — *see* Dependence,
      drug, hallucinogen
Baelz's disease (cheilitis glandularis
  apostematosa) K13.0
Baerensprung's disease (eczema
  marginatum) B35.6
Bagasse disease or pneumonitis J67.1
Bagassosis J67.1
Baker's cyst — *see* Cyst, Baker's
Bakwin-Krida syndrome (metaphyseal
  dysplasia) Q78.5
Balancing side interference M26.56
Balanitis (circinata) (erosiva) (gangrenosa)
  (phagedenic) (vulgaris) N48.1
  amebic A06.82
  candidal B37.42
  due to Haemophilus ducreyi A57
  gonococcal (acute) (chronic) A54.09
  xerotica obliterans N48.0
Balanoposthitis N47.6
  gonococcal (acute) (chronic) A54.09
  ulcerative (specific) A63.8
Balanorrhagia — *see* Balanitis
Balantidiasis, balantidiosis A07.0
Bald tongue K14.4
Baldness — *see also* Alopecia
  male-pattern — *see* Alopecia, androgenic
Balkan grippe A78
Balloon disease — *see* Effect, adverse, high
  altitude
Balo's disease (concentric sclerosis) G37.5

Bamberger-Marie disease — *see*
  Osteoarthropathy, hypertrophic, specified
  type NEC
Bancroft's filariasis B74.0
Band(s)
  adhesive — *see* Adhesions, peritoneum
  anomalous or congenital — *see also* Anomaly,
    by site
    heart (atrial) (ventricular) Q24.8
    intestine Q43.3
    omentum Q43.3
  cervix N88.1
  constricting, congenital Q79.8
  gallbladder (congenital) Q44.1
  intestinal (adhesive) — *see* Adhesions,
    peritoneum
  obstructive
    intestine K56.5
    peritoneum K56.5
  periappendiceal, congenital Q43.3
  peritoneal (adhesive) — *see* Adhesions,
    peritoneum
  uterus N73.6
    internal N85.6
  vagina N89.5
Bandemia D72.825
Bandl's ring (contraction), complicating
  delivery O62.4
Bang's disease (brucella abortus) A23.1
Bangkok hemorrhagic fever A91
Bankruptcy, anxiety concerning Z59.8
Bannister's disease T78.3
  hereditary D84.1
Banti's disease or syndrome (with cirrhosis)
  (with portal hypertension) K76.6
Bar, median, prostate — *see* Enlargement,
  enlarged, prostate
Barcoo disease or rot — *see* Ulcer, skin
Barlow's disease E54
Barodontalgia T70.29
Baron Münchausen syndrome — *see*
  Disorder, factitious
Barosinusitis T70.1
Barotitis T70.0
Barotrauma T70.29
  odontalgia T70.29
  otitic T70.0
  sinus T70.1
**Barraquer(-Simons) disease or
  syndrome** (progressive lipodystrophy)
  E88.1
Barrel chest M95.4
Barrett's
  disease — *see* Barrett's, esophagus
  esophagus K22.70
    with dysplasia K22.719
      high grade K22.711
      low grade K22.710
    without dysplasia K22.70
  syndrome — *see* Barrett's, esophagus
  ulcer K22.10
    with bleeding K22.11
    without bleeding K22.10
Barré-Guillain disease or syndrome
  G61.0
Barré-Liéou syndrome (posterior cervical
  sympathetic) M53.0
**Bársony (-Polgár) (-Teschendorf)
  syndrome** (corkscrew esophagus) K22.4
Barth syndrome E78.71
Bartholinitis (suppurating) N75.8
  gonococcal (acute) (chronic) (with abscess)
    A54.1
Barton's fracture S52.56-
Bartonellosis A44.9
  cutaneous A44.1
  mucocutaneous A44.1
  specified NEC A44.8
  systemic A44.0

Bartter's syndrome E26.81
Basal — *see* condition
Basan's (hidrotic) ectodermal dysplasia Q82.4
Baseball finger — *see* Dislocation, finger
Basedow's disease (exophthalmic goiter) — *see* Hyperthyroidism, with, goiter
Basic — *see* condition
Basilar — *see* condition
Bason's (hidrotic) ectodermal dysplasia Q82.4
Basopenia — *see* Agranulocytosis
Basophilia D72.824
Basophilism (cortico-adrenal) (Cushing's) (pituitary) E24.0
Bassen-Kornzweig disease or syndrome E78.6
Bat ear Q17.5
Bateman's
　disease B08.1
　purpura (senile) D69.2
Bathing cramp T75.1
Bathophobia F40.248
Batten(-Mayou) disease E75.4
　retina E75.4 [H36]
Batten-Steinert syndrome G71.11
Battered — *see* Maltreatment
Battey Mycobacterium infection A31.0
Battle exhaustion F43.0
Battledore placenta O43.19-
Baumgarten-Cruveilhier cirrhosis, disease or syndrome K74.69
Bauxite fibrosis (of lung) J63.1
Bayle's disease (general paresis) A52.17
Bazin's disease (primary) (tuberculous) A18.4
Beach ear — *see* Swimmer's, ear
Beaded hair (congenital) Q84.1
Béal conjunctivitis or syndrome B30.2
Beard's disease (neurasthenia) F48.8
Beat(s)
　atrial, premature I49.1
　ectopic I49.49
　elbow — *see* Bursitis, elbow
　escaped, heart I49.49
　hand — *see* Bursitis, hand
　knee — *see* Bursitis, knee
　premature I49.40
　　atrial I49.1
　　auricular I49.1
　　supraventricular I49.1
Beau's
　disease or syndrome — *see* Degeneration, myocardial
　lines (transverse furrows on fingernails) L60.4
Bechterev's syndrome — *see* Spondylitis, ankylosing
Becker's
　cardiomyopathy I42.8
　disease
　　idiopathic mural endomyocardial disease I42.3
　　myotonia congenita, recessive form G71.12
　dystrophy G71.0
　pigmented hairy nevus D22.5
Beck's syndrome (anterior spinal artery occlusion) I65.8
Beckwith-Wiedemann syndrome Q87.3
Bed confinement status Z74.01
Bed sore — *see* Ulcer, pressure, by site
Bedbug bite(s) — *see* Bite(s), by site, superficial, insect
Bedclothes, asphyxiation or suffocation by — *see* Asphyxia, traumatic, due to, mechanical, trapped
Bednar's
　aphthae K12.0
　tumor — *see* Neoplasm, malignant, by site
Bedridden Z74.01
Bedsore — *see* Ulcer, pressure, by site

Bedwetting — *see* Enuresis
Bee sting (with allergic or anaphylactic shock) — *see* Toxicity, venom, arthropod, bee
Beer drinker's heart (disease) I42.6
Begbie's disease (exophthalmic goiter) — *see* Hyperthyroidism, with, goiter
Behavior
　antisocial
　　adult Z72.811
　　child or adolescent Z72.810
　disorder, disturbance — *see* Disorder, conduct
　disruptive — *see* Disorder, conduct
　drug seeking Z76.5
　inexplicable R46.2
　marked evasiveness R46.5
　obsessive-compulsive R46.81
　overactivity R46.3
　poor responsiveness R46.4
　self-damaging (life-style) Z72.89
　sleep-incompatible Z72.821
　slowness R46.4
　specified NEC R46.89
　strange (and inexplicable) R46.2
　suspiciousness R46.5
　type A pattern Z73.1
　undue concern or preoccupation with stressful events R46.6
　verbosity and circumstantial detail obscuring reason for contact R46.7
Behçet's disease or syndrome M35.2
Behr's disease — *see* Degeneration, macula
Beigel's disease or morbus (white piedra) B36.2
Bejel A65
Bekhterev's syndrome — *see* Spondylitis, ankylosing
Belching — *see* Eructation
Bell's
　mania F30.8
　palsy, paralysis G51.0
　　infant or newborn P11.3
　spasm G51.3
Bence Jones albuminuria or proteinuria NEC R80.3
Bends T70.3
Benedikt's paralysis or syndrome G46.3
Benign — *see also* condition
　prostatic hyperplasia — *see* Hyperplasia, prostate
Bennett's fracture (displaced) S62.21-
Benson's disease — *see* Deposit, crystalline
Bent
　back (hysterical) F44.4
　nose M95.0
　　congenital Q67.4
Bereavement (uncomplicated) Z63.4
Berger's disease — *see* Nephropathy, IgA
Bergeron's disease (hysterical chorea) F44.4
Beriberi (dry) E51.11
　heart (disease) E51.12
　polyneuropathy E51.11
　wet E51.12
　　involving circulatory system E51.11
Berlin's disease or edema (traumatic) S05.8x-
Berlock (berloque) dermatitis L56.2
Bernard-Horner syndrome G90.2
Bernard-Soulier disease or thrombopathia D69.1
Bernhardt(-Roth) disease — *see* Mononeuropathy, lower limb, meralgia paresthetica
Bernheim's syndrome — *see* Failure, heart, congestive
Bertielliasis B71.8
Berylliosis (lung) J63.2
Besnier-Boeck(-Schaumann) disease — *see* Sarcoidosis

Besnier's
　lupus pernio D86.3
　prurigo L20.0
Best's disease H35.50
Bestiality F65.89
Betalipoproteinemia, broad or floating E78.2
Beta-mercaptolactate-cysteine disulfiduria E72.09
Betting and gambling Z72.6
　pathological (compulsive) F63.0
Bezoar T18.9
　intestine T18.3
　stomach T18.2
Bezold's abscess — *see* Mastoiditis, acute
Bianchi's syndrome R48.8
Bicornate or bicornis uterus Q51.3
　in pregnancy or childbirth O34.0-
　　causing obstructed labor O65.5
Bicuspid aortic valve Q23.1
Biedl-Bardet syndrome Q87.89
Bielschowsky(-Jansky) disease E75.4
Biermer's (pernicious) anemia or disease D51.0
Biett's disease L93.0
Bifid (congenital)
　apex, heart Q24.8
　clitoris Q52.6
　kidney Q63.8
　nose Q30.2
　patella Q74.1
　scrotum Q55.29
　toe NEC Q74.2
　tongue Q38.3
　ureter Q62.8
　uterus Q51.3
　uvula Q35.7
Biforis uterus (suprasimplex) Q51.3
Bifurcation (congenital)
　gallbladder Q44.1
　kidney pelvis Q63.8
　renal pelvis Q63.8
　rib Q76.6
　tongue, congenital Q38.3
　trachea Q32.1
　ureter Q62.8
　urethra Q64.74
　vertebra Q76.49
Big spleen syndrome D73.1
Bigeminal pulse R00.8
Bilateral — *see* condition
Bile
　duct — *see* condition
　pigments in urine R82.2
Bilharziasis — *see also* Schistosomiasis
　chyluria B65.0
　cutaneous B65.3
　galacturia B65.0
　hematochyluria B65.0
　intestinal B65.1
　lipemia B65.9
　lipuria B65.0
　oriental B65.2
　piarhemia B65.9
　pulmonary NOS B65.9 [J99]
　　pneumonia B65.9 [J17]
　tropical hematuria B65.0
　vesical B65.0
Biliary — *see* condition
Bilirubin metabolism disorder E80.7
　specified NEC E80.6
Bilirubinemia, familial nonhemolytic E80.4
Bilirubinuria R82.2
Biliuria R82.2
Bilocular stomach K31.2
Binswanger's disease I67.3

DISEASE INDEX

Bite(s) (animal) (human) — *continued*
  foot (except toe(s) alone) S91.35-
    superficial NEC S90.87-
      insect S90.86-
    toe — *see* Bite, toe
  forearm S51.85-
    elbow only — *see* Bite, elbow
    superficial NEC S50.87-
      insect S50.86-
  forehead — *see* Bite, head, specified site NEC
  genital organs, external
    female S31.552
      superficial NEC S30.876
        insect S30.866
      vagina and vulva — *see* Bite, vulva
    male S31.551
      penis — *see* Bite, penis
      scrotum — *see* Bite, scrotum
      superficial NEC S30.875
        insect S30.865
      testes — *see* Bite, testis
  groin — *see* Bite, abdomen, wall
  gum — *see* Bite, oral cavity
  hand S61.45-
    finger — *see* Bite, finger
    superficial NEC S60.57-
      insect S60.56-
    thumb — *see* Bite, thumb
  head S01.95
    cheek — *see* Bite, cheek
    ear — *see* Bite, ear
    eyelid — *see* Bite, eyelid
    lip — *see* Bite, lip
    nose — *see* Bite, nose
    oral cavity — *see* Bite, oral cavity
    scalp — *see* Bite, scalp
    specified site NEC S01.85
      superficial NEC S00.87
        insect S00.86
    superficial NEC S00.97
      insect S00.96
    temporomandibular area — *see* Bite, cheek
  heel — *see* Bite, foot
  hip S71.05-
    superficial NEC S70.27-
      insect S70.26-
  hymen S31.45
  hypochondrium — *see* Bite, abdomen, wall
  hypogastric region — *see* Bite, abdomen, wall
  inguinal region — *see* Bite, abdomen, wall
  insect — *see* Bite, by site, superficial, insect
  instep — *see* Bite, foot
  interscapular region — *see* Bite, thorax, back
  jaw — *see* Bite, head, specified site NEC
  knee S81.05-
    superficial NEC S80.27-
      insect S80.26-
  labium (majus) (minus) — *see* Bite, vulva
  lacrimal duct — *see* Bite, eyelid
  larynx S11.015
    superficial NEC S10.17
      insect S10.16
  leg (lower) S81.85-
    ankle — *see* Bite, ankle
    foot — *see* Bite, foot
    knee — *see* Bite, knee
    superficial NEC S80.87-
      insect S80.86-
    toe — *see* Bite, toe
    upper — *see* Bite, thigh
  lip S01.551
    superficial NEC S00.571
      insect S00.561
  lizard (venomous) — *see* Venom, bite, reptile
  loin — *see* Bite, abdomen, wall
  lower back — *see* Bite, back, lower
  lumbar region — *see* Bite, back, lower
  malar region — *see* Bite, head, specified site NEC

Bite(s) (animal) (human) — *continued*
  mammary — *see* Bite, breast
  marine animals (venomous) — *see* Toxicity, venom, marine animal
  mastoid region — *see* Bite, head, specified site NEC
  mouth — *see* Bite, oral cavity
  nail
    finger — *see* Bite, finger
    toe — *see* Bite, toe
  nape — *see* Bite, neck, specified site NEC
  nasal (septum) (sinus) — *see* Bite, nose
  nasopharynx — *see* Bite, head, specified site NEC
  neck S11.95
    involving
      cervical esophagus — *see* Bite, esophagus, cervical
      larynx — *see* Bite, larynx
      pharynx — *see* Bite, pharynx
      thyroid gland S11.15
      trachea — *see* Bite, trachea
    specified site NEC S11.85
      superficial NEC S10.87
        insect S10.86
    superficial NEC S10.97
      insect S10.96
    throat S11.85
      superficial NEC S10.17
        insect S10.16
  nose (septum) (sinus) S01.25
    superficial NEC S00.37
      insect S00.36
  occipital region — *see* Bite, scalp
  oral cavity S01.552
    superficial NEC S00.572
      insect S00.562
  orbital region — *see* Bite, eyelid
  palate — *see* Bite, oral cavity
  palm — *see* Bite, hand
  parietal region — *see* Bite, scalp
  pelvis S31.050
    with penetration into retroperitoneal space S31.051
    superficial NEC S30.870
      insect S30.860
  penis S31.25
    superficial NEC S30.872
      insect S30.862
  perineum
    female — *see* Bite, vulva
    male — *see* Bite, pelvis
  periocular area (with or without lacrimal passages) — *see* Bite, eyelid
  phalanges
    finger — *see* Bite, finger
    toe — *see* Bite, toe
  pharynx S11.25
    superficial NEC S10.17
      insect S10.16
  pinna — *see* Bite, ear
  poisonous — *see* Venom
  popliteal space — *see* Bite, knee
  prepuce — *see* Bite, penis
  pubic region — *see* Bite, abdomen, wall
  rectovaginal septum — *see* Bite, vulva
  red bug B88.0
  reptile NEC — *see also* Venom, bite, reptile
    nonvenomous — *see* Bite, by site
    snake — *see* Venom, bite, snake
  sacral region — *see* Bite, back, lower
  sacroiliac region — *see* Bite, back, lower
  salivary gland — *see* Bite, oral cavity
  scalp S01.05
    superficial NEC S00.07
      insect S00.06
  scapular region — *see* Bite, shoulder

Bite(s) (animal) (human) — *continued*
  scrotum S31.35
    superficial NEC S30.873
      insect S30.863
  sea-snake (venomous) — *see* Toxicity, venom, snake, sea snake
  shin — *see* Bite, leg
  shoulder S41.05-
    superficial NEC S40.27-
      insect S40.26-
  snake — *see also* Venom, bite, snake
    nonvenomous — *see* Bite, by site
  spermatic cord — *see* Bite, testis
  spider (venomous) — *see* Toxicity, venom, spider
    nonvenomous — *see* Bite, by site, superficial, insect
  sternal region — *see* Bite, thorax, front
  submaxillary region — *see* Bite, head, specified site NEC
  submental region — *see* Bite, head, specified site NEC
  subungual
    finger(s) — *see* Bite, finger
    toe — *see* Bite, toe
  superficial — *see* Bite, by site, superficial
  supraclavicular fossa S11.85
  supraorbital — *see* Bite, head, specified site NEC
  temple, temporal region — *see* Bite, head, specified site NEC
  temporomandibular area — *see* Bite, cheek
  testis S31.35
    superficial NEC S30.873
      insect S30.863
  thigh S71.15-
    superficial NEC S70.37-
      insect S70.36-
  thorax, thoracic (wall) S21.95
    back S21.25-
      with penetration into thoracic cavity S21.45-
    breast — *see* Bite, breast
    front S21.15-
      with penetration into thoracic cavity S21.35-
    superficial NEC S20.97
      back S20.47-
      front S20.37-
      insect S20.96
        back S20.46-
        front S20.36-
  throat — *see* Bite, neck, throat
  thumb S61.05-
    with
      damage to nail S61.15-
    superficial NEC S60.37-
      insect S60.36-
  thyroid S11.15
    superficial NEC S10.87
      insect S10.86
  toe(s) S91.15-
    with
      damage to nail S91.25-
    great S91.15-
      with
        damage to nail S91.25-
    lesser S91.15-
      with
        damage to nail S91.25-
    superficial NEC S90.47-
      great S90.47-
      insect S90.46-
        great S90.46-
  tongue S01.552
  trachea S11.025
    superficial NEC S10.17
      insect S10.16
  tunica vaginalis — *see* Bite, testis

Bite(s) (animal) (human) — *continued*
tympanum, tympanic membrane — *see* Bite, ear
umbilical region S31.155
uvula — *see* Bite, oral cavity
vagina — *see* Bite, vulva
venomous — *see* Venom
vocal cords S11.035
superficial NEC S10.17
insect S10.16
vulva S31.45
superficial NEC S30.874
insect S30.864
wrist S61.55-
superficial NEC S60.87-
insect S60.86-
Biting, cheek or lip K13.1
Biventricular failure (heart) I50.9
Björck (-Thorson) syndrome (malignant carcinoid) E34.0
Black
death A20.9
eye S00.1-
hairy tongue K14.3
heel (foot) S90.3-
lung (disease) J60
palm (hand) S60.22-
Blackfan-Diamond anemia or syndrome (congenital hypoplastic anemia) D61.01
Blackhead L70.0
Blackout R55
Bladder — *see* condition
Blast (air) (hydraulic) (immersion) (underwater)
blindness S05.8x-
injury
abdomen or thorax — *see* Injury, by site
ear (acoustic nerve trauma) — *see* Injury, nerve, acoustic, specified type NEC
syndrome NEC T70.8
Blastoma — *see* Neoplasm, malignant, by site
pulmonary — *see* Neoplasm, lung, malignant
Blastomycosis, blastomycotic B40.9
Brazilian — *see* Paracoccidioidomycosis
cutaneous B40.3
disseminated B40.7
European — *see* Cryptococcosis
generalized B40.7
keloidal B48.0
North American B40.9
primary pulmonary B40.0
pulmonary B40.2
acute B40.0
chronic B40.1
skin B40.3
South American — *see* Paracoccidioidomycosis
specified NEC B40.89
Blebitis, postprocedural H59.40
stage 1 H59.41
stage 2 H59.42
stage 3 H59.43
Bleb(s) R23.8
emphysematous (lung) (solitary) J43.9
endophthalmitis H59.43
filtering (vitreous), after glaucoma surgery Z98.83
inflammed (infected), postprocedural H59.40
stage 1 H59.41
stage 2 H59.42
stage 3 H59.43
lung (ruptured) J43.9
congenital — *see* Atelectasis
newborn P25.8
subpleural (emphysematous) J43.9
Bleeder (familial) (hereditary) — *see* Hemophilia

Bleeding — *see also* Hemorrhage
anal K62.5
anovulatory N97.0
atonic, following delivery O72.1
capillary I78.8
puerperal O72.2
contact (postcoital) N93.0
due to uterine subinvolution N85.3
ear — *see* Otorrhagia
excessive, associated with menopausal onset N92.4
familial — *see* Defect, coagulation
following intercourse N93.0
gastrointestinal K92.2
hemorrhoids — *see* Hemorrhoids
intermenstrual (regular) N92.3
irregular N92.1
intraoperative — *see* Complication, intraoperative, hemorrhage
irregular N92.6
menopausal N92.4
newborn, intraventricular — *see* Newborn, affected by, hemorrhage, intraventricular
nipple N64.59
nose R04.0
ovulation N92.3
postclimacteric N95.0
postcoital N93.0
postmenopausal N95.0
postoperative — *see* Complication, postprocedural, hemorrhage
preclimacteric N92.4
pre-pubertal vaginal N93.1
puberty (excessive, with onset of menstrual periods) N92.2
rectum, rectal K62.5
newborn P54.2
tendencies — *see* Defect, coagulation
throat R04.1
tooth socket (post-extraction) K91.840
umbilical stump P51.9
uterus, uterine NEC N93.9
climacteric N92.4
dysfunctional or functional N93.8
menopausal N92.4
preclimacteric or premenopausal N92.4
unrelated to menstrual cycle N93.9
vagina, vaginal (abnormal) N93.9
dysfunctional or functional N93.8
newborn P54.6
pre-pubertal N93.1
vicarious N94.89
Blennorrhagia, blennorrhagic — *see* Gonorrhea
Blennorrhea (acute) (chronic) — *see also* Gonorrhea
inclusion (neonatal) (newborn) P39.1
lower genitourinary tract (gonococcal) A54.00
neonatorum (gonococcal ophthalmia) A54.31
Blepharelosis — *see* Entropion
Blepharitis (angularis) (ciliaris) (eyelid) (marginal) (nonulcerative) H01.009
herpes zoster B02.39
left H01.006
lower H01.005
upper H01.004
right H01.003
lower H01.002
upper H01.001
squamous H01.029
left H01.026
lower H01.025
upper H01.024
right H01.023
lower H01.022
upper H01.021

Blepharitis (angularis) (ciliaris) (eyelid) (marginal) (nonulcerative) H01.009 — *continued*
ulcerative H01.019
left H01.016
lower H01.015
upper H01.014
right H01.013
lower H01.012
upper H01.011
Blepharochalasis H02.30
congenital Q10.0
left H02.36
lower H02.35
upper H02.34
right H02.33
lower H02.32
upper H02.31
Blepharoclonus H02.59
Blepharoconjunctivitis H10.50-
angular H10.52-
contact H10.53-
ligneous H10.51-
Blepharophimosis (eyelid) H02.529
congenital Q10.3
left H02.526
lower H02.525
upper H02.524
right H02.523
lower H02.522
upper H02.521
Blepharoptosis H02.40-
congenital Q10.0
mechanical H02.41-
myogenic H02.42-
neurogenic H02.43-
paralytic H02.43-
Blepharopyorrhea, gonococcal A54.39
Blepharospasm G24.5
drug induced G24.01
Blighted ovum O02.0
Blind — *see also* Blindness
bronchus (congenital) Q32.4
loop syndrome K90.2
congenital Q43.8
sac, fallopian tube (congenital) Q50.6
spot, enlarged — *see* Defect, visual field, localized, scotoma, blind spot area
tract or tube, congenital NEC — *see* Atresia, by site
Blindness (acquired) (congenital) (both eyes) H54.0
blast S05.8x-
color — *see* Deficiency, color vision
concussion S05.8x-
cortical H47.619
left brain H47.612
right brain H47.611
day H53.11
due to injury (current episode) S05.9-
sequelae — *code to* injury with seventh character S
eclipse (total) — *see* Retinopathy, solar
emotional (hysterical) F44.6
face H53.16
hysterical F44.6
legal (both eyes) (USA definition) H54.8
mind R48.8
night H53.60
abnormal dark adaptation curve H53.61
acquired H53.62
congenital H53.63
specified type NEC H53.69
vitamin A deficiency E50.5

Blindness (acquired) (congenital) (both eyes) H54.0 — *continued*
  one eye (other eye normal) H54.40
    left (normal vision on right) H54.42
      low vision on right H54.12
      low vision, other eye H54.10
    right (normal vision on left) H54.41
      low vision on left H54.11
  psychic R48.8
  river B73.01
  snow — *see* Photokeratitis
  sun, solar — *see* Retinopathy, solar
  transient — *see* Disturbance, vision, subjective, loss, transient
  traumatic (current episode) S05.9-
  word (developmental) F81.0
    acquired R48.0
    secondary to organic lesion R48.0
Blister (nonthermal)
  abdominal wall S30.821
  alveolar process S00.522
  ankle S90.52-
  antecubital space — *see* Blister, elbow
  anus S30.827
  arm (upper) S40.82-
  auditory canal — *see* Blister, ear
  auricle — *see* Blister, ear
  axilla — *see* Blister, arm
  back, lower S30.820
  beetle dermatitis L24.89
  breast S20.12-
  brow S00.82
  calf — *see* Blister, leg
  canthus — *see* Blister, eyelid
  cheek S00.82
    internal S00.522
  chest wall — *see* Blister, thorax
  chin S00.82
  costal region — *see* Blister, thorax
  digit(s)
    foot — *see* Blister, toe
    hand — *see* Blister, finger
  due to burn — *see* Burn, by site, second degree
  ear S00.42-
  elbow S50.32-
  epiglottis S10.12
  esophagus, cervical S10.12
  eyebrow — *see* Blister, eyelid
  eyelid S00.22-
  face S00.82
  fever B00.1
  finger(s) S60.429
    index S60.42-
    little S60.42-
    middle S60.42-
    ring S60.42-
  foot (except toe(s) alone) S90.82-
    toe — *see* Blister, toe
  forearm S50.82-
    elbow only — *see* Blister, elbow
  forehead S00.82
  fracture — *omit code*
  genital organ
    female S30.826
    male S30.825
  gum S00.522
  hand S60.52-
  head S00.92
    ear — *see* Blister, ear
    eyelid — *see* Blister, eyelid
    lip S00.521
    nose S00.32
    oral cavity S00.522
    scalp S00.02
    specified site NEC S00.82
  heel — *see* Blister, foot
  hip S70.22-
  interscapular region S20.429

Blister (nonthermal) — *continued*
  jaw S00.82
  knee S80.22-
  larynx S10.12
  leg (lower) S80.82-
    knee — *see* Blister, knee
    upper — *see* Blister, thigh
  lip S00.521
  malar region S00.82
  mammary — *see* Blister, breast
  mastoid region S00.82
  mouth S00.522
  multiple, skin, nontraumatic R23.8
  nail
    finger — *see* Blister, finger
    toe — *see* Blister, toe
  nasal S00.32
  neck S10.92
    specified site NEC S10.82
    throat S10.12
  nose S00.32
  occipital region S00.02
  oral cavity S00.522
  orbital region — *see* Blister, eyelid
  palate S00.522
  palm — *see* Blister, hand
  parietal region S00.02
  pelvis S30.820
  penis S30.822
  periocular area — *see* Blister, eyelid
  phalanges
    finger — *see* Blister, finger
    toe — *see* Blister, toe
  pharynx S10.12
  pinna — *see* Blister, ear
  popliteal space — *see* Blister, knee
  scalp S00.02
  scapular region — *see* Blister, shoulder
  scrotum S30.823
  shin — *see* Blister, leg
  shoulder S40.22-
  sternal region S20.329
  submaxillary region S00.82
  submental region S00.82
  subungual
    finger(s) — *see* Blister, finger
    toe(s) — *see* Blister, toe
  supraclavicular fossa S10.82
  supraorbital S00.82
  temple S00.82
  temporal region S00.82
  testis S30.823
  thermal — *see* Burn, second degree, by site
  thigh S70.32-
  thorax, thoracic (wall) S20.92
    back S20.42-
    front S20.32-
  throat S10.12
  thumb S60.32-
  toe(s) S90.42-
    great S90.42-
  tongue S00.522
  trachea S10.12
  tympanum, tympanic membrane — *see* Blister, ear
  upper arm — *see* Blister, arm (upper)
  uvula S00.522
  vagina S30.824
  vocal cords S10.12
  vulva S30.824
  wrist S60.82-
Bloating R14.0
Bloch-Sulzberger disease or syndrome Q82.3
Block, blocked
  alveolocapillary J84.10
  arborization (heart) I45.5
  arrhythmic I45.9

Block, blocked — *continued*
  atrioventricular (incomplete) (partial) I44.30
    with atrioventricular dissociation I44.2
    complete I44.2
      congenital Q24.6
    congenital Q24.6
    first degree I44.0
    second degree (types I and II) I44.1
    specified NEC I44.39
    third degree I44.2
    types I and II I44.1
  auriculoventricular — *see* Block, atrioventricular
  bifascicular (cardiac) I45.2
  bundle-branch (complete) (false) (incomplete) I45.4
    bilateral I45.2
    left I44.7
      with right bundle branch block I45.2
      hemiblock I44.60
        anterior I44.4
        posterior I44.5
      incomplete I44.7
        with right bundle branch block I45.2
    right I45.10
      with
        left bundle branch block I45.2
        left fascicular block I45.2
      specified NEC I45.19
    Wilson's type I45.19
  cardiac I45.9
  conduction I45.9
    complete I44.2
  fascicular (left) I44.60
    anterior I44.4
    posterior I44.5
    right I45.0
    specified NEC I44.69
  foramen Magendie (acquired) G91.1
    congenital Q03.1
      with spina bifida — *see* Spina bifida, by site, with hydrocephalus
  heart I45.9
    bundle branch I45.4
      bilateral I45.2
    complete (atrioventricular) I44.2
    congenital Q24.6
    first degree (atrioventricular) I44.0
    second degree (atrioventricular) I44.1
    specified type NEC I45.5
    third degree (atrioventricular) I44.2
  hepatic vein I82.0
  intraventricular (nonspecific) I45.4
    bundle branch
      bilateral I45.2
  kidney N28.9
    postcystoscopic or postprocedural N99.0
  Mobitz (types I and II) I44.1
  myocardial — *see* Block, heart
  nodal I45.5
  organ or site, congenital NEC — *see* Atresia, by site
  portal (vein) I81
  second degree (types I and II) I44.1
  sinoatrial I45.5
  sinoauricular I45.5
  third degree I44.2
  trifascicular I45.3
  tubal N97.1
  vein NOS I82.90
  Wenckebach (types I and II) I44.1
Blockage — *see* Obstruction
Blocq's disease F44.4
Blood
  constituents, abnormal R78.9
  disease D75.9
  donor — *see* Donor, blood

Blood — *continued*
dyscrasia D75.9
  with
    abortion — *see* Abortion, by type,
      complicated by, hemorrhage
    ectopic pregnancy O08.1
    molar pregnancy O08.1
    following ectopic or molar pregnancy O08.1
    newborn P61.9
    puerperal, postpartum O72.3
flukes NEC — *see* Schistosomiasis
in
  feces K92.1
    occult R19.5
  urine — *see* Hematuria
mole O02.0
occult in feces R19.5
pressure
  decreased, due to shock following injury
    T79.4
  examination only Z01.30
  fluctuating I99.8
  high — *see* Hypertension
    borderline R03.0
    incidental reading, without diagnosis of
      hypertension R03.0
  low — *see also* Hypotension
    incidental reading, without diagnosis of
      hypotension R03.1
spitting — *see* Hemoptysis
staining cornea — *see* Pigmentation, cornea,
  stromal
transfusion
  reaction or complication — *see*
    Complications, transfusion
type
  A (Rh positive) Z67.10
    Rh negative Z67.11
  AB (Rh positive) Z67.30
    Rh negative Z67.31
  B (Rh positive) Z67.20
    Rh negative Z67.21
  O (Rh positive) Z67.40
    Rh negative Z67.41
  Rh (positive) Z67.90
    negative Z67.91
vessel rupture — *see* Hemorrhage
vomiting — *see* Hematemesis
Blood-forming organs, disease D75.9
Bloodgood's disease — *see* Mastopathy,
  cystic
Bloom(-Machacek)(-Torre) syndrome
  Q82.8
Blount's disease or osteochondrosis —
  see Osteochondrosis, juvenile, tibia
Blue
baby Q24.9
diaper syndrome E72.09
dome cyst (breast) — *see* Cyst, breast
dot cataract Q12.0
nevus D22.9
sclera Q13.5
  with fragility of bone and deafness Q78.0
toe syndrome I75.02-
Blueness — *see* Cyanosis
Blues, postpartal O90.6
baby O90.6
Blurring, visual H53.8
Blushing (abnormal) (excessive) R23.2
BMI — *see* Body, mass index
Boarder, hospital NEC Z76.4
accompanying sick person Z76.3
healthy infant or child Z76.2
foundling Z76.1
Bockhart's impetigo L01.02
Bodechtel-Guttman disease (subacute
  sclerosing panencephalitis) A81.1
Boder-Sedgwick syndrome (ataxia-
  telangiectasia) G11.3

Body, bodies
Aschoff's — *see* Myocarditis, rheumatic
asteroid, vitreous — *see* Deposit, crystalline
cytoid (retina) — *see* Occlusion, artery, retina
drusen (degenerative) (macula) (retinal) — *see
  also* Degeneration, macula, drusen
  optic disc — *see* Drusen, optic disc
foreign — *see* Foreign body
loose
  joint, except knee — *see* Loose, body, joint
    knee M23.4-
  sheath, tendon — *see* Disorder, tendon,
    specified type NEC
mass index (BMI)
  adult
    19 or less Z68.1
    20.0-20.9 Z68.20
    21.0-21.9 Z68.21
    22.0-22.9 Z68.22
    23.0-23.9 Z68.23
    24.0-24.9 Z68.24
    25.0-25.9 Z68.25
    26.0-26.9 Z68.26
    27.0-27.9 Z68.27
    28.0-28.9 Z68.28
    29.0-29.9 Z68.29
    30.0-30.9 Z68.30
    31.0-31.9 Z68.31
    32.0-32.9 Z68.32
    33.0-33.9 Z68.33
    34.0-34.9 Z68.34
    35.0-35.9 Z68.35
    36.0-36.9 Z68.36
    37.0-37.9 Z68.37
    38.0-38.9 Z68.38
    39.0-39.9 Z68.39
    40.0-44.9 Z68.41
    45.0-49.9 Z68.42
    50.0-59.9 Z68.43
    60.0-69.9 Z68.44
    70 and over Z68.45
  pediatric
    5th percentile to less than 85th percentile
      for age Z68.52
    85th percentile to less than 95th percentile
      for age Z68.53
    greater than or equal to ninety-fifth
      percentile for age Z68.54
    less than fifth percentile for age Z68.51
Mooser's A75.2
rice — *see also* Loose, body, joint
  knee M23.4-
rocking F98.4
Boeck's
disease or sarcoid — *see* Sarcoidosis
lupoid (miliary) D86.3
Boerhaave's syndrome (spontaneous
  esophageal rupture) K22.3
Boggy
cervix N88.8
uterus N85.8
Boil — *see also* Furuncle, by site
Aleppo B55.1
Baghdad B55.1
Delhi B55.1
lacrimal
  gland — *see* Dacryoadenitis
  passages (duct) (sac) — *see* Inflammation,
    lacrimal, passages, acute
Natal B55.1
orbit, orbital — *see* Abscess, orbit
tropical B55.1
Bold hives — *see* Urticaria
Bombé, iris — *see* Membrane, pupillary
Bone — *see* condition
Bonnevie-Ullrich syndrome (*see also*
  Turner's syndrome) Q87.1
Bonnier's syndrome — *see* subcategory
  H81.8

Bonvale dam fever T73.3
Bony block of joint — *see* Ankylosis
BOOP (bronchiolitis obliterans organized
  pneumonia) J84.89
Borderline
diabetes mellitus R73.03
hypertension R03.0
osteopenia M85.8-
pelvis, with obstruction during labor O65.1
personality F60.3
Borna disease A83.9
Bornholm disease B33.0
Boston exanthem A88.0
Botalli, ductus (patent) (persistent) Q25.0
Bothriocephalus latus infestation B70.0
Botulism (foodborne intoxication) A05.1
infant A48.51
non-foodborne A48.52
wound A48.52
Bouba — *see* Yaws
Bouchard's nodes (with arthropathy) M15.2
Bouffée délirante F23
Bouillaud's disease or syndrome
  (rheumatic heart disease) I01.9
Bourneville's disease Q85.1
Boutonniere deformity (finger) — *see*
  Deformity, finger, boutonniere
Bouveret(-Hoffmann) syndrome
  (paroxysmal tachycardia) I47.9
Bovine heart — *see* Hypertrophy, cardiac
Bowel — *see* condition
Bowen's
dermatosis (precancerous) — *see* Neoplasm,
  skin, in situ
disease — *see* Neoplasm, skin, in situ
epithelioma — *see* Neoplasm, skin, in situ
type
  epidermoid carcinoma-in-situ — *see*
    Neoplasm, skin, in situ
  intraepidermal squamous cell carcinoma —
    see Neoplasm, skin, in situ
Bowing
femur — *see also* Deformity, limb, specified
  type NEC, thigh
  congenital Q68.3
fibula — *see also* Deformity, limb, specified
  type NEC, lower leg
  congenital Q68.4
forearm — *see* Deformity, limb, specified type
  NEC, forearm
leg(s), long bones, congenital Q68.5
radius — *see* Deformity, limb, specified type
  NEC, forearm
tibia — *see also* Deformity, limb, specified type
  NEC, lower leg
  congenital Q68.4
Bowleg(s) (acquired) M21.16-
congenital Q68.5
rachitic E64.3
Boyd's dysentery A03.2
Brachial — *see* condition
Brachycardia R00.1
Brachycephaly Q75.0
Bradley's disease A08.19
Bradyarrhythmia, cardiac I49.8
Bradycardia (sinoatrial) (sinus) (vagal) R00.1
neonatal P29.12
reflex G90.09
tachycardia syndrome I49.5
Bradykinesia R25.8
Bradypnea R06.89
Bradytachycardia I49.5
Brailsford's disease or osteochondrosis
  — *see* Osteochondrosis, juvenile, radius
Brain — *see also* condition
death G93.82
syndrome — *see* Syndrome, brain
Branched-chain amino-acid disorder
  E71.2

Branchial — *see* condition
  cartilage, congenital Q18.2
Branchiogenic remnant (in neck) Q18.0
Brandt's syndrome (acrodermatitis
  enteropathica) E83.2
Brash (water) R12
Bravais-jacksonian epilepsy — *see*
  Epilepsy, localization-related, symptomatic,
  with simple partial seizures
Braxton Hicks contractions — *see* False,
  labor
Brazilian leishmaniasis B55.2
BRBPR K62.5
Break, retina (without detachment) H33.30-
  with retinal detachment — *see* Detachment,
    retina
  horseshoe tear H33.31-
  multiple H33.33-
  round hole H33.32-
Breakdown
  device, graft or implant (*see also* Complications,
    by site and type, mechanical) T85.618
    arterial graft NEC — *see* Complication,
      cardiovascular device, mechanical,
      vascular
    breast (implant) T85.41
    catheter NEC T85.618
      cystostomy T83.010
      dialysis (renal) T82.41
        intraperitoneal T85.611
      Hopkins T83.018
      ileostomy T83.018
      infusion NEC T82.514
        cranial T85.610
        epidural T85.610
        intrathecal T85.610
        spinal T85.610
        subarachnoid T85.610
        subdural T85.610
      nephrostomy T83.012
      urethral indwelling T83.011
      urinary NEC T83.018
      urostomy T83.018
    electronic (electrode) (pulse generator)
      (stimulator)
      bone T84.310
      cardiac T82.119
        electrode T82.110
        pulse generator T82.111
        specified type NEC T82.118
      nervous system — *see* Complication,
        prosthetic device, mechanical,
        electronic nervous system stimulator
      urinary — *see* Complication,
        genitourinary, device, urinary,
        mechanical
    fixation, internal (orthopedic) NEC — *see*
      Complication, fixation device,
      mechanical
    gastrointestinal — *see* Complications,
      prosthetic device, mechanical,
      gastrointestinal device
    genital NEC T83.418
      intrauterine contraceptive device T83.31
      penile prosthesis (cylinder) (implanted)
        (pump) (resevoir) T83.410
      testicular prosthesis T83.411
    heart NEC — *see* Complication,
      cardiovascular device, mechanical
    intrathecal infusion pump T85.615
    joint prosthesis — *see* Complications, joint
      prosthesis, internal, mechanical, by site
    nervous system, specified device NEC
      T85.615
    ocular NEC — *see* Complications, prosthetic
      device, mechanical, ocular device
    orthopedic NEC — *see* Complication,
      orthopedic, device, mechanical

Breakdown — *continued*
  device, graft or implant (*see also* Complications,
    by site and type, mechanical) T85.618 —
    continued
    specified NEC T85.618
    subcutaneous device pocket
      nervous system prosthetic device, implant,
        or graft T85.890
      other internal prosthetic device, implant,
        or graft T85.898
    sutures, permanent T85.612
      used in bone repair — *see* Complications,
        fixation device, internal (orthopedic),
        mechanical
    urinary NEC T83.118
      graft T83.21
      sphincter, implanted T83.111
      stent (ileal conduit) (nephroureteral)
        T83.113
      ureteral indwelling T83.112
    vascular NEC — *see* Complication,
      cardiovascular device, mechanical
    ventricular intracranial shunt T85.01
  nervous F48.8
  perineum O90.1
  respirator J95.850
    specified NEC J95.859
  ventilator J95.850
    specified NEC J95.859
Breast — *see also* condition
  buds E30.1
    in newborn P96.89
  dense R92.2
  nodule N63
Breath
  foul R19.6
  holder, child R06.89
  holding spell R06.89
  shortness R06.02
Breathing
  labored — *see* Hyperventilation
  mouth R06.5
    causing malocclusion M26.5
  periodic R06.3
    high altitude G47.32
Breathlessness R06.81
Breda's disease — *see* Yaws
Breech presentation (mother) O32.1
  causing obstructed labor O64.1
  footling O32.8
    causing obstructed labor O64.8
  incomplete O32.8
    causing obstructed labor O64.8
Breisky's disease N90.4
Brennemann's syndrome I88.0
Brenner
  tumor (benign) D27.9
    borderline malignancy D39.1-
    malignant C56
    proliferating D39.1-
Bretonneau's disease or angina A36.0
Breus' mole O02.0
Brevicollis Q76.49
Brickmakers' anemia B76.9 *[D63.8]*
Bridge, myocardial Q24.5
Bright red blood per rectum (BRBPR) K62.5
Bright's disease — *see* Nephritis
  arteriosclerotic — *see* Hypertension, kidney
Brill-Symmers' disease C82.90
Brill(-Zinsser) disease (recrudescent typhus)
  A75.1
  flea-borne A75.2
  louse-borne A75.1
Brion-Kayser disease — *see* Fever,
  paratyphoid
Briquet's disorder or syndrome F45.0
Brissaud's
  infantilism or dwarfism E23.0
  motor-verbal tic F95.2

Brittle
  bones disease Q78.0
  nails L60.3
    congenital Q84.6
Broad — *see also* condition
  beta disease E78.2
  ligament laceration syndrome N83.8
Broad- or floating-betalipoproteinemia
  E78.2
Brock's syndrome (atelectasis due to
  enlarged lymph nodes) J98.19
Brocq-Duhring disease (dermatitis
  herpetiformis) L13.0
Brodie's abscess or disease M86.8x-
Broken
  arches — *see also* Deformity, limb, flat foot
  arm (meaning upper limb) — *see* Fracture, arm
  back — *see* Fracture, vertebra
  bone — *see* Fracture
  implant or internal device — *see*
    Complications, by site and type,
    mechanical
  leg (meaning lower limb) — *see* Fracture, leg
  nose S02.2
  tooth, teeth — *see* Fracture, tooth
Bromhidrosis, bromidrosis L75.0
Bromidism, bromism G92
  chronic (dependence) F13.20
  due to
    correct substance properly administered —
      see Table of Drugs and Chemicals, by
      drug, adverse effect
    overdose or wrong substance given or taken
      — *see* Table of Drugs and Chemicals, by
      drug, poisoning
Bromidrosiphobia F40.298
Bronchi, bronchial — *see* condition
Bronchiectasis (cylindrical) (diffuse) (fusiform)
  (localized) (saccular) J47.9
  with
    acute
      bronchitis J47.0
      lower respiratory infection J47.0
    exacerbation (acute) J47.1
  congenital Q33.4
  tuberculous NEC — *see* Tuberculosis,
    pulmonary
Bronchiolectasis — *see* Bronchiectasis
Bronchiolitis (acute) (infective) (subacute)
  J21.9
  with
    bronchospasm or obstruction J21.9
    influenza, flu or grippe — *see* Influenza,
      with, respiratory manifestations NEC
  chemical (chronic) J68.4
    acute J68.0
  chronic (fibrosing) (obliterative) J44.9
  due to
    external agent — *see* Bronchitis, acute, due to
    human metapneumovirus J21.1
    respiratory syncytial virus J21.0
    specified organism NEC J21.8
  fibrosa obliterans J44.9
  influenzal — *see* Influenza, with, respiratory
    manifestations NEC
  obliterans J42
    with organizing pneumonia (BOOP) J84.89
  obliterative (chronic) (subacute) J44.9
    due to chemicals, gases, fumes or vapors
      (inhalation) J68.4
    due to fumes or vapors J68.4
  respiratory, interstitial lung disease J84.115
Bronchitis (diffuse) (fibrinous) (hypostatic)
  (infective) (membranous) J40
  with
    influenza, flu or grippe — *see* Influenza,
      with, respiratory manifestations NEC
    obstruction (airway) (lung) J44.9

Bronchitis (diffuse) (fibrinous) (hypostatic) (infective) (membranous) J40 — *continued*
  with — *continued*
    tracheitis (15 years of age and above) J40
      acute or subacute J20.9
      chronic J42
      under 15 years of age J20.9
  acute or subacute (with bronchospasm or obstruction) J20.9
    with
      bronchiectasis J47.0
      chronic obstructive pulmonary disease J44.0
    chemical (due to gases, fumes or vapors) J68.0
    due to
      fumes or vapors J68.0
      Haemophilus influenzae J20.1
      Mycoplasma pneumoniae J20.0
      radiation J70.0
      specified organism NEC J20.8
      Streptococcus J20.2
      virus
        coxsackie J20.3
        echovirus J20.7
        parainfluenzae J20.4
        respiratory syncytial J20.5
        rhinovirus J20.6
    viral NEC J20.8
  allergic (acute) J45.909
    with
      exacerbation (acute) J45.901
      status asthmaticus J45.902
  arachidic T17.528
  aspiration (due to fumes or vapors) J68.0
  asthmatic J45.9
    chronic J44.9
      with
        acute lower respiratory infection J44.0
        exacerbation (acute) J44.1
  capillary — *see* Pneumonia, broncho
  caseous (tuberculous) A15.5
  Castellani's A69.8
  catarrhal (15 years of age and above) J40
    acute — *see* Bronchitis, acute
    chronic J41.0
    under 15 years of age J20.9
  chemical (acute) (subacute) J68.0
    chronic J68.4
    due to fumes or vapors J68.0
      chronic J68.4
  chronic J42
    with
      airways obstruction J44.9
      tracheitis (chronic) J42
    asthmatic (obstructive) J44.9
    catarrhal J41.0
    chemical (due to fumes or vapors) J68.4
    due to
      chemicals, gases, fumes or vapors (inhalation) J68.4
      radiation J70.1
      tobacco smoking J41.0
    emphysematous J44.9
    mucopurulent J41.1
    non-obstructive J41.0
    obliterans J44.9
    obstructive J44.9
    purulent J41.1
    simple J41.0
  croupous — *see* Bronchitis, acute
  due to gases, fumes or vapors (chemical) J68.0
  emphysematous (obstructive) J44.9
  exudative — *see* Bronchitis, acute
  fetid J41.1
  grippal — *see* Influenza, with, respiratory manifestations NEC

Bronchitis (diffuse) (fibrinous) (hypostatic) (infective) (membranous) J40 — *continued*
  in those under 15 years age — *see* Bronchitis, acute
    chronic — *see* Bronchitis, chronic
  influenzal — *see* Influenza, with, respiratory manifestations NEC
  mixed simple and mucopurulent J41.8
  moulder's J62.8
  mucopurulent (chronic) (recurrent) J41.1
    acute or subacute J20.9
    simple (mixed) J41.8
  obliterans (chronic) J44.9
  obstructive (chronic) (diffuse) J44.9
  pituitous J41.1
  pneumococcal, acute or subacute J20.2
  pseudomembranous, acute or subacute — *see* Bronchitis, acute
  purulent (chronic) (recurrent) J41.1
    acute or subacute — *see* Bronchitis, acute
  putrid J41.1
  senile (chronic) J42
  simple and mucopurulent (mixed) J41.8
  smokers' J41.0
  spirochetal NEC A69.8
  subacute — *see* Bronchitis, acute
  suppurative (chronic) J41.1
    acute or subacute — *see* Bronchitis, acute
  tuberculous A15.5
  under 15 years of age — *see* Bronchitis, acute
    chronic — *see* Bronchitis, chronic
  viral NEC, acute or subacute (*see also* Bronchitis, acute) J20.8
Bronchoalveolitis J18.0
Bronchoaspergillosis B44.1
Bronchocele meaning goiter E04.0
Broncholithiasis J98.09
  tuberculous NEC A15.5
Bronchomalacia J98.09
  congenital Q32.2
Bronchomycosis NOS B49 *[J99]*
  candidal B37.1
Bronchopleuropneumonia — *see* Pneumonia, broncho
Bronchopneumonia — *see* Pneumonia, broncho
Bronchopneumonitis — *see* Pneumonia, broncho
Bronchopulmonary — *see* condition
Bronchopulmonitis — *see* Pneumonia, broncho
Bronchorrhagia (*see* Hemoptysis)
Bronchorrhea J98.09
  acute J20.9
  chronic (infective) (purulent) J42
Bronchospasm (acute) J98.01
  with
    bronchiolitis, acute J21.9
    bronchitis, acute (conditions in J20) — *see* Bronchitis, acute
  due to external agent — *see* condition, respiratory, acute, due to
  exercise induced J45.990
Bronchospirochetosis A69.8
  Castellani A69.8
Bronchostenosis J98.09
Bronchus — *see* condition
Brontophobia F40.220
Bronze baby syndrome P83.8
Brooke's tumor — *see* Neoplasm, skin, benign
Brown enamel of teeth (hereditary) K00.5
Brown-Séquard disease, paralysis or syndrome G83.81
Brown's sheath syndrome H50.61-
Bruce sepsis A23.0
Brucellosis (infection) A23.9
  abortus A23.1
  canis A23.3

Brucellosis (infection) A23.9 — *continued*
  dermatitis A23.9
  melitensis A23.0
  mixed A23.8
  sepsis A23.9
    melitensis A23.0
    specified NEC A23.8
  suis A23.2
Bruck-de Lange disease Q87.1
Bruck's disease — *see* Deformity, limb
Brugsch's syndrome Q82.8
Bruise (skin surface intact) — *see also* Contusion
  with
    open wound — *see* Wound, open
  internal organ — *see* Injury, by site
  newborn P54.5
  scalp, due to birth injury, newborn P12.3
  umbilical cord O69.5
Bruit (arterial) R09.89
  cardiac R01.1
Brush burn — *see* Abrasion, by site
Bruton's X-linked agammaglobulinemia D80.0
Bruxism
  psychogenic F45.8
  sleep related G47.63
Bubbly lung syndrome P27.0
Bubo I88.8
  blennorrhagic (gonococcal) A54.89
  chancroidal A57
  climatic A55
  due to Haemophilus ducreyi A57
  gonococcal A54.89
  indolent (nonspecific) I88.8
  inguinal (nonspecific) I88.8
    chancroidal A57
    climatic A55
    due to H. ducreyi A57
    infective I88.8
  scrofulous (tuberculous) A18.2
  soft chancre A57
  suppurating — *see* Lymphadenitis, acute
  syphilitic (primary) A51.0
    congenital A50.07
  tropical A55
  virulent (chancroidal) A57
Bubonic plague A20.0
Bubonocele — *see* Hernia, inguinal
Buccal — *see* condition
Buchanan's disease or osteochondrosis M91.0
Buchem's syndrome (hyperostosis corticalis) M85.2
Bucket-handle fracture or tear (semilunar cartilage) — *see* Tear, meniscus
Budd-Chiari syndrome (hepatic vein thrombosis) I82.0
Budgerigar fancier's disease or lung J67.2
Buds
  breast E30.1
  in newborn P96.89
Buerger's disease (thromboangiitis obliterans) I73.1
Bulbar — *see* condition
Bulbus cordis (left ventricle) (persistent) Q21.8
Bulimia (nervosa) F50.2
  atypical F50.9
  normal weight F50.9
Bulky
  stools R19.5
  uterus N85.2
Bulla(e) R23.8
  lung (emphysematous) (solitary) J43.9
  newborn P25.8
Bullet wound — *see also* Wound, open
  fracture — *code as* Fracture, by site
  internal organ — *see* Injury, by site

Bundle
  branch block (complete) (false) (incomplete) —
    see Block, bundle-branch
  of His — *see* condition
Bunion M21.61-
  tailor's M21.62-
Bunionette M21.62-
Buphthalmia, buphthalmos (congenital) Q15.0
Burdwan fever B55.0
Bürger-Grütz disease or syndrome E78.3
Buried
  penis (congenital) Q55.64
    acquired N48.83
  roots K08.3
Burke's syndrome K86.89
Burkitt
  cell leukemia C91.0-
  lymphoma (malignant) C83.7-
    small noncleaved, diffuse C83.7-
    spleen C83.77
    undifferentiated C83.7-
  tumor C83.7-
  type
    acute lymphoblastic leukemia C91.0-
    undifferentiated C83.7-
Burn (electricity) (flame) (hot gas, liquid or hot
    object) (radiation) (steam) (thermal) T30.0
  abdomen, abdominal (muscle) (wall) T21.02
    first degree T21.12
    second degree T21.22
    third degree T21.32
  above elbow T22.039
    first degree T22.139
    left T22.032
      first degree T22.132
      second degree T22.232
      third degree T22.332
    right T22.031
      first degree T22.131
      second degree T22.231
      third degree T22.331
    second degree T22.239
    third degree T22.339
  acid (caustic) (external) (internal) — *see*
    Corrosion, by site
  alimentary tract NEC T28.2
    esophagus T28.1
    mouth T28.0
    pharynx T28.0
  alkaline (caustic) (external) (internal) — *see*
    Corrosion, by site
  ankle T25.019
    first degree T25.119
    left T25.012
      first degree T25.112
      second degree T25.212
      third degree T25.312
    multiple with foot — *see* Burn, lower, limb,
      multiple, ankle and foot
    right T25.011
      first degree T25.111
      second degree T25.211
      third degree T25.311
    second degree T25.219
    third degree T25.319
  anus — *see* Burn, buttock
  arm (lower) (upper) — *see* Burn, upper, limb
  axilla T22.049
    first degree T22.149
    left T22.042
      first degree T22.142
      second degree T22.242
      third degree T22.342
    right T22.041
      first degree T22.141
      second degree T22.241
      third degree T22.341
    second degree T22.249
    third degree T22.349

Burn (electricity) (flame) (hot gas, liquid or hot
    object) (radiation) (steam) (thermal) T30.0
  — continued
  back (lower) T21.04
    first degree T21.14
    second degree T21.24
    third degree T21.34
    upper T21.03
      first degree T21.13
      second degree T21.23
      third degree T21.33
  blisters — *code as* Burn, second degree, by site
  breast(s) — *see* Burn, chest wall
  buttock(s) T21.05
    first degree T21.15
    second degree T21.25
    third degree T21.35
  calf T24.039
    first degree T24.139
    left T24.032
      first degree T24.132
      second degree T24.232
      third degree T24.332
    right T24.031
      first degree T24.131
      second degree T24.231
      third degree T24.331
    second degree T24.239
    third degree T24.339
  canthus (eye) — *see* Burn, eyelid
  caustic acid or alkaline — *see* Corrosion, by
    site
  cervix T28.3
  cheek T20.06
    first degree T20.16
    second degree T20.26
    third degree T20.36
  chemical (acids) (alkalines) (caustics) (external)
    (internal) — *see* Corrosion, by site
  chest wall T21.01
    first degree T21.11
    second degree T21.21
    third degree T21.31
  chin T20.03
    first degree T20.13
    second degree T20.23
    third degree T20.33
  colon T28.2
  conjunctiva (and cornea) — *see* Burn, cornea
  cornea (and conjunctiva) T26.1-
    chemical — *see* Corrosion, cornea
  corrosion (external) (internal) — *see* Corrosion,
    by site
  deep necrosis of underlying tissue — *code as*
    Burn, third degree, by site
  dorsum of hand T23.069
    first degree T23.169
    left T23.062
      first degree T23.162
      second degree T23.262
      third degree T23.362
    right T23.061
      first degree T23.161
      second degree T23.261
      third degree T23.361
    second degree T23.269
    third degree T23.369
  due to ingested chemical agent — *see*
    Corrosion, by site
  ear (auricle) (external) (canal) T20.01
    first degree T20.11
    second degree T20.21
    third degree T20.31

Burn (electricity) (flame) (hot gas, liquid or hot
    object) (radiation) (steam) (thermal) T30.0
  — continued
  elbow T22.029
    first degree T22.129
    left T22.022
      first degree T22.122
      second degree T22.222
      third degree T22.322
    right T22.021
      first degree T22.121
      second degree T22.221
      third degree T22.321
    second degree T22.229
    third degree T22.329
  epidermal loss — *code as* Burn, second
    degree, by site
  erythema, erythematous — *code as* Burn, first
    degree, by site
  esophagus T28.1
  extent (percentage of body surface)
    10-19 percent T31.10
      with 0-9 percent third degree burns
        T31.10
      with 10-19 percent third degree burns
        T31.11
    20-29 percent T31.20
      with 0-9 percent third degree burns
        T31.20
      with 10-19 percent third degree burns
        T31.21
      with 20-29 percent third degree burns
        T31.22
    30-39 percent T31.30
      with 0-9 percent third degree burns
        T31.30
      with 10-19 percent third degree burns
        T31.31
      with 20-29 percent third degree burns
        T31.32
      with 30-39 percent third degree burns
        T31.33
    40-49 percent T31.40
      with 0-9 percent third degree burns
        T31.40
      with 10-19 percent third degree burns
        T31.41
      with 20-29 percent third degree burns
        T31.42
      with 30-39 percent third degree burns
        T31.43
      with 40-49 percent third degree burns
        T31.44
    50-59 percent T31.50
      with 0-9 percent third degree burns
        T31.50
      with 10-19 percent third degree burns
        T31.51
      with 20-29 percent third degree burns
        T31.52
      with 30-39 percent third degree burns
        T31.53
      with 40-49 percent third degree burns
        T31.54
      with 50-59 percent third degree burns
        T31.55
    60-69 percent T31.60
      with 0-9 percent third degree burns
        T31.60
      with 10-19 percent third degree burns
        T31.61
      with 20-29 percent third degree burns
        T31.62
      with 30-39 percent third degree burns
        T31.63
      with 40-49 percent third degree burns
        T31.64

Burn (electricity) (flame) (hot gas, liquid or hot object) (radiation) (steam) (thermal) T30.0 — *continued*
- extent (percentage of body surface) — *continued*
  - 60-69 percent T31.60 — *continued*
    - with 50-59 percent third degree burns T31.65
    - with 60-69 percent third degree burns T31.66
  - 70-79 percent T31.70
    - with 0-9 percent third degree burns T31.70
    - with 10-19 percent third degree burns T31.71
    - with 20-29 percent third degree burns T31.72
    - with 30-39 percent third degree burns T31.73
    - with 40-49 percent third degree burns T31.74
    - with 50-59 percent third degree burns T31.75
    - with 60-69 percent third degree burns T31.76
    - with 70-79 percent third degree burns T31.77
  - 80-89 percent T31.80
    - with 0-9 percent third degree burns T31.80
    - with 10-19 percent third degree burns T31.81
    - with 20-29 percent third degree burns T31.82
    - with 30-39 percent third degree burns T31.83
    - with 40-49 percent third degree burns T31.84
    - with 50-59 percent third degree burns T31.85
    - with 60-69 percent third degree burns T31.86
    - with 70-79 percent third degree burns T31.87
    - with 80-89 percent third degree burns T31.88
  - 90 percent or more T31.90
    - with 0-9 percent third degree burns T31.90
    - with 10-19 percent third degree burns T31.91
    - with 20-29 percent third degree burns T31.92
    - with 30-39 percent third degree burns T31.93
    - with 40-49 percent third degree burns T31.94
    - with 50-59 percent third degree burns T31.95
    - with 60-69 percent third degree burns T31.96
    - with 70-79 percent third degree burns T31.97
    - with 80-89 percent third degree burns T31.98
    - with 90 percent or more third degree burns T31.99
  - less than 10 percent T31.0
- extremity — *see* Burn, limb
- eye(s) and adnexa T26.4-
  - with resulting rupture and destruction of eyeball T26.2-
  - conjunctival sac — *see* Burn, cornea
  - cornea — *see* Burn, cornea
  - lid — *see* Burn, eyelid
  - periocular area — *see* Burn, eyelid
  - specified site NEC T26.3-
- eyeball — *see* Burn, eye

Burn (electricity) (flame) (hot gas, liquid or hot object) (radiation) (steam) (thermal) T30.0 — *continued*
- eyelid(s) T26.0-
  - chemical — *see* Corrosion, eyelid
- face — *see* Burn, head
- finger T23.029
  - first degree T23.129
  - left T23.022
    - first degree T23.122
    - second degree T23.222
    - third degree T23.322
  - multiple sites (without thumb) T23.039
    - with thumb T23.049
      - first degree T23.149
      - left T23.042
        - first degree T23.142
        - second degree T23.242
        - third degree T23.342
      - right T23.041
        - first degree T23.141
        - second degree T23.241
        - third degree T23.341
      - second degree T23.249
      - third degree T23.349
    - first degree T23.139
    - left T23.032
      - first degree T23.132
      - second degree T23.232
      - third degree T23.332
    - right T23.031
      - first degree T23.131
      - second degree T23.231
      - third degree T23.331
    - second degree T23.239
    - third degree T23.339
  - right T23.021
    - first degree T23.121
    - second degree T23.221
    - third degree T23.321
  - second degree T23.229
  - third degree T23.329
- flank — *see* Burn, abdominal wall
- foot T25.029
  - first degree T25.129
  - left T25.022
    - first degree T25.122
    - second degree T25.222
    - third degree T25.322
  - multiple with ankle — *see* Burn, lower, limb, multiple, ankle and foot
  - right T25.021
    - first degree T25.121
    - second degree T25.221
    - third degree T25.321
  - second degree T25.229
  - third degree T25.329
- forearm T22.019
  - first degree T22.119
  - left T22.012
    - first degree T22.112
    - second degree T22.212
    - third degree T22.312
  - right T22.011
    - first degree T22.111
    - second degree T22.211
    - third degree T22.311
  - second degree T22.219
  - third degree T22.319
- forehead T20.06
  - first degree T20.16
  - second degree T20.26
  - third degree T20.36
- fourth degree — *code as* Burn, third degree, by site
- friction — *see* Burn, by site
- from swallowing caustic or corrosive substance NEC — *see* Corrosion, by site

Burn (electricity) (flame) (hot gas, liquid or hot object) (radiation) (steam) (thermal) T30.0 — *continued*
- full thickness skin loss — *code as* Burn, third degree, by site
- gastrointestinal tract NEC T28.2
  - from swallowing caustic or corrosive substance T28.7
- genital organs
  - external
    - female T21.07
      - first degree T21.17
      - second degree T21.27
      - third degree T21.37
    - male T21.06
      - first degree T21.16
      - second degree T21.26
      - third degree T21.36
  - internal T28.3
    - from caustic or corrosive substance T28.8
- groin — *see* Burn, abdominal wall
- hand(s) T23.009
  - back — *see* Burn, dorsum of hand
  - finger — *see* Burn, finger
  - first degree T23.109
  - left T23.002
    - first degree T23.102
    - second degree T23.202
    - third degree T23.302
  - multiple sites with wrist T23.099
    - first degree T23.199
    - left T23.092
      - first degree T23.192
      - second degree T23.292
      - third degree T23.392
    - right T23.091
      - first degree T23.191
      - second degree T23.291
      - third degree T23.391
    - second degree T23.299
    - third degree T23.399
  - palm — *see* Burn, palm
  - right T23.001
    - first degree T23.101
    - second degree T23.201
    - third degree T23.301
  - second degree T23.209
  - third degree T23.309
  - thumb — *see* Burn, thumb
- head (and face) (and neck) T20.00
  - cheek — *see* Burn, cheek
  - chin — *see* Burn, chin
  - ear — *see* Burn, ear
  - eye(s) only — *see* Burn, eye
  - first degree T20.10
  - forehead — *see* Burn, forehead
  - lip — *see* Burn, lip
  - multiple sites T20.09
    - first degree T20.19
    - second degree T20.29
    - third degree T20.39
  - neck — *see* Burn, neck
  - nose — *see* Burn, nose
  - scalp — *see* Burn, scalp
  - second degree T20.20
  - third degree T20.30
- hip(s) — *see* Burn, thigh
- inhalation — *see* Burn, respiratory tract
  - caustic or corrosive substance (fumes) — *see* Corrosion, respiratory tract
- internal organ(s) T28.40
  - alimentary tract T28.2
    - esophagus T28.1
  - eardrum T28.41
  - esophagus T28.1
  - from caustic or corrosive substance (swallowing) NEC — *see* Corrosion, by site

Burn (electricity) (flame) (hot gas, liquid or hot object) (radiation) (steam) (thermal) T30.0
— *continued*
  internal organ(s) T28.40 — *continued*
    genitourinary T28.3
    mouth T28.0
    pharynx T28.0
    respiratory tract — *see* Burn, respiratory tract
    specified organ NEC T28.49
  interscapular region — *see* Burn, back, upper
  intestine (large) (small) T28.2
  knee T24.029
    first degree T24.129
    left T24.022
      first degree T24.122
      second degree T24.222
      third degree T24.322
    right T24.021
      first degree T24.121
      second degree T24.221
      third degree T24.321
    second degree T24.229
    third degree T24.329
  labium (majus) (minus) — *see* Burn, genital organs, external, female
  lacrimal apparatus, duct, gland or sac — *see* Burn, eye, specified site NEC
  larynx T27.0
    with lung T27.1
  leg(s) (lower) (upper) — *see* Burn, lower, limb
  lightning — *see* Burn, by site
  limb(s)
    lower (except ankle or foot alone) — *see* Burn, lower, limb
    upper — *see* Burn, upper limb
  lip(s) T20.02
    first degree T20.12
    second degree T20.22
    third degree T20.32
  lower
    back — *see* Burn, back
    limb T24.009
      ankle — *see* Burn, ankle
      calf — *see* Burn, calf
      first degree T24.109
      foot — *see* Burn, foot
      hip — *see* Burn, thigh
      knee — *see* Burn, knee
      left T24.002
        first degree T24.102
        second degree T24.202
        third degree T24.302
      multiple sites, except ankle and foot T24.099
        ankle and foot T25.099
          first degree T25.199
          left T25.092
            first degree T25.192
            second degree T25.292
            third degree T25.392
          right T25.091
            first degree T25.191
            second degree T25.291
            third degree T25.391
          second degree T25.299
          third degree T25.399
        first degree T24.199
        left T24.092
          first degree T24.192
          second degree T24.292
          third degree T24.392
        right T24.091
          first degree T24.191
          second degree T24.291
          third degree T24.391
        second degree T24.299
        third degree T24.399

Burn (electricity) (flame) (hot gas, liquid or hot object) (radiation) (steam) (thermal) T30.0
— *continued*
  lower — *continued*
    limb T24.009 — *continued*
      right T24.001
        first degree T24.101
        second degree T24.201
        third degree T24.301
      second degree T24.209
      thigh — *see* Burn, thigh
      third degree T24.309
      toe — *see* Burn, toe
  lung (with larynx and trachea) T27.1
  mouth T28.0
  neck T20.07
    first degree T20.17
    second degree T20.27
    third degree T20.37
  nose (septum) T20.04
    first degree T20.14
    second degree T20.24
    third degree T20.34
  ocular adnexa — *see* Burn, eye
  orbit region — *see* Burn, eyelid
  palm T23.059
    first degree T23.159
    left T23.052
      first degree T23.152
      second degree T23.252
      third degree T23.352
    right T23.051
      first degree T23.151
      second degree T23.251
      third degree T23.351
    second degree T23.259
    third degree T23.359
  partial thickness — *code as* Burn, unspecified degree, by site
  pelvis — *see* Burn, trunk
  penis — *see* Burn, genital organs, external, male
  perineum
    female — *see* Burn, genital organs, external, female
    male — *see* Burn, genital organs, external, male
  periocular area — *see* Burn, eyelid
  pharynx T28.0
  rectum T28.2
  respiratory tract T27.3
    larynx — *see* Burn, larynx
    specified part NEC T27.2
    trachea — *see* Burn, trachea
  sac, lacrimal — *see* Burn, eye, specified site NEC
  scalp T20.05
    first degree T20.15
    second degree T20.25
    third degree T20.35
  scapular region T22.069
    first degree T22.169
    left T22.062
      first degree T22.162
      second degree T22.262
      third degree T22.362
    right T22.061
      first degree T22.161
      second degree T22.261
      third degree T22.361
    second degree T22.269
    third degree T22.369
  sclera — *see* Burn, eye, specified site NEC
  scrotum — *see* Burn, genital organs, external, male

Burn (electricity) (flame) (hot gas, liquid or hot object) (radiation) (steam) (thermal) T30.0
— *continued*
  shoulder T22.059
    first degree T22.159
    left T22.052
      first degree T22.152
      second degree T22.252
      third degree T22.352
    right T22.051
      first degree T22.151
      second degree T22.251
      third degree T22.351
    second degree T22.259
    third degree T22.359
  stomach T28.2
  temple — *see* Burn, head
  testis — *see* Burn, genital organs, external, male
  thigh T24.019
    first degree T24.119
    left T24.012
      first degree T24.112
      second degree T24.212
      third degree T24.312
    right T24.011
      first degree T24.111
      second degree T24.211
      third degree T24.311
    second degree T24.219
    third degree T24.319
  thorax (external) — *see* Burn, trunk
  throat (meaning pharynx) T28.0
  thumb(s) T23.019
    first degree T23.119
    left T23.012
      first degree T23.112
      second degree T23.212
      third degree T23.312
    multiple sites with fingers T23.049
      first degree T23.149
      left T23.042
        first degree T23.142
        second degree T23.242
        third degree T23.342
      right T23.041
        first degree T23.141
        second degree T23.241
        third degree T23.341
      second degree T23.249
      third degree T23.349
    right T23.011
      first degree T23.111
      second degree T23.211
      third degree T23.311
    second degree T23.219
    third degree T23.319
  toe T25.039
    first degree T25.139
    left T25.032
      first degree T25.132
      second degree T25.232
      third degree T25.332
    right T25.031
      first degree T25.131
      second degree T25.231
      third degree T25.331
    second degree T25.239
    third degree T25.339
  tongue T28.0
  tonsil(s) T28.0
  trachea T27.0
    with lung T27.1
  trunk T21.00
    abdominal wall — *see* Burn, abdominal wall
    anus — *see* Burn, buttock
    axilla — *see* Burn, upper limb
    back — *see* Burn, back

DISEASE INDEX

Burn (electricity) (flame) (hot gas, liquid or hot object) (radiation) (steam) (thermal) T30.0 — *continued*

trunk T21.00 — *continued*
  breast — *see* Burn, chest wall
  buttock — *see* Burn, buttock
  chest wall — *see* Burn, chest wall
  first degree T21.10
  flank — *see* Burn, abdominal wall
  genital
    female — *see* Burn, genital organs, external, female
    male — *see* Burn, genital organs, external, male
  groin — *see* Burn, abdominal wall
  interscapular region — *see* Burn, back, upper
  labia — *see* Burn, genital organs, external, female
  lower back — *see* Burn, back
  penis — *see* Burn, genital organs, external, male
  perineum
    female — *see* Burn, genital organs, external, female
    male — *see* Burn, genital organs, external, male
  scapula region — *see* Burn, scapular region
  scrotum — *see* Burn, genital organs, external, male
  second degree T21.20
  specified site NEC T21.09
    first degree T21.19
    second degree T21.29
    third degree T21.39
  testes — *see* Burn, genital organs, external, male
  third degree T21.30
  upper back — *see* Burn, back, upper
  vulva — *see* Burn, genital organs, external, female
unspecified site with extent of body surface involved specified
  10-19 per cent (0-9 percent third degree) T31.10
    with 10-19 percent third degree T31.11
  20-29 per cent (0-9 percent third degree) T31.20
    with
      10-19 percent third degree T31.21
      20-29 percent third degree T31.22
  30-39 per cent (0-9 percent third degree) T31.30
    with
      10-19 percent third degree T31.31
      20-29 percent third degree T31.32
      30-39 percent third degree T31.33
  40-49 per cent (0-9 percent third degree) T31.40
    with
      10-19 percent third degree T31.41
      20-29 percent third degree T31.42
      30-39 percent third degree T31.43
      40-49 percent third degree T31.44
  50-59 per cent (0-9 percent third degree) T31.50
    with
      10-19 percent third degree T31.51
      20-29 percent third degree T31.52
      30-39 percent third degree T31.53
      40-49 percent third degree T31.54
      50-59 percent third degree T31.55

Burn (electricity) (flame) (hot gas, liquid or hot object) (radiation) (steam) (thermal) T30.0 — *continued*

unspecified site with extent of body surface involved specified — *continued*
  60-69 per cent (0-9 percent third degree) T31.60
    with
      10-19 percent third degree T31.61
      20-29 percent third degree T31.62
      30-39 percent third degree T31.63
      40-49 percent third degree T31.64
      50-59 percent third degree T31.65
      60-69 percent third degree T31.66
  70-79 per cent (0-9 percent third degree) T31.70
    with
      10-19 percent third degree T31.71
      20-29 percent third degree T31.72
      30-39 percent third degree T31.73
      40-49 percent third degree T31.74
      50-59 percent third degree T31.75
      60-69 percent third degree T31.76
      70-79 percent third degree T31.77
  80-89 per cent (0-9 percent third degree) T31.80
    with
      10-19 percent third degree T31.81
      20-29 percent third degree T31.82
      30-39 percent third degree T31.83
      40-49 percent third degree T31.84
      50-59 percent third degree T31.85
      60-69 percent third degree T31.86
      70-79 percent third degree T31.87
      80-89 percent third degree T31.88
  90 per cent or more (0-9 percent third degree) T31.90
    with
      10-19 percent third degree T31.91
      20-29 percent third degree T31.92
      30-39 percent third degree T31.93
      40-49 percent third degree T31.94
      50-59 percent third degree T31.95
      60-69 percent third degree T31.96
      70-79 percent third degree T31.97
      80-89 percent third degree T31.98
      90-99 percent third degree T31.99
  less than 10 per cent T31.0
upper limb T22.00
  above elbow — *see* Burn, above elbow
  axilla — *see* Burn, axilla
  elbow — *see* Burn, elbow
  first degree T22.10
  forearm — *see* Burn, forearm
  hand — *see* Burn, hand
  interscapular region — *see* Burn, back, upper
  multiple sites T22.099
    first degree T22.199
    left T22.092
      first degree T22.192
      second degree T22.292
      third degree T22.392
    right T22.091
      first degree T22.191
      second degree T22.291
      third degree T22.391
    second degree T22.299
    third degree T22.399
  scapular region — *see* Burn, scapular region
  second degree T22.20
  shoulder — *see* Burn, shoulder
  third degree T22.30
  wrist — *see* Burn, wrist
uterus T28.3
vagina T28.3
vulva — *see* Burn, genital organs, external, female

Burn (electricity) (flame) (hot gas, liquid or hot object) (radiation) (steam) (thermal) T30.0 — *continued*

  wrist T23.079
    first degree T23.179
    left T23.072
      first degree T23.172
      second degree T23.272
      third degree T23.372
    multiple sites with hand T23.099
      first degree T23.199
      left T23.092
        first degree T23.192
        second degree T23.292
        third degree T23.392
      right T23.091
        first degree T23.191
        second degree T23.291
        third degree T23.391
      second degree T23.299
      third degree T23.399
    right T23.071
      first degree T23.171
      second degree T23.271
      third degree T23.371
    second degree T23.279
    third degree T23.379
Burnett's syndrome E83.52
Burn-out (state) Z73.0
Burning
  feet syndrome E53.9
  sensation R20.8
  tongue K14.6
Burns' disease or osteochondrosis — *see* Osteochondrosis, juvenile, ulna
Bursa — *see* condition
Bursitis M71.9
  Achilles — *see* Tendinitis, Achilles
  adhesive — *see* Bursitis, specified NEC
  ankle — *see* Enthesopathy, lower limb, ankle, specified type NEC
  calcaneal — *see* Enthesopathy, foot, specified type NEC
  collateral ligament, tibial — *see* Bursitis, tibial collateral
  due to use, overuse, pressure — *see also* Disorder, soft tissue, due to use, specified type NEC
    specified NEC — *see* Disorder, soft tissue, due to use, specified NEC
  Duplay's M75.0
  elbow NEC M70.3-
    olecranon M70.2-
  finger — *see* Disorder, soft tissue, due to use, specified type NEC, hand
  foot — *see* Enthesopathy, foot, specified type NEC
  gonococcal A54.49
  gouty — *see* Gout
  hand M70.1-
  hip NEC M70.7-
    trochanteric M70.6-
  infective NEC M71.10
    abscess — *see* Abscess, bursa
    ankle M71.17-
    elbow M71.12-
    foot M71.17-
    hand M71.14-
    hip M71.15-
    knee M71.16-
    multiple sites M71.19
    shoulder M71.11-
    specified site NEC M71.18
    wrist M71.13-
  ischial — *see* Bursitis, hip
  knee NEC M70.5-
    prepatellar M70.4-
  occupational NEC — *see also* Disorder, soft tissue, due to, use

© 2016 Channel Publishing, Ltd.

Bursitis M71.9 — *continued*
olecranon — *see* Bursitis, elbow, olecranon
pharyngeal J39.1
popliteal — *see* Bursitis, knee
prepatellar M70.4-
radiohumeral M77.8
rheumatoid M06.20
  ankle M06.27-
  elbow M06.22-
  foot joint M06.27-
  hand joint M06.24-
  hip M06.25-
  knee M06.26-
  multiple site M06.29
  shoulder M06.21-
  vertebra M06.28
  wrist M06.23-
scapulohumeral — *see* Bursitis, shoulder
semimembranous muscle (knee) — *see* Bursitis, knee
shoulder M75.5-
  adhesive — *see* Capsulitis, adhesive
specified NEC M71.50
  ankle M71.57-
  due to use, overuse or pressure — *see* Disorder, soft tissue, due to, use
  elbow M71.52-
  foot M71.57-
  hand M71.54-
  hip M71.55-
  knee M71.56-
  shoulder — *see* Bursitis, shoulder
  specified site NEC M71.58
  tibial collateral M76.4-
  wrist M71.53-
subacromial — *see* Bursitis, shoulder
subcoracoid — *see* Bursitis, shoulder
subdeltoid — *see* Bursitis, shoulder
syphilitic A52.78
Thornwaldt, Tornwaldt J39.2
tibial collateral M76.4-
toe — *see* Enthesopathy, foot, specified type NEC
trochanteric (area) — *see* Bursitis, hip, trochanteric
wrist — *see* Bursitis, hand
Bursopathy M71.9
specified type NEC M71.80
  ankle M71.87-
  elbow M71.82-
  foot M71.87-
  hand M71.84-
  hip M71.85-
  knee M71.86-
  multiple sites M71.89
  shoulder M71.81-
  specified site NEC M71.88
  wrist M71.83-
Burst stitches or sutures (complication of surgery) T81.31
external operation wound T81.31
internal operation wound T81.32
Buruli ulcer A31.1
Bury's disease L95.1
Buschke's
disease B45.3
scleredema — *see* Sclerosis, systemic
Busse-Buschke disease B45.3
Buttock — *see* condition
Button
Biskra B55.1
Delhi B55.1
oriental B55.1
Buttonhole deformity (finger) — *see* Deformity, finger, boutonniere
Bwamba fever A92.8
Byssinosis J66.0
Bywaters' syndrome T79.5

C

Cachexia R64
cancerous R64
cardiac — *see* Disease, heart
dehydration E86.0
due to malnutrition R64
exophthalmic — *see* Hyperthyroidism
heart — *see* Disease, heart
hypophyseal E23.0
hypopituitary E23.0
lead — *see* Poisoning, lead
malignant R64
marsh — *see* Malaria
nervous F48.8
old age R54
paludal — *see* Malaria
pituitary E23.0
renal N28.9
saturnine — *see* Poisoning, lead
senile R54
Simmonds' E23.0
splenica D73.0
strumipriva E03.4
tuberculous NEC — *see* Tuberculosis
Café, au lait spots L81.3
Caffeine-induced
anxiety disorder F15.980
sleep disorder F15.982
Caffey's syndrome Q78.8
Caisson disease T70.3
Cake kidney Q63.1
Caked breast (puerperal, postpartum) O92.79
Calabar swelling B74.3
Calcaneal spur — *see* Spur, bone, calcaneal
Calcaneo-apophysitis M92.8
Calcareous — *see* condition
Calcicosis J62.8
Calciferol (vitamin D) deficiency E55.9
with rickets E55.0
Calcification
adrenal (capsule) (gland) E27.49
  tuberculous E35 [B90.8]
aorta I70.0
artery (annular) — *see* Arteriosclerosis
auricle (ear) — *see* Disorder, pinna, specified type NEC
basal ganglia G23.8
bladder N32.89
  due to Schistosoma hematobium B65.0
brain (cortex) — *see* Calcification, cerebral
bronchus J98.09
bursa M71.40
  ankle M71.47-
  elbow M71.42-
  foot M71.47-
  hand M71.44-
  hip M71.45-
  knee M71.46-
  multiple sites M71.49
  shoulder M75.3-
  specified site NEC M71.48
  wrist M71.43-
cardiac — *see* Degeneration, myocardial
cerebral (cortex) G93.89
  artery I67.2
cervix (uteri) N88.8
choroid plexus G93.89
conjunctiva — *see* Concretion, conjunctiva
corpora cavernosa (penis) N48.89
cortex (brain) — *see* Calcification, cerebral
dental pulp (nodular) K04.2
dentinal papilla K00.4
fallopian tube N83.8
falx cerebri G96.19
gallbladder K82.8
general E83.59

Calcification — *continued*
heart — *see also* Degeneration, myocardial
  valve — *see* Endocarditis
idiopathic infantile arterial (IIAC) Q28.8
intervertebral cartilage or disc (postinfective) — *see* Disorder, disc, specified NEC
intracranial — *see* Calcification, cerebral
joint — *see* Disorder, joint, specified type NEC
kidney N28.89
  tuberculous N29 [B90.1]
larynx (senile) J38.7
lens — *see* Cataract, specified NEC
lung (active) (postinfectional) J98.4
  tuberculous B90.9
lymph gland or node (postinfectional) I89.8
  tuberculous (*see also* Tuberculosis, lymph gland) B90.8
mammographic R92.1
massive (paraplegic) — *see* Myositis, ossificans, in, quadriplegia
medial — *see* Arteriosclerosis, extremities
meninges (cerebral) (spinal) G96.19
metastatic E83.59
muscle M61.9
  due to burns — *see* Myositis, ossificans, in, burns
  paralytic — *see* Myositis, ossificans, in, quadriplegia
  specified type NEC M61.40
    ankle M61.47-
    foot M61.47-
    forearm M61.43-
    hand M61.44-
    lower leg M61.46-
    multiple sites M61.49
    pelvic region M61.45-
    shoulder region M61.41-
    specified site NEC M61.48
    thigh M61.45-
    upper arm M61.42-
myocardium, myocardial — *see* Degeneration, myocardial
Mönckeberg's — *see* Arteriosclerosis, extremities
ovary N83.8
pancreas K86.89
penis N48.89
periarticular — *see* Disorder, joint, specified type NEC
pericardium (*see also* Pericarditis) I31.1
pineal gland E34.8
pleura J94.8
  postinfectional J94.8
  tuberculous NEC B90.9
pulpal (dental) (nodular) K04.2
sclera H15.89
spleen D73.89
subcutaneous L94.2
suprarenal (capsule) (gland) E27.49
tendon (sheath) — *see also* Tenosynovitis, specified type NEC
  with bursitis, synovitis or tenosynovitis — *see* Tendinitis, calcific
trachea J39.8
ureter N28.89
uterus N85.8
vitreous — *see* Deposit, crystalline
Calcified — *see* Calcification
Calcinosis (interstitial) (tumoral) (universalis) E83.59
with Raynaud's phenomenon, esophageal dysfunction, sclerodactyly, telangiectasia (CREST syndrome) M34.1
circumscripta (skin) L94.2
cutis L94.2
Calciphylaxis (*see also* Calcification, by site) E83.59

Calcium
- deposits — *see* Calcification, by site
- metabolism disorder E83.50
- salts or soaps in vitreous — *see* Deposit, crystalline

Calciuria R82.99

Calculi — *see* Calculus

Calculosis, intrahepatic — *see* Calculus, bile duct

Calculus, calculi, calculous
- ampulla of Vater — *see* Calculus, bile duct
- anuria (impacted) (recurrent) (*see also* Calculus, urinary) N20.9
- appendix K38.1
- bile duct (common) (hepatic) K80.50
  - with
    - calculus of gallbladder — *see* Calculus, gallbladder and bile duct
    - cholangitis K80.30
      - with
        - cholecystitis — *see* Calculus, bile duct, with cholecystitis
        - obstruction K80.31
      - acute K80.32
        - with
          - chronic cholangitis K80.36
            - with obstruction K80.37
          - obstruction K80.33
      - chronic K80.34
        - with
          - acute cholangitis K80.36
            - with obstruction K80.37
          - obstruction K80.35
    - cholecystitis (with cholangitis) K80.40
      - with obstruction K80.41
      - acute K80.42
        - with
          - chronic cholecystitis K80.46
            - with obstruction K80.47
          - obstruction K80.43
      - chronic K80.44
        - with
          - acute cholecystitis K80.46
            - with obstruction K80.47
          - obstruction K80.45
    - obstruction K80.51
  - biliary — *see also* Calculus, gallbladder
    - specified NEC K80.80
      - with obstruction K80.81
  - bilirubin, multiple — *see* Calculus, gallbladder
- bladder (encysted) (impacted) (urinary) (diverticulum) N21.0
- bronchus J98.09
- calyx (kidney) (renal) — *see* Calculus, kidney
- cholesterol (pure) (solitary) — *see* Calculus, gallbladder
- common duct (bile) — *see* Calculus, bile duct
- conjunctiva — *see* Concretion, conjunctiva
- cystic N21.0
  - duct — *see* Calculus, gallbladder
- dental (subgingival) (supragingival) K03.6
- diverticulum
  - bladder N21.0
  - kidney N20.0
- epididymis N50.89

Calculus, calculi, calculous — *continued*
- gallbladder K80.20
  - with
    - bile duct calculus — *see* Calculus, gallbladder and bile duct
    - cholecystitis K80.10
      - with obstruction K80.11
      - acute K80.00
        - with
          - chronic cholecystitis K80.12
            - with obstruction K80.13
          - obstruction K80.01
      - chronic K80.10
        - with
          - acute cholecystitis K80.12
            - with obstruction K80.13
          - obstruction K80.11
      - specified NEC K80.18
        - with obstruction K80.19
    - obstruction K80.21
- gallbladder and bile duct K80.70
  - with
    - cholecystitis K80.60
      - with obstruction K80.61
      - acute K80.62
        - with
          - chronic cholecystitis K80.66
            - with obstruction K80.67
          - obstruction K80.63
      - chronic K80.64
        - with
          - acute cholecystitis K80.66
            - with obstruction K80.67
          - obstruction K80.65
    - obstruction K80.71
- hepatic (duct) — *see* Calculus, bile duct
- hepatobiliary K80.80
  - with obstruction K80.81
- ileal conduit N21.8
- intestinal (impaction) (obstruction) K56.49
- kidney (impacted) (multiple) (pelvis) (recurrent) (staghorn) N20.0
  - with calculus, ureter N20.2
  - congenital Q63.8
- lacrimal passages — *see* Dacryolith
- liver (impacted) — *see* Calculus, bile duct
- lung J98.4
- mammographic R92.1
- nephritic (impacted) (recurrent) — *see* Calculus, kidney
- nose J34.89
- pancreas (duct) K86.89
- parotid duct or gland K11.5
- pelvis, encysted — *see* Calculus, kidney
- prostate N42.0
- pulmonary J98.4
- pyelitis (impacted) (recurrent) N20.0
  - with hydronephrosis N13.2
- pyelonephritis (impacted) (recurrent) — *see* category N20
  - with hydronephrosis N13.2
- renal (impacted) (recurrent) — *see* Calculus, kidney
- salivary (duct) (gland) K11.5
- seminal vesicle N50.89
- staghorn — *see* Calculus, kidney
- Stensen's duct K11.5
- stomach K31.89
- sublingual duct or gland K11.5
  - congenital Q38.4
- submandibular duct, gland or region K11.5
- submaxillary duct, gland or region K11.5
- suburethral N21.8
- tonsil J35.8
- tooth, teeth (subgingival) (supragingival) K03.6
- tunica vaginalis N50.89

Calculus, calculi, calculous — *continued*
- ureter (impacted) (recurrent) N20.1
  - with calculus, kidney N20.2
    - with hydronephrosis N13.2
      - with infection N13.6
- urethra (impacted) N21.1
- urinary (duct) (impacted) (passage) (tract) N20.9
  - with hydronephrosis N13.2
    - with infection N13.6
  - in (due to)
    - lower N21.9
      - specified NEC N21.8
- vagina N89.8
- vesical (impacted) N21.0
- Wharton's duct K11.5
- xanthine E79.8 *[N22]*

Calicectasis N28.89

Caliectasis N28.89

California
- disease B38.9
- encephalitis A83.5

Caligo cornea — *see* Opacity, cornea, central

Callositas, callosity (infected) L84

Callus (infected) L84
- bone — *see* Osteophyte
- excessive, following fracture — *code as* Sequelae of fracture

CALME (childhood asymmetric labium majus enlargement) N90.61

Calorie deficiency or malnutrition (*see also* Malnutrition) E46

Calvities — *see* Alopecia, androgenic

Calvé-Perthes disease — *see* Legg-Calvé-Perthes disease

Calvé's disease — *see* Osteochondrosis, juvenile, spine

Cameroon fever — *see* Malaria

Camptocormia (hysterical) F44.4

Camurati-Engelmann syndrome Q78.3

Canal — *see also* condition
- atrioventricular common Q21.2

Canaliculitis (lacrimal) (acute) (subacute) H04.33-
- Actinomyces A42.89
- chronic H04.42-

Canavan's disease E75.29

Canceled procedure (surgical) Z53.9
- because of
  - contraindication Z53.09
    - smoking Z53.01
  - left against medical advice (AMA) Z53.21
  - patient's decision Z53.20
    - for reasons of belief or group pressure Z53.1
    - specified reason NEC Z53.29
  - specified reason NEC Z53.8

Cancer — *see also* Neoplasm, by site, malignant
- bile duct type liver C22.1
- blood — *see* Leukemia
- breast (*see also* Neoplasm, breast, malignant) C50.91-
- hepatocellular C22.0
- lung (*see also* Neoplasm, lung, malignant) C34.90-
- ovarian (*see also* Neoplasm ovary, malignant) C56.9-
- unspecified site (primary) C80.1

Cancer (o)phobia F45.29

Cancerous — *see* Neoplasm, malignant, by site

Cancrum oris A69.0

Candidiasis, candidal B37.9
- balanitis B37.42
- bronchitis B37.1
- cheilitis B37.83
- congenital P37.5
- cystitis B37.41
- disseminated B37.7
- endocarditis B37.6

© 2016 Channel Publishing, Ltd.

Candidiasis, candidal B37.9 — *continued*
  enteritis B37.82
  esophagitis B37.81
  intertrigo B37.2
  lung B37.1
  meningitis B37.5
  mouth B37.0
  nails B37.2
  neonatal P37.5
  onychia B37.2
  oral B37.0
  osteomyelitis B37.89
  otitis externa B37.84
  paronychia B37.2
  perionyxis B37.2
  pneumonia B37.1
  proctitis B37.82
  pulmonary B37.1
  pyelonephritis B37.49
  sepsis B37.7
  skin B37.2
  specified site NEC B37.89
  stomatitis B37.0
  systemic B37.7
  urethritis B37.41
  urogenital site NEC B37.49
  vagina B37.3
  vulva B37.3
  vulvovaginitis B37.3
Candidid L30.2
Candidosis — *see* Candidiasis
Candiru infection or infestation B88.8
Canities (premature) L67.1
  congenital Q84.2
Canker (mouth) (sore) K12.0
  rash A38.9
Cannabinosis J66.2
Cannabis-induced
  anxiety disorder F12.980
  psychotic disorder F12.959
  sleep disorder F12.988
Canton fever A75.9
Cantrell's syndrome Q87.89
Capillariasis (intestinal) B81.1
  hepatic B83.8
Capillary — *see* condition
Caplan's syndrome — *see* Rheumatoid, lung
Capsule — *see* condition
Capsulitis (joint) — *see also* Enthesopathy
  adhesive (shoulder) M75.0-
  hepatic K65.8
  labyrinthine — *see* Otosclerosis, specified NEC
  thyroid E06.9
Caput
  crepitus Q75.8
  medusae I86.8
  succedaneum P12.81
Car sickness T75.3
Carapata (disease) A68.0
Carate — *see* Pinta
Carbon lung J60
Carbuncle L02.93
  abdominal wall L02.231
  anus K61.0
  auditory canal, external — *see* Abscess, ear, external
  auricle ear — *see* Abscess, ear, external
  axilla L02.43-
  back (any part) L02.232
  breast N61.1
  buttock L02.33
  cheek (external) L02.03
  chest wall L02.233
  chin L02.03
  corpus cavernosum N48.21
  ear (any part) (external) (middle) — *see* Abscess, ear, external
  external auditory canal — *see* Abscess, ear, external

Carbuncle L02.93 — *continued*
  eyelid — *see* Abscess, eyelid
  face NEC L02.03
  femoral (region) — *see* Carbuncle, lower limb
  finger — *see* Carbuncle, hand
  flank L02.231
  foot L02.63-
  forehead L02.03
  genital — *see* Abscess, genital
  gluteal (region) L02.33
  groin L02.234
  hand L02.53-
  head NEC L02.831
  heel — *see* Carbuncle, foot
  hip — *see* Carbuncle, lower limb
  kidney — *see* Abscess, kidney
  knee — *see* Carbuncle, lower limb
  labium (majus) (minus) N76.4
  lacrimal
    gland — *see* Dacryoadenitis
    passages (duct) (sac) — *see* Inflammation, lacrimal, passages, acute
  leg — *see* Carbuncle, lower limb
  lower limb L02.43-
  malignant A22.0
  navel L02.236
  neck L02.13
  nose (external) (septum) J34.0
  orbit, orbital — *see* Abscess, orbit
  palmar (space) — *see* Carbuncle, hand
  partes posteriores L02.33
  pectoral region L02.233
  penis N48.21
  perineum L02.235
  pinna — *see* Abscess, ear, external
  popliteal — *see* Carbuncle, lower limb
  scalp L02.831
  seminal vesicle N49.0
  shoulder — *see* Carbuncle, upper limb
  specified site NEC L02.838
  temple (region) L02.03
  thumb — *see* Carbuncle, hand
  toe — *see* Carbuncle, foot
  trunk L02.239
    abdominal wall L02.231
    back L02.232
    chest wall L02.233
    groin L02.234
    perineum L02.235
    umbilicus L02.236
  umbilicus L02.236
  upper limb L02.43-
  urethra N34.0
  vulva N76.4
Carbunculus — *see* Carbuncle
Carcinoid (tumor) — *see* Tumor, carcinoid
Carcinoidosis E34.0
Carcinoma (malignant) — *see also* Neoplasm, by site, malignant
  acidophil
    specified site — *see* Neoplasm, malignant, by site
    unspecified site C75.1
  acidophil-basophil, mixed
    specified site — *see* Neoplasm, malignant, by site
    unspecified site C75.1
  adnexal (skin) — *see* Neoplasm, skin, malignant
  adrenal cortical C74.0-
  alveolar — *see* Neoplasm, lung, malignant
    cell — *see* Neoplasm, lung, malignant
  ameloblastic C41.1
    upper jaw (bone) C41.0
  apocrine
    breast — *see* Neoplasm, breast, malignant
    specified site NEC — *see* Neoplasm, skin, malignant
    unspecified site C44.99

Carcinoma (malignant) (*see also* Neoplasm, by site, malignant) — *continued*
  basal cell (pigmented) (*see also* Neoplasm, skin, malignant) C44.91
    fibro-epithelial — *see* Neoplasm, skin, malignant
    morphea — *see* Neoplasm, skin, malignant
    multicentric — *see* Neoplasm, skin, malignant
  basal-squamous cell, mixed — *see* Neoplasm, skin, malignant
  basaloid
  basophil
    specified site — *see* Neoplasm, malignant, by site
    unspecified site C75.1
  basophil-acidophil, mixed
    specified site — *see* Neoplasm, malignant, by site
    unspecified site C75.1
  basosquamous — *see* Neoplasm, skin, malignant
  bile duct
    with hepatocellular, mixed C22.0
    liver C22.1
    specified site NEC — *see* Neoplasm, malignant, by site
    unspecified site C22.1
  branchial or branchiogenic C10.4
  bronchial or bronchogenic — *see* Neoplasm, lung, malignant
  bronchiolar — *see* Neoplasm, lung, malignant
  bronchioloalveolar — *see* Neoplasm, lung, malignant
  C cell
    specified site — *see* Neoplasm, malignant, by site
    unspecified site C73
  ceruminous C44.29-
  cervix uteri
    in situ D06.9
      endocervix D06.0
      exocervix D06.1
      specified site NEC D06.7
  chorionic
    specified site — *see* Neoplasm, malignant, by site
    unspecified site
      female C58
      male C62.90
  chromophobe
    specified site — *see* Neoplasm, malignant, by site
    unspecified site C75.1
  cloacogenic
    specified site — *see* Neoplasm, malignant, by site
    unspecified site C21.2
  diffuse type
    specified site — *see* Neoplasm, malignant, by site
    unspecified site C16.9
  duct (cell)
    with Paget's disease — *see* Neoplasm, breast, malignant
    infiltrating
      with lobular carcinoma (in situ)
        specified site — *see* Neoplasm, malignant, by site
        unspecified site (female) C50.91-
        male C50.92-
      specified site — *see* Neoplasm, malignant, by site
      unspecified site (female) C50.91-
      male C50.92-

Carcinoma (malignant) (*see also* Neoplasm, by site, malignant) — *continued*
- ductal
  - with lobular
    - specified site — *see* Neoplasm, malignant, by site
    - unspecified site (female) C50.91-
      - male C50.92-
- ductular, infiltrating
  - specified site — *see* Neoplasm, malignant, by site
  - unspecified site (female) C50.91-
    - male C50.92-
- embryonal
  - liver C22.7
- endometrioid
  - specified site — *see* Neoplasm, malignant, by site
  - unspecified site
    - female C56.9
    - male C61
- eosinophil
  - specified site — *see* Neoplasm, malignant, by site
  - unspecified site C75.1
- epidermoid — *see also* Neoplasm, skin, malignant
  - in situ, Bowen's type — *see* Neoplasm, skin, in situ
- fibroepithelial, basal cell — *see* Neoplasm, skin, malignant
- follicular
  - with papillary (mixed) C73
  - moderately differentiated C73
  - pure follicle C73
  - specified site — *see* Neoplasm, malignant, by site
  - trabecular C73
  - unspecified site C73
  - well differentiated C73
- generalized, with unspecified primary site C80.0
- glycogen-rich — *see* Neoplasm, breast, malignant
- granulosa cell C56-
- hepatic cell C22.0
- hepatocellular C22.0
  - with bile duct, mixed C22.0
  - fibrolamellar C22.0
- hepatocholangiolitic C22.0
- Hurthle cell C73
- in
  - adenomatous
    - polyposis coli C18.9
  - pleomorphic adenoma — *see* Neoplasm, salivary glands, malignant
  - situ — *see* Carcinoma-in-situ
- infiltrating
  - duct
    - with lobular
      - specified site — *see* Neoplasm, malignant, by site
      - unspecified site (female) C50.91-
        - male C50.92-
    - with Paget's disease — *see* Neoplasm, breast, malignant
    - specified site — *see* Neoplasm, malignant
    - unspecified site (female) C50.91-
      - male C50.92-
  - ductular
    - specified site — *see* Neoplasm, malignant
    - unspecified site (female) C50.91-
      - male C50.92-
  - lobular
    - specified site — *see* Neoplasm, malignant
    - unspecified site (female) C50.91-
      - male C50.92-

Carcinoma (malignant) (*see also* Neoplasm, by site, malignant) — *continued*
- inflammatory
  - specified site — *see* Neoplasm, malignant
  - unspecified site (female) C50.91-
    - male C50.92-
- intestinal type
  - specified site — *see* Neoplasm, malignant, by site
  - unspecified site C16.9
- intracystic
  - noninfiltrating — *see* Neoplasm, in situ, by site
- intraductal (noninfiltrating)
  - with Paget's disease — *see* Neoplasm, breast, malignant
  - breast D05.1-
  - papillary
    - with invasion
      - specified site — *see* Neoplasm, malignant, by site
      - unspecified site (female) C50.91-
        - male C50.92-
    - breast D05.1-
    - specified site NEC — *see* Neoplasm, in situ, by site
    - unspecified site (female) D05.1-
  - specified site NEC — *see* Neoplasm, in situ, by site
  - unspecified site (female) D05.1-
- intraepidermal — *see* Neoplasm, in situ
  - squamous cell, Bowen's type — *see* Neoplasm, skin, in situ
- intraepithelial — *see* Neoplasm, in situ, by site
  - squamous cell — *see* Neoplasm, in situ, by site
- intraosseous C41.1
  - upper jaw (bone) C41.0
- islet cell
  - with exocrine, mixed
    - specified site — *see* Neoplasm, malignant, by site
    - unspecified site C25.9
  - pancreas C25.4
  - specified site NEC — *see* Neoplasm, malignant, by site
  - unspecified site C25.4
- juvenile, breast — *see* Neoplasm, breast, malignant
- large cell
  - small cell
    - specified site — *see* Neoplasm, malignant, by site
    - unspecified site C34.90
- Leydig cell (testis)
  - specified site — *see* Neoplasm, malignant, by site
  - unspecified site
    - female C56.9
    - male C62.90
- lipid-rich (female) C50.91-
  - male C50.92-
- liver cell C22.0
- liver NEC C22.7
- lobular (infiltrating)
  - with intraductal
    - specified site — *see* Neoplasm, malignant, by site
    - unspecified site (female) C50.91-
      - male C50.92-
  - noninfiltrating
    - breast D05.0-
    - specified site NEC — *see* Neoplasm, in situ, by site
    - unspecified site D05.0-
  - specified site — *see* Neoplasm, malignant, by site
  - unspecified site (female) C50.91-
    - male C50.92-

Carcinoma (malignant) (*see also* Neoplasm, by site, malignant) — *continued*
- medullary
  - with
    - amyloid stroma
      - specified site — *see* Neoplasm, malignant, by site
      - unspecified site C73
    - lymphoid stroma
      - specified site — *see* Neoplasm, malignant, by site
      - unspecified site (female) C50.91-
        - male C50.92-
- Merkel cell C4A.9 *(follows C43)*
  - anal margin C4A.51 *(follows C43)*
  - anal skin C4A.51 *(follows C43)*
  - canthus C4A.1- *(follows C43)*
  - ear and external auricular canal C4A.2- *(follows C43)*
  - external auricular canal C4A.2- *(follows C43)*
  - eyelid, including canthus C4A.1- *(follows C43)*
  - face C4A.30 *(follows C43)*
    - specified NEC C4A.39 *(follows C43)*
  - hip C4A.7- *(follows C43)*
  - lip C4A.0 *(follows C43)*
  - lower limb, including hip C4A.7- *(follows C43)*
  - neck C4A.4 *(follows C43)*
  - nodal presentation C7B.1 *(follows C75)*
  - nose C4A.31 *(follows C43)*
  - overlapping sites C4A.8 *(follows C43)*
  - perianal skin C4A.51 *(follows C43)*
  - scalp C4A.4 *(follows C43)*
  - secondary C7B.1 *(follows C75)*
  - shoulder C4A.6- *(follows C43)*
  - skin of breast C4A.52 *(follows C43)*
  - trunk NEC C4A.59 *(follows C43)*
  - upper limb, including shoulder C4A.6- *(follows C43)*
  - visceral metastatic C7B.1 *(follows C75)*
- metastatic — *see* Neoplasm, secondary, by site
- metatypical — *see* Neoplasm, skin, malignant
- morphea, basal cell — *see* Neoplasm, skin, malignant
- mucoid
  - cell
    - specified site — *see* Neoplasm, malignant, by site
    - unspecified site C75.1
- neuroendocrine — *see also* Tumor, neuroendocrine
  - high grade, any site C7A.1 *(follows C75)*
  - poorly differentiated, any site C7A.1 *(follows C75)*
- nonencapsulated sclerosing C73
- noninfiltrating
  - intracystic — *see* Neoplasm, in situ, by site
  - intraductal
    - breast D05.1-
    - papillary
      - breast D05.1-
      - specified site NEC — *see* Neoplasm, in situ, by site
      - unspecified site D05.1-
    - specified site — *see* Neoplasm, in situ, by site
    - unspecified site D05.1-
  - lobular
    - breast D05.0-
    - specified site NEC — *see* Neoplasm, in situ, by site
    - unspecified site (female) D05.0-
- oat cell
  - specified site — *see* Neoplasm, malignant, by site
  - unspecified site C34.90
- odontogenic C41.1
  - upper jaw (bone) C41.0

Carcinoma (malignant) (*see also* Neoplasm, by site, malignant) — *continued*
  papillary
    with follicular (mixed) C73
    follicular variant C73
    intraductal (noninfiltrating)
      with invasion
        specified site — *see* Neoplasm, malignant, by site
        unspecified site (female) C50.91-
          male C50.92-
      breast D05.1-
      specified site NEC — *see* Neoplasm, in situ, by site
      unspecified site D05.1-
    serous
      specified site — *see* Neoplasm, malignant, by site
      surface
        specified site — *see* Neoplasm, malignant, by site
        unspecified site C56.9
      unspecified site C56.9
  papillocystic
    specified site — *see* Neoplasm, malignant, by site
    unspecified site C56.9
  parafollicular cell
    specified site — *see* Neoplasm, malignant, by site
    unspecified site C73
  pilomatrix — *see* Neoplasm, skin, malignant
  pseudomucinous
    specified site — *see* Neoplasm, malignant, by site
    unspecified site C56.9
  renal cell C64-
  Schmincke — *see* Neoplasm, nasopharynx, malignant
  Schneiderian
    specified site — *see* Neoplasm, malignant, by site
    unspecified site C30.0
  sebaceous — *see* Neoplasm, skin, malignant
  secondary — *see also* Neoplasm, secondary, by site
    Merkel cell C7B.1 **(follows C75)**
  secretory, breast — *see* Neoplasm, breast, malignant
  serous
    papillary
      specified site — *see* Neoplasm, malignant, by site
      unspecified site C56.9
    surface, papillary
      specified site — *see* Neoplasm, malignant, by site
      unspecified site C56.9
  Sertoli cell
    specified site — *see* Neoplasm, malignant, by site
    unspecified site C62.90
      female C56.9
      male C62.90
  skin appendage — *see* Neoplasm, skin, malignant
  small cell
    fusiform cell
      specified site — *see* Neoplasm, malignant, by site
      unspecified site C34.90
    intermediate cell
      specified site — *see* Neoplasm, malignant, by site
      unspecified site C34.90
    large cell
      specified site — *see* Neoplasm, malignant, by site
      unspecified site C34.90

Carcinoma (malignant) (*see also* Neoplasm, by site, malignant) — *continued*
  solid
    with amyloid stroma
      specified site — *see* Neoplasm, malignant, by site
      unspecified site C73
    microinvasive
      specified site — *see* Neoplasm, malignant, by site
      unspecified site C53.9
  sweat gland — *see* Neoplasm, skin, malignant
  theca cell C56-
  thymic C37
  unspecified site (primary) C80.1
  water-clear cell C75.0
Carcinoma-in-situ — *see also* Neoplasm, in situ, by site
  breast NOS D05.9-
    specified type NEC D05.8-
  epidermoid — *see also* Neoplasm, in situ, by site
    with questionable stromal invasion
      cervix D06.9
    specified site NEC — *see* Neoplasm, in situ, by site
    unspecified site D06.9
  Bowen's type — *see* Neoplasm, skin, in situ
  intraductal
    breast D05.1-
    specified site NEC — *see* Neoplasm, in situ, by site
    unspecified site D05.1-
  lobular
    with
      infiltrating duct
        breast (female) C50.91-
          male C50.92-
        specified site NEC — *see* Neoplasm, malignant
        unspecified site (female) C50.91-
          male C50.92-
      intraductal
        breast D05.8-
        specified site NEC — *see* Neoplasm, in situ, by site
        unspecified site (female) D05.8-
    breast D05.0-
    specified site NEC — *see* Neoplasm, in situ, by site
    unspecified site D05.0-
  squamous cell — *see also* Neoplasm, in situ, by site
    with questionable stromal invasion
      cervix D06.9
    specified site NEC — *see* Neoplasm, in situ, by site
    unspecified site D06.9
Carcinomaphobia F45.29
Carcinomatosis C80.0
  peritonei C78.6
  unspecified site (primary) (secondary) C80.0
Carcinosarcoma — *see* Neoplasm, malignant, by site
  embryonal — *see* Neoplasm, malignant, by site
Cardia, cardial — *see* condition

Cardiac — *see also* condition
  death, sudden — *see* Arrest, cardiac
  pacemaker
    in situ Z95.0
    management or adjustment Z45.018
  tamponade I31.4
Cardialgia — *see* Pain, precordial
Cardiectasis — *see* Hypertrophy, cardiac
Cardiochalasia K21.9
Cardiomalacia I51.5

Cardiomegalia glycogenica diffusa E74.02 [*I43*]
Cardiomegaly — *see also* Hypertrophy, cardiac
  congenital Q24.8
  glycogen E74.02 [*I43*]
  idiopathic I51.7
Cardiomyoliposis I51.5
Cardiomyopathy (familial) (idiopathic) I42.9
  alcoholic I42.6
  amyloid E85.4 [*I43*]
  arteriosclerotic — *see* Disease, heart, ischemic, atherosclerotic
  beriberi E51.12
  cobalt-beer I42.6
  congenital I42.4
  congestive I42.0
  constrictive NOS I42.5
  dilated I42.0
  due to
    alcohol I42.6
    beriberi E51.12
    cardiac glycogenosis E74.02 [*I43*]
    drugs I42.7
    external agents NEC I42.7
    Friedreich's ataxia G11.1
    myotonia atrophica G71.11 [*I43*]
    progressive muscular dystrophy G71.0
  glycogen storage E74.02 [*I43*]
  hypertensive — *see* Hypertension, heart
  hypertrophic (nonobstructive) I42.2
    obstructive I42.1
    congenital Q24.8
  in
    Chagas' disease (chronic) B57.2
      acute B57.0
    sarcoidosis D86.85
  ischemic I25.5
  metabolic E88.9 [*I43*]
    thyrotoxic E05.90 [*I43*]
      with thyroid storm E05.91 [*I43*]
  newborn I42.8
    congenital I42.4
  nutritional E63.9 [*I43*]
    beriberi E51.12
  obscure of Africa I42.8
  peripartum O90.3
  postpartum O90.3
  restrictive NEC I42.5
  rheumatic I09.0
  secondary I42.9
  stress induced I51.81
  takotsubo I51.81
  thyrotoxic E05.90 [*I43*]
    with thyroid storm E05.91 [*I43*]
  toxic NEC I42.7
  tuberculous A18.84
  viral B33.24
Cardionephritis — *see* Hypertension, cardiorenal
Cardionephropathy — *see* Hypertension, cardiorenal
Cardionephrosis — *see* Hypertension, cardiorenal
Cardiopathia nigra I27.0
Cardiopathy (*see also* Disease, heart) I51.9
  idiopathic I42.9
  mucopolysaccharidosis E76.3 [*I52*]
Cardiopericarditis — *see* Pericarditis
Cardiophobia F45.29
Cardiorenal — *see* condition
Cardiorrhexis — *see* Infarct, myocardium
Cardiosclerosis — *see* Disease, heart, ischemic, atherosclerotic
Cardiosis — *see* Disease, heart
Cardiospasm (esophagus) (reflex) (stomach) K22.0
  congenital Q39.5
    with megaesophagus Q39.5

Cardiostenosis — see Disease, heart
Cardiosymphysis I31.0
Cardiovascular — see condition
Carditis (acute) (bacterial) (chronic) (subacute) I51.89
  meningococcal A39.50
  rheumatic — see Disease, heart, rheumatic
  rheumatoid — see Rheumatoid, carditis
  viral B33.20
Care (of) (for) (following)
  child (routine) Z76.2
  family member (handicapped) (sick)
    creating problem for family Z63.6
    provided away from home for holiday relief Z75.5
    unavailable, due to
      absence (person rendering care) (sufferer) Z74.2
      inability (any reason) of person rendering care Z74.2
  foundling Z76.1
  holiday relief Z75.5
  improper — see Maltreatment
  lack of (at or after birth) (infant) — see Maltreatment, child, neglect
  lactating mother Z39.1
  palliative Z51.5
  postpartum
    immediately after delivery Z39.0
    routine follow-up Z39.2
  respite Z75.5
  unavailable, due to
    absence of person rendering care Z74.2
    inability (any reason) of person rendering care Z74.2
  well-baby Z76.2
Caries
  bone NEC A18.03
  dental (dentino enamel junction) (early childhood) (of dentine) (pre-eruptive) (recurrent) (to the pulp) K02.9
    arrested (coronal) (root) K02.3
    chewing surface
      limited to enamel K02.51
      penetrating into dentin K02.52
      penetrating into pulp K02.53
    coronal surface
      chewing surface
        limited to enamel K02.51
        penetrating into dentin K02.52
        penetrating into pulp K02.53
      pit and fissure surface
        limited to enamel K02.51
        penetrating into dentin K02.52
        penetrating into pulp K02.53
      smooth surface
        limited to enamel K02.61
        penetrating into dentin K02.62
        penetrating into pulp K02.63
    pit and fissure surface
      limited to enamel K02.51
      penetrating into dentin K02.52
      penetrating into pulp K02.53
    primary, cervical origin K02.52
    root K02.7
    smooth surface
      limited to enamel K02.61
      penetrating into dentin K02.62
      penetrating into pulp K02.63
  external meatus — see Disorder, ear, external, specified type NEC
  hip (tuberculous) A18.02
  initial (tooth)
    chewing surface K02.51
    pit and fissure surface K02.51
    smooth surface K02.61
  knee (tuberculous) A18.02
  labyrinth — see subcategory H83.8
  limb NEC (tuberculous) A18.03

Caries — continued
  mastoid process (chronic) — see Mastoiditis, chronic
    tuberculous A18.03
  middle ear — see subcategory H74.8
  nose (tuberculous) A18.03
  orbit (tuberculous) A18.03
  ossicles, ear — see Abnormal, ear ossicles
  petrous bone — see Petrositis
  root (dental) (tooth) K02.7
  sacrum (tuberculous) A18.01
  spine, spinal (column) (tuberculous) A18.01
  syphilitic A52.77
    congenital (early) A50.02 *[M90.80]*
  tooth, teeth — see Caries, dental
  tuberculous A18.03
  vertebra (column) (tuberculous) A18.01
Carious teeth — see Caries, dental
Carneous mole O02.0
Carnitine insufficiency E71.40
Carotid body or sinus syndrome G90.01
Carotidynia G90.01
Carotinemia (dietary) E67.1
Carotinosis (cutis) (skin) E67.1
Carpal tunnel syndrome — see Syndrome, carpal tunnel
Carpenter's syndrome Q87.0
Carpopedal spasm — see Tetany
Carr-Barr-Plunkett syndrome Q97.1
Carrier (suspected) of
  amebiasis Z22.1
  bacterial disease NEC Z22.39
    diphtheria Z22.2
    intestinal infectious NEC Z22.1
      typhoid Z22.0
    meningococcal Z22.31
    sexually transmitted Z22.4
    specified NEC Z22.39
    staphylococcal (Methicillin susceptible) Z22.321
      Methicillin resistant Z22.322
    streptococcal Z22.338
      group B Z22.330
        complicating pregnancy or delivery O99.82-
    typhoid Z22.0
  cholera Z22.1
  diphtheria Z22.2
  gastrointestinal pathogens NEC Z22.1
  genetic Z14.8
    cystic fibrosis Z14.1
    hemophilia A (asymptomatic) Z14.01
      symptomatic Z14.02
  gestational, pregnant Z33.1
  gonorrhea Z22.4
  HAA (hepatitis Australian-antigen) B18.8
  HB(c)(s)-AG B18.1
  hepatitis (viral) B18.9
    Australia-antigen (HAA) B18.8
    B surface antigen (HBsAg) B18.1
      with acute delta-(super)infection B17.0
    C B18.2
    specified NEC B18.8
  human T-cell lymphotropic virus type-1 (HTLV-1) infection Z22.6
  infectious organism Z22.9
    specified NEC Z22.8
  meningococci Z22.31
  Salmonella typhosa Z22.0
  serum hepatitis — see Carrier, hepatitis
  staphylococci (Methicillin susceptible) Z22.321
    Methicillin resistant Z22.322
  streptococci Z22.338
    group B Z22.330
      complicating pregnancy or delivery O99.82-
  syphilis Z22.4
  typhoid Z22.0
  venereal disease NEC Z22.4

Carrion's disease A44.0
Carter's relapsing fever (Asiatic) A68.1
Cartilage — see condition
Caruncle (inflamed)
  conjunctiva (acute) — see Conjunctivitis, acute
  labium (majus) (minus) N90.89
  lacrimal — see Inflammation, lacrimal, passages
  myrtiform N89.8
  urethral (benign) N36.2
Cascade stomach K31.2
Caseation lymphatic gland (tuberculous) A18.2
Cassidy (-Scholte) syndrome (malignant carcinoid) E34.0
Castellani's disease A69.8
Castration, traumatic, male S38.231
Casts in urine R82.99
Cat
  cry syndrome Q93.4
  ear Q17.3
  eye syndrome Q92.8
Catabolism, senile R54
Catalepsy (hysterical) F44.2
  schizophrenic F20.2
Cataplexy (idiopathic) — see Narcolepsy
Cataract (cortical) (immature) (incipient) H26.9
  with
    neovascularization — see Cataract, complicated
  age-related — see Cataract, senile
  anterior
    and posterior axial embryonal Q12.0
    pyramidal Q12.0
  associated with
    galactosemia E74.21 *[H28]*
    myotonic disorders G71.19 *[H28]*
  blue Q12.0
  central Q12.0
  cerulean Q12.0
  complicated H26.20
    with
      neovascularization H26.21-
      ocular disorder H26.22-
      glaucomatous flecks H26.23-
  congenital Q12.0
  coraliform Q12.0
  coronary Q12.0
  crystalline Q12.0
  diabetic — see Diabetes, cataract
  drug-induced H26.3-
  due to
    ocular disorder — see Cataract, complicated
    radiation H26.8
  electric H26.8
  extraction status Z98.4-
  glass-blower's H26.8
  heat ray H26.8
  heterochromic — see Cataract, complicated
  hypermature — see Cataract, senile, morgagnian type
  in (due to)
    chronic iridocyclitis — see Cataract, complicated
    diabetes — see Diabetes, cataract
    endocrine disease E34.9 *[H28]*
    eye disease — see Cataract, complicated
    hypoparathyroidism E20.9 *[H28]*
    malnutrition-dehydration E46 *[H28]*
    metabolic disease E88.9 *[H28]*
    myotonic disorders G71.19 *[H28]*
    nutritional disease E63.9 *[H28]*
  infantile — see Cataract, presenile
  irradiational — see Cataract, specified NEC
  juvenile — see Cataract, presenile
  malnutrition-dehydration E46 *[H28]*
  morgagnian — see Cataract, senile, morgagnian type
  myotonic G71.19 *[H28]*

Cataract (cortical) (immature) (incipient) H26.9
— *continued*
myxedema E03.9 *[H28]*
nuclear
embryonal Q12.0
sclerosis — *see* Cataract, senile, nuclear
presenile H26.00-
combined forms H26.06-
cortical H26.01-
lamellar — *see* Cataract, presenile, cortical
nuclear H26.03-
specified NEC H26.09
subcapsular polar (anterior) H26.04-
posterior H26.05-
zonular — *see* Cataract, presenile, cortical
secondary H26.40
Soemmering's ring H26.41-
specified NEC H26.49-
to eye disease — *see* Cataract, complicated
senile H25.9
brunescens — *see* Cataract, senile, nuclear
combined forms H25.81-
coronary — *see* Cataract, senile, incipient
cortical H25.01-
hypermature — *see* Cataract, senile,
morgagnian type
incipient (mature) (total) H25.09-
cortical — *see* Cataract, senile, cortical
subcapsular — *see* Cataract, senile,
subcapsular
morgagnian type (hypermature) H25.2-
nuclear (sclerosis) H25.1-
polar subcapsular (anterior) (posterior) —
see Cataract, senile, incipient
punctate — *see* Cataract, senile, incipient
specified NEC H25.89
subcapsular polar (anterior) H25.03-
posterior H25.04-
snowflake — *see* Diabetes, cataract
specified NEC H26.8
toxic — *see* Cataract, drug-induced
traumatic H26.10-
localized H26.11-
partially resolved H26.12-
total H26.13-
zonular (perinuclear) Q12.0
Cataracta — *see also* Cataract
brunescens — *see* Cataract, senile, nuclear
centralis pulverulenta Q12.0
cerulea Q12.0
complicata — *see* Cataract, complicated
congenita Q12.0
coralliformis Q12.0
coronaria Q12.0
diabetic — *see* Diabetes, cataract
membranacea
accreta — *see* Cataract, secondary
congenita Q12.0
nigra — *see* Cataract, senile, nuclear
sunflower — *see* Cataract, complicated
Catarrh, catarrhal (acute) (febrile) (infectious)
(inflammation) (*see also* condition) J00
bronchial — *see* Bronchitis
chest — *see* Bronchitis
chronic J31.0
due to congenital syphilis A50.03
enteric — *see* Enteritis
eustachian H68.009
fauces — *see* Pharyngitis
gastrointestinal — *see* Enteritis
gingivitis K05.00
nonplaque induced K05.01
plaque induced K05.00
hay — *see* Fever, hay
intestinal — *see* Enteritis
larynx, chronic J37.0
liver B15.9
with hepatic coma B15.0
lung — *see* Bronchitis

Catarrh, catarrhal (acute) (febrile) (infectious)
(inflammation) (*see also* condition) J00 —
continued
middle ear, chronic — *see* Otitis, media,
nonsuppurative, chronic, serous
mouth K12.1
nasal (chronic) — *see* Rhinitis
nasobronchial J31.1
nasopharyngeal (chronic) J31.1
acute J00
pulmonary — *see* Bronchitis
spring (eye) (vernal) — *see* Conjunctivitis,
acute, atopic
summer (hay) — *see* Fever, hay
throat J31.2
tubotympanal — *see also* Otitis, media,
nonsuppurative
chronic — *see* Otitis, media, nonsuppurative,
chronic, serous
Catatonia (schizophrenic) F20.2
Catatonic
disorder due to known physiologic condition
F06.1
schizophrenia F20.2
stupor R40.1
Cat-scratch — *see also* Abrasion
disease or fever A28.1
Cauda equina — *see* condition
Cauliflower ear M95.1-
Causalgia (upper limb) G56.4-
lower limb G57.7-
Cause
external, general effects T75.89
Caustic burn — *see* Corrosion, by site
Cavare's disease (familial periodic paralysis)
G72.3
Cave-in, injury
crushing (severe) — *see* Crush
suffocation — *see* Asphyxia, traumatic, due to
low oxygen, due to cave-in
Cavernitis (penis) N48.29
Cavernositis N48.29
Cavernous — *see* condition
Cavitation of lung — *see also* Tuberculosis,
pulmonary
nontuberculous J98.4
Cavities, dental — *see* Caries, dental
Cavity
lung — *see* Cavitation of lung
optic papilla Q14.2
pulmonary — *see* Cavitation of lung
Cavovarus foot, congenital Q66.1
Cavus foot (congenital) Q66.7
acquired — *see* Deformity, limb, foot, specified
NEC
Cazenave's disease L10.2
Cecitis K52.9
with perforation, peritonitis, or rupture K65.8
Cecum — *see* condition
Celiac
artery compression syndrome I77.4
disease (with steatorrhea) K90.0
infantilism K90.0
Cell(s), cellular — *see also* condition
in urine R82.99
Cellulitis (diffuse) (phlegmonous) (septic)
(suppurative) L03.90
abdominal wall L03.311
anaerobic A48.0
ankle — *see* Cellulitis, lower limb
anus K61.0
arm — *see* Cellulitis, upper limb
auricle (ear) — *see* Cellulitis, ear
axilla L03.11-
back (any part) L03.312
breast (acute) (nonpuerperal) (subacute)
N61.0
nipple N61.0

Cellulitis (diffuse) (phlegmonous) (septic)
(suppurative) L03.90 — *continued*
broad ligament
acute N73.0
buttock L03.317
cervical (meaning neck) L03.221
cervix (uteri) — *see* Cervicitis
cheek (external) L03.211
internal K12.2
chest wall L03.313
chronic L03.90
clostridial A48.0
corpus cavernosum N48.22
digit
finger — *see* Cellulitis, finger
toe — *see* Cellulitis, toe
Douglas' cul-de-sac or pouch
acute N73.0
drainage site (following operation) T81.48
ear (external) H60.1-
eosinophilic (granulomatous) L98.3
erysipelatous — *see* Erysipelas
external auditory canal — *see* Cellulitis, ear
eyelid — *see* Abscess, eyelid
face NEC L03.211
finger (intrathecal) (periosteal) (subcutaneous)
(subcuticular) L03.01-
foot — *see* Cellulitis, lower limb
gangrenous — *see* Gangrene
genital organ NEC
female (external) N76.4
male N49.9
multiple sites N49.8
specified NEC N49.8
gluteal (region) L03.317
gonococcal A54.89
groin L03.314
hand — *see* Cellulitis, upper limb
head NEC L03.811
face (any part, except ear, eye and nose)
L03.211
heel — *see* Cellulitis, lower limb
hip — *see* Cellulitis, lower limb
jaw (region) L03.211
knee — *see* Cellulitis, lower limb
labium (majus) (minus) — *see* Vulvitis
lacrimal passages — *see* Inflammation,
lacrimal, passages
larynx J38.7
leg — *see* Cellulitis, lower limb
lip K13.0
lower limb L03.11-
toe — *see* Cellulitis, toe
mouth (floor) K12.2
multiple sites, so stated L03.90
nasopharynx J39.1
navel L03.316
newborn P38.9
with mild hemorrhage P38.1
without hemorrhage P38.9
neck (region) L03.221
nipple (acute) (nonpuerperal) (subacute)
N61.0
nose (septum) (external) J34.0
orbit, orbital H05.01-
palate (soft) K12.2
pectoral (region) L03.313
pelvis, pelvic (chronic)
female (*see also* Disease, pelvis,
inflammatory) N73.2
acute N73.0
following ectopic or molar pregnancy O08.0
male K65.0
penis N48.22
perineal, perineum L03.315
periorbital L03.213
perirectal K61.1
peritonsillar J36
periurethral N34.0

DISEASE INDEX

Cellulitis (diffuse) (phlegmonous) (septic) (suppurative) L03.90 — *continued*
  periuterine (*see also* Disease, pelvis, inflammatory) N73.2
    acute N73.0
  pharynx J39.1
  preseptal L03.213
  rectum K61.1
  retroperitoneal K68.9
  round ligament
    acute N73.0
  scalp (any part) L03.811
  scrotum N49.2
  seminal vesicle N49.0
  shoulder — *see* Cellulitis, upper limb
  specified site NEC L03.818
  submandibular (region) (space) (triangle) K12.2
    gland K11.3
  submaxillary (region) K12.2
    gland K11.3
  thigh — *see* Cellulitis, lower limb
  thumb (intrathecal) (periosteal) (subcutaneous) (subcuticular) — *see* Cellulitis, finger
  toe (intrathecal) (periosteal) (subcutaneous) (subcuticular) L03.03-
  tonsil J36
  trunk L03.319
    abdominal wall L03.311
    back (any part) L03.312
    buttock L03.317
    chest wall L03.313
    groin L03.314
    perineal, perineum L03.315
    umbilicus L03.316
  tuberculous (primary) A18.4
  umbilicus L03.316
  upper limb L03.11-
    axilla — *see* Cellulitis, axilla
    finger — *see* Cellulitis, finger
    thumb — *see* Cellulitis, finger
  vaccinal T88.0
  vocal cord J38.3
  vulva — *see* Vulvitis
  wrist — *see* Cellulitis, upper limb
Cementoblastoma, benign — *see* Cyst, calcifying odontogenic
Cementoma — *see* Cyst, calcifying odontogenic
Cementoperiostitis — *see* Periodontitis
Cementosis K03.4
Central auditory processing disorder H93.25
Central pain syndrome G89.0
Cephalematocele, cephal(o)hematocele
  newborn P52.8
    birth injury P10.8
  traumatic — *see* Hematoma, brain
Cephalematoma, cephalhematoma (calcified)
  newborn (birth injury) P12.0
  traumatic — *see* Hematoma, brain
Cephalgia, cephalalgia — *see also* Headache
  histamine G44.009
    intractable G44.001
    not intractable G44.009
  trigeminal autonomic (TAC) NEC G44.099
    intractable G44.091
    not intractable G44.099
Cephalic — *see* condition
Cephalitis — *see* Encephalitis
Cephalocele — *see* Encephalocele
Cephalomenia N94.89
Cephalopelvic — *see* condition
Cerclage (with cervical incompetence) in pregnancy — *see* Incompetence, cervix, in pregnancy

Cerebellitis — *see* Encephalitis
Cerebellum, cerebellar — *see* condition
Cerebral — *see* condition
Cerebritis — *see* Encephalitis
Cerebro-hepato-renal syndrome Q87.89
Cerebromalacia — *see* Softening, brain
  sequelae of cerebrovascular disease I69.398
Cerebroside lipidosis E75.22
Cerebrospasticity (congenital) G80.1
Cerebrospinal — *see* condition
Cerebrum — *see* condition
Ceroid-lipofuscinosis, neuronal E75.4
Cerumen (accumulation) (impacted) H61.2-
Cervical — *see also* condition
  auricle Q18.2
  dysplasia in pregnancy — *see* Abnormal, cervix, in pregnancy or childbirth
  erosion in pregnancy — *see* Abnormal, cervix, in pregnancy or childbirth
  fibrosis in pregnancy — *see* Abnormal, cervix, in pregnancy or childbirth
  fusion syndrome Q76.1
  rib Q76.5
  shortening (complicating pregnancy) O26.87-
Cervicalgia M54.2
Cervicitis (acute) (chronic) (nonvenereal) (senile (atrophic)) (subacute) (with ulceration) N72
  with
    abortion — *see* Abortion, by type complicated by genital tract and pelvic infection
    ectopic pregnancy O08.0
    molar pregnancy O08.0
  chlamydial A56.09
  gonococcal A54.03
  herpesviral A60.03
  puerperal (postpartum) O86.11
  syphilitic A52.76
  trichomonal A59.09
  tuberculous A18.16
Cervicocolpitis (emphysematosa) (*see also* Cervicitis) N72
Cervix — *see* condition
Cesarean delivery, previous, affecting management of pregnancy O34.219
  classical (vertical) scar O34.212
  low transverse scar O34.211
Céstan(-Chenais) paralysis or syndrome G46.3
Céstan-Raymond syndrome I65.8
Cestode infestation B71.9
  specified type NEC B71.8
Cestodiasis B71.9
Chabert's disease A22.9
Chacaleh E53.8
Chafing L30.4
Chagas' (-Mazza) disease (chronic) B57.2
  with
    cardiovascular involvement NEC B57.2
    digestive system involvement B57.30
      megacolon B57.32
      megaesophagus B57.31
      other specified B57.39
    megacolon B57.32
    megaesophagus B57.31
    myocarditis B57.2
    nervous system involvement B57.40
      meningitis B57.41
      meningoencephalitis B57.42
      other specified B57.49
    specified organ involvement NEC B57.5
  acute (with) B57.1
    cardiovascular NEC B57.0
    myocarditis B57.0
Chagres fever B50.9
Chairridden Z74.09
Chalasia (cardiac sphincter) K21.9

Chalazion H00.19
  left H00.16
    lower H00.15
    upper H00.14
  right H00.13
    lower H00.12
    upper H00.11
Chalcosis — *see also* Disorder, globe, degenerative, chalcosis
  cornea — *see* Deposit, cornea
  crystalline lens — *see* Cataract, complicated
  retina H35.89
Chalicosis (pulmonum) J62.8
Chancre (any genital site) (hard) (hunterian) (mixed) (primary) (seronegative) (seropositive) (syphilitic) A51.0
  congenital A50.07
  conjunctiva NEC A51.2
  Ducrey's A57
  extragenital A51.2
  eyelid A51.2
  lip A51.2
  nipple A51.2
  Nisbet's A57
  of
    carate A67.0
    pinta A67.0
    yaws A66.0
  palate, soft A51.2
  phagedenic A57
  simple A57
  soft A57
    bubo A57
    palate A51.2
  urethra A51.0
  yaws A66.0
Chancroid (anus) (genital) (penis) (perineum) (rectum) (urethra) (vulva) A57
Chandler's disease (osteochondritis dissecans, hip) — *see* Osteochondritis, dissecans, hip
Change(s) (in) (of) — *see also* Removal
  arteriosclerotic — *see* Arteriosclerosis
  bone — *see also* Disorder, bone
    diabetic — *see* Diabetes, bone change
  bowel habit R19.4
  cardiorenal (vascular) — *see* Hypertension, cardiorenal
  cardiovascular — *see* Disease, cardiovascular
  circulatory I99.9
  cognitive (mild) (organic) R41.89
  color, tooth, teeth
    during formation K00.8
    posteruptive K03.7
  contraceptive device Z30.433
  corneal membrane H18.30
    Bowman's membrane fold or rupture H18.31-
    Descemet's membrane
      fold H18.32-
      rupture H18.33-
  coronary — *see* Disease, heart, ischemic
  degenerative, spine or vertebra — *see* Spondylosis
  dental pulp, regressive K04.2
  dressing (nonsurgical) Z48.00
    surgical Z48.01
  heart — *see* Disease, heart
  hip joint — *see* Derangement, joint, hip
  hyperplastic larynx J38.7
  hypertrophic
    nasal sinus J34.89
    turbinate, nasal J34.3
    upper respiratory tract J39.8
  indwelling catheter Z46.6
  inflammatory — *see also* Inflammation
    sacroiliac M46.1
  job, anxiety concerning Z56.1
  joint — *see* Derangement, joint

Change(s) (in) (of) (see also Removal) — continued
life — see Menopause
mental status R41.82
minimal (glomerular) (see also N00-N07 with fourth character .0) N05.0
myocardium, myocardial — see Degeneration, myocardial
of life — see Menopause
pacemaker Z45.018
  pulse generator Z45.010
personality (enduring) F68.8
  due to (secondary to)
    general medical condition F07.0
  secondary (nonspecific) F60.89
regressive, dental pulp K04.2
renal — see Disease, renal
retina H35.9
  myopic H44.2-
sacroiliac joint M53.3
senile (see also condition) R54
sensory R20.8
skin R23.9
  acute, due to ultraviolet radiation L56.9
    specified NEC L56.8
  chronic, due to nonionizing radiation L57.9
    specified NEC L57.8
  cyanosis R23.0
  flushing R23.2
  pallor R23.1
  petechiae R23.3
  specified change NEC R23.8
  swelling — see Mass, localized
  texture R23.4
trophic
  arm — see Mononeuropathy, upper limb
  leg — see Mononeuropathy, lower limb
vascular I99.9
vasomotor I73.9
voice R49.9
  psychogenic F44.4
  specified NEC R49.8
Changing sleep-work schedule, affecting sleep G47.26
Changuinola fever A93.1
Chapping skin T69.8
Charcot-Marie-Tooth disease, paralysis or syndrome G60.0
Charcot's
arthropathy — see Arthropathy, neuropathic
cirrhosis K74.3
disease (tabetic arthropathy) A52.16
joint (disease) (tabetic) A52.16
  diabetic — see Diabetes, with, arthropathy
syringomyelic G95.0
syndrome (intermittent claudication) I73.9
CHARGE association Q89.8
Charley-horse (quadriceps) M62.831
traumatic (quadriceps) S76.11-
Charlouis' disease — see Yaws
Cheadle's disease E54
Checking (of)
cardiac pacemaker (battery) (electrode(s)) Z45.018
  pulse generator Z45.010
implantable subdermal contraceptive Z30.46
intrauterine contraceptive device Z30.431
Check-up — see Examination
Chédiak-Higashi(-Steinbrinck) syndrome (congenital gigantism of peroxidase granules) E70.330
Cheek — see condition
Cheese itch B88.0
Cheese-washer's lung J67.8
Cheese-worker's lung J67.8

Cheilitis (acute) (angular) (catarrhal) (chronic) (exfoliative) (gangrenous) (glandular) (infectional) (suppurative) (ulcerative) (vesicular) K13.0
actinic (due to sun) L56.8
  other than from sun L59.8
candidal B37.83
Cheilodynia K13.0
Cheiloschisis — see Cleft, lip
Cheilosis (angular) K13.0
with pellagra E52
due to
  vitamin B2 (riboflavin) deficiency E53.0
Cheiromegaly M79.89
Cheiropompholyx L30.1
Cheloid — see Keloid
Chemical burn — see Corrosion, by site
Chemodectoma — see Paraganglioma, nonchromaffin
Chemosis, conjunctiva — see Edema, conjunctiva
Chemotherapy (session) (for)
cancer Z51.11
neoplasm Z51.11
Cherubism M27.8
Chest — see condition
Cheyne-Stokes breathing (respiration) R06.3
Chiari's
disease or syndrome (hepatic vein thrombosis) I82.0
malformation
  type I G93.5
  type II — see Spina bifida
net Q24.8
Chicago disease B40.9
Chickenpox — see Varicella
Chiclero ulcer or sore B55.1
Chigger (infestation) B88.0
Chignon (disease) B36.8
newborn (from vacuum extraction) (birth injury) P12.1
Chilaiditi's syndrome (subphrenic displacement, colon) Q43.3
Chilblain(s) (lupus) T69.1
Child
custody dispute Z65.3
Childbirth — see Delivery
Childhood
cerebral X-linked adrenoleukodystrophy E71.520
period of rapid growth Z00.2
Chill(s) R68.83
with fever R50.9
congestive in malarial regions B54
without fever R68.83
Chilomastigiasis A07.8
Chimera 46,XX/46,XY Q99.0
Chin — see condition
Chinese dysentery A03.9
Chionophobia F40.228
Chitral fever A93.1
Chlamydia, chlamydial A74.9
cervicitis A56.09
conjunctivitis A74.0
cystitis A56.01
endometritis A56.11
epididymitis A56.19
female
  pelvic inflammatory disease A56.11
  pelviperitonitis A56.11
orchitis A56.19
peritonitis A74.81
pharyngitis A56.4
proctitis A56.3
psittaci (infection) A70
salpingitis A56.11
sexually-transmitted infection NEC A56.8

Chlamydia, chlamydial A74.9 — continued
specified NEC A74.89
urethritis A56.01
vulvovaginitis A56.02
Chlamydiosis — see Chlamydia
Chloasma (skin) (idiopathic) (symptomatic) L81.1
eyelid H02.719
  hyperthyroid E05.90 [H02.719]
    with thyroid storm E05.91 [H02.719]
  left H02.716
    lower H02.715
    upper H02.714
  right H02.713
    lower H02.712
    upper H02.711
Chloroma C92.3-
Chlorosis D50.9
Egyptian B76.9 [D63.8]
miner's B76.9 [D63.8]
Chlorotic anemia D50.8
Chocolate cyst (ovary) N80.1
Choked
disc or disk — see Papilledema
on food, phlegm, or vomitus NOS — see Foreign body, by site
while vomiting NOS — see Foreign body, by site
Chokes (resulting from bends) T70.3
Choking sensation R09.89
Cholangiectasis K83.8
Cholangiocarcinoma
with hepatocellular carcinoma, combined C22.0
liver C22.1
specified site NEC — see Neoplasm, malignant, by site
unspecified site C22.1
Cholangiohepatitis K83.8
due to fluke infestation B66.1
Cholangiohepatoma C22.0
Cholangiolitis (acute) (chronic) (extrahepatic) (gangrenous) (intrahepatic) K83.0
paratyphoidal — see Fever, paratyphoid
typhoidal A01.09
Cholangioma D13.4
malignant — see Cholangiocarcinoma
Cholangitis (ascending) (primary) (recurrent) (sclerosing) (secondary) (stenosing) (suppurative) K83.0
with calculus, bile duct — see Calculus, bile duct, with cholangitis
chronic nonsuppurative destructive K74.3
Cholecystectasia K82.8
Cholecystitis K81.9
with
  calculus, stones in
    bile duct (common) (hepatic) — see Calculus, bile duct, with cholecystitis
    cystic duct — see Calculus, gallbladder, with cholecystitis
    gallbladder — see Calculus, gallbladder, with cholecystitis
    choledocholithiasis — see Calculus, bile duct, with cholecystitis
    cholelithiasis — see Calculus, gallbladder, with cholecystitis
acute (emphysematous) (gangrenous) (suppurative) K81.0
  with
    calculus, stones in
      cystic duct — see Calculus, gallbladder, with cholecystitis, acute
      gallbladder — see Calculus, gallbladder, with cholecystitis, acute
      choledocholithiasis — see Calculus, bile duct, with cholecystitis, acute

Cholecystitis K81.9 — *continued*
 acute (emphysematous) (gangrenous)
  (suppurative) K81.0 — *continued*
  with — *continued*
   cholelithiasis — *see* Calculus, gallbladder,
    with cholecystitis, acute
   chronic cholecystitis K81.2
    with gallbladder calculus K80.12
     with obstruction K80.13
  chronic K81.1
   with acute cholecystitis K81.2
    with gallbladder calculus K80.12
     with obstruction K80.13
  emphysematous (acute) — *see* Cholecystitis,
    acute
  gangrenous — *see* Cholecystitis, acute
  paratyphoidal, current A01.4
  suppurative — *see* Cholecystitis, acute
  typhoidal A01.09
Cholecystolithiasis — *see* Calculus,
  gallbladder
Choledochitis (suppurative) K83.0
Choledocholith — *see* Calculus, bile duct
Choledocholithiasis (common duct) (hepatic
  duct) — *see* Calculus, bile duct
  cystic — *see* Calculus, gallbladder
  typhoidal A01.09
Cholelithiasis (cystic duct) (gallbladder)
  (impacted) (multiple) — *see* Calculus,
  gallbladder
  bile duct (common) (hepatic) — *see* Calculus,
   bile duct
  hepatic duct — *see* Calculus, bile duct
  specified NEC K80.80
   with obstruction K80.81
Cholemia — *see also* Jaundice
  familial (simple) (congenital) E80.4
  Gilbert's E80.4
Choleperitoneum, choleperitonitis K65.3
Cholera (Asiatic) (epidemic) (malignant) A00.9
  antimonial — *see* Poisoning, antimony
  classical A00.0
  due to Vibrio cholerae 01 A00.9
   biovar cholerae A00.0
   biovar el tor A00.1
   el tor A00.1
  el tor A00.1
Cholerine — *see* Cholera
Cholestasis NEC K83.1
  with hepatocyte injury K71.0
  due to total parenteral nutrition (TPN) K76.89
  pure K71.0
Cholesteatoma (ear) (middle) (with reaction)
  H71.9-
  attic H71.0-
  external ear (canal) H60.4-
  mastoid H71.2-
  postmastoidectomy cavity (recurrent) — *see*
   Complications, postmastoidectomy,
   recurrent cholesteatoma
  recurrent (postmastoidectomy) — *see*
   Complications, postmastoidectomy,
   recurrent cholesteatoma
  tympanum H71.1-
Cholesteatosis, diffuse H71.3-
Cholesteremia E78.00
Cholesterin in vitreous — *see* Deposit,
  crystalline
Cholesterol
  deposit
   retina H35.89
   vitreous — *see* Deposit, crystalline
  elevated (high) E78.00
   with elevated (high) triglycerides E78.2
  screening for Z13.220
  imbibition of gallbladder K82.4

Cholesterolemia (essential) (pure) E78.00
  familial E78.01
  hereditary E78.01
Cholesterolosis, cholesterosis (gallbladder)
  K82.4
  cerebrotendinous E75.5
Cholocolic fistula K82.3
Choluria R82.2
Chondritis M94.8x9
  aurical H61.03-
  costal (Tietze's) M94.0
  external ear H61.03-
  patella, posttraumatic — *see* Chondromalacia,
   patella
  pinna H61.03-
  purulent M94.8x-
  tuberculous NEC A18.02
   intervertebral A18.01
Chondroblastoma — *see also* Neoplasm,
  bone, benign
  malignant — *see* Neoplasm, bone, malignant
Chondrocalcinosis M11.20
  ankle M11.27-
  elbow M11.22-
  familial M11.10
   ankle M11.17-
   elbow M11.12-
   foot joint M11.17-
   hand joint M11.14-
   hip M11.15-
   knee M11.16-
   multiple site M11.19
   shoulder M11.11-
   vertebrae M11.18
   wrist M11.13-
  foot joint M11.27-
  hand joint M11.24-
  hip M11.25-
  knee M11.26-
  multiple site M11.29
  shoulder M11.21-
  specified type NEC M11.20
   ankle M11.27-
   elbow M11.22-
   foot joint M11.27-
   hand joint M11.24-
   hip M11.25-
   knee M11.26-
   multiple site M11.29
   shoulder M11.21-
   vertebrae M11.28
   wrist M11.23-
  vertebrae M11.28
  wrist M11.23-
**Chondrodermatitis nodularis helicis or
  anthelicis** — *see* Perichondritis, ear
Chondrodysplasia Q78.9
  with hemangioma Q78.4
  calcificans congenita Q77.3
  fetalis Q77.4
  metaphyseal (Jansen's) (McKusick's) (Schmid's)
   Q78.8
  punctata Q77.3
Chondrodystrophy, chondrodystrophia
  (familial) (fetalis) (hypoplastic) Q78.9
  calcificans congenita Q77.3
  myotonic (congenital) G71.13
  punctata Q77.3
Chondroectodermal dysplasia Q77.6
Chondrogenesis imperfecta Q77.4
Chondrolysis M94.35-
Chondroma — *see also* Neoplasm, cartilage,
  benign
  juxtacortical — *see* Neoplasm, bone, benign
  periosteal — *see* Neoplasm, bone, benign
Chondromalacia (systemic) M94.20
  acromioclavicular joint M94.21-
  ankle M94.27-

Chondromalacia (systemic) M94.20 —
  continued
  elbow M94.22-
  foot joint M94.27-
  glenohumeral joint M94.21-
  hand joint M94.24-
  hip M94.25-
  knee M94.26-
   patella M22.4-
  multiple sites M94.29
  patella M22.4-
  rib M94.28
  sacroiliac joint M94.259
  shoulder M94.21-
  sternoclavicular joint M94.21-
  vertebral joint M94.28
  wrist M94.23-
Chondromatosis — *see also* Neoplasm,
  cartilage, uncertain behavior
  internal Q78.4
Chondromyxosarcoma — *see* Neoplasm,
  cartilage, malignant
Chondro-osteodysplasia (Morquio-
  Brailsford type) E76.219
Chondro-osteodystrophy E76.29
Chondro-osteoma — *see* Neoplasm, bone,
  benign
Chondropathia tuberosa M94.0
Chondrosarcoma — *see* Neoplasm, cartilage,
  malignant
  juxtacortical — *see* Neoplasm, bone,
   malignant
  mesenchymal — *see* Neoplasm, connective
   tissue, malignant
  myxoid — *see* Neoplasm, cartilage, malignant
Chordee (nonvenereal) N48.89
  congenital Q54.4
  gonococcal A54.09
Chorditis (fibrinous) (nodosa) (tuberosa) J38.2
Chordoma — *see* Neoplasm, vertebral
  (column), malignant
Chorea (chronic) (gravis) (posthemiplegic)
  (senile) (spasmodic) G25.5
  with
   heart involvement I02.0
    active or acute (conditions in I01-) I02.0
    rheumatic I02.9
     with valvular disorder I02.0
    rheumatic heart disease (chronic) (inactive)
     (quiescent) — *code to* rheumatic heart
     condition involved
  drug-induced G25.4
  habit F95.8
  hereditary G10
  Huntington's G10
  hysterical F44.4
  minor I02.9
   with heart involvement I02.0
  progressive G25.5
   hereditary G10
  rheumatic (chronic) I02.9
   with heart involvement I02.0
  Sydenham's I02.9
   with heart involvement — *see* Chorea, with
    rheumatic heart disease
  nonrheumatic G25.5
Choreoathetosis (paroxysmal) G25.5
Chorioadenoma (destruens) D39.2
Chorioamnionitis O41.12-
Chorioangioma D26.7
Choriocarcinoma — *see* Neoplasm,
  malignant, by site
  combined with
   embryonal carcinoma — *see* Neoplasm,
    malignant, by site
   other germ cell elements — *see* Neoplasm,
    malignant, by site
   teratoma — *see* Neoplasm, malignant, by
    site

Choriocarcinoma — *see* Neoplasm, malignant, by site — *continued*
  specified site — *see* Neoplasm, malignant, by site
  unspecified site
    female C58
    male C62.90
Chorioencephalitis (acute) (lymphocytic) (serous) A87.2
Chorioepithelioma — *see* Choriocarcinoma
Choriomeningitis (acute) (lymphocytic) (serous) A87.2
Chorionepithelioma — *see* Choriocarcinoma
Chorioretinitis — *see also* Inflammation, chorioretinal
  disseminated — *see also* Inflammation, chorioretinal, disseminated
    in neurosyphilis A52.19
  Egyptian B76.9 [D63.8]
  focal — *see also* Inflammation, chorioretinal, focal
  histoplasmic B39.9 [H32]
  in (due to)
    histoplasmosis B39.9 [H32]
    syphilis (secondary) A51.43
      late A52.71
    toxoplasmosis (acquired) B58.01
      congenital (active) P37.1 [H32]
    tuberculosis A18.53
  juxtapapillary, juxtapapillaris — *see* Inflammation, chorioretinal, focal, juxtapapillary
  leprous A30.9 [H32]
  miner's B76.9 [D63.8]
  progressive myopia (degeneration) H44.2-
  syphilitic (secondary) A51.43
    congenital (early) A50.01 [H32]
      late A50.32
    late A52.71
  tuberculous A18.53
Chorioretinopathy, central serous H35.71-
Choroid — *see* condition
Choroideremia H31.21
Choroiditis — *see* Chorioretinitis
Choroidopathy — *see* Disorder, choroid
Choroidoretinitis — *see* Chorioretinitis
Choroidoretinopathy, central serous — *see* Chorioretinopathy, central serous
Christian-Weber disease M35.6
Christmas disease D67
Chromaffinoma — *see also* Neoplasm, benign, by site
  malignant — *see* Neoplasm, malignant, by site
Chromatopsia — *see* Deficiency, color vision
Chromhidrosis, chromidrosis L75.1
Chromoblastomycosis — *see* Chromomycosis
Chromoconversion R82.91
Chromomycosis B43.9
  brain abscess B43.1
  cerebral B43.1
  cutaneous B43.0
  skin B43.0
  specified NEC B43.8
  subcutaneous abscess or cyst B43.2
Chromophytosis B36.0
Chromosome — *see* condition by chromosome involved
  D(1) — *see* condition, chromosome 13
  E(3) — *see* condition, chromosome 18
  G — *see* condition, chromosome 21
Chromotrichomycosis B36.8
Chronic — *see* condition
  fracture — *see* Fracture, pathological
Churg-Strauss syndrome M30.1
Chyle cyst, mesentery I89.8
Chylocele (nonfilarial) I89.8
  filarial (*see also* Infestation, filarial) B74.9 [N51]
  tunica vaginalis N50.89

Chylocele (nonfilarial) I89.8 — *continued*
  filarial (*see also* Infestation, filarial) B74.9 [N51]
Chylomicronemia (fasting) (with hyperprebetalipoproteinemia) E78.3
Chylopericardium I31.3
  acute I30.9
Chylothorax (nonfilarial) I89.8
  filarial (*see also* Infestation, filarial) B74.9 [J91.8]
Chylous — *see* condition
Chyluria (nonfilarial) R82.0
  due to
    bilharziasis B65.0
    Brugia (malayi) B74.1
      timori B74.2
    schistosomiasis (bilharziasis) B65.0
    Wuchereria (bancrofti) B74.0
  filarial — *see* Infestation, filarial
Cicatricial (deformity) — *see* Cicatrix
Cicatrix (adherent) (contracted) (painful) (vicious) (*see also* Scar) L90.5
  adenoid (and tonsil) J35.8
  alveolar process M26.79
  anus K62.89
  auricle — *see* Disorder, pinna, specified type NEC
  bile duct (common) (hepatic) K83.8
  bladder N32.89
  bone — *see* Disorder, bone, specified type NEC
  brain G93.89
  cervix (postoperative) (postpartal) N88.1
  common duct K83.8
  cornea H17.9
    tuberculous A18.59
  duodenum (bulb), obstructive K31.5
  esophagus K22.2
  eyelid — *see* Disorder, eyelid function
  hypopharynx J39.2
  lacrimal passages — *see* Obstruction, lacrimal
  larynx J38.7
  lung J98.4
  middle ear — *see* subcategory H74.8
  mouth K13.79
  muscle M62.89
    with contracture — *see* Contraction, muscle NEC
  nasopharynx J39.2
  palate (soft) K13.79
  penis N48.89
  pharynx J39.2
  prostate N42.89
  rectum K62.89
  retina — *see* Scar, chorioretinal
  semilunar cartilage — *see* Derangement, meniscus
  seminal vesicle N50.89
  skin L90.5
    infected L08.89
    postinfective L90.5
    tuberculous B90.8
  specified site NEC L90.5
  throat J39.2
  tongue K14.8
  tonsil (and adenoid) J35.8
  trachea J39.8
  tuberculous NEC B90.9
  urethra N36.8
  uterus N85.8
  vagina N89.8
    postoperative N99.2
  vocal cord J38.3
  wrist, constricting (annular) L90.5
CIDP (chronic inflammatory demyelinating polyneuropathy) G61.81
CIN — *see* Neoplasia, intraepithelial, cervix
CINCA (chronic infantile neurological, cutaneous and articular syndrome) M04.2

Cinchonism — *see* Deafness, ototoxic
  correct substance properly administered — *see* Table of Drugs and Chemicals, by drug, adverse effect
  overdose or wrong substance given or taken — *see* Table of Drugs and Chemicals, by drug, poisoning
Circle of Willis — *see* condition
Circular — *see* condition
Circulating anticoagulants (*see also* Disorder, hemorrhagic) D68.318
  due to drugs (*see also* Disorder, hemorrhagic) D68.32
  following childbirth O72.3
Circulation
  collateral, any site I99.8
  defective (lower extremity) I99.8
    congenital Q28.9
  embryonic Q28.9
  failure (peripheral) R57.9
    newborn P29.89
  fetal, persistent P29.3
  heart, incomplete Q28.9
Circulatory system — *see* condition
Circulus senilis (cornea) — *see* Degeneration, cornea, senile
Circumcision (in absence of medical indication) (ritual) (routine) Z41.2
Circumscribed — *see* condition
Circumvallate placenta O43.11-
Cirrhosis, cirrhotic (hepatic) (liver) K74.60
  alcoholic K70.30
    with ascites K70.31
  atrophic — *see* Cirrhosis, liver
  Baumgarten-Cruveilhier K74.69
  biliary (cholangiolitic) (cholangitic) (hypertrophic) (obstructive) (pericholangiolitic) K74.5
    due to
      Clonorchiasis B66.1
      flukes B66.3
    primary K74.3
    secondary K74.4
  cardiac (of liver) K76.1
  Charcot's K74.3
  cholangiolitic, cholangitic, cholostatic (primary) K74.3
  congestive K76.1
  Cruveilhier-Baumgarten K74.69
  cryptogenic (liver) K74.69
  due to
    hepatolenticular degeneration E83.01
    Wilson's disease E83.01
    xanthomatosis E78.2
  fatty K76.0
    alcoholic K70.0
  Hanot's (hypertrophic) K74.3
  hepatic — *see* Cirrhosis, liver
  hypertrophic K74.3
  Indian childhood K74.69
  kidney — *see* Sclerosis, renal
  Laennec's K70.30
    with ascites K70.31
    alcoholic K70.30
      with ascites K70.31
    nonalcoholic K74.69
  liver K74.60
    alcoholic K70.30
      with ascites K70.31
      fatty K70.0
    congenital P78.81
    syphilitic A52.74
  lung (chronic) J84.10
  macronodular K74.69
    alcoholic K70.30
      with ascites K70.31
  micronodular K74.69
    alcoholic K70.30
      with ascites K70.31

D I S E A S E   I N D E X

Cirrhosis, cirrhotic (hepatic) (liver) K74.60 — *continued*
  mixed type K74.69
  monolobular K74.3
  nephritis — *see* Sclerosis, renal
  nutritional K74.69
    alcoholic K70.30
      with ascites K70.31
  obstructive — *see* Cirrhosis, biliary
  ovarian N83.8
  pancreas (duct) K86.89
  pigmentary E83.110
  portal K74.69
    alcoholic K70.30
      with ascites K70.31
  postnecrotic K74.69
    alcoholic K70.30
      with ascites K70.31
  pulmonary J84.10
  renal — *see* Sclerosis, renal
  spleen D73.2
  stasis K76.1
  Todd's K74.3
  unilobar K74.3
  xanthomatous (biliary) K74.5
    due to xanthomatosis (familial) (metabolic) (primary) E78.2
Cistern, subarachnoid R93.0
Citrullinemia E72.23
Citrullinuria E72.23
Civatte's disease or poikiloderma L57.3
Clam digger's itch B65.3
Clammy skin R23.1
Clap — *see* Gonorrhea
Clarke-Hadfield syndrome (pancreatic infantilism) K86.89
Clark's paralysis G80.9
Clastothrix L67.8
Claude Bernard-Horner syndrome G90.2
  traumatic — *see* Injury, nerve, cervical sympathetic
Claude's disease or syndrome G46.3
Claudicatio venosa intermittens I87.8
Claudication (intermittent) I73.9
  cerebral (artery) G45.9
  spinal cord (arteriosclerotic) G95.19
    syphilitic A52.09
  venous (axillary) I87.8
Claustrophobia F40.240
Clavus (infected) L84
Clawfoot (congenital) Q66.89
  acquired — *see* Deformity, limb, clawfoot
Clawhand (acquired) — *see also* Deformity, limb, clawhand
  congenital Q68.1
Clawtoe (congenital) Q66.89
  acquired — *see* Deformity, toe, specified NEC
Clay eating — *see* Pica
Cleansing of artificial opening — *see* Attention to, artificial, opening
Cleft (congenital) — *see also* Imperfect, closure
  alveolar process M26.79
  branchial (cyst) (persistent) Q18.2
  cricoid cartilage, posterior Q31.8
  foot Q72.7
  hand Q71.6
  lip (unilateral) Q36.9
    with cleft palate Q37.9
      hard Q37.1
        with soft Q37.5
      soft Q37.3
        with hard Q37.5
    bilateral Q36.0
      with cleft palate Q37.8
        hard Q37.0
          with soft Q37.4
        soft Q37.2
          with hard Q37.4
    median Q36.1

Cleft (congenital) — *see also* Imperfect, closure — *continued*
  nose Q30.2
  palate Q35.9
    with cleft lip (unilateral) Q37.9
      bilateral Q37.8
    hard Q35.1
      with
        cleft lip (unilateral) Q37.1
          bilateral Q37.0
        soft Q35.5
          with cleft lip (unilateral) Q37.5
            bilateral Q37.4
    medial Q35.5
    soft Q35.3
      with
        cleft lip (unilateral) Q37.3
          bilateral Q37.2
        hard Q35.5
          with cleft lip (unilateral) Q37.5
            bilateral Q37.4
  penis Q55.69
  scrotum Q55.29
  thyroid cartilage Q31.8
  uvula Q35.7
Cleidocranial dysostosis Q74.0
Cleptomania F63.2
Clicking hip (newborn) R29.4
Climacteric (female) — *see also* Menopause
  arthritis (any site) NEC — *see* Arthritis, specified form NEC
  depression (single episode) F32.89
    recurrent episode F33.8
  male (symptoms) (syndrome) NEC N50.89
  melancholia (single episode) F32.89
    recurrent episode F33.8
  paranoid state F22
  polyarthritis NEC — *see* Arthritis, specified form NEC
  symptoms (female) N95.1
Clinical research investigation (clinical trial) (control subject) (normal comparison) (participant) Z00.6
Clitoris — *see* condition
Cloaca (persistent) Q43.7
Clonorchiasis, clonorchis infection (liver) B66.1
Clonus R25.8
Closed bite M26.29
Clostridium (C.) perfringens, as cause of disease classified elsewhere B96.7
Closure
  congenital, nose Q30.0
  cranial sutures, premature Q75.0
  defective or imperfect NEC — *see* Imperfect, closure
  fistula, delayed — *see* Fistula
  foramen ovale, imperfect Q21.1
  hymen N89.6
  interauricular septum, defective Q21.1
  interventricular septum, defective Q21.0
  lacrimal duct — *see also* Stenosis, lacrimal, duct
    congenital Q10.5
  nose (congenital) Q30.0
    acquired M95.0
  of artificial opening — *see* Attention to, artificial, opening
  primary angle, without glaucoma damage H40.06-
  vagina N89.5
  valve — *see* Endocarditis
  vulva N90.5
Clot (blood) — *see also* Embolism
  artery (obstruction) (occlusion) — *see* Embolism
  bladder N32.89
  brain (intradural or extradural) — *see* Occlusion, artery, cerebral
  circulation I74.9

Clot (blood) — *see also* Embolism — *continued*
  heart — *see also* Infarct, myocardium
    not resulting in infarction I51.3
  vein — *see* Thrombosis
Clouded state R40.1
  epileptic — *see* Epilepsy, specified NEC
  paroxysmal — *see* Epilepsy, specified NEC
Cloudy antrum, antra J32.0
Clouston's (hidrotic) ectodermal dysplasia Q82.4
Clubbed nail pachydermoperiostosis M89.40 *[L62]*
Clubbing of finger(s) (nails) R68.3
Clubfinger R68.3
  congenital Q68.1
Clubfoot (congenital) Q66.89
  acquired — *see* Deformity, limb, clubfoot
  equinovarus Q66.0
  paralytic — *see* Deformity, limb, clubfoot
Clubhand (congenital) (radial) Q71.4-
  acquired — *see* Deformity, limb, clubhand
Clubnail R68.3
  congenital Q84.6
Clump, kidney Q63.1
Clumsiness, clumsy child syndrome F82
Cluttering F80.81
Clutton's joints A50.51 *[M12.80]*
Coagulation, intravascular (diffuse) (disseminated) — *see also* Defibrination syndrome
  complicating abortion — *see* Abortion, by type, complicated by, intravascular coagulation
  following ectopic or molar pregnancy O08.1
Coagulopathy — *see also* Defect, coagulation
  consumption D65
  intravascular D65
  newborn P60
Coalition
  calcaneo-scaphoid Q66.89
  tarsal Q66.89
Coalminer's
  elbow — *see* Bursitis, elbow, olecranon
  lung or pneumoconiosis J60
Coalworker's lung or pneumoconiosis J60
Coarctation
  aorta (preductal) (postductal) Q25.1
  pulmonary artery Q25.71
Coated tongue K14.3
Coats' disease (exudative retinopathy) — *see* Retinopathy, exudative
Cocaine-induced
  anxiety disorder F14.980
  bipolar and related disorder F14.94
  depressive disorder F14.94
  obsessive-compulsive and related disorder F14.988
  psychotic disorder F14.959
  sexual dysfunction F14.981
  sleep disorder F14.982
Cocainism — *see* Disorder, cocaine use
Coccidioidomycosis B38.9
  cutaneous B38.3
  disseminated B38.7
  generalized B38.7
  meninges B38.4
  prostate B38.81
  pulmonary B38.2
    acute B38.0
    chronic B38.1
  skin B38.3
  specified NEC B38.89
Coccidioidosis — *see* Coccidioidomycosis
Coccidiosis (intestinal) A07.3
Coccydynia, coccygodynia M53.3
Coccyx — *see* condition
Cochin-China diarrhea K90.1
Cockayne's syndrome Q87.1

Cock's peculiar tumor L72.3
Cocked up toe — *see* Deformity, toe, specified NEC
Codman's tumor — *see* Neoplasm, bone, benign
Coenurosis B71.8
Coffee-worker's lung J67.8
Cogan's syndrome H16.32-
  oculomotor apraxia H51.8
Coitus, painful (female) N94.10
  male N53.12
  psychogenic F52.6
Cold J00
  with influenza, flu, or grippe — *see* Influenza, with, respiratory manifestations NEC
  agglutinin disease or hemoglobinuria (chronic) D59.1
  bronchial — *see* Bronchitis
  chest — *see* Bronchitis
  common (head) J00
  effects of T69.9
    specified effect NEC T69.8
  excessive, effects of T69.9
    specified effect NEC T69.8
  exhaustion from T69.8
  exposure to T69.9
    specified effect NEC T69.8
  head J00
  injury syndrome (newborn) P80.0
  on lung — *see* Bronchitis
  rose J30.1
  sensitivity, auto-immune D59.1
  virus J00
Coldsore B00.1
Colibacillosis A49.8
  as the cause of other disease (*see also* Escherichia coli) B96.20
  generalized A41.50
Colic (bilious) (infantile) (intestinal) (recurrent) (spasmodic) R10.83
  abdomen R10.83
    psychogenic F45.8
  appendix, appendicular K38.8
  bile duct — *see* Calculus, bile duct
  biliary — *see* Calculus, bile duct
  common duct — *see* Calculus, bile duct
  cystic duct — *see* Calculus, gallbladder
  Devonshire NEC — *see* Poisoning, lead
  gallbladder — *see* Calculus, gallbladder
  gallstone — *see* Calculus, gallbladder
    gallbladder or cystic duct — *see* Calculus, gallbladder
  hepatic (duct) — *see* Calculus, bile duct
  hysterical F45.8
  kidney N23
  lead NEC — *see* Poisoning, lead
  mucous K58.9
    with diarrhea K58.0
    psychogenic F54
  nephritic N23
  painter's NEC — *see* Poisoning, lead
  pancreas K86.89
  psychogenic F45.8
  renal N23
  saturnine NEC — *see* Poisoning, lead
  ureter N23
  urethral N36.8
    due to calculus N21.1
  uterus NEC N94.89
    menstrual — *see* Dysmenorrhea
  worm NOS B83.9
Colicystitis — *see* Cystitis

Colitis (acute) (catarrhal) (chronic) (noninfective) (hemorrhagic) (*see also* Enteritis) K52.9
  allergic K52.29
    with
      food protein-induced enterocolitis syndrome K52.21
      proctocolitis K52.82
  amebic (acute) (*see also* Amebiasis) A06.0
    nondysenteric A06.2
  anthrax A22.2
  bacillary — *see* Infection, Shigella
  balantidial A07.0
  Clostridium difficile A04.7
  coccidial A07.3
  collagenous K52.831
  cystica superficialis K52.89
  dietary counseling and surveillance (for) Z71.3
  dietetic (*see also* Colitis, allergic) K52.29
  drug-induced K52.1
  due to radiation K52.0
  eosinophilic K52.82
  food hypersensitivity (*see also* Colitis, allergic) K52.29
  giardial A07.1
  granulomatous — *see* Enteritis, regional, large intestine
  indeterminate, so stated K52.3
  infectious — *see* Enteritis, infectious
  ischemic K55.9
    acute (subacute) (*see also* Ischemia, intestine, acute) K55.039
    chronic K55.1
    due to mesenteric artery insufficiency K55.1
    fulminant (acute) (*see also* Ischemia, intestine, acute) K55.039
  left sided K51.50
    with
      abscess K51.514
      complication K51.519
        specified NEC K51.518
      fistula K51.513
      obstruction K51.512
      rectal bleeding K51.511
  lymphocytic K52.832
  membranous
    psychogenic F54
  microscopic K52.839
    specified NEC K52.838
  mucous — *see* Syndrome, irritable, bowel
    psychogenic F54
  noninfective K52.9
    specified NEC K52.89
  polyposa — *see* Polyp, colon, inflammatory
  protozoal A07.9
  pseudomembranous A04.7
  pseudomucinous — *see* Syndrome, irritable, bowel
  regional — *see* Enteritis, regional, large intestine
  segmental — *see* Enteritis, regional, large intestine
  septic — *see* Enteritis, infectious
  spastic K58.9
    with diarrhea K58.0
    psychogenic F54
  staphylococcal A04.8
    foodborne A05.0
  subacute ischemic (*see also* Ischemia, intestine, acute) K55.039
  thromboulcerative (*see also* Ischemia, intestine, acute) K55.039
  toxic NEC K52.1
    due to Clostridium difficile A04.7
  transmural — *see* Enteritis, regional, large intestine
  trichomonal A07.8
  tuberculous (ulcerative) A18.32

Colitis (acute) (catarrhal) (chronic) (noninfective) (hemorrhagic) (*see also* Enteritis) K52.9 — *continued*
  ulcerative (chronic) K51.90
    with
      complication K51.919
        abscess K51.914
        fistula K51.913
        obstruction K51.912
        rectal bleeding K51.911
        specified complication NEC K51.918
    enterocolitis — *see* Enterocolitis, ulcerative
    ileocolitis — *see* Ileocolitis, ulcerative
    mucosal proctocolitis — *see* Proctocolitis, mucosal
    proctitis — *see* Proctitis, ulcerative
    pseudopolyposis — *see* Polyp, colon, inflammatory
    psychogenic F54
    rectosigmoiditis — *see* Rectosigmoiditis, ulcerative
    specified type NEC K51.80
      with
        complication K51.819
          abscess K51.814
          fistula K51.813
          obstruction K51.812
          rectal bleeding K51.811
          specified complication NEC K51.818
Collagenosis, collagen disease (nonvascular) (vascular) M35.9
  cardiovascular I42.8
  reactive perforating L87.1
  specified NEC M35.8
Collapse R55
  adrenal E27.2
  cardiorespiratory R57.0
  cardiovascular R57.0
    newborn P29.89
  circulatory (peripheral) R57.9
    during or after labor and delivery O75.1
    following ectopic or molar pregnancy O08.3
    newborn P29.89
  during or
    after labor and delivery O75.1
    resulting from a procedure, not elsewhere classified T81.10
  external ear canal — *see* Stenosis, external ear canal
  general R55
  heart — *see* Disease, heart
  heat T67.1
  hysterical F44.89
  labyrinth, membranous (congenital) Q16.5
  lung (massive) (*see also* Atelectasis) J98.19
    pressure due to anesthesia (general) (local) or other sedation T88.2
      during labor and delivery O74.1
      in pregnancy O29.02-
      postpartum, puerperal O89.09
  myocardial — *see* Disease, heart
  nervous F48.8
  neurocirculatory F45.8
  nose M95.0
  postoperative T81.10
  pulmonary (*see also* Atelectasis) J98.19
    newborn — *see* Atelectasis
  trachea J39.8
  tracheobronchial J98.09
  valvular — *see* Endocarditis
  vascular (peripheral) R57.9
    during or after labor and delivery O75.1
    following ectopic or molar pregnancy O08.3
    newborn P29.89

Collapse R55 — *continued*
  vertebra M48.50-
    cervical region M48.52-
    cervicothoracic region M48.53-
    in (due to)
      metastasis — *see* Collapse, vertebra, in, specified disease NEC
      osteoporosis (*see also* Osteoporosis) M80.88
        cervical region M80.88
        cervicothoracic region M80.88
        lumbar region M80.88
        lumbosacral region M80.88
        multiple sites M80.88
        occipito-atlanto-axial region M80.88
        sacrococcygeal region M80.88
        thoracic region M80.88
        thoracolumbar region M80.88
      specified disease NEC M48.50-
        cervical region M48.52-
        cervicothoracic region M48.53-
        lumbar region M48.56-
        lumbosacral region M48.57-
        occipito-atlanto-axial region M48.51-
        sacrococcygeal region M48.58-
        thoracic region M48.54-
        thoracolumbar region M48.55-
    lumbar region M48.56-
    lumbosacral region M48.57-
    occipito-atlanto-axial region M48.51-
    sacrococcygeal region M48.58-
    thoracic region M48.54-
    thoracolumbar region M48.55-
Collateral — *see also* condition
  circulation (venous) I87.8
  dilation, veins I87.8
Colles' fracture S52.53-
Collet(-Sicard) syndrome G52.7
Collier's asthma or lung J60
Collodion baby Q80.2
Colloid nodule (of thyroid) (cystic) E04.1
Coloboma (iris) Q13.0
  eyelid Q10.3
  fundus Q14.8
  lens Q12.2
  optic disc (congenital) Q14.2
    acquired H47.31-
Coloenteritis — *see* Enteritis
Colon — *see* condition
Colonization
  MRSA (Methicillin resistant Staphylococcus aureus) Z22.322
  MSSA (Methicillin susceptible Staphylococcus aureus) Z22.321
  status — *see* Carrier (suspected) of
Coloptosis K63.4
Color blindness — *see* Deficiency, color vision
Colostomy
  attention to Z43.3
  fitting or adjustment Z46.89
  malfunctioning K94.03
  status Z93.3
Colpitis (acute) — *see* Vaginitis
Colpocele N81.5
Colpocystitis — *see* Vaginitis
Colpospasm N94.2
Column, spinal, vertebral — *see* condition
Coma R40.20
  with
    motor response (none) R40.231
      abnormal R40.233
      extension R40.232
      flexion withdrawal R40.234
      localizes pain R40.235
      obeys commands R40.236

Coma R40.20 — *continued*
  with — *continued*
    opening of eyes (never) R40.211
      in response to
        pain R40.212
        sound R40.213
      spontaneous R40.214
    verbal response (none) R40.221
      confused conversation R40.224
      inappropriate words R40.223
      incomprehensible words R40.222
      oriented R40.225
  eclamptic — *see* Eclampsia
  epileptic — *see* Epilepsy
  Glasgow, scale score — *see* Glasgow coma scale
  hepatic — *see* Failure, hepatic, by type, with coma
  hyperglycemic (diabetic) — *see* Diabetes, by type, with hyperosmolarity, with coma
  hyperosmolar (diabetic) — *see* Diabetes, by type, with hyperosmolarity, with coma
  hypoglycemic (diabetic) — *see* Diabetes, by type, with hypoglycemia, with coma
    nondiabetic E15
  in diabetes — *see* Diabetes, coma
  insulin-induced — *see* Coma, hypoglycemic
  myxedematous E03.5
  newborn P91.5
  persistent vegetative state R40.3
  specified NEC, without documented Glasgow coma scale score, or with partial Glasgow coma scale score reported R40.244
Comatose — *see* Coma
Combat fatigue F43.0
Combined — *see* condition
Comedo, comedones (giant) L70.0
Comedocarcinoma — *see also* Neoplasm, breast, malignant
  noninfiltrating
    breast D05.8-
      specified site — *see* Neoplasm, in situ, by site
      unspecified site D05.8-
Comedomastitis — *see* Ectasia, mammary duct
Comminuted fracture — *code as* Fracture, closed
Common
  arterial trunk Q20.0
  atrioventricular canal Q21.2
  atrium Q21.1
  cold (head) J00
  truncus (arteriosus) Q20.0
  variable immunodeficiency — *see* Immunodeficiency, common variable
  ventricle Q20.4
Commotio, commotion (current)
  brain — *see* Injury, intracranial, concussion
  cerebri — *see* Injury, intracranial, concussion
  retinae S05.8x-
  spinal cord — *see* Injury, spinal cord, by region
  spinalis — *see* Injury, spinal cord, by region
Communication
  between
    base of aorta and pulmonary artery Q21.4
    left ventricle and right atrium Q20.5
    pericardial sac and pleural sac Q34.8
    pulmonary artery and pulmonary vein, congenital Q25.72
  congenital between uterus and digestive or urinary tract Q51.7
Compartment syndrome (deep) (posterior) (traumatic) T79.A0 *(follows T79.7)*
  abdomen T79.A3 *(follows T79.7)*
  lower extremity (hip, buttock, thigh, leg, foot, toes) T79.A2 *(follows T79.7)*

Compartment syndrome (deep) (posterior) — *continued*
  nontraumatic
    abdomen M79.A3 *(follows M79.7)*
    lower extremity (hip, buttock, thigh, leg, foot, toes) M79.A2- *(follows M79.7)*
    specified site NEC M79.A9 *(follows M79.7)*
    upper extremity (shoulder, arm, forearm, wrist, hand, fingers) M79.A1- *(follows M79.7)*
  specified site NEC T79.A9 *(follows T79.7)*
  upper extremity (shoulder, arm, forearm, wrist, hand, fingers) T79.A1 *(follows T79.7)*
Compensation
  failure — *see* Disease, heart
  neurosis, psychoneurosis — *see* Disorder, factitious
Complaint — *see also* Disease
  bowel, functional K59.9
    psychogenic F45.8
  intestine, functional K59.9
    psychogenic F45.8
  kidney — *see* Disease, renal
  miners' J60
Complete — *see* condition
Complex
  Addison-Schilder E71.528
  cardiorenal — *see* Hypertension, cardiorenal
  Costen's M26.69
  disseminated mycobacterium avium-intracellulare (DMAC) A31.2
  Eisenmenger's (ventricular septal defect) I27.89
  hypersexual F52.8
  jumped process, spine — *see* Dislocation, vertebra
  primary, tuberculous A15.7
  Schilder-Addison E71.528
  subluxation (vertebral) M99.19
    abdomen M99.19
    acromioclavicular M99.17
    cervical region M99.11
    cervicothoracic M99.11
    costochondral M99.18
    costovertebral M99.18
    head region M99.10
    hip M99.15
    lower extremity M99.16
    lumbar region M99.13
    lumbosacral M99.13
    occipitocervical M99.10
    pelvic region M99.15
    pubic M99.15
    rib cage M99.18
    sacral region M99.14
    sacrococcygeal M99.14
    sacroiliac M99.14
    specified NEC M99.19
    sternochondral M99.18
    sternoclavicular M99.17
    thoracic region M99.12
    thoracolumbar M99.12
    upper extremity M99.17
  Taussig-Bing (transposition, aorta and overriding pulmonary artery) Q20.1
Complication(s) (from) (of)
  accidental puncture or laceration during a procedure (of) — *see* Complications, intraoperative (intraprocedural), puncture or laceration
  amputation stump (surgical) (late) NEC T87.9
    dehiscence T87.81
    infection or inflammation T87.40
      lower limb T87.4-
      upper limb T87.4-
    necrosis T87.50
      lower limb T87.5-
      upper limb T87.5-

Complication(s) (from) (of) — *continued*
  amputation stump (surgical) (late) NEC T87.9
    — *continued*
    neuroma T87.30
      lower limb T87.3-
      upper limb T87.3-
    specified type NEC T87.89
  anastomosis (and bypass) — *see also*
      Complications, prosthetic device or
      implant
    intestinal (internal) NEC K91.89
      involving urinary tract N99.89
    urinary tract (involving intestinal tract)
        N99.89
    vascular — *see* Complications,
      cardiovascular device or implant
  anesthesia, anesthetic (*see also* Anesthesia,
      complication) T88.59
    brain, postpartum, puerperal O89.2
    cardiac
      in
        labor and delivery O74.2
        pregnancy O29.19-
      postpartum, puerperal O89.1
    central nervous system
      in
        labor and delivery O74.3
        pregnancy O29.29-
      postpartum, puerperal O89.2
    difficult or failed intubation T88.4
      in pregnancy O29.6-
    failed sedation (conscious) (moderate)
        during procedure T88.52
    general, unintended awareness during
        procedure T88.53
    hyperthermia, malignant T88.3
    hypothermia T88.51
    intubation failure T88.4
    malignant hyperthermia T88.3
    pulmonary
      in
        labor and delivery O74.1
        pregnancy NEC O29.09-
      postpartum, puerperal O89.09
    shock T88.2
    spinal and epidural
      in
        labor and delivery NEC O74.6
          headache O74.5
        pregnancy NEC O29.5x-
      postpartum, puerperal NEC O89.5
        headache O89.4
    unintended awareness under general
        anesthesia during procedure T88.53
  anti-reflux device — *see* Complications,
      esophageal anti-reflux device
  aortic (bifurcation) graft — *see* Complications,
      graft, vascular
  aortocoronary (bypass) graft — *see*
      Complications, coronary artery (bypass)
      graft
  aortofemoral (bypass) graft — *see*
      Complications, extremity artery (bypass)
      graft
  arteriovenous
    fistula, surgically created T82.9
      embolism T82.818
      fibrosis T82.828
      hemorrhage T82.838
      infection or inflammation T82.7
      mechanical
        breakdown T82.510
        displacement T82.520
        leakage T82.530
        malposition T82.520
        obstruction T82.590
        perforation T82.590
        protrusion T82.590

Complication(s) (from) (of) — *continued*
  arteriovenous — *continued*
    fistula, surgically created T82.9 —
        continued
      pain T82.848
      specified type NEC T82.898
      stenosis T82.858
      thrombosis T82.868
    shunt, surgically created T82.9
      embolism T82.818
      fibrosis T82.828
      hemorrhage T82.838
      infection or inflammation T82.7
      mechanical
        breakdown T82.511
        displacement T82.521
        leakage T82.531
        malposition T82.521
        obstruction T82.591
        perforation T82.591
        protrusion T82.591
      pain T82.848
      specified type NEC T82.898
      stenosis T82.858
      thrombosis T82.868
  arthroplasty — *see* Complications, joint
      prosthesis
  artificial
    fertilization or insemination N98.9
      attempted introduction (of)
        embryo in embryo transfer N98.3
        ovum following in vitro fertilization
            N98.2
      hyperstimulation of ovaries N98.1
      infection N98.0
      specified NEC N98.8
    heart T82.9
      embolism T82.817
      fibrosis T82.827
      hemorrhage T82.837
      infection or inflammation T82.7
      mechanical
        breakdown T82.512
        displacement T82.522
        leakage T82.532
        malposition T82.522
        obstruction T82.592
        perforation T82.592
        protrusion T82.592
      pain T82.847
      specified type NEC T82.897
      stenosis T82.857
      thrombosis T82.867
    opening
      cecostomy — *see* Complications, colostomy
      colostomy — *see* Complications, colostomy
      cystostomy — *see* Complications,
          cystostomy
      enterostomy — *see* Complications,
          enterostomy
      gastrostomy — *see* Complications,
          gastrostomy
      ileostomy — *see* Complications,
          enterostomy
      jejunostomy — *see* Complications,
          enterostomy
      nephrostomy — *see* Complications, stoma,
          urinary tract
      tracheostomy — *see* Complications,
          tracheostomy
      ureterostomy — *see* Complications, stoma,
          urinary tract
      urethrostomy — *see* Complications, stoma,
          urinary tract

Complication(s) (from) (of) — *continued*
  balloon implant or device
    gastrointestinal T85.9
      embolism T85.818
      fibrosis T85.828
      hemorrhage T85.838
      infection and inflammation T85.79
      pain T85.848
      specified type NEC T85.898
      stenosis T85.858
      thrombosis T85.868
    vascular (counterpulsation) T82.9
      embolism T82.818
      fibrosis T82.828
      hemorrhage T82.838
      infection or inflammation T82.7
      mechanical
        breakdown T82.513
        displacement T82.523
        leakage T82.533
        malposition T82.523
        obstruction T82.593
        perforation T82.593
        protrusion T82.593
      pain T82.848
      specified type NEC T82.898
      stenosis T82.858
      thrombosis T82.868
  bariatric procedure
    gastric band procedure K95.09
      infection K95.01
    specified procedure NEC K95.89
      infection K95.81
  bile duct implant (prosthetic) T85.9
    embolism T85.818
    fibrosis T85.828
    hemorrhage T85.838
    infection and inflammation T85.79
    mechanical
      breakdown T85.510
      displacement T85.520
      malfunction T85.510
      malposition T85.520
      obstruction T85.590
      perforation T85.590
      protrusion T85.590
      specified NEC T85.590
    pain T85.848
    specified type NEC T85.898
    stenosis T85.858
    thrombosis T85.868
  bladder device (auxiliary) — *see*
      Complications, genitourinary, device or
      implant, urinary system
  bleeding (postoperative) — *see* Complication,
      postoperative, hemorrhage
    intraoperative — *see* Complication,
        intraoperative, hemorrhage
  blood vessel graft — *see* Complications, graft,
      vascular
  bone
    device NEC T84.9
      embolism T84.81
      fibrosis T84.82
      hemorrhage T84.83
      infection or inflammation T84.7
      mechanical
        breakdown T84.318
        displacement T84.328
        malposition T84.328
        obstruction T84.398
        perforation T84.398
        protrusion T84.398
      pain T84.84
      specified type NEC T84.89
      stenosis T84.85
      thrombosis T84.86
    graft — *see* Complications, graft, bone

Complication(s) (from) (of) — *continued*
bone — *continued*
growth stimulator (electrode) — *see*
Complications, electronic stimulator
device, bone
marrow transplant — *see* Complications,
transplant, bone, marrow
brain neurostimulator (electrode) — *see*
Complications, electronic stimulator
device, brain
breast implant (prosthetic) T85.9
capsular contracture T85.44
embolism T85.818
fibrosis T85.828
hemorrhage T85.838
infection and inflammation T85.79
mechanical
breakdown T85.41
displacement T85.42
leakage T85.43
malposition T85.42
obstruction T85.49
perforation T85.49
protrusion T85.49
specified NEC T85.49
pain T85.848
specified type NEC T85.898
stenosis T85.858
thrombosis T85.868
bypass — *see also* Complications, prosthetic
device or implant
aortocoronary — *see* Complications,
coronary artery (bypass) graft
arterial — *see also* Complications, graft,
vascular
extremity — *see* Complications, extremity
artery (bypass) graft
cardiac — *see also* Disease, heart
device, implant or graft T82.9
embolism T82.817
fibrosis T82.827
hemorrhage T82.837
infection or inflammation T82.7
valve prosthesis T82.6
mechanical
breakdown T82.519
specified device NEC T82.518
displacement T82.529
specified device NEC T82.528
leakage T82.539
specified device NEC T82.538
malposition T82.529
specified device NEC T82.528
obstruction T82.599
specified device NEC T82.598
perforation T82.599
specified device NEC T82.598
protrusion T82.599
specified device NEC T82.598
pain T82.847
specified type NEC T82.897
stenosis T82.857
thrombosis T82.867
cardiovascular device, graft or implant T82.9
aortic graft — *see* Complications, graft,
vascular
arteriovenous
fistula, artificial — *see* Complication,
arteriovenous, fistula, surgically
created
shunt — *see* Complication, arteriovenous,
shunt, surgically created
artificial heart — *see* Complication, artificial,
heart
balloon (counterpulsation) device — *see*
Complication, balloon implant, vascular
carotid artery graft — *see* Complications,
graft, vascular

Complication(s) (from) (of) — *continued*
cardiovascular device, graft or implant T82.9
— *continued*
coronary bypass graft — *see* Complication,
coronary artery (bypass) graft
dialysis catheter (vascular) — *see*
Complication, catheter, dialysis
electronic T82.9
electrode T82.9
embolism T82.817
fibrosis T82.827
hemorrhage T82.837
infection T82.7
mechanical
breakdown T82.110
displacement T82.120
leakage T82.190
obstruction T82.190
perforation T82.190
protrusion T82.190
specified type NEC T82.190
pain T82.847
specified NEC T82.897
stenosis T82.857
thrombosis T82.867
embolism T82.817
fibrosis T82.827
hemorrhage T82.837
infection T82.7
mechanical
breakdown T82.119
displacement T82.129
leakage T82.199
obstruction T82.199
perforation T82.199
protrusion T82.199
specified type NEC T82.199
pain T82.847
pulse generator T82.9
embolism T82.817
fibrosis T82.827
hemorrhage T82.837
infection T82.7
mechanical
breakdown T82.111
displacement T82.121
leakage T82.191
obstruction T82.191
perforation T82.191
protrusion T82.191
specified type NEC T82.191
pain T82.847
specified NEC T82.897
stenosis T82.857
thrombosis T82.867
specified condition NEC T82.897
specified device NEC T82.9
embolism T82.817
fibrosis T82.827
hemorrhage T82.837
infection T82.7
mechanical
breakdown T82.118
displacement T82.128
leakage T82.198
obstruction T82.198
perforation T82.198
protrusion T82.198
specified type NEC T82.198
pain T82.847
specified NEC T82.897
stenosis T82.857
thrombosis T82.867
stenosis T82.857
thrombosis T82.867
extremity artery graft — *see* Complication,
extremity artery (bypass) graft
femoral artery graft — *see* Complication,
extremity artery (bypass) graft

Complication(s) (from) (of) — *continued*
cardiovascular device, graft or implant T82.9
— *continued*
heart
transplant — *see* Complication, transplant,
heart
valve — *see* Complication, prosthetic
device, heart valve
graft — *see* Complication, heart, valve,
graft
heart-lung transplant — *see* Complication,
transplant, heart, with lung
infection or inflammation T82.7
umbrella device — *see* Complication,
umbrella device, vascular
vascular graft (or anastomosis) — *see*
Complication, graft, vascular
carotid artery (bypass) graft — *see*
Complications, graft, vascular
catheter (device) NEC — *see also*
Complications, prosthetic device or
implant
cranial infusion
infection and inflammation T85.735
mechanical
breakdown T85.610
displacement T85.620
leakage T85.630
malfunction T85.690
malposition T85.620
obstruction T85.690
perforation T85.690
protrusion T85.690
specified NEC T85.690
cystostomy T83.9
embolism T83.81
fibrosis T83.82
hemorrhage T83.83
infection and inflammation T83.510
mechanical
breakdown T83.010
displacement T83.020
leakage T83.030
malposition T83.020
obstruction T83.090
perforation T83.090
protrusion T83.090
specified NEC T83.090
pain T83.84
specified type NEC T83.89
stenosis T83.85
thrombosis T83.86
dialysis (vascular) T82.9
embolism T82.818
fibrosis T82.828
hemorrhage T82.838
infection and inflammation T82.7
intraperitoneal — *see* Complications,
catheter, intraperitoneal
mechanical
breakdown T82.41
displacement T82.42
leakage T82.43
malposition T82.42
obstruction T82.49
perforation T82.49
protrusion T82.49
pain T82.848
specified type NEC T82.898
stenosis T82.858
thrombosis T82.868
epidural infusion T85.9
embolism T85.810
fibrosis T85.820
hemorrhage T85.830
infection and inflammation T85.735

Complication(s) (from) (of) — *continued*
  catheter (device) NEC (*see also* Complications, prosthetic device or implant) — *continued*
    epidural infusion T85.9 — *continued*
      mechanical
        breakdown T85.610
        displacement T85.620
        leakage T85.630
        malfunction T85.610
        malposition T85.620
        obstruction T85.690
        perforation T85.690
        protrusion T85.690
        specified NEC T85.690
      pain T85.840
      specified type NEC T85.890
      stenosis T85.850
      thrombosis T85.860
    intraperitoneal dialysis T85.9
      embolism T85.818
      fibrosis T85.828
      hemorrhage T85.838
      infection and inflammation T85.71
      mechanical
        breakdown T85.611
        displacement T85.621
        leakage T85.631
        malfunction T85.611
        malposition T85.621
        obstruction T85.691
        perforation T85.691
        protrusion T85.691
        specified NEC T85.691
      pain T85.848
      specified type NEC T85.898
      stenosis T85.858
      thrombosis T85.868
    intrathecal infusion
      infection and inflammation T85.735
      mechanical
        breakdown T85.610
        displacement T85.620
        leakage T85.630
        malfunction T85.690
        malposition T85.620
        obstruction T85.690
        perforation T85.690
        protrusion T85.690
        specified NEC T85.690
    intravenous infusion T82.9
      embolism T82.818
      fibrosis T82.828
      hemorrhage T82.838
      infection or inflammation T82.7
      mechanical
        breakdown T82.514
        displacement T82.524
        leakage T82.534
        malposition T82.524
        obstruction T82.594
        perforation T82.594
        protrusion T82.594
      pain T82.848
      specified type NEC T82.898
      stenosis T82.858
      thrombosis T82.868
    spinal infusion
      infection and inflammation T85.735
      mechanical
        breakdown T85.610
        displacement T85.620
        leakage T85.630
        malfunction T85.690
        malposition T85.620
        obstruction T85.690
        perforation T85.690
        protrusion T85.690
        specified NEC T85.690

Complication(s) (from) (of) — *continued*
  catheter (device) NEC (*see also* Complications, prosthetic device or implant) — *continued*
    subarachnoid infusion
      infection and inflammation T85.735
      mechanical
        breakdown T85.610
        displacement T85.620
        leakage T85.630
        malfunction T85.690
        malposition T85.620
        obstruction T85.690
        perforation T85.690
        protrusion T85.690
        specified NEC T85.690
    subdural infusion T85.9
      embolism T85.810
      fibrosis T85.820
      hemorrhage T85.830
      infection and inflammation T85.735
      mechanical
        breakdown T85.610
        displacement T85.620
        leakage T85.630
        malfunction T85.610
        malposition T85.620
        obstruction T85.690
        perforation T85.690
        protrusion T85.690
        specified NEC T85.690
      pain T85.840
      specified type NEC T85.890
      stenosis T85.850
      thrombosis T85.860
    urethral T83.9
      displacement T83.028
      embolism T83.81
      fibrosis T83.82
      hemorrhage T83.83
      indwelling
        breakdown T83.011
        displacement T83.021
        infection and inflammation T83.511
        leakage T83.031
        specified complication NEC T83.091
      infection and inflammation T83.511
      leakage T83.038
      malposition T83.028
      mechanical
        breakdown T83.011
      obstruction (mechanical) T83.091
      pain T83.84
      perforation T83.091
      protrusion T83.091
      specified type NEC T83.091
      stenosis T83.85
      thrombosis T83.86
    urinary NEC
      breakdown T83.018
      displacement T83.028
      infection and inflammation T83.518
      leakage T83.038
      specified complication NEC T83.098
  cecostomy (stoma) — *see* Complications, colostomy
  cesarean delivery wound NEC O90.89
    disruption O90.0
    hematoma O90.2
    infection (following delivery) O86.0
  chemotherapy (antineoplastic) NEC T88.7
  chin implant (prosthetic) — *see* Complication, prosthetic device or implant, specified NEC
  circulatory system I99.8
    intraoperative I97.88
    postprocedural I97.89
      following cardiac surgery I97.19-
        postcardiotomy syndrome I97.0
      hypertension I97.3
      lymphedema after mastectomy I97.2

Complication(s) (from) (of) — *continued*
  circulatory system I99.8 — *continued*
    postprocedural I97.89 — *continued*
      postcardiotomy syndrome I97.0
      specified NEC I97.89
  colostomy (stoma) K94.00
    hemorrhage K94.01
    infection K94.02
    malfunction K94.03
    mechanical K94.03
    specified complication NEC K94.09
  contraceptive device, intrauterine — *see* Complications, intrauterine, contraceptive device
  cord (umbilical) — *see* Complications, umbilical cord
  corneal graft — *see* Complications, graft, cornea
  coronary artery (bypass) graft T82.9
    atherosclerosis — *see* Arteriosclerosis, coronary (artery)
    embolism T82.818
    fibrosis T82.828
    hemorrhage T82.838
    infection and inflammation T82.7
    mechanical
      breakdown T82.211
      displacement T82.212
      leakage T82.213
      malposition T82.212
      obstruction T82.218
      perforation T82.218
      protrusion T82.218
      specified NEC T82.218
    pain T82.848
    specified type NEC T82.898
    stenosis T82.858
    thrombosis T82.868
  counterpulsation device (balloon), intra-aortic — *see* Complications, balloon implant, vascular
  cystostomy (stoma) N99.518
    catheter — *see* Complications, catheter, cystostomy
    hemorrhage N99.510
    infection N99.511
    malfunction N99.512
    specified type NEC N99.518
  delivery (*see also* Complications, obstetric) O75.9
    procedure (instrumental) (manual) (surgical) O75.4
    specified NEC O75.89
  dialysis (peritoneal) (renal) — *see also* Complications, infusion
    catheter (vascular) — *see* Complication, catheter, dialysis
    peritoneal, intraperitoneal — *see* Complications, catheter, intraperitoneal
  dorsal column (spinal) neurostimulator — *see* Complications, electronic stimulator device, spinal cord
  drug NEC T88.7
  ear procedure — *see also* Disorder, ear
    intraoperative H95.88
      hematoma — *see* Complications, intraoperative, hemorrhage (hematoma) (of), ear
      hemorrhage — *see* Complications, intraoperative, hemorrhage (hematoma) (of), ear
      laceration — *see* Complications, intraoperative, puncture or laceration, ear
    specified NEC H95.88

Complication(s) (from) (of) — *continued*
  ear procedure — *see also* Disorder, ear — *continued*
    postoperative H95.89
      external ear canal stenosis H95.81-
      hematoma — *see* Complications, postprocedural, hematoma (of), ear
      hemorrhage — *see* Complications, postprocedural, hemorrhage (of), ear
      postmastoidectomy — *see* Complications, postmastoidectomy
      seroma — *see* Complications, postprocedural, seroma (of), mastoid process
      specified NEC H95.89
  ectopic pregnancy O08.9
    damage to pelvic organs O08.6
    embolism O08.2
    genital infection O08.0
    hemorrhage (delayed) (excessive) O08.1
    metabolic disorder O08.5
    renal failure O08.4
    shock O08.3
    specified type NEC O08.0
    venous complication NEC O08.7
  electronic stimulator device
    bladder (urinary) — *see* Complications, electronic stimulator device, urinary
    bone T84.9
      breakdown T84.310
      displacement T84.320
      embolism T84.81
      fibrosis T84.82
      hemorrhage T84.83
      infection or inflammation T84.7
      malfunction T84.310
      malposition T84.320
      mechanical NEC T84.390
      obstruction T84.390
      pain T84.84
      perforation T84.390
      protrusion T84.390
      specified type NEC T84.89
      stenosis T84.85
      thrombosis T84.86
    brain T85.9
      embolism T85.810
      fibrosis T85.820
      hemorrhage T85.830
      infection and inflammation T85.731
      mechanical
        breakdown T85.110
        displacement T85.120
        leakage T85.190
        malposition T85.120
        obstruction T85.190
        perforation T85.190
        protrusion T85.190
        specified NEC T85.190
      pain T85.840
      specified type NEC T85.890
      stenosis T85.850
      thrombosis T85.860
    cardiac (defibrillator) (pacemaker) — *see* Complications, cardiovascular device or implant, electronic
    generator (brain) (gastric) (peripheral) (sacral) (spinal)
      breakdown T85.113
      displacement T85.123
      leakage T85.193
      malposition T85.123
      obstruction T85.193
      perforation T85.193
      protrusion T85.193
      specified type NEC T85.193

Complication(s) (from) (of) — *continued*
  electronic stimulator device — *continued*
    muscle T84.9
      breakdown T84.418
      displacement T84.428
      embolism T84.81
      fibrosis T84.82
      hemorrhage T84.83
      infection or inflammation T84.7
      mechanical NEC T84.498
      pain T84.84
      specified type NEC T84.89
      stenosis T84.85
      thrombosis T84.86
    nervous system T85.9
      brain — *see* Complications, electronic stimulator device, brain
      cranial nerve — *see* Complications, electronic stimulator device, peripheral nerve
      embolism T85.810
      fibrosis T85.820
      gastric nerve — *see* Complications, electronic stimulator device, peripheral nerve
      hemorrhage T85.830
      infection and inflammation T85.738
      mechanical
        breakdown T85.118
        displacement T85.128
        leakage T85.199
        malposition T85.128
        obstruction T85.199
        perforation T85.199
        protrusion T85.199
        specified NEC T85.199
      pain T85.840
      peripheral nerve — *see* Complications, electronic stimulator device, peripheral nerve
      sacral nerve — *see* Complications, electronic stimulator device, peripheral nerve
      specified type NEC T85.890
      spinal cord — *see* Complications, electronic stimulator device, spinal cord
      stenosis T85.850
      thrombosis T85.860
      vagal nerve — *see* Complications, electronic stimulator device, peripheral nerve
    peripheral nerve T85.9
      embolism T85.810
      fibrosis T85.820
      hemorrhage T85.830
      infection and inflammation T85.732
      mechanical
        breakdown T85.111
        displacement T85.121
        leakage T85.191
        malposition T85.121
        obstruction T85.191
        perforation T85.191
        protrusion T85.191
        specified NEC T85.191
      pain T85.840
      specified type NEC T85.890
      stenosis T85.850
      thrombosis T85.860
    spinal cord T85.9
      embolism T85.810
      fibrosis T85.820
      hemorrhage T85.830
      infection and inflammation T85.733

Complication(s) (from) (of) — *continued*
  electronic stimulator device — *continued*
    spinal cord T85.9 — *continued*
      mechanical
        breakdown T85.112
        displacement T85.122
        leakage T85.192
        malposition T85.122
        obstruction T85.192
        perforation T85.192
        protrusion T85.192
        specified NEC T85.192
      pain T85.840
      specified type NEC T85.890
      stenosis T85.850
      thrombosis T85.860
    urinary T83.9
      embolism T83.81
      fibrosis T83.82
      hemorrhage T83.83
      infection and inflammation T83.598
      mechanical
        breakdown T83.110
        displacement T83.120
        malposition T83.120
        perforation T83.190
        protrusion T83.190
        specified NEC T83.190
      pain T83.84
      specified type NEC T83.89
      stenosis T83.85
      thrombosis T83.86
  electroshock therapy T88.9
    specified NEC T88.8
  endocrine E34.9
    postprocedural
      adrenal hypofunction E89.6
      hypoinsulinemia E89.1
      hypoparathyroidism E89.2
      hypopituitarism E89.3
      hypothyroidism E89.0
      ovarian failure E89.40
        asymptomatic E89.40
        symptomatic E89.41
      specified NEC E89.89
      testicular hypofunction E89.5
  endodontic treatment NEC M27.59
  enterostomy (stoma) K94.10
    hemorrhage K94.11
    infection K94.12
    malfunction K94.13
    mechanical K94.13
    specified complication NEC K94.19
  episiotomy, disruption O90.1
  esophageal anti-reflux device T85.9
    embolism T85.818
    fibrosis T85.828
    hemorrhage T85.838
    infection and inflammation T85.79
    mechanical
      breakdown T85.511
      displacement T85.521
      malfunction T85.511
      malposition T85.521
      obstruction T85.591
      perforation T85.591
      protrusion T85.591
      specified NEC T85.591
    pain T85.848
    specified type NEC T85.898
    stenosis T85.858
    thrombosis T85.868
  esophagostomy K94.30
    hemorrhage K94.31
    infection K94.32
    malfunction K94.33
    mechanical K94.33
    specified complication NEC K94.39
  extracorporeal circulation T80.90

Complication(s) (from) (of) — *continued*
extremity artery (bypass) graft T82.9
  arteriosclerosis — *see* Arteriosclerosis,
    extremities, bypass graft
  embolism T82.818
  fibrosis T82.828
  hemorrhage T82.838
  infection and inflammation T82.7
  mechanical
    breakdown T82.318
      femoral artery T82.312
    displacement T82.328
      femoral artery T82.322
    leakage T82.338
      femoral artery T82.332
    malposition T82.328
      femoral artery T82.322
    obstruction T82.398
      femoral artery T82.392
    perforation T82.398
      femoral artery T82.392
    protrusion T82.398
      femoral artery T82.392
  pain T82.848
  specified type NEC T82.898
  stenosis T82.858
  thrombosis T82.868
eye H57.9
  corneal graft — *see* Complications, graft,
    cornea
  implant (prosthetic) T85.9
    embolism T85.818
    fibrosis T85.828
    hemorrhage T85.838
    infection and inflammation T85.79
    mechanical
      breakdown T85.318
      displacement T85.328
      leakage T85.398
      malposition T85.328
      obstruction T85.398
      perforation T85.398
      protrusion T85.398
      specified NEC T85.398
    pain T85.848
    specified type NEC T85.898
    stenosis T85.858
    thrombosis T85.868
  intraocular lens — *see* Complications,
    intraocular lens
  orbital prosthesis — *see* Complications,
    orbital prosthesis
female genital N94.9
  device, implant or graft NEC — *see*
    Complications, genitourinary, device or
    implant, genital tract
femoral artery (bypass) graft — *see*
  Complication, extremity artery (bypass)
  graft
fixation device, internal (orthopedic) T84.9
  infection and inflammation T84.60
    arm T84.61-
      humerus T84.61-
      radius T84.61-
      ulna T84.61-
    leg T84.629
      femur T84.62-
      fibula T84.62-
      tibia T84.62-
    specified site NEC T84.69
    spine T84.63

Complication(s) (from) (of) — *continued*
fixation device, internal (orthopedic) T84.9 —
  continued
  mechanical
    breakdown
      limb T84.119
        carpal T84.210
        femur T84.11-
        fibula T84.11-
        humerus T84.11-
        metacarpal T84.210
        metatarsal T84.213
        phalanx
          foot T84.213
          hand T84.210
        radius T84.11-
        tarsal T84.213
        tibia T84.11-
        ulna T84.11-
      specified bone NEC T84.218
      spine T84.216
    displacement
      limb T84.129
        carpal T84.220
        femur T84.12-
        fibula T84.12-
        humerus T84.12-
        metacarpal T84.220
        metatarsal T84.223
        phalanx
          foot T84.223
          hand T84.220
        radius T84.12-
        tarsal T84.223
        tibia T84.12-
        ulna T84.12-
      specified bone NEC T84.228
      spine T84.226
    malposition — *see* Complications, fixation
      device, internal, mechanical,
      displacement
    obstruction — *see* Complications, fixation
      device, internal, mechanical, specified
      type NEC
    perforation — *see* Complications, fixation
      device, internal, mechanical, specified
      type NEC
    protrusion — *see* Complications, fixation
      device, internal, mechanical, specified
      type NEC
    specified type NEC
      limb T84.199
        carpal T84.290
        femur T84.19-
        fibula T84.19-
        humerus T84.19-
        metacarpal T84.290
        metatarsal T84.293
        phalanx
          foot T84.293
          hand T84.290
        radius T84.19-
        tarsal T84.293
        tibia T84.19-
        ulna T84.19-
      specified bone NEC T84.298
      vertebra T84.296
  specified type NEC T84.89
    embolism T84.81
    fibrosis T84.82
    hemorrhage T84.83
    pain T84.84
    specified complication NEC T84.89
    stenosis T84.85
    thrombosis T84.86

Complication(s) (from) (of) — *continued*
following
  acute myocardial infarction NEC I23.8
    aneurysm (false) (of cardiac wall) (of heart
      wall) (ruptured) I23.3
    angina I23.7
    atrial
      septal defect I23.1
      thrombosis I23.6
    cardiac wall rupture I23.3
    chordae tendinae rupture I23.4
    defect
      septal
        atrial (heart) I23.1
        ventricular (heart) I23.2
    hemopericardium I23.0
    papillary muscle rupture I23.5
    rupture
      cardiac wall I23.3
        with hemopericardium I23.0
      chordae tendineae I23.4
      papillary muscle I23.5
    specified NEC I23.8
    thrombosis
      atrium I23.6
      auricular appendage I23.6
      ventricle (heart) I23.6
    ventricular
      septal defect I23.2
      thrombosis I23.6
  ectopic or molar pregnancy O08.9
    cardiac arrest O08.81
    sepsis O08.82
    specified type NEC O08.89
    urinary tract infection O08.83
  termination of pregnancy — *see* Abortion
gastrointestinal K92.9
  bile duct prosthesis — *see* Complications,
    bile duct implant
  esophageal anti-reflux device — *see*
    Complications, esophageal anti-reflux
    device
  postoperative
    colostomy — *see* Complications, colostomy
    dumping syndrome K91.1
    enterostomy — *see* Complications,
      enterostomy
    gastrostomy — *see* Complications,
      gastrostomy
    malabsorption NEC K91.2
    obstruction K91.3
    postcholecystectomy syndrome K91.5
    specified NEC K91.89
    vomiting after GI surgery K91.0
  prosthetic device or implant
    bile duct prosthesis — *see* Complications,
      bile duct implant
    esophageal anti-reflux device — *see*
      Complications, esophageal anti-reflux
      device
    specified type NEC
      embolism T85.818
      fibrosis T85.828
      hemorrhage T85.838
      mechanical
        breakdown T85.518
        displacement T85.528
        malfunction T85.518
        malposition T85.528
        obstruction T85.598
        perforation T85.598
        protrusion T85.598
        specified NEC T85.598
      pain T85.848
      specified complication NEC T85.898
      stenosis T85.858
      thrombosis T85.868

DISEASE INDEX

Complication(s) (from) (of) — *continued*
  gastrostomy (stoma) K94.20
    hemorrhage K94.21
    infection K94.22
    malfunction K94.23
    mechanical K94.23
    specified complication NEC K94.29
  genitourinary
    device or implant T83.9
      genital tract T83.9
        infection or inflammation T83.69
        intrauterine contraceptive device — *see* Complications, intrauterine, contraceptive device
        mechanical — *see* Complications, by device, mechanical
        mesh — *see* Complications, mesh
        penile prosthesis — *see* Complications, prosthetic device, penile
        specified type NEC T83.89
          embolism T83.81
          fibrosis T83.82
          hemorrhage T83.83
          pain T83.84
          specified complication NEC T83.89
          stenosis T83.85
          thrombosis T83.86
        vaginal mesh — *see* Complications, mesh
      urinary system T83.9
        cystostomy catheter — *see* Complication, catheter, cystostomy
        electronic stimulator — *see* Complications, electronic stimulator device, urinary
        indwelling urethral catheter — *see* Complications, catheter, urethral, indwelling
        infection or inflammation T83.598
          indwelling urethral catheter T83.511
        kidney transplant — *see* Complication, transplant, kidney
        organ graft — *see* Complication, graft, urinary organ
        specified type NEC T83.89
          embolism T83.81
          fibrosis T83.82
          hemorrhage T83.83
          mechanical T83.198
            breakdown T83.118
            displacement T83.128
            malfunction T83.118
            malposition T83.128
            obstruction T83.198
            perforation T83.198
            protrusion T83.198
            specified NEC T83.198
        sphincter implant — *see* Complications, implant, urinary sphincter
        sphincter, implanted T83.191
        stent (ileal conduit) (nephroureteral) T83.193
          pain T83.84
          specified complication NEC T83.89
          stenosis T83.85
          thrombosis T83.86
          ureteral indwelling T83.192
  postprocedural
    pelvic peritoneal adhesions N99.4
    renal failure N99.0
    specified NEC N99.89
    stoma — *see* Complications, stoma, urinary tract
    urethral stricture — *see* Stricture, urethra, postprocedural
    vaginal
      adhesions N99.2
      vault prolapse N99.3

Complication(s) (from) (of) — *continued*
  graft (bypass) (patch) — *see also* Complications, prosthetic device or implant
    aorta — *see* Complications, graft, vascular
    arterial — *see* Complication, graft, vascular
    bone T86.839
      failure T86.831
      infection T86.832
      mechanical T84.318
        breakdown T84.318
        displacement T84.328
        protrusion T84.398
        specified type NEC T84.398
      rejection T86.830
      specified type NEC T86.838
    carotid artery — *see* Complications, graft, vascular
    cornea T86.849
      failure T86.841
      infection T86.842
      mechanical T85.398
        breakdown T85.318
        displacement T85.328
        protrusion T85.398
        specified type NEC T85.398
      rejection T86.840
      retroprosthetic membrane T85.398
      specified type NEC T86.848
    femoral artery (bypass) — *see* Complication, extremity artery (bypass) graft
    genital organ or tract — *see* Complications, genitourinary, device or implant, genital tract
    muscle T84.9
      breakdown T84.410
      displacement T84.420
      embolism T84.81
      fibrosis T84.82
      hemorrhage T84.83
      infection and inflammation T84.7
      mechanical NEC T84.490
      pain T84.84
      specified type NEC T84.89
      stenosis T84.85
      thrombosis T84.86
    nerve — *see* Complication, prosthetic device or implant, specified NEC
    skin — *see* Complications, prosthetic device or implant, skin graft
    tendon T84.9
      breakdown T84.410
      displacement T84.420
      embolism T84.81
      fibrosis T84.82
      hemorrhage T84.83
      infection and inflammation T84.7
      mechanical NEC T84.490
      pain T84.84
      specified type NEC T84.89
      stenosis T84.85
      thrombosis T84.86
    urinary organ T83.9
      embolism T83.81
      fibrosis T83.82
      hemorrhage T83.83
      infection and inflammation T83.598
        indwelling urinary catheter T83.511
      mechanical
        breakdown T83.21
        displacement T83.22
        erosion T83.24
        exposure T83.25
        leakage T83.23
        malposition T83.22
        obstruction T83.29
        perforation T83.29
        protrusion T83.29
        specified NEC T83.29

Complication(s) (from) (of) — *continued*
  graft (bypass) (patch) (*see also* Complications, prosthetic device or implant) — *continued*
    urinary organ T83.9 — *continued*
      pain T83.84
      specified type NEC T83.89
      stenosis T83.85
      thrombosis T83.86
    vascular T82.9
      embolism T82.818
      femoral artery — *see* Complication, extremity artery (bypass) graft
      fibrosis T82.828
      hemorrhage T82.838
      mechanical
        breakdown T82.319
          aorta (bifurcation) T82.310
          carotid artery T82.311
          specified vessel NEC T82.318
        displacement T82.329
          aorta (bifurcation) T82.320
          carotid artery T82.321
          specified vessel NEC T82.328
        leakage T82.339
          aorta (bifurcation) T82.330
          carotid artery T82.331
          specified vessel NEC T82.338
        malposition T82.329
          aorta (bifurcation) T82.320
          carotid artery T82.321
          specified vessel NEC T82.328
        obstruction T82.399
          aorta (bifurcation) T82.390
          carotid artery T82.391
          specified vessel NEC T82.398
        perforation T82.399
          aorta (bifurcation) T82.390
          carotid artery T82.391
          specified vessel NEC T82.398
        protrusion T82.399
          aorta (bifurcation) T82.390
          carotid artery T82.391
          specified vessel NEC T82.398
      pain T82.848
      specified complication NEC T82.898
      stenosis T82.858
      thrombosis T82.868
  heart I51.9
    assist device
      infection and inflammation T82.7
    following acute myocardial infarction — *see* Complications, following, acute myocardial infarction
    postoperative — *see* Complications, circulatory system
    transplant — *see* Complication, transplant, heart
      and lung(s) — *see* Complications, transplant, heart, with lung
    valve
      graft (biological) T82.9
        embolism T82.817
        fibrosis T82.827
        hemorrhage T82.837
        infection and inflammation T82.7
        mechanical T82.228
          breakdown T82.221
          displacement T82.222
          leakage T82.223
          malposition T82.222
          obstruction T82.228
          perforation T82.228
          protrusion T82.228
        pain T82.847
        specified type NEC T82.897
        stenosis T82.857
        thrombosis T82.867

Complication(s) (from) (of) — *continued*
valve — *continued*
  heart I51.9 — *continued*
    prosthesis T82.9
      embolism T82.817
      fibrosis T82.827
      hemorrhage T82.837
      infection or inflammation T82.6
      mechanical T82.09
        breakdown T82.01
        displacement T82.02
        leakage T82.03
        malposition T82.02
        obstruction T82.09
        perforation T82.09
        protrusion T82.09
      pain T82.847
      specified type NEC T82.897
        mechanical T82.09
      stenosis T82.857
      thrombosis T82.867
hematoma
  intraoperative — *see* Complication,
    intraoperative, hemorrhage
  postprocedural — *see* Complication,
    postprocedural, hematoma
hemodialysis — *see* Complications, dialysis
hemorrhage
  intraoperative — *see* Complication,
    intraoperative, hemorrhage
  postprocedural — *see* Complication,
    postprocedural, hemorrhage
ileostomy (stoma) — *see* Complications,
  enterostomy
immunization (procedure) — *see*
  Complications, vaccination
implant — *see also* Complications, by site and
  type
  urinary sphincter T83.9
    embolism T83.81
    fibrosis T83.82
    hemorrhage T83.83
    infection and inflammation T83.591
    mechanical
      breakdown T83.111
      displacement T83.121
      leakage T83.191
      malposition T83.121
      obstruction T83.191
      perforation T83.191
      protrusion T83.191
      specified NEC T83.191
    pain T83.84
    specified type NEC T83.89
    stenosis T83.85
    thrombosis T83.86
infusion (procedure) T80.90
  air embolism T80.0
  blood — *see* Complications, transfusion
  catheter — *see* Complications, catheter
  infection T80.29
  pump — *see* Complications, cardiovascular,
    device or implant
  sepsis T80.29
  serum reaction (*see also* Reaction, serum)
    T80.69
    anaphylactic shock (*see also* Shock,
      anaphylactic) T80.59
  specified type NEC T80.89
inhalation therapy NEC T81.81
injection (procedure) T80.90
  drug reaction — *see* Reaction, drug
  infection T80.29
  sepsis T80.29
  serum (prophylactic) (therapeutic) — *see*
    Complications, vaccination
  specified type NEC T80.89
  vaccine (any) — *see* Complications,
    vaccination

Complication(s) (from) (of) — *continued*
inoculation (any) — *see* Complications,
  vaccination
insulin pump
  infection and inflammation T85.72
  mechanical
    breakdown T85.614
    displacement T85.624
    leakage T85.633
    malposition T85.624
    obstruction T85.694
    perforation T85.694
    protrusion T85.694
    specified NEC T85.694
intestinal pouch NEC K91.858
intraocular lens (prosthetic) T85.9
  embolism T85.818
  fibrosis T85.828
  hemorrhage T85.838
  infection and inflammation T85.79
  mechanical
    breakdown T85.21
    displacement T85.22
    malposition T85.22
    obstruction T85.29
    perforation T85.29
    protrusion T85.29
    specified NEC T85.29
  pain T85.848
  specified type NEC T85.898
  stenosis T85.858
  thrombosis T85.868
intraoperative (intraprocedural)
  cardiac arrest
    during cardiac surgery I97.710
    during other surgery I97.711
  cardiac functional disturbance NEC
    during cardiac surgery I97.790
    during other surgery I97.791
  hemorrhage (hematoma) (of)
    circulatory system organ or structure
      during cardiac bypass I97.411
      during cardiac catheterization I97.410
      during other circulatory system
        procedure I97.418
      during other procedure I97.42
    digestive system organ
      during procedure on digestive system
        K91.61
      during procedure on other organ
        K91.62
    ear
      during procedure on ear and mastoid
        process H95.21
      during procedure on other organ
        H95.22
    endocrine system organ or structure
      during procedure on endocrine system
        organ or structure E36.01
      during procedure on other organ
        E36.02
    eye and adnexa
      during ophthalmic procedure H59.11-
      during other procedure H59.12-
    genitourinary organ or structure
      during procedure on genitourinary
        organ or structure N99.61
      during procedure on other organ
        N99.62
    mastoid process
      during procedure on ear and mastoid
        process H95.21
      during procedure on other organ
        H95.22

Complication(s) (from) (of) — *continued*
intraoperative (intraprocedural) — *continued*
  hemorrhage (hematoma) (of) — *continued*
    musculoskeletal structure
      during musculoskeletal surgery
        M96.810
      during non-orthopedic surgery
        M96.811
      during orthopedic surgery M96.810
    nervous system
      during a nervous system procedure
        G97.31
      during other procedure G97.32
    respiratory system
      during other procedure J95.62
      during procedure on respiratory system
        organ or structure J95.61
    skin and subcutaneous tissue
      during a dermatologic procedure
        L76.01
      during a procedure on other organ
        L76.02
    spleen
      during a procedure on other organ
        D78.02
      during a procedure on the spleen
        D78.01
  puncture or laceration (accidental)
    (unintentional) (of)
    brain
      during a nervous system procedure
        G97.48
      during other procedure G97.49
    circulatory system organ or structure
      during circulatory system procedure
        I97.51
      during other procedure I97.52
    digestive system
      during procedure on digestive system
        K91.71
      during procedure on other organ
        K91.72
    ear
      during procedure on ear and mastoid
        process H95.31
      during procedure on other organ
        H95.32
    endocrine system organ or structure
      during procedure on endocrine system
        organ or structure E36.11
      during procedure on other organ
        E36.12
    eye and adnexa
      during ophthalmic procedure H59.21-
      during other procedure H59.22-
    genitourinary organ or structure
      during procedure on genitourinary
        organ or structure N99.71
      during procedure on other organ
        N99.72
    mastoid process
      during procedure on ear and mastoid
        process H95.31
      during procedure on other organ
        H95.32
    musculoskeletal structure
      during musculoskeletal surgery
        M96.820
      during non-orthopedic surgery
        M96.821
      during orthopedic surgery M96.820
    nervous system
      during a nervous system procedure
        G97.48
      during other procedure G97.49

Complication(s) (from) (of) — *continued*
  intraoperative (intraprocedural) — *continued*
    puncture or laceration (accidental)
        (unintentional) (of) — *continued*
      respiratory system
        during other procedure J95.72
        during procedure on respiratory system
            organ or structure J95.71
      skin and subcutaneous tissue
        during a dermatologic procedure
            L76.11
        during a procedure on other organ
            L76.12
      spleen
        during a procedure on other organ
            D78.12
        during a procedure on the spleen
            D78.11
    specified NEC
      circulatory system I97.88
      digestive system K91.81
      ear H95.88
      endocrine system E36.8
      eye and adnexa H59.88
      genitourinary system N99.81
      mastoid process H95.88
      musculoskeletal structure M96.89
      nervous system G97.81
      respiratory system J95.88
      skin and subcutaneous tissue L76.81
      spleen D78.81
  intraperitoneal catheter (dialysis) (infusion) —
      see Complications, catheter, intraperitoneal
  intrathecal infusion pump
    infection and inflammation T85.738
    mechanical
      breakdown T85.615
      displacement T85.625
      leakage T85.635
      malfunction T85.695
      malposition T85.625
      obstruction T85.695
      perforation T85.695
      protrusion T85.695
      specified NEC T85.695
  intrauterine
    contraceptive device
      embolism T83.81
      fibrosis T83.82
      hemorrhage T83.83
      infection and inflammation T83.69
      mechanical
        breakdown T83.31
        displacement T83.32
        malposition T83.32
        obstruction T83.39
        perforation T83.39
        protrusion T83.39
        specified NEC T83.39
      pain T83.84
      specified type NEC T83.89
      stenosis T83.85
      thrombosis T83.86
    procedure (fetal), to newborn P96.5
  jejunostomy (stoma) — *see* Complications,
      enterostomy
  joint prosthesis, internal T84.9
    breakage (fracture) T84.01-
    dislocation T84.02-
    fracture T84.01-
    infection or inflammation T84.50
      hip T84.5-
      knee T84.5-
      specified joint NEC T84.59
    instability T84.02-
    malposition — *see* Complications, joint
        prosthesis, mechanical, displacement

Complication(s) (from) (of) — *continued*
  joint prosthesis, internal T84.9 — *continued*
    mechanical
      breakage, broken T84.01-
      dislocation T84.02-
      fracture T84.01-
      instability T84.02-
      leakage — *see* Complications, joint
          prosthesis, mechanical, specified NEC
      loosening T84.039
        hip T84.03-
        knee T84.03-
        specified joint NEC T84.038
      obstruction — *see* Complications, joint
          prosthesis, mechanical, specified NEC
      perforation — *see* Complications, joint
          prosthesis, mechanical, specified NEC
      osteolysis T84.059
        hip T84.05-
        knee T84.05-
        other specified joint T84.058
      protrusion — *see* Complications, joint
          prosthesis, mechanical, specified NEC
      specified complication NEC T84.099
        hip T84.09-
        knee T84.09-
        other specified joint T84.098
      subluxation T84.02-
      wear of articular bearing surface T84.069
        hip T84.06-
        knee T84.06-
        other specified joint T84.068
    specified joint NEC T84.89
      embolism T84.81
      fibrosis T84.82
      hemorrhage T84.83
      pain T84.84
      specified complication NEC T84.89
      stenosis T84.85
      thrombosis T84.86
    subluxation T84.02-
  kidney transplant — *see* Complications,
      transplant, kidney
  labor O75.9
    specified NEC O75.89
  liver transplant (immune or nonimmune) — *see*
      Complications, transplant, liver
  lumbar puncture G97.1
    cerebrospinal fluid leak G97.0
    headache or reaction G97.1
  lung transplant — *see* Complications,
      transplant, lung
    and heart — *see* Complications, transplant,
        lung, with heart
  male genital N50.9
    device, implant or graft — *see*
        Complications, genitourinary, device or
        implant, genital tract
    postprocedural or postoperative — *see*
        Complications, genitourinary,
        postprocedural
    specified NEC N99.89
  mastoid (process) procedure
    intraoperative H95.88
      hematoma — *see* Complications,
          intraoperative, hematoma (of),
          mastoid process
      hemorrhage — *see* Complications,
          intraoperative, hemorrhage (of),
          mastoid process
      laceration — *see* Complications,
          intraoperative, puncture or laceration,
          mastoid process
      seroma - see Complications,
          postprocedural, seroma (of), mastoid
          process
    specified NEC H95.88

Complication(s) (from) (of) — *continued*
  mastoid (process) procedure — *continued*
    postmastoidectomy — *see* Complications,
        postmastoidectomy
    postoperative H95.89
      external ear canal stenosis H95.81-
      hematoma — *see* Complications,
          postprocedural, hematoma (of),
          mastoid process
      hemorrhage — *see* Complications,
          postprocedural, hemorrhage (of),
          mastoid process
      postmastoidectomy — *see* Complications,
          postmastoidectomy
      seroma — *see* Complications,
          postprocedural, seroma (of), mastoid
          process
      specified NEC H95.89
  mastoidectomy cavity — *see* Complications,
      postmastoidectomy
  mechanical — *see* Complications, by site and
      type, mechanical
  medical procedures (*see also* Complication(s),
      intraoperative) T88.9
  metabolic E88.9
    postoperative E89.89
    specified NEC E89.89
  molar pregnancy NOS O08.9
    damage to pelvic organs O08.6
    embolism O08.2
    genital infection O08.0
    hemorrhage (delayed) (excessive) O08.1
    metabolic disorder O08.5
    renal failure O08.4
    shock O08.3
    specified type NEC O08.0
    venous complication NEC O08.7
  musculoskeletal system — *see also*
      Complication, intraoperative
      (intraprocedural), by site
    device, implant or graft NEC — *see*
        Complications, orthopedic, device or
        implant
    internal fixation (nail) (plate) (rod) — *see*
        Complications, fixation device, internal
    joint prosthesis — *see* Complications, joint
        prosthesis
    post radiation M96.89
      kyphosis M96.2
      scoliosis M96.5
      specified complication NEC M96.89
    postoperative (postprocedural) M96.89
      with osteoporosis — *see* Osteoporosis
      fracture following insertion of device — *see*
          Fracture, following insertion of
          orthopedic implant, joint prosthesis or
          bone plate
      joint instability after prosthesis removal
          M96.89
      lordosis M96.4
      postlaminectomy syndrome NEC M96.1
        kyphosis M96.3
      pseudarthrosis M96.0
      specified complication NEC M96.89
  nephrostomy (stoma) — *see* Complications,
      stoma, urinary tract, external NEC

Complication(s) (from) (of) — *continued*
nervous system G98.8
  central G96.9
  device, implant or graft — *see also*
    Complication, prosthetic device or
    implant, specified NEC
    electronic stimulator (electrode(s)) — *see*
      Complications, electronic stimulator
      device
    specified NEC
      infection and inflammation T85.738
      mechanical T85.695
        breakdown T85.615
        displacement T85.625
        leakage T85.635
        malfunction T85.695
        malposition T85.625
        obstruction T85.695
        perforation T85.695
        protrusion T85.695
        specified NEC T85.695
    ventricular shunt — *see* Complications,
      ventricular shunt
    electronic stimulator (electrode(s)) — *see*
      Complications, electronic stimulator
      device
  postprocedural G97.82
    intracranial hypotension G97.2
    specified NEC G97.82
    spinal fluid leak G97.0
newborn, due to intrauterine (fetal) procedure
  P96.5
nonabsorbable (permanent) sutures — *see*
  Complication, sutures, permanent
obstetric O75.9
  procedure (instrumental) (manual) (surgical)
    specified NEC O75.4
  specified NEC O75.89
  surgical wound NEC O90.89
    hematoma O90.2
    infection O86.0
ocular lens implant — *see* Complications,
  intraocular lens
ophthalmologic
  postprocedural bleb — *see* Blebitis
orbital prosthesis T85.9
  embolism T85.818
  fibrosis T85.828
  hemorrhage T85.838
  infection and inflammation T85.79
  mechanical
    breakdown T85.31-
    displacement T85.32-
    malposition T85.32-
    obstruction T85.39-
    perforation T85.39-
    protrusion T85.39-
    specified NEC T85.39-
  pain T85.848
  specified type NEC T85.898
  stenosis T85.858
  thrombosis T85.868
organ or tissue transplant (partial) (total) — *see*
  Complications, transplant
orthopedic — *see also* Disorder, soft tissue
  device or implant T84.9
    bone
      device or implant — *see* Complication,
        bone, device NEC
      graft — *see* Complication, graft, bone
    breakdown T84.418
    displacement T84.428
    electronic bone stimulator — *see*
      Complications, electronic stimulator
      device, bone
    embolism T84.81
    fibrosis T84.82
    fixation device — *see* Complication,
      fixation device, internal

Complication(s) (from) (of) — *continued*
orthopedic — *see also* Disorder, soft tissue —
  continued
  device or implant T84.9 — *continued*
    hemorrhage T84.83
    infection or inflammation T84.7
    joint prosthesis — *see* Complication, joint
      prosthesis, internal
    malfunction T84.418
    malposition T84.428
    mechanical NEC T84.498
    muscle graft — *see* Complications, graft,
      muscle
    obstruction T84.498
    pain T84.84
    perforation T84.498
    protrusion T84.498
    specified complication NEC T84.89
    stenosis T84.85
    tendon graft — *see* Complications, graft,
      tendon
    thrombosis T84.86
  fracture (following insertion of device) — *see*
    Fracture, following insertion of
    orthopedic implant, joint prosthesis or
    bone plate
  postprocedural M96.89
    fracture — *see* Fracture, following insertion
      of orthopedic implant, joint prosthesis
      or bone plate
    postlaminectomy syndrome NEC M96.1
      kyphosis M96.3
      lordosis M96.4
    postradiation
      kyphosis M96.2
      scoliosis M96.5
    pseudarthrosis post-fusion M96.0
    specified type NEC M96.89
pacemaker (cardiac) — *see* Complications,
  cardiovascular device or implant,
  electronic
pancreas transplant — *see* Complications,
  transplant, pancreas
penile prosthesis (implant) — *see*
  Complications, prosthetic device, penile
perfusion NEC T80.90
perineal repair (obstetrical) NEC O90.89
  disruption O90.1
  hematoma O90.2
  infection (following delivery) O86.0
phototherapy T88.9
  specified NEC T88.8
postmastoidectomy NEC H95.19-
  cyst, mucosal H95.13-
  granulation H95.12-
  inflammation, chronic H95.11-
  recurrent cholesteatoma H95.0-
postoperative — *see* Complications,
  postprocedural
  circulatory — *see* Complications, circulatory
    system
  ear — *see* Complications, ear
  endocrine — *see* Complications, endocrine
  eye — *see* Complications, eye
  lumbar puncture G97.1
    cerebrospinal fluid leak G97.0
  nervous system (central) (peripheral) — *see*
    Complications, nervous system
  respiratory system — *see* Complications,
    respiratory system
postprocedural — *see also* Complications,
  surgical procedure
  cardiac arrest
    following cardiac surgery I97.120
    following other surgery I97.121
  cardiac functional disturbance NEC
    following cardiac surgery I97.190
    following other surgery I97.191

Complication(s) (from) (of) — *continued*
postprocedural — *see also* Complications,
  surgical procedure — *continued*
  cardiac insufficiency
    following cardiac surgery I97.110
    following other surgery I97.111
  chorioretinal scars following retinal surgery
    H59.81-
  following cataract surgery
    cataract (lens) fragments H59.02-
    cystoid macular edema H59.03-
    specified NEC H59.09-
    vitreous (touch) syndrome H59.01-
  heart failure
    following cardiac surgery I97.130
    following other surgery I97.131
  hematoma (of)
    circulatory system organ or structure
      following cardiac bypass I97.631
      following cardiac catheterization
        I97.630
      following other circulatory system
        procedure I97.638
      following other procedure I97.621
    digestive system
      following procedure on digestive system
        K91.870
      following procedure on other organ
        K91.871
    ear
      following other procedure H95.52
      following procedure on ear and mastoid
        process H95.51
    endocrine system
      following endocrine system procedure
        E89.820
      following other procedure E89.821
    eye and adnexa
      following ophthalmic procedure
        H59.33-
      following other procedure H59.34-
    genitourinary organ or structure
      following procedure on genitourinary
        organ or structure N99.840
      following procedure on other organ
        N99.841
    mastoid process
      following other procedure H95.52
      following procedure on ear and mastoid
        process H95.51
    musculoskeletal structure
      following musculoskeletal surgery
        M96.840
      following non-orthopedic surgery
        M96.841
      following orthopedic surgery M96.840
    nervous system
      following nervous system procedure
        G97.61
      following other procedure G97.62
    respiratory system
      following other procedure J95.861
      following procedure on respiratory
        system organ or structure J95.860
    skin and subcutaneous tissue
      following dermatologic procedure
        L76.31
      following procedure on other organ
        L76.32
    spleen
      following procedure on other organ
        D78.32
      following procedure on the spleen
        D78.31

Complication(s) (from) (of) — *continued*
postprocedural — *see also* Complications,
　surgical procedure — *continued*
　hemorrhage (of)
　　circulatory system organ or structure
　　　following cardiac bypass I97.611
　　　following cardiac catheterization
　　　　I97.610
　　　following other circulatory system
　　　　procedure I97.618
　　　following other procedure I97.620
　　digestive system
　　　following procedure on digestive system
　　　　K91.840
　　　following procedure on other organ
　　　　K91.841
　　ear
　　　following other procedure H95.42
　　　following procedure on ear and mastoid
　　　　process H95.41
　　endocrine system
　　　following endocrine system procedure
　　　　E89.810
　　　following other procedure E89.811
　　eye and adnexa
　　　following ophthalmic procedure
　　　　H59.31-
　　　following other procedure H59.32-
　　genitourinary organ or structure
　　　following procedure on genitourinary
　　　　organ or structure N99.820
　　　following procedure on other organ
　　　　N99.821
　　mastoid process
　　　following other procedure H95.42
　　　following procedure on ear and mastoid
　　　　process H95.41
　　musculoskeletal structure
　　　following musculoskeletal surgery
　　　　M96.830
　　　following non-orthopedic surgery
　　　　M96.831
　　　following orthopedic surgery M96.830
　　nervous system
　　　following nervous system procedure
　　　　G97.51
　　　following other procedure G97.52
　　respiratory system
　　　following other procedure J95.831
　　　following procedure on respiratory
　　　　system organ or structure J95.830
　　skin and subcutaneous tissue
　　　following dermatologic procedure
　　　　L76.21
　　　following a procedure on other organ
　　　　L76.22
　　spleen
　　　following procedure on other organ
　　　　D78.22
　　　following procedure on the spleen
　　　　D78.21
　seroma (of)
　　circulatory system organ or structure
　　　following cardiac bypass I97.641
　　　following cardiac catheterization
　　　　I97.640
　　　following other circulatory system
　　　　procedure I97.648
　　　following other procedure I97.622
　　digestive system
　　　following procedure on digestive system
　　　　K91.872
　　　following procedure on other organ
　　　　K91.873
　　ear
　　　following other procedure H95.54
　　　following procedure on ear and mastoid
　　　　process H95.53

Complication(s) (from) (of) — *continued*
postprocedural (*see also* Complications, surgical
　procedure) — *continued*
　seroma (of) — *continued*
　　endocrine system
　　　following endocrine system procedure
　　　　E89.822
　　　following other procedure E89.823
　　eye and adnexa
　　　following ophthalmic procedure
　　　　H59.35-
　　　following other procedure H59.36-
　　genitourinary organ or structure
　　　following procedure on genitourinary
　　　　organ or structure N99.842
　　　following procedure on other organ
　　　　N99.843
　　mastoid process
　　　following other procedure H95.54
　　　following procedure on ear and mastoid
　　　　process H95.53
　　musculoskeletal structure
　　　following musculoskeletal surgery
　　　　M96.842
　　　following non-orthopedic surgery
　　　　M96.843
　　　following orthopedic surgery M96.842
　　nervous system
　　　following nervous system procedure
　　　　G97.63
　　　following other procedure G97.64
　　respiratory system
　　　following other procedure J95.863
　　　following procedure on respiratory
　　　　system organ or structure J95.862
　　skin and subcutaneous tissue
　　　following dermatologic procedure
　　　　L76.33
　　　following procedure on other organ
　　　　L76.34
　　spleen
　　　following procedure on other organ
　　　　D78.34
　　　following procedure on the spleen
　　　　D78.33
　specified NEC
　　circulatory system I97.89
　　digestive K91.89
　　ear H95.89
　　endocrine E89.89
　　eye and adnexa H59.89
　　genitourinary N99.89
　　mastoid process H95.89
　　metabolic E89.89
　　musculoskeletal structure M96.89
　　nervous system G97.82
　　respiratory system J95.89
　　skin and subcutaneous tissue L76.82
　　spleen D78.89
pregnancy NEC — *see* Pregnancy, complicated
　by
prosthetic device or implant T85.9
　bile duct — *see* Complications, bile duct
　　implant
　breast — *see* Complications, breast implant
　bulking agent
　　ureteral
　　　erosion T83.714
　　　exposure T83.724
　　urethral
　　　erosion T83.713
　　　exposure T83.723
　cardiac and vascular NEC — *see*
　　Complications, cardiovascular device or
　　implant
　corneal transplant — *see* Complications,
　　graft, cornea

Complication(s) (from) (of) — *continued*
prosthetic device or implant T85.9 —
　continued
　electronic nervous system stimulator — *see*
　　Complications, electronic stimulator
　　device
　epidural infusion catheter — *see*
　　Complications, catheter, epidural
　esophageal anti-reflux device — *see*
　　Complications, esophageal anti-reflux
　　device
　genital organ or tract — *see* Complications,
　　genitourinary, device or implant, genital
　　tract
　specified NEC T83.79
　heart valve — *see* Complications, heart,
　　valve, prosthesis
　infection or inflammation T85.79
　　intestine transplant T86.892
　　liver transplant T86.43
　　lung transplant T86.812
　　pancreas transplant T86.892
　　skin graft T86.822
　intraocular lens — *see* Complications,
　　intraocular lens
　intraperitoneal (dialysis) catheter — *see*
　　Complications, catheter, intraperitoneal
　joint — *see* Complications, joint prosthesis,
　　internal
　mechanical NEC T85.698
　　dialysis catheter (vascular) — *see also*
　　　Complication, catheter, dialysis,
　　　mechanical
　　　peritoneal — *see* Complication, catheter,
　　　　intraperitoneal, mechanical
　　gastrointestinal device T85.598
　　ocular device T85.398
　　subdural (infusion) catheter T85.690
　　suture, permanent T85.692
　　　that for bone repair — *see*
　　　　Complications, fixation device,
　　　　internal (orthopedic), mechanical
　　ventricular shunt
　　　breakdown T85.01
　　　displacement T85.02
　　　leakage T85.03
　　　malposition T85.02
　　　obstruction T85.09
　　　perforation T85.09
　　　protrusion T85.09
　　　specified NEC T85.09
　mesh
　　erosion (to surrounding organ or tissue)
　　　T83.717
　　　urethral (into pelvic floor muscles)
　　　　T83.712
　　　vaginal (into pelvic floor muscles)
　　　　T83.711
　　exposure (into surrounding organ or
　　　tissue) T83.727
　　　urethral (through urethral wall) T83.722
　　　vaginal (into vagina) (through vaginal
　　　　wall) T83.721
　orbital — *see* Complications, orbital
　　prosthesis
　penile T83.9
　　embolism T83.81
　　fibrosis T83.82
　　hemorrhage T83.83
　　infection and inflammation T83.61
　　mechanical
　　　breakdown T83.410
　　　displacement T83.420
　　　leakage T83.490
　　　malposition T83.420
　　　obstruction T83.490
　　　perforation T83.490
　　　protrusion T83.490
　　　specified NEC T83.490

DISEASE INDEX

Complication(s) (from) (of) — *continued*
prosthetic device or implant T85.9 — *continued*
  penile T83.9 — *continued*
    pain T83.84
    specified type NEC T83.89
    stenosis T83.85
    thrombosis T83.86
  prosthetic materials NEC
    erosion (to surrounding organ or tissue) T83.718
    exposure (into surrounding organ or tissue) T83.728
  skin graft T86.829
    artificial skin or decellularized allodermis
      embolism T85.818
      fibrosis T85.828
      hemorrhage T85.838
      infection and inflammation T85.79
      mechanical
        breakdown T85.613
        displacement T85.623
        malfunction T85.613
        malposition T85.623
        obstruction T85.693
        perforation T85.693
        protrusion T85.693
        specified NEC T85.693
      pain T85.848
      specified type NEC T85.898
      stenosis T85.858
      thrombosis T85.868
    failure T86.821
    infection T86.822
    rejection T86.820
    specified NEC T86.828
  sling
    urethral (female) (male)
      erosion T83.712
      exposure T83.722
  specified NEC T85.9
    embolism T85.818
    fibrosis T85.828
    hemorrhage T85.838
    infection and inflammation T85.79
    mechanical
      breakdown T85.618
      displacement T85.628
      leakage T85.638
      malfunction T85.618
      malposition T85.628
      obstruction T85.698
      perforation T85.698
      protrusion T85.698
      specified NEC T85.698
    pain T85.848
    specified type NEC T85.898
    stenosis T85.858
    thrombosis T85.868
  subdural infusion catheter — *see* Complications, catheter, subdural
  sutures — *see* Complications, sutures
  urinary organ or tract NEC — *see* Complications, genitourinary, device or implant, urinary system
  vascular — *see* Complications, cardiovascular device or implant
  ventricular shunt — *see* Complications, ventricular shunt (device)
puerperium — *see* Puerperal
puncture, spinal G97.1
  cerebrospinal fluid leak G97.0
  headache or reaction G97.1
pyelogram N99.89
radiation
  kyphosis M96.2
  scoliosis M96.5

Complication(s) (from) (of) — *continued*
reattached
  extremity (infection) (rejection)
    lower T87.1x-
    upper T87.0x-
  specified body part NEC T87.2
reconstructed breast
  asymmetry between native and reconstructed breast N65.1
  deformity N65.0
  disproportion between native and reconstructed breast N65.1
  excess tissue N65.0
  misshappen N65.0
reimplant NEC — *see also* Complications, prosthetic device or implant
  limb (infection) (rejection) — *see* Complications, reattached, extremity
  organ (partial) (total) — *see* Complications, transplant
  prosthetic device NEC — *see* Complications, prosthetic device
renal N28.9
  allograft — *see* Complications, transplant, kidney
  dialysis — *see* Complications, dialysis
respirator
  mechanical J95.850
    specified NEC J95.859
respiratory system J98.9
  device, implant or graft — *see* Complication, prosthetic device or implant, specified NEC
  lung transplant — *see* Complications, prosthetic device or implant, lung transplant
  postoperative J95.89
    air leak J95.812
    Mendelson's syndrome (chemical pneumonitis) J95.4
    pneumothorax J95.811
    pulmonary insufficiency (acute) (after nonthoracic surgery) J95.2
      chronic J95.3
      following thoracic surgery J95.1
    respiratory failure (acute) J95.821
      acute and chronic J95.822
    specified NEC J95.89
    subglottic stenosis J95.5
    tracheostomy complication — *see* Complications, tracheostomy
  therapy T81.89
sedation during labor and delivery O74.9
  cardiac O74.2
  central nervous system O74.3
  pulmonary NEC O74.1
shunt — *see also* Complications, prosthetic device or implant
  arteriovenous — *see* Complications, arteriovenous, shunt
  ventricular (communicating) — *see* Complications, ventricular shunt
skin
  graft T86.829
    failure T86.821
    infection T86.822
    rejection T86.820
    specified type NEC T86.828
spinal
  anesthesia — *see* Complications, anesthesia, spinal
  catheter (epidural) (subdural) — *see* Complications, catheter
  puncture or tap G97.1
    cerebrospinal fluid leak G97.0
    headache or reaction G97.1

Complication(s) (from) (of) — *continued*
stent
  bile duct — *see* Complications, bile duct prosthesis
  ureteral indwelling
    breakdown T83.112
    displacement T83.122
    leakage T83.192
    malposition T83.122
    obstruction T83.192
    perforation T83.192
    protrusion T83.192
    specified NEC T83.192
  urinary NEC (ileal conduit) (nephroureteral) T83.193
    embolism T83.81
    fibrosis T83.82
    hemorrhage T83.83
    infection and inflammation T83.593
    mechanical
      breakdown T83.113
      displacement T83.123
      leakage T83.193
      malposition T83.123
      obstruction T83.193
      perforation T83.193
      protrusion T83.193
      specified NEC T83.193
    pain T83.84
    specified type NEC T83.89
    stenosis T83.85
    thrombosis T83.86
  vascular
    end stent stenosis — *see* Restenosis, stent
    in stent stenosis — *see* Restenosis, stent
stoma
  digestive tract
    colostomy — *see* Complications, colostomy
    enterostomy — *see* Complications, enterostomy
    esophagostomy — *see* Complications, esophagostomy
    gastrostomy — *see* Complications, gastrostomy
  urinary tract N99.528
    continent N99.538
      hemorrhage N99.530
      herniation N99.533
      infection N99.531
      malfunction N99.532
      specified type NEC N99.538
      stenosis N99.534
    cystostomy — *see* Complications, cystostomy
    external NOS N99.528
    hemorrhage N99.520
    herniation N99.523
    incontinent N99.528
      hemorrhage N99.520
      herniation N99.523
      infection N99.521
      malfunction N99.522
      specified type NEC N99.528
      stenosis N99.524
    infection N99.521
    malfunction N99.522
    specified type NEC N99.528
    stenosis N99.524
stomach banding — *see* Complication(s), bariatric procedure
stomach stapling — *see* Complication(s), bariatric procedure
surgical material, nonabsorbable — *see* Complication, suture, permanent
surgical procedure (on) T81.9
  amputation stump (late) — *see* Complications, amputation stump
  cardiac — *see* Complications, circulatory system

Complication(s) (from) (of) — *continued*
  surgical procedure (on) T81.9 — *continued*
    cholesteatoma, recurrent — *see* Complications, postmastoidectomy, recurrent cholesteatoma
    circulatory (early) — *see* Complications, circulatory system
    digestive system — *see* Complications, gastrointestinal
    dumping syndrome (postgastrectomy) K91.1
    ear — *see* Complications, ear
    elephantiasis or lymphedema I97.89
      postmastectomy I97.2
    emphysema (surgical) T81.82
    endocrine — *see* Complications, endocrine
    eye — *see* Complications, eye
    fistula (persistent postoperative) T81.83
    foreign body inadvertently left in wound (sponge) (suture) (swab) — *see* Foreign body, accidentally left during a procedure
    gastrointestinal — *see* Complications, gastrointestinal
    genitourinary NEC N99.89
    hematoma
      intraoperative — *see* Complication, intraoperative, hemorrhage
      postprocedural — *see* Complication, postprocedural, hematoma
    hemorrhage
      intraoperative — *see* Complication, intraoperative, hemorrhage
      postprocedural — *see* Complication, postprocedural, hemorrhage
    hepatic failure K91.82
    hyperglycemia (postpancreatectomy) E89.1
    hypoinsulinemia (postpancreatectomy) E89.1
    hypoparathyroidism (postparathyroidectomy) E89.2
    hypopituitarism (posthypophysectomy) E89.3
    hypothyroidism (post-thyroidectomy) E89.0
    intestinal obstruction K91.3
    intracranial hypotension following ventricular shunting (ventriculostomy) G97.2
    lymphedema I97.89
      postmastectomy I97.2
    malabsorption (postsurgical) NEC K91.2
      osteoporosis — *see* Osteoporosis, postsurgical malabsorption
    mastoidectomy cavity NEC — *see* Complications, postmastoidectomy
    metabolic E89.89
      specified NEC E89.89
    musculoskeletal — *see* Complications, musculoskeletal system
    nervous system (central) (peripheral) — *see* Complications, nervous system
    ovarian failure E89.40
      asymptomatic E89.40
      symptomatic E89.41
    peripheral vascular — *see* Complications, surgical procedure, vascular
    postcardiotomy syndrome I97.0
    postcholecystectomy syndrome K91.5
    postcommissurotomy syndrome I97.0
    postgastrectomy dumping syndrome K91.1
    postlaminectomy syndrome NEC M96.1
      kyphosis M96.3
    postmastectomy lymphedema syndrome I97.2
    postmastoidectomy cholesteatoma — *see* Complications, postmastoidectomy, recurrent cholesteatoma
    postvagotomy syndrome K91.1
    postvalvulotomy syndrome I97.0

Complication(s) (from) (of) — *continued*
  surgical procedure (on) T81.9 — *continued*
    pulmonary insufficiency (acute) J95.2
      chronic J95.3
      following thoracic surgery J95.1
    reattached body part — *see* Complications, reattached
    respiratory — *see* Complications, respiratory system
    shock (hypovolemic) T81.19
    spleen (postoperative) D78.89
      intraoperative D78.81
    stitch abscess T81.48
    subglottic stenosis (postsurgical) J95.5
    testicular hypofunction E89.5
    transplant — *see* Complications, organ or tissue transplant
    urinary NEC N99.89
    vaginal vault prolapse (posthysterectomy) N99.3
    vascular (peripheral)
      artery T81.719
        mesenteric T81.710
        renal T81.711
        specified NEC T81.718
      vein T81.72
    wound infection T81.40
  suture, permanent (wire) NEC T85.9
    with repair of bone — *see* Complications, fixation device, internal
    embolism T85.818
    fibrosis T85.828
    hemorrhage T85.838
    infection and inflammation T85.79
    mechanical
      breakdown T85.612
      displacement T85.622
      malfunction T85.612
      malposition T85.622
      obstruction T85.692
      perforation T85.692
      protrusion T85.692
      specified NEC T85.692
    pain T85.848
    specified type NEC T85.898
    stenosis T85.858
    thrombosis T85.868
  tracheostomy J95.00
    granuloma J95.09
    hemorrhage J95.01
    infection J95.02
    malfunction J95.03
    mechanical J95.03
    obstruction J95.03
    specified type NEC J95.09
    tracheo-esophageal fistula J95.04
  transfusion (blood) (lymphocytes) (plasma) T80.92
    air embolism T80.0
    circulatory overload E87.71
    febrile nonhemolytic transfusion reaction R50.84
    hemochromatosis E83.111
    hemolysis T80.89
    hemolytic reaction (antigen unspecified) T80.919
    incompatibility reaction (antigen unspecified) T80.919
      ABO T80.30
        delayed serologic (DSTR) T80.39
        hemolytic transfusion reaction (HTR) (unspecified time after transfusion) T80.319
          acute (AHTR) (less than 24 hours after transfusion) T80.310
          delayed (DHTR) (24 hours or more after transfusion) T80.311
        specified NEC T80.39

Complication(s) (from) (of) — *continued*
  transfusion (blood) (lymphocytes) (plasma) T80.92 — *continued*
    incompatibility reaction (antigen unspecified) T80.919 — *continued*
      acute (antigen unspecified) T80.910
      delayed (antigen unspecified) T80.911
      delayed serologic (DSTR) T80.89
      Non-ABO (minor antigens (Duffy) (Kell) (Kidd) (Lewis) (M) (N) (P) (S)) T80.A0
        delayed serologic (DSTR) T80.A9
        hemolytic transfusion reaction (HTR) (unspecified time after transfusion) T80.A19
          acute (AHTR) (less than 24 hours after transfusion) T80.A10
          delayed (DHTR) (24 hours or more after transfusion) T80.A11
        specified NEC T80.A9
      Rh (antigens (C) (c) (D) (E) (e)) (factor) T80.40
        delayed serologic (DSTR) T80.49
        hemolytic transfusion reaction (HTR) (unspecified time after transfusion) T80.419
          acute (AHTR) (less than 24 hours after transfusion) T80.410
          delayed (DHTR) (24 hours or more after transfusion) T80.411
        specified NEC T80.49
    infection T80.29
      acute T80.22
    reaction NEC T80.89
    sepsis T80.29
    shock T80.89
  transplant T86.90
    bone T86.839
      failure T86.831
      infection T86.832
      rejection T86.830
      specified type NEC T86.838
    bone marrow T86.00
      failure T86.02
      infection T86.03
      rejection T86.01
      specified type NEC T86.09
    cornea T86.849
      failure T86.841
      infection T86.842
      rejection T86.840
      specified type NEC T86.848
    failure T86.92
    heart T86.20
      with lung T86.30
      cardiac allograft vasculopathy T86.290
        failure T86.32
        infection T86.33
        rejection T86.31
        specified type NEC T86.39
      failure T86.22
      infection T86.23
      rejection T86.21
      specified type NEC T86.298
    infection T86.93
    intestine T86.859
      failure T86.851
      infection T86.852
      rejection T86.850
      specified type NEC T86.858
    kidney T86.10
      failure T86.12
      infection T86.13
      rejection T86.11
      specified type NEC T86.19
    liver T86.40
      failure T86.42
      infection T86.43
      rejection T86.41
      specified type NEC T86.49

Complication(s) (from) (of) — *continued*
  transplant T86.90 — *continued*
    lung T86.819
      with heart T86.30
        failure T86.32
        infection T86.33
        rejection T86.31
        specified type NEC T86.39
      failure T86.811
      infection T86.812
      rejection T86.810
      specified type NEC T86.818
    malignant neoplasm C80.2
    pancreas T86.899
      failure T86.891
      infection T86.892
      rejection T86.890
      specified type NEC T86.898
    peripheral blood stem cells T86.5
    post-transplant lymphoproliferative disorder (PTLD) D47.Z1
    rejection T86.91
    skin T86.829
      failure T86.821
      infection T86.822
      rejection T86.820
      specified type NEC T86.828
    specified
      tissue T86.899
        failure T86.891
        infection T86.892
        rejection T86.890
        specified type NEC T86.898
      type NEC T86.99
    stem cell (from peripheral blood) (from umbilical cord) T86.5
    umbilical cord stem cells T86.5
  trauma (early) T79.9
    specified NEC T79.8
  ultrasound therapy NEC T88.9
  umbilical cord NEC
    complicating delivery O69.9
      specified NEC O69.89
  umbrella device, vascular T82.9
    embolism T82.818
    fibrosis T82.828
    hemorrhage T82.838
    infection or inflammation T82.7
    mechanical
      breakdown T82.515
      displacement T82.525
      leakage T82.535
      malposition T82.525
      obstruction T82.595
      perforation T82.595
      protrusion T82.595
    pain T82.848
    specified type NEC T82.898
    stenosis T82.858
    thrombosis T82.868
  urethral catheter — *see* Complications, catheter, urethral, indwelling
  vaccination T88.1
    anaphylaxis NEC T80.52
    arthropathy — *see* Arthropathy, postimmunization
    cellulitis T88.0
    encephalitis or encephalomyelitis G04.02
    infection (general) (local) NEC T88.0
    meningitis G03.8
    myelitis G04.02
    protein sickness T80.62
    rash T88.1
    reaction (allergic) T88.1
      serum T80.62
    sepsis T88.0

Complication(s) (from) (of) — *continued*
  vaccination T88.1 — *continued*
    serum intoxication, sickness, rash, or other serum reaction NEC T80.62
    anaphylactic shock T80.52
    shock (allergic) (anaphylactic) T80.52
    vaccinia (generalized) (localized) T88.1
  vas deferens device or implant — *see* Complications, genitourinary, device or implant, genital tract
  vascular I99.9
    device or implant T82.9
      embolism T82.818
      fibrosis T82.828
      hemorrhage T82.838
      infection or inflammation T82.7
      mechanical
        breakdown T82.519
          specified device NEC T82.518
        displacement T82.529
          specified device NEC T82.528
        leakage T82.539
          specified device NEC T82.538
        malposition T82.529
          specified device NEC T82.528
        obstruction T82.599
          specified device NEC T82.598
        perforation T82.599
          specified device NEC T82.598
        protrusion T82.599
          specified device NEC T82.598
      pain T82.848
      specified type NEC T82.898
      stenosis T82.858
      thrombosis T82.868
  dialysis catheter — *see* Complication, catheter, dialysis
  following infusion, therapeutic injection or transfusion T80.1
  graft T82.9
    embolism T82.818
    fibrosis T82.828
    hemorrhage T82.838
    mechanical
      breakdown T82.319
        aorta (bifurcation) T82.310
        carotid artery T82.311
        specified vessel NEC T82.318
      displacement T82.329
        aorta (bifurcation) T82.320
        carotid artery T82.321
        specified vessel NEC T82.328
      leakage T82.339
        aorta (bifurcation) T82.330
        carotid artery T82.331
        specified vessel NEC T82.338
      malposition T82.329
        aorta (bifurcation) T82.320
        carotid artery T82.321
        specified vessel NEC T82.328
      obstruction T82.399
        aorta (bifurcation) T82.390
        carotid artery T82.391
        specified vessel NEC T82.398
      perforation T82.399
        aorta (bifurcation) T82.390
        carotid artery T82.391
        specified vessel NEC T82.398
      protrusion T82.399
        aorta (bifurcation) T82.390
        carotid artery T82.391
        specified vessel NEC T82.398
    pain T82.848
    specified complication NEC T82.898
    stenosis T82.858
    thrombosis T82.868
  postoperative — *see* Complications, postoperative, circulatory

Complication(s) (from) (of) — *continued*
  vena cava device (filter) (sieve) (umbrella) — *see* Complications, umbrella device, vascular
  ventilation therapy NEC T81.81
  ventilator
    mechanical J95.850
      specified NEC J95.859
  ventricular (communicating) shunt (device) T85.9
    embolism T85.810
    fibrosis T85.820
    hemorrhage T85.830
    infection and inflammation T85.730
    mechanical
      breakdown T85.01
      displacement T85.02
      leakage T85.03
      malposition T85.02
      obstruction T85.09
      perforation T85.09
      protrusion T85.09
      specified NEC T85.09
    pain T85.840
    specified type NEC T85.890
    stenosis T85.850
    thrombosis T85.860
  wire suture, permanent (implanted) — *see* Complications, suture, permanent

Compressed air disease T70.3
Compression
  with injury — *code by* nature of injury
  artery I77.1
    celiac, syndrome I77.4
  brachial plexus G54.0
  brain (stem) G93.5
    due to
      contusion (diffuse) — *see* Injury, intracranial, diffuse
        focal — *see* Injury, intracranial, focal
      injury NEC — *see* Injury, intracranial, diffuse
      traumatic — *see* Injury, intracranial, diffuse
  bronchus J98.09
  cauda equina G83.4
  celiac (artery) (axis) I77.4
  cerebral — *see* Compression, brain
  cervical plexus G54.2
  cord
    spinal — *see* Compression, spinal
    umbilical — *see* Compression, umbilical cord
  cranial nerve G52.9
    eighth — *see* subcategory H93.3
    eleventh G52.8
    fifth G50.8
    first G52.0
    fourth — *see* Strabismus, paralytic, fourth nerve
    ninth G52.1
    second — *see* Disorder, nerve, optic
    seventh G52.8
    sixth — *see* Strabismus, paralytic, sixth nerve
    tenth G52.2
    third — *see* Strabismus, paralytic, third nerve
    twelfth G52.3
  diver's squeeze T70.3
  during birth (newborn) P15.9
  esophagus K22.2
  eustachian tube — *see* Obstruction, eustachian tube, cartilaginous
  facies Q67.1
  fracture
    nontraumatic NOS — *see* Collapse, vertebra
    pathological — *see* Fracture, pathological
    traumatic — *see* Fracture, traumatic
  heart — *see* Disease, heart
  intestine — *see* Obstruction, intestine

DISEASE INDEX

Compression — *continued*
  laryngeal nerve, recurrent G52.2
    with paralysis of vocal cords and larynx J38.00
      bilateral J38.02
      unilateral J38.01
  lumbosacral plexus G54.1
  lung J98.4
  lymphatic vessel I89.0
  medulla — *see* Compression, brain
  nerve (*see also* Disorder, nerve) G58.9
    arm NEC — *see* Mononeuropathy, upper limb
    axillary G54.0
    cranial — *see* Compression, cranial nerve
    leg NEC — *see* Mononeuropathy, lower limb
    median (in carpal tunnel) — *see* Syndrome, carpal tunnel
    optic — *see* Disorder, nerve, optic
    plantar — *see* Lesion, nerve, plantar
    posterior tibial (in tarsal tunnel) — *see* Syndrome, tarsal tunnel
    root or plexus NOS (in) G54.9
      intervertebral disc disorder NEC — *see* Disorder, disc, with, radiculopathy
      with myelopathy — *see* Disorder, disc, with, myelopathy
      neoplastic disease (*see also* Neoplasm) D49.9 [G55]
      spondylosis — *see* Spondylosis, with radiculopathy
    sciatic (acute) — *see* Lesion, nerve, sciatic
    sympathetic G90.8
    traumatic — *see* Injury, nerve
    ulnar — *see* Lesion, nerve, ulnar
    upper extremity NEC — *see* Mononeuropathy, upper limb
  spinal (cord) G95.20
    by displacement of intervertebral disc NEC — *see also* Disorder, disc, with, myelopathy
    nerve root NOS G54.9
      due to displacement of intervertebral disc NEC — *see* Disorder, disc, with, radiculopathy
      with myelopathy — *see* Disorder, disc, with, myelopathy
    specified NEC G95.29
    spondylogenic (cervical) (lumbar, lumbosacral) (thoracic) — *see* Spondylosis, with myelopathy NEC
      anterior — *see* Syndrome, anterior, spinal artery, compression
    traumatic — *see* Injury, spinal cord, by region
  subcostal nerve (syndrome) — *see* Mononeuropathy, upper limb, specified NEC
  sympathetic nerve NEC G90.8
  syndrome T79.5
  trachea J39.8
  ulnar nerve (by scar tissue) — *see* Lesion, nerve, ulnar
  umbilical cord
    complicating delivery O69.2
      cord around neck O69.1
      prolapse O69.0
      specified NEC O69.2
  ureter N13.5
  vein I87.1
  vena cava (inferior) (superior) I87.1
Compulsion, compulsive
  gambling F63.0
  neurosis F42.8
  personality F60.5
  states F42.8
  swearing F42.8
    in Gilles de la Tourette's syndrome F95.2
  tics and spasms F95.9

Concato's disease (pericardial polyserositis) A19.9
  nontubercular I31.1
  pleural — *see* Pleurisy, with effusion
Concavity chest wall M95.4
Concealed penis Q55.69
Concern (normal) about sick person in family Z63.6
Concrescence (teeth) K00.2
Concretio cordis I31.1
  rheumatic I09.2
Concretion — *see also* Calculus
  appendicular K38.1
  canaliculus — *see* Dacryolith
  clitoris N90.89
  conjunctiva H11.12-
  eyelid — *see* Disorder, eyelid, specified type NEC
  lacrimal passages — *see* Dacryolith
  prepuce (male) N47.8
  salivary gland (any) K11.5
  seminal vesicle N50.89
  tonsil J35.8
Concussion (brain) (cerebral) (current) S06.0x9
  with
    loss of consciousness of 30 minutes or less S06.0x1
    loss of consciousness of unspecified duration S06.0x9
  blast (air) (hydraulic) (immersion) (underwater)
    abdomen or thorax — *see* Injury, blast, by site
    ear with acoustic nerve injury — *see* Injury, nerve, acoustic, specified type NEC
  cauda equina S34.3
  conus medullaris S34.02
  ocular S05.8x-
  spinal (cord)
    cervical S14.0
    lumbar S34.01
    sacral S34.02
    thoracic S24.0
  syndrome F07.81
  without loss of consciousness S06.0x0
Condition — *see* Disease
Conditions arising in the perinatal period — *see* Newborn, affected by
Conduct disorder — *see* Disorder, conduct
Condyloma A63.0
  acuminatum A63.0
  gonorrheal A54.09
  latum A51.31
  syphilitic A51.31
    congenital A50.07
  venereal, syphilitic A51.31
Conflagration — *see also* Burn
  asphyxia (by inhalation of gases, fumes or vapors) (*see also* Table of Drugs and Chemicals) T59.9-
Conflict (with) — *see also* Discord
  family Z73.9
  marital Z63.0
    involving divorce or estrangement Z63.5
  parent-child Z62.820
    parent-adopted child Z62.821
    parent-biological child Z62.820
    parent-foster child Z62.822
  social role NEC Z73.5
Confluent — *see* condition
Confusion, confused R41.0
  epileptic F05
  mental state (psychogenic) F44.89
  psychogenic F44.89
  reactive (from emotional stress, psychological trauma) F44.89
Confusional arousals G47.51
Congelation T69.9

Congenital — *see also* condition
  aortic septum Q25.49
  intrinsic factor deficiency D51.0
  malformation — *see* Anomaly
Congestion, congestive
  bladder N32.89
  bowel K63.89
  brain G93.89
  breast N64.59
  bronchial J98.09
  catarrhal J31.0
  chest R09.89
  chill, malarial — *see* Malaria
  circulatory NEC I99.8
  duodenum K31.89
  eye — *see* Hyperemia, conjunctiva
  facial, due to birth injury P15.4
  general R68.89
  glottis J37.0
  heart — *see* Failure, heart, congestive
  hepatic K76.1
  hypostatic (lung) — *see* Edema, lung
  intestine K63.89
  kidney N28.89
  labyrinth — *see* subcategory H83.8
  larynx J37.0
  liver K76.1
  lung R09.89
    active or acute — *see* Pneumonia
  malaria, malarial — *see* Malaria
  nasal R09.81
  nose R09.81
  orbit, orbital — *see also* Exophthalmos
    inflammatory (chronic) — *see* Inflammation, orbit
  ovary N83.8
  pancreas K86.89
  pelvic, female N94.89
  pleural J94.8
  prostate (active) N42.1
  pulmonary — *see* Congestion, lung
  renal N28.89
  retina H35.81
  seminal vesicle N50.1
  spinal cord G95.19
  spleen (chronic) D73.2
  stomach K31.89
  trachea — *see* Tracheitis
  urethra N36.8
  uterus N85.8
    with subinvolution N85.3
  venous (passive) I87.8
  viscera R68.89
Congestive — *see* Congestion
Conical
  cervix (hypertrophic elongation) N88.4
  cornea — *see* Keratoconus
  teeth K00.2
Conjoined twins Q89.4
Conjugal maladjustment Z63.0
  involving divorce or estrangement Z63.5
Conjunctiva — *see* condition
Conjunctivitis (staphylococcal) (streptococcal) NOS H10.9
  Acanthamoeba B60.12
  acute H10.3-
    atopic H10.1-
    chemical (*see also* Corrosion, cornea) H10.21-
    mucopurulent H10.2-
      follicular H10.01-
      pseudomembranous H10.22-
    serous except viral H10.23-
    viral — *see* Conjunctivitis, viral
    toxic H10.21-
  adenoviral (acute) (follicular) B30.1
  allergic (acute) — *see* Conjunctivitis, acute, atopic
    chronic H10.45
      vernal H10.44

Conjunctivitis (staphylococcal) (streptococcal) NOS H10.9 — *continued*
- anaphylactic — *see* Conjunctivitis, acute, atopic
- Apollo B30.3
- atopic (acute) — *see* Conjunctivitis, acute, atopic
- blennorrhagic (gonococcal) (neonatorum) A54.31
- Béal's B30.2
- chemical (acute) (*see also* Corrosion, cornea) H10.21-
- chlamydial A74.0
  - due to trachoma A71.1
  - neonatal P39.1
- chronic (nodosa) (petrificans) (phlyctenular) H10.40-
  - allergic H10.45
    - vernal H10.44
  - follicular H10.43-
  - giant papillary H10.41-
  - simple H10.42-
  - vernal H10.44
- coxsackievirus 24 B30.3
- diphtheritic A36.86
- due to
  - dust — *see* Conjunctivitis, acute, atopic
  - filariasis B74.9
  - mucocutaneous leishmaniasis B55.2
- enterovirus type 70 (hemorrhagic) B30.3
- epidemic (viral) B30.9
  - hemorrhagic B30.3
- gonococcal (neonatorum) A54.31
- granular (trachomatous) A71.1
  - sequelae (late effect) B94.0
- hemorrhagic (acute) (epidemic) B30.3
- herpes zoster B02.31
- in (due to)
  - Acanthamoeba B60.12
  - adenovirus (acute) (follicular) B30.1
  - Chlamydia A74.0
  - coxsackievirus 24 B30.3
  - diphtheria A36.86
  - enterovirus type 70 (hemorrhagic) B30.3
  - filariasis B74.9
  - gonococci A54.31
  - herpes (simplex) virus B00.53
    - zoster B02.31
  - infectious disease NEC B99
  - meningococci A39.89
  - mucocutaneous leishmaniasis B55.2
  - rosacea L71.9
  - syphilis (late) A52.71
  - zoster B02.31
- inclusion A74.0
- infantile P39.1
  - gonococcal A54.31
- Koch-Weeks' — *see* Conjunctivitis, acute, mucopurulent
- light — *see* Conjunctivitis, acute, atopic
- ligneous — *see* Blepharoconjunctivitis, ligneous
- meningococcal A39.89
- mucopurulent — *see* Conjunctivitis, acute, mucopurulent
- neonatal P39.1
  - gonococcal A54.31
- Newcastle B30.8
- of Béal B30.2
- parasitic
  - filariasis B74.9
  - mucocutaneous leishmaniasis B55.2
- Parinaud's H10.89
- petrificans H10.89
- rosacea L71.9
- specified NEC H10.89
- swimming-pool B30.1
- trachomatous A71.1
  - acute A71.0
  - sequelae (late effect) B94.0

Conjunctivitis (staphylococcal) (streptococcal) NOS H10.9 — *continued*
- traumatic NEC H10.89
- tuberculous A18.59
- tularemic A21.1
- tularensis A21.1
- viral B30.9
  - due to
    - adenovirus B30.1
    - enterovirus B30.3
  - specified NEC B30.8

Conjunctivochalasis H11.82-
Connective tissue — *see* condition
Conn's syndrome E26.01
Conradi(-Hunermann) disease Q77.3
Consanguinity Z84.3
- counseling Z71.89
Conscious simulation (of illness) Z76.5
Consecutive — *see* condition
Consolidation lung (base) — *see* Pneumonia, lobar
Constipation (atonic) (neurogenic) (simple) (spastic) K59.00
- chronic K59.09
  - idiopathic K59.04
- drug-induced K59.03
- functional K59.04
- outlet dysfunction K59.02
- psychogenic F45.8
- slow transit K59.01
- specified NEC K59.09
Constitutional — *see also* condition
- substandard F60.7
Constitutionally substandard F60.7
Constriction — *see also* Stricture
- auditory canal — *see* Stenosis, external ear canal
- bronchial J98.09
- duodenum K31.5
- esophagus K22.2
- external
  - abdomen, abdominal (wall) S30.841
  - alveolar process S00.542
  - ankle S90.54-
  - antecubital space — *see* Constriction, external, forearm
  - arm (upper) S40.84-
  - auricle — *see* Constriction, external, ear
  - axilla — *see* Constriction, external, arm
  - back, lower S30.840
  - breast S20.14-
  - brow S00.84
  - buttock S30.840
  - calf — *see* Constriction, external, leg
  - canthus — *see* Constriction, external, eyelid
  - cheek S00.84
    - internal S00.542
  - chest wall — *see* Constriction, external, thorax
  - chin S00.84
  - clitoris S30.844
  - costal region — *see* Constriction, external, thorax
  - digit(s)
    - foot — *see* Constriction, external, toe
    - hand — *see* Constriction, external, finger
  - ear S00.44-
  - elbow S50.34-
  - epididymis S30.843
  - epigastric region S30.841
  - esophagus, cervical S10.14
  - eyebrow — *see* Constriction, external, eyelid
  - eyelid S00.24-
  - face S00.84
  - finger(s) S60.44-
    - index S60.44-
    - little S60.44-
    - middle S60.44-
    - ring S60.44-

Constriction (*see also* Stricture) — *continued*
- external — *continued*
  - flank S30.841
  - foot (except toe(s) alone) S90.84-
    - toe — *see* Constriction, external, toe
  - forearm S50.84-
    - elbow only — *see* Constriction, external, elbow
  - forehead S00.84
  - genital organs, external
    - female S30.846
    - male S30.845
  - groin S30.841
  - gum S00.542
  - hand S60.54-
  - head S00.94
    - ear — *see* Constriction, external, ear
    - eyelid — *see* Constriction, external, eyelid
    - lip S00.541
    - nose S00.34
    - oral cavity S00.542
    - scalp S00.04
    - specified site NEC S00.84
  - heel — *see* Constriction, external, foot
  - hip S70.24-
  - inguinal region S30.841
  - interscapular region S20.449
  - jaw S00.84
  - knee S80.24-
  - labium (majus) (minus) S30.844
  - larynx S10.14
  - leg (lower) S80.84-
    - knee — *see* Constriction, external, knee
    - upper — *see* Constriction, external, thigh
  - lip S00.541
  - lower back S30.840
  - lumbar region S30.840
  - malar region S00.84
  - mammary — *see* Constriction, external, breast
  - mastoid region S00.84
  - mouth S00.542
  - nail
    - finger — *see* Constriction, external, finger
    - toe — *see* Constriction, external, toe
  - nasal S00.34
  - neck S10.94
    - specified site NEC S10.84
    - throat S10.14
  - nose S00.34
  - occipital region S00.04
  - oral cavity S00.542
  - orbital region — *see* Constriction, external, eyelid
  - palate S00.542
  - palm — *see* Constriction, external, hand
  - parietal region S00.04
  - pelvis S30.840
  - penis S30.842
  - perineum
    - female S30.844
    - male S30.840
  - periocular area — *see* Constriction, external, eyelid
  - phalanges
    - finger — *see* Constriction, external, finger
    - toe — *see* Constriction, external, toe
  - pharynx S10.14
  - pinna — *see* Constriction, external, ear
  - popliteal space — *see* Constriction, external, knee
  - prepuce S30.842
  - pubic region S30.840
  - pudendum
    - female S30.846
    - male S30.845
  - sacral region S30.840
  - scalp S00.04

DISEASE INDEX

Constriction (see also Stricture) — continued
  external — continued
    scapular region — see Constriction, external, shoulder
    scrotum S30.843
    shin — see Constriction, external, leg
    shoulder S40.24-
    sternal region S20.349
    submaxillary region S00.84
    submental region S00.84
    subungual
      finger(s) — see Constriction, external, finger
      toe(s) — see Constriction, external, toe
    supraclavicular fossa S10.84
    supraorbital S00.84
    temple S00.84
    temporal region S00.84
    testis S30.843
    thigh S70.34-
    thorax, thoracic (wall) S20.94
      back S20.44-
      front S20.34-
    throat S10.14
    thumb S60.34-
    toe(s) (lesser) S90.44-
      great S90.44-
    tongue S00.542
    trachea S10.14
    tunica vaginalis S30.843
    uvula S00.542
    vagina S30.844
    vulva S30.844
    wrist S60.84-
  gallbladder — see Obstruction, gallbladder
  intestine — see Obstruction, intestine
  larynx J38.6
    congenital Q31.8
      specified NEC Q31.8
      subglottic Q31.1
  organ or site, congenital NEC — see Atresia, by site
  prepuce (acquired) (congenital) N47.1
  pylorus (adult hypertrophic) K31.1
    congenital or infantile Q40.0
    newborn Q40.0
  ring dystocia (uterus) O62.4
  spastic — see also Spasm
    ureter N13.5
  ureter N13.5
    with infection N13.6
  urethra — see Stricture, urethra
  visual field (peripheral) (functional) — see Defect, visual field
Constrictive — see condition
Consultation
  medical — see Counseling, medical
  religious Z71.81
  specified reason NEC Z71.89
  spiritual Z71.81
  without complaint or sickness Z71.9
    feared complaint unfounded Z71.1
    specified reason NEC Z71.89
Consumption — see Tuberculosis
Contact (with) — see also Exposure (to)
  acariasis Z20.7
  AIDS virus Z20.6
  air pollution Z77.110
  algae and algae toxins Z77.121
  algae bloom Z77.121
  anthrax Z20.810
  aromatic (hazardous) compounds NEC Z77.028
  aromatic amines Z77.020
  aromatic dyes NOS Z77.028
  arsenic Z77.010
  asbestos Z77.090
  bacterial disease NEC Z20.818
  benzene Z77.021

Contact (with) (see also Exposure (to)) — continued
  blue-green algae bloom Z77.121
  body fluids (potentially hazardous) Z77.21
  brown tide Z77.121
  chemicals (chiefly nonmedicinal) (hazardous) NEC Z77.098
  cholera Z20.09
  chromium compounds Z77.018
  communicable disease Z20.9
    bacterial NEC Z20.818
    specified NEC Z20.89
    viral NEC Z20.828
  cyanobacteria bloom Z77.121
  dyes Z77.098
  Escherichia coli (E. coli) Z20.01
  fiberglass — see Table of Drugs and Chemicals, fiberglass
  German measles Z20.4
  gonorrhea Z20.2
  hazardous metals NEC Z77.018
  hazardous substances NEC Z77.29
  hazards in the physical environment NEC Z77.128
  hazards to health NEC Z77.9
  HIV Z20.6
  HTLV-III/LAV Z20.6
  human immunodeficiency virus (HIV) Z20.6
  infection Z20.9
    specified NEC Z20.89
  infestation (parasitic) NEC Z20.7
  intestinal infectious disease NEC Z20.09
    Escherichia coli (E. coli) Z20.01
  lead Z77.011
  meningococcus Z20.811
  mold (toxic) Z77.120
  nickel dust Z77.018
  noise Z77.122
  parasitic disease Z20.7
  pediculosis Z20.7
  pfiesteria piscicida Z77.121
  poliomyelitis Z20.89
  pollution
    air Z77.110
    environmental NEC Z77.118
    soil Z77.112
    water Z77.111
  polycyclic aromatic hydrocarbons Z77.028
  rabies Z20.3
  radiation, naturally occurring NEC Z77.123
  radon Z77.123
  red tide (Florida) Z77.121
  rubella Z20.4
  sexually-transmitted disease Z20.2
  smallpox (laboratory) Z20.89
  syphilis Z20.2
  tuberculosis Z20.1
  uranium Z77.012
  varicella Z20.820
  venereal disease Z20.2
  viral disease NEC Z20.828
  viral hepatitis Z20.5
  water pollution Z77.111
Contamination, food — see Intoxication, foodborne
Contraception, contraceptive
  advice Z30.09
  counseling Z30.09
  device (intrauterine) (in situ) Z97.5
    causing menorrhagia T83.83
    checking Z30.431
    complications — see Complications, intrauterine, contraceptive device
    in place Z97.5
    initial prescription Z30.014
    reinsertion Z30.433
    removal Z30.432
    replacement Z30.433
  emergency (postcoital) Z30.012

Contraception, contraceptive — continued
  initial prescription Z30.019
    barrier Z30.018
    diaphragm Z30.018
    injectable Z30.013
    intrauterine device Z30.014
    pills Z30.011
    postcoital (emergency) Z30.012
    specified type NEC Z30.018
    subdermal implantable Z30.017
    transdermal patch hormonal Z30.016
    vaginal ring hormonal Z30.015
  maintenance Z30.40
    barrier Z30.49
    diaphragm Z30.49
    examination Z30.8
    injectable Z30.42
    intrauterine device Z30.431
    pills Z30.41
    specified type NEC Z30.49
    subdermal implantable Z30.46
    transdermal patch hormonal Z30.45
    vaginal ring hormonal Z30.44
  management Z30.9
    specified NEC Z30.8
  postcoital (emergency) Z30.012
  prescription Z30.019
    repeat Z30.40
  sterilization Z30.2
  surveillance (drug) — see Contraception, maintenance
Contraction(s), contracture, contracted
  Achilles tendon — see also Short, tendon, Achilles
    congenital Q66.89
  amputation stump (surgical) (flexion) (late) (next proximal joint) T87.89
  anus K59.8
  bile duct (common) (hepatic) K83.8
  bladder N32.89
    neck or sphincter N32.0
  bowel, cecum, colon or intestine, any part — see Obstruction, intestine
  Braxton Hicks — see False, labor
  breast implant, capsular T85.44
  bronchial J98.09
  burn (old) — see Cicatrix
  cervix — see Stricture, cervix
  cicatricial — see Cicatrix
  conjunctiva, trachomatous, active A71.1
    sequelae (late effect) B94.0
  Dupuytren's M72.0
  eyelid — see Disorder, eyelid function
  fascia (lata) (postural) M72.8
    Dupuytren's M72.0
    palmar M72.0
    plantar M72.2
  finger NEC — see also Deformity, finger
    congenital Q68.1
    joint — see Contraction, joint, hand
  flaccid — see Contraction, paralytic
  gallbladder K82.0
  heart valve — see Endocarditis
  hip — see Contraction, joint, hip
  hourglass
    bladder N32.89
      congenital Q64.79
    gallbladder K82.0
      congenital Q44.1
    stomach K31.89
      congenital Q40.2
      psychogenic F45.8
  uterus (complicating delivery) O62.4
  hysterical F44.4
  internal os — see Stricture, cervix

Contraction(s), contracture, contracted — *continued*
- joint (abduction) (acquired) (adduction) (flexion) (rotation) M24.50
  - ankle M24.57-
  - congenital NEC Q68.8
    - hip Q65.89
  - elbow M24.52-
  - foot joint M24.57-
  - hand joint M24.54-
  - hip M24.55-
    - congenital Q65.89
  - hysterical F44.4
  - knee M24.56-
  - shoulder M24.51-
  - wrist M24.53-
- kidney (granular) (secondary) N26.9
  - congenital Q63.8
  - hydronephritic — *see* Hydronephrosis Page N26.2
  - pyelonephritic — *see* Pyelitis, chronic
  - tuberculous A18.11
- ligament — *see also* Disorder, ligament
  - congenital Q79.8
- muscle (postinfective) (postural) NEC M62.40
  - with contracture of joint — *see* Contraction, joint
  - ankle M62.47-
  - congenital Q79.8
    - sternocleidomastoid Q68.0
  - extraocular — *see* Strabismus
  - eye (extrinsic) — *see* Strabismus
  - foot M62.47-
  - forearm M62.43-
  - hand M62.44-
  - hysterical F44.4
  - ischemic (Volkmann's) T79.6
  - lower leg M62.46-
  - multiple sites M62.49
  - pelvic region M62.45-
  - posttraumatic — *see* Strabismus, paralytic
  - psychogenic F45.8
    - conversion reaction F44.4
  - shoulder region M62.41-
  - specified site NEC M62.48
  - thigh M62.45-
  - upper arm M62.42-
- neck — *see* Torticollis
- ocular muscle — *see* Strabismus
- organ or site, congenital NEC — *see* Atresia, by site
- outlet (pelvis) — *see* Contraction, pelvis
- palmar fascia M72.0
- paralytic
  - joint — *see* Contraction, joint
  - muscle — *see also* Contraction, muscle NEC
    - ocular — *see* Strabismus, paralytic
- pelvis (acquired) (general) M95.5
  - with disproportion (fetopelvic) O33.1
    - causing obstructed labor O65.1
  - inlet O33.2
  - mid-cavity O33.3
  - outlet O33.3
- plantar fascia M72.2
- premature
  - atrium I49.1
  - auriculoventricular I49.49
  - heart I49.49
  - junctional I49.2
  - supraventricular I49.1
  - ventricular I49.3
- prostate N42.89
- pylorus NEC — *see also* Pylorospasm
  - psychogenic F45.8
- rectum, rectal (sphincter) K59.8
- ring (Bandl's) (complicating delivery) O62.4
- scar — *see* Cicatrix
- spine — *see* Dorsopathy, deforming

Contraction(s), contracture, contracted — *continued*
- sternocleidomastoid (muscle), congenital Q68.0
- stomach K31.89
  - hourglass K31.89
    - congenital Q40.2
    - psychogenic F45.8
  - psychogenic F45.8
- tendon (sheath) M62.40
  - with contracture of joint — *see* Contraction, joint
  - Achilles — *see* Short, tendon, Achilles
  - ankle M62.47-
    - Achilles — *see* Short, tendon, Achilles
  - foot M62.47-
  - forearm M62.43-
  - hand M62.44-
  - lower leg M62.46-
  - multiple sites M62.49
  - neck M62.48
  - pelvic region M62.45-
  - shoulder region M62.41-
  - specified site NEC M62.48
  - thigh M62.45-
  - thorax M62.48
  - trunk M62.48
  - upper arm M62.42-
- toe — *see* Deformity, toe, specified NEC
- ureterovesical orifice (postinfectional) N13.5
  - with infection N13.6
- urethra — *see also* Stricture, urethra
  - orifice N32.0
- uterus N85.8
  - abnormal NEC O62.9
  - clonic (complicating delivery) O62.4
  - dyscoordinate (complicating delivery) O62.4
  - hourglass (complicating delivery) O62.4
  - hypertonic O62.4
  - hypotonic NEC O62.2
  - inadequate
    - primary O62.0
    - secondary O62.1
  - incoordinate (complicating delivery) O62.4
  - poor O62.2
  - tetanic (complicating delivery) O62.4
- vagina (outlet) N89.5
- vesical N32.89
  - neck or urethral orifice N32.0
- visual field — *see* Defect, visual field, generalized
- Volkmann's (ischemic) T79.6

Contusion (skin surface intact) T14.8
- abdomen, abdominal (muscle) (wall) S30.1
- adnexa, eye NEC S05.8x-
- adrenal gland S37.812
- alveolar process S00.532
- ankle S90.0-
- antecubital space — *see* Contusion, forearm
- anus S30.3
- arm (upper) S40.02-
  - lower (with elbow) — *see* Contusion, forearm
- auditory canal — *see* Contusion, ear
- auricle — *see* Contusion, ear
- axilla — *see* Contusion, arm, upper
- back — *see also* Contusion, thorax, back
  - lower S30.0
- bile duct S36.13
- bladder S37.22
- bone NEC T14.8
- brain (diffuse) — *see* Injury, intracranial, diffuse
  - focal — *see* Injury, intracranial, focal
- brainstem S06.38-
- breast S20.0-
- broad ligament S37.892
- brow S00.83
- buttock S30.0
- canthus, eye S00.1-
- cauda equina S34.3

Contusion (skin surface intact) T14.8 — *continued*
- cerebellar, traumatic S06.37-
- cerebral S06.33-
  - left side S06.32-
  - right side S06.31-
- cheek S00.83
  - internal S00.532
- chest (wall) — *see* Contusion, thorax
- chin S00.83
- clitoris S30.23
- colon — *see* Injury, intestine, large, contusion
- common bile duct S36.13
- conjunctiva S05.1-
  - with foreign body (in conjunctival sac) — *see* Foreign body, conjunctival sac
- conus medullaris (spine) S34.139
- cornea — *see* Contusion, eyeball
  - with foreign body — *see* Foreign body, cornea
- corpus cavernosum S30.21
- cortex (brain) (cerebral) — *see* Injury, intracranial, diffuse
  - focal — *see* Injury, intracranial, focal
- costal region — *see* Contusion, thorax
- cystic duct S36.13
- diaphragm S27.802
- duodenum S36.420
- ear S00.43-
- elbow S50.0-
  - with forearm — *see* Contusion, forearm
- epididymis S30.22
- epigastric region S30.1
- epiglottis S10.0
- esophagus (thoracic) S27.812
  - cervical S10.0
- eyeball S05.1-
- eyebrow S00.1-
- eyelid (and periocular area) S00.1-
- face NEC S00.83
- fallopian tube S37.529
  - bilateral S37.522
  - unilateral S37.521
- femoral triangle S30.1
- finger(s) S60.00
  - with damage to nail (matrix) S60.10
  - index S60.02-
    - with damage to nail S60.12-
  - little S60.05-
    - with damage to nail S60.15-
  - middle S60.03-
    - with damage to nail S60.13-
  - ring S60.04-
    - with damage to nail S60.14-
  - thumb — *see* Contusion, thumb
- flank S30.1
- foot (except toe(s) alone) S90.3-
  - toe — *see* Contusion, toe
- forearm S50.1-
  - elbow only — *see* Contusion, elbow
- forehead S00.83
- gallbladder S36.122
- genital organs, external
  - female S30.202
  - male S30.201
- globe (eye) — *see* Contusion, eyeball
- groin S30.1
- gum S00.532
- hand S60.22-
  - finger(s) — *see* Contusion, finger
  - wrist — *see* Contusion, wrist
- head S00.93
  - ear — *see* Contusion, ear
  - eyelid — *see* Contusion, eyelid
  - lip S00.531
  - nose S00.33
  - oral cavity S00.532
  - scalp S00.03
  - specified part NEC S00.83

Contusion (skin surface intact) T14.8 — *continued*
- heart (*see also* Injury, heart) S26.91
- heel — *see* Contusion, foot
- hepatic duct S36.13
- hip S70.0-
- ileum S36.428
- iliac region S30.1
- inguinal region S30.1
- interscapular region S20.229
- intra-abdominal organ S36.92
  - colon — *see* Injury, intestine, large, contusion
  - liver S36.112
  - pancreas — *see* Contusion, pancreas
  - rectum S36.62
  - small intestine — *see* Injury, intestine, small, contusion
  - specified organ NEC S36.892
  - spleen — *see* Contusion, spleen
  - stomach S36.32
- iris (eye) — *see* Contusion, eyeball
- jaw S00.83
- jejunum S36.428
- kidney S37.01-
  - major (greater than 2 cm) S37.02-
  - minor (less than 2 cm) S37.01-
- knee S80.0-
- labium (majus) (minus) S30.23
- lacrimal apparatus, gland or sac S05.8x-
- larynx S10.0
- leg (lower) S80.1-
  - knee — *see* Contusion, knee
- lens — *see* Contusion, eyeball
- lip S00.531
- liver S36.112
- lower back S30.0
- lumbar region S30.0
- lung S27.329
  - bilateral S27.322
  - unilateral S27.321
- malar region S00.83
- mastoid region S00.83
- membrane, brain — *see* Injury, intracranial, diffuse
  - focal — *see* Injury, intracranial, focal
- mesentery S36.892
- mesosalpinx S37.892
- mouth S00.532
- muscle — *see* Contusion, by site
- nail
  - finger — *see* Contusion, finger, with damage to nail
  - toe — *see* Contusion, toe, with damage to nail
- nasal S00.33
- neck S10.93
  - specified site NEC S10.83
  - throat S10.0
- nerve — *see* Injury, nerve
- newborn P54.5
- nose S00.33
- occipital
  - lobe (brain) — *see* Injury, intracranial, diffuse
    - focal — *see* Injury, intracranial, focal
  - region (scalp) S00.03
- orbit (region) (tissues) S05.1-
- ovary S37.429
  - bilateral S37.422
  - unilateral S37.421
- palate S00.532
- pancreas S36.229
  - body S36.221
  - head S36.220
  - tail S36.222

Contusion (skin surface intact) T14.8 — *continued*
- parietal
  - lobe (brain) — *see* Injury, intracranial, diffuse
    - focal — *see* Injury, intracranial, focal
  - region (scalp) S00.03
- pelvic organ S37.92
  - adrenal gland S37.812
  - bladder S37.22
  - fallopian tube — *see* Contusion, fallopian tube
  - kidney — *see* Contusion, kidney
  - ovary — *see* Contusion, ovary
  - prostate S37.822
  - specified organ NEC S37.892
  - ureter S37.12
  - urethra S37.32
  - uterus S37.62
- pelvis S30.0
- penis S30.21
- perineum
  - female S30.23
  - male S30.0
- periocular area S00.1-
- peritoneum S36.81
- periurethral tissue — *see* Contusion, urethra
- pharynx S10.0
- pinna — *see* Contusion, ear
- popliteal space — *see* Contusion, knee
- prepuce S30.21
- prostate S37.822
- pubic region S30.1
- pudendum
  - female S30.202
  - male S30.201
- quadriceps femoris — *see* Contusion, thigh
- rectum S36.62
- retroperitoneum S36.892
- round ligament S37.892
- sacral region S30.0
- scalp S00.03
  - due to birth injury P12.3
- scapular region — *see* Contusion, shoulder
- sclera — *see* Contusion, eyeball
- scrotum S30.22
- seminal vesicle S37.892
- shoulder S40.01-
- skin NEC T14.8
- small intestine — *see* Injury, intestine, small, contusion
- spermatic cord S30.22
- spinal cord — *see* Injury, spinal cord, by region
  - cauda equina S34.3
  - conus medullaris S34.139
- spleen S36.029
  - major S36.021
  - minor S36.020
- sternal region S20.219
- stomach S36.32
- subconjunctival S05.1-
- subcutaneous NEC T14.8
- submaxillary region S00.83
- submental region S00.83
- subperiosteal NEC T14.8
- subungual
  - finger — *see* Contusion, finger, with damage to nail
  - toe — *see* Contusion, toe, with damage to nail
- supraclavicular fossa S10.83
- supraorbital S00.83
- suprarenal gland S37.812
- temple (region) S00.83
- temporal
  - lobe (brain) — *see* Injury, intracranial, diffuse
    - focal — *see* Injury, intracranial, focal
  - region S00.83

Contusion (skin surface intact) T14.8 — *continued*
- testis S30.22
- thigh S70.1-
- thorax (wall) S20.20
  - back S20.22-
  - front S20.21-
- throat S10.0
- thumb S60.01-
  - with damage to nail S60.11-
- toe(s) (lesser) S90.12-
  - with damage to nail S90.22-
  - great S90.11-
    - with damage to nail S90.21-
    - specified type NEC S90.221
- tongue S00.532
- trachea (cervical) S10.0
  - thoracic S27.52
- tunica vaginalis S30.22
- tympanum, tympanic membrane — *see* Contusion, ear
- ureter S37.12
- urethra S37.32
- urinary organ NEC S37.892
- uterus S37.62
- uvula S00.532
- vagina S30.23
- vas deferens S37.892
- vesical S37.22
- vocal cord(s) S10.0
- vulva S30.23
- wrist S60.21-

Conus (congenital) (any type) Q14.8
- cornea — *see* Keratoconus
- medullaris syndrome G95.81

Conversion hysteria, neurosis or reaction F44.9

Converter, tuberculosis (test reaction) R76.11

Conviction (legal), anxiety concerning Z65.0
- with imprisonment Z65.1

Convulsions (idiopathic) (*see also* Seizure(s)) R56.9
- apoplectiform (cerebral ischemia) I67.82
- dissociative F44.5
- epileptic — *see* Epilepsy
- epileptiform, epileptoid — *see* Seizure, epileptiform
- ether (anesthetic) — *see* Table of Drugs and Chemicals, by drug
- febrile R56.00
  - with status epilepticus G40.901
  - complex R56.01
    - with status epilepticus G40.901
  - simple R56.00
- hysterical F44.5
- infantile P90
  - epilepsy — *see* Epilepsy
- jacksonian — *see* Epilepsy, localization-related, symptomatic, with simple partial seizures
- myoclonic G25.3
- newborn P90
- obstetrical (nephritic) (uremic) — *see* Eclampsia
- paretic A52.17
- post traumatic R56.1
- psychomotor — *see* Epilepsy, localization-related, symptomatic, with complex partial seizures
- recurrent R56.9
- reflex R25.8
- scarlatinal A38.8
- tetanus, tetanic — *see* Tetanus
- thymic E32.8

Convulsive — *see also* Convulsions

Cooley's anemia D56.1

Coolie itch B76.9

DISEASE INDEX

Cooper's
  disease — *see* Mastopathy, cystic
  hernia — *see* Hernia, abdomen, specified site
    NEC
Copra itch B88.0
Coprophagy F50.89
Coprophobia F40.298
Coproporphyria, hereditary E80.29
Cor
  biloculare Q20.8
  bovis, bovinum — *see* Hypertrophy, cardiac
  pulmonale (chronic) I27.81
    acute I26.09
  triatriatum, triatrium Q24.2
  triloculare Q20.8
    biatrium Q20.4
    biventriculare Q21.1
Corbus' disease (gangrenous balanitis) N48.1
Cord — *see also* condition
  around neck (tightly) (with compression)
    complicating delivery O69.1
  bladder G95.89
    tabetic A52.19
Cordis ectopia Q24.8
Corditis (spermatic) N49.1
Corectopia Q13.2
Cori's disease (glycogen storage) E74.03
Corkhandler's disease or lung J67.3
Corkscrew esophagus K22.4
Corkworker's disease or lung J67.3
Corn (infected) L84
Cornea — *see also* condition
  donor Z52.5
  plana Q13.4
Cornelia de Lange syndrome Q87.1
Cornu cutaneum L85.8
Cornual gestation or pregnancy O00.80
  with intrauterine pregnancy O00.81
Coronary (artery) — *see* condition
Coronavirus, as cause of disease classified elsewhere B97.29
  SARS-associated B97.21
Corpora — *see also* condition
  amylacea, prostate N42.89
  cavernosa — *see* condition
Corpulence — *see* Obesity
Corpus — *see* condition
Corrected transposition Q20.5
Corrosion (injury) (acid) (caustic) (chemical) (lime) (external) (internal) T30.4
  abdomen, abdominal (muscle) (wall) T21.42
    first degree T21.52
    second degree T21.62
    third degree T21.72
  above elbow T22.439
    first degree T22.539
    left T22.432
      first degree T22.532
      second degree T22.632
      third degree T22.732
    right T22.431
      first degree T22.531
      second degree T22.631
      third degree T22.731
    second degree T22.639
    third degree T22.739
  alimentary tract NEC T28.7
  ankle T25.419
    first degree T25.519
    left T25.412
      first degree T25.512
      second degree T25.612
      third degree T25.712
    multiple with foot — *see* Corrosion, lower, limb, multiple, ankle and foot

Corrosion (injury) (acid) (caustic) (chemical) (lime) (external) (internal) T30.4 — *continued*
  ankle T25.419 — *continued*
    right T25.411
      first degree T25.511
      second degree T25.611
      third degree T25.711
    second degree T25.619
    third degree T25.719
  anus — *see* Corrosion, buttock
  arm(s) (meaning upper limb(s)) — *see* Corrosion, upper limb
  axilla T22.449
    first degree T22.549
    left T22.442
      first degree T22.542
      second degree T22.642
      third degree T22.742
    right T22.441
      first degree T22.541
      second degree T22.641
      third degree T22.741
    second degree T22.649
    third degree T22.749
  back (lower) T21.44
    first degree T21.54
    second degree T21.64
    third degree T21.74
    upper T21.43
      first degree T21.53
      second degree T21.63
      third degree T21.73
  blisters — *code as* Corrosion, second degree, by site
  breast(s) — *see* Corrosion, chest wall
  buttock(s) T21.45
    first degree T21.55
    second degree T21.65
    third degree T21.75
  calf T24.439
    first degree T24.539
    left T24.432
      first degree T24.532
      second degree T24.632
      third degree T24.732
    right T24.431
      first degree T24.531
      second degree T24.631
      third degree T24.731
    second degree T24.639
    third degree T24.739
  canthus (eye) — *see* Corrosion, eyelid
  cervix T28.8
  cheek T20.46
    first degree T20.56
    second degree T20.66
    third degree T20.76
  chest wall T21.41
    first degree T21.51
    second degree T21.61
    third degree T21.71
  chin T20.43
    first degree T20.53
    second degree T20.63
    third degree T20.73
  colon T28.7
  conjunctiva (and cornea) — *see* Corrosion, cornea
  cornea (and conjunctiva) T26.6-
  deep necrosis of underlying tissue — *code as* Corrosion, third degree, by site
  dorsum of hand T23.469
    first degree T23.569
    left T23.462
      first degree T23.562
      second degree T23.662
      third degree T23.762

Corrosion (injury) (acid) (caustic) (chemical) (lime) (external) (internal) T30.4 — *continued*
  dorsum of hand T23.469 — *continued*
    right T23.461
      first degree T23.561
      second degree T23.661
      third degree T23.761
    second degree T23.669
    third degree T23.769
  ear (auricle) (external) (canal) T20.41
    drum T28.91
    first degree T20.51
    second degree T20.61
    third degree T20.71
  elbow T22.429
    first degree T22.529
    left T22.422
      first degree T22.522
      second degree T22.622
      third degree T22.722
    right T22.421
      first degree T22.521
      second degree T22.621
      third degree T22.721
    second degree T22.629
    third degree T22.729
  entire body — *see* Corrosion, multiple body regions
  epidermal loss — *code as* Corrosion, second degree, by site
  epiglottis T27.4
  erythema, erythematous — *code as* Corrosion, first degree, by site
  esophagus T28.6
  extent (percentage of body surface)
    10-19 per cent (0-9 percent third degree) T32.10
      with 10-19 percent third degree T32.11
    20-29 per cent (0-9 percent third degree) T32.20
      with
        10-19 percent third degree T32.21
        20-29 percent third degree T32.22
    30-39 per cent (0-9 percent third degree) T32.30
      with
        10-19 percent third degree T32.31
        20-29 percent third degree T32.32
        30-39 percent third degree T32.33
    40-49 per cent (0-9 percent third degree) T32.40
      with
        10-19 percent third degree T32.41
        20-29 percent third degree T32.42
        30-39 percent third degree T32.43
        40-49 percent third degree T32.44
    50-59 per cent (0-9 percent third degree) T32.50
      with
        10-19 percent third degree T32.51
        20-29 percent third degree T32.52
        30-39 percent third degree T32.53
        40-49 percent third degree T32.54
        50-59 percent third degree T32.55
    60-69 per cent (0-9 percent third degree) T32.60
      with
        10-19 percent third degree T32.61
        20-29 percent third degree T32.62
        30-39 percent third degree T32.63
        40-49 percent third degree T32.64
        50-59 percent third degree T32.65
        60-69 percent third degree T32.66

Corrosion (injury) (acid) (caustic) (chemical) (lime) (external) (internal) T30.4 — *continued*
  extent (percentage of body surface) — *continued*
    70-79 per cent (0-9 percent third degree) T32.70
     with
      10-19 percent third degree T32.71
      20-29 percent third degree T32.72
      30-39 percent third degree T32.73
      40-49 percent third degree T32.74
      50-59 percent third degree T32.75
      60-69 percent third degree T32.76
      70-79 percent third degree T32.77
    80-89 per cent (0-9 percent third degree) T32.80
     with
      10-19 percent third degree T32.81
      20-29 percent third degree T32.82
      30-39 percent third degree T32.83
      40-49 percent third degree T32.84
      50-59 percent third degree T32.85
      60-69 percent third degree T32.86
      70-79 percent third degree T32.87
      80-89 percent third degree T32.88
    90 per cent or more (0-9 percent third degree) T32.90
     with
      10-19 percent third degree T32.91
      20-29 percent third degree T32.92
      30-39 percent third degree T32.93
      40-49 percent third degree T32.94
      50-59 percent third degree T32.95
      60-69 percent third degree T32.96
      70-79 percent third degree T32.97
      80-89 percent third degree T32.98
      90-99 percent third degree T32.99
    less than 10 per cent T32.0
  extremity — *see* Corrosion, limb
  eye(s) and adnexa T26.9-
    with resulting rupture and destruction of eyeball T26.7-
    conjunctival sac — *see* Corrosion, cornea
    cornea — *see* Corrosion, cornea
    lid — *see* Corrosion, eyelid
    periocular area — *see* Corrosion eyelid
    specified site NEC T26.8-
  eyeball — *see* Corrosion, eye
  eyelid(s) T26.5-
  face — *see* Corrosion, head
  finger T23.429
    first degree T23.529
    left T23.422
     first degree T23.522
     second degree T23.622
     third degree T23.722
    multiple sites (without thumb) T23.439
     with thumb T23.449
      first degree T23.549
      left T23.442
       first degree T23.542
       second degree T23.642
       third degree T23.742
      right T23.441
       first degree T23.541
       second degree T23.641
       third degree T23.741
      second degree T23.649
      third degree T23.749
     first degree T23.539
     left T23.432
      first degree T23.532
      second degree T23.632
      third degree T23.732

Corrosion (injury) (acid) (caustic) (chemical) (lime) (external) (internal) T30.4 — *continued*
  finger T23.429 — *continued*
    multiple sites (without thumb) T23.439 — *continued*
     right T23.431
      first degree T23.531
      second degree T23.631
      third degree T23.731
     second degree T23.639
     third degree T23.739
    right T23.421
     first degree T23.521
     second degree T23.621
     third degree T23.721
    second degree T23.629
    third degree T23.729
  flank — *see* Corrosion, abdomen
  foot T25.429
    first degree T25.529
    left T25.422
     first degree T25.522
     second degree T25.622
     third degree T25.722
    multiple with ankle — *see* Corrosion, lower, limb, multiple, ankle and foot
    right T25.421
     first degree T25.521
     second degree T25.621
     third degree T25.721
    second degree T25.629
    third degree T25.729
  forearm T22.419
    first degree T22.519
    left T22.412
     first degree T22.512
     second degree T22.612
     third degree T22.712
    right T22.411
     first degree T22.511
     second degree T22.611
     third degree T22.711
    second degree T22.619
    third degree T22.719
  forehead T20.46
    first degree T20.56
    second degree T20.66
    third degree T20.76
  fourth degree — *code as* Corrosion, third degree, by site
  full thickness skin loss — *code as* Corrosion, third degree, by site
  gastrointestinal tract NEC T28.7
  genital organs
    external
     female T21.47
      first degree T21.57
      second degree T21.67
      third degree T21.77
     male T21.46
      first degree T21.56
      second degree T21.66
      third degree T21.76
    internal T28.8
  groin — *see* Corrosion, abdominal wall
  hand(s) T23.409
    back — *see* Corrosion, dorsum of hand
    finger — *see* Corrosion, finger
    first degree T23.509
    left T23.402
     first degree T23.502
     second degree T23.602
     third degree T23.702

Corrosion (injury) (acid) (caustic) (chemical) (lime) (external) (internal) T30.4 — *continued*
  hand(s) T23.409 — *continued*
    multiple sites with wrist T23.499
     first degree T23.599
     left T23.492
      first degree T23.592
      second degree T23.692
      third degree T23.792
     right T23.491
      first degree T23.591
      second degree T23.691
      third degree T23.791
     second degree T23.699
     third degree T23.799
    palm — *see* Corrosion, palm
    right T23.401
     first degree T23.501
     second degree T23.601
     third degree T23.701
    second degree T23.609
    third degree T23.709
    thumb — *see* Corrosion, thumb
  head (and face) (and neck) T20.40
    cheek — *see* Corrosion, cheek
    chin — *see* Corrosion, chin
    ear — *see* Corrosion, ear
    eye(s) only — *see* Corrosion, eye
    first degree T20.50
    forehead — *see* Corrosion, forehead
    lip — *see* Corrosion, lip
    multiple sites T20.49
     first degree T20.59
     second degree T20.69
     third degree T20.79
    neck — *see* Corrosion, neck
    nose — *see* Corrosion, nose
    scalp — *see* Corrosion, scalp
    second degree T20.60
    third degree T20.70
  hip(s) — *see* Corrosion, lower, limb
  inhalation — *see* Corrosion, respiratory tract
  internal organ(s) (*see also* Corrosion, by site) T28.90
    alimentary tract T28.7
     esophagus T28.6
    esophagus T28.6
    genitourinary T28.8
    mouth T28.5
    pharynx T28.5
    specified organ NEC T28.99
  interscapular region — *see* Corrosion, back, upper
  intestine (large) (small) T28.7
  knee T24.429
    first degree T24.529
    left T24.422
     first degree T24.522
     second degree T24.622
     third degree T24.722
    right T24.421
     first degree T24.521
     second degree T24.621
     third degree T24.721
    second degree T24.629
    third degree T24.729
  labium (majus) (minus) — *see* Corrosion, genital organs, external, female
  lacrimal apparatus, duct, gland or sac — *see* Corrosion, eye, specified site NEC
  larynx T27.4
    with lung T27.5
  leg(s) (meaning lower limb(s)) — *see* Corrosion, lower limb
  limb(s)
    lower — *see* Corrosion, lower, limb
    upper — *see* Corrosion, upper limb

Corrosion (injury) (acid) (caustic) (chemical) (lime) (external) (internal) T30.4 — *continued*
lip(s) T20.42
  first degree T20.52
  second degree T20.62
  third degree T20.72
lower
  back — *see* Corrosion, back
  limb T24.409
    ankle — *see* Corrosion, ankle
    calf — *see* Corrosion, calf
    first degree T24.509
    foot — *see* Corrosion, foot
    hip — *see* Corrosion, thigh
    knee — *see* Corrosion, knee
    left T24.402
      first degree T24.502
      second degree T24.602
      third degree T24.702
    multiple sites, except ankle and foot T24.499
      ankle and foot T25.499
        first degree T25.599
        left T25.492
          first degree T25.592
          second degree T25.692
          third degree T25.792
        right T25.491
          first degree T25.591
          second degree T25.691
          third degree T25.791
        second degree T25.699
        third degree T25.799
    first degree T24.599
    left T24.492
      first degree T24.592
      second degree T24.692
      third degree T24.792
    right T24.491
      first degree T24.591
      second degree T24.691
      third degree T24.791
    second degree T24.699
    third degree T24.799
    right T24.401
      first degree T24.501
      second degree T24.601
      third degree T24.701
    second degree T24.609
    thigh — *see* Corrosion, thigh
    third degree T24.709
lung (with larynx and trachea) T27.5
mouth T28.5
neck T20.47
  first degree T20.57
  second degree T20.67
  third degree T20.77
nose (septum) T20.44
  first degree T20.54
  second degree T20.64
  third degree T20.74
ocular adnexa — *see* Corrosion, eye
orbit region — *see* Corrosion, eyelid
palm T23.459
  first degree T23.559
  left T23.452
    first degree T23.552
    second degree T23.652
    third degree T23.752
  right T23.451
    first degree T23.551
    second degree T23.651
    third degree T23.751
  second degree T23.659
  third degree T23.759
partial thickness — *code as* Corrosion, unspecified degree, by site

Corrosion (injury) (acid) (caustic) (chemical) (lime) (external) (internal) T30.4 — *continued*
pelvis — *see* Corrosion, trunk
penis — *see* Corrosion, genital organs, external, male
perineum
  female — *see* Corrosion, genital organs, external, female
  male — *see* Corrosion, genital organs, external, male
periocular area — *see* Corrosion, eyelid
pharynx T28.5
rectum T28.7
respiratory tract T27.7
  larynx — *see* Corrosion, larynx
  specified part NEC T27.6
  trachea — *see* Corrosion, larynx
sac, lacrimal — *see* Corrosion, eye, specified site NEC
scalp T20.45
  first degree T20.55
  second degree T20.65
  third degree T20.75
scapular region T22.469
  first degree T22.569
  left T22.462
    first degree T22.562
    second degree T22.662
    third degree T22.762
  right T22.461
    first degree T22.561
    second degree T22.661
    third degree T22.761
  second degree T22.669
  third degree T22.769
sclera — *see* Corrosion, eye, specified site NEC
scrotum — *see* Corrosion, genital organs, external, male
shoulder T22.459
  first degree T22.559
  left T22.452
    first degree T22.552
    second degree T22.652
    third degree T22.752
  right T22.451
    first degree T22.551
    second degree T22.651
    third degree T22.751
  second degree T22.659
  third degree T22.759
stomach T28.7
temple — *see* Corrosion, head
testis — *see* Corrosion, genital organs, external, male
thigh T24.419
  first degree T24.519
  left T24.412
    first degree T24.512
    second degree T24.612
    third degree T24.712
  right T24.411
    first degree T24.511
    second degree T24.611
    third degree T24.711
  second degree T24.619
  third degree T24.719
thorax (external) — *see* Corrosion, trunk
throat (meaning pharynx) T28.5
thumb(s) T23.419
  first degree T23.519
  left T23.412
    first degree T23.512
    second degree T23.612
    third degree T23.712

Corrosion (injury) (acid) (caustic) (chemical) (lime) (external) (internal) T30.4 — *continued*
thumb(s) T23.419 — *continued*
  multiple sites with fingers T23.449
    first degree T23.549
    left T23.442
      first degree T23.542
      second degree T23.642
      third degree T23.742
    right T23.441
      first degree T23.541
      second degree T23.641
      third degree T23.741
    second degree T23.649
    third degree T23.749
  right T23.411
    first degree T23.511
    second degree T23.611
    third degree T23.711
  second degree T23.619
  third degree T23.719
toe T25.439
  first degree T25.539
  left T25.432
    first degree T25.532
    second degree T25.632
    third degree T25.732
  right T25.431
    first degree T25.531
    second degree T25.631
    third degree T25.731
  second degree T25.639
  third degree T25.739
tongue T28.5
tonsil(s) T28.5
total body — *see* Corrosion, multiple body regions
trachea T27.4
  with lung T27.5
trunk T21.40
  abdominal wall — *see* Corrosion, abdominal wall
  anus — *see* Corrosion, buttock
  axilla — *see* Corrosion, upper limb
  back — *see* Corrosion, back
  breast — *see* Corrosion, chest wall
  buttock — *see* Corrosion, buttock
  chest wall — *see* Corrosion, chest wall
  first degree T21.50
  flank — *see* Corrosion, abdominal wall
  genital
    female — *see* Corrosion, genital organs, external, female
    male — *see* Corrosion, genital organs, external, male
  groin — *see* Corrosion, abdominal wall
  interscapular region — *see* Corrosion, back, upper
  labia — *see* Corrosion, genital organs, external, female
  lower back — *see* Corrosion, back
  penis — *see* Corrosion, genital organs, external, male
  perineum
    female — *see* Corrosion, genital organs, external, female
    male — *see* Corrosion, genital organs, external, male
  scapular region — *see* Corrosion, upper limb
  scrotum — *see* Corrosion, genital organs, external, male
  second degree T21.60
  shoulder — *see* Corrosion, upper limb
  specified site NEC T21.49
    first degree T21.59
    second degree T21.69
    third degree T21.79

DISEASE INDEX

Corrosion (injury) (acid) (caustic) (chemical) (lime) (external) (internal) T30.4 — *continued*
  trunk T21.40 — *continued*
    testes — *see* Corrosion, genital organs, external, male
    third degree T21.70
    upper back — *see* Corrosion, back, upper
    vagina T28.8
    vulva — *see* Corrosion, genital organs, external, female
  unspecified site with extent of body surface involved specified
    10-19 per cent (0-9 percent third degree) T32.10
      with 10-19 percent third degree T32.11
    20-29 per cent (0-9 percent third degree) T32.20
      with
        10-19 percent third degree T32.21
        20-29 percent third degree T32.22
    30-39 per cent (0-9 percent third degree) T32.30
      with
        10-19 percent third degree T32.31
        20-29 percent third degree T32.32
        30-39 percent third degree T32.33
    40-49 per cent (0-9 percent third degree) T32.40
      with
        10-19 percent third degree T32.41
        20-29 percent third degree T32.42
        30-39 percent third degree T32.43
        40-49 percent third degree T32.44
    50-59 per cent (0-9 percent third degree) T32.50
      with
        10-19 percent third degree T32.51
        20-29 percent third degree T32.52
        30-39 percent third degree T32.53
        40-49 percent third degree T32.54
        50-59 percent third degree T32.55
    60-69 per cent (0-9 percent third degree) T32.60
      with
        10-19 percent third degree T32.61
        20-29 percent third degree T32.62
        30-39 percent third degree T32.63
        40-49 percent third degree T32.64
        50-59 percent third degree T32.65
        60-69 percent third degree T32.66
    70-79 per cent (0-9 percent third degree) T32.70
      with
        10-19 percent third degree T32.71
        20-29 percent third degree T32.72
        30-39 percent third degree T32.73
        40-49 percent third degree T32.74
        50-59 percent third degree T32.75
        60-69 percent third degree T32.76
        70-79 percent third degree T32.77
    80-89 per cent (0-9 percent third degree) T32.80
      with
        10-19 percent third degree T32.81
        20-29 percent third degree T32.82
        30-39 percent third degree T32.83
        40-49 percent third degree T32.84
        50-59 percent third degree T32.85
        60-69 percent third degree T32.86
        70-79 percent third degree T32.87
        80-89 percent third degree T32.88

Corrosion (injury) (acid) (caustic) (chemical) (lime) (external) (internal) T30.4 — *continued*
  unspecified site with extent of body surface involved specified — *continued*
    90 per cent or more (0-9 percent third degree) T32.90
      with
        10-19 percent third degree T32.91
        20-29 percent third degree T32.92
        30-39 percent third degree T32.93
        40-49 percent third degree T32.94
        50-59 percent third degree T32.95
        60-69 percent third degree T32.96
        70-79 percent third degree T32.97
        80-89 percent third degree T32.98
        90-99 percent third degree T32.99
    less than 10 per cent T32.0
  upper limb (axilla) (scapular region) T22.40
    above elbow — *see* Corrosion, above elbow
    axilla — *see* Corrosion, axilla
    elbow — *see* Corrosion, elbow
    first degree T22.50
    forearm — *see* Corrosion, forearm
    hand — *see* Corrosion, hand
    interscapular region — *see* Corrosion, back, upper
    multiple sites T22.499
      first degree T22.599
      left T22.492
        first degree T22.592
        second degree T22.692
        third degree T22.792
      right T22.491
        first degree T22.591
        second degree T22.691
        third degree T22.791
      second degree T22.699
      third degree T22.799
    scapular region — *see* Corrosion, scapular region
    second degree T22.60
    shoulder — *see* Corrosion, shoulder
    third degree T22.70
    wrist — *see* Corrosion, hand
  uterus T28.8
  vagina T28.8
  vulva — *see* Corrosion, genital organs, external, female
  wrist T23.479
    first degree T23.579
    left T23.472
      first degree T23.572
      second degree T23.672
      third degree T23.772
    multiple sites with hand T23.499
      first degree T23.599
      left T23.492
        first degree T23.592
        second degree T23.692
        third degree T23.792
      right T23.491
        first degree T23.591
        second degree T23.691
        third degree T23.791
      second degree T23.699
      third degree T23.799
    right T23.471
      first degree T23.571
      second degree T23.671
      third degree T23.771
    second degree T23.679
    third degree T23.779

Corrosive burn — *see* Corrosion
Corsican fever — *see* Malaria
Cortical — *see* condition
Cortico-adrenal — *see* condition

Coryza (acute) J00
  with grippe or influenza — *see* Influenza, with, respiratory manifestations NEC
  syphilitic
    congenital (chronic) A50.05
Costen's syndrome or complex M26.69
Costiveness — *see* Constipation
Costochondritis M94.0
Cot death R99
Cotard's syndrome F22
Cotia virus B08.8
Cotton wool spots (retinal) H35.81
Cotungo's disease — *see* Sciatica
Cough (affected) (chronic) (epidemic) (nervous) R05
  with hemorrhage — *see* Hemoptysis
  bronchial R05
    with grippe or influenza — *see* Influenza, with, respiratory manifestations NEC
  functional F45.8
  hysterical F45.8
  laryngeal, spasmodic R05
  psychogenic F45.8
  smokers' J41.0
  tea taster's B49
Counseling (for) Z71.9
  abuse NEC
    perpetrator Z69.82
    victim Z69.81
  alcohol abuser Z71.41
    family Z71.42
  child abuse
    nonparental
      perpetrator Z69.021
      victim Z69.020
    parental
      perpetrator Z69.011
      victim Z69.010
  consanguinity Z71.89
  contraceptive Z30.09
  dietary Z71.3
  drug abuser Z71.51
    family member Z71.52
  family Z71.89
  fertility preservation (prior to cancer therapy) (prior to removal of gonads) Z31.62
  for non-attending third party Z71.0
    related to sexual behavior or orientation Z70.2
  genetic NEC Z31.5
  gestational carrier Z31.7
  health (advice) (education) (instruction) — *see* Counseling, medical
  human immunodeficiency virus (HIV) Z71.7
  impotence Z70.1
  insulin pump use Z46.81
  medical (for) Z71.9
    boarding school resident Z59.3
    consanguinity Z71.89
    feared complaint and no disease found Z71.1
    human immunodeficiency virus (HIV) Z71.7
    institutional resident Z59.3
    on behalf of another Z71.0
      related to sexual behavior or orientation Z70.2
    person living alone Z60.2
    specified reason NEC Z71.89
  natural family planning
    procreative Z31.61
    to avoid pregnancy Z30.02
  perpetrator (of)
    abuse NEC Z69.82
    child abuse
      non-parental Z69.021
      parental Z69.011
    rape NEC Z69.82
    spousal abuse Z69.12

Counseling (for) Z71.9 — continued
  procreative NEC Z31.69
    fertility preservation (prior to cancer therapy)
      (prior to removal of gonads) Z31.62
    using natural family planning Z31.61
  promiscuity Z70.1
  rape victim Z69.81
  religious Z71.81
  sex, sexual (related to) Z70.9
    attitude(s) Z70.0
    behavior or orientation Z70.1
    combined concerns Z70.3
    non-responsiveness Z70.1
    on behalf of third party Z70.2
    specified reason NEC Z70.8
  specified reason NEC Z71.89
  spiritual Z71.81
  spousal abuse (perpetrator) Z69.12
    victim Z69.11
  substance abuse Z71.89
    alcohol Z71.41
    drug Z71.51
    tobacco Z71.6
  tobacco use Z71.6
  use (of)
    insulin pump Z46.81
  victim (of)
    abuse Z69.81
    child abuse
      by parent Z69.010
      non-parental Z69.020
    rape NEC Z69.81
Coupled rhythm R00.8
Couvelaire syndrome or uterus
  (complicating delivery) O45.8x-
Cowper's gland — *see* condition
Cowperitis — *see* Urethritis
Cowpox B08.010
  due to vaccination T88.1
Coxa
  magna M91.4-
  plana M91.2-
  valga (acquired) — *see also* Deformity, limb,
    specified type NEC, thigh
    congenital Q65.81
    sequelae (late effect) of rickets E64.3
  vara (acquired) — *see also* Deformity, limb,
    specified type NEC, thigh
    congenital Q65.82
    sequelae (late effect) of rickets E64.3
Coxalgia, coxalgic (nontuberculous) — *see also*
  Pain, joint, hip
  tuberculous A18.02
Coxitis — *see* Monoarthritis, hip
Coxsackie (virus) (infection) B34.1
  as cause of disease classified elsewhere
    B97.11
  carditis B33.20
  central nervous system NEC A88.8
  endocarditis B33.21
  enteritis A08.39
  meningitis (aseptic) A87.0
  myocarditis B33.22
  pericarditis B33.23
  pharyngitis B08.5
  pleurodynia B33.0
  specific disease NEC B33.8
Crabs, meaning pubic lice B85.3
Crack baby P04.41
Cracked nipple N64.0
  associated with
    lactation O92.13
    pregnancy O92.11-
    puerperium O92.12
Cracked tooth K03.81
Cradle cap L21.0
Craft neurosis F48.8

Cramp(s) R25.2
  abdominal — *see* Pain, abdominal
  bathing T75.1
  colic R10.83
    psychogenic F45.8
  due to immersion T75.1
  fireman T67.2
  heat T67.2
  immersion T75.1
  intestinal — *see* Pain, abdominal
    psychogenic F45.8
  leg, sleep related G47.62
  limb (lower) (upper) NEC R25.2
    sleep related G47.62
  linotypist's F48.8
    organic G25.89
  muscle (limb) (general) R25.2
    due to immersion T75.1
    psychogenic F45.8
  occupational (hand) F48.8
    organic G25.89
  salt-depletion E87.1
  sleep related, leg G47.62
  stoker's T67.2
  swimmer's T75.1
  telegrapher's F48.8
    organic G25.89
  typist's F48.8
    organic G25.89
  uterus N94.89
    menstrual — *see* Dysmenorrhea
  writer's F48.8
    organic G25.89
Cranial — *see* condition
Craniocleidodysostosis Q74.0
Craniofenestria (skull) Q75.8
Craniolacunia (skull) Q75.8
Craniopagus Q89.4
Craniopathy, metabolic M85.2
Craniopharyngeal — *see* condition
Craniopharyngioma D44.4
Craniorachischisis (totalis) Q00.1
Cranioschisis Q75.8
Craniostenosis Q75.0
Craniosynostosis Q75.0
Craniotabes (cause unknown) M83.8
  neonatal P96.3
  rachitic E64.3
  syphilitic A50.56
Cranium — *see* condition
Craw-craw — *see* Onchocerciasis
Creaking joint — *see* Derangement, joint,
  specified type NEC
Creeping
  eruption B76.9
  palsy or paralysis G12.22
Crenated tongue K14.8
Creotoxism A05.9
Crepitus
  caput Q75.8
  joint — *see* Derangement, joint, specified type
    NEC
Crescent or conus choroid, congenital
  Q14.3
CREST syndrome M34.1
Cretin, cretinism (congenital) (endemic)
  (nongoitrous) (sporadic) E00.9
  pelvis
    with disproportion (fetopelvic) O33.0
      causing obstructed labor O65.0
  type
    hypothyroid E00.1
    mixed E00.2
    myxedematous E00.1
    neurological E00.0

Creutzfeldt-Jakob disease or syndrome
  (with dementia) A81.00
  familial A81.09
  iatrogenic A81.09
  specified NEC A81.09
  sporadic A81.09
  variant (vCJD) A81.01
Cri-du-chat syndrome Q93.4
Crib death R99
Cribriform hymen Q52.3
Crigler-Najjar disease or syndrome
  E80.5
Crime, victim of Z65.4
Crimean hemorrhagic fever A98.0
Criminalism F60.2
Crisis
  abdomen R10.0
  acute reaction F43.0
  addisonian E27.2
  adrenal (cortical) E27.2
  celiac K90.0
  Dietl's N13.8
  emotional — *see also* Disorder, adjustment
    acute reaction to stress F43.0
    specific to childhood and adolescence F93.8
  glaucomatocyclitic — *see* Glaucoma,
    secondary, inflammation
  heart — *see* Failure, heart
  nitritoid I95.2
    correct substance properly administered —
      see Table of Drugs and Chemicals, by
      drug, adverse effect
    overdose or wrong substance given or taken
      — *see* Table of Drugs and Chemicals, by
      drug, poisoning
  oculogyric H51.8
    psychogenic F45.8
  Pel's (tabetic) A52.11
  psychosexual identity F64.2
  renal N28.0
  sickle-cell D57.00
    with
      acute chest syndrome D57.01
      splenic sequestration D57.02
  state (acute reaction) F43.0
  tabetic A52.11
  thyroid — *see* Thyrotoxicosis with thyroid storm
  thyrotoxic — *see* Thyrotoxicosis with thyroid
    storm
Crocq's disease (acrocyanosis) I73.89
Crohn's disease — *see* Enteritis, regional
Crooked septum, nasal J34.2
Cross syndrome E70.328
Crossbite (anterior) (posterior) M26.24
Cross-eye — *see* Strabismus, convergent
  concomitant
Croup, croupous (catarrhal) (infectious)
  (inflammatory) (nondiphtheritic) J05.0
  bronchial J20.9
  diphtheritic A36.2
  false J38.5
  spasmodic J38.5
    diphtheritic A36.2
  stridulous J38.5
    diphtheritic A36.2
Crouzon's disease Q75.1
Crowding, tooth, teeth, fully erupted
  M26.31
CRST syndrome M34.1
Cruchet's disease A85.8
Cruelty in children — *see also* Disorder,
  conduct
Crural ulcer — *see* Ulcer, lower limb
Crush, crushed, crushing T14.8
  abdomen S38.1
  ankle S97.0-
  arm (upper) (and shoulder) S47-
  axilla — *see* Crush, arm

Crush, crushed, crushing — *continued*
back, lower S38.1
buttock S38.1
cheek S07.0
chest S28.0
cranium S07.1
ear S07.0
elbow S57.0-
extremity
 lower
  ankle — *see* Crush, ankle
  below knee — *see* Crush, leg
  foot — *see* Crush, foot
  hip — *see* Crush, hip
  knee — *see* Crush, knee
  thigh — *see* Crush, thigh
  toe — *see* Crush, toe
 upper
  below elbow S67.9-
  elbow — *see* Crush, elbow
  finger — *see* Crush, finger
  forearm — *see* Crush, forearm
  hand — *see* Crush, hand
  thumb — *see* Crush, thumb
  upper arm — *see* Crush, arm
  wrist — *see* Crush, wrist
face S07.0
finger(s) S67.1-
 with hand (and wrist) — *see* Crush, hand,
   specified site NEC
 index S67.19-
 little S67.19-
 middle S67.19-
 ring S67.19-
 thumb — *see* Crush, thumb
foot S97.8-
 toe — *see* Crush, toe
forearm S57.8-
genitalia, external
 female S38.002
  vagina S38.03
  vulva S38.03
 male S38.001
  penis S38.01
  scrotum S38.02
  testis S38.02
hand (except fingers alone) S67.2-
 with wrist S67.4-
head S07.9
 specified NEC S07.8
heel — *see* Crush, foot
hip S77.0-
 with thigh S77.2-
internal organ (abdomen, chest, or pelvis)
  NEC T14.8
knee S87.0-
labium (majus) (minus) S38.03
larynx S17.0
leg (lower) S87.8-
 knee — *see* Crush, knee
lip S07.0
lower
 back S38.1
 leg — *see* Crush, leg
neck S17.9
nerve — *see* Injury, nerve
nose S07.0
pelvis S38.1
penis S38.01
scalp S07.8
scapular region — *see* Crush, arm
scrotum S38.02
severe, unspecified site T14.8
shoulder (and upper arm) — *see* Crush, arm
skull S07.1
syndrome (complication of trauma) T79.5
testis S38.02

Crush, crushed, crushing — *continued*
thigh S77.1-
 with hip S77.2-
throat S17.8
thumb S67.0-
 with hand (and wrist) — *see* Crush, hand,
   specified site NEC
toe(s) S97.10-
 great S97.11-
 lesser S97.12-
trachea S17.0
vagina S38.03
vulva S38.03
wrist S67.3-
 with hand S67.4-
Crusta lactea L21.0
Crusts R23.4
Crutch paralysis — *see* Injury, brachial plexus
Cruveilhier's atrophy or disease G12.8
**Cruveilhier-Baumgarten cirrhosis,
 disease or syndrome** K74.69
Crying (constant) (continuous) (excessive)
 child, adolescent, or adult R45.83
 infant (baby) (newborn) R68.11
Cryofibrinogenemia D89.2
Cryoglobulinemia (essential) (idiopathic)
  (mixed) (primary) (purpura) (secondary)
  (vasculitis) D89.1
 with lung involvement D89.1 *[J99]*
Cryptitis (anal) (rectal) K62.89
Cryptococcosis, cryptococcus (infection)
  (neoformans) B45.9
 bone B45.3
 cerebral B45.1
 cutaneous B45.2
 disseminated B45.7
 generalized B45.7
 meningitis B45.1
 meningocerebralis B45.1
 osseous B45.3
 pulmonary B45.0
 skin B45.2
 specified NEC B45.8
Cryptopapillitis (anus) K62.89
Cryptophthalmos Q11.2
 syndrome Q87.0
**Cryptorchid, cryptorchism,
 cryptorchidism** Q53.9
 bilateral Q53.20
  abdominal Q53.21
  perineal Q53.22
 unilateral Q53.10
  abdominal Q53.11
  perineal Q53.12
Cryptosporidiosis A07.2
 hepatobiliary B88.8
 respiratory B88.8
Cryptostromosis J67.6
Crystalluria R82.99
Cubitus
 congenital Q68.8
 valgus (acquired) M21.0-
  congenital Q68.8
  sequelae (late effect) of rickets E64.3
 varus (acquired) M21.1-
  congenital Q68.8
  sequelae (late effect) of rickets E64.3
Cultural deprivation or shock Z60.3
Curling esophagus K22.4
Curling's ulcer — *see* Ulcer, peptic, acute
**Curschmann (-Batten) (-Steinert) disease
 or syndrome** G71.11
Curse, Ondine's — *see* Apnea, sleep
Curvature
 organ or site, congenital NEC — *see* Distortion
 penis (lateral) Q55.61
 Pott's (spinal) A18.01
 radius, idiopathic, progressive (congenital)
  Q74.0

Curvature — *continued*
 spine (acquired) (angular) (idiopathic)
   (incorrect) (postural) — *see* Dorsopathy,
   deforming
  congenital Q67.5
  due to or associated with
   Charcot-Marie-Tooth disease (*see also*
     subcategory M49.8) G60.0
   osteitis
    deformans M88.88
    fibrosa cystica (*see also* subcategory
      M49.8) E21.0
   tuberculosis (Pott's curvature) A18.01
  sequelae (late effect) of rickets E64.3
  tuberculous A18.01
Cushing's
 syndrome or disease E24.9
  drug-induced E24.2
  iatrogenic E24.2
  pituitary-dependent E24.0
  specified NEC E24.8
 ulcer — *see* Ulcer, peptic, acute
Cushingoid due to steroid therapy E24.2
 correct substance properly administered — *see*
   Table of Drugs and Chemicals, by drug,
   adverse effect
 overdose or wrong substance given or taken
   — *see* Table of Drugs and Chemicals, by
   drug, poisoning
Cusp, Carabelli — *omit code*
Cut (external) — *see also* Laceration
 muscle — *see* Injury, muscle
Cutaneous — *see also* condition
 hemorrhage R23.3
 larva migrans B76.9
Cutis — *see also* condition
 hyperelastica Q82.8
  acquired L57.4
 laxa (hyperelastica) — *see* Dermatolysis
 marmorata R23.8
 osteosis L94.2
 pendula — *see* Dermatolysis
 rhomboidalis nuchae L57.2
 verticis gyrata Q82.8
  acquired L91.8
Cyanosis R23.0
 due to
  patent foramen botalli Q21.1
  persistent foramen ovale Q21.1
 enterogenous D74.8
 paroxysmal digital — *see* Raynaud's disease
  with gangrene I73.01
 retina, retinal H35.89
Cyanotic heart disease I24.9
 congenital Q24.9
Cycle
 anovulatory N97.0
 menstrual, irregular N92.6
Cyclencephaly Q04.9
Cyclical vomiting (*see also* Vomiting, cyclical)
  G43.A0 *(follows G43.7)*
 psychogenic F50.89
Cyclitis (*see also* Iridocyclitis) H20.9
 chronic — *see* Iridocyclitis, chronic
 Fuchs' heterochromic H20.81-
 granulomatous — *see* Iridocyclitis, chronic
 lens-induced — *see* Iridocyclitis, lens-induced
 posterior H30.2-
Cycloid personality F34.0
Cyclophoria H50.54
Cyclopia, cyclops Q87.0
Cyclopism Q87.0
Cyclosporiasis A07.4
Cyclothymia F34.0
Cyclothymic personality F34.0
Cyclotropia H50.41-

Cylindroma — *see also* Neoplasm, malignant, by site
  eccrine dermal — *see* Neoplasm, skin, benign
  skin — *see* Neoplasm, skin, benign
Cylindruria R82.99
Cynanche
  diphtheritic A36.2
  tonsillaris J36
Cynophobia F40.218
Cynorexia R63.2
Cyphosis — *see* Kyphosis
Cyprus fever — *see* Brucellosis
Cyst (colloid) (mucous) (simple) (retention)
  adenoid (infected) J35.8
  adrenal gland E27.8
    congenital Q89.1
  air, lung J98.4
  allantoic Q64.4
  alveolar process (jaw bone) M27.40
  amnion, amniotic O41.8x-
  aneurysmal M27.49
  anterior
    chamber (eye) — *see* Cyst, iris
    nasopalatine K09.1
  antrum J34.1
  anus K62.89
  apical (tooth) (periodontal) K04.8
  appendix K38.8
  arachnoid, brain (acquired) G93.0
    congenital Q04.6
  arytenoid J38.7
  Baker's M71.2-
    ruptured M66.0
    tuberculous A18.02
  Bartholin's gland N75.0
  bile duct (common) (hepatic) K83.5
  bladder (multiple) (trigone) N32.89
  blue dome (breast) — *see* Cyst, breast
  bone (local) NEC M85.60
    aneurysmal M85.50
      ankle M85.57-
      foot M85.57-
      forearm M85.53-
      hand M85.54-
      jaw M27.49
      lower leg M85.56-
      multiple site M85.59
      neck M85.58
      rib M85.58
      shoulder M85.51-
      skull M85.58
      specified site NEC M85.58
      thigh M85.55-
      toe M85.57-
      upper arm M85.52-
      vertebra M85.58
    solitary M85.40
      ankle M85.47-
      fibula M85.46-
      foot M85.47-
      hand M85.44-
      humerus M85.42-
      jaw M27.49
      neck M85.48
      pelvis M85.45-
      radius M85.43-
      rib M85.48
      shoulder M85.41-
      skull M85.48
      specified site NEC M85.48
      tibia M85.46-
      toe M85.47-
      ulna M85.43-
      vertebra M85.48

Cyst (colloid) (mucous) (simple) (retention) — *continued*
  bone (local) NEC M85.60 — *continued*
    specified type NEC M85.60
      ankle M85.67-
      foot M85.67-
      forearm M85.63-
      hand M85.64-
      jaw M27.40
        developmental (nonodontogenic) K09.1
          odontogenic K09.0
        latent M27.0
      lower leg M85.66-
      multiple site M85.69
      neck M85.68
      rib M85.68
      shoulder M85.61-
      skull M85.68
      specified site NEC M85.68
      thigh M85.65-
      toe M85.67-
      upper arm M85.62-
      vertebra M85.68
  brain (acquired) G93.0
    congenital Q04.6
    hydatid B67.99 [G94]
    third ventricle (colloid), congenital Q04.6
  branchial (cleft) Q18.0
  branchiogenic Q18.0
  breast (benign) (blue dome) (pedunculated) (solitary) N60.0-
    involution — *see* Dysplasia, mammary, specified type NEC
    sebaceous — *see* Dysplasia, mammary, specified type NEC
  broad ligament (benign) N83.8
  bronchogenic (mediastinal) (sequestration) J98.4
    congenital Q33.0
  buccal K09.8
  bulbourethral gland N36.8
  bursa, bursal NEC M71.30
    with rupture — *see* Rupture, synovium
    ankle M71.37-
    elbow M71.32-
    foot M71.37-
    hand M71.34-
    hip M71.35-
    multiple sites M71.39
    pharyngeal J39.2
    popliteal space — *see* Cyst, Baker's
    shoulder M71.31-
    specified site NEC M71.38
    wrist M71.33-
  calcifying odontogenic D16.5
    upper jaw (bone) (maxilla) D16.4
  canal of Nuck (female) N94.89
    congenital Q52.4
  canthus — *see* Cyst, conjunctiva
  carcinomatous — *see* Neoplasm, malignant, by site
  cauda equina G95.89
  cavum septi pellucidi — *see* Cyst, brain
  celomic (pericardium) Q24.8
  cerebellopontine (angle) — *see* Cyst, brain
  cerebellum — *see* Cyst, brain
  cerebral — *see* Cyst, brain
  cervical lateral Q18.0
  cervix NEC N88.8
    embryonic Q51.6
    nabothian N88.8
  chiasmal optic NEC — *see* Disorder, optic, chiasm
  chocolate (ovary) N80.1
  choledochus, congenital Q44.4
  chorion O41.8x-
  choroid plexus G93.0
  ciliary body — *see* Cyst, iris
  clitoris N90.7

Cyst (colloid) (mucous) (simple) (retention) — *continued*
  colon K63.89
  common (bile) duct K83.5
  congenital NEC Q89.8
    adrenal gland Q89.1
    epiglottis Q31.8
    esophagus Q39.8
    fallopian tube Q50.4
    kidney Q61.00
      more than one (multiple) Q61.02
        specified as polycystic Q61.3
          adult type Q61.2
          infantile type NEC Q61.19
            collecting duct dilation Q61.11
      solitary Q61.01
    larynx Q31.8
    liver Q44.6
    lung Q33.0
    mediastinum Q34.1
    ovary Q50.1
    oviduct Q50.4
    periurethral (tissue) Q64.79
    prepuce Q55.69
    salivary gland (any) Q38.4
    sublingual Q38.6
    submaxillary gland Q38.6
    thymus (gland) Q89.2
    tongue Q38.3
    ureterovesical orifice Q62.8
    vulva Q52.79
  conjunctiva H11.44-
  cornea H18.89-
  corpora quadrigemina G93.0
  corpus
    albicans N83.29-
    luteum (hemorrhagic) (ruptured) N83.1-
  Cowper's gland (benign) (infected) N36.8
  cranial meninges G93.0
  craniobuccal pouch E23.6
  craniopharyngeal pouch E23.6
  cystic duct K82.8
  Cysticercus — *see* Cysticercosis
  Dandy-Walker Q03.1
    with spina bifida — *see* Spina bifida
  dental (root) K04.8
    developmental K09.0
    eruption K09.0
    primordial K09.0
  dentigerous (mandible) (maxilla) K09.0
  dermoid — *see* Neoplasm, benign, by site
    with malignant transformation C56-
    implantation
      external area or site (skin) NEC L72.0
      iris — *see* Cyst, iris, implantation
      vagina N89.8
      vulva N90.7
    mouth K09.8
    oral soft tissue K09.8
    sacrococcygeal — *see* Cyst, pilonidal
  developmental K09.1
    odontogenic K09.0
    oral region (nonodontogenic) K09.1
    ovary, ovarian Q50.1
  dura (cerebral) G93.0
    spinal G96.19
  ear (external) Q18.1
  echinococcal — *see* Echinococcus
  embryonic
    cervix uteri Q51.6
    fallopian tube Q50.4
    vagina Q51.6
  endometrium, endometrial (uterus) N85.8
    ectopic — *see* Endometriosis
  enterogenous Q43.8
  epidermal, epidermoid (inclusion) (*see also* Cyst, skin) L72.0
    mouth K09.8
    oral soft tissue K09.8

Cyst (colloid) (mucous) (simple) (retention) — *continued*
- epididymis N50.3
- epiglottis J38.7
- epiphysis cerebri E34.8
- epithelial (inclusion) L72.0
- epoophoron Q50.5
- eruption K09.0
- esophagus K22.8
- ethmoid sinus J34.1
- external female genital organs NEC N90.7
- eye NEC H57.8
  - congenital Q15.8
- eyelid (sebaceous) H02.829
  - infected — *see* Hordeolum
  - left H02.826
    - lower H02.825
    - upper H02.824
  - right H02.823
    - lower H02.822
    - upper H02.821
- fallopian tube N83.8
  - congenital Q50.4
- fimbrial (twisted) Q50.4
- fissural (oral region) K09.1
- follicle (graafian) (hemorrhagic) N83.0-
  - nabothian N88.8
- follicular (atretic) (hemorrhagic) (ovarian) N83.0-
  - dentigerous K09.0
  - odontogenic K09.0
  - skin L72.9
    - specified NEC L72.8
- frontal sinus J34.1
- gallbladder K82.8
- ganglion — *see* Ganglion
- Gartner's duct Q52.4
- gingiva K09.0
- gland of Moll — *see* Cyst, eyelid
- globulomaxillary K09.1
- graafian follicle (hemorrhagic) N83.0-
- granulosal lutein (hemorrhagic) N83.1-
- hemangiomatous D18.00
  - intra-abdominal D18.03
  - intracranial D18.02
  - skin D18.01
  - specified site NEC D18.09
- hemorrhagic M27.49
- hydatid (*see also* Echinococcus) B67.90
  - brain B67.99 *[G94]*
  - liver (*see also* Cyst, liver, hydatid) B67.8
  - lung NEC B67.99 *[J99]*
  - Morgagni
    - female Q50.5
    - male (epididymal) Q55.4
      - testicular Q55.29
  - specified site NEC B67.99
- hymen N89.8
  - embryonic Q52.4
- hypopharynx J39.2
- hypophysis, hypophyseal (duct) (recurrent) E23.6
  - cerebri E23.6
- implantation (dermoid)
  - external area or site (skin) NEC L72.0
  - iris — *see* Cyst, iris, implantation
  - vagina N89.8
  - vulva N90.7
- incisive canal K09.1
- inclusion (epidermal) (epithelial) (epidermoid) (squamous) L72.0
  - not of skin — *code under* Cyst, by site
- intestine (large) (small) K63.89
- intracranial — *see* Cyst, brain
- intraligamentous — *see also* Disorder, ligament
  - knee — *see* Derangement, knee
- intrasellar E23.6

Cyst (colloid) (mucous) (simple) (retention) — *continued*
- iris H21.309
  - exudative H21.31-
  - idiopathic H21.30-
  - implantation H21.32-
  - parasitic H21.33-
  - pars plana (primary) H21.34-
    - exudative H21.35-
- jaw (bone) M27.40
  - aneurysmal M27.49
  - developmental (odontogenic) K09.0
  - fissural K09.1
  - hemorrhagic M27.49
  - traumatic M27.49
- joint NEC — *see* Disorder, joint, specified type NEC
- kidney (acquired) N28.1
  - calyceal — *see* Hydronephrosis
  - congenital Q61.00
  - more than one (multiple) Q61.02
    - specified as polycystic Q61.3
      - adult type (autosomal dominant) Q61.2
      - infantile type (autosomal recessive) NEC Q61.19
        - collecting duct dilation Q61.11
  - pyelogenic — *see* Hydronephrosis
  - simple N28.1
  - solitary (single) Q61.01
    - acquired N28.1
- labium (majus) (minus) N90.7
  - sebaceous N90.7
- lacrimal — *see also* Disorder, lacrimal system, specified NEC
  - gland H04.13-
  - passages or sac — *see* Disorder, lacrimal system, specified NEC
- larynx J38.7
- lateral periodontal K09.0
- lens H27.8
  - congenital Q12.8
- lip (gland) K13.0
- liver (idiopathic) (simple) K76.89
  - congenital Q44.6
  - hydatid B67.8
    - granulosus B67.0
    - multilocularis B67.5
- lung J98.4
  - congenital Q33.0
  - giant bullous J43.9
- lutein N83.1-
- lymphangiomatous D18.1
- lymphoepithelial, oral soft tissue K09.8
- macula — *see* Degeneration, macula, hole
- malignant — *see* Neoplasm, malignant, by site
- mammary gland — *see* Cyst, breast
- mandible M27.40
  - dentigerous K09.0
  - radicular K04.8
- maxilla M27.40
  - dentigerous K09.0
  - radicular K04.8
- medial, face and neck Q18.8
- median
  - anterior maxillary K09.1
  - palatal K09.1
- mediastinum, congenital Q34.1
- meibomian (gland) — *see* Chalazion
  - infected — *see* Hordeolum
- membrane, brain G93.0
- meninges (cerebral) G93.0
  - spinal G96.19
- meniscus, knee — *see* Derangement, knee, meniscus, cystic
- mesentery, mesenteric K66.8
  - chyle I89.8
- mesonephric duct
  - female Q50.5
  - male Q55.4

Cyst (colloid) (mucous) (simple) (retention) — *continued*
- milk N64.89
- Morgagni (hydatid)
  - female Q50.5
  - male (epididymal) Q55.4
    - testicular Q55.29
- mouth K09.8
- Müllerian duct Q50.4
  - appendix testis Q55.29
  - cervix Q51.6
  - fallopian tube Q50.4
  - female Q50.4
  - male Q55.29
  - prostatic utricle Q55.4
  - vagina (embryonal) Q52.4
- multilocular (ovary) D39.10
  - benign — *see* Neoplasm, benign, by site
- myometrium N85.8
- nabothian (follicle) (ruptured) N88.8
- nasoalveolar K09.1
- nasolabial K09.1
- nasopalatine (anterior) (duct) K09.1
- nasopharynx J39.2
- neoplastic — *see* Neoplasm, uncertain behavior, by site
  - benign — *see* Neoplasm, benign, by site
- nervous system NEC G96.8
- neuroenteric (congenital) Q06.8
- nipple — *see* Cyst, breast
- nose (turbinates) J34.1
  - sinus J34.1
- odontogenic, developmental K09.0
- omentum (lesser) K66.8
  - congenital Q45.8
- ora serrata — *see* Cyst, retina, ora serrata
- oral
  - region K09.9
    - developmental (nonodontogenic) K09.1
    - specified NEC K09.8
  - soft tissue K09.9
    - specified NEC K09.8
- orbit H05.81-
- ovary, ovarian (twisted) N83.20-
  - adherent N83.20-
  - chocolate N80.1
  - corpus
    - albicans N83.29-
    - luteum (hemorrhagic) N83.1-
  - dermoid D27.9
  - developmental Q50.1
  - due to failure of involution NEC N83.20-
  - endometrial N80.1
  - follicular (graafian) (hemorrhagic) N83.0-
  - hemorrhagic N83.20-
  - in pregnancy or childbirth O34.8-
    - with obstructed labor O65.5
  - multilocular D39.10
  - pseudomucinous D27.9
  - retention N83.29-
  - serous N83.20-
  - specified NEC N83.29-
  - theca lutein (hemorrhagic) N83.1-
  - tuberculous A18.18
- oviduct N83.8
- palate (median) (fissural) K09.1
- palatine papilla (jaw) K09.1
- pancreas, pancreatic (hemorrhagic) (true) K86.2
  - congenital Q45.2
  - false K86.3
- paralabral
  - hip M24.85-
  - shoulder S43.43-
- paramesonephric duct Q50.4
  - female Q50.4
  - male Q55.29
- paranephric N28.1
- paraphysis, cerebri, congenital Q04.6

Cyst (colloid) (mucous) (simple) (retention) — *continued*
- parasitic B89
- parathyroid (gland) E21.4
- paratubal N83.8
- paraurethral duct N36.8
- paroophoron Q50.5
- parotid gland K11.6
- parovarian Q50.5
- pelvis, female N94.89
  - in pregnancy or childbirth O34.8-
    - causing obstructed labor O65.5
- penis (sebaceous) N48.89
- periapical K04.8
- pericardial, congenital Q24.8
  - acquired (secondary) I31.8
- pericoronal K09.0
- periodontal K04.8
  - lateral K09.0
- peripelvic (lymphatic) N28.1
- peritoneum K66.8
  - chylous I89.8
- periventricular, acquired, newborn P91.1
- pharynx (wall) J39.2
- pilar L72.11
- pilonidal (infected) (rectum) L05.91
  - with abscess L05.01
  - malignant C44.59-
- pituitary (duct) (gland) E23.6
- placenta O43.19-
- pleura J94.8
- popliteal — *see* Cyst, Baker's
- porencephalic Q04.6
  - acquired G93.0
- postanal (infected) — *see* Cyst, pilonidal
- postmastoidectomy cavity (mucosal) — *see* Complications, postmastoidectomy, cyst
- preauricular Q18.1
- prepuce N47.4
  - congenital Q55.69
- primordial (jaw) K09.0
- prostate N42.83
- pseudomucinous (ovary) D27.9
- pupillary, miotic H21.27-
- radicular (residual) K04.8
- radiculodental K04.8
- ranular K11.8
- Rathke's pouch E23.6
- rectum (epithelium) (mucous) K62.89
- renal — *see* Cyst, kidney
- residual (radicular) K04.8
- retention (ovary) N83.29-
  - salivary gland K11.6
- retina H33.19-
  - ora serrata H33.11-
  - parasitic H33.12-
- retroperitoneal K68.9
- sacrococcygeal (dermoid) — *see* Cyst, pilonidal
- salivary gland or duct (mucous extravasation or retention) K11.6
- Sampson's N80.1
- sclera H15.89
- scrotum L72.9
  - sebaceous L72.3
- sebaceous (duct) (gland) L72.3
  - breast — *see* Dysplasia, mammary, specified type NEC
  - eyelid — *see* Cyst, eyelid
  - genital organ NEC
    - female N94.89
    - male N50.89
  - scrotum L72.3
- semilunar cartilage (knee) (multiple) — *see* Derangement, knee, meniscus, cystic
- seminal vesicle N50.89
- serous (ovary) N83.20-
- sinus (accessory) (nasal) J34.1
- Skene's gland N36.8

Cyst (colloid) (mucous) (simple) (retention) — *continued*
- skin L72.9
  - breast — *see* Dysplasia, mammary, specified type NEC
  - epidermal, epidermoid L72.0
  - epithelial L72.0
  - eyelid — *see* Cyst, eyelid
  - genital organ NEC
    - female N90.7
    - male N50.89
  - inclusion L72.0
  - scrotum L72.9
  - sebaceous L72.3
  - sweat gland or duct L74.8
- solitary
  - bone — *see* Cyst, bone, solitary
  - jaw M27.40
  - kidney N28.1
- spermatic cord N50.89
- sphenoid sinus J34.1
- spinal meninges G96.19
- spleen NEC D73.4
  - congenital Q89.09
  - hydatid (*see also* Echinococcus) B67.99 [D77]
- Stafne's M27.0
- subarachnoid intrasellar R93.0
- subcutaneous, pheomycotic (chromomycotic) B43.2
- subdural (cerebral) G93.0
  - spinal cord G96.19
- sublingual gland K11.6
- submandibular gland K11.6
- submaxillary gland K11.6
- suburethral N36.8
- suprarenal gland E27.8
- suprasellar — *see* Cyst, brain
- sweat gland or duct L74.8
- synovial — *see also* Cyst, bursa
  - ruptured — *see* Rupture, synovium
- tarsal — *see* Chalazion
- tendon (sheath) — *see* Disorder, tendon, specified type NEC
- testis N44.2
  - tunica albuginea N44.1
- theca lutein (ovary) N83.1-
- Thornwaldt's J39.2
- thymus (gland) E32.8
- thyroglossal duct (infected) (persistent) Q89.2
- thyroid (gland) E04.1
- thyrolingual duct (infected) (persistent) Q89.2
- tongue K14.8
- tonsil J35.8
- tooth — *see* Cyst, dental
- Tornwaldt's J39.2
- trichilemmal (proliferating) L72.12
- trichodermal L72.12
- tubal (fallopian) N83.8
  - inflammatory — *see* Salpingitis, chronic
- tubo-ovarian N83.8
  - inflammatory N70.13
- tunica
  - albuginea testis N44.1
  - vaginalis N50.89
- turbinate (nose) J34.1
- Tyson's gland N48.89
- urachus, congenital Q64.4
- ureter N28.89
- ureterovesical orifice N28.89
- urethra, urethral (gland) N36.8
- uterine ligament N83.8
- uterus (body) (corpus) (recurrent) N85.8
  - embryonic Q51.818
  - cervix Q51.6
- vagina, vaginal (implantation) (inclusion) (squamous cell) (wall) N89.8
  - embryonic Q52.4
- vallecula, vallecular (epiglottis) J38.7

Cyst (colloid) (mucous) (simple) (retention) — *continued*
- vesical (orifice) N32.89
- vitreous body H43.89
- vulva (implantation) (inclusion) N90.7
  - congenital Q52.79
  - sebaceous gland N90.7
- vulvovaginal gland N90.7
- wolffian
  - female Q50.5
  - male Q55.4

Cystadenocarcinoma — *see* Neoplasm, malignant, by site
- bile duct C22.1
- endometrioid — *see* Neoplasm, malignant, by site
  - specified site — *see* Neoplasm, malignant, by site
  - unspecified site
    - female C56.9
    - male C61
- mucinous
  - papillary
    - specified site — *see* Neoplasm, malignant, by site
    - unspecified site C56.9
  - specified site — *see* Neoplasm, malignant, by site
  - unspecified site C56.9
- papillary
  - mucinous
    - specified site — *see* Neoplasm, malignant, by site
    - unspecified site C56.9
  - pseudomucinous
    - specified site — *see* Neoplasm, malignant, by site
    - unspecified site C56.9
  - serous
    - specified site — *see* Neoplasm, malignant, by site
    - unspecified site C56.9
  - specified site — *see* Neoplasm, malignant, by site
  - unspecified site C56.9
- pseudomucinous
  - papillary
    - specified site — *see* Neoplasm, malignant, by site
    - unspecified site C56.9
  - specified site — *see* Neoplasm, malignant, by site
  - unspecified site C56.9
- serous
  - papillary
    - specified site — *see* Neoplasm, malignant, by site
    - unspecified site C56.9
  - specified site — *see* Neoplasm, malignant, by site
  - unspecified site C56.9

Cystadenofibroma
- clear cell — *see* Neoplasm, benign, by site
- endometrioid D27.9
  - borderline malignancy D39.1-
  - malignant C56-
- mucinous
  - specified site — *see* Neoplasm, benign, by site
  - unspecified site D27.9
- serous
  - specified site — *see* Neoplasm, benign, by site
  - unspecified site D27.9
- specified site — *see* Neoplasm, benign, by site
- unspecified site D27.9

Cystadenoma — *see also* Neoplasm, benign, by site
bile duct D13.4
endometrioid — *see* Neoplasm, benign, by site
   borderline malignancy — *see* Neoplasm, uncertain behavior, by site
malignant — *see* Neoplasm, malignant, by site
mucinous
  borderline malignancy
    ovary C56-
      specified site NEC — *see* Neoplasm, uncertain behavior, by site
      unspecified site C56.9
  papillary
    borderline malignancy
      ovary C56-
        specified site NEC — *see* Neoplasm, uncertain behavior, by site
        unspecified site C56.9
    specified site — *see* Neoplasm, benign, by site
    unspecified site D27.9
  specified site — *see* Neoplasm, benign, by site
  unspecified site D27.9
papillary
  borderline malignancy
    ovary C56-
      specified site NEC — *see* Neoplasm, uncertain behavior, by site
      unspecified site C56.9
  lymphomatosum
    specified site — *see* Neoplasm, benign, by site
    unspecified site D11.9
  mucinous
    borderline malignancy
      ovary C56-
        specified site NEC — *see* Neoplasm, uncertain behavior, by site
        unspecified site C56.9
    specified site — *see* Neoplasm, benign, by site
    unspecified site D27.9
  pseudomucinous
    borderline malignancy
      ovary C56-
        specified site NEC — *see* Neoplasm, uncertain behavior, by site
        unspecified site C56.9
    specified site — *see* Neoplasm, benign, by site
    unspecified site D27.9
  serous
    borderline malignancy
      ovary C56-
        specified site NEC — *see* Neoplasm, uncertain behavior, by site
        unspecified site C56.9
    specified site — *see* Neoplasm, benign, by site
    unspecified site D27.9
  specified site — *see* Neoplasm, benign, by site
  unspecified site D27.9

Cystadenoma — *see also* Neoplasm, benign, by site — *continued*
pseudomucinous
  borderline malignancy
    ovary C56-
      specified site NEC — *see* Neoplasm, uncertain behavior, by site
      unspecified site C56.9
  papillary
    borderline malignancy
      ovary C56-
        specified site NEC — *see* Neoplasm, uncertain behavior, by site
        unspecified site C56.9
    specified site — *see* Neoplasm, benign, by site
    unspecified site D27.9
  specified site — *see* Neoplasm, benign, by site
  unspecified site D27.9
serous
  borderline malignancy
    ovary C56-
      specified site NEC — *see* Neoplasm, uncertain behavior, by site
      unspecified site C56.9
  papillary
    borderline malignancy
      ovary C56-
        specified site NEC — *see* Neoplasm, uncertain behavior, by site
        unspecified site C56.9
    specified site — *see* Neoplasm, benign, by site
    unspecified site D27.9
  specified site — *see* Neoplasm, benign, by site
  unspecified site D27.9

Cystathionine synthase deficiency E72.11
Cystathioninemia E72.19
Cystathioninuria E72.19
Cystic — *see also* condition
breast (chronic) — *see* Mastopathy, cystic
corpora lutea (hemorrhagic) N83.1-
duct — *see* condition
eyeball (congenital) Q11.0
fibrosis — *see* Fibrosis, cystic
kidney (congenital) Q61.9
  adult type Q61.2
  infantile type NEC Q61.19
    collecting duct dilatation Q61.11
  medullary Q61.5
liver, congenital Q44.6
lung disease J98.4
  congenital Q33.0
mastitis, chronic — *see* Mastopathy, cystic
medullary, kidney Q61.5
meniscus — *see* Derangement, knee, meniscus, cystic
ovary N83.20-
Cysticercosis, cysticerciasis B69.9
with
  epileptiform fits B69.0
  myositis B69.81
brain B69.0
central nervous system B69.0
cerebral B69.0
ocular B69.1
specified NEC B69.89
Cysticercus cellulose infestation — *see* Cysticercosis
Cystinosis (malignant) E72.04
Cystinuria E72.01

Cystitis (exudative) (hemorrhagic) (septic) (suppurative) N30.90
with
  fibrosis — *see* Cystitis, chronic, interstitial
  hematuria N30.91
  leukoplakia — *see* Cystitis, chronic, interstitial
  malakoplakia — *see* Cystitis, chronic, interstitial
  metaplasia — *see* Cystitis, chronic, interstitial
  prostatitis N41.3
acute N30.00
  with hematuria N30.01
  of trigone N30.30
    with hematuria N30.31
allergic — *see* Cystitis, specified type NEC
amebic A06.81
bilharzial B65.9 *[N33]*
blennorrhagic (gonococcal) A54.01
bullous — *see* Cystitis, specified type NEC
calculous N21.0
chlamydial A56.01
chronic N30.20
  with hematuria N30.21
  interstitial N30.10
    with hematuria N30.11
  of trigone N30.30
    with hematuria N30.31
  specified NEC N30.20
    with hematuria N30.21
cystic(a) — *see* Cystitis, specified type NEC
diphtheritic A36.85
echinococcal
  granulosus B67.39
  multilocularis B67.69
emphysematous — *see* Cystitis, specified type NEC
encysted — *see* Cystitis, specified type NEC
eosinophilic — *see* Cystitis, specified type NEC
follicular — *see* Cystitis, of trigone
gangrenous — *see* Cystitis, specified type NEC
glandularis — *see* Cystitis, specified type NEC
gonococcal A54.01
incrusted — *see* Cystitis, specified type NEC
interstitial (chronic) — *see* Cystitis, chronic, interstitial
irradiation N30.40
  with hematuria N30.41
irritation — *see* Cystitis, specified type NEC
malignant — *see* Cystitis, specified type NEC
of trigone N30.30
  with hematuria N30.31
panmural — *see* Cystitis, chronic, interstitial
polyposa — *see* Cystitis, specified type NEC
prostatic N41.3
puerperal (postpartum) O86.22
radiation — *see* Cystitis, irradiation
specified type NEC N30.80
  with hematuria N30.81
subacute — *see* Cystitis, chronic
submucous — *see* Cystitis, chronic, interstitial
syphilitic (late) A52.76
trichomonal A59.03
tuberculous A18.12
ulcerative — *see* Cystitis, chronic, interstitial
Cystocele(-urethrocele)
female N81.10
  with prolapse of uterus — *see* Prolapse, uterus
  lateral N81.12
  midline N81.11
  paravaginal N81.12
in pregnancy or childbirth O34.8-
  causing obstructed labor O65.5
male N32.89
Cystolithiasis N21.0

Cystoma — *see also* Neoplasm, benign, by site
endometrial, ovary N80.1
mucinous
specified site — *see* Neoplasm, benign, by site
unspecified site D27.9
serous
specified site — *see* Neoplasm, benign, by site
unspecified site D27.9
simple (ovary) N83.29-
Cystoplegia N31.2
Cystoptosis N32.89
Cystopyelitis — *see* Pyelonephritis
Cystorrhagia N32.89
Cystosarcoma phyllodes D48.6-
benign D24-
malignant — *see* Neoplasm, breast, malignant
Cystostomy
attention to Z43.5
complication — *see* Complications, cystostomy
status Z93.50
appendico-vesicostomy Z93.52
cutaneous Z93.51
specified NEC Z93.59
Cystourethritis — *see* Urethritis
Cystourethrocele — *see also* Cystocele
female N81.10
with uterine prolapse — *see* Prolapse, uterus
lateral N81.12
midline N81.11
paravaginal N81.12
male N32.89
Cytomegalic inclusion disease
congenital P35.1
Cytomegalovirus infection B25.9
Cytomycosis (reticuloendothelial) B39.4
Cytopenia D75.9
refractory
with multilineage dysplasia D46.A *(follows D46.2)*
and ring sideroblasts (RCMD RS) D46.B *(follows D46.2)*
Czerny's disease (periodic hydrarthrosis of the knee) — *see* Effusion, joint, knee

D

Da Costa's syndrome F45.8
Daae (-Finsen) disease (epidemic pleurodynia) B33.0
Dabney's grip B33.0
Dacryoadenitis, dacryadenitis H04.00-
acute H04.01-
chronic H04.02-
Dacryocystitis H04.30-
acute H04.32-
chronic H04.41-
neonatal P39.1
phlegmonous H04.31-
syphilitic A52.71
congenital (early) A50.01
trachomatous, active A71.1
sequelae (late effect) B94.0
Dacryocystoblennorrhea — *see* Inflammation, lacrimal, passages, chronic
Dacryocystocele — *see* Disorder, lacrimal system, changes
Dacryolith, dacryolithiasis H04.51-
Dacryoma — *see* Disorder, lacrimal system, changes
Dacryopericystitis — *see* Dacryocystitis
Dacryops H04.11-
Dacryostenosis — *see also* Stenosis, lacrimal
congenital Q10.5
Dactylitis
bone — *see* Osteomyelitis
sickle-cell D57.00
Hb C D57.219
Hb SS D57.00
specified NEC D57.819
skin L08.9
syphilitic A52.77
tuberculous A18.03
Dactylolysis spontanea (ainhum) L94.6
Dactylosymphysis Q70.9
fingers — *see* Syndactylism, complex, fingers
toes — *see* Syndactylism, complex, toes
Damage
arteriosclerotic — *see* Arteriosclerosis
brain (nontraumatic) G93.9
anoxic, hypoxic G93.1
resulting from a procedure G97.82
child NEC G80.9
due to birth injury P11.2
cardiorenal (vascular) — *see* Hypertension, cardiorenal
cerebral NEC — *see* Damage, brain
coccyx, complicating delivery O71.6
coronary — *see* Disease, heart, ischemic
eye, birth injury P15.3
liver (nontraumatic) K76.9
alcoholic K70.9
due to drugs — *see* Disease, liver, toxic
toxic — *see* Disease, liver, toxic
medication T88.7
pelvic
joint or ligament, during delivery O71.6
organ NEC
during delivery O71.5
following ectopic or molar pregnancy O08.6
renal — *see* Disease, renal
subendocardium, subendocardial — *see* Degeneration, myocardial
vascular I99.9
Dana-Putnam syndrome (subacute combined sclerosis with pernicious anemia) — *see* Degeneration, combined
Danbolt (-Cross) syndrome (acrodermatitis enteropathica) E83.2
Dandruff L21.0
Dandy-Walker syndrome Q03.1
with spina bifida — *see* Spina bifida

Danlos' syndrome Q79.6
Darier-Roussy sarcoid D86.3
Darier(-White) disease (congenital) Q82.8
meaning erythema annulare centrifugum L53.1
Darling's disease or histoplasmosis B39.4
Darwin's tubercle Q17.8
Dawson's (inclusion body) encephalitis A81.1
De Beurmann(-Gougerot) disease B42.1
De la Tourette's syndrome F95.2
De Lange's syndrome Q87.1
De Morgan's spots (senile angiomas) I78.1
De Quervain's
disease (tendon sheath) M65.4
syndrome E34.51
thyroiditis (subacute granulomatous thyroiditis) E06.1
De Toni-Fanconi(-Debré) syndrome E72.09
with cystinosis E72.04
Dead
fetus, retained (mother) O36.4
early pregnancy O02.1
labyrinth — *see* subcategory H83.2
ovum, retained O02.0
Deaf nonspeaking NEC H91.3
Deafmutism (acquired) (congenital) NEC H91.3
hysterical F44.6
syphilitic, congenital (*see also* subcategory H94.8) A50.09
Deafness (acquired) (complete) (hereditary) (partial) H91.9-
with blue sclera and fragility of bone Q78.0
auditory fatigue — *see* Deafness, specified type NEC
aviation T70.0
nerve injury — *see* Injury, nerve, acoustic, specified type NEC
boilermaker's — *see* subcategory H83.3
central — *see* Deafness, sensorineural
conductive H90.2
and sensorineural
mixed H90.8
bilateral H90.6
bilateral H90.0
unilateral H90.1-
with restricted hearing on the contralateral side H90.A- *(follows H90.8)*
congenital H90.5
with blue sclera and fragility of bone Q78.0
due to toxic agents — *see* Deafness, ototoxic
emotional (hysterical) F44.6
functional (hysterical) F44.6
high frequency H91.9-
hysterical F44.6
low frequency H91.9-
mental R48.8
mixed conductive and sensorineural H90.8
bilateral H90.6
unilateral H90.7-
nerve — *see* Deafness, sensorineural
neural — *see* Deafness, sensorineural
noise-induced (*see also* subcategory) H83.3
nerve injury — *see* Injury, nerve, acoustic, specified type NEC
nonspeaking H91.3
ototoxic — *see* subcategory H91.0
perceptive — *see* Deafness, sensorineural
psychogenic (hysterical) F44.6
sensorineural H90.5
and conductive
mixed H90.8
bilateral H90.6
bilateral H90.3
unilateral H90.4-
with restricted hearing on the contralateral side H90.A- *(follows H90.8)*
sensory — *see* Deafness, sensorineural

Deafness (acquired) (complete) (hereditary) (partial) H91.9- — *continued*
  specified type NEC — *see* subcategory H91.8
  sudden (idiopathic) H91.2-
  syphilitic A52.15
  transient ischemic H93.01-
  traumatic — *see* Injury, nerve, acoustic, specified type NEC
  word (developmental) H93.25
Death (cause unknown) (of) (unexplained) (unspecified cause) R99
  brain G93.82
  cardiac (sudden) (with successful resuscitation) — *code to* underlying disease
    family history of Z82.41
    personal history of Z86.74
  family member (assumed) Z63.4
Debility (chronic) (general) (nervous) R53.81
  congenital or neonatal NOS P96.9
  nervous R53.81
  old age R54
  senile R54
Débove's disease (splenomegaly) R16.1
Decalcification
  bone — *see* Osteoporosis
  teeth K03.89
Decapsulation, kidney N28.89
Decay
  dental — *see* Caries, dental
  senile R54
  tooth, teeth — *see* Caries, dental
Deciduitis (acute)
  following ectopic or molar pregnancy O08.0
Decline (general) — *see* Debility
  cognitive, age-associated R41.81
Decompensation
  cardiac (acute) (chronic) — *see* Disease, heart
  cardiovascular — *see* Disease, cardiovascular
  heart — *see* Disease, heart
  hepatic — *see* Failure, hepatic
  myocardial (acute) (chronic) — *see* Disease, heart
  respiratory J98.8
Decompression sickness T70.3
Decrease(d)
  absolute neutrophile count — *see* Neutropenia
  blood
    platelets — *see* Thrombocytopenia
    pressure R03.1
      due to shock following
        injury T79.4
        operation T81.19
  estrogen E28.39
    postablative E89.40
      asymptomatic E89.40
      symptomatic E89.41
  fragility of erythrocytes D58.8
  function
    lipase (pancreatic) K90.3
    ovary in hypopituitarism E23.0
    parenchyma of pancreas K86.89
    pituitary (gland) (anterior) (lobe) E23.0
      posterior (lobe) E23.0
  functional activity R68.89
  glucose R73.09
  hematocrit R71.0
  hemoglobin R71.0
  leukocytes D72.819
    specified NEC D72.818
  libido R68.82
  lymphocytes D72.810
  platelets D69.6
  respiration, due to shock following injury T79.4
  sexual desire R68.82
  tear secretion NEC — *see* Syndrome, dry eye

Decrease(d) — *continued*
  tolerance
    fat K90.49
    glucose R73.09
    pancreatic K90.3
    salt and water E87.8
  vision NEC H54.7
  white blood cell count D72.819
    specified NEC D72.818
Decubitus (ulcer) — *see* Ulcer, pressure, by site
  cervix N86
Deepening acetabulum — *see* Derangement, joint, specified type NEC, hip
Defect, defective Q89.9
  3-beta-hydroxysteroid dehydrogenase E25.0
  11-hydroxylase E25.0
  21-hydroxylase E25.0
  abdominal wall, congenital Q79.59
  antibody immunodeficiency D80.9
  aorticopulmonary septum Q21.4
  atrial septal (ostium secundum type) Q21.1
    following acute myocardial infarction (current complication) I23.1
    ostium primum type Q21.2
  atrioventricular
    canal Q21.2
    septum Q21.2
  auricular septal Q21.1
  bilirubin excretion NEC E80.6
  biosynthesis, androgen (testicular) E29.1
  bulbar septum Q21.0
  catalase E80.3
  cell membrane receptor complex (CR3) D71
  circulation I99.9
    congenital Q28.9
    newborn Q28.9
  coagulation (factor) (*see also* Deficiency, factor) D68.9
    with
      ectopic pregnancy O08.1
      molar pregnancy O08.1
    acquired D68.4
    antepartum with hemorrhage — *see* Hemorrhage, antepartum, with coagulation defect
    due to
      liver disease D68.4
      vitamin K deficiency D68.4
    hereditary NEC D68.2
    intrapartum O67.0
    newborn, transient P61.6
    postpartum O72.3
    specified type NEC D68.8
  complement system D84.1
  conduction (heart) I45.9
    bone — *see* Deafness, conductive
  congenital, organ or site not listed — *see* Anomaly, by site
  coronary sinus Q21.1
  cushion, endocardial Q21.2
  degradation, glycoprotein E77.1
  dental bridge, crown, fillings — *see* Defect, dental restoration
  dental restoration K08.50
    specified NEC K08.59
  dentin (hereditary) K00.5
  Descemet's membrane, congenital Q13.89
  developmental — *see also* Anomaly
    cauda equina Q06.3
  diaphragm
    with elevation, eventration or hernia — *see* Hernia, diaphragm
    congenital Q79.1
      with hernia Q79.0
      gross (with hernia) Q79.0
  ectodermal, congenital Q82.9
  Eisenmenger's Q21.8

Defect, defective Q89.9 — *continued*
  enzyme
    catalase E80.3
    peroxidase E80.3
  esophagus, congenital Q39.9
  extensor retinaculum M62.89
  fibrin polymerization D68.2
  filling
    bladder R93.41
    kidney R93.42-
    renal pelvis R93.41
    stomach R93.3
    ureter R93.41
    urinary organs, specified NEC R93.49
  Gerbode Q21.0
  glycoprotein degradation E77.1
  Hageman (factor) D68.2
  hearing — *see* Deafness
  high grade F70
  interatrial septal Q21.1
  interauricular septal Q21.1
  interventricular septal Q21.0
    with dextroposition of aorta, pulmonary stenosis and hypertrophy of right ventricle Q21.3
    in tetralogy of Fallot Q21.3
  learning (specific) — *see* Disorder, learning
  lymphocyte function antigen-1 (LFA-1) D84.0
  lysosomal enzyme, post-translational modification E77.0
  major osseous M89.70
    ankle M89.77-
    carpus M89.74-
    clavicle M89.71-
    femur M89.75-
    fibula M89.76-
    fingers M89.74-
    foot M89.77-
    forearm M89.73-
    hand M89.74-
    humerus M89.72-
    lower leg M89.76-
    metacarpus M89.74-
    metatarsus M89.77-
    multiple sites M89.79
    pelvic region M89.75-
    pelvis M89.75-
    radius M89.73-
    scapula M89.71-
    shoulder region M89.71-
    specified NEC M89.78
    tarsus M89.77-
    thigh M89.75-
    tibia M89.76-
    toes M89.77-
    ulna M89.73-
  mental — *see* Disability, intellectual
  modification, lysosomal enzymes, post-translational E77.0
  obstructive, congenital
    renal pelvis Q62.39
    ureter Q62.39
      atresia — *see* Atresia, ureter
      cecoureterocele Q62.32
      megaureter Q62.2
      orthotopic ureterocele Q62.31
  osseous, major M89.70
    ankle M89.77-
    carpus M89.74-
    clavicle M89.71-
    femur M89.75-
    fibula M89.76-
    fingers M89.74-
    foot M89.77-
    forearm M89.73-
    hand M89.74-
    humerus M89.72-
    lower leg M89.76-
    metacarpus M89.74-

Defect, defective Q89.9 — *continued*
  osseous, major M89.70 — *continued*
    metatarsus M89.77-
    multiple sites M89.9
    pelvic region M89.75-
    pelvis M89.75-
    radius M89.73-
    scapula M89.71-
    shoulder region M89.71-
    specified NEC M89.78
    tarsus M89.77-
    thigh M89.75-
    tibia M89.76-
    toes M89.77-
    ulna M89.73-
  osteochondral NEC (*see also* Deformity) M95.8
  ostium
    primum Q21.2
    secundum Q21.1
  peroxidase E80.3
  placental blood supply — *see* Insufficiency,
    placental
  platelets, qualitative D69.1
    constitutional D68.0
  postural NEC, spine — *see* Dorsopathy,
    deforming
  reduction
    limb Q73.8
      lower Q72.9-
        absence — *see* Agenesis, leg
          foot — *see* Agenesis, foot
        longitudinal
          femur Q72.4-
          fibula Q72.6-
          tibia Q72.5-
        specified type NEC Q72.89-
        split foot Q72.7-
      specified type NEC Q73.8
      upper Q71.9-
        absence — *see* Agenesis, arm
          forearm — *see* Agenesis, forearm
          hand — *see* Agenesis, hand
        lobster-claw hand Q71.6-
        longitudinal
          radius Q71.4-
          ulna Q71.5-
        specified type NEC Q71.89-
  renal pelvis Q63.8
    obstructive Q62.39
  respiratory system, congenital Q34.9
  restoration, dental K08.50
    specified NEC K08.59
  retinal nerve bundle fibers H35.89
  septal (heart) NOS Q21.9
    acquired (atrial) (auricular) (ventricular) (old)
      I51.0
    atrial Q21.1
      concurrent with acute myocardial
        infarction — *see* Infarct, myocardium
      following acute myocardial infarction
        (current complication) I23.1
    ventricular (*see also* Defect, ventricular septal)
      Q21.0
  sinus venosus Q21.1
  speech R47.9
    developmental F80.9
    specified NEC R47.89
  Taussig-Bing (aortic transposition and
    overriding pulmonary artery) Q20.1
  teeth, wedge K03.1
  vascular (local) I99.9
    congenital Q27.9
  ventricular septal Q21.0
    concurrent with acute myocardial infarction
      — *see* Infarct, myocardial
    following acute myocardial infarction
      (current complication) I23.2
    in tetralogy of Fallot Q21.3
  vision NEC H54.7

Defect, defective Q89.9 — *continued*
  visual field H53.40
    bilateral
      heteronymous H53.47
      homonymous H53.46-
    generalized contraction H53.48-
    localized
      arcuate H53.43-
      scotoma (central area) H53.41-
        blind spot area H53.42-
      sector H53.43-
      specified type NEC H53.45-
  voice R49.9
    specified NEC R49.8
  wedge, tooth, teeth (abrasion) K03.1
Deferentitis N49.1
  gonorrheal (acute) (chronic) A54.23
Defibrination (syndrome) D65
  antepartum — *see* Hemorrhage, antepartum,
    with coagulation defect, disseminated
    intravascular coagulation
  following ectopic or molar pregnancy O08.1
  intrapartum O67.0
  newborn P60
  postpartum O72.3
Deficiency, deficient
  3-beta hydroxysteroid dehydrogenase E25.0
  5-alpha reductase (with male
    pseudohermaphroditism) E29.1
  11-hydroxylase E25.0
  21-hydroxylase E25.0
  abdominal muscle syndrome Q79.4
  AC globulin (congenital) (hereditary) D68.2
    acquired D68.4
  accelerator globulin (Ac G) (blood) D68.2
  acid phosphatase E83.39
  activating factor (blood) D68.2
  adenosine deaminase (ADA) D81.3
  aldolase (hereditary) E74.19
  alpha-1-antitrypsin E88.01
  amino-acids E72.9
  anemia — *see* Anemia
  aneurin E51.9
  anti-hemophilic
    factor (A) D66
      B D67
      C D68.1
    globulin (AHG) NEC D66
  antibody with
    hyperimmunoglobulinemia D80.6
    near-normal immunoglobins D80.6
  antidiuretic hormone E23.2
  antithrombin (antithrombin III) D68.59
  ascorbic acid E54
  attention (disorder) (syndrome) F98.8
    with hyperactivity — *see* Disorder, attention-
      deficit hyperactivity
  autoprothrombin
    C D68.2
    I D68.2
    II D67
  beta-glucuronidase E76.29
  biotin E53.8
  biotin-dependent carboxylase D81.819
  biotinidase D81.810
  brancher enzyme (amylopectinosis) E74.03
  C1 esterase inhibitor (C1-INH) D84.1
  calciferol E55.9
    with
      adult osteomalacia M83.8
      rickets — *see* Rickets
  calcium (dietary) E58
  calorie, severe E43
    with marasmus E41
      and kwashiorkor E42
  cardiac — *see* Insufficiency, myocardial

Deficiency, deficient — *continued*
  carnitine E71.40
    due to
      hemodialysis E71.43
      inborn errors of metabolism E71.42
      Valproic acid therapy E71.43
    iatrogenic E71.43
    muscle palmityltransferase E71.314
    primary E71.41
    secondary E71.448
  carotene E50.9
  central nervous system G96.8
  ceruloplasmin (Wilson) E83.01
  choline E53.8
  Christmas factor D67
  chromium E61.4
  clotting (blood) (*see also* Deficiency,
    coagulation factor) D68.9
  clotting factor NEC (hereditary) (*see also*
    Deficiency, factor) D68.2
  coagulation NOS D68.9
    with
      ectopic pregnancy O08.1
      molar pregnancy O08.1
    acquired (any) D68.4
    antepartum hemorrhage — *see* Hemorrhage,
      antepartum, with coagulation defect
    clotting factor NEC (*see also* Deficiency,
      factor) D68.2
    due to
      hyperprothrombinemia D68.4
      liver disease D68.4
      vitamin K deficiency D68.4
    newborn, transient P61.6
    postpartum O72.3
    specified NEC D68.8
  cognitive F09
  color vision H53.50
    achromatopsia H53.51
    acquired H53.52
    deuteranomaly H53.53
    protanomaly H53.54
    specified type NEC H53.59
    tritanomaly H53.55
  combined glucocorticoid and mineralocorticoid
    E27.49
  contact factor D68.2
  copper (nutritional) E61.0
  corticoadrenal E27.40
    primary E27.1
  craniofacial axis Q75.0
  cyanocobalamin E53.8
  debrancher enzyme (limit dextrinosis) E74.03
  dehydrogenase
    long chain/very long chain acyl CoA
      E71.310
    medium chain acyl CoA E71.311
    short chain acyl CoA E71.312
  diet E63.9
  dihydropyrimidine dehydrogenase (DPD)
    E88.89
  disaccharidase E73.9
  edema — *see* Malnutrition, severe
  endocrine E34.9
  energy-supply — *see* Malnutrition
  enzymes, circulating NEC E88.09
  ergosterol E55.9
    with
      adult osteomalacia M83.8
      rickets — *see* Rickets
  essential fatty acid (EFA) E63.0
  factor — *see also* Deficiency, coagulation
    I (congenital) (hereditary) D68.2
    II (congenital) (hereditary) D68.2
    V (congenital) (hereditary) D68.2
    VII (congenital) (hereditary) D68.2
    VIII (congenital) (functional) (hereditary)
      (with functional defect) D66
      with vascular defect D68.0

Deficiency, deficient — *continued*

factor — *see also* Deficiency, coagulation — *continued*
  IX (congenital) (functional) (hereditary) (with functional defect) D67
  X (congenital) (hereditary) D68.2
  XI (congenital) (hereditary) D68.1
  XII (congenital) (hereditary) D68.2
  XIII (congenital) (hereditary) D68.2
  Hageman D68.2
  multiple (congenital) D68.8
    acquired D68.4
femoral, proximal focal (congenital) — *see* Defect, reduction, lower limb, longitudinal, femur
fibrin-stabilizing factor (congenital) (hereditary) D68.2
  acquired D68.4
fibrinase D68.2
fibrinogen (congenital) (hereditary) D68.2
  acquired D65
folate E53.8
folic acid E53.8
foreskin N47.3
fructokinase E74.11
fructose 1,6-diphosphatase E74.19
fructose-1-phosphate aldolase E74.19
galactokinase E74.29
galactose-1-phosphate uridyl transferase E74.29
gammaglobulin in blood D80.1
  hereditary D80.0
glass factor D68.2
glucocorticoid E27.49
  mineralocorticoid E27.49
glucose-6-phosphatase E74.01
glucose-6-phosphate dehydrogenase anemia D55.0
glucuronyl transferase E80.5
glycogen synthetase E74.09
gonadotropin (isolated) E23.0
growth hormone (idiopathic) (isolated) E23.0
Hageman factor D68.2
hemoglobin D64.9
hepatophosphorylase E74.09
homogentisate 1,2-dioxygenase E70.29
hormone
  anterior pituitary (partial) NEC E23.0
    growth E23.0
  growth (isolated) E23.0
  pituitary E23.0
  testicular E29.1
hypoxanthine-(guanine)-phosphoribosyltransferase (HG-PRT) (total H-PRT) E79.1
immunity D84.9
  cell-mediated D84.8
    with thrombocytopenia and eczema D82.0
  combined D81.9
  humoral D80.9
  IgA (secretory) D80.2
  IgG D80.3
  IgM D80.4
immuno — *see* Immunodeficiency
immunoglobulin, selective
  A (IgA) D80.2
  G (IgG) (subclasses) D80.3
  M (IgM) D80.4
inositol (B complex) E53.8
intrinsic
  factor (congenital) D51.0
  sphincter N36.42
    with urethral hypermobility N36.43
iodine E61.8
  congenital syndrome — *see* Syndrome, iodine-deficiency, congenital
iron E61.1
  anemia D50.9
kalium E87.6
kappa-light chain D80.8

labile factor (congenital) (hereditary) D68.2
  acquired D68.4
lacrimal fluid (acquired) — *see also* Syndrome, dry eye
  congenital Q10.6
lactase
  congenital E73.0
  secondary E73.1
Laki-Lorand factor D68.2
lecithin cholesterol acyltransferase E78.6
lipocaic K86.89
lipoprotein (familial) (high density) E78.6
liver phosphorylase E74.09
lysosomal alpha-1, 4 glucosidase E74.02
magnesium E61.2
major histocompatibility complex
  class I D81.6
  class II D81.7
manganese E61.3
menadione (vitamin K) E56.1
  newborn P53
mental (familial) (hereditary) — *see* Disability, intellectual
methylenetetrahydrofolate reductase (MTHFR) E72.12
mevalonate kinase M04.1
mineral NEC E61.8
mineralocorticoid E27.49
  with glucocorticoid E27.49
molybdenum (nutritional) E61.5
moral F60.2
multiple nutrient elements E61.7
muscle
  carnitine (palmityltransferase) E71.314
  phosphofructokinase E74.09
myoadenylate deaminase E79.2
myocardial — *see* Insufficiency, myocardial
myophosphorylase E74.04
NADH diaphorase or reductase (congenital) D74.0
NADH-methemoglobin reductase (congenital) D74.0
natrium E87.1
niacin (amide) (-tryptophan) E52
nicotinamide E52
nicotinic acid E52
number of teeth — *see* Anodontia
nutrient element E61.9
  multiple E61.7
  specified NEC E61.8
nutrition, nutritional E63.9
  sequelae — *see* Sequelae, nutritional deficiency
  specified NEC E63.8
of interleukin 1 receptor antagonist [DIRA] M04.8
ornithine transcarbamylase E72.4
ovarian E28.39
oxygen — *see* Anoxia
pantothenic acid E53.8
parathyroid (gland) E20.9
perineum (female) N81.89
phenylalanine hydroxylase E70.1
phosphoenolpyruvate carboxykinase E74.4
phosphofructokinase E74.19
phosphomannomutase E74.8
phosphomannose isomerase E74.8
phosphomannosyl mutase E74.8
phosphorylase kinase, liver E74.09
pituitary hormone (isolated) E23.0
plasma thromboplastin
  antecedent (PTA) D68.1
  component (PTC) D67
platelet NEC D69.1
  constitutional D68.0
polyglandular E31.8
  autoimmune E31.0
potassium (K) E87.6

prepuce N47.3
proaccelerin (congenital) (hereditary) D68.2
  acquired D68.4
proconvertin factor (congenital) (hereditary) D68.2
  acquired D68.4
protein (*see also* Malnutrition) E46
  anemia D53.0
  C D68.59
  S D68.59
prothrombin (congenital) (hereditary) D68.2
  acquired D68.4
Prower factor D68.2
pseudocholinesterase E88.09
PTA (plasma thromboplastin antecedent) D68.1
PTC (plasma thromboplastin component) D67
purine nucleoside phosphorylase (PNP) D81.5
pyracin (alpha) (beta) E53.1
pyridoxal E53.1
pyridoxamine E53.1
pyridoxine (derivatives) E53.1
pyruvate
  carboxylase E74.4
  dehydrogenase E74.4
riboflavin (vitamin B2) E53.0
salt E87.1
secretion
  ovary E28.39
  salivary gland (any) K11.7
  urine R34
selenium (dietary) E59
serum antitrypsin, familial E88.01
short stature homeobox gene (SHOX)
  with
    dyschondrosteosis Q78.8
    short stature (idiopathic) E34.3
    Turner's syndrome Q96.9
sodium (Na) E87.1
SPCA (factor VII) D68.2
sphincter, intrinsic N36.42
  with urethral hypermobility N36.43
stable factor (congenital) (hereditary) D68.2
  acquired D68.4
Stuart-Prower (factor X) D68.2
sucrase E74.39
sulfatase E75.29
sulfite oxidase E72.19
thiamin, thiaminic (chloride) E51.9
  beriberi (dry) E51.11
    wet E51.12
thrombokinase D68.2
  newborn P53
thyroid (gland) — *see* Hypothyroidism
tocopherol E56.0
tooth bud K00.0
transcobalamine II (anemia) D51.2
vanadium E61.6
vascular I99.9
vasopressin E23.2
vertical ridge K06.8
viosterol — *see* Deficiency, calciferol
vitamin (multiple) NOS E56.9
  A E50.9
    with
      Bitot's spot (corneal) E50.1
      follicular keratosis E50.8
      keratomalacia E50.4
      manifestations NEC E50.8
      night blindness E50.5
      scar of cornea, xerophthalmic E50.6
      xeroderma E50.8
      xerophthalmia E50.7
      xerosis
        conjunctival E50.0
          and Bitot's spot E50.1
        cornea E50.2
          and ulceration E50.3
      sequelae E64.1

Deficiency, deficient — *continued*
- vitamin (multiple) NOS E56.9 — *continued*
  - B (complex) NOS E53.9
    - with
      - beriberi (dry) E51.11
        - wet E51.12
      - pellagra E52
  - B1 NOS E51.9
    - beriberi (dry) E51.11
      - with circulatory system manifestations E51.11
      - wet E51.12
  - B12 E53.8
  - B2 (riboflavin) E53.0
  - B6 E53.1
  - C E54
    - sequelae E64.2
  - D E55.9
    - with
      - adult osteomalacia M83.8
      - rickets — *see* Rickets
    - 25-hydroxylase E83.32
  - E E56.0
  - folic acid E53.8
  - G E53.0
  - group B E53.9
    - specified NEC E53.8
  - H (biotin) E53.8
  - K E56.1
    - of newborn P53
  - nicotinic E52
  - P E56.8
  - PP (pellagra-preventing) E52
  - specified NEC E56.8
  - thiamin E51.9
    - beriberi — *see* Beriberi
- zinc, dietary E60

Deficit — *see also* Deficiency
- attention and concentration R41.840
  - disorder — *see* Attention, deficit
  - following
    - cerebral infarction I69.310
    - cerebrovascular disease I69.910
      - specified disease NEC I69.810
    - nontraumatic
      - intracerebral hemorrhage I69.110
      - specified intracranial hemorrhage NEC I69.210
      - subarachnoid hemorrhage I69.010
- cognitive
  - communication R41.841
  - emotional
    - following
      - cerebral infarction I69.315
      - cerebrovascular disease I69.915
        - specified disease NEC I69.815
      - nontraumatic
        - intracerebral hemorrhage I69.115
        - specified intracranial hemorrhage NEC I69.215
        - subarachnoid hemorrhage I69.015
  - following
    - cerebral infarction I69.319
    - cerebrovascular disease I69.919
      - specified disease NEC I69.819
    - nontraumatic
      - intracerebral hemorrhage I69.119
      - specified intracranial hemorrhage NEC I69.219
      - subarachnoid hemorrhage I69.019
  - social
    - following
      - cerebral infarction I69.315
      - cerebrovascular disease I69.915
        - specified disease NEC I69.815
      - nontraumatic
        - intracerebral hemorrhage I69.115
        - specified intracranial hemorrhage NEC I69.215
        - subarachnoid hemorrhage I69.015

Deficit — *see also* Deficiency — *continued*
- cognitive NEC R41.89
  - following
    - cerebral infarction I69.318
    - cerebrovascular disease I69.918
      - specified disease NEC I69.818
    - nontraumatic
      - intracerebral hemorrhage I69.118
      - specified intracranial hemorrhage NEC I69.218
      - subarachnoid hemorrhage I69.018
- concentration R41.840
- executive function R41.844
  - following
    - cerebral infarction I69.314
    - cerebrovascular disease I69.914
      - specified disease NEC I69.814
    - nontraumatic
      - intracerebral hemorrhage I69.114
      - specified intracranial hemorrhage NEC I69.214
      - subarachnoid hemorrhage I69.014
- frontal lobe R41.844
  - following
    - cerebral infarction I69.314
    - cerebrovascular disease I69.914
      - specified disease NEC I69.814
    - nontraumatic
      - intracerebral hemorrhage I69.114
      - specified intracranial hemorrhage NEC I69.214
      - subarachnoid hemorrhage I69.014
- memory
  - following
    - cerebral infarction I69.311
    - cerebrovascular disease I69.911
      - specified disease NEC I69.811
    - nontraumatic
      - intracerebral hemorrhage I69.111
      - specified intracranial hemorrhage NEC I69.211
      - subarachnoid hemorrhage I69.011
- neurologic NEC R29.818
  - ischemic
    - reversible (RIND) I63.9
    - prolonged (PRIND) I63.9
- oxygen R09.02
- prolonged reversible ischemic neurologic (PRIND) I63.9
- psychomotor R41.843
  - following
    - cerebral infarction I69.313
    - cerebrovascular disease I69.913
      - specified disease NEC I69.813
    - nontraumatic
      - intracerebral hemorrhage I69.113
      - specified intracranial hemorrhage NEC I69.213
      - subarachnoid hemorrhage I69.013
- visuospatial R41.842
  - following
    - cerebral infarction I69.312
    - cerebrovascular disease I69.912
      - specified disease NEC I69.812
    - nontraumatic
      - intracerebral hemorrhage I69.112
      - specified intracranial hemorrhage NEC I69.212
      - subarachnoid hemorrhage I69.012

Deflection
- radius — *see* Deformity, limb, specified type NEC, forearm
- septum (acquired) (nasal) (nose) J34.2
- spine — *see* Curvature, spine
- turbinate (nose) J34.2

Defluvium
- capillorum — *see* Alopecia
- ciliorum — *see* Madarosis
- unguium L60.8

Deformity Q89.9
- abdomen, congenital Q89.9
- abdominal wall
  - acquired M95.8
  - congenital Q79.59
- acquired (unspecified site) M95.9
- adrenal gland Q89.1
- alimentary tract, congenital Q45.9
  - upper Q40.9
- ankle (joint) (acquired) — *see also* Deformity, limb, lower leg
  - abduction — *see* Contraction, joint, ankle
  - congenital Q68.8
  - contraction — *see* Contraction, joint, ankle
  - specified type NEC — *see* Deformity, limb, foot, specified NEC
- anus (acquired) K62.89
  - congenital Q43.9
- aorta (arch) (congenital) Q25.40
  - acquired I77.89
- aortic
  - arch, acquired I77.89
  - cusp or valve (congenital) Q23.8
    - acquired (*see also* Endocarditis, aortic) I35.8
- arm (acquired) (upper) — *see also* Deformity, limb, upper arm
  - congenital Q68.8
  - forearm — *see* Deformity, limb, forearm
- artery (congenital) (peripheral) NOS Q27.9
  - acquired I77.89
  - coronary (acquired) I25.9
    - congenital Q24.5
  - umbilical Q27.0
- atrial septal Q21.1
- auditory canal (external) (congenital) — *see also* Malformation, ear, external
  - acquired — *see* Disorder, ear, external, specified type NEC
- auricle
  - ear (congenital) — *see also* Malformation, ear, external
    - acquired — *see* Disorder, pinna, deformity
- back — *see* Dorsopathy, deforming
- bile duct (common) (congenital) (hepatic) Q44.5
  - acquired K83.8
- biliary duct or passage (congenital) Q44.5
  - acquired K83.8
- bladder (neck) (trigone) (sphincter) (acquired) N32.89
  - congenital Q64.79
- bone (acquired) NOS M95.9
  - congenital Q79.9
  - turbinate M95.0
- brain (congenital) Q04.9
  - acquired G93.89
  - reduction Q04.3
- breast (acquired) N64.89
  - congenital Q83.9
  - reconstructed N65.0
- bronchus (congenital) Q32.4
  - acquired NEC J98.09
- bursa, congenital Q79.9
- canaliculi (lacrimalis) (acquired) — *see also* Disorder, lacrimal system, changes
  - congenital Q10.6
- canthus, acquired — *see* Disorder, eyelid, specified type NEC
- capillary (acquired) I78.8
- cardiovascular system, congenital Q28.9
- caruncle, lacrimal (acquired) — *see also* Disorder, lacrimal system, changes
  - congenital Q10.6
- cascade, stomach K31.2
- cecum (congenital) Q43.9
  - acquired K63.89
- cerebral, acquired G93.89
  - congenital Q04.9

DISEASE INDEX

Deformity Q89.9 — *continued*
  cervix (uterus) (acquired) NEC N88.8
    congenital Q51.9
  cheek (acquired) M95.2
    congenital Q18.9
  chest (acquired) (wall) M95.4
    congenital Q67.8
    sequelae (late effect) of rickets E64.3
  chin (acquired) M95.2
    congenital Q18.9
  choroid (congenital) Q14.3
    acquired H31.8
    plexus Q07.8
      acquired G96.19
  cicatricial — *see* Cicatrix
  cilia, acquired — *see* Disorder, eyelid,
    specified type NEC
  clavicle (acquired) M95.8
    congenital Q68.8
  clitoris (congenital) Q52.6
    acquired N90.89
  clubfoot — *see* Clubfoot
  coccyx (acquired) — *see* subcategory M43.8
  colon (congenital) Q43.9
    acquired K63.89
  concha (ear), congenital — *see also*
    Malformation, ear, external
    acquired — *see* Disorder, pinna, deformity
  cornea (acquired) H18.70
    congenital Q13.4
    descemetocele — *see* Descemetocele
    ectasia — *see* Ectasia, cornea
    specified NEC H18.79-
    staphyloma — *see* Staphyloma, cornea
  coronary artery (acquired) I25.9
    congenital Q24.5
  cranium (acquired) — *see* Deformity, skull
  cricoid cartilage (congenital) Q31.8
    acquired J38.7
  cystic duct (congenital) Q44.5
    acquired K82.8
  Dandy-Walker Q03.1
    with spina bifida — *see* Spina bifida
  diaphragm (congenital) Q79.1
    acquired J98.6
  digestive organ NOS Q45.9
  ductus arteriosus Q25.0
  duodenal bulb K31.89
  duodenum (congenital) Q43.9
    acquired K31.89
  dura — *see* Deformity, meninges
  ear (acquired) — *see also* Disorder, pinna,
    deformity
    congenital (external) Q17.9
      internal Q16.5
      middle Q16.4
        ossicles Q16.3
      ossicles Q16.3
  ectodermal (congenital) NEC Q84.9
  ejaculatory duct (congenital) Q55.4
    acquired N50.89
  elbow (joint) (acquired) — *see also* Deformity,
    limb, upper arm
    congenital Q68.8
    contraction — *see* Contraction, joint, elbow
  endocrine gland NEC Q89.2
  epididymis (congenital) Q55.4
    acquired N50.89
  epiglottis (congenital) Q31.8
    acquired J38.7
  esophagus (congenital) Q39.9
    acquired K22.8
  eustachian tube (congenital) NEC Q17.8
  eye, congenital Q15.9
  eyebrow (congenital) Q18.8
  eyelid (acquired) — *see also* Disorder, eyelid,
    specified type NEC
    congenital Q10.3

Deformity Q89.9 — *continued*
  face (acquired) M95.2
    congenital Q18.9
  fallopian tube, acquired N83.8
  femur (acquired) — *see* Deformity, limb,
    specified type NEC, thigh
  fetal
    with fetopelvic disproportion O33.7
    causing obstructed labor O66.3
  finger (acquired) M20.00-
    boutonniere M20.02-
    congenital Q68.1
    flexion contracture — *see* Contraction, joint,
      hand
    mallet finger M20.01-
    specified NEC M20.09-
    swan-neck M20.03-
  flexion (joint) (acquired) (*see also* Deformity,
    limb, flexion) M21.20
    congenital NOS Q74.9
      hip Q65.89
  foot (acquired) — *see also* Deformity, limb,
    lower leg
    cavovarus (congenital) Q66.1
    congenital NOS Q66.9
      specified type NEC Q66.89
    specified type NEC — *see* Deformity, limb,
      foot, specified NEC
    valgus (congenital) Q66.6
      acquired — *see* Deformity, valgus, ankle
    varus (congenital) NEC Q66.3
      acquired — *see* Deformity, varus, ankle
  forearm (acquired) — *see also* Deformity, limb,
    forearm
    congenital Q68.8
  forehead (acquired) M95.2
    congenital Q75.8
  frontal bone (acquired) M95.2
    congenital Q75.8
  gallbladder (congenital) Q44.1
    acquired K82.8
  gastrointestinal tract (congenital) NOS Q45.9
    acquired K63.89
  genitalia, genital organ(s) or system NEC
    female (congenital) Q52.9
      acquired N94.89
      external Q52.70
    male (congenital) Q55.9
      acquired N50.89
  globe (eye) (congenital) Q15.8
    acquired H44.89
  gum, acquired NEC K06.8
  hand (acquired) — *see* Deformity, limb, hand
    congenital Q68.1
  head (acquired) M95.2
    congenital Q75.8
  heart (congenital) Q24.9
    septum Q21.9
      auricular Q21.1
      ventricular Q21.0
    valve (congenital) NEC Q24.8
      acquired — *see* Endocarditis
  heel (acquired) — *see* Deformity, foot
  hepatic duct (congenital) Q44.5
    acquired K83.8
  hip (joint) (acquired) — *see also* Deformity,
    limb, thigh
    congenital Q65.9
    due to (previous) juvenile osteochondrosis —
      see Coxa, plana
    flexion — *see* Contraction, joint, hip
  hourglass — *see* Contraction, hourglass
  humerus (acquired) M21.82-
    congenital Q74.0
  hypophyseal (congenital) Q89.2
  ileocecal (coil) (valve) (acquired) K63.89
    congenital Q43.9
  ileum (congenital) Q43.9
    acquired K63.89

Deformity Q89.9 — *continued*
  ilium (acquired) M95.5
    congenital Q74.2
  integument (congenital) Q84.9
  intervertebral cartilage or disc (acquired) —
    see Disorder, disc, specified NEC
  intestine (large) (small) (congenital) NOS
    Q43.9
    acquired K63.89
  intrinsic minus or plus (hand) — *see* Deformity,
    limb, specified type NEC, forearm
  iris (acquired) H21.89
    congenital Q13.2
  ischium (acquired) M95.5
    congenital Q74.2
  jaw (acquired) (congenital) M26.9
  joint (acquired) NEC M21.90
    congenital Q68.8
    elbow M21.92-
    hand M21.94-
    hip M21.95-
    knee M21.96-
    shoulder M21.92-
    wrist M21.93-
  kidney(s) (calyx) (pelvis) (congenital) Q63.9
    acquired N28.89
    artery (congenital) Q27.2
      acquired I77.89
  Klippel-Feil (brevicollis) Q76.1
  knee (acquired) NEC — *see also* Deformity,
    limb, lower leg
    congenital Q68.2
  labium (majus) (minus) (congenital) Q52.79
    acquired N90.89
  lacrimal passages or duct (congenital) NEC
    Q10.6
    acquired — *see* Disorder, lacrimal system,
      changes
  larynx (muscle) (congenital) Q31.8
    acquired J38.7
    web (glottic) Q31.0
  leg (upper) (acquired) NEC — *see also*
    Deformity, limb, thigh
    congenital Q68.8
    lower leg — *see* Deformity, limb, lower leg
  lens (acquired) H27.8
    congenital Q12.9
  lid (fold) (acquired) — *see also* Disorder, eyelid,
    specified type NEC
    congenital Q10.3
  ligament (acquired) — *see* Disorder, ligament
    congenital Q79.9
  limb (acquired) M21.90
    clawfoot M21.53-
    clawhand M21.51-
    clubfoot M21.54-
    clubhand M21.52-
    congenital, except reduction deformity
      Q74.9
    flat foot M21.4-
    flexion M21.20
      ankle M21.27-
      elbow M21.22-
      finger M21.24-
      hip M21.25-
      knee M21.26-
      shoulder M21.21-
      toe M21.27-
      wrist M21.23-
    foot
      claw — *see* Deformity, limb, clawfoot
      club — *see* Deformity, limb, clubfoot
      drop M21.37-
      flat — *see* Deformity, limb, flat foot
      specified NEC M21.6x-
    forearm M21.93-
    hand M21.94-
    lower leg M21.96-

Deformity Q89.9 — *continued*
  limb (acquired) M21.90 — *continued*
    specified type NEC M21.80
      forearm M21.83-
      lower leg M21.86-
      thigh M21.85-
      upper arm M21.82-
    thigh M21.95-
    unequal length M21.70
      short site is
        femur M21.75-
        fibula M21.76-
        humerus M21.72-
        radius M21.73-
        tibia M21.76-
        ulna M21.73-
    upper arm M21.92-
    valgus — *see* Deformity, valgus
    varus — *see* Deformity, varus
    wrist drop M21.33-
  lip (acquired) NEC K13.0
    congenital Q38.0
  liver (congenital) Q44.7
    acquired K76.89
  lumbosacral (congenital) (joint) (region) Q76.49
    acquired — *see* subcategory M43.8
    kyphosis — *see* Kyphosis, congenital
    lordosis — *see* Lordosis, congenital
  lung (congenital) Q33.9
    acquired J98.4
  lymphatic system, congenital Q89.9
  Madelung's (radius) Q74.0
  mandible (acquired) (congenital) M26.9
  maxilla (acquired) (congenital) M26.9
  meninges or membrane (congenital) Q07.9
    cerebral Q04.8
      acquired G96.19
    spinal cord (congenital) G96.19
      acquired G96.19
  metacarpus (acquired) — *see* Deformity, limb, forearm
    congenital Q74.0
  metatarsus (acquired) — *see* Deformity, foot
    congenital Q66.9
  middle ear (congenital) Q16.4
    ossicles Q16.3
  mitral (leaflets) (valve) I05.8
    parachute Q23.2
    stenosis, congenital Q23.2
  mouth (acquired) K13.79
    congenital Q38.6
  multiple, congenital NEC Q89.7
  muscle (acquired) M62.89
    congenital Q79.9
      sternocleidomastoid Q68.0
  musculoskeletal system (acquired) M95.9
    congenital Q79.9
    specified NEC M95.8
  nail (acquired) L60.8
    congenital Q84.6
  nasal — *see* Deformity, nose
  neck (acquired) M95.3
    congenital Q18.9
      sternocleidomastoid Q68.0
  nervous system (congenital) Q07.9
  nipple (congenital) Q83.9
    acquired N64.89
  nose (acquired) (cartilage) M95.0
    bone (turbinate) M95.0
    congenital Q30.9
      bent or squashed Q67.4
    saddle M95.0
      syphilitic A50.57
    septum (acquired) J34.2
      congenital Q30.8
    sinus (wall) (congenital) Q30.8
      acquired M95.0

Deformity Q89.9 — *continued*
  nose (acquired) (cartilage) M95.0 — *continued*
    syphilitic (congenital) A50.57
      late A52.73
  ocular muscle (congenital) Q10.3
    acquired — *see* Strabismus, mechanical
  opticociliary vessels (congenital) Q13.2
  orbit (eye) (acquired) H05.30
    atrophy — *see* Atrophy, orbit
    congenital Q10.7
    due to
      bone disease NEC H05.32-
      trauma or surgery H05.33-
    enlargement — *see* Enlargement, orbit
    exostosis — *see* Exostosis, orbit
  organ of Corti (congenital) Q16.5
  ovary (congenital) Q50.39
    acquired N83.8
  oviduct, acquired N83.8
  palate (congenital) Q38.5
    acquired M27.8
    cleft (congenital) — *see* Cleft, palate
  pancreas (congenital) Q45.3
    acquired K86.89
  parathyroid (gland) Q89.2
  parotid (gland) (congenital) Q38.4
    acquired K11.8
  patella (acquired) — *see* Disorder, patella, specified NEC
  pelvis, pelvic (acquired) (bony) M95.5
    with disproportion (fetopelvic) O33.0
      causing obstructed labor O65.0
    congenital Q74.2
    rachitic sequelae (late effect) E64.3
  penis (glans) (congenital) Q55.69
    acquired N48.89
  pericardium (congenital) Q24.8
    acquired — *see* Pericarditis
  pharynx (congenital) Q38.8
    acquired J39.2
  pinna, acquired — *see also* Disorder, pinna, deformity
    congenital Q17.9
  pituitary (congenital) Q89.2
  posture — *see* Dorsopathy, deforming
  prepuce (congenital) Q55.69
    acquired N47.8
  prostate (congenital) Q55.4
    acquired N42.89
  pupil (congenital) Q13.2
    acquired — *see* Abnormality, pupillary
  pylorus (congenital) Q40.3
    acquired K31.89
  rachitic (acquired), old or healed E64.3
  radius (acquired) — *see also* Deformity, limb, forearm
    congenital Q68.8
  rectum (congenital) Q43.9
    acquired K62.89
  reduction (extremity) (limb), congenital (*see also* condition and site) Q73.8
    brain Q04.3
    lower — *see* Defect, reduction, lower limb
    upper — *see* Defect, reduction, upper limb
  renal — *see* Deformity, kidney
  respiratory system (congenital) Q34.9
  rib (acquired) M95.4
    congenital Q76.6
      cervical Q76.5
  rotation (joint) (acquired) — *see* Deformity, limb, specified site NEC
    congenital Q74.9
    hip — *see* Deformity, limb, specified type NEC, thigh
      congenital Q65.89
  sacroiliac joint (congenital) Q74.2
    acquired — *see* subcategory M43.8

Deformity Q89.9 — *continued*
  sacrum (acquired) — *see* subcategory M43.8
  saddle
    back — *see* Lordosis
    nose M95.0
      syphilitic A50.57
  salivary gland or duct (congenital) Q38.4
    acquired K11.8
  scapula (acquired) M95.8
    congenital Q68.8
  scrotum (congenital) — *see also* Malformation, testis and scrotum
    acquired N50.89
  seminal vesicles (congenital) Q55.4
    acquired N50.89
  septum, nasal (acquired) J34.2
  shoulder (joint) (acquired) — *see* Deformity, limb, upper arm
    congenital Q74.0
    contraction — *see* Contraction, joint, shoulder
  sigmoid (flexure) (congenital) Q43.9
    acquired K63.89
  skin (congenital) Q82.9
  skull (acquired) M95.2
    congenital Q75.8
    with
      anencephaly Q00.0
      encephalocele — *see* Encephalocele
      hydrocephalus Q03.9
        with spina bifida — *see* Spina bifida, by site, with hydrocephalus
      microcephaly Q02
  soft parts, organs or tissues (of pelvis)
    in pregnancy or childbirth NEC O34.8-
      causing obstructed labor O65.5
  spermatic cord (congenital) Q55.4
    acquired N50.89
    torsion — *see* Torsion, spermatic cord
  spinal — *see* Dorsopathy, deforming
    column (acquired) — *see* Dorsopathy, deforming
    congenital Q67.5
    cord (congenital) Q06.9
      acquired G95.89
    nerve root (congenital) Q07.9
  spine (acquired) — *see also* Dorsopathy, deforming
    congenital Q67.5
    rachitic E64.3
    specified NEC — *see* Dorsopathy, deforming, specified NEC
  spleen
    acquired D73.89
    congenital Q89.09
  Sprengel's (congenital) Q74.0
  sternocleidomastoid (muscle), congenital Q68.0
  sternum (acquired) M95.4
    congenital NEC Q76.7
  stomach (congenital) Q40.3
    acquired K31.89
  submandibular gland (congenital) Q38.4
  submaxillary gland (congenital) Q38.4
    acquired K11.8
  talipes — *see* Talipes
  testis (congenital) — *see also* Malformation, testis and scrotum
    acquired N44.8
    torsion — *see* Torsion, testis
  thigh (acquired) — *see also* Deformity, limb, thigh
    congenital NEC Q68.8
  thorax (acquired) (wall) M95.4
    congenital Q67.8
    sequelae of rickets E64.3
  thumb (acquired) — *see also* Deformity, finger
    congenital NEC Q68.1

D I S E A S E   I N D E X

Deformity Q89.9 — *continued*
thymus (tissue) (congenital) Q89.2
thyroid (gland) (congenital) Q89.2
  cartilage Q31.8
    acquired J38.7
tibia (acquired) — *see also* Deformity, limb,
    specified type NEC, lower leg
  congenital NEC Q68.8
  saber (syphilitic) A50.56
toe (acquired) M20.6-
  congenital Q66.9
  hallux rigidus M20.2-
  hallux valgus M20.1-
  hallux varus M20.3-
  hammer toe M20.4-
  specified NEC M20.5x-
tongue (congenital) Q38.3
  acquired K14.8
tooth, teeth K00.2
trachea (rings) (congenital) Q32.1
  acquired J39.8
transverse aortic arch (congenital) Q25.49
tricuspid (leaflets) (valve) I07.8
  atresia or stenosis Q22.4
  Ebstein's Q22.5
trunk (acquired) M95.8
  congenital Q89.9
ulna (acquired) — *see also* Deformity, limb,
    forearm
  congenital NEC Q68.8
urachus, congenital Q64.4
ureter (opening) (congenital) Q62.8
  acquired N28.89
urethra (congenital) Q64.79
  acquired N36.8
urinary tract (congenital) Q64.9
  urachus Q64.4
uterus (congenital) Q51.9
  acquired N85.8
uvula (congenital) Q38.5
vagina (acquired) N89.8
  congenital Q52.4
valgus NEC M21.00
  ankle M21.07-
  elbow M21.02-
  hip M21.05-
  knee M21.06-
valve, valvular (congenital) (heart) Q24.8
  acquired — *see* Endocarditis
varus NEC M21.10
  ankle M21.17-
  elbow M21.12-
  hip M21.15-
  knee M21.16-
  tibia — *see* Osteochondrosis, juvenile, tibia
vas deferens (congenital) Q55.4
  acquired N50.89
vein (congenital) Q27.9
  great Q26.9
vertebra — *see* Dorsopathy, deforming
vertical talus (congenital) Q66.80
  left foot Q66.82
  right foot Q66.81
vesicourethral orifice (acquired) N32.89
  congenital NEC Q64.79
vessels of optic papilla (congenital) Q14.2
visual field (contraction) — *see* Defect, visual
    field
vitreous body, acquired H43.89
vulva (congenital) Q52.79
  acquired N90.89
wrist (joint) (acquired) — *see also* Deformity,
    limb, forearm
  congenital Q68.8
  contraction — *see* Contraction, joint, wrist

Degeneration, degenerative
adrenal (capsule) (fatty) (gland) (hyaline)
  (infectional) E27.8
amyloid (*see also* Amyloidosis) E85.9
anterior cornua, spinal cord G12.29
anterior labral S43.49-
aorta, aortic I70.0
  fatty I77.89
aortic valve (heart) — *see* Endocarditis, aortic
arteriovascular — *see* Arteriosclerosis
artery, arterial (atheromatous) (calcareous) —
  see also Arteriosclerosis
  cerebral, amyloid E85.4 [I68.0]
  medial — *see* Arteriosclerosis, extremities
articular cartilage NEC — *see* Derangement,
  joint, articular cartilage, by site
atheromatous — *see* Arteriosclerosis
basal nuclei or ganglia G23.9
  specified NEC G23.8
bone NEC — *see* Disorder, bone, specified
  type NEC
brachial plexus G54.0
brain (cortical) (progressive) G31.9
  alcoholic G31.2
  arteriosclerotic I67.2
  childhood G31.9
    specified NEC G31.89
  cystic G31.89
    congenital Q04.6
  in
    alcoholism G31.2
    beriberi E51.2
    cerebrovascular disease I67.9
    congenital hydrocephalus Q03.9
      with spina bifida — *see also* Spina bifida
    Fabry-Anderson disease E75.21
    Gaucher's disease E75.22
    Hunter's syndrome E76.1
    lipidosis
      cerebral E75.4
      generalized E75.6
    mucopolysaccharidosis — *see*
      Mucopolysaccharidosis
    myxedema E03.9 [G32.89]
    neoplastic disease (*see also* Neoplasm)
      D49.6 [G32.89]
    Niemann-Pick disease E75.249 [G32.89]
    sphingolipidosis E75.3 [G32.89]
    vitamin B12 deficiency E53.8 [G32.89]
  senile NEC G31.1
breast N64.89
Bruch's membrane — *see* Degeneration,
  choroid
capillaries (fatty) I78.8
  amyloid E85.8 [I79.8]
cardiac — *see also* Degeneration, myocardial
  valve, valvular — *see* Endocarditis
cardiorenal — *see* Hypertension, cardiorenal
cardiovascular — *see also* Disease,
  cardiovascular
  renal — *see* Hypertension, cardiorenal
cerebellar NOS G31.9
  alcoholic G31.2
  primary (hereditary) (sporadic) G11.9
cerebral — *see* Degeneration, brain
cerebrovascular I67.9
  due to hypertension I67.4
cervical plexus G54.2
cervix N88.8
  due to radiation (intended effect) N88.8
    adverse effect or misadventure N99.89
chamber angle H21.21-
changes, spine or vertebra — *see* Spondylosis
chorioretinal — *see also* Degeneration, choroid
  hereditary H31.20
choroid (colloid) (drusen) H31.10-
  atrophy — *see* Atrophy, choroidal
  hereditary — *see* Dystrophy, choroidal,
    hereditary

Degeneration, degenerative — *continued*
ciliary body H21.22-
cochlear — *see* subcategory H83.8
combined (spinal cord) (subacute) E53.8
  [G32.0]
  with anemia (pernicious) D51.0 [G32.0]
    due to dietary vitamin B12 deficiency
      D51.3 [G32.0]
  in (due to)
    vitamin B12 deficiency E53.8 [G32.0]
      anemia D51.9 [G32.0]
conjunctiva H11.10
  concretions — *see* Concretion, conjunctiva
  deposits — *see* Deposit, conjunctiva
  pigmentations — *see* Pigmentation,
    conjunctiva
  pinguecula — *see* Pinguecula
  xerosis — *see* Xerosis, conjunctiva
cornea H18.40
  calcerous H18.43
    band keratopathy H18.42-
  familial, hereditary — *see* Dystrophy, cornea
  hyaline (of old scars) H18.49
  keratomalacia — *see* Keratomalacia
  nodular H18.45-
  peripheral H18.46-
  senile H18.41-
  specified type NEC H18.49
cortical (cerebellar) (parenchymatous) G31.89
  alcoholic G31.2
  diffuse, due to arteriopathy I67.2
corticobasal G31.85
cutis L98.8
  amyloid E85.4 [L99]
dental pulp K04.2
disc disease — *see* Degeneration,
  intervertebral disc NEC
dorsolateral (spinal cord) — *see* Degeneration,
  combined
extrapyramidal G25.9
eye, macular — *see also* Degeneration, macula
  congenital or hereditary — *see* Dystrophy,
    retina
facet joints — *see* Spondylosis
fatty
  liver NEC K76.0
    alcoholic K70.0
grey matter (brain) (Alpers') G31.81
heart — *see also* Degeneration, myocardial
  amyloid E85.4 [I43]
  atheromatous — *see* Disease, heart,
    ischemic, atherosclerotic
  ischemic — *see* Disease, heart, ischemic
hepatolenticular (Wilson's) E83.01
hepatorenal K76.7
hyaline (diffuse) (generalized)
  localized — *see* Degeneration, by site
infrapatellar fat pad M79.4
intervertebral disc NOS
  with
    myelopathy — *see* Disorder, disc, with,
      myelopathy
    radiculitis or radiculopathy — *see*
      Disorder, disc, with, radiculopathy
  cervical, cervicothoracic — *see* Disorder,
    disc, cervical, degeneration
    with
      myelopathy — *see* Disorder, disc,
        cervical, with myelopathy
      neuritis, radiculitis or radiculopathy —
        see Disorder, disc, cervical, with
        neuritis
  lumbar region M51.36
    with
      myelopathy M51.06
      neuritis, radiculitis, radiculopathy or
        sciatica M51.16

Degeneration, degenerative — *continued*
intervertebral disc NOS — *continued*
lumbosacral region M51.37
with
neuritis, radiculitis, radiculopathy or
sciatica M51.17
sacrococcygeal region M53.3
thoracic region M51.34
with
myelopathy M51.04
neuritis, radiculitis, radiculopathy
M51.14
thoracolumbar region M51.35
with
myelopathy M51.05
neuritis, radiculitis, radiculopathy
M51.15
intestine, amyloid E85.4
iris (pigmentary) H21.23-
ischemic — *see* Ischemia
joint disease — *see* Osteoarthritis
kidney N28.89
amyloid E85.4 *[N29]*
cystic, congenital Q61.9
fatty N28.89
polycystic Q61.3
adult type (autosomal dominant) Q61.2
infantile type (autosomal recessive) NEC
Q61.19
collecting duct dilatation Q61.11
Kuhnt-Junius (*see also* Degeneration, macula)
H35.32-
lens — *see* Cataract
lenticular (familial) (progressive) (Wilson's)
(with cirrhosis of liver) E83.01
liver (diffuse) NEC K76.89
amyloid E85.4 *[K77]*
cystic K76.89
congenital Q44.6
fatty NEC K76.0
alcoholic K70.0
hypertrophic K76.89
parenchymatous, acute or subacute K72.00
with coma K72.01
pigmentary K76.89
toxic (acute) K71.9
lung J98.4
lymph gland I89.8
hyaline I89.8
macula, macular (acquired) (age-related)
(senile) H35.30
angioid streaks H35.33
atrophic age-related H35.31-
congenital or hereditary — *see* Dystrophy,
retina
cystoid H35.35-
drusen H35.36-
dry age-related H35.31-
exudative H35.32-
hole H35.34-
nonexudative H35.31-
puckering H35.37-
toxic H35.38-
wet age-related H35.32-
membranous labyrinth, congenital (causing
impairment of hearing) Q16.5
meniscus — *see* Derangement, meniscus
mitral — *see* Insufficiency, mitral
Mönckeberg's — *see* Arteriosclerosis,
extremities
motor centers, senile G31.1
multi-system G90.3
mural — *see* Degeneration, myocardial
muscle (fatty) (fibrous) (hyaline) (progressive)
M62.89
heart — *see* Degeneration, myocardial
myelin, central nervous system G37.9

Degeneration, degenerative — *continued*
myocardial, myocardium (fatty) (hyaline)
(senile) I51.5
with rheumatic fever (conditions in I00) I09.0
active, acute or subacute I01.2
with chorea I02.0
inactive or quiescent (with chorea) I09.0
hypertensive — *see* Hypertension, heart
rheumatic — *see* Degeneration, myocardial,
with rheumatic fever
syphilitic A52.06
nasal sinus (mucosa) J32.9
frontal J32.1
maxillary J32.0
nerve — *see* Disorder, nerve
nervous system G31.9
alcoholic G31.2
amyloid E85.4 *[G99.8]*
autonomic G90.9
fatty G31.89
specified NEC G31.89
nipple N64.89
olivopontocerebellar (hereditary) (familial)
G23.8
osseous labyrinth — *see* subcategory H83.8
ovary N83.8
cystic N83.20-
microcystic N83.20-
pallidal pigmentary (progressive) G23.0
pancreas K86.89
tuberculous A18.83
penis N48.89
pigmentary (diffuse) (general)
localized — *see* Degeneration, by site
pallidal (progressive) G23.0
pineal gland E34.8
pituitary (gland) E23.6
popliteal fat pad M79.4
posterolateral (spinal cord) — *see*
Degeneration, combined
pulmonary valve (heart) I37.8
pulp (tooth) K04.2
pupillary margin H21.24-
renal — *see* Degeneration, kidney
retina H35.9
hereditary (cerebroretinal) (congenital)
(juvenile) (macula) (peripheral)
(pigmentary) — *see* Dystrophy, retina
Kuhnt-Junius (*see also* Degeneration, macula)
H35.32-
macula (cystic) (exudative) (hole)
(nonexudative) (pseudohole) (senile)
(toxic) — *see* Degeneration, macula
peripheral H35.40
lattice H35.41-
microcystoid H35.42-
paving stone H35.43-
secondary
pigmentary H35.45-
vitreoretinal H35.46-
senile reticular H35.44-
pigmentary (primary) — *see also* Dystrophy,
retina
secondary — *see* Degeneration, retina,
peripheral, secondary
posterior pole — *see* Degeneration, macula
saccule, congenital (causing impairment of
hearing) Q16.5
senile R54
brain G31.1
cardiac, heart or myocardium — *see*
Degeneration, myocardial
motor centers G31.1
vascular — *see* Arteriosclerosis
sinus (cystic) — *see also* Sinusitis
polypoid J33.1
skin L98.8
amyloid E85.4 *[L99]*
colloid L98.8

Degeneration, degenerative — *continued*
spinal (cord) G31.89
amyloid E85.4 *[G32.89]*
combined (subacute) — *see* Degeneration,
combined
dorsolateral — *see* Degeneration, combined
familial NEC G31.89
fatty G31.89
funicular — *see* Degeneration, combined
posterolateral — *see* Degeneration,
combined
subacute combined — *see* Degeneration,
combined
tuberculous A17.81
spleen D73.0
amyloid E85.4 *[D77]*
stomach K31.89
striatonigral G23.2
suprarenal (capsule) (gland) E27.8
synovial membrane (pulpy) — *see* Disorder,
synovium, specified type NEC
tapetoretinal — *see* Dystrophy, retina
thymus (gland) E32.8
fatty E32.8
thyroid (gland) E07.89
tricuspid (heart) (valve) I07.9
tuberculous NEC — *see* Tuberculosis
turbinate J34.89
uterus (cystic) N85.8
vascular (senile) — *see* Arteriosclerosis
hypertensive — *see* Hypertension
vitreoretinal, secondary — *see* Degeneration,
retina, peripheral, secondary, vitreoretinal
vitreous (body) H43.81-
Wallerian — *see* Disorder, nerve
Wilson's hepatolenticular E83.01
Deglutition
paralysis R13.0
hysterical F44.4
pneumonia J69.0
Degos' disease I77.89
Dehiscence (of)
amputation stump T87.81
cesarean wound O90.0
closure of
cornea T81.31
craniotomy T81.32
fascia (muscular) (superficial) T81.32
internal organ or tissue T81.32
laceration (external) (internal) T81.33
ligament T81.32
mucosa T81.31
muscle or muscle flap T81.32
ribs or rib cage T81.32
skin and subcutaneous tissue (full-thickness)
(superficial) T81.31
skull T81.32
sternum (sternotomy) T81.32
tendon T81.32
traumatic laceration (external) (internal)
T81.33
episiotomy O90.1
operation wound NEC T81.31
external operation wound (superficial)
T81.31
internal operation wound (deep) T81.32
perineal wound (postpartum) O90.1
traumatic injury wound repair T81.33
wound T81.30
traumatic repair T81.33
Dehydration E86.0
newborn P74.1
Déjérine-Roussy syndrome G89.0
Déjérine-Sottas disease or neuropathy
(hypertrophic) G60.0
Déjérine-Thomas atrophy G23.8
Delay, delayed
any plane in pelvis
complicating delivery O66.9

Delay, delayed — *continued*
birth or delivery NOS O63.9
closure, ductus arteriosus (Botalli) P29.3
coagulation — *see* Defect, coagulation
conduction (cardiac) (ventricular) I45.9
delivery, second twin, triplet, etc O63.2
development R62.50
  global F88
  intellectual (specific) F81.9
  language F80.9
    due to hearing loss F80.4
  learning F81.9
  pervasive F84.9
  physiological R62.50
    specified stage NEC R62.0
  reading F81.0
  sexual E30.0
  speech F80.9
    due to hearing loss F80.4
  spelling F81.81
ejaculation F52.32
gastric emptying K30
menarche E30.0
menstruation (cause unknown) N91.0
milestone R62.0
passage of meconium (newborn) P76.0
primary respiration P28.9
puberty (constitutional) E30.0
separation of umbilical cord P96.82
sexual maturation, female E30.0
sleep phase syndrome G47.21
union, fracture — *see* Fracture, by site
vaccination Z28.9

Deletion(s)
autosome Q93.9
  identified by fluorescence in situ
    hybridization (FISH) Q93.89
  identified by in situ hybridization (ISH)
    Q93.89
chromosome
  with complex rearrangements NEC Q93.7
  part of NEC Q93.5
  seen only at prometaphase Q93.89
  short arm
    22q11.2 Q93.81
    4 Q93.3
    5p Q93.4
  specified NEC Q93.89
long arm chromosome 18 or 21 Q93.89
  with complex rearrangements NEC Q93.7
microdeletions NEC Q93.88

Delhi boil or button B55.1
Delinquency (juvenile) (neurotic) F91.8
group Z72.810
Delinquent immunization status Z28.3
Delirium, delirious (acute or subacute) (not
  alcohol- or drug-induced) (with dementia)
  R41.0
alcoholic (acute) (tremens) (withdrawal)
  F10.921
  with intoxication F10.921
    in
      abuse F10.121
      dependence F10.221
due to (secondary to)
  alcohol
    intoxication F10.921
      in
        abuse F10.121
        dependence F10.221
    withdrawal F10.231
  amphetamine intoxication F15.921
    in
      abuse F15.121
      dependence F15.221

Delirium, delirious (acute or subacute) (not
  alcohol- or drug-induced) (with dementia)
  R41.0 — *continued*
due to (secondary to) — *continued*
  anxiolytic
    intoxication F13.921
      in
        abuse F13.121
        dependence F13.221
      withdrawal F13.231
  cannabis intoxication (acute) F12.921
    in
      abuse F12.121
      dependence F12.221
  cocaine intoxication (acute) F14.921
    in
      abuse F14.121
      dependence F14.221
  general medical condition F05
  hallucinogen intoxication F16.921
    in
      abuse F16.121
      dependence F16.221
  hypnotic
    intoxication F13.921
      in
        abuse F13.121
        dependence F13.221
      withdrawal F13.231
  inhalant intoxication (acute) F18.921
    in
      abuse F18.121
      dependence F18.221
  multiple etiologies F05
  opioid intoxication (acute) F11.921
    in
      abuse F11.121
      dependence F11.221
  other (or unknown) substance F19.921
  phencyclidine intoxication (acute) F16.921
    in
      abuse F16.121
      dependence F16.221
  psychoactive substance NEC intoxication
    (acute) F19.921
    in
      abuse F19.121
      dependence F19.221
  sedative
    intoxication F13.921
      in
        abuse F13.121
        dependence F13.221
      withdrawal F13.231
  unknown etiology F05
exhaustion F43.0
hysterical F44.89
postprocedural (postoperative) F05
puerperal F05
thyroid — *see* Thyrotoxicosis with thyroid storm
traumatic — *see* Injury, intracranial
tremens (alcohol-induced) F10.231
  sedative-induced F13.231
Delivery (childbirth) (labor)
arrested active phase O62.1
cesarean (for)
  abnormal
    pelvis (bony) (deformity) (major) NEC with
      disproportion (fetopelvic) O33.0
      with obstructed labor O65.0
    presentation or position O32.9
  abruptio placentae (*see also* Abruptio
    placentae) O45.9-
  acromion presentation O32.2
  atony, uterus O62.2
  breech presentation O32.1
    incomplete O32.8
  brow presentation O32.3
  cephalopelvic disproportion O33.9

Delivery (childbirth) (labor) — *continued*
cesarean (for) — *continued*
  cerclage O34.3-
  chin presentation O32.3
  cicatrix of cervix O34.4-
  contracted pelvis (general)
    inlet O33.2
    outlet O33.3
  cord presentation or prolapse O69.0
  cystocele O34.8-
  deformity (acquired) (congenital)
    pelvic organs or tissues NEC O34.8-
    pelvis (bony) NEC O33.0
  disproportion NOS O33.9
  eclampsia — *see* Eclampsia
  face presentation O32.3
  failed
    forceps O66.5
    induction of labor O61.9
      instrumental O61.1
      mechanical O61.1
      medical O61.0
      specified NEC O61.8
      surgical O61.1
    trial of labor NOS O66.40
      following previous cesarean delivery
        O66.41
    vacuum extraction O66.5
    ventouse O66.5
  fetal-maternal hemorrhage O43.01-
  hemorrhage (intrapartum) O67.9
    with coagulation defect O67.0
    specified cause NEC O67.8
  high head at term O32.4
  hydrocephalic fetus O33.6
  incarceration of uterus O34.51-
  incoordinate uterine action O62.4
  increased size, fetus O33.5
  inertia, uterus O62.2
    primary O62.0
    secondary O62.1
  lateroversion, uterus O34.59-
  mal lie O32.9
  malposition
    fetus O32.9
    pelvic organs or tissues NEC O34.8-
    uterus NEC O34.59-
  malpresentation NOS O32.9
  oblique presentation O32.2
  occurring after 37 completed weeks of
    gestation but before 39 completed
    weeks of gestation due to (spontaneous)
    onset of labor O75.82
  oversize fetus O33.5
  pelvic tumor NEC O34.8-
  placenta previa O44.0-
    complete O44.0-
      with hemorrhage O44.1-
  placental insufficiency O36.51-
  planned, occurring after 37 completed
    weeks of gestation but before 39
    completed weeks of gestation due to
    (spontaneous) onset of labor O75.82
  polyp, cervix O34.4-
    causing obstructed labor O65.5
  poor dilatation, cervix O62.0
  pre-eclampsia O14.94
    mild O14.04
    moderate O14.04
    severe O14.14
      with hemolysis, elevated liver enzymes
        and low platelet count (HELLP)
        O14.24
  previous
    cesarean delivery O34.219
      classical (vertical) scar O34.212
      low transverse scar O34.211

Delivery (childbirth) (labor) — *continued*
　cesarean (for) — *continued*
　　previous — *continued*
　　　surgery (to)
　　　　cervix O34.4-
　　　　gynecological NEC O34.8-
　　　　rectum O34.7-
　　　　uterus O34.29
　　　　vagina O34.6-
　　prolapse
　　　arm or hand O32.2
　　　uterus O34.52-
　　prolonged labor NOS O63.9
　　rectocele O34.8-
　　retroversion
　　　uterus O34.53-
　　rigid
　　　cervix O34.4-
　　　pelvic floor O34.8-
　　　perineum O34.7-
　　　vagina O34.6-
　　　vulva O34.7-
　　sacculation, pregnant uterus O34.59-
　　scar(s)
　　　cervix O34.4-
　　　cesarean delivery O34.219
　　　　classical (vertical) O34.212
　　　　low transverse O34.211
　　　transmural uterine O34.29
　　　uterus O34.29
　　Shirodkar suture in situ O34.3-
　　shoulder presentation O32.2
　　stenosis or stricture, cervix O34.4-
　　streptococcus group B (GBS) carrier state
　　　O99.824
　　transmural uterine scar O34.29
　　transverse presentation or lie O32.2
　　tumor, pelvic organs or tissues NEC O34.8-
　　　cervix O34.4-
　　umbilical cord presentation or prolapse
　　　O69.0
　　without indication O82
　completely normal case O80
　complicated O75.9
　　by
　　　abnormal, abnormality (of)
　　　　forces of labor O62.9
　　　　　specified type NEC O62.8
　　　　glucose O99.814
　　　　uterine contractions NOS O62.9
　　　abruptio placentae (*see also* Abruptio
　　　　placentae) O45.9-
　　　abuse
　　　　physical O9A.32 *(follows O99)*
　　　　psychological O9A.52 *(follows O99)*
　　　　sexual O9A.42 *(follows O99)*
　　　adherent placenta O72.0
　　　　without hemorrhage O73.0
　　　alcohol use O99.314
　　　anemia (pre-existing) O99.02
　　　anesthetic death O74.8
　　　annular detachment of cervix O71.3
　　　atony, uterus O62.2
　　　attempted vacuum extraction and forceps
　　　　O66.5
　　　Bandl's ring O62.4
　　　bariatric surgery status O99.844
　　　biliary tract disorder O26.62
　　　bleeding — *see* Delivery, complicated by,
　　　　hemorrhage
　　　blood disorder NEC O99.12
　　　cervical dystocia (hypotonic) O62.2
　　　　primary O62.0
　　　　secondary O62.1
　　　circulatory system disorder O99.42
　　　compression of cord (umbilical) NEC
　　　　O69.2
　　　condition NEC O99.89
　　　contraction, contracted ring O62.4

Delivery (childbirth) (labor) — *continued*
　complicated O75.9 — *continued*
　　by — *continued*
　　　cord (umbilical)
　　　　around neck
　　　　　with compression O69.1
　　　　　without compression O69.81
　　　　bruising O69.5
　　　　complication O69.9
　　　　　specified NEC O69.89
　　　　compression NEC O69.2
　　　　entanglement O69.2
　　　　　without compression O69.82
　　　　hematoma O69.5
　　　　presentation O69.0
　　　　prolapse O69.0
　　　　short O69.3
　　　　thrombosis (vessels) O69.5
　　　　vascular lesion O69.5
　　　Couvelaire uterus O45.8x-
　　　damage to (injury to) NEC
　　　　perineum O71.82
　　　　periurethral tissue O71.82
　　　　vulva O71.82
　　　delay following rupture of membranes
　　　　(spontaneous) — *see* Pregnancy,
　　　　complicated by, premature rupture of
　　　　membranes
　　　depressed fetal heart tones O76
　　　diabetes O24.92
　　　　gestational O24.429
　　　　　diet controlled O24.420
　　　　　insulin controlled O24.424
　　　　　oral drug controlled (antidiabetic)
　　　　　　(hypoglycemic) O24.425
　　　　pre-existing O24.32
　　　　　specified NEC O24.82
　　　　　type 1 O24.02
　　　　　type 2 O24.12
　　　diastasis recti (abdominis) O71.89
　　　dilatation
　　　　bladder O66.8
　　　　cervix incomplete, poor or slow O62.0
　　　disease NEC O99.89
　　　disruptio uteri — *see* Delivery, complicated
　　　　by, rupture, uterus
　　　drug use O99.324
　　　dysfunction, uterus NOS O62.9
　　　　hypertonic O62.4
　　　　hypotonic O62.2
　　　　　primary O62.0
　　　　　secondary O62.1
　　　　incoordinate O62.4
　　　eclampsia O15.1
　　　embolism (pulmonary) — *see* Embolism,
　　　　obstetric
　　　endocrine, nutritional or metabolic disease
　　　　NEC O99.284
　　　failed
　　　　attempted vaginal birth after previous
　　　　　cesarean delivery O66.41
　　　　induction of labor O61.9
　　　　　instrumental O61.1
　　　　　mechanical O61.1
　　　　　medical O61.0
　　　　　specified NEC O61.8
　　　　　surgical O61.1
　　　　trial of labor O66.40
　　　female genital mutilation O65.5
　　　fetal
　　　　abnormal acid-base balance O68
　　　　acidemia O68
　　　　acidosis O68
　　　　alkalosis O68
　　　　death, early O02.1
　　　　deformity O66.3
　　　　heart rate or rhythm (abnormal) (non-
　　　　　reassuring) O76
　　　　hypoxia O77.8

Delivery (childbirth) (labor) — *continued*
　complicated O75.9 — *continued*
　　by — *continued*
　　　fetal — *continued*
　　　　stress O77.9
　　　　　due to drug administration O77.1
　　　　　electrocardiographic evidence of
　　　　　　O77.8
　　　　　specified NEC O77.8
　　　　　ultrasound evidence of O77.8
　　　fever during labor O75.2
　　　gastric banding status O99.844
　　　gastric bypass status O99.844
　　　gastrointestinal disease NEC O99.62
　　　gestational
　　　　diabetes O24.429
　　　　　diet controlled O24.420
　　　　　insulin (and diet) controlled O24.424
　　　　　oral drug controlled (antidiabetic)
　　　　　　(hypoglycemic) O24.425
　　　　edema O12.04
　　　　　with proteinuria O12.24
　　　　proteinuria O12.14
　　　gonorrhea O98.22
　　　hematoma O71.7
　　　　ischial spine O71.7
　　　　pelvic O71.7
　　　　vagina O71.7
　　　　vulva or perineum O71.7
　　　hemorrhage (uterine) O67.9
　　　　associated with
　　　　　afibrinogenemia O67.0
　　　　　coagulation defect O67.0
　　　　　hyperfibrinolysis O67.0
　　　　　hypofibrinogenemia O67.0
　　　　due to
　　　　　low implantation of placenta O44.5-
　　　　　low-lying placenta O44.5-
　　　　　placenta previa O44.1-
　　　　　　marginal O44.3-
　　　　　　partial O44.3-
　　　　　premature separation of placenta
　　　　　　(normally implanted) (*see also*
　　　　　　Abruptio placentae) O45.9-
　　　　　retained placenta O72.0
　　　　　uterine leiomyoma O67.8
　　　　placenta NEC O67.8
　　　　postpartum NEC (atonic) (immediate)
　　　　　O72.1
　　　　　with retained or trapped placenta
　　　　　　O72.0
　　　　delayed O72.2
　　　　secondary O72.2
　　　　third stage O72.0
　　　hourglass contraction, uterus O62.4
　　　hypertension, hypertensive (pre-existing)
　　　　— *see* Hypertension, complicated by,
　　　　childbirth (labor)
　　　hypotension O26.5-
　　　incomplete dilatation (cervix) O62.0
　　　incoordinate uterus contractions O62.4
　　　inertia, uterus O62.2
　　　　during latent phase of labor O62.0
　　　　primary O62.0
　　　　secondary O62.1
　　　infection (maternal) O98.92
　　　　carrier state NEC O99.834
　　　　gonorrhea O98.22
　　　　human immunodeficiency virus (HIV)
　　　　　O98.72
　　　　sexually transmitted NEC O98.32
　　　　specified NEC O98.82
　　　　syphilis O98.12
　　　　tuberculosis O98.02
　　　　viral hepatitis O98.42
　　　　viral NEC O98.52

DISEASE INDEX

Delivery (childbirth) (labor) — *continued*
complicated O75.9 — *continued*
  by — *continued*
    injury (to mother) (*see also* Delivery,
      complicated, by, damage to) O71.9
      nonobstetric O9A.22 *(follows O99)*
        caused by abuse — *see* Delivery,
          complicated by, abuse
    intrauterine fetal death, early O02.1
    inversion, uterus O71.2
    laceration (perineal) O70.9
      anus (sphincter) O70.4
        with third degree laceration (*see also*
          Delivery, complicated, by,
          laceration, perineum, third
          degree) O70.20
          with mucosa O70.3
        without third degree laceration O70.4
      bladder (urinary) O71.5
      bowel O71.5
      cervix (uteri) O71.3
      fourchette O70.0
      hymen O70.0
      labia O70.0
      pelvic
        floor O70.1
        organ NEC O71.5
      perineum, perineal O70.9
        first degree O70.0
        fourth degree O70.3
        muscles O70.1
        second degree O70.1
        skin O70.0
        slight O70.0
        third degree O70.20
          with
            both external anal sphincter (EAS)
              and internal anal sphincter
              (IAS) torn (IIIc) O70.23
            less than 50% of external anal
              sphincter (EAS) thickness torn
              (IIIa) O70.21
            more than 50% external anal
              sphincter (EAS) thickness torn
              (IIIb) O70.22
          IIIa O70.21
          IIIb O70.22
          IIIc O70.23
      peritoneum (pelvic) O71.5
      rectovaginal (septum) (without perineal
        laceration) O71.4
        with perineum (*see also* Delivery,
          complicated, by, laceration,
          perineum, third degree) O70.20
          with anal or rectal mucosa O70.3
      specified NEC O71.89
      sphincter ani — *see* Delivery,
        complicated, by, laceration, anus
        (sphincter)
      urethra O71.5
      uterus O71.81
        before labor O71.81
      vagina, vaginal (deep) (high) (without
        perineal laceration) O71.4
        with perineum O70.0
        muscles, with perineum O70.1
      vulva O70.0
    liver disorder O26.62
    malignancy O9A.12 *(follows O99)*
    malnutrition O25.2
    malposition, malpresentation
      without obstruction (*see also* Delivery,
        complicated by, obstruction) O32.9
        breech O32.1
        compound O32.6
        face (brow) (chin) O32.3
        footling O32.8
        high head O32.4
        oblique O32.2

Delivery (childbirth) (labor) — *continued*
complicated O75.9 — *continued*
  by — *continued*
    malposition, malpresentation
      — *continued*
      without obstruction (*see also* Delivery,
        complicated by, obstruction) O32.9
      — *continued*
        specified NEC O32.8
        transverse O32.2
        unstable lie O32.0
      placenta O44.0-
        with hemorrhage O44.1-
      uterus or cervix O65.5
    meconium in amniotic fluid O77.0
    mental disorder NEC O99.344
    metrorrhexis — *see* Delivery, complicated
      by, rupture, uterus
    nervous system disorder O99.354
    obesity (pre-existing) O99.214
    obesity surgery status O99.844
    obstetric trauma O71.9
      specified NEC O71.89
    obstructed labor
      due to
        breech (complete) (frank) presentation
          O64.1
          incomplete O64.8
        brow presenation O64.3
        buttock presentation O64.1
        chin presentation O64.2
        compound presentation O64.5
        contracted pelvis O65.1
        deep transverse arrest O64.0
        deformed pelvis O65.0
        dystocia (fetal) O66.9
          due to
            conjoined twins O66.3
            fetal
              abnormality NEC O66.3
              ascites O66.3
              hydrops O66.3
              meningomyelocele O66.3
              sacral teratoma O66.3
              tumor O66.3
            hydrocephalic fetus O66.3
          shoulder O66.0
        face presentation O64.2
        fetopelvic disproportion O65.4
        footling presentation O64.8
        impacted shoulders O66.0
        incomplete rotation of fetal head
          O64.0
        large fetus O66.2
        locked twins O66.1
        malposition O64.9
          specified NEC O64.8
        malpresentation O64.9
          specified NEC O64.8
        multiple fetuses NEC O66.6
        pelvic
          abnormality (maternal) O65.9
            organ O65.5
            specified NEC O65.8
          contraction
            inlet O65.2
            mid-cavity O65.3
            outlet O65.3
        persistent (position)
          occipitoiliac O64.0
          occipitoposterior O64.0
          occipitosacral O64.0
          occipitotransverse O64.0
        prolapsed arm O64.4
        shoulder presentation O64.4
      specified NEC O66.8
    pathological retraction ring, uterus O62.4
    penetration, pregnant uterus by instrument
      O71.1

Delivery (childbirth) (labor) — *continued*
complicated O75.9 — *continued*
  by — *continued*
    perforation — *see* Delivery, complicated
      by, laceration
    placenta, placental
      ablatio (*see also* Abruptio placentae)
        O45.9-
      abnormality O43.9-
        specified NEC O43.89-
      abruptio (*see also* Abruptio placentae)
        O45.9-
      accreta O43.21-
      adherent (with hemorrhage) O72.0
        without hemorrhage O73.0
      detachment (premature) (*see also*
        Abruptio placentae) O45.9-
      disorder O43.9-
        specified NEC O43.89-
      hemorrhage NEC O67.8
      increta O43.22-
      low (implantation) (lying) O44.4-
        with hemorrhage O44.5-
      malformation O43.10-
      malposition O44.0-
        without hemorrhage O44.1-
      percreta O43.23-
      previa (central) (complete) (lateral) (total)
        O44.0-
        with hemorrhage O44.1-
        marginal O44.2-
          with hemorrhage O44.3-
        partial O44.2-
          with hemorrhage O44.3-
      retained (with hemorrhage) O72.0
        without hemorrhage O73.0
      separation (premature) O45.9-
        specified NEC O45.8x-
      vicious insertion O44.1-
    precipitate labor O62.3
    premature rupture, membranes (*see also*
      Pregnancy, complicated by, premature
      rupture of membranes) O42.90
    prolapse
      arm or hand O32.2
      cord (umbilical) O69.0
      foot or leg O32.8
      uterus O34.52-
    prolonged labor O63.9
      first stage O63.0
      second stage O63.1
    protozoal disease (maternal) O98.62
    respiratory disease NEC O99.52
    retained membranes or portions of
      placenta O72.2
      without hemorrhage O73.1
    retarded birth O63.9
    retention of secundines (with hemorrhage)
      O72.0
      without hemorrhage O73.0
      partial O72.2
        without hemorrhage O73.1
    rupture
      bladder (urinary) O71.5
      cervix O71.3
      pelvic organ NEC O71.5
      urethra O71.5
      uterus (during or after labor) O71.1
        before labor O71.0-
    separation, pubic bone (symphysis pubis)
      O71.6
    shock O75.1
    shoulder presentation O64.4
    skin disorder NEC O99.72
    spasm, cervix O62.4
    stenosis or stricture, cervix O65.5
    streptococcus group B (GBS) carrier state
      O99.824
    subluxation of symphysis (pubis) O26.72

Delivery (childbirth) (labor) — *continued*
  complicated O75.9 — *continued*
    by — *continued*
      syphilis (maternal) O98.12
      tear — *see* Delivery, complicated by,
        laceration
      tetanic uterus O62.4
      trauma (obstetrical) (*see also* Delivery,
        complicated, by, damage to) O71.9
        non-obstetric O9A.22 **(follows O99)**
        periurethral O71.82
        specified NEC O71.89
      tuberculosis (maternal) O98.02
      tumor, pelvic organs or tissues NEC O65.5
      umbilical cord around neck
        with compression O69.1
        without compression O69.81
      uterine inertia O62.2
        during latent phase of labor O62.0
        primary O62.0
        secondary O62.1
      vasa previa O69.4
      velamentous insertion of cord O43.12-
    specified complication NEC O75.89
  delayed NOS O63.9
    following rupture of membranes
      artificial O75.5
    second twin, triplet, etc. O63.2
  forceps, low following failed vacuum extraction
    O66.5
  missed (at or near term) O36.4
  normal O80
  obstructed — *see* Delivery, complicated by,
    obstruction
  precipitate O62.3
  preterm (*see also* Pregnancy, complicated by,
    preterm labor) O60.10
  spontaneous O80
  term pregnancy NOS O80
  uncomplicated O80
  vaginal, following previous cesarean delivery
    O34.219
    classical (vertical) scar O34.212
    low transverse scar O34.211

Delusions (paranoid) — *see* Disorder,
  delusional

Dementia (degenerative (primary)) (old age)
  (persisting) F03.90
  with
    aggressive behavior F03.91
    behavioral disturbance F03.91
    combative behavior F03.91
    Lewy bodies G31.83 *[F02.80]*
      with behavioral disturbance G31.83
        [F02.81]
    Parkinsonism G31.83 *[F02.80]*
      with behavioral disturbance G31.83
        [F02.81]
    Parkinson's disease G20 *[F02.80]*
      with behavioral disturbance G20 *[F02.81]*
    violent behavior F03.91
  alcoholic F10.97
    with dependence F10.27
  Alzheimer's type — *see* Disease, Alzheimer's
  arteriosclerotic — *see* Dementia, vascular
  atypical, Alzheimer's type — *see* Disease,
    Alzheimer's, specified NEC
  congenital — *see* Disability, intellectual
  frontal (lobe) G31.09 *[F02.80]*
    with behavioral disturbance G31.09 *[F02.81]*
  frontotemporal G31.09 *[F02.80]*
    with behavioral disturbance G31.09
      [F02.81]
    specified NEC G31.09 *[F02.80]*
      with behavioral disturbance G31.09
        [F02.81]
  in (due to)
    with behavioral disturbance G31.83
      [F02.81]

Dementia (degenerative (primary)) (old age)
  (persisting) F03 — *continued*
  in (due to) — *continued*
    alcohol F10.97
      with dependence F10.27
    Alzheimer's disease — *see* Disease,
      Alzheimer's
    arteriosclerotic brain disease — *see*
      Dementia, vascular
    cerebral lipidoses E75- *[F02.80]*
      with behavioral disturbance E75-*[F02.81]*
    Creutzfeldt-Jakob disease (*see also*
      Creutzfeldt-Jakob disease or syndrome
      (with dementia)) A81.00
    epilepsy G40-*[F02.80]*
      with behavioral disturbance G40-*[F02.81]*
    hepatolenticular degeneration E83.01
      [F02.80]
      with behavioral disturbance E83.01
        [F02.81]
    human immunodeficiency virus (HIV) disease
      B20 *[F02.80]*
      with behavioral disturbance B20 *[F02.81]*
    Huntington's disease or chorea G10
    hypercalcemia E83.52 *[F02.80]*
      with behavioral disturbance E83.52
        [F02.81]
    hypothyroidism, acquired E03.9 *[F02.80]*
      with behavioral disturbance E03.9 *[F02.81]*
      due to iodine deficiency E01.8 *[F02.80]*
        with behavioral disturbance E01.8
          [F02.81]
    inhalants F18.97
      with dependence F18.27
    multiple
      etiologies F03
      sclerosis G35 *[F02.80]*
        with behavioral disturbance G35
          [F02.81]
    neurosyphilis A52.17 *[F02.80]*
      with behavioral disturbance A52.17
        [F02.81]
      juvenile A50.49 *[F02.80]*
        with behavioral disturbance A50.49
          [F02.81]
    niacin deficiency E52 *[F02.80]*
      with behavioral disturbance E52 *[F02.81]*
    paralysis agitans G20 *[F02.80]*
      with behavioral disturbance G20 *[F02.81]*
    Parkinson's disease G20 *[F02.80]*
    pellagra E52 *[F02.80]*
      with behavioral disturbance E52 *[F02.81]*
    Pick's G31.01 *[F02.80]*
      with behavioral disturbance G31.01
        [F02.81]
    polyarteritis nodosa M30.0 *[F02.80]*
      with behavioral disturbance M30.0
        [F02.81]
    psychoactive drug F19.97
      with dependence F19.27
      inhalants F18.97
        with dependence F18.27
      sedatives, hypnotics or anxiolytics F13.97
        with dependence F13.27
    sedatives, hypnotics or anxiolytics F13.97
      with dependence F13.27
    systemic lupus erythematosus M32-*[F02.80]*
      with behavioral disturbance M32-*[F02.81]*
    trypanosomiasis
      African B56.9 *[F02.80]*
        with behavioral disturbance B56.9
          [F02.81]
    unknown etiology F03
    vitamin B12 deficiency E53.8 *[F02.80]*
      with behavioral disturbance E53.8
        [F02.81]
    volatile solvents F18.97
      with dependence F18.27
  infantile, infantilis F84.3

Dementia (degenerative (primary)) (old age)
  (persisting) F03 — *continued*
  Lewy body G31.83 *[F02.80]*
    with behavioral disturbance G31.83
      [F02.81]
  multi-infarct — *see* Dementia, vascular
  paralytica, paralytic (syphilitic) A52.17
    [F02.80]
    with behavioral disturbance A52.17
      [F02.81]
    juvenilis A50.45
  paretic A52.17
  praecox — *see* Schizophrenia
  presenile F03
    Alzheimer's type — *see* Disease,
      Alzheimer's, early onset
  primary degenerative F03
  progressive, syphilitic A52.17
  senile F03
    with acute confusional state F05
    Alzheimer's type — *see* Disease,
      Alzheimer's, late onset
    depressed or paranoid type F03
  vascular (acute onset) (mixed) (multi-infarct)
    (subcortical) F01.50
    with behavioral disturbance F01.51

Demineralization, bone — *see* Osteoporosis
Demodex folliculorum (infestation) B88.0
Demophobia F40.248
Demoralization R45.3
Demyelination, demyelinization
  central nervous system G37.9
    specified NEC G37.8
  corpus callosum (central) G37.1
  disseminated, acute G36.9
    specified NEC G36.8
  global G35
  in optic neuritis G36.0
Dengue (classical) (fever) A90
  hemorrhagic A91
  sandfly A93.1
Dennie-Marfan syphilitic syndrome
  A50.45
**Dens evaginatus, in dente or
  invaginatus** K00.2
Dense breasts R92.2
Density
  increased, bone (disseminated) (generalized)
    (spotted) — *see* Disorder, bone, density
    and structure, specified type NEC
  lung (nodular) J98.4
Dental — *see also* condition
  examination Z01.20
    with abnormal findings Z01.21
  restoration
    aesthetically inadequate or displeasing
      K08.56
    defective K08.50
      specified NEC K08.59
    failure of marginal integrity K08.51
    failure of periodontal anatomical integrity
      K08.54
Dentia praecox K00.6
Denticles (pulp) K04.2
Dentigerous cyst K09.0
Dentin
  irregular (in pulp) K04.3
  opalescent K00.5
  secondary (in pulp) K04.3
  sensitive K03.89
Dentinogenesis imperfecta K00.5
Dentinoma — *see* Cyst, calcifying odontogenic
Dentition (syndrome) K00.7
  delayed K00.6
  difficult K00.7
  precocious K00.6
  premature K00.6
  retarded K00.6

Dependence (on) (syndrome) F19.20
  with remission F19.21
  alcohol (ethyl) (methyl) (without remission) F10.20
    with
      amnestic disorder, persisting F10.26
      anxiety disorder F10.280
      dementia, persisting F10.27
      intoxication F10.229
        with delirium F10.221
        uncomplicated F10.220
      mood disorder F10.24
      psychotic disorder F10.259
        with
          delusions F10.250
          hallucinations F10.251
      remission F10.21
      sexual dysfunction F10.281
      sleep disorder F10.282
      specified disorder NEC F10.288
      withdrawal F10.239
        with
          delirium F10.231
          perceptual disturbance F10.232
        uncomplicated F10.230
    counseling and surveillance Z71.41
  amobarbital — *see* Dependence, drug, sedative
  amphetamine(s) (type) — *see* Dependence, drug, stimulant NEC
  amytal (sodium) — *see* Dependence, drug, sedative
  analgesic NEC F55.8
  anesthetic (agent) (gas) (general) (local) NEC — *see* Dependence, drug, psychoactive NEC
  anxiolytic NEC — *see* Dependence, drug, sedative
  barbital(s) — *see* Dependence, drug, sedative
  barbiturate(s) (compounds) (drugs classifiable to T42) — *see* Dependence, drug, sedative
  benzedrine — *see* Dependence, drug, stimulant NEC
  bhang — *see* Dependence, drug, cannabis
  bromide(s) NEC — *see* Dependence, drug, sedative
  caffeine — *see* Dependence, drug, stimulant NEC
  cannabis (sativa) (indica) (resin) (derivatives) (type) — *see* Dependence, drug, cannabis
  chloral (betaine) (hydrate) — *see* Dependence, drug, sedative
  chlordiazepoxide — *see* Dependence, drug, sedative
  coca (leaf) (derivatives) — *see* Dependence, drug, cocaine
  cocaine — *see* Dependence, drug, cocaine
  codeine — *see* Dependence, drug, opioid
  combinations of drugs F19.20
  dagga — *see* Dependence, drug, cannabis
  demerol — *see* Dependence, drug, opioid
  dexamphetamine — *see* Dependence, drug, stimulant NEC
  dexedrine — *see* Dependence, drug, stimulant NEC
  dextro-nor-pseudo-ephedrine — *see* Dependence, drug, stimulant NEC
  dextromethorphan — *see* Dependence, drug, opioid
  dextromoramide — *see* Dependence, drug, opioid
  dextrorphan — *see* Dependence, drug, opioid
  diazepam — *see* Dependence, drug, sedative
  dilaudid — *see* Dependence, drug, opioid
  D-lysergic acid diethylamide — *see* Dependence, drug, hallucinogen

Dependence (on) (syndrome) F19.20 — *continued*
  drug NEC F19.20
    with sleep disorder F19.282
    cannabis F12.20
      with
        anxiety disorder F12.280
        intoxication F12.229
          with
            delirium F12.221
            perceptual disturbance F12.222
          uncomplicated F12.220
        other specified disorder F12.288
        psychosis F12.259
          delusions F12.250
          hallucinations F12.251
        unspecified disorder F12.29
      in remission F12.21
    cocaine F14.20
      with
        anxiety disorder F14.280
        intoxication F14.229
          with
            delirium F14.221
            perceptual disturbance F14.222
          uncomplicated F14.220
        mood disorder F14.24
        other specified disorder F14.288
        psychosis F14.259
          delusions F14.250
          hallucinations F14.251
        sexual dysfunction F14.281
        sleep disorder F14.282
        unspecified disorder F14.29
        withdrawal F14.23
      in remission F14.21
      withdrawal symptoms in newborn P96.1
    counseling and surveillance Z71.51
    hallucinogen F16.20
      with
        anxiety disorder F16.280
        flashbacks F16.283
        intoxication F16.229
          with delirium F16.221
          uncomplicated F16.220
        mood disorder F16.24
        other specified disorder F16.288
        perception disorder, persisting F16.283
        psychosis F16.259
          delusions F16.250
          hallucinations F16.251
        unspecified disorder F16.29
      in remission F16.21
    in remission F19.21
    inhalant F18.20
      with
        anxiety disorder F18.280
        dementia, persisting F18.27
        intoxication F18.229
          with delirium F18.221
          uncomplicated F18.220
        mood disorder F18.24
        other specified disorder F18.288
        psychosis F18.259
          delusions F18.250
          hallucinations F18.251
        unspecified disorder F18.29
      in remission F18.21
    nicotine F17.200
      with disorder F17.209
      remission F17.201
      specified disorder NEC F17.208
      withdrawal F17.203
      chewing tobacco F17.220
        with disorder F17.229
          remission F17.221
          specified disorder NEC F17.228
          withdrawal F17.223

Dependence (on) (syndrome) F19.20 — *continued*
  drug NEC F19.20 — *continued*
    nicotine F17.200 — *continued*
      cigarettes F17.210
        with disorder F17.219
          remission F17.211
          specified disorder NEC F17.218
          withdrawal F17.213
      specified product NEC F17.290
        with disorder F17.299
          remission F17.291
          specified disorder NEC F17.298
          withdrawal F17.293
    opioid F11.20
      with
        intoxication F11.229
          with
            delirium F11.221
            perceptual disturbance F11.222
          uncomplicated F11.220
        mood disorder F11.24
        other specified disorder F11.288
        psychosis F11.259
          delusions F11.250
          hallucinations F11.251
        sexual dysfunction F11.281
        sleep disorder F11.282
        unspecified disorder F11.29
        withdrawal F11.23
      in remission F11.21
    psychoactive NEC F19.20
      with
        amnestic disorder F19.26
        anxiety disorder F19.280
        dementia F19.27
        intoxication F19.229
          with
            delirium F19.221
            perceptual disturbance F19.222
          uncomplicated F19.220
        mood disorder F19.24
        other specified disorder F19.288
        psychosis F19.259
          delusions F19.250
          hallucinations F19.251
        sexual dysfunction F19.281
        sleep disorder F19.282
        unspecified disorder F19.29
        withdrawal F19.239
          with
            delirium F19.231
            perceptual disturbance F19.232
          uncomplicated F19.230
    sedative, hypnotic or anxiolytic F13.20
      with
        amnestic disorder F13.26
        anxiety disorder F13.280
        dementia, persisting F13.27
        intoxication F13.229
          with delirium F13.221
          uncomplicated F13.220
        mood disorder F13.24
        other specified disorder F13.288
        psychosis F13.259
          delusions F13.250
          hallucinations F13.251
        sexual dysfunction F13.281
        sleep disorder F13.282
        unspecified disorder F13.29
        withdrawal F13.239
          with
            delirium F13.231
            perceptual disturbance F13.232
          uncomplicated F13.230
      in remission F13.21

Dependence (on) (syndrome) F19.20 — *continued*
- drug NEC F19.20 — *continued*
  - stimulant NEC F15.20
    - with
      - anxiety disorder F15.280
      - intoxication F15.229
        - with
          - delirium F15.221
          - perceptual disturbance F15.222
        - uncomplicated F15.220
      - mood disorder F15.24
      - other specified disorder F15.288
      - psychosis F15.259
        - delusions F15.250
        - hallucinations F15.251
      - sexual dysfunction F15.281
      - sleep disorder F15.282
      - unspecified disorder F15.29
      - withdrawal F15.23
    - in remission F15.21
  - ethyl
    - alcohol (without remission) F10.20
      - with remission F10.21
    - bromide — *see* Dependence, drug, sedative
    - carbamate F19.20
    - chloride F19.20
    - morphine — *see* Dependence, drug, opioid
  - ganja — *see* Dependence, drug, cannabis
  - glue (airplane) (sniffing) — *see* Dependence, drug, inhalant
  - glutethimide — *see* Dependence, drug, sedative
  - hallucinogenics — *see* Dependence, drug, hallucinogen
  - hashish — *see* Dependence, drug, cannabis
  - hemp — *see* Dependence, drug, cannabis
  - heroin (salt) (any) — *see* Dependence, drug, opioid
  - hypnotic NEC — *see* Dependence, drug, sedative
  - Indian hemp — *see* Dependence, drug, cannabis
  - inhalants — *see* Dependence, drug, inhalant
  - khat — *see* Dependence, drug, stimulant NEC
  - laudanum — *see* Dependence, drug, opioid
  - LSD(-25) (derivatives) — *see* Dependence, drug, hallucinogen
  - luminal — *see* Dependence, drug, sedative
  - lysergic acid — *see* Dependence, drug, hallucinogen
  - maconha — *see* Dependence, drug, cannabis
  - marihuana — *see* Dependence, drug, cannabis
  - meprobamate — *see* Dependence, drug, sedative
  - mescaline — *see* Dependence, drug, hallucinogen
  - methadone — *see* Dependence, drug, opioid
  - methamphetamine(s) — *see* Dependence, drug, stimulant NEC
  - methaqualone — *see* Dependence, drug, sedative
  - methyl
    - alcohol (without remission) F10.20
      - with remission F10.21
    - bromide — *see* Dependence, drug, sedative
    - morphine — *see* Dependence, drug, opioid
    - phenidate — *see* Dependence, drug, stimulant NEC
  - sulfonal — *see* Dependence, drug, sedative
  - morphine (sulfate) (sulfite) (type) — *see* Dependence, drug, opioid
  - narcotic (drug) NEC — *see* Dependence, drug, opioid
  - nembutal — *see* Dependence, drug, sedative
  - neraval — *see* Dependence, drug, sedative
  - neravan — *see* Dependence, drug, sedative
  - neurobarb — *see* Dependence, drug, sedative
  - nicotine — *see* Dependence, drug, nicotine

Dependence (on) (syndrome) F19.20 — *continued*
- nitrous oxide F19.20
- nonbarbiturate sedatives and tranquilizers with similar effect — *see* Dependence, drug, sedative
- on
  - artificial heart (fully implantable) (mechanical) Z95.812
  - aspirator Z99.0
  - care provider (because of) Z74.9
    - impaired mobility Z74.09
    - need for
      - assistance with personal care Z74.1
      - continuous supervision Z74.3
      - no other household member able to render care Z74.2
      - specified reason NEC Z74.8
  - machine Z99.89
    - enabling NEC Z99.89
    - specified type NEC Z99.89
  - renal dialysis (hemodialysis) (peritoneal) Z99.2
  - respirator Z99.11
  - ventilator Z99.11
  - wheelchair Z99.3
- opiate — *see* Dependence, drug, opioid
- opioids — *see* Dependence, drug, opioid
- opium (alkaloids) (derivatives) (tincture) — *see* Dependence, drug, opioid
- oxygen (long-term) (supplemental) Z99.81
- paraldehyde — *see* Dependence, drug, sedative
- paregoric — *see* Dependence, drug, opioid
- PCP (phencyclidine) (or related substance) — *see* Dependence, drug, hallucinogen
- pentobarbital — *see* Dependence, drug, sedative
- pentobarbitone (sodium) — *see* Dependence, drug, sedative
- pentothal — *see* Dependence, drug, sedative
- peyote — *see* Dependence, drug, hallucinogen
- phencyclidine (PCP) (or related substance) — *see* Dependence, drug, hallucinogen
- phenmetrazine — *see* Dependence, drug, stimulant NEC
- phenobarbital — *see* Dependence, drug, sedative
- polysubstance F19.20
- psilocibin, psilocin, psilocyn, psilocyline — *see* Dependence, drug, hallucinogen
- psychostimulant NEC — *see* Dependence, drug, stimulant NEC
- secobarbital — *see* Dependence, drug, sedative
- seconal — *see* Dependence, drug, sedative
- sedative NEC — *see* Dependence, drug, sedative
- specified drug NEC — *see* Dependence, drug
- stimulant NEC — *see* Dependence, drug, stimulant NEC
- substance NEC — *see* Dependence, drug
- supplemental oxygen Z99.81
- tobacco — *see* Dependence, drug, nicotine
  - counseling and surveillance Z71.6
- tranquilizer NEC — *see* Dependence, drug, sedative
- vitamin B6 E53.1
- volatile solvents — *see* Dependence, drug, inhalant

Dependency
- care-provider Z74.9
- passive F60.7
- reactions (persistent) F60.7

Depersonalization (in neurotic state) (neurotic) (syndrome) F48.1

Depletion
- extracellular fluid E86.9
- plasma E86.1

Depletion — *continued*
- potassium E87.6
  - nephropathy N25.89
- salt or sodium E87.1
  - causing heat exhaustion or prostration T67.4
  - nephropathy N28.9
- volume NOS E86.9

Deployment (current) (military) status Z56.82
- in theater or in support of military war, peacekeeping and humanitarian operations Z56.82
- personal history of Z91.82
  - military war, peacekeeping and humanitarian deployment (current or past conflict) Z91.82
- returned from Z91.82

Depolarization, premature I49.40
- atrial I49.1
- junctional I49.2
- specified NEC I49.49
- ventricular I49.3

Deposit
- bone in Boeck's sarcoid D86.89
- calcareous, calcium — *see* Calcification
- cholesterol
  - retina H35.89
  - vitreous (body) (humor) — *see* Deposit, crystalline
- conjunctiva H11.11-
- cornea H18.00-
  - argentous H18.02-
  - due to metabolic disorder H18.03-
  - Kayser-Fleischer ring H18.04-
  - pigmentation — *see* Pigmentation, cornea
- crystalline, vitreous (body) (humor) H43.2-
- hemosiderin in old scars of cornea — *see* Pigmentation, cornea, stromal
- metallic in lens — *see* Cataract, specified NEC
- skin R23.8
- tooth, teeth (betel) (black) (green) (materia alba) (orange) (tobacco) K03.6
- urate, kidney — *see* Calculus, kidney

Depraved appetite — *see* Pica

Depressed
- HDL cholesterol E78.6

Depression (acute) (mental) F32.9
- agitated (single episode) F32.2
- anaclitic — *see* Disorder, adjustment
- anxiety F41.8
  - persistent F34.1
- arches — *see also* Deformity, limb, flat foot
- atypical (single episode) F32.89
  - recurrent episode F33.8
- basal metabolic rate R94.8
- bone marrow D75.89
- central nervous system R09.2
- cerebral R29.818
  - newborn P91.4
- cerebrovascular I67.9
- chest wall M95.4
- climacteric (single episode) F32.89
  - recurrent episode F33.8
- endogenous (without psychotic symptoms) F33.2
  - with psychotic symptoms F33.3
- functional activity R68.89
- hysterical F44.89
- involutional (single episode) F32.89
  - recurrent episode F33.8
- major F32.9
  - with psychotic symptoms F32.3
  - recurrent — *see* Disorder, depressive, recurrent
- manic-depressive — *see* Disorder, depressive, recurrent
- masked (single episode) F32.8
- medullary G93.89

Depression (acute) (mental) F32.9 — *continued*
  menopausal (single episode) F32.89
    recurrent episode F33.8
  metatarsus — *see* Depression, arches
  monopolar F33.9
  nervous F34.1
  neurotic F34.1
  nose M95.0
  postnatal F53
  postpartum F53
  post-psychotic of schizophrenia F32.89
  post-schizophrenic F32.89
  psychogenic (reactive) (single episode) F32.9
  psychoneurotic F34.1
  psychotic (single episode) F32.3
    recurrent F33.3
  reactive (psychogenic) (single episode) F32.9
    psychotic (single episode) F32.3
  recurrent — *see* Disorder, depressive, recurrent
  respiratory center G93.89
  seasonal — *see* Disorder, depressive, recurrent
  senile F03
  severe, single episode F32.2
  situational F43.21
  skull Q67.4
  specified NEC (single episode) F32.89
  sternum M95.4
  visual field — *see* Defect, visual field
  vital (recurrent) (without psychotic symptoms) F33.2
    with psychotic symptoms F33.3
    single episode F32.2

Deprivation
  cultural Z60.3
  effects NOS T73.9
    specified NEC T73.8
  emotional NEC Z65.8
    affecting infant or child — *see* Maltreatment, child, psychological
  food T73.0
  protein — *see* Malnutrition
  sleep Z72.820
  social Z60.4
    affecting infant or child — *see* Maltreatment, child, psychological
  specified NEC T73.8
  vitamins — *see* Deficiency, vitamin
  water T73.1

Derangement
  ankle (internal) — *see* Derangement, joint, ankle
  cartilage (articular) NEC — *see* Derangement, joint, articular cartilage, by site
    recurrent — *see* Dislocation, recurrent
  cruciate ligament, anterior, current injury — *see* Sprain, knee, cruciate, anterior
  elbow (internal) — *see* Derangement, joint, elbow
  hip (joint) (internal) (old) — *see* Derangement, joint, hip
  joint (internal) M24.9
    ankylosis — *see* Ankylosis
    articular cartilage M24.10
      ankle M24.17-
      elbow M24.12-
      foot M24.17-
      hand M24.14-
      hip M24.15-
      knee NEC M23.9-
      loose body — *see* Loose, body
      shoulder M24.11-
      wrist M24.13-
    contracture — *see* Contraction, joint
    current injury — *see also* Dislocation
      knee, meniscus or cartilage — *see* Tear, meniscus

Derangement — *continued*
  joint (internal) M24.9 — *continued*
    dislocation
      pathological — *see* Dislocation, pathological
      recurrent — *see* Dislocation, recurrent
    knee — *see* Derangement, knee
    ligament — *see* Disorder, ligament
    loose body — *see* Loose, body
    recurrent — *see* Dislocation, recurrent
    specified type NEC M24.80
      ankle M24.87-
      elbow M24.82-
      foot joint M24.87-
      hand joint M24.84-
      hip M24.85-
      shoulder M24.81-
      wrist M24.83-
    temporomandibular M26.69
  knee (recurrent) M23.9-
    ligament disruption, spontaneous M23.60-
      anterior cruciate M23.61-
      capsular M23.67-
      instability, chronic M23.5-
      lateral collateral M23.64-
      medial collateral M23.63-
      posterior cruciate M23.62-
    loose body M23.4-
    meniscus M23.30-
      cystic M23.00-
        lateral M23.002
          anterior horn M23.04-
          posterior horn M23.05-
          specified NEC M23.06-
        medial M23.005
          anterior horn M23.01-
          posterior horn M23.02-
          specified NEC M23.03-
      degenerate — *see* Derangement, knee, meniscus, specified NEC
      detached — *see* Derangement, knee, meniscus, specified NEC
      due to old tear or injury M23.20-
        lateral M23.20-
          anterior horn M23.24-
          posterior horn M23.25-
          specified NEC M23.26-
        medial M23.20-
          anterior horn M23.21-
          posterior horn M23.22-
          specified NEC M23.23-
      retained — *see* Derangement, knee, meniscus, specified NEC
      specified NEC M23.30-
        lateral M23.30-
          anterior horn M23.34-
          posterior horn M23.35-
          specified NEC M23.36-
        medial M23.30-
          anterior horn M23.31-
          posterior horn M23.32-
          specified NEC M23.33-
      old M23.8x-
      specified NEC — *see* subcategory M23.8
    low back NEC — *see* Dorsopathy, specified NEC
    meniscus — *see* Derangement, knee, meniscus
    mental — *see* Psychosis
    patella, specified NEC — *see* Disorder, patella, derangement NEC
    semilunar cartilage (knee) — *see* Derangement, knee, meniscus, specified NEC
  shoulder (internal) — *see* Derangement, joint, shoulder
Dercum's disease E88.2
Derealization (neurotic) F48.1
Dermal — *see* condition
Dermaphytid — *see* Dermatophytosis

Dermatitis (eczematous) L30.9
  ab igne L59.0
  acarine B88.0
  actinic (due to sun) L57.8
    other than from sun L59.8
  allergic — *see* Dermatitis, contact, allergic
  ambustionis, due to burn or scald — *see* Burn
  amebic A06.7
  ammonia L22
  arsenical (ingested) L27.8
  artefacta L98.1
    psychogenic F54
  atopic L20.9
    psychogenic F54
    specified NEC L20.89
  autoimmune progesterone L30.8
  berlock, berloque L56.2
  blastomycotic B40.3
  blister beetle L24.89
  bullous, bullosa L13.9
    mucosynechial, atrophic L12.1
    seasonal L30.8
    specified NEC L13.8
  calorica L59.0
    due to burn or scald — *see* Burn
  caterpillar L24.89
  cercarial B65.3
  combustionis L59.0
    due to burn or scald — *see* Burn
  congelationis T69.1
  contact (occupational) L25.9
    allergic L23.9
      due to
        adhesives L23.1
        cement L23.5
        chemical products NEC L23.5
        chromium L23.0
        cosmetics L23.2
        dander (cat) (dog) L23.81
        drugs in contact with skin L23.3
        dyes L23.4
        food in contact with skin L23.6
        hair (cat) (dog) L23.81
        insecticide L23.5
        metals L23.0
        nickel L23.0
        plants, non-food L23.7
        plastic L23.5
        rubber L23.5
        specified agent NEC L23.89
    due to
      cement L25.3
      chemical products NEC L25.3
      cosmetics L25.0
      dander (cat) (dog) L23.81
      drugs in contact with skin L25.1
      dyes L25.2
      food in contact with skin L25.4
      hair (cat) (dog) L23.81
      plants, non-food L25.5
      specified agent NEC L25.8
    irritant L24.9
      due to
        cement L24.5
        chemical products NEC L24.5
        cosmetics L24.3
        detergents L24.0
        drugs in contact with skin L24.4
        food in contact with skin L24.6
        oils and greases L24.1
        plants, non-food L24.7
        solvents L24.2
        specified agent NEC L24.89
  contusiformis L52
  diabetic — *see* E08-E13 with .620
  diaper L22
  diphtheritica A36.3
  dry skin L85.3

Dermatitis (eczematous) L30.9 — *continued*
  due to
    acetone (contact) (irritant) L24.2
    acids (contact) (irritant) L24.5
    adhesive(s) (allergic) (contact) (plaster) L23.1
      irritant L24.5
    alcohol (irritant) (skin contact) (substances in
        category T51) L24.2
      taken internally L27.8
    alkalis (contact) (irritant) L24.5
    arsenic (ingested) L27.8
    carbon disulfide (contact) (irritant) L24.2
    caustics (contact) (irritant) L24.5
    cement (contact) L25.3
    cereal (ingested) L27.2
    chemical(s) NEC L25.3
      taken internally L27.8
    chlorocompounds L24.2
    chromium (contact) (irritant) L24.81
    coffee (ingested) L27.2
    cold weather L30.8
    cosmetics (contact) L25.0
      allergic L23.2
      irritant L24.3
    cyclohexanes L24.2
    dander (cat) (dog) L23.81
    Demodex species B88.0
    Dermanyssus gallinae B88.0
    detergents (contact) (irritant) L24.0
    dichromate L24.81
    drugs and medicaments (generalized)
        (internal use) L27.0
      external — *see* Dermatitis, due to, drugs,
          in contact with skin
      in contact with skin L25.1
        allergic L23.3
        irritant L24.4
      localized skin eruption L27.1
      specified substance — *see* Table of Drugs
          and Chemicals
    dyes (contact) L25.2
      allergic L23.4
      irritant L24.89
    epidermophytosis — *see* Dermatophytosis
    esters L24.2
    external irritant NEC L24.9
    fish (ingested) L27.2
    flour (ingested) L27.2
    food (ingested) L27.2
      in contact with skin L25.4
    fruit (ingested) L27.2
    furs (allergic) (contact) L23.81
    glues — *see* Dermatitis, due to, adhesives
    glycols L24.2
    greases NEC (contact) (irritant) L24.1
    hair (cat) (dog) L23.81
    hot
      objects and materials — *see* Burn
      weather or places L59.0
    hydrocarbons L24.2
    infrared rays L59.8
    ingestion, ingested substance L27.9
      chemical NEC L27.8
      drugs and medicaments — *see* Dermatitis,
          due to, drugs
      food L27.2
      specified NEC L27.8
    insecticide in contact with skin L24.5
    internal agent L27.9
      drugs and medicaments (generalized) —
          see Dermatitis, due to, drugs
      food L27.2
    irradiation — *see* Dermatitis, due to,
        radioactive substance
    ketones L24.2
    lacquer tree (allergic) (contact) L23.7
    light (sun) NEC L57.8
      acute L56.8
      other L59.8

Dermatitis (eczematous) L30.9 — *continued*
  due to — *continued*
    Liponyssoides sanguineus B88.0
    low temperature L30.8
    meat (ingested) L27.2
    metals, metal salts (contact) (irritant) L24.81
    milk (ingested) L27.2
    nickel (contact) (irritant) L24.81
    nylon (contact) (irritant) L24.5
    oils NEC (contact) (irritant) L24.1
    paint solvent (contact) (irritant) L24.2
    petroleum products (contact) (irritant)
        (substances in T52.0) L24.2
    plants NEC (contact) L25.5
      allergic L23.7
      irritant L24.7
    plasters (adhesive) (any) (allergic) (contact)
        L23.1
      irritant L24.5
    plastic (contact) L25.3
    preservatives (contact) — *see* Dermatitis, due
        to, chemical, in contact with skin
    primrose (allergic) (contact) L23.7
    primula (allergic) (contact) L23.7
    radiation L59.8
      nonionizing (chronic exposure) L57.8
      sun NEC L57.8
        acute L56.8
    radioactive substance L58.9
      acute L58.0
      chronic L58.1
    radium L58.9
      acute L58.0
      chronic L58.1
    ragweed (allergic) (contact) L23.7
    Rhus (allergic) (contact) (diversiloba)
        (radicans) (toxicodendron) (venenata)
        (verniciflua) L23.7
    rubber (contact) L24.5
    Senecio jacobaea (allergic) (contact) L23.7
    solvents (contact) (irritant) (substances in
        category T52) L24.2
    specified agent NEC (contact) L25.8
      allergic L23.89
      irritant L24.89
    sunshine NEC L57.8
      acute L56.8
    tetrachlorethylene (contact) (irritant) L24.2
    toluene (contact) (irritant) L24.2
    turpentine (contact) L24.2
    ultraviolet rays (sun NEC) (chronic exposure)
        L57.8
      acute L56.8
    vaccine or vaccination L27.0
      specified substance — *see* Table of Drugs
          and Chemicals
    varicose veins — *see* Varix, leg, with,
        inflammation
    X-rays L58.9
      acute L58.0
      chronic L58.1
  dyshidrotic L30.1
  dysmenorrheica N94.6
  escharotica — *see* Burn
  exfoliative, exfoliativa (generalized) L26
    neonatorum L00
  eyelid — *see also* Dermatosis, eyelid
    allergic H01.119
      left H01.116
        lower H01.115
        upper H01.114
      right H01.113
        lower H01.112
        upper H01.111
    contact — *see* Dermatitis, eyelid, allergic
    due to
      Demodex species B88.0
      herpes (zoster) B02.39
      simplex B00.59

Dermatitis (eczematous) L30.9 — *continued*
  eyelid — *see also* Dermatosis, eyelid
    — *continued*
    eczematous H01.139
      left H01.136
        lower H01.135
        upper H01.134
      right H01.133
        lower H01.132
        upper H01.131
  facta, factitia, factitial L98.1
    psychogenic F54
  flexural NEC L20.82
  friction L30.4
  fungus B36.9
    specified type NEC B36.8
  gangrenosa, gangrenous infantum L08.0
  harvest mite B88.0
  heat L59.0
  herpesviral, vesicular (ear) (lip) B00.1
  herpetiformis (bullous) (erythematous)
      (pustular) (vesicular) L13.0
    juvenile L12.2
    senile L12.0
  hiemalis L30.8
  hypostatic, hypostatica — *see* Varix, leg, with,
      inflammation
  infectious eczematoid L30.3
  infective L30.3
  irritant — *see* Dermatitis, contact, irritant
  Jacquet's (diaper dermatitis) L22
  Leptus B88.0
  lichenified NEC L28.0
  medicamentosa (generalized) (internal use) —
      see Dermatitis, due to drugs
  mite B88.0
  multiformis L13.0
    juvenile L12.2
  napkin L22
  neurotica L13.0
  nummular L30.0
  papillaris capillitii L73.0
  pellagrous E52
  perioral L71.0
  photocontact L56.2
  polymorpha dolorosa L13.0
  pruriginosa L13.0
  pruritic NEC L30.8
  psychogenic F54
  purulent L08.0
  pustular
    contagious B08.02
    subcorneal L13.1
  pyococcal L08.0
  pyogenica L08.0
  repens L40.2
  Ritter's (exfoliativa) L00
  Schamberg's L81.7
  schistosome B65.3
  seasonal bullous L30.8
  seborrheic L21.9
    infantile L21.1
    specified NEC L21.8
  sensitization NOS L23.9
  septic L08.0
  solare L57.8
  specified NEC L30.8
  stasis I87.2
    with
      varicose ulcer — *see* Varix, leg, with ulcer,
          with inflammation
      varicose veins — *see* Varix, leg, with,
          inflammation
    due to postthrombotic syndrome — *see*
        Syndrome, postthrombotic
  suppurative L08.0
  traumatic NEC L30.4
  trophoneurotica L13.0

DISEASE INDEX

Dermatitis (eczematous) L30.9 — *continued*
ultraviolet (sun) (chronic exposure) L57.8
  acute L56.8
varicose — *see* Varix, leg, with, inflammation
vegetans L10.1
verrucosa B43.0
vesicular, herpesviral B00.1
Dermatoarthritis, lipoid E78.81
Dermatochalasis, eyelid H02.839
left H02.836
  lower H02.835
  upper H02.834
right H02.833
  lower H02.832
  upper H02.831
Dermatofibroma (lenticulare) — *see*
  Neoplasm, skin, benign
protuberans — *see* Neoplasm, skin, uncertain
  behavior
Dermatofibrosarcoma (pigmented)
  (protuberans) — *see* Neoplasm, skin,
  malignant
Dermatographia L50.3
Dermatolysis (exfoliativa) (congenital) Q82.8
acquired L57.4
eyelids — *see* Blepharochalasis
palpebrarum — *see* Blepharochalasis
senile L57.4
Dermatomegaly NEC Q82.8
Dermatomucosomyositis M33.10
with
  myopathy M33.12
  respiratory involvement M33.11
  specified organ involvement NEC M33.19
Dermatomycosis B36.9
furfuracea B36.0
specified type NEC B36.8
Dermatomyositis (acute) (chronic) — *see also*
  Dermatopolymyositis
in (due to) neoplastic disease (*see also*
  Neoplasm) D49.9 [M36.0]
Dermatoneuritis of children — *see*
  Poisoning, mercury
Dermatophilosis A48.8
Dermatophytid L30.2
Dermatophytide — *see* Dermatophytosis
Dermatophytosis (epidermophyton) (infection)
  (Microsporum) (tinea) (Trichophyton) B35.9
beard B35.0
body B35.4
capitis B35.0
corporis B35.4
deep-seated B35.8
disseminated B35.8
foot B35.3
granulomatous B35.8
groin B35.6
hand B35.2
nail B35.1
perianal (area) B35.6
scalp B35.0
specified NEC B35.8
Dermatopolymyositis M33.90
with
  myopathy M33.92
  respiratory involvement M33.91
  specified organ involvement NEC M33.99
in neoplastic disease (*see also* Neoplasm)
  D49.9 [M36.0]
juvenile M33.00
  with
    myopathy M33.02
    respiratory involvement M33.01
    specified organ involvement NEC M33.09
specified NEC M33.10
  myopathy M33.12
  respiratory involvement M33.11
  specified organ involvement NEC M33.19

Dermatopolyneuritis — *see* Poisoning,
  mercury
Dermatorrhexis Q79.6
acquired L57.4
Dermatosclerosis — *see also* Scleroderma
localized L94.0
Dermatosis L98.9
Andrews' L08.89
Bowen's — *see* Neoplasm, skin, in situ
bullous L13.9
  specified NEC L13.8
exfoliativa L26
eyelid (noninfectious)
  dermatitis — *see* Dermatitis, eyelid
  discoid lupus erythematosus — *see* Lupus,
    erythematosus, eyelid
  xeroderma — *see* Xeroderma, acquired,
    eyelid
factitial L98.1
febrile neutrophilic L98.2
gonococcal A54.89
herpetiformis L13.0
  juvenile L12.2
linear IgA L13.8
menstrual NEC L98.8
neutrophilic, febrile L98.2
occupational — *see* Dermatitis, contact
papulosa nigra L82.1
pigmentary L81.9
  progressive L81.7
  Schamberg's L81.7
psychogenic F54
purpuric, pigmented L81.7
pustular, subcorneal L13.1
transient acantholytic L11.1
Dermographia, dermographism L50.3
Dermoid (cyst) — *see also* Neoplasm, benign,
  by site
with malignant transformation C56-
due to radiation (nonionizing) L57.8
Dermopathy
infiltrative with thyrotoxicosis — *see*
  Thyrotoxicosis
nephrogenic fibrosing L90.8
Dermophytosis — *see* Dermatophytosis
Descemet's membrane — *see* condition
Descemetocele H18.73-
Descending — *see* condition
Descensus uteri — *see* Prolapse, uterus
Desert
rheumatism B38.0
sore — *see* Ulcer, skin
Desertion (newborn) — *see* Maltreatment
Desmoid (extra-abdominal) (tumor) — *see*
  Neoplasm, connective tissue, uncertain
  behavior
abdominal D48.1
Despondency F32.9
Desquamation, skin R23.4
Destruction, destructive — *see also* Damage
articular facet — *see also* Derangement, joint,
  specified type NEC
  knee M23.8x-
  vertebra — *see* Spondylosis
bone — *see also* Disorder, bone, specified type
  NEC
  syphilitic A52.77
joint — *see also* Derangement, joint, specified
  type NEC
  sacroiliac M53.3
rectal sphincter K62.89
septum (nasal) J34.89
tuberculous NEC — *see* Tuberculosis
tympanum, tympanic membrane
  (nontraumatic) — *see* Disorder, tympanic
  membrane, specified NEC
vertebral disc — *see* Degeneration,
  intervertebral disc

Destructiveness — *see also* Disorder, conduct
adjustment reaction — *see* Disorder, adjustment
Desultory labor O62.2
Detachment
cartilage — *see* Sprain
cervix, annular N88.8
  complicating delivery O71.3
choroid (old) (postinfectional) (simple)
  (spontaneous) H31.40-
  hemorrhagic H31.41-
  serous H31.42-
ligament — *see* Sprain
meniscus (knee) — *see also* Derangement,
  knee, meniscus, specified NEC
  current injury — *see* Tear, meniscus
  due to old tear or injury — *see*
    Derangement, knee, meniscus, due to
    old tear
retina (without retinal break) (serous) H33.2-
  with retinal:
    break H33.00-
      giant H33.03-
      multiple H33.02-
      single H33.01-
    dialysis H33.04-
  pigment epithelium — *see* Degeneration,
    retina, separation of layers, pigment
    epithelium detachment
  rhegmatogenous — *see* Detachment, retina,
    with retinal, break
  specified NEC H33.8
  total H33.05-
  traction H33.4-
vitreous (body) H43.81
Detergent asthma J69.8
Deterioration
epileptic F06.8
general physical R53.81
heart, cardiac — *see* Degeneration,
  myocardial
mental — *see* Psychosis
myocardial, myocardium — *see* Degeneration,
  myocardial
senile (simple) R54
Deuteranomaly (anomalous trichromat)
  H53.53
Deuteranopia (complete) (incomplete) H53.53
Development
abnormal, bone Q79.9
arrested R62.50
  bone — *see* Arrest, development or growth,
    bone
  child R62.50
  due to malnutrition E45
defective, congenital — *see also* Anomaly, by
  site
  cauda equina Q06.3
  left ventricle Q24.8
    in hypoplastic left heart syndrome Q23.4
  valve Q24.8
    pulmonary Q22.3
delayed (*see also* Delay, development) R62.50
  arithmetical skills F81.2
  language (skills) (expressive) F80.1
  learning skill F81.9
  mixed skills F88
  motor coordination F82
  reading F81.0
  specified learning skill NEC F81.89
  speech F80.9
  spelling F81.81
  written expression F81.81
imperfect, congenital — *see also* Anomaly, by
  site
  heart Q24.9
  lungs Q33.6

DISEASE INDEX

Development — *continued*
- incomplete
  - bronchial tree Q32.4
  - organ or site not listed — *see* Hypoplasia, by site
  - respiratory system Q34.9
- sexual, precocious NEC E30.1
- tardy, mental (*see also* Disability, intellectual) F79

Developmental — *see* condition
- testing, infant or child — *see* Examination, child

Devergie's disease (pityriasis rubra pilaris) L44.0

Deviation (in)
- conjugate palsy (eye) (spastic) H51.0
- esophagus (acquired) K22.8
- eye, skew H51.8
- midline (jaw) (teeth) (dental arch) M26.29
  - specified site NEC — *see* Malposition
- nasal septum J34.2
  - congenital Q67.4
- opening and closing of the mandible M26.53
- organ or site, congenital NEC — *see* Malposition, congenital
- septum (nasal) (acquired) J34.2
  - congenital Q67.4
- sexual F65.9
  - bestiality F65.89
  - erotomania F52.8
  - exhibitionism F65.2
  - fetishism, fetishistic F65.0
    - transvestism F65.1
  - frotteurism F65.81
  - masochism F65.51
  - multiple F65.89
  - necrophilia F65.89
  - nymphomania F52.8
  - pederosis F65.4
  - pedophilia F65.4
  - sadism, sadomasochism F65.52
  - satyriasis F52.8
  - specified type NEC F65.89
  - transvestism F64.1
  - voyeurism F65.3
- teeth, midline M26.29
- trachea J39.8
- ureter, congenital Q62.61

Devic's disease G36.0

Device
- cerebral ventricle (communicating) in situ Z98.2
- contraceptive — *see* Contraceptive, device
- drainage, cerebrospinal fluid, in situ Z98.2

Devil's
- grip B33.0
- pinches (purpura simplex) D69.2

Devitalized tooth K04.99

Devonshire colic — *see* Poisoning, lead

Dextraposition, aorta Q20.3
- in tetralogy of Fallot Q21.3

Dextrinosis, limit (debrancher enzyme deficiency) E74.03

Dextrocardia (true) Q24.0
- with
  - complete transposition of viscera Q89.3
  - situs inversus Q89.3

Dextrotransposition, aorta Q20.3

d-glycericacidemia E72.59

Dhat syndrome F48.8

Dhobi itch B35.6

Diabetes, diabetic (mellitus) (sugar) E11.9
- with
  - amyotrophy E11.44
  - arthropathy NEC E11.618
  - autonomic (poly)neuropathy E11.43
  - cataract E11.36
  - Charcôt's joints E11.610
  - chronic kidney disease E11.22

Diabetes, diabetic (mellitus) (sugar) E11.9 — *continued*
- with — *continued*
  - circulatory complication NEC E11.59
  - complication E11.8
    - specified NEC E11.69
  - dermatitis E11.620
  - foot ulcer E11.621
  - gangrene E11.52
  - gastroparalysis E11.43
  - gastroparesis E11.43
  - glomerulonephrosis, intracapillary E11.21
  - glomerulosclerosis, intercapillary E11.21
  - hyperglycemia E11.65
  - hyperosmolarity E11.00
    - with coma E11.01
  - hypoglycemia E11.649
    - with coma E11.641
  - kidney complications NEC E11.29
  - Kimmelstiel-Wilson disease E11.21
  - loss of protective sensation (LOPS) — *see* Diabetes, by type, with neuropathy
  - mononeuropathy E11.41
  - myasthenia E11.44
  - necrobiosis lipoidica E11.620
  - nephropathy E11.21
  - neuralgia E11.42
  - neurologic complication NEC E11.49
  - neuropathic arthropathy E11.610
  - neuropathy E11.40
  - ophthalmic complication NEC E11.39
  - oral complication NEC E11.638
  - osteomyelitis E11.69
  - periodontal disease E11.630
  - peripheral angiopathy E11.51
    - with gangrene E11.52
  - polyneuropathy E11.42
  - renal complication NEC E11.29
  - renal tubular degeneration E11.29
  - retinopathy E11.319
    - with macular edema E11.311
      - resolved following treatment E11.37
    - nonproliferative E11.329
      - with macular edema E11.321
      - mild E11.329
        - with macular edema E11.321
      - moderate E11.339
        - with macular edema E11.331
      - severe E11.349
        - with macular edema E11.341
    - proliferative E11.359
      - with
        - combined traction retinal detachment and rhegmatogenous retinal detachment E11.354
        - macular edema E11.351
        - stable proliferative diabetic retinopathy E11.355
        - traction retinal detachment involving the macula E11.352
        - traction retinal detachment not involving the macula E11.353
  - skin complication NEC E11.628
  - skin ulcer NEC E11.622
- brittle — *see* Diabetes, type 1
- bronzed E83.110
- complicating pregnancy — *see* Pregnancy, complicated by, diabetes
- dietary counseling and surveillance Z71.3
- due to
  - autoimmune process — *see* Diabetes, type 1
  - immune mediated pancreatic islet beta-cell destruction — *see* Diabetes, type 1
- due to drug or chemical E09.9
  - with
    - amyotrophy E09.44
    - arthropathy NEC E09.618
    - autonomic (poly)neuropathy E09.43
    - cataract E09.36

Diabetes, diabetic (mellitus) (sugar) E11.9 — *continued*
- due to drug or chemical E09.9 — *continued*
  - with — *continued*
    - Charcôt's joints E09.610
    - chronic kidney disease E09.22
    - circulatory complication NEC E09.59
    - complication E09.8
      - specified NEC E09.69
    - dermatitis E09.620
    - foot ulcer E09.621
    - gangrene E09.52
    - gastroparalysis E09.43
    - gastroparesis E09.43
    - glomerulonephrosis, intracapillary E09.21
    - glomerulosclerosis, intercapillary E09.21
    - hyperglycemia E09.65
    - hyperosmolarity E09.00
      - with coma E09.01
    - hypoglycemia E09.649
      - with coma E09.641
    - ketoacidosis E09.10
      - with coma E09.11
    - kidney complications NEC E09.29
    - Kimmelstiel-Wilson disease E09.21
    - mononeuropathy E09.41
    - myasthenia E09.44
    - necrobiosis lipoidica E09.620
    - nephropathy E09.21
    - neuralgia E09.42
    - neurologic complication NEC E09.49
    - neuropathic arthropathy E09.610
    - neuropathy E09.40
    - ophthalmic complication NEC E09.39
    - oral complication NEC E09.638
    - periodontal disease E09.630
    - peripheral angiopathy E09.51
      - with gangrene E09.52
    - polyneuropathy E09.42
    - renal complication NEC E09.29
    - renal tubular degeneration E09.29
    - retinopathy E09.319
      - with macular edema E09.311
        - resolved following treatment E09.37
      - nonproliferative E09.329
        - with macular edema E09.321
        - mild E09.329
          - with macular edema E09.321
        - moderate E09.339
          - with macular edema E09.331
        - severe E09.349
          - with macular edema E09.341
      - proliferative E09.359
        - with
          - combined traction retinal detachment and rhegmatogenous retinal detachment E09.354
          - macular edema E09.351
          - stable proliferative diabetic retinopathy E09.355
          - traction retinal detachment involving the macula E09.352
          - traction retinal detachment not involving the macula E09.353
    - skin complication NEC E09.628
    - skin ulcer NEC E09.622
- due to underlying condition E08.9
  - with
    - amyotrophy E08.44
    - arthropathy NEC E08.618
    - autonomic (poly)neuropathy E08.43
    - cataract E08.36
    - Charcôt's joints E08.610
    - chronic kidney disease E08.22
    - circulatory complication NEC E08.59
    - complication E08.8
      - specified NEC E08.69
    - dermatitis E08.620

D I S E A S E   I N D E X

Diabetes, diabetic (mellitus) (sugar) E11.9 — *continued*
- due to underlying condition E08.9 — *continued*
  - with — *continued*
    - foot ulcer E08.621
    - gangrene E08.52
    - gastroparalysis E08.43
    - gastroparesis E08.43
    - glomerulonephrosis, intracapillary E08.21
    - glomerulosclerosis, intercapillary E08.21
    - hyperglycemia E08.65
    - hyperosmolarity E08.00
      - with coma E08.01
    - hypoglycemia E08.649
      - with coma E08.641
    - ketoacidosis E08.10
      - with coma E08.11
    - kidney complications NEC E08.29
    - Kimmelstiel-Wilson disease E08.21
    - mononeuropathy E08.41
    - myasthenia E08.44
    - necrobiosis lipoidica E08.620
    - nephropathy E08.21
    - neuralgia E08.42
    - neurologic complication NEC E08.49
    - neuropathic arthropathy E08.610
    - neuropathy E08.40
    - ophthalmic complication NEC E08.39
    - oral complication NEC E08.638
    - periodontal disease E08.630
    - peripheral angiopathy E08.51
      - with gangrene E08.52
    - polyneuropathy E08.42
    - renal complication NEC E08.29
    - renal tubular degeneration E08.29
    - retinopathy E08.319
      - with macular edema E08.311
        - resolved following treatment E08.37
      - nonproliferative E08.329
        - with macular edema E08.321
        - mild E08.329
          - with macular edema E08.321
        - moderate E08.339
          - with macular edema E08.331
        - severe E08.349
          - with macular edema E08.341
      - proliferative E08.359
        - with
          - combined traction retinal detachment and rhegmatogenous retinal detachment E08.354
          - macular edema E08.351
          - stable proliferative diabetic retinopathy E08.355
          - traction retinal detachment involving the macula E08.352
          - traction retinal detachment not involving the macula E08.353
    - skin complication NEC E08.628
    - skin ulcer NEC E08.622
- gestational (in pregnancy) O24.419
  - affecting newborn P70.0
  - diet controlled O24.410
  - in childbirth O24.429
    - diet controlled O24.420
    - insulin (and diet) controlled O24.424
    - oral drug controlled (antidiabetic) (hypoglycemic) O24.425
  - insulin (and diet) controlled O24.414
  - oral drug controlled (antidiabetic) (hypoglycemic) O24.415
  - puerperal O24.439
    - diet controlled O24.430
    - insulin (and diet) controlled O24.434
    - oral drug controlled (antidiabetic) (hypoglycemic) O24.435
- hepatogenous E13.9

Diabetes, diabetic (mellitus) (sugar) E11.9 — *continued*
- inadequately controlled — *code to* Diabetes, by type, with hyperglycemia
- idiopathic — *see* Diabetes, type 1
- insipidus E23.2
  - nephrogenic N25.1
  - pituitary E23.2
  - vasopressin resistant N25.1
- insulin dependent — *code to* type of diabetes
- juvenile-onset — *see* Diabetes, type 1
- ketosis-prone — *see* Diabetes, type 1
- latent R73.03
- neonatal (transient) P70.2
- non-insulin dependent — *code to* type of diabetes
- out of control — *code to* Diabetes, by type, with hyperglycemia
- phosphate E83.39
- poorly controlled — *code to* Diabetes, by type, with hyperglycemia
- postpancreatectomy — *see* Diabetes, specified type NEC
- postprocedural — *see* Diabetes, specified type NEC
- secondary diabetes mellitus NEC — *see* Diabetes, specified type NEC
- specified type NEC E13.9
  - with
    - amyotrophy E13.44
    - arthropathy NEC E13.618
    - autonomic (poly)neuropathy E13.43
    - cataract E13.36
    - Charcôt's joints E13.610
    - chronic kidney disease E13.22
    - circulatory complication NEC E13.59
    - complication E13.8
      - specified NEC E13.69
    - dermatitis E13.620
    - foot ulcer E13.621
    - gangrene E13.52
    - gastroparalysis E13.43
    - gastroparesis E13.43
    - glomerulonephrosis, intracapillary E13.21
    - glomerulosclerosis, intercapillary E13.21
    - hyperglycemia E13.65
    - hyperosmolarity E13.00
      - with coma E13.01
    - hypoglycemia E13.649
      - with coma E13.641
    - ketoacidosis E13.10
      - with coma E13.11
    - kidney complications NEC E13.29
    - Kimmelstiel-Wilson disease E13.21
    - mononeuropathy E13.41
    - myasthenia E13.44
    - necrobiosis lipoidica E13.620
    - nephropathy E13.21
    - neuralgia E13.42
    - neurologic complication NEC E13.49
    - neuropathic arthropathy E13.610
    - neuropathy E13.40
    - ophthalmic complication NEC E13.39
    - oral complication NEC E13.638
    - periodontal disease E13.630
    - peripheral angiopathy E13.51
      - with gangrene E13.52
    - polyneuropathy E13.42
    - renal complication NEC E13.29
    - renal tubular degeneration E13.29

Diabetes, diabetic (mellitus) (sugar) E11.9 — *continued*
- specified type NEC E13.9 — *continued*
  - with — *continued*
    - retinopathy E13.319
      - with macular edema E13.311
        - resolved following treatment E13.37
      - nonproliferative E13.329
        - with macular edema E13.321
        - mild E13.329
          - with macular edema E13.321
        - moderate E13.339
          - with macular edema E13.331
        - severe E13.349
          - with macular edema E13.341
      - proliferative E13.359
        - with
          - combined traction retinal detachment and rhegmatogenous retinal detachment E13.354
          - macular edema E13.351
          - stable proliferative diabetic retinopathy E13.355
          - traction retinal detachment involving the macula E13.352
          - traction retinal detachment not involving the macula E13.353
    - skin complication NEC E13.628
    - skin ulcer NEC E13.622
- steroid-induced — *see* Diabetes, due to, drug or chemical
- type 1 E10.9
  - with
    - amyotrophy E10.44
    - arthropathy NEC E10.618
    - autonomic (poly)neuropathy E10.43
    - cataract E10.36
    - Charcôt's joints E10.610
    - chronic kidney disease E10.22
    - circulatory complication NEC E10.59
    - complication E10.8
      - specified NEC E10.69
    - dermatitis E10.620
    - foot ulcer E10.621
    - gangrene E10.52
    - gastroparalysis E10.43
    - gastroparesis E10.43
    - glomerulonephrosis, intracapillary E10.21
    - glomerulosclerosis, intercapillary E10.21
    - hyperglycemia E10.65
    - hypoglycemia E10.649
      - with coma E10.641
    - ketoacidosis E10.10
      - with coma E10.11
    - kidney complications NEC E10.29
    - Kimmelstiel-Wilson disease E10.21
    - mononeuropathy E10.41
    - myasthenia E10.44
    - necrobiosis lipoidica E10.620
    - nephropathy E10.21
    - neuralgia E10.42
    - neurologic complication NEC E10.49
    - neuropathic arthropathy E10.610
    - neuropathy E10.40
    - ophthalmic complication NEC E10.39
    - oral complication NEC E10.638
    - periodontal disease E10.630
    - peripheral angiopathy E10.51
      - with gangrene E10.52
    - polyneuropathy E10.42
    - renal complication NEC E10.29
    - renal tubular degeneration E10.29

Diabetes, diabetic (mellitus) (sugar) E11.9 — *continued*
type 1 E10.9 — *continued*
with — *continued*
retinopathy E10.319
with macular edema E10.311
resolved following treatment E10.37
nonproliferative E10.329
with macular edema E10.321
mild E10.329
with macular edema E10.321
moderate E10.339
with macular edema E10.331
severe E10.349
with macular edema E10.341
proliferative E10.359
with
combined traction retinal detachment and rhegmatogenous retinal detachment E10.354
macular edema E10.351
stable proliferative diabetic retinopathy E10.355
traction retinal detachment involving the macula E10.352
traction retinal detachment not involving the macula E10.353
skin complication NEC E10.628
skin ulcer NEC E10.622
type 2 E11.9
with
amyotrophy E11.44
arthropathy NEC E11.618
autonomic (poly)neuropathy E11.43
cataract E11.36
Charcot's joints E11.610
chronic kidney disease E11.22
circulatory complication NEC E11.59
complication E11.8
specified NEC E11.69
dermatitis E11.620
foot ulcer E11.621
gangrene E11.52
gastroparalysis E11.43
gastroparesis E11.43
glomerulonephrosis, intracapillary E11.21
glomerulosclerosis, intercapillary E11.21
hyperglycemia E11.65
hyperosmolarity E11.00
with coma E11.01
hypoglycemia E11.649
with coma E11.641
kidney complications NEC E11.29
Kimmelstiel-Wilson disease E11.21
mononeuropathy E11.41
myasthenia E11.44
necrobiosis lipoidica E11.620
nephropathy E11.21
neuralgia E11.42
neurologic complication NEC E11.49
neuropathic arthropathy E11.610
neuropathy E11.40
ophthalmic complication NEC E11.39
oral complication NEC E11.638
periodontal disease E11.630
peripheral angiopathy E11.51
with gangrene E11.52
polyneuropathy E11.42
renal complication NEC E11.29
renal tubular degeneration E11.29

Diabetes, diabetic (mellitus) (sugar) E11.9 — *continued*
type 2 E11.9 — *continued*
with — *continued*
retinopathy E11.319
with macular edema E11.311
resolved following treatment E11.37
nonproliferative E11.329
with macular edema E11.321
mild E11.329
with macular edema E11.321
moderate E11.339
with macular edema E11.331
severe E11.349
with macular edema E11.341
proliferative E11.359
with
combined traction retinal detachment and rhegmatogenous retinal detachment E11.354
macular edema E11.351
stable proliferative diabetic retinopathy E11.355
traction retinal detachment involving the macula E11.352
traction retinal detachment not involving the macula E11.353
skin complication NEC E11.628
skin ulcer NEC E11.622
uncontrolled
meaning
hyperglycemia — *see* Diabetes, by type, with, hyperglycemia
hypoglycemia — *see* Diabetes, by type, with, hypoglycemia
Diacyclothrombopathia D69.1
Diagnosis deferred R69
Dialysis (intermittent) (treatment)
noncompliance (with) Z91.15
renal (hemodialysis) (peritoneal), status Z99.2
retina, retinal — *see* Detachment, retina, with retinal, dialysis
Diamond-Blackfan anemia (congenital hypoplastic) D61.01
Diamond-Gardener syndrome (autoerythrocyte sensitization) D69.2
Diaper rash L22
Diaphoresis (excessive) R61
Diaphragm — *see* condition
Diaphragmalgia R07.1
Diaphragmatitis, diaphragmitis J98.6
Diaphysial aclasis Q78.6
Diaphysitis — *see* Osteomyelitis, specified type NEC
Diarrhea, diarrheal (disease) (infantile) (inflammatory) R19.7
achlorhydric K31.83
allergic K52.29
due to
colitis — *see* Colitis, allergic
enteritis — *see* Enteritis, allergic
amebic (*see also* Amebiasis) A06.0
with abscess — *see* Abscess, amebic
acute A06.0
chronic A06.1
nondysenteric A06.2
bacillary — *see* Dysentery, bacillary
balantidial A07.0
cachectic NEC K52.89
Chilomastix A07.8
choleriformis A00.1
chronic (noninfectious) K52.9
coccidial A07.3
Cochin-China K90.1
strongyloidiasis B78.0
Dientamoeba A07.8
dietetic (*see also* Diarrhea, allergic) K52.29
drug-induced K52.1

Diarrhea, diarrheal (disease) (infantile) (inflammatory) R19.7 — *continued*
due to
bacteria A04.9
specified NEC A04.8
Campylobacter A04.5
Capillaria philippinensis B81.1
Clostridium difficile A04.7
Clostridium perfringens (C) (F) A04.8
Cryptosporidium A07.2
drugs K52.1
Escherichia coli A04.4
enteroaggregative A04.4
enterohemorrhagic A04.3
enteroinvasive A04.2
enteropathogenic A04.0
enterotoxigenic A04.1
specified NEC A04.4
food hypersensitivity (*see also* Diarrhea, allergic) K52.29
Necator americanus B76.1
S. japonicum B65.2
specified organism NEC A08.8
bacterial A04.8
viral A08.39
Staphylococcus A04.8
Trichuris trichiuria B79
virus — *see* Enteritis, viral
Yersinia enterocolitica A04.6
dysenteric A09
endemic A09
epidemic A09
flagellate A07.9
Flexner's (ulcerative) A03.1
functional K59.1
following gastrointestinal surgery K91.89
psychogenic F45.8
Giardia lamblia A07.1
giardial A07.1
hill K90.1
infectious A09
malarial — *see* Malaria
mite B88.0
mycotic NEC B49
neonatal (noninfectious) P78.3
nervous F45.8
neurogenic K59.1
noninfectious K52.9
postgastrectomy K91.1
postvagotomy K91.1
protozoal A07.9
specified NEC A07.8
psychogenic F45.8
specified
bacterium NEC A04.8
virus NEC A08.39
strongyloidiasis B78.0
toxic K52.1
trichomonal A07.8
tropical K90.1
tuberculous A18.32
viral — *see* Enteritis, viral

Diastasis
cranial bones M84.88
congenital NEC Q75.8
joint (traumatic) — *see* Dislocation
muscle M62.00
ankle M62.07-
congenital Q79.8
foot M62.07-
forearm M62.03-
hand M62.04-
lower leg M62.06-
pelvic region M62.05-
shoulder region M62.01-
specified site NEC M62.08
thigh M62.05-
upper arm M62.02-

© 2016 Channel Publishing, Ltd.

DISEASE INDEX

Diastasis — *continued*
recti (abdomen)
  complicating delivery O71.89
  congenital Q79.59
Diastema, tooth, teeth, fully erupted
  M26.32
Diastematomyelia Q06.2
Diataxia, cerebral G80.4
Diathesis
allergic — *see* History, allergy
bleeding (familial) D69.9
cystine (familial) E72.00
gouty — *see* Gout
hemorrhagic (familial) D69.9
  newborn NEC P53
spasmophilic R29.0
Diaz's disease or osteochondrosis
  (juvenile) (talus) — *see* Osteochondrosis,
  juvenile, tarsus
Dibothriocephalus, dibothriocephaliasis
  (latus) (infection) (infestation) B70.0
  larval B70.1
Dicephalus, dicephaly Q89.4
Dichotomy, teeth K00.2
Dichromat, dichromatopsia (congenital) —
  see Deficiency, color vision
Dichuchwa A65
Dicroceliasis B66.2
Didelphia, didelphys — *see* Double uterus
Didymytis N45.1
with orchitis N45.3
Dietary
inadequacy or deficiency E63.9
surveillance and counseling Z71.3
Dietl's crisis N13.8
Dieulafoy lesion (hemorrhagic)
duodenum K31.82
esophagus K22.8
intestine (colon) K63.81
stomach K31.82
Difficult, difficulty (in)
acculturation Z60.3
feeding R63.3
  newborn P92.9
    breast P92.5
    specified NEC P92.8
  nonorganic (infant or child) F98.29
intubation, in anesthesia T88.4
mechanical, gastroduodenal stoma K91.89
  causing obstruction K91.3
micturition
  need to immediately re-void R39.191
  position dependent R39.192
  specified NEC R39.198
reading (developmental) F81.0
  secondary to emotional disorders F93.9
spelling (specific) F81.81
  with reading disorder F81.89
  due to inadequate teaching Z55.8
swallowing — *see* Dysphagia
walking R26.2
work
  conditions NEC Z56.5
  schedule Z56.3
Diffuse — *see* condition
Di George's syndrome (thymic hypoplasia)
  D82.1
Di Guglielmo's disease C94.0-
Digestive — *see* condition
Dihydropyrimidine dehydrogenase
  disease (DPD) E88.89
Diktyoma — *see* Neoplasm, malignant, by site
Dilaceration, tooth K00.4
Dilatation
anus K59.8
  venule — *see* Hemorrhoids
aorta (focal) (general) — *see* Ectasia, aorta
  with aneurysm — *see* Aneurysm, aorta
  congenital Q25.44

Dilatation — *continued*
artery — *see* Aneurysm
bladder (sphincter) N32.89
  congenital Q64.79
blood vessel I99.8
bronchial J47.9
  with
    exacerbation (acute) J47.1
    lower respiratory infection J47.0
calyx (due to obstruction) — *see*
  Hydronephrosis
capillaries I78.8
cardiac (acute) (chronic) — *see also*
  Hypertrophy, cardiac
  congenital Q24.8
    valve NEC Q24.8
      pulmonary Q22.3
  valve — *see* Endocarditis
cavum septi pellucidi Q06.8
cervix (uteri) — *see also* Incompetency, cervix
  incomplete, poor, slow complicating delivery
    O62.0
colon K59.39
  congenital Q43.1
  psychogenic F45.8
  toxic K59.31
common duct (acquired) K83.8
  congenital Q44.5
cystic duct (acquired) K82.8
  congenital Q44.5
duct, mammary — *see* Ectasia, mammary duct
duodenum K59.8
esophagus K22.8
  congenital Q39.5
  due to achalasia K22.0
eustachian tube, congenital Q17.8
gallbladder K82.8
gastric — *see* Dilatation, stomach
heart (acute) (chronic) — *see also* Hypertrophy,
  cardiac
  congenital Q24.8
  valve — *see* Endocarditis
ileum K59.8
  psychogenic F45.8
jejunum K59.8
  psychogenic F45.8
kidney (calyx) (collecting structures) (cystic)
  (parenchyma) (pelvis) (idiopathic) N28.89
lacrimal passages or duct — *see* Disorder,
  lacrimal system, changes
lymphatic vessel I89.0
mammary duct — *see* Ectasia, mammary duct
Meckel's diverticulum (congenital) Q43.0
  malignant — *see* Table of Neoplasms, small
    intestine, malignant
myocardium (acute) (chronic) — *see*
  Hypertrophy, cardiac
organ or site, congenital NEC — *see* Distortion
pancreatic duct K86.89
pericardium — *see* Pericarditis
pharynx J39.2
prostate N42.89
pulmonary
  artery (idiopathic) I28.8
  valve, congenital Q22.3
pupil H57.04
rectum K59.39
saccule, congenital Q16.5
salivary gland (duct) K11.8
sphincter ani K62.89
stomach K31.89
  acute K31.0
  psychogenic F45.8
submaxillary duct K11.8
trachea, congenital Q32.1
ureter (idiopathic) N28.82
  congenital Q62.2
  due to obstruction N13.4
urethra (acquired) N36.8

Dilatation — *continued*
vasomotor I73.9
vein I86.8
ventricular, ventricle (acute) (chronic) — *see*
  also Hypertrophy, cardiac
  cerebral, congenital Q04.8
venule NEC I86.8
vesical orifice N32.89
Dilated, dilation — *see* Dilatation
Diminished, diminution
hearing (acuity) — *see* Deafness
sense or sensation (cold) (heat) (tactile)
  (vibratory) R20.8
vision NEC H54.7
vital capacity R94.2
Diminuta taenia B71.0
Dimitri-Sturge-Weber disease Q85.8
Dimple
congenital sacral Q82.6
parasacral Q82.6
pilonidal or postanal — *see* Cyst, pilonidal
Dioctophyme renalis (infection) (infestation)
  B83.8
Dipetalonemiasis B74.4
Diphallus Q55.69
Diphtheria, diphtheritic (gangrenous)
  (hemorrhagic) A36.9
carrier (suspected) Z22.2
cutaneous A36.3
faucial A36.0
infection of wound A36.3
laryngeal A36.2
myocarditis A36.81
nasal, anterior A36.89
nasopharyngeal A36.1
neurological complication A36.89
pharyngeal A36.0
specified site NEC A36.89
tonsillar A36.0
Diphyllobothriasis (intestine) B70.0
larval B70.1
Diplacusis H93.22-
Diplegia (upper limbs) G83.0
congenital (cerebral) G80.8
facial G51.0
lower limbs G82.20
spastic G80.1
Diplococcus, diplococcal — *see* condition
Dipsomania F10.20
  with
    psychosis — *see* Psychosis, alcoholic
    remission F10.21
Dipylidiasis B71.1
Diplopia H53.2
DIRA (deficiency of interleukin 1 receptor
  antagonist) M04.8
Direction, teeth, abnormal, fully erupted
  M26.30
Dirofilariasis B74.8
Dirt-eating child F98.3
Disability, disabilities
heart — *see* Disease, heart
intellectual F79
  with
    autistic features F84.9
  mild (I.Q. 50-69) F70
  moderate (I.Q. 35-49) F71
  profound (I.Q. under 20) F73
  severe (I.Q. 20-34) F72
  specified level NEC F78
knowledge acquisition F81.9
learning F81.9
limiting activities Z73.6
spelling, specific F81.81
Disappearance of family member Z63.4
Disarticulation — *see* Amputation
meaning traumatic amputation — *see*
  Amputation, traumatic

Discharge (from)
  abnormal finding in — *see* Abnormal,
    specimen
  breast (female) (male) N64.52
  diencephalic autonomic idiopathic — *see*
    Epilepsy, specified NEC
  ear — *see also* Otorrhea
    blood — *see* Otorrhagia
  excessive urine R35.8
  nipple N64.52
  penile R36.9
  postnasal R09.82
  prison, anxiety concerning Z65.2
  urethral R36.9
    hematospermia R36.1
    without blood R36.0
  vaginal N89.8

Discitis, diskitis M46.40
  cervical region M46.42
  cervicothoracic region M46.43
  lumbar region M46.46
  lumbosacral region M46.47
  multiple sites M46.49
  occipito-atlanto-axial region M46.41
  pyogenic — *see* Infection, intervertebral disc,
    pyogenic
  sacrococcygeal region M46.48
  thoracic region M46.44
  thoracolumbar region M46.45

Discoid
  meniscus (congenital) Q68.6
  semilunar cartilage (congenital) — *see*
    Derangement, knee, meniscus, specified
    NEC

Discoloration
  nails L60.8
  teeth (posteruptive) K03.7
    during formation K00.8

Discomfort
  chest R07.89
  visual H53.14-

Discontinuity, ossicles, ear H74.2-

Discord (with)
  boss Z56.4
  classmates Z55.4
  counselor Z64.4
  employer Z56.4
  family Z63.8
  fellow employees Z56.4
  in-laws Z63.1
  landlord Z59.2
  lodgers Z59.2
  neighbors Z59.2
  probation officer Z64.4
  social worker Z64.4
  teachers Z55.4
  workmates Z56.4

Discordant connection
  atrioventricular (congenital) Q20.5
  ventriculoarterial Q20.3

Discrepancy
  centric occlusion maximum intercuspation
    M26.55
  leg length (acquired) — *see* Deformity, limb,
    unequal length
    congenital — *see* Defect, reduction, lower
      limb
  uterine size date O26.84-

Discrimination
  ethnic Z60.5
  political Z60.5
  racial Z60.5
  religious Z60.5
  sex Z60.5

Disease, diseased — *see also* Syndrome
  absorbent system I87.8
  acid-peptic K30
  Acosta's T70.29
  Adams-Stokes (-Morgagni) (syncope with heart
    block) I45.9
  Addison's anemia (pernicious) D51.0
  adenoids (and tonsils) J35.9
  adrenal (capsule) (cortex) (gland) (medullary)
    E27.9
    hyperfunction E27.0
    specified NEC E27.8
  ainhum L94.6
  airway
    obstructive, chronic J44.9
      due to
        cotton dust J66.0
        specific organic dusts NEC J66.8
    reactive — *see* Asthma
  akamushi (scrub typhus) A75.3
  Albers-Schönberg (marble bones) Q78.2
  Albert's — *see* Tendinitis, Achilles
  alimentary canal K63.9
  alligator-skin Q80.9
    acquired L85.0
  alpha heavy chain C88.3
  alpine T70.29
  altitude T70.20
  alveolar ridge
    edentulous K06.9
      specified NEC K06.8
  alveoli, teeth K08.9
  Alzheimer's G30.9 *[F02.80]*
    with behavioral disturbance G30.9 *[F02.81]*
    early onset G30.0 *[F02.80]*
      with behavioral disturbance G30.0
        [F02.81]
    late onset G30.1 *[F02.80]*
      with behavioral disturbance G30.1
        [F02.81]
    specified NEC G30.8 *[F02.80]*
      with behavioral disturbance G30.8
        [F02.81]
  amyloid — *see* Amyloidosis
  Andersen's (glycogenosis IV) E74.09
  Andes T70.29
  Andrews' (bacterid) L08.89
  angiospastic I73.9
    cerebral G45.9
    vein I87.8
  anterior
    chamber H21.9
    horn cell G12.29
  antiglomerular basement membrane (anti-
    GBM) antibody M31.0
    tubulo-interstitial nephritis N12
  antral — *see* Sinusitis, maxillary
  anus K62.9
    specified NEC K62.89
  aorta (nonsyphilitic) I77.9
    syphilitic NEC A52.02
  aortic (heart) (valve) I35.9
    rheumatic I06.9
  Apollo B30.3
  aponeuroses — *see* Enthesopathy
  appendix K38.9
    specified NEC K38.8
  aqueous (chamber) H21.9
  Arnold-Chiari — *see* Arnold-Chiari disease
  arterial I77.9
    occlusive — *see* Occlusion, by site
      due to stricture or stenosis I77.1
  arteriocardiorenal — *see* Hypertension,
    cardiorenal
  arteriolar (generalized) (obliterative) I77.9
  arteriorenal — *see* Hypertension, kidney

Disease, diseased (*see also* Syndrome) —
continued
  arteriosclerotic — *see also* Arteriosclerosis
    cardiovascular — *see* Disease, heart,
      ischemic, atherosclerotic
    coronary (artery) — *see* Disease, heart,
      ischemic, atherosclerotic
    heart — *see* Disease, heart, ischemic,
      atherosclerotic
  artery I77.9
    cerebral I67.9
    coronary I25.10
      with angina pectoris — *see*
        Arteriosclerosis, coronary (artery)
  arthropod-borne NOS (viral) A94
    specified type NEC A93.8
  atticoantral, chronic H66.20
    left H66.22
      with right H66.23
    right H66.21
      with left H66.23
  auditory canal — *see* Disorder, ear, external
  auricle, ear NEC — *see* Disorder, pinna
  Australian X A83.4
  autoimmune (systemic) NOS M35.9
    hemolytic (cold type) (warm type) D59.1
      drug-induced D59.0
    thyroid E06.3
  aviator's — *see* Effect, adverse, high altitude
  Ayerza's (pulmonary artery sclerosis with
    pulmonary hypertension) I27.0
  Babington's (familial hemorrhagic
    telangiectasia) I78.0
  bacterial A49.9
    specified NEC A48.8
    zoonotic A28.9
      specified type NEC A28.8
  Baelz's (cheilitis glandularis apostematosa)
    K13.0
  bagasse J67.1
  balloon — *see* Effect, adverse, high altitude
  Bang's (brucella abortus) A23.1
  Bannister's T78.3
  barometer makers' — *see* Poisoning, mercury
  Barraquer (-Simons') (progressive
    lipodystrophy) E88.1
  Barrett's — *see* Barrett's, esophagus
  Bartholin's gland N75.9
  basal ganglia G25.9
    degenerative G23.9
      specified NEC G23.8
    specified NEC G25.89
  Basedow's (exophthalmic goiter) — *see*
    Hyperthyroidism, with, goiter (diffuse)
  Bateman's B08.1
  Batten-Steinert G71.11
  Battey A31.0
  Beard's (neurasthenia) F48.8
  Becker
    idiopathic mural endomyocardial I42.3
    myotonia congenita G71.12
  Begbie's (exophthalmic goiter) — *see*
    Hyperthyroidism, with, goiter (diffuse)
  behavioral, organic F07.9
  Beigel's (white piedra) B36.2
  Benson's — *see* Deposit, crystalline
  Bernard-Soulier (thrombopathy) D69.1
  Bernhardt (-Roth) — *see* Mononeuropathy,
    lower limb, meralgia paresthetica
  Biermer's (pernicious anemia) D51.0
  bile duct (common) (hepatic) K83.9
    with calculus, stones — *see* Calculus, bile
      duct
    specified NEC K83.8
  biliary (tract) K83.9
    specified NEC K83.8
  Billroth's — *see* Spina bifida
  bird fancier's J67.2

Disease, diseased (*see also* Syndrome) — *continued*
black lung J60
bladder N32.9
  in (due to)
    schistosomiasis (bilharziasis) B65.0 [N33]
  specified NEC N32.89
bleeder's D66
blood D75.9
  forming organs D75.9
  vessel I99.9
Bloodgood's — *see* Mastopathy, cystic
Bodechtel-Guttmann (subacute sclerosing panencephalitis) A81.1
bone — *see also* Disorder, bone
  aluminum M83.4
  fibrocystic NEC
    jaw M27.49
bone-marrow D75.9
Borna A83.9
Bornholm (epidemic pleurodynia) B33.0
Bouchard's (myopathic dilatation of the stomach) K31.0
Bouillaud's (rheumatic heart disease) I01.9
Bourneville (-Brissaud) (tuberous sclerosis) Q85.1
Bouveret (-Hoffmann) (paroxysmal tachycardia) I47.9
bowel K63.9
  functional K59.9
    psychogenic F45.8
brain G93.9
  arterial, artery I67.9
  arteriosclerotic I67.2
  congenital Q04.9
  degenerative — *see* Degeneration, brain
  inflammatory — *see* Encephalitis
  organic G93.9
    arteriosclerotic I67.2
  parasitic NEC B71.9 [G94]
  senile NEC G31.1
  specified NEC G93.89
breast (*see also* Disorder, breast) N64.9
  cystic (chronic) — *see* Mastopathy, cystic
  fibrocystic — *see* Mastopathy, cystic
  Paget's
    female, unspecified side C50.91-
    male, unspecified side C50.92-
  specified NEC N64.89
Breda's — *see* Yaws
Bretonneau's (diphtheritic malignant angina) A36.0
Bright's — *see* Nephritis
  arteriosclerotic — *see* Hypertension, kidney
Brill's (recrudescent typhus) A75.1
Brill-Zinsser (recrudescent typhus) A75.1
Brion-Kayser — *see* Fever, paratyphoid
broad
  beta E78.2
  ligament (noninflammatory) N83.9
    inflammatory — *see* Disease, pelvis, inflammatory
    specified NEC N83.8
Brocq's
  meaning
    dermatitis herpetiformis L13.0
    prurigo L28.2
Brocq-Duhring (dermatitis herpetiformis) L13.0
bronchopulmonary J98.4
bronchus NEC J98.09
bronze Addison's E27.1
  tuberculous A18.7
budgerigar fancier's J67.2
Buerger's (thromboangiitis obliterans) I73.1
bullous L13.9
  chronic of childhood L12.2
  specified NEC L13.8
Bürger-Grütz (essential familial hyperlipemia) E78.3

Disease, diseased (*see also* Syndrome) — *continued*
bursa — *see* Bursopathy
caisson T70.3
California — *see* Coccidioidomycosis
capillaries I78.9
  specified NEC I78.8
Carapata A68.0
cardiac — *see* Disease, heart
cardiopulmonary, chronic I27.9
cardiorenal (hepatic) (hypertensive) (vascular) — *see* Hypertension, cardiorenal
cardiovascular (atherosclerotic) I25.10
  with angina pectoris — *see* Arteriosclerosis, coronary (artery),
  congenital Q28.9
  hypertensive — *see* Hypertension, heart
  newborn P29.9
    specified NEC P29.89
  renal (hypertensive) — *see* Hypertension, cardiorenal
  syphilitic (asymptomatic) A52.00
cartilage — *see* Disorder, cartilage
Castellani's A69.8
Castleman (unicentric) (multicentric) D47.Z2
  HHV-8-associated (*see also* Herpesvirus, human, 8) D47.Z2
cat-scratch A28.1
Cavare's (familial periodic paralysis) G72.3
cecum K63.9
celiac (adult) (infantile) (with steatorrhea) K90.0
cellular tissue L98.9
central core G71.2
cerebellar, cerebellum — *see* Disease, brain
cerebral — *see also* Disease, brain
  degenerative — *see* Degeneration, brain
cerebrospinal G96.9
cerebrovascular I67.9
  acute I67.89
    embolic I63.4-
    thrombotic I63.3-
  arteriosclerotic I67.2
  specified NEC I67.89
cervix (uteri) (noninflammatory) N88.9
  inflammatory — *see* Cervicitis
  specified NEC N88.8
Chabert's A22.9
Chandler's (osteochondritis dissecans, hip) — *see* Osteochondritis, dissecans, hip
Charlouis — *see* Yaws
Chédiak-Steinbrinck (-Higashi) (congenital gigantism of peroxidase granules) E70.330
chest J98.9
Chiari's (hepatic vein thrombosis) I82.0
Chicago B40.9
Chignon B36.8
chigo, chigoe B88.1
childhood granulomatous D71
Chinese liver fluke B66.1
chlamydial A74.9
  specified NEC A74.89
cholecystic K82.9
choroid H31.9
  specified NEC H31.8
Christmas D67
chronic bullous of childhood L12.2
chylomicron retention E78.3
ciliary body H21.9
  specified NEC H21.89
circulatory (system) NEC I99.8
  newborn P29.9
  syphilitic A52.00
    congenital A50.54
coagulation factor deficiency (congenital) — *see* Defect, coagulation
coccidioidal — *see* Coccidioidomycosis

Disease, diseased (*see also* Syndrome) — *continued*
cold
  agglutinin or hemoglobinuria D59.1
    paroxysmal D59.6
  hemagglutinin (chronic) D59.1
collagen NOS (nonvascular) (vascular) M35.9
  specified NEC M35.8
colon K63.9
  functional K59.9
    congenital Q43.2
  ischemic (*see also* Ischemia, intestine, acute) K55.039
colonic inflammatory bowel, unclassified (IBDU) K52.3
combined system — *see* Degeneration, combined
compressed air T70.3
Concato's (pericardial polyserositis) A19.9
  nontubercular I31.1
  pleural — *see* Pleurisy, with effusion
conjunctiva H11.9
  chlamydial A74.0
  specified NEC H11.89
  viral B30.9
    specified NEC B30.8
connective tissue, systemic (diffuse) M35.9
  in (due to)
    hypogammaglobulinemia D80.1 [M36.8]
    ochronosis E70.29 [M36.8]
  specified NEC M35.8
Conor and Bruch's (boutonneuse fever) A77.1
Cooper's — *see* Mastopathy, cystic
Cori's (glycogenosis III) E74.03
corkhandler's or corkworker's J67.3
cornea H18.9
  specified NEC H18.89-
coronary (artery) — *see* Disease, heart, ischemic, atherosclerotic
  congenital Q24.5
  ostial, syphilitic (aortic) (mitral) (pulmonary) A52.03
corpus cavernosum N48.9
  specified NEC N48.89
Cotugno's — *see* Sciatica
coxsackie (virus) NEC B34.1
cranial nerve NOS G52.9
Creutzfeldt-Jakob — *see* Creutzfeldt-Jakob disease or syndrome
Crocq's (acrocyanosis) I73.89
Crohn's — *see* Enteritis, regional
Curschmann G71.11
cystic
  breast (chronic) — *see* Mastopathy, cystic
  kidney, congenital Q61.9
  liver, congenital Q44.6
  lung J98.4
    congenital Q33.0
cytomegalic inclusion (generalized) B25.9
  with pneumonia B25.0
  congenital P35.1
cytomegaloviral B25.9
  specified NEC B25.8
Czerny's (periodic hydrarthrosis of the knee) — *see* Effusion, joint, knee
Daae (-Finsen) (epidemic pleurodynia) B33.0
Darling's — *see* Histoplasmosis capsulati
de Quervain's (tendon sheath) M65.4
  thyroid (subacute granulomatous thyroiditis) E06.1
Débove's (splenomegaly) R16.1
deer fly — *see* Tularemia
Degos' I77.89
demyelinating, demyelinizating (nervous system) G37.9
  multiple sclerosis G35
  specified NEC G37.8
dense deposit (*see also* N00-N07 with fourth character .6) N05.6

Disease, diseased (*see also* Syndrome) — *continued*

deposition, hydroxyapatite — *see* Disease, hydroxyapatite deposition
Devergie's (pityriasis rubra pilaris) L44.0
Devic's G36.0
diaphorase deficiency D74.0
diaphragm J98.6
diarrheal, infectious NEC A09
digestive system K92.9
    specified NEC K92.89
disc, degenerative — *see* Degeneration, intervertebral disc
discogenic — *see also* Displacement, intervertebral disc NEC
    with myelopathy — *see* Disorder, disc, with, myelopathy
diverticular — *see* Diverticula
Dubois (thymus) A50.59 *[E35]*
Duchenne's
    muscular dystrophy G71.0
    pseudohypertrophy, muscles G71.0
Duchenne-Griesinger G71.0
ductless glands E34.9
Duhring's (dermatitis herpetiformis) L13.0
duodenum K31.9
    specified NEC K31.89
Dupré's (meningism) R29.1
Dupuytren's (muscle contracture) M72.0
Durand-Nicholas-Favre (climatic bubo) A55
Duroziez's (congenital mitral stenosis) Q23.2
ear — *see* Disorder, ear
Eberth's — *see* Fever, typhoid
Ebola (virus) A98.4
Ebstein's heart Q22.5
Echinococcus — *see* Echinococcus
echovirus NEC B34.1
Eddowes' (brittle bones and blue sclera) Q78.0
edentulous (alveolar) ridge K06.9
    specified NEC K06.8
Edsall's T67.2
Eichstedt's (pityriasis versicolor) B36.0
Ellis-van Creveld (chondroectodermal dysplasia) Q77.6
end stage renal (ESRD) N18.6
    due to hypertension I12.0
endocrine glands or system NEC E34.9
endomyocardial (eosinophilic) I42.3
English (rickets) E55.0
enteroviral, enterovirus NEC B34.1
    central nervous system NEC A88.8
epidemic B99.9
    specified NEC B99.8
epididymis N50.9
Erb (-Landouzy) G71.0
Erdheim-Chester (ECD) E88.89
esophagus K22.9
    functional K22.4
    psychogenic F45.8
    specified NEC K22.8
Eulenburg's (congenital paramyotonia) G71.19
eustachian tube — *see* Disorder, eustachian tube
external
    auditory canal — *see* Disorder, ear, external
    ear — *see* Disorder, ear, external
extrapyramidal G25.9
    specified NEC G25.89
eye H57.9
    anterior chamber H21.9
    inflammatory NEC H57.8
    muscle (external) — *see* Strabismus
    specified NEC H57.8
    syphilitic — *see* Oculopathy, syphilitic
eyeball H44.9
    specified NEC H44.89

Disease, diseased (*see also* Syndrome) — *continued*

eyelid — *see* Disorder, eyelid
    specified NEC — *see* Disorder, eyelid, specified type NEC
eyeworm of Africa B74.3
facial nerve (seventh) G51.9
    newborn (birth injury) P11.3
Fahr (of brain) G23.8
Fahr Volhard (of kidney) I12-
fallopian tube (noninflammatory) N83.9
    inflammatory — *see* Salpingo-oophoritis
    specified NEC N83.8
familial periodic paralysis G72.3
Fanconi's (congenital pancytopenia) D61.09
fascia NEC — *see also* Disorder, muscle
    inflammatory — *see* Myositis
    specified NEC M62.89
Fauchard's (periodontitis) — *see* Periodontitis
Favre-Durand-Nicolas (climatic bubo) A55
Fede's K14.0
Feer's — *see* Poisoning, mercury
female pelvic inflammatory (*see also* Disease, pelvis, inflammatory) N73.9
    syphilitic (secondary) A51.42
    tuberculous A18.17
Fernels' (aortic aneurysm) I71.9
fibrocaseous of lung — *see* Tuberculosis, pulmonary
fibrocystic — *see* Fibrocystic disease
Fiedler's (leptospiral jaundice) A27.0
fifth B08.3
file-cutter's — *see* Poisoning, lead
fish-skin Q80.9
    acquired L85.0
Flajani (-Basedow) (exophthalmic goiter) — *see* Hyperthyroidism, with, goiter (diffuse)
flax-dresser's J66.1
fluke — *see* Infestation, fluke
foot-and-mouth B08.8
foot process N04.9
Forbes' (glycogenosis III) E74.03
Fordyce's (ectopic sebaceous glands) (mouth) Q38.6
Fordyce-Fox (apocrine miliaria) L75.2
Forestier's (rhizomelic pseudopolyarthritis) M35.3
    meaning ankylosing hyperostosis — *see* Hyperostosis, ankylosing
Fothergill's
    neuralgia — *see* Neuralgia, trigeminal
    scarlatina anginosa A38.9
Fournier (gangrene) N49.3
    female N76.89
fourth B08.8
Fox (-Fordyce) (apocrine miliaria) L75.2
Francis' — *see* Tularemia
Franklin C88.2
Frei's (climatic bubo) A55
Friedreich's
    combined systemic or ataxia G11.1
    myoclonia G25.3
frontal sinus — *see* Sinusitis, frontal
fungus NEC B49
Gaisböck's (polycythemia hypertonica) D75.1
gallbladder K82.9
    calculus — *see* Calculus, gallbladder
    cholecystitis — *see* Cholecystitis
    cholesterolosis K82.4
    fistula — *see* Fistula, gallbladder
    hydrops K82.1
    obstruction — *see* Obstruction, gallbladder
    perforation K82.2
    specified NEC K82.8
gamma heavy chain C88.2
Gamna's (siderotic splenomegaly) D73.2
Gamstorp's (adynamia episodica hereditaria) G72.3
Gandy-Nanta (siderotic splenomegaly) D73.2

Disease, diseased (*see also* Syndrome) — *continued*

ganister J62.8
gastric — *see* Disease, stomach
gastroesophageal reflux (GERD) K21.9
    with esophagitis K21.0
gastrointestinal (tract) K92.9
    amyloid E85.4
    functional K59.9
      psychogenic F45.8
    specified NEC K92.89
Gee (-Herter) (-Heubner) (-Thaysen) (nontropical sprue) K90.0
genital organs
    female N94.9
    male N50.9
Gerhardt's (erythromelalgia) I73.81
Gibert's (pityriasis rosea) L42
Gierke's (glycogenosis I) E74.01
Gilles de la Tourette's (motor-verbal tic) F95.2
gingiva K06.9
    plaque induced K05.00
    specified NEC K06.8
gland (lymph) I89.9
Glanzmann's (hereditary hemorrhagic thrombasthenia) D69.1
glass-blower's (cataract) — *see* Cataract, specified NEC
salivary gland hypertrophy K11.1
Glisson's — *see* Rickets
globe H44.9
    specified NEC H44.89
glomerular — *see also* Glomerulonephritis
    with edema — *see* Nephrosis
    acute — *see* Nephritis, acute
    chronic — *see* Nephritis, chronic
    minimal change N05.0
    rapidly progressive N01.9
glycogen storage E74.00
    Andersen's E74.09
    Cori's E74.03
    Forbes' E74.03
    generalized E74.00
    glucose-6-phosphatase deficiency E74.01
    heart E74.02 *[I43]*
    hepatorenal E74.09
    Hers' E74.09
    liver and kidney E74.09
    McArdle's E74.04
    muscle phosphofructokinase E74.09
    myocardium E74.02 *[I43]*
    Pompe's E74.02
    Tauri's E74.09
    type 0 E74.09
    type I E74.01
    type II E74.02
    type III E74.03
    type IV E74.09
    type V E74.04
    type VI-XI E74.09
    Von Gierke's E74.01
Goldstein's (familial hemorrhagic telangiectasia) I78.0
gonococcal NOS A54.9
graft-versus-host (GVH) D89.813
    acute D89.810
    acute on chronic D89.812
    chronic D89.811
grainhandler's J67.8
granulomatous (childhood) (chronic) D71
Graves' (exophthalmic goiter) — *see* Hyperthyroidism, with, goiter (diffuse)
Griesinger's — *see* Ancylostomiasis
Grisel's M43.6
Gruby's (tinea tonsurans) B35.0
Guillain-Barré G61.0
Guinon's (motor-verbal tic) F95.2
gum K06.9
gynecological N94.9

DISEASE INDEX

Disease, diseased (*see also* Syndrome) — continued

H (Hartnup's) E72.02
Haff — *see* Poisoning, mercury
Hageman (congenital factor XII deficiency) D68.2
hair (color) (shaft) L67.9
  follicles L73.9
    specified NEC L73.8
Hamman's (spontaneous mediastinal emphysema) J98.2
hand, foot and mouth B08.4
Hansen's — *see* Leprosy
Hantavirus, with pulmonary manifestations B33.4
  with renal manifestations A98.5
Harada's H30.81-
Hart's (pellagra-cerebellar ataxia-renal aminoaciduria) E72.02
Hartnup (pellagra-cerebellar ataxia-renal aminoaciduria) E72.02
Hashimoto's (struma lymphomatosa) E06.3
Hb — *see* Disease, hemoglobin
heart (organic) I51.9
  with
    pulmonary edema (acute) (*see also* Failure, ventricular, left) I50.1
    rheumatic fever (conditions in I00)
      active I01.9
        with chorea I02.0
        specified NEC I01.8
      inactive or quiescent (with chorea) I09.9
        specified NEC I09.89
  amyloid E85.4 [*I43*]
  aortic (valve) I35.9
  arteriosclerotic or sclerotic (senile) — *see* Disease, heart, ischemic, atherosclerotic
  artery, arterial — *see* Disease, heart, ischemic, atherosclerotic
  beer drinkers' I42.6
  beriberi (wet) E51.12
  black I27.0
  congenital Q24.9
    cyanotic Q24.9
    specified NEC Q24.8
  coronary — *see* Disease, heart, ischemic
  cryptogenic I51.9
  fibroid — *see* Myocarditis
  functional I51.89
    psychogenic F45.8
  glycogen storage E74.02 [*I43*]
  gonococcal A54.83
  hypertensive — *see* Hypertension, heart
  hyperthyroid (*see also* Hyperthyroidism) E05.90 [*I43*]
    with thyroid storm E05.91 [*I43*]
  ischemic (chronic or with a stated duration of over 4 weeks) I25.9
    atherosclerotic (of) I25.10
      with angina pectoris — *see* Arteriosclerosis, coronary (artery)
      coronary artery bypass graft — *see* Arteriosclerosis, coronary (artery), cardiomyopathy I25.5
    diagnosed on ECG or other special investigation, but currently presenting no symptoms I25.6
    silent I25.6
    specified form NEC I25.89
  kyphoscoliotic I27.1
  meningococcal A39.50
    endocarditis A39.51
    myocarditis A39.52
    pericarditis A39.53
  mitral I05.9
    specified NEC I05.8
  muscular — *see* Degeneration, myocardial
  psychogenic (functional) F45.8

Disease, diseased (*see also* Syndrome) — continued

heart (organic) I51.9 — continued
  pulmonary (chronic) I27.9
    in schistosomiasis B65.9 [*I52*]
    specified NEC I27.89
  rheumatic (chronic) (inactive) (old) (quiescent) (with chorea) I09.9
    active or acute I01.9
      with chorea (acute) (rheumatic) (Sydenham's) I02.0
    specified NEC I09.89
  senile — *see* Myocarditis
  syphilitic A52.06
    aortic A52.03
      aneurysm A52.01
    congenital A50.54 [*I52*]
  thyrotoxic (*see also* Thyrotoxicosis) E05.90 [*I43*]
    with thyroid storm E05.91 [*I43*]
  valve, valvular (obstructive) (regurgitant) — *see also* Endocarditis
    congenital NEC Q24.8
      pulmonary Q22.3
  vascular — *see* Disease, cardiovascular
heavy chain NEC C88.2
  alpha C88.3
  gamma C88.2
  mu C88.2
Hebra's
  pityriasis
    maculata et circinata L42
    rubra pilaris L44.0
  prurigo L28.2
hematopoietic organs D75.9
hemoglobin or Hb
  abnormal (mixed) NEC D58.2
    with thalassemia D56.9
  AS genotype D57.3
  Bart's D56.0
  C (Hb-C) D58.2
    with other abnormal hemoglobin NEC D58.2
    elliptocytosis D58.1
    Hb-S D57.2-
    sickle-cell D57.2-
    thalassemia D56.8
  Constant Spring D58.2
  D (Hb-D) D58.2
  E (Hb-E) D58.2
  E-beta thalassemia D56.5
  elliptocytosis D58.1
  H (Hb-H) (thalassemia) D56.0
    with other abnormal hemoglobin NEC D56.9
    Constant Spring D56.0
  I thalassemia D56.9
  M D74.0
  S or SS D57.1
  SC D57.2-
  SD D57.8-
  SE D57.8-
  spherocytosis D58.0
  unstable, hemolytic D58.2
hemolytic (newborn) P55.9
  autoimmune (cold type) (warm type) D59.1
  drug-induced D59.0
  due to or with
    incompatibility
      ABO (blood group) P55.1
      blood (group) (Duffy) (K(ell)) (Kidd) (Lewis) (M) (S) NEC P55.8
      Rh (blood group) (factor) P55.0
      Rh negative mother P55.0
  specified type NEC P55.8
  unstable hemoglobin D58.2
hemorrhagic D69.9
  newborn P53
Henoch (-Schönlein) (purpura nervosa) D69.0

Disease, diseased (*see also* Syndrome) — continued

hepatic — *see* Disease, liver
hepatobiliary K83.9
  toxic K71.9
hepatolenticular E83.01
heredodegenerative NEC
  spinal cord G95.89
herpesviral, disseminated B00.7
Hers' (glycogenosis VI) E74.09
Herter (-Gee) (-Heubner) (nontropical sprue) K90.9
Heubner-Herter (nontropical sprue) K90.0
high fetal gene or hemoglobin thalassemia D56.9
Hildenbrand's — *see* Typhus
hip (joint) M25.9
  congenital Q65.89
  suppurative M00.9
  tuberculous A18.02
His (-Werner) (trench fever) A79.0
Hodgson's I71.2
  ruptured I71.1
Holla — *see* Spherocytosis
hookworm B76.9
  specified NEC B76.8
host-versus-graft D89.813
  acute D89.810
  acute on chronic D89.812
  chronic D89.811
human immunodeficiency virus (HIV) B20
Huntington's G10
Hutchinson's (cheiropompholyx) — *see* Hutchinson's disease
hyaline (diffuse) (generalized)
  membrane (lung) (newborn) P22.0
  adult J80
hydatid — *see* Echinococcus
hydroxyapatite deposition M11.00
  ankle M11.07-
  elbow M11.02-
  foot joint M11.07-
  hand joint M11.04-
  hip M11.05-
  knee M11.06-
  multiple site M11.09
  shoulder M11.01-
  vertebra M11.08
  wrist M11.03-
hyperkinetic — *see* Hyperkinesia
hypertensive — *see* Hypertension
hypophysis E23.7
I-cell E77.0
Iceland G93.3
immune D89.9
immunoproliferative (malignant) C88.9
  small intestinal C88.3
  specified NEC C88.8
inclusion B25.9
  salivary gland B25.9
infectious, infective B99.9
  congenital P37.9
    specified NEC P37.8
    viral P35.9
      specified type NEC P35.8
  specified NEC B99.8
inflammatory
  penis N48.29
    abscess N48.21
    cellulitis N48.22
  prepuce N47.7
    balanoposthitis N47.6
  tubo-ovarian — *see* Salpingo-oophoritis

Disease, diseased (*see also* Syndrome) — *continued*

intervertebral disc — *see also* Disorder, disc
  with myelopathy — *see* Disorder, disc, with, myelopathy
  cervical, cervicothoracic — *see* Disorder, disc, cervical
  with
    myelopathy — *see* Disorder, disc, cervical, with myelopathy
    neuritis, radiculitis or radiculopathy — *see* Disorder, disc, cervical, with neuritis
    specified NEC — *see* Disorder, disc, cervical, specified type NEC
  lumbar (with)
    myelopathy M51.06
    neuritis, radiculitis, radiculopathy or sciatica M51.16
    specified NEC M51.86
  lumbosacral (with)
    neuritis, radiculitis, radiculopathy or sciatica M51.17
    specified NEC M51.87
  specified NEC — *see* Disorder, disc, specified NEC
  thoracic (with)
    myelopathy M51.04
    neuritis, radiculitis or radiculopathy M51.14
    specified NEC M51.84
  thoracolumbar (with)
    myelopathy M51.05
    neuritis, radiculitis or radiculopathy M51.15
    specified NEC M51.85
intestine K63.9
  functional K59.9
    psychogenic F45.8
    specified NEC K59.8
  organic K63.9
  protozoal A07.9
  specified NEC K63.89
iris H21.9
  specified NEC H21.89
iron metabolism or storage E83.10
island (scrub typhus) A75.3
itai-itai — *see* Poisoning, cadmium
Jakob-Creutzfeldt — *see* Creutzfeldt-Jakob disease or syndrome
jaw M27.9
  fibrocystic M27.49
  specified NEC M27.8
jigger B88.1
joint — *see also* Disorder, joint
  Charcot's — *see* Arthropathy, neuropathic (Charcot)
  degenerative — *see* Osteoarthritis
    multiple M15.9
    spine — *see* Spondylosis
  hypertrophic — *see* Osteoarthritis
  sacroiliac M53.3
  specified NEC — *see* Disorder, joint, specified type NEC
  spine NEC — *see* Dorsopathy
  suppurative — *see* Arthritis, pyogenic or pyemic
Jourdain's (acute gingivitis) K05.00
  nonplaque induced K05.01
  plaque induced K05.00
Kaschin-Beck (endemic polyarthritis) M12.10
  ankle M12.17-
  elbow M12.12-
  foot joint M12.17-
  hand joint M12.14-
  hip M12.15-
  knee M12.16-
  multiple site M12.19
  shoulder M12.11-
  vertebra M12.18
  wrist M12.13-

Disease, diseased (*see also* Syndrome) — *continued*

Katayama B65.2
Kedani (scrub typhus) A75.3
Keshan E59
kidney (functional) (pelvis) N28.9
  chronic N18.9
    hypertensive — *see* Hypertension, kidney
    stage 1 N18.1
    stage 2 (mild) N18.2
    stage 3 (moderate) N18.3
    stage 4 (severe) N18.4
    stage 5 N18.5
  complicating pregnancy — *see* Pregnancy, complicated by, renal disease
  cystic (congenital) Q61.9
  diabetic — *see* E08-E13 with .22
  fibrocystic (congenital) Q61.8
  hypertensive — *see* Hypertension, kidney
  in (due to)
    schistosomiasis (bilharziasis) B65.9 *[N29]*
  multicystic Q61.4
  polycystic Q61.3
    adult type Q61.2
    childhood type NEC Q61.19
    collecting duct dilatation Q61.11
Kimmelstiel (-Wilson) (intercapillary polycystic (congenital) glomerulosclerosis) — *see* E08-E13 with .21
Kimura D21.9
  specified site — *see* Neoplasm, connective tissue, benign
Kinnier Wilson's (hepatolenticular degeneration) E83.01
kissing — *see* Mononucleosis, infectious
Klebs' (*see also* Glomerulonephritis) N05-
Klippel-Feil (brevicollis) Q76.1
Köhler-Pellegrini-Stieda (calcification, knee joint) — *see* Bursitis, tibial collateral
Kok Q89.8
König's (osteochondritis dissecans) — *see* Osteochondritis, dissecans
Korsakoff's (nonalcoholic) F04
  alcoholic F10.96
    with dependence F10.26
Kostmann's (infantile genetic agranulocytosis) D70.0
kuru A81.81
Kyasanur Forest A98.2
labyrinth, ear — *see* Disorder, ear, inner
lacrimal system — *see* Disorder, lacrimal system
Lafora's — *see* Epilepsy, generalized, idiopathic
Lancereaux-Mathieu (leptospiral jaundice) A27.0
Landry's G61.0
Larrey-Weil (leptospiral jaundice) A27.0
larynx J38.7
legionnaires' A48.1
  nonpneumonic A48.2
Lenegre's I44.2
lens H27.9
  specified NEC H27.8
Lev's (acquired complete heart block) I44.2
Lewy body (dementia) G31.83 *[F02.80]*
  with behavioral disturbance G31.83 *[F02.81]*
Lichtheim's (subacute combined sclerosis with pernicious anemia) D51.0
Lightwood's (renal tubular acidosis) N25.89
Lignac's (cystinosis) E72.04
lip K13.0
lipid-storage E75.6
  specified NEC E75.5
Lipschütz's N76.6

Disease, diseased (*see also* Syndrome) — *continued*

liver (chronic) (organic) K76.9
  alcoholic (chronic) K70.9
    acute — *see* Disease, liver, alcoholic, hepatitis
    cirrhosis K70.30
      with ascites K70.31
    failure K70.40
      with coma K70.41
    fatty liver K70.0
    fibrosis K70.2
    hepatitis K70.10
      with ascites K70.11
    sclerosis K70.2
  cystic, congenital Q44.6
  drug-induced (idiosyncratic) (toxic) (predictable) (unpredictable) — *see* Disease, liver, toxic
  end stage K72.90
    due to hepatitis — *see* Hepatitis
  fatty, nonalcoholic (NAFLD) K76.0
    alcoholic K70.0
  fibrocystic (congenital) Q44.6
  fluke
    Chinese B66.1
    oriental B66.1
    sheep B66.3
  glycogen storage E74.09 *[K77]*
  in (due to)
    schistosomiasis (bilharziasis) B65.9 *[K77]*
  inflammatory K75.9
    alcoholic K70.1
    specified NEC K75.89
  polycystic (congenital) Q44.6
  toxic K71.9
    with
      cholestasis K71.0
      cirrhosis (liver) K71.7
      fibrosis (liver) K71.7
      focal nodular hyperplasia K71.8
      hepatic granuloma K71.8
      hepatic necrosis K71.10
        with coma K71.11
      hepatitis NEC K71.6
        acute K71.2
        chronic
          active K71.50
            with ascites K71.51
          lobular K71.4
          persistent K71.3
          lupoid K71.50
            with ascites K71.51
      peliosis hepatis K71.8
      veno-occlusive disease (VOD) of liver K71.8
  veno-occlusive K76.5
Lobo's (keloid blastomycosis) B48.0
Lobstein's (brittle bones and blue sclera) Q78.0
Ludwig's (submaxillary cellulitis) K12.2
lumbosacral region M53.87
lung J98.4
  black J60
  congenital Q33.9
  cystic J98.4
    congenital Q33.0
  fibroid (chronic) — *see* Fibrosis, lung
  fluke B66.4
    oriental B66.4
  in
    amyloidosis E85.4 *[J99]*
    sarcoidosis D86.0
    Sjögren's syndrome M35.02
    systemic
      lupus erythematosus M32.13
      sclerosis M34.81

DISEASE INDEX

Disease, diseased (*see also* Syndrome) — *continued*
  lung J98.4 — *continued*
    interstitial J84.9
      of childhood, specified NEC J84.848
      respiratory bronchiolitis J84.115
      specified NEC J84.89
    obstructive (chronic) J44.9
      with
        acute
          bronchitis J44.0
          exacerbation NEC J44.1
          lower respiratory infection J44.0
        alveolitis, allergic J67.9
        asthma J44.9
        bronchiectasis J47.9
          with
            exacerbation (acute) J47.1
            lower respiratory infection J47.0
        bronchitis J44.9
          with
            exacerbation (acute) J44.1
            lower respiratory infection J44.0
        emphysema J44.9
        hypersensitivity pneumonitis J67.9
      decompensated J44.1
        with
          exacerbation (acute) J44.1
    polycystic J98.4
      congenital Q33.0
    rheumatoid (diffuse) (interstitial) — *see* Rheumatoid, lung
  Lutembacher's (atrial septal defect with mitral stenosis) Q21.1
  Lyme A69.20
  lymphatic (gland) (system) (channel) (vessel) I89.9
  lymphoproliferative D47.9
    specified NEC D47.Z9
    T-gamma D47.Z9
    X-linked D82.3
  Magitot's M27.2
  malarial — *see* Malaria
  malignant — *see also* Neoplasm, malignant, by site
  Manson's B65.1
  maple bark J67.6
  maple-syrup-urine E71.0
  Marburg (virus) A98.3
  Marion's (bladder neck obstruction) N32.0
  Marsh's (exophthalmic goiter) — *see* Hyperthyroidism, with, goiter (diffuse)
  mastoid (process) — *see* Disorder, ear, middle
  Mathieu's (leptospiral jaundice) A27.0
  Maxcy's A75.2
  McArdle (-Schmid-Pearson) (glycogenosis V) E74.04
  mediastinum J98.59
  medullary center (idiopathic) (respiratory) G93.89
  Meige's (chronic hereditary edema) Q82.0
  meningococcal — *see* Infection, meningococcal
  mental F99
    organic F09
  mesenchymal M35.9
  mesenteric embolic (*see also* Ischemia, intestine, acute) K55.039
  metabolic, metabolism E88.9
    bilirubin E80.7
  metal-polisher's J62.8
  metastatic (*see also* Neoplasm, secondary, by site) C79.9
  microvascular — *code to* condition
  microvillus
    atrophy Q43.8
    inclusion (MVD) Q43.8
  middle ear — *see* Disorder, ear, middle
  Mikulicz' (dryness of mouth, absent or decreased lacrimation) K11.8

Disease, diseased (*see also* Syndrome) — *continued*
  Milroy's (chronic hereditary edema) Q82.0
  Minamata — *see* Poisoning, mercury
  minicore G71.2
  Minor's G95.19
  Minot's (hemorrhagic disease, newborn) P53
  Minot-von Willebrand-Jürgens (angiohemophilia) D68.0
  Mitchell's (erythromelalgia) I73.81
  mitral (valve) I05.9
    nonrheumatic I34.9
  mixed connective tissue M35.1
  moldy hay J67.0
  Monge's T70.29
  Morgagni's (syndrome) (hyperostosis frontalis interna) M85.2
  Morgagni-Adams-Stokes (syncope with heart block) I45.9
  Morton's (with metatarsalgia) — *see* Lesion, nerve, plantar
  Morvan's G60.8
  motor neuron (bulbar) (familial) (mixed type) (spinal) G12.20
    amyotrophic lateral sclerosis G12.21
    progressive bulbar palsy G12.22
    specified NEC G12.29
  moyamoya I67.5
  mu heavy chain disease C88.2
  multicore G71.2
  muscle — *see also* Disorder, muscle
    inflammatory — *see* Myositis
    ocular (external) — *see* Strabismus
  musculoskeletal system, soft tissue — *see also* Disorder, soft tissue
    specified NEC — *see* Disorder, soft tissue, specified type NEC
  mushroom workers' J67.5
  mycotic B49
  myelodysplastic, not classified C94.6
  myeloproliferative, not classified C94.6
    chronic D47.1
  myocardium, myocardial (*see also* Degeneration, myocardial) I51.5
    primary (idiopathic) I42.9
  myoneural G70.9
  Naegeli's D69.1
  nails L60.9
    specified NEC L60.8
  Nairobi (sheep virus) A93.8
  nasal J34.9
  nemaline body G71.2
  nerve — *see* Disorder, nerve
  nervous system G98.8
    autonomic G90.9
    central G96.9
      specified NEC G96.8
    congenital Q07.9
    parasympathetic G90.9
    specified NEC G98.8
    sympathetic G90.9
    vegetative G90.9
  neuromuscular system G70.9
  Newcastle B30.8
  Nicolas (-Durand)-Favre (climatic bubo) A55
  nipple N64.9
    Paget's C50.01-
      female C50.01-
      male C50.02-
  Nishimoto (-Takeuchi) I67.5
  nonarthropod-borne NOS (viral) B34.9
    enterovirus NEC B34.1
  nonautoimmune hemolytic D59.4
    drug-induced D59.2
  Nonne-Milroy-Meige (chronic hereditary edema) Q82.0
  nose J34.9
  nucleus pulposus — *see* Disorder, disc
  nutritional E63.9

Disease, diseased (*see also* Syndrome) — *continued*
  oast-house-urine E72.19
  ocular
    herpesviral B00.50
    zoster B02.30
  obliterative vascular I77.1
  Ohara's — *see* Tularemia
  Opitz's (congestive splenomegaly) D73.2
  Oppenheim-Urbach (necrobiosis lipoidica diabeticorum) — *see* E08-E13 with .620
  optic nerve NEC — *see* Disorder, nerve, optic
  orbit — *see* Disorder, orbit
  Oriental liver fluke B66.1
  Oriental lung fluke B66.4
  Ormond's N13.5
  Oropouche virus A93.0
  Osler-Rendu (familial hemorrhagic telangiectasia) I78.0
  osteofibrocystic E21.0
  Otto's M24.7
  outer ear — *see* Disorder, ear, external
  ovary (noninflammatory) N83.9
    cystic N83.20-
    inflammatory — *see* Salpingo-oophoritis
    polycystic E28.2
    specified NEC N83.8
  Owren's (congenital) — *see* Defect, coagulation
  pancreas K86.9
    cystic K86.2
    fibrocystic E84.9
    specified NEC K86.89
  panvalvular I08.9
    specified NEC I08.8
  parametrium (noninflammatory) N83.9
  parasitic B89
    cerebral NEC B71.9 *[G94]*
    intestinal NOS B82.9
    mouth B37.0
    skin NOS B88.9
    specified type — *see* Infestation
    tongue B37.0
  parathyroid (gland) E21.5
    specified NEC E21.4
  Parkinson's G20
  parodontal K05.6
  Parrot's (syphilitic osteochondritis) A50.02
  Parry's (exophthalmic goiter) — *see* Hyperthyroidism, with, goiter (diffuse)
  Parson's (exophthalmic goiter) — *see* Hyperthyroidism, with, goiter (diffuse)
  Paxton's (white piedra) B36.2
  pearl-worker's — *see* Osteomyelitis, specified type NEC
  Pellegrini-Stieda (calcification, knee joint) — *see* Bursitis, tibial collateral
  pelvis, pelvic
    female NOS N94.9
      specified NEC N94.89
    gonococcal (acute) (chronic) A54.24
    inflammatory (female) N73.9
      acute N73.0
      chlamydial A56.11
      chronic N73.1
      specified NEC N73.8
      syphilitic (secondary) A51.42
        late A52.76
      tuberculous A18.17
    organ, female N94.9
    peritoneum, female NEC N94.89
  penis N48.9
    inflammatory N48.29
      abscess N48.21
      cellulitis N48.22
      specified NEC N48.89
  periapical tissues NOS K04.90
  periodontal K05.6
    specified NEC K05.5

Disease, diseased (*see also* Syndrome) — *continued*
- periosteum — *see* Disorder, bone, specified type NEC
- peripheral
  - arterial I73.9
  - autonomic nervous system G90.9
  - nerves — *see* Polyneuropathy
  - vascular NOS I73.9
- peritoneum K66.9
  - pelvic, female NEC N94.89
  - specified NEC K66.8
- persistent mucosal (middle ear) H66.20
  - left H66.22
    - with right H66.23
  - right H66.21
    - with left H66.23
- Petit's — *see* Hernia, abdomen, specified site NEC
- pharynx J39.2
  - specified NEC J39.2
- Phocas' — *see* Mastopathy, cystic
- photochromogenic (acid-fast bacilli) (pulmonary) A31.0
  - nonpulmonary A31.9
- Pick's G31.01 *[F02.80]*
  - with behavioral disturbance G31.01 *[F02.81]*
  - brain G31.01 [F02.80]
    - with behavioral disturbance G31.01 [F02.81]
  - of pericardium (pericardial pseudocirrhosis of liver) I31.1
- pigeon fancier's J67.2
- pineal gland E34.8
- pink — *see* Poisoning, mercury
- Pinkus' (lichen nitidus) L44.1
- pinworm B80
- Piry virus A93.8
- pituitary (gland) E23.7
- pituitary-snuff-taker's J67.8
- pleura (cavity) J94.9
  - specified NEC J94.8
- pneumatic drill (hammer) T75.21
- Pollitzer's (hidradenitis suppurativa) L73.2
- polycystic
  - kidney or renal Q61.3
    - adult type Q61.2
    - childhood type NEC Q61.19
      - collecting duct dilatation Q61.11
  - liver or hepatic Q44.6
  - lung or pulmonary J98.4
    - congenital Q33.0
  - ovary, ovaries E28.2
  - spleen Q89.09
- polyethylene T84.05-
- Pompe's (glycogenosis II) E74.02
- Posadas-Wernicke B38.9
- Potain's (pulmonary edema) — *see* Edema, lung
- prepuce N47.8
  - inflammatory N47.7
    - balanoposthitis N47.6
- Pringle's (tuberous sclerosis) Q85.1
- prion, central nervous system A81.9
  - specified NEC A81.89
- prostate N42.9
  - specified NEC N42.89
- protozoal B64
  - acanthamebiasis — *see* Acanthamebiasis
  - African trypanosomiasis — *see* African trypanosomiasis
  - babesiosis B60.0
  - Chagas disease — *see* Chagas disease
  - intestine, intestinal A07.9
  - leishmaniasis — *see* Leishmaniasis
  - malaria — *see* Malaria
  - naegleriasis B60.2
  - pneumocystosis B59

Disease, diseased (*see also* Syndrome) — *continued*
- protozoal B64 — *continued*
  - specified organism NEC B60.8
  - toxoplasmosis — *see* Toxoplasmosis
- pseudo-Hurler's E77.0
- psychiatric F99
- psychotic — *see* Psychosis
- Puente's (simple glandular cheilitis) K13.0
- puerperal (*see also* Puerperal) O90.89
- pulmonary — *see also* Disease, lung
  - artery I28.9
  - chronic obstructive J44.9
    - with
      - acute bronchitis J44.0
      - exacerbation (acute) J44.1
      - lower respiratory infection (acute) J44.0
    - decompensated J44.1
      - with
        - exacerbation (acute) J44.1
  - heart I27.9
    - specified NEC I27.89
  - hypertensive (vascular) I27.0
  - valve I37.9
    - rheumatic I09.89
- pulp (dental) NOS K04.90
- pulseless M31.4
- Putnam's (subacute combined sclerosis with pernicious anemia) D51.0
- Pyle (-Cohn) (metaphyseal dysplasia) Q78.5
- ragpicker's or ragsorter's A22.1
- Raynaud's — *see* Raynaud's disease
- reactive airway — *see* Asthma
- Reclus' (cystic) — *see* Mastopathy, cystic
- rectum K62.9
  - specified NEC K62.89
- Refsum's (heredopathia atactica polyneuritiformis) G60.1
- renal (functional) (pelvis) (*see also* Disease, kidney) N28.9
  - with
    - edema — *see* Nephrosis
    - glomerular lesion — *see* Glomerulonephritis
      - with edema — *see* Nephrosis
    - interstitial nephritis N12
  - acute N28.9
  - chronic (*see also* Disease, kidney, chronic) N18.9
  - cystic, congenital Q61.9
  - diabetic — *see* E08-E13 with .22
  - end-stage (failure) N18.6
    - due to hypertension I12.0
  - fibrocystic (congenital) Q61.8
  - hypertensive — *see* Hypertension, kidney
  - lupus M32.14
  - phosphate-losing (tubular) N25.0
  - polycystic (congenital) Q61.3
    - adult type Q61.2
    - childhood type NEC Q61.19
      - collecting duct dilatation Q61.11
  - rapidly progressive N01.9
  - subacute N01.9
- Rendu-Osler-Weber (familial hemorrhagic telangiectasia) I78.0
- renovascular (arteriosclerotic) — *see* Hypertension, kidney
- respiratory (tract) J98.9
  - acute or subacute NOS J06.9
    - due to
      - chemicals, gases, fumes or vapors (inhalation) J68.3
      - external agent J70.9
        - specified NEC J70.8
      - radiation J70.0
      - smoke inhalation J70.5
  - noninfectious J39.8

Disease, diseased (*see also* Syndrome) — *continued*
- respiratory (tract) J98.9 — *continued*
  - chronic NOS J98.9
    - due to
      - chemicals, gases, fumes or vapors J68.4
      - external agent J70.9
        - specified NEC J70.8
      - radiation J70.1
    - newborn P27.9
      - specified NEC P27.8
  - due to
    - chemicals, gases, fumes or vapors J68.9
      - acute or subacute NEC J68.3
      - chronic J68.4
    - external agent J70.9
      - specified NEC J70.8
    - newborn P28.9
      - specified type NEC P28.89
  - upper J39.9
    - acute or subacute J06.9
    - noninfectious NEC J39.8
    - specified NEC J39.8
    - streptococcal J06.9
- retina, retinal H35.9
  - Batten's or Batten-Mayou E75.4 *[H36]*
  - specified NEC H35.89
- rheumatoid — *see* Arthritis, rheumatoid
- rickettsial NOS A79.9
  - specified type NEC A79.89
- Riga (-Fede) (cachectic aphthae) K14.0
- Riggs' (compound periodontitis) — *see* Periodontitis
- Ritter's L00
- Rivalta's (cervicofacial actinomycosis) A42.2
- Robles' (onchocerciasis) B73.01
- Roger's (congenital interventricular septal defect) Q21.0
- Rosenthal's (factor XI deficiency) D68.1
- Ross River B33.1
- Rossbach's (hyperchlorhydria) K30
- Rotes Quérol — *see* Hyperostosis, ankylosing
- Roth (-Bernhardt) — *see* Mononeuropathy, lower limb, meralgia paresthetica
- Runeberg's (progressive pernicious anemia) D51.0
- sacroiliac NEC M53.3
- salivary gland or duct K11.9
  - inclusion B25.9
  - specified NEC K11.8
  - virus B25.9
- sandworm B76.9
- Schimmelbusch's — *see* Mastopathy, cystic
- Schmorl's — *see* Schmorl's disease or nodes
- Schönlein (-Henoch) (purpura rheumatica) D69.0
- Schottmüller's — *see* Fever, paratyphoid
- Schultz's (agranulocytosis) — *see* Agranulocytosis
- Schwalbe-Ziehen-Oppenheim G24.1
- Schwartz-Jampel G71.13
- sclera H15.9
  - specified NEC H15.89
- scrofulous (tuberculous) A18.2
- scrotum N50.9
- sebaceous glands L73.9
- semilunar cartilage, cystic — *see also* Derangement, knee, meniscus, cystic
- seminal vesicle N50.9
- serum NEC (*see also* Reaction, serum) T80.69
- sexually transmitted A64
  - anogenital
    - herpesviral infection — *see* Herpes, anogenital
    - warts A63.0
  - chancroid A57
  - chlamydial infection — *see* Chlamydia
  - gonorrhea — *see* Gonorrhea
  - granuloma inguinale A58

DISEASE INDEX

Disease, diseased (*see also* Syndrome) — *continued*

sexually transmitted A64 — *continued*
  specified organism NEC A63.8
  syphilis — *see* Syphilis
  trichomoniasis — *see* Trichomoniasis
Sézary C84.1-
shimamushi (scrub typhus) A75.3
shipyard B30.0
sickle-cell D57.1
  with crisis (vasoocclusive pain) D57.00
    with
      acute chest syndrome D57.01
      splenic sequestration D57.02
  elliptocytosis D57.8-
  Hb-C D57.20
    with crisis (vasoocclusive pain) D57.219
      with
        acute chest syndrome D57.211
        splenic sequestration D57.212
    without crisis D57.20
  Hb-SD D57.80
    with crisis D57.819
      with
        acute chest syndrome D57.811
        splenic sequestration D57.812
  Hb-SE D57.80
    with crisis D57.819
      with
        acute chest syndrome D57.811
        splenic sequestration D57.812
  specified NEC D57.80
    with crisis D57.819
      with
        acute chest syndrome D57.811
        splenic sequestration D57.812
  spherocytosis D57.80
    with crisis D57.819
      with
        acute chest syndrome D57.811
        splenic sequestration D57.812
  thalassemia D57.40
    with crisis (vasoocclusive pain) D57.419
      with
        acute chest syndrome D57.411
        splenic sequestration D57.412
    without crisis D57.40
silo-filler's J68.8
  bronchitis J68.0
  pneumonitis J68.0
  pulmonary edema J68.1
simian B B00.4
Simons' (progressive lipodystrophy) E88.1
sin nombre virus B33.4
sinus — *see* Sinusitis
Sirkari's B55.0
sixth B08.20
  due to human herpesvirus 6 B08.21
  due to human herpesvirus 7 B08.22
skin L98.9
  due to metabolic disorder NEC E88.9 *[L99]*
  specified NEC L98.8
slim (HIV) B20
small vessel I73.9
Sneddon-Wilkinson (subcorneal pustular dermatosis) L13.1
South African creeping B88.0
spinal (cord) G95.9
  congenital Q06.9
  specified NEC G95.89
spine — *see also* Spondylopathy
  joint — *see* Dorsopathy
  tuberculous A18.01
spinocerebellar (hereditary) G11.9
  specified NEC G11.8

Disease, diseased (*see also* Syndrome) — *continued*

spleen D73.9
  amyloid E85.4 *[D77]*
  organic D73.9
  polycystic Q89.09
  postinfectional D73.89
sponge-diver's — *see* Toxicity, venom, marine animal, sea anemone
Startle Q89.8
Steinert's G71.11
Sticker's (erythema infectiosum) B08.3
Stieda's (calcification, knee joint) — *see* Bursitis, tibial collateral
Stokes' (exophthalmic goiter) — *see* Hyperthyroidism, with, goiter (diffuse)
Stokes-Adams (syncope with heart block) I45.9
stomach K31.9
  functional, psychogenic F45.8
  specified NEC K31.89
stonemason's J62.8
storage
  glycogen — *see* Disease, glycogen storage
  mucopolysaccharide — *see* Mucopolysaccharidosis
striatopallidal system NEC G25.89
Stuart's (congenital factor X deficiency) D68.2
Stuart-Prower (congenital factor X deficiency) D68.2
subcutaneous tissue — *see* Disease, skin
supporting structures of teeth K08.9
  specified NEC K08.89
suprarenal (capsule) (gland) E27.9
  hyperfunction E27.0
  specified NEC E27.8
sweat glands L74.9
  specified NEC L74.8
Sweeley-Klionsky E75.21
Swift (-Feer) — *see* Poisoning, mercury
swimming-pool granuloma A31.1
Sylvest's (epidemic pleurodynia) B33.0
sympathetic nervous system G90.9
synovium — *see* Disorder, synovium
syphilitic — *see* Syphilis
systemic tissue mast cell C96.2
tanapox (virus) B08.71
Tangier E78.6
Tarral-Besnier (pityriasis rubra pilaris) L44.0
Tauri's E74.09
tear duct — *see* Disorder, lacrimal system
tendon, tendinous — *see also* Disorder, tendon
  nodular — *see* Trigger finger
terminal vessel I73.9
testis N50.9
thalassemia Hb-S — *see* Disease, sickle-cell, thalassemia
Thaysen-Gee (nontropical sprue) K90.0
Thomsen G71.12
throat J39.2
  septic J02.0
thromboembolic — *see* Embolism
thymus (gland) E32.9
  specified NEC E32.8
thyroid (gland) E07.9
  heart (*see also* Hyperthyroidism) E05.90 *[I43]*
    with thyroid storm E05.91 *[I43]*
  specified NEC E07.89
Tietze's M94.0
tongue K14.9
  specified NEC K14.8
tonsils, tonsillar (and adenoids) J35.9
tooth, teeth K08.9
  hard tissues K03.9
    specified NEC K03.89
  pulp NEC K04.99
  specified NEC K08.89
Tourette's F95.2
trachea NEC J39.8

Disease, diseased (*see also* Syndrome) — *continued*

tricuspid I07.9
  nonrheumatic I36.9
triglyceride-storage E75.5
trophoblastic — *see* Mole, hydatidiform
tsutsugamushi A75.3
tube (fallopian) (noninflammatory) N83.9
  inflammatory — *see* Salpingitis
  specified NEC N83.8
tuberculous NEC — *see* Tuberculosis
tubo-ovarian (noninflammatory) N83.9
  inflammatory — *see* Salpingo-oophoritis
  specified NEC N83.8
tubotympanic, chronic — *see* Otitis, media, suppurative, chronic, tubotympanic
tubulo-interstitial N15.9
  specified NEC N15.8
tympanum — *see* Disorder, tympanic membrane
Uhl's Q24.8
Underwood's (sclerema neonatorum) P83.0
Unverricht (-Lundborg) — *see* Epilepsy, generalized, idiopathic
Urbach-Oppenheim (necrobiosis lipoidica diabeticorum) — *see* E08-E13 with .620
ureter N28.9
  in (due to)
    schistosomiasis (bilharziasis) B65.0 *[N29]*
urethra N36.9
  specified NEC N36.8
urinary (tract) N39.9
  bladder N32.9
    specified NEC N32.89
  specified NEC N39.8
uterus (noninflammatory) N85.9
  infective — *see* Endometritis
  inflammatory — *see* Endometritis
  specified NEC N85.8
uveal tract (anterior) H21.9
  posterior H31.9
vagabond's B85.1
vagina, vaginal (noninflammatory) N89.9
  inflammatory NEC N76.89
  specified NEC N89.8
valve, valvular I38
  multiple I08.9
  specified NEC I08.8
van Creveld-von Gierke (glycogenosis I) E74.01
vas deferens N50.9
vascular I99.9
  arteriosclerotic — *see* Arteriosclerosis
  ciliary body NEC — *see* Disorder, iris, vascular
  hypertensive — *see* Hypertension
  iris NEC — *see* Disorder, iris, vascular
  obliterative I77.1
    peripheral I73.9
  occlusive I99.8
  peripheral (occlusive) I73.9
    in diabetes mellitus — *see* E08-E13 with .51
vasomotor I73.9
vasospastic I73.9
vein I87.9
venereal (*see also* Disease, sexually transmitted) A64
  chlamydial NEC A56.8
    anus A56.3
    genitourinary NOS A56.2
    pharynx A56.4
    rectum A56.3
  fifth A55
  sixth A55
  specified nature or type NEC A63.8
vertebra, vertebral — *see also* Spondylopathy
  disc — *see* Disorder, disc
vibration — *see* Vibration, adverse effects

Disease, diseased (see also Syndrome) — continued
  viral, virus (see also Disease, by type of virus) B34.9
    arbovirus NOS A94
    arthropod-borne NOS A94
    congenital P35.9
      specified NEC P35.8
    Hanta (with renal manifestations) (Dobrava) (Puumala) (Seoul) A98.5
      with pulmonary manifestations (Andes) (Bayou) (Bermejo) (Black Creek Canal) (Choclo) (Juquitiba) (Laguna negra) (Lechiguanas) (New York) (Oran) (Sin nombre) B33.4
    Hantaan (Korean hemorrhagic fever) A98.5
    human immunodeficiency (HIV) B20
    Kunjin A83.4
    nonarthropod-borne NOS B34.9
    Powassan A84.8
    Rocio (encephalitis) A83.6
    Sin nombre (Hantavirus) (cardio)-pulmonary syndrome) B33.4
    Tahyna B33.8
    vesicular stomatitis A93.8
  vitreous H43.9
    specified NEC H43.89
  vocal cord J38.3
  Volkmann's, acquired T79.6
  von Eulenburg's (congenital paramyotonia) G71.19
  von Gierke's (glycogenosis I) E74.01
  von Graefe's — see Strabismus, paralytic, ophthalmoplegia, progressive
  von Willebrand (-Jürgens) (angiohemophilia) D68.0
  Vrolik's (osteogenesis imperfecta) Q78.0
  vulva (noninflammatory) N90.9
    inflammatory NEC N76.89
    specified NEC N90.89
  Wallgren's (obstruction of splenic vein with collateral circulation) I87.8
  Wassilieff's (leptospiral jaundice) A27.0
  wasting NEC R64
    due to malnutrition E41
  Waterhouse-Friderichsen A39.1
  Wegner's (syphilitic osteochondritis) A50.02
  Weil's (leptospiral jaundice of lung) A27.0
  Weir Mitchell's (erythromelalgia) I73.81
  Werdnig-Hoffmann G12.0
  Wermer's E31.21
  Werner-His (trench fever) A79.0
  Werner-Schultz (neutropenic splenomegaly) D73.81
  Wernicke-Posadas B38.9
  whipworm B79
  white blood cells D72.9
    specified NEC D72.89
  white matter R90.82
  white-spot, meaning lichen sclerosus et atrophicus L90.0
    penis N48.0
    vulva N90.4
  Wilkie's K55.1
  Wilkinson-Sneddon (subcorneal pustular dermatosis) L13.1
  Willis' — see Diabetes
  Wilson's (hepatolenticular degeneration) E83.01
  woolsorter's A22.1
  yaba monkey tumor B08.72
  yaba pox (virus) B08.72
  Zika virus A92.5
  zoonotic, bacterial A28.9
    specified type NEC A28.8
Disfigurement (due to scar) L90.5
Disgerminoma — see Dysgerminoma
DISH (diffuse idiopathic skeletal hyperostosis) — see Hyperostosis, ankylosing

Disinsertion, retina — see Detachment, retina
Dislocatable hip, congenital Q65.6
Dislocation (articular)
  with fracture — see Fracture
  acromioclavicular (joint) S43.10-
    with displacement
      100%-200% S43.12-
      more than 200% S43.13-
    inferior S43.14-
    posterior S43.15-
  ankle S93.0-
  astragalus — see Dislocation, ankle
  atlantoaxial S13.121
  atlantooccipital S13.111
  atloidooccipital S13.111
  breast bone S23.29
  capsule, joint — code by site under Dislocation
  carpal (bone) — see Dislocation, wrist
  carpometacarpal (joint) NEC S63.05-
    thumb S63.04-
  cartilage (joint) — code by site under Dislocation
  cervical spine (vertebra) — see Dislocation, vertebra, cervical
  chronic — see Dislocation, recurrent
  clavicle — see Dislocation, acromioclavicular joint
  coccyx S33.2
  congenital NEC Q68.8
  coracoid — see Dislocation, shoulder
  costal cartilage S23.29
  costochondral S23.29
  cricoarytenoid articulation S13.29
  cricothyroid articulation S13.29
  dorsal vertebra — see Dislocation, vertebra, thoracic
  ear ossicle — see Discontinuity, ossicles, ear
  elbow S53.10-
    congenital Q68.8
    pathological — see Dislocation, pathological NEC, elbow
    radial head alone — see Dislocation, radial head
    recurrent — see Dislocation, recurrent, elbow
    traumatic S53.10-
      anterior S53.11-
      lateral S53.14-
      medial S53.13-
      posterior S53.12-
      specified type NEC S53.19-
  eye, nontraumatic — see Luxation, globe
  eyeball, nontraumatic — see Luxation, globe
  femur
    distal end — see Dislocation, knee
    proximal end — see Dislocation, hip
  fibula
    distal end — see Dislocation, ankle
    proximal end — see Dislocation, knee
  finger S63.25-
    index S63.25-
    interphalangeal S63.27-
      distal S63.29-
        index S63.29-
        little S63.29-
        middle S63.29-
        ring S63.29-
      index S63.27-
      little S63.27-
      middle S63.27-
      proximal S63.28-
        index S63.28-
        little S63.28-
        middle S63.28-
        ring S63.28-
      ring S63.27-
    little S63.25-

Dislocation (articular) — continued
  finger S63.25- — continued
    metacarpophalangeal S63.26-
      index S63.26-
      little S63.26-
      middle S63.26-
      ring S63.26-
    middle S63.25-
    recurrent — see Dislocation, recurrent, finger
    ring S63.25-
    thumb — see Dislocation, thumb
  foot S93.30-
    recurrent — see Dislocation, recurrent, foot
    specified site NEC S93.33-
    tarsal joint S93.31-
    tarsometatarsal joint S93.32-
    toe — see Dislocation, toe
  fracture — see Fracture
  glenohumeral (joint) — see Dislocation, shoulder
  glenoid — see Dislocation, shoulder
  habitual — see Dislocation, recurrent
  hip S73.00-
    anterior S73.03-
      obturator S73.02-
    central S73.04-
    congenital (total) Q65.2
      bilateral Q65.1
      partial Q65.5
        bilateral Q65.4
        unilateral Q65.3-
      unilateral Q65.0-
    developmental M24.85-
    pathological — see Dislocation, pathological NEC, hip
    posterior S73.01-
    recurrent — see Dislocation, recurrent, hip
  humerus, proximal end — see Dislocation, shoulder
  incomplete — see Subluxation, by site
  incus — see Discontinuity, ossicles, ear
  infracoracoid — see Dislocation, shoulder
  innominate (pubic junction) (sacral junction) S33.39
    acetabulum — see Dislocation, hip
  interphalangeal (joint(s))
    finger S63.279
      distal S63.29-
        index S63.29-
        little S63.29-
        middle S63.29-
        ring S63.29-
      index S63.27-
      little S63.27-
      middle S63.27-
      proximal S63.28-
        index S63.28-
        little S63.28-
        middle S63.28-
        ring S63.28-
      ring S63.27-
    foot or toe — see Dislocation, toe
    thumb S63.12-
      distal joint S63.14-
      proximal joint S63.13-
  jaw (cartilage) (meniscus) S03.0-
  joint prosthesis — see Complications, joint prosthesis, mechanical, displacement, by site
  knee S83.106
    cap — see Dislocation, patella
    congenital Q68.2
    old M23.8x-
    patella — see Dislocation, patella
    pathological — see Dislocation, pathological NEC, knee

Dislocation (articular) — *continued*
  knee S83.106 — *continued*
    proximal tibia
      anteriorly S83.11-
      laterally S83.14-
      medially S83.13-
      posteriorly S83.12-
    recurrent — *see also* Derangement, knee,
      specified NEC
    specified type NEC S83.19-
  lacrimal gland H04.16-
  lens (complete) H27.10
    anterior H27.12-
    congenital Q12.1
    ocular implant — *see* Complications,
      intraocular lens
    partial H27.11-
    posterior H27.13-
    traumatic S05.8x-
  ligament — *code by* site under Dislocation
  lumbar (vertebra) — *see* Dislocation, vertebra,
    lumbar
  lumbosacral (vertebra) — *see also* Dislocation,
    vertebra, lumbar
    congenital Q76.49
  mandible S03.0-
  meniscus (knee) — *see* Tear, meniscus
    other sites — *code by* site under Dislocation
  metacarpal (bone)
    distal end — *see* Dislocation, finger
    proximal end S63.06-
  metacarpophalangeal (joint)
    finger S63.26-
      index S63.26-
      little S63.26-
      middle S63.26-
      ring S63.26-
      thumb S63.11-
  metatarsal (bone) — *see* Dislocation, foot
  metatarsophalangeal (joint(s)) — *see*
    Dislocation, toe
  midcarpal (joint) S63.03-
  midtarsal (joint) — *see* Dislocation, foot
  neck S13.20
    specified site NEC S13.29
    vertebra — *see* Dislocation, vertebra,
      cervical
  nose (septal cartilage) S03.1
  occipitoatloid S13.111
  old — *see* Derangement, joint, specified type
    NEC
  ossicles, ear — *see* Discontinuity, ossicles, ear
  partial — *see* Subluxation, by site
  patella S83.006
    congenital Q74.1
    lateral S83.01-
    recurrent (nontraumatic) M22.0-
      incomplete M22.1-
    specified type NEC S83.09-
  pathological NEC M24.30
    ankle M24.37-
    elbow M24.32-
    foot joint M24.37-
    hand joint M24.34-
    hip M24.35-
    knee M24.36-
    lumbosacral joint — *see* subcategory M53.2
    pelvic region — *see* Dislocation,
      pathological, hip
    sacroiliac — *see* subcategory M53.2
    shoulder M24.31-
    wrist M24.33-
  pelvis NEC S33.30
    specified NEC S33.39
  phalanx
    finger or hand — *see* Dislocation, finger
    foot or toe — *see* Dislocation, toe
  prosthesis, internal — *see* Complications,
    prosthetic device, by site, mechanical

Dislocation (articular) — *continued*
  radial head S53.006
    anterior S53.01-
    posterior S53.02-
    specified type NEC S53.09-
  radiocarpal (joint) S63.02-
  radiohumeral (joint) — *see* Dislocation, radial
    head
  radioulnar (joint)
    distal S63.01-
    proximal — *see* Dislocation, elbow
  radius
    distal end — *see* Dislocation, wrist
    proximal end — *see* Dislocation, radial head
  recurrent M24.40
    ankle M24.47-
    elbow M24.42-
    finger M24.44-
    foot joint M24.47-
    hand joint M24.44-
    hip M24.45-
    knee M24.46-
      patella — *see* Dislocation, patella,
        recurrent
    patella — *see* Dislocation, patella, recurrent
    sacroiliac — *see* subcategory M53.2
    shoulder M24.41-
    toe M24.47-
    vertebra (*see also* subcategory) M43.5
      atlantoaxial M43.4
        with myelopathy M43.3
    wrist M24.43-
  rib (cartilage) S23.29
  sacrococcygeal S33.2
  sacroiliac (joint) (ligament) S33.2
    congenital Q74.2
    recurrent — *see* subcategory M53.2
  sacrum S33.2
  scaphoid (bone) (hand) (wrist) — *see*
    Dislocation, wrist
    foot — *see* Dislocation, foot
  scapula — *see* Dislocation, shoulder, girdle,
    scapula
  semilunar cartilage, knee — *see* Tear, meniscus
  septal cartilage (nose) S03.1
  septum (nasal) (old) J34.2
  sesamoid bone — *code by* site under
    Dislocation
  shoulder (blade) (ligament) (joint) (traumatic)
    S43.006
    acromioclavicular — *see* Dislocation,
      acromioclavicular
    chronic — *see* Dislocation, recurrent,
      shoulder
    congenital Q68.8
    girdle S43.30-
      scapula S43.31-
      specified site NEC S43.39-
    humerus S43.00-
      anterior S43.01-
      inferior S43.03-
      posterior S43.02-
    pathological — *see* Dislocation, pathological
      NEC, shoulder
    recurrent — *see* Dislocation, recurrent,
      shoulder
    specified type NEC S43.08-
  spine
    cervical — *see* Dislocation, vertebra, cervical
    congenital Q76.49
    due to birth trauma P11.5
    lumbar — *see* Dislocation, vertebra, lumbar
    thoracic — *see* Dislocation, vertebra,
      thoracic
  spontaneous — *see* Dislocation, pathological
  sternoclavicular (joint) S43.206
    anterior S43.21-
    posterior S43.22-
  sternum S23.29

Dislocation (articular) — *continued*
  subglenoid — *see* Dislocation, shoulder
  symphysis pubis S33.4
  talus — *see* Dislocation, ankle
  tarsal (bone(s)) (joint(s)) — *see* Dislocation, foot
  tarsometatarsal (joint(s)) — *see* Dislocation, foot
  temporomandibular (joint) S03.0-
  thigh, proximal end — *see* Dislocation, hip
  thorax S23.20
    specified site NEC S23.29
    vertebra — *see* Dislocation, vertebra
  thumb S63.10-
    interphalangeal joint — *see* Dislocation,
      interphalangeal (joint), thumb
    metacarpophalangeal joint — *see*
      Dislocation, metacarpophalangeal
      (joint), thumb
  thyroid cartilage S13.29
  tibia
    distal end — *see* Dislocation, ankle
    proximal end — *see* Dislocation, knee
  tibiofibular (joint)
    distal — *see* Dislocation, ankle
    superior — *see* Dislocation, knee
  toe(s) S93.106
    great S93.10-
      interphalangeal joint S93.11-
      metatarsophalangeal joint S93.12-
    interphalangeal joint S93.119
    lesser S93.106
      interphalangeal joint S93.11-
      metatarsophalangeal joint S93.12-
    metatarsophalangeal joint S93.12-
  tooth S03.2
  trachea S23.29
  ulna
    distal end S63.07-
    proximal end — *see* Dislocation, elbow
  ulnohumeral (joint) — *see* Dislocation, elbow
  vertebra (articular process) (body) (traumatic)
    cervical S13.101
      atlantoaxial joint S13.121
      atlantooccipital joint S13.111
      atloidooccipital joint S13.111
      joint between
        C0 and C1 S13.111
        C1 and C2 S13.121
        C2 and C3 S13.131
        C3 and C4 S13.141
        C4 and C5 S13.151
        C5and C6 S13.161
        C6and C7 S13.171
        C7and T1 S13.181
      occipitoatloid joint S13.111
    congenital Q76.49
    lumbar S33.101
      joint between
        L1and L2 S33.111
        L2and L3 S33.121
        L3 and L4 S33.131
        L4and L5 S33.141
    nontraumatic — *see* Displacement,
      intervertebral disc
    partial — *see* Subluxation, by site
    recurrent NEC — *see* subcategory M43.5
    thoracic S23.101
      joint between
        T1 and T2 S23.111
        T10 and T11 S23.161
        T11 and T12 S23.163
        T12 and L1 S23.171
        T2 and T3 S23.121
        T3 and T4 S23.123
        T4 and T5 S23.131
        T5 and T6 S23.133
        T6 and T7 S23.141
        T7 and T8 S23.143
        T8 and T9 S23.151
        T9 and T10 S23.153

DISEASE INDEX

Dislocation (articular) — *continued*
wrist (carpal bone) S63.006
carpometacarpal joint — *see* Dislocation, carpometacarpal (joint)
distal radioulnar joint — *see* Dislocation, radioulnar (joint), distal
metacarpal bone, proximal — *see* Dislocation, metacarpal (bone), proximal end
midcarpal — *see* Dislocation, midcarpal (joint)
radiocarpal joint — *see* Dislocation, radiocarpal (joint)
recurrent — *see* Dislocation, recurrent, wrist
specified site NEC S63.09-
ulna — *see* Dislocation, ulna, distal end
xiphoid cartilage S23.29
Disorder (of) — *see also* Disease
acantholytic L11.9
specified NEC L11.8
acute
psychotic — *see* Psychosis, acute
stress F43.0
adjustment (grief) F43.20
with
anxiety F43.22
with depressed mood F43.23
conduct disturbance F43.24
with emotional disturbance F43.25
depressed mood F43.21
with anxiety F43.23
other specified symptom F43.29
adrenal (capsule) (gland) (medullary) E27.9
specified NEC E27.8
adrenogenital E25.9
drug-induced E25.8
iatrogenic E25.8
idiopathic E25.8
adult personality (and behavior) F69
specified NEC F68.8
affective (mood) — *see* Disorder, mood
aggressive, unsocialized F91.1
alcohol-related F10.99
with
amnestic disorder, persisting F10.96
anxiety disorder F10.980
dementia, persisting F10.97
intoxication F10.929
with delirium F10.921
uncomplicated F10.920
mood disorder F10.94
other specified F10.988
psychotic disorder F10.959
with
delusions F10.950
hallucinations F10.951
sexual dysfunction F10.981
sleep disorder F10.982
alcohol use
mild F10.10
with
alcohol-induced
anxiety disorder F10.180
bipolar and related disorder F10.14
depressive disorder F10.14
psychotic disorder F10.159
sexual dysfunction F10.181
sleep disorder F10.182
alcohol intoxication F10.129
delirium F10.121

Disorder (of) (*see also* Disease) — *continued*
alcohol use — *continued*
moderate or severe F10.20
with
alcohol-induced
anxiety disorder F10.280
bipolar and related disorder F10.24
depressive disorder F10.24
major neurocognitive disorder, amnestic-confabulatory type F10.26
major neurocognitive disorder, nonamnestic-confabulatory type F10.27
mild neurocognitive disorder F10.288
psychotic disorder F10.259
sexual dysfunction F10.281
sleep disorder F10.282
alcohol intoxication F10.229
delirium F10.221
allergic — *see* Allergy
alveolar NEC J84.09
amino-acid
cystathioninuria E72.19
cystinosis E72.04
cystinuria E72.01
glycinuria E72.09
homocystinuria E72.11
metabolism — *see* Disturbance, metabolism, amino-acid
specified NEC E72.8
neonatal, transitory P74.8
renal transport NEC E72.09
transport NEC E72.09
amnesic, amnestic
alcohol-induced F10.96
with dependence F10.26
due to (secondary to) general medical condition F04
psychoactive NEC-induced F19.96
with
abuse F19.16
dependence F19.26
sedative, hypnotic or anxiolytic-induced F13.96
with dependence F13.26
amphetamine-type substance use
mild F15.10
moderate F15.20
severe F15.20
amphetamine (or other stimulant) use
mild
with
amphetamine- (or other stimulant) induced
anxiety disorder F15.180
bipolar and related disorder F15.14
depressive disorder F15.14
obsessive-compulsive and related disorder F15.188
psychotic disorder F15.159
sexual dysfunction F15.181
amphetamine, cocaine, or other stimulant intoxication
with perceptual disturbances F15.122
without perceptual disturbances F15.129
intoxication delirium F15.121
moderate or severe
with
amphetamine- (or other stimulant) induced
anxiety disorder F15.280
obsessive-compulsive and related disorder F15.288
sexual dysfunction F15.281
bipolar and related disorder F15.24
depressive disorder F15.24
psychotic disorder F15.259

Disorder (of) (*see also* Disease) — *continued*
amphetamine (or other stimulant) use — *continued*
moderate or severe — *continued*
with — *continued*
amphetamine, cocaine, or other stimulant intoxication
with perceptual disturbances F15.222
without perceptual disturbances F15.229
intoxication delirium F15.221
anaerobic glycolysis with anemia D55.2
anxiety F41.9
due to (secondary to)
alcohol F10.980
amphetamine F15.980
in
abuse F15.180
dependence F15.280
anxiolytic F13.980
in
abuse F13.180
dependence F13.280
caffeine F15.980
in
abuse F15.180
dependence F15.280
cannabis F12.980
in
abuse F12.180
dependence F12.280
cocaine F14.980
in
abuse F14.180
dependence F14.180
general medical condition F06.4
hallucinogen F16.980
in
abuse F16.180
dependence F16.280
hypnotic F13.980
in
abuse F13.180
dependence F13.280
inhalant F18.980
in
abuse F18.180
dependence F18.280
phencyclidine F16.980
in
abuse F16.180
dependence F16.280
psychoactive substance NEC F19.980
in
abuse F19.180
dependence F19.280
sedative F13.980
in
abuse F13.180
dependence F13.280
volatile solvents F18.980
in
abuse F18.180
dependence F18.280
generalized F41.1
illness F45.21
mixed
with depression (mild) F41.8
specified NEC F41.3
organic F06.4
phobic F40.9
of childhood F40.8
specified NEC F41.8
aortic valve — *see* Endocarditis, aortic
aromatic amino-acid metabolism E70.9
specified NEC E70.8
arteriole NEC I77.89
artery NEC I77.89
articulation — *see* Disorder, joint

Disorder (of) (*see also* Disease) — *continued*
  attachment (childhood)
    disinhibited F94.2
    reactive F94.1
  attention-deficit hyperactivity (adolescent)
    (adult) (child) F90.9
    combined type F90.2
    hyperactive type F90.1
    inattentive type F90.0
    specified type NEC F90.8
  attention-deficit without hyperactivity
    (adolescent) (adult) (child) F98.8
  auditory processing (central) H93.25
  autism spectrum F84.0
  autistic F84.0
  autonomic nervous system G90.9
    specified NEC G90.8
  avoidant
    child or adolescent F40.10
    restrictive food intake F50.89
  balance
    acid-base E87.8
      mixed E87.4
    electrolyte E87.8
    fluid NEC E87.8
  behavioral (disruptive) — *see* Disorder, conduct
  beta-amino-acid metabolism E72.8
  bile acid and cholesterol metabolism E78.70
    Barth syndrome E78.71
    other specified E78.79
    Smith-Lemli-Opitz syndrome E78.72
  bilirubin excretion E80.6
  binge eating F50.81
  binocular
    movement H51.9
      convergence
        excess H51.12
        insufficiency H51.11
      internuclear ophthalmoplegia — *see*
        Ophthalmoplegia, internuclear
      palsy of conjugate gaze H51.0
      specified type NEC H51.8
    vision NEC — *see* Disorder, vision, binocular
  bipolar (I) F31.9
    current episode
      depressed F31.9
        with psychotic features F31.5
        without psychotic features F31.30
          mild F31.31
          moderate F31.32
          severe (without psychotic features)
            F31.4
            with psychotic features F31.5
      hypomanic F31.0
      manic F31.9
        with psychotic features F31.2
        without psychotic features F31.10
          mild F31.11
          moderate F31.12
          severe (without psychotic features)
            F31.13
            with psychotic features F31.2
      mixed F31.60
        mild F31.61
        moderate F31.62
        severe (without psychotic features)
          F31.63
          with psychotic features F31.64
      severe depression (without psychotic
        features) F31.4
        with psychotic features F31.5
    in remission (currently) F31.70
      in full remission
        most recent episode
          depressed F31.76
          hypomanic F31.72
          manic F31.74
          mixed F31.78

Disorder (of) (*see also* Disease) — *continued*
  bipolar (I) F31.9 — *continued*
    in remission (currently) F31.70 — *continued*
      in partial remission
        most recent episode
          depressed F31.75
          hypomanic F31.71
          manic F31.73
          mixed F31.77
  bipolar (II) F31.81
    organic F06.30
    single manic episode F30.9
      mild F30.11
      moderate F30.12
      severe (without psychotic symptoms)
        F30.13
        with psychotic symptoms F30.2
    specified NEC F31.89
  bladder N32.9
    functional NEC N31.9
    in schistosomiasis B65.0 *[N33]*
    specified NEC N32.89
  bleeding D68.9
  blood D75.9
    in congenital early syphilis A50.09 *[D77]*
  body dysmorphic F45.22
  bone M89.9
    continuity M84.9
      specified type NEC M84.80
        ankle M84.87-
        fibula M84.86-
        foot M84.87-
        hand M84.84-
        humerus M84.82-
        neck M84.88
        pelvis M84.859
        radius M84.83-
        rib M84.88
        shoulder M84.81-
        skull M84.88
        thigh M84.85-
        tibia M84.86-
        ulna M84.83-
        vertebra M84.88
    density and structure M85.9
      cyst — *see also* Cyst, bone, specified type
        NEC
      aneurysmal — *see* Cyst, bone,
        aneurysmal
      solitary — *see* Cyst, bone, solitary
      diffuse idiopathic skeletal hyperostosis —
        see Hyperostosis, ankylosing
      fibrous dysplasia (monostotic) — *see*
        Dysplasia, fibrous, bone
      fluorosis — *see* Fluorosis, skeletal
      hyperostosis of skull M85.2
      osteitis condensans — *see* Osteitis,
        condensans
      specified type NEC M85.8-
        ankle M85.87-
        foot M85.87-
        forearm M85.83-
        hand M85.84-
        lower leg M85.86-
        multiple sites M85.89
        neck M85.88
        rib M85.88
        shoulder M85.81-
        skull M85.88
        thigh M85.85-
        upper arm M85.82-
        vertebra M85.88
    development and growth NEC M89.20
      carpus M89.24-
      clavicle M89.21-
      femur M89.25-
      fibula M89.26-
      finger M89.24-
      humerus M89.22-

Disorder (of) (*see also* Disease) — *continued*
  bone M89.9 — *continued*
    development and growth NEC M89.20 —
      continued
      ilium M89.259
      ischium M89.259
      metacarpus M89.24-
      metatarsus M89.27-
      multiple sites M89.29
      neck M89.28
      radius M89.23-
      rib M89.28
      scapula M89.21-
      skull M89.28
      tarsus M89.27-
      tibia M89.26-
      toe M89.27-
      ulna M89.23-
      vertebra M89.28
    specified type NEC M89.8x-
  brachial plexus G54.0
  branched-chain amino-acid metabolism E71.2
    specified NEC E71.19
  breast N64.9
    agalactia — *see* Agalactia
    associated with
      lactation O92.70
        specified NEC O92.79
      pregnancy O92.20
        specified NEC O92.29
      puerperium O92.20
        specified NEC O92.29
    cracked nipple — *see* Cracked nipple
    galactorrhea — *see* Galactorrhea
    hypogalactia O92.4
    lactation disorder NEC O92.79
    mastitis — *see* Mastitis
    nipple infection — *see* Infection, nipple
    retracted nipple — *see* Retraction, nipple
    specified type NEC N64.89
  Briquet's F45.0
  bullous, in diseases classified elsewhere L14
  caffeine use
    mild
      with
        caffeine-induced
          anxiety disorder F15.180
          sleep disorder F15.182
    moderate or severe
      with
        caffeine-induced
          anxiety disorder F15.280
          sleep disorder F15.282
  cannabis use
    mild F12.10
      with
        cannabis-induced
          anxiety disorder F12.180
          psychotic disorder F12.159
          sleep disorder F12.188
        cannabis intoxication delirium F12.121
          with perceptual disturbances F12.122
          without perceptual disturbances
            F12.129
    moderate or severe F12.20
      with
        cannabis-induced
          anxiety disorder F12.280
          psychotic disorder F12.259
          sleep disorder F12.288
        cannabis intoxication
          with perceptual disturbances F12.222
          without perceptual disturbances
            F12.229
        delirium F12.221
  carbohydrate
    absorption, intestinal NEC E74.39
    metabolism (congenital) E74.9
      specified NEC E74.8

Disorder (of) (*see also* Disease) — *continued*
cardiac, functional I51.89
carnitine metabolism E71.40
cartilage M94.9
 articular NEC — *see* Derangement, joint,
  articular cartilage
 chondrocalcinosis — *see* Chondrocalcinosis
 specified type NEC M94.8x-
  articular — *see* Derangement, joint,
   articular cartilage
  multiple sites M94.8x0
catatonia (due to known physiological
 condition) (with another mental disorder)
 F06.1
catatonic
 due to (secondary to) known physiological
  condition F06.1
 organic F06.1
central auditory processing H93.25
cervical
 region NEC M53.82
 root (nerve) NEC G54.2
character NOS F60.9
childhood disintegrative NEC F84.3
cholesterol and bile acid metabolism E78.70
 Barth syndrome E78.71
 other specified E78.79
 Smith-Lemli-Opitz syndrome E78.72
choroid H31.9
 atrophy — *see* Atrophy, choroid
 degeneration — *see* Degeneration, choroid
 detachment — *see* Detachment, choroid
 dystrophy — *see* Dystrophy, choroid
 hemorrhage — *see* Hemorrhage, choroid
 rupture — *see* Rupture, choroid
 scar — *see* Scar, chorioretinal
 solar retinopathy — *see* Retinopathy, solar
 specified type NEC H31.8
ciliary body — *see* Disorder, iris
 degeneration — *see* Degeneration, ciliary
  body
coagulation (factor) (*see also* Defect,
 coagulation) D68.9
 newborn, transient P61.6
cocaine use
 mild F14.10
  with
   amphetamine, cocaine, or other
    stimulant intoxication
    with perceptual disturbances F14.122
    without perceptual disturbances
     F14.129
   cocaine-induced
    anxiety disorder F14.180
    bipolar and related disorder F14.14
    depressive disorder F14.14
    obsessive-compulsive and related
     disorder F14.188
    psychotic disorder F14.159
    sexual dysfunction F14.181
    sleep disorder F14.182
   cocaine intoxication delirium F14.121
 moderate or severe F14.20
  with
   amphetamine, cocaine, or other
    stimulant intoxication
    with perceptual disturbances F14.222
    without perceptual disturbances
     F14.229
   cocaine-induced
    anxiety disorder F14.280
    bipolar and related disorder F14.24
    depressive disorder F14.24
    obsessive-compulsive and related
     disorder F14.288
    psychotic disorder F14.259
    sexual dysfunction F14.281
    sleep disorder F14.282
   cocaine intoxication delirium F14.221

Disorder (of) (*see also* Disease) — *continued*
coccyx NEC M53.3
cognitive F09
 due to (secondary to) general medical
  condition F09
 persisting R41.89
  due to
   alcohol F10.97
    with dependence F10.27
   anxiolytics F13.97
    with dependence F13.27
   hypnotics F13.97
    with dependence F13.27
   sedatives F13.97
    with dependence F13.27
   specified substance NEC F19.97
    with
     abuse F19.17
     dependence F19.27
communication F80.9
 social pragmatic F80.82
conduct (childhood) F91.9
 adjustment reaction — *see* Disorder,
  adjustment
 adolescent onset type F91.2
 childhood onset type F91.1
 compulsive F63.9
 confined to family context F91.0
 depressive F91.8
 group type F91.2
 hyperkinetic — *see* Disorder, attention-deficit
  hyperactivity
 oppositional defiance F91.3
 socialized F91.2
 solitary aggressive type F91.1
 specified NEC F91.8
 unsocialized (aggressive) F91.1
conduction, heart I45.9
congenital glycosylation (CDG) E74.8
conjunctiva H11.9
 infection — *see* Conjunctivitis
connective tissue, localized L94.9
 specified NEC L94.8
conversion (functional neurological symptom
 disorder)
 with
  abnormal movement F44.4
  anesthesia or sensory loss F44.6
  attacks or seizures F44.5
  mixed symptoms F44.7
  special sensory symptoms F44.6
  speech symptoms F44.4
  swallowing symptoms F44.4
  weakness or paralysis F44.4
convulsive (secondary) — *see* Convulsions
cornea H18.9
 deformity — *see* Deformity, cornea
 degeneration — *see* Degeneration, cornea
 deposits — *see* Deposit, cornea
 due to contact lens H18.82-
  specified as edema — *see* Edema, cornea
 edema — *see* Edema, cornea
 keratitis — *see* Keratitis
 keratoconjunctivitis — *see*
  Keratoconjunctivitis
 membrane change — *see* Change, corneal
  membrane
 neovascularization — *see*
  Neovascularization, cornea
 scar — *see* Opacity, cornea
 specified type NEC H18.89-
 ulcer — *see* Ulcer, cornea
corpus cavernosum N48.9
cranial nerve — *see* Disorder, nerve, cranial
cyclothymic F34.0
defiant oppositional F91.3
delusional (persistent) (systematized) F22
 induced F24
depersonalization F48.1

Disorder (of) (*see also* Disease) — *continued*
depressive F32.9
 major F32.9
  with psychotic symptoms F32.3
  in remission (full) F32.5
   partial F32.4
  recurrent F33.9
  single episode F32.9
   mild F32.0
   moderate F32.1
   severe (without psychotic symptoms)
    F32.2
   with psychotic symptoms F32.3
 organic F06.31
 persistent F34.1
 recurrent F33.9
  current episode
   mild F33.0
   moderate F33.1
   severe (without psychotic symptoms)
    F33.2
   with psychotic symptoms F33.3
  in remission F33.40
   full F33.42
   partial F33.41
  specified NEC F33.8
 single episode — *see* Episode, depressive
 specified NEC F32.89
developmental F89
 arithmetical skills F81.2
 coordination (motor) F82
 expressive writing F81.81
 language F80.9
  expressive F80.1
  mixed receptive and expressive F80.2
  receptive type F80.2
  specified NEC F80.89
 learning F81.9
  arithmetical F81.2
  reading F81.0
 mixed F88
 motor coordination or function F82
 pervasive F84.9
  specified NEC F84.8
 phonological F80.0
 reading F81.0
 scholastic skills — *see also* Disorder, learning
  mixed F81.89
 specified NEC F88
 speech F80.9
  articulation F80.0
  specified NEC F80.89
 written expression F81.81
diaphragm J98.6
digestive (system) K92.9
 newborn P78.9
  specified NEC P78.89
 postprocedural — *see* Complication,
  gastrointestinal
psychogenic F45.8
disc (intervertebral) M51.9
 with
  myelopathy
   cervical region M50.00
   cervicothoracic region M50.03
   high cervical region M50.01
   lumbar region M51.06
   mid-cervical region M50.020
   sacrococcygeal region M53.3
   thoracic region M51.04
   thoracolumbar region M51.05
  radiculopathy
   cervical region M50.10
   cervicothoracic region M50.13
   high cervical region M50.11
   lumbar region M51.16
   lumbosacral region M51.17
   mid-cervical region M50.120
   sacrococcygeal region M53.3

DISEASE INDEX

Disorder (of) (*see also* Disease) — *continued*
disc (intervertebral) M51.9 — *continued*
  with — *continued*
    radiculopathy — *continued*
      thoracic region M51.14
      thoracolumbar region M51.15
  cervical M50.90
    with
      myelopathy M50.00
        C2-C3 M50.01
        C3-C4 M50.01
        C4-C5 M50.021
        C5-C6 M50.022
        C6-C7 M50.023
        C7-T1 M50.03
        cervicothoracic region M50.03
        high cervical region M50.01
        mid-cervical region M50.020
      neuritis, radiculitis or radiculopathy
        M50.10
        C2-C3 M50.11
        C3-C4 M50.11
        C4-C5 M50.121
        C5-C6 M50.122
        C6-C7 M50.123
        C7-T1 M50.13
        cervicothoracic region M50.13
        high cervical region M50.11
        mid-cervical region M50.120
    C2-C3 M50.91
    C3-C4 M50.91
    C4-C5 M50.921
    C5-C6 M50.922
    C6-C7 M50.923
    C7-T1 M50.93
    cervicothoracic region M50.93
    degeneration M50.30
      C2-C3 M50.31
      C3-C4 M50.31
      C4-C5 M50.321
      C5-C6 M50.322
      C6-C7 M50.323
      C7-T1 M50.33
      cervicothoracic region M50.33
      high cervical region M50.31
      mid-cervical region M50.320
    displacement M50.20
      C2-C3 M50.21
      C3-C4 M50.21
      C4-C5 M50.221
      C5-C6 M50.222
      C6-C7 M50.223
      C7-T1 M50.23
      cervicothoracic region M50.23
      high cervical region M50.21
      mid-cervical region M50.220
    high cervical region M50.91
    mid-cervical region M50.920
    specified type NEC M50.80
      C2-C3 M50.81
      C3-C4 M50.81
      C4-C5 M50.821
      C5-C6 M50.822
      C6-C7 M50.823
      C7-T1 M50.83
      cervicothoracic region M50.83
      high cervical region M50.81
      mid-cervical region M50.820
  specified NEC
    lumbar region M51.86
    lumbosacral region M51.87
    sacrococcygeal region M53.3
    thoracic region M51.84
    thoracolumbar region M51.85
disinhibited attachment (childhood) F94.2
disintegrative, childhood NEC F84.3
disruptive F91.9
  mood dysregulation F34.81
  specified NEC F91.8

disruptive behavior F91.9
dissocial personality F60.2
dissociative F44.9
  affecting
    motor function F44.4
      and sensation F44.7
    sensation F44.6
      and motor function F44.7
  brief reactive F43.0
  due to (secondary to) general medical
    condition F06.8
  mixed F44.7
  organic F06.8
  other specified NEC F44.89
double heterozygous sickling — *see* Disease,
  sickle-cell
dream anxiety F51.5
drug induced hemorrhagic D68.32
drug related F19.99
  abuse — *see* Abuse, drug
  dependence — *see* Dependence, drug
dysmorphic body F45.22
dysthymic F34.1
ear H93.9-
  bleeding — *see* Otorrhagia
  deafness — *see* Deafness
  degenerative H93.09-
  discharge — *see* Otorrhea
  external H61.9-
    auditory canal stenosis — *see* Stenosis,
      external ear canal
    exostosis — *see* Exostosis, external ear
      canal
    impacted cerumen — *see* Impaction,
      cerumen
    otitis — *see* Otitis, externa
    perichondritis — *see* Perichondritis, ear
    pinna — *see* Disorder, pinna
    specified type NEC H61.89-
      in diseases classified elsewhere H62.8x-
  inner H83.9-
    vestibular dysfunction — *see* Disorder,
      vestibular function
  middle H74.9-
    adhesive H74.1-
    ossicle — *see* Abnormal, ear ossicles
    polyp — *see* Polyp, ear (middle)
    specified NEC, in diseases classified
      elsewhere H75.8-
    postprocedural — *see* Complications, ear,
      procedure
  specified NEC, in diseases classified
    elsewhere H94.8-
eating (adult) (psychogenic) F50.9
  anorexia — *see* Anorexia
  binge F50.81
  bulimia F50.2
  child F98.29
    pica F98.3
    rumination disorder F98.21
  pica F50.89
    childhood F98.3
electrolyte (balance) NEC E87.8
  with
    abortion — *see* Abortion by type
      complicated by specified condition
      NEC
    ectopic pregnancy O08.5
    molar pregnancy O08.5
  acidosis (metabolic) (respiratory) E87.2
  alkalosis (metabolic) (respiratory) E87.3
elimination, transepidermal L87.9
  specified NEC L87.8
emotional (persistent) F34.9
  of childhood F93.9
    specified NEC F93.8

endocrine E34.9
  postprocedural E89.89
  specified NEC E89.89
erectile (male) (organic) (*see also* Dysfunction,
  sexual, male, erectile) N52.9
  nonorganic F52.21
erythematous — *see* Erythema
esophagus K22.9
  functional K22.4
  psychogenic F45.8
eustachian tube H69.9-
  infection — *see* Salpingitis, eustachian
  obstruction — *see* Obstruction, eustachian
    tube
  patulous — *see* Patulous, eustachian tube
  specified NEC H69.8-
extrapyramidal G25.9
  in diseases classified elsewhere — *see*
    category G26
  specified type NEC G25.89
eye H57.9
  postprocedural — *see* Complication,
    postprocedural, eye
eyelid H02.9
  cyst — *see* Cyst, eyelid
  degenerative H02.70
    chloasma — *see* Chloasma, eyelid
    madarosis — *see* Madarosis
    specified type NEC H02.79
    vitiligo — *see* Vitiligo, eyelid
    xanthelasma — *see* Xanthelasma
  dermatochalasis — *see* Dermatochalasis
  edema — *see* Edema, eyelid
  elephantiasis — *see* Elephantiasis, eyelid
  foreign body, retained — *see* Foreign body,
    retained, eyelid
  function H02.59
    abnormal innervation syndrome — *see*
      Syndrome, abnormal innervation
    blepharochalasis — *see* Blepharochalasis
    blepharoclonus — *see* Blepharoclonus
    blepharophimosis — *see* Blepharophimosis
    blepharoptosis — *see* Blepharoptosis
    lagophthalmos — *see* Lagophthalmos
    lid retraction — *see* Retraction, lid
    hypertrichosis — *see* Hypertrichosis, eyelid
  specified type NEC H02.89
  vascular H02.879
    left H02.876
      lower H02.875
      upper H02.874
    right H02.873
      lower H02.872
      upper H02.871
factitious F68.10
  with predominantly
    physical symptoms F68.12
      with psychological symptoms F68.13
    psychological symptoms F68.11
      with physical symptoms F68.13
factor, coagulation — *see* Defect, coagulation
fatty acid
  metabolism E71.30
    specified NEC E71.39
  oxidation
    LCAD E71.310
    MCAD E71.311
    SCAD E71.312
    specified deficiency NEC E71.318
feeding (infant or child) (*see also* Disorder,
  eating) R63.3
feigned (with obvious motivation) Z76.5
  without obvious motivation — *see* Disorder,
    factitious
female
  hypoactive sexual desire F52.0
  orgasmic F52.31
  sexual arousal F52.22

Disorder (of) (see also Disease) — continued
fibroblastic M72.9
  specified NEC M72.8
fluency
  adult onset F98.5
  childhood onset F80.81
  following
    cerebral infarction I69.323
    cerebrovascular disease I69.923
      specified disease NEC I69.823
    intracerebral hemorrhage I69.123
    nontraumatic intracranial hemorrhage
      NEC I69.223
    subarachnoid hemorrhage I69.023
  in conditions classified elsewhere R47.82
fluid balance E87.8
follicular (skin) L73.9
  specified NEC L73.8
fructose metabolism E74.10
  essential fructosuria E74.11
  fructokinase deficiency E74.11
  fructose-1, 6-diphosphatase deficiency
    E74.19
  hereditary fructose intolerance E74.12
  other specified E74.19
functional polymorphonuclear neutrophils D71
gallbladder, biliary tract and pancreas in
    diseases classified elsewhere K87
gamma-glutamyl cycle E72.8
gastric (functional) K31.9
  motility K30
  psychogenic F45.8
  secretion K30
gastrointestinal (functional) NOS K92.9
  newborn P78.9
  psychogenic F45.8
gender-identity or -role F64.9
  childhood F64.2
  effect on relationship F66
  of adolescence or adulthood F64.0
    nontranssexual F64.8
  specified NEC F64.8
  uncertainty F66
genito-pelvic pain penetration F52.6
genitourinary system
  female N94.9
  male N50.9
  psychogenic F45.8
globe H44.9
  degenerated condition H44.50
    absolute glaucoma H44.51-
    atrophy H44.52-
    leucocoria H44.53-
  degenerative H44.30
    chalcosis H44.31-
    myopia H44.2-
    siderosis H44.32-
    specified type NEC H44.39-
  endophthalmitis — see Endophthalmitis
  foreign body, retained — see Foreign body,
    intraocular, old, retained
  hemophthalmos — see Hemophthalmos
  hypotony H44.40
    due to
      ocular fistula H44.42-
      specified disorder NEC H44.43-
    flat anterior chamber H44.41-
    primary H44.44-
  luxation — see Luxation, globe
  specified type NEC H44.89
glomerular (in) N05.9
  amyloidosis E85.4 [N08]
  cryoglobulinemia D89.1 [N08]
  disseminated intravascular coagulation D65
    [N08]
  Fabry's disease E75.21 [N08]
  familial lecithin cholesterol acyltransferase
    deficiency E78.6 [N08]
  Goodpasture's syndrome M31.0

Disorder (of) (see also Disease) — continued
glomerular (in) N05.9 — continued
  hemolytic-uremic syndrome D59.3
  Henoch (-Schönlein) purpura D69.0 [N08]
  malariae malaria B52.0
  microscopic polyangiitis M31.7 [N08]
  multiple myeloma C90.0- [N08]
  mumps B26.83
  schistosomiasis B65.9 [N08]
  sepsis NEC A41.- [N08]
    streptococcal A40.- [N08]
  sickle-cell disorders D57- [N08]
  strongyloidiasis B78.9 [N08]
  subacute bacterial endocarditis I33.0 [N08]
  syphilis A52.75
  systemic lupus erythematosus M32.14
  thrombotic thrombocytopenic purpura
    M31.1 [N08]
  Waldenström macroglobulinemia C88.0 [N08]
  Wegener's granulomatosis M31.31
gluconeogenesis E74.4
glucosaminoglycan metabolism — see
    Disorder, metabolism, glucosaminoglycan
glycine metabolism E72.50
  d-glycericacidemia E72.59
  hyperhydroxyprolinemia E72.59
  hyperoxaluria E72.53
  hyperprolinemia E72.59
  non-ketotic hyperglycinemia E72.51
  oxalosis E72.53
  oxaluria E72.53
  sarcosinemia E72.59
  trimethylaminuria E72.52
glycoprotein metabolism E77.9
  specified NEC E77.8
habit (and impulse) F63.9
  involving sexual behavior NEC F65.9
  specified NEC F63.89
hallucinogen use
  mild F16.10
    with
      hallucinogen-induced
        anxiety disorder F16.180
        bipolar and related disorder F16.14
        depressive disorder F16.14
        psychotic disorder F16.159
      hallucinogen intoxication delirium
        F16.121
      other hallucinogen intoxication F16.129
  moderate or severe F16.20
    with
      hallucinogen-induced
        anxiety disorder F16.280
        bipolar and related disorder F16.24
        depressive disorder F16.24
        psychotic disorder F16.259
      hallucinogen intoxication delirium
        F16.221
      other hallucinogen intoxication F16.229
heart action I49.9
hematological D75.9
  newborn (transient) P61.9
    specified NEC P61.8
hematopoietic organs D75.9
hemorrhagic NEC D69.9
  drug-induced D68.32
  due to
    extrinsic circulating anticoagulants D68.32
    increase in
      anti-IIa D68.32
      anti-Xa D68.32
    intrinsic
      circulating anticoagulants D68.318
      increase in
        antithrombin D68.318
        anti-VIIIa D68.318
        anti-IXa D68.318
        anti-XIa D68.318
  following childbirth O72.3

Disorder (of) (see also Disease) — continued
hemostasis — see Defect, coagulation
histidine metabolism E70.40
  histidinemia E70.41
  other specified E70.49
hoarding F42.3
hyperkinetic — see Disorder, attention-deficit
    hyperactivity
hyperleucine-isoleucinemia E71.19
hypervalinemia E71.19
hypoactive sexual desire F52.0
hypochondriacal F45.20
  body dysmorphic F45.22
  neurosis F45.21
  other specified F45.29
identity
  dissociative F44.81
  illness anxiety F45.21
  of childhood F93.8
immune mechanism (immunity) D89.9
  specified type NEC D89.89
impaired renal tubular function N25.9
  specified NEC N25.89
impulse (control) F63.9
inflammatory
  pelvic, in diseases classified elsewhere — see
    category N74
  penis N48.29
    abscess N48.21
    cellulitis N48.22
inhalant use
  mild F18.10
    with
      inhalant-induced
        anxiety disorder F18.180
        depressive disorder F18.14
        major neurocognitive disorder F18.17
        mild neurocognitive disorder F18.188
        psychotic disorder F18.159
      inhalant intoxication F18.129
      inhalant intoxication delirium F18.121
  moderate or severe F18.20
    with
      inhalant-induced
        anxiety disorder F18.280
        depressive disorder F18.24
        major neurocognitive disorder F18.27
        mild neurocognitive disorder F18.288
        psychotic disorder F18.259
      inhalant intoxication F18.229
      inhalant intoxication delirium F18.221
integument, newborn P83.9
  specified NEC P83.8
intermittent explosive F63.81
internal secretion pancreas — see Increased,
    secretion, pancreas, endocrine
intestine, intestinal
  carbohydrate absorption NEC E74.39
    postoperative K91.2
  functional NEC K59.9
    postoperative K91.89
    psychogenic F45.8
  vascular K55.9
    chronic K55.1
    specified NEC K55.8
intraoperative (intraprocedural) — see
    Complications, intraoperative
involuntary emotional expression (IEED) F48.2
iris H21.9
  adhesions — see Adhesions, iris
  atrophy — see Atrophy, iris
  chamber angle recession — see Recession,
    chamber angle
  cyst — see Cyst, iris
  degeneration — see Degeneration, iris
  in diseases classified elsewhere H22
  iridodialysis — see Iridodialysis
  iridoschisis — see Iridoschisis
  miotic pupillary cyst — see Cyst, pupillary

Disorder (of) (*see also* Disease) — *continued*
iris H21.9 — *continued*
  pupillary
    abnormality — *see* Abnormality, pupillary
    membrane — *see* Membrane, pupillary
  specified type NEC H21.89
  vascular NEC H21.1x-
iron metabolism E83.10
  specified NEC E83.19
isovaleric acidemia E71.110
jaw, developmental M27.0
  temporomandibular (*see also* Anomaly,
    dentofacial, temporomandibular joint)
    M26.60-
joint M25.9
  derangement — *see* Derangement, joint
  effusion — *see* Effusion, joint
  fistula — *see* Fistula, joint
  hemarthrosis — *see* Hemarthrosis
  instability — *see* Instability, joint
  osteophyte — *see* Osteophyte
  pain — *see* Pain, joint
  psychogenic F45.8
  specified type NEC M25.80
    ankle M25.87-
    elbow M25.82-
    foot joint M25.87-
    hand joint M25.84-
    hip M25.85-
    knee M25.86-
    shoulder M25.81-
    wrist M25.83-
  stiffness — *see* Stiffness, joint
ketone metabolism E71.32
kidney N28.9
  functional (tubular) N25.9
  in
    schistosomiasis B65.9 [N29]
  tubular function N25.9
  specified NEC N25.89
lacrimal system H04.9
  changes H04.69
  fistula — *see* Fistula, lacrimal
  gland H04.19
    atrophy — *see* Atrophy, lacrimal gland
    cyst — *see* Cyst, lacrimal, gland
    dacryops — *see* Dacryops
    dislocation — *see* Dislocation, lacrimal
      gland
    dry eye syndrome — *see* Syndrome, dry
      eye
    infection — *see* Dacryoadenitis
    granuloma — *see* Granuloma, lacrimal
    inflammation — *see* Inflammation, lacrimal
    obstruction — *see* Obstruction, lacrimal
    specified NEC H04.89
lactation NEC O92.79
language (developmental) F80.9
  expressive F80.1
  mixed receptive and expressive F80.2
  receptive F80.2
late luteal phase dysphoric N94.89
learning (specific) F81.9
  acalculia R48.8
  alexia R48.0
  mathematics F81.2
  reading F81.0
  specified NEC F81.89
  spelling F81.81
  written expression F81.81
lens H27.9
  aphakia — *see* Aphakia
  cataract — *see* Cataract
  dislocation — *see* Dislocation, lens
  specified type NEC H27.8

Disorder (of) (*see also* Disease) — *continued*
ligament M24.20
  ankle M24.27-
  attachment, spine — *see* Enthesopathy,
    spinal
  elbow M24.22-
  foot joint M24.27-
  hand joint M24.24-
  hip M24.25-
  knee — *see* Derangement, knee, specified
    NEC
  shoulder M24.21-
  vertebra M24.28
  wrist M24.23-
ligamentous attachments — *see also*
  Enthesopathy
  spine — *see* Enthesopathy, spinal
lipid
  metabolism, congenital E78.9
  storage E75.6
  specified NEC E75.5
lipoprotein
  deficiency (familial) E78.6
  metabolism E78.9
  specified NEC E78.89
liver K76.9
  malarial B54 [K77]
low back — *see also* Dorsopathy, specified
  NEC
lumbosacral
  plexus G54.1
  root (nerve) NEC G54.4
lung, interstitial, drug-induced J70.4
  acute J70.2
  chronic J70.3
lymphoproliferative, post-transplant (PTLD)
  D47.Z1 **(follows D47.4)**
lysine and hydroxylysine metabolism E72.3
major neurocognitive — *see* Dementia, in (due
  to)
male
  erectile (organic) (*see also* Dysfunction,
    sexual, male, erectile) N52.9
    nonorganic F52.21
  hypoactive sexual desire F52.0
  orgasmic F52.32
manic F30.9
  organic F06.33
mast cell activation — *see* Activation, mast cell
mastoid — *see also* Disorder, ear, middle
  postprocedural — *see* Complications, ear,
    procedure
meniscus — *see* Derangement, knee, meniscus
menopausal N95.9
  specified NEC N95.8
menstrual N92.6
  psychogenic F45.8
  specified NEC N92.5
mental (or behavioral) (nonpsychotic) F99
  due to (secondary to)
    amphetamine
      due to drug abuse — *see* Abuse, drug,
        stimulant
      due to drug dependence — *see*
        Dependence, drug, stimulant
    brain disease, damage and dysfunction
      F09
    caffeine use
      due to drug abuse — *see* Abuse, drug,
        stimulant
      due to drug dependence — *see*
        Dependence, drug, stimulant
    cannabis use
      due to drug abuse — *see* Abuse, drug,
        cannabis
      due to drug dependence — *see*
        Dependence, drug, cannabis
    general medical condition F09

Disorder (of) (*see also* Disease) — *continued*
mental (or behavioral) (nonpsychotic) F99 —
  continued
  due to (secondary to) — *continued*
    sedative or hypnotic use
      due to drug abuse — *see* Abuse, drug,
        sedative
      due to drug dependence — *see*
        Dependence, drug, sedative
    tobacco (nicotine) use — *see* Dependence,
      drug, nicotine
  following organic brain damage F07.9
    frontal lobe syndrome F07.0
    personality change F07.0
    postconcussional syndrome F07.81
    specified NEC F07.89
  infancy, childhood or adolescence F98.9
  neurotic — *see* Neurosis
  organic or symptomatic F09
  presenile, psychotic F03
  problem NEC
  psychoneurotic — *see* Neurosis
  psychotic — *see* Psychosis
  puerperal F53
  senile, psychotic NEC F03
metabolic, amino acid, transitory, newborn
  P74.8
metabolism NOS E88.9
  amino-acid E72.9
    aromatic E70.9
      albinism — *see* Albinism
      histidine E70.40
        histidinemia E70.41
        other specified E70.49
      hyperphenylalaninemia E70.1
        classical phenylketonuria E70.0
      other specified E70.8
      tryptophan E70.5
      tyrosine E70.20
        hypertyrosinemia E70.21
        other specified E70.29
    branched chain E71.2
      3-methylglutaconic aciduria E71.111
      hyperleucine-isoleucinemia E71.19
      hypervalinemia E71.19
      isovaleric acidemia E71.110
      maple syrup urine disease E71.0
      methylmalonic acidemia E71.120
      organic aciduria NEC E71.118
      other specified E71.19
      proprionate NEC E71.128
      proprionic acidemia E71.121
    glycine E72.50
      d-glycericacidemia E72.59
      hyperhydroxyprolinemia E72.59
      hyperoxaluria E72.53
      hyperprolinemia E72.59
      non-ketotic hyperglycinemia E72.51
      other specified E72.59
      sarcosinemia E72.59
      trimethylaminuria E72.52
    hydroxylysine E72.3
    lysine E72.3
    ornithine E72.4
    other specified E72.8
      beta-amino acid E72.8
      gamma-glutamyl cycle E72.8
    straight-chain E72.8
    sulfur-bearing E72.10
      homocystinuria E72.11
      methylenetetrahydrofolate reductase
        deficiency E72.12
      other specified E72.19
  bile acid and cholesterol metabolism E78.70
  bilirubin E80.7
    specified NEC E80.6

DISEASE INDEX

Disorder (of) (see also Disease) — *continued*
metabolism NOS E88.9 — *continued*
calcium E83.50
hypercalcemia E83.52
hypocalcemia E83.51
other specified E83.59
carbohydrate E74.9
specified NEC E74.8
cholesterol and bile acid metabolism E78.70
congenital E88.9
copper E83.00
specified type NEC E83.09
Wilson's disease E83.01
cystinuria E72.01
fructose E74.10
galactose E74.20
glucosaminoglycan E76.9
mucopolysaccharidosis — *see*
Mucopolysaccharidosis
specified NEC E76.8
glutamine E72.8
glycine E72.50
glycogen storage (hepatorenal) E74.09
glycoprotein E77.9
specified NEC E77.8
glycosaminoglycan E76.9
specified NEC E76.8
in labor and delivery O75.89
iron E83.10
isoleucine E71.19
leucine E71.19
lipoid E78.9
lipoprotein E78.9
specified NEC E78.89
magnesium E83.40
hypermagnesemia E83.41
hypomagnesemia E83.42
other specified E83.49
mineral E83.9
specified NEC E83.89
mitochondrial E88.40
MELAS syndrome E88.41
MERRF syndrome (myoclonic epilepsy
associated with ragged-red fibers)
E88.42
other specified E88.49
ornithine E72.4
phosphatases E83.30
phosphorus E83.30
acid phosphatase deficiency E83.39
hypophosphatasia E83.39
hypophosphatemia E83.39
familial E83.31
other specified E83.39
pseudovitamin D deficiency E83.32
plasma protein NEC E88.09
porphyrin — *see* Porphyria
postprocedural E89.89
specified NEC E89.89
purine E79.9
specified NEC E79.8
pyrimidine E79.9
specified NEC E79.8
pyruvate E74.4
serine E72.8
sodium E87.8
specified NEC E88.89
threonine E72.8
valine E71.19
zinc E83.2
methylmalonic acidemia E71.120
micturition NEC (see also Difficulty, micturition)
R39.198
feeling of incomplete emptying R39.14
hesitancy R39.11
poor stream R39.12
psychogenic F45.8
split stream R39.13
straining R39.16

Disorder (of) (see also Disease) — *continued*
micturition NEC R39.19 — *continued*
urgency R39.15
mild neurocognitive G31.84
mitochondrial metabolism E88.40
mitral (valve) — *see* Endocarditis, mitral
mixed
anxiety and depressive F41.8
of scholastic skills (developmental) F81.89
receptive expressive language F80.2
mood F39
bipolar — *see* Disorder, bipolar
depressive — *see* Disorder, depressive
due to (secondary to)
alcohol F10.94
amphetamine F15.94
in
abuse F15.14
dependence F15.24
anxiolytic F13.94
in
abuse F13.14
dependence F13.24
cocaine F14.94
in
abuse F14.14
dependence F14.24
general medical condition F06.30
hallucinogen F16.94
in
abuse F16.14
dependence F16.24
hypnotic F13.94
in
abuse F13.14
dependence F13.24
inhalant F18.94
in
abuse F18.14
dependence F18.24
opioid F11.94
in
abuse F11.14
dependence F11.24
phencyclidine (PCP) F16.94
in
abuse F16.14
dependence F16.24
physiological condition F06.30
with
depressive features F06.31
major depressive-like episode F06.32
manic features F06.33
mixed features F06.34
psychoactive substance NEC F19.94
in
abuse F19.14
dependence F19.24
sedative F13.94
in
abuse F13.14
dependence F13.24
volatile solvents F18.94
in
abuse F18.14
dependence F18.24
manic episode F30.9
with psychotic symptoms F30.2
in remission (full) F30.4
partial F30.3
specified type NEC F30.8
without psychotic symptoms F30.10
mild F30.11
moderate F30.12
severe F30.13
organic F06.30
right hemisphere F07.89

Disorder (of) (see also Disease) — *continued*
mood F39 — *continued*
persistent F34.9
cyclothymia F34.0
dysthymia F34.1
specified type NEC F34.89
recurrent F39
right hemisphere organic F07.89
movement G25.9
drug-induced G25.70
akathisia G25.71
specified NEC G25.79
hysterical F44.4
in diseases classified elsewhere — *see*
category G26
periodic limb G47.61
sleep related G47.61
sleep related NEC G47.69
specified NEC G25.89
stereotyped F98.4
treatment-induced G25.9
multiple personality F44.81
muscle M62.9
attachment, spine — *see* Enthesopathy, spinal
in trichinellosis — *see* Trichinellosis, with
muscle disorder
psychogenic F45.8
specified type NEC M62.89
tone, newborn P94.9
specified NEC P94.8
muscular
attachments — *see also* Enthesopathy
spine — *see* Enthesopathy, spinal
urethra N36.44
musculoskeletal system, soft tissue — *see*
Disorder, soft tissue
postprocedural M96.89
psychogenic F45.8
myoneural G70.9
due to lead G70.1
specified NEC G70.89
toxic G70.1
myotonic NEC G71.19
nail, in diseases classified elsewhere L62
neck region NEC — *see* Dorsopathy, specified
NEC
neonatal onset multisystemic inflammatory
(NOMID) M04.2
nerve G58.9
abducent NEC — *see* Strabismus, paralytic,
sixth nerve
accessory G52.8
acoustic — *see* subcategory H93.3
auditory — *see* subcategory H93.3
auriculotemporal G50.8
axillary G54.0
cerebral — *see* Disorder, nerve, cranial
cranial G52.9
eighth — *see* subcategory H93.3
eleventh G52.8
fifth G50.9
first G52.0
fourth NEC — *see* Strabismus, paralytic,
fourth nerve
multiple G52.7
ninth G52.1
second NEC — *see* Disorder, nerve, optic
seventh NEC G51.8
sixth NEC — *see* Strabismus, paralytic,
sixth nerve
specified NEC G52.8
tenth G52.2
third NEC — *see* Strabismus, paralytic,
third nerve
twelfth G52.3
entrapment — *see* Neuropathy, entrapment
facial G51.9
specified NEC G51.8
femoral — *see* Lesion, nerve, femoral

Disorder (of) (*see also* Disease) — *continued*
nerve G58.9 — *continued*
glossopharyngeal NEC G52.1
hypoglossal G52.3
intercostal G58.0
lateral
cutaneous of thigh — *see*
Mononeuropathy, lower limb,
meralgia paresthetica
popliteal — *see* Lesion, nerve, popliteal
lower limb — *see* Mononeuropathy, lower
limb
medial popliteal — *see* Lesion, nerve,
popliteal, medial
median NEC — *see* Lesion, nerve, median
multiple G58.7
oculomotor NEC — *see* Strabismus,
paralytic, third nerve
olfactory G52.0
optic NEC H47.09-
hemorrhage into sheath — *see*
Hemorrhage, optic nerve
ischemic H47.01-
peroneal — *see* Lesion, nerve, popliteal
phrenic G58.8
plantar — *see* Lesion, nerve, plantar
pneumogastric G52.2
posterior tibial — *see* Syndrome, tarsal
tunnel
radial — *see* Lesion, nerve, radial
recurrent laryngeal G52.2
root G54.9
cervical G54.2
lumbosacral G54.1
specified NEC G54.8
thoracic G54.3
sciatic NEC — *see* Lesion, nerve, sciatic
specified NEC G58.8
lower limb — *see* Mononeuropathy, lower
limb, specified NEC
upper limb — *see* Mononeuropathy, upper
limb, specified NEC
sympathetic G90.9
tibial — *see* Lesion, nerve, popliteal, medial
trigeminal G50.9
specified NEC G50.8
trochlear NEC — *see* Strabismus, paralytic,
fourth nerve
ulnar — *see* Lesion, nerve, ulnar
upper limb — *see* Mononeuropathy, upper
limb
vagus G52.2
nervous system G98.8
autonomic (peripheral) G90.9
specified NEC G90.8
central G96.9
specified NEC G96.8
parasympathetic G90.9
specified NEC G98.8
sympathetic G90.9
vegetative G90.9
neurocognitive
major
with
aggressive behavior F01.51
combative behavior F01.51
violent behavior F01.51
due to vascular disease, with behavioral
disturbance F01.51
in (due to) (other diseases classified
elsewhere) (*see also* Dementia, in (due
to)) F02.80
with
aggressive behavior F02.81
combative behavior F02.81
violent behavior F02.81
without behavioral disturbance F01.50
mild G31.84

Disorder (of) (*see also* Disease) — *continued*
neurodevelopmental F89
specified NEC F88
neurohypophysis NEC E23.3
neurological NEC R29.818
neuromuscular G70.9
hereditary NEC G71.9
specified NEC G70.89
toxic G70.1
neurotic F48.9
specified NEC F48.8
neutrophil, polymorphonuclear D71
nicotine use — *see* Dependence, drug, nicotine
nightmare F51.5
nose J34.9
specified NEC J34.89
obsessive-compulsive F42.9
odontogenesis NOS K00.9
opioid use
with
opiod-induced psychotic disorder F11.959
with
delusions F11.950
hallucinations F11.951
due to drug abuse — *see* Abuse, drug, opioid
due to drug dependence — *see* Dependence,
drug, opioid
mild F11.10
with
opioid-induced
anxiety disorder F11.188
depressive disorder F11.14
sexual dysfunction F11.181
opioid intoxication
with perceptual disturbances F11.122
delirium F11.121
without perceptual disturbances
F11.129
moderate or severe F11.20
with
opioid-induced
anxiety disorder F11.288
anxiety disorder F11.988
depressive disorder F11.24
depressive disorder F11.94
sexual dysfunction F11.281
sexual dysfunction F11.981
opioid intoxication
with perceptual disturbances F11.222
delirium F11.221
without perceptual disturbances
F11.229
oppositional defiant F91.3
optic
chiasm H47.49
due to
inflammatory disorder H47.41
neoplasm H47.42
vascular disorder H47.43
disc H47.39-
coloboma — *see* Coloboma, optic disc
drusen — *see* Drusen, optic disc
pseudopapilledema — *see*
Pseudopapilledema
radiations — *see* Disorder, visual, pathway
tracts — *see* Disorder, visual, pathway
orbit H05.9
cyst — *see* Cyst, orbit
deformity — *see* Deformity, orbit
edema — *see* Edema, orbit
enophthalmos — *see* Enophthalmos
exophthalmos — *see* Exophthalmos
hemorrhage — *see* Hemorrhage, orbit
inflammation — *see* Inflammation, orbit
myopathy — *see* Myopathy, extraocular
muscles
retained foreign body — *see* Foreign body,
orbit, old
specified type NEC H05.89

Disorder (of) (*see also* Disease) — *continued*
organic
anxiety F06.4
catatonic F06.1
delusional F06.2
dissociative F06.8
emotionally labile (asthenic) F06.8
mood (affective) F06.30
schizophrenia-like F06.2
orgasmic (female) F52.31
male F52.32
ornithine metabolism E72.4
overanxious F41.1
of childhood F93.8
pain
with related psychological factors F45.42
exclusively related to psychological factors
F45.41
genito-pelvic penetration disorder F52.6
pancreatic internal secretion E16.9
specified NEC E16.8
panic F41.0
with agoraphobia F40.01
papulosquamous L44.9
in diseases classified elsewhere L45
specified NEC L44.8
paranoid F22
induced F24
shared F24
parathyroid (gland) E21.5
specified NEC E21.4
parietoalveolar NEC J84.09
paroxysmal, mixed R56.9
patella M22.9-
chondromalacia — *see* Chondromalacia,
patella
derangement NEC M22.3x-
recurrent
dislocation — *see* Dislocation, patella,
recurrent
subluxation — *see* Dislocation, patella,
recurrent, incomplete
specified NEC M22.8x-
patellofemoral M22.2x-
pentose phosphate pathway with anemia
D55.1
perception, due to hallucinogens F16.983
in
abuse F16.183
dependence F16.283
peripheral nervous system NEC G64
peroxisomal E71.50
biogenesis
neonatal adrenoleukodystrophy E71.511
specified disorder NEC E71.518
Zellweger syndrome E71.510
rhizomelic chondrodysplasia punctata
E71.540
specified form NEC E71.548
group 1 E71.518
group 2 E71.53
group 3 E71.542
X-linked adrenoleukodystrophy E71.529
adolescent E71.521
adrenomyeloneuropathy E71.522
childhood E71.520
specified form NEC E71.528
Zellweger-like syndrome E71.541
persistent
(somatoform) pain F45.41
affective (mood) F34.9
personality (*see also* Personality) F60.9
affective F34.0
aggressive F60.3
amoral F60.2
anankastic F60.5
antisocial F60.2
anxious F60.6
asocial F60.2

Disorder (of) (*see also* Disease) — *continued*
personality (*see also* Personality) F60.9 —
   continued
  asthenic F60.7
  avoidant F60.6
  borderline F60.3
  change (secondary) due to general medical
    condition F07.0
  compulsive F60.5
  cyclothymic F34.0
  dependent (passive) F60.7
  depressive F34.1
  dissocial F60.2
  emotional instability F60.3
  expansive paranoid F60.0
  explosive F60.3
  following organic brain damage F07.9
  histrionic F60.4
  hyperthymic F34.0
  hypothymic F34.1
  hysterical F60.4
  immature F60.89
  inadequate F60.7
  labile F60.3
  mixed (nonspecific) F60.89
  moral deficiency F60.2
  narcissistic F60.81
  negativistic F60.89
  obsessional F60.5
  obsessive(-compulsive) F60.5
  organic F07.9
  overconscientious F60.5
  paranoid F60.0
  passive(-dependent) F60.7
  passive-aggressive F60.89
  pathological NEC F60.9
  pseudosocial F60.2
  psychopathic F60.2
  schizoid F60.1
  schizotypal F21
  self-defeating F60.7
  specified NEC F60.89
  type A F60.5
  unstable (emotional) F60.3
pervasive, developmental F84.9
phencyclidine use
  mild F16.10
    with
      phencyclidine-induced
        anxiety disorder F16.180
        bipolar and related disorder F16.14
        depressive disorder F16.14
        psychotic disorder F16.159
      phencyclidine intoxication F16.129
      phencyclidine intoxication delirium
        F16.121
  moderate or severe F16.20
    with
      phencyclidine-induced
        anxiety disorder F16.280
        bipolar and related disorder F16.24
        depressive disorder F16.24
        psychotic disorder F16.259
      phencyclidine intoxication F16.229
      phencyclidine intoxication delirium
        F16.221
phobic anxiety, childhood F40.8
phosphate-losing tubular N25.0
pigmentation L81.9
  choroid, congenital Q14.3
  diminished melanin formation L81.6
  iron L81.8
  specified NEC L81.8
pinna (noninfective) H61.10-
  deformity, acquired H61.11-
  hematoma H61.12-
  perichondritis — *see* Perichondritis, ear
  specified type NEC H61.19-

Disorder (of) (*see also* Disease) — *continued*
pituitary gland E23.7
  iatrogenic (postprocedural) E89.3
  specified NEC E23.6
platelets D69.1
plexus G54.9
  specified NEC G54.8
polymorphonuclear neutrophils D71
porphyrin metabolism — *see* Porphyria
post-transplant lymphoproliferative D47.Z1
  (follows D47.4)
post-traumatic stress (PTSD) F43.10
  acute F43.11
  chronic F43.12
postconcussional F07.81
posthallucinogen perception F16.983
  in
    abuse F16.183
    dependence F16.283
postmenopausal N95.9
  specified NEC N95.8
postprocedural (postoperative) — *see*
  Complications, postprocedural
premenstrual dysphoric (PMDD) N94.81
prepuce N47.8
propionic acidemia E71.121
prostate N42.9
  specified NEC N42.89
psychogenic NOS (*see also* condition) F45.9
  anxiety F41.8
  appetite F50.9
  asthenic F48.8
  cardiovascular (system) F45.8
  compulsive F42.8
  cutaneous F54
  depressive F32.9
  digestive (system) F45.8
  dysmenorrheic F45.8
  dyspneic F45.8
  endocrine (system) F54
  eye NEC F45.8
  feeding — *see* Disorder, eating
  functional NEC F45.8
  gastric F45.8
  gastrointestinal (system) F45.8
  genitourinary (system) F45.8
  heart (function) (rhythm) F45.8
  hyperventilatory F45.8
  hypochondriacal — *see* Disorder,
    hypochondriacal
  intestinal F45.8
  joint F45.8
  learning F81.9
  limb F45.8
  lymphatic (system) F45.8
  menstrual F45.8
  micturition F45.8
  monoplegic NEC F44.4
  motor F44.4
  muscle F45.8
  musculoskeletal F45.8
  neurocirculatory F45.8
  obsessive F42.8
  occupational F48.8
  organ or part of body NEC F45.8
  paralytic NEC F44.4
  phobic F40.9
  physical NEC F45.8
  rectal F45.8
  respiratory (system) F45.8
  rheumatic F45.8
  sexual (function) F52.9
  skin (allergic) (eczematous) F54
  sleep F51.9
  specified part of body NEC F45.8
  stomach F45.8

Disorder (of) (*see also* Disease) — *continued*
psychological F99
  associated with
    disease classified elsewhere F54
  sexual
    development F66
    relationship F66
  uncertainty about gender identity F64.9
psychomotor NEC F44.4
  hysterical F44.4
psychoneurotic — *see also* Neurosis
  mixed NEC F48.8
psychophysiologic — *see* Disorder, somatoform
psychosexual F65.9
  development F66
  identity of childhood F64.2
psychosomatic NOS — *see* Disorder,
  somatoform
  multiple F45.0
  undifferentiated F45.1
psychotic — *see* Psychosis
  transient (acute) F23
puberty E30.9
  specified NEC E30.8
pulmonary (valve) — *see* Endocarditis,
  pulmonary
purine metabolism E79.9
pyrimidine metabolism E79.9
pyruvate metabolism E74.4
reactive attachment (childhood) F94.1
reading R48.0
  developmental (specific) F81.0
receptive language F80.2
receptor, hormonal, peripheral (*see also*
  Syndrome, androgen insensitivity) E34.50
recurrent brief depressive F33.8
reflex R29.2
refraction H52.7
  aniseikonia H52.32
  anisometropia H52.31
  astigmatism — *see* Astigmatism
  hypermetropia — *see* Hypermetropia
  myopia — *see* Myopia
  presbyopia H52.4
  specified NEC H52.6
relationship F68.8
  due to sexual orientation F66
REM sleep behavior G47.52
renal function, impaired (tubular) N25.9
resonance R49.9
  specified NEC R49.8
respiratory function, impaired — *see also*
  Failure, respiration
  postprocedural — *see* Complication,
    postoperative, respiratory system
  psychogenic F45.8
retina H35.9
  angioid streaks H35.33
  changes in vascular appearance H35.01-
  degeneration — *see* Degeneration, retina
  dystrophy (hereditary) — *see* Dystrophy,
    retina
  edema H35.81
  hemorrhage — *see* Hemorrhage, retina
  ischemia H35.82
  macular degeneration — *see* Degeneration,
    macula
  microaneurysms H35.04-
  microvascular abnormality NEC H35.09
  neovascularization — *see*
    Neovascularization, retina
  retinopathy — *see* Retinopathy
  separation of layers H35.70
    central serous chorioretinopathy H35.71-
    pigment epithelium detachment (serous)
      H35.72-
    hemorrhagic H35.73-
  specified type NEC H35.89
  telangiectasis — *see* Telangiectasis, retina

Disorder (of) (*see also* Disease) — *continued*
retina H35.9 — *continued*
  vasculitis — *see* Vasculitis, retina
retroperitoneal K68.9
right hemisphere organic affective F07.89
rumination (infant or child) F98.21
sacrum, sacrococcygeal NEC M53.3
schizoaffective F25.9
  bipolar type F25.0
  depressive type F25.1
  manic type F25.0
  mixed type F25.0
  specified NEC F25.8
schizoid of childhood F84.5
schizophreniform F20.81
  brief F23
schizotypal (personality) F21
secretion, thyrocalcitonin E07.0
sedative, hypnotic, or anxiolytic use
  mild F13.10
    with
      sedative, hypnotic, or anxiolytic-induced
        anxiety disorder F13.180
        bipolar and related disorder F13.14
        depressive disorder F13.14
        psychotic disorder F13.159
        sexual dysfunction F13.181
      sedative, hypnotic, or anxiolytic
        intoxication F13.129
      sedative, hypnotic, or anxiolytic
        intoxication delirium F13.121
  moderate or severe F13.20
    with
      sedative, hypnotic, or anxiolytic-induced
        anxiety disorder F13.280
        bipolar and related disorder F13.24
        depressive disorder F13.24
        major neurocognitive disorder F13.27
        mild neurocognitive disorder F13.288
        psychotic disorder F13.259
        sexual dysfunction F13.281
      sedative, hypnotic, or anxiolytic
        intoxication F13.229
      sedative, hypnotic, or anxiolytic
        intoxication delirium F13.221
seizure (*see also* Epilepsy) G40.909
  intractable G40.919
    with status epilepticus G40.911
semantic pragmatic F80.89
  with autism F84.0
sense of smell R43.1
  psychogenic F45.8
separation anxiety, of childhood F93.0
sexual
  arousal, female F52.22
  aversion F52.1
  function, psychogenic F52.9
  maturation F66
  nonorganic F52.9
  preference (*see also* Deviation, sexual) F65.9
    fetishistic transvestism F65.1
  relationship F66
shyness, of childhood and adolescence F40.10
sibling rivalry F93.8
sickle-cell (sickling) (homozygous) — *see*
    Disease, sickle-cell
  heterozygous D57.3
  specified type NEC D57.8-
  trait D57.3
sinus (nasal) J34.9
  specified NEC J34.89
skin L98.9
  atrophic L90.9
    specified NEC L90.8
  granulomatous L92.9
    specified NEC L92.8
  hypertrophic L91.9
    specified NEC L91.8
  infiltrative NEC L98.6

Disorder (of) (*see also* Disease) — *continued*
skin L98.9 — *continued*
  newborn P83.9
    specified NEC P83.8
  picking F42.4
  psychogenic (allergic) (eczematous) F54
sleep G47.9
  breathing-related — *see* Apnea, sleep
  circadian rhythm G47.20
    advance sleep phase type G47.22
    delayed sleep phase type G47.21
    due to
      alcohol
        abuse F10.182
        dependence F10.282
        use F10.982
      amphetamines
        abuse F15.182
        dependence F15.282
        use F15.982
      caffeine
        abuse F15.182
        dependence F15.282
        use F15.982
      cocaine
        abuse F14.182
        dependence F14.282
        use F14.982
      drug NEC
        abuse F19.182
        dependence F19.282
        use F19.982
      opioid
        abuse F11.182
        dependence F11.282
        use F11.982
      psychoactive substance NEC
        abuse F19.182
        dependence F19.282
        use F19.982
      sedative, hypnotic, or anxiolytic
        abuse F13.182
        dependence F13.282
        use F13.982
      stimulant NEC
        abuse F15.182
        dependence F15.282
        use F15.982
    free running type G47.24
    in conditions classified elsewhere G47.27
    irregular sleep wake type G47.23
    jet lag type G47.25
    shift work type G47.26
    specified NEC G47.29
  due to
    alcohol
      abuse F10.182
      dependence F10.282
      use F10.982
    amphetamine
      abuse F15.182
      dependence F15.282
      use F15.982
    anxiolytic
      abuse F13.182
      dependence F13.282
      use F13.982
    caffeine
      abuse F15.182
      dependence F15.282
      use F15.982
    cocaine
      abuse F14.182
      dependence F14.282
      use F14.982
    drug NEC
      abuse F19.182
      dependence F19.282
      use F19.982

Disorder (of) (*see also* Disease) — *continued*
sleep G47.9 — *continued*
  due to — *continued*
    hypnotic
      abuse F13.182
      dependence F13.282
      use F13.982
    opioid
      abuse F11.182
      dependence F11.282
      use F11.982
    psychoactive substance NEC
      abuse F19.182
      dependence F19.282
      use F19.982
    sedative
      abuse F13.182
      dependence F13.282
      use F13.982
    stimulant NEC
      abuse F15.182
      dependence F15.282
      use F15.982
  emotional F51.9
  excessive somnolence — *see* Hypersomnia
  hypersomnia type — *see* Hypersomnia
  initiating or maintaining — *see* Insomnia
  nightmares F51.5
  nonorganic F51.9
    specified NEC F51.8
  parasomnia type G47.50
  specified NEC G47.8
  terrors F51.4
  walking F51.3
sleep-wake pattern or schedule — *see*
    Disorder, sleep, circadian rhythm
social
  anxiety of childhood F40.10
  functioning in childhood F94.9
    specified NEC F94.8
  pragmatic F80.82
soft tissue M79.9
  ankle M79.9
  due to use, overuse and pressure M70.90
    ankle M70.97-
    bursitis — *see* Bursitis
    foot M70.97-
    forearm M70.93-
    hand M70.94-
    lower leg M70.96-
    multiple sites M70.99
    pelvic region M70.95-
    shoulder region M70.91-
    specified site NEC M70.98
    specified type NEC M70.80
      ankle M70.87-
      foot M70.87-
      forearm M70.83-
      hand M70.84-
      lower leg M70.86-
      multiple sites M70.89
      pelvic region M70.85-
      shoulder region M70.81-
      specified site NEC M70.88
      thigh M70.85-
      upper arm M70.82-
    thigh M70.95-
    upper arm M70.92-
  foot M79.9
  forearm M79.9
  hand M79.9
  lower leg M79.9
  multiple sites M79.9
  occupational — *see* Disorder, soft tissue, due
    to use, overuse and pressure
  pelvic region M79.9
  shoulder region M79.9
  specified type NEC M79.89
  thigh M79.9

Disorder (of) (see also Disease) — continued
  soft tissue M79.9 — continued
    upper arm M79.9
  somatic symptom F45.1
  somatization F45.0
  somatoform F45.9
    pain (persistent) F45.41
    somatization (multiple) (long-lasting) F45.0
    specified NEC F45.8
    undifferentiated F45.1
  somnolence, excessive — see Hypersomnia
  specific
    arithmetical F81.2
    developmental, of motor F82
    reading F81.0
    speech and language F80.9
    spelling F81.81
    written expression F81.81
  speech R47.9
    articulation (functional) (specific) F80.0
    developmental F80.9
    specified NEC R47.89
  speech-sound F80.0
  spelling (specific) F81.81
  spine — see also Dorsopathy
    ligamentous or muscular attachments,
        peripheral — see Enthesopathy, spinal
    specified NEC — see Dorsopathy, specified
        NEC
  stereotyped, habit or movement F98.4
  stimulant use (other) (unspecified)
    mild F15.10
    moderate or severe F15.20
  stomach (functional) — see Disorder, gastric
  stress F43.9
    acute F43.0
    post-traumatic F43.10
      acute F43.11
      chronic F43.12
  substance use (other) (unknown)
    mild F19.10
      with substance-induced
        anxiety disorder F19.180
        bipolar and related disorder F19.14
        depressive disorder F19.14
        major neurocognitive disorder F19.17
        mild neurocognitive disorder F19.188
        obsessive-compulsive and related
            disorder F19.188
        sexual dysfunction F19.181
        substance intoxication F19.129
        substance intoxication delirium F19.121
    moderate or severe F19.20
      with substance-induced
        anxiety disorder F19.280
        bipolar and related disorder F19.24
        depressive disorder F19.24
        major neurocognitive disorder F19.27
        mild neurocognitive disorder F19.288
        obsessive-compulsive and related
            disorder F19.288
        sexual dysfunction F19.281
        substance intoxication F19.229
        substance intoxication delirium F19.221
  sulfur-bearing amino-acid metabolism E72.10
  sweat gland (eccrine) L74.9
    apocrine L75.9
      specified NEC L75.8
    specified NEC L74.8
  synovium M67.90
    acromioclavicular M67.91-
    ankle M67.97-
    elbow M67.92-
    foot M67.97-
    forearm M67.93-
    hand M67.94-
    hip M67.95-
    knee M67.96-
    multiple sites M67.99

Disorder (of) (see also Disease) — continued
  synovium M67.90 — continued
    rupture — see Rupture, synovium
    shoulder M67.91-
    specified type NEC M67.80
      acromioclavicular M67.81-
      ankle M67.87-
      elbow M67.82-
      foot M67.87-
      hand M67.84-
      hip M67.85-
      knee M67.86-
      multiple sites M67.89
      wrist M67.83-
    synovitis — see Synovitis
    upper arm M67.92-
    wrist M67.93-
  temperature regulation, newborn P81.9
    specified NEC P81.8
  temporomandibular joint M26.60-
  tendon M67.90
    acromioclavicular M67.91-
    ankle M67.97-
    contracture — see Contracture, tendon
    elbow M67.92-
    foot M67.97-
    forearm M67.93-
    hand M67.94-
    hip M67.95-
    knee M67.96-
    multiple sites M67.99
    rupture — see Rupture, tendon
    shoulder M67.91-
    specified type NEC M67.80
      acromioclavicular M67.81-
      ankle M67.87-
      elbow M67.82-
      foot M67.87-
      hand M67.84-
      hip M67.85-
      knee M67.86-
      multiple sites M67.89
      trunk M67.88
      wrist M67.83-
    synovitis — see Synovitis
    tendinitis — see Tendinitis
    tenosynovitis — see Tenosynovitis
    trunk M67.98
    upper arm M67.92-
    wrist M67.93-
  thoracic root (nerve) NEC G54.3
  thyrocalcitonin hypersecretion E07.0
  thyroid (gland) E07.9
    function NEC, neonatal, transitory P72.2
    iodine-deficiency related E01.8
    specified NEC E07.89
  tic — see Tic
  tobacco use
    mild Z72.0
    moderate F17.200
    severe F17.200
  tooth K08.9
    development K00.9
      specified NEC K00.8
    eruption K00.6
  Tourette's F95.2
  trance and possession F44.89
  trauma and stressor-related F43.9
    other specified F43.8
  tricuspid (valve) — see Endocarditis, tricuspid
  tryptophan metabolism E70.5
  tubular, phosphate-losing N25.0
  tubulo-interstitial (in)
    brucellosis A23.9 [N16]
    cystinosis E72.04
    diphtheria A36.84
    glycogen storage disease E74.00 [N16]
    leukemia NEC C95.9- [N16]
    lymphoma NEC C85.9- [N16]

Disorder (of) (see also Disease) — continued
  tubulo-interstitial (in) — continued
    mixed cryoglobulinemia D89.1 [N16]
    multiple myeloma C90.0- [N16]
    Salmonella infection A02.25
    sarcoidosis D86.84
    sepsis A41.9 [N16]
      streptococcal A40.9 [N16]
    systemic lupus erythematosus M32.15
    toxoplasmosis B58.83
    transplant rejection T86.91 [N16]
    Wilson's disease E83.01 [N16]
  tubulo-renal function, impaired N25.9
    specified NEC N25.89
  tympanic membrane H73.9-
    atrophy — see Atrophy, tympanic membrane
    infection — see Myringitis
    perforation — see Perforation, tympanum
    specified NEC H73.89-
  unsocialized aggressive F91.1
  urea cycle metabolism E72.20
    argininemia E72.21
    arginosuccinic aciduria E72.22
    citrullinemia E72.23
    ornithine transcarbamylase deficiency E72.4
    other specified E72.29
  ureter (in) N28.9
    schistosomiasis B65.0 [N29]
    tuberculosis A18.11
  urethra N36.9
    specified NEC N36.8
  urinary system N39.9
    specified NEC N39.8
  valve, heart
    aortic — see Endocarditis, aortic
    mitral — see Endocarditis, mitral
    pulmonary — see Endocarditis, pulmonary
    rheumatic
      aortic — see Endocarditis, aortic,
          rheumatic
      mitral — see Endocarditis, mitral
      pulmonary — see Endocarditis,
          pulmonary, rheumatic
      tricuspid — see Endocarditis, tricuspid
    tricuspid — see Endocarditis, tricuspid
  vestibular function H81.9-
    specified NEC — see subcategory H81.8-
    in diseases classified elsewhere H82-
    vertigo — see Vertigo
  vision, binocular H53.30
    abnormal retinal correspondence H53.31
    diplopia H53.2
    fusion with defective stereopsis H53.32
    simultaneous perception H53.33
    suppression H53.34
  visual
    cortex
      blindness H47.619
        left brain H47.612
        right brain H47.611
      due to
        inflammatory disorder H47.629
          left brain H47.622
          right brain H47.621
        neoplasm H47.639
          left brain H47.632
          right brain H47.631
        vascular disorder H47.649
          left brain H47.642
          right brain H47.641
    pathway H47.9
      due to
        inflammatory disorder H47.51-
        neoplasm H47.52-
        vascular disorder H47.53-
        optic chiasm — see Disorder, optic, chiasm

Disorder (of) (see also Disease) — continued
vitreous body H43.9
  crystalline deposits — see Deposit, crystalline
  degeneration — see Degeneration, vitreous
  hemorrhage — see Hemorrhage, vitreous
  opacities — see Opacity, vitreous
  prolapse — see Prolapse, vitreous
  specified type NEC H43.89
voice R49.9
  specified type NEC R49.8
volatile solvent use
  due to drug abuse — see Abuse, drug, inhalant
  due to drug dependence — see Dependence, drug, inhalant
white blood cells D72.9
  specified NEC D72.89
withdrawing, child or adolescent F40.10

Disorientation R41.0

Displacement, displaced
acquired traumatic of bone, cartilage, joint, tendon NEC — see Dislocation
adrenal gland (congenital) Q89.1
appendix, retrocecal (congenital) Q43.8
auricle (congenital) Q17.4
bladder (acquired) N32.89
  congenital Q64.19
brachial plexus (congenital) Q07.8
brain stem, caudal (congenital) Q04.8
canaliculus (lacrimalis), congenital Q10.6
cardia through esophageal hiatus (congenital) Q40.1
cerebellum, caudal (congenital) Q04.8
cervix — see Malposition, uterus
colon (congenital) Q43.3
device, implant or graft (see also Complications, by site and type, mechanical) T85.628
  arterial graft NEC — see Complication, cardiovascular device, mechanical, vascular
  breast (implant) T85.42
  catheter NEC T85.628
    dialysis (renal) T82.42
      intraperitoneal T85.621
    infusion NEC T82.524
      spinal (epidural) (subdural) T85.620
    urinary
      cystostomy T83.020
      Hopkins T83.028
      ileostomy T83.028
      indwelling T83.021
      nephrostomy T83.022
      specified NEC T83.028
      urostomy T83.028
  electronic (electrode) (pulse generator) (stimulator) — see Complication, electronic stimulator
  fixation, internal (orthopedic) NEC — see Complication, fixation device, mechanical
  gastrointestinal — see Complications, prosthetic device, mechanical, gastrointestinal device
  genital NEC T83.428
    intrauterine contraceptive device (string) T83.32
    penile prosthesis (cylinder) (implanted) (pump) (resevoir) T83.420
    testicular prosthesis T83.421
  heart NEC — see Complication, cardiovascular device, mechanical
  joint prosthesis — see Complications, joint prosthesis, mechanical
  ocular — see Complications, prosthetic device, mechanical, ocular device
  orthopedic NEC — see Complication, orthopedic, device or graft, mechanical
  specified NEC T85.628

Displacement, displaced — continued
device, implant or graft (see also Complications, by site and type, mechanical) T85.628 — continued
  urinary NEC T83.128
    graft T83.22
    sphincter, implanted T83.121
    stent (ileal conduit) (nephroureteral) T83.123
    ureteral indwelling T83.122
  vascular NEC — see Complication, cardiovascular device, mechanical
  ventricular intracranial shunt T85.02
electronic stimulator
  bone T84.320
  cardiac — see Complications, cardiac device, electronic
  nervous system — see Complication, prosthetic device, mechanical, electronic nervous system stimulator
  urinary — see Complications, electronic stimulator, urinary
esophageal mucosa into cardia of stomach, congenital Q39.8
esophagus (acquired) K22.8
  congenital Q39.8
eyeball (acquired) (lateral) (old) — see Displacement, globe
  congenital Q15.8
  current — see Avulsion, eye
fallopian tube (acquired) N83.4-
  congenital Q50.6
  opening (congenital) Q50.6
gallbladder (congenital) Q44.1
gastric mucosa (congenital) Q40.2
globe (acquired) (old) (lateral) H05.21-
  current — see Avulsion, eye
heart (congenital) Q24.8
  acquired I51.89
hymen (upward) (congenital) Q52.4
intervertebral disc NEC
  with myelopathy — see Disorder, disc, with, myelopathy
  cervical, cervicothoracic (with) M50.20
    myelopathy — see Disorder, disc, cervical, with myelopathy
    neuritis, radiculitis or radiculopathy — see Disorder, disc, cervical, with neuritis
  due to trauma — see Dislocation, vertebra
  lumbar region M51.26
    with
      myelopathy M51.06
      neuritis, radiculitis, radiculopathy or sciatica M51.16
  lumbosacral region M51.27
    with
      neuritis, radiculitis, radiculopathy or sciatica M51.17
  sacrococcygeal region M53.3
  thoracic region M51.24
    with
      myelopathy M51.04
      neuritis, radiculitis, radiculopathy M51.14
  thoracolumbar region M51.25
    with
      myelopathy M51.05
      neuritis, radiculitis, radiculopathy M51.15
intrauterine device (string) T83.32
kidney (acquired) N28.83
  congenital Q63.2
lachrymal, lacrimal apparatus or duct (congenital) Q10.6
lens, congenital Q12.1
macula (congenital) Q14.1
Meckel's diverticulum Q43.0
  malignant — see Table of Neoplasms, small intestine, malignant

Displacement, displaced — continued
nail (congenital) Q84.6
  acquired L60.8
opening of Wharton's duct in mouth Q38.4
organ or site, congenital NEC — see Malposition, congenital
ovary (acquired) N83.4-
  congenital Q50.39
  free in peritoneal cavity (congenital) Q50.39
  into hernial sac N83.4-
oviduct (acquired) N83.4-
  congenital Q50.6
parathyroid (gland) E21.4
parotid gland (congenital) Q38.4
punctum lacrimale (congenital) Q10.6
sacro-iliac (joint) (congenital) Q74.2
  current injury S33.2
  old — see subcategory M53.2
salivary gland (any) (congenital) Q38.4
spleen (congenital) Q89.09
stomach, congenital Q40.2
sublingual duct Q38.4
tongue (downward) (congenital) Q38.3
tooth, teeth, fully erupted M26.30
  horizontal M26.33
  vertical M26.34
trachea (congenital) Q32.1
ureter or ureteric opening or orifice (congenital) Q62.62
uterine opening of oviducts or fallopian tubes Q50.6
uterus, uterine — see Malposition, uterus
ventricular septum Q21.0
  with rudimentary ventricle Q20.4

Disproportion
between native and reconstructed breast N65.1
fiber-type G71.2

Disruptio uteri — see Rupture, uterus

Disruption (of)
ciliary body NEC H21.89
closure of
  cornea T81.31
  craniotomy T81.32
  fascia (muscular) (superficial) T81.32
  internal organ or tissue T81.32
  laceration (external) (internal) T81.33
  ligament T81.32
  mucosa T81.31
  muscle or muscle flap T81.32
  ribs or rib cage T81.32
  skin and subcutaneous tissue (full-thickness) (superficial) T81.31
  skull T81.32
  sternum (sternotomy) T81.32
  tendon T81.32
  traumatic laceration (external) (internal) T81.33
family Z63.8
  due to
    absence of family member due to military deployment Z63.31
    absence of family member NEC Z63.32
    alcoholism and drug addiction in family Z63.72
    bereavement Z63.4
    death (assumed) or disappearance of family member Z63.4
    divorce or separation Z63.5
    drug addiction in family Z63.72
    return of family member from military deployment (current or past conflict) Z63.71
    stressful life events NEC Z63.79
iris NEC H21.89

Disruption (of) — *continued*
  ligament(s) — *see also* Sprain
    knee
      current injury — *see* Dislocation, knee
      old (chronic) — *see* Derangement, knee,
        ligament, instability, chronic
      spontaneous NEC — *see* Derangement,
        knee, disruption ligament
    ossicular chain — *see* Discontinuity, ossicles,
      ear
  pelvic ring (stable) S32.810
    unstable S32.811
  traumatic injury wound repair T81.33
  wound T81.30
    episiotomy O90.1
    operation T81.31
      cesarean O90.0
      external operation wound (superficial)
        T81.31
      internal operation wound (deep) T81.32
    perineal (obstetric) O90.1
    traumatic injury repair T81.33

Dissatisfaction with
  employment Z56.9
  school environment Z55.4

Dissecting — *see* condition

Dissection
  aorta I71.00
    abdominal I71.02
    thoracic I71.01
    thoracoabdominal I71.03
  artery I77.70
    basilar (trunk) I77.75
    carotid I77.71
    cerebral (nonruptured) I67.0
      ruptured — *see* Hemorrhage, intracranial,
        subarachnoid
    coronary I25.42
    extremity
      lower I77.77
      upper I77.76
    iliac I77.72
    precerebral
      congenital (nonruptured) Q28.1
      specified site NEC I77.75
    renal I77.73
    specified NEC I77.79
    vertebral I77.74
  traumatic — *see* Wound, open, by site
  vascular I99.8
  wound — *see* Wound, open

Disseminated — *see* condition

Dissociation
  auriculoventricular or atrioventricular (AV)
    (any degree) (isorhythmic) I45.89
    with heart block I44.2
  interference I45.89

Dissociative reaction, state F44.9

Dissolution, vertebra — *see* Osteoporosis

Distension, distention
  abdomen R14.0
  bladder N32.89
  cecum K63.89
  colon K63.89
  gallbladder K82.8
  intestine K63.89
  kidney N28.89
  liver K76.89
  seminal vesicle N50.89
  stomach K31.89
    acute K31.0
    psychogenic F45.8
  ureter — *see* Dilatation, ureter
  uterus N85.8

Disto-occlusion (Division I) (Division II)
  M26.212

Distoma hepaticum infestation B66.3

Distomiasis B66.9
  bile passages B66.3
  hemic B65.9
  hepatic B66.3
    due to Clonorchis sinensis B66.1
  intestinal B66.5
  liver B66.3
    due to Clonorchis sinensis B66.1
  lung B66.4
  pulmonary B66.4

Distomolar (fourth molar) K00.1

Distortion(s) (congenital)
  adrenal (gland) Q89.1
  arm NEC Q68.8
  bile duct or passage Q44.5
  bladder Q64.79
  brain Q04.9
  cervix (uteri) Q51.9
  chest (wall) Q67.8
    bones Q76.8
  clavicle Q74.0
  clitoris Q52.6
  coccyx Q76.49
  common duct Q44.5
  coronary Q24.5
  cystic duct Q44.5
  ear (auricle) (external) Q17.3
    inner Q16.5
    middle Q16.4
      ossicles Q16.3
  endocrine NEC Q89.2
  eustachian tube Q17.8
  eye (adnexa) Q15.8
  face bone(s) NEC Q75.8
  fallopian tube Q50.6
  femur NEC Q68.8
  fibula NEC Q68.8
  finger(s) Q68.1
  foot Q66.9
  genitalia, genital organ(s)
    female Q52.8
      external Q52.79
      internal NEC Q52.8
  gyri Q04.8
  hand bone(s) Q68.1
  heart (auricle) (ventricle) Q24.8
    valve (cusp) Q24.8
  hepatic duct Q44.5
  humerus NEC Q68.8
  hymen Q52.4
  intrafamilial communications Z63.8
  jaw NEC M26.89
  labium (majus) (minus) Q52.79
  leg NEC Q68.8
  lens Q12.8
  liver Q44.7
  lumbar spine Q76.49
    with disproportion O33.8
      causing obstructed labor O65.0
  lumbosacral (joint) (region) Q76.49
    kyphosis — *see* Kyphosis, congenital
    lordosis — *see* Lordosis, congenital
  nerve Q07.8
  nose Q30.8
  organ
    of Corti Q16.5
    or site not listed — *see* Anomaly, by site
  ossicles, ear Q16.3
  oviduct Q50.6
  pancreas Q45.3
  parathyroid (gland) Q89.2
  pituitary (gland) Q89.2
  radius NEC Q68.8
  sacroiliac joint Q74.2
  sacrum Q76.49
  scapula Q74.0
  shoulder girdle Q74.0

Distortion(s) (congenital) — *continued*
  skull bone(s) NEC Q75.8
    with
      anencephalus Q00.0
      encephalocele — *see* Encephalocele
      hydrocephalus Q03.9
        with spina bifida — *see* Spina bifida,
          with hydrocephalus
      microcephaly Q02
  spinal cord Q06.8
  spine Q76.49
    kyphosis — *see* Kyphosis, congenital
    lordosis — *see* Lordosis, congenital
  spleen Q89.09
  sternum NEC Q76.7
  thorax (wall) Q67.8
    bony Q76.8
  thymus (gland) Q89.2
  thyroid (gland) Q89.2
  tibia NEC Q68.8
  toe(s) Q66.9
  tongue Q38.3
  trachea (cartilage) Q32.1
  ulna NEC Q68.8
  ureter Q62.8
  urethra Q64.79
    causing obstruction Q64.39
  uterus Q51.9
  vagina Q52.4
  vertebra Q76.49
    kyphosis — *see* Kyphosis, congenital
    lordosis — *see* Lordosis, congenital
  visual — *see also* Disturbance, vision
    shape and size H53.15
  vulva Q52.79
  wrist (bones) (joint) Q68.8

Distress
  abdomen — *see* Pain, abdominal
  acute respiratory R06.00
    syndrome (adult) (child) J80
  epigastric R10.13
  fetal P84
    complicating pregnancy — *see* Stress, fetal
  gastrointestinal (functional) K30
    psychogenic F45.8
  intestinal (functional) NOS K59.9
    psychogenic F45.8
  maternal, during labor and delivery O75.0
  respiratory (adult) (child) R06.00
    newborn P22.9
      specified NEC P22.8
    orthopnea R06.01
    psychogenic F45.8
    shortness of breath R06.02
    specified type NEC R06.09

Distribution vessel, atypical Q27.9
  coronary artery Q24.5
  precerebral Q28.1

Districhiasis L68.8

Disturbance(s) — *see also* Disease
  absorption K90.9
    calcium E58
    carbohydrate K90.49
    fat K90.49
      pancreatic K90.3
    protein K90.49
    starch K90.49
    vitamin — *see* Deficiency, vitamin
  acid-base equilibrium E87.8
    mixed E87.4
  activity and attention (with hyperkinesis) — *see*
    Disorder, attention-deficit hyperactivity
  amino acid transport E72.00
  assimilation, food K90.9
  auditory nerve, except deafness — *see*
    subcategory H93.3
  behavior — *see* Disorder, conduct
  blood clotting (mechanism) (*see also* Defect,
    coagulation) D68.9

Disturbance(s) (*see also* Disease) — *continued*
cerebral
  nerve — *see* Disorder, nerve, cranial
  status, newborn P91.9
    specified NEC P91.8
circulatory I99.9
conduct (*see also* Disorder, conduct) F91.9
  adjustment reaction — *see* Disorder,
    adjustment
  compulsive F63.9
  disruptive F91.9
  hyperkinetic — *see* Disorder, attention-deficit
    hyperactivity
  socialized F91.2
  specified NEC F91.8
  unsocialized F91.1
coordination R27.8
cranial nerve — *see* Disorder, nerve, cranial
deep sensibility — *see* Disturbance, sensation
digestive K30
  psychogenic F45.8
electrolyte — *see also* Imbalance, electrolyte
  newborn, transitory P74.4
    hyperammonemia P74.6
    potassium balance P74.3
    sodium balance P74.2
    specified type NEC P74.4
emotions specific to childhood and
  adolescence F93.9
  with
    anxiety and fearfulness NEC F93.8
    elective mutism F94.0
    oppositional disorder F91.3
    sensitivity (withdrawal) F40.10
    shyness F40.10
    social withdrawal F40.10
  involving relationship problems F93.8
  mixed F93.8
  specified NEC F93.8
endocrine (gland) E34.9
  neonatal, transitory P72.9
    specified NEC P72.8
equilibrium R42
fructose metabolism E74.10
gait — *see* Gait
  hysterical F44.4
  psychogenic F44.4
gastrointestinal (functional) K30
  psychogenic F45.8
habit, child F98.9
hearing, except deafness and tinnitus — *see*
  Abnormal, auditory perception
heart, functional (conditions in I44-I50)
  due to presence of (cardiac) prosthesis
    I97.19-
  postoperative I97.89
    cardiac surgery I97.19-
hormones E34.9
innervation uterus (parasympathetic)
  (sympathetic) N85.8
keratinization NEC
  gingiva K05.10
    nonplaque induced K05.11
    plaque induced K05.10
  lip K13.0
  oral (mucosa) (soft tissue) K13.29
  tongue K13.29
learning (specific) — *see* Disorder, learning
memory — *see* Amnesia
  mild, following organic brain damage F06.8
mental F99
  associated with diseases classified elsewhere
    F54
metabolism E88.9
  with
    abortion — *see* Abortion, by type with
      other specified complication
    ectopic pregnancy O08.5
    molar pregnancy O08.5

Disturbance(s) (*see also* Disease) — *continued*
metabolism E88.9 — *continued*
  amino-acid E72.9
    aromatic E70.9
    branched-chain E71.2
    straight-chain E72.8
    sulfur-bearing E72.10
  ammonia E72.20
  arginine E72.21
  arginosuccinic acid E72.22
  carbohydrate E74.9
  cholesterol E78.9
  citrulline E72.23
  cystathionine E72.19
  general E88.9
  glutamine E72.8
  histidine E70.40
  homocystine E72.19
  hydroxylysine E72.3
  in labor or delivery O75.89
  iron E83.10
  lipoid E78.9
  lysine E72.3
  methionine E72.19
  neonatal, transitory P74.9
    calcium and magnesium P71.9
      specified type NEC P71.8
    carbohydrate metabolism P70.9
      specified type NEC P70.8
    specified NEC P74.8
  ornithine E72.4
  phosphate E83.39
  sodium NEC E87.8
  threonine E72.8
  tryptophan E70.5
  tyrosine E70.20
  urea cycle E72.20
motor R29.2
nervous, functional R45.0
neuromuscular mechanism (eye), due to
  syphilis A52.15
nutritional E63.9
  nail L60.3
ocular motion H51.9
  psychogenic F45.8
oculogyric H51.8
  psychogenic F45.8
oculomotor H51.9
  psychogenic F45.8
olfactory nerve R43.1
optic nerve NEC — *see* Disorder, nerve, optic
oral epithelium, including tongue NEC K13.29
perceptual due to
  alcohol withdrawal F10.232
  amphetamine intoxication F15.922
    in
      abuse F15.122
      dependence F15.222
  anxiolytic withdrawal F13.232
  cannabis intoxication (acute) F12.922
    in
      abuse F12.122
      dependence F12.222
  cocaine intoxication (acute) F14.922
    in
      abuse F14.122
      dependence F14.222
  hypnotic withdrawal F13.232
  opioid intoxication (acute) F11.922
    in
      abuse F11.122
      dependence F11.222
  phencyclidine intoxication (acute) F16.122
  sedative withdrawal F13.232
personality (pattern) (trait) (*see also* Disorder,
  personality) F60.9
  following organic brain damage F07.9
polyglandular E31.9
  specified NEC E31.8

Disturbance(s) (*see also* Disease) — *continued*
potassium balance, newborn P74.3
psychogenic F45.9
psychomotor F44.4
psychophysical visual H53.16
pupillary — *see* Anomaly, pupil, function
reflex R29.2
rhythm, heart I49.9
salivary secretion K11.7
sensation (cold) (heat) (localization) (tactile
  discrimination) (texture) (vibratory) NEC
  R20.9
  hysterical F44.6
  skin R20.9
    anesthesia R20.0
    hyperesthesia R20.3
    hypoesthesia R20.1
    paresthesia R20.2
    specified type NEC R20.8
  smell R43.9
    and taste (mixed) R43.8
    anosmia R43.0
    parosmia R43.1
    specified NEC R43.8
  taste R43.9
    and smell (mixed) R43.8
    parageusia R43.2
    specified NEC R43.8
sensory — *see* Disturbance, sensation
situational (transient) — *see also* Disorder,
  adjustment
  acute F43.0
sleep G47.9
  nonorganic origin F51.9
smell — *see* Disturbance, sensation, smell
sociopathic F60.2
sodium balance, newborn P74.2
speech R47.9
  developmental F80.9
  specified NEC R47.89
stomach (functional) K31.9
sympathetic (nerve) G90.9
taste — *see* Disturbance, sensation, taste
temperature
  regulation, newborn P81.9
    specified NEC P81.8
  sense R20.8
    hysterical F44.6
tooth
  eruption K00.6
  formation K00.4
  structure, hereditary NEC K00.5
touch — *see* Disturbance, sensation
vascular I99.9
  arteriosclerotic — *see* Arteriosclerosis
vasomotor I73.9
vasospastic I73.9
vision, visual H53.9
  following
    cerebral infarction I69.398
    cerebrovascular disease I69.998
    intracerebral hemorrhage I69.198
    nontraumatic intracranial hemorrhage
      NEC I69.298
    specified disease NEC I69.898
    specified NEC I69.898
    subarachnoid hemorrhage I69.098
  psychophysical H53.16
  specified NEC H53.8
  subjective H53.10
    day blindness H53.11
    discomfort H53.14-
    distortions of shape and size H53.15
    loss
      sudden H53.13-
      transient H53.12-
    specified type NEC H53.19

Disturbance(s) (*see also* Disease) — *continued*
  voice R49.9
    psychogenic F44.4
    specified NEC R49.8
Diuresis R35.8
Diver's palsy, paralysis or squeeze T70.3
Diverticulitis (acute) K57.92
  bladder — *see* Cystitis
  ileum — *see* Diverticulitis, intestine, small
  intestine K57.92
    with
      abscess, perforation or peritonitis K57.80
        with bleeding K57.81
      bleeding K57.93
    congenital Q43.8
    large K57.32
      with
        abscess, perforation or peritonitis
          K57.20
          with bleeding K57.21
        bleeding K57.33
        small intestine K57.52
          with
            abscess, perforation or peritonitis
              K57.40
              with bleeding K57.41
            bleeding K57.53
    small K57.12
      with
        abscess, perforation or peritonitis
          K57.00
          with bleeding K57.01
        bleeding K57.13
        large intestine K57.52
          with
            abscess, perforation or peritonitis
              K57.40
              with bleeding K57.41
            bleeding K57.53
Diverticulosis K57.90
  with bleeding K57.91
  large intestine K57.30
    with
      bleeding K57.31
      small intestine K57.50
        with bleeding K57.51
  small intestine K57.10
    with
      bleeding K57.11
      large intestine K57.50
        with bleeding K57.51
Diverticulum, diverticula (multiple) K57.90
  appendix (noninflammatory) K38.2
  bladder (sphincter) N32.3
    congenital Q64.6
  bronchus (congenital) Q32.4
    acquired J98.09
  calyx, calyceal (kidney) N28.89
  cardia (stomach) K31.4
  cecum — *see* Diverticulosis, intestine, large
    congenital Q43.8
  colon — *see* Diverticulosis, intestine, large
    congenital Q43.8
  duodenum — *see* Diverticulosis, intestine, small
    congenital Q43.8
  epiphrenic (esophagus) K22.5
  esophagus (congenital) Q39.6
    acquired (epiphrenic) (pulsion) (traction)
      K22.5
  eustachian tube — *see* Disorder, eustachian
    tube, specified NEC
  fallopian tube N83.8
  gastric K31.4
  heart (congenital) Q24.8
  ileum — *see* Diverticulosis, intestine, small
  jejunum — *see* Diverticulosis, intestine, small
  kidney (pelvis) (calyces) N28.89
    with calculus — *see* Calculus, kidney

Diverticulum, diverticula (multiple) K57.90
  — *continued*
  Meckel's (displaced) (hypertrophic) Q43.0
    malignant — *see* Table of Neoplasms, small
      intestine, malignant
  midthoracic K22.5
  organ or site, congenital NEC — *see* Distortion
  pericardium (congenital) (cyst) Q24.8
    acquired I31.8
  pharyngoesophageal (congenital) Q39.6
    acquired K22.5
  pharynx (congenital) Q38.7
  rectosigmoid — *see* Diverticulosis, intestine,
    large
    congenital Q43.8
  rectum — *see* Diverticulosis, intestine, large
  Rokitansky's K22.5
  seminal vesicle N50.89
  sigmoid — *see* Diverticulosis, intestine, large
    congenital Q43.8
  stomach (acquired) K31.4
    congenital Q40.2
  trachea (acquired) J39.8
  ureter (acquired) N28.89
    congenital Q62.8
  ureterovesical orifice N28.89
  urethra (acquired) N36.1
    congenital Q64.79
  ventricle, left (congenital) Q24.8
  vesical N32.3
    congenital Q64.6
  Zenker's (esophagus) K22.5
Division
  cervix uteri (acquired) N88.8
  glans penis Q55.69
  labia minora (congenital) Q52.79
  ligament (partial or complete) (current) — *see*
    also Sprain
    with open wound — *see* Wound, open
  muscle (partial or complete) (current) — *see*
    also Injury, muscle
    with open wound — *see* Wound, open
  nerve (traumatic) — *see* Injury, nerve
  spinal cord — *see* Injury, spinal cord, by
    region
  vein I87.8
Divorce, causing family disruption Z63.5
Dix-Hallpike neurolabyrinthitis — *see*
  Neuronitis, vestibular
Dizziness R42
  hysterical F44.89
  psychogenic F45.8
DMAC (disseminated mycobacterium
  aviumintracellulare complex) A31.2
DNR (do not resuscitate) Z66
Doan-Wiseman syndrome (primary splenic
  neutropenia) — *see* Agranulocytosis
Doehle-Heller aortitis A52.02
Dog bite — *see* Bite
Dohle body panmyelopathic syndrome
  D72.0
Dolichocephaly Q67.2
Dolichocolon Q43.8
Dolichostenomelia — *see* Syndrome,
  Marfan's
Donohue's syndrome E34.8
Donor (organ or tissue) Z52.9
  blood (whole) Z52.000
    autologous Z52.010
    specified component (lymphocytes) (platelets)
      NEC Z52.008
      autologous Z52.018
      specified donor NEC Z52.098
    specified donor NEC Z52.090
  stem cells Z52.001
    autologous Z52.011
    specified donor NEC Z52.091

Donor (organ or tissue) Z52.9 — *continued*
  bone Z52.20
    autologous Z52.21
    marrow Z52.3
    specified type NEC Z52.29
  cornea Z52.5
  egg (Oocyte) Z52.819
    age 35 and over Z52.812
      anonymous recipient Z52.812
      designated recipient Z52.813
    under age 35 Z52.810
      anonymous recipient Z52.810
      designated recipient Z52.811
  kidney Z52.4
  liver Z52.6
  lung Z52.89
  lymphocyte — *see* Donor, blood, specified
    components NEC
  Oocyte — *see* Donor, egg
  platelets Z52.008
  potential, examination of Z00.5
  semen Z52.89
  skin Z52.10
    autologous Z52.11
    specified type NEC Z52.19
  specified organ or tissue NEC Z52.89
  sperm Z52.89
Donovanosis A58
Dorsalgia M54.9
  psychogenic F45.41
  specified NEC M54.89
Dorsopathy M53.9
  deforming M43.9
    specified NEC — *see* subcategory M43.8
  specified NEC M53.80
    cervical region M53.82
    cervicothoracic region M53.83
    lumbar region M53.86
    lumbosacral region M53.87
    occipito-atlanto-axial region M53.81
    sacrococcygeal region M53.88
    thoracic region M53.84
    thoracolumbar region M53.85
Double
  albumin E88.09
  aortic arch Q25.45
  auditory canal Q17.8
  auricle (heart) Q20.8
  bladder Q64.79
  cervix Q51.820
    with doubling of uterus (and vagina)
      Q51.10
      with obstruction Q51.11
  inlet ventricle Q20.4
  kidney with double pelvis (renal) Q63.0
  meatus urinarius Q64.75
  monster Q89.4
  outlet
    left ventricle Q20.2
    right ventricle Q20.1
  pelvis (renal) with double ureter Q62.5
  tongue Q38.3
  ureter (one or both sides) Q62.5
    with double pelvis (renal) Q62.5
  urethra Q64.74
  urinary meatus Q64.75
  uterus Q51.2
    with
      doubling of cervix (and vagina) Q51.10
        with obstruction Q51.11
      in pregnancy or childbirth O34.59-
        causing obstructed labor O65.5
  vagina Q52.10
    with doubling of uterus (and cervix) Q51.10
      with obstruction Q51.11
  vision H53.2
  vulva Q52.79
Douglas' pouch, cul-de-sac — *see* condition

Down syndrome Q90.9
  meiotic nondisjunction Q90.0
  mitotic nondisjunction Q90.1
  mosaicism Q90.1
  translocation Q90.2
DPD (dihydropyrimidine dehydrogenase deficiency) E88.89
Dracontiasis B72
Dracunculiasis, dracunculosis B72
Dream state, hysterical F44.89
Drepanocytic anemia — *see* Disease, sickle-cell
Dresbach's syndrome (elliptocytosis) D58.1
Dreschlera (hawaiiensis) (infection) B43.8
Dressler's syndrome I24.1
Drift, ulnar — *see* Deformity, limb, specified type NEC, forearm
Drinking (alcohol)
  excessive, to excess NEC (without dependence) F10.10
    habitual (continual) (without remission) F10.20
      with remission F10.21
Drip, postnasal (chronic) R09.82
  due to
    allergic rhinitis — *see* Rhinitis, allergic
    common cold J00
    gastroesophageal reflux — *see* Reflux, gastroesophageal
    nasopharyngitis — *see* Nasopharyngitis
    other know condition — *code to* condition
    sinusitis — *see* Sinusitis
Droop
  facial R29.810
    cerebrovascular disease I69.992
      cerebral infarction I69.392
      intracerebral hemorrhage I69.192
      nontraumatic intracranial hemorrhage NEC I69.292
      specified disease NEC I69.892
      subarachnoid hemorrhage I69.092
Drop (in)
  attack NEC R55
  finger — *see* Deformity, finger
  foot — *see* Deformity, limb, foot, drop
  hematocrit (precipitous) R71.0
  hemoglobin R71.0
  toe — *see* Deformity, toe, specified NEC
  wrist — *see* Deformity, limb, wrist drop
Dropped heart beats I45.9
Dropsy, dropsical — *see also* Hydrops
  abdomen R18.8
  brain — *see* Hydrocephalus
  cardiac, heart — *see* Failure, heart, congestive
  gangrenous — *see* Gangrene
  heart — *see* Failure, heart, congestive
  kidney — *see* Nephrosis
  lung — *see* Edema, lung
  newborn due to isoimmunization P56.0
  pericardium — *see* Pericarditis
Drowned, drowning (near) T75.1
Drowsiness R40.0
Drug
  abuse counseling and surveillance Z71.51
  addiction — *see* Dependence
  dependence — *see* Dependence
  habit — *see* Dependence
  harmful use — *see* Abuse, drug
  induced fever R50.2
  overdose — *see* Table of Drugs and Chemicals, by drug, poisoning
  poisoning — *see* Table of Drugs and Chemicals, by drug, poisoning
  resistant organism infection (*see also* Resistant, organism, to, drug) Z16.30

Drug — *continued*
  therapy
    long term (current) (prophylactic) — *see* Therapy, drug long-term (current) (prophylactic)
    short term — *omit code*
  wrong substance given or taken in error — *see* Table of Drugs and Chemicals, by drug, poisoning
Drunkenness (without dependence) F10.129
  acute in alcoholism F10.229
  chronic (without remission) F10.20
    with remission F10.21
  pathological (without dependence) F10.129
    with dependence F10.229
  sleep F51.9
Drusen
  macula (degenerative) (retina) — *see* Degeneration, macula, drusen
  optic disc H47.32-
Dry, dryness — *see also* condition
  larynx J38.7
  mouth R68.2
    due to dehydration E86.0
  nose J34.89
  socket (teeth) M27.3
  throat J39.2
DSAP L56.5
Duane's syndrome H50.81-
Dubin-Johnson disease or syndrome E80.6
Dubois' disease (thymus gland) A50.59 *[E35]*
Dubowitz' syndrome Q87.1
Duchenne-Aran muscular atrophy G12.21
Duchenne-Griesinger disease G71.0
Duchenne's
  disease or syndrome
    motor neuron disease G12.22
    muscular dystrophy G71.0
  locomotor ataxia (syphilitic) A52.11
  paralysis
    birth injury P14.0
    due to or associated with
      motor neuron disease G12.22
      muscular dystrophy G71.0
Ducrey's chancre A57
Duct, ductus — *see* condition
Duhring's disease (dermatitis herpetiformis) L13.0
Dullness, cardiac (decreased) (increased) R01.2
Dumb ague — *see* Malaria
Dumbness — *see* Aphasia
Dumdum fever B55.0
Dumping syndrome (postgastrectomy) K91.1
Duodenitis (nonspecific) (peptic) K29.80
  with bleeding K29.81
Duodenocholangitis — *see* Cholangitis
Duodenum, duodenal — *see* condition
Duplay's bursitis or periarthritis — *see* Tendinitis, calcific, shoulder
Duplication, duplex — *see also* Accessory
  alimentary tract Q45.8
  anus Q43.4
  appendix (and cecum) Q43.4
  biliary duct (any) Q44.5
  bladder Q64.79
  cecum (and appendix) Q43.4
  cervix Q51.820
  chromosome NEC
    with complex rearrangements NEC Q92.5
    seen only at prometaphase Q92.8
  cystic duct Q44.5
  digestive organs Q45.8
  esophagus Q39.8
  frontonasal process Q75.8
  intestine (large) (small) Q43.4
  kidney Q63.0

Duplication, duplex — *see also* Accessory — *continued*
  liver Q44.7
  pancreas Q45.3
  penis Q55.69
  respiratory organs NEC Q34.8
  salivary duct Q38.4
  spinal cord (incomplete) Q06.2
  stomach Q40.2
Dupré's disease (meningism) R29.1
Dupuytren's contraction or disease M72.0
Durand-Nicolas-Favre disease A55
Durotomy (inadvertent) (incidental) G97.41
Duroziez's disease (congenital mitral stenosis) Q23.2
Dutton's relapsing fever (West African) A68.1
Dwarfism E34.3
  achondroplastic Q77.4
  congenital E34.3
  constitutional E34.3
  hypochondroplastic Q77.4
  hypophyseal E23.0
  infantile E34.3
  Laron-type E34.3
  Lorain(-Levi) type E23.0
  metatropic Q77.8
  nephrotic-glycosuric (with hypophosphatemic rickets) E72.09
  nutritional E45
  pancreatic K86.89
  pituitary E23.0
  renal N25.0
  thanatophoric Q77.1
Dyke-Young anemia (secondary) (symptomatic) D59.1
Dysacusis — *see* Abnormal, auditory perception
Dysadrenocortism E27.9
  hyperfunction E27.0
Dysarthria R47.1
  following
    cerebral infarction I69.322
    cerebrovascular disease I69.922
      specified disease NEC I69.822
    intracerebral hemorrhage I69.122
    nontraumatic intracranial hemorrhage NEC I69.222
    subarachnoid hemorrhage I69.022
Dysautonomia (familial) G90.1
Dysbarism T70.3
Dysbasia R26.2
  angiosclerotica intermittens I73.9
  hysterical F44.4
  lordotica (progressiva) G24.1
  nonorganic origin F44.4
  psychogenic F44.4
Dysbetalipoproteinemia (familial) E78.2
Dyscalculia R48.8
  developmental F81.2
Dyschezia K59.00
Dyschondroplasia (with hemangiomata) Q78.4
Dyschromia (skin) L81.9
Dyscollagenosis M35.9
Dyscranio-pygo-phalangy Q87.0
Dyscrasia
  blood (with) D75.9
    antepartum hemorrhage — *see* Hemorrhage, antepartum, with coagulation defect
    intrapartum hemorrhage O67.0
    newborn P61.9
      specified type NEC P61.8
    puerperal, postpartum O72.3
  polyglandular, pluriglandular E31.9
Dysendocrinism E34.9

Dysentery, dysenteric (catarrhal) (diarrhea) (epidemic) (hemorrhagic) (infectious) (sporadic) (tropical) A09
  abscess, liver A06.4
  amebic (see also Amebiasis) A06.0
    with abscess — see Abscess, amebic
    acute A06.0
    chronic A06.1
  arthritis (see also category M01) A09
    bacillary (see also category M01) A03.9
  bacillary A03.9
    arthritis (see also category M01) A03.9
    Boyd A03.2
    Flexner A03.1
    Schmitz(-Stutzer) A03.0
    Shiga(-Kruse) A03.0
    Shigella A03.9
      boydii A03.2
      dysenteriae A03.0
      flexneri A03.1
      group A A03.0
      group B A03.1
      group C A03.2
      group D A03.3
      sonnei A03.3
      specified type NEC A03.8
    Sonne A03.3
    specified type NEC A03.8
  balantidial A07.0
  Balantidium coli A07.0
  Boyd's A03.2
  candidal B37.82
  Chilomastix A07.8
  Chinese A03.9
  coccidial A07.3
  Dientamoeba (fragilis) A07.8
  Embadomonas A07.8
  Entamoeba, entamebic — see Dysentery, amebic
  Flexner's A03.1
  Flexner-Boyd A03.2
  Giardia lamblia A07.1
  Hiss-Russell A03.1
  Lamblia A07.1
  leishmanial B55.0
  malarial — see Malaria
  metazoal B82.0
  monilial B37.82
  protozoal A07.9
  Salmonella A02.0
  schistosomal B65.1
  Schmitz(-Stutzer) A03.0
  Shiga(-Kruse) A03.0
  Shigella NOS — see Dysentery, bacillary
  Sonne A03.3
  strongyloidiasis B78.0
  trichomonal A07.8
  viral (see also Enteritis, viral) A08.4
Dysequilibrium R42
Dysesthesia R20.8
  hysterical F44.6
Dysfibrinogenemia (congenital) D68.2
Dysfunction
  adrenal E27.9
    hyperfunction E27.0
  autonomic
    due to alcohol G31.2
    somatoform F45.8
  bladder N31.9
    neurogenic NOS — see Dysfunction, bladder, neuromuscular
    neuromuscular NOS N31.9
      atonic (motor) (sensory) N31.2
      autonomous N31.2
      flaccid N31.2
      nonreflex N31.2
      reflex N31.1
      specified NEC N31.8
      uninhibited N31.0

Dysfunction — continued
  bleeding, uterus N93.8
  cerebral G93.89
  colon K59.9
    psychogenic F45.8
  colostomy K94.03
  cystic duct K82.8
  cystostomy (stoma) — see Complications, cystostomy
  ejaculatory N53.19
    anejaculatory orgasm N53.13
    painful N53.12
    premature F52.4
    retarded N53.11
  endocrine NOS E34.9
  endometrium N85.8
  enterostomy K94.13
  erectile — see Dysfunction, sexual, male, erectile
  gallbladder K82.8
  gastrostomy (stoma) K94.23
  gland, glandular NOS E34.9
  heart I51.89
  hemoglobin D75.89
  hepatic K76.89
  hypophysis E23.7
  hypothalamic NEC E23.3
  ileostomy (stoma) K94.13
  jejunostomy (stoma) K94.13
  kidney — see Disease, renal
  labyrinthine — see subcategory H83.2
  left ventricular, following sudden emotional stress I51.81
  liver K76.89
  male — see Dysfunction, sexual, male
  orgasmic (female) F52.31
    male F52.32
  ovary E28.9
    specified NEC E28.8
  papillary muscle I51.89
  parathyroid E21.4
  physiological NEC R68.89
    psychogenic F59
  pineal gland E34.8
  pituitary (gland) E23.3
  platelets D69.1
  polyglandular E31.9
    specified NEC E31.8
  psychophysiologic F59
  psychosexual F52.9
    with
      dyspareunia F52.6
      premature ejaculation F52.4
      vaginismus F52.5
  pylorus K31.9
  rectum K59.9
    psychogenic F45.8
  reflex (sympathetic) — see Syndrome, pain, complex regional I
  segmental — see Dysfunction, somatic
  senile R54
  sexual (due to) R37
    alcohol F10.981
    amphetamine F15.981
      in
        abuse F15.181
        dependence F15.281
    anxiolytic F13.981
      in
        abuse F13.181
        dependence F13.281
    cocaine F14.981
      in
        abuse F14.181
        dependence F14.281
    excessive sexual drive F52.8
    failure of genital response (male) F52.21
      female F52.22

Dysfunction — continued
  sexual (due to) R37 — continued
    female N94.9
      aversion F52.1
      dyspareunia N94.10
        psychogenic F52.6
      frigidity F52.22
      nymphomania F52.8
      orgasmic F52.31
      psychogenic F52.9
        aversion F52.1
        dyspareunia F52.6
        frigidity F52.22
        nymphomania F52.8
        orgasmic F52.31
        vaginismus F52.5
      vaginismus N94.2
        psychogenic F52.5
    hypnotic F13.981
      in
        abuse F13.181
        dependence F13.281
    inhibited orgasm (female) F52.31
      male F52.32
    lack
      of sexual enjoyment F52.1
      or loss of sexual desire F52.0
    male N53.9
      anejaculatory orgasm N53.13
      ejaculatory N53.19
        painful N53.12
        premature F52.4
        retarded N53.11
      erectile N52.9
        drug induced N52.2
        due to
          disease classified elsewhere N52.1
          drug N52.2
        postoperative (postprocedural) N52.39
          following
            cryotherapy N52.37
            interstitial seed therapy N52.36
            prostate ablative therapy N52.37
            prostatectomy N52.34
              radical N52.31
            radiation therapy N52.35
            radical cystectomy N52.32
            ultrasound ablative therapy N52.37
            urethral surgery N52.33
        psychogenic F52.21
        specified cause NEC N52.8
        vasculogenic
          arterial insufficiency N52.01
            with corporo-venous occlusive N52.03
          corporo-venous occlusive N52.02
            with arterial insufficiency N52.03
      impotence — see Dysfunction, sexual, male, erectile
      psychogenic F52.9
        aversion F52.1
        erectile F52.21
        orgasmic F52.32
        premature ejaculation F52.4
        satyriasis F52.8
        specified type NEC F52.8
      specified type NEC N53.8
    nonorganic F52.9
      specified NEC F52.8
    opioid F11.981
      in
        abuse F11.181
        dependence F11.281
    orgasmic dysfunction (female) F52.31
      male F52.32
    premature ejaculation F52.4

Dysfunction — *continued*
  sexual (due to) R37 — *continued*
    psychoactive substances NEC F19.981
      in
        abuse F19.181
        dependence F19.281
    psychogenic F52.9
    sedative F13.981
      in
        abuse F13.181
        dependence F13.281
    sexual aversion F52.1
    vaginismus (nonorganic) (psychogenic)
      F52.5
  sinoatrial node I49.5
  somatic M99.09
    abdomen M99.09
    acromioclavicular M99.07
    cervical region M99.01
    cervicothoracic M99.01
    costochondral M99.08
    costovertebral M99.08
    head region M99.00
    hip M99.05
    lower extremity M99.06
    lumbar region M99.03
    lumbosacral M99.03
    occipitocervical M99.00
    pelvic region M99.05
    pubic M99.05
    rib cage M99.08
    sacral region M99.04
    sacrococcygeal M99.04
    sacroiliac M99.04
    specified NEC M99.09
    sternochondral M99.08
    sternoclavicular M99.07
    thoracic region M99.02
    thoracolumbar M99.02
    upper extremity M99.07
  somatoform autonomic F45.8
  stomach K31.89
    psychogenic F45.8
  suprarenal E27.9
    hyperfunction E27.0
  symbolic R48.9
    specified type NEC R48.8
  temporomandibular (joint) M26.69
    joint-pain syndrome M26.62-
  testicular (endocrine) E29.9
    specified NEC E29.8
  thymus E32.9
  thyroid E07.9
  ureterostomy (stoma) — *see* Complications,
    stoma, urinary tract
  urethrostomy (stoma) — *see* Complications,
    stoma, urinary tract
  uterus, complicating delivery O62.9
    hypertonic O62.4
    hypotonic O62.2
      primary O62.0
      secondary O62.1
  ventricular I51.9
    with congestive heart failure I50.9
    left, reversible, following sudden emotional
      stress I51.81

Dysgenesis
  gonadal (due to chromosomal anomaly)
    Q96.9
    pure Q99.1
  renal Q60.5
    bilateral Q60.4
    unilateral Q60.3
  reticular D72.0
  tidal platelet D69.3

Dysgerminoma
  specified site — *see* Neoplasm, malignant, by
    site
  unspecified site
    female C56.9
    male C62.90
Dysgeusia R43.2
Dysgraphia R27.8
Dyshidrosis, dysidrosis L30.1
Dyskaryotic cervical smear R87.619
Dyskeratosis L85.8
  cervix — *see* Dysplasia, cervix
  congenital Q82.8
  uterus NEC N85.8
Dyskinesia G24.9
  biliary (cystic duct or gallbladder) K82.8
  drug induced
    orofacial G24.01
  esophagus K22.4
  hysterical F44.4
  intestinal K59.8
  nonorganic origin F44.4
  orofacial (idiopathic) G24.4
    drug induced G24.01
  psychogenic F44.4
  subacute, drug induced G24.01
  tardive G24.01
    neuroleptic induced G24.01
  trachea J39.8
  tracheobronchial J98.09
Dyslalia (developmental) F80.0
Dyslexia R48.0
  developmental F81.0
Dyslipidemia E78.5
  depressed HDL cholesterol E78.6
  elevated fasting triglycerides E78.1
Dysmaturity — *see also* Light for dates
  pulmonary (newborn) (Wilson-Mikity) P27.0
Dysmenorrhea (essential) (exfoliative) N94.6
  congestive (syndrome) N94.6
  primary N94.4
  psychogenic F45.8
  secondary N94.5
Dysmetabolic syndrome X E88.81
Dysmetria R27.8
Dysmorphism (due to)
  alcohol Q86.0
  exogenous cause NEC Q86.8
  hydantoin Q86.1
  warfarin Q86.2
Dysmorphophobia (nondelusional) F45.22
  delusional F22
Dysnomia R47.01
Dysorexia R63.0
  psychogenic F50.89
Dysostosis
  cleidocranial, cleidocranialis Q74.0
  craniofacial Q75.1
  Fairbank's (idiopathic familial generalized
    osteophytosis) Q78.9
  mandibulofacial (incomplete) Q75.4
  multiplex E76.01
  oculomandibular Q75.5
Dyspareunia (female) N94.10
  deep N94.12
  male N53.12
  nonorganic F52.6
  psychogenic F52.6
  secondary N94.19
  specified NEC N94.19
  superficial (introital) N94.11
Dyspepsia R10.13
  atonic K30
  functional (allergic) (congenital)
    (gastrointestinal) (occupational) (reflex) K30
  intestinal K59.8
  nervous F45.8
  neurotic F45.8
  psychogenic F45.8

Dysphagia R13.10
  cervical R13.19
  following
    cerebral infarction I69.391
    cerebrovascular disease I69.991
    intracerebral hemorrhage I69.191
    nontraumatic intracranial hemorrhage NEC
      I69.291
    specified disease NEC I69.891
    specified NEC I69.891
    subarachnoid hemorrhage I69.091
  functional (hysterical) F45.8
  hysterical F45.8
  nervous (hysterical) F45.8
  neurogenic R13.19
  oral phase R13.11
  oropharyngeal phase R13.12
  pharyneal phase R13.13
  pharyngoesophageal phase R13.14
  psychogenic F45.8
  sideropenic D50.1
  spastica K22.4
  specified NEC R13.19
Dysphagocytosis, congenital D71
Dysphasia R47.02
  developmental
    expressive type F80.1
    receptive type F80.2
  following
    cerebrovascular disease I69.921
      cerebral infarction I69.321
      intracerebral hemorrhage I69.121
      nontraumatic intracranial hemorrhage
        NEC I69.221
      specified disease NEC I69.821
      subarachnoid hemorrhage I69.021
Dysphonia R49.0
  functional F44.4
  hysterical F44.4
  psychogenic F44.4
  spastica J38.3
Dysphoria
  gender
    in
      adolescence and adulthood F64.0
      children F64.2
  postpartal O90.6
Dyspituitarism E23.3
Dysplasia — *see also* Anomaly
  acetabular, congenital Q65.89
  alveolar capillary, with vein misalignment
    J84.843
  anus (histologically confirmed) (mild)
    (moderate) K62.82
    severe D01.3
  arrhythmogenic right ventricular I42.8
  arterial, fibromuscular I77.3
  asphyxiating thoracic (congenital) Q77.2
  brain Q07.9
  bronchopulmonary, perinatal P27.1
  cervix (uteri) N87.9
    mild N87.0
    moderate N87.1
    severe D06.9
  chondroectodermal Q77.6
  colon D12.6
  craniometaphyseal Q78.8
  dentinal K00.5
  diaphyseal, progressive Q78.3
  dystrophic Q77.5
  ectodermal (anhidrotic) (congenital)
    (hereditary) Q82.4
    hydrotic Q82.8
  epithelial, uterine cervix — *see* Dysplasia,
    cervix
  eye (congenital) Q11.2

Dysplasia (see also Anomaly) — continued
fibrous
  bone NEC (monostotic) M85.00
    ankle M85.07-
    foot M85.07-
    forearm M85.03-
    hand M85.04-
    lower leg M85.06-
    multiple site M85.09
    neck M85.08
    rib M85.08
    shoulder M85.01-
    skull M85.08
    specified site NEC M85.08
    thigh M85.05-
    toe M85.07-
    upper arm M85.02-
    vertebra M85.08
  diaphyseal, progressive Q78.3
  jaw M27.8
  polyostotic Q78.1
florid osseous — see also Cyst, calcifying
  odontogenic
high grade, focal D12.6
hip, congenital Q65.89
joint, congenital Q74.8
kidney Q61.4
  multicystic Q61.4
leg Q74.2
lung, congenital (not associated with short
  gestation) Q33.6
mammary (gland) (benign) N60.9-
  cyst (solitary) — see Cyst, breast
  cystic — see Mastopathy, cystic
  duct ectasia — see Ectasia, mammary duct
  fibroadenosis — see Fibroadenosis, breast
  fibrosclerosis — see Fibrosclerosis, breast
  specified type NEC N60.8-
metaphyseal Q78.5
muscle Q79.8
oculodentodigital Q87.0
periapical (cemental) (cemento-osseous) — see
  Cyst, calcifying odontogenic
periosteum — see Disorder, bone, specified
  type NEC
polyostotic fibrous Q78.1
prostate (see also Neoplasia, intraepithelial,
  prostate) N42.30
  severe D07.5
  specified NEC N42.39
renal Q61.4
  multicystic Q61.4
retinal, congenital Q14.1
right ventricular, arrhythmogenic I42.8
septo-optic Q04.4
skin L98.8
spinal cord Q06.1
spondyloepiphyseal Q77.7
thymic, with immunodeficiency D82.1
vagina N89.3
  mild N89.0
  moderate N89.1
  severe NEC D07.2
vulva N90.3
  mild N90.0
  moderate N90.1
  severe NEC D07.1
Dyspnea (nocturnal) (paroxysmal) R06.00
asthmatic (bronchial) J45.909
  with
    bronchitis J45.909
     with
      exacerbation (acute) J45.901
       status asthmaticus J45.902
     chronic J44.9
    exacerbation (acute) J45.901
    status asthmaticus J45.902
  cardiac — see Failure, ventricular, left
cardiac — see Failure, ventricular, left

Dyspnea (nocturnal) (paroxysmal) R06.00 —
continued
functional F45.8
hyperventilation R06.4
hysterical F45.8
newborn P28.89
orthopnea R06.01
psychogenic F45.8
shortness of breath R06.02
specified type NEC R06.09
Dyspraxia R27.8
developmental (syndrome) F82
Dysproteinemia E88.09
Dysreflexia, autonomic G90.4
Dysrhythmia
cardiac I49.9
  newborn
    bradycardia P29.12
     occurring before birth P03.819
      before onset of labor P03.810
      during labor P03.811
    tachycardia P29.11
  postoperative I97.89
cerebral or cortical — see Epilepsy
Dyssomnia — see Disorder, sleep
Dyssynergia
biliary K83.8
bladder sphincter N36.44
cerebellaris myoclonica (Hunt's ataxia) G11.1
Dysthymia F34.1
Dysthyroidism E07.9
Dystocia O66.9
affecting newborn P03.1
cervical (hypotonic) O62.2
  affecting newborn P03.6
  primary O62.0
  secondary O62.1
contraction ring O62.4
fetal O66.9
  abnormality NEC O66.3
  conjoined twins O66.3
  oversize O66.2
maternal O66.9
positional O64.9
shoulder (girdle) O66.0
  causing obstructed labor O66.0
uterine NEC O62.4
Dystonia G24.9
deformans progressiva G24.1
drug induced NEC G24.09
  acute G24.02
  specified NEC G24.09
familial G24.1
idiopathic G24.1
  familial G24.1
  nonfamilial G24.2
  orofacial G24.4
lenticularis G24.8
musculorum deformans G24.1
neuroleptic induced (acute) G24.02
orofacial (idiopathic) G24.4
oromandibular G24.4
  due to drug G24.01
specified NEC G24.8
torsion (familial) (idiopathic) G24.1
  acquired G24.8
  genetic G24.1
  symptomatic (nonfamilial) G24.2
Dystonic movements R25.8
Dystrophy, dystrophia
adiposogenital E23.6
Becker's type G71.0
cervical sympathetic G90.2
choroid (hereditary) H31.20
  central areolar H31.22
  choroideremia H31.21
  gyrate atrophy H31.23
  specified type NEC H31.29

Dystrophy, dystrophia — continued
cornea (hereditary) H18.50
  endothelial H18.51
  epithelial H18.52
  granular H18.53
  lattice H18.54
  macular H18.55
  specified type NEC H18.59
Duchenne's type G71.0
due to malnutrition E45
Erb's G71.0
Fuchs' H18.51
Gower's muscular G71.0
hair L67.8
infantile neuraxonal G31.89
Landouzy-Déjérine G71.0
Leyden-Möbius G71.0
muscular G71.0
  benign (Becker type) G71.0
  congenital (hereditary) (progressive) (with
    specific morphological abnormalities of
    the muscle fiber) G71.0
    myotonic G71.11
  distal G71.0
  Duchenne type G71.0
  Emery-Dreifuss G71.0
  Erb type G71.0
  facioscapulohumeral G71.0
  Gower's G71.0
  hereditary (progressive) G71.0
  Landouzy-Déjérine type G71.0
  limb-girdle G71.0
  myotonic G71.11
  progressive (hereditary) G71.0
    Charcot-Marie(-Tooth) type G60.0
  pseudohypertrophic (infantile) G71.0
  severe (Duchenne type) G71.0
myocardium, myocardial — see Degeneration,
  myocardial
myotonic, myotonica G71.11
nail L60.3
  congenital Q84.6
nutritional E45
ocular G71.0
oculocerebrorenal E72.03
oculopharyngeal G71.0
ovarian N83.8
polyglandular E31.8
reflex (neuromuscular) (sympathetic) — see
  Syndrome, pain, complex regional I
retinal (hereditary) H35.50
  in
    lipid storage disorders E75.6 [H36]
    systemic lipidoses E75.6 [H36]
  involving
    pigment epithelium H35.54
    sensory area H35.53
  pigmentary H35.52
  vitreoretinal H35.51
Salzmann's nodular — see Degeneration,
  cornea, nodular
scapuloperoneal G71.0
skin NEC L98.8
sympathetic (reflex) — see Syndrome, pain,
  complex regional I
  cervical G90.2
tapetoretinal H35.54
thoracic, asphyxiating Q77.2
unguium L60.3
  congenital Q84.6
vitreoretinal H35.51
vulva N90.4
yellow (liver) — see Failure, hepatic
Dysuria R30.0
psychogenic F45.8

E

Eales' disease H35.06-
Ear — *see also* condition
  piercing Z41.3
  tropical NEC B36.9 *[H62.40]*
    in
      aspergillosis B44.89
      candidiasis B37.84
      moniliasis B37.84
  wax (impacted) H61.20
    left H61.22
      with right H61.23
    right H61.21
      with left H61.23
Earache — *see* subcategory H92.0
Early satiety R68.81
Eaton-Lambert syndrome — *see* Syndrome,
  Lambert-Eaton
Eberth's disease (typhoid fever) A01.00
Ebola virus disease A98.4
Ebstein's anomaly or syndrome (heart)
  Q22.5
Eccentro-osteochondrodysplasia E76.29
Ecchondroma — *see* Neoplasm, bone, benign
Ecchondrosis D48.0
Ecchymosis R58
  conjunctiva — *see* Hemorrhage, conjunctiva
  eye (traumatic) — *see* Contusion, eyeball
  eyelid (traumatic) — *see* Contusion, eyelid
  newborn P54.5
  spontaneous R23.3
  traumatic — *see* Contusion
Echinococciasis — *see* Echinococcus
Echinococcosis — *see* Echinococcus
Echinococcus (infection) B67.90
  granulosus B67.4
    bone B67.2
    liver B67.0
    lung B67.1
    multiple sites B67.32
    specified site NEC B67.39
    thyroid B67.31
  liver NOS B67.8
    granulosus B67.0
    multilocularis B67.5
  lung NEC B67.99
    granulosus B67.1
    multilocularis B67.69
  multilocularis B67.7
    liver B67.5
    multiple sites B67.61
    specified site NEC B67.69
  specified site NEC B67.99
    granulosus B67.39
    multilocularis B67.69
  thyroid NEC B67.99
    granulosus B67.31
    multilocularis B67.69 *[E35]*
Echinorhynchiasis B83.8
Echinostomiasis B66.8
Echolalia R48.8
Echovirus, as cause of disease classified
  elsewhere B97.12
Eclampsia, eclamptic (coma) (convulsions)
  (delirium) (with hypertension) NEC O15.9
  complicating
    labor and delivery O15.1
    postpartum O15.2
    pregnancy O15.0-
    puerperium O15.2
Economic circumstances affecting care
  Z59.9
Economo's disease A85.8

Ectasia, ectasis
  annuloaortic I35.8
  aorta I77.819
    with aneurysm — *see* Aneurysm, aorta
    abdominal I77.811
    thoracic I77.810
    thoracoabdominal I77.812
  breast — *see* Ectasia, mammary duct
  capillary I78.8
  cornea H18.71-
  gastric antral vascular (GAVE) K31.819
    with hemorrhage K31.811
    without hemorrhage K31.819
  mammary duct N60.4-
  salivary gland (duct) K11.8
  sclera — *see* Sclerectasia
Ecthyma L08.0
  contagiosum B08.02
  gangrenosum L08.0
  infectiosum B08.02
Ectocardia Q24.8
Ectodermal dysplasia (anhidrotic) Q82.4
Ectodermosis erosiva pluriorificialis L51.1
Ectopic, ectopia (congenital)
  abdominal viscera Q45.8
    due to defect in anterior abdominal wall
      Q79.59
  ACTH syndrome E24.3
  adrenal gland Q89.1
  anus Q43.5
  atrial beats I49.1
  beats I49.49
    atrial I49.1
    ventricular I49.3
  bladder Q64.10
  bone and cartilage in lung Q33.5
  brain Q04.8
  breast tissue Q83.8
  cardiac Q24.8
  cerebral Q04.8
  cordis Q24.8
  endometrium — *see* Endometriosis
  gastric mucosa Q40.2
  gestation — *see* Pregnancy, by site
  heart Q24.8
  hormone secretion NEC E34.2
  kidney (crossed) (pelvis) Q63.2
  lens, lentis Q12.1
  mole — *see* Pregnancy, by site
  organ or site NEC — *see* Malposition,
    congenital
  pancreas Q45.3
  pregnancy — *see* Pregnancy, ectopic
  pupil — *see* Abnormality, pupillary
  renal Q63.2
  sebaceous glands of mouth Q38.6
  spleen Q89.09
  testis Q53.00
    bilateral Q53.02
    unilateral Q53.01
  thyroid Q89.2
  tissue in lung Q33.5
  ureter Q62.63
  ventricular beats I49.3
  vesicae Q64.10
Ectromelia Q73.8
  lower limb — *see* Defect, reduction, limb,
    lower, specified type NEC
  upper limb — *see* Defect, reduction, limb,
    upper, specified type NEC

Ectropion H02.109
  cervix N86
    with cervicitis N72
  congenital Q10.1
  eyelid (paralytic) H02.109
    cicatricial H02.119
      left H02.116
        lower H02.115
        upper H02.114
      right H02.113
        lower H02.112
        upper H02.111
    congenital Q10.1
    left H02.106
      lower H02.105
      upper H02.104
    mechanical H02.129
      left H02.126
        lower H02.125
        upper H02.124
      right H02.123
        lower H02.122
        upper H02.121
    right H02.103
      lower H02.102
      upper H02.101
    senile H02.139
      left H02.136
        lower H02.135
        upper H02.134
      right H02.133
        lower H02.132
        upper H02.131
    spastic H02.149
      left H02.146
        lower H02.145
        upper H02.144
      right H02.143
        lower H02.142
        upper H02.141
  iris H21.89
  lip (acquired) K13.0
    congenital Q38.0
  urethra N36.8
  uvea H21.89
Eczema (acute) (chronic) (erythematous)
  (fissum) (rubrum) (squamous) (*see also*
  Dermatitis) L30.9
  contact — *see* Dermatitis, contact
  dyshydrotic L30.1
  external ear — *see* Otitis, externa, acute,
    eczematoid
  flexural L20.82
  herpeticum B00.0
  hypertrophicum L28.0
  hypostatic — *see* Varix, leg, with, inflammation
  impetiginous L01.1
  infantile (due to any substance) L20.83
    intertriginous L21.1
    seborrheic L21.1
  intertriginous NEC L30.4
    infantile L21.1
  intrinsic (allergic) L20.84
  lichenified NEC L28.0
  marginatum (hebrae) B35.6
  pustular L30.3
  stasis I87.2
    with varicose veins — *see* Varix, leg, with,
      inflammation
  vaccination, vaccinatum T88.1
  varicose — *see* Varix, leg, with, inflammation
Eczematid L30.2
Eddowes(-Spurway) syndrome Q78.0
Edema, edematous (infectious) (pitting)
  (toxic) R60.9
  with nephritis — *see* Nephrosis
  allergic T78.3
  amputation stump (surgical) (sequelae (late
    effect)) T87.89

DISEASE INDEX

Edema, edematous (infectious) (pitting) (toxic) R60.9 — *continued*
- angioneurotic (allergic) (any site) (with urticaria) T78.3
  - hereditary D84.1
- angiospastic I73.9
- Berlin's (traumatic) S05.8x-
- brain (cytotoxic) (vasogenic) G93.6
  - due to birth injury P11.0
    - newborn (anoxia or hypoxia) P52.4
      - birth injury P11.0
  - traumatic — *see* Injury, intracranial, cerebral edema
- cardiac — *see* Failure, heart, congestive
- cardiovascular — *see* Failure, heart, congestive
- cerebral — *see* Edema, brain
- cerebrospinal — *see* Edema, brain
- cervix (uteri) (acute) N88.8
  - puerperal, postpartum O90.89
- chronic hereditary Q82.0
- circumscribed, acute T78.3
  - hereditary D84.1
- conjunctiva H11.42-
- cornea H18.2-
  - idiopathic H18.22-
  - secondary H18.23-
    - due to contact lens H18.21-
- due to
  - lymphatic obstruction I89.0
  - salt retention E87.0
- epiglottis — *see* Edema, glottis
- essential, acute T78.3
  - hereditary D84.1
- extremities, lower — *see* Edema, legs
- eyelid NEC H02.849
  - left H02.846
    - lower H02.845
    - upper H02.844
  - right H02.843
    - lower H02.842
    - upper H02.841
- familial, hereditary Q82.0
- famine — *see* Malnutrition, severe
- generalized R60.1
- glottis, glottic, glottidis (obstructive) (passive) J38.4
  - allergic T78.3
    - hereditary D84.1
- heart — *see* Failure, heart, congestive
- heat T67.7
- hereditary Q82.0
- inanition — *see* Malnutrition, severe
- intracranial G93.6
- iris H21.89
- joint — *see* Effusion, joint
- larynx — *see* Edema, glottis
- legs R60.0
  - due to venous obstruction I87.1
  - hereditary Q82.0
- localized R60.0
  - due to venous obstruction I87.1
- lower limbs — *see* Edema, legs
- lung J81.1
  - with heart condition or failure — *see* Failure, ventricular, left
  - acute J81.0
  - chemical (acute) J68.1
    - chronic J68.1
  - chronic J81.1
    - due to
      - chemicals, gases, fumes or vapors (inhalation) J68.1
      - external agent J70.9
        - specified NEC J70.8
      - radiation J70.1

Edema, edematous (infectious) (pitting) (toxic) R60.9 — *continued*
- lung J81.1 — *continued*
  - due to
    - chemicals, fumes or vapors (inhalation) J68.1
    - external agent J70.9
      - specified NEC J70.8
    - high altitude T70.29
    - near drowning T75.1
    - radiation J70.0
  - meaning failure, left ventricle I50.1
- lymphatic I89.0
  - due to mastectomy I97.2
- macula H35.81
  - cystoid, following cataract surgery — *see* Complications, postprocedural, following cataract surgery
  - diabetic — *see* Diabetes, by type, with, retinopathy, with macular edema
- malignant — *see* Gangrene, gas
- Milroy's Q82.0
- nasopharynx J39.2
- newborn P83.30
  - hydrops fetalis — *see* Hydrops, fetalis
  - specified NEC P83.39
- nutritional — *see also* Malnutrition, severe
  - with dyspigmentation, skin and hair E40
- optic disc or nerve — *see* Papilledema
- orbit H05.22-
- pancreas K86.89
- papilla, optic — *see* Papilledema
- penis N48.89
- periodic T78.3
  - hereditary D84.1
- pharynx J39.2
- pulmonary — *see* Edema, lung
- Quincke's T78.3
  - hereditary D84.1
- renal — *see* Nephrosis
- retina H35.81
  - diabetic — *see* Diabetes, by type, with, retinopathy, with macular edema
- salt E87.0
- scrotum N50.89
- seminal vesicle N50.89
- spermatic cord N50.89
- spinal (cord) (vascular) (nontraumatic) G95.19
- starvation — *see* Malnutrition, severe
- stasis — *see* Hypertension, venous, (chronic)
- subglottic — *see* Edema, glottis
- supraglottic — *see* Edema, glottis
- testis N44.8
- tunica vaginalis N50.89
- vas deferens N50.89
- vulva (acute) N90.89

Edentulism — *see* Absence, teeth, acquired
Edsall's disease T67.2
Educational handicap Z55.9
- specified NEC Z55.8
Edward's syndrome — *see* Trisomy, 18
Effect(s) (of) (from) — *see* Effect, adverse NEC
Effect, adverse
- abnormal gravitational (G) forces or states T75.81
- abuse — *see* Maltreatment
- air pressure T70.9
  - specified NEC T70.8
- altitude (high) — *see* Effect, adverse, high altitude
- anesthesia (*see also* Anesthesia) T88.59
  - in labor and delivery O74.9
  - local, toxic
    - in labor and delivery O74.4
    - in pregnancy NEC O29.3-
    - postpartum, puerperal O89.3
  - postpartum, puerperal O89.9

Effect, adverse — *continued*
- anesthesia (*see also* Anesthesia) T88.59 — *continued*
  - specified NEC T88.59
    - in labor and delivery O74.8
    - postpartum, puerperal O89.8
  - spinal and epidural T88.59
    - headache T88.59
      - in labor and delivery O74.5
      - postpartum, puerperal O89.4
    - specified NEC
      - in labor and delivery O74.6
      - postpartum, puerperal O89.5
- antitoxin — *see* Complications, vaccination
- atmospheric pressure T70.9
  - due to explosion T70.8
  - high T70.3
  - low — *see* Effect, adverse, high altitude
  - specified effect NEC T70.8
- biological, correct substance properly administered — *see* Effect, adverse, drug
- blood (derivatives) (serum) (transfusion) — *see* Complications, transfusion
- chemical substance — *see* Table of Drugs and Chemicals
- cold (temperature) (weather) T69.9
  - chilblains T69.1
  - frostbite — *see* Frostbite
  - specified effect NEC T69.8
- drugs and medicaments T88.7
  - specified drug — *see* Table of Drugs and Chemicals, by drug, adverse effect
  - specified effect — *code to* condition
- electric current, electricity (shock) T75.4
  - burn — *see* Burn
- exertion (excessive) T73.3
- exposure — *see* Exposure
- external cause NEC T75.89
- foodstuffs T78.1
  - allergic reaction — *see* Allergy, food
  - causing anaphylaxis — *see* Shock, anaphylactic, due to, food
  - noxious — *see* Poisoning, food, noxious
- gases, fumes, or vapors T59.9-
  - specified agent — *see* Table of Drugs and Chemicals
- glue (airplane) sniffing
  - due to drug abuse — *see* Abuse, drug, inhalant
  - due to drug dependence — *see* Dependence, drug, inhalant
- heat — *see* Heat
- high altitude NEC T70.29
  - anoxia T70.29
  - on
    - ears T70.0
    - sinuses T70.1
  - polycythemia D75.1
- high pressure fluids T70.4
- hot weather — *see* Heat
- hunger T73.0
- immersion, foot — *see* Immersion
- immunization — *see* Complications, vaccination
- immunological agents — *see* Complications, vaccination
- infrared (radiation) (rays) NOS T66
  - dermatitis or eczema L59.8
- infusion — *see* Complications, infusion
- lack of care of infants — *see* Maltreatment, child
- lightning — *see* Lightning
- medical care T88.9
  - specified NEC T88.8
- medicinal substance, correct, properly administered — *see* Effect, adverse, drug
- motion T75.3
- noise, on inner ear — *see* subcategory H83.3
- overheated places — *see* Heat

Effect, adverse — *continued*
  psychosocial, of work environment Z56.5
  radiation (diagnostic) (infrared) (natural source) (therapeutic) (ultraviolet) (X-ray) NOS T66
    dermatitis or eczema — *see* Dermatitis, due to, radiation
    fibrosis of lung J70.1
    pneumonitis J70.0
    pulmonary manifestations
      acute J70.0
      chronic J70.1
    skin L59.9
  radioactive substance NOS
  reduced temperature T69.9
    immersion foot or hand — *see* Immersion
    specified effect NEC T69.8
  serum NEC (*see also* Reaction, serum) T80.69
  specified NEC T78.8
    external cause NEC T75.89
  strangulation — *see* Asphyxia, traumatic
  submersion T75.1
  thirst T73.1
  toxic — *see* Toxicity
  transfusion — *see* Complications, transfusion
  ultraviolet (radiation) (rays) NOS T66
    burn — *see* Burn
    dermatitis or eczema — *see* Dermatitis, due to, ultraviolet rays
      acute L56.8
  vaccine (any) — *see* Complications, vaccination
  vibration — *see* Vibration, adverse effects
  water pressure NEC T70.9
    specified NEC T70.8
  weightlessness T75.82
  whole blood — *see* Complications, transfusion
  work environment Z56.5
Effects, late — *see* Sequelae
Effluvium
  anagen L65.1
  telogen L65.0
Effort syndrome (psychogenic) F45.8
Effusion
  amniotic fluid — *see* Pregnancy, complicated by, prematue rupture of membranes
  brain (serous) G93.6
  bronchial — *see* Bronchitis
  cerebral G93.6
  cerebrospinal — *see also* Meningitis
    vessel G93.6
  chest — *see* Effusion, pleura
  chylous, chyliform (pleura) J94.0
  intracranial G93.6
  joint M25.40
    ankle M25.47-
    elbow M25.42-
    foot joint M25.47-
    hand joint M25.44-
    hip M25.45-
    knee M25.46-
    shoulder M25.41-
    specified joint NEC M25.48
    wrist M25.43-
  malignant pleural J91.0
  meninges — *see* Meningitis
  pericardium, pericardial (noninflammatory) I31.3
  acute — *see* Pericarditis, acute
  peritoneal (chronic) R18.8
  pleura, pleurisy, pleuritic, pleuropericardial J90
    chylous, chyliform J94.0
    due to systemic lupus erythematosis M32.13
    influenzal — *see* Influenza, with, respiratory manifestations NEC
    malignant J91.0
    newborn P28.89

Effusion — *continued*
  pleura, pleurisy, pleuritic, pleuropericardial J90 — *continued*
    tuberculous NEC A15.6
      primary (progressive) A15.7
    spinal — *see* Meningitis
    thorax, thoracic — *see* Effusion, pleura
Egg shell nails L60.3
  congenital Q84.6
Egyptian splenomegaly B65.1
Ehlers-Danlos syndrome Q79.6
Ehrlichiosis A77.40
  due to
    E. chafeensis A77.41
    E. sennetsu A79.81
    specified organism NEC A77.49
Eichstedt's disease B36.0
Eisenmenger's
  complex or syndrome I27.89
  defect Q21.8
Ejaculation
  delayed F52.32
  painful N53.12
  premature F52.4
  retarded N53.11
  retrograde N53.14
  semen, painful N53.12
  psychogenic F52.6
Ekbom's syndrome (restless legs) G25.81
Ekman's syndrome (brittle bones and blue sclera) Q78.0
Elastic skin Q82.8
  acquired L57.4
Elastofibroma — *see* Neoplasm, connective tissue, benign
Elastoma (juvenile) Q82.8
  Miescher's L87.2
Elastomyofibrosis I42.4
Elastosis
  actinic, solar L57.8
  atrophicans (senile) L57.4
  perforans serpiginosa L87.2
  senilis L57.4
Elbow — *see* condition
Electric current, electricity, effects (concussion) (fatal) (nonfatal) (shock) T75.4
  burn — *see* Burn
Electric feet syndrome E53.8
Electrocution T75.4
  from electroshock gun (taser) T75.4
Electrolyte imbalance E87.8
  with
    abortion — *see* Abortion, by type, complicated by, electrolyte imbalance
    ectopic pregnancy O08.5
    molar pregnancy O08.5
Elephantiasis (nonfilarial) I89.0
  arabicum — *see* Infestation, filarial
  bancroftian B74.0
  congenital (any site) (hereditary) Q82.0
  due to
    Brugia (malayi) B74.1
      timori B74.2
    mastectomy I97.2
    Wuchereria (bancrofti) B74.0
  eyelid H02.859
    left H02.856
      lower H02.855
      upper H02.854
    right H02.853
      lower H02.852
      upper H02.851
  filarial, filariensis — *see* Infestation, filarial
  glandular I89.0
  graecorum A30.9
  lymphangiectatic I89.0
  lymphatic vessel I89.0
    due to mastectomy I97.2
  scrotum (nonfilarial) I89.0

Elephantiasis (nonfilarial) I89.0 — *continued*
  streptococcal I89.0
  surgical I97.89
    postmastectomy I97.2
  telangiectodes I89.0
  vulva (nonfilarial) N90.89
Elevated, elevation
  antibody titer R76.0
  basal metabolic rate R94.8
  blood pressure — *see also* Hypertension
    reading (incidental) (isolated) (nonspecific), no diagnosis of hypertension R03.0
  blood sugar R73.9
  body temperature (of unknown origin) R50.9
  cancer antigen 125 [CA 125] R97.1
  carcinoembryonic antigen [CEA] R97.0
  cholesterol E78.00
    with high triglycerides E78.2
  conjugate, eye H51.0
  C-reactive protein (CRP) R79.82
  diaphragm, congenital Q79.1
  erythrocyte sedimentation rate R70.0
  fasting glucose R73.01
  fasting triglycerides E78.1
  finding on laboratory examination — *see* Findings, abnormal, inconclusive, without diagnosis, by type of exam
  GFR (glomerular filtration rate) — *see* Findings, abnormal, inconclusive, without diagnosis, by type of exam
  glucose tolerance (oral) R73.02
  immunoglobulin level R76.8
  indoleacetic acid R82.5
  lactic acid dehydrogenase (LDH) level R74.0
  leukocytes D72.829
  lipoprotein a level E78.8
  liver function
    study R94.5
    test R79.89
      alkaline phosphatase R74.8
      aminotransferase R74.0
      bilirubin R17
      hepatic enzyme R74.8
      lactate dehydrogenase R74.0
  lymphocytes D72.820
  prostate specific antigen [PSA] R97.20
  Rh titer — *see* Complication(s), transfusion, incompatibility reaction, Rh (factor)
  scapula, congenital Q74.0
  sedimentation rate R70.0
  SGOT R74.0
  SGPT R74.0
  transaminase level R74.0
  triglycerides E78.1
    with high cholesterol E78.2
  tumor associated antigens [TAA] NEC R97.8
  tumor specific antigens [TSA] NEC R97.8
  urine level of
    17-ketosteroids R82.5
    catecholamine R82.5
    indoleacetic acid R82.5
    steroids R82.5
    vanillylmandelic acid (VMA) R82.5
  venous pressure I87.8
  white blood cell count D72.829
    specified NEC D72.828
Elliptocytosis (congenital) (hereditary) D58.1
  Hb C (disease) D58.1
  hemoglobin disease D58.1
  sickle-cell (disease) D57.8-
    trait D57.3
Ellison-Zollinger syndrome E16.4
Ellis-van Creveld syndrome (chondroectodermal dysplasia) Q77.6

Elongated, elongation (congenital) — *see also* Distortion
  bone Q79.9
  cervix (uteri) Q51.828
    acquired N88.4
    hypertrophic N88.4
  colon Q43.8
  common bile duct Q44.5
  cystic duct Q44.5
  frenulum, penis Q55.69
  labia minora (acquired) N90.69
  ligamentum patellae Q74.1
  petiolus (epiglottidis) Q31.8
  tooth, teeth K00.2
  uvula Q38.6
Eltor cholera A00.1
Emaciation (due to malnutrition) E41
Embadomoniasis A07.8
Embedded tooth, teeth K01.0
  root only K08.3
Embolic — *see* condition
Embolism (multiple) (paradoxical) I74.9
  air (any site) (traumatic) T79.0
    following
      abortion — *see* Abortion by type complicated by embolism
      ectopic pregnancy O08.2
      infusion, therapeutic injection or transfusion T80.0
      molar pregnancy O08.2
      procedure NEC
        artery T81.719
          mesenteric T81.710
          renal T81.711
          specified NEC T81.718
        vein T81.72
    in pregnancy, childbirth or puerperium — *see* Embolism, obstetric
  amniotic fluid (pulmonary) — *see also* Embolism, obstetric
    following
      abortion — *see* Abortion by type complicated by embolism
      ectopic pregnancy O08.2
      molar pregnancy O08.2
  aorta, aortic I74.10
    abdominal I74.09
      saddle I74.01
    bifurcation I74.09
    saddle I74.01
    thoracic I74.11
  artery I74.9
    auditory, internal I65.8
    basilar — *see* Occlusion, artery, basilar
    carotid (common) (internal) — *see* Occlusion, artery, carotid
    cerebellar (anterior inferior) (posterior inferior) (superior) I66.3
    cerebral — *see* Occlusion, artery, cerebral
    choroidal (anterior) I66.8
    communicating posterior I66.8
    coronary — *see also* Infarct, myocardium
      not resulting in infarction I24.0
    extremity I74.4
      lower I74.3
      upper I74.2
    hypophyseal I66.8
    iliac I74.5
    limb I74.4
      lower I74.3
      upper I74.2
    mesenteric (with gangrene) (*see also* Ischemia, intestine, acute) K55.059
    ophthalmic — *see* Occlusion, artery, retina
    peripheral I74.4
    pontine I66.8
    precerebral — *see* Occlusion, artery, precerebral
    pulmonary — *see* Embolism, pulmonary

Embolism (multiple) (paradoxical) I74.9 — *continued*
  artery I74.9 — *continued*
    renal N28.0
    retinal — *see* Occlusion, artery, retina
    septic I76
    specified NEC I74.8
    vertebral — *see* Occlusion, artery, vertebral
  basilar (artery) I65.1
  blood clot
    following
      abortion — *see* Abortion by type complicated by embolism
      ectopic or molar pregnancy O08.2
    in pregnancy, childbirth or puerperium — *see* Embolism, obstetric
  brain — *see also* Occlusion, artery, cerebral
    following
      abortion — *see* Abortion by type complicated by embolism
      ectopic or molar pregnancy O08.2
      puerperal, postpartum, childbirth — *see* Embolism, obstetric
  capillary I78.8
  cardiac — *see also* Infarct, myocardium
    not resulting in infarction I51.3
  carotid (artery) (common) (internal) — *see* Occlusion, artery, carotid
  cavernous sinus (venous) — *see* Embolism, intracranial venous sinus
  cerebral — *see* Occlusion, artery, cerebral
  cholesterol — *see* Atheroembolism
  coronary (artery or vein) (systemic) — *see* Occlusion, coronary
  due to device, implant or graft — *see also* Complications, by site and type, specified NEC
    arterial graft NEC T82.818
    breast (implant) T85.818
    catheter NEC T85.818
      dialysis (renal) T82.818
        intraperitoneal T85.818
      infusion NEC T82.818
        spinal (epidural) (subdural) T85.810
      urinary (indwelling) T83.81
    electronic (electrode) (pulse generator) (stimulator)
      bone T84.81
      cardiac T82.817
      nervous system (brain) (peripheral nerve) (spinal) T85.810
      urinary T83.81
    fixation, internal (orthopedic) NEC T84.81
    gastrointestinal (bile duct) (esophagus) T85.818
    genital NEC T83.81
    heart (graft) (valve) T82.817
    joint prosthesis T84.81
    ocular (corneal graft) (orbital implant) T85.818
    orthopedic (bone graft) NEC T86.838
    specified NEC T85.818
    urinary (graft) NEC T83.81
    vascular NEC T82.818
    ventricular intracranial shunt T85.810
  extremities
    lower — *see* Embolism, vein, lower extremity arterial I74.3
    upper I74.2
  eye H34.9
  fat (cerebral) (pulmonary) (systemic) T79.1
    complicating delivery — *see* Embolism, obstetric
    following
      abortion — *see* Abortion by type complicated by embolism
      ectopic or molar pregnancy O08.2

Embolism (multiple) (paradoxical) I74.9 — *continued*
  following
    abortion — *see* Abortion by type complicated by embolism
    ectopic or molar pregnancy O08.2
    infusion, therapeutic injection or transfusion air T80.0
  heart (fatty) — *see also* Infarct, myocardium
    not resulting in infarction I51.3
  hepatic (vein) I82.0
  in pregnancy, childbirth or puerperium — *see* Embolism, obstetric
  intestine (artery) (vein) (with gangrene) (with gangrene) (*see also* Ischemia, intestine, acute) K55.039
  intracranial — *see also* Occlusion, artery, cerebral
    venous sinus (any) G08
      nonpyogenic I67.6
  intraspinal venous sinuses or veins G08
    nonpyogenic G95.19
  kidney (artery) N28.0
  lateral sinus (venous) — *see* Embolism, intracranial, venous sinus
  leg — *see* Embolism, vein, lower extremity arterial I74.3
  longitudinal sinus (venous) — *see* Embolism, intracranial, venous sinus
  lung (massive) — *see* Embolism, pulmonary
  meninges I66.8
  mesenteric (artery) (vein) (with gangrene) (*see also* Ischemia, intestine, acute) K55.059
  obstetric (in) (pulmonary)
    childbirth O88.22
      air O88.02
      amniotic fluid O88.12
      blood clot O88.22
      fat O88.82
      pyemic O88.32
      septic O88.32
      specified type NEC O88.82
    pregnancy O88.21-
      air O88.01-
      amniotic fluid O88.11-
      blood clot O88.21-
      fat O88.81-
      pyemic O88.31-
      septic O88.31-
      specified type NEC O88.81-
    puerperal O88.23
      air O88.03
      amniotic fluid O88.13
      blood clot O88.23
      fat O88.83
      pyemic O88.33
      septic O88.33
      specified type NEC O88.83
  ophthalmic — *see* Occlusion, artery, retina
  penis N48.81
  peripheral artery NOS I74.4
  pituitary E23.6
  popliteal (artery) I74.3
  portal (vein) I81
  postoperative, postrpocedural
    artery T81.719
      mesenteric T81.710
      renal T81.711
      specified NEC T81.718
    vein T81.72
  precerebral artery — *see* Occlusion, artery, precerebral
  puerperal — *see* Embolism, obstetric

Embolism (multiple) (paradoxical) I74.9 — *continued*
  pulmonary (acute) (artery) (vein) I26.99
    with acute cor pulmonale I26.09
    chronic I27.82
    following
      abortion — *see* Abortion by type
        complicated by embolism
      ectopic or molar pregnancy O08.2
    healed or old Z86.711
    in pregnancy, childbirth or puerperium — *see* Embolism, obstetric
    personal history of Z86.711
    saddle I26.92
      with acute cor pulmonale I26.02
    septic I26.90
      with acute cor pulmonale I26.01
  pyemic (multiple) I76
    following
      abortion — *see* Abortion by type
        complicated by embolism
      ectopic or molar pregnancy O08.2
    Hemophilus influenzae A41.3
    pneumococcal A40.3
      with pneumonia J13
    puerperal, postpartum, childbirth (any organism) — *see* Embolism, obstetric
    specified organism NEC A41.89
    staphylococcal A41.2
    streptococcal A40.9
  renal (artery) N28.0
    vein I82.3
  retina, retinal — *see* Occlusion, artery, retina
  saddle
    abdominal aorta I74.01
    pulmonary artery I26.92
      with acute cor pulmonale I26.02
  septic (arterial) I76
    complicating abortion — *see* Abortion, by type, complicated by, embolism
  sinus — *see* Embolism, intracranial, venous sinus
  soap complicating abortion — *see* Abortion, by type, complicated by, embolism
  spinal cord G95.19
    pyogenic origin G06.1
  spleen, splenic (artery) I74.8
  upper extremity I74.2
  vein (acute) I82.90
    antecubital I82.61-
      chronic I82.71-
    axillary I82.A1-
      chronic I82.A2-
    basilic I82.61-
      chronic I82.71-
    brachial I82.62-
      chronic I82.72-
    brachiocephalic (innominate) I82.290
      chronic I82.291
    cephalic I82.61-
      chronic I82.71-
    chronic I82.91
    deep (DVT) I82.40-
      calf I82.4Z-
        chronic I82.5Z-
      lower leg I82.4Z-
        chronic I82.5Z-
      thigh I82.4Y-
        chronic I82.5Y-
      upper leg I82.4Y
        chronic I82.5Y-
    femoral I82.41-
      chronic I82.51-
    iliac (iliofemoral) I82.42-
      chronic I82.52-
    innominate I82.290
      chronic I82.291
    internal jugular I82.C1-
      chronic I82.C2-

Embolism (multiple) (paradoxical) I74.9 — *continued*
  vein (acute) I82.90 — *continued*
    lower extremity
      deep I82.40-
        chronic I82.50-
        specified NEC I82.49-
          chronic NEC I82.59-
        distal
          deep I82.4Z-
        proximal
          deep I82.4Y-
            chronic I82.5Y-
        superficial I82.81-
      popliteal I82.43-
        chronic I82.53-
    radial I82.62-
      chronic I82.72-
    renal I82.3
    saphenous (greater) (lesser) I82.81-
    specified NEC I82.890
      chronic NEC I82.891
    subclavian I82.B1-
      chronic I82.B2-
    thoracic NEC I82.290
      chronic I82.291
    tibial I82.44-
      chronic I82.54-
    ulnar I82.62-
      chronic I82.72-
    upper extremity I82.60-
      chronic I82.70-
      deep I82.62-
        chronic I82.72-
      superficial I82.61-
        chronic I82.71-
    vena cava
      inferior (acute) I82.220
        chronic I82.221
      superior (acute) I82.210
        chronic I82.211
    venous sinus G08
    vessels of brain — *see* Occlusion, artery, cerebral
Embolus — *see* Embolism
Embryoma — *see also* Neoplasm, uncertain behavior, by site
  benign — *see* Neoplasm, benign, by site
  kidney C64-
  liver C22.0
  malignant — *see also* Neoplasm, malignant, by site
    kidney C64-
    liver C22.0
    testis C62.9-
      descended (scrotal) C62.1-
      undescended C62.0-
  testis C62.9-
    descended (scrotal) C62.1-
    undescended C62.0-
Embryonic
  circulation Q28.9
  heart Q28.9
  vas deferens Q55.4
Embryopathia NOS Q89.9
Embryotoxon Q13.4
Emesis — *see* Vomiting
Emotional lability R45.86
Emotionality, pathological F60.3
Emotogenic disease — *see* Disorder, psychogenic
Emphysema (atrophic) (bullous) (chronic) (interlobular) (lung) (obstructive) (pulmonary) (senile) (vesicular) J43.9
  cellular tissue (traumatic) T79.7
    surgical T81.82
  centrilobular J43.2
  compensatory J98.3
  congenital (interstitial) P25.0

Emphysema (atrophic) (bullous) (chronic) (interlobular) (lung) (obstructive) (pulmonary) (senile) (vesicular) J43.9 — *continued*
  conjunctiva H11.89
  connective tissue (traumatic) T79.7
    surgical T81.82
  due to chemicals, gases, fumes or vapors J68.4
  eyelid(s) — *see* Disorder, eyelid, specified type NEC
    surgical T81.82
    traumatic T79.7
  interstitial J98.2
    congenital P25.0
    perinatal period P25.0
  laminated tissue T79.7
    surgical T81.82
  mediastinal J98.2
    newborn P25.2
  orbit, orbital — *see* Disorder, orbit, specified type NEC
  panacinar J43.1
  panlobular J43.1
  specified NEC J43.8
  subcutaneous (traumatic) T79.7
    nontraumatic J98.2
    postprocedural T81.82
    surgical T81.82
  surgical T81.82
  thymus (gland) (congenital) E32.8
  traumatic (subcutaneous) T79.7
  unilateral J43.0
Empty nest syndrome Z60.0
Empyema (acute) (chest) (double) (pleura) (supradiaphragmatic) (thorax) J86.9
  with fistula J86.0
  accessory sinus (chronic) — *see* Sinusitis
  antrum (chronic) — *see* Sinusitis, maxillary
  brain (any part) — *see* Abscess, brain
  ethmoidal (chronic) (sinus) — *see* Sinusitis, ethmoidal
  extradural — *see* Abscess, extradural
  frontal (chronic) (sinus) — *see* Sinusitis, frontal
  gallbladder K81.0
  mastoid (process) (acute) — *see* Mastoiditis, acute
  maxilla, maxillary M27.2
    sinus (chronic) — *see* Sinusitis, maxillary
  nasal sinus (chronic) — *see* Sinusitis
  sinus (accessory) (chronic) (nasal) — *see* Sinusitis
  sphenoidal (sinus) (chronic) — *see* Sinusitis, sphenoidal
  subarachnoid — *see* Abscess, extradural
  subdural — *see* Abscess, subdural
  tuberculous A15.6
  ureter — *see* Ureteritis
  ventricular — *see* Abscess, brain
En coup de sabre lesion L94.1
Enamel pearls K00.2
Enameloma K00.2
Enanthema, viral B09
Encephalitis (chronic) (hemorrhagic) (idiopathic) (nonepidemic) (spurious) (subacute) G04.90
  acute (*see also* Encephalitis, viral) A86
    disseminated G04.00
      infectious G04.01
      noninfectious G04.81
      postimmunization (postvaccination) G04.02
      postinfectious G04.01
    inclusion body A85.8
    necrotizing hemorrhagic G04.30
      postimmunization G04.32
      postinfectious G04.31
      specified NEC G04.39
  arboviral, arbovirus NEC A85.2
  arthropod-borne NEC (viral) A85.2

Encephalitis (chronic) (hemorrhagic) (idiopathic) (nonepidemic) (spurious) (subacute) G04.90 — *continued*
Australian A83.4
California (virus) A83.5
Central European (tick-borne) A84.1
Czechoslovakian A84.1
Dawson's (inclusion body) A81.1
diffuse sclerosing A81.1
disseminated, acute G04.00
due to
  cat scratch disease A28.1
  human immunodeficiency virus (HIV) disease B20 *[G05.3]*
  malaria — *see* Malaria
  rickettsiosis — *see* Rickettsiosis
  smallpox inoculation G04.02
  typhus — *see* Typhus
Eastern equine A83.2
endemic (viral) A86
epidemic NEC (viral) A86
equine (acute) (infectious) (viral) A83.9
  Eastern A83.2
  Venezuelan A92.2
  Western A83.1
Far Eastern (tick-borne) A84.0
following vaccination or other immunization procedure G04.02
herpes zoster B02.0
herpesviral B00.4
  due to herpesvirus 6 B10.01
  due to herpesvirus 7 B10.09
  specified NEC B10.09
Ilheus (virus) A83.8
in (due to)
  actinomycosis A42.82
  adenovirus A85.1
  African trypanosomiasis B56.9 *[G05.3]*
  Chagas' disease (chronic) B57.42
  cytomegalovirus B25.8
  enterovirus A85.0
  herpes (simplex) virus B00.4
    due to herpesvirus 6 B10.01
    due to herpesvirus 7 B10.09
    specified NEC B10.09
  infectious disease NEC B99 *[G05.3]*
  influenza — *see* Influenza, with, encephalopathy
  listeriosis A32.12
  measles B05.0
  mumps B26.2
  naegleriasis B60.2
  parasitic disease NEC B89 *[G05.3]*
  poliovirus A80.9 *[G05.3]*
  rubella B06.01
  syphilis
    congenital A50.42
    late A52.14
  systemic lupus erythematosus M32.19
  toxoplasmosis (acquired) B58.2
    congenital P37.1
  tuberculosis A17.82
  zoster B02.0
inclusion body A81.1
infectious (acute) (virus) NEC A86
Japanese (B type) A83.0
La Crosse A83.5
lead — *see* Poisoning, lead
lethargica (acute) (infectious) A85.8
louping ill A84.8
lupus erythematosus, systemic M32.19
lymphatica A87.2
Mengo A85.8
meningococcal A39.81
Murray Valley A83.4
otitic NEC H66.40 *[G05.3]*
parasitic NOS B71.9
periaxial G37.0
periaxialis (concentrica) (diffuse) G37.5

Encephalitis (chronic) (hemorrhagic) (idiopathic) (nonepidemic) (spurious) (subacute) G04.90 — *continued*
postchickenpox B01.11
postexanthematous NEC B09
postimmunization G04.02
postinfectious NEC G04.01
postmeasles B05.0
postvaccinal G04.02
postvaricella B01.11
postviral NEC A86
Powassan A84.8
Rasmussen G04.81
Rio Bravo A85.8
Russian
  autumnal A83.0
  spring-summer (taiga) A84.0
saturnine — *see* Poisoning, lead
specified NEC G04.81
St. Louis A83.3
subacute sclerosing A81.1
summer A83.0
suppurative G04.81
tick-borne A84.9
Torula, torular (cryptococcal) B45.1
toxic NEC G92
trichinosis B75 *[G05.3]*
type
  B A83.0
  C A83.3
van Bogaert's A81.1
Venezuelan equine A92.2
Vienna A85.8
viral, virus A86
  arthropod-borne NEC A85.2
    mosquito-borne A83.9
      Australian X disease A83.4
      California virus A83.5
      Eastern equine A83.2
      Japanese (B type) A83.0
      Murray Valley A83.4
      specified NEC A83.8
      St. Louis A83.3
      type B A83.0
      type C A83.3
      Western equine A83.1
    tick-borne A84.9
      biundulant A84.1
      central European A84.1
      Czechoslovakian A84.1
      diphasic meningoencephalitis A84.1
      Far Eastern A84.0
      Russian spring-summer (taiga) A84.0
      specified NEC A84.8
    specified type NEC A85.8
  Western equine A83.1

Encephalocele Q01.9
frontal Q01.0
nasofrontal Q01.1
occipital Q01.2
specified NEC Q01.8

Encephalocystocele — *see* Encephalocele

Encephaloduroarteriomyosynangiosis (EDAMS) I67.5

Encephalomalacia (brain) (cerebellar) (cerebral) — *see* Softening, brain

Encephalomeningitis — *see* Meningoencephalitis

Encephalomeningocele — *see* Encephalocele

Encephalomeningomyelitis — *see* Meningoencephalitis

Encephalomyelitis (*see also* Encephalitis) G04.90
acute disseminated G04.00
  infectious G04.01
  noninfectious G04.81
  postimmunization G04.02
  postinfectious G04.01

Encephalomyelitis (*see also* Encephalitis) G04.90 — *continued*
acute necrotizing hemorrhagic G04.30
  postimmunization G04.32
  postinfectious G04.31
  specified NEC G04.39
benign myalgic G93.3
equine A83.9
  Eastern A83.2
  Venezuelan A92.2
  Western A83.1
in diseases classified elsewhere G05.3
myalgic, benign G93.3
postchickenpox B01.11
postinfectious NEC G04.01
postmeasles B05.0
postvaccinal G04.02
postvaricella B01.11
rubella B06.01
specified NEC G04.81
Venezuelan equine A92.2

Encephalomyelocele — *see* Encephalocele

Encephalomyelomeningitis — *see* Meningoencephalitis

Encephalomyelopathy G96.9

Encephalomyeloradiculitis (acute) G61.0

Encephalomyeloradiculoneuritis (acute) (Guillain-Barré) G61.0

Encephalomyeloradiculopathy G96.9

Encephalopathia hyperbilirubinemica, newborn P57.9
due to isoimmunization (conditions in P55) P57.0

Encephalopathy (acute) G93.40
acute necrotizing hemorrhagic G04.30
  postimmunization G04.32
  postinfectious G04.31
  specified NEC G04.39
alcoholic G31.2
anoxic — *see* Damage, brain, anoxic
arteriosclerotic I67.2
centrolobar progressive (Schilder) G37.0
congenital Q07.9
degenerative, in specified disease NEC G32.89
demyelinating callosal G37.1
due to
  drugs (*see also* Table of drugs and chemicals) G92
hepatic — *see* Failure, hepatic
hyperbilirubinemic, newborn P57.9
  due to isoimmunization (conditions in P55) P57.0
hypertensive I67.4
hypoglycemic E16.2
hypoxic — *see* Damage, brain, anoxic
hypoxic ischemic P91.60
  mild P91.61
  moderate P91.62
  severe P91.63
in (due to) (with)
  birth injury P11.1
  hyperinsulinism E16.1 *[G94]*
  influenza — *see* Influenza, with, encephalopathy
  lack of vitamin (*see also* Deficiency, vitamin) E56.9 *[G32.89]*
  neoplastic disease (*see also* Neoplasm) D49.9 *[G13.1]*
  serum (*see also* Reaction, serum) T80.69
  syphilis A52.17
  trauma (postconcussional) F07.81
    current injury — *see* Injury, intracranial
  vaccination G04.02
lead — *see* Poisoning, lead
metabolic G93.41
  drug-induced G92
  toxic G92

DISEASE INDEX

Encephalopathy (acute) G93.40 —
continued
    myoclonic, early, symptomatic — *see* Epilepsy,
        generalized, specified NEC
    necrotizing, subacute (Leigh) G31.82
    pellagrous E52 *[G32.89]*
    portosystemic — *see* Failure, hepatic
    postcontusional F07.81
        current injury — *see* Injury, intracranial,
            diffuse
    posthypoglycemic (coma) E16.1 *[G94]*
    postradiation G93.89
    saturnine — *see* Poisoning, lead
    septic G93.41
    specified NEC G93.49
    spongiform, subacute (viral) A81.09
    toxic G92
        metabolic G92
    traumatic (postconcussional) F07.81
        current injury — *see* Injury, intracranial
    vitamin B deficiency NEC E53.9 *[G32.89]*
        vitamin B1 E51.2
        Wernicke's E51.2
Encephalorrhagia — *see* Hemorrhage,
    intracranial, intracerebral
Encephalosis, posttraumatic F07.81
Enchondroma — *see also* Neoplasm, bone,
    benign
Enchondromatosis (cartilaginous) (multiple)
    Q78.4
Encopresis R15.9
    functional F98.1
    nonorganic origin F98.1
    psychogenic F98.1
Encounter (with health service) (for) Z76.89
    adjustment and management (of)
        breast implant Z45.81
        implanted device NEC Z45.89
        myringotomy device (stent) (tube) Z45.82
    administrative purpose only Z02.9
        examination for
            adoption Z02.82
            armed forces Z02.3
            disability determination Z02.71
            driving license Z02.4
            employment Z02.1
            insurance Z02.6
            medical certificate NEC Z02.79
            paternity testing Z02.81
            residential institution admission Z02.2
            school admission Z02.0
            sports Z02.5
            specified reason NEC Z02.89
    aftercare — *see* Aftercare
    antenatal screening Z36
    assisted reproductive fertility procedure cycle
        Z31.83
    blood typing Z01.83
        Rh typing Z01.83
    breast augmentation or reduction Z41.1
    breast implant exchange (different material)
        (different size) Z45.81
    breast reconstruction following mastectomy
        Z42.1
    check-up — *see* Examination
    chemotherapy for neoplasm Z51.11
    colonoscopy, screening Z12.11
    counseling — *see* Counseling
    delivery, full-term, uncomplicated O80
        cesarean, without indication O82
    desensitization to allergens Z51.6
    ear piercing Z41.3
    examination — *see* Examination
    expectant parent(s) (adoptive) pre-birth
        pediatrician visit Z76.81
    fertility preservation procedure (prior to cancer
        therapy) (prior to removal of gonads)
        Z31.84
    fitting (of) — *see* Fitting (and adjustment) (of)

Encounter (with health service) (for) Z76.89 —
continued
    genetic
        counseling Z31.5
        testing — *see* Test, genetic
    hearing conservation and treatment Z01.12
    immunotherapy for neoplasm Z51.12
    in vitro fertilization cycle Z31.83
    instruction (in)
        child care (postpartal) (prenatal) Z32.3
        childbirth Z32.2
        natural family planning
            procreative Z31.61
            to avoid pregnancy Z30.02
    insulin pump titration Z46.81
    joint prosthesis insertion following prior
        explantation of joint prosthesis (staged
        procedure)
        hip Z47.32
        knee Z47.33
        shoulder Z47.31
    laboratory (as part of a general medical
        examination) Z00.00
        with abnormal findings Z00.01
    mental health services (for)
        abuse NEC
            perpetrator Z69.82
            victim Z69.81
        child abuse
            nonparental
                perpetrator Z69.021
                victim Z69.020
            parental
                perpetrator Z69.011
                victim Z69.010
        spousal or partner abuse
            perpetrator Z69.12
            victim Z69.11
    observation (for) (ruled out)
        exposure to (suspected)
            anthrax Z03.810
            biological agent NEC Z03.818
    pediatrician visit, by expectant parent(s)
        (adoptive) Z76.81
    plastic and reconstructive surgery following
        medical procedure or healed injury NEC
        Z42.8
    pregnancy
        supervision of — *see* Pregnancy, supervision
            of
        test Z32.00
            result negative Z32.02
            result positive Z32.01
    procreative management and counseling for
        gestational carrier Z31.7
    prophylactic measures Z29.9
        antivenin Z29.12
        fluoride administration Z29.3
        immunotherapy for respiratory syncytial
            virus (RSV) Z29.11
        rabies immune globin Z29.14
        Rho (D) immune globulin Z29.13
        specified NEC Z29.8
    radiation therapy (antineoplastic) Z51.0
    radiological (as part of a general medical
        examination) Z00.00
        with abnormal findings Z00.01
    reconstructive surgery following medical
        procedure or healed injury NEC Z42.8
    removal (of) — *see also* Removal
        artificial
            arm Z44.00-
                complete Z44.01-
                partial Z44.02-
            eye Z44.2-
            leg Z44.10-
                complete Z44.11-
                partial Z44.12-

Encounter (with health service) (for) Z76.89 —
continued
    removal (of) — *see also* Removal — *continued*
        breast implant Z45.81
            tissue expander (without synchronous
                insertion of permanent implant)
                Z45.81
        device Z46.9
            specified NEC Z46.89
        external
            fixation device — *code to* fracture with
                seventh character D
            prosthesis, prosthetic device Z44.9
                breast Z44.3-
                specified NEC Z44.8
        implanted device NEC Z45.89
        insulin pump Z46.81
        internal fixation device Z47.2
        myringotomy device (stent) (tube) Z45.82
        nervous system device NEC Z46.2
            brain neuropacemaker Z46.2
            visual substitution device Z46.2
                implanted Z45.31
        non-vascular catheter Z46.82
        orthodontic device Z46.4
        stent
            ureteral Z46.6
        urinary device Z46.6
    repeat cervical smear to confirm findings of
        recent normal smear following initial
        abnormal smear Z01.42
    respirator [ventilator] use during power failure
        Z99.12
    Rh typing Z01.83
    screening — *see* Screening
    specified NEC Z76.89
    sterilization Z30.2
    suspected condition, ruled out
        amniotic cavity and membrane Z03.71
        cervical shortening Z03.75
        fetal anomaly Z03.73
        fetal growth Z03.74
        maternal and fetal conditions NEC Z03.79
        oligohydramnios Z03.71
        placental problem Z03.72
        polyhydramnios Z03.71
    suspected exposure (to), ruled out
        anthrax Z03.810
        biological agents NEC Z03.818
    termination of pregnancy, elective Z33.2
    testing — *see* Test
    therapeutic drug level monitoring Z51.81
    titration, insulin pump Z46.81
    to determine fetal viability of pregnancy
        O36.80
    training
        insulin pump Z46.81
    X-ray of chest (as part of a general medical
        examination) Z00.00
        with abnormal findings Z00.01
Encystment — *see* Cyst
Endarteritis (bacterial, subacute) (infective)
    I77.6
    brain I67.7
    cerebral or cerebrospinal I67.7
    deformans — *see* Arteriosclerosis
    embolic — *see* Embolism
    obliterans — *see also* Arteriosclerosis
        pulmonary I28.8
    pulmonary I28.8
    retina — *see* Vasculitis, retina
    senile — *see* Arteriosclerosis
    syphilitic A52.09
        brain or cerebral A52.04
        congenital A50.54 *[I79.8]*
    tuberculous A18.89
Endemic — *see* condition

Endocarditis (chronic) (marantic)
(nonbacterial) (thrombotic) (valvular) I38
　with rheumatic fever (conditions in I00)
　　active — *see* Endocarditis, acute, rheumatic
　　inactive or quiescent (with chorea) I09.1
　acute or subacute I33.9
　　infective I33.0
　　rheumatic (aortic) (mitral) (pulmonary)
　　　(tricuspid) I01.1
　　　with chorea (acute) (rheumatic)
　　　　(Sydenham's) I02.0
　aortic (heart) (nonrheumatic) (valve) I35.8
　　with
　　　mitral disease I08.0
　　　　with tricuspid (valve) disease I08.3
　　　　active or acute I01.1
　　　　　with chorea (acute) (rheumatic)
　　　　　　(Sydenham's) I02.0
　　　rheumatic fever (conditions in I00)
　　　　active — *see* Endocarditis, acute,
　　　　　rheumatic
　　　　inactive or quiescent (with chorea) I06.9
　　　tricuspid (valve) disease I08.2
　　　　with mitral (valve) disease I08.3
　　acute or subacute I33.9
　　arteriosclerotic I35.8
　　rheumatic I06.9
　　　with mitral disease I08.0
　　　　with tricuspid (valve) disease I08.3
　　　　active or acute I01.1
　　　　　with chorea (acute) (rheumatic)
　　　　　　(Sydenham's) I02.0
　　　active or acute I01.1
　　　　with chorea (acute) (rheumatic)
　　　　　(Sydenham's) I02.0
　　　specified NEC I06.8
　　specified cause NEC I35.8
　　syphilitic A52.03
　arteriosclerotic I38
　atypical verrucous (Libman-Sacks) M32.11
　bacterial (acute) (any valve) (subacute) I33.0
　candidal B37.6
　congenital Q24.8
　constrictive I33.0
　Coxiella burnetii A78 *[I39]*
　Coxsackie B33.21
　due to
　　prosthetic cardiac valve T82.6
　　Q fever A78 *[I39]*
　　Serratia marcescens I33.0
　　typhoid (fever) A01.02
　gonococcal A54.83
　infectious or infective (acute) (any valve)
　　(subacute) I33.0
　lenta (acute) (any valve) (subacute) I33.0
　Libman-Sacks M32.11
　listerial A32.82
　Löffler's I42.3
　malignant (acute) (any valve) (subacute) I33.0
　meningococcal A39.51
　mitral (chronic) (double) (fibroid) (heart)
　　(inactive) (valve) (with chorea) I05.9
　　with
　　　aortic (valve) disease I08.0
　　　　with tricuspid (valve) disease I08.3
　　　　active or acute I01.1
　　　　　with chorea (acute) (rheumatic)
　　　　　　(Sydenham's) I02.0
　　　rheumatic fever (conditions in I00)
　　　　active — *see* Endocarditis, acute,
　　　　　rheumatic
　　　　inactive or quiescent (with chorea) I05.9
　　　tricuspid (valve) disease I08.1
　　　　with aortic (valve) disease I08.3
　　active or acute I01.1
　　　with chorea (acute) (rheumatic)
　　　　(Sydenham's) I02.0
　　bacterial I33.0

Endocarditis (chronic) (marantic)
(nonbacterial) (thrombotic) (valvular) I38 —
continued
　mitral (chronic) (double) (fibroid) (heart)
　　(inactive) (valve) (with chorea) I05.9 —
　　continued
　　arteriosclerotic I34.8
　　nonrheumatic I34.8
　　　acute or subacute I33.9
　　specified NEC I05.8
　monilial B37.6
　multiple valves I08.9
　　specified disorders I08.8
　mycotic (acute) (any valve) (subacute) I33.0
　pneumococcal (acute) (any valve) (subacute)
　　I33.0
　pulmonary (chronic) (heart) (valve) I37.8
　　with rheumatic fever (conditions in I00)
　　　active — *see* Endocarditis, acute,
　　　　rheumatic
　　　inactive or quiescent (with chorea) I09.89
　　　　with aortic, mitral or tricuspid disease
　　　　　I08.8
　　acute or subacute I33.9
　　　rheumatic I01.1
　　　　with chorea (acute) (rheumatic)
　　　　　(Sydenham's) I02.0
　　arteriosclerotic I37.8
　　congenital Q22.2
　　rheumatic (chronic) (inactive) (with chorea)
　　　I09.89
　　　active or acute I01.1
　　　　with chorea (acute) (rheumatic)
　　　　　(Sydenham's) I02.0
　　syphilitic A52.03
　purulent (acute) (any valve) (subacute) I33.0
　Q fever A78 *[I39]*
　rheumatic (chronic) (inactive) (with chorea)
　　I09.1
　　active or acute (aortic) (mitral) (pulmonary)
　　　(tricuspid) I01.1
　　　with chorea (acute) (rheumatic)
　　　　(Sydenham's) I02.0
　rheumatoid — *see* Rheumatoid, carditis
　septic (acute) (any valve) (subacute) I33.0
　streptococcal (acute) (any valve) (subacute)
　　I33.0
　subacute — *see* Endocarditis, acute
　suppurative (acute) (any valve) (subacute)
　　I33.0
　syphilitic A52.03
　toxic I33.9
　tricuspid (chronic) (heart) (inactive) (rheumatic)
　　(valve) (with chorea) I07.9
　　with
　　　aortic (valve) disease I08.2
　　　　mitral (valve) disease I08.3
　　　mitral (valve) disease I08.1
　　　　aortic (valve) disease I08.3
　　　rheumatic fever (conditions in I00)
　　　　active — *see* Endocarditis, acute,
　　　　　rheumatic
　　　　inactive or quiescent (with chorea) I07.8
　　active or acute I01.1
　　　with chorea (acute) (rheumatic)
　　　　(Sydenham's) I02.0
　　arteriosclerotic I36.8
　　nonrheumatic I36.8
　　　acute or subacute I33.9
　　specified cause, except rheumatic I36.8
　tuberculous — *see* Tuberculosis, endocarditis
　typhoid A01.02
　ulcerative (acute) (any valve) (subacute) I33.0
　vegetative (acute) (any valve) (subacute) I33.0
　verrucous (atypical) (nonbacterial)
　　(nonrheumatic) M32.11
Endocardium, endocardial — *see also*
　condition
　cushion defect Q21.2

Endocervicitis — *see also* Cervicitis
　due to intrauterine (contraceptive) device
　　T83.69
　hyperplastic N72
Endocrine — *see* condition
Endocrinopathy, pluriglandular E31.9
Endodontic
　overfill M27.52
　underfill M27.53
Endodontitis K04.01
　irreversible K04.02
　reversible K04.01
Endomastoiditis — *see* Mastoiditis
Endometrioma N80.9
Endometriosis N80.9
　appendix N80.5
　bladder N80.8
　bowel N80.5
　broad ligament N80.3
　cervix N80.0
　colon N80.5
　cul-de-sac (Douglas') N80.3
　exocervix N80.0
　fallopian tube N80.2
　female genital organ NEC N80.8
　gallbladder N80.8
　in scar of skin N80.6
　internal N80.0
　intestine N80.5
　lung N80.8
　myometrium N80.0
　ovary N80.1
　parametrium N80.3
　pelvic peritoneum N80.3
　peritoneal (pelvic) N80.3
　rectovaginal septum N80.4
　rectum N80.5
　round ligament N80.3
　skin (scar) N80.6
　specified site NEC N80.8
　stromal D39.0
　umbilicus N80.8
　uterus (internal) N80.0
　vagina N80.4
　vulva N80.8
Endometritis (decidual) (nonspecific) (purulent)
　(senile) (atrophic) (suppurative) N71.9
　with ectopic pregnancy O08.0
　acute N71.0
　blenorrhagic (gonococcal) (acute) (chronic)
　　A54.24
　cervix, cervical (with erosion or ectropion) —
　　see also Cervicitis
　　hyperplastic N72
　chlamydial A56.11
　chronic N71.1
　following
　　abortion — *see* Abortion by type
　　　complicated by genital infection
　　ectopic or molar pregnancy O08.0
　gonococcal, gonorrheal (acute) (chronic)
　　A54.24
　hyperplastic (*see also* Hyperplasia, endometrial)
　　N85.00-
　　cervix N72
　puerperal, postpartum, childbirth O86.12
　subacute N71.0
　tuberculous A18.17
Endometrium — *see* condition
Endomyocardiopathy, South African I42.3
Endomyocarditis — *see* Endocarditis
Endomyofibrosis I42.3
Endomyometritis — *see* Endometritis
Endopericarditis — *see* Endocarditis
Endoperineuritis — *see* Disorder, nerve
Endophlebitis — *see* Phlebitis
Endophthalmia — *see* Endophthalmitis,
　purulent

Endophthalmitis (acute) (infective) (metastatic) (subacute) H44.009
  bleb associated H59.4 — *see also* Bleb, inflammed (infected), postprocedural
  gonorrheal A54.39
  in (due to)
    cysticercosis B69.1
    onchocerciasis B73.01
    toxocariasis B83.0
  panuveitis — *see* Panuveitis
  parasitic H44.12-
  purulent H44.00-
    panophthalmitis — *see* Panophthalmitis
    vitreous abscess H44.02-
  specified NEC H44.19
  sympathetic — *see* Uveitis, sympathetic
Endosalpingioma D28.2
Endosalpingiosis N94.89
Endosteitis — *see* Osteomyelitis
Endothelioma, bone — *see* Neoplasm, bone, malignant
Endotheliosis (hemorrhagic infectional) D69.8
Endotoxemia — *code to* condition
Endotrachelitis — *see* Cervicitis
Engelmann(-Camurati) syndrome Q78.3
English disease — *see* Rickets
Engman's disease L30.3
Engorgement
  breast N64.59
    newborn P83.4
    puerperal, postpartum O92.79
  lung (passive) — *see* Edema, lung
  pulmonary (passive) — *see* Edema, lung
  stomach K31.89
  venous, retina — *see* Occlusion, retina, vein, engorgement
Enlargement, enlarged — *see also* Hypertrophy
  adenoids J35.2
    with tonsils J35.3
  alveolar ridge K08.89
    congenital — *see* Anomaly, alveolar
  apertures of diaphragm (congenital) Q79.1
  gingival K06.1
  heart, cardiac — *see* Hypertrophy, cardiac
  labium majus, childhood asymmetric (CALME) N90.61
  lacrimal gland, chronic H04.03-
  liver — *see* Hypertrophy, liver
  lymph gland or node R59.9
    generalized R59.1
    localized R59.0
  orbit H05.34-
  organ or site, congenital NEC — *see* Anomaly, by site
  parathyroid (gland) E21.0
  pituitary fossa R93.0
  prostate N40.0
    with lower urinary tract symptoms (LUTS) N40.1
    without lower urinary tract symtpoms (LUTS) N40.0
  sella turcica R93.0
  spleen — *see* Splenomegaly
  thymus (gland) (congenital) E32.0
  thyroid (gland) — *see* Goiter
  tongue K14.8
  tonsils J35.1
    with adenoids J35.3
  uterus N85.2
Enophthalmos H05.40-
  due to
    orbital tissue atrophy H05.41-
    trauma or surgery H05.42-
Enostosis M27.8
Entamebic, entamebiasis — *see* Amebiasis

Entanglement
  umbilical cord(s) O69.2
    with compression O69.2
      without compression O69.82
    around neck (with compression) O69.1
      without compression O69.81
    of twins in monoamniotic sac O69.2
Enteralgia — *see* Pain, abdominal
Enteric — *see* condition
Enteritis (acute) (diarrheal) (hemorrhagic) (noninfective) K52.9
  adenovirus A08.2
  aertrycke infection A02.0
  allergic K52.29
    with
      eosinophilic gastritis or gastroenteritis K52.81
      food protein-induced enterocolitis syndrome K52.21
      food protein-induced enteropathy K52.22
  amebic (acute) A06.0
    with abscess — *see* Abscess, amebic
    chronic A06.1
      with abscess — *see* Abscess, amebic
      nondysenteric A06.2
    nondysenteric A06.2
  astrovirus A08.32
  bacillary NOS A03.9
  bacterial A04.9
    specified NEC A04.8
  calicivirus A08.31
  candidal B37.82
  Chilomastix A07.8
  choleriformis A00.1
  chronic (noninfectious) K52.9
    ulcerative — *see* Colitis, ulcerative
  cicatrizing (chronic) — *see* Enteritis, regional, small intestine
  Clostridium
    botulinum (food poisoning) A05.1
    difficile A04.7
  coccidial A07.3
  coxsackie virus A08.39
  dietetic (*see also* Enteritis, allergic) K52.29
  drug-induced K52.1
  due to
    astrovirus A08.32
    calicivirus A08.31
    coxsackie virus A08.39
    drugs K52.1
    echovirus A08.39
    enterovirus NEC A08.39
    food hypersensitivity (*see also* Enteritis, allergic) K52.29
    infectious organism (bacterial) (viral) — *see* Enteritis, infectious
    torovirus A08.39
    Yersinia enterocolitica A04.6
  echovirus A08.39
  eltor A00.1
  enterovirus NEC A08.39
  eosinophilic K52.81
  epidemic (infectious) A09
  fulminant (*see also* Ischemia, intestine, acute) K55.019
  gangrenous — *see* Enteritis, infectious
  giardial A07.1
  infectious NOS A09
    due to
      adenovirus A08.2
      Aerobacter aerogenes A04.8
      Arizona (bacillus) A02.0
      bacteria NOS A04.9
        specified NEC A04.8
      Campylobacter A04.5
      Clostridium difficile A04.7
      Clostridium perfringens A04.8
      Enterobacter aerogenes A04.8
      enterovirus A08.39

Enteritis (acute) (diarrheal) (hemorrhagic) (noninfective) K52.9 — *continued*
  infectious NOS A09 — *continued*
    due to — *continued*
      Escherichia coli A04.4
        enteroaggregative A04.4
        enterohemorrhagic A04.3
        enteroinvasive A04.2
        enteropathogenic A04.0
        enterotoxigenic A04.1
        specified NEC A04.4
      specified
        bacteria NEC A04.8
        virus NEC A08.39
      Staphylococcus A04.8
      virus NEC A08.4
        specified type NEC A08.39
      Yersinia enterocolitica A04.6
      specified organism NEC A08.8
  influenzal — *see* Influenza, with, digestive manifestations
  ischemic K55.9
    acute (*see also* Ischemia, intestine, acute) K55.019
    chronic K55.1
  microsporidial A07.8
  mucomembranous, myxomembranous — *see* Syndrome, irritable bowel
  mucous — *see* Syndrome, irritable bowel
  necroticans A05.2
  necrotizing of newborn — *see* Enterocolitis, necrotizing, in newborn
  neurogenic — *see* Syndrome, irritable bowel
  newborn necrotizing — *see* Enterocolitis, necrotizing, in newborn
  noninfectious K52.9
  norovirus A08.11
  parasitic NEC B82.9
  paratyphoid (fever) — *see* Fever, paratyphoid
  protozoal A07.9
    specified NEC A07.8
  radiation K52.0
  regional (of) K50.90
    with
      complication K50.919
        abscess K50.914
        fistula K50.913
        intestinal obstruction K50.912
        rectal bleeding K50.911
        specified complication NEC K50.918
    colon — *see* Enteritis, regional, large intestine
    duodenum — *see* Enteritis, regional, small intestine
    ileum — *see* Enteritis, regional, small intestine
    jejunum — *see* Enteritis, regional, small intestine
    large bowel — *see* Enteritis, regional, large intestine
    large intestine (colon) (rectum) K50.10
      with
        complication K50.119
          abscess K50.114
          fistula K50.113
          intestinal obstruction K50.112
          rectal bleeding K50.111
          small intestine (duodenum) (ileum) (jejunum) involvement K50.80
          with
            complication K50.819
              abscess K50.814
              fistula K50.813
              intestinal obstruction K50.812
              rectal bleeding K50.811
              specified complication NEC K50.818
        specified complication NEC K50.118

Enteritis (acute) (diarrheal) (hemorrhagic)
(noninfective) K52.9 — *continued*
  regional (of) K50.90 — *continued*
    rectum — *see* Enteritis, regional, large
      intestine
    small intestine (duodenum) (ileum) (jejunum)
      K50.00
      with
        complication K50.019
          abscess K50.014
          fistula K50.013
          intestinal obstruction K50.012
          large intestine (colon) (rectum)
            involvement K50.80
            with
              complication K50.819
                abscess K50.814
                fistula K50.813
                intestinal obstruction K50.812
                rectal bleeding K50.811
                specified complication NEC
                  K50.818
          rectal bleeding K50.011
          specified complication NEC K50.018
  rotaviral A08.0
  Salmonella, salmonellosis (arizonae)
    (cholerae-suis) (enteritidis) (typhimurium)
    A02.0
  segmental — *see* Enteritis, regional
  septic A09
  Shigella — *see* Infection, Shigella
  small round structured NEC A08.19
  spasmodic, spastic — *see* Syndrome, irritable
    bowel
  staphylococcal A04.8
    due to food A05.0
  torovirus A08.39
  toxic NEC K52.1
    due to Clostridium difficile A04.7
  trichomonal A07.8
  tuberculous A18.32
  typhosa A01.00
  ulcerative (chronic) — *see* Colitis, ulcerative
  viral A08.4
    adenovirus A08.2
    enterovirus A08.39
    Rotavirus A08.0
    small round structured NEC A08.19
    specified NEC A08.39
    virus specified NEC A08.39
Enterobiasis B80
Enterobius vermicularis (infection)
(infestation) B80
Enterocele — *see also* Hernia, abdomen
  pelvic, pelvis (acquired) (congenital) N81.5
  vagina, vaginal (acquired) (congenital) NEC
    N81.5
Enterocolitis (*see also* Enteritis) K52.9
  due to Clostridium difficile A04.7
  fulminant ischemic (*see also* Ischemia, intestine,
    acute) K55.059
  granulomatous — *see* Enteritis, regional
  hemorrhagic (acute) (*see also* Ischemia,
    intestine, acute) K55.059
    chronic K55.1
  infectious NEC A09
  ischemic K55.9
  necrotizing
    with
      perforation K55.33
      pneumatosis K55.32
        and perforation K55.33
    due to Clostridium difficile A04.7
    in newborn P77.9
      stage 1 (without pneumatosis, without
        perforation) P77.1
      stage 2 (with pneumatosis, without
        perforation) P77.2

Enterocolitis (*see also* Enteritis) K52.9 —
continued
  necrotizing — *continued*
    in newborn P77.9 — *continued*
      stage 3 (with pneumatosis, with
        perforation) P77.3
    in non-newborn K55.30
      stage 1 (without pneumatosis, without
        perforation) K55.31
      stage 2 (with pneumatosis, without
        perforation) K55.32
      stage 3 (with pneumatosis, with
        perforation) K55.33
    without pneumatosis or perforation K55.31
  noninfectious K52.9
    newborn — *see* Enterocolitis, necrotizing, in
      newborn
  pseudomembranous (newborn) A04.7
  radiation K52.0
    newborn — *see* Enterocolitis, necrotizing, in
      newborn
  ulcerative (chronic) — *see* Pancolitis, ulcerative
    (chronic)
Enterogastritis — *see* Enteritis
Enteropathy K63.9
  food protein-induced enterocolitis K52.22
  gluten-sensitive K90.0
    non-celiac K90.41
  hemorrhagic, terminal (*see also* Ischemia,
    intestine, acute) K55.059
  protein-losing K90.49
Enteroperitonitis — *see* Peritonitis
Enteroptosis K63.4
Enterorrhagia K92.2
Enterospasm — *see also* Syndrome, irritable,
  bowel
  psychogenic F45.8
Enterostenosis — *see also* Obstruction,
  intestine K56.69
Enterostomy
  complication — *see* Complication, enterostomy
  status Z93.4
Enterovirus, as cause of disease
  classified elsewhere B97.10
  coxsackievirus B97.11
  echovirus B97.12
  other specified B97.19
Enthesopathy (peripheral) M77.9
  Achilles tendinitis — *see* Tendinitis, Achilles
  ankle and tarsus M77.9
    specified type NEC — *see* Enthesopathy,
      foot, specified type NEC
  anterior tibial syndrome M76.81-
  calcaneal spur — *see* Spur, bone, calcaneal
  elbow region M77.8
    lateral epicondylitis — *see* Epicondylitis,
      lateral
    medial epicondylitis — *see* Epicondylitis,
      medial
  foot NEC M77.9
    metatarsalgia — *see* Metatarsalgia
    specified type NEC M77.5-
  forearm M77.9
  gluteal tendinitis — *see* Tendinitis, gluteal
  hand M77.9
  hip — *see* Enthesopathy, lower limb, specified
    type NEC
  iliac crest spur — *see* Spur, bone, iliac crest
  iliotibial band syndrome — *see* Syndrome,
    iliotibial band
  knee — *see* Enthesopathy, lower limb, lower
    leg, specified type NEC
  lateral epicondylitis — *see* Epicondylitis, lateral
  lower limb (excluding foot) M76.9
    Achilles tendinitis — *see* Tendinitis, Achilles
    anterior tibial syndrome M76.81-
    gluteal tendinitis — *see* Tendinitis, gluteal
    iliac crest spur — *see* Spur, bone, iliac crest

Enthesopathy (peripheral) M77.9 —
continued
  lower limb (excluding foot) M76.9 —
    continued
    iliotibial band syndrome — *see* Syndrome,
      iliotibial band
    patellar tendinitis — *see* Tendinitis, patellar
    pelvic region — *see* Enthesopathy, lower
      limb, specified type NEC
    peroneal tendinitis — *see* Tendinitis, peroneal
    posterior tibial syndrome M76.82-
    psoas tendinitis — *see* Tendinitis, psoas
    specified type NEC M76.89-
    tibial collateral bursitis — *see* Bursitis, tibial
      collateral
  medial epicondylitis — *see* Epicondylitis,
    medial
  metatarsalgia — *see* Metatarsalgia
  multiple sites M77.9
  patellar tendinitis — *see* Tendinitis, patellar
  pelvis M77.9
  periarthritis of wrist — *see* Periarthritis, wrist
  peroneal tendinitis — *see* Tendinitis, peroneal
  posterior tibial syndrome M76.82-
  psoas tendinitis — *see* Tendinitis, psoas
  shoulder M77.9
  shoulder region — *see* Lesion, shoulder
  specified site NEC M77.9
  specified type NEC M77.8
  spinal M46.00
    cervical region M46.02
    cervicothoracic region M46.03
    lumbar region M46.06
    lumbosacral region M46.07
    multiple sites M46.09
    occipito-atlanto-axial region M46.01
    sacrococcygeal region M46.08
    thoracic region M46.04
    thoracolumbar region M46.05
  tibial collateral bursitis — *see* Bursitis, tibial
    collateral
  upper arm M77.9
  wrist and carpus NEC M77.8
    calcaneal spur — *see* Spur, bone, calcaneal
    periarthritis of wrist — *see* Periarthritis, wrist
Entomophobia F40.218
Entomophthoromycosis B46.8
Entrance, air into vein — *see* Embolism, air
Entrapment, nerve — *see* Neuropathy,
  entrapment
Entropion (eyelid) (paralytic) H02.009
  cicatricial H02.019
    left H02.016
      lower H02.015
      upper H02.014
    right H02.013
      lower H02.012
      upper H02.011
  congenital Q10.2
  left H02.006
    lower H02.005
    upper H02.004
  mechanical H02.029
    left H02.026
      lower H02.025
      upper H02.024
    right H02.023
      lower H02.022
      upper H02.021
  right H02.003
    lower H02.002
    upper H02.001
  senile H02.039
    left H02.036
      lower H02.035
      upper H02.034
    right H02.033
      lower H02.032
      upper H02.031

Entropion (eyelid) (paralytic) H02.009 — *continued*
  spastic H02.049
    left H02.046
      lower H02.045
      upper H02.044
    right H02.043
      lower H02.042
      upper H02.041
Enucleated eye (traumatic, current) S05.7-
Enuresis R32
  functional F98.0
  habit disturbance F98.0
  nocturnal N39.44
    psychogenic F98.0
  nonorganic origin F98.0
  psychogenic F98.0
Eosinopenia — *see* Agranulocytosis
Eosinophilia (allergic) (hereditary) (idiopathic) (secondary) D72.1
  with
    angiolymphoid hyperplasia (ALHE) D18.01
  infiltrative J82
  Löffler's J82
  peritoneal — *see* Peritonitis, eosinophilic
  pulmonary NEC J82
  tropical (pulmonary) J82
Eosinophilia-myalgia syndrome M35.8
Ependymitis (acute) (cerebral) (chronic) (granular) — *see* Encephalomyelitis
Ependymoblastoma
  specified site — *see* Neoplasm, malignant, by site
  unspecified site C71.9
Ependymoma (epithelial) (malignant)
  anaplastic
    specified site — *see* Neoplasm, malignant, by site
    unspecified site C71.9
  benign
    specified site — *see* Neoplasm, benign, by site
    unspecified site D33.2
  myxopapillary D43.2
    specified site — *see* Neoplasm, uncertain behavior, by site
    unspecified site D43.2
  papillary D43.2
    specified site — *see* Neoplasm, uncertain behavior, by site
    unspecified site D43.2
  specified site — *see* Neoplasm, malignant, by site
  unspecified site C71.9
Ependymopathy G93.89
Ephelis, ephelides L81.2
Epiblepharon (congenital) Q10.3
Epicanthus, epicanthic fold (eyelid) (congenital) Q10.3
Epicondylitis (elbow)
  lateral M77.1-
  medial M77.0-
Epicystitis — *see* Cystitis
Epidemic — *see* condition
Epidermidalization, cervix — *see* Dysplasia, cervix
Epidermis, epidermal — *see* condition
Epidermodysplasia verruciformis B07.8
Epidermolysis
  bullosa (congenital) Q81.9
    acquired L12.30
      drug-induced L12.31
      specified cause NEC L12.35
    dystrophica Q81.2
    letalis Q81.1
    simplex Q81.0
    specified NEC Q81.8
  necroticans combustiformis L51.2

Epidermolysis — *continued*
  due to drug — *see* Table of Drugs and Chemicals, by drug
Epidermophytid — *see* Dermatophytosis
Epidermophytosis (infected) — *see* Dermatophytosis
Epididymis — *see* condition
Epididymitis (acute) (nonvenereal) (recurrent) (residual) N45.1
  with orchitis N45.3
  blennorrhagic (gonococcal) A54.23
  caseous (tuberculous) A18.15
  chlamydial A56.19
  filarial (*see also* Infestation, filarial) B74.9 [N51]
  gonococcal A54.23
  syphilitic A52.76
  tuberculous A18.15
Epididymo-orchitis (*see also* Epididymitis) N45.3
Epidural — *see* condition
Epigastrium, epigastric — *see* condition
Epigastrocele — *see* Hernia, ventral
Epiglottis — *see* condition
Epiglottitis, epiglottiditis (acute) J05.10
  with obstruction J05.11
  chronic J37.0
Epignathus Q89.4
Epilepsia partialis continua (*see also* Kozhevnikof's epilepsy) G40.1-
Epilepsy, epileptic, epilepsia (attack) (cerebral) (convulsion) (fit) (seizure) G40.909
Note: The following terms are to be considered equivalent to intractable: pharmacoresistant (pharmacologically resistant), treatment resistant, refractory (medically) and poorly controlled
  with
    complex partial seizures — *see* Epilepsy, localization-related, symptomatic, with complex partial seizures
    grand mal seizures on awakening — *see* Epilepsy, generalized, specified NEC
    myoclonic absences — *see* Epilepsy, generalized, specified NEC
    myoclonic-astatic seizures — *see* Epilepsy, generalized, specified NEC
    simple partial seizures — *see* Epilepsy, localization-related, symptomatic, with simple partial seizures
  akinetic — *see* Epilepsy, generalized, specified NEC
  benign childhood with centrotemporal EEG spikes — *see* Epilepsy, localization-related, idiopathic
  benign myoclonic in infancy G40.80-
  Bravais-jacksonian — *see* Epilepsy, localization-related, symptomatic, with simple partial seizures
  childhood
    with occipital EEG paroxysms — *see* Epilepsy, localization-related, idiopathic
    absence G40.A09 *(follows G40.3)*
      intractable G40.A19 *(follows G40.3)*
        with status epilepticus G40.A11 *(follows G40.3)*
        without status epilepticus G40.A19 *(follows G40.3)*
      not intractable G40.A09 *(follows G40.3)*
        with status epilepticus G40.A01 *(follows G40.3)*
        without status epilepticus G40.A09 *(follows G40.3)*
  climacteric — *see* Epilepsy, specified NEC
  cysticercosis B69.0
  deterioration (mental) F06.8
  due to syphilis A52.19

Epilepsy, epileptic, epilepsia (attack) (cerebral) (convulsion) (fit) (seizure) G40.909 — *continued*
  focal — *see* Epilepsy, localization-related, symptomatic, with simple partial seizures
  generalized
    idiopathic G40.309
      intractable G40.319
        with status epilepticus G40.311
        without status epilepticus G40.319
      not intractable G40.309
        with status epilepticus G40.301
        without status epilepticus G40.309
    specified NEC G40.409
      intractable G40.419
        with status epilepticus G40.411
        without status epilepticus G40.419
      not intractable G40.409
        with status epilepticus G40.401
        without status epilepticus G40.409
  impulsive petit mal — *see* Epilepsy, juvenile myoclonic
  intractable G40.919
    with status epilepticus G40.911
    without status epilepticus G40.919
  juvenile absence G40.A09 *(follows G40.3)*
    intractable G40.A19 *(follows G40.3)*
      with status epilepticus G40.A11 *(follows G40.3)*
      without status epilepticus G40.A19 *(follows G40.3)*
    not intractable G40.A09 *(follows G40.3)*
      with status epilepticus G40.A01 *(follows G40.3)*
      without status epilepticus G40.A09 *(follows G40.3)*
  juvenile myoclonic G40.B09 *(follows G40.3)*
    intractable G40.B19 *(follows G40.3)*
      with status epilepticus G40.B11 *(follows G40.3)*
      without status epilepticus G40.B19 *(follows G40.3)*
    not intractable G40.B09 *(follows G40.3)*
      with status epilepticus G40.B01 *(follows G40.3)*
      without status epilepticus G40.B09 *(follows G40.3)*
  localization-related (focal) (partial)
    idiopathic G40.009
      with seizures of localized onset G40.009
        intractable G40.019
          with status epilepticus G40.011
          without status epilepticus G40.019
        not intractable G40.009
          with status epilepticus G40.001
          without status epilepticus G40.009
    symptomatic
      with complex partial seizures G40.209
        intractable G40.219
          with status epilepticus G40.211
          without status epilepticus G40.219
        not intractable G40.209
          with status epilepticus G40.201
          without status epilepticus G40.209
      with simple partial seizures G40.109
        intractable G40.119
          with status epilepticus G40.111
          without status epilepticus G40.119
        not intractable G40.109
          with status epilepticus G40.101
          without status epilepticus G40.109
  myoclonus, myoclonic — *see* Epilepsy, generalized, specified NEC
  progressive — *see* Epilepsy, generalized, idiopathic
  not intractable G40.909
    with status epilepticus G40.901
    without status epilepticus G40.909

Epilepsy, epileptic, epilepsia (attack) (cerebral) (convulsion) (fit) (seizure) G40.909 — *continued*
on awakening — *see* Epilepsy, generalized, specified NEC
parasitic NOS B71.9 *[G94]*
partialis continua (*see also* Kozhevnikof's epilepsy) G40.1-
peripheral — *see* Epilepsy, specified NEC
procursiva — *see* Epilepsy, localization-related, symptomatic, with simple partial seizures
progressive (familial) myoclonic — *see* Epilepsy, generalized, idiopathic
reflex — *see* Epilepsy, specified NEC
related to
  alcohol G40.509
    not intractable G40.509
      with status epilepticus G40.501
      without status epilepticus G40.509
  drugs G40.509
    not intractable G40.509
      with status epilepticus G40.501
      without status epilepticus G40.509
  external causes G40.509
    not intractable G40.509
      with status epilepticus G40.501
      without status epilepticus G40.509
  hormonal changes G40.509
    not intractable G40.509
      with status epilepticus G40.501
      without status epilepticus G40.509
  sleep deprivation G40.509
    not intractable G40.509
      with status epilepticus G40.501
      without status epilepticus G40.509
  stress G40.509
    not intractable G40.509
      with status epilepticus G40.501
      without status epilepticus G40.509
somatomotor — *see* Epilepsy, localization-related, symptomatic, with simple partial seizures
somatosensory — *see* Epilepsy, localization-related, symptomatic, with simple partial seizures
spasms G40.822
  intractable G40.824
    with status epilepticus G40.823
    without status epilepticus G40.824
  not intractable G40.822
    with status epilepticus G40.821
    without status epilepticus G40.822
specified NEC G40.802
  intractable G40.804
    with status epilepticus G40.803
    without status epilepticus G40.804
  not intractable G40.802
    with status epilepticus G40.801
    without status epilepticus G40.802
syndromes
  generalized
    idiopathic G40.309
      intractable G40.319
        with status epilepticus G40.311
        without status epilepticus G40.319
      not intractable G40.309
        with status epilepticus G40.301
        without status epilepticus G40.309
    specified NEC G40.409
      intractable G40.419
        with status epilepticus G40.411
        without status epilepticus G40.419
      not intractable G40.409
        with status epilepticus G40.401
        without status epilepticus G40.409

Epilepsy, epileptic, epilepsia (attack) (cerebral) (convulsion) (fit) (seizure) G40.909 — *continued*
syndromes — *continued*
  localization-related (focal) (partial)
    idiopathic G40.009
      with seizures of localized onset G40.009
        intractable G40.019
          with status epilepticus G40.011
          without status epilepticus G40.019
        not intractable G40.009
          with status epilepticus G40.001
          without status epilepticus G40.009
    symptomatic
      with complex partial seizures G40.209
        intractable G40.219
          with status epilepticus G40.211
          without status epilepticus G40.219
        not intractable G40.209
          with status epilepticus G40.201
          without status epilepticus G40.209
      with simple partial seizures G40.109
        intractable G40.119
          with status epilepticus G40.111
          without status epilepticus G40.119
        not intractable G40.109
          with status epilepticus G40.101
          without status epilepticus G40.109
  specified NEC G40.802
    intractable G40.804
      with status epilepticus G40.803
      without status epilepticus G40.804
    not intractable G40.802
      with status epilepticus G40.801
      without status epilepticus G40.802
tonic(-clonic) — *see* Epilepsy, generalized, specified NEC
twilight F05
uncinate (gyrus) — *see* Epilepsy, localization-related, symptomatic, with complex partial seizures
Unverricht (-Lundborg) (familial myoclonic) — *see* Epilepsy, generalized, idiopathic
visceral — *see* Epilepsy, specified NEC
visual — *see* Epilepsy, specified NEC
Epiloia Q85.1
Epimenorrhea N92.0
Epipharyngitis — *see* Nasopharyngitis
Epiphora H04.20-
due to
  excess lacrimation H04.21-
  insufficient drainage H04.22-
Epiphyseal arrest — *see* Arrest, epiphyseal
Epiphyseolysis, epiphysiolysis — *see* Osteochondropathy
Epiphysitis — *see also* Osteochondropathy
juvenile M92.9
syphilitic (congenital) A50.02
Epiplocele — *see* Hernia, abdomen
Epiploitis — *see* Peritonitis
Epiplosarcomphalocele — *see* Hernia, umbilicus
Episcleritis (suppurative) H15.10-
in (due to)
  syphilis A52.71
  tuberculosis A18.51
nodular H15.12-
periodica fugax H15.11-
  angioneurotic — *see* Edema, angioneurotic
syphilitic (late) A52.71
tuberculous A18.51
Episode
affective, mixed F39
depersonalization (in neurotic state) F48.1

Episode — *continued*
depressive F32.9
  major F32.9
    mild F32.0
    moderate F32.1
    severe (without psychotic symptoms) F32.2
      with psychotic symptoms F32.3
  recurrent F33.9
    brief F33.8
  specified NEC F32.89
hypomanic F30.8
manic F30.9
  with
    psychotic symptoms F30.2
    remission (full) F30.4
      partial F30.3
  other specified F30.8
  recurrent F31.89
  without psychotic symptoms F30.10
    mild F30.11
    moderate F30.12
    severe (without psychotic symptoms) F30.13
      with psychotic symptoms F30.2
psychotic F23
  organic F06.8
schizophrenic (acute) NEC, brief F23
Epispadias (female) (male) Q64.0
Episplenitis D73.89
Epistaxis (multiple) R04.0
hereditary I78.0
vicarious menstruation N94.89
Epithelioma (malignant) — *see also* Neoplasm, malignant, by site
adenoides cysticum — *see* Neoplasm, skin, benign
basal cell — *see* Neoplasm, skin, malignant
benign — *see* Neoplasm, benign, by site
Bowen's — *see* Neoplasm, skin, in situ
calcifying, of Malherbe — *see* Neoplasm, skin, benign
external site — *see* Neoplasm, skin, malignant
intraepidermal, Jadassohn — *see* Neoplasm, skin, benign
squamous cell — *see* Neoplasm, malignant, by site
Epitheliomatosis pigmented Q82.1
Epitheliopathy, multifocal placoid pigment H30.14-
Epithelium, epithelial — *see* condition
Epituberculosis (with atelectasis) (allergic) A15.7
Eponychia Q84.6
Epstein's
nephrosis or syndrome — *see* Nephrosis
pearl K09.8
Epulis (gingiva) (fibrous) (giant cell) K06.8
Equinia A24.0
Equinovarus (congenital) (talipes) Q66.0
acquired — *see* Deformity, limb, clubfoot
Equivalent
convulsive (abdominal) — *see* Epilepsy, specified NEC
epileptic (psychic) — *see* Epilepsy, localization-related, symptomatic, with complex partial seizures
Erb(-Duchenne) paralysis (birth injury) (newborn) P14.0
Erb-Goldflam disease or syndrome G70.00
with exacerbation (acute) G70.01
in crisis G70.01
Erb's
disease G71.0
palsy, paralysis (brachial) (birth) (newborn) P14.0
spinal (spastic) syphilitic A52.17
pseudohypertrophic muscular dystrophy G71.0

Erdheim's syndrome (acromegalic macrospondylitis) E22.0
Erection, painful (persistent) — *see* Priapism
Ergosterol deficiency (vitamin D) E55.9
  with
    adult osteomalacia M83.8
    rickets — *see* Rickets
Ergotism — *see also* Poisoning, food, noxious, plant
  from ergot used as drug (migraine therapy) — *see* Table of Drugs and Chemicals
Erosio interdigitalis blastomycetica B37.2
Erosion
  artery I77.2
    without rupture I77.89
  bone — *see* Disorder, bone, density and structure, specified NEC
  bronchus J98.09
  cartilage (joint) — *see* Disorder, cartilage, specified type NEC
  cervix (uteri) (acquired) (chronic) (congenital) N86
    with cervicitis N72
  cornea (nontraumatic) — *see* Ulcer, cornea
    recurrent H18.83-
    traumatic — *see* Abrasion, cornea
  dental (idiopathic) (occupational) (due to diet, drugs or vomiting) K03.2
  duodenum, postpyloric — *see* Ulcer, duodenum
  esophagus K22.10
    with bleeding K22.11
  gastric — *see* Ulcer, stomach
  gastrojejunal — *see* Ulcer, gastrojejunal
  implanted mesh — *see* Complications, mesh
  intestine K63.3
  lymphatic vessel I89.8
  pylorus, pyloric (ulcer) — *see* Ulcer, stomach
  spine, aneurysmal A52.09
  stomach — *see* Ulcer, stomach
  subcutaneous device pocket
    nervous system prosthetic device, implant, or graft T85.890
    other internal prosthetic device, implant, or graft T85.898
  teeth (idiopathic) (occupational) (due to diet, drugs or vomiting) K03.2
  urethra N36.8
  uterus N85.8
Erotomania F52.8
Error
  metabolism, inborn — *see* Disorder, metabolism
  refractive — *see* Disorder, refraction
Eructation R14.2
  nervous or psychogenic F45.8
Eruption
  creeping B76.9
  drug (generalized) (taken internally) L27.0
    fixed L27.1
    in contact with skin — *see* Dermatitis, due to drugs
    localized L27.1
  Hutchinson, summer L56.4
  Kaposi's varicelliform B00.0
  napkin L22
  polymorphous light (sun) L56.4
  recalcitrant pustular L13.8
  ringed R23.8
  skin (nonspecific) R21
    creeping (meaning hookworm) B76.9
    due to inoculation/vaccination (generalized) (*see also* Dermatitis, due to, vaccine) L27.0
      localized L27.1
    erysipeloid A26.0
    feigned L98.1
    Kaposi's varicelliform B00.0
    lichenoid L28.0
    meaning dermatitis — *see* Dermatitis
    toxic NEC L53.0

Eruption — *continued*
  tooth, teeth, abnormal (incomplete) (late) (premature) (sequence) K00.6
  vesicular R23.8
Erysipelas (gangrenous) (infantile) (newborn) (phlegmonous) (suppurative) A46
  external ear A46 *[H62.40]*
  puerperal, postpartum O86.89
Erysipeloid A26.9
  cutaneous (Rosenbach's) A26.0
  disseminated A26.8
  sepsis A26.7
  specified NEC A26.8
Erythema, erythematous (infectional) (inflammation) L53.9
  ab igne L59.0
  annulare (centrifugum) (rheumaticum) L53.1
  arthriticum epidemicum A25.1
  brucellum — *see* Brucellosis
  chronic figurate NEC L53.3
  chronicum migrans (Borrelia burgdorferi) A69.20
  diaper L22
  due to
    chemical NEC L53.0
      in contact with skin L24.5
    drug (internal use) — *see* Dermatitis, due to, drugs
  elevatum diutinum L95.1
  endemic E52
  epidemic, arthritic A25.1
  figuratum perstans L53.3
  gluteal L22
  heat — *code by* site under Burn, first degree
  ichthyosiforme congenitum bullous Q80.3
  in diseases classified elsewhere L54
  induratum (nontuberculous) L52
    tuberculous A18.4
  infectiosum B08.3
  intertrigo L30.4
  iris L51.9
  marginatum L53.2
    in (due to) acute rheumatic fever I00
  medicamentosum — *see* Dermatitis, due to, drugs
  migrans A26.0
    chronicum A69.20
    tongue K14.1
  multiforme (major) (minor) L51.9
    bullous, bullosum L51.1
    conjunctiva L51.1
    nonbullous L51.0
    pemphigoides L12.0
    specified NEC L51.8
  napkin L22
  neonatorum P83.8
    toxic P83.1
  nodosum L52
    tuberculous A18.4
  palmar L53.8
  pernio T69.1
  rash, newborn P83.8
  scarlatiniform (recurrent) (exfoliative) L53.8
  solare L55.0
  specified NEC L53.8
  toxic, toxicum NEC L53.0
    newborn P83.1
  tuberculous (primary) A18.4
Erythematous, erythematosus — *see* condition
Erythermalgia (primary) I73.81
Erythralgia I73.81
Erythrasma L08.1
Erythredema (polyneuropathy) — *see* Poisoning, mercury
Erythremia (acute) C94.0-
  chronic D45
  secondary D75.1

Erythroblastopenia (*see also* Aplasia, red cell) D60.9
  congenital D61.01
Erythroblastophthisis D61.09
Erythroblastosis (fetalis) (newborn) P55.9
  due to
    ABO (antibodies) (incompatibility) (isoimmunization) P55.1
    Rh (antibodies) (incompatibility) (isoimmunization) P55.0
Erythrocyanosis (crurum) I73.89
Erythrocythemia — *see* Erythremia
Erythrocytosis (megalosplenic) (secondary) D75.1
  familial D75.0
  oval, hereditary — *see* Elliptocytosis
  secondary D75.1
  stress D75.1
Erythroderma (secondary) (*see also* Erythema) L53.9
  bullous ichthyosiform, congenital Q80.3
  desquamativum L21.1
  ichthyosiform, congenital (bullous) Q80.3
  neonatorum P83.8
  psoriaticum L40.8
Erythrodysesthesia, palmar plantar (PPE) L27.1
Erythrogenesis imperfecta D61.09
Erythroleukemia C94.0-
Erythromelalgia I73.81
Erythrophagocytosis D75.89
Erythrophobia F40.298
Erythroplakia, oral epithelium, and tongue K13.29
Erythroplasia (Queyrat) D07.4
  specified site — *see* Neoplasm, skin, in situ
  unspecified site D07.4
Escherichia coli (E. coli), as cause of disease classified elsewhere B96.20
  non-O157 Shiga toxin-producing (with known O group) B96.22
  non-Shiga toxin-producing B96.29
  O157 with confirmation of Shiga toxin when H antigen is unknown, or is not H7 B96.21
  O157:H- (nonmotile) with confirmation of Shiga toxin B96.21
  O157:H7 with or without confirmation of Shiga toxin-production B96.21
  Shiga toxin-producing (with unspecified O group) (STEC) B96.23
    O157 B96.21
    O157:H7 with or without confirmation of Shiga toxin-production B96.21
    specified NEC B96.22
  specified NEC B96.29
Esophagismus K22.4
Esophagitis (acute) (alkaline) (chemical) (chronic) (infectional) (necrotic) (peptic) (postoperative) K20.9
  candidal B37.81
  due to gastrointestinal reflux disease K21.0
  eosinophilic K20.0
  reflux K21.0
  specified NEC K20.8
  tuberculous A18.83
  ulcerative K22.10
    with bleeding K22.11
Esophagocele K22.5
Esophagomalacia K22.8
Esophagospasm K22.4
Esophagostenosis K22.2
Esophagostomiasis B81.8
Esophagotracheal — *see* condition
Esophagus — *see* condition
Esophoria H50.51
  convergence, excess H51.12
  divergence, insufficiency H51.8
Esotropia — *see* Strabismus, convergent concomitant

Espundia B55.2
Essential — *see* condition
Esthesioneuroblastoma C30.0
Esthesioneurocytoma C30.0
Esthesioneuroepithelioma C30.0
Esthiomene A55
Estivo-autumnal malaria (fever) B50.9
Estrangement (marital) Z63.5
  parent-child NEC Z62.890
Estriasis — *see* Myiasis
Ethanolism — *see* Alcoholism
Etherism — *see* Dependence, drug, inhalant
Ethmoid, ethmoidal — *see* condition
Ethmoiditis (chronic) (nonpurulent) (purulent)
  — *see also* Sinusitis, ethmoidal
  influenzal — *see* Influenza, with, respiratory
    manifestations NEC
  Woakes' J33.1
Ethylism — *see* Alcoholism
Eulenburg's disease (congenital
    paramyotonia) G71.19
Eumycetoma B47.0
Eunuchoidism E29.1
  hypogonadotropic E23.0
European blastomycosis — *see*
    Cryptococcosis
Eustachian — *see* condition
Evaluation (for) (of)
  development state
    adolescent Z00.3
    period of
      delayed growth in childhood Z00.70
        with abnormal findings Z00.71
      rapid growth in childhood Z00.2
    puberty Z00.3
  growth and developmental state (period of
      rapid growth) Z00.2
  delayed growth Z00.70
    with abnormal findings Z00.71
  mental health (status) Z00.8
    requested by authority Z04.6
  period of
    delayed growth in childhood Z00.70
      with abnormal findings Z00.71
    rapid growth in childhood Z00.2
  suspected condition — *see* Observation
Evans syndrome D69.41
**Event, apparent life threatening in
    newborn and infant** (ALTE) R68.13
Eventration — *see also* Hernia, ventral
  colon into chest — *see* Hernia, diaphragm
  diaphragm (congenital) Q79.1
Eversion
  bladder N32.89
  cervix (uteri) N86
    with cervicitis N72
  foot NEC — *see also* Deformity, valgus, ankle
    congenital Q66.6
  punctum lacrimale (postinfectional) (senile)
    H04.52-
  ureter (meatus) N28.89
  urethra (meatus) N36.8
  uterus N81.4
Evidence
  cytologic
    of malignancy on anal smear R85.614
    of malignancy on cervical smear R87.614
    of malignancy on vaginal smear R87.624
Evisceration
  birth injury P15.8
  traumatic NEC
    eye — *see* Enucleated eye
Evulsion — *see* Avulsion
Ewing's sarcoma or tumor — *see*
    Neoplasm, bone, malignant

Examination (for) (following) (general) (of)
    (routine) Z00.00
  with abnormal findings Z00.01
  abuse, physical (alleged), ruled out
    adult Z04.71
    child Z04.72
  adolescent (development state) Z00.3
  alleged rape or sexual assault (victim), ruled
      out
    adult Z04.41
    child Z04.42
  allergy Z01.82
  annual (adult) (periodic) (physical) Z00.00
    with abnormal findings Z00.01
    gynecological Z01.419
      with abnormal findings Z01.411
  antibody response Z01.84
  blood — *see* Examination, laboratory
  blood pressure Z01.30
    with abnormal findings Z01.31
  cancer staging — *see* Neoplasm, malignant,
      by site
  cervical Papanicolaou smear Z12.4
    as part of routine gynecological examination
      Z01.419
      with abnormal findings Z01.411
  child (over 28 days old) Z00.129
    with abnormal findings Z00.121
    under 28 days old — *see* Newborn,
        examination
  clinical research control or normal comparison
      (control) (participant) Z00.6
  contraceptive (drug) maintenance (routine)
      Z30.8
    device (intrauterine) Z30.431
  dental Z01.20
    with abnormal findings Z01.21
  developmental — *see* Examination, child
  donor (potential) Z00.5
  ear Z01.10
    with abnormal findings NEC Z01.118
  eye Z01.00
    with abnormal findings Z01.01
  follow-up (routine) (following) Z09
    chemotherapy NEC Z09
      malignant neoplasm Z08
    fracture Z09
    malignant neoplasm Z08
    postpartum Z39.2
    psychotherapy Z09
    radiotherapy NEC Z09
      malignant neoplasm Z08
    surgery NEC Z09
      malignant neoplasm Z08
  following
    accident NEC Z04.3
      transport Z04.1
      work Z04.2
    assault, alleged, ruled out
      adult Z04.71
      child Z04.72
    motor vehicle accident Z04.1
    treatment (for) Z09
      combined NEC Z09
        fracture Z09
        malignant neoplasm Z08
      malignant neoplasm Z08
      mental disorder Z09
      specified condition NEC Z09
  gynecological Z01.419
    with abnormal findings Z01.411
    for contraceptive maintenance Z30.8
  health — *see* Examination, medical
  hearing Z01.10
    with abnormal findings NEC Z01.118
    following failed hearing screening Z01.110
  immunity status testing Z01.84

Examination (for) (following) (general) (of)
    (routine) Z00.00 — *continued*
  laboratory (as part of a general medical
      examination) Z00.00
    with abnormal findings Z00.01
    preprocedural Z01.812
  lactating mother Z39.1
  medical (adult) (for) (of) Z00.00
    with abnormal findings Z00.01
    administrative purpose only Z02.9
      specified NEC Z02.89
    admission to
      armed forces Z02.3
      old age home Z02.2
      prison Z02.89
      residential institution Z02.2
      school Z02.0
        following illness or medical treatment
          Z02.0
      summer camp Z02.89
    adoption Z02.82
    blood alcohol or drug level Z02.83
    camp (summer) Z02.89
    clinical research, normal subject (control)
        (participant) Z00.6
    control subject in clinical research (normal
        comparison) (participant) Z00.6
    donor (potential) Z00.5
    driving license Z02.4
    general (adult) Z00.00
      with abnormal findings Z00.01
    immigration Z02.89
    insurance purposes Z02.6
    marriage Z02.89
    medicolegal reasons NEC Z04.8
    naturalization Z02.89
    participation in sport Z02.5
    paternity testing Z02.81
    population survey Z00.8
    pre-employment Z02.1
    pre-operative — *see* Examination, pre-
        procedural
    pre-procedural
      cardiovascular Z01.810
      respiratory Z01.811
      specified NEC Z01.818
    preschool children
      for admission to school Z02.0
    prisoners
      for entrance into prison Z02.89
    recruitment for armed forces Z02.3
    specified NEC Z00.8
    sport competition Z02.5
  medicolegal reason NEC Z04.8
  newborn — *see* Newborn, examination
  pelvic (annual) (periodic) Z01.419
    with abnormal findings Z01.411
  period of rapid growth in childhood Z00.2
  periodic (adult) (annual) (routine) Z00.00
    with abnormal findings Z00.01
  physical (adult) — *see also* Examination,
      medical Z00.00
    sports Z02.5
  postpartum
    immediately after delivery Z39.0
    routine follow-up Z39.2
  pre-chemotherapy (antineoplastic) Z01.818
  prenatal (normal pregnancy) (*see also*
      Pregnancy, normal) Z34.9-
  pre-procedural (pre-operative)
    cardiovascular Z01.810
    laboratory Z01.812
    respiratory Z01.811
    specified NEC Z01.818
  prior to chemotherapy (antineoplastic)
      Z01.818
  psychiatric NEC Z00.8
    follow-up not needing further care Z09
    requested by authority Z04.6

Examination (for) (following) (general) (of) (routine) Z00.00 — *continued*
  radiological (as part of a general medical examination) Z00.00
    with abnormal findings Z00.01
  repeat cervical smear to confirm findings of recent normal smear following initial abnormal smear Z01.42
  skin (hypersensitivity) Z01.82
  special (*see also* Examination, by type) Z01.89
    specified type NEC Z01.89
  specified type or reason NEC Z04.8
  teeth Z01.20
    with abnormal findings Z01.21
  urine — *see* Examination, laboratory
  vision Z01.00
    with abnormal findings Z01.01

Exanthem, exanthema — *see also* Rash
  with enteroviral vesicular stomatitis B08.4
  Boston A88.0
  epidemic with meningitis A88.0 *[G02]*
  subitum B08.20
    due to human herpesvirus 6 B08.21
    due to human herpesvirus 7 B08.22
  viral, virus B09
    specified type NEC B08.8

Excess, excessive, excessively
  alcohol level in blood R78.0
  androgen (ovarian) E28.1
  attrition, tooth, teeth K03.0
  carotene, carotin (dietary) E67.1
  cold, effects of T69.9
    specified effect NEC T69.8
  convergence H51.12
  crying
    in child, adolescent, or adult R45.83
    in infant R68.11
  development, breast N62
  divergence H51.8
  drinking (alcohol) NEC (without dependence) F10.10
    habitual (continual) (without remission) F10.20
  eating R63.2
  estrogen E28.0
  fat — *see also* Obesity
    in heart — *see* Degeneration, myocardial
    localized E65
  foreskin N47.8
  gas R14.0
  glucagon E16.3
  heat — *see* Heat
  intermaxillary vertical dimension of fully erupted teeth M26.37
  interocclusal distance of fully erupted teeth M26.37
  kalium E87.5
  large
    colon K59.39
      congenital Q43.8
    infant P08.0
    organ or site, congenital NEC — *see* Anomaly, by site
  long
    organ or site, congenital NEC — *see* Anomaly, by site
  menstruation (with regular cycle) N92.0
    with irregular cycle N92.1
  napping Z72.821
  natrium E87.0
  number of teeth K00.1
  nutrient (dietary) NEC R63.2
  potassium (K) E87.5
  salivation K11.7
  secretion — *see also* Hypersecretion
    milk O92.6
    sputum R09.3
    sweat R61
  sexual drive F52.8

Excess, excessive, excessively — *continued*
  short
    organ or site, congenital NEC — *see* Anomaly, by site
    umbilical cord in labor or delivery O69.3
  skin L98.7
    and subcutaneous tissue L98.7
    eyelid (acquired) — *see* Blepharochalasis
      congenital Q10.3
  sodium (Na) E87.0
  spacing of fully erupted teeth M26.32
  sputum R09.3
  sweating R61
  thirst R63.1
    due to deprivation of water T73.1
  tuberosity of jaw M26.07
  vitamin
    A (dietary) E67.0
      administered as drug (prolonged intake) — *see* Table of Drugs and Chemicals, vitamins, adverse effect
      overdose or wrong substance given or taken — *see* Table of Drugs and Chemicals, vitamins, poisoning
    D (dietary) E67.3
      administered as drug (prolonged intake) — *see* Table of Drugs and Chemicals, vitamins, adverse effect
      overdose or wrong substance given or taken — *see* Table of Drugs and Chemicals, vitamins, poisoning
  weight
    gain R63.5
    loss R63.4

Excitability, abnormal, under minor stress (personality disorder) F60.3

Excitation
  anomalous atrioventricular I45.6
  psychogenic F30.8
  reactive (from emotional stress, psychological trauma) F30.8

Excitement
  hypomanic F30.8
  manic F30.9
  mental, reactive (from emotional stress, psychological trauma) F30.8
  state, reactive (from emotional stress, psychological trauma) F30.8

Excoriation (traumatic) — *see also* Abrasion
  neurotic L98.1
  skin picking disorder F42.4

Exfoliation
  due to erythematous conditions according to extent of body surface involved L49.0
    10-19 percent of body surface L49.1
    20-29 percent of body surface L49.2
    30-39 percent of body surface L49.3
    40-49 percent of body surface L49.4
    50-59 percent of body surface L49.5
    60-69 percent of body surface L49.6
    70-79 percent of body surface L49.7
    80-89 percent of body surface L49.8
    90-99 percent of body surface L49.9
    less than 10 percent of body surface L49.0
  teeth, due to systemic causes K08.0

Exfoliative — *see* condition

Exhaustion, exhaustive (physical NEC) R53.83
  battle F43.0
  cardiac — *see* Failure, heart
  delirium F43.0
  due to
    cold T69.8
    excessive exertion T73.3
    exposure T73.2
    neurasthenia F48.8
  heart — *see* Failure, heart

Exhaustion, exhaustive (physical NEC) R53.83 — *continued*
  heat (*see also* Heat, exhaustion) T67.5
    due to
      salt depletion T67.4
      water depletion T67.3
  maternal, complicating delivery O75.81
  mental F48.8
  myocardium, myocardial — *see* Failure, heart
  nervous F48.8
  old age R54
  psychogenic F48.8
  psychosis F43.0
  senile R54
  vital NEC Z73.0

Exhibitionism F65.2

Exocervicitis — *see* Cervicitis

Exomphalos Q79.2
  meaning hernia — *see* Hernia, umbilicus

Exophoria H50.52
  convergence, insufficiency H51.11
  divergence, excess H51.8

Exophthalmos H05.2-
  congenital Q15.8
  constant NEC H05.24-
  displacement, globe — *see* Displacement, globe
  due to thyrotoxicosis (hyperthyroidism) — *see* Hyperthyroidism, with, goiter (diffuse)
  dysthyroid — *see* Hyperthyroidism, with, goiter (diffuse)
  goiter — *see* Hyperthyroidism, with, goiter (diffuse)
  intermittent NEC H05.25-
  malignant — *see* Hyperthyroidism, with, goiter (diffuse)
  orbital
    edema — *see* Edema, orbit
    hemorrhage — *see* Hemorrhage, orbit
  pulsating NEC H05.26-
  thyrotoxic, thyrotropic — *see* Hyperthyroidism, with, goiter (diffuse)

Exostosis — *see also* Disorder, bone
  cartilaginous — *see* Neoplasm, bone, benign
  congenital (multiple) Q78.6
  external ear canal H61.81-
  gonococcal A54.49
  jaw (bone) M27.8
  multiple, congenital Q78.6
  orbit H05.35-
  osteocartilaginous — *see* Neoplasm, bone, benign
  syphilitic A52.77

Exotropia — *see* Strabismus, divergent concomitant

Explanation of
  investigation finding Z71.2
  medication Z71.89

Exposure (to) (*see also* Contact, with) T75.89
  acariasis Z20.7
  AIDS virus Z20.6
  air pollution Z77.110
  algae and algae toxins Z77.121
  algae bloom Z77.121
  anthrax Z20.810
  aromatic (hazardous) compounds NEC Z77.028
  aromatic amines Z77.020
  aromatic dyes NOS Z77.028
  arsenic Z77.010
  asbestos Z77.090
  bacterial disease NEC Z20.818
  benzene Z77.021
  blue-green algae bloom Z77.121
  body fluids (potentially hazardous) Z77.21
  brown tide Z77.121
  chemicals (chiefly nonmedicinal) (hazardous) NEC Z77.098
  cholera Z20.09

Exposure (to) (see also Contact, with) T75.89 — continued
  chromium compounds Z77.018
  cold, effects of T69.9
    specified effect NEC T69.8
  communicable disease Z20.9
    bacterial NEC Z20.818
    specified NEC Z20.89
    viral NEC Z20.828
  cyanobacteria bloom Z77.121
  disaster Z65.5
  discrimination Z60.5
  dyes Z77.098
  effects of T73.9
  environmental tobacco smoke (acute) (chronic) Z77.22
  Escherichia coli (E. coli) Z20.01
  exhaustion due to T73.2
  fiberglass — see Table of Drugs and Chemicals, fiberglass
  German measles Z20.4
  gonorrhea Z20.2
  hazardous metals NEC Z77.018
  hazardous substances NEC Z77.29
  hazards in the physical environment NEC Z77.128
  hazards to health NEC Z77.9
  human immunodeficiency virus (HIV) Z20.6
  human T-lymphotropic virus type-1 (HTLV-1) Z20.89
  implanted
    mesh — see Complications, mesh
    prosthetic materials NEC — see Complications, prosthetic materials NEC
  infestation (parasitic) NEC Z20.7
  intestinal infectious disease NEC Z20.09
    Escherichia coli (E. coli) Z20.01
  lead Z77.011
  meningococcus Z20.811
  mold (toxic) Z77.120
  nickel dust Z77.018
  noise Z77.122
  occupational
    air contaminants NEC Z57.39
    dust Z57.2
    environmental tobacco smoke Z57.31
    extreme temperature Z57.6
    noise Z57.0
    radiation Z57.1
    risk factors Z57.9
      specified NEC Z57.8
    toxic agents (gases) (liquids) (solids) (vapors) in agriculture Z57.4
    toxic agents (gases) (liquids) (solids) (vapors) in industry NEC Z57.5
    vibration Z57.7
  parasitic disease NEC Z20.7
  pediculosis Z20.7
  persecution Z60.5
  pfiesteria piscicida Z77.121
  poliomyelitis Z20.89
  pollution
    air Z77.110
    environmental NEC Z77.118
    soil Z77.112
    water Z77.111
  polycyclic aromatic hydrocarbons Z77.028
  prenatal (drugs) (toxic chemicals) — see Newborn, affected by, noxious substances transmitted via placenta or breast milk
  rabies Z20.3
  radiation, naturally occurring NEC Z77.123
  radon Z77.123
  red tide (Florida) Z77.121
  rubella Z20.4
  second hand tobacco smoke (acute) (chronic) Z77.22
    in the perinatal period P96.81
  sexually-transmitted disease Z20.2

Exposure (to) (see also Contact, with) T75.89 — continued
  smallpox (laboratory) Z20.89
  syphilis Z20.2
  terrorism Z65.4
  torture Z65.4
  tuberculosis Z20.1
  uranium Z77.012
  varicella Z20.820
  venereal disease Z20.2
  viral disease NEC Z20.828
  war Z65.5
  water pollution Z77.111
Exsanguination — see Hemorrhage
Exstrophy
  abdominal contents Q45.8
  bladder Q64.10
    cloacal Q64.12
    specified type NEC Q64.19
    supravesical fissure Q64.11
Extensive — see condition
Extra — see also Accessory
  marker chromosomes (normal individual) Q92.61
    in abnormal individual Q92.62
  rib Q76.6
    cervical Q76.5
Extrasystoles (supraventricular) I49.49
  atrial I49.1
  auricular I49.1
  junctional I49.2
  ventricular I49.3
Extrauterine gestation or pregnancy — see Pregnancy, by site
Extravasation
  blood R58
  chyle into mesentery I89.8
  pelvicalyceal N13.8
  pyelosinus N13.8
  urine (from ureter) R39.0
  vesicant agent
    antineoplastic chemotherapy T80.810
    other agent NEC T80.818
Extremity — see condition, limb
Extrophy — see Exstrophy
Extroversion
  bladder Q64.19
  uterus N81.4
    complicating delivery O71.2
    postpartal (old) N81.4
Extruded tooth (teeth) M26.34
Extrusion
  breast implant (prosthetic) T85.42
  eye implant (globe) (ball) T85.328
  intervertebral disc — see Displacement, intervertebral disc
  ocular lens implant (prosthetic) — see Complications, intraocular lens
  vitreous — see Prolapse, vitreous
Exudate
  pleural — see Effusion, pleura
  retina H35.89
Exudative — see condition
Eye, eyeball, eyelid — see condition
Eyestrain — see Disturbance, vision, subjective
Eyeworm disease of Africa B74.3

F

Faber's syndrome (achlorhydric anemia) D50.9
Fabry(-Anderson) disease E75.21
Faciocephalalgia, autonomic (see also Neuropathy, peripheral, autonomic) G90.09
Factor(s)
  psychic, associated with diseases classified elsewhere F54
  psychological
    affecting physical conditions F54
    or behavioral
      affecting general medical condition F54
      associated with disorders or diseases classified elsewhere F54
Fahr disease (of brain) G23.8
Fahr Volhard disease (of kidney) I12-
Failure, failed
  abortion — see Abortion, attempted
  aortic (valve) I35.8
    rheumatic I06.8
  attempted abortion — see Abortion, attempted
  biventricular I50.9
  bone marrow — see Anemia, aplastic
  cardiac — see Failure, heart
  cardiorenal (chronic) I50.9
    hypertensive I13.2
  cardiorespiratory (see also Failure, heart) R09.2
  cardiovascular (chronic) — see Failure, heart
  cerebrovascular I67.9
  cervical dilatation in labor O62.0
  circulation, circulatory (peripheral) R57.9
    newborn P29.89
  compensation — see Disease, heart
  compliance with medical treatment or regimen — see Noncompliance
  congestive — see Failure, heart, congestive
  dental implant (endosseous) M27.69
    due to
      failure of dental prosthesis M27.63
      lack of attached gingiva M27.62
      occlusal trauma (poor prosthetic design) M27.62
      parafunctional habits M27.62
      periodontal infection (peri-implantitis) M27.62
      poor oral hygiene M27.62
    osseointegration M27.61
      due to
        complications of systemic disease M27.61
        poor bone quality M27.61
      iatrogenic M27.61
      post-osseointegration
        biological M27.62
        due to complications of systemic disease M27.62
        iatrogenic M27.62
        mechanical M27.63
      pre-integration M27.61
      pre-osseointegration M27.61
    specified NEC M27.69
  descent of head (at term) of pregnancy (mother) O32.4
  endosseous dental implant — see Failure, dental implant
  engagement of head (term of pregnancy) (mother) O32.4
  erection (penile) (see also Dysfunction, sexual, male, erectile) N52.9
    nonorganic F52.21
  examination(s), anxiety concerning Z55.2
  expansion terminal respiratory units (newborn) (primary) P28.0
  forceps NOS (with subsequent cesarean delivery) O66.5

DISEASE INDEX

Failure, failed — *continued*

gain weight (child over 28 days old) R62.51
  adult R62.7
  newborn P92.6
genital response (male) F52.21
  female F52.22
heart (acute) (senile) (sudden) I50.9
  with
    acute pulmonary edema — *see* Failure,
      ventricular, left
    decompensation — *see* Failure, heart,
      congestive
    dilatation — *see* Disease, heart
  arteriosclerotic I70.90
  biventricular I50.9
  combined left-right sided I50.9
  compensated I50.9
  complicating
    anesthesia (general) (local) or other
      sedation
      in labor and delivery O74.2
      in pregnancy O29.12-
      postpartum, puerperal O89.1
    delivery (cesarean) (instrumental) O75.4
  congestive (compensated) (decompensated)
    I50.9
    with rheumatic fever (conditions in I00)
      active I01.8
      inactive or quiescent (with chorea)
        I09.81
    newborn P29.0
    rheumatic (chronic) (inactive) (with chorea)
      I09.81
      active or acute I01.8
        with chorea I02.0
  decompensated I50.9
  degenerative — *see* Degeneration,
    myocardial
  diastolic (congestive) I50.30
    acute (congestive) I50.31
      and (on) chronic (congestive) I50.33
    chronic (congestive) I50.32
      and (on) acute (congestive) I50.33
    combined with systolic (congestive) I50.40
      acute (congestive) I50.41
        and (on) chronic (congestive) I50.43
      chronic (congestive) I50.42
        and (on) acute (congestive) I50.43
  due to presence of cardiac prosthesis
    I97.13-
  following cardiac surgery I97.13-
  high output NOS I50.9
  hypertensive — *see* Hypertension, heart
  left (ventricular) — *see* Failure, ventricular,
    left
  low output (syndrome) NOS I50.9
  newborn P29.0
  organic — *see* Disease, heart
  peripartum O90.3
  postprocedural I97.13-
  rheumatic (chronic) (inactive) I09.9
  right (ventricular) (secondary to left heart
    failure) — *see* Failure, heart, congestive
  systolic (congestive) I50.20
    acute (congestive) I50.21
      and (on) chronic (congestive) I50.23
    chronic (congestive) I50.22
      and (on) acute (congestive) I50.23
    combined with diastolic (congestive)
      I50.40
      acute (congestive) I50.41
        and (on) chronic (congestive) I50.43
      chronic (congestive) I50.42
        and (on) acute (congestive) I50.43
  thyrotoxic (*see also* Thyrotoxicosis) E05.90
    [I43]
    with thyroid storm E05.91 *[I43]*
  valvular — *see* Endocarditis

Failure, failed — *continued*

hepatic K72.90
  with coma K72.91
  acute or subacute K72.00
    with coma K72.01
    due to drugs K71.10
      with coma K71.11
  alcoholic (acute) (chronic) (subacute) K70.40
    with coma K70.41
  chronic K72.10
    with coma K72.11
    due to drugs (acute) (subacute) (chronic)
      K71.10
      with coma K71.11
    due to drugs (acute) (subacute) (chronic)
      K71.10
      with coma K71.11
  postprocedural K91.82
hepatorenal K76.7
induction (of labor) O61.9
  abortion — *see* Abortion, attempted
  by
    oxytocic drugs O61.0
    prostaglandins O61.0
  instrumental O61.1
  mechanical O61.1
  medical O61.0
  specified NEC O61.8
  surgical O61.1
intubation during anesthesia T88.4
  in pregnancy O29.6-
  labor and delivery O74.7
  postpartum, puerperal O89.6
involution, thymus (gland) E32.0
kidney (*see also* Disease, kidney, chronic) N19
  acute (*see also* Failure, renal, acute) N17.9
  diabetic — *see* E08-E13 with .22
lactation (complete) O92.3
  partial O92.4
Leydig's cell, adult E29.1
liver — *see* Failure, hepatic
menstruation at puberty N91.0
mitral I05.8
myocardial, myocardium (*see also* Failure,
  heart) I50.9
  chronic (*see also* Failure, heart, congestive)
    I50.9
  congestive (*see also* Failure, heart, congestive)
    I50.9
orgasm (female) (psychogenic) F52.31
  male F52.32
ovarian (primary) E28.39
  iatrogenic E89.40
    asymptomatic E89.40
    symptomatic E89.41
  postprocedural (postablative)
    (postirradiation) (postsurgical) E89.40
    asymptomatic E89.40
    symptomatic E89.41
ovulation causing infertility N97.0
polyglandular, autoimmune E31.0
prosthetic joint implant — *see* Complications,
  joint prosthesis, mechanical, breakdown,
  by site
renal N19
  with
    tubular necrosis (acute) N17.0
  acute N17.9
    with
      cortical necrosis N17.1
      medullary necrosis N17.2
      tubular necrosis N17.0
      specified NEC N17.8
  chronic N18.9
    hypertensive — *see* Hypertension, kidney
    congenital P96.0
  end stage (chronic) N18.6
    due to hypertension I12.0

Failure, failed — *continued*

renal N19 — *continued*
  following
    abortion — *see* Abortion by type
      complicated by specified condition
      NEC
    crushing T79.5
    ectopic or molar pregnancy O08.4
    labor and delivery (acute) O90.4
  hypertensive — *see* Hypertension, kidney
  postprocedural N99.0
respiration, respiratory J96.90
  with
    hypercapnia J96.92
    hypoxia J96.91
  acute J96.00
    with
      hypercapnia J96.02
      hypoxia J96.01
  acute and (on) chronic J96.20
    with
      hypercapnia J96.22
      hypoxia J96.21
  center G93.89
  chronic J96.10
    with
      hypercapnia J96.12
      hypoxia J96.11
  newborn P28.5
  postprocedural (acute) J95.821
    acute and chronic J95.822
rotation
  cecum Q43.3
  colon Q43.3
  intestine Q43.3
  kidney Q63.2
sedation (conscious) (moderate) during
  procedure T88.52
  history of Z92.83
segmentation — *see also* Fusion
  fingers — *see* Syndactylism, complex, fingers
  vertebra Q76.49
    with scoliosis Q76.3
seminiferous tubule, adult E29.1
senile (general) R54
sexual arousal (male) F52.21
  female F52.22
testicular endocrine function E29.1
to thrive (child over 28 days old) R62.51
  adult R62.7
  newborn P92.6
transplant T86.92
  bone T86.831
    marrow T86.02
  cornea T86.841
  heart T86.22
    with lung(s) T86.32
  intestine T86.851
  kidney T86.12
  liver T86.42
  lung(s) T86.811
    with heart T86.32
  pancreas T86.891
  skin (allograft) (autograft) T86.821
  specified organ or tissue NEC T86.891
  stem cell (peripheral blood) (umbilical cord)
    T86.5
trial of labor (with subsequent cesarean
  delivery) O66.40
  following previous cesarean delivery
    O66.41
tubal ligation N99.89
urinary — *see* Disease, kidney, chronic
vacuum extraction NOS (with subsequent
  cesarean delivery) O66.5
vasectomy N99.89
ventouse NOS (with subsequent cesarean
  delivery) O66.5

Failure, failed — *continued*
  ventricular (*see also* Failure, heart) I50.9
    left I50.1
      with rheumatic fever (conditions in I00)
        active I01.8
          with chorea I02.0
        inactive or quiescent (with chorea)
            I09.81
        rheumatic (chronic) (inactive) (with chorea)
            I09.81
          active or acute I01.8
            with chorea I02.0
    right (*see also* Failure, heart, congestive)
        I50.9
  vital centers, newborn P91.8
Fainting (fit) R55
Fallen arches — *see* Deformity, limb, flat foot
Falling, falls (repeated) R29.6
  any organ or part — *see* Prolapse
Fallopian
  insufflation Z31.41
  tube — *see* condition
Fallot's
  pentalogy Q21.8
  tetrad or tetralogy Q21.3
  triad or trilogy Q22.3
False — *see also* condition
  croup J38.5
  joint — *see* Nonunion, fracture
  labor (pains) O47.9
    at or after 37 completed weeks of gestation
        O47.1
    before 37 completed weeks of gestation
        O47.0-
  passage, urethra (prostatic) N36.5
  pregnancy F45.8
Family, familial — *see also* condition
  disruption Z63.8
    involving divorce or separation Z63.5
  Li-Fraumeni (syndrome) Z15.01
  planning advice Z30.09
  problem Z63.9
    specified NEC Z63.8
  retinoblastoma C69.2-
Famine (effects of) T73.0
  edema — *see* Malnutrition, severe
Fanconi (-de Toni) (-Debré) syndrome
    E72.09
  with cystinosis E72.04
Fanconi's anemia (congenital pancytopenia)
    D61.09
Farber's disease or syndrome E75.29
Farcy A24.0
Farmer's
  lung J67.0
  skin L57.8
Farsightedness — *see* Hypermetropia
Fascia — *see* condition
Fasciculation R25.3
Fasciitis M72.9
  diffuse (eosinophilic) M35.4
  infective M72.8
    necrotizing M72.6
  necrotizing M72.6
  nodular M72.4
  perirenal (with ureteral obstruction) N13.5
    with infection N13.6
  plantar M72.2
  specified NEC M72.8
  traumatic (old) M72.8
    current — *code by* site under Sprain
Fascioliasis B66.3
Fasciolopsis, fasciolopsiasis (intestinal)
    B66.5
Fascioscapulohumeral myopathy G71.0
Fast pulse R00.0

Fat
  embolism — *see* Embolism, fat
  excessive — *see also* Obesity
    in heart — *see* Degeneration, myocardial
  in stool R19.5
  localized (pad) E65
    heart — *see* Degeneration, myocardial
    knee M79.4
    retropatellar M79.4
  necrosis
    breast N64.1
    mesentery K65.4
    omentum K65.4
  pad E65
    knee M79.4
Fatigue R53.83
  auditory deafness — *see* Deafness
  chronic R53.82
  combat F43.0
  general R53.83
    psychogenic F48.8
  heat (transient) T67.6
  muscle M62.89
  myocardium — *see* Failure, heart
  neoplasm-related R53.0
  nervous, neurosis F48.8
  operational F48.8
  psychogenic (general) F48.8
  senile R54
  voice R49.8
Fatness — *see* Obesity
Fatty — *see also* condition
  apron E65
  degeneration — *see* Degeneration, fatty
  heart (enlarged) — *see* Degeneration,
      myocardial
  liver NEC K76.0
    alcoholic K70.0
    nonalcoholic K76.0
  necrosis — *see* Degeneration, fatty
Fauces — *see* condition
Fauchard's disease (periodontitis) — *see*
      Periodontitis
Faucitis J02.9
Favism (anemia) D55.0
Favus — *see* Dermatophytosis
Fazio-Londe disease or syndrome G12.1
Fear complex or reaction F40.9
Fear of — *see* Phobia
Feared complaint unfounded Z71.1
Febris, febrile — *see also* Fever
  flava (*see also* Fever, yellow) A95.9
  melitensis A23.0
  pestis — *see* Plague
  recurrens — *see* Fever, relapsing
  rubra A38.9
Fecal
  incontinence R15.9
  smearing R15.1
  soiling R15.1
  urgency R15.2
Fecalith (impaction) K56.41
  appendix K38.1
  congenital P76.8
Fede's disease K14.0
**Feeble rapid pulse due to shock
    following injury** T79.4
Feeble-minded F70
Feeding
  difficulties R63.3
  problem R63.3
    newborn P92.9
      specified NEC P92.8
    nonorganic (adult) — *see* Disorder, eating
Feeling (of)
  foreign body in throat R09.89
Feer's disease — *see* Poisoning, mercury
Feet — *see* condition
Feigned illness Z76.5

Feil-Klippel syndrome (brevicollis) Q76.1
**Feinmesser's (hidrotic) ectodermal
    dysplasia** Q82.4
Felinophobia F40.218
Felon — *see also* Cellulitis, digit
  with lymphangitis — *see* Lymphangitis, acute,
      digit
Felty's syndrome M05.00
  ankle M05.07-
  elbow M05.02-
  foot joint M05.07-
  hand joint M05.04-
  hip M05.05-
  knee M05.06-
  multiple site M05.09
  shoulder M05.01-
  vertebra — *see* Spondylitis, ankylosing
  wrist M05.03-
Female genital mutilation status (FGM)
    N90.810
  specified NEC N90.818
  type I (clitorectomy status) N90.811
  type II (clitorectomy with excision of labia
      minora status) N90.812
  type III (infibulation status) N90.813
  type IV N90.818
Female genital cutting status — *see* Female
      genital mutilation status (FGM)
Femur, femoral — *see* condition
Fenestration, fenestrated — *see also*
      Imperfect, closure
  aortico-pulmonary Q21.4
  cusps, heart valve NEC Q24.8
    pulmonary Q22.3
  pulmonic cusps Q22.3
Fernell's disease (aortic aneurysm) I71.9
Fertile eunuch syndrome E23.0
Fetid
  breath R19.6
  sweat L75.0
Fetishism F65.0
  transvestic F65.1
Fetus, fetal — *see also* condition
  alcohol syndrome (dysmorphic) Q86.0
  compressus O31.0-
  hydantoin syndrome Q86.1
  lung tissue P28.0
  papyraceous O31.0-
Fever (inanition) (of unknown origin) (persistent)
    (with chills) (with rigor) R50.9
  abortus A23.1
  Aden (dengue) A90
  African tick-borne A68.1
  American
    mountain (tick) A93.2
    spotted A77.0
  aphthous B08.8
  arbovirus, arboviral A94
    hemorrhagic A94
    specified NEC A93.8
  Argentinian hemorrhagic A96.0
  Assam B55.0
  Australian Q A78
  Bangkok hemorrhagic A91
  Barmah forest A92.8
  Bartonella A44.0
  bilious, hemoglobinuric B50.8
  blackwater B50.8
  blister B00.1
  Bolivian hemorrhagic A96.1
  Bonvale dam T73.3
  boutonneuse A77.1
  brain — *see* Encephalitis
  Brazilian purpuric A48.4
  breakbone A90
  Bullis A77.0
  Bunyamwera A92.8

© 2016 Channel Publishing, Ltd.

Fever (inanition) (of unknown origin) (persistent) (with chills) (with rigor) R50.9 — *continued*
- Burdwan B55.0
- Bwamba A92.8
- Cameroon — *see* Malaria
- Canton A75.9
- catarrhal (acute) J00
  - chronic J31.0
- cat-scratch A28.1
- Central Asian hemorrhagic A98.0
- cerebral — *see* Encephalitis
- cerebrospinal meningococcal A39.0
- Chagres B50.9
- Chandipura A92.8
- Changuinola A93.1
- Charcot's (biliary) (hepatic) (intermittent) — *see* Calculus, bile duct
- Chikungunya (viral) (hemorrhagic) A92.0
- Chitral A93.1
- Colombo — *see* Fever, paratyphoid
- Colorado tick (virus) A93.2
- congestive (remittent) — *see* Malaria
- Congo virus A98.0
- continued malarial B50.9
- Corsican — *see* Malaria
- Crimean-Congo hemorrhagic A98.0
- Cyprus — *see* Brucellosis
- dandy A90
- deer fly — *see* Tularemia
- dengue (virus) A90
  - hemorrhagic A91
  - sandfly A93.1
- desert B38.0
- drug induced R50.2
- due to
  - conditions classified elsewhere R50.81
  - heat T67.0
- enteric A01.00
- enteroviral exanthematous (Boston exanthem) A88.0
- ephemeral (of unknown origin) R50.9
- epidemic hemorrhagic A98.5
- erysipelatous — *see* Erysipelas
- estivo-autumnal (malarial) B50.9
- famine A75.0
- five day A79.0
- following delivery O86.4
- Fort Bragg A27.89
- gastroenteric A01.00
- gastromalarial — *see* Malaria
- Gibraltar — *see* Brucellosis
- glandular — *see* Mononucleosis, infectious
- Guama (viral) A92.8
- Haverhill A25.1
- hay (allergic) J30.1
  - with asthma (bronchial) J45.909
    - with
      - exacerbation (acute) J45.901
      - status asthmaticus J45.902
    - due to
      - allergen other than pollen J30.89
      - pollen, any plant or tree J30.1
- heat (effects) T67.0
- hematuric, bilious B50.8
- hemoglobinuric (malarial) (bilious) B50.8
- hemorrhagic (arthropod-borne) NOS A94
  - with renal syndrome A98.5
  - arenaviral A96.9
    - specified NEC A96.8
  - Argentinian A96.0
  - Bangkok A91
  - Bolivian A96.1
  - Central Asian A98.0
  - Chikungunya A92.0
  - Crimean-Congo A98.0
  - dengue (virus) A91
  - epidemic A98.5
  - Junin (virus) A96.0

Fever (inanition) (of unknown origin) (persistent) (with chills) (with rigor) R50.9 — *continued*
- hemorrhagic (arthropod-borne) NOS A94 — *continued*
  - Korean A98.5
  - Kyasanur forest A98.2
  - Machupo (virus) A96.1
  - mite-borne A93.8
  - mosquito-borne A92.8
  - Omsk A98.1
  - Philippine A91
  - Russian A98.5
  - Singapore A91
  - Southeast Asia A91
  - Thailand A91
  - tick-borne NEC A93.8
  - viral A99
    - specified NEC A98.8
- hepatic — *see* Cholecystitis
- herpetic — *see* Herpes
- icterohemorrhagic A27.0
- Indiana A93.8
- infective B99.9
  - specified NEC B99.8
- intermittent (bilious) — *see also* Malaria
  - of unknown origin R50.9
  - pernicious B50.9
- iodide R50.2
- Japanese river A75.3
- jungle — *see also* Malaria
  - yellow A95.0
- Junin (virus) hemorrhagic A96.0
- Katayama B65.2
- kedani A75.3
- Kenya (tick) A77.1
- Kew Garden A79.1
- Korean hemorrhagic A98.5
- Lassa A96.2
- Lone Star A77.0
- Machupo (virus) hemorrhagic A96.1
- malaria, malarial — *see* Malaria
- Malta A23.9
- Marseilles A77.1
- marsh — *see* Malaria
- Mayaro (viral) A92.8
- Mediterranean (*see also* Brucellosis) A23.9
  - familial M04.1
  - tick A77.1
- meningeal — *see* Meningitis
- Meuse A79.0
- Mexican A75.2
- mianeh A68.1
- miasmatic — *see* Malaria
- mosquito-borne (viral) A92.9
  - hemorrhagic A92.8
- mountain — *see also* Brucellosis
  - meaning Rocky Mountain spotted fever A77.0
  - tick (American) (Colorado) (viral) A93.2
- Mucambo (viral) A92.8
- mud A27.9
- Neapolitan — *see* Brucellosis
- neutropenic D70.9
- newborn P81.9
  - environmental P81.0
- Nine-Mile A78
- non-exanthematous tick A93.2
- North Asian tick-borne A77.2
- O'nyong-nyong (viral) A92.1
- Omsk hemorrhagic A98.1
- Oropouche (viral) A93.0
- Oroya A44.0
- paludal — *see* Malaria
- Panama (malarial) B50.9
- Pappataci A93.1
- paratyphoid A01.4
  - A A01.1
  - B A01.2
  - C A01.3

Fever (inanition) (of unknown origin) (persistent) (with chills) (with rigor) R50.9 — *continued*
- parrot A70
- periodic (Mediterranean) M04.1
- persistent (of unknown origin) R50.9
- petechial A39.0
- pharyngoconjunctival B30.2
- Philippine hemorrhagic A91
- phlebotomus A93.1
- Piry (virus) A93.8
- Pixuna (viral) A92.8
- Plasmodium ovale B53.0
- polioviral (nonparalytic) A80.4
- Pontiac A48.2
- postimmunization R50.83
- postoperative R50.82
  - due to infection T81.40
- posttransfusion R50.84
- postvaccination R50.83
- presenting with conditions classified elsewhere R50.81
- pretibial A27.89
- puerperal O86.4
- Q A78
- quadrilateral A78
- quartan (malaria) B52.9
- Queensland (coastal) (tick) A77.3
- quintan A79.0
- rabbit — *see* Tularemia
- rat-bite A25.9
  - due to
    - Spirillum A25.0
    - Streptobacillus moniliformis A25.1
- recurrent — *see* Fever, relapsing
- relapsing (Borrelia) A68.9
  - Carter's (Asiatic) A68.1
  - Dutton's (West African) A68.1
  - Koch's A68.9
  - louse-borne A68.0
  - Novy's
    - louse-borne A68.0
    - tick-borne A68.1
  - Obermeyer's (European) A68.0
  - tick-borne A68.1
- remittent (bilious) (congestive) (gastric) — *see* Malaria
- rheumatic (active) (acute) (chronic) (subacute) I00
  - with central nervous system involvement I02.9
  - active with heart involvement — *see* category I01
  - inactive or quiescent with
    - cardiac hypertrophy I09.89
    - carditis I09.9
    - endocarditis I09.1
      - aortic (valve) I06.9
        - with mitral (valve) disease I08.0
      - mitral (valve) I05.9
        - with aortic (valve) disease I08.0
      - pulmonary (valve) I09.89
      - tricuspid (valve) I07.8
    - heart disease NEC I09.89
    - heart failure (congestive) (conditions in I50.9) I09.81
    - left ventricular failure (conditions in I50.1) I09.81
    - myocarditis, myocardial degeneration (conditions in I51.4) I09.0
    - pancarditis I09.9
    - pericarditis I09.2
- Rift Valley (viral) A92.4
- Rocky Mountain spotted A77.0
- rose J30.1
- Ross River B33.1
- Russian hemorrhagic A98.5
- San Joaquin (Valley) B38.0
- sandfly A93.1
- Sao Paulo A77.0

Fever (inanition) (of unknown origin) (persistent) (with chills) (with rigor) R50.9 — *continued*
scarlet A38.9
seven day (leptospirosis) (autumnal) (Japanese) A27.89
dengue A90
shin-bone A79.0
Singapore hemorrhagic A91
solar A90
Songo A98.5
sore B00.1
South African tick-bite A68.1
Southeast Asia hemorrhagic A91
spinal — *see* Meningitis
spirillary A25.0
splenic — *see* Anthrax
spotted A77.9
  American A77.0
  Brazilian A77.0
  cerebrospinal meningitis A39.0
  Colombian A77.0
  due to Rickettsia
    australis A77.3
    conorii A77.1
    rickettsii A77.0
    sibirica A77.2
    specified type NEC A77.8
  Ehrlichiosis A77.40
    due to
      E. chafeensis A77.41
      specified organism NEC A77.49
  Rocky Mountain A77.0
steroid R50.2
streptobacillary A25.1
subtertian B50.9
Sumatran mite A75.3
sun A90
swamp A27.9
swine A02.8
sylvatic, yellow A95.0
Tahyna B33.8
tertian — *see* Malaria, tertian
Thailand hemorrhagic A91
thermic T67.0
three-day A93.1
tick
  American mountain A93.2
  Colorado A93.2
  Kemerovo A93.8
  Mediterranean A77.1
  mountain A93.2
  nonexanthematous A93.2
  Quaranfil A93.8
tick-bite NEC A93.8
tick-borne (hemorrhagic) NEC A93.8
trench A79.0
tsutsugamushi A75.3
typhogastric A01.00
typhoid (abortive) (hemorrhagic) (intermittent) (malignant) A01.00
  complicated by
    arthritis A01.04
    heart involvement A01.02
    meningitis A01.01
    osteomyelitis A01.05
    pneumonia A01.03
    specified NEC A01.09
typhomalarial — *see* Malaria
typhus — *see* Typhus (fever)
undulant — *see* Brucellosis
unknown origin R50.9
uveoparotid D86.89
valley B38.0
Venezuelan equine A92.2
vesicular stomatitis A93.8
viral hemorrhagic — *see* Fever, hemorrhagic, by type of virus
Volhynian A79.0
Wesselsbron (viral) A92.8

Fever (inanition) (of unknown origin) (persistent) (with chills) (with rigor) R50.9 — *continued*
West
  African B50.8
  Nile (viral) A92.30
    with
      complications NEC A92.39
      cranial nerve disorders A92.32
      encephalitis A92.31
      encephalomyelitis A92.31
      neurologic manifestation NEC A92.32
      optic neuritis A92.32
      polyradiculitis A92.32
Whitmore's — *see* Melioidosis
Wolhynian A79.0
worm B83.9
yellow A95.9
  jungle A95.0
  sylvatic A95.0
  urban A95.1
Zika virus A92.5
Fibrillation
atrial or auricular (established) I48.91
  chronic I48.2
  paroxysmal I48.0
  permanent I48.2
  persistent I48.1
cardiac I49.8
heart I49.8
muscular M62.89
ventricular I49.01
Fibrin
ball or bodies, pleural (sac) J94.1
chamber, anterior (eye) (gelatinous exudate) — *see* Iridocyclitis, acute
Fibrinogenolysis — *see* Fibrinolysis
Fibrinogenopenia D68.8
acquired D65
congenital D68.2
Fibrinolysis (hemorrhagic) (acquired) D65
antepartum hemorrhage — *see* Hemorrhage, antepartum, with coagulation defect
following
  abortion — *see* Abortion by type complicated by hemorrhage
  ectopic or molar pregnancy O08.1
intrapartum O67.0
newborn, transient P60
postpartum O72.3
Fibrinopenia (hereditary) D68.2
acquired D68.4
Fibrinopurulent — *see* condition
Fibrinous — *see* condition
Fibroadenoma
cellular intracanalicular D24-
giant D24-
intracanalicular
  cellular D24-
  giant D24-
  specified site — *see* Neoplasm, benign, by site
  unspecified site D24-
juvenile D24-
pericanalicular
  specified site — *see* Neoplasm, benign, by site
  unspecified site D24-
phyllodes D24-
prostate D29.1
specified site NEC — *see* Neoplasm, benign, by site
unspecified site D24-
Fibroadenosis, breast (chronic) (cystic) (diffuse) (periodic) (segmental) N60.2-
Fibroangioma — *see also* Neoplasm, benign, by site
juvenile
  specified site — *see* Neoplasm, benign, by site
  unspecified site D10.6

Fibrochondrosarcoma — *see* Neoplasm, cartilage, malignant
Fibrocystic
disease — *see also* Fibrosis, cystic
  breast — *see* Mastopathy, cystic
  jaw M27.49
  kidney (congenital) Q61.8
  liver Q44.6
  pancreas E84.9
kidney (congenital) Q61.8
Fibrodysplasia ossificans progressiva — *see* Myositis, ossificans, progressiva
Fibroelastosis (cordis) (endocardial) (endomyocardial) I42.4
Fibroid (tumor) — *see also* Neoplasm, connective tissue, benign
disease, lung (chronic) — *see* Fibrosis, lung
heart (disease) — *see* Myocarditis
in pregnancy or childbirth O34.1-
  causing obstructed labor O65.5
induration, lung (chronic) — *see* Fibrosis, lung
lung — *see* Fibrosis, lung
pneumonia (chronic) — *see* Fibrosis, lung
uterus D25.9
Fibrolipoma — *see* Lipoma
Fibroliposarcoma — *see* Neoplasm, connective tissue, malignant
Fibroma — *see also* Neoplasm, connective tissue, benign
ameloblastic — *see* Cyst, calcifying odontogenic
bone (nonossifying) — *see* Disorder, bone, specified type NEC
  ossifying — *see* Neoplasm, bone, benign
cementifying — *see* Neoplasm, bone, benign
chondromyxoid — *see* Neoplasm, bone, benign
desmoplastic — *see* Neoplasm, connective tissue, uncertain behavior
durum — *see* Neoplasm, connective tissue, benign
fascial — *see* Neoplasm, connective tissue, benign
invasive — *see* Neoplasm, connective tissue, uncertain behavior
molle — *see* Lipoma
myxoid — *see* Neoplasm, connective tissue, benign
nasopharynx, nasopharyngeal (juvenile) D10.6
nonosteogenic (nonossifying) — *see* Dysplasia, fibrous
odontogenic (central) — *see* Cyst, calcifying odontogenic
ossifying — *see* Neoplasm, bone, benign
periosteal — *see* Neoplasm, bone, benign
soft — *see* Lipoma
Fibromatosis M72.9
abdominal — *see* Neoplasm, connective tissue, uncertain behavior
aggressive — *see* Neoplasm, connective tissue, uncertain behavior
congenital generalized — *see* Neoplasm, connective tissue, uncertain behavior
Dupuytren's M72.0
gingival K06.1
palmar (fascial) M72.0
plantar (fascial) M72.2
pseudosarcomatous (proliferative) (subcutaneous) M72.4
retroperitoneal D48.3
specified NEC M72.8
Fibromyalgia M79.7
Fibromyoma — *see also* Neoplasm, connective tissue, benign
uterus (corpus) — *see also* Leiomyoma, uterus
in pregnancy or childbirth — *see* Fibroid, in pregnancy or childbirth
  causing obstructed labor O65.5

DISEASE INDEX

Fibromyositis M79.7
Fibromyxolipoma D17.9
Fibromyxoma — see Neoplasm, connective tissue, benign
Fibromyxosarcoma — see Neoplasm, connective tissue, malignant
Fibro-odontoma, ameloblastic — see Cyst, calcifying odontogenic
Fibro-osteoma — see Neoplasm, bone, benign
Fibroplasia, retrolental H35.17-
Fibropurulent — see condition
Fibrosarcoma — see also Neoplasm, connective tissue, malignant
  ameloblastic C41.1
    upper jaw (bone) C41.0
  congenital — see Neoplasm, connective tissue, malignant
  fascial — see Neoplasm, connective tissue, malignant
  infantile — see Neoplasm, connective tissue, malignant
  odontogenic C41.1
    upper jaw (bone) C41.0
  periosteal — see Neoplasm, bone, malignant
Fibrosclerosis
  breast N60.3-
  multifocal M35.5
  penis (corpora cavernosa) N48.6
Fibrosis, fibrotic
  adrenal (gland) E27.8
  amnion O41.8x-
  anal papillae K62.89
  arteriocapillary — see Arteriosclerosis
  bladder N32.89
    interstitial — see Cystitis, chronic, interstitial
    localized submucosal — see Cystitis, chronic, interstitial
    panmural — see Cystitis, chronic, interstitial
  breast — see Fibrosclerosis, breast
  capillary (see also Arteriosclerosis) I70.90
    lung (chronic) — see Fibrosis, lung
  cardiac — see Myocarditis
  cervix N88.8
  chorion O41.8x-
  corpus cavernosum (sclerosing) N48.6
  cystic (of pancreas) E84.9
    with
      distal intestinal obstruction syndrome E84.19
      fecal impaction E84.19
      intestinal manifestations NEC E84.19
      pulmonary manifestations E84.0
      specified manifestations NEC E84.8
  due to device, implant or graft (see also Complications, by site and type, specified NEC) T85.828
    arterial graft NEC T82.828
    breast (implant) T85.828
    catheter NEC T85.828
      dialysis (renal) T82.828
        intraperitoneal T85.828
      infusion NEC T82.828
        spinal (epidural) (subdural) T85.820
      urinary (indwelling) T83.82
    electronic (electrode) (pulse generator) (stimulator)
      bone T84.82
      cardiac T82.827
      nervous system (brain) (peripheral nerve) (spinal) T85.820
      urinary T83.82
    fixation, internal (orthopedic) NEC T84.82
    gastrointestinal (bile duct) (esophagus) T85.828
    genital NEC T83.82
    heart NEC T82.827
    joint prosthesis T84.82

Fibrosis, fibrotic — continued
  due to device, implant or graft (see also Complications, by site and type, specified NEC) T85.82 — continued
    ocular (corneal graft) (orbital implant) NEC T85.828
    orthopedic NEC T84.82
    specified NEC T85.828
    urinary NEC T83.82
    vascular NEC T82.828
    ventricular intracranial shunt T85.820
  ejaculatory duct N50.89
  endocardium — see Endocarditis
  endomyocardial (tropical) I42.3
  epididymis N50.89
  eye muscle — see Strabismus, mechanical
  heart — see Myocarditis
  hepatic — see Fibrosis, liver
  hepatolienal (portal hypertension) K76.6
  hepatosplenic (portal hypertension) K76.6
  infrapatellar fat pad M79.4
  intrascrotal N50.89
  kidney N26.9
  liver K74.0
    with sclerosis K74.2
    alcoholic K70.2
  lung (atrophic) (chronic) (confluent) (massive) (perialveolar) (peribronchial) J84.10
    with
      anthracosilicosis J60
      anthracosis J60
      asbestosis J61
      bagassosis J67.1
      bauxite J63.1
      berylliosis J63.2
      byssinosis J66.0
      calcicosis J62.8
      chalicosis J62.8
      dust reticulation J64
      farmer's lung J67.0
      ganister disease J62.8
      graphite J63.3
      pneumoconiosis NOS J64
      siderosis J63.4
      silicosis J62.8
    capillary J84.10
    congenital P27.8
    diffuse (idiopathic) J84.10
      chemicals, gases, fumes or vapors (inhalation) J68.4
      interstitial J84.10
        acute J84.114
        talc J62.0
    following radiation J70.1
    idiopathic J84.112
    postinflammatory J84.10
    silicotic J62.8
    tuberculous — see Tuberculosis, pulmonary
  lymphatic gland I89.8
  median bar — see Hyperplasia, prostate
  mediastinum (idiopathic) J98.59
  meninges G96.19
  myocardium, myocardial — see Myocarditis
  ovary N83.8
  oviduct N83.8
  pancreas K86.89
  penis NEC N48.6
  pericardium I31.0
  perineum, in pregnancy or childbirth O34.7-
    causing obstructed labor O65.5
  pleura J94.1
  popliteal fat pad M79.4
  prostate (chronic) — see Hyperplasia, prostate
  pulmonary (see also Fibrosis, lung) J84.10
    congenital P27.8
    idiopathic J84.112
  rectal sphincter K62.89

Fibrosis, fibrotic — continued
  retroperitoneal, idiopathic (with ureteral obstruction) N13.5
    with infection N13.6
  sclerosing mesenteric (idiopathic) K65.4
  scrotum N50.89
  seminal vesicle N50.89
  senile R54
  skin L90.5
  spermatic cord N50.89
  spleen D73.89
    in schistosomiasis (bilharziasis) B65.9 [D77]
  subepidermal nodular — see Neoplasm, skin, benign
  submucous (oral) (tongue) K13.5
  testis N44.8
    chronic, due to syphilis A52.76
  thymus (gland) E32.8
  tongue, submucous K13.5
  tunica vaginalis N50.89
  uterus (non-neoplastic) N85.8
  vagina N89.8
  valve, heart — see Endocarditis
  vas deferens N50.89
  vein I87.8
Fibrositis (periarticular) M79.7
  nodular, chronic (Jaccoud's) (rheumatoid) — see Arthropathy, postrheumatic, chronic
Fibrothorax J94.1
Fibrotic — see Fibrosis
Fibrous — see condition
Fibroxanthoma — see also Neoplasm, connective tissue, benign
  atypical — see Neoplasm, connective tissue, uncertain behavior
  malignant — see Neoplasm, connective tissue, malignant
Fibroxanthosarcoma — see Neoplasm, connective tissue, malignant
Fiedler's
  disease (icterohemorrhagic leptospirosis) A27.0
  myocarditis (acute) I40.1
Fifth disease B08.3
  venereal A55
Filaria, filarial, filariasis — see Infestation, filarial
Filatov's disease — see Mononucleosis, infectious
File-cutter's disease — see Poisoning, lead
Filling defect
  biliary tract R93.2
  bladder R93.41
  duodenum R93.3
  gallbladder R93.2
  gastrointestinal tract R93.3
  intestine R93.3
  kidney R93.42-
  stomach R93.3
  ureter R93.41
  urinary organs, specified NEC R93.49
Fimbrial cyst Q50.4
Financial problem affecting care NOS Z59.9
  bankruptcy Z59.8
  foreclosure on loan Z59.8
Findings, abnormal, inconclusive, without diagnosis — see also Abnormal
  17-ketosteroids, elevated R82.5
  acetonuria R82.4
  alcohol in blood R78.0
  anisocytosis R71.8
  antenatal screening of mother O28.9
    biochemical O28.1
    chromosomal O28.5
    cytological O28.2
    genetic O28.5
    hematological O28.0
    radiological O28.4

DISEASE INDEX

Findings, abnormal, inconclusive, without diagnosis (*see also* Abnormal) — *continued*
antenatal screening of mother O28.9 — *continued*
  specified NEC O28.8
  ultrasonic O28.3
antibody titer, elevated R76.0
anticardiolipin antibody R76.0
antiphosphatidylglycerol antibody R76.0
antiphosphatidylinositol antibody R76.0
antiphosphatidylserine antibody R76.0
antiphospholipid antibody R76.0
bacteriuria R82.71
bicarbonate E87.8
bile in urine R82.2
blood sugar R73.09
  high R73.9
  low (transient) E16.2
body fluid or substance, specified NEC R88.8
casts, urine R82.99
catecholamines R82.5
cells, urine R82.99
chloride E87.8
cholesterol E78.9
  high E78.00
    with high triglycerides E78.2
chyluria R82.0
cloudy
  dialysis effluent R88.0
  urine R82.90
creatinine clearance R94.4
crystals, urine R82.99
culture
  blood R78.81
  positive — *see* Positive, culture
echocardiogram R93.1
electrolyte level, urinary R82.99
function study NEC R94.8
  bladder R94.8
  endocrine NEC R94.7
    thyroid R94.6
  kidney R94.4
  liver R94.5
  pancreas R94.8
  placenta R94.8
  pulmonary R94.2
  spleen R94.8
gallbladder, nonvisualization R93.2
glucose (tolerance test) (non-fasting) R73.09
glycosuria R81
heart
  shadow R93.1
  sounds R01.2
hematinuria R82.3
hematocrit drop (precipitous) R71.0
hemoglobinuria R82.3
human papillomavirus (HPV) DNA test positive
  cervix
    high risk R87.810
    low risk R87.820
  vagina
    high risk R87.811
    low risk R87.821
in blood (of substance not normally found in blood) R78.9
  addictive drug NEC R78.4
  alcohol (excessive level) R78.0
  cocaine R78.2
  hallucinogen R78.3
  heavy metals (abnormal level) R78.79
  lead R78.71
  lithium (abnormal level) R78.89
  opiate drug R78.1
  psychotropic drug R78.5
  specified substance NEC R78.89
  steroid agent R78.6
indoleacetic acid, elevated R82.5
ketonuria R82.4

Findings, abnormal, inconclusive, without diagnosis (*see also* Abnormal) — *continued*
lactic acid dehydrogenase (LDH) R74.0
liver function test R79.89
mammogram NEC R92.8
  calcification (calculus) R92.1
  inconclusive result (due to dense breasts) R92.2
  microcalcification R92.0
mediastinal shift R93.8
melanin, urine R82.99
myoglobinuria R82.1
neonatal screening P09
nonvisualization of gallbladder R93.2
odor of urine NOS R82.90
Papanicolaou cervix R87.619
  non-atypical endometrial cells R87.618
pneumoencephalogram R93.0
poikilocytosis R71.8
potassium (deficiency) E87.6
  excess E87.5
PPD R76.11
radiologic (X-ray) R93.8
  abdomen R93.5
  biliary tract R93.2
  breast R92.8
  gastrointestinal tract R93.3
  genitourinary organs R93.8
  head R93.0
  inconclusive due to excess body fat of patient R93.9
  intrathoracic organs NEC R93.1
  placenta R93.8
  retroperitoneum R93.5
  skin R93.8
  skull R93.0
  subcutaneous tissue R93.8
red blood cell (count) (morphology) (sickling) (volume) R71.8
scan NEC R94.8
  bladder R94.8
  bone R94.8
  kidney R94.4
  liver R93.2
  lung R94.2
  pancreas R94.8
  placental R94.8
  spleen R94.8
  thyroid R94.6
sedimentation rate, elevated R70.0
SGOT R74.0
SGPT R74.0
sodium (deficiency) E87.1
  excess E87.0
specified body fluid NEC R88.8
stress test R94.39
thyroid (function) (metabolic rate) (scan) (uptake) R94.6
transaminase (level) R74.0
triglycerides E78.9
  high E78.1
    with high cholesterol E78.2
tuberculin skin test (without active tuberculosis) R76.11
urine R82.90
  acetone R82.4
  bacteria R82.71
  bile R82.2
  casts or cells R82.99
  chyle R82.0
  culture positive R82.79
  glucose R81
  hemoglobin R82.3
  ketone R82.4
  sugar R81
vanillylmandelic acid (VMA), elevated R82.5
vectorcardiogram (VCG) R94.39
ventriculogram R93.0

Findings, abnormal, inconclusive, without diagnosis (*see also* Abnormal) — *continued*
white blood cell (count) (differential) (morphology) D72.9
xerography R92.8
Finger — *see* condition
Fire, Saint Anthony's — *see* Erysipelas
Fire-setting
pathological (compulsive) F63.1
Fish hook stomach K31.89
Fishmeal-worker's lung J67.8
Fissure, fissured
anus, anal K60.2
  acute K60.0
  chronic K60.1
  congenital Q43.8
ear, lobule, congenital Q17.8
epiglottis (congenital) Q31.8
larynx J38.7
  congenital Q31.8
lip K13.0
  congenital — *see* Cleft, lip
nipple N64.0
  associated with
    lactation O92.13
    pregnancy O92.11-
  puerperium O92.12
nose Q30.2
palate (congenital) — *see* Cleft, palate
skin R23.4
spine (congenital) — *see also* Spina bifida
  with hydrocephalus — *see* Spina bifida, by site, with hydrocephalus
tongue (acquired) K14.5
  congenital Q38.3
Fistula (cutaneous) L98.8
abdomen (wall) K63.2
  bladder N32.2
  intestine NEC K63.2
  ureter N28.89
  uterus N82.5
abdominorectal K63.2
abdominosigmoidal K63.2
abdominothoracic J86.0
abdominouterine N82.5
  congenital Q51.7
abdominovesical N32.2
accessory sinuses — *see* Sinusitis
actinomycotic — *see* Actinomycosis
alveolar antrum — *see* Sinusitis, maxillary
alveolar process K04.6
anorectal K60.5
antrobuccal — *see* Sinusitis, maxillary
antrum — *see* Sinusitis, maxillary
anus, anal (recurrent) (infectional) K60.3
  congenital Q43.6
    with absence, atresia and stenosis Q42.2
  tuberculous A18.32
aorta-duodenal I77.2
appendix, appendicular K38.3
arteriovenous (acquired) (nonruptured) I77.0
  brain I67.1
    congenital Q28.2
      ruptured I60.8
    ruptured I60.8
  cerebral — *see* Fistula, arteriovenous, brain
  congenital (peripheral) — *see also* Malformation, arteriovenous
    brain Q28.2
      ruptured I60.8
    coronary Q24.5
    pulmonary Q25.72
  coronary I25.41
    congenital Q24.5
  pulmonary I28.0
    congenital Q25.72

Fistula (cutaneous) L98.8 — *continued*
  arteriovenous (acquired) (nonruptured) I77.0 — *continued*
    surgically created (for dialysis) Z99.2
      complication — *see* Complication, arteriovenous, fistula, surgically created
    traumatic — *see* Injury, blood vessel
  artery I77.2
  aural (mastoid) — *see* Mastoiditis, chronic
  auricle — *see also* Disorder, pinna, specified type NEC
    congenital Q18.1
  Bartholin's gland N82.8
  bile duct (common) (hepatic) K83.3
    with calculus, stones — *see* Calculus, bile duct
  biliary (tract) — *see* Fistula, bile duct
  bladder (sphincter) NEC (*see also* Fistula, vesico-) N32.2
    into seminal vesicle N32.2
  bone — *see also* Disorder, bone, specified type NEC
    with osteomyelitis, chronic — *see* Osteomyelitis, chronic, with draining sinus
  brain G93.89
    arteriovenous (acquired) I67.1
      congenital Q28.2
  branchial (cleft) Q18.0
  branchiogenous Q18.0
  breast N61.0
    puerperal, postpartum or gestational, due to mastitis (purulent) — *see* Mastitis, obstetric, purulent
  bronchial J86.0
  bronchocutaneous, bronchomediastinal, bronchopleural, bronchopleuromediastinal (infective) J86.0
    tuberculous NEC A15.5
  bronchoesophageal J86.0
    congenital Q39.2
      with atresia of esophagus Q39.1
  bronchovisceral J86.0
  buccal cavity (infective) K12.2
  cecosigmoidal K63.2
  cecum K63.2
  cerebrospinal (fluid) G96.0
  cervical, lateral Q18.1
  cervicoaural Q18.1
  cervicosigmoidal N82.4
  cervicovesical N82.1
  cervix N82.8
  chest (wall) J86.0
  cholecystenteric — *see* Fistula, gallbladder
  cholecystocolic — *see* Fistula, gallbladder
  cholecystocolonic — *see* Fistula, gallbladder
  cholecystoduodenal — *see* Fistula, gallbladder
  cholecystogastric — *see* Fistula, gallbladder
  cholecystointestinal — *see* Fistula, gallbladder
  choledochoduodenal — *see* Fistula, bile duct
  cholocolic K82.3
  coccyx — *see* Sinus, pilonidal
  colon K63.2
  colostomy K94.09
  common duct — *see* Fistula, bile duct
  congenital, site not listed — *see* Anomaly, by site
  coronary, arteriovenous I25.41
    congenital Q24.5
  costal region J86.0
  cul-de-sac, Douglas' N82.8
  cystic duct — *see also* Fistula, gallbladder
    congenital Q44.5
  dental K04.6
  diaphragm J86.0
  duodenum K31.6
  ear (external) (canal) — *see* Disorder, ear, external, specified type NEC

Fistula (cutaneous) L98.8 — *continued*
  enterocolic K63.2
  enterocutaneous K63.2
  enterouterine N82.4
    congenital Q51.7
  enterovaginal N82.4
    congenital Q52.2
    large intestine N82.3
    small intestine N82.2
  enterovesical N32.1
  epididymis N50.89
    tuberculous A18.15
  esophagobronchial J86.0
    congenital Q39.2
      with atresia of esophagus Q39.1
  esophagocutaneous K22.8
  esophagopleural-cutaneous J86.0
  esophagotracheal J86.0
    congenital Q39.2
      with atresia of esophagus Q39.1
  esophagus K22.8
    congenital Q39.2
      with atresia of esophagus Q39.1
  ethmoid — *see* Sinusitis, ethmoidal
  eyeball (cornea) (sclera) — *see* Disorder, globe, hypotony
  eyelid H01.8
  fallopian tube, external N82.5
  fecal K63.2
    congenital Q43.6
  from periapical abscess K04.6
  frontal sinus — *see* Sinusitis, frontal
  gallbladder K82.3
    with calculus, cholelithiasis, stones — *see* Calculus, gallbladder
  gastric K31.6
  gastrocolic K31.6
    congenital Q40.2
    tuberculous A18.32
  gastroenterocolic K31.6
  gastroesophageal K31.6
  gastrojejunal K31.6
  gastrojejunocolic K31.6
  genital tract (female) N82.9
    specified NEC N82.8
    to intestine NEC N82.4
    to skin N82.5
  hepatic artery-portal vein, congenital Q26.6
  hepatopleural J86.0
  hepatopulmonary J86.0
  ileorectal or ileosigmoidal K63.2
  ileovaginal N82.2
  ileovesical N32.1
  ileum K63.2
  in ano K60.3
    tuberculous A18.32
  inner ear (labyrinth) — *see* subcategory H83.1
  intestine NEC K63.2
  intestinocolonic (abdominal) K63.2
  intestinoureteral N28.89
  intestinouterine N82.4
  intestinovaginal N82.4
    large intestine N82.3
    small intestine N82.2
  intestinovesical N32.1
  ischiorectal (fossa) K61.3
  jejunum K63.2
  joint M25.10
    ankle M25.17-
    elbow M25.12-
    foot joint M25.17-
    hand joint M25.14-
    hip M25.15-
    knee M25.16-
    shoulder M25.11-
    specified joint NEC M25.18
    tuberculous — *see* Tuberculosis, joint
    vertebrae M25.18
    wrist M25.13-

Fistula (cutaneous) L98.8 — *continued*
  kidney N28.89
  labium (majus) (minus) N82.8
  labyrinth — *see* subcategory H83.1
  lacrimal (gland) (sac) H04.61-
  lacrimonasal duct — *see* Fistula, lacrimal
  laryngotracheal, congenital Q34.8
  larynx J38.7
  lip K13.0
    congenital Q38.0
  lumbar, tuberculous A18.01
  lung J86.0
  lymphatic I89.8
  mammary (gland) N61.0
  mastoid (process) (region) — *see* Mastoiditis, chronic
  maxillary J32.0
  medial, face and neck Q18.8
  mediastinal J86.0
  mediastinobronchial J86.0
  mediastinocutaneous J86.0
  middle ear — *see* subcategory H74.8
  mouth K12.2
  nasal J34.89
    sinus — *see* Sinusitis
  nasopharynx J39.2
  nipple N64.0
  nose J34.89
  oral (cutaneous) K12.2
    maxillary J32.0
    nasal (with cleft palate) — *see* Cleft, palate
  orbit, orbital — *see* Disorder, orbit, specified type NEC
  oroantral J32.0
  oviduct, external N82.5
  palate (hard) M27.8
  pancreatic K86.89
  pancreaticoduodenal K86.89
  parotid (gland) K11.4
    region K12.2
  penis N48.89
  perianal K60.3
  pericardium (pleura) (sac) — *see* Pericarditis
  pericecal K63.2
  perineorectal K60.4
  perineosigmoidal K63.2
  perineum, perineal (with urethral involvement) NEC N36.0
    tuberculous A18.13
    ureter N28.89
  perirectal K60.4
    tuberculous A18.32
  peritoneum K65.9
  pharyngoesophageal J39.2
  pharynx J39.2
    branchial cleft (congenital) Q18.0
  pilonidal (infected) (rectum) — *see* Sinus, pilonidal
  pleura, pleural, pleurocutaneous, pleuroperitoneal J86.0
    tuberculous NEC A15.6
  pleuropericardial I31.8
  portal vein-hepatic artery, congenital Q26.6
  postauricular H70.81-
  postoperative, persistent T81.83
    specified site — *see* Fistula, by site
  preauricular (congenital) Q18.1
  prostate N42.89
  pulmonary J86.0
    arteriovenous I28.0
      congenital Q25.72
    tuberculous — *see* Tuberculosis, pulmonary
  pulmonoperitoneal J86.0
  rectolabial N82.4
  rectosigmoid (intercommunicating) K63.2
  rectoureteral N28.89
  rectourethral N36.0
    congenital Q64.73

Fistula (cutaneous) L98.8 — *continued*
    rectouterine N82.4
        congenital Q51.7
    rectovaginal N82.3
        congenital Q52.2
        tuberculous A18.18
    rectovesical N32.1
        congenital Q64.79
    rectovesicovaginal N82.3
    rectovulval N82.4
        congenital Q52.79
    rectum (to skin) K60.4
        congenital Q43.6
            with absence, atresia and stenosis Q42.0
        tuberculous A18.32
    renal N28.89
    retroauricular — *see* Fistula, postauricular
    salivary duct or gland (any) K11.4
        congenital Q38.4
    scrotum (urinary) N50.89
        tuberculous A18.15
    semicircular canals — *see* subcategory H83.1
    sigmoid K63.2
        to bladder N32.1
    sinus — *see* Sinusitis
    skin L98.8
        to genital tract (female) N82.5
    splenocolic D73.89
    stercoral K63.2
    stomach K31.6
    sublingual gland K11.4
    submandibular gland K11.4
    submaxillary (gland) K11.4
        region K12.2
    thoracic J86.0
        duct I89.8
    thoracoabdominal J86.0
    thoracogastric J86.0
    thoracointestinal J86.0
    thorax J86.0
    thyroglossal duct Q89.2
    thyroid E07.89
    trachea, congenital (external) (internal) Q32.1
    tracheoesophageal J86.0
        congenital Q39.2
            with atresia of esophagus Q39.1
        following tracheostomy J95.04
    traumatic arteriovenous — *see* Injury, blood
        vessel, by site
    tuberculous — *code by* site under Tuberculosis
    typhoid A01.09
    umbilicourinary Q64.8
    urachus, congenital Q64.4
    ureter (persistent) N28.89
    ureteroabdominal N28.89
    ureterorectal N28.89
    ureterosigmoido-abdominal N28.89
    ureterovaginal N82.1
    ureterovesical N32.2
    urethra N36.0
        congenital Q64.79
        tuberculous A18.13
    urethroperineal N36.0
    urethroperineovesical N32.2
    urethrorectal N36.0
        congenital Q64.73
    urethroscrotal N50.89
    urethrovaginal N82.1
    urethrovesical N32.2
    urinary (tract) (persistent) (recurrent) N36.0
    uteroabdominal N82.5
        congenital Q51.7
    uteroenteric, uterointestinal N82.4
        congenital Q51.7
    uterorectal N82.4
        congenital Q51.7
    uteroureteric N82.1
    uterourethral Q51.7
    uterovaginal N82.8

Fistula (cutaneous) L98.8 — *continued*
    uterovesical N82.1
        congenital Q51.7
    uterus N82.8
    vagina (postpartal) (wall) N82.8
    vaginocutaneous (postpartal) N82.5
    vaginointestinal NEC N82.4
        large intestine N82.3
        small intestine N82.2
    vaginoperineal N82.5
    vasocutaneous, congenital Q55.7
    vesical NEC N32.2
    vesicoabdominal N32.2
    vesicocervicovaginal N82.1
    vesicocolic N32.1
    vesicocutaneous N32.2
    vesicoenteric N32.1
    vesicointestinal N32.1
    vesicometrorectal N82.4
    vesicoperineal N32.2
    vesicorectal N32.1
        congenital Q64.79
    vesicosigmoidal N32.1
    vesicosigmoidovaginal N82.3
    vesicoureteral N32.2
    vesicoureterovaginal N82.1
    vesicourethral N32.2
    vesicourethrorectal N32.1
    vesicouterine N82.1
        congenital Q51.7
    vesicovaginal N82.0
    vulvorectal N82.4
        congenital Q52.79
Fit R56.9
    epileptic — *see* Epilepsy
    fainting R55
    hysterical F44.5
    newborn P90
Fitting (and adjustment) (of)
    artificial
        arm — *see* Admission, adjustment, artificial,
            arm
        breast Z44.3
        eye Z44.2
        leg — *see* Admission, adjustment, artificial,
            leg
    automatic implantable cardiac defibrillator
        (with synchronous cardiac pacemaker)
        Z45.02
    brain neuropacemaker Z46.2
        implanted Z45.42
    cardiac defibrillator — *see* Fitting (and
        adjustment) (of), automatic implantable
        cardiac defibrillator
    catheter, non-vascular Z46.82
    colostomy belt Z46.89
    contact lenses Z46.0
    CRT-D (resynchronization therapy defibrillator)
        Z45.02
    CRT-P (cardiac resynchronization therapy
        pacemaker) Z45.018
        pulse generator Z45.010
    cystostomy device Z46.6
    defibrillator, cardiac — *see* Fitting (and
        adjustment) (of), automatic implantable
        cardiac defibrillator
    dentures Z46.3
    device NOS Z46.9
        abdominal Z46.89
        gastrointestinal NEC Z46.59
        implanted NEC Z45.89
        nervous system Z46.2
            implanted — *see* Admission, adjustment,
                device, implanted, nervous system
        orthodontic Z46.4
        orthoptic Z46.0
        orthotic Z46.89

Fitting (and adjustment) (of) — *continued*
    device NOS Z46.9 — *continued*
        prosthetic (external) Z44.9
            breast Z44.3
            dental Z46.3
            eye Z44.2
            specified NEC Z44.8
        specified NEC Z46.89
        substitution
            auditory Z46.2
                implanted — *see* Admission, adjustment,
                    device, implanted, hearing device
            nervous system Z46.2
                implanted — *see* Admission, adjustment,
                    device, implanted, nervous system
            visual Z46.2
                implanted Z45.31
            urinary Z46.6
    gastric lap band Z46.51
    gastrointestinal appliance NEC Z46.59
    glasses (reading) Z46.0
    hearing aid Z46.1
    ileostomy device Z46.89
    insulin pump Z46.81
    intestinal appliance NEC Z46.89
    myringotomy device (stent) (tube) Z45.82
    neuropacemaker Z46.2
        implanted Z45.42
    non-vascular catheter Z46.82
    orthodontic device Z46.4
    orthopedic device (brace) (cast) (corset) (shoes)
        Z46.89
    pacemaker (cardiac) (cardiac
        resynchronization therapy (CRT-P))
        Z45.018
        nervous system (brain) (peripheral nerve)
            (spinal cord) Z46.2
            implanted Z45.42
        pulse generator Z45.010
    portacath (port-a-cath) Z45.2
    prosthesis (external) Z44.9
        arm — *see* Admission, adjustment, artificial,
            arm
        breast Z44.3
        dental Z46.3
        eye Z44.2
        leg — *see* Admission, adjustment, artificial,
            leg
        specified NEC Z44.8
    spectacles Z46.0
    wheelchair Z46.89
Fitz's syndrome (acute hemorrhagic
    pancreatitis) (*see also* Pancreatitis, acute)
    K85.80
Fitzhugh-Curtis syndrome
    due to
        Chlamydia trachomatis A74.81
        Neisseria gonorrhorea (gonococcal
            peritonitis) A54.85
Fixation
    joint — *see* Ankylosis
    larynx J38.7
    stapes — *see* Ankylosis, ear ossicles
        deafness — *see* Deafness, conductive
    uterus (acquired) — *see* Malposition, uterus
    vocal cord J38.3
Flabby ridge K06.8

Flaccid — *see also* condition
    palate, congenital Q38.5
Flail
    chest S22.5
        newborn (birth injury) P13.8
    joint (paralytic) M25.20
        ankle M25.27-
        elbow M25.22-
        foot joint M25.27-
        hand joint M25.24-
        hip M25.25-

DISEASE INDEX

Flail — *continued*
  joint (paralytic) M25.20 — *continued*
    knee M25.26-
    shoulder M25.21-
    specified joint NEC M25.28
    wrist M25.23-
Flajani's disease — *see* Hyperthyroidism, with, goiter (diffuse)
Flap, liver K71.3
Flashbacks (residual to hallucinogen use) F16.283
Flat
  chamber (eye) — *see* Disorder, globe, hypotony, flat anterior chamber
  chest, congenital Q67.8
  foot (acquired) (fixed type) (painful) (postural) — *see also* Deformity, limb, flat foot
    congenital (rigid) (spastic (everted)) Q66.5-
    rachitic sequelae (late effect) E64.3
  organ or site, congenital NEC — *see* Anomaly, by site
  pelvis M95.5
    with disproportion (fetopelvic) O33.0
      causing obstructed labor O65.0
    congenital Q74.2
Flatau-Schilder disease G37.0
Flatback syndrome M40.30
  lumbar region M40.36
  lumbosacral region M40.37
  thoracolumbar region M40.35
Flattening
  head, femur M89.8x5
  hip — *see* Coxa, plana
  lip (congenital) Q18.8
  nose (congenital) Q67.4
    acquired M95.0
Flatulence R14.3
  psychogenic F45.8
Flatus R14.3
  vaginalis N89.8
Flax-dresser's disease J66.1
Flea bite — *see* Injury, bite, by site, superficial, insect
Flecks, glaucomatous (subcapsular) — *see* Cataract, complicated
Fleischer(-Kayser) ring (cornea) H18.04-
Fleshy mole O02.0
Flexibilitas cerea — *see* Catalepsy
Flexion
  amputation stump (surgical) T87.89
  cervix — *see* Malposition, uterus
  contracture, joint — *see* Contraction, joint
  deformity, joint (*see also* Deformity, limb, flexion) M21.20
    hip, congenital Q65.89
  uterus — *see also* Malposition, uterus
    lateral — *see* Lateroversion, uterus
Flexner's dysentery A03.1
Flexner-Boyd dysentery A03.2
Flexure — *see* Flexion
Flint murmur (aortic insufficiency) I35.1
Floater, vitreous — *see* Opacity, vitreous
Floating
  cartilage (joint) — *see also* Loose, body, joint
    knee — *see* Derangement, knee, loose body
  gallbladder, congenital Q44.1
  kidney N28.89
    congenital Q63.8
  spleen D73.89
Flooding N92.0
Floor — *see* condition
Floppy
  baby syndrome (nonspecific) P94.2
  iris syndrome (intraoperative) (IFIS) H21.81
  nonrheumatic mitral valve syndrome I34.1

Flu — *see also* Influenza
  avian (*see also* Influenza, due to, identified novel influenza A virus) J09.x2
  bird (*see also* Influenza, due to, identified novel influenza A virus) J09.x2
  intestinal NEC A08.4
  swine (viruses that normally cause infections in pigs) (*see also* Influenza, due to, identified novel influenza A virus) J09.x2
Fluctuating blood pressure I99.8
Fluid
  abdomen R18.8
  chest J94.8
  heart — *see* Failure, heart, congestive
  joint — *see* Effusion, joint
  loss (acute) E86.9
  lung — *see* Edema, lung
  overload E87.70
    specified NEC E87.79
  peritoneal cavity R18.8
  pleural cavity J94.8
  retention R60.9
Flukes NEC — *see also* Infestation, fluke
  blood NEC — *see* Schistosomiasis
  liver B66.3
Fluor (vaginalis) N89.8
  trichomonal or due to Trichomonas (vaginalis) A59.00
Fluorosis
  dental K00.3
  skeletal M85.10
    ankle M85.17-
    foot M85.17-
    forearm M85.13-
    hand M85.14-
    lower leg M85.16-
    multiple site M85.19
    neck M85.18
    rib M85.18
    shoulder M85.11-
    skull M85.18
    specified site NEC M85.18
    thigh M85.15-
    toe M85.17-
    upper arm M85.12-
    vertebra M85.18
Flush syndrome E34.0
Flushing R23.2
  menopausal N95.1
Flutter
  atrial or auricular I48.92
    atypical I48.4
    type I I48.3
    type II I48.4
    typical I48.3
  heart I49.8
    atrial or auricular I48.92
      atypical I48.4
      type I I48.3
      type II I48.4
      typical I48.3
    ventricular I49.02
  ventricular I49.02
FNHTR (febrile nonhemolytic transfusion reaction) R50.84
Fochier's abscess — *code by* site under Abscess
Focus, Assmann's — *see* Tuberculosis, pulmonary
Fogo selvagem L10.3
Foix-Alajouanine syndrome G95.19
Fold, folds (anomalous) — *see also* Anomaly, by site
  Descemet's membrane — *see* Change, corneal membrane, Descemet's, fold
  epicanthic Q10.3
  heart Q24.8

Folie à deux F24
Follicle
  cervix (nabothian) (ruptured) N88.8
  graafian, ruptured, with hemorrhage N83.0-
  nabothian N88.8
Follicular — *see* condition
Folliculitis (superficial) L73.9
  abscedens et suffodiens L66.3
  cyst N83.0-
  decalvans L66.2
  deep — *see* Furuncle, by site
  gonococcal (acute) (chronic) A54.01
  keloid, keloidalis L73.0
  pustular L01.02
  ulerythematosa reticulata L66.4
Folliculome lipidique
  specified site — *see* Neoplasm, benign, by site
  unspecified site
    female D27.9
    male D29.20
Følling's disease E70.0
Follow-up — *see* Examination, follow-up
Fong's syndrome (hereditary osteo-onychodysplasia) Q87.2
Food
  allergy L27.2
  asphyxia (from aspiration or inhalation) — *see* Foreign body, by site
  choked on — *see* Foreign body, by site
  deprivation T73.0
    specified kind of food NEC E63.8
  intoxication — *see* Poisoning, food
  lack of T73.0
  poisoning — *see* Poisoning, food
  rejection NEC — *see* Disorder, eating
  strangulation or suffocation — *see* Foreign body, by site
  toxemia — *see* Poisoning, food
Foot — *see* condition
Foramen ovale (nonclosure) (patent) (persistent) Q21.1
Forbes' glycogen storage disease E74.03
Fordyce's disease (mouth) Q38.6
Fordyce-Fox disease L75.2
Forearm — *see* condition
Foreign body
  with
    laceration — *see* Laceration, by site, with foreign body
    puncture wound — *see* Puncture, by site, with foreign body
  accidentally left following a procedure T81.509
    aspiration T81.506
      resulting in
        adhesions T81.516
        obstruction T81.526
        perforation T81.536
        specified complication NEC T81.596
    cardiac catheterization T81.505
      resulting in
        acute reaction T81.60
          aseptic peritonitis T81.61
          specified NEC T81.69
        adhesions T81.515
        obstruction T81.525
        perforation T81.535
        specified complication NEC T81.595
    causing
      acute reaction T81.60
        aseptic peritonitis T81.61
        specified complication NEC T81.69
      adhesions T81.519
      aseptic peritonitis T81.61
      obstruction T81.529
      perforation T81.539
      specified complication NEC T81.599

Foreign body — *continued*
  accidentally left following a procedure
    T81.509 — *continued*
    endoscopy T81.504
      resulting in
        adhesions T81.514
        obstruction T81.524
        perforation T81.534
        specified complication NEC T81.594
    immunization T81.503
      resulting in
        adhesions T81.513
        obstruction T81.523
        perforation T81.533
        specified complication NEC T81.593
    infusion T81.501
      resulting in
        adhesions T81.511
        obstruction T81.521
        perforation T81.531
        specified complication NEC T81.591
    injection T81.503
      resulting in
        adhesions T81.513
        obstruction T81.523
        perforation T81.533
        specified complication NEC T81.593
    kidney dialysis T81.502
      resulting in
        adhesions T81.512
        obstruction T81.522
        perforation T81.532
        specified complication NEC T81.592
    packing removal T81.507
      resulting in
        acute reaction T81.60
          aseptic peritonitis T81.61
          specified NEC T81.69
        adhesions T81.517
        obstruction T81.527
        perforation T81.537
        specified complication NEC T81.597
    puncture T81.506
      resulting in
        adhesions T81.516
        obstruction T81.526
        perforation T81.536
        specified complication NEC T81.596
    specified procedure NEC T81.508
      resulting in
        acute reaction T81.60
          aseptic peritonitis T81.61
          specified NEC T81.69
        adhesions T81.518
        obstruction T81.528
        perforation T81.538
        specified complication NEC T81.598
    surgical operation T81.500
      resulting in
        acute reaction T81.60
          aseptic peritonitis T81.61
          specified NEC T81.69
        adhesions T81.510
        obstruction T81.520
        perforation T81.530
        specified complication NEC T81.590
    transfusion T81.501
      resulting in
        adhesions T81.511
        obstruction T81.521
        perforation T81.531
        specified complication NEC T81.591
  alimentary tract T18.9
    anus T18.5
    colon T18.4
    esophagus — *see* Foreign body, esophagus
    mouth T18.0
    multiple sites T18.8
    rectosigmoid (junction) T18.5

Foreign body — *continued*
  alimentary tract T18.9 — *continued*
    rectum T18.5
    small intestine T18.3
    specified site NEC T18.8
    stomach T18.2
  anterior chamber (eye) S05.5-
  auditory canal — *see* Foreign body, entering
      through orifice, ear
  bronchus T17.508
    causing
      asphyxiation T17.500
        food (bone) (seed) T17.520
        gastric contents (vomitus) T17.510
        specified type NEC T17.590
      injury NEC T17.508
        food (bone) (seed) T17.528
        gastric contents (vomitus) T17.518
        specified type NEC T17.598
  canthus — *see* Foreign body, conjunctival sac
  ciliary body (eye) S05.5-
  conjunctival sac T15.1-
  cornea T15.0-
  entering through orifice
    accessory sinus T17.0
    alimentary canal T18.9
      multiple parts T18.8
      specified part NEC T18.8
    alveolar process T18.0
    antrum (Highmore's) T17.0
    anus T18.5
    appendix T18.4
    auditory canal — *see* Foreign body, entering
        through orifice, ear
    auricle — *see* Foreign body, entering
        through orifice, ear
    bladder T19.1
    bronchioles — *see* Foreign body, respiratory
        tract, specified site NEC
    bronchus (main) — *see* Foreign body,
        bronchus
    buccal cavity T18.0
    canthus (inner) — *see* Foreign body,
        conjunctival sac
    cecum T18.4
    cervix (canal) (uteri) T19.3
    colon T18.4
    conjunctival sac — *see* Foreign body,
        conjunctival sac
    cornea — *see* Foreign body, cornea
    digestive organ or tract NOS T18.9
      multiple parts T18.8
      specified part NEC T18.8
    duodenum T18.3
    ear (external) T16-
    esophagus — *see* Foreign body, esophagus
    eye (external) NOS T15.9-
      conjunctival sac — *see* Foreign body,
          conjunctival sac
      cornea — *see* Foreign body, cornea
      specified part NEC T15.8-
    eyeball — *see also* Foreign body, entering
        through orifice, eye, specified part NEC
      with penetrating wound — *see* Puncture,
          eyeball
    eyelid — *see also* Foreign body, conjunctival
        sac
      with
        laceration — *see* Laceration, eyelid, with
            foreign body
        puncture — *see* Puncture, eyelid, with
            foreign body
        superficial injury — *see* Foreign body,
            superficial, eyelid
    gastrointestinal tract T18.9
      multiple parts T18.8
      specified part NEC T18.8

Foreign body — *continued*
  entering through orifice — *continued*
    genitourinary tract T19.9
      multiple parts T19.8
      specified part NEC T19.8
    globe — *see* Foreign body, entering through
        orifice, eyeball
    gum T18.0
    Highmore's antrum T17.0
    hypopharynx — *see* Foreign body, pharynx
    ileum T18.3
    intestine (small) T18.3
      large T18.4
    lacrimal apparatus (punctum) — *see* Foreign
        body, entering through orifice, eye,
        specified part NEC
    large intestine T18.4
    larynx — *see* Foreign body, larynx
    lung — *see* Foreign body, respiratory tract,
        specified site NEC
    maxillary sinus T17.0
    mouth T18.0
    nasal sinus T17.0
    nasopharynx — *see* Foreign body, pharynx
    nose (passage) T17.1
    nostril T17.1
    oral cavity T18.0
    palate T18.0
    penis T19.4
    pharynx — *see* Foreign body, pharynx
    piriform sinus — *see* Foreign body, pharynx
    rectosigmoid (junction) T18.5
    rectum T18.5
    respiratory tract — *see* Foreign body,
        respiratory tract
    sinus (accessory) (frontal) (maxillary) (nasal)
        T17.0
      piriform — *see* Foreign body, pharynx
    small intestine T18.3
    stomach T18.2
    suffocation by — *see* Foreign body, by site
    tear ducts or glands — *see* Foreign body,
        entering through orifice, eye, specified
        part NEC
    throat — *see* Foreign body, pharynx
    tongue T18.0
    tonsil, tonsillar (fossa) — *see* Foreign body,
        pharynx
    trachea — *see* Foreign body, trachea
    ureter T19.8
    urethra T19.0
    uterus (any part) T19.3
    vagina T19.2
    vulva T19.2
  esophagus T18.108
    causing
      injury NEC T18.108
        food (bone) (seed) T18.128
        gastric contents (vomitus) T18.118
        specified type NEC T18.198
      tracheal compression T18.100
        food (bone) (seed) T18.120
        gastric contents (vomitus) T18.110
        specified type NEC T18.190
  felling of, in throat R09.89
  fragment — *see* Retained, foreign body
      fragments (type of)
  genitourinary tract T19.9
    bladder T19.1
    multiple parts T19.8
    penis T19.4
    specified site NEC T19.8
    urethra T19.0
    uterus T19.3
    IUD Z97.5
    vagina T19.2
      contraceptive device Z97.5
    vulva T19.2

Foreign body — *continued*
  granuloma (old) (soft tissue) — *see also*
      Granuloma, foreign body
    skin L92.3
  in
    laceration — *see* Laceration, by site, with
        foreign body
    puncture wound — *see* Puncture, by site,
        with foreign body
    soft tissue (residual) M79.5
  inadvertently left in operation wound — *see*
      Foreign body, accidentally left during a
      procedure
  ingestion, ingested NOS T18.9
  inhalation or inspiration — *see* Foreign body,
      by site
  internal organ, not entering through a natural
      orifice — *code as* specific injury with
      foreign body
  intraocular S05.5-
    old, retained (nonmagnetic) H44.70-
      anterior chamber H44.71-
      ciliary body H44.72-
      iris H44.72-
      lens H44.73-
      magnetic H44.60-
        anterior chamber H44.61-
        ciliary body H44.62-
        iris H44.62-
        lens H44.63-
        posterior wall H44.64-
        specified site NEC H44.69-
        vitreous body H44.65-
      posterior wall H44.74-
      specified site NEC H44.79-
      vitreous body H44.75-
    iris — *see* Foreign body, intraocular
  lacrimal punctum — *see* Foreign body,
      entering through orifice, eye, specified
      part NEC
  larynx T17.308
    causing
      asphyxiation T17.300
        food (bone) (seed) T17.320
        gastric contents (vomitus) T17.310
        specified type NEC T17.390
      injury NEC T17.308
        food (bone) (seed) T17.328
        gastric contents (vomitus) T17.318
        specified type NEC T17.398
  lens — *see* Foreign body, intraocular
  ocular muscle S05.4-
    old, retained — *see* Foreign body, orbit, old
  old or residual
    soft tissue (residual) M79.5
  operation wound, left accidentally — *see*
      Foreign body, accidentally left during a
      procedure
  orbit S05.4-
    old, retained H05.5-
  pharynx T17.208
    causing
      asphyxiation T17.200
        food (bone) (seed) T17.220
        gastric contents (vomitus) T17.210
        specified type NEC T17.290
      injury NEC T17.208
        food (bone) (seed) T17.228
        gastric contents (vomitus) T17.218
        specified type NEC T17.298
  respiratory tract T17.908
    bronchioles — *see* Foreign body, respiratory
        tract, specified site NEC
    bronchus — *see* Foreign body, bronchus
    causing
      asphyxiation T17.900
        food (bone) (seed) T17.920
        gastric contents (vomitus) T17.910
        specified type NEC T17.990

Foreign body — *continued*
  respiratory tract T17.908 — *continued*
    causing — *continued*
      injury NEC T17.908
        food (bone) (seed) T17.928
        gastric contents (vomitus) T17.918
        specified type NEC T17.998
    larynx — *see* Foreign body, larynx
    lung — *see* Foreign body, respiratory tract,
        specified site NEC
    multiple parts — *see* Foreign body,
        respiratory tract, specified site NEC
    nasal sinus T17.0
    nasopharynx — *see* Foreign body, pharynx
    nose T17.1
    nostril T17.1
    pharynx — *see* Foreign body, pharynx
    specified site NEC T17.808
      causing
        asphyxiation T17.800
          food (bone) (seed) T17.820
          gastric contents (vomitus) T17.810
          specified type NEC T17.890
        injury NEC T17.808
          food (bone) (seed) T17.828
          gastric contents (vomitus) T17.818
          specified type NEC T17.898
    throat — *see* Foreign body, pharynx
    trachea — *see* Foreign body, trachea
  retained (old) (nonmagnetic) (in)
    anterior chamber (eye) — *see* Foreign body,
        intraocular, old, retained, anterior
        chamber
      magnetic — *see* Foreign body, intraocular,
          old, retained, magnetic, anterior
          chamber
    ciliary body — *see* Foreign body,
        intraocular, old, retained, ciliary body
      magnetic — *see* Foreign body, intraocular,
          old, retained, magnetic, ciliary body
    eyelid H02.819
      left H02.816
        lower H02.815
        upper H02.814
      right H02.813
        lower H02.812
        upper H02.811
    fragments — *see* Retained, foreign body
        fragments (type of)
    globe — *see* Foreign body, intraocular, old,
        retained
      magnetic — *see* Foreign body, intraocular,
          old, retained, magnetic
    intraocular — *see* Foreign body, intraocular,
        old, retained
      magnetic — *see* Foreign body, intraocular,
          old, retained, magnetic
    iris — *see* Foreign body, intraocular, old,
        retained, iris
      magnetic — *see* Foreign body, intraocular,
          old, retained, magnetic, iris
    lens — *see* Foreign body, intraocular, old,
        retained, lens
      magnetic — *see* Foreign body, intraocular,
          old, retained, magnetic, lens
    muscle — *see* Foreign body, retained, soft
        tissue
    orbit — *see* Foreign body, orbit, old
    posterior wall of globe — *see* Foreign body,
        intraocular, old, retained, posterior wall
      magnetic — *see* Foreign body, intraocular,
          old, retained, magnetic, posterior wall
    retrobulbar — *see* Foreign body, orbit, old,
        retrobulbar
    soft tissue M79.5
    vitreous — *see* Foreign body, intraocular,
        old, retained, vitreous body
      magnetic — *see* Foreign body, intraocular,
          old, retained, magnetic, vitreous body

Foreign body — *continued*
  retina S05.5-
  superficial, without open wound
    abdomen, abdominal (wall) S30.851
    alveolar process S00.552
    ankle S90.55-
    antecubital space — *see* Foreign body,
        superficial, forearm
    anus S30.857
    arm (upper) S40.85-
    auditory canal — *see* Foreign body,
        superficial, ear
    auricle — *see* Foreign body, superficial, ear
    axilla — *see* Foreign body, superficial, arm
    back, lower S30.850
    breast S20.15-
    brow S00.85
    buttock S30.850
    calf — *see* Foreign body, superficial, leg
    canthus — *see* Foreign body, superficial,
        eyelid
    cheek S00.85
      internal S00.552
    chest wall — *see* Foreign body, superficial,
        thorax
    chin S00.85
    clitoris S30.854
    costal region — *see* Foreign body,
        superficial, thorax
    digit(s)
      foot — *see* Foreign body, superficial, toe
      hand — *see* Foreign body, superficial,
          finger
    ear S00.45-
    elbow S50.35-
    epididymis S30.853
    epigastric region S30.851
    epiglottis S10.15
    esophagus, cervical S10.15
    eyebrow — *see* Foreign body, superficial,
        eyelid
    eyelid S00.25-
    face S00.85
    finger(s) S60.459
      index S60.45-
      little S60.45-
      middle S60.45-
      ring S60.45-
    flank S30.851
    foot (except toe(s) alone) S90.85-
      toe — *see* Foreign body, superficial, toe
    forearm S50.85-
      elbow only — *see* Foreign body,
          superficial, elbow
    forehead S00.85
    genital organs, external
      female S30.856
      male S30.855
    groin S30.851
    gum S00.552
    hand S60.55-
    head S00.95
      ear — *see* Foreign body, superficial, ear
      eyelid — *see* Foreign body, superficial,
          eyelid
      lip S00.551
      nose S00.35
      oral cavity S00.552
      scalp S00.05
      specified site NEC S00.85
    heel — *see* Foreign body, superficial, foot
    hip S70.25-
    inguinal region S30.851
    interscapular region S20.459
    jaw S00.85
    knee S80.25-
    labium (majus) (minus) S30.854
    larynx S10.15

Foreign body — *continued*
  superficial, without open wound — *continued*
    leg (lower) S80.85-
      knee — *see* Foreign body, superficial, knee
      upper — *see* Foreign body, superficial, thigh
    lip S00.551
    lower back S30.850
    lumbar region S30.850
    malar region S00.85
    mammary — *see* Foreign body, superficial, breast
    mastoid region S00.85
    mouth S00.552
    nail
      finger — *see* Foreign body, superficial, finger
      toe — *see* Foreign body, superficial, toe
    nape S10.85
    nasal S00.35
    neck S10.95
      specified site NEC S10.85
      throat S10.15
    nose S00.35
    occipital region S00.05
    oral cavity S00.552
    orbital region — *see* Foreign body, superficial, eyelid
    palate S00.552
    palm — *see* Foreign body, superficial, hand
    parietal region S00.05
    pelvis S30.850
    penis S30.852
    perineum
      female S30.854
      male S30.850
    periocular area — *see* Foreign body, superficial, eyelid
    phalanges
      finger — *see* Foreign body, superficial, finger
      toe — *see* Foreign body, superficial, toe
    pharynx S10.15
    pinna — *see* Foreign body, superficial, ear
    popliteal space — *see* Foreign body, superficial, knee
    prepuce S30.852
    pubic region S30.850
    pudendum
      female S30.856
      male S30.855
    sacral region S30.850
    scalp S00.05
    scapular region — *see* Foreign body, superficial, shoulder
    scrotum S30.853
    shin — *see* Foreign body, superficial, leg
    shoulder S40.25-
    sternal region S20.359
    submaxillary region S00.85
    submental region S00.85
    subungual
      finger(s) — *see* Foreign body, superficial, finger
      toe(s) — *see* Foreign body, superficial, toe
    supraclavicular fossa S10.85
    supraorbital S00.85
    temple S00.85
    temporal region S00.85
    testis S30.853
    thigh S70.35-
    thorax, thoracic (wall) S20.95
      back S20.45-
      front S20.35-
    throat S10.15
    thumb S60.35-
    toe(s) (lesser) S90.456
      great S90.45-
    tongue S00.552

Foreign body — *continued*
  superficial, without open wound — *continued*
    trachea S10.15
    tunica vaginalis S30.853
    tympanum, tympanic membrane — *see* Foreign body, superficial, ear
    uvula S00.552
    vagina S30.854
    vocal cords S10.15
    vulva S30.854
    wrist S60.85-
  swallowed T18.9
  trachea T17.408
    causing
      asphyxiation T17.400
        food (bone) (seed) T17.420
        gastric contents (vomitus) T17.410
        specified type NEC T17.490
      injury NEC T17.408
        food (bone) (seed) T17.428
        gastric contents (vomitus) T17.418
        specified type NEC T17.498
  type of fragment — *see* Retained, foreign body fragments (type of)
  vitreous (humor) S05.5-
Forestier's disease (rhizomelic pseudopolyarthritis) M35.3
  meaning ankylosing hyperostosis — *see* Hyperostosis, ankylosing
Formation
  hyalin in cornea — *see* Degeneration, cornea
  sequestrum in bone (due to infection) — *see* Osteomyelitis, chronic
  valve
    colon, congenital Q43.8
    ureter (congenital) Q62.39
Formication R20.2
Fort Bragg fever A27.89
Fossa — *see also* condition
  pyriform — *see* condition
Foster-Kennedy syndrome H47.14-
Fothergill's
  disease (trigeminal neuralgia) — *see also* Neuralgia, trigeminal
  scarlatina anginosa A38.9
Foul breath R19.6
Foundling Z76.1
Fournier disease or gangrene N49.3
  female N76.89
Fourth
  cranial nerve — *see* condition
  molar K00.1
Foville's (peduncular) disease or syndrome G46.3
Fox(-Fordyce) disease (apocrine miliaria) L75.2
Fracture, burst — *see* Fracture, traumatic, by site
Fracture, chronic — *see* Fracture, pathological
Fracture, insufficiency — *see* Fracture, pathologic, by site
Fracture, nontraumatic, NEC
  atypical
    femur M84.750-
      complete
        oblique M84.759
          left side M84.758
          right side M84.757
        transverse M84.756
          left side M84.755
          right side M84.754
      incomplete M84.753
        left side M84.752
        right side M84.751
Fracture, pathological (pathologic) — (*see also* **Fracture, traumatic**) M84.40
  ankle M84.47-
  carpus M84.44-
  clavicle M84.41-

Fracture, pathological (pathologic) — (*see also* **Fracture, traumatic**) M84.40 — *continued*
  compression (not due to trauma) (*see also* Collapse, vertebra) M48.50-
  dental implant M27.63
  dental restorative material K08.539
    with loss of material K08.531
    without loss of material K08.530
  due to
    neoplastic disease NEC (*see also* Neoplasm) M84.50
      ankle M84.57-
      carpus M84.54-
      clavicle M84.51-
      femur M84.55-
      fibula M84.56-
      finger M84.54-
      hip M84.559
      humerus M84.52-
      ilium M84.550
      ischium M84.550
      metacarpus M84.54-
      metatarsus M84.57-
      neck M84.58
      pelvis M84.550
      radius M84.53-
      rib M84.58
      scapula M84.51-
      skull M84.58
      specified site NEC M84.58
      tarsus M84.57-
      tibia M84.56-
      toe M84.57-
      ulna M84.53-
      vertebra M84.58
    osteoporosis M80.00
      disuse — *see* Osteoporosis, specified type NEC, with pathological fracture
      drug-induced — *see* Osteoporosis, drug induced, with pathological fracture
      idiopathic — *see* Osteoporosis, specified type NEC, with pathological fracture
      postmenopausal — *see* Osteoporosis, postmenopausal, with pathological fracture
      postoophorectomy — *see* Osteoporosis, postoophorectomy, with pathological fracture
      postsurgical malabsorption — *see* Osteoporosis, specified type NEC, with pathological fracture
      specified cause NEC — *see* Osteoporosis, specified type NEC, with pathological fracture
  specified disease NEC M84.60
    ankle M84.67-
    carpus M84.64-
    clavicle M84.61-
    femur M84.65-
    fibula M84.66-
    finger M84.64-
    hip M84.65-
    humerus M84.62-
    ilium M84.650
    ischium M84.650
    metacarpus M84.64-
    metatarsus M84.67-
    neck M84.68
    radius M84.63-
    rib M84.68
    scapula M84.61-
    skull M84.68
    tarsus M84.67-
    tibia M84.66-
    toe M84.67-
    ulna M84.63-
    vertebra M84.68

Fracture, pathological (pathologic) — (*see also* **Fracture, traumatic**) M84.40 — *continued*
femur M84.45-
fibula M84.46-
finger M84.44-
hip M84.459
humerus M84.42-
ilium M84.454
ischium M84.454
joint prosthesis — *see* Complications, joint prosthesis, mechanical, breakdown, by site
  periprosthetic — *see* Fracture, pathological, periprosthetic
metacarpus M84.44-
metatarsus M84.47-
neck M84.48
pelvis M84.454
periprosthetic M97.9
  ankle M97.2-
  elbow M97.4-
  finger M97.8
  hip M97.0-
  knee M97.1-
  other specified joint M97.8
  shoulder M97.3-
  spinal joint M97.8
  toe joint M97.8
  wrist joint M97.8
radius M84.43-
restorative material (dental) K08.539
  with loss of material K08.531
  without loss of material K08.530
rib M84.48
scapula M84.41-
skull M84.48
tarsus M84.47-
tibia M84.46-
toe M84.47-
ulna M84.43-
vertebra M84.48

Fracture, traumatic (abduction) (adduction) (separation) (*see also* **Fracture, pathological**) T14.8
acetabulum S32.40-
  column
    anterior (displaced) (iliopubic) S32.43-
      nondisplaced S32.436
    posterior (displaced) (ilioischial) S32.443
      nondisplaced S32.44-
  dome (displaced) S32.48-
    nondisplaced S32.48
  specified NEC S32.49-
  transverse (displaced) S32.45-
    with associated posterior wall fracture (displaced) S32.46-
      nondisplaced S32.46-
    nondisplaced S32.45-
  wall
    anterior (displaced) S32.41-
      nondisplaced S32.41-
    medial (displaced) S32.47-
      nondisplaced S32.47-
    posterior (displaced) S32.42-
      with associated transverse fracture (displaced) S32.46-
        nondisplaced S32.46-
      nondisplaced S32.42-
acromion — *see* Fracture, scapula, acromial process
ankle S82.899
  bimalleolar (displaced) S82.84-
    nondisplaced S82.84-
  lateral malleolus only (displaced) S82.6-
    nondisplaced S82.6-

Fracture, traumatic (abduction) (adduction) (separation) (*see also* **Fracture, pathological**) T14.8 — *continued*
ankle S82.899 — *continued*
  medial malleolus (displaced) S82.5-
    associated with Maisonneuve's fracture — *see* Fracture, Maisonneuve's
    nondisplaced S82.5-
  talus — *see* Fracture, tarsal, talus
  trimalleolar (displaced) S82.85-
    nondisplaced S82.85-
arm (upper) — *see also* Fracture, humerus, shaft
  humerus — *see* Fracture, humerus
  radius — *see* Fracture, radius
  ulna — *see* Fracture, ulna
astragalus — *see* Fracture, tarsal, talus
atlas — *see* Fracture, neck, cervical vertebra, first
axis — *see* Fracture, neck, cervical vertebra, second
back — *see* Fracture, vertebra
Barton's — *see* Barton's fracture
base of skull — *see* Fracture, skull, base
basicervical (basal) (femoral) S72.0
Bennett's — *see* Bennett's fracture
bimalleolar — *see* Fracture, ankle, bimalleolar
blow-out S02.3-
bone NEC T14.8
  birth injury P13.9
  following insertion of orthopedic implant, joint prosthesis or bone plate — *see* Fracture, following insertion of orthopedicimplant, joint prosthesis or bone plate
  in (due to) neoplastic disease NEC — *see* Fracture, pathological, due to, neoplastic disease
  pathological (cause unknown) — *see* Fracture, pathological
breast bone — *see* Fracture, sternum
bucket handle (semilunar cartilage) — *see* Tear, meniscus
burst — *see* Fracture, traumatic, by site
calcaneus — *see* Fracture, tarsal, calcaneus
carpal bone(s) S62.10-
  capitate (displaced) S62.13-
    nondisplaced S62.13-
  cuneiform — *see* Fracture, carpal bone, triquetrum
  hamate (body) (displaced) S62.143
    hook process (displaced) S62.15-
      nondisplaced S62.15-
    nondisplaced S62.14-
  larger multangular — *see* Fracture, carpal bones, trapezium
  lunate (displaced) S62.12-
    nondisplaced S62.12-
  navicular S62.00-
    distal pole (displaced) S62.01-
      nondisplaced S62.01-
    middle third (displaced) S62.02-
      nondisplaced S62.02-
    proximal third (displaced) S62.03-
      nondisplaced S62.03-
    volar tuberosity — *see* Fracture, carpal bones, navicular, distal pole
  os magnum — *see* Fracture, carpal bones, capitate
  pisiform (displaced) S62.16-
    nondisplaced S62.16-
  semilunar — *see* Fracture, carpal bones, lunate
  smaller multangular — *see* Fracture, carpal bones, trapezoid
  trapezium (displaced) S62.17-
    nondisplaced S62.17-
  trapezoid (displaced) S62.18-
    nondisplaced S62.18-

Fracture, traumatic (abduction) (adduction) (separation) (*see also* **Fracture, pathological**) T14.8 — *continued*
carpal bone(s) S62.10- — *continued*
  triquetrum (displaced) S62.11-
    nondisplaced S62.11-
  unciform — *see* Fracture, carpal bones, hamate
cervical — *see* Fracture, vertebra, cervical
clavicle S42.00-
  acromial end (displaced) S42.03-
    nondisplaced S42.03-
  birth injury P13.4
  lateral end — *see* Fracture, clavicle, acromial end
  shaft (displaced) S42.02-
    nondisplaced S42.02-
  sternal end (anterior) (displaced) S42.01-
    nondisplaced S42.01-
    posterior S42.01-
coccyx S32.2
collapsed — *see* Collapse, vertebra
collar bone — *see* Fracture, clavicle
Colles' — *see* Colles' fracture
coronoid process — *see* Fracture, ulna, upper end, coronoid process
corpus cavernosum penis S39.840
costochondral cartilage S23.41
costochondral, costosternal junction — *see* Fracture, rib
cranium — *see* Fracture, skull
cricoid cartilage S12.8
cuboid (ankle) — *see* Fracture, tarsal, cuboid
cuneiform
  foot — *see* Fracture, tarsal, cuneiform
  wrist — *see* Fracture, carpal, triquetrum
delayed union — *see* Delay, union, fracture
dental restorative material K08.539
  with loss of material K08.531
  without loss of material K08.530
due to
  birth injury — *see* Birth, injury, fracture
  osteoporosis — *see* Osteoporosis, with fracture
Dupuytren's — *see* Fracture, ankle, lateral malleolus
elbow S42.40-
ethmoid (bone) (sinus) — *see* Fracture, skull, base
face bone S02.92
fatigue — *see also* Fracture, stress
  vertebra M48.40
    cervical region M48.42
    cervicothoracic region M48.43
    lumbar region M48.46
    lumbosacral region M48.47
    occipito-atlanto-axial region M48.41
    sacrococcygeal region M48.48
    thoracic region M48.44
    thoracolumbar region M48.45
femur, femoral S72.9-
  basicervical (basal) S72.0
  birth injury P13.2
  capital epiphyseal S79.01-
  condyles, epicondyles — *see* Fracture, femur, lower end
  distal end — *see* Fracture, femur, lower end
  epiphysis
    head — *see* Fracture, femur, upper end, epiphysis
    lower — *see* Fracture, femur, lower end, epiphysis
    upper — *see* Fracture, femur, upper end, epiphysis
  following insertion of implant, prosthesis or plate M96.66-

Fracture, traumatic (abduction) (adduction) (separation) (*see also* **Fracture, pathological**) T14.8 — *continued*
femur, femoral S72.9- — *continued*
  head — *see* Fracture, femur, upper end, head
  intertrochanteric — *see* Fracture, femur, trochanteric
  intratrochanteric — *see* Fracture, femur, trochanteric
  lower end S72.40-
    condyle (displaced) S72.41-
      lateral (displaced) S72.42-
        nondisplaced S72.42-
      medial (displaced) S72.43-
        nondisplaced S72.43-
      nondisplaced S72.41-
    epiphysis (displaced) S72.44-
      nondisplaced S72.44-
    physeal S79.10-
      Salter-Harris
        Type I S79.11-
        Type II S79.12-
        Type III S79.13-
        Type IV S79.14-
      specified NEC S79.19-
    specified NEC S72.49-
    supracondylar (displaced) S72.45-
      with intracondylar extension (displaced) S72.46-
        nondisplaced S72.46-
      nondisplaced S72.45-
    torus S72.47-
  neck — *see* Fracture, femur, upper end, neck
  pertrochanteric — *see* Fracture, femur, trochanteric
  shaft (lower third) (middle third) (upper third) S72.30-
    comminuted (displaced) S72.35-
      nondisplaced S72.35-
    oblique (displaced) S72.33-
      nondisplaced S72.33-
    segmental (displaced) S72.36-
      nondisplaced S72.36-
    specified NEC S72.39-
    spiral (displaced) S72.34-
      nondisplaced S72.34-
    transverse (displaced) S72.32-
      nondisplaced S72.32-
  specified site NEC — *see* subcategory S72.8
  subcapital (displaced) S72.01-
  subtrochanteric (region) (section) (displaced) S72.2-
    nondisplaced S72.2-
  transcervical — *see* Fracture, femur, upper end, neck
  transtrochanteric — *see* Fracture, femur, trochanteric
  trochanteric S72.10-
    apophyseal (displaced) S72.13-
      nondisplaced S72.13-
    greater trochanter (displaced) S72.11-
      nondisplaced S72.11-
    intertrochanteric (displaced) S72.14-
      nondisplaced S72.14-
    lesser trochanter (displaced) S72.12-
      nondisplaced S72.12-
  upper end S72.00-
    apophyseal (displaced) S72.13-
      nondisplaced S72.13-
    cervicotrochanteric — *see* Fracture, femur, upper end, neck, base
    epiphysis (displaced) S72.02-
      nondisplaced S72.02-
    head S72.05-
      articular (displaced) S72.06-
        nondisplaced S72.06-
      specified NEC S72.09-

Fracture, traumatic (abduction) (adduction) (separation) (*see also* **Fracture, pathological**) T14.8 — *continued*
femur, femoral S72.9- — *continued*
  upper end S72.00- — *continued*
    intertrochanteric (displaced) S72.14-
      nondisplaced S72.14-
    intracapsular S72.01-
    midcervical (displaced) S72.03-
      nondisplaced S72.03-
    neck S72.00-
      base (displaced) S72.04-
        nondisplaced S72.04-
      specified NEC S72.09-
    pertrochanteric — *see* Fracture, femur, upper end, trochanteric
    physeal S79.00-
      Salter-Harris type I S79.01-
      specified NEC S79.09-
    subcapital (displaced) S72.01-
    subtrochanteric (displaced) S72.2-
      nondisplaced S72.2-
    transcervical — *see* Fracture, femur, upper end, midcervical
    trochanteric S72.10-
      greater (displaced) S72.11-
        nondisplaced S72.11-
      lesser (displaced) S72.12-
        nondisplaced S72.12-
fibula (shaft) (styloid) S82.40-
  comminuted (displaced) S82.45-
    nondisplaced S82.45-
  following insertion of implant, prosthesis or plate M96.67-
  involving ankle or malleolus — *see* Fracture, fibula, lateral malleolus
  lateral malleolus (displaced) S82.6-
    nondisplaced S82.6-
  lower end
    physeal S89.30-
      Salter-Harris
        Type I S89.31-
        Type II S89.32-
      specified NEC S89.39-
    specified NEC S82.83-
    torus S82.82-
  oblique (displaced) S82.43-
    nondisplaced S82.43-
  segmental (displaced) S82.46-
    nondisplaced S82.46-
  specified NEC S82.49-
  spiral (displaced) S82.44-
    nondisplaced S82.44-
  transverse (displaced) S82.42-
    nondisplaced S82.42-
  upper end
    physeal S89.20-
      Salter-Harris
        Type I S89.21-
        Type II S89.22-
      specified NEC S89.29-
    specified NEC S82.83-
    torus S82.81-
finger (except thumb) S62.60-
  distal phalanx (displaced) S62.63-
    nondisplaced S62.66-
  index S62.60-
    distal phalanx (displaced) S62.63-
      nondisplaced S62.66-
    medial phalanx (displaced) S62.62-
      nondisplaced S62.65-
    proximal phalanx (displaced) S62.61-
      nondisplaced S62.64-
  little S62.60-
    distal phalanx (displaced) S62.63-
      nondisplaced S62.66-
    medial phalanx (displaced) S62.62-
      nondisplaced S62.65-

Fracture, traumatic (abduction) (adduction) (separation) (*see also* **Fracture, pathological**) T14.8 — *continued*
finger (except thumb) S62.60- — *continued*
  little S62.60- — *continued*
    proximal phalanx (displaced) S62.61-
      nondisplaced S62.64-
  medial phalanx (displaced) S62.62-
    nondisplaced S62.65-
  middle S62.60-
    distal phalanx (displaced) S62.63-
      nondisplaced S62.66-
    medial phalanx (displaced) S62.62-
      nondisplaced S62.65-
    proximal phalanx (displaced) S62.61-
      nondisplaced S62.64-
  proximal phalanx (displaced) S62.61-
    nondisplaced S62.64-
  ring S62.60-
    distal phalanx (displaced) S62.63-
      nondisplaced S62.66-
    medial phalanx (displaced) S62.62-
      nondisplaced S62.65-
    proximal phalanx (displaced) S62.61-
      nondisplaced S62.64-
  thumb — *see* Fracture, thumb
following insertion (intraoperative) (postoperative) of orthopedic implant, joint prosthesis or bone plate M96.69
  femur M96.66-
  fibula M96.67-
  humerus M96.62-
  pelvis M96.65
  radius M96.63-
  specified bone NEC M96.69
  tibia M96.67-
  ulna M96.63-
foot S92.90-
  astragalus — *see* Fracture, tarsal, talus
  calcaneus — *see* Fracture, tarsal, calcaneus
  cuboid — *see* Fracture, tarsal, cuboid
  cuneiform — *see* Fracture, tarsal, cuneiform
  metatarsal — *see* Fracture, metatarsal
  navicular — *see* Fracture, tarsal, navicular
  sesamoid S92.81-
  specified NEC S92.81-
  talus — *see* Fracture, tarsal, talus
  tarsal — *see* Fracture, tarsal
  toe — *see* Fracture, toe
forearm S52.9-
  radius — *see* Fracture, radius
  ulna — *see* Fracture, ulna
fossa (anterior) (middle) (posterior) S02.19
frontal (bone) (skull) S02.0
  sinus S02.19
glenoid (cavity) (scapula) — *see* Fracture, scapula, glenoid cavity
greenstick — *see* Fracture, by site
hallux — *see* Fracture, toe, great
hand S62.9-
  carpal — *see* Fracture, carpal bone
  finger (except thumb) — *see* Fracture, finger
  metacarpal — *see* Fracture, metacarpal
  navicular (scaphoid) (hand) — *see* Fracture, carpal bone, navicular
  thumb — *see* Fracture, thumb
healed or old
  with complications — code by Nature of the complication
heel bone — *see* Fracture, tarsal, calcaneus
Hill-Sachs S42.29-
hip — *see* Fracture, femur, neck
humerus S42.30-
  anatomical neck — *see* Fracture, humerus, upper end
  articular process — *see* Fracture, humerus, lower end
  capitellum — *see* Fracture, humerus, lower end, condyle, lateral

DISEASE INDEX

DISEASE INDEX

Fracture, traumatic (abduction) (adduction) (separation) (*see also* **Fracture, pathological**) T14.8 — *continued*
humerus S42.30- — *continued*
distal end — *see* Fracture, humerus, lower end
epiphysis
lower — *see* Fracture, humerus, lower end, physeal
upper — *see* Fracture, humerus, upper end, physeal
external condyle — *see* Fracture, humerus, lower end, condyle, lateral
following insertion of implant, prosthesis or plate M96.62-
great tuberosity — *see* Fracture, humerus, upper end, greater tuberosity
intercondylar — *see* Fracture, humerus, lower end
internal epicondyle — *see* Fracture, humerus, lower end, epicondyle, medial
lesser tuberosity — *see* Fracture, humerus, upper end, lesser tuberosity
lower end S42.40-
condyle
lateral (displaced) S42.45-
nondisplaced S42.45-
medial (displaced) S42.46-
nondisplaced S42.46-
epicondyle
lateral (displaced) S42.43-
nondisplaced S42.43-
medial (displaced) S42.44-
incarcerated S42.44-
nondisplaced S42.44-
physeal S49.10-
Salter-Harris
Type I S49.11-
Type II S49.12-
Type III S49.13-
Type IV S49.14-
specified NEC S49.19-
specified NEC (displaced) S42.49-
nondisplaced S42.49-
supracondylar (simple) (displaced) S42.41-
with intercondylar fracture — *see* Fracture, humerus, lower end
comminuted (displaced) S42.42-
nondisplaced S42.41-
torus S42.48-
transcondylar (displaced) S42.47-
nondisplaced S42.47-
proximal end — *see* Fracture, humerus, upper end
shaft S42.30-
comminuted (displaced) S42.35-
nondisplaced S42.35-
greenstick S42.31-
oblique (displaced) S42.33-
nondisplaced S42.33-
segmental (displaced) S42.36-
nondisplaced S42.36-
specified NEC S42.39-
spiral (displaced) S42.34-
nondisplaced S42.34-
transverse (displaced) S42.32-
nondisplaced S42.32-
supracondylar — *see* Fracture, humerus, lower end
surgical neck — *see* Fracture, humerus, upper end, surgical neck
trochlea — *see* Fracture, humerus, lower end, condyle, medial
tuberosity — *see* Fracture, humerus, upper end

Fracture, traumatic (abduction) (adduction) (separation) (*see also* **Fracture, pathological**) T14.8 — *continued*
humerus S42.30- — *continued*
upper end S42.20-
anatomical neck — *see* Fracture, humerus, upper end, specified NEC
articular head — *see* Fracture, humerus, upper end, specified NEC
epiphysis — *see* Fracture, humerus, upper end, physeal
greater tuberosity (displaced) S42.25-
nondisplaced S42.25-
lesser tuberosity (displaced) S42.26-
nondisplaced S42.26-
physeal S49.00-
Salter-Harris
Type I S49.01-
Type II S49.02-
Type III S49.03-
Type IV S49.04-
specified NEC S49.09-
specified NEC (displaced) S42.29-
nondisplaced S42.29-
surgical neck (displaced) S42.21-
four-part S42.24-
nondisplaced S42.21-
three-part S42.23-
two-part (displaced) S42.22-
nondisplaced S42.22-
torus S42.27-
transepiphyseal — *see* Fracture, humerus, upper end, physeal
hyoid bone S12.8
ilium S32.30-
with disruption of pelvic ring — *see* Disruption, pelvic ring
avulsion (displaced) S32.31-
nondisplaced S32.31-
specified NEC S32.39-
impaction, impacted — *code as* Fracture, by site
innominate bone — *see* Fracture, ilium
instep — *see* Fracture, foot
ischium S32.60-
with disruption of pelvic ring — *see* Disruption, pelvic ring
avulsion (displaced) S32.61-
nondisplaced S32.61-
specified NEC S32.69-
jaw (bone) (lower) — *see* Fracture, mandible
upper — *see* Fracture, maxilla
joint prosthesis — *see* Complications, joint prosthesis, mechanical, breakdown, by site
periprosthetic — *see* Fracture, traumatic, periprosthetic
knee cap — *see* Fracture, patella
larynx S12.8
late effects — *see* Sequelae, fracture
leg (lower) S82.9-
ankle — *see* Fracture, ankle
femur — *see* Fracture, femur
fibula — *see* Fracture, fibula
malleolus — *see* Fracture, ankle
patella — *see* Fracture, patella
specified site NEC S82.89-
tibia — *see* Fracture, tibia
lumbar spine — *see* Fracture, vertebra, lumbar
lumbosacral spine S32.9
Maisonneuve's (displaced) S82.86-
nondisplaced S82.86-
malar bone (*see also* Fracture, maxilla) S02.400
left side S02.40B *(follows S02.402)*
right side S02.40A *(follows S02.402)*
malleolus — *see* Fracture, ankle
malunion — *see* Fracture, by site

Fracture, traumatic (abduction) (adduction) (separation) (*see also* **Fracture, pathological**) T14.8 — *continued*
mandible (lower jaw (bone)) S02.609
alveolus S02.67-
angle (of jaw) S02.65-
body, unspecified S02.600
left side S02.602
right side S02.601
condylar process S02.61-
coronoid process S02.63-
ramus, unspecified S02.64-
specified site NEC S02.69-
subcondylar process S02.62-
symphysis S02.66
manubrium (sterni) S22.21
dissociation from sternum S22.23
march — *see* Fracture, traumatic, stress, by site
maxilla, maxillary (bone) (sinus) (superior) (upper jaw) S02.401
alveolus S02.42
inferior — *see* Fracture, mandible
LeFort I S02.411
LeFort II S02.412
LeFort III S02.413
left side S02.40D *(follows S02.402)*
right side S02.40C *(follows S02.402)*
metacarpal S62.309
base (displaced) S62.319
nondisplaced S62.349
fifth S62.30-
base (displaced) S62.31-
nondisplaced S62.34-
neck (displaced) S62.33-
nondisplaced S62.36-
shaft (displaced) S62.32-
nondisplaced S62.35-
specified NEC S62.398
first S62.20-
base NEC (displaced) S62.23-
nondisplaced S62.23-
Bennett's — *see* Bennett's fracture
neck (displaced) S62.25-
nondisplaced S62.25-
shaft (displaced) S62.24-
nondisplaced S62.24-
specified NEC S62.29-
fourth S62.30-
base (displaced) S62.31-
nondisplaced S62.34-
neck (displaced) S62.33-
nondisplaced S62.36-
shaft (displaced) S62.32-
nondisplaced S62.35-
specified NEC S62.39-
neck (displaced) S62.33-
nondisplaced S62.36-
Rolando's — *see* Rolando's fracture
second S62.30-
base (displaced) S62.31-
nondisplaced S62.34-
neck (displaced) S62.33-
nondisplaced S62.36-
shaft (displaced) S62.32-
nondisplaced S62.35-
specified NEC S62.39-
shaft (displaced) S62.32-
nondisplaced S62.35-
specified NEC S62.399
third S62.30-
base (displaced) S62.31-
nondisplaced S62.34-
neck (displaced) S62.33-
nondisplaced S62.36-
shaft (displaced) S62.32-
nondisplaced S62.35-
specified NEC S62.39-

Fracture, traumatic (abduction) (adduction) (separation) (*see also* **Fracture, pathological**) T14.8 — *continued*
- metastatic — *see* Fracture, pathological, due to, neoplastic disease — *see also* Neoplasm
- metatarsal bone S92.30-
  - fifth (displaced) S92.35-
    - nondisplaced S92.35-
  - first (displaced) S92.31-
    - nondisplaced S92.31-
  - fourth (displaced) S92.34-
    - nondisplaced S92.34-
  - physeal S99.10-
    - Salter-Harris
      - Type I S99.11-
      - Type II S99.12-
      - Type III S99.13-
      - Type IV S99.14-
    - specified NEC S99.19-
  - second (displaced) S92.32-
    - nondisplaced S92.32-
  - third (displaced) S92.33-
    - nondisplaced S92.33-
- Monteggia's — *see* Monteggia's fracture
- multiple
  - hand (and wrist) NEC — *see* Fracture, by site
  - ribs — *see* Fracture, rib, multiple
- nasal (bone(s)) S02.2
- navicular (scaphoid) (foot) — *see also* Fracture, tarsal, navicular
  - hand — *see* Fracture, carpal, navicular
- neck S12.9
  - cervical vertebra S12.9
    - fifth (displaced) S12.400
      - nondisplaced S12.401
      - specified type NEC (displaced) S12.490
        - nondisplaced S12.491
    - first (displaced) S12.000
      - burst (stable) S12.01
        - unstable S12.02
      - lateral mass (displaced) S12.040
        - nondisplaced S12.041
      - nondisplaced S12.001
      - posterior arch (displaced) S12.030
        - nondisplaced S12.031
      - specified type NEC (displaced) S12.090
        - nondisplaced S12.091
    - fourth (displaced) S12.300
      - nondisplaced S12.301
      - specified type NEC (displaced) S12.390
        - nondisplaced S12.391
    - second (displaced) S12.100
      - dens (anterior) (displaced) (type II) S12.110
        - nondisplaced S12.112
        - posterior S12.111
      - specified type NEC (displaced) S12.120
        - nondisplaced S12.121
      - nondisplaced S12.101
      - specified type NEC (displaced) S12.190
        - nondisplaced S12.191
    - seventh (displaced) S12.600
      - nondisplaced S12.601
      - specified type NEC (displaced) S12.690
        - nondisplaced S12.691
    - sixth (displaced) S12.500
      - nondisplaced S12.501
      - specified type NEC (displaced) S12.590
        - nondisplaced S12.591
    - third (displaced) S12.200
      - nondisplaced S12.201
      - specified type NEC (displaced) S12.290
        - nondisplaced S12.291
  - hyoid bone S12.8
  - larynx S12.8
  - specified site NEC S12.8
  - thyroid cartilage S12.8
  - trachea S12.8

Fracture, traumatic (abduction) (adduction) (separation) (*see also* **Fracture, pathological**) T14.8 — *continued*
- neoplastic NEC — *see* Fracture, pathological, due to, neoplastic disease
- neural arch — *see* Fracture, vertebra
- newborn — *see* Birth, injury, fracture
- nontraumatic — *see* Fracture, pathological
- nonunion — *see* Nonunion, fracture
- nose, nasal (bone) (septum) S02.2
- occiput — *see* Fracture, skull, base, occiput
- odontoid process — *see* Fracture, neck, cervical vertebra, second
- olecranon (process) (ulna) — *see* Fracture, ulna, upper end, olecranon process
- orbit, orbital (bone) (region) S02.8-
  - floor (blow-out) S02.3-
  - roof S02.19
- os
  - calcis — *see* Fracture, tarsal, calcaneus
  - magnum — *see* Fracture, carpal, capitate
  - pubis — *see* Fracture, pubis
- palate S02.8-
- parietal bone (skull) S02.0
- patella S82.00-
  - comminuted (displaced) S82.04-
    - nondisplaced S82.04-
  - longitudinal (displaced) S82.02-
    - nondisplaced S82.02-
  - osteochondral (displaced) S82.01-
    - nondisplaced S82.01-
  - specified NEC S82.09-
  - transverse (displaced) S82.03-
    - nondisplaced S82.03-
- pedicle (of vertebral arch) — *see* Fracture, vertebra
- pelvis, pelvic (bone) S32.9
  - acetabulum — *see* Fracture, acetabulum
  - circle — *see* Disruption, pelvic ring
  - following insertion of implant, prosthesis or plate M96.65
  - ilium — *see* Fracture, ilium
  - ischium — *see* Fracture, ischium
  - multiple
    - with disruption of pelvic ring (circle) — *see* Disruption, pelvic ring
    - without disruption of pelvic ring (circle) S32.82
  - pubis — *see* Fracture, pubis
  - sacrum — *see* Fracture, sacrum
  - specified site NEC S32.89
- periprosthetic, around internal prosthetic joint M97.9
  - ankle M97.2-
  - elbow M97.4-
  - finger M97.8
  - hip M97.0-
  - knee M97.1-
  - shoulder M97.3-
  - specified joint NEC M97.8
  - spine M97.8
  - toe M97.8
  - wrist M97.8
- phalanx
  - foot — *see* Fracture, toe
  - hand — *see* Fracture, finger
- pisiform — *see* Fracture, carpal, pisiform
- pond — *see* Fracture, skull
- prosthetic device, internal — *see* Complications, prosthetic device, by site, mechanical
- pubis S32.50-
  - with disruption of pelvic ring — *see* Disruption, pelvic ring
  - specified site NEC S32.59-
  - superior rim S32.51-
- radius S52.9-
  - distal end — *see* Fracture, radius, lower end

Fracture, traumatic (abduction) (adduction) (separation) (*see also* **Fracture, pathological**) T14.8 — *continued*
- radius S52.9- — *continued*
  - following insertion of implant, prosthesis or plate M96.63-
  - head — *see* Fracture, radius, upper end, head
  - lower end S52.50-
    - Barton's — *see* Barton's fracture
    - Colles' — *see* Colles' fracture
    - extraarticular NEC S52.55-
    - intraarticular NEC S52.57-
    - physeal S59.20-
      - Salter-Harris
        - Type I S59.21-
        - Type II S59.22-
        - Type III S59.23-
        - Type IV S59.24-
      - specified NEC S59.29-
    - Smith's — *see* Smith's fracture
    - specified NEC S52.59-
    - styloid process (displaced) S52.51-
      - nondisplaced S52.51-
    - torus S52.52-
  - neck — *see* Fracture, radius, upper end
  - proximal end — *see* Fracture, radius, upper end
  - shaft S52.30-
    - bent bone S52.38-
    - comminuted (displaced) S52.35-
      - nondisplaced S52.35-
    - Galeazzi's — *see* Galeazzi's fracture
    - greenstick S52.31-
    - oblique (displaced) S52.33-
      - nondisplaced S52.33-
    - segmental (displaced) S52.36-
      - nondisplaced S52.36-
    - specified NEC S52.39-
    - spiral (displaced) S52.34-
      - nondisplaced S52.34-
    - transverse (displaced) S52.32-
      - nondisplaced S52.32-
  - upper end S52.10-
    - head (displaced) S52.12-
      - nondisplaced S52.12-
    - neck (displaced) S52.13-
      - nondisplaced S52.13-
    - physeal S59.10-
      - Salter-Harris
        - Type I S59.11-
        - Type II S59.12-
        - Type III S59.13-
        - Type IV S59.14-
      - specified NEC S59.19-
    - specified NEC S52.18-
    - torus S52.11-
- ramus
  - inferior or superior, pubis — *see* Fracture, pubis
  - mandible — *see* Fracture, mandible
- restorative material (dental) K08.539
  - with loss of material K08.531
  - without loss of material K08.530
- rib S22.3-
  - with flail chest — *see* Flail, chest
  - multiple S22.4-
    - with flail chest — *see* Flail, chest
- root, tooth — *see* Fracture, tooth
- sacrum S32.10
  - specified NEC S32.19
  - Type
    - 1 S32.14
    - 2 S32.15
    - 3 S32.16
    - 4 S32.17

Fracture, traumatic (abduction) (adduction) (separation) (*see also* **Fracture, pathological**) T14.8 — *continued*
- sacrum S32.10 — *continued*
  - Zone
    - I S32.119
      - displaced (minimally) S32.111
        - severely S32.112
      - nondisplaced S32.110
    - II S32.129
      - displaced (minimally) S32.121
        - severely S32.122
      - nondisplaced S32.120
    - III S32.139
      - displaced (minimally) S32.131
        - severely S32.132
      - nondisplaced S32.130
- scaphoid (hand) — *see also* Fracture, carpal, navicular
  - foot — *see* Fracture, tarsal, navicular
- scapula S42.10-
  - acromial process (displaced) S42.12-
    - nondisplaced S42.12-
  - body (displaced) S42.11-
    - nondisplaced S42.11-
  - coracoid process (displaced) S42.13-
    - nondisplaced S42.13-
  - glenoid cavity (displaced) S42.14-
    - nondisplaced S42.14-
  - neck (displaced) S42.15-
    - nondisplaced S42.15-
  - specified NEC S42.19-
- semilunar bone, wrist — *see* Fracture, carpal, lunate
- sequelae — *see* Sequelae, fracture
- sesamoid bone
  - hand — *see* Fracture, carpal
  - foot S92.81-
  - other — *see* Fracture, traumatic, by site
- shepherd's — *see* Fracture, tarsal, talus
- shoulder (girdle) S42.9-
  - blade — *see* Fracture, scapula
- sinus (ethmoid) (frontal) S02.19
- skull S02.91
  - base S02.10-
    - occiput S02.119
      - condyle S02.113
      - type I S02.110
        - left side S02.11B *(follows S02.119)*
        - right side S02.11A *(follows S02.119)*
      - type II S02.111
        - left side S02.11D *(follows S02.119)*
        - right side S02.11C *(follows S02.119)*
      - type III S02.112
        - left side S02.11F *(follows S02.119)*
        - right side S02.11E *(follows S02.119)*
      - specified NEC S02.118
        - left side S02.11H *(follows S02.119)*
        - right side S02.11G *(follows S02.119)*
    - specified NEC S02.19
  - birth injury P13.0
  - frontal bone S02.0
  - parietal bone S02.0
  - specified site NEC S02.8-
  - temporal bone S02.19
  - vault S02.0
- Smith's — *see* Smith's fracture
- sphenoid (bone) (sinus) S02.19
- spine — *see* Fracture, vertebra
- spinous process — *see* Fracture, vertebra
- spontaneous (cause unknown) — *see* Fracture, pathological
- stave (of thumb) — *see* Fracture, metacarpal, first
- sternum S22.20
  - with flail chest — *see* Flail, chest
  - body S22.22
  - manubrium S22.21
  - xiphoid (process) S22.24

Fracture, traumatic (abduction) (adduction) (separation) (*see also* **Fracture, pathological**) T14.8 — *continued*
- stress M84.30
  - ankle M84.37-
  - carpus M84.34-
  - clavicle M84.31-
  - femoral neck M84.359
  - femur M84.35-
  - fibula M84.36-
  - finger M84.34-
  - hip M84.359
  - humerus M84.32-
  - ilium M84.350
  - ischium M84.350
  - metacarpus M84.34-
  - metatarsus M84.37-
  - neck — *see* Fracture, fatigue, vertebra
  - pelvis M84.350
  - radius M84.33-
  - rib M84.38
  - scapula M84.31-
  - skull M84.38
  - tarsus M84.37-
  - tibia M84.36-
  - toe M84.37-
  - ulna M84.33-
  - vertebra — *see* Fracture, fatigue, vertebra
- supracondylar, elbow — *see* Fracture, humerus, lower end, supracondylar
- symphysis pubis — *see* Fracture, pubis
- talus (ankle bone) — *see* Fracture, tarsal, talus
- tarsal bone(s) S92.20-
  - astragalus — *see* Fracture, tarsal, talus
  - calcaneus S92.00-
    - anterior process (displaced) S92.02-
      - nondisplaced S92.02-
    - body (displaced) S92.01-
      - nondisplaced S92.01-
    - extraarticular NEC (displaced) S92.05-
      - nondisplaced S92.05-
    - intraarticular (displaced) S92.06-
      - nondisplaced S92.06-
    - physeal S99.00-
      - Salter-Harris
        - Type I S99.01-
        - Type II S99.02-
        - Type III S99.03-
        - Type IV S99.04-
      - specified NEC S99.09-
    - tuberosity (displaced) S92.04-
      - avulsion (displaced) S92.03-
        - nondisplaced S92.03-
      - nondisplaced S92.04-
  - cuboid (displaced) S92.21-
    - nondisplaced S92.21-
  - cuneiform
    - intermediate (displaced) S92.23-
      - nondisplaced S92.23-
    - lateral (displaced) S92.22-
      - nondisplaced S92.22-
    - medial (displaced) S92.24-
      - nondisplaced S92.24-
  - navicular (displaced) S92.25-
    - nondisplaced S92.25-
  - scaphoid — *see* Fracture, tarsal, navicular
  - talus S92.10-
    - avulsion (displaced) S92.15-
      - nondisplaced S92.15-
    - body (displaced) S92.12-
      - nondisplaced S92.12-
    - dome (displaced) S92.14-
      - nondisplaced S92.14-
    - head (displaced) S92.12-
      - nondisplaced S92.12-
    - lateral process (displaced) S92.14-
      - nondisplaced S92.14-
    - neck (displaced) S92.11-
      - nondisplaced S92.11-

Fracture, traumatic (abduction) (adduction) (separation) (*see also* **Fracture, pathological**) T14.8 — *continued*
- tarsal bone(s) S92.20- — *continued*
  - talus S92.10- — *continued*
    - posterior process (displaced) S92.13-
      - nondisplaced S92.13-
    - specified NEC S92.19-
- temporal bone (styloid) S02.19
- thorax (bony) S22.9
  - with flail chest — *see* Flail, chest
  - rib S22.3-
    - multiple S22.4-
      - with flail chest — *see* Flail, chest
  - sternum S22.20
    - body S22.22
    - manubrium S22.21
    - xiphoid process S22.24
  - vertebra (displaced) S22.009
    - burst (stable) S22.001
      - unstable S22.002
    - eighth S22.069
      - burst (stable) S22.061
        - unstable S22.062
      - specified type NEC S22.068
      - wedge compression S22.060
    - eleventh S22.089
      - burst (stable) S22.081
        - unstable S22.082
      - specified type NEC S22.088
      - wedge compression S22.080
    - fifth S22.059
      - burst (stable) S22.051
        - unstable S22.052
      - specified type NEC S22.058
      - wedge compression S22.050
    - first S22.019
      - burst (stable) S22.011
        - unstable S22.012
      - specified type NEC S22.018
      - wedge compression S22.010
    - fourth S22.049
      - burst (stable) S22.041
        - unstable S22.042
      - specified type NEC S22.048
      - wedge compression S22.040
    - ninth S22.079
      - burst (stable) S22.071
        - unstable S22.072
      - specified type NEC S22.078
      - wedge compression S22.070
    - nondisplaced S22.001
    - second S22.029
      - burst (stable) S22.021
        - unstable S22.022
      - specified type NEC S22.028
      - wedge compression S22.020
    - seventh S22.069
      - burst (stable) S22.061
        - unstable S22.062
      - specified type NEC S22.068
      - wedge compression S22.060
    - sixth S22.059
      - burst (stable) S22.051
        - unstable S22.052
      - specified type NEC S22.058
      - wedge compression S22.050
    - specified type NEC S22.008
    - tenth S22.079
      - burst (stable) S22.071
        - unstable S22.072
      - specified type NEC S22.078
      - wedge compression S22.070
    - third S22.039
      - burst (stable) S22.031
        - unstable S22.032
      - specified type NEC S22.038
      - wedge compression S22.030

DISEASE INDEX

Fracture, traumatic (abduction) (adduction) (separation) (*see also* **Fracture, pathological**) T14.8 — *continued*
  thorax (bony) S22.9 — *continued*
    vertebra (displaced) S22.009 — *continued*
      twelfth S22.089
        burst (stable) S22.081
          unstable S22.082
        specified type NEC S22.088
        wedge compression S22.080
      wedge compression S22.000
  thumb S62.50-
    distal phalanx (displaced) S62.52-
      nondisplaced S62.52-
    proximal phalanx (displaced) S62.51-
      nondisplaced S62.51-
  thyroid cartilage S12.8
  tibia (shaft) S82.20-
    comminuted (displaced) S82.25-
      nondisplaced S82.25-
    condyles — *see* Fracture, tibia, upper end
    distal end — *see* Fracture, tibia, lower end
    epiphysis
      lower — *see* Fracture, tibia, lower end
      upper — *see* Fracture, tibia, upper end
    following insertion of implant, prosthesis or plate M96.67-
    head (involving knee joint) — *see* Fracture, tibia, upper end
    intercondyloid eminence — *see* Fracture, tibia, upper end
    involving ankle or malleolus — *see* Fracture, ankle, medial malleolus
    lower end S82.30-
      physeal S89.10-
        Salter-Harris
          Type I S89.11-
          Type II S89.12-
          Type III S89.13-
          Type IV S89.14-
          specified NEC S89.19-
      pilon (displaced) S82.87-
        nondisplaced S82.87-
      specified NEC S82.39-
      torus S82.31-
    malleolus — *see* Fracture, ankle, medial malleolus
    oblique (displaced) S82.23-
      nondisplaced S82.23-
    pilon — *see* Fracture, tibia, lower end, pilon
    proximal end — *see* Fracture, tibia, upper end
    segmental (displaced) S82.26-
      nondisplaced S82.26-
    specified NEC S82.29-
    spine — *see* Fracture, upper end, spine
    spiral (displaced) S82.24-
      nondisplaced S82.24-
    transverse (displaced) S82.22-
      nondisplaced S82.22-
    tuberosity — *see* Fracture, tibia, upper end, tuberosity
    upper end S82.10-
      bicondylar (displaced) S82.14-
        nondisplaced S82.14-
      lateral condyle (displaced) S82.12-
        nondisplaced S82.12-
      medial condyle (displaced) S82.13-
        nondisplaced S82.13-
      physeal S89.00-
        Salter-Harris
          Type I S89.01-
          Type II S89.02-
          Type III S89.03-
          Type IV S89.04-
          specified NEC S89.09-
      plateau — *see* Fracture, tibia, upper end, bicondylar

Fracture, traumatic (abduction) (adduction) (separation) (*see also* **Fracture, pathological**) T14.8 — *continued*
  tibia (shaft) S82.20- — *continued*
    upper end S82.10- — *continued*
      specified NEC S82.19-
      spine (displaced) S82.11-
        nondisplaced S82.11-
      torus S82.16-
      tuberosity (displaced) S82.15-
        nondisplaced S82.15-
  toe S92.91-
    great (displaced) S92.40-
      distal phalanx (displaced) S92.42-
        nondisplaced S92.42-
      nondisplaced S92.40-
      proximal phalanx (displaced) S92.41-
        nondisplaced S92.41-
      specified NEC S92.49-
    lesser (displaced) S92.50-
      distal phalanx (displaced) S92.53-
        nondisplaced S92.53-
      medial phalanx (displaced) S92.52-
        nondisplaced S92.52-
      nondisplaced S92.50-
      proximal phalanx (displaced) S92.51-
        nondisplaced S92.51-
      specified NEC S92.59-
    physeal
      phalanx S99.20-
        Salter-Harris
          Type I S99.21-
          Type II S99.22-
          Type III S99.23-
          Type IV S99.24-
          specified NEC S99.29-
  tooth (root) S02.5
  trachea (cartilage) S12.8
  transverse process — *see* Fracture, vertebra
  trapezium or trapezoid bone — *see* Fracture, carpal
  trimalleolar — *see* Fracture, ankle, trimalleolar
  triquetrum (cuneiform of carpus) — *see* Fracture, carpal, triquetrum
  trochanter — *see* Fracture, femur, trochanteric
  tuberosity (external) — *see* Fracture, traumatic, by site
  ulna (shaft) S52.20-
    bent bone S52.28-
    coronoid process — *see* Fracture, ulna, upper end, coronoid process
    distal end — *see* Fracture, ulna, lower end
    following insertion of implant, prosthesis or plate M96.63-
    head S52.00-
    lower end S52.60-
      physeal S59.00-
        Salter-Harris
          Type I S59.01-
          Type II S59.02-
          Type III S59.03-
          Type IV S59.04-
          specified NEC S59.09-
      specified NEC S52.69-
      styloid process (displaced) S52.61-
        nondisplaced S52.61-
      torus S52.62-
    proximal end — *see* Fracture, ulna, upper end
    shaft S52.20-
      comminuted (displaced) S52.25-
        nondisplaced S52.25-
      greenstick S52.21-
      Monteggia's — *see* Monteggia's fracture
      oblique (displaced) S52.23-
        nondisplaced S52.23-
      segmental (displaced) S52.26-
        nondisplaced S52.26-

Fracture, traumatic (abduction) (adduction) (separation) (*see also* **Fracture, pathological**) T14.8 — *continued*
  ulna (shaft) S52.20- — *continued*
    shaft S52.20- — *continued*
      specified NEC S52.29-
      spiral (displaced) S52.24-
        nondisplaced S52.24-
      transverse (displaced) S52.22-
        nondisplaced S52.22-
    upper end S52.00-
      coronoid process (displaced) S52.04-
        nondisplaced S52.04-
      olecranon process (displaced) S52.02-
        with intraarticular extension S52.03-
        nondisplaced S52.02-
        with intraarticular extension S52.03-
      specified NEC S52.09-
      torus S52.01-
  unciform — *see* Fracture, carpal, hamate
  vault of skull S02.0
  vertebra, vertebral (arch) (body) (column) (neural arch) (pedicle) (spinous process) (transverse process)
    atlas — *see* Fracture, neck, cervical vertebra, first
    axis — *see* Fracture, neck, cervical vertebra, second
    cervical (teardrop) S12.9
      axis — *see* Fracture, neck, cervical vertebra, second
      first (atlas) — *see* Fracture, neck, cervical vertebra, first
      second (axis) — *see* Fracture, neck, cervical vertebra, second
    chronic M84.48
    coccyx S32.2
    dorsal — *see* Fracture, thorax, vertebra
    lumbar S32.009
      burst (stable) S32.001
        unstable S32.002
      fifth S32.059
        burst (stable) S32.051
          unstable S32.052
        specified type NEC S32.058
        wedge compression S32.050
      first S32.019
        burst (stable) S32.011
          unstable S32.012
        specified type NEC S32.018
        wedge compression S32.010
      fourth S32.049
        burst (stable) S32.041
          unstable S32.042
        specified type NEC S32.048
        wedge compression S32.040
      second S32.029
        burst (stable) S32.021
          unstable S32.022
        specified type NEC S32.028
        wedge compression S32.020
      specified type NEC S32.008
      third S32.039
        burst (stable) S32.031
          unstable S32.032
        specified type NEC S32.038
        wedge compression S32.030
      wedge compression S32.000
    metastatic — *see* Collapse, vertebra, in, specified disease NEC — *see also* Neoplasm
    newborn (birth injury) P11.5
    sacrum S32.10
      specified NEC S32.19
      Type
        1 S32.14
        2 S32.15
        3 S32.16
        4 S32.17

Fracture, traumatic (abduction) (adduction) (separation) (*see also* **Fracture, pathological**) T14.8 — *continued*
- vertebra, vertebral (arch) (body) (column) (neural arch) (pedicle) (spinous process) (transverse process) — *continued*
  - sacrum S32.10 — *continued*
    - Zone
      - I S32.119
        - displaced (minimally) S32.111
          - severely S32.112
        - nondisplaced S32.110
      - II S32.129
        - displaced (minimally) S32.121
          - severely S32.122
        - nondisplaced S32.120
      - III S32.139
        - displaced (minimally) S32.131
          - severely S32.132
        - nondisplaced S32.130
  - thoracic — *see* Fracture, thorax, vertebra
- vertex S02.0
- vomer (bone) S02.2
- wrist S62.10-
  - carpal — *see* Fracture, carpal bone
  - navicular (scaphoid) (hand) — *see* Fracture, carpal, navicular
- xiphisternum, xiphoid (process) S22.24
- zygoma S02.402
  - left side S02.40F *(follows S02.402)*
  - right side S02.40E *(follows S02.402)*

Fragile, fragility
- autosomal site Q95.5
- bone, congenital (with blue sclera) Q78.0
- capillary (hereditary) D69.8
- hair L67.8
- nails L60.3
- non-sex chromosome site Q95.5
- X chromosome Q99.2

Fragilitas
- crinium L67.8
- ossium (with blue sclerae) (hereditary) Q78.0
- unguium L60.3
  - congenital Q84.6

Fragments, cataract (lens), following cataract surgery H59.02-
- retained foreign body — *see* Retained, foreign body fragments (type of)

Frailty (frail) R54
- mental R41.81

Frambesia, frambesial (tropica) — *see also* Yaws
- initial lesion or ulcer A66.0
- primary A66.0

Frambeside
- gummatous A66.4
- of early yaws A66.2

Frambesioma A66.1

Franceschetti-Klein(-Wildervanck) disease or syndrome Q75.4

Francis' disease — *see* Tularemia

Frank's essential thrombocytopenia D69.3

Franklin disease C88.2

Fraser's syndrome Q87.0

Freckle(s) L81.2
- malignant melanoma in — *see* Melanoma
- melanotic (Hutchinson's) — *see* Melanoma, in situ
- retinal D49.81

Frederickson's hyperlipoproteinemia, type
- I and V E78.3
- IIA E78.00
- IIB and III E78.2
- IV E78.1

Freeman Sheldon syndrome Q87.0

Freezing (*see also* Effect, adverse, cold) T69.9

Frei's disease A55

Freiberg's disease (infraction of metatarsal head or osteochondrosis) — *see* Osteochondrosis, juvenile, metatarsus

Fremitus, friction, cardiac R01.2

Frenum, frenulum
- external os Q51.828
- tongue (shortening) (congenital) Q38.1

Frequency micturition (nocturnal) R35.0
- psychogenic F45.8

Frey's syndrome
- auriculotemporal G50.8
- hyperhidrosis L74.52

Friction
- burn — *see* Burn, by site
- fremitus, cardiac R01.2
- precordial R01.2
- sounds, chest R09.89

Friderichsen-Waterhouse syndrome or disease A39.1

Friedländer's B (bacillus) NEC (*see also* condition) A49.8

Friedreich's
- ataxia G11.1
- combined systemic disease G11.1
- facial hemihypertrophy Q67.4
- sclerosis (cerebellum) (spinal cord) G11.1

Frigidity F52.22

Fröhlich's syndrome E23.6

Frontal — *see also* condition
- lobe syndrome F07.0

Frostbite (superficial) T33.90
- with
  - partial thickness skin loss — *see* Frostbite (superficial), by site
  - tissue necrosis T34.90
- abdominal wall T33.3
  - with tissue necrosis T34.3
- ankle T33.81-
  - with tissue necrosis T34.81-
- arm T33.4-
  - with tissue necrosis T34.4-
  - finger(s) — *see* Frostbite, finger
  - hand — *see* Frostbite, hand
  - wrist — *see* Frostbite, wrist
- ear T33.01-
  - with tissue necrosis T34.01-
- face T33.09
  - with tissue necrosis T34.09
- finger T33.53-
  - with tissue necrosis T34.53-
- foot T33.82-
  - with tissue necrosis T34.82-
- hand T33.52-
  - with tissue necrosis T34.52-
- head T33.09
  - with tissue necrosis T34.09
  - ear — *see* Frostbite, ear
  - nose — *see* Frostbite, nose
- hip (and thigh) T33.6-
  - with tissue necrosis T34.6-
- knee T33.7-
  - with tissue necrosis T34.7-
- leg T33.9-
  - with tissue necrosis T34.9-
  - ankle — *see* Frostbite, ankle
  - foot — *see* Frostbite, foot
  - knee — *see* Frostbite, knee
  - lower T33.7-
    - with tissue necrosis T34.7-
  - thigh — *see* Frostbite, hip
  - toe — *see* Frostbite, toe
- limb
  - lower T33.99
    - with tissue necrosis T34.99
  - upper — *see* Frostbite, arm
- neck T33.1
  - with tissue necrosis T34.1
- nose T33.02
  - with tissue necrosis T34.02

Frostbite (superficial) T33.90 — *continued*
- pelvis T33.3
  - with tissue necrosis T34.3
- specified site NEC T33.99
  - with tissue necrosis T34.99
- thigh — *see* Frostbite, hip
- thorax T33.2
  - with tissue necrosis T34.2
- toes T33.83-
  - with tissue necrosis T34.83-
- trunk T33.99
  - with tissue necrosis T34.99
- wrist T33.51-
  - with tissue necrosis T34.51-

Frotteurism F65.81

Frozen (*see also* Effect, adverse, cold) T69.9
- pelvis (female) N94.89
  - male K66.8
- shoulder — *see* Capsulitis, adhesive

Fructokinase deficiency E74.11

Fructose 1,6 diphosphatase deficiency E74.19

Fructosemia (benign) (essential) E74.12

Fructosuria (benign) (essential) E74.11

Fuchs'
- black spot (myopic) H44.2-
- dystrophy (corneal endothelium) H18.51
- heterochromic cyclitis — *see* Cyclitis, Fuchs' heterochromic

Fucosidosis E77.1

Fugue R68.89
- dissociative F44.1
- hysterical (dissociative) F44.1
- postictal in epilepsy — *see* Epilepsy
- reaction to exceptional stress (transient) F43.0

Fulminant, fulminating — *see* condition

Functional — *see also* condition
- bleeding (uterus) N93.8

Functioning, intellectual, borderline R41.83

Fundus — *see* condition

Fungemia NOS B49

Fungus, fungous
- cerebral G93.89
- disease NOS B49
- infection — *see* Infection, fungus

Funiculitis (acute) (chronic) (endemic) N49.1
- gonococcal (acute) (chronic) A54.23
- tuberculous A18.15

Funnel
- breast (acquired) M95.4
  - congenital Q67.6
  - sequelae (late effect) of rickets E64.3
- chest (acquired) M95.4
  - congenital Q67.6
  - sequelae (late effect) of rickets E64.3
- pelvis (acquired) M95.5
  - with disproportion (fetopelvic) O33.3
    - causing obstructed labor O65.3
  - congenital Q74.2

FUO (fever of unknown origin) R50.9

Furfur L21.0
- microsporon B36.0

Furrier's lung J67.8

Furrowed K14.5
- nail(s) (transverse) L60.4
  - congenital Q84.6
- tongue K14.5
  - congenital Q38.3

Furuncle L02.92
- abdominal wall L02.221
- ankle — *see* Furuncle, lower limb
- antecubital space — *see* Furuncle, upper limb
- anus K61.0
- arm — *see* Furuncle, upper limb
- auditory canal, external — *see* Abscess, ear, external
- auricle (ear) — *see* Abscess, ear, external
- axilla (region) L02.42-

Furuncle L02.92 — *continued*
  back (any part) L02.222
  breast N61.1
  buttock L02.32
  cheek (external) L02.02
  chest wall L02.223
  chin L02.02
  corpus cavernosum N48.21
  ear, external — *see* Abscess, ear, external
  external auditory canal — *see* Abscess, ear, external
  eyelid — *see* Abscess, eyelid
  face L02.02
  femoral (region) — *see* Furuncle, lower limb
  finger — *see* Furuncle, hand
  flank L02.221
  foot L02.62-
  forehead L02.02
  gluteal (region) L02.32
  groin L02.224
  hand L02.52-
  head L02.821
    face L02.02
  hip — *see* Furuncle, lower limb
  kidney — *see* Abscess, kidney
  knee — *see* Furuncle, lower limb
  labium (majus) (minus) N76.4
  lacrimal
    gland — *see* Dacryoadenitis
    passages (duct) (sac) — *see* Inflammation, lacrimal, passages, acute
  leg (any part) — *see* Furuncle, lower limb
  lower limb L02.42-
  malignant A22.0
  mouth K12.2
  navel L02.226
  neck L02.12
  nose J34.0
  orbit, orbital — *see* Abscess, orbit
  palmar (space) — *see* Furuncle, hand
  partes posteriores L02.32
  pectoral region L02.223
  penis N48.21
  perineum L02.225
  pinna — *see* Abscess, ear, external
  popliteal — *see* Furuncle, lower limb
  prepatellar — *see* Furuncle, lower limb
  scalp L02.821
  seminal vesicle N49.0
  shoulder — *see* Furuncle, upper limb
  specified site NEC L02.828
  submandibular K12.2
  temple (region) L02.02
  thumb — *see* Furuncle, hand
  toe — *see* Furuncle, foot
  trunk L02.229
    abdominal wall L02.221
    back L02.222
    chest wall L02.223
    groin L02.224
    perineum L02.225
    umbilicus L02.226
  umbilicus L02.226
  upper limb L02.42-
  vulva N76.4
Furunculosis — *see* Furuncle
Fused — *see* Fusion, fused
Fusion, fused (congenital)
  astragaloscaphoid Q74.2
  atria Q21.1
  auditory canal Q16.1
  auricles, heart Q21.1
  binocular with defective stereopsis H53.32
  bone Q79.8
  cervical spine M43.22
  choanal Q30.0
  commissure, mitral valve Q23.2

Fusion, fused (congenital) — *continued*
  cusps, heart valve NEC Q24.8
    mitral Q23.2
    pulmonary Q22.1
    tricuspid Q22.4
  ear ossicles Q16.3
  fingers Q70.0-
  hymen Q52.3
  joint (acquired) — *see also* Ankylosis
    congenital Q74.8
  kidneys (incomplete) Q63.1
  labium (majus) (minus) Q52.5
  larynx and trachea Q34.8
  limb, congenital Q74.8
    lower Q74.2
    upper Q74.0
  lobes, lung Q33.8
  lumbosacral (acquired) M43.27
    arthrodesis status Z98.1
    congenital Q76.49
    postprocedural status Z98.1
  nares, nose, nasal, nostril(s) Q30.0
  organ or site not listed — *see* Anomaly, by site
  ossicles Q79.9
    auditory Q16.3
  pulmonic cusps Q22.1
  ribs Q76.6
  sacroiliac (joint) (acquired) M43.28
    arthrodesis status Z98.1
    congenital Q74.2
    postprocedural status Z98.1
  spine (acquired) NEC M43.20
    arthrodesis status Z98.1
    cervical region M43.22
    cervicothoracic region M43.23
    congenital Q76.49
    lumbar M43.26
    lumbosacral region M43.27
    occipito-atlanto-axial region M43.21
    postoperative status Z98.1
    sacrococcygeal region M43.28
    thoracic region M43.24
    thoracolumbar region M43.25
  sublingual duct with submaxillary duct at opening in mouth Q38.4
  testes Q55.1
  toes Q70.2-
  tooth, teeth K00.2
  trachea and esophagus Q39.8
  twins Q89.4
  vagina Q52.4
  ventricles, heart Q21.0
  vertebra (arch) — *see* Fusion, spine
  vulva Q52.5
Fusospirillosis (mouth) (tongue) (tonsil) A69.1
Fussy baby R68.12

G

Gain in weight (abnormal) (excessive) — *see also* Weight, gain
Gaisböck's disease (polycythemia hypertonica) D75.1
Gait abnormality R26.9
  ataxic R26.0
  falling R29.6
  hysterical (ataxic) (staggering) F44.4
  paralytic R26.1
  spastic R26.1
  specified type NEC R26.89
  staggering R26.0
  unsteadiness R26.81
  walking difficulty NEC R26.2
Galactocele (breast) N64.89
  puerperal, postpartum O92.79
Galactokinase deficiency E74.29
Galactophoritis N61.0
  gestational, puerperal, postpartum O91.2-
Galactorrhea O92.6
  not associated with childbirth N64.3
Galactosemia (classic) (congenital) E74.21
Galactosuria E74.29
Galacturia R82.0
  schistosomiasis (bilharziasis) B65.0
Galeazzi's fracture S52.37-
Galen's vein — *see* condition
Galeophobia F40.218
Gall duct — *see* condition
Gallbladder — *see also* condition
  acute K81.0
Gallop rhythm R00.8
Gallstone (colic) (cystic duct) (gallbladder) (impacted) (multiple) — *see also* Calculus, gallbladder
  with
    cholecystitis — *see* Calculus, gallbladder, with cholecystitis
  bile duct (common) (hepatic) — *see* Calculus, bile duct
  causing intestinal obstruction K56.3
  specified NEC K80.80
    with obstruction K80.81
Gambling Z72.6
  pathological (compulsive) F63.0
Gammopathy (of undetermined significance [MGUS]) D47.2
  associated with lymphoplasmacytic dyscrasia D47.2
  monoclonal D47.2
  polyclonal D89.0
Gamna's disease (siderotic splenomegaly) D73.1
Gamophobia F40.298
Gampsodactylia (congenital) Q66.7
Gamstorp's disease (adynamia episodica hereditaria) G72.3
Gandy-Nanta disease (siderotic splenomegaly) D73.1
Gang
  membership offenses Z72.810
Gangliocytoma D36.10
Ganglioglioma — *see* Neoplasm, uncertain behavior, by site
Ganglion (compound) (diffuse) (joint) (tendon (sheath)) M67.40
  ankle M67.47-
  foot M67.47-
  forearm M67.43-
  hand M67.44-
  lower leg M67.46-
  multiple sites M67.49
  of yaws (early) (late) A66.6
  pelvic region M67.45-
  periosteal — *see* Periostitis

D I S E A S E   I N D E X

Ganglion (compound) (diffuse) (joint) (tendon (sheath)) M67.40 — *continued*
shoulder region M67.41-
specified site NEC M67.48
thigh region M67.45-
tuberculous A18.09
upper arm M67.42-
wrist M67.43-
Ganglioneuroblastoma — *see* Neoplasm, nerve, malignant
Ganglioneuroma D36.10
malignant — *see* Neoplasm, nerve, malignant
Ganglioneuromatosis D36.10
Ganglionitis
fifth nerve — *see* Neuralgia, trigeminal
gasserian (postherpetic) (postzoster) B02.21
geniculate G51.1
newborn (birth injury) P11.3
postherpetic, postzoster B02.21
herpes zoster B02.21
postherpetic geniculate B02.21
Gangliosidosis E75.10
GM1 E75.19
GM2 E75.00
other specified E75.09
Sandhoff disease E75.01
Tay-Sachs disease E75.02
GM3 E75.19
mucolipidosis IV E75.11
Gangosa A66.5
Gangrene, gangrenous (connective tissue) (dropsical) (dry) (moist) (skin) (ulcer) (*see also* Necrosis) I96
with diabetes (mellitus) — *see* Diabetes, gangrene
abdomen (wall) I96
alveolar M27.3
appendix K35.80
with
perforation or rupture K35.2
peritoneal abscess K35.3
peritonitis NEC K35.3
generalized (with perforation or rupture) K35.2
localized (with perforation or rupture) K35.3
arteriosclerotic (general) (senile) — *see* Arteriosclerosis, extremities, with, gangrene
auricle I96
Bacillus welchii A48.0
bladder (infectious) — *see* Cystitis, specified type NEC
bowel, cecum, or colon — *see* Gangrene, intestine
Clostridium perfringens or welchii A48.0
cornea H18.89-
corpora cavernosa N48.29
noninfective N48.89
cutaneous, spreading I96
decubital — *see* Ulcer, pressure, by site
diabetic (any site) — *see* Diabetes, gangrene
emphysematous — *see* Gangrene, gas
epidemic — *see* Poisoning, food, noxious, plant
epididymis (infectional) N45.1
erysipelas — *see* Erysipelas
extremity (lower) (upper) I96
Fournier N49.3
female N76.89
fusospirochetal A69.0
gallbladder — *see* Cholecystitis, acute
gas (bacillus) A48.0
following
abortion — *see* Abortion by type complicated by infection
ectopic or molar pregnancy O08.0
glossitis K14.0

Gangrene, gangrenous (connective tissue) (dropsical) (dry) (moist) (skin) (ulcer) (*see also* Necrosis) I96 — *continued*
hernia — *see* Hernia, by site, with gangrene
intestine, intestinal (hemorrhagic) (massive) (*see also* Infarct, intestine) K55.069
with
mesenteric embolism (*see also* Infarct, intestine) K55.069
obstruction — *see* Obstruction, intestine
laryngitis J04.0
limb (lower) (upper) I96
lung J85.0
spirochetal A69.8
lymphangitis I89.1
Meleney's (synergistic) — *see* Ulcer, skin
mesentery (*see also* Infarct, intestine) K55.069
with
embolism (*see also* Infarct, intestine) K55.069
intestinal obstruction — *see* Obstruction, intestine
mouth A69.0
ovary — *see* Oophoritis
pancreas — *see* Pancreatitis, acute
penis N48.29
noninfective N48.89
perineum I96
pharynx — *see also* Pharyngitis
Vincent's A69.1
presenile I73.1
progressive synergistic — *see* Ulcer, skin
pulmonary J85.0
pulpal (dental) K04.1
quinsy J36
Raynaud's (symmetric gangrene) I73.01
retropharyngeal J39.2
scrotum N49.3
noninfective N50.89
senile (atherosclerotic) — *see* Arteriosclerosis, extremities, with, gangrene
spermatic cord N49.1
noninfective N50.89
spine I96
spirochetal NEC A69.8
spreading cutaneous I96
stomatitis A69.0
symmetrical I73.01
testis (infectional) N45.2
noninfective N44.8
throat — *see also* Pharyngitis
diphtheritic A36.0
Vincent's A69.1
thyroid (gland) E07.89
tooth (pulp) K04.1
tuberculous NEC — *see* Tuberculosis
tunica vaginalis N49.1
noninfective N50.89
umbilicus I96
uterus — *see* Endometritis
uvulitis K12.2
vas deferens N49.1
noninfective N50.89
vulva N76.89
Ganister disease J62.8
Ganser's syndrome (hysterical) F44.89
Gardner-Diamond syndrome (autoerythrocyte sensitization) D69.2
Gargoylism E76.01
Garré's disease, osteitis (sclerosing), osteomyelitis — *see* Osteomyelitis, specified type NEC
Garrod's pad, knuckle M72.1
Gartner's duct
cyst Q52.4
persistent Q50.6

Gas R14.3
asphyxiation, inhalation, poisoning, suffocation NEC — *see* Table of Drugs and Chemicals
excessive R14.0
gangrene A48.0
following
abortion — *see* Abortion by type complicated by infection
ectopic or molar pregnancy O08.0
on stomach R14.0
pains R14.1
Gastralgia — *see also* Pain, abdominal
Gastrectasis K31.0
psychogenic F45.8
Gastric — *see* condition
Gastrinoma
malignant
pancreas C25.4
specified site NEC — *see* Neoplasm, malignant, by site
unspecified site C25.4
specified site — *see* Neoplasm, uncertain behavior
unspecified site D37.9
Gastritis (simple) K29.70
with bleeding K29.71
acute (erosive) K29.00
with bleeding K29.01
alcoholic K29.20
with bleeding K29.21
allergic K29.60
with bleeding K29.61
atrophic (chronic) K29.40
with bleeding K29.41
chronic (antral) (fundal) K29.50
with bleeding K29.51
atrophic K29.40
with bleeding K29.41
superficial K29.30
with bleeding K29.31
dietary counseling and surveillance Z71.3
due to diet deficiency E63.9
eosinophilic K52.81
giant hypertrophic K29.60
with bleeding K29.61
granulomatous K29.60
with bleeding K29.61
hypertrophic (mucosa) K29.60
with bleeding K29.61
nervous F54
spastic K29.60
with bleeding K29.61
specified NEC K29.60
with bleeding K29.61
superficial chronic K29.30
with bleeding K29.31
tuberculous A18.83
viral NEC A08.4
Gastrocarcinoma — *see* Neoplasm, malignant, stomach
Gastrocolic — *see* condition
Gastrodisciasis, gastrodiscoidiasis B66.8
Gastroduodenitis K29.90
with bleeding K29.91
virus, viral A08.4
specified type NEC A08.39
Gastrodynia — *see* Pain, abdominal
Gastroenteritis (acute) (chronic) (noninfectious) (*see also* Enteritis) K52.9
allergic K52.29
with
eosinophilic gastritis or gastroenteritis K52.81
food protein-induced enterocolitis syndrome K52.21
food protein-induced enteropathy K52.22
dietetic (*see also* Gastroenteritis, allergic) K52.29

Gastroenteritis (acute) (chronic)
(noninfectious) (*see also* Enteritis) K52.9 —
continued
drug-induced K52.1
due to
Cryptosporidium A07.2
drugs K52.1
food poisoning — *see* Intoxication,
foodborne
radiation K52.0
eosinophilic K52.81
epidemic (infectious) A09
food hypersensitivity (*see also* Gastroenteritis,
allergic) K52.29
infectious — *see* Enteritis, infectious
influenzal — *see* Influenza, with gastroenteritis
noninfectious K52.9
specified NEC K52.89
rotaviral A08.0
Salmonella A02.0
toxic K52.1
viral NEC A08.4
acute infectious A08.39
type Norwalk A08.11
infantile (acute) A08.39
Norwalk agent A08.11
rotaviral A08.0
severe of infants A08.39
specified type NEC A08.39
Gastroenteropathy (*see also* Gastroenteritis)
K52.9
acute, due to Norovirus A08.11
acute, due to Norwalk agent A08.11
infectious A09
Gastroenteroptosis K63.4
**Gastroesophageal laceration-
hemorrhage syndrome** K22.6
Gastrointestinal — *see* condition
Gastrojejunal — *see* condition
Gastrojejunitis (*see also* Enteritis) K52.9
Gastrojejunocolic — *see* condition
Gastroliths K31.89
Gastromalacia K31.89
Gastroparalysis K31.84
diabetic — *see* Diabetes, gastroparalysis
Gastroparesis K31.84
diabetic — *see* Diabetes, by type, with
gastroparesis
Gastropathy K31.9
congestive portal K31.89
erythematous K29.70
exudative K90.89
portal hypertensive K31.89
Gastroptosis K31.89
Gastrorrhagia K92.2
psychogenic F45.8
Gastroschisis (congenital) Q79.3
Gastrospasm (neurogenic) (reflex) K31.89
neurotic F45.8
psychogenic F45.8
Gastrostaxis — *see* Gastritis, with bleeding
Gastrostenosis K31.89
Gastrostomy
attention to Z43.1
status Z93.1
Gastrosuccorrhea (continuous) (intermittent)
K31.89
neurotic F45.8
psychogenic F45.8
Gatophobia F40.218
Gaucher's disease or splenomegaly
(adult) (infantile) E75.22
Gee(-Herter)(-Thaysen) disease
(nontropical sprue) K90.0
Gélineau's syndrome G47.419
with cataplexy G47.411
Gemination, tooth, teeth K00.2

Gemistocytoma
specified site — *see* Neoplasm, malignant, by
site
unspecified site C71.9
General, generalized — *see* condition
Genetic
carrier (status)
cystic fibrosis Z14.1
hemophilia A (asymptomatic) Z14.01
symptomatic Z14.02
specified NEC Z14.8
susceptibility to disease NEC Z15.89
malignant neoplasm Z15.09
breast Z15.01
endometrium Z15.04
ovary Z15.02
prostate Z15.03
specified NEC Z15.09
multiple endocrine neoplasia Z15.81
Genital — *see* condition
Genito-anorectal syndrome A55
Genitourinary system — *see* condition
Genu
congenital Q74.1
extrorsum (acquired) — *see also* Deformity,
varus, knee
congenital Q74.1
sequelae (late effect) of rickets E64.3
introrsum (acquired) — *see also* Deformity,
valgus, knee
congenital Q74.1
sequelae (late effect) of rickets E64.3
rachitic (old) E64.3
recurvatum (acquired) — *see also* Deformity,
limb, specified type NEC, lower leg
congenital Q68.2
sequelae (late effect) of rickets E64.3
valgum (acquired) (knock-knee) M21.06-
congenital Q74.1
sequelae (late effect) of rickets E64.3
varum (acquired) (bowleg) M21.16-
congenital Q74.1
sequelae (late effect) of rickets E64.3
Geographic tongue K14.1
Geophagia — *see* Pica
Geotrichosis B48.3
stomatitis B48.3
Gephyrophobia F40.242
Gerbode defect Q21.0
GERD (gastroesophageal reflux disease) K21.9
Gerhardt's
disease (erythromelalgia) I73.81
syndrome (vocal cord paralysis) J38.00
bilateral J38.02
unilateral J38.01
German measles — *see also* Rubella
exposure to Z20.4
Germinoblastoma (diffuse) C85.9-
follicular C82.9-
Germinoma — *see* Neoplasm, malignant, by
site
Gerontoxon — *see* Degeneration, cornea,
senile
Gerstmann's syndrome R48.8
developmental F81.2
**Gerstmann-Sträussler-Scheinker
syndrome** (GSS) A81.82
Gestation (period) — *see also* Pregnancy
ectopic — *see* Pregnancy, by site
multiple O30.9-
greater than quadruplets — *see* Pregnancy,
multiple (gestation), specified NEC
specified NEC — *see* Pregnancy, multiple
(gestation), specified NEC
Gestational
mammary abscess O91.11-
purulent mastitis O91.11-
subareolar abscess O91.11-

Ghon tubercle, primary infection A15.7
Ghost
teeth K00.4
vessels (cornea) H16.41-
Ghoul hand A66.3
Gianotti-Crosti disease L44.4
Giant
cell
epulis K06.8
peripheral granuloma K06.8
esophagus, congenital Q39.5
kidney, congenital Q63.3
urticaria T78.3
hereditary D84.1
Giardiasis A07.1
Gibert's disease or pityriasis L42
Giddiness R42
hysterical F44.89
psychogenic F45.8
Gierke's disease (glycogenosis I) E74.01
Gigantism (cerebral) (hypophyseal) (pituitary)
E22.0
constitutional E34.4
Gilbert's disease or syndrome E80.4
Gilchrist's disease B40.9
Gilford-Hutchinson disease E34.8
**Gilles de la Tourette's disease or
syndrome** (motor-verbal tic) F95.2
Gingivitis K05.10
acute (catarrhal) K05.00
necrotizing A69.1
nonplaque induced K05.01
plaque induced K05.00
chronic (desquamative) (hyperplastic) (simple
marginal) (pregnancy associated)
(ulcerative) K05.10
nonplaque induced K05.11
plaque induced K05.10
expulsiva — *see* Periodontitis
necrotizing ulcerative (acute) A69.1
pellagrous E52
acute necrotizing A69.1
Vincent's A69.1
Gingivoglossitis K14.0
Gingivopericementitis — *see* Periodontitis
Gingivosis — *see* Gingivitis, chronic
Gingivostomatitis K05.10
herpesviral B00.2
necrotizing ulcerative (acute) A69.1
Gland, glandular — *see* condition
Glanders A24.0
**Glanzmann (-Naegeli) disease or
thrombasthenia** D69.1
Glasgow coma scale
total score
3-8 R40.243
9-12 R40.242
13-15 R40.241
Glass-blower's disease (cataract) — *see*
Cataract, specified NEC
Glaucoma H40.9
with
increased episcleral venous pressure
H40.81-
pseudoexfoliation of lens — *see* Glaucoma,
open angle, primary, capsular
absolute H44.51-
angle-closure (primary) H40.20-
acute (attack) (crisis) H40.21-
chronic H40.22-
intermittent H40.23-
residual stage H40.24-
borderline H40.00-
capsular (with pseudoexfoliation of lens) — *see*
Glaucoma, open angle, primary, capsular
childhood Q15.0
closed angle — *see* Glaucoma, angle-closure
congenital Q15.0

Glaucoma H40.9 — *continued*
  corticosteroid-induced — *see* Glaucoma, secondary, drugs
  hypersecretion H40.82-
  in (due to)
    amyloidosis E85.4 *[H42]*
    aniridia Q13.1 *[H42]*
    concussion of globe — *see* Glaucoma, secondary, trauma
    dislocation of lens — *see* Glaucoma, secondary
    disorder of lens NEC — *see* Glaucoma, secondary
    drugs — *see* Glaucoma, secondary, drugs
    endocrine disease NOS E34.9 *[H42]*
    eye
      inflammation — *see* Glaucoma, secondary, inflammation
      trauma — *see* Glaucoma, secondary, trauma
    hypermature cataract — *see* Glaucoma, secondary
    iridocyclitis — *see* Glaucoma, secondary, inflammation
    lens disorder — *see* Glaucoma, secondary,
    Lowe's syndrome E72.03 *[H42]*
    metabolic disease NOS E88.9 *[H42]*
    ocular disorders NEC — *see* Glaucoma, secondary
    onchocerciasis B73.02
    pupillary block — *see* Glaucoma, secondary
    retinal vein occlusion — *see* Glaucoma, secondary
    Rieger's anomaly Q13.81 *[H42]*
    rubeosis of iris — *see* Glaucoma, secondary
    tumor of globe — *see* Glaucoma, secondary
  infantile Q15.0
  low tension — *see* Glaucoma, open angle, primary, low-tension
  malignant H40.83-
  narrow angle — *see* Glaucoma, angle-closure
  newborn Q15.0
  noncongestive (chronic) — *see* Glaucoma, open angle
  nonobstructive — *see* Glaucoma, open angle
  obstructive — *see also* Glaucoma, angle-closure
    due to lens changes — *see* Glaucoma, secondary
  open angle H40.10-
    primary H40.11-
      capsular (with pseudoexfoliation of lens) H40.14-
      low-tension H40.12-
      pigmentary H40.13-
      residual stage H40.15-
    phacolytic — *see* Glaucoma, secondary
    pigmentary — *see* Glaucoma, open angle, primary, pigmentary
  postinfectious — *see* Glaucoma, secondary, inflammation
  secondary (to) H40.5-
    drugs H40.6-
    inflammation H40.4-
    trauma H40.3-
  simple (chronic) H40.11-
  simplex H40.11-
  specified type NEC H40.89
  suspect H40.00-
  syphilitic A52.71
  traumatic — *see also* Glaucoma, secondary, trauma
    newborn (birth injury) P15.3
  tuberculous A18.59
Glaucomatous flecks (subcapsular) — *see* Cataract, complicated
Glazed tongue K14.4
Gleet (gonococcal) A54.01
Glénard's disease K63.4

Glioblastoma (multiforme)
  with sarcomatous component
    specified site — *see* Neoplasm, malignant, by site
    unspecified site C71.9
  giant cell
    specified site — *see* Neoplasm, malignant, by site
    unspecified site C71.9
  specified site — *see* Neoplasm, malignant, by site
  unspecified site C71.9
Glioma (malignant)
  astrocytic
    specified site — *see* Neoplasm, malignant, by site
    unspecified site C71.9
  mixed
    specified site — *see* Neoplasm, malignant, by site
    unspecified site C71.9
  nose Q30.8
  specified site NEC — *see* Neoplasm, malignant, by site
  subependymal D43.2
    specified site — *see* Neoplasm, uncertain behavior, by site
    unspecified site D43.2
  unspecified site C71.9
Gliomatosis cerebri C71.0
Glioneuroma — *see* Neoplasm, uncertain behavior, by site
Gliosarcoma
  specified site — *see* Neoplasm, malignant, by site
  unspecified site C71.9
Gliosis (cerebral) G93.89
  spinal G95.89
Glisson's disease — *see* Rickets
Globinuria R82.3
Globus (hystericus) F45.8
Glomangioma D18.00
  intra-abdominal D18.03
  intracranial D18.02
  skin D18.01
  specified site NEC D18.09
Glomangiomyoma D18.00
  intra-abdominal D18.03
  intracranial D18.02
  skin D18.01
  specified site NEC D18.09
Glomangiosarcoma — *see* Neoplasm, connective tissue, malignant
Glomerular
  disease in syphilis A52.75
  nephritis — *see* Glomerulonephritis
Glomerulitis — *see* Glomerulonephritis
Glomerulonephritis (*see also* Nephritis) N05.9
  with
    edema — *see* Nephrosis
    minimal change N05.0
    minor glomerular abnormality N05.0
  acute N00.9
  chronic N03.9
  crescentic (diffuse) NEC (*see also* N00-N07 with fourth character .7) N05.7
  dense deposit (*see also* N00-N07 with fourth character .6) N05.6
  diffuse
    crescentic (*see also* N00-N07 with fourth character .7) N05.7
    endocapillary proliferative (*see also* N00-N07 with fourth character .4) N05.4
    membranous (*see also* N00-N07 with fourth character .2) N05.2
    mesangial proliferative (*see also* N00-N07 with fourth character .3) N05.3

Glomerulonephritis (*see also* Nephritis) N05.9 — *continued*
  diffuse — *continued*
    mesangiocapillary (*see also* N00-N07 with fourth character .5) N05.5
    sclerosing N05.8
  endocapillary proliferative (diffuse) NEC (*see also* N00-N07 with fourth character .4) N05.4
  extracapillary NEC (*see also* N00-N07 with fourth character .7) N05.7
  focal (and segmental) (*see also* N00-N07 with fourth character .1) N05.1
  hypocomplementemic — *see* Glomerulonephritis, membranoproliferative
  IgA — *see* Nephropathy, IgA
  immune complex (circulating) NEC N05.8
  in (due to)
    amyloidosis E85.4 *[N08]*
    bilharziasis B65.9 *[N08]*
    cryoglobulinemia D89.1 *[N08]*
    defibrination syndrome D65 *[N08]*
    diabetes mellitus — *see* Diabetes, glomerulosclerosis
    disseminated intravascular coagulation D65 *[N08]*
    Fabry(-Anderson) disease E75.21 *[N08]*
    Goodpasture's syndrome M31.0
    hemolytic-uremic syndrome D59.3
    Henoch(-Schönlein) purpura D69.0 *[N08]*
    lecithin cholesterol acyltransferase deficiency E78.6 *[N08]*
    microscopic polyangiitis M31.7 *[N08]*
    multiple myeloma C90.0- *[N08]*
    Plasmodium malariae B52.0
    schistosomiasis B65.9 *[N08]*
    sepsis A41.9 *[N08]*
      streptococcal A40- *[N08]*
    sickle-cell disorders D57- *[N08]*
    strongyloidiasis B78.9 *[N08]*
    subacute bacterial endocarditis I33.0 *[N08]*
    syphilis (late) congenital A50.59 *[N08]*
    systemic lupus erythematosus M32.14
    thrombotic thrombocytopenic purpura M31.1 *[N08]*
    typhoid fever A01.09
    Waldenström macroglobulinemia C88.0 *[N08]*
    Wegener's granulomatosis M31.31
  latent or quiescent N03.9
  lobular, lobulonodular — *see* Glomerulonephritis, membranoproliferative
  membranoproliferative (diffuse) (type 1 or 3) (*see also* N00-N07 with fourth character .5) N05.5
    dense deposit (type 2) NEC (*see also* N00-N07 with fourth character .6) N05.6
  membranous (diffuse) NEC (*see also* N00-N07 with fourth character .2) N05.2
  mesangial
    IgA/IgG — *see* Nephropathy, IgA
    proliferative (diffuse) NEC (*see also* N00-N07 with fourth character .3) N05.3
  mesangiocapillary (diffuse) NEC (*see also* N00-N07 with fourth character .5) N05.5
  necrotic, necrotizing NEC (*see also* N00-N07 with fourth character .8) N05.8
  nodular — *see* Glomerulonephritis, membranoproliferative
  poststreptococcal NEC N05.9
    acute N00.9
    chronic N03.9
    rapidly progressive N01.9
  proliferative NEC (*see also* N00-N07 with fourth character .8) N05.8
    diffuse (lupus) M32.14

Glomerulonephritis (*see also* Nephritis)
　N05.9 — *continued*
　rapidly progressive N01.9
　sclerosing, diffuse N05.8
　specified pathology NEC (*see also* N00-N07
　　with fourth character .8) N05.8
　subacute N01.9
Glomerulopathy — *see* Glomerulonephritis
Glomerulosclerosis — *see also* Sclerosis, renal
　intercapillary (nodular) (with diabetes) — *see*
　　Diabetes, glomerulosclerosis
　intracapillary — *see* Diabetes,
　　glomerulosclerosis
Glossagra K14.6
Glossalgia K14.6
Glossitis (chronic superficial) (gangrenous)
　　(Moeller's) K14.0
　areata exfoliativa K14.1
　atrophic K14.4
　benign migratory K14.1
　cortical superficial, sclerotic K14.0
　Hunter's D51.0
　interstitial, sclerous K14.0
　median rhomboid K14.2
　pellagrous E52
　superficial, chronic K14.0
Glossocele K14.8
Glossodynia K14.6
　exfoliativa K14.4
Glossoncus K14.8
Glossopathy K14.9
Glossophytia K14.3
Glossoplegia K14.8
Glossoptosis K14.8
Glossopyrosis K14.6
Glossotrichia K14.3
Glossy skin L90.8
Glottis — *see* condition
Glottitis (*see also* Laryngitis) J04.0
Glucagonoma
　pancreas
　　benign D13.7
　　malignant C25.4
　　uncertain behavior D37.8
　specified site NEC
　　benign — *see* Neoplasm, benign, by site
　　malignant — *see* Neoplasm, malignant, by
　　　site
　　uncertain behavior — *see* Neoplasm,
　　　uncertain behavior, by site
　unspecified site
　　benign D13.7
　　malignant C25.4
　　uncertain behavior D37.8
Glucoglycinuria E72.51
Glucose-galactose malabsorption E74.39
Glue
　ear — *see* Otitis, media, nonsuppurative,
　　chronic, mucoid
　sniffing (airplane) — *see* Abuse, drug, inhalant
　　dependence — *see* Dependence, drug,
　　　inhalant
Glutaric aciduria E72.3
Glycinemia E72.51
Glycinuria (renal) (with ketosis) E72.09
Glycogen
　infiltration — *see* Disease, glycogen storage
　storage disease — *see* Disease, glycogen
　　storage
Glycogenosis (diffuse) (generalized) — *see also*
　　Disease, glycogen storage
　cardiac E74.02 [*I43*]
　diabetic, secondary — *see* Diabetes,
　　glycogenosis, secondary
　pulmonary interstitial J84.842
Glycopenia E16.2
Glycosuria R81
　renal E74.8

Gnathostoma spinigerum (infection)
　(infestation), gnathostomiasis
　　(wandering swelling) B83.1
Goiter (plunging) (substernal) E04.9
　with
　　hyperthyroidism (recurrent) — *see*
　　　Hyperthyroidism, with, goiter
　　thyrotoxicosis — *see* Hyperthyroidism, with,
　　　goiter
　adenomatous — *see* Goiter, nodular
　cancerous C73
　congenital (nontoxic) E03.0
　　diffuse E03.0
　　parenchymatous E03.0
　　transitory, with normal functioning P72.0
　cystic E04.2
　　due to iodine-deficiency E01.1
　due to
　　enzyme defect in synthesis of thyroid
　　　hormone E07.1
　　iodine-deficiency (endemic) E01.2
　dyshormonogenetic (familial) E07.1
　endemic (iodine-deficiency) E01.2
　　diffuse E01.0
　　multinodular E01.1
　exophthalmic — *see* Hyperthyroidism, with,
　　goiter
　iodine-deficiency (endemic) E01.2
　　diffuse E01.0
　　multinodular E01.1
　　nodular E01.1
　lingual Q89.2
　lymphadenoid E06.3
　malignant C73
　multinodular (cystic) (nontoxic) E04.2
　　toxic or with hyperthyroidism E05.20
　　　with thyroid storm E05.21
　neonatal NEC P72.0
　nodular (nontoxic) (due to) E04.9
　　with
　　　hyperthyroidism E05.20
　　　　with thyroid storm E05.21
　　　thyrotoxicosis E05.20
　　　　with thyroid storm E05.21
　　endemic E01.1
　　iodine-deficiency E01.1
　　sporadic E04.9
　　toxic E05.20
　　　with thyroid storm E05.21
　nontoxic E04.9
　　diffuse (colloid) E04.0
　　multinodular E04.2
　　simple E04.0
　　specified NEC E04.8
　　uninodular E04.1
　simple E04.0
　toxic — *see* Hyperthyroidism, with, goiter
　uninodular (nontoxic) E04.1
　　toxic or with hyperthyroidism E05.10
　　　with thyroid storm E05.11
Goiter-deafness syndrome E07.1
Goldberg syndrome Q89.8
Goldberg-Maxwell syndrome E34.51
Goldblatt's hypertension or kidney I70.1
Goldenhar(-Gorlin) syndrome Q87.0
Goldflam-Erb disease or syndrome
　　G70.00
　with exacerbation (acute) G70.01
　in crisis G70.01
Goldscheider's disease Q81.8
Goldstein's disease (familial hemorrhagic
　　telangiectasia) I78.0
Golfer's elbow — *see* Epicondylitis, medial
Gonadoblastoma
　specified site — *see* Neoplasm, uncertain
　　behavior, by site
　unspecified site
　　female D39.10
　　male D40.10

Gonecystitis — *see* Vesiculitis
Gongylonemiasis B83.8
Goniosynechiae — *see* Adhesions, iris,
　goniosynechiae
Gonococcemia A54.86
Gonococcus, gonococcal (disease) (infection)
　　(*see also* condition) A54.9
　anus A54.6
　bursa, bursitis A54.49
　conjunctiva, conjunctivitis (neonatorum)
　　A54.31
　endocardium A54.83
　eye A54.30
　　conjunctivitis A54.31
　　iridocyclitis A54.32
　　keratitis A54.33
　　newborn A54.31
　　other specified A54.39
　fallopian tubes (acute) (chronic) A54.24
　genitourinary (organ) (system) (tract) (acute)
　　A54.00
　　lower A54.00
　　　with abscess (accessory gland)
　　　　(periurethral) A54.1
　　upper (*see also* condition) A54.29
　heart A54.83
　iridocyclitis A54.32
　joint A54.42
　lymphatic (gland) (node) A54.89
　meninges, meningitis A54.81
　musculoskeletal A54.40
　　arthritis A54.42
　　osteomyelitis A54.43
　　other specified A54.49
　　spondylopathy A54.41
　pelviperitonitis A54.24
　pelvis (acute) (chronic) A54.24
　pharynx A54.5
　proctitis A54.6
　pyosalpinx (acute) (chronic) A54.24
　rectum A54.6
　skin A54.89
　specified site NEC A54.89
　tendon sheath A54.49
　throat A54.5
　urethra (acute) (chronic) A54.01
　　with abscess (accessory gland) (periurethral)
　　　A54.1
　vulva (acute) (chronic) A54.02
Gonocytoma
　specified site — *see* Neoplasm, uncertain
　　behavior, by site
　unspecified site
　　female D39.10
　　male D40.10
Gonorrhea (acute) (chronic) A54.9
　Bartholin's gland (acute) (chronic) (purulent)
　　A54.02
　　with abscess (accessory gland) (periurethral)
　　　A54.1
　bladder A54.01
　cervix A54.03
　conjunctiva, conjunctivitis (neonatorum)
　　A54.31
　contact Z20.2
　Cowper's gland (with abscess) A54.1
　exposure to Z20.2
　fallopian tube (acute) (chronic) A54.24
　kidney (acute) (chronic) A54.21
　lower genitourinary tract A54.00
　　with abscess (accessory gland) (periurethral)
　　　A54.1
　ovary (acute) (chronic) A54.24
　pelvis (acute) (chronic) A54.24
　　female pelvic inflammatory disease A54.24
　penis A54.09
　prostate (acute) (chronic) A54.22
　seminal vesicle (acute) (chronic) A54.23
　specified site not listed (*see also* Gonococcus)
　　A54.89

Gonorrhea (acute) (chronic) A54.9 — continued
- spermatic cord (acute) (chronic) A54.23
- urethra A54.01
  - with abscess (accessory gland) (periurethral) A54.1
- vagina A54.02
- vas deferens (acute) (chronic) A54.23
- vulva A54.02

Goodall's disease A08.19

Goodpasture's syndrome M31.0

Gopalan's syndrome (burning feet) E53.0

Gorlin-Chaudry-Moss syndrome Q87.0

Gottron's papules L94.4

Gougerot-Blum syndrome (pigmented purpuric lichenoid dermatitis) L81.7

Gougerot-Carteaud disease or syndrome (confluent reticulate papillomatosis) L83

Gougerot's syndrome (trisymptomatic) L81.7

Gouley's syndrome (constrictive pericarditis) I31.1

Goundou A66.6

Gout, chronic (see also Gout, gouty) M1A.9 (follows M08)
- drug-induced M1A.20 (follows M08)
  - ankle M1A.27- (follows M08)
  - elbow M1A.22- (follows M08)
  - foot joint M1A.27- (follows M08)
  - hand joint M1A.24- (follows M08)
  - hip M1A.25- (follows M08)
  - knee M1A.26- (follows M08)
  - multiple site M1A.29- (follows M08)
  - shoulder M1A.21- (follows M08)
  - vertebrae M1A.28 (follows M08)
  - wrist M1A.23- (follows M08)
- idiopathic M1A.00 (follows M08)
  - ankle M1A.07- (follows M08)
  - elbow M1A.02- (follows M08)
  - foot joint M1A.07- (follows M08)
  - hand joint M1A.04- (follows M08)
  - hip M1A.05- (follows M08)
  - knee M1A.06- (follows M08)
  - multiple site M1A.09 (follows M08)
  - shoulder M1A.01- (follows M08)
  - vertebrae M1A.08 (follows M08)
  - wrist M1A.03- (follows M08)
- in (due to) renal impairment M1A.30 (follows M08)
  - ankle M1A.37- (follows M08)
  - elbow M1A.32- (follows M08)
  - foot joint M1A.37- (follows M08)
  - hand joint M1A.34- (follows M08)
  - hip M1A.35- (follows M08)
  - knee M1A.36- (follows M08)
  - multiple site M1A.39 (follows M08)
  - shoulder M1A.31- (follows M08)
  - vertebrae M1A.38 (follows M08)
  - wrist M1A.33- (follows M08)
- lead-induced M1A.10 (follows M08)
  - ankle M1A.17- (follows M08)
  - elbow M1A.12- (follows M08)
  - foot joint M1A.17- (follows M08)
  - hand joint M1A.14- (follows M08)
  - hip M1A.15- (follows M08)
  - knee M1A.16- (follows M08)
  - multiple site M1A.19 (follows M08)
  - shoulder M1A.11- (follows M08)
  - vertebrae M1A.18 (follows M08)
  - wrist M1A.13- (follows M08)
- primary — see Gout, chronic, idiopathic
- saturnine — see Gout, chronic, lead-induced
- secondary NEC M1A.40 (follows M08)
  - ankle M1A.47- (follows M08)
  - elbow M1A.42- (follows M08)
  - foot joint M1A.47- (follows M08)
  - hand joint M1A.44- (follows M08)
  - hip M1A.45- (follows M08)
  - knee M1A.46- (follows M08)
  - multiple site M1A.49 (follows M08)

Gout, chronic (see also Gout, gouty) M1A.9 (follows M08) — continued
- secondary NEC M1A.40 (follows M08) — continued
  - shoulder M1A.41- (follows M08)
  - vertebrae M1A.48 (follows M08)
  - wrist M1A.43- (follows M08)
- syphilitic (see also subcategory M14.8-) A52.77
- tophi M1A.9 (follows M08)

Gout, gouty (acute) (attack) (flare) (see also Gout, chronic) M10.9
- drug-induced M10.20
  - ankle M10.27-
  - elbow M10.22-
  - foot joint M10.27-
  - hand joint M10.24-
  - hip M10.25-
  - knee M10.26-
  - multiple site M10.29
  - shoulder M10.21-
  - vertebrae M10.28
  - wrist M10.23-
- idiopathic M10.00
  - ankle M10.07-
  - elbow M10.02-
  - foot joint M10.07-
  - hand joint M10.04-
  - hip M10.05-
  - knee M10.06-
  - multiple site M10.09
  - shoulder M10.01-
  - vertebrae M10.08
  - wrist M10.03-
- in (due to) renal impairment M10.30
  - ankle M10.37-
  - elbow M10.32-
  - foot joint M10.37-
  - hand joint M10.34-
  - hip M10.35-
  - knee M10.36-
  - multiple site M10.39
  - shoulder M10.31-
  - vertebrae M10.38
  - wrist M10.33-
- lead-induced M10.10
  - ankle M10.17-
  - elbow M10.12-
  - foot joint M10.17-
  - hand joint M10.14-
  - hip M10.15-
  - knee M10.16-
  - multiple site M10.19
  - shoulder M10.11-
  - vertebrae M10.18
  - wrist M10.13-
- primary — see Gout, idiopathic
- saturnine — see Gout, lead-induced
- secondary NEC M10.40
  - ankle M10.47-
  - elbow M10.42-
  - foot joint M10.47-
  - hand joint M10.44-
  - hip M10.45-
  - knee M10.46-
  - multiple site M10.49
  - shoulder M10.41-
  - vertebrae M10.48
  - wrist M10.43-
- syphilitic (see also subcategory M14.8-) A52.77
- tophi — see Gout, chronic

Gower's
- muscular dystrophy G71.0
- syndrome (vasovagal attack) R55

Gradenigo's syndrome — see Otitis, media, suppurative, acute

Graefe's disease — see Strabismus, paralytic, ophthalmoplegia, progressive

Graft-versus-host disease D89.813
- acute D89.810
- acute on chronic D89.812
- chronic D89.811

Grain mite (itch) B88.0

Grainhandler's disease or lung J67.8

Grand mal — see Epilepsy, generalized, specified NEC

Grand multipara status only (not pregnant) Z64.1
- pregnant — see Pregnancy, complicated by, grand multiparity

Granite worker's lung J62.8

Granular — see also condition
- inflammation, pharynx J31.2
- kidney (contracting) — see Sclerosis, renal
- liver K74.69

Granulation tissue (abnormal) (excessive) L92.9
- postmastoidectomy cavity — see Complications, postmastoidectomy, granulation

Granulocytopenia (primary) (malignant) — see Agranulocytosis

Granuloma L92.9
- abdomen K66.8
  - from residual foreign body L92.3
  - pyogenicum L98.0
- actinic L57.5
- annulare (perforating) L92.0
- apical K04.5
- aural — see Otitis, externa, specified NEC
- beryllium (skin) L92.3
- bone
  - eosinophilic C96.6
  - from residual foreign body — see Osteomyelitis, specified type NEC
  - lung C96.6
- brain (any site) G06.0
  - schistosomiasis B65.9 [G07]
- canaliculus lacrimalis — see Granuloma, lacrimal
- candidal (cutaneous) B37.2
- cerebral (any site) G06.0
- coccidioidal (primary) (progressive) B38.7
  - lung B38.1
  - meninges B38.4
- colon K63.89
- conjunctiva H11.22-
- dental K04.5
- ear, middle — see Cholesteatoma
- eosinophilic C96.6
  - bone C96.6
  - lung C96.6
  - oral mucosa K13.4
  - skin L92.2
- eyelid H01.8
- facial(e) L92.2
- foreign body (in soft tissue) NEC M60.20
  - ankle M60.27-
  - foot M60.27-
  - forearm M60.23-
  - hand M60.24-
  - in operation wound — see Foreign body, accidentally left during a procedure
  - lower leg M60.26-
  - pelvic region M60.25-
  - shoulder region M60.21-
  - skin L92.3
  - specified site NEC M60.28
  - subcutaneous tissue L92.3
  - thigh M60.25-
  - upper arm M60.22-
- gangraenescens M31.2
- genito-inguinale A58
- giant cell (central) (reparative) (jaw) M27.1
  - gingiva (peripheral) K06.8
- gland (lymph) I88.8

Granuloma L92.9 — continued
hepatic NEC K75.3
  in (due to)
    berylliosis J63.2 [K77]
    sarcoidosis D86.89
Hodgkin C81.9
ileum K63.89
infectious B99.9
  specified NEC B99.8
inguinale (Donovan) (venereal) A58
intestine NEC K63.89
intracranial (any site) G06.0
intraspinal (any part) G06.1
iridocyclitis — see Iridocyclitis, chronic
jaw (bone) (central) M27.1
  reparative giant cell M27.1
kidney (see also Infection, kidney) N15.8
lacrimal H04.81-
larynx J38.7
lethal midline (faciale(e)) M31.2
liver NEC — see Granuloma, hepatic
lung (infectious) — see also Fibrosis, lung
  coccidioidal B38.1
  eosinophilic C96.6
Majocchi's B35.8
malignant (facial(e)) M31.2
mandible (central) M27.1
midline (lethal) M31.2
monilial (cutaneous) B37.2
nasal sinus — see Sinusitis
operation wound T81.89
  foreign body — see Foreign body,
    accidentally left during a procedure
  stitch T81.89
  talc — see Foreign body, accidentally left
    during a procedure
oral mucosa K13.4
orbit, orbital H05.11-
paracoccidioidal B41.8
penis, venereal A58
periapical K04.5
peritoneum K66.8
  due to ova of helminths NOS (see also
    Helminthiasis) B83.9 [K67]
postmastoidectomy cavity — see
    Complications, postmastoidectomy,
    recurrent cholesteatoma
prostate N42.89
pudendi (ulcerating) A58
pulp, internal (tooth) K03.3
pyogenic, pyogenicum (of) (skin) L98.0
  gingiva K06.8
  maxillary alveolar ridge K04.5
  oral mucosa K13.4
rectum K62.89
reticulohistiocytic D76.3
rubrum nasi L74.8
Schistosoma — see Schistosomiasis
septic (skin) L98.0
silica (skin) L92.3
sinus (accessory) (infective) (nasal) — see
    Sinusitis
skin L92.9
  from residual foreign body L92.3
  pyogenicum L98.0
spine
  syphilitic (epidural) A52.19
  tuberculous A18.01
stitch (postoperative) T81.89
suppurative (skin) L98.0
swimming pool A31.1
talc — see also Granuloma, foreign body
  in operation wound — see Foreign body,
    accidentally left during a procedure
telangiectaticum (skin) L98.0
tracheostomy J95.09
trichophyticum B35.8
tropicum A66.4
umbilicus L92.9

Granuloma L92.9 — continued
urethra N36.8
uveitis — see Iridocyclitis, chronic
vagina A58
venereum A58
vocal cord J38.3
Granulomatosis L92.9
lymphoid C83.8-
miliary (listerial) A32.89
necrotizing, respiratory M31.30
progressive septic D71
specified NEC L92.8
Wegener's M31.30
  with renal involvement M31.31
Granulomatous tissue (abnormal)
  (excessive) L92.9
Granulosis rubra nasi L74.8
Graphite fibrosis (of lung) J63.3
Graphospasm F48.8
organic G25.89
Grating scapula M89.8x1
Gravel (urinary) — see Calculus, urinary
Graves' disease — see Hyperthyroidism, with,
  goiter
Gravis — see condition
Grawitz tumor C64-
Gray syndrome (newborn) P93.0
Grayness, hair (premature) L67.1
congenital Q84.2
Green sickness D50.8
Greenfield's disease
meaning
  concentric sclerosis (encephalitis periaxialis
    concentrica) G37.5
  metachromatic leukodystrophy E75.25
Greenstick fracture — code as Fracture, by
  site
Grey syndrome (newborn) P93.0
Grief F43.21
prolonged F43.29
reaction (see also Disorder, adjustment) F43.20
Griesinger's disease B76.9
Grinder's lung or pneumoconiosis J62.8
Grinding, teeth
psychogenic F45.8
sleep related G47.63
Grip
Dabney's B33.0
devil's B33.0
Grippe, grippal — see also Influenza
Balkan A78
summer, of Italy A93.1
Grisel's disease M43.6
Groin — see condition
Grooved tongue K14.5
Ground itch B76.9
Grover's disease or syndrome L11.1
Growing pains, children R29.898
Growth (fungoid) (neoplastic) (new) — see also
  Neoplasm
adenoid (vegetative) J35.8
benign — see Neoplasm, benign, by site
malignant — see Neoplasm, malignant, by site
rapid, childhood Z00.2
secondary — see Neoplasm, secondary, by
  site
Gruby's disease B35.0
Gubler-Millard paralysis or syndrome
  G46.3
Guerin-Stern syndrome Q74.3
Guidance, insufficient anterior (occlusal)
  M26.54
Guillain-Barré disease or syndrome
  G61.0
sequelae G65.0
Guinea worms (infection) (infestation) B72
Guinon's disease (motor-verbal tic) F95.2
Gull's disease E03.4
Gum — see condition

Gumboil K04.7
with sinus K04.6
Gumma (syphilitic) A52.79
artery A52.09
  cerebral A52.04
bone A52.77
  of yaws (late) A66.6
brain A52.19
cauda equina A52.19
central nervous system A52.3
ciliary body A52.71
congenital A50.59
eyelid A52.71
heart A52.06
intracranial A52.19
iris A52.71
kidney A52.75
larynx A52.73
leptomeninges A52.19
liver A52.74
meninges A52.19
myocardium A52.06
nasopharynx A52.73
neurosyphilitic A52.3
nose A52.73
orbit A52.71
palate (soft) A52.79
penis A52.76
pericardium A52.06
pharynx A52.73
pituitary A52.79
scrofulous (tuberculous) A18.4
skin A52.79
specified site NEC A52.79
spinal cord A52.19
tongue A52.79
tonsil A52.73
trachea A52.73
tuberculous A18.4
ulcerative due to yaws A66.4
ureter A52.75
yaws A66.4
  bone A66.6
Gunn's syndrome Q07.8
Gunshot wound — see also Wound, open
fracture — code as Fracture, by site
internal organs — see Injury, by site
Gynandrism Q56.0
Gynandroblastoma
specified site — see Neoplasm, uncertain
    behavior, by site
unspecified site
  female D39.10
  male D40.10
Gynecological examination (periodic)
  (routine) Z01.419
with abnormal findings Z01.411
Gynecomastia N62
Gynephobia F40.291
Gyrate scalp Q82.8

H

H (Hartnup's) disease E72.02
Haas' disease or osteochondrosis
(juvenile) (head of humerus) — *see*
Osteochondrosis, juvenile, humerus
Habit, habituation
bad sleep Z72.821
chorea F95.8
disturbance, child F98.9
drug — *see* Dependence, drug
irregular sleep Z72.821
laxative F55.2
spasm — *see* Tic
tic — *see* Tic
**Haemophilus (H.) influenzae, as cause of
disease classified elsewhere** B96.3
Haff disease — *see* Poisoning, mercury
**Hageman's factor defect, deficiency or
disease** D68.2
Haglund's disease or osteochondrosis
(juvenile) (os tibiale externum) — *see*
Osteochondrosis, juvenile, tarsus
Hailey-Hailey disease Q82.8
Hair — *see also* condition
plucking F63.3
in stereotyped movement disorder F98.4
tourniquet syndrome — *see also* Constriction,
external, by site
finger S60.44-
penis S30.842
thumb S60.34-
toe S90.44-
Hairball in stomach T18.2
Hair-pulling, pathological (compulsive) F63.3
Hairy black tongue K14.3
Half vertebra Q76.49
Halitosis R19.6
Hallerman-Streiff syndrome Q87.0
Hallervorden-Spatz disease G23.0
Hallopeau's acrodermatitis or disease
L40.2
Hallucination R44.3
auditory R44.0
gustatory R44.2
olfactory R44.2
specified NEC R44.2
tactile R44.2
visual R44.1
Hallucinosis (chronic) F28
alcoholic (acute) F10.951
in
abuse F10.151
dependence F10.251
drug-induced F19.951
cannabis F12.951
cocaine F14.951
hallucinogen F16.151
in
abuse F19.151
cannabis F12.151
cocaine F14.151
hallucinogen F16.151
inhalant F18.151
opioid F11.151
sedative, anxiolytic or hypnotic F13.151
stimulant NEC F15.151
dependence F19.251
cannabis F12.251
cocaine F14.251
hallucinogen F16.251
inhalant F18.251
opioid F11.251
sedative, anxiolytic or hypnotic F13.251
stimulant NEC F15.251
inhalant F18.951
opioid F11.951

Hallucinosis (chronic) F28 — *continued*
drug-induced F19.951 — *continued*
sedative, anxiolytic or hypnotic F13.951
stimulant NEC F15.951
organic F06.0
Hallux
deformity (acquired) NEC M20.5x-
limitus M20.5x-
malleus (acquired) NEC M20.3-
rigidus (acquired) M20.2-
congenital Q74.2
sequelae (late effect) of rickets E64.3
valgus (acquired) M20.1-
congenital Q66.6
varus (acquired) M20.3-
congenital Q66.3
Halo, visual H53.19
Hamartoma, hamartoblastoma Q85.9
epithelial (gingival), odontogenic, central or
peripheral — *see* Cyst, calcifying
odontogenic
Hamartosis Q85.9
Hamman-Rich syndrome J84.114
Hammer toe (acquired) NEC — *see also*
Deformity, toe, hammer toe
congenital Q66.89
sequelae (late effect) of rickets E64.3
Hand — *see* condition
Hand-foot syndrome L27.1
Handicap, handicapped
educational Z55.9
specified NEC Z55.8
**Hand-Schüller-Christian disease or
syndrome** C96.5
Hanging (asphyxia) (strangulation)
(suffocation) — *see* Asphyxia, traumatic, due
to mechanical threat
Hangnail — *see also* Cellulitis, digit
with lymphangitis — *see* Lymphangitis, acute,
digit
Hangover (alcohol) F10.129
Hanhart's syndrome Q87.0
Hanot's cirrhosis or disease K74.3
Hanot-Chauffard(-Troisier) syndrome
E83.19
Hansen's disease — *see* Leprosy
Hantaan virus disease (Korean hemorrhagic
fever) A98.5
Hantavirus disease (with renal
manifestations) (Dobrava) (Puumala) (Seoul)
A98.5
with pulmonary manifestations (Andes)
(Bayou) (Bermejo) (Black Creek Canal)
(Choclo) (Juquitiba) (Laguna negra)
(Lechiguanas) (New York) (Oran) (Sin
nombre) B33.4
Happy puppet syndrome Q93.5
Harada's disease or syndrome H30.81-
Hardening
artery — *see* Arteriosclerosis
brain G93.89
Harelip (complete) (incomplete) — *see* Cleft, lip
Harlequin (newborn) Q80.4
Harley's disease D59.6
Harmful use (of)
alcohol F10.10
anxiolytics — *see* Abuse, drug, sedative
cannabinoids — *see* Abuse, drug, cannabis
cocaine — *see* Abuse, drug, cocaine
drug — *see* Abuse, drug
hallucinogens — *see* Abuse, drug,
hallucinogen
hypnotics — *see* Abuse, drug, sedative
opioids — *see* Abuse, drug, opioid
PCP (phencyclidine) — *see* Abuse, drug,
hallucinogen
sedatives — *see* Abuse, drug, sedative
stimulants NEC — *see* Abuse, drug, stimulant
Harris' lines — *see* Arrest, epiphyseal

Hartnup's disease E72.02
Harvester's lung J67.0
Harvesting ovum for in vitro fertilization
Z31.83
Hashimoto's disease or thyroiditis E06.3
Hashitoxicosis (transient) E06.3
Hassal-Henle bodies or warts (cornea)
H18.49
Haut mal — *see* Epilepsy, generalized,
specified NEC
Haverhill fever A25.1
Hay fever (*see also* Fever, hay) J30.1
Hayem-Widal syndrome D59.8
Haygarth's nodes M15.8
Haymaker's lung J67.0
Hb (abnormal)
Bart's disease D56.0
disease — *see* Disease, hemoglobin
trait — *see* Trait
Head — *see* condition
Headache R51
allergic NEC G44.89
associated with sexual activity G44.82
chronic daily R51
cluster G44.009
chronic G44.029
intractable G44.021
not intractable G44.029
episodic G44.019
intractable G44.011
not intractable G44.019
intractable G44.001
not intractable G44.009
cough (primary) G44.83
daily chronic R51
drug-induced NEC G44.40
intractable G44.41
not intractable G44.40
exertional (primary) G44.84
histamine G44.009
intractable G44.001
not intractable G44.009
hypnic G44.81
lumbar puncture G97.1
medication overuse G44.40
intractable G44.41
not intractable G44.40
menstrual — *see* Migraine, menstrual
migraine (type) (*see also* Migraine) G43.909
nasal septum R51
neuralgiform, short lasting unilateral, with
conjunctival injection and tearing (SUNCT)
G44.059
intractable G44.051
not intractable G44.059
new daily persistent (NDPH) G44.52
orgasmic G44.82
periodic syndromes in adults and children
G43.C0 *(follows G43.7)*
with refractory migraine G43.C1 *(follows
G43.7)*
intractable G43.C19 *(follows G43.7)*
not intractable G43.C09 *(follows G43.7)*
without refractory migraine G43.C0 *(follows
G43.7)*
post-traumatic G44.309
acute G44.319
intractable G44.311
not intractable G44.319
chronic G44.329
intractable G44.321
not intractable G44.329
intractable G44.301
not intractable G44.309
postspinal puncture G97.1
pre-menstrual — *see* Migraine, menstrual
preorgasmic G44.82

Headache R51 — *continued*
  primary
    cough G44.83
    exertional G44.84
    stabbing G44.85
    thunderclap G44.53
  rebound G44.40
    intractable G44.41
    not intractable G44.40
  short lasting unilateral neuralgiform, with
      conjunctival injection and tearing (SUNCT)
      G44.059
    intractable G44.051
    not intractable G44.059
  specified syndrome NEC G44.89
  spinal and epidural anesthesia-induced
      T88.59
    in labor and delivery O74.5
    in pregnancy O29.4-
    postpartum, puerperal O89.4
  spinal fluid loss (from puncture) G97.1
  stabbing (primary) G44.85
  tension(-type) G44.209
    chronic G44.229
      intractable G44.221
      not intractable G44.229
    episodic G44.219
      intractable G44.211
      not intractable G44.219
    intractable G44.201
    not intractable G44.209
  thunderclap (primary) G44.53
  vascular NEC G44.1
Healthy
  infant
    accompanying sick mother Z76.3
    receiving care Z76.2
  person accompanying sick person Z76.3
Hearing examination Z01.10
  with abnormal findings NEC Z01.118
  following failed hearing screening Z01.110
  for hearing conservation and treatment
      Z01.12
Heart — *see* condition
Heart beat
  abnormality R00.9
    specified NEC R00.8
  awareness R00.2
  rapid R00.0
  slow R00.1
Heartburn R12
  psychogenic F45.8
Heat (effects) T67.9
  apoplexy T67.0
  burn (*see also* Burn) L55.9
  collapse T67.1
  cramps T67.2
  dermatitis or eczema L59.0
  edema T67.7
  erythema — *code by* site under Burn, first
      degree
  excessive T67.9
    specified effect NEC T67.8
  exhaustion T67.5
    anhydrotic T67.3
    due to
      salt (and water) depletion T67.4
      water depletion T67.3
        with salt depletion T67.4
  fatigue (transient) T67.6
  fever T67.0
  hyperpyrexia T67.0
  prickly L74.0
  prostration — *see* Heat, exhaustion
  pyrexia T67.0
  rash L74.0
  specified effect NEC T67.8
  stroke T67.0

Heat (effects) T67.9 — *continued*
  sunburn — *see* Sunburn
  syncope T67.1
Heavy-for-dates NEC (infant) (4000g to
    4499g) P08.1
  exceptionally (4500g or more) P08.0
Hebephrenia, hebephrenic (schizophrenia)
    F20.1
Heberden's disease or nodes (with
    arthropathy) M15.1
Hebra's
  pityriasis L26
  prurigo L28.2
Heel — *see* condition
Heerfordt's disease D86.89
Hegglin's anomaly or syndrome D72.0
Heilmeyer-Schoner disease D45
Heine-Medin disease A80.9
Heinz body anemia, congenital D58.2
Heliophobia F40.228
Heller's disease or syndrome F84.3
HELLP syndrome (hemolysis, elevated liver
    enzymes and low platelet count) O14.2-
  complicating
    childbirth O14.24
    puerperium O14.25
Helminthiasis — *see also* Infestation, helminth
  Ancylostoma B76.0
  intestinal B82.0
    mixed types (types classifiable to more than
        one of the titles B65.0-B81.3 and
        B81.8) B81.4
    specified type NEC B81.8
  mixed types (intestinal) (types classifiable to
      more than one of the titles B65.0-B81.3
      and B81.8) B81.4
  Necator (americanus) B76.1
  specified type NEC B83.8
Heloma L84
Hemangioblastoma — *see* Neoplasm,
    connective tissue, uncertain behavior
  malignant — *see* Neoplasm, connective tissue,
      malignant
Hemangioendothelioma — *see also*
    Neoplasm, uncertain behavior, by site
  benign D18.00
    intra-abdominal D18.03
    intracranial D18.02
    skin D18.01
    specified site NEC D18.09
  bone (diffuse) — *see* Neoplasm, bone,
      malignant
  epithelioid — *see also* Neoplasm, uncertain
      behavior, by site
    malignant — *see* Neoplasm, malignant, by
        site
  malignant — *see* Neoplasm, connective tissue,
      malignant
Hemangiofibroma — *see* Neoplasm, benign,
    by site
Hemangiolipoma — *see* Lipoma
Hemangioma D18.00
  arteriovenous D18.00
    intra-abdominal D18.03
    intracranial D18.02
    skin D18.01
    specified site NEC D18.09
  capillary D18.00
    intra-abdominal D18.03
    intracranial D18.02
    skin D18.01
    specified site NEC D18.09
  cavernous D18.00
    intra-abdominal D18.03
    intracranial D18.02
    skin D18.01
    specified site NEC D18.09

Hemangioma D18.00 — *continued*
  epithelioid D18.00
    intra-abdominal D18.03
    intracranial D18.02
    skin D18.01
    specified site NEC D18.09
  histiocytoid D18.00
    intra-abdominal D18.03
    intracranial D18.02
    skin D18.01
    specified site NEC D18.09
  infantile D18.00
    intra-abdominal D18.03
    intracranial D18.02
    skin D18.01
    specified site NEC D18.09
  intra-abdominal D18.03
  intracranial D18.02
  intramuscular D18.00
    intra-abdominal D18.03
    intracranial D18.02
    skin D18.01
    specified site NEC D18.09
  intrathoracic structures D18.09
  juvenile D18.00
  malignant — *see* Neoplasm,connective tissue,
      malignant
  plexiform D18.00
    intra-abdominal D18.03
    intracranial D18.02
    skin D18.01
    specified site NEC D18.09
  racemose D18.00
    intra-abdominal D18.03
    intracranial D18.02
    skin D18.01
    specified site NEC D18.09
  sclerosing — *see* Neoplasm,skin, benign
  simplex D18.00
    intra-abdominal D18.03
    intracranial D18.02
    skin D18.01
    specified site NEC D18.09
  skin D18.01
  specified site NEC D18.09
  venous D18.00
    intra-abdominal D18.03
    intracranial D18.02
    skin D18.01
    specified site NEC D18.09
  verrucous keratotic D18.00
    intra-abdominal D18.03
    intracranial D18.02
    skin D18.01
    specified site NEC D18.09
Hemangiomatosis (systemic) I78.8
  involving single site — *see* Hemangioma
Hemangiopericytoma — *see also* Neoplasm,
    connective tissue, uncertain behavior
  benign — *see* Neoplasm, connective tissue,
      benign
  malignant — *see* Neoplasm, connective tissue,
      malignant
Hemangiosarcoma — *see* Neoplasm,
    connective tissue, malignant
Hemarthrosis (nontraumatic) M25.00
  ankle M25.07-
  elbow M25.02-
  foot joint M25.07-
  hand joint M25.04-
  hip M25.05-
  in hemophilic arthropathy — *see* Arthropathy,
      hemophilic
  knee M25.06-
  shoulder M25.01-
  specified joint NEC M25.08
  traumatic — *see* Sprain, by site
  vertebrae M25.08
  wrist M25.03-

Hematemesis K92.0
- with ulcer — *code by* site under Ulcer, with hemorrhage K27.4
- newborn, neonatal P54.0
  - due to swallowed maternal blood P78.2

Hematidrosis L74.8

Hematinuria — *see also* Hemoglobinuria
- malarial B50.8

Hematobilia K83.8

Hematocele
- female NEC N94.89
  - with ectopic pregnancy O00.90
    - with intrauterine pregnancy O00.91
  - ovary N83.8
- male N50.1

Hematochezia (*see also* Melena) K92.1

Hematochyluria — *see also* Infestation, filarial
- schistosomiasis (bilharziasis) B65.0

Hematocolpos (with hematometra or hematosalpinx) N89.7

Hematocornea — *see* Pigmentation, cornea, stromal

Hematogenous — *see* condition

Hematoma (traumatic) (skin surface intact) — *see also* Contusion
- with
  - injury of internal organs — *see* Injury, by site
  - open wound — *see* Wound, open
- amputation stump (surgical) (late) T87.89
- aorta, dissecting I71.00
  - abdominal I71.02
  - thoracic I71.01
  - thoracoabdominal I71.03
- aortic intramural — *see* Dissection, aorta
- arterial (complicating trauma) — *see* Injury, blood vessel, by site
- auricle — *see* Contusion, ear
  - nontraumatic — *see* Disorder, pinna, hematoma
- birth injury NEC P15.8
- brain (traumatic)
  - with
    - cerebral laceration or contusion (diffuse) — *see* Injury, intracranial, diffuse
    - focal — *see* Injury, intracranial, focal
  - cerebellar, traumatic S06.37-
  - intracerebral, traumatic — *see* Injury, intracranial, intracerebral hemorrhage
  - newborn NEC P52.4
    - birth injury P10.1
  - nontraumatic — *see* Hemorrhage, intracranial
  - subarachnoid, arachnoid, traumatic — *see* Injury, intracranial, subarachnoid hemorrhage
  - subdural, traumatic — *see* Injury, intracranial, subdural hemorrhage
- breast (nontraumatic) N64.89
- broad ligament (nontraumatic) N83.7
  - traumatic S37.892
- cerebellar, traumatic S06.37-
- cerebral — *see* Hematoma, brain
- cerebrum S06.36-
  - left S06.35-
  - right S06.34-
- cesarean delivery wound O90.2
- complicating delivery (perineal) (pelvic) (vagina) (vulva) O71.7
- corpus cavernosum (nontraumatic) N48.89
- epididymis (nontraumatic) N50.1
- epidural (traumatic) — *see* Injury, intracranial, epidural hemorrhage
  - spinal — *see* Injury, spinal cord, by region
- episiotomy O90.2
- face, birth injury P15.4

Hematoma (traumatic) (skin surface intact) (*see also* Contusion) — *continued*
- genital organ NEC (nontraumatic)
  - female (nonobstetric) N94.89
    - traumatic S30.202
  - male N50.1
    - traumatic S30.201
- internal organs — *see* Injury, by site
- intracerebral, traumatic — *see* Injury, intracranial, intracerebral hemorrhage
- intraoperative — *see* Complications, intraoperative, hemorrhage
- labia (nontraumatic) (nonobstetric) N90.89
- liver (subcapsular) (nontraumatic) K76.89
  - birth injury P15.0
- mediastinum — *see* Injury, intrathoracic
- mesosalpinx (nontraumatic) N83.7
  - traumatic S37.898
- muscle — *code by* site under Contusion
- nontraumatic
  - muscle M79.81
  - soft tissue M79.81
- obstetrical surgical wound O90.2
- orbit, orbital (nontraumatic) — *see also* Hemorrhage, orbit
  - traumatic — *see* Contusion, orbit
- pelvis (female) (nontraumatic) (nonobstetric) N94.89
  - obstetric O71.7
  - traumatic — *see* Injury, by site
- penis (nontraumatic) N48.89
  - birth injury P15.5
- perianal (nontraumatic) K64.5
- perineal S30.23
  - complicating delivery O71.7
- perirenal — *see* Injury, kidney
- pinna — *see* Contusion, ear
  - nontraumatic — *see* Disorder, pinna, hematoma
- placenta O43.89-
- postoperative (postprocedural) — *see* Complication, postprocedural, hematoma
- retroperitoneal (nontraumatic) K66.1
  - traumatic S36.892
- scrotum, superficial S30.22
  - birth injury P15.5
- seminal vesicle (nontraumatic) N50.1
  - traumatic S37.892
- spermatic cord (traumatic) S37.892
  - nontraumatic N50.1
- spinal (cord) (meninges) — *see also* Injury, spinal cord, by region
  - newborn (birth injury) P11.5
- spleen D73.5
  - intraoperative — *see* Complications, intraoperative, hemorrhage, spleen
  - postprocedural (postoperative) — *see* Complications, postprocedural, hemorrhage, spleen
- sternocleidomastoid, birth injury P15.2
- sternomastoid, birth injury P15.2
- subarachnoid (traumatic) — *see* Injury, intracranial, subarachnoid hemorrhage
  - newborn (nontraumatic) P52.5
    - due to birth injury P10.3
  - nontraumatic — *see* Hemorrhage, intracranial, subarachnoid
- subdural (traumatic) — *see* Injury, intracranial, subdural hemorrhage
  - newborn (localized) P52.8
    - birth injury P10.0
  - nontraumatic — *see* Hemorrhage, intracranial, subdural
- superficial, newborn P54.5
- testis (nontraumatic) N50.1
  - birth injury P15.5
- tunica vaginalis (nontraumatic) N50.1

Hematoma (traumatic) (skin surface intact) (*see also* Contusion) — *continued*
- umbilical cord, complicating delivery O69.5
- uterine ligament (broad) (nontraumatic) N83.7
  - traumatic S37.892
- vagina (ruptured) (nontraumatic) N89.8
  - complicating delivery O71.7
- vas deferens (nontraumatic) N50.1
  - traumatic S37.892
- vitreous — *see* Hemorrhage, vitreous
- vulva (nontraumatic) (nonobstetric) N90.89
  - complicating delivery O71.7
  - newborn (birth injury) P15.5

Hematometra N85.7
- with hematocolpos N89.7

Hematomyelia (central) G95.19
- newborn (birth injury) P11.5
- traumatic T14.8

Hematomyelitis G04.90

Hematoperitoneum — *see* Hemoperitoneum

Hematophobia F40.230

Hematopneumothorax — *see* Hemothorax

Hematopoiesis, cyclic D70.4

Hematoporphyria — *see* Porphyria

Hematorachis, hematorrhachis G95.19
- newborn (birth injury) P11.5

Hematosalpinx N83.6
- with
  - hematocolpos N89.7
  - hematometra N85.7
    - with hematocolpos N89.7
- infectional — *see* Salpingitis

Hematospermia R36.1

Hematothorax — *see* Hemothorax

Hematuria R31.9
- benign (familial) (of childhood) — *see also* Hematuria, idiopathic
  - essential microscopic R31.1
- due to sulphonamide, sulfonamide — *see* Table of Drugs and Chemicals, by drug
- endemic (*see also* Schistosomiasis) B65.0
- gross R31.0
- idiopathic N02.9
  - with glomerular lesion
    - crescentic (diffuse) glomerulonephritis N02.7
    - dense deposit disease N02.6
    - endocapillary proliferative glomerulonephritis N02.4
    - focal and segmental hyalinosis or sclerosis N02.1
    - membranoproliferative (diffuse) N02.5
    - membranous (diffuse) N02.2
    - mesangial proliferative (diffuse) N02.3
    - mesangiocapillary (diffuse) N02.5
    - minor abnormality N02.0
    - proliferative NEC N02.8
    - specified pathology NEC N02.8
- intermittent — *see* Hematuria, idiopathic
- malarial B50.8
- microscopic NEC (with symptoms) R31.29
  - asymptomatic R31.21
  - benign essential R31.1
- paroxysmal — *see also* Hematuria, idiopathic
  - nocturnal D59.5
- persistent — *see* Hematuria, idiopathic
- recurrent — *see* Hematuria, idiopathic
- tropical (*see also* Schistosomiasis) B65.0
- tuberculous A18.13

Hemeralopia (day blindness) H53.11
- vitamin A deficiency E50.5

Hemi-akinesia R41.4

Hemianalgesia R20.0

Hemianencephaly Q00.0

Hemianesthesia R20.0

Hemianopia, hemianopsia (heteronymous) H53.47
- homonymous H53.46-
- syphilitic A52.71

Hemiathetosis R25.8
Hemiatrophy R68.89
 cerebellar G31.9
 face, facial, progressive (Romberg) G51.8
 tongue K14.8
Hemiballism(us) G25.5
Hemicardia Q24.8
Hemicephalus, hemicephaly Q00.0
Hemichorea G25.5
Hemicolitis, left — *see* Colitis, left sided
Hemicrania
 congenital malformation Q00.0
 continua G44.51
 meaning migraine (*see also* Migraine)
  G43.909
 paroxysmal G44.039
  chronic G44.049
   intractable G44.041
   not intractable G44.049
  episodic G44.039
   intractable G44.031
   not intractable G44.039
  intractable G44.031
  not intractable G44.039
Hemidystrophy — *see* Hemiatrophy
Hemiectromelia Q73.8
Hemihypalgesia R20.8
Hemihypesthesia R20.1
Hemi-inattention R41.4
Hemimelia Q73.8
 lower limb — *see* Defect, reduction, lower limb,
  specified type NEC
 upper limb — *see* Defect, reduction, upper
  limb, specified type NEC
Hemiparalysis — *see* Hemiplegia
Hemiparesis — *see* Hemiplegia
Hemiparesthesia R20.2
Hemiparkinsonism G20
Hemiplegia G81.9-
 alternans facialis G83.89
 ascending NEC G81.90
  spinal G95.89
 congenital (cerebral) G80.8
  spastic G80.2
 embolic (current episode) I63.4-
 flaccid G81.0-
 following
  cerebrovascular disease I69.959
   cerebral infarction I69.35-
   intracerebral hemorrhage I69.15-
   nontraumatic intracranial hemorrhage
    NEC I69.25-
   specified disease NEC I69.85-
   stroke NOS I69.35-
   subarachnoid hemorrhage I69.05-
 hysterical F44.4
 newborn NEC P91.8
  birth injury P11.9
 spastic G81.1-
  congenital G80.2
 thrombotic (current episode) I63.3-
Hemisection, spinal cord — *see* Injury,
 spinal cord, by region
Hemispasm (facial) R25.2
Hemisporosis B48.8
Hemitremor R25.1
Hemivertebra Q76.49
 failure of segmentation with scoliosis Q76.3
 fusion with scoliosis Q76.3
Hemochromatosis E83.119
 with refractory anemia D46.1
 due to repeated red blood cell transfusion
  E83.111
 hereditary (primary) E83.110
 primary E83.110
 specified NEC E83.118

Hemoglobin — *see also* condition
 abnormal (disease) — *see* Disease,
  hemoglobin
 AS genotype D57.3
 Constant Spring D58.2
 E-beta thalassemia D56.5
 fetal, hereditary persistence (HPFH) D56.4
 H Constant Spring D56.0
 low NOS D64.9
 S (Hb S), heterozygous D57.3
Hemoglobinemia D59.9
 due to blood transfusion T80.89
 paroxysmal D59.6
  nocturnal D59.5
Hemoglobinopathy (mixed) D58.2
 with thalassemia D56.8
 sickle-cell D57.1
  with thalassemia D57.40
   with crisis (vasoocclusive pain) D57.419
    with
     acute chest syndrome D57.411
     splenic sequestration D57.412
   without crisis D57.40
Hemoglobinuria R82.3
 with anemia, hemolytic, acquired (chronic)
  NEC D59.6
 cold (agglutinin) (paroxysmal) (with Raynaud's
  syndrome) D59.6
 due to exertion or hemolysis NEC D59.6
 intermittent D59.6
 malarial B50.8
 march D59.6
 nocturnal (paroxysmal) D59.5
 paroxysmal (cold) D59.6
  nocturnal D59.5
Hemolymphangioma D18.1
Hemolysis
 intravascular
  with
   abortion — *see* Abortion, by type,
    complicated by, hemorrhage
   ectopic or molar pregnancy O08.1
   hemorrhage
    antepartum — *see* Hemorrhage,
     antepartum, with coagulation defect
    intrapartum (*see also* Hemorrhage,
     complicating, delivery) O67.0
   postpartum O72.3
 neonatal (excessive) P58.9
  specified NEC P58.8
Hemolytic — *see* condition
Hemopericardium I31.2
 following acute myocardial infarction (current
  complication) I23.0
 newborn P54.8
 traumatic — *see* Injury, heart, with
  hemopericardium
Hemoperitoneum K66.1
 infectional K65.9
 traumatic S36.899
  with open wound — *see* Wound, open, with
   penetration into peritoneal cavity
Hemophilia (classical) (familial) (hereditary)
 D66
 A D66
 acquired D68.311
 autoimmune D68.311
 B D67
 C D68.1
 calcipriva (*see also* Defect, coagulation) D68.4
 nonfamilial (*see also* Defect, coagulation)
  D68.4
 secondary D68.311
 vascular D68.0
Hemophthalmos H44.81-
Hemopneumothorax — *see also* Hemothorax
 traumatic S27.2

Hemoptysis R04.2
 newborn P26.9
 tuberculous — *see* Tuberculosis, pulmonary
Hemorrhage, hemorrhagic (concealed) R58
 abdomen R58
 accidental antepartum — *see* Hemorrhage,
  antepartum
 acute idiopathic pulmonary, in infants R04.81
 adenoid J35.8
 adrenal (capsule) (gland) E27.49
  medulla E27.8
  newborn P54.4
 after delivery — *see* Hemorrhage, postpartum
 alveolar
  lung, newborn P26.8
  process K08.89
 alveolus K08.89
 amputation stump (surgical) T87.89
 anemia (chronic) D50.0
  acute D62
 antepartum (with) O46.90
  with coagulation defect O46.00-
   afibrinogenemia O46.01-
   disseminated intravascular coagulation
    O46.02-
   hypofibrinogenemia O46.01-
   specified defect NEC O46.09-
  before 20 weeks gestation O20.9
   specified type NEC O20.8
   threatened abortion O20.0
  due to
   abruptio placenta (*see also* Abruptio
    placentae) O45.9-
   leiomyoma, uterus — *see* Hemorrhage,
    antepartum, specified cause NEC
   placenta previa O44.1-
  specified cause NEC — *see* subcategory
   O46.8x-
 anus (sphincter) K62.5
 apoplexy (stroke) — *see* Hemorrhage,
  intracranial, intracerebral
 arachnoid — *see* Hemorrhage, intracranial,
  subarachnoid
 artery R58
  brain — *see* Hemorrhage, intracranial,
   intracerebral
 basilar (ganglion) I61.0
 bladder N32.89
 bowel K92.2
  newborn P54.3
 brain (miliary) (nontraumatic) — *see*
  Hemorrhage, intracranial, intracerebral
  due to
   birth injury P10.1
   syphilis A52.05
  epidural or extradural (traumatic) — *see*
   Injury, intracranial, epidural
   hemorrhage
  newborn P52.4
   birth injury P10.1
  subarachnoid — *see* Hemorrhage,
   intracranial, subarachnoid
  subdural — *see* Hemorrhage, intracranial,
   subdural
 brainstem (nontraumatic) I61.3
  traumatic S06.38-
 breast N64.59
 bronchial tube — *see* Hemorrhage, lung
 bronchopulmonary — *see* Hemorrhage, lung
 bronchus — *see* Hemorrhage, lung
 bulbar I61.5
 capillary I78.8
  primary D69.8
 cecum K92.2
 cerebellar, cerebellum (nontraumatic) I61.4
  newborn P52.6
  traumatic S06.37-

DISEASE INDEX

Hemorrhage, hemorrhagic (concealed) R58
— continued
- cerebral, cerebrum — see also Hemorrhage, intracranial, intracerebral
  - lobe I61.1
  - newborn (anoxic) P52.4
    - birth injury P10.1
- cerebromeningeal I61.8
- cerebrospinal — see Hemorrhage, intracranial, intracerebral
- cervix (uteri) (stump) NEC N88.8
- chamber, anterior (eye) — see Hyphema
- childbirth — see Hemorrhage, complicating, delivery
- choroid H31.30-
  - expulsive H31.31-
- ciliary body — see Hyphema
- cochlea — see subcategory H83.8
- colon K92.2
- complicating
  - abortion — see Abortion, by type, complicated by, hemorrhage
  - delivery O67.9
    - associated with coagulation defect (afibrinogenemia) (DIC) (hyperfibrinolysis) O67.0
    - specified cause NEC O67.8
  - surgical procedure — see Hemorrhage, intraoperative
- conjunctiva H11.3-
  - newborn P54.8
- cord, newborn (stump) P51.9
- corpus luteum (ruptured) cyst N83.1-
- cortical (brain) I61.1
- cranial — see Hemorrhage, intracranial
- cutaneous R23.3
  - due to autosensitivity, erythrocyte D69.2
  - newborn P54.5
- delayed
  - following ectopic or molar pregnancy O08.1
  - postpartum O72.2
- diathesis (familial) D69.9
- disease D69.9
  - newborn P53
  - specified type NEC D69.8
- due to or associated with
  - afibrinogenemia or other coagulation defect (conditions in categories D65-D69)
    - antepartum — see Hemorrhage, antepartum, with coagulation defect
    - intrapartum O67.0
  - dental implant M27.61
  - device, implant or graft (see also Complications, by site and type, specified NEC) T85.838
    - arterial graft NEC T82.838
    - breast T85.838
    - catheter NEC T85.838
      - dialysis (renal) T82.838
        - intraperitoneal T85.838
      - infusion NEC T82.838
        - spinal (epidural) (subdural) T85.830
      - urinary (indwelling) T83.83
    - electronic (electrode) (pulse generator) (stimulator)
      - bone T84.83
      - cardiac T82.837
      - nervous system (brain) (peripheral nerve) (spinal) T85.830
      - urinary T83.83
    - fixation, internal (orthopedic) NEC T84.83
    - gastrointestinal (bile duct) (esophagus) T85.838
    - genital NEC T83.83
    - heart T82.837
    - joint prosthesis T84.83
    - ocular (corneal graft) (orbital implant) NEC T85.838

Hemorrhage, hemorrhagic (concealed) R58
— continued
- due to or associated with — continued
  - device, implant or graft (see also Complications, by site and type, specified NEC) T85.83 — continued
    - orthopedic NEC T84.83
      - bone graft T86.838
    - specified NEC T85.838
    - urinary NEC T83.83
    - vascular NEC T82.838
    - ventricular intracranial shunt T85.830
- duodenum, duodenal K92.2
  - ulcer — see Ulcer, duodenum, with hemorrhage
- dura mater — see Hemorrhage, intracranial, subdural
- endotracheal — see Hemorrhage, lung
- epicranial subaponeurotic (massive), birth injury P12.2
- epidural (traumatic) — see also Injury, intracranial, epidural hemorrhage
  - nontraumatic I62.1
- esophagus K22.8
  - varix I85.01
    - secondary I85.11
- excessive, following ectopic gestation (subsequent episode) O08.1
- extradural (traumatic) — see Injury, intracranial, epidural hemorrhage
  - birth injury P10.8
  - newborn (anoxic) (nontraumatic) P52.8
  - nontraumatic I62.1
- eye NEC H57.8
  - fundus — see Hemorrhage, retina
  - lid — see Disorder, eyelid, specified type NEC
- fallopian tube N83.6
- fibrinogenolysis — see Fibrinolysis
- fibrinolytic (acquired) — see Fibrinolysis
- from
  - ear (nontraumatic) — see Otorrhagia
  - tracheostomy stoma J95.01
- fundus, eye — see Hemorrhage, retina
- funis — see Hemorrhage, umbilicus, cord
- gastric — see Hemorrhage, stomach
- gastroenteric K92.2
  - newborn P54.3
- gastrointestinal (tract) K92.2
  - newborn P54.3
- genital organ, male N50.1
- genitourinary (tract) NOS R31.9
- gingiva K06.8
- globe (eye) — see Hemophthalmos
- graafian follicle cyst (ruptured) N83.0-
- gum K06.8
- heart I51.89
- hypopharyngeal (throat) R04.1
- intermenstrual (regular) N92.3
  - irregular N92.1
- internal (organs) NEC R58
  - capsule I61.0
  - ear — see subcategory H83.8
  - newborn P54.8
- intestine K92.2
  - newborn P54.3
- intra-abdominal R58
- intra-alveolar (lung), newborn P26.8
- intracerebral (nontraumatic) — see Hemorrhage, intracranial, intracerebral
- intracranial (nontraumatic) I62.9
  - birth injury P10.9
  - epidural, nontraumatic I62.1
  - extradural, nontraumatic I62.1

Hemorrhage, hemorrhagic (concealed) R58
— continued
- intracranial (nontraumatic) I62.9 — continued
  - intracerebral (nontraumatic) (in) I61.9
    - brain stem I61.3
    - cerebellum I61.4
    - hemisphere I61.2
      - cortical (superficial) I61.1
      - subcortical (deep) I61.0
    - intraoperative
      - during a nervous system procedure G97.31
      - during other procedure G97.32
    - intraventricular I61.5
    - multiple localized I61.6
    - newborn P52.4
      - birth injury P10.1
    - postprocedural
      - following a nervous system procedure G97.51
      - following other procedure G97.52
    - specified NEC I61.8
    - superficial I61.1
    - traumatic (diffuse) — see Injury, intracranial, diffuse
      - focal — see Injury, intracranial, focal
  - newborn P52.9
    - specified NEC P52.8
  - subarachnoid (nontraumatic) (from) I60.9
    - intracranial (cerebral) artery I60.7
      - anterior communicating I60.2
      - basilar I60.4
      - carotid siphon and bifurcation I60.0-
      - communicating I60.7
        - anterior I60.2
        - posterior I60.3-
      - middle cerebral I60.1-
      - posterior communicating I60.3-
      - specified artery NEC I60.6
      - vertebral I60.5-
    - newborn P52.5
      - birth injury P10.3
    - specified NEC I60.8
    - traumatic S06.6x-
  - subdural (nontraumatic) I62.00
    - acute I62.01
    - birth injury P10.0
    - chronic I62.03
    - newborn (anoxic) (hypoxic) P52.8
      - birth injury P10.0
    - spinal G95.19
    - subacute I62.02
    - traumatic — see Injury, intracranial, subdural hemorrhage
  - subgaleal P12.1
  - traumatic — see Injury, intracranial, focal brain injury
- intramedullary NEC G95.19
- intraocular — see Hemophthalmos
- intraoperative, intraprocedural — see Complication, hemorrhage (hematoma), intraoperative (intraprocedural), by site
- intrapartum — see Hemorrhage, complicating, delivery
- intrapelvic
  - female N94.89
  - male K66.1
- intraperitoneal K66.1
- intrapontine I61.3
- intraprocedural — see Complication, hemorrhage (hematoma), intraoperative (intraprocedural), by site
- intrauterine N85.7
  - complicating delivery (see also Hemorrhage, complicating, delivery) O67.9
  - postpartum — see Hemorrhage, postpartum

Hemorrhage, hemorrhagic (concealed) R58
— continued
intraventricular I61.5
  newborn (nontraumatic) (see also Newborn, affected by, hemorrhage) P52.3
    due to birth injury P10.2
    grade
      1 P52.0
      2 P52.1
      3 P52.21
      4 P52.22
intravesical N32.89
iris (postinfectional) (postinflammatory) (toxic) — see Hyphema
joint (nontraumatic) — see Hemarthrosis
kidney N28.89
knee (joint) (nontraumatic) — see Hemarthrosis, knee
labyrinth — see subcategory H83.8
lenticular striate artery I61.0
ligature, vessel — see Hemorrhage, postoperative
liver K76.89
lung R04.89
  newborn P26.9
    massive P26.1
    specified NEC P26.8
  tuberculous — see Tuberculosis, pulmonary
massive umbilical, newborn P51.0
mediastinum — see Hemorrhage, lung
medulla I61.3
membrane (brain) I60.8
  spinal cord — see Hemorrhage, spinal cord
meninges, meningeal (brain) (middle) I60.8
  spinal cord — see Hemorrhage, spinal cord
mesentery K66.1
metritis — see Endometritis
mouth K13.79
mucous membrane NEC R58
  newborn P54.8
muscle M62.89
nail (subungual) L60.8
nasal turbinate R04.0
  newborn P54.8
navel, newborn P51.9
newborn P54.9
  specified NEC P54.8
nipple N64.59
nose R04.0
  newborn P54.8
omentum K66.1
optic nerve (sheath) H47.02-
orbit, orbital H05.23-
ovary NEC N83.8
oviduct N83.6
pancreas K86.89
parathyroid (gland) (spontaneous) E21.4
parturition — see Hemorrhage, complicating, delivery
penis N48.89
pericardium, pericarditis I31.2
peritoneum, peritoneal K66.1
peritonsillar tissue J35.8
  due to infection J36
petechial R23.3
  due to autosensitivity, erythrocyte D69.2
pituitary (gland) E23.6
pleura — see Hemorrhage, lung
polioencephalitis, superior E51.2
polymyositis — see Polymyositis
pons, pontine I61.3
posterior fossa (nontraumatic) I61.8
  newborn P52.6
postmenopausal N95.0
postnasal R04.0
postoperative — see Complications, postprocedural, hemorrhage, by site

Hemorrhage, hemorrhagic (concealed) R58
— continued
postpartum NEC (following delivery of placenta) O72.1
  delayed or secondary O72.2
  retained placenta O72.0
  third stage O72.0
pregnancy — see Hemorrhage, antepartum
preretinal — see Hemorrhage, retina
prostate N42.1
puerperal — see Hemorrhage, postpartum
  delayed or secondary O72.2
pulmonary R04.89
  newborn P26.9
    massive P26.1
    specified NEC P26.8
  tuberculous — see Tuberculosis, pulmonary
purpura (primary) D69.3
rectum (sphincter) K62.5
  newborn P54.2
recurring, following initial hemorrhage at time of injury T79.2
renal N28.89
respiratory passage or tract R04.9
  specified NEC R04.89
retina, retinal (vessels) H35.6-
  diabetic — see Diabetes, retinal, hemorrhage
retroperitoneal R58
scalp R58
scrotum N50.1
secondary (nontraumatic) R58
  following initial hemorrhage at time of injury T79.2
seminal vesicle N50.1
skin R23.3
  newborn P54.5
slipped umbilical ligature P51.8
spermatic cord N50.1
spinal (cord) G95.19
  newborn (birth injury) P11.5
spleen D73.5
  intraoperative — see Complications, intraoperative, hemorrhage, spleen
  postprocedural — see Complications, postprocedural, hemorrhage, spleen
stomach K92.2
  newborn P54.3
  ulcer — see Ulcer, stomach, with hemorrhage
subarachnoid (nontraumatic) — see Hemorrhage, intracranial, subarachnoid
subconjunctival — see also Hemorrhage, conjunctiva
  birth injury P15.3
subcortical (brain) I61.0
subcutaneous R23.3
subdiaphragmatic R58
subdural (acute) (nontraumatic) — see Hemorrhage, intracranial, subdural
subependymal
  newborn P52.0
    with intraventricular extension P52.1
      and intracerebral extension P52.22
subgaleal P12.2
subhyaloid — see Hemorrhage, retina
subperiosteal — see Disorder, bone, specified type NEC
subretinal — see Hemorrhage, retina
subtentorial — see Hemorrhage, intracranial, subdural
subungual L60.8
suprarenal (capsule) (gland) E27.49
  newborn P54.4
tentorium (traumatic) NEC — see Hemorrhage, brain
  newborn (birth injury) P10.4
testis N50.1
third stage (postpartum) O72.0
thorax — see Hemorrhage, lung

Hemorrhage, hemorrhagic (concealed) R58
— continued
throat R04.1
thymus (gland) E32.8
thyroid (cyst) (gland) E07.89
tongue K14.8
tonsil J35.8
trachea — see Hemorrhage, lung
tracheobronchial R04.89
  newborn P26.0
traumatic — code to specific injury
  cerebellar — see Hemorrhage, brain
  intracranial — see Hemorrhage, brain
  recurring or secondary (following initial hemorrhage at time of injury) T79.2
tuberculous NEC (see also Tuberculosis, pulmonary) A15.0
tunica vaginalis N50.1
ulcer — code by site under Ulcer, with hemorrhage K27.4
umbilicus, umbilical
  cord
    after birth, newborn P51.9
    complicating delivery O69.5
  newborn P51.9
    massive P51.0
    slipped ligature P51.8
    stump P51.9
urethra (idiopathic) N36.8
uterus, uterine (abnormal) N93.9
  climacteric N92.4
  complicating delivery — see Hemorrhage, complicating, delivery
  dysfunctional or functional N93.8
  intermenstrual (regular) N92.3
    irregular N92.1
  postmenopausal N95.0
  postpartum — see Hemorrhage, postpartum
  preclimacteric or premenopausal N92.4
  prepubertal N93.8
  pubertal N92.2
vagina (abnormal) N93.9
  newborn P54.6
vas deferens N50.1
vasa previa O69.4
ventricular I61.5
vesical N32.89
viscera NEC R58
  newborn P54.8
vitreous (humor) (intraocular) H43.1-
vulva N90.89

Hemorrhoids (bleeding) (without mention of degree) K64.9
1st degree (grade/stage I) (without prolapse outside of anal canal) K64.0
2nd degree (grade/stage II) (that with prolapse with straining but retract spontaneously) K64.1
3rd degree (grade/stage III) (that with prolapse with straining and require manual replacement back inside anal canal) K64.2
4th degree (grade/stage IV) (with prolapsed tissue that cannot be manually replaced) K64.3
complicating
  pregnancy O22.4
  puerperium O87.2
external K64.4
  with
    thrombosis K64.5
internal (without mention of degree) K64.8
prolapsed K64.8
skin tags
  anus K64.4
  residual K64.4
specified NEC K64.8

DISEASE INDEX

Hemorrhoids (bleeding) (without mention of degree) K64.9 — *continued*
  strangulated (*see also* Hemorrhoids, by degree) K64.8
  thrombosed (*see also* Hemorrhoids, by degree) K64.5
  ulcerated (*see also* Hemorrhoids, by degree) K64.8
Hemosalpinx N83.6
  with
    hematocolpos N89.7
    hematometra N85.7
      with hematocolpos N89.7
Hemosiderosis (dietary) E83.19
  pulmonary, idiopathic E83.1- *[J84.03]*
  transfusion T80.89
Hemothorax (bacterial) (nontuberculous) J94.2
  newborn P54.8
  traumatic S27.1
    with pneumothorax S27.2
  tuberculous NEC A15.6
Henoch(-Schönlein) disease or syndrome (purpura) D69.0
Henpue, henpuye A66.6
Hepar lobatum (syphilitic) A52.74
Hepatalgia K76.89
Hepatitis K75.9
  acute B17.9
    with coma K72.01
    with hepatic failure — *see* Failure, hepatic
    alcoholic — *see* Hepatitis, alcoholic
    infectious B17.9
    non-viral K72.0
    viral B17.9
  alcoholic (acute) (chronic) K70.10
    with ascites K70.11
  amebic — *see* Abscess, liver, amebic
  anicteric, (viral) — *see* Hepatitis, viral
  antigen-associated (HAA) — *see* Hepatitis, B
  Australia-antigen (positive) — *see* Hepatitis, B
  autoimmune K75.4
  B B19.10
    with hepatic coma B19.11
    acute B16.9
      with
        delta-agent (coinfection) (without hepatic coma) B16.1
          with hepatic coma B16.0
        hepatic coma (without delta-agent coinfection) B16.2
    chronic B18.1
      with delta-agent B18.0
  bacterial NEC K75.89
  C (viral) B19.20
    with hepatic coma B19.21
    acute B17.10
      with hepatic coma B17.11
    chronic B18.2
  catarrhal (acute) B15.9
    with hepatic coma B15.0
  cholangiolitic K75.89
  cholestatic K75.89
  chronic K73.9
    active NEC K73.2
    lobular NEC K73.1
    persistent NEC K73.0
    specified NEC K73.8
  cytomegaloviral B25.1
  due to ethanol (acute) (chronic) — *see* Hepatitis, alcoholic
  epidemic B15.9
    with hepatic coma B15.0
  fulminant NEC (viral) — *see* Hepatitis, viral
  granulomatous NEC K75.3
  herpesviral B00.81
  history of
    B Z86.19
    C Z86.19

Hepatitis K75.9 — *continued*
  homologous serum — *see* Hepatitis, viral, type B
  in (due to)
    mumps B26.81
    toxoplasmosis (acquired) B58.1
      congenital (active) P37.1 *[K77]*
  infectious, infective B15.9
    acute (subacute) B17.9
    chronic B18.9
  inoculation — *see* Hepatitis, viral, type B
  interstitial (chronic) K74.69
  lupoid NEC K75.4
  malignant NEC (with hepatic failure) K72.90
    with coma K72.91
  neonatal giant cell P59.29
  neonatal (idiopathic) (toxic) P59.29
  newborn P59.29
  post-transfusion — *see* Hepatitis, viral, type B
  postimmunization — *see* Hepatitis, viral, type B
  reactive, nonspecific K75.2
  serum — *see* Hepatitis, viral, type B
  specified type NEC
    with hepatic failure — *see* Failure, hepatic
  syphilitic (late) A52.74
    congenital (early) A50.08 *[K77]*
      late A50.59 *[K77]*
    secondary A51.45
  toxic (*see also* Disease, liver, toxic) K71.6
  tuberculous A18.83
  viral, virus B19.9
    with hepatic coma B19.0
    acute B17.9
    chronic B18.9
      specified NEC B18.8
      type
        B B18.1
          with delta-agent B18.0
        C B18.2
    congenital P35.3
    coxsackie B33.8 *[K77]*
    cytomegalic inclusion B25.1
    in remission, any type — *code to* Hepatitis, chronic, by type
    non-A, non-B B17.8
    specified type NEC (with or without coma) B17.8
    type
      A B15.9
        with hepatic coma B15.0
      B B19.10
        with hepatic coma B19.11
        acute B16.9
          with
            delta-agent (coinfection) (without hepatic coma) B16.1
              with hepatic coma B16.0
            hepatic coma (without delta-agent coinfection) B16.2
        chronic B18.1
          with delta-agent B18.0
      C B19.20
        with hepatic coma B19.21
        acute B17.10
          with hepatic coma B17.11
        chronic B18.2
      E B17.2
      non-A, non-B B17.8
Hepatization lung (acute) — *see* Pneumonia, lobar
Hepatoblastoma C22.2
Hepatocarcinoma C22.0
Hepatocholangiocarcinoma C22.0
Hepatocholangioma, benign D13.4
Hepatocholangitis K75.89
Hepatolenticular degeneration E83.01
Hepatoma (malignant) C22.0
  benign D13.4
  embryonal C22.0

Hepatomegaly — *see also* Hypertrophy, liver
  with splenomegaly R16.2
  congenital Q44.7
  in mononucleosis
    gammaherpesviral B27.09
    infectious specified NEC B27.89
Hepatoptosis K76.89
Hepatorenal syndrome following labor and delivery O90.4
Hepatosis K76.89
Hepatosplenomegaly R16.2
  hyperlipemic (Bürger-Grütz type) E78.3 *[K77]*
Hereditary — *see* condition
Heredodegeneration, macular — *see* Dystrophy, retina
Heredopathia atactica polyneuritiformis G60.1
Heredosyphilis — *see* Syphilis, congenital
Herlitz' syndrome Q81.1
Hermansky-Pudlak syndrome E70.331
Hermaphrodite, hermaphroditism (true) Q56.0
  46,XX with streak gonads Q99.1
  46,XX/46,XY Q99.0
  46,XY with streak gonads Q99.1
  chimera 46,XX/46,XY Q99.0
Hernia, hernial (acquired) (recurrent) K46.9
  with
    gangrene — *see* Hernia, by site, with, gangrene
    incarceration — *see* Hernia, by site, with, obstruction
    irreducible — *see* Hernia, by site, with, obstruction
    obstruction — *see* Hernia, by site, with, obstruction
    strangulation — *see* Hernia, by site, with, obstruction
  abdomen, abdominal K46.9
    with
      gangrene (and obstruction) K46.1
      obstruction K46.0
    femoral — *see* Hernia, femoral
    incisional — *see* Hernia, incisional
    inguinal — *see* Hernia, inguinal
    specified site NEC K45.8
      with
        gangrene (and obstruction) K45.1
        obstruction K45.0
    umbilical — *see* Hernia, umbilical
    wall — *see* Hernia, ventral
  appendix — *see* Hernia, abdomen
  bladder (mucosa) (sphincter)
    congenital (female) (male) Q79.51
    female — *see* Cystocele
    male N32.89
  brain, congenital — *see* Encephalocele
  cartilage, vertebra — *see* Displacement, intervertebral disc
  cerebral, congenital — *see also* Encephalocele
    endaural Q01.8
  ciliary body (traumatic) S05.2-
  colon — *see* Hernia, abdomen
  Cooper's — *see* Hernia, abdomen, specified site NEC
  crural — *see* Hernia, femoral
  diaphragm, diaphragmatic K44.9
    with
      gangrene (and obstruction) K44.1
      obstruction K44.0
    congenital Q79.0
  direct (inguinal) — *see* Hernia, inguinal
  diverticulum, intestine — *see* Hernia, abdomen
  double (inguinal) — *see* Hernia, inguinal, bilateral
  due to adhesions (with obstruction) K56.5
  epigastric (*see also* Hernia, ventral) K43.9
  esophageal hiatus — *see* Hernia, hiatal
  external (inguinal) — *see* Hernia, inguinal

Hernia, hernial (acquired) (recurrent) K46.9
— *continued*
   fallopian tube N83.4-
   fascia M62.89
   femoral K41.90
      with
         gangrene (and obstruction) K41.40
            not specified as recurrent K41.40
            recurrent K41.41
         obstruction K41.30
            not specified as recurrent K41.30
            recurrent K41.31
      bilateral K41.20
         with
            gangrene (and obstruction) K41.10
               not specified as recurrent K41.10
               recurrent K41.11
            obstruction K41.00
               not specified as recurrent K41.00
               recurrent K41.01
         not specified as recurrent K41.20
         recurrent K41.21
      not specified as recurrent K41.90
      recurrent K41.91
      unilateral K41.90
         with
            gangrene (and obstruction) K41.40
               not specified as recurrent K41.40
               recurrent K41.41
            obstruction K41.30
               not specified as recurrent K41.30
               recurrent K41.31
         not specified as recurrent K41.90
         recurrent K41.91
   foramen magnum G93.5
      congenital Q01.8
   funicular (umbilical) — *see also* **Hernia,**
      umbilicus
      spermatic (cord) — *see* **Hernia, inguinal**
   gastrointestinal tract — *see* **Hernia, abdomen**
   Hesselbach's — *see* **Hernia, femoral, specified**
      site NEC
   hiatal (esophageal) (sliding) K44.9
      with
         gangrene (and obstruction) K44.1
         obstruction K44.0
      congenital Q40.1
   hypogastric — *see* **Hernia, ventral**
   incarcerated — *see also* **Hernia, by site, with**
      obstruction
      with gangrene — *see* **Hernia, by site, with**
         gangrene
   incisional K43.2
      with
         gangrene (and obstruction) K43.1
         obstruction K43.0
   indirect (inguinal) — *see* **Hernia, inguinal**
   inguinal (direct) (external) (funicular) (indirect)
      (internal) (oblique) (scrotal) (sliding)
      K40.90
      with
         gangrene (and obstruction) K40.40
            not specified as recurrent K40.40
            recurrent K40.41
         obstruction K40.30
            not specified as recurrent K40.30
            recurrent K40.31
      bilateral K40.20
         with
            gangrene (and obstruction) K40.10
               not specified as recurrent K40.10
               recurrent K40.11
            obstruction K40.00
               not specified as recurrent K40.00
               recurrent K40.01
         not specified as recurrent K40.20
         recurrent K40.21
      not specified as recurrent K40.90
      recurrent K40.91

Hernia, hernial (acquired) (recurrent) K46.9
— *continued*
   inguinal (direct) (external) (funicular) (indirect)
      (internal) (oblique) (scrotal) (sliding)
      K40.90 — *continued*
      unilateral K40.90
         with
            gangrene (and obstruction) K40.40
               not specified as recurrent K40.40
               recurrent K40.41
            obstruction K40.30
               not specified as recurrent K40.30
               recurrent K40.31
         not specified as recurrent K40.90
         recurrent K40.91
   internal — *see also* **Hernia, abdomen**
      inguinal — *see* **Hernia, inguinal**
   interstitial — *see* **Hernia, abdomen**
   intervertebral cartilage or disc — *see*
      Displacement, intervertebral disc
   intestine, intestinal — *see* **Hernia, by site**
   intra-abdominal — *see* **Hernia, abdomen**
   iris (traumatic) S05.2-
   irreducible — *see also* **Hernia, by site, with**
      obstruction
      with gangrene — *see* **Hernia, by site, with**
         gangrene
   ischiatic — *see* **Hernia, abdomen, specified site**
      NEC
   ischiorectal — *see* **Hernia, abdomen, specified**
      site NEC
   lens (traumatic) S05.2-
   linea (alba) (semilunaris) — *see* **Hernia, ventral**
   Littre's — *see* **Hernia, abdomen**
   lumbar — *see* **Hernia, abdomen, specified site**
      NEC
   lung (subcutaneous) J98.4
   mediastinum J98.59
   mesenteric (internal) — *see* **Hernia, abdomen**
   midline — *see* **Hernia, ventral**
   muscle (sheath) M62.89
   nucleus pulposus — *see* **Displacement,**
      intervertebral disc
   oblique (inguinal) — *see* **Hernia, inguinal**
   obstructive — *see also* **Hernia, by site, with**
      obstruction
      with gangrene — *see* **Hernia, by site, with**
         gangrene
   obturator — *see* **Hernia, abdomen, specified**
      site NEC
   omental — *see* **Hernia, abdomen**
   ovary N83.4-
   oviduct N83.4-
   paraesophageal — *see also* **Hernia, diaphragm**
      congenital Q40.1
   parastomal K43.5
      with
         gangrene (and obstruction) K43.4
         obstruction K43.3
   paraumbilical — *see* **Hernia, umbilicus**
   perineal — *see* **Hernia, abdomen, specified**
      site NEC
   Petit's — *see* **Hernia, abdomen, specified site**
      NEC
   postoperative — *see* **Hernia, incisional**
   pregnant uterus — *see* **Abnormal, uterus in**
      pregnancy or childbirth
   prevesical N32.89
   properitoneal — *see* **Hernia, abdomen,**
      specified site NEC
   pudendal — *see* **Hernia, abdomen, specified**
      site NEC
   rectovaginal N81.6
   retroperitoneal — *see* **Hernia, abdomen,**
      specified site NEC
   Richter's — *see* **Hernia, abdomen, with**
      obstruction
   Rieux's, Riex's — *see* **Hernia, abdomen,**
      specified site NEC

Hernia, hernial (acquired) (recurrent) K46.9
— *continued*
   sac condition (adhesion) (dropsy)
      (inflammation) (laceration) (suppuration)
      — *code by* site under **Hernia**
   sciatic — *see* **Hernia, abdomen, specified site**
      NEC
   scrotum, scrotal — *see* **Hernia, inguinal**
   sliding (inguinal) — *see also* **Hernia, inguinal**
      hiatus — *see* **Hernia, hiatal**
   spigelian — *see* **Hernia, ventral**
   spinal — *see* **Spina bifida**
   strangulated — *see also* **Hernia, by site, with**
      obstruction
      with gangrene — *see* **Hernia, by site, with**
         gangrene
   subxiphoid — *see* **Hernia, ventral**
   supra-umbilicus — *see* **Hernia, ventral**
   tendon — *see* **Disorder, tendon, specified type**
      NEC
   Treitz's (fossa) — *see* **Hernia, abdomen,**
      specified site NEC
   tunica vaginalis Q55.29
   umbilicus, umbilical K42.9
      with
         gangrene (and obstruction) K42.1
         obstruction K42.0
   ureter N28.89
   urethra, congenital Q64.79
   urinary meatus, congenital Q64.79
   uterus N81.4
      pregnant — *see* **Abnormal, uterus in**
         pregnancy or childbirth
   vaginal (anterior) (wall) — *see* **Cystocele**
   Velpeau's — *see* **Hernia, femoral**
   ventral K43.9
      with
         gangrene (and obstruction) K43.7
         obstruction K43.6
      incisional K43.2
         with
            gangrene (and obstruction) K43.1
            obstruction K43.0
         recurrent — *see* **Hernia, incisional**
      specified NEC K43.9
         with
            gangrene (and obstruction) K43.7
            obstruction K43.6
   vesical
      congenital (female) (male) Q79.51
      female — *see* **Cystocele**
      male N32.89
   vitreous (into wound) S05.2-
      into anterior chamber — *see* **Prolapse,**
         vitreous
Herniation — *see also* **Hernia**
   brain (stem) G93.5
   cerebral G93.5
   mediastinum J98.59
   nucleus pulposus — *see* **Displacement,**
      intervertebral disc
Herpangina B08.5
Herpes, herpesvirus, herpetic B00.9
   anogenital A60.9
      perianal skin A60.1
      rectum A60.1
      urogenital tract A60.00
         cervix A60.03
         male genital organ NEC A60.02
         penis A60.01
         specified site NEC A60.09
         vagina A60.04
         vulva A60.04
   blepharitis (zoster) B02.39
      simplex B00.59
   circinatus B35.4
      bullosus L12.0
   conjunctivitis (simplex) B00.53
      zoster B02.31

Herpes, herpesvirus, herpetic B00.9 — *continued*
  cornea B02.33
  encephalitis B00.4
    due to herpesvirus 6 B10.01
    due to herpesvirus 7 B10.09
    specified NEC B10.09
  eye (zoster) B02.30
    simplex B00.50
  eyelid (zoster) B02.39
    simplex B00.59
  facialis B00.1
  febrilis B00.1
  geniculate ganglionitis B02.21
  genital, genitalis A60.00
    female A60.09
    male A60.02
  gestational, gestationis O26.4-
  gingivostomatitis B00.2
  human B00.9
    1 — *see* Herpes, simplex
    2 — *see* Herpes, simplex
    3 — *see* Varicella
    4 — *see* Mononucleosis, Epstein-Barr (virus)
    5 — *see* Disease, cytomegalic inclusion (generalized)
    6
      encephalitis B10.01
      specified NEC B10.81
    7
      encephalitis B10.09
      specified NEC B10.82
    8 B10.89
  infection NEC B10.89
    Kaposi's sarcoma associated B10.89
  iridocyclitis (simplex) B00.51
    zoster B02.32
  iris (vesicular erythema multiforme) L51.9
  iritis (simplex) B00.51
  Kaposi's sarcoma associated B10.89
  keratitis (simplex) (dendritic) (disciform) (interstitial) B00.52
    zoster (interstitial) B02.33
  keratoconjunctivitis (simplex) B00.52
    zoster B02.33
  labialis B00.1
  lip B00.1
  meningitis (simplex) B00.3
    zoster B02.1
  ophthalmicus (zoster) NEC B02.30
    simplex B00.50
  penis A60.01
  perianal skin A60.1
  pharyngitis, pharyngotonsillitis B00.2
  rectum A60.1
  scrotum A60.02
  sepsis B00.7
  simplex B00.9
    complicated NEC B00.89
    congenital P35.2
    conjunctivitis B00.53
    external ear B00.1
    eyelid B00.59
    hepatitis B00.81
    keratitis (interstitial) B00.52
    myelitis B00.82
    specified complication NEC B00.89
    visceral B00.89
  stomatitis B00.2
  tonsurans B35.0
  visceral B00.89
  vulva A60.04
  whitlow B00.89
  zoster (*see also* condition) B02.9
    auricularis B02.21
    complicated NEC B02.8
    conjunctivitis B02.31
    disseminated B02.7
    encephalitis B02.0

Herpes, herpesvirus, herpetic B00.9 — *continued*
  zoster (*see also* condition) B02.9 — *continued*
    eye(lid) B02.39
    geniculate ganglionitis B02.21
    keratitis (interstitial) B02.33
    meningitis B02.1
    myelitis B02.24
    neuritis, neuralgia B02.29
    ophthalmicus NEC B02.30
    oticus B02.21
    polyneuropathy B02.23
    specified complication NEC B02.8
    trigeminal neuralgia B02.22
Herpesvirus (human) — *see* Herpes
Herpetophobia F40.218
Herrick's anemia — *see* Disease, sickle-cell
Hers' disease E74.09
Herter-Gee syndrome K90.0
Herxheimer's reaction R68.89
Hesitancy
  of micturition R39.11
  urinary R39.11
Hesselbach's hernia — *see* Hernia, femoral, specified site NEC
Heterochromia (congenital) Q13.2
  cataract — *see* Cataract, complicated
  cyclitis (Fuchs) — *see* Cyclitis, Fuchs' heterochromic
  hair L67.1
  iritis — *see* Cyclitis, Fuchs' heterochromic
  retained metallic foreign body (nonmagnetic) — *see* Foreign body, intraocular, old, retained
    magnetic — *see* Foreign body, intraocular, old, retained, magnetic
  uveitis — *see* Cyclitis, Fuchs' heterochromic
Heterophoria — *see* Strabismus, heterophoria
Heterophyes, heterophyiasis (small intestine) B66.8
Heterotopia, heterotopic — *see also* Malposition, congenital
  cerebralis Q04.8
Heterotropia — *see* Strabismus
Heubner-Herter disease K90.0
Hexadactylism Q69.9
HGSIL (cytology finding) (high grade squamous intraepithelial lesion on cytologic smear) (Pap smear finding)
  anus R85.613
  cervix R87.613
    biopsy (histology) finding — *see* Neoplasia, intraepithelial, cervix, grade II or grade III
  vagina R87.623
    biopsy (histology) finding — *see* Neoplasia, intraepithelial, vagina, grade II or grade III
Hibernoma — *see* Lipoma
Hiccup, hiccough R06.6
  epidemic B33.0
  psychogenic F45.8
Hidden penis (congenital) Q55.64
  acquired N48.83
Hidradenitis (axillaris) (suppurative) L73.2
Hidradenoma (nodular) — *see also* Neoplasm, skin, benign
  clear cell — *see* Neoplasm, skin, benign
  papillary — *see* Neoplasm, skin, benign
Hidrocystoma — *see* Neoplasm, skin, benign
High
  altitude effects T70.20
    anoxia T70.29
    on
      ears T70.0
      sinuses T70.1
  polycythemia D75.1

High — *continued*
  arch
    foot Q66.7
    palate, congenital Q38.5
  arterial tension — *see* Hypertension
  basal metabolic rate R94.8
  blood pressure — *see also* Hypertension
    borderline R03.0
    reading (incidental) (isolated) (nonspecific), without diagnosis of hypertension R03.0
  cholesterol E78.00
    with high triglycerides E78.2
  diaphragm (congenital) Q79.1
  expressed emotional level within family Z63.8
  head at term O32.4
  palate, congenital Q38.5
  risk
    infant NEC Z76.2
    sexual behavior (heterosexual) Z72.51
      bisexual Z72.53
      homosexual Z72.52
  temperature (of unknown origin) R50.9
  thoracic rib Q76.6
  triglycerides E78.1
    with high cholesterol E78.2
Hildenbrand's disease A75.0
Hilum — *see* condition
Hip — *see* condition
Hippel's disease Q85.8
Hippophobia F40.218
Hippus H57.09
Hirschsprung's disease or megacolon Q43.1
Hirsutism, hirsuties L68.0
Hirudiniasis
  external B88.3
  internal B83.4
Hiss-Russell dysentery A03.1
His-Werner disease A79.0
Histidinemia, histidinuria E70.41
Histiocytoma — *see also* Neoplasm, skin, benign
  fibrous — *see also* Neoplasm, skin, benign
    atypical — *see* Neoplasm, connective tissue, uncertain behavior
    malignant — *see* Neoplasm, connective tissue, malignant
Histiocytosis D76.3
  acute differentiated progressive C96.0
  Langerhans' cell NEC C96.6
    multifocal X
      multisystemic (disseminated) C96.0
      unisystemic C96.5
    pulmonary, adult (adult PLCH) J84.82
    unifocal (X) C96.6
  lipid, lipoid D76.3
    essential E75.29
  malignant C96.A
  mononuclear phagocytes NEC D76.1
    Langerhans' cells C96.6
  non-Langerhans cell D76.3
  polyostotic sclerosing D76.3
  sinus, with massive lymphadenopathy D76.3
  syndrome NEC D76.3
  X NEC C96.6
    acute (progressive) C96.0
    chronic C96.6
    multifocal C96.5
    multisystemic C96.0
    unifocal C96.6
Histoplasmosis B39.9
  with pneumonia NEC B39.2
  African B39.5
  American — *see* Histoplasmosis, capsulati
  capsulati B39.4
    disseminated B39.3
    generalized B39.3

Histoplasmosis B39.9 — *continued*
  capsulati B39.4 — *continued*
    pulmonary B39.2
      acute B39.0
      chronic B39.1
  Darling's B39.4
  duboisii B39.5
  lung NEC B39.2
History
  family (of) — *see also* History, personal (of)
    alcohol abuse Z81.1
    allergy NEC Z84.89
    anemia Z83.2
    arthritis Z82.61
    asthma Z82.5
    blindness Z82.1
    cardiac death (sudden) Z82.41
    carrier of genetic disease Z84.81
    chromosomal anomaly Z82.79
    chronic
      disabling disease NEC Z82.8
      lower respiratory disease Z82.5
    colonic polyps Z83.71
    congenital malformations and deformations Z82.79
      polycystic kidney Z82.71
    consanguinity Z84.3
    deafness Z82.2
    diabetes mellitus Z83.3
    disability NEC Z82.8
    disease or disorder (of)
      allergic NEC Z84.89
      behavioral NEC Z81.8
      blood and blood-forming organs Z83.2
      cardiovascular NEC Z82.49
      chronic disabling NEC Z82.8
      digestive Z83.79
      ear NEC Z83.52
      endocrine NEC Z83.49
      eye NEC Z83.518
        glaucoma Z83.511
      familial hypercholesterolemia Z83.42
      genitourinary NEC Z84.2
      glaucoma Z83.511
      hematological Z83.2
      immune mechanism Z83.2
      infectious NEC Z83.1
      ischemic heart Z82.49
      kidney Z84.1
      mental NEC Z81.8
      metabolic Z83.49
      musculoskeletal NEC Z82.69
      neurological NEC Z82.0
      nutritional Z83.49
      parasitic NEC Z83.1
      psychiatric NEC Z81.8
      respiratory NEC Z83.6
      skin and subcutaneous tissue NEC Z84.0
      specified NEC Z84.89
    drug abuse NEC Z81.3
    epilepsy Z82.0
    familial hypercholesterolemia Z83.42
    genetic disease carrier Z84.81
    glaucoma Z83.511
    hearing loss Z82.2
    human immunodeficiency virus (HIV) infection Z83.0
    Huntington's chorea Z82.0
    intellectual disability Z81.0
    leukemia Z80.6
    malignant neoplasm (of) NOS Z80.9
      bladder Z80.52
      breast Z80.3
      bronchus Z80.1
      digestive organ Z80.0
      gastrointestinal tract Z80.0

History — *continued*
  family (of) (*see also* History, personal (of)) — *continued*
    malignant neoplasm (of) NOS Z80.9 — *continued*
      genital organ Z80.49
        ovary Z80.41
        prostate Z80.42
        specified organ NEC Z80.49
        testis Z80.43
      hematopoietic NEC Z80.7
      intrathoracic organ NEC Z80.2
      kidney Z80.51
      lung Z80.1
      lymphatic NEC Z80.7
      ovary Z80.41
      prostate Z80.42
      respiratory organ NEC Z80.2
      specified site NEC Z80.8
      testis Z80.43
      trachea Z80.1
      urinary organ or tract Z80.59
        bladder Z80.52
        kidney Z80.51
    mental
      disorder NEC Z81.8
    multiple endocrine neoplasia (MEN) syndrome Z83.41
    osteoporosis Z82.62
    polycystic kidney Z82.71
    polyps (colon) Z83.71
    psychiatric disorder Z81.8
    psychoactive substance abuse NEC Z81.3
    respiratory condition NEC Z83.6
      asthma and other lower respiratory conditions Z82.5
    self-harmful behavior Z81.8
    SIDS (sudden infant death syndrome) Z84.82
    skin condition Z84.0
    specified condition NEC Z84.89
    stroke (cerebrovascular) Z82.3
    substance abuse NEC Z81.4
      alcohol Z81.1
      drug NEC Z81.3
      psychoactive NEC Z81.3
      tobacco Z81.2
    sudden
      cardiac death Z82.41
      infant death syndrome (SIDS) Z84.82
    tobacco abuse Z81.2
    violence, violent behavior Z81.8
    visual loss Z82.1
  personal (of) — *see also* History, family (of)
    abuse
      adult Z91.419
        physical and sexual Z91.410
        psychological Z91.411
      childhood Z62.819
        physical Z62.810
        psychological Z62.811
        sexual Z62.810
    alcohol dependence F10.21
    allergy (to) Z88.9
      analgesic agent NEC Z88.6
      anesthetic Z88.4
      anti-infective agent NEC Z88.3
      antibiotic agent NEC Z88.1
      contrast media Z91.041
      drugs, medicaments and biological substances Z88.9
        specified NEC Z88.8
      food Z91.018
        additives Z91.02
        eggs Z91.012
        milk products Z91.011
        peanuts Z91.010
        seafood Z91.013
        specified food NEC Z91.018

History — *continued*
  personal (of) (*see also* History, family (of)) — *continued*
    allergy (to) Z88.9 — *continued*
      insect Z91.038
        bee Z91.030
      latex Z91.040
      medicinal agents Z88.9
        specified NEC Z88.8
      narcotic agent NEC Z88.5
      nonmedicinal agents Z91.048
      penicillin Z88.0
      serum Z88.7
      specified NEC Z91.09
      sulfonamides Z88.2
      vaccine Z88.7
    anaphylactic shock Z87.892
    anaphylaxis Z87.892
    behavioral disorders Z86.59
    benign carcinoid tumor Z86.012
    benign neoplasm Z86.018
      brain Z86.011
      carcinoid Z86.012
      colonic polyps Z86.010
    brain injury (traumatic) Z87.820
    breast implant removal Z98.86
    calculi, renal Z87.442
    cancer — *see* History, personal (of), malignant neoplasm (of)
    cardiac arrest (death), successfully resuscitated Z86.74
    cerebral infarction without residual deficit Z86.73
    cervical dysplasia Z87.410
    chemotherapy for neoplastic condition Z92.21
    childhood abuse — *see* History, personal (of), abuse
    cleft lip (corrected) Z87.730
    cleft palate (corrected) Z87.730
    collapsed vertebra (healed) Z87.311
      due to osteoporosis Z87.310
    combat and operational stress reaction Z86.51
    congenital malformation (corrected) Z87.798
      circulatory system (corrected) Z87.74
      digestive system (corrected) NEC Z87.738
      ear (corrected) Z87.720
      eye (corrected) Z87.721
      face and neck (corrected) Z87.790
      genitourinary system (corrected) NEC Z87.718
      heart (corrected) Z87.74
      integument (corrected) Z87.76
      limb(s) (corrected) Z87.76
      musculoskeletal system (corrected) Z87.76
      neck (corrected) Z87.790
      nervous system (corrected) NEC Z87.728
      respiratory system (corrected) Z87.75
      sense organs (corrected) NEC Z87.728
      specified NEC Z87.798
    contraception Z92.0
    deployment (military) Z91.82
    diabetic foot ulcer Z86.31
    disease or disorder (of) Z87.898
      anaphylaxis Z87.892
      blood and blood-forming organs Z86.2
      circulatory system Z86.79
        specified condition NEC Z86.79
      connective tissue NEC Z87.39
      digestive system Z87.19
        colonic polyp Z86.010
        peptic ulcer disease Z87.11
        specified condition NEC Z87.19
      ear Z86.69
      endocrine Z86.39
        diabetic foot ulcer Z86.31
        gestational diabetes Z86.32
        specified type NEC Z86.39

History — *continued*
  personal (of) (*see also* History, family (of)) — *continued*
    disease or disorder (of) Z87.898 — *continued*
      eye Z86.69
      genital (track) system NEC
        female Z87.42
        male Z87.438
      hematological Z86.2
      Hodgkin Z85.71
      immune mechanism Z86.2
      infectious Z86.19
        malaria Z86.13
        methicillin resistant Staphylococcus aureus (MRSA) Z86.14
        poliomyelitis Z86.12
        specified NEC Z86.19
        tuberculosis Z86.11
      mental NEC Z86.59
      metabolic Z86.39
        diabetic foot ulcer Z86.31
        gestational diabetes Z86.32
        specified type NEC Z86.39
      musculoskeletal NEC Z87.39
      nervous system Z86.69
      nutritional Z86.39
      parasitic Z86.19
      respiratory system NEC Z87.09
      sense organs Z86.69
      skin Z87.2
      specified site or type NEC Z87.898
      subcutaneous tissue Z87.2
      trophoblastic Z87.59
      urinary system NEC Z87.448
    drug dependence — *see* Dependence, drug, by type, in remission
    drug therapy
      antineoplastic chemotherapy Z92.21
      estrogen Z92.23
      immunosupression Z92.25
      inhaled steroids Z92.240
      monoclonal drug Z92.22
      specified NEC Z92.29
      steroid Z92.241
      systemic steroids Z92.241
    dysplasia
      cervical (mild) (moderate) Z87.410
        severe (grade III) Z86.001
      prostatic Z87.430
      vaginal (mild) (moderate) Z87.411
        severe (grade III) Z86.008
      vulvar (mild) (moderate) Z87.412
        severe (grade III) Z86.008
    embolism (venous) Z86.718
      pulmonary Z86.711
    encephalitis Z86.61
    estrogen therapy Z92.23
    extracorporeal membrane oxygenation (ECMO) Z92.81
    failed conscious sedation Z92.83
    failed moderate sedation Z92.83
    fall, falling Z91.81
    fracture (healed)
      fatigue Z87.312
      fragility Z87.310
      osteoporosis Z87.310
      pathological NEC Z87.311
      stress Z87.312
      traumatic Z87.81
    gestational diabetes Z86.32
    hepatitis
      B Z86.19
      C Z86.19
    Hodgkin disease Z85.71
    hyperthermia, malignant Z88.4
    hypospadias (corrected) Z87.710
    hysterectomy Z90.710
    immunosupression therapy Z92.25

History — *continued*
  personal (of) (*see also* History, family (of)) — *continued*
    in situ neoplasm
      breast Z86.000
      cervix uteri Z86.001
      specified NEC Z86.008
    in utero procedure during pregnancy Z98.870
    in utero procedure while a fetus Z98.871
    infection NEC Z86.19
      central nervous system Z86.61
      methicillin resistant Staphylococcus aureus (MRSA) Z86.14
      urinary (recurrent) (tract) Z87.440
    injury NEC Z87.828
    irradiation Z92.3
    kidney stones Z87.442
    leukemia Z85.6
    lymphoma (non-Hodgkin) Z85.72
    malignant melanoma (skin) Z85.820
    malignant neoplasm (of) Z85.9
      accessory sinuses Z85.22
      anus NEC Z85.048
        carcinoid Z85.040
      bladder Z85.51
      bone Z85.830
      brain Z85.841
      breast Z85.3
      bronchus NEC Z85.118
        carcinoid Z85.110
      carcinoid — *see* History, personal (of), malignant neoplasm, by site, carcinoid
      cervix Z85.41
      colon NEC Z85.038
        carcinoid Z85.030
      digestive organ Z85.00
        specified NEC Z85.09
      endocrine gland NEC Z85.858
      epididymis Z85.48
      esophagus Z85.01
      eye Z85.840
      gastrointestinal tract — *see* History, malignant neoplasm, digestive organ
      genital organ
        female Z85.40
          specified NEC Z85.44
        male Z85.45
          specified NEC Z85.49
      hematopoietic NEC Z85.79
      intrathoracic organ Z85.20
      kidney NEC Z85.528
        carcinoid Z85.520
      large intestine NEC Z85.038
        carcinoid Z85.030
      larynx Z85.21
      liver Z85.05
      lung NEC Z85.118
        carcinoid Z85.110
      mediastinum Z85.29
      Merkel cell Z85.821
      middle ear Z85.22
      nasal cavities Z85.22
      nervous system NEC Z85.848
      oral cavity Z85.819
        specified site NEC Z85.818
      ovary Z85.43
      pancreas Z85.07
      pelvis Z85.53
      pharynx Z85.819
        specified site NEC Z85.818
      pleura Z85.29
      prostate Z85.46
      rectosigmoid junction NEC Z85.048
        carcinoid Z85.040
      rectum NEC Z85.048
        carcinoid Z85.040
      respiratory organ Z85.20

History — *continued*
  personal (of) (*see also* History, family (of)) — *continued*
    malignant neoplasm (of) Z85.9 — *continued*
      sinuses, accessory Z85.22
      skin NEC Z85.828
        melanoma Z85.820
        Merkel cell Z85.821
      small intestine NEC Z85.068
        carcinoid Z85.060
      soft tissue Z85.831
      specified site NEC Z85.89
      stomach NEC Z85.028
        carcinoid Z85.020
      testis Z85.47
      thymus NEC Z85.238
        carcinoid Z85.230
      thyroid Z85.850
      tongue Z85.810
      trachea Z85.12
      ureter Z85.54
      urinary organ or tract Z85.50
        specified NEC Z85.59
      uterus Z85.42
    maltreatment Z91.89
    medical treatment NEC Z92.89
    melanoma (malignant) (skin) Z85.820
    meningitis Z86.61
    mental disorder Z86.59
    Merkel cell carcinoma (skin) Z85.821
    Methicillin resistant Staphylococcus aureus (MRSA) Z86.14
    military deployment Z91.82
    military war, peacekeeping and humanitarian deployment (current or past conflict) Z91.82
    myocardial infarction (old) I25.2
    neglect (in)
      adult Z91.412
      childhood Z62.812
    neoplasm
      benign Z86.018
        brain Z86.011
        colon polyp Z86.010
      in situ
        breast Z86.000
        cervix uteri Z86.001
        specified NEC Z86.008
      malignant — *see* History of, malignant neoplasm
      uncertain behavior Z86.03
    nephrotic syndrome Z87.441
    nicotine dependence Z87.891
    noncompliance with medical treatment or regimen — *see* Noncompliance
    nutritional deficiency Z86.39
    obstetric complications Z87.59
      childbirth Z87.59
      pre-term labor Z87.51
      pregnancy Z87.59
      puerperium Z87.59
    osteoporosis fractures Z87.31
    parasuicide (attempt) Z91.5
    physical trauma NEC Z87.828
    self-harm or suicide attempt Z91.5
    pneumonia (recurrent) Z87.01
    poisoning NEC Z91.89
      self-harm or suicide attempt Z91.5
    poor personal hygiene Z91.89
    preterm labor Z87.51
    procedure during pregnancy Z98.870
    procedure while a fetus Z98.871
    prolonged reversible ischemic neurologic deficit (PRIND) Z86.73
    prostatic dysplasia Z87.430

DISEASE INDEX

History — *continued*
  personal (of) (*see also* History, family (of)) — *continued*
    psychological
      abuse
        adult Z91.411
        child Z62.811
        trauma, specified NEC Z91.49
    radiation therapy Z92.3
    removal
      implant
        breast Z98.86
      renal calculi Z87.442
    respiratory condition NEC Z87.09
    retained foreign body fully removed Z87.821
    risk factors NEC Z91.89
    self-harm Z91.5
    self-poisoning attempt Z91.5
    sex reassignment Z87.890
    sleep-wake cycle problem Z72.821
    specified NEC Z87.898
    steroid therapy (systemic) Z92.241
      inhaled Z92.240
    stroke without residual deficits Z86.73
    substance abuse NEC F10-F19 with fifth character 1
    sudden cardiac arrest Z86.74
    sudden cardiac death successfully resuscitated Z86.74
    suicide attempt Z91.5
    surgery NEC Z98.890
      with uterine scar Z98.891
      sex reassignment Z87.890
      transplant — *see* Transplant
    thrombophlebitis Z86.72
    thrombosis (venous) Z86.718
      pulmonary Z86.711
    tobacco dependence Z87.891
    transient ischemic attack (TIA) without residual deficits Z86.73
    trauma (physical) NEC Z87.828
      psychological NEC Z91.49
      self-harm Z91.5
    traumatic brain injury Z87.820
    unhealthy sleep-wake cycle Z72.821
    unintended awareness under general anesthesia Z92.84
    urinary (recurrent) (tract) infection(s) Z87.440
    urinary calculi Z87.442
    uterine scar from previous surgery Z98.891
    vaginal dysplasia Z87.411
    venous thrombosis or embolism Z86.718
      pulmonary Z86.711
    vulvar dysplasia Z87.412
HIV (*see also* Human, immunodeficiency virus) B20
  laboratory evidence (nonconclusive) R75
  nonconclusive test (in infants) R75
  positive, seropositive Z21
Hives (bold) — *see* Urticaria
Hoarseness R49.0
Hobo Z59.0
Hodgkin disease — *see* Lymphoma, Hodgkin
Hodgson's disease I71.2
  ruptured I71.1
Hoffa-Kastert disease E88.89
Hoffa's disease E88.89
Hoffmann's syndrome E03.9 *[G73.7]*
Hoffmann-Bouveret syndrome I47.9
Hole (round)
  macula H35.34-
  retina (without detachment) — *see* Break, retina, round hole
    with detachment — *see* Detachment, retina, with retinal, break
Holiday relief care Z75.5

Hollenhorst's plaque — *see* Occlusion, artery, retina
Hollow foot (congenital) Q66.7
  acquired — *see* Deformity, limb, foot, specified NEC
Holoprosencephaly Q04.2
Holt-Oram syndrome Q87.2
Homelessness Z59.0
Homesickness — *see* Disorder, adjustment
Homocystinemia, homocystinuria E72.11
Homogentisate 1,2-dioxygenase deficiency E70.29
Homologous serum hepatitis (prophylactic) (therapeutic) — *see* Hepatitis, viral, type B
Honeycomb lung J98.4
  congenital Q33.0
Hooded
  clitoris Q52.6
  penis Q55.69
Hookworm (anemia) (disease) (infection) (infestation) B76.9
  specified NEC B76.8
Hordeolum (eyelid) (externum) (recurrent) H00.019
  internum H00.029
    left H00.026
      lower H00.025
      upper H00.024
    right H00.023
      lower H00.022
      upper H00.021
    left H00.016
      lower H00.015
      upper H00.014
    right H00.013
      lower H00.012
      upper H00.011
Horn
  cutaneous L85.8
  nail L60.2
    congenital Q84.6
Horner(-Claude Bernard) syndrome G90.2
  traumatic — *see* Injury, nerve, cervical sympathetic
Horseshoe kidney (congenital) Q63.1
Horton's headache or neuralgia G44.099
  intractable G44.091
  not intractable G44.099
Hospital hopper syndrome — *see* Disorder, factitious
Hospitalism in children — *see* Disorder, adjustment
Hostility R45.5
  towards child Z62.3
Hot flashes
  menopausal N95.1
Hourglass (contracture) — *see also* Contraction, hourglass
  stomach K31.89
    congenital Q40.2
    stricture K31.2
Household, housing circumstance affecting care Z59.9
  specified NEC Z59.8
Housemaid's knee — *see* Bursitis, prepatellar
Hudson(-Stähli) line (cornea) — *see* Pigmentation, cornea, anterior
Human
  bite (open wound) — *see also* Bite
    intact skin surface — *see* Bite, superficial
  herpesvirus — *see* Herpes
  immunodeficiency virus (HIV) disease (infection) B20
    asymptomatic status Z21
    contact Z20.6
    counseling Z71.7

Human — *continued*
  immunodeficiency virus (HIV) disease (infection) B20 — *continued*
    dementia B20 *[F02.80]*
      with behavioral disturbance B20 *[F02.81]*
    exposure to Z20.6
    laboratory evidence R75
    type-2 (HIV 2) as cause of disease classified elsewhere B97.35
  papillomavirus (HPV)
    DNA test positive
      high risk
        cervix R87.810
        vagina R87.811
      low risk
        cervix R87.820
        vagina R87.821
    screening for Z11.51
  T-cell lymphotropic virus
    type-1 (HTLV-I) infection B33.3
      as cause of disease classified elsewhere B97.33
      carrier Z22.6
    type-2 (HTLV-II) as cause of disease classified elsewhere B97.34
Humidifier lung or pneumonitis J67.7
Humiliation (experience) in childhood Z62.898
Humpback (acquired) — *see* Kyphosis
Hunchback (acquired) — *see* Kyphosis
Hunger T73.0
  air, psychogenic F45.8
Hungry bone syndrome E83.81
Hunner's ulcer — *see* Cystitis, chronic, interstitial
Hunter's
  glossitis D51.0
  syndrome E76.1
Huntington's disease or chorea G10
  with dementia G10 *[F02.80]*
    with behavioral disturbance G10 *[F02.81]*
Hunt's
  disease or syndrome (herpetic geniculate ganglionitis) B02.21
  dyssynergia cerebellaris myoclonica G11.1
  neuralgia B02.21
Hurler(-Scheie) disease or syndrome E76.02
Hurst's disease G36.1
Hurthle cell
  adenocarcinoma C73
  adenoma D34
  carcinoma C73
  tumor D34
Hutchinson's
  disease, meaning
    angioma serpiginosum L81.7
    pompholyx (cheiropompholyx) L30.1
    prurigo estivalis L56.4
    summer eruption or summer prurigo L56.4
  melanotic freckle — *see* Melanoma, in situ
    malignant melanoma in — *see* Melanoma
  teeth or incisors (congenital syphilis) A50.52
  triad (congenital syphilis) A50.53
Hutchinson-Boeck disease or syndrome — *see* Sarcoidosis
Hutchinson-Gilford disease or syndrome E34.8
Hyalin plaque, sclera, senile H15.89
Hyaline membrane (disease) (lung) (pulmonary) (newborn) P22.0
Hyalinosis
  cutis (et mucosae) E78.89
  focal and segmental (glomerular) (*see also* N00-N07 with fourth character .1) N05.1
Hyalitis, hyalosis, asteroid — *see also* Deposit, crystalline
  syphilitic (late) A52.71

Hydatid
- cyst or tumor — *see* Echinococcus
- mole — *see* Hydatidiform mole
- Morgagni
  - female Q50.5
  - male (epididymal) Q55.4
  - testicular Q55.29

Hydatidiform mole (benign) (complicating pregnancy) (delivered) (undelivered) O01.9
- classical O01.0
- complete O01.0
- incomplete O01.1
- invasive D39.2
- malignant D39.2
- partial O01.1

Hydatidosis — *see* Echinococcus
Hydradenitis (axillaris) (suppurative) L73.2
Hydradenoma — *see* Hidradenoma
Hydramnios O40-
Hydrancephaly, hydranencephaly Q04.3
- with spina bifida — *see* Spina bifida, with hydrocephalus

Hydrargyrism NEC — *see* Poisoning, mercury
Hydrarthrosis — *see also* Effusion, joint
- gonococcal A54.42
- intermittent M12.40
  - ankle M12.47-
  - elbow M12.42-
  - foot joint M12.47-
  - hand joint M12.44-
  - hip M12.45-
  - knee M12.46-
  - multiple site M12.49
  - shoulder M12.41-
  - specified joint NEC M12.48
  - wrist M12.43-
- of yaws (early) (late) (*see also* subcategory M14.8-) A66.6
- syphilitic (late) A52.77
  - congenital A50.55 [M12.80]

Hydremia D64.89
Hydrencephalocele (congenital) — *see* Encephalocele
Hydrencephalomeningocele (congenital) — *see* Encephalocele
Hydroa R23.8
- aestivale L56.4
- vacciniforme L56.4

Hydroadenitis (axillaris) (suppurative) L73.2
Hydrocalycosis — *see* Hydronephrosis
Hydrocele (spermatic cord) (testis) (tunica vaginalis) N43.3
- canal of Nuck N94.89
- communicating N43.2
  - congenital P83.5
- congenital P83.5
- encysted N43.0
- female NEC N94.89
- infected N43.1
- newborn P83.5
- round ligament N94.89
- specified NEC N43.2
- spinalis — *see* Spina bifida
- vulva N90.89

Hydrocephalus (acquired) (external) (internal) (malignant) (recurrent) G91.9
- aqueduct Sylvius stricture Q03.0
- causing disproportion O33.6
  - with obstructed labor O66.3
- communicating G91.0
- congenital (external) (internal) Q03.9
  - with spina bifida Q05.4
    - cervical Q05.0
    - dorsal Q05.1
    - lumbar Q05.2
    - lumbosacral Q05.2
    - sacral Q05.3
    - thoracic Q05.1
    - thoracolumbar Q05.1

Hydrocephalus (acquired) (external) (internal) (malignant) (recurrent) G91.9 — *continued*
- congenital (external) (internal) Q03.9 — *continued*
  - specified NEC Q03.8
- due to toxoplasmosis (congenital) P37.1
- foramen Magendie block (acquired) G91.1
  - congenital (*see also* Hydrocephalus, congenital) Q03.1
- in (due to)
  - infectious disease NEC B89 [*G91.4*]
  - neoplastic disease NEC (*see also* Neoplasm) G91.4
  - parasitic disease B89 [*G91.4*]
- newborn Q03.9
  - with spina bifida — *see* Spina bifida, with hydrocephalus
- noncommunicating G91.1
- normal pressure G91.2
  - secondary G91.0
- obstructive G91.1
- otitic G93.2
- post-traumatic NEC G91.3
- secondary G91.4
  - post-traumatic G91.3
- specified NEC G91.8
- syphilitic, congenital A50.49

Hydrocolpos (congenital) N89.8
Hydrocystoma — *see* Neoplasm, skin, benign
Hydroencephalocele (congenital) — *see* Encephalocele
Hydroencephalomeningocele (congenital) — *see* Encephalocele
Hydrohematopneumothorax — *see* Hemothorax
Hydromeningitis — *see* Meningitis
Hydromeningocele (spinal) — *see also* Spina bifida
- cranial — *see* Encephalocele
Hydrometra N85.8
Hydrometrocolpos N89.8
Hydromicrocephaly Q02
Hydromphalos (since birth) Q45.8
Hydromyelia Q06.4
Hydromyelocele — *see* Spina bifida
Hydronephrosis (atrophic) (early) (functionless) (intermittent) (primary) (secondary) NEC N13.30
- with
  - infection N13.6
  - obstruction (by) (of)
    - renal calculus N13.2
      - with infection N13.6
    - ureteral NEC N13.1
      - with infection N13.6
      - calculus N13.2
        - with infection N13.6
    - ureteropelvic junction (congenital) Q62.0
      - acquired N13.0
        - with infection N13.6
    - ureteral stricture NEC N13.1
      - with infection N13.6
- congenital Q62.0
- due to acquired occlusion of ureteropelvic junction N13.0
- specified type NEC N13.39
- tuberculous A18.11

Hydropericarditis — *see* Pericarditis
Hydropericardium — *see* Pericarditis
Hydroperitoneum R18.8
Hydrophobia — *see* Rabies
Hydrophthalmos Q15.0
Hydropneumohemothorax — *see* Hemothorax
Hydropneumopericarditis — *see* Pericarditis
Hydropneumopericardium — *see* Pericarditis

Hydropneumothorax J94.8
- traumatic — *see* Injury, intrathoracic, lung
- tuberculous NEC A15.6

Hydrops R60.9
- abdominis R18.8
- articulorum intermittens — *see* Hydrarthrosis, intermittent
- cardiac — *see* Failure, heart, congestive
- causing obstructed labor (mother) O66.3
- endolymphatic H81.0-
- fetal — *see* Pregnancy, complicated by, hydrops, fetalis
- fetalis P83.2
  - due to
    - ABO isoimmunization P56.0
    - alpha thalassemia D56.0
    - hemolytic disease D56.90
      - specified NEC P56.99
    - isoimmunization (ABO) (Rh) P56.0
    - other specified nonhemolytic disease NEC P83.2
    - Rh incompatibility P56.0
  - during pregnancy — *see* Pregnancy, complicated by, hydrops, fetalis
- gallbladder K82.1
- joint — *see* Effusion, joint
- labyrinth H81.0-
- newborn (idiopathic) P83.2
  - due to
    - ABO isoimmunization P56.0
    - alpha thalassemia D56.0
    - hemolytic disease P56.90
    - specified NEC P56.99
    - isoimmunization (ABO) (Rh) P56.0
    - Rh incompatibility P56.0
- nutritional — *see* Malnutrition, severe
- pericardium — *see* Pericarditis
- pleura — *see* Hydrothorax
- spermatic cord — *see* Hydrocele

Hydropyonephrosis N13.6
Hydrorachis Q06.4
Hydrorrhea (nasal) J34.89
- pregnancy — *see* Rupture, membranes, premature
Hydrosadenitis (axillaris) (suppurative) L73.2
Hydrosalpinx (fallopian tube) (follicularis) N70.11
Hydrothorax (double) (pleura) J94.8
- chylous (nonfilarial) I89.8
  - filarial (*see also* Infestation, filarial) B74.9 [*J91.8*]
- traumatic — *see* Injury, intrathoracic
- tuberculous NEC (non primary) A15.6
Hydroureter (*see also* Hydronephrosis) N13.4
- with infection N13.6
- congenital Q62.39
Hydroureteronephrosis — *see* Hydronephrosis
Hydrourethra N36.8
Hydroxykynureninuria E70.8
Hydroxylysinemia E72.3
Hydroxyprolinemia E72.59
Hygiene, sleep
- abuse Z72.821
- inadequate Z72.821
- poor Z72.821
Hygroma (congenital) (cystic) D18.1
- praepatellare, prepatellar — *see* Bursitis, prepatellar
Hymen — *see* condition
Hymenolepis, hymenolepiasis (diminuta) (infection) (infestation) (nana) B71.0
Hypalgesia R20.8
Hyperacidity (gastric) K31.89
- psychogenic F45.8

Hyperactive, hyperactivity F90.9
basal cell, uterine cervix — *see* Dysplasia, cervix
bowel sounds R19.12
cervix epithelial (basal) — *see* Dysplasia, cervix
child F90.9
attention deficit — *see* Disorder, attention-deficit hyperactivity
detrusor muscle N32.81
gastrointestinal K31.89
psychogenic F45.8
nasal mucous membrane J34.3
stomach K31.89
thyroid (gland) — *see* Hyperthyroidism
Hyperacusis H93.23-
Hyperadrenalism E27.5
Hyperadrenocorticism E24.9
congenital E25.0
iatrogenic E24.2
correct substance properly administered — *see* Table of Drugs and Chemicals, by drug, adverse effect
overdose or wrong substance given or taken — *see* Table of Drugs and Chemicals, by drug, poisoning
not associated with Cushing's syndrome E27.0
pituitary-dependent E24.0
Hyperaldosteronism E26.9
familial (type I) E26.02
glucocorticoid-remediable E26.02
primary (due to (bilateral) adrenal hyperplasia) E26.09
primary NEC E26.09
secondary E26.1
specified NEC E26.89
Hyperalgesia R20.8
Hyperalimentation R63.2
carotene, carotin E67.1
specified NEC E67.8
vitamin
A E67.0
D E67.3
Hyperaminoaciduria
arginine E72.21
cystine E72.01
lysine E72.3
ornithine E72.4
Hyperammonemia (congenital) E72.20
Hyperazotemia — *see* Uremia
Hyperbetalipoproteinemia (familial) E78.00
with prebetalipoproteinemia E78.2
Hyperbilirubinemia
constitutional E80.6
familial conjugated E80.6
neonatal (transient) — *see* Jaundice, newborn
Hypercalcemia, hypocalciuric, familial E83.52
Hypercalciuria, idiopathic E83.52
Hypercapnia R06.89
newborn P84
Hypercarotenemia, hypercarotinemia (dietary) E67.1
Hypercementosis K03.4
Hyperchloremia E87.8
Hyperchlorhydria K31.89
neurotic F45.8
psychogenic F45.8
Hypercholesterinemia — *see* Hypercholesterolemia
Hypercholesterolemia (essential) (primary) (pure) E78.00
with hyperglyceridemia, endogenous E78.2
dietary counseling and surveillance Z71.3
familial E78.01
hereditary E78.01
Hyperchylia gastrica, psychogenic F45.8

Hyperchylomicronemia (familial) (primary) E78.3
with hyperbetalipoproteinemia E78.3
Hypercoagulable (state) D68.59
activated protein C resistance D68.51
antithrombin (III) deficiency D68.59
factor V Leiden mutation D68.51
primary NEC D68.59
protein C deficiency D68.59
protein S deficiency D68.59
prothrombin gene mutation D68.52
secondary D68.69
specified NEC D68.69
Hypercoagulation (state) D68.59
Hypercorticalism, pituitary-dependent E24.0
Hypercorticosolism — *see* Cushing's, syndrome
Hypercorticosteronism E24.2
correct substance properly administered — *see* Table of Drugs and Chemicals, by drug, adverse effect
overdose or wrong substance given or taken — *see* Table of Drugs and Chemicals, by drug, poisoning
Hypercortisonism E24.2
correct substance properly administered — *see* Table of Drugs and Chemicals, by drug, adverse effect
overdose or wrong substance given or taken — *see* Table of Drugs and Chemicals, by drug, poisoning
Hyperekplexia Q89.8
Hyperelectrolytemia E87.8
Hyperemesis R11.10
with nausea R11.2
gravidarum (mild) O21.0
with
carbohydrate depletion O21.1
dehydration O21.1
electrolyte imbalance O21.1
metabolic disturbance O21.1
severe (with metabolic disturbance) O21.1
projectile R11.12
psychogenic F45.8
Hyperemia (acute) (passive) R68.89
anal mucosa K62.89
bladder N32.89
cerebral I67.89
conjunctiva H11.43-
ear internal, acute — *see* subcategory H83.0
enteric K59.8
eye — *see* Hyperemia, conjunctiva
eyelid (active) (passive) — *see* Disorder, eyelid, specified type NEC
intestine K59.8
iris — *see* Disorder, iris, vascular
kidney N28.89
labyrinth — *see* subcategory H83.0
liver (active) K76.89
lung (passive) — *see* Edema, lung
pulmonary (passive) — *see* Edema, lung
renal N28.89
retina H35.89
stomach K31.89
Hyperesthesia (body surface) R20.3
larynx (reflex) J38.7
hysterical F44.89
pharynx (reflex) J39.2
hysterical F44.89
Hyperestrogenism (drug-induced) (iatrogenic) E28.0
Hyperexplexia Q89.8
Hyperfibrinolysis — *see* Fibrinolysis
Hyperfructosemia E74.19

Hyperfunction
adrenal cortex, not associated with Cushing's syndrome E27.0
medulla E27.5
adrenomedullary E27.5
virilism E25.9
congenital E25.0
ovarian E28.8
pancreas K86.89
parathyroid (gland) E21.3
pituitary (gland) (anterior) E22.9
specified NEC E22.8
polyglandular E31.1
testicular E29.0
Hypergammaglobulinemia D89.2
polyclonal D89.0
Waldenström D89.0
Hypergastrinemia E16.4
Hyperglobulinemia R77.1
Hyperglycemia, hyperglycemic (transient) R73.9
coma — *see* Diabetes, by type, with coma
postpancreatectomy E89.1
Hyperglyceridemia (endogenous) (essential) (familial) (hereditary) (pure) E78.1
mixed E78.3
Hyperglycinemia (non-ketotic) E72.51
Hypergonadism
ovarian E28.8
testicular (primary) (infantile) E29.0
Hyperheparinemia D68.32
Hyperhidrosis, hyperidrosis R61
focal
primary L74.519
axilla L74.510
face L74.511
palms L74.512
soles L74.513
secondary L74.52
generalized R61
localized
primary L74.519
axilla L74.510
face L74.511
palms L74.512
soles L74.513
secondary L74.52
psychogenic F45.8
secondary R61
focal L74.52
Hyperhistidinemia E70.41
Hyperhomocysteinemia E72.11
Hyperhydroxyprolinemia E72.59
Hyperinsulinism (functional) E16.1
with
coma (hypoglycemic) E15
encephalopathy E16.1 *[G94]*
ectopic E16.1
therapeutic misadventure (from administration of insulin) — *see* subcategory T38.3
Hyperkalemia E87.5
Hyperkeratosis (*see also* Keratosis) L85.9
cervix N88.0
due to yaws (early) (late) (palmar or plantar) A66.3
follicularis Q82.8
penetrans (in cutem) L87.0
palmoplantaris climacterica L85.1
pinta A67.1
senile (with pruritus) L57.0
universalis congenita Q80.8
vocal cord J38.3
vulva N90.4
Hyperkinesia, hyperkinetic (disease) (reaction) (syndrome) (childhood) (adolescence) — *see also* Disorder, attention-deficit hyperactivity
heart I51.89

Hyperleucine-isoleucinemia E71.19
Hyperlipemia, hyperlipidemia E78.5
- combined E78.2
  - familial E78.4
- group
  - A E78.00
  - B E78.1
  - C E78.2
  - D E78.3
  - mixed E78.2
  - specified NEC E78.4
Hyperlipidosis E75.6
- hereditary NEC E75.5
Hyperlipoproteinemia E78.5
- Fredrickson's type
  - I E78.3
  - IIa E78.00
  - IIb E78.2
  - III E78.2
  - IV E78.1
  - V E78.3
- low-density-lipoprotein-type (LDL) E78.00
- very-low-density-lipoprotein-type (VLDL) E78.1
Hyperlucent lung, unilateral J43.0
Hyperlysinemia E72.3
Hypermagnesemia E83.41
- neonatal P71.8
Hypermenorrhea N92.0
Hypermethioninemia E72.19
Hypermetropia (congenital) H52.0-
Hypermobility, hypermotility
- cecum — see Syndrome, irritable bowel
- coccyx — see subcategory M53.2
- colon — see Syndrome, irritable bowel
  - psychogenic F45.8
- ileum K58.9
- intestine (see also Syndrome, irritable bowel) K58.9
  - psychogenic F45.8
- meniscus (knee) — see Derangement, knee, meniscus
- scapula — see Instability, joint, shoulder
- stomach K31.89
  - psychogenic F45.8
- syndrome M35.7
- urethra N36.41
  - with intrinsic sphincter deficiency N36.43
Hypernasality R49.21
Hypernatremia E87.0
Hypernephroma C64-
Hyperopia — see Hypermetropia
Hyperorexia nervosa F50.2
Hyperornithinemia E72.4
Hyperosmia R43.1
Hyperosmolality E87.0
Hyperostosis (monomelic) — see also Disorder, bone, density and structure, specified NEC
- ankylosing (spine) M48.10
  - cervical region M48.12
  - cervicothoracic region M48.13
  - lumbar region M48.16
  - lumbosacral region M48.17
  - multiple sites M48.19
  - occipito-atlanto-axial region M48.11
  - sacrococcygeal region M48.18
  - thoracic region M48.14
  - thoracolumbar region M48.15
- cortical (skull) M85.2
  - infantile M89.8x-
- frontal, internal of skull M85.2
- interna frontalis M85.2
- skeletal, diffuse idiopathic — see Hyperostosis, ankylosing
- skull M85.2
  - congenital Q75.8
- vertebral, ankylosing — see Hyperostosis, ankylosing
Hyperovarism E28.8
Hyperoxaluria (primary) E72.53

Hyperparathyroidism E21.3
- primary E21.0
- secondary (renal) N25.81
  - non-renal E21.1
- specified NEC E21.2
- tertiary E21.2
Hyperpathia R20.8
Hyperperistalsis R19.2
- psychogenic F45.8
Hyperpermeability, capillary I78.8
Hyperphagia R63.2
Hyperphenylalaninemia NEC E70.1
Hyperphoria (alternating) H50.53
Hyperphosphatemia E83.39
Hyperpiesis, hyperpiesia — see Hypertension
Hyperpigmentation — see also Pigmentation
- melanin NEC L81.4
- postinflammatory L81.0
Hyperpinealism E34.8
Hyperpituitarism E22.9
Hyperplasia, hyperplastic
- adenoids J35.2
- adrenal (capsule) (cortex) (gland) E27.8
  - with
    - sexual precocity (male) E25.9
      - congenital E25.0
    - virilism, adrenal E25.9
      - congenital E25.0
    - virilization (female) E25.9
      - congenital E25.0
  - congenital E25.0
  - salt-losing E25.0
- adrenomedullary E27.5
- angiolymphoid, eosinophilia (ALHE) D18.01
- appendix (lymphoid) K38.0
- artery, fibromuscular I77.3
- bone — see Hypertrophy, bone
  - marrow D75.89
- breast — see also Hypertrophy, breast
  - ductal (atypical) N60.9-
- C-cell, thyroid E07.0
- cementation (tooth) (teeth) K03.4
- cervical gland R59.0
- cervix (uteri) (basal cell) (endometrium) (polypoid) — see also Dysplasia, cervix
  - congenital Q51.828
- clitoris, congenital Q52.6
- denture K06.2
- endocervicitis N72
- endometrium, endometrial (adenomatous) (benign) (cystic) (glandular) (glandular-cystic) (polypoid) N85.00
  - with atypia N85.02
  - cervix — see Dysplasia, cervix
  - complex (without atypia) N85.01
  - simple (without atypia) N85.01
- epithelial L85.9
  - focal, oral, including tongue K13.29
  - nipple N62
  - skin L85.9
  - tongue K13.29
  - vaginal wall N89.3
- erythroid D75.89
- fibromuscular of artery (carotid) (renal) I77.3
- genital
  - female NEC N94.89
  - male N50.89
- gingiva K06.1
- glandularis cystica uteri (interstitialis) (see also Hyperplasia, endometrial) N85.00-
- gum K06.1
- hymen, congenital Q52.4
- irritative, edentulous (alveolar) K06.2

Hyperplasia, hyperplastic — continued
- jaw M26.09
  - alveolar M26.79
  - lower M26.03
    - alveolar M26.72
  - upper M26.01
    - alveolar M26.71
- kidney (congenital) Q63.3
- labia N90.69
  - epithelial N90.3
- liver (congenital) Q44.7
  - nodular, focal K76.89
- lymph gland or node R59.9
- mandible, mandibular M26.03
  - alveolar M26.72
  - unilateral condylar M27.8
- maxilla, maxillary M26.01
  - alveolar M26.71
- myometrium, myometrial N85.2
- neuroendocrine cell, of infancy J84.841
- nose
  - lymphoid J34.89
  - polypoid J33.9
- oral mucosa (irritative) K13.6
- organ or site, congenital NEC — see Anomaly, by site
- ovary N83.8
- palate, papillary (irritative) K13.6
- pancreatic islet cells E16.9
  - alpha E16.8
    - with excess
      - gastrin E16.4
      - glucagon E16.3
  - beta E16.1
- parathyroid (gland) E21.0
- pharynx (lymphoid) J39.2
- prostate (adenofibromatous) (nodular) N40.0
  - with lower urinary tract symptoms (LUTS) N40.1
  - without lower urinary tract symtpoms (LUTS) N40.0
- renal artery I77.89
- reticulo-endothelial (cell) D75.89
- salivary gland (any) K11.1
- Schimmelbusch's — see Mastopathy, cystic
- suprarenal capsule (gland) E27.8
- thymus (gland) (persistent) E32.0
- thyroid (gland) — see Goiter
- tonsils (faucial) (infective) (lingual) (lymphoid) J35.1
  - with adenoids J35.3
- unilateral condylar M27.8
- uterus, uterine N85.2
  - endometrium (glandular) (see also Hyperplasia, endometrial) N85.00-
- vulva N90.69
  - epithelial N90.3
Hyperpnea — see Hyperventilation
Hyperpotassemia E87.5
Hyperprebetalipoproteinemia (familial) E78.1
Hyperprolactinemia E22.1
Hyperprolinemia (type I) (type II) E72.59
Hyperproteinemia E88.09
Hyperprothrombinemia, causing coagulation factor deficiency D68.4
Hyperpyrexia R50.9
- heat (effects) T67.0
- malignant, due to anesthetic T88.3
- rheumatic — see Fever, rheumatic
- unknown origin R50.9
Hyper-reflexia R29.2
Hypersalivation K11.7
Hypersecretion
- ACTH (not associated with Cushing's syndrome) E27.0
  - pituitary E24.0
- adrenaline E27.5

Hypersecretion — *continued*
  adrenomedullary E27.5
  androgen (testicular) E29.0
    ovarian (drug-induced) (iatrogenic) E28.1
  calcitonin E07.0
  catecholamine E27.5
  corticoadrenal E24.9
  cortisol E24.9
  epinephrine E27.5
  estrogen E28.0
  gastric K31.89
    psychogenic F45.8
  gastrin E16.4
  glucagon E16.3
  hormone(s)
    ACTH (not associated with Cushing's
        syndrome) E27.0
      pituitary E24.0
    antidiuretic E22.2
    growth E22.0
    intestinal NEC E34.1
    ovarian androgen E28.1
    pituitary E22.9
    testicular E29.0
    thyroid stimulating E05.80
      with thyroid storm E05.81
  insulin — *see* Hyperinsulinism
  lacrimal glands — *see* Epiphora
  medulloadrenal E27.5
  milk O92.6
  ovarian androgens E28.1
  salivary gland (any) K11.7
  thyrocalcitonin E07.0
  upper respiratory J39.8
Hypersegmentation, leukocytic,
  hereditary D72.0
Hypersensitive, hypersensitiveness,
  hypersensitivity — *see also* Allergy
  carotid sinus G90.01
  colon — *see* Irritable, colon
  drug T88.7
  gastrointestinal K52.29
    immediate K52.29
    psychogenic F45.8
  labyrinth — *see* subcategory H83.2
  pain R20.8
  pneumonitis — *see* Pneumonitis, allergic
  reaction T78.40
  upper respiratory tract NEC J39.3
Hypersomnia (organic) G47.10
  due to
    alcohol
      abuse F10.182
      dependence F10.282
      use F10.982
    amphetamines
      abuse F15.182
      dependence F15.282
      use F15.982
    caffeine
      abuse F15.182
      dependence F15.282
      use F15.982
    cocaine
      abuse F14.182
      dependence F14.282
      use F14.982
    drug NEC
      abuse F19.182
      dependence F19.282
      use F19.982
    medical condition G47.14
    mental disorder F51.13
    opioid
      abuse F11.182
      dependence F11.282
      use F11.982

Hypersomnia (organic) G47.10 — *continued*
  due to — *continued*
    psychoactive substance NEC
      abuse F19.182
      dependence F19.282
      use F19.982
    sedative, hypnotic, or anxiolytic
      abuse F13.182
      dependence F13.282
      use F13.982
    stimulant NEC
      abuse F15.182
      dependence F15.282
      use F15.982
  idiopathic G47.11
    with long sleep time G47.11
    without long sleep time G47.12
  menstrual related G47.13
  nonorganic origin F51.11
    specified NEC F51.19
  not due to a substance or known physiological
      condition F51.11
    specified NEC F51.19
  primary F51.11
  recurrent G47.13
  specified NEC G47.19
Hypersplenia, hypersplenism D73.1
Hyperstimulation, ovaries (associated with
  induced ovulation) N98.1
Hypersusceptibility — *see* Allergy
Hypertelorism (ocular) (orbital) Q75.2
Hypertension, hypertensive (accelerated)
  (benign) (essential) (idiopathic) (malignant)
  (systemic) I10
  with
    heart involvement (conditions in I51.4 –
        I51.9 due to hypertension) — *see*
        Hypertension, heart
    kidney involvement — *see* Hypertension,
        kidney
  benign, intracranial G93.2
  borderline R03.0
  cardiorenal (disease) I13.10
    with heart failure I13.0
      with stage 1 through stage 4 chronic
          kidney disease I13.0
      with stage 5 or end stage renal disease
          I13.2
    without heart failure I13.10
      with stage 1 through stage 4 chronic
          kidney disease I13.10
      with stage 5 or end stage renal disease
          I13.11
  cardiovascular
    disease (arteriosclerotic) (sclerotic) — *see*
        Hypertension, heart
    renal (disease) — *see* Hypertension,
        cardiorenal
  chronic venous — *see* Hypertension, venous
      (chronic)
  complicating
    childbirth (labor) O16.4
      pre-existing O10.92
        with
          heart disease O10.12
            with renal disease O10.32
          pre-eclampsia O11.4
          renal disease O10.22
            with heart disease O10.32
          essential O10.02
          secondary O10.42

Hypertension, hypertensive (accelerated)
  (benign) (essential) (idiopathic) (malignant)
  (systemic) I10 — *continued*
  complicating — *continued*
    pregnancy O16-
      with edema (*see also* Pre-eclampsia)
          O14.9-
      gestational (pregnancy induced) (without
          proteinuria) O13-
        with proteinuria O14.9-
          mild pre-eclampsia O14.0-
          moderate pre-eclampsia O14.0-
          severe pre-eclampsia O14.1-
            with hemolysis, elevated liver
                enzymes and low platelet count
                (HELLP) O14.2-
      pre-existing O10.91-
        with
          heart disease O10.11-
            with renal disease O10.31-
          pre-eclampsia — *see* category O11
          renal disease O10.21-
            with heart disease O10.31-
          essential O10.01-
          secondary O10.41-
      transient O13.-
    puerperium, pre-existing O16.5
      pre-existing
        with
          heart disease O10.13
            with renal disease O10.33
          pre-eclampsia O11.5
          renal disease O10.23
            with heart disease O10.33
          essential O10.03
      pregnancy-induced O13.9
      secondary O10.43
  crisis I16.9
  due to
    endocrine disorders I15.2
    pheochromocytoma I15.2
    renal disorders NEC I15.1
      arterial I15.0
    renovascular disorders I15.0
    specified disease NEC I15.8
  emergency I16.2
  encephalopathy I67.4
  gestational (without significant proteinuria)
      (pregnancy-induced) (transient) O13-
    with significant proteinuria — *see* Pre-
        eclampsia
    complicating
      delivery O13.4
      puerperium O13.5
  Goldblatt's I70.1
  heart (disease) (conditions in I51.4-I51.9 due
      to hypertension) I11.9
    with
      heart failure (congestive) I11.0
      kidney disease (chronic) — *see*
          Hypertension, cardiorenal
  intracranial (benign) G93.2
  kidney I12.9
    with
      heart disease — *see* Hypertension,
          cardiorenal
      stage 1 through stage 4 chronic kidney
          disease I12.9
      stage 5 chronic kidney disease (CKD) or
          end stage renal disease (ESRD) I12.0
  lesser circulation I27.0
  maternal O16.-
  newborn P29.2
    pulmonary (persistent) P29.3
  ocular H40.05-
  pancreatic duct — *code to* underlying
      condition
    with chronic pancreatitis K86.1

Hypertension, hypertensive (accelerated) (benign) (essential) (idiopathic) (malignant) (systemic) I10 — *continued*
  portal (due to chronic liver disease) (idiopathic) K76.6
    gastropathy K31.89
  in (due to) schistosomiasis (bilharziasis) B65.9 *[K77]*
  postoperative I97.3
  psychogenic F45.8
  pulmonary (artery) (secondary) NEC I27.2
    with
      cor pulmonale (chronic) I27.2
        acute I26.09
      right heart ventricular strain/failure I27.2
        acute I26.09
    of newborn (persistent) P29.3
    primary (idiopathic) I27.0
  renal — *see* Hypertension, kidney
  renovascular I15.0
  secondary NEC I15.9
    due to
      endocrine disorders I15.2
      pheochromocytoma I15.2
      renal disorders NEC I15.1
        arterial I15.0
      renovascular disorders I15.0
    specified NEC I15.8
  transient, of pregnancy O13.-
  urgency I16.0
  venous (chronic)
    due to
      deep vein thrombosis — *see* Syndrome, postthrombotic
    idiopathic I87.309
      with
        inflammation I87.32-
          with ulcer I87.33-
        specified complication NEC I87.39-
        ulcer I87.31-
          with inflammation I87.33-
      asymptomatic I87.30-

Hypertensive urgency — *see* Hypertension
Hyperthecosis ovary E28.8
Hyperthermia (of unknown origin) — *see also* Hyperpyrexia
  malignant, due to anesthesia T88.3
  newborn P81.9
    environmental P81.0
Hyperthyroid (recurrent) — *see* Hyperthyroidism
Hyperthyroidism (latent) (pre-adult) (recurrent) E05.90
  with
    goiter (diffuse) E05.00
      with thyroid storm E05.01
      nodular (multinodular) E05.20
        with thyroid storm E05.21
        uninodular E05.10
          with thyroid storm E05.11
    storm E05.91
  due to ectopic thyroid tissue E05.30
    with thyroid storm E05.31
  neonatal, transitory P72.1
  specified NEC E05.80
    with thyroid storm E05.81
Hypertony, hypertonia, hypertonicity
  bladder N31.8
  congenital P94.1
  stomach K31.89
    psychogenic F45.8
  uterus, uterine (contractions) (complicating delivery) O62.4

Hypertrichosis L68.9
  congenital Q84.2
  eyelid H02.869
    left H02.866
      lower H02.865
      upper H02.864
    right H02.863
      lower H02.862
      upper H02.861
  lanuginosa Q84.2
    acquired L68.1
  localized L68.2
  specified NEC L68.8
Hypertriglyceridemia, essential E78.1
Hypertrophy, hypertrophic
  adenofibromatous, prostate — *see* Enlargement, enlarged, prostate
  adenoids (infective) J35.2
    with tonsils J35.3
  adrenal cortex E27.8
  alveolar process or ridge — *see* Anomaly, alveolar
  anal papillae K62.89
  artery I77.89
    congenital NEC Q27.8
      digestive system Q27.8
      lower limb Q27.8
      specified site NEC Q27.8
      upper limb Q27.8
  auricular — *see* Hypertrophy, cardiac
  Bartholin's gland N75.8
  bile duct (common) (hepatic) K83.8
  bladder (sphincter) (trigone) N32.89
  bone M89.30
    carpus M89.34-
    clavicle M89.31-
    femur M89.35-
    fibula M89.36-
    finger M89.34-
    humerus M89.32-
    ilium M89.359
    ischium M89.359
    metacarpus M89.34-
    metatarsus M89.37-
    multiple sites M89.39
    neck M89.38
    radius M89.33-
    rib M89.38
    scapula M89.31-
    skull M89.38
    tarsus M89.37-
    tibia M89.36-
    toe M89.37-
    ulna M89.33-
    vertebra M89.38
  brain G93.89
  breast N62
    cystic — *see* Mastopathy, cystic
    newborn P83.4
    pubertal, massive N62
    puerperal, postpartum — *see* Disorder, breast, specified type NEC
    senile (parenchymatous) N62
  cardiac (chronic) (idiopathic) I51.7
    with rheumatic fever (conditions in I00)
      active I01.8
      inactive or quiescent (with chorea) I09.89
    congenital NEC Q24.8
    fatty — *see* Degeneration, myocardial
    hypertensive — *see* Hypertension, heart
    rheumatic (with chorea) I09.89
      active or acute I01.8
        with chorea I02.0
    valve — *see* Endocarditis
  cartilage — *see* Disorder, cartilage, specified type NEC
  cecum — *see* Megacolon

Hypertrophy, hypertrophic — *continued*
  cervix (uteri) N88.8
    congenital Q51.828
    elongation N88.4
  clitoris (cirrhotic) N90.89
    congenital Q52.6
  colon — *see also* Megacolon
    congenital Q43.2
  conjunctiva, lymphoid H11.89
  corpora cavernosa N48.89
  cystic duct K82.8
  duodenum K31.89
  endometrium (glandular) (*see also* Hyperplasia, endometrial) N85.00-
    cervix N88.8
  epididymis N50.89
  esophageal hiatus (congenital) Q79.1
    with hernia — *see* Hernia, hiatal
  eyelid — *see* Disorder, eyelid, specified type NEC
  fat pad E65
    knee (infrapatellar) (popliteal) (prepatellar) (retropatellar) M79.4
  foot (congenital) Q74.2
  frenulum, frenum (tongue) K14.8
    lip K13.0
  gallbladder K82.8
  gastric mucosa K29.60
    with bleeding K29.61
  gland, glandular R59.9
    generalized R59.1
    localized R59.0
  gum (mucous membrane) K06.1
  heart (idiopathic) — *see also* Hypertrophy, cardiac
    valve (*see also* Endocarditis) I38
  hemifacial Q67.4
  hepatic — *see* Hypertrophy, liver
  hiatus (esophageal) Q79.1
  hilus gland R59.0
  hymen, congenital Q52.4
  ileum K63.89
  intestine NEC K63.89
  jejunum K63.89
  kidney (compensatory) N28.81
    congenital Q63.3
  labium (majus) (minus) N90.60
  ligament — *see* Disorder, ligament
  lingual tonsil (infective) J35.1
    with adenoids J35.3
  lip K13.0
    congenital Q18.6
  liver R16.0
    acute K76.89
    cirrhotic — *see* Cirrhosis, liver
    congenital Q44.7
    fatty — *see* Fatty, liver
  lymph, lymphatic gland R59.9
    generalized R59.1
    localized R59.0
    tuberculous — *see* Tuberculosis, lymph gland
  mammary gland — *see* Hypertrophy, breast
  Meckel's diverticulum (congenital) Q43.0
    malignant — *see* Table of Neoplasms, small intestine, malignant
  median bar — *see* Hyperplasia, prostate
  meibomian gland — *see* Chalazion
  meniscus, knee, congenital Q74.1
  metatarsal head — *see* Hypertrophy, bone, metatarsus
  metatarsus — *see* Hypertrophy, bone, metatarsus
  mucous membrane
    alveolar ridge K06.2
    gum K06.1
    nose (turbinate) J34.3
  muscle M62.89
  muscular coat, artery I77.89

Hypertrophy, hypertrophic — *continued*
- myocardium — *see also* Hypertrophy, cardiac
  - idiopathic I42.2
- myometrium N85.2
- nail L60.2
  - congenital Q84.5
- nasal J34.89
  - alae J34.89
  - bone J34.89
  - cartilage J34.89
  - mucous membrane (septum) J34.3
  - sinus J34.89
  - turbinate J34.3
- nasopharynx, lymphoid (infectional) (tissue) (wall) J35.2
- nipple N62
- organ or site, congenital NEC — *see* Anomaly, by site
- ovary N83.8
- palate (hard) M27.8
  - soft K13.79
- pancreas, congenital Q45.3
- parathyroid (gland) E21.0
- parotid gland K11.1
- penis N48.89
- pharyngeal tonsil J35.2
- pharynx J39.2
  - lymphoid (infectional) (tissue) (wall) J35.2
- pituitary (anterior) (fossa) (gland) E23.6
- prepuce (congenital) N47.8
  - female N90.89
- prostate — *see* Enlargement, enlarged, prostate
  - congenital Q55.4
- pseudomuscular G71.0
- pylorus (adult) (muscle) (sphincter) K31.1
  - congenital or infantile Q40.0
- rectal, rectum (sphincter) K62.89
- rhinitis (turbinate) J31.0
- salivary gland (any) K11.1
  - congenital Q38.4
- scaphoid (tarsal) — *see* Hypertrophy, bone, tarsus
- scar L91.0
- scrotum N50.89
- seminal vesicle N50.89
- sigmoid — *see* Megacolon
- skin L91.9
  - specified NEC L91.8
- spermatic cord N50.89
- spleen — *see* Splenomegaly
- spondylitis — *see* Spondylosis
- stomach K31.89
- sublingual gland K11.1
- submandibular gland K11.1
- suprarenal cortex (gland) E27.8
- synovial NEC M67.20
  - acromioclavicular M67.21-
  - ankle M67.27-
  - elbow M67.22-
  - foot M67.27-
  - hand M67.24-
  - hip M67.25-
  - knee M67.26-
  - multiple sites M67.29
  - specified site NEC M67.28
  - wrist M67.23-
- tendon — *see* Disorder, tendon, specified type NEC
- testis N44.8
  - congenital Q55.29
- thymic, thymus (gland) (congenital) E32.0
- thyroid (gland) — *see* Goiter
- toe (congenital) Q74.2
  - acquired — *see also* Deformity, toe, specified NEC
- tongue K14.8
  - congenital Q38.2
  - papillae (foliate) K14.3

Hypertrophy, hypertrophic — *continued*
- tonsils (faucial) (infective) (lingual) (lymphoid) J35.1
  - with adenoids J35.3
- tunica vaginalis N50.89
- ureter N28.89
- urethra N36.8
- uterus N85.2
  - neck (with elongation) N88.4
  - puerperal O90.89
- uvula K13.79
- vagina N89.8
- vas deferens N50.89
- vein I87.8
- ventricle, ventricular (heart) — *see also* Hypertrophy, cardiac
  - congenital Q24.8
  - in tetralogy of Fallot Q21.3
- verumontanum N36.8
- vocal cord J38.3
- vulva N90.60
  - stasis (nonfilarial) N90.69

Hypertropia H50.2-
Hypertyrosinemia E70.21
Hyperuricemia (asymptomatic) E79.0
Hypervalinemia E71.19
Hyperventilation (tetany) R06.4
- hysterical F45.8
- psychogenic F45.8
- syndrome F45.8
Hypervitaminosis (dietary) NEC E67.8
- A E67.0
  - administered as drug (prolonged intake) — *see* Table of Drugs and Chemicals, vitamins, adverse effect
  - overdose or wrong substance given or taken — *see* Table of Drugs and Chemicals, vitamins, poisoning
- B6 E67.2
- D E67.3
  - administered as drug (prolonged intake) — *see* Table of Drugs and Chemicals, vitamins, adverse effect
  - overdose or wrong substance given or taken — *see* Table of Drugs and Chemicals, vitamins, poisoning
- K E67.8
  - administered as drug (prolonged intake) — *see* Table of Drugs and Chemicals, vitamins, adverse effect
  - overdose or wrong substance given or taken — *see* Table of Drugs and Chemicals, vitamins, poisoning
Hypervolemia E87.70
- specified NEC E87.79
Hypesthesia R20.1
- cornea — *see* Anesthesia, cornea
Hyphema H21.0-
- traumatic S05.1-
Hypo-osmolality E87.1
Hypo-ovarianism, hypo-ovarism E28.39
Hypoacidity, gastric K31.89
- psychogenic F45.8
Hypoadrenalism, hypoadrenia E27.40
- primary E27.1
- tuberculous A18.7
Hypoadrenocorticism E27.40
- pituitary E23.0
- primary E27.1
Hypoalbuminemia E88.09
Hypoaldosteronism E27.40
Hypoalphalipoproteinemia E78.6
Hypobarism T70.29
Hypobaropathy T70.29
Hypobetalipoproteinemia (familial) E78.6

Hypocalcemia E83.51
- dietary E58
- neonatal P71.1
  - due to cow's milk P71.0
- phosphate-loading (newborn) P71.1
Hypochloremia E87.8
Hypochlorhydria K31.89
- neurotic F45.8
- psychogenic F45.8
Hypochondria, hypochondriac, hypochondriasis (reaction) F45.21
- sleep F51.03
Hypochondrogenesis Q77.0
Hypochondroplasia Q77.4
Hypochromasia, blood cells D50.8
Hypodontia — *see* Anodontia
Hypoeosinophilia D72.89
Hypoesthesia R20.1
Hypofibrinogenemia D68.8
- acquired D65
- congenital (hereditary) D68.2
Hypofunction
- adrenocortical E27.40
  - drug-induced E27.3
  - postprocedural E89.6
  - primary E27.1
- adrenomedullary, postprocedural E89.6
- cerebral R29.818
- corticoadrenal NEC E27.40
- intestinal K59.8
- labyrinth — *see* subcategory H83.2
- ovary E28.39
- pituitary (gland) (anterior) E23.0
- testicular E29.1
  - postprocedural (postsurgical) (postirradiation) (iatrogenic) E89.5
Hypogalactia O92.4
Hypogammaglobulinemia (*see also* Agammaglobulinemia) D80.1
- hereditary D80.0
- nonfamilial D80.1
- transient, of infancy D80.7
Hypogenitalism (congenital) — *see* Hypogonadism
Hypoglossia Q38.3
Hypoglycemia (spontaneous) E16.2
- coma E15
  - diabetic — *see* Diabetes, coma
- diabetic — *see* Diabetes, hypoglycemia
- dietary counseling and surveillance Z71.3
- drug-induced E16.0
  - with coma (nondiabetic) E15
- due to insulin E16.0
  - with coma (nondiabetic) E15
  - therapeutic misadventure — *see* subcategory T38.3
- functional, nonhyperinsulinemic E16.1
- iatrogenic E16.0
  - with coma (nondiabetic) E15
- in infant of diabetic mother P70.1
  - gestational diabetes P70.0
- infantile E16.1
- leucine-induced E71.19
- neonatal (transitory) P70.4
  - iatrogenic P70.3
- reactive (not drug-induced) E16.1
- transitory neonatal P70.4
Hypogonadism
- female E28.39
- hypogonadotropic E23.0
- male E29.1
- ovarian (primary) E28.39
- pituitary E23.0
- testicular (primary) E29.1
Hypohidrosis, hypoidrosis L74.4
Hypoinsulinemia, postprocedural E89.1
Hypokalemia E87.6
Hypoleukocytosis — *see* Agranulocytosis
Hypolipoproteinemia (alpha) (beta) E78.6

Hypomagnesemia E83.42
neonatal P71.2
Hypomania, hypomanic reaction F30.8
Hypomenorrhea — see Oligomenorrhea
Hypometabolism R63.8
Hypomotility
gastrointestinal (tract) K31.89
psychogenic F45.8
intestine K59.8
psychogenic F45.8
stomach K31.89
psychogenic F45.8
Hyponasality R49.22
Hyponatremia E87.1
Hypoparathyroidism E20.9
familial E20.8
idiopathic E20.0
neonatal, transitory P71.4
postprocedural E89.2
specified NEC E20.8
Hypoperfusion (in)
newborn P96.89
Hypopharyngitis — see Laryngopharyngitis
Hypophoria H50.53
Hypophosphatemia, hypophosphatasia
(acquired) (congenital) (renal) E83.39
familial E83.31
Hypophyseal, hypophysis — see also
condition
dwarfism E23.0
gigantism E22.0
Hypopiesis — see Hypotension
Hypopinealism E34.8
Hypopituitarism (juvenile) E23.0
drug-induced E23.1
due to
hypophysectomy E89.3
radiotherapy E89.3
iatrogenic NEC E23.1
postirradiation E89.3
postpartum O99.285
postprocedural E89.3
Hypoplasia, hypoplastic
adrenal (gland), congenital Q89.1
alimentary tract, congenital Q45.8
upper Q40.8
anus, anal (canal) Q42.3
with fistula Q42.2
aorta, aortic Q25.42
ascending, in hypoplastic left heart
syndrome Q23.4
valve Q23.1
in hypoplastic left heart syndrome Q23.4
areola, congenital Q83.8
arm (congenital) — see Defect, reduction,
upper limb
artery (peripheral) Q27.8
brain (congenital) Q28.3
coronary Q24.5
digestive system Q27.8
lower limb Q27.8
pulmonary Q25.79
functional, unilateral J43.0
retinal (congenital) Q14.1
specified site NEC Q27.8
umbilical Q27.0
upper limb Q27.8
auditory canal Q17.8
causing impairment of hearing Q16.9
biliary duct or passage Q44.5
bone NOS Q79.9
face Q75.8
marrow D61.9
megakaryocytic D69.49
skull — see Hypoplasia, skull
brain Q02
gyri Q04.3
part of Q04.3
breast (areola) N64.82

Hypoplasia, hypoplastic — continued
bronchus Q32.4
cardiac Q24.8
carpus — see Defect, reduction, upper limb,
specified type NEC
cartilage hair Q78.8
cecum Q42.8
cementum K00.4
cephalic Q02
cerebellum Q04.3
cervix (uteri), congenital Q51.821
clavicle (congenital) Q74.0
coccyx Q76.49
colon Q42.9
specified NEC Q42.8
corpus callosum Q04.0
cricoid cartilage Q31.2
digestive organ(s) or tract NEC Q45.8
upper (congenital) Q40.8
ear (auricle) (lobe) Q17.2
middle Q16.4
enamel of teeth (neonatal) (postnatal)
(prenatal) K00.4
endocrine (gland) NEC Q89.2
endometrium N85.8
epididymis (congenital) Q55.4
epiglottis Q31.2
erythroid, congenital D61.01
esophagus (congenital) Q39.8
eustachian tube Q17.8
eye Q11.2
eyelid (congenital) Q10.3
face Q18.8
bone(s) Q75.8
femur (congenital) — see Defect, reduction,
lower limb, specified type NEC
fibula (congenital) — see Defect, reduction,
lower limb, specified type NEC
finger (congenital) — see Defect, reduction,
upper limb, specified type NEC
focal dermal Q82.8
foot — see Defect, reduction, lower limb,
specified type NEC
gallbladder Q44.0
genitalia, genital organ(s)
female, congenital Q52.8
external Q52.79
internal NEC Q52.8
in adiposogenital dystrophy E23.6
glottis Q31.2
hair Q84.2
hand (congenital) — see Defect, reduction,
upper limb, specified type NEC
heart Q24.8
humerus (congenital) — see Defect, reduction,
upper limb, specified type NEC
intestine (small) Q41.9
large Q42.9
specified NEC Q42.8
jaw M26.09
alveolar M26.79
lower M26.04
alveolar M26.74
upper M26.02
alveolar M26.73
kidney(s) Q60.5
bilateral Q60.4
unilateral Q60.3
labium (majus) (minus), congenital Q52.79
larynx Q31.2
left heart syndrome Q23.4
leg (congenital) — see Defect, reduction, lower
limb
limb Q73.8
lower (congenital) — see Defect, reduction,
lower limb
upper (congenital) — see Defect, reduction,
upper limb
liver Q44.7

Hypoplasia, hypoplastic — continued
lung (lobe) (not associated with short gestation)
Q33.6
associated with immaturity, low birth weight,
prematurity, or short gestation P28.0
mammary (areola), congenital Q83.8
mandible, mandibular M26.04
alveolar M26.74
unilateral condylar M27.8
maxillary M26.02
alveolar M26.73
medullary D61.9
megakaryocytic D69.49
metacarpus — see Defect, reduction, upper
limb, specified type NEC
metatarsus — see Defect, reduction, lower
limb, specified type NEC
muscle Q79.8
nail(s) Q84.6
nose, nasal Q30.1
optic nerve H47.03-
osseous meatus (ear) Q17.8
ovary, congenital Q50.39
pancreas Q45.0
parathyroid (gland) Q89.2
parotid gland Q38.4
patella Q74.1
pelvis, pelvic girdle Q74.2
penis (congenital) Q55.62
peripheral vascular system Q27.8
digestive system Q27.8
lower limb Q27.8
specified site NEC Q27.8
upper limb Q27.8
pituitary (gland) (congenital) Q89.2
pulmonary (not associated with short
gestation) Q33.6
artery, functional J43.0
associated with short gestation P28.0
radioulnar — see Defect, reduction, upper
limb, specified type NEC
radius — see Defect, reduction, upper limb
rectum Q42.1
with fistula Q42.0
respiratory system NEC Q34.8
rib Q76.6
right heart syndrome Q22.6
sacrum Q76.49
scapula Q74.0
scrotum Q55.1
shoulder girdle Q74.0
skin Q82.8
skull (bone) Q75.8
with
anencephaly Q00.0
encephalocele — see Encephalocele
hydrocephalus Q03.9
with spina bifida — see Spina bifida, by
site, with hydrocephalus
microcephaly Q02
spinal (cord) (ventral horn cell) Q06.1
spine Q76.49
sternum Q76.7
tarsus — see Defect, reduction, lower limb,
specified type NEC
testis Q55.1
thymic, with immunodeficiency D82.1
thymus (gland) Q89.2
with immunodeficiency D82.1
thyroid (gland) E03.1
cartilage Q31.2
tibiofibular (congenital) — see Defect,
reduction, lower limb, specified type NEC
toe — see Defect, reduction, lower limb,
specified type NEC
tongue Q38.3
Turner's K00.4
ulna (congenital) — see Defect, reduction,
upper limb

Hypoplasia, hypoplastic — *continued*
umbilical artery Q27.0
unilateral condylar M27.8
ureter Q62.8
uterus, congenital Q51.811
vagina Q52.4
vascular NEC peripheral Q27.8
brain Q28.3
digestive system Q27.8
lower limb Q27.8
specified site NEC Q27.8
upper limb Q27.8
vein(s) (peripheral) Q27.8
brain Q28.3
digestive system Q27.8
great Q26.8
lower limb Q27.8
specified site NEC Q27.8
upper limb Q27.8
vena cava (inferior) (superior) Q26.8
vertebra Q76.49
vulva, congenital Q52.79
zonule (ciliary) Q12.8
Hypopotassemia E87.6
Hypoproconvertinemia, congenital
(hereditary) D68.2
Hypoproteinemia E77.8
Hypoprothrombinemia (congenital)
(hereditary) (idiopathic) D68.2
acquired D68.4
newborn, transient P61.6
Hypoptyalism K11.7
Hypopyon (eye) (anterior chamber) — *see*
Iridocyclitis, acute, hypopyon
Hypopyrexia R68.0
Hyporeflexia R29.2
Hyposecretion
ACTH E23.0
antidiuretic hormone E23.2
ovary E28.39
salivary gland (any) K11.7
vasopressin E23.2
Hyposegmentation, leukocytic,
hereditary D72.0
Hyposiderinemia D50.9
Hypospadias Q54.9
balanic Q54.0
coronal Q54.0
glandular Q54.0
penile Q54.1
penoscrotal Q54.2
perineal Q54.3
specified NEC Q54.8
Hypospermatogenesis — *see* Oligospermia
Hyposplenism D73.0
Hypostasis pulmonary, passive — *see*
Edema, lung
Hypostatic — *see* condition
Hyposthenuria N28.89
Hypotension (arterial) (constitutional) I95.9
chronic I95.89
drug-induced I95.2
due to (of) hemodialysis I95.3
iatrogenic I95.89
idiopathic (permanent) I95.0
intra-dialytic I95.3
intracranial, following ventricular shunting
(ventriculostomy) G97.2
maternal, syndrome (following labor and
delivery) O26.5-
neurogenic, orthostatic G90.3
orthostatic (chronic) I95.1
due to drugs I95.2
neurogenic G90.3
postoperative I95.81
postural I95.1
specified NEC I95.89

Hypothermia (accidental) T68
due to anesthesia, anesthetic T88.51
low environmental temperature T68
neonatal P80.9
environmental (mild) NEC P80.8
mild P80.8
severe (chronic) (cold injury syndrome)
P80.0
specified NEC P80.8
not associated with low environmental
temperature R68.0
Hypothyroidism (acquired) E03.9
congenital (without goiter) E03.1
with goiter (diffuse) E03.0
due to
exogenous substance NEC E03.2
iodine-deficiency, acquired E01.8
subclinical E02
irradiation therapy E89.0
medicament NEC E03.2
P-aminosalicylic acid (PAS) E03.2
phenylbutazone E03.2
resorcinol E03.2
sulfonamide E03.2
surgery E89.0
thiourea group drugs E03.2
iatrogenic NEC E03.2
iodine-deficiency (acquired) E01.8
congenital — *see* Syndrome, iodine-
deficiency, congenital
subclinical E02
neonatal, transitory P72.2
postinfectious E03.3
postirradiation E89.0
postprocedural E89.0
postsurgical E89.0
specified NEC E03.8
subclinical, iodine-deficiency related E02
Hypotonia, hypotonicity, hypotony
bladder N31.2
congenital (benign) P94.2
eye — *see* Disorder, globe, hypotony
Hypotrichosis — *see* Alopecia
Hypotropia H50.2-
Hypoventilation R06.89
congenital central alveolar G47.35
sleep related
idiopathic nonobstructive alveolar G47.34
in conditions classified elsewhere G47.36
Hypovitaminosis — *see* Deficiency, vitamin
Hypovolemia E86.1
surgical shock T81.19
traumatic (shock) T79.4
Hypoxemia R09.02
newborn P84
sleep related, in conditions classified elsewhere
G47.36
Hypoxia (see also Anoxia) R09.02
cerebral, during a procedure NEC G97.81
postprocedural NEC G97.82
intrauterine P84
myocardial — *see* Insufficiency, coronary
newborn P84
sleep-related G47.34
Hypsarhythmia — *see* Epilepsy, generalized,
specified NEC
Hysteralgia, pregnant uterus O26.89-
Hysteria, hysterical (conversion) (dissociative
state) F44.9
anxiety F41.8
convulsions F44.5
psychosis, acute F44.9
Hysteroepilepsy F44.5

I

IBDU (colonic inflammatory bowel dissease
unclassified) K52.3
Ichthyoparasitism due to Vandellia
cirrhosa B88.8
Ichthyosis (congenital) Q80.9
acquired L85.0
fetalis Q80.4
hystrix Q80.8
lamellar Q80.2
lingual K13.29
palmaris and plantaris Q82.8
simplex Q80.0
vera Q80.8
vulgaris Q80.0
X-linked Q80.1
Ichthyotoxism — *see* Poisoning, fish
bacterial — *see* Intoxication, foodborne
Icteroanemia, hemolytic (acquired) D59.9
congenital — *see* Spherocytosis
Icterus — *see also* Jaundice
conjunctiva R17
gravis, newborn P55.0
hematogenous (acquired) D59.9
hemolytic (acquired) D59.9
congenital — *see* Spherocytosis
hemorrhagic (acute) (leptospiral) (spirochetal)
A27.0
newborn P53
infectious B15.9
with hepatic coma B15.0
leptospiral A27.0
spirochetal A27.0
neonatorum — *see* Jaundice, newborn
newborn P59.9
spirochetal A27.0
Ictus solaris, solis T67.0
Id reaction (due to bacteria) L30.2
Ideation
homicidal R45.850
suicidal R45.851
Identity disorder (child) F64.9
gender role F64.2
psychosexual F64.2
Idioglossia F80.0
Idiopathic — *see* condition
Idiot, idiocy (congenital) F73
amaurotic (Bielschowsky(-Jansky)) (family)
(infantile (late)) (juvenile (late)) (Vogt-
Spielmeyer) E75.4
microcephalic Q02
IgE asthma J45.909
IIAC (idiopathic infantile arterial calcification)
Q28.8
Ileitis (chronic) (noninfectious) (*see also* Enteritis)
K52.9
backwash — *see* Pancolitis, ulcerative (chronic)
infectious A09
regional (ulcerative) — *see* Enteritis, regional,
small intestine
segmental — *see* Enteritis, regional
terminal (ulcerative) — *see* Enteritis, regional,
small intestine
Ileocolitis (*see also* Enteritis) K52.9
infectious A09
regional — *see* Enteritis, regional
Ileostomy
attention to Z43.2
malfunctioning K94.13
status Z93.2
with complication — *see* Complications,
enterostomy
Ileotyphus — *see* Typhoid
Ileum — *see* condition

Ileus (bowel) (colon) (inhibitory) (intestine) K56.7
  adynamic K56.0
  due to gallstone (in intestine) K56.3
  duodenal (chronic) K31.5
  gallstone K56.3
  mechanical NEC K56.69
  meconium P76.0
    in cystic fibrosis E84.11
    meaning meconium plug (without cystic
      fibrosis) P76.0
  myxedema K59.8
  neurogenic K56.0
    Hirschsprung's disease or megacolon Q43.1
  newborn
    due to meconium P76.0
      in cystic fibrosis E84.11
      meaning meconium plug (without cystic
        fibrosis) P76.0
    transitory P76.1
  obstructive K56.69
  paralytic K56.0
Iliac — see condition
Iliotibial band syndrome M76.3-
Illiteracy Z55.0
Illness (see also Disease) R69
  manic-depressive — see Disorder, bipolar
Imbalance R26.89
  autonomic G90.8
  constituents of food intake E63.1
  electrolyte E87.8
    with
      abortion — see Abortion, by type,
        complicated by, electrolyte imbalance
      molar pregnancy O08.5
    due to hyperemesis gravidarum O21.1
    following ectopic or molar pregnancy O08.5
    neonatal, transitory NEC P74.4
      potassium P74.3
      sodium P74.2
  endocrine E34.9
  eye muscle NOS H50.9
  hormone E34.9
  hysterical F44.4
  labyrinth — see subcategory H83.2
  posture R29.3
  protein-energy — see Malnutrition
  sympathetic G90.8
Imbecile, imbecility (I.Q. 35-49) F71
Imbedding, intrauterine device T83.39
Imbibition, cholesterol (gallbladder) K82.4
Imbrication, teeth, fully erupted M26.30
Imerslund(-Gräsbeck) syndrome D51.1
Immature — see also Immaturity
  birth (less than 37 completed weeks) — see
    Preterm, newborn
    extremely (less than 28 completed weeks) —
      see Immaturity, extreme
  personality F60.89
Immaturity (less than 37 completed weeks) —
    see also Preterm, newborn
  extreme of newborn (less than 28 completed
    weeks of gestation) (less than 196
    completed days of gestation) (unspecified
    weeks of gestation) P07.20
    gestational age
      23 completed weeks (23 weeks, 0 days
        through 23 weeks, 6 days) P07.22
      24 completed weeks (24 weeks, 0 days
        through 24 weeks, 6 days) P07.23
      25 completed weeks (25 weeks, 0 days
        through 25 weeks, 6 days) P07.24
      26 completed weeks (26 weeks, 0 days
        through 26 weeks, 6 days) P07.25
      27 completed weeks (27 weeks, 0 days
        through 27 weeks, 6 days) P07.26
      less than 23 completed weeks P07.21
  fetus or infant light-for-dates — see Light-for-
    dates

Immaturity (less than 37 completed weeks) —
    see also Preterm, newborn — continued
  lung, newborn P28.0
  organ or site NEC — see Hypoplasia
  pulmonary, newborn P28.0
  reaction F60.89
  sexual (female) (male), after puberty E30.0
Immersion T75.1
  foot T69.02-
  hand T69.01-
Immobile, immobility
  complete, due to severe physical disability or
    frailty R53.2
  intestine K59.8
  syndrome (paraplegic) M62.3
Immune reconstitution (inflammatory)
  syndrome [IRIS] D89.3
Immunization — see also Vaccination
  ABO — see Incompatibility, ABO
    in newborn P55.1
  complication — see Complications, vaccination
  encounter for Z23
  not done (not carried out) Z28.9
    because (of)
      acute illness of patient Z28.01
      allergy to vaccine (or component) Z28.04
      caregiver refusal Z28.82
      chronic illness of patient Z28.02
      contraindication NEC Z28.09
      group pressure Z28.1
      guardian refusal Z28.82
      immune compromised state of patient
        Z28.03
      parent refusal Z28.82
      patient's belief Z28.1
      patient had disease being vaccinated
        against Z28.81
      patient refusal Z28.21
      religious beliefs of patient Z28.1
      specified reason NEC Z28.89
        of patient Z28.29
      unspecified patient reason Z28.20
    Rh factor
      affecting management of pregnancy NEC
        O36.09-
        anti-D antibody O36.01-
      from transfusion — see Complication(s),
        transfusion, incompatibility reaction, Rh
        (factor)
Immunocytoma C83.0-
Immunodeficiency D84.9
  with
    adenosine-deaminase deficiency D81.3
    antibody defects D80.9
      specified type NEC D80.8
    hyperimmunoglobulinemia D80.6
    increased immunoglobulin M (IgM) D80.5
    major defect D82.9
      specified type NEC D82.8
    partial albinism D82.8
    short-limbed stature D82.2
    thrombocytopenia and eczema D82.0
  antibody with
    hyperimmunoglobulinemia D80.6
    near-normal immunoglobulins D80.6
  autosomal recessive, Swiss type D80.0
  combined D81.9
    biotin-dependent carboxylase D81.819
      biotinidase D81.810
      holocarboxylase synthetase D81.818
      specified type NEC D81.818
    severe (SCID) D81.9
      with
        low or normal B-cell numbers D81.2
        low T-and B-cell numbers D81.1
        reticular dysgenesis D81.0
    specified type NEC D81.89

Immunodeficiency D84.9 — continued
  common variable D83.9
    with
      abnormalities of B-cell numbers and
        function D83.0
      autoantibodies to B-or T-cells D83.2
      immunoregulatory T-cell disorders D83.1
      specified type NEC D83.8
  following hereditary defective response to
    Epstein-Barr virus (EBV) D82.3
  selective, immunoglobulin
    A (IgA) D80.2
    G (IgG) (subclasses) D80.3
    M (IgM) D80.4
  severe combined (SCID) D81.9
  specified type NEC D84.8
  X-linked, with increased IgM D80.5
Immunotherapy (encounter for)
  antineoplastic Z51.12
Impaction, impacted
  bowel, colon, rectum (see also Impaction, fecal)
    K56.49
    by gallstone K56.3
  calculus — see Calculus
  cerumen (ear) (external) H61.2-
  cuspid — see Impaction, tooth
  dental (same or adjacent tooth) K01.1
  fecal, feces K56.41
  fracture — see Fracture, by site
  gallbladder — see Calculus, gallbladder
  gallstone(s) — see Calculus, gallbladder
    bile duct (common) (hepatic) — see Calculus,
      bile duct
    cystic duct — see Calculus, gallbladder
    in intestine, with obstruction (any part)
      K56.3
  intestine (calculous) NEC (see also Impaction,
    fecal) K56.49
    gallstone, with ileus K56.3
  intrauterine device (IUD) T83.39
  molar — see Impaction, tooth
  shoulder, causing obstructed labor O66.0
  tooth, teeth K01.1
  turbinate J34.89
Impaired, impairment (function)
  auditory discrimination — see Abnormal,
    auditory perception
  cognitive, mild, so stated G31.84
  dual sensory Z73.82
  fasting glucose R73.01
  glucose tolerance (oral) R73.02
  hearing — see Deafness
  heart — see Disease, heart
  kidney N28.9
    disorder resulting from N25.9
      specified NEC N25.89
  liver K72.90
    with coma K72.91
  mastication K08.89
  mild cognitive, so stated G31.84
  mobility
    ear ossicles — see Ankylosis, ear ossicles
    requiring care provider Z74.09
  myocardium, myocardial — see Insufficiency,
    myocardial
  rectal sphincter R19.8
  renal (acute) (chronic) N28.9
    disorder resulting from N25.9
      specified NEC N25.89
  vision NEC H54.7
    both eyes H54.3
Impediment, speech R47.9
  psychogenic (childhood) F98.8
  slurring R47.81
  specified NEC R47.89
Impending
  coronary syndrome I20.0
  delirium tremens F10.239
  myocardial infarction I20.0

Imperception auditory (acquired) — *see also*
Deafness
congenital H93.25
Imperfect
aeration, lung (newborn) NEC — *see*
Atelectasis
closure (congenital)
alimentary tract NEC Q45.8
lower Q43.8
upper Q40.8
atrioventricular ostium Q21.2
atrium (secundum) Q21.1
branchial cleft or sinus Q18.0
choroid Q14.3
cricoid cartilage Q31.8
cusps, heart valve NEC Q24.8
pulmonary Q22.3
ductus
arteriosus Q25.0
Botalli Q25.0
ear drum (causing impairment of hearing)
Q16.4
esophagus with communication to bronchus
or trachea Q39.1
eyelid Q10.3
foramen
botalli Q21.1
ovale Q21.1
genitalia, genital organ(s) or system
female Q52.8
external Q52.79
internal NEC Q52.8
male Q55.8
glottis Q31.8
interatrial ostium or septum Q21.1
interauricular ostium or septum Q21.1
interventricular ostium or septum Q21.0
larynx Q31.8
lip — *see* Cleft, lip
nasal septum Q30.3
nose Q30.2
omphalomesenteric duct Q43.0
optic nerve entry Q14.2
organ or site not listed — *see* Anomaly, by
site
ostium
interatrial Q21.1
interauricular Q21.1
interventricular Q21.0
palate — *see* Cleft, palate
preauricular sinus Q18.1
retina Q14.1
roof of orbit Q75.8
sclera Q13.5
septum
aorticopulmonary Q21.4
atrial (secundum) Q21.1
between aorta and pulmonary artery
Q21.4
heart Q21.9
interatrial (secundum) Q21.1
interauricular (secundum) Q21.1
interventricular Q21.0
in tetralogy of Fallot Q21.3
nasal Q30.3
ventricular Q21.0
with pulmonary stenosis or atresia,
dextraposition of aorta, and
hypertrophy of right ventricle Q21.3
in tetralogy of Fallot Q21.3
skull Q75.0
with
anencephaly Q00.0
encephalocele — *see* Encephalocele
hydrocephalus Q03.9
with spina bifida — *see* Spina bifida,
by site, with hydrocephalus
microcephaly Q02

Imperfect — *continued*
closure (congenital) — *continued*
spine (with meningocele) — *see* Spina bifida
trachea Q32.1
tympanic membrane (causing impairment of
hearing) Q16.4
uterus Q51.818
vitelline duct Q43.0
erection — *see* Dysfunction, sexual, male,
erectile
fusion — *see* Imperfect, closure
inflation, lung (newborn) — *see* Atelectasis
posture R29.3
rotation, intestine Q43.3
septum, ventricular Q21.0
Imperfectly descended testis — *see*
Cryptorchid
Imperforate (congenital) — *see also* Atresia
anus Q42.3
with fistula Q42.2
cervix (uteri) Q51.828
esophagus Q39.0
with tracheoesophageal fistula Q39.1
hymen Q52.3
jejunum Q41.1
pharynx Q38.8
rectum Q42.1
with fistula Q42.0
urethra Q64.39
vagina Q52.4
Impervious (congenital) — *see also* Atresia
anus Q42.3
with fistula Q42.2
bile duct Q44.2
esophagus Q39.0
with tracheoesophageal fistula Q39.1
intestine (small) Q41.9
large Q42.9
rectum Q42.1
with fistula Q42.0
ureter — *see* Atresia, ureter
urethra Q64.39
Impetiginization of dermatoses L01.1
Impetigo (any organism) (any site) (circinate)
(contagiosa) (simplex) (vulgaris) L01.00
Bockhart's L01.02
bullous, bullosa L01.03
external ear L01.00 [H62.40]
follicularis L01.02
furfuracea L30.5
herpetiformis L40.1
nonobstetrical L40.1
neonatorum L01.03
nonbullous L01.01
specified type NEC L01.09
ulcerative L01.09
Impingement (on teeth)
soft tissue
anterior M26.81
posterior M26.82
Implant, endometrial N80.9
Implantation
anomalous — *see* Anomaly, by site
ureter Q62.63
cyst
external area or site (skin) NEC L72.0
iris — *see* Cyst, iris, implantation
vagina N89.8
vulva N90.7
dermoid (cyst) — *see* Implantation, cyst
Impotence (sexual) N52.9
counseling Z70.1
organic origin (*see also* Dysfunction, sexual,
male, erectile) N52.9
psychogenic F52.21
Impression, basilar Q75.8
Imprisonment, anxiety concerning Z65.1

Improper care (child) (newborn) — *see*
Maltreatment
Improperly tied umbilical cord (causing
hemorrhage) P51.8
Impulsiveness (impulsive) R45.87
Inability to swallow — *see* Aphagia
Inaccessible, inaccessibility
health care NEC Z75.3
due to
waiting period Z75.2
for admission to facility elsewhere Z75.1
other helping agencies Z75.4
Inactive — *see* condition
Inadequate, inadequacy
aesthetics of dental restoration K08.56
biologic, constitutional, functional, or social
F60.7
development
child R62.50
genitalia
after puberty NEC E30.0
congenital
female Q52.8
external Q52.79
internal Q52.8
male Q55.8
lungs Q33.6
associated with short gestation P28.0
organ or site not listed — *see* Anomaly, by
site
diet (causing nutritional deficiency) E63.9
eating habits Z72.4
environment, household Z59.1
family support Z63.8
food (supply) NEC Z59.4
hunger effects T73.0
functional F60.7
household care, due to
family member
handicapped or ill Z74.2
on vacation Z75.5
temporarily away from home Z74.2
technical defects in home Z59.1
temporary absence from home of person
rendering care Z74.2
housing (heating) (space) Z59.1
income (financial) Z59.6
intrafamilial communication Z63.8
material resources Z59.9
mental — *see* Disability, intellectual
parental supervision or control of child Z62.0
personality F60.7
pulmonary
function R06.89
newborn P28.5
ventilation, newborn P28.5
sample of cytologic smear
anus R85.615
cervix R87.615
vagina R87.625
social F60.7
insurance Z59.7
skills NEC Z73.4
supervision of child by parent Z62.0
teaching affecting education Z55.8
welfare support Z59.7
Inanition R64
with edema — *see* Malnutrition, severe
due to
deprivation of food T73.0
malnutrition — *see* Malnutrition
fever R50.9
Inappropriate
change in quantitative human chorionic
gonadotropin (hCG) in early pregnancy
O02.81
diet or eating habits Z72.4

Inappropriate — *continued*
  level of quantitative human chorionic
      gonadotropin (hCG) for gestational age in
      early pregnancy O02.81
  secretion
      antidiuretic hormone (ADH) (excessive) E22.2
      deficiency E23.2
      pituitary (posterior) E22.2
Inattention at or after birth — *see* Neglect
Incarceration, incarcerated
  enterocele K46.0
      gangrenous K46.1
  epiplocele K46.0
      gangrenous K46.1
  exomphalos K42.0
      gangrenous K42.1
  hernia — *see also* Hernia, by site, with
      obstruction
      with gangrene — *see* Hernia, by site, with
          gangrene
  iris, in wound — *see* Injury, eye, laceration,
      with prolapse
  lens, in wound — *see* Injury, eye, laceration,
      with prolapse
  omphalocele K42.0
  prison, anxiety concerning Z65.1
  rupture — *see* Hernia, by site
  sarcoepiplocele K46.0
      gangrenous K46.1
  sarcoepiplomphalocele K42.0
      with gangrene K42.1
  uterus N85.8
      gravid O34.51-
          causing obstructed labor O65.5
Incised wound
  external — *see* Laceration
  internal organs — *see* Injury, by site
Incision, incisional
  hernia K43.2
      with
          gangrene (and obstruction) K43.1
          obstruction K43.0
      surgical, complication — *see* Complications,
          surgical procedure
      traumatic
          external — *see* Laceration
          internal organs — *see* Injury, by site
Inclusion
  azurophilic leukocytic D72.0
  blennorrhea (neonatal) (newborn) P39.1
  gallbladder in liver (congenital) Q44.1
Incompatibility
  ABO
      affecting management of pregnancy O36.11-
          anti-A sensitization O36.11-
          anti-B sensitization O36.19-
          specified NEC O36.19-
      infusion or transfusion reaction — *see*
          Complication(s), transfusion,
          incompatibility reaction, ABO
      newborn P55.1
  blood (group) (Duffy) (K(ell)) (Kidd) (Lewis) (M)
      (S) NEC
      affecting management of pregnancy
          O36.11-
          anti-A sensitization O36.11-
          anti-B sensitization O36.19-
      infusion or transfusion reaction T80.89
      newborn P55.8
  divorce or estrangement Z63.5
  Rh (blood group) (factor) Z31.82
      affecting management of pregnancy NEC
          O36.09-
          anti-D antibody O36.01-
      infusion or transfusion reaction — *see*
          Complication(s), transfusion,
          incompatibility reaction, Rh (factor)
      newborn P55.0
  rhesus — *see* Incompatibility, Rh

Incompetency, incompetent,
  incompetence
  annular
      aortic (valve) — *see* Insufficiency, aortic
      mitral (valve) I34.0
      pulmonary valve (heart) I37.1
  aortic (valve) — *see* Insufficiency, aortic
  cardiac valve — *see* Endocarditis
  cervix, cervical (os) N88.3
      in pregnancy O34.3-
  chronotropic I45.89
      with
          autonomic dysfunction G90.8
          ischemic heart disease I25.89
          left ventricular dysfunction I51.89
          sinus node dysfunction I49.8
  esophagogastric (junction) (sphincter) K22.0
  mitral (valve) — *see* Insufficiency, mitral
  pelvic fundus N81.89
  pubocervical tissue N81.82
  pulmonary valve (heart) I37.1
      congenital Q22.3
  rectovaginal tissue N81.83
  tricuspid (annular) (valve) — *see* Insufficiency,
      tricuspid
  valvular — *see* Endocarditis
      congenital Q24.8
  vein, venous (saphenous) (varicose) — *see*
      Varix, leg
Incomplete — *see also* condition
  bladder, emptying R33.9
  defecation R15.0
  expansion lungs (newborn) NEC — *see*
      Atelectasis
  rotation, intestine Q43.3
Inconclusive
  diagnostic imaging due to excess body fat of
      patient R93.9
  findings on diagnostic imaging of breast NEC
      R92.8
  mammogram (due to dense breasts) R92.2
Incontinence R32
  anal sphincter R15.9
  coital N39.491
  feces R15.9
      nonorganic origin F98.1
  insensible (urinary) N39.42
  overflow N39.490
  postural (urinary) N39.492
  psychogenic F45.8
  rectal R15.9
  reflex N39.498
  stress (female) (male) N39.3
      and urge N39.46
  urethral sphincter R32
  urge N39.41
      and stress (female) (male) N39.46
  urine (urinary) R32
      continuous N39.45
      due to cognitive impairment, or severe
          physical disability or immobility R39.81
      functional R39.81
      insensible N39.42
      mixed (stress and urge) N39.46
      nocturnal N39.44
      nonorganic origin F98.0
      overflow N39.490
      post dribbling N39.43
      postural N39.492
      reflex N39.498
      specified NEC N39.498
      stress (female) (male) N39.3
          and urge N39.46
      total N39.498
      unaware N39.42
      urge N39.41
          and stress (female) (male) N39.46
Incontinentia pigmenti Q82.3

Incoordinate, incoordination
  esophageal-pharyngeal (newborn) — *see*
      Dysphagia
  muscular R27.8
  uterus (action) (contractions) (complicating
      delivery) O62.4
Increase, increased
  abnormal, in development R63.8
  androgens (ovarian) E28.1
  anticoagulants (antithrombin) (anti-VIIIa) (anti-
      IXa) (anti-Xa) (anti-XIa) — *see* Circulating
      anticoagulants
  cold sense R20.8
  estrogen E28.0
  function
      adrenal
          cortex — *see* Cushing's, syndrome
          medulla E27.5
      pituitary (gland) (anterior) (lobe) E22.9
          posterior E22.2
  heat sense R20.8
  intracranial pressure (benign) G93.2
  permeability, capillaries I78.8
  pressure, intracranial G93.2
  secretion
      gastrin E16.4
      glucagon E16.3
      pancreas, endocrine E16.9
          growth hormone-releasing hormone E16.8
          pancreatic polypeptide E16.8
          somatostatin E16.8
          vasoactive-intestinal polypeptide E16.8
  sphericity, lens Q12.4
  splenic activity D73.1
  venous pressure I87.8
      portal K76.6
Increta placenta O43.22-
Incrustation, cornea, foreign body (lead)
  (zinc) — *see* Foreign body, cornea
Incyclophoria H50.54
Incyclotropia — *see* Cyclotropia
Indeterminate sex Q56.4
India rubber skin Q82.8
Indigestion (acid) (bilious) (functional) K30
  catarrhal K31.89
  due to decomposed food NOS A05.9
  nervous F45.8
  psychogenic F45.8
Indirect — *see* condition
Induratio penis plastica N48.6
Induration, indurated
  brain G93.89
  breast (fibrous) N64.51
      puerperal, postpartum O92.29
  broad ligament N83.8
  chancre
      anus A51.1
      congenital A50.07
      extragenital NEC A51.2
  corpora cavernosa (penis) (plastic) N48.6
  liver (chronic) K76.89
  lung (black) (chronic) (fibroid) (*see also* Fibrosis,
      lung) J84.10
      essential brown J84.03
  penile (plastic) N48.6
  phlebitic — *see* Phlebitis
  skin R23.4
Inebriety (without dependence) — *see* Alcohol,
  intoxication
Inefficiency, kidney N28.9
Inelasticity, skin R23.4
Inequality, leg (length) (acquired) — *see also*
  Deformity, limb, unequal length
  congenital — *see* Defect, reduction, lower limb
  lower leg — *see* Deformity, limb, unequal
      length

Inertia
  bladder (neurogenic) N31.2
  stomach K31.89
    psychogenic F45.8
  uterus, uterine during labor O62.2
    during latent phase of labor O62.0
    primary O62.0
    secondary O62.1
  vesical (neurogenic) N31.2
Infancy, infantile, infantilism — *see also* condition
  celiac K90.0
  genitalia, genitals (after puberty) E30.0
  Herter's (nontropical sprue) K90.0
  intestinal K90.0
  Lorain E23.0
  pancreatic K86.89
  pelvis M95.5
    with disproportion (fetopelvic) O33.1
      causing obstructed labor O65.1
  pituitary E23.0
  renal N25.0
  uterus — *see* Infantile, genitalia
Infant(s) — *see also* Infancy
  excessive crying R68.11
  irritable child R68.12
  lack of care — *see* Neglect
  liveborn (singleton) Z38.2
    born in hospital Z38.00
      by cesarean Z38.01
    born outside hospital Z38.1
    multiple NEC Z38.8
      born in hospital Z38.68
        by cesarean Z38.69
      born outside hospital Z38.7
    quadruplet Z38.8
      born in hospital Z38.63
        by cesarean Z38.64
      born outside hospital Z38.7
    quintuplet Z38.8
      born in hospital Z38.65
        by cesarean Z38.66
      born outside hospital Z38.7
    triplet Z38.8
      born in hospital Z38.61
        by cesarean Z38.62
      born outside hospital Z38.7
    twin Z38.5
      born in hospital Z38.30
        by cesarean Z38.31
      born outside hospital Z38.4
  of diabetic mother (syndrome of) P70.1
    gestational diabetes P70.0
Infantile — *see also* condition
  genitalia, genitals E30.0
  os, uterine E30.0
  penis E30.0
  testis E29.1
  uterus E30.0
Infantilism — *see* Infancy
Infarct, infarction
  adrenal (capsule) (gland) E27.49
  appendices epiploicae (*see also* Infarct, intestine) K55.069
  bowel (*see also* Infarct, intestine) K55.069
  brain (stem) — *see* Infarct, cerebral
  breast N64.89
  brewer's (kidney) N28.0
  cardiac — *see* Infarct, myocardium
  cerebellar — *see* Infarct, cerebral
  cerebral (*see also* Occlusion, artery cerebral or precerebral, with infarction) I63.9
    aborted I63.9
    cortical I63.9

Infarct, infarction — *continued*
  cerebral (*see also* Occlusion, artery cerebral or precerebral, with infarction) I63.9 — *continued*
    due to
      cerebral venous thrombosis, nonpyogenic I63.6
      embolism
        cerebral arteries I63.4-
        precerebral arteries I63.1-
      occlusion NEC
        cerebral arteries I63.5-
        precerebral arteries I63.2-
      stenosis NEC
        cerebral arteries I63.5-
        precerebral arteries I63.2-
      thrombosis
        cerebral artery I63.3-
        precerebral artery I63.0-
    intraoperative
      during cardiac surgery I97.810
      during other surgery I97.811
    postprocedural
      following cardiac surgery I97.820
      following other surgery I97.821
    specified NEC I63.8
  colon (acute) (agnogenic) (embolic) (hemorrhagic) (nonocclusive) (nonthrombotic) (occlusive) (segmental) (thrombotic) (with gangrene) (*see also* Infarct, intestine) K55.049
  coronary artery — *see* Infarct, myocardium
  embolic — *see* Embolism
  fallopian tube N83.8
  gallbladder K82.8
  heart — *see* Infarct, myocardium
  hepatic K76.3
  hypophysis (anterior lobe) E23.6
  impending (myocardium) I20.0
  intestine (acute) (agnogenic) (embolic) (hemorrhagic) (nonocclusive) (nonthrombotic) (occlusive) (thrombotic) (with gangrene) K55.069
    diffuse K55.062
    focal K55.061
    large K55.049
      diffuse K55.042
      focal K55.041
    small K55.029
      diffuse K55.022
      focal K55.021
  kidney N28.0
  liver K76.3
  lung (embolic) (thrombotic) — *see* Embolism, pulmonary
  lymph node I89.8
  mesentery, mesenteric (embolic) (thrombotic) (with gangrene) (*see also* Infarct, intestine) K55.069
  muscle (ischemic) M62.20
    ankle M62.27-
    foot M62.27-
    forearm M62.23-
    hand M62.24-
    lower leg M62.26-
    pelvic region M62.25-
    shoulder region M62.21-
    specified site NEC M62.28
    thigh M62.25-
    upper arm M62.22-
  myocardium, myocardial (acute) (with stated duration of 4 weeks or less) I21.3
    diagnosed on ECG, but presenting no symptoms I25.2
    healed or old I25.2
    intraoperative
      during cardiac surgery I97.790
      during other surgery I97.791
    non-Q wave I21.4

Infarct, infarction — *continued*
  myocardium, myocardial (acute) (with stated duration of 4 weeks or less) I21.3 — *continued*
    non-ST elevation (NSTEMI) I21.4
      subsequent I22.2
    nontransmural I21.4
    past (diagnosed on ECG or other investigation, but currently presenting no symptoms) I25.2
    postprocedural
      following cardiac surgery I97.190
      following other surgery I97.191
    Q wave (*see also* Infarct, myocardium, by site) I21.3
    ST elevation (STEMI) I21.3
      anterior (anteroapical) (anterolateral) (anteroseptal) (Q wave) (wall) I21.09
        subsequent I22.0
      inferior (diaphragmatic) (inferolateral) (inferoposterior) (wall) NEC I21.19
        subsequent I22.1
      inferoposterior transmural (Q wave) I21.11
      involving
        coronary artery of anterior wall NEC I21.09
        coronary artery of inferior wall NEC I21.19
        diagonal coronary artery I21.02
        left anterior descending coronary artery I21.02
        left circumflex coronary artery I21.21
        left main coronary artery I21.01
        oblique marginal coronary artery I21.21
        right coronary artery I21.11
      lateral (apical-lateral) (basal-lateral) (high) I21.29
        subsequent I22.8
      posterior (posterobasal) (posterolateral) (posteroseptal) (true) I21.29
        subsequent I22.8
      septal I21.29
        subsequent I22.8
      specified NEC I21.29
        subsequent I22.8
      subsequent I22.9
    subsequent (recurrent) (reinfarction) I22.9
      anterior (anteroapical) (anterolateral) (anteroseptal) (wall) I22.0
      diaphragmatic (wall) I22.1
      inferior (diaphragmatic) (inferolateral) (inferoposterior) (wall) I22.1
      lateral (apical-lateral) (basal-lateral) (high) I22.8
      non-ST elevation (NSTEMI) I22.2
      posterior (posterobasal) (posterolateral) (posteroseptal) (true) I22.8
      septal I22.8
      specified NEC I22.8
      ST elevation I22.9
        anterior (anteroapical) (anterolateral) (anteroseptal) (wall) I22.0
        inferior (diaphragmatic) (inferolateral) (inferoposterior) (wall) I22.1
        specified NEC I22.8
    subendocardial I22.2
    transmural I22.9
      anterior (anteroapical) (anterolateral) (anteroseptal) (wall) I22.0
      diaphragmatic (wall) I22.1
      inferior (diaphragmatic) (inferolateral) (inferoposterior) (wall) I22.1
      lateral (apical-lateral) (basal-lateral) (high) I22.8
      posterior (posterobasal) (posterolateral) (posteroseptal) (true) I22.8
      specified NEC I22.8

DISEASE INDEX

Infarct, infarction — *continued*
  myocardium, myocardial (acute) (with stated duration of 4 weeks or less) I21.3 — *continued*
    syphilitic A52.06
    transmural I21.3
      anterior (anteroapical) (anterolateral) (anteroseptal) (Q wave) (wall) NEC I21.09
      inferior (diaphragmatic) (inferolateral) (inferoposterior) (Q wave) (wall) NEC I21.19
      inferoposterior (Q wave) I21.11
      lateral (apical-lateral) (basal-lateral) (high) NEC I21.29
      posterior (posterobasal) (posterolateral) (posteroseptal) (true) NEC I21.29
      septal NEC I21.29
      specified NEC I21.29
  nontransmural I21.4
  omentum (*see also* Infarct, intestine) K55.069
  ovary N83.8
  pancreas K86.89
  papillary muscle — *see* Infarct, myocardium
  parathyroid gland E21.4
  pituitary (gland) E23.6
  placenta O43.81-
  prostate N42.89
  pulmonary (artery) (vein) (hemorrhagic) — *see* Embolism, pulmonary
  renal (embolic) (thrombotic) N28.0
  retina, retinal (artery) — *see* Occlusion, artery, retina
  spinal (cord) (acute) (embolic) (nonembolic) G95.11
  spleen D73.5
    embolic or thrombotic I74.8
  subendocardial (acute) (nontransmural) I21.4
  suprarenal (capsule) (gland) E27.49
  testis N50.1
  thrombotic — *see also* Thrombosis
    artery, arterial — *see* Embolism
  thyroid (gland) E07.89
  ventricle (heart) — *see* Infarct, myocardium
Infecting — *see* condition
Infection, infected, infective (opportunistic) B99.9
  with
    drug resistant organism — *see* Resistance (to), drug — *see also* specific organism
    lymphangitis — *see* Lymphangitis
    organ dysfunction (acute) R65.20
      with septic shock R65.21
  abscess (skin) — *code by* site under Abscess
  Absidia — *see* Mucormycosis
  Acanthamoeba — *see* Acanthamebiasis
  Acanthocheilonema (perstans) (streptocerca) B74.4
  accessory sinus (chronic) — *see* Sinusitis
  achorion — *see* Dermatophytosis
  Acremonium falciforme B47.0
  acromioclavicular M00.9
  Actinobacillus (actinomycetem-comitans) A28.8
    mallei A24.0
    muris A25.1
  Actinomadura B47.1
  Actinomyces (israelii) (*see also* Actinomycosis) A42.9
  Actinomycetales — *see* Actinomycosis
  actinomycotic NOS — *see* Actinomycosis
  adenoid (and tonsil) J03.90
    chronic J35.02
  adenovirus NEC
    as cause of disease classified elsewhere B97.0
    unspecified nature or site B34.0
  aerogenes capsulatus A48.0
  aertrycke — *see* Infection, salmonella

Infection, infected, infective (opportunistic) B99.9 — *continued*
  alimentary canal NOS — *see* Enteritis, infectious
  Allescheria boydii B48.2
  Alternaria B48.8
  alveolus, alveolar (process) K04.7
  Ameba, amebic (histolytica) — *see* Amebiasis
  amniotic fluid, sac or cavity O41.10-
    chorioamnionitis O41.12-
    placentitis O41.14-
  amputation stump (surgical) — *see* Complication, amputation stump, infection
  Ancylostoma (duodenalis) B76.0
  Anisakiasis, Anisakis larvae B81.0
  anthrax — *see* Anthrax
  antrum (chronic) — *see* Sinusitis, maxillary
  anus, anal (papillae) (sphincter) K62.89
  arbovirus (arbor virus) A94
    specified type NEC A93.8
  artificial insemination N98.0
  Ascaris lumbricoides — *see* Ascariasis
  Ascomycetes B47.0
  Aspergillus (flavus) (fumigatus) (terreus) — *see* Aspergillosis
  atypical
    acid-fast (bacilli) — *see* Mycobacterium, atypical
    mycobacteria — *see* Mycobacterium, atypical
    virus A81.9
      specified type NEC A81.89
  auditory meatus (external) — *see* Otitis, externa, infective
  auricle (ear) — *see* Otitis, externa, infective
  axillary gland (lymph) L04.2
  Bacillus A49.9
    abortus A23.1
    anthracis — *see* Anthrax
    Ducrey's (any location) A57
    Flexner's A03.1
    Friedländer's NEC A49.8
    gas (gangrene) A48.0
    mallei A24.0
    melitensis A23.0
    paratyphoid, paratyphosus A01.4
      A A01.1
      B A01.2
      C A01.3
    Shiga(-Kruse) A03.0
    suipestifer — *see* Infection, salmonella
    swimming pool A31.1
    typhosa A01.00
    welchii — *see* Gangrene, gas
  bacterial NOS A49.9
    as cause of disease classified elsewhere B96.89
      Bacteroides fragilis [B. fragilis] B96.6
      Clostridium perfringens [C. perfringens] B96.7
      Enterobacter sakazakii B96.89
      Enterococcus B95.2
      Escherichia coli [E. coli] (*see also* Escherichia coli) B96.20
      Helicobacter pylori [H.pylori] B96.81
      Hemophilus influenzae [H. influenzae] B96.3
      Klebsiella pneumoniae [K. pneumoniae] B96.1
      Mycoplasma pneumoniae [M. pneumoniae] B96.0
      Proteus (mirabilis) (morganii) B96.4
      Pseudomonas (aeruginosa) (mallei) (pseudomallei) B96.5
      Staphylococcus B95.8
        aureus (methicillin susceptible) (MSSA) B95.61
        methicillin resistant (MRSA) B95.62
        specified NEC B95.7

Infection, infected, infective (opportunistic) B99.9 — *continued*
  bacterial NOS A49.9 — *continued*
    as cause of disease classified elsewhere B96.89 — *continued*
      Streptococcus B95.5
      group A B95.0
      group B B95.1
      pneumoniae B95.3
      specified NEC B95.4
      Vibrio vulnificus B96.82
    specified NEC A48.8
  Bacterium
    paratyphosum A01.4
      A A01.1
      B A01.2
      C A01.3
    typhosum A01.00
  Bacteroides NEC A49.8
    fragilis, as cause of disease classified elsewhere B96.6
  Balantidium coli A07.0
  Bartholin's gland N75.8
  Basidiobolus B46.8
  bile duct (common) (hepatic) — *see* Cholangitis
  bladder — *see* Cystitis
  Blastomyces, blastomycotic — *see also* Blastomycosis
    brasiliensis — *see* Paracoccidioidomycosis
    dermatitidis — *see* Blastomycosis
    European — *see* Cryptococcosis
    Loboi B48.0
    North American B40.9
    South American — *see* Paracoccidioidomycosis
  bleb, postprocedure — *see* Blebitis
  bone — *see* Osteomyelitis
  Bordetella — *see* Whooping cough
  Borrelia bergdorfi A69.20
  brain (*see also* Encephalitis) G04.90
    membranes — *see* Meningitis
    septic G06.0
    meninges — *see* Meningitis, bacterial
  branchial cyst Q18.0
  breast — *see* Mastitis
  bronchus — *see* Bronchitis
  Brucella A23.9
    abortus A23.1
    canis A23.3
    melitensis A23.0
    mixed A23.8
    specified NEC A23.8
    suis A23.2
  Brugia (malayi) B74.1
    timori B74.2
  bursa — *see* Bursitis, infective
  buttocks (skin) L08.9
  Campylobacter, intestinal A04.5
    as cause of disease classified elsewhere B96.81
  Candida (albicans) (tropicalis) — *see* Candidiasis
  candiru B88.8
  Capillaria (intestinal) B81.1
    hepatica B83.8
    philippinensis B81.1
  cartilage — *see* Disorder, cartilage, specified type NEC
  cat liver fluke B66.0
  catheter-related bloodstream (CRBSI) T80.211
  cellulitis — *code by* site under Cellulitis
  central line-associated T80.219
    bloodstream (CLABSI) T80.211
    specified NEC T80.218
  Cephalosporium falciforme B47.0
  cerebrospinal — *see* Meningitis
  cervical gland (lymph) L04.0
  cervix — *see* Cervicitis
  cesarean delivery wound (puerperal) O86.0

Infection, infected, infective (opportunistic)
B99.9 — *continued*
cestodes — *see* Infestation, cestodes
chest J22
Chilomastix (intestinal) A07.8
Chlamydia, chlamydial A74.9
  anus A56.3
  genitourinary tract A56.2
    lower A56.00
    specified NEC A56.19
  lymphogranuloma A55
  pharynx A56.4
  psittaci A70
  rectum A56.3
  sexually transmitted NEC A56.8
cholera — *see* Cholera
Cladosporium
  bantianum (brain abscess) B43.1
  carrionii B43.0
  castellanii B36.1
  trichoides (brain abscess) B43.1
  werneckii B36.1
Clonorchis (sinensis) (liver) B66.1
Clostridium NEC
  bifermentans A48.0
  botulinum (food poisoning) A05.1
    infant A48.51
    wound A48.52
  difficile
    as cause of disease classified elsewhere B96.89
    foodborne (disease) A04.7
    gas gangrene A48.0
    necrotizing enterocolitis A04.7
    sepsis A41.4
  gas-forming NEC A48.0
  histolyticum A48.0
  novyi, causing gas gangrene A48.0
  oedematiens A48.0
  perfringens
    as cause of disease classified elsewhere B96.7
    due to food A05.2
    foodborne (disease) A05.2
    gas gangrene A48.0
    sepsis A41.4
  septicum, causing gas gangrene A48.0
  sordellii, causing gas gangrene A48.0
  welchii
    as cause of disease classified elsewhere B96.7
    foodborne (disease) A05.2
    gas gangrene A48.0
    necrotizing enteritis A05.2
    sepsis A41.4
Coccidioides (immitis) — *see* Coccidioidomycosis
colon — *see* Enteritis, infectious
colostomy K94.02
common duct — *see* Cholangitis
congenital P39.9
  Candida (albicans) P37.5
  cytomegalovirus P35.1
  hepatitis, viral P35.3
  herpes simplex P35.2
  infectious or parasitic disease P37.9
    specified NEC P37.8
  listeriosis (disseminated) P37.2
  malaria NEC P37.4
    falciparum P37.3
  Plasmodium falciparum P37.3
  poliomyelitis P35.8
  rubella P35.0
  skin P39.4
  toxoplasmosis (acute) (subacute) (chronic) P37.1
  tuberculosis P37.0
  urinary (tract) P39.3
  vaccinia P35.8

Infection, infected, infective (opportunistic)
B99.9 — *continued*
congenital P39.9 — *continued*
  virus P35.9
    specified type NEC P35.8
Conidiobolus B46.8
coronavirus NEC B34.2
  as cause of disease classified elsewhere B97.29
  severe acute respiratory syndrome (SARS associated) B97.21
corpus luteum — *see* Salpingo-oophoritis
Corynebacterium diphtheriae — *see* Diphtheria
cotia virus B08.8
Coxiella burnetii A78
coxsackie — *see* Coxsackie
Cryptococcus neoformans — *see* Cryptococcosis
Cryptosporidium A07.2
Cunninghamella — *see* Mucormycosis
cyst — *see* Cyst
cystic duct (*see also* Cholecystitis) K81.9
Cysticercus cellulosae — *see* Cysticercosis
cytomegalovirus, cytomegaloviral B25.9
  congenital P35.1
  maternal, maternal care for (suspected) damage to fetus O35.3
  mononucleosis B27.10
    with
      complication NEC B27.19
      meningitis B27.12
      polyneuropathy B27.11
delta-agent (acute), in hepatitis B carrier B17.0
dental (pulpal origin) K04.7
Deuteromycetes B47.0
Dicrocoelium dendriticum B66.2
Dipetalonema (perstans) (streptocerca) B74.4
diphtherial — *see* Diphtheria
Diphyllobothrium (adult) (latum) (pacificum) B70.0
  larval B70.1
Diplogonoporus (grandis) B71.8
Dipylidium caninum B67.4
Dirofilaria B74.8
Dracunculus medinensis B72
Drechslera (hawaiiensis) B43.8
Ducrey Haemophilus (any location) A57
due to or resulting from
  artificial insemination N98.0
  central venous catheter T80.219
    bloodstream T80.211
    exit or insertion site T80.212
    localized T80.212
    port or reservoir T80.212
    specified NEC T80.218
    tunnel T80.212
  device, implant or graft (*see also* Complications, by site and type, infection or inflammation) T85.79
    arterial graft NEC T82.7
    breast (implant) T85.79
    catheter NEC T85.79
      dialysis (renal) T82.7
        intraperitoneal T85.71
      infusion NEC T82.7
        cranial T85.735
        intrathecal T85.735
        spinal (epidural) (subdural) T85.735
        subarachnoid T85.735
      urinary T83.518
        cystostomy T83.510
        Hopkins T83.518
        ileostomy T83.518
        nephrostomy T83.512
        specified NEC T83.518
        urethral indwelling T83.511
        urostomy T83.518

Infection, infected, infective (opportunistic)
B99.9 — *continued*
due to or resulting from — *continued*
  device, implant or graft (*see also* Complications, by site and type, infection or inflammation) T85.79 — *continued*
    electronic (electrode) (pulse generator) (stimulator)
      bone T84.7
      cardiac T82.7
      nervous system T85.738
        brain T85.731
        cranial nerve T85.732
        gastric nerve T85.732
        generator pocket T85.734
        neurostimulator generator T85.734
        peripheral nerve T85.732
        sacral nerve T85.732
        spinal cord T85.733
        vagal nerve T85.732
      urinary T83.590
    fixation, internal (orthopedic) NEC — *see* Complication, fixation device, infection
    gastrointestinal (bile duct) (esophagus) T85.79
      neurostimulator electrode (lead) T85.732
    genital NEC T83.69
    heart NEC T82.7
      valve (prosthesis) T82.6
      graft T82.7
    joint prosthesis — *see* Complication, joint prosthesis, infection
    ocular (corneal graft) (orbital implant) NEC T85.79
    orthopedic NEC T84.7
    penile (cylinder) (pump) (resevoir) T83.61
    specified NEC T85.79
    testicular T83.62
    urinary NEC T83.598
      ileal conduit stent T83.593
      implanted neurostimulation T83.590
      implanted sphincter T83.591
      indwelling ureteral stent T83.592
      nephroureteral stent T83.593
      specified stent NEC T83.593
    vascular NEC T82.7
    ventricular intracranial (communicating) shunt T85.730
  Hickman catheter T80.219
    bloodstream T80.211
    localized T80.212
    specified NEC T80.218
  immunization or vaccination T88.0
  infusion, injection or transfusion NEC T80.29
    acute T80.22
  injury NEC — *code by* site under Wound, open
  peripherally inserted central catheter (PICC) T80.219
    bloodstream T80.211
    localized T80.212
    specified NEC T80.218
  portacath (port-a-cath) T80.219
    bloodstream T80.211
    localized T80.212
    specified NEC T80.218
  pulmonary artery catheter — *see* Infection, due to or resulting from, central venous catheter
  surgery T81.40
  Swan Ganz catheter — *see* Infection, due to or resulting from, central venous catheter
  triple lumen catheter T80.219
    bloodstream T80.211
    localized T80.212
    specified NEC T80.218

Infection, infected, infective (opportunistic)
B99.9 — *continued*
due to or resulting from — *continued*
umbilical venous catheter T80.219
bloodstream T80.211
localized T80.212
specified NEC T80.218
during labor NEC O75.3
ear (middle) — *see also* Otitis media
external — *see* Otitis, externa, infective
inner — *see* subcategory H83.0
Eberthella typhosa A01.00
Echinococcus — *see* Echinococcus
echovirus
as cause of disease classified elsewhere
B97.12
unspecified nature or site B34.1
endocardium I33.0
endocervix — *see* Cervicitis
Entamoeba — *see* Amebiasis
enteric — *see* Enteritis, infectious
Enterobacter sakazakii B96.89
Enterobius vermicularis B80
enterostomy K94.12
enterovirus B34.1
as cause of disease classified elsewhere
B97.10
coxsackievirus B97.11
echovirus B97.12
specified NEC B97.19
Entomophthora B46.8
Epidermophyton — *see* Dermatophytosis
epididymis — *see* Epididymitis
episiotomy (puerperal) O86.0
Erysipelothrix (insidiosa) (rhusiopathiae) — *see*
Erysipeloid
erythema infectiosum B08.3
Escherichia (E.) coli NEC A49.8
as cause of disease classified elsewhere (*see
also* Escherichia coli) B96.20
congenital P39.8
sepsis P36.4
generalized A41.51
intestinal — *see* Enteritis, infectious, due to,
Escherichia coli
ethmoidal (chronic) (sinus) — *see* Sinusitis,
ethmoidal
eustachian tube (ear) — *see* Salpingitis,
eustachian
external auditory canal (meatus) NEC — *see*
Otitis, externa, infective
eye (purulent) — *see* Endophthalmitis, purulent
eyelid — *see* Inflammation, eyelid
fallopian tube — *see* Salpingo-oophoritis
Fasciola (gigantica) (hepatica) (indica) B66.3
Fasciolopsis (buski) B66.5
filarial — *see* Infestation, filarial
finger (skin) L08.9
nail L03.01-
fungus B35.1
fish tapeworm B70.0
larval B70.1
flagellate, intestinal A07.9
fluke — *see* Infestation, fluke
focal
teeth (pulpal origin) K04.7
tonsils J35.01
Fonsecaea (compactum) (pedrosoi) B43.0
food — *see* Intoxication, foodborne
foot (skin) L08.9
dermatophytic fungus B35.3
Francisella tularensis — *see* Tularemia
frontal (sinus) (chronic) — *see* Sinusitis, frontal
fungus NOS B49
beard B35.0
dermatophytic — *see* Dermatophytosis
foot B35.3
groin B35.6
hand B35.2

Infection, infected, infective (opportunistic)
B99.9 — *continued*
fungus NOS B49 — *continued*
nail B35.1
pathogenic to compromised host only B48.8
perianal (area) B35.6
scalp B35.0
skin B36.9
foot B35.3
hand B35.2
toenails B35.1
Fusarium B48.8
gallbladder — *see* Cholecystitis
gas bacillus — *see* Gangrene, gas
gastrointestinal — *see* Enteritis, infectious
generalized NEC — *see* Sepsis
generator pocket, implanted electronic
neurostimulator T85.734
genital organ or tract
female — *see* Disease, pelvis, inflammatory
male N49.9
multiple sites N49.8
specified NEC N49.8
Ghon tubercle, primary A15.7
Giardia lamblia A07.1
gingiva (chronic) K05.10
acute K05.00
nonplaque induced K05.01
plaque induced K05.00
nonplaque induced K05.11
plaque induced K05.10
glanders A24.0
glenosporopsis B48.0
Gnathostoma (spinigerum) B83.1
Gongylonema B83.8
gonococcal — *see* Gonococcus
gram-negative bacilli NOS A49.9
guinea worm B72
gum (chronic) K05.10
acute K05.00
nonplaque induced K05.01
plaque induced K05.00
nonplaque induced K05.11
plaque induced K05.10
Haemophilus — *see* Infection, Hemophilus
heart — *see* Carditis
Helicobacter pylori A04.8
as cause of disease classified elsewhere
B96.81
helminths B83.9
intestinal B82.0
mixed (types classifiable to more than one
of the titles B65.0-B81.3 and B81.8)
B81.4
specified type NEC B81.8
specified type NEC B83.8
Hemophilus
aegyptius, systemic A48.4
ducrey (any location) A57
generalized A41.3
influenzae NEC A49.2
as cause of disease classified elsewhere
B96.3
herpes (simplex) — *see also* Herpes
congenital P35.2
disseminated B00.7
zoster B02.9
herpesvirus, herpesviral — *see* Herpes
Heterophyes (heterophyes) B66.8
hip (joint) NEC M00.9
due to internal joint prosthesis
left T84.52
right T84.51
skin NEC L08.9
Histoplasma — *see* Histoplasmosis
American B39.4
capsulatum B39.4
hookworm B76.9

Infection, infected, infective (opportunistic)
B99.9 — *continued*
human
papilloma virus A63.0
T-cell lymphotropic virus type-1 (HTLV-1)
B33.3
hydrocele N43.0
Hymenolepis B71.0
hypopharynx — *see* Pharyngitis
inguinal (lymph) glands L04.1
due to soft chancre A57
intervertebral disc, pyogenic M46.30
cervical region M46.32
cervicothoracic region M46.33
lumbar region M46.36
lumbosacral region M46.37
multiple sites M46.39
occipito-atlanto-axial region M46.31
sacrococcygeal region M46.38
thoracic region M46.34
thoracolumbar region M46.35
intestine, intestinal — *see* Enteritis, infectious
specified NEC A08.8
intra-amniotic affecting newborn NEC P39.2
Isospora belli or hominis A07.3
Japanese B encephalitis A83.0
jaw (bone) (lower) (upper) M27.2
joint NEC M00.9
due to internal joint prosthesis T84.50
kidney (cortex) (hematogenous) N15.9
with calculus N20.0
with hydronephrosis N13.6
following ectopic gestation O08.83
pelvis and ureter (cystic) N28.85
puerperal (postpartum) O86.21
specified NEC N15.8
Klebsiella (K.) pneumoniae NEC A49.8
as cause of disease classified elsewhere
B96.1
knee (joint) NEC M00.9
due to internal joint prosthesis
left T84.54
right T84.53
skin NEC L08.9
Koch's — *see* Tuberculosis
labia (majora) (minora) (acute) — *see* Vulvitis
lacrimal
gland — *see* Dacryoadenitis
passages (duct) (sac) — *see* Inflammation,
lacrimal, passages
lancet fluke B66.2
larynx NEC J38.7
leg (skin) NOS L08.9
Legionella pneumophila A48.1
nonpneumonic A48.2
Leishmania — *see also* Leishmaniasis
aethiopica B55.1
braziliensis B55.2
chagasi B55.0
donovani B55.0
infantum B55.0
major B55.1
mexicana B55.1
tropica B55.1
lentivirus, as cause of disease classified
elsewhere B97.31
Leptosphaeria senegalensis B47.0
Leptospira interrogans A27.9
autumnalis A27.89
canicola A27.89
hebdomadis A27.89
icterohaemorrhagiae A27.0
pomona A27.89
specified type NEC A27.89
leptospirochetal NEC — *see* Leptospirosis
Listeria monocytogenes — *see also* Listeriosis
congenital P37.2

Infection, infected, infective (opportunistic)
  B99.9 — *continued*
  Loa loa B74.3
    with conjunctival infestation B74.3
    eyelid B74.3
  Loboa loboi B48.0
  local, skin (staphylococcal) (streptococcal)
      L08.9
    abscess — *code by* site under Abscess
    cellulitis — *code by* site under Cellulitis
    specified NEC L08.89
    ulcer — *see* Ulcer, skin
  Loefflerella mallei A24.0
  lung (*see also* Pneumonia) J18.9
    atypical Mycobacterium A31.0
    spirochetal A69.8
    tuberculous — *see* Tuberculosis, pulmonary
    virus — *see* Pneumonia, viral
  lymph gland — *see also* Lymphadenitis, acute
    mesenteric I88.0
  lymphoid tissue, base of tongue or posterior
      pharynx, NEC (chronic) J35.03
  Madurella (grisea) (mycetomii) B47.0
  major
    following ectopic or molar pregnancy O08.0
    puerperal, postpartum, childbirth O85
  Malassezia furfur B36.0
  Malleomyces
    mallei A24.0
    pseudomallei (whitmori) — *see* Melioidosis
  mammary gland N61.0
  Mansonella (ozzardi) (perstans) (streptocerca)
      B74.4
  mastoid — *see* Mastoiditis
  maxilla, maxillary M27.2
    sinus (chronic) — *see* Sinusitis, maxillary
  mediastinum J98.51
  Medina (worm) B72
  meibomian cyst or gland — *see* Hordeolum
  meninges — *see* Meningitis, bacterial
  meningococcal (*see also* condition) A39.9
    adrenals A39.1
    brain A39.81
    cerebrospinal A39.0
    conjunctiva A39.89
    endocardium A39.51
    heart A39.50
      endocardium A39.51
      myocardium A39.52
      pericardium A39.53
    joint A39.83
    meninges A39.0
    meningococcemia A39.4
      acute A39.2
      chronic A39.3
    myocardium A39.52
    pericardium A39.53
    retrobulbar neuritis A39.82
    specified site NEC A39.89
  mesenteric lymph nodes or glands NEC I88.0
  Metagonimus B66.8
  metatarsophalangeal M00.9
  methicillin
    resistant Staphylococcus aureus (MRSA)
        A49.02
    susceptible Staphylococcus aureus (MSSA)
        A49.01
  Microsporum, microsporic — *see*
      Dermatophytosis
  mixed flora (bacterial) NEC A49.8
  Monilia — *see* Candidiasis
  Monosporium apiospermum B48.2
  mouth, parasitic B37.0
  Mucor — *see* Mucormycosis
  muscle NEC — *see* Myositis, infective
  mycelium NOS B49
  mycetoma B47.9
    actinomycotic NEC B47.1
    mycotic NEC B47.0

Infection, infected, infective (opportunistic)
  B99.9 — *continued*
  Mycobacterium, mycobacterial — *see*
      Mycobacterium
  Mycoplasma NEC A49.3
    pneumoniae, as cause of disease classified
        elsewhere B96.0
  mycotic NOS B49
    pathogenic to compromised host only B48.8
    skin NOS B36.9
  myocardium NEC I40.0
  nail (chronic)
    with lymphangitis — *see* Lymphangitis,
        acute, digit
    finger L03.01-
      fungus B35.1
    ingrowing L60.0
    toe L03.03-
      fungus B35.1
  nasal sinus (chronic) — *see* Sinusitis
  nasopharynx — *see* Nasopharyngitis
  navel L08.82
  Necator americanus B76.1
  Neisseria — *see* Gonococcus
  Neotestudina rosatii B47.0
  newborn P39.9
    intra-amniotic NEC P39.2
    skin P39.4
    specified type NEC P39.8
  nipple N61.0
    associated with
      lactation O91.03
      pregnancy O91.01-
      puerperium O91.02
  Nocardia — *see* Nocardiosis
  obstetrical surgical wound (puerperal) O86.0
  Oesophagostomum (apiostomum) B81.8
  Oestrus ovis — *see* Myiasis
  Oidium albicans B37.9
  Onchocerca (volvulus) — *see* Onchocerciasis
  oncovirus, as cause of disease classified
      elsewhere B97.32
  operation wound T81.40
  Opisthorchis (felineus) (viverrini) B66.0
  orbit, orbital — *see* Inflammation, orbit
  orthopoxvirus NEC B08.09
  ovary — *see* Salpingo-oophoritis
  Oxyuris vermicularis B80
  pancreas (acute) — *see* Pancreatitis, acute
    abscess — *see* Pancreatitis, acute
    specified NEC (*see also* Pancreatitis, acute)
        K85.80
  papillomavirus, as cause of disease classified
      elsewhere B97.7
  papovavirus NEC B34.4
  Paracoccidioides brasiliensis — *see*
      Paracoccidioidomycosis
  Paragonimus (westermani) B66.4
  parainfluenza virus B34.8
  parameningococcus NOS A39.9
  parapoxvirus B08.60
    specified NEC B08.69
  parasitic B89
  Parastrongylus
    cantonensis B83.2
    costaricensis B81.3
    paratyphoid A01.4
      Type A A01.1
      Type B A01.2
      Type C A01.3
  paraurethral ducts N34.2
  parotid gland — *see* Sialoadenitis
  parvovirus NEC B34.3
    as cause of disease classified elsewhere
        B97.6
  Pasteurella NEC A28.0
    multocida A28.0
    pestis — *see* Plague
    pseudotuberculosis A28.0

Infection, infected, infective (opportunistic)
  B99.9 — *continued*
  Pasteurella NEC A28.0 — *continued*
    septica (cat bite) (dog bite) A28.0
    tularensis — *see* Tularemia
  pelvic, female — *see* Disease, pelvis,
      inflammatory
  Penicillium (marneffei) B48.4
  penis (glans) (retention) NEC N48.29
  periapical K04.5
  peridental, periodontal K05.20
    generalized — *see* Peridontitis, aggressive,
        generalized
    localized — *see* Peridontitis, aggressive,
        localized
  perinatal period P39.9
    specified type NEC P39.8
  perineal repair (puerperal) O86.0
  periorbital — *see* Inflammation, orbit
  perirectal K62.89
  perirenal — *see* Infection, kidney
  peritoneal — *see* Peritonitis
  periureteral N28.89
  Petriellidium boydii B48.2
  pharynx — *see also* Pharyngitis
    coxsackievirus B08.5
    posterior, lymphoid (chronic) J35.03
  Phialophora
    gougerotii (subcutaneous abscess or cyst)
        B43.2
    jeanselmei (subcutaneous abscess or cyst)
        B43.2
    verrucosa (skin) B43.0
  Piedraia hortae B36.3
  pinta A67.9
    intermediate A67.1
    late A67.2
    mixed A67.3
    primary A67.0
  pinworm B80
  pityrosporum furfur B36.0
  pleuro-pneumonia-like organism (PPLO) NEC
      A49.3
    as cause of disease classified elsewhere
        B96.0
  pneumococcus, pneumococcal NEC A49.1
    as cause of disease classified elsewhere
        B95.3
    generalized (purulent) A40.3
      with pneumonia J13
  Pneumocystis carinii (pneumonia) B59
  Pneumocystis jiroveci (pneumonia) B59
  port or reservoir T80.212
  postoperative T81.40
  postoperative wound T81.40
  postprocedural T81.40
    deep incisional surgical site T81.42
    organ and space surgical site T81.43
    sepsis T81.49
    specified surgical site NEC T81.48
    superficial incisional surgical site T81.41
  postvaccinal T88.0
  prepuce NEC N47.7
    with penile inflammation N47.6
  prion — *see* Disease, prion, central nervous
      system
  prostate (capsule) — *see* Prostatitis
  Proteus (mirabilis) (morganii) (vulgaris) NEC
      A49.8
    as cause of disease classified elsewhere
        B96.4
  protozoal NEC B64
    intestinal A07.9
      specified NEC A07.8
    specified NEC B60.8
  Pseudoallescheria boydii B48.2

Infection, infected, infective (opportunistic)
B99.9 — *continued*
Pseudomonas NEC A49.8
as cause of disease classified elsewhere
B96.5
mallei A24.0
pneumonia J15.1
pseudomallei — *see* Melioidosis
puerperal O86.4
genitourinary tract NEC O86.89
major or generalized O85
minor O86.4
specified NEC O86.89
pulmonary — *see* Infection, lung
purulent — *see* Abscess
Pyrenochaeta romeroi B47.0
Q fever A78
rectum (sphincter) K62.89
renal — *see also* Infection, kidney
pelvis and ureter (cystic) N28.85
reovirus, as cause of disease classified
elsewhere B97.5
respiratory (tract) NEC J98.8
acute J22
chronic J98.8
influenzal (upper) (acute) — *see* Influenza,
with, respiratory manifestations NEC
lower (acute) J22
chronic — *see* Bronchitis, chronic
rhinovirus J00
syncytial virus, as cause of disease classified
elsewhere B97.4
upper (acute) NOS J06.9
chronic J39.8
streptococcal J06.9
viral NOS J06.9
resulting from
presence of internal prosthesis, implant, graft
— *see* Complications, by site and type,
infection
retortamoniasis A07.8
retroperitoneal NEC K68.9
retrovirus B33.3
as cause of disease classified elsewhere
B97.30
human
immunodeficiency, type 2 (HIV 2)
B97.35
T-cell lymphotropic
type I (HTLV-I) B97.33
type II (HTLV-II) B97.34
lentivirus B97.31
oncovirus B97.32
specified NEC B97.39
Rhinosporidium (seeberi) B48.1
rhinovirus
as cause of disease classified elsewhere
B97.89
unspecified nature or site B34.8
Rhizopus — *see* Mucormycosis
rickettsial NOS A79.9
roundworm (large) NEC B82.0
Ascariasis (*see also* Ascariasis) B77.9
rubella — *see* Rubella
Saccharomyces — *see* Candidiasis
salivary duct or gland (any) — *see*
Sialoadenitis
Salmonella (aertrycke) (arizonae) (callinarum)
(cholerae-suis) (enteritidis) (suipestifer)
(typhimurium) A02.9
with
(gastro)enteritis A02.0
sepsis A02.1
specified manifestation NEC A02.8
due to food (poisoning) A02.9
hirschfeldii A01.3
localized A02.20
arthritis A02.23
meningitis A02.21

Infection, infected, infective (opportunistic)
B99.9 — *continued*
Salmonella (aertrycke) (arizonae) (callinarum)
(cholerae-suis) (enteritidis) (suipestifer)
(typhimurium) A02.9 — *continued*
localized A02.20 — *continued*
osteomyelitis A02.24
pneumonia A02.22
pyelonephritis A02.25
specified NEC A02.29
paratyphi A01.4
A A01.1
B A01.2
C A01.3
schottmuelleri A01.2
typhi, typhosa — *see* Typhoid
Sarcocystis A07.8
scabies B86
Schistosoma — *see* Infestation, Schistosoma
scrotum (acute) NEC N49.2
seminal vesicle — *see* Vesiculitis
septic
localized, skin — *see* Abscess
sheep liver fluke B66.3
Shigella A03.9
boydii A03.2
dysenteriae A03.0
flexneri A03.1
group
A A03.0
B A03.1
C A03.2
D A03.3
Schmitz (-Stutzer) A03.0
schmitzii A03.0
shigae A03.0
sonnei A03.3
specified NEC A03.8
shoulder (joint) NEC M00.9
due to internal joint prosthesis T84.59
skin NEC L08.9
sinus (accessory) (chronic) (nasal) — *see also*
Sinusitis
pilonidal — *see* Sinus, pilonidal
skin NEC L08.89
Skene's duct or gland — *see* Urethritis
skin (local) (staphylococcal) (streptococcal)
L08.9
abscess — *code by* site under Abscess
cellulitis — *code by* site under Cellulitis
due to fungus B36.9
specified type NEC B36.8
mycotic B36.9
specified type NEC B36.8
newborn P39.4
ulcer — *see* Ulcer, skin
slow virus A81.9
specified NEC A81.89
Sparganum (mansoni) (proliferum) (baxteri)
B70.1
specific — *see also* Syphilis
to perinatal period — *see* Infection,
congenital
specified NEC B99.8
spermatic cord NEC N49.1
sphenoidal (sinus) — *see* Sinusitis, sphenoidal
spinal cord NOS (*see also* Myelitis) G04.91
abscess G06.1
meninges — *see* Meningitis
streptococcal G04.89
Spirillum A25.0
spirochetal NOS A69.9
lung A69.8
specified NEC A69.8
Spirometra larvae B70.1
spleen D73.89
Sporotrichum, Sporothrix (schenckii) — *see*
Sporotrichosis

Infection, infected, infective (opportunistic)
B99.9 — *continued*
staphylococcal, unspecified site
as cause of disease classified elsewhere
B95.8
aureus (methicillin susceptible) (MSSA)
B95.61
methicillin resistant (MRSA) B95.62
specified NEC B95.7
aureus (methicillin susceptible) (MSSA)
A49.01
methicillin resistant (MRSA) A49.02
food poisoning A05.0
generalized (purulent) A41.2
pneumonia — *see* Pneumonia,
staphylococcal
Stellantchasmus falcatus B66.8
streptobacillus moniliformis A25.1
streptococcal NEC A49.1
as cause of disease classified elsewhere
B95.5
B genitourinary complicating
childbirth O98.82
pregnancy O98.81-
puerperium O98.83
congenital
sepsis P36.10
group B P36.0
specified NEC P36.19
generalized (purulent) A40.9
Streptomyces B47.1
Strongyloides (stercoralis) — *see*
Strongyloidiasis
stump (amputation) (surgical) — *see*
Complication, amputation stump, infection
subcutaneous tissue, local L08.9
suipestifer — *see* Infection, salmonella
swimming pool bacillus A31.1
Taenia — *see* Infestation, Taenia
Taeniarhynchus saginatus B68.1
tapeworm — *see* Infestation, tapeworm
tendon (sheath) — *see* Tenosynovitis, infective
NEC
Ternidens diminutus B81.8
testis — *see* Orchitis
threadworm B80
throat — *see* Pharyngitis
thyroglossal duct K14.8
toe (skin) L08.9
cellulitis L03.03-
fungus B35.1
nail L03.03-
fungus B35.1
tongue NEC K14.0
parasitic B37.0
tonsil (and adenoid) (faucial) (lingual)
(pharyngeal) — *see* Tonsillitis
tooth, teeth K04.7
periapical K04.7
peridental, periodontal K05.20
generalized — *see* Periodontitis, aggressive,
generalized
localized — *see* Periodontitis, aggressive,
localized
pulp K04.01
irreversible K04.02
reversible K04.01
socket M27.3
TORCH — *see* Infection, congenital
without active infection P00.2
Torula histolytica — *see* Cryptococcosis
Toxocara (canis) (cati) (felis) B83.0
Toxoplasma gondii — *see* Toxoplasma
trachea, chronic J42
trematode NEC — *see* Infestation, fluke
trench fever A79.0
Treponema pallidum — *see* Syphilis
Trichinella (spiralis) B75

Infection, infected, infective (opportunistic)
B99.9 — *continued*
Trichomonas A59.9
cervix A59.09
intestine A07.8
prostate A59.02
specified site NEC A59.8
urethra A59.03
urogenitalis A59.00
vagina A59.01
vulva A59.01
Trichophyton, trichophytic — *see* Dermatophytosis
Trichosporon (beigelii) cutaneum B36.2
Trichostrongylus B81.2
Trichuris (trichiura) B79
Trombicula (irritans) B88.0
Trypanosoma
brucei
gambiense B56.0
rhodesiense B56.1
cruzi — *see* Chagas' disease
tubal — *see* Salpingo-oophoritis
tuberculous NEC — *see* Tuberculosis
tubo-ovarian — *see* Salpingo-oophoritis
tunica vaginalis N49.1
tunnel T80.212
tympanic membrane NEC — *see* Myringitis
typhoid (abortive) (ambulant) (bacillus) — *see* Typhoid
typhus A75.9
flea-borne A75.2
mite-borne A75.3
recrudescent A75.1
tick-borne A77.9
African A77.1
North Asian A77.2
umbilicus L08.82
ureter N28.86
urethra — *see* Urethritis
urinary (tract) N39.0
bladder — *see* Cystitis
complicating
pregnancy O23.4-
specified type NEC O23.3-
kidney — *see* Infection, kidney
newborn P39.3
puerperal (postpartum) O86.20
tuberculous A18.13
urethra — *see* Urethritis
uterus, uterine — *see* Endometritis
vaccination T88.0
vaccinia not from vaccination B08.011
vagina (acute) — *see* Vaginitis
varicella B01.9
varicose veins — *see* Varix
vas deferens NEC N49.1
vesical — *see* Cystitis
Vibrio
cholerae A00.0
El Tor A00.1
parahaemolyticus (food poisoning) A05.3
vulnificus
as cause of disease classified elsewhere B96.82
foodborne intoxication A05.5
Vincent's (gum) (mouth) (tonsil) A69.1
virus, viral NOS B34.9
adenovirus
as cause of disease classified elsewhere B97.0
unspecified nature or site B34.0
arborvirus, arbovirus arthropod-borne A94
as cause of disease classified elsewhere B97.89
adenovirus B97.0
coronavirus B97.29
SARS-associated B97.21
coxsackievirus B97.11

Infection, infected, infective (opportunistic)
B99.9 — *continued*
virus, viral NOS B34.9 — *continued*
as cause of disease classified elsewhere
B97.89 — *continued*
echovirus B97.12
enterovirus B97.10
coxsackievirus B97.11
echovirus B97.12
specified NEC B97.19
human
immunodeficiency, type 2 (HIV 2) B97.35
metapneumovirus B97.81
T-cell lymphotropic,
type I (HTLV-I) B97.33
type II (HTLV-II) B97.34
papillomavirus B97.7
parvovirus B97.6
reovirus B97.5
respiratory syncytial B97.4
retrovirus B97.30
human
immunodeficiency, type 2 (HIV 2) B97.35
T-cell lymphotropic,
type I (HTLV-I) B97.33
type II (HTLV-II) B97.34
lentivirus B97.31
oncovirus B97.32
specified NEC B97.39
specified NEC B97.89
central nervous system A89
atypical A81.9
specified NEC A81.89
enterovirus NEC A88.8
meningitis A87.0
slow virus A81.9
specified NEC A81.89
specified NEC A88.8
chest J98.8
cotia B08.8
coxsackie (*see also* Infection, coxsackie) B34.1
as cause of disease classified elsewhere B97.11
ECHO
as cause of disease classified elsewhere B97.12
unspecified nature or site B34.1
encephalitis, tick-borne A84.9
enterovirus, as cause of disease classified elsewhere B97.10
coxsackievirus B97.11
echovirus B97.12
specified NEC B97.19
exanthem NOS B09
human metapneumovirus as cause of disease classified elsewhere B97.81
human papilloma as cause of disease classified elsewhere B97.7
intestine — *see* Enteritis, viral
respiratory syncytial
as cause of disease classified elsewhere B97.4
bronchopneumonia J12.1
common cold syndrome J00
nasopharyngitis (acute) J00
rhinovirus
as cause of disease classified elsewhere B97.89
unspecified nature or site B34.8
slow A81.9
specified NEC A81.89
specified type NEC B33.8
as cause of disease classified elsewhere B97.89
unspecified nature or site B34.8
unspecified nature or site B34.9
West Nile — *see* Virus, West Nile

Infection, infected, infective (opportunistic)
B99.9 — *continued*
vulva (acute) — *see* Vulvitis
West Nile — *see* Virus, West Nile
whipworm B79
worms B83.9
specified type NEC B83.8
Wuchereria (bancrofti) B74.0
malayi B74.1
yatapoxvirus B08.70
specified NEC B08.79
yeast (*see also* Candidiasis) B37.9
yellow fever — *see* Fever, yellow
Yersinia
enterocolitica (intestinal) A04.6
pestis — *see* Plague
pseudotuberculosis A28.2
Zeis' gland — *see* Hordeolum
Zika virus A92.5
zoonotic bacterial NOS A28.9
Zopfia senegalensis B47.0
Infective, infectious — *see* condition
Infertility
female N97.9
age-related N97.8
associated with
anovulation N97.0
cervical (mucus) disease or anomaly N88.3
congenital anomaly
cervix N88.3
fallopian tube N97.1
uterus N97.2
vagina N97.8
dysmucorrhea N88.3
fallopian tube disease or anomaly N97.1
pituitary-hypothalamic origin E23.0
specified origin NEC N97.8
Stein-Leventhal syndrome E28.2
uterine disease or anomaly N97.2
vaginal disease or anomaly N97.8
due to
cervical anomaly N88.3
fallopian tube anomaly N97.1
ovarian failure E28.39
Stein-Leventhal syndrome E28.2
uterine anomaly N97.2
vaginal anomaly N97.8
nonimplantation N97.2
origin
cervical N88.3
tubal (block) (occlusion) (stenosis) N97.1
uterine N97.2
vaginal N97.8
male N46.9
azoospermia N46.01
extratesticular cause N46.029
drug therapy N46.021
efferent duct obstruction N46.023
infection N46.022
radiation N46.024
specified cause NEC N46.029
systemic disease N46.025
oligospermia N46.11
extratesticular cause N46.129
drug therapy N46.121
efferent duct obstruction N46.123
infection N46.122
radiation N46.124
specified cause NEC N46.129
systemic disease N46.125
specified type NEC N46.8
Infestation B88.9
Acanthocheilonema (perstans) (streptocerca) B74.4
Acariasis B88.0
demodex folliculorum B88.0
sarcoptes scabiei B86
trombiculae B88.0

DISEASE INDEX

Infestation B88.9 — *continued*
- Agamofilaria streptocerca B74.4
- Ancylostoma, ankylostoma (braziliense) (caninum) (ceylanicum) (duodenale) B76.0
  - americanum B76.1
  - new world B76.1
- Anisakis larvae, anisakiasis B81.0
- arthropod NEC B88.2
- Ascaris lumbricoides — *see* Ascariasis
- Balantidium coli A07.0
- beef tapeworm B68.1
- Bothriocephalus (latus) B70.0
  - larval B70.1
- broad tapeworm B70.0
  - larval B70.1
- Brugia (malayi) B74.1
  - timori B74.2
- candiru B88.8
- Capillaria
  - hepatica B83.8
  - philippinensis B81.1
- cat liver fluke B66.0
- cestodes B71.9
  - diphyllobothrium — *see* Infestation, diphyllobothrium
  - dipylidiasis B71.1
  - hymenolepiasis B71.0
  - specified type NEC B71.8
- chigger B88.0
- chigo, chigoe B88.1
- Clonorchis (sinensis) (liver) B66.1
- coccidial A07.3
- crab-lice B85.3
- Cysticercus cellulosae — *see* Cysticercosis
- Demodex (folliculorum) B88.0
- Dermanyssus gallinae B88.0
- Dermatobia (hominis) — *see* Myiasis
- Dibothriocephalus (latus) B70.0
  - larval B70.1
- Dicrocoelium dendriticum B66.2
- Diphyllobothrium (adult) (latum) (intestinal) (pacificum) B70.0
  - larval B70.1
- Diplogonoporus (grandis) B71.8
- Dipylidium caninum B67.4
- Distoma hepaticum B66.3
- dog tapeworm B67.4
- Dracunculus medinensis B72
- dragon worm B72
- dwarf tapeworm B71.0
- Echinococcus — *see* Echinococcus
- Echinostomum ilocanum B66.8
- Entamoeba (histolytica) — *see* Infection, Ameba
- Enterobius vermicularis B80
- eyelid
  - in (due to)
    - leishmaniasis B55.1
    - loiasis B74.3
    - onchocerciasis B73.09
    - phthiriasis B85.3
  - parasitic NOS B89
- eyeworm B74.3
- Fasciola (gigantica) (hepatica) (indica) B66.3
- Fasciolopsis (buski) (intestine) B66.5
- filarial B74.9
  - bancroftian B74.0
  - conjunctiva B74.9
  - due to
    - Acanthocheilonema (perstans) (streptocerca) B74.4
    - Brugia (malayi) B74.1
      - timori B74.2
    - Dracunculus medinensis B72
    - guinea worm B72
    - loa loa B74.3
    - Mansonella (ozzardi) (perstans) (streptocerca) B74.4

Infestation B88.9 — *continued*
- filarial B74.9 — *continued*
  - due to — *continued*
    - Onchocerca volvulus B73.00
      - eye B73.00
      - eyelid B73.09
    - Wuchereria (bancrofti) B74.0
  - Malayan B74.1
  - ozzardi B74.4
  - specified type NEC B74.8
- fish tapeworm B70.0
  - larval B70.1
- fluke B66.9
  - blood NOS — *see* Schistosomiasis
  - cat liver B66.0
  - intestinal B66.5
  - lancet B66.2
  - liver (sheep) B66.3
    - cat B66.0
    - Chinese B66.1
    - due to clonorchiasis B66.1
    - oriental B66.1
  - lung (oriental) B66.4
  - sheep liver B66.3
  - specified type NEC B66.8
- fly larvae — *see* Myiasis
- Gasterophilus (intestinalis) — *see* Myiasis
- Gastrodiscoides hominis B66.8
- Giardia lamblia A07.1
- Gnathostoma (spinigerum) B83.1
- Gongylonema B83.8
- guinea worm B72
- helminth B83.9
  - angiostrongyliasis B83.2
    - intestinal B81.3
  - gnathostomiasis B83.1
  - hirudiniasis, internal B83.4
  - intestinal B82.0
    - angiostrongyliasis B81.3
    - anisakiasis B81.0
    - ascariasis — *see* Ascariasis
    - capillariasis B81.1
    - cysticercosis — *see* Cysticercosis
    - diphyllobothriasis — *see* Infestation, diphyllobothriasis
    - dracunculiasis B72
    - echinococcus — *see* Echinococcosis
    - enterobiasis B80
    - filariasis — *see* Infestation, filarial
    - fluke — *see* Infestation, fluke
    - hookworm — *see* Infestation, hookworm
    - mixed (types classifiable to more than one of the titles B65.0-B81.3 and B81.8) B81.4
    - onchocerciasis — *see* Onchocerciasis
    - schistosomiasis — *see* Infestation, schistosoma
    - specified
      - cestode NEC — *see* Infestation, cestode
      - type NEC B81.8
    - strongyloidiasis — *see* Strongyloidiasis
    - taenia — *see* Infestation, taenia
    - trichinellosis B75
    - trichostrongyliasis B81.2
    - trichuriasis B79
  - specified type NEC B83.8
  - syngamiasis B83.3
  - visceral larva migrans B83.0
- Heterophyes (heterophyes) B66.8
- hookworm B76.9
  - ancylostomiasis B76.0
  - necatoriasis B76.1
  - specified type NEC B76.8
- Hymenolepis (diminuta) (nana) B71.0
- intestinal NEC B82.9
- leeches (aquatic) (land) — *see* Hirudiniasis
- Leishmania — *see* Leishmaniasis
- lice, louse — *see* Infestation, Pediculus
- Linguatula B88.8

Infestation B88.9 — *continued*
- Liponyssoides sanguineus B88.0
- Loa loa B74.3
  - conjunctival B74.3
  - eyelid B74.3
- louse — *see* Infestation, Pediculus
- maggots — *see* Myiasis
- Mansonella (ozzardi) (perstans) (streptocerca) B74.4
- Medina (worm) B72
- Metagonimus (yokogawai) B66.8
- microfilaria streptocerca — *see* Onchocerciasis
  - eye B73.00
  - eyelid B73.09
- mites B88.9
  - scabic B86
- Monilia (albicans) — *see* Candidiasis
- mouth B37.0
- Necator americanus B76.1
- nematode NEC (intestinal) B82.0
  - Ancylostoma B76.0
  - conjunctiva NEC B83.9
  - Enterobius vermicularis B80
  - Gnathostoma spinigerum B83.1
  - physaloptera B80
  - specified NEC B81.8
  - trichostrongylus B81.2
  - trichuris (trichuria) B79
- Oesophagostomum (apiostomum) B81.8
- Oestrus ovis (*see also* Myiasis) B87.9
- Onchocerca (volvulus) — *see* Onchocerciasis
- Opisthorchis (felineus) (viverrini) B66.0
- orbit, parasitic NOS B89
- Oxyuris vermicularis B80
- Paragonimus (westermani) B66.4
- parasite, parasitic B89
  - eyelid B89
  - intestinal NOS B82.9
  - mouth B37.0
  - skin B88.9
  - tongue B37.0
- Parastrongylus
  - cantonensis B83.2
  - costaricensis B81.3
- Pediculus B85.2
  - body B85.1
  - capitis (humanus) (any site) B85.0
  - corporis (humanus) (any site) B85.1
  - head B85.0
  - mixed (classifiable to more than one of the titles B85.0-B85.3) B85.4
  - pubis (any site) B85.3
- Pentastoma B88.8
- Phthirus (pubis) (any site) B85.3
  - with any infestation classifiable to B85.0-B85.2 B85.4
- pinworm B80
- pork tapeworm (adult) B68.0
- protozoal NEC B64
  - intestinal A07.9
    - specified NEC A07.8
  - specified NEC B60.8
- pubic, louse B85.3
- rat tapeworm B71.0
- red bug B88.0
- roundworm (large) NEC B82.0
  - Ascariasis (*see also* Ascariasis) B77.9
- sandflea B88.1
- Sarcoptes scabiei B86
- scabies B86
- Schistosoma B65.9
  - bovis B65.8
  - cercariae B65.3
  - haematobium B65.0
  - intercalatum B65.8
  - japonicum B65.2
  - mansoni B65.1
  - mattheei B65.8
  - mekongi B65.8

Infestation B88.9 — *continued*
  Schistosoma B65.9 — *continued*
    specified type NEC B65.8
    spindale B65.8
  screw worms — *see* Myiasis
  skin NOS B88.9
  Sparganum (mansoni) (proliferum) (baxteri)
    B70.1
    larval B70.1
  specified type NEC B88.8
  Spirometra larvae B70.1
  Stellantchasmus falcatus B66.8
  Strongyloides stercoralis — *see* Strongyloidiasis
  Taenia B68.9
    diminuta B71.0
    echinococcus — *see* Echinococcus
    mediocanellata B68.1
    nana B71.0
    saginata B68.1
    solium (intestinal form) B68.0
      larval form — *see* Cysticercosis
  Taeniarhynchus saginatus B68.1
  tapeworm B71.9
    beef B68.1
    broad B70.0
      larval B70.1
    dog B67.4
    dwarf B71.0
    fish B70.0
      larval B70.1
    pork B68.0
    rat B71.0
  Ternidens diminutus B81.8
  Tetranychus molestissimus B88.0
  threadworm B80
  tongue B37.0
  Toxocara (canis) (cati) (felis) B83.0
  trematode(s) NEC — *see* Infestation, fluke
  Trichinella (spiralis) B75
  Trichocephalus B79
  Trichomonas — *see* Trichomoniasis
  Trichostrongylus B81.2
  Trichuris (trichiura) B79
  Trombicula (irritans) B88.0
  Tunga penetrans B88.1
  Uncinaria americana B76.1
  Vandellia cirrhosa B88.8
  whipworm B79
  worms B83.9
    intestinal B82.0
  Wuchereria (bancrofti) B74.0

Infiltrate, infiltration
  amyloid (generalized) (localized) — *see*
    Amyloidosis
  calcareous NEC R89.7
    localized — *see* Degeneration, by site
  calcium salt R89.7
  cardiac
    fatty — *see* Degeneration, myocardial
    glycogenic E74.02 *[I43]*
  corneal — *see* Edema, cornea
  eyelid — *see* Inflammation, eyelid
  glycogen, glycogenic — *see* Disease, glycogen
    storage
  heart, cardiac
    fatty — *see* Degeneration, myocardial
    glycogenic E74.02 *[I43]*
  inflammatory in vitreous H43.89
  kidney N28.89
  leukemic — *see* Leukemia
  liver K76.89
    fatty — *see* Fatty, liver NEC
    glycogen (*see also* Disease, glycogen storage)
      E74.03 *[K77]*
  lung R91.8
    eosinophilic J82
  lymphatic (*see also* Leukemia, lymphatic)
    C91.9-
    gland I88.9

Infiltrate, infiltration — *continued*
  muscle, fatty M62.89
  myocardium, myocardial
    fatty — *see* Degeneration, myocardial
    glycogenic E74.02 *[I43]*
  on chest x-ray R91.8
  pulmonary R91.8
    with eosinophilia J82
  skin (lymphocytic) L98.6
  thymus (gland) (fatty) E32.8
  urine R39.0
  vesicant agent
    antineoplastic chemotherapy T80.810
    other agent NEC T80.818
  vitreous body H43.89
Infirmity R68.89
  senile R54
Inflammation, inflamed, inflammatory
  (with exudation)
  abducent (nerve) — *see* Strabismus, paralytic,
    sixth nerve
  accessory sinus (chronic) — *see* Sinusitis
  adrenal (gland) E27.8
  alveoli, teeth M27.3
    scorbutic E54
  anal canal, anus K62.89
  antrum (chronic) — *see* Sinusitis, maxillary
  appendix — *see* Appendicitis
  arachnoid — *see* Meningitis
  areola N61.0
    puerperal, postpartum or gestational — *see*
      Infection, nipple
  areolar tissue NOS L08.9
  artery — *see* Arteritis
  auditory meatus (external) — *see* Otitis,
    externa
  Bartholin's gland N75.8
  bile duct (common) (hepatic) or passage — *see*
    Cholangitis
  bladder — *see* Cystitis
  bone — *see* Osteomyelitis
  brain — *see also* Encephalitis
    membrane — *see* Meningitis
  breast N61.0
    puerperal, postpartum, gestational — *see*
      Mastitis, obstetric
  broad ligament — *see* Disease, pelvis,
    inflammatory
  bronchi — *see* Bronchitis
  catarrhal J00
  cecum — *see* Appendicitis
  cerebral — *see also* Encephalitis
    membrane — *see* Meningitis
  cerebrospinal
    meningococcal A39.0
  cervix (uteri) — *see* Cervicitis
  chest J98.8
  chorioretinal H30.9-
    cyclitis — *see* Cyclitis
    disseminated H30.10-
      generalized H30.13-
      peripheral H30.12-
      posterior pole H30.11-
    epitheliopathy — *see* Epitheliopathy
    focal H30.00-
      juxtapapillary H30.01-
      macular H30.04-
      paramacular — *see* Inflammation,
        chorioretinal, focal, macular
      peripheral H30.03-
      posterior pole H30.02-
    specified type NEC H30.89-
  choroid — *see* Inflammation, chorioretinal
  chronic, postmastoidectomy cavity — *see*
    Complications, postmastoidectomy,
    inflammation
  colon — *see* Enteritis
  connective tissue (diffuse) NEC — *see* Disorder,
    soft tissue, specified type NEC

Inflammation, inflamed, inflammatory
  (with exudation) — *continued*
  cornea — *see* Keratitis
  corpora cavernosa N48.29
  cranial nerve — *see* Disorder, nerve, cranial
  Douglas' cul-de-sac or pouch (chronic) N73.0
  due to device, implant or graft — *see also*
    Complications, by site and type, infection
    or inflammation
    arterial graft T82.7
    breast (implant) T85.79
    catheter T85.79
      dialysis (renal) T82.7
        intraperitoneal T85.71
      infusion T82.7
        cranial T85.735
        intrathecal T85.735
        spinal (epidural) (subdural) T85.735
        subarachnoid T85.735
      urinary T83.518
        cystostomy T83.510
        Hopkins T83.518
        ileostomy T83.518
        nephrostomy T83.512
        specified NEC T83.518
        urethral indwelling T83.511
        urostomy T83.518
    electronic (electrode) (pulse generator)
      (stimulator)
      bone T84.7
      cardiac T82.7
      nervous system T85.738
        brain T85.731
        cranial nerve T85.732
        gastric nerve T85.732
        neurostimulator generator T85.734
        peripheral nerve T85.732
        sacral nerve T85.732
        spinal cord T85.733
        vagal nerve T85.732
      urinary T83.590
    fixation, internal (orthopedic) NEC — *see*
      Complication, fixation device, infection
    gastrointestinal (bile duct) (esophagus)
      T85.79
    neurostimulator electrode (lead) T85.732
    genital NEC T83.69
    heart NEC T82.7
      valve (prosthesis) T82.6
        graft T82.7
    joint prosthesis — *see* Complication, joint
      prosthesis, infection
    ocular (corneal graft) (orbital implant) NEC
      T85.79
    orthopedic NEC T84.7
    penile (cylinder) (pump) (resevoir) T83.61
    specified NEC T85.79
    testicular T83.62
    urinary NEC T83.598
      ileal conduit stent T83.593
      implanted neurostimulation T83.590
      implanted sphincter T83.591
      indwelling ureteral stent T83.592
      nephroureteral stent T83.593
      specified stent NEC T83.593
    vascular NEC T82.7
    ventricular intracranial (communicating)
      shunt T85.730
  duodenum K29.80
    with bleeding K29.81
  dura mater — *see* Meningitis
  ear (middle) — *see also* Otitis, media
    external — *see* Otitis, externa
    inner — *see* subcategory H83.0
  epididymis — *see* Epididymitis
  esophagus K20.9
  ethmoidal (sinus) (chronic) — *see* Sinusitis,
    ethmoidal

Inflammation, inflamed, inflammatory (with exudation) — *continued*
  eustachian tube (catarrhal) — *see* Salpingitis, eustachian
  eyelid H01.9
    abscess — *see* Abscess, eyelid
    blepharitis — *see* Blepharitis
    chalazion — *see* Chalazion
    dermatosis (noninfectious) — *see* Dermatosis, eyelid
    hordeolum — *see* Hordeolum
    specified NEC H01.8
  fallopian tube — *see* Salpingo-oophoritis
  fascia — *see* Myositis
  follicular, pharynx J31.2
  frontal (sinus) (chronic) — *see* Sinusitis, frontal
  gallbladder — *see* Cholecystitis
  gastric — *see* Gastritis
  gastrointestinal — *see* Enteritis
  genital organ (internal) (diffuse)
    female — *see* Disease, pelvis, inflammatory
    male N49.9
      multiple sites N49.8
      specified NEC N49.8
  gland (lymph) — *see* Lymphadenitis
  glottis — *see* Laryngitis
  granular, pharynx J31.2
  gum K05.10
    nonplaque induced K05.11
    plaque induced K05.10
  heart — *see* Carditis
  hepatic duct — *see* Cholangitis
  ileoanal (internal) pouch K91.850
  ileum — *see also* Enteritis
    regional or terminal — *see* Enteritis, regional
  intestinal pouch K91.850
  intestine (any part) — *see* Enteritis
  jaw (acute) (bone) (chronic) (lower) (suppurative) (upper) M27.2
  joint NEC — *see* Arthritis
    sacroiliac M46.1
  kidney — *see* Nephritis
  knee (joint) M13.169
    tuberculous A18.02
  labium (majus) (minus) — *see* Vulvitis
  lacrimal
    gland — *see* Dacryoadenitis
    passages (duct) (sac) — *see also* Dacryocystitis
      canaliculitis — *see* Canaliculitis, lacrimal
  larynx — *see* Laryngitis
  leg NOS L08.9
  lip K13.0
  liver (capsule) — *see also* Hepatitis
    chronic K73.9
    suppurative K75.0
  lung (acute) — *see also* Pneumonia
    chronic J98.4
  lymph gland or node — *see* Lymphadenitis
  lymphatic vessel — *see* Lymphangitis
  maxilla, maxillary M27.2
    sinus (chronic) — *see* Sinusitis, maxillary
  membranes of brain or spinal cord — *see* Meningitis
  meninges — *see* Meningitis
  mouth K12.1
  muscle — *see* Myositis
  myocardium — *see* Myocarditis
  nasal sinus (chronic) — *see* Sinusitis
  nasopharynx — *see* Nasopharyngitis
  navel L08.82
  nerve NEC — *see* Neuralgia
  nipple N61.0
    puerperal, postpartum or gestational — *see* Infection, nipple
  nose — *see* Rhinitis
  oculomotor (nerve) — *see* Strabismus, paralytic, third nerve
  optic nerve — *see* Neuritis, optic

Inflammation, inflamed, inflammatory (with exudation) — *continued*
  orbit (chronic) H05.10
    acute H05.00
      abscess — *see* Abscess, orbit
      cellulitis — *see* Cellulitis, orbit
      osteomyelitis — *see* Osteomyelitis, orbit
      periostitis — *see* Periostitis, orbital
      tenonitis — *see* Tenonitis, eye
    granuloma — *see* Granuloma, orbit
    myositis — *see* Myositis, orbital
  ovary — *see* Salpingo-oophoritis
  oviduct — *see* Salpingo-oophoritis
  pancreas (acute) — *see* Pancreatitis
  parametrium N73.0
  parotid region L08.9
  pelvis, female — *see* Disease, pelvis, inflammatory
  penis (corpora cavernosa) N48.29
  perianal K62.89
  pericardium — *see* Pericarditis
  perineum (female) (male) L08.9
  perirectal K62.89
  peritoneum — *see* Peritonitis
  periuterine — *see* Disease, pelvis, inflammatory
  perivesical — *see* Cystitis
  petrous bone (acute) (chronic) — *see* Petrositis
  pharynx (acute) — *see* Pharyngitis
  pia mater — *see* Meningitis
  pleura — *see* Pleurisy
  polyp, colon (*see also* Polyp, colon, inflammatory) K51.40
  prostate — *see also* Prostatitis
    specified type NEC N41.8
  rectosigmoid — *see* Rectosigmoiditis
  rectum (*see also* Proctitis) K62.89
  respiratory, upper (*see also* Infection, respiratory, upper) J06.9
    acute, due to radiation J70.0
    chronic, due to external agent — *see* condition, respiratory, chronic, due to
    due to
      chemicals, gases, fumes or vapors (inhalation) J68.2
      radiation J70.1
  retina — *see* Chorioretinitis
  retrocecal — *see* Appendicitis
  retroperitoneal — *see* Peritonitis
  salivary duct or gland (any) (suppurative) — *see* Sialoadenitis
  scorbutic, alveoli, teeth E54
  scrotum N49.2
  seminal vesicle — *see* Vesiculitis
  sigmoid — *see* Enteritis
  sinus — *see* Sinusitis
  Skene's duct or gland — *see* Urethritis
  skin L08.9
  spermatic cord N49.1
  sphenoidal (sinus) — *see* Sinusitis, sphenoidal
  spinal
    cord — *see* Encephalitis
    membrane — *see* Meningitis
    nerve — *see* Disorder, nerve
  spine — *see* Spondylopathy, inflammatory
  spleen (capsule) D73.89
  stomach — *see* Gastritis
  subcutaneous tissue L08.9
  suprarenal (gland) E27.8
  synovial — *see* Tenosynovitis
  tendon (sheath) NEC — *see* Tenosynovitis
  testis — *see* Orchitis
  throat (acute) — *see* Pharyngitis
  thymus (gland) E32.8
  thyroid (gland) — *see* Thyroiditis
  tongue K14.0
  tonsil — *see* Tonsillitis
  trachea — *see* Tracheitis

Inflammation, inflamed, inflammatory (with exudation) — *continued*
  trochlear (nerve) — *see* Strabismus, paralytic, fourth nerve
  tubal — *see* Salpingo-oophoritis
  tuberculous NEC — *see* Tuberculosis
  tubo-ovarian — *see* Salpingo-oophoritis
  tunica vaginalis N49.1
  tympanic membrane — *see* Tympanitis
  umbilicus, umbilical L08.82
  uterine ligament — *see* Disease, pelvis, inflammatory
  uterus (catarrhal) — *see* Endometritis
  uveal tract (anterior) NOS — *see also* Iridocyclitis
    posterior — *see* Chorioretinitis
  vagina — *see* Vaginitis
  vas deferens N49.1
  vein — *see also* Phlebitis
    intracranial or intraspinal (septic) G08
    thrombotic I80.9
      leg — *see* Phlebitis, leg
      lower extremity — *see* Phlebitis, leg
  vocal cord J38.3
  vulva — *see* Vulvitis
  Wharton's duct (suppurative) — *see* Sialoadenitis
Inflation, lung, imperfect (newborn) — *see* Atelectasis
Influenza (bronchial) (epidemic) (respiratory (upper)) (unidentified influenza virus) J11.1
  with
    digestive manifestations J11.2
    encephalopathy J11.81
    enteritis J11.2
    gastroenteritis J11.2
    gastrointestinal manifestations J11.2
    laryngitis J11.1
    myocarditis J11.82
    otitis media J11.83
    pharyngitis J11.1
    pneumonia J11.00
      specified type J11.08
    respiratory manifestations NEC J11.1
    specified manifestation NEC J11.89
  A/H5N1 (*see also* Influenza, due to, identified novel influenza A virus) J09.x2
  avian (*see also* Influenza, due to, identified novel influenza A virus) J09.x2
  bird (*see also* Influenza, due to, identified novel influenza A virus) J09.x2
  due to
    avian (*see also* Influenza, due to, identified novel influenza A virus) J09.x2
    identified influenza virus NEC J10.1
      with
        digestive manifestations J10.2
        encephalopathy J10.81
        enteritis J10.2
        gastroenteritis J10.2
        gastrointestinal manifestations J10.2
        laryngitis J10.1
        myocarditis J10.82
        otitis media J10.83
        pharyngitis J10.1
        pneumonia (unspecified type) J10.00
          with same identified influenza virus J10.01
          specified type NEC J10.08
        respiratory manifestations NEC J10.1
        specified manifestation NEC J10.89
    identified novel influenza A virus J09.x2
      with
        digestive manifestations J09.x3
        encephalopathy J09.x9
        enteritis J09.x3
        gastroenteritis J09.x3
        gastrointestinal manifestations J09.x3
        laryngitis J09.x2

Influenza (bronchial) (epidemic) (respiratory
(upper)) (unidentified influenza virus) J11.1
due to — *continued*
  identified novel influenza A virus J09.x2 —
    continued
    with — *continued*
      myocarditis J09.x9
      otitis media J09.x9
      pharyngitis J09.x2
      pneumonia J09.x1
      respiratory manifestations NEC J09.x2
      specified manifestation NEC J09.x9
      upper respiratory symptoms J09.x2
  novel (2009) H1N1 influenza (*see also*
    Influenza, due to, identified influenza
    virus NEC) J10.1
  novel influenza A/H1N1 (*see also* Influenza,
    due to, identified influenza virus NEC)
    J10.1
  of other animal origin, not bird or swine (*see
    also* Influenza, due to, identified novel
    influenza A virus) J09.x2
  swine (viruses that normally cause infections in
    pigs) (*see also* Influenza, due to, identified
    novel influenza A virus) J09.x2
Influenzal — *see* Influenza
Influenza-like disease — *see* Influenza
Infraction, Freiberg's (metatarsal head) —
  see Osteochondrosis, juvenile, metatarsus
Infraeruption of tooth (teeth) M26.34
**Infusion complication, misadventure, or
  reaction** — *see* Complications, infusion
Ingestion
  chemical — *see* Table of Drugs and Chemicals,
    by substance, poisoning
  drug or medicament
    correct substance properly administered —
      see Table of Drugs and Chemicals, by
      drug, adverse effect
    overdose or wrong substance given or taken
      — *see* Table of Drugs and Chemicals, by
      drug, poisoning
  foreign body — *see* Foreign body, alimentary
    tract
  tularemia A21.3
Ingrowing
  hair (beard) L73.1
  nail (finger) (toe) L60.0
Inguinal — *see also* condition
  testicle Q53.9
    bilateral Q53.21
    unilateral Q53.11
Inhalant-induced
  anxiety disorder F18.980
  depressive disorder F18.94
  major neurocognitive disorder F18.97
  mild neurocognitive disorder F18.988
  psychotic disorder F18.959
Inhalation
  anthrax A22.1
  flame T27.3
  food or foreign body — *see* Foreign body, by
    site
  gases, fumes, or vapors NEC T59.9-
    specified agent — *see* Table of Drugs and
      Chemicals, by substance
  liquid or vomitus — *see* Asphyxia
  meconium (newborn) P24.00
    with
      with respiratory symptoms P24.01
      pneumonia (pneumonitis) P24.01
  mucus — *see* Asphyxia, mucus
  oil or gasoline (causing suffocation) — *see*
    Foreign body, by site
  smoke J70.5
    due to chemicals, gases, fumes and vapors
      J68.9
  steam — *see* Toxicity, vapors

Inhalation — *continued*
  stomach contents or secretions — *see* Foreign
    body, by site
    due to anesthesia (general) (local) or other
      sedation T88.59
    in labor and delivery O74.0
    in pregnancy O29.01-
    postpartum, puerperal O89.01
Inhibition, orgasm
  female F52.31
  male F52.32
Inhibitor, systemic lupus erythematosus
  (presence of) D68.62
Iniencephalus, iniencephaly Q00.2
Injection, traumatic jet (air) (industrial)
  (water) (paint or dye) T70.4
Injury (*see also* specified injury type) T14.90
  abdomen, abdominal S39.91
    blood vessel — *see* Injury, blood vessel,
      abdomen
    cavity — *see* Injury, intra-abdominal
    contusion S30.1
    internal — *see* Injury, intra-abdominal
    intra-abdominal organ — *see* Injury, intra-
      abdominal
    nerve — *see* Injury, nerve, abdomen
    open — *see* Wound, open, abdomen
    specified NEC S39.81
    superficial — *see* Injury, superficial,
      abdomen
  Achilles tendon S86.00-
    laceration S86.02-
    specified type NEC S86.09-
    strain S86.01-
  acoustic, resulting in deafness — *see* Injury,
    nerve, acoustic
  adrenal (gland) S37.819
    contusion S37.812
    laceration S37.813
    specified type NEC S37.818
  alveolar (process) S09.93
  ankle S99.91-
    contusion — *see* Contusion, ankle
    dislocation — *see* Dislocation, ankle
    fracture — *see* Fracture, ankle
    nerve — *see* Injury, nerve, ankle
    open — *see* Wound, open, ankle
    specified type NEC S99.81-
    sprain — *see* Sprain, ankle
    superficial — *see* Injury, superficial, ankle
  anterior chamber, eye — *see* Injury, eye,
    specified site NEC
  anus — *see* Injury, abdomen
  aorta (thoracic) S25.00
    abdominal S35.00
      laceration (minor) (superficial) S35.01
        major S35.02
      specified type NEC S35.09
    laceration (minor) (superficial) S25.01
      major S25.02
    specified type NEC S25.09
  arm (upper) S49.9-
    blood vessel — *see* Injury, blood vessel, arm
    contusion — *see* Contusion, arm, upper
    fracture — *see* Fracture, humerus
    lower — *see* Injury, forearm
    muscle — *see* Injury, muscle, shoulder
    nerve — *see* Injury, nerve, arm
    open — *see* Wound, open, arm
    specified type NEC S49.8-
    superficial — *see* Injury, superficial, arm
  artery (complicating trauma) — *see also* Injury,
    blood vessel, by site
    cerebral or meningeal — *see* Injury,
      intracranial
  auditory canal (external) (meatus) S09.91
  auricle, auris, ear S09.91
  axilla — *see* Injury, shoulder
  back — *see* Injury, back, lower

Injury (*see also* specified injury type) T14.90 —
  continued
  bile duct S36.13
  birth (*see also* Birth, injury) P15.9
  bladder (sphincter) S37.20
    at delivery O71.5
    contusion S37.22
    laceration S37.23
    obstetrical trauma O71.5
    specified type NEC S37.29
  blast (air) (hydraulic) (immersion) (underwater)
    NEC T14.8
    acoustic nerve trauma — *see* Injury, nerve,
      acoustic
    bladder — *see* Injury, bladder
    brain — *see* Concussion
    colon — *see* Injury, intestine, large, blast
      injury
    ear (primary) S09.31-
      secondary S09.39-
    generalized T70.8
    lung — *see* Injury, intrathoracic, lung, blast
      injury
    multiple body organs T70.8
    peritoneum S36.81
    rectum S36.61
    retroperitoneum S36.898
    small intestine S36.419
      duodenum S36.410
      specified site NEC S36.418
    specified
      intra-abdominal organ NEC S36.898
      pelvic organ NEC S37.899
  blood vessel NEC T14.8
    abdomen S35.9-
      aorta — *see* Injury, aorta, abdominal
      celiac artery — *see* Injury, blood vessel,
        celiac artery
      iliac vessel — *see* Injury, blood vessel, iliac
      laceration S35.91
      mesenteric vessel — *see* Injury, mesenteric
      portal vein — *see* Injury, blood vessel,
        portal vein
      renal vessel — *see* Injury, blood vessel,
        renal
      specified vessel NEC S35.8x-
      splenic vessel — *see* Injury, blood vessel,
        splenic
      vena cava — *see* Injury, vena cava,
        inferior
    ankle — *see* Injury, blood vessel, foot
    aorta (abdominal) (thoracic) — *see* Injury,
      aorta
    arm (upper) NEC S45.90-
      forearm — *see* Injury, blood vessel,
        forearm
      laceration S45.91-
      specified
        site NEC S45.80-
          laceration S45.81-
          specified type NEC S45.89-
        type NEC S45.99-
      superficial vein S45.30-
        laceration S45.31-
        specified type NEC S45.39-
    axillary
      artery S45.00-
        laceration S45.01-
        specified type NEC S45.09-
      vein S45.20-
        laceration S45.21-
        specified type NEC S45.29-
    azygos vein — *see* Injury, blood vessel,
      thoracic, specified site NEC
    brachial
      artery S45.10-
        laceration S45.11-
        specified type NEC S45.19-

DISEASE INDEX

Injury (*see also* specified injury type) T14.90 — continued
  blood vessel NEC T14.8 — *continued*
    brachial — *continued*
      vein S45.20-
        laceration S45.219
        specified type NEC S45.29-
    carotid artery (common) (external) (internal, extracranial) S15.00-
      internal, intracranial S06.8-
      laceration (minor) (superficial) S15.01-
        major S15.02-
      specified type NEC S15.09-
    celiac artery S35.219
      branch S35.299
        laceration (minor) (superficial) S35.291
          major S35.292
        specified NEC S35.298
      laceration (minor) (superficial) S35.211
        major S35.212
      specified type NEC S35.218
    cerebral — *see* Injury, intracranial
    deep plantar — *see* Injury, blood vessel, plantar artery
    digital (hand) — *see* Injury, blood vessel, finger
    dorsal
      artery (foot) S95.00-
        laceration S95.01-
        specified type NEC S95.09-
      vein (foot) S95.20-
        laceration S95.21-
        specified type NEC S95.29-
    due to accidental laceration during procedure — *see* Laceration, accidental complicating surgery
    extremity — *see* Injury, blood vessel, limb
    femoral
      artery (common) (superficial) S75.00-
        laceration (minor) (superficial) S75.01-
          major S75.02-
        specified type NEC S75.09-
      vein (hip level) (thigh level) S75.10-
        laceration (minor) (superficial) S75.11-
          major S75.12-
        specified type NEC S75.19-
    finger S65.50-
      index S65.50-
        laceration S65.51-
        specified type NEC S65.59-
      laceration S65.51-
      little S65.50-
        laceration S65.51-
        specified type NEC S65.59-
      middle S65.50-
      specified type NEC S65.59-
      thumb — *see* Injury, blood vessel, thumb
    foot S95.90-
      dorsal
        artery — *see* Injury, blood vessel, dorsal, artery
        vein — *see* Injury, blood vessel, dorsal, vein
      laceration S95.91-
      plantar artery — *see* Injury, blood vessel, plantar artery
      specified
        site NEC S95.80-
          laceration S95.81-
          specified type NEC S95.89-
        specified type NEC S95.99-
    forearm S55.90-
      laceration S55.91-
      radial artery — *see* Injury, blood vessel, radial artery

Injury (*see also* specified injury type) T14.90 — continued
  blood vessel NEC T14.8 — *continued*
    forearm S55.90- — *continued*
      specified
        site NEC S55.80-
          laceration S55.81-
          specified type NEC S55.89-
        type NEC S55.99-
      ulnar artery — *see* Injury, blood vessel, ulnar artery
      vein S55.20-
        laceration S55.21-
        specified type NEC S55.29-
    gastric
      artery — *see* Injury, mesenteric, artery, branch
      vein — *see* Injury, blood vessel, abdomen
    gastroduodenal artery — *see* Injury, mesenteric, artery, branch
    greater saphenous vein (lower leg level) S85.30-
      hip (and thigh) level S75.20-
        laceration (minor) (superficial) S75.21-
          major S75.22-
        specified type NEC S75.29-
      laceration S85.31-
      specified type NEC S85.39-
    hand (level) S65.90-
      finger — *see* Injury, blood vessel, finger
      laceration S65.91-
      palmar arch — *see* Injury, blood vessel, palmar arch
      radial artery — *see* Injury, blood vessel, radial artery, hand
      specified
        site NEC S65.80-
          laceration S65.81-
          specified type NEC S65.89-
        type NEC S65.99-
      thumb — *see* Injury, blood vessel, thumb
      ulnar artery — *see* Injury, blood vessel, ulnar artery, hand
    head S09.0
      intracranial — *see* Injury, intracranial
      multiple S09.0
    hepatic
      artery — *see* Injury, mesenteric, artery
      vein — *see* Injury, vena cava, inferior
    hip S75.90-
      femoral artery — *see* Injury, blood vessel, femoral, artery
      femoral vein — *see* Injury, blood vessel, femoral, vein
      greater saphenous vein — *see* Injury, blood vessel, greater saphenous, hip level
      laceration S75.91-
      specified
        site NEC S75.80-
          laceration S75.81-
          specified type NEC S75.89-
        type NEC S75.99-
    hypogastric (artery) (vein) — *see* Injury, blood vessel, iliac
    iliac S35.5-
      artery S35.51-
      specified vessel NEC S35.5-
      uterine vessel — *see* Injury, blood vessel, uterine
      vein S35.51-
    innominate — *see* Injury, blood vessel, thoracic, innominate
    intercostal (artery) (vein) — *see* Injury, blood vessel, thoracic, intercostal

Injury (*see also* specified injury type) T14.90 — continued
  blood vessel NEC T14.8 — *continued*
    jugular vein (external) S15.20-
      internal S15.30-
        laceration (minor) (superficial) S15.31-
          major S15.32-
        specified type NEC S15.39-
      laceration (minor) (superficial) S15.21-
        major S15.22-
      specified type NEC S15.29-
    leg (level) (lower) S85.90-
      greater saphenous — *see* Injury, blood vessel, greater saphenous
      laceration S85.91-
      lesser saphenous — *see* Injury, blood vessel, lesser saphenous
      peroneal artery — *see* Injury, blood vessel, peroneal artery
      popliteal
        artery — *see* Injury, blood vessel, popliteal, artery
        vein — *see* Injury, blood vessel, popliteal, vein
      specified
        site NEC S85.80-
          laceration S85.81-
          specified type NEC S85.89-
        type NEC S85.99-
      thigh — *see* Injury, blood vessel, hip
      tibial artery — *see* Injury, blood vessel, tibial artery
    lesser saphenous vein (lower leg level) S85.40-
      laceration S85.41-
      specified type NEC S85.49-
    limb
      lower — *see* Injury, blood vessel, leg
      upper — *see* Injury, blood vessel, arm
    lower back — *see* Injury, blood vessel, abdomen
      specified NEC — *see* Injury, blood vessel, abdomen, specified, site NEC
    mammary (artery) (vein) — *see* Injury, blood vessel, thoracic, specified site NEC
    mesenteric (inferior) (superior)
      artery — *see* Injury, mesenteric, artery
      vein — *see* Injury, mesenteric, vein
    neck S15.9
      specified site NEC S15.8
    ovarian (artery) (vein) — *see* subcategory S35.8
    palmar arch (superficial) S65.20-
      deep S65.30-
        laceration S65.31-
        specified type NEC S65.39-
      laceration S65.21-
      specified type NEC S65.29-
    pelvis — *see* Injury, blood vessel, abdomen
      specified NEC — *see* Injury, blood vessel, abdomen, specified, site NEC
    peroneal artery S85.20-
      laceration S85.21-
      specified type NEC S85.29-
    plantar artery (deep) (foot) S95.10-
      laceration S95.11-
      specified type NEC S95.19-
    popliteal
      artery S85.00-
        laceration S85.01-
        specified type NEC S85.09-
      vein S85.50-
        laceration S85.51-
        specified type NEC S85.59-
    portal vein S35.319
      laceration S35.311
      specified type NEC S35.318
    precerebral — *see* Injury, blood vessel, neck

Injury (*see also* specified injury type) T14.90 — *continued*
  blood vessel NEC T14.8 — *continued*
    pulmonary (artery) (vein) — *see* Injury, blood vessel, thoracic, pulmonary
    radial artery (forearm level) S55.10-
      hand and wrist (level) S65.10-
        laceration S65.11-
        specified type NEC S65.19-
      laceration S55.11-
      specified type NEC S55.19-
    renal
      artery S35.40-
        laceration S35.41-
        specified NEC S35.49-
      vein S35.40-
        laceration S35.41-
        specified NEC S35.49-
    saphenous vein (greater) (lower leg level) — *see* Injury, blood vessel, greater saphenous
      hip and thigh level — *see* Injury, blood vessel, greater saphenous, hip level
      lesser — *see* Injury, blood vessel, lesser saphenous
    shoulder
      specified NEC — *see* Injury, blood vessel, arm, specified site NEC
      superficial vein — *see* Injury, blood vessel, arm, superficial vein
    specified NEC T14.8
    splenic
      artery — *see* Injury, blood vessel, celiac artery, branch
      vein S35.329
        laceration S35.321
        specified NEC S35.328
    subclavian — *see* Injury, blood vessel, thoracic, innominate
    thigh — *see* Injury, blood vessel, hip
    thoracic S25.90
      aorta S25.00
        laceration (minor) (superficial) S25.01
          major S25.02
        specified type NEC S25.09
      azygos vein — *see* Injury, blood vessel, thoracic, specified, site NEC
      innominate
        artery S25.10-
          laceration (minor) (superficial) S25.11-
            major S25.12-
          specified type NEC S25.19-
        vein S25.30-
          laceration (minor) (superficial) S25.31-
            major S25.32-
          specified type NEC S25.39-
      intercostal S25.50-
        laceration S25.51-
        specified type NEC S25.59-
      laceration S25.91
      mammary vessel — *see* Injury, blood vessel, thoracic, specified, site NEC
      pulmonary S25.40-
        laceration (minor) (superficial) S25.41-
          major S25.42-
        specified type NEC S25.49-
      specified
        site NEC S25.80-
          laceration S25.81-
          specified type NEC S25.89-
        type NEC S25.99
      subclavian — *see* Injury, blood vessel, thoracic, innominate
      vena cava (superior) S25.20
        laceration (minor) (superficial) S25.21
          major S25.22
        specified type NEC S25.29

Injury (*see also* specified injury type) T14.90 — *continued*
  blood vessel NEC T14.8 — *continued*
    thumb S65.40-
      laceration S65.41-
      specified type NEC S65.49-
    tibial artery S85.10-
      anterior S85.13-
        laceration S85.14-
        specified injury NEC S85.15-
      laceration S85.11-
      posterior S85.16-
        laceration S85.17-
        specified injury NEC S85.18-
      specified injury NEC S85.12-
    ulnar artery (forearm level) S55.00-
      hand and wrist (level) S65.00-
        laceration S65.01-
        specified type NEC S65.09-
      laceration S55.01-
      specified type NEC S55.09-
    upper arm (level) — *see* Injury, blood vessel, arm
    superficial vein — *see* Injury, blood vessel, arm, superficial vein
    uterine S35.5-
      artery S35.53-
      vein S35.53-
    vena cava — *see* Injury, vena cava
    vertebral artery S15.10-
      laceration (minor) (superficial) S15.11-
        major S15.12-
      specified type NEC S15.19-
    wrist (level) — *see* Injury, blood vessel, hand
  brachial plexus S14.3
    newborn P14.3
  brain (traumatic) S06.9-
    diffuse (axonal) S06.2x-
    focal S06.30-
  brainstem S06.38-
  breast NOS S29.9
  broad ligament — *see* Injury, pelvic organ, specified site NEC
  bronchus, bronchi — *see* Injury, intrathoracic, bronchus
  brow S09.90
  buttock S39.92
  canthus, eye S05.90
  cardiac plexus — *see* Injury, nerve, thorax, sympathetic
  cauda equina S34.3
  cavernous sinus — *see* Injury, intracranial
  cecum — *see* Injury, colon
  celiac ganglion or plexus — *see* Injury, nerve, lumbosacral, sympathetic
  cerebellum — *see* Injury, intracranial
  cerebral — *see* Injury, intracranial
  cervix (uteri) — *see* Injury, uterus
  cheek (wall) S09.93
  chest — *see* Injury, thorax
  childbirth (newborn) — *see also* Birth, injury maternal NEC O71.9
  chin S09.93
  choroid (eye) — *see* Injury, eye, specified site NEC
  clitoris S39.94
  coccyx — *see also* Injury, back, lower complicating delivery O71.6
  colon — *see* Injury, intestine, large
  common bile duct — *see* Injury, liver
  conjunctiva (superficial) — *see* Injury, eye, conjunctiva
  conus medullaris — *see* Injury, spinal, sacral cord
    spermatic (pelvic region) S37.898
      scrotal region S39.848
  spinal — *see* Injury, spinal cord, by region

Injury (*see also* specified injury type) T14.90 — *continued*
  cornea — *see* Injury, eye, specified site NEC
    abrasion — *see* Injury, eye, cornea, abrasion
  cortex (cerebral) — *see also* Injury, intracranial
    visual — *see* Injury, nerve, optic
  costal region NEC S29.9
  costochondral NEC S29.9
  cranial
    cavity — *see* Injury, intracranial
    nerve — *see* Injury, nerve, cranial
  crushing — *see* Crush
  cutaneous sensory nerve
  cystic duct — *see* Injury, liver
  deep tissue — *see* Contusion, by site
    meaning pressure ulcer — *see* Ulcer, pressure, unstageable, by site
  delivery (newborn) P15.9
    maternal NEC O71.9
  Descemet's membrane — *see* Injury, eyeball, penetrating
  diaphragm — *see* Injury, intrathoracic, diaphragm
  duodenum — *see* Injury, intestine, small, duodenum
  ear (auricle) (external) (canal) S09.91
    abrasion — *see* Abrasion, ear
    bite — *see* Bite, ear
    blister — *see* Blister, ear
    bruise — *see* Contusion, ear
    contusion — *see* Contusion, ear
    external constriction — *see* Constriction, external, ear
    hematoma — *see* Hematoma, ear
    inner — *see* Injury, ear, middle
    laceration — *see* Laceration, ear
    middle S09.30-
      blast — *see* Injury, blast, ear
      specified NEC S09.39-
    puncture — *see* Puncture, ear
    superficial — *see* Injury, superficial, ear
  eighth cranial nerve (acoustic or auditory) — *see* Injury, nerve, acoustic
  elbow S59.90-
    contusion — *see* Contusion, elbow
    dislocation — *see* Dislocation, elbow
    fracture — *see* Fracture, ulna, upper end
    open — *see* Wound, open, elbow
    specified NEC S59.80-
    sprain — *see* Sprain, elbow
    superficial — *see* Injury, superficial, elbow
  eleventh cranial nerve (accessory) — *see* Injury, nerve, accessory
  epididymis S39.94
  epigastric region S39.91
  epiglottis NEC S19.89
  esophageal plexus — *see* Injury, nerve, thorax, sympathetic
  esophagus (thoracic part) — *see also* Injury, intrathoracic, esophagus
    cervical NEC S19.85
  eustachian tube S09.30-
  eye S05.9-
    avulsion S05.7-
    ball — *see* Injury, eyeball
    conjunctiva S05.0-
    cornea
      abrasion S05.0-
      laceration S05.3-
        with prolapse S05.2-
    lacrimal apparatus S05.8x-
    orbit penetration S05.4-
    specified site NEC S05.8x-

Injury (*see also* specified injury type) T14.90 — *continued*
- eyeball S05.8x-
  - contusion S05.1-
  - penetrating S05.6-
    - with
      - foreign body S05.5-
        - prolapse or loss of intraocular tissue S05.2-
      - without prolapse or loss of intraocular tissue S05.3-
    - specified type NEC S05.8-
- eyebrow S09.93
- eyelid S09.93
  - abrasion — *see* Abrasion, eyelid
  - contusion — *see* Contusion, eyelid
  - open — *see* Wound, open, eyelid
- face S09.93
- fallopian tube S37.509
  - bilateral S37.502
    - blast injury S37.512
    - contusion S37.522
    - laceration S37.532
    - specified type NEC S37.592
  - blast injury (primary) S37.519
    - bilateral S37.512
    - secondary — *see* Injury, fallopian tube, specified type NEC
    - unilateral S37.511
  - contusion S37.529
    - bilateral S37.522
    - unilateral S37.521
  - laceration S37.539
    - bilateral S37.532
    - unilateral S37.531
  - specified type NEC S37.599
    - bilateral S37.592
    - unilateral S37.591
  - unilateral S37.501
    - blast injury S37.511
    - contusion S37.521
    - laceration S37.531
    - specified type NEC S37.591
- fascia — *see* Injury, muscle
- fifth cranial nerve (trigeminal) — *see* Injury, nerve, trigeminal
- finger (nail) S69.9-
  - blood vessel — *see* Injury, blood vessel, finger
  - contusion — *see* Contusion, finger
  - dislocation — *see* Dislocation, finger
  - fracture — *see* Fracture, finger
  - muscle — *see* Injury, muscle, finger
  - nerve — *see* Injury, nerve, digital, finger
  - open — *see* Wound, open, finger
  - specified NEC S69.8-
  - sprain — *see* Sprain, finger
  - superficial — *see* Injury, superficial, finger
- first cranial nerve (olfactory) — *see* Injury, nerve, olfactory
- flank — *see* Injury, abdomen
- foot S99.92-
  - blood vessel — *see* Injury, blood vessel, foot
  - contusion — *see* Contusion, foot
  - dislocation — *see* Dislocation, foot
  - fracture — *see* Fracture, foot
  - muscle — *see* Injury, muscle, foot
  - open — *see* Wound, open, foot
  - specified type NEC S99.82-
  - sprain — *see* Sprain, foot
  - superficial — *see* Injury, superficial, foot
- forceps NOS P15.9
- forearm S59.91-
  - blood vessel — *see* Injury, blood vessel, forearm
  - contusion — *see* Contusion, forearm
  - fracture — *see* Fracture, forearm
  - muscle — *see* Injury, muscle, forearm
  - nerve — *see* Injury, nerve, forearm

Injury (*see also* specified injury type) T14.90 — *continued*
- forearm S59.91- — *continued*
  - open — *see* Wound, open, forearm
  - specified NEC S59.81-
  - superficial — *see* Injury, superficial, forearm
- forehead S09.90
- fourth cranial nerve (trochlear) — *see* Injury, nerve, trochlear
- gallbladder S36.129
  - contusion S36.122
  - laceration S36.123
  - specified NEC S36.128
- ganglion
  - celiac, coeliac — *see* Injury, nerve, lumbosacral, sympathetic
  - gasserian — *see* Injury, nerve, trigeminal
  - stellate — *see* Injury, nerve, thorax, sympathetic
  - thoracic sympathetic — *see* Injury, nerve, thorax, sympathetic
- gasserian ganglion — *see* Injury, nerve, trigeminal
- gastric artery — *see* Injury, blood vessel, celiac artery, branch
- gastroduodenal artery — *see* Injury, blood vessel, celiac artery, branch
- gastrointestinal tract — *see* Injury, intra-abdominal
  - with open wound into abdominal cavity — *see* Wound, open, with penetration into peritoneal cavity
  - colon — *see* Injury, intestine, large
  - rectum — *see* Injury, intestine, large, rectum
    - with open wound into abdominal cavity S36.61
  - small intestine — *see* Injury, intestine, small
  - specified site NEC — *see* Injury, intra-abdominal, specified, site NEC
  - stomach — *see* Injury, stomach
- genital organ(s)
  - external S39.94
    - specified NEC S39.848
  - internal S37.90
    - fallopian tube — *see* Injury, fallopian tube
    - ovary — *see* Injury, ovary
    - prostate — *see* Injury, prostate
    - seminal vesicle — *see* Injury, pelvis, organ, specified site NEC
    - uterus — *see* Injury, uterus
    - vas deferens — *see* Injury, pelvis, organ, specified site NEC
  - obstetrical trauma O71.9
- gland
  - lacrimal laceration — *see* Injury, eye, specified site NEC
  - salivary S09.93
  - thyroid NEC S19.84
- globe (eye) S05.90
  - specified NEC S05.8x-
- groin — *see* Injury, abdomen
- gum S09.90
- hand S69.9-
  - blood vessel — *see* Injury, blood vessel, hand
  - contusion — *see* Contusion, hand
  - fracture — *see* Fracture, hand
  - muscle — *see* Injury, muscle, hand
  - nerve — *see* Injury, nerve, hand
  - open — *see* Wound, open, hand
  - specified NEC S69.8-
  - sprain — *see* Sprain, hand
  - superficial — *see* Injury, superficial, hand
- head S09.90
  - with loss of consciousness S06.9-
  - specified NEC S09.8

Injury (*see also* specified injury type) T14.90 — *continued*
- heart S26.90
  - with hemopericardium S26.00
    - contusion S26.01
    - laceration (mild) S26.020
      - major S26.022
      - moderate S26.021
    - specified type NEC S26.09
  - contusion S26.91
  - laceration S26.92
  - specified type NEC S26.99
  - without hemopericardium S26.10
    - contusion S26.11
    - laceration S26.12
    - specified type NEC S26.19
- heel — *see* Injury, foot
- hepatic
  - artery — *see* Injury, blood vessel, celiac artery, branch
  - duct — *see* Injury, liver
  - vein — *see* Injury, vena cava, inferior
- hip S79.91-
  - blood vessel — *see* Injury, blood vessel, hip
  - contusion — *see* Contusion, hip
  - dislocation — *see* Dislocation, hip
  - fracture — *see* Fracture, femur, neck
  - muscle — *see* Injury, muscle, hip
  - nerve — *see* Injury, nerve, hip
  - open — *see* Wound, open, hip
  - specified NEC S79.81-
  - sprain — *see* Sprain, hip
  - superficial — *see* Injury, superficial, hip
- hymen S39.94
- hypogastric
  - blood vessel — *see* Injury, blood vessel, iliac
  - plexus — *see* Injury, nerve, lumbosacral, sympathetic
- ileum — *see* Injury, intestine, small
- iliac region S39.91
- instrumental (during surgery) — *see* Laceration, accidental complicating surgery
  - birth injury — *see* Birth, injury
  - nonsurgical — *see* Injury, by site
  - obstetrical O71.9
    - bladder O71.5
    - cervix O71.3
    - high vaginal O71.4
    - perineal NOS O70.9
    - urethra O71.5
    - uterus O71.5
      - with rupture or perforation O71.1
- internal T14.8
  - aorta — *see* Injury, aorta
  - bladder (sphincter) — *see* Injury, bladder
    - with
      - ectopic or molar pregnancy O08.6
      - following ectopic or molar pregnancy O08.6
      - obstetrical trauma O71.5
  - bronchus, bronchi — *see* Injury, intrathoracic, bronchus
  - cecum — *see* Injury, intestine, large
  - cervix (uteri) — *see also* Injury, uterus
    - with ectopic or molar pregnancy O08.6
    - following ectopic or molar pregnancy O08.6
    - obstetrical trauma O71.3
  - chest — *see* Injury, intrathoracic
  - gastrointestinal tract — *see* Injury, intra-abdominal
  - heart — *see* Injury, heart
  - intestine NEC — *see* Injury, intestine
  - intrauterine — *see* Injury, uterus
  - mesentery — *see* Injury, intra-abdominal, specified, site NEC

Injury (*see also* specified injury type) T14.90 — *continued*
  internal T14.8 — *continued*
    pelvis, pelvic (organ) S37.90
      following ectopic or molar pregnancy (subsequent episode) O08.6
      obstetrical trauma NEC O71.5
      rupture or perforation O71.1
      specified NEC S39.83
    rectum — *see* Injury, intestine, large, rectum
    stomach — *see* Injury, stomach
    ureter — *see* Injury, ureter
    urethra (sphincter) following ectopic or molar pregnancy O08.6
    uterus — *see* Injury, uterus
  interscapular area — *see* Injury, thorax
  intestine
    large S36.509
      ascending (right) S36.500
        blast injury (primary) S36.510
          secondary S36.590
        contusion S36.520
        laceration S36.530
        specified type NEC S36.590
      blast injury (primary) S36.519
        ascending (right) S36.510
        descending (left) S36.512
        rectum S36.61
        sigmoid S36.513
        specified site NEC S36.518
        transverse S36.511
      contusion S36.529
        ascending (right) S36.520
        descending (left) S36.522
        rectum S36.62
        sigmoid S36.523
        specified site NEC S36.528
        transverse S36.521
      descending (left) S36.502
        blast injury (primary) S36.512
          secondary S36.592
        contusion S36.522
        laceration S36.532
        specified type NEC S36.592
      laceration S36.539
        ascending (right) S36.530
        descending (left) S36.532
        rectum S36.63
        sigmoid S36.533
        specified site NEC S36.538
        transverse S36.531
      rectum S36.60
        blast injury (primary) S36.61
          secondary S36.69
        contusion S36.62
        laceration S36.63
        specified type NEC S36.69
      sigmoid S36.503
        blast injury (primary) S36.513
          secondary S36.593
        contusion S36.523
        laceration S36.533
        specified type NEC S36.593
      specified
        site NEC S36.508
          blast injury (primary) S36.518
            secondary S36.598
          contusion S36.528
          laceration S36.538
          specified type NEC S36.598
        type NEC S36.599
          ascending (right) S36.590
          descending (left) S36.592
          rectum S36.69
          sigmoid S36.593
          specified site NEC S36.598
          transverse S36.591

Injury (*see also* specified injury type) T14.90 — *continued*
  intestine — *continued*
    large S36.509 — *continued*
      transverse S36.501
        blast injury (primary) S36.511
          secondary S36.591
        contusion S36.521
        laceration S36.531
        specified type NEC S36.591
    small S36.409
      blast injury (primary) S36.419
        duodenum S36.410
        secondary S36.499
          duodenum S36.490
          specified site NEC S36.498
        specified site NEC S36.418
      contusion S36.429
        duodenum S36.420
        specified site NEC S36.428
      duodenum S36.400
        blast injury (primary) S36.410
          secondary S36.490
        contusion S36.420
        laceration S36.430
        specified NEC S36.490
      laceration S36.439
        duodenum S36.430
        specified site NEC S36.438
      specified
        site NEC S36.408
        type NEC S36.499
          duodenum S36.490
          specified site NEC S36.498
    intra-abdominal S36.90
      adrenal gland — *see* Injury, adrenal gland
      bladder — *see* Injury, bladder
      colon — *see* Injury, intestine, large
      contusion S36.92
      fallopian tube — *see* Injury, fallopian tube
      gallbladder — *see* Injury, gallbladder
      intestine — *see* Injury, intestine
      kidney — *see* Injury, kidney
      laceration S36.93
      liver — *see* Injury, liver
      ovary — *see* Injury, ovary
      pancreas — *see* Injury, pancreas
      pelvic NOS S37.90
      peritoneum — *see* Injury, intra-abdominal, specified, site NEC
      prostate — *see* Injury, prostate
      rectum — *see* Injury, intestine, large, rectum
      retroperitoneum — *see* Injury, intra-abdominal, specified, site NEC
      seminal vesicle — *see* Injury, pelvis, organ, specified site NEC
      small intestine — *see* Injury, intestine, small
      specified
        pelvic S37.90
          specified
            site NEC S37.899
              specified type NEC S37.898
            type NEC S37.99
          site NEC S36.899
            contusion S36.892
            laceration S36.893
            specified type NEC S36.898
          type NEC S36.99
        spleen — *see* Injury, spleen
        stomach — *see* Injury, stomach
        ureter — *see* Injury, ureter
        urethra — *see* Injury, urethra
        uterus — *see* Injury, uterus
        vas deferens — *see* Injury, pelvis, organ, specified site NEC

Injury (*see also* specified injury type) T14.90 — *continued*
  intracranial (traumatic) S06.9-
    cerebellar hemorrhage, traumatic — *see* Injury, intracranial, focal
    cerebral edema, traumatic S06.1x-
      diffuse S06.1x-
      focal S06.1x-
    diffuse (axonal) S06.2x-
    epidural hemorrhage (traumatic) S06.4x-
    focal brain injury S06.30-
      contusion — *see* Contusion, cerebral
      laceration — *see* Laceration, cerebral
    intracerebral hemorrhage, traumatic S06.36-
      left side S06.35-
      right side S06.34-
    subarachnoid hemorrhage, traumatic S06.6x-
    subdural hemorrhage, traumatic S06.5x-
  intraocular — *see* Injury, eyeball, penetrating
  intrathoracic S27.9
    bronchus S27.409
      bilateral S27.402
      blast injury (primary) S27.419
        bilateral S27.412
        secondary — *see* Injury, intrathoracic, bronchus, specified type NEC
        unilateral S27.411
      contusion S27.429
        bilateral S27.422
        unilateral S27.421
      laceration S27.439
        bilateral S27.432
        unilateral S27.431
      specified type NEC S27.499
        bilateral S27.492
        unilateral S27.491
      unilateral S27.401
    diaphragm S27.809
      contusion S27.802
      laceration S27.803
      specified type NEC S27.808
    esophagus (thoracic) S27.819
      contusion S27.812
      laceration S27.813
      specified type NEC S27.818
    heart — *see* Injury, heart
    hemopneumothorax S27.2
    hemothorax S27.1
    lung S27.309
      aspiration J69.0
      bilateral S27.302
      blast injury (primary) S27.319
        bilateral S27.312
        secondary — *see* Injury, intrathoracic, lung, specified type NEC
        unilateral S27.311
      contusion S27.329
        bilateral S27.322
        unilateral S27.321
      laceration S27.339
        bilateral S27.332
        unilateral S27.331
      specified type NEC S27.399
        bilateral S27.392
        unilateral S27.391
      unilateral S27.301
    pleura S27.60
      laceration S27.63
      specified type NEC S27.69
    pneumothorax S27.0
    specified organ NEC S27.899
      contusion S27.892
      laceration S27.893
      specified type NEC S27.898
    thoracic duct — *see* Injury, intrathoracic, specified organ NEC

Injury (see also specified injury type) T14.90 — continued
- intrathoracic S27.9 — continued
  - thymus gland — see Injury, intrathoracic, specified organ NEC
  - trachea, thoracic S27.50
    - blast (primary) S27.51
    - contusion S27.52
    - laceration S27.53
    - specified type NEC S27.59
- iris — see Injury, eye, specified site NEC
  - penetrating — see Injury, eyeball, penetrating
- jaw S09.93
- jejunum — see Injury, intestine, small
- joint NOS T14.8
  - old or residual — see Disorder, joint, specified type NEC
- kidney S37.00-
  - acute (nontraumatic) N17.9
  - contusion — see Contusion, kidney
  - laceration — see Laceration, kidney
  - specified NEC S37.09-
- knee S89.9-
  - contusion — see Contusion, knee
  - dislocation — see Dislocation, knee
  - meniscus (lateral) (medial) — see Sprain, knee, specified site NEC
    - old injury or tear — see Derangement, knee, meniscus, due to old injury
  - open — see Wound, open, knee
  - specified NEC S89.8-
  - sprain — see Sprain, knee
  - superficial — see Injury, superficial, knee
- labium (majus) (minus) S39.94
- labyrinth, ear S09.30-
- lacrimal apparatus, duct, gland, or sac — see Injury, eye, specified site NEC
- larynx NEC S19.81
- leg (lower) S89.9-
  - blood vessel — see Injury, blood vessel, leg
  - contusion — see Contusion, leg
  - fracture — see Fracture, leg
  - muscle — see Injury, muscle, leg
  - nerve — see Injury, nerve, leg
  - open — see Wound, open, leg
  - specified NEC S89.8-
  - superficial — see Injury, superficial, leg
- lens, eye — see Injury, eye, specified site NEC
  - penetrating — see Injury, eyeball, penetrating
- limb NEC T14.8
- lip S09.93
- liver S36.119
  - contusion S36.112
  - laceration S36.113
    - major (stellate) S36.116
    - minor S36.114
    - moderate S36.115
  - specified NEC S36.118
- lower back S39.92
  - specified NEC S39.82
- lumbar, lumbosacral (region) S39.92
  - plexus — see Injury, lumbosacral plexus
- lumbosacral plexus S34.4
- lung — see also Injury, intrathoracic, lung
  - aspiration J69.0
  - transfusion-related (TRALI) J95.84
- lymphatic thoracic duct — see Injury, intrathoracic, specified organ NEC
- malar region S09.93
- mastoid region S09.90
- maxilla S09.93
- mediastinum — see Injury, intrathoracic, specified organ NEC
- membrane, brain — see Injury, intracranial
- meningeal artery — see Injury, intracranial, subdural hemorrhage
- meninges (cerebral) — see Injury, intracranial

Injury (see also specified injury type) T14.90 — continued
- mesenteric
  - artery
    - branch S35.299
      - laceration (minor) (superficial) S35.291
        - major S35.292
      - specified NEC S35.298
    - inferior S35.239
      - laceration (minor) (superficial) S35.231
        - major S35.232
      - specified NEC S35.238
    - superior S35.229
      - laceration (minor) (superficial) S35.221
        - major S35.222
      - specified NEC S35.228
  - plexus (inferior) (superior) — see Injury, nerve, lumbosacral, sympathetic
  - vein
    - inferior S35.349
      - laceration S35.341
      - specified NEC S35.348
    - superior S35.339
      - laceration S35.331
      - specified NEC S35.338
- mesentery — see Injury, intra-abdominal, specified site NEC
- mesosalpinx — see Injury, pelvic organ, specified site NEC
- middle ear S09.30-
- midthoracic region NOS S29.9
- mouth S09.93
- multiple NOS T07
- muscle (and fascia) (and tendon)
  - abdomen S39.001
    - laceration S39.021
    - specified type NEC S39.091
    - strain S39.011
  - abductor
    - thumb, forearm level — see Injury, muscle, thumb, abductor
  - adductor
    - thigh S76.20-
      - laceration S76.22-
      - specified type NEC S76.29-
      - strain S76.21-
    - ankle — see Injury, muscle, foot
  - anterior muscle group, at leg level (lower) S86.20-
    - laceration S86.22-
    - specified type NEC S86.29-
    - strain S86.21-
  - arm (upper) — see Injury, muscle, shoulder
  - biceps (parts NEC) S46.20-
    - laceration S46.22-
    - long head S46.10-
      - laceration S46.12-
      - specified type NEC S46.19-
      - strain S46.11-
    - specified type NEC S46.29-
    - strain S46.21-
  - extensor
    - finger(s) (other than thumb) — see Injury, muscle, finger by site, extensor
    - forearm level, specified NEC — see Injury, muscle, forearm, extensor
    - thumb — see Injury, muscle, thumb, extensor
    - toe (large) (ankle level) (foot level) — see Injury, muscle, toe, extensor
  - finger
    - extensor (forearm level) S56.40-
      - hand level S66.309
        - laceration S66.329
        - specified type NEC S66.399
        - strain S66.319
      - laceration S56.429
      - specified type NEC S56.499
      - strain S56.419

Injury (see also specified injury type) T14.90 — continued
- muscle (and fascia) (and tendon) — continued
  - finger — continued
    - flexor (forearm level) S56.10-
      - hand level S66.109
        - laceration S66.129
        - specified type NEC S66.199
        - strain S66.119
      - laceration S56.129
      - specified type NEC S56.199
      - strain S56.119
    - index
      - extensor (forearm level)
        - hand level S66.308
          - laceration S66.32-
          - specified type NEC S66.39-
          - strain S66.31-
        - specified type NEC S56.492-
      - flexor (forearm level)
        - hand level S66.108
          - laceration S66.12-
          - specified type NEC S66.19-
          - strain S66.11-
        - specified type NEC S56.19-
        - strain S56.11-
      - intrinsic S66.50-
        - laceration S66.52-
        - specified type NEC S66.59-
        - strain S66.51-
    - intrinsic S66.509
      - laceration S66.529
      - specified type NEC S66.599
      - strain S66.519
    - little
      - extensor (forearm level)
        - hand level S66.30-
          - laceration S66.32-
          - specified type NEC S66.39-
          - strain S66.31-
        - laceration S56.42-
        - specified type NEC S56.49-
        - strain S56.41-
      - flexor (forearm level)
        - hand level S66.10-
          - laceration S66.12-
          - specified type NEC S66.19-
          - strain S66.11-
        - laceration S56.12-
        - specified type NEC S56.19-
        - strain S56.11-
      - intrinsic S66.50-
        - laceration S66.52-
        - specified type NEC S66.59-
        - strain S66.51-
    - middle
      - extensor (forearm level)
        - hand level S66.30-
          - laceration S66.32-
          - specified type NEC S66.39-
          - strain S66.31-
        - laceration S56.42-
        - specified type NEC S56.49-
        - strain S56.41-
      - flexor (forearm level)
        - hand level S66.10-
          - laceration S66.12-
          - specified type NEC S66.19-
          - strain S66.11-
        - laceration S56.12-
        - specified type NEC S56.19-
        - strain S56.11-
      - intrinsic S66.50-
        - laceration S66.52-
        - specified type NEC S66.59-
        - strain S66.51-

Injury (*see also* specified injury type) T14.90 — *continued*
muscle (and fascia) (and tendon) — *continued*
  finger — *continued*
    ring
      extensor (forearm level)
        hand level S66.30-
          laceration S66.32-
          specified type NEC S66.39-
          strain S66.31-
        laceration S56.42-
        specified type NEC S56.49-
        strain S56.41-
      flexor (forearm level)
        hand level S66.10-
          laceration S66.12-
          specified type NEC S66.19-
          strain S66.11-
        laceration S56.12-
        specified type NEC S56.19-
        strain S56.11-
      intrinsic S66.50-
        laceration S66.52-
        specified type NEC S66.59-
        strain S66.51-
  flexor
    finger(s) (other than thumb) — *see* Injury, muscle, finger
    forearm level, specified NEC — *see* Injury, muscle, forearm, flexor
    thumb — *see* Injury, muscle, thumb, flexor
    toe (long) (ankle level) (foot level) — *see* Injury, muscle, toe, flexor
  foot S96.90-
    intrinsic S96.20-
      laceration S96.22-
      specified type NEC S96.29-
      strain S96.21-
    laceration S96.92-
    long extensor, toe — *see* Injury, muscle, toe, extensor
    long flexor, toe — *see* Injury, muscle, toe, flexor
    specified
      site NEC S96.80-
        laceration S96.82-
        specified type NEC S96.89-
        strain S96.81-
      type NEC S96.99-
    strain S96.91-
  forearm (level) S56.90-
    extensor S56.50-
      laceration S56.52-
      specified type NEC S56.59-
      strain S56.51-
    flexor S56.20-
      laceration S56.22-
      specified type NEC S56.29-
      strain S56.21-
    laceration S56.92-
    specified S56.99-
      site NEC S56.80-
        laceration S56.82-
        strain S56.81-
        type NEC S56.89-
      strain S56.91-
  hand (level) S66.90-
    laceration S66.92-
    specified
      site NEC S66.80-
        laceration S66.82-
        specified type NEC S66.89-
        strain S66.81-
      type NEC S66.99-
    strain S66.91-

Injury (*see also* specified injury type) T14.90 — *continued*
muscle (and fascia) (and tendon) — *continued*
  head S09.10
    laceration S09.12
    specified type NEC S09.19
    strain S09.11
  hip NEC S76.00-
    laceration S76.02-
    specified type NEC S76.09-
    strain S76.01-
  intrinsic
    ankle and foot level — *see* Injury, muscle, foot, intrinsic
    finger (other than thumb) — *see* Injury, muscle, finger by site, intrinsic
    foot (level) — *see* Injury, muscle, foot, intrinsic
    thumb — *see* Injury, muscle, thumb, intrinsic
  leg (level) (lower) S86.90-
    Achilles tendon — *see* Injury, Achilles tendon
    anterior muscle group — *see* Injury, muscle, anterior muscle group
    laceration S86.92-
    peroneal muscle group — *see* Injury, muscle, peroneal muscle group
    posterior muscle group — *see* Injury, muscle, posterior muscle group, leg level
    specified
      site NEC S86.80-
        laceration S86.82-
        specified type NEC S86.89-
        strain S86.81-
      type NEC S86.99-
    strain S86.91-
  long
    extensor toe, at ankle and foot level — *see* Injury, muscle, toe, extensor
    flexor, toe, at ankle and foot level — *see* Injury, muscle, toe, flexor
    head, biceps — *see* Injury, muscle, biceps, long head
  lower back S39.002
    laceration S39.022
    specified type NEC S39.092
    strain S39.012
  neck (level) S16.9
    laceration S16.2
    specified type NEC S16.8
    strain S16.1
  pelvis S39.003
    laceration S39.023
    specified type NEC S39.093
    strain S39.013
  peroneal muscle group, at leg level (lower) S86.30-
    laceration S86.32-
    specified type NEC S86.39-
    strain S86.31-
  posterior muscle (group)
    leg level (lower) S86.10-
      laceration S86.12-
      specified type NEC S86.19-
      strain S86.11-
    thigh level S76.30-
      laceration S76.32-
      specified type NEC S76.39-
      strain S76.31-
  quadriceps (thigh) S76.10-
    laceration S76.12-
    specified type NEC S76.19-
    strain S76.11-
  shoulder S46.90-
    laceration S46.92-
    rotator cuff — *see* Injury, rotator cuff

Injury (*see also* specified injury type) T14.90 — *continued*
muscle (and fascia) (and tendon) — *continued*
  shoulder S46.90- — *continued*
    specified site NEC S46.80-
      laceration S46.82-
      specified type NEC S46.89-
      strain S46.81-
    specified type NEC S46.99-
    strain S46.91-
  thigh NEC (level) S76.90-
    adductor — *see* Injury, muscle, adductor, thigh
    laceration S76.92-
    posterior muscle (group) — *see* Injury, muscle, posterior muscle, thigh level
    quadriceps — *see* Injury, muscle, quadriceps
    specified
      site NEC S76.80-
        laceration S76.82-
        specified type NEC S76.89-
        strain S76.81-
      type NEC S76.99-
    strain S76.91-
  thorax (level) S29.009
    back wall S29.002
    front wall S29.001
    laceration S29.029
      back wall S29.022
      front wall S29.021
    specified type NEC S29.099
      back wall S29.092
      front wall S29.091
    strain S29.019
      back wall S29.012
      front wall S29.011
  thumb
    abductor (forearm level) S56.30-
      laceration S56.32-
      specified type NEC S56.39-
      strain S56.31-
    extensor (forearm level) S56.30-
      hand level S66.20-
        laceration S66.22-
        specified type NEC S66.29-
        strain S66.21-
      laceration S56.32-
      specified type NEC S56.39-
      strain S56.31-
    flexor (forearm level) S56.00-
      hand level S66.00-
        laceration S66.02-
        specified type NEC S66.09-
        strain S66.01-
      laceration S56.02-
      specified type NEC S56.09-
      strain S56.01-
      wrist level — *see* Injury, muscle, thumb, flexor, hand level
    intrinsic S66.40-
      laceration S66.42-
      specified type NEC S66.49-
      strain S66.41-
  toe — *see also* Injury, muscle, foot
    extensor, long S96.10-
      laceration S96.12-
      specified type NEC S96.19-
      strain S96.11-
    flexor, long S96.00-
      laceration S96.02-
      specified type NEC S96.09-
      strain S96.01-
  triceps S46.30-
    laceration S46.32-
    specified type NEC S46.39-
    strain S46.31-
  wrist (and hand) level — *see* Injury, muscle, hand

Injury (*see also* specified injury type) T14.90 — *continued*

musculocutaneous nerve — *see* Injury, nerve, musculocutaneous
myocardium — *see* Injury, heart
nape — *see* Injury, neck
nasal (septum) (sinus) S09.92
nasopharynx S09.92
neck S19.9
  specified NEC S19.80
    specified site NEC S19.89
nerve NEC T14.8
  abdomen S34.9
    peripheral S34.6
    specified site NEC S34.8
  abducens S04.4-
    contusion S04.4-
    laceration S04.4-
    specified type NEC S04.4-
  abducent — *see* Injury, nerve, abducens
  accessory S04.7-
    contusion S04.7-
    laceration S04.7-
    specified type NEC S04.7-
  acoustic S04.6-
    contusion S04.6-
    laceration S04.6-
    specified type NEC S04.6-
  ankle S94.9-
    cutaneous sensory S94.3-
    specified site NEC — *see* subcategory S94.8
  anterior crural, femoral — *see* Injury, nerve, femoral
  arm (upper) S44.9-
    axillary — *see* Injury, nerve, axillary
    cutaneous — *see* Injury, nerve, cutaneous, arm
    median — *see* Injury, nerve, median, upper arm
    musculocutaneous — *see* Injury, nerve, musculocutaneous
    radial — *see* Injury, nerve, radial, upper arm
    specified site NEC — *see* subcategory S44.8
    ulnar — *see* Injury, nerve, ulnar, arm
  auditory — *see* Injury, nerve, acoustic
  axillary S44.3-
  brachial plexus — *see* Injury, brachial plexus
  cervical sympathetic S14.5
  cranial S04.9
    contusion S04.9
    eighth (acoustic or auditory) — *see* Injury, nerve, acoustic
    eleventh (accessory) — *see* Injury, nerve, accessory
    fifth (trigeminal) — *see* Injury, nerve, trigeminal
    first (olfactory) — *see* Injury, nerve, olfactory
    fourth (trochlear) — *see* Injury, nerve, trochlear
    laceration S04.9
    ninth (glossopharyngeal) — *see* Injury, nerve, glossopharyngeal
    second (optic) — *see* Injury, nerve, optic
    seventh (facial) — *see* Injury, nerve, facial
    sixth (abducent) — *see* Injury, nerve, abducens
    specified
      nerve NEC S04.89-
        contusion S04.89-
        laceration S04.89-
        specified type NEC S04.89-
      type NEC S04.9
    tenth (pneumogastric or vagus) — *see* Injury, nerve, vagus

Injury (*see also* specified injury type) T14.90 — *continued*

nerve NEC T14.8 — *continued*
  cranial S04.9 — *continued*
    third (oculomotor) — *see* Injury, nerve, oculomotor
    twelfth (hypoglossal) — *see* Injury, nerve, hypoglossal
  cutaneous sensory
    ankle (level) S94.3-
    arm (upper) (level) S44.5-
    foot (level) — *see* Injury, nerve, cutaneous sensory, ankle
    forearm (level) S54.3-
    hip (level) S74.2-
    leg (lower level) S84.2-
    shoulder (level) — *see* Injury, nerve, cutaneous sensory, arm
    thigh (level) — *see* Injury, nerve, cutaneous sensory, hip
  deep peroneal — *see* Injury, nerve, peroneal, foot
  digital
    finger S64.4-
      index S64.49-
      little S64.49-
      middle S64.49-
      ring S64.49-
    thumb S64.3-
    toe — *see* Injury, nerve, ankle, specified site NEC
  eighth cranial (acoustic or auditory) — *see* Injury, nerve, acoustic
  eleventh cranial (accessory) — *see* Injury, nerve, accessory
  facial S04.5-
    contusion S04.5-
    laceration S04.5-
    newborn P11.3
    specified type NEC S04.5-
  femoral (hip level) (thigh level) S74.1-
  fifth cranial (trigeminal) — *see* Injury, nerve, trigeminal
  finger (digital) — *see* Injury, nerve, digital, finger
  first cranial (olfactory) — *see* Injury, nerve, olfactory
  foot S94.9-
    cutaneous sensory S94.3-
    deep peroneal S94.2-
    lateral plantar S94.0-
    medial plantar S94.1-
    specified site NEC — *see* subcategory S94.8
  forearm (level) S54.9-
    cutaneous sensory — *see* Injury, nerve, cutaneous sensory, forearm
    median — *see* Injury, nerve, median
    radial — *see* Injury, nerve, radial
    specified site NEC — *see* subcategory S54.8
    ulnar — *see* Injury, nerve, ulnar
  fourth cranial (trochlear) — *see* Injury, nerve, trochlear
  glossopharyngeal S04.89-
    specified type NEC S04.89-
  hand S64.9-
    median — *see* Injury, nerve, median, hand
    radial — *see* Injury, nerve, radial, hand
    specified NEC — *see* subcategory S64.8
    ulnar — *see* Injury, nerve, ulnar, hand
  hip (level) S74.9-
    cutaneous sensory — *see* Injury, nerve, cutaneous sensory, hip
    femoral — *see* Injury, nerve, femoral
    sciatic — *see* Injury, nerve, sciatic
    specified site NEC — *see* subcategory S74.8

Injury (*see also* specified injury type) T14.90 — *continued*

nerve NEC T14.8 — *continued*
  hypoglossal S04.89-
    specified type NEC S04.89-
  lateral plantar S94.0-
  leg (lower) S84.9-
    cutaneous sensory — *see* Injury, nerve, cutaneous sensory, leg
    peroneal — *see* Injury, nerve, peroneal
    specified site NEC — *see* subcategory S84.8
    tibial — *see* Injury, nerve, tibial
    upper — *see* Injury, nerve, thigh
  lower
    back — *see* Injury, nerve, abdomen, specified site NEC
    peripheral — *see* Injury, nerve, abdomen, peripheral
    limb — *see* Injury, nerve, leg
  lumbar plexus — *see* Injury, nerve, lumbosacral, sympathetic
  lumbar spinal — *see* Injury, nerve, spinal, lumbar
  lumbosacral
    plexus — *see* Injury, nerve, lumbosacral, sympathetic
    sympathetic S34.5
  medial plantar S94.1-
  median (forearm level) S54.1-
    hand (level) S64.1-
    upper arm (level) S44.1-
    wrist (level) — *see* Injury, nerve, median, hand
  musculocutaneous S44.4-
  musculospiral (upper arm level) — *see* Injury, nerve, radial, upper arm
  neck S14.9
    peripheral S14.4
    specified site NEC S14.8
    sympathetic S14.5
  ninth cranial (glossopharyngeal) — *see* Injury, nerve, glossopharyngeal
  oculomotor S04.1-
    contusion S04.1-
    laceration S04.1-
    specified type NEC S04.1-
  olfactory S04.81-
    specified type NEC S04.81-
  optic S04.01-
    contusion S04.01-
    laceration S04.01-
    specified type NEC S04.01-
  pelvic girdle — *see* Injury, nerve, hip
  pelvis — *see* Injury, nerve, abdomen, specified site NEC
  peripheral — *see* Injury, nerve, abdomen, peripheral
  peripheral NEC T14.8
    abdomen — *see* Injury, nerve, abdomen, peripheral
    lower back — *see* Injury, nerve, abdomen, peripheral
    neck — *see* Injury, nerve, neck, peripheral
    pelvis — *see* Injury, nerve, abdomen, peripheral
    specified NEC T14.8
  peroneal (lower leg level) S84.1-
    foot S94.2-
  plexus
    brachial — *see* Injury, brachial plexus
    celiac, coeliac — *see* Injury, nerve, lumbosacral, sympathetic
    mesenteric, inferior — *see* Injury, nerve, lumbosacral, sympathetic
    sacral — *see* Injury, lumbosacral plexus

Injury (see also specified injury type) T14.90 — continued
- nerve NEC T14.8 — continued
  - plexus — continued
    - spinal
      - brachial — see Injury, brachial plexus
      - lumbosacral — see Injury, lumbosacral plexus
  - pneumogastric — see Injury, nerve, vagus
  - radial (forearm level) S54.2-
    - hand (level) S64.2-
    - upper arm (level) S44.2-
    - wrist (level) — see Injury, nerve, radial, hand
  - root — see Injury, nerve, spinal, root
  - sacral plexus — see Injury, lumbosacral plexus
  - sacral spinal — see Injury, nerve, spinal, sacral
  - sciatic (hip level) (thigh level) S74.0-
  - second cranial (optic) — see Injury, nerve, optic
  - seventh cranial (facial) — see Injury, nerve, facial
  - shoulder — see Injury, nerve, arm
  - sixth cranial (abducent) — see Injury, nerve, abducens
  - spinal
    - plexus — see Injury, nerve, plexus, spinal
    - root
      - cervical S14.2
      - dorsal S24.2
      - lumbar S34.21
      - sacral S34.22
      - thoracic — see Injury, nerve, spinal, root, dorsal
  - splanchnic — see Injury, nerve, lumbosacral, sympathetic
  - sympathetic NEC — see Injury, nerve, lumbosacral, sympathetic
    - cervical — see Injury, nerve, cervical sympathetic
  - tenth cranial (pneumogastric or vagus) — see Injury, nerve, vagus
  - thigh (level) — see Injury, nerve, hip
    - cutaneous sensory — see Injury, nerve, cutaneous sensory, hip
    - femoral — see Injury, nerve, femoral
    - sciatic — see Injury, nerve, sciatic
    - specified NEC — see Injury, nerve, hip
  - third cranial (oculomotor) — see Injury, nerve, oculomotor
  - thorax S24.9
    - peripheral S24.3
    - specified site NEC S24.8
    - sympathetic S24.4
  - thumb, digital — see Injury, nerve, digital, thumb
  - tibial (lower leg level) (posterior) S84.0-
  - toe — see Injury, nerve, ankle
  - trigeminal S04.3-
    - contusion S04.3-
    - laceration S04.3-
    - specified type NEC S04.3-
  - trochlear S04.2-
    - contusion S04.2-
    - laceration S04.2-
    - specified type NEC S04.2-
  - twelfth cranial (hypoglossal) — see Injury, nerve, hypoglossal
  - ulnar (forearm level) S54.0-
    - arm (upper) (level) S44.0-
    - hand (level) S64.0-
    - wrist (level) — see Injury, nerve, ulnar, hand
  - vagus S04.89-
    - specified type NEC S04.89-
  - wrist (level) — see Injury, nerve, hand

Injury (see also specified injury type) T14.90 — continued
- ninth cranial nerve (glossopharyngeal) — see Injury, nerve, glossopharyngeal
- nose (septum) S09.92
- obstetrical O71.9
  - specified NEC O71.89
- occipital (region) (scalp) S09.90
  - lobe — see Injury, intracranial
- optic chiasm S04.02
- optic radiation S04.03-
- optic tract and pathways S04.03-
- orbit, orbital (region) — see Injury, eye
  - penetrating (with foreign body) — see Injury, eye, orbit, penetrating
  - specified NEC — see Injury, eye, specified site NEC
- ovary, ovarian S37.409
  - bilateral S37.402
    - contusion S37.422
    - laceration S37.432
    - specified type NEC S37.492
  - blood vessel — see Injury, blood vessel, ovarian
  - contusion S37.429
    - bilateral S37.422
    - unilateral S37.421
  - laceration S37.439
    - bilateral S37.432
    - unilateral S37.431
  - specified type NEC S37.499
    - bilateral S37.492
    - unilateral S37.491
  - unilateral S37.401
    - contusion S37.421
    - laceration S37.431
    - specified type NEC S37.491
- palate (hard) (soft) S09.93
- pancreas S36.209
  - body S36.201
    - contusion S36.221
    - laceration S36.231
      - major S36.261
      - minor S36.241
      - moderate S36.251
    - specified type NEC S36.291
  - contusion S36.229
  - head S36.200
    - contusion S36.220
    - laceration S36.230
      - major S36.260
      - minor S36.240
      - moderate S36.250
    - specified type NEC S36.290
  - laceration S36.239
    - major S36.269
    - minor S36.249
    - moderate S36.259
  - specified type NEC S36.299
  - tail S36.202
    - contusion S36.222
    - laceration S36.232
      - major S36.262
      - minor S36.242
      - moderate S36.252
    - specified type NEC S36.292
- parietal (region) (scalp) S09.90
  - lobe — see Injury, intracranial
- patellar ligament (tendon) S76.10-
  - laceration S76.12-
  - specified NEC S76.19-
  - strain S76.11-
- pelvis, pelvic (floor) S39.93
  - complicating delivery O70.1
  - joint or ligament, complicating delivery O71.6
  - organ S37.90
    - with ectopic or molar pregnancy O08.6
    - complication of abortion — see Abortion

Injury (see also specified injury type) T14.90 — continued
- pelvis, pelvic (floor) S39.93 — continued
  - organ S37.90 — continued
    - contusion S37.92
      - following ectopic or molar pregnancy O08.6
    - laceration S37.93
    - obstetrical trauma NEC O71.5
    - specified
      - site NEC S37.899
        - contusion S37.892
        - laceration S37.893
        - specified type NEC S37.898
      - type NEC S37.99
  - specified NEC S39.83
- penis S39.94
- perineum S39.94
- peritoneum S36.81
  - laceration S36.893
- periurethral tissue — see Injury, urethra
  - complicating delivery O71.82
- phalanges
  - foot — see Injury, foot
  - hand — see Injury, hand
- pharynx NEC S19.85
- pleura — see Injury, intrathoracic, pleura
- plexus
  - brachial — see Injury, brachial plexus
  - cardiac — see Injury, nerve, thorax, sympathetic
  - celiac, coeliac — see Injury, nerve, lumbosacral, sympathetic
  - esophageal — see Injury, nerve, thorax, sympathetic
  - hypogastric — see Injury, nerve, lumbosacral, sympathetic
  - lumbar, lumbosacral — see Injury, lumbosacral plexus
  - mesenteric — see Injury, nerve, lumbosacral, sympathetic
  - pulmonary — see Injury, nerve, thorax, sympathetic
- postcardiac surgery (syndrome) I97.0
- prepuce S39.94
- prostate S37.829
  - contusion S37.822
  - laceration S37.823
  - specified type NEC S37.828
- pubic region S39.94
- pudendum S39.94
- pulmonary plexus — see Injury, nerve, thorax, sympathetic
- rectovaginal septum NEC S39.83
- rectum — see Injury, intestine, large, rectum
- retina — see Injury, eye, specified site NEC
  - penetrating — see Injury, eyeball, penetrating
- retroperitoneal — see Injury, intra-abdominal, specified site NEC
- rotator cuff (muscle(s)) (tendon(s)) S46.00-
  - laceration S46.02-
  - specified type NEC S46.09-
  - strain S46.01-
- round ligament — see Injury, pelvic organ, specified site NEC
- sacral plexus — see Injury, lumbosacral plexus
- salivary duct or gland S09.93
- scalp S09.90
  - newborn (birth injury) P12.9
    - due to monitoring (electrode) (sampling incision) P12.4
    - specified NEC P12.89
      - caput succedaneum P12.81
- scapular region — see Injury, shoulder
- sclera — see Injury, eye, specified site NEC
  - penetrating — see Injury, eyeball, penetrating
- scrotum S39.94

0

Injury (see also specified injury type) T14.90 — continued
- second cranial nerve (optic) — see Injury, nerve, optic
- seminal vesicle — see Injury, pelvic organ, specified site NEC
- seventh cranial nerve (facial) — see Injury, nerve, facial
- shoulder S49.9-
  - blood vessel — see Injury, blood vessel, arm
  - contusion — see Contusion, shoulder
  - dislocation — see Dislocation, shoulder
  - fracture — see Fracture, shoulder
  - muscle — see Injury, muscle, shoulder
  - nerve — see Injury, nerve, shoulder
  - open — see Wound, open, shoulder
  - specified type NEC S49.8-
  - sprain — see Sprain, shoulder girdle
  - superficial — see Injury, superficial, shoulder
- sinus
  - cavernous — see Injury, intracranial
  - nasal S09.92
- sixth cranial nerve (abducent) — see Injury, nerve, abducens
- skeleton, birth injury P13.9
  - specified part NEC P13.8
- skin NEC T14.8
  - surface intact — see Injury, superficial
- skull NEC S09.90
- specified NEC T14.8
- spermatic cord (pelvic region) S37.898
  - scrotal region S39.848
- spinal (cord)
  - cervical (neck) S14.109
    - anterior cord syndrome S14.139
      - C1 level S14.131
      - C2 level S14.132
      - C3 level S14.133
      - C4 level S14.134
      - C5 level S14.135
      - C6 level S14.136
      - C7 level S14.137
      - C8 level S14.138
    - Brown-Séquard syndrome S14.149
      - C1 level S14.141
      - C2 level S14.142
      - C3 level S14.143
      - C4 level S14.144
      - C5 level S14.145
      - C6 level S14.146
      - C7 level S14.147
      - C8 level S14.148
    - C1 level S14.101
    - C2 level S14.102
    - C3 level S14.103
    - C4 level S14.104
    - C5 level S14.105
    - C6 level S14.106
    - C7 level S14.107
    - C8 level S14.108
    - central cord syndrome S14.129
      - C1 level S14.121
      - C2 level S14.122
      - C3 level S14.123
      - C4 level S14.124
      - C5 level S14.125
      - C6 level S14.126
      - C7 level S14.127
      - C8 level S14.128
    - complete lesion S14.119
      - C1 level S14.111
      - C2 level S14.112
      - C3 level S14.113
      - C4 level S14.114
      - C5 level S14.115
      - C6 level S14.116
      - C7 level S14.117
      - C8 level S14.118
    - concussion S14.0

Injury (see also specified injury type) T14.90 — continued
- spinal (cord) — continued
  - cervical (neck) S14.109 — continued
    - edema S14.0
    - incomplete lesion specified NEC S14.159
      - C1 level S14.151
      - C2 level S14.152
      - C3 level S14.153
      - C4 level S14.154
      - C5 level S14.155
      - C6 level S14.156
      - C7 level S14.157
      - C8 level S14.158
    - posterior cord syndrome S14.159
      - C1 level S14.151
      - C2 level S14.152
      - C3 level S14.153
      - C4 level S14.154
      - C5 level S14.155
      - C6 level S14.156
      - C7 level S14.157
      - C8 level S14.158
  - dorsal — see Injury, spinal, thoracic
  - lumbar S34.109
    - complete lesion S34.119
      - L1 level S34.111
      - L2 level S34.112
      - L3 level S34.113
      - L4 level S34.114
      - L5 level S34.115
    - concussion S34.01
    - edema S34.01
    - incomplete lesion S34.129
      - L1 level S34.121
      - L2 level S34.122
      - L3 level S34.123
      - L4 level S34.124
      - L5 level S34.125
    - L1 level S34.101
    - L2 level S34.102
    - L3 level S34.103
    - L4 level S34.104
    - L5 level S34.105
  - nerve root NEC
    - cervical — see Injury, nerve, spinal, root, cervical
    - dorsal — see Injury, nerve, spinal, root, dorsal
    - lumbar S34.21
    - sacral S34.22
    - thoracic — see Injury, nerve, spinal, root, dorsal
  - plexus
    - brachial — see Injury, brachial plexus
    - lumbosacral — see Injury, lumbosacral plexus
  - sacral S34.139
    - complete lesion S34.131
    - incomplete lesion S34.132
  - thoracic S24.109
    - anterior cord syndrome S24.139
      - T1 level S24.131
      - T11-T12 level S24.134
      - T2-T6 level S24.132
      - T7-T10 level S24.133
    - Brown-Séquard syndrome S24.149
      - T1 level S24.141
      - T11-T12 level S24.144
      - T2-T6 level S24.142
      - T7-T10 level S24.143
    - complete lesion S24.119
      - T1 level S24.111
      - T11-T12 level S24.114
      - T2-T6 level S24.112
      - T7-T10 level S24.113
    - concussion S24.0
    - edema S24.0

Injury (see also specified injury type) T14.90 — continued
- spinal (cord) — continued
  - thoracic S24.109 — continued
    - incomplete lesion specified NEC S24.159
      - T1 level S24.151
      - T11-T12 level S24.154
      - T2-T6 level S24.152
      - T7-T10 level S24.153
    - posterior cord syndrome S24.159
      - T1 level S24.151
      - T11-T12 level S24.154
      - T2-T6 level S24.152
      - T7-T10 level S24.153
    - T1 level S24.101
    - T11-T12 level S24.104
    - T2-T6 level S24.102
    - T7-T10 level S24.103
- splanchnic nerve — see Injury, nerve, lumbosacral, sympathetic
- spleen S36.00
  - contusion S36.029
    - major S36.021
    - minor S36.020
  - laceration S36.039
    - major (massive) (stellate) S36.032
    - moderate S36.031
    - superficial (capsular) (minor) S36.030
  - specified type NEC S36.09
- splenic artery — see Injury, blood vessel, celiac artery, branch
- stellate ganglion — see Injury, nerve, thorax, sympathetic
- sternal region S29.9
- stomach S36.30
  - contusion S36.32
  - laceration S36.33
  - specified type NEC S36.39
- subconjunctival — see Injury, eye, conjunctiva
- subcutaneous NEC T14.8
- submaxillary region S09.93
- submental region S09.93
- subungual
  - fingers — see Injury, hand
  - toes — see Injury, foot
- superficial NEC T14.8
  - abdomen, abdominal (wall) S30.92
    - abrasion S30.811
    - bite S30.871
      - insect S30.861
    - contusion S30.1
    - external constriction S30.841
    - foreign body S30.851
  - abrasion — see Abrasion, by site
  - adnexa, eye NEC — see Injury, eye, specified site NEC
  - alveolar process — see Injury, superficial, oral cavity
  - ankle S90.91-
    - abrasion — see Abrasion, ankle
    - bite — see Bite, ankle
    - blister — see Blister, ankle
    - contusion — see Contusion, ankle
    - external constriction — see Constriction, external, ankle
    - foreign body — see Foreign body, superficial, ankle
  - anus S30.98
  - arm (upper) S40.92-
    - abrasion — see Abrasion, arm
    - bite — see Bite, superficial, arm
    - blister — see Blister, arm (upper)
    - contusion — see Contusion, arm
    - external constriction — see Constriction, external, arm
    - foreign body — see Foreign body, superficial, arm

Injury (see also specified injury type) T14.90 — continued

superficial NEC T14.8 — continued

auditory canal (external) (meatus) — see Injury, superficial, ear

auricle — see Injury, superficial, ear

axilla — see Injury, superficial, arm

back — see also Injury, superficial, thorax, back

  lower S30.91

    abrasion S30.810

    contusion S30.0

    external constriction S30.840

    superficial

      bite NEC S30.870

        insect S30.860

      foreign body S30.850

bite NEC — see Bite, superficial NEC, by site

blister — see Blister, by site

breast S20.10-

  abrasion — see Abrasion, breast

  bite — see Bite, superficial, breast

  contusion — see Contusion, breast

  external constriction — see Constriction, external, breast

  foreign body — see Foreign body, superficial, breast

brow — see Injury, superficial, head, specified NEC

buttock S30.91

calf — see Injury, superficial, leg

canthus, eye — see Injury, superficial, periocular area

cheek (external) — see Injury, superficial, head, specified NEC

  internal — see Injury, superficial, oral cavity

chest wall — see Injury, superficial, thorax

chin — see Injury, superficial, head NEC

clitoris S30.95

conjunctiva — see Injury, eye, conjunctiva

  with foreign body (in conjunctival sac) — see Foreign body, conjunctival sac

contusion — see Contusion, by site

costal region — see Injury, superficial, thorax

digit(s)

  hand — see Injury, superficial, finger

ear (auricle) (canal) (external) S00.40-

  abrasion — see Abrasion, ear

  bite — see Bite, superficial, ear

  contusion — see Contusion, ear

  external constriction — see Constriction, external, ear

  foreign body — see Foreign body, superficial, ear

elbow S50.90-

  abrasion — see Abrasion, elbow

  bite — see Bite, superficial, elbow

  blister — see Blister, elbow

  contusion — see Contusion, elbow

  external constriction — see Constriction, external, elbow

  foreign body — see Foreign body, superficial, elbow

epididymis S30.94

epigastric region S30.92

epiglottis — see Injury, superficial, throat

esophagus

  cervical — see Injury, superficial, throat

external constriction — see Constriction, external, by site

extremity NEC T14.8

eyeball NEC — see Injury, eye, specified site NEC

eyebrow — see Injury, superficial, periocular area

Injury (see also specified injury type) T14.90 — continued

superficial NEC T14.8 — continued

eyelid S00.20-

  abrasion — see Abrasion, eyelid

  bite — see Bite, superficial, eyelid

  contusion — see Contusion, eyelid

  external constriction — see Constriction, external, eyelid

  foreign body — see Foreign body, superficial, eyelid

face NEC — see Injury, superficial, head, specified NEC

finger(s) S60.949

  abrasion — see Abrasion, finger

  bite — see Bite, superficial, finger

  blister — see Blister, finger

  contusion — see Contusion, finger

  external constriction — see Constriction, external, finger

  foreign body — see Foreign body, superficial, finger

  index S60.94-

  insect bite — see Bite, by site, superficial, insect

  little S60.94-

  middle S60.94-

  ring S60.94-

flank S30.92

foot S90.92-

  abrasion — see Abrasion, foot

  bite — see Bite, foot

  blister — see Blister, foot

  contusion — see Contusion, foot

  external constriction — see Constriction, external, foot

  foreign body — see Foreign body, superficial, foot

forearm S50.91-

  abrasion — see Abrasion, forearm

  bite — see Bite, forearm, superficial

  blister — see Blister, forearm

  contusion — see Contusion, forearm

  elbow only — see Injury, superficial, elbow

  external constriction — see Constriction, external, forearm

  foreign body — see Foreign body, superficial, forearm

forehead — see Injury, superficial, head NEC

foreign body — see Foreign body, superficial

genital organs, external

  female S30.97

  male S30.96

globe (eye) — see Injury, eye, specified site NEC

groin S30.92

gum — see Injury, superficial, oral cavity

hand S60.92-

  abrasion — see Abrasion, hand

  bite — see Bite, superficial, hand

  contusion — see Contusion, hand

  external constriction — see Constriction, external, hand

  foreign body — see Foreign body, superficial, hand

head S00.90

  ear — see Injury, superficial, ear

  eyelid — see Injury, superficial, eyelid

  nose S00.30

  oral cavity S00.502

  scalp S00.00

  specified site NEC S00.80

heel — see Injury, superficial, foot

Injury (see also specified injury type) T14.90 — continued

superficial NEC T14.8 — continued

hip S70.91-

  abrasion — see Abrasion, hip

  bite — see Bite, superficial, hip

  blister — see Blister, hip

  contusion — see Contusion, hip

  external constriction — see Constriction, external, hip

  foreign body — see Foreign body, superficial, hip

iliac region — see Injury, superficial, abdomen

inguinal region — see Injury, superficial, abdomen

insect bite — see Bite, by site, superficial, insect

interscapular region — see Injury, superficial, thorax, back

jaw — see Injury, superficial, head, specified NEC

knee S80.91-

  abrasion — see Abrasion, knee

  bite — see Bite, superficial, knee

  blister — see Blister, knee

  contusion — see Contusion, knee

  external constriction — see Constriction, external, knee

  foreign body — see Foreign body, superficial, knee

labium (majus) (minus) S30.95

lacrimal (apparatus) (gland) (sac) — see Injury, eye, specified site NEC

larynx — see Injury, superficial, throat

leg (lower) S80.92-

  abrasion — see Abrasion, leg

  bite — see Bite, superficial, leg

  contusion — see Contusion, leg

  external constriction — see Constriction, external, leg

  foreign body — see Foreign body, superficial, leg

  knee — see Injury, superficial, knee

limb NEC T14.8

lip S00.501

lower back S30.91

lumbar region S30.91

malar region — see Injury, superficial, head, specified NEC

mammary — see Injury, superficial, breast

mastoid region — see Injury, superficial, head, specified NEC

mouth — see Injury, superficial, oral cavity

muscle NEC T14.8

nail NEC T14.8

  finger — see Injury, superficial, finger

  toe — see Injury, superficial, toe

nasal (septum) — see Injury, superficial, nose

neck S10.90

  specified site NEC S10.80

nose (septum) S00.30

occipital region — see Injury, superficial, scalp

oral cavity S00.502

orbital region — see Injury, superficial, periocular area

palate — see Injury, superficial, oral cavity

palm — see Injury, superficial, hand

parietal region — see Injury, superficial, scalp

pelvis S30.91

  girdle — see Injury, superficial, hip

penis S30.93

perineum

  female S30.95

  male S30.91

Injury (see also specified injury type) T14.90 — continued
superficial NEC T14.8 — continued
  periocular area S00.20-
    abrasion — see Abrasion, eyelid
    bite — see Bite, superficial, eyelid
    contusion — see Contusion, eyelid
    external constriction — see Constriction, external, eyelid
    foreign body — see Foreign body, superficial, eyelid
  phalanges
    finger — see Injury, superficial, finger
    toe — see Injury, superficial, toe
  pharynx — see Injury, superficial, throat
  pinna — see Injury, superficial, ear
  popliteal space — see Injury, superficial, knee
  prepuce S30.93
  pubic region S30.91
  pudendum
    female S30.97
    male S30.96
  sacral region S30.91
  scalp S00.00
  scapular region — see Injury, superficial, shoulder
  sclera — see Injury, eye, specified site NEC
  scrotum S30.94
  shin — see Injury, superficial, leg
  shoulder S40.91-
    abrasion — see Abrasion, shoulder
    bite — see Bite, superficial, shoulder
    blister — see Blister, shoulder
    contusion — see Contusion, shoulder
    external constriction — see Constriction, external, shoulder
    foreign body — see Foreign body, superficial, shoulder
  skin NEC T14.8
  sternal region — see Injury, superficial, thorax, front
  subconjunctival — see Injury, eye, specified site NEC
  subcutaneous NEC T14.8
  submaxillary region — see Injury, superficial, head, specified NEC
  submental region — see Injury, superficial, head, specified NEC
  subungual
    finger(s) — see Injury, superficial, finger
    toe(s) — see Injury, superficial, toe
  supraclavicular fossa — see Injury, superficial, neck
  supraorbital — see Injury, superficial, head, specified NEC
  temple — see Injury, superficial, head, specified NEC
  temporal region — see Injury, superficial, head, specified NEC
  testis S30.94
  thigh S70.92-
    abrasion — see Abrasion, thigh
    bite — see Bite, superficial, thigh
    blister — see Blister, thigh
    contusion — see Contusion, thigh
    external constriction — see Constriction, external, thigh
    foreign body — see Foreign body, superficial, thigh
  thorax, thoracic (wall) S20.90
    abrasion — see Abrasion, thorax
    back S20.40-
    bite — see Bite, thorax, superficial
    blister — see Blister, thorax
    contusion — see Contusion, thorax
    external constriction — see Constriction, external, thorax

Injury (see also specified injury type) T14.90 — continued
superficial NEC T14.8 — continued
  thorax, thoracic (wall) S20.90 — continued
    foreign body — see Foreign body, superficial, thorax
    front S20.30-
    throat S10.10
      abrasion S10.11
      bite S10.17
        insect S10.16
      blister S10.12
      contusion S10.0
      external constriction S10.14
      foreign body S10.15
    thumb S60.93-
      abrasion — see Abrasion, thumb
      bite — see Bite, superficial, thumb
      blister — see Blister, thumb
      contusion — see Contusion, thumb
      external constriction — see Constriction, external, thumb
      foreign body — see Foreign body, superficial, thumb
      insect bite — see Bite, by site, superficial, insect
      specified type NEC S60.39-
    toe(s) S90.93-
      abrasion — see Abrasion, toe
      bite — see Bite, toe
      blister — see Blister, toe
      contusion — see Contusion, toe
      external constriction — see Constriction, external, toe
      foreign body — see Foreign body, superficial, toe
      great S90.93-
    tongue — see Injury, superficial, oral cavity
    tooth, teeth — see Injury, superficial, oral cavity
    trachea S10.10
    tunica vaginalis S30.94
    tympanum, tympanic membrane — see Injury, superficial, ear
    uvula — see Injury, superficial, oral cavity
    vagina S30.95
    vocal cords — see Injury, superficial, throat
    vulva S30.95
    wrist S60.91-
  supraclavicular region — see Injury, neck
  supraorbital S09.93
  suprarenal gland (multiple) — see Injury, adrenal
  surgical complication (external or internal site) — see Laceration, accidental complicating surgery
  temple S09.90
  temporal region S09.90
  tendon — see also Injury, muscle, by site
    abdomen — see Injury, muscle, abdomen
    Achilles — see Injury, Achilles tendon
    lower back — see Injury, muscle, lower back
    pelvic organs — see Injury, muscle, pelvis
  tenth cranial nerve (pneumogastric or vagus) — see Injury, nerve, vagus
  testis S39.94
  thigh S79.92-
    blood vessel — see Injury, blood vessel, hip
    contusion — see Contusion, thigh
    fracture — see Fracture, femur
    muscle — see Injury, muscle, thigh
    nerve — see Injury, nerve, thigh
    open — see Wound, open, thigh
    specified NEC S79.82-
    superficial — see Injury, superficial, thigh
  third cranial nerve (oculomotor) — see Injury, nerve, oculomotor

Injury (see also specified injury type) T14.90 — continued
  thorax, thoracic S29.9
    blood vessel — see Injury, blood vessel, thorax
    cavity — see Injury, intrathoracic
    dislocation — see Dislocation, thorax
    external (wall) S29.9
      contusion — see Contusion, thorax
      nerve — see Injury, nerve, thorax
      open — see Wound, open, thorax
      specified NEC S29.8
      sprain — see Sprain, thorax
      superficial — see Injury, superficial, thorax
    fracture — see Fracture, thorax
    internal — see Injury, intrathoracic
    intrathoracic organ — see Injury, intrathoracic
    sympathetic ganglion — see Injury, nerve, thorax, sympathetic
  throat (see also Injury, neck) S19.9
  thumb S69.9-
    blood vessel — see Injury, blood vessel, thumb
    contusion — see Contusion, thumb
    dislocation — see Dislocation, thumb
    fracture — see Fracture, thumb
    muscle — see Injury, muscle, thumb
    nerve — see Injury, nerve, digital, thumb
    open — see Wound, open, thumb
    specified NEC S69.8-
    sprain — see Sprain, thumb
    superficial — see Injury, superficial, thumb
  thymus (gland) — see Injury, intrathoracic, specified organ NEC
  thyroid (gland) NEC S19.84
  toe S99.92-
    contusion — see Contusion, toe
    dislocation — see Dislocation, toe
    fracture — see Fracture, toe
    muscle — see Injury, muscle, toe
    open — see Wound, open, toe
    specified type NEC S99.82-
    sprain — see Sprain, toe
    superficial — see Injury, superficial, toe
  tongue S09.93
  tonsil S09.93
  tooth S09.93
  trachea (cervical) NEC S19.82
    thoracic — see Injury, intrathoracic, trachea, thoracic
  transfusion-related acute lung (TRALI) J95.84
  tunica vaginalis S39.94
  twelfth cranial nerve (hypoglossal) — see Injury, nerve, hypoglossal
  ureter S37.10
    contusion S37.12
    laceration S37.13
    specified type NEC S37.19
  urethra (sphincter) S37.30
    at delivery O71.5
    contusion S37.32
    laceration S37.33
    specified type NEC S37.39
  urinary organ S37.90
    contusion S37.92
    laceration S37.93
    specified
      site NEC S37.899
        contusion S37.892
        laceration S37.893
        specified type NEC S37.898
      type NEC S37.99
  uterus, uterine S37.60
    with ectopic or molar pregnancy O08.6
    blood vessel — see Injury, blood vessel, iliac
    contusion S37.62

DISEASE INDEX

Injury (see also specified injury type) T14.90 —
— continued
  uterus, uterine S37.60 — continued
    laceration S37.63
      cervix at delivery O71.3
    rupture associated with obstetrics — see
      Rupture, uterus
    specified type NEC S37.69
  uvula S09.93
  vagina S39.93
    abrasion S30.814
    bite S31.45
      insect S30.864
      superficial NEC S30.874
    contusion S30.23
    crush S38.03
    during delivery — see Laceration, vagina,
      during delivery
    external constriction S30.844
    insect bite S30.864
    laceration S31.41
      with foreign body S31.42
    open wound S31.40
    puncture S31.43
      with foreign body S31.44
    superficial S30.95
      foreign body S30.854
  vas deferens — see Injury, pelvic organ,
    specified site NEC
  vascular NEC T14.8
  vein — see Injury, blood vessel
  vena cava (superior) S25.20
    inferior S35.10
      laceration (minor) (superficial) S35.11
        major S35.12
      specified type NEC S35.19
    laceration (minor) (superficial) S25.21
      major S25.22
    specified type NEC S25.29
  vesical (sphincter) — see Injury, bladder
  visual cortex S04.04-
  vitreous (humor) S05.90
    specified NEC S05.8x-
  vocal cord NEC S19.83
  vulva S39.94
    abrasion S30.814
    bite S31.45
      insect S30.864
      superficial NEC S30.874
    contusion S30.23
    crush S38.03
    during delivery — see Laceration, perineum,
      female, during delivery
    external constriction S30.844
    insect bite S30.864
    laceration S31.41
      with foreign body S31.42
    open wound S31.40
    puncture S31.43
      with foreign body S31.44
    superficial S30.95
      foreign body S30.854
  whiplash (cervical spine) S13.4
  wrist S69.9-
    blood vessel — see Injury, blood vessel,
      hand
    contusion — see Contusion, wrist
    dislocation — see Dislocation, wrist
    fracture — see Fracture, wrist
    muscle — see Injury, muscle, hand
    nerve — see Injury, nerve, hand
    open — see Wound, open, wrist
    specified NEC S69.8-
    sprain — see Sprain, wrist
    superficial — see Injury, superficial, wrist
Inoculation — see also Vaccination
  complication or reaction — see Complications,
    vaccination

Insanity, insane — see also Psychosis
  adolescent — see Schizophrenia
  confusional F28
    acute or subacute F05
  delusional F22
  senile F03
Insect
  bite — see Bite, by site, superficial, insect
  venomous, poisoning NEC (by) — see Venom,
    arthropod
Insensitivity
  adrenocorticotropin hormone (ACTH) E27.49
  androgen E34.50
    complete E34.51
    partial E34.52
Insertion
  cord (umbilical) lateral or velamentous
    O43.12-
  intrauterine contraceptive device (encounter
    for) — see Intrauterine contraceptive
    device
Insolation (sunstroke) T67.0
Insomnia (organic) G47.00
  adjustment F51.02
  adjustment disorder F51.02
  behavioral, of childhood Z73.819
    combined type Z73.812
    limit setting type Z73.811
    sleep-onset association type Z73.810
  childhood Z73.819
  chronic F51.04
    somatized tension F51.04
  conditioned F51.04
  due to
    alcohol
      abuse F10.182
      dependence F10.282
      use F10.982
    amphetamines
      abuse F15.182
      dependence F15.282
      use F15.982
    anxiety disorder F51.05
    caffeine
      abuse F15.182
      dependence F15.282
      use F15.982
    cocaine
      abuse F14.182
      dependence F14.282
      use F14.982
    depression F51.05
    drug NEC
      abuse F19.182
      dependence F19.282
      use F19.982
    medical condition G47.01
    mental disorder NEC F51.05
    opioid
      abuse F11.182
      dependence F11.282
      use F11.982
    psychoactive substance NEC
      abuse F19.182
      dependence F19.282
      use F19.982
    sedative, hypnotic, or anxiolytic
      abuse F13.182
      dependence F13.282
      use F13.982
    stimulant NEC
      abuse F15.182
      dependence F15.282
      use F15.982
  fatal familial (FFI) A81.83
  idiopathic F51.01
  learned F51.3
  nonorganic origin F51.01

Insomnia (organic) G47.00 — continued
  not due to a substance or known physiological
    condition F51.01
    specified NEC F51.09
  paradoxical F51.03
  primary F51.01
  psychiatric F51.05
  psychophysiologic F51.04
  related to psychopathology F51.05
  short-term F51.02
  specified NEC G47.09
  stress-related F51.02
  transient F51.02
  without objective findings F51.02
Inspiration
  food or foreign body — see Foreign body, by
    site
  mucus — see Asphyxia, mucus
Inspissated bile syndrome (newborn) P59.1
Instability
  emotional (excessive) F60.3
  joint (post-traumatic) M25.30
    ankle M25.37-
    due to old ligament injury — see Disorder,
      ligament
    elbow M25.32-
    flail — see Flail, joint
    foot M25.37-
    hand M25.34-
    hip M25.35-
    knee M25.36-
    lumbosacral — see subcategory M53.2
    prosthesis — see Complications, joint
      prosthesis, mechanical, displacement, by
      site
    sacroiliac — see subcategory M53.2
    secondary to
      old ligament injury — see Disorder,
        ligament
      removal of joint prosthesis M96.89
    shoulder (region) M25.31-
    spine — see subcategory M53.2
    wrist M25.33-
  knee (chronic) M23.5-
  lumbosacral — see subcategory M53.2
  nervous F48.8
  personality (emotional) F60.3
  spine — see Instability, joint, spine
  vasomotor R55
Institutional syndrome (childhood) F94.2
Institutionalization, affecting child
  Z62.22
  disinhibited attachment F94.2
Insufficiency, insufficient
  accommodation, old age H52.4
  adrenal (gland) E27.40
    primary E27.1
  adrenocortical E27.40
    drug-induced E27.3
    iatrogenic E27.3
    primary E27.1
  anatomic crown height K08.89
  anterior (occlusal) guidance M26.54
  anus K62.89
  aortic (valve) I35.1
    with
      mitral (valve) disease I08.0
        with tricuspid (valve) disease I08.3
      stenosis I35.2
      tricuspid (valve) disease I08.2
        with mitral (valve) disease I08.3
    congenital Q23.1

Insufficiency, insufficient — *continued*
aortic (valve) I35.1 — *continued*
  rheumatic I06.1
    with
      mitral (valve) disease I08.0
        with tricuspid (valve) disease I08.3
      stenosis I06.2
        with mitral (valve) disease I08.0
          with tricuspid (valve) disease I08.3
      tricuspid (valve) disease I08.2
        with mitral (valve) disease I08.3
  specified cause NEC I35.1
  syphilitic A52.03
arterial I77.1
  basilar G45.0
  carotid (hemispheric) G45.1
  cerebral I67.81
  coronary (acute or subacute) I24.8
  mesenteric K55.1
  peripheral I73.9
  precerebral (multiple) (bilateral) G45.2
  vertebral G45.0
arteriovenous I99.8
biliary K83.8
cardiac — *see also* Insufficiency, myocardial
  due to presence of (cardiac) prosthesis
    I97.11-
  postprocedural I97.11-
cardiorenal, hypertensive I13.2
cardiovascular — *see* Disease, cardiovascular
cerebrovascular (acute) I67.81
  with transient focal neurological signs and
    symptoms G45.8
circulatory NEC I99.8
  newborn P29.89
clinical crown length K08.89
convergence H51.11
coronary (acute or subacute) I24.8
  chronic or with a stated duration of over 4
    weeks I25.89
corticoadrenal E27.40
  primary E27.1
dietary E63.9
divergence H51.8
food T73.0
gastroesophageal K22.8
gonadal
  ovary E28.39
  testis E29.1
heart — *see also* Insufficiency, myocardial
  newborn P29.0
  valve — *see* Endocarditis
hepatic — *see* Failure, hepatic
idiopathic autonomic G90.09
interocclusal distance of fully erupted teeth
  (ridge) M26.36
kidney N28.9
  acute N28.9
  chronic N18.9
lacrimal (secretion) H04.12-
  passages — *see* Stenosis, lacrimal
liver — *see* Failure, hepatic
lung — *see* Insufficiency, pulmonary
mental (congenital) — *see* Disability,
  intellectual
mesenteric K55.1
mitral (valve) I34.0
  with
    aortic valve disease I08.0
      with tricuspid (valve) disease I08.3
    obstruction or stenosis I05.2
      with aortic valve disease I08.0
    tricuspid (valve) disease I08.1
      with aortic (valve) disease I08.3
  congenital Q23.3

Insufficiency, insufficient — *continued*
mitral (valve) I34.0 — *continued*
  rheumatic I05.1
    with
      aortic valve disease I08.0
        with tricuspid (valve) disease I08.3
      obstruction or stenosis I05.2
        with aortic valve disease I08.0
          with tricuspid (valve) disease
          I08.3
      tricuspid (valve) disease I08.1
        with aortic (valve) disease I08.3
    active or acute I01.1
      with chorea, rheumatic (Sydenham's)
      I02.0
  specified cause, except rheumatic I34.0
muscle — *see also* Disease, muscle
  heart — *see* Insufficiency, myocardial
  ocular NEC H50.9
myocardial, myocardium (with arteriosclerosis)
  I50.9
  with
    rheumatic fever (conditions in I00) I09.0
      active, acute or subacute I01.2
        with chorea I02.0
      inactive or quiescent (with chorea) I09.0
  congenital Q24.8
  hypertensive — *see* Hypertension, heart
  newborn P29.0
  rheumatic I09.0
    active, acute, or subacute I01.2
  syphilitic A52.06
nourishment T73.0
pancreatic K86.89
  exocrine K86.81
parathyroid (gland) E20.9
peripheral vascular (arterial) I73.9
pituitary E23.0
placental (mother) O36.51-
platelets D69.6
prenatal care affecting management of
  pregnancy O09.3-
progressive pluriglandular E31.0
pulmonary J98.4
  acute, following surgery (nonthoracic) J95.2
    thoracic J95.1
  chronic, following surgery J95.3
  following
    shock J98.4
    trauma J98.4
  newborn P28.5
  valve I37.1
    with stenosis I37.2
    congenital Q22.2
    rheumatic I09.89
      with aortic, mitral or tricuspid (valve)
        disease I08.8
pyloric K31.89
renal (acute) N28.9
  chronic N18.9
respiratory R06.89
  newborn P28.5
rotation — *see* Malrotation
sleep syndrome F51.12
social insurance Z59.7
suprarenal E27.40
  primary E27.1
tarso-orbital fascia, congenital Q10.3
testis E29.1
thyroid (gland) (acquired) E03.9
  congenital E03.1

Insufficiency, insufficient — *continued*
tricuspid (valve) (rheumatic) I07.1
  with
    aortic (valve) disease I08.2
      with mitral (valve) disease I08.3
    mitral (valve) disease I08.1
      with aortic (valve) disease I08.3
    obstruction or stenosis I07.2
      with aortic (valve) disease I08.2
        with mitral (valve) disease I08.3
  congenital Q22.8
  nonrheumatic I36.1
    with stenosis I36.2
urethral sphincter R32
valve, valvular (heart) — *see* Endocarditis
  congenital Q24.8
vascular I99.8
  intestine K55.9
    acute (*see also* Ischemia, intestine, acute)
      K55.059
  mesenteric K55.1
  peripheral I73.9
  renal — *see* Hypertension, kidney
velopharyngeal
  acquired K13.79
  congenital Q38.8
venous (chronic) (peripheral) I87.2
ventricular — *see* Insufficiency, myocardial
welfare support Z59.7
Insufflation, fallopian Z31.41
Insular — *see* condition
Insulinoma
pancreas
  benign D13.7
  malignant C25.4
  uncertain behavior D37.8
specified site
  benign — *see* Neoplasm, by site, benign
  malignant — *see* Neoplasm, by site,
    malignant
  uncertain behavior — *see* Neoplasm, by site,
    uncertain behavior
unspecified site
  benign D13.7
  malignant C25.4
  uncertain behavior D37.8
Insuloma — *see* Insulinoma
Interference
balancing side M26.56
non-working side M26.56
Intermenstrual — *see* condition
Intermittent — *see* condition
Internal — *see* condition
Interrogation
cardiac defibrillator (automatic) (implantable)
  Z45.02
cardiac pacemaker Z45.018
cardiac (event) (loop) recorder Z45.09
infusion pump (implanted) (intrathecal) Z45.1
neurostimulator Z46.2
Interruption
aortic arch Q25.21
bundle of His I44.30
phase-shift, sleep cycle — *see* Disorder, sleep,
  circadian rhythm
sleep phase-shift, or 24 hour sleep-wake cycle
  — *see* Disorder, sleep, circadian rhythm
Interstitial — *see* condition
Intertrigo L30.4
labialis K13.0
Intervertebral disc — *see* condition
Intestine, intestinal — *see* condition
Intolerance
carbohydrate K90.49
disaccharide, hereditary E73.0
fat NEC K90.49
  pancreatic K90.3
food K90.49
  dietary counseling and surveillance Z71.3

DISEASE INDEX

Intolerance — *continued*
  fructose E74.10
    hereditary E74.12
  glucose(-galactose) E74.39
  gluten K90.41
  lactose E73.9
    specified NEC E73.8
  lysine E72.3
  milk NEC K90.49
    lactose E73.9
  protein K90.49
  starch NEC K90.49
  sucrose(-isomaltose) E74.31
Intoxicated NEC (without dependence) — *see* Alcohol, intoxication
Intoxication
  acid E87.2
  alcoholic (acute) (without dependence) — *see* Alcohol, intoxication
  alimentary canal K52.1
  amphetamine (without dependence) — *see* Abuse, drug, stimulant, with intoxication
    with dependence — *see* Dependence, drug, stimulant, with intoxication
  anxiolytic (acute) (without dependence) — *see* Abuse, drug, sedative, with intoxication
    with dependence — *see* Dependence, drug, sedative, with intoxication
  caffeine F15.929
    with dependence — *see* Dependence, drug, stimulant, with intoxication
  cannabinoids (acute) (without dependence) — *see* Use, cannabis, with intoxication
    with
      abuse — *see* Abuse, drug, cannabis, with intoxication
      dependence — *see* Dependence, drug, cannabis, with intoxication
  chemical — *see* Table of Drugs and Chemicals
    via placenta or breast milk — *see* Absorption, chemical, through placenta
  cocaine (acute) (without dependence) — *see* Abuse, drug, cocaine, with intoxication
    with dependence — *see* Dependence, drug, cocaine, with intoxication
  drug
    acute (without dependence) — *see* Abuse, drug, by type with intoxication
      with dependence — *see* Dependence, drug, by type with intoxication
    addictive
      via placenta or breast milk — *see* Absorption, drug, addictive, through placenta
    newborn P93.8
      gray baby syndrome P93.0
    overdose or wrong substance given or taken — *see* Table of Drugs and Chemicals, by drug, poisoning
  enteric K52.1
  foodborne A05.9
    bacterial A05.9
    classical (Clostridium botulinum) A05.1
    due to
      Bacillus cereus A05.4
      bacterium A05.9
        specified NEC A05.8
      Clostridium
        botulinum A05.1
        perfringens A05.2
        welchii A05.2
      Salmonella A02.9
        with
          (gastro)enteritis A02.0
          localized infection(s) A02.20
            arthritis A02.23
            meningitis A02.21
            osteomyelitis A02.24
            pneumonia A02.22

Intoxication — *continued*
  foodborne A05.9 — *continued*
    due to — *continued*
      Salmonella A02.9 — *continued*
        with — *continued*
          localized infection(s) A02.20 — *continued*
            pyelonephritis A02.25
            specified NEC A02.29
          sepsis A02.1
          specified manifestation NEC A02.8
      Staphylococcus A05.0
      Vibrio
        parahaemolyticus A05.3
        vulnificus A05.5
    enterotoxin, staphylococcal A05.0
    noxious — *see* Poisoning, food, noxious
  gastrointestinal K52.1
  hallucinogenic (without dependence) — *see* Abuse, drug, hallucinogen, with intoxication
    with dependence — *see* Dependence, drug, hallucinogen, with intoxication
  hypnotic (acute) (without dependence) — *see* Abuse, drug, sedative, with intoxication
    with dependence — *see* Dependence, drug, sedative, with intoxication
  inhalant (acute) (without dependence) — *see* Abuse, drug, inhalant, with intoxication
    with dependence — *see* Dependence, drug, inhalant, with intoxication
  meaning
    inebriation — *see* category F10
    poisoning — *see* Table of Drugs and Chemicals
  methyl alcohol (acute) (without dependence) — *see* Alcohol, intoxication
  opioid (acute) (without dependence) — *see* Abuse, drug, opioid, with intoxication
    with dependence — *see* Dependence, drug, opioid, with intoxication
  pathologic NEC (without dependence) — *see* Alcohol, intoxication
  phencyclidine (without dependence) — *see* Abuse, drug, hallucinogen NEC, with intoxication
    with dependence — *see* Dependence, drug, hallucinogen, with intoxication
  potassium (K) E87.5
  psychoactive substance NEC (without dependence) — *see* Abuse, drug, hallucinogen, with intoxication
    with dependence — *see* Dependence, drug, hallucinogen, with intoxication
  sedative (acute) (without dependence) — *see* Abuse, drug, sedative, with intoxication
    with dependence — *see* Dependence, drug, sedative, with intoxication
  serum (*see also* Reaction, serum) T80.69
  uremic — *see* Uremia
  volatile solvents (acute) (without dependence) — *see* Abuse, drug, inhalant, with intoxication
    with dependence — *see* Dependence, drug, inhalant, with intoxication
  water E87.79
Intracranial — *see* condition
Intrahepatic gallbladder Q44.1
Intraligamentous — *see* condition
Intrathoracic — *see also* condition
  kidney Q63.2
Intrauterine contraceptive device
  checking Z30.431
  in situ Z97.5
  insertion Z30.430
    immediately following removal Z30.433
  management Z30.431
  reinsertion Z30.433

Intrauterine contraceptive device — *continued*
  removal Z30.432
  replacement Z30.433
  retention in pregnancy O26.3-
Intraventricular — *see* condition
Intrinsic deformity — *see* Deformity
Intubation, difficult or failed T88.4
Intumescence, lens (eye) (cataract) — *see* Cataract
Intussusception (bowel) (colon) (enteric) (ileocecal) (ileocolic) (intestine) (rectum) K56.1
  appendix K38.8
  congenital Q43.8
  ureter (with obstruction) N13.5
Invagination (bowel, colon, intestine or rectum) K56.1
Inversion
  albumin-globulin (A-G) ratio E88.09
  bladder N32.89
  cecum — *see* Intussusception
  cervix N88.8
  chromosome in normal individual Q95.1
  circadian rhythm — *see* Disorder, sleep, circadian rhythm
  nipple N64.59
    congenital Q83.8
    gestational — *see* Retraction, nipple
    puerperal, postpartum — *see* Retraction, nipple
  nyctohemeral rhythm — *see* Disorder, sleep, circadian rhythm
  optic papilla Q14.2
  organ or site, congenital NEC — *see* Anomaly, by site
  sleep rhythm — *see* Disorder, sleep, circadian rhythm
  testis (congenital) Q55.29
  uterus (chronic) (postinfectional) (postpartal, old) N85.5
    postpartum O71.2
  vagina (posthysterectomy) N99.3
  ventricular Q20.5
Investigation (*see also* Examination) Z04.9
  clinical research subject (control) (normal comparison) (participant) Z00.6
Involuntary movement, abnormal R25.9
Involution, involutional — *see also* condition
  breast, cystic — *see* Dysplasia, mammary, specified type NEC
  depression (single episode) F32.89
    recurrent episode F33.9
  melancholia (single episode) F32.89
    recurrent episode F33.8
  ovary, senile — *see* Atrophy, ovary
  thymus failure E32.8
I.Q.
  20-34 F72
  35-49 F71
  50-69 F70
  under 20 F73
IRDS (type I) P22.0
  type II P22.1
Irideremia Q13.1
Iridis rubeosis — *see* Disorder, iris, vascular
Iridochoroiditis (panuveitis) — *see* Panuveitis
Iridocyclitis H20.9
  acute H20.0-
    hypopyon H20.05-
    primary H20.01-
    recurrent H20.02-
    secondary (noninfectious) H20.04-
      infectious H20.03-
  chronic H20.1-
  due to allergy — *see* Iridocyclitis, acute, secondary
  endogenous — *see* Iridocyclitis, acute, primary

Iridocyclitis H20.9- — *continued*
  Fuchs' — *see* Cyclitis, Fuchs' heterochromic
  gonococcal A54.32
  granulomatous — *see* Iridocyclitis, chronic
  herpes, herpetic (simplex) B00.51
    zoster B02.32
  hypopyon — *see* Iridocyclitis, acute, hypopyon
  in (due to)
    ankylosing spondylitis M45.9
    gonococcal infection A54.32
    herpes (simplex) virus B00.51
      zoster B02.32
    infectious disease NOS B99
    parasitic disease NOS B89 *[H22]*
    sarcoidosis D86.83
    syphilis A51.43
    tuberculosis A18.54
    zoster B02.32
  lens-induced H20.2-
  nongranulomatous — *see* Iridocyclitis, acute
  recurrent — *see* Iridocyclitis, acute, recurrent
  rheumatic — *see* Iridocyclitis, chronic
  subacute — *see* Iridocyclitis, acute
  sympathetic — *see* Uveitis, sympathetic
  syphilitic (secondary) A51.43
  tuberculous (chronic) A18.54
  Vogt-Koyanagi H20.82-
Iridocyclochoroiditis (panuveitis) — *see*
  Panuveitis
Iridodialysis H21.53-
Iridodonesis H21.89
Iridoplegia (complete) (partial) (reflex) H57.09
Iridoschisis H21.25-
Iris — *see also* condition
  bombé — *see* Membrane, pupillary
Iritis — *see also* Iridocyclitis
  chronic — *see* Iridocyclitis, chronic
  diabetic — *see* E08-E13 with .39
  due to
    herpes simplex B00.51
    leprosy A30.9 *[H22]*
  gonococcal A54.32
  gouty (*see also* Gout, by type) M10.9 *[H22]*
  granulomatous — *see* Iridocyclitis, chronic
  lens induced — *see* Iridocyclitis, lens-induced
  papulosa (syphilitic) A52.71
  rheumatic — *see* Iridocyclitis, chronic
  syphilitic (secondary) A51.43
    congenital (early) A50.01
    late A52.71
  tuberculous A18.54
Iron — *see* condition
Iron-miner's lung J63.4
Irradiated enamel (tooth, teeth) K03.89
Irradiation effects, adverse T66
Irreducible, irreducibility — *see* condition
Irregular, irregularity
  action, heart I49.9
  alveolar process K08.89
  bleeding N92.6
  breathing R06.89
  contour of cornea (acquired) — *see* Deformity,
    cornea
    congenital Q13.4
  contour, reconstructed breast N65.0
  dentin (in pulp) K04.3
  eye movements H55.89
    nystagmus — *see* Nystagmus
    saccadic H55.81
  labor O62.2
  menstruation (cause unknown) N92.6
  periods N92.6
  prostate N42.9
  pupil — *see* Abnormality, pupillary
  reconstructed breast N65.0
  respiratory R06.89
  septum (nasal) J34.2

Irregular, irregularity — *continued*
  shape, organ or site, congenital NEC — *see*
    Distortion
  sleep-wake pattern (rhythm) G47.23
Irritable, irritability R45.4
  bladder N32.89
  bowel (syndrome) K58.9
    with
      constipation K58.1
      diarrhea K58.0
    mixed K58.2
    psychogenic F45.8
    specified NEC K58.8
  bronchial — *see* Bronchitis
  cerebral, in newborn P91.3
  colon (*see also* Irritable, bowel) K58.9
    with diarrhea K58.0
    psychogenic F45.8
  duodenum K59.8
  heart (psychogenic) F45.8
  hip — *see* Derangement, joint, specified type
    NEC, hip
  ileum K59.8
  infant R68.12
  jejunum K59.8
  rectum K59.8
  stomach K31.89
    psychogenic F45.8
  sympathetic G90.8
  urethra N36.8
Irritation
  anus K62.89
  axillary nerve G54.0
  bladder N32.89
  brachial plexus G54.0
  bronchial — *see* Bronchitis
  cervical plexus G54.2
  cervix — *see* Cervicitis
  choroid, sympathetic — *see* Endophthalmitis
  cranial nerve — *see* Disorder, nerve, cranial
  gastric K31.89
    psychogenic F45.8
  globe, sympathetic — *see* Uveitis, sympathetic
  labyrinth — *see* subcategory H83.2
  lumbosacral plexus G54.1
  meninges (traumatic) — *see* Injury, intracranial
    nontraumatic — *see* Meningismus
  nerve — *see* Disorder, nerve
  nervous R45.0
  penis N48.89
  perineum NEC L29.3
  peripheral autonomic nervous system G90.8
  peritoneum — *see* Peritonitis
  pharynx J39.2
  plantar nerve — *see* Lesion, nerve, plantar
  spinal (cord) (traumatic) — *see also* Injury,
    spinal cord, by region
    nerve G58.9
      root NEC — *see* Radiculopathy
    nontraumatic — *see* Myelopathy
  stomach K31.89
    psychogenic F45.8
  sympathetic nerve NEC G90.8
  ulnar nerve — *see* Lesion, nerve, ulnar
  vagina N89.8
Ischemia, ischemic I99.8
  bowel (transient)
    acute (*see also* Ischemia, intestine, acute)
      K55.059
    chronic K55.1
    due to mesenteric artery insufficiency K55.1
  brain — *see* Ischemia, cerebral
  cardiac (*see* Disease, heart, ischemic)
  cardiomyopathy I25.5

Ischemia, ischemic I99.8 — *continued*
  cerebral (chronic) (generalized) I67.82
    arteriosclerotic I67.2
    intermittent G45.9
    newborn P91.0
    recurrent focal G45.8
    transient G45.9
  colon chronic (due to mesenteric artery
    insufficiency) K55.1
  coronary — *see* Disease, heart, ischemic
  demand (coronary) (*see also* Angina) I24.8
  heart (chronic or with a stated duration of over
    4 weeks) I25.9
    acute or with a stated duration of 4 weeks or
      less I24.9
    subacute I24.9
  infarction, muscle — *see* Infarct, muscle
  intestine (large) (small) (transient) K55.9
    acute K55.059
      diffuse K55.052
      focal K55.051
      large K55.039
        diffuse K55.032
        focal K55.031
      small K55.019
        diffuse K55.012
        focal K55.011
    chronic K55.1
    due to mesenteric artery insufficiency K55.1
  kidney N28.0
  mesenteric, acute (*see also* Ischemia, intestine,
    acute) K55.059
  muscle, traumatic T79.6
  myocardium, myocardial (chronic or with a
    stated duration of over 4 weeks) I25.9
    acute, without myocardial infarction I51.3
    silent (asymptomatic) I25.6
    transient of newborn P29.4
  renal N28.0
  retina, retinal — *see* Occlusion, artery, retina
  small bowel
    acute K55.019
      diffuse K55.012
      focal K55.011
    chronic K55.1
    due to mesenteric artery insufficiency K55.1
  spinal cord G95.11
  subendocardial — *see* Insufficiency, coronary
  supply (coronary) (*see also* Angina) I25.9
    due to vasospasm I20.1
Ischial spine — *see* condition
Ischialgia — *see* Sciatica
Ischiopagus Q89.4
Ischium, ischial — *see* condition
Ischuria R34
Iselin's disease or osteochondrosis — *see*
  Osteochondrosis, juvenile, metatarsus
Islands of
  parotid tissue in
    lymph nodes Q38.6
    neck structures Q38.6
  submaxillary glands in
    fascia Q38.6
    lymph nodes Q38.6
    neck muscles Q38.6
Islet cell tumor, pancreas D13.7

Isoimmunization NEC — *see also*
  Incompatibility
  affecting management of pregnancy (ABO)
      (with hydrops fetalis) O36.11-
    anti-A sensitization O36.11-
    anti-B sensitization O36.19-
    anti-c sensitization O36.09-
    anti-C sensitization O36.09-
    anti-e sensitization O36.09-
    anti-E sensitization O36.09-
    Rh NEC O36.09-
      anti-D antibody O36.01-
    specified NEC O36.19-
  newborn P55.9
    with
      hydrops fetalis P56.0
      kernicterus P57.0
    ABO (blood groups) P55.1
    Rhesus (Rh) factor P55.0
    specified type NEC P55.8
Isolation, isolated
  dwelling Z59.8
  family Z63.79
  social Z60.4
Isoleucinosis E71.19
Isomerism atrial appendages (with
    asplenia or polysplenia) Q20.6
Isosporiasis, isosporosis A07.3
Isovaleric acidemia E71.110
Issue of
  medical certificate Z02.79
    for disability determination Z02.71
  repeat prescription (appliance) (glasses)
      (medicinal substance, medicament,
      medicine) Z76.0
  contraception — *see* Contraception
Itch, itching — *see also* Pruritus
  baker's L23.6
  barber's B35.0
  bricklayer's L24.5
  cheese B88.0
  clam digger's B65.3
  coolie B76.9
  copra B88.0
  dew B76.9
  dhobi B35.6
  filarial — *see* Infestation, filarial
  grain B88.0
  grocer's B88.0
  ground B76.9
  harvest B88.0
  jock B35.6
  Malabar B35.5
    beard B35.0
    foot B35.3
    scalp B35.0
  meaning scabies B86
  Norwegian B86
  perianal L29.0
  poultrymen's B88.0
  sarcoptic B86
  scabies B86
  scrub B88.0
  straw B88.0
  swimmer's B65.3
  water B76.9
  winter L29.8
Ivemark's syndrome (asplenia with
    congenital heart disease) Q89.01
Ivory bones Q78.2
Ixodiasis NEC B88.8

J

Jaccoud's syndrome — *see* Arthropathy,
    postrheumatic, chronic
Jackson's
  membrane Q43.3
  paralysis or syndrome G83.89
  veil Q43.3
Jacquet's dermatitis (diaper dermatitis) L22
Jadassohn's
  blue nevus — *see* Nevus
  intraepidermal epithelioma — *see* Neoplasm,
    skin, benign
**Jadassohn-Pellizari's disease or
  anetoderma** L90.2
**Jaffe-Lichtenstein (-Uehlinger)
  syndrome** — *see* Dysplasia, fibrous, bone
  NEC
Jakob-Creutzfeldt disease or syndrome
    — *see* Creutzfeldt-Jakob disease or
    syndrome
Jaksch-Luzet disease D64.89
Jamaican
  neuropathy G92
  paraplegic tropical ataxic-spastic syndrome
    G92
Janet's disease F48.8
Janiceps Q89.4
Jansky-Bielschowsky amaurotic idiocy
    E75.4
Japanese
  B-type encephalitis A83.0
  river fever A75.3
Jaundice (yellow) R17
  acholuric (familial) (splenomegalic) — *see also*
    Spherocytosis
    acquired D59.8
  breast-milk (inhibitor) P59.3
  catarrhal (acute) B15.9
    with hepatic coma B15.0
  cholestatic (benign) R17
  due to or associated with
    delayed conjugation P59.8
      associated with (due to) preterm delivery
        P59.0
    preterm delivery P59.0
  epidemic (catarrhal) B15.9
    with hepatic coma B15.0
    leptospiral A27.0
    spirochetal A27.0
  familial nonhemolytic (congenital) (Gilbert)
    E80.4
    Crigler-Najjar E80.5
  febrile (acute) B15.9
    with hepatic coma B15.0
    leptospiral A27.0
    spirochetal A27.0
  hematogenous D59.9
  hemolytic (acquired) D59.9
    congenital — *see* Spherocytosis
  hemorrhagic (acute) (leptospiral) (spirochetal)
    A27.0
  infectious (acute) (subacute) B15.9
    with hepatic coma B15.0
    leptospiral A27.0
    spirochetal A27.0
  leptospiral (hemorrhagic) A27.0
  malignant (without coma) K72.90
    with coma K72.91
  neonatal — *see* Jaundice, newborn

Jaundice (yellow) R17 — *continued*
  newborn P59.9
    due to or associated with
      ABO
        antibodies P55.1
        incompatibility, maternal/fetal P55.1
        isoimmunization P55.1
      absence or deficiency of enzyme system
        for bilirubin conjugation (congenital)
        P59.8
      bleeding P58.1
      breast milk inhibitors to conjugation P59.3
        associated with preterm delivery P59.0
      bruising P58.0
      Crigler-Najjar syndrome E80.5
      delayed conjugation P59.8
        associated with preterm delivery P59.0
      drugs or toxins
        given to newborn P58.42
        transmitted from mother P58.41
      excessive hemolysis P58.9
        due to
          bleeding P58.1
          bruising P58.0
          drugs or toxins
            given to newborn P58.42
            transmitted from mother P58.41
          infection P58.2
          polycythemia P58.3
          swallowed maternal blood P58.5
        specified type NEC P58.8
      galactosemia E74.21
      Gilbert syndrome E80.4
      hemolytic disease P55.9
        ABO isoimmunization P55.1
        Rh isoimmunization P55.0
        specified NEC P55.8
      hepatocellular damage P59.20
        specified NEC P59.29
      hereditary hemolytic anemia P58.8
      hypothyroidism, congenital E03.1
      incompatibility, maternal/fetal NOS P55.9
      infection P58.2
      inspissated bile syndrome P59.1
      isoimmunization NOS P55.9
      mucoviscidosis E84.9
      polycythemia P58.3
      preterm delivery P59.0
      Rh
        antibodies P55.0
        incompatibility, maternal/fetal P55.0
        isoimmunization P55.0
      specified cause NEC P59.8
      swallowed maternal blood P58.5
    spherocytosis (congenital) D58.0
  nonhemolytic congenital familial (Gilbert)
    E80.4
  nuclear, newborn (*see also* Kernicterus of
    newborn) P57.9
  obstructive (*see also* Obstruction, bile duct)
    K83.1
  post-immunization — *see* Hepatitis, viral, type,
    B
  post-transfusion — *see* Hepatitis, viral, type, B
  regurgitation (*see also* Obstruction, bile duct)
    K83.1
  serum (homologous) (prophylactic)
    (therapeutic) — *see* Hepatitis, viral, type, B
  spirochetal (hemorrhagic) A27.0
  symptomatic R17
    newborn P59.9
Jaw — *see* condition
Jaw-winking phenomenon or syndrome
    Q07.8

Jealousy
  alcoholic F10.988
  childhood F93.8
  sibling F93.8
Jejunitis — *see* Enteritis
Jejunostomy status Z93.4
Jejunum, jejunal — *see* condition
Jensen's disease — *see* Inflammation,
  chorioretinal, focal, juxtapapillary
Jerks, myoclonic G25.3
Jervell-Lange-Nielsen syndrome I45.81
Jeune's disease Q77.2
Jigger disease B88.1
Job's syndrome (chronic granulomatous
  disease) D71
Joint — *see also* condition
  mice — *see* Loose, body, joint
    knee M23.4-
Jordan's anomaly or syndrome D72.0
Joseph-Diamond-Blackfan anemia
  (congenital hypoplastic) D61.01
Jungle yellow fever A95.0
Jüngling's disease — *see* Sarcoidosis
Juvenile — *see* condition

K

Kahler's disease C90.0-
Kakke E51.11
Kala-azar B55.0
Kallmann's syndrome E23.0
Kanner's syndrome (autism) — *see* Psychosis,
  childhood
Kaposi's
  dermatosis (xeroderma pigmentosum) Q82.1
  lichen ruber L44.0
    acuminatus L44.0
  sarcoma
    colon C46.4
    connective tissue C46.1
    gastrointestinal organ C46.4
    lung C46.5-
    lymph node (multiple) C46.3
    palate (hard) (soft) C46.2
    rectum C46.4
    skin (multiple sites) C46.0
    specified site NEC C46.7
    stomach C46.4
    unspecified site C46.9
  varicelliform eruption B00.0
  vaccinia T88.1
Kartagener's syndrome or triad (sinusitis,
  bronchiectasis, situs inversus) Q89.3
Karyotype
  with abnormality except iso (Xq) Q96.2
  45,X Q96.0
  46,X
    iso (Xq) Q96.1
  46,XX Q98.3
    with streak gonads Q50.32
    hermaphrodite (true) Q99.1
    male Q98.3
  46,XY
    with streak gonads Q56.1
    female Q97.3
    hermaphrodite (true) Q99.1
  47,XXX Q97.0
  47,XXY Q98.0
  47,XYY Q98.5
Kaschin-Beck disease — *see* Disease,
  Kaschin-Beck
Katayama's disease or fever B65.2
Kawasaki's syndrome M30.3
Kayser-Fleischer ring (cornea)
  (pseudosclerosis) H18.04-
Kaznelson's syndrome (congenital
  hypoplastic anemia) D61.01
Kearns-Sayre syndrome H49.81-
Kedani fever A75.3
Kelis L91.0
Kelly (-Patterson) syndrome (sideropenic
  dysphagia) D50.1
Keloid, cheloid L91.0
  acne L73.0
  Addison's L94.0
  cornea — *see* Opacity, cornea
  Hawkin's L91.0
  scar L91.0
Keloma L91.0
Kenya fever A77.1
Keratectasia — *see also* Ectasia, cornea
  congenital Q13.4
Keratinization of alveolar ridge mucosa
  excessive K13.23
  minimal K13.22
Keratinized residual ridge mucosa
  excessive K13.23
  minimal K13.22

Keratitis (nodular) (nonulcerative) (simple)
  (zonular) H16.9
  with ulceration (central) (marginal) (perforated)
    (ring) — *see* Ulcer, cornea
  actinic — *see* Photokeratitis
  arborescens (herpes simplex) B00.52
  areolar H16.11-
  bullosa H16.8
  deep H16.309
    specified type NEC H16.399
  dendritic(a) (herpes simplex) B00.52
  disciform(is) (herpes simplex) B00.52
    varicella B01.81
  filamentary H16.12-
  gonococcal (congenital or prenatal) A54.33
  herpes, herpetic (simplex) B00.52
    zoster B02.33
  in (due to)
    acanthamebiasis B60.13
    adenovirus B30.0
    exanthema (*see also* Exanthem) B09
    herpes (simplex) virus B00.52
    measles B05.81
    syphilis A50.31
    tuberculosis A18.52
    zoster B02.33
  interstitial (nonsyphilitic) H16.30-
    diffuse H16.32-
    herpes, herpetic (simplex) B00.52
      zoster B02.33
    sclerosing H16.33-
    specified type NEC H16.39-
    syphilitic (congenital) (late) A50.31
    tuberculous A18.52
  macular H16.11-
  nummular H16.11-
  oyster shuckers' H16.8
  parenchymatous — *see* Keratitis, interstitial
  petrificans H16.8
  postmeasles B05.81
  punctata
    leprosa A30.9 *[H16.14-]*
    syphilitic (profunda) A50.31
  punctate H16.14-
  purulent H16.8
  rosacea L71.8
  sclerosing H16.33-
  specified type NEC H16.8
  stellate H16.11-
  striate H16.11-
  superficial H16.10-
    with conjunctivitis — *see* Keratoconjunctivitis
    due to light — *see* Photokeratitis
  suppurative H16.8
  syphilitic (congenital) (prenatal) A50.31
  trachomatous A71.1
    sequelae B94.0
  tuberculous A18.52
  vesicular H16.8
  xerotic (*see also* Keratomalacia) H16.8
    vitamin A deficiency E50.4
Kerato-uveitis — *see* Iridocyclitis
Keratoacanthoma L85.8
Keratocele — *see* Descemetocele
Keratoconjunctivitis H16.20-
  Acanthamoeba B60.13
  adenoviral B30.0
  epidemic B30.0
  exposure H16.21-
  herpes, herpetic (simplex) B00.52
    zoster B02.33
  in exanthema (*see also* Exanthem) B09
  infectious B30.0
  lagophthalmic — *see* Keratoconjunctivitis,
    specified type NEC
  neurotrophic H16.23-
  phlyctenular H16.25-
  postmeasles B05.81
  shipyard B30.0

Keratoconjunctivitis H16.20- — *continued*
sicca (Sjogren's) M35.0-
not Sjogren's H16.22-
specified type NEC H16.29-
tuberculous (phlyctenular) A18.52
vernal H16.26-
Keratoconus H18.60-
congenital Q13.4
stable H18.61-
unstable H18.62-
Keratocyst (dental) (odontogenic) — *see* Cyst, calcifying odontogenic
Keratoderma, keratodermia (congenital) (palmaris et plantaris) (symmetrical) Q82.8
acquired L85.1
in diseases classified elsewhere L86
climactericum L85.1
gonococcal A54.89
gonorrheal A54.89
punctata L85.2
Reiter's — *see* Reiter's disease
Keratodermatocele — *see* Descemetocele
Keratoglobus H18.79
congenital Q15.8
with glaucoma Q15.0
Keratohemia — *see* Pigmentation, cornea, stromal
Keratoiritis — *see also* Iridocyclitis
syphilitic A50.39
tuberculous A18.54
Keratoma L57.0
palmaris and plantaris hereditarium Q82.8
senile L57.0
Keratomalacia H18.44-
vitamin A deficiency E50.4
Keratomegaly Q13.4
Keratomycosis B49
nigrans, nigricans (palmaris) B36.1
Keratopathy H18.9
band H18.42-
bullous H18.1-
bullous (aphakic), following cataract surgery H59.01-
Keratoscleritis, tuberculous A18.52
Keratosis L57.0
actinic L57.0
arsenical L85.8
congenital, specified NEC Q80.8
female genital NEC N94.89
follicularis Q82.8
acquired L11.0
congenita Q82.8
et parafollicularis in cutem penetrans L87.0
spinulosa (decalvans) Q82.8
vitamin A deficiency E50.8
gonococcal A54.89
male genital (external) N50.89
nigricans L83
obturans, external ear (canal) — *see* Cholesteatoma, external ear
palmaris et plantaris (inherited) (symmetrical) Q82.8
acquired L85.1
penile N48.89
pharynx J39.2
pilaris, acquired L85.8
punctata (palmaris et plantaris) L85.2
scrotal N50.89
seborrheic L82.1
inflamed L82.0
senile L57.0
solar L57.0
tonsillaris J35.8
vagina N89.4
vegetans Q82.8
vitamin A deficiency E50.8
vocal cord J38.3
Kerion (celsi) B35.0

Kernicterus of newborn (not due to isoimmunization) P57.9
due to isoimmunization (conditions in P55.0-P55.9) P57.0
specified type NEC P57.8
Kerunoparalysis T75.09
Keshan disease E59
Ketoacidosis E87.2
diabetic — *see* Diabetes, by type, with ketoacidosis
Ketonuria R82.4
Ketosis NEC E88.89
diabetic — *see* Diabetes, by type, with ketoacidosis
Kew Garden fever A79.1
Kidney — *see* condition
Kienböck's disease — *see also* Osteochondrosis, juvenile, hand, carpal lunate
adult M93.1
Kimmelstiel (-Wilson) disease — *see* Diabetes, Kimmelstiel (-Wilson) disease
Kimura disease D21.9
specified site — *see* Neoplasm, connective tissue, benign
Kink, kinking
artery I77.1
hair (acquired) L67.8
ileum or intestine — *see* Obstruction, intestine
Lane's — *see* Obstruction, intestine
organ or site, congenital NEC — *see* Anomaly, by site
ureter (pelvic junction) N13.5
with
hydronephrosis N13.1
with infection N13.6
pyelonephritis (chronic) N11.1
congenital Q62.39
vein(s) I87.8
caval I87.1
peripheral I87.1
Kinnier Wilson's disease (hepatolenticular degeneration) E83.01
Kissing spine M48.20
cervical region M48.22
cervicothoracic region M48.23
lumbar region M48.26
lumbosacral region M48.27
occipito-atlanto-axial region M48.21
thoracic region M48.24
thoracolumbar region M48.25
Klatskin's tumor C24.0
Klauder's disease A26.8
Klebs' disease (*see also* Glomerulonephritis) N05-
Klebsiella (K.) pneumoniae, as cause of disease classified elsewhere B96.1
Klein(e)-Levin syndrome G47.13
Kleptomania F63.2
Klinefelter's syndrome Q98.4
karyotype 47,XXY Q98.0
male with more than two X chromosomes Q98.1
Klippel-Feil deficiency, disease, or syndrome (brevicollis) Q76.1
Klippel's disease I67.2
Klippel-Trenaunay (-Weber) syndrome Q87.2
Klumpke(-Déjerine) palsy, paralysis (birth) (newborn) P14.1
Knee — *see* condition
Knock knee (acquired) M21.06-
congenital Q74.1
Knot(s)
intestinal, syndrome (volvulus) K56.2
surfer S89.8-
umbilical cord (true) O69.2
Knotting (of)
hair L67.8
intestine K56.2

Knuckle pad (Garrod's) M72.1
Koch's
infection — *see* Tuberculosis
relapsing fever A68.9
Koch-Weeks' conjunctivitis — *see* Conjunctivitis, acute, mucopurulent
Köebner's syndrome Q81.8
Köenig's disease (osteochondritis dissecans) — *see* Osteochondritis, dissecans
Köhler's disease
patellar — *see* Osteochondrosis, juvenile, patella
tarsal navicular — *see* Osteochondrosis, juvenile, tarsus
Köhler-Pellegrini-Steida disease or syndrome (calcification, knee joint) — *see* Bursitis, tibial collateral
Koilonychia L60.3
congenital Q84.6
Kojevnikov's, epilepsy — *see* Kozhevnikof's epilepsy
Kozhevnikof's epilepsy G40.109
intractable G40.119
with status epilepticus G40.111
without status epilepticus G40.119
not intractable G40.109
with status epilepticus G40.101
without status epilepticus G40.109
Koplik's spots B05.9
Kopp's asthma E32.8
Korsakoff's (Wernicke) disease, psychosis or syndrome (alcoholic) F10.96
with dependence F10.26
drug-induced
due to drug abuse — *see* Abuse, drug, by type, with amnestic disorder
due to drug dependence — *see* Dependence, drug, by type, with amnestic disorder
nonalcoholic F04
Korsakov's disease, psychosis or syndrome — *see* Korsakoff's disease
Korsakow's disease, psychosis or syndrome — *see* Korsakoff's disease
Kostmann's disease or syndrome (infantile genetic agranulocytosis) — *see* Agranulocytosis
Krabbe's
disease E75.23
syndrome, congenital muscle hypoplasia Q79.8
Kraepelin-Morel disease — *see* Schizophrenia
Kraft-Weber-Dimitri disease Q85.8
Kraurosis
ani K62.89
penis N48.0
vagina N89.8
vulva N90.4
Kreotoxism A05.9
Krukenberg's
spindle — *see* Pigmentation, cornea, posterior
tumor C79.6-
Kufs' disease E75.4
Kugelberg-Welander disease G12.1
Kuhnt-Junius degeneration (*see also* Degeneration, macula) H35.32-
Kümmell's disease or spondylitis — *see* Spondylopathy, traumatic
Kupffer cell sarcoma C22.3
Kuru A81.81
Kussmaul's
disease M30.0
respiration E87.2
in diabetic acidosis — *see* Diabetes, by type, with ketoacidosis
Kwashiorkor E40
marasmic, marasmus type E42

Kyasanur Forest disease A98.2
Kyphoscoliosis, kyphoscoliotic (acquired)
    (*see also* Scoliosis) M41.9
    congenital Q67.5
    heart (disease) I27.1
    sequelae of rickets E64.3
    tuberculous A18.01
Kyphosis, kyphotic (acquired) M40.209
    cervical region M40.202
    cervicothoracic region M40.203
    congenital Q76.419
        cervical region Q76.412
        cervicothoracic region Q76.413
        occipito-atlanto-axial region Q76.411
        thoracic region Q76.414
        thoracolumbar region Q76.415
    Morquio-Brailsford type (spinal) (*see also*
        subcategory M49.8) E76.219
    postlaminectomy M96.3
    postradiation therapy M96.2
    postural (adolescent) M40.00
        cervicothoracic region M40.03
        thoracic region M40.04
        thoracolumbar region M40.05
    secondary NEC M40.10
        cervical region M40.12
        cervicothoracic region M40.13
        thoracic region M40.14
        thoracolumbar region M40.15
    sequelae of rickets E64.3
    specified type NEC M40.299
        cervical region M40.292
        cervicothoracic region M40.293
        thoracic region M40.294
        thoracolumbar region M40.295
    syphilitic, congenital A50.56
    thoracic region M40.204
    thoracolumbar region M40.205
    tuberculous A18.01
Kyrle disease L87.0

L

Labia, labium — *see* condition
Labile
    blood pressure R09.89
    vasomotor system I73.9
Labioglossal paralysis G12.29
Labium leporinum — *see* Cleft, lip
Labor — *see* Delivery
Labored breathing — *see* Hyperventilation
Labyrinthitis (circumscribed) (destructive)
    (diffuse) (inner ear) (latent) (purulent)
    (suppurative) (*see also* subcategory) H83.0
    syphilitic A52.79
Laceration
    with abortion — *see* Abortion, by type,
        complicated by laceration of pelvic organs
    abdomen, abdominal
        wall S31.119
            with
                foreign body S31.129
                penetration into peritoneal cavity
                    S31.619
                    with foreign body S31.629
        epigastric region S31.112
            with
                foreign body S31.122
                penetration into peritoneal cavity
                    S31.612
                    with foreign body S31.622
        left
            lower quadrant S31.114
                with
                    foreign body S31.124
                    penetration into peritoneal cavity
                      S31.614
                      with foreign body S31.624
            upper quadrant S31.111
                with
                    foreign body S31.121
                    penetration into peritoneal cavity
                      S31.611
                      with foreign body S31.621
        periumbilic region S31.115
            with
                foreign body S31.125
                penetration into peritoneal cavity
                    S31.615
                    with foreign body S31.625
        right
            lower quadrant S31.113
                with
                    foreign body S31.123
                    penetration into peritoneal cavity
                      S31.613
                    with foreign body S31.623
            upper quadrant S31.110
                with
                    foreign body S31.120
                  penetration into peritoneal cavity
                    S31.610
                    with foreign body S31.620
    accidental, complicating surgery — *see*
        Complications, surgical, accidental
        puncture or laceration
    Achilles tendon S86.02-
    adrenal gland S37.813
    alveolar (process) — *see* Laceration, oral cavity
    ankle S91.01-
        with
            foreign body S91.02-
    antecubital space — *see* Laceration, elbow
    anus (sphincter) S31.831
        with
            ectopic or molar pregnancy O08.6
            foreign body S31.832

Laceration — *continued*
    anus (sphincter) S31.831 — *continued*
        complicating delivery — *see* Delivery,
            complicated, by, laceration, anus
            (sphincter)
        following ectopic or molar pregnancy O08.6
        nontraumatic, nonpuerperal — *see* Fissure,
            anus
    arm (upper) S41.11-
        with foreign body S41.12-
        lower — *see* Laceration, forearm
    auditory canal (external) (meatus) — *see*
        Laceration, ear
    auricle, ear — *see* Laceration, ear
    axilla — *see* Laceration, arm
    back — *see also* Laceration, thorax, back
        lower S31.010
            with
                foreign body S31.020
                  with penetration into retroperitoneal
                    space S31.021
                penetration into retroperitoneal space
                  S31.011
    bile duct S36.13
    bladder S37.23
        with ectopic or molar pregnancy O08.6
        following ectopic or molar pregnancy O08.6
        obstetrical trauma O71.5
    blood vessel — *see* Injury, blood vessel
    bowel — *see also* Laceration, intestine
        with ectopic or molar pregnancy O08.6
        complicating abortion — *see* Abortion, by
            type, complicated by, specified
            condition NEC
        following ectopic or molar pregnancy O08.6
        obstetrical trauma O71.5
    brain (any part) (cortex) (diffuse) (membrane)
        — *see also* Injury, intracranial, diffuse
        during birth P10.8
            with hemorrhage P10.1
        focal — *see* Injury, intracranial, focal brain
            injury
    brainstem S06.38-
    breast S21.01-
        with foreign body S21.02-
    broad ligament S37.893
        with ectopic or molar pregnancy O08.6
        following ectopic or molar pregnancy O08.6
        laceration syndrome N83.8
        obstetrical trauma O71.6
        syndrome (laceration) N83.8
    buttock S31.801
        with foreign body S31.802
        left S31.821
            with foreign body S31.822
        right S31.811
            with foreign body S31.812
    calf — *see* Laceration, leg
    canaliculus lacrimalis — *see* Laceration, eyelid
    canthus, eye — *see* Laceration, eyelid
    capsule, joint — *see* Sprain
    causing eversion of cervix uteri (old) N86
    central (perineal), complicating delivery O70.9
    cerebellum, traumatic S06.37-
    cerebral S06.33-
        during birth P10.8
            with hemorrhage P10.1
        left side S06.32-
        right side S06.31-
    cervix (uteri)
        with ectopic or molar pregnancy O08.6
        following ectopic or molar pregnancy O08.6
        nonpuerperal, nontraumatic N88.1
        obstetrical trauma (current) O71.3
        old (postpartal) N88.1
        traumatic S37.63
    cheek (external) S01.41-
        with foreign body S01.42-
        internal — *see* Laceration, oral cavity

Laceration — continued
  chest wall — see Laceration, thorax
  chin — see Laceration, head, specified site NEC
  chordae tendinae NEC I51.1
    concurrent with acute myocardial infarction — see Infarct, myocardium
    following acute myocardial infarction (current complication) I23.4
  clitoris — see Laceration, vulva
  colon — see Laceration, intestine, large, colon
  common bile duct S36.13
  cortex (cerebral) — see Injury, intracranial, diffuse
  costal region — see Laceration, thorax
  cystic duct S36.13
  diaphragm S27.803
  digit(s)
    foot — see Laceration, toe
    hand — see Laceration, finger
  duodenum S36.430
  ear (canal) (external) S01.31-
    with foreign body S01.32-
    drum S09.2-
  elbow S51.01-
    with
      foreign body S51.02-
  epididymis — see Laceration, testis
  epigastric region — see Laceration, abdomen, wall, epigastric region
  esophagus K22.8
    traumatic
      cervical S11.21
        with foreign body S11.22
      thoracic S27.813
  eye(ball) S05.3-
    with prolapse or loss of intraocular tissue S05.2-
    penetrating S05.6-
  eyebrow — see Laceration, eyelid
  eyelid S01.11-
    with foreign body S01.12-
  face NEC — see Laceration, head, specified site NEC
  fallopian tube S37.539
    bilateral S37.532
    unilateral S37.531
  finger(s) S61.219
    with
      damage to nail S61.319
        with
          foreign body S61.329
      foreign body S61.229
    index S61.218
      with
        damage to nail S61.318
          with
            foreign body S61.328
        foreign body S61.228
    left S61.211
      with
        damage to nail S61.311
          with
            foreign body S61.321
        foreign body S61.221
    right S61.210
      with
        damage to nail S61.310
          with
            foreign body S61.320
        foreign body S61.220
    little S61.218
      with
        damage to nail S61.318
          with
            foreign body S61.328
        foreign body S61.228

Laceration — continued
  finger(s) S61.219 — continued
    little S61.218 — continued
      left S61.217
        with
          damage to nail S61.317
            with
              foreign body S61.327
            foreign body S61.227
      right S61.216
        with
          damage to nail S61.316
            with
              foreign body S61.326
            foreign body S61.226
    middle S61.218
      with
        damage to nail S61.318
          with
            foreign body S61.328
        foreign body S61.228
      left S61.213
        with
          damage to nail S61.313
            with
              foreign body S61.323
            foreign body S61.223
      right S61.212
        with
          damage to nail S61.312
            with
              foreign body S61.322
            foreign body S61.222
    ring S61.218
      with
        damage to nail S61.318
          with
            foreign body S61.328
        foreign body S61.228
      left S61.215
        with
          damage to nail S61.315
            with
              foreign body S61.325
            foreign body S61.225
      right S61.214
        with
          damage to nail S61.314
            with
              foreign body S61.324
            foreign body S61.224
  flank S31.119
    with foreign body S31.129
  foot (except toe(s) alone) S91.319
    with foreign body S91.329
    left S91.312
      with foreign body S91.322
    right S91.311
      with foreign body S91.321
    toe — see Laceration, toe
  forearm S51.819
    with
      foreign body S51.829
    elbow only — see Laceration, elbow
    left S51.812
      with
        foreign body S51.822
    right S51.811
      with
        foreign body S51.821
  forehead S01.81
    with foreign body S01.82
  fourchette O70.0
    with ectopic or molar pregnancy O08.6
    complicating delivery O70.0
    following ectopic or molar pregnancy O08.6
  gallbladder S36.123

Laceration — continued
  genital organs, external
    female S31.512
      with foreign body S31.522
      vagina — see Laceration, vagina
      vulva — see Laceration, vulva
    male S31.511
      with foreign body S31.521
      penis — see Laceration, penis
      scrotum — see Laceration, scrotum
      testis — see Laceration, testis
  groin — see Laceration, abdomen, wall
  gum — see Laceration, oral cavity
  hand S61.419
    with
      foreign body S61.429
    finger — see Laceration, finger
    left S61.412
      with
        foreign body S61.422
    right S61.411
      with
        foreign body S61.421
    thumb — see Laceration, thumb
  head S01.91
    with foreign body S01.92
    cheek — see Laceration, cheek
    ear — see Laceration, ear
    eyelid — see Laceration, eyelid
    lip — see Laceration, lip
    nose — see Laceration, nose
    oral cavity — see Laceration, oral cavity
    scalp S01.01
      with foreign body S01.02
    specified site NEC S01.81
      with foreign body S01.82
    temporomandibular area — see Laceration, cheek
  heart — see Injury, heart, laceration
  heel — see Laceration, foot
  hepatic duct S36.13
  hip S71.019
    with foreign body S71.029
    left S71.012
      with foreign body S71.022
    right S71.011
      with foreign body S71.021
  hymen — see Laceration, vagina
  hypochondrium — see Laceration, abdomen, wall
  hypogastric region — see Laceration, abdomen, wall
  ileum S36.438
  inguinal region — see Laceration, abdomen, wall
  instep — see Laceration, foot
  internal organ — see Injury, by site
  interscapular region — see Laceration, thorax, back
  intestine
    large
      colon S36.539
        ascending S36.530
        descending S36.532
        sigmoid S36.533
        specified site NEC S36.538
      rectum S36.63
      transverse S36.531
    small S36.439
      duodenum S36.430
      specified site NEC S36.438
  intra-abdominal organ S36.93
    intestine — see Laceration, intestine
    liver — see Laceration, liver
    pancreas — see Laceration, pancreas
    peritoneum S36.81
    specified site NEC S36.893
    spleen — see Laceration, spleen
    stomach — see Laceration, stomach

Laceration — *continued*
intracranial NEC — *see also* Injury,
　intracranial, diffuse
　birth injury P10.9
jaw — *see* Laceration, head, specified site NEC
jejunum S36.438
joint capsule — *see* Sprain, by site
kidney S37.03-
　major (greater than 3 cm) (massive) (stellate)
　　S37.06-
　minor (less than 1 cm) S37.04-
　moderate (1 to 3 cm) S37.05-
　multiple S37.06-
knee S81.01-
　with foreign body S81.02-
labium (majus) (minus) — *see* Laceration, vulva
lacrimal duct — *see* Laceration, eyelid
large intestine — *see* Laceration, intestine,
　large
larynx S11.011
　with foreign body S11.012
leg (lower) S81.819
　with foreign body S81.829
　foot — *see* Laceration, foot
　knee — *see* Laceration, knee
　left S81.812
　　with foreign body S81.822
　right S81.811
　　with foreign body S81.821
　upper — *see* Laceration, thigh
ligament — *see* Sprain
lip S01.511
　with foreign body S01.521
liver S36.113
　major (stellate) S36.116
　minor S36.114
　moderate S36.115
loin — *see* Laceration, abdomen, wall
lower back — *see* Laceration, back, lower
lumbar region — *see* Laceration, back, lower
lung S27.339
　bilateral S27.332
　unilateral S27.331
malar region — *see* Laceration, head, specified
　site NEC
mammary — *see* Laceration, breast
mastoid region — *see* Laceration, head,
　specified site NEC
meninges — *see* Injury, intracranial, diffuse
meniscus — *see* Tear, meniscus
mesentery S36.893
mesosalpinx S37.893
mouth — *see* Laceration, oral cavity
muscle — *see* Injury, muscle, by site, laceration
nail
　finger — *see* Laceration, finger, with damage
　　to nail
　toe — *see* Laceration, toe, with damage to
　　nail
nasal (septum) (sinus) — *see* Laceration, nose
nasopharynx — *see* Laceration, head,
　specified site NEC
neck S11.91
　with foreign body S11.92
　involving
　　cervical esophagus S11.21
　　　with foreign body S11.22
　　larynx — *see* Laceration, larynx
　　pharynx — *see* Laceration, pharynx
　　thyroid gland — *see* Laceration, thyroid
　　　gland
　　trachea — *see* Laceration, trachea
　specified site NEC S11.81
　　with foreign body S11.82
nerve — *see* Injury, nerve
nose (septum) (sinus) S01.21
　with foreign body S01.22
ocular NOS S05.3-
　adnexa NOS S01.11-

Laceration — *continued*
oral cavity S01.512
　with foreign body S01.522
orbit (eye) — *see* Wound, open, ocular, orbit
ovary S37.439
　bilateral S37.432
　unilateral S37.431
palate — *see* Laceration, oral cavity
palm — *see* Laceration, hand
pancreas S36.239
　body S36.231
　　major S36.261
　　minor S36.241
　　moderate S36.251
　head S36.230
　　major S36.260
　　minor S36.240
　　moderate S36.250
　major S36.269
　minor S36.249
　moderate S36.259
　tail S36.232
　　major S36.262
　　minor S36.242
　　moderate S36.252
pelvic S31.010
　with
　　foreign body S31.020
　　　penetration into retroperitoneal cavity
　　　　S31.021
　　penetration into retroperitoneal cavity
　　　S31.011
　floor — *see also* Laceration, back, lower
　　with ectopic or molar pregnancy O08.6
　　complicating delivery O70.1
　　following ectopic or molar pregnancy
　　　O08.6
　　old (postpartal) N81.89
　organ S37.93
　　with ectopic or molar pregnancy O08.6
　　adrenal gland S37.813
　　bladder S37.23
　　fallopian tube — *see* Laceration, fallopian
　　　tube
　　following ectopic or molar pregnancy
　　　O08.6
　　kidney — *see* Laceration, kidney
　　obstetrical trauma O71.5
　　ovary — *see* Laceration, ovary
　　prostate S37.823
　　specified site NEC S37.893
　　ureter S37.13
　　urethra S37.33
　　uterus S37.63
penis S31.21
　with foreign body S31.22
perineum
　female S31.41
　　with
　　　ectopic or molar pregnancy O08.6
　　　foreign body S31.42
　　during delivery O70.9
　　　first degree O70.0
　　　fourth degree O70.3
　　　second degree O70.1
　　　third degree (*see also* Delivery,
　　　　complicated, by, laceration,
　　　　perineum, third degree) O70.20
　　old (postpartal) N81.89
　　postpartal N81.89
　　secondary (postpartal) O90.1
　male S31.119
　　with foreign body S31.129
periocular area (with or without lacrimal
　passages) — *see* Laceration, eyelid
peritoneum S36.893
periumbilic region — *see* Laceration,
　abdomen, wall, periumbilic
periurethral tissue — *see* Laceration, urethra

Laceration — *continued*
phalanges
　finger — *see* Laceration, finger
　toe — *see* Laceration, toe
pharynx S11.21
　with foreign body S11.22
pinna — *see* Laceration, ear
popliteal space — *see* Laceration, knee
prepuce — *see* Laceration, penis
prostate S37.823
pubic region S31.119
　with foreign body S31.129
pudendum — *see* Laceration, genital organs,
　external
rectovaginal septum — *see* Laceration, vagina
rectum S36.63
retroperitoneum S36.893
round ligament S37.893
sacral region — *see* Laceration, back, lower
sacroiliac region — *see* Laceration, back,
　lower
salivary gland — *see* Laceration, oral cavity
scalp S01.01
　with foreign body S01.02
scapular region — *see* Laceration, shoulder
scrotum S31.31
　with foreign body S31.32
seminal vesicle S37.893
shin — *see* Laceration, leg
shoulder S41.019
　with foreign body S41.029
　left S41.012
　　with foreign body S41.022
　right S41.011
　　with foreign body S41.021
small intestine — *see* Laceration, intestine,
　small
spermatic cord — *see* Laceration, testis
spinal cord (meninges) — *see also* Injury, spinal
　cord, by region
　due to injury at birth P11.5
　newborn (birth injury) P11.5
spleen S36.039
　major (massive) (stellate) S36.032
　moderate S36.031
　superficial (minor) S36.030
sternal region — *see* Laceration, thorax, front
stomach S36.33
submaxillary region — *see* Laceration, head,
　specified site NEC
submental region — *see* Laceration, head,
　specified site NEC
subungual
　finger(s) — *see* Laceration, finger, with
　　damage to nail
　toe(s) — *see* Laceration, toe, with damage to
　　nail
suprarenal gland — *see* Laceration, adrenal
　gland
temple, temporal region — *see* Laceration,
　head, specified site NEC
temporomandibular area — *see* Laceration,
　cheek
tendon — *see* Injury, muscle, by site, laceration
　Achilles S86.02-
tentorium cerebelli — *see* Injury, intracranial,
　diffuse
testis S31.31
　with foreign body S31.32
thigh S71.11-
　with foreign body S71.12-
thorax, thoracic (wall) S21.91
　with foreign body S21.92
　　back S21.22-
　　　with penetration into thoracic cavity
　　　　S21.42-
　　front S21.12-
　　　with penetration into thoracic cavity
　　　　S21.32-

DISEASE INDEX

Laki-Lorand factor deficiency — see Defect, coagulation, specified type NEC
Lalling F80.0
Lambert-Eaton syndrome — see Syndrome, Lambert-Eaton
Lambliasis, lambliosis A07.1
Landau-Kleffner syndrome — see Epilepsy, specified NEC
Landouzy-Déjérine dystrophy or facioscapulohumeral atrophy G71.0
Landouzy's disease (icterohemorrhagic leptospirosis) A27.0
Landry-Guillain-Barré, syndrome or paralysis G61.0
Landry's disease or paralysis G61.0
Lane's
  band Q43.3
  kink — see Obstruction, intestine
  syndrome K90.2
Langdon Down syndrome — see Trisomy, 21
Lapsed immunization schedule status Z28.3
Large
  baby (regardless of gestational age) (4000g to 4499g) P08.1
  ear, congenital Q17.1
  physiological cup Q14.2
  stature R68.89
Large-for-dates NEC (infant) (4000g to 4499g) P08.1
  affecting management of pregnancy O36.6-
  exceptionally (4500g or more) P08.0
Larsen-Johansson disease orosteochondrosis — see Osteochondrosis, juvenile, patella
Larsen's syndrome (flattened facies and multiple congenital dislocations) Q74.8
Larva migrans
  cutaneous B76.9
    Ancylostoma B76.0
  visceral B83.0
Laryngeal — see condition
Laryngismus (stridulus) J38.5
  congenital P28.89
  diphtheritic A36.2
Laryngitis (acute) (edematous) (fibrinous) (infective) (infiltrative) (malignant) (membranous) (phlegmonous) (pneumococcal) (pseudomembranous) (septic) (subglottic) (suppurative) (ulcerative) J04.0
  with
    influenza, flu, or grippe — see Influenza, with, laryngitis
    tracheitis (acute) — see Laryngotracheitis
  atrophic J37.0
  catarrhal J37.0
  chronic J37.0
    with tracheitis (chronic) J37.1
  diphtheritic A36.2
  due to external agent — see Inflammation, respiratory, upper, due to
  H. influenzae J04.0
  Hemophilus influenzae J04.0
  hypertrophic J37.0
  influenzal — see Influenza, with, respiratory manifestations NEC
  obstructive J05.0
  sicca J37.0
  spasmodic J05.0
    acute J04.0
  streptococcal J04.0
  stridulous J05.0
  syphilitic (late) A52.73
    congenital A50.59 [J99]
    early A50.03 [J99]
  tuberculous A15.5
  Vincent's A69.1

Laryngocele (congenital) (ventricular) Q31.3
Laryngofissure J38.7
  congenital Q31.8
Laryngomalacia (congenital) Q31.5
Laryngopharyngitis (acute) J06.0
  chronic J37.0
  due to external agent — see Inflammation, respiratory, upper, due to
Laryngoplegia J38.00
  bilateral J38.02
  unilateral J38.01
Laryngoptosis J38.7
Laryngospasm J38.5
Laryngostenosis J38.6
Laryngotracheitis (acute) (Infectional) (infective) (viral) J04.2
  atrophic J37.1
  catarrhal J37.1
  chronic J37.1
  diphtheritic A36.2
  due to external agent — see Inflammation, respiratory, upper, due to
  Hemophilus influenzae J04.2
  hypertrophic J37.1
  influenzal — see Influenza, with, respiratory manifestations NEC
  pachydermic J38.7
  sicca J37.1
  spasmodic J38.5
    acute J05.0
  streptococcal J04.2
  stridulous J38.5
  syphilitic (late) A52.73
    congenital A50.59 [J99]
    early A50.03 [J99]
  tuberculous A15.5
  Vincent's A69.1
Laryngotracheobronchitis — see Bronchitis
Larynx, laryngeal — see condition
Lassa fever A96.2
Lassitude — see Weakness
Late
  talker R62.0
  walker R62.0
Late effect(s) — see Sequelae
Latent — see condition
Laterocession — see Lateroversion
Lateroflexion — see Lateroversion
Lateroversion
  cervix — see Lateroversion, uterus
  uterus, uterine (cervix) (postinfectional) (postpartal, old) N85.4
    congenital Q51.818
    in pregnancy or childbirth O34.59-
Lathyrism — see Poisoning, food, noxious, plant
Launois' syndrome (pituitary gigantism) E22.0
Launois-Bensaude adenolipomatosis E88.89
Laurence-Moon(-Bardet)-Biedl syndrome Q87.89
Lax, laxity — see also Relaxation
  ligament(ous) — see also Disorder, ligament
    familial M35.7
    knee — see Derangement, knee
  skin (acquired) L57.4
    congenital Q82.8
Laxative habit F55.2
Lazy leukocyte syndrome D70.8
Lead miner's lung J63.6
Leak, leakage
  air NEC J93.82
    postprocedural J95.812
  amniotic fluid — see Rupture, membranes, premature

Leak, leakage — continued
  blood (microscopic), fetal, into maternal circulation affecting management of pregnancy — see Pregnancy, complicated by
  cerebrospinal fluid G96.0
    from spinal (lumbar) puncture G97.0
  device, implant or graft — see also Complications, by site and type, mechanical
    arterial graft NEC — see Complication, cardiovascular device, mechanical, vascular
    breast (implant) T85.43
    catheter NEC T85.638
      dialysis (renal) T82.43
        intraperitoneal T85.631
      infusion NEC T82.534
        spinal (epidural) (subdural) T85.630
      urinary T83.038
        cystostomy T83.030
        Hopkins T83.038
        ileostomy T83.038
        indwelling T83.031
        nephrostomy T83.032
        specified NEC T83.038
        urostomy T83.038
    gastrointestinal — see Complications, prosthetic device, mechanical, gastrointestinal device
    genital NEC T83.498
      penile prosthesis (cylinder) (implanted) (pump) (resevoir) T83.490
      testicular prosthesis T83.491
    heart NEC — see Complication, cardiovascular device, mechanical
    ocular NEC — see Complications, prosthetic device, mechanical, ocular device
    orthopedic NEC — see Complication, orthopedic, device, mechanical
    persistent air J93.82
    specified NEC T85.638
    urinary NEC — see also Complication, genitourinary, device, urinary, mechanical
      graft T83.23
    vascular NEC — see Complication, cardiovascular device, mechanical
    ventricular intracranial shunt T85.03
  urine — see Incontinence
Leaky heart — see Endocarditis
Learning defect (specific) F81.9
Leather bottle stomach C16.9
Leber's
  congenital amaurosis H35.50
  optic atrophy (hereditary) H47.22
Lederer's anemia D59.1
Leeches (external) — see Hirudiniasis
Leg — see condition
Legg(-Calvé)-Perthes disease, syndrome or osteochondrosis M91.1-
Legionellosis A48.1
  nonpneumonic A48.2
Legionnaires'
  disease A48.1
    nonpneumonic A48.2
  pneumonia A48.1
Leigh's disease G31.82
Leiner's disease L21.1
Leiofibromyoma — see Leiomyoma
Leiomyoblastoma — see Neoplasm, connective tissue, benign
Leiomyofibroma — see also Neoplasm, connective tissue, benign
  uterus (cervix) (corpus) D25.9

Leiomyoma — *see also* Neoplasm, connective tissue, benign
  bizarre — *see* Neoplasm, connective tissue, benign
  cellular — *see* Neoplasm, connective tissue, benign
  epithelioid — *see* Neoplasm, connective tissue, benign
  uterus (cervix) (corpus) D25.9
    intramural D25.1
    submucous D25.0
    subserosal D25.2
  vascular — *see* Neoplasm, connective tissue, benign
Leiomyoma, leiomyomatosis (intravascular) — *see* Neoplasm, connective tissue, uncertain behavior
Leiomyosarcoma — *see also* Neoplasm, connective tissue, malignant
  epithelioid — *see* Neoplasm, connective tissue, malignant
  myxoid — *see* Neoplasm, connective tissue, malignant
Leishmaniasis B55.9
  American (mucocutaneous) B55.2
    cutaneous B55.1
  Asian Desert B55.1
  Brazilian B55.2
  cutaneous (any type) B55.1
  dermal — *see also* Leishmaniasis, cutaneous
    post-kala-azar B55.0
  eyelid B55.1
  infantile B55.0
  Mediterranean B55.0
  mucocutaneous (American) (New World) B55.2
  naso-oral B55.2
  nasopharyngeal B55.2
  old world B55.1
  tegumentaria diffusa B55.1
  visceral B55.0
Leishmanoid, dermal — *see also* Leishmaniasis, cutaneous
  post-kala-azar B55.0
Lenegre's disease I44.2
Lengthening, leg — *see* Deformity, limb, unequal length
Lennert's lymphoma — *see* Lymphoma, Lennert's
Lennox-Gastaut syndrome G40.812
  intractable G40.814
    with status epilepticus G40.813
    without status epilepticus G40.814
  not intractable G40.812
    with status epilepticus G40.811
    without status epilepticus G40.812
Lens — *see* condition
Lenticonus (anterior) (posterior) (congenital) Q12.8
Lenticular degeneration, progressive E83.01
Lentiglobus (posterior) (congenital) Q12.8
Lentigo (congenital) L81.4
  maligna — *see also* Melanoma, in situ
  melanoma — *see* Melanoma
Lentivirus, as cause of disease classified elsewhere B97.31
Leontiasis
  ossium M85.2
  syphilitic (late) A52.78
    congenital A50.59
Lepothrix A48.8
Lepra — *see* Leprosy
Leprechaunism E34.8
Leprosy A30-
  with muscle disorder A30.9 *[M63.80]*
    ankle A30.9 *[M63.8-]*
    foot A30.9 *[M63.8-]*
    forearm A30.9 *[M63.8-]*

Leprosy A30- — *continued*
  with muscle disorder A30.9 *[M63.80]* — *continued*
    hand A30.9 *[M63.8-]*
    lower leg A30.9 *[M63.8-]*
    multiple sites A30.9 *[M63.8-]*
    pelvic region A30.9 *[M63.8-]*
    shoulder region A30.9 *[M63.8-]*
    specified site NEC A30.9 *[M63.8-]*
    thigh A30.9 *[M63.8-]*
    upper arm A30.9 *[M63.8-]*
  anesthetic A30.9
  BB A30.3
  BL A30.4
  borderline (infiltrated) (neuritic) A30.3
    lepromatous A30.4
    tuberculoid A30.2
  BT A30.2
  dimorphous (infiltrated) (neuritic) A30.3
  I A30.0
  indeterminate (macular) (neuritic) A30.0
  lepromatous (diffuse) (infiltrated) (macular) (neuritic) (nodular) A30.5
  LL A30.5
  macular (early) (neuritic) (simple) A30.9
  maculoanesthetic A30.9
  mixed A30.3
  neural A30.9
  nodular A30.5
  primary neuritic A30.3
  specified type NEC A30.8
  TT A30.1
  tuberculoid (major) (minor) A30.1
Leptocytosis, hereditary D56.9
Leptomeningitis (chronic) (circumscribed) (hemorrhagic) (nonsuppurative) — *see* Meningitis
Leptomeningopathy G96.19
Leptospiral — *see* condition
Leptospirochetal — *see* condition
Leptospirosis A27.9
  canicola A27.89
  due to Leptospira interrogans serovar icterohaemorrhagiae A27.0
  icterohemorrhagica A27.0
  pomona A27.89
  Weil's disease A27.0
Leptus dermatitis B88.0
Leri's pleonosteosis Q78.8
Leri-Weill syndrome Q77.8
Leriche's syndrome (aortic bifurcation occlusion) I74.09
Lermoyez' syndrome — *see* Vertigo, peripheral NEC
Lesch-Nyhan syndrome E79.1
Leser-Trélat disease L82.1
  inflamed L82.0
Lesion(s) (nontraumatic)
  abducens nerve — *see* Strabismus, paralytic, sixth nerve
  alveolar process K08.9
  angiocentric immunoproliferative D47.Z9
  anorectal K62.9
  aortic (valve) I35.9
  auditory nerve — *see* subcategory H93.3
  basal ganglion G25.9
  bile duct — *see* Disease, bile duct
  biomechanical M99.9
    specified type NEC M99.89
      abdomen M99.89
      acromioclavicular M99.87
      cervical region M99.81
      cervicothoracic M99.81
      costochondral M99.88
      costovertebral M99.88
      head region M99.80
      hip M99.85
      lower extremity M99.86
      lumbar region M99.83

Lesion(s) (nontraumatic) — *continued*
  biomechanical M99.9 — *continued*
    specified type NEC M99.89 — *continued*
      lumbosacral M99.83
      occipitocervical M99.80
      pelvic region M99.85
      pubic M99.85
      rib cage M99.88
      sacral region M99.84
      sacrococcygeal M99.84
      sacroiliac M99.84
      specified NEC M99.89
      sternochondral M99.88
      sternoclavicular M99.87
      thoracic region M99.82
      thoracolumbar M99.82
      upper extremity M99.87
  bladder N32.9
  bone — *see* Disorder, bone
  brachial plexus G54.0
  brain G93.9
    congenital Q04.9
    vascular I67.9
      degenerative I67.9
      hypertensive I67.4
  buccal cavity K13.79
  calcified — *see* Calcification
  canthus — *see* Disorder, eyelid
  carate — *see* Pinta, lesions
  cardia K31.9
  cardiac (*see also* Disease, heart) I51.9
    congenital Q24.9
    valvular — *see* Endocarditis
  cauda equina G83.4
  cecum K63.9
  cerebral — *see* Lesion, brain
  cerebrovascular I67.9
    degenerative I67.9
    hypertensive I67.4
  cervical (nerve) root NEC G54.2
  chiasmal — *see* Disorder, optic, chiasm
  chorda tympani G51.8
  coin, lung R91.1
  colon K63.9
  combined periodontic-endodontic K05.5
  congenital — *see* Anomaly, by site
  conjunctiva H11.9
  conus medullaris — *see* Injury, conus medullaris
  coronary artery — *see* Ischemia, heart
  cranial nerve G52.9
    eighth — *see* Disorder, ear
    eleventh G52.9
    fifth G50.9
    first G52.0
    fourth — *see* Strabismus, paralytic, fourth nerve
    seventh G51.9
    sixth — *see* Strabismus, paralytic, sixth nerve
    tenth G52.2
    twelfth G52.3
  cystic — *see* Cyst
  degenerative — *see* Degeneration
  duodenum K31.9
  edentulous (alveolar) ridge, associated with trauma, due to traumatic occlusion K06.2
  en coup de sabre L94.1
  eyelid — *see* Disorder, eyelid
  gasserian ganglion G50.8
  gastric K31.9
  gastroduodenal K31.9
  gastrointestinal K63.9
  gingiva, associated with trauma K06.2
  glomerular
    focal and segmental (*see also* N00-N07 with fourth character .1) N05.1
    minimal change (*see also* N00-N07 with fourth character .0) N05.0
  heart (organic) — *see* Disease, heart

Lesion(s) (nontraumatic) — *continued*
  hyperchromic, due to pinta (carate) A67.1
  hyperkeratotic — *see* Hyperkeratosis
  hypothalamic E23.7
  ileocecal K63.9
  ileum K63.9
  iliohypogastric nerve G57.8-
  inflammatory — *see* Inflammation
  intestine K63.9
  intracerebral — *see* Lesion, brain
  intrachiasmal (optic) — *see* Disorder, optic,
    chiasm
  intracranial, space-occupying R90.0
  joint — *see* Disorder, joint
    sacroiliac (old) M53.3
  keratotic — *see* Keratosis
  kidney — *see* Disease, renal
  laryngeal nerve (recurrent) G52.2
  lip K13.0
  liver K76.9
  lumbosacral
    plexus G54.1
    root (nerve) NEC G54.4
  lung (coin) R91.1
  maxillary sinus J32.0
  mitral I05.9
  Morel-Lavallée — *see* Hematoma, by site
  motor cortex NEC G93.89
  mouth K13.79
  nerve G58.9
    femoral G57.2-
    median G56.1-
      carpal tunnel syndrome — *see* Syndrome,
        carpal tunnel
    plantar G57.6-
    popliteal (lateral) G57.3-
      medial G57.4-
    radial G56.3-
    sciatic G57.0-
    spinal — *see* Injury, nerve, spinal
    ulnar G56.2-
  nervous system, congenital Q07.9
  nonallopathic — *see* Lesion, biomechanical
  nose (internal) J34.89
  obstructive — *see* Obstruction
  obturator nerve G57.8-
  oral mucosa K13.70
  organ or site NEC — *see* Disease, by site
  osteolytic — *see* Osteolysis
  peptic K27.9
  periodontal, due to traumatic occlusion K05.5
  pharynx J39.2
  pigment, pigmented (skin) L81.9
  pinta — *see* Pinta, lesions
  polypoid — *see* Polyp
  prechiasmal (optic) — *see* Disorder, optic,
    chiasm
  primary (*see also* Syphilis, primary) A51.0
    carate A67.0
    pinta A67.0
    yaws A66.0
  pulmonary J98.4
    valve I37.9
  pylorus K31.9
  rectosigmoid K63.9
  retina, retinal H35.9
  sacroiliac (joint) (old) M53.3
  salivary gland K11.9
    benign lymphoepithelial K11.8
  saphenous nerve G57.8-
  sciatic nerve G57.0-
  secondary — *see* Syphilis, secondary
  shoulder (region) M75.9-
    specified NEC M75.8-
  sigmoid K63.9
  sinus (accessory) (nasal) J34.89
  skin L98.9
    suppurative L08.0
  SLAP S43.43-

Lesion(s) (nontraumatic) — *continued*
  spinal cord G95.9
  congenital Q06.9
  spleen D73.89
  stomach K31.9
  superior glenoid labrum S43.43-
  syphilitic — *see* Syphilis
  tertiary — *see* Syphilis, tertiary
  thoracic root (nerve) NEC G54.3
  tonsillar fossa J35.9
  tooth, teeth K08.9
    white spot
      chewing surface K02.51
      pit and fissure surface K02.51
      smooth surface K02.61
  traumatic — *see* specific type of injury by site
  tricuspid (valve) I07.9
    nonrheumatic I36.9
  trigeminal nerve G50.9
  ulcerated or ulcerative — *see* Ulcer, skin
  uterus N85.9
  vagus nerve G52.2
  valvular — *see* Endocarditis
  vascular I99.9
    affecting central nervous system I67.9
    following trauma NEC T14.8
    umbilical cord, complicating delivery O69.5
  warty — *see* Verruca
  white spot (tooth)
    chewing surface K02.51
    pit and fissure surface K02.51
    smooth surface K02.61
Lethargic — *see* condition
Lethargy R53.83
Letterer-Siwe's disease C96.0
Leukemia, leukemic C95.9-
  acute basophilic C94.8-
  acute bilineal C95.0-
  acute erythroid C94.0-
  acute lymphoblastic C91.0-
  acute megakaryoblastic C94.2-
  acute megakaryocytic C94.2-
  acute mixed lineage C95.0-
  acute monoblastic (monoblastic/monocytic)
    C93.0-
  acute monocytic (monoblastic/monocytic)
    C93.0-
  acute myeloblastic (minimal differentiation)
    (with maturation) C92.0-
  acute myeloid
    with
      11q23-abnormality C92.6-
      dysplasia of remaining hematopoesis
        and/or myelodysplastic disease in its
        history C92.A- *(follows C92.6)*
      multilineage dysplasia C92.A- *(follows*
        C92.6)
      variation of MLL-gene C92.6-
    M6(a)(b) C94.0-
    M7 C94.2-
  acute myelomonocytic C92.5-
  acute promyelocytic C92.4-
  adult T-cell (HTLV-1-associated) (acute variant)
    (chronic variant) (lymphomatoid variant)
    (smouldering variant) C91.5-
  aggressive NK-cell C94.8-
  AML (1/ETO) (M0) (M1) (M2) (without a FAB
    classification) C92.0-
  AML M3 C92.4-
  AML M4 (Eo with inv(16) or t(16;16)) C92.5-
  AML M5 C93.0-
  AML M5a C93.0-
  AML M5b C93.0-
  AML Me with t(15;17) and variants C92.4-
  atypical chronic myeloid, BCR/ABL-negative
    C92.2-
  biphenotypic acute C95.0-
  blast cell C95.0-
  Burkitt-type, mature B-cell C91.A- *(follows C91.6)*

Leukemia, leukemic C95.9- — *continued*
  chronic lymphocytic, of B-cell type C91.1-
  chronic monocytic C93.1-
  chronic myelogenous (Philadelphia
    chromosome (Ph1) positive) (t(9;22))
    (q34;q11) (with crisis of blast cells) C92.1-
  chronic myeloid, BCR/ABL-positive C92.1-
    atypical, BCR/ABL-negative C92.2-
  chronic myelomonocytic C93.1-
  chronic neutrophilic D47.1
  CMML (-1) (-2) (with eosinophilia) C93.1-
  granulocytic (*see also* Category C92) C92.9-
  hairy cell C91.4-
  juvenile myelomonocytic C93.3-
  lymphoid C91.9-
    specified NEC C91.Z- *(follows C91.6)*
  mast cell C94.3-
  mature B-cell, Burkitt-type C91.A- *(follows C91.6)*
  monocytic (subacute) C93.9-
    specified NEC C93.Z- *(follows C93.3)*
  myelogenous (*see also* Category C92) C92.9-
  myeloid C92.9-
    specified NEC C92.Z- *(follows C92.6)*
  plasma cell C90.1-
  plasmacytic C90.1-
  prolymphocytic
    of B-cell type C91.3-
    of T-cell type C91.6-
  specified NEC C94.8-
  stem cell, of unclear lineage C95.0-
  subacute lymphocytic C91.9-
  T-cell large granular lymphocytic C91.Z-
    (follows C91.6)
  unspecified cell type C95.9-
    acute C95.0-
    chronic C95.1-
Leukemoid reaction (*see also* Reaction,
  leukemoid) D72.823-
Leukoaraiosis (hypertensive) I67.81
Leukoariosis — *see* Leukoaraiosis
Leukocoria — *see* Disorder, globe,
  degenerated condition, leucocoria
Leukocytopenia D72.819
Leukocytosis D72.829
  eosinophilic D72.1
Leukoderma, leukodermia NEC L81.5
  syphilitic A51.39
    late A52.79
Leukodystrophy E75.29
Leukoedema, oral epithelium K13.29
Leukoencephalitis G04.81
  acute (subacute) hemorrhagic G36.1
    postimmunization or postvaccinal G04.02
  postinfectious G04.01
  subacute sclerosing A81.1
  van Bogaert's (sclerosing) A81.1
Leukoencephalopathy (*see also*
  Encephalopathy) G93.49
  Binswanger's I67.3
  heroin vapor G92
  metachromatic E75.25
  multifocal (progressive) A81.2
  postimmunization and postvaccinal G04.02
  progressive multifocal A81.2
  reversible, posterior G93.6
  van Bogaert's (sclerosing) A81.1
  vascular, progressive I67.3
Leukoerythroblastosis D75.9
Leukokeratosis — *see also* Leukoplakia
  mouth K13.21
  nicotina palati K13.24
  oral mucosa K13.21
  tongue K13.21
  vocal cord J38.3
Leukokraurosis vulva(e) N90.4
Leukoma (cornea) — *see also* Opacity, cornea
  adherent H17.0-
  interfering with central vision — *see* Opacity,
    cornea, central

Leukomalacia, cerebral, newborn P91.2
  periventricular P91.2
Leukomelanopathy, hereditary D72.0
Leukonychia (punctata) (striata) L60.8
  congenital Q84.4
Leukopathia unguium L60.8
  congenital Q84.4
Leukopenia D72.819
  basophilic D72.818
  chemotherapy (cancer) induced D70.1
  congenital D70.0
  cyclic D70.0
  drug induced NEC D70.2
    due to cytoreductive cancer chemotherapy
      D70.1
  eosinophilic D72.818
  familial D70.0
  infantile genetic D70.0
  malignant D70.9
  periodic D70.0
  transitory neonatal P61.5
Leukopenic — *see* condition
Leukoplakia
  anus K62.89
  bladder (postinfectional) N32.89
  buccal K13.21
  cervix (uteri) N88.0
  esophagus K22.8
  gingiva K13.21
  hairy (oral mucosa) (tongue) K13.3
  kidney (pelvis) N28.89
  larynx J38.7
  lip K13.21
  mouth K13.21
  oral epithelium, including tongue (mucosa)
    K13.21
  palate K13.21
  pelvis (kidney) N28.89
  penis (infectional) N48.0
  rectum K62.89
  syphilitic (late) A52.79
  tongue K13.21
  ureter (postinfectional) N28.89
  urethra (postinfectional) N36.8
  uterus N85.8
  vagina N89.4
  vocal cord J38.3
  vulva N90.4
Leukorrhea N89.8
  due to Trichomonas (vaginalis) A59.00
  trichomonal A59.00
Leukosarcoma C85.9-
Levocardia (isolated) Q24.1
  with situs inversus Q89.3
Levotransposition Q20.5
Lev's disease or syndrome (acquired
    complete heart block) I44.2
Levulosuria — *see* Fructosuria
Levurid L30.2
Lewy body(ies) (dementia) (disease) G31.83
Leyden-Moebius dystrophy G71.0
Leydig cell
  carcinoma
    specified site — *see* Neoplasm, malignant,
      by site
    unspecified site
      female C56.9
      male C62.9-
  tumor
    benign
      specified site — *see* Neoplasm, benign, by
        site
      unspecified site
        female D27-
        male D29.2-

Leydig cell — *continued*
  tumor — *continued*
    malignant
      specified site — *see* Neoplasm, malignant,
        by site
      unspecified site
        female C56-
        male C62.9-
    specified site — *see* Neoplasm, uncertain
      behavior, by site
    unspecified site
      female D39.1-
      male D40.1-
Leydig-Sertoli cell tumor
  specified site — *see* Neoplasm, benign, by site
  unspecified site
    female D27-
    male D29.2-
LGSIL (low grade squamous intraepithelial
  lesion on cytologic smear of)
  anus R85.612
  cervix R87.612
  vagina R87.622
Liar, pathologic F60.2
Libido
  decreased R68.82
Libman-Sacks disease M32.11
Lice (infestation) B85.2
  body (Pediculus corporis) B85.1
  crab B85.3
  head (Pediculus capitis) B85.0
  mixed (classifiable to more than one of the
    titles B85.0-B85.3) B85.4
  pubic (Phthirus pubis) B85.3
Lichen L28.0
  albus L90.0
    penis N48.0
    vulva N90.4
  amyloidosis E85.4 *[L99]*
  atrophicus L90.0
    penis N48.0
    vulva N90.4
  congenital Q82.8
  myxedematosus L98.5
  nitidus L44.1
  pilaris Q82.8
    acquired L85.8
  planopilaris L66.1
  planus (chronicus) L43.9
    annularis L43.8
    bullous L43.1
    follicular L66.1
    hypertrophic L43.0
    moniliformis L44.3
    of Wilson L43.9
    specified NEC L43.8
    subacute (active) L43.3
    tropicus L43.3
  ruber
    acuminatus L44.0
    moniliformis L44.3
    planus L43.9
  sclerosus (et atrophicus) L90.0
    penis N48.0
    vulva N90.4
  scrofulosus (primary) (tuberculous) A18.4
  simplex (chronicus) (circumscriptus) L28.0
  striatus L44.2
  urticatus L28.2
Lichenification L28.0
Lichenoides tuberculosis (primary) A18.4
Lichtheim's disease or syndrome — *see*
  Degeneration, combined
Lien migrans D73.89
Ligament — *see* condition
Light
  for gestational age — *see* Light for dates
  headedness R42

Light-for-dates (infant) P05.00
  with weight of
    499 grams or less P05.01
    500-749 grams P05.02
    750-999 grams P05.03
    1000-1249 grams P05.04
    1250-1499 grams P05.05
    1500-1749 grams P05.06
    1750-1999 grams P05.07
    2000-2499 grams P05.08
    2500 grams and over P05.09
  affecting management of pregnancy O36.59-
  and small-for-dates — *see* Small for dates
  specified NEC P05.09
Lightning (effects) (stroke) (struck by) T75.00
  burn — *see* Burn
  foot E53.8
  shock T75.01
  specified effect NEC T75.09
Lightwood-Albright syndrome N25.89
Lightwood's disease or syndrome (renal
    tubular acidosis) N25.89
**Lignac(-de Toni) (-Fanconi) (-Debré)
    disease or syndrome** E72.09
  with cystinosis E72.04
Ligneous thyroiditis E06.5
Likoff's syndrome I20.8
Limb — *see* condition
Limbic epilepsy personality syndrome
  F07.0
Limitation, limited
  activities due to disability Z73.6
  cardiac reserve — *see* Disease, heart
  eye muscle duction, traumatic — *see*
    Strabismus, mechanical
  mandibular range of motion M26.52
Lindau(-von Hippel) disease Q85.8
Line(s)
  Beau's L60.4
  Harris' — *see* Arrest, epiphyseal
  Hudson's (cornea) — *see* Pigmentation, cornea,
    anterior
  Stähli's (cornea) — *see* Pigmentation, cornea,
    anterior
Linea corneae senilis — *see* Change,
  cornea, senile
Lingua
  geographica K14.1
  nigra (villosa) K14.3
  plicata K14.5
  tylosis K13.29
Lingual — *see* condition
Linguatulosis B88.8
Linitis (gastric) plastica C16.9
Lip — *see* condition
Lipedema — *see* Edema
Lipemia — *see also* Hyperlipidemia
  retina, retinalis E78.3
Lipidosis E75.6
  cerebral (infantile) (juvenile) (late) E75.4
  cerebroretinal E75.4
  cerebroside E75.22
  cholesterol (cerebral) E75.5
  glycolipid E75.21
  hepatosplenomegalic E78.3
  sphingomyelin — *see* Niemann-Pick disease or
    syndrome
  sulfatide E75.29
Lipoadenoma — *see* Neoplasm, benign, by
  site
Lipoblastoma — *see* Lipoma
Lipoblastomatosis — *see* Lipoma
Lipochondrodystrophy E76.01
Lipochrome histiocytosis (familial) D71
Lipodermatosclerosis — *see* Varix, leg, with,
    inflammation
  ulcerated — *see* Varix, leg, with, ulcer, with
    inflammation by site
Lipodystrophia progressiva E88.1

DISEASE INDEX

Lipodystrophy (progressive) E88.1
 insulin E88.1
 intestinal K90.81
 mesenteric K65.4
Lipofibroma — *see* Lipoma
Lipofuscinosis, neuronal (with ceroidosis)
 E75.4
Lipogranuloma, sclerosing L92.8
Lipogranulomatosis E78.89
Lipoid — *see also* condition
 histiocytosis D76.3
  essential E75.29
 nephrosis N04.9
 proteinosis of Urbach E78.89
Lipoidemia — *see* Hyperlipidemia
Lipoidosis — *see* Lipidosis
Lipoma D17.9
 fetal D17.9
  fat cell D17.9
 infiltrating D17.9
 intramuscular D17.9
 pleomorphic D17.9
 site classification
  arms (skin) (subcutaneous) D17.2-
  connective tissue D17.30
   intra-abdominal D17.5
   intrathoracic D17.4
   peritoneum D17.79
   retroperitoneum D17.79
   specified site NEC D17.39
   spermatic cord D17.6
  face (skin) (subcutaneous) D17.0
  genitourinary organ NEC D17.72
  head (skin) (subcutaneous) D17.0
  intra-abdominal D17.5
  intrathoracic D17.4
  kidney D17.71
  legs (skin) (subcutaneous) D17.2-
  neck (skin) (subcutaneous) D17.0
  peritoneum D17.79
  retroperitoneum D17.79
  skin D17.30
   specified site NEC D17.39
  specified site NEC D17.79
  spermatic cord D17.6
  subcutaneous D17.30
   specified site NEC D17.39
  trunk (skin) (subcutaneous) D17.1
  unspecified D17.9
 spindle cell D17.9
Lipomatosis E88.2
 dolorosa (Dercum) E88.2
 fetal — *see* Lipoma
 Launois-Bensaude E88.89
Lipomyoma — *see* Lipoma
Lipomyxoma — *see* Lipoma
Lipomyxosarcoma — *see* Neoplasm,
 connective tissue, malignant
Lipoprotein metabolism disorder E78.9
Lipoproteinemia E78.5
 broad-beta E78.2
 floating-beta E78.2
 hyper-pre-beta E78.1
Liposarcoma — *see also* Neoplasm, connective
 tissue, malignant
 dedifferentiated — *see* Neoplasm, connective
  tissue, malignant
 differentiated type — *see* Neoplasm,
  connective tissue, malignant
 embryonal — *see* Neoplasm, connective tissue,
  malignant
 mixed type — *see* Neoplasm, connective tissue,
  malignant
 myxoid — *see* Neoplasm, connective tissue,
  malignant
 pleomorphic — *see* Neoplasm, connective
  tissue, malignant
 round cell — *see* Neoplasm, connective tissue,
  malignant

Liposarcoma — *see also* Neoplasm, connective
 tissue, malignant — *continued*
 well differentiated type — *see* Neoplasm,
  connective tissue, malignant
Liposynovitis prepatellaris E88.89
Lipping, cervix N86
Lipschütz disease or ulcer N76.6
Lipuria R82.0
 schistosomiasis (bilharziasis) B65.0
Lisping F80.0
Lissauer's paralysis A52.17
Lissencephalia, lissencephaly Q04.3
Listeriosis, listerellosis A32.9
 congenital (disseminated) P37.2
 cutaneous A32.0
 neonatal, newborn (disseminated) P37.2
 oculoglandular A32.81
 specified NEC A32.89
Lithemia E79.0
Lithiasis — *see* Calculus
Lithosis J62.8
Lithuria R82.99
Litigation, anxiety concerning Z65.3
Little leaguer's elbow — *see* Epicondylitis,
 medial
Little's disease G80.9
Littre's
 gland — *see* condition
 hernia — *see* Hernia, abdomen
Littritis — *see* Urethritis
Livedo (annularis) (racemosa) (reticularis)
 R23.1
Liver — *see* condition
Living alone (problems with) Z60.2
 with handicapped person Z74.2
Lloyd's syndrome — *see* Adenomatosis,
 endocrine
Loa loa, loaiasis, loasis B74.3
Lobar — *see* condition
Lobomycosis B48.0
Lobo's disease B48.0
Lobotomy syndrome F07.0
Lobstein(-Ekman) disease or syndrome
 Q78.0
Lobster-claw hand Q71.6-
Lobulation (congenital) — *see also* Anomaly,
 by site
 kidney, Q63.1
 liver, abnormal Q44.7
 spleen Q89.09
Lobule, lobular — *see* condition
Local, localized — *see* condition
Locked twins causing obstructed labor
 O66.1
Locked-in state G83.5
Locking
 joint — *see* Derangement, joint, specified type
  NEC
 knee — *see* Derangement, knee
Lockjaw — *see* Tetanus
Löffler's
 endocarditis I42.3
 eosinophilia J82
 pneumonia J82
 syndrome (eosinophilic pneumonitis) J82
Loiasis (with conjunctival infestation) (eyelid)
 B74.3
Lone Star fever A77.0
Long
 labor O63.9
  first stage O63.0
  second stage O63.1
 QT syndrome I45.81

Long-term (current) (prophylactic) drug
 therapy (use of)
 agents affecting estrogen receptors and
  estrogen levels NEC Z79.818
 anastrozole (Arimidex) Z79.811
 anti-inflammatory, non-steroidal (NSAID)
  Z79.1
 antibiotics Z79.2
  short-term use — *omit code*
 anticoagulants Z79.01
 antiplatelet Z79.02
 antithrombotics Z79.02
 aromatase inhibitors Z79.811
 aspirin Z79.82
 birth control pill or patch Z79.3
 bisphosphonates Z79.83
 contraceptive, oral Z79.3
 drug, specified NEC Z79.899
 estrogen receptor downregulators Z79.818
 Evista Z79.810
 exemestane (Aromasin) Z79.811
 Fareston Z79.810
 fulvestrant (Faslodex) Z79.818
 gonadotropin-releasing hormone (GnRH)
  agonist Z79.818
 goserelin acetate (Zoladex) Z79.818
 hormone replacement (postmenopausal)
  Z79.890
 insulin Z79.4
 letrozole (Femara) Z79.811
 leuprolide acetate (leuprorelin) (Lupron)
  Z79.818
 megestrol acetate (Megace) Z79.818
 methadone for pain management Z79.891
 Nolvadex Z79.810
 non-steroidal anti-inflammatories (NSAID)
  Z79.1
 opiate analgesic Z79.891
 oral
  antidiabetic Z79.84
  contraceptive Z79.3
  hypoglycemic Z79.84
 raloxifene (Evista) Z79.810
 selective estrogen receptor modulators (SERMs)
  Z79.810
 steroids
  inhaled Z79.51
  systemic Z79.52
 tamoxifen (Nolvadex) Z79.810
 toremifene (Fareston) Z79.810
Longitudinal stripes or grooves, nails
 L60.8
 congenital Q84.6
Loop
 intestine — *see* Volvulus
 vascular on papilla (optic) Q14.2
Loose — *see also* condition
 body
  joint M24.00
   ankle M24.07-
   elbow M24.02-
   hand M24.04-
   hip M24.05-
   knee M23.4-
   shoulder (region) M24.01-
   specified site NEC M24.08
   toe M24.07-
   vertebra M24.08
   wrist M24.03-
  knee M23.4-
  sheath, tendon — *see* Disorder, tendon,
   specified type NEC
 cartilage — *see* Loose, body, joint
 skin and subcutaneous tissue (following
  bariatric surgery weight loss) (following
  dietary weight loss) L98.7
 tooth, teeth K08.89

Loosening
aseptic
joint prosthesis — *see* Complications, joint prosthesis, mechanical, loosening, by site
epiphysis — *see* Osteochondropathy
mechanical
joint prosthesis — *see* Complications, joint prosthesis, mechanical, loosening, by site
Looser-Milkman(-Debray) syndrome M83.8
Lop ear (deformity) Q17.3
Lorain(-Levi) short stature syndrome E23.0
Lordosis M40.50
acquired — *see* Lordosis, specified type NEC
congenital Q76.429
lumbar region Q76.426
lumbosacral region Q76.427
sacral region Q76.428
sacrococcygeal region Q76.428
thoracolumbar region Q76.425
lumbar region M40.56
lumbosacral region M40.57
postsurgical M96.4
postural — *see* Lordosis, specified type NEC
rachitic (late effect) (sequelae) E64.3
sequelae of rickets E64.3
specified type NEC M40.40
lumbar region M40.46
lumbosacral region M40.47
thoracolumbar region M40.45
thoracolumbar region M40.55
tuberculous A18.01
Loss (of)
appetite (*see also* Anorexia) R63.0
hysterical F50.89
nonorganic origin F50.89
psychogenic F50.89
blood — *see* Hemorrhage
bone — *see* Loss, substance of, bone
consciousness, transient R55
traumatic — *see* Injury, intracranial
control, sphincter, rectum R15.9
nonorganic origin F98.1
elasticity, skin R23.4
family (member) in childhood Z62.898
fluid (acute) E86.9
function of labyrinth — *see* subcategory H83.2
hair, nonscarring — *see* Alopecia
hearing — *see also* Deafness
central NOS H90.5
conductive H90.2
bilateral H90.0
unilateral
with
restricted hearing on the contralateral side H90.A1- *(follows H90.8)*
unrestricted hearing on the contralateral side H90.1-
mixed conductive and sensorineural hearing loss H90.8
bilateral H90.6
unilateral
with
restricted hearing on the contralateral side H90.A3- *(follows H90.8)*
unrestricted hearing on the contralateral side H90.7-
neural NOS H90.5
perceptive NOS H90.5

Loss (of) — *continued*
hearing — *see also* Deafness — *continued*
sensorineural NOS H90.5
bilateral H90.3
unilateral
with
restricted hearing on the contralateral side H90.A2- *(follows H90.8)*
unrestricted hearing on the contralateral side H90.4-
sensory NOS H90.5
height R29.890
limb or member, traumatic, current — *see* Amputation, traumatic
love relationship in childhood Z62.898
memory — *see also* Amnesia
mild, following organic brain damage F06.8
mind — *see* Psychosis
occlusal vertical dimension of fully erupted teeth M26.37
organ or part — *see* Absence, by site, acquired
ossicles, ear (partial) H74.32-
parent in childhood Z63.4
pregnancy, recurrent N96
care in current pregnancy O26.2-
without current pregnancy N96
recurrent pregnancy — *see* Loss, pregnancy, recurrent
self-esteem, in childhood Z62.898
sense of
smell — *see* Disturbance, sensation, smell
taste — *see* Disturbance, sensation, taste
touch R20.8
sensory R44.9
dissociative F44.6
sexual desire F52.0
sight (acquired) (complete) (congenital) — *see* Blindness
substance of
bone — *see* Disorder, bone, density and structure, specified NEC
horizontal alveolar K06.3
cartilage — *see* Disorder, cartilage, specified type NEC
auricle (ear) — *see* Disorder, pinna, specified type NEC
vitreous (humor) H15.89
tooth, teeth — *see* Absence, teeth, acquired
vision, visual H54.7
both eyes H54.3
one eye H54.60
left (normal vision on right) H54.62
right (normal vision on left) H54.61
specified as blindness — *see* Blindness
subjective
sudden H53.13-
transient H53.12-
vitreous — *see* Prolapse, vitreous
voice — *see* Aphonia
weight (abnormal) (cause unknown) R63.4
Louis-Bar syndrome (ataxia-telangiectasia) G11.3
Louping ill (encephalitis) A84.8
Louse, lousiness — *see* Lice
Low
achiever, school Z55.3
back syndrome M54.5
basal metabolic rate R94.8
birthweight (2499 grams or less) P07.10
with weight of
1000-1249 grams P07.14
1250-1499 grams P07.15
1500-1749 grams P07.16
1750-1999 grams P07.17
2000-2499 grams P07.18

Low — *continued*
birthweight (2499 grams or less) P07.10 — *continued*
extreme (999 grams or less) P07.00
with weight of
499 grams or less P07.01
500-749 grams P07.02
750-999 grams P07.03
for gestational age — *see* Light for dates
blood pressure — *see also* Hypotension
reading (incidental) (isolated) (nonspecific) R03.1
cardiac reserve — *see* Disease, heart
function — *see also* Hypofunction
kidney N28.9
hematocrit D64.9
hemoglobin D64.9
income Z59.6
level of literacy Z55.0
lying
kidney N28.89
organ or site, congenital — *see* Malposition, congenital
output syndrome (cardiac) — *see* Failure, heart
platelets (blood) — *see* Thrombocytopenia
reserve, kidney N28.89
salt syndrome E87.1
self esteem R45.81
set ears Q17.4
vision H54.2
one eye (other eye normal) H54.50
left (normal vision on right) H54.52
other eye blind — *see* Blindness
right (normal vision on left) H54.51
Low-density-lipoprotein-type (LDL) hyperlipoproteinemia E78.00
Lowe's syndrome E72.03
Lown-Ganong-Levine syndrome I45.6
LSD reaction (acute) (without dependence) F16.90
with dependence F16.20
L-shaped kidney Q63.8
Ludwig's angina or disease K12.2
Lues (venerea), luetic — *see* Syphilis
Luetscher's syndrome (dehydration) E86.0
Lumbago, lumbalgia M54.5
with sciatica M54.4-
due to intervertebral disc disorder M51.17
due to displacement, intervertebral disc M51.27
with sciatica M51.17
Lumbar — *see* condition
Lumbarization, vertebra, congenital Q76.49
Lumbermen's itch B88.0
Lump — *see* Mass
Lunacy — *see* Psychosis
Lung — *see* condition
Lupoid (miliary) of Boeck D86.3
Lupus
anticoagulant D68.62
with
hemorrhagic disorder D68.312
hypercoagulable state D68.62
finding without diagnosis R76.0
discoid (local) L93.0
erythematosus (discoid) (local) L93.0
disseminated — *see* Lupus, erythematosus, systemic
eyelid H01.129
left H01.126
lower H01.125
upper H01.124
right H01.123
lower H01.122
upper H01.121
profundus L93.2
specified NEC L93.2
subacute cutaneous L93.1

Lupus — *continued*
　erythematosus (discoid) (local) L93.0 — *continued*
　　systemic M32.9
　　　with organ or system involvement M32.10
　　　　endocarditis M32.11
　　　　lung M32.13
　　　　pericarditis M32.12
　　　　renal (glomerular) M32.14
　　　　　tubulo-interstitial M32.15
　　　　specified organ or system NEC M32.19
　　　drug-induced M32.0
　　　inhibitor (presence of) D68.62
　　　　with
　　　　　hemorrhagic disorder D68.312
　　　　　hypercoagulable state D68.62
　　　　finding without diagnosis R76.0
　　　specified NEC M32.8
　exedens A18.4
　hydralazine M32.0
　　correct substance properly administered — *see* Table of Drugs and Chemicals, by drug, adverse effect
　　overdose or wrong substance given or taken — *see* Table of Drugs and Chemicals, by drug, poisoning
　nephritis (chronic) M32.14
　nontuberculous, not disseminated L93.0
　panniculitis L93.2
　pernio (Besnier) D86.3
　systemic — *see* Lupus, erythematosus, systemic
　tuberculous A18.4
　　eyelid A18.4
　vulgaris A18.4
　　eyelid A18.4
Luteinoma D27-
Lutembacher's disease or syndrome (atrial septal defect with mitral stenosis) Q21.1
Luteoma D27-
Lutz(-Splendore-de Almeida) disease — *see* Paracoccidioidomycosis
Luxation — *see also* Dislocation
　eyeball (nontraumatic) — *see* Luxation, globe
　　birth injury P15.3
　globe, nontraumatic H44.82-
　lacrimal gland — *see* Dislocation, lacrimal gland
　lens (old) (partial) (spontaneous)
　　congenital Q12.1
　　syphilitic A50.39
Lycanthropy F22
Lyell's syndrome L51.2
　due to drug L51.2
　　correct substance properly administered — *see* Table of Drugs and Chemicals, by drug, adverse effect
　　overdose or wrong substance given or taken — *see* Table of Drugs and Chemicals, by drug, poisoning
Lyme disease A69.20
Lymph
　gland or node — *see* condition
　scrotum — *see* Infestation, filarial
Lymphadenitis I88.9
　with ectopic or molar pregnancy O08.0
　acute L04.9
　　axilla L04.2
　　face L04.0
　　head L04.0
　　hip L04.3
　　limb
　　　lower L04.3
　　　upper L04.2
　　neck L04.0
　　shoulder L04.2
　　specified site NEC L04.8
　　trunk L04.1
　anthracosis (occupational) J60

Lymphadenitis I88.9 — *continued*
　any site, except mesenteric I88.9
　　chronic I88.1
　　subacute I88.1
　breast
　　gestational — *see* Mastitis, obstetric
　　puerperal, postpartum (nonpurulent) O91.22
　chancroidal (congenital) A57
　chronic I88.1
　　mesenteric I88.0
　due to
　　Brugia (malayi) B74.1
　　　timori B74.2
　　chlamydial lymphogranuloma A55
　　diphtheria (toxin) A36.89
　　lymphogranuloma venereum A55
　　Wuchereria bancrofti B74.0
　following ectopic or molar pregnancy O08.0
　gonorrheal A54.89
　infective — *see* Lymphadenitis, acute
　mesenteric (acute) (chronic) (nonspecific) (subacute) I88.0
　　due to Salmonella typhi A01.09
　　tuberculous A18.39
　mycobacterial A31.8
　purulent — *see* Lymphadenitis, acute
　pyogenic — *see* Lymphadenitis, acute
　regional, nonbacterial I88.8
　septic — *see* Lymphadenitis, acute
　subacute, unspecified site I88.1
　suppurative — *see* Lymphadenitis, acute
　syphilitic (early) (secondary) A51.49
　　late A52.79
　tuberculous — *see* Tuberculosis, lymph gland
　venereal (chlamydial) A55
Lymphadenoid goiter E06.3
Lymphadenopathy (generalized) R59.1
　angioimmunoblastic, with dysproteinemia (AILD) C86.5
　due to toxoplasmosis (acquired) B58.89
　　congenital (acute) (subacute) (chronic) P37.1
　localized R59.0
　syphilitic (early) (secondary) A51.49
Lymphadenosis R59.1
Lymphangiectasis I89.0
　conjunctiva H11.89
　postinfectional I89.0
　scrotum I89.0
Lymphangiectatic elephantiasis, nonfilarial I89.0
Lymphangioendothelioma D18.1
　malignant — *see* Neoplasm, connective tissue, malignant
Lymphangioleiomyomatosis J84.81
Lymphangioma D18.1
　capillary D18.1
　cavernous D18.1
　cystic D18.1
　malignant — *see* Neoplasm, connective tissue, malignant
Lymphangiomyoma D18.1
Lymphangiomyomatosis J84.81
Lymphangiosarcoma — *see* Neoplasm, connective tissue, malignant
Lymphangitis I89.1
　with
　　abscess — *code by* site under Abscess
　　cellulitis — *code by* site under Cellulitis
　　ectopic or molar pregnancy O08.0
　acute L03.91
　　abdominal wall L03.321
　　ankle — *see* Lymphangitis, acute, lower limb
　　arm — *see* Lymphangitis, acute, upper limb
　　auricle (ear) — *see* Lymphangitis, acute, ear
　　axilla L03.12-
　　back (any part) L03.322
　　buttock L03.327
　　cervical (meaning neck) L03.222

Lymphangitis I89.1 — *continued*
　acute L03.91 — *continued*
　　cheek (external) L03.212
　　chest wall L03.323
　　digit
　　　finger — *see* Lymphangitis, acute, finger
　　　toe — *see* Lymphangitis, acute, toe
　　ear (external) H60.1-
　　external auditory canal — *see* Lymphangitis, acute, ear
　　eyelid — *see* Abscess, eyelid
　　face NEC L03.212
　　finger (intrathecal) (periosteal) (subcutaneous) (subcuticular) L03.02-
　　foot — *see* Lymphangitis, acute, lower limb
　　gluteal (region) L03.327
　　groin L03.324
　　hand — *see* Lymphangitis, acute, upper limb
　　head NEC L03.891
　　　face (any part, except ear, eye and nose) L03.212
　　heel — *see* Lymphangitis, acute, lower limb
　　hip — *see* Lymphangitis, acute, lower limb
　　jaw (region) L03.212
　　knee — *see* Lymphangitis, acute, lower limb
　　leg — *see* Lymphangitis, acute, lower limb
　　lower limb L03.12-
　　　toe — *see* Lymphangitis, acute, toe
　　navel L03.326
　　neck (region) L03.222
　　orbit, orbital — *see* Cellulitis, orbit
　　pectoral (region) L03.323
　　perineal, perineum L03.325
　　scalp (any part) L03.891
　　shoulder — *see* Lymphangitis, acute, upper limb
　　specified site NEC L03.898
　　thigh — *see* Lymphangitis, acute, lower limb
　　thumb (intrathecal) (periosteal) (subcutaneous) (subcuticular) — *see* Lymphangitis, acute, finger
　　toe (intrathecal) (periosteal) (subcutaneous) (subcuticular) L03.04-
　　trunk L03.329
　　　abdominal wall L03.321
　　　back (any part) L03.322
　　　buttock L03.327
　　　chest wall L03.323
　　　groin L03.324
　　　perineal, perineum L03.325
　　　umbilicus L03.326
　　umbilicus L03.326
　　upper limb L03.12-
　　　axilla — *see* Lymphangitis, acute, axilla
　　　finger — *see* Lymphangitis, acute, finger
　　　thumb — *see* Lymphangitis, acute, finger
　　　wrist — *see* Lymphangitis, acute, upper limb
　breast
　　gestational — *see* Mastitis, obstetric
　chancroidal A57
　chronic (any site) I89.1
　due to
　　Brugia (malayi) B74.1
　　　timori B74.2
　　Wuchereria bancrofti B74.0
　following ectopic or molar pregnancy O08.89
　penis
　　acute N48.29
　　gonococcal (acute) (chronic) A54.09
　puerperal, postpartum, childbirth O86.89
　strumous, tuberculous A18.2
　subacute (any site) I89.1
　tuberculous — *see* Tuberculosis, lymph gland
Lymphatic (vessel) — *see* condition
Lymphatism E32.8
Lymphectasia I89.0

Lymphedema (acquired) — *see also*
  Elephantiasis
  congenital Q82.0
  hereditary (chronic) (idiopathic) Q82.0
  postmastectomy I97.2
  praecox I89.0
  secondary I89.0
  surgical NEC I97.89
    postmastectomy (syndrome) I97.2
Lymphoblastic — *see* condition
Lymphoblastoma (diffuse) — *see* Lymphoma,
    lymphoblastic (diffuse)
  giant follicular — *see* Lymphoma,
    lymphoblastic (diffuse)
  macrofollicular — *see* Lymphoma,
    lymphoblastic (diffuse)
Lymphocele I89.8
Lymphocytic
  chorioencephalitis (acute) (serous) A87.2
  choriomeningitis (acute) (serous) A87.2
  meningoencephalitis A87.2
Lymphocytoma, benign cutis L98.8
Lymphocytopenia D72.810
Lymphocytosis (symptomatic) D72.820
  infectious (acute) B33.8
Lymphoepithelioma — *see* Neoplasm,
    malignant, by site
Lymphogranuloma (malignant) — *see also*
    Lymphoma, Hodgkin
  chlamydial A55
  inguinale A55
  venereum (any site) (chlamydial) (with stricture
    of rectum) A55
Lymphogranulomatosis (malignant) — *see*
    also Lymphoma, Hodgkin
  benign (Boeck's sarcoid) (Schaumann's) D86.1
Lymphohistiocytosis, hemophagocytic
    (familial) D76.1
Lymphoid — *see* condition
Lymphoma (of) (malignant) C85.90
  adult T-cell (HTLV-1-associated) (acute variant)
    (chronic variant) (lymphomatoid variant)
    (smouldering variant) C91.5-
  anaplastic large cell
    ALK-negative C84.7-
    ALK-positive C84.6-
    CD30-positive C84.6-
    primary cutaneous C86.6
  angioimmunoblastic T-cell C86.5
  BALT C88.4
  B-cell C85.1-
  blastic NK-cell C86.4
  B-precursor C83.5-
  bronchial-associated lymphoid tissue [BALT-
    lymphoma] C88.4
  Burkitt (atypical) C83.7-
  Burkitt-like C83.7-
  centrocytic C83.1-
  cutaneous follicle center C82.6-
  cutaneous T-cell C84.A- *(follows C84.7)*
  diffuse follicle center C82.5-
  diffuse large cell C83.3-
    anaplastic C83.3-
    B-cell C83.3-
    CD30-positive C83.3-
    centroblastic C83.3-
    immunoblastic C83.3-
    plasmablastic C83.3-
    subtype not specified C83.3-
    T-cell rich C83.3-
  enteropathy-type (associated) (intestinal) T-cell
    C86.2
  extranodal marginal zone B-cell lymphoma of
    mucosa-associated lymphoid tissue [MALT-
    lymphoma] C88.4
  extranodal NK/T-cell, nasal type C86.0

Lymphoma (of) (malignant) C85.90 —
    continued
  follicular C82.9-
    grade
      I C82.0-
      II C82.1-
      III C82.2-
      IIIa C82.3-
      IIIb C82.4-
    specified NEC C82.8-
  hepatosplenic T-cell (alpha-beta) (gamma-
    delta) C86.1
  histiocytic C85.9-
    true C96.A *(follows C96.6)*
  Hodgkin C81.9
    lymphocyte depleted (classical) C81.3-
    lymphocyte-rich (classical) C81.4-
    mixed cellularity (classical) C81.2-
    nodular
      lymphocyte predominant C81.0-
      sclerosis (classical) C81.1-
    specified NEC (classical) C81.7-
  intravascular large B-cell C83.8-
  Lennert's C84.4-
  lymphoblastic (diffuse) C83.5-
  lymphoblastic B-cell C83.5-
  lymphoblastic T-cell C83.5-
  lymphoepithelioid C84.4-
  lymphoplasmacytic C83.0-
    with IgM-production C88.0
  MALT C88.4
  mantle cell C83.1-
  mature T-cell NEC C84.4-
  mature T/NK-cell C84.9-
    specified NEC C84.Z- *(follows C84.7)*
  mediastinal (thymic) large B-cell C85.2-
  Mediterranean C88.3
  mucosa-associated lymphoid tissue [MALT-
    lymphoma] C88.4
  NK/T cell C84.9-
  nodal marginal zone C83.0-
  non-follicular (diffuse) C83.9-
    specified NEC C83.8-
  non-Hodgkin (*see also* Lymphoma, by type)
    C85.9-
    specified NEC C85.8-
  non-leukemic variant of B-CLL C83.0-
  peripheral T-cell, not classified C84.4-
  primary cutaneous
    anaplastic large cell C86.6
    CD30-positive large T-cell C86.6
  primary effusion B-cell C83.8-
  SALT C88.4
  skin-associated lymphoid tissue [SALT-
    lymphoma] C88.4
  small cell B-cell C83.0-
  splenic marginal zone C83.0-
  subcutaneous panniculitis-like T-cell C86.3
  T-precursor C83.5-
  true histiocytic C96.A *(follows C96.6)*
Lymphomatosis — *see* Lymphoma
Lymphopathia venereum, veneris A55
Lymphopenia D72.810
Lymphoplasmacytic leukemia — *see*
    Leukemia, chronic lymphocytic, B-cell type
Lymphoproliferation, X-linked disease
    D82.3
Lymphoreticulosis, benign (of inoculation)
    A28.1
Lymphorrhea I89.8
Lymphosarcoma (diffuse) (*see also* Lymphoma)
    C85.9-
Lymphostasis I89.8
Lypemania — *see* Melancholia
Lysine and hydroxylysine metabolism
    disorder E72.3
Lyssa — *see* Rabies

M

Macacus ear Q17.3
Maceration, wet feet, tropical (syndrome)
    T69.02-
MacLeod's syndrome J43.0
Macrocephalia, macrocephaly Q75.3
Macrocheilia, macrochilia (congenital)
    Q18.6
Macrocolon (*see also* Megacolon) Q43.1
Macrocornea Q15.8
  with glaucoma Q15.0
Macrocytic — *see* condition
Macrocytosis D75.89
Macrodactylia, macrodactylism (fingers)
    (thumbs) Q74.0
  toes Q74.2
Macrodontia K00.2
Macrogenia M26.05
Macrogenitosomia (adrenal) (male) (praecox)
    E25.9
  congenital E25.0
Macroglobulinemia (idiopathic) (primary)
    C88.0
  monoclonal (essential) D47.2
  Waldenström C88.0
Macroglossia (congenital) Q38.2
  acquired K14.8
Macrognathia, macrognathism
    (congenital) (mandibular) (maxillary)
    M26.09
Macrogyria (congenital) Q04.8
Macrohydrocephalus — *see* Hydrocephalus
Macromastia — *see* Hypertrophy, breast
Macrophthalmos Q11.3
  in congenital glaucoma Q15.0
Macropsia H53.15
Macrosigmoid K59.39
  congenital Q43.2
Macrospondylitis , acromegalic E22.0
Macrostomia (congenital) Q18.4
Macrotia (external ear) (congenital) Q17.1
Macula
  cornea, corneal — *see* Opacity, cornea
  degeneration (atrophic) (exudative) (senile) —
    see also Degeneration, macula
  hereditary — *see* Dystrophy, retina
Maculae ceruleae B85.1
Maculopathy, toxic — *see* Degeneration,
    macula, toxic
Madarosis (eyelid) H02.729
  left H02.726
    lower H02.725
    upper H02.724
  right H02.723
    lower H02.722
    upper H02.721
Madelung's
  deformity (radius) Q74.0
  disease
    radial deformity Q74.0
    symmetrical lipomas, neck E88.89
Madness — *see* Psychosis
Madura
  foot B47.9
    actinomycotic B47.1
    mycotic B47.0
Maduromycosis B47.0
Maffucci's syndrome Q78.4
Magnesium metabolism disorder — *see*
    Disorder, metabolism, magnesium
Main en griffe (acquired) — *see also*
    Deformity, limb, clawhand
  congenital Q74.0

Maintenance (encounter for)
  antineoplastic chemotherapy Z51.11
  antineoplastic radiation therapy Z51.0
  methadone F11.20
Majocchi's
  disease L81.7
  granuloma B35.8
Major — *see* condition
Mal de los pintos — *see* Pinta
Mal de mer T75.3
Malabar itch (any site) B35.5
Malabsorption K90.9
  calcium K90.89
  carbohydrate K90.49
  disaccharide E73.9
  fat K90.49
  galactose E74.20
  glucose(-galactose) E74.39
  intestinal K90.9
    specified NEC K90.89
  isomaltose E74.31
  lactose E73.9
  methionine E72.19
  monosaccharide E74.39
  postgastrectomy K91.2
  postsurgical K91.2
  protein K90.49
  starch K90.49
  sucrose E74.39
  syndrome K90.9
    postsurgical K91.2
Malacia, bone (adult) M83.9
  juvenile — *see* Rickets
Malacoplakia
  bladder N32.89
  pelvis (kidney) N28.89
  ureter N28.89
  urethra N36.8
Malacosteon, juvenile — *see* Rickets
Maladaptation — *see* Maladjustment
Maladie de Roger Q21.0
Maladjustment
  conjugal Z63.0
    involving divorce or estrangement Z63.5
  educational Z55.4
  family Z63.9
  marital Z63.0
    involving divorce or estrangement Z63.5
  occupational NEC Z56.89
  simple, adult — *see* Disorder, adjustment
  situational — *see* Disorder, adjustment
  social Z60.9
    due to
      acculturation difficulty Z60.3
      discrimination and persecution (perceived) Z60.5
      exclusion and isolation Z60.4
      life-cycle (phase of life) transition Z60.0
      rejection Z60.4
      specified reason NEC Z60.8
Malaise R53.81
Malakoplakia — *see* Malacoplakia
Malaria, malarial (fever) B54
  with
    blackwater fever B50.8
      hemoglobinuric (bilious) B50.8
    hemoglobinuria B50.8
  accidentally induced (therapeutically) — *code by type under* Malaria
  algid B50.9
  cerebral B50.0 *[G94]*
  clinically diagnosed (without parasitological confirmation) B54
  congenital NEC P37.4
    falciparum P37.3
  congestion, congestive B54
  continued (fever) B50.9
  estivo-autumnal B50.9

Malaria, malarial (fever) B54 — *continued*
  falciparum B50.9
    with complications NEC B50.8
      cerebral B50.0 *[G94]*
    severe B50.8
  hemorrhagic B54
  malariae B52.9
    with
      complications NEC B52.8
      glomerular disorder B52.0
  malignant (tertian) — *see* Malaria, falciparum
  mixed infections — *code to* first listed type in B50-B53
  ovale B53.0
  parasitologically confirmed NEC B53.8
  pernicious, acute — *see* Malaria, falciparum
  Plasmodium (P.)
    falciparum NEC — *see* Malaria, falciparum
    malariae NEC B52.9
      with Plasmodium
        falciparum (and or vivax) — *see* Malaria, falciparum
        vivax — *see also* Malaria, vivax
        and falciparum — *see* Malaria, falciparum
    ovale B53.0
      with Plasmodium malariae — *see also* Malaria, malariae
      and vivax — *see also* Malaria, vivax
      and falciparum — *see* Malaria, falciparum
    simian B53.1
      with Plasmodium malariae — *see also* Malaria, malariae
      and vivax — *see also* Malaria, vivax
      and falciparum — *see* Malaria, falciparum
    vivax NEC B51.9
      with Plasmodium falciparum — *see* Malaria, falciparum
  quartan — *see* Malaria, malariae
  quotidian — *see* Malaria, falciparum
  recurrent B54
  remittent B54
  specified type NEC (parasitologically confirmed) B53.8
  spleen B54
  subtertian (fever) — *see* Malaria, falciparum
  tertian (benign) — *see also* Malaria, vivax
    malignant B50.9
  tropical B50.9
  typhoid B54
  vivax B51.9
    with
      complications NEC B51.8
      ruptured spleen B51.0
Malassez's disease (cystic) N50.89
Malassimilation K90.9
Maldescent, testis Q53.9
  bilateral Q53.20
    abdominal Q53.21
    perineal Q53.22
  unilateral Q53.10
    abdominal Q53.11
    perineal Q53.12
Maldevelopment — *see also* Anomaly
  brain Q07.9
  colon Q43.9
  hip Q74.2
    congenital dislocation Q65.2
      bilateral Q65.1
      unilateral Q65.0-
  mastoid process Q75.8
  middle ear Q16.4
    except ossicles Q16.4
    ossicles Q16.3
  ossicles Q16.3
  spine Q76.49
  toe Q74.2

Male type pelvis Q74.2
  with disproportion (fetopelvic) O33.3
    causing obstructed labor O65.3
Malformation (congenital) — *see also* Anomaly
  adrenal gland Q89.1
  affecting multiple systems with skeletal changes NEC Q87.5
  alimentary tract Q45.9
    specified type NEC Q45.8
    upper Q40.9
      specified type NEC Q40.8
  aorta Q25.40
    absence Q25.41
    aneurysm, congenital Q25.43
    aplasia Q25.41
    atresia Q25.29
      aortic arch Q25.21
    coarctation (preductal) (postductal) Q25.1
    dilatation, congenital Q25.44
    hypoplasia Q25.42
    patent ductus arteriosus Q25.0
    specified type NEC Q25.49
    stenosis Q25.1
      supravalvular Q25.3
  aortic valve Q23.9
    specified NEC Q23.8
  arteriovenous, aneurysmatic (congenital) Q27.30
    brain Q28.2
    cerebral Q28.2
    peripheral Q27.30
      digestive system Q27.33
      lower limb Q27.32
      other specified site Q27.39
      renal vessel Q27.34
      upper limb Q27.31
    precerebral vessels (nonruptured) Q28.0
  auricle
    ear (congenital) Q17.3
      acquired H61.119
        left H61.112
          with right H61.113
        right H61.111
          with left H61.113
  bile duct Q44.5
  bladder Q64.79
    aplasia Q64.5
    diverticulum Q64.6
    exstrophy — *see* Exstrophy, bladder
    neck obstruction Q64.31
  bone Q79.9
    face Q75.9
      specified type NEC Q75.8
    skull Q75.9
      specified type NEC Q75.8
  brain (multiple) Q04.9
    arteriovenous Q28.2
    specified type NEC Q04.8
  branchial cleft Q18.2
  breast Q83.9
    specified type NEC Q83.8
  broad ligament Q50.6
  bronchus Q32.4
  bursa Q79.9
  cardiac
    chambers Q20.9
      specified type NEC Q20.8
    septum Q21.9
      specified type NEC Q21.8
  cerebral Q04.9
    vessels Q28.3
  cervix uteri Q51.9
    specified type NEC Q51.828
  Chiari
    Type I G93.5
    Type II Q07.01
  choroid (congenital) Q14.3
    plexus Q07.8
  circulatory system Q28.9

DISEASE INDEX

Malformation (congenital) (*see also* Anomaly)
— continued
cochlea Q16.5
cornea Q13.4
coronary vessels Q24.5
corpus callosum (congenital) Q04.0
diaphragm Q79.1
digestive system NEC, specified type NEC
   Q45.8
dura Q07.9
   brain Q04.9
   spinal Q06.9
ear Q17.9
   causing impairment of hearing Q16.9
   external Q17.9
      accessory auricle Q17.0
      causing impairment of hearing Q16.9
         absence of
            auditory canal Q16.1
            auricle Q16.0
      macrotia Q17.1
      microtia Q17.2
      misplacement Q17.4
      misshapen NEC Q17.3
      prominence Q17.5
      specified type NEC Q17.8
   inner Q16.5
   middle Q16.4
      absence of eustachian tube Q16.2
      ossicles (fusion) Q16.3
   ossicles Q16.3
   specified type NEC Q17.8
epididymis Q55.4
esophagus Q39.9
   specified type NEC Q39.8
eye Q15.9
   lid Q10.3
   specified NEC Q15.8
fallopian tube Q50.6
genital organ — *see* Anomaly, genitalia
great
   artery Q25.9
      aorta — *see* Malformation, aorta
      pulmonary artery — *see* Malformation,
         pulmonary, artery
      specified type NEC Q25.8
   vein Q26.9
      anomalous
         portal venous connection Q26.5
         pulmonary venous connection Q26.4
            partial Q26.3
            total Q26.2
      persistent left superior vena cava Q26.1
      portal vein-hepatic artery fistula Q26.6
      specified type NEC Q26.8
      vena cava stenosis, congenital Q26.0
gum Q38.6
hair Q84.2
heart Q24.9
   specified type NEC Q24.8
integument Q84.9
   specified type NEC Q84.8
internal ear Q16.5
intestine Q43.9
   specified type NEC Q43.8
iris Q13.2
joint Q74.9
   ankle Q74.2
   lumbosacral Q76.49
   sacroiliac Q74.2
   specified type NEC Q74.8
kidney Q63.9
   accessory Q63.0
   giant Q63.3
   horseshoe Q63.1
   hydronephrosis Q62.0
   malposition Q63.2
   specified type NEC Q63.8
lacrimal apparatus Q10.6

Malformation (congenital) (*see also* Anomaly)
— continued
lingual Q38.3
lip Q38.0
liver Q44.7
lung Q33.9
meninges or membrane (congenital) Q07.9
   cerebral Q04.8
   spinal (cord) Q06.9
middle ear Q16.4
   ossicles Q16.3
mitral valve Q23.9
   specified NEC Q23.8
Mondini's (congenital) (malformation, cochlea)
   Q16.5
mouth (congenital) Q38.6
multiple types NEC Q89.7
musculoskeletal system Q79.9
myocardium Q24.8
nail Q84.6
nervous system (central) Q07.9
nose Q30.9
   specified type NEC Q30.8
optic disc Q14.2
orbit Q10.7
ovary Q50.39
palate Q38.5
parathyroid gland Q89.2
pelvic organs or tissues NEC
   in pregnancy or childbirth O34.8-
      causing obstructed labor O65.5
penis Q55.69
   aplasia Q55.5
   curvature (lateral) Q55.61
   hypoplasia Q55.62
pericardium Q24.8
peripheral vascular system Q27.9
   specified type NEC Q27.8
pharynx Q38.8
precerebral vessels Q28.1
prostate Q55.4
pulmonary
   arteriovenous Q25.72
   artery Q25.9
      atresia Q25.5
      specified type NEC Q25.79
      stenosis Q25.6
   valve Q22.3
renal artery Q27.2
respiratory system Q34.9
retina Q14.1
scrotum — *see* Malformation, testis and
   scrotum
seminal vesicles Q55.4
sense organs NEC Q07.9
skin Q82.9
specified NEC Q89.8
spinal
   cord Q06.9
   nerve root Q07.8
spine Q76.49
   kyphosis — *see* Kyphosis, congenital
   lordosis — *see* Lordosis, congenital
spleen Q89.09
stomach Q40.3
   specified type NEC Q40.2
teeth, tooth K00.9
tendon Q79.9
testis and scrotum Q55.20
   aplasia Q55.0
   hypoplasia Q55.1
   polyorchism Q55.21
   retractile testis Q55.22
   scrotal transposition Q55.23
   specified NEC Q55.29
thorax, bony Q76.9
throat Q38.8
thyroid gland Q89.2

Malformation (congenital) (*see also* Anomaly)
— continued
tongue (congenital) Q38.3
   hypertrophy Q38.2
   tie Q38.1
trachea Q32.1
tricuspid valve Q22.9
   specified type NEC Q22.8
umbilical cord NEC (complicating delivery)
   O69.89
umbilicus Q89.9
ureter Q62.8
   agenesis Q62.4
   duplication Q62.5
   malposition — *see* Malposition, congenital,
      ureter
   obstructive defect — *see* Defect, obstructive,
      ureter
   vesico-uretero-renal reflux Q62.7
urethra Q64.79
   aplasia Q64.5
   duplication Q64.74
   posterior valves Q64.2
   prolapse Q64.71
   stricture Q64.32
urinary system Q64.9
uterus Q51.9
   specified type NEC Q51.818
vagina Q52.4
vas deferens Q55.4
   atresia Q55.3
vascular system, peripheral Q27.9
venous — *see* Anomaly, vein(s)
vulva Q52.70
Malfunction — *see also* Dysfunction
cardiac electronic device T82.119
   electrode T82.110
   pulse generator T82.111
   specified type NEC T82.118
catheter device NEC T85.618
   cystostomy T83.010
   dialysis (renal) (vascular) T82.41
      intraperitoneal T85.611
   infusion NEC T82.514
      cranial T85.610
      epidural T85.610
      intrathecal T85.610
      spinal T85.610
      subarachnoid T85.610
      subdural T85.610
   urinary (*see also* Breakdown, device,
      catheter) T83.018
colostomy K94.03
   valve K94.03
cystostomy (stoma) N99.512
   catheter T83.010
enteric stoma K94.13
enterostomy K94.13
esophagostomy K94.33
gastroenteric K31.89
gastrostomy K94.23
ileostomy K94.13
   valve K94.13
intrathecal infusion pump T85.615
jejunostomy K94.13
nervous system device, implant or graft,
   specified NEC T85.615
pacemaker — *see* Malfunction, cardiac
   electronic device
prosthetic device, internal — *see*
   Complications, prosthetic device, by site,
   mechanical
tracheostomy J95.03
urinary device NEC — *see* Complication,
   genitourinary, device, urinary, mechanical
valve
   colostomy K94.03
   heart T82.09
      ileostomy K94.13

Malfunction — *see also* Dysfunction — *continued*
  vascular graft or shunt NEC — *see* Complication, cardiovascular device, mechanical, vascular
  ventricular (communicating shunt) T85.01
Malherbe's tumor — *see* Neoplasm, skin, benign
Malibu disease L98.8
Malignancy — *see also* Neoplasm, malignant, by site
  unspecified site (primary) C80.1
Malignant — *see* condition
Malingerer, malingering Z76.5
Mallet finger (acquired) — *see* Deformity, finger, mallet finger
  congenital Q74.0
  sequelae of rickets E64.3
Malleus A24.0
Mallory's bodies R89.7
Mallory-Weiss syndrome K22.6
Malnutrition E46
  degree
    first E44.1
    mild (protein) E44.1
    moderate (protein) E44.0
    second E44.0
    severe (protein-energy) E43
      intermediate form E42
        with
          kwashiorkor (and marasmus) E42
          marasmus E41
      third E43
  following gastrointestinal surgery K91.2
  intrauterine
    light-for-dates — *see* Light for dates
    small-for-dates — *see* Small for dates
  lack of care, or neglect (child) (infant) T76.02
    confirmed T74.02
  malignant E40
  protein E46
    calorie E46
      mild E44.1
      moderate E44.0
      severe E43
        intermediate form E42
          with
            kwashiorkor (and marasmus) E42
            marasmus E41
    energy E46
      mild E44.1
      moderate E44.0
      severe E43
        intermediate form E42
          with
            kwashiorkor (and marasmus) E42
            marasmus E41
  severe (protein-energy) E43
    with
      kwashiorkor (and marasmus) E42
      marasmus E41
Malocclusion (teeth) M26.4
  Angle's M26.219
    class I M26.211
    class II M26.212
    class III M26.213
  due to
    abnormal swallowing M26.59
    mouth breathing M26.59
    tongue, lip or finger habits M26.59
  temporomandibular (joint) M26.69
Malposition
  cervix — *see* Malposition, uterus
  congenital
    adrenal (gland) Q89.1
    alimentary tract Q45.8
      lower Q43.8
      upper Q40.8
    aorta Q25.49

Malposition — *continued*
  congenital — *continued*
    appendix Q43.8
    arterial trunk Q20.0
    artery (peripheral) Q27.8
      coronary Q24.5
      digestive system Q27.8
      lower limb Q27.8
      pulmonary Q25.79
      specified site NEC Q27.8
      upper limb Q27.8
    auditory canal Q17.8
      causing impairment of hearing Q16.9
    auricle (ear) Q17.4
      causing impairment of hearing Q16.9
      cervical Q18.2
    biliary duct or passage Q44.5
    bladder (mucosa) — *see* Exstrophy, bladder
    brachial plexus Q07.8
    brain tissue Q04.8
    breast Q83.8
    bronchus Q32.4
    cecum Q43.8
    clavicle Q74.0
    colon Q43.8
    digestive organ or tract NEC Q45.8
      lower Q43.8
      upper Q40.8
    ear (auricle) (external) Q17.4
      ossicles Q16.3
    endocrine (gland) NEC Q89.2
    epiglottis Q31.8
    eustachian tube Q17.8
    eye Q15.8
    facial features Q18.8
    fallopian tube Q50.6
    finger(s) Q68.1
      supernumerary Q69.0
    foot Q66.9
    gallbladder Q44.1
    gastrointestinal tract Q45.8
    genitalia, genital organ(s) or tract
      female Q52.8
        external Q52.79
        internal NEC Q52.8
      male Q55.8
    glottis Q31.8
    hand Q68.1
    heart Q24.8
      dextrocardia Q24.0
      with complete transposition of viscera Q89.3
    hepatic duct Q44.5
    hip (joint) Q65.89
    intestine (large) (small) Q43.8
      with anomalous adhesions, fixation or malrotation Q43.3
    joint NEC Q68.8
    kidney Q63.2
    larynx Q31.8
    limb Q68.8
      lower Q68.8
      upper Q68.8
    liver Q44.7
    lung (lobe) Q33.8
    nail(s) Q84.6
    nerve Q07.8
    nervous system NEC Q07.8
    nose, nasal (septum) Q30.8
    organ or site not listed — *see* Anomaly, by site
    ovary Q50.39
    pancreas Q45.3
    parathyroid (gland) Q89.2
    patella Q74.1
    peripheral vascular system Q27.8
    pituitary (gland) Q89.2
    respiratory organ or system NEC Q34.8

Malposition — *continued*
  congenital — *continued*
    rib (cage) Q76.6
      supernumerary in cervical region Q76.5
    scapula Q74.0
    shoulder Q74.0
    spinal cord Q06.8
    spleen Q89.09
    sternum NEC Q76.7
    stomach Q40.2
    symphysis pubis Q74.2
    thymus (gland) Q89.2
    thyroid (gland) (tissue) Q89.2
      cartilage Q31.8
    toe(s) Q66.9
      supernumerary Q69.2
    tongue Q38.3
    trachea Q32.1
    ureter Q62.60
      deviation Q62.61
      displacement Q62.62
      ectopia Q62.63
      specified type NEC Q62.69
    uterus Q51.818
    vein(s) (peripheral) Q27.8
      great Q26.8
    vena cava (inferior) (superior) Q26.8
  device, implant or graft (*see also* Complications, by site and type, mechanical) T85.628
    arterial graft NEC — *see* Complication, cardiovascular device, mechanical, vascular
    breast (implant) T85.42
    catheter NEC T85.628
      cystostomy T83.020
      dialysis (renal) T82.42
        intraperitoneal T85.621
      infusion NEC T82.524
        spinal (epidural) (subdural) T85.620
      urinary (*see also* Displacement, device, catheter, urinary) T83.028
    electronic (electrode) (pulse generator) (stimulator)
      bone T84.320
      cardiac T82.129
      electrode T82.120
      pulse generator T82.121
      specified type NEC T82.128
      nervous system — *see* Complication, prosthetic device, mechanical, electronic nervous system stimulator
      urinary — *see* Complication, genitourinary, device, urinary, mechanical
    fixation, internal (orthopedic) NEC — *see* Complication, fixation device, mechanical
    gastrointestinal — *see* Complications, prosthetic device, mechanical, gastrointestinal device
    genital NEC T83.428
      intrauterine contraceptive device (string) T83.32
      penile prosthesis (cylinder) (implanted) (pump) (resevoir) T83.420
      testicular prosthesis T83.421
    heart NEC — *see* Complication, cardiovascular device, mechanical
    joint prosthesis — *see* Complication, joint prosthesis, mechanical
    ocular NEC — *see* Complications, prosthetic device, mechanical, ocular device
    orthopedic NEC — *see* Complication, orthopedic, device, mechanical
    specified NEC T85.628
    urinary NEC — *see also* Complication, genitourinary, device, urinary, mechanical
      graft T83.22

Malposition — *continued*
  device, implant or graft (*see also* Complications, by site and type, mechanical) T85.628 — *continued*
    vascular NEC — *see* Complication, cardiovascular device, mechanical
    ventricular intracranial shunt T85.02
  fetus — *see* Pregnancy, complicated by (management affected by), presentation, fetal
  gallbladder K82.8
  gastrointestinal tract, congenital Q45.8
  heart, congenital NEC Q24.8
  joint prosthesis — *see* Complications, joint prosthesis, mechanical, displacement, by site
  stomach K31.89
    congenital Q40.2
  tooth, teeth, fully erupted M26.30
  uterus (acute) (acquired) (adherent) (asymptomatic) (postinfectional) (postpartal, old) N85.4
    anteflexion or anteversion N85.4
      congenital Q51.818
    flexion N85.4
      lateral — *see* Lateroversion, uterus
    inversion N85.5
    lateral (flexion) (version) — *see* Lateroversion, uterus
      in pregnancy or childbirth — *see* subcategory O34.5
    retroflexion or retroversion — *see* Retroversion, uterus
Malposture R29.3
Malrotation
  cecum Q43.3
  colon Q43.3
  intestine Q43.3
  kidney Q63.2
Malta fever — *see* Brucellosis
Maltreatment
  adult
    abandonment
      confirmed T74.01
      suspected T76.01
    confirmed T74.91
    history of Z91.419
    neglect
      confirmed T74.01
      suspected T76.01
    physical abuse
      confirmed T74.11
      suspected T76.11
    psychological abuse
      confirmed T74.31
      history of Z91.411
      suspected T76.31
    sexual abuse
      confirmed T74.21
      suspected T76.21
    suspected T76.91
  child
    abandonment
      confirmed T74.02
      suspected T76.02
    confirmed T74.92
    history of — *see* History, personal (of), abuse
    neglect
      confirmed T74.02
      history of — *see* History, personal (of), abuse
      suspected T76.02
    physical abuse
      confirmed T74.12
      history of — *see* History, personal (of), abuse
      suspected T76.12

Maltreatment — *continued*
  child — *continued*
    psychological abuse
      confirmed T74.32
      history of — *see* History, personal (of), abuse
      suspected T76.32
    sexual abuse
      confirmed T74.22
      history of — *see* History, personal (of), abuse
      suspected T76.22
    suspected T76.92
  personal history of Z91.89
Maltworker's lung J67.4
Malunion, fracture — *see* Fracture, by site
Mammillitis N61.0
  puerperal, postpartum O91.02
Mammitis — *see* Mastitis
Mammogram (examination) Z12.39
  routine Z12.31
Mammoplasia N62
Management (of)
  bone conduction hearing device (implanted) Z45.320
  cardiac pacemaker NEC Z45.018
  cerebrospinal fluid drainage device Z45.41
  cochlear device (implanted) Z45.321
  contraceptive Z30.9
    specified NEC Z30.8
  implanted device Z45.9
    specified NEC Z45.89
  infusion pump Z45.1
  procreative Z31.9
    male factor infertility in female Z31.81
    specified NEC Z31.89
  prosthesis (external) (*see also* Fitting) Z44.9
    implanted Z45.9
      specified NEC Z45.89
  renal dialysis catheter Z49.01
  vascular access device Z45.2
Mangled — *see* specified injury by site
Mania (monopolar) — *see also* Disorder, mood, manic episode
  with psychotic symptoms F30.2
  Bell's F30.8
  chronic (recurrent) F31.89
  hysterical F44.89
  puerperal F30.8
  recurrent F31.89
  without psychotic symptoms F30.10
    mild F30.11
    moderate F30.12
    severe F30.13
Manic-depressive insanity, psychosis, or syndrome — *see* Disorder, bipolar
Mannosidosis E77.1
Manson's
  disease B65.1
  schistosomiasis B65.1
Mansonelliasis, mansonellosis B74.4
Manual — *see* condition
Maple-bark-stripper's lung (disease) J67.6
Maple-syrup-urine disease E71.0
Marable's syndrome (celiac artery compression) O77.4
Marasmus E41
  due to malnutrition E41
  intestinal E41
  nutritional E41
  senile R54
  tuberculous NEC — *see* Tuberculosis
Marble
  bones Q78.2
  skin R23.8
Marburg virus disease A98.3

March
  fracture — *see* Fracture, traumatic, stress, by site
  hemoglobinuria D59.6
Marchesani(-Weill) syndrome Q87.0
Marchiafava(-Bignami) syndrome or disease G37.1
Marchiafava-Micheli syndrome D59.5
Marcus Gunn's syndrome Q07.8
Marfan's syndrome — *see* Syndrome, Marfan's
Marie-Bamberger disease — *see* Osteoarthropathy, hypertrophic, specified NEC
Marie-Charcot-Tooth neuropathic muscular atrophy G60.0
Marie's
  cerebellar ataxia (late-onset) G11.2
  disease or syndrome (acromegaly) E22.0
Marie-Strümpell arthritis, disease or spondylitis — *see* Spondylitis, ankylosing
Marion's disease (bladder neck obstruction) N32.0
Marital conflict Z63.0
Mark
  port wine Q82.5
  raspberry Q82.5
  strawberry Q82.5
  stretch L90.6
  tattoo L81.8
Marker heterochromatin — *see* Extra, marker chromosomes
Maroteaux-Lamy syndrome (mild) (severe) E76.29
Marrow (bone)
  arrest D61.9
  poor function D75.89
Marseilles fever A77.1
Marsh fever — *see* Malaria
Marsh's disease (exophthalmic goiter) E05.00
  with storm E05.01
Marshall's (hidrotic) ectodermal dysplasia Q82.4
Masculinization (female) with adrenal hyperplasia E25.9
  congenital E25.0
Masculinovoblastoma D27-
Masochism (sexual) F65.51
Mason's lung J62.8
Mass
  abdominal R19.00
    epigastric R19.06
    generalized R19.07
    left lower quadrant R19.04
    left upper quadrant R19.02
    periumbilic R19.05
    right lower quadrant R19.03
    right upper quadrant R19.01
    specified site NEC R19.09
  breast N63
  chest R22.2
  cystic — *see* Cyst
  ear H93.8-
  head R22.0
  intra-abdominal (diffuse) (generalized) — *see* Mass, abdominal
  kidney N28.89
  liver R16.0
  localized (skin) R22.9
    chest R22.2
    head R22.0
    limb
      lower R22.4-
      upper R22.3-
    neck R22.1
    trunk R22.2
  lung R91.8
  malignant — *see* Neoplasm, malignant, by site
  neck R22.1

DISEASE INDEX

Mass — *continued*
  pelvic (diffuse) (generalized) — *see* Mass, abdominal
  specified organ NEC — *see* Disease, by site
  splenic R16.1
  substernal thyroid — *see* Goiter
  superficial (localized) R22.9
  umbilical (diffuse) (generalized) R19.09
Massive — *see* condition
Mast cell
  disease, systemic tissue D47.0
  leukemia C94.3-
  sarcoma C96.2
  tumor D47.0
    malignant C96.2
Mastalgia N64.4
Masters-Allen syndrome N83.8
Mastitis (acute) (diffuse) (nonpuerperal) (subacute) N61.0
  with abscess N61.1
  chronic (cystic) — *see* Mastopathy, cystic
  cystic (Schimmelbusch's type) — *see* Mastopathy, cystic
  fibrocystic — *see* Mastopathy, cystic
  infective N61.0
    newborn P39.0
  interstitial, gestational or puerperal — *see* Mastitis, obstetric
  neonatal (noninfective) P83.4
    infective P39.0
  obstetric (interstitial) (nonpurulent)
    associated with
      lactation O91.23
      pregnancy O91.21-
      puerperium O91.22
    purulent
      associated with
        lactation O91.13
        pregnancy O91.11-
        puerperium O91.12
  periductal — *see* Ectasia, mammary duct
  phlegmonous — *see* Mastopathy, cystic
  plasma cell — *see* Ectasia, mammary duct
  without abscess N61.0
Mastocytoma D47.0
  malignant C96.2
Mastocytosis Q82.2
  aggressive systemic C96.2
  indolent systemic D47.0
  malignant C96.2
  systemic, associated with clonal hematopoetic non-mast-cell disease (SM-AHNMD) D47.0
Mastodynia N64.4
Mastoid — *see* condition
Mastoidalgia — *see* subcategory H92.0
Mastoiditis (coalescent) (hemorrhagic) (suppurative) H70.9-
  acute, subacute H70.00-
    complicated NEC H70.09-
    subperiosteal H70.01-
  chronic (necrotic) (recurrent) H70.1-
  in (due to)
    infectious disease NEC B99 [H75.-]
    parasitic disease NEC B89 [H75.-]
    tuberculosis A18.03
  petrositis — *see* Petrositis
  postauricular fistula — *see* Fistula, postauricular
  specified NEC H70.89-
  tuberculous A18.03
Mastopathy, mastopathia N64.9
  chronica cystica — *see* Mastopathy, cystic
  cystic (chronic) (diffuse) N60.1-
    with epithelial proliferation N60.3-
  diffuse cystic — *see* Mastopathy, cystic
  estrogenic, oestrogenica N64.89
  ovarian origin N64.89
Mastoplasia, mastoplastia N62

Masturbation (excessive) F98.8
Maternal care (for) — *see* Pregnancy (complicated by) (management affected by)
Matheiu's disease (leptospiral jaundice) A27.0
Mauclaire's disease or osteochondrosis — *see* Osteochondrosis, juvenile, hand, metacarpal
Maxcy's disease A75.2
Maxilla, maxillary — *see* condition
May(-Hegglin) anomaly or syndrome D72.0
McArdle(-Schmid)(-Pearson) disease (glycogen storage) E74.04
McCune-Albright syndrome Q78.1
McQuarrie's syndrome (idiopathic familial hypoglycemia) E16.2
Meadow's syndrome Q86.1
Measles (black) (hemorrhagic) (suppressed) B05.9
  with
    complications NEC B05.89
    encephalitis B05.0
    intestinal complications B05.4
    keratitis (keratoconjunctivitis) B05.81
    meningitis B05.1
    otitis media B05.3
    pneumonia B05.2
  French — *see* Rubella
  German — *see* Rubella
  Liberty — *see* Rubella
Meat-wrappers' asthma J68.9
Meatitis, urethral — *see* Urethritis
Meatus, meatal — *see* condition
Meckel's diverticulitis, diverticulum (displaced) (hypertrophic) Q43.0
  malignant — *see* Table of Neoplasms, small intestine, malignant
Meckel-Gruber syndrome Q61.9
Meconium
  ileus, newborn P76.0
    in cystic fibrosis E84.11
    meaning meconium plug (without cystic fibrosis) P76.0
  obstruction, newborn P76.0
    due to fecaliths P76.0
    in mucoviscidosis E84.11
  peritonitis P78.0
  plug syndrome (newborn) NEC P76.0
Median — *see also* condition
  arcuate ligament syndrome I77.4
  bar (prostate) (vesical orifice) — *see* Hyperplasia, prostate
  rhomboid glossitis K14.2
Mediastinal shift R93.8
Mediastinitis (acute) (chronic) J98.51
  syphilitic A52.73
  tuberculous A15.8
Mediastinopericarditis — *see also* Pericarditis
  acute I30.9
  adhesive I31.0
  chronic I31.8
  rheumatic I09.2
Mediastinum, mediastinal — *see* condition
Medicine poisoning — *see* Table of Drugs and Chemicals, by drug, poisoning
Mediterranean
  fever — *see* Brucellosis
    familial M04.1
    tick A77.1
  kala-azar B55.0
  leishmaniasis B55.0
  tick fever A77.1
Medulla — *see* condition
Medullary cystic kidney Q61.5
Medullated fibers
  optic (nerve) Q14.8
  retina Q14.1

Medulloblastoma
  desmoplastic C71.6
  specified site — *see* Neoplasm, malignant, by site
  unspecified site C71.6
Medulloepithelioma — *see also* Neoplasm, malignant, by site
  teratoid — *see* Neoplasm, malignant, by site
Medullomyoblastoma
  specified site — *see* Neoplasm, malignant, by site
  unspecified site C71.6
Meekeren-Ehlers-Danlos syndrome Q79.6
Megacolon (acquired) (functional) (not Hirschsprung's disease) (in) K59.39
  Chagas' disease B57.32
  congenital, congenitum (aganglionic) Q43.1
  Hirschsprung's (disease) Q43.1
  toxic NEC K59.31
    due to Clostridium difficile A04.7
Megaesophagus (functional) K22.0
  congenital Q39.5
  in (due to) Chagas' disease B57.31
Megalencephaly Q04.5
Megalerythema (epidemic) B08.3
Megaloappendix Q43.8
Megalocephalus, megalocephaly NEC Q75.3
Megalocornea Q15.8
  with glaucoma Q15.0
Megalocytic anemia D53.91
Megalodactylia (fingers) (thumbs) (congenital) Q74.0
  toes Q74.2
Megaloduodenum Q43.8
Megaloesophagus (functional) K22.0
  congenital Q39.5
Megalogastria (acquired) K31.89
  congenital Q40.2
Megalophthalmos Q11.3
Megalopsia H53.15
Megalosplenia — *see* Splenomegaly
Megaloureter N28.82
  congenital Q62.2
Megarectum K62.89
Megasigmoid K59.39
  congenital Q43.2
Megaureter N28.82
  congenital Q62.2
Megavitamin-B6 syndrome E67.2
Megrim — *see* Migraine
Meibomian
  cyst, infected — *see* Hordeolum
  gland — *see* condition
  sty, stye — *see* Hordeolum
Meibomitis — *see* Hordeolum
Meige's syndrome Q82.0
Meige-Milroy disease (chronic hereditary edema) Q82.0
Melalgia, nutritional E53.8
Melancholia F32.9
  climacteric (single episode) F32.89
    recurrent episode F33.8
  hypochondriac F45.29
  intermittent (single episode) F32.89
    recurrent episode F33.8
  involutional (single episode) F32.89
    recurrent episode F33.8
  menopausal (single episode) F32.89
    recurrent episode F33.8
  puerperal F32.89
  reactive (emotional stress or trauma) F32.3
  recurrent F33.9
  senile F03
  stuporous (single episode) F32.89
    recurrent episode F33.8
Melanemia R79.89

Melanoameloblastoma — *see* Neoplasm, bone, benign
Melanoblastoma — *see* Melanoma
Melanocarcinoma — *see* Melanoma
Melanocytoma, eyeball D31.9-
Melanocytosis, neurocutaneous Q82.8
Melanoderma, melanodermia L81.4
Melanodontia, infantile K03.89
Melanodontoclasia K03.89
Melanoepithelioma — *see* Melanoma
Melanoma (malignant) C43.9
  acral lentiginous, malignant — *see* Melanoma, skin, by site
  amelanotic — *see* Melanoma, skin, by site
  balloon cell — *see* Melanoma, skin, by site
  benign — *see* Nevus
  desmoplastic, malignant — *see* Melanoma, skin, by site
  epithelioid cell — *see* Melanoma, skin, by site
    with spindle cell, mixed — *see* Melanoma, skin, by site
  in
    giant pigmented nevus — *see* Melanoma, skin, by site
    Hutchinson's melanotic freckle — *see* Melanoma, skin, by site
    junctional nevus — *see* Melanoma, skin, by site
    precancerous melanosis — *see* Melanoma, skin, by site
  in situ D03.9
    abdominal wall D03.59
    ala nasi D03.39
    ankle D03.7-
    anus, anal (margin) (skin) D03.51
    arm D03.6-
    auditory canal D03.2-
    auricle (ear) D03.2-
    auricular canal (external) D03.2-
    axilla, axillary fold D03.59
    back D03.59
    breast D03.52
    brow D03.39
    buttock D03.59
    canthus (eye) D03.1-
    cheek (external) D03.39
    chest wall D03.59
    chin D03.39
    choroid D03.8
    conjunctiva D03.8
    ear (external) D03.2-
    external meatus (ear) D03.2-
    eye D03.8
    eyebrow D03.39
    eyelid (lower) (upper) D03.1-
    face D03.30
      specified NEC D03.39
    female genital organ (external) NEC D03.8
    finger D03.6-
    flank D03.59
    foot D03.7-
    forearm D03.6-
    forehead D03.39
    foreskin D03.8
    gluteal region D03.59
    groin D03.59
    hand D03.6-
    heel D03.7-
    helix D03.2-
    hip D03.7-
    interscapular region D03.59
    iris D03.8
    jaw D03.39
    knee D03.7-
    labium (majus) (minus) D03.8
    lacrimal gland D03.8
    leg D03.7-
    lip (lower) (upper) D03.0
    lower limb NEC D03.7-

Melanoma (malignant) C43.9 — *continued*
  in situ D03.9 — *continued*
    male genital organ (external) NEC D03.8
    nail D03.9
      finger D03.6-
      toe D03.7-
    neck D03.4
    nose (external) D03.39
    orbit D03.8
    penis D03.8
    perianal skin D03.51
    perineum D03.51
    pinna D03.2-
    popliteal fossa or space D03.7-
    prepuce D03.8
    pudendum D03.8
    retina D03.8
    retrobulbar D03.8
    scalp D03.4
    scrotum D03.8
    shoulder D03.6-
    specified site NEC D03.8
    submammary fold D03.52
    temple D03.39
    thigh D03.7-
    toe D03.7-
    trunk NEC D03.59
    umbilicus D03.59
    upper limb NEC D03.6-
    vulva D03.8
  juvenile — *see* Nevus
  malignant, of soft parts except skin — *see* Neoplasm, connective tissue, malignant
  metastatic
    breast C79.81
    genital organ C79.82
    specified site NEC C79.89
  neurotropic, malignant — *see* Melanoma, skin, by site
  nodular — *see* Melanoma, skin, by site
  regressing, malignant — *see* Melanoma, skin, by site
  skin C43.9
    abdominal wall C43.59
    ala nasi C43.31
    ankle C43.7-
    anus, anal (skin) C43.51
    arm C43.6-
    auditory canal (external) C43.2-
    auricle (ear) C43.2-
    auricular canal (external) C43.2-
    axilla, axillary fold C43.59
    back C43.59
    breast (female) (male) C43.52
    brow C43.39
    buttock C43.59
    canthus (eye) C43.1-
    cheek (external) C43.39
    chest wall C43.59
    chin C43.39
    ear (external) C43.2-
    elbow C43.6-
    external meatus (ear) C43.2-
    eyebrow C43.39
    eyelid (lower) (upper) C43.1-
    face C43.30
      specified NEC C43.39
    female genital organ (external) NEC C51.9
    finger C43.6-
    flank C43.59
    foot C43.7-
    forearm C43.6-
    forehead C43.39
    foreskin C60.0
    glabella C43.39
    gluteal region C43.59
    groin C43.59
    hand C43.6-
    heel C43.7-

Melanoma (malignant) C43.9 — *continued*
  skin C43.9 — *continued*
    helix C43.2-
    hip C43.7-
    interscapular region C43.59
    jaw (external) C43.39
    knee C43.7-
    labium C51.9
      majus C51.0
      minus C51.1
    leg C43.7-
    lip (lower) (upper) C43.0
    lower limb NEC C43.7-
    male genital organ (external) NEC C63.9
    nail
      finger C43.6-
      toe C43.7-
    nasolabial groove C43.39
    nates C43.59
    neck C43.4
    nose (external) C43.31
    overlapping site C43.8
    palpebra C43.1-
    penis C60.9
    perianal skin C43.51
    perineum C43.51
    pinna C43.2-
    popliteal fossa or space C43.7-
    prepuce C60.0
    pudendum C51.9
    scalp C43.4
    scrotum C63.2
    shoulder C43.6-
    skin NEC C43.9
    submammary fold C43.52
    temple C43.39
    thigh C43.7-
    toe C43.7-
    trunk NEC C43.59
    umbilicus C43.59
    upper limb NEC C43.6-
    vulva C51.9
      overlapping sites C51.8
    spindle cell
      with epithelioid, mixed — *see* Melanoma, skin, by site
      type A C69.4-
      type B C69.4-
    superficial spreading — *see* Melanoma, skin, by site
Melanosarcoma — *see also* Melanoma
  epithelioid cell — *see* Melanoma
Melanosis L81.4
  addisonian E27.1
    tuberculous A18.7
  adrenal E27.1
  colon K63.89
  conjunctiva — *see* Pigmentation, conjunctiva
    congenital Q13.89
  cornea (presenile) (senile) — *see also* Pigmentation, cornea
    congenital Q13.4
  eye NEC H57.8
    congenital Q15.8
  lenticularis progressiva Q82.1
  liver K76.89
  precancerous — *see also* Melanoma, in situ
    malignant melanoma in — *see* Melanoma
  Riehl's L81.4
  sclera H15.89
    congenital Q13.89
  suprarenal E27.1
  tar L81.4
  toxic L81.4
Melanuria R82.99
MELAS syndrome E88.41
Melasma L81.1
  adrenal (gland) E27.1
  suprarenal (gland) E27.1

Melena K92.1
  with ulcer — *code by* site under Ulcer, with
    hemorrhage K27.4
  due to swallowed maternal blood P78.2
  newborn, neonatal P54.1
    due to swallowed maternal blood P78.2
Meleney's
  gangrene (cutaneous) — *see* Ulcer, skin
  ulcer (chronic undermining) — *see* Ulcer, skin
Melioidosis A24.9
  acute A24.1
  chronic A24.2
  fulminating A24.1
  pneumonia A24.1
  pulmonary (chronic) A24.2
    acute A24.1
    subacute A24.2
  sepsis A24.1
  specified NEC A24.3
  subacute A24.2
Melitensis, febris A23.0
Melkersson(-Rosenthal) syndrome G51.2
Mellitus, diabetes — *see* Diabetes
Melorheostosis (bone) — *see* Disorder, bone,
  density and structure, specified NEC
Meloschisis Q18.4
Melotia Q17.4
Membrana
  capsularis lentis posterior Q13.89
  epipapillaris Q14.2
Membranacea placenta O43.19-
Membranaceous uterus N85.8
Membrane(s), membranous — *see also*
  condition
  cyclitic — *see* Membrane, pupillary
  folds, congenital — *see* Web
  Jackson's Q43.3
  over face of newborn P28.9
  premature rupture — *see* Rupture, membranes,
    premature
  pupillary H21.4-
    persistent Q13.89
  retained (with hemorrhage) (complicating
    delivery) O72.2
    without hemorrhage O73.1
  secondary cataract — *see* Cataract, secondary
  unruptured (causing asphyxia) — *see*
    Asphyxia, newborn
  vitreous — *see* Opacity, vitreous, membranes
    and strands
Membranitis — *see* Chorioamnionitis
Memory disturbance, lack or loss — *see*
  also Amnesia
  mild, following organic brain damage F06.8
Menadione deficiency E56.1
Menarche
  delayed E30.0
  precocious E30.1
Mendacity, pathologic F60.2
Mendelson's syndrome (due to anesthesia)
  J95.4
  in labor and delivery O74.0
  in pregnancy O29.01-
  obstetric O74.0
  postpartum, puerperal O89.01
Ménétrier's disease or syndrome K29.60
  with bleeding K29.61
Ménière's disease, syndrome or vertigo
  H81.0-
Meninges, meningeal — *see* condition
Meningioma — *see also* Neoplasm, meninges,
  benign
  angioblastic — *see* Neoplasm, meninges,
    benign
  angiomatous — *see* Neoplasm, meninges,
    benign
  endotheliomatous — *see* Neoplasm, meninges,
    benign

Meningioma — *see also* Neoplasm, meninges,
  benign — *continued*
  fibroblastic — *see* Neoplasm, meninges,
    benign
  fibrous — *see* Neoplasm, meninges, benign
  hemangioblastic — *see* Neoplasm, meninges,
    benign
  hemangiopericytic — *see* Neoplasm,
    meninges, benign
  malignant — *see* Neoplasm, meninges,
    malignant
  meningiothelial — *see* Neoplasm, meninges,
    benign
  meningotheliomatous — *see* Neoplasm,
    meninges, benign
  mixed — *see* Neoplasm, meninges, benign
  multiple — *see* Neoplasm, meninges, uncertain
    behavior
  papillary — *see* Neoplasm, meninges,
    uncertain behavior
  psammomatous — *see* Neoplasm, meninges,
    benign
  syncytial — *see* Neoplasm, meninges, benign
  transitional — *see* Neoplasm, meninges,
    benign
Meningiomatosis (diffuse) — *see* Neoplasm,
  meninges, uncertain behavior
Meningism — *see* Meningismus
Meningismus (infectional) (pneumococcal)
  R29.1
  due to serum or vaccine R29.1
  influenzal — *see* Influenza, with,
    manifestations NEC
Meningitis (basal) (basic) (brain) (cerebral)
  (cervical) (congestive) (diffuse) (hemorrhagic)
  (infantile) (membranous)(metastatic)
  (nonspecific) (pontine) (progressive) (simple)
  (spinal) (subacute) (sympathetic) (toxic)
  G03.9
  abacterial G03.0
  actinomycotic A42.81
  adenoviral A87.1
  arbovirus A87.8
  aseptic (acute) G03.0
  bacterial G00.9
    Escherichia coli (E. coli) G00.8
    Friedländer (bacillus) G00.8
    gram-negative G00.9
    H. influenzae G00.0
    Klebsiella G00.8
    pneumococcal G00.1
    specified organism NEC G00.8
    staphylococcal G00.3
    streptococcal (acute) G00.2
  benign recurrent (Mollaret) G03.2
  candidal B37.5
  caseous (tuberculous) A17.0
  cerebrospinal A39.0
  chronic NEC G03.1
  clear cerebrospinal fluid NEC G03.0
  coxsackievirus A87.0
  cryptococcal B45.1
  diplococcal (gram positive) A39.0
  echovirus A87.0
  enteroviral A87.0
  eosinophilic B83.2
  epidemic NEC A39.0
  Escherichia coli (E. coli) G00.8
  fibrinopurulent G00.9
    specified organism NEC G00.8
  Friedländer (bacillus) G00.8
  gonococcal A54.81
  gram-negative cocci G00.9
  gram-positive cocci G00.9
  H. influenzae G00.0
  Haemophilus (influenzae) G00.0

Meningitis (basal) (basic) (brain) (cerebral)
  (cervical) (congestive) (diffuse) (hemorrhagic)
  (infantile) (membranous)(metastatic)
  (nonspecific) (pontine) (progressive) (simple)
  (spinal) (subacute) (sympathetic) (toxic)
  G03.9 — *continued*
  in (due to)
    adenovirus A87.1
    African trypanosomiasis B56.9 *[G02]*
    anthrax A22.8
    bacterial disease NEC A48.8 *[G01]*
    Chagas' disease (chronic) B57.41
    chickenpox B01.0
    coccidioidomycosis B38.4
    Diplococcus pneumoniae G00.1
    enterovirus A87.0
    herpes (simplex) virus B00.3
      zoster B02.1
    infectious mononucleosis B27.92
    leptospirosis A27.81
    Listeria monocytogenes A32.11
    Lyme disease A69.21
    measles B05.1
    mumps (virus) B26.1
    neurosyphilis (late) A52.13
    parasitic disease NEC B89 *[G02]*
    poliovirus A80.9 *[G02]*
    preventive immunization, inoculation or
      vaccination G03.8
    rubella B06.02
    Salmonella infection A02.21
    specified cause NEC G03.8
    Streptococcal pneumoniae G00.1
    typhoid fever A01.01
    varicella B01.0
    viral disease NEC A87.8
    whooping cough A37.90
    zoster B02.1
  infectious G00.9
  influenzal (H. influenzae) G00.0
  Klebsiella G00.8
  leptospiral (aseptic) A27.81
  lymphocytic (acute) (benign) (serous) A87.2
  meningococcal A39.0
  Mima polymorpha G00.8
  Mollaret (benign recurrent) G03.2
  monilial B37.5
  mycotic NEC B49 *[G02]*
  Neisseria A39.0
  nonbacterial G03.0
  nonpyogenic NEC G03.0
  ossificans G96.19
  pneumococcal streptococcus pneumoniae
    G00.1
  poliovirus A80.9 *[G02]*
  postmeasles B05.1
  purulent G00.9
    specified organism NEC G00.8
  pyogenic G00.9
    specified organism NEC G00.8
  Salmonella (arizonae) (Cholerae-Suis)
    (enteritidis) (typhimurium) A02.21
  septic G00.9
    specified organism NEC G00.8
  serosa circumscripta NEC G03.0
  serous NEC G93.2
  specified organism NEC G00.8
  sporotrichosis B42.81
  staphylococcal G00.3
  sterile G03.0
  Streptococcal (acute) G00.2
    pneumoniae G00.1
  suppurative G00.9
    specified organism NEC G00.8
  syphilitic (late) (tertiary) A52.13
    acute A51.41
    congenital A50.41
    secondary A51.41
  Torula histolytica (cryptococcal) B45.1

Meningitis (basal) (basic) (brain) (cerebral) (cervical) (congestive) (diffuse) (hemorrhagic) (infantile) (membranous)(metastatic) (nonspecific) (pontine) (progressive) (simple) (spinal) (subacute) (sympathetic) (toxic) G03.9 — *continued*
  traumatic (complication of injury) T79.8
  tuberculous A17.0
  typhoid A01.01
  viral NEC A87.9
  Yersinia pestis A20.3
Meningocele (spinal) — *see also* Spina bifida
  with hydrocephalus — *see* Spina bifida, by site, with hydrocephalus
  acquired (traumatic) G96.19
  cerebral — *see* Encephalocele
Meningocerebritis — *see* Meningoencephalitis
Meningococcemia A39.4
  acute A39.2
  chronic A39.3
Meningococcus, meningococcal (*see also* condition) A39.9
  adrenalitis, hemorrhagic A39.1
  carrier (suspected) of Z22.31
  meningitis (cerebrospinal) A39.0
Meningoencephalitis (*see also* Encephalitis) G04.90
  acute NEC (*see also* Encephalitis, viral) A86
  bacterial NEC G04.2
  California A83.5
  diphasic A84.1
  eosinophilic B83.2
  epidemic A39.81
  herpesviral, herpetic B00.4
    due to herpesvirus 6 B10.01
    due to herpesvirus 7 B10.09
    specified NEC B10.09
  in (due to)
    blastomycosis NEC B40.81
    diseases classified elsewhere G05.3
    free-living amebae B60.2
    H. influenzae G00.0
    Hemophilus influenzae (H .influenzae) G00.0
    herpes B00.4
      due to herpesvirus 6 B10.01
      due to herpesvirus 7 B10.09
      specified NEC B10.09
    Lyme disease A69.22
    mercury — *see* subcategory T56.1
    mumps B26.2
    Naegleria (amebae) (organisms) (fowleri) B60.2
    Parastrongylus cantonensis B83.2
    toxoplasmosis (acquired) B58.2
      congenital P37.1
  infectious (acute) (viral) A86
  influenzal (H. influenzae) G00.0
  Listeria monocytogenes A32.12
  lymphocytic (serous) A87.2
  mumps B26.2
  parasitic NEC B89 *[G05.3]*
  pneumococcal G04.2
  primary amebic B60.2
  specific (syphilitic) A52.14
  specified organism NEC G04.81
  staphylococcal G04.2
  streptococcal G04.2
  syphilitic A52.14
  toxic NEC G92
    due to mercury — *see* subcategory T56.1
  tuberculous A17.82
  virus NEC A86
Meningoencephalocele — *see also* Encephalocele
  syphilitic A52.19
    congenital A50.49

Meningoencephalomyelitis — *see also* Meningoencephalitis
  acute NEC (viral) A86
    disseminated G04.00
      postimmunization or postvaccination G04.02
      postinfectious G04.01
  due to
    actinomycosis A42.82
    Torula B45.1
    Toxoplasma or toxoplasmosis (acquired) B58.2
      congenital P37.1
  postimmunization or postvaccination G04.02
Meningoencephalomyelopathy G96.9
Meningoencephalopathy G96.9
Meningomyelitis — *see also* Meningoencephalitis
  bacterial NEC G04.2
  blastomycotic NEC B40.81
  cryptococcal B45.1
  in diseases classified elsewhere G05.4
  meningococcal A39.81
  syphilitic A52.14
  tuberculous A17.82
Meningomyelocele — *see also* Spina bifida
  syphilitic A52.19
Meningomyeloneuritis — *see* Meningoencephalitis
Meningoradiculitis — *see* Meningitis
Meningovascular — *see* condition
Menkes' disease or syndrome E83.09
  meaning maple-syrup-urine disease E71.0
Menometrorrhagia N92.1
Menopause, menopausal (asymptomatic) (state) Z78.0
  arthritis (any site) NEC — *see* Arthritis, specified form NEC
  bleeding N92.4
  depression (single episode) F32.89
    agitated (single episode) F32.2
      recurrent episode F33.9
    psychotic (single episode) F32.89
      recurrent episode F33.9
    recurrent episode F33.8
  melancholia (single episode) F32.89
    recurrent episode F33.8
  paranoid state F22
  premature E28.319
    asymptomatic E28.319
      postirradiation E89.40
      postsurgical E89.40
    symptomatic E28.310
      postirradiation E89.41
      postsurgical E89.41
  psychosis NEC F28
  symptomatic N95.1
  toxic polyarthritis NEC — *see* Arthritis, specified form NEC
Menorrhagia (primary) N92.0
  climacteric N92.4
    menopausal N92.4
  menopausal N92.4
  postclimacteric N95.0
  postmenopausal N95.0
  preclimacteric or premenopausal N92.4
  pubertal (menses retained) N92.2
Menostaxis N92.0
Menses, retention N94.89
Menstrual — *see* Menstruation
Menstruation
  absent — *see* Amenorrhea
  anovulatory N97.0
  cycle, irregular N92.6
  delayed N91.0
  disorder N93.9
    psychogenic F45.8
  during pregnancy O20.8

Menstruation — *continued*
  excessive (with regular cycle) N92.0
    with irregular cycle N92.1
    at puberty N92.2
  frequent N92.0
  infrequent — *see* Oligomenorrhea
  irregular N92.6
    specified NEC N92.5
  latent N92.5
  membranous N92.5
  painful (*see also* Dysmenorrhea) N94.6
    primary N94.4
    psychogenic F45.8
    secondary N94.5
  passage of clots N92.0
  precocious E30.1
  protracted N92.5
  rare — *see* Oligomenorrhea
  retained N94.89
  retrograde N92.5
  scanty — *see* Oligomenorrhea
  suppression N94.89
  vicarious (nasal) N94.89
Mental — *see also* condition
  deficiency — *see* Disability, intellectual
  deterioration — *see* Psychosis
  disorder — *see* Disorder, mental
  exhaustion F48.8
  insufficiency (congenital) — *see* Disability, intellectual
  observation without need for further medical care Z03.89
  retardation — *see* Disability, intellectual
  subnormality — *see* Disability, intellectual
  upset — *see* Disorder, mental
Meralgia paresthetica G57.1-
Mercurial — *see* condition
Mercurialism — *see* subcategory T56.1
MERFF syndrome (myoclonic epilepsy associated with ragged-red fiber) E88.42
Merkel cell tumor — *see* Carcinoma, Merkel cell
Merocele — *see* Hernia, femoral
Meromelia
  lower limb — *see* Defect, reduction, lower limb
    intercalary
      femur — *see* Defect, reduction, lower limb, specified type NEC
        tibiofibular (complete) (incomplete) — *see* Defect, reduction, lower limb
  upper limb — *see* Defect, reduction, upper limb
    intercalary, humeral, radioulnar — *see* Agenesis, arm, with hand present
Merzbacher-Pelizaeus disease E75.29
Mesaortitis — *see* Aortitis
Mesarteritis — *see* Arteritis
Mesencephalitis — *see* Encephalitis
Mesenchymoma — *see also* Neoplasm, connective tissue, uncertain behavior
  benign — *see* Neoplasm, connective tissue, benign
  malignant — *see* Neoplasm, connective tissue, malignant
Mesenteritis
  retractile K65.4
  sclerosing K65.4
Mesentery, mesenteric — *see* condition
Mesio-occlusion M26.213
Mesiodens, mesiodentes K00.1
Mesocolon — *see* condition
Mesonephroma (malignant) — *see* Neoplasm, malignant, by site
  benign — *see* Neoplasm, benign, by site
Mesophlebitis — *see* Phlebitis
Mesostromal dysgenesia Q13.89

Mesothelioma (malignant) C45.9
  benign
    mesentery D19.1
    mesocolon D19.1
    omentum D19.1
    peritoneum D19.1
    pleura D19.0
    specified site NEC D19.7
    unspecified site D19.9
  biphasic C45.9
    benign
      mesentery D19.1
      mesocolon D19.1
      omentum D19.1
      peritoneum D19.1
      pleura D19.0
      specified site NEC D19.7
      unspecified site D19.9
  cystic D48.4
  epithelioid C45.9
    benign
      mesentery D19.1
      mesocolon D19.1
      omentum D19.1
      peritoneum D19.1
      pleura D19.0
      specified site NEC D19.7
      unspecified site D19.9
  fibrous C45.9
    benign
      mesentery D19.1
      mesocolon D19.1
      omentum D19.1
      peritoneum D19.1
      pleura D19.0
      specified site NEC D19.7
      unspecified site D19.9
  site classification
    liver C45.7
    lung C45.7
    mediastinum C45.7
    mesentery C45.1
    mesocolon C45.1
    omentum C45.1
    pericardium C45.2
    peritoneum C45.1
    pleura C45.0
      parietal C45.0
    retroperitoneum C45.7
    specified site NEC C45.7
    unspecified C45.9
Metabolic syndrome E88.81
Metagonimiasis B66.8
Metagonimus infestation (intestine) B66.8
Metal
  pigmentation L81.8
  polisher's disease J62.8
Metamorphopsia H53.15
Metaplasia
  apocrine (breast) — see Dysplasia, mammary,
    specified type NEC
  cervix (squamous) — see Dysplasia, cervix
  endometrium (squamous) (uterus) N85.8
  esophagus K22.7-
  kidney (pelvis) (squamous) N28.89
  myelogenous D73.1
  myeloid (agnogenic) (megakaryocytic) D73.1
  spleen D73.1
  squamous cell, bladder N32.89
Metastasis, metastatic
  abscess — see Abscess
  calcification E83.59
  cancer
    from specified site — see Neoplasm,
      malignant, by site
    to specified site — see Neoplasm,
      secondary, by site
  deposits (in) — see Neoplasm, secondary, by
    site

Metastasis, metastatic — continued
  disease (see also Neoplasm, secondary, by site)
    C79.9
  spread (to) — see Neoplasm, secondary, by
    site
Metastrongyliasis B83.8
Metatarsalgia M77.4-
  anterior G57.6-
  Morton's G57.6-
Metatarsus, metatarsal — see also condition
  adductus, congenital Q66.22
  valgus (abductus), congenital Q66.6
  varus (congenital) Q66.22
    primus Q66.21
Methadone use — see Use, opioid
Methemoglobinemia D74.9
  acquired (with sulfhemoglobinemia) D74.8
  congenital D74.0
  enzymatic (congenital) D74.0
  Hb M disease D74.0
  hereditary D74.0
  toxic D74.8
Methemoglobinuria — see Hemoglobinuria
Methioninemia E72.19
Methylmalonic acidemia E71.120
Metritis (catarrhal) (hemorrhagic) (septic)
  (suppurative) — see also Endometritis
  cervical — see Cervicitis
Metropathia hemorrhagica N93.8
Metroperitonitis — see Peritonitis, pelvic,
  female
Metrorrhagia N92.1
  climacteric N92.4
  menopausal N92.4
  postpartum NEC (atonic) (following delivery of
    placenta) O72.1
    delayed or secondary O72.2
  preclimacteric or premenopausal N92.4
  psychogenic F45.8
Metrorrhexis — see Rupture, uterus
Metrosalpingitis N70.91
Metrostaxis N93.8
Metrovaginitis — see Endometritis
**Meyer-Schwickerath and Weyers
  syndrome** Q87.0
Meynert's amentia (nonalcoholic) F04
  alcoholic F10.96
    with dependence F10.26
Mibelli's disease (porokeratosis) Q82.8
Mice, joint — see Loose, body, joint
  knee M23.4-
Micrencephalon, micrencephaly Q02
Microalbuminuria R80.9
Microaneurysm, retinal — see also Disorder,
  retina, microaneurysms
  diabetic — see E08-E13 with .31
Microangiopathy (peripheral) I73.9
  thrombotic M31.1
Microcalcifications, breast R92.0
**Microcephalus, microcephalic,
  microcephaly** Q02
  due to toxoplasmosis (congenital) P37.1
Microcheilia Q18.7
Microcolon (congenital) Q43.8
Microcornea (congenital) Q13.4
Microcytic — see condition
Microdeletions NEC Q93.88
Microdontia K00.2
Microdrepanocytosis D57.40
  with crisis (vasoocclusive pain) D57.419
    with
      acute chest syndrome D57.411
      splenic sequestration D57.412
Microembolism
  atherothrombotic — see Atheroembolism
  retinal — see Occlusion, artery, retina
Microencephalon Q02
Microfilaria streptocerca infestation —
  see Onchocerciasis

Microgastria (congenital) Q40.2
Microgenia M26.06
Microgenitalia, congenital
  female Q52.8
  male Q55.8
Microglioma — see Lymphoma, non-Hodgkin,
  specified NEC
Microglossia (congenital) Q38.3
Micrognathia, micrognathism (congenital)
  (mandibular) (maxillary) M26.09
Microgyria (congenital) Q04.3
Microinfarct of heart — see Insufficiency,
  coronary
Microlentia (congenital) Q12.8
Microlithiasis, alveolar, pulmonary
  J84.02
Micromastia N64.82
Micromyelia (congenital) Q06.8
Micropenis Q55.62
Microphakia (congenital) Q12.8
Microphthalmos, microphthalmia
  (congenital) Q11.2
  due to toxoplasmosis P37.1
Micropsia H53.15
Microscopic polyangiitis (polyarteritis)
  M31.7
Microsporidiosis B60.8
  intestinal A07.8
Microsporon furfur infestation B36.0
Microsporosis — see also Dermatophytosis
  nigra B36.1
Microstomia (congenital) Q18.5
Microtia (congenital) (external ear) Q17.2
Microtropia H50.40
Microvillus inclusion disease (MVD) (MVID)
  Q43.8
Micturition
  disorder NEC (see also Difficulty, micturition)
    R39.198
    psychogenic F45.8
  frequency R35.0
    psychogenic F45.8
  hesitancy R39.11
  incomplete emptying R39.14
  nocturnal R35.1
  painful R30.9
    dysuria R30.0
    psychogenic F45.8
    tenesmus R30.1
  poor stream R39.12
  position dependent R39.192
  split stream R39.13
  straining R39.16
  urgency R39.15
Mid plane — see condition
Middle
  ear — see condition
  lobe (right) syndrome J98.19
Miescher's elastoma L87.2
Mietens' syndrome Q87.2
Migraine (idiopathic) G43.909
  with aura (acute-onset) (prolonged) (typical)
    (without headache) G43.109
    with refractory migraine G43.119
      with status migrainosus G43.111
      without status migrainosus G43.919
    intractable G43.119
      with status migrainosus G43.111
      without status migrainosus G43.119
    not intractable G43.109
      with status migrainosus G43.101
      without status migrainosus G43.109

Migraine (idiopathic) G43.909 — *continued*
with aura (acute-onset) (prolonged) (typical)
(without headache) G43.109 —
continued
persistent G43.509
with cerebral infarction G43.609
with refractory migraine G43.619
with status migrainosus G43.611
without status migrainosus G43.619
intractable G43.619
with status migrainosus G43.611
without status migrainosus G43.619
not intractable G43.609
with status migrainosus G43.601
without status migrainosus G43.609
without refractory migraine G43.609
with status migrainosus G43.601
without status migrainosus G43.609
without cerebral infarction G43.509
with refractory migraine G43.519
with status migrainosus G43.511
without status migrainosus G43.519
intractable G43.519
with status migrainosus G43.511
without status migrainosus G43.519
not intractable G43.509
with status migrainosus G43.501
without status migrainosus G43.509
without refractory migraine G43.509
with status migrainosus G43.501
without status migrainosus G43.509
without mention of refractory migraine
G43.109
with status migrainosus G43.101
without status migrainosus G43.109
with refractory migraine G43.919
with status migrainosus G43.911
without status migrainosus G43.919
abdominal G43.D0 *(follows G43.7)*
with refractory migraine G43.D1 *(follows G43.7)*
intractable G43.D1 *(follows G43.7)*
not intractable G43.D0 *(follows G43.7)*
without refractory migraine G43.D0 *(follows G43.7)*
basilar — *see* Migraine, with aura
classical — *see* Migraine, with aura
common — *see* Migraine, without aura
complicated G43.109
equivalents — *see* Migraine, with aura
familiar — *see* Migraine, hemiplegic
hemiplegic G43.409
with refractory migraine G43.419
with status migrainosus G43.411
without status migrainosus G43.419
intractable G43.419
with status migrainosus G43.411
without status migrainosus G43.419
not intractable G43.409
with status migrainosus G43.401
without status migrainosus G43.409
without refractory migraine G43.409
with status migrainosus G43.401
without status migrainosus G43.409
intractable G43.919
with status migrainosus G43.911
without status migrainosus G43.919
menstrual G43.829
with refractory migraine G43.839
with status migrainosus G43.831
without status migrainosus G43.839
intractable G43.839
with status migrainosus G43.831
without status migrainosus G43.839
not intractable G43.829
with status migrainosus G43.821
without status migrainosus G43.829

Migraine (idiopathic) G43.909 — *continued*
menstrual G43.829 — *continued*
without refractory migraine G43.829
with status migrainosus G43.821
without status migrainosus G43.829
menstrually related — *see* Migraine, menstrual
not intractable G43.909
with status migrainosus G43.901
without status migrainosus G43.919
ophthalmoplegic G43.B0 *(follows G43.7)*
with refractory migraine G43.B1 *(follows G43.7)*
intractable G43.B1 *(follows G43.7)*
not intractable G43.B0 *(follows G43.7)*
without refractory migraine G43.B0 *(follows G43.7)*
persistent aura (with, without) cerebral
infarction — *see* Migraine, with aura,
persistent
preceded or accompanied by transient focal
neurological phenomena — *see* Migraine,
with aura
pre-menstrual — *see* Migraine, menstrual
pure menstrual — *see* Migraine, menstrual
retinal — *see* Migraine, with aura
specified NEC G43.809
intractable G43.819
with status migrainosus G43.811
without status migrainosus G43.819
not intractable G43.809
with status migrainosus G43.801
without status migrainosus G43.809
sporadic — *see* Migraine, hemiplegic
transformed — *see* Migraine, without aura,
chronic
triggered seizures — *see* Migraine, with aura
without aura G43.009
with refractory migraine G43.019
with status migrainosus G43.011
without status migrainosus G43.019
chronic G43.709
with refractory migraine G43.719
with status migrainosus G43.711
without status migrainosus G43.719
intractable
with status migrainosus G43.711
without status migrainosus G43.719
not intractable
with status migrainosus G43.701
without status migrainosus G43.709
without refractory migraine G43.709
with status migrainosus G43.701
without status migrainosus G43.709
intractable
with status migrainosus G43.011
without status migrainosus G43.019
not intractable
with status migrainosus G43.001
without status migrainosus G43.009
without mention of refractory migraine
G43.009
with status migrainosus G43.001
without status migrainosus G43.009
without refractory migraine G43.909
with status migrainosus G43.901
without status migrainosus G43.909
Migrant, social Z59.0
Migration, anxiety concerning Z60.3
Migratory, migrating — *see also* condition
person Z59.0
testis Q55.29
Mikity-Wilson disease or syndrome P27.0
Mikulicz' disease or syndrome K11.8

Miliaria L74.3
alba L74.1
apocrine L75.2
crystallina L74.1
profunda L74.2
rubra L74.0
tropicalis L74.2
Miliary — *see* condition
Milium L72.0
colloid L57.8
Milk
crust L21.0
excessive secretion O92.6
poisoning — *see* Poisoning, food, noxious
retention O92.79
sickness — *see* Poisoning, food, noxious
spots I31.0
Milk-alkali disease or syndrome E83.52
Milk-leg (deep vessels) (nonpuerperal) — *see*
Embolism, vein, lower extremity
complicating pregnancy O22.3-
puerperal, postpartum, childbirth O87.1
Milkman's disease or syndrome M83.8
Milky urine — *see* Chyluria
Millar's asthma J38.5
**Millard-Gubler(-Foville) paralysis or
syndrome** G46.3
Miller Fisher syndrome G61.0
Mills' disease — *see* Hemiplegia
Millstone maker's pneumoconiosis J62.8
Milroy's disease (chronic hereditary edema)
Q82.0
Minamata disease T56.1-
Miners' asthma or lung J60
Minkowski-Chauffard syndrome — *see*
Spherocytosis
Minor — *see* condition
Minor's disease (hematomyelia) G95.19
Minot's disease (hemorrhagic disease),
newborn P53
**Minot-von Willebrand-Jurgens disease
or syndrome** (angiohemophilia) D68.0
Minus (and plus) hand (intrinsic) — *see*
Deformity, limb, specified type NEC,
forearm
Miosis (pupil) H57.03
Mirizzi's syndrome (hepatic duct stenosis)
K83.1
Mirror writing F81.0
Misadventure (of) (prophylactic) (therapeutic)
(*see also* Complications) T88.9
administration of insulin (by accident) — *see*
subcategory T38.3
infusion — *see* Complications, infusion
local applications (of fomentations, plasters,
etc.) T88.9
burn or scald — *see* Burn
specified NEC T88.8
medical care (early) (late) T88.9
adverse effect of drugs or chemicals — *see*
Table of Drugs and Chemicals
specified NEC T88.8
surgical procedure (early) (late) — *see*
Complications, surgical procedure
transfusion — *see* Complications, transfusion
vaccination or other immunological procedure
— *see* Complications, vaccination
Miscarriage O03.9
Misdirection, aqueous H40.83-
Misperception, sleep state F51.02
Misplaced, misplacement
ear Q17.4
kidney (acquired) N28.89
congenital Q63.2
organ or site, congenital NEC — *see*
Malposition, congenital
Missed
abortion O02.1
delivery O36.4

Missing — *see also* Absence
  string of intrauterine contraceptive device
    T83.32
Misuse of drugs F19.99
Mitchell's disease (erythromelalgia) I73.81
Mite(s) (infestation) B88.9
  diarrhea B88.0
  grain (itch) B88.0
  hair follicle (itch) B88.0
  in sputum B88.0
Mitral — *see* condition
Mittelschmerz N94.0
Mixed — *see* condition
MNGIE (mitochondrial neurogastrointestinal
  encephalopathy) syndrome E88.49
MNN (multifocal motor neuropathy) G61.82
Mobile, mobility
  cecum Q43.3
  excessive — *see* Hypermobility
  gallbladder, congenital Q44.1
  kidney N28.89
  organ or site, congenital NEC — *see*
    Malposition, congenital
Mobitz heart block (atrioventricular) I44.1
Moebius, Möbius
  disease (ophthalmoplegic migraine) — *see*
    Migraine, ophthalmoplegic
  syndrome Q87.0
    congenital oculofacial paralysis (with other
      anomalies) Q87.0
    ophthalmoplegic migraine — *see* Migraine,
      ophthalmoplegic
Moeller's glossitis K14.0
Mohr's syndrome (Types I and II) Q87.0
Mola destruens D39.2
Molar pregnancy O02.0
Molarization of premolars K00.2
Molding, head (during birth) — *omit code*
Mole (pigmented) — *see also* Nevus
  blood O02.0
  Breus' O02.0
  cancerous — *see* Melanoma
  carneous O02.0
  destructive D39.2
  fleshy O02.0
  hydatid, hydatidiform (benign) (complicating
    pregnancy) (delivered) (undelivered)
    O01.9
    classical O01.0
    complete O01.0
    incomplete O01.1
    invasive D39.2
    malignant D39.2
    partial O01.1
  intrauterine O02.0
  invasive (hydatidiform) D39.2
  malignant
    meaning
      malignant hydatidiform mole D39.2
      melanoma — *see* Melanoma
  nonhydatidiform O02.0
  nonpigmented — *see* Nevus
  pregnancy NEC O02.0
  skin — *see* Nevus
  tubal O00.10
    with intrauterine pregnancy O00.11
  vesicular — *see* Mole, hydatidiform
Molimen, molimina (menstrual) N94.3
Molluscum contagiosum (epitheliale) B08.1
**Mönckeberg's arteriosclerosis, disease,
  or sclerosis** — *see* Arteriosclerosis,
  extremities
Mondini's malformation (cochlea) Q16.5
Mondor's disease I80.8
Monge's disease T70.29
Monilethrix (congenital) Q84.1
Moniliasis (*see also* Candidiasis) B37.9
  neonatal P37.5

Monitoring (encounter for)
  therapeutic drug level Z51.81
Monkey malaria B53.1
Monkeypox B04
Monoarthritis M13.10
  ankle M13.17-
  elbow M13.12-
  foot joint M13.17-
  hand joint M13.14-
  hip M13.15-
  knee M13.16-
  shoulder M13.11-
  wrist M13.13-
Monoblastic — *see* condition
Monochromat(ism), monochromatopsia
  (acquired) (congenital) H53.51
Monocytic — *see* condition
Monocytopenia D72.818
Monocytosis (symptomatic) D72.821
Monomania — *see* Psychosis
Mononeuritis G58.9
  cranial nerve — *see* Disorder, nerve, cranial
  femoral nerve G57.2-
  lateral
    cutaneous nerve of thigh G57.1-
    popliteal nerve G57.3-
  lower limb G57.9-
    specified nerve NEC G57.8-
  medial popliteal nerve G57.4-
  median nerve G56.1-
  multiplex G58.7
  plantar nerve G57.6-
  posterior tibial nerve G57.5-
  radial nerve G56.3-
  sciatic nerve G57.0-
  specified NEC G58.8
  tibial nerve G57.4-
  ulnar nerve G56.2-
  upper limb G56.9-
    specified nerve NEC G56.8-
  vestibular — *see* subcategory H93.3
Mononeuropathy G58.9
  carpal tunnel syndrome — *see* Syndrome,
    carpal tunnel
  diabetic NEC — *see* E08-E13 with .41
  femoral nerve — *see* Lesion, nerve, femoral
  ilioinguinal nerve G57.8-
  in diseases classified elsewhere — *see*
    category G59
  intercostal G58.0
  lower limb G57.9-
    causalgia — *see* Causalgia, lower limb
    femoral nerve — *see* Lesion, nerve, femoral
    meralgia paresthetica G57.1-
    plantar nerve — *see* Lesion, nerve, plantar
    popliteal nerve — *see* Lesion, nerve,
      popliteal
    sciatic nerve — *see* Lesion, nerve, sciatic
    specified NEC G57.8-
    tarsal tunnel syndrome — *see* Syndrome,
      tarsal tunnel
  median nerve — *see* Lesion, nerve, median
  multiplex G58.7
  obturator nerve G57.8-
  popliteal nerve — *see* Lesion, nerve, popliteal
  radial nerve — *see* Lesion, nerve, radial
  saphenous nerve G57.8-
  specified NEC G58.8
  tarsal tunnel syndrome — *see* Syndrome, tarsal
    tunnel
  tuberculous A17.83
  ulnar nerve — *see* Lesion, nerve, ulnar
  upper limb G56.9-
    carpal tunnel syndrome — *see* Syndrome,
      carpal tunnel
    causalgia — *see* Causalgia
    median nerve — *see* Lesion, nerve, median
    radial nerve — *see* Lesion, nerve, radial
    specified site NEC G56.8-

Mononeuropathy G58.9 — *continued*
  upper limb G56.9- — *continued*
    ulnar nerve — *see* Lesion, nerve, ulnar
Mononucleosis, infectious B27.90
  with
    complication NEC B27.99
    meningitis B27.92
    polyneuropathy B27.91
  cytomegaloviral B27.10
    with
      complication NEC B27.19
      meningitis B27.12
      polyneuropathy B27.11
  Epstein-Barr (virus) B27.00
    with
      complication NEC B27.09
      meningitis B27.02
      polyneuropathy B27.01
  gammaherpesviral B27.00
    with
      complication NEC B27.09
      meningitis B27.02
      polyneuropathy B27.01
  specified NEC B27.80
    with
      complication NEC B27.89
      meningitis B27.82
      polyneuropathy B27.81
Monoplegia G83.3-
  congenital (cerebral) G80.8
    spastic G80.1
  embolic (current episode) I63.4-
  following
    cerebrovascular disease
      cerebral infarction
        lower limb I69.34-
        upper limb I69.33-
      intracerebral hemorrhage
        lower limb I69.14-
        upper limb I69.13-
      lower limb I69.94-
      nontraumatic intracranial hemorrhage NEC
        lower limb I69.24-
        upper limb I69.23-
      specified disease NEC
        lower limb I69.84-
        upper limb I69.83-
      stroke NOS
        lower limb I69.34-
        upper limb I69.33-
      subarachnoid hemorrhage
        lower limb I69.04-
        upper limb I69.03-
      upper limb I69.93-
  hysterical (transient) F44.4
  lower limb G83.1-
  psychogenic (conversion reaction) F44.4
  thrombotic (current episode) I63.3-
  transient R29.818
  upper limb G83.2-
Monorchism, monorchidism Q55.0
Monosomy (*see also* Deletion, chromosome)
  Q93.9
  specified NEC Q93.89
  whole chromosome
    meiotic nondisjunction Q93.0
    mitotic nondisjunction Q93.1
    mosaicism Q93.1
  X Q96.9
Monster, monstrosity (single) Q89.7
  acephalic Q00.0
  twin Q89.4
Monteggia's fracture(-dislocation)
  S52.27-
Moore's syndrome — *see* Epilepsy, specified
  NEC
Mooren's ulcer (cornea) — *see* Ulcer, cornea,
  Mooren's
Mooser's bodies A75.2

Mooser-Neill reaction A75.2
Morbidity not stated or unknown R69
Morbilli — *see* Measles
Morbus — *see also* Disease
  angelicus, anglorum E55.0
  Beigel B36.2
  caducus — *see* Epilepsy
  celiacus K90.0
  comitialis — *see* Epilepsy
  cordis (*see also* Disease, heart) I51.9
    valvulorum — *see* Endocarditis
  coxae senilis M16.9
    tuberculous A18.02
  hemorrhagicus neonatorum P53
  maculosus neonatorum P54.5
Morel-Kraepelin disease — *see*
  Schizophrenia
Morel-Moore syndrome M85.2
Morel(-Stewart)(-Morgagni) syndrome
  M85.2
Morgagni's
  cyst, organ, hydatid, or appendage
    female Q50.5
    male (epididymal) Q55.4
      testicular Q55.29
  syndrome M85.2
Morgagni-Stewart-Morel syndrome
  M85.2
Morgagni-Stokes-Adams syndrome I45.9
Morgagni-Turner(-Albright) syndrome
  Q96.9
Moria F07.0
Moron (I.Q. 50-69) F70
Morphea L94.0
Morphinism (without remission) F11.20
  with remission F11.21
Morphinomania (without remission) F11.20
  with remission F11.21
Morquio(-Ullrich)(-Brailsford) disease or
  syndrome — *see* Mucopolysaccharidosis
Mortification (dry) (moist) — *see* Gangrene
Morton's metatarsalgia (neuralgia)
  (neuroma) (syndrome) G57.6-
Morvan's disease or syndrome G60.8
Mosaicism, mosaic (autosomal)
  (chromosomal)
  45,X/46,XX Q96.3
  45,X/other cell lines NEC with abnormal sex
    chromosome Q96.4
  sex chromosome
    female Q97.8
    lines with various numbers of X
      chromosomes Q97.2
    male Q98.7
  XY Q96.3
Moschowitz' disease M31.1
Mother yaw A66.0
Motion sickness (from travel, any vehicle)
  (from roundabouts or swings) T75.3
Mottled, mottling, teeth (enamel) (endemic)
  (nonendemic) K00.3
Mounier-Kuhn syndrome Q32.4
  with bronchiectasis J47.9
    exacerbation (acute) J47.1
    lower respiratory infection J47.0
  acquired J98.09
    with bronchiectasis J47.9
      with
        exacerbation (acute) J47.1
        lower respiratory infection J47.0
Mountain
  sickness T70.29
    with polycythemia , acquired (acute) D75.1
  tick fever A93.2
Mouse, joint — *see* Loose, body, joint
  knee M23.4-
Mouth — *see* condition

Movable
  coccyx — *see* subcategory M53.2
  kidney N28.89
    congenital Q63.8
  spleen D73.89
Movements, dystonic R25.8
Moyamoya disease I67.5
MRSA (methacillin resistant Staphylococcus
  aureus)
  infection A49.02
    as the cause of diseases classified elsewhere
      B95.62
  sepsis A41.02
MSSA (methacillin susceptible Staphylococcus
  aureus)
  infection A49.01
    as the cause of diseases classified elsewhere
      B95.61
  sepsis A41.01
Mucha-Habermann disease L41.0
Mucinosis (cutaneous) (focal) (papular)
  (reticular erythematous) (skin) L98.5
  oral K13.79
Mucocele
  appendix K38.8
  buccal cavity K13.79
  gallbladder K82.1
  lacrimal sac, chronic H04.43-
  nasal sinus J34.1
  nose J34.1
  salivary gland (any) K11.6
  sinus (accessory) (nasal) J34.1
  turbinate (bone) (middle) (nasal) J34.1
  uterus N85.8
Mucolipidosis
  I E77.1
  II, III E77.0
  IV E75.11
Mucopolysaccharidosis E76.3
  beta-gluduronidase deficiency E76.29
  cardiopathy E76.3 *[I52]*
  Hunter's syndrome E76.1
  Hurler's syndrome E76.01
  Hurler-Scheie syndrome E76.02
  Maroteaux-Lamy syndrome E76.29
  Morquio syndrome E76.219
    A E76.210
    B E76.211
    classic E76.210
  Sanfilippo syndrome E76.22
  Scheie's syndrome E76.03
  specified NEC E76.29
  type
    I
      Hurler's syndrome E76.01
      Hurler-Scheie syndrome E76.02
      Scheie's syndrome E76.03
    II E76.1
    III E76.22
    IV E76.219
    IVA E76.210
    IVB E76.211
    VI E76.29
    VII E76.29
Mucormycosis B46.5
  cutaneous B46.3
  disseminated B46.4
  gastrointestinal B46.2
  generalized B46.4
  pulmonary B46.0
  rhinocerebral B46.1
  skin B46.3
  subcutaneous B46.3

Mucositis (ulcerative) K12.30
  due to drugs NEC K12.32
  gastrointestinal K92.81
  mouth (oral) (oropharyngeal) K12.30
    due to antineoplastic therapy K12.31
    due to drugs NEC K12.32
    due to radiation K12.33
    specified NEC K12.39
    viral K12.39
  nasal J34.81
  oral cavity — *see* Mucositis, mouth
  oral soft tissues — *see* Mucositis, mouth
  vagina and vulva N76.81
Mucositis necroticans agranulocytica —
  see Agranulocytosis
Mucous — *see also* condition
  patches (syphilitic) A51.39
    congenital A50.07
Mucoviscidosis E84.9
  with meconium obstruction E84.11
Mucus
  asphyxia or suffocation — *see* Asphyxia,
    mucus
  in stool R19.5
  plug — *see* Asphyxia, mucus
Muguet B37.0
Mulberry molars (congenital syphilis) A50.52
Müllerian mixed tumor
  specified site — *see* Neoplasm, malignant, by
    site
  unspecified site C54.9
Multicystic kidney (development) Q61.4
Multiparity (grand) Z64.1
  affecting management of pregnancy, labor
    and delivery (supervision only) O09.4-
  requiring contraceptive management — *see*
    Contraception
Multipartita placenta O43.19-
Multiple, multiplex — *see also* condition
  digits (congenital) Q69.9
  endocrine neoplasia — *see* Neoplasia,
    endocrine, multiple (MEN)
  personality F44.81
Mumps B26.9
  arthritis B26.85
  complication NEC B26.89
  encephalitis B26.2
  hepatitis B26.81
  meningitis (aseptic) B26.1
  meningoencephalitis B26.2
  myocarditis B26.82
  oophoritis B26.89
  orchitis B26.0
  pancreatitis B26.3
  polyneuropathy B26.84
Mumu (*see also* Infestation, filarial) B74.9 *[N51]*
Münchhausen's syndrome — *see* Disorder,
  factitious
Münchmeyer's syndrome — *see* Myositis,
  ossificans, progressiva
Mural — *see* condition
Murmur (cardiac) (heart) (organic) R01.1
  abdominal R19.15
  aortic (valve) — *see* Endocarditis, aortic
  benign R01.0
  diastolic — *see* Endocarditis
  Flint I35.1
  functional R01.0
  Graham Steell I37.1
  innocent R01.0
  mitral (valve) — *see* Insufficiency, mitral
  nonorganic R01.0
  presystolic, mitral — *see* Insufficiency, mitral
  pulmonic (valve) I37.8
  systolic R01.1
  tricuspid (valve) I07.9
  valvular — *see* Endocarditis
Murri's disease (intermittent hemoglobinuria)
  D59.6

Muscle, muscular — *see also* condition
  carnitine (palmityltransferase) deficiency
    E71.314
Musculoneuralgia — *see* Neuralgia
Mushroom-workers' (pickers') disease or
  lung J67.5
Mushrooming hip — *see* Derangement, joint,
  specified NEC, hip
Mutation(s)
  factor V Leiden D68.51
  prothrombin gene D68.52
  surfactant, of lung J84.83
Mutism — *see also* Aphasia
  deaf (acquired) (congenital) NEC H91.3
  elective (adjustment reaction) (childhood)
    F94.0
  hysterical F44.4
  selective (childhood) F94.0
MVD (microvillus inclusion disease) Q43.8
MVID (microvillus inclusion disease) Q43.8
Myalgia M79.1
  epidemic (cervical) B33.0
  traumatic NEC T14.8
Myasthenia G70.9
  congenital G70.2
  cordis — *see* Failure, heart
  developmental G70.2
  gravis G70.00
    with exacerbation (acute) G70.01
    in crisis G70.01
    neonatal, transient P94.0
    pseudoparalytica G70.00
      with exacerbation (acute) G70.01
      in crisis G70.01
  stomach, psychogenic F45.8
  syndrome
    in
      diabetes mellitus — *see* E08-E13 with .44
      neoplastic disease (*see also* Neoplasm)
        D49.9 *[G73.3]*
      pernicious anemia D51.0 *[G73.3]*
      thyrotoxicosis E05.90 *[G73.3]*
        with thyroid storm E05.91 *[G73.3]*
Myasthenic M62.81
Mycelium infection B49
Mycetismus — *see* Poisoning, food, noxious,
  mushroom
Mycetoma B47.9
  actinomycotic B47.1
  bone (mycotic) B47.9 *[M90.80]*
  eumycotic B47.0
  foot B47.9
    actinomycotic B47.1
    mycotic B47.0
  madurae NEC B47.9
    mycotic B47.0
  maduromycotic B47.0
  mycotic B47.0
  nocardial B47.1
Mycobacteriosis — *see* Mycobacterium
Mycobacterium, mycobacterial (infection)
  A31.9
  anonymous A31.9
  atypical A31.9
    cutaneous A31.1
    pulmonary A31.0
      tuberculous — *see* Tuberculosis, pulmonary
    specified site NEC A31.8
  avium (intracellulare complex) A31.0
  balnei A31.1
  Battey A31.0
  chelonei A31.8
  cutaneous A31.1
  extrapulmonary systemic A31.8
  fortuitum A31.8
  intracellulare (Battey bacillus) A31.0
  kakaferifu A31.8
  kansasii (yellow bacillus) A31.0
  kasongo A31.8

Mycobacterium, mycobacterial (infection)
  A31.9 — *continued*
  leprae (*see also* Leprosy) A30.9
  luciflavum A31.1
  marinum (M. balnei) A31.1
  nonspecific — *see* Mycobacterium, atypical
  pulmonary (atypical) A31.0
    tuberculous — *see* Tuberculosis, pulmonary
  scrofulaceum A31.8
  simiae A31.8
  systemic, extrapulmonary A31.8
  szulgai A31.8
  terrae A31.8
  triviale A31.8
  tuberculosis (human, bovine) —
    seeTuberculosis
  ulcerans A31.1
  xenopi A31.8
**Mycoplasma (M.) pneumoniae, as cause
  of disease classified elsewhere** B96.0
Mycosis, mycotic B49
  cutaneous NEC B36.9
  ear B36.9
    in
      aspergillosis B44.89
      candidiasis B37.84
      moniliasis B37.84
  fungoides (extranodal) (solid organ) C84.0-
  mouth B37.0
  nails B35.1
  opportunistic B48.8
  skin NEC B36.9
  specified NEC B48.8
  stomatitis B37.0
  vagina, vaginitis (candidal) B37.3
Mydriasis (pupil) H57.04
Myelatelia Q06.1
Myelinolysis, pontine, central G37.2
Myelitis (acute) (ascending) (childhood)
  (chronic) (descending) (diffuse)
  (disseminated) (idiopathic) (pressure)
  (progressive) (spinal cord) (subacute) (*see
  also* Encephalitis) G04.91
  herpes simplex B00.82
  herpes zoster B02.24
  in diseases classified elsewhere G05.4
  necrotizing, subacute G37.4
  optic neuritis in G36.0
  postchickenpox B01.12
  postherpetic B02.24
  postimmunization G04.02
  postinfectious NEC G04.89
  postvaccinal G04.02
  specified NEC G04.89
  syphilitic (transverse) A52.14
  toxic G92
  transverse (in demyelinating diseases of central
    nervous system) G37.3
  tuberculous A17.82
  varicella B01.12
**Myelo-osteo-musculodysplasia
  hereditaria** Q79.8
Myeloblastic — *see* condition
Myeloblastoma
  granular cell — *see also* Neoplasm, connective
    tissue
    malignant — *see* Neoplasm, connective
      tissue, malignant
    tongue D10.1
Myelocele — *see* Spina bifida
Myelocystocele — *see* Spina bifida
Myelocytic — *see* condition
Myelodysplasia D46.9
  specified NEC D46.Z
  spinal cord (congenital) Q06.1

Myelodysplastic syndrome D46.9
  with
    5q deletion D46.C
    isolated del(5q) chromosomal abnormality
      D46.C
  specified NEC D46.Z
Myeloencephalitis — *see* Encephalitis
Myelofibrosis D75.81
  with myeloid metaplasia D47.4
  acute C94.4-
  idiopathic (chronic) D47.4
  primary D47.1
  secondary D75.81
    in myeloproliferative disease D47.4
Myelogenous — *see* condition
Myeloid — *see* condition
Myelokathexis D70.9
Myeloleukodystrophy E75.29
Myelolipoma — *see* Lipoma
Myeloma (multiple) C90.0-
  monostatic C90.3
    plasma cell C90.0-
  plasma cell C90.0-
  solitary (*see also* Plasmacytoma, solitary)
    C90.3-
Myelomalacia G95.89
Myelomatosis C90.0-
Myelomeningitis — *see* Meningoencephalitis
Myelomeningocele (spinal cord) — *see* Spina
  bifida
Myelopathic
  anemia D64.89
  muscle atrophy — *see* Atrophy, muscle, spinal
  pain syndrome G89.0
Myelopathy (spinal cord) G95.9
  drug-induced G95.89
  in (due to)
    degeneration or displacement, intervertebral
      disc NEC — *see* Disorder, disc, with,
      myelopathy
    infection — *see* Encephalitis
    intervertebral disc disorder — *see also*
      Disorder, disc, with, myelopathy
    mercury — *see* subcategory T56.1
    neoplastic disease (*see also* Neoplasm)
      D49.9 *[G99.2]*
    pernicious anemia D51.0 *[G99.2]*
    spondylosis — *see* Spondylosis, with
      myelopathy NEC
  necrotic (subacute) (vascular) G95.19
  radiation-induced G95.89
  spondylogenic NEC — *see* Spondylosis, with
    myelopathy NEC
  toxic G95.89
  transverse, acute G37.3
  vascular G95.19
  vitamin B12 E53.8 *[G32.0]*
Myelophthisis D61.82
Myeloradiculitis G04.91
Myeloradiculodysplasia (spinal) Q06.1
Myelosarcoma C92.3-
Myelosclerosis D75.89
  with myeloid metaplasia D47.4
  disseminated, of nervous system G35
  megakaryocytic D47.4
    with myeloid metaplasia D47.4
Myelosis
  acute C92.0-
  aleukemic C92.9-
  chronic D47.1
  erythremic (acute) C94.0-
  megakaryocytic C94.2-
  nonleukemic D72.828
  subacute C92.9-

Myiasis (cavernous) B87.9
  aural B87.4
  creeping B87.0
  cutaneous B87.0
  dermal B87.0
  ear (external) (middle) B87.4
  eye B87.2
  genitourinary B87.81
  intestinal B87.82
  laryngeal B87.3
  nasopharyngeal B87.3
  ocular B87.2
  orbit B87.2
  skin B87.0
  specified site NEC B87.89
  traumatic B87.1
  wound B87.1
Myoadenoma, prostate — *see* Hyperplasia, prostate
Myoblastoma
  granular cell — *see also* Neoplasm, connective tissue, benign
    malignant — *see* Neoplasm, connective tissue, malignant
  tongue D10.1
Myocardial — *see* condition
Myocardiopathy (congestive) (constrictive) (familial) (hypertrophic nonobstructive) (idiopathic) (infiltrative) (obstructive) (primary) (restrictive) (sporadic) (*see also* Cardiomyopathy) I42.9
  alcoholic I42.6
  cobalt-beer I42.6
  glycogen storage E74.02 *[I43]*
  hypertrophic obstructive I42.1
  in (due to)
    beriberi E51.12
    cardiac glycogenosis E74.02 *[I43]*
    Friedreich's ataxia G11.1 *[I43]*
    myotonia atrophica G71.11 *[I43]*
    progressive muscular dystrophy G71.0 *[I43]*
  obscure (African) I42.8
  secondary I42.9
  thyrotoxic E05.90 *[I43]*
    with storm E05.91 *[I43]*
  toxic NEC I42.7
Myocarditis (with arteriosclerosis) (chronic) (fibroid) (interstitial) (old) (progressive) (senile) I51.4
  with
    rheumatic fever (conditions in I00) I09.0
      active — *see* Myocarditis, acute, rheumatic
      inactive or quiescent (with chorea) I09.0
  active I40.9
    rheumatic I01.2
      with chorea (acute) (rheumatic) (Sydenham's) I02.0
  acute or subacute (interstitial) I40.9
    due to
      streptococcus (beta-hemolytic) I01.2
    idiopathic I40.1
    rheumatic I01.2
      with chorea (acute) (rheumatic) (Sydenham's) I02.0
    specified NEC I40.8
  aseptic of newborn B33.22
  bacterial (acute) I40.0
  Coxsackie (virus) B33.22
  diphtheritic A36.81
  eosinophilic I40.1
  epidemic of newborn (Coxsackie) B33.22
  Fiedler's (acute) (isolated) I40.1
  giant cell (acute) (subacute) I40.1
  gonococcal A54.83
  granulomatous (idiopathic) (isolated) (nonspecific) I40.1
  hypertensive — *see* Hypertension, heart
  idiopathic (granulomatous) I40.1

Myocarditis (with arteriosclerosis) (chronic) (fibroid) (interstitial) (old) (progressive) (senile) I51.4 — *continued*
  in (due to)
    diphtheria A36.81
    epidemic louse-borne typhus A75.0 *[I41]*
    Lyme disease A69.29
    sarcoidosis D86.85
    scarlet fever A38.1
    toxoplasmosis (acquired) B58.81
    typhoid A01.02
    typhus NEC A75.9 *[I41]*
  infective I40.0
  influenzal — *see* Influenza, with, myocarditis
  isolated (acute) I40.1
  meningococcal A39.52
  mumps B26.82
  nonrheumatic, active I40.9
  parenchymatous I40.9
  pneumococcal I40.0
  rheumatic (chronic) (inactive) (with chorea) I09.0
    active or acute I01.2
      with chorea (acute) (rheumatic) (Sydenham's) I02.0
  rheumatoid — *see* Rheumatoid, carditis
  septic I40.0
  staphylococcal I40.0
  suppurative I40.0
  syphilitic (chronic) A52.06
  toxic I40.8
    rheumatic — *see* Myocarditis, acute, rheumatic
  tuberculous A18.84
  typhoid A01.02
  valvular — *see* Endocarditis
  virus, viral I40.0
    of newborn (Coxsackie) B33.22
Myocardium, myocardial — *see* condition
Myocardosis — *see* Cardiomyopathy
Myoclonus, myoclonic, myoclonia (familial) (essential) (multifocal) (simplex) G25.3
  drug-induced G25.3
  epilepsy (*see also* Epilepsy, generalized, specified NEC) G40.4-
    familial (progressive) G25.3
  epileptica G40.409
    with status epilepticus G40.401
  facial G51.3
  familial progressive G25.3
  Friedreich's G25.3
  jerks G25.3
  massive G25.3
  palatal G25.3
  pharyngeal G25.3
Myocytolysis I51.5
Myodiastasis — *see* Diastasis, muscle
Myoendocarditis — *see* Endocarditis
Myoepithelioma — *see* Neoplasm, benign, by site
Myofasciitis (acute) — *see* Myositis
Myofibroma — *see also* Neoplasm, connective tissue, benign
  uterus (cervix) (corpus) — *see* Leiomyoma
Myofibromatosis D48.1
  infantile Q89.8
Myofibrosis M62.89
  heart — *see* Myocarditis
  scapulohumeral — *see* Lesion, shoulder, specified NEC
Myofibrositis M79.7
  scapulohumeral — *see* Lesion, shoulder, specified NEC
Myoglobulinuria, myoglobinuria (primary) R82.1
Myokymia, facial G51.4
Myolipoma — *see* Lipoma

Myoma — *see also* Neoplasm, connective tissue, benign
  malignant — *see* Neoplasm, connective tissue, malignant
  prostate D29.1
  uterus (cervix) (corpus) — *see* Leiomyoma
Myomalacia M62.89
Myometritis — *see* Endometritis
Myometrium — *see* condition
Myonecrosis, clostridial A48.0
Myopathy G72.9
  acute
    necrotizing G72.81
    quadriplegic G72.81
  alcoholic G72.1
  benign congenital G71.2
  central core G71.2
  centronuclear G71.2
  congenital (benign) G71.2
  critical illness G72.81
  distal G71.0
  drug-induced G72.0
  endocrine NEC E34.9 *[G73.7]*
  extraocular muscles H05.82-
  facioscapulohumeral G71.0
  hereditary G71.9
    specified NEC G71.8
  immune NEC G72.49
  in (due to)
    Addison's disease E27.1 *[G73.7]*
    alcohol G72.1
    amyloidosis E85.0 *[G73.7]*
    cretinism E00.9 *[G73.7]*
    Cushing's syndrome E24.9 *[G73.7]*
    drugs G72.0
    endocrine disease NEC E34.9 *[G73.7]*
    giant cell arteritis M31.6 *[G73.7]*
    glycogen storage disease E74.00 *[G73.7]*
    hyperadrenocorticism E24.9 *[G73.7]*
    hyperparathyroidism NEC E21.3 *[G73.7]*
    hypoparathyroidism E20.9 *[G73.7]*
    hypopituitarism E23.0 *[G73.7]*
    hypothyroidism E03.9 *[G73.7]*
    infectious disease NEC B99 *[G73.7]*
    lipid storage disease E75.6 *[G73.7]*
    metabolic disease NEC E88.9 *[G73.7]*
    myxedema E03.9 *[G73.7]*
    parasitic disease NEC B89 *[G73.7]*
    polyarteritis nodosa M30.0 *[G73.7]*
    rheumatoid arthritis — *see* Rheumatoid, myopathy
    sarcoidosis D86.87
    scleroderma M34.82
    sicca syndrome M35.03
    Sjögren's syndrome M35.03
    systemic lupus erythematosus M32.19
    thyrotoxicosis (hyperthyroidism) E05.90 *[G73.7]*
      with thyroid storm E05.91 *[G73.7]*
    toxic agent NEC G72.2
  inflammatory NEC G72.49
  intensive care (ICU) G72.81
  limb-girdle G71.0
  mitochondrial NEC G71.3
  myotubular G71.2
  mytonic, proximal (PROMM) G71.11
  nemaline G71.2
  ocular G71.0
  oculopharyngeal G71.0
  of critical illness G72.81
  primary G71.9
    specified NEC G71.8
  progressive NEC G72.89
  proximal myotonic (PROMM) G71.11
  rod G71.2
  scapulohumeral G71.0
  specified NEC G72.89
  toxic G72.2

DISEASE INDEX

Myopericarditis — *see also* Pericarditis
  chronic rheumatic I09.2
Myopia (axial) (congenital) H52.1-
  degenerative (malignant) H44.2-
  malignant H44.2-
  pernicious H44.2-
  progressive high (degenerative) H44.2-
Myosarcoma — *see* Neoplasm, connective
  tissue, malignant
Myosis (pupil) H57.03
  stromal (endolymphatic) D39.0
Myositis M60.9
  clostridial A48.0
  due to posture — *see* Myositis, specified type
    NEC
  epidemic B33.0
  fibrosa or fibrous (chronic), Volkmann's T79.6
  foreign body granuloma — *see* Granuloma,
    foreign body
  in (due to)
    bilharziasis B65.9 *[M63.8-]*
    cysticercosis B69.81
    leprosy A30.9 *[M63.8-]*
    mycosis B49 *[M63.8-]*
    sarcoidosis D86.87
    schistosomiasis B65.9 *[M63.8-]*
    syphilis
      late A52.78
      secondary A51.49
    toxoplasmosis (acquired) B58.82
    trichinellosis B75 *[M63.8-]*
    tuberculosis A18.09
  inclusion body [IBM] G72.41
  infective M60.009
    arm M60.002
      left M60.001
      right M60.000
    leg M60.005
      left M60.004
      right M60.003
    lower limb M60.005
      ankle M60.07-
      foot M60.07-
      lower leg M60.06-
      thigh M60.05-
      toe M60.07-
    multiple sites M60.09
    specified site NEC M60.08
    upper limb M60.002
      finger M60.04-
      forearm M60.03-
      hand M60.04-
      shoulder region M60.01-
      upper arm M60.02-
  interstitial M60.10
    ankle M60.17-
    foot M60.17-
    forearm M60.13-
    hand M60.14-
    lower leg M60.16-
    multiple sites M60.19
    shoulder region M60.11-
    specified site NEC M60.18
    thigh M60.15-
    upper arm M60.12-
  mycotic B49 *[M63.8-]*
  orbital, chronic H05.12-

Myositis M60.9 — *continued*
  ossificans or ossifying (circumscripta) — *see
    also* Ossification, muscle, specified NEC
    in (due to)
      burns M61.30
        ankle M61.37-
        foot M61.37-
        forearm M61.33-
        hand M61.34-
        lower leg M61.36-
        multiple sites M61.39
        pelvic region M61.35-
        shoulder region M61.31-
        specified site NEC M61.38
        thigh M61.35-
        upper arm M61.32-
      quadriplegia or paraplegia M61.20
        ankle M61.27-
        foot M61.27-
        forearm M61.23-
        hand M61.24-
        lower leg M61.26-
        multiple sites M61.29
        pelvic region M61.25-
        shoulder region M61.21-
        specified site NEC M61.28
        thigh M61.25-
        upper arm M61.22-
  progressiva M61.10
    ankle M61.17-
    finger M61.14-
    foot M61.17-
    forearm M61.13-
    hand M61.14-
    lower leg M61.16-
    multiple sites M61.19
    pelvic region M61.15-
    shoulder region M61.11-
    specified site NEC M61.18
    thigh M61.15-
    toe M61.17-
    upper arm M61.12-
  traumatica M61.00
    ankle M61.07-
    foot M61.07-
    forearm M61.03-
    hand M61.04-
    lower leg M61.06-
    multiple sites M61.09
    pelvic region M61.05-
    shoulder region M61.01-
    specified site NEC M61.08
    thigh M61.05-
    upper arm M61.02-
  purulent — *see* Myositis, infective
  specified type NEC M60.80
    ankle M60.87-
    foot M60.87-
    forearm M60.83-
    hand M60.84-
    lower leg M60.86-
    multiple sites M60.89
    pelvic region M60.85-
    shoulder region M60.81-
    specified site NEC M60.88
    thigh M60.85-
    upper arm M60.82-
  suppurative — *see* Myositis, infective
  traumatic (old) — *see* Myositis, specified type
    NEC

Myospasia impulsiva F95.2
Myotonia (acquisita) (intermittens) M62.89
  atrophica G71.11
  chondrodystrophic G71.13
  congenita (acetazolamide responsive)
    (dominant) (recessive) G71.12
  drug-induced G71.14
  dystrophica G71.11
  fluctuans G71.19
  levior G71.12
  permanens G71.19
  symptomatic G71.19
Myotonic pupil — *see* Anomaly, pupil,
  function, tonic pupil
Myriapodiasis B88.2
Myringitis H73.2-
  with otitis media — *see* Otitis, media
  acute H73.00-
    bullous H73.01-
    specified NEC H73.09-
  bullous — *see* Myringitis, acute, bullous
  chronic H73.1-
Mysophobia F40.228
Mytilotoxism — *see* Poisoning, fish
Myxadenitis labialis K13.0
Myxedema (adult) (idiocy) (infantile) (juvenile)
  (*see also* Hypothyroidism) E03.9
  circumscribed E05.90
    with storm E05.91
  coma E03.5
  congenital E00.1
  cutis L98.5
  localized (pretibial) E05.90
    with storm E05.91
  papular L98.5
Myxochondrosarcoma — *see* Neoplasm,
  cartilage, malignant
Myxofibroma — *see* Neoplasm, connective
  tissue, benign
  odontogenic — *see* Cyst, calcifying
    odontogenic
Myxofibrosarcoma — *see* Neoplasm,
  connective tissue, malignant
Myxolipoma D17.9
Myxoliposarcoma — *see* Neoplasm,
  connective tissue, malignant
Myxoma — *see also* Neoplasm, connective
  tissue, benign
  nerve sheath — *see* Neoplasm, nerve, benign
  odontogenic — *see* Cyst, calcifying
    odontogenic
Myxosarcoma — *see* Neoplasm, connective
  tissue, malignant

N

Naegeli's
  disease Q82.8
  leukemia, monocytic C93.1-
Naegleriasis (with meningoencephalitis)
  B60.2
Naffziger's syndrome G54.0
Naga sore — see Ulcer, skin
Nägele's pelvis M95.5
  with disproportion (fetopelvic) O33.0
    causing obstructed labor O65.0
Nail — see also condition
  biting F98.8
  patella syndrome Q87.2
Nanism, nanosomia — see Dwarfism
Nanophyetiasis B66.8
Nanukayami A27.89
Napkin rash L22
Narcolepsy G47.419
  with cataplexy G47.411
  in conditions classified elsewhere G47.429
    with cataplexy G47.421
Narcosis R06.89
Narcotism — see Dependence
NARP (neuropathy, ataxia and retinitis
  pigmentosa) syndrome E88.49
Narrow
  anterior chamber angle H40.03-
  gingival width (of periodontal soft tissue)
    K05.5
  pelvis — see Contraction, pelvis
Narrowing — see also Stenosis
  artery I77.1
    auditory, internal I65.8
    basilar — see Occlusion, artery, basilar
    carotid — see Occlusion, artery, carotid
    cerebellar — see Occlusion, artery,
      cerebellar
    cerebral — see Occlusion artery, cerebral
    choroidal — see Occlusion, artery, cerebral,
      specified NEC
    communicating posterior — see Occlusion,
      artery, cerebral, specified NEC
    coronary — see also Disease, heart,
      ischemic, atherosclerotic
      congenital Q24.5
        syphilitic A50.54 [I52]
      due to syphilis NEC A52.06
    hypophyseal — see Occlusion, artery,
      cerebral, specified NEC
    pontine — see Occlusion, artery, cerebral,
      specified NEC
    precerebral — see Occlusion, artery,
      precerebral
    vertebral — see Occlusion, artery, vertebral
  auditory canal (external) — see Stenosis,
    external ear canal
  eustachian tube — see Obstruction, eustachian
    tube
  eyelid — see Disorder, eyelid function
  larynx J38.6
  mesenteric artery (see also Ischemia, intestine,
    acute) K55.059
  palate M26.89
  palpebral fissure — see Disorder, eyelid
    function
  ureter N13.5
    with infection N13.6
  urethra — see Stricture, urethra
Narrowness, abnormal, eyelid Q10.3
Nasal — see condition
Nasolachrymal, nasolacrimal — see
  condition
Nasopharyngeal — see also condition
  pituitary gland Q89.2
  torticollis M43.6

Nasopharyngitis (acute) (infective)
  (streptococcal) (subacute) J00
  chronic (suppurative) (ulcerative) J31.1
Nasopharynx, nasopharyngeal — see
  condition
Natal tooth, teeth K00.6
Nausea (without vomiting) R11.0
  with vomiting R11.2
  gravidarum — see Hyperemesis, gravidarum
  marina T75.3
  navalis T75.3
Navel — see condition
Neapolitan fever — see Brucellosis
Near drowning T75.1
Near-syncope R55
Nearsightedness — see Myopia
Nebula, cornea — see Opacity, cornea
Necator americanus infestation B76.1
Necatoriasis B76.1
Neck — see condition
Necrobiosis R68.89
  lipoidica NEC L92.1
  with diabetes — see E08-E13 with .620
Necrolysis, toxic epidermal L51.2
  due to drug
    correct substance properly administered —
      see Table of Drugs and Chemicals, by
      drug, adverse effect
    overdose or wrong substance given or taken
      — see Table of Drugs and Chemicals, by
      drug, poisoning
Necrophilia F65.89
Necrosis, necrotic (ischemic) — see also
  Gangrene
  adrenal (capsule) (gland) E27.49
  amputation stump (surgical) (late) T87.50
    arm T87.5-
    leg T87.5-
  antrum J32.0
  aorta (hyaline) — see also Aneurysm, aorta
    cystic medial — see Dissection, aorta
  artery I77.5
  bladder (aseptic) (sphincter) N32.89
  bone (see also Osteonecrosis) M87.9
    aseptic or avascular — see Osteonecrosis
      idiopathic M87.00
    ethmoid J32.2
    jaw M27.2
    tuberculous — see Tuberculosis, bone
  brain I67.89
  breast (aseptic) (fat) (segmental) N64.1
  bronchus J98.09
  central nervous system NEC I67.89
  cerebellar I67.89
  cerebral I67.89
  colon (see also Infarct, intestine) K55.049
  cornea H18.89-
  cortical (acute) (renal) N17.1
  cystic medial (aorta) — see Dissection, aorta
  dental pulp K04.1
  esophagus K22.8
  ethmoid (bone) J32.2
  eyelid — see Disorder, eyelid, degenerative
  fat, fatty (generalized) — see also Disorder, soft
    tissue, specified type NEC
    abdominal wall K65.4
    breast (aseptic) (segmental) N64.1
    localized — see Degeneration, by site, fatty
    mesentery K65.4
    omentum K65.4
    pancreas K86.89
    peritoneum K65.4
    skin (subcutaneous), newborn P83.0
    subcutaneous, due to birth injury P15.6
  gallbladder — see Cholecystitis, acute
  heart — see Infarct, myocardium
  hip, aseptic or avascular — see Osteonecrosis,
    by type, femur

Necrosis, necrotic (ischemic) — see also
  Gangrene — continued
  intestine (acute) (hemorrhagic) (massive) (see
    also Infarct, intestine) K55.069
  jaw M27.2
  kidney (bilateral) N28.0
    acute N17.9
    cortical (acute) (bilateral) N17.1
      with ectopic or molar pregnancy O08.4
    medullary (bilateral) (in acute renal failure)
      (papillary) N17.2
    papillary (bilateral) (in acute renal failure)
      N17.2
    tubular N17.0
      with ectopic or molar pregnancy O08.4
      complicating
        abortion — see Abortion, by type,
          complicated by, tubular necrosis
        ectopic or molar pregnancy O08.4
        pregnancy — see Pregnancy,
          complicated by, diseases of,
          specified type or system NEC
      following ectopic or molar pregnancy
        O08.4
      traumatic T79.5
  larynx J38.7
  liver (with hepatic failure) (cell) — see Failure,
    hepatic
    hemorrhagic, central K76.2
  lung J85.0
  lymphatic gland — see Lymphadenitis, acute
  mammary gland (fat) (segmental) N64.1
  mastoid (chronic) — see Mastoiditis, chronic
  medullary (acute) (renal) N17.2
  mesentery (see also Infarct, intestine) K55.069
    fat K65.4
  mitral valve — see Insufficiency, mitral
  myocardium, myocardial — see Infarct,
    myocardium
  nose J34.0
  omentum (with mesenteric infarction) (see also
    Infarct, intestine) K55.069
    fat K65.4
  orbit, orbital — see Osteomyelitis, orbit
  ossicles, ear — see Abnormal, ear ossicles
  ovary N70.92
  pancreas (aseptic) (duct) (fat) K86.89
    acute (infective) — see Pancreatitis, acute
    infective — see Pancreatitis, acute
  papillary (acute) (renal) N17.2
  perineum N90.89
  peritoneum (with mesenteric infarction) (see also
    Infarct, intestine) K55.069
    fat K65.4
  pharynx J02.9
    in granulocytopenia — see Neutropenia
      Vincent's A69.1
  phosphorus — see subcategory T54.2
  pituitary (gland) E23.0
    postpartum O99.285
    Sheehan O99.285
  pressure — see Ulcer, pressure, by site
  pulmonary J85.0
  pulp (dental) K04.1
  radiation — see Necrosis, by site
  radium — see Necrosis, by site
  renal — see Necrosis, kidney
  sclera H15.89
  scrotum N50.89
  skin or subcutaneous tissue NEC I96
  spine, spinal (column) — see also
    Osteonecrosis, by type, vertebra
    cord G95.19
  spleen D73.5
  stomach K31.89
  stomatitis (ulcerative) A69.0
  subcutaneous fat, newborn P83.8
  subendocardial (acute) I21.4
    chronic I25.89

Necrosis, necrotic (ischemic) — *see also*
    Gangrene — *continued*
  suprarenal (capsule) (gland) E27.49
  testis N50.89
  thymus (gland) E32.8
  tonsil J35.8
  trachea J39.8
  tuberculous NEC — *see* Tuberculosis
  tubular (acute) (anoxic) (renal) (toxic) N17.0
    postprocedural N99.0
  vagina N89.8
  vertebra — *see also* Osteonecrosis, by type,
    vertebra
    tuberculous A18.01
  vulva N90.89
  X-ray — *see* Necrosis, by site
Necrospermia — *see* Infertility, male
Need (for)
  care provider because (of)
    assistance with personal care Z74.1
    continuous supervision required Z74.3
    impaired mobility Z74.09
    no other household member able to render
      care Z74.2
    specified reason NEC Z74.8
  immunization — *see* Vaccination
  vaccination — *see* Vaccination
Neglect
  adult
    confirmed T74.01
    history of Z91.412
    suspected T76.01
  child (childhood)
    confirmed T74.02
    history of Z62.812
    suspected T76.02
  emotional, in childhood Z62.898
  hemispatial R41.4
  left-sided R41.4
  sensory R41.4
  visuospatial R41.4
Neisserian infection NEC — *see* Gonococcus
Nelaton's syndrome G60.8
Nelson's syndrome E24.1
Nematodiasis (intestinal) B82.0
  Ancylostoma B76.0
Neonatal — *see also* Newborn
  acne L70.4
  bradycardia P29.12
  screening, abnormal findings on P09
  tachycardia P29.11
  tooth, teeth K00.6
Neonatorum — *see* condition
Neoplasia
  endocrine, multiple (MEN) E31.20
    type I E31.21
    type IIA E31.22
    type IIB E31.23
  intraepithelial (histologically confirmed)
    anal (AIN) (histologically confirmed) K62.82
      grade I K62.82
      grade II K62.82
      severe D01.3
    cervical glandular (histologically confirmed)
      D06.9
    cervix (uteri) (CIN) (histologically confirmed)
      N87.9
      glandular D06.9
      grade I N87.0
      grade II N87.1
      grade III (severe dysplasia) (*see also*
        Carcinoma, cervix uteri, in situ) D06.9
    prostate (histologically confirmed) (PIN)
      N42.31
      grade I N42.31
      grade II N42.31
      grade III (severe dysplasia) D07.5

Neoplasia — *continued*
  intraepithelial (histologically confirmed) —
    continued
    vagina (histologically confirmed) (VAIN)
      N89.3
      grade I N89.0
      grade II N89.1
      grade III (severe dysplasia) D07.2
    vulva (histologically confirmed) (VIN) N90.3
      grade I N90.0
      grade II N90.1
      grade III (severe dysplasia) D07.1
Neoplasm, neoplastic — *see also* Table of
  Neoplasms
  lipomatous, benign — *see* Lipoma

Neoplasm Table	Malignant Primary	Malignant Secondary	Ca in situ	Benign	Uncertain Behavior	Unspecified Behavior

NEOPLASM TABLE

ICD-10-CM Table of Neoplasms

The list below gives the code numbers for neoplasms by anatomical site. For each site there are six possible code numbers according to whether the neoplasm in question is malignant, benign, in situ, of uncertain behavior, or of unspecified nature. The description of the neoplasm will often indicate which of the six columns is appropriate; e.g., malignant melanoma of skin, benign fibroadenoma of breast, carcinoma in situ of cervix uteri.

Where such descriptors are not present, the remainder of the Index should be consulted where guidance is given to the appropriate column for each morphological (histological) variety listed; e.g., Mesonephroma — *see* Neoplasm, malignant; Embryoma — *see also* Neoplasm, uncertain behavior; Disease, Bowen's — *see* Neoplasm, skin, in situ. However, the guidance in the Index can be overridden if one of the descriptors mentioned above is present; e.g., malignant adenoma of colon is coded to C18.9 and not to D12.6 as the adjective "malignant" overrides the Index entry "Adenoma — *see also* Neoplasm, benign."

Codes listed with a dash -, following the code have a required additional character for laterality. The tabular list must be reviewed for the complete code.

Neoplasm Table	Malignant Primary	Malignant Secondary	Ca in situ	Benign	Uncertain Behavior	Unspecified Behavior
Neoplasm, neoplastic	C80.1	C79.9	D09.9	D36.9	D48.9	D49.9
abdomen, abdominal	C76.2	C79.8-	D09.8	D36.7	D48.7	D49.89
cavity	C76.2	C79.8-	D09.8	D36.7	D48.7	D49.89
organ	C76.2	C79.8-	D09.8	D36.7	D48.7	D49.89
viscera	C76.2	C79.8-	D09.8	D36.7	D48.7	D49.89
wall — *see also* Neoplasm,						
abdomen, wall, skin	C44.509	C79.2-	D04.5	D23.5	D48.5	D49.2
connective tissue	C49.4	C79.8-	—	D21.4	D48.1	D49.2
skin	C44.509	—	—	—	—	—
basal cell carcinoma	C44.519	—	—	—	—	—
specified type NEC	C44.599	—	—	—	—	—
squamous cell						
carcinoma	C44.529	—	—	—	—	—
abdominopelvic	C76.8	C79.8-	—	D36.7	D48.7	D49.89
accessory sinus — *see*						
Neoplasm, sinus						
acoustic nerve	C72.4-	C79.49	—	D33.3	D43.3	D49.7
adenoid (pharynx) (tissue)	C11.1	C79.89	D00.08	D10.6	D37.05	D49.0
adipose tissue — *see also*						
Neoplasm, connective						
tissue	C49.4	C79.89	—	D21.9	D48.1	D49.2
adnexa (uterine)	C57.4	C79.89	D07.39	D28.7	D39.8	D49.59
adrenal	C74.9-	C79.7-	D09.3	D35.0-	D44.1-	D49.7
capsule	C74.9-	C79.7-	D09.3	D35.0-	D44.1-	D49.7
cortex	C74.0-	C79.7-	D09.3	D35.0-	D44.1-	D49.7
gland	C74.9-	C79.7-	D09.3	D35.0-	D44.1-	D49.7
medulla	C74.1-	C79.7-	D09.3	D35.0-	D44.1-	D49.7
ala nasi (external) — *see also*						
Neoplasm, skin, nose	C44.301	C79.2	D04.39	D23.39	D48.5	D49.2
alimentary canal or tract NEC	C26.9	C78.80	D01.9	D13.9	D37.9	D49.0
alveolar	C03.9	C79.89	D00.03	D10.39	D37.09	D49.0
mucosa	C03.9	C79.89	D00.03	D10.39	D37.09	D49.0
lower	C03.1	C79.89	D00.03	D10.39	D37.09	D49.0
upper	C03.0	C79.89	D00.03	D10.39	D37.09	D49.0

Neoplasm Table	Malignant Primary	Malignant Secondary	Ca in situ	Benign	Uncertain Behavior	Unspecified Behavior
Neoplasm, neoplastic - *continued*						
alveolar - *continued*	C03.9	C79.89	D00.03	D10.39	D37.09	D49.0
ridge or process	C41.1	C79.51	—	D16.5-	D48.0	D49.2
carcinoma	C03.9	C79.8-	—	—	—	—
lower	C03.1	C79.8-	—	—	—	—
upper	C03.0	C79.8-	—	—	—	—
lower	C41.1	C79.51	—	D16.5-	D48.0	D49.2
mucosa	C03.9	C79.89	D00.03	D10.39	D37.09	D49.0
lower	C03.1	C79.89	D00.03	D10.39	D37.09	D49.0
upper	C03.0	C79.89	D00.03	D10.39	D37.09	D49.0
upper	C41.0	C79.51	—	D16.4-	D48.0	D49.2
sulcus	C06.1	C79.89	D00.02	D10.39	D37.09	D49.0
alveolus	C03.9	C79.89	D00.03	D10.39	D37.09	D49.0
lower	C03.1	C79.89	D00.03	D10.39	D37.09	D49.0
upper	C03.0	C79.89	D00.03	D10.39	D37.09	D49.0
ampulla of Vater	C24.1	C78.89	D01.5	D13.5	D37.6	D49.0
ankle NEC	C76.5-	C79.89	D04.7-	D36.7	D48.7	D49.89
anorectum, anorectal						
(junction)	C21.8	C78.5	D01.3	D12.9	D37.8	D49.0
antecubital fossa or space	C76.4-	C79.89	D04.6-	D36.7	D48.7	D49.89
antrum (Highmore)						
(maxillary)	C31.0	C78.39	D02.3	D14.0	D38.5	D49.1
pyloric	C16.3	C78.89	D00.2	D13.1	D37.1	D49.0
tympanicum	C30.1	C78.39	D02.3	D14.0	D38.5	D49.1
anus, anal	C21.0	C78.5	D01.3	D12.9	D37.8	D49.0
canal	C21.1	C78.5	D01.3	D12.9	D37.8	D49.0
cloacogenic zone	C21.2	C78.5	D01.3	D12.9	D37.8	D49.0
margin — *see also*						
Neoplasm, anus, skin	C44.500	C79.2	D04.5	D23.5	D48.5	D49.2
overlapping lesion with						
rectosigmoid junction						
or rectum	C21.8	—	—	—	—	—
skin	C44.500	C79.2	D04.5	D23.5	D48.5	D49.2
basal cell carcinoma	C44.510	—	—	—	—	—
specified type NEC	C44.590	—	—	—	—	—
squamous cell						
carcinoma	C44.520	—	—	—	—	—
sphincter	C21.1	C78.5	D01.3	D12.9	D37.8	D49.0
aorta (thoracic)	C49.3	C79.89	—	D21.3	D48.1	D49.2
abdominal	C49.4	C79.89	—	D21.4	D48.1	D49.2
aortic body	C75.5	C79.89	—	D35.6	D44.7	D49.7
aponeurosis	C49.9	C79.89	—	D21.9	D48.1	D49.2
palmar	C49.1-	C79.89	—	D21.1-	D48.1	D49.2
plantar	C49.2-	C79.89	—	D21.2-	D48.1	D49.2
appendix	C18.1	C78.5	D01.0	D12.1	D37.3	D49.0
arachnoid	C70.9	C79.49	—	D32.9	D42.9	D49.7
cerebral	C70.0	C79.32	—	D32.0	D42.0	D49.7
spinal	C70.1	C79.49	—	D32.1	D42.1	D49.7
areola	C50.0-	C79.81	D05.-	D24.-	D48.6-	D49.3
arm NEC	C76.4-	C79.89	D04.6-	D36.7	D48.7	D49.89
artery — *see* Neoplasm,						
connective tissue						
aryepiglottic fold	C13.1	C79.89	D00.08	D10.7	D37.05	D49.0
hypopharyngeal aspect	C13.1	C79.89	D00.08	D10.7	D37.05	D49.0
laryngeal aspect	C32.1	C78.39	D02.0	D14.1	D38.0	D49.1
marginal zone	C13.1	C79.89	D00.08	D10.7	D37.05	D49.0
arytenoid (cartilage)	C32.3	C78.39	D02.0	D14.1	D38.0	D49.1
fold — *see* Neoplasm,						
aryepiglottic						
associated with transplanted						
organ	C80.2	—	—	D16.6	D48.0	D49.2
atlas	C41.2	C79.51	—	D16.6	D48.0	D49.2
atrium, cardiac	C38.0	C79.89	—	D15.1	D48.7	D49.89

NEOPLASM TABLE

Neoplasm Table	Malignant Primary	Malignant Secondary	Ca In situ	Benign	Uncertain Behavior	Unspecified Behavior
Neoplasm, neoplastic - *continued*						
auditory						
canal (external) (skin)	C44.20-	C79.2	D04.2-	D23.2-	D48.5	D49.2
internal	C30.1	C78.39	D02.3	D14.0	D38.5	D49.1
nerve	C72.4-	C79.49	—	D33.3	D43.3	D49.7
tube	C30.1	C78.39	D02.3	D14.0	D38.5	D49.1
opening	C11.2	C79.89	D00.08	D10.6	D37.05	D49.0
auricle, ear — *see also*						
Neoplasm, skin, ear	C44.20-	C79.2	D04.2-	D23.2-	D48.5	D49.2
auricular canal (external) —						
see also Neoplasm, skin,						
ear	C44.20-	C79.2	D04.2-	D23.2-	D48.5	D49.2
internal	C30.1	C78.39	D02.3	D14.0	D38.5	D49.2
autonomic nerve or nervous						
system NEC (*see*						
Neoplasm, nerve,						
peripheral)						
axilla, axillary	C76.1	C79.89	D09.8	D36.7	D48.7	D49.89
fold — *see also*						
Neoplasm, skin, trunk	C44.509	C79.2	D04.5	D23.5	D48.5	D49.2
back NEC	C76.8	C79.89	D04.5	D36.7	D48.7	D49.89
Bartholin's gland	C51.0	C79.82	D07.1	D28.0	D39.8	D49.59
basal ganglia	C71.0	C79.31	—	D33.0	D43.0	D49.6
basis pedunculi	C71.7	C79.31	—	D33.1	D43.1	D49.6
bile or biliary (tract)	C24.9	C78.89	D01.5	D13.5	D37.6	D49.0
canaliculi (biliferi)						
(intrahepatic)	C22.1	C78.7	D01.5	D13.4	D37.6	D49.0
canals, interlobular	C22.1	C78.89	D01.5	D13.4	D37.6	D49.0
duct or passage (common)						
(cystic) (extrahepatic)	C24.0	C78.89	D01.5	D13.5	D37.6	D49.0
interlobular	C22.1	C78.89	D01.5	D13.4	D37.6	D49.0
intrahepatic	C22.1	C78.7	D01.5	D13.4	D37.6	D49.0
and extrahepatic	C24.8	C78.89	D01.5	D13.5	D37.6	D49.0
bladder (urinary)	C67.9	C79.11	D09.0	D30.3	D41.4	D49.4
dome	C67.1	C79.11	D09.0	D30.3	D41.4	D49.4
neck	C67.5	C79.11	D09.0	D30.3	D41.4	D49.4
orifice	C67.9	C79.11	D09.0	D30.3	D41.4	D49.4
ureteric	C67.6	C79.11	D09.0	D30.3	D41.4	D49.4
urethral	C67.5	C79.11	D09.0	D30.3	D41.4	D49.4
overlapping lesion	C67.8	—	—	—	—	—
sphincter	C67.8	C79.11	D09.0	D30.3	D41.4	D49.4
trigone	C67.0	C79.11	D09.0	D30.3	D41.4	D49.4
urachus	C67.7	C79.11	D09.0	D30.3	D41.4	D49.4
wall	C67.9	C79.11	D09.0	D30.3	D41.4	D49.4
anterior	C67.3	C79.11	D09.0	D30.3	D41.4	D49.4
lateral	C67.2	C79.11	D09.0	D30.3	D41.4	D49.4
posterior	C67.4	C79.11	D09.0	D30.3	D41.4	D49.4
blood vessel — *see* Neoplasm,						
connective tissue						
bone (periosteum)	C41.9	C79.51	—	D16.9-	D48.0	D49.2
acetabulum	C41.4	C79.51	—	D16.8-	D48.0	D49.2
ankle	C40.3-	C79.51	—	D16.3-	—	—
arm NEC	C40.0-	C79.51	—	D16.0-	—	—
astragalus	C40.3-	C79.51	—	D16.3-	—	—
atlas	C41.2	C79.51	—	D16.6-	D48.0	D49.2
axis	C41.2	C79.51	—	D16.6-	D48.0	D49.2
back NEC	C41.2	C79.51	—	D16.6-	D48.0	D49.2
calcaneus	C40.3-	C79.51	—	D16.3-	—	—
calvarium	C41.0	C79.51	—	D16.4-	D48.0	D49.2
carpus (any)	C40.1-	C79.51	—	D16.1-	—	—
cartilage NEC	C41.9	C79.51	—	D16.9-	D48.0	D49.2
clavicle	C41.3	C79.51	—	D16.7-	D48.0	D49.2
clivus	C41.0	C79.51	—	D16.4-	D48.0	D49.2
coccygeal vertebra	C41.4	C79.51	—	D16.8-	D48.0	D49.2
Neoplasm, neoplastic - *continued*						
bone (periosteum) - *continued*	C41.9	C79.51	—	D16.9-	D48.0	D49.2
coccyx	C41.4	C79.51	—	D16.8-	D48.0	D49.2
costal cartilage	C41.3	C79.51	—	D16.7-	D48.0	D49.2
costovertebral joint	C41.3	C79.51	—	D16.7-	D48.0	D49.2
cranial	C41.0	C79.51	—	D16.4-	D48.0	D49.2
cuboid	C40.3-	C79.51	—	D16.3-		
cuneiform	C41.9	C79.51	—	D16.9-	D48.0	D49.2
elbow	C40.0-	C79.51	—	D16.0-		
ethmoid (labyrinth)	C41.0	C79.51	—	D16.4-	D48.0	D49.2
face	C41.0	C79.51	—	D16.4-	D48.0	D49.2
femur (any part)	C40.2-	C79.51	—	D16.2-		
fibula (any part)	C40.2-	C79.51	—	D16.2-		
finger (any)	C40.1-	C79.51	—	D16.1-		
foot	C40.3-	C79.51	—	D16.3-		
forearm	C40.0-	C79.51	—	D16.0-		
frontal	C41.0	C79.51	—	D16.4-	D48.0	D49.2
hand	C40.1-	C79.51	—	D16.1-		
heel	C40.3-	C79.51	—	D16.3-		
hip	C41.4	C79.51	—	D16.8-	D48.0	D49.2
humerus (any part)	C40.0-	C79.51	—	D16.0-		
hyoid	C41.0	C79.51	—	D16.4-	D48.0	D49.2
ilium	C41.4	C79.51	—	D16.8-	D48.0	D49.2
innominate	C41.4	C79.51	—	D16.8-	D48.0	D49.2
intervertebral cartilage or						
disc	C41.2	C79.51	—	D16.6-	D48.0	D49.2
ischium	C41.4	C79.51	—	D16.8-	D48.0	D49.2
jaw (lower)	C41.1	C79.51	—	D16.5-	D48.0	D49.2
knee	C40.2-	C79.51	—	D16.2-		
leg NEC	C40.2-	C79.51	—	D16.2-		
limb NEC	C40.9-	C79.51	—	D16.9-		
lower (long bones)	C40.2-	C79.51	—	D16.2-		
short bones	C40.3-	C79.51	—	D16.3-		
upper (long bones)	C40.0-	C79.51	—	D16.0-		
short bones	C40.1-	C79.51	—	D16.1-		
malar	C41.0	C79.51	—	D16.4-	D48.0	D49.2
mandible	C41.1	C79.51	—	D16.5-	D48.0	D49.2
marrow NEC (any bone)	C96.9	C79.52	—	—	D47.9	D49.89
mastoid	C41.0	C79.51	—	D16.4-	D48.0	D49.2
maxilla, maxillary						
(superior)	C41.0	C79.51	—	D16.4-	D48.0	D49.2
inferior	C41.1	C79.51	—	D16.5-	D48.0	D49.2
metacarpus (any)	C40.1-	C79.51	—	D16.1-		
metatarsus (any)	C40.3-	C79.51	—	D16.3-		
overlapping sites	C40.8-	—	—	—		
navicular						
ankle	C40.3-	C79.51	—			
hand	C40.1-	C79.51	—			
nose, nasal	C41.0	C79.51	—	D16.4-	D48.0	D49.2
occipital	C41.0	C79.51	—	D16.4-	D48.0	D49.2
orbit	C41.0	C79.51	—	D16.4-	D48.0	D49.2
parietal	C41.0	C79.51	—	D16.4-	D48.0	D49.2
patella	C40.2-	C79.51	—	D16.2-		
pelvic	C41.4	C79.51	—	D16.8	D48.0	D49.2
phalanges						
foot	C40.3-	C79.51	—	D16.3-		
hand	C40.1-	C79.51	—			
pubic	C41.4	C79.51	—	D16.8	D48.0	D49.2
radius (any part)	C40.0-	C79.51	—	D16.0-		
rib	C41.3	C79.51	—	D16.7	D48.0	D49.2
sacral vertebra	C41.4	C79.51	—	D16.8	D48.0	D49.2
sacrum	C41.4	C79.51	—	D16.8	D48.0	D49.2

Neoplasm, neoplastic - *continued*

Neoplasm Table	Malignant Primary	Malignant Secondary	Ca In situ	Benign	Uncertain Behavior	Unspecified Behavior
bone (periosteum) - *continued*	C41.9	C79.51	—	D16.9-	D48.0	D49.2
scaphoid	—					
of ankle	C40.3-	C79.51	—	—	—	—
of hand	C40.1-	C79.51		—	—	—
scapula (any part)	C40.0-	C79.51	—	D16.0-	—	—
sella turcica	C41.0	C79.51	—	D16.4-	D48.0	D49.2
shoulder	C40.0-	C79.51	—	D16.0-	—	—
skull	C41.0	C79.51	—	D16.4-	D48.0	D49.2
sphenoid	C41.0	C79.51	—	D16.4-	D48.0	D49.2
spine, spinal (column)	C41.2	C79.51	—	D16.6	D48.0	D49.2
coccyx	C41.4	C79.51	—	D16.8	D48.0	D49.2
sacrum	C41.4	C79.51	—	D16.8	D48.0	D49.2
sternum	C41.3	C79.51	—	D16.7	D48.0	D49.2
tarsus (any)	C40.3-	C79.51	—	—	—	—
temporal	C41.0	C79.51	—	D16.4-	D48.0	D49.2
thumb	C40.1-	C79.51				
tibia (any part)	C40.2-	C79.51				
toe (any)	C40.3-	C79.51				
trapezium	C40.1-	C79.51				
trapezoid	C40.1-	C79.51				
turbinate	C41.0	C79.51	—	D16.4-	D48.0	D49.2
ulna (any part)	C40.0-	C79.51	—	D16.0-		
unciform	C40.1-	C79.51		—	—	—
vertebra (column)	C41.2	C79.51	—	D16.6	D48.0	D49.2
coccyx	C41.4	C79.51	—	D16.8	D48.0	D49.2
sacrum	C41.4	C79.51	—	D16.8	D48.0	D49.2
vomer	C41.0	C79.51	—	D16.4-	D48.0	D49.2
wrist	C40.1-	C79.51	—	—	—	—
xiphoid process	C41.3	C79.51	—	D16.7	D48.0	D49.2
zygomatic	C41.0	C79.51	—	D16.4-	D48.0	D49.2
book-leaf (mouth) [ventral surface of tongue and floor of mouth]	C06.89	C79.89	D00.00	D10.39	D37.09	D49.0
bowel — *see* Neoplasm, intestine						
brachial plexus	C47.1-	C79.89	—	D36.12	D48.2	D49.2
brain NEC	C71.9	C79.31	—	D33.2	D43.2	D49.6
basal ganglia	C71.0	C79.31	—	D33.0	D43.0	D49.6
cerebellopontine angle	C71.6	C79.31	—	D33.1	D43.1	D49.6
cerebellum NOS	C71.6	C79.31	—	D33.1	D43.1	D49.6
cerebrum	C71.0	C79.31	—	D33.0	D43.0	D49.6
choroid plexus	C71.7	C79.31	—	D33.1	D43.1	D49.6
corpus callosum	C71.8	C79.31	—	D33.2	D43.2	D49.6
corpus striatum	C71.0	C79.31	—	D33.0	D43.0	D49.6
cortex (cerebral)	C71.0	C79.31	—	D33.0	D43.0	D49.6
frontal lobe	C71.1	C79.31	—	D33.0	D43.0	D49.6
globus pallidus	C71.0	C79.31	—	D33.0	D43.0	D49.6
hippocampus	C71.2	C79.31	—	D33.0	D43.0	D49.6
hypothalamus	C71.0	C79.31	—	D33.0	D43.0	D49.6
internal capsule	C71.0	C79.31	—	D33.0	D43.0	D49.6
medulla oblongata	C71.7	C79.31	—	D33.1	D43.1	D49.6
meninges	C70.0	C79.32	—	D32.0	D42.0	D49.7
midbrain	C71.7	C79.31	—	D33.1	D43.1	D49.6
occipital lobe	C71.4	C79.31	—	D33.0	D43.0	D49.6
overlapping lesion	C71.8	C79.31	—	—	—	—
parietal lobe	C71.3	C79.31	—	D33.0	D43.0	D49.6
peduncle	C71.7	C79.31	—	D33.1	D43.1	D49.6
pons	C71.7	C79.31	—	D33.1	D43.1	D49.6
stem	C71.7	C79.31	—	D33.1	D43.1	D49.6
tapetum	C71.8	C79.31	—	D33.2	D43.2	D49.6
temporal lobe	C71.2	C79.31	—	D33.0	D43.0	D49.6
thalamus	C71.0	C79.31	—	D33.0	D43.0	D49.6
uncus	C71.2	C79.31	—	D33.0	D43.0	D49.6

Neoplasm, neoplastic - *continued*

Neoplasm Table	Malignant Primary	Malignant Secondary	Ca In situ	Benign	Uncertain Behavior	Unspecified Behavior
brain NEC - *continued*	C71.9	C79.31	—	D33.2	D43.2	D49.6
ventricle (floor)	C71.5	C79.31	—	D33.0	D43.0	D49.6
fourth	C71.7	C79.31	—	D33.1	D43.1	D49.6
branchial (cleft) (cyst) (vestiges)	C10.4	C79.89	D00.08	D10.5	D37.05	D49.0
breast (connective tissue) (glandular tissue) (soft parts)	C50.9-	C79.81	D05.-	D24.-	D48.6-	D49.3
areola	C50.0-	C79.81	D05.-	D24.-	D48.6-	D49.3
axillary tail	C50.6-	C79.81	D05.-	D24.-	D48.6-	D49.3
central portion	C50.1-	C79.81	D05.-	D24.-	D48.6-	D49.3
inner	C50.8-	C79.81	D05.-	D24.-	D48.6-	D49.3
lower	C50.8-	C79.81	D05.-	D24.-	D48.6-	D49.3
lower-inner quadrant	C50.3-	C79.81	D05.-	D24.-	D48.6-	D49.3
lower-outer quadrant	C50.5-	C79.81	D05.-	D24.-	D48.6-	D49.3
mastectomy site (skin) — *see also* Neoplasm, breast, skin	C44.501	C79.2	—	—	—	—
specified as breast tissue	C50.8-	C79.81	—	—	—	—
midline	C50.8-	C79.81	D05.-	D24.-	D48.6-	D49.3
nipple	C50.0-	C79.81	D05.-	D24.-	D48.6-	D49.3
outer	C50.8-	C79.81	D05.-	D24.-	D48.6-	D49.3
overlapping lesion	C50.8-	—	—	—	—	—
skin	C44.501	C79.2	D04.5	D23.5	D48.5	D49.2
basal cell carcinoma	C44.511	—	—	—	—	—
specified type NEC	C44.591	—	—	—	—	—
squamous cell carcinoma	C44.521	—	—	—	—	—
tail (axillary)	C50.6-	C79.81	D05.-	D24.-	D48.6-	D49.3
upper	C50.8-	C79.81	D05.-	D24.-	D48.6-	D49.3
upper-inner quadrant	C50.2-	C79.81	D05.-	D24.-	D48.6-	D49.3
upper-outer quadrant	C50.4-	C79.81	D05.-	D24.-	D48.6-	D49.3
broad ligament	C57.1	C79.82	D07.39	D28.2	D39.8	D49.59
bronchiogenic, bronchogenic (lung)	C34.9-	C78.0-	D02.2-	D14.3-	D38.1	D49.1
bronchiole	C34.9-	C78.0-	D02.2-	D14.3-	D38.1	D49.1
bronchus	C34.9-	C78.0-	D02.2-	D14.3-	D38.1	D49.1
carina	C34.0-	C78.0-	D02.2-	D14.3-	D38.1	D49.1
lower lobe of lung	C34.3-	C78.0-	D02.2-	D14.3-	D38.1	D49.1
main	C34.0-	C78.0-	D02.2-	D14.3-	D38.1	D49.1
middle lobe of lung	C34.2	C78.0-	D02.21	D14.31	D38.1	D49.1
overlapping lesion	C34.8-	—	—	—	—	—
upper lobe of lung	C34.1-	C78.0-	D02.2-	D14.3-	D38.1	D49.1
brow	C44.309	C79.2	D04.39	D23.39	D48.5	D49.2
basal cell carcinoma	C44.319	—	—	—	—	—
specified type NEC	C44.399	—	—	—	—	—
squamous cell carcinoma	C44.329	—	—	—	—	—
buccal (cavity)	C06.9	C79.89	D00.00	D10.39	D37.09	D49.0
commissure	C06.0	C79.89	D00.02	D10.39	D37.09	D49.0
groove (lower) (upper)	C06.1	C79.89	D00.02	D10.39	D37.09	D49.0
mucosa	C06.0	C79.89	D00.02	D10.39	D37.09	D49.0
sulcus (lower) (upper)	C06.1	C79.89	D00.02	D10.39	D37.09	D49.0
bulbourethral gland	C68.0	C79.19	D09.19	D30.4	D41.3	D49.59
bursa — *see* Neoplasm, connective tissue						
buttock NEC	C76.3	C79.89	D04.5	D36.7	D48.7	D49.89
calf	C76.5-	C79.89	D04.7-	D36.7	D48.7	D49.89
calvarium	C41.0	C79.51	—	D16.4-	D48.0	D49.2
calyx, renal	C65.-	C79.0	D09.19	D30.1-	D41.1-	D49.51

NEOPLASM TABLE

NEOPLASM TABLE

Neoplasm Table	Malignant Primary	Malignant Secondary	Ca In situ	Benign	Uncertain Behavior	Unspecified Behavior
Neoplasm, neoplastic - *continued*						
canal						
anal	C21.1	C78.5	D01.3	D12.9	D37.8	D49.0
auditory (external) — *see also* Neoplasm, skin,						
ear	C44.20-	C79.2	D04.2-	D23.2-	D48.5	D49.2
auricular (external) — *see also* Neoplasm, skin,						
ear	C44.20-	C79.2	D04.2-	D23.2-	D48.5	D49.2
canaliculi, biliary (biliferi) (intrahepatic)	C22.1	C78.7	D01.5	D13.4	D37.6	D49.0
canthus (eye) (inner) (outer)	C44.10-	C79.2	D04.1-	D23.1-	D48.5	D49.2
basal cell carcinoma	C44.11-	—	—	—	—	—
specified type NEC	C44.19-	—	—	—	—	—
squamous cell carcinoma	C44.12-	—	—	—	—	—
capillary — *see* Neoplasm, connective tissue						
caput coli	C18.0	C78.5	D01.0	D12.0	D37.4	D49.0
carcinoid — *see* Tumor, carcinoid						
cardia (gastric)	C16.0	C78.89	D00.2	D13.1	D37.1	D49.0
cardiac orifice (stomach)	C16.0	C78.89	D00.2	D13.1	D37.1	D49.0
cardio-esophageal junction	C16.0	C78.89	D00.2	D13.1	D37.1	D49.0
cardio-esophagus	C16.0	C78.89	D00.2	D13.1	D37.1	D49.0
carina (bronchus)	C34.0-	C78.0-	D02.2-	D14.3-	D38.1	D49.1
carotid (artery)	C49.0	C79.89	—	D21.0	D48.1	D49.2
body	C75.4	C79.89	—	D35.5	D44.6	D49.7
carpus (any bone)	C40.1-	C79.51	—	D16.1-	—	—
cartilage (articular) (joint) NEC — *see also* Neoplasm, bone	C41.9	C79.51	—	D16.9-	D48.0	D49.2
arytenoid	C32.3	C78.39	D02.0	D14.1	D38.0	D49.1
auricular	C49.0	C79.89	—	D21.0	D48.1	D49.2
bronchi	C34.0-	C78.39	—	D14.3-	D38.1	D49.1
costal	C41.3	C79.51	—	D16.7	D48.0	D49.2
cricoid	C32.3	C78.39	D02.0	D14.1	D38.0	D49.1
cuneiform	C32.3	C78.39	D02.0	D14.1	D38.0	D49.1
ear (external)	C49.0	C79.89	—	D21.0	D48.1	D49.2
ensiform	C41.3	C79.51	—	D16.7	D48.0	D49.2
epiglottis	C32.1	C78.39	D02.0	D14.1	D38.0	D49.1
anterior surface	C10.1	C79.89	D00.08	D10.5	D37.05	D49.0
eyelid	C49.0	C79.89	—	D21.0	D48.1	D49.2
intervertebral	C41.2	C79.51	—	D16.6	D48.0	D49.2
larynx, laryngeal	C32.3	C78.39	D02.0	D14.1	D38.0	D49.1
nose, nasal	C30.0	C78.39	D02.3	D14.0	D38.5	D49.1
pinna	C49.0	C79.89	—	D21.0	D48.1	D49.2
rib	C41.3	C79.51	—	D16.7	D48.0	D49.2
semilunar (knee)	C40.2-	C79.51	—	D16.2-	D48.0	D49.2
thyroid	C32.3	C78.39	D02.0	D14.1	D38.0	D49.1
trachea	C33	C78.39	D02.1	D14.2	D38.1	D49.1
cauda equina	C72.1	C79.49	—	D33.4	D43.4	D49.7
cavity						
buccal	C06.9	C79.89	D00.00	D10.30	D37.09	D49.0
nasal	C30.0	C78.39	D02.3	D14.0	D38.5	D49.1
oral	C06.9	C79.89	D00.00	D10.30	D37.09	D49.0
peritoneal	C48.2	C78.6	—	D20.1	D48.4	D49.0
tympanic	C30.1	C78.39	D02.3	D14.0	D38.5	D49.1
cecum	C18.0	C78.5	D01.0	D12.0	D37.4	D49.0
central nervous system	C72.9	C79.40	—	—	—	—

Neoplasm Table	Malignant Primary	Malignant Secondary	Ca In situ	Benign	Uncertain Behavior	Unspecified Behavior
Neoplasm, neoplastic - *continued*						
cerebellopontine (angle)	C71.6	C79.31	—	D33.1	D43.1	D49.6
cerebellum, cerebellar	C71.6	C79.31	—	D33.1	D43.1	D49.6
cerebrum, cerebral (cortex) (hemisphere)						
(white matter)	C71.0	C79.31	—	D33.0	D43.0	D49.6
meninges	C70.0	C79.32	—	D32.0	D42.0	D49.7
peduncle	C71.7	C79.31	—	D33.1	D43.1	D49.6
ventricle	C71.5	C79.31	—	D33.0	D43.0	D49.6
fourth	C71.7	C79.31	—	D33.1	D43.1	D49.6
cervical region	C76.0	C79.89	D09.8	D36.7	D48.7	D49.89
cervix (cervical) (uteri)						
(uterus)	C53.9	C79.82	D06.9	D26.0	D39.0	D49.59
canal	C53.0	C79.82	D06.0	D26.0	D39.0	D49.59
endocervix (canal) (gland)	C53.0	C79.82	D06.0	D26.0	D39.0	D49.59
exocervix	C53.1	C79.82	D06.1	D26.0	D39.0	D49.59
external os	C53.1	C79.82	D06.1	D26.0	D39.0	D49.59
internal os	C53.0	C79.82	D06.0	D26.0	D39.0	D49.59
nabothian gland	C53.0	C79.82	D06.0	D26.0	D39.0	D49.59
overlapping lesion	C53.8	—	—	—	—	—
squamocolumnar junction	C53.8	C79.82	D06.7	D26.0	D39.0	D49.59
stump	C53.8	C79.82	D06.7	D26.0	D39.0	D49.59
cheek	C76.0	C79.89	D09.8	D36.7	D48.7	D49.89
external	C44.309	C79.2	D04.39	D23.39	D48.5	D49.2
basal cell carcinoma	C44.319	—	—	—	—	—
specified type NEC	C44.399	—	—	—	—	—
squamous cell carcinoma	C44.329	—	—	—	—	—
inner aspect	C06.0	C79.89	D00.02	D10.39	D37.09	D49.0
internal	C06.0	C79.89	D00.02	D10.39	D37.09	D49.0
mucosa	C06.0	C79.89	D00.02	D10.39	D37.09	D49.0
chest (wall) NEC	C76.1	C79.89	D09.8	D36.7	D48.7	D49.89
chiasma opticum	C72.3-	C79.49	—	D33.3	D43.3	D49.7
chin	C44.309	C79.2	D04.39	D23.39	D48.5	D49.2
basal cell carcinoma	C44.319	—	—	—	—	—
specified type NEC	C44.399	—	—	—	—	—
squamous cell carcinoma	C44.329	—	—	—	—	—
choana	C11.3	C79.89	D00.08	D10.6	D37.05	D49.0
cholangiole	C22.1	C78.89	D01.5	D13.4	D37.6	D49.0
choledochal duct	C24.0	C78.89	D01.5	D13.5	D37.6	D49.0
choroid	C69.3-	C79.49	D09.2-	D31.3	D48.7	D49.81
plexus	C71.5	C79.31	—	D33.0	D43.0	D49.6
ciliary body	C69.4-	C79.49	D09.2-	D31.4-	D48.7	D49.89
clavicle	C41.3	C79.51	—	D16.7	D48.0	D49.2
clitoris	C51.2	C79.82	D07.1	D28.0	D39.8	D49.59
clivus	C41.0	C79.51	—	D16.4-	D48.0	D49.2
cloacogenic zone	C21.2	C78.5	D01.3	D12.9	D37.8	D49.0
coccygeal						
body or glomus	C49.5	C79.89	—	D21.5	D48.1	D49.2
vertebra	C41.4	C79.51	—	D16.8	D48.0	D49.2
coccyx	C41.4	C79.51	—	D16.8	D48.0	D49.2
colon — *see also* Neoplasm, intestine, large	C18.9	C78.5	—	—	—	—
with rectum	C19	C78.5	D01.1	D12.7	D37.5	D49.0
column, spinal — *see* Neoplasm, spine						
columnella — *see also* Neoplasm, skin, face	C44.390	C79.2	D04.39	D23.39	D48.5	D49.2
commissure						
labial, lip	C00.6	C79.89	D00.01	D10.39	D37.01	D49.0
laryngeal	C32.0	C78.39	D02.0	D14.1	D38.0	D49.1

NEOPLASM TABLE

Neoplasm Table	Malignant Primary	Malignant Secondary	Ca In situ	Benign	Uncertain Behavior	Unspecified Behavior
Neoplasm, neoplastic - *continued*						
common (bile) duct	C24.0	C78.89	D01.5	D13.5	D37.6	D49.0
concha — *see also*						
Neoplasm, skin, ear	C44.20-	C79.2	D04.2-	D23.2-	D48.5	D49.2
nose	C30.0	C78.39	D02.3	D14.0	D38.5	D49.1
conjunctiva	C69.0-	C79.49	D09.2-	D31.0-	D48.7	D49.89
connective tissue NEC	C49.9	C79.89	—	D21.9	D48.1	D49.2

Connective tissue Notes:

Note: For neoplasms of connective tissue (blood vessel, bursa, fascia, ligament, muscle, peripheral nerves, sympathetic and parasympathetic nerves and ganglia, synovia, tendon, etc.) or of morphological types that indicate connective tissue, code according to the list under "Neoplasm, connective tissue". For sites that do not appear in this list, code to neoplasm of that site; e.g., fibrosarcoma, pancreas (C25.9)

Note: Morphological types that indicate connective tissue appear in their proper place in the alphabetic index with the instruction "see Neoplasm, connective tissue ...."

Neoplasm Table	Malignant Primary	Malignant Secondary	Ca In situ	Benign	Uncertain Behavior	Unspecified Behavior
abdomen	C49.4	C79.89	—	D21.4	D48.1	D49.2
abdominal wall	C49.4	C79.89	—	D21.4	D48.1	D49.2
ankle	C49.2-	C79.89	—	D21.2-	D48.1	D49.2
antecubital fossa or space	C49.1-	C79.89	—	D21.1-	D48.1	D49.2
arm	C49.1-	C79.89	—	D21.1-	D48.1	D49.2
auricle (ear)	C49.0	C79.89	—	D21.0	D48.1	D49.2
axilla	C49.3	C79.89	—	D21.3	D48.1	D49.2
back	C49.6	C79.89	—	D21.6	D48.1	D49.2
breast — *see* Neoplasm, breast						
buttock	C49.5	C79.89	—	D21.5	D48.1	D49.2
calf	C49.2-	C79.89	—	D21.2-	D48.1	D49.2
cervical region	C49.0	C79.89	—	D21.0	D48.1	D49.2
cheek	C49.0	C79.89	—	D21.0	D48.1	D49.2
chest (wall)	C49.3	C79.89	—	D21.3	D48.1	D49.2
chin	C49.0	C79.89	—	D21.0	D48.1	D49.2
diaphragm	C49.3	C79.89	—	D21.3	D48.1	D49.2
ear (external)	C49.0	C79.89	—	D21.0	D48.1	D49.2
elbow	C49.1-	C79.89	—	D21.1-	D48.1	D49.2
extrarectal	C49.5	C79.89	—	D21.5	D48.1	D49.2
extremity	C49.9	C79.89	—	D21.9	D48.1	D49.2
lower	C49.2-	C79.89	—	D21.2-	D48.1	D49.2
upper	C49.1-	C79.89	—	D21.1-	D48.1	D49.2
eyelid	C49.0	C79.89	—	D21.0	D48.1	D49.2
face	C49.0	C79.89	—	D21.0	D48.1	D49.2
finger	C49.1-	C79.89	—	D21.1-	D48.1	D49.2
flank	C49.6	C79.89	—	D21.6	D48.1	D49.2
foot	C49.2-	C79.89	—	D21.2-	D48.1	D49.2
forearm	C49.1-	C79.89	—	D21.1-	D48.1	D49.2
forehead	C49.0	C79.89	—	D21.0	D48.1	D49.2
gastric	C49.4	C79.89	—	D21.4	D48.1	D49.2
gastrointestinal	C49.4	C79.89	—	D21.4	D48.1	D49.2
gluteal region	C49.5	C79.89	—	D21.5	D48.1	D49.2
great vessels NEC	C49.3	C79.89	—	D21.3	D48.1	D49.2
groin	C49.5	C79.89	—	D21.5	D48.1	D49.2
hand	C49.1-	C79.89	—	D21.1-	D48.1	D49.2
head	C49.0	C79.89	—	D21.0	D48.1	D49.2
heel	C49.2-	C79.89	—	D21.2-	D48.1	D49.2
hip	C49.2-	C79.89	—	D21.2-	D48.1	D49.2
hypochondrium	C49.4	C79.89	—	D21.4	D48.1	D49.2
iliopsoas muscle	C49.5	C79.89	—	D21.5	D48.1	D49.2

Neoplasm Table	Malignant Primary	Malignant Secondary	Ca In situ	Benign	Uncertain Behavior	Unspecified Behavior
Neoplasm, neoplastic - *continued*						
connective tissue NEC - *continued*						
infraclavicular region	C49.3	C79.89	—	D21.3	D48.1	D49.2
inguinal (canal) (region)	C49.5	C79.89	—	D21.5	D48.1	D49.2
intestinal	C49.4	C79.89	—	D21.4	D48.1	D49.2
intrathoracic	C49.3	C79.89	—	D21.3	D48.1	D49.2
ischiorectal fossa	C49.5	C79.89	—	D21.5	D48.1	D49.2
jaw	C03.9	C79.89	D00.03	D10.39	D48.1	D49.0
knee	C49.2-	C79.89	—	D21.2-	D48.1	D49.2
leg	C49.2-	C79.89	—	D21.2-	D48.1	D49.2
limb NEC	C49.9	C79.89	—	D21.9	D48.1	D49.2
lower	C49.2-	C79.89	—	D21.2-	D48.1	D49.2
upper	C49.1-	C79.89	—	D21.1-	D48.1	D49.2
nates	C49.5	C79.89	—	D21.5	D48.1	D49.2
neck	C49.0	C79.89	—	D21.0	D48.1	D49.2
orbit	C69.6-	C79.49	D09.2-	D31.6-	D48.1	D49.89
overlapping lesion	C49.8	—	—	—	—	—
pararectal	C49.5	C79.89	—	D21.5	D48.1	D49.2
para-urethral	C49.5	C79.89	—	D21.5	D48.1	D49.2
paravaginal	C49.5	C79.89	—	D21.5	D48.1	D49.2
pelvis (floor)	C49.5	C79.89	—	D21.5	D48.1	D49.2
pelvo-abdominal	C49.8	C79.89	—	D21.6	D48.1	D49.2
perineum	C49.5	C79.89	—	D21.5	D48.1	D49.2
perirectal (tissue)	C49.5	C79.89	—	D21.5	D48.1	D49.2
periurethral (tissue)	C49.5	C79.89	—	D21.5	D48.1	D49.2
popliteal fossa or space	C49.2-	C79.89	—	D21.2-	D48.1	D49.2
presacral	C49.5	C79.89	—	D21.5	D48.1	D49.2
psoas muscle	C49.4	C79.89	—	D21.4	D48.1	D49.2
pterygoid fossa	C49.0	C79.89	—	D21.0	D48.1	D49.2
rectovaginal septum or wall	C49.5	C79.89	—	D21.5	D48.1	D49.2
rectovesical	C49.5	C79.89	—	D21.5	D48.1	D49.2
retroperitoneum	C48.0	C78.6	—	D20.0	D48.3	D49.0
sacrococcygeal region	C49.5	C79.89	—	D21.5	D48.1	D49.2
scalp	C49.0	C79.89	—	D21.0	D48.1	D49.2
scapular region	C49.3	C79.89	—	D21.3	D48.1	D49.2
shoulder	C49.1-	C79.89	—	D21.1-	D48.1	D49.2
skin (dermis) NEC — *see also* Neoplasm, skin, by site	C44.90	C79.2	D04.9	D23.9	D48.5	D49.2
stomach	C49.4	C79.89	—	D21.4	D48.1	D49.2
submental	C49.0	C79.89	—	D21.0	D48.1	D49.2
supraclavicular region	C49.0	C79.89	—	D21.0	D48.1	D49.2
temple	C49.0	C79.89	—	D21.0	D48.1	D49.2
temporal region	C49.0	C79.89	—	D21.0	D48.1	D49.2
thigh	C49.2-	C79.89	—	D21.2-	D48.1	D49.2
thoracic (duct) (wall)	C49.3	C79.89	—	D21.3	D48.1	D49.2
thorax	C49.3	C79.89	—	D21.3	D48.1	D49.2
thumb	C49.1-	C79.89	—	D21.1-	D48.1	D49.2
toe	C49.2-	C79.89	—	D21.2-	D48.1	D49.2
trunk	C49.6	C79.89	—	D21.6	D48.1	D49.2
umbilicus	C49.4	C79.89	—	D21.4	D48.1	D49.2
vesicorectal	C49.5	C79.89	—	D21.5	D48.1	D49.2
wrist	C49.1-	C79.89	—	D21.1-	D48.1	D49.2
conus medullaris	C72.0	C79.49	—	D33.4	D43.4	D49.7
cord (true) (vocal)	C32.0	C78.39	D02.0	D14.1	D38.0	D49.1
false	C32.1	C78.39	D02.0	D14.1	D38.0	D49.1
spermatic	C63.1-	C79.82	D07.69	D29.8	D40.8	D49.59
spinal (cervical) (lumbar) (thoracic)	C72.0	C79.49	—	D33.4	D43.4	D49.7
cornea (limbus)	C69.1-	C79.49	D09.2-	D31.1-	D48.7	D49.89

Neoplasm Table	Malignant Primary	Malignant Secondary	Ca In situ	Benign	Uncertain Behavior	Unspecified Behavior
Neoplasm, neoplastic - *continued*						
corpus						
albicans	C56.-	C79.6-	D07.39	D27.-	D39.1-	D49.59
callosum, brain	C71.0	C79.31	—	D33.2	D43.2	D49.6
cavernosum	C60.2	C79.82	D07.4	D29.0	D40.8	D49.59
gastric	C16.2	C78.89	D00.2	D13.1	D37.1	D49.0
overlapping sites	C54.8	—	—	—	—	—
penis	C60.2	C79.82	D07.4	D29.0	D40.8	D49.59
striatum, cerebrum	C71.0	C79.31	—	D33.0	D43.0	D49.6
uteri	C54.9	C79.82	D07.0	D26.1	D39.0	D49.59
isthmus	C54.0	C79.82	D07.0	D26.1	D39.0	D49.59
cortex						
adrenal	C74.0-	C79.7-	D09.3	D35.0-	D44.1-	D49.7
cerebral	C71.0	C79.31	—	D33.0	D43.0	D49.6
costal cartilage	C41.3	C79.51	—	D16.7	D48.0	D49.2
costovertebral joint	C41.3	C79.51	—	D16.7	D48.0	D49.2
Cowper's gland	C68.0	C79.19	D09.19	D30.4	D41.3	D49.59
cranial (fossa, any)	C71.9	C79.31	—	D33.2	D43.2	D49.6
meninges	C70.0	C79.32	—	D32.0	D42.0	D49.7
nerve	C72.50	C79.49	—	D33.3	D43.3	D49.7
specified NEC	C72.59	C79.49	—	D33.3	D43.3	D49.7
craniobuccal pouch	C75.2	C79.89	D09.3	D35.2	D44.3	D49.7
craniopharyngeal (duct) (pouch)	C75.2	C79.89	D09.3	D35.3	D44.4	D49.7
cricoid	C13.0	C79.89	D00.08	D10.7	D37.05	D49.0
cartilage	C32.3	C78.39	D02.0	D14.1	D38.0	D49.1
cricopharynx	C13.0	C79.89	D00.08	D10.7	D37.05	D49.0
crypt of Morgagni	C21.8	C78.5	D01.3	D12.9	D37.8	D49.0
crystalline lens	C69.4-	C79.49	D09.2-	D31.4-	D48.7	D49.89
cul-de-sac (Douglas')	C48.1	C78.6	—	D20.1	D48.4	D49.0
cuneiform cartilage	C32.3	C78.39	D02.0	D14.1	D38.0	D49.1
cutaneous — *see* Neoplasm, skin						
cutis — *see* Neoplasm, skin						
cystic (bile) duct (common)	C24.0	C78.89	D01.5	D13.5	D37.6	D49.0
dermis — *see* Neoplasm, skin						
diaphragm	C49.3	C79.89	—	D21.3	D48.1-	D49.2
digestive organs, system, tube, or tract NEC	C26.9	C78.89	D01.9	D13.9	D37.9	D49.0
disc, intervertebral	C41.2	C79.51	—	D16.6	D48.0	D49.2
disease, generalized	C80.0	—	—	—	—	—
disseminated	C80.0	—	—	—	—	—
Douglas' cul-de-sac or pouch	C48.1	C78.6	—	D20.1	D48.4	D49.0
duodenojejunal junction	C17.8	C78.4	D01.49	D13.39	D37.2	D49.0
duodenum	C17.0	C78.4	D01.49	D13.2	D37.2	D49.0
dura (cranial) (mater)	C70.9	C79.49	—	D32.9	D42.9	D49.7
cerebral	C70.0	C79.32	—	D32.0	D42.0	D49.7
spinal	C70.1	C79.49	—	D32.1	D42.1	D49.7
ear (external) — *see also* Neoplasm, skin, ear	C44.20-	C79.2	D04.2-	D23.2-	D48.5	D49.2
auricle or auris — *see also* Neoplasm, skin, ear	C44.20-	C79.2	D04.2-	D23.2-	D48.5	D49.2
canal, external — *see also* Neoplasm, skin, ear	C44.20-	C79.2	D04.2-	D23.2-	D48.5	D49.2
cartilage	C49.0	C79.89	—	D21.0	D48.1	D49.2
external meatus — *see also* Neoplasm, skin, ear	C44.20-	C79.2	D04.2-	D23.2-	D48.5	D49.2
inner	C30.1	C78.39	D02.3	D14.0	D38.5	D49.1
lobule — *see also* Neoplasm, skin, ear	C44.20-	C79.2	D04.2-	D23.2-	D48.5	D49.2
middle	C30.1	C78.39	D02.3	D14.0	D38.5	D49.1
overlapping lesion with accessory sinuses	C31.8	—	—	—	—	—

Neoplasm Table	Malignant Primary	Malignant Secondary	Ca In situ	Benign	Uncertain Behavior	Unspecified Behavior
Neoplasm, neoplastic - *continued*						
ear (external) — *see also* Neoplasm, skin, ear - *continued*	C44.20-	C79.2	D04.2-	D23.2-	D48.5	D49.2
skin	C44.20-	C79.2	D04.2-	D23.2-	D48.5	D49.2
basal cell carcinoma	C44.21-	—	—	—	—	—
specified type NEC	C44.29-	—	—	—	—	—
squamous cell carcinoma	C44.22-	—	—	—	—	—
earlobe	C44.20-	C79.2	D04.2-	D23.2-	D48.5	D49.2
basal cell carcinoma	C44.21-	—	—	—	—	—
specified type NEC	C44.29-	—	—	—	—	—
squamous cell carcinoma	C44.22-	—	—	—	—	—
ejaculatory duct	C63.7	C79.82	D07.69	D29.8	D40.8	D49.59
elbow NEC	C76.4-	C79.89	D04.6-	D36.7	D48.7	D49.89
endocardium	C38.0	C79.89	—	D15.1	D48.7	D49.89
endocervix (canal) (gland)	C53.0	C79.82	D06.0	D26.0	D39.0	D49.59
endocrine gland NEC	C75.9	C79.89	D09.3	D35.9	D44.9	D49.7
pluriglandular	C75.8	C79.89	D09.3	D35.7	D44.9	D49.7
endometrium (gland) (stroma)	C54.1	C79.82	D07.0	D26.1	D39.0	D49.59
ensiform cartilage	C41.3	C79.51	—	D16.7	D48.0	D49.2
enteric — *see* Neoplasm, intestine						
ependyma (brain)	C71.5	C79.31	—	D33.0	D43.0	D49.6
fourth ventricle	C71.7	C79.31	—	D33.1	D43.1	D49.6
epicardium	C38.0	C79.89	—	D15.1	D48.7	D49.89
epididymis	C63.0-	C79.82	D07.69	D29.3-	D40.8	D49.59
epidural	C72.9	C79.49	—	D33.9	D43.9	D49.7
epiglottis	C32.1	C78.39	D02.0	D14.1	D38.0	D49.1
anterior aspect or surface	C10.1	C79.89	D00.08	D10.5	D37.05	D49.0
cartilage	C32.3	C78.39	D02.0	D14.1	D38.0	D49.1
free border (margin)	C10.1	C79.89	D00.08	D10.5	D37.05	D49.0
junctional region	C10.8	C79.89	D00.08	D10.5	D37.05	D49.0
posterior (laryngeal) surface	C32.1	C78.39	D02.0	D14.1	D38.0	D49.1
suprahyoid portion	C32.1	C78.39	D02.0	D14.1	D38.0	D49.1
esophagogastric junction	C16.0	C78.89	D00.2	D13.1	D37.1	D49.0
esophagus	C15.9	C78.89	D00.1	D13.0	D37.8	D49.0
abdominal	C15.5	C78.89	D00.1	D13.0	D37.8	D49.0
cervical	C15.3	C78.89	D00.1	D13.0	D37.8	D49.0
distal (third)	C15.5	C78.89	D00.1	D13.0	D37.8	D49.0
lower (third)	C15.5	C78.89	D00.1	D13.0	D37.8	D49.0
middle (third)	C15.4	C78.89	D00.1	D13.0	D37.8	D49.0
overlapping lesion	C15.8	—	—	—	—	—
proximal (third)	C15.3	C78.89	D00.1	D13.0	D37.8	D49.0
thoracic	C15.4	C78.89	D00.1	D13.0	D37.8	D49.0
upper (third)	C15.3	C78.89	D00.1	D13.0	D37.8	D49.0
ethmoid (sinus)	C31.1	C78.39	D02.3	D14.0	D38.5	D49.1
bone or labyrinth	C41.0	C79.51	—	D16.4-	D48.0	D49.2
eustachian tube	C30.1	C78.39	D02.3	D14.0	D38.5	D49.1
exocervix	C53.1	C79.82	D06.1	D26.0	D39.0	D49.59
external						
meatus (ear) — *see also* Neoplasm, skin, ear	C44.20-	C79.2	D04.2-	D23.2-	D48.5	D49.2
os, cervix uteri	C53.1	C79.82	D06.1	D26.0	D39.0	D49.59
extradural	C72.9	C79.49	—	D33.9	D43.9	D49.7
extrahepatic (bile) duct	C24.0	C78.89	D01.5	D13.5	D37.6	D49.0
overlapping lesion with gallbladder	C24.8	—	—	—	—	—
extraocular muscle	C69.6-	C79.49	D09.2-	D31.6-	D48.7	D49.89
extrarectal	C76.3	C79.89	D09.8	D36.7	D48.7	D49.89

NEOPLASM TABLE

Neoplasm, neoplastic - continued

Neoplasm Table	Malignant Primary	Malignant Secondary	Ca In situ	Benign	Uncertain Behavior	Unspecified Behavior
extremity	C76.8	C79.89	D04.8	D36.7	D48.7	D49.89
lower	C76.5-	C79.89	D04.7-	D36.7	D48.7	D49.89
upper	C76.4-	C79.89	D04.6-	D36.7	D48.7	D49.89
eye NEC	C69.9-	C79.49	D09.2	D31.9-	D48.7	D49.89
overlapping sites	C69.8	—	—	—	—	—
eyeball	C69.9-	C79.49	D09.2-	D31.9-	D48.7	D49.89
eyebrow	C44.309	C79.2	D04.39	D23.39	D48.5	D49.2
basal cell carcinoma	C44.319	—	—	—	—	—
specified type NEC	C44.399	—	—	—	—	—
squamous cell carcinoma	C44.329	—	—	—	—	—
eyelid (lower) (skin) (upper)	C44.10-	—	—	—	—	—
basal cell carcinoma	C44.11-	—	—	—	—	—
cartilage	C49.0	C79.89	—	D21.0	D48.1	D49.2
specified type NEC	C44.19-	—	—	—	—	—
squamous cell carcinoma	C44.12-	—	—	—	—	—
face NEC	C76.0	C79.89	D04.39	D36.7	D48.7	D49.89
fallopian tube (accessory)	C57.0-	C79.82	D07.39	D28.2	D39.8	D49.59
falx (cerebella) (cerebri)	C70.0	C79.32	—	D32.0	D42.0	D49.7
fascia — see also Neoplasm, connective tissue						
palmar	C49.1-	C79.89	—	D21.1-	D48.1	D49.2
plantar	C49.2-	C79.89	—	D21.2-	D48.1	D49.2
fatty tissue — see Neoplasm, connective tissue						
fauces, faucial NEC	C10.9	C79.89	D00.08	D10.5	D37.05	D49.0
pillars	C09.1	C79.89	D00.08	D10.5	D37.05	D49.0
tonsil	C09.9	C79.89	D00.08	D10.4	D37.05	D49.0
femur (any part)	C40.2-	—	—	D16.2-	—	—
fetal membrane	C58	C79.82	D07.0	D26.7	D39.2	D49.59
fibrous tissue — see Neoplasm, connective tissue						
fibula (any part)	C40.2-	C79.51	—	D16.2-	—	—
filum terminale	C72.0	C79.49	—	D33.4	D43.4	D49.7
finger NEC	C76.4-	C79.89	D04.6-	D36.7	D48.7	D49.89
flank NEC	C76.8	C79.89	D04.5	D36.7	D48.7	D49.89
follicle, nabothian	C53.0	C79.82	D06.0	D26.0	D39.0	D49.59
foot NEC	C76.5-	C79.89	D04.7-	D36.7	D48.7	D49.89
forearm NEC	C76.4-	C79.89	D04.6-	D36.7	D48.7	D49.89
forehead (skin)	C44.309	C79.2	D04.39	D23.39	D48.5	D49.2
basal cell carcinoma	C44.319	—	—	—	—	—
specified type NEC	C44.399	—	—	—	—	—
squamous cell carcinoma	C44.329	—	—	—	—	—
foreskin	C60.0	C79.82	D07.4	D29.0	D40.8	D49.59
fornix						
pharyngeal	C11.3	C79.89	D00.08	D10.6	D37.05	D49.0
vagina	C52	C79.82	D07.2	D28.1	D39.8	D49.59
fossa (of)						
anterior (cranial)	C71.9	C79.31	—	D33.2	D43.2	D49.6
cranial	C71.9	C79.31	—	D33.2	D43.2	D49.6
ischiorectal	C76.3	C79.89	D09.8	D36.7	D48.7	D49.89
middle (cranial)	C71.9	C79.31	—	D33.2	D43.2	D49.6
piriform	C12	C79.89	D00.08	D10.7	D37.05	D49.0
pituitary	C75.1	C79.89	D09.3	D35.2	D44.3	D49.7
posterior (cranial)	C71.9	C79.31	—	D33.2	D43.2	D49.6
pterygoid	C49.0	C79.89	—	D21.0	D48.1	D49.2
pyriform	C12	C79.89	D00.08	D10.7	D37.05	D49.0
Rosenmüller	C11.2	C79.89	D00.08	D10.6	D37.05	D49.0
tonsillar	C09.0	C79.89	D00.08	D10.5	D37.05	D49.0
fourchette	C51.9	C79.82	D07.1	D28.0	D39.8	D49.59

Neoplasm, neoplastic - continued

Neoplasm Table	Malignant Primary	Malignant Secondary	Ca In situ	Benign	Uncertain Behavior	Unspecified Behavior
frenulum						
labii — see Neoplasm, lip, internal						
linguae	C02.2	C79.89	D00.07	D10.1	D37.02	D49.0
frontal						
bone	C41.0	C79.51	—	D16.4-	D48.0	D49.2
lobe, brain	C71.1	C79.31	—	D33.0	D43.0	D49.6
pole	C71.1	C79.31	—	D33.0	D43.0	D49.6
sinus	C31.2	C78.39	D02.3	D14.0	D38.5	D49.1
fundus						
stomach	C16.1	C78.89	D00.2	D13.1	D37.1	D49.0
uterus	C54.3	C79.82	D07.0	D26.1	D39.0	D49.59
gall duct (extrahepatic)	C24.0	C78.89	D01.5	D13.5	D37.6	D49.0
intrahepatic	C22.1	C78.7	D01.5	D13.4	D37.6	D49.0
gallbladder	C23	C78.89	D01.5	D13.5	D37.6	D49.0
overlapping lesion with extrahepatic bile ducts	C24.8	—	—	—	—	—
ganglia — see also Neoplasm, nerve, peripheral	C47.9	C79.89	—	D36.10	D48.2	D49.2
basal	C71.0	C79.31	—	D33.0	D43.0	D49.6
cranial nerve	C72.50	C79.49	—	D33.3	D43.3	D49.7
Gartner's duct	C52	C79.82	D07.2	D28.1	D39.8	D49.59
gastric — see Neoplasm, stomach						
gastrocolic	C26.9	C78.89	D01.9	D13.9	D37.9	D49.0
gastroesophageal junction	C16.0	C78.89	D00.2	D13.1	D37.1	D49.0
gastrointestinal (tract) NEC	C26.9	C78.89	D01.9	D13.9	D37.9	D49.0
generalized	C80.0	—	—	—	—	—
genital organ or tract						
female NEC	C57.9	C79.82	D07.30	D28.9	D39.9	D49.59
overlapping lesion	C57.8	—	—	—	—	—
specified site NEC	C57.7	C79.82	D07.39	D28.7	D39.8	D49.59
male NEC	C63.9	C79.82	D07.60	D29.9	D40.9	D49.59
overlapping lesion	C63.8	—	—	—	—	—
specified site NEC	C63.7	C79.82	D07.69	D29.8	D40.8	D49.59
genitourinary tract						
female	C57.9	C79.82	D07.30	D28.9	D39.9	D49.59
male	C63.9	C79.82	D07.60	D29.9	D40.9	D49.59
gingiva (alveolar) (marginal)	C03.9	C79.89	D00.03	D10.39	D37.09	D49.0
lower	C03.1	C79.89	D00.03	D10.39	D37.09	D49.0
mandibular	C03.1	C79.89	D00.03	D10.39	D37.09	D49.0
maxillary	C03.0	C79.89	D00.03	D10.39	D37.09	D49.0
upper	C03.0	C79.89	D00.03	D10.39	D37.09	D49.0
gland, glandular (lymphatic) (system) — see also Neoplasm, lymph gland						
endocrine NEC	C75.9	C79.89	D09.3	D35.9	D44.9	D49.7
salivary — see Neoplasm, salivary gland						
glans penis	C60.1	C79.82	D07.4	D29.0	D40.8	D49.59
globus pallidus	C71.0	C79.31	—	D33.0	D43.0	D49.6
glomus						
coccygeal	C49.5	C79.89	—	D21.5	D48.1	D49.2
jugularis	C75.5	C79.89	—	D35.6	D44.7	D49.7
glosso-epiglottic fold (s)	C10.1	C79.89	D00.08	D10.5	D37.05	D49.0
glossopalatine fold	C09.1	C79.89	D00.08	D10.5	D37.05	D49.0
glossopharyngeal sulcus	C09.0	C79.89	D00.08	D10.5	D37.05	D49.0
glottis	C32.0	C78.39	D02.0	D14.1	D38.0	D49.1
gluteal region	C76.3	C79.89	D04.5	D36.7	D48.7	D49.89
great vessels NEC	C49.3	C79.89	—	D21.3	D48.1	D49.2
groin NEC	C76.3	C79.89	D04.5	D36.7	D48.7	D49.89

NEOPLASM TABLE

Neoplasm Table	Malignant Primary	Malignant Secondary	Ca In situ	Benign	Uncertain Behavior	Unspecified Behavior
Neoplasm, neoplastic - *continued*						
gum	C03.9	C79.89	D00.03	D10.39	D37.09	D49.0
lower	C03.1	C79.89	D00.03	D10.39	D37.09	D49.0
upper	C03.0	C79.89	D00.03	D10.39	D37.09	D49.0
hand NEC	C76.4-	C79.89	D04.6-	D36.7	D48.7	D49.89
head NEC	C76.0	C79.89	D04.4	D36.7	D48.7	D49.89
heart	C38.0	C79.89	—	D15.1	D48.7	D49.89
heel NEC	C76.5-	C79.89	D04.7-	D36.7	D48.7	D49.89
helix — *see also* Neoplasm, skin, ear	C44.20-	C79.2	D04.2-	D23.2-	D48.5	D49.2
hematopoietic, hemopoietic tissue NEC	C96.9	—	—	—	—	—
specified NEC	C96.Z	—	—	—	—	—
hemisphere, cerebral	C71.0	C79.31	—	D33.0	D43.0	D49.6
hemorrhoidal zone	C21.1	C78.5	D01.3	D12.9	D37.8	D49.0
hepatic — *see also* Index to disease, by histology	C22.9	C78.7	D01.5	D13.4	D37.6	D49.0
duct (bile)	C24.0	C78.89	D01.5	D13.5	D37.6	D49.0
flexure (colon)	C18.3	C78.5	D01.0	D12.3	D37.4	D49.0
primary	C22.8	C78.7	D01.5	D13.4	D37.6	D49.0
hepatobiliary	C24.9	C78.89	D01.5	D13.5	D37.6	D49.0
hepatoblastoma	C22.2	C78.7	D01.5	D13.4	D37.6	D49.0
hepatoma	C22.0	C78.7	D01.5	D13.4	D37.6	D49.0
hilus of lung	C34.0-	C78.0-	D02.2-	D14.3-	D38.1	D49.1
hip NEC	C76.5-	C79.89	D04.7-	D36.7	D48.7	D49.89
hippocampus, brain	C71.2	C79.31	—	D33.0	D43.0	D49.6
humerus (any part)	C40.0-	C79.51	—	D16.0-	—	—
hymen	C52	C79.82	D07.2	D28.1	D39.8	D49.59
hypopharynx, hypopharyngeal NEC	C13.9	C79.89	D00.08	D10.7	D37.05	D49.0
overlapping lesion	C13.8	—	—	—	—	—
postcricoid region	C13.0	C79.89	D00.08	D10.7	D37.05	D49.0
posterior wall	C13.2	C79.89	D00.08	D10.7	D37.05	D49.0
pyriform fossa (sinus)	C12	C79.89	D00.08	D10.7	D37.05	D49.0
hypophysis	C75.1	C79.89	D09.3	D35.2	D44.3	D49.7
hypothalamus	C71.0	C79.31	—	D33.0	D43.0	D49.6
ileocecum, ileocecal (coil) (junction) (valve)	C18.0	C78.5	D01.0	D12.0	D37.4	D49.0
ileum	C17.2	C78.4	D01.49	D13.39	D37.2	D49.0
ilium	C41.4	C79.51	—	D16.8	D48.0	D49.2
immunoproliferative NEC	C88.9	—	—	—	—	—
infraclavicular (region)	C76.1	C79.89	D04.5	D36.7	D48.7	D49.89
inguinal (region)	C76.3	C79.89	D04.5	D36.7	D48.7	D49.89
insula	C71.0	C79.31	—	D33.0	D43.0	D49.6
insular tissue (pancreas)	C25.4	C78.89	D01.7	D13.7	D37.8	D49.0
brain	C71.0	C79.31	—	D33.0	D43.0	D49.6
interarytenoid fold	C13.1	C79.89	D00.08	D10.7	D37.05	D49.0
hypopharyngeal aspect	C13.1	C79.89	D00.08	D10.7	D37.05	D49.0
laryngeal aspect	C32.1	C78.39	D02.0	D14.1	D38.0	D49.1
marginal zone	C13.1	C79.89	D00.08	D10.7	D37.05	D49.0
interdental papillae	C03.9	C79.89	D00.03	D10.39	D37.09	D49.0
lower	C03.1	C79.89	D00.03	D10.39	D37.09	D49.0
upper	C03.0	C79.89	D00.03	D10.39	D37.09	D49.0
internal						
capsule	C71.0	C79.31	—	D33.0	D43.0	D49.6
os (cervix)	C53.0	C79.82	D06.0	D26.0	D39.0	D49.59
intervertebral cartilage or disc	C41.2	C79.51	—	D16.6	D48.0	D49.2
Neoplasm, neoplastic - *continued*						
intestine, intestinal	C26.0	C78.80	D01.40	D13.9	D37.8	D49.0
large	C18.9	C78.5	D01.0	D12.6	D37.4	D49.0
appendix	C18.1	C78.5	D01.0	D12.1	D37.3	D49.0
caput coli	C18.0	C78.5	D01.0	D12.0	D37.4	D49.0
cecum	C18.0	C78.5	D01.0	D12.0	D37.4	D49.0
colon	C18.9	C78.5	D01.0	D12.6	D37.4	D49.0
and rectum	C19	C78.5	D01.1	D12.7	D37.5	D49.0
ascending	C18.2	C78.5	D01.0	D12.2	D37.4	D49.0
caput	C18.0	C78.5	D01.0	D12.0	D37.4	D49.0
descending	C18.6	C78.5	D01.0	D12.4	D37.4	D49.0
distal	C18.6	C78.5	D01.0	D12.4	D37.4	D49.0
left	C18.6	C78.5	D01.0	D12.4	D37.4	D49.0
overlapping lesion	C18.8	—	—	—	—	—
pelvic	C18.7	C78.5	D01.0	D12.5	D37.4	D49.0
right	C18.2	C78.5	D01.0	D12.2	D37.4	D49.0
sigmoid (flexure)	C18.7	C78.5	D01.0	D12.5	D37.4	D49.0
transverse	C18.4	C78.5	D01.0	D12.3	D37.4	D49.0
hepatic flexure	C18.3	C78.5	D01.0	D12.3	D37.4	D49.0
ileocecum, ileocecal (coil) (valve)	C18.0	C78.5	D01.0	D12.0	D37.4	D49.0
overlapping lesion	C18.8	—	—	—	—	—
sigmoid flexure (lower) (upper)	C18.7	C78.5	D01.0	D12.5	D37.4	D49.0
splenic flexure	C18.5	C78.5	D01.0	D12.3	D37.4	D49.0
small	C17.9	C78.4	D01.40	D13.30	D37.2	D49.0
duodenum	C17.0	C78.4	D01.49	D13.2	D37.2	D49.0
ileum	C17.2	C78.4	D01.49	D13.39	D37.2	D49.0
jejunum	C17.1	C78.4	D01.49	D13.39	D37.2	D49.0
overlapping lesion	C17.8	—	—	—	—	—
tract NEC	C26.0	C78.89	D01.40	D13.9	D37.8	D49.0
intra-abdominal	C76.2	C79.89	D09.8	D36.7	D48.7	D49.89
intracranial NEC	C71.9	C79.31	—	D33.2	D43.2	D49.6
intrahepatic (bile) duct	C22.1	C78.7	D01.5	D13.4	D37.6	D49.0
intraocular	C69.9-	C79.49	D09.2-	D31.9-	D48.7	D49.89
intraorbital	C69.6-	C79.49	D09.2-	D31.6-	D48.7	D49.89
intrasellar	C75.1	C79.89	D09.3	D35.2	D44.3	D49.7
intrathoracic (cavity) (organs)	C76.1	C79.89	D09.8	D15.9	D48.7	D49.89
specified NEC	C76.1	C79.89	D09.8	D15.7	—	—
iris	C69.4-	C79.49	D09.2-	D31.4-	D48.7	D49.89
ischiorectal (fossa)	C76.3	C79.89	D09.8	D36.7	D48.7	D49.89
ischium	C41.4	C79.51	—	D16.8	D48.0	D49.2
island of Reil	C71.0	C79.31	—	D33.0	D43.0	D49.6
islands or islets of Langerhans	C25.4	C78.89	D01.7	D13.7	D37.8	D49.0
isthmus uteri	C54.0	C79.82	D07.0	D26.1	D39.0	D49.59
jaw	C76.0	C79.89	D09.8	D36.7	D48.7	D49.89
bone	C41.1	C79.51	—	D16.5-	D48.0	D49.2
lower	C41.1	C79.51	—	D16.5-	—	—
upper	C41.0	C79.51	—	D16.4-	—	—
carcinoma (any type) (lower) (upper)	C76.0	C79.89	—	—	—	—
skin — *see also* Neoplasm, skin, face	C44.309	C79.2	D04.39	D23.39	D48.5	D49.2
soft tissues	C03.9	C79.89	D00.03	D10.39	D37.09	D49.0
lower	C03.1	C79.89	D00.03	D10.39	D37.09	D49.0
upper	C03.0	C79.89	D00.03	D10.39	D37.09	D49.0
jejunum	C17.1	C78.4	D01.49	D13.39	D37.2	D49.0

NEOPLASM TABLE

Neoplasm Table	Malignant Primary	Malignant Secondary	Ca In situ	Benign	Uncertain Behavior	Unspecified Behavior
Neoplasm, neoplastic - *continued*						
joint NEC — *see also*						
Neoplasm, bone	C41.9	C79.51	—	D16.9-	D48.0	D49.2
acromioclavicular	C40.0-	C79.51	—	D16.0-	—	—
bursa or synovial membrane — *see* Neoplasm, connective tissue						
costovertebral	C41.3	C79.51	—	D16.7	D48.0	D49.2
sternocostal	C41.3	C79.51	—	D16.7	D48.0	D49.2
temporomandibular	C41.1	C79.51	—	D16.5-	D48.0	D49.2
junction						
anorectal	C21.8	C78.5	D01.3	D12.9	D37.8	D49.0
cardioesophageal	C16.0	C78.89	D00.2	D13.1	D37.1	D49.0
esophagogastric	C16.0	C78.89	D00.2	D13.1	D37.1	D49.0
gastroesophageal	C16.0	C78.89	D00.2	D13.1	D37.1	D49.0
hard and soft palate	C05.9	C79.89	D00.00	D10.39	D37.09	D49.0
ileocecal	C18.0	C78.5	D01.0	D12.0	D37.4	D49.0
pelvirectal	C19	C78.5	D01.1	D12.7	D37.5	D49.0
pelviureteric	C65.-	C79.0-	D09.19	D30.1-	D41.1-	D49.59
rectosigmoid	C19	C78.5	D01.1	D12.7	D37.5	D49.0
squamocolumnar, of cervix	C53.8	C79.82	D06.7	D26.0	D39.0	D49.59
Kaposi's sarcoma — *see* Kaposi's, sarcoma						
kidney (parenchymal)	C64.-	C79.0-	D09.19	D30.0-	D41.0-	D49.51-
calyx	C65.-	C79.0-	D09.19	D30.1-	D41.1-	D49.51-
hilus	C65.-	C79.0-	D09.19	D30.1-	D41.1-	D49.51-
pelvis	C65.-	C79.0-	D09.19	D30.1-	D41.1-	D49.51-
knee NEC	C76.5-	C79.89	D04.7-	D36.7	D48.7	D49.89
labia (skin)	C51.9	C79.82	D07.1	D28.0	D39.8	D49.59
majora	C51.0	C79.82	D07.1	D28.0	D39.8	D49.59
minora	C51.1	C79.82	D07.1	D28.0	D39.8	D49.59
labial — *see also* Neoplasm, lip	C00.9	C79.89	D00.01	D10.0	D37.01	D49.0
sulcus (lower) (upper)	C06.1	C79.89	D00.02	D10.39	D37.09	D49.0
labium (skin)	C51.9	C79.82	D07.1	D28.0	D39.8	D49.59
majus	C51.0	C79.82	D07.1	D28.0	D39.8	D49.59
minus	C51.1	C79.82	D07.1	D28.0	D39.8	D49.59
lacrimal						
canaliculi	C69.5-	C79.49	D09.2-	D31.5-	D48.7	D49.89
duct (nasal)	C69.5-	C79.49	D09.2-	D31.5-	D48.7	D49.89
gland	C69.5-	C79.49	D09.2-	D31.5-	D48.7	D49.89
punctum	C69.5-	C79.49	D09.2-	D31.5-	D48.7	D49.89
sac	C69.5-	C79.49	D09.2-	D31.5-	D48.7	D49.89
Langerhans, islands or islets	C25.4	C78.89	D01.7	D13.7	D37.8	D49.0
laryngopharynx	C13.9	C79.89	D00.08	D10.7	D37.05	D49.0
larynx, laryngeal NEC	C32.9	C78.39	D02.0	D14.1	D38.0	D49.1
aryepiglottic fold	C32.1	C78.39	D02.0	D14.1	D38.0	D49.1
cartilage (arytenoid) (cricoid) (cuneiform) (thyroid)	C32.3	C78.39	D02.0	D14.1	D38.0	D49.1
commissure (anterior) (posterior)	C32.0	C78.39	D02.0	D14.1	D38.0	D49.1
extrinsic NEC	C32.1	C78.39	D02.0	D14.1	D38.0	D49.1
meaning hypopharynx	C13.9	C79.89	D00.08	D10.7	D37.05	D49.0
interarytenoid fold	C32.1	C78.39	D02.0	D14.1	D38.0	D49.1
intrinsic	C32.0	C78.39	D02.0	D14.1	D38.0	D49.1
overlapping lesion	C32.8	—	—	—	—	—
ventricular band	C32.1	C78.39	D02.0	D14.1	D38.0	D49.1
leg NEC	C76.5-	C79.89	D04.7-	D36.7	D48.7	D49.89
lens, crystalline	C69.4-	C79.49	D09.2-	D31.4-	D48.7	D49.89
lid (lower) (upper)	C44.10-	C79.2	D04.1-	D23.1-	D48.5	D49.2
basal cell carcinoma	C44.11-	—	—	—	—	—
specified type NEC	C44.19-	—	—	—	—	—
squamous cell carcinoma	C44.12-	—	—	—	—	—

Neoplasm Table	Malignant Primary	Malignant Secondary	Ca In situ	Benign	Uncertain Behavior	Unspecified Behavior
Neoplasm, neoplastic - *continued*						
ligament — *see also* Neoplasm, connective tissue						
broad	C57.1	C79.82	D07.39	D28.2	D39.8	D49.59
Mackenrodt's	C57.7	C79.82	D07.39	D28.7	D39.8	D49.59
non-uterine — *see* Neoplasm, connective tissue						
round	C57.2	C79.82	—	D28.2	D39.8	D49.59
sacro-uterine	C57.3	C79.82	—	D28.2	D39.8	D49.59
uterine	C57.3	C79.82	—	D28.2	D39.8	D49.59
utero-ovarian	C57.7	C79.82	D07.39	D28.2	D39.8	D49.59
uterosacral	C57.3	C79.82	—	D28.2	D39.8	D49.59
limb	C76.8	C79.89	D04.8	D36.7	D48.7	D49.89
lower	C76.5-	C79.89	D04.7-	D36.7	D48.7	D49.89
upper	C76.4-	C79.89	D04.6-	D36.7	D48.7	D49.89
limbus of cornea	C69.1-	C79.49	D09.2-	D31.1-	D48.7	D49.89
lingual NEC — *see also* Neoplasm, tongue	C02.9	C79.89	D00.07	D10.1	D37.02	D49.0
lingula, lung	C34.1-	C78.0-	D02.2-	D14.3-	D38.1	D49.1
lip	C00.9	C79.89	D00.01	D10.0	D37.01	D49.0
buccal aspect — *see* Neoplasm, lip, internal						
commissure	C00.6	C79.89	D00.01	D10.0	D37.01	D49.0
external	C00.2	C79.89	D00.01	D10.0	D37.01	D49.0
lower	C00.1	C79.89	D00.01	D10.0	D37.01	D49.0
upper	C00.0	C79.89	D00.01	D10.0	D37.01	D49.0
frenulum — *see* Neoplasm, lip, internal						
inner aspect — *see* Neoplasm, lip, internal						
internal	C00.5	C79.89	D00.01	D10.0	D37.01	D49.0
lower	C00.4	C79.89	D00.01	D10.0	D37.01	D49.0
upper	C00.3	C79.89	D00.01	D10.0	D37.01	D49.0
lipstick area	C00.2	C79.89	D00.01	D10.0	D37.01	D49.0
lower	C00.1	C79.89	D00.01	D10.0	D37.01	D49.0
upper	C00.0	C79.89	D00.01	D10.0	D37.01	D49.0
lower	C00.1	C79.89	D00.01	D10.0	D37.01	D49.0
internal	C00.4	C79.89	D00.01	D10.0	D37.01	D49.0
mucosa — *see* Neoplasm, lip, internal						
oral aspect — *see* Neoplasm, lip, internal						
overlapping lesion	C00.8	—	—	—	—	—
with oral cavity or pharynx	C14.8	—	—	—	—	—
skin (commissure) (lower) (upper)	C44.00	C79.2	D04.0	D23.0	D48.5	D49.2
basal cell carcinoma	C44.01	—	—	—	—	—
specified type NEC	C44.09	—	—	—	—	—
squamous cell carcinoma	C44.02	—	—	—	—	—
upper	C00.0	C79.89	D00.01	D10.0	D37.01	D49.0
internal	C00.3	C79.89	D00.01	D10.0	D37.01	D49.0
vermilion border	C00.2	C79.89	D00.01	D10.0	D37.01	D49.0
lower	C00.1	C79.89	D00.01	D10.0	D37.01	D49.0
upper	C00.0	C79.89	D00.01	D10.0	D37.01	D49.0
lipomatous — *see* Lipoma, by site						
liver — *see also* Index to disease, by histology	C22.9	C78.7	D01.5	D13.4	D37.6	D49.0
primary ICD-10-CM	C22.8	C78.7	D01.5	D13.4	D37.6	D49.0

NEOPLASM TABLE

Neoplasm Table	Malignant Primary	Malignant Secondary	Ca In situ	Benign	Uncertain Behavior	Unspecified Behavior
Neoplasm, neoplastic - *continued*						
lumbosacral plexus	C47.5	C79.89	—	D36.16	D48.2	D49.2
lung	C34.9-	C78.0-	D02.2-	D14.3-	D38.1	D49.1
azygos lobe	C34.1-	C78.0-	D02.2-	D14.3-	D38.1	D49.1
carina	C34.0-	C78.0-	D02.2-	D14.3-	D38.1	D49.1
hilus	C34.0-	C78.0-	D02.2-	D14.3-	D38.1	D49.1
lingula	C34.1-	C78.0-	D02.2-	D14.3-	D38.1	D49.1
lobe NEC	C34.9-	C78.0-	D02.2-	D14.3-	D38.1	D49.1
lower lobe	C34.3-	C78.0-	D02.2-	D14.3-	D38.1	D49.1
main bronchus	C34.0-	C78.0-	D02.2-	D14.3-	D38.1	D49.1
mesothelioma — *see* Mesothelioma						
middle lobe	C34.2	C78.0-	D02.21	D14.31	D38.1	D49.1
overlapping lesion	C34.8-	—	—	—	—	—
upper lobe	C34.1-	C78.0-	D02.2-	D14.3-	D38.1	D49.1
lymph, lymphatic channel						
NEC	C49.9	C79.89	—	D21.9	D48.1	D49.2
gland (secondary)	—	C77.9	—	D36.0	D48.7	D49.89
abdominal	—	C77.2	—	D36.0	D48.7	D49.89
aortic	—	C77.2	—	D36.0	D48.7	D49.89
arm	—	C77.3	—	D36.0	D48.7	D49.89
auricular (anterior) (posterior)	—	C77.0	—	D36.0	D48.7	D49.89
axilla, axillary	—	C77.3	—	D36.0	D48.7	D49.89
brachial	—	C77.3	—	D36.0	D48.7	D49.89
bronchial	—	C77.1	—	D36.0	D48.7	D49.89
bronchopulmonary	—	C77.1	—	D36.0	D48.7	D49.89
celiac	—	C77.2	—	D36.0	D48.7	D49.89
cervical	—	C77.0	—	D36.0	D48.7	D49.89
cervicofacial	—	C77.0	—	D36.0	D48.7	D49.89
Cloquet	—	C77.4	—	D36.0	D48.7	D49.89
colic	—	C77.2	—	D36.0	D48.7	D49.89
common duct	—	C77.2	—	D36.0	D48.7	D49.89
cubital	—	C77.3	—	D36.0	D48.7	D49.89
diaphragmatic	—	C77.1	—	D36.0	D48.7	D49.89
epigastric, inferior	—	C77.1	—	D36.0	D48.7	D49.89
epitrochlear	—	C77.3	—	D36.0	D48.7	D49.89
esophageal	—	C77.1	—	D36.0	D48.7	D49.89
face	—	C77.0	—	D36.0	D48.7	D49.89
femoral	—	C77.4	—	D36.0	D48.7	D49.89
gastric	—	C77.2	—	D36.0	D48.7	D49.89
groin	—	C77.4	—	D36.0	D48.7	D49.89
head	—	C77.0	—	D36.0	D48.7	D49.89
hepatic	—	C77.2	—	D36.0	D48.7	D49.89
hilar (pulmonary)	—	C77.1	—	D36.0	D48.7	D49.89
splenic	—	C77.2	—	D36.0	D48.7	D49.89
hypogastric	—	C77.5	—	D36.0	D48.7	D49.89
ileocolic	—	C77.2	—	D36.0	D48.7	D49.89
iliac	—	C77.5	—	D36.0	D48.7	D49.89
infraclavicular	—	C77.3	—	D36.0	D48.7	D49.89
inguina, inguinal	—	C77.4	—	D36.0	D48.7	D49.89
innominate	—	C77.1	—	D36.0	D48.7	D49.89
intercostal	—	C77.1	—	D36.0	D48.7	D49.89
intestinal	—	C77.2	—	D36.0	D48.7	D49.89
intrabdominal	—	C77.2	—	D36.0	D48.7	D49.89
intrapelvic	—	C77.5	—	D36.0	D48.7	D49.89
intrathoracic	—	C77.1	—	D36.0	D48.7	D49.89
jugular	—	C77.0	—	D36.0	D48.7	D49.89
leg	—	C77.4	—	D36.0	D48.7	D49.89
limb						
lower	—	C77.4	—	D36.0	D48.7	D49.89
upper	—	C77.3	—	D36.0	D48.7	D49.89
lower limb	—	C77.4	—	D36.0	D48.7	D49.89
Neoplasm, neoplastic - *continued*						
lymph, lymphatic channel						
NEC - *continued*	C49.9	C79.89	—	D21.9	D48.1	D49.2
gland (secondary) - *continued*	—	C77.9	—	D36.0	D48.7	D49.89
lumbar	—	C77.2	—	D36.0	D48.7	D49.89
mandibular	—	C77.0	—	D36.0	D48.7	D49.89
mediastinal	—	C77.1	—	D36.0	D48.7	D49.89
mesenteric (inferior) (superior)	—	C77.2	—	D36.0	D48.7	D49.89
midcolic	—	C77.2	—	D36.0	D48.7	D49.89
multiple sites in categories C77.0-C77.5	—	C77.8	—	D36.0	D48.7	D49.89
neck	—	C77.0	—	D36.0	D48.7	D49.89
obturator	—	C77.5	—	D36.0	D48.7	D49.89
occipital	—	C77.0	—	D36.0	D48.7	D49.89
pancreatic	—	C77.2	—	D36.0	D48.7	D49.89
para-aortic	—	C77.2	—	D36.0	D48.7	D49.89
paracervical	—	C77.5	—	D36.0	D48.7	D49.89
parametrial	—	C77.5	—	D36.0	D48.7	D49.89
parasternal	—	C77.1	—	D36.0	D48.7	D49.89
parotid	—	C77.0	—	D36.0	D48.7	D49.89
pectoral	—	C77.3	—	D36.0	D48.7	D49.89
pelvic	—	C77.5	—	D36.0	D48.7	D49.89
peri-aortic	—	C77.2	—	D36.0	D48.7	D49.89
peripancreatic	—	C77.2	—	D36.0	D48.7	D49.89
popliteal	—	C77.4	—	D36.0	D48.7	D49.89
porta hepatis	—	C77.2	—	D36.0	D48.7	D49.89
portal	—	C77.2	—	D36.0	D48.7	D49.89
preauricular	—	C77.0	—	D36.0	D48.7	D49.89
prelaryngeal	—	C77.0	—	D36.0	D48.7	D49.89
presymphysial	—	C77.5	—	D36.0	D48.7	D49.89
pretracheal	—	C77.0	—	D36.0	D48.7	D49.89
primary (any site) NEC	C96.9	—	—	—	—	—
pulmonary (hiler)	—	C77.1	—	D36.0	D48.7	D49.89
pyloric	—	C77.2	—	D36.0	D48.7	D49.89
retroperitoneal	—	C77.2	—	D36.0	D48.7	D49.89
retropharyngeal	—	C77.0	—	D36.0	D48.7	D49.89
Rosenmüller's	—	C77.4	—	D36.0	D48.7	D49.89
sacral	—	C77.5	—	D36.0	D48.7	D49.89
scalene	—	C77.0	—	D36.0	D48.7	D49.89
site NEC	—	C77.9	—	D36.0	D48.7	D49.89
splenic (hilar)	—	C77.2	—	D36.0	D48.7	D49.89
subclavicular	—	C77.3	—	D36.0	D48.7	D49.89
subinguinal	—	C77.4	—	D36.0	D48.7	D49.89
sublingual	—	C77.0	—	D36.0	D48.7	D49.89
submandibular	—	C77.0	—	D36.0	D48.7	D49.89
submaxillary	—	C77.0	—	D36.0	D48.7	D49.89
submental	—	C77.0	—	D36.0	D48.7	D49.89
subscapular	—	C77.3	—	D36.0	D48.7	D49.89
supraclavicular	—	C77.0	—	D36.0	D48.7	D49.89
thoracic	—	C77.1	—	D36.0	D48.7	D49.89
tibial	—	C77.4	—	D36.0	D48.7	D49.89
tracheal	—	C77.1	—	D36.0	D48.7	D49.89
tracheobronchial	—	C77.1	—	D36.0	D48.7	D49.89
upper limb	—	C77.3	—	D36.0	D48.7	D49.89
Virchow's	—	C77.0	—	D36.0	D48.7	D49.89
node — *see also* Neoplasm, lymph gland						
primary NEC	C96.9	—	—	—	—	—
vessel — *see also* Neoplasm, connective tissue	C49.9	C79.89	—	D21.9	D48.1	D49.2

Neoplasm Table	Malignant Primary	Malignant Secondary	Ca In situ	Benign	Uncertain Behavior	Unspecified Behavior
Neoplasm, neoplastic - *continued*						
Mackenrodt's ligament	C57.7	C79.82	D07.39	D28.7	D39.8	D49.59
malar	C41.0	C79.51	—	D16.4-	D48.0	D49.2
region — *see* Neoplasm, cheek						
mammary gland — *see* Neoplasm, breast						
mandible	C41.1	C79.51	—	D16.5-	D48.0	D49.2
alveolar						
mucosa (carcinoma)	C03.1	C79.89	D00.03	D10.39	D37.09	D49.0
ridge or process	C41.1	C79.51	—	D16.5-	D48.0	D49.2
marrow (bone) NEC	C96.9	C79.52	—	—	D47.9	D49.89
mastectomy site (skin) — *see also* Neoplasm, breast, skin	C44.501	C79.2	—	—	—	—
specified as breast tissue	C50.8	C79.81	—	—	—	—
mastoid (air cells) (antrum) (cavity)	C30.1	C78.39	D02.3	D14.0	D38.5	D49.1
bone or process	C41.0	C79.51	—	D16.4-	D48.0	D49.2
maxilla, maxillary (superior)	C41.0	C79.51	—	D16.4-	D48.0	D49.2
alveolar						
mucosa	C03.0	C79.89	D00.03	D10.39	D37.09	D49.0
ridge or process (carcinoma)	C41.0	C79.51	—	D16.4-	D48.0	D49.2
antrum	C31.0	C78.39	D02.3	D14.0	D38.5	D49.1
carcinoma	C03.0	C79.51	—	—	—	—
inferior — *see* Neoplasm, mandible						
sinus	C31.0	C78.39	D02.3	D14.0	D38.5	D49.1
meatus external (ear) — *see also* Neoplasm, skin, ear	C44.20-	C79.2	D04.2-	D23.2-	D48.5	D49.2
Meckel diverticulum, malignant	C17.3	C78.4	D01.49	D13.39	D37.2	D49.0
mediastinum, mediastinal	C38.3	C78.1	—	D15.2	D38.3	D49.89
anterior	C38.1	C78.1	—	D15.2	D38.3	D49.89
posterior	C38.2	C78.1	—	D15.2	D38.3	D49.89
medulla						
adrenal	C74.1-	C79.7-	D09.3	D35.0-	D44.1-	D49.7
oblongata	C71.7	C79.31	—	D33.1	D43.1	D49.6
meibomian gland	C44.10-	C79.2	D04.1-	D23.1-	D48.5	D49.2
basal cell carcinoma	C44.11-	—	—	—	—	—
specified type NEC	C44.19-	—	—	—	—	—
squamous cell carcinoma	C44.12-	—	—	—	—	—
melanoma — *see* Melanoma						
meninges	C70.9	C79.49	—	D32.9	D42.9	D49.7
brain	C70.0	C79.32	—	D32.0	D42.0	D49.7
cerebral	C70.0	C79.32	—	D32.0	D42.0	D49.7
crainial	C70.0	C79.32	—	D32.0	D42.0	D49.7
intracranial	C70.0	C79.32	—	D32.0	D42.0	D49.7
spinal (cord)	C70.1	C79.49	—	D32.1	D42.1	D49.7
meniscus, knee joint (lateral) (medial)	C40.2-	C79.51	—	D16.2-	D48.0	D49.2
Merkel cell — *see* Carcinoma, Merkel cell						
mesentery, mesenteric	C48.1	C78.6	—	D20.1	D48.4	D49.0
mesoappendix	C48.1	C78.6	—	D20.1	D48.4	D49.0
mesocolon	C48.1	C78.6	—	D20.1	D48.4	D49.0
mesopharynx — *see* Neoplasm, oropharynx						
mesosalpinx	C57.1	C79.82	D07.39	D28.2	D39.8	D49.59

Neoplasm Table	Malignant Primary	Malignant Secondary	Ca In situ	Benign	Uncertain Behavior	Unspecified Behavior
Neoplasm, neoplastic - *continued*						
mesothelial tissue — *see* Mesothelioma						
mesothelioma — *see* Mesothelioma						
mesovarium	C57.1	C79.82	D07.39	D28.2	D39.8	D49.59
metacarpus (any bone)	C40.1-	C79.51	—	D16.1-	—	—
metastatic NEC — *see also* Neoplasm, by site, secondary	—	C79.9	—	—	—	—
metatarsus (any bone)	C40.3-	C79.51	—	D16.3-	—	—
midbrain	C71.7	C79.31	—	D33.1	D43.1	D49.6
milk duct — *see* Neoplasm, breast						
mons						
pubis	C51.9	C79.82	D07.1	D28.0	D39.8	D49.59
veneris	C51.9	C79.82	D07.1	D28.0	D39.8	D49.59
motor tract	C72.9	C79.49	—	D33.9	D43.9	D49.7
brain	C71.9	C79.31	—	D33.2	D43.2	D49.6
cauda equina	C72.1	C79.49	—	D33.4	D43.4	D49.7
spinal	C72.0	C79.49	—	D33.4	D43.4	D49.7
mouth	C06.9	C79.89	D00.00	D10.30	D37.09	D49.0
book-leaf	C06.89	C79.89				
floor	C04.9	C79.89	D00.06	D10.2	D37.09	D49.0
anterior portion	C04.0	C79.89	D00.06	D10.2	D37.09	D49.0
lateral portion	C04.1	C79.89	D00.06	D10.2	D37.09	D49.0
overlapping lesion	C04.8	—	—	—	—	—
overlapping NEC	C06.80	—	—	—	—	—
roof	C05.9	C79.89	D00.00	D10.39	D37.09	D49.0
specified part NEC	C06.89	C79.89	D00.00	D10.39	D37.09	D49.0
vestibule	C06.1	C79.89	D00.00	D10.39	D37.09	D49.0
mucosa						
alveolar (ridge or process)	C03.9	C79.89	D00.03	D10.39	D37.09	D49.0
lower	C03.1	C79.89	D00.03	D10.39	D37.09	D49.0
upper	C03.0	C79.89	D00.03	D10.39	D37.09	D49.0
buccal	C06.0	C79.89	D00.02	D10.39	D37.09	D49.0
cheek	C06.0	C79.89	D00.02	D10.39	D37.09	D49.0
lip — *see* Neoplasm, lip, internal						
nasal	C30.0	C78.39	D02.3	D14.0	D38.5	D49.1
oral	C06.0	C79.89	D00.02	D10.39	D37.09	D49.0
Müllerian duct						
female	C57.7	C79.82	D07.39	D28.7	D39.8	D49.59
male	C63.7	C79.82	D07.69	D29.8	D40.8	D49.59
muscle — *see also* Neoplasm, connective tissue						
extraocular	C69.6-	C79.49	D09.2-	D31.6-	D48.7	D49.89
myocardium	C38.0	C79.89	—	D15.1	D48.7	D49.89
myometrium	C54.2	C79.82	D07.0	D26.1	D39.0	D49.59
myopericardium	C38.0	C79.89	—	D15.1	D48.7	D49.89
nabothian gland (follicle)	C53.0	C79.82	D06.0	D26.0	D39.0	D49.59
nail — *see also* Neoplasm, skin, limb	C44.90	C79.2	D04.9	D23.9	D48.5	D49.2
finger — *see also* Neoplasm, skin, limb, upper	C44.60-	C79.2	D04.6-	D23.6-	D48.5	D49.2
toe — *see also* Neoplasm, skin, limb, lower	C44.70-	C79.2	D04.7-	D23.7-	D48.5	D49.2
nares, naris (anterior) (posterior)	C30.0	C78.39	D02.3	D14.0	D38.5	D49.1

NEOPLASM TABLE

NEOPLASM TABLE

Neoplasm, neoplastic - continued

Neoplasm Table	Malignant Primary	Malignant Secondary	Ca In situ	Benign	Uncertain Behavior	Unspecified Behavior
nasal — see Neoplasm, nose						
nasolabial groove — see also Neoplasm, skin, face	C44.309	C79.2	D04.39	D23.39	D48.5	D49.2
nasolacrimal duct	C69.5-	C79.49	D09.2-	D31.5-	D48.7	D49.89
nasopharynx, nasopharyngeal	C11.9	C79.89	D00.08	D10.6	D37.05	D49.0
floor	C11.3	C79.89	D00.08	D10.6	D37.05	D49.0
overlapping lesion	C11.8	—	—	—	—	—
roof	C11.0	C79.89	D00.08	D10.6	D37.05	D49.0
wall	C11.9	C79.89	D00.08	D10.6	D37.05	D49.0
anterior	C11.3	C79.89	D00.08	D10.6	D37.05	D49.0
lateral	C11.2	C79.89	D00.08	D10.6	D37.05	D49.0
posterior	C11.1	C79.89	D00.08	D10.6	D37.05	D49.0
superior	C11.0	C79.89	D00.08	D10.6	D37.05	D49.0
nates — see also Neoplasm, skin, trunk	C44.509	C79.2	D04.5	D23.5	D48.5	D49.2
neck NEC	C76.0	C79.89	D09.8	D36.7	D48.7	D49.89
skin	C44.40	—	—	—	—	—
basal cell carcinoma	C44.41	—	—	—	—	—
specified type NEC	C44.49	—	—	—	—	—
squamous cell carcinoma	C44.42	—	—	—	—	—
nerve (ganglion)	C47.9	C79.89	—	D36.10	D48.2	D49.2
abducens	C72.59	C79.49	—	D33.3	D43.3	D49.7
accessory (spinal)	C72.59	C79.49	—	D33.3	D43.3	D49.7
acoustic	C72.4-	C79.49	—	D33.3	D43.3	D49.7
auditory	C72.4-	C79.49	—	D33.3	D43.3	D49.7
autonomic NEC — see also Neoplasm, nerve, peripheral	C47.9	C79.89	—	D36.10	D48.2	D49.2
brachial	C47.1-	C79.89	—	D36.12	D48.2	D49.2
cranial	C72.50	C79.49	—	D33.3	D43.3	D49.7
specified NEC	C72.59	C79.49	—	D33.3	D43.3	D49.7
facial	C72.59	C79.49	—	D33.3	D43.3	D49.7
femoral	C47.2-	C79.89	—	D36.13	D48.2	D49.2
ganglion NEC — see also Neoplasm, nerve, peripheral	C47.9	C79.89	—	D36.10	D48.2	D49.2
glossopharyngeal	C72.59	C79.49	—	D33.3	D43.3	D49.7
hypoglossal	C72.59	C79.49	—	D33.3	D43.3	D49.7
intercostal	C47.3	C79.89	—	D36.14	D48.2	D49.2
lumbar	C47.6	C79.89	—	D36.17	D48.2	D49.2
median	C47.1-	C79.89	—	D36.12	D48.2	D49.2
obturator	C47.2-	C79.89	—	D36.13	D48.2	D49.2
oculomotor	C72.59	C79.49	—	D33.3	D43.3	D49.7
olfactory	C47.2-	C79.49	—	D33.3	D43.3	D49.7
optic	C72.3-	C79.49	—	D33.3	D43.3	D49.7
parasympathetic NEC	C47.9	C79.89	—	D36.10	D48.2	D49.2
peripheral NEC	C47.9	C79.89	—	D36.10	D48.2	D49.2
abdomen	C47.4	C79.89	—	D36.15	D48.2	D49.2
abdominal wall	C47.4	C79.89	—	D36.15	D48.2	D49.2
ankle	C47.2-	C79.89	—	D36.13	D48.2	D49.2
antecubital fossa or space	C47.1-	C79.89	—	D36.12	D48.2	D49.2
arm	C47.1-	C79.89	—	D36.12	D48.2	D49.2
auricle (ear)	C47.0	C79.89	—	D36.11	D48.2	D49.2
axilla	C47.3	C79.89	—	D36.12	D48.2	D49.2
back	C47.6	C79.89	—	D36.17	D48.2	D49.2
buttock	C47.5	C79.89	—	D36.16	D48.2	D49.2
calf	C47.2-	C79.89	—	D36.13	D48.2	D49.2
cervical region	C47.0	C79.89	—	D36.11	D48.2	D49.2
cheek	C47.0	C79.89	—	D36.11	D48.2	D49.2
chest (wall)	C47.3	C79.89	—	D36.14	D48.2	D49.2
chin	C47.0	C79.89	—	D36.11	D48.2	D49.2
ear (external)	C47.0	C79.89	—	D36.11	D48.2	D49.2
elbow	C47.1-	C79.89	—	D36.12	D48.2	D49.2

Neoplasm, neoplastic - continued

Neoplasm Table	Malignant Primary	Malignant Secondary	Ca In situ	Benign	Uncertain Behavior	Unspecified Behavior
nerve (ganglion) - continued	C47.9	C79.89	—	D36.10	D48.2	D49.2
peripheral NEC - continued	C47.9	C79.89	—	D36.10	D48.2	D49.2
extrarectal	C47.5	C79.89	—	D36.16	D48.2	D49.2
extremity	C47.9	C79.89	—	D36.10	D48.2	D49.2
lower	C47.2-	C79.89	—	D36.13	D48.2	D49.2
upper	C47.1-	C79.89	—	D36.12	D48.2	D49.2
eyelid	C47.0	C79.89	—	D36.11	D48.2	D49.2
face	C47.0	C79.89	—	D36.11	D48.2	D49.2
finger	C47.1-	C79.89	—	D36.12	D48.2	D49.2
flank	C47.6	C79.89	—	D36.17	D48.2	D49.2
foot	C47.2-	C79.89	—	D36.13	D48.2	D49.2
forearm	C47.1-	C79.89	—	D36.12	D48.2	D49.2
forehead	C47.0	C79.89	—	D36.11	D48.2	D49.2
gluteal region	C47.5	C79.89	—	D36.16	D48.2	D49.2
groin	C47.5	C79.89	—	D36.16	D48.2	D49.2
hand	C47.1-	C79.89	—	D36.12	D48.2	D49.2
head	C47.0	C79.89	—	D36.11	D48.2	D49.2
heel	C47.2-	C79.89	—	D36.13	D48.2	D49.2
hip	C47.2-	C79.89	—	D36.13	D48.2	D49.2
infraclavicular region	C47.3	C79.89	—	D36.14	D48.2	D49.2
inguinal (canal) (region)	C47.5	C79.89	—	D36.16	D48.2	D49.2
intrathoracic	C47.3	C79.89	—	D36.14	D48.2	D49.2
ischiorectal fossa	C47.5	C79.89	—	D36.16	D48.2	D49.2
knee	C47.2-	C79.89	—	D36.13	D48.2	D49.2
leg	C47.2-	C79.89	—	D36.13	D48.2	D49.2
limb NEC	C47.9	C79.89	—	D36.10	D48.2	D49.2
lower	C47.2	C79.89	—	D36.13	D48.2	D49.2
upper	C47.1	C79.89	—	D36.12	D48.2	D49.2
nates	C47.5	C79.89	—	D36.16	D48.2	D49.2
neck	C47.0	C79.89	—	D36.11	D48.2	D49.2
orbit	C69.6-	C79.49	—	D31.6-	D48.7	D49.2
pararectal	C47.5	C79.89	—	D36.16	D48.2	D49.2
paraurethral	C47.5	C79.89	—	D36.16	D48.2	D49.2
paravaginal	C47.5	C79.89	—	D36.16	D48.2	D49.2
pelvis (floor)	C47.5	C79.89	—	D36.16	D48.2	D49.2
pelvoabdominal	C47.8	C79.89	—	D36.17	D48.2	D49.2
perineum	C47.5	C79.89	—	D36.16	D48.2	D49.2
perirectal (tissue)	C47.5	C79.89	—	D36.16	D48.2	D49.2
periurethral (tissue)	C47.5	C79.89	—	D36.16	D48.2	D49.2
popliteal fossa or space	C47.2-	C79.89	—	D36.13	D48.2	D49.2
presacral	C47.5	C79.89	—	D36.16	D48.2	D49.2
pterygoid fossa	C47.0	C79.89	—	D36.11	D48.2	D49.2
rectovaginal septum or wall	C47.5	C79.89	—	D36.16	D48.2	D49.2
rectovesical	C47.5	C79.89	—	D36.16	D48.2	D49.2
sacrococcygeal region	C47.5	C79.89	—	D36.16	D48.2	D49.2
scalp	C47.0	C79.89	—	D36.11	D48.2	D49.2
scapular region	C47.3	C79.89	—	D36.14	D48.2	D49.2
shoulder	C47.1-	C79.89	—	D36.12	D48.2	D49.2
submental	C47.0	C79.89	—	D36.11	D48.2	D49.2
supraclavicular region	C47.0	C79.89	—	D36.11	D48.2	D49.2
temple	C47.0	C79.89	—	D36.11	D48.2	D49.2
temporal region	C47.0	C79.89	—	D36.11	D48.2	D49.2
thigh	C47.2-	C79.89	—	D36.13	D48.2	D49.2
thoracic (duct) (wall)	C47.3	C79.89	—	D36.14	D48.2	D49.2
thorax	C47.3	C79.89	—	D36.14	D48.2	D49.2
thumb	C47.1-	C79.89	—	D36.12	D48.2	D49.2
toe	C47.2-	C79.89	—	D36.13	D48.2	D49.2
trunk	C47.6	C79.89	—	D36.17	D48.2	D49.2
umbilicus	C47.4	C79.89	—	D36.15	D48.2	D49.2
vesicorectal	C47.5	C79.89	—	D36.16	D48.2	D49.2
wrist	C47.1-	C79.89	—	D36.12	D48.2	D49.2

NEOPLASM TABLE

Neoplasm Table	Malignant Primary	Malignant Secondary	Ca In situ	Benign	Uncertain Behavior	Unspecified Behavior
Neoplasm, neoplastic - *continued*						
nerve (ganglion) - *continued* ..	C47.9	C79.89	—	D36.10	D48.2	D49.2
radial	C47.1-	C79.89	—	D36.12	D48.2	D49.2
sacral	C47.5	C79.89	—	D36.16	D48.2	D49.2
sciatic	C47.2-	C79.89	—	D36.13	D48.2	D49.2
spinal NEC	C47.9	C79.89	—	D36.10	D48.2	D49.2
accessory	C72.59	C79.49	—	D33.3	D43.3	D49.7
sympathetic NEC — *see also* Neoplasm, nerve, peripheral	C47.9	C79.89	—	D36.10	D48.2	D49.2
trigeminal	C72.59	C79.49	—	D33.3	D43.3	D49.7
trochlear	C72.59	C79.49	—	D33.3	D43.3	D49.7
ulnar	C47.1-	C79.89	—	D36.12	D48.2	D49.2
vagus	C72.59	C79.49	—	D33.3	D43.3	D49.7
nervous system (central)	C72.9	C79.40	—	D33.9	D43.9	D49.7
autonomic — *see* Neoplasm, nerve, peripheral						
parasympathetic — *see* Neoplasm, nerve, peripheral						
specified site NEC	—	C79.49	—	D33.7	D43.8	—
sympathetic — *see* Neoplasm, nerve, peripheral						
nevus — *see* Nevus						
nipple	C50.0-	C79.81	D05.-	D24.-	—	—
nose, nasal	C76.0	C79.89	D09.8	D36.7	D48.7	D49.89
ala (external) (nasi) — *see also* Neoplasm, nose, skin	C44.301	C79.2	D04.39	D23.39	D48.5	D49.2
bone	C41.0	C79.51	—	D16.4-	D48.0	D49.2
cartilage	C30.0	C78.39	D02.3	D14.0	D38.5	D49.1
cavity	C30.0	C78.39	D02.3	D14.0	D38.5	D49.1
choana	C11.3	C79.89	D00.08	D10.6	D37.05	D49.0
external (skin) — *see also* Neoplasm, nose, skin	C44.301	C79.2	D04.39	D23.39	D48.5	D49.2
fossa	C30.0	C78.39	D02.3	D14.0	D38.5	D49.1
internal	C30.0	C78.39	D02.3	D14.0	D38.5	D49.1
mucosa	C30.0	C78.39	D02.3	D14.0	D38.5	D49.1
septum	C30.0	C78.39	D02.3	D14.0	D38.5	D49.1
posterior margin	C11.3	C79.89	D00.08	D10.6	D37.05	D49.0
sinus — *see* Neoplasm, sinus						
skin	C44.301	C79.2	D04.39	D23.39	D48.5	D49.2
basal cell carcinoma	C44.311	—	—	—	—	—
specified type NEC	C44.391	—	—	—	—	—
squamous cell carcinoma	C44.321	—	—	—	—	—
turbinate (mucosa)	C30.0	C78.39	D02.3	D14.0	D38.5	D49.1
bone	C41.0	C79.51	—	D16.4-	D48.0	D49.2
vestibule	C30.0	C78.39	D02.3	D14.0	D38.5	D49.1
nostril	C30.0	C78.39	D02.3	D14.0	D38.5	D49.1
nucleus pulposus	C41.2	C79.51	—	D16.6	D48.0	D49.2
occipital						
bone	C41.0	C79.51	—	D16.4-	D48.0	D49.2
lobe or pole, brain	C71.4	C79.31	—	D33.0	D43.0	D49.6
odontogenic — *see* Neoplasm, jaw bone						
olfactory nerve or bulb	C72.2-	C79.49	—	D33.3	D43.3	D49.7
olive (brain)	C71.7	C79.31	—	D33.1	D43.1	D49.6
omentum	C48.1	C78.6	—	D20.1	D48.4	D49.0

Neoplasm Table	Malignant Primary	Malignant Secondary	Ca In situ	Benign	Uncertain Behavior	Unspecified Behavior
Neoplasm, neoplastic - *continued*						
operculum (brain)	C71.0	C79.31	—	D33.0	D43.0	D49.6
optic nerve, chiasm, or tract	C72.3-	C79.49	—	D33.3	D43.3	D49.7
oral (cavity)	C06.9	C79.89	D00.00	D10.30	D37.09	D49.0
ill-defined	C14.8	C79.89	D00.00	D10.30	D37.09	D49.0
mucosa	C06.0	C79.89	D00.02	D10.39	D37.09	D49.0
orbit	C69.6-	C79.49	D09.2-	D31.6-	D48.7	D49.89
autonomic nerve	C69.6-	C79.49	—	D31.6-	D48.7	D49.2
bone	C41.0	C79.51	—	D16.4-	D48.0	D49.2
eye	C69.6-	C79.49	D09.2-	D31.6-	D48.7	D49.89
peripheral nerves	C69.6-	C79.49	—	D31.6-	D48.7	D49.2
soft parts	C69.6-	C79.49	D09.2-	D31.6-	D48.7	D49.89
organ of Zuckerkandl	C75.5	C79.89	—	D35.6	D44.7	D49.7
oropharynx	C10.9	C79.89	D00.08	D10.5	D37.05	D49.0
branchial cleft (vestige)	C10.4	C79.89	D00.08	D10.5	D37.05	D49.0
junctional region	C10.8	C79.89	D00.08	D10.5	D37.05	D49.0
lateral wall	C10.2	C79.89	D00.08	D10.5	D37.05	D49.0
overlapping lesion	C10.8	—	—	—	—	—
pillars or fauces	C09.1	C79.89	D00.08	D10.5	D37.05	D49.0
posterior wall	C10.3	C79.89	D00.08	D10.5	D37.05	D49.0
vallecula	C10.0	C79.89	D00.08	D10.5	D37.05	D49.0
os						
external	C53.1	C79.82	D06.1	D26.0	D39.0	D49.59
internal	C53.0	C79.82	D06.0	D26.0	D39.0	D49.59
ovary	C56.-	C79.6-	D07.39	D27.-	D39.1-	D49.59
oviduct	C57.0-	C79.82	D07.39	D28.2	D39.8	D49.59
palate	C05.9	C79.89	D00.00	D10.39	D37.09	D49.0
hard	C05.0	C79.89	D00.05	D10.39	D37.09	D49.0
junction of hard and soft palate	C05.9	C79.89	D00.00	D10.39	D37.09	D49.0
overlapping lesions	C05.8	—	—	—	—	—
soft	C05.1	C79.89	D00.04	D10.39	D37.09	D49.0
nasopharyngeal surface	C11.3	C79.89	D00.08	D10.6	D37.05	D49.0
posterior surface	C11.3	C79.89	D00.08	D10.6	D37.05	D49.0
superior surface	C11.3	C79.89	D00.08	D10.6	D37.05	D49.0
palatoglossal arch	C09.1	C79.89	D00.00	D10.5	D37.09	D49.0
palatopharyngeal arch	C09.1	C79.89	D00.00	D10.5	D37.09	D49.0
pallium	C71.0	C79.31	—	D33.0	D43.0	D49.6
palpebra	C44.10-	C79.2	D04.1-	D23.1-	D48.5	D49.2
basal cell carcinoma	C44.11-	—	—	—	—	—
specified type NEC	C44.19-	—	—	—	—	—
squamous cell carcinoma	C44.12-	—	—	—	—	—
pancreas	C25.9	C78.89	D01.7	D13.6	D37.8	D49.0
body	C25.1	C78.89	D01.7	D13.6	D37.8	D49.0
duct (of Santorini) (of Wirsung)	C25.3	C78.89	D01.7	D13.6	D37.8	D49.0
ectopic tissue	C25.7	C78.89	—	D13.6	D37.8	D49.0
head	C25.0	C78.89	D01.7	D13.6	D37.8	D49.0
islet cells	C25.4	C78.89	D01.7	D13.7	D37.8	D49.0
neck	C25.7	C78.89	D01.7	D13.6	D37.8	D49.0
overlapping lesion	C25.8	—	—	—	—	—
tail	C25.2	C78.89	D01.7	D13.6	D37.8	D49.0
para-aortic body	C75.5	C79.89	—	D35.6	D44.7	D49.7
paraganglion NEC	C75.5	C79.89	—	D35.6	D44.7	D49.7
parametrium	C57.3	C79.82	—	D28.2	D39.8	D49.59
paranephric	C48.0	C78.6	—	D20.0	D48.3	D49.0
pararectal	C76.3	C79.89	—	D36.7	D48.7	D49.89
parasagittal (region)	C76.0	C79.89	D09.8	D36.7	D48.7	D49.89
parasellar	C72.9	C79.49	—	D33.9	D43.8	D49.7
parathyroid (gland)	C75.0	C79.89	D09.3	D35.1	D44.2	D49.7
paraurethral	C76.3	C79.89	—	D36.7	D48.7	D49.89
gland	C68.1	C79.19	D09.19	D30.8	D41.8	D49.59

© 2016 Channel Publishing, Ltd.

NEOPLASM TABLE

Neoplasm Table	Malignant Primary	Malignant Secondary	Ca In situ	Benign	Uncertain Behavior	Unspecified Behavior
Neoplasm, neoplastic - *continued*						
paravaginal	C76.3	C79.89	—	D36.7	D48.7	D49.89
parenchyma, kidney	C64.-	C79.0-	D09.19	D30.0-	D41.0-	D49.51-
parietal						
bone	C41.0	C79.51	—	D16.4-	D48.0	D49.2
lobe, brain	C71.3	C79.31	—	D33.0	D43.0	D49.6
paroophoron	C57.1	C79.82	D07.39	D28.2	D39.8	D49.59
parotid (duct) (gland)	C07	C79.89	D00.00	D11.0	D37.030	D49.0
parovarium	C57.1	C79.82	D07.39	D28.2	D39.8	D49.59
patella	C40.20	C79.51	—	—	—	—
peduncle, cerebral	C71.7	C79.31	—	D33.1	D43.1	D49.6
pelvirectal junction	C19	C78.5	D01.1	D12.7	D37.5	D49.0
pelvis, pelvic	C76.3	C79.89	D09.8	D36.7	D48.7	D49.89
bone	C41.4	C79.51	—	D16.8	D48.0	D49.2
floor	C76.3	C79.89	D09.8	D36.7	D48.7	D49.89
renal	C65.-	C79.0-	D09.19	D30.1-	D41.1-	D49.51-
viscera	C76.3	C79.89	D09.8	D36.7	D48.7	D49.89
wall	C76.3	C79.89	D09.8	D36.7	D48.7	D49.89
pelvo-abdominal	C76.8	C79.89	D09.8	D36.7	D48.7	D49.89
penis	C60.9	C79.82	D07.4	D29.0	D40.8	D49.59
body	C60.2	C79.82	D07.4	D29.0	D40.8	D49.59
corpus (cavernosum)	C60.2	C79.82	D07.4	D29.0	D40.8	D49.59
glans	C60.1	C79.82	D07.4	D29.0	D40.8	D49.59
overlapping sites	C60.8	—	—	—	—	—
skin NEC	C60.9	C79.82	D07.4	D29.0	D40.8	D49.59
periadrenal (tissue)	C48.0	C78.6	—	D20.0	D48.3	D49.0
perianal (skin) — *see also*						
Neoplasm, anus, skin	C44.500	C79.2	D04.5	D23.5	D48.5	D49.2
pericardium	C38.0	C79.89	—	D15.1	D48.7	D49.89
perinephric	C48.0	C78.6	—	D20.0	D48.3	D49.0
perineum	C76.3	C79.89	D09.8	D36.7	D48.7	D49.89
periodontal tissue NEC	C03.9	C79.89	D00.03	D10.39	D37.09	D49.0
periosteum — *see Neoplasm, bone*						
peripancreatic	C48.0	C78.6	—	D20.0	D48.3	D49.0
peripheral nerve NEC	C47.9	C79.89	—	D36.10	D48.2	D49.2
perirectal (tissue)	C76.3	C79.89	—	D36.7	D48.7	D49.89
perirenal (tissue)	C48.0	C78.6	—	D20.0	D48.3	D49.0
peritoneum, peritoneal (cavity)	C48.2	C78.6	—	D20.1	D48.4	D49.0
benign mesothelial tissue — *see Mesothelioma, benign*						
overlapping lesion	C48.8	—	—	—	—	—
with digestive organs	C26.9	—	—	—	—	—
parietal	C48.1	C78.6	—	D20.1	D48.4	D49.0
pelvic	C48.1	C78.6	—	D20.1	D48.4	D49.0
specified part NEC	C48.1	C78.6	—	D20.1	D48.4	D49.0
peritonsillar (tissue)	C76.0	C79.89	D09.8	D36.7	D48.7	D49.89
periurethral tissue	C76.3	C79.89	—	D36.7	D48.7	D49.89
phalanges						
foot	C40.3-	C79.51	—	D16.3-	—	—
hand	C40.1-	C79.51	—	D16.1-	—	—
pharynx, pharyngeal	C14.0	C79.89	D00.08	D10.9	D37.05	D49.0
bursa	C11.1	C79.89	D00.08	D10.6	D37.05	D49.0
fornix	C11.3	C79.89	D00.08	D10.6	D37.05	D49.0
recess	C11.2	C79.89	D00.08	D10.6	D37.05	D49.0
region	C14.0	C79.89	D00.08	D10.9	D37.05	D49.0
tonsil	C11.1	C79.89	D00.08	D10.6	D37.05	D49.0
wall (lateral) (posterior)	C14.0	C79.89	D00.08	D10.9	D37.05	D49.0

Neoplasm Table	Malignant Primary	Malignant Secondary	Ca In situ	Benign	Uncertain Behavior	Unspecified Behavior
Neoplasm, neoplastic - *continued*						
pia mater	C70.9	C79.40	—	D32.9	D42.9	D49.7
cerebral	C70.0	C79.32	—	D32.0	D42.0	D49.7
cranial	C70.0	C79.32	—	D32.0	D42.0	D49.7
spinal	C70.1	C79.49	—	D32.1	D42.1	D49.7
pillars of fauces	C09.1	C79.89	D00.08	D10.5	D37.05	D49.0
pineal (body) (gland)	C75.3	C79.89	D09.3	D35.4	D44.5	D49.7
pinna (ear) NEC — *see also*						
Neoplasm, skin, ear	C44.20-	C79.2	D04.2-	D23.2-	D48.5	D49.2
piriform fossa or sinus	C12	C79.89	D00.08	D10.7	D37.05	D49.0
pituitary (body) (fossa) (gland) (lobe)	C75.1	C79.89	D09.3	D35.2	D44.3	D49.7
placenta	C58	C79.82	D07.0	D26.7	D39.2	D49.59
pleura, pleural (cavity)	C38.4	C78.2	—	D19.0	D38.2	D49.1
overlapping lesion with heart or mediastinum	C38.8	—	—	—	—	—
parietal	C38.4	C78.2	—	D19.0	D38.2	D49.1
visceral	C38.4	C78.2	—	D19.0	D38.2	D49.1
plexus						
brachial	C47.1-	C79.89	—	D36.12	D48.2	D49.2
cervical	C47.0	C79.89	—	D36.11	D48.2	D49.2
choroid	C71.5	C79.31	—	D33.0	D43.0	D49.6
lumbosacral	C47.5	C79.89	—	D36.16	D48.2	D49.2
sacral	C47.5	C79.89	—	D36.16	D48.2	D49.2
pluriendocrine	C75.8	C79.89	D09.3	D35.7	D44.9	D49.7
pole						
frontal	C71.1	C79.31	—	D33.0	D43.0	D49.6
occipital	C71.4	C79.31	—	D33.0	D43.0	D49.6
pons (varolii)	C71.7	C79.31	—	D33.1	D43.1	D49.6
popliteal fossa or space	C76.5-	C79.89	D04.7-	D36.7	D48.7	D49.89
postcricoid (region)	C13.0	C79.89	D00.08	D10.7	D37.05	D49.0
posterior fossa (cranial)	C71.9	C79.31	—	D33.2	D43.2	D49.6
postnasal space	C11.9	C79.89	D00.08	D10.6	D37.05	D49.0
prepuce	C60.0	C79.82	D07.4	D29.0	D40.8	D49.59
prepylorus	C16.4	C78.89	D00.2	D13.1	D37.1	D49.0
presacral (region)	C76.3	C79.89	—	D36.7	D48.7	D49.89
prostate (gland)	C61	C79.82	D07.5	D29.1	D40.0	D49.59
utricle	C68.0	C79.19	D09.19	D30.4	D41.3	D49.59
pterygoid fossa	C49.0	C79.89	—	D21.0	D48.1	D49.2
pubic bone	C41.4	C79.51	—	D16.8	D48.0	D49.2
pudenda, pudendum (female)	C51.9	C79.82	D07.1	D28.0	D39.8	D49.59
pulmonary — *see also*						
Neoplasm, lung	C34.9-	C78.0-	D02.2-	D14.3-	D38.1	D49.1
putamen	C71.0	C79.31	—	D33.0	D43.0	D49.6
pyloric						
antrum	C16.3	C78.89	D00.2	D13.1	D37.1	D49.0
canal	C16.4	C78.89	D00.2	D13.1	D37.1	D49.0
pylorus	C16.4	C78.89	D00.2	D13.1	D37.1	D49.0
pyramid (brain)	C71.7	C79.31	—	D33.1	D43.1	D49.6
pyriform fossa or sinus	C12	C79.89	D00.08	D10.7	D37.05	D49.0
radius (any part)	C40.0-	C79.51	—	D16.0-	—	—
Rathke's pouch	C75.1	C79.89	D09.3	D35.2	D44.3	D49.7
rectosigmoid (junction)	C19	C78.5	D01.1	D12.7	D37.5	D49.0
overlapping lesion with anus or rectum	C21.8	—	—	—	—	—
rectouterine pouch	C48.1	C78.6	—	D20.1	D48.4	D49.0
rectovaginal septum or wall	C76.3	C79.89	D09.8	D36.7	D48.7	D49.89
rectovesical septum	C76.3	C79.89	D09.8	D36.7	D48.7	D49.89

NEOPLASM TABLE

Neoplasm Table	Malignant Primary	Malignant Secondary	Ca In situ	Benign	Uncertain Behavior	Unspecified Behavior
Neoplasm, neoplastic - *continued*						
rectum (ampulla)	C20	C78.5	D01.2	D12.8	D37.5	D49.0
and colon	C19	C78.5	D01.1	D12.7	D37.5	D49.0
overlapping lesion with anus or rectosigmoid junction	C21.8	—	—	—	—	—
renal	C64.-	C79.0-	D09.19	D30.0-	D41.0-	D49.51-
calyx	C65.-	C79.0-	D09.19	D30.1-	D41.1-	D49.51-
hilus	C65.-	C79.0-	D09.19	D30.1-	D41.1-	D49.51-
parenchyma	C64.-	C79.0-	D09.19	D30.0-	D41.0-	D49.51-
pelvis	C65.-	C79.0-	D09.19	D30.1-	D41.1-	D49.51-
respiratory						
organs or system NEC	C39.9	C78.30	D02.4	D14.4	D38.6	D49.1
tract NEC	C39.9	C78.30	D02.4	D14.4	D38.5	D49.1
upper	C39.0	C78.30	D02.4	D14.4	D38.5	D49.1
retina	C69.2-	C79.49	D09.2-	D31.2-	D48.7	D49.81
retrobulbar	C69.6-	C79.49	—	D31.6-	D48.7	D49.89
retrocecal	C48.0	C78.6	—	D20.0	D48.3	D49.0
retromolar (area) (triangle) (trigone)	C06.2	C79.89	D00.00	D10.39	D37.09	D49.0
retro-orbital	C76.0	C79.89	D09.8	D36.7	D48.7	D49.89
retroperitoneal (space) (tissue)	C48.0	C78.6	—	D20.0	D48.3	D49.0
retroperitoneum	C48.0	C78.6	—	D20.0	D48.3	D49.0
retropharyngeal	C14.0	C79.89	D00.08	D10.9	D37.05	D49.0
retrovesical (septum)	C76.3	C79.89	D09.8	D36.7	D48.7	D49.89
rhinencephalon	C71.0	C79.31	—	D33.0	D43.0	D49.6
rib	C41.3	C79.51	—	D16.7	D48.0	D49.2
Rosenmüller's fossa	C11.2	C79.89	D00.08	D10.6	D37.05	D49.0
round ligament	C57.2	C79.82	—	D28.2	D39.8	D49.59
sacrococcyx, sacrococcygeal	C41.4	C79.51	—	D16.8	D48.0	D49.2
region	C76.3	C79.89	D09.8	D36.7	D48.7	D49.89
sacrouterine ligament	C57.3	C79.82	—	D28.2	D39.8	D49.59
sacrum, sacral (vertebra)	C41.4	C79.51	—	D16.8	D48.0	D49.2
salivary gland or duct (major)	C08.9	C79.89	D00.00	D11.9	D37.039	D49.0
minor NEC	C06.9	C79.89	D00.00	D10.39	D37.04	D49.0
overlapping lesion	C08.9	—	—	—	—	—
parotid	C07	C79.89	D00.00	D11.0	D37.030	D49.0
pluriglandular	C08.9	C79.89	D00.00	D11.9	D37.039	D49.0
sublingual	C08.1	C79.89	D00.00	D11.7	D37.031	D49.0
submandibular	C08.0	C79.89	D00.00	D11.7	D37.032	D49.0
submaxillary	C08.0	C79.89	D00.00	D11.7	D37.032	D49.0
salpinx (uterine)	C57.0-	C79.82	D07.39	D28.2	D39.8	D49.59
Santorini's duct	C25.3	C78.89	D01.7	D13.6	D37.8	D49.0
scalp	C44.40	C79.2	D04.4	D23.4	D48.5	D49.2
basal cell carcinoma	C44.41	—	—	—	—	—
specified type NEC	C44.49	—	—	—	—	—
squamous cell carcinoma	C44.42	—	—	—	—	—
scapula (any part)	C40.0-	C79.51	—	D16.0-	—	—
scapular region	C76.1	C79.89	D09.8	D36.7	D48.7	D49.89
scar NEC — *see also* Neoplasm, skin, by site	C44.90	C79.2	D04.9	D23.9	D48.5	D49.2
sciatic nerve	C47.2-	C79.89	—	D36.13	D48.2	D49.2
sclera	C69.4-	C79.49	D09.2-	D31.4-	D48.7	D49.89
scrotum (skin)	C63.2	C79.82	D07.61	D29.4	D40.8	D49.59
sebaceous gland — *see* Neoplasm, skin						
sella turcica	C75.1	C79.89	D09.3	D35.2	D44.3	D49.7
bone	C41.0	C79.51	—	D16.4-	D48.0	D49.2
semilunar cartilage (knee)	C40.2-	C79.51	—	D16.2-	D48.0	D49.2
seminal vesicle	C63.7	C79.82	D07.69	D29.8	D40.8	D49.59
septum						
nasal	C30.0	C78.39	D02.3	D14.0	D38.5	D49.1
posterior margin	C11.3	C79.89	D00.08	D10.6	D37.05	D49.0
rectovaginal	C76.3	C79.89	D09.8	D36.7	D48.7	D49.89
rectovesical	C76.3	C79.89	D09.8	D36.7	D48.7	D49.89
urethrovaginal	C57.9	C79.82	D07.30	D28.9	D39.9	D49.59
vesicovaginal	C57.9	C79.82	D07.30	D28.9	D39.9	D49.59
shoulder NEC	C76.4-	C79.89	D04.6-	D36.7	D48.7	D49.89
sigmoid flexure (lower) (upper)	C18.7	C78.5	D01.0	D12.5	D37.4	D49.0
sinus (accessory)	C31.9	C78.39	D02.3	D14.0	D38.5	D49.1
bone (any)	C41.0	C79.51	—	D16.4-	D48.0	D49.2
ethmoidal	C31.1	C78.39	D02.3	D14.0	D38.5	D49.1
frontal	C31.2	C78.39	D02.3	D14.0	D38.5	D49.1
maxillary	C31.0	C78.39	D02.3	D14.0	D38.5	D49.1
nasal, paranasal NEC	C31.9	C78.39	D02.3	D14.0	D38.5	D49.1
overlapping lesion	C31.8	—	—	—	—	—
pyriform	C12	C79.89	D00.08	D10.7	D37.05	D49.0
sphenoid	C31.3	C78.39	D02.3	D14.0	D38.5	D49.1
skeleton, skeletal NEC	C41.9	C79.51	—	D16.9-	D48.0	D49.2
Skene's gland	C68.1	C79.19	D09.19	D30.8	D41.8	D49.59
skin NOS	C44.90	C79.2	D04.9	D23.9	D48.5	D49.2
abdominal wall	C44.509	C79.2	D04.5	D23.5	D48.5	D49.2
basal cell carcinoma	C44.519	—	—	—	—	—
specified type NEC	C44.599	—	—	—	—	—
squamous cell carcinoma	C44.529	—	—	—	—	—
ala nasi — *see also* Neoplasm, nose, skin	C44.301	C79.2	D04.39	D23.39	D48.5	D49.2
ankle — *see also* Neoplasm, skin, limb, lower	C44.70-	C79.2	D04.7-	D23.7-	D48.5	D49.2
antecubital space — *see also* Neoplasm, skin, limb, upper	C44.60-	C79.2	D04.6-	D23.6-	D48.5	D49.2
anus	C44.500	C79.2	D04.5	D23.5	D48.5	D49.2
basal cell carcinoma	C44.510	—	—	—	—	—
specified type NEC	C44.590	—	—	—	—	—
squamous cell carcinoma	C44.520	—	—	—	—	—
arm — *see also* Neoplasm, skin, limb, upper	C44.60-	C79.2	D04.6-	D23.6-	D48.5	D49.2
auditory canal (external) — *see also* Neoplasm, skin, ear	C44.20-	C79.2	D04.2-	D23.2-	D48.5	D49.2
auricle (ear) — *see also* Neoplasm, skin, ear	C44.20-	C79.2	D04.2-	D23.2-	D48.5	D49.2
auricular canal (external) — *see also* Neoplasm, skin, ear	C44.20-	C79.2	D04.2-	D23.2-	D48.5	D49.2
axilla, axillary fold — *see also* Neoplasm, skin, trunk	C44.509	C79.2	D04.5	D23.5	D48.5	D49.2
back — *see also* Neoplasm, skin, trunk	C44.509	C79.2	D04.5	D23.5	D48.5	D49.2
basal cell carcinoma	C44.91	—	—	—	—	—
breast	C44.501	C79.2	D04.5	D23.5	D48.5	D49.2
basal cell carcinoma	C44.511	—	—	—	—	—
specified type NEC	C44.591	—	—	—	—	—
squamous cell carcinoma	C44.521	—	—	—	—	—
brow — *see also* Neoplasm, skin, face	C44.309	C79.2	D04.39	D23.39	D48.5	D49.2
buttock — *see also* Neoplasm, skin, trunk	C44.509	C79.2	D04.5	D23.5	D48.5	D49.2

NEOPLASM TABLE

Neoplasm Table	Malignant Primary	Malignant Secondary	Ca In situ	Benign	Uncertain Behavior	Unspecified Behavior
Neoplasm, neoplastic - *continued*						
skin NOS - *continued*	C44.90	C79.2	D04.9	D23.9	D48.5	D49.2
calf — *see also* Neoplasm, skin, limb, lower	C44.70-	C79.2	D04.7-	D23.7-	D48.5	D49.2
canthus (eye) (inner) (outer)	C44.10-	C79.2	D04.1-	D23.1-	D48.5	D49.2
basal cell carcinoma	C44.11-	—	—	—	—	—
specified type NEC	C44.19-	—	—	—	—	—
squamous cell carcinoma	C44.12-	—	—	—	—	—
cervical region — *see also* Neoplasm, skin, neck	C44.40	C79.2	D04.4	D23.4	D48.5	D49.2
cheek (external) — *see also* Neoplasm, skin, face	C44.309	C79.2	D04.39	D23.39	D48.5	D49.2
chest (wall) — *see also* Neoplasm, trunk	C44.509	C79.2	D04.5	D23.5	D48.5	D49.2
chin — *see also* Neoplasm, skin, face	C44.309	C79.2	D04.39	D23.39	D48.5	D49.2
clavicular area — *see also* Neoplasm, skin, trunk	C44.509	C79.2	D04.5	D23.5	D48.5	D49.2
clitoris	C51.2	C79.82	D07.1	D28.0	D39.8	D49.59
columnella — *see also* Neoplasm, skin, face	C44.309	C79.2	D04.39	D23.39	D48.5	D49.2
concha — *see also* Neoplasm, skin, ear	C44.20-	C79.2	D04.2-	D23.2-	D48.5	D49.2
ear (external)	C44.20-	C79.2	D04.2-	D23.2-	D48.5	D49.2
basal cell carcinoma	C44.21-	—	—	—	—	—
specified type NEC	C44.29-	—	—	—	—	—
squamous cell carcinoma	C44.22-	—	—	—	—	—
elbow — *see also* Neoplasm, skin, limb, upper	C44.60-	C79.2	D04.6-	D23.6-	D48.5	D49.2
eyebrow — *see also* Neoplasm, skin, face	C44.309	C79.2	D04.39	D23.39	D48.5	D49.2
eyelid	C44.10-	C79.2	D04.1-	D23.1-	D48.5	D49.2
basal cell carcinoma	C44.11-	—	—	—	—	—
specified type NEC	C44.19-	—	—	—	—	—
squamous cell carcinoma	C44.12-	—	—	—	—	—
face NOS	C44.300	C79.2	D04.30	D23.30	D48.5	D49.2
basal cell carcinoma	C44.310	—	—	—	—	—
specified type NEC	C44.390	—	—	—	—	—
squamous cell carcinoma	C44.320	—	—	—	—	—
female genital organs (external)	C51.9	C79.82	D07.1	D28.0	D39.8	D49.59
clitoris	C51.2	C79.82	D07.1	D28.0	D39.8	D49.59
labium NEC	C51.9	C79.82	D07.1	D28.0	D39.8	D49.59
majus	C51.0	C79.82	D07.1	D28.0	D39.8	D49.59
minus	C51.1	C79.82	D07.1	D28.0	D39.8	D49.59
pudendum	C51.9	C79.82	D07.1	D28.0	D39.8	D49.59
vulva	C51.9	C79.82	D07.1	D28.0	D39.8	D49.59
finger — *see also* Neoplasm, skin, limb, upper	C44.60-	C79.2	D04.6-	D23.6-	D48.5	D49.2
flank — *see also* Neoplasm, skin, trunk	C44.509	C79.2	D04.5	D23.5	D48.5	D49.2
foot — *see also* Neoplasm, skin, limb, lower	C44.70-	C79.2	D04.7-	D23.7-	D48.5	D49.2
forearm — *see also* Neoplasm, skin, limb, upper	C44.60-	C79.2	D04.6-	D23.6-	D48.5	D49.2
forehead — *see also* Neoplasm, skin, face	C44.309	C79.2	D04.39	D23.39	D48.5	D49.2
glabella — *see also* Neoplasm, skin, face	C44.309	C79.2	D04.39	D23.39	D48.5	D49.2
gluteal region — *see also* Neoplasm, skin, trunk	C44.509	C79.2	D04.5	D23.5	D48.5	D49.2

Neoplasm Table	Malignant Primary	Malignant Secondary	Ca In situ	Benign	Uncertain Behavior	Unspecified Behavior
Neoplasm, neoplastic - *continued*						
skin NOS - *continued*	C44.90	C79.2	D04.9	D23.9	D48.5	D49.2
groin — *see also* Neoplasm, skin, trunk	C44.509	C79.2	D04.5	D23.5	D48.5	D49.2
hand — *see also* Neoplasm, skin, limb, upper	C44.60-	C79.2	D04.6-	D23.6-	D48.5	D49.2
head NEC — *see also* Neoplasm, skin, scalp	C44.40	C79.2	D04.4	D23.4	D48.5	D49.2
heel — *see also* Neoplasm, skin, limb, lower	C44.70-	C79.2	D04.7-	D23.7-	D48.5	D49.2
helix — *see also* Neoplasm, skin, ear	C44.20-	C79.2	D04.2-	D23.2-	D48.5	D49.2
hip — *see also* Neoplasm, skin, limb, lower	C44.70-	C79.2	D04.7-	D23.7-	D48.5	D49.2
infraclavicular region — *see also* Neoplasm, skin, trunk	C44.509	C79.2	D04.5	D23.5	D48.5	D49.2
inguinal region — *see also* Neoplasm, skin, trunk	C44.509	C79.2	D04.5	D23.5	D48.5	D49.2
jaw — *see also* Neoplasm, skin, face	C44.309	C79.2	D04.39	D23.39	D48.5	D49.2
Kaposi's sarcoma — *see* Kaposi's, sarcoma, skin						
knee — *see also* Neoplasm, skin, limb, lower	C44.70-	C79.2	D04.7-	D23.7-	D48.5	D49.2
labia						
majora	C51.0	C79.82	D07.1	D28.0	D39.8	D49.59
minora	C51.1	C79.82	D07.1	D28.0	D39.8	D49.59
leg — *see also* Neoplasm, skin, limb, lower	C44.70-	C79.2	D04.7-	D23.7-	D48.5	D49.2
lid (lower) (upper)	C44.10-	C79.2	D04.1-	D23.1-	D48.5	D49.2
basal cell carcinoma	C44.11-	—	—	—	—	—
specified type NEC	C44.19-	—	—	—	—	—
squamous cell carcinoma	C44.12-	—	—	—	—	—
limb NEC	C44.90	C79.2	D04.9	D23.9	D48.5	D49.2
basal cell carcinoma	C44.91	—	—	—	—	—
lower	C44.70-	C79.2	D04.7-	D23.7-	D48.5	D49.2
basal cell carcinoma	C44.71-	—	—	—	—	—
specified type NEC	C44.79-	—	—	—	—	—
squamous cell carcinoma	C44.72-	—	—	—	—	—
upper	C44.60-	C79.2	D04.6-	D23.6-	D48.5	D49.2
basal cell carcinoma	C44.61-	—	—	—	—	—
specified type NEC	C44.69-	—	—	—	—	—
squamous cell carcinoma	C44.62-	—	—	—	—	—
lip (lower) (upper)	C44.00	C79.2	D04.0	D23.0	D48.5	D49.2
basal cell carcinoma	C44.01	—	—	—	—	—
specified type NEC	C44.09	—	—	—	—	—
squamous cell carcinoma	C44.02	—	—	—	—	—
male genital organs	C63.9	C79.82	D07.60	D29.9	D40.8	D49.59
penis	C60.9	C79.82	D07.4	D29.0	D40.8	D49.59
prepuce	C60.0	C79.82	D07.4	D29.0	D40.8	D49.59
scrotum	C63.2	C79.82	D07.61	D29.4	D40.8	D49.59
mastectomy site (skin) — *see also* Neoplasm, skin, breast	C44.501	C79.2	—	—	—	—
specified as breast tissue	C50.8-	C79.81	—	—	—	—
meatus, acoustic (external) — *see also* Neoplasm, skin, ear	C44.20-	C79.2	D04.2-	D23.2-	D48.5	D49.2

© 2016 Channel Publishing, Ltd.

Neoplasm Table	Malignant Primary	Malignant Secondary	Ca In situ	Benign	Uncertain Behavior	Unspecified Behavior
Neoplasm, neoplastic - *continued*						
skin NOS - *continued*	C44.90	C79.2	D04.9	D23.9	D48.5	D49.2
melanotic — *see* Melanoma						
Merkel cell — *see* Carcinoma, Merkel cell						
nates — *see also* Neoplasm, skin, trunk	C44.509	C79.2	D04.5	D23.5	D48.5	D49.2
neck	C44.40	C79.2	D04.4	D23.4	D48.5	D49.2
basal cell carcinoma	C44.41	—	—	—	—	—
specified type NEC	C44.49	—	—	—	—	—
squamous cell carcinoma	C44.42	—	—	—	—	—
nevus — *see* Nevus, skin						
nose (external) — *see also* Neoplasm, nose, skin	C44.301	C79.2	D04.39	D23.39	D48.5	D49.2
overlapping lesion	C44.80	—	—	—	—	—
basal cell carcinoma	C44.81	—	—	—	—	—
specified type NEC	C44.89	—	—	—	—	—
squamous cell carcinoma	C44.82	—	—	—	—	—
palm — *see also* Neoplasm, skin, limb, upper	C44.60-	C79.2	D04.6-	D23.6-	D48.5	D49.2
palpebra	C44.10-	C79.2	D04.1-	D23.1-	D48.5	D49.2
basal cell carcinoma	C44.11-	—	—	—	—	—
specified type NEC	C44.19-	—	—	—	—	—
squamous cell carcinoma	C44.12-	—	—	—	—	—
penis NEC	C60.9	C79.82	D07.4	D29.0	D40.8	D49.59
perianal — *see also* Neoplasm, skin, anus	C44.500	C79.2	D04.5	23.5	D48.5	D49.2
perineum — *see also* Neoplasm, skin, anus	C44.500	C79.2	D04.5	D23.5	D48.5	D49.2
pinna — *see also* Neoplasm, skin, ear	C44.20-	C79.2	D04.2-	D23.2-	D48.5	D49.2
plantar — *see also* Neoplasm, skin, limb, lower	C44.70-	C79.2	D04.7-	D23.7-	D48.5	D49.2
popliteal fossa or space — *see also* Neoplasm, skin, limb, lower	C44.70-	C79.2	D04.7-	D23.7-	D48.5	D49.2
prepuce	C60.0	C79.82	D07.4	D29.0	D40.8	D49.59
pubes — *see also* Neoplasm, skin, trunk	C44.509	C79.2	D04.5	D23.5	D48.5	D49.2
sacrococcygeal region — *see also* Neoplasm, skin, trunk	C44.509	C79.2	D04.5	D23.5	D48.5	D49.2
scalp	C44.40	C79.2	D04.4	D23.4	D48.5	D49.2
basal cell carcinoma	C44.41	—	—	—	—	—
specified type NEC	C44.49	—	—	—	—	—
squamous cell carcinoma	C44.42	—	—	—	—	—
scapular region — *see also* Neoplasm, skin, trunk	C44.509	C79.2	D04.5	D23.5	D48.5	D49.2
scrotum	C63.2	C79.82	D07.61	D29.4	D40.8	D49.59
shoulder — *see also* Neoplasm, skin, limb, upper	C44.60-	C79.2	D04.6-	D23.6-	D48.5	D49.2
sole (foot) — *see also* Neoplasm, skin, limb, lower	C44.70-	C79.2	D04.7-	D23.7-	D48.5	D49.2
specified sites NEC	C44.80	C79.2	D04.8	D23.9	D48.5	D49.2
basal cell carcinoma	C44.81	—	—	—	—	—
specified type NEC	C44.89	—	—	—	—	—
squamous cell carcinoma	C44.82	—	—	—	—	—
specified type NEC	C44.99	—	—	—	—	—

Neoplasm Table	Malignant Primary	Malignant Secondary	Ca In situ	Benign	Uncertain Behavior	Unspecified Behavior
Neoplasm, neoplastic - *continued*						
skin NOS - *continued*	C44.90	C79.2	D04.9	D23.9	D48.5	D49.2
squamous cell carcinoma	C44.92	—	—	—	—	—
submammary fold — *see also* Neoplasm, skin, trunk	C44.509	C79.2	D04.5	D23.5	D48.5	D49.2
supraclavicular region — *see also* Neoplasm, skin, neck	C44.40	C79.2	D04.4	D23.4	D48.5	D49.2
temple — *see also* Neoplasm, skin, face	C44.309	C79.2	D04.39	D23.39	D48.5	D49.2
thigh — *see also* Neoplasm, skin, limb, lower	C44.70-	C79.2	D04.7-	D23.7-	D48.5	D49.2
thoracic wall — *see also* Neoplasm, skin, trunk	C44.509	C79.2	D04.5	D23.5	D48.5	D49.2
thumb — *see also* Neoplasm, skin, limb, upper	C44.60-	C79.2	D04.6-	D23.6-	D48.5	D49.2
toe — *see also* Neoplasm, skin, limb, lower	C44.70-	C79.2	D04.7-	D23.7-	D48.5	D49.2
tragus — *see also* Neoplasm, skin, ear	C44.20-	C79.2	D04.2-	D23.2-	D48.5	D49.2
trunk	C44.509	C79.2	D04.5	D23.5	D48.5	D49.2
basal cell carcinoma	C44.519	—	—	—	—	—
specified type NEC	C44.599	—	—	—	—	—
squamous cell carcinoma	C44.529	—	—	—	—	—
umbilicus — *see also* Neoplasm, skin, trunk	C44.509	C79.2	D04.5	D23.5	D48.5	D49.2
vulva	C51.9	C79.82	D07.1	D28.0	D39.8	D49.59
overlapping lesion	C51.8	—	—	—	—	—
wrist — *see also* Neoplasm, skin, limb, upper	C44.60-	C79.2	D04.6-	D23.6-	D48.5	D49.2
skull	C41.0	C79.51	—	D16.4-	D48.0	D49.2
soft parts or tissues — *see* Neoplasm, connective tissue						
specified site NEC	C76.8	C79.89	D09.8	D36.7	D48.7	D49.89
spermatic cord	C63.1-	C79.82	D07.69	D29.8	D40.8	D49.59
sphenoid	C31.3	C78.39	D02.3	D14.0	D38.5	D49.1
bone	C41.0	C79.51	—	D16.4-	D48.0	D49.2
sinus	C31.3	C78.39	D02.3	D14.0	D38.5	D49.1
sphincter						
anal	C21.1	C78.5	D01.3	D12.9	D37.8	D49.0
of Oddi	C24.0	C78.89	D01.5	D13.5	D37.6	D49.0
spine, spinal (column)	C41.2	C79.51	—	D16.6	D48.0	D49.2
bulb	C71.7	C79.31	—	D33.1	D43.1	D49.6
coccyx	C41.4	C79.51	—	D16.8	D48.0	D49.2
cord (cervical) (lumbar) (sacral) (thoracic)	C72.0	C79.49	—	D33.4	D43.4	D49.7
dura mater	C70.1	C79.49	—	D32.1	D42.1	D49.7
lumbosacral	C41.2	C79.51	—	D16.6	D48.0	D49.2
marrow NEC	C96.9	C79.52	—	—	D47.9	D49.89
membrane	C70.1	C79.49	—	D32.1	D42.1	D49.7
meninges	C70.1	C79.49	—	D32.1	D42.1	D49.7
nerve (root)	C47.9	C79.89	—	D36.10	D48.2	D49.2
pia mater	C70.1	C79.49	—	D32.1	D42.1	D49.7
root	C47.9	C79.89	—	D36.10	D48.2	D49.2
sacrum	C41.4	C79.51	—	D16.8	D48.0	D49.2
spleen, splenic NEC	C26.1	C78.89	D01.7	D13.9	D37.8	D49.0
flexure (colon)	C18.5	C78.5	D01.0	D12.3	D37.4	D49.0
stem, brain	C71.7	C79.31	—	D33.1	D43.1	D49.6
Stensen's duct	C07	C79.89	D00.00	D11.0	D37.030	D49.0
sternum	C41.3	C79.51	—	D16.7	D48.0	D49.2

NEOPLASM TABLE

Neoplasm Table	Malignant Primary	Malignant Secondary	Ca In situ	Benign	Uncertain Behavior	Unspecified Behavior
Neoplasm, neoplastic - *continued*						
stomach	C16.9	C78.89	D00.2	D13.1	D37.1	D49.0
antrum (pyloric)	C16.3	C78.89	D00.2	D13.1	D37.1	D49.0
body	C16.2	C78.89	D00.2	D13.1	D37.1	D49.0
cardia	C16.0	C78.89	D00.2	D13.1	D37.1	D49.0
cardiac orifice	C16.0	C78.89	D00.2	D13.1	D37.1	D49.0
corpus	C16.2	C78.89	D00.2	D13.1	D37.1	D49.0
fundus	C16.1	C78.89	D00.2	D13.1	D37.1	D49.0
greater curvature NEC	C16.6	C78.89	D00.2	D13.1	D37.1	D49.0
lesser curvature NEC	C16.5	C78.89	D00.2	D13.1	D37.1	D49.0
overlapping lesion	C16.8	—	—	—	—	—
prepylorus	C16.4	C78.89	D00.2	D13.1	D37.1	D49.0
pylorus	C16.4	C78.89	D00.2	D13.1	D37.1	D49.0
wall NEC	C16.9	C78.89	D00.2	D13.1	D37.1	D49.0
anterior NEC	C16.8	C78.89	D00.2	D13.1	D37.1	D49.0
posterior NEC	C16.8	C78.89	D00.2	D13.1	D37.1	D49.0
stroma, endometrial	C54.1	C79.82	D07.0	D26.1	D39.0	D49.59
stump, cervical	C53.8	C79.82	D06.7	D26.0	D39.0	D49.59
subcutaneous (nodule) (tissue) NEC — *see* Neoplasm, connective tissue						
subdural	C70.9	C79.32	—	D32.9	D42.9	D49.7
subglottis, subglottic	C32.2	C78.39	D02.0	D14.1	D38.0	D49.1
sublingual	C04.9	C79.89	D00.06	D10.2	D37.09	D49.0
gland or duct	C08.1	C79.89	D00.00	D11.7	D37.031	D49.0
submandibular gland	C08.0	C79.89	D00.00	D11.7	D37.032	D49.0
submaxillary gland or duct	C08.0	C79.89	D00.00	D11.7	D37.032	D49.0
submental	C76.0	C79.89	D09.8	D36.7	D48.7	D49.89
subpleural	C34.9-	C78.0-	D02.2-	D14.3-	D38.1	D49.1
substernal	C38.1	C78.1	—	D15.2	D38.3	D49.89
sudoriferous, sudoriparous gland, site unspecified	C44.90	C79.2	D04.9	D23.9	D48.5	D49.2
specified site — *see* Neoplasm, skin						
supraclavicular region	C76.0	C79.89	D09.8	D36.7	D48.7	D49.89
supraglottis	C32.1	C78.39	D02.0	D14.1	D38.0	D49.1
suprarenal	C74.9-	C79.7-	D09.3	D35.0-	D44.1-	D49.7
capsule	C74.9-	C79.7-	D09.3	D35.0-	D44.1-	D49.7
cortex	C74.0-	C79.7-	D09.3	D35.0-	D44.1-	D49.7
gland	C74.9-	C79.7-	D09.3	D35.0-	D44.1-	D49.7
medulla	C74.1-	C79.7-	D09.3	D35.0-	D44.1-	D49.7
suprasellar (region)	C71.9	C79.31	—	D33.2	D43.2	D49.6
supratentorial (brain) NEC	C71.0	C79.31	—	D33.0	D43.0	D49.6
sweat gland (apocrine) (eccrine), site unspecified	C44.90	C79.2	D04.9	D23.9	D48.5	D49.2
specified site — *see* Neoplasm, skin						
sympathetic nerve or nervous system NEC	C47.9	C79.89	—	D36.10	D48.2	D49.2
symphysis pubis	C41.4	C79.51	—	D16.8	D48.0	D49.2
synovial membrane — *see* Neoplasm, connective tissue						
tapetum, brain	C71.8	C79.31	—	D33.2	D43.2	D49.6
tarsus (any bone)	C40.3-	C79.51	—	D16.3-	—	—
temple (skin) — *see also* Neoplasm, skin, face	C44.309	C79.2	D04.39	D23.39	D48.5	D49.2

Neoplasm Table	Malignant Primary	Malignant Secondary	Ca In situ	Benign	Uncertain Behavior	Unspecified Behavior
Neoplasm, neoplastic - *continued*						
temporal						
bone	C41.0	C79.51	—	D16.4-	D48.0	D49.2
lobe or pole	C71.2	C79.31	—	D33.0	D43.0	D49.6
region	C76.0	C79.89	D09.8	D36.7	D48.7	D49.89
skin — *see also* Neoplasm, skin, face	C44.309	C79.2	D04.39	D23.39	D48.5	D49.2
tendon (sheath) — *see* Neoplasm, connective tissue						
tentorium (cerebelli)	C70.0	C79.32	—	D32.0	D42.0	D49.7
testis, testes	C62.9-	C79.82	D07.69	D29.2-	D40.1-	D49.59
descended	C62.1-	C79.82	D07.69	D29.2-	D40.1-	D49.59
ectopic	C62.0-	C79.82	D07.69	D29.2-	D40.1-	D49.59
retained	C62.0-	C79.82	D07.69	D29.2-	D40.1-	D49.59
scrotal	C62.1-	C79.82	D07.69	D29.2-	D40.1-	D49.59
undescended	C62.0-	C79.82	D07.69	D29.2-	D40.1-	D49.59
unspecified whether descended or undescended	C62.9-	C79.82	D07.69	D29.2-	D40.1-	D49.59
thalamus	C71.0	C79.31	—	D33.0	D43.0	D49.6
thigh NEC	C76.5-	C79.89	D04.7-	D36.7	D48.7	D49.89
thorax, thoracic (cavity) (organs NEC)	C76.1	C79.89	D09.8	D36.7	D48.7	D49.89
duct	C49.3	C79.89	—	D21.3	D48.1	D49.2
wall NEC	C76.1	C79.89	D09.8	D36.7	D48.7	D49.89
throat	C14.0	C79.89	D00.08	D10.9	D37.05	D49.0
thumb NEC	C76.4-	C79.89	D04.6-	D36.7	D48.7	D49.89
thymus (gland)	C37	C79.89	D09.3	D15.0	D38.4	D49.89
thyroglossal duct	C73	C79.89	D09.3	D34	D44.0	D49.7
thyroid (gland)	C73	C79.89	D09.3	D34	D44.0	D49.7
cartilage	C32.3	C78.39	D02.0	D14.1	D38.0	D49.1
tibia (any part)	C40.2-	C79.51	—	D16.2-	—	—
toe NEC	C76.5-	C79.89	D04.7-	D36.7	D48.7	D49.89
tongue	C02.9	C79.89	D00.07	D10.1	D37.02	D49.0
anterior (two-thirds) NEC	C02.3	C79.89	D00.07	D10.1	D37.02	D49.0
dorsal surface	C02.0	C79.89	D00.07	D10.1	D37.02	D49.0
ventral surface	C02.2	C79.89	D00.07	D10.1	D37.02	D49.0
base (dorsal surface)	C01	C79.89	D00.07	D10.1	D37.02	D49.0
border (lateral)	C02.1	C79.89	D00.07	D10.1	D37.02	D49.0
dorsal surface NEC	C02.0	C79.89	D00.07	D10.1	D37.02	D49.0
fixed part NEC	C01	C79.89	D00.07	D10.1	D37.02	D49.0
foreamen cecum	C02.0	C79.89	D00.07	D10.1	D37.02	D49.0
frenulum linguae	C02.2	C79.89	D00.07	D10.1	D37.02	D49.0
junctional zone	C02.8	C79.89	D00.07	D10.1	D37.02	D49.0
margin (lateral)	C02.1	C79.89	D00.07	D10.1	D37.02	D49.0
midline NEC	C02.0	C79.89	D00.07	D10.1	D37.02	D49.0
mobile part NEC	C02.3	C79.89	D00.07	D10.1	D37.02	D49.0
overlapping lesion	C02.8	—	—	—	—	—
posterior (third)	C01	C79.89	D00.07	D10.1	D37.02	D49.0
root	C01	C79.89	D00.07	D10.1	D37.02	D49.0
surface (dorsal)	C02.0	C79.89	D00.07	D10.1	D37.02	D49.0
base	C01	C79.89	D00.08	D10.1	D37.02	D49.0
ventral	C02.2	C79.89	D00.07	D10.1	D37.02	D49.0
tip	C02.1	C79.89	D00.07	D10.1	D37.02	D49.0
tonsil	C02.4	C79.89	D00.07	D10.1	D37.02	D49.0
tonsil	C09.9	C79.89	D00.08	D10.4	D37.05	D49.0
fauces, faucial	C09.9	C79.89	D00.08	D10.4	D37.05	D49.0
lingual	C02.4	C79.89	D00.07	D10.1	D37.02	D49.0
overlapping sites	C09.8	—	—	—	—	—
palatine	C09.9	C79.89	D00.08	D10.4	D37.05	D49.0
pharyngeal	C11.1	C79.89	D00.08	D10.6	D37.05	D49.0
pillar (anterior) (posterior)	C09.1	C79.89	D00.08	D10.5	D37.05	D49.0

Neoplasm, neoplastic - *continued*

Neoplasm Table	Malignant Primary	Malignant Secondary	Ca In situ	Benign	Uncertain Behavior	Unspecified Behavior
tonsillar fossa	C09.0	C79.89	D00.08	D10.5	D37.05	D49.0
tooth socket NEC	C03.9	C79.89	D00.03	D10.39	D37.09	D49.0
trachea (cartilage) (mucosa)	C33	C78.39	D02.1	D14.2	D38.1	D49.1
overlapping lesion with bronchus or lung	C34.8-	—	—	—	—	—
tracheobronchial	C34.8-	C78.39	D02.1	D14.2	D38.1	D49.1
overlapping lesion with lung	C34.8-	—	—	—	—	—
tragus — *see also* Neoplasm, skin, ear	C44.20-	C79.2	D04.2-	D23.2-	D48.5	D49.2
trunk NEC	C76.8	C79.89	D04.5	D36.7	D48.7	D49.89
tubo-ovarian	C57.8	C79.82	D07.39	D28.7	D39.8	D49.59
tunica vaginalis	C63.7	C79.82	D07.69	D29.8	D40.8	D49.59
turbinate (bone)	C41.0	C79.51	—	D16.4-	D48.0	D49.2
nasal	C30.0	C78.39	D02.3	D14.0	D38.5	D49.1
tympanic cavity	C30.1	C78.39	D02.3	D14.0	D38.5	D49.1
ulna (any part)	C40.0-	C79.51	—	D16.0-	—	—
umbilicus, umbilical — *see also* Neoplasm, skin, trunk	C44.509	C79.2	D04.5	D23.5	D48.5	D49.2
uncus, brain	C71.2	C79.31	—	D33.0	D43.0	D49.6
unknown site or unspecified	C80.1	C79.9	D09.9	D36.9	D48.9	D49.9
urachus	C67.7	C79.11	D09.0	D30.3	D41.4	D49.4
ureter, ureteral	C66.-	C79.19	D09.19	D30.2-	D41.2-	D49.59
orifice (bladder)	C67.6	C79.11	D09.0	D30.3	D41.4	D49.4
ureter-bladder (junction)	C67.6	C79.11	D09.0	D30.3	D41.4	D49.4
urethra, urethral (gland)	C68.0	C79.19	D09.19	D30.4	D41.3	D49.59
orifice, internal	C67.5	C79.11	D09.0	D30.3	D41.4	D49.4
urethrovaginal (septum)	C57.9	C79.82	D07.30	D28.9	D39.8	D49.59
urinary organ or system	C68.9	C79.10	D09.10	D30.9	D41.9	D49.59
bladder — *see* Neoplasm, bladder						
overlapping lesion	C68.8	—	—	—	—	—
specified sites NEC	C68.8	C79.19	D09.19	D30.8	D41.8	D49.59
utero-ovarian	C57.8	C79.82	D07.39	D28.7	D39.8	D49.59
ligament	C57.1	C79.82	D07.39	D28.2	D39.8	D49.59
uterosacral ligament	C57.3	C79.82	—	D28.2	D39.8	D49.59
uterus, uteri, uterine	C55	C79.82	D07.0	D26.9	D39.0	D49.59
adnexa NEC	C57.4	C79.82	D07.39	D28.7	D39.8	D49.59
body	C54.9	C79.82	D07.0	D26.1	D39.0	D49.59
cervix	C53.9	C79.82	D06.9	D26.0	D39.0	D49.59
cornu	C54.9	C79.82	D07.0	D26.1	D39.0	D49.59
corpus	C54.9	C79.82	D07.0	D26.1	D39.0	D49.59
endocervix (canal) (gland)	C53.0	C79.82	D06.0	D26.0	D39.0	D49.59
endometrium	C54.1	C79.82	D07.0	D26.1	D39.0	D49.59
exocervix	C53.1	C79.82	D06.1	D26.0	D39.0	D49.59
external os	C53.1	C79.82	D06.1	D26.0	D39.0	D49.59
fundus	C54.3	C79.82	D07.0	D26.1	D39.0	D49.59
internal os	C53.0	C79.82	D06.0	D26.0	D39.0	D49.59
isthmus	C54.0	C79.82	D07.0	D26.1	D39.0	D49.59
ligament	C57.3	C79.82	—	D28.2	D39.8	D49.59
broad	C57.1	C79.82	D07.39	D28.2	D39.8	D49.59
round	C57.2	C79.82	—	D28.2	D39.8	D49.59
lower segment	C54.0	C79.82	D07.0	D26.1	D39.0	D49.59
myometrium	C54.2	C79.82	D07.0	D26.1	D39.0	D49.59
overlapping sites	C54.8	—				
squamocolumnar junction	C53.8	C79.82	D06.7	D26.0	D39.0	D49.59
tube	C57.0-	C79.82	D07.39	D28.2	D39.8	D49.59
utricle, prostatic	C68.0	C79.19	D09.19	D30.4	D41.3	D49.59
uveal tract	C69.4-	C79.49	D09.2-	D31.4-	D48.7	D49.89
uvula	C05.2	C79.89	D00.04	D10.39	D37.09	D49.09

Neoplasm Table	Malignant Primary	Malignant Secondary	Ca In situ	Benign	Uncertain Behavior	Unspecified Behavior
vagina, vaginal (fornix) (vault) (wall)	C52	C79.82	D07.2	D28.1	D39.8	D49.59
vaginovesical	C57.9	C79.82	D07.30	D28.9	D39.9	D49.59
septum	C57.9	C79.82	D07.30	D28.9	D39.9	D49.59
vallecula (epigiottis)	C10.0	C79.89	D00.08	D10.5	D37.05	D49.0
vas deferens	C63.1-	C79.82	D07.69	D29.8	D40.8	D49.59
vascular — *see* Neoplasm, connective tissue						
Vater's ampulla	C24.1	C78.89	D01.5	D13.5	D37.6	D49.0
vein, venous — *see* Neoplasm, connective tissue						
vena cava (abdominal) (inferior)	C49.4	C79.89	—	D21.4	D48.1	D49.2
superior	C49.3	C79.89	—	D21.3	D48.1	D49.2
ventricle (cerebral) (floor) (lateral) (third)	C71.5	C79.31	—	D33.0	D43.0	D49.6
cardiac (left) (right)	C38.0	C79.89	—	D15.1	D48.7	D49.89
fourth	C71.7	C79.31	—	D33.1	D43.1	D49.6
ventricular band of larynx	C32.1	C78.39	D02.0	D14.1	D38.0	D49.1
ventriculus — *see* Neoplasm, stomach						
vermillion border — *see* Neoplasm, lip						
vermis, cerebellum	C71.6	C79.31	—	D33.1	D43.1	D49.6
vertebra (column)	C41.2	C79.51	—	D16.6	D48.0	D49.2
coccyx	C41.4	C79.51	—	D16.8-	D48.0	D49.2
marrow NEC	C96.9	C79.52	—	—	D47.9	D49.89
sacrum	C41.4	C79.51	—	D16.8-	D48.0	D49.2
vesical — *see* Neoplasm, bladder						
vesicle, seminal	C63.7	C79.82	D07.69	D29.8	D40.8	D49.59
vesicocervical tissue	C57.9	C79.82	D07.30	D28.9	D39.9	D49.59
vesicorectal	C76.3	C79.82	D09.8	D36.7	D48.7	D49.89
vesicovaginal	C57.9	C79.82	D07.30	D28.9	D39.9	D49.59
septum	C57.9	C79.82	D07.30	D28.9	D39.8	D49.59
vessel (blood) — *see* Neoplasm, connective tissue						
vestibular gland, greater	C51.0	C79.82	D07.1	D28.0	D39.8	D49.59
vestibule						
mouth	C06.1	C79.89	D00.00	D10.39	D37.09	D49.0
nose	C30.0	C78.39	D02.3	D14.0	D38.5	D49.1
Virchow's gland	C77.0	C77.0	—	D36.0	D48.7	D49.89
viscera NEC	C76.8	C79.89	D09.8	D36.7	D48.7	D49.89
vocal cords (true)	C32.0	C78.39	D02.0	D14.1	D38.0	D49.1
false	C32.1	C78.39	D02.0	D14.1	D38.0	D49.1
vomer	C41.0	C79.51	—	D16.4-	D48.0	D49.2
vulva	C51.9	C79.82	D07.1	D28.0	D39.8	D49.59
vulvovaginal gland	C51.0	C79.82	D07.1	D28.0	D39.8	D49.59
Waldeyer's ring	C14.2	C79.89	D00.08	D10.9	D37.05	D49.0
Wharton's duct	C08.0	C79.89	D00.00	D11.7	D37.032	D49.0
white matter (central) (cerebral)	C71.0	C79.31	—	D33.0	D43.0	D49.6
windpipe	C33	C78.39	D02.1	D14.2	D38.1	D49.1
Wirsung's duct	C25.3	C78.89	D01.7	D13.6	D37.8	D49.0
wolffian (body) (duct)						
female	C57.7	C79.82	D07.39	D28.7	D39.8	D49.59
male	C63.7	C79.82	D07.69	D29.8	D40.8	D49.59
womb — *see* Neoplasm, uterus						
wrist NEC	C76.4-	C79.89	D04.6-	D36.7	D48.7	D49.89
xiphoid process	C41.3	C79.51	—	D16.7	D48.0	D49.2
Zuckerkandl organ	C75.5	C79.89	—	D35.6	D44.7	D49.7

NOTES

Neovascularization
ciliary body — *see* Disorder, iris, vascular
cornea H16.40-
  deep H16.44-
  ghost vessels — *see* Ghost, vessels
  localized H16.43-
  pannus — *see* Pannus
iris — *see* Disorder, iris, vascular
retina H35.05-
Nephralgia N23
Nephritis, nephritic (albuminuric) (azotemic)
(congenital) (disseminated) (epithelial)
(familial) (focal) (granulomatous)
(hemorrhagic) (infantile) (nonsuppurative,
excretory) (uremic) N05.9
with
  dense deposit disease N05.6
  diffuse
    crescentic glomerulonephritis N05.7
    endocapillary proliferative
      glomerulonephritis N05.4
    membranous glomerulonephritis N05.2
    mesangial proliferative glomerulonephritis
      N05.3
    mesangiocapillary glomerulonephritis
      N05.5
  edema — *see* Nephrosis
  focal and segmental glomerular lesions
    N05.1
  foot process disease N04.9
  glomerular lesion
    diffuse sclerosing N05.8
    hypocomplementemic — *see* Nephritis,
      membranoproliferative
    IgA — *see* Nephropathy, IgA
    lobular, lobulonodular — *see* Nephritis,
      membranoproliferative
    nodular — *see* Nephritis,
      membranoproliferative
  lesion of
    glomerulonephritis, proliferative N05.8
    renal necrosis N05.9
  minor glomerular abnormality N05.0
  specified morphological changes NEC
    N05.8
acute N00.9
  with
    dense deposit disease N00.6
    diffuse
      crescentic glomerulonephritis N00.7
      endocapillary proliferative
        glomerulonephritis N00.4
      membranous glomerulonephritis N00.2
      mesangial proliferative
        glomerulonephritis N00.3
      mesangiocapillary glomerulonephritis
        N00.5
    focal and segmental glomerular lesions
      N00.1
    minor glomerular abnormality N00.0
    specified morphological changes NEC
      N00.8
amyloid E85.4 *[N08]*
antiglomerular basement membrane (anti-
  GBM) antibody NEC
  in Goodpasture's syndrome M31.0
antitubular basement membrane (tubulo-
  interstitial) NEC N12
  toxic — *see* Nephropathy, toxic
arteriolar — *see* Hypertension, kidney
arteriosclerotic — *see* Hypertension, kidney
ascending — *see* Nephritis, tubulo-interstitial
atrophic N03.9
Balkan (endemic) N15.0
calculous, calculus — *see* Calculus, kidney
cardiac — *see* Hypertension, kidney
cardiovascular — *see* Hypertension, kidney

Nephritis, nephritic (albuminuric) (azotemic)
(congenital) (disseminated) (epithelial)
(familial) (focal) (granulomatous)
(hemorrhagic) (infantile) (nonsuppurative,
excretory) (uremic) N05.9 — *continued*
chronic N03.9
  with
    dense deposit disease N03.6
    diffuse
      crescentic glomerulonephritis N03.7
      endocapillary proliferative
        glomerulonephritis N03.4
      membranous glomerulonephritis N03.2
      mesangial proliferative
        glomerulonephritis N03.3
      mesangiocapillary glomerulonephritis
        N03.5
    focal and segmental glomerular lesions
      N03.1
    minor glomerular abnormality N03.0
    specified morphological changes NEC
      N03.8
  arteriosclerotic — *see* Hypertension, kidney
cirrhotic N26.9
complicating pregnancy O26.83-
croupous N00.9
degenerative — *see* Nephrosis
diffuse sclerosing N05.8
due to
  diabetes mellitus — *see* E08-E13 with .21
  subacute bacterial endocarditis I33.0
  systemic lupus erythematosus (chronic)
    M32.14
  typhoid fever A01.09
gonococcal (acute) (chronic) A54.21
hypocomplementemic — *see* Nephritis,
  membranoproliferative
IgA — *see* Nephropathy, IgA
immune complex (circulating) NEC N05.8
infective — *see* Nephritis, tubulo-interstitial
interstitial — *see* Nephritis, tubulo-interstitial
lead N14.3
membranoproliferative (diffuse) (type 1 or 3)
  (*see also* N00-N07 with fourth character
    .5) N05.5
  type 2 (*see also* N00-N07 with fourth
    character .6) N05.6
minimal change N05.0
necrotic, necrotizing NEC (*see also* N00-N07
  with fourth character .8) N05.8
nephrotic — *see* Nephrosis
nodular — *see* Nephritis,
  membranoproliferative
polycystic Q61.3
  adult type Q61.2
  autosomal
    dominant Q61.2
    recessive NEC Q61.19
  childhood type NEC Q61.19
  infantile type NEC Q61.19
poststreptococcal N05.9
  acute N00.9
  chronic N03.9
  rapidly progressive N01.9
proliferative NEC (*see also* N00-N07 with
  fourth character .8) N05.8
purulent — *see* Nephritis, tubulo-interstitial
rapidly progressive N01.9
  with
    dense deposit disease N01.6
    diffuse
      crescentic glomerulonephritis N01.7
      endocapillary proliferative
        glomerulonephritis N01.4
      membranous glomerulonephritis N01.2
      mesangial proliferative
        glomerulonephritis N01.3
      mesangiocapillary glomerulonephritis
        N01.5

Nephritis, nephritic (albuminuric) (azotemic)
(congenital) (disseminated) (epithelial)
(familial) (focal) (granulomatous)
(hemorrhagic) (infantile) (nonsuppurative,
excretory) (uremic) N05.9 — *continued*
rapidly progressive N01.9 — *continued*
  with — *continued*
    focal and segmental glomerular lesions
      N01.1
    minor glomerular abnormality N01.0
    specified morphological changes NEC
      N01.8
salt losing or wasting NEC N28.89
saturnine N14.3
sclerosing, diffuse N05.8
septic — *see* Nephritis, tubulo-interstitial
specified pathology NEC (*see also* N00-N07
  with fourth character .8) N05.8
subacute N01.9
suppurative — *see* Nephritis, tubulo-interstitial
syphilitic (late) A52.75
  congenital A50.59 *[N08]*
  early (secondary) A51.44
toxic — *see* Nephropathy, toxic
tubal, tubular — *see* Nephritis, tubulo-
  interstitial
tuberculous A18.11
tubulo-interstitial (in) N12
  acute (infectious) N10
  chronic (infectious) N11.9
    nonobstructive N11.8
      reflux-associated N11.0
    obstructive N11.1
    specified NEC N11.8
  due to
    brucellosis A23.9 *[N16]*
    cryoglobulinemia D89.1 *[N16]*
    glycogen storage disease E74.00 *[N16]*
    Sjögren's syndrome M35.04
vascular — *see* Hypertension, kidney
war N00.9
Nephroblastoma (epithelial) (mesenchymal)
C64-
Nephrocalcinosis E83.59 *[N29]*
Nephrocystitis, pustular — *see* Nephritis,
  tubulo-interstitial
Nephrolithiasis (congenital) (pelvis)
(recurrent) — *see also* Calculus, kidney
Nephroma C64-
  mesoblastic D41.0-
Nephronephritis — *see* Nephrosis
Nephronophthisis Q61.5
Nephropathia epidemica A98.5
Nephropathy (*see also* Nephritis) N28.9
  with
    edema — *see* Nephrosis
    glomerular lesion — *see* Glomerulonephritis
  amyloid, hereditary E85.0
  analgesic N14.0
    with medullary necrosis, acute N17.2
  Balkan (endemic) N15.0
  chemical — *see* Nephropathy, toxic
  diabetic — *see* E08-E13 with .21
  drug-induced N14.2
    specified NEC N14.1
  focal and segmental hyalinosis or sclerosis
    N02.1
  heavy metal-induced N14.3
  hereditary NEC N07.9
    with
      dense deposit disease N07.6
      diffuse
        crescentic glomerulonephritis N07.7
        endocapillary proliferative
          glomerulonephritis N07.4
        membranous glomerulonephritis N07.2
        mesangial proliferative
          glomerulonephritis N07.3

DISEASE INDEX

Nephropathy (see also Nephritis) N28.9 — continued
  hereditary NEC N07.9 — continued
    with — continued
      diffuse — continued
        mesangiocapillary glomerulonephritis N07.5
      focal and segmental glomerular lesions N07.1
      minor glomerular abnormality N07.0
      specified morphological changes NEC N07.8
  hypercalcemic N25.89
  hypertensive — see Hypertension, kidney
  hypokalemic (vacuolar) N25.89
  IgA N02.8
    with glomerular lesion N02.9
      focal and segmental hyalinosis or sclerosis N02.1
      membranoproliferative (diffuse) N02.5
      membranous (diffuse) N02.2
      mesangial proliferative (diffuse) N02.3
      mesangiocapillary (diffuse) N02.5
      proliferative NEC N02.8
      specified pathology NEC N02.8
  lead N14.3
  membranoproliferative (diffuse) N02.5
  membranous (diffuse) N02.2
  mesangial (IgA/IgG) — see Nephropathy, IgA
    proliferative (diffuse) N02.3
  mesangiocapillary (diffuse) N02.5
  obstructive N13.8
  phenacetin N17.2
  phosphate-losing N25.0
  potassium depletion N25.89
  pregnancy-related O26.83-
  proliferative NEC (see also N00-N07 with fourth character .8) N05.8
  protein-losing N25.89
  saturnine N14.3
  sickle-cell D57- [N08]
  toxic NEC N14.4
    due to
      drugs N14.2
        analgesic N14.0
        specified NEC N14.1
      heavy metals N14.3
  vasomotor N17.0
  water-losing N25.89
Nephroptosis N28.83
Nephropyosis — see Abscess, kidney
Nephrorrhagia N28.89
Nephrosclerosis (arteriolar) (arteriosclerotic) (chronic) (hyaline) — see also Hypertension, kidney
  hyperplastic — see Hypertension, kidney
  senile N26.9
Nephrosis, nephrotic (Epstein's) (syndrome) (congenital) N04.9
  with
    foot process disease N04.9
    glomerular lesion N04.1
    hypocomplementemic N04.5
  acute N04.9
  anoxic — see Nephrosis, tubular
  chemical — see Nephrosis, tubular
  cholemic K76.7
  diabetic — see E08-E13 with .21
  Finnish type (congenital) Q89.8
  hemoglobin N10
  hemoglobinuric — see Nephrosis, tubular
  in
    amyloidosis E85.4 [N08]
    diabetes mellitus — see E08-E13 with .21
    epidemic hemorrhagic fever A98.5
    malaria (malariae) B52.0
  ischemic — see Nephrosis, tubular
  lipoid N04.9
  lower nephron — see Nephrosis, tubular

Nephrosis, nephrotic (Epstein's) (syndrome) (congenital) N04.9 — continued
  malarial (malariae) B52.0
  minimal change N04.0
  myoglobin N10
  necrotizing — see Nephrosis, tubular
  osmotic (sucrose) N25.89
  radiation N04.9
  syphilitic (late) A52.75
  toxic — see Nephrosis, tubular
  tubular (acute) N17.0
    postprocedural N99.0
    radiation N04.9
Nephrosonephritis, hemorrhagic (endemic) A98.5
Nephrostomy
  attention to Z43.6
  status Z93.6
Nerve — see also condition
  injury — see Injury, nerve, by body site
Nerves R45.0
Nervous (see also condition) R45.0
  heart F45.8
  stomach F45.8
  tension R45.0
Nervousness R45.0
Nesidioblastoma
  pancreas D13.7
  specified site NEC — see Neoplasm, benign, by site
  unspecified site D13.7
Nettleship's syndrome Q82.2
Neumann's disease or syndrome L10.1
Neuralgia, neuralgic (acute) M79.2
  accessory (nerve) G52.8
  acoustic (nerve) — see subcategory H93.3
  auditory (nerve) — see subcategory H93.3
  ciliary G44.009
    intractable G44.001
    not intractable G44.009
  cranial
    nerve — see also Disorder, nerve, cranial
      fifth or trigeminal — see Neuralgia, trigeminal
    postherpetic, postzoster B02.29
  ear — see subcategory H92.0
  facialis vera G51.1
  Fothergill's — see Neuralgia, trigeminal
  glossopharyngeal (nerve) G52.1
  Horton's G44.099
    intractable G44.091
    not intractable G44.099
  Hunt's B02.21
  hypoglossal (nerve) G52.3
  infraorbital — see Neuralgia, trigeminal
  malarial — see Malaria
  migrainous G44.009
    intractable G44.001
    not intractable G44.009
  Morton's G57.6-
  nerve, cranial — see Disorder, nerve, cranial
  nose G52.0
  occipital M54.81
  olfactory G52.0
  penis N48.9
  perineum R10.2
  postherpetic NEC B02.29
    trigeminal B02.22
  pubic region R10.2
  scrotum R10.2
  Sluder's G44.89
  specified nerve NEC G58.8
  spermatic cord R10.2
  sphenopalatine (ganglion) G90.09
  trifacial — see Neuralgia, trigeminal
  trigeminal G50.0
    postherpetic, postzoster B02.22
  vagus (nerve) G52.2

Neuralgia, neuralgic (acute) M79.2 — continued
  writer's F48.8
  organic G25.89
Neurapraxia — see Injury, nerve
Neurasthenia F48.8
  cardiac F45.8
  gastric F45.8
  heart F45.8
Neurilemmoma — see also Neoplasm, nerve, benign
  acoustic (nerve) D33.3
  malignant — see also Neoplasm, nerve, malignant
    acoustic (nerve) C72.4-
Neurilemmosarcoma — see Neoplasm, nerve, malignant
Neurinoma — see Neoplasm, nerve, benign
Neurinomatosis — see Neoplasm, nerve, uncertain behavior
Neuritis (rheumatoid) M79.2
  abducens (nerve) — see Strabismus, paralytic, sixth nerve
  accessory (nerve) G52.8
  acoustic (nerve) (see also subcategory) H93.3
    in (due to)
      infectious disease NEC B99 [H94.-]
      parasitic disease NEC B89 [H94.-]
    syphilitic A52.15
  alcoholic G62.1
    with psychosis — see Psychosis, alcoholic
  amyloid, any site E85.4 [G63]
  auditory (nerve) — see subcategory H93.3
  brachial — see Radiculopathy
    due to displacement, intervertebral disc — see Disorder, disc, cervical, with neuritis
  cranial nerve
    due to Lyme disease A69.22
    eighth or acoustic or auditory — see subcategory H93.3
    eleventh or accessory G52.8
    fifth or trigeminal G51.0
    first or olfactory G52.0
    fourth or trochlear — see Strabismus, paralytic, fourth nerve
    second or optic — see Neuritis, optic
    seventh or facial G51.8
      newborn (birth injury) P11.3
    sixth or abducent — see Strabismus, paralytic, sixth nerve
    tenth or vagus G52.2
    third or oculomotor — see Strabismus, paralytic, third nerve
    twelfth or hypoglossal G52.3
  Déjérine-Sottas G60.0
  diabetic (mononeuropathy) — see E08-E13 with .41
    polyneuropathy — see E08-E13 with .42
  due to
    beriberi E51.11
    displacement, prolapse or rupture, intervertebral disc — see Disorder, disc, with, radiculopathy
    herniation, nucleus pulposus M51.9 [G55]
  endemic E51.11
  facial G51.8
    newborn (birth injury) P11.3
  general — see Polyneuropathy
  geniculate ganglion G51.1
    due to herpes (zoster) B02.21
  gouty (see also Gout, by type) M10.9 [G63]
  hypoglossal (nerve) G52.3
  ilioinguinal (nerve) G57.9-
  infectious (multiple) NEC G61.0
  interstitial hypertrophic progressive G60.0
  lumbar M54.16
  lumbosacral M54.17

Neuritis (rheumatoid) M79.2 — *continued*
  multiple — *see also* Polyneuropathy
    endemic E51.11
    infective, acute G61.0
  multiplex endemica E51.11
  nerve root — *see* Radiculopathy
  oculomotor (nerve) — *see* Strabismus,
    paralytic, third nerve
  olfactory nerve G52.0
  optic (nerve) (hereditary) (sympathetic) H46.9
    with demyelination G36.0
    in myelitis G36.0
    nutritional H46.2
    papillitis — *see* Papillitis, optic
    retrobulbar H46.1-
    specified type NEC H46.8
    toxic H46.3
  peripheral (nerve) G62.9
    multiple — *see* Polyneuropathy
    single — *see* Mononeuritis
  pneumogastric (nerve) G52.2
  postherpetic, postzoster B02.29
  progressive hypertrophic interstitial G60.0
  retrobulbar — *see also* Neuritis, optic,
    retrobulbar
    in (due to)
      late syphilis A52.15
      meningococcal infection A39.82
    meningococcal A39.82
    syphilitic A52.15
  sciatic (nerve) — *see also* Sciatica
    due to displacement of intervertebral disc —
      see Disorder, disc, with, radiculopathy
  serum (*see also* Reaction, serum) T80.69
  shoulder-girdle G54.5
  specified nerve NEC G58.8
  spinal (nerve) root — *see* Radiculopathy
  syphilitic A52.15
  thenar (median) G56.1-
  thoracic M54.14
  toxic NEC G62.2
  trochlear (nerve) — *see* Strabismus, paralytic,
    fourth nerve
  vagus (nerve) G52.2
Neuroastrocytoma — *see* Neoplasm,
  uncertain behavior, by site
Neuroavitaminosis E56.9 *[G99.8]*
Neuroblastoma
  olfactory C30.0
  specified site — *see* Neoplasm, malignant, by
    site
  unspecified site C74.90
Neurochorioretinitis — *see* Chorioretinitis
Neurocirculatory asthenia F45.8
Neurocysticercosis B69.0
Neurocytoma — *see* Neoplasm, benign, by
  site
Neurodermatitis (circumscribed)
  (circumscripta) (local) L28.0
  atopic L20.81
  diffuse (Brocq) L20.81
  disseminated L20.81
Neuroencephalomyelopathy, optic G36.0
Neuroepithelioma — *see also* Neoplasm,
  malignant, by site
  olfactory C30.0
Neurofibroma — *see also* Neoplasm, nerve,
  benign
  melanotic — *see* Neoplasm, nerve, benign
  multiple — *see* Neurofibromatosis
  plexiform — *see* Neoplasm, nerve, benign
Neurofibromatosis (multiple) (nonmalignant)
  Q85.00
  acoustic Q85.02
  malignant — *see* Neoplasm, nerve, malignant
  specified NEC Q85.09
  type 1 (von Recklinghausen) Q85.01
  type 2 Q85.02

Neurofibrosarcoma — *see* Neoplasm, nerve,
  malignant
Neurogenic — *see also* condition
  bladder (*see also* Dysfunction, bladder,
    neuromuscular) N31.9
    cauda equina syndrome G83.4
  bowel NEC K59.2
  heart F45.8
Neuroglioma — *see* Neoplasm, uncertain
  behavior, by site
Neurolabyrinthitis (of Dix and Hallpike) —
  see Neuronitis, vestibular
Neurolathyrism — *see* Poisoning, food,
  noxious, plant
Neuroleprosy A30.9
Neuroma — *see also* Neoplasm, nerve, benign
  acoustic (nerve) D33.3
  amputation (stump) (traumatic) (surgical
    complication) (late) T87.3-
    arm T87.3-
    leg T87.3-
  digital (toe) G57.6-
  interdigital G58.8
    lower limb (toe) G57.8-
    upper limb G56.8-
  intermetatarsal G57.8-
  Morton's G57.6-
  nonneoplastic
    arm G56.9-
    leg G57.9-
    lower extremity G57.9-
    upper extremity G56.9-
  optic (nerve) D33.3
  plantar G57.6-
  plexiform — *see* Neoplasm, nerve, benign
  surgical (nonneoplastic)
    arm G56.9-
    leg G57.9-
    lower extremity G57.9-
    upper extremity G56.9-
Neuromyalgia — *see* Neuralgia
Neuromyasthenia (epidemic) (postinfectious)
  G93.3
Neuromyelitis G36.9
  ascending G61.0
  optica G36.0
Neuromyopathy G70.9
  paraneoplastic D49.9 *[G13.0]*
Neuromyotonia (Isaacs) G71.19
Neuronevus — *see* Nevus
Neuronitis G58.9
  ascending (acute) G57.2-
  vestibular H81.2-
Neuroparalytic — *see* condition
Neuropathy, neuropathic G62.9
  acute motor G62.81
  alcoholic G62.1
    with psychosis — *see* Psychosis, alcoholic
  arm G56.9-
  autonomic, peripheral — *see* Neuropathy,
    peripheral, autonomic
  axillary G56.9-
  bladder N31.9
    atonic (motor) (sensory) N31.2
    autonomous N31.2
    flaccid N31.2
    nonreflex N31.2
    reflex N31.1
    uninhibited N31.0
  brachial plexus G54.0
  cervical plexus G54.2
  chronic
    progressive segmentally demyelinating
      G62.89
    relapsing demyelinating G62.89
  Déjérine-Sottas G60.0
  diabetic — *see* E08-E13 with .40
    mononeuropathy — *see* E08-E13 with .41
    polyneuropathy — *see* E08-E13 with .42

Neuropathy, neuropathic G62.9 —
  continued
  entrapment G58.9
    iliohypogastric nerve G57.8-
    ilioinguinal nerve G57.8-
    lateral cutaneous nerve of thigh G57.1-
    median nerve G56.0-
    obturator nerve G57.8-
    peroneal nerve G57.3-
    posterior tibial nerve G57.5-
    saphenous nerve G57.8-
    ulnar nerve G56.2-
  facial nerve G51.9
  hereditary G60.9
    motor and sensory (types I-IV) G60.0
    sensory G60.8
    specified NEC G60.8
  hypertrophic G60.0
    Charcot-Marie-Tooth G60.0
    Déjérine-Sottas G60.0
    interstitial progressive G60.0
    of infancy G60.0
    Refsum G60.1
  idiopathic G60.9
    progressive G60.3
    specified NEC G60.8
  in association with hereditary ataxia G60.2
  intercostal G58.0
  ischemic — *see* Disorder, nerve
  Jamaica (ginger) G62.2
  leg NEC G57.9-
  lower extremity G57.9-
  lumbar plexus G54.1
  median nerve G56.1-
  motor and sensory — *see also* Polyneuropathy
    hereditary (types I-IV) G60.0
  multifocal motor (MMN) G61.82
  multiple (acute) (chronic) — *see* Polyneuropathy
  optic (nerve) — *see also* Neuritis, optic
    ischemic H47.01-
  paraneoplastic (sensorial) (Denny Brown)
    D49.9 *[G13.0]*
  peripheral (nerve) (*see also* Polyneuropathy)
    G62.9
    autonomic G90.9
      idiopathic G90.09
      in (due to)
        amyloidosis E85.4 *[G99.0]*
        diabetes mellitus — *see* E08-E13 with
          .43
        endocrine disease NEC E34.9 *[G99.0]*
        gout M10.00 *[G99.0]*
        hyperthyroidism E05.90 *[G99.0]*
          with thyroid storm E05.91 *[G99.0]*
        metabolic disease NEC E88.9 *[G99.0]*
    idiopathic G60.9
      progressive G60.3
    in (due to)
      antitetanus serum G62.0
      arsenic G62.2
      drugs NEC G62.0
      lead G62.2
      organophosphate compounds G62.2
      toxic agent NEC G62.2
  plantar nerves G57.6-
  progressive
    hypertrophic interstitial G60.0
    inflammatory G62.81
  radicular NEC — *see* Radiculopathy
  sacral plexus G54.1
  sciatic G57.0-
  serum G61.1
  toxic NEC G62.2
  trigeminal sensory G50.8
  ulnar nerve G56.2-
  uremic N18.9 *[G63]*
  vitamin B12 E53.8 *[G63]*
    with anemia (pernicious) D51.0 *[G63]*
      due to dietary deficiency D51.3 *[G63]*

Neurophthisis — see also Disorder, nerve
  peripheral, diabetic — see E08-E13 with .42
Neuroretinitis — see Chorioretinitis
Neuroretinopathy, hereditary optic
  H47.22
Neurosarcoma — see Neoplasm, nerve,
  malignant
Neurosclerosis — see Disorder, nerve
Neurosis, neurotic F48.9
  anankastic F42.8
  anxiety (state) F41.1
    panic type F41.0
  asthenic F48.8
  bladder F45.8
  cardiac (reflex) F45.8
  cardiovascular F45.8
  character F60.9
  colon F45.8
  compensation F68.1
  compulsive, compulsion F42.8
  conversion F44.9
  craft F48.8
  cutaneous F45.8
  depersonalization F48.1
  depressive (reaction) (type) F34.1
  environmental F48.8
  excoriation L98.1
  fatigue F48.8
  functional — see Disorder, somatoform
  gastric F45.8
  gastrointestinal F45.8
  heart F45.8
  hypochondriacal F45.21
  hysterical F44.9
  incoordination F45.8
    larynx F45.8
    vocal cord F45.8
  intestine F45.8
  larynx (sensory) F45.8
    hysterical F44.4
  mixed NEC F48.8
  musculoskeletal F45.8
  obsessional F42.8
  obsessive-compulsive F42.8
  occupational F48.8
  ocular NEC F45.8
  organ — see Disorder, somatoform
  pharynx F45.8
  phobic F40.9
  posttraumatic (situational) F43.10
    acute F43.11
    chronic F43.12
  psychasthenic (type) F48.8
  railroad F48.8
  rectum F45.8
  respiratory F45.8
  rumination F45.8
  sexual F65.9
  situational F48.8
  social F40.10
    generalized F40.11
  specified type NEC F48.8
  state F48.9
    with depersonalization episode F48.1
  stomach F45.8
  traumatic F43.10
    acute F43.11
    chronic F43.12
  vasomotor F45.8
  visceral F45.8
  war F48.8
Neurospongioblastosis diffusa Q85.1
Neurosyphilis (arrested) (early) (gumma) (late)
  (latent) (recurrent) (relapse) A52.3
  with ataxia (cerebellar) (locomotor) (spastic)
    (spinal) A52.19
  aneurysm (cerebral) A52.05
  arachnoid (adhesive) A52.13
  arteritis (any artery) (cerebral) A52.04

Neurosyphilis (arrested) (early) (gumma) (late)
  (latent) (recurrent) (relapse) A52.3 —
  continued
  asymptomatic A52.2
  congenital A50.40
  dura (mater) A52.13
  general paresis A52.17
  hemorrhagic A52.05
  juvenile (asymptomatic) (meningeal) A50.40
  leptomeninges (aseptic) A52.13
  meningeal, meninges (adhesive) A52.13
  meningitis A52.13
  meningovascular (diffuse) A52.13
  optic atrophy A52.15
  parenchymatous (degenerative) A52.19
  paresis, paretic A52.17
    juvenile A50.45
  remission in (sustained) A52.3
  serological (without symptoms) A52.2
  specified nature or site NEC A52.19
  tabes, tabetic (dorsalis) A52.11
    juvenile A50.45
  taboparesis A52.17
    juvenile A50.45
  thrombosis (cerebral) A52.05
  vascular (cerebral) NEC A52.05
Neurothekeoma — see Neoplasm, nerve,
  benign
Neurotic — see Neurosis
Neurotoxemia — see Toxemia
Neutroclusion M26.211
Neutropenia, neutropenic (chronic)
  (genetic) (idiopathic) (immune) (infantile)
  (malignant) (pernicious) (splenic) D70.9
  congenital (primary) D70.0
  cyclic D70.4
  cytoreductive cancer chemotherapy sequela
    D70.1
  drug-induced D70.2
    due to cytoreductive cancer chemotherapy
      D70.1
  due to infection D70.3
  fever D70.9
  neonatal, transitory (isoimmune) (maternal
    transfer) P61.5
  periodic D70.4
  secondary (cyclic) (periodic) (splenic) D70.4
    drug-induced D70.2
      due to cytoreductive cancer chemotherapy
        D70.1
  toxic D70.8
Neutrophilia, hereditary giant D72.0
Nevocarcinoma — see Melanoma
Nevus D22.9
  achromic — see Neoplasm, skin, benign
  amelanotic — see Neoplasm, skin, benign
  angiomatous D18.00
    intra-abdominal D18.03
    intracranial D18.02
    skin D18.01
    specified site NEC D18.09
  araneus I78.1
  balloon cell — see Neoplasm, skin, benign
  bathing trunk D48.5
  blue — see Neoplasm, skin, benign
    cellular — see Neoplasm, skin, benign
    giant — see Neoplasm, skin, benign
    Jadassohn's — see Neoplasm, skin, benign
    malignant — see Melanoma
  capillary D18.00
    intra-abdominal D18.03
    intracranial D18.02
    skin D18.01
    specified site NEC D18.09
  cavernous D18.00
    intra-abdominal D18.03
    intracranial D18.02
    skin D18.01
    specified site NEC D18.09

Nevus D22.9 — continued
  cellular — see Neoplasm, skin, benign
    blue — see Neoplasm, skin, benign
  choroid D31.3-
  comedonicus Q82.5
  conjunctiva D31.0-
  dermal — see Neoplasm, skin, benign
    with epidermal nevus — see Neoplasm, skin,
      benign
  dysplastic — see Neoplasm, skin, benign
  eye D31.9-
  flammeus Q82.5
  hemangiomatous D18.00
    intra-abdominal D18.03
    intracranial D18.02
    skin D18.01
    specified site NEC D18.09
  iris D31.4-
  lacrimal gland D31.5-
  lymphatic D18.1
  magnocellular
    specified site — see Neoplasm, benign, by
      site
    unspecified site D31.40
  malignant — see Melanoma
  meaning hemangioma D18.00
    intra-abdominal D18.03
    intracranial D18.02
    skin D18.01
    specified site NEC D18.09
  mouth (mucosa) D10.30
    specified site NEC D10.39
    white sponge Q38.6
  multiplex Q85.1
  non-neoplastic I78.1
  oral mucosa D10.30
    specified site NEC D10.39
    white sponge Q38.6
  orbit D31.6-
  pigmented
    giant (see also Neoplasm, skin, uncertain
      behavior) D48.5
      malignant melanoma in — see Melanoma
  portwine Q82.5
  retina D31.2-
  retrobulbar D31.6-
  sanguineous Q82.5
  senile I78.1
  skin D22.9
    abdominal wall D22.5
    ala nasi D22.39
    ankle D22.7-
    anus, anal D22.5
    arm D22.6-
    auditory canal (external) D22.2-
    auricle (ear) D22.2-
    auricular canal (external) D22.2-
    axilla, axillary fold D22.5
    back D22.5
    breast D22.5
    brow D22.39
    buttock D22.5
    canthus (eye) D22.1-
    cheek (external) D22.39
    chest wall D22.5
    chin D22.39
    ear (external) D22.2-
    external meatus (ear) D22.2-
    eyebrow D22.39
    eyelid (lower) (upper) D22.1-
    face D22.30
      specified NEC D22.39
    female genital organ (external) NEC D28.0
    finger D22.6-
    flank D22.5
    foot D22.7-
    forearm D22.6-
    forehead D22.39
    foreskin D29.0

Nevus D22.9 — *continued*
  skin D22.9 — *continued*
    genital organ (external) NEC
      female D28.0
      male D29.9
    gluteal region D22.5
    groin D22.5
    hand D22.6-
    heel D22.7-
    helix D22.2-
    hip D22.7-
    interscapular region D22.5
    jaw D22.39
    knee D22.7-
    labium (majus) (minus) D28.0
    leg D22.7-
    lip (lower) (upper) D22.0
    lower limb D22.7-
    male genital organ (external) D29.9
    nail D22.9
      finger D22.6-
      toe D22.7-
    nasolabial groove D22.39
    nates D22.5
    neck D22.4
    nose (external) D22.39
    palpebra D22.1-
    penis D29.0
    perianal skin D22.5
    perineum D22.5
    pinna D22.2-
    popliteal fossa or space D22.7-
    prepuce D29.0
    pudendum D28.0
    scalp D22.4
    scrotum D29.4
    shoulder D22.6-
    submammary fold D22.5
    temple D22.39
    thigh D22.7-
    toe D22.7-
    trunk NEC D22.5
    umbilicus D22.5
    upper limb D22.6-
    vulva D28.0
  specified site NEC — *see* Neoplasm, by site, benign
  spider I78.1
  stellar I78.1
  strawberry Q82.5
  Sutton's — *see* Neoplasm, skin, benign
  unius lateris Q82.5
  Unna's Q82.5
  vascular Q82.5
  verrucous Q82.5

Newborn (infant) (liveborn) (singleton) Z38.2
  abstinence syndrome P96.1
  acne L70.4
  affected by
    abnormalities of membranes P02.9
      specified NEC P02.8
    abruptio placenta P02.1
    amino-acid metabolic disorder, transitory P74.8
    amniocentesis (while in utero) P00.6
    amnionitis P02.7
    apparent life threatening event (ALTE) R68.13
    bleeding (into)
      cerebral cortex P52.22
      germinal matrix P52.0
      ventricles P52.1
    breech delivery P03.0
    cardiac arrest P29.81
    cardiomyopathy I42.8
      congenital I42.4
    cerebral ischemia P91.0
    cesarean delivery P03.4
    chemotherapy agents P04.1

Newborn (infant) (liveborn) (singleton) Z38.2
  — *continued*
  affected by — *continued*
    chorioamnionitis P02.7
    cocaine (crack) P04.41
    complications of labor and delivery P03.9
      specified NEC P03.89
    compression of umbilical cord NEC P02.5
    contracted pelvis P03.1
    delivery P03.9
      cesarean P03.4
      forceps P03.2
      vacuum extractor P03.3
    entanglement (knot) in umbilical cord P02.5
    environmental chemicals P04.6
    fetal (intrauterine)
      growth retardation P05.9
      malnutrition not light or small for gestational age P05.2
    forceps delivery P03.2
    heart rate abnormalities
      bradycardia P29.12
      intrauterine P03.819
        before onset of labor P03.810
        during labor P03.811
      tachycardia P29.11
    hemorrhage (antepartum) P02.1
      cerebellar (nontraumatic) P52.6
      intracerebral (nontraumatic) P52.4
      intracranial (nontraumatic) P52.9
        specified NEC P52.8
      intraventricular (nontraumatic) P52.3
        grade 1 P52.0
        grade 2 P52.1
        grade 3 P52.21
        grade 4 P52.22
      posterior fossa (nontraumatic) P52.6
      subarachnoid (nontraumatic) P52.5
      subependymal P52.0
        with intracerebral extension P52.22
        with intraventricular extension P52.1
          with enlargment of ventricles P52.21
        without intraventricular extension P52.0
    hypoxic ischemic encephalopathy [HIE] P91.60
      mild P91.61
      moderate P91.62
      severe P91.63
    induction of labor P03.89
    intestinal perforation P78.0
    intrauterine (fetal) blood loss P50.9
      due to (from)
        cut end of co-twin cord P50.5
        hemorrhage into
          co-twin P50.3
          maternal circulation P50.4
        placenta P50.2
        ruptured cord blood P50.1
        vasa previa P50.0
      specified NEC P50.8
    intrauterine (fetal) hemorrhage P50.9
    intrauterine (in utero) procedure P96.5
    malpresentation (malposition) NEC P03.1
    maternal (complication of) (use of)
      alcohol P04.3
      analgesia (maternal) P04.0
      anesthesia (maternal) P04.0
      blood loss P02.1
      circulatory disease P00.3
      condition P00.9
        specified NEC P00.89
      delivery P03.9
        Cesarean P03.4
        forceps P03.2
        vacuum extractor P03.3
      diabetes mellitus (pre-existing) P70.1
      disorder P00.9
        specified NEC P00.89
      drugs (addictive) (illegal) NEC P04.49

Newborn (infant) (liveborn) (singleton) Z38.2
  — *continued*
  affected by — *continued*
    maternal (complication of) (use of) — *continued*
      ectopic pregnancy P01.4
      gestational diabetes P70.0
      hemorrhage P02.1
      hypertensive disorder P00.0
      incompetent cervix P01.0
      infectious disease P00.2
      injury P00.5
      labor and delivery P03.9
      malpresentation before labor P01.7
      maternal death P01.6
      medical procedure P00.7
      medication P04.1
      multiple pregnancy P01.5
      nutritional disorder P00.4
      oligohydramnios P01.2
      parasitic disease P00.2
      periodontal disease P00.81
      placenta previa P02.0
      polyhydramnios P01.3
      precipitate delivery P03.5
      pregnancy P01.9
        specified P01.8
      premature rupture of membranes P01.1
      renal disease P00.1
      respiratory disease P00.3
      surgical procedure P00.6
      urinary tract disease P00.1
      uterine contraction (abnormal) P03.6
    meconium peritonitis P78.0
    medication (legal) (maternal use) (prescribed) P04.1
    membrane abnormalities P02.9
      specified NEC P02.8
    membranitis P02.7
    methamphetamine(s) P04.49
    mixed metabolic and respiratory acidosis P84
    neonatal abstinence syndrome P96.1
    noxious substances transmitted via placenta or breast milk P04.9
      specified NEC P04.8
    nutritional supplements P04.5
    placenta previa P02.0
    placental
      abnormality (functional) (morphological) P02.20
        specified NEC P02.29
      dysfunction P02.29
      infarction P02.29
      insufficiency P02.29
      separation NEC P02.1
      transfusion syndromes P02.3
    placentitis P02.7
    precipitate delivery P03.5
    prolapsed cord P02.4
    respiratory arrest P28.81
    slow intrauterine growth P05.9
    tobacco P04.2
    twin to twin transplacental transfusion P02.3
    umbilical cord (tightly) around neck P02.5
    umbilical cord condition P02.60
      short cord P02.69
      specified NEC P02.69
    uterine contractions (abnormal) P03.6
    vasa previa P02.69
      from intrauterine blood loss P50.0
  apnea P28.4
    obstructive P28.4
    primary P28.3
    sleep (central) (obstructive) (primary) P28.3
  born in hospital Z38.00
    by cesarean Z38.01
  born outside hospital Z38.1
  breast buds P96.89

DISEASE INDEX

Newborn (infant) (liveborn) (singleton) Z38.2
— *continued*
  breast engorgement P83.4
  check-up — *see* Newborn, examination
  convulsion P90
  dehydration P74.1
  examination
    8 to 28 days old Z00.111
    under 8 days old Z00.110
  fever P81.9
    environmentally-induced P81.0
  hyperbilirubinemia P59.9
    of prematurity P59.0
  hypernatremia P74.2
  hyponatremia P74.2
  infection P39.9
    candidal P37.5
    specified NEC P39.8
    urinary tract P39.3
  jaundice P59.9
    due to
      breast milk inhibitor P59.3
      hepatocellular damage P59.20
        specified NEC P59.29
      preterm delivery P59.0
    of prematurity P59.0
    specified NEC P59.8
  late metabolic acidosis P74.0
  mastitis P39.0
    infective P39.0
    noninfective P83.4
  multiple born NEC Z38.8
    born in hospital Z38.68
      by cesarean Z38.69
    born outside hospital Z38.7
  omphalitis P38.9
    with mild hemorrhage P38.1
    without hemorrhage P38.9
  post-term P08.21
  prolonged gestation (over 42 completed
    weeks) P08.22
  quadruplet Z38.8
    born in hospital Z38.63
      by cesarean Z38.64
    born outside hospital Z38.7
  quintuplet Z38.8
    born in hospital Z38.65
      by cesarean Z38.66
    born outside hospital Z38.7
  seizure P90
  sepsis (congenital) P36.9
    due to
      anaerobes NEC P36.5
      Escherichia coli P36.4
      Staphylococcus P36.30
        aureus P36.2
        specified NEC P36.39
      Streptococcus P36.10
        group B P36.0
        specified NEC P36.19
    specified NEC P36.8
  triplet Z38.8
    born in hospital Z38.61
      by cesarean Z38.62
    born outside hospital Z38.7
  twin Z38.5
    born in hospital Z38.30
      by cesarean Z38.31
    born outside hospital Z38.4
  vomiting P92.09
    bilious P92.01
  weight check Z00.111
Newcastle conjunctivitis or disease B30.8
Nezelof's syndrome (pure alymphocytosis)
  D81.4
Niacin(amide) deficiency E52
Nicolas(-Durand)-Favre disease A55
Nicotine — *see* Tobacco
Nicotinic acid deficiency E52

Niemann-Pick disease or syndrome
  E75.249
  specified NEC E75.248
  type
    A E75.240
    B E75.241
    C E75.242
    D E75.243
Night
  blindness — *see* Blindness, night
  sweats R61
  terrors (child) F51.4
Nightmares (REM sleep type) F51.5
NIHSS (National Institutes of Health Stroke
  Scale) score R29.7-
Nipple — *see* condition
Nisbet's chancre A57
Nishimoto (-Takeuchi) disease I67.5
Nitritoid crisis or reaction — *see* Crisis,
  nitritoid
Nitrosohemoglobinemia D74.8
Njovera A65
Nocardiosis, nocardiasis A43.9
  cutaneous A43.1
  lung A43.0
  pneumonia A43.0
  pulmonary A43.0
  specified site NEC A43.8
Nocturia R35.1
  psychogenic F45.8
Nocturnal — *see* condition
Nodal rhythm I49.8
Node(s) — *see also* Nodule
  Bouchard's (with arthropathy) M15.2
  Haygarth's M15.8
  Heberden's (with arthropathy) M15.1
  larynx J38.7
  lymph — *see* condition
  milker's B08.03
  Osler's I33.0
  Schmorl's — *see* Schmorl's disease
  singer's J38.2
  teacher's J38.2
  tuberculous — *see* Tuberculosis, lymph gland
  vocal cord J38.2
Nodule(s), nodular
  actinomycotic — *see* Actinomycosis
  breast NEC N63
  colloid (cystic), thyroid E04.1
  cutaneous — *see* Swelling, localized
  endometrial (stromal) D26.1
  Haygarth's M15.8
  inflammatory — *see* Inflammation
  juxta-articular
    syphilitic A52.77
    yaws A66.7
  larynx J38.7
  lung, solitary (subsegmental branch of the
    bronchial tree) R91.1
    multiple R91.8
  milker's B08.03
  prostate N40.2
    with lower urinary tract symptoms (LUTS)
      N40.3
    without lower urinary tract symptoms (LUTS)
      N40.2
  pulmonary, solitary (subsegmental branch of
    the bronchial tree) R91.1
  retrocardiac R09.89
  rheumatoid M06.30
    ankle M06.37-
    elbow M06.32-
    foot joint M06.37-
    hand joint M06.34-
    hip M06.35-
    knee M06.36-
    multiple site M06.39
    shoulder M06.31-
    vertebra M06.38

Nodule(s), nodular — *continued*
  rheumatoid M06.30 — *continued*
    wrist M06.33-
  scrotum (inflammatory) N49.2
  singer's J38.2
  solitary, lung (subsegmental branch of the
    bronchial tree) R91.1
    multiple R91.8
  subcutaneous — *see* Swelling, localized
  teacher's J38.2
  thyroid (cold) (gland) (nontoxic) E04.1
    with thyrotoxicosis E05.20
      with thyroid storm E05.21
    toxic or with hyperthyroidism E05.20
      with thyroid storm E05.21
  vocal cord J38.2
Noma (gangrenous) (hospital) (infective) A69.0
  auricle I96
  mouth A69.0
  pudendi N76.89
  vulvae N76.89
Nomad, nomadism Z59.0
NOMID (neonatal onset multisystemic
  inflammatory disorder) M04.2
Nonautoimmune hemolytic anemia
  D59.4
  drug-induced D59.2
Nonclosure — *see also* Imperfect, closure
  ductus arteriosus (Botallo's) Q25.0
  foramen
    botalli Q21.1
    ovale Q21.1
Noncompliance Z91.19
  with
    dialysis Z91.15
    dietary regimen Z91.11
    medical treatment Z91.19
    medication regimen NEC Z91.14
      underdosing (*see also* Table of Drugs and
        Chemicals, categories T36-T50, with
        final character 6) Z91.14
        intentional NEC Z91.128
          due to financial hardship of patient
            Z91.120
        unintentional NEC Z91.138
          due to patient's age related debility
            Z91.130
    renal dialysis Z91.15
Nondescent (congenital) — *see also*
  Malposition, congenital
  cecum Q43.3
  colon Q43.3
  testicle Q53.9
    bilateral Q53.20
      abdominal Q53.21
      perineal Q53.22
    unilateral Q53.10
      abdominal Q53.11
      perineal Q53.12
Nondevelopment
  brain Q02
    part of Q04.3
  organ or site, congenital NEC — *see*
    Hypoplasia
Nonengagement
  head NEC O32.4
  in labor, causing obstructed labor O64.8
Nonexanthematous tick fever A93.2
Nonexpansion, lung (newborn) P28.0
Nonfunctioning
  cystic duct (*see also* Disease, gallbladder)
    K82.8
  gallbladder (*see also* Disease, gallbladder)
    K82.8
  kidney N28.9
  labyrinth — *see* subcategory H83.2
Non-Hodgkin lymphoma NEC — *see*
  Lymphoma, non-Hodgkin
Nonimplantation, ovum N97.2

DISEASE INDEX

Noninsufflation, fallopian tube N97.1
Non-ketotic hyperglycinemia E72.51
Nonne-Milroy syndrome Q82.0
Nonovulation N97.0
Nonpatent fallopian tube N97.1
Nonpneumatization, lung NEC P28.0
Nonrotation — *see* Malrotation
Nonsecretion, urine — *see* Anuria
Nonunion
  fracture — *see* Fracture, by site
  joint, following fusion or arthrodesis M96.0
  organ or site, congenital NEC — *see* Imperfect,
    closure
  symphysis pubis, congenital Q74.2
Nonvisualization, gallbladder R93.2
Nonvital, nonvitalized tooth K04.99
Non-working side interference M26.56
Noonan's syndrome Q87.1
**Normocytic anemia (infectional) due to
  blood loss** (chronic) D50.0
  acute D62
Norrie's disease (congenital) Q15.8
North American blastomycosis B40.9
Norwegian itch B86
Nose, nasal — *see* condition
Nosebleed R04.0
Nosomania F45.21
Nosophobia F45.22
Nose-picking F98.8
Nostalgia F43.20
Notch of iris Q13.2
Notching nose, congenital (tip) Q30.2
Nothnagel's
  syndrome — *see* Strabismus, paralytic, third
    nerve
  vasomotor acroparesthesia I73.89
Novy's relapsing fever A68.9
  louse-borne A68.0
  tick-borne A68.1
Noxious
  foodstuffs, poisoning by — *see* Poisoning,
    food, noxious, plant
  substances transmitted through placenta or
    breast milk P04.9
Nucleus pulposus — *see* condition
Numbness R20.0
Nuns' knee — *see* Bursitis, prepatellar
Nursemaid's elbow S53.03-
Nutcracker esophagus K22.4
Nutmeg liver K76.1
Nutrient element deficiency E61.9
  specified NEC E61.8
Nutrition deficient or insufficient (*see also*
  Malnutrition) E46
  due to
    insufficient food T73.0
    lack of
      care (child) T76.02
        adult T76.01
      food T73.0
Nutritional stunting E45
Nyctalopia (night blindness) — *see* Blindness,
  night
Nycturia R35.1
  psychogenic F45.8
Nymphomania F52.8
Nystagmus H55.00
  benign paroxysmal — *see* Vertigo, benign
    paroxysmal
  central positional H81.4-
  congenital H55.01
  dissociated H55.04
  latent H55.02
  miners' H55.09
  positional
    benign paroxysmal H81.4-
    central H81.4-
  specified form NEC H55.09
  visual deprivation H55.03

Obermeyer's relapsing fever (European)
  A68.0
Obesity E66.9
  with alveolar hypoventilation E66.2
  adrenal E27.8
  complicating
    childbirth O99.214
    pregnancy O99.21-
    puerperium O99.215
  constitutional E66.8
  dietary counseling and surveillance Z71.3
  drug-induced E66.1
  due to
    drug E66.1
    excess calories E66.09
      morbid E66.01
      severe E66.01
  endocrine E66.8
  endogenous E66.8
  exogenous E66.09
  familial E66.8
  glandular E66.8
  hypothyroid — *see* Hypothyroidism
  hypoventilation syndrome (OHS) E66.2
  morbid E66.01
    with
      alveolar hypoventilation E66.2
      obesity hypoventilation syndrome (OHS)
        E66.2
    due to excess calories E66.01
  nutritional E66.09
  pituitary E23.6
  severe E66.01
  specified type NEC E66.8
Oblique — *see* condition
Obliteration
  appendix (lumen) K38.8
  artery I77.1
  bile duct (noncalculous) K83.1
  common duct (noncalculous) K83.1
  cystic duct — *see* Obstruction, gallbladder
  disease, arteriolar I77.1
  endometrium N85.8
  eye, anterior chamber — *see* Disorder, globe,
    hypotony
  fallopian tube N97.1
  lymphatic vessel I89.0
    due to mastectomy I97.2
  organ or site, congenital NEC — *see* Atresia,
    by site
  ureter N13.5
    with infection N13.6
  urethra — *see* Stricture, urethra
  vein I87.8
  vestibule (oral) K08.89
Observation (following) (for) (without need for
  further medical care) Z04.9
  accident NEC Z04.3
    at work Z04.2
    transport Z04.1
  adverse effect of drug Z03.6
  alleged rape or sexual assault (victim), ruled
    out
    adult Z04.41
    child Z04.42
  criminal assault Z04.8
  development state
    adolescent Z00.3
    period of rapid growth in childhood Z00.2
    puberty Z00.3
  disease, specified NEC Z03.89
  following work accident Z04.2
  growth and development state — *see*
    Observation, development state
  injuries (accidental) NEC — *see also*
    Observation, accident

Observation (following) (for) (without need for
  further medical care) Z04.9 — *continued*
  newborn (for)
    suspected condition, related to exposure
      from the mother or birth process — *see*
      Newborn, affected by, maternal
      ruled out Z05.9
        cardiac Z05.0
        connective tissue Z05.73
        gastrointestinal Z05.5
        genetic Z05.41
        genitourinary Z05.6
        immunologic Z05.43
        infectious Z05.1
        metabolic Z05.42
        musculoskeletal Z05.72
        neurological Z05.2
        respiratory Z05.3
        skin and subcutaneous tissue Z05.71
        specified condition NEC Z05.8
  postpartum
    immediately after delivery Z39.0
    routine follow-up Z39.2
  pregnancy (normal) (without complication)
    Z34.9-
    high risk O09.9-
  suicide attempt, alleged NEC Z03.89
    self-poisoning Z03.6
  suspected, ruled out — *see also* Suspected
    condition, ruled out
    abuse, physical
      adult Z04.71
      child Z04.72
    accident at work Z04.2
    adult battering victim Z04.71
    child battering victim Z04.72
    condition NEC Z03.89
      newborn (*see also* Observation, newborn
        (for), suspected condition, ruled out)
        Z05.9
    drug poisoning or adverse effect Z03.6
    exposure (to)
      anthrax Z03.810
      biological agent NEC Z03.818
    inflicted injury NEC Z04.8
    suicide attempt, alleged Z03.89
      self-poisoning Z03.6
    toxic effects from ingested substance (drug)
      (poison) Z03.6
  toxic effects from ingested substance (drug)
    (poison) Z03.6
Obsession, obsessional state F42.8
  mixed thoughts and acts F42.2
**Obsessive-compulsive neurosis or
  reaction** F42.8
Obstetric embolism, septic — *see* Embolism,
  obstetric, septic
Obstetrical trauma (complicating delivery)
  O71.9
  with or following ectopic or molar pregnancy
    O08.6
  specified type NEC O71.89
Obstipation — *see* Constipation
Obstruction, obstructed, obstructive
  airway J98.8
    with
      allergic alveolitis J67.9
      asthma J45.909
        with
          exacerbation (acute) J45.901
          status asthmaticus J45.902
      bronchiectasis J47.9
        with
          exacerbation (acute) J47.1
          lower respiratory infection J47.0
      bronchitis (chronic) J44.9
      emphysema J43.9

Obstruction, obstructed, obstructive — *continued*
  airway J98.8 — *continued*
    chronic J44.9
      with
        allergic alveolitis — *see* Pneumonitis, hypersensitivity
        bronchiectasis J47.9
          with
            exacerbation (acute) J47.1
            lower respiratory infection J47.0
      due to
        foreign body — *see* Foreign body, by site, causing asphyxia
        inhalation of fumes or vapors J68.9
        laryngospasm J38.5
  ampulla of Vater K83.1
  aortic (heart) (valve) — *see* Stenosis, aortic
  aortoiliac I74.09
  aqueduct of Sylvius G91.1
    congenital Q03.0
      with spina bifida — *see* Spina bifida, by site, with hydrocephalus
  Arnold-Chiari — *see* Arnold-Chiari disease
  artery (*see also* Embolism, artery) I74.9
    basilar (complete) (partial) — *see* Occlusion, artery, basilar
    carotid (complete) (partial) — *see* Occlusion, artery, carotid
    cerebellar — *see* Occlusion, artery, cerebellar
    cerebral (anterior) (middle) (posterior) — *see* Occlusion, artery, cerebral
    precerebral — *see* Occlusion, artery, precerebral
    renal N28.0
    retinal NEC — *see* Occlusion, artery, retina
    stent — *see* Restenosis, stent
    vertebral (complete) (partial) — *see* Occlusion, artery, vertebral
  band (intestinal) K56.69
  bile duct or passage (common) (hepatic) (noncalculous) K83.1
    with calculus K80.51
    congenital (causing jaundice) Q44.3
  biliary (duct) (tract) K83.1
    gallbladder K82.0
  bladder-neck (acquired) N32.0
    congenital Q64.31
    due to hyperplasia (hypertrophy) of prostate — *see* Hyperplasia, prostate
  bowel — *see* Obstruction, intestine
  bronchus J98.09
  canal, ear — *see* Stenosis, external ear canal
  cardia K22.2
  caval veins (inferior) (superior) I87.1
  cecum — *see* Obstruction, intestine
  circulatory I99.8
  colon — *see* Obstruction, intestine
  common duct (noncalculous) K83.1
  coronary (artery) — *see* Occlusion, coronary
  cystic duct — *see also* Obstruction, gallbladder
    with calculus K80.21
  device, implant or graft (*see also* Complications, by site and type, mechanical) T85.698
    arterial graft NEC — *see* Complication, cardiovascular device, mechanical, vascular
    catheter NEC T85.628
      cystostomy T83.090
      dialysis (renal) T82.49
        intraperitoneal T85.691
      Hopkins T83.098
      ileostomy T83.098
      infusion NEC T82.594
        spinal (epidural) (subdural) T85.690
      nephrostomy T83.092
      urethral indwelling T83.091
      urinary T83.098

Obstruction, obstructed, obstructive — *continued*
  device, implant or graft (*see also* Complications, by site and type, mechanical) T85.698 — *continued*
    catheter NEC T85.628 — *continued*
      urostomy T83.098
    due to infection T85.79
    gastrointestinal — *see* Complications, prosthetic device, mechanical, gastrointestinal device
    genital NEC T83.498
      intrauterine contraceptive device T83.39
      penile prosthesis (cylinder) (implanted) (pump) (resevoir) T83.490
      testicular prosthesis T83.491
    heart NEC — *see* Complication, cardiovascular device, mechanical
    joint prosthesis — *see* Complications, joint prosthesis, mechanical, specified NEC, by site
    orthopedic NEC — *see* Complication, orthopedic, device, mechanical
    specified NEC T85.628
    urinary NEC — *see also* Complication, genitourinary, device, urinary, mechanical
      graft T83.29
    vascular NEC — *see* Complication, cardiovascular device, mechanical
    ventricular intracranial shunt T85.09
  due to foreign body accidentally left in operative wound T81.529
  duodenum K31.5
  ejaculatory duct N50.89
  esophagus K22.2
  eustachian tube (complete) (partial) H68.10-
    cartilagenous (extrinsic) H68.13-
      intrinsic H68.12-
    osseous H68.11-
  fallopian tube (bilateral) N97.1
  fecal K56.41
    with hernia — *see* Hernia, by site, with obstruction
  foramen of Monro (congenital) Q03.8
    with spina bifida — *see* Spina bifida, by site, with hydrocephalus
  foreign body — *see* Foreign body
  gallbladder K82.0
    with calculus, stones K80.21
    congenital Q44.1
  gastric outlet K31.1
  gastrointestinal — *see* Obstruction, intestine
  hepatic K76.89
    duct (noncalculous) K83.1
  hepatobiliary K83.1
  ileum — *see* Obstruction, intestine
  iliofemoral (artery) I74.5
  intestine K56.60
    with
      adhesions (intestinal) (peritoneal) K56.5
    adynamic K56.0
    by gallstone K56.3
    congenital (small) Q41.9
      large Q42.9
        specified part NEC Q42.8
    neurogenic K56.0
      Hirschsprung's disease or megacolon Q43.1
    newborn P76.9
      due to
        fecaliths P76.8
        inspissated milk P76.2
        meconium (plug) P76.0
          in mucoviscidosis E84.11
      specified NEC P76.8
    postoperative K91.3
    reflex K56.0
    specified NEC K56.69
    volvulus K56.2

Obstruction, obstructed, obstructive — *continued*
  intracardiac ball valve prosthesis T82.09
  jejunum — *see* Obstruction, intestine
  joint prosthesis — *see* Complications, joint prosthesis, mechanical, specified NEC, by site
  kidney (calices) N28.89
  labor — *see* Delivery
  lacrimal (passages) (duct)
    by
      dacryolith — *see* Dacryolith
      stenosis — *see* Stenosis, lacrimal
    congenital Q10.5
    neonatal H04.53-
  lacrimonasal duct — *see* Obstruction, lacrimal
  lacteal, with steatorrhea K90.2
  laryngitis — *see* Laryngitis
  larynx NEC J38.6
    congenital Q31.8
  lung J98.4
    disease, chronic J44.9
  lymphatic I89.0
  meconium (plug)
    newborn P76.0
      due to fecaliths P76.0
      in mucoviscidosis E84.11
  mitral — *see* Stenosis, mitral
  nasal J34.89
  nasolacrimal duct — *see also* Obstruction, lacrimal
    congenital Q10.5
  nasopharynx J39.2
  nose J34.89
  organ or site, congenital NEC — *see* Atresia, by site
  pancreatic duct K86.89
  parotid duct or gland K11.8
  pelviureteral junction N13.5
    with hydronephrosis N13.0
    congenital Q62.39
  pharynx J39.2
  portal (circulation) (vein) I81
  prostate — *see also* Hyperplasia, prostate
    valve (urinary) N32.0
  pulmonary valve (heart) I37.0
  pyelonephritis (chronic) N11.1
  pylorus
    adult K31.1
    congenital or infantile Q40.0
  rectosigmoid — *see* Obstruction, intestine
  rectum K62.4
  renal N28.89
    outflow N13.8
    pelvis, congenital Q62.39
  respiratory J98.8
    chronic J44.9
  retinal (vessels) H34.9
  salivary duct (any) K11.8
    with calculus K11.5
  sigmoid — *see* Obstruction, intestine
  sinus (accessory) (nasal) J34.89
  Stensen's duct K11.8
  stomach NEC K31.89
    acute K31.0
    congenital Q40.2
    due to pylorospasm K31.3
  submandibular duct K11.8
  submaxillary gland K11.8
    with calculus K11.5
  thoracic duct I89.0
  thrombotic — *see* Thrombosis
  trachea J39.8
  tracheostomy airway J95.03
  tricuspid (valve) — *see* Stenosis, tricuspid
  upper respiratory, congenital Q34.8

Obstruction, obstructed, obstructive — *continued*
ureter (functional) (pelvic junction) NEC N13.5
  with
    hydronephrosis N13.1
      with infection N13.6
    pyelonephritis (chronic) N11.1
  congenital Q62.39
  due to calculus — *see* Calculus, ureter
urethra NEC N36.8
  congenital Q64.39
urinary (moderate) N13.9
  due to hyperplasia (hypertrophy) of prostate
    — *see* Hyperplasia, prostate
  organ or tract (lower) N13.9
  prostatic valve N32.0
  specified NEC N13.8
uropathy N13.9
uterus N85.8
vagina N89.5
valvular — *see* Endocarditis
vein, venous I87.1
  caval (inferior) (superior) I87.1
  thrombotic — *see* Thrombosis
vena cava (inferior) (superior) I87.1
vesical NEC N32.0
vesicourethral orifice N32.0
  congenital Q64.31
vessel NEC I99.8
  stent — *see* Restenosis, stent
Obturator — *see* condition
Occlusal wear, teeth K03.0
Occlusio pupillae — *see* Membrane, pupillary
Occlusion, occluded
anus K62.4
  congenital Q42.3
    with fistula Q42.2
aortoiliac (chronic) I74.09
aqueduct of Sylvius G91.1
  congenital Q03.0
    with spina bifida — *see* Spina bifida, by
      site, with hydrocephalus
artery (*see also* Embolism, artery) I74.9
  auditory, internal I65.8
  basilar I65.1
    with
      infarction I63.22
        due to
          embolism I63.12
          thrombosis I63.02
  brain or cerebral I66.9
    with infarction (due to) I63.5-
      embolism I63.4-
      thrombosis I63.3-
  carotid I65.2-
    with
      infarction I63.23-
        due to
          embolism I63.13-
          thrombosis I63.03-
  cerebellar (anterior inferior) (posterior
    inferior) (superior) I66.3
    with infarction I63.54-
      due to
        embolism I63.44-
        thrombosis I63.34-
  cerebral I66.9
    with infarction I63.50
      due to
        embolism I63.40
          specified NEC I63.49
        thrombosis I63.30
          specified NEC I63.39
    anterior I66.1-
      with infarction I63.52-
        due to
          embolism I63.42-
          thrombosis I63.32-

Occlusion, occluded — *continued*
artery (*see also* Embolism, artery) I74.9 —
  continued
  cerebral I66.9 — *continued*
    middle I66.0-
      with infarction I63.51-
        due to
          embolism I63.41-
          thrombosis I63.31-
    posterior I66.2-
      with infarction I63.53-
        due to
          embolism I63.43-
          thrombosis I63.33-
    specified NEC I66.8
      with infarction I63.59
        due to
          embolism I63.4-
          thrombosis I63.3-
  choroidal (anterior) — *see* Occlusion, artery,
    precerebral, specified NEC
  communicating posterior — *see* Occlusion,
    artery, cerebral, specified NEC
  complete
    coronary I25.82
    extremities I70.92
  coronary (acute) (thrombotic) (without
    myocardial infarction) I24.0
    with myocardial infarction — *see*
      Infarction, myocardium
    chronic total I25.82
    complete I25.82
    healed or old I25.2
    total (chronic) I25.82
  hypophyseal — *see* Occlusion, artery,
    precerebral, specified NEC
  iliac I74.5
  lower extremities due to stenosis or stricture
    I77.1
  mesenteric (embolic) (thrombotic) (*see also*
    Infarct, intestine) K55.069
  perforating — *see* Occlusion, artery,
    cerebral, specified NEC
  peripheral I77.9
    thrombotic or embolic I74.4
  pontine — *see* Occlusion, artery, cerebral,
    specified NEC
  precerebral I65.9
    with infarction I63.20
      due to
        embolism I63.10
          specified NEC I63.19
        thrombosis I63.00
          specified NEC I63.09
      specified NEC I63.29
    basilar — *see* Occlusion, artery, basilar
    carotid — *see* Occlusion, artery, carotid
    puerperal O88.23
    specified NEC I65.8
      with infarction I63.29
        due to
          embolism I63.19
          thrombosis I63.00
    vertebral — *see* Occlusion, artery,
      vertebral
  renal N28.0
  retinal
    branch H34.23-
    central H34.1-
    partial H34.21-
    transient H34.0-
  spinal — *see* Occlusion, artery, precerebral,
    vertebral
  total (chronic)
    coronary I25.82
    extremities I70.92

Occlusion, occluded — *continued*
artery (*see also* Embolism, artery) I74.9 —
  continued
  vertebral I65.0-
    with
      infarction I63.21-
        due to
          embolism I63.11-
          thrombosis I63.01-
basilar artery — *see* Occlusion, artery, basilar
bile duct (common) (hepatic) (noncalculous)
  K83.1
bowel — *see* Obstruction, intestine
carotid (artery) (common) (internal) — *see*
  Occlusion, artery, carotid
centric (of teeth) M26.59
  maximum intercuspation discrepancy
    M26.55
cerebellar (artery) — *see* Occlusion, artery,
  cerebellar
cerebral (artery) — *see* Occlusion, artery,
  cerebral
cerebrovascular — *see also* Occlusion, artery,
  cerebral
  with infarction I63.5-
cervical canal — *see* Stricture, cervix
cervix (uteri) — *see* Stricture, cervix
choanal Q30.0
choroidal (artery) — *see* Occlusion, artery,
  precerebral, specified NEC
colon — *see* Obstruction, intestine
communicating posterior artery — *see*
  Occlusion, artery, precerebral, specified
  NEC
coronary (artery) (vein) (thrombotic) — *see also*
  Infarct, myocardium
  chronic total I25.82
  healed or old I25.2
  not resulting in infarction I24.0
  total (chronic) I25.82
cystic duct — *see* Obstruction, gallbladder
embolic — *see* Embolism
fallopian tube N97.1
  congenital Q50.6
gallbladder — *see also* Obstruction,
  gallbladder
  congenital (causing jaundice) Q44.1
gingiva, traumatic K06.2
hymen N89.6
  congenital Q52.3
hypophyseal (artery) — *see* Occlusion, artery,
  precerebral, specified NEC
iliac artery I74.5
intestine — *see* Obstruction, intestine
lacrimal passages — *see* Obstruction, lacrimal
lung J98.4
lymph or lymphatic channel I89.0
mammary duct N64.89
mesenteric artery (embolic) (thrombotic) (*see*
  also Infarct, intestine) K55.069
nose J34.89
  congenital Q30.0
organ or site, congenital NEC — *see* Atresia,
  by site
oviduct N97.1
  congenital Q50.6
peripheral arteries
  due to stricture or stenosis I77.1
  upper extremity I74.2
pontine (artery) — *see* Occlusion, artery,
  precerebral, specified NEC
posterior lingual, of mandibular teeth M26.29
precerebral artery — *see* Occlusion, artery,
  precerebral
punctum lacrimale — *see* Obstruction, lacrimal
pupil — *see* Membrane, pupillary
pylorus, adult (*see also* Stricture, pylorus) K31.1
renal artery N28.0

Occlusion, occluded — *continued*
  retina, retinal
    artery — *see* Occlusion, artery, retinal
    vein (central) H34.81-
      engorgement H34.82-
      tributary H34.83-
      vessels H34.9
  spinal artery — *see* Occlusion, artery,
    precerebral, vertebral
  teeth (mandibular) (posterior lingual) M26.29
  thoracic duct I89.0
  thrombotic — *see* Thrombosis, artery
  traumatic
    edentulous (alveolar) ridge K06.2
    gingiva K06.2
    periodontal K05.5
  tubal N97.1
  ureter (complete) (partial) N13.5
    congenital Q62.10
  ureteropelvic junction N13.5
    congenital Q62.11
  ureterovesical orifice N13.5
    congenital Q62.12
  urethra — *see* Stricture, urethra
  uterus N85.8
  vagina N89.5
  vascular NEC I99.8
  vein — *see* Thrombosis
    retinal — *see* Occlusion, retinal, vein
  vena cava (inferior) (superior) — *see*
    Embolism, vena cava
  ventricle (brain) NEC G91.1
  vertebral (artery) — *see* Occlusion, artery,
    vertebral
  vessel (blood) I99.8
  vulva N90.5
Occult
  blood in feces (stools) R19.5
Occupational
  problems NEC Z56.89
Ochlophobia — *see* Agoraphobia
Ochronosis (endogenous) E70.29
Ocular muscle — *see* condition
Oculogyric crisis or disturbance H51.8
  psychogenic F45.8
Oculomotor syndrome H51.9
Oculopathy
  syphilitic NEC A52.71
    congenital
      early A50.01
      late A50.30
    early (secondary) A51.43
    late A52.71
Oddi's sphincter spasm K83.4
Odontalgia K08.89
Odontoameloblastoma — *see* Cyst,
  calcifying odontogenic
Odontoclasia K03.89
Odontodysplasia, regional K00.4
Odontogenesis imperfecta K00.5
Odontoma (ameloblastic) (complex)
  (compound) (fibroameloblastic) — *see* Cyst,
  calcifying odontogenic
Odontomyelitis (closed) (open) K04.01
  irreversible K04.02
  reversible K04.01
Odontorrhagia K08.89
Odontosarcoma, ameloblastic C41.1
  upper jaw (bone) C41.0
Oestriasis — *see* Myiasis
Oguchi's disease H53.63
Ohara's disease — *see* Tularemia
OHS (obesity hypoventilation syndrome) E66.2
Oidiomycosis — *see* Candidiasis
Oidium albicans infection — *see*
  Candidiasis
Old age (without mention of debility) R54
  dementia F03

Old (previous) myocardial infarction
  I25.2
Olfactory — *see* condition
Oligemia — *see* Anemia
Oligoastrocytoma
  specified site — *see* Neoplasm, malignant, by
    site
  unspecified site C71.9
Oligocythemia D64.9
Oligodendroblastoma
  specified site — *see* Neoplasm, malignant
  unspecified site C71.9
Oligodendroglioma
  anaplastic type
    specified site — *see* Neoplasm, malignant,
      by site
    unspecified site C71.9
  specified site — *see* Neoplasm, malignant, by
    site
  unspecified site C71.9
Oligodontia — *see* Anodontia
Oligoencephalon Q02
Oligohidrosis L74.4
Oligohydramnios O41.0-
Oligohydrosis L74.4
Oligomenorrhea N91.5
  primary N91.3
  secondary N91.4
Oligophrenia — *see also* Disability, intellectual
  phenylpyruvic E70.0
Oligospermia N46.11
  due to
    drug therapy N46.121
    efferent duct obstruction N46.123
    infection N46.122
    radiation N46.124
    specified cause NEC N46.129
    systemic disease N46.125
Oligotrichia — *see* Alopecia
Oliguria R34
  postprocedural N99.0
  with, complicating or following ectopic or
    molar pregnancy O08.4
Ollier's disease Q78.4
Omenotocele — *see* Hernia, abdomen,
  specified site NEC
Omentitis — *see* Peritonitis
Omentum, omental — *see* condition
Omphalitis (congenital) (newborn) P38.9
  with mild hemorrhage P38.1
  not of newborn L08.82
  tetanus A33
  without hemorrhage P38.9
Omphalocele Q79.2
Omphalomesenteric duct, persistent
  Q43.0
Omphalorrhagia, newborn P51.9
Omsk hemorrhagic fever A98.1
Onanism (excessive) F98.8
Onchocerciasis, onchocercosis B73.1
  with
    eye disease B73.00
      endophthalmitis B73.01
      eyelid B73.09
      glaucoma B73.02
      specified NEC B73.09
    eye NEC B73.00
    eyelid B73.09
Oncocytoma — *see* Neoplasm, benign, by site
Oncovirus, as cause of disease classified
  elsewhere B97.32
Ondine's curse — *see* Apnea, sleep
Oneirophrenia F23
Onychauxis L60.2
  congenital Q84.5

Onychia — *see also* Cellulitis, digit
  with lymphangitis — *see* Lymphangitis, acute,
    digit
  candidal B37.2
  dermatophytic B35.1
Onychitis — *see also* Cellulitis, digit
  with lymphangitis — *see* Lymphangitis, acute,
    digit
Onychocryptosis L60.0
Onychodystrophy L60.3
  congenital Q84.6
Onychogryphosis, onychogryposis L60.2
Onycholysis L60.1
Onychomadesis L60.8
Onychomalacia L60.3
Onychomycosis (finger) (toe) B35.1
Onycho-osteodysplasia Q87.2
Onychophagia F98.8
Onychophosis L60.8
Onychoptosis L60.8
Onychorrhexis L60.3
  congenital Q84.6
Onychoschizia L60.3
Onyxis (finger) (toe) L60.0
Onyxitis — *see also* Cellulitis, digit
  with lymphangitis — *see* Lymphangitis, acute,
    digit
Oophoritis (cystic) (infectional) (interstitial)
  N70.92
  with salpingitis N70.93
  acute N70.02
    with salpingitis N70.03
  chronic N70.12
    with salpingitis N70.13
  complicating abortion — *see* Abortion, by
    type, complicated by, oophoritis
Oophorocele N83.4-
Opacity, opacities
  cornea H17-
    central H17.1-
    congenital Q13.3
    degenerative — *see* Degeneration, cornea
    hereditary — *see* Dystrophy, cornea
    inflammatory — *see* Keratitis
    minor H17.81-
    peripheral H17.82-
    sequelae of trachoma (healed) B94.0
    specified NEC H17.89
  enamel (teeth) (fluoride) (nonfluoride) K00.3
  lens — *see* Cataract
  snowball — *see* Deposit, crystalline
  vitreous (humor) NEC H43.39-
    congenital Q14.0
    membranes and strands H43.31-
Opalescent dentin (hereditary) K00.5
Open, opening
  abnormal, organ or site, congenital — *see*
    Imperfect, closure
  angle with
    borderline
      findings
        high risk H40.02-
        low risk H40.01-
      intraocular pressure H40.00-
    cupping of discs H40.01-
    glaucoma (primary) — *see* Glaucoma, open
      angle
  bite
    anterior M26.220
    posterior M26.221
  false — *see* Imperfect, closure
  margin on tooth restoration K08.51
  restoration margins of tooth K08.51
  wound — *see* Wound, open
Operational fatigue F48.8
Operative — *see* condition
Operculitis — *see* Periodontitis
Operculum — *see* Break, retina
Ophiasis L63.2

Ophthalmia (see also Conjunctivitis) H10.9
  actinic rays — see Photokeratitis
  allergic (acute) — see Conjunctivitis, acute,
    atopic
  blennorrhagic (gonococcal) (neonatorum)
    A54.31
  diphtheritic A36.86
  Egyptian A71.1
  electrica — see Photokeratitis
  gonococcal (neonatorum) A54.31
  metastatic — see Endophthalmitis, purulent
  migraine — see Migraine, ophthalmoplegic
  neonatorum, newborn P39.1
    gonococcal A54.31
  nodosa H16.24-
  purulent — see Conjunctivitis, acute,
    mucopurulent
  spring — see Conjunctivitis, acute, atopic
  sympathetic — see Uveitis, sympathetic
Ophthalmitis — see Ophthalmia
Ophthalmocele (congenital) Q15.8
Ophthalmoneuromyelitis G36.0
Ophthalmoplegia — see also Strabismus,
  paralytic
  anterior internuclear — see Ophthalmoplegia,
    internuclear
  ataxia-areflexia G61.0
  diabetic — see E08-E13 with .39
  exophthalmic E05.00
    with thyroid storm E05.01
  external H49.88-
    progressive H49.4-
      with pigmentary retinopathy — see
        Kearns-Sayre syndrome
    total H49.3-
  internal (complete) (total) H52.51-
  internuclear H51.2-
  migraine — see Migraine, ophthalmoplegic
  Parinaud's H49.88-
  progressive external — see Ophthalmoplegia,
    external, progressive
  supranuclear, progressive G23.1
  total (external) — see Ophthalmoplegia,
    external, total
Opioid(s)
  abuse — see Abuse, drug, opioids
  dependence — see Dependence, drug, opioids
  induced, without use disorder
    anxiety disorder F11.988
    delirium F11.921
    depressive disorder F11.94
    sexual dysfunction F11.981
    sleep disorder F11.982
Opisthognathism M26.09
Opisthorchiasis (felineus) (viverrini) B66.0
Opitz' disease D73.2
Opiumism — see Dependence, drug, opioid
Oppenheim's disease G70.2
Oppenheim-Urbach disease (necrobiosis
  lipoidica diabeticorum) — see E08-E13 with
  .620
Optic nerve — see condition
Orbit — see condition
Orchioblastoma C62.9-
Orchitis (gangrenous) (nonspecific) (septic)
  (suppurative) N45.2
  blennorrhagic (gonococcal) (acute) (chronic)
    A54.23
  chlamydial A56.19
  filarial (see also Infestation, filarial) B74.9
    [N51]
  gonococcal (acute) (chronic) A54.23
  mumps B26.0
  syphilitic A52.76
  tuberculous A18.15
Orf (virus disease) B08.02

Organic — see also condition
  brain syndrome F09
  heart — see Disease, heart
  mental disorder F09
  psychosis F09
Orgasm
  anejaculatory N53.13
Oriental
  bilharziasis B65.2
  schistosomiasis B65.2
Orifice — see condition
**Origin of both great vessels from right
  ventricle** Q20.1
Ormond's disease (with ureteral obstruction)
  N13.5
  with infection N13.6
Ornithine metabolism disorder E72.4
Ornithinemia (Type I) (Type II) E72.4
Ornithosis A70
Orotaciduria, oroticaciduria (congenital)
  (hereditary) (pyrimidine deficiency) E79.8
  anemia D53.0
Orthodontics
  adjustment Z46.4
  fitting Z46.4
Orthopnea R06.01
Orthopoxvirus B08.09
  specified NEC B08.09
Os, uterus — see condition
**Osgood-Schlatter disease or
  osteochondrosis** — see Osteochondrosis,
  juvenile, tibia
Osler's nodes I33.0
Osler(-Weber)-Rendu disease I78.0
Osmidrosis L75.0
Osseous — see condition
Ossification
  artery — see Arteriosclerosis
  auricle (ear) — see Disorder, pinna, specified
    type NEC
  bronchial J98.09
  cardiac — see Degeneration, myocardial
  cartilage (senile) — see Disorder, cartilage,
    specified type NEC
  coronary (artery) — see Disease, heart,
    ischemic, atherosclerotic
  diaphragm J98.6
  ear, middle — see Otosclerosis
  falx cerebri G96.19
  fontanel, premature Q75.0
  heart — see also Degeneration, myocardial
    valve — see Endocarditis
  larynx J38.7
  ligament — see Disorder, tendon, specified
    type NEC
    posterior longitudinal — see Spondylopathy,
      specified NEC
  meninges (cerebral) (spinal) G96.19
  multiple, eccentric centers — see Disorder,
    bone, development or growth
  muscle — see also Calcification, muscle
    due to burns — see Myositis, ossificans, in,
      burns
    paralytic — see Myositis, ossificans, in,
      quadriplegia
    progressive — see Myositis, ossificans,
      progressiva
    specified NEC M61.50
      ankle M61.57-
      foot M61.57-
      forearm M61.53-
      hand M61.54-
      lower leg M61.56-
      multiple sites M61.59
      pelvic region M61.55-
      shoulder region M61.51-
      specified site NEC M61.58
      thigh M61.55-
      upper arm M61.52-

Ossification — continued
  muscle — see also Calcification, muscle —
    continued
    traumatic — see Myositis, ossificans,
      traumatica
  myocardium, myocardial — see Degeneration,
    myocardial
  penis N48.89
  periarticular — see Disorder, joint, specified
    type NEC
  pinna — see Disorder, pinna, specified type
    NEC
  rider's bone — see Ossification, muscle,
    specified NEC
  sclera H15.89
  subperiosteal, post-traumatic M89.8x-
  tendon — see Disorder, tendon, specified type
    NEC
  trachea J39.8
  tympanic membrane — see Disorder, tympanic
    membrane, specified NEC
  vitreous (humor) — see Deposit, crystalline
Osteitis — see also Osteomyelitis
  alveolar M27.3
  condensans M85.30
    ankle M85.37- ·
    foot M85.37-
    forearm M85.33-
    hand M85.34-
    lower leg M85.36-
    multiple site M85.39
    neck M85.38
    rib M85.38
    shoulder M85.31-
    skull M85.38
    specified site NEC M85.38
    thigh M85.35-
    toe M85.37-
    upper arm M85.32-
    vertebra M85.38
  deformans M88.9
    in (due to)
      malignant neoplasm of bone C41.9
        [M90.60]
      neoplastic disease (see also Neoplasm)
        D49.9 [M90.60]
        carpus D49.9 [M90.6-]
        clavicle D49.9 [M90.6-]
        femur D49.9 [M90.6-]
        fibula D49.9 [M90.6-]
        finger D49.9 [M90.6-]
        humerus D49.9 [M90.6-]
        ilium D49.9 [M90.6-]
        ischium D49.9 [M90.6-]
        metacarpus D49.9 [M90.6-]
        metatarsus D49.9 [M90.6-]
        multiple sites D49.9 [M90.69]
        neck D49.9 [M90.68]
        radius D49.9 [M90.6-]
        rib D49.9 [M90.68]
        scapula D49.9 [M90.6-]
        skull D49.9 [M90.68]
        tarsus D49.9 [M90.6-]
        tibia D49.9 [M90.6-]
        toe D49.9 [M90.6-]
        ulna D49.9 [M90.6-]
        vertebra D49.9 [M90.68]
    skull M88.0
    specified NEC — see Paget's disease, bone,
      by site
    vertebra M88.1
  due to yaws A66.6
  fibrosa NEC — see Cyst, bone, by site
    circumscripta — see Dysplasia, fibrous, bone
      NEC
    cystica (generalisata) E21.0
    disseminata Q78.1
    osteoplastica E21.0
  fragilitans Q78.0

Osteitis (see also Osteomyelitis) — continued
Garr's (sclerosing) — see Osteomyelitis, specified type NEC
jaw (acute) (chronic) (lower) (suppurative) (upper) M27.2
parathyroid E21.0
petrous bone (acute) (chronic) — see Petrositis
sclerotic, nonsuppurative — see Osteomyelitis, specified type NEC
tuberculosa A18.09
cystica D86.89
multiplex cystoides D86.89
Osteoarthritis M19.90
ankle M19.07-
elbow M19.02-
foot joint M19.07-
generalized M15.9
erosive M15.4
primary M15.0
specified NEC M15.8
hand joint M19.04-
first carpometacarpal joint M18.9
hip M16.1-
bilateral M16.0
due to hip dysplasia (unilateral) M16.3-
bilateral M16.2
interphalangeal
distal (Heberden) M15.1
proximal (Bouchard) M15.2
knee M17.9
bilateral M17.0
post-traumatic NEC M19.92
ankle M19.17-
elbow M19.12-
foot joint M19.17-
hand joint M19.14-
first carpometacarpal joint M18.3-
bilateral M18.2
hip M16.5-
bilateral M16.4
knee M17.3-
bilateral M17.2
shoulder M19.11-
wrist M19.13-
primary M19.91
ankle M19.07-
elbow M19.02-
foot joint M19.07-
hand joint M19.04-
first carpometacarpal joint M18.1-
bilateral M18.0
hip M16.1-
bilateral M16.0
knee M17.1-
bilateral M17.0
shoulder M19.01-
spine — see Spondylosis
wrist M19.03-
secondary M19.93
ankle M19.27-
elbow M19.22-
foot joint M19.27-
hand joint M19.24-
first carpometacarpal joint M18.5-
bilateral M18.4
hip M16.7
bilateral M16.6
knee M17.5
bilateral M17.4
multiple M15.3
shoulder M19.21-
spine — see Spondylosis
wrist M19.23-
shoulder M19.01-
spine — see Spondylosis
wrist M19.03-
Osteoarthropathy (hypertrophic) M19.90
ankle — see Osteoarthritis, primary, ankle
elbow — see Osteoarthritis, primary, elbow

Osteoarthropathy (hypertrophic) M19.90 — continued
foot joint — see Osteoarthritis, primary, foot
hand joint — see Osteoarthritis, primary, hand joint
knee joint — see Osteoarthritis, primary, knee
multiple site — see Osteoarthritis, primary, multiple joint
pulmonary — see also Osteoarthropathy, specified type NEC
hypertrophic — see Osteoarthropathy, hypertrophic, specified type NEC
secondary — see Osteoarthropathy, specified type NEC
secondary hypertrophic — see Osteoarthropathy, specified type NEC
shoulder — see Osteoarthritis, primary, shoulder
specified joint NEC — see Osteoarthritis, primary, specified joint NEC
specified type NEC M89.40
carpus M89.44-
clavicle M89.41-
femur M89.45-
fibula M89.46-
finger M89.44-
humerus M89.42-
ilium M89.459
ischium M89.459
metacarpus M89.44-
metatarsus M89.47-
multiple sites M89.49
neck M89.48
radius M89.43-
rib M89.48
scapula M89.41-
skull M89.48
tarsus M89.47-
tibia M89.46-
toe M89.47-
ulna M89.43-
vertebra M89.48
spine — see Spondylosis
wrist — see Osteoarthritis, primary, wrist
Osteoarthrosis (degenerative) (hypertrophic) (joint) — see also Osteoarthritis
deformans alkaptonurica E70.29 [M36.8]
erosive M15.4
generalized M15.9
primary M15.0
polyarticular M15.9
spine — see Spondylosis
Osteoblastoma — see Neoplasm, bone, benign
aggressive — see Neoplasm, bone, uncertain behavior
Osteochondritis — see also Osteochondropathy, by site
Brailsford's — see Osteochondrosis, juvenile, radius
dissecans M93.20
ankle M93.27-
elbow M93.22-
foot M93.27-
hand M93.24-
hip M93.25-
knee M93.26-
multiple sites M93.29
shoulder joint M93.21-
specified site NEC M93.28
wrist M93.23-
juvenile M92.9
patellar — see Osteochondrosis, juvenile, patella
syphilitic (congenital) (early) A50.02 [M90.80]
ankle A50.02 [M90.8-]
elbow A50.02 [M90.8-]
foot A50.02 [M90.8-]
forearm A50.02 [M90.8-]

Osteochondritis — see also Osteochondropathy, by site — continued
syphilitic (congenital) (early) A50.02 [M90.80] — continued
hand A50.02 [M90.8-]
hip A50.02 [M90.8-]
knee A50.02 [M90.8-]
multiple sites A50.02 [M90.89]
shoulder joint A50.02 [M90.8-]
specified site NEC A50.02 [M90.88]
Osteochondroarthrosis deformans endemica — see Disease, Kaschin-Beck
Osteochondrodysplasia Q78.9
with defects of growth of tubular bones and spine Q77.9
specified NEC Q77.8
specified NEC Q78.8
Osteochondrodystrophy E78.9
Osteochondrolysis — see Osteochondritis, dissecans
Osteochondroma — see Neoplasm, bone, benign
Osteochondromatosis D48.0
syndrome Q78.4
Osteochondromyxosarcoma — see Neoplasm, bone, malignant
Osteochondropathy M93.90
ankle M93.97-
elbow M93.92-
foot M93.97-
hand M93.94-
hip M93.95-
Kienböck's disease of adults M93.1
knee M93.96-
multiple joints M93.99
osteochondritis dissecans — see Osteochondritis, dissecans
osteochondrosis — see Osteochondrosis
shoulder region M93.91-
slipped upper femoral epiphysis — see Slipped, epiphysis, upper femoral
specified joint NEC M93.98
specified type NEC M93.80
ankle M93.87-
elbow M93.82-
foot M93.87-
hand M93.84-
hip M93.85-
knee M93.86-
multiple joints M93.89
shoulder region M93.81-
specified joint NEC M93.88
wrist M93.83-
syphilitic, congenital
early A50.02 [M90.80]
late A50.56 [M90.80]
wrist M93.93-
Osteochondrosarcoma — see Neoplasm, bone, malignant
Osteochondrosis — see also Osteochondropathy, by site
acetabulum (juvenile) M91.0
adult — see Osteochondropathy, specified type NEC, by site
astragalus (juvenile) — see Osteochondrosis, juvenile, tarsus
Blount's — see Osteochondrosis, juvenile, tibia
Buchanan's M91.0
Burns' — see Osteochondrosis, juvenile, ulna
calcaneus (juvenile) — see Osteochondrosis, juvenile, tarsus
capitular epiphysis (femur) (juvenile) — see Legg-Calvé-Perthes disease
carpal (juvenile) (lunate) (scaphoid) — see Osteochondrosis, juvenile, hand, carpal lunate
adult M93.1
coxae juvenilis — see Legg-Calvé-Perthes disease

Osteochondrosis (see also Osteochondropathy, by site) — continued
- deformans juvenilis, coxae — see Legg-Calvé-Perthes disease
- Diaz's — see Osteochondrosis, juvenile, tarsus
- dissecans (knee) (shoulder) — see Osteochondritis, dissecans
- femoral capital epiphysis (juvenile) — see Legg-Calvé-Perthes disease
- femur (head), juvenile — see Legg-Calvé-Perthes disease
- fibula (juvenile) — see Osteochondrosis, juvenile, fibula
- foot NEC (juvenile) M92.8
- Freiberg's — see Osteochondrosis, juvenile, metatarsus
- Haas' (juvenile) — see Osteochondrosis, juvenile, humerus
- Haglund's — see Osteochondrosis, juvenile, tarsus
- hip (juvenile) — see Legg-Calvé-Perthes disease
- humerus (capitulum) (head) (juvenile) — see Osteochondrosis, juvenile, humerus
- ilium, iliac crest (juvenile) M91.0
- ischiopubic synchondrosis M91.0
- Iselin's — see Osteochondrosis, juvenile, metatarsus
- juvenile, juvenilis M92.9
  - after congenital dislocation of hip reduction — see Osteochondrosis, juvenile, hip, specified NEC
  - arm — see Osteochondrosis, juvenile, upper limb NEC
  - capitular epiphysis (femur) — see Legg-Calvé-Perthes disease
  - clavicle, sternal epiphysis — see Osteochondrosis, juvenile, upper limb NEC
  - coxae — see Legg-Calvé-Perthes disease
  - deformans M92.9
  - fibula M92.5-
  - foot NEC M92.8
  - hand M92.20-
    - carpal lunate M92.21-
    - metacarpal head M92.22-
    - specified site NEC M92.29-
  - head of femur — see Legg-Calvé-Perthes disease
  - hip and pelvis M91.9-
    - coxa plana — see Coxa, plana
    - femoral head — see Legg-Calvé-Perthes disease
    - pelvis M91.0
    - pseudocoxalgia — see Pseudocoxalgia
    - specified NEC M91.8-
  - humerus M92.0-
  - limb
    - lower NEC M92.8
    - upper NEC — see Osteochondrosis, juvenile, upper limb NEC
  - medial cuneiform bone — see Osteochondrosis, juvenile, tarsus
  - metatarsus M92.7-
  - patella M92.4-
  - radius M92.1-
  - specified site NEC M92.8
  - spine M42.00
    - cervical region M42.02
    - cervicothoracic region M42.03
    - lumbar region M42.06
    - lumbosacral region M42.07
    - multiple sites M42.09
    - occipito-atlanto-axial region M42.01
    - sacrococcygeal region M42.08
    - thoracic region M42.04
    - thoracolumbar region M42.05
  - tarsus M92.6-
  - tibia M92.5-
  - ulna M92.1-

Osteochondrosis (see also Osteochondropathy, by site) — continued
- juvenile, juvenilis M92.9 — continued
  - upper limb NEC M92.3-
  - vertebra (body) (epiphyseal plates) (Calvé's) (Scheuermann's) — see Osteochondrosis, juvenile, spine
- Kienböck's — see Osteochondrosis, juvenile, hand, carpal lunate
  - adult M93.1
- Köhler's
  - patellar — see Osteochondrosis, juvenile, patella
  - tarsal navicular — see Osteochondrosis, juvenile, tarsus
- Legg-Perthes(-Calvé)(-Waldenström) — see Legg-Calvé-Perthes disease
- limb
  - lower NEC (juvenile) M92.8
  - upper NEC (juvenile) — see Osteochondrosis, juvenile, upper limb NEC
- lunate bone (carpal) (juvenile) — see also Osteochondrosis, juvenile, hand, carpal lunate
  - adult M93.1
- Mauclaire's — see Osteochondrosis, juvenile, hand, metacarpal
- metacarpal (head) (juvenile) — see Osteochondrosis, juvenile, hand, metacarpal
- metatarsus (fifth) (head) (juvenile) (second) — see Osteochondrosis, juvenile, metatarsus
- navicular (juvenile) — see Osteochondrosis, juvenile, tarsus
- os
  - calcis (juvenile) — see Osteochondrosis, juvenile, tarsus
  - tibiale externum (juvenile) — see Osteochondrosis, juvenile, tarsus
- Osgood-Schlatter — see Osteochondrosis, juvenile, tibia
- Panner's — see Osteochondrosis, juvenile, humerus
- patellar center (juvenile) (primary) (secondary) — see Osteochondrosis, juvenile, patella
- pelvis (juvenile) M91.0
- Pierson's M91.0
- radius (head) (juvenile) — see Osteochondrosis, juvenile, radius
- Scheuermann's — see Osteochondrosis, juvenile, spine
- Sever's — see Osteochondrosis, juvenile, tarsus
- Sinding-Larsen — see Osteochondrosis, juvenile, patella
- spine M42.9
  - adult M42.10
    - cervical region M42.12
    - cervicothoracic region M42.13
    - lumbar region M42.16
    - lumbosacral region M42.17
    - multiple sites M42.19
    - occipito-atlanto-axial region M42.11
    - sacrococcygeal region M42.18
    - thoracic region M42.14
    - thoracolumbar region M42.15
  - juvenile — see Osteochondrosis, juvenile, spine
- symphysis pubis (juvenile) M91.0
- syphilitic (congenital) A50.02
- talus (juvenile) — see Osteochondrosis, juvenile, tarsus
- tarsus (navicular) (juvenile) — see Osteochondrosis, juvenile, tarsus
- tibia (proximal) (tubercle) (juvenile) — see Osteochondrosis, juvenile, tibia
- tuberculous — see Tuberculosis, bone
- ulna (lower) (juvenile) — see Osteochondrosis, juvenile, ulna

Osteochondrosis (see also Osteochondropathy, by site) — continued
- van Neck's M91.0
- vertebral — see Osteochondrosis, spine

Osteoclastoma D48.0
- malignant — see Neoplasm, bone, malignant

Osteodynia — see Disorder, bone, specified type NEC

Osteodystrophy Q78.9
- azotemic N25.0
- congenital Q78.9
- parathyroid, secondary E21.1
- renal N25.0

Osteofibroma — see Neoplasm, bone, benign

Osteofibrosarcoma — see Neoplasm, bone, malignant

Osteogenesis imperfecta Q78.0

Osteogenic — see condition

Osteolysis M89.50
- carpus M89.54-
- clavicle M89.51-
- femur M89.55-
- fibula M89.56-
- finger M89.54-
- humerus M89.52-
- ilium M89.559
- ischium M89.559
- joint prosthesis (periprosthetic) — see Complications, joint prosthesis, mechanical, periprosthetic, osteolysis, by site
- metacarpus M89.54-
- metatarsus M89.57-
- multiple sites M89.59
- neck M89.58
- periprosthetic — see Complications, joint prosthesis, mechanical, periprosthetic, osteolysis, by site
- radius M89.53-
- rib M89.58
- scapula M89.51-
- skull M89.58
- tarsus M89.57-
- tibia M89.56-
- toe M89.57-
- ulna M89.53-
- vertebra M89.58

Osteoma — see also Neoplasm, bone, benign
- osteoid — see also Neoplasm, bone, benign
- giant — see Neoplasm, bone, benign

Osteomalacia M83.9
- adult M83.9
  - drug-induced NEC M83.5
  - due to
    - malabsorption (postsurgical) M83.2
    - malnutrition M83.3
  - specified NEC M83.8
- aluminium-induced M83.4
- infantile — see Rickets
- juvenile — see Rickets
- oncogenic E83.89
- pelvis M83.8
- puerperal M83.0
- senile M83.1
- vitamin-D-resistant in adults E83.31 [M90.-]
  - carpus E83.31 [M90.8-]
  - clavicle E83.31 [M90.8-]
  - femur E83.31 [M90.8-]
  - fibula E83.31 [M90.8-]
  - finger E83.31 [M90.8-]
  - humerus E83.31 [M90.8-]
  - ilium E83.31 [M90.859]
  - ischium E83.31 [M90.859]
  - metacarpus E83.31 [M90.8-]
  - metatarsus E83.31 [M90.8-]
  - multiple sites E83.31 [M90.89]
  - neck E83.31 [M90.88]
  - radius E83.31 [M90.8-]
  - rib E83.31 [M90.88]

D I S E A S E   I N D E X

Osteomalacia M83.9 — *continued*
  vitamin-D-resistant in adults E83.31 *[M90.-]*
    — *continued*
    scapula E83.31 *[M90.819]*
    skull E83.31 *[M90.88]*
    tarsus E83.31 *[M90.879]*
    tibia E83.31 *[M90.869]*
    toe E83.31 *[M90.879]*
    ulna E83.31 *[M90.839]*
    vertebra E83.31 *[M90.88]*
Osteomyelitis (general) (infective) (localized)
  (neonatal) (purulent) (septic) (staphylococcal)
  (streptococcal) (suppurative) (with periostitis)
  M86.9
  acute M86.10
    carpus M86.14-
    clavicle M86.11-
    femur M86.15-
    fibula M86.16-
    finger M86.14-
    hematogenous M86.00
      carpus M86.04-
      clavicle M86.01-
      femur M86.05-
      fibula M86.06-
      finger M86.04-
      humerus M86.02-
      ilium M86.059
      ischium M86.059
      mandible M27.2
      metacarpus M86.04-
      metatarsus M86.07-
      multiple sites M86.09
      neck M86.08
      orbit H05.02-
      petrous bone — *see* Petrositis
      radius M86.03-
      rib M86.08
      scapula M86.01-
      skull M86.08
      tarsus M86.07-
      tibia M86.06-
      toe M86.07-
      ulna M86.03-
      vertebra — *see* Osteomyelitis, vertebra
    humerus M86.12-
    ilium M86.159
    ischium M86.159
    mandible M27.2
    metacarpus M86.14-
    metatarsus M86.17-
    multiple sites M86.19
    neck M86.18
    orbit H05.02-
    petrous bone — *see* Petrositis
    radius M86.13-
    rib M86.18
    scapula M86.11-
    skull M86.18
    tarsus M86.17-
    tibia M86.16-
    toe M86.17-
    ulna M86.13-
    vertebra — *see* Osteomyelitis, vertebra
  chronic (or old) M86.60
    with draining sinus M86.40
      carpus M86.44-
      clavicle M86.41-
      femur M86.45-
      fibula M86.46-
      finger M86.44-
      humerus M86.42-
      ilium M86.459
      ischium M86.459
      mandible M27.2
      metacarpus M86.44-
      metatarsus M86.47-
      multiple sites M86.49
      neck M86.48

Osteomyelitis (general) (infective) (localized)
  (neonatal) (purulent) (septic) (staphylococcal)
  (streptococcal) (suppurative) (with periostitis)
  M86.9 — *continued*
  chronic (or old) M86.60 — *continued*
    with draining sinus M86.40 — *continued*
      orbit H05.02-
      petrous bone — *see* Petrositis
      radius M86.43-
      rib M86.48
      scapula M86.41-
      skull M86.48
      tarsus M86.47-
      tibia M86.46-
      toe M86.47-
      ulna M86.43-
      vertebra — *see* Osteomyelitis, vertebra
    carpus M86.64-
    clavicle M86.61-
    femur M86.65-
    fibula M86.66-
    finger M86.64-
    hematogenous NEC M86.50
      carpus M86.54-
      clavicle M86.51-
      femur M86.55-
      fibula M86.56-
      finger M86.54-
      humerus M86.52-
      ilium M86.559
      ischium M86.559
      mandible M27.2
      metacarpus M86.54-
      metatarsus M86.57-
      multifocal M86.30
        carpus M86.34-
        clavicle M86.31-
        femur M86.35-
        fibula M86.36-
        finger M86.34-
        humerus M86.32-
        ilium M86.359
        ischium M86.359
        metacarpus M86.34-
        metatarsus M86.37-
        multiple sites M86.39
        neck M86.38
        radius M86.33-
        rib M86.38
        scapula M86.31-
        skull M86.38
        tarsus M86.37-
        tibia M86.36-
        toe M86.37-
        ulna M86.33-
        vertebra — *see* Osteomyelitis, vertebra
      multiple sites M86.59
      neck M86.58
      orbit H05.02-
      petrous bone — *see* Petrositis
      radius M86.53-
      rib M86.58
      scapula M86.51-
      skull M86.58
      tarsus M86.57-
      tibia M86.56-
      toe M86.57-
      ulna M86.53-
      vertebra — *see* Osteomyelitis, vertebra
    humerus M86.62-
    ilium M86.659
    ischium M86.659
    mandible M27.2
    metacarpus M86.64-
    metatarsus M86.67-
    multifocal — *see* Osteomyelitis, chronic,
      hematogenous, multifocal
    multiple sites M86.69
    neck M86.68

Osteomyelitis (general) (infective) (localized)
  (neonatal) (purulent) (septic) (staphylococcal)
  (streptococcal) (suppurative) (with periostitis)
  M86.9 — *continued*
  chronic (or old) M86.60 — *continued*
    orbit H05.02-
    petrous bone — *see* Petrositis
    radius M86.63-
    rib M86.68
    scapula M86.61-
    skull M86.68
    tarsus M86.67-
    tibia M86.66-
    toe M86.67-
    ulna M86.63-
    vertebra — *see* Osteomyelitis, vertebra
  echinococcal B67.2
  Garr's — *see* Osteomyelitis, specified type
    NEC
  in diabetes mellitus — *see* E08-E13 with .69
  jaw (acute) (chronic) (lower) (neonatal)
    (suppurative) (upper) M27.2
  nonsuppurating — *see* Osteomyelitis, specified
    type NEC
  orbit H05.02-
  petrous bone — *see* Petrositis
  Salmonella (arizonae) (cholerae-suis)
    (enteritidis) (typhimurium) A02.24
  sclerosing, nonsuppurative — *see*
    Osteomyelitis, specified type NEC
  specified type NEC (*see also* subcategory)
    M86.8x-
    mandible M27.2
    orbit H05.02-
    petrous bone — *see* Petrositis
    vertebra — *see* Osteomyelitis, vertebra
  subacute M86.20
    carpus M86.24-
    clavicle M86.21-
    femur M86.25-
    fibula M86.26-
    finger M86.24-
    humerus M86.22-
    mandible M27.2
    metacarpus M86.24-
    metatarsus M86.27-
    multiple sites M86.29
    neck M86.28
    orbit H05.02-
    petrous bone — *see* Petrositis
    radius M86.23-
    rib M86.28
    scapula M86.21-
    skull M86.28
    tarsus M86.27-
    tibia M86.26-
    toe M86.27-
    ulna M86.23-
    vertebra — *see* Osteomyelitis, vertebra
  syphilitic A52.77
    congenital (early) A50.02 *[M90.80]*
  tuberculous — *see* Tuberculosis, bone
  typhoid A01.05
  vertebra M46.20
    cervical region M46.22
    cervicothoracic region M46.23
    lumbar region M46.26
    lumbosacral region M46.27
    occipito-atlanto-axial region M46.21
    sacrococcygeal region M46.28
    thoracic region M46.24
    thoracolumbar region M46.25
Osteomyelofibrosis D47.4
Osteomyelosclerosis D75.89
Osteonecrosis M87.9
  due to
    drugs — *see* Osteonecrosis, secondary, due
      to, drugs

Osteonecrosis M87.9 — *continued*
  due to — *continued*
    trauma — *see* Osteonecrosis, secondary,
      due to, trauma
  idiopathic aseptic M87.00
    ankle M87.07-
    carpus M87.03-
    clavicle M87.01-
    femur M87.05-
    fibula M87.06-
    finger M87.04-
    humerus M87.02-
    ilium M87.050
    ischium M87.050
    metacarpus M87.04-
    metatarsus M87.07-
    multiple sites M87.09
    neck M87.08
    pelvis M87.050
    radius M87.03-
    rib M87.08
    scapula M87.01-
    skull M87.08
    tarsus M87.07-
    tibia M87.06-
    toe M87.07-
    ulna M87.03-
    vertebra M87.08
  secondary NEC M87.30
    carpus M87.33-
    clavicle M87.31-
    due to
      drugs M87.10
        carpus M87.13-
        clavicle M87.11-
        femur M87.15-
        fibula M87.16-
        finger M87.14-
        humerus M87.12-
        ilium M87.159
      drugs M87.10
        ischium M87.159
        jaw M87.180
        metacarpus M87.14-
        metatarsus M87.17-
        multiple sites M87.19
        neck M87.18
        radius M87.13-
        rib M87.18
        scapula M87.11-
        skull M87.18
        tarsus M87.17-
        tibia M87.16-
        toe M87.17-
        ulna M87.13-
        vertebra M87.18
      hemoglobinopathy NEC D58.2 *[M90.50]*
        carpus D58.2 *[M90.5-]*
        clavicle D58.2 *[M90.5-]*
        femur D58.2 *[M90.5-]*
        fibula D58.2 *[M90.5-]*
        finger D58.2 *[M90.5-]*
        humerus D58.2 *[M90.5-]*
        ilium D58.2 *[M90.5-]*
        ischium D58.2 *[M90.5-]*
        metacarpus D58.2 *[M90.5-]*
        metatarsus D58.2 *[M90.5-]*
        multiple sites D58.2 *[M90.58]*
        neck D58.2 *[M90.5-]*
        radius D58.2 *[M90.5-]*
        rib D58.2 *[M90.58]*
        scapula D58.2 *[M90.5-]*
        skull D58.2 *[M90.58]*
        tarsus D58.2 *[M90.5-]*
        tibia D58.2 *[M90.5-]*
        toe D58.2 *[M90.5-]*
        ulna D58.2 *[M90.5-]*
        vertebra D58.2 *[M90.58]*

Osteonecrosis M87.9 — *continued*
  secondary NEC M87.30 — *continued*
    due to — *continued*
      trauma (previous) M87.20
        carpus M87.23-
        clavicle M87.21-
        femur M87.25-
        fibula M87.26-
        finger M87.24-
        humerus M87.22-
        ilium M87.25-
        ischium M87.25-
        metacarpus M87.24-
        metatarsus M87.27-
        multiple sites M87.29
        neck M87.28
        radius M87.23-
        rib M87.28
        scapula M87.21-
        skull M87.28
        tarsus M87.27-
        tibia M87.26-
        toe M87.27-
        ulna M87.23-
        vertebra M87.28
    femur M87.35-
    fibula M87.36-
    finger M87.34-
    humerus M87.32-
    ilium M87.350
    in
      caisson disease T70.3 *[M90.50]*
        carpus T70.3 *[M90.5-]*
        clavicle T70.3 *[M90.5-]*
        femur T70.3 *[M90.5-]*
        fibula T70.3 *[M90.5-]*
        finger T70.3 *[M90.5-]*
        humerus T70.3 *[M90.5-]*
        ilium T70.3 *[M90.5-]*
        ischium T70.3 *[M90.5-]*
        metacarpus T70.3 *[M90.5-]*
        metatarsus T70.3 *[M90.5-]*
        multiple sites T70.3 *[M90.59]*
        neck T70.3 *[M90.58]*
        radius T70.3 *[M90.5-]*
        rib T70.3 *[M90.58]*
        scapula T70.3 *[M90.5-]*
        skull T70.3 *[M90.58]*
        tarsus T70.3 *[M90.5-]*
        tibia T70.3 *[M90.5-]*
        toe T70.3 *[M90.5-]*
        ulna T70.3 *[M90.5-]*
        vertebra T70.3 *[M90.58]*
    ischium M87.350
    metacarpus M87.34-
    metatarsus M87.37-
    multiple site M87.39
    neck M87.38
    radius M87.33-
    rib M87.38
    scapula M87.319
    skull M87.38
    tarsus M87.379
    tibia M87.366
    toe M87.379
    ulna M87.33-
    vertebra M87.38
  specified type NEC M87.80
    carpus M87.83-
    clavicle M87.81-
    femur M87.85-
    fibula M87.86-
    finger M87.84-
    humerus M87.82-
    ilium M87.85-
    ischium M87.85-
    metacarpus M87.84-
    metatarsus M87.87-
    multiple sites M87.89

Osteonecrosis M87.9 — *continued*
  specified type NEC M87.80 — *continued*
    neck M87.88
    radius M87.83-
    rib M87.88
    scapula M87.81-
    skull M87.88
    tarsus M87.87-
    tibia M87.86-
    toe M87.87-
    ulna M87.83-
    vertebra M87.88
Osteo-onycho-arthro-dysplasia Q87.2
Osteo-onychodysplasia, hereditary Q87.2
Osteopathia condensans disseminata
  Q78.8
Osteopathy — *see also* Osteomyelitis,
  Osteonecrosis, Osteoporosis
  after poliomyelitis M89.60
    carpus M89.64-
    clavicle M89.61-
    femur M89.65-
    fibula M89.66-
    finger M89.64-
    humerus M89.62-
    ilium M89.659
    ischium M89.659
    metacarpus M89.64-
    metatarsus M89.67-
    multiple sites M89.69
    neck M89.68
    radius M89.63-
    rib M89.68
    scapula M89.61-
    skull M89.68
    tarsus M89.67-
    tibia M89.66-
    toe M89.67-
    ulna M89.63-
    vertebra M89.68
  in (due to)
    renal osteodystrophy N25.0
    specified diseases classified elsewhere — *see*
      subcategory M90.8
Osteopenia M85.8-
  borderline M85.8-
Osteoperiostitis — *see* Osteomyelitis,
  specified type NEC
Osteopetrosis (familial) Q78.2
Osteophyte M25.70
  ankle M25.77-
  elbow M25.72-
  foot joint M25.77-
  hand joint M25.74-
  hip M25.75-
  knee M25.76-
  shoulder M25.71-
  spine M25.78
  vertebrae M25.78
  wrist M25.73-
Osteopoikilosis Q78.8
Osteoporosis (female) (male) M81.0
  with current pathological fracture M80.00
  age-related M81.0
    with current pathologic fracture M80.00
      carpus M80.04-
      clavicle M80.01-
      fibula M80.06-
      finger M80.04-
      humerus M80.02-
      ilium M80.05-
      ischium M80.05-
      metacarpus M80.04-
      metatarsus M80.07-
      pelvis M80.05-
      radius M80.03-
      scapula M80.01-
      tarsus M80.07-
      tibia M80.06-

Osteoporosis (female) (male) M81.0 — *continued*
  age-related M81.0 — *continued*
    with current pathologic fracture M80.00 — *continued*
      toe M80.07-
      ulna M80.03-
      vertebra M80.08
  disuse M81.8
    with current pathological fracture M80.80
      carpus M80.84-
      clavicle M80.81-
      fibula M80.86-
      finger M80.84-
      humerus M80.82-
      ilium M80.85-
      ischium M80.85-
      metacarpus M80.84-
      metatarsus M80.87-
      pelvis M80.85-
      radius M80.83-
      scapula M80.81-
      tarsus M80.87-
      tibia M80.86-
      toe M80.87-
      ulna M80.83-
      vertebra M80.88
  drug-induced — *see* Osteoporosis, specified type NEC
  idiopathic — *see* Osteoporosis, specified type NEC
  involutional — *see* Osteoporosis, age-related
  Lequesne M81.6
  localized M81.6
  post-traumatic — *see* Osteoporosis, specified type NEC
  postmenopausal M81.0
    with pathological fracture M80.00
      carpus M80.04-
      clavicle M80.01-
      fibula M80.06-
      finger M80.04-
      humerus M80.02-
      ilium M80.05-
      ischium M80.05-
      metacarpus M80.04-
      metatarsus M80.07-
      pelvis M80.05-
      radius M80.03-
      scapula M80.01-
      tarsus M80.07-
      tibia M80.06-
      toe M80.07-
      ulna M80.03-
      vertebra M80.08
  postoophorectomy — *see* Osteoporosis, specified type NEC
  postsurgical malabsorption — *see* Osteoporosis, specified type NEC
  senile — *see* Osteoporosis, age-related
  specified type NEC M81.8
    with pathological fracture M80.80
      carpus M80.84-
      clavicle M80.81-
      fibula M80.86-
      finger M80.84-
      humerus M80.82-
      ilium M80.85-
      ischium M80.85-
      metacarpus M80.84-
      metatarsus M80.87-
      pelvis M80.85-
      radius M80.83-
      scapula M80.81-
      tarsus M80.87-
      tibia M80.86-
      toe M80.87-
      ulna M80.83-
      vertebra M80.88

Osteopsathyrosis (idiopathica) Q78.0
Osteoradionecrosis, jaw (acute) (chronic) (lower) (suppurative) (upper) M27.2
Osteosarcoma (any form) — *see* Neoplasm, bone, malignant
Osteosclerosis Q78.2
  acquired M85.8-
  congenita Q77.4
  fragilitas (generalisata) Q78.2
  myelofibrosis D75.81
Osteosclerotic anemia D64.89
Osteosis
  cutis L94.2
  renal fibrocystic N25.0
Österreicher-Turner syndrome Q87.2
Ostium
  atrioventriculare commune Q21.2
  primum (arteriosum) (defect) (persistent) Q21.2
  secundum (arteriosum) (defect) (patent) (persistent) Q21.1
Ostrum-Furst syndrome Q75.8
Otalgia — *see* subcategory H92.0
Otitis (acute) H66.90
  with effusion — *see also* Otitis, media, nonsuppurative
    purulent — *see* Otitis, media, suppurative
  adhesive — *see* subcategory H74.1
  chronic — *see also* Otitis, media, chronic
    with effusion — *see also* Otitis, media, nonsuppurative, chronic
  externa H60.9-
    abscess — *see* Abscess, ear, external
    acute (noninfective) H60.50-
      actinic H60.51-
      chemical H60.52-
      contact H60.53-
      eczematoid H60.54-
      infective — *see* Otitis, externa, infective
      reactive H60.55-
      specified NEC H60.59-
    cellulitis — *see* Cellulitis, ear
    chronic H60.6-
    diffuse — *see* Otitis, externa, infective, diffuse
    hemorrhagic — *see* Otitis, externa, infective, hemorrhagic
    in (due to)
      aspergillosis B44.89
      candidiasis B37.84
      erysipelas A46 *[H62.40]*
      herpes (simplex) virus infection B00.1
        zoster B02.8
      impetigo L01.00 *[H62.40]*
      infectious disease NEC B99 *[H62.-]*
      mycosis NEC B36.9 *[H62.40]*
      parasitic disease NEC B89 *[H62.40]*
      viral disease NEC B34.9 *[H62.40]*
      zoster B02.8
    infective NEC H60.39-
      abscess — *see* Abscess, ear, external
      cellulitis — *see* Cellulitis, ear
      diffuse H60.31-
      hemorrhagic H60.32-
      swimmer's ear — *see* Swimmer's, ear
    malignant H60.2-
    mycotic NEC B36.9 *[H62.40]*
      in
        aspergillosis B44.89
        candidiasis B37.84
        moniliasis B37.84
    necrotizing — *see* Otitis, externa, malignant
    Pseudomonas aeruginosa — *see* Otitis, externa, malignant
    reactive — *see* Otitis, externa, acute, reactive
    specified NEC — *see* subcategory H60.8

Otitis (acute) H66.90 — *continued*
  externa H60.9- — *continued*
    tropical NEC B36.9 *[H62.40]*
      in
        aspergillosis B44.89
        candidiasis B37.84
        moniliasis B37.84
  insidiosa — *see* Otosclerosis
  interna — *see* subcategory H83.0
  media (hemorrhagic) (staphylococcal) (streptococcal) H66.9-
    with effusion (nonpurulent) — *see* Otitis, media, nonsuppurative
    acute, subacute H66.90
      allergic — *see* Otitis, media, nonsuppurative, acute, allergic
      exudative — *see* Otitis, media, suppurative, acute
      mucoid — *see* Otitis, media, nonsuppurative, acute
      necrotizing — *see also* Otitis, media, suppurative, acute
      in
        measles B05.3
        scarlet fever A38.0
      nonsuppurative NEC — *see* Otitis, media, nonsuppurative, acute
      purulent — *see* Otitis, media, suppurative, acute
      sanguinous — *see* Otitis, media, nonsuppurative, acute
      secretory — *see* Otitis, media, nonsuppurative, acute, serous
      seromucinous — *see* Otitis, media, nonsuppurative, acute
      serous — *see* Otitis, media, nonsuppurative, acute, serous
      suppurative — *see* Otitis, media, suppurative, acute
    allergic — *see* Otitis, media, nonsuppurative
    catarrhal — *see* Otitis, media, nonsuppurative
    chronic H66.90
      with effusion (nonpurulent) — *see* Otitis, media, nonsuppurative, chronic
      allergic — *see* Otitis, media, nonsuppurative, chronic, allergic
      benign suppurative — *see* Otitis, media, suppurative, chronic, tubotympanic
      catarrhal — *see* Otitis, media, nonsuppurative, chronic, serous
      exudative — *see* Otitis, media, nonsuppurative, chronic
      mucinous — *see* Otitis, media, nonsuppurative, chronic, mucoid
      mucoid — *see* Otitis, media, nonsuppurative, chronic, mucoid
      nonsuppurative NEC — *see* Otitis, media, nonsuppurative, chronic
      purulent — *see* Otitis, media, suppurative, chronic
      secretory — *see* Otitis, media, nonsuppurative, chronic, mucoid
      seromucinous — *see* Otitis, media, nonsuppurative, chronic
      serous — *see* Otitis, media, nonsuppurative, chronic, serous
      suppurative — *see* Otitis, media, suppurative, chronic
      transudative — *see* Otitis, media, nonsuppurative, chronic, mucoid
    exudative — *see* Otitis, media, suppurative
    in (due to) (with)
      influenza — *see* Influenza, with, otitis media
      measles B05.3
      scarlet fever A38.0
      tuberculosis A18.6
      viral disease NEC B34- *[H67-]*

Otitis (acute) H66.90 — *continued*
  media (hemorrhagic) (staphylococcal)
    (streptococcal) H66.9- — *continued*
    mucoid — *see* Otitis, media, nonsuppurative
    nonsuppurative H65.9-
      acute or subacute NEC H65.19-
        allergic H65.11-
          recurrent H65.11-
        recurrent H65.19-
        secretory — *see* Otitis, media,
          nonsuppurative, serous
        serous H65.0-
          recurrent H65.0-
      chronic H65.49-
        allergic H65.41-
        mucoid H65.3-
        serous H65.2-
    postmeasles B05.3
    purulent — *see* Otitis, media, suppurative
    secretory — *see* Otitis, media,
      nonsuppurative
    seromucinous — *see* Otitis, media,
      nonsuppurative
    serous — *see* Otitis, media, nonsuppurative
    suppurative H66.4-
      acute H66.00-
        with rupture of ear drum H66.01-
        recurrent H66.00-
          with rupture of ear drum H66.01-
      chronic (*see also* subcategory) H66.3
        atticoantral H66.2-
        benign — *see* Otitis, media, suppurative,
          chronic, tubotympanic
        tubotympanic H66.1-
    transudative — *see* Otitis, media,
      nonsuppurative
  tuberculous A18.6
Otocephaly Q18.2
Otolith syndrome — *see* subcategory H81.8
Otomycosis (diffuse) NEC B36.9 *[H62.40]*
  in
    aspergillosis B44.89
    candidiasis B37.84
    moniliasis B37.84
Otoporosis — *see* Otosclerosis
Otorrhagia (nontraumatic) H92.2-
  traumatic — *code by* Type of injury
Otorrhea H92.1-
  cerebrospinal G96.0
Otosclerosis (general) H80.9-
  cochlear (endosteal) H80.2-
  involving
    otic capsule — *see* Otosclerosis, cochlear
    oval window
      nonobliterative H80.0-
      obliterative H80.1-
    round window — *see* Otosclerosis, cochlear
  nonobliterative — *see* Otosclerosis, involving,
    oval window, nonobliterative
  obliterative — *see* Otosclerosis, involving, oval
    window, obliterative
  specified NEC H80.8-
Otospongiosis — *see* Otosclerosis
Otto's disease or pelvis M24.7
Outcome of delivery Z37.9
  multiple births Z37.9
    all liveborn Z37.50
      quadruplets Z37.52
      quintuplets Z37.53
      sextuplets Z37.54
      specified number NEC Z37.59
      triplets Z37.51
    all stillborn Z37.7
    some liveborn Z37.60
      quadruplets Z37.62
      quintuplets Z37.63
      sextuplets Z37.64
      specified number NEC Z37.69
      triplets Z37.61

Outcome of delivery Z37.9 — *continued*
  single NEC Z37.9
    liveborn Z37.0
    stillborn Z37.1
  twins NEC Z37.9
    both liveborn Z37.2
    both stillborn Z37.4
    one liveborn, one stillborn Z37.3
Outlet — *see* condition
Ovalocytosis (congenital) (hereditary) — *see*
  Elliptocytosis
Ovarian — *see* condition
Ovariocele N83.4-
Ovaritis (cystic) — *see* Oophoritis
Ovary, ovarian — *see also* condition
  resistant syndrome E28.39
  vein syndrome N13.8
Overactive — *see also* Hyperfunction
  adrenal cortex NEC E27.0
  bladder N32.81
  hypothalamus E23.3
  thyroid — *see* Hyperthyroidism
Overactivity R46.3
  child — *see* Disorder, attention-deficit
    hyperactivity
Overbite (deep) (excessive) (horizontal)
  (vertical) M26.29
Overbreathing — *see* Hyperventilation
Overconscientious personality F60.5
Overdevelopment — *see* Hypertrophy
Overdistension — *see* Distension
Overdose, overdosage (drug) — *see* Table of
  Drugs and Chemicals, by drug, poisoning
Overeating R63.2
  nonorganic origin F50.89
  psychogenic F50.89
Overexertion (effects) (exhaustion) T73.3
Overexposure (effects) T73.9
  exhaustion T73.2
Overfeeding — *see* Overeating
  newborn P92.4
Overfill, endodontic M27.52
Overgrowth, bone — *see* Hypertrophy, bone
**Overhanging of dental restorative
  material** (unrepairable) K08.52
Overheated (places) (effects) — *see* Heat
Overjet (excessive horizontal) M26.23
Overlaid, overlying (suffocation) — *see*
  Asphyxia, traumatic, due to mechanical
  threat
Overlap, excessive horizontal (teeth)
  M26.23
Overlapping toe (acquired) — *see also*
  Deformity, toe, specified NEC
  congenital (fifth toe) Q66.89
Overload
  circulatory, due to transfusion (blood) (blood
    components) (TACO) E87.71
  fluid E87.70
    due to transfusion (blood) (blood
      components) E87.71
    specified NEC E87.79
  iron, due to repeated red blood cell
    transfusions E83.111
  potassium (K) E87.5
  sodium (Na) E87.0
Overnutrition — *see* Hyperalimentation
Overproduction — *see also* Hypersecretion
  ACTH E27.0
  catecholamine E27.5
  growth hormone E22.0
Overprotection, child by parent Z62.1
Overriding
  aorta Q25.49
  finger (acquired) — *see* Deformity, finger
    congenital Q68.1
  toe (acquired) — *see also* Deformity, toe,
    specified NEC
    congenital Q66.89

Overstrained R53.83
  heart — *see* Hypertrophy, cardiac
Overuse, muscle NEC M70.8-
Overweight E66.3
Overworked R53.83
Oviduct — *see* condition
Ovotestis Q56.0
Ovulation (cycle)
  failure or lack of N97.0
  pain N94.0
Ovum — *see* condition
Owren's disease or syndrome
  (parahemophilia) D68.2
Ox heart — *see* Hypertrophy, cardiac
Oxalosis E72.53
Oxaluria E72.53
Oxycephaly, oxycephalic Q75.0
  syphilitic, congenital A50.02
Oxyuriasis B80
Oxyuris vermicularis (infestation) B80
Ozena J31.0

DISEASE INDEX

P

Pachyderma, pachydermia L85.9
　larynx (verrucosa) J38.7
Pachydermatocele (congenital) Q82.8
Pachydermoperiostosis — see also
　　Osteoarthropathy, hypertrophic, specified
　　type NEC
　clubbed nail M89.40 [L62]
Pachygyria Q04.3
Pachymeningitis (adhesive) (basal) (brain)
　　(cervical) (chronic) (circumscribed) (external)
　　(fibrous) (hemorrhagic) (hypertrophic)
　　(internal) (purulent) (spinal) (suppurative) —
　　see Meningitis
Pachyonychia (congenital) Q84.5
Pacinian tumor — see Neoplasm, skin, benign
Pad, knuckle or Garrod's M72.1
Paget's disease
　with infiltrating duct carcinoma — see
　　　Neoplasm, breast, malignant
　bone M88.9
　　carpus M88.84-
　　clavicle M88.81-
　　femur M88.85-
　　fibula M88.86-
　　finger M88.84-
　　humerus M88.82-
　　ilium M88.85-
　　in neoplastic disease — see Osteitis,
　　　　deformans, in neoplastic disease
　　ischium M88.85-
　　metacarpus M88.84-
　　metatarsus M88.87-
　　multiple sites M88.89
　　neck M88.88
　　radius M88.83-
　　rib M88.88
　　scapula M88.81-
　　skull M88.0
　　tarsus M88.87-
　　tibia M88.86-
　　toe M88.87-
　　ulna M88.83-
　　vertebra M88.88
　breast (female) C50.01-
　　male C50.02-
　extramammary — see also Neoplasm, skin,
　　　malignant
　　anus C21.0
　　margin C44.590
　　skin C44.590
　intraductal carcinoma — see Neoplasm,
　　　breast, malignant
　malignant — see Neoplasm, skin, malignant
　　breast (female) C50.01-
　　　male C50.02-
　　unspecified site (female) C50.01-
　　　male C50.02-
　mammary — see Paget's disease, breast
　nipple — see Paget's disease, breast
　osteitis deformans — see Paget's disease, bone
Paget-Schroetter syndrome I82.890
Pain(s) (see also Painful) R52
　abdominal R10.9
　　colic R10.83
　　generalized R10.84
　　　with acute abdomen R10.0
　　lower R10.30
　　　left quadrant R10.32
　　　pelvic or perineal R10.2
　　　periumbilical R10.33
　　　right quadrant R10.31
　　rebound — see Tenderness, abdominal,
　　　　rebound
　　severe with abdominal rigidity R10.0
　　tenderness — see Tenderness, abdominal

Pain(s) (see also Painful) R52 — continued
　abdominal R10.9 — continued
　　upper R10.10
　　　epigastric R10.13
　　　left quadrant R10.12
　　　right quadrant R10.11
　acute R52
　　due to trauma G89.11
　　neoplasm related G89.3
　　post-thoracotomy G89.12
　　postprocedural NEC G89.18
　　specified by site — code to Pain, by site
　adnexa (uteri) R10.2
　anginoid — see Pain, precordial
　anus K62.89
　arm — see Pain, limb, upper
　axillary (axilla) M79.62-
　back (postural) M54.9
　bladder R39.89
　　associated with micturition — see Micturition,
　　　painful
　　chronic R39.82
　bone — see Disorder, bone, specified type
　　　NEC
　breast N64.4
　broad ligament R10.2
　cancer associated (acute) (chronic) G89.3
　cecum — see Pain, abdominal
　cervicobrachial M53.1
　chest (central) R07.9
　　anterior wall R07.89
　　atypical R07.89
　　ischemic I20.9
　　musculoskeletal R07.89
　　non-cardiac R07.89
　　on breathing R07.1
　　pleurodynia R07.81
　　precordial R07.2
　　wall (anterior) R07.89
　chronic G89.29
　　associated with significant psychosocial
　　　dysfunction G89.4
　　due to trauma G89.21
　　neoplasm related G89.3
　　post-thoracotomy G89.22
　　postoperative NEC G89.28
　　postprocedural NEC G89.28
　　specified NEC G89.29
　coccyx M53.3
　colon — see Pain, abdominal
　coronary — see Angina
　costochondral R07.1
　diaphragm R07.1
　due to cancer G89.3
　due to device, implant or graft (see also
　　　Complications, by site and type, specified
　　　NEC) T85.848
　　arterial graft NEC T82.848
　　breast (implant) T85.848
　　catheter NEC T85.848
　　　dialysis (renal) T82.848
　　　　intraperitoneal T85.848
　　　infusion NEC T82.848
　　　　spinal (epidural) (subdural) T85.840
　　　urinary (indwelling) T83.84
　　electronic (electrode) (pulse generator)
　　　(stimulator)
　　　bone T84.84
　　　cardiac T82.847
　　　nervous system (brain) (peripheral nerve)
　　　　(spinal) T85.840
　　　urinary T83.84
　　fixation, internal (orthopedic) NEC T84.84
　　gastrointestinal (bile duct) (esophagus)
　　　T85.848
　　genital NEC T83.84
　　heart NEC T82.847
　　infusion NEC T85.848
　　joint prosthesis T84.84

Pain(s) (see also Painful) R52 — continued
　due to device, implant or graft (see also
　　　Complications, by site and type, specified
　　　NEC) T85.848 — continued
　　ocular (corneal graft) (orbital implant) NEC
　　　T85.848
　　orthopedic NEC T84.84
　　specified NEC T85.848
　　urinary NEC T83.84
　　vascular NEC T82.848
　　ventricular intracranial shunt T85.840
　due to malignancy (primary) (secondary)
　　　G89.3
　ear — see subcategory H92.0
　epigastric, epigastrium R10.13
　eye — see Pain, ocular
　face, facial R51
　　atypical G50.1
　female genital organs NEC N94.89
　finger — see Pain, limb, upper
　flank — see Pain, abdominal
　foot — see Pain, limb, lower
　gallbladder K82.9
　gas (intestinal) R14.1
　gastric — see Pain, abdominal
　generalized NOS R52
　genital organ
　　female N94.89
　　male N50.89
　groin — see Pain, abdominal, lower
　hand — see Pain, limb, upper
　head — see Headache
　heart — see Pain, precordial
　infra-orbital — see Neuralgia, trigeminal
　intercostal R07.82
　intermenstrual N94.0
　jaw R68.84
　joint M25.50
　　ankle M25.57-
　　elbow M25.52-
　　finger M25.54-
　　foot M25.57-
　　hand M25.54-
　　hip M25.55-
　　knee M25.56-
　　shoulder M25.51-
　　toe M25.57-
　　wrist M25.53-
　kidney N23
　laryngeal R07.0
　leg — see Pain, limb, lower
　limb M79.609
　　lower M79.60-
　　　foot M79.67-
　　　lower leg M79.66-
　　　thigh M79.65-
　　　toe M79.67-
　　upper M79.60-
　　　axilla M79.62-
　　　finger M79.64-
　　　forearm M79.63-
　　　hand M79.64-
　　　upper arm M79.62-
　loin M54.5
　low back M54.5
　lumbar region M54.5
　mandibular R68.84
　mastoid — see subcategory H92.0
　maxilla R68.84
　menstrual (see also Dysmenorrhea) N94.6
　metacarpophalangeal (joint) — see Pain, joint,
　　　hand
　metatarsophalangeal (joint) — see Pain, joint,
　　　foot
　mouth K13.79
　muscle — see Myalgia
　musculoskeletal (see also Pain, by site) M79.1
　myofascial M79.1

Pain(s) (see also Painful) R52 — *continued*
nasal J34.89
nasopharynx J39.2
neck NEC M54.2
nerve NEC — see Neuralgia
neuromuscular — see Neuralgia
nose J34.89
ocular H57.1-
ophthalmic — see Pain, ocular
orbital region — see Pain, ocular
ovary N94.89
over heart — see Pain, precordial
ovulation N94.0
pelvic (female) R10.2
penis N48.89
pericardial — see Pain, precordial
perineal, perineum R10.2
pharynx J39.2
pleura, pleural, pleuritic R07.81
post-thoracotomy G89.12
postoperative NOS G89.18
postprocedural NOS G89.18
precordial (region) R07.2
premenstrual N94.3
psychogenic (persistent) (any site) F45.41
radicular (spinal) — see Radiculopathy
rectum K62.89
respiration R07.1
retrosternal R07.2
rheumatoid, muscular — see Myalgia
rib R07.81
root (spinal) — see Radiculopathy
round ligament (stretch) R10.2
sacroiliac M53.3
sciatic — see Sciatica
scrotum N50.82
seminal vesicle N50.89
shoulder M25.51-
spermatic cord N50.89
spinal root — see Radiculopathy
spine M54.9
   cervical M54.2
   low back M54.5
      with sciatica M54.4-
   thoracic M54.6
stomach — see Pain, abdominal
substernal R07.2
temporomandibular (joint) M26.62-
testis N50.81-
thoracic spine M54.6
   with radicular and visceral pain M54.14
throat R07.0
tibia — see Pain, limb, lower
toe — see Pain, limb, lower
tongue K14.6
tooth K08.89
trigeminal — see Neuralgia, trigeminal
tumor associated G89.3
ureter N23
urinary (organ) (system) N23
uterus NEC N94.89
vagina R10.2
vertebrogenic (syndrome) M54.89
vesical R39.89
   associated with micturition — see Micturition, painful
vulva R10.2
Painful — see also Pain
coitus
   female N94.10
   male N53.12
      psychogenic F52.6
ejaculation (semen) N53.12
      psychogenic F52.6
erection — see Priapism
feet syndrome E53.8
joint replacement (hip) (knee) T84.84
menstruation — see Dysmenorrhea
   psychogenic F45.8

Painful — see also Pain — *continued*
micturition — see Micturition, painful
respiration R07.1
scar NEC L90.5
wire sutures T81.89
Painter's colic — see subcategory T56.0
Palate — see condition
Palatoplegia K13.79
Palatoschisis — see Cleft, palate
Palilalia R48.8
Palliative care Z51.5
Pallor R23.1
optic disc, temporal — see Atrophy, optic
Palmar — see also condition
fascia — see condition
Palpable
cecum K63.89
kidney N28.89
ovary N83.8
prostate N42.9
spleen — see Splenomegaly
Palpitations (heart) R00.2
psychogenic F45.8
Palsy (see also Paralysis) G83.9
atrophic diffuse (progressive) G12.22
Bell's — see also Palsy, facial
   newborn P11.3
brachial plexus NEC G54.0
   newborn (birth injury) P14.3
brain — see Palsy, cerebral
bulbar (progressive) (chronic) G12.22
   of childhood (Fazio-Londe) G12.1
   pseudo NEC G12.29
   supranuclear (progressive) G23.1
cerebral (congenital) G80.9
   ataxic G80.4
   athetoid G80.3
   choreathetoid G80.3
   diplegic G80.8
      spastic G80.1
   dyskinetic G80.3
      athetoid G80.3
      choreathetoid G80.3
      distonic G80.3
   dystonic G80.3
   hemiplegic G80.8
      spastic G80.2
   mixed G80.8
   monoplegic G80.8
      spastic G80.1
   paraplegic G80.8
      spastic G80.1
   quadriplegic G80.8
      spastic G80.0
   spastic G80.1
      diplegic G80.1
      hemiplegic G80.2
      monoplegic G80.1
      quadriplegic G80.0
      specified NEC G80.1
      tetrapelgic G80.0
   specified NEC G80.8
   syphilitic A52.12
      congenital A50.49
   tetraplegic G80.8
      spastic G80.0
cranial nerve — see also Disorder, nerve, cranial
   multiple G52.7
      in
         infectious disease B99 [G53]
         neoplastic disease (see also Neoplasm)
            D49.9 [G53]
         parasitic disease B89 [G53]
         sarcoidosis D86.82
creeping G12.22
diver's T70.3
Erb's P14.0

Palsy (see also Paralysis) G83.9 — *continued*
facial G51.0
   newborn (birth injury) P11.3
glossopharyngeal G52.1
Klumpke(-Déjérine) P14.1
lead — see subcategory T56.0
median nerve (tardy) G56.1-
nerve G58.9
   specified NEC G58.8
peroneal nerve (acute) (tardy) G57.3-
progressive supranuclear G23.1
pseudobulbar NEC G12.29
radial nerve (acute) G56.3-
seventh nerve — see also Palsy, facial
   newborn P11.3
shaking — see Parkinsonism
spastic (cerebral) (spinal) G80.1
ulnar nerve (tardy) G56.2-
wasting G12.29
Paludism — see Malaria
Panangiitis M30.0
Panaris, panaritium — see also Cellulitis, digit
with lymphangitis — see Lymphangitis, acute, digit
Panarteritis nodosa M30.0
brain or cerebral I67.7
Pancake heart R93.1
with cor pulmonale (chronic) I27.81
Pancarditis (acute) (chronic) I51.89
rheumatic I09.89
   active or acute I01.8
Pancoast's syndrome or tumor C34.1-
Pancolitis, ulcerative (chronic) K51.00
with
   abscess K51.014
   complication K51.019
   fistula K51.013
   obstruction K51.012
   rectal bleeding K51.011
   specified complication NEC K51.018
Pancreas, pancreatic — see condition
Pancreatitis (annular) (apoplectic) (calcareous) (edematous) (hemorrhagic) (malignant) (recurrent) (subacute) (suppurative) K85.90
with necrosis (uninfected) K85.91
   infected K85.92
acute (without necrosis or infection) K85.90
   with necrosis (uninfected) K85.91
      infected K85.92
   alcohol-induced (without necrosis or infection) K85.20
      with necrosis (uninfected) K85.21
         infected K85.22
   biliary (without necrosis or infection) K85.10
      with necrosis (uninfected) K85.11
         infected K85.12
   drug-induced (without necrosis or infection) K85.30
      with necrosis (uninfected) K85.31
         infected K85.32
   gallstone (without necrosis or infection) K85.10
      with necrosis (uninfected) K85.11
         infected K85.12
   idiopathic (without necrosis or infection) K85.00
      with necrosis (uninfected) K85.01
         infected K85.02
   specified NEC (without necrosis or infection) K85.80
      with necrosis (uninfected) K85.81
         infected K85.82
chronic (infectious) K86.1
   alcohol-induced K86.0
   recurrent K86.1
   relapsing K86.1
cystic (chronic) K86.1
cytomegaloviral B25.2

Pancreatitis (annular) (apoplectic) (calcareous) (edematous) (hemorrhagic) (malignant) (recurrent) (subacute) (suppurative) K85.9 — *continued*
fibrous (chronic) K86.1
gallstone (without necrosis or infection) K85.10
with necrosis (uninfected) K85.11
infected K85.12
gangrenous — *see* Pancreatitis, acute
interstitial (chronic) K86.1
acute (*see also* Pancreatitis, acute) K85.80
mumps B26.3
recurrent (chronic) K86.1
relapsing, chronic K86.1
syphilitic A52.74
Pancreatoblastoma — *see* Neoplasm, pancreas, malignant
Pancreolithiasis K86.89
Pancytolysis D75.89
Pancytopenia (acquired) D61.818
with
malformations D61.09
myelodysplastic syndrome — *see* Syndrome, myelodysplastic
antineoplastic chemotherapy induced D61.810
congenital D61.09
drug-induced NEC D61.811
Panencephalitis, subacute, sclerosing A81.1
Panhematopenia D61.9
congenital D61.09
constitutional D61.09
splenic, primary D73.1
Panhemocytopenia D61.9
congenital D61.09
constitutional D61.09
Panhypogonadism E29.1
Panhypopituitarism E23.0
prepubertal E23.0
Panic (attack) (state) F41.0
reaction to exceptional stress (transient) F43.0
Panmyelopathy, familial, constitutional D61.09
Panmyelophthisis D61.82
congenital D61.09
Panmyelosis (acute) (with myelofibrosis) C94.4-
Panner's disease — *see* Osteochondrosis, juvenile, humerus
Panneuritis endemica E51.11
Panniculitis (nodular) (nonsuppurative) M79.3
back M54.00
cervical region M54.02
cervicothoracic region M54.03
lumbar region M54.06
lumbosacral region M54.07
multiple sites M54.09
occipito-atlanto-axial region M54.01
sacrococcygeal region M54.08
thoracic region M54.04
thoracolumbar region M54.05
lupus L93.2
mesenteric K65.4
neck M54.02
cervicothoracic region M54.03
occipito-atlanto-axial region M54.01
relapsing M35.6
Panniculus adiposus (abdominal) E65
Pannus (allergic) (cornea) (degenerativus) (keratic) H16.42-
abdominal (symptomatic) E65
trachomatosus, trachomatous (active) A71.1
Panophthalmitis H44.01-
Pansinusitis (chronic) (hyperplastic) (nonpurulent) (purulent) J32.4
acute J01.40
recurrent J01.41
tuberculous A15.8
Panuveitis (sympathetic) H44.11-

Panvalvular disease I08.9
specified NEC I08.8
PAPA (pyogenic arthritis, pyoderma gangrenosum, and acne syndrome) M04.8
Papanicolaou smear, cervix Z12.4
as part of routine gynecological examination Z01.419
with abnormal findings Z01.411
for suspected neoplasm Z12.4
nonspecific abnormal finding R87.619
routine Z01.419
with abnormal findings Z01.411
Papilledema (choked disc) H47.10
associated with
decreased ocular pressure H47.12
increased intracranial pressure H47.11
retinal disorder H47.13
Foster-Kennedy syndrome H47.14-
Papillitis H46.00
anus K62.89
chronic lingual K14.4
necrotizing, kidney N17.2
optic H46.0-
rectum K62.89
renal, necrotizing N17.2
tongue K14.0
Papilloma — *see also* Neoplasm, benign, by site
acuminatum (female) (male) (anogenital) A63.0
basal cell L82.1
inflamed L82.0
benign pinta (primary) A67.0
bladder (urinary) (transitional cell) D41.4
choroid plexus (lateral ventricle) (third ventricle) D33.0
anaplastic C71.5
fourth ventricle D33.1
malignant C71.5
renal pelvis (transitional cell) D41.1-
benign D30.1-
Schneiderian
specified site — *see* Neoplasm, benign, by site
unspecified site D14.0
serous surface
borderline malignancy
specified site — *see* Neoplasm, uncertain behavior, by site
unspecified site D39.10
specified site — *see* Neoplasm, benign, by site
unspecified site D27.9
transitional (cell)
bladder (urinary) D41.4
inverted type — *see* Neoplasm, uncertain behavior, by site
renal pelvis D41.1-
ureter D41.2-
ureter (transitional cell) D41.2-
benign D30.2-
urothelial — *see* Neoplasm, uncertain behavior, by site
villous — *see* Neoplasm, uncertain behavior, by site
adenocarcinoma in — *see* Neoplasm, malignant, by site
in situ — *see* Neoplasm, in situ
yaws, plantar or palmar A66.1
Papillomata, multiple, of yaws A66.1
Papillomatosis — *see also* Neoplasm, benign, by site
confluent and reticulated L83
cystic, breast — *see* Mastopathy, cystic
ductal, breast — *see* Mastopathy, cystic
intraductal (diffuse) — *see* Neoplasm, benign, by site
subareolar duct D24-

Papillomavirus, as cause of disease classified elsewhere B97.7
Papillon-Léage and Psaume syndrome Q87.0
Papule(s) R23.8
carate (primary) A67.0
fibrous, of nose D22.39
Gottron's L94.4
pinta (primary) A67.0
Papulosis
lymphomatoid C86.6
malignant I77.89
Papyraceous fetus O31.0-
Para-albuminemia E88.09
Paracephalus Q89.7
Parachute mitral valve Q23.2
Paracoccidioidomycosis B41.9
disseminated B41.7
generalized B41.7
mucocutaneous-lymphangitic B41.8
pulmonary B41.0
specified NEC B41.8
visceral B41.8
Paradentosis K05.4
Paraffinoma T88.8
Paraganglioma D44.7
adrenal D35.0-
malignant C74.1-
aortic body D44.7
malignant C75.5
carotid body D44.6
malignant C75.4
chromaffin — *see also* Neoplasm, benign, by site
malignant — *see* Neoplasm, malignant, by site
extra-adrenal D44.7
malignant C75.5
specified site — *see* Neoplasm, malignant, by site
unspecified site C75.5
specified site — *see* Neoplasm, uncertain behavior, by site
unspecified site D44.7
gangliocytic D13.2
specified site — *see* Neoplasm, benign, by site
unspecified site D13.2
glomus jugulare D44.7
malignant C75.5
jugular D44.7
malignant C75.5
specified site — *see* Neoplasm, malignant, by site
unspecified site C75.5
nonchromaffin D44.7
malignant C75.5
specified site — *see* Neoplasm, malignant, by site
unspecified site C75.5
specified site — *see* Neoplasm, uncertain behavior, by site
unspecified site D44.7
parasympathetic D44.7
specified site — *see* Neoplasm, uncertain behavior, by site
unspecified site D44.7
specified site — *see* Neoplasm, uncertain behavior, by site
sympathetic D44.7
specified site — *see* Neoplasm, uncertain behavior, by site
unspecified site D44.7
unspecified site D44.7
Parageusia R43.2
psychogenic F45.8
Paragonimiasis B66.4

Paragranuloma, Hodgkin — *see*
    Lymphoma, Hodgkin, classical, specified
    type NEC
Parahemophilia (*see also* Defect, coagulation)
    D68.2
Parakeratosis R23.4
    variegata L41.0
Paralysis, paralytic (complete) (incomplete)
    G83.9
    with
       syphilis A52.17
    abducens, abducent (nerve) — *see* Strabismus,
       paralytic, sixth nerve
    abductor, lower extremity G57.9-
    accessory nerve G52.8
    accommodation — *see also* Paresis, of
       accommodation
       hysterical F44.89
    acoustic nerve (except Deafness) — *see*
       subcategory H93.3
    agitans (*see also* Parkinsonism) G20
       arteriosclerotic G21.4
    alternating (oculomotor) G83.89
    amyotrophic G12.21
    ankle G57.9-
    anus (sphincter) K62.89
    arm — *see* Monoplegia, upper limb
    ascending (spinal), acute G61.0
    association G12.29
    asthenic bulbar G70.00
       with exacerbation (acute) G70.01
       in crisis G70.01
    ataxic (hereditary) G11.9
       general (syphilitic) A52.17
    atrophic G58.9
       infantile, acute — *see* Poliomyelitis, paralytic
       progressive G12.22
       spinal (acute) — *see* Poliomyelitis, paralytic
    axillary G54.0
    Babinski-Nageotte's G83.89
    Bell's G51.0
       newborn P11.3
    Benedikt's G46.3
    birth injury P14.9
       spinal cord P11.5
    bladder (neurogenic) (sphincter) N31.2
    bowel, colon or intestine K56.0
    brachial plexus G54.0
       birth injury P14.3
       newborn (birth injury) P14.3
    brain G83.9
       diplegia G83.0
       triplegia G83.89
    bronchial J98.09
    Brown-Séquard G83.81
    bulbar (chronic) (progressive) G12.22
       infantile — *see* Poliomyelitis, paralytic
       poliomyelitic — *see* Poliomyelitis, paralytic
       pseudo G12.29
    bulbospinal G70.00
       with exacerbation (acute) G70.01
       in crisis G70.01
    cardiac (*see also* Failure, heart) I50.9
    cerebrocerebellar, diplegic G80.1
    cervical
       plexus G54.2
       sympathetic G90.09
    Céstan-Chenais G46.3
    Charcot-Marie-Tooth type G60.0
    Clark's G80.9
    colon K56.0
    compressed air T70.3
    compression
       arm G56.9-
       leg G57.9-
       lower extremity G57.9-
       upper extremity G56.9-
    congenital (cerebral) — *see* Palsy, cerebral

Paralysis, paralytic (complete) (incomplete)
    G83.9 — *continued*
    conjugate movement (gaze) (of eye) H51.0
       cortical (nuclear) (supranuclear) H51.0
    cordis — *see* Failure, heart
    cranial or cerebral nerve G52.9
    creeping G12.22
    crossed leg G83.89
    crutch — *see* Injury, brachial plexus
    deglutition R13.0
       hysterical F44.4
    dementia A52.17
    descending (spinal) NEC G12.29
    diaphragm (flaccid) J98.6
       due to accidental dissection of phrenic nerve
          during procedure — *see* Puncture,
          accidental complicating surgery
    digestive organs NEC K59.8
    diplegic — *see* Diplegia
    diver's T70.3
    divergence (nuclear) H51.8
    Duchenne's
       birth injury P14.0
       due to or associated with
          motor neuron disease G12.22
          muscular dystrophy G71.0
       due to intracranial or spinal birth injury — *see*
          Palsy, cerebral
    embolic (current episode) I63.4-
    Erb's syphilitic spastic spinal A52.17
    Erb(-Duchenne) (birth) (newborn) P14.0
    esophagus K22.8
    eye muscle (extrinsic) H49.9
       intrinsic — *see also* Paresis, of
          accommodation
    facial (nerve) G51.0
       birth injury P11.3
       congenital P11.3
       following operation NEC — *see* Puncture,
          accidental complicating surgery
       newborn (birth injury) P11.3
    familial (recurrent) (periodic) G72.3
       spastic G11.4
    fauces J39.2
    finger G56.9-
    gait R26.1
    gastric nerve (nondiabetic) G52.2
    gaze, conjugate H51.0
    general (progressive) (syphilitic) A52.17
       juvenile A50.45
    glottis J38.00
       bilateral J38.02
       unilateral J38.01
    gluteal G54.1
    Gubler(-Millard) G46.3
    hand — *see* Monoplegia, upper limb
    heart — *see* Arrest, cardiac
    hemiplegic — *see* Hemiplegia
    hyperkalemic periodic (familial) G72.3
    hypoglossal (nerve) G52.3
    hypokalemic periodic G72.3
    hysterical F44.4
    ileus K56.0
    infantile (*see also* Poliomyelitis, paralytic)
       A80.30
       bulbar — *see* Poliomyelitis, paralytic
       cerebral — *see* Palsy, cerebral
       spastic — *see* Palsy, cerebral, spastic
    infective — *see* Poliomyelitis, paralytic
    inferior nuclear G83.9
    internuclear — *see* Ophthalmoplegia,
       internuclear
    intestine K56.0
    iris H57.09
       due to diphtheria (toxin) A36.89
    ischemic, Volkmann's (complicating trauma)
       T79.6
    Jackson's G83.89
    jake — *see* Poisoning, food, noxious, plant

Paralysis, paralytic (complete) (incomplete)
    G83.9 — *continued*
    Jamaica ginger (jake) G62.2
    juvenile general A50.45
    Klumpke(-Déjérine) (birth) (newborn) P14.1
    labioglossal (laryngeal) (pharyngeal) G12.29
    Landry's G61.0
    laryngeal nerve (recurrent) (superior)
       (unilateral) J38.00
       bilateral J38.02
       unilateral J38.01
    larynx J38.00
       bilateral J38.02
       due to diphtheria (toxin) A36.2
       unilateral J38.01
    lateral G12.21
    lead — *see* subcategory T56.0
    left side — *see* Hemiplegia
    leg G83.1-
       both — *see* Paraplegia
       crossed G83.89
       hysterical F44.4
       psychogenic F44.4
       transient or transitory R29.818
          traumatic NEC — *see* Injury, nerve, leg
    levator palpebrae superioris — *see*
       Blepharoptosis, paralytic
    limb — *see* Monoplegia
    lip K13.0
    Lissauer's A52.17
    lower limb — *see* Monoplegia, lower limb
       both — *see* Paraplegia
    lung J98.4
    median nerve G56.1-
    medullary (tegmental) G83.89
    mesencephalic NEC G83.89
       tegmental G83.89
    middle alternating G83.89
    Millard-Gubler-Foville G46.3
    monoplegic — *see* Monoplegia
    motor G83.9
    muscle, muscular NEC G72.89
       due to nerve lesion G58.9
       eye (extrinsic) H49.9
          intrinsic — *see* Paresis, of accommodation
          oblique — *see* Strabismus, paralytic, fourth
            nerve
       iris sphincter H21.9
       ischemic (Volkmann's) (complicating trauma)
          T79.6
       progressive G12.21
       pseudohypertrophic G71.0
    musculocutaneous nerve G56.9-
    musculospiral G56.9-
    nerve — *see also* Disorder, nerve
       abducent — *see* Strabismus, paralytic, sixth
          nerve
       accessory G52.8
       auditory (except Deafness) — *see*
          subcategory H93.3
       birth injury P14.9
       cranial or cerebral G52.9
       facial G51.0
          birth injury P11.3
          congenital P11.3
          newborn (birth injury) P11.3
       fourth or trochlear — *see* Strabismus,
          paralytic, fourth nerve
       newborn (birth injury) P14.9
       oculomotor — *see* Strabismus, paralytic,
          third nerve
       phrenic (birth injury) P14.2
       radial G56.3-
       seventh or facial G51.0
          newborn (birth injury) P11.3
       sixth or abducent — *see* Strabismus,
          paralytic, sixth nerve
       syphilitic A52.15

Paralysis, paralytic (complete) (incomplete) G83.9 — *continued*
nerve — *see also* Disorder, nerve — *continued*
third or oculomotor — *see* Strabismus, paralytic, third nerve
trigeminal G50.9
trochlear — *see* Strabismus, paralytic, fourth nerve
ulnar G56.2-
normokalemic periodic G72.3
ocular H49.9
alternating G83.89
oculofacial, congenital (Moebius) Q87.0
oculomotor (external bilateral) (nerve) — *see* Strabismus, paralytic, third nerve
palate (soft) K13.79
paratrigeminal G50.9
periodic (familial) (hyperkalemic) (hypokalemic) (myotonic) (normokalemic) (potassium sensitive) (secondary) G72.3
peripheral autonomic nervous system — *see* Neuropathy, peripheral, autonomic
peroneal (nerve) G57.3-
pharynx J39.2
phrenic nerve G56.8-
plantar nerve(s) G57.6-
pneumogastric nerve G52.2
poliomyelitis (current) — *see* Poliomyelitis, paralytic
popliteal nerve G57.3-
postepileptic transitory G83.84
progressive (atrophic) (bulbar) (spinal) G12.22
general A52.17
infantile acute — *see* Poliomyelitis, paralytic
supranuclear G23.1
pseudobulbar G12.29
pseudohypertrophic (muscle) G71.0
psychogenic F44.4
quadriceps G57.9-
quadriplegic — *see* Tetraplegia
radial nerve G56.3-
rectus muscle (eye) H49.9
recurrent isolated sleep G47.53
respiratory (muscle) (system) (tract) R06.81
center NEC G93.89
congenital P28.89
newborn P28.89
right side — *see* Hemiplegia
saturnine — *see* subcategory T56.0
sciatic nerve G57.0-
senile G83.9
shaking — *see* Parkinsonism
shoulder G56.9-
sleep, recurrent isolated G47.53
spastic G83.9
cerebral — *see* Palsy, cerebral, spastic
congenital (cerebral) — *see* Palsy, cerebral, spastic
familial G11.4
hereditary G11.4
quadriplegic G80.0
syphilitic (spinal) A52.17
sphincter, bladder — *see* Paralysis, bladder
spinal (cord) G83.9
accessory nerve G52.8
acute — *see* Poliomyelitis, paralytic
ascending acute G61.0
atrophic (acute) — *see also* Poliomyelitis, paralytic
spastic, syphilitic A52.17
congenital NEC — *see* Palsy, cerebral
hereditary G95.89
infantile — *see* Poliomyelitis, paralytic
progressive G12.21
sequelae NEC G83.89
sternomastoid G52.8

Paralysis, paralytic (complete) (incomplete) G83.9 — *continued*
stomach K31.84
diabetic — *see* Diabetes, by type, with gastroparesis
nerve G52.2
diabetic — *see* Diabetes, by type, with gastroparesis
stroke — *see* Infarct, brain
subcapsularis G56.8-
supranuclear (progressive) G23.1
sympathetic G90.8
cervical G90.09
nervous system — *see* Neuropathy, peripheral, autonomic
syndrome G83.9
specified NEC G83.89
syphilitic spastic spinal (Erb's) A52.17
thigh G57.9-
throat J39.2
diphtheritic A36.0
muscle J39.2
thrombotic (current episode) I63.3-
thumb G56.9-
tick — *see* Toxicity, venom, arthropod, specified NEC
Todd's (postepileptic transitory paralysis) G83.84
toe G57.6-
tongue K14.8
transient R29.5
arm or leg NEC R29.818
traumatic NEC — *see* Injury, nerve
trapezius G52.8
traumatic, transient NEC — *see* Injury, nerve
trembling — *see* Parkinsonism
triceps brachii G56.9-
trigeminal nerve G50.9
trochlear (nerve) — *see* Strabismus, paralytic, fourth nerve
ulnar nerve G56.2-
upper limb — *see* Monoplegia, upper limb
uremic N18.9 *[G99.8]*
uveoparotitic D86.89
uvula K13.79
postdiphtheritic A36.0
vagus nerve G52.2
vasomotor NEC G90.8
velum palati K13.79
vesical — *see* Paralysis, bladder
vestibular nerve (except Vertigo) — *see* subcategory H93.3
vocal cords J38.00
bilateral J38.02
unilateral J38.01
Volkmann's (complicating trauma) T79.6
wasting G12.29
Weber's G46.3
wrist G56.9-
Paramedial urethrovesical orifice Q64.79
Paramenia N92.6
Parametritis (*see also* Disease, pelvis, inflammatory) N73.2
acute N73.0
complicating abortion — *see* Abortion, by type, complicated by, parametritis
Parametrium, parametric — *see* condition
Paramnesia — *see* Amnesia
Paramolar K00.1
Paramyloidosis E85.8
Paramyoclonus multiplex G25.3
Paramyotonia (congenita) G71.19
Parangi — *see* Yaws
Paranoia (querulans) F22
senile F03
Paranoid
dementia (senile) F03
praecox — *see* Schizophrenia
personality F60.0

Paranoid — *continued*
psychosis (climacteric) (involutional) (menopausal) F22
psychogenic (acute) F23
senile F03
reaction (acute) F23
chronic F22
schizophrenia F20.0
state (climacteric) (involutional) (menopausal) (simple) F22
senile F03
tendencies F60.0
traits F60.0
trends F60.0
type, psychopathic personality F60.0
Paraparesis — *see* Paraplegia
Paraphasia R47.02
Paraphilia F65.9
Paraphimosis (congenital) N47.2
chancroidal A57
Paraphrenia, paraphrenic (late) F22
schizophrenia F20.0
Paraplegia (lower) G82.20
ataxic — *see* Degeneration, combined, spinal cord
complete G82.21
congenital (cerebral) G80.8
spastic G80.1
familial spastic G11.4
functional (hysterical) F44.4
hereditary, spastic G11.4
hysterical F44.4
incomplete G82.22
Pott's A18.01
psychogenic F44.4
spastic
Erb's spinal, syphilitic A52.17
hereditary G11.4
tropical G04.1
syphilitic (spastic) A52.17
tropical spastic G04.1
Parapoxvirus B08.60
specified NEC B08.69
Paraproteinemia D89.2
benign (familial) D89.2
monoclonal D47.2
secondary to malignant disease D47.2
Parapsoriasis L41.9
en plaques L41.4
guttata L41.1
large plaque L41.4
retiform, retiformis L41.5
small plaque L41.3
specified NEC L41.8
varioliformis (acuta) L41.0
Parasitic — *see also* condition
disease NEC B89
stomatitis B37.0
sycosis (beard) (scalp) B35.0
twin Q89.4
Parasitism B89
intestinal B82.9
skin B88.9
specified — *see* Infestation
Parasitophobia F40.218
Parasomnia G47.50
due to
alcohol
abuse F10.182
dependence F10.282
use F10.982
amphetamines
abuse F15.182
dependence F15.282
use F15.982
caffeine
abuse F15.182
dependence F15.282
use F15.982

Parasomnia G47.50 — *continued*
  due to — *continued*
    cocaine
      abuse F14.182
      dependence F14.282
      use F14.982
    drug NEC
      abuse F19.182
      dependence F19.282
      use F19.982
    opioid
      abuse F11.182
      dependence F11.282
      use F11.982
    psychoactive substance NEC
      abuse F19.182
      dependence F19.282
      use F19.982
    sedative, hypnotic, or anxiolytic
      abuse F13.182
      dependence F13.282
      use F13.982
    stimulant NEC
      abuse F15.182
      dependence F15.282
      use F15.982
  in conditions classified elsewhere G47.54
  nonorganic origin F51.8
  organic G47.50
  specified NEC G47.59
Paraspadias Q54.9
Paraspasmus facialis G51.8
Parasuicide (attempt)
  history of (personal) Z91.5
  in family Z81.8
Parathyroid gland — *see* condition
Parathyroid tetany E20.9
Paratrachoma A74.0
Paratyphilitis — *see* Appendicitis
Paratyphoid (fever) — *see* Fever, paratyphoid
Paratyphus — *see* Fever, paratyphoid
Paraurethral duct Q64.79
  nonorganic origin F51.5
Paraurethritis — *see also* Urethritis
  gonococcal (acute) (chronic) (with abscess) A54.1
Paravaccinia NEC B08.04
Paravaginitis — *see* Vaginitis
Parencephalitis — *see also* Encephalitis
  sequelae G09
Parent-child conflict — *see* Conflict, parent-child
  estrangement NEC Z62.890
Paresis — *see also* Paralysis
  accommodation — *see* Paresis, of accommodation
  Bernhardt's G57.1-
  bladder (sphincter) — *see also* Paralysis, bladder
    tabetic A52.17
  bowel, colon or intestine K56.0
  extrinsic muscle, eye H49.9
  general (progressive) (syphilitic) A52.17
    juvenile A50.45
  heart — *see* Failure, heart
  insane (syphilitic) A52.17
  juvenile (general) A50.45
  of accommodation H52.52-
  peripheral progressive (idiopathic) G60.3
  pseudohypertrophic G71.0
  senile G83.9
  syphilitic (general) A52.17
    congenital A50.45
  vesical NEC N31.2
Paresthesia — *see also* Disturbance, sensation
  Bernhardt G57.1-
Paretic — *see* condition

Parinaud's
  conjunctivitis H10.89
  oculoglandular syndrome H10.89
  ophthalmoplegia H49.88-
Parkinson's disease, syndrome or tremor — *see* Parkinsonism
Parkinsonism (idiopathic) (primary) G20
  with neurogenic orthostatic hypotension (symptomatic) G90.3
  arteriosclerotic G21.4
  dementia G31.83 *[F02.80]*
    with behavioral disturbance G31.83 *[F02.81]*
  due to
    drugs NEC G21.19
      neuroleptic G21.11
  neuroleptic induced G21.11
  postencephalitic G21.3
  secondary G21.9
    due to
      arteriosclerosis G21.4
      drugs NEC G21.19
        neuroleptic G21.11
      encephalitis G21.3
      external agents NEC G21.2
      syphilis A52.19
    specified NEC G21.8
  syphilitic A52.19
  treatment-induced NEC G21.19
  vascular G21.4
Parodontitis — *see* Periodontitis
Parodontosis K05.4
Paronychia — *see also* Cellulitis, digit
  with lymphangitis — *see* Lymphangitis, acute, digit
  candidal (chronic) B37.2
  tuberculous (primary) A18.4
Parorexia (psychogenic) F50.89
Parosmia R43.1
  psychogenic F45.8
Parotid gland — *see* condition
Parotitis, parotiditis (allergic) (nonspecific toxic) (purulent) (septic) (suppurative) — *see also* Sialoadenitis
  epidemic — *see* Mumps
  infectious — *see* Mumps
  postoperative K91.89
  surgical K91.89
Parrot fever A70
Parrot's disease (early congenital syphilitic pseudoparalysis) A50.02
Parry-Romberg syndrome G51.8
Parry's disease or syndrome E05.00
  with thyroid storm E05.01
Pars planitis — *see* Cyclitis
Parson's disease (exophthalmic goiter) E05.00
  with thyroid storm E05.01
Parsonage(-Aldren)-Turner syndrome G54.5
Particolored infant Q82.8
Parturition — *see* Delivery
Parulis K04.7
  with sinus K04.6
Parvovirus, as cause of disease classified elsewhere B97.6
Pasini and Pierini's atrophoderma L90.3
Passage
  false, urethra N36.5
  meconium (newborn) during delivery P03.82
  of sounds or bougies — *see* Attention to, artificial, opening
Passive — *see* condition
  smoking Z77.22
Pasteurella septica A28.0
Pasteurellosis — *see* Infection, Pasteurella
PAT (paroxysmal atrial tachycardia) I47.1
Patau's syndrome — *see* Trisomy, 13

Patches
  mucous (syphilitic) A51.39
    congenital A50.07
  smokers' (mouth) K13.24
Patellar — *see* condition
Patent — *see also* Imperfect, closure
  canal of Nuck Q52.4
  cervix N88.3
  ductus arteriosus or Botallo's Q25.0
  foramen
    botalli Q21.1
    ovale Q21.1
  interauricular septum Q21.1
  interventricular septum Q21.0
  omphalomesenteric duct Q43.0
  os (uteri) — *see* Patent, cervix
  ostium secundum Q21.1
  urachus Q64.4
  vitelline duct Q43.0
Paterson(-Brown)(-Kelly) syndrome or web D50.1
Pathologic, pathological — *see also* condition
  asphyxia R09.01
  fire-setting F63.1
  gambling F63.0
  ovum O02.0
  resorption, tooth K03.3
  stealing F63.2
Pathology (of) — *see* Disease
  periradicular, associated with previous endodontic treatment NEC M27.59
Pattern, sleep-wake, irregular G47.23
Patulous — *see also* Imperfect, closure (congenital)
  alimentary tract Q45.8
    lower Q43.8
    upper Q40.8
  eustachian tube H69.0-
Pause, sinoatrial I49.5
Paxton's disease B36.2
Pearl(s)
  enamel K00.2
  Epstein's K09.8
Pearl-worker's disease — *see* Osteomyelitis, specified type NEC
Pectenosis K62.4
Pectoral — *see* condition
Pectus
  carinatum (congenital) Q67.7
    acquired M95.4
    rachitic sequelae (late effect) E64.3
  excavatum (congenital) Q67.6
    acquired M95.4
    rachitic sequelae (late effect) E64.3
  recurvatum (congenital) Q67.6
Pedatrophia E41
Pederosis F65.4
Pediculosis (infestation) B85.2
  capitis (head-louse) (any site) B85.0
  corporis (body-louse) (any site) B85.1
  eyelid B85.0
  mixed (classifiable to more than one of the titles B85.0-B85.3) B85.4
  pubis (pubic louse) (any site) B85.3
  vestimenti B85.1
  vulvae B85.3
Pediculus (infestation) — *see* Pediculosis
Pedophilia F65.4
Peg-shaped teeth K00.2
Pelade — *see* Alopecia, areata
Pelger-Huët anomaly or syndrome D72.0
Peliosis (rheumatica) D69.0
  hepatis K76.4
    with toxic liver disease K71.8
Pelizaeus-Merzbacher disease E75.29
Pellagra (alcoholic) (with polyneuropathy) E52
Pellagra-cerebellar-ataxia-renal aminoaciduria syndrome E72.02

Pellegrini (-Stieda) disease or syndrome — *see* Bursitis, tibial collateral
Pellizzi's syndrome E34.8
Pel's crisis A52.11
Pelvic — *see also* condition
  examination (periodic) (routine) Z01.419
    with abnormal findings Z01.411
  kidney, congenital Q63.2
Pelviolithiasis — *see* Calculus, kidney
Pelviperitonitis — *see also* Peritonitis, pelvic
  gonococcal A54.24
  puerperal O85
Pelvis — *see* condition or type
Pemphigoid L12.9
  benign, mucous membrane L12.1
  bullous L12.0
  cicatricial L12.1
  juvenile L12.2
  ocular L12.1
  specified NEC L12.8
Pemphigus L10.9
  benign familial (chronic) Q82.8
  Brazilian L10.3
  circinatus L13.0
  conjunctiva L12.1
  drug-induced L10.5
  erythematosus L10.4
  foliaceous L10.2
  gangrenous — *see* Gangrene
  neonatorum L01.03
  ocular L12.1
  paraneoplastic L10.81
  specified NEC L10.89
  syphilitic (congenital) A50.06
  vegetans L10.1
  vulgaris L10.0
  wildfire L10.3
Pendred's syndrome E07.1
Pendulous
  abdomen, in pregnancy — *see* Pregnancy, complicated by, abnormal, pelvic organs or tissues NEC
  breast N64.89
Penetrating wound — *see also* Puncture
  with internal injury — *see* Injury, by site
  eyeball — *see* Puncture, eyeball
  orbit (with or without foreign body) — *see* Puncture, orbit
  uterus by instrument with or following ectopic or molar pregnancy O08.6
Penicillosis B48.4
Penis — *see* condition
Penitis N48.29
Pentalogy of Fallot Q21.8
Pentasomy X syndrome Q97.1
Pentosuria (essential) E74.8
Percreta placenta O43.23-
Peregrinating patient — *see* Disorder, factitious
Perforation, perforated (nontraumatic) (of)
  accidental during procedure (blood vessel) (nerve) (organ) — *see* Complication, accidental puncture or laceration
  antrum — *see* Sinusitis, maxillary
  appendix K35.2
    with localized peritonitis K35.3
  atrial septum, multiple Q21.1
  attic, ear — *see* Perforation, tympanum, attic
  bile duct (common) (hepatic) K83.2
    cystic K82.2
  bladder (urinary)
    with or following ectopic or molar pregnancy O08.6
    obstetrical trauma O71.5
    traumatic S37.29
      at delivery O71.5

Perforation, perforated (nontraumatic) (of) — *continued*
  bowel K63.1
    with or following ectopic or molar pregnancy O08.6
    newborn P78.0
    obstetrical trauma O71.5
    traumatic — *see* Laceration, intestine
  broad ligament N83.8
    with or following ectopic or molar pregnancy O08.6
    obstetrical trauma O71.6
  by
    device, implant or graft (*see also* Complications, by site and type, mechanical) T85.628
      arterial graft NEC — *see* Complication, cardiovascular device, mechanical, vascular
      breast (implant) T85.49
      catheter NEC T85.698
        cystostomy T83.090
        dialysis (renal) T82.49
          intraperitoneal T85.691
        infusion NEC T82.594
          spinal (epidural) (subdural) T85.690
        urinary (see also Complications, catheter, urinary) T83.098
      electronic (electrode) (pulse generator) (stimulator)
        bone T84.390
        cardiac T82.199
          electrode T82.190
          pulse generator T82.191
          specified type NEC T82.198
        nervous system — *see* Complication, prosthetic device, mechanical, electronic nervous system stimulator
        urinary — *see* Complication, genitourinary, device, urinary, mechanical
      fixation, internal (orthopedic) NEC — *see* Complication, fixation device, mechanical
      gastrointestinal — *see* Complications, prosthetic device, mechanical, gastrointestinal device
      genital NEC T83.498
        intrauterine contraceptive device T83.39
        penile prosthesis T83.490
      heart NEC — *see* Complication, cardiovascular device, mechanical
      joint prosthesis — *see* Complications, joint prosthesis, mechanical, specified NEC, by site
      ocular NEC — *see* Complications, prosthetic device, mechanical, ocular device
      orthopedic NEC — *see* Complication, orthopedic, device, mechanical
      specified NEC T85.628
      urinary NEC — *see also* Complication, genitourinary, device, urinary, mechanical
        graft T83.29
      vascular NEC — *see* Complication, cardiovascular device, mechanical
      ventricular intracranial shunt T85.09
    foreign body left accidentally in operative wound T81.539
    instrument (any) during a procedure, accidental — *see* Puncture, accidental complicating surgery
  cecum K35.2
    with localized peritonitis K35.3
  cervix (uteri) N88.8
    with or following ectopic or molar pregnancy O08.6
    obstetrical trauma O71.3

Perforation, perforated (nontraumatic) (of) — *continued*
  colon K63.1
    newborn P78.0
    obstetrical trauma O71.5
    traumatic — *see* Laceration, intestine, large
  common duct (bile) K83.2
  cornea (due to ulceration) — *see* Ulcer, cornea, perforated
  cystic duct K82.2
  diverticulum (intestine) K57.80
    with bleeding K57.81
    large intestine K57.20
      with
        bleeding K57.21
        small intestine K57.40
          with bleeding K57.41
    small intestine K57.00
      with
        bleeding K57.01
        large intestine K57.40
          with bleeding K57.41
  ear drum — *see* Perforation, tympanum
  esophagus K22.3
  ethmoidal sinus — *see* Sinusitis, ethmoidal
  frontal sinus — *see* Sinusitis, frontal
  gallbladder K82.2
  heart valve — *see* Endocarditis
  ileum K63.1
    newborn P78.0
    obstetrical trauma O71.5
    traumatic — *see* Laceration, intestine, small
  instrumental, surgical (accidental) (blood vessel) (nerve) (organ) — *see* Puncture, accidental complicating surgery
  intestine NEC K63.1
    with ectopic or molar pregnancy O08.6
    newborn P78.0
    obstetrical trauma O71.5
    traumatic — *see* Laceration, intestine
    ulcerative NEC K63.1
      newborn P78.0
  jejunum, jejunal K63.1
    obstetrical trauma O71.5
    traumatic — *see* Laceration, intestine, small
    ulcer — *see* Ulcer, gastrojejunal, with perforation
  joint prosthesis — *see* Complications, joint prosthesis, mechanical, specified NEC, by site
  mastoid (antrum) (cell) — *see* Disorder, mastoid, specified NEC
  maxillary sinus — *see* Sinusitis, maxillary
  membrana tympani — *see* Perforation, tympanum
  nasal
    septum J34.89
      congenital Q30.3
      syphilitic A52.73
    sinus J34.89
      congenital Q30.8
      due to sinusitis — *see* Sinusitis
  palate (*see also* Cleft, palate) Q35.9
    syphilitic A52.79
  palatine vault (*see also* Cleft, palate, hard) Q35.1
    syphilitic A52.79
    congenital A50.59
  pars flaccida (ear drum) — *see* Perforation, tympanum, attic
  pelvic
    floor S31.030
      with
        ectopic or molar pregnancy O08.6
        penetration into retroperitoneal space S31.031
        retained foreign body S31.040
          with penetration into retroperitoneal space S31.041

Perforation, perforated (nontraumatic) (of)
— *continued*
pelvic — *continued*
  floor S31.030 — *continued*
    following ectopic or molar pregnancy
      O08.6
    obstetrical trauma O70.1
  organ S37.99
    adrenal gland S37.818
    bladder — *see* Perforation, bladder
    fallopian tube S37.599
      bilateral S37.592
      unilateral S37.591
    kidney S37.09-
    obstetrical trauma O71.5
    ovary S37.499
      bilateral S37.492
      unilateral S37.491
    prostate S37.828
    specified organ NEC S37.898
    ureter — *see* Perforation, ureter
    urethra — *see* Perforation, urethra
    uterus — *see* Perforation, uterus
  perineum — *see* Laceration, perineum
pharynx J39.2
rectum K63.1
  newborn P78.0
  obstetrical trauma O71.5
  traumatic S36.63
root canal space due to endodontic treatment
  M27.51
sigmoid K63.1
  newborn P78.0
  obstetrical trauma O71.5
  traumatic S36.533
sinus (accessory) (chronic) (nasal) J34.89
sphenoidal sinus — *see* Sinusitis, sphenoidal
surgical (accidental) (by instrument) (blood
  vessel) (nerve) (organ) — *see* Puncture,
  accidental complicating surgery
traumatic
  external — *see* Puncture
  eye — *see* Puncture, eyeball
  internal organ — *see* Injury, by site
tympanum, tympanic (membrane) (persistent
  post-traumatic) (postinflammatory) H72.9-
  attic H72.1-
    multiple — *see* Perforation, tympanum,
      multiple
    total — *see* Perforation, tympanum, total
  central H72.0-
    multiple — *see* Perforation, tympanum,
      multiple
    total — *see* Perforation, tympanum, total
  marginal NEC — *see* subcategory H72.2
  multiple H72.81-
  pars flaccida — *see* Perforation, tympanum,
    attic
  total H72.82-
  traumatic, current episode S09.2-
typhoid, gastrointestinal — *see* Typhoid
ulcer — *see* Ulcer, by site, with perforation
ureter N28.89
  traumatic S37.19
urethra N36.8
  with ectopic or molar pregnancy O08.6
  following ectopic or molar pregnancy O08.6
  obstetrical trauma O71.5
  traumatic S37.39
    at delivery O71.5
uterus
  with ectopic or molar pregnancy O08.6
  by intrauterine contraceptive device T83.39
  following ectopic or molar pregnancy O08.6
  obstetrical trauma O71.1
  traumatic S37.69
    obstetric O71.1
uvula K13.79
  syphilitic A52.79

Perforation, perforated (nontraumatic) (of)
— *continued*
vagina
  obstetrical trauma O71.4
  other trauma — *see* Puncture, vagina
Periadenitis mucosa necrotica recurrens
  K12.0
Periappendicitis (acute) — *see* Appendicitis
Periarteritis nodosa (disseminated)
  (infectious) (necrotizing) M30.0
Periarthritis (joint) — *see also* Enthesopathy
  Duplay's M75.0-
  gonococcal A54.42
  humeroscapularis — *see* Capsulitis, adhesive
  scapulohumeral — *see* Capsulitis, adhesive
  shoulder — *see* Capsulitis, adhesive
  wrist M77.2-
Periarthrosis (angioneural) — *see*
  Enthesopathy
Pericapsulitis, adhesive (shoulder) — *see*
  Capsulitis, adhesive
Pericarditis (with decompensation) (with
  effusion) I31.9
  with rheumatic fever (conditions in I00)
    active — *see* Pericarditis, rheumatic
    inactive or quiescent I09.2
  acute (hemorrhagic) (nonrheumatic) (Sicca)
    I30.9
    with chorea (acute) (rheumatic) (Sydenham's)
      I02.0
    benign I30.8
    nonspecific I30.0
    rheumatic I01.0
      with chorea (acute) (Sydenham's) I02.0
  adhesive or adherent (chronic) (external)
    (internal) I31.0
    acute — *see* Pericarditis, acute
    rheumatic I09.2
  bacterial (acute) (subacute) (with serous or
    seropurulent effusion) I30.1
  calcareous I31.1
  cholesterol (chronic) I31.8
    acute I30.9
  chronic (nonrheumatic) I31.9
    rheumatic I09.2
  constrictive (chronic) I31.1
  coxsackie B33.23
  fibrinocaseous (tuberculous) A18.84
  fibrinopurulent I30.1
  fibrinous I30.8
  fibrous I31.0
  gonococcal A54.83
  idiopathic I30.0
  in systemic lupus erythematosus M32.12
  infective I30.1
  meningococcal A39.53
  neoplastic (chronic) I31.8
    acute I30.9
  obliterans, obliterating I31.0
  plastic I31.0
  pneumococcal I30.1
  postinfarction I24.1
  purulent I30.1
  rheumatic (active) (acute) (with effusion) (with
    pneumonia) I01.0
    with chorea (acute) (rheumatic) (Sydenham's)
      I02.0
    chronic or inactive (with chorea) I09.2
  rheumatoid — *see* Rheumatoid, carditis
  septic I30.1
  serofibrinous I30.8
  staphylococcal I30.1
  streptococcal I30.1
  suppurative I30.1
  syphilitic A52.06
  tuberculous A18.84
  uremic N18.9 *[I32]*
  viral I30.1
Pericardium, pericardial — *see* condition

Pericellulitis — *see* Cellulitis
Pericementitis (chronic) (suppurative) — *see*
  also Periodontitis
  acute K05.20
    generalized — *see* Peridontitis, aggressive,
      generalized
    localized — *see* Peridontitis, aggressive,
      localized
Perichondritis
  auricle — *see* Perichondritis, ear
  bronchus J98.09
  ear (external) H61.00-
    acute H61.01-
    chronic H61.02-
  external auditory canal — *see* Perichondritis,
    ear
  larynx J38.7
    syphilitic A52.73
    typhoid A01.09
  nose J34.89
  pinna — *see* Perichondritis, ear
  trachea J39.8
Periclasia K05.4
Pericoronitis — *see* Periodontitis
Pericystitis N30.90
  with hematuria N30.91
Peridiverticulitis (intestine) K57.92
  cecum — *see* Diverticulitis, intestine, large
  colon — *see* Diverticulitis, intestine, large
  duodenum — *see* Diverticulitis, intestine, small
  intestine — *see* Diverticulitis, intestine
  jejunum — *see* Diverticulitis, intestine, small
  rectosigmoid — *see* Diverticulitis, intestine,
    large
  rectum — *see* Diverticulitis, intestine, large
  sigmoid — *see* Diverticulitis, intestine, large
Periendocarditis — *see* Endocarditis
Periepididymitis N45.1
Perifolliculitis L01.02
  abscedens, caput, scalp L66.3
  capitis, abscedens (et suffodiens) L66.3
  superficial pustular L01.02
Perihepatitis K65.8
Perilabyrinthitis (acute) — *see* subcategory
  H83.0
Perimeningitis — *see* Meningitis
Perimetritis — *see* Endometritis
Perimetrosalpingitis — *see* Salpingo-
  oophoritis
Perineocele N81.81
Perinephric, perinephritic — *see* condition
Perinephritis — *see also* Infection, kidney
  purulent — *see* Abscess, kidney
Perineum, perineal — *see* condition
Perineuritis NEC — *see* Neuralgia
Periodic — *see* condition
Periodontitis (chronic) (complex) (compound)
  (local) (simplex) K05.30
  acute K05.20
    generalized K05.229
      moderate K05.222
      severe K05.223
      slight K05.221
    localized K05.219
      moderate K05.212
      severe K05.213
      slight K05.211
  apical K04.5
    acute (pulpal origin) K04.4
  generalized K05.329
    moderate K05.322
    severe K05.323
    slight K05.321
  localized K05.319
    moderate K05.312
    severe K05.313
    slight K05.311
Periodontoclasia K05.4
Periodontosis (juvenile) K05.4

Periods — *see also* Menstruation
  heavy N92.0
  irregular N92.6
  shortened intervals (irregular) N92.1
Perionychia — *see also* Cellulitis, digit
  with lymphangitis — *see* Lymphangitis, acute,
    digit
Perioophoritis — *see* Salpingo-oophoritis
Periorchitis N45.2
Periosteum, periosteal — *see* condition
Periostitis (albuminosa) (circumscribed)
  (diffuse) (infective) (monomelic) — *see also*
  Osteomyelitis
  alveolar M27.3
  alveolodental M27.3
  dental M27.3
  gonorrheal A54.43
  jaw (lower) (upper) M27.2
  orbit H05.03-
  syphilitic A52.77
    congenital (early) A50.02 [M90.80]
    secondary A51.46
  tuberculous — *see* Tuberculosis, bone
  yaws (hypertrophic) (early) (late) A66.6
    [M90.80]
Periostosis (hyperplastic) — *see also* Disorder,
  bone, specified type NEC
  with osteomyelitis — *see* Osteomyelitis,
    specified type NEC
Peripartum
  cardiomyopathy O90.3
Periphlebitis — *see* Phlebitis
Periproctitis K62.89
Periprostatitis — *see* Prostatitis
Perirectal — *see* condition
Perirenal — *see* condition
Perisalpingitis — *see* Salpingo-oophoritis
Perisplenitis (infectional) D73.89
Peristalsis, visible or reversed R19.2
Peritendinitis — *see* Enthesopathy
Peritoneum, peritoneal — *see* condition
Peritonitis (adhesive) (bacterial) (fibrinous)
  (hemorrhagic) (idiopathic) (localized)
  (perforative) (primary) (with adhesions) (with
  effusion) K65.9
  with or following
    abscess K65.1
    appendicitis K35.3
      with perforation or rupture K35.2
      generalized K35.2
      localized K35.3
    diverticular disease (intestine) K57.80
      with bleeding K57.81
    ectopic or molar pregnancy O08.0
    large intestine K57.20
      with
        bleeding K57.21
        small intestine K57.40
          with bleeding K57.41
    small intestine K57.00
      with
        bleeding K57.01
        large intestine K57.40
          with bleeding K57.41
  acute (generalized) K65.0
  aseptic T81.61
  bile, biliary K65.3
  chemical T81.61
  chlamydial A74.81
  chronic proliferative K65.8
  complicating abortion — *see* Abortion, by
    type, complicated by, pelvic peritonitis
  congenital P78.1
  diaphragmatic K65.0
  diffuse K65.0
  diphtheritic A36.89
  disseminated K65.0

Peritonitis (adhesive) (bacterial) (fibrinous)
  (hemorrhagic) (idiopathic) (localized)
  (perforative) (primary) (with adhesions) (with
  effusion) K65.9 — *continued*
  due to
    bile K65.3
    foreign
      body or object accidentally left during a
        procedure (instrument) (sponge)
        (swab) T81.599
      substance accidentally left during a
        procedure (chemical) (powder) (talc)
        T81.61
      talc T81.61
    urine K65.8
  eosinophilic K65.8
    acute K65.0
  fibrocaseous (tuberculous) A18.31
  fibropurulent K65.0
  following ectopic or molar pregnancy O08.0
  general(ized) K65.0
  gonococcal A54.85
  meconium (newborn) P78.0
  neonatal P78.1
    meconium P78.0
  pancreatic K65.0
  paroxysmal, familial E85.0
    benign E85.0
  pelvic
    female N73.5
      acute N73.3
      chronic N73.4
        with adhesions N73.6
    male K65.0
  periodic, familial E85.0
  proliferative, chronic K65.8
  puerperal, postpartum, childbirth O85
  purulent K65.0
  septic K65.0
  specified NEC K65.8
  spontaneous bacterial K65.2
  subdiaphragmatic K65.0
  subphrenic K65.0
  suppurative K65.0
  syphilitic A52.74
    congenital (early) A50.08 [K67]
  talc T81.61
  tuberculous A18.31
  urine K65.8
Peritonsillar — *see* condition
Peritonsillitis J36
Perityphlitis K37
Periureteritis N28.89
Periurethral — *see* condition
Periurethritis (gangrenous) — *see* Urethritis
Periuterine — *see* condition
Perivaginitis — *see* Vaginitis
Perivasculitis, retinal H35.06-
Perivasitis (chronic) N49.1
Perivesiculitis (seminal) — *see* Vesiculitis
Perlèche NEC K13.0
  due to
    candidiasis B37.83
    moniliasis B37.83
    riboflavin deficiency E53.0
    vitamin B2 (riboflavin) deficiency E53.0
Pernicious — *see* condition
Pernio, perniosis T69.1
Perpetrator (of abuse) — *see* Index to External
  Causes of Injury, Perpetrator
Persecution
  delusion F22
  social Z60.5
Perseveration (tonic) R48.8
Persistence, persistent (congenital)
  anal membrane Q42.3
    with fistula Q42.2
  arteria stapedia Q16.3
  atrioventricular canal Q21.2

Persistence, persistent (congenital) —
  continued
  branchial cleft Q18.0
  bulbus cordis in left ventricle Q21.8
  canal of Cloquet Q14.0
  capsule (opaque) Q12.8
  cilioretinal artery or vein Q14.8
  cloaca Q43.7
  communication — *see* Fistula, congenital
  convolutions
    aortic arch Q25.46
    fallopian tube Q50.6
    oviduct Q50.6
    uterine tube Q50.6
  double aortic arch Q25.45
  ductus arteriosus (Botalli) Q25.0
  fetal
    circulation P29.3
    form of cervix (uteri) Q51.828
    hemoglobin, hereditary (HPFH) D56.4
  foramen
    Botalli Q21.1
    ovale Q21.1
  Gartner's duct Q52.4
  hemoglobin, fetal (hereditary) (HPFH) D56.4
  hyaloid
    artery (generally incomplete) Q14.0
    system Q14.8
  hymen, in pregnancy or childbirth — *see*
    Pregnancy, complicated by, abnormal,
    vulva
  lanugo Q84.2
  left
    posterior cardinal vein Q26.8
    root with right arch of aorta Q25.49
    superior vena cava Q26.1
  Meckel's diverticulum Q43.0
    malignant — *see* Table of Neoplasms, small
      intestine, malignant
  mucosal disease (middle ear) — *see* Otitis,
    media, suppurative, chronic, tubotympanic
  nail(s), anomalous Q84.6
  omphalomesenteric duct Q43.0
  organ or site not listed — *see* Anomaly, by site
  ostium
    atrioventriculare commune Q21.2
    primum Q21.2
    secundum Q21.1
  ovarian rests in fallopian tube Q50.6
  pancreatic tissue in intestinal tract Q43.8
  primary (deciduous)
    teeth K00.6
    vitreous hyperplasia Q14.0
  pupillary membrane Q13.89
  rhesus (Rh) titer — *see* Complication(s),
    transfusion, incompatibility reaction, Rh
    (factor)
  right aortic arch Q25.47
  sinus
    urogenitalis
      female Q52.8
      male Q55.8
    venosus with imperfect incorporation in right
      auricle Q26.8
  thymus (gland) (hyperplasia) E32.0
  thyroglossal duct Q89.2
  thyrolingual duct Q89.2
  truncus arteriosus or communis Q20.0
  tunica vasculosa lentis Q12.2
  umbilical sinus Q64.4
  urachus Q64.4
  vitelline duct Q43.0
Person (with)
  admitted for clinical research, as a control
    subject (normal comparison) (participant)
    Z00.6
  awaiting admission to adequate facility
    elsewhere Z75.1

Person (with) — *continued*
concern (normal) about sick person in family
Z63.6
consulting on behalf of another Z71.0
feigning illness Z76.5
living (in)
alone Z60.2
boarding school Z59.3
residential institution Z59.3
without
adequate housing (heating) (space) Z59.1
housing (permanent) (temporary) Z59.0
person able to render necessary care
Z74.2
shelter Z59.0
on waiting list Z75.1
sick or handicapped in family Z63.6
Personality (disorder) F60.9
accentuation of traits (type A pattern) Z73.1
affective F34.0
aggressive F60.3
amoral F60.2
anacastic, anankastic F60.5
antisocial F60.2
anxious F60.6
asocial F60.2
asthenic F60.7
avoidant F60.6
borderline F60.3
change due to organic condition (enduring)
F07.0
compulsive F60.5
cycloid F34.0
cyclothymic F34.0
dependent F60.7
depressive F34.1
dissocial F60.2
dual F44.81
eccentric F60.89
emotionally unstable F60.3
expansive paranoid F60.0
explosive F60.3
fanatic F60.0
haltose type F60.89
histrionic F60.4
hyperthymic F34.0
hypothymic F34.1
hysterical F60.4
immature F60.89
inadequate F60.7
labile (emotional) F60.3
mixed (nonspecific) F60.89
morally defective F60.2
multiple F44.81
narcissistic F60.81
obsessional F60.5
obsessive(-compulsive) F60.5
organic F07.0
overconscientious F60.5
paranoid F60.0
passive-aggressive F60.89
passive(-dependent) F60.7
pathologic F60.9
pattern defect or disturbance F60.9
pseudopsychopathic (organic) F07.0
pseudoretarded (organic) F07.0
psychoinfantile F60.4
psychoneurotic NEC F60.89
psychopathic F60.2
querulant F60.0
sadistic F60.89
schizoid F60.1
self-defeating F60.7
sensitive paranoid F60.0
sociopathic (amoral) (antisocial) (asocial)
(dissocial) F60.2
specified NEC F60.89
type A Z73.1
unstable (emotional) F60.3

Perthes' disease — *see* Legg-Calvé-Perthes
disease
Pertussis (*see also* Whooping cough) A37.90
Perversion, perverted
appetite F50.89
psychogenic F50.89
function
pituitary gland E23.2
posterior lobe E22.2
sense of smell and taste R43.8
psychogenic F45.8
sexual — *see* Deviation, sexual
Pervious, congenital — *see also* Imperfect,
closure
ductus arteriosus Q25.0
Pes (congenital) — *see also* Talipes
acquired — *see also* Deformity, limb, foot,
specified NEC
planus — *see* Deformity, limb, flat foot
adductus Q66.89
cavus Q66.7
deformity NEC, acquired — *see* Deformity,
limb, foot, specified NEC
planus (acquired) (any degree) — *see also*
Deformity, limb, flat foot
rachitic sequelae (late effect) E64.3
valgus Q66.6
Pest, pestis — *see* Plague
Petechia, petechiae R23.3
newborn P54.5
Petechial typhus A75.9
Peter's anomaly Q13.4
Petit mal seizure — *see* Epilepsy,
generalized, specified NEC
Petit's hernia — *see* Hernia, abdomen,
specified site NEC
Petrellidosis B48.2
Petrositis H70.20-
acute H70.21-
chronic H70.22-
Peutz-Jeghers disease or syndrome
Q85.8
Peyronie's disease N48.6
PFAPA (periodic fever, aphthous stomatitis,
pharyngitis, and adenopathy syndrome)
M04.8
Pfeiffer's disease — *see* Mononucleosis,
infectious
Phagedena (dry) (moist) (sloughing) — *see also*
Gangrene
geometric L88
penis N48.29
tropical — *see* Ulcer, skin
vulva N76.6
Phagedenic — *see* condition
Phakoma H35.89
Phakomatosis (*see also* specific eponymous
syndromes) Q85.9
Bourneville's Q85.1
specified NEC Q85.8
Phantom limb syndrome (without pain)
G54.7
with pain G54.6
Pharyngeal pouch syndrome D82.1
Pharyngitis (acute) (catarrhal) (gangrenous)
(infective) (malignant) (membranous)
(phlegmonous) (pseudomembranous)
(simple) (subacute) (suppurative) (ulcerative)
(viral) J02.9
with influenza, flu, or grippe — *see* Influenza,
with, pharyngitis
aphthous B08.5
atrophic J31.2
chlamydial A56.4
chronic (atrophic) (granular) (hypertrophic)
J31.2
coxsackievirus B08.5
diphtheritic A36.0
enteroviral vesicular B08.5

Pharyngitis (acute) (catarrhal) (gangrenous)
(infective) (malignant) (membranous)
(phlegmonous) (pseudomembranous)
(simple) (subacute) (suppurative) (ulcerative)
(viral) J02.9 — *continued*
follicular (chronic) J31.2
fusospirochetal A69.1
gonococcal A54.5
granular (chronic) J31.2
herpesviral B00.2
hypertrophic J31.2
infectional, chronic J31.2
influenzal — *see* Influenza, with, respiratory
manifestations NEC
lymphonodular, acute (enteroviral) B08.8
pneumococcal J02.8
purulent J02.9
putrid J02.9
septic J02.0
sicca J31.2
specified organism NEC J02.8
staphylococcal J02.8
streptococcal J02.0
syphilitic, congenital (early) A50.03
tuberculous A15.8
vesicular, enteroviral B08.5
viral NEC J02.8
Pharyngoconjunctivitis, viral B30.2
Pharyngolaryngitis (acute) J06.0
chronic J37.0
Pharyngoplegia J39.2
Pharyngotonsillitis, herpesviral B00.2
Pharyngotracheitis, chronic J42
Pharynx, pharyngeal — *see* condition
Phencyclidine-induced
anxiety disorder F16.980
bipolar and related disorder F16.94
depressive disorder F16.94
psychotic disorder F16.959
Phenomenon
Arthus' — *see* Arthus' phenomenon
jaw-winking Q07.8
lupus erythematosus (LE) cell M32.9
Raynaud's (secondary) I73.00
with gangrene I73.01
vasomotor R55
vasospastic I73.9
vasovagal R55
Wenckebach's I44.1
Phenylketonuria E70.1
classical E70.0
maternal E70.1
Pheochromoblastoma
specified site — *see* Neoplasm, malignant, by
site
unspecified site C74.10
Pheochromocytoma
malignant
specified site — *see* Neoplasm, malignant,
by site
unspecified site C74.10
specified site — *see* Neoplasm, benign, by site
unspecified site D35.00
Pheohyphomycosis — *see* Chromomycosis
Pheomycosis — *see* Chromomycosis
Phimosis (congenital) (due to infection) N47.1
chancroidal A57
Phlebectasia — *see also* Varix
congenital Q27.4
Phlebitis (infective) (pyemic) (septic)
(suppurative) I80.9
antepartum — *see* Thrombophlebitis,
antepartum
blue — *see* Phlebitis, leg, deep
breast, superficial I80.8
cavernous (venous) sinus — *see* Phlebitis,
intracranial (venous) sinus
cerebral (venous) sinus — *see* Phlebitis,
intracranial (venous) sinus

Phlebitis (infective) (pyemic) (septic) (suppurative) I80.9 — *continued*
  chest wall, superficial I80.8
  cranial (venous) sinus — *see* Phlebitis, intracranial (venous) sinus
  deep (vessels) — *see* Phlebitis, leg, deep
  due to implanted device — *see* Complications, by site and type, specified NEC
  during or resulting from a procedure T81.72
  femoral vein (superficial) I80.1-
  femoropopliteal vein I80.0-
  gestational — *see* Phlebopathy, gestational
  hepatic veins I80.8
  iliofemoral — *see* Phlebitis, femoral vein
  intracranial (venous) sinus (any) G08
    nonpyogenic I67.6
  intraspinal venous sinuses and veins G08
    nonpyogenic G95.19
  lateral (venous) sinus — *see* Phlebitis, intracranial (venous) sinus
  leg I80.3
    antepartum — *see* Thrombophlebitis, antepartum
    deep (vessels) NEC I80.20-
      iliac I80.21-
      popliteal vein I80.22-
      specified vessel NEC I80.29-
      tibial vein I80.23-
    femoral vein (superficial) I80.1-
    superficial (vessels) I80.0-
  longitudinal sinus — *see* Phlebitis, intracranial (venous) sinus
  lower limb — *see* Phlebitis, leg
  migrans, migrating (superficial) I82.1
  pelvic
    with ectopic or molar pregnancy O08.0
    following ectopic or molar pregnancy O08.0
    puerperal, postpartum O87.1
  popliteal vein — *see* Phlebitis, leg, deep, popliteal
  portal (vein) K75.1
  postoperative T81.72
  pregnancy — *see* Thrombophlebitis, antepartum
  puerperal, postpartum, childbirth O87.0
    deep O87.1
    pelvic O87.1
    superficial O87.0
  retina — *see* Vasculitis, retina
  saphenous (accessory) (great) (long) (small) — *see* Phlebitis, leg, superficial
  sinus (meninges) — *see* Phlebitis, intracranial (venous) sinus
  specified site NEC I80.8
  syphilitic A52.09
  tibial vein — *see* Phlebitis, leg, deep, tibial
  ulcerative I80.9
    leg — *see* Phlebitis, leg
  umbilicus I80.8
  uterus (septic) — *see* Endometritis
  varicose (leg) (lower limb) — *see* Varix, leg, with, inflammation
Phlebofibrosis I87.8
Pheboliths I87.8
Phlebopathy
  gestational O22.9-
  puerperal O87.9
Phlebosclerosis I87.8
Phlebothrombosis — *see also* Thrombosis
  antepartum — *see* Thrombophlebitis, antepartum
  pregnancy — *see* Thrombophlebitis, antepartum
  puerperal — *see* Thrombophlebitis, puerperal
Phlebotomus fever A93.1
Phlegmasia
  alba dolens O87.1
    nonpuerperal — *see* Phlebitis, femoral vein
  cerulea dolens — *see* Phlebitis, leg, deep

Phlegmon — *see* Abscess
Phlegmonous — *see* condition
Phlyctenulosis (allergic) (keratoconjunctivitis) (nontuberculous) — *see also* Keratoconjunctivitis
  cornea — *see* Keratoconjunctivitis
  tuberculous A18.52
Phobia, phobic F40.9
  animal F40.218
    spiders F40.210
  examination F40.298
  reaction F40.9
  simple F40.298
  social F40.10
    generalized F40.11
  specific (isolated) F40.298
    animal F40.218
      spiders F40.210
    blood F40.230
    injection F40.231
    injury F40.233
    men F40.290
    natural environment F40.228
      thunderstorms F40.220
    situational F40.248
      bridges F40.242
      closed in spaces F40.240
      flying F40.243
      heights F40.241
    specified focus NEC F40.298
    transfusion F40.231
    women F40.291
  specified NEC F40.8
    medical care NEC F40.232
  state F40.9
Phocas' disease — *see* Mastopathy, cystic
Phocomelia Q73.1
  lower limb — *see* Agenesis, leg, with foot present
  upper limb — *see* Agenesis, arm, with hand present
Phoria H50.50
Phosphate-losing tubular disorder N25.0
Phosphatemia E83.39
Phosphaturia E83.39
Photodermatitis (sun) L56.8
  chronic L57.8
  due to drug L56.8
  light other than sun L59.8
Photokeratitis H16.13-
Photophobia H53.14
Photophthalmia — *see* Photokeratitis
Photopsia H53.19
Photoretinitis — *see* Retinopathy, solar
Photosensitivity, photosensitization (sun) skin L56.8
  light other than sun L59.8
Phrenitis — *see* Encephalitis
Phrynoderma (vitamin A deficiency) E50.8
Phthiriasis (pubis) B85.3
  with any infestation classifiable to B85.0-B85.2 B85.4
Phthirus infestation — *see* Phthiriasis
Phthisis — *see also* Tuberculosis
  bulbi (infectional) — *see* Disorder, globe, degenerated condition, atrophy
  eyeball (due to infection) — *see* Disorder, globe, degenerated condition, atrophy
Phycomycosis — *see* Zygomycosis
Physalopteriasis B81.8
Physical restraint status Z78.1
Phytobezoar T18.9
  intestine T18.3
  stomach T18.2
Pian — *see* Yaws
Pianoma A66.1
Pica F50.89
  in adults F50.89
  infant or child F98.3

Picking, nose F98.8
Pick-Niemann disease — *see* Niemann-Pick disease or syndrome
Pick's
  cerebral atrophy G31.01 *[F02.80]*
    with behavioral disturbance G31.01 *[F02.81]*
  disease or syndrome (brain) G31.01 *[F02.80]*
    with behavioral disturbance G31.01 *[F02.81]*
    brain G31.01 *[F02.80]*
      with behavioral disturbance G31.01 *[F02.81]*
    pericardium (pericardial pseudocirrhosis of liver) I31.1
  syndrome
    brain G31.01 *[F02.80]*
      with behavioral disturbance G31.01 *[F02.81]*
    of heart (pericardial pseudocirrhosis of liver) I31.1
Pickwickian syndrome E66.2
Piebaldism E70.39
Piedra (beard) (scalp) B36.8
  black B36.3
  white B36.2
Pierre Robin deformity or syndrome Q87.0
Pierson's disease or osteochondrosis M91.0
Pig-bel A05.2
Pigeon
  breast or chest (acquired) M95.4
    congenital Q67.7
    rachitic sequelae (late effect) E64.3
  breeder's disease or lung J67.2
  fancier's disease or lung J67.2
  toe — *see* Deformity, toe, specified NEC
Pigmentation (abnormal) (anomaly) L81.9
  conjunctiva H11.13-
  cornea (anterior) H18.01-
    posterior H18.05-
    stromal H18.06-
  diminished melanin formation NEC L81.6
  iron L81.8
  lids, congenital Q82.8
  limbus corneae — *see* Pigmentation, cornea
  metals L81.8
  optic papilla, congenital Q14.2
  retina, congenital (grouped) (nevoid) Q14.1
  scrotum, congenital Q82.8
  tattoo L81.8
Piles (see also Hemorrhoids) K64.9
Pili
  annulati or torti (congenital) Q84.1
  incarnati L73.1
Pill roller hand (intrinsic) — *see* Parkinsonism
Pilomatrixoma — *see* Neoplasm, skin, benign
  malignant — *see* Neoplasm, skin, malignant
Pilonidal — *see* condition
Pimple R23.8
PIN — *see* Neoplasia, intraepithelial, prostate
Pinched nerve — *see* Neuropathy, entrapment
Pindborg tumor — *see* Cyst, calcifying odontogenic
Pineal body or gland — *see* condition
Pinealoblastoma C75.3
Pinealoma D44.5
  malignant C75.3
Pineoblastoma C75.3
Pineocytoma D44.5
Pinguecula H11.15-
Pingueculitis H10.81-
Pinhole meatus (see also Stricture, urethra) N35.9
Pink
  disease — *see* subcategory T56.1
  eye — *see* Conjunctivitis, acute, mucopurulent
Pinkus' disease (lichen nitidus) L44.1

Pinpoint
 meatus — *see* Stricture, urethra
 os (uteri) — *see* Stricture, cervix
Pins and needles R20.2
Pinta A67.9
 cardiovascular lesions A67.2
 chancre (primary) A67.0
 erythematous plaques A67.1
 hyperchromic lesions A67.1
 hyperkeratosis A67.1
 lesions A67.9
  cardiovascular A67.2
  hyperchromic A67.1
  intermediate A67.1
  late A67.2
  mixed A67.3
  primary A67.0
  skin (achromic) (cicatricial) (dyschromic)
   A67.2
   hyperchromic A67.1
   mixed (achromic and hyperchromic)
    A67.3
 papule (primary) A67.0
 skin lesions (achromic) (cicatricial)
  (dyschromic) A67.2
  hyperchromic A67.1
  mixed (achromic and hyperchromic) A67.3
 vitiligo A67.2
Pintids A67.1
Pinworm (disease) (infection) (infestation) B80
Piroplasmosis B60.0
Pistol wound — *see* Gunshot wound
Pitchers' elbow — *see* Derangement, joint,
  specified type NEC, elbow
Pithecoid pelvis Q74.2
 with disproportion (fetopelvic) O33.0
  causing obstructed labor O65.0
Pithiatism F48.8
Pitted — *see* Pitting
Pitting (*see also* Edema) R60.9
 lip R60.0
 nail L60.8
 teeth K00.4
Pituitary gland — *see* condition
Pituitary-snuff-taker's disease J67.8
Pityriasis (capitis) L21.0
 alba L30.5
 circinata (et maculata) L42
 furfuracea L21.0
 Hebra's L26
 lichenoides L41.0
  chronica L41.1
  et varioliformis (acuta) L41.0
 maculata (et circinata) L30.5
 nigra B36.1
 pilaris, Hebra's L44.0
 rosea L42
 rotunda L44.8
 rubra (Hebra) pilaris L44.0
 simplex L30.5
 specified type NEC L30.5
 streptogenes L30.5
 versicolor (scrotal) B36.0
Placenta, placental — *see* Pregnancy,
  complicated by (care of) (management
  affected by), specified condition
Placentitis O41.14-
Plagiocephaly Q67.3
Plague A20.9
 abortive A20.8
 ambulatory A20.8
 asymptomatic A20.8
 bubonic A20.0
 cellulocutaneous A20.1
 cutaneobubonic A20.1
 lymphatic gland A20.0
 meningitis A20.3
 pharyngeal A20.8
 pneumonic (primary) (secondary) A20.2

Plague A20.9 — *continued*
 pulmonary, pulmonic A20.2
 septicemic A20.7
 tonsillar A20.8
  septicemic A20.7
Planning, family
 contraception Z30.9
 procreation Z31.69
Plaque(s)
 artery, arterial — *see* Arteriosclerosis
 calcareous — *see* Calcification
 coronary, lipid rich I25.83
 epicardial I31.8
 erythematous, of pinta A67.1
 Hollenhorst's — *see* Occlusion, artery, retina
 lipid rich, coronary I25.83
 pleural (without asbestos) J92.9
  with asbestos J92.0
 tongue K13.29
Plasmacytoma C90.3-
 extramedullary C90.2-
 medullary C90.0-
 solitary C90.3-
Plasmacytopenia D72.818
Plasmacytosis D72.822
Plaster ulcer — *see* Ulcer, pressure, by site
Plateau iris syndrome (post-iridectomy)
  (postprocedural) (without glaucoma) H21.82
 with glaucoma H40.22-
Platybasia Q75.8
Platyonychia (congenital) Q84.6
 acquired L60.8
Platypelloid pelvis M95.5
 with disproportion (fetopelvic) O33.0
  causing obstructed labor O65.0
 congenital Q74.2
Platyspondylisis Q76.49
Plaut(-Vincent) disease (*see also* Vincent's)
  A69.1
Plethora R23.2
 newborn P61.1
Pleura, pleural — *see* condition
Pleuralgia R07.81
Pleurisy (acute) (adhesive) (chronic) (costal)
  (diaphragmatic) (double) (dry) (fibrinous)
  (fibrous) (interlobar) (latent) (plastic)
  (primary) (residual) (sicca) (sterile)
  (subacute) (unresolved) R09.1
 with
  adherent pleura J86.0
  effusion J90
   chylous, chyliform J94.0
   tuberculous (non primary) A15.6
    primary (progressive) A15.7
   tuberculosis — *see* Pleurisy, tuberculous (non
     primary)
 encysted — *see* Pleurisy, with effusion
 exudative — *see* Pleurisy, with effusion
 fibrinopurulent, fibropurulent — *see* Pyothorax
 hemorrhagic — *see* Hemothorax
 pneumococcal J90
 purulent — *see* Pyothorax
 septic — *see* Pyothorax
 serofibrinous — *see* Pleurisy, with effusion
 seropurulent — *see* Pyothorax
 serous — *see* Pleurisy, with effusion
 staphylococcal J86.9
 streptococcal J90
 suppurative — *see* Pyothorax
 traumatic (post) (current) — *see* Injury,
   intrathoracic, pleura
 tuberculous (with effusion) (non primary) A15.6
  primary (progressive) A15.7
Pleuritis sicca — *see* Pleurisy
Pleurobronchopneumonia — *see*
  Pneumonia, broncho-
Pleurodynia R07.81
 epidemic B33.0
 viral B33.0

Pleuropericarditis — *see also* Pericarditis
 acute I30.9
Pleuropneumonia (acute) (bilateral) (double)
  (septic) (*see also* Pneumonia) J18.8
 chronic — *see* Fibrosis, lung
**Pleuro-pneumonia-like-organism
  (PPLO), as cause of disease classified
  elsewhere** B96.0
Pleurorrhea — *see* Pleurisy, with effusion
Plexitis, brachial G54.0
Plica
 polonica B85.0
 syndrome, knee M67.5-
 tonsil J35.8
Plicated tongue K14.5
Plug
 bronchus NEC J98.09
 meconium (newborn) NEC syndrome P76.0
 mucus — *see* Asphyxia, mucus
Plumbism — *see* subcategory T56.0
Plummer's disease E05.20
 with thyroid storm E05.21
Plummer-Vinson syndrome D50.1
Pluricarential syndrome of infancy E40
Plus (and minus) hand (intrinsic) — *see*
  Deformity, limb, specified type NEC,
  forearm
Pneumathemia — *see* Air, embolism
Pneumatic hammer (drill) syndrome
  T75.21
Pneumatocele (lung) J98.4
 intracranial G93.89
 tension J44.9
Pneumatosis
 cystoides intestinalis K63.89
 intestinalis K63.89
 peritonei K66.8
Pneumaturia R39.89
Pneumoblastoma — *see* Neoplasm, lung,
  malignant
Pneumocephalus G93.89
Pneumococcemia A40.3
Pneumococcus, pneumococcal — *see*
  condition
Pneumoconiosis (due to) (inhalation of) J64
 with tuberculosis (any type in A15) J65
 aluminum J63.0
 asbestos J61
 bagasse, bagassosis J67.1
 bauxite J63.1
 beryllium J63.2
 coal miners' (simple) J60
 coalworkers' (simple) J60
 collier's J60
 cotton dust J66.0
 diatomite (diatomaceous earth) J62.8
 dust
  inorganic NEC J63.6
  lime J62.8
  marble J62.8
  organic NEC J66.8
 fumes or vapors (from silo) J68.9
 graphite J63.3
 grinder's J62.8
 kaolin J62.8
 mica J62.8
 millstone maker's J62.8
 miner's J60
 mineral fibers NEC J61
 moldy hay J67.0
 potter's J62.8
 rheumatoid — *see* Rheumatoid, lung
 sandblaster's J62.8
 silica, silicate NEC J62.8
  with carbon J60
 stonemason's J62.8
 talc (dust) J62.0
Pneumocystis carinii pneumonia B59
Pneumocystis jiroveci (pneumonia) B59

Pneumocystosis (with pneumonia) B59
Pneumohemopericardium I31.2
Pneumohemothorax J94.2
  traumatic S27.2
Pneumohydropericardium — see
  Pericarditis
Pneumohydrothorax — see Hydrothorax
Pneumomediastinum J98.2
  congenital or perinatal P25.2
Pneumomycosis B49 [J99]
Pneumonia (acute) (double) (migratory)
  (purulent) (septic) (unresolved) J18.9
  with
    influenza — see Influenza, with, pneumonia
    lung abscess J85.1
      due to specified organism — see
        Pneumonia, in (due to)
  adenoviral J12.0
  adynamic J18.2
  alba A50.04
  allergic (eosinophilic) J82
  alveolar — see Pneumonia, lobar
  anaerobes J15.8
  anthrax A22.1
  apex, apical — see Pneumonia, lobar
  Ascaris B77.81
  aspiration J69.0
    due to
      aspiration of microorganisms
        bacterial J15.9
        viral J12.9
      food (regurgitated) J69.0
      gastric secretions J69.0
      milk (regurgitated) J69.0
      oils, essences J69.1
      solids, liquids NEC J69.8
      vomitus J69.0
    newborn P24.81
      amniotic fluid (clear) P24.11
      blood P24.21
      food (regurgitated) P24.31
      liquor (amnii) P24.11
      meconium P24.01
      milk P24.31
      mucus P24.11
      specified NEC P24.81
      stomach contents P24.31
    postprocedural J95.4
  atypical NEC J18.9
  bacillus J15.9
    specified NEC J15.8
  bacterial J15.9
    specified NEC J15.8
  Bacteroides (fragilis) (oralis) (melaninogenicus)
    J15.8
  basal, basic, basilar — see Pneumonia, by
    type
  bronchiolitis obliterans organized (BOOP)
    J84.89
  broncho-, bronchial (confluent) (croupous)
    (diffuse) (disseminated) (hemorrhagic)
    (involving lobes) (lobar) (terminal) J18.0
    allergic (eosinophilic) J82
    aspiration — see Pneumonia, aspiration
    bacterial J15.9
      specified NEC J15.8
    chronic — see Fibrosis, lung
    diplococcal J13
    Eaton's agent J15.7
    Escherichia coli (E. coli) J15.5
    Friedländer's bacillus J15.0
    Hemophilus influenzae J14
    hypostatic J18.2
    inhalation — see also Pneumonia, aspiration
      due to fumes or vapors (chemical) J68.0
      of oils or essences J69.1
    Klebsiella (pneumoniae) J15.0
  lipid, lipoid J69.1
    endogenous J84.89

Pneumonia (acute) (double) (migratory)
  (purulent) (septic) (unresolved) J18.9 —
  continued
  broncho-, bronchial (confluent) (croupous)
    (diffuse) (disseminated) (hemorrhagic)
    (involving lobes) (lobar) (terminal) J18.0
    — continued
    Mycoplasma (pneumoniae) J15.7
    pleuro-pneumonia-like-organisms (PPLO)
      J15.7
    pneumococcal J13
    Proteus J15.6
    Pseudomonas J15.1
    Serratia marcescens J15.6
    specified organism NEC J16.8
    staphylococcal — see Pneumonia,
      staphylococcal
    streptococcal NEC J15.4
      group B J15.3
      pneumoniae J13
    viral, virus — see Pneumonia, viral
  Butyrivibrio (fibriosolvens) J15.8
  Candida B37.1
  caseous — see Tuberculosis, pulmonary
  catarrhal — see Pneumonia, broncho
  chlamydial J16.0
    congenital P23.1
  cholesterol J84.89
  cirrhotic (chronic) — see Fibrosis, lung
  Clostridium (haemolyticum) (novyi) J15.8
  confluent — see Pneumonia, broncho
  congenital (infective) P23.9
    due to
      bacterium NEC P23.6
      Chlamydia P23.1
      Escherichia coli P23.4
      Haemophilus influenzae P23.6
      infective organism NEC P23.8
      Klebsiella pneumoniae P23.6
      Mycoplasma P23.6
      Pseudomonas P23.5
      Staphylococcus P23.2
      Streptococcus (except group B) P23.6
        group B P23.3
      viral agent P23.0
    specified NEC P23.8
  croupous — see Pneumonia, lobar
  cryptogenic organizing J84.116
  cytomegalic inclusion B25.0
  cytomegaloviral B25.0
  deglutition — see Pneumonia, aspiration
  desquamative interstitial J84.117
  diffuse — see Pneumonia, broncho
  diplococcal, diplococcus (broncho-) (lobar) J13
  disseminated (focal) — see Pneumonia,
    broncho
  Eaton's agent J15.7
  embolic, embolism — see Embolism,
    pulmonary
  Enterobacter J15.6
  eosinophilic J82
  Escherichia coli (E. coli) J15.5
  Eubacterium J15.8
  fibrinous — see Pneumonia, lobar
  fibroid, fibrous (chronic) — see Fibrosis, lung
  Friedländer's bacillus J15.0
  Fusobacterium (nucleatum) J15.8
  gangrenous J85.0
  giant cell (measles) B05.2
  gonococcal A54.84
  gram-negative bacteria NEC J15.6
    anaerobic J15.8
  Hemophilus influenzae (broncho) (lobar) J14
  human metapneumovirus J12.3
  hypostatic (broncho) (lobar) J18.2
  in (due to)
    actinomycosis A42.0
    adenovirus J12.0
    anthrax A22.1

Pneumonia (acute) (double) (migratory)
  (purulent) (septic) (unresolved) J18.9 —
  continued
  in (due to) — continued
    ascariasis B77.81
    aspergillosis B44.9
    Bacillus anthracis A22.1
    Bacterium anitratum J15.6
    candidiasis B37.1
    chickenpox B01.2
    Chlamydia J16.0
      neonatal P23.1
    coccidioidomycosis B38.2
      acute B38.0
      chronic B38.1
    cytomegalovirus disease B25.0
    Diplococcus (pneumoniae) J13
    Eaton's agent J15.7
    Enterobacter J15.6
    Escherichia coli (E. coli) J15.5
    Friedländer's bacillus J15.0
    fumes and vapors (chemical) (inhalation)
      J68.0
    gonorrhea A54.84
    Hemophilus influenzae (H. influenzae) J14
    Herellea J15.6
    histoplasmosis B39.2
      acute B39.0
      chronic B39.1
    human metapneumovirus J12.3
    Klebsiella (pneumoniae) J15.0
    measles B05.2
    Mycoplasma (pneumoniae) J15.7
    nocardiosis, nocardiasis A43.0
    ornithosis A70
    parainfluenza virus J12.2
    pleuro-pneumonia-like-organism (PPLO)
      J15.7
    pneumococcus J13
    pneumocystosis (Pneumocystis carinii)
      (Pneumocystis jiroveci) B59
    Proteus J15.6
    Pseudomonas NEC J15.1
      pseudomallei A24.1
    psittacosis A70
    Q fever A78
    respiratory syncytial virus J12.1
    rheumatic fever I00 [J17]
    rubella B06.81
    Salmonella (infection) A02.22
      typhi A01.03
    schistosomiasis B65.9 [J17]
    Serratia marcescens J15.6
    specified
      bacterium NEC J15.8
      organism NEC J16.8
    spirochetal NEC A69.8
    Staphylococcus J15.20
      aureus (methicillin susceptible) (MSSA)
        J15.211
        methicillin resistant (MRSA) J15.212
      specified NEC J15.29
    Streptococcus J15.4
      group B J15.3
      pneumoniae J13
      specified NEC J15.4
    toxoplasmosis B58.3
    tularemia A21.2
    typhoid (fever) A01.03
    varicella B01.2
    virus — see Pneumonia, viral
    whooping cough A37.91
      due to
        Bordetella parapertussis A37.11
        Bordetella pertussis A37.01
        specified NEC A37.81
  Yersinia pestis A20.2
  inhalation of food or vomit — see Pneumonia,
    aspiration

Pneumonia (acute) (double) (migratory) (purulent) (septic) (unresolved) J18.9 — *continued*
interstitial J84.9
  chronic J84.111
  desquamative J84.117
  due to
    collagen vascular disease J84.17
    known underlying cause J84.17
  idiopathic NOS J84.111
  in diseases classified elsewhere J84.17
  lymphocytic (due to collagen vacular disease) (in diseases classified elsewhere) J84.17
  lymphoid J84.2
  non-specific J84.89
    due to
      collagen vascular disease J84.17
      known underlying cause J84.17
    idiopathic J84.113
    in diseases classified elsewhere J84.17
  plasma cell B59
  pseudomonas J15.1
  usual J84.112
    due to collagen vascular disease J84.17
    idiopathic J84.112
    in diseases classified elsewhere J84.17
Klebsiella (pneumoniae) J15.0
lipid, lipoid (exogenous) J69.1
  endogenous J84.89
lobar (disseminated) (double) (interstitial) J18.1
  bacterial J15.9
    specified NEC J15.8
  chronic — *see* Fibrosis, lung
  Escherichia coli (E. coli) J15.5
  Friedländer's bacillus J15.0
  Hemophilus influenzae J14
  hypostatic J18.2
  Klebsiella (pneumoniae) J15.0
  pneumococcal J13
  Proteus J15.6
  Pseudomonas J15.1
  specified organism NEC J16.8
  staphylococcal — *see* Pneumonia, staphylococcal
  streptococcal NEC J15.4
  Streptococcus pneumoniae J13
  viral, virus — *see* Pneumonia, viral
lobular — *see* Pneumonia, broncho
lymphoid interstitial J84.2
Löffler's J82
massive — *see* Pneumonia, lobar
meconium P24.01
MRSA (Methicillin resistant Staphylococcus aureus) J15.212
MSSA (methicillin susceptible Staphylococcus aureus) J15.211
Mycoplasma (pneumoniae) J15.7
necrotic J85.0
neonatal P23.9
  aspiration — *see* Aspiration, by substance, with pneumonia
nitrogen dioxide J68.0
organizing J84.89
  due to
    collagen vascular disease J84.17
    known underlying cause J84.17
  in diseases classified elsewhere J84.17
orthostatic J18.2
parainfluenza virus J12.2
parenchymatous — *see* Fibrosis, lung
passive J18.2
patchy — *see* Pneumonia, broncho
Peptococcus J15.8
Peptostreptococcus J15.8
plasma cell (of infants) B59
pleurolobar — *see* Pneumonia, lobar
pleuro-pneumonia-like organism (PPLO) J15.7

Pneumonia (acute) (double) (migratory) (purulent) (septic) (unresolved) J18.9 — *continued*
pneumococcal (broncho) (lobar) J13
Pneumocystis (carinii) (jiroveci) B59
postinfectional NEC B99 *[J17]*
postmeasles B05.2
Proteus J15.6
Pseudomonas J15.1
psittacosis A70
radiation J70.0
respiratory syncytial virus J12.1
resulting from a procedure J95.89
rheumatic I00 *[J17]*
Salmonella (arizonae) (cholerae-suis) (enteritidis) (typhimurium) A02.22
  typhi A01.03
  typhoid fever A01.03
SARS-associated coronavirus J12.81
segmented, segmental — *see* Pneumonia, broncho-
Serratia marcescens J15.6
specified NEC J18.8
  bacterium NEC J15.8
  organism NEC J16.8
  virus NEC J12.89
spirochetal NEC A69.8
staphylococcal (broncho) (lobar) J15.20
  aureus (methicillin susceptible) (MSSA) J15.211
    methicillin resistant (MRSA) J15.212
  specified NEC J15.29
static, stasis J18.2
streptococcal NEC (broncho) (lobar) J15.4
  group
    A J15.4
    B J15.3
    specified NEC J15.4
Streptococcus pneumoniae J13
syphilitic, congenital (early) A50.04
traumatic (complication) (early) (secondary) T79.8
tuberculous (any) — *see* Tuberculosis, pulmonary
tularemic A21.2
varicella B01.2
Veillonella J15.8
ventilator associated J95.851
viral, virus (broncho) (interstitial) (lobar) J12.9
  adenoviral J12.0
  congenital P23.0
  human metapneumovirus J12.3
  parainfluenza J12.2
  respiratory syncytial J12.1
  SARS-associated coronavirus J12.81
  specified NEC J12.89
white (congenital) A50.04
Pneumonic — *see* condition
Pneumonitis (acute) (primary) — *see also* Pneumonia
air-conditioner J67.7
allergic (due to) J67.9
  organic dust NEC J67.8
  red cedar dust J67.8
  sequoiosis J67.8
  wood dust J67.8
aspiration J69.0
  due to
    anesthesia J95.4
      during
        labor and delivery O74.0
        pregnancy O29.01-
        puerperium O89.01
    fumes or gases J68.0
  obstetric O74.0
chemical (due to gases, fumes or vapors) (inhalation) J68.0
  due to anesthesia J95.4
cholesterol J84.89

Pneumonitis (acute) (primary) — *see also* Pneumonia — *continued*
chronic — *see* Fibrosis, lung
congenital rubella P35.0
crack (cocaine) J68.0
due to
  beryllium J68.0
  cadmium J68.0
  crack (cocaine) J68.0
  detergent J69.8
  fluorocarbon-polymer J68.0
  food, vomit (aspiration) J69.0
  fumes or vapors J68.0
  gases, fumes or vapors (inhalation) J68.0
  inhalation
    blood J69.8
    essences J69.1
    food (regurgitated), milk, vomit J69.0
    oils, essences J69.1
    saliva J69.0
    solids, liquids NEC J69.8
  manganese J68.0
  nitrogen dioxide J68.0
  oils, essences J69.1
  solids, liquids NEC J69.8
  toxoplasmosis (acquired) B58.3
    congenital P37.1
  vanadium J68.0
  ventilator J95.851
eosinophilic J82
hypersensitivity J67.9
  air conditioner lung J67.7
  bagassosis J67.1
  bird fancier's lung J67.2
  farmer's lung J67.0
  maltworker's lung J67.4
  maple bark-stripper's lung J67.6
  mushroom worker's lung J67.5
  specified organic dust NEC J67.8
  suberosis J67.3
interstitial (chronic) J84.89
  acute J84.114
  lymphoid J84.2
  non-specific J84.89
    idiopathic J84.113
lymphoid, interstitial J84.2
meconium P24.01
postanesthetic J95.4
  correct substance properly administered — *see* Table of Drugs and Chemcials, by drug, adverse effect
  in labor and delivery O74.0
  in pregnancy O29.01-
  obstetric O74.0
  overdose or wrong substance given or taken (by accident) — *see* Table of Drugs and Chemicals, by drug, poisoning
  postpartum, puerperal O89.01
postoperative J95.4
  obstetric O74.0
radiation J70.0
rubella, congenital P35.0
ventilation (air-conditioning) J67.7
ventilator associated J95.851
wood-dust J67.8
Pneumonoconiosis — *see* Pneumoconiosis
Pneumoparotid K11.8
Pneumopathy NEC J98.4
alveolar J84.09
due to organic dust NEC J66.8
parietoalveolar J84.09
Pneumopericarditis — *see also* Pericarditis
acute I30.9
Pneumopericardium — *see also* Pericarditis
congenital P25.3
newborn P25.3
traumatic (post) — *see* Injury, heart
Pneumophagia (psychogenic) F45.8

Pneumopleurisy, pneumopleuritis (see also Pneumonia) J18.8
Pneumopyopericardium I30.1
Pneumopyothorax — see Pyopneumothorax
with fistula J86.0
Pneumorrhagia — see also Hemorrhage, lung
tuberculous — see Tuberculosis, pulmonary
Pneumothorax NOS J93.9
acute J93.8
chronic J93.81
congenital P25.1
perinatal period P25.1
postprocedural J95.811
specified NEC J93.83
spontaneous NOS J93.83
newborn P25.1
primary J93.11
secondary J93.12
tension J93.0
tense valvular, infectional J93.0
tension (spontaneous) J93.0
traumatic S27.0
with hemothorax S27.2
tuberculous — see Tuberculosis, pulmonary
Podagra (see also Gout) M10.9
Podencephalus Q01.9
Poikilocytosis R71.8
Poikiloderma L81.6
Civatte's L57.3
congenital Q82.8
vasculare atrophicans L94.5
Poikilodermatomyositis M33.10
with
myopathy M33.12
respiratory involvement M33.11
specified organ involvement NEC M33.19
Pointed ear (congenital) Q17.3
Poison ivy, oak, sumac or other plant dermatitis (allergic) (contact) L23.7
Poisoning (acute) — see also Table of Drugs and Chemicals
algae and toxins T65.82-
Bacillus B (aertrycke) (cholerae (suis)) (paratyphosus) (suipestifer) A02.9
botulinus A05.1
bacterial toxins A05.9
berries, noxious — see Poisoning, food, noxious, berries
botulism A05.1
ciguatera fish T61.0-
Clostridium botulinum A05.1
death-cap (Amanita phalloides) (Amanita verna) — see Poisoning, food, noxious, mushrooms
drug — see Table of Drugs and Chemicals, by drug, poisoning
epidemic, fish (noxious) — see Poisoning, seafood
bacterial A05.9
fava bean D55.0
fish (noxious) T61.9-
bacterial — see Intoxication, foodborne, by agent
ciguatera fish — see Poisoning, ciguatera fish
scombroid fish — see Poisoning, scombroid fish
specified type NEC T61.77-
food (acute) (diseased) (infected) (noxious) NEC T62.9-
bacterial — see Intoxication, foodborne, by agent
due to
Bacillus (aertrycke) (choleraesuis) (paratyphosus) (suipestifer) A02.9
botulinus A05.1
Clostridium (perfringens) (Welchii) A05.2

Poisoning (acute) (see also Table of Drugs and Chemicals) — continued
food (acute) (diseased) (infected) (noxious) NEC T62.9- — continued
due to — continued
salmonella (aertrycke) (callinarum) (choleraesuis) (enteritidis) (paratyphi) (suipestifer) A02.9
with
gastroenteritis A02.0
sepsis A02.1
staphylococcus A05.0
Vibrio
parahaemolyticus A05.3
vulnificus A05.5
noxious or naturally toxic T62.9-
berries — see subcategory T62.1-
fish — see Poisoning, seafood
mushrooms — see subcategory T62.0x-
plants NEC — see subcategory T62.2x-
seafood — see Poisoning, seafood
specified NEC — see subcategory T62.8x-
ichthyotoxism — see Poisoning, seafood
kreotoxism, food A05.9
latex T65.81-
lead T56.0-
mushroom — see Poisoning, food, noxious, mushroom
mussels — see also Poisoning, shellfish
bacterial — see Intoxication, foodborne, by agent
nicotine (tobacco) T65.2-
noxious foodstuffs — see Poisoning, food, noxious
plants, noxious — see Poisoning, food, noxious, plants NEC
ptomaine — see Poisoning, food
radiation J70.0
Salmonella (arizonae) (cholerae-suis) (enteritidis) (typhimurium) A02.9
scombroid fish T61.1-
seafood (noxious) T61.9-
bacterial — see Intoxication, foodborne, by agent
fish — see Poisoning, fish
shellfish — see Poisoning, shellfish
specified NEC — see subcategory T61.8x-
shellfish (amnesic) (azaspiracid) (diarrheic) (neurotoxic) (noxious) (paralytic) T61.78-
bacterial — see Intoxication, foodborne, by agent
ciguatera mollusk — see Poisoning, ciguatera fish
specified substance NEC T65.891
Staphylococcus, food A05.0
tobacco (nicotine) T65.2-
water E87.79
Poker spine — see Spondylitis, ankylosing
Poland syndrome Q79.8
Polioencephalitis (acute) (bulbar) A80.9
inferior G12.22
influenzal — see Influenza, with, encephalopathy
superior hemorrhagic (acute) (Wernicke's) E51.2
Wernicke's E51.2
Polioencephalomyelitis (acute) (anterior) A80.9
with beriberi E51.2
Polioencephalopathy, superior hemorrhagic E51.2
with
beriberi E51.11
pellagra E52
Poliomeningoencephalitis — see Meningoencephalitis

Poliomyelitis (acute) (anterior) (epidemic) A80.9
with paralysis (bulbar) — see Poliomyelitis, paralytic
abortive A80.4
ascending (progressive) — see Poliomyelitis, paralytic
bulbar (paralytic) — see Poliomyelitis, paralytic
congenital P35.8
nonepidemic A80.9
nonparalytic A80.4
paralytic A80.30
specified NEC A80.39
vaccine-associated A80.0
wild virus
imported A80.1
indigenous A80.2
spinal, acute A80.9
Poliosis (eyebrow) (eyelashes) L67.1
circumscripta, acquired L67.1
Pollakiuria R35.0
psychogenic F45.8
Pollinosis J30.1
Pollitzer's disease L73.2
Polyadenitis — see also Lymphadenitis
malignant A20.0
Polyalgia M79.89
Polyangiitis M30.0
microscopic M31.7
overlap syndrome M30.8
Polyarteritis
microscopic M31.7
nodosa M30.0
with lung involvement M30.1
juvenile M30.2
related condition NEC M30.8
Polyarthralgia — see Pain, joint
Polyarthritis, polyarthropathy (see also Arthritis) M13.0
due to or associated with other specified conditions — see Arthritis
epidemic (Australian) (with exanthema) B33.1
infective — see Arthritis, pyogenic or pyemic
inflammatory M06.4
juvenile (chronic) (seronegative) M08.3
migratory — see Fever, rheumatic
rheumatic, acute — see Fever, rheumatic
Polyarthrosis M15.9
post-traumatic M15.3
primary M15.0
specified NEC M15.8
Polycarential syndrome of infancy E40
Polychondritis (atrophic) (chronic) — see also Disorder, cartilage, specified type NEC
relapsing M94.1
Polycoria Q13.2
Polycystic (disease)
degeneration, kidney Q61.3
autosomal dominant (adult type) Q61.2
autosomal recessive (infantile type) NEC Q61.19
kidney Q61.3
autosomal
dominant Q61.2
recessive NEC Q61.19
autosomal dominant (adult type) Q61.2
autosomal recessive (childhood type) NEC Q61.19
infantile type NEC Q61.19
liver Q44.6
lung J98.4
congenital Q33.0
ovary, ovaries E28.2
spleen Q89.09
Polycythemia (secondary) D75.1
acquired D75.1
benign (familial) D75.0

Polycythemia (secondary) D75.1— *continued*
- due to
  - donor twin P61.1
  - erythropoietin D75.1
  - fall in plasma volume D75.1
  - high altitude D75.1
  - maternal-fetal transfusion P61.1
  - stress D75.1
- emotional D75.1
- erythropoietin D75.1
- familial (benign) D75.0
- Gaisböck's (hypertonica) D75.1
- high altitude D75.1
- hypertonica D75.1
- hypoxemic D75.1
- neonatorum P61.1
- nephrogenous D75.1
- relative D75.1
- secondary D75.1
- spurious D75.1
- stress D75.1
- vera D45

Polycytosis cryptogenica D75.1

Polydactylism, polydactyly Q69.9
- toes Q69.2

Polydipsia R63.1

Polydystrophy, pseudo-Hurler E77.0

Polyembryoma — *see* Neoplasm, malignant, by site

Polyglandular
- deficiency E31.0
- dyscrasia E31.9
- dysfunction E31.9
- syndrome E31.8

Polyhydramnios O40-

Polymastia Q83.1

Polymenorrhea N92.0

Polymyalgia M35.3
- arteritica, giant cell M31.5
- rheumatica M35.3
  - with giant cell arteritis M31.5

Polymyositis (acute) (chronic) (hemorrhagic) M33.20
- with
  - myopathy M33.22
  - respiratory involvement M33.21
  - skin involvement — *see* Dermatopolymyositis
  - specified organ involvement NEC M33.29
- ossificans (generalisata) (progressiva) — *see* Myositis, ossificans, progressiva

Polyneuritis, polyneuritic — *see also* Polyneuropathy
- acute (post-)infective G61.0
- alcoholic G62.1
- cranialis G52.7
- demyelinating, chronic inflammatory (CIDP) G61.81
- diabetic — *see* Diabetes, polyneuropathy
- diphtheritic A36.83
- due to lack of vitamin NEC E56.9 *[G63]*
- endemic E51.11
- erythredema — *see* subcategory T56.1
- febrile, acute G61.0
- hereditary ataxic G60.1
- idiopathic, acute G61.0
- infective (acute) G61.0
- inflammatory, chronic demyelinating (CIDP) G61.81
- nutritional E63.9 *[G63]*
- postinfective (acute) G61.0
- specified NEC G62.89

Polyneuropathy (peripheral) G62.9
- alcoholic G62.1
- amyloid (Portuguese) E85.1 *[G63]*
- arsenical G62.2
- critical illness G62.81
- demyelinating, chronic inflammatory (CIDP) G61.81
- diabetic — *see* Diabetes, polyneuropathy

Polyneuropathy (peripheral) G62.9 — *continued*
- drug-induced G62.0
- hereditary G60.9
  - specified NEC G60.8
- idiopathic G60.9
  - progressive G60.3
- in (due to)
  - alcohol G62.1
    - sequelae G65.2
  - amyloidosis, familial (Portuguese) E85.1 *[G63]*
  - antitetanus serum G61.1
  - arsenic G62.2
    - sequelae G65.2
  - avitaminosis NEC E56.9 *[G63]*
  - beriberi E51.11
  - collagen vascular disease NEC M35.9 *[G63]*
  - deficiency (of)
    - B(-complex) vitamins E53.9 *[G63]*
    - vitamin B6 E53.1 *[G63]*
  - diabetes — *see* Diabetes, polyneuropathy
  - diphtheria A36.83
  - drug or medicament G62.0
    - correct substance properly administered — *see* Table of Drugs and Chemicals, by drug, adverse effect
    - overdose or wrong substance given or taken — *see* Table of Drugs and Chemicals, by drug, poisoning
  - endocrine disease NEC E34.9 *[G63]*
  - herpes zoster B02.23
  - hypoglycemia E16.2 *[G63]*
  - infectious
    - disease NEC B99 *[G63]*
    - mononucleosis B27.91
  - lack of vitamin NEC E56.9 *[G63]*
  - lead G62.2
    - sequelae G65.2
  - leprosy A30.9 *[G63]*
  - Lyme disease A69.22
  - metabolic disease NEC E88.9 *[G63]*
  - microscopic polyangiitis M31.7 *[G63]*
  - mumps B26.84
  - neoplastic disease (*see also* Neoplasm) D49.9 *[G63]*
  - nutritional deficiency NEC E63.9 *[G63]*
  - organophosphate compounds G62.2
    - sequelae G65.2
  - parasitic disease NEC B89 *[G63]*
  - pellagra E52 *[G63]*
  - polyarteritis nodosa M30.0
  - porphyria E80.20 *[G63]*
  - radiation G62.82
  - rheumatoid arthritis — *see* Rheumatoid, polyneuropathy
  - sarcoidosis D86.89
  - serum G61.1
  - syphilis (late) A52.15
    - congenital A50.43
  - systemic
    - connective tissue disorder M35.9 *[G63]*
    - lupus erythematosus M32.19
  - toxic agent NEC G62.2
    - sequelae G65.2
  - triorthocresyl phosphate G62.2
    - sequelae G65.2
  - tuberculosis A17.89
  - uremia N18.9 *[G63]*
  - vitamin B12 deficiency E53.8 *[G63]*
    - with anemia (pernicious) D51.0 *[G63]*
      - due to dietary deficiency D51.3 *[G63]*
  - zoster B02.23
- inflammatory G61.9
  - chronic demyelinating (CIDP) G61.81
  - sequelae G65.1
  - specified NEC G61.89

Polyneuropathy (peripheral) G62.9 — *continued*
- lead G62.2
  - sequelae G65.2
- nutritional NEC E63.9 *[G63]*
- postherpetic (zoster) B02.23
- progressive G60.3
- radiation-induced G62.82
- sensory (hereditary) (idiopathic) G60.8
- specified NEC G62.89
- syphilitic (late) A52.15
  - congenital A50.43

Polyopia H53.8

Polyorchism, polyorchidism Q55.21

Polyosteoarthritis (*see also* Osteoarthritis, generalized) M15.9-
- post-traumatic M15.3
- specified NEC M15.8

Polyostotic fibrous dysplasia Q78.1

Polyotia Q17.0

Polyp, polypus
- accessory sinus J33.8
- adenocarcinoma in — *see* Neoplasm, malignant, by site
- adenocarcinoma in situ in — *see* Neoplasm, in situ, by site
- adenoid tissue J33.0
- adenomatous — *see also* Neoplasm, benign, by site
  - adenocarcinoma in — *see* Neoplasm, malignant, by site
  - adenocarcinoma in situ in — *see* Neoplasm, in situ, by site
  - carcinoma in — *see* Neoplasm, malignant, by site
  - carcinoma in situ in — *see* Neoplasm, in situ, by site
  - multiple — *see* Neoplasm, benign
    - adenocarcinoma in — *see* Neoplasm, malignant, by site
    - adenocarcinoma in situ in — *see* Neoplasm, in situ, by site
- antrum J33.8
- anus, anal (canal) K62.0
- Bartholin's gland N84.3
- bladder D41.4
- carcinoma in — *see* Neoplasm, malignant, by site
- carcinoma in situ in — *see* Neoplasm, in situ, by site
- cecum D12.0
- cervix (uteri) N84.1
  - in pregnancy or childbirth — *see* Pregnancy, complicated by, abnormal, cervix
  - mucous N84.1
  - nonneoplastic N84.1
- choanal J33.0
- cholesterol K82.4
- clitoris N84.3
- colon K63.5
  - adenomatous D12.6
  - ascending D12.2
  - cecum D12.0
  - descending D12.4
  - inflammatory K51.40
    - with
      - abscess K51.414
      - complication K51.419
        - specified NEC K51.418
      - fistula K51.413
      - intestinal obstruction K51.412
      - rectal bleeding K51.411
  - sigmoid D12.5
  - transverse D12.3
- corpus uteri N84.0
- dental K04.01
  - irreversible K04.02
  - reversible K04.01
- duodenum K31.7

DISEASE INDEX

Polyp, polypus — *continued*
  ear (middle) H74.4-
  endometrium N84.0
  ethmoidal (sinus) J33.8
  fallopian tube N84.8
  female genital tract N84.9
    specified NEC N84.8
  frontal (sinus) J33.8
  gallbladder K82.4
  gingiva, gum K06.8
  labia, labium (majus) (minus) N84.3
  larynx (mucous) J38.1
    adenomatous D14.1
  malignant — *see* Neoplasm, malignant, by site
  maxillary (sinus) J33.8
  middle ear — *see* Polyp, ear (middle)
  myometrium N84.0
  nares
    anterior J33.9
    posterior J33.0
  nasal (mucous) J33.9
    cavity J33.0
    septum J33.0
  nasopharyngeal J33.0
  nose (mucous) J33.9
  oviduct N84.8
  pharynx J39.2
  placenta O90.89
  prostate — *see* Enlargement, enlarged,
    prostate
  pudenda, pudendum N84.3
  pulpal (dental) K04.01
    irreversible K04.02
    reversible K04.01
  rectum (nonadenomatous) K62.1
    adenomatous — *see* Polyp, adenomatous
  septum (nasal) J33.0
  sinus (accessory) (ethmoidal) (frontal)
    (maxillary) (sphenoidal) J33.8
  sphenoidal (sinus) J33.8
  stomach K31.7
    adenomatous D13.1
  tube, fallopian N84.8
  turbinate, mucous membrane J33.8
  umbilical, newborn P83.6
  ureter N28.89
  urethra N36.2
  uterus (body) (corpus) (mucous) N84.0
    cervix N84.1
    in pregnancy or childbirth — *see* Pregnancy,
      complicated by, tumor, uterus
  vagina N84.2
  vocal cord (mucous) J38.1
  vulva N84.3
Polyphagia R63.2
Polyploidy Q92.7
Polypoid — *see* condition
Polyposis — *see also* Polyp
  coli (adenomatous) D12.6
    adenocarcinoma in C18.9
    adenocarcinoma in situ in — *see* Neoplasm,
      in situ, by site
    carcinoma in C18.9
  colon (adenomatous) D12.6
  familial D12.6
    adenocarcinoma in situ in — *see* Neoplasm,
      in situ, by site
  intestinal (adenomatous) D12.6
  malignant lymphomatous C83.1-
  multiple, adenomatous (*see also* Neoplasm,
    benign) D36.9
Polyradiculitis — *see* Polyneuropathy
Polyradiculoneuropathy (acute)
  (postinfective) (segmentally demyelinating)
  G61.0
Polyserositis
  due to pericarditis I31.1
  pericardial I31.1
  periodic, familial E85.0

Polyserositis — *continued*
  tuberculous A19.9
    acute A19.1
    chronic A19.8
Polysplenia syndrome Q89.09
Polysyndactyly (*see also* Syndactylism,
  syndactyly) Q70.4
Polytrichia L68.3
Polyunguia Q84.6
Polyuria R35.8
  nocturnal R35.1
  psychogenic F45.8
Pompe's disease (glycogen storage) E74.02
Pompholyx L30.1
Poncet's disease (tuberculous rheumatism)
  A18.09
Pond fracture — *see* Fracture, skull
Ponos B55.0
Pons, pontine — *see* condition
Poor
  aesthetic of existing restoration of tooth K08.56
  contractions, labor O62.2
  gingival margin to tooth restoration K08.51
  personal hygiene R46.0
  prenatal care, affecting management of
    pregnancy — *see* Pregnancy, complicated
    by, insufficient, prenatal care
  sucking reflex (newborn) R29.2
  urinary stream R39.12
  vision NEC H54.7
Poradenitis, nostras inguinalis or
  venerea A55
Porencephaly (congenital) (developmental)
  (true) Q04.6
  acquired G93.0
  nondevelopmental G93.0
  traumatic (post) F07.89
Porocephaliasis B88.8
Porokeratosis Q82.8
Poroma, eccrine — *see* Neoplasm, skin,
  benign
Porphyria (South African) E80.20
  acquired E80.20
  acute intermittent (hepatic) (Swedish) E80.21
  cutanea tarda (hereditary) (symptomatic)
    E80.1
  due to drugs E80.20
    correct substance properly administered —
      see Table of Drugs and Chemicals, by
      drug, adverse effect
    overdose or wrong substance given or taken
      — *see* Table of Drugs and Chemicals, by
      drug, poisoning
  erythropoietic (congenital) (hereditary) E80.0
  hepatocutaneous type E80.1
  secondary E80.20
  toxic NEC E80.20
  variegata E80.20
Porphyrinuria — *see* Porphyria
Porphyruria — *see* Porphyria
Port wine nevus, mark, or stain Q82.5
Portal — *see* condition
Posadas-Wernicke disease B38.9
Positive
  culture (nonspecific)
    blood R78.81
    bronchial washings R84.5
    cerebrospinal fluid R83.5
    cervix uteri R87.5
    nasal secretions R84.5
    nipple discharge R89.5
    nose R84.5
      staphylococcus (methicillin susceptible)
        Z22.321
        methicillin resistant Z22.322
    peritoneal fluid R85.5
    pleural fluid R84.5
    prostatic secretions R86.5
    saliva R85.5

Positive — *continued*
  culture (nonspecific) — *continued*
    seminal fluid R86.5
    sputum R84.5
    synovial fluid R89.5
    throat scrapings R84.5
    urine R82.79
    vagina R87.5
    vulva R87.5
    wound secretions R89.5
  PPD (skin test) R76.11
  serology for syphilis A53.0
    with signs or symptoms — *code as* Syphilis,
      by site and stage
    false R76.8
  skin test, tuberculin (without active tuberculosis)
    R76.11
  test, human immunodeficiency virus (HIV) R75
  VDRL A53.0
    with signs or symptoms — *code by* site and
      stage under Syphilis A53.9
  Wassermann reaction A53.0
Postcardiotomy syndrome I97.0
Postcaval ureter Q62.62
Postcholecystectomy syndrome K91.5
Postclimacteric bleeding N95.0
Postcommissurotomy syndrome I97.0
Postconcussional syndrome F07.81
Postcontusional syndrome F07.81
Postcricoid region — *see* condition
Post-dates (40-42 weeks) (pregnancy)
  (mother) O48.0
  more than 42 weeks gestation O48.1
Postencephalitic syndrome F07.89
Posterior — *see* condition
Posterolateral sclerosis (spinal cord) — *see*
  Degeneration, combined
Postexanthematous — *see* condition
Postfebrile — *see* condition
Postgastrectomy dumping syndrome
  K91.1
Posthemiplegic chorea — *see* Monoplegia
Posthemorrhagic anemia (chronic) D50.0
  acute D62
  newborn P61.3
Postherpetic neuralgia (zoster) B02.29
  trigeminal B02.22
Posthitis N47.7
Postimmunization complication or
  reaction — *see* Complications, vaccination
Postinfectious — *see* condition
Postlaminectomy syndrome NEC M96.1
Postleukotomy syndrome F07.0
Postmastectomy lymphedema (syndrome)
  I97.2
Postmaturity, postmature (over 42 weeks)
  maternal (over 42 weeks gestation) O48.1
  newborn P08.22
Postmeasles complication NEC (*see also*
  condition) B05.89
Postmenopausal
  endometrium (atrophic) N95.8
    suppurative (*see also* Endometritis) N71.9
  osteoporosis — *see* Osteoporosis,
    postmenopausal
Postnasal drip R09.82
  due to
    allergic rhinitis — *see* Rhinitis, allergic
    common cold J00
    gastroesophageal reflux — *see* Reflux,
      gastroesophageal
    nasopharyngitis — *see* Nasopharyngitis
    other know condition — *code to* condition
    sinusitis — *see* Sinusitis
Postnatal — *see* condition
Postoperative (postprocedural) — *see*
  Complication, postoperative
  pneumothorax, therapeutic Z98.3
  state NEC Z98.890

Postpancreatectomy hyperglycemia E89.1
Postpartum — *see* Puerperal
Postphlebitic syndrome — *see* Syndrome, postthrombotic
Postpolio (myelitic) syndrome G14
Postpoliomyelitic — *see also* condition
  osteopathy — *see* Osteopathy, after poliomyelitis
Postprocedural — *see also* Postoperative
  hypoinsulinemia E89.1
Postschizophrenic depression F32.89
Postsurgery status — *see also* Status (post)
  pneumothorax, therapeutic Z98.3
Post-term (40-42 weeks) (pregnancy) (mother) O48.0
  infant P08.21
  more than 42 weeks gestation (mother) O48.1
Post-traumatic brain syndrome, nonpsychotic F07.81
Post-typhoid abscess A01.09
Postures, hysterical F44.2
Postvaccinal reaction or complication — *see* Complications, vaccination
Postvalvulotomy syndrome I97.0
Potain's
  disease (pulmonary edema) — *see* Edema, lung
  syndrome (gastrectasis with dyspepsia) K31.0
Potter's
  asthma J62.8
  facies Q60.6
  lung J62.8
  syndrome (with renal agenesis) Q60.6
Pott's
  curvature (spinal) A18.01
  disease or paraplegia A18.01
  spinal curvature A18.01
  tumor, puffy — *see* Osteomyelitis, specified type NEC
Pouch
  bronchus Q32.4
  Douglas' — *see* condition
  esophagus, esophageal, congenital Q39.6
    acquired K22.5
  gastric K31.4
  Hartmann's K82.8
  pharynx, pharyngeal (congenital) Q38.7
Pouchitis K91.850
Poultrymen's itch B88.0
Poverty NEC Z59.6
  extreme Z59.5
Poxvirus NEC B08.8
Prader-Willi syndrome Q87.1
Preauricular appendage or tag Q17.0
Prebetalipoproteinemia (acquired) (essential) (familial) (hereditary) (primary) (secondary) E78.1
  with chylomicronemia E78.3
Precipitate labor or delivery O62.3
Preclimacteric bleeding (menorrhagia) N92.4
Precocious
  adrenarche E30.1
  menarche E30.1
  menstruation E30.1
  pubarche E30.1
  puberty E30.1
    central E22.8
  sexual development NEC E30.1
  thelarche E30.8
Precocity, sexual (constitutional) (cryptogenic) (female) (idiopathic) (male) E30.1
  with adrenal hyperplasia E25.9
    congenital E25.0
Precordial pain R07.2
Predeciduous teeth K00.2

Prediabetes, prediabetic R73.03
  complicating
    pregnancy — *see* Pregnancy, complicated by, diseases of, specified type or system NEC
    puerperium O99.89
Predislocation status of hip at birth Q65.6
Pre-eclampsia O14.9-
  with pre-existing hypertension — *see* Hypertension, complicating pregnancy, pre-existing, with, pre-eclampsia
  complicating
    childbirth O14.94
    puerperium O14.95
  mild O14.0-
    complicating
      childbirth O14.04
      puerperium O14.05
  moderate O14.0-
    complicating
      childbirth O14.04
      puerperium O14.05
  severe O14.1-
    with hemolysis, elevated liver enzymes and low platelet count (HELLP) O14.2-
      complicating
        childbirth O14.24
        puerperium O14.25
    complicating
      childbirth O14.14
      puerperium O14.15
Pre-eruptive color change, teeth, tooth K00.8
Pre-excitation atrioventricular conduction I45.6
Pre-glaucoma H40.00-
Pregnancy (childbirth) (labor) (puerperium) — *see also* Delivery and Puerperal
Note — *The tabular must be reviewed for assignment of the appropriate character indicating the trimester of the pregnancy*
Note — *The tabular must be reviewed for assignment of the appropriate seventh character for multiple gestation codes in Chapter 15*
  abdominal (ectopic) O00.00
    with intrauterine pregnancy O00.01
    with viable fetus O36.7-
  ampullar O00.10
    with intrauterine pregnancy O00.11
  biochemical O02.81
  broad ligament O00.80
    with intrauterine pregnancy O00.81
  cervical O00.80
    with intrauterine pregnancy O00.81
  chemical O02.81
  complicated by (care of) (management affected by)
    abnormal, abnormality
      cervix O34.4-
        causing obstructed labor O65.5
      cord (umbilical) O69.9
      findings on antenatal screening of mother O28.9
        biochemical O28.1
        chromosomal O28.5
        cytological O28.2
        genetic O28.5
        hematological O28.0
        radiological O28.4
        specified NEC O28.8
        ultrasonic O28.3
      glucose (tolerance) NEC O99.810
      pelvic organs O34.9-
        specified NEC O34.8-
          causing obstructed labor O65.5
      pelvis (bony) (major) NEC O33.0
      perineum O34.7-

Pregnancy (childbirth) (labor) (puerperium) (*see also* Delivery and Puerperal) — *continued*
  complicated by (care of) (management affected by) — *continued*
    abnormal, abnormality — *continued*
      position
        placenta O44.0-
          with hemorrhage O44.1-
        uterus O34.59-
      uterus O34.59-
        causing obstructed labor O65.5
        congenital O34.0-
      vagina O34.6-
        causing obstructed labor O65.5
      vulva O34.7-
        causing obstructed labor O65.5
    abruptio placentae — *see* Abruptio placentae
    abscess or cellulitis
      bladder O23.1-
      breast O91.11-
      genital organ or tract O23.9-
    abuse
      physical O9A.31- *(follows O99)*
      psychological O9A.51- *(follows O99)*
      sexual O9A.41- *(follows O99)*
    adverse effect anesthesia O29.9-
      aspiration pneumonitis O29.01-
      cardiac arrest O29.11-
      cardiac complication NEC O29.19-
      cardiac failure O29.12-
      central nervous system complication NEC O29.29-
      cerebral anoxia O29.21-
      failed or difficult intubation O29.6-
      inhalation of stomach contents or secretions NOS O29.01-
      local, toxic reaction O29.3x
      Mendelson's syndrome O29.01-
      pressure collapse of lung O29.02-
      pulmonary complications NEC O29.09-
      specified NEC O29.8x-
      spinal and epidural type NEC O29.5x
        induced headache O29.4-
    albuminuria (*see also* Proteinuria, gestational) O12.1-
    alcohol use O99.31-
    amnionitis O41.12-
    anaphylactoid syndrome of pregnancy O88.01-
    anemia (conditions in D50-D64) (pre-existing) O99.01-
      complicating the puerperium O99.03
    antepartum hemorrhage O46.9-
      with coagulation defect — *see* Hemorrhage, antepartum, with coagulation defect
      specified NEC O46.8x-
    appendicitis O99.61-
    atrophy (yellow) (acute) liver (subacute) O26.61-
    bariatric surgery status O99.84-
    bicornis or bicornuate uterus O34.0-
    biliary tract problems O26.61-
    breech presentation O32.1
    cardiovascular diseases (conditions in I00-I09, I20-I52, I70-I99) O99.41-
    cerebrovascular disorders (conditions in I60-I69) O99.41-
    cervical shortening O26.87-
    cervicitis O23.51-
    chloasma (gravidarum) O26.89-
    cholecystitis O99.61-
    cholestasis (intrahepatic) O26.61-
    chorioamnionitis O41.12-
    circulatory system disorder (conditions in I00-I09, I20-I99) O99.41-
    compound presentation O32.6
    conjoined twins O30.02-

Pregnancy (childbirth) (labor) (puerperium) (*see also* Delivery and Puerperal) — *continued*
complicated by (care of) (management affected by) — *continued*
connective system disorders (conditions in M00-M99) O99.89
contracted pelvis (general) O33.1
  inlet O33.2
  outlet O33.3
convulsions (eclamptic) (uremic) (*see also* Eclampsia) O15.9-
cracked nipple O92.11-
cystitis O23.1-
cystocele O34.8-
death of fetus (near term) O36.4
  early pregnancy O02.1
  of one fetus or more in multiple gestation O31.2-
deciduitis O41.14-
decreased fetal movement O36.81-
dental problems O99.61-
diabetes (mellitus) O24.91-
  gestational (pregnancy induced) — *see* Diabetes, gestational
  pre-existing O24.31-
    specified NEC O24.81-
    type 1 O24.01-
    type 2 O24.11-
digestive system disorders (conditions in K00-K93) O99.61-
diseases of — *see* Pregnancy, complicated by, specified body system disease
  biliary tract O26.61-
  blood NEC (conditions in D65-D77) O99.11-
  liver O26.61-
  specified NEC O99.89
disorders of — *see* Pregnancy, complicated by, specified body system disorder
  amniotic fluid and membranes O41.9-
    specified NEC O41.8x-
  biliary tract O26.61-
  ear and mastoid process (conditions in H60-H95) O99.89
  eye and adnexa (conditions in H00-H59) O99.89
  liver O26.61-
  skin (conditions in L00-L99) O99.71-
  specified NEC O99.89
displacement, uterus NEC O34.59-
  causing obstructed labor O65.5
disproportion (due to) O33.9
  fetal (ascites) (hydrops) (meningomyelocele) (sacral teratoma) (tumor) deformities NEC O33.7
  generally contracted pelvis O33.1
  hydrocephalic fetus O33.6
  inlet contraction of pelvis O33.2
  mixed maternal and fetal origin O33.4
  specified NEC O33.8
double uterus O34.0-
  causing obstructed labor O65.5
drug use (conditions in F11-F19) O99.32-
eclampsia, eclamptic (coma) (convulsions) (delirium) (nephritis) (uremia) (*see also* Eclampsia) O15-
ectopic pregnancy — *see* Pregnancy, ectopic
edema O12.0-
  with
    gestational hypertension, mild (*see also* Pre-eclampsia) O14.0-
    proteinuria O12.2-
effusion, amniotic fluid — *see* Pregnancy, complicated by, premature rupture of membranes
elderly
  multigravida O09.52-
  primigravida O09.51-

Pregnancy (childbirth) (labor) (puerperium) (*see also* Delivery and Puerperal) — *continued*
complicated by (care of) (management affected by) — *continued*
embolism (*see also* Embolism, obstetric, pregnancy) O88.-
endocrine diseases NEC O99.28-
endometritis O86.12
excessive weight gain O26.0-
exhaustion O26.81-
  during labor and delivery O75.81
face presentation O32.3
failed induction of labor O61.9
  instrumental O61.1
  mechanical O61.1
  medical O61.0
  specified NEC O61.8
  surgical O61.1
failed or difficult intubation for anesthesia O29.6-
false labor (pains) O47.9
  at or after 37 completed weeks of pregnancy O47.1
  before 37 completed weeks of pregnancy O47.0-
fatigue O26.81-
  during labor and delivery O75.81
fatty metamorphosis of liver O26.61-
female genital mutilation O34.8- [N90.8-]
fetal (maternal care for)
  abnormality or damage O35.9
    acid-base balance O68
    specified type NEC O35.8
  acidemia O68
  acidosis O68
  alkalosis O68
  anemia and thrombocytopenia O36.82-
  anencephaly O35.0
  chromosomal abnormality (conditions in Q90-Q99) O35.1
  conjoined twins O30.02-
  damage from
    amniocentesis O35.7
    biopsy procedures O35.7
    drug addiction O35.5
    hematological investigation O35.7
    intrauterine contraceptive device O35.7
    maternal
      alcohol addiction O35.4
      cytomegalovirus infection O35.3
      disease NEC O35.8
      drug addiction O35.5
      listeriosis O35.8
      rubella O35.3
      toxoplasmosis O35.8
      viral infection O35.3
    medical procedure NEC O35.7
    radiation O35.6
  death (near term) O36.4
    early pregnancy O02.1
  decreased movement O36.81-
  disproportion due to deformity (fetal) O33.7
  excessive growth (large for dates) O36.6-
  growth retardation O36.59-
    light for dates O36.59-
    small for dates O36.59-
  heart rate irregularity (bradycardia) (decelerations) (tachycardia) O76
  hereditary disease O35.2
  hydrocephalus O35.0
  intrauterine death O36.4
  poor growth O36.59-
    light for dates O36.59-
    small for dates O36.59-
  problem O36.9-
    specified NEC O36.89-
  reduction (elective) O31.3-
  selective termination O31.3-

Pregnancy (childbirth) (labor) (puerperium) (*see also* Delivery and Puerperal) — *continued*
complicated by (care of) (management affected by) — *continued*
fetal (maternal care for) — *continued*
  spina bifida O35.0
  thrombocytopenia O36.82-
fibroid (tumor) (uterus) O34.1-
fissure of nipple O92.11-
gallstones O99.61-
gastric banding status O99.84-
gastric bypass status O99.84-
genital herpes (asymptomatic) (history of) (inactive) O98.51-
genital tract infection O23.9-
glomerular diseases (conditions in N00-N07) O26.83-
  with hypertension, pre-existing — *see* Hypertension, complicating, pregnancy, pre-existing, with, renal disease
gonorrhea O98.21-
grand multiparity O09.4
habitual aborter — *see* Pregnancy, complicated by, recurrent pregnancy loss
HELLP syndrome (hemolysis, elevated liver enzymes and low platelet count) O14.2-
hemorrhage
  antepartum — *see* Hemorrhage, antepartum
  before 20 completed weeks gestation O20.9
    specified NEC O20.8
  due to premature separation, placenta (*see also* Abruptio placentae) O45.9-
  early O20.9
    specified NEC O20.8
  threatened abortion O20.0
hemorrhoids O22.4-
hepatitis (viral) O98.41-
herniation of uterus O34.59-
high
  head at term O32.4
  risk — *see* Supervision (of) (for), high-risk
history of in utero procedure during previous pregnancy O09.82-
HIV O98.71-
human immunodeficiency virus (HIV) disease O98.71-
hydatidiform mole (*see also* Mole, hydatidiform) O01.9-
hydramnios O40-
hydrocephalic fetus (disproportion) O33.6
hydrops
  amnii O40-
  fetalis O36.2-
    associated with isoimmunization (*see also* Pregnancy, complicated by, isoimmunization) O36.11-
hydrorrhea O42.90
hyperemesis (gravidarum) (mild) (*see also* Hyperemesis, gravidarum) O21.0-
hypertension — *see* Hypertension, complicating pregnancy
hypertensive
  heart and renal disease, pre-existing — *see* Hypertension, complicating, pregnancy, pre-existing, with, heart disease, with renal disease
  heart disease, pre-existing — *see* Hypertension, complicating, pregnancy, pre-existing, with, heart disease
  renal disease, pre-existing — *see* Hypertension, complicating, pregnancy, pre-existing, with, renal disease
hypotension O26.5-

Pregnancy (childbirth) (labor) (puerperium) (*see also* Delivery and Puerperal) — *continued*
  complicated by (care of) (management affected by) — *continued*
    immune disorders NEC (conditions in D80-D89) O99.11-
    incarceration, uterus O34.51-
    incompetent cervix O34.3-
    inconclusive fetal viability O36.80
    infection(s) O98.91-
      amniotic fluid or sac O41.10-
      bladder O23.1-
      carrier state NEC O99.830
        streptococcus B O99.820
      genital organ or tract O23.9-
        specified NEC O23.59-
      genitourinary tract O23.9-
      gonorrhea O98.21-
      hepatitis (viral) O98.41-
      HIV O98.71-
      human immunodeficiency virus (HIV) O98.71-
      kidney O23.0-
      nipple O91.01-
      parasitic disease O98.91-
        specified NEC O98.81-
      protozoal disease O98.61-
      sexually transmitted NEC O98.31-
      specified type NEC O98.81-
      syphilis O98.11-
      tuberculosis O98.01-
      urethra O23.2-
      urinary (tract) O23.4-
        specified NEC O23.3-
      viral disease O98.51-
    injury or poisoning (conditions in S00-T88) O9A.21- *(follows O99)*
      due to abuse
        physical O9A.31- *(follows O99)*
        psychological O9A.51- *(follows O99)*
        sexual O9A.41- *(follows O99)*
    insufficient
      prenatal care O09.3-
      weight gain O26.1-
    insulin resistance O26.89-
    intrauterine fetal death (near term) O36.4
      early pregnancy O02.1
      multiple gestation (one fetus or more) O31.2-
    isoimmunization O36.11-
      anti-A sensitization O36.11-
      anti-B sensitization O36.19-
      Rh O36.09-
        anti-D antibody O36.01-
        specified NEC O36.19-
    laceration of uterus NEC O71.81
    malformation
      placenta, placental (vessel) O43.10-
        specified NEC O43.19-
      uterus (congenital) O34.0-
    malnutrition (conditions in E40-E46) O25.1-
    maternal hypotension syndrome O26.5-
    mental disorders (conditions in F01-F09, F20-F99) O99.34-
      alcohol use O99.31-
      drug use O99.32-
      smoking O99.33-
    mentum presentation O32.3
    metabolic disorders O99.28-
    missed
      abortion O02.1
      delivery O36.4
    multiple gestations O30.9-
      conjoined twins O30.02-
      quadruplet — *see* Pregnancy, quadruplet
      specified complication NEC O31.8x-
      specified number of multiples NEC — *see* Pregnancy, multiple (gestation), specified NEC

Pregnancy (childbirth) (labor) (puerperium) (*see also* Delivery and Puerperal) — *continued*
  complicated by (care of) (management affected by) — *continued*
    multiple gestations O30.9- — *continued*
      triplet — *see* Pregnancy, triplet
      twin — *see* Pregnancy, twin
    musculoskeletal condition (conditions is M00-M99) O99.89
    necrosis, liver (conditions in K72) O26.61-
    neoplasm
      benign
        cervix O34.4-
        corpus uteri O34.1-
        uterus O34.1-
      malignant O9A.11- *(follows O99)*
    nephropathy NEC O26.83-
    nervous system condition (conditions in G00-G99) O99.35-
    nutritional diseases NEC O99.28-
    obesity (pre-existing) O99.21-
    obesity surgery status O99.84-
    oblique lie or presentation O32.2
    older mother — *see* Pregnancy, complicated by, elderly
    oligohydramnios O41.0-
      with premature rupture of membranes (*see also* Pregnancy, complicated by, premature rupture of membranes) O42-
    onset (spontaneous) of labor after 37 completed weeks of gestation but before 39 completed weeks gestation, with delivery by (planned) cesarean section O75.82
    oophoritis O23.52-
    overdose, drug (*see also* Table of Drugs and Chemicals, by drug, poisoning) O9A.21- *(follows O99)*
    oversize fetus O33.5
    papyraceous fetus O31.0-
    pelvic inflammatory disease O99.89
    periodontal disease O99.61-
    peripheral neuritis O26.82-
    peritoneal (pelvic) adhesions O99.89
    phlebitis O22.9-
    phlebopathy O22.9-
    phlebothrombosis (superficial) O22.2-
      deep O22.3-
    placenta accreta O43.21-
    placenta increta O43.22-
    placenta percreta O43.23-
    placenta previa O44.0-
      complete O44.0-
        with hemorrhage O44.1-
      marginal O44.2-
        with hemorrhage O44.3-
      partial O44.2-
        with hemorrhage O44.3-
    placental disorder O43.9-
      specified NEC O43.89-
    placental dysfunction O43.89-
    placental infarction O43.81-
    placental insufficiency O36.51-
    placental transfusion syndromes
      fetomaternal O43.01-
      fetus to fetus O43.02-
      maternofetal O43.01-
    placentitis O41.14-
    pneumonia O99.51-
    poisoning (*see also* Table of Drugs and Chemicals) O9A.21- *(follows O99)*
    polyhydramnios O40-
    polymorphic eruption of pregnancy O26.86
    poor obstetric history NEC O09.29-
    postmaturity (post-term) (40 to 42 weeks) O48.0
      more than 42 completed weeks gestation (prolonged) O48.1

Pregnancy (childbirth) (labor) (puerperium) (*see also* Delivery and Puerperal) — *continued*
  complicated by (care of) (management affected by) — *continued*
    pre-eclampsia O14.9-
      mild O14.0-
      moderate O14.0-
      severe O14.1-
        with hemolysis, elevated liver enzymes and low platelet count (HELLP) O14.2-
    premature labor — *see* Pregnancy, complicated by, preterm labor
    premature rupture of membranes O42.90
      with onset of labor
        after 24 hours O42.10
          at or after 37 weeks gestation, onset of labor more than 24 hours following rupture O42.12
          pre-term (before 37 completed weeks of gestation) O42.11-
        within 24 hours O42.00
          at or after 37 weeks gestation, onset of labor within 24 hours of rupture O42.02
          pre-term (before 37 completed weeks of gestation) O42.01-
      at or after 37 weeks gestation, unspecified as to length of time between rupture and onset of labor O42.92
      full-term, unspecified as to length of time between rupture and onset of labor O42.92
      pre-term (before 37 completed weeks of gestation) O42.91-
    premature separation of placenta (*see also* Abruptio placentae) O45.9-
    presentation, fetal — *see* Delivery, complicated by, malposition
    preterm delivery O60.10
    preterm labor
      with delivery O60.10
        preterm O60.10
        term O60.20
      without delivery O60.00
        second trimester O60.02
        third trimester O60.03
      second trimester
        with preterm delivery
          second trimester O60.12
          third trimester O60.13
        with term delivery O60.22
        without delivery O60.02
      third trimester
        with term delivery O60.23
        with third trimester preterm delivery O60.14
        without delivery O60.03
    previous history of — *see* Pregnancy, supervision of, high-risk
    prolapse, uterus O34.52-
    proteinuria (gestational) (*see also* Proteinuria, gestational) O12.1-
      with edema O12.2-
    pruritic urticarial papules and plaques of pregnancy (PUPPP) O26.86
    pruritus (neurogenic) O26.89-
    psychosis or psychoneurosis (puerperal) F53
    ptyalism O26.89-
    PUPPP (pruritic urticarial papules and plaques of pregnancy) O26.86
    pyelitis O23.0-
    recurrent pregnancy loss O26.2-
    renal disease or failure NEC O26.83-
      with secondary hypertension, pre-existing — *see* Hypertension, complicating, pregnancy, pre-existing, secondary

D I S E A S E   I N D E X

3

Pregnancy (childbirth) (labor) (puerperium) (*see also* Delivery and Puerperal) — *continued*
complicated by (care of) (management affected by) — *continued*
  renal disease or failure NEC O26.83- — *continued*
    hypertensive, pre-existing — *see* Hypertension, complicating, pregnancy, pre-existing, with, renal disease
  respiratory condition (conditions in J00-J99) O99.51-
  retained, retention
    dead ovum O02.0
    intrauterine contraceptive device O26.3-
  retroversion, uterus O34.53-
  Rh immunization, incompatibility or sensitization NEC O36.09-
    anti-D antibody O36.01-
  rupture
    amnion (premature) (*see also* Pregnancy, complicated by, premature rupture of membranes) O42-
    membranes (premature) (*see also* Pregnancy, complicated by, premature rupture of membranes) O42-
    uterus (during labor) O71.1
      before onset of labor O71.0-
  salivation (excessive) O26.89-
  salpingitis O23.52-
  salpingo-oophoritis O23.52-
  sepsis (conditions in A40, A41) O98.81-
  size date discrepancy (uterine) O26.84-
  skin condition (conditions in L00-L99) O99.71-
  smoking (tobacco) O99.33-
  social problem O09.7-
  specified condition NEC O26.89-
  spotting O26.85-
  streptococcus group B (GBS) carrier state O99.820
  subluxation of symphysis (pubis) O26.71-
  syphilis (conditions in A50-A53) O98.11-
  threatened
    abortion O20.0
    labor O47.9
      at or after 37 completed weeks of gestation O47.1
      before 37 completed weeks of gestation O47.0-
  thrombophlebitis (superficial) O22.2-
  thrombosis O22.9-
    cerebral venous O22.5-
    cerebrovenous sinus O22.5-
    deep O22.3-
  tobacco use disorder (smoking) O99.33-
  torsion of uterus O34.59-
  toxemia O14.9-
  transverse lie or presentation O32.2
  tuberculosis (conditions in A15-A19) O98.01-
  tumor (benign)
    cervix O34.4-
      malignant O9A.11- *(follows O99)*
    uterus O34.1-
  unstable lie O32.0
  upper respiratory infection O99.51-
  urethritis O23.2-
  uterine size date discrepancy O26.84-
  vaginitis or vulvitis O23.59-
  varicose veins (lower extremities) O22.0-
    genitals O22.1-
    legs O22.0-
    perineal O22.1-
    vaginal or vulval O22.1-
  venereal disease NEC (conditions in A63.8) O98.31-
  venous disorders O22.9-
    specified NEC O22.8x-

Pregnancy (childbirth) (labor) (puerperium) (*see also* Delivery and Puerperal) — *continued*
complicated by (care of) (management affected by) — *continued*
  very young mother — *see* Pregnancy, complicated by, young mother
  viral diseases (conditions in A80-B09, B25-B34) O98.51-
  vomiting O21.9
    due to diseases classified elsewhere O21.8
    hyperemesis gravidarum (mild) (*see also* Hyperemesis, gravidarum) O21.0-
    late (occurring after 20 weeks of gestation) O21.2
  young mother
    multigravida O09.62-
    primigravida O09.61-
complicated NOS O26.9-
concealed O09.3-
continuing following
  elective fetal reduction of one or more fetus O31.3-
  intrauterine death of one or more fetus O31.2-
  spontaneous abortion of one or more fetus O31.1-
cornual O00.80
  with intrauterine pregnancy O00.81
ectopic (ruptured) O00.90
  with intrauterine pregnancy O00.91
  abdominal O00.00
    with
      intrauterine pregnancy O00.01
      viable fetus O36.7-
    cervical O00.80
      with intrauterine pregnancy O00.81
    complicated (by) O08.9
      afibrinogenemia O08.1
      cardiac arrest O08.81
      chemical damage of pelvic organ(s) O08.6
      circulatory collapse O08.3
      defibrination syndrome O08.1
      electrolyte imbalance O08.5
      embolism (amniotic fluid) (blood clot) (pulmonary) (septic) O08.2
      endometritis O08.0
      genital tract and pelvic infection O08.0
      hemorrhage (delayed) (excessive) O08.1
      infection
        genital tract or pelvic O08.0
        kidney O08.83
        urinary tract O08.83
      intravascular coagulation O08.1
      laceration of pelvic organ(s) O08.6
      metabolic disorder O08.5
      oliguria O08.4
      oophoritis O08.0
      parametritis O08.0
      pelvic peritonitis O08.0
      perforation of pelvic organ(s) O08.6
      renal failure or shutdown O08.4
      salpingitis or salpingo-oophoritis O08.0
      sepsis O08.82
      shock O08.83
        septic O08.82
      specified condition NEC O08.89
      tubular necrosis (renal) O08.4
      uremia O08.4
      urinary infection O08.83
      venous complication NEC O08.7
        embolism O08.2
    cornual O00.80
      with intrauterine pregnancy O00.81
    intraligamentous O00.80
      with intrauterine pregnancy O00.81
    mural O00.80
      with intrauterine pregnancy O00.81

Pregnancy (childbirth) (labor) (puerperium) (*see also* Delivery and Puerperal) — *continued*
ectopic (ruptured) O00.90 — *continued*
  ovarian O00.20
    with intrauterine pregnancy O00.21
  specified site NEC O00.80
    with intrauterine pregnancy O00.81
  tubal (ruptured) O00.10
    with intrauterine pregnancy O00.11
examination (normal) Z34.9-
  first Z34.0-
  high-risk — *see* Pregnancy, supervision of, high-risk
  specified Z34.8-
extrauterine — *see* Pregnancy, ectopic
fallopian O00.10
  with intrauterine pregnancy O00.11
false F45.8
gestational carrier Z33.3
hidden O09.3-
high-risk — *see* Pregnancy, supervision of, high-risk
incidental finding Z33.1
interstitial O00.80
  with intrauterine pregnancy O00.81
intraligamentous O00.80
  with intrauterine pregnancy O00.81
intramural O00.80
  with intrauterine pregnancy O00.81
intraperitoneal O00.00
  with intrauterine pregnancy O00.01
isthmian O00.10
  with intrauterine pregnancy O00.11
mesometric (mural) O00.80
  with intrauterine pregnancy O00.81
molar NEC O02.0
  complicated (by) O08.9
    afibrinogenemia O08.1
    cardiac arrest O08.81
    chemical damage of pelvic organ(s) O08.6
    circulatory collapse O08.3
    defibrination syndrome O08.1
    electrolyte imbalance O08.5
    embolism (amniotic fluid) (blood clot) (pulmonary) (septic) O08.2
    endometritis O08.0
    genital tract and pelvic infection O08.0
    hemorrhage (delayed) (excessive) O08.1
    infection
      genital tract or pelvic O08.0
      kidney O08.83
      urinary tract O08.83
    intravascular coagulation O08.1
    laceration of pelvic organ(s) O08.6
    metabolic disorder O08.5
    oliguria O08.4
    oophoritis O08.0
    parametritis O08.0
    pelvic peritonitis O08.0
    perforation of pelvic organ(s) O08.6
    renal failure or shutdown O08.4
    salpingitis or salpingo-oophoritis O08.0
    sepsis O08.82
    shock O08.3
      septic O08.82
    specified condition NEC O08.89
    tubular necrosis (renal) O08.4
    uremia O08.4
    urinary infection O08.83
    venous complication NEC O08.7
      embolism O08.2
  hydatidiform (*see also* Mole, hydatidiform) O01.9-
multiple (gestation) O30.9-
  greater than quadruplets — *see* Pregnancy, multiple (gestation), specified NEC

Pregnancy (childbirth) (labor) (puerperium) (*see also* Delivery and Puerperal) — *continued*
multiple (gestation) O30.9- — *continued*
  specified NEC O30.80-
    with
      two or more monoamniotic fetuses O30.82-
      two or more monochorionic fetuses O30.81-
    two or more monoamniotic fetuses O30.82-
    two or more monochorionic fetuses O30.81-
    unable to determine number of placenta and number of amniotic sacs O30.89-
    unspecified number of placenta and unspecified number of amniotic sacs O30.80-
  mural O00.80
    with intrauterine pregnancy O00.81
  normal (supervision of) Z34.9-
    first Z34.0-
    high-risk — *see* Pregnancy, supervision of, high-risk
    specified Z34.8-
  ovarian O00.20
    with intrauterine pregnancy O00.21
  postmature (40 to 42 weeks) O48.0
    more than 42 weeks gestation O48.1
  post-term (40 to 42 weeks) O48.0
  prenatal care only Z34.9-
    first Z34.0-
    high-risk — *see* Pregnancy, supervision of, high-risk
    specified Z34.8-
  prolonged (more than 42 weeks gestation) O48.1
  quadruplet O30.20-
    with
      two or more monoamniotic fetuses O30.22-
      two or more monochorionic fetuses O30.21-
    two or more monoamniotic fetuses O30.22-
    two or more monochorionic fetuses O30.21-
    unable to determine number of placenta and number of amniotic sacs O30.29-
    unspecified number of placenta and unspecified number of amniotic sacs O30.20-
  quintuplet — *see* Pregnancy, multiple (gestation), specified NEC
  sextuplet — *see* Pregnancy, multiple (gestation), specified NEC
  supervision of
    concealed pregnancy O09.3-
    elderly mother
      multigravida O09.52-
      primigravida O09.51-
    hidden pregnancy O09.3-
    high-risk O09.9-
      due to (history of)
        ectopic pregnancy O09.1-
        elderly — *see* Pregnancy, supervision of, elderly mother
        grand multiparity O09.4
        in utero procedure during previous pregnancy O09.82-
        in vitro fertilization O09.81-
        infertility O09.0-
        insufficient prenatal care O09.3-
        molar pregnancy O09.A- *(follows O09.1)*
        multiple previous pregnancies O09.4-
        older mother — *see* Pregnancy, supervision of, elderly mother
        poor reproductive or obstetric history NEC O09.29-
        pre-term labor O09.21-

Pregnancy (childbirth) (labor) (puerperium) (*see also* Delivery and Puerperal) — *continued*
supervision of — *continued*
  high-risk O09.9- — *continued*
    due to (history of) — *continued*
      previous
        neonatal death O09.29-
        social problems O09.7-
      specified NEC O09.89-
      very young mother — *see* Pregnancy, supervision of, young mother
    resulting from in vitro fertilization O09.81-
  normal Z34.9-
    first Z34.0-
    specified NEC Z34.8-
  young mother
    multigravida O09.62-
    primigravida O09.61-
triplet O30.10-
  with
    two or more monoamniotic fetuses O30.12-
    two or more monochrorionic fetuses O30.11-
  two or more monoamniotic fetuses O30.12-
  two or more monochrorionic fetuses O30.11-
  unable to determine number of placenta and number of amniotic sacs O30.19-
  unspecified number of placenta and unspecified number of amniotic sacs O30.10-
tubal (with abortion) (with rupture) O00.10
  with intrauterine pregnancy O00.11
twin O30.00-
  conjoined O30.02-
  dichorionic/diamniotic (two placenta, two amniotic sacs) O30.04-
  monochorionic/diamniotic (one placenta, two amniotic sacs) O30.03-
  monochorionic/monoamniotic (one placenta, one amniotic sac) O30.01-
  unable to determine number of placenta and number of amniotic sacs O30.09-
  unspecified number of placenta and unspecified number of amniotic sacs O30.00-
unwanted Z64.0
weeks of gestation
  8 weeks Z3A.08 *(follows Z36)*
  9 weeks Z3A.09 *(follows Z36)*
  10 weeks Z3A.10 *(follows Z36)*
  11 weeks Z3A.11 *(follows Z36)*
  12 weeks Z3A.12 *(follows Z36)*
  13 weeks Z3A.13 *(follows Z36)*
  14 weeks Z3A.14 *(follows Z36)*
  15 weeks Z3A.15 *(follows Z36)*
  16 weeks Z3A.16 *(follows Z36)*
  17 weeks Z3A.17 *(follows Z36)*
  18 weeks Z3A.18 *(follows Z36)*
  19 weeks Z3A.19 *(follows Z36)*
  20 weeks Z3A.20 *(follows Z36)*
  21 weeks Z3A.21 *(follows Z36)*
  22 weeks Z3A.22 *(follows Z36)*
  23 weeks Z3A.23 *(follows Z36)*
  24 weeks Z3A.24 *(follows Z36)*
  25 weeks Z3A.25 *(follows Z36)*
  26 weeks Z3A.26 *(follows Z36)*
  27 weeks Z3A.27 *(follows Z36)*
  28 weeks Z3A.28 *(follows Z36)*
  29 weeks Z3A.29 *(follows Z36)*
  30 weeks Z3A.30 *(follows Z36)*
  31 weeks Z3A.31 *(follows Z36)*
  32 weeks Z3A.32 *(follows Z36)*
  33 weeks Z3A.33 *(follows Z36)*
  34 weeks Z3A.34 *(follows Z36)*
  35 weeks Z3A.35 *(follows Z36)*
  36 weeks Z3A.36 *(follows Z36)*
  37 weeks Z3A.37 *(follows Z36)*

Pregnancy (childbirth) (labor) (puerperium) (*see also* Delivery and Puerperal) — *continued*
weeks of gestation — *continued*
  38 weeks Z3A.38 *(follows Z36)*
  39 weeks Z3A.39 *(follows Z36)*
  40 weeks Z3A.40 *(follows Z36)*
  41 weeks Z3A.41 *(follows Z36)*
  42 weeks Z3A.42 *(follows Z36)*
  greater than 42 weeks Z3A.49 *(follows Z36)*
  less than 8 weeks Z3A.01 *(follows Z36)*
  not specified Z3A.00 *(follows Z36)*
Preiser's disease — *see* Osteonecrosis, secondary, due to, trauma, metacarpus
Pre-kwashiorkor — *see* Malnutrition, severe
Preleukemia (syndrome) D46.9
Preluxation, hip, congenital Q65.6
Premature — *see also* condition
  adrenarche E27.0
  aging E34.8
  beats I49.40
    atrial I49.1
    auricular I49.1
    supraventricular I49.1
  birth NEC — *see* Preterm, newborn
  closure, foramen ovale Q21.8
  contraction
    atrial I49.1
    atrioventricular I49.2
    auricular I49.1
    auriculoventricular I49.49
    heart (extrasystole) I49.49
    junctional I49.2
    ventricular I49.3
  delivery (*see also* Pregnancy, complicated by, preterm labor) O60.10
  ejaculation F52.4
  infant NEC — *see* Preterm, newborn
    light-for-dates — *see* Light for dates
  labor — *see* Pregnancy, complicated by, preterm labor
  lungs P28.0
  menopause E28.319
    asymptomatic E28.319
    symptomatic E28.310
  newborn
    extreme (less than 28 completed weeks) — *see* Immaturity, extreme
    less than 37 completed weeks — *see* Preterm, newborn
  puberty E30.1
  rupture membranes or amnion — *see* Pregnancy, complicated by, premature rupture of membranes
  senility E34.8
  thelarche E30.8
  ventricular systole I49.3
Prematurity NEC (less than 37 completed weeks) — *see* Preterm, newborn
  extreme (less than 28 completed weeks) — *see* Immaturity, extreme
Premenstrual
  dysphoric disorder (PMDD) F32.81
  tension (syndrome) N94.3
Premolarization, cuspids K00.2
Prenatal
  care, normal pregnancy — *see* Pregnancy, normal
  screening of mother Z36
  teeth K00.6
Preparatory care for subsequent treatment NEC
  for dialysis Z49.01
    peritoneal Z49.02
Prepartum — *see* condition
Preponderance, left or right ventricular I51.7
Prepuce — *see* condition
PRES (posterior reversible encephalopathy syndrome) I67.83

DISEASE INDEX

Presbycardia R54
Presbycusis, presbyacusia H91.1-
Presbyesophagus K22.8
Presbyophrenia F03
Presbyopia H52.4
Prescription of contraceptives (initial)
Z30.019
  barrier Z30.018
  diaphragm Z30.018
  emergency (postcoital) Z30.012
  implantable subdermal Z30.017
  injectable Z30.013
  intrauterine contraceptive device Z30.014
  pills Z30.011
  postcoital (emergency) Z30.012
  repeat Z30.40
    barrier Z30.49
    diaphragm Z30.49
    implantable subdermal Z30.46
    injectable Z30.42
    pills Z30.41
    specified type NEC Z30.49
    transdermal patch hormonal Z30.45
    vaginal ring hormonal Z30.44
  specified type NEC Z30.018
    transdermal patch hormonal Z30.016
    vaginal ring hormonal Z30.015
Presence (of)
  ankle-joint implant (functional) (prosthesis)
    Z96.66-
  aortocoronary (bypass) graft Z95.1
  arterial-venous shunt (dialysis) Z99.2
  artificial
    eye (globe) Z97.0
    heart (fully implantable) (mechanical)
      Z95.812
      valve Z95.2
    larynx Z96.3
    lens (intraocular) Z96.1
    limb (complete) (partial) Z97.1-
      arm Z97.1-
        bilateral Z97.15
      leg Z97.1-
        bilateral Z97.16
  audiological implant (functional) Z96.29
  bladder implant (functional) Z96.0
  bone
    conduction hearing device Z96.29
    implant (functional) NEC Z96.7
    joint (prosthesis) — see Presence, joint
      implant
  cardiac
    defibrillator (functional) (with synchronous
      cardiac pacemaker) Z95.810
    implant or graft Z95.9
      specified type NEC Z95.818
    pacemaker Z95.0
    resynchronization therapy
      defibrillator Z95.810
      pacemaker Z95.0
  cardioverter-defibrillator (ICD) Z95.810
  cerebrospinal fluid drainage device Z98.2
  cochlear implant (functional) Z96.21
  contact lens(es) Z97.3
  coronary artery graft or prosthesis Z95.5
  CRT-D (cardiac resynchronization therapy
    defibrillator) Z95.810
  CRT-P (cardiac resynchronization therapy
    pacemaker) Z95.0
  CSF shunt Z98.2
  dental prosthesis device Z97.2
  dentures Z97.2
  device (external) NEC Z97.8
    cardiac NEC Z95.818
    heart assist Z95.811
    implanted (functional) Z96.9
      specified NEC Z96.89
    prosthetic Z97.8

Presence (of) — continued
  ear implant Z96.20
    cochlear implant Z96.21
    myringotomy tube Z96.22
    specified type NEC Z96.29
  elbow-joint implant (functional) (prosthesis)
    Z96.62-
  endocrine implant (functional) NEC Z96.49
  eustachian tube stent or device (functional)
    Z96.29
  external hearing-aid or device Z97.4
  finger-joint implant (functional) (prosthetic)
    Z96.69-
  functional implant Z96.9
    specified NEC Z96.89
  graft
    cardiac NEC Z95.818
    vascular NEC Z95.828
  hearing-aid or device (external) Z97.4
    implant (bone) (cochlear) (functional)
      Z96.21
  heart assist device Z95.811
  heart valve implant (functional) Z95.2
    prosthetic Z95.2
    specified type NEC Z95.4
    xenogenic Z95.3
  hip-joint implant (functional) (prosthesis)
    Z96.64-
  ICD (cardioverter-defibrillator) Z95.810
  implanted device (artificial) (functional)
    (prosthetic) Z96.9
    automatic cardiac defibrillator (with
      synchronous cardiac pacemaker)
      Z95.810
    cardiac pacemaker Z95.0
    cochlear Z96.21
    dental Z96.5
    heart Z95.812
    heart valve Z95.2
      prosthetic Z95.2
      specified NEC Z95.4
      xenogenic Z95.3
    insulin pump Z96.41
    intraocular lens Z96.1
    joint Z96.60
      ankle Z96.66-
      elbow Z96.62-
      finger Z96.69-
      hip Z96.64-
      knee Z96.65-
      shoulder Z96.61-
      specified NEC Z96.698
      wrist Z96.63-
    larynx Z96.3
    myringotomy tube Z96.22
    otological Z96.20
      cochlear Z96.21
      eustachian stent Z96.29
      myringotomy Z96.22
      specified NEC Z96.29
      stapes Z96.29
    skin Z96.81
    skull plate Z96.7
    specified NEC Z96.89
    urogenital Z96.0
  insulin pump (functional) Z96.41
  intestinal bypass or anastomosis Z98.0
  intraocular lens (functional) Z96.1
  intrauterine contraceptive device (IUD) Z97.5
  intravascular implant (functional) (prosthetic)
    NEC Z95.9
    coronary artery Z95.5
    defibrillator (with synchronous cardiac
      pacemaker) Z95.810
    peripheral vessel (with angioplasty) Z95.820
  joint implant (prosthetic) (any) Z96.60
    ankle — see Presence, ankle joint implant
    elbow — see Presence, elbow joint implant
    finger — see Presence, finger joint implant

Presence (of) — continued
  joint implant (prosthetic) (any) Z96.60 —
    continued
    hip — see Presence, hip joint implant
    knee — see Presence, knee joint implant
    shoulder — see Presence, shoulder joint
      implant
    specified joint NEC Z96.698
    wrist — see Presence, wrist joint implant
  knee-joint implant (functional) (prosthesis)
    Z96.65-
  laryngeal implant (functional) Z96.3
  mandibular implant (dental) Z96.5
  myringotomy tube(s) Z96.22
  orthopedic-joint implant (prosthetic) (any) —
    see Presence, joint implant
  otological implant (functional) Z96.29
  shoulder-joint implant (functional) (prosthesis)
    Z96.61-
  skull-plate implant Z96.7
  spectacles Z97.3
  stapes implant (functional) Z96.29
  systemic lupus erythematosus [SLE] inhibitor
    D68.62
  tendon implant (functional) (graft) Z96.7
  tooth root(s) implant Z96.5
  ureteral stent Z96.0
  urethral stent Z96.0
  urogenital implant (functional) Z96.0
  vascular implant or device Z95.9
    access port device Z95.828
    specified type NEC Z95.828
  wrist-joint implant (functional) (prosthesis)
    Z96.63-
Presenile — see also condition
  dementia F03
  premature aging E34.8
Presentation, fetal — see Delivery,
  complicated by, malposition
Prespondylolisthesis (congenital) Q76.2
Pressure
  area, skin — see Ulcer, pressure, by site
  brachial plexus G54.0
  brain G93.5
    injury at birth NEC P11.1
  cerebral — see Pressure, brain
  chest R07.89
  cone, tentorial G93.5
  hyposystolic — see also Hypotension
    incidental reading, without diagnosis of
      hypotension R03.1
  increased
    intracranial (benign) G93.2
      injury at birth P11.0
    intraocular H40.05-
  lumbosacral plexus G54.1
  mediastinum J98.59
  necrosis (chronic) — see Ulcer, pressure, by site
  parental, inappropriate (excessive) Z62.6
  sore (chronic) — see Ulcer, pressure, by site
  spinal cord G95.20
  ulcer (chronic) — see Ulcer, pressure, by site
  venous, increased I87.8
Pre-syncope R55
Preterm
  delivery (see also Pregnancy, complicated by,
    preterm labor) O60.10
  labor — see Pregnancy, complicated by,
    preterm labor
  newborn (infant) P07.30
    gestational age
      28 completed weeks (28 weeks, 0 days
        through 28 weeks, 6 days) P07.31
      29 completed weeks (29 weeks, 0 days
        through 29 weeks, 6 days) P07.32
      30 completed weeks (30 weeks, 0 days
        through 30 weeks, 6 days) P07.33
      31 completed weeks (31 weeks, 0 days
        through 31 weeks, 6 days) P07.34

Preterm — *continued*
  newborn (infant) P07.30 — *continued*
    gestational age — *continued*
      32 completed weeks (32 weeks, 0 days
        through 32 weeks, 6 days) P07.35
      33 completed weeks (33 weeks, 0 days
        through 33 weeks, 6 days) P07.36
      34 completed weeks (34 weeks, 0 days
        through 34 weeks, 6 days) P07.37
      35 completed weeks (35 weeks, 0 days
        through 35 weeks, 6 days) P07.38
      36 completed weeks (36 weeks, 0 days
        through 36 weeks, 6 days) P07.39

Previa
  placenta (total) (with hemorrhage) O44.0-
    with hemorrhage O44.1-
    complete O44.0-
      with hemorrhage O44.1-
    low (see also Delivery, complicated, by,
      placenta, low) O44.4-
      with hemorrhage O44.5-
    marginal O44.2-
      with hemorrhage O44.3-
    partial O44.2-
      with hemorrhage O44.3-
  vasa O69.4

Priapism N48.30
  due to
    disease classified elsewhere N48.32
    drug N48.33
    specified cause NEC N48.39
    trauma N48.31

Prickling sensation (skin) R20.2
Prickly heat L74.0
Primary — *see* condition
Primigravida
  elderly, affecting management of pregnancy,
    labor and delivery (supervision only) —
    see Pregnancy, complicated by, elderly,
    primigravida
  older, affecting management of pregnancy,
    labor and delivery (supervision only) —
    see Pregnancy, complicated by, elderly,
    primigravida
  very young, affecting management of
    pregnancy, labor and delivery
    (supervision only) — *see* Pregnancy,
    complicated by, young mother,
    primigravida

Primipara
  elderly, affecting management of pregnancy,
    labor and delivery (supervision only) —
    see Pregnancy, complicated by, elderly,
    primigravida
  older, affecting management of pregnancy,
    labor and delivery (supervision only) —
    see Pregnancy, complicated by, elderly,
    primigravida
  very young, affecting management of
    pregnancy, labor and delivery
    (supervision only) — *see* Pregnancy,
    complicated by, young mother,
    primigravida

Primus varus (bilateral) Q66.2
PRIND (prolonged reversible ischemic
  neurologic deficit) I63.9
Pringle's disease (tuberous sclerosis) Q85.1
Prinzmetal angina I20.1
Prizefighter ear — *see* Cauliflower ear
Problem (with) (related to)
  academic Z55.8
  acculturation Z60.3
  adjustment (to)
    change of job Z56.1
    life-cycle transition Z60.0
    pension Z60.0
    retirement Z60.0
  adopted child Z62.821
  alcoholism in family Z63.72

Problem (with) (related to) — *continued*
  atypical parenting situation Z62.9
  bankruptcy Z59.8
  behavioral (adult) F69
    drug seeking Z76.5
  birth of sibling affecting child Z62.898
  care (of)
    provider dependency Z74.9
      specified NEC Z74.8
    sick or handicapped person in family or
      household Z63.6
  child
    abuse (affecting the child) — *see*
      Maltreatment, child
    custody or support proceedings Z65.3
    in care of non-parental family member
      Z62.21
    in foster care Z62.21
    in welfare custody Z62.21
    living in orphanage or group home Z62.22
  child-rearing Z62.9
    specified NEC Z62.898
  communication (developmental) F80.9
  conflict or discord (with)
    boss Z56.4
    classmates Z55.4
    counselor Z64.4
    employer Z56.4
    family Z63.9
      specified NEC Z63.8
    probation officer Z64.4
    social worker Z64.4
    teachers Z55.4
    workmates Z56.4
  conviction in legal proceedings Z65.0
    with imprisonment Z65.1
  counselor Z64.4
  creditors Z59.8
  digestive K92.9
  drug addict in family Z63.72
  ear — *see* Disorder, ear
  economic Z59.9
    affecting care Z59.9
    specified NEC Z59.8
  education Z55.9
    specified NEC Z55.8
  employment Z56.9
    change of job Z56.1
    discord Z56.4
    environment Z56.5
    sexual harassment Z56.81
    specified NEC Z56.89
    stress NEC Z56.6
    stressful schedule Z56.3
    threat of job loss Z56.2
    unemployment Z56.0
  enuresis, child F98.0
  eye H57.9
  failed examinations (school) Z55.2
  falling Z91.81
  family (*see also* Disruption, family) Z63.9-
    specified NEC Z63.8
  feeding (elderly) (infant) R63.3
    newborn P92.9
      breast P92.5
      overfeeding P92.4
      slow P92.2
      specified NEC P92.8
      underfeeding P92.3
    nonorganic F50.89
  finance Z59.9
    specified NEC Z59.8
  foreclosure on loan Z59.8
  foster child Z62.822
  frightening experience(s) in childhood
    Z62.898
  genital NEC
    female N94.9
    male N50.9

Problem (with) (related to) — *continued*
  health care Z75.9
    specified NEC Z75.8
  hearing — *see* Deafness
  homelessness Z59.0
  housing Z59.9
    inadequate Z59.1
    isolated Z59.8
    specified NEC Z59.8
  identity (of childhood) F93.8
  illegitimate pregnancy (unwanted) Z64.0
  illiteracy Z55.0
  impaired mobility Z74.09
  imprisonment or incarceration Z65.1
  inadequate teaching affecting education Z55.8
  inappropriate (excessive) parental pressure
    Z62.6
  influencing health status NEC Z78.9
  in-law Z63.1
  institutionalization, affecting child Z62.22
  intrafamilial communication Z63.8
  jealousy, child F93.8
  landlord Z59.2
  language (developmental) F80.9
  learning (developmental) F81.9
  legal Z65.3
    conviction without imprisonment Z65.0
    imprisonment Z65.1
    release from prison Z65.2
  life-management Z73.9
    specified NEC Z73.89
  life-style Z72.9
    gambling Z72.6
    high-risk sexual behavior (heterosexual)
      Z72.51
      bisexual Z72.53
      homosexual Z72.52
    inappropriate eating habits Z72.4
    self-damaging behavior NEC Z72.89
    specified NEC Z72.89
    tobacco use Z72.0
  literacy Z55.9
    low level Z55.0
    specified NEC Z55.8
  living alone Z60.2
  lodgers Z59.2
  loss of love relationship in childhood Z62.898
  marital Z63.0
    involving
      divorce Z63.5
      estrangement Z63.5
      gender identity F66
  mastication K08.89
  medical
    care, within family Z63.6
    facilities Z75.9
      specified NEC Z75.8
  mental F48.9
  multiparity Z64.1
  negative life events in childhood Z62.9
    altered pattern of family relationships
      Z62.898
    frightening experience Z62.898
    loss of
      love relationship Z62.898
      self-esteem Z62.898
    physical abuse (alleged) — *see*
      Maltreatment, child
    removal from home Z62.29
    specified event NEC Z62.898
  neighbor Z59.2
  neurological NEC R29.818
  new step-parent affecting child Z62.898
  none (feared complaint unfounded) Z71.1
  occupational NEC Z56.89
  parent-child — *see* Conflict, parent-child
  personal hygiene Z91.89
  personality F69
  phase-of-life transition, adjustment Z60.0

Problem (with) (related to) — *continued*
  presence of sick or disabled person in family
    or household Z63.79
    needing care Z63.6
  primary support group (family) Z63.9
    specified NEC Z63.8
  probation officer Z64.4
  psychiatric F99
  psychosexual (development) F66
  psychosocial Z65.9
    specified NEC Z65.8
  relationship Z63.9
    childhood F93.8
  release from prison Z65.2
  removal from home affecting child Z62.29
  seeking and accepting known hazardous and
    harmful
    behavioral or psychological interventions
      Z65.8
    chemical, nutritional or physical
      interventions Z65.8
  sexual function (nonorganic) F52.9
  sight H54.7
  sleep disorder, child F51.9
  smell — *see* Disturbance, sensation, smell
  social
    environment Z60.9
      specified NEC Z60.8
    exclusion and rejection Z60.4
    worker Z64.4
  speech R47.9
    developmental F80.9
    specified NEC R47.89
  swallowing — *see* Dysphagia
  taste — *see* Disturbance, sensation, taste
  tic, child F95.0
  underachievement in school Z55.3
  unemployment Z56.0
    threatened Z56.2
  unwanted pregnancy Z64.0
  upbringing Z62.9
    specified NEC Z62.898
  urinary N39.9
  voice production R47.89
  work schedule (stressful) Z56.3
Procedure (surgical)
  converted
    arthroscopic to open Z53.33
    laparoscopic to open Z53.31
    specified procedure NEC to open Z53.39
    thoracoscopic to open Z53.32
  for purpose other than remedying health state
    Z41.9
    specified NEC Z41.8
  not done Z53.9
    because of
      administrative reasons Z53.8
      contraindication Z53.09
        smoking Z53.01
      patient's decision Z53.20
        for reasons of belief or group pressure
          Z53.1
        left against medical advice (AMA)
          Z53.21
        specified reason NEC Z53.29
      specified reason NEC Z53.8
Procidentia (uteri) N81.3
Proctalgia K62.89
  fugax K59.4
  spasmodic K59.4
Proctitis K62.89
  amebic (acute) A06.0
  chlamydial A56.3
  gonococcal A54.6
  granulomatous — *see* Enteritis, regional, large
    intestine
  herpetic A60.1
  radiation K62.7
  tuberculous A18.32

Proctitis K62.89 — *continued*
  ulcerative (chronic) K51.20
    with
      complication K51.219
        abscess K51.214
        fistula K51.213
        obstruction K51.212
        rectal bleeding K51.211
        specified NEC K51.218
Proctocele
  female (without uterine prolapse) N81.6
    with uterine prolapse N81.2
      complete N81.3
  male K62.3
Proctocolitis
  food-induced eosinophilic K52.82
  food protein-induced K52.82
  milk protein-induced K52.82
  mucosal — *see* Rectosigmoiditis, ulcerative
Proctocolitis, mucosal — *see*
  Rectosigmoiditis, ulcerative
Proctoptosis K62.3
Proctorrhagia K62.5
Proctosigmoiditis K63.89
  ulcerative (chronic) — *see* Rectosigmoiditis,
    ulcerative
Proctospasm K59.4
  psychogenic F45.8
Profichet's disease — *see* Disorder, soft
  tissue, specified type NEC
Progeria E34.8
Prognathism (mandibular) (maxillary)
  M26.19
Progonoma (melanotic) — *see* Neoplasm,
  benign, by site
Progressive — *see* condition
Prolactinoma
  specified site — *see* Neoplasm, benign, by site
  unspecified site D35.2
Prolapse, prolapsed
  anus, anal (canal) (sphincter) K62.2
  arm or hand O32.2
    causing obstructed labor O64.4
  bladder (mucosa) (sphincter) (acquired)
    congenital Q79.4
    female — *see* Cystocele
    male N32.89
  breast implant (prosthetic) T85.49
  cecostomy K94.09
  cecum K63.4
  cervix, cervical (hypertrophied) N81.2
    anterior lip, obstructing labor O65.5
    congenital Q51.828
    postpartal, old N81.2
    stump N81.85
  ciliary body (traumatic) — *see* Laceration,
    eye(ball), with prolapse or loss of
    interocular tissue
  colon (pedunculated) K63.4
  colostomy K94.09
  disc (intervertebral) — *see* Displacement,
    intervertebral disc
  eye implant (orbital) T85.398
    lens (ocular) — *see* Complications,
      intraocular lens
  fallopian tube N83.4-
  gastric (mucosa) K31.89
  genital, female N81.9
    specified NEC N81.89
  globe, nontraumatic — *see* Luxation, globe
  ileostomy bud K94.19
  intervertebral disc — *see* Displacement,
    intervertebral disc
  intestine (small) K63.4
  iris (traumatic) — *see* Laceration, eye(ball),
    with prolapse or loss of interocular tissue
    nontraumatic H21.89
  kidney N28.83
    congenital Q63.2

Prolapse, prolapsed — *continued*
  laryngeal muscles or ventricle J38.7
  liver K76.89
  meatus urinarius N36.8
  mitral (valve) I34.1
  ocular lens implant — *see* Complications,
    intraocular lens
  organ or site, congenital NEC — *see*
    Malposition, congenital
  ovary N83.4-
  pelvic floor, female N81.89
  perineum, female N81.89
  rectum (mucosa) (sphincter) K62.3
    due to trichuris trichuria B79
  spleen D73.89
  stomach K31.89
  umbilical cord
    complicating delivery O69.0
  urachus, congenital Q64.4
  ureter N28.89
    with obstruction N13.5
      with infection N13.6
  ureterovesical orifice N28.89
  urethra (acquired) (infected) (mucosa) N36.8
    congenital Q64.71
  urinary meatus N36.8
    congenital Q64.72
  uterovaginal N81.4
    complete N81.3
    incomplete N81.2
  uterus (with prolapse of vagina) N81.4
    complete N81.3
    congenital Q51.818
    first degree N81.2
    in pregnancy or childbirth — *see* Pregnancy,
      complicated by, abnormal, uterus
    incomplete N81.2
    postpartal (old) N81.4
    second degree N81.2
    third degree N81.3
  uveal (traumatic) — *see* Laceration, eye(ball),
    with prolapse or loss of interocular tissue
  vagina (anterior) (wall) — *see* Cystocele
    with prolapse of uterus N81.4
      complete N81.3
      incomplete N81.2
    posterior wall N81.6
    posthysterectomy N99.3
  vitreous (humor) H43.0-
    in wound — *see* Laceration, eye(ball), with
      prolapse or loss of interocular tissue
  womb — *see* Prolapse, uterus
Prolapsus, female N81.9
  specified NEC N81.89
Proliferation(s)
  primary cutaneous CD30-positive large T-cell
    C86.6
  prostate, atypical small acinar N42.32
Proliferative — *see* condition
Prolonged, prolongation (of)
  bleeding (time) (idiopathic) R79.1
  coagulation (time) R79.1
  gestation (over 42 completed weeks)
    mother O48.1
    newborn P08.22
  interval I44.0
  labor O63.9
    first stage O63.0
    second stage O63.1
  partial thromboplastin time (PTT) R79.1
  pregnancy (more than 42 weeks gestation)
    O48.1
  prothrombin time R79.1
  QT interval I45.81
  uterine contractions in labor O62.4

Prominence, prominent
with disproportion (fetopelvic) O33.0
  causing obstructed labor O65.0
auricle (congenital) (ear) Q17.5
ischial spine or sacral promontory
nose (congenital) acquired M95.0
Promiscuity — *see* High, risk, sexual behavior
Pronation
ankle — *see* Deformity, limb, foot, specified NEC
foot — *see also* Deformity, limb, foot, specified NEC
  congenital Q74.2
Prophylactic
administration of
  antibiotics, long-term Z79.2
    short-term use — *omit code*
  drug (*see also* Long-term (current) drug therapy (use of)) Z79.899-
medication Z79.899
organ removal (for neoplasia management) Z40.00
  breast Z40.01
  ovary Z40.02
  specified site NEC Z40.09
surgery Z40.9
  for risk factors related to malignant neoplasm — *see* Prophylactic, organ removal
  specified NEC Z40.8
vaccination Z23
Propionic acidemia E71.121
Proptosis (ocular) — *see also* Exophthalmos
thyroid — *see* Hyperthyroidism, with goiter
Prosecution, anxiety concerning Z65.3
Prosopagnosia R48.3
Prostadynia N42.81
Prostate, prostatic — *see* condition
Prostatism — *see* Hyperplasia, prostate
Prostatitis (congestive) (suppurative) (with cystitis) N41.9
acute N41.0
cavitary N41.8
chronic N41.1
diverticular N41.8
due to Trichomonas (vaginalis) A59.02
fibrous N41.1
gonococcal (acute) (chronic) A54.22
granulomatous N41.4
hypertrophic N41.1
subacute N41.1
trichomonal A59.02
tuberculous A18.14
Prostatocystitis N41.3
Prostatorrhea N42.89
Prostatosis N42.82
Prostration R53.83
heat — *see also* Heat, exhaustion
  anhydrotic T67.3
  due to
    salt (and water) depletion T67.4
    water depletion T67.3
nervous F48.8
senile R54
Protanomaly (anomalous trichromat) H53.54
Protanopia (complete) (incomplete) H53.54
Protection (against) (from) — *see* Prophylactic
Protein
deficiency NEC — *see* Malnutrition
malnutrition — *see* Malnutrition
sickness (*see also* Reaction, serum) T80.69
Proteinemia R77.9
Proteinosis
alveolar (pulmonary) J84.01
lipid or lipoid (of Urbach) E78.89
Proteinuria R80.9
Bence Jones R80.3
complicating pregnancy — *see* Proteinuria, gestational

Proteinuria R80.9 — *continued*
gestational
complicating
  childbirth O12.14
  pregnancy O12.1-
    with edema O12.2-
  puerperium O12.15
idiopathic R80.0
isolated R80.0
with glomerular lesion N06.9
  dense deposit disease N06.6
  diffuse
    crescentic glomerulonephritis N06.7
    endocapillary proliferative glomerulonephritis N06.4
    mesangiocapillary glomerulonephritis N06.5
  focal and segmental hyalinosis or sclerosis N06.1
  membranous (diffuse) N06.2
  mesangial proliferative (diffuse) N06.3
  minimal change N06.0
  specified pathology NEC N06.8
orthostatic R80.2
with glomerular lesion — *see* Proteinuria, isolated, with glomerular lesion
persistent R80.1
with glomerular lesion — *see* Proteinuria, isolated, with glomerular lesion
postural R80.2
with glomerular lesion — *see* Proteinuria, isolated, with glomerular lesion
pre-eclamptic — *see* Pre-eclampsia
puerperal O12.15
specified type NEC R80.8
Proteolysis, pathologic D65
Proteus (mirabilis) (morganii), as cause of disease classified elsewhere B96.4
Prothrombin gene mutation D68.52
Protoporphyria, erythropoietic E80.0
Protozoal — *see also* condition
disease B64
  specified NEC B60.8
Protrusion, protrusio
acetabuli M24.7
acetabulum (into pelvis) M24.7
device, implant or graft (*see also* Complications, by site and type, mechanical) T85.698
  arterial graft NEC — *see* Complication, cardiovascular device, mechanical, vascular
  breast (implant) T85.49
  catheter NEC T85.698
    cystostomy T83.090
    dialysis (renal) T82.49
      intraperitoneal T85.691
    infusion NEC T82.594
      spinal (epidural) (subdural) T85.690
    urinary (*see also* Complications, catheter, urinary) T83.098
  electronic (electrode) (pulse generator) (stimulator)
    bone T84.390
    nervous system — *see* Complication, prosthetic device, mechanical, electronic nervous system stimulator
  fixation, internal (orthopedic) NEC — *see* Complication, fixation device, mechanical
  gastrointestinal — *see* Complications, prosthetic device, mechanical, gastrointestinal device
  genital NEC T83.498
    intrauterine contraceptive device T83.39
    penile prosthesis (cylinder) (implanted) (pump) (resevoir) T83.490
    testicular prosthesis T83.491

Protrusion, protrusio — *continued*
heart NEC — *see* Complication, cardiovascular device, mechanical
joint prosthesis — *see* Complications, joint prosthesis, mechanical, specified NEC, by site
ocular NEC — *see* Complications, prosthetic device, mechanical, ocular device
orthopedic NEC — *see* Complication, orthopedic, device, mechanical
specified NEC T85.628
urinary NEC — *see also* Complication, genitourinary, device, urinary, mechanical
  graft T83.29
vascular NEC — *see* Complication, cardiovascular device, mechanical
ventricular intracranial shunt T85.09
intervertebral disc — *see* Displacement, intervertebral disc
joint prosthesis — *see* Complications, joint prosthesis, mechanical, specified NEC, by site
nucleus pulposus — *see* Displacement, intervertebral disc
Prune belly (syndrome) Q79.4
Prurigo (ferox) (gravis) (Hebrae) (Hebra's) (mitis) (simplex) L28.2
Besnier's L20.0
estivalis L56.4
nodularis L28.1
psychogenic F45.8
Pruritus, pruritic (essential) L29.9
ani, anus L29.0
  psychogenic F45.8
anogenital L29.3
  psychogenic F45.8
due to onchocerca volvulus B73.1
gravidarum — *see* Pregnancy, complicated by, specified pregnancy-related condition NEC
hiemalis L29.8
neurogenic (any site) F45.8
perianal L29.0
psychogenic (any site) F45.8
scroti, scrotum L29.1
  psychogenic F45.8
senile, senilis L29.8
specified NEC L29.8
  psychogenic F45.8
Trichomonas A59.9
vulva, vulvae L29.2
  psychogenic F45.8
Pseudarthrosis, pseudoarthrosis (bone) — *see* Nonunion, fracture
clavicle, congenital Q74.0
joint, following fusion or arthrodesis M96.0
Pseudoaneurysm — *see* Aneurysm
Pseudoangina (pectoris) — *see* Angina
Pseudoangioma I81
Pseudoarteriosus Q28.8
Pseudoarthrosis — *see* Pseudarthrosis
Pseudobulbar affect (PBA) F48.2
Pseudochromhidrosis L67.8
Pseudocirrhosis, liver, pericardial I31.1
Pseudocowpox B08.03
Pseudocoxalgia M91.3-
Pseudocroup J38.5
Pseudo-Cushing's syndrome, alcohol-induced E24.4
Pseudocyesis F45.8
Pseudocyst
lung J98.4
pancreas K86.3
retina — *see* Cyst, retina
Pseudoelephantiasis neuroarthritica Q82.0
Pseudoexfoliation, capsule (lens) — *see* Cataract, specified NEC

Pseudofolliculitis barbae L73.1
Pseudoglioma H44.89
Pseudohemophilia (Bernuth's) (hereditary)
    (type B) D68.0
    Type A D69.8
    vascular D69.8
Pseudohermaphroditism Q56.3
    adrenal E25.8
    female Q56.2
        with adrenocortical disorder E25.8
        without adrenocortical disorder Q56.2
        adrenal (congenital) E25.0
    male Q56.1
        with
            5-alpha-reductase deficiency E29.1
            adrenocortical disorder E25.8
            androgen resistance E34.51
            cleft scrotum Q56.1
            feminizing testis E34.51
        without gonadal disorder Q56.1
        adrenal E25.8
Pseudo-Hurler's polydystrophy E77.0
Pseudohydrocephalus G93.2
Pseudohypertrophic muscular dystrophy
    (Erb's) G71.0
Pseudohypertrophy, muscle G71.0
Pseudohypoparathyroidism E20.1
Pseudoinsomnia F51.03
Pseudoleukemia, infantile D64.89
Pseudo-obstruction intestine (acute)
    (chronic) (idiopathic) (intermittent secondary)
    (primary) K59.8
Pseudomembranous — see condition
Pseudomeningocele (cerebral) (infective)
    (post-traumatic) G96.19
    postprocedural (spinal) G97.82
Pseudomenses (newborn) P54.6
Pseudomenstruation (newborn) P54.6
Pseudomonas
    aeruginosa, as cause of disease classified
        elsewhere B96.5
    mallei infection A24.0
        as cause of disease classified elsewhere
            B96.5
    pseudomallei, as cause of disease classified
        elsewhere B96.5
Pseudomyotonia G71.19
Pseudomyxoma peritonei C78.6
Pseudoneuritis, optic (nerve) (disc) (papilla),
    congenital Q14.2
Pseudopapilledema H47.33-
    congenital Q14.2
Pseudoparalysis
    arm or leg R29.818
    atonic, congenital P94.2
Pseudopelade L66.0
Pseudophakia Z96.1
Pseudopolyarthritis, rhizomelic M35.3
Pseudopolycythemia D75.1
Pseudopseudohypoparathyroidism E20.1
Pseudopterygium H11.81-
Pseudoptosis (eyelid) — see Blepharochalasis
Pseudopuberty, precocious
    female heterosexual E25.8
    male isosexual E25.8
Pseudorickets (renal) N25.0
Pseudorubella B08.20
Pseudosclerema, newborn P83.8
Pseudosclerosis (brain)
    Jakob's — see Creutzfeldt-Jakob disease or
        syndrome
    of Westphal (Strümpell) E83.01
    spastic — see Creutzfeldt-Jakob disease or
        syndrome
Pseudotetanus — see Convulsions
Pseudotetany R29.0
    hysterical F44.5
Pseudotruncus arteriosus Q25.49

Pseudotuberculosis A28.2
    enterocolitis A04.8
    pasteurella (infection) A28.0
Pseudotumor
    cerebri G93.2
    orbital H05.11-
Pseudoxanthoma elasticum Q82.8
Psilosis (sprue) (tropical) K90.1
    nontropical K90.0
Psittacosis A70
Psoitis M60.88
Psoriasis L40.9
    arthropathic L40.50
        arthritis mutilans L40.52
        distal interphalangeal L40.51
        juvenile L40.54
        other specified L40.59
        spondylitis L40.53
    buccal K13.29
    flexural L40.8
    guttate L40.4
    mouth K13.29
    nummular L40.0
    plaque L40.0
    psychogenic F54
    pustular (generalized) L40.1
        palmaris et plantaris L40.3
    specified NEC L40.8
    vulgaris L40.0
Psychasthenia F48.8
Psychiatric disorder or problem F99
Psychogenic — see also condition
    factors associated with physical conditions F54
Psychological and behavioral factors
    affecting medical condition F59
Psychoneurosis, psychoneurotic — see also
    Neurosis
    anxiety (state) F41.1
    depersonalization F48.1
    hypochondriacal F45.21
    hysteria F44.9
    neurasthenic F48.8
    personality NEC F60.89
Psychopathy, psychopathic
    affectionless F94.2
    autistic F84.5
    constitution, post-traumatic F07.81
    personality — see Disorder, personality
    sexual — see Deviation, sexual
    state F60.2
Psychosexual identity disorder of
    childhood F64.2
Psychosis, psychotic F29
    acute (transient) F23
        hysterical F44.9
    affective — see Disorder, mood
    alcoholic F10.959
        with
            abuse F10.159
            anxiety disorder F10.980
                with
                    abuse F10.180
                    dependence F10.280
            delirium tremens F10.231
            delusions F10.950
                with
                    abuse F10.150
                    dependence F10.250
            dementia F10.97
                with dependence F10.27
            dependence F10.259
            hallucinosis F10.951
                with
                    abuse F10.151
                    dependence F10.251
            mood disorder F10.94
                with
                    abuse F10.14
                    dependence F10.24

Psychosis, psychotic F29 — continued
    alcoholic F10.959 — continued
        with — continued
            paranoia F10.950
                with
                    abuse F10.150
                    dependence F10.250
            persisting amnesia F10.96
                with dependence F10.26
        amnestic confabulatory F10.96
            with dependence F10.26
        delirium tremens F10.231
        Korsakoff's, Korsakov's, Korsakow's F10.26
        paranoid type F10.950
            with
                abuse F10.150
                dependence F10.250
    anergastic — see Psychosis, organic
    arteriosclerotic (simple type) (uncomplicated)
        F01.50
        with behavioral disturbance F01.51
    childhood F84.0
        atypical F84.8
    climacteric — see Psychosis, involutional
    confusional F29
        acute or subacute F05
        reactive F23
    cycloid F23
    depressive — see Disorder, depressive
    disintegrative (childhood) F84.3
    drug-induced — see F11-F19 with .x59
        paranoid and hallucinatory states — see
            F11-F19 with .x50 or .x51
    due to or associated with
        addiction, drug — see F11-F19 with .x59
        dependence
            alcohol F10.259
            drug — see F11-F19 with .x59
        epilepsy F06.8
        Huntington's chorea F06.8
        ischemia, cerebrovascular (generalized)
            F06.8
        multiple sclerosis F06.8
        physical disease F06.8
        presenile dementia F03
        senile dementia F03
        vascular disease (arteriosclerotic) (cerebral)
            F01.50
            with behavioral disturbance F01.51
    epileptic F06.8
    episode F23
        due to or associated with physical condition
            F06.8
    exhaustive F43.0
    hallucinatory, chronic F28
    hypomanic F30.8
    hysterical (acute) F44.9
    induced F24
    infantile F84.0
        atypical F84.8
    infective (acute) (subacute) F05
    involutional F28
        depressive — see Disorder, depressive
        melancholic — see Disorder, depressive
        paranoid (state) F22
    Korsakoff's, Korsakov's, Korsakow's
        (nonalcoholic) F04
        alcoholic F10.96
            in dependence F10.26
        induced by other psychoactive substance —
            see categories F11-F19 with .x5x
    mania, manic (single episode) F30.2
        recurrent type F31.89
    manic-depressive — see Disorder, bipolar
    menopausal — see Psychosis, involutional
    mixed schizophrenic and affective F25.8
    multi-infarct (cerebrovascular) F01.50
        with behavioral disturbance F01.51

Psychosis, psychotic F29 — *continued*
- nonorganic F29
  - specified NEC F28
- organic F09
  - due to or associated with
    - arteriosclerosis (cerebral) — *see* Psychosis, arteriosclerotic
    - cerebrovascular disease, arteriosclerotic — *see* Psychosis, arteriosclerotic
    - childbirth — *see* Psychosis, puerperal
    - Creutzfeldt-Jakob disease or syndrome — *see* Creutzfeldt-Jakob disease or syndrome
    - dependence, alcohol F10.259
    - disease
      - alcoholic liver F10.259
      - brain, arteriosclerotic — *see* Psychosis, arteriosclerotic
      - cerebrovascular F01.50
        - with behavioral disturbance F01.51
        - Creutzfeldt-Jakob — *see* Creutzfeldt-Jakob disease or syndrome
        - endocrine or metabolic F06.8
          - acute or subacute F05
      - liver, alcoholic F10.259
    - epilepsy transient (acute) F05
    - infection
      - brain (intracranial) F06.8
        - acute or subacute F05
    - intoxication
      - alcoholic (acute) F10.259
      - drug F19 with .x59 F11-
    - ischemia, cerebrovascular (generalized) — *see* Psychosis, arteriosclerotic
    - puerperium — *see* Psychosis, puerperal
    - trauma, brain (birth) (from electric current) (surgical) F06.8
      - acute or subacute F05
  - infective F06.8
    - acute or subacute F05
  - post-traumatic F06.8
    - acute or subacute F05
- paranoiac F22
- paranoid (climacteric) (involutional) (menopausal) F22
  - psychogenic (acute) F23
  - schizophrenic F20.0
  - senile F03
- postpartum F53
- presbyophrenic (type) F03
- presenile F03
- psychogenic (paranoid) F23
  - depressive F32.3
- puerperal F53
  - specified type — *see* Psychosis, by type
- reactive (brief) (transient) (emotional stress) (psychological trauma) F23
  - depressive F32.3
    - recurrent F33.3
  - excitative type F30.8
- schizoaffective F25.9
  - depressive type F25.1
  - manic type F25.0
- schizophrenia, schizophrenic — *see* Schizophrenia
- schizophrenia-like, in epilepsy F06.2
- schizophreniform F20.81
  - affective type F25.9
  - brief F23
  - confusional type F23
  - depressive type F25.1
  - manic type F25.0
  - mixed type F25.0
- senile NEC F03
  - depressed or paranoid type F03
  - simple deterioration F03
  - specified type — *code to* condition
- shared F24
- situational (reactive) F23

Psychosis, psychotic F29 — *continued*
- symbiotic (childhood) F84.3
- symptomatic F09

Psychosomatic — *see* Disorder, psychosomatic

Psychosyndrome, organic F07.9

Psychotic episode due to or associated with physical condition F06.8

Pterygium (eye) H11.00-
- amyloid H11.01-
- central H11.02-
- colli Q18.3
- double H11.03-
- peripheral
  - progressive H11.05-
  - stationary H11.04-
- recurrent H11.06-

Ptilosis (eyelid) — *see* Madarosis

Ptomaine (poisoning) — *see* Poisoning, food

Ptosis — *see also* Blepharoptosis
- adiposa (false) — *see* Blepharoptosis
- breast N64.81
- cecum K63.4
- colon K63.4
- congenital (eyelid) Q10.0
  - specified site NEC — *see* Anomaly, by site
- eyelid — *see* Blepharoptosis
  - congenital Q10.0
- gastric K31.89
- intestine K63.4
- kidney N28.83
- liver K76.89
- renal N28.83
- splanchnic K63.4
- spleen D73.89
- stomach K31.89
- viscera K63.4

PTP D69.51

Ptyalism (periodic) K11.7
- hysterical F45.8
- pregnancy — *see* Pregnancy, complicated by, specified pregnancy-related condition NEC
- psychogenic F45.8

Ptyalolithiasis K11.5

Pubarche, precocious E30.1

Pubertas praecox E30.1

Puberty (development state) Z00.3
- bleeding (excessive) N92.2
- delayed E30.0
- precocious (constitutional) (cryptogenic) (idiopathic) E30.1
  - central E22.8
  - due to
    - ovarian hyperfunction E28.1
      - estrogen E28.0
    - testicular hyperfunction E29.0
- premature E30.1
  - due to
    - adrenal cortical hyperfunction E25.8
    - pineal tumor E34.8
    - pituitary (anterior) hyperfunction E22.8

Puckering, macula — *see* Degeneration, macula, puckering

Pudenda, pudendum — *see* condition

Puente's disease (simple glandular cheilitis) K13.0

Puerperal, puerperium (complicated by, complications)
- abnormal glucose (tolerance test) O99.815
- abscess
  - areola O91.02
    - associated with lactation O91.03
  - Bartholin's gland O86.19
  - breast O91.12
    - associated with lactation O91.13
  - cervix (uteri) O86.11
  - genital organ NEC O86.19
  - kidney O86.21

Puerperal, puerperium (complicated by, complications) — *continued*
- abscess — *continued*
  - mammary O91.12
    - associated with lactation O91.13
  - nipple O91.02
    - associated with lactation O91.03
  - peritoneum O85
  - subareolar O91.12
    - associated with lactation O91.13
  - urinary tract — *see* Puerperal, infection, urinary
  - uterus O86.12
  - vagina (wall) O86.13
  - vaginorectal O86.13
  - vulvovaginal gland O86.13
- adnexitis O86.19
- afibrinogenemia, or other coagulation defect O72.3
- albuminuria (acute) (subacute) — *see* Proteinuria, gestational
- alcohol use O99.315
- anemia O90.81
  - pre-existing (pre-pregnancy) O99.03
- anesthetic death O89.8
- apoplexy O99.43
- bariatric surgery status O99.845
- blood disorder NEC O99.13
- blood dyscrasia O72.3
- cardiomyopathy O90.3
- cerebrovascular disorder (conditions in I60-I69) O99.43
- cervicitis O86.11
- circulatory system disorder O99.43
- coagulopathy (any) O72.3
- complications O90.9
  - specified NEC O90.89
- convulsions — *see* Eclampsia
- cystitis O86.22
- cystopyelitis O86.29
- delirium NEC F05
- diabetes O24.93
  - gestational — *see* Puerperal, gestational diabetes
  - pre-existing O24.33
    - specified NEC O24.83
    - type 1 O24.03
    - type 2 O24.13
- digestive system disorder O99.63
- disease O90.9
  - breast NEC O92.29
  - cerebrovascular (acute) O99.43
  - nonobstetric NEC O99.89
  - tubo-ovarian O86.19
  - Valsuani's O99.03
- disorder O90.9
  - biliary tract O26.63
  - lactation O92.70
  - liver O26.63
  - nonobstetric NEC O99.89
- disruption
  - cesarean wound O90.0
  - episiotomy wound O90.1
  - perineal laceration wound O90.1
- drug use O99.325
- eclampsia (with pre-existing hypertension) O15.2
- embolism (pulmonary) (blood clot) — *see* Embolism, obstetric, puerperal
- endocrine, nutritional or metabolic disease NEC O99.285
- endophlebitis — *see* Puerperal, phlebitis
- endotrachelitis O86.11
- failure
  - lactation (complete) O92.3
    - partial O92.4
  - renal, acute O90.4
- fever (of unknown origin) O86.4
  - septic O85

Puerperal, puerperium (complicated by, complications) — *continued*
fissure, nipple O92.12
  associated with lactation O92.13
fistula
  breast (due to mastitis) O91.12
    associated with lactation O91.13
  nipple O91.02
    associated with lactation O91.03
galactophoritis O91.22
  associated with lactation O91.23
galactorrhea O92.6
gastric banding status O99.845
gastric bypass status O99.845
gastrointestinal disease NEC O99.63
gestational
  diabetes O24.439
    diet controlled O24.430
    insulin (and diet) controlled O24.434
    oral drug controlled (antidiabetic) (hypoglycemic) O24.435
  edema O12.05
    with proteinuria O12.25
  proteinuria O12.15
gonorrhea O98.23
hematoma, subdural O99.43
hemiplegia, cerebral O99.355
  due to cerbrovascular disorder O99.43
hemorrhage O72.1
  brain O99.43
  bulbar O99.43
  cerebellar O99.43
  cerebral O99.43
  cortical O99.43
  delayed or secondary O72.2
  extradural O99.43
  internal capsule O99.43
  intracranial O99.43
  intrapontine O99.43
  meningeal O99.43
  pontine O99.43
  retained placenta O72.0
  subarachnoid O99.43
  subcortical O99.43
  subdural O99.43
  third stage O72.0
  uterine, delayed O72.2
  ventricular O99.43
hemorrhoids O87.2
hepatorenal syndrome O90.4
hypertension — *see* Hypertension, complicating, puerperium
hypertrophy, breast O92.29
induration breast (fibrous) O92.29
infection O86.4
  cervix O86.11
  generalized O85
  genital tract NEC O86.19
    obstetric surgical wound O86.0
  kidney (bacillus coli) O86.21
  maternal O98.93
    carrier state NEC O99.835
    gonorrhea O98.23
    human immunodeficiency virus (HIV) O98.73
    protozoal O98.63
    sexually transmitted NEC O98.33
    specified NEC O98.83
    streptococcus group B (GBS) carrier state O99.825
    syphilis O98.13
    tuberculosis O98.03
    viral hepatitis O98.43
    viral NEC O98.53
  nipple O91.02
    associated with lactation O91.03
  peritoneum O85
  renal O86.21
  specified NEC O86.89

Puerperal, puerperium (complicated by, complications) — *continued*
infection O86.4 — *continued*
  urinary (asymptomatic) (tract) NEC O86.20
    bladder O86.22
    kidney O86.21
    specified site NEC O86.29
    urethra O86.22
  vagina O86.13
  vein — *see* Puerperal, phlebitis
ischemia, cerebral O99.43
lymphangitis O86.89
  breast O91.22
    associated with lactation O91.23
malignancy O9A.13 *(follows O99)*
malnutrition O25.3
mammillitis O91.02
  associated with lactation O91.03
mammitis O91.22
  associated with lactation O91.23
mania F30.8
mastitis O91.22
  associated with lactation O91.23
  purulent O91.12
    associated with lactation O91.13
melancholia — *see* Disorder, depressive
mental disorder NEC O99.345
metroperitonitis O85
metrorrhagia — *see* Hemorrhage, postpartum
metrosalpingitis O86.19
metrovaginitis O86.13
milk leg O87.1
monoplegia, cerebral O99.43
mood disturbance O90.6
necrosis, liver (acute) (subacute) (conditions in subcategory K72.0) O26.63
  with renal failure O90.4
nervous system disorder O99.355
neuritis O90.89
obesity (pre-existing prior to pregnancy) O99.215
obesity surgery status O99.845
occlusion, precerebral artery O99.43
paralysis
  bladder (sphincter) O90.89
  cerebral O99.43
paralytic stroke O99.43
parametritis O85
paravaginitis O86.13
pelviperitonitis O85
perimetritis O86.12
perimetrosalpingitis O86.19
perinephritis O86.21
periphlebitis — *see* Puerperal phlebitis
peritoneal infection O85
peritonitis (pelvic) O85
perivaginitis O86.13
phlebitis O87.0
  deep O87.1
  pelvic O87.1
  superficial O87.0
phlebothrombosis, deep O87.1
phlegmasia alba dolens O87.1
placental polyp O90.89
pneumonia, embolic — *see* Embolism, obstetric, puerperal
pre-eclampsia — *see* Pre-eclampsia
psychosis F53
pyelitis O86.21
pyelocystitis O86.29
pyelonephritis O86.21
pyelonephrosis O86.21
pyemia O85
pyocystitis O86.29
pyohemia O85
pyometra O86.12
pyonephritis O86.21
pyosalpingitis O86.19
pyrexia (of unknown origin) O86.4

Puerperal, puerperium (complicated by, complications) — *continued*
renal
  disease NEC O90.89
  failure O90.4
respiratory disease NEC O99.53
retention
  decidua — *see* Retention, decidua
  placenta O72.0
  secundines — *see* Retention, secundines
retrated nipple O92.02
salpingo-ovaritis O86.19
salpingoperitonitis O85
secondary perineal tear O90.1
sepsis O85
sepsis (pelvic) O85
septic thrombophlebitis O86.81
skin disorder NEC O99.73
specified condition NEC O99.89
stroke O99.43
subinvolution (uterus) O90.89
subluxation of symphysis (pubis) O26.73
suppuration — *see* Puerperal, abscess
tetanus A34
thelitis O91.02
  associated with lactation O91.03
thrombocytopenia O72.3
thrombophlebitis (superficial) O87.0
  deep O87.1
  pelvic O87.1
  septic O86.81
thrombosis (venous) — *see* Thrombosis, puerperal
thyroiditis O90.5
toxemia (eclamptic) (pre-eclamptic) (with convulsions) O15.2
trauma, non-obstetric O9A.23 *(follows O99)*
  caused by abuse (physical) (suspected) O9A.33 *(follows O99)*
    confirmed O9A.33 *(follows O99)*
    psychological (suspected) O9A.53 *(follows O99)*
      confirmed O9A.53 *(follows O99)*
    sexual (suspected) O9A.43 *(follows O99)*
      confirmed O9A.43 *(follows O99)*
uremia (due to renal failure) O90.4
urethritis O86.22
vaginitis O86.13
varicose veins (legs) O87.4
  vulva or perineum O87.8
venous O87.9
vulvitis O86.19
vulvovaginitis O86.13
white leg O87.1
Puerperium — *see* Puerperal
Pulmolithiasis J98.4
Pulmonary — *see* condition
Pulpitis (acute) (anachoretic) (chronic) (hyperplastic) (putrescent) (suppurative) (ulcerative) K04.01
irreversible K04.02
reversible K04.01
Pulpless tooth K04.99
Pulse
alternating R00.8
bigeminal R00.8
fast R00.0
feeble, rapid due to shock following injury T79.4
rapid R00.0
weak R09.89
Pulsus alternans or trigeminus R00.8
Punch drunk F07.81
Punctum lacrimale occlusion — *see* Obstruction, lacrimal

Puncture
- abdomen, abdominal
  - wall S31.139
    - with
      - foreign body S31.149
      - penetration into peritoneal cavity S31.639
        - with foreign body S31.649
  - epigastric region S31.132
    - with
      - foreign body S31.142
      - penetration into peritoneal cavity S31.632
        - with foreign body S31.642
  - left
    - lower quadrant S31.134
      - with
        - foreign body S31.144
        - penetration into peritoneal cavity S31.634
          - with foreign body S31.644
    - upper quadrant S31.131
      - with
        - foreign body S31.141
        - penetration into peritoneal cavity S31.631
          - with foreign body S31.641
  - periumbilic region S31.135
    - with
      - foreign body S31.145
      - penetration into peritoneal cavity S31.635
        - with foreign body S31.645
  - right
    - lower quadrant S31.133
      - with
        - foreign body S31.143
        - penetration into peritoneal cavity S31.633
          - with foreign body S31.643
    - upper quadrant S31.130
      - with
        - foreign body S31.140
        - penetration into peritoneal cavity S31.630
          - with foreign body S31.640
- accidental, complicating surgery — see Complication, accidental puncture or laceration
- alveolar (process) — see Puncture, oral cavity
- ankle S91.039
  - with
    - foreign body S91.049
  - left S91.032
    - with
      - foreign body S91.042
  - right S91.031
    - with
      - foreign body S91.041
- anus S31.833
  - with foreign body S31.834
- arm (upper) S41.139
  - with foreign body S41.149
  - left S41.132
    - with foreign body S41.142
  - lower — see Puncture, forearm
  - right S41.131
    - with foreign body S41.141
- auditory canal (external) (meatus) — see Puncture, ear
- auricle, ear — see Puncture, ear
- axilla — see Puncture, arm

Puncture — continued
- back — see also Puncture, thorax, back
  - lower S31.030
    - with
      - foreign body S31.040
        - with penetration into retroperitoneal space S31.041
      - penetration into retroperitoneal space S31.031
- bladder (traumatic) S37.29
  - nontraumatic N32.89
- breast S21.039
  - with foreign body S21.049
  - left S21.032
    - with foreign body S21.042
  - right S21.031
    - with foreign body S21.041
- buttock S31.803
  - with foreign body S31.804
  - left S31.823
    - with foreign body S31.824
  - right S31.813
    - with foreign body S31.814
- by
  - device, implant or graft — see Complications, by site and type, mechanical
  - foreign body left accidentally in operative wound T81.539
  - instrument (any) during a procedure, accidental — see Puncture, accidental complicating surgery
- calf — see Puncture, leg
- canaliculus lacrimalis — see Puncture, eyelid
- canthus, eye — see Puncture, eyelid
- cervical esophagus S11.23
  - with foreign body S11.24
- cheek (external) S01.439
  - with foreign body S01.449
  - internal — see Puncture, oral cavity
  - left S01.432
    - with foreign body S01.442
  - right S01.431
    - with foreign body S01.441
- chest wall — see Puncture, thorax
- chin — see Puncture, head, specified site NEC
- clitoris — see Puncture, vulva
- costal region — see Puncture, thorax
- digit(s)
  - foot — see Puncture, toe
  - hand — see Puncture, finger
- ear (canal) (external) S01.339
  - with foreign body S01.349
  - drum S09.2-
  - left S01.332
    - with foreign body S01.342
  - right S01.331
    - with foreign body S01.341
- elbow S51.039
  - with
    - foreign body S51.049
  - left S51.032
    - with
      - foreign body S51.042
  - right S51.031
    - with
      - foreign body S51.041
- epididymis — see Puncture, testis
- epigastric region — see Puncture, abdomen, wall, epigastric
- epiglottis S11.83
  - with foreign body S11.84
- esophagus
  - cervical S11.23
    - with foreign body S11.24
  - thoracic S27.818
- eyeball S05.6-
  - with foreign body S05.5-
- eyebrow — see Puncture, eyelid

Puncture — continued
- eyelid S01.13-
  - with foreign body S01.14-
  - left S01.132
    - with foreign body S01.142
  - right S01.131
    - with foreign body S01.141
- face NEC — see Puncture, head, specified site NEC
- finger(s) S61.239
  - with
    - damage to nail S61.339
      - with
        - foreign body S61.349
    - foreign body S61.249
  - index S61.238
    - with
      - damage to nail S61.338
        - with
          - foreign body S61.348
      - foreign body S61.248
    - left S61.231
      - with
        - damage to nail S61.331
          - with
            - foreign body S61.341
        - foreign body S61.241
    - right S61.230
      - with
        - damage to nail S61.330
          - with
            - foreign body S61.340
        - foreign body S61.240
  - little S61.238
    - with
      - damage to nail S61.338
        - with
          - foreign body S61.348
      - foreign body S61.248
    - left S61.237
      - with
        - damage to nail S61.337
          - with
            - foreign body S61.347
        - foreign body S61.247
    - right S61.236
      - with
        - damage to nail S61.336
          - with
            - foreign body S61.346
        - foreign body S61.246
  - middle S61.238
    - with
      - damage to nail S61.338
        - with
          - foreign body S61.348
      - foreign body S61.248
    - left S61.233
      - with
        - damage to nail S61.333
          - with
            - foreign body S61.343
        - foreign body S61.243
    - right S61.232
      - with
        - damage to nail S61.332
          - with
            - foreign body S61.342
        - foreign body S61.242
  - ring S61.238
    - with
      - damage to nail S61.338
        - with
          - foreign body S61.348
      - foreign body S61.248

Puncture — *continued*
- finger(s) S61.239 — *continued*
  - ring S61.238 — *continued*
    - left S61.235
      - with
        - damage to nail S61.335
          - with
            - foreign body S61.345
        - foreign body S61.245
    - right S61.234
      - with
        - damage to nail S61.334
          - with
            - foreign body S61.344
        - foreign body S61.244
- flank S31.139
  - with foreign body S31.149
- foot (except toe(s) alone) S91.339
  - with foreign body S91.349
  - left S91.332
    - with foreign body S91.342
  - right S91.331
    - with foreign body S91.341
  - toe — *see* Puncture, toe
- forearm S51.839
  - with
    - foreign body S51.849
  - elbow only — *see* Puncture, elbow
  - left S51.832
    - with
      - foreign body S51.842
  - right S51.831
    - with
      - foreign body S51.841
- forehead — *see* Puncture, head, specified site NEC
- genital organs, external
  - female S31.532
    - with foreign body S31.542
    - vagina — *see* Puncture, vagina
    - vulva — *see* Puncture, vulva
  - male S31.531
    - with foreign body S31.541
    - penis — *see* Puncture, penis
    - scrotum — *see* Puncture, scrotum
    - testis — *see* Puncture, testis
- groin — *see* Puncture, abdomen, wall
- gum — *see* Puncture, oral cavity
- hand S61.439
  - with
    - foreign body S61.449
  - finger — *see* Puncture, finger
  - left S61.432
    - with
      - foreign body S61.442
  - right S61.431
    - with
      - foreign body S61.441
  - thumb — *see* Puncture, thumb
- head S01.93
  - with foreign body S01.94
  - cheek — *see* Puncture, cheek
  - ear — *see* Puncture, ear
  - eyelid — *see* Puncture, eyelid
  - lip — *see* Puncture, oral cavity
  - nose — *see* Puncture, nose
  - oral cavity — *see* Puncture, oral cavity
  - scalp S01.03
    - with foreign body S01.04
  - specified site NEC S01.83
    - with foreign body S01.84
  - temporomandibular area — *see* Puncture, cheek
- heart S26.99
  - with hemopericardium S26.09
  - without hemopericardium S26.19
- heel — *see* Puncture, foot

Puncture — *continued*
- hip S71.039
  - with foreign body S71.049
  - left S71.032
    - with foreign body S71.042
  - right S71.031
    - with foreign body S71.041
- hymen — *see* Puncture, vagina
- hypochondrium — *see* Puncture, abdomen, wall
- hypogastric region — *see* Puncture, abdomen, wall
- inguinal region — *see* Puncture, abdomen, wall
- instep — *see* Puncture, foot
- internal organs — *see* Injury, by site
- interscapular region — *see* Puncture, thorax, back
- intestine
  - large
    - colon S36.599
      - ascending S36.590
      - descending S36.592
      - sigmoid S36.593
      - specified site NEC S36.598
      - transverse S36.591
    - rectum S36.69
  - small S36.499
    - duodenum S36.490
    - specified site NEC S36.498
- intra-abdominal organ S36.99
  - gallbladder S36.128
  - intestine — *see* Puncture, intestine
  - liver S36.118
  - pancreas — *see* Puncture, pancreas
  - peritoneum S36.81
  - specified site NEC S36.898
  - spleen S36.09
  - stomach S36.39
- jaw — *see* Puncture, head, specified site NEC
- knee S81.039
  - with foreign body S81.049
  - left S81.032
    - with foreign body S81.042
  - right S81.031
    - with foreign body S81.041
- labium (majus) (minus) — *see* Puncture, vulva
- lacrimal duct — *see* Puncture, eyelid
- larynx S11.013
  - with foreign body S11.014
- leg (lower) S81.839
  - with foreign body S81.849
  - foot — *see* Puncture, foot
  - knee — *see* Puncture, knee
  - left S81.832
    - with foreign body S81.842
  - right S81.831
    - with foreign body S81.841
  - upper — *see* Puncture, thigh
- lip S01.531
  - with foreign body S01.541
- loin — *see* Puncture, abdomen, wall
- lower back — *see* Puncture, back, lower
- lumbar region — *see* Puncture, back, lower
- malar region — *see* Puncture, head, specified site NEC
- mammary — *see* Puncture, breast
- mastoid region — *see* Puncture, head, specified site NEC
- mouth — *see* Puncture, oral cavity
- nail
  - finger — *see* Puncture, finger, with damage to nail
  - toe — *see* Puncture, toe, with damage to nail
- nasal (septum) (sinus) — *see* Puncture, nose
- nasopharynx — *see* Puncture, head, specified site NEC

Puncture — *continued*
- neck S11.93
  - with foreign body S11.94
  - involving
    - cervical esophagus — *see* Puncture, cervical esophagus
    - larynx — *see* Puncture, larynx
    - pharynx — *see* Puncture, pharynx
    - thyroid gland — *see* Puncture, thyroid gland
    - trachea — *see* Puncture, trachea
  - specified site NEC S11.83
    - with foreign body S11.84
- nose (septum) (sinus) S01.23
  - with foreign body S01.24
- ocular — *see* Puncture, eyeball
- oral cavity S01.532
  - with foreign body S01.542
- orbit S05.4-
- palate — *see* Puncture, oral cavity
- palm — *see* Puncture, hand
- pancreas S36.299
  - body S36.291
  - head S36.290
  - tail S36.292
- pelvis — *see* Puncture, back, lower
- penis S31.23
  - with foreign body S31.24
- perineum
  - female S31.43
    - with foreign body S31.44
  - male S31.139
    - with foreign body S31.149
- periocular area (with or without lacrimal passages) — *see* Puncture, eyelid
- phalanges
  - finger — *see* Puncture, finger
  - toe — *see* Puncture, toe
- pharynx S11.23
  - with foreign body S11.24
- pinna — *see* Puncture, ear
- popliteal space — *see* Puncture, knee
- prepuce — *see* Puncture, penis
- pubic region S31.139
  - with foreign body S31.149
- pudendum — *see* Puncture, genital organs, external
- rectovaginal septum — *see* Puncture, vagina
- sacral region — *see* Puncture, back, lower
- sacroiliac region — *see* Puncture, back, lower
- salivary gland — *see* Puncture, oral cavity
- scalp S01.03
  - with foreign body S01.04
- scapular region — *see* Puncture, shoulder
- scrotum S31.33
  - with foreign body S31.34
- shin — *see* Puncture, leg
- shoulder S41.039
  - with foreign body S41.049
  - left S41.032
    - with foreign body S41.042
  - right S41.031
    - with foreign body S41.041
- spermatic cord — *see* Puncture, testis
- sternal region — *see* Puncture, thorax, front
- submaxillary region — *see* Puncture, head, specified site NEC
- submental region — *see* Puncture, head, specified site NEC
- subungual
  - finger(s) — *see* Puncture, finger, with damage to nail
  - toe — *see* Puncture, toe, with damage to nail
- supraclavicular fossa — *see* Puncture, neck, specified site NEC
- temple, temporal region — *see* Puncture, head, specified site NEC
- temporomandibular area — *see* Puncture, cheek

Puncture — *continued*
  testis S31.33
    with foreign body S31.34
  thigh S71.139
    with foreign body S71.149
    left S71.132
      with foreign body S71.142
    right S71.131
      with foreign body S71.141
  thorax, thoracic (wall) S21.93
    with foreign body S21.94
    back S21.23-
      with
        foreign body S21.24-
          with penetration S21.44
        penetration S21.43
    breast — *see* Puncture, breast
    front S21.13-
      with
        foreign body S21.14-
          with penetration S21.34
        penetration S21.33
  throat — *see* Puncture, neck
  thumb S61.039
    with
      damage to nail S61.139
        with
          foreign body S61.149
      foreign body S61.049
    left S61.032
      with
        damage to nail S61.132
          with
            foreign body S61.142
        foreign body S61.042
    right S61.031
      with
        damage to nail S61.131
          with
            foreign body S61.141
        foreign body S61.041
  thyroid gland S11.13
    with foreign body S11.14
  toe(s) S91.139
    with
      damage to nail S91.239
        with
          foreign body S91.249
      foreign body S91.149
    great S91.133
      with
        damage to nail S91.233
          with
            foreign body S91.243
        foreign body S91.143
      left S91.132
        with
          damage to nail S91.232
            with
              foreign body S91.242
          foreign body S91.142
      right S91.131
        with
          damage to nail S91.231
            with
              foreign body S91.241
          foreign body S91.141
    lesser S91.136
      with
        damage to nail S91.236
          with
            foreign body S91.246
        foreign body S91.146
      left S91.135
        with
          damage to nail S91.235
            with
              foreign body S91.245
          foreign body S91.145

Puncture — *continued*
  toe(s) S91.139 — *continued*
    lesser S91.136 — *continued*
      right S91.134
        with
          damage to nail S91.234
            with
              foreign body S91.244
          foreign body S91.144
  tongue — *see* Puncture, oral cavity
  trachea S11.023
    with foreign body S11.024
  tunica vaginalis — *see* Puncture, testis
  tympanum, tympanic membrane S09.2-
  umbilical region S31.135
    with foreign body S31.145
  uvula — *see* Puncture, oral cavity
  vagina S31.43
    with foreign body S31.44
  vocal cords S11.033
    with foreign body S11.034
  vulva S31.43
    with foreign body S31.44
  wrist S61.539
    with
      foreign body S61.549
    left S61.532
      with
        foreign body S61.542
    right S61.531
      with
        foreign body S61.541
PUO (pyrexia of unknown origin) R50.9
Pupillary membrane (persistent) Q13.89
Pupillotonia — *see* Anomaly, pupil, function,
  tonic pupil
Purpura D69.2
  abdominal D69.0
  allergic D69.0
  anaphylactoid D69.0
  annularis telangiectodes L81.7
  arthritic D69.0
  autoerythrocyte sensitization D69.2
  autoimmune D69.0
  bacterial D69.0
  Bateman's (senile) D69.2
  capillary fragility (hereditary) (idiopathic)
    D69.8
  cryoglobulinemic D89.1
  Devil's pinches D69.2
  fibrinolytic — *see* Fibrinolysis
  fulminans, fulminous D65
  gangrenous D65
  hemorrhagic, hemorrhagica D69.3
    not due to thrombocytopenia D69.0
  Henoch(-Schönlein) (allergic) D69.0
  hypergammaglobulinemic (benign)
    (Waldenström) D89.0
  idiopathic (thrombocytopenic) D69.3
    nonthrombocytopenic D69.0
  immune thrombocytopenic D69.3
  infectious D69.0
  malignant D69.0
  neonatorum P54.5
  nervosa D69.0
  newborn P54.5
  nonthrombocytopenic D69.2
    hemorrhagic D69.0
    idiopathic D69.0
  nonthrombopenic D69.2
  peliosis rheumatica D69.0
  posttransfusion (post-transfusion) (from (fresh)
    whole blood or blood products) D69.51
  primary D69.49
  red cell membrane sensitivity D69.2
  rheumatica D69.0
  Schönlein(-Henoch) (allergic) D69.0
  scorbutic E54 *[D77]*
  senile D69.2

Purpura D69.2 — *continued*
  simplex D69.2
  symptomatica D69.0
  telangiectasia annularis L81.7
  thrombocytopenic D69.49
    congenital D69.42
    hemorrhagic D69.3
    hereditary D69.42
    idiopathic D69.3
    immune D69.3
    neonatal, transitory P61.0
    thrombotic M31.1
  thrombohemolytic — *see* Fibrinolysis
  thrombolytic — *see* Fibrinolysis
  thrombopenic D69.49
  thrombotic, thrombocytopenic M31.1
  toxic D69.0
  vascular D69.0
  visceral symptoms D69.0
Purpuric spots R23.3
Purulent — *see* condition
Pus
  in
    stool R19.5
    urine N39.0
  tube (rupture) — *see* Salpingo-oophoritis
Pustular rash L08.0
Pustule (nonmalignant) L08.9
  malignant A22.0
Pustulosis palmaris et plantaris L40.3
Putnam(-Dana) disease or syndrome —
  see Degeneration, combined
Putrescent pulp (dental) K04.1
Pyarthritis, pyarthrosis — *see* Arthritis,
  pyogenic or pyemic
  tuberculous — *see* Tuberculosis, joint
Pyelectasis — *see* Hydronephrosis
Pyelitis (congenital) (uremic) — *see also*
  Pyelonephritis
  with
    calculus — *see* category N20
      with hydronephrosis N13.2
    contracted kidney N11.9
  acute N10
  chronic N11.9
    with calculus — *see* category N20
      with hydronephrosis N13.2
  cystica N28.84
  puerperal (postpartum) O86.21
  tuberculous A18.11
Pyelocystitis — *see* Pyelonephritis
Pyelonephritis — *see also* Nephritis, tubulo-
  interstitial
  with
    calculus — *see* category N20
      with hydronephrosis N13.2
    contracted kidney N11.9
  acute N10
  calculous — *see* category N20
    with hydronephrosis N13.2
  chronic N11.9
    with calculus — *see* category N20
      with hydronephrosis N13.2
    associated with ureteral obstruction or
      stricture N11.1
    nonobstructive N11.8
      with reflux (vesicoureteral) N11.0
    obstructive N11.1
    specified NEC N11.8
  in (due to)
    brucellosis A23.9 *[N16]*
    cryoglobulinemia (mixed) D89.1 *[N16]*
    cystinosis E72.04
    diphtheria A36.84
    glycogen storage disease E74.09 *[N16]*
    leukemia NEC C95.9- *[N16]*
    lymphoma NEC C85.90 *[N16]*
    multiple myeloma C90.0- *[N16]*
    obstruction N11.1

Pyelonephritis — *see also* Nephritis, tubulo-
   interstitial — *continued*
  in (due to) — *continued*
    Salmonella infection A02.25
    sarcoidosis D86.84
    sepsis A41.9 *[N16]*
    Sjögren's disease M35.04
    toxoplasmosis B58.83
    transplant rejection T86.91 *[N16]*
    Wilson's disease E83.01 *[N16]*
   nonobstructive N12
    with reflux (vesicoureteral) N11.0
    chronic N11.8
   syphilitic A52.75
Pyelonephrosis (obstructive) N11.1
  chronic N11.9
Pyelophlebitis I80.8
Pyeloureteritis cystica N28.85
Pyemia, pyemic (fever) (infection) (purulent)
  — *see also* Sepsis
  joint — *see* Arthritis, pyogenic or pyemic
  liver K75.1
  pneumococcal A40.3
  portal K75.1
  postvaccinal T88.0
  puerperal, postpartum, childbirth O85
  specified organism NEC A41.89
  tuberculous — *see* Tuberculosis, miliary
Pygopagus Q89.4
Pyknoepilepsy (idiopathic) — *see* Pyknolepsy
Pyknolepsy
  intractable G40.A19
   with status epilepticus G40.A11
   without status epilepticus G40.A19
  not intractable G40.A09
   with status epilepticus G40.A01
   without status epilepticus G40.A09
Pylephlebitis K75.1
Pyle's syndrome Q78.5
Pylethrombophlebitis K75.1
Pylethrombosis K75.1
Pyloritis K29.90
  with bleeding K29.91
Pylorospasm (reflex) NEC K31.3
  congenital or infantile Q40.0
  neurotic F45.8
  newborn Q40.0
  psychogenic F45.8
Pylorus, pyloric — *see* condition
Pyoarthrosis — *see* Arthritis, pyogenic or
  pyemic
Pyocele
  mastoid — *see* Mastoiditis, acute
  sinus (accessory) — *see* Sinusitis
  turbinate (bone) J32.9
  urethra (*see also* Urethritis) N34.0
Pyocolpos — *see* Vaginitis
Pyocystitis N30.80
  with hematuria N30.81
Pyoderma, pyodermia L08.0
  gangrenosum L88
  newborn P39.4
  phagedenic L88
  vegetans L08.81
Pyodermatitis L08.0
  vegetans L08.81
Pyogenic — *see* condition
Pyohydronephrosis N13.6
Pyometra, pyometrium, pyometritis — *see*
  Endometritis
Pyomyositis (tropical) — *see* Myositis, infective
Pyonephritis N12
Pyonephrosis N13.6
  tuberculous A18.11
Pyo-oophoritis — *see* Salpingo-oophoritis
Pyo-ovarium — *see* Salpingo-oophoritis
Pyopericarditis, pyopericardium I30.1
Pyophlebitis — *see* Phlebitis
Pyopneumopericardium I30.1

Pyopneumothorax (infective) J86.9
  with fistula J86.0
  tuberculous NEC A15.6
Pyosalpinx, pyosalpingitis — *see also*
  Salpingo-oophoritis
Pyothorax J86.9
  with fistula J86.0
  tuberculous NEC A15.6
Pyoureter N28.89
  tuberculous A18.11
Pyramidopallidonigral syndrome G20
Pyrexia (of unknown origin) R50.9
  atmospheric T67.0
  during labor NEC O75.2
  heat T67.0
  newborn P81.9
   environmentally-induced P81.0
  persistent R50.9
  puerperal O86.4
Pyroglobulinemia NEC E88.09
Pyromania F63.1
Pyrosis R12
Pyuria (bacterial) N39.0

Q

Q fever A78
  with pneumonia A78
Quadricuspid aortic valve Q23.8
Quadrilateral fever A78
Quadriparesis — *see* Quadriplegia
  meaning muscle weakness M62.81
Quadriplegia G82.50
  complete
   C1-C4 level G82.51
   C5-C7 level G82.53
  congenital (cerebral) (spinal) G80.8
   spastic G80.0
  embolic (current episode) I63.4-
  incomplete
   C1-C4 level G82.52
   C5-C7 level G82.54
  thrombotic (current episode) I63.3-
  traumatic — *code to* injury with seventh
   character S
   current episode — *see* Injury, spinal (cord),
    cervical
Quadruplet, pregnancy — *see* Pregnancy,
  quadruplet
Quarrelsomeness F60.3
Queensland fever A77.3
Quervain's disease M65.4
  thyroid E06.1
Queyrat's erythroplasia D07.4
  penis D07.4
  specified site — *see* Neoplasm, skin, in situ
  unspecified site D07.4
Quincke's disease or edema T78.3
  hereditary D84.1
Quinsy (gangrenous) J36
Quintan fever A79.0
Quintuplet, pregnancy — *see* Pregnancy,
  quintuplet

R

Rabbit fever — *see* Tularemia
Rabies A82.9
  contact Z20.3
  exposure to Z20.3
  inoculation reaction — *see* Complications, vaccination
  sylvatic A82.0
  urban A82.1
Rachischisis — *see* Spina bifida
Rachitic — *see also* condition
  deformities of spine (late effect) (sequelae) E64.3
  pelvis (late effect) (sequelae) E64.3
    with disproportion (fetopelvic) O33.0
      causing obstructed labor O65.0
Rachitis, rachitism (acute) (tarda) — *see also* Rickets
  renalis N25.0
  sequelae E64.3
Radial nerve — *see* condition
Radiation
  burn — *see* Burn
  effects NOS T66
  sickness NOS T66
  therapy, encounter for Z51.0
Radiculitis (pressure) (vertebrogenic) — *see* Radiculopathy
Radiculomyelitis — *see also* Encephalitis
  toxic, due to
    Clostridium tetani A35
    Corynebacterium diphtheriae A36.82
Radiculopathy M54.10
  cervical region M54.12
  cervicothoracic region M54.13
  due to
    disc disorder
      C3 M50.11
      C4 M50.11
      C5 M50.121
      C6 M50.122
      C7 M50.123
      C8 M50.13
    displacement of intervertebral disc — *see* Disorder, disc, with, radiculopathy
  leg M54.1-
  lumbar region M54.16
  lumbosacral region M54.17
  occipito-atlanto-axial region M54.11
  postherpetic B02.29
  sacrococcygeal region M54.18
  syphilitic A52.11
  thoracic region (with visceral pain) M54.14
  thoracolumbar region M54.15
Radiodermal burns (acute, chronic, or occupational) — *see* Burn
Radiodermatitis L58.9
  acute L58.0
  chronic L58.1
Radiotherapy session Z51.0
RAEB (refractory anemia with excess blasts) D46.2-
Rage, meaning rabies — *see* Rabies
Ragpicker's disease A22.1
Ragsorter's disease A22.1
Raillietiniasis B71.8
Railroad neurosis F48.8
Railway spine F48.8
Raised — *see also* Elevated
  antibody titer R76.0
Rake teeth, tooth M26.39
Rales R09.89
Ramifying renal pelvis Q63.8
Ramsay-Hunt disease or syndrome (*see also* Hunt's disease) B02.21
  meaning dyssynergia cerebellaris myoclonica G11.1

Ranula K11.6
  congenital Q38.4
Rape
  adult
    confirmed T74.21
    suspected T76.21
  alleged, observation or examination, ruled out
    adult Z04.41
    child Z04.42
  child
    confirmed T74.22
    suspected T76.22
Rapid
  feeble pulse, due to shock, following injury T79.4
  heart (beat) R00.0
    psychogenic F45.8
  second stage (delivery) O62.3
  time-zone change syndrome — *see* Disorder, sleep, circadian rhythm, psychogenic
Rarefaction, bone — *see* Disorder, bone, density and structure, specified NEC
Rash (toxic) R21
  canker A38.9
  diaper L22
  drug (internal use) L27.0
    contact (*see also* Dermatitis, due to, drugs, external) L25.1
  following immunization T88.1
  food — *see* Dermatitis, due to, food
  heat L74.0
  napkin (psoriasiform) L22
  nettle — *see* Urticaria
  pustular L08.0
  rose R21
    epidemic B06.9
  scarlet A38.9
  serum (*see also* Reaction, serum) T80.69
  wandering tongue K14.1
Rasmussen aneurysm — *see* Tuberculosis, pulmonary
Rasmussen encephalitis G04.81
Rat-bite fever A25.9
  due to Streptobacillus moniliformis A25.1
  spirochetal (morsus muris) A25.0
Rathke's pouch tumor D44.3
Raymond (-Céstan) syndrome I65.8
Raynaud's disease, phenomenon or syndrome (secondary) I73.00
  with gangrene (symmetric) I73.01
RDS (newborn) (type I) P22.0
  type II P22.1
Reaction — *see also* Disorder
  adaptation — *see* Disorder, adjustment
  adjustment (anxiety) (conduct disorder) (depressiveness) (distress) — *see* Disorder, adjustment
    with
      mutism, elective (child) (adolescent) F94.0
  adverse
    food (any) (ingested) NEC T78.1
      anaphylactic — *see* Shock, anaphylactic, due to food
  affective — *see* Disorder, mood
  allergic — *see* Allergy
  anaphylactic — *see* Shock, anaphylactic
  anaphylactoid — *see* Shock, anaphylactic
  anesthesia — *see* Anesthesia, complication
  antitoxin (prophylactic) (therapeutic) — *see* Complications, vaccination
  anxiety F41.1
  Arthus — *see* Arthus' phenomenon
  asthenic F48.8
  combat and operational stress F43.0
  compulsive F42.8
  conversion F44.9
  crisis, acute F43.0
  deoxyribonuclease (DNA) (DNase) hypersensitivity D69.2

Reaction (*see also* Disorder) — *continued*
  depressive (single episode) F32.9
    affective (single episode) F31.4
      recurrent episode F33.9
    neurotic F34.1
    psychoneurotic F34.1
    psychotic F32.3
    recurrent — *see* Disorder, depressive, recurrent
  dissociative F44.9
  drug NEC T88.7
    addictive — *see* Dependence, drug
      transmitted via placenta or breast milk — *see* Absorption, drug, addictive, through placenta
    allergic — *see* Allergy, drug
    lichenoid L43.2
    newborn P93.8
      gray baby syndrome P93.0
    overdose or poisoning (by accident) — *see* Table of Drugs and Chemicals, by drug, poisoning
    photoallergic L56.1
    phototoxic L56.0
    withdrawal — *see* Dependence, by drug, with, withdrawal
      infant of dependent mother P96.1
      newborn P96.1
    wrong substance given or taken (by accident) — *see* Table of Drugs and Chemicals, by drug, poisoning
  fear F40.9
    child (abnormal) F93.8
  febrile nonhemolytic transfusion (FNHTR) R50.84
  fluid loss, cerebrospinal G97.1
  foreign
    body NEC — *see* Granuloma, foreign body
      in operative wound (inadvertently left) — *see* Foreign body, accidentally left during a procedure
    substance accidentally left during a procedure (chemical) (powder) (talc) T81.60
      aseptic peritonitis T81.61
      body or object (instrument) (sponge) (swab) — *see* Foreign body, accidentally left during a procedure
      specified reaction NEC T81.69
  grief — *see* Disorder, adjustment
  Herxheimer's R68.89
  hyperkinetic — *see* Hyperkinesia
  hypochondriacal F45.20
  hypoglycemic, due to insulin E16.0
    with coma (diabetic) — *see* Diabetes, coma nondiabetic E15
    therapeutic misadventure — *see* subcategory T38.3
  hypomanic F30.8
  hysterical F44.9
  immunization — *see* Complications, vaccination
  incompatibility
    ABO blood group (infusion) (transfusion) — *see* Complication(s), transfusion, incompatibility reaction, ABO
    delayed serologic T80.39
    minor blood group (Duffy) (E) (K(ell)) (Kidd) (Lewis) (M) (N) (P) (S) T80.89
    Rh (factor) (infusion) (transfusion) — *see* Complication(s), transfusion, incompatibility reaction, Rh (factor)
  inflammatory — *see* Infection
  infusion — *see* Complications, infusion
  inoculation (immune serum) — *see* Complications, vaccination
  insulin T38.3-
  involutional psychotic — *see* Disorder, depressive

Reaction (see also Disorder) — continued
leukemoid D72.823
basophilic D72.823
lymphocytic D72.823
monocytic D72.823
myelocytic D72.823
neutrophilic D72.823
LSD (acute)
due to drug abuse — see Abuse, drug, hallucinogen
due to drug dependence — see Dependence, drug, hallucinogen
lumbar puncture G97.1
manic-depressive — see Disorder, bipolar
neurasthenic F48.8
neurogenic — see Neurosis
neurotic F48.9
neurotic-depressive F34.1
nitritoid — see Crisis, nitritoid
nonspecific
to
cell mediated immunity measurement of gamma interferon anitgen response without active tuberculosis R76.12
Quanti-FERON-TB test (QFT) without active tuberculosis R76.12
tuberculin test (see also Reaction, tuberculin skin test) R76.11
obsessive-compulsive F42.8
organic, acute or subacute — see Delirium
paranoid (acute) F23
chronic F22
senile F03
passive dependency F60.7
phobic F40.9
post-traumatic stress, uncomplicated Z73.3
psychogenic F99
psychoneurotic — see also Neurosis
compulsive F42.8
depersonalization F48.1
depressive F34.1
hypochondriacal F45.20
neurasthenic F48.8
obsessive F42.8
psychophysiologic — see Disorder, somatoform
psychosomatic — see Disorder, somatoform
psychotic — see Psychosis
scarlet fever toxin — see Complications, vaccination
schizophrenic F23
acute (brief) (undifferentiated) F23
latent F21
undifferentiated (acute) (brief) F23
serological for syphilis — see Serology for syphilis
serum T80.69
anaphylactic (immediate) (see also Shock, anaphylactic) T80.59
specified reaction NEC
due to
administration of blood and blood products T80.61
immunization T80.62
serum specified NEC T80.69
vaccination T80.62
situational — see Disorder, adjustment
somatization — see Disorder, somatoform
spinal puncture G97.1
stress (severe) F43.9
acute (agitation) ("daze") (disorientation) (disturbance of consciousness) (flight reaction) (fugue) F43.0
specified NEC F43.8
surgical procedure — see Complications, surgical procedure
tetanus antitoxin — see Complications, vaccination

Reaction (see also Disorder) — continued
toxic, to local anesthesia T88.59
in labor and delivery O74.4
in pregnancy O29.3x-
postpartum, puerperal O89.3
toxin-antitoxin — see Complications, vaccination
transfusion (blood) (bone marrow) (lymphocytes) (allergic) — see Complications, transfusion
tuberculin skin test, abnormal R76.11
vaccination (any) — see Complications, vaccination
withdrawing, child or adolescent F93.8
Reactive airway disease — see Asthma
Reactive depression — see Reaction, depressive
Rearrangement
chromosomal
balanced (in) Q95.9
abnormal individual (autosomal) Q95.2
non-sex (autosomal) chromosomes Q95.2
sex/non-sex chromosomes Q95.3
specified NEC Q95.8
Recalcitrant patient — see Noncompliance
Recanalization, thrombus — see Thrombosis
Recession, receding
chamber angle (eye) H21.55-
chin M26.09
gingival (generalized) (localized) (postinfective) (postoperative) K06.00
Miller Class I K06.01
Miller Class II K06.02
Miller Class III K06.03
Miller Class IV K06.04
Recklinghausen disease Q85.01
bones E21.0
Reclus' disease (cystic) — see Mastopathy, cystic
Recrudescent typhus (fever) A75.1
Recruitment, auditory H93.21-
Rectalgia K62.89
Rectitis K62.89
Rectocele
female (without uterine prolapse) N81.6
with uterine prolapse N81.4
incomplete N81.2
in pregnancy — see Pregnancy, complicated by, abnormal, pelvic organs or tissues NEC
male K62.3
Rectosigmoid junction — see condition
Rectosigmoiditis K63.89
ulcerative (chronic) K51.30
with
complication K51.319
abscess K51.314
fistula K51.313
obstruction K51.312
rectal bleeding K51.311
specified NEC K51.318
Rectourethral — see condition
Rectovaginal — see condition
Rectovesical — see condition
Rectum, rectal — see condition
Recurrent — see condition
pregnancy loss — see Loss (of), pregnancy, recurrent
Red bugs B88.0
Red-cedar lung or pneumonitis J67.8
Red tide (see also Table of Drugs and Chemicals) T65.82-
Reduced
mobility Z74.09
ventilatory or vital capacity R94.2

Redundant, redundancy
anus (congenital) Q43.8
clitoris N90.89
colon (congenital) Q43.8
foreskin (congenital) N47.8
intestine (congenital) Q43.8
labia N90.69
organ or site, congenital NEC — see Accessory
panniculus (abdominal) E65
prepuce (congenital) N47.8
pylorus K31.89
rectum (congenital) Q43.8
scrotum N50.89
sigmoid (congenital) Q43.8
skin L98.7
and subcutaneous tissue L98.7
of face L57.4
eyelids — see Blepharochalasis
stomach K31.89
Reduplication — see Duplication
Reflex R29.2
hyperactive gag J39.2
pupillary, abnormal — see Anomaly, pupil, function
vasoconstriction I73.9
vasovagal R55
Reflux K21.9
acid K21.9
esophageal K21.9
with esophagitis K21.0
newborn P78.83
gastroesophageal K21.9
with esophagitis K21.0
mitral — see Insufficiency, mitral
ureteral — see Reflux, vesicoureteral
vesicoureteral (with scarring) N13.70
with
nephropathy N13.729
with hydroureter N13.739
bilateral N13.732
unilateral N13.731
bilateral N13.722
unilateral N13.721
without hydroureter N13.729
bilateral N13.722
unilateral N13.721
pyelonephritis (chronic) N11.0
congenital Q62.7
without nephropathy N13.71
Reforming, artificial openings — see Attention to, artificial, opening
Refractive error — see Disorder, refraction
Refsum's disease or syndrome G60.1
Refusal of
food, psychogenic F50.89
treatment (because of) Z53.20
left against medical advice (AMA) Z53.21
patient's decision NEC Z53.29
reasons of belief or group pressure Z53.1
Regional — see condition
Regurgitation R11.10
aortic (valve) — see Insufficiency, aortic
food — see also Vomiting
with reswallowing — see Rumination
newborn P92.1
gastric contents — see Vomiting
heart — see Endocarditis
mitral (valve) — see Insufficiency, mitral
congenital Q23.3
myocardial — see Endocarditis
pulmonary (valve) (heart) I37.1
congenital Q22.2
syphilitic A52.03
tricuspid — see Insufficiency, tricuspid
valve, valvular — see Endocarditis
congenital Q24.8
vesicoureteral — see Reflux, vesicoureteral
Reichmann's disease or syndrome K31.89
Reifenstein syndrome E34.52

Reinsertion
  implantable subdermal contraceptive Z30.46
  intrauterine contraceptive device Z30.433
Reiter's disease, syndrome, or urethritis
  M02.30
  ankle M02.37-
  elbow M02.32-
  foot joint M02.37-
  hand joint M02.34-
  hip M02.35-
  knee M02.36-
  multiple site M02.39
  shoulder M02.31-
  vertebra M02.38
  wrist M02.33-
Rejection
  food, psychogenic F50.89
  transplant T86.91
    bone T86.830
      marrow T86.01
    cornea T86.840
    heart T86.21
      with lung(s) T86.31
    intestine T86.850
    kidney T86.11
    liver T86.41
    lung(s) T86.810
      with heart T86.31
    organ (immune or nonimmune cause)
        T86.91
    pancreas T86.890
    skin (allograft) (autograft) T86.820
    specified NEC T86.890
    stem cell (peripheral blood) (umbilical cord)
        T86.5
Relapsing fever A68.9
  Carter's (Asiatic) A68.1
  Dutton's (West African) A68.1
  Koch's A68.9
  louse-borne (epidemic) A68.0
  Novy's (American) A68.1
  Obermeyers's (European) A68.0
  Spirillum A68.9
  tick-borne (endemic) A68.1
Relationship
  occlusal
    open anterior M26.220
    open posterior M26.221
Relaxation
  anus (sphincter) K62.89
    psychogenic F45.8
  arch (foot) — see also Deformity, limb, flat foot
  back ligaments — see Instability, joint, spine
  bladder (sphincter) N31.2
  cardioesophageal K21.9
  cervix — see Incompetency, cervix
  diaphragm J98.6
  joint (capsule) (ligament) (paralytic) — see
      Flail, joint
    congenital NEC Q74.8
  lumbosacral (joint) — see subcategory M53.2
  pelvic floor N81.89
  perineum N81.89
  posture R29.3
  rectum (sphincter) K62.89
  sacroiliac (joint) — see subcategory M53.2
  scrotum N50.89
  urethra (sphincter) N36.44
  vesical N31.2
Release from prison, anxiety concerning
  Z65.2
Remains
  canal of Cloquet Q14.0
  capsule (opaque) Q14.8
Remittent fever (malarial) B54
Remnant
  canal of Cloquet Q14.0
  capsule (opaque) Q14.8

Remnant — continued
  cervix, cervical stump (acquired)
      (postoperative) N88.8
  cystic duct, postcholecystectomy K91.5
  fingernail L60.8
    congenital Q84.6
  meniscus, knee — see Derangement, knee,
      meniscus, specified NEC
  thyroglossal duct Q89.2
  tonsil J35.8
    infected (chronic) J35.01
  urachus Q64.4
Removal (from) (of)
  artificial
    arm Z44.00-
      complete Z44.01-
      partial Z44.02-
    eye Z44.2-
    leg Z44.10-
      complete Z44.11-
      partial Z44.12-
  breast implant Z45.81
  cardiac pulse generator (battery) (end-of-life)
      Z45.010
  catheter (urinary) (indwelling) Z46.6
    from artificial opening — see Attention to,
        artificial, opening
    non-vascular Z46.82
    vascular NEC Z45.2
  device Z46.9
    contraceptive Z30.432
      implantable subdermal Z30.46
    implanted NEC Z45.89
    specified NEC Z46.89
  drains Z48.03
  dressing (nonsurgical) Z48.00
    surgical Z48.01
  external
    fixation device — code to fracture with
        seventh character D
    prosthesis, prosthetic device Z44.9
      breast Z44.3-
      specified NEC Z44.8
  home in childhood (to foster home or
      institution) Z62.29
  ileostomy Z43.2
  insulin pump Z46.81
  myringotomy device (stent) (tube) Z45.82
  nervous system device NEC Z46.2
    brain neuropacemaker Z46.2
    visual substitution device Z46.2
      implanted Z45.31
  non-vascular catheter Z46.82
  organ, prophylactic (for neoplasia manage-
      ment) — see Prophylactic, organ removal
  orthodontic device Z46.4
  staples Z48.02
  stent
    ureteral Z46.6
  suture Z48.02
  urinary device Z46.6
  vascular access device or catheter Z45.2
Ren
  arcuatus Q63.1
  mobile, mobilis N28.89
    congenital Q63.8
  unguliformis Q63.1
Renal — see condition
Rendu-Osler-Weber disease or
  syndrome I78.0
Reninoma D41.0-
Renon-Delille syndrome E23.3
Reovirus, as cause of disease classified
  elsewhere B97.5
Repeated falls NEC R29.6
Replaced chromosome by dicentric ring
  Q93.2

Replacement by artificial or mechanical
  device or prosthesis of
  bladder Z96.0
  blood vessel NEC Z95.828
  bone NEC Z96.7
  cochlea Z96.21
  coronary artery Z95.5
  eustachian tube Z96.29
  eye globe Z97.0
  heart Z95.812
    valve Z95.2
      prosthetic Z95.2
      specified NEC Z95.4
      xenogenic Z95.3
  intestine Z96.89
  joint Z96.60
    hip — see Presence, hip joint implant
    knee — see Presence, knee joint implant
    specified site NEC Z96.698
  larynx Z96.3
  lens Z96.1
  limb(s) — see Presence, artificial, limb
  mandible NEC (for tooth root implant(s)) Z96.5
  organ NEC Z96.89
  peripheral vessel NEC Z95.828
  stapes Z96.29
  teeth Z97.2
  tendon Z96.7
  tissue NEC Z96.89
  tooth root(s) Z96.5
  vessel NEC Z95.828
    coronary (artery) Z95.5
Request for expert evidence Z04.8
Reserve, decreased or low
  cardiac — see Disease, heart
  kidney N28.89
Residual — see also condition
  ovary syndrome N99.83
  state, schizophrenic F20.5
  urine R39.198
Resistance, resistant (to)
  activated protein C D68.51
  complicating pregnancy O26.89
  insulin E88.81
  organism(s)
    to
      drug Z16.30
        aminoglycosides Z16.29
        amoxicillin Z16.11
        ampicillin Z16.11
        antibiotic(s) Z16.20
          multiple Z16.24
          specified NEC Z16.29
        antifungal Z16.32
        antimicrobial (single) Z16.30
          multiple Z16.35
          specified NEC Z16.39
        antimycobacterial (single) Z16.341
          multiple Z16.342
        antiparasitic Z16.31
        antiviral Z16.33
        beta lactam antibiotics Z16.10
          specified NEC Z16.19
        cephalosporins Z16.19
        extended beta lactamase (ESBL) Z16.12
        fluoroquinolones Z16.23
        macrolides Z16.29
        methicillin — see MRSA
        multiple drugs (MDRO)
          antibiotics Z16.24
          antimicrobial Z16.35
          antimycobacterial (single) Z16.341
        penicillins Z16.11
        quinine (and related compounds)
            Z16.31
        quinolones Z16.23
        sulfonamides Z16.29
        tetracyclines Z16.29

DISEASE INDEX

D I S E A S E   I N D E X

Resistance, resistant (to) — *continued*
  organism(s) — *continued*
    to — *continued*
      drug Z16.30 — *continued*
        tuberculostatics (single) Z16.341
          multiple Z16.342
        vancomycin Z16.21
          related antibiotics Z16.22
  thyroid hormone E07.89
Resorption
  dental (roots) K03.3
    alveoli M26.79
  teeth (external) (internal) (pathological) (roots)
    K03.3
Respiration
  Cheyne-Stokes R06.3
  decreased due to shock, following injury T79.4
  disorder of, psychogenic F45.8
  insufficient, or poor R06.89
    newborn P28.5
  painful R07.1
  sighing, psychogenic F45.8
Respiratory — *see also* condition
  distress syndrome (newborn) (type I) P22.0
    type II P22.1
  syncytial virus, as cause of disease classified
    elsewhere B97.4
Respite care Z75.5
Response (drug)
  photoallergic L56.1
  phototoxic L56.0
Restenosis
  stent
    vascular
      end stent
        adjacent to stent — *see* Arteriosclerosis
        within the stent
          coronary T82.855
          peripheral T82.856
      in stent
        coronary vessel T82.855
        peripheral vessel T82.856
Restless legs (syndrome) G25.81
Restlessness R45.1
Restoration (of)
  dental
    aesthetically inadequate or displeasing
      K08.56
    defective K08.50
      specified NEC K08.59
    failure of marginal integrity K08.51
    failure of periodontal anatomical intergrity
      K08.54
  organ continuity from previous sterilization
    (tuboplasty) (vasoplasty) Z31.0
    aftercare Z31.42
  tooth (existing)
    contours biologically incompatible with oral
      health K08.54
    open margins K08.51
    overhanging K08.52
    poor aesthetic K08.56
    poor gingival margins K08.51
  unsatisfactory, of tooth K08.50
    specified NEC K08.59
Restorative material (dental)
  allergy to K08.55
  fractured K08.539
    with loss of material K08.531
    without loss of material K08.530
  unrepairable overhanging of K08.52
Restriction of housing space Z59.1
Rests, ovarian, in fallopian tube Q50.6
Restzustand (schizophrenic) F20.5
Retained — *see also* Retention
  cholelithiasis following cholecystectomy
    K91.86

Retained — *see also* Retention — *continued*
  foreign body fragments (type of) Z18.9
    acrylics Z18.2
    animal quill(s) or spines Z18.31
    cement Z18.83
    concrete Z18.83
    crystalline Z18.83
    depleted isotope Z18.09
    depleted uranium Z18.01
    diethylhexylphthalates Z18.2
    glass Z18.81
    isocyanate Z18.2
    magnetic metal Z18.11
    metal Z18.10
    nonmagnectic metal Z18.12
    nontherapeutic radioactive Z18.09
    organic NEC Z18.39
    plastic Z18.2
    quill(s) (animal) Z18.31
    radioactive (nontherapeutic) NEC Z18.09
    specified NEC Z18.89
    spine(s) (animal) Z18.31
    stone Z18.83
    tooth (teeth) Z18.32
    wood Z18.33
  fragments (type of) Z18.9
    acrylics Z18.2
    animal quill(s) or spines Z18.31
    cement Z18.83
    concrete Z18.83
    crystalline Z18.83
    depleted isotope Z18.09
    depleted uranium Z18.01
    diethylhexylphthalates Z18.2
    glass Z18.81
    isocyanate Z18.2
    magnetic metal Z18.11
    metal Z18.10
    nonmagnectic metal Z18.12
    nontherapeutic radioactive Z18.09
    organic NEC Z18.39
    plastic Z18.2
    quill(s) (animal) Z18.31
    radioactive (nontherapeutic) NEC Z18.09
    specified NEC Z18.89
    spine(s) (animal) Z18.31
    stone Z18.83
    tooth (teeth) Z18.32
    wood Z18.33
  gallstones, following cholecystectomy K91.86
Retardation
  development, developmental, specific — *see*
    Disorder, developmental
  endochondral bone growth — *see* Disorder,
    bone, development or growth
  growth R62.50
    due to malnutrition E45
  mental — *see* Disability, intellectual
  motor function, specific F82
  physical (child) R62.52
    due to malnutrition E45
  reading (specific) F81.0
  spelling (specific) (without reading disorder)
    F81.81
Retching — *see* Vomiting
Retention — *see also* Retained
  bladder — *see* Retention, urine
  carbon dioxide E87.2
  cholelithiasis following cholecystectomy
    K91.86
  cyst — *see* Cyst
  dead
    fetus (at or near term) (mother) O36.4
      early fetal death O02.1
    ovum O02.0
  decidua (fragments) (following delivery) (with
    hemorrhage) O72.2
    without hemorrhage O73.1
  deciduous tooth K00.6

Retention (*see also* Retained) — *continued*
  dental root K08.3
  fecal — *see* Constipation
  fetus
    dead O36.4
      early O02.1
  fluid R60.9
  foreign body — *see also* Foreign body, retained
    current trauma — *code as* Foreign body, by
      site or type
  gallstones, following cholecystectomy K91.86
  gastric K31.89
  intrauterine contraceptive device, in pregnancy
    — *see* Pregnancy, complicated by,
      retention, intrauterine device
  membranes (complicating delivery) (with
    hemorrhage) O72.2
    with abortion — *see* Abortion, by type
    without hemorrhage O73.1
  meniscus — *see* Derangement, meniscus
  menses N94.89
  milk (puerperal, postpartum) O92.79
  nitrogen, extrarenal R39.2
  ovary syndrome N99.83
  placenta (total) (with hemorrhage) O72.0
    portions or fragments (with hemorrhage)
      O72.2
      without hemorrhage O73.1
    without hemorrhage O73.0
  products of conception
    early pregnancy (dead fetus) O02.1
    following
      delivery (with hemorrhage) O72.2
        without hemorrhage O73.1
  secundines (following delivery) (with
    hemorrhage) O72.0
  complicating puerperium (delayed
    hemorrhage) O72.2
  partial O72.2
    without hemorrhage O73.1
    without hemorrhage O73.0
  smegma, clitoris N90.89
  urine R33.9
    drug-induced R33.0
    due to hyperplasia (hypertrophy) of prostate
      — *see* Hyperplasia, prostate
    organic R33.8
      drug-induced R33.0
    psychogenic F45.8
    specified NEC R33.8
  water (in tissues) — *see* Edema
Reticular erythematous mucinosis L98.5
Reticulation, dust — *see* Pneumoconiosis
Reticulocytosis R70.1
Reticuloendotheliosis
  acute infantile C96.0
  leukemic C91.4-
  nonlipid C96.0
Reticulohistiocytoma (giant-cell) D76.3
Reticuloid, actinic L57.1
Reticulosis (skin)
  acute of infancy C96.0
  hemophagocytic, familial D76.1
  histiocytic medullary C96.A
  lipomelanotic I89.8
  malignant (midline) C86.0
  polymorphic C86.0
  Sézary — *see* Sézary disease
Retina, retinal — *see also* condition
  dark area D49.81
Retinitis — *see also* Inflammation, chorioretinal
  albuminurica N18.9 *[H32]*
  diabetic — *see* Diabetes, retinitis
  disciformis — *see* Degeneration, macula
  focal — *see* Inflammation, chorioretinal, focal
  gravidarum — *see* Pregnancy, complicated by,
    specified pregnancy-related condition
    NEC

Retinitis — *see also* Inflammation, chorioretinal
— *continued*
  juxtapapillaris — *see* Inflammation,
    chorioretinal, focal, juxtapapillary
  luetic — *see* Retinitis, syphilitic
  pigmentosa H35.52
  proliferans — *see* Disorder, globe,
    degenerative, specified type NEC
  proliferating — *see* Disorder, globe,
    degenerative, specified type NEC
  renal N18.9 *[H32]*
  syphilitic (early) (secondary) A51.43
    central, recurrent A52.71
    congenital (early) A50.01 *[H32]*
    late A52.71
  tuberculous A18.53
Retinoblastoma C69.2-
  differentiated C69.2-
  undifferentiated C69.2-
Retinochoroiditis — *see also* Inflammation,
  chorioretinal
  disseminated — *see* Inflammation,
    chorioretinal, disseminated
    syphilitic A52.71
  focal — *see* Inflammation, chorioretinal
  juxtapapillaris — *see* Inflammation,
    chorioretinal, focal, juxtapapillary
Retinopathy (background) H35.00
  arteriosclerotic I70.8 *[H35.0-]*
  atherosclerotic I70.8 *[H35.0-]*
  central serous — *see* Chorioretinopathy, central
    serous
  Coats H35.02-
  diabetic — *see* Diabetes, retinopathy
  exudative H35.02-
  hypertensive H35.03-
  in (due to)
    diabetes — *see* Diabetes, retinopathy
    sickle-cell disorders D57-*[H36]*
  of prematurity H35.10-
    stage 0 H35.11-
    stage 1 H35.12-
    stage 2 H35.13-
    stage 3 H35.14-
    stage 4 H35.15-
    stage 5 H35.16-
  pigmentary, congenital — *see* Dystrophy,
    retina
  proliferative NEC H35.2-
    diabetic — *see* Diabetes, retinopathy,
      proliferative
    sickle-cell D57-*[H36]*
  solar H31.02-
Retinoschisis H33.10-
  congenital Q14.1
  specified type NEC H33.19-
Retortamoniasis A07.8
Retractile testis Q55.22
Retraction
  cervix — *see* Retroversion, uterus
  drum (membrane) — *see* Disorder, tympanic
    membrane, specified NEC
  finger — *see* Deformity, finger
  lid H02.539
    left H02.536
      lower H02.535
      upper H02.534
    right H02.533
      lower H02.532
      upper H02.531
  lung J98.4
  mediastinum J98.59
  nipple N64.53
    associated with
      lactation O92.03
      pregnancy O92.01-
      puerperium O92.02
    congenital Q83.8
  palmar fascia M72.0

Retraction — *continued*
  pleura — *see* Pleurisy
  ring, uterus (Bandl's) (pathological) O62.4
  sternum (congenital) Q76.7
    acquired M95.4
  uterus — *see* Retroversion, uterus
  valve (heart) — *see* Endocarditis
Retrobulbar — *see* condition
Retrocecal — *see* condition
Retrocession — *see* Retroversion
Retrodisplacement — *see* Retroversion
Retroflection, retroflexion — *see*
  Retroversion
Retrognathia, retrognathism (mandibular)
  (maxillary) M26.19
Retrograde menstruation N92.5
Retroperineal — *see* condition
Retroperitoneal — *see* condition
Retroperitonitis K68.9
Retropharyngeal — *see* condition
Retroplacental — *see* condition
Retroposition — *see* Retroversion
Retroprosthetic membrane T85.398
Retrosternal thyroid (congenital) Q89.2
Retroversion, retroverted
  cervix — *see* Retroversion, uterus
  female NEC — *see* Retroversion, uterus
  iris H21.89
  testis (congenital) Q55.29
  uterus (acquired) (acute) (any degree)
    (asymptomatic) (cervix) (postinfectional)
    (postpartal, old) N85.4
    congenital Q51.818
    in pregnancy O34.53-
Retrovirus, as cause of disease classified
  elsewhere B97.30
  human
    immunodeficiency, type 2 (HIV 2) B97.35
    T-cell lymphotropic
      type I (HTLV-I) B97.33
      type II (HTLV-II) B97.34
  lentivirus B97.31
  oncovirus B97.32
  specified NEC B97.39
Retrusion, premaxilla (developmental)
  M26.09
Rett's disease or syndrome F84.2
Reverse peristalsis R19.2
Reye's syndrome G93.7
Rh (factor)
  hemolytic disease (newborn) P55.0
  incompatibility, immunization or sensitization
    affecting management of pregnancy NEC
    O36.09-
    anti-D antibody O36.01-
    newborn P55.0
    transfusion reaction — *see* Complication(s),
      transfusion, incompatibility reaction, Rh
      (factor)
  negative mother affecting newborn P55.0
  titer elevated — *see* Complication(s),
    transfusion, incompatibility reaction, Rh
    (factor)
  transfusion reaction — *see* Complication(s),
    transfusion, incompatibility reaction, Rh
    (factor)
Rhabdomyolysis (idiopathic) NEC M62.82
  traumatic T79.6
Rhabdomyoma — *see also* Neoplasm,
  connective tissue, benign
  adult — *see* Neoplasm, connective tissue,
    benign
  fetal — *see* Neoplasm, connective tissue,
    benign
  glycogenic — *see* Neoplasm, connective tissue,
    benign
Rhabdomyosarcoma (any type) — *see*
  Neoplasm, connective tissue, malignant
Rhabdosarcoma — *see* Rhabdomyosarcoma

Rhesus (factor) incompatibility — *see* Rh,
  incompatibility
Rheumatic (acute) (subacute) (chronic)
  adherent pericardium I09.2
  coronary arteritis I01.9
  degeneration, myocardium I09.0
  fever (acute) — *see* Fever, rheumatic
  heart — *see* Disease, heart, rheumatic
  myocardial degeneration — *see* Degeneration,
    myocardium
  myocarditis (chronic) (inactive) (with chorea)
    I09.0
    with chorea (acute) (rheumatic) (Sydenham's)
      I02.0
    active or acute I01.2
  pancarditis, acute I01.8
    with chorea (acute (rheumatic) Sydenham's)
      I02.0
  pericarditis (active) (acute) (with effusion) (with
    pneumonia) I01.0
    with chorea (acute) (rheumatic) (Sydenham's)
      I02.0
    chronic or inactive I09.2
  pneumonia I00 *[J17]*
  torticollis M43.6
  typhoid fever A01.09
Rheumatism (articular) (neuralgic)
  (nonarticular) M79.0
  gout — *see* Arthritis, rheumatoid
  intercostal, meaning Tietze's disease M94.0
  palindromic (any site) M12.30
    ankle M12.37-
    elbow M12.32-
    foot joint M12.37-
    hand joint M12.34-
    hip M12.35-
    knee M12.36-
    multiple site M12.39
    shoulder M12.31-
    specified joint NEC M12.38
    vertebrae M12.38
    wrist M12.33-
  sciatic M54.4-
Rheumatoid — *see also* condition
  arthritis — *see also* Arthritis, rheumatoid
    with involvement of organs NEC M05.60
      ankle M05.67-
      elbow M05.62-
      foot joint M05.67-
      hand joint M05.64-
      hip M05.65-
      knee M05.66-
      multiple site M05.69
      shoulder M05.61-
      vertebra — *see* Spondylitis, ankylosing
      wrist M05.63-
    seronegative — *see* Arthritis, rheumatoid,
      seronegative
    seropositive — *see* Arthritis, rheumatoid,
      seropositive
  carditis M05.30
    ankle M05.37-
    elbow M05.32-
    foot joint M05.37-
    hand joint M05.34-
    hip M05.35-
    knee M05.36-
    multiple site M05.39
    shoulder M05.31-
    vertebra — *see* Spondylitis, ankylosing
    wrist M05.33-
  endocarditis — *see* Rheumatoid, carditis
  lung (disease) M05.10
    ankle M05.17-
    elbow M05.12-
    foot joint M05.17-
    hand joint M05.14-
    hip M05.15-
    knee M05.16-

Rheumatoid (see also condition) — continued
  lung (disease) M05.10 — continued
    multiple site M05.19
    shoulder M05.11-
    vertebra — see Spondylitis, ankylosing
    wrist M05.13-
  myocarditis — see Rheumatoid, carditis
  myopathy M05.40
    ankle M05.47-
    elbow M05.42-
    foot joint M05.47-
    hand joint M05.44-
    hip M05.45-
    knee M05.46-
    multiple site M05.49
    shoulder M05.41-
    vertebra — see Spondylitis, ankylosing
    wrist M05.43-
  pericarditis — see Rheumatoid, carditis
  polyarthritis — see Arthritis, rheumatoid
  polyneuropathy M05.50
    ankle M05.57-
    elbow M05.52-
    foot joint M05.57-
    hand joint M05.54-
    hip M05.55-
    knee M05.56-
    multiple site M05.59
    shoulder M05.51-
    vertebra — see Spondylitis, ankylosing
    wrist M05.53-
  vasculitis M05.20
    ankle M05.27-
    elbow M05.22-
    foot joint M05.27-
    hand joint M05.24-
    hip M05.25-
    knee M05.26-
    multiple site M05.29
    shoulder M05.21-
    vertebra — see Spondylitis, ankylosing
    wrist M05.23-
Rhinitis (atrophic) (catarrhal) (chronic)
  (croupous) (fibrinous) (granulomatous)
  (hyperplastic) (hypertrophic) (membranous)
  (obstructive) (purulent) (suppurative)
  (ulcerative) J31.0
  with
    sore throat — see Nasopharyngitis
  acute J00
  allergic J30.9
    with asthma J45.909
      with
        exacerbation (acute) J45.901
        status asthmaticus J45.902
      due to
        food J30.5
        pollen J30.1
      nonseasonal J30.89
      perennial J30.89
      seasonal NEC J30.2
      specified NEC J30.89
  infective J00
  pneumococcal J00
  syphilitic A52.73
    congenital A50.05 [J99]
  tuberculous A15.8
  vasomotor J30.0
Rhinoantritis (chronic) — see Sinusitis,
  maxillary
Rhinodacryolith — see Dacryolith
Rhinolith (nasal sinus) J34.89
Rhinomegaly J34.89
Rhinopharyngitis (acute) (subacute) — see
  also Nasopharyngitis
  chronic J31.1
  destructive ulcerating A66.5
  mutilans A66.5
Rhinophyma L71.1

Rhinorrhea J34.89
  cerebrospinal (fluid) G96.0
  paroxysmal — see Rhinitis, allergic
  spasmodic — see Rhinitis, allergic
Rhinosalpingitis — see Salpingitis, eustachian
Rhinoscleroma A48.8
Rhinosporidiosis B48.1
Rhinovirus infection NEC B34.8
Rhizomelic chondrodysplasia punctata
  E71.540
Rhythm
  atrioventricular nodal I49.8
  disorder I49.9
    coronary sinus I49.8
    ectopic I49.8
    nodal I49.8
  escape I49.9
  heart, abnormal I49.9
  idioventricular I44.2
  nodal I49.8
  sleep, inversion G47.2-
    nonorganic origin — see Disorder, sleep,
      circadian rhythm, psychogenic
Rhytidosis facialis L98.8
Rib — see also condition
  cervical Q76.5
Riboflavin deficiency E53.0
Rice bodies — see also Loose, body, joint
  knee M23.4-
Richter syndrome — see Leukemia, chronic
  lymphocytic, B-cell type
Richter's hernia — see Hernia, abdomen,
  with obstruction
Ricinism — see Poisoning, food, noxious, plant
Rickets (active) (acute) (adolescent) (chest wall)
  (congenital) (current) (infantile) (intestinal)
  E55.0
  adult — see Osteomalacia
  celiac K90.0
  hypophosphatemic with nephrotic-glycosuric
    dwarfism E72.09
  inactive E64.3
  kidney N25.0
  renal N25.0
  sequelae, any E64.3
  vitamin-D-resistant E83.31 [M90.80]
Rickettsial disease A79.9
  specified type NEC A79.89
Rickettsialpox (Rickettsia akari) A79.1
Rickettsiosis A79.9
  due to
    Ehrlichia sennetsu A79.81
    Rickettsia akari (rickettsialpox) A79.1
  specified type NEC A79.89
  tick-borne A77.9
  vesicular A79.1
Rider's bone — see Ossification, muscle,
  specified NEC
Ridge, alveolus — see also condition
  flabby K06.8
Ridged ear, congenital Q17.3
Riedel's
  lobe, liver Q44.7
  struma, thyroiditis or disease E06.5
Rieger's anomaly or syndrome Q13.81
Riehl's melanosis L81.4
Rietti-Greppi-Micheli anemia D56.9
Rieux's hernia — see Hernia, abdomen,
  specified site NEC
Riga (-Fede) disease K14.0
Riggs' disease — see Periodontitis
Right aortic arch Q25.47
Right middle lobe syndrome J98.11
Rigid, rigidity — see also condition
  abdominal R19.30
    with severe abdominal pain R10.0
      epigastric R19.36
      generalized R19.37
      left lower quadrant R19.34

Rigid, rigidity — see also condition —
  continued
  abdominal R19.30 — continued
    left upper quadrant R19.32
    periumbilic R19.35
    right lower quadrant R19.33
    right upper quadrant R19.31
  articular, multiple, congenital Q68.8
  cervix (uteri) in pregnancy — see Pregnancy,
    complicated by, abnormal, cervix
  hymen (acquired) (congenital) N89.6
  nuchal R29.1
  pelvic floor in pregnancy — see Pregnancy,
    complicated by, abnormal, pelvic organs
    or tissues NEC
  perineum or vulva in pregnancy — see
    Pregnancy, complicated by, abnormal,
    vulva
  spine — see Dorsopathy, specified NEC
  vagina in pregnancy — see Pregnancy,
    complicated by, abnormal, vagina
Rigors R68.89
  with fever R50.9
Riley-Day syndrome G90.1
RIND (reversible ischemic neurologic deficit)
  I63.9
Ring(s)
  aorta (vascular) Q25.45
  Bandl's O62.4
  contraction, complicating delivery O62.4
  esophageal, lower (muscular) K22.2
  Fleischer's (cornea) H18.04-
  hymenal, tight (acquired) (congenital) N89.6
  Kayser-Fleischer (cornea) H18.04-
  retraction, uterus, pathological O62.4
  Schatzki's (esophagus) (lower) K22.2
    congenital Q39.3
  Soemmerring's — see Cataract, secondary
  vascular (congenital) Q25.8
    aorta Q25.45
Ringed hair (congenital) Q84.1
Ringworm B35.9
  beard B35.0
  black dot B35.0
  body B35.4
  Burmese B35.5
  corporeal B35.4
  foot B35.3
  groin B35.6
  hand B35.2
  honeycomb B35.0
  nails B35.1
  perianal (area) B35.6
  scalp B35.0
  specified NEC B35.8
  Tokelau B35.5
Rise, venous pressure I87.8
Rising, PSA following treatment for
  malignant neoplasm of prostate
  R97.21
Risk, suicidal
  meaning personal history of attempted suicide
    Z91.5
  meaning suicidal ideation — see Ideation,
    suicidal
Ritter's disease L00
Rivalry, sibling Z62.891
Rivalta's disease A42.2
River blindness B73.01
Robert's pelvis Q74.2
  with disproportion (fetopelvic) O33.0
    causing obstructed labor O65.0
Robin(-Pierre) syndrome Q87.0
Robinow-Silvermann-Smith syndrome
  Q87.1
Robinson's (hidrotic) ectodermal
  dysplasia or syndrome Q82.4
Robles' disease B73.01
Rocky Mountain (spotted) fever A77.0

DISEASE INDEX

Roetheln — *see* Rubella
Roger's disease Q21.0
Rokitansky-Aschoff sinuses (gallbladder) K82.8
Rolando's fracture (displaced) S62.22-
  nondisplaced S62.22-
Romano-Ward (prolonged QT interval) syndrome I45.81
Romberg's disease or syndrome G51.8
Roof, mouth — *see* condition
Rosacea L71.9
  acne L71.9
  keratitis L71.8
  specified NEC L71.8
Rosary, rachitic E55.0
Rose
  cold J30.1
  fever J30.1
  rash R21
    epidemic B06.9
Rosenbach's erysipeloid A26.0
Rosenthal's disease or syndrome D68.1
Roseola B09
  infantum B08.20
    due to human herpesvirus 6 B08.21
    due to human herpesvirus 7 B08.22
Ross River disease or fever B33.1
Rossbach's disease K31.89
  psychogenic F45.8
Rostan's asthma (cardiac) — *see* Failure, ventricular, left
Rotation
  anomalous, incomplete or insufficient, intestine Q43.3
  cecum (congenital) Q43.3
  colon (congenital) Q43.3
  spine, incomplete or insufficient — *see* Dorsopathy, deforming, specified NEC
  tooth, teeth, fully erupted M26.35
  vertebra, incomplete or insufficient — *see* Dorsopathy, deforming, specified NEC
Rotes Quérol disease or syndrome — *see* Hyperostosis, ankylosing
Roth(-Bernhardt) disease or syndrome — *see* Meralgia paraesthetica
Rothmund(-Thomson) syndrome Q82.8
Rotor's disease or syndrome E80.6
Round
  back (with wedging of vertebrae) — *see* Kyphosis
  sequelae (late effect) of rickets E64.3
  worms (large) (infestation) NEC B82.0
    Ascariasis (*see also* Ascariasis) B77.9
Roussy-Lévy syndrome G60.0
Rubella (German measles) B06.9
  complication NEC B06.09
    neurological B06.00
  congenital P35.0
  contact Z20.4
  exposure to Z20.4
  maternal
    care for (suspected) damage to fetus O35.3
    manifest rubella in infant P35.0
    suspected damage to fetus affecting management of pregnancy O35.3
  specified complications NEC B06.89
Rubeola (meaning measles) — *see* Measles
  meaning rubella — *see* Rubella
Rubeosis, iris — *see* Disorder, iris, vascular
Rubinstein-Taybi syndrome Q87.2
Rudimentary (congenital) — *see also* Agenesis
  arm — *see* Defect, reduction, upper limb
  bone Q79.9
  cervix uteri Q51.828
  eye Q11.2
  lobule of ear Q17.3
  patella Q74.1
  respiratory organs in thoracopagus Q89.4
  tracheal bronchus Q32.4

Rudimentary (congenital) — *see also* Agenesis — *continued*
  uterus Q51.818
    in male Q56.1
  vagina Q52.0
Ruled out condition — *see* Observation, suspected
Rumination R11.10
  with nausea R11.2
  disorder of infancy F98.21
  neurotic F42.8
  newborn P92.1
  obsessional F42.8
  psychogenic F42.8
Runeberg's disease D51.0
Runny nose R09.89
Rupia (syphilitic) A51.39
  congenital A50.06
  tertiary A52.79
Rupture, ruptured
  abscess (spontaneous) — *code by site under* Abscess
  aneurysm — *see* Aneurysm
  anus (sphincter) — *see* Laceration, anus
  aorta, aortic I71.8
    abdominal I71.3
    arch I71.1
    ascending I71.1
    descending I71.8
      abdominal I71.3
      thoracic I71.1
    syphilitic A52.01
    thoracoabdominal I71.5
    thorax, thoracic I71.1
    transverse I71.1
    traumatic — *see* Injury, aorta, laceration, major
    valve or cusp (*see also* Endocarditis, aortic) I35.8
  appendix (with peritonitis) K35.2
    with localized peritonitis K35.3
  arteriovenous fistula, brain I60.8
  artery I77.2
    brain — *see* Hemorrhage, intracranial, intracerebral
    coronary — *see* Infarct, myocardium
    heart — *see* Infarct, myocardium
    pulmonary I28.8
    traumatic (complication) — *see* Injury, blood vessel
  bile duct (common) (hepatic) K83.2
    cystic K82.2
  bladder (sphincter) (nontraumatic) (spontaneous) N32.89
    following ectopic or molar pregnancy O08.6
    obstetrical trauma O71.5
    traumatic S37.29
  blood vessel — *see also* Hemorrhage
    brain — *see* Hemorrhage, intracranial, intracerebral
    heart — *see* Infarct, myocardium
    traumatic (complication) — *see* Injury, blood vessel, laceration, major, by site
  bone — *see* Fracture
  bowel (nontraumatic) K63.1
  brain
    aneurysm (congenital) — *see also* Hemorrhage, intracranial, subarachnoid
      syphilitic A52.05
    hemorrhagic — *see* Hemorrhage, intracranial, intracerebral
  capillaries I78.8
  cardiac (auricle) (ventricle) (wall) I23.3
    with hemopericardium I23.0
    infectional I40.9
    traumatic — *see* Injury, heart
  cartilage (articular) (current) — *see also* Sprain
    knee S83.3-
    semilunar — *see* Tear, meniscus

Rupture, ruptured — *continued*
  cecum (with peritonitis) K65.0
    with peritoneal abscess K35.3
    traumatic S36.598
  celiac artery, traumatic — *see* Injury, blood vessel, celiac artery, laceration, major
  cerebral aneurysm (congenital) (*see* Hemorrhage, intracranial, subarachnoid)
  cervix (uteri)
    with ectopic or molar pregnancy O08.6
    following ectopic or molar pregnancy O08.6
    obstetrical trauma O71.3
    traumatic S37.69
  chordae tendineae NEC I51.1
    concurrent with acute myocardial infarction — *see* Infarct, myocardium
    following acute myocardial infarction (current complication) I23.4
  choroid (direct) (indirect) (traumatic) H31.32-
  circle of Willis I60.6
  colon (nontraumatic) K63.1
    traumatic — *see* Injury, intestine, large
  cornea (traumatic) — *see* Injury, eye, laceration
  coronary (artery) (thrombotic) — *see* Infarct, myocardium
  corpus luteum (infected) (ovary) N83.1-
  cyst — *see* Cyst
  cystic duct K82.2
  Descemet's membrane — *see* Change, corneal membrane, Descemet's, rupture
    traumatic — *see* Injury, eye, laceration
  diaphragm, traumatic — *see* Injury, intrathoracic, diaphragm
  disc — *see* Rupture, intervertebral disc
  diverticulum (intestine) K57.80
    with bleeding K57.81
    bladder N32.3
    large intestine K57.20
      with
        bleeding K57.21
        small intestine K57.40
          with bleeding K57.41
    small intestine K57.00
      with
        bleeding K57.01
        large intestine K57.40
          with bleeding K57.41
  duodenal stump K31.89
  ear drum (nontraumatic) — *see also* Perforation, tympanum
    traumatic S09.2-
    due to blast injury — *see* Injury, blast, ear
  esophagus K22.3
  eye (without prolapse or loss of intraocular tissue) — *see* Injury, eye, laceration
  fallopian tube NEC (nonobstetric) (nontraumatic) N83.8
    due to pregnancy O00.10
      with intrauterine pregnancy O00.11
  fontanel P13.1
  gallbladder K82.2
    traumatic S36.128
  gastric — *see also* Rupture, stomach
    vessel K92.2
  globe (eye) (traumatic) — *see* Injury, eye, laceration
  graafian follicle (hematoma) N83.0-
  heart — *see* Rupture, cardiac
  hymen (nontraumatic) (nonintentional) N89.8
  internal organ, traumatic — *see* Injury, by site
  intervertebral disc — *see* Displacement, intervertebral disc
    traumatic — *see* Rupture, traumatic, intervertebral disc
  intestine NEC (nontraumatic) K63.1
    traumatic — *see* Injury, intestine
  iris — *see also* Abnormality, pupillary
    traumatic — *see* Injury, eye, laceration

Rupture, ruptured — *continued*
- joint capsule, traumatic — *see* Sprain
- kidney (traumatic) S37.06-
  - birth injury P15.8
  - nontraumatic N28.89
- lacrimal duct (traumatic) — *see* Injury, eye, specified site NEC
- lens (cataract) (traumatic) — *see* Cataract, traumatic
- ligament, traumatic — *see* Rupture, traumatic, ligament, by site
- liver S36.116
  - birth injury P15.0
- lymphatic vessel I89.8
- marginal sinus (placental) (with hemorrhage) — *see* Hemorrhage, antepartum, specified cause NEC
- membrana tympani (nontraumatic) — *see* Perforation, tympanum
- membranes (spontaneous)
  - artificial
    - delayed delivery following O75.5
  - delayed delivery following — *see* Pregnancy, complicated by, premature rupture of membranes
- meningeal artery I60.8
- meniscus (knee) — *see also* Tear, meniscus
  - old — *see* Derangement, meniscus
  - site other than knee — *code as* Sprain
- mesenteric artery, traumatic — *see* Injury, mesenteric, artery, laceration, major
- mesentery (nontraumatic) K66.8
  - traumatic — *see* Injury, intra-abdominal, specified, site NEC
- mitral (valve) I34.8
- muscle (traumatic) — *see also* Strain
  - diastasis — *see* Diastasis, muscle
  - nontraumatic M62.10
    - ankle M62.17-
    - foot M62.17-
    - forearm M62.13-
    - hand M62.14-
    - lower leg M62.16-
    - pelvic region M62.15-
    - shoulder region M62.11-
    - specified site NEC M62.18
    - thigh M62.15-
    - upper arm M62.12-
  - traumatic — *see* Strain, by site
- musculotendinous junction NEC, nontraumatic — *see* Rupture, tendon, spontaneous
- mycotic aneurysm causing cerebral hemorrhage — *see* Hemorrhage, intracranial, subarachnoid
- myocardium, myocardial — *see* Rupture, cardiac
  - traumatic — *see* Injury, heart
- nontraumatic, meaning hernia — *see* Hernia
- obstructed — *see* Hernia, by site, obstructed
- operation wound — *see* Disruption, wound, operation
- ovary, ovarian N83.8
  - corpus luteum cyst N83.1-
  - follicle (graafian) N83.0-
- oviduct (nonobstetric) (nontraumatic) N83.8
  - due to pregnancy O00.10
    - with intrauterine pregnancy O00.11
- pancreas (nontraumatic) K86.89
  - traumatic S36.299
- papillary muscle NEC I51.2
  - following acute myocardial infarction (current complication) I23.5
- pelvic
  - floor, complicating delivery O70.1
  - organ NEC, obstetrical trauma O71.5
- perineum (nonobstetric) (nontraumatic) N90.89
  - complicating delivery — *see* Delivery, complicated, by, laceration, anus (sphincter)

Rupture, ruptured — *continued*
- postoperative wound — *see* Disruption, wound, operation
- prostate (traumatic) S37.828
- pulmonary
  - artery I28.8
  - valve (heart) I37.8
  - vein I28.8
  - vessel I28.8
- pus tube — *see* Salpingitis
- pyosalpinx — *see* Salpingitis
- rectum (nontraumatic) K63.1
  - traumatic S36.69
- retina, retinal (traumatic) (without detachment) — *see also* Break, retina
  - with detachment — *see* Detachment, retina, with retinal, break
- rotator cuff (nontraumatic) M75.10-
  - complete M75.12-
  - incomplete M75.11-
- sclera — *see* Injury, eye, laceration
- sigmoid (nontraumatic) K63.1
  - traumatic S36.593
- spinal cord — *see also* Injury, spinal cord, by region
  - due to injury at birth P11.5
  - newborn (birth injury) P11.5
- spleen (traumatic) S36.09
  - birth injury P15.1
  - congenital (birth injury) P15.1
  - due to P. vivax malaria B51.0
  - nontraumatic D73.5
  - spontaneous D73.5
- splenic vein R58
  - traumatic — *see* Injury, blood vessel, splenic vein
- stomach (nontraumatic) (spontaneous) K31.89
  - traumatic S36.39
- supraspinatus (complete) (incomplete) (nontraumatic) — *see* Tear, rotator cuff
- symphysis pubis
  - obstetric O71.6
  - traumatic S33.4
- synovium (cyst) M66.10
  - ankle M66.17-
  - elbow M66.12-
  - finger M66.14-
  - foot M66.17-
  - forearm M66.13-
  - hand M66.14-
  - pelvic region M66.15-
  - shoulder region M66.11-
  - specified site NEC M66.18
  - thigh M66.15-
  - toe M66.17-
  - upper arm M66.12-
  - wrist M66.13-
- tendon (traumatic) — *see* Strain
  - nontraumatic (spontaneous) M66.9
    - ankle M66.87-
    - extensor M66.20
      - ankle M66.27-
      - foot M66.27-
      - forearm M66.23-
      - hand M66.24-
      - lower leg M66.26-
      - multiple sites M66.29
      - pelvic region M66.25-
      - shoulder region M66.21-
      - specified site NEC M66.28
      - thigh M66.25-
      - upper arm M66.22-
    - flexor M66.30
      - ankle M66.37-
      - foot M66.37-
      - forearm M66.33-
      - hand M66.34-
      - lower leg M66.36-
      - multiple sites M66.39

Rupture, ruptured — *continued*
- tendon (traumatic) — *see* Strain — *continued*
  - nontraumatic (spontaneous) M66.9 — *continued*
    - flexor M66.30 — *continued*
      - pelvic region M66.35-
      - shoulder region M66.31-
      - specified site NEC M66.38
      - thigh M66.35-
      - upper arm M66.32-
    - foot M66.87-
    - forearm M66.83-
    - hand M66.84-
    - lower leg M66.86-
    - multiple sites M66.89
    - pelvic region M66.85-
    - shoulder region M66.81-
    - specified
      - site NEC M66.88
      - tendon M66.80
    - thigh M66.85-
    - upper arm M66.82-
- thoracic duct I89.8
- tonsil J35.8
- traumatic
  - aorta — *see* Injury, aorta, laceration, major
  - diaphragm — *see* Injury, intrathoracic, diaphragm
  - external site — *see* Wound, open, by site
  - eye — *see* Injury, eye, laceration
  - internal organ — *see* Injury, by site
  - intervertebral disc
    - cervical S13.0
    - lumbar S33.0
    - thoracic S23.0
  - kidney S37.06-
  - ligament — *see also* Sprain
    - ankle — *see* Sprain, ankle
    - carpus — *see* Rupture, traumatic, ligament, wrist
    - collateral (hand) — *see* Rupture, traumatic, ligament, finger, collateral
    - finger (metacarpophalangeal) (interphalangeal) S63.40-
      - collateral S63.41-
        - index S63.41-
        - little S63.41-
        - middle S63.41-
        - ring S63.41-
      - index S63.40-
      - little S63.40-
      - middle S63.40-
      - palmar S63.42-
        - index S63.42-
        - little S63.42-
        - middle S63.42-
        - ring S63.42-
      - ring S63.40-
      - specified site NEC S63.499
        - index S63.49-
        - little S63.49-
        - middle S63.49-
        - ring S63.49-
      - volar plate S63.43-
        - index S63.43-
        - little S63.43-
        - middle S63.43-
        - ring S63.43-
    - foot — *see* Sprain, foot
    - radial collateral S53.2-
    - radiocarpal — *see* Rupture, traumatic, ligament, wrist, radiocarpal
    - ulnar collateral S53.3-
    - ulnocarpal — *see* Rupture, traumatic, ligament, wrist, ulnocarpal

DISEASE INDEX

Rupture, ruptured — *continued*
> traumatic — *continued*
>> wrist S63.30-
>>> collateral S63.31-
>>> radiocarpal S63.32-
>>> specified site NEC S63.39-
>>> ulnocarpal (palmar) S63.33-
>> liver S36.116
>> membrana tympani — *see* Rupture, ear drum, traumatic
>> muscle or tendon — *see* Strain
>> myocardium — *see* Injury, heart
>> pancreas S36.299
>> rectum S36.69
>> sigmoid S36.593
>> spleen S36.09
>> stomach S36.39
>> symphysis pubis S33.4
>> tympanum, tympanic (membrane) — *see* Rupture, ear drum, traumatic
>> ureter S37.19
>> uterus S37.69
>> vagina — *see* Injury, vagina
>> vena cava — *see* Injury, vena cava, laceration, major
> tricuspid (heart) (valve) I07.8
> tube, tubal (nonobstetric) (nontraumatic) N83.8
>> abscess — *see* Salpingitis
>> due to pregnancy O00.10
>>> with intrauterine pregnancy O00.11
> tympanum, tympanic (membrane) (nontraumatic) (*see also* Perforation, tympanic membrane) H72.9-
>> traumatic — *see* Rupture, ear drum, traumatic
> umbilical cord, complicating delivery O69.89
> ureter (traumatic) S37.19
>> nontraumatic N28.89
> urethra (nontraumatic) N36.8
>> with ectopic or molar pregnancy O08.6
>> following ectopic or molar pregnancy O08.6
>> obstetrical trauma O71.5
>> traumatic S37.39
> uterosacral ligament (nonobstetric) (nontraumatic) N83.8
> uterus (traumatic) S37.69
>> before labor O71.0-
>> during or after labor O71.1
>> nonpuerperal, nontraumatic N85.8
>> pregnant (during labor) O71.1
>>> before labor O71.0-
> vagina — *see* Injury, vagina
> valve, valvular (heart) — *see* Endocarditis
> varicose vein — *see* Varix
> varix — *see* Varix
> vena cava R58
>> traumatic — *see* Injury, vena cava, laceration, major
> vesical (urinary) N32.89
> vessel (blood) R58
>> pulmonary I28.8
>> traumatic — *see* Injury, blood vessel
> viscus R19.8
> vulva complicating delivery O70.0

Russell-Silver syndrome Q87.1
Russian spring-summer type encephalitis A84.0
Rust's disease (tuberculous cervical spondylitis) A18.01
Ruvalcaba-Myhre-Smith syndrome E71.440
Rytand-Lipsitch syndrome I44.2

S

Saber, sabre shin or tibia (syphilitic) A50.56 *[M90.-]*
Sac lacrimal — *see* condition
Saccharomyces infection B37.9
Saccharopinuria E72.3
Saccular — *see* condition
Sacculation
> aorta (nonsyphilitic) — *see* Aneurysm, aorta
> bladder N32.3
> intralaryngeal (congenital) (ventricular) Q31.3
> larynx (congenital) (ventricular) Q31.3
> organ or site, congenital — *see* Distortion
> pregnant uterus — *see* Pregnancy, complicated by, abnormal, uterus
> ureter N28.89
> urethra N36.1
> vesical N32.3
Sachs' amaurotic familial idiocy or disease E75.02
Sachs-Tay disease E75.02
Sacks-Libman disease M32.11
Sacralgia M53.3
Sacralization Q76.49
Sacrodynia M53.3
Sacroiliac joint — *see* condition
Sacroiliitis NEC M46.1
Sacrum — *see* condition
Saddle
> back — *see* Lordosis
> embolus
>> abdominal aorta I74.01
>> pulmonary artery I26.92
>>> with acute cor pulmonale I26.02
> injury — *code to* condition
> nose M95.0
>> due to syphilis A50.57
Sadism (sexual) F65.52
Sadness, postpartal O90.6
Sadomasochism F65.50
Saemisch's ulcer (cornea) — *see* Ulcer, cornea, central
Sagging
> skin and subcutaneous tissue (following bariatric surgery weight loss) (following dietary weight loss) L98.7
Sahib disease B55.0
Sailors' skin L57.8
Saint
> Anthony's fire — *see* Erysipelas
> triad — *see* Hernia, diaphragm
> Vitus' dance — *see* Chorea, Sydenham's
Salaam
> attack(s) — *see* Epilepsy, spasms
> tic R25.8
Salicylism
> abuse F55.8
> overdose or wrong substance given — *see* Table of Drugs and Chemicals, by drug, poisoning
Salivary duct or gland — *see* condition
Salivation, excessive K11.7
Salmonella — *see* Infection, Salmonella
Salmonellosis A02.0
Salpingitis (catarrhal) (fallopian tube) (nodular) (pseudofollicular) (purulent) (septic) N70.91
> with oophoritis N70.93
> acute N70.01
>> with oophoritis N70.03
> chlamydial A56.11
> chronic N70.11
>> with oophoritis N70.13
> complicating abortion — *see* Abortion, by type, complicated by, salpingitis
> ear — *see* Salpingitis, eustachian

Salpingitis (catarrhal) (fallopian tube) (nodular) (pseudofollicular) (purulent) (septic) N70.91 — *continued*
> eustachian (tube) H68.00-
>> acute H68.01-
>> chronic H68.02-
> follicularis N70.11
>> with oophoritis N70.13
> gonococcal (acute) (chronic) A54.24
> interstitial, chronic N70.11
>> with oophoritis N70.13
> isthmica nodosa N70.11
>> with oophoritis N70.13
> specific (gonococcal) (acute) (chronic) A54.24
> tuberculous (acute) (chronic) A18.17
> venereal (gonococcal) (acute) (chronic) A54.24
Salpingocele N83.4-
Salpingo-oophoritis (catarrhal) (purulent) (ruptured) (septic) (suppurative) N70.93
> acute N70.03
>> with ectopic or molar pregnancy O08.0
>> following ectopic or molar pregnancy O08.0
>> gonococcal A54.24
> chronic N70.13
> following ectopic or molar pregnancy O08.0
> gonococcal (acute) (chronic) A54.24
> puerperal O86.19
> specific (gonococcal) (acute) (chronic) A54.24
> subacute N70.03
> tuberculous (acute) (chronic) A18.17
> venereal (gonococcal) (acute) (chronic) A54.24
Salpingo-ovaritis — *see* Salpingo-oophoritis
Salpingoperitonitis — *see* Salpingo-oophoritis
Salzmann's nodular dystrophy — *see* Degeneration, cornea, nodular
Sampson's cyst or tumor N80.1
San Joaquin (Valley) fever B38.0
Sandblaster's asthma, lung or pneumoconiosis J62.8
Sander's disease (paranoia) F22
Sandfly fever A93.1
Sandhoff's disease E75.01
Sanfilippo (Type B) (Type C) (Type D) syndrome E76.22
Sanger-Brown ataxia G11.2
Sao Paulo fever or typhus A77.0
Saponification, mesenteric K65.8
Sarcocele (benign)
> syphilitic A52.76
>> congenital A50.59
Sarcocystosis A07.8
Sarcoepiplocele — *see* Hernia
Sarcoepiplomphalocele Q79.2
Sarcoid — *see also* Sarcoidosis
> arthropathy D86.86
> Boeck's D86.9
> Darier-Roussy D86.3
> iridocyclitis D86.83
> meningitis D86.81
> myocarditis D86.85
> myositis D86.87
> pyelonephritis D86.84
> Spiegler-Fendt L08.89
Sarcoidosis D86.9
> with
>> cranial nerve palsies D86.82
>> hepatic granuloma D86.89
>> polyarthritis D86.86
>> tubulo-interstitial nephropathy D86.84
> combined sites NEC D86.89
> lung D86.0
>> and lymph nodes D86.2
> lymph nodes D86.1
>> and lung D86.2
> meninges D86.81
> skin D86.3
> specified type NEC D86.89

Sarcoma (of) — see also Neoplasm, connective tissue, malignant
  alveolar soft part — see Neoplasm, connective tissue, malignant
  ameloblastic C41.1
    upper jaw (bone) C41.0
  botryoid — see Neoplasm, connective tissue, malignant
  botryoides — see Neoplasm, connective tissue, malignant
  cerebellar C71.6
    circumscribed (arachnoidal) C71.6
  circumscribed (arachnoidal) cerebellar C71.6
  clear cell — see also Neoplasm, connective tissue, malignant
    kidney C64-
  dendritic cells (accessory cells) C96.4
  embryonal — see Neoplasm, connective tissue, malignant
  endometrial (stromal) C54.1
    isthmus C54.0
  epithelioid (cell) — see Neoplasm, connective tissue, malignant
  Ewing's — see Neoplasm, bone, malignant
  follicular dendritic cell C96.4
  germinoblastic (diffuse) — see Lymphoma, diffuse large cell
    follicular — see Lymphoma, follicular, specified NEC
  giant cell (except of bone) — see also Neoplasm, connective tissue, malignant
    bone — see Neoplasm, bone, malignant
  glomoid — see Neoplasm, connective tissue, malignant
  granulocytic C92.3-
  hemangioendothelial — see Neoplasm, connective tissue, malignant
  hemorrhagic, multiple — see Sarcoma, Kaposi's
  histiocytic C96.A (follows C96.6)
  Hodgkin — see Lymphoma, Hodgkin
  immunoblastic (diffuse) — see Lymphoma, diffuse large cell
  interdigitating dendritic cell C96.4
  Kaposi's
    colon C46.4
    connective tissue C46.1
    gastrointestinal organ C46.4
    lung C46.5-
    lymph node(s) C46.3
    palate (hard) (soft) C46.2
    rectum C46.4
    skin C46.0
    specified site NEC C46.7
    stomach C46.4
    unspecified site C46.9
  Kupffer cell C22.3
  Langerhans cell C96.4
  leptomeningeal — see Neoplasm, meninges, malignant
  liver NEC C22.4
  lymphangioendothelial — see Neoplasm, connective tissue, malignant
  lymphoblastic — see Lymphoma, lymphoblastic (diffuse)
  lymphocytic — see Lymphoma, small cell B-cell
  mast cell C96.2
  melanotic — see Melanoma
  meningeal — see Neoplasm, meninges, malignant
  meningothelial — see Neoplasm, meninges, malignant
  mesenchymal — see also Neoplasm, connective tissue, malignant
    mixed — see Neoplasm, connective tissue, malignant
  mesothelial — see Mesothelioma

Sarcoma (of) (see also Neoplasm, connective tissue, malignant) — continued
  monstrocellular
    specified site — see Neoplasm, malignant, by site
    unspecified site C71.9
  myeloid C92.3-
  neurogenic — see Neoplasm, nerve, malignant
  odontogenic C41.1
    upper jaw (bone) C41.0
  osteoblastic — see Neoplasm, bone, malignant
  osteogenic — see also Neoplasm, bone, malignant
    juxtacortical — see Neoplasm, bone, malignant
    periosteal — see Neoplasm, bone, malignant
  periosteal — see also Neoplasm, bone, malignant
    osteogenic — see Neoplasm, bone, malignant
  pleomorphic cell — see Neoplasm, connective tissue, malignant
  reticulum cell (diffuse) — see Lymphoma, diffuse large cell
  nodular — see Lymphoma, follicular
  pleomorphic cell type — see Lymphoma, diffuse large cell
  rhabdoid — see Neoplasm, malignant, by site
  round cell — see Neoplasm, connective tissue, malignant
  small cell — see Neoplasm, connective tissue, malignant
  soft tissue — see Neoplasm, connective tissue, malignant
  spindle cell — see Neoplasm, connective tissue, malignant
  stromal (endometrial) C54.1
    isthmus C54.0
  synovial — see also Neoplasm, connective tissue, malignant
    biphasic — see Neoplasm, connective tissue, malignant
    epithelioid cell — see Neoplasm, connective tissue, malignant
    spindle cell — see Neoplasm, connective tissue, malignant

Sarcomatosis
  meningeal — see Neoplasm, meninges, malignant
  specified site NEC — see Neoplasm, connective tissue, malignant
  unspecified site C80.1
Sarcopenia (age-related) M62.84
Sarcosinemia E72.59
Sarcosporidiosis (intestinal) A07.8
Satiety, early R68.81
Saturnine — see condition
Saturnism
  overdose or wrong substance given or taken — see Table of Drugs and Chemicals, by drug, poisoning
Satyriasis F52.8
Sauriasis — see Ichthyosis
SBE (subacute bacterial endocarditis) I33.0
Scabies (any site) B86
Scabs R23.4
Scaglietti-Dagnini syndrome E22.0
Scald — see Burn
Scalenus anticus (anterior) syndrome G54.0
Scales R23.4
Scaling, skin R23.4
Scalp — see condition
Scapegoating affecting child Z62.3
Scaphocephaly Q75.0
Scapulalgia M89.8x1
Scapulohumeral myopathy G71.0

Scar, scarring (see also Cicatrix) L90.5
  adherent L90.5
  atrophic L90.5
  cervix
    in pregnancy or childbirth — see Pregnancy, complicated by, abnormal cervix
  cheloid L91.0
  chorioretinal H31.00-
    posterior pole macula H31.01-
    postsurgical H59.81-
    solar retinopathy H31.02-
    specified type NEC H31.09-
  choroid — see Scar, chorioretinal
  conjunctiva H11.24-
  cornea H17.9
    xerophthalmic — see also Opacity, cornea vitamin A deficiency E50.6
  duodenum, obstructive K31.5
  hypertrophic L91.0
  keloid L91.0
  labia N90.89
  lung (base) J98.4
  macula — see Scar, chorioretinal, posterior pole
  muscle M62.89
  myocardium, myocardial I25.2
  painful L90.5
  posterior pole (eye) — see Scar, chorioretinal, posterior pole
  retina — see Scar, chorioretinal
  trachea J39.8
  transmural uterine, in pregnancy O34.29
  uterus N85.8
    in pregnancy O34.29
  vagina N89.8
    postoperative N99.2
  vulva N90.89
Scarabiasis B88.2
Scarlatina (anginosa) (maligna) (ulcerosa) A38.9
  myocarditis (acute) A38.1
  old — see Myocarditis
  otitis media A38.0
Scarlet fever (albuminuria) (angina) A38.9
Schamberg's disease (progressive pigmentary dermatosis) L81.7
Schatzki's ring (acquired) (esophagus) (lower) K22.2
  congenital Q39.3
Schaufenster krankheit I20.8
Schaumann's
  benign lymphogranulomatosis D86.1
  disease or syndrome — see Sarcoidosis
Scheie's syndrome E76.03
Schenck's disease B42.1
Scheuermann's disease or osteochondrosis — see Osteochondrosis, juvenile, spine
Schilder(-Flatau) disease G37.0
Schilling-type monocytic leukemia C93.0-
Schimmelbusch's disease, cystic mastitis, or hyperplasia — see Mastopathy, cystic
Schistosoma infestation — see Infestation, Schistosoma
Schistosomiasis B65.9
  with muscle disorder B65.9 [M63.80]
    ankle B65.9 [M63.8-]
    foot B65.9 [M63.8-]
    forearm B65.9 [M63.8-]
    hand B65.9 [M63.8-]
    lower leg B65.9 [M63.8-]
    multiple sites B65.9 [M63.89]
    pelvic region B65.9 [M63.8-]
    shoulder region B65.9 [M63.8-]
    specified site NEC B65.9 [M63.88]
    thigh B65.9 [M63.8-]
    upper arm B65.9 [M63.8-]
  Asiatic B65.2
  bladder B65.0

Schistosomiasis B65.9 — *continued*
  chestermani B65.8
  colon B65.1
  cutaneous B65.3
  due to
    S. haematobium B65.0
    S. japonicum B65.2
    S. mansoni B65.1
    S. mattheii B65.8
  Eastern B65.2
  genitourinary tract B65.0
  intestinal B65.1
  lung NEC B65.9 *[J99]*
    pneumonia B65.9 *[J17]*
  Manson's (intestinal) B65.1
  oriental B65.2
  pulmonary NEC B65.9 *[J99]*
    pneumonia B65.9
  Schistosoma
    haematobium B65.0
    japonicum B65.2
    mansoni B65.1
  specified type NEC B65.8
  urinary B65.0
  vesical B65.0
Schizencephaly Q04.6
Schizoaffective psychosis F25.9
Schizodontia K00.2
Schizoid personality F60.1
Schizophrenia, schizophrenic F20.9
  acute (brief) (undifferentiated) F23
  atypical (form) F20.3
  borderline F21
  catalepsy F20.2
  catatonic (type) (excited) (withdrawn) F20.2
  cenesthopathic, cenesthesiopathic F20.89
  childhood type F84.5
  chronic undifferentiated F20.5
  cyclic F25.0
  disorganized (type) F20.1
  flexibilitas cerea F20.2
  hebephrenic (type) F20.1
  incipient F21
  latent F21
  negative type F20.5
  paranoid (type) F20.0
  paraphrenic F20.0
  post-psychotic depression F32.89
  prepsychotic F21
  prodromal F21
  pseudoneurotic F21
  pseudopsychopathic F21
  reaction F23
  residual (state) (type) F20.5
  restzustand F20.5
  schizoaffective (type) — *see* Psychosis, schizoaffective
  simple (type) F20.89
  simplex F20.89
  specified type NEC F20.89
  stupor F20.2
  syndrome of childhood F84.5
  undifferentiated (type) F20.3
    chronic F20.5
Schizothymia (persistent) F60.1
Schlatter-Osgood disease or osteochondrosis — *see* Osteochondrosis, juvenile, tibia
Schlatter's tibia — *see* Osteochondrosis, juvenile, tibia
Schmidt's syndrome (polyglandular, autoimmune) E31.0
Schmincke's carcinoma or tumor — *see* Neoplasm, nasopharynx, malignant
Schmitz(-Stutzer) dysentery A03.0

Schmorl's disease or nodes
  lumbar region M51.46
  lumbosacral region M51.47
  sacrococcygeal region M53.3
  thoracic region M51.44
  thoracolumbar region M51.45
Schneiderian
  papilloma — *see* Neoplasm, nasopharynx, benign
    specified site — *see* Neoplasm, benign, by site
    unspecified site D14.0
  specified site — *see* Neoplasm, malignant, by site
  unspecified site C30.0
Scholte's syndrome (malignant carcinoid) E34.0
Scholz(-Bielchowsky-Henneberg) disease or syndrome E75.25
Schönlein(-Henoch) disease or purpura (primary) (rheumatic) D69.0
Schottmuller's disease A01.4
Schroeder's syndrome (endocrine hypertensive) E27.0
Schüller-Christian disease or syndrome C96.5
Schultze's type acroparesthesia, simple I73.89
Schultz's disease or syndrome — *see* Agranulocytosis
Schwalbe-Ziehen-Oppenheim disease G24.1
Schwannoma — *see also* Neoplasm, nerve, benign
  malignant — *see also* Neoplasm, nerve, malignant
    with rhabdomyoblastic differentiation — *see* Neoplasm, nerve, malignant
  melanocytic (9560/0) — *see* Neoplasm, nerve, benign
  pigmented — *see* Neoplasm, nerve, benign
Schwannomatosis Q85.03
Schwartz-Bartter syndrome E22.2
Schwartz(-Jampel) syndrome G71.13
Schweniger-Buzzi anetoderma L90.1
Sciatic — *see* condition
Sciatica (infective)
  with lumbago M54.4-
    due to intervertebral disc disorder — *see* Disorder, disc, with, radiculopathy
  due to displacement of intervertebral disc (with lumbago) — *see* Disorder, disc, with, radiculopathy
  wallet M54.3-
Scimitar syndrome Q26.8
Sclera — *see* condition
Sclerectasia H15.84-
Scleredema
  adultorum — *see* Sclerosis, systemic
  Buschke's — *see* Sclerosis, systemic
  newborn P83.0
Sclerema (adiposum) (edematosum) (neonatorum) (newborn) P83.0
  adultorum — *see* Sclerosis, systemic
Scleriasis — *see* Scleroderma
Scleritis H15.00-
  with corneal involvement H15.04-
  anterior H15.01-
  brawny H15.02-
  in (due to) zoster B02.34
  posterior H15.03-
  specified type NEC H15.09-
  syphilitic A52.71
  tuberculous (nodular) A18.51
Sclerochoroiditis H31.8
Scleroconjunctivitis — *see* Scleritis
Sclerocystic ovary syndrome E28.2
Sclerodactyly, sclerodactylia L94.3

Scleroderma, sclerodermia (acrosclerotic) (diffuse) (generalized) (progressive) (pulmonary) (*see also* Sclerosis, systemic) M34.9-
  circumscribed L94.0
  linear L94.1
  localized L94.0
  newborn P83.8
  systemic M34.9
Sclerokeratitis H16.8
  tuberculous A18.52
Scleroma nasi A48.8
Scleromalacia (perforans) H15.05-
Scleromyxedema L98.5
Sclérose en plaques G35
Sclerosis, sclerotic
  adrenal (gland) E27.8
  Alzheimer's — *see* Disease, Alzheimer's
  amyotrophic (lateral) G12.21
  aorta, aortic I70.0
    valve — *see* Endocarditis, aortic
  artery, arterial, arteriolar, arteriovascular — *see* Arteriosclerosis
  ascending multiple G35
  brain (generalized) (lobular) G37.9
    artery, arterial I67.2
    diffuse G37.0
    disseminated G35
    insular G35
    Krabbe's E75.23
    miliary G35
    multiple G35
    presenile (Alzheimer's) — *see* Disease, Alzheimer's, early onset
    senile (arteriosclerotic) I67.2
    stem, multiple G35
    tuberous Q85.1
  bulbar, multiple G35
  bundle of His I44.39
  cardiac — *see* Disease, heart, ischemic, atherosclerotic
  cardiorenal — *see* Hypertension, cardiorenal
  cardiovascular — *see also* Disease, cardiovascular
    renal — *see* Hypertension, cardiorenal
  cerebellar — *see* Sclerosis, brain
  cerebral — *see* Sclerosis, brain
  cerebrospinal (disseminated) (multiple) G35
  cerebrovascular I67.2
  choroid — *see* Degeneration, choroid
  combined (spinal cord) — *see also* Degeneration, combined
    multiple G35
  concentric (Balo) G37.5
  cornea — *see* Opacity, cornea
  coronary (artery) I25.10
    with angina pectoris — *see* Arteriosclerosis, coronary (artery),
  corpus cavernosum
    female N90.89
    male N48.6
  diffuse (brain) (spinal cord) G37.0
  disseminated G35
  dorsal G35
  dorsolateral (spinal cord) — *see* Degeneration, combined
  endometrium N85.5
  extrapyramidal G25.9
  eye, nuclear (senile) — *see* Cataract, senile, nuclear
  focal and segmental (glomerular) (*see also* N00-N07 with fourth character .1) N05.1
  Friedreich's (spinal cord) G11.1
  funicular (spermatic cord) N50.89
  general (vascular) — *see* Arteriosclerosis
  gland (lymphatic) I89.8
  hepatic K74.1
    alcoholic K70.2

DISEASE INDEX

Sclerosis, sclerotic — *continued*
  hereditary
    cerebellar G11.9
    spinal (Friedreich's ataxia) G11.1
  hippocampal G93.81
  insular G35
  kidney — *see* Sclerosis, renal
  larynx J38.7
  lateral (amyotrophic) (descending) (primary)
    (spinal) G12.21
  lens, senile nuclear — *see* Cataract, senile,
    nuclear
  liver K74.1
    with fibrosis K74.2
      alcoholic K70.2
    alcoholic K70.2
    cardiac K76.1
  lung — *see* Fibrosis, lung
  mastoid — *see* Mastoiditis, chronic
  mesial temporal G93.81
  mitral I05.8
  Mönckeberg's (medial) — *see* Arteriosclerosis,
    extremities
  multiple (brain stem) (cerebral) (generalized)
    (spinal cord) G35
  myocardium, myocardial — *see* Disease,
    heart, ischemic, atherosclerotic
  nuclear (senile), eye — *see* Cataract, senile,
    nuclear
  ovary N83.8
  pancreas K86.89
  penis N48.6
  peripheral arteries — *see* Arteriosclerosis,
    extremities
  plaques G35
  pluriglandular E31.8
  polyglandular E31.8
  posterolateral (spinal cord) — *see*
    Degeneration, combined
  presenile (Alzheimer's) — *see* Disease,
    Alzheimer's, early onset
  primary, lateral G12.29
  progressive, systemic M34.0
  pulmonary — *see* Fibrosis, lung
    artery I27.0
    valve (heart) — *see* Endocarditis, pulmonary
  renal N26.9
    with
      cystine storage disease E72.09
      hypertensive heart disease (conditions in
        I11) — *see* Hypertension, cardiorenal
    arteriolar (hyaline) (hyperplastic) — *see*
      Hypertension, kidney
  retina (senile) (vascular) H35.00
  senile (vascular) — *see* Arteriosclerosis
  spinal (cord) (progressive) G95.89
    ascending G61.0
    combined — *see also* Degeneration,
      combined
      multiple G35
      syphilitic A52.11
    disseminated G35
    dorsolateral — *see* Degeneration, combined
    hereditary (Friedreich's) (mixed form) G11.1
    lateral (amyotrophic) G12.21
    multiple G35
    posterior (syphilitic) A52.11
  stomach K31.89
  subendocardial, congenital I42.4
  systemic M34.9
    with
      lung involvement M34.81
      myopathy M34.82
      polyneuropathy M34.83
    drug-induced M34.2
    due to chemicals NEC M34.2
    progressive M34.0
    specified NEC M34.89

Sclerosis, sclerotic — *continued*
  temporal (mesial) G93.81
  tricuspid (heart) (valve) I07.8
  tuberous (brain) Q85.1
  tympanic membrane — *see* Disorder, tympanic
    membrane, specified NEC
  valve, valvular (heart) — *see* Endocarditis
  vascular — *see* Arteriosclerosis
  vein I87.8
Scoliosis (acquired) (postural) M41.9
  adolescent (idiopathic) — *see* Scoliosis,
    idiopathic, adolescent
  congenital Q67.5
    due to bony malformation Q76.3
    failure of segmentation (hemivertebra)
      Q76.3
    hemivertebra fusion Q76.3
    postural Q67.5
  idiopathic M41.20
    adolescent M41.129
      cervical region M41.122
      cervicothoracic region M41.123
      lumbar region M41.126
      lumbosacral region M41.127
      thoracic region M41.124
      thoracolumbar region M41.125
    cervical region M41.22
    cervicothoracic region M41.23
    infantile M41.00
      cervical region M41.02
      cervicothoracic region M41.03
      lumbar region M41.06
      lumbosacral region M41.07
      sacrococcygeal region M41.08
      thoracic region M41.04
      thoracolumbar region M41.05
    juvenile M41.119
      cervical region M41.112
      cervicothoracic region M41.113
      lumbar region M41.116
      lumbosacral region M41.117
      thoracic region M41.114
      thoracolumbar region M41.115
    lumbar region M41.26
    lumbosacral region M41.27
    thoracic region M41.24
    thoracolumbar region M41.25
  infantile — *see* Scoliosis, idiopathic, infantile
  neuromuscular M41.40
    cervical region M41.42
    cervicothoracic region M41.43
    lumbar region M41.46
    lumbosacral region M41.47
    occipito-atlanto-axial region M41.41
    thoracic region M41.44
    thoracolumbar region M41.45
  paralytic — *see* Scoliosis, neuromuscular
  postradiation therapy M96.5
  rachitic (late effect or sequelae) E64.3
    [M49.80]
    cervical region E64.3 *[M49.82]*
    cervicothoracic region E64.3 *[M49.83]*
    lumbar region E64.3 *[M49.86]*
    lumbosacral region E64.3 *[M49.87]*
    multiple sites E64.3 *[M49.89]*
    occipito-atlanto-axial region E64.3
      [M49.81]
    sacrococcygeal region E64.3 *[M49.88]*
    thoracic region E64.3 *[M49.84]*
    thoracolumbar region E64.3 *[M49.85]*
  sciatic M54.4-
  secondary (to) NEC M41.50
    cerebral palsy, Friedreich's ataxia,
      poliomyelitis, neuromuscular disorders
      — *see* Scoliosis, neuromuscular
    cervical region M41.52
    cervicothoracic region M41.53
    lumbar region M41.56
    lumbosacral region M41.57

Scoliosis (acquired) (postural) M41.9 —
  continued
  secondary (to) NEC M41.50 — *continued*
    thoracic region M41.54
    thoracolumbar region M41.55
    specified form NEC M41.80
      cervical region M41.82
      cervicothoracic region M41.83
      lumbar region M41.86
      lumbosacral region M41.87
      thoracic region M41.84
      thoracolumbar region M41.85
    thoracogenic M41.30
      thoracic region M41.34
      thoracolumbar region M41.35
    tuberculous A18.01
Scoliotic pelvis
  with disproportion (fetopelvic) O33.0
    causing obstructed labor O65.0
Scorbutus, scorbutic — *see also* Scurvy
  anemia D53.2
Score, NIHSS (National Institutes of Health
  Stroke Scale) R29.7-
Scotoma (arcuate) (Bjerrum) (central) (ring) —
  see also Defect, visual field, localized,
  scotoma
  scintillating H53.19
Scratch — *see* Abrasion
Scratchy throat R09.89
Screening (for) Z13.9
  alcoholism Z13.89
  anemia Z13.0
  anomaly, congenital Z13.89
  antenatal, of mother Z36
  arterial hypertension Z13.6
  arthropod-borne viral disease NEC Z11.59
  bacteriuria, asymptomatic Z13.89
  behavioral disorder Z13.89
  brain injury, traumatic Z13.850
  bronchitis, chronic Z13.83
  brucellosis Z11.2
  cardiovascular disorder Z13.6
  cataract Z13.5
  chlamydial diseases Z11.8
  cholera Z11.0
  chromosomal abnormalities (nonprocreative)
    NEC Z13.79
  colonoscopy Z12.11
  congenital
    dislocation of hip Z13.89
    eye disorder Z13.5
    malformation or deformation Z13.89
  contamination NEC Z13.88
  cystic fibrosis Z13.228
  dengue fever Z11.59
  dental disorder Z13.84
  depression Z13.89
  developmental handicap Z13.42
    in early childhood Z13.42
    infant Z13.41
  diabetes mellitus Z13.1
  diphtheria Z11.2
  disability, intellectual Z13.42
    infant Z13.41
  disease or disorder Z13.9
    bacterial NEC Z11.2
      intestinal infectious Z11.0
      respiratory tuberculosis Z11.1
    blood or blood-forming organ Z13.0
    cardiovascular Z13.6
    Chagas' Z11.6
    chlamydial Z11.8
    dental Z13.89
    developmental Z13.42
      in child Z13.42
      infant Z13.41
    digestive tract NEC Z13.818
      lower GI Z13.811
      upper GI Z13.810

Screening (for) Z13.9 — *continued*
  disease or disorder Z13.9 — *continued*
    ear Z13.5
    endocrine Z13.29
    eye Z13.5
    genitourinary Z13.89
    heart Z13.6
    human immunodeficiency virus (HIV)
      infection Z11.4
    immunity Z13.0
    infection
      intestinal Z11.0
        specified NEC Z11.6
    infectious Z11.9
    mental Z13.89
    metabolic Z13.228
    neurological Z13.89
    nutritional Z13.21
      metabolic Z13.228
        lipoid disorders Z13.220
    protozoal Z11.6
      intestinal Z11.0
    respiratory Z13.83
    rheumatic Z13.828
    rickettsial Z11.8
    sexually-transmitted NEC Z11.3
      human immunodeficiency virus (HIV)
        Z11.4
    sickle-cell (trait) Z13.0
    skin Z13.89
    specified NEC Z13.89
    spirochetal Z11.8
    thyroid Z13.29
    vascular Z13.6
    venereal Z11.3
    viral NEC Z11.59
      human immunodeficiency virus (HIV)
        Z11.4
      intestinal Z11.0
  elevated titer Z13.89
  emphysema Z13.83
  encephalitis, viral (mosquito-or tick-borne)
    Z11.59
  exposure to contaminants (toxic) Z13.88
  fever
    dengue Z11.59
    hemorrhagic Z11.59
    yellow Z11.59
  filariasis Z11.6
  galactosemia Z13.228
  gastrointestinal condition Z13.818
  genetic (nonprocreative)
    disease carrier status (nonprocreative)
      Z13.71
    for procreative management — *see* Testing,
      genetic, for procreative management
    specified NEC (nonprocreative) Z13.79
  genitourinary condition Z13.89
  glaucoma Z13.5
  gonorrhea Z11.3
  gout Z13.89
  helminthiasis (intestinal) Z11.6
  hematopoietic malignancy Z12.89
  hemoglobinopathies NEC Z13.0
  hemorrhagic fever Z11.59
  Hodgkin disease Z12.89
  human immunodeficiency virus (HIV) Z11.4
  human papillomavirus Z11.51
  hypertension Z13.6
  immunity disorders Z13.0
  infection
    mycotic Z11.8
    parasitic Z11.8
  ingestion of radioactive substance Z13.88
  intellectual disability Z13.42
    infant Z13.41
  intestinal
    helminthiasis Z11.6
    infectious disease Z11.0

Screening (for) Z13.9 — *continued*
  leishmaniasis Z11.6
  leprosy Z11.2
  leptospirosis Z11.8
  leukemia Z12.89
  lymphoma Z12.89
  malaria Z11.6
  malnutrition Z13.29
    metabolic Z13.228
    nutritional Z13.21
  measles Z11.59
  mental disorder Z13.89
  metabolic errors, inborn Z13.228
  multiphasic Z13.89
  musculoskeletal disorder Z13.828
    osteoporosis Z13.820
  mycoses Z11.8
  myocardial infarction (acute) Z13.6
  neoplasm (malignant) (of) Z12.9
    bladder Z12.6
    blood Z12.89
    breast Z12.39
      routine mammogram Z12.31
    cervix Z12.4
    colon Z12.11
    genitourinary organs NEC Z12.79
      bladder Z12.6
      cervix Z12.4
      ovary Z12.73
      prostate Z12.5
      testis Z12.71
      vagina Z12.72
    hematopoietic system Z12.89
    intestinal tract Z12.10
      colon Z12.11
      rectum Z12.12
      small intestine Z12.13
    lung Z12.2
    lymph (glands) Z12.89
    nervous system Z12.82
    oral cavity Z12.81
    prostate Z12.5
    rectum Z12.12
    respiratory organs Z12.2
    skin Z12.83
    small intestine Z12.13
    specified site NEC Z12.89
    stomach Z12.0
  nephropathy Z13.89
  nervous system disorders NEC Z13.858
  neurological condition Z13.89
  osteoporosis Z13.820
  parasitic infestation Z11.9
    specified NEC Z11.8
  phenylketonuria Z13.228
  plague Z11.2
  poisoning (chemical) (heavy metal) Z13.88
  poliomyelitis Z11.59
  postnatal, chromosomal abnormalities Z13.89
  prenatal, of mother Z36
  protozoal disease Z11.6
    intestinal Z11.0
  pulmonary tuberculosis Z11.1
  radiation exposure Z13.88
  respiratory condition Z13.83
  respiratory tuberculosis Z11.1
  rheumatoid arthritis Z13.828
  rubella Z11.59
  schistosomiasis Z11.6
  sexually-transmitted disease NEC Z11.3
    human immunodeficiency virus (HIV) Z11.4
  sickle-cell disease or trait Z13.0
  skin condition Z13.89
  sleeping sickness Z11.6
  special Z13.9
    specified NEC Z13.89
  syphilis Z11.3
  tetanus Z11.2
  trachoma Z11.8

Screening (for) Z13.9 — *continued*
  traumatic brain injury Z13.850
  trypanosomiasis Z11.6
  tuberculosis, respiratory Z11.1
  venereal disease Z11.3
  viral encephalitis (mosquito-or tick-borne)
    Z11.59
  whooping cough Z11.2
  worms, intestinal Z11.6
  yaws Z11.8
  yellow fever Z11.59
Scrofula, scrofulosis (tuberculosis of cervical
  lymph glands) A18.2
Scrofulide (primary) (tuberculous) A18.4
Scrofuloderma, scrofulodermia (any site)
  (primary) A18.4
Scrofulosus lichen (primary) (tuberculous)
  A18.4
Scrofulous — *see* condition
Scrotal tongue K14.5
Scrotum — *see* condition
Scurvy, scorbutic E54
  anemia D53.2
  gum E54
  infantile E54
  rickets E55.0 *[M90.80]*
Sealpox B08.62
Seasickness T75.3
Seatworm (infection) (infestation) B80
Sebaceous — *see also* condition
  cyst — *see* Cyst, sebaceous
Seborrhea, seborrheic L21.9
  capillitii R23.8
  capitis L21.0
  dermatitis L21.9
    infantile L21.1
  eczema L21.9
    infantile L21.1
  sicca L21.0
Seckel's syndrome Q87.1
Seclusion, pupil — *see* Membrane, pupillary
Second hand tobacco smoke exposure
  (acute) (chronic) Z77.22
  in the perinatal period P96.81
Secondary
  dentin (in pulp) K04.3
  neoplasm, secondaries — *see* Table of
    Neoplasms, secondary
Secretion
  antidiuretic hormone, inappropriate E22.2
  catecholamine, by pheochromocytoma E27.5
  hormone
    antidiuretic, inappropriate (syndrome) E22.2
    by
      carcinoid tumor E34.0
      pheochromocytoma E27.5
    ectopic NEC E34.2
  urinary
    excessive R35.8
    suppression R34
Section
  nerve, traumatic — *see* Injury, nerve
Sedative, hypnotic, or anxiolytic-induced
  anxiety disorder F13.980
  bipolar and related disorder F13.94
  delirium F13.921
  depressive disorder F13.94
  major neurocognitive disorder F13.97
  mild neurocognitive disorder F13.988
  psychotic disorder F13.959
  sexual dysfunction F13.981
  sleep disorder F13.982
Segmentation, incomplete (congenital) —
  see also Fusion
  bone NEC Q78.8
  lumbosacral (joint) (vertebra) Q76.49
Seitelberger's syndrome (infantile
  neuraxonal dystrophy) G31.89

Seizure(s) (see also Convulsions) R56.9
  akinetic — see Epilepsy, generalized, specified NEC
  atonic — see Epilepsy, generalized, specified NEC
  autonomic (hysterical) F44.5
  convulsive — see Convulsions
  cortical (focal) (motor) — see Epilepsy, localization-related, symptomatic, with simple partial seizures
  disorder (see also Eplepsy) G40.909
  due to stroke — see Sequelae (of), disease, cerebrovascular, by type, specified NEC
  epileptic — see Epilepsy
  febrile (simple) R56.00
    with status epilepticus G40.901
    complex (atypical) (complicated) R56.01
      with status epilepticus G40.901
  grand mal G40.409
    intractable G40.419
      with status epilepticus G40.411
      without status epilepticus G40.419
    not intractable G40.409
      with status epilepticus G40.401
      without status epilepticus G40.409
  heart — see Disease, heart
  hysterical F44.5
  intractable G40.919
    with status epilepticus G40.911
  Jacksonian (focal) (motor type) (sensory type) — see Epilepsy, localization-related, symptomatic, with simple partial seizures
  newborn P90
  nonspecific epileptic
    atonic — see Epilepsy, generalized, specified NEC
    clonic — see Epilepsy, generalized, specified NEC
    myoclonic — see Epilepsy, generalized, specified NEC
    tonic — see Epilepsy, generalized, specified NEC
    tonic-clonic — see Epilepsy, generalized, specified NEC
  partial, developing into secondarily generalized seizures
    complex — see Epilepsy, localization-related, symptomatic, with complex partial seizures
    simple — see Epilepsy, localization-related, symptomatic, with simple partial seizures
  petit mal G40.409
    intractable G40.419
      with status epilepticus G40.411
      without status epilepticus G40.419
    not intractable G40.409
      with status epilepticus G40.401
      without status epilepticus G40.409
  post traumatic R56.1
  recurrent G40.909
  specified NEC G40.89
  uncinate — see Epilepsy, localization-related, symptomatic, with complex partial seizures
Selenium deficiency, dietary E59
Self-damaging behavior (life-style) Z72.89
Self-harm (attempted)
  history (personal) Z91.5
    in family Z81.8
Self-mutilation (attempted)
  history (personal) Z91.5
    in family Z81.8
Self-poisoning
  history (personal) Z91.5
    in family Z81.8
  observation following (alleged) attempt Z03.6
Semicoma R40.1
Seminal vesiculitis N49.0

Seminoma C62.9-
  specified site — see Neoplasm, malignant, by site
Senear-Usher disease or syndrome L10.4
Senectus R54
Senescence (without mention of psychosis) R54
Senile, senility (see also condition) R41.81
  with
    acute confusional state F05
    mental changes NOS F03
    psychosis NEC — see Psychosis, senile
  asthenia R54
  cervix (atrophic) N88.8
  debility R54
  endometrium (atrophic) N85.8
  fallopian tube (atrophic) — see Atrophy, fallopian tube
  heart (failure) R54
  ovary (atrophic) — see Atrophy, ovary
  premature E34.8
  vagina, vaginitis (atrophic) N95.2
  wart L82.1
Sensation
  burning (skin) R20.8
    tongue K14.6
  loss of R20.8
  prickling (skin) R20.2
  tingling (skin) R20.2
Sense loss
  smell — see Disturbance, sensation, smell
  taste — see Disturbance, sensation, taste
  touch R20.8
Sensibility disturbance (cortical) (deep) (vibratory) R20.9
Sensitive, sensitivity — see also Allergy
  carotid sinus G90.01
  child (excessive) F93.8
  cold, autoimmune D59.1
  dentin K03.89
  gluten (non-celiac) K90.41
  latex Z91.040
  methemoglobin D74.8
  tuberculin, without clinical or radiological symptoms R76.11
  visual
    glare H53.71
    impaired contrast H53.72
Sensitiver Beziehungswahn F22
Sensitization, auto-erythrocytic D69.2
Separation
  anxiety, abnormal (of childhood) F93.0
  apophysis, traumatic — code as Fracture, by site
  choroid — see Detachment, choroid
  epiphysis, epiphyseal
    nontraumatic — see also Osteochondropathy, specified type NEC
      upper femoral — see Slipped, epiphysis, upper femoral
    traumatic — code as Fracture, by site
  fracture — see Fracture
  infundibulum cardiac from right ventricle by a partition Q24.3
  joint (traumatic) (current) — code by site under Dislocation
  pubic bone, obstetrical trauma O71.6
  retina, retinal — see Detachment, retina
  symphysis pubis, obstetrical trauma O71.6
  tracheal ring, incomplete, congenital Q32.1
Sepsis (generalized) (unspecified organism) A41.9
  with
    organ dysfunction (acute) (multiple) R65.20
      with septic shock R65.21
  actinomycotic A42.7
  adrenal hemorrhage syndrome (meningococcal) A39.1
  anaerobic A41.4
  Bacillus anthracis A22.7

Sepsis (generalized) (unspecified organism) A41.9 — continued
  Brucella (see also Brucellosis) A23.9
  candidal B37.7
  cryptogenic A41.9
  due to device, implant or graft T85.79
    arterial graft NEC T82.7
    breast (implant) T85.79
    catheter NEC T85.79
      dialysis (renal) T82.7
        intraperitoneal T85.71
      infusion NEC T82.7
        spinal (cranial) (epidural) (intrathecal) (spinal) (subarachnoid) (subdural) T85.735
      urethral indwelling T83.511
      urinary T83.518
    ectopic or molar pregnancy O08.82
    electronic (electrode) (pulse generator) (stimulator)
      bone T84.7
      cardiac T82.7
      nervous system T85.738
        brain T85.731
        neurostimulator generator T85.734
        peripheral nerve T85.732
        spinal cord T85.733
      urinary T83.590
    fixation, internal (orthopedic) — see Complication, fixation device, infection
    gastrointestinal (bile duct) (esophagus) T85.79
      neurostimulator electrode (lead) T85.732
    genital T83.69
    heart NEC T82.7
      valve (prosthesis) T82.6
      graft T82.7
    joint prosthesis — see Complication, joint prosthesis, infection
    ocular (corneal graft) (orbital implant) T85.79
    orthopedic NEC T84.7
      fixation device, internal — see Complication, fixation device, infection
    specified NEC T85.79
    vascular T82.7
    ventricular intracranial (communicating) shunt T85.730
  during labor O75.3
  Enterococcus A41.81
  Erysipelothrix (rhusiopathiae) (erysipeloid) A26.7
  Escherichia coli (E. coli) A41.5
  extraintestinal yersiniosis A28.2
  following
    abortion (subsequent episode) O08.0
      current episode — see Abortion
    ectopic or molar pregnancy O08.82
    immunization T88.0
    infusion, therapeutic injection or transfusion NEC T80.29
  gangrenous A41.9
  gonococcal A54.86
  Gram-negative (organism) A41.5
    anaerobic A41.4
  Haemophilus influenzae A41.3
  herpesviral B00.7
  intra-abdominal K65.1
  intraocular — see Endophthalmitis, purulent
  Listeria monocytogenes A32.7
  localized — code to specific localized infection
    in operation wound T81.49
    skin — see Abscess
  malleus A24.0
  melioidosis A24.1
  meningeal — see Meningitis

Sepsis (generalized) (unspecified organism)
A41.9 — *continued*
  meningococcal A39.4
    acute A39.2
    chronic A39.3
  MSSA (methicillin susceptible Staphylococcus
    aureus) A41.01
  newborn P36.9
    due to
      anaerobes NEC P36.5
      Escherichia coli P36.4
      Staphylococcus P36.30
        aureus P36.2
        specified NEC P36.39
      Streptococcus P36.10
        group B P36.0
        specified NEC P36.19
      specified NEC P36.8
  Pasteurella multocida A28.0
  pelvic, puerperal, postpartum, childbirth O85
  pneumococcal A40.3
  postprocedural T81.49
  puerperal, postpartum, childbirth (pelvic) O85
  Salmonella (arizonae) (cholerae-suis)
    (enteritidis) (typhimurium) A02.1
  severe R65.20
    with septic shock R65.21
  Shigella (*see also* Dysentery, bacillary) A03.9
  skin, localized — *see* Abscess
  specified organism NEC A41.89
  Staphylococcus, staphylococcal A41.2
    aureus (methicillin susceptible) (MSSA)
      A41.01
      methicillin resistant (MRSA) A41.02
    coagulase-negative A41.1
    specified NEC A41.1
  Streptococcus, streptococcal A40.9
    agalactiae A40.1
    group
      A A40.0
      B A40.1
      D A41.81
    neonatal P36.10
      group B P36.0
      specified NEC P36.19
    pneumoniae A40.3
    pyogenes A40.0
    specified NEC A40.8
  tracheostomy stoma J95.02
  tularemic A21.7
  umbilical, umbilical cord (newborn) — *see*
    Sepsis, newborn
  Yersinia pestis A20.7
Septate — *see* Septum
Septic — *see* condition
  arm — *see* Cellulitis, upper limb
    with lymphangitis — *see* Lymphangitis,
      acute, upper limb
  embolus — *see* Embolism
  finger — *see* Cellulitis, digit
    with lymphangitis — *see* Lymphangitis,
      acute, digit
  foot — *see* Cellulitis, lower limb
    with lymphangitis — *see* Lymphangitis,
      acute, lower limb
  gallbladder (acute) K81.0
  hand — *see* Cellulitis, upper limb
    with lymphangitis — *see* Lymphangitis,
      acute, upper limb
  joint — *see* Arthritis, pyogenic or pyemic
  leg — *see* Cellulitis, lower limb
    with lymphangitis — *see* Lymphangitis,
      acute, lower limb
  nail — *see also* Cellulitis, digit
    with lymphangitis — *see* Lymphangitis,
      acute, digit
  sore — *see also* Abscess
    throat J02.0
      streptococcal J02.0

Septic — *see* condition — *continued*
  spleen (acute) D73.89
  teeth, tooth (pulpal origin) K04.4
  throat — *see* Pharyngitis
  thrombus — *see* Thrombosis
  toe — *see* Cellulitis, digit
    with lymphangitis — *see* Lymphangitis,
      acute, digit
  tonsils, chronic J35.01
    with adenoiditis J35.03
  uterus — *see* Endometritis
Septicemia A41.9
  meaning sepsis — *see* Sepsis
Septum, septate (congenital) — *see also*
  Anomaly, by site
  anal Q42.3
    with fistula Q42.2
  aqueduct of Sylvius Q03.0
    with spina bifida — *see* Spina bifida, by site,
      with hydrocephalus
  uterus (complete) (partial) Q51.2
  vagina Q52.10
    in pregnancy — *see* Pregnancy, complicated
      by, abnormal vagina
      causing obstructed labor O65.5
    longitudinal Q52.129
      microperforate
        left side Q52.124
        right side Q52.123
      nonobstruction Q52.120
      obstructing Q52.129
        left side Q52.122
        right side Q52.121
    transverse Q52.11
Sequelae (of) — *see also* condition
  abscess, intracranial or intraspinal (conditions
    in G06) G09
  amputation — *code to* injury with seventh
    character S
  burn and corrosion — *code to* injury with
    seventh character S
  calcium deficiency E64.8
  cerebrovascular disease — *see* Sequelae,
    disease, cerebrovascular
  childbirth O94
  contusion — *code to* injury with seventh
    character S
  corrosion — *see* Sequelae, burn and corrosion
  crushing injury — *code to* injury with seventh
    character S
  disease
    cerebrovascular I69.90
      alteration of sensation I69.998
      aphasia I69.920
      apraxia I69.990
      ataxia I69.993
      cognitive deficits I69.91
      disturbance of vision I69.998
      dysarthria I69.922
      dysphagia I69.991
      dysphasia I69.921
      facial droop I69.992
      facial weakness I69.992
      fluency disorder I69.923
      hemiplegia I69.95-
      hemorrhage
        intracerebral — *see* Sequelae,
          hemorrhage, intracerebral
        intracranial, nontraumatic NEC — *see*
          Sequelae, hemorrhage, intracranial,
          nontraumatic
        subarachnoid — *see* Sequelae,
          hemorrhage, subarachnoid
      language deficit I69.928
      monoplegia
        lower limb I69.84-
        upper limb I69.93-
      paralytic syndrome I69.96-
      specified effect NEC I69.998

Sequelae (of) (*see also* condition) — *continued*
  disease — *continued*
    cerebrovascular I69.90 — *continued*
      specified type NEC I69.80
        alteration of sensation I69.898
        aphasia I69.820
        apraxia I69.890
        ataxia I69.893
        cognitive deficits I69.81
        disturbance of vision I69.898
        dysarthria I69.822
        dysphagia I69.891
        dysphasia I69.821
        facial droop I69.892
        facial weakness I69.892
        fluency disorder I69.823
        hemiplegia I69.85-
        language deficit I69.828
        monoplegia
          lower limb I69.84-
          upper limb I69.83-
        paralytic syndrome I69.86-
        specified effect NEC I69.898
      speech deficit I69.928
        speech deficit I69.828
      stroke NOS — *see* Sequelae, stroke NOS
  dislocation — *code to* injury with seventh
    character S
  encephalitis or encephalomyelitis (conditions in
    G04) G09
    in infectious disease NEC B94.8
    viral B94.1
  external cause — *code to* injury with seventh
    character S
  foreign body entering natural orifice — *code to*
    injury with seventh character S
  fracture — *code to* injury with seventh
    character S
  frostbite — *code to* injury with seventh
    character S
  Hansen's disease B92
  hemorrhage
    intracerebral I69.10
      alteration of sensation I69.198
      aphasia I69.120
      apraxia I69.190
      ataxia I69.193
      cognitive deficits I69.11
      disturbance of vision I69.198
      dysarthria I69.122
      dysphagia I69.191
      dysphasia I69.121
      facial droop I69.192
      facial weakness I69.192
      fluency disorder I69.123
      hemiplegia I69.15-
      language deficit NEC I69.128
      monoplegia
        lower limb I69.14-
        upper limb I69.13-
      paralytic syndrome I69.16-
      specified effect NEC I69.198
      speech deficit NEC I69.128
    intracranial, nontraumatic NEC I69.20
      alteration of sensation I69.298
      aphasia I69.220
      apraxia I69.290
      ataxia I69.293
      cognitive deficits I69.21
      disturbance of vision I69.298
      dysarthria I69.222
      dysphagia I69.291
      dysphasia I69.221
      facial droop I69.292
      facial weakness I69.292
      fluency disorder I69.223
      hemiplegia I69.25-
      language deficit NEC I69.228

Sequelae (of) (*see also* condition) — *continued*
  hemorrhage — *continued*
    intracranial, nontraumatic NEC I69.20 — *continued*
      monoplegia
        lower limb I69.24-
        upper limb I69.23-
      paralytic syndrome I69.26-
      specified effect NEC I69.298
      speech deficit NEC I69.228
    subarachnoid I69.00
      alteration of sensation I69.098
      aphasia I69.020
      apraxia I69.090
      ataxia I69.093
      cognitive deficits — *see* subcategory I69.01-
      disturbance of vision I69.098
      dysarthria I69.022
      dysphagia I69.091
      dysphasia I69.021
      facial droop I69.092
      facial weakness I69.092
      fluency disorder I69.023
      hemiplegia I69.05-
      language deficit NEC I69.028
      monoplegia
        lower limb I69.04-
        upper limb I69.03-
      paralytic syndrome I69.06-
      specified effect NEC I69.098
      speech deficit NEC I69.028
  hepatitis, viral B94.2
  hyperalimentation E68
  infarction
    cerebral I69.30
      alteration of sensation I69.398
      aphasia I69.320
      apraxia I69.390
      ataxia I69.393
      cognitive deficits I69.31
      disturbance of vision I69.398
      dysarthria I69.322
      dysphagia I69.391
      dysphasia I69.321
      facial droop I69.392
      facial weakness I69.392
      fluency disorder I69.323
      hemiplegia I69.35-
      language deficit NEC I69.328
      monoplegia
        lower limb I69.34-
        upper limb I69.33-
      paralytic syndrome I69.36-
      specified effect NEC I69.398
      speech deficit NEC I69.328
  infection, pyogenic, intracranial or intraspinal G09
  infectious disease B94.9
    specified NEC B94.8
  injury — *code to* injury with seventh character S
  leprosy B92
  meningitis
    bacterial (conditions in G00) G09
    other or unspecified cause (conditions in G03) G09
  muscle (and tendon) injury — *code to* injury with seventh character S
  myelitis — *see* Sequelae, encephalitis
  niacin deficiency E64.8
  nutritional deficiency E64.9
    specified NEC E64.8
  obstetrical condition O94
  parasitic disease B94.9
  phlebitis or thrombophlebitis of intracranial or intraspinal venous sinuses and veins (conditions in G08) G09

Sequelae (of) (*see also* condition) — *continued*
  poisoning — *code to* poisoning with seventh character S
    nonmedicinal substance — *see* Sequelae, toxic effect, nonmedicinal substance
  poliomyelitis (acute) B91
  pregnancy O94
  protein-energy malnutrition E64.0
  puerperium O94
  rickets E64.3
  selenium deficiency E64.8
  sprain and strain — *code to* injury with seventh character S
  stroke NOS I69.30
    alteration in sensation I69.398
    aphasia I69.320
    apraxia I69.390
    ataxia I69.393
    cognitive deficits I69.31
    disturbance of vision I69.398
    dysarthria I69.322
    dysphagia I69.391
    dysphasia I69.321
    facial droop I69.392
    facial weakness I69.392
    hemiplegia I69.35-
    language deficit NEC I69.328
    monoplegia
      lower limb I69.34-
      upper limb I69.33-
    paralytic syndrome I69.36-
    specified effect NEC I69.398
    speech deficit NEC I69.328
  tendon and muscle injury — *code to* injury with seventh character S
  thiamine deficiency E64.8
  trachoma B94.0
  tuberculosis B90.9
    bones and joints B90.2
    central nervous system B90.0
    genitourinary B90.1
    pulmonary (respiratory) B90.9
    specified organs NEC B90.8
  viral
    encephalitis B94.1
    hepatitis B94.2
  vitamin deficiency NEC E64.8
    A E64.1
    B E64.8
    C E64.2
  wound, open — *code to* injury with seventh character S
Sequestration — *see also* Sequestrum
  disk — *see* Displacement, intervertebral disk
  lung, congenital Q33.2
Sequestrum
  bone — *see* Osteomyelitis, chronic
  dental M27.2
  jaw bone M27.2
  orbit — *see* Osteomyelitis, orbit
  sinus (accessory) (nasal) — *see* Sinusitis
Sequoiosis lung or pneumonitis J67.8
Serology for syphilis
  doubtful
    with signs or symptoms — *code by* site and stage under Syphilis
    follow-up of latent syphilis — *see* Syphilis, latent
  negative, with signs or symptoms — *code by* site and stage under Syphilis
  positive A53.0
    with signs or symptoms — *code by* site and stage under Syphilis
  reactivated A53.0
Seroma — *see also* Hematoma
  postprocedural — *see* Complication, postprocedural, seroma
  traumatic, secondary and recurrent T79.2
Seropurulent — *see* condition

Serositis, multiple K65.8
  pericardial I31.1
  peritoneal K65.8
Serous — *see* condition
Sertoli cell
  adenoma
    specified site — *see* Neoplasm, benign, by site
    unspecified site
      female D27.9
      male D29.20
  carcinoma
    specified site — *see* Neoplasm, malignant, by site
    unspecified site (male) C62.9-
      female C56.9
  tumor
    with lipid storage
      specified site — *see* Neoplasm, benign, by site
      unspecified site
        female D27.9
        male D29.20
    specified site — *see* Neoplasm, benign, by site
    unspecified site
      female D27.9
      male D29.20
Sertoli-Leydig cell tumor — *see* Neoplasm, benign, by site
  specified site — *see* Neoplasm, benign, by site
  unspecified site
    female D27.9
    male D29.20
Serum
  allergy, allergic reaction (*see also* Reaction, serum) T80.69
  shock (*see also* Shock, anaphylactic) T80.59
  arthritis T80.6
  complication or reaction NEC (*see also* Reaction, serum) T80.69
  disease NEC (*see also* Reaction, serum) T80.69
  hepatitis — *see also* Hepatitis, viral, type B
    carrier (suspected) of B18.1
  intoxication (*see also* Reaction, serum) T80.69
  neuritis (*see also* Reaction, serum) T80.69
  neuropathy G61.1
  poisoning NEC (*see also* Reaction, serum) T80.69
  rash NEC (*see also* Reaction, serum) T80.69
  reaction NEC (*see also* Reaction, serum) T80.69
  sickness NEC (*see also* Reaction, serum) T80.69
  urticaria (*see also* Reaction, serum) T80.69
Sesamoiditis M25.8-
Sever's disease or osteochondrosis — *see* Osteochondrosis, juvenile, tarsus
Severe sepsis R65.20
  with septic shock R65.21
Sex
  chromosome mosaics Q97.8
    lines with various numbers of X chromosomes Q97.2
  education Z70.8
  reassignment surgery status Z87.890
Sextuplet pregnancy — *see* Pregnancy, sextuplet
Sexual
  function, disorder of (psychogenic) F52.9
  immaturity (female) (male) E30.0
  impotence (psychogenic) organic origin NEC — *see* Dysfunction, sexual, male
  precocity (constitutional) (cryptogenic) (female) (idiopathic) (male) E30.1
Sexuality, pathologic — *see* Deviation, sexual
Sézary disease C84.1-
Shadow, lung R91.8
Shaking palsy or paralysis — *see* Parkinsonism

© 2016 Channel Publishing, Ltd.

DISEASE INDEX

Shallowness, acetabulum — *see*
 Derangement, joint, specified type NEC, hip
Shaver's disease J63.1
Sheath (tendon) — *see* condition
Sheathing, retinal vessels H35.01
Shedding
 nail L60.8
 premature, primary (deciduous) teeth K00.6
Sheehan's disease or syndrome E23.0
Shelf, rectal K62.89
Shell teeth K00.5
Shellshock (current) F43.0
 lasting state — *see* Disorder, post-traumatic
 stress
Shield kidney Q63.1
Shift
 auditory threshold (temporary) H93.24-
 mediastinal R93.8
Shifting sleep-work schedule (affecting
 sleep) G47.26
Shiga(-Kruse) dysentery A03.0
Shiga's bacillus A03.0
Shigella (dysentery) — *see* Dysentery, bacillary
Shigellosis A03.9
 Group A A03.0
 Group B A03.1
 Group C A03.2
 Group D A03.3
Shin splints S86.89
Shingles — *see* Herpes, zoster
Shipyard disease or eye B30.0
Shirodkar suture, in pregnancy — *see*
 Pregnancy, complicated by, incompetent
 cervix
Shock R57.9
 with ectopic or molar pregnancy O08.3
 adrenal (cortical) (Addisonian) E27.2
 adverse food reaction (anaphylactic) — *see*
  Shock, anaphylactic, due to food
 allergic — *see* Shock, anaphylactic
 anaphylactic T78.2
  chemical — *see* Table of Drugs and
   Chemicals
  due to drug or medicinal substance
   correct substance properly administered
    T88.6
   overdose or wrong substance given or
    taken (by accident) — *see* Table of
    Drugs and Chemicals, by drug,
    poisoning
  due to food (nonpoisonous) T78.00
   additives T78.06
   dairy products T78.07
   eggs T78.08
   fish T78.03
    shellfish T78.02
   fruit T78.04
   milk T78.07
   nuts T78.05
    multiple types T78.05
    peanuts T78.01
   peanuts T78.01
   seeds T78.05
   specified type NEC T78.09
   vegetable T78.04
  following sting(s) — *see* Venom
  immunization T80.52
  serum T80.59
   blood and blood products T80.51
   immunization T80.52
   specified NEC T80.59
   vaccination T80.52
 anaphylactoid — *see* Shock, anaphylactic
 anesthetic
  correct substance properly administered
   T88.2

Shock R57.9 — *continued*
 anesthetic — *continued*
  overdose or wrong substance given or taken
   — *see* Table of Drugs and Chemicals, by
   drug, poisoning
   specified anesthetic — *see* Table of Drugs
    and Chemicals, by drug, poisoning
 cardiogenic R57.0
 chemical substance — *see* Table of Drugs and
  Chemicals
 complicating ectopic or molar pregnancy
  O08.3
 culture — *see* Disorder, adjustment
 drug
  due to correct substance properly
   administered T88.6
  overdose or wrong substance given or taken
   (by accident) — *see* Table of Drugs and
   Chemicals, by drug, poisoning
 during or after labor and delivery O75.1
 electric T75.4
  (taser) T75.4
 endotoxic R65.21
  postprocedural (resulting from a procedure,
   not elsewhere classified) T81.12
 following
  ectopic or molar pregnancy O08.3
  injury (immediate) (delayed) T79.4
  labor and delivery O75.1
 food (anaphylactic) — *see* Shock,
  anaphylactic, due to food
 from electroshock gun (taser) T75.4
 gram-negative R65.21
  postprocedural (resulting from a procedure,
   not elsewhere classified) T81.12
 hematologic R57.8
 hemorrhagic
  surgery (intraoperative) (postoperative)
   T81.19
  trauma T79.4
 hypovolemic R57.1
  surgical T81.19
  traumatic T79.4
 insulin E15
  therapeutic misadventure — *see* subcategory
   T38.3
 kidney N17.0
  traumatic (following crushing) T79.5
 lightning T75.01
 liver K72.00
 lung J80
 obstetric O75.1
  with ectopic or molar pregnancy O08.3
  following ectopic or molar pregnancy O08.3
 pleural (surgical) T81.19
  due to trauma T79.4
 postprocedural (postoperative) T81.10
  with ectopic or molar pregnancy O08.3
  cardiogenic T81.11
  endotoxic T81.12
  following ectopic or molar pregnancy O08.3
  gram-negative T81.12
  hypovolemic T81.19
  septic T81.12
  specified type NEC T81.19
 psychic F43.0
 septic (due to severe sepsis) R65.21
 specified NEC R57.8
 surgical T81.10
 taser gun (taser) T75.4
 therapeutic misadventure NEC T81.10
 thyroxin
  overdose or wrong substance given or taken
   — *see* Table of Drugs and Chemicals, by
   drug, poisoning
 toxic, syndrome A48.3
 transfusion — *see* Complications, transfusion
 traumatic (immediate) (delayed) T79.4
Shoemaker's chest M95.4

Short, shortening, shortness
 arm (acquired) — *see also* Deformity, limb,
  unequal length
  congenital Q71.81-
  forearm — *see* Deformity, limb, unequal
   length
 bowel syndrome K91.2
 breath R06.02
 cervical (complicating pregnancy) O26.87-
  non-gravid uterus N88.3
 common bile duct, congenital Q44.5
 cord (umbilical), complicating delivery O69.3
 cystic duct, congenital Q44.5
 esophagus (congenital) Q39.8
 femur (acquired) — *see* Deformity, limb,
  unequal length, femur
  congenital — *see* Defect, reduction, lower
   limb, longitudinal, femur
 frenum, frenulum, linguae (congenital) Q38.1
 hip (acquired) — *see also* Deformity, limb,
  unequal length
  congenital Q65.89
 leg (acquired) — *see also* Deformity, limb,
  unequal length
  congenital Q72.81-
  lower leg — *see also* Deformity, limb,
   unequal length
 limbed stature, with immunodeficiency D82.2
 lower limb (acquired) — *see also* Deformity,
  limb, unequal length
  congenital Q72.81-
 organ or site, congenital NEC — *see* Distortion
 palate, congenital Q38.5
 radius (acquired) — *see also* Deformity, limb,
  unequal length
  congenital — *see* Defect, reduction, upper
   limb, longitudinal, radius
 rib syndrome Q77.2
 stature (child) (hereditary) (idiopathic) NEC
  R62.52
  constitutional E34.3
  due to endocrine disorder E34.3
  Laron-type E34.3
 tendon — *see also* Contraction, tendon
  with contracture of joint — *see* Contraction,
   joint
  Achilles (acquired) M67.0-
   congenital Q66.89
  congenital Q79.8
 thigh (acquired) — *see also* Deformity, limb,
  unequal length, femur
  congenital — *see* Defect, reduction, lower
   limb, longitudinal, femur
 tibialis anterior (tendon) — *see* Contraction,
  tendon
 umbilical cord
  complicating delivery O69.3
 upper limb, congenital — *see* Defect,
  reduction, upper limb, specified type NEC
 urethra N36.8
 uvula, congenital Q38.5
 vagina (congenital) Q52.4
Shortsightedness — *see* Myopia
Shoshin (acute fulminating beriberi) E51.11
Shoulder — *see* condition
Shovel-shaped incisors K00.2
Shower, thromboembolic — *see* Embolism
Shunt
 arterial-venous (dialysis) Z99.2
 arteriovenous, pulmonary (acquired) I28.0
  congenital Q25.72
 cerebral ventricle (communicating) in situ
  Z98.2
 surgical, prosthetic, with complications — *see*
  Complications, cardiovascular, device or
  implant
Shutdown, renal N28.9
Shy-Drager syndrome G90.3

DISEASE INDEX

Sialadenitis, sialadenosis (any gland) (chronic) (periodic) (suppurative) — *see* Sialoadenitis
Sialectasia K11.8
Sialidosis E77.1
Sialitis, silitis (any gland) (chronic) (suppurative) — *see* Sialoadenitis
Sialoadenitis (any gland) (periodic) (suppurative) K11.20
  acute K11.21
    recurrent K11.22
  chronic K11.23
Sialoadenopathy K11.9
Sialoangitis — *see* Sialoadenitis
Sialodochitis (fibrinosa) — *see* Sialoadenitis
Sialodocholithiasis K11.5
Sialolithiasis K11.5
Sialometaplasia, necrotizing K11.8
Sialorrhea — *see also* Ptyalism
  periodic — *see* Sialoadenitis
Sialosis K11.7
Siamese twin Q89.4
Sibling rivalry Z62.891
Sicard's syndrome G52.7
Sicca syndrome M35.00
  with
    keratoconjunctivitis M35.01
    lung involvement M35.02
    myopathy M35.03
    renal tubulo-interstitial disorders M35.04
  specified organ involvement NEC M35.09
Sick R69
  or handicapped person in family Z63.79
    needing care at home Z63.6
  sinus (syndrome) I49.5
Sick-euthyroid syndrome E07.81
Sickle-cell
  anemia — *see* Disease, sickle-cell
  trait D57.3
Sicklemia — *see also* Disease, sickle-cell
  trait D57.3
Sickness
  air (travel) T75.3
  airplane T75.3
  alpine T70.29
  altitude T70.20
  Andes T70.29
  aviator's T70.29
  balloon T70.29
  car T75.3
  compressed air T70.3
  decompression T70.3
  green D50.8
  milk — *see* Poisoning, food, noxious
  motion T75.3
  mountain T70.29
    acute D75.1
  protein (*see also* Reaction, serum) T80.69
  radiation T66
  roundabout (motion) T75.3
  sea T75.3
  serum NEC (*see also* Reaction, serum) T80.69
  sleeping (African) B56.9
    by Trypanosoma B56.9
      brucei
        gambiense B56.0
        rhodesiense B56.1
    East African B56.1
    Gambian B56.0
    Rhodesian B56.1
    West African B56.0
  swing (motion) T75.3
  train (railway) (travel) T75.3
  travel (any vehicle) T75.3
Sideropenia — *see* Anemia, iron deficiency
Siderosilicosis J62.8
Siderosis (lung) J63.4
  eye (globe) — *see* Disorder, globe, degenerative, siderosis

Siemens' syndrome (ectodermal dysplasia) Q82.8
Sighing R06.89
  psychogenic F45.8
Sigmoid — *see also* condition
  flexure — *see* condition
  kidney Q63.1
Sigmoiditis (*see also* Enteritis) K52.9
  infectious A09
  noninfectious K52.9
Silfversköld's syndrome Q78.9
Silicosiderosis J62.8
Silicosis, silicotic (simple) (complicated) J62.8
  with tuberculosis J65
Silicotuberculosis J65
Silo-fillers' disease J68.8
  bronchitis J68.0
  pneumonitis J68.0
  pulmonary edema J68.1
Silver's syndrome Q87.1
Simian malaria B53.1
Simmonds' cachexia or disease E23.0
Simons' disease or syndrome (progressive lipodystrophy) E88.1
Simple, simplex — *see* condition
Simulation, conscious (of illness) Z76.5
Simultanagnosia (asimultagnosia) R48.3
Sin Nombre virus disease (Hantavirus) (cardio)-pulmonary syndrome) B33.4
Sinding-Larsen disease or osteochondrosis — *see* Osteochondrosis, juvenile, patella
Singapore hemorrhagic fever A91
Singer's node or nodule J38.2
Single
  atrium Q21.2
  coronary artery Q24.5
  umbilical artery Q27.0
  ventricle Q20.4
Singultus R06.6
  epidemicus B33.0
Sinus — *see also* Fistula
  abdominal K63.89
  arrest I45.5
  arrhythmia I49.8
  bradycardia R00.1
  branchial cleft (internal) (external) Q18.0
  coccygeal — *see* Sinus, pilonidal
  dental K04.6
  dermal (congenital) Q06.8
    with abscess Q06.8
    coccygeal, pilonidal — *see* Sinus, coccygeal
    infected, skin NEC L08.89
  marginal, ruptured or bleeding — *see* Hemorrhage, antepartum, specified cause NEC
  medial, face and neck Q18.8
  pause I45.5
  pericranii Q01.9
  pilonidal (infected) (rectum) L05.92
    with abscess L05.02
  preauricular Q18.1
  rectovaginal N82.3
  Rokitansky-Aschoff (gallbladder) K82.8
  sacrococcygeal (dermoid) (infected) — *see* Sinus, pilonidal
  tachycardia R00.0
    paroxysmal I47.1
  tarsi syndrome M25.57-
  testis N50.89
  tract (postinfective) — *see* Fistula
  urachus Q64.4
Sinusitis (accessory) (chronic) (hyperplastic) (nasal) (nonpurulent) (purulent) J32.9
  acute J01.90
    ethmoidal J01.20
      recurrent J01.21
    frontal J01.10
      recurrent J01.11

Sinusitis (accessory) (chronic) (hyperplastic) (nasal) (nonpurulent) (purulent) J32.9 — *continued*
  acute J01.90 — *continued*
    involving more than one sinus, other than pansinusitis J01.80
      recurrent J01.81
    maxillary J01.00
      recurrent J01.01
    pansinusitis J01.40
      recurrent J01.41
    recurrent J01.91
    specified NEC J01.80
      recurrent J01.81
    sphenoidal J01.30
      recurrent J01.31
  allergic — *see* Rhinitis, allergic
  due to high altitude T70.1
  ethmoidal J32.2
    acute J01.20
      recurrent J01.21
  frontal J32.1
    acute J01.10
      recurrent J01.11
  influenzal — *see* Influenza, with, respiratory manifestations NEC
  involving more than one sinus but not pansinusitis J32.8
    acute J01.80
      recurrent J01.81
  maxillary J32.0
    acute J01.00
      recurrent J01.01
  sphenoidal J32.3
    acute J01.30
      recurrent J01.31
  tuberculous, any sinus A15.8
Sinusitis-bronchiectasis-situs inversus (syndrome) (triad) Q89.3
Sipple's syndrome E31.22
Sirenomelia (syndrome) Q87.2
Siriasis T67.0
Sirkari's disease B55.0
Siti A65
Situation, psychiatric F99
Situational
  disturbance (transient) — *see* Disorder, adjustment
    acute F43.0
  maladjustment — *see* Disorder, adjustment
  reaction — *see* Disorder, adjustment
    acute F43.0
Situs inversus or transversus (abdominalis) (thoracis) Q89.3
Sixth disease B08.20
  due to human herpesvirus 6 B08.21
  due to human herpesvirus 7 B08.22
Sjögren-Larsson syndrome Q87.1
Sjögren's syndrome or disease — *see* Sicca syndrome
Skeletal — *see* condition
Skene's gland — *see* condition
Skenitis — *see* Urethritis
Skerljevo A65
Skevas-Zerfus disease — *see* Toxicity, venom, marine animal, sea anemone
Skin — *see also* condition
  clammy R23.1
  donor — *see* Donor, skin
  hidebound M35.9
Slate-dressers' or slate-miners' lung J62.8
Sleep
  apnea — *see* Apnea, sleep
  deprivation Z72.820
  disorder or disturbance G47.9
    child F51.9
      nonorganic origin F51.9
    specified NEC G47.8

Sleep — *continued*
disturbance G47.9
nonorganic origin F51.9
drunkenness F51.9
rhythm inversion G47.2-
terrors F51.4
walking F51.3
hysterical F44.89
Sleep hygiene
abuse Z72.821
inadequate Z72.821
poor Z72.821
Sleeping sickness — *see* Sickness, sleeping
Sleeplessness — *see* Insomnia
menopausal N95.1
Sleep-wake schedule disorder G47.20
Slim disease (in HIV infection) B20
Slipped, slipping
epiphysis (traumatic) — *see also*
Osteochondropathy, specified type NEC
capital femoral (traumatic)
acute (on chronic) S79.01-
current traumatic — *code as* Fracture, by site
upper femoral (nontraumatic) M93.00-
acute M93.01-
on chronic M93.03-
chronic M93.02-
intervertebral disc — *see* Displacement,
intervertebral disc
ligature, umbilical P51.8
patella — *see* Disorder, patella, derangement
NEC
rib M89.8x8
sacroiliac joint — *see* subcategory M53.2
tendon — *see* Disorder, tendon
ulnar nerve, nontraumatic — *see* Lesion, nerve,
ulnar
vertebra NEC — *see* Spondylolisthesis
Slocumb's syndrome E27.0
Sloughing (multiple) (phagedena) (skin) — *see*
also Gangrene
abscess — *see* Abscess
appendix K38.8
fascia — *see* Disorder, soft tissue, specified
type NEC
scrotum N50.89
tendon — *see* Disorder, tendon
transplanted organ — *see* Rejection, transplant
ulcer — *see* Ulcer, skin
Slow
feeding, newborn P92.2
flow syndrome, coronary I20.8
heart(beat) R00.1
Slowing, urinary stream R39.198
Sluder's neuralgia (syndrome) G44.89
Slurred, slurring speech R47.81
Small(ness)
for gestational age — *see* Small for dates
introitus, vagina N89.6
kidney (unknown cause) N27.9
bilateral N27.1
unilateral N27.0
ovary (congenital) Q50.39
pelvis
with disproportion (fetopelvic) O33.1
causing obstructed labor O65.1
uterus N85.8
white kidney N03.9
Small-and-light-for-dates — *see* Small for
dates
Small-for-dates (infant) P05.10
with weight of
99 grams or less P05.11
500-749 grams P05.12
4750-999 grams P05.13
1000-1249 grams P05.14
1250-1499 grams P05.15
1500-1749 grams P05.16
1750-1999 grams P05.17

Small-for-dates (infant) P05.10 — *continued*
with weight of — *continued*
2000-2499 grams P05.18
2500 grams and over P05.19
specified NEC P05.19
Smallpox B03
Smearing, fecal R15.1
Smith-Lemli-Opitz syndrome E78.72
Smith's fracture S52.54-
Smoker — *see* Dependence, drug, nicotine
Smoker's
bronchitis J41.0
cough J41.0
palate K13.24
throat J31.2
tongue K13.24
Smoking
passive Z77.22
Smothering spells R06.81
Snaggle teeth, tooth M26.39
Snapping
finger — *see* Trigger finger
hip — *see* Derangement, joint, specified type
NEC, hip
involving the iliotibial band M76.3-
knee — *see* Derangement, knee
involving the iliotibial band M76.3-
Sneddon-Wilkinson disease or syndrome
(sub-corneal pustular dermatosis) L13.1
Sneezing (intractable) R06.7
Sniffing
cocaine
abuse — *see* Abuse, drug, cocaine
dependence — *see* Dependence, drug,
cocaine
gasoline
abuse — *see* Abuse, drug, inhalant
dependence — *see* Dependence, drug,
inhalant
glue (airplane)
abuse — *see* Abuse, drug, inhalant
drug dependence — *see* Dependence, drug,
inhalant
Sniffles
newborn P28.89
Snoring R06.83
Snow blindness — *see* Photokeratitis
Snuffles (non-syphilitic) R06.5
newborn P28.89
syphilitic (infant) A50.05 *[J99]*
Social
exclusion Z60.4
due to discrimination or persecution
(perceived) Z60.5
migrant Z59.0
acculturation difficulty Z60.3
rejection Z60.4
due to discrimination or persecution Z60.5
role conflict NEC Z73.5
skills inadequacy NEC Z73.4
transplantation Z60.3
Sodoku A25.0
Soemmerring's ring — *see* Cataract,
secondary
Soft — *see also* condition
nails L60.3
Softening
bone — *see* Osteomalacia
brain (necrotic) (progressive) G93.89
congenital Q04.8
embolic I63.4-
hemorrhagic — *see* Hemorrhage,
intracranial, intracerebral
occlusive I63.5-
thrombotic I63.3-
cartilage M94.2-
patella M22.4-
cerebellar — *see* Softening, brain
cerebral — *see* Softening, brain

Softening — *continued*
cerebrospinal — *see* Softening, brain
myocardial, heart — *see* Degeneration,
myocardial
spinal cord G95.89
stomach K31.89
Soldier's
heart F45.8
patches I31.0
Solitary
cyst, kidney N28.1
kidney, congenital Q60.0
Solvent abuse — *see* Abuse, drug, inhalant
dependence — *see* Dependence, drug,
inhalant
Somatization reaction, somatic reaction
— *see* Disorder, somatoform
Somnambulism F51.3
hysterical F44.89
Somnolence R40.0
nonorganic origin F51.11
Sonne dysentery A03.3
Soor B37.0
Sore
bed — *see* Ulcer, pressure, by site
chiclero B55.1
Delhi B55.1
desert — *see* Ulcer, skin
eye H57.1-
Lahore B55.1
mouth K13.79
canker K12.0
muscle M79.1
Naga — *see* Ulcer, skin
of skin — *see* Ulcer, skin
oriental B55.1
pressure — *see* Ulcer, pressure, by site
skin L98.9
soft A57
throat (acute) — *see also* Pharyngitis
with influenza, flu, or grippe — *see*
Influenza, with, respiratory
manifestations NEC
chronic J31.2
coxsackie (virus) B08.5
diphtheritic A36.0
herpesviral B00.2
influenzal — *see* Influenza, with, respiratory
manifestations NEC
septic J02.0
streptococcal (ulcerative) J02.0
viral NEC J02.8
coxsackie B08.5
tropical — *see* Ulcer, skin
veldt — *see* Ulcer, skin
Soto's syndrome (cerebral gigantism) Q87.3
South African cardiomyopathy syndrome
I42.8
Southeast Asian hemorrhagic fever A91
Spacing
abnormal, tooth, teeth, fully erupted M26.30
excessive, tooth, fully erupted M26.32
Spade-like hand (congenital) Q68.1
Spading nail L60.8
congenital Q84.6
Spanish collar N47.1
Sparganosis B70.1
Spasm(s), spastic, spasticity (*see also*
condition) R25.2
accommodation — *see* Spasm, of
accommodation
ampulla of Vater K83.4
anus, ani (sphincter) (reflex) K59.4
psychogenic F45.8
artery I73.9
cerebral G45.9
Bell's G51.3

Spasm(s), spastic, spasticity (see also condition) R25.2 — continued
bladder (sphincter, external or internal) N32.89
  psychogenic F45.8
bronchus, bronchiole J98.01
cardia K22.0
cardiac I20.1
carpopedal — see Tetany
cerebral (arteries) (vascular) G45.9
cervix, complicating delivery O62.4
ciliary body (of accommodation) — see Spasm, of accommodation
colon (see also Irritable, bowel) K58.9
  with diarrhea K58.0
  psychogenic F45.8
common duct K83.8
compulsive — see Tic
conjugate H51.8
coronary (artery) I20.1
diaphragm (reflex) R06.6
  epidemic B33.0
  psychogenic F45.8
duodenum K59.8
epidemic diaphragmatic (transient) B33.0
esophagus (diffuse) K22.4
  psychogenic F45.8
facial G51.3
fallopian tube N83.8
gastrointestinal (tract) K31.89
  psychogenic F45.8
glottis J38.5
  hysterical F44.4
  psychogenic F45.8
    conversion reaction F44.4
  reflex through recurrent laryngeal nerve J38.5
habit — see Tic
heart I20.1
hemifacial (clonic) G51.3
hourglass — see Contraction, hourglass
hysterical F44.4
infantile — see Epilepsy, spasms
inferior oblique, eye H51.8
intestinal (see also Syndrome, irritable bowel) K58.9
  psychogenic F45.8
larynx, laryngeal J38.5
  hysterical F44.4
  psychogenic F45.8
    conversion reaction F44.4
levator palpebrae superioris — see Disorder, eyelid function
muscle NEC M62.838
  back M62.830
nerve, trigeminal G51.0
nervous F45.8
nodding F98.4
occupational F48.8
oculogyric H51.8
  psychogenic F45.8
of accommodation H52.53-
ophthalmic artery — see Occlusion, artery, retina
perineal, female N94.89
peroneo-extensor — see also Deformity, limb, flat foot
pharynx (reflex) J39.2
  hysterical F45.8
  psychogenic F45.8
psychogenic F45.8
pylorus NEC K31.3
  adult hypertrophic K31.89
  congenital or infantile Q40.0
  psychogenic F45.8
rectum (sphincter) K59.4
  psychogenic F45.8
retinal (artery) — see Occlusion, artery, retina

Spasm(s), spastic, spasticity (see also condition) R25.2 — continued
sigmoid (see also Syndrome, irritable bowel) K58.9
  psychogenic F45.8
sphincter of Oddi K83.4
stomach K31.89
  neurotic F45.8
throat J39.2
  hysterical F45.8
  psychogenic F45.8
tic F95.9
  chronic F95.1
  transient of childhood F95.0
tongue K14.8
torsion (progressive) G24.1
trigeminal nerve — see Neuralgia, trigeminal
ureter N13.5
urethra (sphincter) N35.9
uterus N85.8
  complicating labor O62.4
vagina N94.2
  psychogenic F52.5
vascular I73.9
vasomotor I73.9
vein NEC I87.8
viscera — see Pain, abdominal
Spasmodic — see condition
Spasmophilia — see Tetany
Spasmus nutans F98.4
Spastic, spasticity — see also Spasm
child (cerebral) (congenital) (paralysis) G80.1
Speaker's throat R49.8
Specific, specified — see condition
Speech
defect, disorder, disturbance, impediment R47.9
  psychogenic, in childhood and adolescence F98.8
  slurring R47.81
  specified NEC R47.89
Spencer's disease A08.19
Spens' syndrome (syncope with heart block) I45.9
Sperm counts (fertility testing) Z31.41
postvasectomy Z30.8
  reversal Z31.42
Spermatic cord — see condition
Spermatocele N43.40
congenital Q55.4
multiple N43.42
single N43.41
Spermatocystitis N49.0
Spermatocytoma C62.9-
specified site — see Neoplasm, malignant, by site
Spermatorrhea N50.89
Sphacelus — see Gangrene
Sphenoidal — see condition
Sphenoiditis (chronic) — see Sinusitis, sphenoidal
Sphenopalatine ganglion neuralgia G90.09
Sphericity, increased, lens (congenital) Q12.4
Spherocytosis (congenital) (familial) (hereditary) D58.0
hemoglobin disease D58.0
sickle-cell (disease) D57.8-
Spherophakia Q12.4
Sphincter — see condition
Sphincteritis, sphincter of Oddi — see Cholangitis
Sphingolipidosis E75.3
specified NEC E75.29
Sphingomyelinosis E75.3
Spicule tooth K00.2

Spider
bite — see Toxicity, venom, spider
fingers — see Syndrome, Marfan's
nevus I78.1
toes — see Syndrome, Marfan's
vascular I78.1
Spiegler-Fendt
benign lymphocytoma L98.8
sarcoid L08.89
Spielmeyer-Vogt disease E75.4
Spina bifida (aperta) Q05.9
with hydrocephalus NEC Q05.4
cervical Q05.5
  with hydrocephalus Q05.0
dorsal Q05.6
  with hydrocephalus Q05.1
lumbar Q05.7
  with hydrocephalus Q05.2
lumbosacral Q05.7
  with hydrocephalus Q05.2
occulta Q76.0
sacral Q05.8
  with hydrocephalus Q05.3
thoracic Q05.6
  with hydrocephalus Q05.1
thoracolumbar Q05.6
  with hydrocephalus Q05.1
Spindle, Krukenberg's — see Pigmentation, cornea, posterior
Spine, spinal — see condition
Spiradenoma (eccrine) — see Neoplasm, skin, benign
Spirillosis A25.0
Spirillum
minus A25.0
obermeieri infection A68.0
Spirochetal — see condition
Spirochetosis A69.9
arthritic, arthritica A69.9
bronchopulmonary A69.8
icterohemorrhagic A27.0
lung A69.8
Spirometrosis B70.1
Spitting blood — see Hemoptysis
Splanchnoptosis K63.4
Spleen, splenic — see condition
Splenectasis — see Splenomegaly
Splenitis (interstitial) (malignant) (nonspecific) D73.89
malarial (see also Malaria) B54 [D77]
tuberculous A18.85
Splenocele D73.89
Splenomegaly, splenomegalia (Bengal) (cryptogenic) (idiopathic) (tropical) R16.1
with hepatomegaly R16.2
cirrhotic D73.2
congenital Q89.09
congestive, chronic D73.2
Egyptian B65.1
Gaucher's E75.22
malarial (see also Malaria) B54 [D77]
neutropenic D73.81
Niemann-Pick — see Niemann-Pick disease or syndrome
siderotic D73.2
syphilitic A52.79
  congenital (early) A50.08 [D77]
Splenopathy D73.9
Splenoptosis D73.89
Splenosis D73.89
Splinter — see Foreign body, superficial, by site
Split, splitting
foot Q72.7-
hand Q71.6
heart sounds R01.2
lip, congenital — see Cleft, lip
nails L60.3
urinary stream R39.13
Spondylarthrosis — see Spondylosis

Spondylitis (chronic) — *see also*
Spondylopathy, inflammatory
ankylopoietica — *see* Spondylitis, ankylosing
ankylosing (chronic) M45.9
  with lung involvement M45.9 *[J99]*
  cervical region M45.2
  cervicothoracic region M45.3
  juvenile M08.1
  lumbar region M45.6
  lumbosacral region M45.7
  multiple sites M45.0
  occipito-atlanto-axial region M45.1
  sacrococcygeal region M45.8
  thoracic region M45.4
  thoracolumbar region M45.5
atrophic (ligamentous) — *see* Spondylitis, ankylosing
deformans (chronic) — *see* Spondylosis
gonococcal A54.41
gouty (*see also* Gout, by type, vertebrae) M10.08
in (due to)
  brucellosis A23.9 *[M49.80]*
    cervical region A23.9 *[M49.82]*
    cervicothoracic region A23.9 *[M49.83]*
    lumbar region A23.9 *[M49.86]*
    lumbosacral region A23.9 *[M49.87]*
    multiple sites A23.9 *[M49.89]*
    occipito-atlanto-axial region A23.9 *[M49.81]*
    sacrococcygeal region A23.9 *[M49.88]*
    thoracic region A23.9 *[M49.84]*
    thoracolumbar region A23.9 *[M49.85]*
  enterobacteria (*see also* subcategory M49.8) A04.9
  tuberculosis A18.01
infectious NEC — *see* Spondylopathy, infective
juvenile ankylosing (chronic) M08.1
Kümmell's — *see* Spondylopathy, traumatic
Marie-Strümpell — *see* Spondylitis, ankylosing
muscularis — *see* Spondylopathy, specified NEC
psoriatic L40.53
rheumatoid — *see* Spondylitis, ankylosing
rhizomelica — *see* Spondylitis, ankylosing
sacroiliac NEC M46.1
senescent, senile — *see* Spondylosis
traumatic (chronic) or post-traumatic — *see* Spondylopathy, traumatic
tuberculous A18.01
typhosa A01.05
Spondylolisthesis (acquired) (degenerative) M43.10
with disproportion (fetopelvic) O33.0
  causing obstructed labor O65.0
cervical region M43.12
cervicothoracic region M43.13
congenital Q76.2
lumbar region M43.16
lumbosacral region M43.17
multiple sites M43.19
occipito-atlanto-axial region M43.11
sacrococcygeal region M43.18
thoracic region M43.14
thoracolumbar region M43.15
traumatic (old) M43.10
  acute
    fifth cervical (displaced) S12.430
      nondisplaced S12.431
      specified type NEC (displaced) S12.450
        nondisplaced S12.451
      type III S12.44
    fourth cervical (displaced) S12.330
      nondisplaced S12.331
      specified type NEC (displaced) S12.350
        nondisplaced S12.351
      type III S12.34

Spondylolisthesis (acquired) (degenerative) M43.10 — *continued*
traumatic (old) M43.10 — *continued*
  acute — *continued*
    second cervical (displaced) S12.130
      nondisplaced S12.131
      specified type NEC (displaced) S12.150
        nondisplaced S12.151
      type III S12.14
    seventh cervical (displaced) S12.630
      nondisplaced S12.631
      specified type NEC (displaced) S12.650
        nondisplaced S12.651
      type III S12.64
    sixth cervical (displaced) S12.530
      nondisplaced S12.531
      specified type NEC (displaced) S12.550
        nondisplaced S12.551
      type III S12.54
    third cervical (displaced) S12.230
      nondisplaced S12.231
      specified type NEC (displaced) S12.250
        nondisplaced S12.251
      type III S12.24
Spondylolysis (acquired) M43.00
cervical region M43.02
cervicothoracic region M43.03
congenital Q76.2
lumbar region M43.06
lumbosacral region M43.07
  with disproportion (fetopelvic) O33.0
    causing obstructed labor O65.8
multiple sites M43.09
occipito-atlanto-axial region M43.01
sacrococcygeal region M43.08
thoracic region M43.04
thoracolumbar region M43.05
Spondylopathy M48.9
infective NEC M46.50
  cervical region M46.52
  cervicothoracic region M46.53
  lumbar region M46.56
  lumbosacral region M46.57
  multiple sites M46.59
  occipito-atlanto-axial region M46.51
  sacrococcygeal region M46.58
  thoracic region M46.54
  thoracolumbar region M46.55
inflammatory M46.90
  cervical region M46.92
  cervicothoracic region M46.93
  lumbar region M46.96
  lumbosacral region M46.97
  multiple sites M46.99
  occipito-atlanto-axial region M46.91
  sacrococcygeal region M46.98
  specified type NEC M46.80
    cervical region M46.82
    cervicothoracic region M46.83
    lumbar region M46.86
    lumbosacral region M46.87
    multiple sites M46.89
    occipito-atlanto-axial region M46.81
    sacrococcygeal region M46.88
    thoracic region M46.84
    thoracolumbar region M46.85
  thoracic region M46.94
  thoracolumbar region M46.95
neuropathic, in
  syringomyelia and syringobulbia G95.0
  tabes dorsalis A52.11
specified NEC — *see* subcategory M48.8
traumatic M48.30
  cervical region M48.32
  cervicothoracic region M48.33
  lumbar region M48.36
  lumbosacral region M48.37
  occipito-atlanto-axial region M48.31
  sacrococcygeal region M48.38

Spondylopathy M48.9 — *continued*
traumatic M48.30 — *continued*
  thoracic region M48.34
  thoracolumbar region M48.35
Spondylosis M47.9
with
  disproportion (fetopelvic) O33.0
    causing obstructed labor O65.0
  myelopathy NEC M47.10
    cervical region M47.12
    cervicothoracic region M47.13
    lumbar region M47.16
    occipito-atlanto-axial region M47.11
    thoracic region M47.14
    thoracolumbar region M47.15
  radiculopathy M47.20
    cervical region M47.22
    cervicothoracic region M47.23
    lumbar region M47.26
    lumbosacral region M47.27
    occipito-atlanto-axial region M47.21
    sacrococcygeal region M47.28
    thoracic region M47.24
    thoracolumbar region M47.25
specified NEC M47.899
  cervical region M47.892
  cervicothoracic region M47.893
  lumbar region M47.896
  lumbosacral region M47.897
  occipito-atlanto-axial region M47.891
  sacrococcygeal region M47.898
  thoracic region M47.894
  thoracolumbar region M47.895
traumatic — *see* Spondylopathy, traumatic
without myelopathy or radiculopathy M47.819
  cervical region M47.812
  cervicothoracic region M47.813
  lumbar region M47.816
  lumbosacral region M47.817
  occipito-atlanto-axial region M47.811
  sacrococcygeal region M47.818
  thoracic region M47.814
  thoracolumbar region M47.815
Sponge
inadvertently left in operation wound — *see* Foreign body, accidentally left during a procedure
kidney (medullary) Q61.5
Sponge-diver's disease — *see* Toxicity, venom, marine animal, sea anemone
Spongioblastoma (any type) — *see* Neoplasm, malignant, by site
specified site — *see* Neoplasm, malignant, by site
unspecified site C71.9
Spongioneuroblastoma — *see* Neoplasm, malignant, by site
Spontaneous — *see also* condition
fracture (cause unknown) — *see* Fracture, pathological
Spoon nail L60.3
congenital Q84.6
Sporadic — *see* condition
Sporothrix schenckii infection — *see* Sporotrichosis
Sporotrichosis B42.9
arthritis B42.82
disseminated B42.7
generalized B42.7
lymphocutaneous (fixed) (progressive) B42.1
pulmonary B42.0
specified NEC B42.89
Spots, spotting (in) (of)
Bitot's — *see also* Pigmentation, conjunctiva
  in the young child E50.1
  vitamin A deficiency E50.1
café, au lait L81.3
Cayenne pepper I78.1

Spots, spotting (in) (of) — *continued*
  cotton wool, retina — *see* Occlusion, artery, retina
  de Morgan's (senile angiomas) I78.1
  Fuchs' black (myopic) H44.2-
  intermenstrual (regular) N92.0
    irregular N92.1
  Koplik's B05.9
  liver L81.4
  pregnancy O26.85-
  purpuric R23.3
  ruby I78.1
Spotted fever — *see* Fever, spotted N92.3
Sprain (joint) (ligament)
  acromioclavicular joint or ligament S43.5-
  ankle S93.40-
    calcaneofibular ligament S93.41-
    deltoid ligament S93.42-
    internal collateral ligament — *see* Sprain, ankle, specified ligament NEC
    specified ligament NEC S93.49-
    talofibular ligament — *see* Sprain, ankle, specified ligament NEC
    tibiofibular ligament S93.43-
  anterior longitudinal, cervical S13.4
  atlas, atlanto-axial, atlanto-occipital S13.4
  breast bone — *see* Sprain, sternum
  calcaneofibular — *see* Sprain, ankle
  carpal — *see* Sprain, wrist
  carpometacarpal — *see* Sprain, hand, specified site NEC
  cartilage
    costal S23.41
    semilunar (knee) — *see* Sprain, knee, specified site NEC
      with current tear — *see* Tear, meniscus
    thyroid region S13.5
    xiphoid — *see* Sprain, sternum
  cervical, cervicodorsal, cervicothoracic S13.4
  chondrosternal S23.421
  coracoclavicular S43.8-
  coracohumeral S43.41-
  coronary, knee — *see* Sprain, knee, specified site NEC
  costal cartilage S23.41
  cricoarytenoid articulation or ligament S13.5
  cricothyroid articulation S13.5
  cruciate, knee — *see* Sprain, knee, cruciate
  deltoid, ankle — *see* Sprain, ankle
  dorsal (spine) S23.3
  elbow S53.40-
    radial collateral ligament S53.43-
    radiohumeral S53.41-
    rupture
      radial collateral ligament — *see* Rupture, traumatic, ligament, radial collateral
      ulnar collateral ligament — *see* Rupture, traumatic, ligament, ulnar collateral
    specified type NEC S53.49-
    ulnar collateral ligament S53.44-
    ulnohumeral S53.42-
  femur, head — *see* Sprain, hip
  fibular collateral, knee — *see* Sprain, knee, collateral
  fibulocalcaneal — *see* Sprain, ankle
  finger(s) S63.61-
    index S63.61-
    interphalangeal (joint) S63.63-
      index S63.63-
      little S63.63-
      middle S63.63-
      ring S63.63-
    little S63.61-
    metacarpophalangeal (joint) S63.65-
    middle S63.61-
    ring S63.61-
    specified site NEC S63.69-
      index S63.69-
      little S63.69-

Sprain (joint) (ligament) — *continued*
  finger(s) S63.61- — *continued*
    specified site NEC S63.69- — *continued*
      middle S63.69-
      ring S63.69-
  foot S93.60-
    specified ligament NEC S93.69-
    tarsal ligament S93.61-
    tarsometatarsal ligament S93.62-
    toe — *see* Sprain, toe
  hand S63.9-
    finger — *see* Sprain, finger
    specified site NEC — *see* subcategory S63.8
    thumb — *see* Sprain, thumb
  head S03.9
  hip S73.10-
    iliofemoral ligament S73.11-
    ischiocapsular (ligament) S73.12-
    specified NEC S73.19-
  iliofemoral — *see* Sprain, hip
  innominate
    acetabulum — *see* Sprain, hip
    sacral junction S33.6
  internal
    collateral, ankle — *see* Sprain, ankle
    semilunar cartilage — *see* Sprain, knee, specified site NEC
  interphalangeal
    finger — *see* Sprain, finger, interphalangeal (joint)
    toe — *see* Sprain, toe, interphalangeal joint
  ischiocapsular — *see* Sprain, hip
  ischiofemoral — *see* Sprain, hip
  jaw (articular disc) (cartilage) (meniscus) S03.4-
    old M26.69
  knee S83.9-
    collateral ligament S83.40-
      lateral (fibular) S83.42-
      medial (tibial) S83.41-
    cruciate ligament S83.50-
      anterior S83.51-
      posterior S83.52-
    lateral (fibular) collateral ligament S83.42-
    medial (tibial) collateral ligament S83.41-
    patellar ligament S76.11-
    specified site NEC S83.8x-
    superior tibiofibular joint (ligament) S83.6-
  lateral collateral, knee — *see* Sprain, knee, collateral
  lumbar (spine) S33.5
  lumbosacral S33.9
  mandible (articular disc) S03.4-
    old M26.69
  medial collateral, knee — *see* Sprain, knee, collateral
  meniscus
    jaw S03.4-
      old M26.69
    knee — *see* Sprain, knee, specified site NEC
      with current tear — *see* Tear, meniscus
      old — *see* Derangement, knee, meniscus, due to old tear
    mandible S03.4-
      old M26.69
  metacarpal (distal) (proximal) — *see* Sprain, hand, specified site NEC
  metacarpophalangeal — *see* Sprain, finger, metacarpophalangeal (joint)
  metatarsophalangeal — *see* Sprain, toe, metatarsophalangeal joint
  midcarpal — *see* Sprain, hand, specified site NEC
  midtarsal — *see* Sprain, foot, specified site NEC
  neck S13.9
    anterior longitudinal cervical ligament S13.4
    atlanto-axial joint S13.4
    atlanto-occipital joint S13.4

Sprain (joint) (ligament) — *continued*
  neck S13.9 — *continued*
    cervical spine S13.4
    cricoarytenoid ligament S13.5
    cricothyroid ligament S13.5
    specified site NEC S13.8
    thyroid region (cartilage) S13.5
  nose S03.8
  orbicular, hip — *see* Sprain, hip
  patella — *see* Sprain, knee, specified site NEC
  patellar ligament S76.11-
  pelvis NEC S33.8
  phalanx
    finger — *see* Sprain, finger
    toe — *see* Sprain, toe
  pubofemoral — *see* Sprain, hip
  radiocarpal — *see* Sprain, wrist
  radiohumeral — *see* Sprain, elbow
  radius, collateral — *see* Rupture, traumatic, ligament, radial collateral
  rib (cage) S23.41
  rotator cuff (capsule) S43.42-
  sacroiliac (region)
    chronic or old — *see* subcategory M53.2
    joint S33.6
  scaphoid (hand) — *see* Sprain, hand, specified site NEC
  scapula(r) — *see* Sprain, shoulder girdle, specified site NEC
  semilunar cartilage (knee) — *see* Sprain, knee, specified site NEC
    with current tear — *see* Tear, meniscus
    old — *see* Derangement, knee, meniscus, due to old tear
  shoulder joint S43.40-
    acromioclavicular joint (ligament) — *see* Sprain, acromioclavicular joint
    blade — *see* Sprain, shoulder, girdle, specified site NEC
    coracoclavicular joint (ligament) — *see* Sprain, coracoclavicular joint
    coracohumeral ligament — *see* Sprain, coracohumeral joint
    girdle S43.9-
      specified site NEC S43.8-
    rotator cuff — *see* Sprain, rotator cuff
    specified site NEC S43.49-
    sternoclavicular joint (ligament) — *see* Sprain, sternoclavicular joint
  spine
    cervical S13.4
    lumbar S33.5
    thoracic S23.3
  sternoclavicular joint S43.6-
  sternum S23.429
    chondrosternal joint S23.421
    specified site NEC S23.428
    sternoclavicular (joint) (ligament) S23.420
  symphysis
    jaw S03.4-
      old M26.69
    mandibular S03.4-
      old M26.69
  talofibular — *see* Sprain, ankle
  tarsal — *see* Sprain, foot, specified site NEC
  tarsometatarsal — *see* Sprain, foot, specified site NEC
  temporomandibular S03.4-
    old M26.69
  thorax S23.9
    ribs S23.41
    specified site NEC S23.8
    spine S23.3
    sternum — *see* Sprain, sternum
  thumb S63.60-
    interphalangeal (joint) S63.62-
    metacarpophalangeal (joint) S63.64-
    specified site NEC S63.68-
  thyroid cartilage or region S13.5

DISEASE INDEX

Sprain (joint) (ligament) — *continued*
  tibia (proximal end) — *see* Sprain, knee, specified site NEC
  tibial collateral, knee — *see* Sprain, knee, collateral
  tibiofibular
    distal — *see* Sprain, ankle
    superior — *see* Sprain, knee, specified site NEC
  toe(s) S93.50-
    great S93.50-
    interphalangeal joint S93.51-
      great S93.51-
      lesser S93.51-
    lesser S93.50-
    metatarsophalangeal joint S93.52-
      great S93.52-
      lesser S93.52-
  ulna, collateral — *see* Rupture, traumatic, ligament, ulnar collateral
  ulnohumeral — *see* Sprain, elbow
  wrist S63.50-
    carpal S63.51-
    radiocarpal S63.52-
    specified site NEC S63.59-
  xiphoid cartilage — *see* Sprain, sternum
Sprengel's deformity (congenital) Q74.0
Sprue (tropical) K90.1
  celiac K90.0
  idiopathic K90.49
  meaning thrush B37.0
  nontropical K90.0
Spur, bone — *see also* Enthesopathy
  calcaneal M77.3-
  iliac crest M76.2-
  nose (septum) J34.89
Spurway's syndrome Q78.0
Sputum
  abnormal (amount) (color) (odor) (purulent) R09.3
  blood-stained R04.2
  excessive (cause unknown) R09.3
Squamous — *see also* condition
  epithelium in
    cervical canal (congenital) Q51.828
    uterine mucosa (congenital) Q51.818
Squashed nose M95.0
  congenital Q67.4
Squeeze, diver's T70.3
Squint — *see also* Strabismus
  accommodative — *see* Strabismus, convergent concomitant
St. Hubert's disease A82.9
Stab — *see also* Laceration
  internal organs — *see* Injury, by site
Stafne's cyst or cavity M27.0
Staggering gait R26.0
  hysterical F44.4
Staghorn calculus — *see* Calculus, kidney
Stähli's line (cornea) (pigment) — *see* Pigmentation, cornea, anterior
Stain, staining
  meconium (newborn) P96.83
  port wine Q82.5
  tooth, teeth (hard tissues) (extrinsic) K03.6
    due to
      accretions K03.6
      deposits (betel) (black) (green) (materia alba) (orange) (soft) (tobacco) K03.6
      metals (copper) (silver) K03.7
      nicotine K03.6
      pulpal bleeding K03.7
      tobacco K03.6
    intrinsic K00.8
Stammering (*see also* Disorder, fluency) F80.81

Standstill
  auricular I45.5
  cardiac — *see* Arrest, cardiac
  sinoatrial I45.5
  ventricular — *see* Arrest, cardiac
Stannosis J63.5
Stanton's disease — *see* Melioidosis
Staphylitis (acute) (catarrhal) (chronic) (gangrenous) (membranous) (suppurative) (ulcerative) K12.2
Staphylococcal scalded skin syndrome L00
Staphylococcemia A41.2
Staphylococcus, staphylococcal — *see also* condition
  as cause of disease classified elsewhere B95.8
    aureus (methicillin susceptible) (MSSA) B95.61
      methicillin resistant (MRSA) B95.62
    specified NEC, as cause of disease classified elsewhere B95.7
Staphyloma (sclera)
  cornea H18.72-
  equatorial H15.81-
  localized (anterior) H15.82-
  posticum H15.83-
  ring H15.85-
Stargardt's disease — *see* Dystrophy, retina
Starvation (inanition) (due to lack of food) T73.0
  edema — *see* Malnutrition, severe
Stasis
  bile (noncalculous) K83.1
  bronchus J98.09
    with infection — *see* Bronchitis
  cardiac — *see* Failure, heart, congestive
  cecum K59.8
  colon K59.8
  dermatitis I87.2
    with
      varicose ulcer — *see* Varix, leg, with ulcer, with inflammation
      varicose veins — *see* Varix, leg, with, inflammation
      due to postthrombotic syndrome — *see* Syndrome, postthrombotic
  duodenal K31.5
  eczema — *see* Varix, leg, with, inflammation
  edema — *see* Hypertension, venous (chronic), idiopathic
  foot T69.0-
  ileocecal coil K59.8
  ileum K59.8
  intestinal K59.8
  jejunum K59.8
  kidney N19
  liver (cirrhotic) K76.1
  lymphatic I89.8
  pneumonia J18.2
  pulmonary — *see* Edema, lung
  rectal K59.8
  renal N19
    tubular N17.0
  ulcer — *see* Varix, leg, with, ulcer
    without varicose veins I87.2
  urine — *see* Retention, urine
  venous I87.8
State (of)
  affective and paranoid, mixed, organic psychotic F06.8
  agitated R45.1
    acute reaction to stress F43.0
  anxiety (neurotic) F41.1
  apprehension F41.1
  burn-out Z73.0
  climacteric, female Z78.0
    symptomatic N95.1
  compulsive F42.8
    mixed with obsessional thoughts F42.2

State (of) — *continued*
  confusional (psychogenic) F44.89
    acute — *see also* Delirium
      with
        arteriosclerotic dementia F01.50
          with behavioral disturbance F01.51
        senility or dementia F05
    alcoholic F10.231
    epileptic F05
    reactive (from emotional stress, psychological trauma) F44.89
    subacute — *see* Delirium
  convulsive — *see* Convulsions
  crisis F43.0
  depressive F32.9
    neurotic F34.1
  dissociative F44.9
  emotional shock (stress) R45.7
  hypercoagulation — *see* Hypercoagulable
  locked-in G83.5
  menopausal Z78.0
    symptomatic N95.1
  neurotic F48.9
    with depersonalization F48.1
  obsessional F42.8
  oneiroid (schizophrenia-like) F23
  organic
    hallucinatory (nonalcoholic) F06.0
    paranoid(-hallucinatory) F06.2
  panic F41.0
  paranoid F22
    climacteric F22
    involutional F22
    menopausal F22
    organic F06.2
    senile F03
    simple F22
  persistent vegetative R40.3
  phobic F40.9
  postleukotomy F07.0
  pregnant
    gestational carrier Z33.3
    incidental Z33.1
  psychogenic, twilight F44.89
  psychopathic (constitutional) F60.2
  psychotic, organic — *see also* Psychosis, organic
    mixed paranoid and affective F06.8
    senile or presenile F03
    transient NEC F06.8
      with
        depression F06.31
        hallucinations F06.0
  residual schizophrenic F20.5
  restlessness R45.1
  stress (emotional) R45.7
  tension (mental) F48.9
    specified NEC F48.8
  transient organic psychotic NEC F06.8
    depressive type F06.31
    hallucinatory type F06.0
  twilight
    epileptic F05
    psychogenic F44.89
  vegetative, persistent R40.3
  vital exhaustion Z73.0
  withdrawal — *see* Withdrawal, state
Status (post) — *see also* Presence (of)
  absence, epileptic — *see* Epilepsy, by type, with status epilepticus
  administration of tPA (rtPA) in a different facility within the last 24 hours prior to admission to current facility Z92.82
  adrenalectomy (unilateral) (bilateral) E89.6
  anastomosis Z98.0
  anginosus I20.9

363

Status (post) (*see also* Presence (of)) — *continued*
- angioplasty (peripheral) Z98.62
  - with implant Z95.820
  - coronary artery Z98.61
    - with implant Z95.5
- aortocoronary bypass Z95.1
- arthrodesis Z98.1
- artificial opening (of) Z93.9
  - gastrointestinal tract Z93.4
  - specified NEC Z93.8
  - urinary tract Z93.6
  - vagina Z93.8
- asthmaticus — *see* Asthma, by type, with status asthmaticus
- awaiting organ transplant Z76.82
- bariatric surgery Z98.84
- bed confinement Z74.01
- bleb, filtering (vitreous), after glaucoma surgery Z98.83
- breast implant Z98.82
  - removal Z98.86
- cataract extraction Z98.4-
- cholecystectomy Z90.49
- clitorectomy N90.811
  - with excision of labia minora N90.812
- colectomy (complete) (partial) Z90.49
- colonization — *see* Carrier (suspected) of
- colostomy Z93.3
- convulsivus idiopathicus — *see* Epilepsy, by type, with status epilepticus
- coronary artery angioplasty — *see* Status, angioplasty, coronary artery
- cystectomy (urinary bladder) Z90.6
- cystostomy Z93.50
  - appendico-vesicostomy Z93.52
  - cutaneous Z93.51
  - specified NEC Z93.59
- delinquent immunization Z28.3
- dental Z98.818
  - crown Z98.811
  - fillings Z98.811
  - restoration Z98.811
  - sealant Z98.810
  - specified NEC Z98.818
- deployment (current) (military) Z56.82
- dialysis (hemodialysis) (peritoneal) Z99.2
- do not resuscitate (DNR) Z66
- donor — *see* Donor
- embedded fragments — *see* Retained, foreign body fragments (type of)
- embedded splinter — *see* Retained, foreign body fragments (type of)
- enterostomy Z93.4
- epileptic, epilepticus (*see also* Epilepsy, by type, with status epilepticus) G40.901
- estrogen receptor
  - negative Z17.1
  - positive Z17.0
- female genital cutting — *see* Female genital mutilation status
- female genital mutilation — *see* Female genital mutilation status
- filtering (vitreous) bleb after glaucoma surgery Z98.83
- gastrectomy (complete) (partial) Z90.3
- gastric banding Z98.84
- gastric bypass for obesity Z98.84
- gastrostomy Z93.1
- human immunodeficiency virus (HIV) infection, asymptomatic Z21
- hysterectomy (complete) (total) Z90.710
  - partial (with remaining cervial stump) Z90.711
- ileostomy Z93.2
- implant
  - breast Z98.82
- infibulation N90.813
- intestinal bypass Z98.0

Status (post) (*see also* Presence (of)) — *continued*
- jejunostomy Z93.4
- lapsed immunization schedule Z28.3
- laryngectomy Z90.02
- lymphaticus E32.8
- malignancy
  - castrate resistant prostate Z19.2
  - hormone resistant Z19.2
  - hormone sensitive Z19.1
- marmoratus G80.3
- mastectomy (unilateral) (bilateral) Z90.1-
- military deployment status (current) Z56.82
  - in theater or in support of military war, peacekeeping and humanitarian operations Z56.82
- nephrectomy (unilateral) (bilateral) Z90.5
- nephrostomy Z93.6
- obesity surgery Z98.84
- oophorectomy
  - bilateral Z90.722
  - unilateral Z90.721
- organ replacement
  - by artificial or mechanical device or prosthesis of
    - artery Z95.828
    - bladder Z96.0
    - blood vessel Z95.828
    - breast Z97.8
    - eye globe Z97.0
    - heart Z95.812
      - valve Z95.2
    - intestine Z97.8
    - joint Z96.60
      - hip — *see* Presence, hip joint implant
      - knee — *see* Presence, knee joint implant
      - specified site NEC Z96.698
    - kidney Z97.8
    - larynx Z96.3
    - lens Z96.1
    - limbs — *see* Presence, artificial, limb
    - liver Z97.8
    - lung Z97.8
    - pancreas Z97.8
  - by organ transplant (heterologous) (homologous) — *see* Transplant
- pacemaker
  - brain Z96.89
  - cardiac Z95.0
  - specified NEC Z96.89
- pancreatectomy Z90.410
  - complete Z90.410
  - partial Z90.411
  - total Z90.410
- physical restraint Z78.1
- pneumonectomy (complete) (partial) Z90.2
- pneumothorax, therapeutic Z98.3
- postcommotio cerebri F07.81
- postoperative (postprocedural) NEC Z98.890
  - breast implant Z98.82
  - dental Z98.818
    - crown Z98.811
    - fillings Z98.811
    - restoration Z98.811
    - sealant Z98.810
    - specified NEC Z98.818
  - pneumothorax, therapeutic Z98.3
  - uterine scar Z98.891
- postpartum (routine follow-up) Z39.2
  - care immediately after delivery Z39.0
- postsurgical (postprocedural) NEC Z98.890
  - pneumothorax, therapeutic Z98.3
- pregnancy, incidental Z33.1
- prosthesis coronary angioplasty Z95.5
- pseudophakia Z96.1
- renal dialysis (hemodialysis) (peritoneal) Z99.2
- retained foreign body — *see* Retained, foreign body fragments (type of)

Status (post) (*see also* Presence (of)) — *continued*
- reversed jejunal transposition (for bypass) Z98.0
- salpingo-oophorectomy
  - bilateral Z90.722
  - unilateral Z90.721
- sex reassignment surgery status Z87.890
- shunt
  - arteriovenous (for dialysis) Z99.2
  - cerebrospinal fluid Z98.2
  - ventricular (communicating) (for drainage) Z98.2
- splenectomy Z90.81
- thymicolymphaticus E32.8
- thymicus E32.8
- thymolymphaticus E32.8
- thyroidectomy (hypothyroidism) E89.0
- tooth (teeth) extraction (*see also* Absence, teeth, acquired) K08.409
- tPA (rtPA) administration in a different facility within the last 24 hours prior to admission to current facility Z92.82
- tracheostomy Z93.0
- transplant — *see* Transplant
  - organ removed Z98.85
- tubal ligation Z98.51
- underimmunization Z28.3
- ureterostomy Z93.6
- urethrostomy Z93.6
- vagina, artificial Z93.8
- vasectomy Z98.52
- wheelchair confinement Z99.3

Stealing
- child problem F91.8
  - in company with others Z72.810
- pathological (compulsive) F63.2

Steam burn — *see* Burn

Steatocystoma multiplex L72.2

Steatohepatitis (nonalcoholic) (NASH) K75.81

Steatoma L72.3
- eyelid (cystic) — *see* Dermatosis, eyelid
  - infected — *see* Hordeolum

Steatorrhea (chronic) K90.9
- with lacteal obstruction K90.2
- idiopathic (adult) (infantile) K90.9
- pancreatic K90.3
- primary K90.0
- tropical K90.1

Steatosis E88.89
- heart — *see* Degeneration, myocardial
- kidney N28.89
- liver NEC K76.0

Steele-Richardson-Olszewski disease or syndrome G23.1

Stein-Leventhal syndrome E28.2

Stein's syndrome E28.2

Steinbrocker's syndrome G90.8

Steinert's disease G71.11

STEMI (*see also* Infarct, myocardium, ST elevation) I21.3

Stenocardia I20.8

Stenocephaly Q75.8

Stenosis, stenotic (cicatricial) — *see also* Stricture
- ampulla of Vater K83.1
- anus, anal (canal) (sphincter) K62.4
  - and rectum K62.4
  - congenital Q42.3
    - with fistula Q42.2
- aorta (ascending) (supraventricular) (congenital) Q25.1
  - arteriosclerotic I70.0
  - calcified I70.0
  - supravalvular Q25.3

Stenosis, stenotic (cicatricial) (*see also* Stricture) — *continued*
 aortic (valve) I35.0
  with insufficiency I35.2
  congenital Q23.0
  rheumatic I06.0
   with
    incompetency, insufficiency or regurgitation I06.2
     with mitral (valve) disease I08.0
      with tricuspid (valve) disease I08.3
     mitral (valve) disease I08.0
      with tricuspid (valve) disease I08.3
     tricuspid (valve) disease I08.2
      with mitral (valve) disease I08.3
  specified cause NEC I35.0
  syphilitic A52.03
 aqueduct of Sylvius (congenital) Q03.0
  with spina bifida — *see* Spina bifida, by site, with hydrocephalus
  acquired G91.1
 artery NEC (*see also* Arteriosclerosis) I77.1
  celiac I77.4
  cerebral — *see* Occlusion, artery, cerebral
  extremities — *see* Arteriosclerosis, extremities
  precerebral — *see* Occlusion, artery, precerebral
  pulmonary (congenital) Q25.6
   acquired I28.8
  renal I70.1
  stent
   coronary T82.855
   peripheral T82.856
 bile duct (common) (hepatic) K83.1
  congenital Q44.3
 bladder-neck (acquired) N32.0
  congenital Q64.31
 brain G93.89
 bronchus J98.09
  congenital Q32.3
  syphilitic A52.72
 cardia (stomach) K22.2
  congenital Q39.3
 cardiovascular — *see* Disease, cardiovascular
 caudal M48.08
 cervix, cervical (canal) N88.2
  congenital Q51.828
  in pregnancy or childbirth — *see* Pregnancy, complicated by, abnormal cervix
 colon — *see also* Obstruction, intestine
  congenital Q42.9
   specified NEC Q42.8
 colostomy K94.03
 common (bile) duct K83.1
  congenital Q44.3
 coronary (artery) — *see* Disease, heart, ischemic, atherosclerotic
 cystic duct — *see* Obstruction, gallbladder
 due to presence of device, implant or graft (*see also* Complications, by site and type, specified NEC) T85.858
  arterial graft NEC T82.858
  breast (implant) T85.858
  catheter T85.858
   dialysis (renal) T82.858
    intraperitoneal T85.858
   infusion NEC T82.858
    spinal (epidural) (subdural) T85.858
   urinary (indwelling) T83.85
  fixation, internal (orthopedic) NEC T84.85
  gastrointestinal (bile duct) (esophagus) T85.858
  genital NEC T83.85
  heart NEC T82.857
  joint prosthesis T84.85
  ocular (corneal graft) (orbital implant) NEC T85.858
  orthopedic NEC T84.85
  specified NEC T85.858

Stenosis, stenotic (cicatricial) (*see also* Stricture) — *continued*
 due to presence of device, implant or graft (*see also* Complications, by site and type, specified NEC) T85.858 — *continued*
  urinary NEC T83.85
  vascular NEC T82.858
  ventricular intracranial shunt T85.850
 duodenum K31.5
  congenital Q41.0
 ejaculatory duct NEC N50.89
 endocervical os — *see* Stenosis, cervix
 enterostomy K94.13
 esophagus K22.2
  congenital Q39.3
  syphilitic A52.79
   congenital A50.59 [K23]
 eustachian tube — *see* Obstruction, eustachian tube
 external ear canal (acquired) H61.30-
  congenital Q16.1
  due to
   inflammation H61.32-
   trauma H61.31-
  postprocedural H95.81-
  specified cause NEC H61.39-
 gallbladder — *see* Obstruction, gallbladder
 glottis J38.6
 heart valve (congenital) Q24.8
  aortic Q23.0
  mitral Q23.2
  pulmonary Q22.1
  tricuspid Q22.4
 hepatic duct K83.1
 hymen N89.6
 hypertrophic subaortic (idiopathic) I42.1
 ileum K56.69
  congenital Q41.2
 infundibulum cardia Q24.3
 intervertebral foramina — *see also* Lesion, biomechanical, specified NEC
  connective tissue M99.79
   abdomen M99.79
   cervical region M99.71
   cervicothoracic M99.71
   head region M99.70
   lumbar region M99.73
   lumbosacral M99.73
   occipitocervical M99.70
   sacral region M99.74
   sacrococcygeal M99.74
   sacroiliac M99.74
   specified NEC M99.79
   thoracic region M99.72
   thoracolumbar M99.72
  disc M99.79
   abdomen M99.79
   cervical region M99.71
   cervicothoracic M99.71
   head region M99.70
   lower extremity M99.76
   lumbar region M99.73
   lumbosacral M99.73
   occipitocervical M99.70
   pelvic M99.75
   rib cage M99.78
   sacral region M99.74
   sacrococcygeal M99.74
   sacroiliac M99.74
   specified NEC M99.79
   thoracic region M99.72
   thoracolumbar M99.72
   upper extremity M99.77
  osseous M99.69
   abdomen M99.69
   cervical region M99.61
   cervicothoracic M99.61
   head region M99.60
   lower extremity M99.66

Stenosis, stenotic (cicatricial) (*see also* Stricture) — *continued*
 intervertebral foramina — *see also* Lesion, biomechanical, specified NEC — *continued*
  osseous M99.69 — *continued*
   lumbar region M99.63
   lumbosacral M99.63
   occipitocervical M99.60
   pelvic M99.65
   rib cage M99.68
   sacral region M99.64
   sacrococcygeal M99.64
   sacroiliac M99.64
   specified NEC M99.69
   thoracic region M99.62
   thoracolumbar M99.62
   upper extremity M99.67
  subluxation — *see* Stenosis, intervertebral foramina, osseous
 intestine — *see also* Obstruction, intestine
  congenital (small) Q41.9
   large Q42.9
    specified NEC Q42.8
   specified NEC Q41.8
 jejunum K56.69
  congenital Q41.1
 lacrimal (passage)
  canaliculi H04.54-
  congenital Q10.5
  duct H04.55-
  punctum H04.56-
  sac H04.57-
 lacrimonasal duct — *see* Stenosis, lacrimal, duct
  congenital Q10.5
 larynx J38.6
  congenital NEC Q31.8
   subglottic Q31.1
  syphilitic A52.73
   congenital A50.59 [J99]
 mitral (chronic) (inactive) (valve) I05.0
  with
   aortic valve disease I08.0
   incompetency, insufficiency or regurgitation I05.2
  active or acute I01.1
   with rheumatic or Sydenham's chorea I02.0
  congenital Q23.2
  specified cause, except rheumatic I34.2
  syphilitic A52.03
 myocardium, myocardial — *see also* Degeneration, myocardial
  hypertrophic subaortic (idiopathic) I42.1
 nares (anterior) (posterior) J34.89
  congenital Q30.0
 nasal duct — *see also* Stenosis, lacrimal, duct
  congenital Q10.5
 nasolacrimal duct — *see also* Stenosis, lacrimal, duct
  congenital Q10.5
 neural canal — *see also* Lesion, biomechanical, specified NEC
  connective tissue M99.49
   abdomen M99.49
   cervical region M99.41
   cervicothoracic M99.41
   head region M99.40
   lower extremity M99.46
   lumbar region M99.43
   lumbosacral M99.43
   occipitocervical M99.40
   pelvic M99.45
   rib cage M99.48
   sacral region M99.44
   sacrococcygeal M99.44
   sacroiliac M99.44
   specified NEC M99.49

Stenosis, stenotic (cicatricial) (*see also* Stricture) — *continued*
neural canal — *see also* Lesion, biomechanical, specified NEC — *continued*
  connective tissue M99.49 — *continued*
    thoracic region M99.42
    thoracolumbar M99.42
    upper extremity M99.47
  intervertebral disc M99.59
    abdomen M99.59
    cervical region M99.51
    cervicothoracic M99.51
    head region M99.50
    lower extremity M99.56
    lumbar region M99.53
    lumbosacral M99.53
    occipitocervical M99.50
    pelvic M99.55
    rib cage M99.58
    sacral region M99.54
    sacrococcygeal M99.54
    sacroiliac M99.54
    specified NEC M99.59
    thoracic region M99.52
    thoracolumbar M99.52
    upper extremity M99.57
  osseous M99.39
    abdomen M99.39
    cervical region M99.31
    cervicothoracic M99.31
    head region M99.30
    lower extremity M99.36
    lumbar region M99.33
    lumbosacral M99.33
    occipitocervical M99.30
    pelvic M99.35
    rib cage M99.38
    sacral region M99.34
    sacrococcygeal M99.34
    sacroiliac M99.34
    specified NEC M99.39
    thoracic region M99.32
    thoracolumbar M99.32
    upper extremity M99.37
  subluxation M99.29
    cervical region M99.21
    cervicothoracic M99.21
    head region M99.20
    lower extremity M99.26
    lumbar region M99.23
    lumbosacral M99.23
    occipitocervical M99.20
    pelvic M99.25
    rib cage M99.28
    sacral region M99.24
    sacrococcygeal M99.24
    sacroiliac M99.24
    specified NEC M99.29
    thoracic region M99.22
    thoracolumbar M99.22
    upper extremity M99.27
organ or site, congenital NEC — *see* Atresia, by site
papilla of Vater K83.1
pulmonary (artery) (congenital) Q25.6
  with ventricular septal defect, transposition of aorta, and hypertrophy of right ventricle Q21.3
  acquired I28.8
  in tetralogy of Fallot Q21.3
  infundibular Q24.3
  subvalvular Q24.3
  supravalvular Q25.6
  valve I37.0
    with insufficiency I37.2
    congenital Q22.1
    rheumatic I09.89
      with aortic, mitral or tricuspid (valve) disease I08.8

Stenosis, stenotic (cicatricial) (*see also* Stricture) — *continued*
pulmonary (artery) (congenital) Q25.6 — *continued*
  vein, acquired I28.8
  vessel NEC I28.8
pulmonic (congenital) Q22.1
  infundibular Q24.3
  subvalvular Q24.3
pylorus (hypertrophic) (acquired) K31.1
  adult K31.1
  congenital Q40.0
  infantile Q40.0
rectum (sphincter) — *see* Stricture, rectum
renal artery I70.1
  congenital Q27.1
salivary duct (any) K11.8
sphincter of Oddi K83.1
spinal M48.00
  cervical region M48.02
  cervicothoracic region M48.03
  lumbar region M48.06
  lumbosacral region M48.07
  occipito-atlanto-axial region M48.01
  sacrococcygeal region M48.08
  thoracic region M48.04
  thoracolumbar region M48.05
stent
  vascular
    end stent
      adjacent to stent — *see* Arteriosclerosis
      within the stent
        coronary T82.855
        peripheral T82.856
    in stent
      coronary vessel T82.855
      peripheral vessel T82.856
stomach, hourglass K31.2
subaortic (congenital) Q24.4
  hypertrophic (idiopathic) I42.1
subglottic J38.6
  congenital Q31.1
  postprocedural J95.5
trachea J39.8
  congenital Q32.1
  syphilitic A52.73
  tuberculous NEC A15.5
tracheostomy J95.03
tricuspid (valve) I07.0
  with
    aortic (valve) disease I08.2
    incompetency, insufficiency or regurgitation I07.2
      with aortic (valve) disease I08.2
        with mitral (valve) disease I08.3
    mitral (valve) disease I08.1
      with aortic (valve) disease I08.3
  congenital Q22.4
  nonrheumatic I36.0
    with insufficiency I36.2
tubal N97.1
ureter — *see* Atresia, ureter
ureteropelvic junction, congenital Q62.11
ureterovesical orifice, congenital Q62.12
urethra (valve) — *see also* Stricture, urethra
  congenital Q64.32
urinary meatus, congenital Q64.33
vagina N89.5
  congenital Q52.4
  in pregnancy — *see* Pregnancy, complicated by, abnormal vagina
    causing obstructed labor O65.5
valve (cardiac) (heart) (*see also* Endocarditis) I38
  congenital Q24.8
    aortic Q23.0
    mitral Q23.2
    pulmonary Q22.1
    tricuspid Q22.4

Stenosis, stenotic (cicatricial) (*see also* Stricture) — *continued*
vena cava (inferior) (superior) I87.1
  congenital Q26.0
vesicourethral orifice Q64.31
vulva N90.5
Stent jail T82.897
Stercolith (impaction) K56.41
  appendix K38.1
Stercoraceous, stercoral ulcer K63.3
  anus or rectum K62.6
Stereotypies NEC F98.4
Sterility — *see* Infertility
Sterilization — *see* Encounter (for), sterilization
Sternalgia — *see* Angina
Sternopagus Q89.4
Sternum bifidum Q76.7
Steroid
  effects (adverse) (adrenocortical) (iatrogenic)
    cushingoid E24.2
      correct substance properly administered — *see* Table of Drugs and Chemicals, by drug, adverse effect
      overdose or wrong substance given or taken — *see* Table of Drugs and Chemicals, by drug, poisoning
    diabetes — *see* category E09
      correct substance properly administered — *see* Table of Drugs and Chemicals, by drug, adverse effect
      overdose or wrong substance given or taken — *see* Table of Drugs and Chemicals, by drug, poisoning
    fever R50.2
    insufficiency E27.3
      correct substance properly administered — *see* Table of Drugs and Chemicals, by drug, adverse effect
      overdose or wrong substance given or taken — *see* Table of Drugs and Chemicals, by drug, poisoning
  responder H40.04-
Stevens-Johnson disease or syndrome L51.1
  toxic epidermal necrolysis overlap L51.3
Stewart-Morel syndrome M85.2
Sticker's disease B08.3
Sticky eye — *see* Conjunctivitis, acute, mucopurulent
Stieda's disease — *see* Bursitis, tibial collateral
Stiff neck — *see* Torticollis
Stiff-man syndrome G25.82
Stiffness, joint NEC M25.60-
  ankle M25.67-
  ankylosis — *see* Ankylosis, joint
  contracture — *see* Contraction, joint
  elbow M25.62-
  foot M25.67-
  hand M25.64-
  hip M25.65-
  knee M25.66-
  shoulder M25.61-
  wrist M25.63-
Stigmata congenital syphilis A50.59
Still's disease or syndrome (juvenile) M08.20
  adult-onset M06.1
  ankle M08.27-
  elbow M08.22-
  foot joint M08.27-
  hand joint M08.24-
  hip M08.25-
  knee M08.26-
  multiple site M08.29
  shoulder M08.21-
  vertebra M08.28
  wrist M08.23-
Still-Felty syndrome — *see* Felty's syndrome

Stillbirth P95
Stimulation, ovary E28.1
Sting (venomous) (with allergic or anaphylactic shock) — *see* Table of Drugs and Chemicals, by animal or substance, poisoning
Stippled epiphyses Q78.8
Stitch
  abscess T81.48
  burst (in operation wound) — *see* Disruption, wound, operation
Stokes' disease E05.00
  with thyroid storm E05.01
Stokes-Adams disease or syndrome I45.9
Stokvis(-Talma) disease D74.8
Stoma malfunction
  colostomy K94.03
  enterostomy K94.13
  gastrostomy K94.23
  ileostomy K94.13
  tracheostomy J95.03
Stomach — *see* condition
Stomatitis (denture) (ulcerative) K12.1
  angular K13.0
    due to dietary or vitamin deficiency E53.0
  aphthous K12.0
  bovine B08.61
  candidal B37.0
  catarrhal K12.1
  diphtheritic A36.89
  due to
    dietary deficiency E53.0
    thrush B37.0
    vitamin deficiency
      B group NEC E53.9
      B2 (riboflavin) E53.0
  epidemic B08.8
  epizootic B08.8
  follicular K12.1
  gangrenous A69.0
  Geotrichum B48.3
  herpesviral, herpetic B00.2
  herpetiformis K12.0
  malignant K12.1
  membranous acute K12.1
  monilial B37.0
  mycotic B37.0
  necrotizing ulcerative A69.0
  parasitic B37.0
  septic K12.1
  spirochetal A69.1
  suppurative (acute) K12.2
  ulceromembranous A69.1
  vesicular K12.1
    with exanthem (enteroviral) B08.4
    virus disease A93.8
  Vincent's A69.1
Stomatocytosis D58.8
Stomatomycosis B37.0
Stomatorrhagia K13.79
Stone(s) — *see also* Calculus
  bladder (diverticulum) N21.0
  cystine E72.09
  heart syndrome I50.1
  kidney N20.0
  prostate N42.0
  pulpal (dental) K04.2
  renal N20.0
  salivary gland or duct (any) K11.5
  urethra (impacted) N21.1
  urinary (duct) (impacted) (passage) N20.9
    bladder (diverticulum) N21.0
    lower tract N21.9
    specified NEC N21.8
  xanthine E79.8 *[N22]*
Stonecutter's lung J62.8
Stonemason's asthma, disease, lung or pneumoconiosis J62.8

Stoppage
  heart — *see* Arrest, cardiac
  urine — *see* Retention, urine
Storm, thyroid — *see* Thyrotoxicosis
Strabismus (congenital) (nonparalytic) H50.9
  concomitant H50.40
    convergent — *see* Strabismus, convergent concomitant
    divergent — *see* Strabismus, divergent concomitant
  convergent concomitant H50.00
    accommodative component H50.43
    alternating H50.05
      with
        A pattern H50.06
        specified nonconcomitances NEC H50.08
        V pattern H50.07
    monocular H50.01-
      with
        A pattern H50.02-
        specified nonconcomitances NEC H50.04-
        V pattern H50.03-
      intermittent H50.31-
        alternating H50.32
  cyclotropia H50.41
  divergent concomitant H50.10
    alternating H50.15
      with
        A pattern H50.16
        specified noncomitances NEC H50.18
        V pattern H50.17
    monocular H50.11-
      with
        A pattern H50.12-
        specified noncomitances NEC H50.14-
        V pattern H50.13-
      intermittent H50.33
        alternating H50.34
  Duane's syndrome H50.81-
  due to adhesions, scars H50.69
  heterophoria H50.50
    alternating H50.55
    cyclophoria H50.54
    esophoria H50.51
    exophoria H50.52
    vertical H50.53
  heterotropia H50.40
    intermittent H50.30
  hypertropia H50.2-
  hypotropia — *see* Hypertropia
  latent H50.50
  mechanical H50.60
    Brown's sheath syndrome H50.61-
    specified type NEC H50.69
  monofixation syndrome H50.42
  paralytic H49.9
    abducens nerve H49.2-
    fourth nerve H49.1-
    Kearns-Sayre syndrome H49.81-
    ophthalmoplegia (external)
      progressive H49.4-
        with pigmentary retinopathy H49.81-
      total H49.3-
    sixth nerve H49.2-
    specified type NEC H49.88-
    third nerve H49.0-
    trochlear nerve H49.1-
  specified type NEC H50.89
  vertical H50.2-
Strain
  back S39.012
  cervical S16.1
  eye NEC — *see* Disturbance, vision, subjective
  heart — *see* Disease, heart
  low back S39.012
  mental NOS Z73.3
    work-related Z56.6

Strain — *continued*
  muscle (tendon) — *see* Injury, muscle, by site, strain
  neck S16.1
  physical NOS Z73.3
    work-related Z56.6
  postural — *see also* Disorder, soft tissue, due to use
  psychological NEC Z73.3
  tendon — *see* Injury, muscle, by site, strain
Straining, on urination R39.16
Strand, vitreous — *see* Opacity, vitreous, membranes and strands
Strangulation, strangulated — *see also* Asphyxia, traumatic
  appendix K38.8
  bladder-neck N32.0
  bowel or colon K56.2
  food or foreign body — *see* Foreign body, by site
  hemorrhoids — *see* Hemorrhoids, with complication
  hernia — *see also* Hernia, by site, with obstruction
    with gangrene — *see* Hernia, by site, with gangrene
  intestine (large) (small) K56.2
    with hernia — *see also* Hernia, by site, with obstruction
      with gangrene — *see* Hernia, by site, with gangrene
  mesentery K56.2
  mucus — *see* Asphyxia, mucus
  omentum K56.2
  organ or site, congenital NEC — *see* Atresia, by site
  ovary — *see* Torsion, ovary
  penis N48.89
    foreign body T19.4
  rupture — *see* Hernia, by site, with obstruction
  stomach due to hernia — *see also* Hernia, by site, with obstruction
    with gangrene — *see* Hernia, by site, with gangrene
  vesicourethral orifice N32.0
Strangury R30.0
Straw itch B88.0
Strawberry
  gallbladder K82.4
  mark Q82.5
  tongue (red) (white) K14.3
Streak(s)
  macula, angioid H35.33
  ovarian Q50.32
Strephosymbolia F81.0
  secondary to organic lesion R48.8
Streptobacillary fever A25.1
Streptobacillosis A25.1
Streptobacillus moniliformis A25.1
Streptococcus, streptococcal — *see also* condition
  as cause of disease classified elsewhere B95.5
  group
    A, as cause of disease classified elsewhere B95.0
    B, as cause of disease classified elsewhere B95.1
    D, as cause of disease classified elsewhere B95.2
  pneumoniae, as cause of disease classified elsewhere B95.3
  specified NEC, as cause of disease classified elsewhere B95.4
Streptomycosis B47.1
Streptotrichosis A48.8

Stress F43.9
  family — *see* Disruption, family
  fetal P84
    complicating pregnancy O77.9
      due to drug administration O77.1
  mental NEC Z73.3
    work-related Z56.6
  physical NEC Z73.3
    work-related Z56.6
  polycythemia D75.1
  reaction (*see also* Reaction, stress) F43.9
  work schedule Z56.3
Stretching, nerve — *see* Injury, nerve
Striae albicantes, atrophicae or
  distensae (cutis) L90.6
Stricture — *see also* Stenosis
  ampulla of Vater K83.1
  anus (sphincter) K62.4
    congenital Q42.3
      with fistula Q42.2
    infantile Q42.3
      with fistula Q42.2
  aorta (ascending) (congenital) Q25.1
    arteriosclerotic I70.0
    calcified I70.0
    supravalvular, congenital Q25.3
  aortic (valve) — *see* Stenosis, aortic
  aqueduct of Sylvius (congenital) Q03.0
    with spina bifida — *see* Spina bifida, by site,
      with hydrocephalus
    acquired G91.1
  artery I77.1
    basilar — *see* Occlusion, artery, basilar
    carotid — *see* Occlusion, artery, carotid
    celiac I77.4
    congenital (peripheral) Q27.8
      cerebral Q28.3
      coronary Q24.5
      digestive system Q27.8
      lower limb Q27.8
      retinal Q14.1
      specified site NEC Q27.8
      umbilical Q27.0
      upper limb Q27.8
    coronary — *see* Disease, heart, ischemic,
      atherosclerotic
      congenital Q24.5
    precerebral — *see* Occlusion, artery,
      precerebral
    pulmonary (congenital) Q25.6
      acquired I28.8
    renal I70.1
    vertebral — *see* Occlusion, artery, vertebral
  auditory canal (external) (congenital)
    acquired — *see* Stenosis, external ear canal
  bile duct (common) (hepatic) K83.1
    congenital Q44.3
    postoperative K91.89
  bladder N32.89
    neck N32.0
  bowel — *see* Obstruction, intestine
  brain G93.89
  bronchus J98.09
    congenital Q32.3
    syphilitic A52.72
  cardia (stomach) K22.2
    congenital Q39.3
  cardiac — *see also* Disease, heart
    orifice (stomach) K22.2
  cecum — *see* Obstruction, intestine
  cervix, cervical (canal) N88.2
    congenital Q51.828
    in pregnancy — *see* Pregnancy, complicated
      by, abnormal cervix
      causing obstructed labor O65.5
  colon — *see also* Obstruction, intestine
    congenital Q42.9
      specified NEC Q42.8
  colostomy K94.03

Stricture (*see also* Stenosis) — *continued*
  common (bile) duct K83.1
  coronary (artery) — *see* Disease, heart,
    ischemic, atherosclerotic
  cystic duct — *see* Obstruction, gallbladder
  digestive organs NEC, congenital Q45.8
  duodenum K31.5
    congenital Q41.0
  ear canal (external) (congenital) Q16.1
    acquired — *see* Stricture, auditory canal,
      acquired
  ejaculatory duct N50.89
  enterostomy K94.13
  esophagus K22.2
    congenital Q39.3
    syphilitic A52.79
      congenital A50.59 *[K23]*
  eustachian tube — *see also* Obstruction,
    eustachian tube
    congenital Q17.8
  fallopian tube N97.1
    gonococcal A54.24
    tuberculous A18.17
  gallbladder — *see* Obstruction, gallbladder
  glottis J38.6
  heart — *see also* Disease, heart
    valve (*see also* Endocarditis) I38
      aortic Q23.0
      mitral Q23.4
      pulmonary Q22.1
      tricuspid Q22.4
  hepatic duct K83.1
  hourglass, of stomach K31.2
  hymen N89.6
  hypopharynx J39.2
  ileum K56.69
    congenital Q41.2
  intestine — *see also* Obstruction, intestine
    congenital (small) Q41.9
      large Q42.9
        specified NEC Q42.8
      specified NEC Q41.8
    ischemic K55.1
  jejunum K56.69
    congenital Q41.1
  lacrimal passages — *see also* Stenosis, lacrimal
    congenital Q10.5
  larynx J38.6
    congenital NEC Q31.8
      subglottic Q31.1
    syphilitic A52.73
      congenital A50.59 *[J99]*
  meatus
    ear (congenital) Q16.1
      acquired — *see* Stricture, auditory canal,
        acquired
    osseous (ear) (congenital) Q16.1
      acquired — *see* Stricture, auditory canal,
        acquired
    urinarius — *see also* Stricture, urethra
      congenital Q64.33
  mitral (valve) — *see* Stenosis, mitral
  myocardium, myocardial I51.5
    hypertrophic subaortic (idiopathic) I42.1
  nares (anterior) (posterior) J34.89
    congenital Q30.0
  nasal duct — *see also* Stenosis, lacrimal, duct
    congenital Q10.5
  nasolacrimal duct — *see also* Stenosis, lacrimal,
    duct
    congenital Q10.5
  nasopharynx J39.2
    syphilitic A52.73
  nose J34.89
    congenital Q30.0
  nostril (anterior) (posterior) J34.89
    congenital Q30.0
    syphilitic A52.73
      congenital A50.59 *[J99]*

Stricture (*see also* Stenosis) — *continued*
  organ or site, congenital NEC — *see* Atresia,
    by site
  os uteri — *see* Stricture, cervix
  osseous meatus (ear) (congenital) Q16.1
    acquired — *see* Stricture, auditory canal,
      acquired
  oviduct — *see* Stricture, fallopian tube
  pelviureteric junction (congenital) Q62.11
    acquired, with hydronephrosis N13.0
  penis, by foreign body T19.4
  pharynx J39.2
  prostate N42.89
  pulmonary, pulmonic
    artery (congenital) Q25.6
      acquired I28.8
      noncongenital I28.8
    infundibulum (congenital) Q24.3
    valve I37.0
      congenital Q22.1
    vein, acquired I28.8
    vessel NEC I28.8
  punctum lacrimale — *see also* Stenosis,
    lacrimal, punctum
    congenital Q10.5
  pylorus (hypertrophic) K31.1
    adult K31.1
    congenital Q40.0
    infantile Q40.0
  rectosigmoid K56.69
  rectum (sphincter) K62.4
    congenital Q42.1
      with fistula Q42.0
    due to
      chlamydial lymphogranuloma A55
      irradiation K91.89
      lymphogranuloma venereum A55
    gonococcal A54.6
    inflammatory (chlamydial) A55
    syphilitic A52.74
    tuberculous A18.32
  renal artery I70.1
    congenital Q27.1
  salivary duct or gland (any) K11.8
  sigmoid (flexure) — *see* Obstruction, intestine
  spermatic cord N50.89
  stoma (following) (of)
    colostomy K94.03
    enterostomy K94.13
    gastrostomy K94.23
    ileostomy K94.13
    tracheostomy J95.03
  stomach K31.89
    congenital Q40.2
    hourglass K31.2
  subaortic Q24.4
    hypertrophic (acquired) (idiopathic) I42.1
  subglottic J38.6
  syphilitic NEC A52.79
  trachea J39.8
    congenital Q32.1
    syphilitic A52.73
    tuberculous NEC A15.5
  tracheostomy J95.03
  tricuspid (valve) — *see* Stenosis, tricuspid
  tunica vaginalis N50.89
  ureter (postoperative) N13.5
    with
      hydronephrosis N13.1
        with infection N13.6
      pyelonephritis (chronic) N11.1
    congenital — *see* Atresia, ureter
    tuberculous A18.11
  ureteropelvic junction (congenital) Q62.11
    acquired, with hydronephrosis N13.0
  ureterovesical orifice N13.5
    with infection N13.6

DISEASE INDEX

Stricture (*see also* Stenosis) — *continued*
  urethra (organic) (spasmodic) N35.9
    associated with schistosomiasis B65.0 [N37]
    congenital Q64.39
      valvular (posterior) Q64.2
    due to
      infection — *see* Stricture, urethra,
        postinfective
      trauma — *see* Stricture, urethra, post-
        traumatic
    gonococcal, gonorrheal A54.01
    infective NEC — *see* Stricture, urethra,
      postinfective
    late effect (sequelae) of injury — *see*
      Stricture, urethra, post-traumatic
    post-traumatic
      female N35.028
        due to childbirth N35.021
      male N35.014
        anterior urethra N35.013
        bulbous urethra N35.011
        meatal N35.010
        membranous urethra N35.012
    postcatheterization — *see* Stricture, urethra,
      postprocedural
    postinfective NEC
      female N35.12
      male N35.119
        anterior urethra N35.114
        bulbous urethra N35.112
        meatal N35.111
        membranous urethra N35.113
    postobstetric N35.021
    postoperative — *see* Stricture, urethra,
      postprocedural
    postprocedural
      female N99.12
      male N99.114
        anterior bulbous urethra N99.113
        bulbous urethra N99.111
        fossa navicularis N99.115
        meatal N99.110
        membranous urethra N99.112
    sequela (late effect) of
      childbirth N35.021
      injury — *see* Stricture, urethra, post-
        traumatic
    specified cause NEC N35.8
    syphilitic A52.76
    traumatic — *see* Stricture, urethra, post-
      traumatic
    valvular (posterior), congenital Q64.2
  urinary meatus — *see* Stricture, urethra
  uterus, uterine (synechiae) N85.6
    os (external) (internal) — *see* Stricture, cervix
  vagina (outlet) — *see* Stenosis, vagina
  valve (cardiac) (heart) — *see also* Endocarditis
    congenital
      aortic Q23.0
      mitral Q23.2
      pulmonary Q22.1
      tricuspid Q22.4
  vas deferens N50.89
    congenital Q55.4
  vein I87.1
  vena cava (inferior) (superior) NEC I87.1
    congenital Q26.0
  vesicourethral orifice N32.0
    congenital Q64.31
  vulva (acquired) N90.5
Stridor R06.1
  congenital (larynx) P28.89
Stridulous — *see* condition
Stroke (apoplectic) (brain) (embolic) (ischemic)
  (paralytic) (thrombotic) I63.9
  epileptic — *see* Epilepsy
  heat T67.0
  in evolution I63.9

Stroke (apoplectic) (brain) (embolic) (ischemic)
  (paralytic) (thrombotic) I63.9 — *continued*
  intraoperative
    during cardiac surgery I97.810
    during other surgery I97.811
  lightning — *see* Lightning
  meaning
    cerebral hemorrhage — *code to*
      Hemorrhage, intracranial
    cerebral infarction — *code to* Infarction,
      cerebral
  postprocedural
    following cardiac surgery I97.820
    following other surgery I97.821
  unspecified (NOS) I63.9
Stromatosis, endometrial D39.0
Strongyloidiasis, strongyloidosis B78.9
  cutaneous B78.1
  disseminated B78.7
  intestinal B78.0
Strophulus pruriginosus L28.2
Struck by lightning — *see* Lightning
Struma — *see also* Goiter
  Hashimoto E06.3
  lymphomatosa E06.3
  nodosa (simplex) E04.9
    endemic E01.2
      multinodular E01.1
    multinodular E04.2
      iodine-deficiency related E01.1
    toxic or with hyperthyroidism E05.20
      with thyroid storm E05.21
      multinodular E05.20
        with thyroid storm E05.21
      uninodular E05.10
        with thyroid storm E05.11
    toxicosa E05.20
      with thyroid storm E05.21
      multinodular E05.20
        with thyroid storm E05.21
      uninodular E05.10
        with thyroid storm E05.11
    uninodular E04.1
  ovarii D27-
  Riedel's E06.5
Strumipriva cachexia E03.4
Strümpell-Marie spine — *see* Spondylitis,
  ankylosing
Strümpell-Westphal pseudosclerosis
  E83.01
Stuart deficiency disease (factor X) D68.2
Stuart-Prower factor deficiency (factor X)
  D68.2
Student's elbow — *see* Bursitis, elbow,
  olecranon
Stump — *see* Amputation
Stunting, nutritional E45
Stupor (catatonic) R40.1
  depressive (single episode) F32.89
    recurrent episode F33.8
  dissociative F44.2
  manic F30.2
  manic-depressive F31.89
  psychogenic (anergic) F44.2
  reaction to exceptional stress (transient) F43.0
Sturge (-Weber) (-Dimitri) (-Kalischer)
  disease or syndrome Q85.8
Stuttering F80.81
  adult onset F98.5
  childhood onset F80.81
  following cerebrovascular disease — *see*
    Disorder, fluency, following
    cerebrovascular disease
  in conditions classified elsewhere R47.82
Sty, stye (external) (internal) (meibomian)
  (zeisian) — *see* Hordeolum
Subacidity, gastric K31.89
  psychogenic F45.8
Subacute — *see* condition

Subarachnoid — *see* condition
Subcortical — *see* condition
Subcostal syndrome, nerve compression
  — *see* Mononeuropathy, upper limb,
  specified site NEC
Subcutaneous, subcuticular — *see* condition
Subdural — *see* condition
Subendocardium — *see* condition
Subependymoma
  specified site — *see* Neoplasm, uncertain
    behavior, by site
  unspecified site D43.2
Suberosis J67.3
Subglossitis — *see* Glossitis
Subhemophilia D66
Subinvolution
  breast (postlactational) (postpuerperal)
    N64.89
  puerperal O90.89
  uterus (chronic) (nonpuerperal) N85.3
    puerperal O90.89
Sublingual — *see* condition
Sublinguitis — *see* Sialoadenitis
Subluxatable hip Q65.6
Subluxation — *see also* Dislocation
  acromioclavicular S43.11-
  ankle S93.0-
  atlantoaxial, recurrent M43.4
    with myelopathy M43.3
  carpometacarpal (joint) NEC S63.05-
    thumb S63.04-
  complex, vertebral — *see* Complex,
    subluxation
  congenital — *see also* Malposition, congenital
    hip — *see* Dislocation, hip, congenital,
      partial
    joint (excluding hip)
      lower limb Q68.8
      shoulder Q68.8
      upper limb Q68.8
  elbow (traumatic) S53.10-
    anterior S53.11-
    lateral S53.14-
    medial S53.13-
    posterior S53.12-
    specified type NEC S53.19-
  finger S63.20-
    index S63.20-
    interphalangeal S63.22-
      distal S63.24-
        index S63.24-
        little S63.24-
        middle S63.24-
        ring S63.24-
      index S63.22-
      little S63.22-
      middle S63.22-
      proximal S63.23-
        index S63.23-
        little S63.23-
        middle S63.23-
        ring S63.23-
      ring S63.22-
    little S63.20-
    metacarpophalangeal S63.21-
      index S63.21-
      little S63.21-
      middle S63.21-
      ring S63.21-
    middle S63.20-
    ring S63.20-
  foot S93.30-
    specified site NEC S93.33-
    tarsal joint S93.31-
    tarsometatarsal joint S93.32-
    toe — *see* Subluxation, toe

Subluxation (see also Dislocation) — continued
  hip S73.00-
    anterior S73.03-
      obturator S73.02-
    central S73.04-
    posterior S73.01-
  interphalangeal (joint)
    finger S63.22-
      distal joint S63.24-
        index S63.24-
        little S63.24-
        middle S63.24-
        ring S63.24-
      index S63.22-
      little S63.22-
      middle S63.22-
      proximal joint S63.23-
        index S63.23-
        little S63.23-
        middle S63.23-
        ring S63.23-
      ring S63.22-
    thumb S63.12-
      distal joint S63.14-
      proximal joint S63.13-
    toe S93.13-
      great S93.13-
      lesser S93.13-
  joint prosthesis — see Complications, joint
    prosthesis, mechanical, displacement, by
    site
  knee S83.10-
    cap — see Subluxation, patella
    patella — see Subluxation, patella
    proximal tibia
      anteriorly S83.11-
      laterally S83.14-
      medially S83.13-
      posteriorly S83.12-
    specified type NEC S83.19-
  lens — see Dislocation, lens, partial
  ligament, traumatic — see Sprain, by site
  metacarpal (bone)
    proximal end S63.06-
  metacarpophalangeal (joint)
    finger S63.21-
      index S63.21-
      little S63.21-
      middle S63.21-
      ring S63.21-
    thumb S63.11-
  metatarsophalangeal joint S93.14-
    great toe S93.14-
    lesser toe S93.14-
  midcarpal (joint) S63.03-
  patella S83.00-
    lateral S83.01-
    recurrent (nontraumatic) — see Dislocation,
      patella, recurrent, incomplete
    specified type NEC S83.09-
  pathological — see Dislocation, pathological
  radial head S53.00-
    anterior S53.01-
    nursemaid's elbow S53.03-
    posterior S53.02-
    specified type NEC S53.09-
  radiocarpal (joint) S63.02-
  radioulnar (joint)
    distal S63.01-
    proximal — see Subluxation, elbow
  shoulder
    congenital Q68.8
    girdle S43.30-
      scapula S43.31-
      specified site NEC S43.39-
    traumatic S43.00-
      anterior S43.01-
      inferior S43.03-
      posterior S43.02-

Subluxation (see also Dislocation) — continued
  shoulder — continued
    traumatic S43.00- — continued
      specified type NEC S43.08-
  sternoclavicular (joint) S43.20-
    anterior S43.21-
    posterior S43.22-
  symphysis (pubis)
  thumb S63.103
    interphalangeal joint — see Subluxation,
      interphalangeal (joint), thumb
    metacarpophalangeal joint — see
      Subluxation, metacarpophalangeal
      (joint), thumb
  toe(s) S93.10-
    great S93.10-
      interphalangeal joint S93.13-
      metatarsophalangeal joint S93.14-
    interphalangeal joint S93.13-
    lesser S93.10-
      interphalangeal joint S93.13-
      metatarsophalangeal joint S93.14-
    metatarsophalangeal joint S93.149
  ulna
    distal end S63.07-
    proximal end — see Subluxation, elbow
  ulnohumeral joint — see Subluxation, elbow
  vertebral
    recurrent NEC — see subcategory M43.5
    traumatic
      cervical S13.100
        atlantoaxial joint S13.120
        atlantooccipital joint S13.110
        atloidooccipital joint S13.110
        joint between
          C0 and C1 S13.110
          C1 and C2 S13.120
          C2 and C3 S13.130
          C3 and C4 S13.140
          C4 and C5 S13.150
          C5and C6 S13.160
          C6and C7 S13.170
          C7and T1 S13.180
        occipitoatloid joint S13.110
      lumbar S33.100
        joint between
          L1and L2 S33.110
          L2and L3 S33.120
          L3 and L4 S33.130
          L4and L5 S33.140
      thoracic S23.100
        joint between
          T10 and T11 S23.160
          T11 and T12 S23.162
          T12 and L1 S23.170
          T1and T2 S23.110
          T2and T3 S23.120
          T3 and T4 S23.122
          T4 and T5 S23.130
          T5 and T6 S23.132
          T6 and T7 S23.140
          T7 and T8 S23.142
          T8 and T9 S23.150
          T9 and T10 S23.152
  wrist (carpal bone) S63.00-
    carpometacarpal joint — see Subluxation,
      carpometacarpal (joint)
    distal radioulnar joint — see Subluxation,
      radioulnar (joint), distal
    metacarpal bone, proximal — see
      Subluxation, metacarpal (bone),
      proximal end
    midcarpal — see Subluxation, midcarpal
      (joint)
    radiocarpal joint — see Subluxation,
      radiocarpal (joint)
    recurrent — see Dislocation, recurrent, wrist
    specified site NEC S63.09-
    ulna — see Subluxation, ulna, distal end

Submaxillary — see condition
Submersion (fatal) (nonfatal) T75.1
Submucous — see condition
Subnormal, subnormality
  accommodation (old age) H52.4
  mental — see Disability, intellectual
  temperature (accidental) T68
Subphrenic — see condition
Subscapular nerve — see condition
Subseptus uterus Q51.2
Subsiding appendicitis K36
Substance (other psychoactive) -induced
  anxiety disorder F19.980
  bipolar and related disorder F19.94
  delirium F19.921
  depressive disorder F19.94
  major neurocognitive disorder F19.97
  mild neurocognitive disorder F19.988
  obsessive-compulsive and related disorder
    F19.988
  psychotic disorder F19.959
  sexual dysfunction F19.981
  sleep disorder F19.982
Substernal thyroid E04.9
  congenital Q89.2
Substitution disorder F44.9
Subtentorial — see condition
Subthyroidism (acquired) — see also
  Hypothyroidism
  congenital E03.1
Succenturiate placenta O43.19-
Sucking thumb, child (excessive) F98.8
Sudamen, sudamina L74.1
Sudanese kala-azar B55.0
Sudden
  hearing loss — see Deafness, sudden
  heart failure — see Failure, heart
Sudeck's atrophy, disease, or syndrome
  — see Algoneurodystrophy
Suffocation — see Asphyxia, traumatic
Sugar
  blood
    high (transient) R73.9
    low (transient) E16.2
  in urine R81
Suicide, suicidal (attempted) T14.91
  by poisoning — see Table of Drugs and
    Chemicals
  history of (personal) Z91.5
    in family Z81.8
  ideation — see Ideation, suicidal
  risk
    meaning personal history of attempted
      suicide Z91.5
    meaning suicidal ideation — see Ideation,
      suicidal
  tendencies
    meaning personal history of attempted
      suicide Z91.5
    meaning suicidal ideation — see Ideation,
      suicidal
  trauma — see nature of injury by site
Suipestifer infection — see Infection,
  salmonella
Sulfhemoglobinemia,
  sulphemoglobinemia (acquired) (with
  methemoglobinemia) D74.8
Sumatran mite fever A75.3
Summer — see condition
Sunburn L55.9
  due to
    tanning bed (acute) L56.8
      chronic L57.8
    ultraviolet radiation (acute) L56.8
      chronic L57.8
  first degree L55.0
  second degree L55.1
  third degree L55.2

SUNCT (short lasting unilateral neuralgiform headache with conjunctival injection and tearing) G44.059
  intractable G44.051
  not intractable G44.059
Sunken acetabulum — *see* Derangement, joint, specified type NEC, hip
Sunstroke T67.0
Superfecundation — *see* Pregnancy, multiple
Superfetation — *see* Pregnancy, multiple
Superinvolution (uterus) N85.8
Supernumerary (congenital)
  aortic cusps Q23.8
  auditory ossicles Q16.3
  bone Q79.8
  breast Q83.1
  carpal bones Q74.0
  cusps, heart valve NEC Q24.8
    aortic Q23.8
    mitral Q23.2
    pulmonary Q22.3
  digit(s) Q69.9
  ear (lobule) Q17.0
  fallopian tube Q50.6
  finger Q69.0
  hymen Q52.4
  kidney Q63.0
  lacrimonasal duct Q10.6
  lobule (ear) Q17.0
  mitral cusps Q23.2
  muscle Q79.8
  nipple(s) Q83.3
  organ or site not listed — *see* Accessory
  ossicles, auditory Q16.3
  ovary Q50.31
  oviduct Q50.6
  pulmonary, pulmonic cusps Q22.3
  rib Q76.6
    cervical or first (syndrome) Q76.5
  roots (of teeth) K00.2
  spleen Q89.09
  tarsal bones Q74.2
  teeth K00.1
  testis Q55.29
  thumb Q69.1
  toe Q69.2
  uterus Q51.2
  vagina Q52.1
  vertebra Q76.49
Supervision (of)
  contraceptive — *see* Prescription, contraceptives
  dietary (for) Z71.3
    allergy (food) Z71.3
    colitis Z71.3
    diabetes mellitus Z71.3
    food allergy or intolerance Z71.3
    gastritis Z71.3
    hypercholesterolemia Z71.3
    hypoglycemia Z71.3
    intolerance (food) Z71.3
    obesity Z71.3
    specified NEC Z71.3
  healthy infant or child Z76.2
    foundling Z76.1
  high-risk pregnancy — *see* Pregnancy, complicated by, high, risk
  lactation Z39.1
  pregnancy — *see* Pregnancy, supervision of
Supplemental teeth K00.1
Suppression
  binocular vision H53.34
  lactation O92.5
  menstruation N94.89
  ovarian secretion E28.39
  renal N28.9
  urine, urinary secretion R34

Suppuration, suppurative — *see also* condition
  accessory sinus (chronic) — *see* Sinusitis
  adrenal gland
  antrum (chronic) — *see* Sinusitis, maxillary
  bladder — *see* Cystitis
  brain G06.0
    sequelae G09
  breast N61.1
    puerperal, postpartum or gestational — *see* Mastitis, obstetric, purulent
  dental periosteum M27.3
  ear (middle) — *see also* Otitis, media
    external NEC — *see* Otitis, externa, infective
    internal — *see* subcategory H83.0
  ethmoidal (chronic) (sinus) — *see* Sinusitis, ethmoidal
  fallopian tube — *see* Salpingo-oophoritis
  frontal (chronic) (sinus) — *see* Sinusitis, frontal
  gallbladder (acute) K81.0
  gum K05.20
    generalized — *see* Peridontitis, aggressive, generalized
    localized — *see* Peridontitis, aggressive, localized
  intracranial G06.0
  joint — *see* Arthritis, pyogenic or pyemic
  labyrinthine — *see* subcategory H83.0
  lung — *see* Abscess, lung
  mammary gland N61.1
    puerperal, postpartum O91.12
      associated with lactation O91.13
  maxilla, maxillary M27.2
    sinus (chronic) — *see* Sinusitis, maxillary
  muscle — *see* Myositis, infective
  nasal sinus (chronic) — *see* Sinusitis
  pancreas, acute (*see also* Pancreatitis, acute) K85.80
  parotid gland — *see* Sialoadenitis
  pelvis, pelvic
    female — *see* Disease, pelvis, inflammatory
    male K65.0
  pericranial — *see* Osteomyelitis
  salivary duct or gland (any) — *see* Sialoadenitis
  sinus (accessory) (chronic) (nasal) — *see* Sinusitis
  sphenoidal sinus (chronic) — *see* Sinusitis, sphenoidal
  thymus (gland) E32.1
  thyroid (gland) E06.0
  tonsil — *see* Tonsillitis
  uterus — *see* Endometritis
Supraeruption of tooth (teeth) M26.34
Supraglottitis J04.30
  with obstruction J04.31
Suprarenal (gland) — *see* condition
Suprascapular nerve — *see* condition
Suprasellar — *see* condition
Surfer's knots or nodules S89.8-
Surgical
  emphysema T81.82
  procedures, complication or misadventure — *see* Complications, surgical procedures
  shock T81.10
Surveillance (of) (for) — *see also* Observation
  alcohol abuse Z71.41
  contraceptive — *see* Prescription, contraceptives
  dietary Z71.3
  drug abuse Z71.51
Susceptibility to disease, genetic Z15.89
  malignant neoplasm Z15.09
    breast Z15.01
    endometrium Z15.04
    ovary Z15.02
    prostate Z15.03
    specified NEC Z15.09
  multiple endocrine neoplasia Z15.81

Suspected condition, ruled out — *see also* Observation, suspected
  amniotic cavity and membrane Z03.71
  cervical shortening Z03.75
  fetal anomaly Z03.73
  fetal growth Z03.74
  maternal and fetal conditions NEC Z03.79
  newborn (*see also* Observation, newborn, suspected condition ruled out) Z05.9
  oligohydramnios Z03.71
  placental problem Z03.72
  polyhydramnios Z03.71
Suspended uterus
  in pregnancy or childbirth — *see* Pregnancy, complicated by, abnormal uterus
Sutton's nevus D22.9
Suture
  burst (in operation wound) T81.31
    external operation wound T81.31
    internal operation wound T81.32
  inadvertently left in operation wound — *see* Foreign body, accidentally left during a procedure
  removal Z48.02
Swab inadvertently left in operation wound — *see* Foreign body, accidentally left during a procedure
Swallowed, swallowing
  difficulty — *see* Dysphagia
  foreign body — *see* Foreign body, alimentary tract
Swan-neck deformity (finger) — *see* Deformity, finger, swan-neck
Swearing, compulsive F42.8
  in Gilles de la Tourette's syndrome F95.2
Sweat, sweats
  fetid L75.0
  night R61
Sweating, excessive R61
Sweeley-Klionsky disease E75.21
Sweet's disease or dermatosis L98.2
Swelling (of) R60.9
  abdomen, abdominal (not referable to any particular organ) — *see* Mass, abdominal
  ankle — *see* Effusion, joint, ankle
  arm M79.89
    forearm M79.89
  breast N63
  Calabar B74.3
  cervical gland R59.0
  chest, localized R22.2
  ear H93.8-
  extremity (lower) (upper) — *see* Disorder, soft tissue, specified type NEC
  finger M79.89
  foot M79.89
  glands R59.9
    generalized R59.1
    localized R59.0
  hand M79.89
  head (localized) R22.0
  inflammatory — *see* Inflammation
  intra-abdominal — *see* Mass, abdominal
  joint — *see* Effusion, joint
  leg M79.89
    lower M79.89
  limb — *see* Disorder, soft tissue, specified type NEC
  localized (skin) R22.9
    chest R22.2
    head R22.0
    limb
      lower — *see* Mass, localized, limb, lower
      upper — *see* Mass, localized, limb, upper
    neck R22.1
    trunk R22.2
  neck (localized) R22.1
  pelvic — *see* Mass, abdominal
  scrotum N50.89

Swelling (of) R60.9 — *continued*
- splenic — *see* Splenomegaly
- testis N50.89
- toe M79.89
- umbilical R19.09
- wandering, due to Gnathostoma (spinigerum) B83.1
- white — *see* Tuberculosis, arthritis

Swift(-Feer) disease
- overdose or wrong substance given or taken — *see* Table of Drugs and Chemicals, by drug, poisoning

Swimmer's
- cramp T75.1
- ear H60.33-
- itch B65.3

Swimming in the head R42
Swollen — *see* Swelling
Swyer syndrome Q99.1
Sycosis L73.8
- barbae (not parasitic) L73.8
- contagiosa (mycotic) B35.0
- lupoides L73.8
- mycotic B35.0
- parasitic B35.0
- vulgaris L73.8

Sydenham's chorea — *see* Chorea, Sydenham's
Sylvatic yellow fever A95.0
Sylvest's disease B33.0
Symblepharon H11.23-
- congenital Q10.3

Symond's syndrome G93.2
Sympathetic — *see* condition
Sympatheticotonia G90.8
Sympathicoblastoma
- specified site — *see* Neoplasm, malignant, by site
- unspecified site C74.90

Sympathogonioma — *see* Sympathicoblastoma
Symphalangy (fingers) (toes) Q70.9
Symptoms NEC R68.89
- breast NEC N64.59
- development NEC R63.8
- factitious, self-induced — *see* Disorder, factitious
- genital organs, female R10.2
- involving
  - abdomen NEC R19.8
  - appearance NEC R46.89
  - awareness R41.9
    - altered mental status R41.82
    - amnesia — *see* Amnesia
    - borderline intellectual functioning R41.83
    - coma — *see* Coma
    - disorientation R41.0
    - neurologic neglect syndrome R41.4
    - senile cognitive decline R41.81
    - specified symptom NEC R41.89
  - behavior NEC R46.89
  - cardiovascular system NEC R09.89
  - chest NEC R09.89
  - circulatory system NEC R09.89
  - cognitive functions R41.9
    - altered mental status R41.82
    - amnesia — *see* Amnesia
    - borderline intellectual functioning R41.83
    - coma — *see* Coma
    - disorientation R41.0
    - neurologic neglect syndrome R41.4
    - senile cognitive decline R41.81
    - specified symptom NEC R41.89
  - development NEC R62.50
  - digestive system NEC R19.8
  - emotional state NEC R45.89
    - emotional lability R45.86
  - food and fluid intake R63.8

Symptoms NEC R68.89 — *continued*
- involving — *continued*
  - general perceptions and sensations R44.9
    - specified NEC R44.8
  - musculoskeletal system R29.91
    - specified NEC R29.898
  - nervous system R29.90
    - specified NEC R29.818
  - pelvis NEC R19.8
  - respiratory system NEC R09.89
  - skin and integument R23.9
  - urinary system R39.9
- menopausal N95.1
- metabolism NEC R63.8
- neurotic F48.8
- of infancy R68.19
- pelvis NEC, female R10.2
- skin and integument NEC R23.9
- subcutaneous tissue NEC R23.9

Sympus Q74.2
Syncephalus Q89.4
Synchondrosis
- abnormal (congenital) Q78.8
- ischiopubic M91.0

Synchysis (scintillans) (senile) (vitreous body) H43.89
Syncope (near) (pre-) R55
- anginosa I20.8
- bradycardia R00.1
- cardiac R55
- carotid sinus G90.01
- due to spinal (lumbar) puncture G97.1
- heart R55
- heat T67.1
- laryngeal R05
- psychogenic F48.8
- tussive R05
- vasoconstriction R55
- vasodepressor R55
- vasomotor R55
- vasovagal R55

Syndactylism, syndactyly Q70.9
- complex (with synostosis)
  - fingers Q70.0-
  - toes Q70.2-
- simple (without synostosis)
  - fingers Q70.1-
  - toes Q70.3-

Syndrome — *see also* Disease
- 48,XXXX Q97.1
- 49,XXXXX Q97.1
- 5q minus NOS D46.C
- abdominal
  - acute R10.0
  - muscle deficiency Q79.4
- abnormal innervation H02.519
  - left H02.516
    - lower H02.515
    - upper H02.514
  - right H02.513
    - lower H02.512
    - upper H02.511
- abstinence, neonatal P96.1
- acid pulmonary aspiration, obstetric O74.0
- acquired immunodeficiency — *see* Human, immunodeficiency virus (HIV) disease
- acute abdominal R10.0
- acute respiratory distress (adult) (child) J80
  - idiopathic J84.114
- Adair-Dighton Q78.0
- Adams-Stokes(-Morgagni) I45.9
- adiposogenital E23.6
- adrenal
  - hemorrhage (meningococcal) A39.1
  - meningococcic A39.1
- adrenocortical — *see* Cushing's, syndrome
- adrenogenital E25.9
  - congenital, associated with enzyme deficiency E25.0

Syndrome (*see also* Disease) — *continued*
- afferent loop NEC K91.89
- Alagille's Q44.7
- alcohol withdrawal (without convulsions) — *see* Dependence, alcohol, with, withdrawal
- Alder's D72.0
- Aldrich(-Wiskott) D82.0
- alien hand R41.4
- Alport Q87.81
- alveolar hypoventilation E66.2
- alveolocapillary block J84.10
- amnesic, amnestic (confabulatory) (due to) — *see* Disorder, amnesic
- amyostatic (Wilson's disease) E83.01
- androgen insensitivity E34.50
  - complete E34.51
  - partial E34.52
- androgen resistance (*see also* Syndrome, androgen insensitivity) E34.50
- Angelman Q93.5
- anginal — *see* Angina
- ankyloglossia superior Q38.1
- anterior
  - chest wall R07.89
  - cord G83.82
  - spinal artery G95.19
    - compression M47.019
      - cervical region M47.012
      - cervicothoracic region M47.013
      - lumbar region M47.016
      - occipito-atlanto-axial region M47.011
      - thoracic region M47.014
      - thoracolumbar region M47.015
  - tibial M76.81-
- antibody deficiency D80.9
  - agammaglobulinemic D80.1
    - hereditary D80.0
  - congenital D80.0
  - hypogammaglobulinemic D80.1
    - hereditary D80.0
- anticardiolipin (-antibody) D68.61
- antiphospholipid (-antibody) D68.61
- aortic
  - arch M31.4
  - bifurcation I74.09
- aortomesenteric duodenum occlusion K31.5
- apical ballooning (transient left ventricular) I51.81
- arcuate ligament I77.4
- argentaffin, argintaffinoma E34.0
- Arnold-Chiari — *see* Arnold-Chiari disease
- Arrillaga-Ayerza I27.0
- arterial tortuosity Q87.82
- arteriovenous steal T82.898-
- Asherman's N85.6
- aspiration, of newborn — *see* Aspiration, by substance, with pneumonia
  - meconium P24.01
- ataxia-telangiectasia G11.3
- auriculotemporal G50.8
- autoerythrocyte sensitization (Gardner-Diamond) D69.2
- autoimmune lymphoproliferative [ALPS] D89.82
- autoimmune polyglandular E31.0
- autoinflammatory M04.9
  - specified type NEC M04.8
- autosomal — *see* Abnormal, autosomes
- Avellis' G46.8
- Ayerza(-Arrillaga) I27.0
- Babinski-Nageotte G83.89
- Bakwin-Krida Q78.5
- bare lymphocyte D81.6
- Barrett's — *see* Barrett's, esophagus
- Barré-Guillain G61.0
- Barré-Liéou M53.0
- Barsony-Polgar K22.4
- Barsony-Teschendorf K22.4
- Barth E78.71

Syndrome (see also Disease) — continued
Bartter's E26.81
basal cell nevus Q87.89
Basedow's E05.00
  with thyroid storm E05.01
basilar artery G45.0
Batten-Steinert G71.11
battered
  baby or child — see Maltreatment, child,
    physical abuse
  spouse — see Maltreatment, adult, physical
    abuse
Beals Q87.40
Beau's I51.5
Beck's I65.8
Benedikt's G46.3
Béquez César (-Steinbrinck-Chédiak-Higashi)
  E70.330
Bernhardt-Roth — see Meralgia paresthetica
Bernheim's I50.9
big spleen D73.1
bilateral polycystic ovarian E28.2
Bing-Horton's — see Horton's headache
Birt-Hogg-Dube syndrome Q87.89
Björck(-Thorsen) E34.0
black
  lung J60
  widow spider bite — see Toxicity, venom,
    spider, black widow
Blackfan-Diamond D61.01
Blau M04.8
blind loop K90.2
  congenital Q43.8
  postsurgical K91.2
blue sclera Q78.0
blue toe I75.02-
Boder-Sedgewick G11.3
Boerhaave's K22.3
Borjeson Forssman Lehmann Q89.8
Bouillaud's I01.9
Bourneville(-Pringle) Q85.1
Bouveret(-Hoffman) I47.9
brachial plexus G54.0
bradycardia-tachycardia I49.5
brain (nonpsychotic) F09
  with psychosis, psychotic reaction F09
  acute or subacute — see Delirium
  congenital — see Disability, intellectual
  organic F09
    post-traumatic (nonpsychotic) F07.81
      psychotic F09
    personality change F07.0
    post-traumatic, nonpsychotic F07.81
    postcontusional F07.81
    psycho-organic F09
    psychotic F06.8
brain stem stroke G46.3
Brandt's (acrodermatitis enteropathica) E83.2
broad ligament laceration N83.8
Brock's J98.11
bronze baby P83.8
Brown-Sequard G83.81
bubbly lung P27.0
Buchem's M85.2
Budd-Chiari I82.0
bulbar (progressive) G12.22
Bürger-Grütz E78.3
Burke's K86.89
Burnett's (milk-alkali) E83.52
burning feet E53.9
Bywaters' T79.5
Call-Fleming I67.841
carbohydrate-deficient glycoprotein (CDGS)
  E77.8
carcinogenic thrombophlebitis I82.1
carcinoid E34.0
cardiac asthma I50.1
cardiacos negros I27.0
cardiofaciocutaneous Q87.89

Syndrome (see also Disease) — continued
cardiopulmonary-obesity E66.2
cardiorenal — see Hypertension, cardiorenal
cardiorespiratory distress (idiopathic),
  newborn P22.0
cardiovascular renal — see Hypertension,
  cardiorenal
carotid
  artery (hemispheric) (internal) G45.1
  body G90.01
  sinus G90.01
carpal tunnel G56.0-
Cassidy(-Scholte) E34.0
cat cry Q93.4
cat eye Q92.8
cauda equina G83.4
causalgia — see Causalgia
celiac K90.0
  artery compression I77.4
  axis I77.4
central pain G89.0
cerebellar
  hereditary G11.9
  stroke G46.4
cerebellomedullary malformation — see Spina
  bifida
cerebral
  artery
    anterior G46.1
    middle G46.0
    posterior G46.2
  gigantism E22.0
cervical (root) M53.1
  disc — see Disorder, disc, cervical, with
    neuritis
  fusion Q76.1
  posterior, sympathicus M53.0
  rib Q76.5
  sympathetic paralysis G90.2
cervicobrachial (diffuse) M53.1
cervicocranial M53.0
cervicodorsal outlet G54.2
cervicothoracic outlet G54.0
Céstan(-Raymond) I65.8
Charcot's (angina cruris) (intermittent
  claudication) I73.9
Charcot-Weiss-Baker G90.09
CHARGE Q89.8
Chédiak-Higashi(-Steinbrinck) E70.330
chest wall R07.1
Chiari's (hepatic vein thrombosis) I82.0
Chilaiditi's Q43.3
child maltreatment — see Maltreatment, child
chondrocostal junction M94.0
chondroectodermal dysplasia Q77.6
chromosome 4 short arm deletion Q93.3
chromosome 5 short arm deletion Q93.4
chronic
  infantile neurological, cutaneous and
    articular (CINCA) M04.2
  pain G89.4
    personality F68.8
Clarke-Hadfield K86.89
Clerambault's automatism G93.89
Clouston's (hidrotic ectodermal dysplasia)
  Q82.4
clumsiness, clumsy child F82
cluster headache G44.009
  intractable G44.001
  not intractable G44.009
Coffin-Lowry Q89.8
cold injury (newborn) P80.0
combined immunity deficiency D81.9
compartment (deep) (posterior) (traumatic)
  T79.A0 *(follows T79.7)*
  abdomen T79.A3 *(follows T79.7)*
  lower extremity (hip, buttock, thigh, leg, foot,
    toes) T79.A2 *(follows T79.7)*

Syndrome (see also Disease) — continued
compartment (deep) (posterior) (traumatic)
  T79.A0 *(follows T79.7)* — continued
  nontraumatic
    abdomen M79.A3 *(follows M79.7)*
    lower extremity (hip, buttock, thigh, leg,
      foot, toes) M79.A2- *(follows M79.7)*
    specified site NEC M79.A9 *(follows M79.7)*
    upper extremity (shoulder, arm, forearm,
      wrist, hand, fingers) M79.A1- *(follows
      M79.7)*
  postprocedural — see Syndrome,
    compartment, nontraumatic
  specified site NEC T79.A9 *(follows T79.7)*
  upper extremity (shoulder, arm, forearm,
    wrist, hand, fingers) T79.A1 *(follows
    T79.7)*
complex regional pain — see Syndrome, pain,
  complex regional
compression T79.5
  anterior spinal — see Syndrome, anterior,
    spinal artery, compression
  cauda equina G83.4
  celiac artery I77.4
  vertebral artery M47.029
    cervical region M47.022
    occipito-atlanto-axial region M47.021
concussion F07.81
congenital
  affecting multiple systems NEC Q87.89
  central alveolar hypoventilation G47.35
  facial diplegia Q87.0
  muscular hypertrophy-cerebral Q87.89
  oculo-auriculovertebral Q87.0
  oculofacial diplegia (Moebius) Q87.0
  rubella (manifest) P35.0
congestion-fibrosis (pelvic), female N94.89
congestive dysmenorrhea N94.6
Conn's E26.01
connective tissue M35.9
  overlap NEC M35.1
conus medullaris G95.81
cord
  anterior G83.82
  posterior G83.83
coronary
  acute NEC I24.9
  insufficiency or intermediate I20.0
  slow flow I20.8
Costen's (complex) M26.69
costochondral junction M94.0
costoclavicular G54.0
costovertebral E22.0
Cowden Q85.8
craniovertebral M53.0
Creutzfeldt-Jakob — see Creutzfeldt-Jakob
  disease or syndrome
crib death R99
cricopharyngeal — see Dysphagia
cri-du-chat Q93.4
croup J05.0
CRPS I — see Syndrome, pain, complex
  regional I
crush T79.5
cryopyrin-associated periodic M04.2
cryptophthalmos Q87.0
cubital tunnel — see Lesion, nerve, ulnar
Curschmann (-Batten) (-Steinert) G71.11
Cushing's E24.9
  alcohol-induced E24.4
  drug-induced E24.2
  due to
    alcohol
    drugs E24.2
    ectopic ACTH E24.3
    overproduction of pituitary ACTH E24.0
  overdose or wrong substance given or taken
    — see Table of Drugs and Chemicals, by
    drug, poisoning

Syndrome (see also Disease) — continued
Cushing's E24.9 — continued
  pituitary-dependent E24.0
  specified type NEC E24.8
cystic duct stump K91.5
Dana-Putnam D51.0
Danbolt (-Cross) (acrodermatitis enteropathica) E83.2
Dandy-Walker Q03.1
  with spina bifida Q07.01
Danlos' Q79.6
De Quervain E34.51
de Toni-Fanconi (-Debré) E72.09
  with cystinosis E72.04
defibrination — see also Fibrinolysis
  with
    antepartum hemorrhage — see
      Hemorrhage, antepartum, with
      coagulation defect
    intrapartum hemorrhage — see
      Hemorrhage, complicating, delivery
  newborn P60
  postpartum O72.3
Degos' I77.89
Déjérine-Roussy G89.0
delayed sleep phase G47.21
demyelinating G37.9
dependence — see F10-F19 with fourth character .2
depersonalization(-derealization) F48.1
diabetes mellitus in newborn infant P70.2
diabetes mellitus-hypertension-nephrosis — see Diabetes, nephrosis
diabetes-nephrosis — see Diabetes, nephrosis
diabetic amyotrophy — see Diabetes, amyotrophy
dialysis associated steal T82.898-
Diamond-Blackfan D61.01
Diamond-Gardener D69.2
DIC (diffuse or disseminated intravascular coagulopathy) D65
di George's D82.1
Dighton's Q78.0
disequilibrium E87.8
Döhle body-panmyelopathic D72.0
dorsolateral medullary G46.4
double athetosis G80.3
Down (see also Down syndrome) Q90.9
Dresbach's (elliptocytosis) D58.1
Dressler's (postmyocardial infarction) I24.1
  postcardiotomy I97.0
drug withdrawal, infant of dependent mother P96.1
dry eye H04.12-
due to abnormality
  chromosomal Q99.9
    sex
      female phenotype Q97.9
      male phenotype Q98.9
    specified NEC Q99.8
dumping (postgastrectomy) K91.1
  nonsurgical K31.89
Dupré's (meningism) R29.1
dysmetabolic X E88.81
dyspraxia, developmental F82
Eagle-Barrett Q79.4
Eaton-Lambert — see Syndrome, Lambert-Eaton
Ebstein's Q22.5
ectopic ACTH E24.3
eczema-thrombocytopenia D82.0
Eddowes' Q78.0
effort (psychogenic) F45.8
Ehlers-Danlos Q79.6
Eisenmenger's I27.89
Ekman's Q78.0
electric feet E53.8
Ellis-van Creveld Q77.6
empty nest Z60.0

Syndrome (see also Disease) — continued
endocrine-hypertensive E27.0
entrapment — see Neuropathy, entrapment
eosinophilia-myalgia M35.8
epileptic — see also Epilepsy, by type
  absence G40.A09 (follows G40.3)
    intractable G40.A19 (follows G40.3)
      with status epilepticus G40.A11 (follows G40.3)
      without status epilepticus G40.A19 (follows G40.3)
    not intractable G40.A09 (follows G40.3)
      with status epilepticus G40.A01 (follows G40.3)
      without status epilepticus G40.A09 (follows G40.3)
Erdheim-Chester (ECD) E88.89
Erdheim's E22.0
erythrocyte fragmentation D59.4
Evans D69.41
exhaustion F48.8
extrapyramidal G25.9
  specified NEC G25.89
eye retraction — see Strabismus
eyelid-malar-mandible Q87.0
Faber's D50.9
facial pain, paroxysmal G50.0
Fallot's Q21.3
familial cold autoinflammatory M04.2
familial eczema-thrombocytopenia (Wiskott-Aldrich) D82.0
Fanconi (-de Toni) (-Debré) E72.09
  with cystinosis E72.04
Fanconi's (anemia) (congenital pancytopenia) D61.09
fatigue
  chronic R53.82
  psychogenic F48.8
faulty bowel habit K59.39
Feil-Klippel (brevicollis) Q76.1
Felty's — see Felty's syndrome
fertile eunuch E23.0
fetal
  alcohol (dysmorphic) Q86.0
  hydantoin Q86.1
Fiedler's I40.1
first arch Q87.0
fish odor E72.8
Fisher's G61.0
Fitz's (see also Pancreatitis, acute) K85.80
Fitzhugh-Curtis
  due to
    Chlamydia trachomatis A74.81
    Neisseria gonorrhorea (gonococcal peritonitis) A54.85
Flajani (-Basedow) E05.00
  with thyroid storm E05.01
flatback — see Flatback syndrome
floppy
  baby P94.2
  iris (intraoeprative) (IFIS) H21.81
  mitral valve I34.1
flush E34.0
Foix-Alajouanine G95.19
Fong's Q87.2
food protein-induced enterocolitis K52.21
foramen magnum G93.5
Foster-Kennedy H47.14-
Foville's (peduncular) G46.3
fragile X Q99.2
Franceschetti Q75.4
Frey's
  auriculotemporal G50.8
  hyperhidrosis L74.52
Friderichsen-Waterhouse A39.1
Froin's G95.89
frontal lobe F07.0
Fukuhara E88.49

Syndrome (see also Disease) — continued
functional
  bowel K59.9
  prepubertal castrate E29.1
Gaisböck's D75.1
ganglion (basal ganglia brain) G25.9
  geniculi G51.1
Gardner-Diamond D69.2
gastroesophageal
  junction K22.0
  laceration-hemorrhage K22.6
gastrojejunal loop obstruction K91.89
Gee-Herter-Heubner K90.0
Gelineau's G47.419
  with cataplexy G47.411
genito-anorectal A55
Gerstmann-Sträussler-Scheinker (GSS) A81.82
giant platelet (Bernard-Soulier) D69.1
Gilles de la Tourette's F95.2
goiter-deafness E07.1
Goldberg Q89.8
Goldberg-Maxwell E34.51
Good's D83.8
Gopalan' (burning feet) E53.8
Gorlin's Q87.89
Gougerot-Blum L81.7
Gouley's I31.1
Gower's R55
gray or grey (newborn) P93.0
  platelet D69.1
Gubler-Millard G46.3
Guillain-Barré (-Strohl) G61.0
gustatory sweating G50.8
Hadfield-Clarke K86.89
hair tourniquet — see Constriction, external, by site
Hamman's J98.19
hand-foot L27.1
hand-shoulder G90.8
hantavirus (cardio)-pulmonary (HPS) (HCPS) B33.4
happy puppet Q93.5
Harada's H30.81-
Hayem-Faber D50.9
headache NEC G44.89
  complicated NEC G44.59
Heberden's I20.8
Hedinger's E34.0
Hegglin's D72.0
HELLP (hemolysis, elevated liver enzymes and low platelet count) O14.2-
  complicating
    childbirth O14.24
    puerperium O14.25
hemolytic-uremic D59.3
hemophagocytic, infection-associated D76.2
Henoch-Schönlein D69.0
hepatic flexure K59.8
hepatopulmonary K76.81
hepatorenal K76.7
  following delivery O90.4
  postoperative or postprocedural K91.83
  postpartum, puerperal O90.4
hepatourologic K76.7
Herter (-Gee) (nontropical sprue) K90.0
Heubner-Herter K90.0
Heyd's K76.7
Hilger's G90.09
histamine-like (fish poisoning) — see Poisoning, fish
histiocytic D76.3
histiocytosis NEC D76.3
HIV infection, acute B20
Hoffmann-Werdnig G12.0
Hollander-Simons E88.1
Hoppe-Goldflam G70.00
  with exacerbation (acute) G70.01
  in crisis G70.01

Syndrome (*see also* Disease) — *continued*
Horner's G90.2
hungry bone E83.81
hunterian glossitis D51.0
Hutchinson's triad A50.53
hyperabduction G54.0
hyperammonemia-hyperornithinemia-
    homocitrullinemia E72.4
hypereosinophilic (idiopathic) D72.1
hyperimmunoglobulin D M04.1
hyperimmunoglobulin E (IgE) D82.4
hyperkalemic E87.5
hyperkinetic — *see* Hyperkinesia
hypermobility M35.7
hypernatremia E87.0
hyperosmolarity E87.0
hyperperfusion G97.82
hypersplenic D73.1
hypertransfusion, newborn P61.1
hyperventilation F45.8
hyperviscosity (of serum)
    polycythemic D75.1
    sclerothymic D58.8
hypoglycemic (familial) (neonatal) E16.2
hypokalemic E87.6
hyponatremic E87.1
hypopituitarism E23.0
hypoplastic left-heart Q23.4
hypopotassemia E87.6
hyposmolality E87.1
hypotension, maternal O26.5-
hypothenar hammer I73.89
hypoventilation, obesity (OHS) E66.2
ICF (intravascular coagulation-fibrinolysis) D65
idiopathic
    cardiorespiratory distress, newborn P22.0
    nephrotic (infantile) N04.9
iliotibial band M76.3-
immobility, immobilization (paraplegic) M62.3
immune reconstitution D89.3
immune reconstitution inflammatory [IRIS]
    D89.3
immunity deficiency, combined D81.9
immunodeficiency
    acquired — *see* Human, immunodeficiency
        virus (HIV) disease
    combined D81.9
impending coronary I20.0
impingement, shoulder M75.4-
inappropriate secretion of antidiuretic
        hormone E22.2
infant
    gestational diabetes P70.0
    of diabetic mother P70.1
infantilism (pituitary) E23.0
inferior vena cava I87.1
inspissated bile (newborn) P59.1
institutional (childhood) F94.2
insufficient sleep F51.12
intermediate coronary (artery) I20.0
interspinous ligament — *see* Spondylopathy,
        specified NEC
intestinal
    carcinoid E34.0
    knot K56.2
intravascular coagulation-fibrinolysis (ICF) D65
iodine-deficiency, congenital E00.9
    type
        mixed E00.2
        myxedematous E00.1
        neurological E00.0
IRDS (idiopathic respiratory distress, newborn)
    P22.0

Syndrome (*see also* Disease) — *continued*
irritable
    bowel K58.9
        with
            constipation K58.1
            diarrhea K58.0
        mixed K58.2
        psychogenic F45.8
        specified NEC K58.8
    heart (psychogenic) F45.8
    weakness F48.8
ischemic
    bowel (transient) K55.9
        chronic K55.1
        due to mesenteric artery insufficiency
            K55.1
    steal T82.898
IVC (intravascular coagulopathy) D65
Ivemark's Q89.01
Jaccoud's — *see* Arthropathy, postrheumatic,
        chronic
Jackson's G83.89
Jakob-Creutzfeldt — *see* Creutzfeldt-Jakob
        disease or syndrome
jaw-winking Q07.8
Jervell-Lange-Nielsen I45.81
jet lag G47.25
Job's D71
Joseph-Diamond-Blackfan D61.01
jugular foramen G52.7
Kabuki Q89.8
Kanner's (autism) F84.0
Kartagener's Q89.3
Kelly's D50.1
Kimmelstiel-Wilson — *see* Diabetes, specified
        type, with Kimmelstiel-Wilson disease
Klein(e)-Levine G47.13
Klippel-Feil (brevicollis) Q76.1
Köhler-Pellegrini-Steida — *see* Bursitis, tibial
        collateral
König's K59.8
Korsakoff (-Wernicke) (nonalcoholic) F04
    alcoholic F10.26
Kostmann's D70.0
Krabbe's congenital muscle hypoplasia Q79.8
labyrinthine — *see* subcategory H83.2
lacunar NEC G46.7
Lambert-Eaton G70.80
    in
        neoplastic disease G73.1
        specified disease NEC G70.81
Landau-Kleffner — *see* Epilepsy, specified NEC
Larsen's Q74.8
lateral
    cutaneous nerve of thigh G57.1-
    medullary G46.4
Launois' E22.0
lazy
    leukocyte D70.8
    posture M62.3
Lemiere I80.8
Lennox-Gastaut G40.812
    intractable G40.814
        with status epilepticus G40.813
        without status epilepticus G40.814
    not intractable G40.812
        with status epilepticus G40.811
        without status epilepticus G40.812
lenticular, progressive E83.01
Leopold-Levi's E05.90
Lev's I44.2
Li-Fraumeni Z15.01
Lichtheim's D51.0
Lightwood's N25.89
Lignac (de Toni) (-Fanconi) (-Debré) E72.09
    with cystinosis E72.04
Likoff's I20.8
limbic epilepsy personality F07.0
liver-kidney K76.7

Syndrome (*see also* Disease) — *continued*
lobotomy F07.0
Loffler's J82
long arm 18 or 21 deletion Q93.89
long QT I45.81
Louis-Barré G11.3
low
    atmospheric pressure T70.29
    back M54.5
    output (cardiac) I50.9
lower radicular, newborn (birth injury) P14.8
Luetscher's (dehydration) E86.0
Lupus anticoagulant D68.62
Lutembacher's Q21.1
macrophage activation D76.1
    due to infection D76.2
magnesium-deficiency R29.0
Majeed M04.8
Mal de Debarquement R42
malformation, congenital, due to
    alcohol Q86.0
    exogenous cause NEC Q86.8
    hydantoin Q86.1
    warfarin Q86.2
malignant
    carcinoid E34.0
    neuroleptic G21.0
Mallory-Weiss K22.6
mandibulofacial dysostosis Q75.4
manic-depressive — *see* Disorder, bipolar
maple-syrup-urine E71.0
Marable's I77.4
Marfan's Q87.40
    with
        cardiovascular manifestations Q87.418
            aortic dilation Q87.410
        ocular manifestations Q87.42
        skeletal manifestations Q87.43
Marie's (acromegaly) E22.0
mast cell activation — *see* Activation, mast cell
maternal hypotension — *see* Syndrome,
        hypotension, maternal
May (-Hegglin) D72.0
McArdle (-Schmidt) (-Pearson) E74.04
McQuarrie's E16.2
meconium plug (newborn) P76.0
median arcuate ligament I77.4
Meekeren-Ehlers-Danlos Q79.6
megavitamin-B6 E67.2
Meige G24.4
MELAS E88.41
Mendelson's O74.0
MERFF (myoclonic epilepsy associated with
        ragged-red fibers) E88.42
mesenteric
    artery (superior) K55.1
    vascular insufficiency K55.1
metabolic E88.81
metastatic carcinoid E34.0
micrognathia-glossoptosis Q87.0
midbrain NEC G93.89
middle lobe (lung) J98.19
middle radicular G54.0
migraine (*see also* Migraine) G43.909-
Mikulicz' K11.8
milk-alkali E83.52
Millard-Gubler G46.3
Miller-Dieker Q93.88
Miller-Fisher G61.0
Minkowski-Chauffard D58.0
Mirizzi's K83.1
MNGIE (mitochondrial neurogastrointestinal
        encephalopathy) E88.49
Möbius, ophthalmoplegic migraine — *see*
        Migraine, ophthalmoplegic
monofixation H50.42
Morel-Moore M85.2
Morel-Morgagni M85.2
Morgagni (-Morel) (-Stewart) M85.2

Syndrome (*see also* Disease) — *continued*
Morgagni-Adams-Stokes I45.9
Mounier-Kuhn Q32.4
　with bronchiectasis J47.9
　　with
　　　exacerbation (acute) J47.1
　　　lower respiratory infection J47.0
　acquired J98.09
　　with bronchiectasis J47.9
　　　with
　　　　exacerbation (acute) J47.1
　　　　lower respiratory infection J47.0
Muckle-Wells M04.2
mucocutaneous lymph node (acute febrile)
　　(MCLS) M30.3
multiple endocrine neoplasia (MEN) — *see*
　　Neoplasia, endocrine, multiple (MEN)
multiple operations — *see* Disorder, factitious
myasthenic G70.9
　in
　　diabetes mellitus — *see* Diabetes,
　　　amyotrophy
　　endocrine disease NEC E34.9 *[G73.3]*
　　neoplastic disease (*see also* Neoplasm)
　　　D49.9 *[G73.3]*
　　thyrotoxicosis (hyperthyroidism) E05.90
　　　[G73.3]
　　　with thyroid storm E05.91 *[G73.3]*
myelodysplastic D46.9
　with
　　5q deletion D46.C *(follows D46.2)*
　　isolated del(5q) chromosomal abnormality
　　　D46.C *(follows D46.2)*
　　lesions, low grade D46.20
　　specified NEC D46.Z *(follows D46.4)*
myelopathic pain G89.0
myeloproliferative (chronic) D47.1
myofascial pain M79.1
Naffziger's G54.0
nail patella Q87.2
NARP (Neuropathy, Ataxia and Retinitis
　　pigmentosa) E88.49
neonatal abstinence P96.1
nephritic — *see also* Nephritis
　with edema — *see* Nephrosis
　acute N00.9
　chronic N03.9
　rapidly progressive N01.9
nephrotic (congenital) (*see also* Nephrosis)
　　N04.9
　with
　　dense deposit disease N04.6
　　diffuse
　　　crescentic glomerulonephritis N04.7
　　　endocapillary proliferative
　　　　glomerulonephritis N04.4
　　　membranous glomerulonephritis N04.2
　　　mesangial proliferative
　　　　glomerulonephritis N04.3
　　　mesangiocapillary glomerulonephritis
　　　　N04.5
　　focal and segmental glomerular lesions
　　　N04.1
　　minor glomerular abnormality N04.0
　　specified morphological changes NEC
　　　N04.8
　diabetic — *see* Diabetes, nephrosis
neurologic neglect R41.4
Nezelof's D81.4
Nonne-Milroy-Meige Q82.0
Nothnagel's vasomotor acroparesthesia I73.89
obesity hypoventilation (OHS) E66.2
oculomotor H51.9
ophthalmoplegia-cerebellar ataxia — *see*
　　Strabismus, paralytic, third nerve
oral allergy T78.1
oral-facial-digital Q87.0

Syndrome (*see also* Disease) — *continued*
organic
　affective F06.30
　amnesic (not alcohol-or drug-induced) F04
　brain F09
　depressive F06.31
　hallucinosis F06.0
　personality F07.0
Ormond's N13.5
oro-facial-digital Q87.0
os trigonum Q68.8
Osler-Weber-Rendu I78.0
osteoporosis-osteomalacia M83.8
Osterreicher-Turner Q87.2
oto-palatal-digital Q87.0
otolith — *see* subcategory H81.8
outlet (thoracic) G54.0
ovary
　polycystic E28.2
　resistant E28.39
　sclerocystic E28.2
Owren's D68.2
Paget-Schroetter I82.890
pain — *see also* Pain
　complex regional I G90.50
　　lower limb G90.52-
　　specified site NEC G90.59
　　upper limb G90.51-
　complex regional II — *see* Causalgia
painful
　bruising D69.2
　feet E53.8
　prostate N42.81
paralysis agitans — *see* Parkinsonism
paralytic G83.9
　specified NEC G83.89
Parinaud's H51.0
Parkinson's — *see* Parkinsonism
parkinsonian — *see* Parkinsonism
paroxysmal facial pain G50.0
Parry's E05.00
　with thyroid storm E05.01
Parsonage(-Aldren)-Turner G54.5
patella clunk M25.86-
Paterson(-Brown) (-Kelly) D50.1
pectoral girdle I77.89
pectoralis minor I77.89
Pelger-Huet D72.0
pellagra-cerebellar ataxia-renal aminoaciduria
　　E72.02
pellagroid E52
Pellegrini-Stieda — *see* Bursitis, tibial collateral
pelvic congestion-fibrosis, female N94.89
penta X Q97.1
peptic ulcer — *see* Ulcer, peptic
perabduction I77.89
periodic fever M04.1
periodic fever, aphthous stomatitis,
　　pharyngitis, and adenopathy [PFAPA]
　　M04.8
periodic headache, in adults and children —
　　see Headache, periodic syndromes in
　　adults and children
periurethral fibrosis N13.5
phantom limb (without pain) G54.7
　with pain G54.6
pharyngeal pouch D82.1
Pick's — *see* Disease, Pick's
Pickwickian E66.2
PIE (pulmonary infiltration with eosinophilia)
　　J82
pigmentary pallidal degeneration (progressive)
　　G23.0
pineal E34.8
pituitary E22.0
placental transfusion — *see* Pregnancy,
　　complicated by, placental transfusion
　　syndromes
plantar fascia M72.2

Syndrome (*see also* Disease) — *continued*
plateau iris (post-iridectomy) (postprocedural)
　　H21.82
Plummer-Vinson D50.1
pluricarential of infancy E40
plurideficiency E40
pluriglandular (compensatory) E31.8
　autoimmune E31.0
pneumatic hammer T75.21
polyangiitis overlap M30.8
polycarential of infancy E40
polyglandular E31.8
　autoimmune E31.0
polysplenia Q89.09
pontine NEC G93.89
popliteal
　artery entrapment I77.89
　web Q87.89
post chemoembolization — *code to* associated
　　conditions
postcardiac injury
　postcardiotomy I97.0
　postmyocardial infarction I24.1
postcardiotomy I97.0
postcholecystectomy K91.5
postcommissurotomy I97.0
postconcussional F07.81
postcontusional F07.81
postencephalitic F07.89
posterior
　cervical sympathetic M53.0
　cord G83.83
　fossa compression G93.5
　reversible encephalopathy (PRES) I67.83
postgastrectomy (dumping) K91.1
postgastric surgery K91.1
postinfarction I24.1
postlaminectomy NEC M96.1
postleukotomy F07.0
postmastectomy lymphedema I97.2
postmyocardial infarction I24.1
postoperative NEC T81.9
　blind loop K90.2
postpartum panhypopituitary (Sheehan) E23.0
postpolio (myelitic) G14
postthrombotic I87.009
　with
　　inflammation I87.02-
　　　with ulcer I87.03-
　　specified complication NEC I87.09-
　　ulcer I87.01-
　　　with inflammation I87.03-
　asymptomatic I87.00-
postvagotomy K91.1
postvalvulotomy I97.0
postviral NEC G93.3
　fatigue G93.3
Potain's K31.0
potassium intoxication E87.5
precerebral artery (multiple) (bilateral) G45.2
preinfarction I20.0
preleukemic D46.9
premature senility E34.8
premenstrual dysphoric F32.89
premenstrual tension N94.3
Prinzmetal-Massumi R07.1
prune belly Q79.4
pseudocarpal tunnel (sublimis) — *see*
　　Syndrome, carpal tunnel
pseudoparalytica G70.00
　with exacerbation (acute) G70.01
　in crisis G70.01
pseudo-Turner's Q87.1
psycho-organic (nonpsychotic severity) F07.9
　acute or subacute F05
　depressive type F06.31
　hallucinatory type F06.0
　nonpsychotic severity F07.0
　specified NEC F07.89

Syndrome (see also Disease) — continued
- pulmonary
  - arteriosclerosis I27.0
  - dysmaturity (Wilson-Mikity) P27.0
  - hypoperfusion (idiopathic) P22.0
  - renal (hemorrhagic) (Goodpasture's) M31.0
- pure
  - motor lacunar G46.5
  - sensory lacunar G46.6
- Putnam-Dana D51.0
- pyogenic arthritis, pyoderma gangrenosum, and acne [PAPA] M04.8
- pyramidopallidonigral G20
- pyriformis — see Lesion, nerve, sciatic
- QT interval prolongation I45.81
- radicular NEC — see Radiculopathy
  - upper limbs, newborn (birth injury) P14.3
- rapid time-zone change G47.25
- Rasmussen G04.81
- Raymond (-Céstan) I65.8
- Raynaud's I73.00
  - with gangrene I73.01
- RDS (respiratory distress syndrome, newborn) P22.0
- reactive airways dysfunction J68.3
- Refsum's G60.1
- Reifenstein E34.52
- renal glomerulohyalinosis-diabetic — see Diabetes, nephrosis
- Rendu-Osler-Weber I78.0
- residual ovary N99.83
- resistant ovary E28.39
- respiratory
  - distress
    - acute J80
      - adult J80
      - child J80
      - idiopathic J84.114
    - newborn (idiopathic) (type I) P22.0
      - type II P22.1
- restless legs G25.81
- retinoblastoma (familial) C69.2
- retroperitoneal fibrosis N13.5
- retroviral seroconversion (acute) Z21
- Reye's G93.7
- Richter — see Leukemia, chronic lymphocytic, B-cell type
- Ridley's I50.1
- right
  - heart, hypoplastic Q22.6
  - ventricular obstruction — see Failure, heart, congestive
- Romano-Ward (prolonged QT interval) I45.81
- rotator cuff, shoulder (see also Tear, rotator cuff) M75.10-
- Rotes Quérol — see Hyperostosis, ankylosing
- Roth — see Meralgia paresthetica
- rubella (congenital) P35.0
- Ruvalcaba-Myhre-Smith E71.440
- Rytand-Lipsitch I44.2
- salt
  - depletion E87.1
    - due to heat NEC T67.8
      - causing heat exhaustion or prostration T67.4
  - low E87.1
- salt-losing N28.89
- Scaglietti-Dagnini E22.0
- scalenus anticus (anterior) G54.0
- scapulocostal — see Mononeuropathy, upper limb, specified site NEC
- scapuloperoneal G71.0
- schizophrenic, of childhood NEC F84.5
- Schnitzler D47.2
- Scholte's E34.0
- Schroeder's E27.0
- Schüller-Christian C96.5
- Schwachman's — see Syndrome, Shwachman's
- Schwartz (-Jampel) G71.13

Syndrome (see also Disease) — continued
- Schwartz-Bartter E22.2
- scimitar Q26.8
- sclerocystic ovary E28.2
- Seitelberger's G31.89
- septicemic adrenal hemorrhage A39.1
- seroconversion, retroviral (acute) Z21
- serous meningitis G93.2
- severe acute respiratory (SARS) J12.81
- shaken infant T74.4
- shock (traumatic) T79.4
  - kidney N17.0
    - following crush injury T79.5
  - toxic A48.3
- shock-lung J80
- Shone's — code to specific anomalies
- short
  - bowel K91.2
  - rib Q77.2
- shoulder-hand — see Algoneurodystrophy
- Shwachman's D70.4
- sicca — see Sicca syndrome
- sick
  - cell E87.1
  - sinus I49.5
- sick-euthyroid E07.81
- sideropenic D50.1
- Siemens' ectodermal dysplasia Q82.4
- Silfversköld's Q78.9
- Simons' E88.1
- sinus tarsi M25.57-
- sinusitis-bronchiectasis-situs inversus Q89.3
- Sipple's E31.22
- sirenomelia Q87.2
- Slocumb's E27.0
- slow flow, coronary I20.8
- Sluder's G44.89
- Smith-Magenis Q93.88
- Sneddon-Wilkinson L13.1
- Soto's Q87.3
- South African cardiomyopathy I42.8
- spasmodic
  - upward movement, eyes H51.8
  - winking F95.8
- Spen's I45.9
- splenic
  - agenesis Q89.01
  - flexure K59.8
  - neutropenia D73.81
- Spurway's Q78.0
- staphylococcal scalded skin L00
- steal
  - arteriovenous T82.898-
  - ischemic T82.898-
  - subclavian G45.8
- Stein-Leventhal E28.2
- Stein's E28.2
- Stevens-Johnson syndrome L51.1
  - toxic epidermal necrolysis overlap L51.3
- Stewart-Morel M85.2
- Stickler Q89.8
- stiff baby Q89.8
- stiff man G25.82
- Still-Felty — see Felty's syndrome
- Stokes (-Adams) I45.9
- stone heart I50.1
- straight back, congenital Q76.49
- subclavian steal G45.8
- subcoracoid-pectoralis minor G54.0
- subcostal nerve compression I77.89
- subphrenic interposition Q43.3
- superior
  - cerebellar artery I63.8
  - mesenteric artery K55.1
  - semi-circular canal dehiscence H83.8x-
  - vena cava I87.1
- supine hypotensive (maternal) — see Syndrome, hypotension, maternal
- suprarenal cortical E27.0

Syndrome (see also Disease) — continued
- supraspinatus (see also Tear, rotator cuff) M75.10-
- Susac G93.49
- swallowed blood P78.2
- sweat retention L74.0
- Swyer Q99.1
- Symond's G93.2
- sympathetic
  - cervical paralysis G90.2
  - pelvic, female N94.89
- systemic inflammatory response (SIRS), of non-infectious origin (without organ dysfunction) R65.10
  - with acute organ dysfunction R65.11
- tachycardia-bradycardia I49.5
- takotsubo I51.81
- TAR (thrombocytopenia with absent radius) Q87.2
- tarsal tunnel G57.5-
- teething K00.7
- tegmental G93.89
- telangiectasic-pigmentation-cataract Q82.8
- temporal pyramidal apex — see Otitis, media, suppurative, acute
- temporomandibular joint-pain-dysfunction M26.62-
- Terry's H44.2-
- testicular feminization (see also Syndrome, androgen insensitivity) E34.51
- thalamic pain (hyperesthetic) G89.0
- thoracic outlet (compression) G54.0
- Thorson-Björck E34.0
- thrombocytopenia with absent radius (TAR) Q87.2
- thyroid-adrenocortical insufficiency E31.0
- tibial
  - anterior M76.81-
  - posterior M76.82-
- Tietze's M94.0
- time-zone (rapid) G47.25
- Toni-Fanconi E72.09
  - with cystinosis E72.04
- Touraine's Q79.8
- tourniquet — see Constriction, external, by site
- toxic shock A48.3
- transient left ventricular apical ballooning I51.81
- traumatic vasospastic T75.22
- Treacher Collins Q75.4
- triple X, female Q97.0
- trisomy Q92.9
  - 13 Q91.7
    - meiotic nondisjunction Q91.4
    - mitotic nondisjunction Q91.5
    - mosaicism Q91.5
    - translocation Q91.6
  - 18 Q91.3
    - meiotic nondisjunction Q91.0
    - mitotic nondisjunction Q91.1
    - mosaicism Q91.1
    - translocation Q91.2
  - 20(q) (p) Q92.8
  - 21 Q90.9
    - meiotic nondisjunction Q90.0
    - mitotic nondisjunction Q90.1
    - mosaicism Q90.1
    - translocation Q90.2
  - 22 Q92.8
- tropical wet feet T69.0-
- Trousseau's I82.1
- tumor lysis (following antineoplastic chemotherapy) (spontaneous) NEC E88.3
- tumor necrosis factor receptor associated periodic (TRAPS) M04.1
- Twiddler's (due to)
  - automatic implantable defibrillator T82.198
  - cardiac pacemaker T82.198

Syndrome (*see also* Disease) — *continued*
  Unverricht (-Lundborg) — *see* Epilepsy,
    generalized, idiopathic
  upward gaze H51.8
  uremia, chronic (*see also* Disease, kidney,
    chronic) N18.9
  urethral N34.3
  urethro-oculo-articular — *see* Reiter's disease
  urohepatic K76.7
  vago-hypoglossal G52.7
  van Buchem's M85.2
  van der Hoeve's Q78.0
  vascular NEC in cerebrovascular disease
    G46.8
  vasoconstriction, reversible cerebrovascular
    I67.841
  vasomotor I73.9
  vasospastic (traumatic) T75.22
  vasovagal R55
  VATER Q87.2
  velo-cardio-facial Q93.81
  vena cava (inferior) (superior) (obstruction)
    I87.1
  vertebral
    artery G45.0
      compression — *see* Syndrome, anterior,
        spinal artery, compression
    steal G45.0
  vertebro-basilar artery G45.0
  vertebrogenic (pain) M54.89
  vertiginous — *see* Disorder, vestibular function
  Vinson-Plummer D50.1
  virus B34.9
  visceral larva migrans B83.0
  visual disorientation H53.8
  vitamin B6 deficiency E53.1
  vitreal corneal H59.01-
  vitreous (touch) H59.01-
  Vogt-Koyanagi H20.82-
  Volkmann's T79.6
  von Schroetter's I82.890
  von Willebrand (-Jürgen) D68.0
  Waldenström-Kjellberg D50.1
  Wallenberg's G46.3
  water retention E87.79
  Waterhouse (-Friderichsen) A39.1
  Weber-Gubler G46.3
  Weber-Leyden G46.3
  Weber's G46.3
  Wegener's M31.30
    with
      kidney involvement M31.31
      lung involvement M31.30
        with kidney involvement M31.31
  Weingarten's (tropical eosinophilia) J82
  Weiss-Baker G90.09
  Werdnig-Hoffman G12.0
  Wermer's E31.21
  Werner's E34.8
  Wernicke-Korsakoff (nonalcoholic) F04
    alcoholic F10.26
  West's — *see* Epilepsy, spasms
  Westphal-Strümpell E83.01
  wet
    feet (maceration) (tropical) T69.0-
    lung, newborn P22.1
  whiplash S13.4
  whistling face Q87.0
  Wilkie's K55.1
  Wilkinson-Sneddon L13.1
  Willebrand (-Jürgens) D68.0
  Wilson's (hepatolenticular degeneration)
    E83.01
  Wiskott-Aldrich D82.0
  withdrawal — *see* Withdrawal, state
    drug
      infant of dependent mother P96.1
      therapeutic use, newborn P96.2
  Woakes' (ethmoiditis) J33.1

Syndrome (*see also* Disease) — *continued*
  Wright's (hyperabduction) I77.89
  X I20.9
  XXXX Q97.1
  XXXXX Q97.1
  XXXXY Q98.1
  XXY Q98.0
  yellow nail L60.5
  Zahorsky's B08.5
  Zellweger syndrome E71.510
  Zellweger-like syndrome E71.541
Synechia (anterior) (iris) (posterior) (pupil) —
  see also Adhesions, iris
  intra-uterine (traumatic) N85.6
Synesthesia R20.8
Syngamiasis, syngamosis B83.3
Synodontia K00.2
Synorchidism, synorchism Q55.1
Synostosis (congenital) Q78.8
  astragalo-scaphoid Q74.2
  radioulnar Q74.0
Synovial sarcoma — *see* Neoplasm,
  connective tissue, malignant
Synovioma (malignant) — *see also* Neoplasm,
  connective tissue, malignant
  benign — *see* Neoplasm, connective tissue,
    benign
Synoviosarcoma — *see* Neoplasm, connective
  tissue, malignant
Synovitis (*see also* Tenosynovitis) M65.9
  crepitant
    hand M70.0-
    wrist M70.03-
  gonococcal A54.49
  gouty — *see* Gout
  in (due to)
    crystals M65.8-
    gonorrhea A54.49
    syphilis (late) A52.78
    use, overuse, pressure — *see* Disorder, soft
      tissue, due to use
  infective NEC — *see* Tenosynovitis, infective
    NEC
  specified NEC — *see* Tenosynovitis, specified
    type NEC
  syphilitic A52.78
    congenital (early) A50.02
  toxic — *see* Synovitis, transient
  transient M67.3-
    ankle M67.37-
    elbow M67.32-
    foot joint M67.37-
    hand joint M67.34-
    hip M67.35-
    knee M67.36-
    multiple site M67.39
    pelvic region M67.35-
    shoulder M67.31-
    specified joint NEC M67.38
    wrist M67.33-
  traumatic, current — *see* Sprain
  tuberculous — *see* Tuberculosis, synovitis
  villonodular (pigmented) M12.2-
    ankle M12.27-
    elbow M12.22-
    foot joint M12.27-
    hand joint M12.24-
    hip M12.25-
    knee M12.26-
    multiple site M12.29
    pelvic region M12.25-
    shoulder M12.21-
    specified joint NEC M12.28
    vertebrae M12.28
    wrist M12.23-
Syphilid A51.39
  congenital A50.06
  newborn A50.06
  tubercular (late) A52.79

Syphilis, syphilitic (acquired) A53.9
  abdomen (late) A52.79
  acoustic nerve A52.15
  adenopathy (secondary) A51.49
  adrenal (gland) (with cortical hypofunction)
    A52.79
  age under 2 years NOS — *see also* Syphilis,
    congenital, early
    acquired A51.9
  alopecia (secondary) A51.32
  anemia (late) A52.79 [D63.8]
  aneurysm (aorta) (ruptured) A52.01
    central nervous system A52.05
    congenital A50.54 [I79.0]
  anus (late) A52.74
    primary A51.1
    secondary A51.39
  aorta (arch) (abdominal) (thoracic) A52.02
    aneurysm A52.01
  aortic (insufficiency) (regurgitation) (stenosis)
    A52.03
    aneurysm A52.01
  arachnoid (adhesive) (cerebral) (spinal)
    A52.13
  asymptomatic — *see* Syphilis, latent
  ataxia (locomotor) A52.11
  atrophoderma maculatum A51.39
  auricular fibrillation A52.06
  bladder (late) A52.76
  bone A52.77
    secondary A51.46
  brain A52.17
  breast (late) A52.79
  bronchus (late) A52.72
  bubo (primary) A51.0
  bulbar palsy A52.19
  bursa (late) A52.78
  cardiac decompensation A52.06
  cardiovascular A52.00
  central nervous system (late) (recurrent)
    (relapse) (tertiary) A52.3
    with
      ataxia A52.11
      general paralysis A52.17
        juvenile A50.45
      paresis (general) A52.17
        juvenile A50.45
      tabes (dorsalis) A52.11
        juvenile A50.45
      taboparesis A52.17
        juvenile A50.45
    aneurysm A52.05
    congenital A50.40
    juvenile A50.40
    remission in (sustained) A52.3
    serology doubtful, negative, or positive
      A52.3
    specified nature or site NEC A52.19
    vascular A52.05
  cerebral A52.17
    meningovascular A52.13
    nerves (multiple palsies) A52.15
    sclerosis A52.17
    thrombosis A52.05
  cerebrospinal (tabetic type) A52.12
  cerebrovascular A52.05
  cervix (late) A52.76
  chancre (multiple) A51.0
    extragenital A51.2
    Rollet's A51.0
  Charcôt's joint A52.16
  chorioretinitis A51.43
    congenital A50.01
    late A52.71
    prenatal A50.01
  choroiditis — *see* Syphilitic chorioretinitis
  choroidoretinitis — *see* Syphilitic chorioretinitis
  ciliary body (secondary) A51.43
    late A52.71

Syphilis, syphilitic (acquired) A53.9 — *continued*
  colon (late) A52.74
  combined spinal sclerosis A52.11
  condyloma (latum) A51.31
  congenital A50.9
    with
      paresis (general) A50.45
      tabes (dorsalis) A50.45
      taboparesis A50.45
    chorioretinitis, choroiditis A50.01 *[H32]*
    early, or less than 2 years after birth NEC A50.2
      with manifestations — *see* Syphilis, congenital, early, symptomatic
      latent (without manifestations) A50.1
        negative spinal fluid test A50.1
        serology positive A50.1
      symptomatic A50.09
        cutaneous A50.06
        mucocutaneous A50.07
        oculopathy A50.01
        osteochondropathy A50.02
        pharyngitis A50.03
        pneumonia A50.04
        rhinitis A50.05
        visceral A50.08
    interstitial keratitis A50.31
    juvenile neurosyphilis A50.45
    late, or 2 years or more after birth NEC A50.7
      chorioretinitis, choroiditis A50.32
      interstitial keratitis A50.31
      juvenile neurosyphilis A50.45
      latent (without manifestations) A50.6
        negative spinal fluid test A50.6
        serology positive A50.6
      symptomatic or with manifestations NEC A50.59
        arthropathy A50.55
        cardiovascular A50.54
        Clutton's joints A50.51
        Hutchinson's teeth A50.52
        Hutchinson's triad A50.53
        osteochondropathy A50.56
        saddle nose A50.57
  conjugal A53.9
    tabes A52.11
  conjunctiva (late) A52.71
  contact Z20.2
  cord bladder A52.19
  cornea, late A52.71
  coronary (artery) (sclerosis) A52.06
  coryza, congenital A50.05
  cranial nerve A52.15
    multiple palsies A52.15
  cutaneous — *see* Syphilis, skin
  dacryocystitis (late) A52.71
  degeneration, spinal cord A52.12
  dementia paralytica A52.17
    juvenilis A50.45
  destruction of bone A52.77
  dilatation, aorta A52.01
  due to blood transfusion A53.9
  dura mater A52.13
  ear A52.79
    inner A52.79
      nerve (eighth) A52.15
      neurorecurrence A52.15
  early A51.9
    cardiovascular A52.00
    central nervous system A52.3
    latent (without manifestations) (less than 2 years after infection) A51.5
      negative spinal fluid test A51.5
      serological relapse after treatment A51.5
      serology positive A51.5
    relapse (treated, untreated) A51.9
    skin A51.39

Syphilis, syphilitic (acquired) A53.9 — *continued*
  early A51.9 — *continued*
    symptomatic A51.9
      extragenital chancre A51.2
      primary, except extragenital chancre A51.0
      secondary (*see also* Syphilis, secondary) A51.39
        relapse (treated, untreated) A51.49
      ulcer A51.39
  eighth nerve (neuritis) A52.15
  endemic A65
  endocarditis A52.03
    aortic A52.03
    pulmonary A52.03
  epididymis (late) A52.76
  epiglottis (late) A52.73
  epiphysitis (congenital) (early) A50.02
  episcleritis (late) A52.71
  esophagus A52.79
  eustachian tube A52.73
  exposure to Z20.2
  eye A52.71
  eyelid (late) (with gumma) A52.71
  fallopian tube (late) A52.76
  fracture A52.77
  gallbladder (late) A52.74
  gastric (polyposis) (late) A52.74
  general A53.9
    paralysis A52.17
      juvenile A50.45
    genital (primary) A51.0
    glaucoma A52.71
    gumma NEC A52.79
      cardiovascular system A52.00
      central nervous system A52.3
      congenital A50.59
    heart (block) (decompensation) (disease) (failure) A52.06 *[I52]*
      valve NEC A52.03
    hemianesthesia A52.19
    hemianopsia A52.71
    hemiparesis A52.17
    hemiplegia A52.17
    hepatic artery A52.09
    hepatis A52.74
    hepatomegaly, congenital A50.08
    hereditaria tarda — *see* Syphilis, congenital, late
    hereditary — *see* Syphilis, congenital
    Hutchinson's teeth A50.52
    hyalitis A52.71
    inactive — *see* Syphilis, latent
    infantum — *see* Syphilis, congenital
    inherited — *see* Syphilis, congenital
    internal ear A52.79
    intestine (late) A52.74
    iris, iritis (secondary) A51.43
      late A52.71
    joint (late) A52.77
    keratitis (congenital) (interstitial) (late) A50.31
    kidney (late) A52.75
    lacrimal passages (late) A52.71
    larynx (late) A52.73
    late A52.9
      cardiovascular A52.00
      central nervous system A52.3
      kidney A52.75
      latent or 2 years or more after infection (without manifestations) A52.8
        negative spinal fluid test A52.8
        serology positive A52.8
      paresis A52.17
      specified site NEC A52.79
      symptomatic or with manifestations A52.79
      tabes A52.11

Syphilis, syphilitic (acquired) A53.9 — *continued*
  latent A53.0
    with signs or symptoms — *code by* site and stage under Syphilis
    central nervous system A52.2
    date of infection unspecified A53.0
    early, or less than 2 years after infection A51.5
    follow-up of latent syphilis A53.0
      date of infection unspecified A53.0
      late, or 2 years or more after infection A52.8
    late, or 2 years or more after infection A52.8
    positive serology (only finding) A53.0
      date of infection unspecified A53.0
      early, or less than 2 years after infection A51.5
      late, or 2 years or more after infection A52.8
  lens (late) A52.71
  leukoderma A51.39
    late A52.79
  lienitis A52.79
  lip A51.39
    chancre (primary) A51.2
    late A52.79
  Lissauer's paralysis A52.17
  liver A52.74
  locomotor ataxia A52.11
  lung A52.72
  lymph gland (early) (secondary) A51.49
    late A52.79
  lymphadenitis (secondary) A51.49
  macular atrophy of skin A51.39
    striated A52.79
  mediastinum (late) A52.73
  meninges (adhesive) (brain) (spinal cord) A52.13
  meningitis A52.13
    acute (secondary) A51.41
    congenital A50.41
  meningoencephalitis A52.14
  meningovascular A52.13
    congenital A50.41
  mesarteritis A52.09
    brain A52.04
  middle ear A52.77
  mitral stenosis A52.03
  monoplegia A52.17
  mouth (secondary) A51.39
    late A52.79
  mucocutaneous (secondary) A51.39
    late A52.79
  mucous
    membrane (secondary) A51.39
      late A52.79
    patches A51.39
      congenital A50.07
  mulberry molars A50.52
  muscle A52.78
  myocardium A52.06
  nasal sinus (late) A52.73
  neonatorum — *see* Syphilis, congenital
  nephrotic syndrome (secondary) A51.44
  nerve palsy (any cranial nerve) A52.15
    multiple A52.15
  nervous system, central A52.3
  neuritis A52.15
    acoustic A52.15
  neurorecidive of retina A52.19
  neuroretinitis A52.19
  newborn — *see* Syphilis, congenital
  nodular superficial (late) A52.79
  nonvenereal A65
  nose (late) A52.73
    saddle back deformity A50.57
  occlusive arterial disease A52.09

Syphilis, syphilitic (acquired) A53.9 — *continued*
  oculopathy A52.71
  ophthalmic (late) A52.71
  optic nerve (atrophy) (neuritis) (papilla) A52.15
  orbit (late) A52.71
  organic A53.9
  osseous (late) A52.77
  osteochondritis (congenital) (early) A50.02 *[M90.80]*
  osteoporosis A52.77
  ovary (late) A52.76
  oviduct (late) A52.76
  palate (late) A52.79
  pancreas (late) A52.74
  paralysis A52.17
    general A52.17
      juvenile A50.45
  paresis (general) A52.17
    juvenile A50.45
  paresthesia A52.19
  Parkinson's disease or syndrome A52.19
  paroxysmal tachycardia A52.06
  pemphigus (congenital) A50.06
  penis (chancre) A51.0
    late A52.76
  pericardium A52.06
  perichondritis, larynx (late) A52.73
  periosteum (late) A52.77
    congenital (early) A50.02 *[M90.80]*
    early (secondary) A51.46
  peripheral nerve A52.79
  petrous bone (late) A52.77
  pharynx (late) A52.73
    secondary A51.39
  pituitary (gland) A52.79
  pleura (late) A52.73
  pneumonia, white A50.04
  pontine lesion A52.17
  portal vein A52.09
  primary A51.0
    anal A51.1
    and secondary — *see* Syphilis, secondary
    central nervous system A52.3
    extragenital chancre NEC A51.2
    fingers A51.2
    genital A51.0
    lip A51.2
    specified site NEC A51.2
    tonsils A51.2
  prostate (late) A52.76
  ptosis (eyelid) A52.71
  pulmonary (late) A52.72
    artery A52.09
  pyelonephritis (late) A52.75
  recently acquired, symptomatic A51.9
  rectum (late) A52.74
  respiratory tract (late) A52.73
  retina, late A52.71
  retrobulbar neuritis A52.15
  salpingitis A52.76
  sclera (late) A52.71
  sclerosis
    cerebral A52.17
    coronary A52.06
    multiple A52.11
  scotoma (central) A52.71
  scrotum (late) A52.76
  secondary (and primary) A51.49
    adenopathy A51.49
    anus A51.39
    bone A51.46
    chorioretinitis, choroiditis A51.43
    hepatitis A51.45
    liver A51.45
    lymphadenitis A51.49
    meningitis (acute) A51.41
    mouth A51.39

Syphilis, syphilitic (acquired) A53.9 — *continued*
  secondary (and primary) A51.49 — *continued*
    mucous membranes A51.39
    periosteum, periostitis A51.46
    pharynx A51.39
    relapse (treated, untreated) A51.49
    skin A51.39
    specified form NEC A51.49
    tonsil A51.39
    ulcer A51.39
    viscera NEC A51.49
    vulva A51.39
  seminal vesicle (late) A52.76
  seronegative with signs or symptoms — *code by* site and stage under Syphilis
  seropositive
    with signs or symptoms — *code by* site and stage under Syphilis
    follow-up of latent syphilis — *see* Syphilis, latent
    only finding — *see* Syphilis, latent
  seventh nerve (paralysis) A52.15
  sinus, sinusitis (late) A52.73
  skeletal system A52.77
  skin (with ulceration) (early) (secondary) A51.39
    late or tertiary A52.79
  small intestine A52.74
  spastic spinal paralysis A52.17
  spermatic cord (late) A52.76
  spinal (cord) A52.12
  spleen A52.79
  splenomegaly A52.79
  spondylitis A52.77
  staphyloma A52.71
  stigmata (congenital) A50.59
  stomach A52.74
  synovium A52.78
  tabes dorsalis (late) A52.11
    juvenile A50.45
  tabetic type A52.11
    juvenile A50.45
  taboparesis A52.17
    juvenile A50.45
  tachycardia A52.06
  tendon (late) A52.78
  tertiary A52.9
    with symptoms NEC A52.79
    cardiovascular A52.00
    central nervous system A52.3
    multiple NEC A52.79
    specified site NEC A52.79
  testis A52.76
  thorax A52.73
  throat A52.73
  thymus (gland) (late) A52.79
  thyroid (late) A52.79
  tongue (late) A52.79
  tonsil (lingual) (late) A52.73
    primary A51.2
    secondary A51.39
  trachea (late) A52.73
  tunica vaginalis (late) A52.76
  ulcer (any site) (early) (secondary) A51.39
    late A52.79
    perforating A52.79
      foot A52.11
  urethra (late) A52.76
  urogenital (late) A52.76
  uterus (late) A52.76
  uveal tract (secondary) A51.43
    late A52.71
  uveitis (secondary) A51.43
    late A52.71
  uvula (late) (perforated) A52.79
  vagina A51.0
    late A52.76

Syphilis, syphilitic (acquired) A53.9 — *continued*
  valvulitis NEC A52.03
  vascular A52.00
    brain (cerebral) A52.05
  ventriculi A52.74
  vesicae urinariae (late) A52.76
  viscera (abdominal) (late) A52.74
    secondary A51.49
  vitreous (opacities) (late) A52.71
    hemorrhage A52.71
  vulva A51.0
    late A52.76
    secondary A51.39
Syphiloma A52.79
  cardiovascular system A52.00
  central nervous system A52.3
  circulatory system A52.00
  congenital A50.59
Syphilophobia F45.29
Syringadenoma — *see also* Neoplasm, skin, benign
  papillary — *see* Neoplasm, skin, benign
Syringobulbia G95.0
Syringocystadenoma — *see* Neoplasm, skin, benign
  papillary — *see* Neoplasm, skin, benign
Syringoma — *see also* Neoplasm, skin, benign
  chondroid — *see* Neoplasm, skin, benign
Syringomyelia G95.0
Syringomyelitis — *see* Encephalitis
Syringomyelocele — *see* Spina bifida
Syringopontia G95.0
System, systemic — *see also* condition
  disease, combined — *see* Degeneration, combined
  inflammatory response syndrome (SIRS) of non-infectious origin (without organ dysfunction) R65.10
    with acute organ dysfunction R65.11
  lupus erythematosus M32.9
    inhibitor present D68.62

T

Tabacism, tabacosis, tabagism — *see also* Poisoning, tobacco
meaning dependence (without remission) F17.200
with
disorder F17.299
remission F17.211
specified disorder NEC F17.298
withdrawal F17.203
Tabardillo A75.9
flea-borne A75.2
louse-borne A75.0
Tabes, tabetic A52.10
with
central nervous system syphilis A52.10
Charcot's joint A52.16
cord bladder A52.19
crisis, viscera (any) A52.19
paralysis, general A52.17
paresis (general) A52.17
perforating ulcer (foot) A52.19
arthropathy (Charcot) A52.16
bladder A52.19
bone A52.11
cerebrospinal A52.12
congenital A50.45
conjugal A52.10
dorsalis A52.11
juvenile A50.49
juvenile A50.49
latent A52.19
mesenterica A18.39
paralysis, insane, general A52.17
spasmodic A52.17
syphilis (cerebrospinal) A52.12
Taboparalysis A52.17
Taboparesis (remission) A52.17
juvenile A50.45
TAC (trigeminal autonomic cephalgia) NEC G44.099
intractable G44.091
not intractable G44.099
Tache noir S60.22-
Tachyalimentation K91.2
Tachyarrhythmia, tachyrhythmia — *see* Tachycardia
Tachycardia R00.0
atrial (paroxysmal) I47.1
auricular I47.1
AV nodal re-entry (re-entrant) I47.1
junctional (paroxysmal) I47.1
newborn P29.11
nodal (paroxysmal) I47.1
non-paroxysmal AV nodal I45.89
paroxysmal (sustained) (nonsustained) I47.9
with sinus bradycardia I49.5
atrial (PAT) I47.1
atrioventricular (AV) (re-entrant) I47.1
psychogenic F54
junctional I47.1
ectopic I47.1
nodal I47.1
psychogenic (atrial) (supraventricular) (ventricular) F54
supraventricular (sustained) I47.1
psychogenic F54
ventricular I47.2
psychogenic F54
psychogenic F45.8
sick sinus I49.5
sinoauricular NOS R00.0
paroxysmal I47.1
sinus [sinusal] NOS R00.0
paroxysmal I47.1
supraventricular I47.1

Tachycardia R00.0 — *continued*
ventricular (paroxysmal) (sustained) I47.2
psychogenic F54
Tachygastria K31.89
Tachypnea R06.82
hysterical F45.8
newborn (idiopathic) (transitory) P22.1
psychogenic F45.8
transitory, of newborn P22.1
TACO (transfusion associated circulatory overload) E87.71
Taenia (infection) (infestation) B68.9
diminuta B71.0
echinococcal infestation B67.90
mediocanellata B68.1
nana B71.0
saginata B68.1
solium (intestinal form) B68.0
larval form — *see* Cysticercosis
Taeniasis (intestine) — *see* Taenia
Tag (hypertrophied skin) (infected) L91.8
adenoid J35.8
anus K64.4
hemorrhoidal K64.4
hymen N89.8
perineal N90.89
preauricular Q17.0
sentinel K64.4
skin L91.8
accessory (congenital) Q82.8
anus K64.4
congenital Q82.8
preauricular Q17.0
tonsil J35.8
urethra, urethral N36.8
vulva N90.89
Tahyna fever B33.8
Takahara's disease E80.3
Takayasu's disease or syndrome M31.4
Talcosis (pulmonary) J62.0
Talipes (congenital) Q66.89
acquired, planus — *see* Deformity, limb, flat foot
asymmetric Q66.89
calcaneovalgus Q66.4
calcaneovarus Q66.1
calcaneus Q66.89
cavus Q66.7
equinovalgus Q66.6
equinovarus Q66.0
equinus Q66.89
percavus Q66.7
planovalgus Q66.6
planus (acquired) (any degree) — *see also* Deformity, limb, flat foot
congenital Q66.5-
due to rickets (sequelae) E64.3
valgus Q66.6
varus Q66.3
Tall stature, constitutional E34.4
Talma's disease M62.89
Talon noir S90.3-
hand S60.22-
heel S90.3-
toe S90.1-
Tamponade, heart I31.4
Tanapox (virus disease) B08.71
Tangier disease E78.6
Tantrum, child problem F91.8
Tapeworm (infection) (infestation) — *see* Infestation, tapeworm
Tapia's syndrome G52.7
TAR (thrombocytopenia with absent radius) syndrome Q87.2
Tarral-Besnier disease L44.0
Tarsal tunnel syndrome — *see* Syndrome, tarsal tunnel
Tarsalgia — *see* Pain, limb, lower

Tarsitis (eyelid) H01.8
syphilitic A52.71
tuberculous A18.4
Tartar (teeth) (dental calculus) K03.6
Tattoo (mark) L81.8
Tauri's disease E74.09
Taurodontism K00.2
Taussig-Bing syndrome Q20.1
Taybi's syndrome Q87.2
Tay-Sachs amaurotic familial idiocy or disease E75.02
TBI (traumatic brain injury) S06.9
Teacher's node or nodule J38.2
Tear, torn (traumatic) — *see also* Laceration
with abortion — *see* Abortion
annular fibrosis M51.35
anus, anal (sphincter) S31.831
complicating delivery
with third degree perineal laceration (*see also* Delivery, complicated, by, laceration, perineum, third degree) O70.20
with mucosa O70.3
without third degree perineal laceration O70.4
nontraumatic (healed) (old) K62.81
articular cartilage, old — *see* Derangement, joint, articular cartilage, by site
bladder
with ectopic or molar pregnancy O08.6
following ectopic or molar pregnancy O08.6
obstetrical O71.5
traumatic — *see* Injury, bladder
bowel
with ectopic or molar pregnancy O08.6
following ectopic or molar pregnancy O08.6
obstetrical trauma O71.5
broad ligament
with ectopic or molar pregnancy O08.6
following ectopic or molar pregnancy O08.6
obstetrical trauma O71.6
bucket handle (knee) (meniscus) — *see* Tear, meniscus
capsule, joint — *see* Sprain
cartilage — *see also* Sprain
articular, old — *see* Derangement, joint, articular cartilage, by site
cervix
with ectopic or molar pregnancy O08.6
following ectopic or molar pregnancy O08.6
obstetrical trauma (current) O71.3
old N88.1
traumatic — *see* Injury, uterus
dural G97.41
nontraumatic G96.11
internal organ — *see* Injury, by site
knee cartilage
articular (current) S83.3-
old — *see* Derangement, knee, meniscus, due to old tear
ligament — *see* Sprain
meniscus (knee) (current injury) S83.209
bucket-handle S83.20-
lateral
bucket-handle S83.25-
complex S83.27-
peripheral S83.26-
specified type NEC S83.28-
medial
bucket-handle S83.21-
complex S83.23-
peripheral S83.22-
specified type NEC S83.24-
old — *see* Derangement, knee, meniscus, due to old tear
site other than knee — *code as* Sprain
specified type NEC S83.20-
muscle — *see* Strain

Tear, torn (traumatic) (see also Laceration) — continued
  pelvic
    floor, complicating delivery O70.1
    organ NEC, obstetrical trauma O71.5
      with ectopic or molar pregnancy O08.6
      following ectopic or molar pregnancy O08.6
  perineal, secondary O90.1
  periurethral tissue, obstetrical trauma O71.82
    with ectopic or molar pregnancy O08.6
    following ectopic or molar pregnancy O08.6
  rectovaginal septum — see Laceration, vagina
  retina, retinal (without detachment) (horseshoe) — see also Break, retina, horseshoe
    with detachment — see Detachment, retina, with retinal, break
  rotator cuff (nontraumatic) M75.10-
    complete M75.12-
    incomplete M75.11-
    traumatic S46.01-
    capsule S43.42-
  semilunar cartilage, knee — see Tear, meniscus
  supraspinatus (complete) (incomplete) (nontraumatic) (see also Tear, rotator cuff) M75.10-
  tendon — see Strain
  tentorial, at birth P10.4
  umbilical cord
    complicating delivery O69.89
  urethra
    with ectopic or molar pregnancy O08.6
    following ectopic or molar pregnancy O08.6
    obstetrical trauma O71.5
  uterus — see Injury, uterus
  vagina — see Laceration, vagina
  vessel, from catheter — see Puncture, accidental complicating surgery
  vulva, complicating delivery O70.0
Tear-stone — see Dacryolith
Teeth — see also condition
  grinding
    psychogenic F45.8
    sleep related G47.63
Teething (syndrome) K00.7
Telangiectasia, telangiectasis (verrucous) I78.1
  ataxic (cerebellar) (Louis-Bar) G11.3
  familial I78.0
  hemorrhagic, hereditary (congenital) (senile) I78.0
  hereditary, hemorrhagic (congenital) (senile) I78.0
  juxtafoveal H35.07-
  macular H35.07-
  parafoveal H35.07-
  retinal (idiopathic) (juxtafoveal) (macular) (parafoveal) H35.07-
  spider I78.1
Telephone scatologia F65.89
Telescoped bowel or intestine K56.1
  congenital Q43.8
Temperature
  body, high (of unknown origin) R50.9
  cold, trauma from T69.9
    newborn P80.0
    specified effect NEC T69.8
Temple — see condition
Temporal — see condition
Temporomandibular joint pain-dysfunction syndrome M26.62-
Temporosphenoidal — see condition
Tendency
  bleeding — see Defect, coagulation
  suicide
    meaning personal history of attempted suicide Z91.5
    meaning suicidal ideation — see Ideation, suicidal

Tendency — continued
  to fall R29.6
Tenderness, abdominal R10.819
  epigastric R10.816
  generalized R10.817
  left lower quadrant R10.814
  left upper quadrant R10.812
  periumbilic R10.815
  rebound R10.829
    epigastric R10.826
    generalized R10.827
    left lower quadrant R10.824
    left upper quadrant R10.822
    periumbilic R10.825
    right lower quadrant R10.823
    right upper quadrant R10.821
  right lower quadrant R10.813
  right upper quadrant R10.811
Tendinitis, tendonitis — see also Enthesopathy
  Achilles M76.6-
  adhesive — see Tenosynovitis, specified type NEC
    shoulder — see Capsulitis, adhesive
  bicipital M75.2-
  calcific M65.2-
    ankle M65.27-
    foot M65.27-
    forearm M65.23-
    hand M65.24-
    lower leg M65.26-
    multiple sites M65.29
    pelvic region M65.25-
    shoulder M75.3-
    specified site NEC M65.28
    thigh M65.25-
    upper arm M65.22-
  due to use, overuse, pressure — see also Disorder, soft tissue, due to use
    specified NEC — see Disorder, soft tissue, due to use, specified NEC
  gluteal M76.0-
  patellar M76.5-
  peroneal M76.7-
  psoas M76.1-
  tibial (posterior) M76.82-
    anterior M76.81-
  trochanteric — see Bursitis, hip, trochanteric
Tendon — see condition
Tendosynovitis — see Tenosynovitis
Tenesmus (rectal) R19.8
  vesical R30.1
Tennis elbow — see Epicondylitis, lateral
Tenonitis — see also Tenosynovitis
  eye (capsule) H05.04-
Tenontosynovitis — see Tenosynovitis
Tenontothecitis — see Tenosynovitis
Tenophyte — see Disorder, synovium, specified type NEC
Tenosynovitis (see also Synovitis) M65.9
  adhesive — see Tenosynovitis, specified type NEC
    shoulder — see Capsulitis, adhesive
  bicipital (calcifying) — see Tendinitis, bicipital
  gonococcal A54.49
  in (due to)
    crystals M65.8-
    gonorrhea A54.49
    syphilis (late) A52.78
    use, overuse, pressure — see also Disorder, soft tissue, due to use
      specified NEC — see Disorder, soft tissue, due to use, specified NEC
  infective NEC M65.1-
    ankle M65.17-
    foot M65.17-
    forearm M65.13-
    hand M65.14-
    lower leg M65.16-

Tenosynovitis (see also Synovitis) M65.9 — continued
  infective NEC M65.1- — continued
    multiple sites M65.19
    pelvic region M65.15-
    shoulder region M65.11-
    specified site NEC M65.18
    thigh M65.15-
    upper arm M65.12-
  radial styloid M65.4
  shoulder region M65.81-
    adhesive — see Capsulitis, adhesive
  specified type NEC M65.88
    ankle M65.87-
    foot M65.87-
    forearm M65.83-
    hand M65.84-
    lower leg M65.86-
    multiple sites M65.89
    pelvic region M65.85-
    shoulder region M65.81-
    specified site NEC M65.88
    thigh M65.85-
    upper arm M65.82-
  tuberculous — see Tuberculosis, tenosynovitis
Tenovaginitis — see Tenosynovitis
Tension
  arterial, high — see also Hypertension
    without diagnosis of hypertension R03.0
  headache G44.209
    intractable G44.201
    not intractable G44.209
  nervous R45.0
  pneumothorax J93.0
  premenstrual N94.3
  state (mental) F48.9
Tentorium — see condition
Teratencephalus Q89.8
Teratism Q89.7
Teratoblastoma (malignant) — see Neoplasm, malignant, by site
Teratocarcinoma — see also Neoplasm, malignant, by site
  liver C22.7
Teratoma (solid) — see also Neoplasm, uncertain behavior, by site
  with embryonal carcinoma, mixed — see Neoplasm, malignant, by site
  with malignant transformation — see Neoplasm, malignant, by site
  adult (cystic) — see Neoplasm, benign, by site
  benign — see Neoplasm, benign, by site
  combined with choriocarcinoma — see Neoplasm, malignant, by site
  cystic (adult) — see Neoplasm, benign, by site
  differentiated — see Neoplasm, benign, by site
  embryonal — see also Neoplasm, malignant, by site
    liver C22.7
  immature — see Neoplasm, malignant, by site
  liver C22.7
    adult, benign, cystic, differentiated type or mature D13.4
  malignant — see also Neoplasm, malignant, by site
    anaplastic — see Neoplasm, malignant, by site
    intermediate — see Neoplasm, malignant, by site
    specified site — see Neoplasm, malignant, by site
    unspecified site C62.90
    undifferentiated — see Neoplasm, malignant, by site
  mature — see Neoplasm, uncertain behavior, by site
    malignant — see Neoplasm, by site, malignant, by site

Teratoma (solid) (*see also* Neoplasm, uncertain behavior, by site) — *continued*
- ovary D27-
  - embryonal, immature or malignant C56-
  - solid — *see* Neoplasm, uncertain behavior, by site
- testis C62.9-
  - adult, benign, cystic, differentiated type or mature D29.2-
  - scrotal C62.1-
  - undescended C62.0-

Termination
- anomalous — *see also* Malposition, congenital
  - right pulmonary vein Q26.3
- pregnancy, elective Z33.2

Ternidens diminutus infestation B81.8
Ternidensiasis B81.8
Terror(s) night (child) F51.4
Terrorism, victim of Z65.4
Terry's syndrome H44.2-
Tertiary — *see* condition
Test, tests, testing (for)
- adequacy (for dialysis)
  - hemodialysis Z49.31
  - peritoneal Z49.32
- blood pressure Z01.30
  - abnormal reading — *see* Blood, pressure
- blood typing Z01.83
  - Rh typing Z01.83
- blood-alcohol Z04.8
  - positive — *see* Findings, abnormal, in blood
- blood-drug Z04.8
  - positive — *see* Findings, abnormal, in blood
- cardiac pulse generator (battery) Z45.010
- fertility Z31.41
- genetic
  - disease carrier status for procreative management
    - female Z31.430
    - male Z31.440
  - male partner of patient with recurrent pregnancy loss Z31.441
  - procreative management NEC
    - female Z31.438
    - male Z31.448
- hearing Z01.10
  - with abnormal findings NEC Z01.118
- HIV (human immunodeficiency virus)
  - nonconclusive (in infants) R75
  - positive Z21
  - seropositive Z21
- immunity status Z01.84
- intelligence NEC Z01.89
- laboratory (as part of a general medical examination) Z00.00
  - with abnormal finding Z00.01
  - for medicolegal reason NEC Z04.8
- male partner of patient with recurrent pregnancy loss Z31.441
- Mantoux (for tuberculosis) Z11.1
  - abnormal result R76.11
- pregnancy, positive first pregnancy — *see* Pregnancy, normal, first
- procreative Z31.49
  - fertility Z31.41
- skin, diagnostic
  - allergy Z01.82
    - special screening examination — *see* Screening, by name of disease
  - Mantoux Z11.1
  - tuberculin Z11.1
- specified NEC Z01.89
- tuberculin Z11.1
  - abnormal result R76.11
- vision Z01.00
  - with abnormal findings Z01.01
- Wassermann Z11.3
  - positive — *see* Serology for syphilis, positive

Testicle, testicular, testis — *see also* condition
- feminization syndrome (*see also* Syndrome, androgen insensitivity) E34.51
- migrans Q55.29

Tetanus, tetanic (cephalic) (convulsions) A35
- with
  - abortion A34
  - ectopic or molar pregnancy O08.0
- following ectopic or molar pregnancy O08.0
- inoculation reaction (due to serum) — *see* Complications, vaccination
- neonatorum A33
- obstetrical A34
- puerperal, postpartum, childbirth A34

Tetany (due to) R29.0
- alkalosis E87.3
- associated with rickets E55.0
- convulsions R29.0
  - hysterical F44.5
- functional (hysterical) F44.5
- hyperkinetic R29.0
  - hysterical F44.5
- hyperpnea R06.4
  - hysterical F44.5
  - psychogenic F45.8
- hyperventilation (*see also* Hyperventilation) R06.4
  - hysterical F44.5
- neonatal (without calcium or magnesium deficiency) P71.3
- parathyroid (gland) E20.9
- parathyroprival E89.2
- post- (para)thyroidectomy E89.2
- postoperative E89.2
- pseudotetany R29.0
- psychogenic (conversion reaction) F44.5

Tetralogy of Fallot Q21.3
Tetraplegia (chronic) (*see also* Quadriplegia) G82.50
Thailand hemorrhagic fever A91
Thalassanemia — *see* Thalassemia
Thalassemia (anemia) (disease) D56.9
- with other hemoglobinopathy D56.8
- alpha (major) (severe) (triple gene defect) D56.0
  - minor D56.3
  - silent carrier D56.3
  - trait D56.3
- beta (severe) D56.1
  - homozygous D56.1
  - major D56.1
  - minor D56.3
  - trait D56.3
- delta-beta (homozygous) D56.2
  - minor D56.3
  - trait D56.3
- dominant D56.8
- hemoglobin
  - C D56.8
  - E-beta D56.5
- intermedia D56.1
- major D56.1
- minor D56.3
- mixed D56.8
- sickle-cell — *see* Disease, sickle-cell, thalassemia
- specified type NEC D56.8
- trait D56.3
- variants D56.8

Thanatophoric dwarfism or short stature Q77.1
Thaysen-Gee disease (nontropical sprue) K90.0
Thaysen's disease K90.0
Thecoma D27-
- luteinized D27-
- malignant C56-
Thelarche, premature E30.8
Thelaziasis B83.8

Thelitis N61.0
- puerperal, postpartum or gestational — *see* Infection, nipple
Therapeutic — *see* condition
Therapy
- drug, long-term (current) (prophylactic)
  - agents affecting estrogen receptors and estrogen levels NEC Z79.818
  - anastrozole (Arimidex) Z79.811
  - anti-inflammatory Z79.1
  - antibiotics Z79.2
    - short-term use — *omit code*
  - anticoagulants Z79.01
  - antiplatelet Z79.02
  - antithrombotics Z79.02
  - aromatase inhibitors Z79.811
  - aspirin Z79.82
  - birth control pill or patch Z79.3
  - bisphosphonates Z79.83
  - contraceptive, oral Z79.3
  - drug, specified NEC Z79.899
  - estrogen receptor downregulators Z79.818
  - Evista Z79.810
  - exemestane (Aromasin) Z79.811
  - Fareston Z79.810
  - fulvestrant (Faslodex) Z79.818
  - gonadotropin-releasing hormone (GnRH) agonist Z79.818
  - goserelin acetate (Zoladex) Z79.818
  - hormone replacement (postmenopausal) Z79.890
  - insulin Z79.4
  - letrozole (Femara) Z79.811
  - leuprolide acetate (leuprorelin) (Lupron) Z79.818
  - megestrol acetate (Megace) Z79.818
  - methadone
    - for pain management Z79.891
    - maintenance therapy F11.20
  - Nolvadex Z79.810
  - opiate analgesic Z79.891
  - oral contraceptive Z79.3
  - raloxifene (Evista) Z79.810
  - selective estrogen receptor modulators (SERMs) Z79.810
  - short term — *omit code*
  - steroids
    - inhaled Z79.51
    - systemic Z79.52
  - tamoxifen (Nolvadex) Z79.810
  - toremifene (Fareston) Z79.810

Thermic — *see* condition
Thermography (abnormal) (*see also* Abnormal, diagnostic imaging) R93.8
- breast R92.8
Thermoplegia T67.0
Thesaurismosis, glycogen — *see* Disease, glycogen storage
Thiamin deficiency E51.9
- specified NEC E51.8
Thiaminic deficiency with beriberi E51.11
Thibierge-Weissenbach syndrome — *see* Sclerosis, systemic
Thickening
- bone — *see* Hypertrophy, bone
- breast N64.59
- endometrium R93.8
- epidermal L85.9
  - specified NEC L85.8
- hymen N89.6
- larynx J38.7
- nail L60.2
  - congenital Q84.5
- periosteal — *see* Hypertrophy, bone
- pleura J92.9
  - with asbestos J92.0
- skin R23.4
- subepiglottic J38.7
- tongue K14.8

DISEASE INDEX

Thickening — *continued*
  valve, heart — *see* Endocarditis
Thigh — *see* condition
Thinning vertebra — *see* Spondylopathy,
  specified NEC
Thirst, excessive R63.1
  due to deprivation of water T73.1
Thomsen disease G71.12
Thoracic — *see also* condition
  kidney Q63.2
  outlet syndrome G54.0
Thoracogastroschisis (congenital) Q79.8
Thoracopagus Q89.4
Thorax — *see* condition
Thorn's syndrome N28.89
Thorson-Björck syndrome E34.0
Threadworm (infection) (infestation) B80
Threatened
  abortion O20.0
    with subsequent abortion O03.9
  job loss, anxiety concerning Z56.2
  labor (without delivery) O47.9
    at or after 37 completed weeks of gestation
      O47.1
    before 37 completed weeks of gestation
      O47.0-
  loss of job, anxiety concerning Z56.2
  miscarriage O20.0
  unemployment, anxiety concerning Z56.2
Three-day fever A93.1
Threshers' lung J67.0
Thrix annulata (congenital) Q84.1
Throat — *see* condition
Thrombasthenia (Glanzmann) (hemorrhagic)
  (hereditary) D69.1
Thromboangiitis I73.1
  obliterans (general) I73.1
    cerebral I67.89
    vessels
      brain I67.89
      spinal cord I67.89
Thromboarteritis — *see* Arteritis
Thromboasthenia (Glanzmann)
  (hemorrhagic) (hereditary) D69.1
Thrombocytasthenia (Glanzmann) D69.1
Thrombocythemia (essential) (hemorrhagic)
  (idiopathic) (primary) D47.3
Thrombocytopathy (dystrophic)
  (granulopenic) D69.1
Thrombocytopenia, thrombocytopenic
  D69.6
  with absent radius (TAR) Q87.2
  congenital D69.42
  dilutional D69.59
  due to
    drugs D69.59
    extracorporeal circulation of blood D69.59
    (massive) blood transfusion D69.59
    platelet alloimmunization D69.59
  essential D69.3
  heparin induced (HIT) D75.82
  hereditary D69.42
  idiopathic D69.3
  neonatal, transitory P61.0
    due to
      exchange transfusion P61.0
      idiopathic maternal thrombocytopenia
        P61.0
      isoimmunization P61.0
  primary NEC D69.49
    idiopathic D69.3
  puerperal, postpartum O72.3
  secondary D69.59
  transient neonatal P61.0
Thrombocytosis, essential D47.3
  primary D47.3
Thromboembolism — *see* Embolism

Thrombopathy (Bernard-Soulier) D69.1
  constitutional D68.0
  Willebrand-Jurgens D68.0
Thrombopenia — *see* Thrombocytopenia
Thrombophilia D68.59
  primary NEC D68.59
  secondary NEC D68.69
  specified NEC D68.69
Thrombophlebitis I80.9
  antepartum O22.2-
    deep O22.3-
    superficial O22.2-
  cavernous (venous) sinus G08
    complicating pregnancy O22.5-
    nonpyogenic I67.6
  cerebral (sinus) (vein) G08
    nonpyogenic I67.6
    sequelae G09
  due to implanted device — *see* Complications,
    by site and type, specified NEC
  during or resulting from a procedure NEC
    T81.72
  femoral vein (superficial) I80.1-
  femoropopliteal vein I80.0-
  hepatic (vein) I80.8
  idiopathic, recurrent I82.1
  iliofemoral I80.1-
  intracranial venous sinus (any) G08
    nonpyogenic I67.6
    sequelae G09
  intraspinal venous sinuses and veins G08
    nonpyogenic G95.19
  lateral (venous) sinus G08
    nonpyogenic I67.6
  leg I80.299
    superficial I80.0-
  longitudinal (venous) sinus G08
    nonpyogenic I67.6
  lower extremity I80.299
  migrans, migrating I82.1
  pelvic
    with ectopic or molar pregnancy O08.0
    following ectopic or molar pregnancy O08.0
    puerperal O87.1
  popliteal vein — *see* Phlebitis, leg, deep,
    popliteal
  portal (vein) K75.1
  postoperative T81.72
  pregnancy — *see* Thrombophlebitis,
    antepartum
  puerperal, postpartum, childbirth O87.0
    deep O87.1
    pelvic O87.1
    septic O86.81
    superficial O87.0
  saphenous (greater) (lesser) I80.0-
  sinus (intracranial) G08
    nonpyogenic I67.6
  specified site NEC I80.8
  tibial vein I80.23-
Thrombosis, thrombotic (bland) (multiple)
  (progressive) (silent) (vessel) I82.90
  anal K64.5
  antepartum — *see* Thrombophlebitis,
    antepartum
  aorta, aortic I74.10
    abdominal I74.09
      saddle I74.01
    bifurcation I74.09
    saddle I74.09
    specified site NEC I74.19
    terminal I74.09
    thoracic I74.11
    valve — *see* Endocarditis, aortic
  apoplexy I63.3-
  artery, arteries (postinfectional) I74.9
    auditory, internal — *see* Occlusion, artery,
      precerebral, specified NEC
    basilar — *see* Occlusion, artery, basilar

Thrombosis, thrombotic (bland) (multiple)
  (progressive) (silent) (vessel) I82.90 —
  continued
  artery, arteries (postinfectional) I74.9 —
    continued
    carotid (common) (internal) — *see* Occlusion,
      artery, carotid
    cerebellar (anterior inferior) (posterior
      inferior) (superior) — *see* Occlusion,
      artery, cerebellar
    cerebral — *see* Occlusion, artery, cerebral
    choroidal (anterior) — *see* Occlusion, artery,
      cerebral, specified NEC
    communicating, posterior — *see* Occlusion,
      artery, cerebral, specified NEC
    coronary — *see also* Infarct, myocardium
      not resulting in infarction I24.0
    hepatic I74.8
    hypophyseal — *see* Occlusion, artery,
      cerebral, specified NEC
    iliac I74.5
    limb I74.4
      lower I74.3
      upper I74.2
    meningeal, anterior or posterior — *see*
      Occlusion, artery, cerebral, specified
      NEC
    mesenteric (with gangrene) (*see also* Infarct,
      intestine) K55.069
    ophthalmic — *see* Occlusion, artery, retina
    pontine — *see* Occlusion, artery, cerebral,
      specified NEC
    precerebral — *see* Occlusion, artery,
      precerebral
    pulmonary (iatrogenic) — *see* Embolism,
      pulmonary
    renal N28.0
    retinal — *see* Occlusion, artery, retina
    spinal, anterior or posterior G95.11
    traumatic NEC T14.8
    vertebral — *see* Occlusion, artery, vertebral
  atrium, auricular — *see also* Infarct,
    myocardium
    following acute myocardial infarction
      (current complication) I23.6
    not resulting in infarction I51.3
  basilar (artery) — *see* Occlusion, artery,
    basilar
  brain (artery) (stem) — *see also* Occlusion,
    artery, cerebral
    due to syphilis A52.05
    puerperal O99.43
    sinus — *see* Thrombosis, intracranial venous
      sinus
  capillary I78.8
  cardiac — *see also* Infarct, myocardium
    not resulting in infarction I51.3
    valve — *see* Endocarditis
  carotid (artery) (common) (internal) — *see*
    Occlusion, artery, carotid
  cavernous (venous) sinus — *see* Thrombosis,
    intracranial venous sinus
  cerebellar artery (anterior inferior) (posterior
    inferior) (superior) I66.3
  cerebral (artery) — *see* Occlusion, artery,
    cerebral
  cerebrovenous sinus — *see also* Thrombosis,
    intracranial venous sinus
    puerperium O87.3
  chronic I82.91
  coronary (artery) (vein) — *see also* Infarct,
    myocardium
    not resulting in infarction I24.0
  corpus cavernosum N48.89
  cortical I66.9
  deep — *see* Embolism, vein, lower extremity

Thrombosis, thrombotic (bland) (multiple) (progressive) (silent) (vessel) I82.90 — *continued*
- due to device, implant or graft (*see also* Complications, by site and type, specified NEC) T85.868
  - arterial graft NEC T82.868
  - breast (implant) T85.868
  - catheter NEC T85.868
    - dialysis (renal) T82.868
      - intraperitoneal T85.868
    - infusion NEC T82.868
      - spinal (epidural) (subdural) T85.860
    - urinary (indwelling) T83.86
  - electronic (electrode) (pulse generator) (stimulator)
    - bone T84.86
    - cardiac T82.867
    - nervous system (brain) (peripheral nerve) (spinal) T85.860
    - urinary T83.86
  - fixation, internal (orthopedic) NEC T84.86
  - gastrointestinal (bile duct) (esophagus) T85.868
  - genital NEC T83.86
  - heart T82.867
  - joint prosthesis T84.86
  - ocular (corneal graft) (orbital implant) NEC T85.868
  - orthopedic NEC T84.868
  - specified NEC T85.868
  - urinary NEC T83.86
  - vascular NEC T82.868
  - ventricular intracranial shunt T85.860
- during the puerperium — *see* Thrombosis, puerperal
- endocardial — *see also* Infarct, myocardium
  - not resulting in infarction I51.3
- eye — *see* Occlusion, retina
- genital organ
  - female NEC N94.89
    - pregnancy — *see* Thrombophlebitis, antepartum
  - male N50.1
- gestational — *see* Phlebopathy, gestational
- heart (chamber) — *see also* Infarct, myocardium
  - not resulting in infarction I51.3
- hepatic (vein) I82.0
  - artery I74.8
- history (of) Z86.718
- intestine (with gangrene) (*see also* Infarct, intestine) K55.069
- intracardiac NEC (apical) (atrial) (auricular) (ventricular) (old) I51.3
- intracranial (arterial) I66.9
  - venous sinus (any) G08
    - nonpyogenic origin I67.6
    - puerperium O87.3
- intramural — *see also* Infarct, myocardium
  - not resulting in infarction I51.3
- intraspinal venous sinuses and veins G08
  - nonpyogenic G95.19
- kidney (artery) N28.0
- lateral (venous) sinus — *see* Thrombosis, intracranial venous sinus
- leg — *see* Thrombosis, vein, lower extremity
  - arterial I74.3
- liver (venous) I82.0
  - artery I74.8
  - portal vein I81
- longitudinal (venous) sinus — *see* Thrombosis, intracranial venous sinus
- lower limb — *see* Thrombosis, vein, lower extremity
- lung (iatrogenic) (postoperative) — *see* Embolism, pulmonary
- meninges (brain) (arterial) I66.8

Thrombosis, thrombotic (bland) (multiple) (progressive) (silent) (vessel) I82.90 — *continued*
- mesenteric (artery) (with gangrene) (*see also* Infarct, intestine) K55.069
  - vein (inferior) (superior) I81
- mitral I34.8
- mural — *see also* Infarct, myocardium
  - due to syphilis A52.06
  - not resulting in infarction I51.3
- omentum (with gangrene) (*see also* Infarct, intestine) K55.069
- ophthalmic — *see* Occlusion, retina
- pampiniform plexus (male) N50.1
- parietal — *see also* Infarct, myocardium
  - not resulting in infarction I24.0
- penis, superficial vein N48.81
- perianal venous K64.5
- peripheral arteries I74.4
  - upper I74.2
- personal history (of) Z86.718
- portal I81
  - due to syphilis A52.09
- precerebral artery — *see* Occlusion, artery, precerebral
- puerperal, postpartum O87.0
  - brain (artery) O99.43
    - venous (sinus) O87.3
  - cardiac O99.43
  - cerebral (artery) O99.43
    - venous (sinus) O87.3
  - superficial O87.0
- pulmonary (artery) (iatrogenic) (postoperative) (vein) — *see* Embolism, pulmonary
- renal (artery) N28.0
  - vein I82.3
- resulting from presence of device, implant or graft — *see* Complications, by site and type, specified NEC
- retina, retinal — *see* Occlusion, retina
- scrotum N50.1
- seminal vesicle N50.1
- sigmoid (venous) sinus — *see* Thrombosis, intracranial venous sinus
- sinus, intracranial (any) — *see* Thrombosis, intracranial venous sinus
- specified site NEC I82.890
  - chronic I82.891
- spermatic cord N50.1
- spinal cord (arterial) G95.11
  - due to syphilis A52.09
  - pyogenic origin G06.1
- spleen, splenic D73.5
  - artery I74.8
- testis N50.1
- traumatic NEC T14.8
- tricuspid I07.8
- tumor — *see* Neoplasm, unspecified behavior, by site
- tunica vaginalis N50.1
- umbilical cord (vessels), complicating delivery O69.5
- vas deferens N50.1
- vein (acute) I82.90
  - antecubital I82.61-
    - chronic I82.71-
  - axillary I82.A1- *(follows I82.7)*
    - chronic I82.A2- *(follows I82.7)*
  - basilic I82.61-
    - chronic I82.71-
  - brachial I82.62-
    - chronic I82.72-
  - brachiocephalic (innominate) I82.290
    - chronic I82.291
  - cephalic I82.61-
    - chronic I82.71-
  - cerebral, nonpyogenic I67.6
  - chronic I82.91

Thrombosis, thrombotic (bland) (multiple) (progressive) (silent) (vessel) I82.90 — *continued*
- vein (acute) I82.90 — *continued*
  - deep (DVT) I82.40-
    - calf I82.4Z- *(follows I82.49)*
      - chronic I82.5Z- *(follows I82.59)*
    - lower leg I82.4Z- *(follows I82.49)*
      - chronic I82.5Z- *(follows I82.59)*
    - thigh I82.4Y- *(follows I82.49)*
      - chronic I82.5Y- *(follows I82.59)*
    - upper leg I82.4Y- *(follows I82.49)*
      - chronic I82.5Y- *(follows I82.59)*
  - femoral I82.41-
    - chronic I82.51-
  - iliac (iliofemoral) I82.42-
    - chronic I82.52-
  - innominate I82.290
    - chronic I82.291
  - internal jugular I82.C1- *(follows I82.7)*
    - chronic I82.C2- *(follows I82.7)*
  - lower extremity
    - deep I82.40-
      - chronic I82.50-
      - specified NEC I82.49-
        - chronic NEC I82.59-
    - distal
      - deep I82.4Z- *(follows I82.49)*
    - proximal
      - deep I82.4Y- *(follows I82.49)*
        - chronic I82.5Y- *(follows I82.59)*
    - superficial I82.81-
  - perianal K64.5
  - popliteal I82.43-
    - chronic I82.53-
  - radial I82.62-
    - chronic I82.72-
  - renal I82.3
  - saphenous (greater) (lesser) I82.81-
  - specified NEC I82.890
    - chronic NEC I82.891
  - subclavian I82.B1- *(follows I82.7)*
    - chronic I82.B2- *(follows I82.7)*
  - thoracic NEC I82.290
    - chronic I82.291
  - tibial I82.44-
    - chronic I82.54-
  - ulnar I82.62-
    - chronic I82.72-
  - upper extremity I82.60-
    - chronic I82.70-
    - deep I82.62-
      - chronic I82.72-
    - superficial I82.61-
      - chronic I82.71-
- vena cava
  - inferior I82.220
    - chronic I82.221
  - superior I82.210
    - chronic I82.211
- ventricle — *see also* Infarct, myocardium
  - following acute myocardial infarction (current complication) I23.6
  - not resulting in infarction I24.0
- venous, perianal K64.5

Thrombus — *see* Thrombosis

Thrush — *see also* Candidiasis
- newborn P37.5
- oral B37.0
- vaginal B37.3

Thumb — *see also* condition
- sucking (child problem) F98.8

Thymitis E32.8

Thymoma (benign) D15.0
- malignant C37

Thymus, thymic (gland) — *see* condition

Thyrocele — *see* Goiter

Thyroglossal — see also condition
  cyst Q89.2
  duct, persistent Q89.2
Thyroid (gland) (body) — see also condition
  hormone resistance E07.89
  lingual Q89.2
  nodule (cystic) (nontoxic) (single) E04.1
Thyroiditis E06.9
  acute (nonsuppurative) (pyogenic)
    (suppurative) E06.0
  autoimmune E06.3
  chronic (nonspecific) (sclerosing) E06.5
    with thyrotoxicosis, transient E06.2
    fibrous E06.5
    lymphadenoid E06.3
    lymphocytic E06.3
    lymphoid E06.3
  de Quervain's E06.1
  drug-induced E06.4
  fibrous (chronic) E06.5
  giant-cell (follicular) E06.1
  granulomatous (de Quervain) (subacute)
    E06.1
  Hashimoto's (struma lymphomatosa) E06.3
  iatrogenic E06.4
  ligneous E06.5
  lymphocytic (chronic) E06.3
  lymphoid E06.3
  lymphomatous E06.3
  nonsuppurative E06.1
  postpartum, puerperal O90.5
  pseudotuberculous E06.1
  pyogenic E06.0
  radiation E06.4
  Riedel's E06.5
  subacute (granulomatous) E06.1
  suppurative E06.0
  tuberculous A18.81
  viral E06.1
  woody E06.5
Thyrolingual duct, persistent Q89.2
Thyromegaly E01.0
Thyrotoxic
  crisis — see Thyrotoxicosis
  heart disease or failure (see also Thyrotoxicosis)
    E05.90 [I43]
    with thyroid storm E05.91 [I43]
  storm — see Thyrotoxicosis
Thyrotoxicosis (recurrent) E05.90
  with
    goiter (diffuse) E05.00
      with thyroid storm E05.01
      adenomatous uninodular E05.10
        with thyroid storm E05.11
      multinodular E05.20
        with thyroid storm E05.21
      nodular E05.20
        with thyroid storm E05.21
      uninodular E05.10
        with thyroid storm E05.11
    infiltrative
      dermopathy E05.00
        with thyroid storm E05.01
      ophthalmopathy E05.00
        with thyroid storm E05.01
    single thyroid nodule E05.10
      with thyroid storm E05.11
  due to
    ectopic thyroid nodule or tissue E05.30
      with thyroid storm E05.31
    ingestion of (excessive) thyroid material
      E05.40
      with thyroid storm E05.41
    overproduction of thyroid-stimulating
      hormone E05.80
      with thyroid storm E05.81
    specified cause NEC E05.80
      with thyroid storm E05.81

Thyrotoxicosis (recurrent) E05.90 —
  continued
  factitia E05.40
    with thyroid storm E05.41
  heart E05.90 [I43]
    with thyroid storm E05.91 [I43]
    failure E05.90 [I43]
  neonatal (transient) P72.1
  transient with chronic thyroiditis E06.2
Tibia vara — see Osteochondrosis, juvenile,
  tibia
Tic (disorder) F95.9
  breathing F95.8
  child problem F95.0
  compulsive F95.1
  de la Tourette F95.2
  degenerative (generalized) (localized) G25.69
    facial G25.69
  disorder
    chronic
      motor F95.1
      vocal F95.1
    combined vocal and multiple motor F95.2
    transient F95.0
  douloureux G50.0
    atypical G50.1
    postherpetic, postzoster B02.22
  drug-induced G25.61
  eyelid F95.8
  habit F95.9
    chronic F95.1
    transient of childhood F95.0
  lid, transient of childhood F95.0
  motor-verbal F95.2
  occupational F48.8
  orbicularis F95.8
    transient of childhood F95.0
  organic origin G25.69
  postchoreic G25.69
  provisional F95.0
  psychogenic, compulsive F95.1
  salaam R25.8
  spasm (motor or vocal) F95.9
    chronic F95.1
    transient of childhood F95.0
  specified NEC F95.8
Tick-borne — see condition
Tietze's disease or syndrome M94.0
Tight, tightness
  anus K62.89
  chest R07.89
  fascia (lata) M62.89
  foreskin (congenital) N47.1
  hymen, hymenal ring N89.6
  introitus (acquired) (congenital) N89.6
  rectal sphincter K62.89
  tendon — see Short, tendon
  urethral sphincter N35.9
Tilting vertebra — see Dorsopathy,
  deforming, specified NEC
Timidity, child F93.8
Tin-miner's lung J63.5
Tinea (intersecta) (tarsi) B35.9
  amiantacea L44.8
  asbestina B35.0
  barbae B35.0
  beard B35.0
  black dot B35.0
  blanca B36.2
  capitis B35.0
  corporis B35.4
  cruris B35.6
  flava B36.0
  foot B35.3
  furfuracea B36.0
  imbricata (Tokelau) B35.5
  kerion B35.0
  manuum B35.2
  microsporic — see Dermatophytosis

Tinea (intersecta) (tarsi) B35.9 — continued
  nigra B36.1
  nodosa — see Piedra
  pedis B35.3
  scalp B35.0
  specified site NEC B35.8
  sycosis B35.0
  tonsurans B35.0
  trichophytic — see Dermatophytosis
  unguium B35.1
  versicolor B36.0
Tingling sensation (skin) R20.2
Tinnitus NOS H93.1-
  audible H93.1-
  aurium H93.1-
  pulsatile H93.A- *(follows H93.1)*
  subjective H93.1-
Tipped tooth (teeth) M26.33
Tipping
  pelvis M95.5
    with disproportion (fetopelvic) O33.0
      causing obstructed labor O65.0
  tooth (teeth), fully erupted M26.33
Tiredness R53.83
Tissue — see condition
Tobacco (nicotine)
  abuse — see Tobacco, use
  dependence — see Dependence, drug, nicotine
  harmful use Z72.0
  heart — see Tobacco, toxic effect
  maternal use, affecting newborn P04.2
  toxic effect — see Table of Drugs and
    Chemicals, by substance, poisoning
    chewing tobacco — see Table of Drugs and
      Chemicals, by substance, poisoning
    cigarettes — see Table of Drugs and
      Chemicals, by substance, poisoning
  use Z72.0
    complicating
      childbirth O99.334
      pregnancy O99.33-
      puerperium O99.335
    counseling and surveillance Z71.6
    history Z87.891
  withdrawal state (see also Dependence, drug,
    nicotine) F17.203
Tocopherol deficiency E56.0
Todd's
  cirrhosis K74.3
  paralysis (postepileptic) (transitory) G83.84
Toe — see condition
Toilet, artificial opening — see Attention to,
  artificial, opening
Tokelau (ringworm) B35.5
Tollwut — see Rabies
Tommaselli's disease R31.9
  correct substance properly administered — see
    Table of Drugs and Chemicals, by drug,
    adverse effect
  overdose or wrong substance given or taken
    — see Table of Drugs and Chemicals, by
    drug, poisoning
Tongue — see also condition
  tie Q38.1
Tonic pupil — see Anomaly, pupil, function,
  tonic pupil
Toni-Fanconi syndrome (cystinosis) E72.09
  with cystinosis E72.04
Tonsil — see condition

Tonsillitis (acute) (catarrhal) (croupous) (follicular) (gangrenous) (infective) (lacunar) (lingual) (malignant) (membranous) (parenchymatous) (phlegmonous) (pseudomembranous) (purulent) (septic) (subacute) (suppurative) (toxic) (ulcerative) (vesicular) (viral) J03.90
  chronic J35.01
    with adenoiditis J35.03
  diphtheritic A36.0
  hypertrophic J35.01
    with adenoiditis J35.03
  recurrent J03.91
  specified organism NEC J03.80
    recurrent J03.81
  staphylococcal J03.80
    recurrent J03.81
  streptococcal J03.00
    recurrent J03.01
  tuberculous A15.8
  Vincent's A69.1
Tooth, teeth — see condition
Toothache K08.89
Topagnosis R20.8
Tophi — see Gout, chronic
TORCH infection — see Infection, congenital
  without active infection P00.2
Torn — see Tear
Tornwaldt's cyst or disease J39.2
Torsion
  accessory tube — see Torsion, fallopian tube
  adnexa (female) — see Torsion, fallopian tube
  aorta, acquired I77.1
  appendix epididymis N44.04
  appendix testis N44.03
  bile duct (common) (hepatic) K83.8
    congenital Q44.5
  bowel, colon or intestine K56.2
  cervix — see Malposition, uterus
  cystic duct K82.8
  dystonia — see Dystonia, torsion
  epididymis (appendix) N44.04
  fallopian tube N83.52-
    with ovary N83.53
  gallbladder K82.8
    congenital Q44.1
  hydatid of Morgagni
    female N83.52-
    male N44.03
  kidney (pedicle) (leading to infarction) N28.0
  Meckel's diverticulum (congenital) Q43.0
    malignant — see Table of Neoplasms, small intestine, malignant
  mesentery K56.2
  omentum K56.2
  organ or site, congenital NEC — see Anomaly, by site
  ovary (pedicle) N83.51-
    with fallopian tube N83.53
    congenital Q50.2
  oviduct — see Torsion, fallopian tube
  penis (acquired) N48.82
    congenital Q55.69
  spasm — see Dystonia, torsion
  spermatic cord N44.02
    extravaginal N44.01
    intravaginal N44.02
  spleen D73.5
  testis, testicle N44.00
    appendix N44.03
  tibia — see Deformity, limb, specified type NEC, lower leg
  uterus — see Malposition, uterus
Torticollis (intermittent) (spastic) M43.6
  congenital (sternomastoid) Q68.0
  due to birth injury P15.8
  hysterical F44.4
  ocular R29.891

Torticollis (intermittent) (spastic) M43.6 — continued
  psychogenic F45.8
    conversion reaction F44.4
  rheumatic M43.6
  rheumatoid M06.88
  spasmodic G24.3
  traumatic, current S13.4
Tortipelvis G24.1
Tortuous
  aortic arch Q25.46
  artery I77.1
  organ or site, congenital NEC — see Distortion
  retinal vessel, congenital Q14.1
  ureter N13.8
  urethra N36.8
  vein — see Varix
Torture, victim of Z65.4
Torula, torular (histolytica) (infection) — see Cryptococcosis
Torulosis — see Cryptococcosis
Torus (mandibularis) (palatinus) M27.0
  fracture — see Fracture, by site, torus
Touraine's syndrome Q79.8
Tourette's syndrome F95.2
Tourniquet syndrome — see Constriction, external, by site
Tower skull Q75.0
  with exophthalmos Q87.0
Toxemia R68.89
  bacterial — see Sepsis
  burn — see Burn
  eclamptic (with pre-existing hypertension) — see Eclampsia
  erysipelatous — see Erysipelas
  fatigue R68.89
  food — see Poisoning, food
  gastrointestinal K52.1
  intestinal K52.1
  kidney — see Uremia
  malarial — see Malaria
  myocardial — see Myocarditis, toxic
  of pregnancy — see Pre-eclampsia
  pre-eclamptic — see Pre-eclampsia
  small intestine K52.1
  staphylococcal, due to food A05.0
  stasis R68.89
  uremic — see Uremia
  urinary — see Uremia
Toxemica cerebropathia psychica (nonalcoholic) F04
  alcoholic — see Alcohol, amnestic disorder
Toxic (poisoning) (see also condition) T65.91
  effect — see Table of Drugs and Chemicals, by substance, poisoning
  shock syndrome A48.3
  thyroid (gland) — see Thyrotoxicosis
Toxicemia — see Toxemia
Toxicity — see Table of Drugs and Chemicals, by substance, poisoning
  fava bean D55.0
  food, noxious — see Poisoning, food
  from drug or nonmedicinal substance — see Table of Drugs and Chemicals, by drug
Toxicosis — see also Toxemia
  capillary, hemorrhagic D69.0
Toxinfection, gastrointestinal K52.1
Toxocariasis B83.0
Toxoplasma, toxoplasmosis (acquired) B58.9
  with
    hepatitis B58.1
    meningoencephalitis B58.2
    ocular involvement B58.00
    other organ involvement B58.89
    pneumonia, pneumonitis B58.3
  congenital (acute) (subacute) (chronic) P37.1
  maternal, manifest toxoplasmosis in infant (acute) (subacute) (chronic) P37.1

tPA (rtPA) administation in a different facility within the last 24 hours prior to admission to current facility Z92.82
Trabeculation, bladder N32.89
Trachea — see condition
Tracheitis (catarrhal) (infantile) (membranous) (plastic) (septal) (suppurative) (viral) J04.10
  with
    bronchitis (15 years of age and above) J40
      acute or subacute — see Bronchitis, acute
      chronic J42
      tuberculous NEC A15.5
      under 15 years of age J20.9
    laryngitis (acute) J04.2
      chronic J37.1
      tuberculous NEC A15.5
  acute J04.10
    with obstruction J04.11
  chronic J42
    with
      bronchitis (chronic) J42
      laryngitis (chronic) J37.1
  diphtheritic (membranous) A36.89
  due to external agent — see Inflammation, respiratory, upper, due to
  syphilitic A52.73
  tuberculous A15.5
Trachelitis (nonvenereal) — see Cervicitis
Tracheobronchial — see condition
Tracheobronchitis (15 years of age and above) — see also Bronchitis
  due to
    Bordetella bronchiseptica A37.80
      with pneumonia A37.81
    Francisella tularensis A21.8
Tracheobronchomegaly Q32.4
  with bronchiectasis J47.9
    with
      exacerbation (acute) J47.1
      lower respiratory infection J47.0
  acquired J98.09
    with bronchiectasis J47.9
      with
        exacerbation (acute) J47.1
        lower respiratory infection J47.0
Tracheobronchopneumonitis — see Pneumonia, broncho-
Tracheocele (external) (internal) J39.8
  congenital Q32.1
Tracheomalacia J39.8
  congenital Q32.0
Tracheopharyngitis (acute) J06.9
  chronic J42
  due to external agent — see Inflammation, respiratory, upper, due to
Tracheostenosis J39.8
Tracheostomy
  complication — see Complication, tracheostomy
  status Z93.0
    attention to Z43.0
    malfunctioning J95.03
Trachoma, trachomatous A71.9
  active (stage) A71.1
  contraction of conjunctiva A71.1
  dubium A71.0
  healed or sequelae B94.0
  initial (stage) A71.0
  pannus A71.1
  Türck's J37.0
Traction, vitreomacular H43.82-
Train sickness T75.3
Trait(s)
  Hb-S D57.3
  hemoglobin
    abnormal NEC D58.2
      with thalassemia D56.3
    C — see Disease, hemoglobin C
    S (Hb-S) D57.3

Trait(s) — *continued*
Lepore D56.3
personality, accentuated Z73.1
sickle-cell D57.3
with elliptocytosis or spherocytosis D57.3
type A personality Z73.1
Tramp Z59.0
Trance R41.89
hysterical F44.89
Transaminasemia R74.0
Transection
abdomen (partial) S38.3
aorta (incomplete) — *see also* Injury, aorta
complete — *see* Injury, aorta, laceration, major
carotid artery (incomplete) — *see also* Injury, blood vessel, carotid, laceration
complete — *see* Injury, blood vessel, carotid, laceration, major
celiac artery (incomplete) S35.211
branch (incomplete) S35.291
complete S35.292
complete S35.212
innominate
artery (incomplete) — *see also* Injury, blood vessel, thoracic, innominate, artery, laceration
complete — *see* Injury, blood vessel, thoracic, innominate, artery, laceration, major
vein (incomplete) — *see also* Injury, blood vessel, thoracic, innominate, vein, laceration
complete — *see* Injury, blood vessel, thoracic, innominate, vein, laceration, major
jugular vein (external) (incomplete) — *see also* Injury, blood vessel, jugular vein, laceration
complete — *see* Injury, blood vessel, jugular vein, laceration, major
internal (incomplete) — *see also* Injury, blood vessel, jugular vein, internal, laceration
complete — *see* Injury, blood vessel, jugular vein, internal, laceration, major
mesenteric artery (incomplete) — *see also* Injury, mesenteric, artery, laceration
complete — *see* Injury, mesenteric artery, laceration, major
pulmonary vessel (incomplete) — *see also* Injury, blood vessel, thoracic, pulmonary, laceration
complete — *see* Injury, blood vessel, thoracic, pulmonary, laceration, major
subclavian — *see* Transection, innominate
vena cava (incomplete) — *see also* Injury, vena cava
complete — *see* Injury, vena cava, laceration, major
vertebral artery (incomplete) — *see also* Injury, blood vessel, vertebral, laceration
complete — *see* Injury, blood vessel, vertebral, laceration, major
Transfusion
associated (red blood cell) hemochromatosis E83.111
blood
ABO incompatible — *see* Complication(s), transfusion, incompatibility reaction, ABO
minor blood group (Duffy) (E) (K(ell)) (Kidd) (Lewis) (M) (N) (P) (S) T80.89
reaction or complication — *see* Complications, transfusion
fetomaternal (mother) — *see* Pregnancy, complicated by, placenta, transfusion syndrome

Transfusion — *continued*
maternofetal (mother) — *see* Pregnancy, complicated by, placenta, transfusion syndrome
placental (syndrome) (mother) — *see* Pregnancy, complicated by, placenta, transfusion syndrome
reaction (adverse) — *see* Complications, transfusion
related acute lung injury (TRALI) J95.84
twin-to-twin — *see* Pregnancy, complicated by, placenta, transfusion syndrome, fetus to fetus
Transient (meaning homeless) (*see also* condition) Z59.0
Translocation
balanced autosomal Q95.9
in normal individual Q95.0
chromosomes NEC Q99.8
balanced and insertion in normal individual Q95.0
Down syndrome Q90.2
trisomy
13 Q91.6
18 Q91.2
21 Q90.2
Translucency, iris — *see* Degeneration, iris
Transmission of chemical substances through the placenta — *see* Absorption, chemical, through placenta
Transparency, lung, unilateral J43.0
Transplant(ed) (status) Z94.9
awaiting organ Z76.82
bone Z94.6
marrow Z94.81
candidate Z76.82
complication — *see* Complication, transplant
cornea Z94.7
heart Z94.1
and lung(s) Z94.3
valve Z95.2
prosthetic Z95.2
specified NEC Z95.4
xenogenic Z95.3
intestine Z94.82
kidney Z94.0
liver Z94.4
lung(s) Z94.2
and heart Z94.3
organ (failure) (infection) (rejection) Z94.9
removal status Z98.85
pancreas Z94.83
skin Z94.5
social Z60.3
specified organ or tissue NEC Z94.89
stem cells Z94.84
tissue Z94.9
Transplants, ovarian, endometrial N80.1
Transposed — *see* Transposition
Transposition (congenital) — *see also* Malposition, congenital
abdominal viscera Q89.3
aorta (dextra) Q20.3
appendix Q43.8
colon Q43.8
corrected Q20.5
great vessels (complete) (partial) Q20.3
heart Q24.0
with complete transposition of viscera Q89.3
intestine (large) (small) Q43.8
reversed jejunal (for bypass) (status) Z98.0
scrotum Q55.23
stomach Q40.2
with general transposition of viscera Q89.3
tooth, teeth, fully erupted M26.30
vessels, great (complete) (partial) Q20.3
viscera (abdominal) (thoracic) Q89.3
Transsexualism F64.0

Transverse — *see also* condition
arrest (deep), in labor O64.0
lie (mother) O32.2
causing obstructed labor O64.8
Transvestism, transvestitism (dual-role) F64.1
fetishistic F65.1
Trapped placenta (with hemorrhage) O72.0
without hemorrhage O73.0
TRAPS (tumor necrosis factor receptor associated periodic syndrome) M04.1
Trauma, traumatism — *see also* Injury
acoustic — *see* subcategory H83.3
birth — *see* Birth, injury
complicating ectopic or molar pregnancy O08.6
during delivery O71.9
following ectopic or molar pregnancy O08.6
obstetric O71.9
specified NEC O71.89
occlusal
primary K08.81
secondary K08.82
Traumatic — *see also* condition
brain injury S06.9
Treacher Collins syndrome Q75.4
Treitz's hernia — *see* Hernia, abdomen, specified site NEC
Trematode infestation — *see* Infestation, fluke
Trematodiasis — *see* Infestation, fluke
Trembling paralysis — *see* Parkinsonism
Tremor(s) R25.1
drug induced G25.1
essential (benign) G25.0
familial G25.0
hereditary G25.0
hysterical F44.4
intention G25.2
medication induced postural G25.1
mercurial — *see* subcategory T56.1
Parkinson's — *see* Parkinsonism
psychogenic (conversion reaction) F44.4
senilis R54
specified type NEC G25.2
Trench
fever A79.0
foot — *see* Immersion, foot
mouth A69.1
Treponema pallidum infection — *see* Syphilis
Treponematosis
due to
T. pallidum — *see* Syphilis
T. pertenue — *see* Yaws
Triad
Hutchinson's (congenital syphilis) A50.53
Kartagener's Q89.3
Saint's — *see* Hernia, diaphragm
Trichiasis (eyelid) H02.059
with entropion — *see* Entropion
left H02.056
lower H02.055
upper H02.054
right H02.053
lower H02.052
upper H02.051
Trichinella spiralis (infection) (infestation) B75
Trichinellosis, trichiniasis, trichinelliasis, trichinosis B75
with muscle disorder B75 [M63.80]
ankle B75 [M63.8-]
foot B75 [M63.8-]
forearm B75 [M63.8-]
hand B75 [M63.8-]
lower leg B75 [M63.8-]
multiple sites B75 [M63.89]
pelvic region B75 [M63.8-]

Trichinellosis, trichiniasis, trichinelliasis, trichinosis B75 — *continued*
  with muscle disorder B75 *[M63.80]* — *continued*
    shoulder region B75 *[M63.8-]*
    specified site NEC B75 *[M63.88]*
    thigh B75 *[M63.8-]*
    upper arm B75 *[M63.8-]*
Trichobezoar T18.9
  intestine T18.3
  stomach T18.2
Trichocephaliasis, trichocephalosis B79
Trichocephalus infestation B79
Trichoclasis L67.8
Trichoepithelioma — *see also* Neoplasm, skin, benign
  malignant — *see* Neoplasm, skin, malignant
Trichofolliculoma — *see* Neoplasm, skin, benign
Tricholemmoma — *see* Neoplasm, skin, benign
Trichomoniasis A59.9
  bladder A59.03
  cervix A59.09
  intestinal A07.8
  prostate A59.02
  seminal vesicles A59.09
  specified site NEC A59.8
  urethra A59.03
  urogenitalis A59.00
  vagina A59.01
  vulva A59.01
Trichomycosis
  axillaris A48.8
  nodosa, nodularis B36.8
Trichonodosis L67.8
Trichophytid, trichophyton infection — *see* Dermatophytosis
Trichophytobezoar T18.9
  intestine T18.3
  stomach T18.2
Trichophytosis — *see* Dermatophytosis
Trichoptilosis L67.8
Trichorrhexis (nodosa) (invaginata) L67.0
Trichosis axillaris A48.8
Trichosporosis nodosa B36.2
Trichostasis spinulosa (congenital) Q84.1
Trichostrongyliasis, trichostrongylosis (small intestine) B81.2
Trichostrongylus infection B81.2
Trichotillomania F63.3
Trichromat, trichromatopsia, anomalous (congenital) H53.55
Trichuriasis B79
Trichuris trichiura (infection) (infestation) (any site) B79
Tricuspid (valve) — *see* condition
Trifid — *see also* Accessory
  kidney (pelvis) Q63.8
  tongue Q38.3
Trigeminal neuralgia — *see* Neuralgia, trigeminal
Trigeminy R00.8
Trigger finger (acquired) M65.30
  congenital Q74.0
  index finger M65.32-
  little finger M65.35-
  middle finger M65.33-
  ring finger M65.34-
  thumb M65.31-
Trigonitis (bladder) (chronic) (pseudomembranous) N30.30
  with hematuria N30.31
Trigonocephaly Q75.0
Trilocular heart — *see* Cor triloculare
Trimethylaminuria E72.52
Tripartite placenta O43.19-
Triphalangeal thumb Q74.0

Triple — *see also* Accessory
  kidneys Q63.0
  uteri Q51.818
  X, female Q97.0
Triplegia G83.89
  congenital G80.8
Triplet (newborn) — *see also* Newborn, triplet
  complicating pregnancy — *see* Pregnancy, triplet
Triplication — *see* Accessory
Triploidy Q92.7
Trismus R25.2
  neonatorum A33
  newborn A33
Trisomy (syndrome) Q92.9
  13 (partial) Q91.7
    meiotic nondisjunction Q91.4
    mitotic nondisjunction Q91.5
    mosaicism Q91.5
    translocation Q91.6
  18 (partial) Q91.3
    meiotic nondisjunction Q91.0
    mitotic nondisjunction Q91.1
    mosaicism Q91.1
    translocation Q91.2
  20 Q92.8
  21 (partial) Q90.9
    meiotic nondisjunction Q90.0
    mitotic nondisjunction Q90.1
    mosaicism Q90.1
    translocation Q90.2
  22 Q92.8
  autosomes Q92.9
  chromosome specified NEC Q92.8
    partial Q92.2
      due to unbalanced translocation Q92.5
    specified NEC Q92.8
    whole (nonsex chromosome)
      meiotic nondisjunction Q92.0
      mitotic nondisjunction Q92.1
      mosaicism Q92.1
  due to
    dicentrics — *see* Extra, marker chromosomes
    extra rings — *see* Extra, marker chromosomes
    isochromosomes — *see* Extra, marker chromosomes
  specified NEC Q92.8
  whole chromosome Q92.9
    meiotic nondisjunction Q92.0
    mitotic nondisjunction Q92.1
    mosaicism Q92.1
    partial Q92.9
    specified NEC Q92.8
Tritanomaly, tritanopia H53.55
Trombiculosis, trombiculiasis, trombidiosis B88.0
Trophedema (congenital) (hereditary) Q82.0
Trophoblastic disease (*see also* Mole, hydatidiform) O01.9
Tropholymphedema Q82.0
Trophoneurosis NEC G96.8
  disseminated M34.9
Tropical — *see* condition
Trouble — *see also* Disease
  heart — *see* Disease, heart
  kidney — *see* Disease, renal
  nervous R45.0
  sinus — *see* Sinusitis
Trousseau's syndrome (thrombophlebitis migrans) I82.1
Truancy, childhood
  from school Z72.810
Truncus
  arteriosus (persistent) Q20.0
  communis Q20.0
Trunk — *see* condition

Trypanosomiasis
  African B56.9
    by Trypanosoma brucei
      gambiense B56.0
      rhodesiense B56.1
  American — *see* Chagas' disease
  Brazilian — *see* Chagas' disease
  by Trypanosoma
    brucei gambiense B56.0
    brucei rhodesiense B56.1
    cruzi — *see* Chagas' disease
  gambiensis, Gambian B56.0
  rhodesiensis, Rhodesian B56.1
  South American — *see* Chagas' disease
  where
    African trypanosomiasis is prevalent B56.9
    Chagas' disease is prevalent B57.2
T-shaped incisors K00.2
Tsutsugamushi (disease) (fever) A75.3
Tube, tubal, tubular — *see* condition
Tubercle — *see also* Tuberculosis
  brain, solitary A17.81
  Darwin's Q17.8
  Ghon, primary infection A15.7
Tuberculid, tuberculide (indurating, subcutaneous) (lichenoid) (miliary) (papulonecrotic) (primary) (skin) A18.4
Tuberculoma — *see also* Tuberculosis
  brain A17.81
  meninges (cerebral) (spinal) A17.1
  spinal cord A17.81
Tuberculosis, tubercular, tuberculous (calcification) (calcified) (caseous) (chromogenic acid-fast bacilli) (degeneration) (fibrocaseous) (fistula) (interstitial) (isolated circumscribed lesions) (necrosis) (parenchymatous) (ulcerative) A15.9
  with pneumoconiosis (any condition in J60-J64) J65
  abdomen (lymph gland) A18.39
  abscess (respiratory) A15.9
    bone A18.03
      hip A18.02
      knee A18.02
      sacrum A18.01
      specified site NEC A18.03
      spinal A18.01
      vertebra A18.01
    brain A17.81
    breast A18.89
    Cowper's gland A18.15
    dura (mater) (cerebral) (spinal) A17.81
    epidural (cerebral) (spinal) A17.81
    female pelvis A18.17
    frontal sinus A15.8
    genital organs NEC A18.10
    genitourinary A18.10
    gland (lymphatic) — *see* Tuberculosis, lymph gland
    hip A18.02
    intestine A18.32
    ischiorectal A18.32
    joint NEC A18.02
      hip A18.02
      knee A18.02
      specified NEC A18.02
      vertebral A18.01
    kidney A18.11
    knee A18.02
    latent R76.11
    lumbar (spine) A18.01
    lung — *see* Tuberculosis, pulmonary
    meninges (cerebral) (spinal) A17.0
    muscle A18.09
    perianal (fistula) A18.32
    perinephritic A18.11
    perirectal A18.32
    rectum A18.32

Tuberculosis, tubercular, tuberculous
(calcification) (calcified) (caseous)
(chromogenic acid-fast bacilli)
(degeneration) (fibrocaseous) (fistula)
(interstitial) (isolated circumscribed lesions)
(necrosis) (parenchymatous) (ulcerative)
A15.9 — *continued*
abscess (respiratory) A15.9 — *continued*
  retropharyngeal A15.8
  sacrum A18.01
  scrofulous A18.2
  scrotum A18.15
  skin (primary) A18.4
  spinal cord A17.81
  spine or vertebra (column) A18.01
  subdiaphragmatic A18.31
  testis A18.15
  urinary A18.13
  uterus A18.17
accessory sinus — *see* Tuberculosis, sinus
Addison's disease A18.7
adenitis — *see* Tuberculosis, lymph gland
adenoids A15.8
adenopathy — *see* Tuberculosis, lymph gland
adherent pericardium A18.84
adnexa (uteri) A18.17
adrenal (capsule) (gland) A18.7
alimentary canal A18.32
anemia A18.89
ankle (joint) (bone) A18.02
anus A18.32
apex, apical — *see* Tuberculosis, pulmonary
appendicitis, appendix A18.32
arachnoid A17.0
artery, arteritis A18.89
  cerebral A18.89
arthritis (chronic) (synovial) A18.02
  spine or vertebra (column) A18.01
articular — *see* Tuberculosis, joint
ascites A18.31
asthma — *see* Tuberculosis, pulmonary
axilla, axillary (gland) A18.2
bladder A18.12
bone A18.03
  hip A18.02
  knee A18.02
  limb NEC A18.03
  sacrum A18.01
  spine or vertebral column A18.01
bowel (miliary) A18.32
brain A17.81
breast A18.89
broad ligament A18.17
bronchi, bronchial, bronchus A15.5
  ectasia, ectasis (bronchiectasis) — *see*
    Tuberculosis, pulmonary
  fistula A15.5
    primary (progressive) A15.7
  gland or node A15.4
    primary (progressive) A15.7
  lymph gland or node A15.4
    primary (progressive) A15.7
bronchiectasis — *see* Tuberculosis, pulmonary
bronchitis A15.5
bronchopleural A15.6
bronchopneumonia, bronchopneumonic — *see*
  Tuberculosis, pulmonary
bronchorrhagia A15.5
bronchotracheal A15.5
bronze disease A18.7
buccal cavity A18.83
bulbourethral gland A18.15
bursa A18.09
cachexia A15.9
cardiomyopathy A18.84
caries — *see* Tuberculosis, bone
cartilage A18.02
  intervertebral A18.01
catarrhal — *see* Tuberculosis, respiratory

Tuberculosis, tubercular, tuberculous
(calcification) (calcified) (caseous)
(chromogenic acid-fast bacilli)
(degeneration) (fibrocaseous) (fistula)
(interstitial) (isolated circumscribed lesions)
(necrosis) (parenchymatous) (ulcerative)
A15.9 — *continued*
cecum A18.32
cellulitis (primary) A18.4
cerebellum A17.81
cerebral, cerebrum A17.81
cerebrospinal A17.81
  meninges A17.0
cervical (lymph gland or node) A18.2
cervicitis, cervix (uteri) A18.16
chest — *see* Tuberculosis, respiratory
chorioretinitis A18.53
choroid, choroiditis A18.53
ciliary body A18.54
colitis A18.32
collier's J65
colliquativa (primary) A18.4
colon A18.32
complex, primary A15.7
congenital P37.0
conjunctiva A18.59
connective tissue (systemic) A18.89
contact Z20.1
cornea (ulcer) A18.52
Cowper's gland A18.15
coxae A18.02
coxalgia A18.02
cul-de-sac of Douglas A18.17
curvature, spine A18.01
cutis (colliquativa) (primary) A18.4
cyst, ovary A18.18
cystitis A18.12
dactylitis A18.03
diarrhea A18.32
diffuse — *see* Tuberculosis, miliary
digestive tract A18.32
disseminated — *see* Tuberculosis, miliary
duodenum A18.32
dura (mater) (cerebral) (spinal) A17.0
  abscess (cerebral) (spinal) A17.81
dysentery A18.32
ear (inner) (middle) A18.6
  bone A18.03
  external (primary) A18.4
  skin (primary) A18.4
elbow A18.02
emphysema — *see* Tuberculosis, pulmonary
empyema A15.6
encephalitis A17.82
endarteritis A18.89
endocarditis A18.84
  aortic A18.84
  mitral A18.84
  pulmonary A18.84
  tricuspid A18.84
endocrine glands NEC A18.82
endometrium A18.17
enteric, enterica, enteritis A18.32
enterocolitis A18.32
epididymis, epididymitis A18.15
epidural abscess (cerebral) (spinal) A17.81
epiglottis A15.5
episcleritis A18.51
erythema (induratum) (nodosum) (primary)
  A18.4
esophagus A18.83
eustachian tube A18.6
exposure (to) Z20.1
exudative — *see* Tuberculosis, pulmonary
eye A18.50
eyelid (primary) (lupus) A18.4
fallopian tube (acute) (chronic) A18.17
fascia A18.09
fauces A15.8

Tuberculosis, tubercular, tuberculous
(calcification) (calcified) (caseous)
(chromogenic acid-fast bacilli)
(degeneration) (fibrocaseous) (fistula)
(interstitial) (isolated circumscribed lesions)
(necrosis) (parenchymatous) (ulcerative)
A15.9 — *continued*
female pelvic inflammatory disease A18.17
finger A18.03
first infection A15.7
gallbladder A18.83
ganglion A18.09
gastritis A18.83
gastrocolic fistula A18.32
gastroenteritis A18.32
gastrointestinal tract A18.32
general, generalized — *see* Tuberculosis,
  miliary
genital organs A18.10
genitourinary A18.10
genu A18.02
glandula suprarenalis A18.7
glandular, general A18.2
glottis A15.5
grinder's J65
gum A18.83
hand A18.03
heart A18.84
hematogenous — *see* Tuberculosis, miliary
hemoptysis — *see* Tuberculosis, pulmonary
hemorrhage NEC — *see* Tuberculosis,
  pulmonary
hemothorax A15.6
hepatitis A18.83
hilar lymph nodes A15.4
  primary (progressive) A15.7
hip (joint) (disease) (bone) A18.02
hydropneumothorax A15.6
hydrothorax A15.6
hypoadrenalism A18.7
hypopharynx A15.8
ileocecal (hyperplastic) A18.32
ileocolitis A18.32
ileum A18.32
iliac spine (superior) A18.03
immunological findings only A15.7
indurativa (primary) A18.4
infantile A15.7
infection A15.9
  without clinical manifestations A15.7
infraclavicular gland A18.2
inguinal gland A18.2
inguinalis A18.2
intestine (any part) A18.32
iridocyclitis A18.54
iris, iritis A18.54
ischiorectal A18.32
jaw A18.03
jejunum A18.32
joint A18.02
  vertebral A18.01
keratitis (interstitial) A18.52
keratoconjunctivitis A18.52
kidney A18.11
knee (joint) A18.02
kyphosis, kyphoscoliosis A18.01
laryngitis A15.5
larynx A15.5
latent R76.11
leptomeninges, leptomeningitis (cerebral)
  (spinal) A17.0
lichenoides (primary) A18.4
linguae A18.83
lip A18.83
liver A18.83
lordosis A18.01
lung — *see* Tuberculosis, pulmonary
lupus vulgaris A18.4

Tuberculosis, tubercular, tuberculous
  (calcification) (calcified) (caseous)
  (chromogenic acid-fast bacilli)
  (degeneration) (fibrocaseous) (fistula)
  (interstitial) (isolated circumscribed lesions)
  (necrosis) (parenchymatous) (ulcerative)
  A15.9 — continued
  lymph gland or node (peripheral) A18.2
    abdomen A18.39
    bronchial A15.4
      primary (progressive) A15.7
    cervical A18.2
    hilar A15.4
      primary (progressive) A15.7
    intrathoracic A15.4
      primary (progressive) A15.7
    mediastinal A15.4
      primary (progressive) A15.7
    mesenteric A18.39
    retroperitoneal A18.39
    tracheobronchial A15.4
      primary (progressive) A15.7
  lymphadenitis — see Tuberculosis, lymph gland
  lymphangitis — see Tuberculosis, lymph gland
  lymphatic (gland) (vessel) — see Tuberculosis,
    lymph gland
  mammary gland A18.89
  marasmus A15.9
  mastoiditis A18.03
  mediastinal lymph gland or node A15.4
    primary (progressive) A15.7
  mediastinitis A15.8
    primary (progressive) A15.7
  mediastinum A15.8
    primary (progressive) A15.7
  medulla A17.81
  melanosis, Addisonian A18.7
  meninges, meningitis (basilar) (cerebral)
    (cerebrospinal) (spinal) A17.0
  meningoencephalitis A17.82
  mesentery, mesenteric (gland or node) A18.39
  miliary A19.9
    acute A19.2
      multiple sites A19.1
      single specified site A19.0
    chronic A19.8
    specified NEC A19.8
  millstone makers' J65
  miner's J65
  molder's J65
  mouth A18.83
  multiple A19.9
    acute A19.1
    chronic A19.8
  muscle A18.09
  myelitis A17.82
  myocardium, myocarditis A18.84
  nasal (passage) (sinus) A15.8
  nasopharynx A15.8
  neck gland A18.2
  nephritis A18.11
  nerve (mononeuropathy) A17.83
  nervous system A17.9
  nose (septum) A15.8
  ocular A18.50
  omentum A18.31
  oophoritis (acute) (chronic) A18.17
  optic (nerve trunk) (papilla) A18.59
  orbit A18.59
  orchitis A18.15
  organ, specified NEC A18.89
  osseous — see Tuberculosis, bone
  osteitis — see Tuberculosis, bone
  osteomyelitis — see Tuberculosis, bone
  otitis media A18.6
  ovary, ovaritis (acute) (chronic) A18.17
  oviduct (acute) (chronic) A18.17
  pachymeningitis A17.0
  palate (soft) A18.83

Tuberculosis, tubercular, tuberculous
  (calcification) (calcified) (caseous)
  (chromogenic acid-fast bacilli)
  (degeneration) (fibrocaseous) (fistula)
  (interstitial) (isolated circumscribed lesions)
  (necrosis) (parenchymatous) (ulcerative)
  A15.9 — continued
  pancreas A18.83
  papulonecrotic(a) (primary) A18.4
  parathyroid glands A18.82
  paronychia (primary) A18.4
  parotid gland or region A18.83
  pelvis (bony) A18.03
  penis A18.15
  peribronchitis A15.5
  pericardium, pericarditis A18.84
  perichondritis, larynx A15.5
  periostitis — see Tuberculosis, bone
  perirectal fistula A18.32
  peritoneum NEC A18.31
  peritonitis A18.31
  pharynx, pharyngitis A15.8
  phlyctenulosis (keratoconjunctivitis) A18.52
  phthisis NEC — see Tuberculosis, pulmonary
  pituitary gland A18.82
  pleura, pleural, pleurisy, pleuritis (fibrinous)
    (obliterative) (purulent) (simple plastic)
    (with effusion) A15.6
    primary (progressive) A15.7
  pneumonia, pneumonic — see Tuberculosis,
    pulmonary
  pneumothorax (spontaneous) (tense valvular)
    — see Tuberculosis, pulmonary
  polyneuropathy A17.89
  polyserositis A19.9
    acute A19.1
    chronic A19.8
  potter's J65
  prepuce A18.15
  primary (complex) A15.7
  proctitis A18.32
  prostate, prostatitis A18.14
  pulmonalis — see Tuberculosis, pulmonary
  pulmonary (cavitated) (fibrotic) (infiltrative)
    (nodular) A15.0
    childhood type or first infection A15.7
    primary (complex) A15.7
  pyelitis A18.11
  pyelonephritis A18.11
  pyemia — see Tuberculosis, miliary
  pyonephrosis A18.11
  pyopneumothorax A15.6
  pyothorax A15.6
  rectum (fistula) (with abscess) A18.32
  reinfection stage — see Tuberculosis,
    pulmonary
  renal A18.11
  renis A18.11
  respiratory A15.9
    primary A15.7
    specified site NEC A15.8
  retina, retinitis A18.53
  retroperitoneal (lymph gland or node) A18.39
  rheumatism NEC A18.09
  rhinitis A15.8
  sacroiliac (joint) A18.01
  sacrum A18.01
  salivary gland A18.83
  salpingitis (acute) (chronic) A18.17
  sandblaster's J65
  sclera A18.51
  scoliosis A18.01
  scrofulous A18.2
  scrotum A18.15
  seminal tract or vesicle A18.15
  senile A15.9
  septic — see Tuberculosis, miliary
  shoulder (joint) A18.02
    blade A18.03

Tuberculosis, tubercular, tuberculous
  (calcification) (calcified) (caseous)
  (chromogenic acid-fast bacilli)
  (degeneration) (fibrocaseous) (fistula)
  (interstitial) (isolated circumscribed lesions)
  (necrosis) (parenchymatous) (ulcerative)
  A15.9 — continued
  sigmoid A18.32
  sinus (any nasal) A15.8
    bone A18.03
    epididymis A18.15
  skeletal NEC A18.03
  skin (any site) (primary) A18.4
  small intestine A18.32
  soft palate A18.83
  spermatic cord A18.15
  spine, spinal (column) A18.01
    cord A17.81
    medulla A17.81
    membrane A17.0
    meninges A17.0
  spleen, splenitis A18.85
  spondylitis A18.01
  sternoclavicular joint A18.02
  stomach A18.83
  stonemason's J65
  subcutaneous tissue (cellular) (primary) A18.4
  subcutis (primary) A18.4
  subdeltoid bursa A18.83
  submaxillary (region) A18.83
  supraclavicular gland A18.2
  suprarenal (capsule) (gland) A18.7
  swelling, joint (see also category M01) (see also
    Tuberculosis, joint) A18.02
  symphysis pubis A18.02
  synovitis A18.09
    articular A18.02
    spine or vertebra A18.01
  systemic — see Tuberculosis, miliary
  tarsitis A18.4
  tendon (sheath) — see Tuberculosis,
    tenosynovitis
  tenosynovitis A18.09
    spine or vertebra A18.01
  testis A18.15
  throat A15.8
  thymus gland A18.82
  thyroid gland A18.81
  tongue A18.83
  tonsil, tonsillitis A15.8
  trachea, tracheal A15.5
    lymph gland or node A15.4
      primary (progressive) A15.7
  tracheobronchial A15.5
    lymph gland or node A15.4
      primary (progressive) A15.7
  tubal (acute) (chronic) A18.17
  tunica vaginalis A18.15
  ulcer (skin) (primary) A18.4
    bowel or intestine A18.32
    specified NEC — code under Tuberculosis,
      by site
  unspecified site A15.9
  ureter A18.11
  urethra, urethral (gland) A18.13
  urinary organ or tract A18.13
  uterus A18.17
  uveal tract A18.54
  uvula A18.83
  vagina A18.18
  vas deferens A18.15
  verruca, verrucosa (cutis) (primary) A18.4
  vertebra (column) A18.01
  vesiculitis A18.15
  vulva A18.18
  wrist (joint) A18.02

Tuberculum
Carabelli — *see* Note at K00.2
occlusal — *see* Note at K00.2
paramolare K00.2
Tuberosity, enitre maxillary M26.07
Tuberous sclerosis (brain) Q85.1
Tubo-ovarian — *see* condition
Tuboplasty, after previous sterilization
Z31.0
aftercare Z31.42
Tubotympanitis, catarrhal (chronic) — *see*
Otitis, media, nonsuppurative, chronic,
serous
Tularemia A21.9
with
conjunctivitis A21.1
pneumonia A21.2
abdominal A21.3
bronchopneumonic A21.2
conjunctivitis A21.1
cryptogenic A21.3
enteric A21.3
gastrointestinal A21.3
generalized A21.7
ingestion A21.3
intestinal A21.3
oculoglandular A21.1
ophthalmic A21.1
pneumonia (any), pneumonic A21.2
pulmonary A21.2
sepsis A21.7
specified NEC A21.8
typhoidal A21.7
ulceroglandular A21.0
Tularensis conjunctivitis A21.1
Tumefaction — *see also* Swelling
liver — *see* Hypertrophy, liver
Tumor — *see also* Neoplasm, unspecified
behavior, by site
acinar cell — *see* Neoplasm, uncertain
behavior, by site
acinic cell — *see* Neoplasm, uncertain
behavior, by site
adenocarcinoid — *see* Neoplasm, malignant,
by site
adenomatoid — *see also* Neoplasm, benign, by
site
odontogenic — *see* Cyst, calcifying
odontogenic
adnexal (skin) — *see* Neoplasm, skin, benign,
by site
adrenal
cortical (benign) D35.0-
malignant C74.0-
rest — *see* Neoplasm, benign, by site
alpha-cell
malignant
pancreas C25.4
specified site NEC — *see* Neoplasm,
malignant, by site
unspecified site C25.4
pancreas D13.7
specified site NEC — *see* Neoplasm, benign,
by site
unspecified site D13.7
aneurysmal — *see* Aneurysm
aortic body D44.7
malignant C75.5
Askin's — *see* Neoplasm, connective tissue,
malignant
basal cell (*see also* Neoplasm, skin, uncertain
behavior) D48.5
Bednar — *see* Neoplasm, skin, malignant
benign (unclassified) — *see* Neoplasm, benign,
by site

Tumor (*see also* Neoplasm, unspecified behavior,
by site) — *continued*
beta-cell
malignant
pancreas C25.4
specified site NEC — *see* Neoplasm,
malignant, by site
unspecified site C25.4
pancreas D13.7
specified site NEC — *see* Neoplasm, benign,
by site
unspecified site D13.7
Brenner D27.9
borderline malignancy D39.1-
malignant C56-
proliferating D39.1-
bronchial alveolar, intravascular D38.1
Brooke's — *see* Neoplasm, skin, benign
brown fat — *see* Lipoma
Burkitt — *see* Lymphoma, Burkitt
calcifying epithelial odontogenic — *see* Cyst,
calcifying odontogenic
carcinoid
benign D3A.00 *(follows D36)*
appendix D3A.020 *(follows D36)*
ascending colon D3A.022 *(follows D36)*
bronchus (lung) D3A.090 *(follows D36)*
cecum D3A.021 *(follows D36)*
colon D3A.029 *(follows D36)*
descending colon D3A.024 *(follows D36)*
duodenum D3A.010 *(follows D36)*
foregut NOS D3A.094 *(follows D36)*
hindgut NOS D3A.096 *(follows D36)*
ileum D3A.012 *(follows D36)*
jejunum D3A.011 *(follows D36)*
kidney D3A.093 *(follows D36)*
large intestine D3A.029 *(follows D36)*
lung (bronchus) D3A.090 *(follows D36)*
midgut NOS D3A.095 *(follows D36)*
rectum D3A.026 *(follows D36)*
sigmoid colon D3A.025 *(follows D36)*
small intestine D3A.019 *(follows D36)*
specified NEC D3A.098 *(follows D36)*
stomach D3A.092 *(follows D36)*
thymus D3A.091 *(follows D36)*
transverse colon D3A.023 *(follows D36)*
malignant C7A.00 *(follows C75)*
appendix C7A.020 *(follows C75)*
ascending colon C7A.022 *(follows C75)*
bronchus (lung) C7A.090 *(follows C75)*
cecum C7A.021 *(follows C75)*
colon C7A.029 *(follows C75)*
descending colon C7A.024 *(follows C75)*
duodenum C7A.010 *(follows C75)*
foregut NOS C7A.094 *(follows C75)*
hindgut NOS C7A.096 *(follows C75)*
ileum C7A.012 *(follows C75)*
jejunum C7A.011 *(follows C75)*
kidney C7A.093 *(follows C75)*
large intestine C7A.029 *(follows C75)*
lung (bronchus) C7A.090 *(follows C75)*
midgut NOS C7A.095 *(follows C75)*
rectum C7A.026 *(follows C75)*
sigmoid colon C7A.025 *(follows C75)*
small intestine C7A.019 *(follows C75)*
specified NEC C7A.098 *(follows C75)*
stomach C7A.092 *(follows C75)*
thymus C7A.091 *(follows C75)*
transverse colon C7A.023 *(follows C75)*
mesentary metastasis C7B.04 *(follows C75)*
secondary C7B.00 *(follows C75)*
bone C7B.03 *(follows C75)*
distant lymph nodes C7B.01 *(follows C75)*
liver C7B.02 *(follows C75)*
peritoneum C7B.04 *(follows C75)*
specified NEC C7B.09 *(follows C75)*
carotid body D44.6
malignant C75.4

Tumor (*see also* Neoplasm, unspecified behavior,
by site) — *continued*
cells — *see also* Neoplasm, unspecified
behavior, by site
benign — *see* Neoplasm, benign, by site
malignant — *see* Neoplasm, malignant, by
site
uncertain whether benign or malignant —
see Neoplasm, uncertain behavior, by
site
cervix, in pregnancy or childbirth — *see*
Pregnancy, complicated by, tumor, cervix
chondromatous giant cell — *see* Neoplasm,
bone, benign
chromaffin — *see also* Neoplasm, benign, by
site
malignant — *see* Neoplasm, malignant, by
site
Cock's peculiar L72.3
Codman's — *see* Neoplasm, bone, benign
dentigerous, mixed — *see* Cyst, calcifying
odontogenic
dermoid — *see* Neoplasm, benign, by site
with malignant transformation C56-
desmoid (extra-abdominal) — *see also*
Neoplasm, connective tissue, uncertain
behavior
abdominal — *see* Neoplasm, connective
tissue, uncertain behavior
embolus — *see* Neoplasm, secondary, by site
embryonal (mixed) — *see also* Neoplasm,
uncertain behavior, by site
liver C22.7
endodermal sinus
specified site — *see* Neoplasm, malignant,
by site
unspecified site
female C56-
male C62.90
epithelial
benign — *see* Neoplasm, benign, by site
malignant — *see* Neoplasm, malignant, by
site
Ewing's — *see* Neoplasm, bone, malignant, by
site
fatty — *see* Lipoma
fibroid — *see* Leiomyoma
G cell
malignant
pancreas C25.4
specified site NEC — *see* Neoplasm,
malignant, by site
unspecified site C25.4
specified site — *see* Neoplasm, uncertain
behavior, by site
unspecified site D37.8
germ cell — *see also* Neoplasm, malignant, by
site
mixed — *see* Neoplasm, malignant, by site
ghost cell, odontogenic — *see* Cyst, calcifying
odontogenic
giant cell — *see also* Neoplasm, uncertain
behavior, by site
bone D48.0
malignant — *see* Neoplasm, bone,
malignant
chondromatous — *see* Neoplasm, bone,
benign
malignant — *see* Neoplasm, malignant, by
site
soft parts — *see* Neoplasm, connective
tissue, uncertain behavior
malignant — *see* Neoplasm, connective
tissue, malignant

Tumor (*see also* Neoplasm, unspecified behavior, by site) — *continued*
- glomus D18.00
  - intra-abdominal D18.03
  - intracranial D18.02
  - jugulare D44.7
    - malignant C75.5
  - skin D18.01
  - specified site NEC D18.09
- gonadal stromal — *see* Neoplasm, uncertain behavior, by site
- granular cell — *see also* Neoplasm, connective tissue, benign
  - malignant — *see* Neoplasm, connective tissue, malignant
- granulosa cell D39.1-
  - juvenile D39.1-
    - malignant C56-
- granulosa cell-theca cell D39.1-
  - malignant C56-
- Grawitz's C64-
- hemorrhoidal — *see* Hemorrhoids
- hilar cell D27-
- hilus cell D27-
- Hurthle cell (benign) D34
  - malignant C73
- hydatid — *see* Echinococcus
- hypernephroid — *see also* Neoplasm, uncertain behavior, by site
- interstitial cell — *see also* Neoplasm, uncertain behavior, by site
  - benign — *see* Neoplasm, benign, by site
  - malignant — *see* Neoplasm, malignant, by site
- intravascular bronchial alveolar D38.1
- islet cell — *see* Neoplasm, benign, by site
  - malignant — *see* Neoplasm, malignant, by site
    - pancreas C25.4
    - specified site NEC — *see* Neoplasm, malignant, by site
    - unspecified site C25.4
  - pancreas D13.7
  - specified site NEC — *see* Neoplasm, benign, by site
  - unspecified site D13.7
- juxtaglomerular D41.0-
- Klatskin's C24.0
- Krukenberg's C79.6-
- Leydig cell — *see* Neoplasm, uncertain behavior, by site
  - benign — *see* Neoplasm, benign, by site
    - specified site — *see* Neoplasm, benign, by site
    - unspecified site
      - female D27.9
      - male D29.20
  - malignant — *see* Neoplasm, malignant, by site
    - specified site — *see* Neoplasm, malignant, by site
    - unspecified site
      - female C56.9
      - male C62.90
  - specified site — *see* Neoplasm, uncertain behavior, by site
  - unspecified site
    - female D39.10
    - male D40.10
- lipid cell, ovary D27-
- lipoid cell, ovary D27-
- malignant (*see also* Neoplasm, malignant, by site) C80.1
  - fusiform cell (type) C80.1
  - giant cell (type) C80.1
  - localized, plasma cell — *see* Plasmacytoma, solitary
  - mixed NEC C80.1
  - small cell (type) C80.1

Tumor (*see also* Neoplasm, unspecified behavior, by site) — *continued*
- malignant (*see also* Neoplasm, malignant, by site) C80.1 — *continued*
  - spindle cell (type) C80.1
  - unclassified C80.1
- mast cell D47.0
  - malignant C96.2
- melanotic, neuroectodermal — *see* Neoplasm, benign, by site
- Merkel cell — *see* Carcinoma, Merkel cell
- mesenchymal
  - malignant — *see* Neoplasm, connective tissue, malignant
  - mixed — *see* Neoplasm, connective tissue, uncertain behavior
- mesodermal, mixed — *see also* Neoplasm, malignant, by site
  - liver C22.4
- mesonephric — *see also* Neoplasm, uncertain behavior, by site
  - malignant — *see* Neoplasm, malignant, by site
- metastatic
  - from specified site — *see* Neoplasm, malignant, by site
  - of specified site — *see* Neoplasm, malignant, by site
  - to specified site — *see* Neoplasm, secondary, by site
- mixed NEC — *see also* Neoplasm, benign, by site
  - malignant — *see* Neoplasm, malignant, by site
- mucinous of low malignant potential
  - specified site — *see* Neoplasm, malignant, by site
  - unspecified site C56.9
- mucocarcinoid
  - specified site — *see* Neoplasm, malignant, by site
  - unspecified site C18.1
- mucoepidermoid — *see* Neoplasm, uncertain behavior, by site
- Müllerian, mixed
  - specified site — *see* Neoplasm, malignant, by site
  - unspecified site C54.9
- myoepithelial — *see* Neoplasm, benign, by site
- neuroectodermal (peripheral) — *see* Neoplasm, malignant, by site
  - primitive
    - specified site — *see* Neoplasm, malignant, by site
    - unspecified site C71.9
- neuroendocrine D3A.8 *(follows D36)*
  - malignant poorly differentiated C7A.1 *(follows C75)*
  - secondary NEC C7B.8 *(follows C75)*
  - specified NEC C7A.8 *(follows C75)*
- neurogenic olfactory C30.0
- nonencapsulated sclerosing C73
- odontogenic (adenomatoid) (benign) (calcifying epithelial) (keratocystic) (squamous) — *see* Cyst, calcifying odontogenic
  - malignant C41.1
    - upper jaw (bone) C41.0
- ovarian stromal D39.1-
- ovary, in pregnancy — *see* Pregnancy, complicated by
- pacinian — *see* Neoplasm, skin, benign
- Pancoast's — *see* Pancoast's syndrome
- papillary — *see also* Papilloma
  - cystic D37.9
  - mucinous of low malignant potential C56-
    - specified site — *see* Neoplasm, malignant, by site
    - unspecified site C56.9

Tumor (*see also* Neoplasm, unspecified behavior, by site) — *continued*
- papillary — *see also* Papilloma — *continued*
  - serous of low malignant potential
    - specified site — *see* Neoplasm, malignant, by site
    - unspecified site C56.9
- pelvic, in pregnancy or childbirth — *see* Pregnancy, complicated by
- phantom F45.8
- phyllodes D48.6-
  - benign D24-
  - malignant — *see* Neoplasm, breast, malignant
- Pindborg — *see* Cyst, calcifying odontogenic
- placental site trophoblastic D39.2
- plasma cell (malignant) (localized) — *see* Plasmacytoma, solitary
- polyvesicular vitelline
  - specified site — *see* Neoplasm, malignant, by site
  - unspecified site
    - female C56.9
    - male C62.90
- Pott's puffy — *see* Osteomyelitis, specified NEC
- Rathke's pouch D44.3
- retinal anlage — *see* Neoplasm, benign, by site
- salivary gland type, mixed — *see* Neoplasm, salivary gland, benign
  - malignant — *see* Neoplasm, salivary gland, malignant
- Sampson's N80.1
- Schmincke's — *see* Neoplasm, nasopharynx, malignant
- sclerosing stromal D27-
- sebaceous — *see* Cyst, sebaceous
- secondary — *see* Neoplasm, secondary, by site
  - carcinoid C7B.00 *(follows C75)*
    - bone C7B.03 *(follows C75)*
    - distant lymph nodes C7B.01 *(follows C75)*
    - liver C7B.02 *(follows C75)*
    - peritoneum C7B.04 *(follows C75)*
    - specified NEC C7B.09 *(follows C75)*
  - neuroendocrine NEC C7B.8 *(follows C75)*
- serous of low malignant potential
  - specified site — *see* Neoplasm, malignant, by site
  - unspecified site C56.9
- Sertoli cell — *see* Neoplasm, benign, by site
  - with lipid storage
    - specified site — *see* Neoplasm, benign, by site
    - unspecified site
      - female D27.9
      - male D29.20
  - specified site — *see* Neoplasm, benign, by site
  - unspecified site
    - female D27.9
    - male D29.20
- Sertoli-Leydig cell — *see* Neoplasm, benign, by site
  - specified site — *see* Neoplasm, benign, by site
  - unspecified site
    - female D27.9
    - male D29.20
- sex cord(-stromal) — *see* Neoplasm, uncertain behavior, by site
  - with annular tubules D39.1-
- skin appendage — *see* Neoplasm, skin, benign
- smooth muscle — *see* Neoplasm, connective tissue, uncertain behavior

D I S E A S E   I N D E X

Tumor (see also Neoplasm, unspecified behavior, by site) — continued
- soft tissue
  - benign — see Neoplasm, connective tissue, benign
  - malignant — see Neoplasm, connective tissue, malignant
- sternomastoid (congenital) Q68.0
- stromal
  - endometrial D39.0
  - gastric D48.1
    - benign D21.4
    - malignant C16.9
    - uncertain behavior D48.1
  - gastrointestinal C49.A- (follows C49.9)
    - benign D21.4
    - esophagus C49.A1 (follows C49.9)
    - large intestine C49.A4 (follows C49.9)
    - malignant C49.A0 (follows C49.9)
      - colon C49.A4 (follows C49.9)
      - duodenum C49.A3 (follows C49.9)
      - esophagus C49.A1 (follows C49.9)
      - ileum C49.A3 (follows C49.9)
      - jejunum C49.A3 (follows C49.9)
      - Meckel diverticulum C49.A3 (follows C49.9)
      - large intestine C49.A4 (follows C49.9)
      - omentum C49.A9 (follows C49.9)
      - peritoneum C49.A9 (follows C49.9)
      - rectum C49.A5 (follows C49.9)
      - small intestine C49.A3 (follows C49.9)
      - specified site NEC C49.A9 (follows C49.9)
      - stomach C49.A2 (follows C49.9)
    - large intestine C49.A4 (follows C49.9)
    - rectum C49.A5 (follows C49.9)
    - small intestine C49.A3 (follows C49.9)
    - specified site NEC C49.A9 (follows C49.9)
    - stomach C49.A2 (follows C49.9)
    - uncertain behavior D48.1
  - intestine
    - benign D21.4
    - malignant
      - large C49.A4 (follows C49.9)
      - small C49.A3 (follows C49.9)
    - uncertain behavior D48.1
  - ovarian D39.1-
  - stomach C49.A2 (follows C49.9)
    - benign D21.4
    - malignant C49.A2 (follows C49.9)
    - uncertain behavior D48.1
- sweat gland — see also Neoplasm, skin, uncertain behavior
  - benign — see Neoplasm, skin, benign
  - malignant — see Neoplasm, skin, malignant
- syphilitic, brain A52.17
- testicular D40.10
- testicular stromal D40.1-
- theca cell D27-
- theca cell-granulosa cell D39.1-
- Triton, malignant — see Neoplasm, nerve, malignant
- trophoblastic, placental site D39.2
- turban D23.4
- uterus (body), in pregnancy or childbirth — see Pregnancy, complicated by, tumor, uterus
- vagina, in pregnancy or childbirth — see Pregnancy, complicated by
- varicose — see Varix
- von Recklinghausen's — see Neurofibromatosis
- vulva or perineum, in pregnancy or childbirth — see Pregnancy, complicated by
  - causing obstructed labor O65.5
- Warthin's — see Neoplasm, salivary gland, benign
- Wilms' C64-

Tumor (see also Neoplasm, unspecified behavior, by site) — continued
- yolk sac — see Neoplasm, malignant, by site
  - specified site — see Neoplasm, malignant, by site
  - unspecified site
    - female C56.9
    - male C62.90

Tumor lysis syndrome (following antineoplastic chemotherapy) (spontaneous) NEC E88.3

Tumorlet — see Neoplasm, uncertain behavior, by site

Tungiasis B88.1

Tunica vasculosa lentis Q12.2

Turban tumor D23.4

Türck's trachoma J37.0

Turner's
- hypoplasia (tooth) K00.4
- syndrome Q96.9
  - specified NEC Q96.8
- tooth K00.4

Turner-Kieser syndrome Q87.2

Turner-like syndrome Q87.1

Turner-Ullrich syndrome Q96.9

Tussis convulsiva — see Whooping cough

Twiddler's syndrome (due to)
- automatic implantable defibrillator T82.198
- cardiac pacemaker T82.198

Twilight state
- epileptic F05
- psychogenic F44.89

Twin (newborn) — see also Newborn, twin
- conjoined Q89.4
- pregnancy — see Pregnancy, twin, conjoined

Twinning, teeth K00.2

Twist, twisted
- bowel, colon or intestine K56.2
- hair (congenital) Q84.1
- mesentery K56.2
- omentum K56.2
- organ or site, congenital NEC — see Anomaly, by site
- ovarian pedicle — see Torsion, ovary

Twitching R25.3

Tylosis (acquired) L84
- buccalis K13.29
- linguae K13.29
- palmaris et plantaris (congenital) (inherited) Q82.8
- acquired L85.1

Tympanism R14.0

Tympanites (abdominal) (intestinal) R14.0

Tympanitis — see Myringitis

Tympanosclerosis — see subcategory H74.0

Tympanum — see condition

Tympany
- abdomen R14.0
- chest R09.89

Type A behavior pattern Z73.1

Typhlitis — see Appendicitis

Typhoenteritis — see Typhoid

Typhoid (abortive) (ambulant) (any site) (clinical) (fever) (hemorrhagic) (infection) (intermittent) (malignant) (rheumatic) (Widal negative) A01.00
- with pneumonia A01.03
- abdominal A01.09
- arthritis A01.04
- carrier (suspected) of Z22.0
- cholecystitis (current) A01.09
- endocarditis A01.02
- heart involvement A01.02
- inoculation reaction — see Complications, vaccination

Typhoid (abortive) (ambulant) (any site) (clinical) (fever) (hemorrhagic) (infection) (intermittent) (malignant) (rheumatic) (Widal negative) A01.00 — continued
- meningitis A01.01
- mesenteric lymph nodes A01.09
- myocarditis A01.02
- osteomyelitis A01.05
- perichondritis, larynx A01.09
- pneumonia A01.03
- specified NEC A01.09
- spine A01.05
- ulcer (perforating) A01.09

Typhomalaria (fever) — see Malaria

Typhomania A01.00

Typhoperitonitis A01.09

Typhus (fever) A75.9
- abdominal, abdominalis — see Typhoid
- African tick A77.1
- amarillic A95.9
- brain A75.9 [G94]
- cerebral A75.9 [G94]
- classical A75.0
- due to Rickettsia
  - prowazekii A75.0
    - recrudescent A75.1
  - tsutsugamushi A75.3
  - typhi A75.2
- endemic (flea-borne) A75.2
- epidemic (louse-borne) A75.0
- exanthematic NEC A75.0
- exanthematicus SAI A75.0
  - brillii SAI A75.1
  - mexicanus SAI A75.2
  - typhus murinus A75.2
- flea-borne A75.2
- India tick A77.1
- Kenya (tick) A77.1
- louse-borne A75.0
- Mexican A75.2
- mite-borne A75.3
- murine A75.2
- North Asian tick-borne A77.2
- petechial A75.9
- Queensland tick A77.3
- rat A75.2
- recrudescent A75.1
- recurrens — see Fever, relapsing
- Sao Paulo A77.0
- scrub (China) (India) (Malaysia) (New Guinea) A75.3
- shop (of Malaysia) A75.2
- Siberian tick A77.2
- tick-borne A77.9
- tropical (mite-borne) A75.3

Tyrosinemia E70.21
- newborn, transitory P74.5

Tyrosinosis E70.21

Tyrosinuria E70.29

U

Uhl's anomaly or disease Q24.8
Ulcer, ulcerated, ulcerating, ulceration, ulcerative
alveolar process M27.3
amebic (intestine) A06.1
skin A06.7
anastomotic — see Ulcer, gastrojejunal
anorectal K62.6
antral — see Ulcer, stomach
anus (sphincter) (solitary) K62.6
aorta — see Aneurysm
aphthous (oral) (recurrent) K12.0
genital organ(s)
female N76.6
male N50.89
artery I77.2
atrophic — see Ulcer, skin
decubitus — see Ulcer, pressure, by site
back L98.429
with
bone necrosis L98.424
exposed fat layer L98.422
muscle necrosis L98.423
skin breakdown only L98.421
Barrett's (esophagus) K22.10
with bleeding K22.11
bile duct (common) (hepatic) K83.8
bladder (solitary) (sphincter) NEC N32.89
bilharzial B65.9 [N33]
in schistosomiasis (bilharzial) B65.9 [N33]
submucosal — see Cystitis, interstitial
tuberculous A18.12
bleeding K27.4
bone — see Osteomyelitis, specified type NEC
bowel — see Ulcer, intestine
breast N61.1
bronchus J98.09
buccal (cavity) (traumatic) K12.1
Buruli A31.1
buttock L98.419
with
bone necrosis L98.414
exposed fat layer L98.412
muscle necrosis L98.413
skin breakdown only L98.411
cancerous — see Neoplasm, malignant, by site
cardia K22.10
with bleeding K22.11
cardioesophageal (peptic) K22.10
with bleeding K22.11
cecum — see Ulcer, intestine
cervix (uteri) (decubitus) (trophic) N86
with cervicitis N72
chancroidal A57
chiclero B55.1
chronic (cause unknown) — see Ulcer, skin
Cochin-China B55.1
colon — see Ulcer, intestine
conjunctiva H10.89
cornea H16.00-
with hypopyon H16.03-
central H16.01-
dendritic (herpes simplex) B00.52
marginal H16.04-
Mooren's H16.05-
mycotic H16.06-
perforated H16.07-
ring H16.02-
tuberculous (phlyctenular) A18.52
corpus cavernosum (chronic) N48.5
crural — see Ulcer, lower limb
Curling's — see Ulcer, peptic, acute
Cushing's — see Ulcer, peptic, acute
cystic duct K82.8
cystitis (interstitial) — see Cystitis, interstitial

Ulcer, ulcerated, ulcerating, ulceration, ulcerative — continued
decubitus — see Ulcer, pressure, by site
dendritic, cornea (herpes simplex) B00.52
diabetes, diabetic — see Diabetes, ulcer
Dieulafoy's K25.0
due to
infection NEC — see Ulcer, skin
radiation NEC L59.8
trophic disturbance (any region) — see Ulcer, skin
X-ray L58.1
duodenum, duodenal (eroded) (peptic) K26.9
with
hemorrhage K26.4
and perforation K26.6
perforation K26.5
acute K26.3
with
hemorrhage K26.0
and perforation K26.2
perforation K26.1
chronic K26.7
with
hemorrhage K26.4
and perforation K26.6
perforation K26.5
dysenteric A09
elusive — see Cystitis, interstitial
endocarditis (acute) (chronic) (subacute) I28.8
epiglottis J38.7
esophagus (peptic) K22.10
with bleeding K22.11
due to
aspirin K22.10
with bleeding K22.11
gastrointestinal reflux disease K21.0
ingestion of chemical or medicament K22.10
with bleeding K22.11
fungal K22.10
with bleeding K22.11
infective K22.10
with bleeding K22.11
varicose — see Varix, esophagus
eyelid (region) H01.8
fauces J39.2
Fenwick (-Hunner) (solitary) — see Cystitis, interstitial
fistulous — see Ulcer, skin
foot (indolent) (trophic) — see Ulcer, lower limb
frambesial, initial A66.0
frenum (tongue) K14.0
gallbladder or duct K82.8
gangrenous — see Gangrene
gastric — see Ulcer, stomach
gastrocolic — see Ulcer, gastrojejunal
gastroduodenal — see Ulcer, peptic
gastroesophageal — see Ulcer, stomach
gastrointestinal — see Ulcer, gastrojejunal
gastrojejunal (peptic) K28.9
with
hemorrhage K28.4
and perforation K28.6
perforation K28.5
acute K28.3
with
hemorrhage K28.0
and perforation K28.2
perforation K28.1
chronic K28.7
with
hemorrhage K28.4
and perforation K28.6
perforation K28.5
gastrojejunocolic — see Ulcer, gastrojejunal
gingiva K06.8

Ulcer, ulcerated, ulcerating, ulceration, ulcerative — continued
gingivitis K05.10
nonplaque induced K05.11
plaque induced K05.10
glottis J38.7
granuloma of pudenda A58
gum K06.8
gumma, due to yaws A66.4
heel — see Ulcer, lower limb
hemorrhoid (see also Hemorrhoids, by degree) K64.8
Hunner's — see Cystitis, interstitial
hypopharynx J39.2
hypopyon (chronic) (subacute) — see Ulcer, cornea, with hypopyon
hypostaticum — see Ulcer, varicose
ileum — see Ulcer, intestine
intestine, intestinal K63.3
with perforation K63.1
amebic A06.1
duodenal — see Ulcer, duodenum
granulocytopenic (with hemorrhage) — see Neutropenia
marginal — see Ulcer, gastrojejunal
perforating K63.1
newborn P78.0
primary, small intestine K63.3
rectum K62.6
stercoraceous, stercoral K63.3
tuberculous A18.32
typhoid (fever) — see Typhoid
varicose I86.8
jejunum, jejunal — see Ulcer, gastrojejunal
keratitis — see Ulcer, cornea
knee — see Ulcer, lower limb
labium (majus) (minus) N76.6
laryngitis — see Laryngitis
larynx (aphthous) (contact) J38.7
diphtheritic A36.2
leg — see Ulcer, lower limb
lip K13.0
Lipschütz's N76.6
lower limb (atrophic) (chronic) (neurogenic) (perforating) (pyogenic) (trophic) (tropical) L97.909
with
bone necrosis L97.904
exposed fat layer L97.902
muscle necrosis L97.903
skin breakdown only L97.901
ankle L97.309
with
bone necrosis L97.304
exposed fat layer L97.302
muscle necrosis L97.303
skin breakdown only L97.301
left L97.329
with
bone necrosis L97.324
exposed fat layer L97.322
muscle necrosis L97.323
skin breakdown only L97.321
right L97.319
with
bone necrosis L97.314
exposed fat layer L97.312
muscle necrosis L97.313
skin breakdown only L97.311
calf L97.209
with
bone necrosis L97.204
exposed fat layer L97.202
muscle necrosis L97.203
skin breakdown only L97.201

Ulcer, ulcerated, ulcerating, ulceration, ulcerative — *continued*
 lower limb (atrophic) (chronic) (neurogenic) (perforating) (pyogenic) (trophic) (tropical) L97.909 — *continued*
  calf L97.209 — *continued*
   left L97.229
    with
     bone necrosis L97.224
     exposed fat layer L97.222
     muscle necrosis L97.223
     skin breakdown only L97.221
   right L97.219
    with
     bone necrosis L97.214
     exposed fat layer L97.212
     muscle necrosis L97.213
     skin breakdown only L97.211
  decubitus — *see* Ulcer, pressure, by site
  foot specified NEC L97.509
   with
    bone necrosis L97.504
    exposed fat layer L97.502
    muscle necrosis L97.503
    skin breakdown only L97.501
   left L97.529
    with
     bone necrosis L97.524
     exposed fat layer L97.522
     muscle necrosis L97.523
     skin breakdown only L97.521
   right L97.519
    with
     bone necrosis L97.514
     exposed fat layer L97.512
     muscle necrosis L97.513
     skin breakdown only L97.511
  heel L97.409
   with
    bone necrosis L97.404
    exposed fat layer L97.402
    muscle necrosis L97.403
    skin breakdown only L97.401
   left L97.429
    with
     bone necrosis L97.424
     exposed fat layer L97.422
     muscle necrosis L97.423
     skin breakdown only L97.421
   right L97.419
    with
     bone necrosis L97.414
     exposed fat layer L97.412
     muscle necrosis L97.413
     skin breakdown only L97.411
  left L97.929
   with
    bone necrosis L97.924
    exposed fat layer L97.922
    muscle necrosis L97.923
    skin breakdown only L97.921
  leprous A30.1
  lower leg NOS L97.909
   with
    bone necrosis L97.904
    exposed fat layer L97.902
    muscle necrosis L97.903
    skin breakdown only L97.901
   left L97.929
    with
     bone necrosis L97.924
     exposed fat layer L97.922
     muscle necrosis L97.923
     skin breakdown only L97.921

Ulcer, ulcerated, ulcerating, ulceration, ulcerative — *continued*
 lower limb (atrophic) (chronic) (neurogenic) (perforating) (pyogenic) (trophic) (tropical) L97.909 — *continued*
  lower leg NOS L97.909 — *continued*
   right L97.919
    with
     bone necrosis L97.914
     exposed fat layer L97.912
     muscle necrosis L97.913
     skin breakdown only L97.911
  specified site NEC L97.809
   with
    bone necrosis L97.804
    exposed fat layer L97.802
    muscle necrosis L97.803
    skin breakdown only L97.801
   left L97.829
    with
     bone necrosis L97.824
     exposed fat layer L97.822
     muscle necrosis L97.823
     skin breakdown only L97.821
   right L97.819
    with
     bone necrosis L97.814
     exposed fat layer L97.812
     muscle necrosis L97.813
     skin breakdown only L97.811
  midfoot L97.409
   with
    bone necrosis L97.404
    exposed fat layer L97.402
    muscle necrosis L97.403
    skin breakdown only L97.401
   left L97.429
    with
     bone necrosis L97.424
     exposed fat layer L97.422
     muscle necrosis L97.423
     skin breakdown only L97.421
   right L97.419
    with
     bone necrosis L97.414
     exposed fat layer L97.412
     muscle necrosis L97.413
     skin breakdown only L97.411
  right L97.919
   with
    bone necrosis L97.914
    exposed fat layer L97.912
    muscle necrosis L97.913
    skin breakdown only L97.911
  syphilitic A52.19
  thigh L97.109
   with
    bone necrosis L97.104
    exposed fat layer L97.102
    muscle necrosis L97.103
    skin breakdown only L97.101
   left L97.129
    with
     bone necrosis L97.124
     exposed fat layer L97.122
     muscle necrosis L97.123
     skin breakdown only L97.121
   right L97.119
    with
     bone necrosis L97.114
     exposed fat layer L97.112
     muscle necrosis L97.113
     skin breakdown only L97.111

Ulcer, ulcerated, ulcerating, ulceration, ulcerative — *continued*
 lower limb (atrophic) (chronic) (neurogenic) (perforating) (pyogenic) (trophic) (tropical) L97.909 — *continued*
  toe L97.509
   with
    bone necrosis L97.504
    exposed fat layer L97.502
    muscle necrosis L97.503
    skin breakdown only L97.501
   left L97.529
    with
     bone necrosis L97.524
     exposed fat layer L97.522
     muscle necrosis L97.523
     skin breakdown only L97.521
   right L97.519
    with
     bone necrosis L97.514
     exposed fat layer L97.512
     muscle necrosis L97.513
     skin breakdown only L97.511
  varicose — *see* Varix, leg, with, ulcer
 luetic — *see* Ulcer, syphilitic
 lung J98.4
  tuberculous — *see* Tuberculosis, pulmonary
 malignant — *see* Neoplasm, malignant, by site
 marginal NEC — *see* Ulcer, gastrojejunal
 meatus (urinarius) N34.2
 Meckel's diverticulum Q43.0
  malignant — *see* Table of Neoplasms, small intestine, malignant
 Meleney's (chronic undermining) — *see* Ulcer, skin
 Mooren's (cornea) — *see* Ulcer, cornea, Mooren's
 mycobacterial (skin) A31.1
 nasopharynx J39.2
 neck, uterus N86
 neurogenic NEC — *see* Ulcer, skin
 nose, nasal (passage) (infective) (septum) J34.0
  skin — *see* Ulcer, skin
  spirochetal A69.8
  varicose (bleeding) I86.8
 oral mucosa (traumatic) K12.1
 palate (soft) K12.1
 penis (chronic) N48.5
 peptic (site unspecified) K27.9
  with
   hemorrhage K27.4
    and perforation K27.6
   perforation K27.5
  acute K27.3
   with
    hemorrhage K27.0
     and perforation K27.2
    perforation K27.1
  chronic K27.7
   with
    hemorrhage K27.4
     and perforation K27.6
    perforation K27.5
  esophagus K22.10
   with bleeding K22.11
  newborn P78.82
  perforating K27.5
 skin — *see* Ulcer, skin
 peritonsillar J35.8
 phagedenic (tropical) — *see* Ulcer, skin
 pharynx J39.2
 phlebitis — *see* Phlebitis
 plaster — *see* Ulcer, pressure, by site
 popliteal space — *see* Ulcer, lower limb
 postpyloric — *see* Ulcer, duodenum
 prepuce N47.7
 prepyloric — *see* Ulcer, stomach

© 2016 Channel Publishing, Ltd.

Ulcer, ulcerated, ulcerating, ulceration, ulcerative — *continued*
  pressure (pressure area) L89.9-
    ankle L89.5-
    back L89.1-
    buttock L89.3-
    coccyx L89.15-
    contiguous site of back, buttock, hip L89.4-
    elbow L89.0-
    face L89.81-
    head L89.81-
    heel L89.6-
    hip L89.2-
    sacral region (tailbone) L89.15-
    specified site NEC L89.89-
    stage 1 (healing) (pre-ulcer skin changes limited to persistent focal edema)
      ankle L89.5-
      back L89.1-
      buttock L89.3-
      coccyx L89.15-
      contiguous site of back, buttock, hip L89.4-
      elbow L89.0-
      face L89.81-
      head L89.81-
      heel L89.6-
      hip L89.2-
      sacral region (tailbone) L89.15-
      specified site NEC L89.89-
    stage 2 (healing) (abrasion, blister, partial thickness skin loss involving epidermis and/or dermis)
      ankle L89.5-
      back L89.1-
      buttock L89.3-
      coccyx L89.15-
      contiguous site of back, buttock, hip L89.4-
      elbow L89.0-
      face L89.81-
      head L89.81-
      heel L89.6-
      hip L89.2-
      sacral region (tailbone) L89.15-
      specified site NEC L89.89-
    stage 3 (healing) (full thickness skin loss involving damage or necrosis of subcutaneous tissue)
      ankle L89.5-
      back L89.1-
      buttock L89.3-
      coccyx L89.15-
      contiguous site of back, buttock, hip L89.4-
      elbow L89.0-
      face L89.81-
      head L89.81-
      heel L89.6-
      hip L89.2-
      sacral region (tailbone) L89.15-
      specified site NEC L89.89-
    stage 4 (healing) (necrosis of soft tissues through to underlying muscle, tendon, or bone)
      ankle L89.5-
      back L89.1-
      buttock L89.3-
      coccyx L89.15-
      contiguous site of back, buttock, hip L89.4-
      elbow L89.0-
      face L89.81-
      head L89.81-
      heel L89.6-
      hip L89.2-
      sacral region (tailbone) L89.15-
      specified site NEC L89.89-

Ulcer, ulcerated, ulcerating, ulceration, ulcerative — *continued*
  pressure (pressure area) L89.9- — *continued*
    unspecified stage
      ankle L89.5-
      back L89.1-
      buttock L89.3-
      coccyx L89.15-
      contiguous site of back, buttock, hip L89.4-
      elbow L89.0-
      face L89.81-
      head L89.81-
      heel L89.6-
      hip L89.2-
      sacral region (tailbone) L89.15-
      specified site NEC L89.89-
    unstageable
      ankle L89.5-
      back L89.1-
      buttock L89.3-
      coccyx L89.15-
      contiguous site of back, buttock, hip L89.4-
      elbow L89.0-
      face L89.81-
      head L89.81-
      heel L89.6-
      hip L89.2-
      sacral region (tailbone) L89.15-
      specified site NEC L89.89-
  primary of intestine K63.3
    with perforation K63.1
  prostate N41.9
  pyloric — *see* Ulcer, stomach
  rectosigmoid K63.3
    with perforation K63.1
  rectum (sphincter) (solitary) K62.6
    stercoraceous, stercoral K62.6
  retina — *see* Inflammation, chorioretinal
  rodent — *see also* Neoplasm, skin, malignant
  sclera — *see* Scleritis
  scrofulous (tuberculous) A18.2
  scrotum N50.89
    tuberculous A18.15
    varicose I86.1
  seminal vesicle N50.89
  sigmoid — *see* Ulcer, intestine
  skin (atrophic) (chronic) (neurogenic) (non-healing) (perforating) (pyogenic) (trophic) (tropical) L98.499
    with gangrene — *see* Gangrene
    amebic A06.7
    back — *see* Ulcer, back
    buttock — *see* Ulcer, buttock
    decubitus — *see* Ulcer, pressure
    lower limb — *see* Ulcer, lower limb
    mycobacterial A31.1
    specified site NEC L98.499
      with
        bone necrosis L98.494
        exposed fat layer L98.492
        muscle necrosis L98.493
        skin breakdown only L98.491
    tuberculous (primary) A18.4
    varicose — *see* Ulcer, varicose
  sloughing — *see* Ulcer, skin
  solitary, anus or rectum (sphincter) K62.6
  sore throat J02.9
    streptococcal J02.0
  spermatic cord N50.89
  spine (tuberculous) A18.01
  stasis (venous) — *see* Varix, leg, with, ulcer
    without varicose veins I87.2
  stercoraceous, stercoral K63.3
    with perforation K63.1
    anus or rectum K62.6
  stoma, stomal — *see* Ulcer, gastrojejunal

Ulcer, ulcerated, ulcerating, ulceration, ulcerative — *continued*
  stomach (eroded) (peptic) (round) K25.9
    with
      hemorrhage K25.4
        and perforation K25.6
      perforation K25.5
    acute K25.3
      with
        hemorrhage K25.0
          and perforation K25.2
        perforation K25.1
    chronic K25.7
      with
        hemorrhage K25.4
          and perforation K25.6
        perforation K25.5
  stomal — *see* Ulcer, gastrojejunal
  stomatitis K12.1
  stress — *see* Ulcer, peptic
  strumous (tuberculous) A18.2
  submucosal, bladder — *see* Cystitis, interstitial
  syphilitic (any site) (early) (secondary) A51.39
    late A52.79
      perforating A52.79
        foot A52.11
  testis N50.89
  thigh — *see* Ulcer, lower limb
  throat J39.2
    diphtheritic A36.0
  toe — *see* Ulcer, lower limb
  tongue (traumatic) K14.0
  tonsil J35.8
    diphtheritic A36.0
  trachea J39.8
  trophic — *see* Ulcer, skin
  tropical — *see* Ulcer, skin
  tuberculous — *see* Tuberculosis, ulcer
  tunica vaginalis N50.89
  turbinate J34.89
  typhoid (perforating) — *see* Typhoid
  unspecified site — *see* Ulcer, skin
  urethra (meatus) — *see* Urethritis
  uterus N85.8
    cervix N86
      with cervicitis N72
    neck N86
      with cervicitis N72
  vagina N76.5
    in Behçet's disease M35.2 [N77.0]
    pessary N89.8
  valve, heart I33.0
  varicose (lower limb, any part) — *see also* Varix, leg, with, ulcer
    broad ligament I86.2
    esophagus — *see* Varix, esophagus
    inflamed or infected — *see* Varix, leg, with, ulcer, with inflammation
    nasal septum I86.8
    perineum I86.3
    scrotum I86.1
    specified site NEC I86.8
    sublingual I86.0
    vulva I86.3
  vas deferens N50.89
  vulva (acute) (infectional) N76.6
    in (due to)
      Behçet's disease M35.2 [N77.0]
      herpesviral (herpes simplex) infection A60.04
      tuberculosis A18.18
  vulvobuccal, recurring N76.6
  X-ray L58.1
  yaws A66.4

Ulcerosa scarlatina A38.8
Ulcus — *see also* Ulcer
  cutis tuberculosum A18.4
  duodeni — *see* Ulcer, duodenum
  durum (syphilitic) A51.0
    extragenital A51.2
  gastrojejunale — *see* Ulcer, gastrojejunal
  hypostaticum — *see* Ulcer, varicose
  molle (cutis) (skin) A57
  serpens corneae — *see* Ulcer, cornea, central
  ventriculi — *see* Ulcer, stomach
Ulegyria Q04.8
Ulerythema
  ophryogenes, congenital Q84.2
  sycosiforme L73.8
Ullrich(-Bonnevie)(-Turner) syndrome (*see also* Turner's syndrome) Q87.1
Ullrich-Feichtiger syndrome Q87.0
Ulnar — *see* condition
Ulorrhagia, ulorrhea K06.8
Umbilicus, umbilical — *see* condition
Unacceptable
  contours of tooth K08.54
  morphology of tooth K08.54
Unavailability (of)
  bed at medical facility Z75.1
  health service-related agencies Z75.4
  medical facilities (at) Z75.3
    due to
      investigation by social service agency Z75.2
      lack of services at home Z75.0
      remoteness from facility Z75.3
      waiting list Z75.1
    home Z75.0
    outpatient clinic Z75.3
  schooling Z55.1
  social service agencies Z75.4
Uncinaria americana infestation B76.1
Uncinariasis B76.9
Uncongenial work Z56.5
Unconscious(ness) — *see* Coma
Under observation — *see* Observation
Underachievement in school Z55.3
Underdevelopment — *see also* Undeveloped
  nose Q30.1
  sexual E30.0
Underdosing (*see also* Table of Drugs and Chemicals, categories T36-T50, with final character 6) Z91.14
  intentional NEC Z91.128
    due to financial hardship of patient Z91.120
  unintentional NEC Z91.138
    due to patient's age related debility Z91.130
Underfeeding, newborn P92.3
Underfill, endodontic M27.53
Underimmunization status Z28.3
Undernourishment — *see* Malnutrition
Undernutrition — *see* Malnutrition
Underweight R63.6
  for gestational age — *see* Light for dates
Underwood's disease P83.0
Undescended — *see also* Malposition, congenital
  cecum Q43.3
  colon Q43.3
  testicle — *see* Cryptorchid
Undeveloped, undevelopment — *see also* Hypoplasia
  brain (congenital) Q02
  cerebral (congenital) Q02
  heart Q24.8
  lung Q33.6
  testis E29.1
  uterus E30.0
Undiagnosed (disease) R69
Undulant fever — *see* Brucellosis
Unemployment, anxiety concerning Z56.0
  threatened Z56.2

Unequal length (acquired) (limb) — *see also* Deformity, limb, unequal length
  leg — *see also* Deformity, limb, unequal length
  congenital Q72.9-
Unextracted dental root K08.3
Unguis incarnatus L60.0
Unhappiness R45.2
Unicornate uterus Q51.4
Unilateral — *see also* condition
  development, breast N64.89
  organ or site, congenital NEC — *see* Agenesis, by site
Unilocular heart Q20.8
Union, abnormal — *see also* Fusion
  larynx and trachea Q34.8
Universal mesentery Q43.3
Unrepairable overhanging of dental restorative materials K08.52
Unsatisfactory
  restoration of tooth K08.50
    specified NEC K08.59
  sample of cytologic smear
    anus R85.615
    cervix R87.615
    vagina R87.625
  surroundings Z59.1
  work Z56.5
Unsoundness of mind — *see* Psychosis
Unstable
  back NEC — *see* Instability, joint, spine
  hip (congenital) Q65.6
    acquired — *see* Derangement, joint, specified type NEC, hip
  joint — *see* Instability, joint
    secondary to removal of joint prosthesis M96.89
  lie (mother) O32.0
  lumbosacral joint (congenital)
    acquired — *see* subcategory M53.2
  sacroiliac — *see* subcategory M53.2
  spine NEC — *see* Instability, joint, spine
Unsteadiness on feet R26.81
Untruthfulness, child problem F91.8
Unverricht(-Lundborg) disease or epilepsy — *see* Epilepsy, generalized, idiopathic
Unwanted pregnancy Z64.0
Upbringing, institutional Z62.22
  away from parents NEC Z62.29
  in care of non-parental family member Z62.21
  in foster care Z62.21
  in orphanage or group home Z62.22
  in welfare custody Z62.21
Upper respiratory — *see* condition
Upset
  gastric K30
  gastrointestinal K30
    psychogenic F45.8
  intestinal (large) (small) K59.9
    psychogenic F45.8
  menstruation N93.9
  mental F48.9
  stomach K30
    psychogenic F45.8
Urachus — *see also* condition
  patent or persistent Q64.4
Urbach-Oppenheim disease (necrobiosis lipoidica diabeticorum) — *see* E08-E13 with .620
Urbach's lipoid proteinosis E78.89
Urbach-Wiethe disease E78.89
Urban yellow fever A95.1
Urea
  blood, high — *see* Uremia
  cycle metabolism disorder — *see* Disorder, urea cycle metabolism

Uremia, uremic N19
  with
    ectopic or molar pregnancy O08.4
    polyneuropathy N18.9 *[G63]*
  chronic (*see also* Disease, kidney, chronic) N18.9
    due to hypertension — *see* Hypertensive, kidney
  complicating
    ectopic or molar pregnancy O08.4
  congenital P96.0
  extrarenal R39.2
  following ectopic or molar pregnancy O08.4
  newborn P96.0
  prerenal R39.2
Ureter, ureteral — *see* condition
Ureteralgia N23
Ureterectasis — *see* Hydroureter
Ureteritis N28.89
  cystica N28.86
  due to calculus N20.1
    with calculus, kidney N20.2
      with hydronephrosis N13.2
  gonococcal (acute) (chronic) A54.21
  nonspecific N28.89
Ureterocele N28.89
  congenital (orthotopic) Q62.31
  ectopic Q62.32
Ureterolith, ureterolithiasis — *see* Calculus, ureter
Ureterostomy
  attention to Z43.6
  status Z93.6
Urethra, urethral — *see* condition
Urethralgia R39.89
Urethritis (anterior) (posterior) N34.2
  calculous N21.1
  candidal B37.41
  chlamydial A56.01
  diplococcal (gonococcal) A54.01
    with abscess (accessory gland) (periurethral) A54.1
  gonococcal A54.01
    with abscess (accessory gland) (periurethral) A54.1
  nongonococcal N34.1
    Reiter's — *see* Reiter's disease
  nonspecific N34.1
  nonvenereal N34.1
  postmenopausal N34.2
  puerperal O86.22
  Reiter's — *see* Reiter's disease
  specified NEC N34.2
  trichomonal or due to Trichomonas (vaginalis) A59.03
Urethrocele N81.0
  with
    cystocele — *see* Cystocele
    prolapse of uterus — *see* Prolapse, uterus
Urethrolithiasis (with colic or infection) N21.1
Urethrorectal — *see* condition
Urethrorrhagia N36.8
Urethrorrhea R36.9
Urethrostomy
  attention to Z43.6
  status Z93.6
Urethrotrigonitis — *see* Trigonitis
Urethrovaginal — *see* condition
Urgency
  fecal R15.2
  hypertensive — *see* Hypertension
  urinary R39.15
Urhidrosis, uridrosis L74.8
Uric acid in blood (increased) E79.0
Uricacidemia (asymptomatic) E79.0
Uricemia (asymptomatic) E79.0
Uricosuria R82.99
Urinary — *see* condition

DISEASE INDEX

Urination
  frequent R35.0
  painful R30.9
Urine
  blood in — *see* Hematuria
  discharge, excessive R35.8
  enuresis, nonorganic origin F98.0
  extravasation R39.0
  frequency R35.0
  incontinence R32
    nonorganic origin F98.0
  intermittent stream R39.198
  pus in N39.0
  retention or stasis R33.9
    organic R33.8
      drug-induced R33.0
    psychogenic F45.8
  secretion
    deficient R34
    excessive R35.8
    frequency R35.0
  stream
    intermittent R39.198
    slowing R39.198
    splitting R39.13
    weak R39.12
Urinemia — *see* Uremia
Urinoma, urethra N36.8
Uroarthritis, infectious (Reiter's) — *see*
  Reiter's disease
Urodialysis R34
Urolithiasis — *see* Calculus, urinary
Uronephrosis — *see* Hydronephrosis
Uropathy N39.9
  obstructive N13.9
    specified NEC N13.8
  reflux N13.9
    specified NEC N13.8
  vesicoureteral reflux-associated — *see* Reflux,
    vesicoureteral
Urosepsis — *code to* condition
Urticaria L50.9
  with angioneurotic edema T78.3
    hereditary D84.1
  allergic L50.0
  cholinergic L50.5
  chronic L50.8
  cold, familial L50.2
  contact L50.6
  dermatographic L50.3
  due to
    cold or heat L50.2
    drugs L50.0
    food L50.0
    inhalants L50.0
    plants L50.6
    serum (*see also* Reaction, serum) T80.69
  factitial L50.3
  familial cold M04.2
  giant T78.3
    hereditary D84.1
  gigantea T78.3
  idiopathic L50.1
  larynx T78.3
    hereditary D84.1
  neonatorum P83.8
  nonallergic L50.1
  papulosa (Hebra) L28.2
  pigmentosa Q82.2
  recurrent periodic L50.8
  serum (*see also* Reaction, serum) T80.69
  solar L56.3
  specified type NEC L50.8
  thermal (cold) (heat) L50.2
  vibratory L50.4
  xanthelasmoidea Q82.2

Use (of)
  alcohol Z72.89
    with
      intoxication F10.929
      sleep disorder F10.982
    harmful — *see* Abuse, alcohol
  amphetamines — *see* Use, stimulant NEC
  caffeine — *see* Use, stimulant NEC
  cannabis F12.90
    with
      anxiety disorder F12.980
      intoxication F12.929
        with
          delirium F12.921
          perceptual disturbance F12.922
          uncomplicated F12.920
      other specified disorder F12.988
      psychosis F12.959
        delusions F12.950
        hallucinations F12.951
      unspecified disorder F12.99
  cocaine F14.90
    with
      anxiety disorder F14.980
      intoxication F14.929
        with
          delirium F14.921
          perceptual disturbance F14.922
          uncomplicated F14.920
      other specified disorder F14.988
      psychosis F14.959
        delusions F14.950
        hallucinations F14.951
      sexual dysfunction F14.981
      sleep disorder F14.982
      unspecified disorder F14.99
    harmful — *see* Abuse, drug, cocaine
  drug(s) NEC F19.90
    with sleep disorder F19.982
    harmful — *see* Abuse, drug, by type
  hallucinogen NEC F16.90
    with
      anxiety disorder F16.980
      intoxication F16.929
        with
          delirium F16.921
          uncomplicated F16.920
      mood disorder F16.94
      other specified disorder F16.988
      perception disorder (flashbacks) F16.983
      psychosis F16.959
        delusions F16.950
        hallucinations F16.951
      unspecified disorder F16.99
    harmful — *see* Abuse, drug, hallucinogen
      NEC
  inhalants F18.90
    with
      anxiety disorder F18.980
      intoxication F18.929
        with delirium F18.921
        uncomplicated F18.920
      mood disorder F18.94
      other specified disorder F18.988
      persisting dementia F18.97
      psychosis F18.959
        delusions F18.950
        hallucinations F18.951
      unspecified disorder F18.99
    harmful — *see* Abuse, drug, inhalant
  methadone — *see* Use, opioid
  nonprescribed drugs F19.90
    harmful — *see* Abuse, non-psychoactive
      substance

Use (of) — *continued*
  opioid F11.90
    with
      disorder F11.99
      mood F11.94
      sleep F11.982
      specified type NEC F11.988
    intoxication F11.929
      with
        delirium F11.921
        perceptual disturbance F11.922
        uncomplicated F11.920
    withdrawal F11.93
    harmful — *see* Abuse, drug, opioid
  patent medicines F19.90
    harmful — *see* Abuse, non-psychoactive
      substance
  psychoactive drug NEC F19.90
    with
      anxiety disorder F19.980
      intoxication F19.929
        with
          delirium F19.921
          perceptual disturbance F19.922
          uncomplicated F19.920
      mood disorder F19.94
      other specified disorder F19.988
      persisting
        amnestic disorder F19.96
        dementia F19.97
      psychosis F19.959
        delusions F19.950
        hallucinations F19.951
      sexual dysfunction F19.981
      sleep disorder F19.982
      unspecified disorder F19.99
    withdrawal F19.939
      with
        delirium F19.931
        perceptual disturbance F19.932
        uncomplicated F19.930
    harmful — *see* Abuse, drug NEC,
      psychoactive NEC
  sedative, hypnotic, or anxiolytic F13.90
    with
      anxiety disorder F13.980
      intoxication F13.929
        with
          delirium F13.921
          uncomplicated F13.920
      other specified disorder F13.988
      persisting
        amnestic disorder F13.96
        dementia F13.97
      psychosis F13.959
        delusions F13.950
        hallucinations F13.951
      sexual dysfunction F13.981
      sleep disorder F13.982
      unspecified disorder F13.99
    harmful — *see* Abuse, drug, sedative,
      hypnotic, or anxiolytic
  stimulant NEC F15.90
    with
      anxiety disorder F15.980
      intoxication F15.929
        with
          delirium F15.921
          perceptual disturbance F15.922
          uncomplicated F15.920
      mood disorder F15.94
      other specified disorder F15.988
      psychosis F15.959
        delusions F15.950
        hallucinations F15.951
      sexual dysfunction F15.981
      sleep disorder F15.982
      unspecified disorder F15.99

Use (of) — *continued*
  stimulant NEC F15.90 — *continued*
    with — *continued*
      withdrawal F15.93
    harmful — *see* Abuse, drug, stimulant NEC
  tobacco Z72.0
    with dependence — *see* Dependence, drug, nicotine
  volatile solvents (*see also* Use, inhalant) F18.90
    harmful — *see* Abuse, drug, inhalant
Usher-Senear disease or syndrome L10.4
Uta B55.1
Uteromegaly N85.2
Uterovaginal — *see* condition
Uterovesical — *see* condition
Uveal — *see* condition
Uveitis (anterior) — *see also* Iridocyclitis
  acute — *see* Iridocyclitis, acute
  chronic — *see* Iridocyclitis, chronic
  due to toxoplasmosis (acquired) B58.09
    congenital P37.1
  granulomatous — *see* Iridocyclitis, chronic
  heterochromic — *see* Cyclitis, Fuchs' heterochromic
  lens-induced — *see* Iridocyclitis, lens-induced
  posterior — *see* Chorioretinitis
  sympathetic H44.13-
  syphilitic (secondary) A51.43
    congenital (early) A50.01
    late A52.71
  tuberculous A18.54
Uveoencephalitis — *see* Inflammation, chorioretinal
Uveokeratitis — *see* Iridocyclitis
Uveoparotitis D86.89
Uvula — *see* condition
Uvulitis (acute) (catarrhal) (chronic) (membranous) (suppurative) (ulcerative) K12.2

V

Vaccination (prophylactic)
  complication or reaction — *see* Complications, vaccination
  delayed Z28.9
  encounter for Z23
  not done — *see* Immunization, not done, because (of)
Vaccinia (generalized) (localized) T88.1
  congenital P35.8
  without vaccination B08.011
Vacuum, in sinus (accessory) (nasal) J34.89
Vagabond's disease B85.1
Vagabond, vagabondage Z59.0
Vagina, vaginal — *see* condition
Vaginalitis (tunica) (testis) N49.1
Vaginismus (reflex) N94.2
  functional F52.5
  nonorganic F52.5
  psychogenic F52.5
  secondary N94.2
Vaginitis (acute) (circumscribed) (diffuse) (emphysematous) (nonvenereal) (ulcerative) N76.0
  with ectopic or molar pregnancy O08.0
  amebic A06.82
  atrophic, postmenopausal N95.2
  bacterial N76.0
  blennorrhagic (gonococcal) A54.02
  candidal B37.3
  chlamydial A56.02
  chronic N76.1
  due to Trichomonas (vaginalis) A59.01
  following ectopic or molar pregnancy O08.0
  gonococcal A54.02
    with abscess (accessory gland) (periurethral) A54.1
  granuloma A58
  in (due to)
    candidiasis B37.3
    herpesviral (herpes simplex) infection A60.04
    pinworm infection B80 [*N77.1*]
  monilial B37.3
  mycotic (candidal) B37.3
  postmenopausal atrophic N95.2
  puerperal (postpartum) O86.13
  senile (atrophic) N95.2
  subacute or chronic N76.1
  syphilitic (early) A51.0
    late A52.76
  trichomonal A59.01
  tuberculous A18.18
Vaginosis — *see* Vaginitis
Vagotonia G52.2
Vagrancy Z59.0
VAIN — *see* Neoplasia, intraepithelial, vagina
Vallecula — *see* condition
Valley fever B38.0
Valsuani's disease — *see* Anemia, obstetric
Valve, valvular (formation) — *see also* condition
  cerebral ventricle (communicating) in situ Z98.2
  cervix, internal os Q51.828
  congenital NEC — *see* Atresia, by site
  ureter (pelvic junction) (vesical orifice) Q62.39
  urethra (congenital) (posterior) Q64.2
Valvulitis (chronic) — *see* Endocarditis
Valvulopathy — *see* Endocarditis
Van Bogaert's leukoencephalopathy (sclerosing) (subacute) A81.1
Van Bogaert-Scherer-Epstein disease or syndrome E75.5
Van Buchem's syndrome M85.2
Van Creveld-von Gierke disease E74.01

Van der Hoeve(-de Kleyn) syndrome Q78.0
Van der Woude's syndrome Q38.0
Van Neck's disease or osteochondrosis M91.0
Vanishing lung J44.9
Vapor asphyxia or suffocation T59.9
  specified agent — *see* Table of Drugs and Chemicals
Variance, lethal ball, prosthetic heart valve T82.09
Variants, thalassemic D56.8
Variations in hair color L67.1
Varicella B01.9
  with
    complications NEC B01.89
    encephalitis B01.11
    encephalomyelitis B01.11
    meningitis B01.0
    myelitis B01.12
    pneumonia B01.2
  congenital P35.8
Varices — *see* Varix
Varicocele (scrotum) (thrombosed) I86.1
  ovary I86.2
  perineum I86.3
  spermatic cord (ulcerated) I86.1
Varicose
  aneurysm (ruptured) I77.0
  dermatitis — *see* Varix, leg, with, inflammation
  eczema — *see* Varix, leg, with, inflammation
  phlebitis — *see* Varix, with, inflammation
  tumor — *see* Varix
  ulcer (lower limb, any part) — *see also* Varix, leg, with, ulcer
    anus (*see also* Hemorrhoids) K64.8
    esophagus — *see* Varix, esophagus
    inflamed or infected — *see* Varix, leg, with ulcer, with inflammation
    nasal septum I86.8
    perineum I86.3
    scrotum I86.1
    specified site NEC I86.8
  vein — *see* Varix
  vessel — *see* Varix, leg
Varicosis, varicosities, varicosity — *see* Varix
Variola (major) (minor) B03
Varioloid B03
Varix (lower limb) (ruptured) I83.90
  with
    edema I83.899
    inflammation I83.10
      with ulcer (venous) I83.209
    pain I83.819
    specified complication NEC I83.899
    stasis dermatitis I83.10
      with ulcer (venous) I83.209
    swelling I83.899
    ulcer I83.009
      with inflammation I83.209
  aneurysmal I77.0
  asymptomatic I83.9-
  bladder I86.2
  broad ligament I86.2
  complicating
    childbirth (lower extremity) O87.4
      anus or rectum O87.2
      genital (vagina, vulva or perineum) O87.8
    pregnancy (lower extremity) O22.0-
      anus or rectum O22.4-
      genital (vagina, vulva or perineum) O22.1-
    puerperium (lower extremity) O87.4
      anus or rectum O87.2
      genital (vagina, vulva, perineum) O87.8
  congenital (any site) Q27.8

Varix (lower limb) (ruptured) I83.90 — *continued*
  esophagus (idiopathic) (primary) (ulcerated) I85.00
    bleeding I85.01
    congenital Q27.8
    in (due to)
      alcoholic liver disease I85.10
        bleeding I85.11
      cirrhosis of liver I85.10
        bleeding I85.11
      portal hypertension I85.10
        bleeding I85.11
      schistosomiasis I85.10
        bleeding I85.11
      toxic liver disease I85.10
        bleeding I85.11
    secondary I85.10
      bleeding I85.11
  gastric I86.4
  inflamed or infected I83.10
    ulcerated I83.209
  labia (majora) I86.3
  leg (asymptomatic) I83.90
    with
      edema I83.899
      inflammation I83.10
        with ulcer — *see* Varix, leg, with, ulcer, with inflammation by site
      pain I83.819
      specified complication NEC I83.899
      swelling I83.899
      ulcer I83.009
        with inflammation I83.209
        ankle I83.003
          with inflammation I83.203
        calf I83.002
          with inflammation I83.202
        foot NEC I83.005
          with inflammation I83.205
        heel I83.004
          with inflammation I83.204
        lower leg NEC I83.008
          with inflammation I83.208
        midfoot I83.004
          with inflammation I83.204
        thigh I83.001
          with inflammation I83.201
    bilateral (asymptomatic) I83.93
      with
        edema I83.893
        pain I83.813
        specified complication NEC I83.893
        swelling I83.893
        ulcer I83.009
          with inflammation I83.209
    left (asymptomatic) I83.92
      with
        edema I83.892
        inflammation I83.12
          with ulcer — *see* Varix, leg, with, ulcer, with inflammation by site
        pain I83.812
        specified complication NEC I83.892
        swelling I83.892
        ulcer I83.029
          with inflammation I83.229
          ankle I83.023
            with inflammation I83.223
          calf I83.022
            with inflammation I83.222
          foot NEC I83.025
            with inflammation I83.225
          heel I83.024
            with inflammation I83.224
          lower leg NEC I83.028
            with inflammation I83.228

Varix (lower limb) (ruptured) I83.90 — *continued*
  leg (asymptomatic) I83.90 — *continued*
    left (asymptomatic) I83.92 — *continued*
      with — *continued*
        ulcer I83.029 — *continued*
          midfoot I83.024
            with inflammation I83.224
          thigh I83.021
            with inflammation I83.221
    right (asymptomatic) I83.91
      with
        edema I83.891
        inflammation I83.11
          with ulcer — *see* Varix, leg, with, ulcer, with inflammation by site
        pain I83.811
        specified complication NEC I83.891
        swelling I83.891
        ulcer I83.019
          with inflammation I83.219
          ankle I83.013
            with inflammation I83.213
          calf I83.012
            with inflammation I83.212
          foot NEC I83.015
            with inflammation I83.215
          heel I83.014
            with inflammation I83.214
          lower leg NEC I83.018
            with inflammation I83.218
          midfoot I83.014
            with inflammation I83.214
          thigh I83.011
            with inflammation I83.211
  nasal septum I86.8
  orbit I86.8
    congenital Q27.8
  ovary I86.2
  papillary I78.1
  pelvis I86.2
  perineum I86.3
  pharynx I86.8
  placenta O43.89-
  renal papilla I86.8
  retina H35.09
  scrotum (ulcerated) I86.1
  sigmoid colon I86.8
  specified site NEC I86.8
  spinal (cord) (vessels) I86.8
  spleen, splenic (vein) (with phlebolith) I86.8
  stomach I86.4
  sublingual I86.0
  ulcerated I83.009
    inflamed or infected I83.209
  uterine ligament I86.2
  vagina I86.8
  vocal cord I86.8
  vulva I86.3
Vas deferens — *see* condition
Vas deferentitis N49.1
Vasa previa O69.4
  hemorrhage from, affecting newborn P50.0
Vascular — *see also* condition
  loop on optic papilla Q14.2
  spasm I73.9
  spider I78.1
Vascularization, cornea — *see* Neovascularization, cornea
Vasculitis I77.6
  allergic D69.0
  cryoglobulinemic D89.1
  disseminated I77.6
  hypocomplementemic M31.8
  kidney I77.89
  livedoid L95.0
  nodular L95.8
  retina H35.06-

Vasculitis I77.6 — *continued*
  rheumatic — *see* Fever, rheumatic
  rheumatoid — *see* Rheumatoid, vasculitis
  skin (limited to) L95.9
    specified NEC L95.8
Vasculopathy, necrotizing M31.9
  cardiac allograft T86.290
  specified NEC M31.8
Vasitis (nodosa) N49.1
  tuberculous A18.15
Vasodilation I73.9
Vasomotor — *see* condition
Vasoplasty, after previous sterilization Z31.0
  aftercare Z31.42
Vasospasm (vasoconstriction) I73.9
  cerebral (artery) (cerebrovascular) I67.848
    reversible I67.841
  coronary I20.1
  nerve
    arm — *see* Mononeuropathy, upper limb
    brachial plexus G54.0
    cervical plexus G54.2
    leg — *see* Mononeuropathy, lower limb
  peripheral NOS I73.9
  retina (artery) — *see* Occlusion, artery, retina
Vasospastic — *see* condition
Vasovagal attack (paroxysmal) R55
  psychogenic F45.8
VATER syndrome Q87.2
Vater's ampulla — *see* condition
Vegetation, vegetative
  adenoid (nasal fossa) J35.8
  endocarditis (acute) (any valve) (subacute) I33.0
  heart (mycotic) (valve) I33.0
Veil
  Jackson's Q43.3
Vein, venous — *see* condition
Veldt sore — *see* Ulcer, skin
Velpeau's hernia — *see* Hernia, femoral
Venereal
  bubo A55
  disease A64
  granuloma inguinale A58
  lymphogranuloma (Durand-Nicolas-Favre) A55
Venofibrosis I87.8
Venom, venomous — *see* Table of Drugs and Chemicals, by animal or substance, poisoning
Venous — *see* condition
Ventilator lung, newborn P27.8
Ventral — *see* condition
Ventricle, ventricular — *see also* condition
  escape I49.3
  inversion Q20.5
Ventriculitis (cerebral) (*see also* Encephalitis) G04.90
Ventriculostomy status Z98.2
Vernet's syndrome G52.7
Verneuil's disease (syphilitic bursitis) A52.78
Verruca (due to HPV) (filiformis) (simplex) (viral) (vulgaris) B07.9
  acuminata A63.0
  necrogenica (primary) (tuberculosa) A18.4
  plana B07.8
  plantaris B07.0
  seborrheica L82.1
    inflamed L82.0
  senile (seborrheic) L82.1
    inflamed L82.0
  tuberculosa (primary) A18.4
  venereal A63.0
Verrucosities — *see* Verruca
Verruga peruana, peruviana A44.1

Version
  with extraction
    cervix — *see* Malposition, uterus
    uterus (postinfectional) (postpartal, old) — *see* Malposition, uterus
Vertebra, vertebral — *see* condition
Vertical talus (congenital) Q66.80
  left foot Q66.82
  right foot Q66.81
Vertigo R42
  auditory — *see* Vertigo, aural
  aural H81.31-
  benign paroxysmal (positional) H81.1-
  central (origin) H81.4-
  cerebral H81.4-
  Dix and Hallpike (epidemic) — *see* Neuronitis, vestibular
  due to infrasound T75.23
  epidemic A88.1
    Dix and Hallpike — *see* Neuronitis, vestibular
    Pedersen's — *see* Neuronitis, vestibular
    vestibular neuronitis — *see* Neuronitis, vestibular
  hysterical F44.89
  infrasound T75.23
  labyrinthine — *see* subcategory H81.0
  laryngeal R05
  malignant positional H81.4-
  menopausal N95.1
  Ménière's — *see* subcategory H81.0
  otogenic — *see* Vertigo, aural
  paroxysmal positional, benign — *see* Vertigo, benign paroxysmal
  Pedersen's (epidemic) — *see* Neuronitis, vestibular
  peripheral NEC H81.39-
  positional
    benign paroxysmal — *see* Vertigo, benign paroxysmal
    malignant H81.4-
Very-low-density-lipoprotein-type (VLDL) hyperlipoproteinemia E78.1
Vesania — *see* Psychosis
Vesical — *see* condition
Vesicle
  cutaneous R23.8
  seminal — *see* condition
  skin R23.8
Vesicocolic — *see* condition
Vesicoperineal — *see* condition
Vesicorectal — *see* condition
Vesicourethrorectal — *see* condition
Vesicovaginal — *see* condition
Vesicular — *see* condition
Vesiculitis (seminal) N49.0
  amebic A06.82
  gonorrheal (acute) (chronic) A54.23
  trichomonal A59.09
  tuberculous A18.15
Vestibulitis (ear) (*see also* subcategory) H83.0
  nose (external) J34.89
  vulvar N94.810
Vestibulopathy, acute peripheral (recurrent) — *see* Neuronitis, vestibular
Vestige, vestigial — *see also* Persistence
  branchial Q18.0
  structures in vitreous Q14.0
Vibration
  adverse effects T75.20
    pneumatic hammer syndrome T75.21
    specified effect NEC T75.29
    vasospastic syndrome T75.22
    vertigo from infrasound T75.23
  exposure (occupational) Z57.7
  vertigo T75.23
Vibriosis A28.9

Victim (of)
  crime Z65.4
  disaster Z65.5
  terrorism Z65.4
  torture Z65.4
  war Z65.5
Vidal's disease L28.0
Villaret's syndrome G52.7
Villous — *see* condition
VIN — *see* Neoplasia, intraepithelial, vulva
Vincent's infection (angina) (gingivitis) A69.1
  stomatitis NEC A69.1
Vinson-Plummer syndrome D50.1
Violence, physical R45.6
Viosterol deficiency — *see* Deficiency, calciferol
Vipoma — *see* Neoplasm, malignant, by site
Viremia B34.9
Virilism (adrenal) E25.9
  congenital E25.0
Virilization (female) (suprarenal) E25.9
  congenital E25.0
  isosexual E28.2
Virulent bubo A57
Virus, viral — *see also* condition
  as cause of disease classified elsewhere B97.89
  cytomegalovirus B25.9
  human immunodeficiency (HIV) — *see* Human, immunodeficiency virus (HIV) disease
  infection — *see* Infection, virus
  specified NEC B34.8
  swine influenza (viruses that normally cause infections in pigs) (*see also* Influenza, due to, identified novel influenza A virus) J09.x2
  West Nile (fever) A92.30
    with
      complications NEC A92.39
      cranial nerve disorders A92.32
      encephalitis A92.31
      encephalomyelitis A92.31
      neurologic manifestation NEC A92.32
      optic neuritis A92.32
      polyradiculitis A92.32
Viscera, visceral — *see* condition
Visceroptosis K63.4
Visible peristalsis R19.2
Vision, visual
  binocular, suppression H53.34
  blurred, blurring H53.8
    hysterical F44.6
  defect, defective NEC H54.7
  disorientation (syndrome) H53.8
  disturbance H53.9
    hysterical F44.6
  double H53.2
  examination Z01.00
    with abnormal findings Z01.01
  field, limitation (defect) — *see* Defect, visual field
  hallucinations R44.1
  halos H53.19
  loss — *see* Loss, vision
    sudden — *see* Disturbance, vision, subjective, loss, sudden
  low (both eyes) — *see* Low, vision
  perception, simultaneous without fusion H53.33
Vitality, lack or want of R53.83
  newborn P96.89
Vitamin deficiency — *see* Deficiency, vitamin
Vitelline duct, persistent Q43.0

Vitiligo L80
  eyelid H02.739
    left H02.736
      lower H02.735
      upper H02.734
    right H02.733
      lower H02.732
      upper H02.731
  pinta A67.2
  vulva N90.89
Vitreal corneal syndrome H59.01-
Vitreoretinopathy, proliferative — *see also* Retinopathy, proliferative
  with retinal detachment — *see* Detachment, retina, traction
Vitreous — *see also* condition
  touch syndrome — *see* Complication, postprocedural, following cataract surgery
Vocal cord — *see* condition
Vogt-Koyanagi syndrome H20.82-
Vogt's disease or syndrome G80.3
Vogt-Spielmeyer amaurotic idiocy or disease E75.4
Voice
  change R49.9
    specified NEC R49.8
  loss — *see* Aphonia
Volhynian fever A79.0
Volkmann's ischemic contracture or paralysis (complicating trauma) T79.6
Volvulus (bowel) (colon) (intestine) K56.2
  with perforation K56.2
  congenital Q43.8
  duodenum K31.5
  fallopian tube — *see* Torsion, fallopian tube
  oviduct — *see* Torsion, fallopian tube
  stomach (due to absence of gastrocolic ligament) K31.89
Vomiting R11.10
  with nausea R11.2
  asphyxia — *see* Foreign body, by site, causing asphyxia, gastric contents
  bilious (cause unknown) R11.14
    following gastro-intestinal surgery K91.0
    in newborn P92.01
  blood — *see* Hematemesis
  causing asphyxia, choking, or suffocation — *see* Foreign body, by site
  cyclical G43.A0 *(follows G43.7)*
    with refractory migraine G43.A1 *(follows G43.7)*
    intractable G43.A1 *(follows G43.7)*
    not intractable G43.A0 *(follows G43.7)*
    psychogenic F50.89
    without refractory migraine G43.A0 *(follows G43.7)*
  fecal mater R11.13
  following gastrointestinal surgery K91.0
    psychogenic F50.89
  functional K31.89
  hysterical F50.89
  nervous F50.89
  neurotic F50.89
  newborn NEC P92.09
    bilious P92.01
  periodic R11.10
    psychogenic F50.89
  projectile R11.12
  psychogenic F50.89
  uremic — *see* Uremia
  without nausea R11.11
Vomito negro — *see* Fever, yellow
Von Bezold's abscess — *see* Mastoiditis, acute
Von Economo-Cruchet disease A85.8
Von Eulenburg's disease G71.19
Von Gierke's disease E74.01

W

Von Hippel(-Lindau) disease or syndrome Q85.8
Von Jaksch's anemia or disease D64.89
Von Recklinghausen
  disease (neurofibromatosis) Q85.01
    bones E21.0
Von Schroetter's syndrome I82.890
Von Willebrand(-Jurgens)(-Minot) disease or syndrome D68.0
Von Zumbusch's disease L40.1
Voyeurism F65.3
Vrolik's disease Q78.0
Vulva — see condition
Vulvismus N94.2
Vulvitis (acute) (allergic) (atrophic) (hypertrophic) (intertriginous) (senile) N76.2
  with ectopic or molar pregnancy O08.0
  adhesive, congenital Q52.79
  blennorrhagic (gonococcal) A54.02
  candidal B37.3
  chlamydial A56.02
  due to Haemophilus ducreyi A57
  following ectopic or molar pregnancy O08.0
  gonococcal A54.02
    with abscess (accessory gland) (periurethral) A54.1
  herpesviral A60.04
  leukoplakia N90.4
  monilial B37.3
  puerperal (postpartum) O86.19
  subacute or chronic N76.3
  syphilitic (early) A51.0
    late A52.76
  trichomonal A59.01
  tuberculous A18.18
Vulvodynia N94.819
  specified NEC N94.818
Vulvorectal — see condition
Vulvovaginitis (acute) — see Vaginitis

Waiting list, person on Z75.1
  for organ transplant Z76.82
  undergoing social agency investigation Z75.2
Waldenström
  hypergammaglobulinemia D89.0
  syndrome or macroglobulinemia C88.0
Waldenström-Kjellberg syndrome D50.1
Walking
  difficulty R26.2
    psychogenic F44.4
  sleep F51.3
    hysterical F44.89
Wall, abdominal — see condition
Wallenberg's disease or syndrome G46.3
Wallgren's disease I87.8
Wandering
  gallbladder, congenital Q44.1
  in diseases classified elsewhere Z91.83
  kidney, congenital Q63.8
  organ or site, congenital NEC — see Malposition, congenital, by site
  pacemaker (heart) I49.8
  spleen D73.89
War neurosis F48.8
Wart (due to HPV) (filiform) (infectious) (viral) B07.9
  anogenital region (venereal) A63.0
  common B07.8
  external genital organs (venereal) A63.0
  flat B07.8
  Hassal-Henle's (of cornea) H18.49
  Peruvian A44.1
  plantar B07.0
  prosector (tuberculous) A18.4
  seborrheic L82.1
    inflamed L82.0
  senile (seborrheic) L82.1
    inflamed L82.0
  tuberculous A18.4
  venereal A63.0
Warthin's tumor — see Neoplasm, salivary gland, benign
Wassilieff's disease A27.0
Wasting
  disease R64
    due to malnutrition E41
  extreme (due to malnutrition) E41
  muscle NEC — see Atrophy, muscle
Water
  clefts (senile cataract) — see Cataract, senile, incipient
  deprivation of T73.1
  intoxication E87.79
  itch B76.9
  lack of T73.1
  loading E87.70
  on
    brain — see Hydrocephalus
    chest J94.8
  poisoning E87.79
Waterbrash R12
Water-losing nephritis N25.89
Waterhouse(-Friderichsen) syndrome or disease (meningococcal) A39.1
Watermelon stomach K31.819
  with hemorrhage K31.811
  without hemorrhage K31.819
Watsoniasis B66.8
Wax in ear — see Impaction, cerumen
Weak, weakening, weakness (generalized) R53.1
  arches (acquired) — see also Deformity, limb, flat foot
  bladder (sphincter) R32

Weak, weakening, weakness (generalized) R53.1 — continued
  facial R29.810
    following
      cerebrovascular disease I69.992
        cerebral infarction I69.392
        intracerebral hemorrhage I69.192
        nontraumatic intracranial hemorrhage NEC I69.292
        specified disease NEC I69.892
        stroke I69.392
        subarachnoid hemorrhage I69.092
  foot (double) — see Weak, arches
  heart, cardiac — see Failure, heart
  mind F70
  muscle M62.81
  myocardium — see Failure, heart
  newborn P96.89
  pelvic fundus N81.89
  pubocervical tissue N81.82
  rectovaginal tissue N81.83
  senile R54
  urinary stream R39.12
  valvular — see Endocarditis
Wear, worn (with normal or routine use)
  articular bearing surface of internal joint prosthesis — see Complications, joint prosthesis, mechanical, wear of articularbearing surfaces, by site
  device, implant or graft — see Complications, by site, mechanical complication
  tooth, teeth (approximal) (hard tissues) (interproximal) (occlusal) K03.0
Weather, weathered
  effects of
    cold T69.9
      specified effect NEC T69.8
    hot — see Heat
  skin L57.8
Weaver's syndrome Q87.3
Web, webbed (congenital)
  duodenal Q43.8
  esophagus Q39.4
  fingers Q70.1-
  larynx (glottic) (subglottic) Q31.0
  neck (pterygium colli) Q18.3
  Paterson-Kelly D50.1
  popliteal syndrome Q87.89
  toes Q70.3-
Weber-Christian disease M35.6
Weber-Cockayne syndrome (epidermolysis bullosa) Q81.8
Weber-Gubler syndrome G46.3
Weber-Leyden syndrome G46.3
Weber-Osler syndrome I78.0
Weber's paralysis or syndrome G46.3
Wedge-shaped or wedging vertebra — see Collapse, vertebra NEC
Wegener's granulomatosis or syndrome M31.30
  with
    kidney involvement M31.31
    lung involvement M31.30
      with kidney involvement M31.31
Wegner's disease A50.02
Weight
  1000-2499 grams at birth (low) — see Low, birthweight
  999 grams or less at birth (extremely low) — see Low, birthweight, extreme
  and length below 10th percentile for gestational age P05.1-
  below but length above 10th percentile for gestational age P05.0-
  gain (abnormal) (excessive) R63.5
    in pregnancy — see Pregnancy, complicated by, excessive weight gain
    low — see Pregnancy, complicated by, insufficient, weight gain

Weight — *continued*
  loss (abnormal) (cause unknown) R63.4
Weightlessness (effect of) T75.82
Weil (I)-Marchesani syndrome Q87.1
Weil's disease A27.0
Weingarten's syndrome J82
Weir Mitchell's disease I73.81
Weiss-Baker syndrome G90.09
Wells' disease L98.3
Wen — *see* Cyst, sebaceous
Wenckebach's block or phenomenon
  I44.1
Werdnig-Hoffmann syndrome (muscular
  atrophy) G12.0
Werlhof's disease D69.3
Wermer's disease or syndrome E31.21
Werner-His disease A79.0
Werner's disease or syndrome E34.8
Wernicke-Korsakoff's syndrome or
  psychosis (alcoholic) F10.96
  with dependence F10.26
  drug-induced
    due to drug abuse — *see* Abuse, drug, by
      type, with amnestic disorder
    due to drug dependence — *see* Dependence,
      drug, by type, with amnestic disorder
  nonalcoholic F04
Wernicke-Posadas disease B38.9
Wernicke's
  developmental aphasia F80.2
  disease or syndrome E51.2
  encephalopathy E51.2
  polioencephalitis, superior E51.2
West African fever B50.8
Westphal-Strümpell syndrome E83.01
West's syndrome — *see* Epilepsy, spasms
Wet
  feet, tropical (maceration) (syndrome) — *see*
    Immersion, foot
  lung (syndrome), newborn P22.1
Wharton's duct — *see* condition
Wheal — *see* Urticaria
Wheezing R06.2
Whiplash injury S13.4
Whipple's disease (*see also* subcategory
  M14.8-) K90.81
Whipworm (disease) (infection) (infestation)
  B79
Whistling face Q87.0
White — *see also* condition
  kidney, small N03.9
  leg, puerperal, postpartum, childbirth O87.1
  mouth B37.0
  patches of mouth K13.29
  spot lesions, teeth
    chewing surface K02.51
    pit and fissure surface K02.51
    smooth surface K02.61
Whitehead L70.0
Whitlow — *see also* Cellulitis, digit
  with lymphangitis — *see* Lymphangitis, acute,
    digit
  herpesviral B00.89
Whitmore's disease or fever — *see*
  Melioidosis
Whooping cough A37.90
  with pneumonia A37.91
  due to Bordetella
    bronchiseptica A37.81
    parapertussis A37.11
    pertussis A37.01
    specified organism NEC A37.81
  due to
    Bordetella
      bronchiseptica A37.80
        with pneumonia A37.81
      parapertussis A37.10
        with pneumonia A37.11

Whooping cough A37.90 — *continued*
  due to — *continued*
    Bordetella — *continued*
      pertussis A37.00
        with pneumonia A37.01
      specified NEC A37.80
        with pneumonia A37.81
Wichman's asthma J38.5
Wide cranial sutures, newborn P96.3
Widening aorta — *see* Ectasia, aorta
  with aneurysm — *see* Aneurysm, aorta
Wilkie's disease or syndrome K55.1
Wilkinson-Sneddon disease or syndrome
  L13.1
Willebrand (-Jürgens) thrombopathy
  D68.0
Willige-Hunt disease or syndrome G23.1
Wilms' tumor C64-
Wilson-Mikity syndrome P27.0
Wilson's
  disease or syndrome E83.01
  hepatolenticular degeneration E83.01
  lichen ruber L43.9
Window — *see also* Imperfect, closure
  aorticopulmonary Q21.4
Winter — *see* condition
Wiskott-Aldrich syndrome D82.0
Withdrawal state — *see also* Dependence,
  drug by type, with withdrawal
  alcohol
    with perceptual disturbances F10.232
    without perceptual disturbances F10.239
  caffeine F15.93
  cannabis F12.288
  newborn
    correct therapeutic substance properly
      administered P96.2
    infant of dependent mother P96.1
  therapeutic substance, neonatal P96.2
Witts' anemia D50.8
Witzelsucht F07.0
Woakes' ethmoiditis or syndrome J33.1
Wolff-Hirschorn syndrome Q93.3
Wolff-Parkinson-White syndrome I45.6
Wolhynian fever A79.0
Wolman's disease E75.5
Wood lung or pneumonitis J67.8
Woolly, wooly hair (congenital) (nevus)
  Q84.1
Woolsorter's disease A22.1
Word
  blindness (congenital) (developmental) F81.0
  deafness (congenital) (developmental) H93.25
Worm-eaten soles A66.3
Worm(s) (infection) (infestation) — *see also*
  Infestation, helminth
  guinea B72
  in intestine NEC B82.0
Worn out — *see* Exhaustion
  cardiac
    defibrillator (with synchronous cardiac
      pacemaker) Z45.02
    pacemaker
      battery Z45.010
      lead Z45.018
  device, implant or graft — *see* Complications,
    by site, mechanical
Worried well Z71.1
Worries R45.82

Wound, open
  abdomen, abdominal
    wall S31.109
      with penetration into peritoneal cavity
        S31.609
      bite — *see* Bite, abdomen, wall
      epigastric region S31.102
        with penetration into peritoneal cavity
          S31.602
        bite — *see* Bite, abdomen, wall,
          epigastric region
        laceration — *see* Laceration, abdomen,
          wall, epigastric region
        puncture — *see* Puncture, abdomen,
          wall, epigastric region
      laceration — *see* Laceration, abdomen,
        wall
      left
        lower quadrant S31.104
          with penetration into peritoneal cavity
            S31.604
          bite — *see* Bite, abdomen, wall, left,
            lower quadrant
          laceration — *see* Laceration,
            abdomen, wall, left, lower
            quadrant
          puncture — *see* Puncture, abdomen,
            wall, left, lower quadrant
        upper quadrant S31.101
          with penetration into peritoneal cavity
            S31.601
          bite — *see* Bite, abdomen, wall, left,
            upper quadrant
          laceration — *see* Laceration,
            abdomen, wall, left, upper
            quadrant
          puncture — *see* Puncture, abdomen,
            wall, left, upper quadrant
      periumbilic region S31.105
        with penetration into peritoneal cavity
          S31.605
        bite — *see* Bite, abdomen, wall,
          periumbilic region
        laceration — *see* Laceration, abdomen,
         wall, periumbilic region
        puncture — *see* Puncture, abdomen,
         wall, periumbilic region
      puncture — *see* Puncture, abdomen, wall
      right
        lower quadrant S31.103
          with penetration into peritoneal cavity
            S31.603
          bite — *see* Bite, abdomen, wall, right,
            lower quadrant
          laceration — *see* Laceration,
            abdomen, wall, right, lower
            quadrant
          puncture — *see* Puncture, abdomen,
            wall, right, lower quadrant
        upper quadrant S31.100
          with penetration into peritoneal cavity
            S31.600
          bite — *see* Bite, abdomen, wall, right,
            upper quadrant
          laceration — *see* Laceration,
            abdomen, wall, right, upper
            quadrant
          puncture — *see* Puncture, abdomen,
            wall, right, upper quadrant
  alveolar (process) — *see* Wound, open, oral
    cavity
  ankle S91.00-
    bite — *see* Bite, ankle
    laceration — *see* Laceration, ankle
    puncture — *see* Puncture, ankle
  antecubital space — *see* Wound, open, elbow
  anterior chamber, eye — *see* Wound, open,
    ocular

Wound, open — *continued*
- anus S31.839
  - bite S31.835
  - laceration — *see* Laceration, anus
  - puncture — *see* Puncture, anus
- arm (upper) S41.10-
  - with amputation — *see* Amputation, traumatic, arm
  - bite — *see* Bite, arm
  - forearm — *see* Wound, open, forearm
  - laceration — *see* Laceration, arm
  - puncture — *see* Puncture, arm
- auditory canal (external) (meatus) — *see* Wound, open, ear
- auricle, ear — *see* Wound, open, ear
- axilla — *see* Wound, open, arm
- back — *see also* Wound, open, thorax, back
  - lower S31.000
    - with penetration into retroperitoneal space S31.001
    - bite — *see* Bite, back, lower
    - laceration — *see* Laceration, back, lower
    - puncture — *see* Puncture, back, lower
- bite — *see* Bite
- blood vessel — *see* Injury, blood vessel
- breast S21.00-
  - with amputation — *see* Amputation, traumatic, breast
  - bite — *see* Bite, breast
  - laceration — *see* Laceration, breast
  - puncture — *see* Puncture, breast
- buttock S31.809
  - bite — *see* Bite, buttock
  - laceration — *see* Laceration, buttock
  - left S31.829
  - puncture — *see* Puncture, buttock
  - right S31.819
- calf — *see* Wound, open, leg
- canaliculus lacrimalis — *see* Wound, open, eyelid
- canthus, eye — *see* Wound, open, eyelid
- cervical esophagus S11.20
  - bite S11.25
  - laceration — *see* Laceration, esophagus, traumatic, cervical
  - puncture — *see* Puncture, cervical esophagus
- cheek (external) S01.40-
  - bite — *see* Bite, cheek
  - internal — *see* Wound, open, oral cavity
  - laceration — *see* Laceration, cheek
  - puncture — *see* Puncture, cheek
- chest wall — *see* Wound, open, thorax
- chin — *see* Wound, open, head, specified site NEC
- choroid — *see* Wound, open, ocular
- ciliary body (eye) — *see* Wound, open, ocular
- clitoris S31.40
  - with amputation — *see* Amputation, traumatic, clitoris
  - bite S31.45
  - laceration — *see* Laceration, vulva
  - puncture — *see* Puncture, vulva
- conjunctiva — *see* Wound, open, ocular
- cornea — *see* Wound, open, ocular
- costal region — *see* Wound, open, thorax
- Descemet's membrane — *see* Wound, open, ocular
- digit(s)
  - foot — *see* Wound, open, toe
  - hand — *see* Wound, open, finger
- ear (canal) (external) S01.30-
  - with amputation — *see* Amputation, traumatic, ear
  - bite — *see* Bite, ear
  - drum S09.2-
  - laceration — *see* Laceration, ear
  - puncture — *see* Puncture, ear

Wound, open — *continued*
- elbow S51.00-
  - bite — *see* Bite, elbow
  - laceration — *see* Laceration, elbow
  - puncture — *see* Puncture, elbow
- epididymis — *see* Wound, open, testis
- epigastric region S31.102
  - with penetration into peritoneal cavity S31.602
  - bite — *see* Bite, abdomen, wall, epigastric region
  - laceration — *see* Laceration, abdomen, wall, epigastric region
  - puncture — *see* Puncture, abdomen, wall, epigastric region
- epiglottis — *see* Wound, open, neck, specified site NEC
- esophagus (thoracic) S27.819
  - cervical — *see* Wound, open, cervical esophagus
  - laceration S27.813
  - specified type NEC S27.818
- eye — *see* Wound, open, ocular
- eyeball — *see* Wound, open, ocular
- eyebrow — *see* Wound, open, eyelid
- eyelid S01.10-
  - bite — *see* Bite, eyelid
  - laceration — *see* Laceration, eyelid
  - puncture — *see* Puncture, eyelid
- face NEC — *see* Wound, open, head, specified site NEC
- finger(s) S61.209
  - with
    - amputation — *see* Amputation, traumatic, finger
    - damage to nail S61.309
  - bite — *see* Bite, finger
  - index S61.208
    - with
      - damage to nail S61.308
    - left S61.201
      - with
        - damage to nail S61.301
    - right S61.200
      - with
        - damage to nail S61.300
  - laceration — *see* Laceration, finger
  - little S61.208
    - with
      - damage to nail S61.308
    - left S61.207
      - with damage to nail S61.307
    - right S61.206
      - with damage to nail S61.306
  - middle S61.208
    - with
      - damage to nail S61.308
    - left S61.203
      - with damage to nail S61.303
    - right S61.202
      - with damage to nail S61.302
  - puncture — *see* Puncture, finger
  - ring S61.208
    - with
      - damage to nail S61.308
    - left S61.205
      - with damage to nail S61.305
    - right S61.204
      - with damage to nail S61.304
- flank — *see* Wound, open, abdomen, wall
- foot (except toe(s) alone) S91.30-
  - with amputation — *see* Amputation, traumatic, foot
  - bite — *see* Bite, foot
  - laceration — *see* Laceration, foot
  - puncture — *see* Puncture, foot
  - toe — *see* Wound, open, toe

Wound, open — *continued*
- forearm S51.80-
  - with
    - amputation — *see* Amputation, traumatic, forearm
  - bite — *see* Bite, forearm
  - elbow only — *see* Wound, open, elbow
  - laceration — *see* Laceration, forearm
  - puncture — *see* Puncture, forearm
- forehead — *see* Wound, open, head, specified site NEC
- genital organs, external
  - with amputation — *see* Amputation, traumatic, genital organs
  - bite — *see* Bite, genital organ
  - female S31.502
    - vagina S31.40
    - vulva S31.40
  - laceration — *see* Laceration, genital organ
  - male S31.501
    - penis S31.20
    - scrotum S31.30
    - testes S31.30
  - puncture — *see* Puncture, genital organ
- globe (eye) — *see* Wound, open, ocular
- groin — *see* Wound, open, abdomen, wall
- gum — *see* Wound, open, oral cavity
- hand S61.40-
  - with
    - amputation — *see* Amputation, traumatic, hand
  - bite — *see* Bite, hand
  - finger(s) — *see* Wound, open, finger
  - laceration — *see* Laceration, hand
  - puncture — *see* Puncture, hand
  - thumb — *see* Wound, open, thumb
- head S01.90
  - bite — *see* Bite, head
  - cheek — *see* Wound, open, cheek
  - ear — *see* Wound, open, ear
  - eyelid — *see* Wound, open, eyelid
  - laceration — *see* Laceration, head
  - lip — *see* Wound, open, lip
  - nose S01.20
  - oral cavity — *see* Wound, open, oral cavity
  - puncture — *see* Puncture, head
  - scalp — *see* Wound, open, scalp
  - specified site NEC S01.80
  - temporomandibular area — *see* Wound, open, cheek
- heel — *see* Wound, open, foot
- hip S71.00-
  - with amputation — *see* Amputation, traumatic, hip
  - bite — *see* Bite, hip
  - laceration — *see* Laceration, hip
  - puncture — *see* Puncture, hip
- hymen S31.40
  - bite — *see* Bite, vulva
  - laceration — *see* Laceration, vagina
  - puncture — *see* Puncture, vagina
- hypochondrium S31.109
  - bite — *see* Bite, hypochondrium
  - laceration — *see* Laceration, hypochondrium
  - puncture — *see* Puncture, hypochondrium
- hypogastric region S31.109
  - bite — *see* Bite, hypogastric region
  - laceration — *see* Laceration, hypogastric region
  - puncture — *see* Puncture, hypogastric region
- iliac (region) — *see* Wound, open, inguinal region
- inguinal region S31.109
  - bite — *see* Bite, abdomen, wall, lower quadrant
  - laceration — *see* Laceration, inguinal region
  - puncture — *see* Puncture, inguinal region
- instep — *see* Wound, open, foot

DISEASE INDEX

Wound, open — *continued*

interscapular region — *see* Wound, open, thorax, back
intraocular — *see* Wound, open, ocular
iris — *see* Wound, open, ocular
jaw — *see* Wound, open, head, specified site NEC
knee S81.00-
   bite — *see* Bite, knee
   laceration — *see* Laceration, knee
   puncture — *see* Puncture, knee
labium (majus) (minus) — *see* Wound, open, vulva
laceration — *see* Laceration, by site
lacrimal duct — *see* Wound, open, eyelid
larynx S11.019
   bite — *see* Bite, larynx
   laceration — *see* Laceration, larynx
   puncture — *see* Puncture, larynx
left
   lower quadrant S31.104
     with penetration into peritoneal cavity S31.604
     bite — *see* Bite, abdomen, wall, left, lower quadrant
     laceration — *see* Laceration, abdomen, wall, left, lower quadrant
     puncture — *see* Puncture, abdomen, wall, left, lower quadrant
   upper quadrant S31.101
     with penetration into peritoneal cavity S31.601
     bite — *see* Bite, abdomen, wall, left, upper quadrant
     laceration — *see* Laceration, abdomen, wall, left, upper quadrant
     puncture — *see* Puncture, abdomen, wall, left, upper quadrant
leg (lower) S81.80-
   with amputation — *see* Amputation, traumatic, leg
   ankle — *see* Wound, open, ankle
   bite — *see* Bite, leg
   foot — *see* Wound, open, foot
   knee — *see* Wound, open, knee
   laceration — *see* Laceration, leg
   puncture — *see* Puncture, leg
   toe — *see* Wound, open, toe
   upper — *see* Wound, open, thigh
lip S01.501
   bite — *see* Bite, lip
   laceration — *see* Laceration, lip
   puncture — *see* Puncture, lip
loin S31.109
   bite — *see* Bite, abdomen, wall
   laceration — *see* Laceration, loin
   puncture — *see* Puncture, loin
lower back — *see* Wound, open, back, lower
lumbar region — *see* Wound, open, back, lower
malar — *see* Wound, open, head, specified site NEC
mammary — *see* Wound, open, breast
mastoid region — *see* Wound, open, head, specified site NEC
mouth — *see* Wound, open, oral cavity
nail
   finger — *see* Wound, open, finger, with damage to nail
   toe — *see* Wound, open, toe, with damage to nail
nape (neck) — *see* Wound, open, neck
nasal (septum) (sinus) — *see* Wound, open, nose
nasopharynx — *see* Wound, open, head, specified site NEC

Wound, open — *continued*

neck S11.90
   bite — *see* Bite, neck
   involving
     cervical esophagus S11.20
     larynx — *see* Wound, open, larynx
     pharynx S11.20
     thyroid S11.10
     trachea (cervical) S11.029
       bite — *see* Bite, trachea
       laceration S11.021
         with foreign body S11.022
       puncture S11.023
         with foreign body S11.024
   laceration — *see* Laceration, neck
   puncture — *see* Puncture, neck
   specified site NEC S11.80
   specified type NEC S11.89
nose (septum) (sinus) S01.20
   with amputation — *see* Amputation, traumatic, nose
   bite — *see* Bite, nose
   laceration — *see* Laceration, nose
   puncture — *see* Puncture, nose
ocular S05.90
   avulsion (traumatic enucleation) S05.7-
   eyeball S05.6-
     with foreign body S05.5-
   eyelid — *see* Wound, open, eyelid
   laceration and rupture S05.3-
     with prolapse or loss of intraocular tissue S05.2-
   orbit (penetrating) (with or without foreign body) S05.4-
   periocular area — *see* Wound, open, eyelid
   specified NEC S05.8x-
oral cavity S01.502
   bite S01.552
   laceration — *see* Laceration, oral cavity
   puncture — *see* Puncture, oral cavity
orbit — *see* Wound, open, ocular, orbit
palate — *see* Wound, open, oral cavity
palm — *see* Wound, open, hand
pelvis, pelvic — *see also* Wound, open, back, lower
   girdle — *see* Wound, open, hip
   penetrating — *see* Puncture, by site
penis S31.20
   with amputation — *see* Amputation, traumatic, penis
   bite S31.25
   laceration — *see* Laceration, penis
   puncture — *see* Puncture, penis
perineum
   bite — *see* Bite, perineum
   female S31.502
   laceration — *see* Laceration, perineum
   male S31.501
   puncture — *see* Puncture, perineum
periocular area (with or without lacrimal passages) — *see* Wound, open, eyelid
periumbilic region S31.105
   with penetration into peritoneal cavity S31.605
   bite — *see* Bite, abdomen, wall, periumbilic region
   laceration — *see* Laceration, abdomen, wall, periumbilic region
   puncture — *see* Puncture, abdomen, wall, periumbilic region
phalanges
   finger — *see* Wound, open, finger
   toe — *see* Wound, open, toe
pharynx S11.20
pinna — *see* Wound, open, ear
popliteal space — *see* Wound, open, knee
prepuce — *see* Wound, open, penis
pubic region — *see* Wound, open, back, lower

Wound, open — *continued*

pudendum — *see* Wound, open, genital organs, external
puncture wound — *see* Puncture
rectovaginal septum — *see* Wound, open, vagina
right
   lower quadrant S31.103
     with penetration into peritoneal cavity S31.603
     bite — *see* Bite, abdomen, wall, right, lower quadrant
     laceration — *see* Laceration, abdomen, wall, right, lower quadrant
     puncture — *see* Puncture, abdomen, wall, right, lower quadrant
   upper quadrant S31.100
     with penetration into peritoneal cavity S31.600
     bite — *see* Bite, abdomen, wall, right, upper quadrant
     laceration — *see* Laceration, abdomen, wall, right, upper quadrant
     puncture — *see* Puncture, abdomen, wall, right, upper quadrant
sacral region — *see* Wound, open, back, lower
sacroiliac region — *see* Wound, open, back, lower
salivary gland — *see* Wound, open, oral cavity
scalp S01.00
   bite S01.05
   laceration — *see* Laceration, scalp
   puncture — *see* Puncture, scalp
scalpel, newborn (birth injury) P15.8
scapular region — *see* Wound, open, shoulder
sclera — *see* Wound, open, ocular
scrotum S31.30
   with amputation — *see* Amputation, traumatic, scrotum
   bite S31.35
   laceration — *see* Laceration, scrotum
   puncture — *see* Puncture, scrotum
shin — *see* Wound, open, leg
shoulder S41.00-
   with amputation — *see* Amputation, traumatic, arm
   bite — *see* Bite, shoulder
   laceration — *see* Laceration, shoulder
   puncture — *see* Puncture, shoulder
skin NOS T14.8
spermatic cord — *see* Wound, open, testis
sternal region — *see* Wound, open, thorax, front wall
submaxillary region — *see* Wound, open, head, specified site NEC
submental region — *see* Wound, open, head, specified site NEC
subungual
   finger(s) — *see* Wound, open, finger
   toe(s) — *see* Wound, open, toe
supraclavicular region — *see* Wound, open, neck, specified site NEC
temple, temporal region — *see* Wound, open, head, specified site NEC
temporomandibular area — *see* Wound, open, cheek
testis S31.30
   with amputation — *see* Amputation, traumatic, testes
   bite S31.35
   laceration — *see* Laceration, testis
   puncture — *see* Puncture, testis
thigh S71.10-
   with amputation — *see* Amputation, traumatic, hip
   bite — *see* Bite, thigh
   laceration — *see* Laceration, thigh
   puncture — *see* Puncture, thigh

Wound, open — *continued*
  thorax, thoracic (wall) S21.90
    back S21.20-
      with penetration S21.40
    bite — *see* Bite, thorax
    breast — *see* Wound, open, breast
    front S21.10-
      with penetration S21.30
    laceration — *see* Laceration, thorax
    puncture — *see* Puncture, thorax
  throat — *see* Wound, open, neck
  thumb S61.009
    with
      amputation — *see* Amputation, traumatic,
        thumb
      damage to nail S61.109
    bite — *see* Bite, thumb
    laceration — *see* Laceration, thumb
    left S61.002
      with
        damage to nail S61.102
    puncture — *see* Puncture, thumb
    right S61.001
      with
        damage to nail S61.101
  thyroid (gland) — *see* Wound, open, neck,
    thyroid
  toe(s) S91.109
    with
      amputation — *see* Amputation, traumatic,
        toe
      damage to nail S91.209
    bite — *see* Bite, toe
    great S91.103
      with
        damage to nail S91.203
      left S91.102
        with
          damage to nail S91.202
      right S91.101
        with
          damage to nail S91.201
    laceration — *see* Laceration, toe
    lesser S91.106
      with
        damage to nail S91.206
      left S91.105
        with
          damage to nail S91.205
      right S91.104
        with
          damage to nail S91.204
    puncture — *see* Puncture, toe
  tongue — *see* Wound, open, oral cavity
  trachea (cervical region) — *see* Wound, open,
    neck, trachea
  tunica vaginalis — *see* Wound, open, testis
  tympanum, tympanic membrane S09.2-
    laceration — *see* Laceration, ear, drum
    puncture — *see* Puncture, tympanum
  umbilical region — *see* Wound, open,
    abdomen, wall, periumbilic region
  uvula — *see* Wound, open, oral cavity
  vagina S31.40
    bite S31.45
    laceration — *see* Laceration, vagina
    puncture — *see* Puncture, vagina
  vitreous (humor) — *see* Wound, open, ocular
  vocal cord S11.039
    bite — *see* Bite, vocal cord
    laceration S11.031
      with foreign body S11.032
    puncture S11.033
      with foreign body S11.034

Wound, open — *continued*
  vulva S31.40
    with amputation — *see* Amputation,
      traumatic, vulva
    bite S31.45
    laceration — *see* Laceration, vulva
    puncture — *see* Puncture, vulva
  wrist S61.50-
    bite — *see* Bite, wrist
    laceration — *see* Laceration, wrist
    puncture — *see* Puncture, wrist
Wound, superficial — *see* Injury — *see also*
  specified injury type
Wright's syndrome G54.0
Wrist — *see* condition
Wrong drug (by accident) (given in error) —
  see Table of Drugs and Chemicals, by drug,
  poisoning
Wry neck — *see* Torticollis
Wuchereria (bancrofti) infestation B74.0
Wuchereriasis B74.0
Wuchernde Struma Langhans C73

X-ray (of)
  abnormal findings — *see* Abnormal,
    diagnostic imaging
  breast (mammogram) (routine) Z12.31
  chest
    routine (as part of a general medical
      examination) Z00.00
      with abnormal findings Z00.01
  routine (as part of a general medical
    examination) Z00.00
    with abnormal findings Z00.01
Xanthelasma (eyelid) (palpebrarum) H02.60
  left H02.66
    lower H02.65
    upper H02.64
  right H02.63
    lower H02.62
    upper H02.61
Xanthelasmatosis (essential) E78.2
Xanthinuria, hereditary E79.8
Xanthoastrocytoma
  specified site — *see* Neoplasm, malignant, by
    site
  unspecified site C71.9
Xanthofibroma — *see* Neoplasm, connective
  tissue, benign
Xanthogranuloma D76.3
Xanthoma(s), xanthomatosis (primary)
  (familial) (hereditary) E75.5
  with
    hyperlipoproteinemia
      Type I E78.3
      Type III E78.2
      Type IV E78.1
      Type V E78.3
  bone (generalisata) C96.5
  cerebrotendinous E75.5
  cutaneotendinous E75.5
  disseminatum (skin) E78.2
  eruptive E78.2
  hypercholesterinemic E78.00
  hypercholesterolemic E78.00
  hyperlipidemic E78.5
  joint E75.5
  multiple (skin) E78.2
  tendon (sheath) E75.5
  tuberosum E78.2
  tuberous E78.2
  tubo-eruptive E78.2
  verrucous, oral mucosa K13.4
Xanthosis R23.8
Xenophobia F40.10
Xeroderma — *see also* Ichthyosis
  acquired L85.0
  eyelid H01.149
    left H01.146
      lower H01.145
      upper H01.144
    right H01.143
      lower H01.142
      upper H01.141
  pigmentosum Q82.1
  vitamin A deficiency E50.8
Xerophthalmia (vitamin A deficiency) E50.7
  unrelated to vitamin A deficiency — *see*
    Keratoconjunctivitis

Xerosis
  conjunctiva H11.14-
    with Bitot's spots — *see also* Pigmentation,
      conjunctiva
      vitamin A deficiency E50.1
    vitamin A deficiency E50.0
  cornea H18.89-
    with ulceration — *see* Ulcer, cornea
      vitamin A deficiency E50.3
    vitamin A deficiency E50.2
  cutis L85.3
  skin L85.3
Xerostomia K11.7
Xiphopagus Q89.4
XO syndrome Q96.9
XXXXY syndrome Q98.1
XXY syndrome Q98.0

Y

Yaba pox (virus disease) B08.72
Yatapoxvirus B08.70
  specified NEC B08.79
Yawning R06.89
  psychogenic F45.8
Yaws A66.9
  bone lesions A66.6
  butter A66.1
  chancre A66.0
  cutaneous, less than five years after infection
    A66.2
  early (cutaneous) (macular) (maculopapular)
    (micropapular) (papular) A66.2
    frambeside A66.2
    skin lesions NEC A66.2
  eyelid A66.2
  ganglion A66.6
  gangosis, gangosa A66.5
  gumma, gummata A66.4
    bone A66.6
  gummatous
    frambeside A66.4
    osteitis A66.6
    periostitis A66.6
  hydrarthrosis (*see also* subcategory M14.8-)
    A66.6
  hyperkeratosis (early) (late) A66.3
  initial lesions A66.0
  joint lesions (*see also* subcategory M14.8-)
    A66.6
  juxta-articular nodules A66.7
  late nodular (ulcerated) A66.4
  latent (without clinical manifestations) (with
    positive serology) A66.8
  mother A66.0
  mucosal A66.7
  multiple papillomata A66.1
  nodular, late (ulcerated) A66.4
  osteitis A66.6
  papilloma, plantar or palmar A66.1
  periostitis (hypertrophic) A66.6
  specified NEC A66.7
  ulcers A66.4
  wet crab A66.1
Yeast infection (*see also* Candidiasis) B37.9
Yellow
  atrophy (liver) — *see* Failure, hepatic
  fever — *see* Fever, yellow
  jack — *see* Fever, yellow
  jaundice — *see* Jaundice
  nail syndrome L60.5
Yersiniosis — *see also* Infection, Yersinia
  extraintestinal A28.2
  intestinal A04.6

Z

Zahorsky's syndrome (herpangina) B08.5
Zellweger's syndrome Q87.89
Zenker's diverticulum (esophagus) K22.5
Ziehen-Oppenheim disease G24.1
Zieve's syndrome K70.0
Zika NOS A92.5
Zinc
  deficiency, dietary E60
  metabolism disorder E83.2
Zollinger-Ellison syndrome E16.4
Zona — *see* Herpes, zoster
Zoophobia F40.218
Zoster (herpes) — *see* Herpes, zoster
Zygomycosis B46.9
  specified NEC B46.8
Zymotic — *see* condition

DRUGS & CHEMICALS

Table of Drugs & Chemicals	POISONING Accidental (Unintentional)	Self-Harm (Intentional)	Assault	Undetermined	Adverse Effect	Underdosing
14-hydroxydihydro- morphinone	T40.2x1-	T40.2x2-	T40.2x3-	T40.2x4-	T40.2x5-	T40.2x6-
1-propanol	T51.3x1-	T51.3x2-	T51.3x3-	T51.3x4-	—	—
2,4,5-T (trichloro- phenoxyacetic acid)	T60.1x1-	T60.1x2-	T60.1x3-	T60.1x4-	—	—
2,4-D (dichlorophen- oxyacetic acid)	T60.3x1-	T60.3x2-	T60.3x3-	T60.3x4-	—	—
2,4-toluene diisocyanate	T65.0x1-	T65.0x2-	T65.0x3-	T65.0x4-	—	—
2-propanol	T51.2x1-	T51.2x2-	T51.2x3-	T51.2x4-	—	—
ABOB	T37.5x1-	T37.5x2-	T37.5x3-	T37.5x4-	T37.5x5-	T37.5x6-
Abrine	T62.2x1-	T62.2x2-	T62.2x3-	T62.2x4-	—	—
Abrus (seed)	T62.2x1-	T62.2x2-	T62.2x3-	T62.2x4-	—	—
Absinthe	T51.0x1-	T51.0x2-	T51.0x3-	T51.0x4-	—	—
beverage	T51.0x1-	T51.0x2-	T51.0x3-	T51.0x4-	—	—
Acaricide	T60.8x1-	T60.8x2-	T60.8x3-	T60.8x4-	—	—
Acebutolol	T44.7x1-	T44.7x2-	T44.7x3-	T44.7x4-	T44.7x5-	T44.7x6-
Acecarbromal	T42.6x1-	T42.6x2-	T42.6x3-	T42.6x4-	T42.6x5-	T42.6x6-
Aceclidine	T44.1x1-	T44.1x2-	T44.1x3-	T44.1x4-	T44.1x5-	T44.1x6-
Acedapsone	T37.0x1-	T37.0x2-	T37.0x3-	T37.0x4-	T37.0x5-	T37.0x6-
Acefylline piperazine	T48.6x1-	T48.6x2-	T48.6x3-	T48.6x4-	T48.6x5-	T48.6x6-
Acemorphan	T40.2x1-	T40.2x2-	T40.2x3-	T40.2x4-	T40.2x5-	T40.2x6-
Acenocoumarin	T45.511-	T45.512-	T45.513-	T45.514-	T45.515-	T45.516-
Acenocoumarol	T45.511-	T45.512-	T45.513-	T45.514-	T45.515-	T45.516-
Acepifylline	T48.6x1-	T48.6x2-	T48.6x3-	T48.6x4-	T48.6x5-	T48.6x6-
Acepromazine	T43.3x1-	T43.3x2-	T43.3x3-	T43.3x4-	T43.3x5-	T43.3x6-
Acesulfamethoxypyridazine	T37.0x1-	T37.0x2-	T37.0x3-	T37.0x4-	T37.0x5-	T37.0x6-
Acetal	T52.8x1-	T52.8x2-	T52.8x3-	T52.8x4-	—	—
Acetaldehyde (vapor)	T52.8x1-	T52.8x2-	T52.8x3-	T52.8x4-	—	—
liquid	T65.891-	T65.892-	T65.893-	T65.894-	—	—
P-Acetamidophenol	T39.1x1-	T39.1x2-	T39.1x3-	T39.1x4-	T39.1x5-	T39.1x6-
Acetaminophen	T39.1x1-	T39.1x2-	T39.1x3-	T39.1x4-	T39.1x5-	T39.1x6-
Acetaminosalol	T39.1x1-	T39.1x2-	T39.1x3-	T39.1x4-	T39.1x5-	T39.1x6-
Acetanilide	T39.1x1-	T39.1x2-	T39.1x3-	T39.1x4-	T39.1x5-	T39.1x6-
Acetarsol	T37.3x1-	T37.3x2-	T37.3x3-	T37.3x4-	T37.3x5-	T37.3x6-
Acetazolamide	T50.2x1-	T50.2x2-	T50.2x3-	T50.2x4-	T50.2x5-	T50.2x6-
Acetiamine	T45.2x1-	T45.2x2-	T45.2x3-	T45.2x4-	T45.2x5-	T45.2x6-
Acetic						
acid	T54.2x1-	T54.2x2-	T54.2x3-	T54.2x4-	—	—
with sodium acetate (ointment)	T49.3x1-	T49.3x2-	T49.3x3-	T49.3x4-	T49.3x5-	T49.3x6-
ester (solvent) (vapor)	T52.8x1-	T52.8x2-	T52.8x3-	T52.8x4-	—	—
irrigating solution	T50.3x1-	T50.3x2-	T50.3x3-	T50.3x4-	T50.3x5-	T50.3x6-
medicinal (lotion)	T49.2x1-	T49.2x2-	T49.2x3-	T49.2x4-	T49.2x5-	T49.2x6-
anhydride	T65.891-	T65.892-	T65.893-	T65.894-	—	—
ether (vapor)	T52.8x1-	T52.8x2-	T52.8x3-	T52.8x4-	—	—
Acetohexamide	T38.3x1-	T38.3x2-	T38.3x3-	T38.3x4-	T38.3x5-	T38.3x6-
Acetohydroxamic acid	T50.991-	T50.992-	T50.993-	T50.994-	T50.995-	T50.996-
Acetomenaphthone	T45.7x1-	T45.7x2-	T45.7x3-	T45.7x4-	T45.7x5-	T45.7x6-
Acetomorphine	T40.1x1-	T40.1x2-	T40.1x3-	T40.1x4-	—	—
Acetone (oils)	T52.4x1-	T52.4x2-	T52.4x3-	T52.4x4-	—	—
chlorinated	T52.4x1-	T52.4x2-	T52.4x3-	T52.4x4-	—	—
vapor	T52.4x1-	T52.4x2-	T52.4x3-	T52.4x4-	—	—
Acetonitrile	T52.8x1-	T52.8x2-	T52.8x3-	T52.8x4-	—	—
Acetophenazine	T43.3x1-	T43.3x2-	T43.3x3-	T43.3x4-	T43.3x5-	T43.3x6-
Acetophenetedin	T39.1x1-	T39.1x2-	T39.1x3-	T39.1x4-	T39.1x5-	T39.1x6-
Acetophenone	T52.4x1-	T52.4x2-	T52.4x3-	T52.4x4-	—	—
Acetorphine	T40.2x1-	T40.2x2-	T40.2x3-	T40.2x4-	—	—
Acetosulfone (sodium)	T37.1x1-	T37.1x2-	T37.1x3-	T37.1x4-	T37.1x5-	T37.1x6-
Acetrizoate (sodium)	T50.8x1-	T50.8x2-	T50.8x3-	T50.8x4-	T50.8x5-	T50.8x6-
Acetrizoic acid	T50.8x1-	T50.8x2-	T50.8x3-	T50.8x4-	T50.8x5-	T50.8x6-
Acetyl						
bromide	T53.6x1-	T53.6x2-	T53.6x3-	T53.6x4-	—	—
chloride	T53.6x1-	T53.6x2-	T53.6x3-	T53.6x4-	—	—

Table of Drugs & Chemicals	POISONING Accidental (Unintentional)	Self-Harm (Intentional)	Assault	Undetermined	Adverse Effect	Underdosing
Acetylcarbromal	T42.6x1-	T42.6x2-	T42.6x3-	T42.6x4-	T42.6x5-	T42.6x6-
Acetylcholine						
chloride	T44.1x1-	T44.1x2-	T44.1x3-	T44.1x4-	T44.1x5-	T44.1x6-
derivative	T44.1x1-	T44.1x2-	T44.1x3-	T44.1x4-	T44.1x5-	T44.1x6-
Acetylcysteine	T48.4x1-	T48.4x2-	T48.4x3-	T48.4x4-	T48.4x5-	T48.4x6-
Acetyldigitoxin	T46.0x1-	T46.0x2-	T46.0x3-	T46.0x4-	T46.0x5-	T46.0x6-
Acetyldigoxin	T46.0x1-	T46.0x2-	T46.0x3-	T46.0x4-	T46.0x5-	T46.0x6-
Acetyldihydrocodeine	T40.2x1-	T40.2x2-	T40.2x3-	T40.2x4-	—	—
Acetyldihydrocodeinone	T40.2x1-	T40.2x2-	T40.2x3-	T40.2x4-	—	—
Acetylene (gas)	T59.891-	T59.892-	T59.893-	T59.894-	—	—
dichloride	T53.6x1-	T53.6x2-	T53.6x3-	T53.6x4-	—	—
incomplete combustion of	T58.11x-	T58.12x-	T58.13x-	T58.14x-	—	—
industrial	T59.891-	T59.892-	T59.893-	T59.894-	—	—
tetrachloride	T53.6x1-	T53.6x2-	T53.6x3-	T53.6x4-	—	—
vapor	T53.6x1-	T53.6x2-	T53.6x3-	T53.6x4-	—	—
Acetylpheneturide	T42.6x1-	T42.6x2-	T42.6x3-	T42.6x4-	T42.6x5-	T42.6x6-
Acetylphenylhydrazine	T39.8x1-	T39.8x2-	T39.8x3-	T39.8x4-	T39.8x5-	T39.8x6-
Acetylsalicylic acid (salts)	T39.011-	T39.012-	T39.013-	T39.014-	T39.015-	T39.016-
enteric coated	T39.011-	T39.012-	T39.013-	T39.014-	T39.015-	T39.016-
Acetylsulfamethoxypyrida- zine	T37.0x1-	T37.0x2-	T37.0x3-	T37.0x4-	T37.0x5-	T37.0x6-
Achromycin	T36.4x1-	T36.4x2-	T36.4x3-	T36.4x4-	T36.4x5-	T36.4x6-
ophthalmic preparation	T49.5x1-	T49.5x2-	T49.5x3-	T49.5x4-	T49.5x5-	T49.5x6-
topical NEC	T49.0x1-	T49.0x2-	T49.0x3-	T49.0x4-	T49.0x5-	T49.0x6-
Aciclovir	T37.5x1-	T37.5x2-	T37.5x3-	T37.5x4-	T37.5x5-	T37.5x6
Acid (corrosive) NEC	T54.2x1-	T54.2x2-	T54.2x3-	T54.2x4-	—	—
Acidifying agent NEC	T50.901-	T50.902-	T50.903-	T50.904-	T50.905-	T50.906-
Acipimox	T46.6x1-	T46.6x2-	T46.6x3-	T46.6x4-	T46.6x5-	T46.6x6-
Acitretin	T50.991-	T50.992-	T50.993-	T50.994-	T50.995-	T50.996-
Aclarubicin	T45.1x1-	T45.1x2-	T45.1x3-	T45.1x4-	T45.1x5-	T45.1x6-
Aclatonium napadisilate	T48.1x1-	T48.1x2-	T48.1x3-	T48.1x4-	T48.1x5-	T48.1x6-
Aconite (wild)	T46.991-	T46.992-	T46.993-	T46.994-	T46.995-	T46.996-
Aconitine	T46.991-	T46.992-	T46.993-	T46.994-	T46.995-	T46.996-
Aconitum ferox	T46.991-	T46.992-	T46.993-	T46.994-	T46.995-	T46.996-
Acridine	T65.6x1-	T65.6x2-	T65.6x3-	T65.6x4-	—	—
vapor	T59.891-	T59.892-	T59.893-	T59.894-	—	—
Acriflavine	T37.91x-	T37.92x-	T37.93x-	T37.94x-	T37.95x-	T37.96x-
Acriflavinium chloride	T49.0x1-	T49.0x2-	T49.0x3-	T49.0x4-	T49.0x5-	T49.0x6-
Acrinol	T49.0x1-	T49.0x2-	T49.0x3-	T49.0x4-	T49.0x5-	T49.0x6-
Acrisorcin	T49.0x1-	T49.0x2-	T49.0x3-	T49.0x4-	T49.0x5-	T49.0x6-
Acrivastine	T45.0x1-	T45.0x2-	T45.0x3-	T45.0x4-	T45.0x5-	T45.0x6-
Acrolein (gas)	T59.891-	T59.892-	T59.893-	T59.894-	—	—
liquid	T54.1x1-	T54.1x2-	T54.1x3-	T54.1x4-	—	—
Acrylamide	T65.891-	T65.892-	T65.893-	T65.894-	—	—
Acrylic resin	T49.3x1-	T49.3x2-	T49.3x3-	T49.3x4-	T49.3x5-	T49.3x6-
Acrylonitrile	T65.891-	T65.892-	T65.893-	T65.894-	—	—
Actaea spicata	T62.2x1-	T62.2x2-	T62.2x3-	T62.2x4-	—	—
berry	T62.1x1-	T62.1x2-	T62.1x3-	T62.1x4-	—	—
Acterol	T37.3x1-	T37.3x2-	T37.3x3-	T37.3x4-	T37.3x5-	T37.3x6-
ACTH	T38.811-	T38.812-	T38.813-	T38.814-	T38.815-	T38.816-
Actinomycin C	T45.1x1-	T45.1x2-	T45.1x3-	T45.1x4-	T45.1x5-	T45.1x6-
Actinomycin D	T45.1x1-	T45.1x2-	T45.1x3-	T45.1x4-	T45.1x5-	T45.1x6-
Activated charcoal — see also Charcoal, medicinal	T47.6x1-	T47.6x2-	T47.6x3-	T47.6x4-	T47.6x5-	T47.6x6-
Acyclovir	T37.5x1-	T37.5x2-	T37.5x3-	T37.5x4-	T37.5x5-	T37.5x6-
Adenine	T45.2x1-	T45.2x2-	T45.2x3-	T45.2x4-	T45.2x5-	T45.2x6-
arabinoside	T37.5x1-	T37.5x2-	T37.5x3-	T37.5x4-	T37.5x5-	T37.5x6-
Adenosine (phosphate)	T46.2x1-	T46.2x2-	T46.2x3-	T46.2x4-	T46.2x5-	T46.2x6-
ADH	T38.891-	T38.892-	T38.893-	T38.894-	T38.895-	T38.896-
Adhesive NEC	T65.891-	T65.892-	T65.893-	T65.894-	—	—
Adicillin	T36.0x1-	T36.0x2-	T36.0x3-	T36.0x4-	T36.0x5-	T36.0x6-

DRUGS & CHEMICALS

Table of Drugs & Chemicals	POISONING Accidental (Unintentional)	POISONING Self-Harm (Intentional)	POISONING Assault	POISONING Undetermined	Adverse Effect	Underdosing
Adiphenine	T44.3x1-	T44.3x2-	T44.3x3-	T44.3x4-	T44.3x5-	T44.3x6-
Adipiodone	T50.8x1-	T50.8x2-	T50.8x3-	T50.8x4-	T50.8x5-	T50.8x6-
Adjunct, pharmaceutical	T50.901-	T50.902-	T50.903-	T50.904-	T50.905-	T50.906-
Adrenal (extract, cortex or medulla) (glucocorticoids) (hormones) (mineralocorticoids)	T38.0x1-	T38.0x2-	T38.0x3-	T38.0x4-	T38.0x5-	T38.0x6-
ENT agent	T49.6x1-	T49.6x2-	T49.6x3-	T49.6x4-	T49.6x5-	T49.6x6-
ophthalmic preparation	T49.5x1-	T49.5x2-	T49.5x3-	T49.5x4-	T49.5x5-	T49.5x6-
topical NEC	T49.0x1-	T49.0x2-	T49.0x3-	T49.0x4-	T49.0x5-	T49.0x6-
Adrenaline	T44.5x1-	T44.5x2-	T44.5x3-	T44.5x4-	T44.5x5-	T44.5x6-
Adrenalin — see Adrenaline						
Adrenergic NEC	T44.901-	T44.902-	T44.903-	T44.904-	T44.905-	T44.906-
blocking agent NEC	T44.8x1-	T44.8x2-	T44.8x3-	T44.8x4-	T44.8x5-	T44.8x6-
beta, heart	T44.7x1-	T44.7x2-	T44.7x3-	T44.7x4-	T44.7x5-	T44.7x6-
specified NEC	T44.991-	T44.992-	T44.993-	T44.994-	T44.995-	T44.996-
Adrenochrome derivative	T46.991-	T46.992-	T46.993-	T46.994-	T46.995-	T46.996-
(mono) semicarbazone	T46.991-	T46.992-	T46.993-	T46.994-	T46.995-	T46.996-
Adrenocorticotrophic hormone	T38.811-	T38.812-	T38.813-	T38.814-	T38.815-	T38.816-
Adrenocorticotrophin	T38.811-	T38.812-	T38.813-	T38.814-	T38.815-	T38.816-
Adriamycin	T45.1x1-	T45.1x2-	T45.1x3-	T45.1x4-	T45.1x5-	T45.1x6-
Aerosol spray NEC	T65.91x-	T65.92x-	T65.93x-	T65.94x-	—	—
Aerosporin	T36.8x1-	T36.8x2-	T36.8x3-	T36.8x4-	T36.8x5-	T36.8x6-
ENT agent	T49.6x1-	T49.6x2-	T49.6x3-	T49.6x4-	T49.6x5-	T49.6x6-
ophthalmic preparation	T49.5x1-	T49.5x2-	T49.5x3-	T49.5x4-	T49.5x5-	T49.5x6-
topical NEC	T49.0x1-	T49.0x2-	T49.0x3-	T49.0x4-	T49.0x5-	T49.0x6-
Aethusa cynapium	T62.2x1-	T62.2x2-	T62.2x3-	T62.2x4-	—	—
Afghanistan black	T40.7x1-	T40.7x2-	T40.7x3-	T40.7x4-	T40.7x5-	T40.7x6-
Aflatoxin	T64.01x-	T64.02x-	T64.03x-	T64.04x-	—	—
Afloqualone	T42.8x1-	T42.8x2-	T42.8x3-	T42.8x4-	T42.8x5-	T42.8x6-
African boxwood	T62.2x1-	T62.2x2-	T62.2x3-	T62.2x4-	—	—
Agar	T47.4x1-	T47.4x2-	T47.4x3-	T47.4x4-	T47.4x5-	T47.4x6-
Agonist predominantly alpha-adrenoreceptor	T44.4x1-	T44.4x2-	T44.4x3-	T44.4x4-	T44.4x5-	T44.4x6-
beta-adrenoreceptor	T44.5x1-	T44.5x2-	T44.5x3-	T44.5x4-	T44.5x5-	T44.5x6-
Agricultural agent NEC	T65.91x-	T65.92x-	T65.93x-	T65.94x-	—	—
Agrypnal	T42.3x1-	T42.3x2-	T42.3x3-	T42.3x4-	T42.3x5-	T42.3x6-
AHLG	T50.Z11-	T50.Z12-	T50.Z13-	T50.Z14-	T50.Z15-	T50.Z16-
Air contaminant(s), source/type NOS	T65.91x-	T65.92x-	T65.93x-	T65.94x-	—	—
Ajmaline	T46.2x1-	T46.2x2-	T46.2x3-	T46.2x4-	T46.2x5-	T46.2x6-
Akee	T62.1x1-	T62.1x2-	T62.1x3-	T62.1x4-	—	—
Akrinol	T49.0x1-	T49.0x2-	T49.0x3-	T49.0x4-	T49.0x5-	T49.0x6-
Akritoin	T37.8x1-	T37.8x2-	T37.8x3-	T37.8x4-	T37.8x5-	T37.8x6-
Alacepril	T46.4x1-	T46.4x2-	T46.4x3-	T46.4x4-	T46.4x5-	T46.4x6-
Alantolactone	T37.4x1-	T37.4x2-	T37.4x3-	T37.4x4-	T37.4x5-	T37.4x6-
Albamycin	T36.8x1-	T36.8x2-	T36.8x3-	T36.8x4-	T36.8x5-	T36.8x6-
Albendazole	T37.4x1-	T37.4x2-	T37.4x3-	T37.4x4-	T37.4x5-	T37.4x6-
Albumin bovine	T45.8x1-	T45.8x2-	T45.8x3-	T45.8x4-	T45.8x5-	T45.8x6-
human serum	T45.8x1-	T45.8x2-	T45.8x3-	T45.8x4-	T45.8x5-	T45.8x6-
salt-poor	T45.8x1-	T45.8x2-	T45.8x3-	T45.8x4-	T45.8x5-	T45.8x6-
normal human serum	T45.8x1-	T45.8x2-	T45.8x3-	T45.8x4-	T45.8x5-	T45.8x6-
Albuterol	T48.6x1-	T48.6x2-	T48.6x3-	T48.6x4-	T48.6x5-	T48.6x6-
Albutoin	T42.0x1-	T42.0x2-	T42.0x3-	T42.0x4-	T42.0x5-	T42.0x6-
Alclometasone	T49.0x1-	T49.0x2-	T49.0x3-	T49.0x4-	T49.0x5-	T49.0x6-
Alcohol	T51.91x-	T51.92x-	T51.93x-	T51.94x-	—	—
absolute	T51.0x1-	T51.0x2-	T51.0x3-	T51.0x4-	—	—
beverage	T51.0x1-	T51.0x2-	T51.0x3-	T51.0x4-	—	—
allyl	T51.8x1-	T51.8x2-	T51.8x3-	T51.8x4-	—	—
antifreeze	T51.1x1-	T51.1x2-	T51.1x3-	T51.1x4-	—	—

Table of Drugs & Chemicals	POISONING Accidental (Unintentional)	POISONING Self-Harm (Intentional)	POISONING Assault	POISONING Undetermined	Adverse Effect	Underdosing
Alcohol - *continued*	T51.91x-	T51.92x-	T51.93x-	T51.94x-	—	—
amyl	T51.3x1-	T51.3x2-	T51.3x3-	T51.3x4-	—	—
beverage	T51.0x1-	T51.0x2-	T51.0x3-	T51.0x4-	—	—
butyl	T51.3x1-	T51.3x2-	T51.3x3-	T51.3x4-	—	—
dehydrated	T51.0x1-	T51.0x2-	T51.0x3-	T51.0x4-	—	—
beverage	T51.0x1-	T51.0x2-	T51.0x3-	T51.0x4-	—	—
denatured	T51.0x1-	T51.0x2-	T51.0x3-	T51.0x4-	—	—
deterrent NEC	T50.6x1-	T50.6x2-	T50.6x3-	T50.6x4-	T50.6x5-	T50.6x6-
diagnostic (gastric function)	T50.8x1-	T50.8x2-	T50.8x3-	T50.8x4-	T50.8x5-	T50.8x6-
ethyl	T51.0x1-	T51.0x2-	T51.0x3-	T51.0x4-	—	—
beverage	T51.0x1-	T51.0x2-	T51.0x3-	T51.0x4-	—	—
grain	T51.0x1-	T51.0x2-	T51.0x3-	T51.0x4-	—	—
beverage	T51.0x1-	T51.0x2-	T51.0x3-	T51.0x4-	—	—
industrial	T51.0x1-	T51.0x2-	T51.0x3-	T51.0x4-	—	—
isopropyl	T51.2x1-	T51.2x2-	T51.2x3-	T51.2x4-	—	—
methyl	T51.1x1-	T51.1x2-	T51.1x3-	T51.1x4-	—	—
preparation for consumption	T51.0x1-	T51.0x2-	T51.0x3-	T51.0x4-	—	—
propyl	T51.3x1-	T51.3x2-	T51.3x3-	T51.3x4-	—	—
secondary	T51.2x1-	T51.2x2-	T51.2x3-	T51.2x4-	—	—
radiator	T51.1x1-	T51.1x2-	T51.1x3-	T51.1x4-	—	—
rubbing	T51.2x1-	T51.2x2-	T51.2x3-	T51.2x4-	—	—
specified type NEC	T51.8x1-	T51.8x2-	T51.8x3-	T51.8x4-	—	—
surgical	T51.0x1-	T51.0x2-	T51.0x3-	T51.0x4-	—	—
vapor (from any type of alcohol)	T59.891-	T59.892-	T59.893-	T59.894-	—	—
wood	T51.1x1-	T51.1x2-	T51.1x3-	T51.1x4-	—	—
Alcuronium (chloride)	T48.1x1-	T48.1x2-	T48.1x3-	T48.1x4-	T48.1x5-	T48.1x6-
Aldactone	T50.0x1-	T50.0x2-	T50.0x3-	T50.0x4-	T50.0x5-	T50.0x6-
Aldesulfone sodium	T37.1x1-	T37.1x2-	T37.1x3-	T37.1x4-	T37.1x5-	T37.1x6-
Aldicarb	T60.0x1-	T60.0x2-	T60.0x3-	T60.0x4-	—	—
Aldomet	T46.5x1-	T46.5x2-	T46.5x3-	T46.5x4-	T46.5x5-	T46.5x6-
Aldosterone	T50.0x1-	T50.0x2-	T50.0x3-	T50.0x4-	T50.0x5-	T50.0x6-
Aldrin (dust)	T60.1x1-	T60.1x2-	T60.1x3-	T60.1x4-	—	—
Aleve — see Naproxen						
Alexitol sodium	T47.1x1-	T47.1x2-	T47.1x3-	T47.1x4-	T47.1x5-	T47.1x6-
Alfacalcidol	T45.2x1-	T45.2x2-	T45.2x3-	T45.2x4-	T45.2x5-	T45.2x6-
Alfadolone	T41.1x1-	T41.1x2-	T41.1x3-	T41.1x4-	T41.1x5-	T41.1x6-
Alfaxalone	T41.1x1-	T41.1x2-	T41.1x3-	T41.1x4-	T41.1x5-	T41.1x6-
Alfentanil	T40.4x1-	T40.4x2-	T40.4x3-	T40.4x4-	T40.4x5-	T40.4x6-
Alfuzosin (hydrochloride)	T44.8x1-	T44.8x2-	T44.8x3-	T44.8x4-	T44.8x5-	T44.8x6-
Algae (harmful) (toxin)	T65.821-	T65.822-	T65.823-	T65.824-	—	—
Algeldrate	T47.1x1-	T47.1x2-	T47.1x3-	T47.1x4-	T47.1x5-	T47.1x6-
Algin	T47.8x1-	T47.8x2-	T47.8x3-	T47.8x4-	T47.8x5-	T47.8x6-
Alglucerase	T45.3x1-	T45.3x2-	T45.3x3-	T45.3x4-	T45.3x5-	T45.3x6-
Alidase	T45.3x1-	T45.3x2-	T45.3x3-	T45.3x4-	T45.3x5-	T45.3x6-
Alimemazine	T43.3x1-	T43.3x2-	T43.3x3-	T43.3x4-	T43.3x5-	T43.3x6-
Aliphatic thiocyanates	T65.0x1-	T65.0x2-	T65.0x3-	T65.0x4-	—	—
Alizapride	T45.0x1-	T45.0x2-	T45.0x3-	T45.0x4-	T45.0x5-	T45.0x6-
Alkali (caustic)	T54.3x1-	T54.3x2-	T54.3x3-	T54.3x4-	—	—
Alkaline antiseptic solution (aromatic)	T49.6x1-	T49.6x2-	T49.6x3-	T49.6x4-	T49.6x5-	T49.6x6-
Alkalinizing agents (medicinal)	T50.901-	T50.902-	T50.903-	T50.904-	T50.905-	T50.906-
Alkalizing agent NEC	T50.901-	T50.902-	T50.903-	T50.904-	T50.905-	T50.906-
Alka-seltzer	T39.011-	T39.012-	T39.013-	T39.014-	T39.015-	T39.016-
Alkavervir	T46.5x1-	T46.5x2-	T46.5x3-	T46.5x4-	T46.5x5-	T46.5x6-
Alkonium (bromide)	T49.0x1-	T49.0x2-	T49.0x3-	T49.0x4-	T49.0x5-	T49.0x6-
Alkylating drug NEC	T45.1x1-	T45.1x2-	T45.1x3-	T45.1x4-	T45.1x5-	T45.1x6-
antimyeloproliferative	T45.1x1-	T45.1x2-	T45.1x3-	T45.1x4-	T45.1x5-	T45.1x6-
lymphatic	T45.1x1-	T45.1x2-	T45.1x3-	T45.1x4-	T45.1x5-	T45.1x6-
Alkylisocyanate	T65.0x1-	T65.0x2-	T65.0x3-	T65.0x4-	—	—
Allantoin	T49.4x1-	T49.4x2-	T49.4x3-	T49.4x4-	T49.4x5-	T49.4x6-
Allegron	T43.011-	T43.012-	T43.013-	T43.014-	T43.015-	T43.016-

DRUGS & CHEMICALS

Table of Drugs & Chemicals	Poisoning Accidental (Unintentional)	Poisoning Self-Harm (Intentional)	Poisoning Assault	Poisoning Undetermined	Adverse Effect	Underdosing
Allethrin	T49.0x1-	T49.0x2-	T49.0x3-	T49.0x4-	T49.0x5-	T49.0x6-
Allobarbital	T42.3x1-	T42.3x2-	T42.3x3-	T42.3x4-	T42.3x5-	T42.3x6-
Allopurinol	T50.4x1-	T50.4x2-	T50.4x3-	T50.4x4-	T50.4x5-	T50.4x6-
Allyl						
alcohol	T51.8x1-	T51.8x2-	T51.8x3-	T51.8x4-	—	—
disulfide	T46.6x1-	T46.6x2-	T46.6x3-	T46.6x4-	T46.6x5-	T46.6x6-
Allylestrenol	T38.5x1-	T38.5x2-	T38.5x3-	T38.5x4-	T38.5x5-	T38.5x6-
Allylisopropylacetylurea	T42.6x1-	T42.6x2-	T42.6x3-	T42.6x4-	T42.6x5-	T42.6x6-
Allylisopropylmalonylurea	T42.3x1-	T42.3x2-	T42.3x3-	T42.3x4-	T42.3x5-	T42.3x6-
Allylthiourea	T49.3x1-	T49.3x2-	T49.3x3-	T49.3x4-	T49.3x5-	T49.3x6-
Allyltribromide	T42.6x1-	T42.6x2-	T42.6x3-	T42.6x4-	T42.6x5-	T42.6x6-
Allypropymal	T42.3x1-	T42.3x2-	T42.3x3-	T42.3x4-	T42.3x5-	T42.3x6-
Almagate	T47.1x1-	T47.1x2-	T47.1x3-	T47.1x4-	T47.1x5-	T47.1x6-
Almasilate	T47.1x1-	T47.1x2-	T47.1x3-	T47.1x4-	T47.1x5-	T47.1x6-
Almitrine	T50.7x1-	T50.7x2-	T50.7x3-	T50.7x4-	T50.7x5-	T50.7x6-
Aloes	T47.2x1-	T47.2x2-	T47.2x3-	T47.2x4-	T47.2x5-	T47.2x6-
Aloglutamol	T47.1x1-	T47.1x2-	T47.1x3-	T47.1x4-	T47.1x5-	T47.1x6-
Aloin	T47.2x1-	T47.2x2-	T47.2x3-	T47.2x4-	T47.2x5-	T47.2x6-
Aloxidone	T42.2x1-	T42.2x2-	T42.2x3-	T42.2x4-	T42.2x5-	T42.2x6-
Alpha						
acetyldigoxin	T46.0x1-	T46.0x2-	T46.0x3-	T46.0x4-	T46.0x5-	T46.0x6-
adrenergic blocking drug	T44.6x1-	T44.6x2-	T44.6x3-	T44.6x4-	T44.6x5-	T44.6x6-
amylase	T45.3x1-	T45.3x2-	T45.3x3-	T45.3x4-	T45.3x5-	T45.3x6-
tocoferol (acetate)	T45.2x1-	T45.2x2-	T45.2x3-	T45.2x4-	T45.2x5-	T45.2x6-
Alphadolone	T41.1x1-	T41.1x2-	T41.1x3-	T41.1x4-	T41.1x5-	T41.1x6-
Alphaprodine	T40.4x1-	T40.4x2-	T40.4x3-	T40.4x4-	T40.4x5-	T40.4x6-
Alphaxalone	T41.1x1-	T41.1x2-	T41.1x3-	T41.1x4-	T41.1x5-	T41.1x6-
Alprazolam	T42.4x1-	T42.4x2-	T42.4x3-	T42.4x4-	T42.4x5-	T42.4x6-
Alprenolol	T44.7x1-	T44.7x2-	T44.7x3-	T44.7x4-	T44.7x5-	T44.7x6-
Alprostadil	T46.7x1-	T46.7x2-	T46.7x3-	T46.7x4-	T46.7x5-	T46.7x6-
Alsactide	T38.811-	T38.812-	T38.813-	T38.814-	T38.815-	T38.816-
Alseroxylon	T46.5x1-	T46.5x2-	T46.5x3-	T46.5x4-	T46.5x5-	T46.5x6-
Alteplase	T45.611-	T45.612-	T45.613-	T45.614-	T45.615-	T45.616-
Altizide	T50.2x1-	T50.2x2-	T50.2x3-	T50.2x4-	T50.2x5-	T50.2x6-
Altretamine	T45.1x1-	T45.1x2-	T45.1x3-	T45.1x4-	T45.1x5-	T45.1x6-
Alum (medicinal)	T49.4x1-	T49.4x2-	T49.4x3-	T49.4x4-	T49.4x5-	T49.4x6-
nonmedicinal						
(ammonium)						
(potassium)	T56.891-	T56.892-	T56.893-	T56.894-	—	—
Aluminium, aluminum						
acetate	T49.2x1-	T49.2x2-	T49.2x3-	T49.2x4-	T49.2x5-	T49.2x6-
solution	T49.0x1-	T49.0x2-	T49.0x3-	T49.0x4-	T49.0x5-	T49.0x6-
aspirin	T39.011-	T39.012-	T39.013-	T39.014-	T39.015-	T39.016-
bis (acetylsalicylate)	T39.011-	T39.012-	T39.013-	T39.014-	T39.015-	T39.016-
carbonate (gel, basic)	T47.1x1-	T47.1x2-	T47.1x3-	T47.1x4-	T47.1x5-	T47.1x6-
chlorhydroxide-complex	T47.1x1-	T47.1x2-	T47.1x3-	T47.1x4-	T47.1x5-	T47.1x6-
chloride	T49.2x1-	T49.2x2-	T49.2x3-	T49.2x4-	T49.2x5-	T49.2x6-
clofibrate	T46.6x1-	T46.6x2-	T46.6x3-	T46.6x4-	T46.6x5-	T46.6x6-
diacetate	T49.2x1-	T49.2x2-	T49.2x3-	T49.2x4-	T49.2x5-	T49.2x6-
glycinate	T47.1x1-	T47.1x2-	T47.1x3-	T47.1x4-	T47.1x5-	T47.1x6-
hydroxide (gel)	T47.1x1-	T47.1x2-	T47.1x3-	T47.1x4-	T47.1x5-	T47.1x6-
hydroxide-magnesium						
carb. gel	T47.1x1-	T47.1x2-	T47.1x3-	T47.1x4-	T47.1x5-	T47.1x6-
magnesium silicate	T47.1x1-	T47.1x2-	T47.1x3-	T47.1x4-	T47.1x5-	T47.1x6-
nicotinate	T46.7x1-	T46.7x2-	T46.7x3-	T46.7x4-	T46.7x5-	T46.7x6-
ointment (surgical)						
(topical)	T49.3x1-	T49.3x2-	T49.3x3-	T49.3x4-	T49.3x5-	T49.3x6-
phosphate	T47.1x1-	T47.1x2-	T47.1x3-	T47.1x4-	T47.1x5-	T47.1x6-
salicylate	T39.091-	T39.092-	T39.093-	T39.094-	T39.095-	T39.096-
silicate	T47.1x1-	T47.1x2-	T47.1x3-	T47.1x4-	T47.1x5-	T47.1x6-
sodium silicate	T47.1x1-	T47.1x2-	T47.1x3-	T47.1x4-	T47.1x5-	T47.1x6-
subacetate	T49.2x1-	T49.2x2-	T49.2x3-	T49.2x4-	T49.2x5-	T49.2x6-
sulfate	T49.0x1-	T49.0x2-	T49.0x3-	T49.0x4-	T49.0x5-	T49.0x6-
tannate	T47.6x1-	T47.6x2-	T47.6x3-	T47.6x4-	T47.6x5-	T47.6x6-
topical NEC	T49.3x1-	T49.3x2-	T49.3x3-	T49.3x4-	T49.3x5-	T49.3x6-

Table of Drugs & Chemicals	Poisoning Accidental (Unintentional)	Poisoning Self-Harm (Intentional)	Poisoning Assault	Poisoning Undetermined	Adverse Effect	Underdosing
Alurate	T42.3x1-	T42.3x2-	T42.3x3-	T42.3x4-	T42.3x5-	T42.3x6-
Alverine	T44.3x1-	T44.3x2-	T44.3x3-	T44.3x4-	T44.3x5-	T44.3x6-
Alvodine	T40.2x1-	T40.2x2-	T40.2x3-	T40.2x4-	T40.2x5-	T40.2x6-
Amanita phalloides	T62.0x1-	T62.0x2-	T62.0x3-	T62.0x4-	—	—
Amanitine	T62.0x1-	T62.0x2-	T62.0x3-	T62.0x4-	—	—
Amantadine	T42.8x1-	T42.8x2-	T42.8x3-	T42.8x4-	T42.8x5-	T42.8x6-
Ambazone	T49.6x1-	T49.6x2-	T49.6x3-	T49.6x4-	T49.6x5-	T49.6x6-
Ambenonium (chloride)	T44.0x1-	T44.0x2-	T44.0x3-	T44.0x4-	T44.0x5-	T44.0x6-
Ambroxol	T48.4x1-	T48.4x2-	T48.4x3-	T48.4x4-	T48.4x5-	T48.4x6-
Ambuphylline	T48.6x1-	T48.6x2-	T48.6x3-	T48.6x4-	T48.6x5-	T48.6x6-
Ambutonium bromide	T44.3x1-	T44.3x2-	T44.3x3-	T44.3x4-	T44.3x5-	T44.3x6-
Amcinonide	T49.0x1-	T49.0x2-	T49.0x3-	T49.0x4-	T49.0x5-	T49.0x6-
Amdinocilline	T36.0x1-	T36.0x2-	T36.0x3-	T36.0x4-	T36.0x5-	T36.0x6-
Ametazole	T50.8x1-	T50.8x2-	T50.8x3-	T50.8x4-	T50.8x5-	T50.8x6-
Amethocaine	T41.3x1-	T41.3x2-	T41.3x3-	T41.3x4-	T41.3x5-	T41.3x6-
regional	T41.3x1-	T41.3x2-	T41.3x3-	T41.3x4-	T41.3x5-	T41.3x6-
spinal	T41.3x1-	T41.3x2-	T41.3x3-	T41.3x4-	T41.3x5-	T41.3x6-
Amethopterin	T45.1x1-	T45.1x2-	T45.1x3-	T45.1x4-	T45.1x5-	T45.1x6-
Amezinium metilsulfate	T44.991-	T44.992-	T44.993-	T44.994-	T44.995-	T44.996-
Amfebutamone	T43.291-	T43.292-	T43.293-	T43.294-	T43.295-	T43.296-
Amfepramone	T50.5x1-	T50.5x2-	T50.5x3-	T50.5x4-	T50.5x5-	T50.5x6-
Amfetamine	T43.621-	T43.622-	T43.623-	T43.624-	T43.625-	T43.626-
Amfetaminil	T43.621-	T43.622-	T43.623-	T43.624-	T43.625-	T43.626-
Amfomycin	T36.8x1-	T36.8x2-	T36.8x3-	T36.8x4-	T36.8x5-	T36.8x6-
Amidefrine mesilate	T48.5x1-	T48.5x2-	T48.5x3-	T48.5x4-	T48.5x5-	T48.5x6-
Amidone	T40.3x1-	T40.3x2-	T40.3x3-	T40.3x4-	T40.3x5-	T40.3x6-
Amidopyrine	T39.2x1-	T39.2x2-	T39.2x3-	T39.2x4-	T39.2x5-	T39.2x6-
Amidotrizoate	T50.8x1-	T50.8x2-	T50.8x3-	T50.8x4-	T50.8x5-	T50.8x6-
Amiflamine	T43.1x1-	T43.1x2-	T43.1x3-	T43.1x4-	T43.1x5-	T43.1x6-
Amikacin	T36.5x1-	T36.5x2-	T36.5x3-	T36.5x4-	T36.5x5-	T36.5x6-
Amikhelline	T46.3x1-	T46.3x2-	T46.3x3-	T46.3x4-	T46.3x5-	T46.3x6-
Amiloride	T50.2x1-	T50.2x2-	T50.2x3-	T50.2x4-	T50.2x5-	T50.2x6-
Aminacrine	T49.0x1-	T49.0x2-	T49.0x3-	T49.0x4-	T49.0x5-	T49.0x6-
Amineptine	T43.011-	T43.012-	T43.013-	T43.014-	T43.015-	T43.016-
Aminitrozole	T37.3x1-	T37.3x2-	T37.3x3-	T37.3x4-	T37.3x5-	T37.3x6-
Amino acids	T50.3x1-	T50.3x2-	T50.3x3-	T50.3x4-	T50.3x5-	T50.3x6-
Aminoacetic acid						
(derivatives)	T50.3x1-	T50.3x2-	T50.3x3-	T50.3x4-	T50.3x5-	T50.3x6-
Aminoacridine	T49.0x1-	T49.0x2-	T49.0x3-	T49.0x4-	T49.0x5-	T49.0x6-
Aminobenzoic acid (-p)	T49.3x1-	T49.3x2-	T49.3x3-	T49.3x4-	T49.3x5-	T49.3x6-
4-Aminobutyric acid	T43.8x1-	T43.8x2-	T43.8x3-	T43.8x4-	T43.8x5-	T43.8x6-
Aminocaproic acid	T45.621-	T45.622-	T45.623-	T45.624-	T45.625-	T45.626-
Aminoethylisothiourium	T45.8x1-	T45.8x2-	T45.8x3-	T45.8x4-	T45.8x5-	T45.8x6-
Aminofenazone	T39.2x1-	T39.2x2-	T39.2x3-	T39.2x4-	T39.2x5-	T39.2x6-
Aminoglutethimide	T45.1x1-	T45.1x2-	T45.1x3-	T45.1x4-	T45.1x5-	T45.1x6-
Aminohippuric acid	T50.8x1-	T50.8x2-	T50.8x3-	T50.8x4-	T50.8x5-	T50.8x6-
Aminomethylbenzoic acid	T45.691-	T45.692-	T45.693-	T45.694-	T45.695-	T45.696-
Aminometradine	T50.2x1-	T50.2x2-	T50.2x3-	T50.2x4-	T50.2x5-	T50.2x6-
Aminopentamide	T44.3x1-	T44.3x2-	T44.3x3-	T44.3x4-	T44.3x5-	T44.3x6-
Aminophenazone	T39.2x1-	T39.2x2-	T39.2x3-	T39.2x4-	T39.2x5-	T39.2x6-
Aminophenol	T54.0x1-	T54.0x2-	T54.0x3-	T54.0x4-	—	—
4-Aminophenol derivatives	T39.1x1-	T39.1x2-	T39.1x3-	T39.1x4-	T39.1x5-	T39.1x6-
Aminophenylpyridone	T43.591-	T43.592-	T43.593-	T43.594-	T43.595-	T43.596-
Aminophylline	T48.6x1-	T48.6x2-	T48.6x3-	T48.6x4-	T48.6x5-	T48.6x6-
Aminopterin sodium	T45.1x1-	T45.1x2-	T45.1x3-	T45.1x4-	T45.1x5-	T45.1x6-
Aminopyrine	T39.2x1-	T39.2x2-	T39.2x3-	T39.2x4-	T39.2x5-	T39.2x6-
8-Aminoquinoline drugs	T37.2x1-	T37.2x2-	T37.2x3-	T37.2x4-	T37.2x5-	T37.2x6-
Aminorex	T50.5x1-	T50.5x2-	T50.5x3-	T50.5x4-	T50.5x5-	T50.5x6-
Aminosalicylic acid	T37.1x1-	T37.1x2-	T37.1x3-	T37.1x4-	T37.1x5-	T37.1x6-
Aminosalylum	T37.1x1-	T37.1x2-	T37.1x3-	T37.1x4-	T37.1x5-	T37.1x6-
Amiodarone	T46.2x1-	T46.2x2-	T46.2x3-	T46.2x4-	T46.2x5-	T46.2x6-

DRUGS & CHEMICALS

Table of Drugs & Chemicals	POISONING Accidental (Unintentional)	Self-Harm (Intentional)	Assault	Undetermined	Adverse Effect	Underdosing
Amiphenazole	T50.7x1-	T50.7x2-	T50.7x3-	T50.7x4-	T50.7x5-	T50.7x6-
Amiquinsin	T46.5x1-	T46.5x2-	T46.5x3-	T46.5x4-	T46.5x5-	T46.5x6-
Amisometradine	T50.2x1-	T50.2x2-	T50.2x3-	T50.2x4-	T50.2x5-	T50.2x6-
Amisulpride	T43.591-	T43.592-	T43.593-	T43.594-	T43.595-	T43.596-
Amitriptyline	T43.011-	T43.012-	T43.013-	T43.014-	T43.015-	T43.016-
Amitriptylinoxide	T43.011-	T43.012-	T43.013-	T43.014-	T43.015-	T43.016-
Amlexanox	T48.6x1-	T48.6x2-	T48.6x3-	T48.6x4-	T48.6x5-	T48.6x6-
Ammonia (fumes) (gas) (vapor)	T59.891-	T59.892-	T59.893-	T59.894-	—	—
aromatic spirit	T48.991-	T48.992-	T48.993-	T48.994-	T48.995-	T48.996-
liquid (household)	T54.3x1-	T54.3x2-	T54.3x3-	T54.3x4-	—	—
Ammoniated mercury	T49.0x1-	T49.0x2-	T49.0x3-	T49.0x4-	T49.0x5-	T49.0x6-
Ammonium						
acid tartrate	T49.5x1-	T49.5x2-	T49.5x3-	T49.5x4-	T49.5x5-	T49.5x6-
bromide	T42.6x1-	T42.6x2-	T42.6x3-	T42.6x4-	T42.6x5-	T42.6x6-
carbonate	T54.3x1-	T54.3x2-	T54.3x3-	T54.3x4-	—	—
chloride	T50.991-	T50.992-	T50.993-	T50.994-	T50.995-	T50.996-
expectorant	T48.4x1-	T48.4x2-	T48.4x3-	T48.4x4-	T48.4x5-	T48.4x6-
compounds (household) NEC	T54.3x1-	T54.3x2-	T54.3x3-	T54.3x4-	—	—
fumes (any usage)	T59.891-	T59.892-	T59.893-	T59.894-	—	—
industrial	T54.3x1-	T54.3x2-	T54.3x3-	T54.3x4-	—	—
ichthyosulronate	T49.4x1-	T49.4x2-	T49.4x3-	T49.4x4-	T49.4x5-	T49.4x6-
mandelate	T37.91x-	T37.92x-	T37.93x-	T37.94x-	T37.95x-	T37.96x-
sulfamate	T60.3x1-	T60.3x2-	T60.3x3-	T60.3x4-	—	—
sulfonate resin	T47.8x1-	T47.8x2-	T47.8x3-	T47.8x4-	T47.8x5-	T47.8x6-
Amobarbital (sodium)	T42.3x1-	T42.3x2-	T42.3x3-	T42.3x4-	T42.3x5-	T42.3x6-
Amodiaquine	T37.2x1-	T37.2x2-	T37.2x3-	T37.2x4-	T37.2x5-	T37.2x6-
Amopyroquin (e)	T37.2x1-	T37.2x2-	T37.2x3-	T37.2x4-	T37.2x5-	T37.2x6-
Amoxapine	T43.011-	T43.012-	T43.013-	T43.014-	T43.015-	T43.016-
Amoxicillin	T36.0x1-	T36.0x2-	T36.0x3-	T36.0x4-	T36.0x5-	T36.0x6-
Amperozide	T43.591-	T43.592-	T43.593-	T43.594-	T43.595-	T43.596-
Amphenidone	T43.591-	T43.592-	T43.593-	T43.594-	T43.595-	T43.596-
Amphetamine NEC	T43.621-	T43.622-	T43.623-	T43.624-	T43.625-	T43.626-
Amphomycin	T36.8x1-	T36.8x2-	T36.8x3-	T36.8x4-	T36.8x5-	T36.8x6-
Amphotalide	T37.4x1-	T37.4x2-	T37.4x3-	T37.4x4-	T37.4x5-	T37.4x6-
Amphotericin B	T36.7x1-	T36.7x2-	T36.7x3-	T36.7x4-	T36.7x5-	T36.7x6-
topical	T49.0x1-	T49.0x2-	T49.0x3-	T49.0x4-	T49.0x5-	T49.0x6-
Ampicillin	T36.0x1-	T36.0x2-	T36.0x3-	T36.0x4-	T36.0x5-	T36.0x6-
Amprotropine	T44.3x1-	T44.3x2-	T44.3x3-	T44.3x4-	T44.3x5-	T44.3x6-
Amsacrine	T45.1x1-	T45.1x2-	T45.1x3-	T45.1x4-	T45.1x5-	T45.1x6-
Amygdaline	T62.2x1-	T62.2x2-	T62.2x3-	T62.2x4-	—	—
Amyl						
acetate	T52.8x1-	T52.8x2-	T52.8x3-	T52.8x4-	—	—
vapor	T59.891-	T59.892-	T59.893-	T59.894-	—	—
alcohol	T51.3x1-	T51.3x2-	T51.3x3-	T51.3x4-	—	—
chloride	T53.6x1-	T53.6x2-	T53.6x3-	T53.6x4-	—	—
formate	T52.8x1-	T52.8x2-	T52.8x3-	T52.8x4-	—	—
nitrite	T46.3x1-	T46.3x2-	T46.3x3-	T46.3x4-	T46.3x5-	T46.3x6-
propionate	T65.891-	T65.892-	T65.893-	T65.894-	—	—
Amylase	T47.5x1-	T47.5x2-	T47.5x3-	T47.5x4-	T47.5x5-	T47.5x6-
Amyleine, regional	T41.3x1-	T41.3x2-	T41.3x3-	T41.3x4-	T41.3x5-	T41.3x6-
Amylene						
dichloride	T53.6x1-	T53.6x2-	T53.6x3-	T53.6x4-	—	—
hydrate	T51.3x1-	T51.3x2-	T51.3x3-	T51.3x4-	—	—
Amylmetacresol	T49.6x1-	T49.6x2-	T49.6x3-	T49.6x4-	T49.6x5-	T49.6x6-
Amylobarbitone	T42.3x1-	T42.3x2-	T42.3x3-	T42.3x4-	T42.3x5-	T42.3x6-
Amylocaine, regional	T41.3x1-	T41.3x2-	T41.3x3-	T41.3x4-	T41.3x5-	T41.3x6-
infiltration (subcutaneous)	T41.3x1-	T41.3x2-	T41.3x3-	T41.3x4-	T41.3x5-	T41.3x6-
nerve block (peripheral) (plexus)	T41.3x1-	T41.3x2-	T41.3x3-	T41.3x4-	T41.3x5-	T41.3x6-
spinal	T41.3x1-	T41.3x2-	T41.3x3-	T41.3x4-	T41.3x5-	T41.3x6-
topical (surface)	T41.3x1-	T41.3x2-	T41.3x3-	T41.3x4-	T41.3x5-	T41.3x6-

Table of Drugs & Chemicals	POISONING Accidental (Unintentional)	Self-Harm (Intentional)	Assault	Undetermined	Adverse Effect	Underdosing
Amylopectin	T47.6x1-	T47.6x2-	T47.6x3-	T47.6x4-	T47.6x5-	T47.6x6-
Amytal (sodium)	T42.3x1-	T42.3x2-	T42.3x3-	T42.3x4-	T42.3x5-	T42.3x6-
Anabolic steroid	T38.7x1-	T38.7x2-	T38.7x3-	T38.7x4-	T38.7x5-	T38.7x6-
Analeptic NEC	T50.7x1-	T50.7x2-	T50.7x3-	T50.7x4-	T50.7x5-	T50.7x6-
Analgesic	T39.91x-	T39.92x-	T39.93x-	T39.94x-	T39.95x-	T39.96x-
anti-inflammatory NEC	T39.91x-	T39.92x-	T39.93x-	T39.94x-	T39.95x-	T39.96x-
propionic acid derivative	T39.311-	T39.312-	T39.313-	T39.314-	T39.315-	T39.316-
antirheumatic NEC	T39.4x1-	T39.4x2-	T39.4x3-	T39.4x4-	T39.4x5-	T39.4x6-
aromatic NEC	T39.1x1-	T39.1x2-	T39.1x3-	T39.1x4-	T39.1x5-	T39.1x6-
narcotic NEC	T40.601-	T40.602-	T40.603-	T40.604-	T40.605-	T40.606-
combination	T40.601-	T40.602-	T40.603-	T40.604-	T40.605-	T40.606-
obstetric	T40.601-	T40.602-	T40.603-	T40.604-	T40.605-	T40.606-
non-narcotic NEC	T39.91x-	T39.92x-	T39.93x-	T39.94x-	T39.95x-	T39.96x-
combination	T39.91x-	T39.92x-	T39.93x-	T39.94x-	T39.95x-	T39.96x-
pyrazole	T39.2x1-	T39.2x2-	T39.2x3-	T39.2x4-	T39.2x5-	T39.2x6-
specified NEC	T39.8x1-	T39.8x2-	T39.8x3-	T39.8x4-	T39.8x5-	T39.8x6-
Analgin	T39.2x1-	T39.2x2-	T39.2x3-	T39.2x4-	T39.2x5-	T39.2x6-
Anamirta cocculus	T62.1x1-	T62.1x2-	T62.1x3-	T62.1x4-	—	—
Ancillin	T36.0x1-	T36.0x2-	T36.0x3-	T36.0x4-	T36.0x5-	T36.0x6-
Ancrod	T45.691-	T45.692-	T45.693-	T45.694-	T45.695-	T45.696-
Androgen	T38.7x1-	T38.7x2-	T38.7x3-	T38.7x4-	T38.7x5-	T38.7x6-
Androgen-estrogen mixture	T38.7x1-	T38.7x2-	T38.7x3-	T38.7x4-	T38.7x5-	T38.7x6-
Androstalone	T38.7x1-	T38.7x2-	T38.7x3-	T38.7x4-	T38.7x5-	T38.7x6-
Androstanolone	T38.7x1-	T38.7x2-	T38.7x3-	T38.7x4-	T38.7x5-	T38.7x6-
Androsterone	T38.7x1-	T38.7x2-	T38.7x3-	T38.7x4-	T38.7x5-	T38.7x6-
Anemone pulsatilla	T62.2x1-	T62.2x2-	T62.2x3-	T62.2x4-	—	—
Anesthesia						
caudal	T41.3x1-	T41.3x2-	T41.3x3-	T41.3x4-	T41.3x5-	T41.3x6-
endotracheal	T41.0x1-	T41.0x2-	T41.0x3-	T41.0x4-	T41.0x5-	T41.0x6-
epidural	T41.3x1-	T41.3x2-	T41.3x3-	T41.3x4-	T41.3x5-	T41.3x6-
inhalation	T41.0x1-	T41.0x2-	T41.0x3-	T41.0x4-	T41.0x5-	T41.0x6-
local	T41.3x1-	T41.3x2-	T41.3x3-	T41.3x4-	T41.3x5-	T41.3x6-
mucosal	T41.3x1-	T41.3x2-	T41.3x3-	T41.3x4-	T41.3x5-	T41.3x6-
muscle relaxation	T48.1x1-	T48.1x2-	T48.1x3-	T48.1x4-	T48.1x5-	T48.1x6-
nerve blocking	T41.3x1-	T41.3x2-	T41.3x3-	T41.3x4-	T41.3x5-	T41.3x6-
plexus blocking	T41.3x1-	T41.3x2-	T41.3x3-	T41.3x4-	T41.3x5-	T41.3x6-
potentiated	T41.201-	T41.202-	T41.203-	T41.204-	T41.205-	T41.206-
rectal	T41.201-	T41.202-	T41.203-	T41.204-	T41.205-	T41.206-
general	T41.201-	T41.202-	T41.203-	T41.204-	T41.205-	T41.206-
local	T41.3x1-	T41.3x2-	T41.3x3-	T41.3x4-	T41.3x5-	T41.3x6-
regional	T41.3x1-	T41.3x2-	T41.3x3-	T41.3x4-	T41.3x5-	T41.3x6-
surface	T41.3x1-	T41.3x2-	T41.3x3-	T41.3x4-	T41.3x5-	T41.3x6-
Anesthetic NEC – see also Anesthesia	T41.41x-	T41.42x-	T41.43x-	T41.44x-	T41.45x-	T41.46x-
with muscle relaxant	T41.201-	T41.202-	T41.203-	T41.204-	T41.205-	T41.206-
general	T41.201-	T41.202-	T41.203-	T41.204-	T41.205-	T41.206-
local	T41.3x1-	T41.3x2-	T41.3x3-	T41.3x4-	T41.3x5-	T41.3x6-
gaseous NEC	T41.0x1-	T41.0x2-	T41.0x3-	T41.0x4-	T41.0x5-	T41.0x6-
general NEC	T41.201-	T41.202-	T41.203-	T41.204-	T41.205-	T41.206-
halogenated hydrocarbon derivatives NEC	T41.0x1-	T41.0x2-	T41.0x3-	T41.0x4-	T41.0x5-	T41.0x6-
infiltration NEC	T41.3x1-	T41.3x2-	T41.3x3-	T41.3x4-	T41.3x5-	T41.3x6-
intravenous NEC	T41.1x1-	T41.1x2-	T41.1x3-	T41.1x4-	T41.1x5-	T41.1x6-
local NEC	T41.3x1-	T41.3x2-	T41.3x3-	T41.3x4-	T41.3x5-	T41.3x6-
rectal	T41.201-	T41.202-	T41.203-	T41.204-	T41.205-	T41.206-
general	T41.201-	T41.202-	T41.203-	T41.204-	T41.205-	T41.206-
local	T41.3x1-	T41.3x2-	T41.3x3-	T41.3x4-	T41.3x5-	T41.3x6-
regional NEC	T41.3x1-	T41.3x2-	T41.3x3-	T41.3x4-	T41.3x5-	T41.3x6-
spinal NEC	T41.3x1-	T41.3x2-	T41.3x3-	T41.3x4-	T41.3x5-	T41.3x6-
thiobarbiturate	T41.1x1-	T41.1x2-	T41.1x3-	T41.1x4-	T41.1x5-	T41.1x6-
topical	T41.3x1-	T41.3x2-	T41.3x3-	T41.3x4-	T41.3x5-	T41.3x6-

Table of Drugs & Chemicals	POISONING Accidental (Unintentional)	Self-Harm (Intentional)	Assault	Undetermined	Adverse Effect	Underdosing
Aneurine	T45.2x1-	T45.2x2-	T45.2x3-	T45.2x4-	T45.2x5-	T45.2x6-
Angio-Conray	T50.8x1-	T50.8x2-	T50.8x3-	T50.8x4-	T50.8x5-	T50.8x6-
Angiotensin	T44.5x1-	T44.5x2-	T44.5x3-	T44.5x4-	T44.5x5-	T44.5x6-
Angiotensinamide	T44.991-	T44.992-	T44.993-	T44.994-	T44.995-	T44.996-
Anhydrohydroxy-progesterone	T38.5x1-	T38.5x2-	T38.5x3-	T38.5x4-	T38.5x5-	T38.5x6-
Anhydron	T50.2x1-	T50.2x2-	T50.2x3-	T50.2x4-	T50.2x5-	T50.2x6-
Anileridine	T40.4x1-	T40.4x2-	T40.4x3-	T40.4x4-	T40.4x5-	T40.4x6-
Aniline (dye) (liquid)	T65.3x1-	T65.3x2-	T65.3x3-	T65.3x4-	—	—
analgesic	T39.1x1-	T39.1x2-	T39.1x3-	T39.1x4-	T39.1x5-	T39.1x6-
derivatives, therapeutic NEC	T39.1x1-	T39.1x2-	T39.1x3-	T39.1x4-	T39.1x5-	T39.1x6-
vapor	T65.3x1-	T65.3x2-	T65.3x3-	T65.3x4-	—	—
Aniscoropine	T44.3x1-	T44.3x2-	T44.3x3-	T44.3x4-	T44.3x5-	T44.3x6-
Anise oil	T47.5x1-	T47.5x2-	T47.5x3-	T47.5x4-	T47.5x5-	T47.5x6-
Anisidine	T65.3x1-	T65.3x2-	T65.3x3-	T65.3x4-	—	—
Anisindione	T45.511-	T45.512-	T45.513-	T45.514-	T45.515-	T45.516-
Anisotropine methyl-bromide	T44.3x1-	T44.3x2-	T44.3x3-	T44.3x4-	T44.3x5-	T44.3x6-
Anistreplase	T45.611-	T45.612-	T45.613-	T45.614-	T45.615-	T45.616-
Anorexiant (central)	T50.5x1-	T50.5x2-	T50.5x3-	T50.5x4-	T50.5x5-	T50.5x6-
Anorexic agents	T50.5x1-	T50.5x2-	T50.5x3-	T50.5x4-	T50.5x5-	T50.5x6-
Ansamycin	T36.6x1-	T36.6x2-	T36.6x3-	T36.6x4-	T36.6x5-	T36.6x6-
Ant (bite) (sting)	T63.421-	T63.422-	T63.423-	T63.424-	—	—
Ant poison — see Insecticide						
Antabuse	T50.6x1-	T50.6x2-	T50.6x3-	T50.6x4-	T50.6x5-	T50.6x6-
Antacid NEC	T47.1x1-	T47.1x2-	T47.1x3-	T47.1x4-	T47.1x5-	T47.1x6-
Antagonist						
aldosterone	T50.0x1-	T50.0x2-	T50.0x3-	T50.0x4-	T50.0x5-	T50.0x6-
alpha-adrenoreceptor	T44.6x1-	T44.6x2-	T44.6x3-	T44.6x4-	T44.6x5-	T44.6x6-
anticoagulant	T45.7x1-	T45.7x2-	T45.7x3-	T45.7x4-	T45.7x5-	T45.7x6-
beta-adrenoreceptor	T44.7x1-	T44.7x2-	T44.7x3-	T44.7x4-	T44.7x5-	T44.7x6-
extrapyramidal NEC	T44.3x1-	T44.3x2-	T44.3x3-	T44.3x4-	T44.3x5-	T44.3x6-
folic acid	T45.1x1-	T45.1x2-	T45.1x3-	T45.1x4-	T45.1x5-	T45.1x6-
heavy metal	T45.8x1-	T45.8x2-	T45.8x3-	T45.8x4-	T45.8x5-	T45.8x6-
H2 receptor	T47.0x1-	T47.0x2-	T47.0x3-	T47.0x4-	T47.0x5-	T47.0x6-
narcotic analgesic	T50.7x1-	T50.7x2-	T50.7x3-	T50.7x4-	T50.7x5-	T50.7x6-
opiate	T50.7x1-	T50.7x2-	T50.7x3-	T50.7x4-	T50.7x5-	T50.7x6-
pyrimidine	T45.1x1-	T45.1x2-	T45.1x3-	T45.1x4-	T45.1x5-	T45.1x6-
serotonin	T46.5x1-	T46.5x2-	T46.5x3-	T46.5x4-	T46.5x5-	T46.5x6-
Antazolin(e)	T45.0x1-	T45.0x2-	T45.0x3-	T45.0x4-	T45.0x5-	T45.0x6-
Anterior pituitary hormone NEC	T38.811-	T38.812-	T38.813-	T38.814-	T38.815-	T38.816-
Anthelmintic NEC	T37.4x1-	T37.4x2-	T37.4x3-	T37.4x4-	T37.4x5-	T37.4x6-
Anthiolimine	T37.4x1-	T37.4x2-	T37.4x3-	T37.4x4-	T37.4x5-	T37.4x6-
Anthralin	T49.4x1-	T49.4x2-	T49.4x3-	T49.4x4-	T49.4x5-	T49.4x6-
Anthramycin	T45.1x1-	T45.1x2-	T45.1x3-	T45.1x4-	T45.1x5-	T45.1x6-
Antiadrenergic NEC	T44.8x1-	T44.8x2-	T44.8x3-	T44.8x4-	T44.8x5-	T44.8x6-
Antiallergic NEC	T45.0x1-	T45.0x2-	T45.0x3-	T45.0x4-	T45.0x5-	T45.0x6-
Antiandrogen NEC	T38.6x1-	T38.6x2-	T38.6x3-	T38.6x4-	T38.6x5-	T38.6x6-
Anti-anemic (drug) (preparation)	T45.8x1-	T45.8x2-	T45.8x3-	T45.8x4-	T45.8x5-	T45.8x6-
Antianxiety drug NEC	T43.501-	T43.502-	T43.503-	T43.504-	T43.505-	T43.506-
Antiaris toxicaria	T65.891-	T65.892-	T65.893-	T65.894-	—	—
Antiarteriosclerotic drug	T46.6x1-	T46.6x2-	T46.6x3-	T46.6x4-	T46.6x5-	T46.6x6-
Antiasthmatic drug NEC	T48.6x1-	T48.6x2-	T48.6x3-	T48.6x4-	T48.6x5-	T48.6x6-
Antibiotic NEC	T36.91x-	T36.92x-	T36.93x-	T36.94x-	T36.95x-	T36.96x-
aminoglycoside	T36.5x1-	T36.5x2-	T36.5x3-	T36.5x4-	T36.5x5-	T36.5x6-
anticancer	T45.1x1-	T45.1x2-	T45.1x3-	T45.1x4-	T45.1x5-	T45.1x6-
antifungal	T36.7x1-	T36.7x2-	T36.7x3-	T36.7x4-	T36.7x5-	T36.7x6-
antimycobacterial	T36.5x1-	T36.5x2-	T36.5x3-	T36.5x4-	T36.5x5-	T36.5x6-
antineoplastic	T45.1x1-	T45.1x2-	T45.1x3-	T45.1x4-	T45.1x5-	T45.1x6-
cephalosporin (group)	T36.1x1-	T36.1x2-	T36.1x3-	T36.1x4-	T36.1x5-	T36.1x6-
chloramphenicol (group)	T36.2x1-	T36.2x2-	T36.2x3-	T36.2x4-	T36.2x5-	T36.2x6-
ENT	T49.6x1-	T49.6x2-	T49.6x3-	T49.6x4-	T49.6x5-	T49.6x6-

Table of Drugs & Chemicals	POISONING Accidental (Unintentional)	Self-Harm (Intentional)	Assault	Undetermined	Adverse Effect	Underdosing
Antibiotic NEC - *continued*						
eye	T49.5x1-	T49.5x2-	T49.5x3-	T49.5x4-	T49.5x5-	T49.5x6-
fungicidal (local)	T49.0x1-	T49.0x2-	T49.0x3-	T49.0x4-	T49.0x5-	T49.0x6-
intestinal	T36.8x1-	T36.8x2-	T36.8x3-	T36.8x4-	T36.8x5-	T36.8x6-
b-lactam NEC	T36.1x1-	T36.1x2-	T36.1x3-	T36.1x4-	T36.1x5-	T36.1x6-
local	T49.0x1-	T49.0x2-	T49.0x3-	T49.0x4-	T49.0x5-	T49.0x6-
macrolides	T36.3x1-	T36.3x2-	T36.3x3-	T36.3x4-	T36.3x5-	T36.3x6-
polypeptide	T36.8x1-	T36.8x2-	T36.8x3-	T36.8x4-	T36.8x5-	T36.8x6-
specified NEC	T36.8x1-	T36.8x2-	T36.8x3-	T36.8x4-	T36.8x5-	T36.8x6-
tetracycline (group)	T36.4x1-	T36.4x2-	T36.4x3-	T36.4x4-	T36.4x5-	T36.4x6-
throat	T49.6x1-	T49.6x2-	T49.6x3-	T49.6x4-	T49.6x5-	T49.6x6-
Anticancer agents NEC	T45.1x1-	T45.1x2-	T45.1x3-	T45.1x4-	T45.1x5-	T45.1x6-
Anticholesterolemic drug NEC	T46.6x1-	T46.6x2-	T46.6x3-	T46.6x4-	T46.6x5-	T46.6x6-
Anticholinergic NEC	T44.3x1-	T44.3x2-	T44.3x3-	T44.3x4-	T44.3x5-	T44.3x6-
Anticholinesterase	T44.0x1-	T44.0x2-	T44.0x3-	T44.0x4-	T44.0x5-	T44.0x6-
organophosphorus	T44.0x1-	T44.0x2-	T44.0x3-	T44.0x4-	T44.0x5-	T44.0x6-
insecticide	T60.0x1-	T60.0x2-	T60.0x3-	T60.0x4-	—	—
nerve gas	T59.891-	T59.892-	T59.893-	T59.894-	—	—
reversible	T44.0x1-	T44.0x2-	T44.0x3-	T44.0x4-	T44.0x5-	T44.0x6-
ophthalmological	T49.5x1-	T49.5x2-	T49.5x3-	T49.5x4-	T49.5x5-	T49.5x6-
Anticoagulant NEC	T45.511-	T45.512-	T45.513-	T45.514-	T45.515-	T45.516-
antagonist	T45.7x1-	T45.7x2-	T45.7x3-	T45.7x4-	T45.7x5-	T45.7x6-
Anti-common-cold drug NEC	T48.5x1-	T48.5x2-	T48.5x3-	T48.5x4-	T48.5x5-	T48.5x6-
Anticonvulsant	T42.71x-	T42.72x-	T42.73x-	T42.74x-	T42.75x-	T42.76x-
barbiturate	T42.3x1-	T42.3x2-	T42.3x3-	T42.3x4-	T42.3x5-	T42.3x6-
combination (with barbiturate)	T42.3x1-	T42.3x2-	T42.3x3-	T42.3x4-	T42.3x5-	T42.3x6-
hydantoin	T42.0x1-	T42.0x2-	T42.0x3-	T42.0x4-	T42.0x5-	T42.0x6-
hypnotic NEC	T42.6x1-	T42.6x2-	T42.6x3-	T42.6x4-	T42.6x5-	T42.6x6-
oxazolidinedione	T42.2x1-	T42.2x2-	T42.2x3-	T42.2x4-	T42.2x5-	T42.2x6-
pyrimidinedione	T42.6x1-	T42.6x2-	T42.6x3-	T42.6x4-	T42.6x5-	T42.6x6-
specified NEC	T42.6x1-	T42.6x2-	T42.6x3-	T42.6x4-	T42.6x5-	T42.6x6-
succinimide	T42.2x1-	T42.2x2-	T42.2x3-	T42.2x4-	T42.2x5-	T42.2x6-
Anti-D immunoglobulin (human)	T50.Z11-	T50.Z12-	T50.Z13-	T50.Z14-	T50.Z15-	T50.Z16-
Antidepressant	T43.201-	T43.202-	T43.203-	T43.204-	T43.205-	T43.206-
monoamine oxidase inhibitor	T43.1x1-	T43.1x2-	T43.1x3-	T43.1x4-	T43.1x5-	T43.1x6-
selective serotonin norepinephrine reuptake inhibitor	T43.211-	T43.212-	T43.213-	T43.214-	T43.215-	T43.216-
selective serotonin reuptake inhibitor	T43.221-	T43.222-	T43.223-	T43.224-	T43.225-	T43.226-
specified NEC	T43.291-	T43.292-	T43.293-	T43.294-	T43.295-	T43.296-
triazolopyridine	T43.211-	T43.212-	T43.213-	T43.214-	T43.215-	T43.216-
tetracyclic	T43.021-	T43.022-	T43.023-	T43.024-	T43.025-	T43.026-
tricyclic	T43.011-	T43.012-	T43.013-	T43.014-	T43.015-	T43.016-
Antidiabetic NEC	T38.3x1-	T38.3x2-	T38.3x3-	T38.3x4-	T38.3x5-	T38.3x6-
biguanide	T38.3x1-	T38.3x2-	T38.3x3-	T38.3x4-	T38.3x5-	T38.3x6-
and sulfonyl combined	T38.3x1-	T38.3x2-	T38.3x3-	T38.3x4-	T38.3x5-	T38.3x6-
combined	T38.3x1-	T38.3x2-	T38.3x3-	T38.3x4-	T38.3x5-	T38.3x6-
sulfonylurea	T38.3x1-	T38.3x2-	T38.3x3-	T38.3x4-	T38.3x5-	T38.3x6-
Antidiarrheal drug NEC	T47.6x1-	T47.6x2-	T47.6x3-	T47.6x4-	T47.6x5-	T47.6x6-
absorbent	T47.6x1-	T47.6x2-	T47.6x3-	T47.6x4-	T47.6x5-	T47.6x6-
Antidiphtheria serum	T50.Z11-	T50.Z12-	T50.Z13-	T50.Z14-	T50.Z15-	T50.Z16-
Antidiuretic hormone	T38.891-	T38.892-	T38.893-	T38.894-	T38.895-	T38.896-
Antidote NEC	T50.6x1-	T50.6x2-	T50.6x3-	T50.6x4-	T50.6x5-	T50.6x6-
heavy metal	T45.8x1-	T45.8x2-	T45.8x3-	T45.8x4-	T45.8x5-	T45.8x6-
Antidysrhythmic NEC	T46.2x1-	T46.2x2-	T46.2x3-	T46.2x4-	T46.2x5-	T46.2x6-

DRUGS & CHEMICALS

Table of Drugs & Chemicals	POISONING Accidental (Unintentional)	Self-Harm (Intentional)	Assault	Undetermined	Adverse Effect	Underdosing
Antiemetic drug	T45.0x1-	T45.0x2-	T45.0x3-	T45.0x4-	T45.0x5-	T45.0x6-
Antiepilepsy agent	T42.71x-	T42.72x-	T42.73x-	T42.74x-	T42.75x-	T42.76x-
combination	T42.5x1-	T42.5x2-	T42.5x3-	T42.5x4-	T42.5x5-	T42.5x6-
mixed	T42.5x1-	T42.5x2-	T42.5x3-	T42.5x4-	T42.5x5-	T42.5x6-
specified, NEC	T42.6x1-	T42.6x2-	T42.6x3-	T42.6x4-	T42.6x5-	T42.6x6-
Antiestrogen NEC	T38.6x1-	T38.6x2-	T38.6x3-	T38.6x4-	T38.6x5-	T38.6x6-
Antifertility pill	T38.4x1-	T38.4x2-	T38.4x3-	T38.4x4-	T38.4x5-	T38.4x6-
Antifibrinolytic drug	T45.621-	T45.622-	T45.623-	T45.624-	T45.625-	T45.626-
Antifilarial drug	T37.4x1-	T37.4x2-	T37.4x3-	T37.4x4-	T37.4x5-	T37.4x6-
Antiflatulent	T47.5x1-	T47.5x2-	T47.5x3-	T47.5x4-	T47.5x5-	T47.5x6-
Antifreeze	T65.91x-	T65.92x-	T65.93x-	T65.94x-	—	—
alcohol	T51.1x1-	T51.1x2-	T51.1x3-	T51.1x4-	—	—
ethylene glycol	T51.8x1-	T51.8x2-	T51.8x3-	T51.8x4-	—	—
Antifungal						
antibiotic (systemic)	T36.7x1-	T36.7x2-	T36.7x3-	T36.7x4-	T36.7x5-	T36.7x6-
anti-infective NEC	T37.91x-	T37.92x-	T37.93x-	T37.94x-	T37.95x-	T37.96x-
disinfectant, local	T49.0x1-	T49.0x2-	T49.0x3-	T49.0x4-	T49.0x5-	T49.0x6-
nonmedicinal (spray)	T60.3x1-	T60.3x2-	T60.3x3-	T60.3x4-	—	—
topical	T49.0x1-	T49.0x2-	T49.0x3-	T49.0x4-	T49.0x5-	T49.0x6-
Anti-gastric-secretion drug NEC	T47.1x1-	T47.1x2-	T47.1x3-	T47.1x4-	T47.1x5-	T47.1x6-
Antigonadotrophin NEC	T38.6x1-	T38.6x2-	T38.6x3-	T38.6x4-	T38.6x5-	T38.6x6-
Antihallucinogen	T43.501-	T43.502-	T43.503-	T43.504-	T43.505-	T43.506-
Antihelmintics	T37.4x1-	T37.4x2-	T37.4x3-	T37.4x4-	T37.4x5-	T37.4x6-
Antihemophilic						
factor	T45.8x1-	T45.8x2-	T45.8x3-	T45.8x4-	T45.8x5-	T45.8x6-
fraction	T45.8x1-	T45.8x2-	T45.8x3-	T45.8x4-	T45.8x5-	T45.8x6-
globulin concentrate	T45.7x1-	T45.7x2-	T45.7x3-	T45.7x4-	T45.7x5-	T45.7x6-
human plasma	T45.8x1-	T45.8x2-	T45.8x3-	T45.8x4-	T45.8x5-	T45.8x6-
plasma, dried	T45.7x1-	T45.7x2-	T45.7x3-	T45.7x4-	T45.7x5-	T45.7x6-
Antihemorrhoidal						
preparation	T49.2x1-	T49.2x2-	T49.2x3-	T49.2x4-	T49.2x5-	T49.2x6-
Antiheparin drug	T45.7x1-	T45.7x2-	T45.7x3-	T45.7x4-	T45.7x5-	T45.7x6-
Antihistamine	T45.0x1-	T45.0x2-	T45.0x3-	T45.0x4-	T45.0x5-	T45.0x6-
Antihookworm drug	T37.4x1-	T37.4x2-	T37.4x3-	T37.4x4-	T37.4x5-	T37.4x6-
Anti-human lymphocytic globulin	T50.Z11-	T50.Z12-	T50.Z13-	T50.Z14-	T50.Z15-	T50.Z16-
Antihyperlipidemic drug	T46.6x1-	T46.6x2-	T46.6x3-	T46.6x4-	T46.6x5-	T46.6x6-
Antihypertensive drug NEC	T46.5x1-	T46.5x2-	T46.5x3-	T46.5x4-	T46.5x5-	T46.5x6-
Anti-infective NEC	T37.91x-	T37.92x-	T37.93x-	T37.94x-	T37.95x-	T37.96x-
antibiotics	T36.91x-	T36.92x-	T36.93x-	T36.94x-	T36.95x-	T36.96x-
specified NEC	T36.8x1-	T36.8x2-	T36.8x3-	T36.8x4-	T36.8x5-	T36.8x6-
anthelmintic	T37.4x1-	T37.4x2-	T37.4x3-	T37.4x4-	T37.4x5-	T37.4x6-
antimalarial	T37.2x1-	T37.2x2-	T37.2x3-	T37.2x4-	T37.2x5-	T37.2x6-
antimycobacterial NEC	T37.1x1-	T37.1x2-	T37.1x3-	T37.1x4-	T37.1x5-	T37.1x6-
antibiotics	T36.5x1-	T36.5x2-	T36.5x3-	T36.5x4-	T36.5x5-	T36.5x6-
antiprotozoal NEC	T37.3x1-	T37.3x2-	T37.3x3-	T37.3x4-	T37.3x5-	T37.3x6-
blood	T37.2x1-	T37.2x2-	T37.2x3-	T37.2x4-	T37.2x5-	T37.2x6-
antiviral	T37.5x1-	T37.5x2-	T37.5x3-	T37.5x4-	T37.5x5-	T37.5x6-
arsenical	T37.8x1-	T37.8x2-	T37.8x3-	T37.8x4-	T37.8x5-	T37.8x6-
bismuth, local	T49.0x1-	T49.0x2-	T49.0x3-	T49.0x4-	T49.0x5-	T49.0x6-
ENT	T49.6x1-	T49.6x2-	T49.6x3-	T49.6x4-	T49.6x5-	T49.6x6-
eye NEC	T49.5x1-	T49.5x2-	T49.5x3-	T49.5x4-	T49.5x5-	T49.5x6-
heavy metals NEC	T37.8x1-	T37.8x2-	T37.8x3-	T37.8x4-	T37.8x5-	T37.8x6-
local NEC	T49.0x1-	T49.0x2-	T49.0x3-	T49.0x4-	T49.0x5-	T49.0x6-
specified NEC	T49.0x1-	T49.0x2-	T49.0x3-	T49.0x4-	T49.0x5-	T49.0x6-
mixed	T37.91x-	T37.92x-	T37.93x-	T37.94x-	T37.95x-	T37.96x-
ophthalmic preparation	T49.5x1-	T49.5x2-	T49.5x3-	T49.5x4-	T49.5x5-	T49.5x6-
topical NEC	T49.0x1-	T49.0x2-	T49.0x3-	T49.0x4-	T49.0x5-	T49.0x6-

Table of Drugs & Chemicals	POISONING Accidental (Unintentional)	Self-Harm (Intentional)	Assault	Undetermined	Adverse Effect	Underdosing
Anti-inflammatory drug						
NEC	T39.391-	T39.392-	T39.393-	T39.394-	T39.395-	T39.396-
local	T49.0x1-	T49.0x2-	T49.0x3-	T49.0x4-	T49.0x5-	T49.0x6-
nonsteroidal NEC	T39.391-	T39.392-	T39.393-	T39.394-	T39.395-	T39.396-
propionic acid derivative	T39.311-	T39.312-	T39.313-	T39.314-	T39.315-	T39.316-
specified NEC	T39.391-	T39.392-	T39.393-	T39.394-	T39.395-	T39.396-
Antikaluretic	T50.3x1-	T50.3x2-	T50.3x3-	T50.3x4-	T50.3x5-	T50.3x6-
Antiknock (tetraethyl lead)	T56.0x1-	T56.0x2-	T56.0x3-	T56.0x4-	—	—
Antilipemic drug NEC	T46.6x1-	T46.6x2-	T46.6x3-	T46.6x4-	T46.6x5-	T46.6x6-
Antimalarial	T37.2x1-	T37.2x2-	T37.2x3-	T37.2x4-	T37.2x5-	T37.2x6-
prophylactic NEC	T37.2x1-	T37.2x2-	T37.2x3-	T37.2x4-	T37.2x5-	T37.2x6-
pyrimidine derivative	T37.2x1-	T37.2x2-	T37.2x3-	T37.2x4-	T37.2x5-	T37.2x6-
Antimetabolite	T45.1x1-	T45.1x2-	T45.1x3-	T45.1x4-	T45.1x5-	T45.1x6-
Antimitotic agent	T45.1x1-	T45.1x2-	T45.1x3-	T45.1x4-	T45.1x5-	T45.1x6-
Antimony (compounds) (vapor) NEC	T56.891-	T56.892-	T56.893-	T56.894-	—	—
anti-infectives	T37.8x1-	T37.8x2-	T37.8x3-	T37.8x4-	T37.8x5-	T37.8x6-
dimercaptosuccinate	T37.3x1-	T37.3x2-	T37.3x3-	T37.3x4-	T37.3x5-	T37.3x6-
hydride	T56.891-	T56.892-	T56.893-	T56.894-	—	—
pesticide (vapor)	T60.8x1-	T60.8x2-	T60.8x3-	T60.8x4-	—	—
potassium (sodium) tartrate	T37.8x1-	T37.8x2-	T37.8x3-	T37.8x4-	T37.8x5-	T37.8x6-
tartrated	T37.8x1-	T37.8x2-	T37.8x3-	T37.8x4-	T37.8x5-	T37.8x6-
sodium dimercapto-succinate	T37.3x1-	T37.3x2-	T37.3x3-	T37.3x4-	T37.3x5-	T37.3x6-
Antimuscarinic NEC	T44.3x1-	T44.3x2-	T44.3x3-	T44.3x4-	T44.3x5-	T44.3x6-
Antimycobacterial drug NEC	T37.1x1-	T37.1x2-	T37.1x3-	T37.1x4-	T37.1x5-	T37.1x6-
antibiotics	T36.5x1-	T36.5x2-	T36.5x3-	T36.5x4-	T36.5x5-	T36.5x6-
combination	T37.1x1-	T37.1x2-	T37.1x3-	T37.1x4-	T37.1x5-	T37.1x6-
Antinausea drug	T45.0x1-	T45.0x2-	T45.0x3-	T45.0x4-	T45.0x5-	T45.0x6-
Antinematode drug	T37.4x1-	T37.4x2-	T37.4x3-	T37.4x4-	T37.4x5-	T37.4x6-
Antineoplastic NEC	T45.1x1-	T45.1x2-	T45.1x3-	T45.1x4-	T45.1x5-	T45.1x6-
antibiotics	T45.1x1-	T45.1x2-	T45.1x3-	T45.1x4-	T45.1x5-	T45.1x6-
alkaloidal	T45.1x1-	T45.1x2-	T45.1x3-	T45.1x4-	T45.1x5-	T45.1x6-
combination	T45.1x1-	T45.1x2-	T45.1x3-	T45.1x4-	T45.1x5-	T45.1x6-
estrogen	T38.5x1-	T38.5x2-	T38.5x3-	T38.5x4-	T38.5x5-	T38.5x6-
steroid	T38.7x1-	T38.7x2-	T38.7x3-	T38.7x4-	T38.7x5-	T38.7x6-
Antiparasitic drug (systemic)	T37.91x-	T37.92x-	T37.93x-	T37.94x-	T37.95x-	T37.96x-
local	T49.0x1-	T49.0x2-	T49.0x3-	T49.0x4-	T49.0x5-	T49.0x6-
specified NEC	T37.8x1-	T37.8x2-	T37.8x3-	T37.8x4-	T37.8x5-	T37.8x6-
Antiparkinsonism drug NEC	T42.8x1-	T42.8x2-	T42.8x3-	T42.8x4-	T42.8x5-	T42.8x6-
Antiperspirant NEC	T49.2x1-	T49.2x2-	T49.2x3-	T49.2x4-	T49.2x5-	T49.2x6-
Antiphlogistic NEC	T39.4x1-	T39.4x2-	T39.4x3-	T39.4x4-	T39.4x5-	T39.4x6-
Antiplatyhelmintic drug	T37.4x1-	T37.4x2-	T37.4x3-	T37.4x4-	T37.4x5-	T37.4x6-
Antiprotozoal drug NEC	T37.3x1-	T37.3x2-	T37.3x3-	T37.3x4-	T37.3x5-	T37.3x6-
blood	T37.2x1-	T37.2x2-	T37.2x3-	T37.2x4-	T37.2x5-	T37.2x6-
local	T49.0x1-	T49.0x2-	T49.0x3-	T49.0x4-	T49.0x5-	T49.0x6-
Antipruritic drug NEC	T49.1x1-	T49.1x2-	T49.1x3-	T49.1x4-	T49.1x5-	T49.1x6-
Antipsychotic drug	T43.501-	T43.502-	T43.503-	T43.504-	T43.505-	T43.506-
specified NEC	T43.591-	T43.592-	T43.593-	T43.594-	T43.595-	T43.596-
Antipyretic	T39.91x-	T39.92x-	T39.93x-	T39.94x-	T39.95x-	T39.96x-
specified NEC	T39.8x1-	T39.8x2-	T39.8x3-	T39.8x4-	T39.8x5-	T39.8x6-
Antipyrine	T39.2x1-	T39.2x2-	T39.2x3-	T39.2x4-	T39.2x5-	T39.2x6-
Antirabies hyperimmune serum	T50.Z11-	T50.Z12-	T50.Z13-	T50.Z14-	T50.Z15-	T50.Z16-
Antirheumatic NEC	T39.4x1-	T39.4x2-	T39.4x3-	T39.4x4-	T39.4x5-	T39.4x6-
Antirigidity drug NEC	T42.8x1-	T42.8x2-	T42.8x3-	T42.8x4-	T42.8x5-	T42.8x6-
Antischistosomal drug	T37.4x1-	T37.4x2-	T37.4x3-	T37.4x4-	T37.4x5-	T37.4x6-
Antiscorpion sera	T50.Z11-	T50.Z12-	T50.Z13-	T50.Z14-	T50.Z15-	T50.Z16-
Antiseborrheics	T49.4x1-	T49.4x2-	T49.4x3-	T49.4x4-	T49.4x5-	T49.4x6-
Antiseptics (external) (medicinal)	T49.0x1-	T49.0x2-	T49.0x3-	T49.0x4-	T49.0x5-	T49.0x6-

DRUGS & CHEMICALS

Table of Drugs & Chemicals	Accidental (Unintentional)	Self-Harm (Intentional)	Assault	Undetermined	Adverse Effect	Underdosing
Antistine	T45.0x1-	T45.0x2-	T45.0x3-	T45.0x4-	T45.0x5-	T45.0x6-
Antitapeworm drug	T37.4x1-	T37.4x2-	T37.4x3-	T37.4x4-	T37.4x5-	T37.4x6-
Antitetanus immunoglobulin	T50.Z11-	T50.Z12-	T50.Z13-	T50.Z14-	T50.Z15-	T50.Z16-
Antithyroid drug NEC	T38.2x1-	T38.2x2-	T38.2x3-	T38.2x4-	T38.2x5-	T38.2x6-
Antitoxin	T50.Z11-	T50.Z12-	T50.Z13-	T50.Z14-	T50.Z15-	T50.Z16-
diphtheria	T50.Z11-	T50.Z12-	T50.Z13-	T50.Z14-	T50.Z15-	T50.Z16-
gas gangrene	T50.Z11-	T50.Z12-	T50.Z13-	T50.Z14-	T50.Z15-	T50.Z16-
tetanus	T50.Z11-	T50.Z12-	T50.Z13-	T50.Z14-	T50.Z15-	T50.Z16-
Antitrichomonal drug	T37.3x1-	T37.3x2-	T37.3x3-	T37.3x4-	T37.3x5-	T37.3x6-
Antituberculars	T37.1x1-	T37.1x2-	T37.1x3-	T37.1x4-	T37.1x5-	T37.1x6-
antibiotics	T36.5x1-	T36.5x2-	T36.5x3-	T36.5x4-	T36.5x5-	T36.5x6-
Antitussive NEC	T48.3x1-	T48.3x2-	T48.3x3-	T48.3x4-	T48.3x5-	T48.3x6-
codeine mixture	T40.2x1-	T40.2x2-	T40.2x3-	T40.2x4-	T40.2x5-	T40.2x6-
opiate	T40.2x1-	T40.2x2-	T40.2x3-	T40.2x4-	T40.2x5-	T40.2x6-
Antivaricose drug	T46.8x1-	T46.8x2-	T46.8x3-	T46.8x4-	T46.8x5-	T46.8x6-
Antivenin, antivenom (sera)	T50.Z11-	T50.Z12-	T50.Z13-	T50.Z14-	T50.Z15-	T50.Z16-
crotaline	T50.Z11-	T50.Z12-	T50.Z13-	T50.Z14-	T50.Z15-	T50.Z16-
spider bite	T50.Z11-	T50.Z12-	T50.Z13-	T50.Z14-	T50.Z15-	T50.Z16-
Antivertigo drug	T45.0x1-	T45.0x2-	T45.0x3-	T45.0x4-	T45.0x5-	T45.0x6-
Antiviral drug NEC	T37.5x1-	T37.5x2-	T37.5x3-	T37.5x4-	T37.5x5-	T37.5x6-
eye	T49.5x1-	T49.5x2-	T49.5x3-	T49.5x4-	T49.5x5-	T49.5x6-
Antiwhipworm drug	T37.4x1-	T37.4x2-	T37.4x3-	T37.4x4-	T37.4x5-	T37.4x6-
Antrol — see also by specific chemical substance	T60.91x-	T60.92x-	T60.93x-	T60.94x-	—	—
fungicide	T60.91x-	T60.92x-	T60.93x-	T60.94x-	—	—
ANTU (alpha naphthylthiourea)	T60.4x1-	T60.4x2-	T60.4x3-	T60.4x4-	—	—
Apalcillin	T36.0x1-	T36.0x2-	T36.0x3-	T36.0x4-	T36.0x5-	T36.0x6-
APC	T48.5x1-	T48.5x2-	T48.5x3-	T48.5x4-	T48.5x5-	T48.5x6-
Aplonidine	T44.4x1-	T44.4x2-	T44.4x3-	T44.4x4-	T44.4x5-	T44.4x6-
Apomorphine	T47.7x1-	T47.7x2-	T47.7x3-	T47.7x4-	T47.7x5-	T47.7x6-
Appetite depressants, central	T50.5x1-	T50.5x2-	T50.5x3-	T50.5x4-	T50.5x5-	T50.5x6-
Apraclonidine (hydrochloride)	T44.4x1-	T44.4x2-	T44.4x3-	T44.4x4-	T44.4x5-	T44.4x6-
Apresoline	T46.5x1-	T46.5x2-	T46.5x3-	T46.5x4-	T46.5x5-	T46.5x6-
Aprindine	T46.2x1-	T46.2x2-	T46.2x3-	T46.2x4-	T46.2x5-	T46.2x6-
Aprobarbital	T42.3x1-	T42.3x2-	T42.3x3-	T42.3x4-	T42.3x5-	T42.3x6-
Apronalide	T42.6x1-	T42.6x2-	T42.6x3-	T42.6x4-	T42.6x5-	T42.6x6-
Aprotinin	T45.621-	T45.622-	T45.623-	T45.624-	T45.625-	T45.626-
Aptocaine	T41.3x1-	T41.3x2-	T41.3x3-	T41.3x4-	T41.3x5-	T41.3x6-
Aqua fortis	T54.2x1-	T54.2x2-	T54.2x3-	T54.2x4-	—	—
Ara-A	T37.5x1-	T37.5x2-	T37.5x3-	T37.5x4-	T37.5x5-	T37.5x6-
Ara-C	T45.1x1-	T45.1x2-	T45.1x3-	T45.1x4-	T45.1x5-	T45.1x6-
Arachis oil	T49.3x1-	T49.3x2-	T49.3x3-	T49.3x4-	T49.3x5-	T49.3x6-
cathartic	T47.4x1-	T47.4x2-	T47.4x3-	T47.4x4-	T47.4x5-	T47.4x6-
Aralen	T37.2x1-	T37.2x2-	T37.2x3-	T37.2x4-	T37.2x5-	T37.2x6-
Arecoline	T44.1x1-	T44.1x2-	T44.1x3-	T44.1x4-	T44.1x5-	T44.1x6-
Arginine	T50.991-	T50.992-	T50.993-	T50.994-	T50.995-	T50.996-
glutamate	T50.991-	T50.992-	T50.993-	T50.994-	T50.995-	T50.996-
Argyrol	T49.0x1-	T49.0x2-	T49.0x3-	T49.0x4-	T49.0x5-	T49.0x6-
ENT agent	T49.6x1-	T49.6x2-	T49.6x3-	T49.6x4-	T49.6x5-	T49.6x6-
ophthalmic preparation	T49.5x1-	T49.5x2-	T49.5x3-	T49.5x4-	T49.5x5-	T49.5x6-
Aristocort	T38.0x1-	T38.0x2-	T38.0x3-	T38.0x4-	T38.0x5-	T38.0x6-
ENT agent	T49.6x1-	T49.6x2-	T49.6x3-	T49.6x4-	T49.6x5-	T49.6x6-
ophthalmic preparation	T49.5x1-	T49.5x2-	T49.5x3-	T49.5x4-	T49.5x5-	T49.5x6-
topical NEC	T49.0x1-	T49.0x2-	T49.0x3-	T49.0x4-	T49.0x5-	T49.0x6-
Aromatics, corrosive	T54.1x1-	T54.1x2-	T54.1x3-	T54.1x4-	—	—
disinfectants	T54.1x1-	T54.1x2-	T54.1x3-	T54.1x4-	—	—
Arsenate of lead	T57.0x1-	T57.0x2-	T57.0x3-	T57.0x4-	—	—
herbicide	T57.0x1-	T57.0x2-	T57.0x3-	T57.0x4-	—	—
Arsenic, arsenicals (compounds) (dust) (vapor) NEC	T57.0x1-	T57.0x2-	T57.0x3-	T57.0x4-	—	—
anti-infectives	T37.8x1-	T37.8x2-	T37.8x3-	T37.8x4-	T37.8x5-	T37.8x6-
pesticide (dust) (fumes)	T57.0x1-	T57.0x2-	T57.0x3-	T57.0x4-	—	—
Arsine (gas)	T57.0x1-	T57.0x2-	T57.0x3-	T57.0x4-	—	—
Arsphenamine (silver)	T37.8x1-	T37.8x2-	T37.8x3-	T37.8x4-	T37.8x5-	T37.8x6-
Arsthinol	T37.3x1-	T37.3x2-	T37.3x3-	T37.3x4-	T37.3x5-	T37.3x6-
Artane	T44.3x1-	T44.3x2-	T44.3x3-	T44.3x4-	T44.3x5-	T44.3x6-
Arthropod (venomous) NEC	T63.481-	T63.482-	T63.483-	T63.484-	—	—
Articaine	T41.3x1-	T41.3x2-	T41.3x3-	T41.3x4-	T41.3x5-	T41.3x6-
Asbestos	T57.8x1-	T57.8x2-	T57.8x3-	T57.8x4-	—	—
Ascaridole	T37.4x1-	T37.4x2-	T37.4x3-	T37.4x4-	T37.4x5-	T37.4x6-
Ascorbic acid	T45.2x1-	T45.2x2-	T45.2x3-	T45.2x4-	T45.2x5-	T45.2x6-
Asiaticoside	T49.0x1-	T49.0x2-	T49.0x3-	T49.0x4-	T49.0x5-	T49.0x6-
Asparaginase	T45.1x1-	T45.1x2-	T45.1x3-	T45.1x4-	T45.1x5-	T45.1x6-
Aspidium (oleoresin)	T37.4x1-	T37.4x2-	T37.4x3-	T37.4x4-	T37.4x5-	T37.4x6-
Aspirin (aluminum) (soluble)	T39.011-	T39.012-	T39.013-	T39.014-	T39.015-	T39.016-
Aspoxicillin	T36.0x1-	T36.0x2-	T36.0x3-	T36.0x4-	T36.0x5-	T36.0x6-
Astemizole	T45.0x1-	T45.0x2-	T45.0x3-	T45.0x4-	T45.0x5-	T45.0x6-
Astringent (local)	T49.2x1-	T49.2x2-	T49.2x3-	T49.2x4-	T49.2x5-	T49.2x6-
specified NEC	T49.2x1-	T49.2x2-	T49.2x3-	T49.2x4-	T49.2x5-	T49.2x6-
Astromicin	T36.5x1-	T36.5x2-	T36.5x3-	T36.5x4-	T36.5x5-	T36.5x6-
Ataractic drug NEC	T43.501-	T43.502-	T43.503-	T43.504-	T43.505-	T43.506-
Atenolol	T44.7x1-	T44.7x2-	T44.7x3-	T44.7x4-	T44.7x5-	T44.7x6-
Atonia drug, intestinal	T47.4x1-	T47.4x2-	T47.4x3-	T47.4x4-	T47.4x5-	T47.4x6-
Atophan	T50.4x1-	T50.4x2-	T50.4x3-	T50.4x4-	T50.4x5-	T50.4x6-
Atracurium besilate	T48.1x1-	T48.1x2-	T48.1x3-	T48.1x4-	T48.1x5-	T48.1x6-
Atropine	T44.3x1-	T44.3x2-	T44.3x3-	T44.3x4-	T44.3x5-	T44.3x6-
derivative	T44.3x1-	T44.3x2-	T44.3x3-	T44.3x4-	T44.3x5-	T44.3x6-
methonitrate	T44.3x1-	T44.3x2-	T44.3x3-	T44.3x4-	T44.3x5-	T44.3x6-
Attapulgite	T47.6x1-	T47.6x2-	T47.6x3-	T47.6x4-	T47.6x5-	T47.6x6-
Auramine	T65.891-	T65.892-	T65.893-	T65.894-	—	—
dye	T65.6x1-	T65.6x2-	T65.6x3-	T65.6x4-	—	—
fungicide	T60.3x1-	T60.3x2-	T60.3x3-	T60.3x4-	—	—
Auranofin	T39.4x1-	T39.4x2-	T39.4x3-	T39.4x4-	T39.4x5-	T39.4x6-
Aurantiin	T46.991-	T46.992-	T46.993-	T46.994-	T46.995-	T46.996-
Aureomycin	T36.4x1-	T36.4x2-	T36.4x3-	T36.4x4-	T36.4x5-	T36.4x6-
ophthalmic preparation	T49.5x1-	T49.5x2-	T49.5x3-	T49.5x4-	T49.5x5-	T49.5x6-
topical NEC	T49.0x1-	T49.0x2-	T49.0x3-	T49.0x4-	T49.0x5-	T49.0x6-
Aurothioglucose	T39.4x1-	T39.4x2-	T39.4x3-	T39.4x4-	T39.4x5-	T39.4x6-
Aurothioglycanide	T39.4x1-	T39.4x2-	T39.4x3-	T39.4x4-	T39.4x5-	T39.4x6-
Aurothiomalate sodium	T39.4x1-	T39.4x2-	T39.4x3-	T39.4x4-	T39.4x5-	T39.4x6-
Aurotioprol	T39.4x1-	T39.4x2-	T39.4x3-	T39.4x4-	T39.4x5-	T39.4x6-
Automobile fuel	T52.0x1-	T52.0x2-	T52.0x3-	T52.0x4-	—	—
Autonomic nervous system agent NEC	T44.901-	T44.902-	T44.903-	T44.904-	T44.905-	T44.906-
Avlosulfon	T37.1x1-	T37.1x2-	T37.1x3-	T37.1x4-	T37.1x5-	T37.1x6-
Avomine	T42.6x1-	T42.6x2-	T42.6x3-	T42.6x4-	T42.6x5-	T42.6x6-
Axerophthol	T45.2x1-	T45.2x2-	T45.2x3-	T45.2x4-	T45.2x5-	T45.2x6-
Azacitidine	T45.1x1-	T45.1x2-	T45.1x3-	T45.1x4-	T45.1x5-	T45.1x6-
Azacyclonol	T43.591-	T43.592-	T43.593-	T43.594-	T43.595-	T43.596-
Azadirachta	T60.2x1-	T60.2x2-	T60.2x3-	T60.2x4-	—	—
Azanidazole	T37.3x1-	T37.3x2-	T37.3x3-	T37.3x4-	T37.3x5-	T37.3x6-
Azapetine	T46.7x1-	T46.7x2-	T46.7x3-	T46.7x4-	T46.7x5-	T46.7x6-
Azapropazone	T39.2x1-	T39.2x2-	T39.2x3-	T39.2x4-	T39.2x5-	T39.2x6-
Azaribine	T45.1x1-	T45.1x2-	T45.1x3-	T45.1x4-	T45.1x5-	T45.1x6-
Azaserine	T45.1x1-	T45.1x2-	T45.1x3-	T45.1x4-	T45.1x5-	T45.1x6-
Azatadine	T45.0x1-	T45.0x2-	T45.0x3-	T45.0x4-	T45.0x5-	T45.0x6-
Azatepa	T45.1x1-	T45.1x2-	T45.1x3-	T45.1x4-	T45.1x5-	T45.1x6-
Azathioprine	T45.1x1-	T45.1x2-	T45.1x3-	T45.1x4-	T45.1x5-	T45.1x6-

DRUGS & CHEMICALS

Table of Drugs & Chemicals	POISONING Accidental (Unintentional)	Self-Harm (Intentional)	Assault	Undetermined	Adverse Effect	Underdosing
Azelaic acid	T49.0x1-	T49.0x2-	T49.0x3-	T49.0x4-	T49.0x5-	T49.0x6-
Azelastine	T45.0x1-	T45.0x2-	T45.0x3-	T45.0x4-	T45.0x5-	T45.0x6-
Azidocillin	T36.0x1-	T36.0x2-	T36.0x3-	T36.0x4-	T36.0x5-	T36.0x6-
Azidothymidine	T37.5x1-	T37.5x2-	T37.5x3-	T37.5x4-	T37.5x5-	T37.5x6-
Azinphos (ethyl) (methyl)	T60.0x1-	T60.0x2-	T60.0x3-	T60.0x4-	—	—
Aziridine (chelating)	T54.1x1-	T54.1x2-	T54.1x3-	T54.1x4-		
Azithromycin	T36.3x1-	T36.3x2-	T36.3x3-	T36.3x4-	T36.3x5-	T36.3x6-
Azlocillin	T36.0x1-	T36.0x2-	T36.0x3-	T36.0x4-	T36.0x5-	T36.0x6-
Azobenzene smoke	T65.3x1-	T65.3x2-	T65.3x3-	T65.3x4-	—	—
acaricide	T60.8x1-	T60.8x2-	T60.8x3-	T60.8x4-	—	—
Azosulfamide	T37.0x1-	T37.0x2-	T37.0x3-	T37.0x4-	T37.0x5-	T37.0x6-
AZT	T37.5x1-	T37.5x2-	T37.5x3-	T37.5x4-	T37.5x5-	T37.5x6-
Aztreonam	T36.1x1-	T36.1x2-	T36.1x3-	T36.1x4-	T36.1x5-	T36.1x6-
Azulfidine	T37.0x1-	T37.0x2-	T37.0x3-	T37.0x4-	T37.0x5-	T37.0x6-
Azuresin	T50.8x1-	T50.8x2-	T50.8x3-	T50.8x4-	T50.8x5-	T50.8x6-
Bacampicillin	T36.0x1-	T36.0x2-	T36.0x3-	T36.0x4-	T36.0x5-	T36.0x6-
b-acetyldigoxin	T46.0x1-	T46.0x2-	T46.0x3-	T46.0x4-	T46.0x5-	T46.0x6-
Bacillus						
lactobacillus	T47.8x1-	T47.8x2-	T47.8x3-	T47.8x4-	T47.8x5-	T47.8x6-
subtilis	T47.6x1-	T47.6x2-	T47.6x3-	T47.6x4-	T47.6x5-	T47.6x6-
Bacimycin	T49.0x1-	T49.0x2-	T49.0x3-	T49.0x4-	T49.0x5-	T49.0x6-
ophthalmic preparation	T49.5x1-	T49.5x2-	T49.5x3-	T49.5x4-	T49.5x5-	T49.5x6-
Bacitracin zinc	T49.0x1-	T49.0x2-	T49.0x3-	T49.0x4-	T49.0x5-	T49.0x6-
with neomycin	T49.0x1-	T49.0x2-	T49.0x3-	T49.0x4-	T49.0x5-	T49.0x6-
ENT agent	T49.6x1-	T49.6x2-	T49.6x3-	T49.6x4-	T49.6x5-	T49.6x6-
ophthalmic preparation	T49.5x1-	T49.5x2-	T49.5x3-	T49.5x4-	T49.5x5-	T49.5x6-
topical NEC	T49.0x1-	T49.0x2-	T49.0x3-	T49.0x4-	T49.0x5-	T49.0x6-
Baclofen	T42.8x1-	T42.8x2-	T42.8x3-	T42.8x4-	T42.8x5-	T42.8x6-
Baking soda	T50.991-	T50.992-	T50.993-	T50.994-	T50.995-	T50.996-
BAL	T45.8x1-	T45.8x2-	T45.8x3-	T45.8x4-	T45.8x5-	T45.8x6-
Bambuterol	T48.6x1-	T48.6x2-	T48.6x3-	T48.6x4-	T48.6x5-	T48.6x6-
Bamethan (sulfate)	T46.7x1-	T46.7x2-	T46.7x3-	T46.7x4-	T46.7x5-	T46.7x6-
Bamifylline	T48.6x1-	T48.6x2-	T48.6x3-	T48.6x4-	T48.6x5-	T48.6x6-
Bamipine	T45.0x1-	T45.0x2-	T45.0x3-	T45.0x4-	T45.0x5-	T45.0x6-
Baneberry — see Actaea spicata						
Banewort — see Belladonna						
Barbenyl	T42.3x1-	T42.3x2-	T42.3x3-	T42.3x4-	T42.3x5-	T42.3x6-
Barbexaclone	T42.6x1-	T42.6x2-	T42.6x3-	T42.6x4-	T42.6x5-	T42.6x6-
Barbital	T42.3x1-	T42.3x2-	T42.3x3-	T42.3x4-	T42.3x5-	T42.3x6-
sodium	T42.3x1-	T42.3x2-	T42.3x3-	T42.3x4-	T42.3x5-	T42.3x6-
Barbitone	T42.3x1-	T42.3x2-	T42.3x3-	T42.3x4-	T42.3x5-	T42.3x6-
Barbiturate NEC	T42.3x1-	T42.3x2-	T42.3x3-	T42.3x4-	T42.3x5-	T42.3x6-
with tranquilizer	T42.3x1-	T42.3x2-	T42.3x3-	T42.3x4-	T42.3x5-	T42.3x6-
anesthetic (intravenous)	T41.1x1-	T41.1x2-	T41.1x3-	T41.1x4-	T41.1x5-	T41.1x6-
Barium (carbonate) (chloride) (sulfite)	T57.8x1-	T57.8x2-	T57.8x3-	T57.8x4-	—	—
diagnostic agent	T50.8x1-	T50.8x2-	T50.8x3-	T50.8x4-	T50.8x5-	T50.8x6-
pesticide	T60.4x1-	T60.4x2-	T60.4x3-	T60.4x4-	—	—
rodenticide	T60.4x1-	T60.4x2-	T60.4x3-	T60.4x4-	—	—
sulfate (medicinal)	T50.8x1-	T50.8x2-	T50.8x3-	T50.8x4-	T50.8x5-	T50.8x6-
Barrier cream	T49.3x1-	T49.3x2-	T49.3x3-	T49.3x4-	T49.3x5-	T49.3x6-
Basic fuchsin	T49.0x1-	T49.0x2-	T49.0x3-	T49.0x4-	T49.0x5-	T49.0x6-
Battery acid or fluid	T54.2x1-	T54.2x2-	T54.2x3-	T54.2x4-		
Bay rum	T51.8x1-	T51.8x2-	T51.8x3-	T51.8x4-	—	—
b-benzalbutyramide	T46.6x1-	T46.6x2-	T46.6x3-	T46.6x4-	T46.6x5-	T46.6x6-
BCG (vaccine)	T50.A91-	T50.A92-	T50.A93-	T50.A94-	T50.A95	T50.A96-
BCNU	T45.1x1-	T45.1x2-	T45.1x3-	T45.1x4-	T45.1x5-	T45.1x6-
Bearsfoot	T62.2x1-	T62.2x2-	T62.2x3-	T62.2x4-	—	—
Beclamide	T42.6x1-	T42.6x2-	T42.6x3-	T42.6x4-	T42.6x5-	T42.6x6-
Beclomethasone	T44.5x1-	T44.5x2-	T44.5x3-	T44.5x4-	T44.5x5-	T44.5x6-
Bee (sting) (venom)	T63.441-	T63.442-	T63.443-	T63.444-	—	—
Befunolol	T49.5x1-	T49.5x2-	T49.5x3-	T49.5x4-	T49.5x5-	T49.5x6-

Table of Drugs & Chemicals	POISONING Accidental (Unintentional)	Self-Harm (Intentional)	Assault	Undetermined	Adverse Effect	Underdosing
Bekanamycin	T36.5x1-	T36.5x2-	T36.5x3-	T36.5x4-	T36.5x5-	T36.5x6-
Belladonna — see also Nightshade						
alkaloids	T44.3x1-	T44.3x2-	T44.3x3-	T44.3x4-	T44.3x5-	T44.3x6-
extract	T44.3x1-	T44.3x2-	T44.3x3-	T44.3x4-	T44.3x5-	T44.3x6-
herb	T44.3x1-	T44.3x2-	T44.3x3-	T44.3x4-	T44.3x5-	T44.3x6-
Bemegride	T50.7x1-	T50.7x2-	T50.7x3-	T50.7x4-	T50.7x5-	T50.7x6-
Benactyzine	T44.3x1-	T44.3x2-	T44.3x3-	T44.3x4-	T44.3x5-	T44.3x6-
Benadryl	T45.0x1-	T45.0x2-	T45.0x3-	T45.0x4-	T45.0x5-	T45.0x6-
Benaprizine	T44.3x1-	T44.3x2-	T44.3x3-	T44.3x4-	T44.3x5-	T44.3x6-
Benazepril	T46.4x1-	T46.4x2-	T46.4x3-	T46.4x4-	T46.4x5-	T46.4x6-
Bencyclane	T46.7x1-	T46.7x2-	T46.7x3-	T46.7x4-	T46.7x5-	T46.7x6-
Bendazol	T46.3x1-	T46.3x2-	T46.3x3-	T46.3x4-	T46.3x5-	T46.3x6-
Bendrofluazide	T50.2x1-	T50.2x2-	T50.2x3-	T50.2x4-	T50.2x5-	T50.2x6-
Bendroflumethiazide	T50.2x1-	T50.2x2-	T50.2x3-	T50.2x4-	T50.2x5-	T50.2x6-
Benemid	T50.4x1-	T50.4x2-	T50.4x3-	T50.4x4-	T50.4x5-	T50.4x6-
Benethamine penicillin	T36.0x1-	T36.0x2-	T36.0x3-	T36.0x4-	T36.0x5-	T36.0x6-
Benexate	T47.1x1-	T47.1x2-	T47.1x3-	T47.1x4-	T47.1x5-	T47.1x6-
Benfluorex	T46.6x1-	T46.6x2-	T46.6x3-	T46.6x4-	T46.6x5-	T46.6x6-
Benfotiamine	T45.2x1-	T45.2x2-	T45.2x3-	T45.2x4-	T45.2x5-	T45.2x6-
Benisone	T49.0x1-	T49.0x2-	T49.0x3-	T49.0x4-	T49.0x5-	T49.0x6-
Benomyl	T60.0x1-	T60.0x2-	T60.0x3-	T60.0x4-	—	—
Benoquin	T49.8x1-	T49.8x2-	T49.8x3-	T49.8x4-	T49.8x5-	T49.8x6-
Benoxinate	T41.3x1-	T41.3x2-	T41.3x3-	T41.3x4-	T41.3x5-	T41.3x6-
Benperidol	T43.4x1-	T43.4x2-	T43.4x3-	T43.4x4-	T43.4x5-	T43.4x6-
Benproperine	T48.3x1-	T48.3x2-	T48.3x3-	T48.3x4-	T48.3x5-	T48.3x6-
Benserazide	T42.8x1-	T42.8x2-	T42.8x3-	T42.8x4-	T42.8x5-	T42.8x6-
Bentazepam	T42.4x1-	T42.4x2-	T42.4x3-	T42.4x4-	T42.4x5-	T42.4x6-
Bentiromide	T50.8x1-	T50.8x2-	T50.8x3-	T50.8x4-	T50.8x5-	T50.8x6-
Bentonite	T49.3x1-	T49.3x2-	T49.3x3-	T49.3x4-	T49.3x5-	T49.3x6-
Benzalbutyramide	T46.6x1-	T46.6x2-	T46.6x3-	T46.6x4-	T46.6x5-	T46.6x6-
Benzalkonium (chloride)	T49.0x1-	T49.0x2-	T49.0x3-	T49.0x4-	T49.0x5-	T49.0x6-
ophthalmic preparation	T49.5x1-	T49.5x2-	T49.5x3-	T49.5x4-	T49.5x5-	T49.5x6-
Benzamidosalicylate (calcium)	T37.1x1-	T37.1x2-	T37.1x3-	T37.1x4-	T37.1x5-	T37.1x6-
Benzamine	T41.3x1-	T41.3x2-	T41.3x3-	T41.3x4-	T41.3x5-	T41.3x6-
lactate	T49.1x1-	T49.1x2-	T49.1x3-	T49.1x4-	T49.1x5-	T49.1x6-
Benzamphetamine	T50.5x1-	T50.5x2-	T50.5x3-	T50.5x4-	T50.5x5-	T50.5x6-
Benzapril hydrochloride	T46.5x1-	T46.5x2-	T46.5x3-	T46.5x4-	T46.5x5-	T46.5x6-
Benzathine benzylpenicillin	T36.0x1-	T36.0x2-	T36.0x3-	T36.0x4-	T36.0x5-	T36.0x6-
Benzathine penicillin	T36.0x1-	T36.0x2-	T36.0x3-	T36.0x4-	T36.0x5-	T36.0x6-
Benzatropine	T42.8x1-	T42.8x2-	T42.8x3-	T42.8x4-	T42.8x5-	T42.8x6-
Benzbromarone	T50.4x1-	T50.4x2-	T50.4x3-	T50.4x4-	T50.4x5-	T50.4x6-
Benzcarbimine	T45.1x1-	T45.1x2-	T45.1x3-	T45.1x4-	T45.1x5-	T45.1x6-
Benzedrex	T44.991-	T44.992-	T44.993-	T44.994-	T44.995-	T44.996-
Benzedrine (amphetamine)	T43.621-	T43.622-	T43.623-	T43.624-	T43.625-	T43.626-
Benzenamine	T65.3x1-	T65.3x2-	T65.3x3-	T65.3x4-	—	—
Benzene	T52.1x1-	T52.1x2-	T52.1x3-	T52.1x4-	—	—
homologues (acetyl) (dimethyl) (methyl) (solvent)	T52.2x1-	T52.2x2-	T52.2x3-	T52.2x4-	—	—
Benzethonium (chloride)	T49.0x1-	T49.0x2-	T49.0x3-	T49.0x4-	T49.0x5-	T49.0x6-
Benzfetamine	T50.5x1-	T50.5x2-	T50.5x3-	T50.5x4-	T50.5x5-	T50.5x6-
Benzhexol	T44.3x1-	T44.3x2-	T44.3x3-	T44.3x4-	T44.3x5-	T44.3x6-
Benzhydramine (chloride)	T45.0x1-	T45.0x2-	T45.0x3-	T45.0x4-	T45.0x5-	T45.0x6-
Benzidine	T65.891-	T65.892-	T65.893-	T65.894-		
Benzilonium bromide	T44.3x1-	T44.3x2-	T44.3x3-	T44.3x4-	T44.3x5-	T44.3x6-
Benzimidazole	T60.3x1-	T60.3x2-	T60.3x3-	T60.3x4-		
Benzin (e) — see Ligroin						
Benziodarone	T46.3x1-	T46.3x2-	T46.3x3-	T46.3x4-	T46.3x5-	T46.3x6-
Benznidazole	T37.3x1-	T37.3x2-	T37.3x3-	T37.3x4-	T37.3x5-	T37.3x6-
Benzocaine	T41.3x1-	T41.3x2-	T41.3x3-	T41.3x4-	T41.3x5-	T41.3x6-
Benzodiapin	T42.4x1-	T42.4x2-	T42.4x3-	T42.4x4-	T42.4x5-	T42.4x6-

DRUGS & CHEMICALS

Table of Drugs & Chemicals	Poisoning Accidental (Unintentional)	Poisoning Self-Harm (Intentional)	Assault	Undetermined	Adverse Effect	Underdosing
Benzodiazepine NEC	T42.4x1-	T42.4x2-	T42.4x3-	T42.4x4-	T42.4x5-	T42.4x6-
Benzoic acid	T49.0x1-	T49.0x2-	T49.0x3-	T49.0x4-	T49.0x5-	T49.0x6-
with salicylic acid	T49.0x1-	T49.0x2-	T49.0x3-	T49.0x4-	T49.0x5-	T49.0x6-
Benzoin (tincture)	T48.5x1-	T48.5x2-	T48.5x3-	T48.5x4-	T48.5x5-	T48.5x6-
Benzol (benzene)	T52.1x1-	T52.1x2-	T52.1x3-	T52.1x4-	—	—
vapor	T52.0x1-	T52.0x2-	T52.0x3-	T52.0x4-	—	—
Benzomorphan	T40.2x1-	T40.2x2-	T40.2x3-	T40.2x4-	T40.2x5-	T40.2x6-
Benzonatate	T48.3x1-	T48.3x2-	T48.3x3-	T48.3x4-	T48.3x5-	T48.3x6-
Benzophenones	T49.3x1-	T49.3x2-	T49.3x3-	T49.3x4-	T49.3x5-	T49.3x6-
Benzopyrone	T46.991-	T46.992-	T46.993-	T46.994-	T46.995-	T46.996-
Benzothiadiazides	T50.2x1-	T50.2x2-	T50.2x3-	T50.2x4-	T50.2x5-	T50.2x6-
Benzoxonium chloride	T49.0x1-	T49.0x2-	T49.0x3-	T49.0x4-	T49.0x5-	T49.0x6-
Benzoyl peroxide	T49.0x1-	T49.0x2-	T49.0x3-	T49.0x4-	T49.0x5-	T49.0x6-
Benzoylpas calcium	T37.1x1-	T37.1x2-	T37.1x3-	T37.1x4-	T37.1x5-	T37.1x6-
Benzperidin	T43.591-	T43.592-	T43.593-	T43.594-	T43.595-	T43.596-
Benzperidol	T43.591-	T43.592-	T43.593-	T43.594-	T43.595-	T43.596-
Benzphetamine	T50.5x1-	T50.5x2-	T50.5x3-	T50.5x4-	T50.5x5-	T50.5x6-
Benzpyrinium bromide	T44.1x1-	T44.1x2-	T44.1x3-	T44.1x4-	T44.1x5-	T44.1x6-
Benzquinamide	T45.0x1-	T45.0x2-	T45.0x3-	T45.0x4-	T45.0x5-	T45.0x6-
Benzthiazide	T50.2x1-	T50.2x2-	T50.2x3-	T50.2x4-	T50.2x5-	T50.2x6-
Benztropine						
anticholinergic	T44.3x1-	T44.3x2-	T44.3x3-	T44.3x4-	T44.3x5-	T44.3x6-
antiparkinson	T42.8x1-	T42.8x2-	T42.8x3-	T42.8x4-	T42.8x5-	T42.8x6-
Benzydamine	T49.0x1-	T49.0x2-	T49.0x3-	T49.0x4-	T49.0x5-	T49.0x6-
Benzyl						
acetate	T52.8x1-	T52.8x2-	T52.8x3-	T52.8x4-	—	—
alcohol	T49.0x1-	T49.0x2-	T49.0x3-	T49.0x4-	T49.0x5-	T49.0x6-
benzoate	T49.0x1-	T49.0x2-	T49.0x3-	T49.0x4-	T49.0x5-	T49.0x6-
Benzoic acid	T49.0x1-	T49.0x2-	T49.0x3-	T49.0x4-	T49.0x5-	T49.0x6-
morphine	T40.2x1-	T40.2x2-	T40.2x3-	T40.2x4-	—	—
nicotinate	T46.6x1-	T46.6x2-	T46.6x3-	T46.6x4-	T46.6x5-	T46.6x6-
penicillin	T36.0x1-	T36.0x2-	T36.0x3-	T36.0x4-	T36.0x5-	T36.0x6-
Benzylhydrochlorthiazide	T50.2x1-	T50.2x2-	T50.2x3-	T50.2x4-	T50.2x5-	T50.2x6-
Benzylpenicillin	T36.0x1-	T36.0x2-	T36.0x3-	T36.0x4-	T36.0x5-	T36.0x6-
Benzylthiouracil	T38.2x1-	T38.2x2-	T38.2x3-	T38.2x4-	T38.2x5-	T38.2x6-
Bephenium hydroxy-naphthoate	T37.4x1-	T37.4x2-	T37.4x3-	T37.4x4-	T37.4x5-	T37.4x6-
Bepridil	T46.1x1-	T46.1x2-	T46.1x3-	T46.1x4-	T46.1x5-	T46.1x6-
Bergamot oil	T65.891-	T65.892-	T65.893-	T65.894-	—	—
Bergapten	T50.991-	T50.992-	T50.993-	T50.994-	T50.995-	T50.996-
Berries, poisonous	T62.1x1-	T62.1x2-	T62.1x3-	T62.1x4-		
Beryllium (compounds)	T56.7x1-	T56.7x2-	T56.7x3-	T56.7x4-	—	—
Beta adrenergic blocking agent, heart	T44.7x1-	T44.7x2-	T44.7x3-	T44.7x4-	T44.7x5-	T44.7x6-
Betacarotene	T45.2x1-	T45.2x2-	T45.2x3-	T45.2x4-	T45.2x5-	T45.2x6-
Beta-Chlor	T42.6x1-	T42.6x2-	T42.6x3-	T42.6x4-	T42.6x5-	T42.6x6-
Betahistine	T46.7x1-	T46.7x2-	T46.7x3-	T46.7x4-	T46.7x5-	T46.7x6-
Betaine	T47.5x1-	T47.5x2-	T47.5x3-	T47.5x4-	T47.5x5-	T47.5x6-
Betamethasone	T49.0x1-	T49.0x2-	T49.0x3-	T49.0x4-	T49.0x5-	T49.0x6-
topical	T49.0x1-	T49.0x2-	T49.0x3-	T49.0x4-	T49.0x5-	T49.0x6-
Betamicin	T36.8x1-	T36.8x2-	T36.8x3-	T36.8x4-	T36.8x5-	T36.8x6-
Betanidine	T46.5x1-	T46.5x2-	T46.5x3-	T46.5x4-	T46.5x5-	T46.5x6-
Betaxolol	T44.7x1-	T44.7x2-	T44.7x3-	T44.7x4-	T44.7x5-	T44.7x6-
Betazole	T50.8x1-	T50.8x2-	T50.8x3-	T50.8x4-	T50.8x5-	T50.8x6-
Bethanechol	T44.1x1-	T44.1x2-	T44.1x3-	T44.1x4-	T44.1x5-	T44.1x6-
chloride	T44.1x1-	T44.1x2-	T44.1x3-	T44.1x4-	T44.1x5-	T44.1x6-
Bethanidine	T46.5x1-	T46.5x2-	T46.5x3-	T46.5x4-	T46.5x5-	T46.5x6-
Betoxycaine	T41.3x1-	T41.3x2-	T41.3x3-	T41.3x4-	T41.3x5-	T41.3x6-
Betula oil	T49.3x1-	T49.3x2-	T49.3x3-	T49.3x4-	T49.3x5-	T49.3x6-
b-eucaine	T49.1x1-	T49.1x2-	T49.1x3-	T49.1x4-	T49.1x5-	T49.1x6-
Bevantolol	T44.7x1-	T44.7x2-	T44.7x3-	T44.7x4-	T44.7x5-	T44.7x6-
Bevonium metilsulfate	T44.3x1-	T44.3x2-	T44.3x3-	T44.3x4-	T44.3x5-	T44.3x6-
Bezafibrate	T46.6x1-	T46.6x2-	T46.6x3-	T46.6x4-	T46.6x5-	T46.6x6-

Table of Drugs & Chemicals	Poisoning Accidental (Unintentional)	Poisoning Self-Harm (Intentional)	Assault	Undetermined	Adverse Effect	Underdosing
Bezitramide	T40.4x1-	T40.4x2-	T40.4x3-	T40.4x4-	T40.4x5-	T40.4x6-
b-galactosidase	T47.5x1-	T47.5x2-	T47.5x3-	T47.5x4-	T47.5x5-	T47.5x6-
BHA	T50.991-	T50.992-	T50.993-	T50.994-	T50.995-	T50.996-
Bhang	T40.7x1-	T40.7x2-	T40.7x3-	T40.7x4-	T40.7x5-	T40.7x6-
BHC (medicinal)	T49.0x1-	T49.0x2-	T49.0x3-	T49.0x4-	T49.0x5-	T49.0x6-
nonmedicinal (vapor)	T53.6x1-	T53.6x2-	T53.6x3-	T53.6x4-	—	—
Bialamicol	T37.3x1-	T37.3x2-	T37.3x3-	T37.3x4-	T37.3x5-	T37.3x6-
Bibenzonium bromide	T48.3x1-	T48.3x2-	T48.3x3-	T48.3x4-	T48.3x5-	T48.3x6-
Bibrocathol	T49.5x1-	T49.5x2-	T49.5x3-	T49.5x4-	T49.5x5-	T49.5x6-
Bichloride of mercury — see Mercury, chloride						
Bichromates (calcium) (potassium) (sodium) (crystals)	T57.8x1-	T57.8x2-	T57.8x3-	T57.8x4-	—	—
fumes	T56.2x1-	T56.2x2-	T56.2x3-	T56.2x4-	—	—
Biclotymol	T49.6x1-	T49.6x2-	T49.6x3-	T49.6x4-	T49.6x5-	T49.6x6-
Bicucculine	T50.7x1-	T50.7x2-	T50.7x3-	T50.7x4-	T50.7x5-	T50.7x6-
Bifemelane	T43.291-	T43.292-	T43.293-	T43.294-	T43.295-	T43.296-
Biguanide derivatives, oral	T38.3x1-	T38.3x2-	T38.3x3-	T38.3x4-	T38.3x5-	T38.3x6-
Bile salts	T47.5x1-	T47.5x2-	T47.5x3-	T47.5x4-	T47.5x5-	T47.5x6-
Biligrafin	T50.8x1-	T50.8x2-	T50.8x3-	T50.8x4-	T50.8x5-	T50.8x6-
Bilopaque	T50.8x1-	T50.8x2-	T50.8x3-	T50.8x4-	T50.8x5-	T50.8x6-
Binifibrate	T46.6x1-	T46.6x2-	T46.6x3-	T46.6x4-	T46.6x5-	T46.6x6-
Binitrobenzol	T65.3x1-	T65.3x2-	T65.3x3-	T65.3x4-	—	—
Bioflavonoid(s)	T46.991-	T46.992-	T46.993-	T46.994-	T46.995-	T46.996-
Biological substance NEC	T50.901-	T50.902-	T50.903-	T50.904-	T50.905-	T50.906-
Biotin	T45.2x1-	T45.2x2-	T45.2x3-	T45.2x4-	T45.2x5-	T45.2x6-
Biperiden	T44.3x1-	T44.3x2-	T44.3x3-	T44.3x4-	T44.3x5-	T44.3x6-
Bisacodyl	T47.2x1-	T47.2x2-	T47.2x3-	T47.2x4-	T47.2x5-	T47.2x6-
Bisbentiamine	T45.2x1-	T45.2x2-	T45.2x3-	T45.2x4-	T45.2x5-	T45.2x6-
Bisbutiamine	T45.2x1-	T45.2x2-	T45.2x3-	T45.2x4-	T45.2x5-	T45.2x6-
Bisdequalinium (salts) (diacetate)	T49.6x1-	T49.6x2-	T49.6x3-	T49.6x4-	T49.6x5-	T49.6x6-
Bishydroxycoumarin	T45.511-	T45.512-	T45.513-	T45.514-	T45.515-	T45.516-
Bismarsen	T37.8x1-	T37.8x2-	T37.8x3-	T37.8x4-	T37.8x5-	T37.8x6-
Bismuth salts	T47.6x1-	T47.6x2-	T47.6x3-	T47.6x4-	T47.6x5-	T47.6x6-
aluminate	T47.1x1-	T47.1x2-	T47.1x3-	T47.1x4-	T47.1x5-	T47.1x6-
anti-infectives	T37.8x1-	T37.8x2-	T37.8x3-	T37.8x4-	T37.8x5-	T37.8x6-
formic iodide	T49.0x1-	T49.0x2-	T49.0x3-	T49.0x4-	T49.0x5-	T49.0x6-
glycolylarsenate	T49.0x1-	T49.0x2-	T49.0x3-	T49.0x4-	T49.0x5-	T49.0x6-
nonmedicinal (compounds) NEC	T65.91x-	T65.92x-	T65.93x-	T65.94x-	—	—
subcarbonate	T47.6x1-	T47.6x2-	T47.6x3-	T47.6x4-	T47.6x5-	T47.6x6-
subsalicylate	T37.8x1-	T37.8x2-	T37.8x3-	T37.8x4-	T37.8x5-	T37.8x6-
sulfarsphenamine	T37.8x1-	T37.8x2-	T37.8x3-	T37.8x4-	T37.8x5-	T37.8x6-
Bisoprolol	T44.7x1-	T44.7x2-	T44.7x3-	T44.7x4-	T44.7x5-	T44.7x6-
Bisoxatin	T47.2x1-	T47.2x2-	T47.2x3-	T47.2x4-	T47.2x5-	T47.2x6-
Bisulepin (hydrochloride)	T45.0x1-	T45.0x2-	T45.0x3-	T45.0x4-	T45.0x5-	T45.0x6-
Bithionol	T37.8x1-	T37.8x2-	T37.8x3-	T37.8x4-	T37.8x5-	T37.8x6-
anthelminthic	T37.4x1-	T37.4x2-	T37.4x3-	T37.4x4-	T37.4x5-	T37.4x6-
Bitolterol	T48.6x1-	T48.6x2-	T48.6x3-	T48.6x4-	T48.6x5-	T48.6x6-
Bitoscanate	T37.4x1-	T37.4x2-	T37.4x3-	T37.4x4-	T37.4x5-	T37.4x6-
Bitter almond oil	T62.8x1-	T62.8x2-	T62.8x3-	T62.8x4-		
Bittersweet	T62.2x1-	T62.2x2-	T62.2x3-	T62.2x4-	—	—
Black						
flag	T60.91x-	T60.92x-	T60.93x-	T60.94x-	—	—
henbane	T62.2x1-	T62.2x2-	T62.2x3-	T62.2x4-		
leaf (40)	T60.91x-	T60.92x-	T60.93x-	T60.94x-	—	—
widow spider (bite)	T63.311-	T63.312-	T63.313-	T63.314-	—	—
antivenin	T50.Z11-	T50.Z12-	T50.Z13-	T50.Z14-	T50.Z15-	T50.Z16-
Blast furnace gas (carbon monoxide from)	T58.8x1-	T58.8x2-	T58.8x3-	T58.8x4-	—	—

Table of Drugs & Chemicals	Poisoning Accidental (Unintentional)	Poisoning Self-Harm (Intentional)	Poisoning Assault	Poisoning Undetermined	Adverse Effect	Underdosing
Bleach	T54.91x-	T54.92x-	T54.93x-	T54.94x-	—	—
Bleaching agent (medicinal)	T49.4x1-	T49.4x2-	T49.4x3-	T49.4x4-	T49.4x5-	T49.4x6-
Bleomycin	T45.1x1-	T45.1x2-	T45.1x3-	T45.1x4-	T45.1x5-	T45.1x6-
Blockain	T41.3x1-	T41.3x2-	T41.3x3-	T41.3x4-	T41.3x5-	T41.3x6-
infiltration (subcutaneous)	T41.3x1-	T41.3x2-	T41.3x3-	T41.3x4-	T41.3x5-	T41.3x6-
nerve block (peripheral) (plexus)	T41.3x1-	T41.3x2-	T41.3x3-	T41.3x4-	T41.3x5-	T41.3x6-
topical (surface)	T41.3x1-	T41.3x2-	T41.3x3-	T41.3x4-	T41.3x5-	T41.3x6-
Blockers, calcium channel	T46.1x1-	T46.1x2-	T46.1x3-	T46.1x4-	T46.1x5-	T46.1x6-
Blood (derivatives) (natural) (plasma) (whole)	T45.8x1-	T45.8x2-	T45.8x3-	T45.8x4-	T45.8x5-	T45.8x6-
dried	T45.8x1-	T45.8x2-	T45.8x3-	T45.8x4-	T45.8x5-	T45.8x6-
drug affecting NEC	T45.91x-	T45.92x-	T45.93x-	T45.94x-	T45.95x-	T45.96x-
expander NEC	T45.8x1-	T45.8x2-	T45.8x3-	T45.8x4-	T45.8x5-	T45.8x6-
fraction NEC	T45.8x1-	T45.8x2-	T45.8x3-	T45.8x4-	T45.8x5-	T45.8x6-
substitute (macromolecular)	T45.8x1-	T45.8x2-	T45.8x3-	T45.8x4-	T45.8x5-	T45.8x6-
Blue velvet	T40.2x1-	T40.2x2-	T40.2x3-	T40.2x4-	—	—
Bone meal	T62.8x1-	T62.8x2-	T62.8x3-	T62.8x4-	—	—
Bonine	T45.0x1-	T45.0x2-	T45.0x3-	T45.0x4-	T45.0x5-	T45.0x6-
Bopindolol	T44.7x1-	T44.7x2-	T44.7x3-	T44.7x4-	T44.7x5-	T44.7x6-
Boracic acid	T49.0x1-	T49.0x2-	T49.0x3-	T49.0x4-	T49.0x5-	T49.0x6-
ENT agent	T49.6x1-	T49.6x2-	T49.6x3-	T49.6x4-	T49.6x5-	T49.6x6-
ophthalmic preparation	T49.5x1-	T49.5x2-	T49.5x3-	T49.5x4-	T49.5x5-	T49.5x6-
Borane complex	T57.8x1-	T57.8x2-	T57.8x3-	T57.8x4-	—	—
Borate (s)	T57.8x1-	T57.8x2-	T57.8x3-	T57.8x4-	—	—
buffer	T50.991-	T50.992-	T50.993-	T50.994-	T50.995-	T50.996-
cleanser	T54.91x-	T54.92x-	T54.93x-	T54.94x-	—	—
sodium	T57.8x1-	T57.8x2-	T57.8x3-	T57.8x4-	—	—
Borax (cleanser)	T54.91x-	T54.92x-	T54.93x-	T54.94x-	—	—
Bordeaux mixture	T60.3x1-	T60.3x2-	T60.3x3-	T60.3x4-	—	—
Boric acid	T49.0x1-	T49.0x2-	T49.0x3-	T49.0x4-	T49.0x5-	T49.0x6-
ENT agent	T49.6x1-	T49.6x2-	T49.6x3-	T49.6x4-	T49.6x5-	T49.6x6-
ophthalmic preparation	T49.5x1-	T49.5x2-	T49.5x3-	T49.5x4-	T49.5x5-	T49.5x6-
Bornaprine	T44.3x1-	T44.3x2-	T44.3x3-	T44.3x4-	T44.3x5-	T44.3x6-
Boron	T57.8x1-	T57.8x2-	T57.8x3-	T57.8x4-	—	—
hydride NEC	T57.8x1-	T57.8x2-	T57.8x3-	T57.8x4-	—	—
fumes or gas	T57.8x1-	T57.8x2-	T57.8x3-	T57.8x4-	—	—
trifluoride	T59.891-	T59.892-	T59.893-	T59.894-	—	—
Botox	T48.291-	T48.292-	T48.293-	T48.294-	T48.295-	T48.296-
Botulinus anti-toxin (type A, B)	T50.Z11-	T50.Z12-	T50.Z13-	T50.Z14-	T50.Z15-	T50.Z16-
Brake fluid vapor	T59.891-	T59.892-	T59.893-	T59.894-	—	—
Brallobarbital	T42.3x1-	T42.3x2-	T42.3x3-	T42.3x4-	T42.3x5-	T42.3x6-
Bran (wheat)	T47.4x1-	T47.4x2-	T47.4x3-	T47.4x4-	T47.4x5-	T47.4x6-
Brass (fumes)	T56.891-	T56.892-	T56.893-	T56.894-	—	—
Brasso	T52.0x1-	T52.0x2-	T52.0x3-	T52.0x4-	—	—
Bretylium tosilate	T46.2x1-	T46.2x2-	T46.2x3-	T46.2x4-	T46.2x5-	T46.2x6-
Brevital (sodium)	T41.1x1-	T41.1x2-	T41.1x3-	T41.1x4-	T41.1x5-	T41.1x6-
Brinase	T45.3x1-	T45.3x2-	T45.3x3-	T45.3x4-	T45.3x5-	T45.3x6-
British antilewisite	T45.8x1-	T45.8x2-	T45.8x3-	T45.8x4-	T45.8x5-	T45.8x6-
Brodifacoum	T60.4x1-	T60.4x2-	T60.4x3-	T60.4x4-	—	—
Bromal (hydrate)	T42.6x1-	T42.6x2-	T42.6x3-	T42.6x4-	T42.6x5-	T42.6x6-
Bromazepam	T42.4x1-	T42.4x2-	T42.4x3-	T42.4x4-	T42.4x5-	T42.4x6-
Bromazine	T45.0x1-	T45.0x2-	T45.0x3-	T45.0x4-	T45.0x5-	T45.0x6-
Brombenzylcyanide	T59.3x1-	T59.3x2-	T59.3x3-	T59.3x4-	—	—
Bromelains	T45.3x1-	T45.3x2-	T45.3x3-	T45.3x4-	T45.3x5-	T45.3x6-
Bromethalin	T60.4x1-	T60.4x2-	T60.4x3-	T60.4x4-	—	—
Bromhexine	T48.4x1-	T48.4x2-	T48.4x3-	T48.4x4-	T48.4x5-	T48.4x6-
Bromide salts	T42.6x1-	T42.6x2-	T42.6x3-	T42.6x4-	T42.6x5-	T42.6x6-
Bromindione	T45.511-	T45.512-	T45.513-	T45.514-	T45.515-	T45.516-
Bromine						
compounds (medicinal)	T42.6x1-	T42.6x2-	T42.6x3-	T42.6x4-	T42.6x5-	T42.6x6-
sedative	T42.6x1-	T42.6x2-	T42.6x3-	T42.6x4-	T42.6x5-	T42.6x6-
vapor	T59.891-	T59.892-	T59.893-	T59.894-	—	—
Bromisoval	T42.6x1-	T42.6x2-	T42.6x3-	T42.6x4-	T42.6x5-	T42.6x6-
Bromisovalum	T42.6x1-	T42.6x2-	T42.6x3-	T42.6x4-	T42.6x5-	T42.6x6-
Bromobenzylcyanide	T59.3x1-	T59.3x2-	T59.3x3-	T59.3x4-	—	—
Bromochlorosalicylanilide	T49.0x1-	T49.0x2-	T49.0x3-	T49.0x4-	T49.0x5-	T49.0x6-
Bromocriptine	T42.8x1-	T42.8x2-	T42.8x3-	T42.8x4-	T42.8x5-	T42.8x6-
Bromodiphenhydramine	T45.0x1-	T45.0x2-	T45.0x3-	T45.0x4-	T45.0x5-	T45.0x6-
Bromoform	T42.6x1-	T42.6x2-	T42.6x3-	T42.6x4-	T42.6x5-	T42.6x6-
Bromophenol blue reagent	T50.991-	T50.992-	T50.993-	T50.994-	T50.995-	T50.996-
Bromopride	T47.8x1-	T47.8x2-	T47.8x3-	T47.8x4-	T47.8x5-	T47.8x6-
Bromosalicylchloranitide	T49.0x1-	T49.0x2-	T49.0x3-	T49.0x4-	T49.0x5-	T49.0x6-
Bromosalicylhydroxamic acid	T37.1x1-	T37.1x2-	T37.1x3-	T37.1x4-	T37.1x5-	T37.1x6-
Bromo-seltzer	T39.1x1-	T39.1x2-	T39.1x3-	T39.1x4-	T39.1x5-	T39.1x6-
Bromoxynil	T60.3x1-	T60.3x2-	T60.3x3-	T60.3x4-	—	—
Bromperidol	T43.4x1-	T43.4x2-	T43.4x3-	T43.4x4-	T43.4x5-	T43.4x6-
Brompheniramine	T45.0x1-	T45.0x2-	T45.0x3-	T45.0x4-	T45.0x5-	T45.0x6-
Bromsulfophthalein	T50.8x1-	T50.8x2-	T50.8x3-	T50.8x4-	T50.8x5-	T50.8x6-
Bromural	T42.6x1-	T42.6x2-	T42.6x3-	T42.6x4-	T42.6x5-	T42.6x6-
Bromvaletone	T42.6x1-	T42.6x2-	T42.6x3-	T42.6x4-	T42.6x5-	T42.6x6-
Bronchodilator NEC	T48.6x1-	T48.6x2-	T48.6x3-	T48.6x4-	T48.6x5-	T48.6x6-
Brotizolam	T42.4x1-	T42.4x2-	T42.4x3-	T42.4x4-	T42.4x5-	T42.4x6-
Brovincamine	T46.7x1-	T46.7x2-	T46.7x3-	T46.7x4-	T46.7x5-	T46.7x6-
Brown recluse spider (bite) (venom)	T63.331-	T63.332-	T63.333-	T63.334-	—	—
Brown spider (bite) (venom)	T63.391-	T63.392-	T63.393-	T63.394-	—	—
Broxaterol	T48.6x1-	T48.6x2-	T48.6x3-	T48.6x4-	T48.6x5-	T48.6x6-
Broxuridine	T45.1x1-	T45.1x2-	T45.1x3-	T45.1x4-	T45.1x5-	T45.1x6-
Broxyquinoline	T37.8x1-	T37.8x2-	T37.8x3-	T37.8x4-	T37.8x5-	T37.8x6-
Bruceine	T48.291-	T48.292-	T48.293-	T48.294-	T48.295-	T48.296-
Brucia	T62.2x1-	T62.2x2-	T62.2x3-	T62.2x4-	—	—
Brucine	T65.1x1-	T65.1x2-	T65.1x3-	T65.1x4-	—	—
Brunswick green — see Copper						
Bruten — see Ibuprofen						
Bryonia	T47.2x1-	T47.2x2-	T47.2x3-	T47.2x4-	T47.2x5-	T47.2x6-
b-sitosterol(s)	T46.6x1-	T46.6x2-	T46.6x3-	T46.6x4-	T46.6x5-	T46.6x6-
Buclizine	T45.0x1-	T45.0x2-	T45.0x3-	T45.0x4-	T45.0x5-	T45.0x6-
Buclosamide	T49.0x1-	T49.0x2-	T49.0x3-	T49.0x4-	T49.0x5-	T49.0x6-
Budesonide	T44.5x1-	T44.5x2-	T44.5x3-	T44.5x4-	T44.5x5-	T44.5x6-
Budralazine	T46.5x1-	T46.5x2-	T46.5x3-	T46.5x4-	T46.5x5-	T46.5x6-
Bufferin	T39.011-	T39.012-	T39.013-	T39.014-	T39.015-	T39.016-
Buflomedil	T46.7x1-	T46.7x2-	T46.7x3-	T46.7x4-	T46.7x5-	T46.7x6-
Buformin	T38.3x1-	T38.3x2-	T38.3x3-	T38.3x4-	T38.3x5-	T38.3x6-
Bufotenine	T40.991-	T40.992-	T40.993-	T40.994-	—	—
Bufrolin	T48.6x1-	T48.6x2-	T48.6x3-	T48.6x4-	T48.6x5-	T48.6x6-
Bufylline	T48.6x1-	T48.6x2-	T48.6x3-	T48.6x4-	T48.6x5-	T48.6x6-
Bulk filler	T50.5x1-	T50.5x2-	T50.5x3-	T50.5x4-	T50.5x5-	T50.5x6-
cathartic	T47.4x1-	T47.4x2-	T47.4x3-	T47.4x4-	T47.4x5-	T47.4x6-
Bumetanide	T50.1x1-	T50.1x2-	T50.1x3-	T50.1x4-	T50.1x5-	T50.1x6-
Bunaftine	T46.2x1-	T46.2x2-	T46.2x3-	T46.2x4-	T46.2x5-	T46.2x6-
Bunamiodyl	T50.8x1-	T50.8x2-	T50.8x3-	T50.8x4-	T50.8x5-	T50.8x6-
Bunazosin	T44.6x1-	T44.6x2-	T44.6x3-	T44.6x4-	T44.6x5-	T44.6x6-
Bunitrolol	T44.7x1-	T44.7x2-	T44.7x3-	T44.7x4-	T44.7x5-	T44.7x6-
Buphenine	T46.7x1-	T46.7x2-	T46.7x3-	T46.7x4-	T46.7x5-	T46.7x6-
Bupivacaine	T41.3x1-	T41.3x2-	T41.3x3-	T41.3x4-	T41.3x5-	T41.3x6-
infiltration (subcutaneous)	T41.3x1-	T41.3x2-	T41.3x3-	T41.3x4-	T41.3x5-	T41.3x6-
nerve block (peripheral) (plexus)	T41.3x1-	T41.3x2-	T41.3x3-	T41.3x4-	T41.3x5-	T41.3x6-
spinal	T41.3x1-	T41.3x2-	T41.3x3-	T41.3x4-	T41.3x5-	T41.3x6-

DRUGS & CHEMICALS

Table of Drugs & Chemicals	POISONING Accidental (Unintentional)	Self-Harm (Intentional)	Assault	Undetermined	Adverse Effect	Underdosing
Bupranolol	T44.7x1-	T44.7x2-	T44.7x3-	T44.7x4-	T44.7x5-	T44.7x6-
Buprenorphine	T40.4x1-	T40.4x2-	T40.4x3-	T40.4x4-	T40.4x5-	T40.4x6-
Bupropion	T43.291-	T43.292-	T43.293-	T43.294-	T43.295-	T43.296-
Burimamide	T47.1x1-	T47.1x2-	T47.1x3-	T47.1x4-	T47.1x5-	T47.1x6-
Buserelin	T38.891-	T38.892-	T38.893-	T38.894-	T38.895-	T38.896-
Buspirone	T43.591-	T43.592-	T43.593-	T43.594-	T43.595-	T43.596-
Busulfan, busulphan	T45.1x1-	T45.1x2-	T45.1x3-	T45.1x4-	T45.1x5-	T45.1x6-
Butabarbital (sodium)	T42.3x1-	T42.3x2-	T42.3x3-	T42.3x4-	T42.3x5-	T42.3x6-
Butabarbitone	T42.3x1-	T42.3x2-	T42.3x3-	T42.3x4-	T42.3x5-	T42.3x6-
Butabarpal	T42.3x1-	T42.3x2-	T42.3x3-	T42.3x4-	T42.3x5-	T42.3x6-
Butacaine	T41.3x1-	T41.3x2-	T41.3x3-	T41.3x4-	T41.3x5-	T41.3x6-
Butalamine	T46.7x1-	T46.7x2-	T46.7x3-	T46.7x4-	T46.7x5-	T46.7x6-
Butalbital	T42.3x1-	T42.3x2-	T42.3x3-	T42.3x4-	T42.3x5-	T42.3x6-
Butallylonal	T42.3x1-	T42.3x2-	T42.3x3-	T42.3x4-	T42.3x5-	T42.3x6-
Butamben	T41.3x1-	T41.3x2-	T41.3x3-	T41.3x4-	T41.3x5-	T41.3x6-
Butamirate	T48.3x1-	T48.3x2-	T48.3x3-	T48.3x4-	T48.3x5-	T48.3x6-
Butane (distributed in mobile container)	T59.891-	T59.892-	T59.893-	T59.894-	—	—
distributed through pipes	T59.891-	T59.892-	T59.893-	T59.894-	—	—
incomplete combustion	T58.11x-	T58.12x-	T58.13x-	T58.14x-	—	—
Butanilicaine	T41.3x1-	T41.3x2-	T41.3x3-	T41.3x4-	T41.3x5-	T41.3x6-
Butanol	T51.3x1-	T51.3x2-	T51.3x3-	T51.3x4-	—	—
Butanone, 2-butanone	T52.4x1-	T52.4x2-	T52.4x3-	T52.4x4-	—	—
Butantrone	T49.4x1-	T49.4x2-	T49.4x3-	T49.4x4-	T49.4x5-	T49.4x6-
Butaperazine	T43.3x1-	T43.3x2-	T43.3x3-	T43.3x4-	T43.3x5-	T43.3x6-
Butazolidin	T39.2x1-	T39.2x2-	T39.2x3-	T39.2x4-	T39.2x5-	T39.2x6-
Butetamate	T48.6x1-	T48.6x2-	T48.6x3-	T48.6x4-	T48.6x5-	T48.6x6-
Butethal	T42.3x1-	T42.3x2-	T42.3x3-	T42.3x4-	T42.3x5-	T42.3x6-
Butethamate	T44.3x1-	T44.3x2-	T44.3x3-	T44.3x4-	T44.3x5-	T44.3x6-
Buthalitone (sodium)	T41.1x1-	T41.1x2-	T41.1x3-	T41.1x4-	T41.1x5-	T41.1x6-
Butisol (sodium)	T42.3x1-	T42.3x2-	T42.3x3-	T42.3x4-	T42.3x5-	T42.3x6-
Butizide	T50.2x1-	T50.2x2-	T50.2x3-	T50.2x4-	T50.2x5-	T50.2x6-
Butobarbital	T42.3x1-	T42.3x2-	T42.3x3-	T42.3x4-	T42.3x5-	T42.3x6-
sodium	T42.3x1-	T42.3x2-	T42.3x3-	T42.3x4-	T42.3x5-	T42.3x6-
Butobarbitone	T42.3x1-	T42.3x2-	T42.3x3-	T42.3x4-	T42.3x5-	T42.3x6-
Butoconazole (nitrate)	T49.0x1-	T49.0x2-	T49.0x3-	T49.0x4-	T49.0x5-	T49.0x6-
Butorphanol	T40.4x1-	T40.4x2-	T40.4x3-	T40.4x4-	T40.4x5-	T40.4x6-
Butriptyline	T43.011-	T43.012-	T43.013-	T43.014-	T43.015-	T43.016-
Butropium bromide	T44.3x1-	T44.3x2-	T44.3x3-	T44.3x4-	T44.3x5-	T44.3x6-
Butter of antimony — see Antimony						
Buttercups	T62.2x1-	T62.2x2-	T62.2x3-	T62.2x4-	—	—
Butyl						
acetate (secondary)	T52.8x1-	T52.8x2-	T52.8x3-	T52.8x4-	—	—
alcohol	T51.3x1-	T51.3x2-	T51.3x3-	T51.3x4-	—	—
aminobenzoate	T41.3x1-	T41.3x2-	T41.3x3-	T41.3x4-	T41.3x5-	T41.3x6-
butyrate	T52.8x1-	T52.8x2-	T52.8x3-	T52.8x4-	—	—
carbinol	T51.3x1-	T51.3x2-	T51.3x3-	T51.3x4-	—	—
carbitol	T52.3x1-	T52.3x2-	T52.3x3-	T52.3x4-	—	—
cellosolve	T52.3x1-	T52.3x2-	T52.3x3-	T52.3x4-	—	—
chloral (hydrate)	T42.6x1-	T42.6x2-	T42.6x3-	T42.6x4-	T42.6x5-	T42.6x6-
formate	T52.8x1-	T52.8x2-	T52.8x3-	T52.8x4-	—	—
lactate	T52.8x1-	T52.8x2-	T52.8x3-	T52.8x4-	—	—
propionate	T52.8x1-	T52.8x2-	T52.8x3-	T52.8x4-	—	—
scopolamine bromide	T44.3x1-	T44.3x2-	T44.3x3-	T44.3x4-	T44.3x5-	T44.3x6-
thiobarbital sodium	T41.1x1-	T41.1x2-	T41.1x3-	T41.1x4-	T41.1x5-	T41.1x6-
Butylated hydroxy-anisole	T50.991-	T50.992-	T50.993-	T50.994-	T50.995-	T50.996-
Butylchloral hydrate	T42.6x1-	T42.6x2-	T42.6x3-	T42.6x4-	T42.6x5-	T42.6x6-
Butyltoluene	T52.2x1-	T52.2x2-	T52.2x3-	T52.2x4-	—	—
Butyn	T41.3x1-	T41.3x2-	T41.3x3-	T41.3x4-	T41.3x5-	T41.3x6-
Butyrophenone (-based tranquilizers)	T43.4x1-	T43.4x2-	T43.4x3-	T43.4x4-	T43.4x5-	T43.4x6-
Cabergoline	T42.8x1-	T42.8x2-	T42.8x3-	T42.8x4-	T42.8x5-	T42.8x6-
Cacodyl, cacodylic acid	T57.0x1-	T57.0x2-	T57.0x3-	T57.0x4-	—	—
Cactinomycin	T45.1x1-	T45.1x2-	T45.1x3-	T45.1x4-	T45.1x5-	T45.1x6-
Cade oil	T49.4x1-	T49.4x2-	T49.4x3-	T49.4x4-	T49.4x5-	T49.4x6-
Cadexomer iodine	T49.0x1-	T49.0x2-	T49.0x3-	T49.0x4-	T49.0x5-	T49.0x6-
Cadmium (chloride) (fumes) (oxide)	T56.3x1-	T56.3x2-	T56.3x3-	T56.3x4-	—	—
sulfide (medicinal) NEC	T49.4x1-	T49.4x2-	T49.4x3-	T49.4x4-	T49.4x5-	T49.4x6-
Cadralazine	T46.5x1-	T46.5x2-	T46.5x3-	T46.5x4-	T46.5x5-	T46.5x6-
Caffeine	T43.611-	T43.612-	T43.613-	T43.614-	T43.615-	T43.616-
Calabar bean	T62.2x1-	T62.2x2-	T62.2x3-	T62.2x4-	—	—
Caladium seguinum	T62.2x1-	T62.2x2-	T62.2x3-	T62.2x4-	—	—
Calamine (lotion)	T49.3x1-	T49.3x2-	T49.3x3-	T49.3x4-	T49.3x5-	T49.3x6-
Calcifediol	T45.2x1-	T45.2x2-	T45.2x3-	T45.2x4-	T45.2x5-	T45.2x6-
Calciferol	T45.2x1-	T45.2x2-	T45.2x3-	T45.2x4-	T45.2x5-	T45.2x6-
Calcitonin	T50.991-	T50.992-	T50.993-	T50.994-	T50.995-	T50.996-
Calcitriol	T45.2x1-	T45.2x2-	T45.2x3-	T45.2x4-	T45.2x5-	T45.2x6-
Calcium	T50.3x1-	T50.3x2-	T50.3x3-	T50.3x4-	T50.3x5-	T50.3x6-
actylsalicylate	T39.011-	T39.012-	T39.013-	T39.014-	T39.015-	T39.016-
benzamidosalicylate	T37.1x1-	T37.1x2-	T37.1x3-	T37.1x4-	T37.1x5-	T37.1x6-
bromide	T42.6x1-	T42.6x2-	T42.6x3-	T42.6x4-	T42.6x5-	T42.6x6-
bromolactobionate	T42.6x1-	T42.6x2-	T42.6x3-	T42.6x4-	T42.6x5-	T42.6x6-
carbaspirin	T39.011-	T39.012-	T39.013-	T39.014-	T39.015-	T39.016-
carbimide	T50.6x1-	T50.6x2-	T50.6x3-	T50.6x4-	T50.6x5-	T50.6x6-
carbonate	T47.1x1-	T47.1x2-	T47.1x3-	T47.1x4-	T47.1x5-	T47.1x6-
chloride	T50.991-	T50.992-	T50.993-	T50.994-	T50.995-	T50.996-
anhydrous	T50.991-	T50.992-	T50.993-	T50.994-	T50.995-	T50.996-
cyanide	T57.8x1-	T57.8x2-	T57.8x3-	T57.8x4-	—	—
dioctyl sulfosuccinate	T47.4x1-	T47.4x2-	T47.4x3-	T47.4x4-	T47.4x5-	T47.4x6-
disodium edathamil	T45.8x1-	T45.8x2-	T45.8x3-	T45.8x4-	T45.8x5-	T45.8x6-
disodium edetate	T45.8x1-	T45.8x2-	T45.8x3-	T45.8x4-	T45.8x5-	T45.8x6-
dobesilate	T46.991-	T46.992-	T46.993-	T46.994-	T46.995-	T46.996-
EDTA	T45.8x1-	T45.8x2-	T45.8x3-	T45.8x4-	T45.8x5-	T45.8x6-
ferrous citrate	T45.4x1-	T45.4x2-	T45.4x3-	T45.4x4-	T45.4x5-	T45.4x6-
folinate	T45.8x1-	T45.8x2-	T45.8x3-	T45.8x4-	T45.8x5-	T45.8x6-
glubionate	T50.3x1-	T50.3x2-	T50.3x3-	T50.3x4-	T50.3x5-	T50.3x6-
gluconate	T50.3x1-	T50.3x2-	T50.3x3-	T50.3x4-	T50.3x5-	T50.3x6-
gluconogalactogluc-onate	T50.3x1-	T50.3x2-	T50.3x3-	T50.3x4-	T50.3x5-	T50.3x6-
hydrate, hydroxide	T54.3x1-	T54.3x2-	T54.3x3-	T54.3x4-	—	—
hypochlorite	T54.3x1-	T54.3x2-	T54.3x3-	T54.3x4-	—	—
iodide	T48.4x1-	T48.4x2-	T48.4x3-	T48.4x4-	T48.4x5-	T48.4x6-
ipodate	T50.8x1-	T50.8x2-	T50.8x3-	T50.8x4-	T50.8x5-	T50.8x6-
lactate	T50.3x1-	T50.3x2-	T50.3x3-	T50.3x4-	T50.3x5-	T50.3x6-
leucovorin	T45.8x1-	T45.8x2-	T45.8x3-	T45.8x4-	T45.8x5-	T45.8x6-
mandelate	T37.91x-	T37.92x-	T37.93x-	T37.94x-	T37.95x-	T37.96x-
oxide	T54.3x1-	T54.3x2-	T54.3x3-	T54.3x4-	—	—
pantothenate	T45.2x1-	T45.2x2-	T45.2x3-	T45.2x4-	T45.2x5-	T45.2x6-
phosphate	T50.3x1-	T50.3x2-	T50.3x3-	T50.3x4-	T50.3x5-	T50.3x6-
salicylate	T39.091-	T39.092-	T39.093-	T39.094-	T39.095-	T39.096-
salts	T50.3x1-	T50.3x2-	T50.3x3-	T50.3x4-	T50.3x5-	T50.3x6-
Calculus-dissolving drug	T50.991-	T50.992-	T50.993-	T50.994-	T50.995-	T50.996-
Calomel	T49.0x1-	T49.0x2-	T49.0x3-	T49.0x4-	T49.0x5-	T49.0x6-
Caloric agent	T50.3x1-	T50.3x2-	T50.3x3-	T50.3x4-	T50.3x5-	T50.3x6-
Calusterone	T38.7x1-	T38.7x2-	T38.7x3-	T38.7x4-	T38.7x5-	T38.7x6-
Camazepam	T42.4x1-	T42.4x2-	T42.4x3-	T42.4x4-	T42.4x5-	T42.4x6-
Camomile	T49.0x1-	T49.0x2-	T49.0x3-	T49.0x4-	T49.0x5-	T49.0x6-
Camoquin	T37.2x1-	T37.2x2-	T37.2x3-	T37.2x4-	T37.2x5-	T37.2x6-
Camphor insecticide	T60.2x1-	T60.2x2-	T60.2x3-	T60.2x4-	—	—
medicinal	T49.8x1-	T49.8x2-	T49.8x3-	T49.8x4-	T49.8x5-	T49.8x6-
Camylofin	T44.3x1-	T44.3x2-	T44.3x3-	T44.3x4-	T44.3x5-	T44.3x6-
Cancer chemotherapy drug regimen	T45.1x1-	T45.1x2-	T45.1x3-	T45.1x4-	T45.1x5-	T45.1x6-

DRUGS & CHEMICALS

Table of Drugs & Chemicals	POISONING Accidental (Unintentional)	Self-Harm (Intentional)	Assault	Undetermined	Adverse Effect	Underdosing
Candeptin	T49.0x1-	T49.0x2-	T49.0x3-	T49.0x4-	T49.0x5-	T49.0x6-
Candicidin	T49.0x1-	T49.0x2-	T49.0x3-	T49.0x4-	T49.0x5-	T49.0x6-
Cannabinol	T40.7x1-	T40.7x2-	T40.7x3-	T40.7x4-	T40.7x5-	T40.7x6-
Cannabis (derivatives)	T40.7x1-	T40.7x2-	T40.7x3-	T40.7x4-	T40.7x5-	T40.7x6-
Canned heat	T51.1x1-	T51.1x2-	T51.1x3-	T51.1x4-	—	—
Canrenoic acid	T50.0x1-	T50.0x2-	T50.0x3-	T50.0x4-	T50.0x5-	T50.0x6-
Canrenone	T50.0x1-	T50.0x2-	T50.0x3-	T50.0x4-	T50.0x5-	T50.0x6-
Cantharides, cantharidin, cantharis	T49.8x1-	T49.8x2-	T49.8x3-	T49.8x4-	T49.8x5-	T49.8x6-
Canthaxanthin	T50.991-	T50.992-	T50.993-	T50.994-	T50.995-	T50.996-
Capillary-active drug NEC	T46.901-	T46.902-	T46.903-	T46.904-	T46.905-	T46.906-
Capreomycin	T36.8x1-	T36.8x2-	T36.8x3-	T36.8x4-	T36.8x5-	T36.8x6-
Capsicum	T49.4x1-	T49.4x2-	T49.4x3-	T49.4x4-	T49.4x5-	T49.4x6-
Captafol	T60.3x1-	T60.3x2-	T60.3x3-	T60.3x4-	—	—
Captan	T60.3x1-	T60.3x2-	T60.3x3-	T60.3x4-	—	—
Captodiame, captodiamine	T43.591-	T43.592-	T43.593-	T43.594-	T43.595-	T43.596-
Captopril	T46.4x1-	T46.4x2-	T46.4x3-	T46.4x4-	T46.4x5-	T46.4x6-
Caramiphen	T44.3x1-	T44.3x2-	T44.3x3-	T44.3x4-	T44.3x5-	T44.3x6-
Carazolol	T44.7x1-	T44.7x2-	T44.7x3-	T44.7x4-	T44.7x5-	T44.7x6-
Carbachol	T44.1x1-	T44.1x2-	T44.1x3-	T44.1x4-	T44.1x5-	T44.1x6-
Carbacrylamine (resin)	T50.3x1-	T50.3x2-	T50.3x3-	T50.3x4-	T50.3x5-	T50.3x6-
Carbamate (insecticide)	T60.0x1-	T60.0x2-	T60.0x3-	T60.0x4-	—	—
Carbamate (sedative)	T42.6x1-	T42.6x2-	T42.6x3-	T42.6x4-	T42.6x5-	T42.6x6-
herbicide	T60.0x1-	T60.0x2-	T60.0x3-	T60.0x4-	—	—
insecticide	T60.0x1-	T60.0x2-	T60.0x3-	T60.0x4-	—	—
Carbamazepine	T42.1x1-	T42.1x2-	T42.1x3-	T42.1x4-	T42.1x5-	T42.1x6-
Carbamide	T47.3x1-	T47.3x2-	T47.3x3-	T47.3x4-	T47.3x5-	T47.3x6-
peroxide	T49.0x1-	T49.0x2-	T49.0x3-	T49.0x4-	T49.0x5-	T49.0x6-
topical	T49.8x1-	T49.8x2-	T49.8x3-	T49.8x4-	T49.8x5-	T49.8x6-
Carbamylcholine chloride	T44.1x1-	T44.1x2-	T44.1x3-	T44.1x4-	T44.1x5-	T44.1x6-
Carbaril	T60.0x1-	T60.0x2-	T60.0x3-	T60.0x4-	—	—
Carbarsone	T37.3x1-	T37.3x2-	T37.3x3-	T37.3x4-	T37.3x5-	T37.3x6-
Carbaryl	T60.0x1-	T60.0x2-	T60.0x3-	T60.0x4-	—	—
Carbaspirin	T39.011-	T39.012-	T39.013-	T39.014-	T39.015-	T39.016-
Carbazochrome (salicylate) (sodium sulfonate)	T49.4x1-	T49.4x2-	T49.4x3-	T49.4x4-	T49.4x5-	T49.4x6-
Carbenicillin	T36.0x1-	T36.0x2-	T36.0x3-	T36.0x4-	T36.0x5-	T36.0x6-
Carbenoxolone	T47.1x1-	T47.1x2-	T47.1x3-	T47.1x4-	T47.1x5-	T47.1x6-
Carbetapentane	T48.3x1-	T48.3x2-	T48.3x3-	T48.3x4-	T48.3x5-	T48.3x6-
Carbethyl salicylate	T39.091-	T39.092-	T39.093-	T39.094-	T39.095-	T39.096-
Carbidopa (with levodopa)	T42.8x1-	T42.8x2-	T42.8x3-	T42.8x4-	T42.8x5-	T42.8x6-
Carbimazole	T38.2x1-	T38.2x2-	T38.2x3-	T38.2x4-	T38.2x5-	T38.2x6-
Carbinol	T51.1x1-	T51.1x2-	T51.1x3-	T51.1x4-	—	—
Carbinoxamine	T45.0x1-	T45.0x2-	T45.0x3-	T45.0x4-	T45.0x5-	T45.0x6-
Carbiphene	T39.8x1-	T39.8x2-	T39.8x3-	T39.8x4-	T39.8x5-	T39.8x6-
Carbitol	T52.3x1-	T52.3x2-	T52.3x3-	T52.3x4-	—	—
Carbo medicinalis	T47.6x1-	T47.6x2-	T47.6x3-	T47.6x4-	T47.6x5-	T47.6x6-
Carbocaine	T41.3x1-	T41.3x2-	T41.3x3-	T41.3x4-	T41.3x5-	T41.3x6-
infiltration (subcutaneous)	T41.3x1-	T41.3x2-	T41.3x3-	T41.3x4-	T41.3x5-	T41.3x6-
nerve block (peripheral) (plexus)	T41.3x1-	T41.3x2-	T41.3x3-	T41.3x4-	T41.3x5-	T41.3x6-
topical (surface)	T41.3x1-	T41.3x2-	T41.3x3-	T41.3x4-	T41.3x5-	T41.3x6-
Carbocisteine	T48.4x1-	T48.4x2-	T48.4x3-	T48.4x4-	T48.4x5-	T48.4x6-
Carbocromen	T46.3x1-	T46.3x2-	T46.3x3-	T46.3x4-	T46.3x5-	T46.3x6-
Carbol fuchsin	T49.0x1-	T49.0x2-	T49.0x3-	T49.0x4-	T49.0x5-	T49.0x6-
Carbolic acid — see also Phenol	T54.0x1-	T54.0x2-	T54.0x3-	T54.0x4-	—	—
Carbolonium (bromide)	T48.1x1-	T48.1x2-	T48.1x3-	T48.1x4-	T48.1x5-	T48.1x6-
Carbomycin	T36.8x1-	T36.8x2-	T36.8x3-	T36.8x4-	T36.8x5-	T36.8x6-

Table of Drugs & Chemicals	POISONING Accidental (Unintentional)	Self-Harm (Intentional)	Assault	Undetermined	Adverse Effect	Underdosing
Carbon						
bisulfide (liquid)	T65.4x1-	T65.4x2-	T65.4x3-	T65.4x4-	—	—
vapor	T65.4x1-	T65.4x2-	T65.4x3-	T65.4x4-	—	—
dioxide (gas)	T59.7x1-	T59.7x2-	T59.7x3-	T59.7x4-	—	—
medicinal	T41.5x1-	T41.5x2-	T41.5x3-	T41.5x4-	T41.5x5-	T41.5x6-
nonmedicinal	T59.7x1-	T59.7x2-	T59.7x3-	T59.7x4-	—	—
snow	T49.4x1-	T49.4x2-	T49.4x3-	T49.4x4-	T49.4x5-	T49.4x6-
disulfide (liquid)	T65.4x1-	T65.4x2-	T65.4x3-	T65.4x4-	—	—
vapor	T65.4x1-	T65.4x2-	T65.4x3-	T65.4x4-	—	—
monoxide (from incomplete combustion)	T58.91x-	T58.92x-	T58.93x-	T58.94x-	—	—
blast furnace gas	T58.8x1-	T58.8x2-	T58.8x3-	T58.8x4-	—	—
butane (distributed in mobile container)	T58.11x-	T58.12x-	T58.13x-	T58.14x-	—	—
distributed through pipes	T58.11x-	T58.12x-	T58.13x-	T58.14x-	—	—
charcoal fumes	T58.2x1-	T58.2x2-	T58.2x3-	T58.2x4-	—	—
coal	T58.2x1-	T58.2x2-	T58.2x3-	T58.2x4-	—	—
gas (piped)	T58.11x-	T58.12x-	T58.13x-	T58.14x-	—	—
solid (in domestic stoves, fireplaces)	T58.2x1-	T58.2x2-	T58.2x3-	T58.2x4-	—	—
coke (in domestic stoves, fireplaces)	T58.2x1-	T58.2x2-	T58.2x3-	T58.2x4-	—	—
exhaust gas (motor) not in transit	T58.01x-	T58.02x-	T58.03x-	T58.04x-	—	—
combustion engine, any not in watercraft	T58.01x-	T58.02x-	T58.03x-	T58.04x-	—	—
farm tractor, not in transit	T58.01x-	T58.02x-	T58.03x-	T58.04x-	—	—
gas engine	T58.01x-	T58.02x-	T58.03x-	T58.04x-	—	—
motor pump	T58.01x-	T58.02x-	T58.03x-	T58.04x-	—	—
motor vehicle, not in transit	T58.01x-	T58.02x-	T58.03x-	T58.04x-	—	—
fuel (in domestic use)	T58.2x1-	T58.2x2-	T58.2x3-	T58.2x4-	—	—
gas (piped)	T58.11x-	T58.12x-	T58.13x-	T58.14x-	—	—
in mobile container	T58.11x-	T58.12x-	T58.13x-	T58.14x-	—	—
utility	T58.11x-	T58.12x-	T58.13x-	T58.14x-	—	—
in mobile container	T58.11x-	T58.12x-	T58.13x-	T58.14x-	—	—
piped (natural)	T58.11x-	T58.12x-	T58.13x-	T58.14x-	—	—
illuminating gas	T58.11x-	T58.12x-	T58.13x-	T58.14x-	—	—
industrial fuels or gases, any	T58.8x1-	T58.8x2-	T58.8x3-	T58.8x4-	—	—
kerosene (in domestic stoves, fireplaces)	T58.2x1-	T58.2x2-	T58.2x3-	T58.2x4-	—	—
kiln gas or vapor	T58.8x1-	T58.8x2-	T58.8x3-	T58.8x4-	—	—
motor exhaust gas, not in transit	T58.01x-	T58.02x-	T58.03x-	T58.04x-	—	—
piped gas (manufactured) (natural)	T58.11x-	T58.12x-	T58.13x-	T58.14x-	—	—
producer gas	T58.8x1-	T58.8x2-	T58.8x3-	T58.8x4-	—	—
propane (distributed in mobile container)	T58.11x-	T58.12x-	T58.13x-	T58.14x-	—	—
distributed through pipes	T58.11x-	T58.12x-	T58.13x-	T58.14x-	—	—
specified source NEC	T58.8x1-	T58.8x2-	T58.8x3-	T58.8x4-	—	—
stove gas	T58.11x-	T58.12x-	T58.13x-	T58.14x-	—	—
piped	T58.11x-	T58.12x-	T58.13x-	T58.14x-	—	—
utility gas	T58.11x-	T58.12x-	T58.13x-	T58.14x-	—	—
piped	T58.11x-	T58.12x-	T58.13x-	T58.14x-	—	—

DRUGS & CHEMICALS

Table of Drugs & Chemicals	POISONING Accidental (Unintentional)	POISONING Self-Harm (Intentional)	POISONING Assault	POISONING Undetermined	Adverse Effect	Underdosing
Carbon - *continued*						
monoxide (from incomplete combustion)						
- *continued*	T58.91x-	T58.92x-	T58.93x-	T58.94x-	—	—
water gas	T58.11x-	T58.12x-	T58.13x-	T58.14x-	—	—
wood (in domestic stoves, fireplaces)	T58.2x1-	T58.2x2-	T58.2x3-	T58.2x4-	—	—
tetrachloride (vapor) NEC	T53.0x1-	T53.0x2-	T53.0x3-	T53.0x4-	—	—
liquid (cleansing agent) NEC	T53.0x1-	T53.0x2-	T53.0x3-	T53.0x4-	—	—
solvent	T53.0x1-	T53.0x2-	T53.0x3-	T53.0x4-	—	—
Carbonic acid gas	T59.7x1-	T59.7x2-	T59.7x3-	T59.7x4-	—	—
anhydrase inhibitor NEC	T50.2x1-	T50.2x2-	T50.2x3-	T50.2x4-	T50.2x5-	T50.2x6-
Carbophenothion	T60.0x1-	T60.0x2-	T60.0x3-	T60.0x4-	—	—
Carboplatin	T45.1x1-	T45.1x2-	T45.1x3-	T45.1x4-	T45.1x5-	T45.1x6-
Carboprost	T48.0x1-	T48.0x2-	T48.0x3-	T48.0x4-	T48.0x5-	T48.0x6-
Carboquone	T45.1x1-	T45.1x2-	T45.1x3-	T45.1x4-	T45.1x5-	T45.1x6-
Carbowax	T49.3x1-	T49.3x2-	T49.3x3-	T49.3x4-	T49.3x5-	T49.3x6-
Carboxymethyl-cellulose	T47.4x1-	T47.4x2-	T47.4x3-	T47.4x4-	T47.4x5-	T47.4x6-
S-Carboxymethyl-cysteine	T48.4x1-	T48.4x2-	T48.4x3-	T48.4x4-	T48.4x5-	T48.4x6-
Carbrital	T42.3x1-	T42.3x2-	T42.3x3-	T42.3x4-	T42.3x5-	T42.3x6-
Carbromal	T42.6x1-	T42.6x2-	T42.6x3-	T42.6x4-	T42.6x5-	T42.6x6-
Carbutamide	T38.3x1-	T38.3x2-	T38.3x3-	T38.3x4-	T38.3x5-	T38.3x6-
Carbuterol	T48.6x1-	T48.6x2-	T48.6x3-	T48.6x4-	T48.6x5-	T48.6x6-
Cardiac						
depressants	T46.2x1-	T46.2x2-	T46.2x3-	T46.2x4-	T46.2x5-	T46.2x6-
rhythm regulator	T46.2x1-	T46.2x2-	T46.2x3-	T46.2x4-	T46.2x5-	T46.2x6-
specified NEC	T46.2x1-	T46.2x2-	T46.2x3-	T46.2x4-	T46.2x5-	T46.2x6-
Cardiografin	T50.8x1-	T50.8x2-	T50.8x3-	T50.8x4-	T50.8x5-	T50.8x6-
Cardio-green	T50.8x1-	T50.8x2-	T50.8x3-	T50.8x4-	T50.8x5-	T50.8x6-
Cardiotonic (glycoside) NEC	T46.0x1-	T46.0x2-	T46.0x3-	T46.0x4-	T46.0x5-	T46.0x6-
Cardiovascular drug NEC	T46.901-	T46.902-	T46.903-	T46.904-	T46.905-	T46.906-
Cardrase	T50.2x1-	T50.2x2-	T50.2x3-	T50.2x4-	T50.2x5-	T50.2x6-
Carfecillin	T36.0x1-	T36.0x2-	T36.0x3-	T36.0x4-	T36.0x5-	T36.0x6-
Carfenazine	T43.3x1-	T43.3x2-	T43.3x3-	T43.3x4-	T43.3x5-	T43.3x6-
Carfusin	T49.0x1-	T49.0x2-	T49.0x3-	T49.0x4-	T49.0x5-	T49.0x6-
Carindacillin	T36.0x1-	T36.0x2-	T36.0x3-	T36.0x4-	T36.0x5-	T36.0x6-
Carisoprodol	T42.8x1-	T42.8x2-	T42.8x3-	T42.8x4-	T42.8x5-	T42.8x6-
Carmellose	T47.4x1-	T47.4x2-	T47.4x3-	T47.4x4-	T47.4x5-	T47.4x6-
Carminative	T47.5x1-	T47.5x2-	T47.5x3-	T47.5x4-	T47.5x5-	T47.5x6-
Carmofur	T45.1x1-	T45.1x2-	T45.1x3-	T45.1x4-	T45.1x5-	T45.1x6-
Carmustine	T45.1x1-	T45.1x2-	T45.1x3-	T45.1x4-	T45.1x5-	T45.1x6-
Carotene	T45.2x1-	T45.2x2-	T45.2x3-	T45.2x4-	T45.2x5-	T45.2x6-
Carphenazine	T43.3x1-	T43.3x2-	T43.3x3-	T43.3x4-	T43.3x5-	T43.3x6-
Carpipramine	T42.4x1-	T42.4x2-	T42.4x3-	T42.4x4-	T42.4x5-	T42.4x6-
Carprofen	T39.311-	T39.312-	T39.313-	T39.314-	T39.315-	T39.316-
Carpronium chloride	T44.3x1-	T44.3x2-	T44.3x3-	T44.3x4-	T44.3x5-	T44.3x6-
Carrageenan	T47.8x1-	T47.8x2-	T47.8x3-	T47.8x4-	T47.8x5-	T47.8x6-
Carteolol	T44.7x1-	T44.7x2-	T44.7x3-	T44.7x4-	T44.7x5-	T44.7x6-
Carter's Little Pills	T47.2x1-	T47.2x2-	T47.2x3-	T47.2x4-	T47.2x5-	T47.2x6-
Cascara (sagrada)	T47.2x1-	T47.2x2-	T47.2x3-	T47.2x4-	T47.2x5-	T47.2x6-
Cassava	T62.2x1-	T62.2x2-	T62.2x3-	T62.2x4-	—	—
Castellani's paint	T49.0x1-	T49.0x2-	T49.0x3-	T49.0x4-	T49.0x5-	T49.0x6-
Castor						
bean	T62.2x1-	T62.2x2-	T62.2x3-	T62.2x4-	—	—
oil	T47.2x1-	T47.2x2-	T47.2x3-	T47.2x4-	T47.2x5-	T47.2x6-
Catalase	T45.3x1-	T45.3x2-	T45.3x3-	T45.3x4-	T45.3x5-	T45.3x6-
Caterpillar (sting)	T63.431-	T63.432-	T63.433-	T63.434-	—	—
Catha (edulis) (tea)	T43.691-	T43.692-	T43.693-	T43.694-	—	—

Table of Drugs & Chemicals	POISONING Accidental (Unintentional)	POISONING Self-Harm (Intentional)	POISONING Assault	POISONING Undetermined	Adverse Effect	Underdosing
Cathartic NEC	T47.4x1-	T47.4x2-	T47.4x3-	T47.4x4-	T47.4x5-	T47.4x6-
anthacene derivative	T47.2x1-	T47.2x2-	T47.2x3-	T47.2x4-	T47.2x5-	T47.2x6-
bulk	T47.4x1-	T47.4x2-	T47.4x3-	T47.4x4-	T47.4x5-	T47.4x6-
contact	T47.2x1-	T47.2x2-	T47.2x3-	T47.2x4-	T47.2x5-	T47.2x6-
emollient NEC	T47.4x1-	T47.4x2-	T47.4x3-	T47.4x4-	T47.4x5-	T47.4x6-
irritant NEC	T47.2x1-	T47.2x2-	T47.2x3-	T47.2x4-	T47.2x5-	T47.2x6-
mucilage	T47.4x1-	T47.4x2-	T47.4x3-	T47.4x4-	T47.4x5-	T47.4x6-
saline	T47.3x1-	T47.3x2-	T47.3x3-	T47.3x4-	T47.3x5-	T47.3x6-
vegetable	T47.2x1-	T47.2x2-	T47.2x3-	T47.2x4-	T47.2x5-	T47.2x6-
Cathine	T50.5x1-	T50.5x2-	T50.5x3-	T50.5x4-	T50.5x5-	T50.5x6-
Cathomycin	T36.8x1-	T36.8x2-	T36.8x3-	T36.8x4-	T36.8x5-	T36.8x6-
Cation exchange resin	T50.3x1-	T50.3x2-	T50.3x3-	T50.3x4-	T50.3x5-	T50.3x6-
Caustic(s) NEC	T54.91x-	T54.92x-	T54.93x-	T54.94x-	—	—
alkali	T54.3x1-	T54.3x2-	T54.3x3-	T54.3x4-	—	—
hydroxide	T54.3x1-	T54.3x2-	T54.3x3-	T54.3x4-	—	—
potash	T54.3x1-	T54.3x2-	T54.3x3-	T54.3x4-	—	—
specified NEC	T54.91x-	T54.92x-	T54.93x-	T54.94x-	—	—
soda	T54.3x1-	T54.3x2-	T54.3x3-	T54.3x4-	—	—
Ceepryn	T49.0x1-	T49.0x2-	T49.0x3-	T49.0x4-	T49.0x5-	T49.0x6-
ENT agent	T49.6x1-	T49.6x2-	T49.6x3-	T49.6x4-	T49.6x5-	T49.6x6-
lozenges	T49.6x1-	T49.6x2-	T49.6x3-	T49.6x4-	T49.6x5-	T49.6x6-
Cefacetrile	T36.1x1-	T36.1x2-	T36.1x3-	T36.1x4-	T36.1x5-	T36.1x6-
Cefaclor	T36.1x1-	T36.1x2-	T36.1x3-	T36.1x4-	T36.1x5-	T36.1x6-
Cefadroxil	T36.1x1-	T36.1x2-	T36.1x3-	T36.1x4-	T36.1x5-	T36.1x6-
Cefalexin	T36.1x1-	T36.1x2-	T36.1x3-	T36.1x4-	T36.1x5-	T36.1x6-
Cefaloglycin	T36.1x1-	T36.1x2-	T36.1x3-	T36.1x4-	T36.1x5-	T36.1x6-
Cefaloridine	T36.1x1-	T36.1x2-	T36.1x3-	T36.1x4-	T36.1x5-	T36.1x6-
Cefalosporins	T36.1x1-	T36.1x2-	T36.1x3-	T36.1x4-	T36.1x5-	T36.1x6-
Cefalotin	T36.1x1-	T36.1x2-	T36.1x3-	T36.1x4-	T36.1x5-	T36.1x6-
Cefamandole	T36.1x1-	T36.1x2-	T36.1x3-	T36.1x4-	T36.1x5-	T36.1x6-
Cefamycin antibiotic	T36.1x1-	T36.1x2-	T36.1x3-	T36.1x4-	T36.1x5-	T36.1x6-
Cefapirin	T36.1x1-	T36.1x2-	T36.1x3-	T36.1x4-	T36.1x5-	T36.1x6-
Cefatrizine	T36.1x1-	T36.1x2-	T36.1x3-	T36.1x4-	T36.1x5-	T36.1x6-
Cefazedone	T36.1x1-	T36.1x2-	T36.1x3-	T36.1x4-	T36.1x5-	T36.1x6-
Cefazolin	T36.1x1-	T36.1x2-	T36.1x3-	T36.1x4-	T36.1x5-	T36.1x6-
Cefbuperazone	T36.1x1-	T36.1x2-	T36.1x3-	T36.1x4-	T36.1x5-	T36.1x6-
Cefetamet	T36.1x1-	T36.1x2-	T36.1x3-	T36.1x4-	T36.1x5-	T36.1x6-
Cefixime	T36.1x1-	T36.1x2-	T36.1x3-	T36.1x4-	T36.1x5-	T36.1x6-
Cefmenoxime	T36.1x1-	T36.1x2-	T36.1x3-	T36.1x4-	T36.1x5-	T36.1x6-
Cefmetazole	T36.1x1-	T36.1x2-	T36.1x3-	T36.1x4-	T36.1x5-	T36.1x6-
Cefminox	T36.1x1-	T36.1x2-	T36.1x3-	T36.1x4-	T36.1x5-	T36.1x6-
Cefonicid	T36.1x1-	T36.1x2-	T36.1x3-	T36.1x4-	T36.1x5-	T36.1x6-
Cefoperazone	T36.1x1-	T36.1x2-	T36.1x3-	T36.1x4-	T36.1x5-	T36.1x6-
Ceforanide	T36.1x1-	T36.1x2-	T36.1x3-	T36.1x4-	T36.1x5-	T36.1x6-
Cefotaxime	T36.1x1-	T36.1x2-	T36.1x3-	T36.1x4-	T36.1x5-	T36.1x6-
Cefotetan	T36.1x1-	T36.1x2-	T36.1x3-	T36.1x4-	T36.1x5-	T36.1x6-
Cefotiam	T36.1x1-	T36.1x2-	T36.1x3-	T36.1x4-	T36.1x5-	T36.1x6-
Cefoxitin	T36.1x1-	T36.1x2-	T36.1x3-	T36.1x4-	T36.1x5-	T36.1x6-
Cefpimizole	T36.1x1-	T36.1x2-	T36.1x3-	T36.1x4-	T36.1x5-	T36.1x6-
Cefpiramide	T36.1x1-	T36.1x2-	T36.1x3-	T36.1x4-	T36.1x5-	T36.1x6-
Cefradine	T36.1x1-	T36.1x2-	T36.1x3-	T36.1x4-	T36.1x5-	T36.1x6-
Cefroxadine	T36.1x1-	T36.1x2-	T36.1x3-	T36.1x4-	T36.1x5-	T36.1x6-
Cefsulodin	T36.1x1-	T36.1x2-	T36.1x3-	T36.1x4-	T36.1x5-	T36.1x6-
Ceftazidime	T36.1x1-	T36.1x2-	T36.1x3-	T36.1x4-	T36.1x5-	T36.1x6-
Cefteram	T36.1x1-	T36.1x2-	T36.1x3-	T36.1x4-	T36.1x5-	T36.1x6-
Ceftezole	T36.1x1-	T36.1x2-	T36.1x3-	T36.1x4-	T36.1x5-	T36.1x6-
Ceftizoxime	T36.1x1-	T36.1x2-	T36.1x3-	T36.1x4-	T36.1x5-	T36.1x6-
Ceftriaxone	T36.1x1-	T36.1x2-	T36.1x3-	T36.1x4-	T36.1x5-	T36.1x6-
Cefuroxime	T36.1x1-	T36.1x2-	T36.1x3-	T36.1x4-	T36.1x5-	T36.1x6-
Cefuzonam	T36.1x1-	T36.1x2-	T36.1x3-	T36.1x4-	T36.1x5-	T36.1x6-
Celestone	T38.0x1-	T38.0x2-	T38.0x3-	T38.0x4-	T38.0x5-	T38.0x6-
topical	T49.0x1-	T49.0x2-	T49.0x3-	T49.0x4-	T49.0x5-	T49.0x6-

Table of Drugs & Chemicals	POISONING Accidental (Unintentional)	Self-Harm (Intentional)	Assault	Undetermined	Adverse Effect	Underdosing
Celiprolol	T44.7x1-	T44.7x2-	T44.7x3-	T44.7x4-	T44.7x5-	T44.7x6-
Cell stimulants and proliferants	T49.8x1-	T49.8x2-	T49.8x3-	T49.8x4-	T49.8x5-	T49.8x6-
Cellosolve	T52.91x-	T52.92x-	T52.93x-	T52.94x-	—	—
Cellulose						
cathartic	T47.4x1-	T47.4x2-	T47.4x3-	T47.4x4-	T47.4x5-	T47.4x6-
hydroxyethyl	T47.4x1-	T47.4x2-	T47.4x3-	T47.4x4-	T47.4x5-	T47.4x6-
nitrates (topical)	T49.3x1-	T49.3x2-	T49.3x3-	T49.3x4-	T49.3x5-	T49.3x6-
oxidized	T49.4x1-	T49.4x2-	T49.4x3-	T49.4x4-	T49.4x5-	T49.4x6-
Centipede (bite)	T63.411-	T63.412-	T63.413-	T63.414-	—	—
Central nervous system						
depressants	T42.71x-	T42.72x-	T42.73x-	T42.74x-	T42.75x-	T42.76x-
anesthetic (general)						
NEC	T41.201-	T41.202-	T41.203-	T41.204-	T41.205-	T41.206-
gases NEC	T41.0x1-	T41.0x2-	T41.0x3-	T41.0x4-	T41.0x5-	T41.0x6-
intravenous	T41.1x1-	T41.1x2-	T41.1x3-	T41.1x4-	T41.1x5-	T41.1x6-
barbiturates	T42.3x1-	T42.3x2-	T42.3x3-	T42.3x4-	T42.3x5-	T42.3x6-
benzodiazepines	T42.4x1-	T42.4x2-	T42.4x3-	T42.4x4-	T42.4x5-	T42.4x6-
bromides	T42.6x1-	T42.6x2-	T42.6x3-	T42.6x4-	T42.6x5-	T42.6x6-
cannabis sativa	T40.7x1-	T40.7x2-	T40.7x3-	T40.7x4-	T40.7x5-	T40.7x6-
chloral hydrate	T42.6x1-	T42.6x2-	T42.6x3-	T42.6x4-	T42.6x5-	T42.6x6-
ethanol	T51.0x1-	T51.0x2-	T51.0x3-	T51.0x4-	—	—
hallucinogenics	T40.901-	T40.902-	T40.903-	T40.904-	T40.905-	T40.906-
hypnotics	T42.71x-	T42.72x-	T42.73x-	T42.74x-	T42.75x-	T42.76x-
specified NEC	T42.6x1-	T42.6x2-	T42.6x3-	T42.6x4-	T42.6x5-	T42.6x6-
muscle relaxants	T42.8x1-	T42.8x2-	T42.8x3-	T42.8x4-	T42.8x5-	T42.8x6-
paraldehyde	T42.6x1-	T42.6x2-	T42.6x3-	T42.6x4-	T42.6x5-	T42.6x6-
sedatives; sedative-hypnotics	T42.71x-	T42.72x-	T42.73x-	T42.74x-	T42.75x-	T42.76x-
mixed NEC	T42.6x1-	T42.6x2-	T42.6x3-	T42.6x4-	T42.6x5-	T42.6x6-
specified NEC	T42.6x1-	T42.6x2-	T42.6x3-	T42.6x4-	T42.6x5-	T42.6x6-
muscle-tone depressants	T42.8x1-	T42.8x2-	T42.8x3-	T42.8x4-	T42.8x5-	T42.8x6-
stimulants	T43.601-	T43.602-	T43.603-	T43.604-	T43.605-	T43.606-
amphetamines	T43.621-	T43.622-	T43.623-	T43.624-	T43.625-	T43.626-
analeptics	T50.7x1-	T50.7x2-	T50.7x3-	T50.7x4-	T50.7x5-	T50.7x6-
antidepressants	T43.201-	T43.202-	T43.203-	T43.204-	T43.205-	T43.206-
opiate antagonists	T50.7x1-	T50.7x2-	T50.7x3-	T50.7x4-	T50.7x5-	T50.7x6-
specified NEC	T43.691-	T43.692-	T43.693-	T43.694-	T43.695-	T43.696-
Cephalexin	T36.1x1-	T36.1x2-	T36.1x3-	T36.1x4-	T36.1x5-	T36.1x6-
Cephaloglycin	T36.1x1-	T36.1x2-	T36.1x3-	T36.1x4-	T36.1x5-	T36.1x6-
Cephaloridine	T36.1x1-	T36.1x2-	T36.1x3-	T36.1x4-	T36.1x5-	T36.1x6-
Cephalosporins	T36.1x1-	T36.1x2-	T36.1x3-	T36.1x4-	T36.1x5-	T36.1x6-
N (adicillin)	T36.0x1-	T36.0x2-	T36.0x3-	T36.0x4-	T36.0x5-	T36.0x6-
Cephalothin	T36.1x1-	T36.1x2-	T36.1x3-	T36.1x4-	T36.1x5-	T36.1x6-
Cephalotin	T36.1x1-	T36.1x2-	T36.1x3-	T36.1x4-	T36.1x5-	T36.1x6-
Cephradine	T36.1x1-	T36.1x2-	T36.1x3-	T36.1x4-	T36.1x5-	T36.1x6-
Cerbera (odallam)	T62.2x1-	T62.2x2-	T62.2x3-	T62.2x4-	—	—
Cerberin	T46.0x1-	T46.0x2-	T46.0x3-	T46.0x4-	T46.0x5-	T46.0x6-
Cerebral stimulants	T43.601-	T43.602-	T43.603-	T43.604-	T43.605-	T43.606-
psychotherapeutic	T43.601-	T43.602-	T43.603-	T43.604-	T43.605-	T43.606-
specified NEC	T43.691-	T43.692-	T43.693-	T43.694-	T43.695-	T43.696-
Cerium oxalate	T45.0x1-	T45.0x2-	T45.0x3-	T45.0x4-	T45.0x5-	T45.0x6-
Cerous oxalate	T45.0x1-	T45.0x2-	T45.0x3-	T45.0x4-	T45.0x5-	T45.0x6-
Ceruletide	T50.8x1-	T50.8x2-	T50.8x3-	T50.8x4-	T50.8x5-	T50.8x6-
Cetalkonium (chloride)	T49.0x1-	T49.0x2-	T49.0x3-	T49.0x4-	T49.0x5-	T49.0x6-
Cethexonium chloride	T49.0x1-	T49.0x2-	T49.0x3-	T49.0x4-	T49.0x5-	T49.0x6-
Cetiedil	T46.7x1-	T46.7x2-	T46.7x3-	T46.7x4-	T46.7x5-	T46.7x6-
Cetirizine	T45.0x1-	T45.0x2-	T45.0x3-	T45.0x4-	T45.0x5-	T45.0x6-
Cetomacrogol	T50.991-	T50.992-	T50.993-	T50.994-	T50.995-	T50.996-
Cetotiamine	T45.2x1-	T45.2x2-	T45.2x3-	T45.2x4-	T45.2x5-	T45.2x6-
Cetoxime	T45.0x1-	T45.0x2-	T45.0x3-	T45.0x4-	T45.0x5-	T45.0x6-
Cetraxate	T47.1x1-	T47.1x2-	T47.1x3-	T47.1x4-	T47.1x5-	T47.1x6-
Cetrimide	T49.0x1-	T49.0x2-	T49.0x3-	T49.0x4-	T49.0x5-	T49.0x6-
Cetrimonium (bromide)	T49.0x1-	T49.0x2-	T49.0x3-	T49.0x4-	T49.0x5-	T49.0x6-
Cetylpyridinium chloride	T49.0x1-	T49.0x2-	T49.0x3-	T49.0x4-	T49.0x5-	T49.0x6-
ENT agent	T49.6x1-	T49.6x2-	T49.6x3-	T49.6x4-	T49.6x5-	T49.6x6-
lozenges	T49.6x1-	T49.6x2-	T49.6x3-	T49.6x4-	T49.6x5-	T49.6x6-
Cevadilla — see Sabadilla						
Cevitamic acid	T45.2x1-	T45.2x2-	T45.2x3-	T45.2x4-	T45.2x5-	T45.2x6-
Ch'an su	T46.0x1-	T46.0x2-	T46.0x3-	T46.0x4-	T46.0x5-	T46.0x6-
Chalk, precipitated	T47.1x1-	T47.1x2-	T47.1x3-	T47.1x4-	T47.1x5-	T47.1x6-
Chamomile	T49.0x1-	T49.0x2-	T49.0x3-	T49.0x4-	T49.0x5-	T49.0x6-
Charcoal	T47.6x1-	T47.6x2-	T47.6x3-	T47.6x4-	T47.6x5-	T47.6x6-
activated — see also						
Charcoal, medicinal	T47.6x1-	T47.6x2-	T47.6x3-	T47.6x4-	T47.6x5-	T47.6x6-
fumes (carbon monoxide)	T58.2x1-	T58.2x2-	T58.2x3-	T58.2x4-	—	—
industrial	T58.8x1-	T58.8x2-	T58.8x3-	T58.8x4-	—	—
medicinal (activated)	T47.6x1-	T47.6x2-	T47.6x3-	T47.6x4-	T47.6x5-	T47.6x6-
antidiarrheal	T47.6x1-	T47.6x2-	T47.6x3-	T47.6x4-	T47.6x5-	T47.6x6-
poison control	T47.8x1-	T47.8x2-	T47.8x3-	T47.8x4-	T47.8x5-	T47.8x6-
specified use other than for diarrhea	T47.8x1-	T47.8x2-	T47.8x3-	T47.8x4-	T47.8x5-	T47.8x6-
topical	T49.8x1-	T49.8x2-	T49.8x3-	T49.8x4-	T49.8x5-	T49.8x6-
Chaulmosulfone	T37.1x1-	T37.1x2-	T37.1x3-	T37.1x4-	T37.1x5-	T37.1x6-
Chelating agent NEC	T50.6x1-	T50.6x2-	T50.6x3-	T50.6x4-	T50.6x5-	T50.6x6-
Chelidonium majus	T62.2x1-	T62.2x2-	T62.2x3-	T62.2x4-	—	—
Chemical substance NEC	T65.91x-	T65.92x-	T65.93x-	T65.94x-	—	—
Chenodeoxycholic acid	T47.5x1-	T47.5x2-	T47.5x3-	T47.5x4-	T47.5x5-	T47.5x6-
Chenodiol	T47.5x1-	T47.5x2-	T47.5x3-	T47.5x4-	T47.5x5-	T47.5x6-
Chenopodium	T37.4x1-	T37.4x2-	T37.4x3-	T37.4x4-	T37.4x5-	T37.4x6-
Cherry laurel	T62.2x1-	T62.2x2-	T62.2x3-	T62.2x4-	—	—
Chinidin(e)	T46.2x1-	T46.2x2-	T46.2x3-	T46.2x4-	T46.2x5-	T46.2x6-
Chiniofon	T37.8x1-	T37.8x2-	T37.8x3-	T37.8x4-	T37.8x5-	T37.8x6-
Chlophedianol	T48.3x1-	T48.3x2-	T48.3x3-	T48.3x4-	T48.3x5-	T48.3x6-
Chloral	T42.6x1-	T42.6x2-	T42.6x3-	T42.6x4-	T42.6x5-	T42.6x6-
derivative	T42.6x1-	T42.6x2-	T42.6x3-	T42.6x4-	T42.6x5-	T42.6x6-
hydrate	T42.6x1-	T42.6x2-	T42.6x3-	T42.6x4-	T42.6x5-	T42.6x6-
Chloralamide	T42.6x1-	T42.6x2-	T42.6x3-	T42.6x4-	T42.6x5-	T42.6x6-
Chloralodol	T42.6x1-	T42.6x2-	T42.6x3-	T42.6x4-	T42.6x5-	T42.6x6-
Chloralose	T60.4x1-	T60.4x2-	T60.4x3-	T60.4x4-	—	—
Chlorambucil	T45.1x1-	T45.1x2-	T45.1x3-	T45.1x4-	T45.1x5-	T45.1x6-
Chloramine	T57.8x1-	T57.8x2-	T57.8x3-	T57.8x4-	—	—
T	T49.0x1-	T49.0x2-	T49.0x3-	T49.0x4-	T49.0x5-	T49.0x6-
topical	T49.0x1-	T49.0x2-	T49.0x3-	T49.0x4-	T49.0x5-	T49.0x6-
Chloramphenicol	T36.2x1-	T36.2x2-	T36.2x3-	T36.2x4-	T36.2x5-	T36.2x6-
ENT agent	T49.6x1-	T49.6x2-	T49.6x3-	T49.6x4-	T49.6x5-	T49.6x6-
ophthalmic preparation	T49.5x1-	T49.5x2-	T49.5x3-	T49.5x4-	T49.5x5-	T49.5x6-
topical NEC	T49.0x1-	T49.0x2-	T49.0x3-	T49.0x4-	T49.0x5-	T49.0x6-
Chlorate (potassium) (sodium) NEC	T60.3x1-	T60.3x2-	T60.3x3-	T60.3x4-	—	—
herbicide	T60.3x1-	T60.3x2-	T60.3x3-	T60.3x4-	—	—
Chlorazanil	T50.2x1-	T50.2x2-	T50.2x3-	T50.2x4-	T50.2x5-	T50.2x6-
Chlorbenzene, chlorbenzol	T53.7x1-	T53.7x2-	T53.7x3-	T53.7x4-	—	—
Chlorbenzoxamine	T44.3x1-	T44.3x2-	T44.3x3-	T44.3x4-	T44.3x5-	T44.3x6-
Chlorbutol	T42.6x1-	T42.6x2-	T42.6x3-	T42.6x4-	T42.6x5-	T42.6x6-
Chlorcyclizine	T45.0x1-	T45.0x2-	T45.0x3-	T45.0x4-	T45.0x5-	T45.0x6-
Chlordan(e) (dust)	T60.1x1-	T60.1x2-	T60.1x3-	T60.1x4-	—	—
Chlordantoin	T49.0x1-	T49.0x2-	T49.0x3-	T49.0x4-	T49.0x5-	T49.0x6-
Chlordiazepoxide	T42.4x1-	T42.4x2-	T42.4x3-	T42.4x4-	T42.4x5-	T42.4x6-
Chlordiethyl benzamide	T49.3x1-	T49.3x2-	T49.3x3-	T49.3x4-	T49.3x5-	T49.3x6-
Chloresium	T49.8x1-	T49.8x2-	T49.8x3-	T49.8x4-	T49.8x5-	T49.8x6-
Chlorethiazol	T42.6x1-	T42.6x2-	T42.6x3-	T42.6x4-	T42.6x5-	T42.6x6-
Chlorethyl — see Ethyl chloride						
Chloretone	T42.6x1-	T42.6x2-	T42.6x3-	T42.6x4-	T42.6x5-	T42.6x6-
Chlorex	T53.6x1-	T53.6x2-	T53.6x3-	T53.6x4-	—	—
insecticide	T60.1x1-	T60.1x2-	T60.1x3-	T60.1x4-	—	—

Table of Drugs & Chemicals	POISONING				Adverse Effect	Underdosing
	Accidental (Unintentional)	Self-Harm (Intentional)	Assault	Undetermined		
Chlorfenvinphos	T60.0x1-	T60.0x2-	T60.0x3-	T60.0x4-	—	—
Chlorhexadol	T42.6x1-	T42.6x2-	T42.6x3-	T42.6x4-	T42.6x5-	T42.6x6-
Chlorhexamide	T45.1x1-	T45.1x2-	T45.1x3-	T45.1x4-	T45.1x5-	T45.1x6-
Chlorhexidine	T49.0x1-	T49.0x2-	T49.0x3-	T49.0x4-	T49.0x5-	T49.0x6-
Chlorhydroxyquinolin	T49.0x1-	T49.0x2-	T49.0x3-	T49.0x4-	T49.0x5-	T49.0x6-
Chloride of lime (bleach)	T54.3x1-	T54.3x2-	T54.3x3-	T54.3x4-	—	—
Chlorimipramine	T43.011-	T43.012-	T43.013-	T43.014-	T43.015-	T43.016-
Chlorinated						
camphene	T53.6x1-	T53.6x2-	T53.6x3-	T53.6x4-	—	—
diphenyl	T53.7x1-	T53.7x2-	T53.7x3-	T53.7x4-	—	—
hydrocarbons NEC	T53.91x-	T53.92x-	T53.93x-	T53.94x-	—	—
solvents	T53.91x-	T53.92x-	T53.93x-	T53.94x-	—	—
lime (bleach)	T54.3x1-	T54.3x2-	T54.3x3-	T54.3x4-	—	—
and boric acid solution	T49.0x1-	T49.0x2-	T49.0x3-	T49.0x4-	T49.0x5-	T49.0x6-
naphthalene (insecticide)	T60.1x1-	T60.1x2-	T60.1x3-	T60.1x4-	—	—
industrial						
(non-pesticide)	T53.7x1-	T53.7x2-	T53.7x3-	T53.7x4-	—	—
pesticide NEC	T60.8x1-	T60.8x2-	T60.8x3-	T60.8x4-	—	—
soda — see also Sodium						
hypochlorite						
solution	T49.0x1-	T49.0x2-	T49.0x3-	T49.0x4-	T49.0x5-	T49.0x6-
Chlorine (fumes) (gas)	T59.4x1-	T59.4x2-	T59.4x3-	T59.4x4-	—	—
bleach	T54.3x1-	T54.3x2-	T54.3x3-	T54.3x4-	—	—
compound gas NEC	T59.4x1-	T59.4x2-	T59.4x3-	T59.4x4-	—	—
disinfectant	T59.4x1-	T59.4x2-	T59.4x3-	T59.4x4-	—	—
releasing agents NEC	T59.4x1-	T59.4x2-	T59.4x3-	T59.4x4-	—	—
Chlorisondamine chloride	T46.991-	T46.992-	T46.993-	T46.994-	T46.995-	T46.996-
Chlormadinone	T38.5x1-	T38.5x2-	T38.5x3-	T38.5x4-	T38.5x5-	T38.5x6-
Chlormephos	T60.0x1-	T60.0x2-	T60.0x3-	T60.0x4-	—	—
Chlormerodrin	T50.2x1-	T50.2x2-	T50.2x3-	T50.2x4-	T50.2x5-	T50.2x6-
Chlormethiazole	T42.6x1-	T42.6x2-	T42.6x3-	T42.6x4-	T42.6x5-	T42.6x6-
Chlormethine	T45.1x1-	T45.1x2-	T45.1x3-	T45.1x4-	T45.1x5-	T45.1x6-
Chlormethylenecycline	T36.4x1-	T36.4x2-	T36.4x3-	T36.4x4-	T36.4x5-	T36.4x6-
Chlormezanone	T42.6x1-	T42.6x2-	T42.6x3-	T42.6x4-	T42.6x5-	T42.6x6-
Chloroacetic acid	T60.3x1-	T60.3x2-	T60.3x3-	T60.3x4-	—	—
Chloroacetone	T59.3x1-	T59.3x2-	T59.3x3-	T59.3x4-	—	—
Chloroacetophenone	T59.3x1-	T59.3x2-	T59.3x3-	T59.3x4-	—	—
Chloroaniline	T53.7x1-	T53.7x2-	T53.7x3-	T53.7x4-	—	—
Chlorobenzene, chlorobenzol	T53.7x1-	T53.7x2-	T53.7x3-	T53.7x4-	—	—
Chlorobromomethane (fire extinguisher)	T53.6x1-	T53.6x2-	T53.6x3-	T53.6x4-	—	—
Chlorobutanol	T49.0x1-	T49.0x2-	T49.0x3-	T49.0x4-	T49.0x5-	T49.0x6-
Chlorocresol	T49.0x1-	T49.0x2-	T49.0x3-	T49.0x4-	T49.0x5-	T49.0x6-
Chlorodehydro-methyltestosterone	T38.7x1-	T38.7x2-	T38.7x3-	T38.7x4-	T38.7x5-	T38.7x6-
Chlorodinitrobenzene	T53.7x1-	T53.7x2-	T53.7x3-	T53.7x4-	—	—
dust or vapor	T53.7x1-	T53.7x2-	T53.7x3-	T53.7x4-	—	—
Chlorodiphenyl	T53.7x1-	T53.7x2-	T53.7x3-	T53.7x4-	—	—
Chloroethane — see Ethyl chloride						
Chloroethylene	T53.6x1-	T53.6x2-	T53.6x3-	T53.6x4-	—	—
Chlorofluorocarbons	T53.5x1-	T53.5x2-	T53.5x3-	T53.5x4-	—	—
Chloroform (fumes) (vapor)	T53.1x1-	T53.1x2-	T53.1x3-	T53.1x4-	—	—
anesthetic	T41.0x1-	T41.0x2-	T41.0x3-	T41.0x4-	T41.0x5-	T41.0x6-
solvent	T53.1x1-	T53.1x2-	T53.1x3-	T53.1x4-	—	—
water, concentrated	T41.0x1-	T41.0x2-	T41.0x3-	T41.0x4-	T41.0x5-	T41.0x6-
Chloroguanide	T37.2x1-	T37.2x2-	T37.2x3-	T37.2x4-	T37.2x5-	T37.2x6-
Chloromycetin	T36.2x1-	T36.2x2-	T36.2x3-	T36.2x4-	T36.2x5-	T36.2x6-
ENT agent	T49.6x1-	T49.6x2-	T49.6x3-	T49.6x4-	T49.6x5-	T49.6x6-
ophthalmic preparation	T49.5x1-	T49.5x2-	T49.5x3-	T49.5x4-	T49.5x5-	T49.5x6-
otic solution	T49.6x1-	T49.6x2-	T49.6x3-	T49.6x4-	T49.6x5-	T49.6x6-
topical NEC	T49.0x1-	T49.0x2-	T49.0x3-	T49.0x4-	T49.0x5-	T49.0x6-

Table of Drugs & Chemicals	POISONING				Adverse Effect	Underdosing
	Accidental (Unintentional)	Self-Harm (Intentional)	Assault	Undetermined		
Chloronitrobenzene	T53.7x1-	T53.7x2-	T53.7x3-	T53.7x4-	—	—
dust or vapor	T53.7x1-	T53.7x2-	T53.7x3-	T53.7x4-	—	—
Chlorophacinone	T60.4x1-	T60.4x2-	T60.4x3-	T60.4x4-	—	—
Chlorophenol	T53.7x1-	T53.7x2-	T53.7x3-	T53.7x4-	—	—
Chlorophenothane	T60.1x1-	T60.1x2-	T60.1x3-	T60.1x4-	—	—
Chlorophyll	T50.991-	T50.992-	T50.993-	T50.994-	T50.995-	T50.996-
Chloropicrin (fumes)	T53.6x1-	T53.6x2-	T53.6x3-	T53.6x4-	—	—
fumigant	T60.8x1-	T60.8x2-	T60.8x3-	T60.8x4-	—	—
fungicide	T60.3x1-	T60.3x2-	T60.3x3-	T60.3x4-	—	—
pesticide	T60.8x1-	T60.8x2-	T60.8x3-	T60.8x4-	—	—
Chloroprocaine	T41.3x1-	T41.3x2-	T41.3x3-	T41.3x4-	T41.3x5-	T41.3x6-
infiltration (subcutaneous)	T41.3x1-	T41.3x2-	T41.3x3-	T41.3x4-	T41.3x5-	T41.3x6-
nerve block (peripheral) (plexus)	T41.3x1-	T41.3x2-	T41.3x3-	T41.3x4-	T41.3x5-	T41.3x6-
spinal	T41.3x1-	T41.3x2-	T41.3x3-	T41.3x4-	T41.3x5-	T41.3x6-
Chloroptic	T49.5x1-	T49.5x2-	T49.5x3-	T49.5x4-	T49.5x5-	T49.5x6-
Chloropurine	T45.1x1-	T45.1x2-	T45.1x3-	T45.1x4-	T45.1x5-	T45.1x6-
Chloropyramine	T45.0x1-	T45.0x2-	T45.0x3-	T45.0x4-	T45.0x5-	T45.0x6-
Chloropyrifos	T60.0x1-	T60.0x2-	T60.0x3-	T60.0x4-	—	—
Chloropyrilene	T45.0x1-	T45.0x2-	T45.0x3-	T45.0x4-	T45.0x5-	T45.0x6-
Chloroquine	T37.2x1-	T37.2x2-	T37.2x3-	T37.2x4-	T37.2x5-	T37.2x6-
Chlorothalonil	T60.3x1-	T60.3x2-	T60.3x3-	T60.3x4-	—	—
Chlorothen	T45.0x1-	T45.0x2-	T45.0x3-	T45.0x4-	T45.0x5-	T45.0x6-
Chlorothiazide	T50.2x1-	T50.2x2-	T50.2x3-	T50.2x4-	T50.2x5-	T50.2x6-
Chlorothymol	T49.4x1-	T49.4x2-	T49.4x3-	T49.4x4-	T49.4x5-	T49.4x6-
Chlorotrianisene	T38.5x1-	T38.5x2-	T38.5x3-	T38.5x4-	T38.5x5-	T38.5x6-
Chlorovinyldichloro-arsine, not in war	T57.0x1-	T57.0x2-	T57.0x3-	T57.0x4-	—	—
Chloroxine	T49.4x1-	T49.4x2-	T49.4x3-	T49.4x4-	T49.4x5-	T49.4x6-
Chloroxylenol	T49.0x1-	T49.0x2-	T49.0x3-	T49.0x4-	T49.0x5-	T49.0x6-
Chlorphenamine	T45.0x1-	T45.0x2-	T45.0x3-	T45.0x4-	T45.0x5-	T45.0x6-
Chlorphenesin	T42.8x1-	T42.8x2-	T42.8x3-	T42.8x4-	T42.8x5-	T42.8x6-
topical (antifungal)	T49.0x1-	T49.0x2-	T49.0x3-	T49.0x4-	T49.0x5-	T49.0x6-
Chlorpheniramine	T45.0x1-	T45.0x2-	T45.0x3-	T45.0x4-	T45.0x5-	T45.0x6-
Chlorphenoxamine	T45.0x1-	T45.0x2-	T45.0x3-	T45.0x4-	T45.0x5-	T45.0x6-
Chlorphentermine	T50.5x1-	T50.5x2-	T50.5x3-	T50.5x4-	T50.5x5-	T50.5x6-
Chlorprocaine — see Chloroprocaine						
Chlorproguanil	T37.2x1-	T37.2x2-	T37.2x3-	T37.2x4-	T37.2x5-	T37.2x6-
Chlorpromazine	T43.3x1-	T43.3x2-	T43.3x3-	T43.3x4-	T43.3x5-	T43.3x6-
Chlorpropamide	T38.3x1-	T38.3x2-	T38.3x3-	T38.3x4-	T38.3x5-	T38.3x6-
Chlorprothixene	T43.4x1-	T43.4x2-	T43.4x3-	T43.4x4-	T43.4x5-	T43.4x6-
Chlorquinaldol	T49.0x1-	T49.0x2-	T49.0x3-	T49.0x4-	T49.0x5-	T49.0x6-
Chlorquinol	T49.0x1-	T49.0x2-	T49.0x3-	T49.0x4-	T49.0x5-	T49.0x6-
Chlortalidone	T50.2x1-	T50.2x2-	T50.2x3-	T50.2x4-	T50.2x5-	T50.2x6-
Chlortetracycline	T36.4x1-	T36.4x2-	T36.4x3-	T36.4x4-	T36.4x5-	T36.4x6-
Chlorthalidone	T50.2x1-	T50.2x2-	T50.2x3-	T50.2x4-	T50.2x5-	T50.2x6-
Chlorthion	T60.0x1-	T60.0x2-	T60.0x3-	T60.0x4-	—	—
Chlorthiophos	T60.0x1-	T60.0x2-	T60.0x3-	T60.0x4-	—	—
Chlortrianisene	T38.5x1-	T38.5x2-	T38.5x3-	T38.5x4-	T38.5x5-	T38.5x6-
Chlor-Trimeton	T45.0x1-	T45.0x2-	T45.0x3-	T45.0x4-	T45.0x5-	T45.0x6-
Chlorzoxazone	T42.8x1-	T42.8x2-	T42.8x3-	T42.8x4-	T42.8x5-	T42.8x6-
Choke damp	T59.7x1-	T59.7x2-	T59.7x3-	T59.7x4-	—	—
Cholagogues	T47.5x1-	T47.5x2-	T47.5x3-	T47.5x4-	T47.5x5-	T47.5x6-
Cholebrine	T50.8x1-	T50.8x2-	T50.8x3-	T50.8x4-	T50.8x5-	T50.8x6-
Cholecalciferol	T45.2x1-	T45.2x2-	T45.2x3-	T45.2x4-	T45.2x5-	T45.2x6-
Cholecystokinin	T50.8x1-	T50.8x2-	T50.8x3-	T50.8x4-	T50.8x5-	T50.8x6-
Cholera vaccine	T50.A91-	T50.A92-	T50.A93-	T50.A94-	T50.A95-	T50.A96-
Choleretic	T47.5x1-	T47.5x2-	T47.5x3-	T47.5x4-	T47.5x5-	T47.5x6-
Cholesterol-lowering agents	T46.6x1-	T46.6x2-	T46.6x3-	T46.6x4-	T46.6x5-	T46.6x6-
Cholestyramine (resin)	T46.6x1-	T46.6x2-	T46.6x3-	T46.6x4-	T46.6x5-	T46.6x6-

DRUGS & CHEMICALS

6

DRUGS & CHEMICALS

Table of Drugs & Chemicals	POISONING				Adverse Effect	Underdosing
	Accidental (Unintentional)	Self-Harm (Intentional)	Assault	Undetermined		
Cholic acid	T47.5x1-	T47.5x2-	T47.5x3-	T47.5x4-	T47.5x5-	T47.5x6-
Choline	T48.6x1-	T48.6x2-	T48.6x3-	T48.6x4-	T48.6x5-	T48.6x6-
chloride	T50.991-	T50.992-	T50.993-	T50.994-	T50.995-	T50.996-
dihydrogen citrate	T50.991-	T50.992-	T50.993-	T50.994-	T50.995-	T50.996-
salicylate	T39.091-	T39.092-	T39.093-	T39.094-	T39.095-	T39.096-
theophyllinate	T48.6x1-	T48.6x2-	T48.6x3-	T48.6x4-	T48.6x5-	T48.6x6-
Cholinergic (drug) NEC	T44.1x1-	T44.1x2-	T44.1x3-	T44.1x4-	T44.1x5-	T44.1x6-
muscle tone enhancer	T44.1x1-	T44.1x2-	T44.1x3-	T44.1x4-	T44.1x5-	T44.1x6-
organophosphorus	T44.0x1-	T44.0x2-	T44.0x3-	T44.0x4-	T44.0x5-	T44.0x6-
insecticide	T60.0x1-	T60.0x2-	T60.0x3-	T60.0x4-	—	—
nerve gas	T59.891-	T59.892-	T59.893-	T59.894-	—	—
trimethyl ammonium propanediol	T44.1x1-	T44.1x2-	T44.1x3-	T44.1x4-	T44.1x5-	T44.1x6-
Cholinesterase reactivator	T50.6x1-	T50.6x2-	T50.6x3-	T50.6x4-	T50.6x5-	T50.6x6-
Cholografin	T50.8x1-	T50.8x2-	T50.8x3-	T50.8x4-	T50.8x5-	T50.8x6-
Chorionic gonadotropin	T38.891-	T38.892-	T38.893-	T38.894-	T38.895-	T38.896-
Chromate	T56.2x1-	T56.2x2-	T56.2x3-	T56.2x4-		
dust or mist	T56.2x1-	T56.2x2-	T56.2x3-	T56.2x4-		
lead — see also Lead	T56.0x1-	T56.0x2-	T56.0x3-	T56.0x4-		
paint	T56.0x1-	T56.0x2-	T56.0x3-	T56.0x4-		
Chromic						
acid	T56.2x1-	T56.2x2-	T56.2x3-	T56.2x4-		
dust or mist	T56.2x1-	T56.2x2-	T56.2x3-	T56.2x4-		
phosphate 32P	T45.1x1-	T45.1x2-	T45.1x3-	T45.1x4-	T45.1x5-	T45.1x6-
Chromium	T56.2x1-	T56.2x2-	T56.2x3-	T56.2x4-		
compounds — see Chromate						
sesquioxide	T50.8x1-	T50.8x2-	T50.8x3-	T50.8x4-	T50.8x5-	T50.8x6-
Chromomycin A3	T45.1x1-	T45.1x2-	T45.1x3-	T45.1x4-	T45.1x5-	T45.1x6-
Chromonar	T46.3x1-	T46.3x2-	T46.3x3-	T46.3x4-	T46.3x5-	T46.3x6-
Chromyl chloride	T56.2x1-	T56.2x2-	T56.2x3-	T56.2x4-	—	—
Chrysarobin	T49.4x1-	T49.4x2-	T49.4x3-	T49.4x4-	T49.4x5-	T49.4x6-
Chrysazin	T47.2x1-	T47.2x2-	T47.2x3-	T47.2x4-	T47.2x5-	T47.2x6-
Chymar	T45.3x1-	T45.3x2-	T45.3x3-	T45.3x4-	T45.3x5-	T45.3x6-
ophthalmic preparation	T49.5x1-	T49.5x2-	T49.5x3-	T49.5x4-	T49.5x5-	T49.5x6-
Chymopapain	T45.3x1-	T45.3x2-	T45.3x3-	T45.3x4-	T45.3x5-	T45.3x6-
Chymotrypsin	T45.3x1-	T45.3x2-	T45.3x3-	T45.3x4-	T45.3x5-	T45.3x6-
ophthalmic preparation	T49.5x1-	T49.5x2-	T49.5x3-	T49.5x4-	T49.5x5-	T49.5x6-
Cianidanol	T50.991-	T50.992-	T50.993-	T50.994-	T50.995-	T50.996-
Cianopramine	T43.011-	T43.012-	T43.013-	T43.014-	T43.015-	T43.016-
Cibenzoline	T46.2x1-	T46.2x2-	T46.2x3-	T46.2x4-	T46.2x5-	T46.2x6-
Ciclacillin	T36.0x1-	T36.0x2-	T36.0x3-	T36.0x4-	T36.0x5-	T36.0x6-
Ciclobarbital — see Hexobarbital						
Ciclonicate	T46.7x1-	T46.7x2-	T46.7x3-	T46.7x4-	T46.7x5-	T46.7x6-
Ciclopirox (olamine)	T49.0x1-	T49.0x2-	T49.0x3-	T49.0x4-	T49.0x5-	T49.0x6-
Ciclosporin	T45.1x1-	T45.1x2-	T45.1x3-	T45.1x4-	T45.1x5-	T45.1x6-
Cicuta maculata or virosa	T62.2x1-	T62.2x2-	T62.2x3-	T62.2x4-	—	—
Cicutoxin	T62.2x1-	T62.2x2-	T62.2x3-	T62.2x4-	—	—
Cigarette lighter fluid	T52.0x1-	T52.0x2-	T52.0x3-	T52.0x4-	—	—
Cigarettes (tobacco)	T65.221-	T65.222-	T65.223-	T65.224-	—	—
Ciguatoxin	T61.01x-	T61.02x-	T61.03x-	T61.04x-	—	—
Cilazapril	T46.4x1-	T46.4x2-	T46.4x3-	T46.4x4-	T46.4x5-	T46.4x6-
Cimetidine	T47.0x1-	T47.0x2-	T47.0x3-	T47.0x4-	T47.0x5-	T47.0x6-
Cimetropium bromide	T44.3x1-	T44.3x2-	T44.3x3-	T44.3x4-	T44.3x5-	T44.3x6-
Cinchocaine	T41.3x1-	T41.3x2-	T41.3x3-	T41.3x4-	T41.3x5-	T41.3x6-
topical (surface)	T41.3x1-	T41.3x2-	T41.3x3-	T41.3x4-	T41.3x5-	T41.3x6-
Cinchona	T37.2x1-	T37.2x2-	T37.2x3-	T37.2x4-	T37.2x5-	T37.2x6-
Cinchonine alkaloids	T37.2x1-	T37.2x2-	T37.2x3-	T37.2x4-	T37.2x5-	T37.2x6-
Cinchophen	T50.4x1-	T50.4x2-	T50.4x3-	T50.4x4-	T50.4x5-	T50.4x6-
Cinepazide	T46.7x1-	T46.7x2-	T46.7x3-	T46.7x4-	T46.7x5-	T46.7x6-
Cinnamedrine	T48.5x1-	T48.5x2-	T48.5x3-	T48.5x4-	T48.5x5-	T48.5x6-
Cinnarizine	T45.0x1-	T45.0x2-	T45.0x3-	T45.0x4-	T45.0x5-	T45.0x6-

Table of Drugs & Chemicals	POISONING				Adverse Effect	Underdosing
	Accidental (Unintentional)	Self-Harm (Intentional)	Assault	Undetermined		
Cinoxacin	T37.8x1-	T37.8x2-	T37.8x3-	T37.8x4-	T37.8x5-	T37.8x6-
Ciprofibrate	T46.6x1-	T46.6x2-	T46.6x3-	T46.6x4-	T46.6x5-	T46.6x6-
Ciprofloxacin	T36.8x1-	T36.8x2-	T36.8x3-	T36.8x4-	T36.8x5-	T36.8x6-
Cisapride	T47.8x1-	T47.8x2-	T47.8x3-	T47.8x4-	T47.8x5-	T47.8x6-
Cisplatin	T45.1x1-	T45.1x2-	T45.1x3-	T45.1x4-	T45.1x5-	T45.1x6-
Citalopram	T43.221-	T43.222-	T43.223-	T43.224-	T43.225-	T43.226-
Citanest	T41.3x1-	T41.3x2-	T41.3x3-	T41.3x4-	T41.3x5-	T41.3x6-
infiltration (subcutaneous)	T41.3x1-	T41.3x2-	T41.3x3-	T41.3x4-	T41.3x5-	T41.3x6-
nerve block (peripheral) (plexus)	T41.3x1-	T41.3x2-	T41.3x3-	T41.3x4-	T41.3x5-	T41.3x6-
Citric acid	T47.5x1-	T47.5x2-	T47.5x3-	T47.5x4-	T47.5x5-	T47.5x6-
Citrovorum (factor)	T45.8x1-	T45.8x2-	T45.8x3-	T45.8x4-	T45.8x5-	T45.8x6-
Claviceps purpurea	T62.2x1-	T62.2x2-	T62.2x3-	T62.2x4-	—	—
Clavulanic acid	T36.1x1-	T36.1x2-	T36.1x3-	T36.1x4-	T36.1x5-	T36.1x6-
Cleaner, cleansing agent, type not specified	T65.891-	T65.892-	T65.893-	T65.894-	—	—
of paint or varnish	T52.91x-	T52.92x-	T52.93x-	T52.94x-	—	—
specified type NEC	T65.891-	T65.892-	T65.893-	T65.894-	—	—
Clebopride	T47.8x1-	T47.8x2-	T47.8x3-	T47.8x4-	T47.8x5-	T47.8x6-
Clefamide	T37.3x1-	T37.3x2-	T37.3x3-	T37.3x4-	T37.3x5-	T37.3x6-
Clemastine	T45.0x1-	T45.0x2-	T45.0x3-	T45.0x4-	T45.0x5-	T45.0x6-
Clematis vitalba	T62.2x1-	T62.2x2-	T62.2x3-	T62.2x4-		
Clemizole	T45.0x1-	T45.0x2-	T45.0x3-	T45.0x4-	T45.0x5-	T45.0x6-
penicillin	T36.0x1-	T36.0x2-	T36.0x3-	T36.0x4-	T36.0x5-	T36.0x6-
Clenbuterol	T48.6x1-	T48.6x2-	T48.6x3-	T48.6x4-	T48.6x5-	T48.6x6-
Clidinium bromide	T44.3x1-	T44.3x2-	T44.3x3-	T44.3x4-	T44.3x5-	T44.3x6-
Clindamycin	T36.8x1-	T36.8x2-	T36.8x3-	T36.8x4-	T36.8x5-	T36.8x6-
Clinofibrate	T46.6x1-	T46.6x2-	T46.6x3-	T46.6x4-	T46.6x5-	T46.6x6-
Clioquinol	T37.8x1-	T37.8x2-	T37.8x3-	T37.8x4-	T37.8x5-	T37.8x6-
Cliradon	T40.2x1-	T40.2x2-	T40.2x3-	T40.2x4-	—	—
Clobazam	T42.4x1-	T42.4x2-	T42.4x3-	T42.4x4-	T42.4x5-	T42.4x6-
Clobenzorex	T50.5x1-	T50.5x2-	T50.5x3-	T50.5x4-	T50.5x5-	T50.5x6-
Clobetasol	T49.0x1-	T49.0x2-	T49.0x3-	T49.0x4-	T49.0x5-	T49.0x6-
Clobetasone	T49.0x1-	T49.0x2-	T49.0x3-	T49.0x4-	T49.0x5-	T49.0x6-
Clobutinol	T48.3x1-	T48.3x2-	T48.3x3-	T48.3x4-	T48.3x5-	T48.3x6-
Clocortolone	T38.0x1-	T38.0x2-	T38.0x3-	T38.0x4-	T38.0x5-	T38.0x6-
Clodantoin	T49.0x1-	T49.0x2-	T49.0x3-	T49.0x4-	T49.0x5-	T49.0x6-
Clodronic acid	T50.991-	T50.992-	T50.993-	T50.994-	T50.995-	T50.996-
Clofazimine	T37.1x1-	T37.1x2-	T37.1x3-	T37.1x4-	T37.1x5-	T37.1x6-
Clofedanol	T48.3x1-	T48.3x2-	T48.3x3-	T48.3x4-	T48.3x5-	T48.3x6-
Clofenamide	T50.2x1-	T50.2x2-	T50.2x3-	T50.2x4-	T50.2x5-	T50.2x6-
Clofenotane	T49.0x1-	T49.0x2-	T49.0x3-	T49.0x4-	T49.0x5-	T49.0x6-
Clofezone	T39.2x1-	T39.2x2-	T39.2x3-	T39.2x4-	T39.2x5-	T39.2x6-
Clofibrate	T46.6x1-	T46.6x2-	T46.6x3-	T46.6x4-	T46.6x5-	T46.6x6-
Clofibride	T46.6x1-	T46.6x2-	T46.6x3-	T46.6x4-	T46.6x5-	T46.6x6-
Cloforex	T50.5x1-	T50.5x2-	T50.5x3-	T50.5x4-	T50.5x5-	T50.5x6-
Clomethiazole	T42.6x1-	T42.6x2-	T42.6x3-	T42.6x4-	T42.6x5-	T42.6x6-
Clometocillin	T36.0x1-	T36.0x2-	T36.0x3-	T36.0x4-	T36.0x5-	T36.0x6-
Clomifene	T38.5x1-	T38.5x2-	T38.5x3-	T38.5x4-	T38.5x5-	T38.5x6-
Clomiphene	T38.5x1-	T38.5x2-	T38.5x3-	T38.5x4-	T38.5x5-	T38.5x6-
Clomipramine	T43.011-	T43.012-	T43.013-	T43.014-	T43.015-	T43.016-
Clomocycline	T36.4x1-	T36.4x2-	T36.4x3-	T36.4x4-	T36.4x5-	T36.4x6-
Clonazepam	T42.4x1-	T42.4x2-	T42.4x3-	T42.4x4-	T42.4x5-	T42.4x6-
Clonidine	T46.5x1-	T46.5x2-	T46.5x3-	T46.5x4-	T46.5x5-	T46.5x6-
Clonixin	T39.8x1-	T39.8x2-	T39.8x3-	T39.8x4-	T39.8x5-	T39.8x6-
Clopamide	T50.2x1-	T50.2x2-	T50.2x3-	T50.2x4-	T50.2x5-	T50.2x6-
Clopenthixol	T43.4x1-	T43.4x2-	T43.4x3-	T43.4x4-	T43.4x5-	T43.4x6-
Cloperastine	T48.3x1-	T48.3x2-	T48.3x3-	T48.3x4-	T48.3x5-	T48.3x6-
Clophedianol	T48.3x1-	T48.3x2-	T48.3x3-	T48.3x4-	T48.3x5-	T48.3x6-
Cloponone	T36.2x1-	T36.2x2-	T36.2x3-	T36.2x4-	T36.2x5-	T36.2x6-
Cloprednol	T38.0x1-	T38.0x2-	T38.0x3-	T38.0x4-	T38.0x5-	T38.0x6-
Cloral betaine	T42.6x1-	T42.6x2-	T42.6x3-	T42.6x4-	T42.6x5-	T42.6x6-

Table of Drugs & Chemicals	POISONING Accidental (Unintentional)	Self-Harm (Intentional)	Assault	Undetermined	Adverse Effect	Underdosing
Cloramfenicol	T36.2x1-	T36.2x2-	T36.2x3-	T36.2x4-	T36.2x5-	T36.2x6-
Clorazepate (dipotassium)	T42.4x1-	T42.4x2-	T42.4x3-	T42.4x4-	T42.4x5-	T42.4x6-
Clorexolone	T50.2x1-	T50.2x2-	T50.2x3-	T50.2x4-	T50.2x5-	T50.2x6-
Clorfenamine	T45.0x1-	T45.0x2-	T45.0x3-	T45.0x4-	T45.0x5-	T45.0x6-
Clorgiline	T43.1x1-	T43.1x2-	T43.1x3-	T43.1x4-	T43.1x5-	T43.1x6-
Clorotepine	T44.3x1-	T44.3x2-	T44.3x3-	T44.3x4-	T44.3x5-	T44.3x6-
Clorox (bleach)	T54.91x-	T54.92x-	T54.93x-	T54.94x-	—	—
Clorprenaline	T48.6x1-	T48.6x2-	T48.6x3-	T48.6x4-	T48.6x5-	T48.6x6-
Clortermine	T50.5x1-	T50.5x2-	T50.5x3-	T50.5x4-	T50.5x5-	T50.5x6-
Clotiapine	T43.591-	T43.592-	T43.593-	T43.594-	T43.595-	T43.596-
Clotiazepam	T42.4x1-	T42.4x2-	T42.4x3-	T42.4x4-	T42.4x5-	T42.4x6-
Clotibric acid	T46.6x1-	T46.6x2-	T46.6x3-	T46.6x4-	T46.6x5-	T46.6x6-
Clotrimazole	T49.0x1-	T49.0x2-	T49.0x3-	T49.0x4-	T49.0x5-	T49.0x6-
Cloxacillin	T36.0x1-	T36.0x2-	T36.0x3-	T36.0x4-	T36.0x5-	T36.0x6-
Cloxazolam	T42.4x1-	T42.4x2-	T42.4x3-	T42.4x4-	T42.4x5-	T42.4x6-
Cloxiquine	T49.0x1-	T49.0x2-	T49.0x3-	T49.0x4-	T49.0x5-	T49.0x6-
Clozapine	T42.4x1-	T42.4x2-	T42.4x3-	T42.4x4-	T42.4x5-	T42.4x6-
Coagulant NEC	T45.7x1-	T45.7x2-	T45.7x3-	T45.7x4-	T45.7x5-	T45.7x6-
Coal (carbon monoxide from) — see also Carbon, monoxide, coal	T58.2x1-	T58.2x2-	T58.2x3-	T58.2x4-	—	—
oil — see Kerosene						
tar	T49.1x1-	T49.1x2-	T49.1x3-	T49.1x4-	T49.1x5-	T49.1x6-
fumes	T59.891-	T59.892-	T59.893-	T59.894-	—	—
medicinal (ointment)	T49.4x1-	T49.4x2-	T49.4x3-	T49.4x4-	T49.4x5-	T49.4x6-
analgesics NEC	T39.2x1-	T39.2x2-	T39.2x3-	T39.2x4-	T39.2x5-	T39.2x6-
naphtha (solvent)	T52.0x1-	T52.0x2-	T52.0x3-	T52.0x4-	—	—
Cobalamine	T45.2x1-	T45.2x2-	T45.2x3-	T45.2x4-	T45.2x5-	T45.2x6-
Cobalt (nonmedicinal) (fumes) (industrial)	T56.891-	T56.892-	T56.893-	T56.894-	—	—
medicinal (trace) (chloride)	T45.8x1-	T45.8x2-	T45.8x3-	T45.8x4-	T45.8x5-	T45.8x6-
Cobra (venom)	T63.041-	T63.042-	T63.043-	T63.044-	—	—
Coca (leaf)	T40.5x1-	T40.5x2-	T40.5x3-	T40.5x4-	T40.5x5-	T40.5x6-
Cocaine	T40.5x1-	T40.5x2-	T40.5x3-	T40.5x4-	T40.5x5-	T40.5x6-
topical anesthetic	T41.3x1-	T41.3x2-	T41.3x3-	T41.3x4-	T41.3x5-	T41.3x6-
Cocarboxylase	T45.3x1-	T45.3x2-	T45.3x3-	T45.3x4-	T45.3x5-	T45.3x6-
Coccidioidin	T50.8x1-	T50.8x2-	T50.8x3-	T50.8x4-	T50.8x5-	T50.8x6-
Cocculus indicus	T62.1x1-	T62.1x2-	T62.1x3-	T62.1x4-	—	—
Cochineal	T65.6x1-	T65.6x2-	T65.6x3-	T65.6x4-	—	—
medicinal products	T50.991-	T50.992-	T50.993-	T50.994-	T50.995-	T50.996-
Codeine	T40.2x1-	T40.2x2-	T40.2x3-	T40.2x4-	T40.2x5-	T40.2x6-
Cod-liver oil	T45.2x1-	T45.2x2-	T45.2x3-	T45.2x4-	T45.2x5-	T45.2x6-
Coenzyme A	T50.991-	T50.992-	T50.993-	T50.994-	T50.995-	T50.996-
Coffee	T62.8x1-	T62.8x2-	T62.8x3-	T62.8x4-	—	—
Cogalactoiso-merase	T50.991-	T50.992-	T50.993-	T50.994-	T50.995-	T50.996-
Cogentin	T44.3x1-	T44.3x2-	T44.3x3-	T44.3x4-	T44.3x5-	T44.3x6-
Coke fumes or gas (carbon monoxide)	T58.2x1-	T58.2x2-	T58.2x3-	T58.2x4-	—	—
industrial use	T58.8x1-	T58.8x2-	T58.8x3-	T58.8x4-	—	—
Colace	T47.4x1-	T47.4x2-	T47.4x3-	T47.4x4-	T47.4x5-	T47.4x6-
Colaspase	T45.1x1-	T45.1x2-	T45.1x3-	T45.1x4-	T45.1x5-	T45.1x6-
Colchicine	T50.4x1-	T50.4x2-	T50.4x3-	T50.4x4-	T50.4x5-	T50.4x6-
Colchicum	T62.2x1-	T62.2x2-	T62.2x3-	T62.2x4-	—	—
Cold cream	T49.3x1-	T49.3x2-	T49.3x3-	T49.3x4-	T49.3x5-	T49.3x6-
Colecalciferol	T45.2x1-	T45.2x2-	T45.2x3-	T45.2x4-	T45.2x5-	T45.2x6-
Colestipol	T46.6x1-	T46.6x2-	T46.6x3-	T46.6x4-	T46.6x5-	T46.6x6-
Colestyramine	T46.6x1-	T46.6x2-	T46.6x3-	T46.6x4-	T46.6x5-	T46.6x6-
Colimycin	T36.8x1-	T36.8x2-	T36.8x3-	T36.8x4-	T36.8x5-	T36.8x6-
Colistimethate	T36.8x1-	T36.8x2-	T36.8x3-	T36.8x4-	T36.8x5-	T36.8x6-
Colistin	T36.8x1-	T36.8x2-	T36.8x3-	T36.8x4-	T36.8x5-	T36.8x6-
sulfate (eye preparation)	T49.5x1-	T49.5x2-	T49.5x3-	T49.5x4-	T49.5x5-	T49.5x6-

Table of Drugs & Chemicals	POISONING Accidental (Unintentional)	Self-Harm (Intentional)	Assault	Undetermined	Adverse Effect	Underdosing
Collagen	T50.991-	T50.992-	T50.993-	T50.994-	T50.995-	T50.996-
Collagenase	T49.4x1-	T49.4x2-	T49.4x3-	T49.4x4-	T49.4x5-	T49.4x6-
Collodion	T49.3x1-	T49.3x2-	T49.3x3-	T49.3x4-	T49.3x5-	T49.3x6-
Colocynth	T47.2x1-	T47.2x2-	T47.2x3-	T47.2x4-	T47.2x5-	T47.2x6-
Colophony adhesive	T49.3x1-	T49.3x2-	T49.3x3-	T49.3x4-	T49.3x5-	T49.3x6-
Colorant — see also Dye	T50.991-	T50.992-	T50.993-	T50.994-	T50.995-	T50.996-
Coloring matter — see Dye(s)						
Combustion gas (after combustion) — see Carbon, monoxide						
prior to combustion	T59.891-	T59.892-	T59.893-	T59.894-	—	—
Compazine	T43.3x1-	T43.3x2-	T43.3x3-	T43.3x4-	T43.3x5-	T43.3x6-
Compound						
1080 (sodium fluoroacetate)	T60.4x1-	T60.4x2-	T60.4x3-	T60.4x4-	—	—
269 (endrin)	T60.1x1-	T60.1x2-	T60.1x3-	T60.1x4-	—	—
497 (dieldrin)	T60.1x1-	T60.1x2-	T60.1x3-	T60.1x4-	—	—
3422 (parathion)	T60.0x1-	T60.0x2-	T60.0x3-	T60.0x4-	—	—
3911 (phorate)	T60.0x1-	T60.0x2-	T60.0x3-	T60.0x4-	—	—
3956 (toxaphene)	T60.1x1-	T60.1x2-	T60.1x3-	T60.1x4-	—	—
4049 (malathion)	T60.0x1-	T60.0x2-	T60.0x3-	T60.0x4-	—	—
4069 (malathion)	T60.0x1-	T60.0x2-	T60.0x3-	T60.0x4-	—	—
4124 (dicapthon)	T60.0x1-	T60.0x2-	T60.0x3-	T60.0x4-	—	—
E (cortisone)	T38.0x1-	T38.0x2-	T38.0x3-	T38.0x4-	T38.0x5-	T38.0x6-
F (hydrocortisone)	T38.0x1-	T38.0x2-	T38.0x3-	T38.0x4-	T38.0x5-	T38.0x6-
Congener, anabolic	T38.7x1-	T38.7x2-	T38.7x3-	T38.7x4-	T38.7x5-	T38.7x6-
Congo red	T50.8x1-	T50.8x2-	T50.8x3-	T50.8x4-	T50.8x5-	T50.8x6-
Coniine, conine	T62.2x1-	T62.2x2-	T62.2x3-	T62.2x4-	—	—
Conium (maculatum)	T62.2x1-	T62.2x2-	T62.2x3-	T62.2x4-	—	—
Conjugated estrogenic substances	T38.5x1-	T38.5x2-	T38.5x3-	T38.5x4-	T38.5x5-	T38.5x6-
Contac	T48.5x1-	T48.5x2-	T48.5x3-	T48.5x4-	T48.5x5-	T48.5x6-
Contact lens solution	T49.5x1-	T49.5x2-	T49.5x3-	T49.5x4-	T49.5x5-	T49.5x6-
Contraceptive (oral)	T38.4x1-	T38.4x2-	T38.4x3-	T38.4x4-	T38.4x5-	T38.4x6-
vaginal	T49.8x1-	T49.8x2-	T49.8x3-	T49.8x4-	T49.8x5-	T49.8x6-
Contrast medium, radiography	T50.8x1-	T50.8x2-	T50.8x3-	T50.8x4-	T50.8x5-	T50.8x6-
Convallaria glycosides	T46.0x1-	T46.0x2-	T46.0x3-	T46.0x4-	T46.0x5-	T46.0x6-
Convallaria majalis	T62.2x1-	T62.2x2-	T62.2x3-	T62.2x4-	—	—
berry	T62.1x1-	T62.1x2-	T62.1x3-	T62.1x4-	—	—
Copper (dust) (fumes) (nonmedicinal) NEC	T56.4x1-	T56.4x2-	T56.4x3-	T56.4x4-	—	—
arsenate, arsenite	T57.0x1-	T57.0x2-	T57.0x3-	T57.0x4-	—	—
insecticide	T60.2x1-	T60.2x2-	T60.2x3-	T60.2x4-	—	—
emetic	T47.7x1-	T47.7x2-	T47.7x3-	T47.7x4-	T47.7x5-	T47.7x6-
fungicide	T60.3x1-	T60.3x2-	T60.3x3-	T60.3x4-	—	—
gluconate	T49.0x1-	T49.0x2-	T49.0x3-	T49.0x4-	T49.0x5-	T49.0x6-
insecticide	T60.2x1-	T60.2x2-	T60.2x3-	T60.2x4-	—	—
medicinal (trace)	T45.8x1-	T45.8x2-	T45.8x3-	T45.8x4-	T45.8x5-	T45.8x6-
oleate	T49.0x1-	T49.0x2-	T49.0x3-	T49.0x4-	T49.0x5-	T49.0x6-
sulfate	T56.4x1-	T56.4x2-	T56.4x3-	T56.4x4-	—	—
cupric	T56.4x1-	T56.4x2-	T56.4x3-	T56.4x4-	—	—
fungicide	T60.3x1-	T60.3x2-	T60.3x3-	T60.3x4-	—	—
medicinal						
ear	T49.6x1-	T49.6x2-	T49.6x3-	T49.6x4-	T49.6x5-	T49.6x6-
emetic	T47.7x1-	T47.7x2-	T47.7x3-	T47.7x4-	T47.7x5-	T47.7x6-
eye	T49.5x1-	T49.5x2-	T49.5x3-	T49.5x4-	T49.5x5-	T49.5x6-
cuprous	T56.4x1-	T56.4x2-	T56.4x3-	T56.4x4-	—	—
fungicide	T60.3x1-	T60.3x2-	T60.3x3-	T60.3x4-	—	—
medicinal						
ear	T49.6x1-	T49.6x2-	T49.6x3-	T49.6x4-	T49.6x5-	T49.6x6-
emetic	T47.7x1-	T47.7x2-	T47.7x3-	T47.7x4-	T47.7x5-	T47.7x6-
eye	T49.5x1-	T49.5x2-	T49.5x3-	T49.5x4-	T49.5x5-	T49.5x6-

DRUGS & CHEMICALS

Table of Drugs & Chemicals	POISONING Accidental (Unintentional)	POISONING Self-Harm (Intentional)	POISONING Assault	POISONING Undetermined	Adverse Effect	Underdosing
Copperhead snake (bite) (venom)	T63.061-	T63.062-	T63.063-	T63.064-	—	—
Coral (sting)	T63.691-	T63.692-	T63.693-	T63.694-	—	—
snake (bite) (venom)	T63.021-	T63.022-	T63.023-	T63.024-	—	—
Corbadrine	T49.6x1-	T49.6x2-	T49.6x3-	T49.6x4-	T49.6x5-	T49.6x6-
Cordite	T65.891-	T65.892-	T65.893-	T65.894-	—	—
vapor	T59.891-	T59.892-	T59.893-	T59.894-	—	—
Cordran	T49.0x1-	T49.0x2-	T49.0x3-	T49.0x4-	T49.0x5-	T49.0x6-
Corn cures	T49.4x1-	T49.4x2-	T49.4x3-	T49.4x4-	T49.4x5-	T49.4x6-
Corn starch	T49.3x1-	T49.3x2-	T49.3x3-	T49.3x4-	T49.3x5-	T49.3x6-
Cornhusker's lotion	T49.3x1-	T49.3x2-	T49.3x3-	T49.3x4-	T49.3x5-	T49.3x6-
Coronary vasodilator NEC	T46.3x1-	T46.3x2-	T46.3x3-	T46.3x4-	T46.3x5-	T46.3x6-
Corrosive NEC	T54.91x-	T54.92x-	T54.93x-	T54.94x-	—	—
acid NEC	T54.2x1-	T54.2x2-	T54.2x3-	T54.2x4-	—	—
aromatics	T54.1x1-	T54.1x2-	T54.1x3-	T54.1x4-	—	—
disinfectant	T54.1x1-	T54.1x2-	T54.1x3-	T54.1x4-	—	—
fumes NEC	T54.91x-	T54.92x-	T54.93x-	T54.94x-	·	—
specified NEC	T54.91x-	T54.92x-	T54.93x-	T54.94x-	—	—
sublimate	T56.1x1-	T56.1x2-	T56.1x3-	T56.1x4-	—	—
Cortate	T38.0x1-	T38.0x2-	T38.0x3-	T38.0x4-	T38.0x5-	T38.0x6-
Cort-Dome	T38.0x1-	T38.0x2-	T38.0x3-	T38.0x4-	T38.0x5-	T38.0x6-
ENT agent	T49.6x1-	T49.6x2-	T49.6x3-	T49.6x4-	T49.6x5-	T49.6x6-
ophthalmic preparation	T49.5x1-	T49.5x2-	T49.5x3-	T49.5x4-	T49.5x5-	T49.5x6-
topical NEC	T49.0x1-	T49.0x2-	T49.0x3-	T49.0x4-	T49.0x5-	T49.0x6-
Cortef	T38.0x1-	T38.0x2-	T38.0x3-	T38.0x4-	T38.0x5-	T38.0x6-
ENT agent	T49.6x1-	T49.6x2-	T49.6x3-	T49.6x4-	T49.6x5-	T49.6x6-
ophthalmic preparation	T49.5x1-	T49.5x2-	T49.5x3-	T49.5x4-	T49.5x5-	T49.5x6-
topical NEC	T49.0x1-	T49.0x2-	T49.0x3-	T49.0x4-	T49.0x5-	T49.0x6-
Corticosteroid	T38.0x1-	T38.0x2-	T38.0x3-	T38.0x4-	T38.0x5-	T38.0x6-
ENT agent	T49.6x1-	T49.6x2-	T49.6x3-	T49.6x4-	T49.6x5-	T49.6x6-
mineral	T50.0x1-	T50.0x2-	T50.0x3-	T50.0x4-	T50.0x5-	T50.0x6-
ophthalmic	T49.5x1-	T49.5x2-	T49.5x3-	T49.5x4-	T49.5x5-	T49.5x6-
topical NEC	T49.0x1-	T49.0x2-	T49.0x3-	T49.0x4-	T49.0x5-	T49.0x6-
Corticotropin	T38.811-	T38.812-	T38.813-	T38.814-	T38.815-	T38.816-
Cortisol	T49.0x1-	T49.0x2-	T49.0x3-	T49.0x4-	T49.0x5-	T49.0x6-
ENT agent	T49.6x1-	T49.6x2-	T49.6x3-	T49.6x4-	T49.6x5-	T49.6x6-
ophthalmic preparation	T49.5x1-	T49.5x2-	T49.5x3-	T49.5x4-	T49.5x5-	T49.5x6-
topical NEC	T49.0x1-	T49.0x2-	T49.0x3-	T49.0x4-	T49.0x5-	T49.0x6-
Cortisone (acetate)	T38.0x1-	T38.0x2-	T38.0x3-	T38.0x4-	T38.0x5-	T38.0x6-
ENT agent	T49.6x1-	T49.6x2-	T49.6x3-	T49.6x4-	T49.6x5-	T49.6x6-
ophthalmic preparation	T49.5x1-	T49.5x2-	T49.5x3-	T49.5x4-	T49.5x5-	T49.5x6-
topical NEC	T49.0x1-	T49.0x2-	T49.0x3-	T49.0x4-	T49.0x5-	T49.0x6-
Cortivazol	T38.0x1-	T38.0x2-	T38.0x3-	T38.0x4-	T38.0x5-	T38.0x6-
Cortogen	T38.0x1-	T38.0x2-	T38.0x3-	T38.0x4-	T38.0x5-	T38.0x6-
ENT agent	T49.6x1-	T49.6x2-	T49.6x3-	T49.6x4-	T49.6x5-	T49.6x6-
ophthalmic preparation	T49.5x1-	T49.5x2-	T49.5x3-	T49.5x4-	T49.5x5-	T49.5x6-
Cortone	T38.0x1-	T38.0x2-	T38.0x3-	T38.0x4-	T38.0x5-	T38.0x6-
ENT agent	T49.6x1-	T49.6x2-	T49.6x3-	T49.6x4-	T49.6x5-	T49.6x6-
ophthalmic preparation	T49.5x1-	T49.5x2-	T49.5x3-	T49.5x4-	T49.5x5-	T49.5x6-
Cortril	T38.0x1-	T38.0x2-	T38.0x3-	T38.0x4-	T38.0x5-	T38.0x6-
ENT agent	T49.6x1-	T49.6x2-	T49.6x3-	T49.6x4-	T49.6x5-	T49.6x6-
ophthalmic preparation	T49.5x1-	T49.5x2-	T49.5x3-	T49.5x4-	T49.5x5-	T49.5x6-
topical NEC	T49.0x1-	T49.0x2-	T49.0x3-	T49.0x4-	T49.0x5-	T49.0x6-
Corynebacterium parvum	T45.1x1-	T45.1x2-	T45.1x3-	T45.1x4-	T45.1x5-	T45.1x6-
Cosmetic preparation	T49.8x1-	T49.8x2-	T49.8x3-	T49.8x4-	T49.8x5-	T49.8x6-
Cosmetics	T49.8x1-	T49.8x2-	T49.8x3-	T49.8x4-	T49.8x5-	T49.8x6-
Cosyntropin	T38.811-	T38.812-	T38.813-	T38.814-	T38.815-	T38.816-
Cotarnine	T45.7x1-	T45.7x2-	T45.7x3-	T45.7x4-	T45.7x5-	T45.7x6-
Co-trimoxazole	T36.8x1-	T36.8x2-	T36.8x3-	T36.8x4-	T36.8x5-	T36.8x6-
Cottonseed oil	T49.3x1-	T49.3x2-	T49.3x3-	T49.3x4-	T49.3x5-	T49.3x6-
Cough mixture (syrup)	T48.4x1-	T48.4x2-	T48.4x3-	T48.4x4-	T48.4x5-	T48.4x6-
containing opiates	T40.2x1-	T40.2x2-	T40.2x3-	T40.2x4-	T40.2x5-	T40.2x6-
expectorants	T48.4x1-	T48.4x2-	T48.4x3-	T48.4x4-	T48.4x5-	T48.4x6-
Coumadin	T45.511-	T45.512-	T45.513-	T45.514-	T45.515-	T45.516-
rodenticide	T60.4x1-	T60.4x2-	T60.4x3-	T60.4x4-	—	—
Coumaphos	T60.0x1-	T60.0x2-	T60.0x3-	T60.0x4-	—	—
Coumarin	T45.511-	T45.512-	T45.513-	T45.514-	T45.515-	T45.516-
Coumetarol	T45.511-	T45.512-	T45.513-	T45.514-	T45.515-	T45.516-
Cowbane	T62.2x1-	T62.2x2-	T62.2x3-	T62.2x4-	—	—
Cozyme	T45.2x1-	T45.2x2-	T45.2x3-	T45.2x4-	T45.2x5-	T45.2x6-
Crack	T40.5x1-	T40.5x2-	T40.5x3-	T40.5x4-	—	—
Crataegus extract	T46.0x1-	T46.0x2-	T46.0x3-	T46.0x4-	T46.0x5-	T46.0x6-
Creolin	T54.1x1-	T54.1x2-	T54.1x3-	T54.1x4-	—	—
disinfectant	T54.1x1-	T54.1x2-	T54.1x3-	T54.1x4-	—	—
Creosol (compound)	T49.0x1-	T49.0x2-	T49.0x3-	T49.0x4-	T49.0x5-	T49.0x6-
Creosote (coal tar) (beechwood)	T49.0x1-	T49.0x2-	T49.0x3-	T49.0x4-	T49.0x5-	T49.0x6-
medicinal (expectorant)	T48.4x1-	T48.4x2-	T48.4x3-	T48.4x4-	T48.4x5-	T48.4x6-
syrup	T48.4x1-	T48.4x2-	T48.4x3-	T48.4x4-	T48.4x5-	T48.4x6-
Cresol(s)	T49.0x1-	T49.0x2-	T49.0x3-	T49.0x4-	T49.0x5-	T49.0x6-
and soap solution	T49.0x1-	T49.0x2-	T49.0x3-	T49.0x4-	T49.0x5-	T49.0x6-
Cresyl acetate	T49.0x1-	T49.0x2-	T49.0x3-	T49.0x4-	T49.0x5-	T49.0x6-
Cresylic acid	T49.0x1-	T49.0x2-	T49.0x3-	T49.0x4-	T49.0x5-	T49.0x6-
Crimidine	T60.4x1-	T60.4x2-	T60.4x3-	T60.4x4-	—	—
Croconazole	T37.8x1-	T37.8x2-	T37.8x3-	T37.8x4-	T37.8x5-	T37.8x6-
Cromoglicic acid	T48.6x1-	T48.6x2-	T48.6x3-	T48.6x4-	T48.6x5-	T48.6x6-
Cromolyn	T48.6x1-	T48.6x2-	T48.6x3-	T48.6x4-	T48.6x5-	T48.6x6-
Cromonar	T46.3x1-	T46.3x2-	T46.3x3-	T46.3x4-	T46.3x5-	T46.3x6-
Cropropamide	T39.8x1-	T39.8x2-	T39.8x3-	T39.8x4-	T39.8x5-	T39.8x6-
with crotethamide	T50.7x1-	T50.7x2-	T50.7x3-	T50.7x4-	T50.7x5-	T50.7x6-
Crotamiton	T49.0x1-	T49.0x2-	T49.0x3-	T49.0x4-	T49.0x5-	T49.0x6-
Crotethamide	T39.8x1-	T39.8x2-	T39.8x3-	T39.8x4-	T39.8x5-	T39.8x6-
with cropropamide	T50.7x1-	T50.7x2-	T50.7x3-	T50.7x4-	T50.7x5-	T50.7x6-
Croton (oil)	T47.2x1-	T47.2x2-	T47.2x3-	T47.2x4-	T47.2x5-	T47.2x6-
chloral	T42.6x1-	T42.6x2-	T42.6x3-	T42.6x4-	T42.6x5-	T42.6x6-
Crude oil	T52.0x1-	T52.0x2-	T52.0x3-	T52.0x4-	—	—
Cryogenine	T39.8x1-	T39.8x2-	T39.8x3-	T39.8x4-	T39.8x5-	T39.8x6-
Cryolite (vapor)	T60.1x1-	T60.1x2-	T60.1x3-	T60.1x4-	—	—
insecticide	T60.1x1-	T60.1x2-	T60.1x3-	T60.1x4-	—	—
Cryptenamine (tannates)	T46.5x1-	T46.5x2-	T46.5x3-	T46.5x4-	T46.5x5-	T46.5x6-
Crystal violet	T49.0x1-	T49.0x2-	T49.0x3-	T49.0x4-	T49.0x5-	T49.0x6-
Cuckoopint	T62.2x1-	T62.2x2-	T62.2x3-	T62.2x4-	—	—
Cumetharol	T45.511-	T45.512-	T45.513-	T45.514-	T45.515-	T45.516-
Cupric						
acetate	T60.3x1-	T60.3x2-	T60.3x3-	T60.3x4-	—	—
acetoarsenite	T57.0x1-	T57.0x2-	T57.0x3-	T57.0x4-	—	—
arsenate	T57.0x1-	T57.0x2-	T57.0x3-	T57.0x4-	—	—
gluconate	T49.0x1-	T49.0x2-	T49.0x3-	T49.0x4-	T49.0x5-	T49.0x6-
oleate	T49.0x1-	T49.0x2-	T49.0x3-	T49.0x4-	T49.0x5-	T49.0x6-
sulfate	T56.4x1-	T56.4x2-	T56.4x3-	T56.4x4-	—	—
Cuprous sulfate — see also Copper sulfate	T56.4x1-	T56.4x2-	T56.4x3-	T56.4x4-	—	—
Curare, curarine	T48.1x1-	T48.1x2-	T48.1x3-	T48.1x4-	T48.1x5-	T48.1x6-
Cyamemazine	T43.3x1-	T43.3x2-	T43.3x3-	T43.3x4-	T43.3x5-	T43.3x6-
Cyamopsis tetragono-loba	T46.6x1-	T46.6x2-	T46.6x3-	T46.6x4-	T46.6x5-	T46.6x6-
Cyanacetyl hydrazide	T37.1x1-	T37.1x2-	T37.1x3-	T37.1x4-	T37.1x5-	T37.1x6-
Cyanic acid (gas)	T59.891-	T59.892-	T59.893-	T59.894-	—	—
Cyanide (s) (compounds) (potassium) (sodium) NEC	T65.0x1-	T65.0x2-	T65.0x3-	T65.0x4-	—	—
dust or gas (inhalation) NEC	T57.3x1-	T57.3x2-	T57.3x3-	T57.3x4-	—	—
fumigant	T65.0x1-	T65.0x2-	T65.0x3-	T65.0x4-	—	—
hydrogen	T57.3x1-	T57.3x2-	T57.3x3-	T57.3x4-	—	—
mercuric — see Mercury						
pesticide (dust) (fumes)	T65.0x1-	T65.0x2-	T65.0x3-	T65.0x4-	—	—

DRUGS & CHEMICALS

Table of Drugs & Chemicals	Accidental (Unintentional)	Self-Harm (Intentional)	Assault	Undetermined	Adverse Effect	Underdosing
Cyanoacrylate adhesive	T49.3x1-	T49.3x2-	T49.3x3-	T49.3x4-	T49.3x5-	T49.3x6-
Cyanocobalamin	T45.8x1-	T45.8x2-	T45.8x3-	T45.8x4-	T45.8x5-	T45.8x6-
Cyanogen (chloride) (gas) NEC	T59.891-	T59.892-	T59.893-	T59.894-	—	—
Cyclacillin	T36.0x1-	T36.0x2-	T36.0x3-	T36.0x4-	T36.0x5-	T36.0x6-
Cyclaine	T41.3x1-	T41.3x2-	T41.3x3-	T41.3x4-	T41.3x5-	T41.3x6-
Cyclamate	T50.991-	T50.992-	T50.993-	T50.994-	T50.995-	T50.996-
Cyclamen europaeum	T62.2x1-	T62.2x2-	T62.2x3-	T62.2x4-	—	—
Cyclandelate	T46.7x1-	T46.7x2-	T46.7x3-	T46.7x4-	T46.7x5-	T46.7x6-
Cyclazocine	T50.7x1-	T50.7x2-	T50.7x3-	T50.7x4-	T50.7x5-	T50.7x6-
Cyclizine	T45.0x1-	T45.0x2-	T45.0x3-	T45.0x4-	T45.0x5-	T45.0x6-
Cyclobarbital	T42.3x1-	T42.3x2-	T42.3x3-	T42.3x4-	T42.3x5-	T42.3x6-
Cyclobarbitone	T42.3x1-	T42.3x2-	T42.3x3-	T42.3x4-	T42.3x5-	T42.3x6-
Cyclobenzaprine	T48.1x1-	T48.1x2-	T48.1x3-	T48.1x4-	T48.1x5-	T48.1x6-
Cyclodrine	T44.3x1-	T44.3x2-	T44.3x3-	T44.3x4-	T44.3x5-	T44.3x6-
Cycloguanil embonate	T37.2x1-	T37.2x2-	T37.2x3-	T37.2x4-	T37.2x5-	T37.2x6-
Cyclohexane	T52.8x1-	T52.8x2-	T52.8x3-	T52.8x4-	—	—
Cyclohexanol	T51.8x1-	T51.8x2-	T51.8x3-	T51.8x4-	—	—
Cyclohexanone	T52.4x1-	T52.4x2-	T52.4x3-	T52.4x4-	—	—
Cycloheximide	T60.3x1-	T60.3x2-	T60.3x3-	T60.3x4-	—	—
Cyclohexyl acetate	T52.8x1-	T52.8x2-	T52.8x3-	T52.8x4-	—	—
Cycloleucin	T45.1x1-	T45.1x2-	T45.1x3-	T45.1x4-	T45.1x5-	T45.1x6-
Cyclomethycaine	T41.3x1-	T41.3x2-	T41.3x3-	T41.3x4-	T41.3x5-	T41.3x6-
Cyclopentamine	T44.4x1-	T44.4x2-	T44.4x3-	T44.4x4-	T44.4x5-	T44.4x6-
Cyclopenthiazide	T50.2x1-	T50.2x2-	T50.2x3-	T50.2x4-	T50.2x5-	T50.2x6-
Cyclopentolate	T44.3x1-	T44.3x2-	T44.3x3-	T44.3x4-	T44.3x5-	T44.3x6-
Cyclophosphamide	T45.1x1-	T45.1x2-	T45.1x3-	T45.1x4-	T45.1x5-	T45.1x6-
Cycloplegic drug	T49.5x1-	T49.5x2-	T49.5x3-	T49.5x4-	T49.5x5-	T49.5x6-
Cyclopropane	T41.291-	T41.292-	T41.293-	T41.294-	T41.295-	T41.296-
Cyclopyrabital	T39.8x1-	T39.8x2-	T39.8x3-	T39.8x4-	T39.8x5-	T39.8x6-
Cycloserine	T37.1x1-	T37.1x2-	T37.1x3-	T37.1x4-	T37.1x5-	T37.1x6-
Cyclosporin	T45.1x1-	T45.1x2-	T45.1x3-	T45.1x4-	T45.1x5-	T45.1x6-
Cyclothiazide	T50.2x1-	T50.2x2-	T50.2x3-	T50.2x4-	T50.2x5-	T50.2x6-
Cycrimine	T44.3x1-	T44.3x2-	T44.3x3-	T44.3x4-	T44.3x5-	T44.3x6-
Cyhalothrin	T60.1x1-	T60.1x2-	T60.1x3-	T60.1x4-	—	—
Cymarin	T46.0x1-	T46.0x2-	T46.0x3-	T46.0x4-	T46.0x5-	T46.0x6-
Cypermethrin	T60.1x1-	T60.1x2-	T60.1x3-	T60.1x4-	—	—
Cyphenothrin	T60.2x1-	T60.2x2-	T60.2x3-	T60.2x4-	—	—
Cyproheptadine	T45.0x1-	T45.0x2-	T45.0x3-	T45.0x4-	T45.0x5-	T45.0x6-
Cyproterone	T38.6x1-	T38.6x2-	T38.6x3-	T38.6x4-	T38.6x5-	T38.6x6-
Cysteamine	T50.6x1-	T50.6x2-	T50.6x3-	T50.6x4-	T50.6x5-	T50.6x6-
Cytarabine	T45.1x1-	T45.1x2-	T45.1x3-	T45.1x4-	T45.1x5-	T45.1x6-
Cytisus laburnum	T62.2x1-	T62.2x2-	T62.2x3-	T62.2x4-	—	—
scoparius	T62.2x1-	T62.2x2-	T62.2x3-	T62.2x4-	—	—
Cytochrome C	T47.5x1-	T47.5x2-	T47.5x3-	T47.5x4-	T47.5x5-	T47.5x6-
Cytomel	T38.1x1-	T38.1x2-	T38.1x3-	T38.1x4-	T38.1x5-	T38.1x6-
Cytosine arabinoside	T45.1x1-	T45.1x2-	T45.1x3-	T45.1x4-	T45.1x5-	T45.1x6-
Cytoxan	T45.1x1-	T45.1x2-	T45.1x3-	T45.1x4-	T45.1x5-	T45.1x6-
Cytozyme	T45.7x1-	T45.7x2-	T45.7x3-	T45.7x4-	T45.7x5-	T45.7x6-
2,4-D	T60.3x1-	T60.3x2-	T60.3x3-	T60.3x4-		
Dacarbazine	T45.1x1-	T45.1x2-	T45.1x3-	T45.1x4-	T45.1x5-	T45.1x6-
Dactinomycin	T45.1x1-	T45.1x2-	T45.1x3-	T45.1x4-	T45.1x5-	T45.1x6-
DADPS	T37.1x1-	T37.1x2-	T37.1x3-	T37.1x4-	T37.1x5-	T37.1x6-
Dakin's solution	T49.0x1-	T49.0x2-	T49.0x3-	T49.0x4-	T49.0x5-	T49.0x6-
Dalapon (sodium)	T60.3x1-	T60.3x2-	T60.3x3-	T60.3x4-	—	—
Dalmane	T42.4x1-	T42.4x2-	T42.4x3-	T42.4x4-	T42.4x5-	T42.4x6-
Danazol	T38.6x1-	T38.6x2-	T38.6x3-	T38.6x4-	T38.6x5-	T38.6x6-
Danilone	T45.511-	T45.512-	T45.513-	T45.514-	T45.515-	T45.516-
Danthron	T47.2x1-	T47.2x2-	T47.2x3-	T47.2x4-	T47.2x5-	T47.2x6-
Dantrolene	T42.8x1-	T42.8x2-	T42.8x3-	T42.8x4-	T42.8x5-	T42.8x6-
Dantron	T47.2x1-	T47.2x2-	T47.2x3-	T47.2x4-	T47.2x5-	T47.2x6-

Table of Drugs & Chemicals	Accidental (Unintentional)	Self-Harm (Intentional)	Assault	Undetermined	Adverse Effect	Underdosing
Daphne (gnidium) (mezereum)	T62.2x1-	T62.2x2-	T62.2x3-	T62.2x4-	—	—
berry	T62.1x1-	T62.1x2-	T62.1x3-	T62.1x4-	—	—
Dapsone	T37.1x1-	T37.1x2-	T37.1x3-	T37.1x4-	T37.1x5-	T37.1x6-
Daraprim	T37.2x1-	T37.2x2-	T37.2x3-	T37.2x4-	T37.2x5-	T37.2x6-
Darnel	T62.2x1-	T62.2x2-	T62.2x3-	T62.2x4-		
Darvon	T39.8x1-	T39.8x2-	T39.8x3-	T39.8x4-	T39.8x5-	T39.8x6-
Daunomycin	T45.1x1-	T45.1x2-	T45.1x3-	T45.1x4-	T45.1x5-	T45.1x6-
Daunorubicin	T45.1x1-	T45.1x2-	T45.1x3-	T45.1x4-	T45.1x5-	T45.1x6-
DBI	T38.3x1-	T38.3x2-	T38.3x3-	T38.3x4-	T38.3x5-	T38.3x6-
D-Con	T60.91x-	T60.92x-	T60.93x-	T60.94x-		
insecticide	T60.2x1-	T60.2x2-	T60.2x3-	T60.2x4-	—	—
rodenticide	T60.4x1-	T60.4x2-	T60.4x3-	T60.4x4-	—	—
DDAVP	T38.891-	T38.892-	T38.893-	T38.894-	T38.895-	T38.896-
DDE (bis(chlorophenyl)-dichloroethylene)	T60.2x1-	T60.2x2-	T60.2x3-	T60.2x4-		
DDS	T37.1x1-	T37.1x2-	T37.1x3-	T37.1x4-	T37.1x5-	T37.1x6-
DDT (dust)	T60.1x1-	T60.1x2-	T60.1x3-	T60.1x4-		
Deadly nightshade — see also Belladonna	T62.2x1-	T62.2x2-	T62.2x3-	T62.2x4-		
berry	T62.1x1-	T62.1x2-	T62.1x3-	T62.1x4-		
Deamino-D-arginine vasopressin	T38.891-	T38.892-	T38.893-	T38.894-	T38.895-	T38.896-
Deanol (aceglumate)	T50.991-	T50.992-	T50.993-	T50.994-	T50.995-	T50.996-
Debrisoquine	T46.5x1-	T46.5x2-	T46.5x3-	T46.5x4-	T46.5x5-	T46.5x6-
Decaborane	T57.8x1-	T57.8x2-	T57.8x3-	T57.8x4-	—	—
fumes	T59.891-	T59.892-	T59.893-	T59.894-	—	—
Decadron	T38.0x1-	T38.0x2-	T38.0x3-	T38.0x4-	T38.0x5-	T38.0x6-
ENT agent	T49.6x1-	T49.6x2-	T49.6x3-	T49.6x4-	T49.6x5-	T49.6x6-
ophthalmic preparation	T49.5x1-	T49.5x2-	T49.5x3-	T49.5x4-	T49.5x5-	T49.5x6-
topical NEC	T49.0x1-	T49.0x2-	T49.0x3-	T49.0x4-	T49.0x5-	T49.0x6-
Decahydronaphthalene	T52.8x1-	T52.8x2-	T52.8x3-	T52.8x4-	—	—
Decalin	T52.8x1-	T52.8x2-	T52.8x3-	T52.8x4-	—	—
Decamethonium (bromide)	T48.1x1-	T48.1x2-	T48.1x3-	T48.1x4-	T48.1x5-	T48.1x6-
Decholin	T47.5x1-	T47.5x2-	T47.5x3-	T47.5x4-	T47.5x5-	T47.5x6-
Declomycin	T36.4x1-	T36.4x2-	T36.4x3-	T36.4x4-	T36.4x5-	T36.4x6-
Decongestant, nasal (mucosa)	T48.5x1-	T48.5x2-	T48.5x3-	T48.5x4-	T48.5x5-	T48.5x6-
combination	T48.5x1-	T48.5x2-	T48.5x3-	T48.5x4-	T48.5x5-	T48.5x6-
Deet	T60.8x1-	T60.8x2-	T60.8x3-	T60.8x4-	—	—
Deferoxamine	T45.8x1-	T45.8x2-	T45.8x3-	T45.8x4-	T45.8x5-	T45.8x6-
Deflazacort	T38.0x1-	T38.0x2-	T38.0x3-	T38.0x4-	T38.0x5-	T38.0x6-
Deglycyrrhizinized extract of licorice	T48.4x1-	T48.4x2-	T48.4x3-	T48.4x4-	T48.4x5-	T48.4x6-
Dehydrocholic acid	T47.5x1-	T47.5x2-	T47.5x3-	T47.5x4-	T47.5x5-	T47.5x6-
Dehydroemetine	T37.3x1-	T37.3x2-	T37.3x3-	T37.3x4-	T37.3x5-	T37.3x6-
Dekalin	T52.8x1-	T52.8x2-	T52.8x3-	T52.8x4-		
Delalutin	T38.5x1-	T38.5x2-	T38.5x3-	T38.5x4-	T38.5x5-	T38.5x6-
Delorazepam	T42.4x1-	T42.4x2-	T42.4x3-	T42.4x4-	T42.4x5-	T42.4x6-
Delphinium	T62.2x1-	T62.2x2-	T62.2x3-	T62.2x4-		
Deltamethrin	T60.1x1-	T60.1x2-	T60.1x3-	T60.1x4-	—	—
Deltasone	T38.0x1-	T38.0x2-	T38.0x3-	T38.0x4-	T38.0x5-	T38.0x6-
Deltra	T38.0x1-	T38.0x2-	T38.0x3-	T38.0x4-	T38.0x5-	T38.0x6-
Delvinal	T42.3x1-	T42.3x2-	T42.3x3-	T42.3x4-	T42.3x5-	T42.3x6-
Demecarium (bromide)	T49.5x1-	T49.5x2-	T49.5x3-	T49.5x4-	T49.5x5-	T49.5x6-
Demeclocycline	T36.4x1-	T36.4x2-	T36.4x3-	T36.4x4-	T36.4x5-	T36.4x6-
Demecolcine	T45.1x1-	T45.1x2-	T45.1x3-	T45.1x4-	T45.1x5-	T45.1x6-
Demegestone	T38.5x1-	T38.5x2-	T38.5x3-	T38.5x4-	T38.5x5-	T38.5x6-
Demelanizing agents	T49.8x1-	T49.8x2-	T49.8x3-	T49.8x4-	T49.8x5-	T49.8x6-
Demephion -O and -S	T60.0x1-	T60.0x2-	T60.0x3-	T60.0x4-	—	—
Demerol	T40.2x1-	T40.2x2-	T40.2x3-	T40.2x4-	T40.2x5-	T40.2x6-
Demethylchlortetracycline	T36.4x1-	T36.4x2-	T36.4x3-	T36.4x4-	T36.4x5-	T36.4x6-
Demethyltetracycline	T36.4x1-	T36.4x2-	T36.4x3-	T36.4x4-	T36.4x5-	T36.4x6-

Table of Drugs & Chemicals	POISONING Accidental (Unintentional)	Self-Harm (Intentional)	Assault	Undetermined	Adverse Effect	Underdosing
Demeton -O and -S	T60.0x1-	T60.0x2-	T60.0x3-	T60.0x4-	—	—
Demulcent (external)	T49.3x1-	T49.3x2-	T49.3x3-	T49.3x4-	T49.3x5-	T49.3x6-
specified NEC	T49.3x1-	T49.3x2-	T49.3x3-	T49.3x4-	T49.3x5-	T49.3x6-
Demulen	T38.4x1-	T38.4x2-	T38.4x3-	T38.4x4-	T38.4x5-	T38.4x6-
Denatured alcohol	T51.0x1-	T51.0x2-	T51.0x3-	T51.0x4-	—	—
Dendrid	T49.5x1-	T49.5x2-	T49.5x3-	T49.5x4-	T49.5x5-	T49.5x6-
Dental drug, topical application NEC	T49.7x1-	T49.7x2-	T49.7x3-	T49.7x4-	T49.7x5-	T49.7x6-
Dentifrice	T49.7x1-	T49.7x2-	T49.7x3-	T49.7x4-	T49.7x5-	T49.7x6-
Deodorant spray (feminine hygiene)	T49.8x1-	T49.8x2-	T49.8x3-	T49.8x4-	T49.8x5-	T49.8x6-
Deoxycortone	T50.0x1-	T50.0x2-	T50.0x3-	T50.0x4-	T50.0x5-	T50.0x6-
2-Deoxy-5-fluorouridine	T45.1x1-	T45.1x2-	T45.1x3-	T45.1x4-	T45.1x5-	T45.1x6-
5-Deoxy-5-fluorouridine	T45.1x1-	T45.1x2-	T45.1x3-	T45.1x4-	T45.1x5-	T45.1x6-
Deoxyribonuclease (pancreatic)	T45.3x1-	T45.3x2-	T45.3x3-	T45.3x4-	T45.3x5-	T45.3x6-
Depilatory	T49.4x1-	T49.4x2-	T49.4x3-	T49.4x4-	T49.4x5-	T49.4x6-
Deprenalin	T42.8x1-	T42.8x2-	T42.8x3-	T42.8x4-	T42.8x5-	T42.8x6-
Deprenyl	T42.8x1-	T42.8x2-	T42.8x3-	T42.8x4-	T42.8x5-	T42.8x6-
Depressant, appetite	T50.5x1-	T50.5x2-	T50.5x3-	T50.5x4-	T50.5x5-	T50.5x6-
Depressant						
appetite, central	T50.5x1-	T50.5x2-	T50.5x3-	T50.5x4-	T50.5x5-	T50.5x6-
cardiac	T46.2x1-	T46.2x2-	T46.2x3-	T46.2x4-	T46.2x5-	T46.2x6-
central nervous system (anesthetic) — see also Central nervous system, depressants	T42.71x-	T42.72x-	T42.73x-	T42.74x-	T42.75x-	T42.76x-
general anesthetic	T41.201-	T41.202-	T41.203-	T41.204-	T41.205-	T41.206-
muscle tone	T42.8x1-	T42.8x2-	T42.8x3-	T42.8x4-	T42.8x5-	T42.8x6-
muscle tone, central	T42.8x1-	T42.8x2-	T42.8x3-	T42.8x4-	T42.8x5-	T42.8x6-
psychotherapeutic	T43.501-	T43.502-	T43.503-	T43.504-	T43.505-	T43.506-
Deptropine	T45.0x1-	T45.0x2-	T45.0x3-	T45.0x4-	T45.0x5-	T45.0x6-
Dequalinium (chloride)	T49.0x1-	T49.0x2-	T49.0x3-	T49.0x4-	T49.0x5-	T49.0x6-
Derris root	T60.2x1-	T60.2x2-	T60.2x3-	T60.2x4-	—	—
Deserpidine	T46.5x1-	T46.5x2-	T46.5x3-	T46.5x4-	T46.5x5-	T46.5x6-
Desferrioxamine	T45.8x1-	T45.8x2-	T45.8x3-	T45.8x4-	T45.8x5-	T45.8x6-
Desipramine	T43.011-	T43.012-	T43.013-	T43.014-	T43.015-	T43.016-
Deslanoside	T46.0x1-	T46.0x2-	T46.0x3-	T46.0x4-	T46.0x5-	T46.0x6-
Desloughing agent	T49.4x1-	T49.4x2-	T49.4x3-	T49.4x4-	T49.4x5-	T49.4x6-
Desmethylimipramine	T43.011-	T43.012-	T43.013-	T43.014-	T43.015-	T43.016-
Desmopressin	T38.891-	T38.892-	T38.893-	T38.894-	T38.895-	T38.896-
Desocodeine	T40.2x1-	T40.2x2-	T40.2x3-	T40.2x4-	T40.2x5-	T40.2x6-
Desogestrel	T38.5x1-	T38.5x2-	T38.5x3-	T38.5x4-	T38.5x5-	T38.5x6-
Desomorphine	T40.2x1-	T40.2x2-	T40.2x3-	T40.2x4-	—	—
Desonide	T49.0x1-	T49.0x2-	T49.0x3-	T49.0x4-	T49.0x5-	T49.0x6-
Desoximetasone	T49.0x1-	T49.0x2-	T49.0x3-	T49.0x4-	T49.0x5-	T49.0x6-
Desoxycorticosteroid	T50.0x1-	T50.0x2-	T50.0x3-	T50.0x4-	T50.0x5-	T50.0x6-
Desoxycortone	T50.0x1-	T50.0x2-	T50.0x3-	T50.0x4-	T50.0x5-	T50.0x6-
Desoxyephedrine	T43.621-	T43.622-	T43.623-	T43.624-	T43.625-	T43.626-
Detaxtran	T46.6x1-	T46.6x2-	T46.6x3-	T46.6x4-	T46.6x5-	T46.6x6-
Detergent	T49.2x1-	T49.2x2-	T49.2x3-	T49.2x4-	T49.2x5-	T49.2x6-
external medication	T49.2x1-	T49.2x2-	T49.2x3-	T49.2x4-	T49.2x5-	T49.2x6-
local	T49.2x1-	T49.2x2-	T49.2x3-	T49.2x4-	T49.2x5-	T49.2x6-
medicinal	T49.2x1-	T49.2x2-	T49.2x3-	T49.2x4-	T49.2x5-	T49.2x6-
nonmedicinal	T55.1x1-	T55.1x2-	T55.1x3-	T55.1x4-	—	—
specified NEC	T55.1x1-	T55.1x2-	T55.1x3-	T55.1x4-	—	—
Deterrent, alcohol	T50.6x1-	T50.6x2-	T50.6x3-	T50.6x4-	T50.6x5-	T50.6x6-
Detoxifying agent	T50.6x1-	T50.6x2-	T50.6x3-	T50.6x4-	T50.6x5-	T50.6x6-
Detrothyronine	T38.1x1-	T38.1x2-	T38.1x3-	T38.1x4-	T38.1x5-	T38.1x6-
Dettol (external medication)	T49.0x1-	T49.0x2-	T49.0x3-	T49.0x4-	T49.0x5-	T49.0x6-
Dexamethasone	T38.0x1-	T38.0x2-	T38.0x3-	T38.0x4-	T38.0x5-	T38.0x6-
ENT agent	T49.6x1-	T49.6x2-	T49.6x3-	T49.6x4-	T49.6x5-	T49.6x6-
ophthalmic preparation	T49.5x1-	T49.5x2-	T49.5x3-	T49.5x4-	T49.5x5-	T49.5x6-
topical NEC	T49.0x1-	T49.0x2-	T49.0x3-	T49.0x4-	T49.0x5-	T49.0x6-

Table of Drugs & Chemicals	POISONING Accidental (Unintentional)	Self-Harm (Intentional)	Assault	Undetermined	Adverse Effect	Underdosing
Dexamfetamine	T43.621-	T43.622-	T43.623-	T43.624-	T43.625-	T43.626-
Dexamphetamine	T43.621-	T43.622-	T43.623-	T43.624-	T43.625-	T43.626-
Dexbrompheniramine	T45.0x1-	T45.0x2-	T45.0x3-	T45.0x4-	T45.0x5-	T45.0x6-
Dexchlorpheniramine	T45.0x1-	T45.0x2-	T45.0x3-	T45.0x4-	T45.0x5-	T45.0x6-
Dexedrine	T43.621-	T43.622-	T43.623-	T43.624-	T43.625-	T43.626-
Dexetimide	T44.3x1-	T44.3x2-	T44.3x3-	T44.3x4-	T44.3x5-	T44.3x6-
Dexfenfluramine	T50.5x1-	T50.5x2-	T50.5x3-	T50.5x4-	T50.5x5-	T50.5x6-
Dexpanthenol	T45.2x1-	T45.2x2-	T45.2x3-	T45.2x4-	T45.2x5-	T45.2x6-
Dextran (40) (70) (150)	T45.8x1-	T45.8x2-	T45.8x3-	T45.8x4-	T45.8x5-	T45.8x6-
Dextriferron	T45.4x1-	T45.4x2-	T45.4x3-	T45.4x4-	T45.4x5-	T45.4x6-
Dextro calcium pantothenate	T45.2x1-	T45.2x2-	T45.2x3-	T45.2x4-	T45.2x5-	T45.2x6-
Dextro pantothenyl alcohol	T45.2x1-	T45.2x2-	T45.2x3-	T45.2x4-	T45.2x5-	T45.2x6-
Dextroamphetamine	T43.621-	T43.622-	T43.623-	T43.624-	T43.625-	T43.626-
Dextromethorphan	T48.3x1-	T48.3x2-	T48.3x3-	T48.3x4-	T48.3x5-	T48.3x6-
Dextromoramide	T40.4x1-	T40.4x2-	T40.4x3-	T40.4x4-	—	—
topical	T49.8x1-	T49.8x2-	T49.8x3-	T49.8x4-	T49.8x5-	T49.8x6-
Dextropropoxyphene	T40.4x1-	T40.4x2-	T40.4x3-	T40.4x4-	T40.4x5-	T40.4x6-
Dextrorphan	T40.2x1-	T40.2x2-	T40.2x3-	T40.2x4-	T40.2x5-	T40.2x6-
Dextrose	T50.3x1-	T50.3x2-	T50.3x3-	T50.3x4-	T50.3x5-	T50.3x6-
concentrated solution, intravenous	T46.8x1-	T46.8x2-	T46.8x3-	T46.8x4-	T46.8x5-	T46.8x6-
Dextrothyroxin	T38.1x1-	T38.1x2-	T38.1x3-	T38.1x4-	T38.1x5-	T38.1x6-
Dextrothyroxine sodium	T38.1x1-	T38.1x2-	T38.1x3-	T38.1x4-	T38.1x5-	T38.1x6-
DFP	T44.0x1-	T44.0x2-	T44.0x3-	T44.0x4-	T44.0x5-	T44.0x6-
DHE	T37.3x1-	T37.3x2-	T37.3x3-	T37.3x4-	T37.3x5-	T37.3x6-
45	T46.5x1-	T46.5x2-	T46.5x3-	T46.5x4-	T46.5x5-	T46.5x6-
Diabinese	T38.3x1-	T38.3x2-	T38.3x3-	T38.3x4-	T38.3x5-	T38.3x6-
Diacetone alcohol	T52.4x1-	T52.4x2-	T52.4x3-	T52.4x4-	—	—
Diacetyl monoxime	T50.991-	T50.992-	T50.993-	T50.994-	—	—
Diacetylmorphine	T40.1x1-	T40.1x2-	T40.1x3-	T40.1x4-	—	—
Diachylon plaster	T49.4x1-	T49.4x2-	T49.4x3-	T49.4x4-	T49.4x5-	T49.4x6-
Diaethylstilboestrolum	T38.5x1-	T38.5x2-	T38.5x3-	T38.5x4-	T38.5x5-	T38.5x6-
Diagnostic agent NEC	T50.8x1-	T50.8x2-	T50.8x3-	T50.8x4-	T50.8x5-	T50.8x6-
Dial (soap)	T49.2x1-	T49.2x2-	T49.2x3-	T49.2x4-	T49.2x5-	T49.2x6-
sedative	T42.3x1-	T42.3x2-	T42.3x3-	T42.3x4-	T42.3x5-	T42.3x6-
Dialkyl carbonate	T52.91x-	T52.92x-	T52.93x-	T52.94x-	—	—
Diallylbarbituric acid	T42.3x1-	T42.3x2-	T42.3x3-	T42.3x4-	T42.3x5-	T42.3x6-
Diallymal	T42.3x1-	T42.3x2-	T42.3x3-	T42.3x4-	T42.3x5-	T42.3x6-
Dialysis solution (intraperitoneal)	T50.3x1-	T50.3x2-	T50.3x3-	T50.3x4-	T50.3x5-	T50.3x6-
Diaminodiphenylsulfone	T37.1x1-	T37.1x2-	T37.1x3-	T37.1x4-	T37.1x5-	T37.1x6-
Diamorphine	T40.1x1-	T40.1x2-	T40.1x3-	T40.1x4-	—	—
Diamox	T50.2x1-	T50.2x2-	T50.2x3-	T50.2x4-	T50.2x5-	T50.2x6-
Diamthazole	T49.0x1-	T49.0x2-	T49.0x3-	T49.0x4-	T49.0x5-	T49.0x6-
Dianthone	T47.2x1-	T47.2x2-	T47.2x3-	T47.2x4-	T47.2x5-	T47.2x6-
Diaphenylsulfone	T37.0x1-	T37.0x2-	T37.0x3-	T37.0x4-	T37.0x5-	T37.0x6-
Diasone (sodium)	T37.1x1-	T37.1x2-	T37.1x3-	T37.1x4-	T37.1x5-	T37.1x6-
Diastase	T47.5x1-	T47.5x2-	T47.5x3-	T47.5x4-	T47.5x5-	T47.5x6-
Diatrizoate	T50.8x1-	T50.8x2-	T50.8x3-	T50.8x4-	T50.8x5-	T50.8x6-
Diazepam	T42.4x1-	T42.4x2-	T42.4x3-	T42.4x4-	T42.4x5-	T42.4x6-
Diazinon	T60.0x1-	T60.0x2-	T60.0x3-	T60.0x4-	—	—
Diazomethane (gas)	T59.891-	T59.892-	T59.893-	T59.894-	—	—
Diazoxide	T46.5x1-	T46.5x2-	T46.5x3-	T46.5x4-	T46.5x5-	T46.5x6-
Dibekacin	T36.5x1-	T36.5x2-	T36.5x3-	T36.5x4-	T36.5x5-	T36.5x6-
Dibenamine	T44.6x1-	T44.6x2-	T44.6x3-	T44.6x4-	T44.6x5-	T44.6x6-
Dibenzepin	T43.011-	T43.012-	T43.013-	T43.014-	T43.015-	T43.016-
Dibenzheptropine	T45.0x1-	T45.0x2-	T45.0x3-	T45.0x4-	T45.0x5-	T45.0x6-
Dibenzyline	T44.6x1-	T44.6x2-	T44.6x3-	T44.6x4-	T44.6x5-	T44.6x6-
Diborane (gas)	T59.891-	T59.892-	T59.893-	T59.894-	—	—
Dibromochloropropane	T60.8x1-	T60.8x2-	T60.8x3-	T60.8x4-	—	—

Table of Drugs & Chemicals	Accidental (Unintentional)	Self-Harm (Intentional)	Assault	Undetermined	Adverse Effect	Underdosing
Dibromodulcitol	T45.1x1-	T45.1x2-	T45.1x3-	T45.1x4-	T45.1x5-	T45.1x6-
Dibromoethane	T53.6x1-	T53.6x2-	T53.6x3-	T53.6x4-	—	—
Dibromomannitol	T45.1x1-	T45.1x2-	T45.1x3-	T45.1x4-	T45.1x5-	T45.1x6-
Dibromopropamidine isethionate	T49.0x1-	T49.0x2-	T49.0x3-	T49.0x4-	T49.0x5-	T49.0x6-
Dibrompropamidine	T49.0x1-	T49.0x2-	T49.0x3-	T49.0x4-	T49.0x5-	T49.0x6-
Dibucaine	T41.3x1-	T41.3x2-	T41.3x3-	T41.3x4-	T41.3x5-	T41.3x6-
topical (surface)	T41.3x1-	T41.3x2-	T41.3x3-	T41.3x4-	T41.3x5-	T41.3x6-
Dibunate sodium	T48.3x1-	T48.3x2-	T48.3x3-	T48.3x4-	T48.3x5-	T48.3x6-
Dibutoline sulfate	T44.3x1-	T44.3x2-	T44.3x3-	T44.3x4-	T44.3x5-	T44.3x6-
Dicamba	T60.3x1-	T60.3x2-	T60.3x3-	T60.3x4-	—	—
Dicapthon	T60.0x1-	T60.0x2-	T60.0x3-	T60.0x4-	—	—
Dichlobenil	T60.3x1-	T60.3x2-	T60.3x3-	T60.3x4-	—	—
Dichlone	T60.3x1-	T60.3x2-	T60.3x3-	T60.3x4-	—	—
Dichloralphenozone	T42.6x1-	T42.6x2-	T42.6x3-	T42.6x4-	T42.6x5-	T42.6x6-
Dichlorbenzidine	T65.3x1-	T65.3x2-	T65.3x3-	T65.3x4-	—	—
Dichlorhydrin	T52.8x1-	T52.8x2-	T52.8x3-	T52.8x4-	—	—
Dichlorhydroxyquinoline	T37.8x1-	T37.8x2-	T37.8x3-	T37.8x4-	T37.8x5-	T37.8x6-
Dichlorobenzene	T53.7x1-	T53.7x2-	T53.7x3-	T53.7x4-	—	—
Dichlorobenzyl alcohol	T49.6x1-	T49.6x2-	T49.6x3-	T49.6x4-	T49.6x5-	T49.6x6-
Dichlorodifluoromethane	T53.5x1-	T53.5x2-	T53.5x3-	T53.5x4-	—	—
Dichloroethane	T52.8x1-	T52.8x2-	T52.8x3-	T52.8x4-	—	—
Sym-Dichloroethyl ether	T53.6x1-	T53.6x2-	T53.6x3-	T53.6x4-	—	—
Dichloroethyl sulfide, not in war	T59.891-	T59.892-	T59.893-	T59.894-	—	—
Dichloroethylene	T53.6x1-	T53.6x2-	T53.6x3-	T53.6x4-	—	—
Dichloroformoxine, not in war	T59.891-	T59.892-	T59.893-	T59.894-	—	—
Dichlorohydrin, alpha-dichlorohydrin	T52.8x1-	T52.8x2-	T52.8x3-	T52.8x4-	—	—
Dichloromethane (solvent)	T53.4x1-	T53.4x2-	T53.4x3-	T53.4x4-	—	—
vapor	T53.4x1-	T53.4x2-	T53.4x3-	T53.4x4-	—	—
Dichloronaphthoquinone	T60.3x1-	T60.3x2-	T60.3x3-	T60.3x4-	—	—
Dichlorophen	T37.4x1-	T37.4x2-	T37.4x3-	T37.4x4-	T37.4x5-	T37.4x6-
2,4-Dichlorophenoxyacetic acid	T60.3x1-	T60.3x2-	T60.3x3-	T60.3x4-	—	—
Dichloropropene	T60.3x1-	T60.3x2-	T60.3x3-	T60.3x4-	—	—
Dichloropropionic acid	T60.3x1-	T60.3x2-	T60.3x3-	T60.3x4-	—	—
Dichlorphenamide	T50.2x1-	T50.2x2-	T50.2x3-	T50.2x4-	T50.2x5-	T50.2x6-
Dichlorvos	T60.0x1-	T60.0x2-	T60.0x3-	T60.0x4-	—	—
Diclofenac	T39.391-	T39.392-	T39.393-	T39.394-	T39.395-	T39.396-
Diclofenamide	T50.2x1-	T50.2x2-	T50.2x3-	T50.2x4-	T50.2x5-	T50.2x6-
Diclofensine	T43.291-	T43.292-	T43.293-	T43.294-	T43.295-	T43.296-
Diclonixine	T39.8x1-	T39.8x2-	T39.8x3-	T39.8x4-	T39.8x5-	T39.8x6-
Dicloxacillin	T36.0x1-	T36.0x2-	T36.0x3-	T36.0x4-	T36.0x5-	T36.0x6-
Dicophane	T49.0x1-	T49.0x2-	T49.0x3-	T49.0x4-	T49.0x5-	T49.0x6-
Dicoumarol, dicoumarin, dicumarol	T45.511-	T45.512-	T45.513-	T45.514-	T45.515-	T45.516-
Dicrotophos	T60.0x1-	T60.0x2-	T60.0x3-	T60.0x4-	—	—
Dicyanogen (gas)	T65.0x1-	T65.0x2-	T65.0x3-	T65.0x4-	—	—
Dicyclomine	T44.3x1-	T44.3x2-	T44.3x3-	T44.3x4-	T44.3x5-	T44.3x6-
Dicycloverine	T44.3x1-	T44.3x2-	T44.3x3-	T44.3x4-	T44.3x5-	T44.3x6-
Dideoxycytidine	T37.5x1-	T37.5x2-	T37.5x3-	T37.5x4-	T37.5x5-	T37.5x6-
Dideoxyinosine	T37.5x1-	T37.5x2-	T37.5x3-	T37.5x4-	T37.5x5-	T37.5x6-
Dieldrin (vapor)	T60.1x1-	T60.1x2-	T60.1x3-	T60.1x4-	—	—
Diemal	T42.3x1-	T42.3x2-	T42.3x3-	T42.3x4-	T42.3x5-	T42.3x6-
Dienestrol	T38.5x1-	T38.5x2-	T38.5x3-	T38.5x4-	T38.5x5-	T38.5x6-
Dienoestrol	T38.5x1-	T38.5x2-	T38.5x3-	T38.5x4-	T38.5x5-	T38.5x6-
Dietetic drug NEC	T50.901-	T50.902-	T50.903-	T50.904-	T50.905-	T50.906-
Diethazine	T42.8x1-	T42.8x2-	T42.8x3-	T42.8x4-	T42.8x5-	T42.8x6-

Table of Drugs & Chemicals	Accidental (Unintentional)	Self-Harm (Intentional)	Assault	Undetermined	Adverse Effect	Underdosing
Diethyl						
barbituric acid	T42.3x1-	T42.3x2-	T42.3x3-	T42.3x4-	T42.3x5-	T42.3x6-
carbamazine	T37.4x1-	T37.4x2-	T37.4x3-	T37.4x4-	T37.4x5-	T37.4x6-
carbinol	T51.3x1-	T51.3x2-	T51.3x3-	T51.3x4-	—	—
carbonate	T52.8x1-	T52.8x2-	T52.8x3-	T52.8x4-	—	—
ether (vapor) — see also Ether	T41.0x1-	T41.0x2-	T41.0x3-	T41.0x4-	T41.0x5-	T41.0x6-
oxide	T52.8x1-	T52.8x2-	T52.8x3-	T52.8x4-	—	—
propion	T50.5x1-	T50.5x2-	T50.5x3-	T50.5x4-	T50.5x5-	T50.5x6-
stilbestrol	T38.5x1-	T38.5x2-	T38.5x3-	T38.5x4-	T38.5x5-	T38.5x6-
toluamide (nonmedicinal)	T60.8x1-	T60.8x2-	T60.8x3-	T60.8x4-	—	—
medicinal	T49.3x1-	T49.3x2-	T49.3x3-	T49.3x4-	T49.3x5-	T49.3x6-
Diethylcarbamazine	T37.4x1-	T37.4x2-	T37.4x3-	T37.4x4-	T37.4x5-	T37.4x6-
Diethylene						
dioxide	T52.8x1-	T52.8x2-	T52.8x3-	T52.8x4-	—	—
glycol (monoacetate) (monobutyl ether) (monoethyl ether)	T52.3x1-	T52.3x2-	T52.3x3-	T52.3x4-	—	—
Diethylhexylphthalate	T65.891-	T65.892-	T65.893-	T65.894-	—	—
Diethylpropion	T50.5x1-	T50.5x2-	T50.5x3-	T50.5x4-	T50.5x5-	T50.5x6-
Diethylstilbestrol	T38.5x1-	T38.5x2-	T38.5x3-	T38.5x4-	T38.5x5-	T38.5x6-
Diethylstilboestrol	T38.5x1-	T38.5x2-	T38.5x3-	T38.5x4-	T38.5x5-	T38.5x6-
Diethylsulfone-diethylmethane	T42.6x1-	T42.6x2-	T42.6x3-	T42.6x4-	T42.6x5-	T42.6x6-
Diethyltoluamide	T49.0x1-	T49.0x2-	T49.0x3-	T49.0x4-	T49.0x5-	T49.0x6-
Diethyltryptamine (DET)	T40.991-	T40.992-	T40.993-	T40.994-	—	—
Difebarbamate	T42.3x1-	T42.3x2-	T42.3x3-	T42.3x4-	T42.3x5-	T42.3x6-
Difencloxazine	T40.2x1-	T40.2x2-	T40.2x3-	T40.2x4-	T40.2x5-	T40.2x6-
Difenidol	T45.0x1-	T45.0x2-	T45.0x3-	T45.0x4-	T45.0x5-	T45.0x6-
Difenoxin	T47.6x1-	T47.6x2-	T47.6x3-	T47.6x4-	T47.6x5-	T47.6x6-
Difetarsone	T37.3x1-	T37.3x2-	T37.3x3-	T37.3x4-	T37.3x5-	T37.3x6-
Diffusin	T45.3x1-	T45.3x2-	T45.3x3-	T45.3x4-	T45.3x5-	T45.3x6-
Diflorasone	T49.0x1-	T49.0x2-	T49.0x3-	T49.0x4-	T49.0x5-	T49.0x6-
Diflos	T44.0x1-	T44.0x2-	T44.0x3-	T44.0x4-	T44.0x5-	T44.0x6-
Diflubenzuron	T60.1x1-	T60.1x2-	T60.1x3-	T60.1x4-	—	—
Diflucortolone	T49.0x1-	T49.0x2-	T49.0x3-	T49.0x4-	T49.0x5-	T49.0x6-
Diflunisal	T39.091-	T39.092-	T39.093-	T39.094-	T39.095-	T39.096-
Difluoromethyldopa	T42.8x1-	T42.8x2-	T42.8x3-	T42.8x4-	T42.8x5-	T42.8x6-
Difluorophate	T44.0x1-	T44.0x2-	T44.0x3-	T44.0x4-	T44.0x5-	T44.0x6-
Digestant NEC	T47.5x1-	T47.5x2-	T47.5x3-	T47.5x4-	T47.5x5-	T47.5x6-
Digitalin(e)	T46.0x1-	T46.0x2-	T46.0x3-	T46.0x4-	T46.0x5-	T46.0x6-
Digitalis (leaf) (glycoside)	T46.0x1-	T46.0x2-	T46.0x3-	T46.0x4-	T46.0x5-	T46.0x6-
lanata	T46.0x1-	T46.0x2-	T46.0x3-	T46.0x4-	T46.0x5-	T46.0x6-
purpurea	T46.0x1-	T46.0x2-	T46.0x3-	T46.0x4-	T46.0x5-	T46.0x6-
Digitoxin	T46.0x1-	T46.0x2-	T46.0x3-	T46.0x4-	T46.0x5-	T46.0x6-
Digitoxose	T46.0x1-	T46.0x2-	T46.0x3-	T46.0x4-	T46.0x5-	T46.0x6-
Digoxin	T46.0x1-	T46.0x2-	T46.0x3-	T46.0x4-	T46.0x5-	T46.0x6-
Digoxine	T46.0x1-	T46.0x2-	T46.0x3-	T46.0x4-	T46.0x5-	T46.0x6-
Dihydralazine	T46.5x1-	T46.5x2-	T46.5x3-	T46.5x4-	T46.5x5-	T46.5x6-
Dihydrazine	T46.5x1-	T46.5x2-	T46.5x3-	T46.5x4-	T46.5x5-	T46.5x6-
Dihydrocodeine	T40.2x1-	T40.2x2-	T40.2x3-	T40.2x4-	T40.2x5-	T40.2x6-
Dihydrocodein-one	T40.2x1-	T40.2x2-	T40.2x3-	T40.2x4-	T40.2x5-	T40.2x6-
Dihydroergocornine	T46.7x1-	T46.7x2-	T46.7x3-	T46.7x4-	T46.7x5-	T46.7x6-
Dihydroergocristine (mesilate)	T46.7x1-	T46.7x2-	T46.7x3-	T46.7x4-	T46.7x5-	T46.7x6-
Dihydroergokryptine	T46.7x1-	T46.7x2-	T46.7x3-	T46.7x4-	T46.7x5-	T46.7x6-
Dihydroergotamine	T46.5x1-	T46.5x2-	T46.5x3-	T46.5x4-	T46.5x5-	T46.5x6-
Dihydroergotoxine	T46.7x1-	T46.7x2-	T46.7x3-	T46.7x4-	T46.7x5-	T46.7x6-
mesilate	T46.7x1-	T46.7x2-	T46.7x3-	T46.7x4-	T46.7x5-	T46.7x6-
Dihydrohydroxycodein-one	T40.2x1-	T40.2x2-	T40.2x3-	T40.2x4-	T40.2x5-	T40.2x6-
Dihydrohydroxymorphinone	T40.2x1-	T40.2x2-	T40.2x3-	T40.2x4-	T40.2x5-	T40.2x6-
Dihydroisocodeine	T40.2x1-	T40.2x2-	T40.2x3-	T40.2x4-	T40.2x5-	T40.2x6-

DRUGS & CHEMICALS

Table of Drugs & Chemicals	POISONING Accidental (Unintentional)	Self-Harm (Intentional)	Assault	Undetermined	Adverse Effect	Underdosing
Dihydromorphine	T40.2x1-	T40.2x2-	T40.2x3-	T40.2x4-	—	—
Dihydromorphinone	T40.2x1-	T40.2x2-	T40.2x3-	T40.2x4-	T40.2x5-	T40.2x6-
Dihydrostreptomycin	T36.5x1-	T36.5x2-	T36.5x3-	T36.5x4-	T36.5x5-	T36.5x6-
Dihydrotachysterol	T45.2x1-	T45.2x2-	T45.2x3-	T45.2x4-	T45.2x5-	T45.2x6-
Dihydroxyaluminum aminoacetate	T47.1x1-	T47.1x2-	T47.1x3-	T47.1x4-	T47.1x5-	T47.1x6-
Dihydroxyaluminum sodium carbonate	T47.1x1-	T47.1x2-	T47.1x3-	T47.1x4-	T47.1x5-	T47.1x6-
Dihydroxyanthraquinone	T47.2x1-	T47.2x2-	T47.2x3-	T47.2x4-	T47.2x5-	T47.2x6-
Dihydroxycodeinone	T40.2x1-	T40.2x2-	T40.2x3-	T40.2x4-	T40.2x5-	T40.2x6-
Dihydroxypropyl theophylline	T50.2x1-	T50.2x2-	T50.2x3-	T50.2x4-	T50.2x5-	T50.2x6-
Diiodohydroxyquin	T37.8x1-	T37.8x2-	T37.8x3-	T37.8x4-	T37.8x5-	T37.8x6-
topical	T49.0x1-	T49.0x2-	T49.0x3-	T49.0x4-	T49.0x5-	T49.0x6-
Diiodohydroxyquinoline	T37.8x1-	T37.8x2-	T37.8x3-	T37.8x4-	T37.8x5-	T37.8x6-
Diiodotyrosine	T38.2x1-	T38.2x2-	T38.2x3-	T38.2x4-	T38.2x5-	T38.2x6-
Diisopromine	T44.3x1-	T44.3x2-	T44.3x3-	T44.3x4-	T44.3x5-	T44.3x6-
Diisopropylamine	T46.3x1-	T46.3x2-	T46.3x3-	T46.3x4-	T46.3x5-	T46.3x6-
Diisopropylfluorophosphonate	T44.0x1-	T44.0x2-	T44.0x3-	T44.0x4-	T44.0x5-	T44.0x6-
Dilantin	T42.0x1-	T42.0x2-	T42.0x3-	T42.0x4-	T42.0x5-	T42.0x6-
Dilaudid	T40.2x1-	T40.2x2-	T40.2x3-	T40.2x4-	T40.2x5-	T40.2x6-
Dilazep	T46.3x1-	T46.3x2-	T46.3x3-	T46.3x4-	T46.3x5-	T46.3x6-
Dill	T47.5x1-	T47.5x2-	T47.5x3-	T47.5x4-	T47.5x5-	T47.5x6-
Diloxanide	T37.3x1-	T37.3x2-	T37.3x3-	T37.3x4-	T37.3x5-	T37.3x6-
Diltiazem	T46.1x1-	T46.1x2-	T46.1x3-	T46.1x4-	T46.1x5-	T46.1x6-
Dimazole	T49.0x1-	T49.0x2-	T49.0x3-	T49.0x4-	T49.0x5-	T49.0x6-
Dimefline	T50.7x1-	T50.7x2-	T50.7x3-	T50.7x4-	T50.7x5-	T50.7x6-
Dimefox	T60.0x1-	T60.0x2-	T60.0x3-	T60.0x4-	—	—
Dimemorfan	T48.3x1-	T48.3x2-	T48.3x3-	T48.3x4-	T48.3x5-	T48.3x6-
Dimenhydrinate	T45.0x1-	T45.0x2-	T45.0x3-	T45.0x4-	T45.0x5-	T45.0x6-
Dimercaprol (British anti-lewisite)	T45.8x1-	T45.8x2-	T45.8x3-	T45.8x4-	T45.8x5-	T45.8x6-
Dimercaptopropanol	T45.8x1-	T45.8x2-	T45.8x3-	T45.8x4-	T45.8x5-	T45.8x6-
Dimestrol	T38.5x1-	T38.5x2-	T38.5x3-	T38.5x4-	T38.5x5-	T38.5x6-
Dimetane	T45.0x1-	T45.0x2-	T45.0x3-	T45.0x4-	T45.0x5-	T45.0x6-
Dimethicone	T47.1x1-	T47.1x2-	T47.1x3-	T47.1x4-	T47.1x5-	T47.1x6-
Dimethindene	T45.0x1-	T45.0x2-	T45.0x3-	T45.0x4-	T45.0x5-	T45.0x6-
Dimethisoquin	T49.1x1-	T49.1x2-	T49.1x3-	T49.1x4-	T49.1x5-	T49.1x6-
Dimethisterone	T38.5x1-	T38.5x2-	T38.5x3-	T38.5x4-	T38.5x5-	T38.5x6-
Dimethoate	T60.0x1-	T60.0x2-	T60.0x3-	T60.0x4-	—	—
Dimethocaine	T41.3x1-	T41.3x2-	T41.3x3-	T41.3x4-	T41.3x5-	T41.3x6-
Dimethoxanate	T48.3x1-	T48.3x2-	T48.3x3-	T48.3x4-	T48.3x5-	T48.3x6-
Dimethyl arsine, arsinic acid	T57.0x1-	T57.0x2-	T57.0x3-	T57.0x4-	—	—
carbinol	T51.2x1-	T51.2x2-	T51.2x3-	T51.2x4-	—	—
carbonate	T52.8x1-	T52.8x2-	T52.8x3-	T52.8x4-	—	—
diguanide	T38.3x1-	T38.3x2-	T38.3x3-	T38.3x4-	T38.3x5-	T38.3x6-
ketone	T52.4x1-	T52.4x2-	T52.4x3-	T52.4x4-	—	—
vapor	T52.4x1-	T52.4x2-	T52.4x3-	T52.4x4-	—	—
meperidine	T40.2x1-	T40.2x2-	T40.2x3-	T40.2x4-	T40.2x5-	T40.2x6-
parathion	T60.0x1-	T60.0x2-	T60.0x3-	T60.0x4-	—	—
phthlate	T49.3x1-	T49.3x2-	T49.3x3-	T49.3x4-	T49.3x5-	T49.3x6-
polysiloxane	T47.8x1-	T47.8x2-	T47.8x3-	T47.8x4-	T47.8x5-	T47.8x6-
sulfate (fumes)	T59.891-	T59.892-	T59.893-	T59.894-	—	—
liquid	T65.891-	T65.892-	T65.893-	T65.894-	—	—
sulfoxide (nonmedicinal)	T52.8x1-	T52.8x2-	T52.8x3-	T52.8x4-	—	—
medicinal	T49.4x1-	T49.4x2-	T49.4x3-	T49.4x4-	T49.4x5-	T49.4x6-
tryptamine	T40.991-	T40.992-	T40.993-	T40.994-	—	—
tubocurarine	T48.1x1-	T48.1x2-	T48.1x3-	T48.1x4-	T48.1x5-	T48.1x6-
Dimethylamine sulfate	T49.4x1-	T49.4x2-	T49.4x3-	T49.4x4-	T49.4x5-	T49.4x6-
Dimethylformamide	T52.8x1-	T52.8x2-	T52.8x3-	T52.8x4-	—	—
Dimethyltubocurarinium chloride	T48.1x1-	T48.1x2-	T48.1x3-	T48.1x4-	T48.1x5-	T48.1x6-

Table of Drugs & Chemicals	POISONING Accidental (Unintentional)	Self-Harm (Intentional)	Assault	Undetermined	Adverse Effect	Underdosing
Dimeticone	T47.1x1-	T47.1x2-	T47.1x3-	T47.1x4-	T47.1x5-	T47.1x6-
Dimetilan	T60.0x1-	T60.0x2-	T60.0x3-	T60.0x4-	—	—
Dimetindene	T45.0x1-	T45.0x2-	T45.0x3-	T45.0x4-	T45.0x5-	T45.0x6-
Dimetotiazine	T43.3x1-	T43.3x2-	T43.3x3-	T43.3x4-	T43.3x5-	T43.3x6-
Dimorpholamine	T50.7x1-	T50.7x2-	T50.7x3-	T50.7x4-	T50.7x5-	T50.7x6-
Dimoxyline	T46.3x1-	T46.3x2-	T46.3x3-	T46.3x4-	T46.3x5-	T46.3x6-
Dinitro (-ortho-)cresol (pesticide) (spray)	T65.3x1-	T65.3x2-	T65.3x3-	T65.3x4-	—	—
Dinitrobenzene	T65.3x1-	T65.3x2-	T65.3x3-	T65.3x4-	—	—
vapor	T59.891-	T59.892-	T59.893-	T59.894-	—	—
Dinitrobenzol	T65.3x1-	T65.3x2-	T65.3x3-	T65.3x4-	—	—
vapor	T59.891-	T59.892-	T59.893-	T59.894-	—	—
Dinitrobutylphenol	T65.3x1-	T65.3x2-	T65.3x3-	T65.3x4-	—	—
Dinitrocyclohexylphenol	T65.3x1-	T65.3x2-	T65.3x3-	T65.3x4-	—	—
Dinitrophenol	T65.3x1-	T65.3x2-	T65.3x3-	T65.3x4-	—	—
Dinoprost	T48.0x1-	T48.0x2-	T48.0x3-	T48.0x4-	T48.0x5-	T48.0x6-
Dinoprostone	T48.0x1-	T48.0x2-	T48.0x3-	T48.0x4-	T48.0x5-	T48.0x6-
Dinoseb	T60.3x1-	T60.3x2-	T60.3x3-	T60.3x4-	—	—
Dioctyl sulfosuccinate (calcium) (sodium)	T47.4x1-	T47.4x2-	T47.4x3-	T47.4x4-	T47.4x5-	T47.4x6-
Diodone	T50.8x1-	T50.8x2-	T50.8x3-	T50.8x4-	T50.8x5-	T50.8x6-
Diodoquin	T37.8x1-	T37.8x2-	T37.8x3-	T37.8x4-	T37.8x5-	T37.8x6-
Dionin	T40.2x1-	T40.2x2-	T40.2x3-	T40.2x4-	T40.2x5-	T40.2x6-
Diosmin	T46.991-	T46.992-	T46.993-	T46.994-	T46.995-	T46.996-
Dioxane	T52.8x1-	T52.8x2-	T52.8x3-	T52.8x4-	—	—
Dioxathion	T60.0x1-	T60.0x2-	T60.0x3-	T60.0x4-	—	—
Dioxin	T53.7x1-	T53.7x2-	T53.7x3-	T53.7x4-	—	—
Dioxopromethazine	T43.3x1-	T43.3x2-	T43.3x3-	T43.3x4-	T43.3x5-	T43.3x6-
Dioxyline	T46.3x1-	T46.3x2-	T46.3x3-	T46.3x4-	T46.3x5-	T46.3x6-
Dipentene	T52.8x1-	T52.8x2-	T52.8x3-	T52.8x4-	—	—
Diperodon	T41.3x1-	T41.3x2-	T41.3x3-	T41.3x4-	T41.3x5-	T41.3x6-
Diphacinone	T60.4x1-	T60.4x2-	T60.4x3-	T60.4x4-	—	—
Diphemanil	T44.3x1-	T44.3x2-	T44.3x3-	T44.3x4-	T44.3x5-	T44.3x6-
metilsulfate	T44.3x1-	T44.3x2-	T44.3x3-	T44.3x4-	T44.3x5-	T44.3x6-
Diphenadione	T45.511-	T45.512-	T45.513-	T45.514-	T45.515-	T45.516-
rodenticide	T60.4x1-	T60.4x2-	T60.4x3-	T60.4x4-	—	—
Diphenhydramine	T45.0x1-	T45.0x2-	T45.0x3-	T45.0x4-	T45.0x5-	T45.0x6-
Diphenidol	T45.0x1-	T45.0x2-	T45.0x3-	T45.0x4-	T45.0x5-	T45.0x6-
Diphenoxylate	T47.6x1-	T47.6x2-	T47.6x3-	T47.6x4-	T47.6x5-	T47.6x6-
Diphenylamine	T65.3x1-	T65.3x2-	T65.3x3-	T65.3x4-	—	—
Diphenylbutazone	T39.2x1-	T39.2x2-	T39.2x3-	T39.2x4-	T39.2x5-	T39.2x6-
Diphenylchloroarsine, not in war	T57.0x1-	T57.0x2-	T57.0x3-	T57.0x4-	—	—
Diphenylhydantoin	T42.0x1-	T42.0x2-	T42.0x3-	T42.0x4-	T42.0x5-	T42.0x6-
Diphenylmethane dye	T52.1x1-	T52.1x2-	T52.1x3-	T52.1x4-	—	—
Diphenylpyraline	T45.0x1-	T45.0x2-	T45.0x3-	T45.0x4-	T45.0x5-	T45.0x6-
Diphtheria antitoxin	T50.Z11-	T50.Z12-	T50.Z13-	T50.Z14-	T50.Z15-	T50.Z16-
toxoid	T50.A91-	T50.A92-	T50.A93-	T50.A94-	T50.A95-	T50.A96-
with tetanus toxoid	T50.A21-	T50.A22-	T50.A23-	T50.A24-	T50.A25-	T50.A26-
with pertussis component	T50.A11-	T50.A12-	T50.A13-	T50.A14-	T50.A15-	T50.A16-
vaccine	T50.A91-	T50.A92-	T50.A93-	T50.A94-	T50.A95-	T50.A96-
combination including pertussis	T50.A11-	T50.A12-	T50.A13-	T50.A14-	T50.A15-	T50.A16-
without pertussis	T50.A21-	T50.A22-	T50.A23-	T50.A24-	T50.A25-	T50.A26-
Diphylline	T50.2x1-	T50.2x2-	T50.2x3-	T50.2x4-	T50.2x5-	T50.2x6-
Dipipanone	T40.4x1-	T40.4x2-	T40.4x3-	T40.4x4-	—	—
Dipivefrine	T49.5x1-	T49.5x2-	T49.5x3-	T49.5x4-	T49.5x5-	T49.5x6-
Diplovax	T50.B91-	T50.B92-	T50.B93-	T50.B94-	T50.B95-	T50.B96-
Diprophylline	T50.2x1-	T50.2x2-	T50.2x3-	T50.2x4-	T50.2x5-	T50.2x6-
Dipropyline	T48.291-	T48.292-	T48.293-	T48.294-	T48.295-	T48.296-
Dipyridamole	T46.3x1-	T46.3x2-	T46.3x3-	T46.3x4-	T46.3x5-	T46.3x6-
Dipyrone	T39.2x1-	T39.2x2-	T39.2x3-	T39.2x4-	T39.2x5-	T39.2x6-

430

DRUGS & CHEMICALS

Table of Drugs & Chemicals	POISONING Accidental (Unintentional)	Self-Harm (Intentional)	Assault	Undetermined	Adverse Effect	Underdosing
Diquat (dibromide)	T60.3x1-	T60.3x2-	T60.3x3-	T60.3x4-	—	—
Disinfectant	T65.891-	T65.892-	T65.893-	T65.894-	—	—
alkaline	T54.3x1-	T54.3x2-	T54.3x3-	T54.3x4-	—	—
aromatic	T54.1x1-	T54.1x2-	T54.1x3-	T54.1x4-	—	—
intestinal	T37.8x1-	T37.8x2-	T37.8x3-	T37.8x4-	T37.8x5-	T37.8x6-
Disipal	T42.8x1-	T42.8x2-	T42.8x3-	T42.8x4-	T42.8x5-	T42.8x6-
Disodium edetate	T50.6x1-	T50.6x2-	T50.6x3-	T50.6x4-	T50.6x5-	T50.6x6-
Disoprofol	T41.291-	T41.292-	T41.293-	T41.294-	T41.295-	T41.296-
Distigmine (bromide)	T44.0x1-	T44.0x2-	T44.0x3-	T44.0x4-	T44.0x5-	T44.0x6-
Disulfamide	T50.2x1-	T50.2x2-	T50.2x3-	T50.2x4-	T50.2x5-	T50.2x6-
Disulfanilamide	T37.0x1-	T37.0x2-	T37.0x3-	T37.0x4-	T37.0x5-	T37.0x6-
Disulfiram	T50.6x1-	T50.6x2-	T50.6x3-	T50.6x4-	T50.6x5-	T50.6x6-
Disulfoton	T60.0x1-	T60.0x2-	T60.0x3-	T60.0x4-	—	—
Dithiazanine iodide	T37.4x1-	T37.4x2-	T37.4x3-	T37.4x4-	T37.4x5-	T37.4x6-
Dithiocarbamate	T60.0x1-	T60.0x2-	T60.0x3-	T60.0x4-	—	—
Dithranol	T49.4x1-	T49.4x2-	T49.4x3-	T49.4x4-	T49.4x5-	T49.4x6-
Diucardin	T50.2x1-	T50.2x2-	T50.2x3-	T50.2x4-	T50.2x5-	T50.2x6-
Diupres	T50.2x1-	T50.2x2-	T50.2x3-	T50.2x4-	T50.2x5-	T50.2x6-
Diuretic NEC	T50.2x1-	T50.2x2-	T50.2x3-	T50.2x4-	T50.2x5-	T50.2x6-
benzothiadiazine	T50.2x1-	T50.2x2-	T50.2x3-	T50.2x4-	T50.2x5-	T50.2x6-
carbonic acid anhydrase inhibitors	T50.2x1-	T50.2x2-	T50.2x3-	T50.2x4-	T50.2x5-	T50.2x6-
furfuryl NEC	T50.2x1-	T50.2x2-	T50.2x3-	T50.2x4-	T50.2x5-	T50.2x6-
loop (high-ceiling)	T50.1x1-	T50.1x2-	T50.1x3-	T50.1x4-	T50.1x5-	T50.1x6-
mercurial NEC	T50.2x1-	T50.2x2-	T50.2x3-	T50.2x4-	T50.2x5-	T50.2x6-
osmotic	T50.2x1-	T50.2x2-	T50.2x3-	T50.2x4-	T50.2x5-	T50.2x6-
purine NEC	T50.2x1-	T50.2x2-	T50.2x3-	T50.2x4-	T50.2x5-	T50.2x6-
saluretic NEC	T50.2x1-	T50.2x2-	T50.2x3-	T50.2x4-	T50.2x5-	T50.2x6-
sulfonamide	T50.2x1-	T50.2x2-	T50.2x3-	T50.2x4-	T50.2x5-	T50.2x6-
thiazide NEC	T50.2x1-	T50.2x2-	T50.2x3-	T50.2x4-	T50.2x5-	T50.2x6-
xanthine	T50.2x1-	T50.2x2-	T50.2x3-	T50.2x4-	T50.2x5-	T50.2x6-
Diurgin	T50.2x1-	T50.2x2-	T50.2x3-	T50.2x4-	T50.2x5-	T50.2x6-
Diuril	T50.2x1-	T50.2x2-	T50.2x3-	T50.2x4-	T50.2x5-	T50.2x6-
Diuron	T60.3x1-	T60.3x2-	T60.3x3-	T60.3x4-	—	—
Divalproex	T42.6x1-	T42.6x2-	T42.6x3-	T42.6x4-	T42.6x5-	T42.6x6-
Divinyl ether	T41.0x1-	T41.0x2-	T41.0x3-	T41.0x4-	T41.0x5-	T41.0x6-
Dixanthogen	T49.0x1-	T49.0x2-	T49.0x3-	T49.0x4-	T49.0x5-	T49.0x6-
Dixyrazine	T43.3x1-	T43.3x2-	T43.3x3-	T43.3x4-	T43.3x5-	T43.3x6-
D-lysergic acid diethylamide	T40.8x1-	T40.8x2-	T40.8x3-	T40.8x4-	—	—
DMCT	T36.4x1-	T36.4x2-	T36.4x3-	T36.4x4-	T36.4x5-	T36.4x6-
DMSO — see Dimethyl sulfoxide						
DNBP	T60.3x1-	T60.3x2-	T60.3x3-	T60.3x4-	—	—
DNOC	T65.3x1-	T65.3x2-	T65.3x3-	T65.3x4-	—	—
Dobutamine	T44.5x1-	T44.5x2-	T44.5x3-	T44.5x4-	T44.5x5-	T44.5x6-
DOCA	T38.0x1-	T38.0x2-	T38.0x3-	T38.0x4-	T38.0x5-	T38.0x6-
Docusate sodium	T47.4x1-	T47.4x2-	T47.4x3-	T47.4x4-	T47.4x5-	T47.4x6-
Dodicin	T49.0x1-	T49.0x2-	T49.0x3-	T49.0x4-	T49.0x5-	T49.0x6-
Dofamium chloride	T49.0x1-	T49.0x2-	T49.0x3-	T49.0x4-	T49.0x5-	T49.0x6-
Dolophine	T40.3x1-	T40.3x2-	T40.3x3-	T40.3x4-	T40.3x5-	T40.3x6-
Doloxene	T39.8x1-	T39.8x2-	T39.8x3-	T39.8x4-	T39.8x5-	T39.8x6-
Domestic gas (after combustion) — see Gas, utility						
prior to combustion	T59.891-	T59.892-	T59.893-	T59.894-	—	—
Domiodol	T48.4x1-	T48.4x2-	T48.4x3-	T48.4x4-	T48.4x5-	T48.4x6-
Domiphen (bromide)	T49.0x1-	T49.0x2-	T49.0x3-	T49.0x4-	T49.0x5-	T49.0x6-
Domperidone	T45.0x1-	T45.0x2-	T45.0x3-	T45.0x4-	T45.0x5-	T45.0x6-
Dopa	T42.8x1-	T42.8x2-	T42.8x3-	T42.8x4-	T42.8x5-	T42.8x6-
Dopamine	T44.991-	T44.992-	T44.993-	T44.994-	T44.995-	T44.996-
Doriden	T42.6x1-	T42.6x2-	T42.6x3-	T42.6x4-	T42.6x5-	T42.6x6-

Table of Drugs & Chemicals	POISONING Accidental (Unintentional)	Self-Harm (Intentional)	Assault	Undetermined	Adverse Effect	Underdosing
Dormiral	T42.3x1-	T42.3x2-	T42.3x3-	T42.3x4-	T42.3x5-	T42.3x6-
Dormison	T42.6x1-	T42.6x2-	T42.6x3-	T42.6x4-	T42.6x5-	T42.6x6-
Dornase	T48.4x1-	T48.4x2-	T48.4x3-	T48.4x4-	T48.4x5-	T48.4x6-
Dorsacaine	T41.3x1-	T41.3x2-	T41.3x3-	T41.3x4-	T41.3x5-	T41.3x6-
Dosulepin	T43.011-	T43.012-	T43.013-	T43.014-	T43.015-	T43.016-
Dothiepin	T43.011-	T43.012-	T43.013-	T43.014-	T43.015-	T43.016-
Doxantrazole	T48.6x1-	T48.6x2-	T48.6x3-	T48.6x4-	T48.6x5-	T48.6x6-
Doxapram	T50.7x1-	T50.7x2-	T50.7x3-	T50.7x4-	T50.7x5-	T50.7x6-
Doxazosin	T44.6x1-	T44.6x2-	T44.6x3-	T44.6x4-	T44.6x5-	T44.6x6-
Doxepin	T43.011-	T43.012-	T43.013-	T43.014-	T43.015-	T43.016-
Doxifluridine	T45.1x1-	T45.1x2-	T45.1x3-	T45.1x4-	T45.1x5-	T45.1x6-
Doxorubicin	T45.1x1-	T45.1x2-	T45.1x3-	T45.1x4-	T45.1x5-	T45.1x6-
Doxycycline	T36.4x1-	T36.4x2-	T36.4x3-	T36.4x4-	T36.4x5-	T36.4x6-
Doxylamine	T45.0x1-	T45.0x2-	T45.0x3-	T45.0x4-	T45.0x5-	T45.0x6-
Dramamine	T45.0x1-	T45.0x2-	T45.0x3-	T45.0x4-	T45.0x5-	T45.0x6-
Drano (drain cleaner)	T54.3x1-	T54.3x2-	T54.3x3-	T54.3x4-	—	—
Dressing, live pulp	T49.7x1-	T49.7x2-	T49.7x3-	T49.7x4-	T49.7x5-	T49.7x6-
Drocode	T40.2x1-	T40.2x2-	T40.2x3-	T40.2x4-	T40.2x5-	T40.2x6-
Dromoran	T40.2x1-	T40.2x2-	T40.2x3-	T40.2x4-	T40.2x5-	T40.2x6-
Dromostanolone	T38.7x1-	T38.7x2-	T38.7x3-	T38.7x4-	T38.7x5-	T38.7x6-
Dronabinol	T40.7x1-	T40.7x2-	T40.7x3-	T40.7x4-	T40.7x5-	T40.7x6-
Droperidol	T43.591-	T43.592-	T43.593-	T43.594-	T43.595-	T43.596-
Dropropizine	T48.3x1-	T48.3x2-	T48.3x3-	T48.3x4-	T48.3x5-	T48.3x6-
Drostanolone	T38.7x1-	T38.7x2-	T38.7x3-	T38.7x4-	T38.7x5-	T38.7x6-
Drotaverine	T44.3x1-	T44.3x2-	T44.3x3-	T44.3x4-	T44.3x5-	T44.3x6-
Drotrecogin alfa	T45.511-	T45.512-	T45.513-	T45.514-	T45.515-	T45.516-
Drug NEC	T50.901-	T50.902-	T50.903-	T50.904-	T50.905-	T50.906-
specified NEC	T50.991-	T50.992-	T50.993-	T50.994-	T50.995-	T50.996-
DTIC	T45.1x1-	T45.1x2-	T45.1x3-	T45.1x4-	T45.1x5-	T45.1x6-
Duboisine	T44.3x1-	T44.3x2-	T44.3x3-	T44.3x4-	T44.3x5-	T44.3x6-
Dulcolax	T47.2x1-	T47.2x2-	T47.2x3-	T47.2x4-	T47.2x5-	T47.2x6-
Duponol (C) (EP)	T49.2x1-	T49.2x2-	T49.2x3-	T49.2x4-	T49.2x5-	T49.2x6-
Durabolin	T38.7x1-	T38.7x2-	T38.7x3-	T38.7x4-	T38.7x5-	T38.7x6-
Dyclone	T41.3x1-	T41.3x2-	T41.3x3-	T41.3x4-	T41.3x5-	T41.3x6-
Dyclonine	T41.3x1-	T41.3x2-	T41.3x3-	T41.3x4-	T41.3x5-	T41.3x6-
Dydrogesterone	T38.5x1-	T38.5x2-	T38.5x3-	T38.5x4-	T38.5x5-	T38.5x6-
Dye NEC	T65.6x1-	T65.6x2-	T65.6x3-	T65.6x4-	—	—
antiseptic	T49.0x1-	T49.0x2-	T49.0x3-	T49.0x4-	T49.0x5-	T49.0x6-
diagnostic agents	T50.8x1-	T50.8x2-	T50.8x3-	T50.8x4-	T50.8x5-	T50.8x6-
pharmaceutical NEC	T50.901-	T50.902-	T50.903-	T50.904-	T50.905-	T50.906-
Dyflos	T44.0x1-	T44.0x2-	T44.0x3-	T44.0x4-	T44.0x5-	T44.0x6-
Dymelor	T38.3x1-	T38.3x2-	T38.3x3-	T38.3x4-	T38.3x5-	T38.3x6-
Dynamite	T65.3x1-	T65.3x2-	T65.3x3-	T65.3x4-	—	—
fumes	T59.891-	T59.892-	T59.893-	T59.894-	—	—
Dyphylline	T44.3x1-	T44.3x2-	T44.3x3-	T44.3x4-	T44.3x5-	T44.3x6-
Ear drug NEC	T49.6x1-	T49.6x2-	T49.6x3-	T49.6x4-	T49.6x5-	T49.6x6-
Ear preparations	T49.6x1-	T49.6x2-	T49.6x3-	T49.6x4-	T49.6x5-	T49.6x6-
Echothiophate, echothiopate, ecothiopate	T49.5x1-	T49.5x2-	T49.5x3-	T49.5x4-	T49.5x5-	T49.5x6-
Econazole	T49.0x1-	T49.0x2-	T49.0x3-	T49.0x4-	T49.0x5-	T49.0x6-
Ecothiopate iodide	T49.5x1-	T49.5x2-	T49.5x3-	T49.5x4-	T49.5x5-	T49.5x6-
Ecstasy	T43.621-	T43.622-	T43.623-	T43.624-	T43.625-	T43.626-
Ectylurea	T42.6x1-	T42.6x2-	T42.6x3-	T42.6x4-	T42.6x5-	T42.6x6-
Edathamil disodium	T45.8x1-	T45.8x2-	T45.8x3-	T45.8x4-	T45.8x5-	T45.8x6-
Edecrin	T50.1x1-	T50.1x2-	T50.1x3-	T50.1x4-	T50.1x5-	T50.1x6-
Edetate, disodium (calcium)	T45.8x1-	T45.8x2-	T45.8x3-	T45.8x4-	T45.8x5-	T45.8x6-
Edoxudine	T49.5x1-	T49.5x2-	T49.5x3-	T49.5x4-	T49.5x5-	T49.5x6-
Edrophonium chloride	T44.0x1-	T44.0x2-	T44.0x3-	T44.0x4-	T44.0x5-	T44.0x6-
EDTA	T50.6x1-	T50.6x2-	T50.6x3-	T50.6x4-	T50.6x5-	T50.6x6-
Eflornithine	T37.2x1-	T37.2x2-	T37.2x3-	T37.2x4-	T37.2x5-	T37.2x6-
Efloxate	T46.3x1-	T46.3x2-	T46.3x3-	T46.3x4-	T46.3x5-	T46.3x6-

DRUGS & CHEMICALS

Table of Drugs & Chemicals	POISONING Accidental (Unintentional)	Self-Harm (Intentional)	Assault	Undetermined	Adverse Effect	Underdosing
Elase	T49.8x1-	T49.8x2-	T49.8x3-	T49.8x4-	T49.8x5-	T49.8x6-
Elastase	T47.5x1-	T47.5x2-	T47.5x3-	T47.5x4-	T47.5x5-	T47.5x6-
Elaterium	T47.2x1-	T47.2x2-	T47.2x3-	T47.2x4-	T47.2x5-	T47.2x6-
Elcatonin	T50.991	T50.992	T50.993	T50.994	T50.995	T50.996
Elder	T62.2x1-	T62.2x2-	T62.2x3-	T62.2x4-	—	—
berry, (unripe)	T62.1x1-	T62.1x2-	T62.1x3-	T62.1x4-	—	—
Electrolyte balance drug	T50.3x1-	T50.3x2-	T50.3x3-	T50.3x4-	T50.3x5-	T50.3x6-
Electrolytes NEC	T50.3x1-	T50.3x2-	T50.3x3-	T50.3x4-	T50.3x5-	T50.3x6-
Electrolytic agent NEC	T50.3x1-	T50.3x2-	T50.3x3-	T50.3x4-	T50.3x5-	T50.3x6-
Elemental diet	T50.901	T50.902	T50.903	T50.904	T50.905	T50.906
Elliptinium acetate	T45.1x1-	T45.1x2-	T45.1x3-	T45.1x4-	T45.1x5-	T45.1x6-
Embramine	T45.0x1-	T45.0x2-	T45.0x3-	T45.0x4-	T45.0x5-	T45.0x6-
Emepronium (salts)	T44.3x1-	T44.3x2-	T44.3x3-	T44.3x4-	T44.3x5-	T44.3x6-
bromide	T44.3x1-	T44.3x2-	T44.3x3-	T44.3x4-	T44.3x5-	T44.3x6-
Emetic NEC	T47.7x1-	T47.7x2-	T47.7x3-	T47.7x4-	T47.7x5-	T47.7x6-
Emetine	T37.3x1-	T37.3x2-	T37.3x3-	T37.3x4-	T37.3x5-	T37.3x6-
Emollient NEC	T49.3x1-	T49.3x2-	T49.3x3-	T49.3x4-	T49.3x5-	T49.3x6-
Emorfazone	T39.8x1-	T39.8x2-	T39.8x3-	T39.8x4-	T39.8x5-	T39.8x6-
Emylcamate	T43.591	T43.592	T43.593	T43.594	T43.595	T43.596
Enalapril	T46.4x1-	T46.4x2-	T46.4x3-	T46.4x4-	T46.4x5-	T46.4x6-
Enalaprilat	T46.4x1-	T46.4x2-	T46.4x3-	T46.4x4-	T46.4x5-	T46.4x6-
Encainide	T46.2x1-	T46.2x2-	T46.2x3-	T46.2x4-	T46.2x5-	T46.2x6-
Endocaine	T41.3x1-	T41.3x2-	T41.3x3-	T41.3x4-	T41.3x5-	T41.3x6-
Endosulfan	T60.2x1-	T60.2x2-	T60.2x3-	T60.2x4-	—	—
Endothall	T60.3x1-	T60.3x2-	T60.3x3-	T60.3x4-	—	—
Endralazine	T46.5x1-	T46.5x2-	T46.5x3-	T46.5x4-	T46.5x5-	T46.5x6-
Endrin	T60.1x1-	T60.1x2-	T60.1x3-	T60.1x4-	—	—
Enflurane	T41.0x1-	T41.0x2-	T41.0x3-	T41.0x4-	T41.0x5-	T41.0x6-
Enhexymal	T42.3x1-	T42.3x2-	T42.3x3-	T42.3x4-	T42.3x5-	T42.3x6-
Enocitabine	T45.1x1-	T45.1x2-	T45.1x3-	T45.1x4-	T45.1x5-	T45.1x6-
Enovid	T38.4x1-	T38.4x2-	T38.4x3-	T38.4x4-	T38.4x5-	T38.4x6-
Enoxacin	T36.8x1-	T36.8x2-	T36.8x3-	T36.8x4-	T36.8x5-	T36.8x6-
Enoxaparin (sodium)	T45.511	T45.512	T45.513	T45.514	T45.515	T45.516
Enpiprazole	T43.591	T43.592	T43.593	T43.594	T43.595	T43.596
Enprofylline	T48.6x1-	T48.6x2-	T48.6x3-	T48.6x4-	T48.6x5-	T48.6x6-
Enprostil	T47.1x1-	T47.1x2-	T47.1x3-	T47.1x4-	T47.1x5-	T47.1x6-
ENT preparations (anti-infectives)	T49.6x1-	T49.6x2-	T49.6x3-	T49.6x4-	T49.6x5-	T49.6x6-
Enterogastrone	T38.891	T38.892	T38.893	T38.894	T38.895	T38.896
Enviomycin	T36.8x1-	T36.8x2-	T36.8x3-	T36.8x4-	T36.8x5-	T36.8x6-
Enzodase	T45.3x1-	T45.3x2-	T45.3x3-	T45.3x4-	T45.3x5-	T45.3x6-
Enzyme NEC	T45.3x1-	T45.3x2-	T45.3x3-	T45.3x4-	T45.3x5-	T45.3x6-
depolymerizing	T49.8x1-	T49.8x2-	T49.8x3-	T49.8x4-	T49.8x5-	T49.8x6-
fibrolytic	T45.3x1-	T45.3x2-	T45.3x3-	T45.3x4-	T45.3x5-	T45.3x6-
gastric	T47.5x1-	T47.5x2-	T47.5x3-	T47.5x4-	T47.5x5-	T47.5x6-
intestinal	T47.5x1-	T47.5x2-	T47.5x3-	T47.5x4-	T47.5x5-	T47.5x6-
local action	T49.4x1-	T49.4x2-	T49.4x3-	T49.4x4-	T49.4x5-	T49.4x6-
proteolytic	T49.4x1-	T49.4x2-	T49.4x3-	T49.4x4-	T49.4x5-	T49.4x6-
thrombolytic	T45.3x1-	T45.3x2-	T45.3x3-	T45.3x4-	T45.3x5-	T45.3x6-
EPAB	T41.3x1-	T41.3x2-	T41.3x3-	T41.3x4-	T41.3x5-	T41.3x6-
Epanutin	T42.0x1-	T42.0x2-	T42.0x3-	T42.0x4-	T42.0x5-	T42.0x6-
Ephedra	T44.991	T44.992	T44.993	T44.994	T44.995	T44.996
Ephedrine	T44.991	T44.992	T44.993	T44.994	T44.995	T44.996
Epichlorhydrin, epichlorohydrin	T52.8x1-	T52.8x2-	T52.8x3-	T52.8x4-	—	—
Epicillin	T36.0x1-	T36.0x2-	T36.0x3-	T36.0x4-	T36.0x5-	T36.0x6-
Epiestriol	T38.5x1-	T38.5x2-	T38.5x3-	T38.5x4-	T38.5x5-	T38.5x6-
Epilim — see Sodium valproate						
Epimestrol	T38.5x1-	T38.5x2-	T38.5x3-	T38.5x4-	T38.5x5-	T38.5x6-
Epinephrine	T44.5x1-	T44.5x2-	T44.5x3-	T44.5x4-	T44.5x5-	T44.5x6-
Epirubicin	T45.1x1-	T45.1x2-	T45.1x3-	T45.1x4-	T45.1x5-	T45.1x6-

Table of Drugs & Chemicals	POISONING Accidental (Unintentional)	Self-Harm (Intentional)	Assault	Undetermined	Adverse Effect	Underdosing
Epitiostanol	T38.7x1-	T38.7x2-	T38.7x3-	T38.7x4-	T38.7x5-	T38.7x6-
Epitizide	T50.2x1-	T50.2x2-	T50.2x3-	T50.2x4-	T50.2x5-	T50.2x6-
EPN	T60.0x1-	T60.0x2-	T60.0x3-	T60.0x4-	—	—
EPO	T45.8x1-	T45.8x2-	T45.8x3-	T45.8x4-	T45.8x5-	T45.8x6-
Epoetin alpha	T45.8x1-	T45.8x2-	T45.8x3-	T45.8x4-	T45.8x5-	T45.8x6-
Epomediol	T50.991	T50.992	T50.993	T50.994	T50.995	T50.996
Epoprostenol	T45.521	T45.522	T45.523	T45.524	T45.525	T45.526
Epoxy resin	T65.891	T65.892	T65.893	T65.894	—	—
Eprazinone	T48.4x1-	T48.4x2-	T48.4x3-	T48.4x4-	T48.4x5-	T48.4x6-
Epsilon amino-caproic acid	T45.621	T45.622	T45.623	T45.624	T45.625	T45.626
Epsom salt	T47.3x1-	T47.3x2-	T47.3x3-	T47.3x4-	T47.3x5-	T47.3x6-
Eptazocine	T40.4x1-	T40.4x2-	T40.4x3-	T40.4x4-	T40.4x5-	T40.4x6-
Equanil	T43.591	T43.592	T43.593	T43.594	T43.595	T43.596
Equisetum	T62.2x1-	T62.2x2-	T62.2x3-	T62.2x4-	—	—
diuretic	T50.2x1-	T50.2x2-	T50.2x3-	T50.2x4-	T50.2x5-	T50.2x6-
Ergobasine	T48.0x1-	T48.0x2-	T48.0x3-	T48.0x4-	T48.0x5-	T48.0x6-
Ergocalciferol	T45.2x1-	T45.2x2-	T45.2x3-	T45.2x4-	T45.2x5-	T45.2x6-
Ergoloid mesylates	T46.7x1-	T46.7x2-	T46.7x3-	T46.7x4-	T46.7x5-	T46.7x6-
Ergometrine	T48.0x1-	T48.0x2-	T48.0x3-	T48.0x4-	T48.0x5-	T48.0x6-
Ergonovine	T48.0x1-	T48.0x2-	T48.0x3-	T48.0x4-	T48.0x5-	T48.0x6-
Ergot NEC	T64.81x-	T64.82x-	T64.83x-	T64.84x-	—	—
derivative	T48.0x1-	T48.0x2-	T48.0x3-	T48.0x4-	T48.0x5-	T48.0x6-
medicinal (alkaloids)	T48.0x1-	T48.0x2-	T48.0x3-	T48.0x4-	T48.0x5-	T48.0x6-
prepared	T48.0x1-	T48.0x2-	T48.0x3-	T48.0x4-	T48.0x5-	T48.0x6-
Ergotamine	T46.5x1-	T46.5x2-	T46.5x3-	T46.5x4-	T46.5x5-	T46.5x6-
Ergotocine	T48.0x1-	T48.0x2-	T48.0x3-	T48.0x4-	T48.0x5-	T48.0x6-
Ergotrate	T48.0x1-	T48.0x2-	T48.0x3-	T48.0x4-	T48.0x5-	T48.0x6-
Eritrityl tetranitrate	T46.3x1-	T46.3x2-	T46.3x3-	T46.3x4-	T46.3x5-	T46.3x6-
Erythrityl tetranitrate	T46.3x1-	T46.3x2-	T46.3x3-	T46.3x4-	T46.3x5-	T46.3x6-
Erythrol tetranitrate	T46.3x1-	T46.3x2-	T46.3x3-	T46.3x4-	T46.3x5-	T46.3x6-
Erythromycin (salts)	T36.3x1-	T36.3x2-	T36.3x3-	T36.3x4-	T36.3x5-	T36.3x6-
ophthalmic preparation	T49.5x1-	T49.5x2-	T49.5x3-	T49.5x4-	T49.5x5-	T49.5x6-
topical NEC	T49.0x1-	T49.0x2-	T49.0x3-	T49.0x4-	T49.0x5-	T49.0x6-
Erythropoietin	T45.8x1-	T45.8x2-	T45.8x3-	T45.8x4-	T45.8x5-	T45.8x6-
human	T45.8x1-	T45.8x2-	T45.8x3-	T45.8x4-	T45.8x5-	T45.8x6-
Escin	T46.991	T46.992	T46.993	T46.994	T46.995	T46.996
Esculin	T45.2x1-	T45.2x2-	T45.2x3-	T45.2x4-	T45.2x5-	T45.2x6-
Esculoside	T45.2x1-	T45.2x2-	T45.2x3-	T45.2x4-	T45.2x5-	T45.2x6-
ESDT (ether-soluble tar distillate)	T49.1x1-	T49.1x2-	T49.1x3-	T49.1x4-	T49.1x5-	T49.1x6-
Eserine	T49.5x1-	T49.5x2-	T49.5x3-	T49.5x4-	T49.5x5-	T49.5x6-
Esflurbiprofen	T39.311	T39.312	T39.313	T39.314	T39.315	T39.316
Eskabarb	T42.3x1-	T42.3x2-	T42.3x3-	T42.3x4-	T42.3x5-	T42.3x6-
Eskalith	T43.8x1-	T43.8x2-	T43.8x3-	T43.8x4-	T43.8x5-	T43.8x6-
Esmolol	T44.7x1-	T44.7x2-	T44.7x3-	T44.7x4-	T44.7x5-	T44.7x6-
Estanozolol	T38.7x1-	T38.7x2-	T38.7x3-	T38.7x4-	T38.7x5-	T38.7x6-
Estazolam	T42.4x1-	T42.4x2-	T42.4x3-	T42.4x4-	T42.4x5-	T42.4x6-
Estradiol	T38.5x1-	T38.5x2-	T38.5x3-	T38.5x4-	T38.5x5-	T38.5x6-
with testosterone	T38.7x1-	T38.7x2-	T38.7x3-	T38.7x4-	T38.7x5-	T38.7x6-
benzoate	T38.5x1-	T38.5x2-	T38.5x3-	T38.5x4-	T38.5x5-	T38.5x6-
Estramustine	T45.1x1-	T45.1x2-	T45.1x3-	T45.1x4-	T45.1x5-	T45.1x6-
Estriol	T38.5x1-	T38.5x2-	T38.5x3-	T38.5x4-	T38.5x5-	T38.5x6-
Estrogen	T38.5x1-	T38.5x2-	T38.5x3-	T38.5x4-	T38.5x5-	T38.5x6-
with progesterone	T38.5x1-	T38.5x2-	T38.5x3-	T38.5x4-	T38.5x5-	T38.5x6-
conjugated	T38.5x1-	T38.5x2-	T38.5x3-	T38.5x4-	T38.5x5-	T38.5x6-
Estrone	T38.5x1-	T38.5x2-	T38.5x3-	T38.5x4-	T38.5x5-	T38.5x6-
Estropipate	T38.5x1-	T38.5x2-	T38.5x3-	T38.5x4-	T38.5x5-	T38.5x6-
Etacrynate sodium	T50.1x1-	T50.1x2-	T50.1x3-	T50.1x4-	T50.1x5-	T50.1x6-
Etacrynic acid	T50.1x1-	T50.1x2-	T50.1x3-	T50.1x4-	T50.1x5-	T50.1x6-
Etafedrine	T48.6x1-	T48.6x2-	T48.6x3-	T48.6x4-	T48.6x5-	T48.6x6-
Etafenone	T46.3x1-	T46.3x2-	T46.3x3-	T46.3x4-	T46.3x5-	T46.3x6-
Etambutol	T37.1x1-	T37.1x2-	T37.1x3-	T37.1x4-	T37.1x5-	T37.1x6-

Table of Drugs & Chemicals	POISONING Accidental (Unintentional)	Self-Harm (Intentional)	Assault	Undetermined	Adverse Effect	Underdosing
Etamiphyllin	T48.6x1-	T48.6x2-	T48.6x3-	T48.6x4-	T48.6x5-	T48.6x6-
Etamivan	T50.7x1-	T50.7x2-	T50.7x3-	T50.7x4-	T50.7x5-	T50.7x6-
Etamsylate	T45.7x1-	T45.7x2-	T45.7x3-	T45.7x4-	T45.7x5-	T45.7x6-
Etebenecid	T50.4x1-	T50.4x2-	T50.4x3-	T50.4x4-	T50.4x5-	T50.4x6-
Ethacridine	T49.0x1-	T49.0x2-	T49.0x3-	T49.0x4-	T49.0x5-	T49.0x6-
Ethacrynic acid	T50.1x1-	T50.1x2-	T50.1x3-	T50.1x4-	T50.1x5-	T50.1x6-
Ethadione	T42.2x1-	T42.2x2-	T42.2x3-	T42.2x4-	T42.2x5-	T42.2x6-
Ethambutol	T37.1x1-	T37.1x2-	T37.1x3-	T37.1x4-	T37.1x5-	T37.1x6-
Ethamide	T50.2x1-	T50.2x2-	T50.2x3-	T50.2x4-	T50.2x5-	T50.2x6-
Ethamivan	T50.7x1-	T50.7x2-	T50.7x3-	T50.7x4-	T50.7x5-	T50.7x6-
Ethamsylate	T45.7x1-	T45.7x2-	T45.7x3-	T45.7x4-	T45.7x5-	
Ethanol	T51.0x1-	T51.0x2-	T51.0x3-	T51.0x4-	—	—
beverage	T51.0x1-	T51.0x2-	T51.0x3-	T51.0x4-	—	—
Ethanolamine oleate	T46.8x1-	T46.8x2-	T46.8x3-	T46.8x4-	T46.8x5-	T46.8x6-
Ethaverine	T44.3x1-	T44.3x2-	T44.3x3-	T44.3x4-	T44.3x5-	T44.3x6-
Ethchlorvynol	T42.6x1-	T42.6x2-	T42.6x3-	T42.6x4-	T42.6x5-	T42.6x6-
Ethebenecid	T50.4x1-	T50.4x2-	T50.4x3-	T50.4x4-	T50.4x5-	T50.4x6-
Ether (vapor)	T41.0x1-	T41.0x2-	T41.0x3-	T41.0x4-	T41.0x5-	T41.0x6-
anesthetic	T41.0x1-	T41.0x2-	T41.0x3-	T41.0x4-	T41.0x5-	T41.0x6-
divinyl	T41.0x1-	T41.0x2-	T41.0x3-	T41.0x4-	T41.0x5-	T41.0x6-
ethyl (medicinal)	T41.0x1-	T41.0x2-	T41.0x3-	T41.0x4-	T41.0x5-	T41.0x6-
nonmedicinal	T52.8x1-	T52.8x2-	T52.8x3-	T52.8x4-	—	—
petroleum — see Ligroin						
solvent	T52.8x1-	T52.8x2-	T52.8x3-	T52.8x4-	—	—
Ethiazide	T50.2x1-	T50.2x2-	T50.2x3-	T50.2x4-	T50.2x5-	T50.2x6-
Ethidium chloride (vapor)	T59.891-	T59.892-	T59.893-	T59.894-	—	—
Ethinamate	T42.6x1-	T42.6x2-	T42.6x3-	T42.6x4-	T42.6x5-	T42.6x6-
Ethinylestradiol, ethinyloestradiol	T38.5x1-	T38.5x2-	T38.5x3-	T38.5x4-	T38.5x5-	T38.5x6-
with						
levonorgestrel	T38.4x1-	T38.4x2-	T38.4x3-	T38.4x4-	T38.4x5-	T38.4x6-
norethisterone	T38.4x1-	T38.4x2-	T38.4x3-	T38.4x4-	T38.4x5-	T38.4x6-
Ethiodized oil (131 I)	T50.8x1-	T50.8x2-	T50.8x3-	T50.8x4-	T50.8x5-	T50.8x6-
Ethion	T60.0x1-	T60.0x2-	T60.0x3-	T60.0x4-	—	—
Ethionamide	T37.1x1-	T37.1x2-	T37.1x3-	T37.1x4-	T37.1x5-	T37.1x6-
Ethioniamide	T37.1x1-	T37.1x2-	T37.1x3-	T37.1x4-	T37.1x5-	T37.1x6-
Ethisterone	T38.5x1-	T38.5x2-	T38.5x3-	T38.5x4-	T38.5x5-	T38.5x6-
Ethobral	T42.3x1-	T42.3x2-	T42.3x3-	T42.3x4-	T42.3x5-	T42.3x6-
Ethocaine (Infiltration) (topical)	T41.3x1-	T41.3x2-	T41.3x3-	T41.3x4-	T41.3x5-	T41.3x6-
nerve block (peripheral) (plexus)	T41.3x1-	T41.3x2-	T41.3x3-	T41.3x4-	T41.3x5-	T41.3x6-
spinal	T41.3x1-	T41.3x2-	T41.3x3-	T41.3x4-	T41.3x5-	T41.3x6-
Ethoheptazine	T40.4x1-	T40.4x2-	T40.4x3-	T40.4x4-	T40.4x5-	T40.4x6-
Ethopropazine	T44.3x1-	T44.3x2-	T44.3x3-	T44.3x4-	T44.3x5-	T44.3x6-
Ethosuximide	T42.2x1-	T42.2x2-	T42.2x3-	T42.2x4-	T42.2x5-	T42.2x6-
Ethotoin	T42.0x1-	T42.0x2-	T42.0x3-	T42.0x4-	T42.0x5-	T42.0x6-
Ethoxazene	T37.91x-	T37.92x-	T37.93x-	T37.94x-	T37.95x-	T37.96x-
Ethoxazorutoside	T46.991-	T46.992-	T46.993-	T46.994-	T46.995-	T46.996-
2-Ethoxyethanol	T52.3x1-	T52.3x2-	T52.3x3-	T52.3x4-	—	—
Ethoxzolamide	T50.2x1-	T50.2x2-	T50.2x3-	T50.2x4-	T50.2x5-	T50.2x6-
Ethyl						
acetate	T52.8x1-	T52.8x2-	T52.8x3-	T52.8x4-	—	—
alcohol	T51.0x1-	T51.0x2-	T51.0x3-	T51.0x4-	—	—
beverage	T51.0x1-	T51.0x2-	T51.0x3-	T51.0x4-	—	—
aldehyde (vapor)	T59.891-	T59.892-	T59.893-	T59.894-	—	—
liquid	T52.8x1-	T52.8x2-	T52.8x3-	T52.8x4-	—	—
aminobenzoate	T41.3x1-	T41.3x2-	T41.3x3-	T41.3x4-	T41.3x5-	T41.3x6-
aminophenothiazine	T43.3x1-	T43.3x2-	T43.3x3-	T43.3x4-	T43.3x5-	T43.3x6-
benzoate	T52.8x1-	T52.8x2-	T52.8x3-	T52.8x4-	—	—
biscoumacetate	T45.511-	T45.512-	T45.513-	T45.514-	T45.515-	T45.516-
bromide (anesthetic)	T41.0x1-	T41.0x2-	T41.0x3-	T41.0x4-	T41.0x5-	T41.0x6-
carbamate	T45.1x1-	T45.1x2-	T45.1x3-	T45.1x4-	T45.1x5-	T45.1x6-
carbinol	T51.3x1-	T51.3x2-	T51.3x3-	T51.3x4-	—	—
carbonate	T52.8x1-	T52.8x2-	T52.8x3-	T52.8x4-	—	—

Table of Drugs & Chemicals	POISONING Accidental (Unintentional)	Self-Harm (Intentional)	Assault	Undetermined	Adverse Effect	Underdosing
Ethyl - *continued*						
chaulmoograte	T37.1x1-	T37.1x2-	T37.1x3-	T37.1x4-	T37.1x5-	T37.1x6-
chloride (anesthetic)	T41.0x1-	T41.0x2-	T41.0x3-	T41.0x4-	T41.0x5-	T41.0x6-
anesthetic (local)	T41.3x1-	T41.3x2-	T41.3x3-	T41.3x4-	T41.3x5-	T41.3x6-
inhaled	T41.0x1-	T41.0x2-	T41.0x3-	T41.0x4-	T41.0x5-	T41.0x6-
local	T49.4x1-	T49.4x2-	T49.4x3-	T49.4x4-	T49.4x5-	T49.4x6-
solvent	T53.6x1-	T53.6x2-	T53.6x3-	T53.6x4-	—	—
dibunate	T48.3x1-	T48.3x2-	T48.3x3-	T48.3x4-	T48.3x5-	T48.3x6-
dichloroarsine (vapor)	T57.0x1-	T57.0x2-	T57.0x3-	T57.0x4-	—	—
estranol	T38.7x1-	T38.7x2-	T38.7x3-	T38.7x4-	T38.7x5-	T38.7x6-
ether — see also Ether	T52.8x1-	T52.8x2-	T52.8x3-	T52.8x4-		
formate NEC (solvent)	T52.0x1-	T52.0x2-	T52.0x3-	T52.0x4-		
fumarate	T49.4x1-	T49.4x2-	T49.4x3-	T49.4x4-	T49.4x5-	T49.4x6-
hydroxyisobutyrate NEC (solvent)	T52.8x1-	T52.8x2-	T52.8x3-	T52.8x4-		
iodoacetate	T59.3x1-	T59.3x2-	T59.3x3-	T59.3x4-		
lactate NEC (solvent)	T52.8x1-	T52.8x2-	T52.8x3-	T52.8x4-		
loflazepate	T42.4x1-	T42.4x2-	T42.4x3-	T42.4x4-	T42.4x5-	T42.4x6-
mercuric chloride	T56.1x1-	T56.1x2-	T56.1x3-	T56.1x4-		
methylcarbinol	T51.8x1-	T51.8x2-	T51.8x3-	T51.8x4-		
morphine	T40.2x1-	T40.2x2-	T40.2x3-	T40.2x4-	T40.2x5-	T40.2x6-
noradrenaline	T48.6x1-	T48.6x2-	T48.6x3-	T48.6x4-	T48.6x5-	T48.6x6-
oxybutyrate NEC (solvent)	T52.8x1-	T52.8x2-	T52.8x3-	T52.8x4-		
Ethylene (gas)	T59.891-	T59.892-	T59.893-	T59.894-		
anesthetic (general)	T41.0x1-	T41.0x2-	T41.0x3-	T41.0x4-	T41.0x5-	T41.0x6-
chlorohydrin	T52.8x1-	T52.8x2-	T52.8x3-	T52.8x4-		
vapor	T53.6x1-	T53.6x2-	T53.6x3-	T53.6x4-		
dichloride	T52.8x1-	T52.8x2-	T52.8x3-	T52.8x4-		
vapor	T53.6x1-	T53.6x2-	T53.6x3-	T53.6x4-		
dinitrate	T52.3x1-	T52.3x2-	T52.3x3-	T52.3x4-		
glycol(s)	T52.8x1-	T52.8x2-	T52.8x3-	T52.8x4-		
dinitrate	T52.3x1-	T52.3x2-	T52.3x3-	T52.3x4-		
monobutyl ether	T52.3x1-	T52.3x2-	T52.3x3-	T52.3x4-		
imine	T54.1x1-	T54.1x2-	T54.1x3-	T54.1x4-		
oxide (fumigant) (nonmedicinal)	T59.891-	T59.892-	T59.893-	T59.894-		
medicinal	T49.0x1-	T49.0x2-	T49.0x3-	T49.0x4-	T49.0x5-	T49.0x6-
Ethylenediamine theophylline	T48.6x1-	T48.6x2-	T48.6x3-	T48.6x4-	T48.6x5-	T48.6x6-
Ethylenediaminetetra-acetic acid	T50.6x1-	T50.6x2-	T50.6x3-	T50.6x4-	T50.6x5-	T50.6x6-
Ethylenedinitrilotetra-acetate	T50.6x1-	T50.6x2-	T50.6x3-	T50.6x4-	T50.6x5-	T50.6x6-
Ethylestrenol	T38.7x1-	T38.7x2-	T38.7x3-	T38.7x4-	T38.7x5-	T38.7x6-
Ethylhydroxycellulose	T47.4x1-	T47.4x2-	T47.4x3-	T47.4x4-	T47.4x5-	T47.4x6-
Ethylidene						
chloride NEC	T53.6x1-	T53.6x2-	T53.6x3-	T53.6x4-		
diacetate	T60.3x1-	T60.3x2-	T60.3x3-	T60.3x4-	—	—
dicoumarin	T45.511-	T45.512-	T45.513-	T45.514-	T45.515-	T45.516-
dicoumarol	T45.511-	T45.512-	T45.513-	T45.514-	T45.515-	T45.516-
diethyl ether	T52.0x1-	T52.0x2-	T52.0x3-	T52.0x4-	—	—
Ethylmorphine	T40.2x1-	T40.2x2-	T40.2x3-	T40.2x4-	T40.2x5-	T40.2x6-
Ethylnorepinephrine	T48.6x1-	T48.6x2-	T48.6x3-	T48.6x4-	T48.6x5-	T48.6x6-
Ethylparachlorophen-oxyisobutyrate	T46.6x1-	T46.6x2-	T46.6x3-	T46.6x4-	T46.6x5-	T46.6x6-
Ethynodiol	T38.4x1-	T38.4x2-	T38.4x3-	T38.4x4-	T38.4x5-	T38.4x6-
with mestranol diacetate	T38.4x1-	T38.4x2-	T38.4x3-	T38.4x4-	T38.4x5-	T38.4x6-
Etidocaine	T41.3x1-	T41.3x2-	T41.3x3-	T41.3x4-	T41.3x5-	T41.3x6-
infiltration (subcutaneous)	T41.3x1-	T41.3x2-	T41.3x3-	T41.3x4-	T41.3x5-	T41.3x6-
nerve (peripheral) (plexus)	T41.3x1-	T41.3x2-	T41.3x3-	T41.3x4-	T41.3x5-	T41.3x6-

DRUGS & CHEMICALS

Table of Drugs & Chemicals	Poisoning Accidental (Unintentional)	Poisoning Self-Harm (Intentional)	Poisoning Assault	Poisoning Undetermined	Adverse Effect	Underdosing
Etidronate	T50.991-	T50.992-	T50.993-	T50.994-	T50.995-	T50.996-
Etidronic acid (disodium salt)	T50.991-	T50.992-	T50.993-	T50.994-	T50.995-	T50.996-
Etifoxine	T42.6x1-	T42.6x2-	T42.6x3-	T42.6x4-	T42.6x5-	T42.6x6-
Etilefrine	T44.4x1-	T44.4x2-	T44.4x3-	T44.4x4-	T44.4x5-	T44.4x6-
Etilfen	T42.3x1-	T42.3x2-	T42.3x3-	T42.3x4-	T42.3x5-	T42.3x6-
Etinodiol	T38.4x1-	T38.4x2-	T38.4x3-	T38.4x4-	T38.4x5-	T38.4x6-
Etiroxate	T46.6x1-	T46.6x2-	T46.6x3-	T46.6x4-	T46.6x5-	T46.6x6-
Etizolam	T42.4x1-	T42.4x2-	T42.4x3-	T42.4x4-	T42.4x5-	T42.4x6-
Etodolac	T39.391-	T39.392-	T39.393-	T39.394-	T39.395-	T39.396-
Etofamide	T37.3x1-	T37.3x2-	T37.3x3-	T37.3x4-	T37.3x5-	T37.3x6-
Etofibrate	T46.6x1-	T46.6x2-	T46.6x3-	T46.6x4-	T46.6x5-	T46.6x6-
Etofylline	T46.7x1-	T46.7x2-	T46.7x3-	T46.7x4-	T46.7x5-	T46.7x6-
clofibrate	T46.6x1-	T46.6x2-	T46.6x3-	T46.6x4-	T46.6x5-	T46.6x6-
Etoglucid	T45.1x1-	T45.1x2-	T45.1x3-	T45.1x4-	T45.1x5-	T45.1x6-
Etomidate	T41.1x1-	T41.1x2-	T41.1x3-	T41.1x4-	T41.1x5-	T41.1x6-
Etomide	T39.8x1-	T39.8x2-	T39.8x3-	T39.8x4-	T39.8x5-	T39.8x6-
Etomidoline	T44.3x1-	T44.3x2-	T44.3x3-	T44.3x4-	T44.3x5-	T44.3x6-
Etoposide	T45.1x1-	T45.1x2-	T45.1x3-	T45.1x4-	T45.1x5-	T45.1x6-
Etorphine	T40.2x1-	T40.2x2-	T40.2x3-	T40.2x4-	T40.2x5-	T40.2x6-
Etoval	T42.3x1-	T42.3x2-	T42.3x3-	T42.3x4-	T42.3x5-	T42.3x6-
Etozolin	T50.1x1-	T50.1x2-	T50.1x3-	T50.1x4-	T50.1x5-	T50.1x6-
Etretinate	T50.991-	T50.992-	T50.993-	T50.994-	T50.995-	T50.996-
Etryptamine	T43.691-	T43.692-	T43.693-	T43.694-	T43.695-	T43.696-
Etybenzatropine	T44.3x1-	T44.3x2-	T44.3x3-	T44.3x4-	T44.3x5-	T44.3x6-
Etynodiol	T38.4x1-	T38.4x2-	T38.4x3-	T38.4x4-	T38.4x5-	T38.4x6-
Eucaine	T41.3x1-	T41.3x2-	T41.3x3-	T41.3x4-	T41.3x5-	T41.3x6-
Eucalyptus oil	T49.7x1-	T49.7x2-	T49.7x3-	T49.7x4-	T49.7x5-	T49.7x6-
Eucatropine	T49.5x1-	T49.5x2-	T49.5x3-	T49.5x4-	T49.5x5-	T49.5x6-
Eucodal	T40.2x1-	T40.2x2-	T40.2x3-	T40.2x4-	T40.2x5-	T40.2x6-
Euneryl	T42.3x1-	T42.3x2-	T42.3x3-	T42.3x4-	T42.3x5-	T42.3x6-
Euphthalmine	T44.3x1-	T44.3x2-	T44.3x3-	T44.3x4-	T44.3x5-	T44.3x6-
Eurax	T49.0x1-	T49.0x2-	T49.0x3-	T49.0x4-	T49.0x5-	T49.0x6-
Euresol	T49.4x1-	T49.4x2-	T49.4x3-	T49.4x4-	T49.4x5-	T49.4x6-
Euthroid	T38.1x1-	T38.1x2-	T38.1x3-	T38.1x4-	T38.1x5-	T38.1x6-
Evans blue	T50.8x1-	T50.8x2-	T50.8x3-	T50.8x4-	T50.8x5-	T50.8x6-
Evipal	T42.3x1-	T42.3x2-	T42.3x3-	T42.3x4-	T42.3x5-	T42.3x6-
sodium	T41.1x1-	T41.1x2-	T41.1x3-	T41.1x4-	T41.1x5-	T41.1x6-
Evipan	T42.3x1-	T42.3x2-	T42.3x3-	T42.3x4-	T42.3x5-	T42.3x6-
sodium	T41.1x1-	T41.1x2-	T41.1x3-	T41.1x4-	T41.1x5-	T41.1x6-
Exalamide	T49.0x1-	T49.0x2-	T49.0x3-	T49.0x4-	T49.0x5-	T49.0x6-
Exalgin	T39.1x1-	T39.1x2-	T39.1x3-	T39.1x4-	T39.1x5-	T39.1x6-
Excipients, pharmaceutical	T50.901-	T50.902-	T50.903-	T50.904-	T50.905-	T50.906-
Exhaust gas (engine) (motor vehicle)	T58.01x-	T58.02x-	T58.03x-	T58.04x-	—	—
Ex-Lax (phenolphthalein)	T47.2x1-	T47.2x2-	T47.2x3-	T47.2x4-	T47.2x5-	T47.2x6-
Expectorant NEC	T48.4x1-	T48.4x2-	T48.4x3-	T48.4x4-	T48.4x5-	T48.4x6-
Extended insulin zinc suspension	T38.3x1-	T38.3x2-	T38.3x3-	T38.3x4-	T38.3x5-	T38.3x6-
External medications (skin) (mucous membrane)	T49.91x-	T49.92x-	T49.93x-	T49.94x-	T49.95x-	T49.96x-
dental agent	T49.7x1-	T49.7x2-	T49.7x3-	T49.7x4-	T49.7x5-	T49.7x6-
ENT agent	T49.6x1-	T49.6x2-	T49.6x3-	T49.6x4-	T49.6x5-	T49.6x6-
ophthalmic preparation	T49.5x1-	T49.5x2-	T49.5x3-	T49.5x4-	T49.5x5-	T49.5x6-
specified NEC	T49.8x1-	T49.8x2-	T49.8x3-	T49.8x4-	T49.8x5-	T49.8x6-
Extrapyramidal antagonist NEC	T44.3x1-	T44.3x2-	T44.3x3-	T44.3x4-	T44.3x5-	T44.3x6-
Eye agents (anti-infective)	T49.5x1-	T49.5x2-	T49.5x3-	T49.5x4-	T49.5x5-	T49.5x6-
Eye drug NEC	T49.5x1-	T49.5x2-	T49.5x3-	T49.5x4-	T49.5x5-	T49.5x6-
FAC (fluorouracil + doxorubicin + cyclophosphamide)	T45.1x1-	T45.1x2-	T45.1x3-	T45.1x4-	T45.1x5-	T45.1x6-
Factor						
I (fibrinogen)	T45.8x1-	T45.8x2-	T45.8x3-	T45.8x4-	T45.8x5-	T45.8x6-
III (thromboplastin)	T45.8x1-	T45.8x2-	T45.8x3-	T45.8x4-	T45.8x5-	T45.8x6-
VIII (antihemophilic Factor) (concentrate)	T45.8x1-	T45.8x2-	T45.8x3-	T45.8x4-	T45.8x5-	T45.8x6-
IX complex	T45.7x1-	T45.7x2-	T45.7x3-	T45.7x4-	T45.7x5-	T45.7x6-
human	T45.8x1-	T45.8x2-	T45.8x3-	T45.8x4-	T45.8x5-	T45.8x6-
Famotidine	T47.0x1-	T47.0x2-	T47.0x3-	T47.0x4-	T47.0x5-	T47.0x6-
Fat suspension, intravenous	T50.991-	T50.992-	T50.993-	T50.994-	T50.995-	T50.996-
Fazadinium bromide	T48.1x1-	T48.1x2-	T48.1x3-	T48.1x4-	T48.1x5-	T48.1x6-
Febarbamate	T42.3x1-	T42.3x2-	T42.3x3-	T42.3x4-	T42.3x5-	T42.3x6-
Fecal softener	T47.4x1-	T47.4x2-	T47.4x3-	T47.4x4-	T47.4x5-	T47.4x6-
Fedrilate	T48.3x1-	T48.3x2-	T48.3x3-	T48.3x4-	T48.3x5-	T48.3x6-
Felodipine	T46.1x1-	T46.1x2-	T46.1x3-	T46.1x4-	T46.1x5-	T46.1x6-
Felypressin	T38.891-	T38.892-	T38.893-	T38.894-	T38.895-	T38.896-
Femoxetine	T43.221-	T43.222-	T43.223-	T43.224-	T43.225-	T43.226-
Fenalcomine	T46.3x1-	T46.3x2-	T46.3x3-	T46.3x4-	T46.3x5-	T46.3x6-
Fenamisole	T37.1x1-	T37.1x2-	T37.1x3-	T37.1x4-	T37.1x5-	T37.1x6-
Fenazone	T39.2x1-	T39.2x2-	T39.2x3-	T39.2x4-	T39.2x5-	T39.2x6-
Fenbendazole	T37.4x1-	T37.4x2-	T37.4x3-	T37.4x4-	T37.4x5-	T37.4x6-
Fenbutrazate	T50.5x1-	T50.5x2-	T50.5x3-	T50.5x4-	T50.5x5-	T50.5x6-
Fencamfamine	T43.691-	T43.692-	T43.693-	T43.694-	T43.695-	T43.696-
Fendiline	T46.1x1-	T46.1x2-	T46.1x3-	T46.1x4-	T46.1x5-	T46.1x6-
Fenetylline	T43.691-	T43.692-	T43.693-	T43.694-	T43.695-	T43.696-
Fenflumizole	T39.391-	T39.392-	T39.393-	T39.394-	T39.395-	T39.396-
Fenfluramine	T50.5x1-	T50.5x2-	T50.5x3-	T50.5x4-	T50.5x5-	T50.5x6-
Fenobarbital	T42.3x1-	T42.3x2-	T42.3x3-	T42.3x4-	T42.3x5-	T42.3x6-
Fenofibrate	T46.6x1-	T46.6x2-	T46.6x3-	T46.6x4-	T46.6x5-	T46.6x6-
Fenoprofen	T39.311-	T39.312-	T39.313-	T39.314-	T39.315-	T39.316-
Fenoterol	T48.6x1-	T48.6x2-	T48.6x3-	T48.6x4-	T48.6x5-	T48.6x6-
Fenoverine	T44.3x1-	T44.3x2-	T44.3x3-	T44.3x4-	T44.3x5-	T44.3x6-
Fenoxazoline	T48.5x1-	T48.5x2-	T48.5x3-	T48.5x4-	T48.5x5-	T48.5x6-
Fenproporex	T50.5x1-	T50.5x2-	T50.5x3-	T50.5x4-	T50.5x5-	T50.5x6-
Fenquizone	T50.2x1-	T50.2x2-	T50.2x3-	T50.2x4-	T50.2x5-	T50.2x6-
Fentanyl	T40.4x1-	T40.4x2-	T40.4x3-	T40.4x4-	T40.4x5-	T40.4x6-
Fentazin	T43.3x1-	T43.3x2-	T43.3x3-	T43.3x4-	T43.3x5-	T43.3x6-
Fenthion	T60.0x1-	T60.0x2-	T60.0x3-	T60.0x4-	—	—
Fenticlor	T49.0x1-	T49.0x2-	T49.0x3-	T49.0x4-	T49.0x5-	T49.0x6-
Fenylbutazone	T39.2x1-	T39.2x2-	T39.2x3-	T39.2x4-	T39.2x5-	T39.2x6-
Feprazone	T39.2x1-	T39.2x2-	T39.2x3-	T39.2x4-	T39.2x5-	T39.2x6-
Fer de lance (bite) (venom)	T63.061-	T63.062-	T63.063-	T63.064-	—	—
Ferric — see also Iron						
chloride	T45.4x1-	T45.4x2-	T45.4x3-	T45.4x4-	T45.4x5-	T45.4x6-
citrate	T45.4x1-	T45.4x2-	T45.4x3-	T45.4x4-	T45.4x5-	T45.4x6-
hydroxide						
colloidal	T45.4x1-	T45.4x2-	T45.4x3-	T45.4x4-	T45.4x5-	T45.4x6-
polymaltose	T45.4x1-	T45.4x2-	T45.4x3-	T45.4x4-	T45.4x5-	T45.4x6-
pyrophosphate	T45.4x1-	T45.4x2-	T45.4x3-	T45.4x4-	T45.4x5-	T45.4x6-
Ferritin	T45.4x1-	T45.4x2-	T45.4x3-	T45.4x4-	T45.4x5-	T45.4x6-
Ferrocholinate	T45.4x1-	T45.4x2-	T45.4x3-	T45.4x4-	T45.4x5-	T45.4x6-
Ferrodextrane	T45.4x1-	T45.4x2-	T45.4x3-	T45.4x4-	T45.4x5-	T45.4x6-
Ferropolimaler	T45.4x1-	T45.4x2-	T45.4x3-	T45.4x4-	T45.4x5-	T45.4x6-
Ferrous — see also Iron						
phosphate	T45.4x1-	T45.4x2-	T45.4x3-	T45.4x4-	T45.4x5-	T45.4x6-
salt	T45.4x1-	T45.4x2-	T45.4x3-	T45.4x4-	T45.4x5-	T45.4x6-
with folic acid	T45.4x1-	T45.4x2-	T45.4x3-	T45.4x4-	T45.4x5-	T45.4x6-
Ferrous fumerate, gluconate, lactate, salt NEC, sulfate (medicinal)	T45.4x1-	T45.4x2-	T45.4x3-	T45.4x4-	T45.4x5-	T45.4x6-
Ferrovanadium (fumes)	T59.891-	T59.892-	T59.893-	T59.894-	—	—
Ferrum — see Iron						
Fertilizers NEC	T65.891-	T65.892-	T65.893-	T65.894-	—	—
with herbicide mixture	T60.3x1-	T60.3x2-	T60.3x3-	T60.3x4-	—	—

Table of Drugs & Chemicals	POISONING Accidental (Unintentional)	Self-Harm (Intentional)	Assault	Undetermined	Adverse Effect	Underdosing
Fetoxilate	T47.6x1-	T47.6x2-	T47.6x3-	T47.6x4-	T47.6x5-	T47.6x6-
Fiber, dietary	T47.4x1-	T47.4x2-	T47.4x3-	T47.4x4-	T47.4x5-	T47.4x6-
Fiberglass	T65.831-	T65.832-	T65.833-	T65.834-	—	—
Fibrinogen (human)	T45.8x1-	T45.8x2-	T45.8x3-	T45.8x4-	T45.8x5-	T45.8x6-
Fibrinolysin (human)	T45.691-	T45.692-	T45.693-	T45.694-	T45.695-	T45.696-
Fibrinolysis						
affecting drug	T45.601-	T45.602-	T45.603-	T45.604-	T45.605-	T45.606-
inhibitor NEC	T45.621-	T45.622-	T45.623-	T45.624-	T45.625-	T45.626-
Fibrinolytic drug	T45.611-	T45.612-	T45.613-	T45.614-	T45.615-	T45.616-
Filix mas	T37.4x1-	T37.4x2-	T37.4x3-	T37.4x4-	T37.4x5-	T37.4x6-
Filtering cream	T49.3x1-	T49.3x2-	T49.3x3-	T49.3x4-	T49.3x5-	T49.3x6-
Fiorinal	T39.011-	T39.012-	T39.013-	T39.014-	T39.015-	T39.016-
Firedamp	T59.891-	T59.892-	T59.893-	T59.894-	—	—
Fish, noxious, nonbacterial	T61.91x-	T61.92x-	T61.93x-	T61.94x-	—	—
ciguatera	T61.01x-	T61.02x-	T61.03x-	T61.04x-	—	—
scombroid	T61.11x-	T61.12x-	T61.13x-	T61.14x-	—	—
shell	T61.781-	T61.782-	T61.783-	T61.784-	—	—
specified NEC	T61.771-	T61.772-	T61.773-	T61.774-	—	—
Flagyl	T37.3x1-	T37.3x2-	T37.3x3-	T37.3x4-	T37.3x5-	T37.3x6-
Flavine adenine						
dinucleotide	T45.2x1-	T45.2x2-	T45.2x3-	T45.2x4-	T45.2x5-	T45.2x6-
Flavodic acid	T46.991-	T46.992-	T46.993-	T46.994-	T46.995-	T46.996-
Flavoxate	T44.3x1-	T44.3x2-	T44.3x3-	T44.3x4-	T44.3x5-	T44.3x6-
Flaxedil	T48.1x1-	T48.1x2-	T48.1x3-	T48.1x4-	T48.1x5-	T48.1x6-
Flaxseed (medicinal)	T49.3x1-	T49.3x2-	T49.3x3-	T49.3x4-	T49.3x5-	T49.3x6-
Flecainide	T46.2x1-	T46.2x2-	T46.2x3-	T46.2x4-	T46.2x5-	T46.2x6-
Fleroxacin	T36.8x1-	T36.8x2-	T36.8x3-	T36.8x4-	T36.8x5-	T36.8x6-
Floctafenine	T39.8x1-	T39.8x2-	T39.8x3-	T39.8x4-	T39.8x5-	T39.8x6-
Flomax	T44.6x1-	T44.6x2-	T44.6x3-	T44.6x4-	T44.6x5-	T44.6x6-
Flomoxef	T36.1x1-	T36.1x2-	T36.1x3-	T36.1x4-	T36.1x5-	T36.1x6-
Flopropione	T44.3x1-	T44.3x2-	T44.3x3-	T44.3x4-	T44.3x5-	T44.3x6-
Florantyrone	T47.5x1-	T47.5x2-	T47.5x3-	T47.5x4-	T47.5x5-	T47.5x6-
Floraquin	T37.8x1-	T37.8x2-	T37.8x3-	T37.8x4-	T37.8x5-	T37.8x6-
Florinef	T38.0x1-	T38.0x2-	T38.0x3-	T38.0x4-	T38.0x5-	T38.0x6-
ENT agent	T49.6x1-	T49.6x2-	T49.6x3-	T49.6x4-	T49.6x5-	T49.6x6-
ophthalmic preparation	T49.5x1-	T49.5x2-	T49.5x3-	T49.5x4-	T49.5x5-	T49.5x6-
topical NEC	T49.0x1-	T49.0x2-	T49.0x3-	T49.0x4-	T49.0x5-	T49.0x6-
Flowers of sulfur	T49.4x1-	T49.4x2-	T49.4x3-	T49.4x4-	T49.4x5-	T49.4x6-
Floxuridine	T45.1x1-	T45.1x2-	T45.1x3-	T45.1x4-	T45.1x5-	T45.1x6-
Fluanisone	T43.4x1-	T43.4x2-	T43.4x3-	T43.4x4-	T43.4x5-	T43.4x6-
Flubendazole	T37.4x1-	T37.4x2-	T37.4x3-	T37.4x4-	T37.4x5-	T37.4x6-
Fluclorolone acetonide	T49.0x1-	T49.0x2-	T49.0x3-	T49.0x4-	T49.0x5-	T49.0x6-
Flucloxacillin	T36.0x1-	T36.0x2-	T36.0x3-	T36.0x4-	T36.0x5-	T36.0x6-
Fluconazole	T37.8x1-	T37.8x2-	T37.8x3-	T37.8x4-	T37.8x5-	T37.8x6-
Flucytosine	T37.8x1-	T37.8x2-	T37.8x3-	T37.8x4-	T37.8x5-	T37.8x6-
Fludeoxyglucose (18F)	T50.8x1-	T50.8x2-	T50.8x3-	T50.8x4-	T50.8x5-	T50.8x6-
Fludiazepam	T42.4x1-	T42.4x2-	T42.4x3-	T42.4x4-	T42.4x5-	T42.4x6-
Fludrocortisone	T50.0x1-	T50.0x2-	T50.0x3-	T50.0x4-	T50.0x5-	T50.0x6-
ENT agent	T49.6x1-	T49.6x2-	T49.6x3-	T49.6x4-	T49.6x5-	T49.6x6-
ophthalmic preparation	T49.5x1-	T49.5x2-	T49.5x3-	T49.5x4-	T49.5x5-	T49.5x6-
topical NEC	T49.0x1-	T49.0x2-	T49.0x3-	T49.0x4-	T49.0x5-	T49.0x6-
Fludroxycortide	T49.0x1-	T49.0x2-	T49.0x3-	T49.0x4-	T49.0x5-	T49.0x6-
Flufenamic acid	T39.391-	T39.392-	T39.393-	T39.394-	T39.395-	T39.396-
Fluindione	T45.511-	T45.512-	T45.513-	T45.514-	T45.515-	T45.516-
Flumequine	T37.8x1-	T37.8x2-	T37.8x3-	T37.8x4-	T37.8x5-	T37.8x6-
Flumethasone	T49.0x1-	T49.0x2-	T49.0x3-	T49.0x4-	T49.0x5-	T49.0x6-
Flumethiazide	T50.2x1-	T50.2x2-	T50.2x3-	T50.2x4-	T50.2x5-	T50.2x6-
Flumidin	T37.5x1-	T37.5x2-	T37.5x3-	T37.5x4-	T37.5x5-	T37.5x6-
Flunarizine	T46.7x1-	T46.7x2-	T46.7x3-	T46.7x4-	T46.7x5-	T46.7x6-
Flunidazole	T37.8x1-	T37.8x2-	T37.8x3-	T37.8x4-	T37.8x5-	T37.8x6-
Flunisolide	T48.6x1-	T48.6x2-	T48.6x3-	T48.6x4-	T48.6x5-	T48.6x6-
Flunitrazepam	T42.4x1-	T42.4x2-	T42.4x3-	T42.4x4-	T42.4x5-	T42.4x6-

Table of Drugs & Chemicals	POISONING Accidental (Unintentional)	Self-Harm (Intentional)	Assault	Undetermined	Adverse Effect	Underdosing
Fluocinolone (acetonide)	T49.0x1-	T49.0x2-	T49.0x3-	T49.0x4-	T49.0x5-	T49.0x6-
Fluocinonide	T49.0x1-	T49.0x2-	T49.0x3-	T49.0x4-	T49.0x5-	T49.0x6-
Fluocortin (butyl)	T49.0x1-	T49.0x2-	T49.0x3-	T49.0x4-	T49.0x5-	T49.0x6-
Fluocortolone	T49.0x1-	T49.0x2-	T49.0x3-	T49.0x4-	T49.0x5-	T49.0x6-
Fluohydrocortisone	T38.0x1-	T38.0x2-	T38.0x3-	T38.0x4-	T38.0x5-	T38.0x6-
ENT agent	T49.6x1-	T49.6x2-	T49.6x3-	T49.6x4-	T49.6x5-	T49.6x6-
ophthalmic preparation	T49.5x1-	T49.5x2-	T49.5x3-	T49.5x4-	T49.5x5-	T49.5x6-
topical NEC	T49.0x1-	T49.0x2-	T49.0x3-	T49.0x4-	T49.0x5-	T49.0x6-
Fluonid	T49.0x1-	T49.0x2-	T49.0x3-	T49.0x4-	T49.0x5-	T49.0x6-
Fluopromazine	T43.3x1-	T43.3x2-	T43.3x3-	T43.3x4-	T43.3x5-	T43.3x6-
Fluoracetate	T60.8x1-	T60.8x2-	T60.8x3-	T60.8x4-	—	—
Fluorescein	T50.8x1-	T50.8x2-	T50.8x3-	T50.8x4-	T50.8x5-	T50.8x6-
Fluorhydrocortisone	T50.0x1-	T50.0x2-	T50.0x3-	T50.0x4-	T50.0x5-	T50.0x6-
Fluoride (nonmedicinal) (pesticide) (sodium)						
NEC	T60.8x1-	T60.8x2-	T60.8x3-	T60.8x4-		
hydrogen — see Hydrofluoric acid						
medicinal NEC	T50.991-	T50.992-	T50.993-	T50.994-	T50.995-	T50.996-
dental use	T49.7x1-	T49.7x2-	T49.7x3-	T49.7x4-	T49.7x5-	T49.7x6-
not pesticide NEC	T54.91x-	T54.92x-	T54.93x-	T54.94x-		
stannous	T49.7x1-	T49.7x2-	T49.7x3-	T49.7x4-	T49.7x5-	T49.7x6-
Fluorinated corticosteroids	T38.0x1-	T38.0x2-	T38.0x3-	T38.0x4-	T38.0x5-	T38.0x6-
Fluorine (gas)	T59.5x1-	T59.5x2-	T59.5x3-	T59.5x4-		
salt — see Fluoride(s)						
Fluoristan	T49.7x1-	T49.7x2-	T49.7x3-	T49.7x4-	T49.7x5-	T49.7x6-
Fluormetholone	T49.0x1-	T49.0x2-	T49.0x3-	T49.0x4-	T49.0x5-	T49.0x6-
Fluoroacetate	T60.8x1-	T60.8x2-	T60.8x3-	T60.8x4-	—	—
Fluorocarbon monomer	T53.6x1-	T53.6x2-	T53.6x3-	T53.6x4-	—	—
Fluorocytosine	T37.8x1-	T37.8x2-	T37.8x3-	T37.8x4-	T37.8x5-	T37.8x6-
Fluorodeoxyuridine	T45.1x1-	T45.1x2-	T45.1x3-	T45.1x4-	T45.1x5-	T45.1x6-
Fluorometholone	T49.0x1-	T49.0x2-	T49.0x3-	T49.0x4-	T49.0x5-	T49.0x6-
ophthalmic preparation	T49.5x1-	T49.5x2-	T49.5x3-	T49.5x4-	T49.5x5-	T49.5x6-
Fluorophosphate insecticide	T60.0x1-	T60.0x2-	T60.0x3-	T60.0x4-	—	—
Fluorosol	T46.3x1-	T46.3x2-	T46.3x3-	T46.3x4-	T46.3x5-	T46.3x6-
Fluorouracil	T45.1x1-	T45.1x2-	T45.1x3-	T45.1x4-	T45.1x5-	T45.1x6-
Fluorphenylalanine	T49.5x1-	T49.5x2-	T49.5x3-	T49.5x4-	T49.5x5-	T49.5x6-
Fluothane	T41.0x1-	T41.0x2-	T41.0x3-	T41.0x4-	T41.0x5-	T41.0x6-
Fluoxetine	T43.221-	T43.222-	T43.223-	T43.224-	T43.225-	T43.226-
Fluoxymesterone	T38.7x1-	T38.7x2-	T38.7x3-	T38.7x4-	T38.7x5-	T38.7x6-
Flupenthixol	T43.4x1-	T43.4x2-	T43.4x3-	T43.4x4-	T43.4x5-	T43.4x6-
Flupentixol	T43.4x1-	T43.4x2-	T43.4x3-	T43.4x4-	T43.4x5-	T43.4x6-
Fluphenazine	T43.3x1-	T43.3x2-	T43.3x3-	T43.3x4-	T43.3x5-	T43.3x6-
Fluprednidene	T49.0x1-	T49.0x2-	T49.0x3-	T49.0x4-	T49.0x5-	T49.0x6-
Fluprednisolone	T38.0x1-	T38.0x2-	T38.0x3-	T38.0x4-	T38.0x5-	T38.0x6-
Fluradoline	T39.8x1-	T39.8x2-	T39.8x3-	T39.8x4-	T39.8x5-	T39.8x6-
Flurandrenolide	T49.0x1-	T49.0x2-	T49.0x3-	T49.0x4-	T49.0x5-	T49.0x6-
Flurandrenolone	T49.0x1-	T49.0x2-	T49.0x3-	T49.0x4-	T49.0x5-	T49.0x6-
Flurazepam	T42.4x1-	T42.4x2-	T42.4x3-	T42.4x4-	T42.4x5-	T42.4x6-
Flurbiprofen	T39.311-	T39.312-	T39.313-	T39.314-	T39.315-	T39.316-
Flurobate	T49.0x1-	T49.0x2-	T49.0x3-	T49.0x4-	T49.0x5-	T49.0x6-
Fluroxene	T41.0x1-	T41.0x2-	T41.0x3-	T41.0x4-	T41.0x5-	T41.0x6-
Fluspirilene	T43.591-	T43.592-	T43.593-	T43.594-	T43.595-	T43.596-
Flutamide	T38.6x1-	T38.6x2-	T38.6x3-	T38.6x4-	T38.6x5-	T38.6x6-
Flutazolam	T42.4x1-	T42.4x2-	T42.4x3-	T42.4x4-	T42.4x5-	T42.4x6-
Fluticasone propionate	T49.1x1-	T49.1x2-	T49.1x3-	T49.1x4-	T49.1x5-	T49.1x6-
Flutoprazepam	T42.4x1-	T42.4x2-	T42.4x3-	T42.4x4-	T42.4x5-	T42.4x6-
Flutropium bromide	T48.6x1-	T48.6x2-	T48.6x3-	T48.6x4-	T48.6x5-	T48.6x6-
Fluvoxamine	T43.221-	T43.222-	T43.223-	T43.224-	T43.225-	T43.226-
Folacin	T45.8x1-	T45.8x2-	T45.8x3-	T45.8x4-	T45.8x5-	T45.8x6-

DRUGS & CHEMICALS

© 2016 Channel Publishing, Ltd.

DRUGS & CHEMICALS

Table of Drugs & Chemicals	POISONING Accidental (Unintentional)	Self-Harm (Intentional)	Assault	Undetermined	Adverse Effect	Underdosing
Folic acid	T45.8x1-	T45.8x2-	T45.8x3-	T45.8x4-	T45.8x5-	T45.8x6-
with ferrous salt	T45.2x1-	T45.2x2-	T45.2x3-	T45.2x4-	T45.2x5-	T45.2x6-
antagonist	T45.1x1-	T45.1x2-	T45.1x3-	T45.1x4-	T45.1x5-	T45.1x6-
Folinic acid	T45.8x1-	T45.8x2-	T45.8x3-	T45.8x4-	T45.8x5-	T45.8x6-
Folium stramoniae	T48.6x1-	T48.6x2-	T48.6x3-	T48.6x4-	T48.6x5-	T48.6x6-
Follicle-stimulating hormone, human	T38.811	T38.812	T38.813	T38.814	T38.815	T38.816
Folpet	T60.3x1-	T60.3x2-	T60.3x3-	T60.3x4-	—	—
Fominoben	T48.3x1-	T48.3x2-	T48.3x3-	T48.3x4-	T48.3x5-	T48.3x6-
Food, foodstuffs, noxious, nonbacterial, NEC	T62.91x-	T62.92x-	T62.93x-	T62.94x-	—	—
berries	T62.1x1-	T62.1x2-	T62.1x3-	T62.1x4-	—	—
fish — see also Fish	T61.91x-	T61.92x-	T61.93x-	T61.94x-	—	—
mushrooms	T62.0x1-	T62.0x2-	T62.0x3-	T62.0x4-	—	—
plants	T62.2x1-	T62.2x2-	T62.2x3-	T62.2x4-	—	—
seafood	T61.91x-	T61.92x-	T61.93x-	T61.94x-	—	—
specified NEC	T61.8x1-	T61.8x2-	T61.8x3-	T61.8x4-	—	—
seeds	T62.2x1-	T62.2x2-	T62.2x3-	T62.2x4-	—	—
shellfish	T61.781	T61.782	T61.783	T61.784	—	—
specified NEC	T62.8x1-	T62.8x2-	T62.8x3-	T62.8x4-	—	—
Fool's parsley	T62.2x1-	T62.2x2-	T62.2x3-	T62.2x4-	—	—
Formaldehyde (solution), gas or vapor	T59.2x1-	T59.2x2-	T59.2x3-	T59.2x4-	—	—
fungicide	T60.3x1-	T60.3x2-	T60.3x3-	T60.3x4-	—	—
Formalin	T59.2x1-	T59.2x2-	T59.2x3-	T59.2x4-	—	—
fungicide	T60.3x1-	T60.3x2-	T60.3x3-	T60.3x4-	—	—
vapor	T59.2x1-	T59.2x2-	T59.2x3-	T59.2x4-	—	—
Formic acid	T54.2x1-	T54.2x2-	T54.2x3-	T54.2x4-	—	—
vapor	T59.891-	T59.892-	T59.893-	T59.894-	—	—
Foscarnet sodium	T37.5x1-	T37.5x2-	T37.5x3-	T37.5x4-	T37.5x5-	T37.5x6-
Fosfestrol	T38.5x1-	T38.5x2-	T38.5x3-	T38.5x4-	T38.5x5-	T38.5x6-
Fosfomycin	T36.8x1-	T36.8x2-	T36.8x3-	T36.8x4-	T36.8x5-	T36.8x6-
Fosfonet sodium	T37.5x1-	T37.5x2-	T37.5x3-	T37.5x4-	T37.5x5-	T37.5x6-
Fosinopril	T46.4x1-	T46.4x2-	T46.4x3-	T46.4x4-	T46.4x5-	T46.4x6-
sodium	T46.4x1-	T46.4x2-	T46.4x3-	T46.4x4-	T46.4x5-	T46.4x6-
Fowler's solution	T57.0x1-	T57.0x2-	T57.0x3-	T57.0x4-	—	—
Foxglove	T62.2x1-	T62.2x2-	T62.2x3-	T62.2x4-	—	—
Framycetin	T36.5x1-	T36.5x2-	T36.5x3-	T36.5x4-	T36.5x5-	T36.5x6-
Frangula	T47.2x1-	T47.2x2-	T47.2x3-	T47.2x4-	T47.2x5-	T47.2x6-
extract	T47.2x1-	T47.2x2-	T47.2x3-	T47.2x4-	T47.2x5-	T47.2x6-
Frei antigen	T50.8x1-	T50.8x2-	T50.8x3-	T50.8x4-	T50.8x5-	T50.8x6-
Freon	T53.5x1-	T53.5x2-	T53.5x3-	T53.5x4-	—	—
Fructose	T50.3x1-	T50.3x2-	T50.3x3-	T50.3x4-	T50.3x5-	T50.3x6-
Frusemide	T50.1x1-	T50.1x2-	T50.1x3-	T50.1x4-	T50.1x5-	T50.1x6-
FSH	T38.811	T38.812	T38.813	T38.814	T38.815	T38.816
Ftorafur	T45.1x1-	T45.1x2-	T45.1x3-	T45.1x4-	T45.1x5-	T45.1x6-
Fuel automobile	T52.0x1-	T52.0x2-	T52.0x3-	T52.0x4-	—	—
exhaust gas, not in transit	T58.01x-	T58.02x-	T58.03x-	T58.04x-	—	—
vapor NEC	T52.0x1-	T52.0x2-	T52.0x3-	T52.0x4-	—	—
gas (domestic use) — see also Carbon, monoxide, fuel, utility	T59.891-	T59.892-	T59.893-	T59.894-	—	—
utility	T59.891-	T59.892-	T59.893-	T59.894-	—	—
incomplete combustion of — see Carbon, monoxide, fuel, utility in mobile container	T59.891-	T59.892-	T59.893-	T59.894-	—	—
piped (natural)	T59.891-	T59.892-	T59.893-	T59.894-	—	—
industrial, incomplete combustion	T58.8x1-	T58.8x2-	T58.8x3-	T58.8x4-	—	—

Table of Drugs & Chemicals	POISONING Accidental (Unintentional)	Self-Harm (Intentional)	Assault	Undetermined	Adverse Effect	Underdosing
Fugillin	T36.8x1-	T36.8x2-	T36.8x3-	T36.8x4-	T36.8x5-	T36.8x6-
Fulminate of mercury	T56.1x1-	T56.1x2-	T56.1x3-	T56.1x4-	—	—
Fulvicin	T36.7x1-	T36.7x2-	T36.7x3-	T36.7x4-	T36.7x5-	T36.7x6-
Fumadil	T36.8x1-	T36.8x2-	T36.8x3-	T36.8x4-	T36.8x5-	T36.8x6-
Fumagillin	T36.8x1-	T36.8x2-	T36.8x3-	T36.8x4-	T36.8x5-	T36.8x6-
Fumaric acid	T49.4x1-	T49.4x2-	T49.4x3-	T49.4x4-	T49.4x5-	T49.4x6-
Fumes (from)	T59.91x-	T59.92x-	T59.93x-	T59.94x-	—	—
carbon monoxide — see Carbon, monoxide						
charcoal (domestic use) — see Charcoal, fumes						
chloroform — see Chloroform						
coke (in domestic stoves, fireplaces) — see Coke fumes						
corrosive NEC	T54.91x-	T54.92x-	T54.93x-	T54.94x-	—	—
ether — see Ether						
freons	T53.5x1-	T53.5x2-	T53.5x3-	T53.5x4-	—	—
hydrocarbons	T59.891-	T59.892-	T59.893-	T59.894-	—	—
petroleum (liquefied) distributed through pipes (pure or mixed with air)	T59.891-	T59.892-	T59.893-	T59.894-	—	—
lead — see Lead						
metal — see Metals, or the specified metal						
nitrogen dioxide	T59.0x1-	T59.0x2-	T59.0x3-	T59.0x4-	—	—
pesticides — see Pesticides						
petroleum (liquefied) distributed through pipes (pure or mixed with air)	T59.891-	T59.892-	T59.893-	T59.894-	—	—
polyester	T59.891-	T59.892-	T59.893-	T59.894-	—	—
specified source NEC — see also substance, specified	T59.891-	T59.892-	T59.893-	T59.894-	—	—
sulfur dioxide	T59.1x1-	T59.1x2-	T59.1x3-	T59.1x4-	—	—
Fumigant NEC	T60.91x-	T60.92x-	T60.93x-	T60.94x-	—	—
Fungi, noxious, used as food	T62.0x1-	T62.0x2-	T62.0x3-	T62.0x4-	—	—
Fungicide NEC (nonmedicinal)	T60.3x1-	T60.3x2-	T60.3x3-	T60.3x4-	—	—
Fungizone	T36.7x1-	T36.7x2-	T36.7x3-	T36.7x4-	T36.7x5-	T36.7x6-
topical	T49.0x1-	T49.0x2-	T49.0x3-	T49.0x4-	T49.0x5-	T49.0x6-
Furacin	T49.0x1-	T49.0x2-	T49.0x3-	T49.0x4-	T49.0x5-	T49.0x6-
Furadantin	T37.91x-	T37.92x-	T37.93x-	T37.94x-	T37.95x-	T37.96x-
Furazolidone	T37.8x1-	T37.8x2-	T37.8x3-	T37.8x4-	T37.8x5-	T37.8x6-
Furazolium chloride	T49.0x1-	T49.0x2-	T49.0x3-	T49.0x4-	T49.0x5-	T49.0x6-
Furfural	T52.8x1-	T52.8x2-	T52.8x3-	T52.8x4-	—	—
Furnace (coal burning) (domestic), gas from	T58.2x1-	T58.2x2-	T58.2x3-	T58.2x4-	—	—
industrial	T58.8x1-	T58.8x2-	T58.8x3-	T58.8x4-	—	—
Furniture polish	T65.891-	T65.892-	T65.893-	T65.894-	—	—
Furosemide	T50.1x1-	T50.1x2-	T50.1x3-	T50.1x4-	T50.1x5-	T50.1x6-
Furoxone	T37.91x-	T37.92x-	T37.93x-	T37.94x-	T37.95x-	T37.96x-
Fursultiamine	T45.2x1-	T45.2x2-	T45.2x3-	T45.2x4-	T45.2x5-	T45.2x6-
Fusafungine	T36.8x1-	T36.8x2-	T36.8x3-	T36.8x4-	T36.8x5-	T36.8x6-
Fusel oil (any) (amyl) (butyl) (propyl), vapor	T51.3x1-	T51.3x2-	T51.3x3-	T51.3x4-	—	—
Fusidate (ethanolamine) (sodium)	T36.8x1-	T36.8x2-	T36.8x3-	T36.8x4-	T36.8x5-	T36.8x6-
Fusidic acid	T36.8x1-	T36.8x2-	T36.8x3-	T36.8x4-	T36.8x5-	T36.8x6-
Fytic acid, nonasodium	T50.6x1-	T50.6x2-	T50.6x3-	T50.6x4-	T50.6x5-	T50.6x6-

DRUGS & CHEMICALS

Table of Drugs & Chemicals	POISONING Accidental (Unintentional)	POISONING Self-Harm (Intentional)	POISONING Assault	POISONING Undetermined	Adverse Effect	Underdosing
GABA	T43.8x1-	T43.8x2-	T43.8x3-	T43.8x4-	T43.8x5-	T43.8x6-
Gadopentetic acid	T50.8x1-	T50.8x2-	T50.8x3-	T50.8x4-	T50.8x5-	T50.8x6-
Galactose	T50.3x1-	T50.3x2-	T50.3x3-	T50.3x4-	T50.3x5-	T50.3x6-
b-Galactosidase	T47.5x1-	T47.5x2-	T47.5x3-	T47.5x4-	T47.5x5-	T47.5x6-
Galantamine	T44.0x1-	T44.0x2-	T44.0x3-	T44.0x4-	T44.0x5-	T44.0x6-
Gallamine (triethiodide)	T48.1x1-	T48.1x2-	T48.1x3-	T48.1x4-	T48.1x5-	T48.1x6-
Gallium citrate	T50.991-	T50.992-	T50.993-	T50.994-	T50.995-	T50.996-
Gallopamil	T46.1x1-	T46.1x2-	T46.1x3-	T46.1x4-	T46.1x5-	T46.1x6-
Gamboge	T47.2x1-	T47.2x2-	T47.2x3-	T47.2x4-	T47.2x5-	T47.2x6-
Gamimune	T50.Z11-	T50.Z12-	T50.Z13-	T50.Z14-	T50.Z15-	T50.Z16-
Gamma globulin	T50.Z11-	T50.Z12-	T50.Z13-	T50.Z14-	T50.Z15-	T50.Z16-
Gamma-aminobutyric acid	T43.8x1-	T43.8x2-	T43.8x3-	T43.8x4-	T43.8x5-	T43.8x6-
Gamma-benzene hexachloride (medicinal)	T49.0x1-	T49.0x2-	T49.0x3-	T49.0x4-	T49.0x5-	T49.0x6-
nonmedicinal, vapor	T53.6x1-	T53.6x2-	T53.6x3-	T53.6x4-	—	—
Gamma-BHC (medicinal) — see also Gamma-benzene hexachloride	T49.0x1-	T49.0x2-	T49.0x3-	T49.0x4-	T49.0x5-	T49.0x6-
Gamulin	T50.Z11-	T50.Z12-	T50.Z13-	T50.Z14-	T50.Z15-	T50.Z16-
Ganciclovir (sodium)	T37.5x1-	T37.5x2-	T37.5x3-	T37.5x4-	T37.5x5-	T37.5x6-
Ganglionic blocking drug NEC	T44.2x1-	T44.2x2-	T44.2x3-	T44.2x4-	T44.2x5-	T44.2x6-
specified NEC	T44.2x1-	T44.2x2-	T44.2x3-	T44.2x4-	T44.2x5-	T44.2x6-
Ganja	T40.7x1-	T40.7x2-	T40.7x3-	T40.7x4-	T40.7x5-	T40.7x6-
Garamycin	T36.5x1-	T36.5x2-	T36.5x3-	T36.5x4-	T36.5x5-	T36.5x6-
ophthalmic preparation	T49.5x1-	T49.5x2-	T49.5x3-	T49.5x4-	T49.5x5-	T49.5x6-
topical NEC	T49.0x1-	T49.0x2-	T49.0x3-	T49.0x4-	T49.0x5-	T49.0x6-
Gardenal	T42.3x1-	T42.3x2-	T42.3x3-	T42.3x4-	T42.3x5-	T42.3x6-
Gardepanyl	T42.3x1-	T42.3x2-	T42.3x3-	T42.3x4-	T42.3x5-	T42.3x6-
Gas	T59.91x-	T59.92x-	T59.93x-	T59.94x-	—	—
acetylene	T59.891-	T59.892-	T59.893-	T59.894-	—	—
incomplete combustion of	T58.11x-	T58.12x-	T58.13x-	T58.14x-	—	—
air contaminants, source or type not specified	T59.91x-	T59.92x-	T59.93x-	T59.94x-		
anesthetic	T41.0x1-	T41.0x2-	T41.0x3-	T41.0x4-	T41.0x5-	T41.0x6-
blast furnace	T58.8x1-	T58.8x2-	T58.8x3-	T58.8x4-	—	—
butane — see Butane						
carbon monoxide — see Carbon, monoxide						
chlorine	T59.4x1-	T59.4x2-	T59.4x3-	T59.4x4-	—	—
coal	T58.2x1-	T58.2x2-	T58.2x3-	T58.2x4-	—	—
cyanide	T57.3x1-	T57.3x2-	T57.3x3-	T57.3x4-	—	—
dicyanogen	T65.0x1-	T65.0x2-	T65.0x3-	T65.0x4-	—	—
domestic — see Domestic gas						
exhaust	T58.01x-	T58.02x-	T58.03x-	T58.04x-	—	—
from utility (for cooking, heating, or lighting) (after combustion) — see Carbon, monoxide, fuel, utility						
prior to combustion	T59.891-	T59.892-	T59.893-	T59.894-	—	—
from wood- or coal-burning stove or fireplace	T58.2x1-	T58.2x2-	T58.2x3-	T58.2x4-	—	—
Gas - continued	T59.91x-	T59.92x-	T59.93x-	T59.94x-	—	—
fuel (domestic use) (after combustion) — see also Carbon, monoxide, fuel						
industrial use	T58.8x1-	T58.8x2-	T58.8x3-	T58.8x4-	—	—
prior to combustion	T59.891-	T59.892-	T59.893-	T59.894-	—	—
utility	T59.891-	T59.892-	T59.893-		—	—
incomplete combustion of — see Carbon, monoxide, fuel, utility						
in mobile container	T59.891-	T59.892-	T59.893-	T59.894-	—	—
piped (natural)	T59.891-	T59.892-	T59.893-	T59.894-	—	—
garage	T58.01x-	T58.02x-	T58.03x-	T58.04x-	—	—
hydrocarbon NEC	T59.891-	T59.892-	T59.893-	T59.894-	—	—
incomplete combustion of — see Carbon, monoxide, fuel, utility						
liquefied — see Butane						
piped	T59.891-	T59.892-	T59.893-	T59.894-	—	—
hydrocyanic acid	T65.0x1-	T65.0x2-	T65.0x3-	T65.0x4-	—	—
illuminating (after combustion)	T58.11x-	T58.12x-	T58.13x-	T58.14x-	—	—
prior to combustion	T59.891-	T59.892-	T59.893-	T59.894-	—	—
incomplete combustion, any — see Carbon, monoxide						
kiln	T58.8x1-	T58.8x2-	T58.8x3-	T58.8x4-	—	—
lacrimogenic	T59.3x1-	T59.3x2-	T59.3x3-	T59.3x4-	—	—
liquefied petroleum — see Butane						
marsh	T59.891-	T59.892-	T59.893-	T59.894-	—	—
motor exhaust, not in transit	T58.01x-	T58.02x-	T58.03x-	T58.04x-	—	—
mustard, not in war	T59.891-	T59.892-	T59.893-	T59.894-	—	—
natural	T59.891-	T59.892-	T59.893-	T59.894-	—	—
nerve, not in war	T59.91x-	T59.92x-	T59.93x-	T59.94x-	—	—
oil	T52.0x1-	T52.0x2-	T52.0x3-	T52.0x4-	—	—
petroleum (liquefied) (distributed in mobile containers)	T59.891-	T59.892-	T59.893-	T59.894-	—	—
piped (pure or mixed with air)	T59.891-	T59.892-	T59.893-	T59.894-	—	—
piped (manufactured) (natural) NEC	T59.891-	T59.892-	T59.893-	T59.894-	—	—
producer	T58.8x1-	T58.8x2-	T58.8x3-	T58.8x4-	—	—
propane — see Propane						
refrigerant (chlorofluoro-carbon)	T53.5x1-	T53.5x2-	T53.5x3-	T53.5x4-	—	—
not chlorofluoro-carbon	T59.891-	T59.892-	T59.893-	T59.894-	—	—
sewer	T59.91x-	T59.92x-	T59.93x-	T59.94x-	—	—
specified source NEC	T59.91x-	T59.92x-	T59.93x-	T59.94x-	—	—
stove (after combustion)	T58.11x-	T58.12x-	T58.13x-	T58.14x-	—	—
prior to combustion	T59.891-	T59.892-	T59.893-	T59.894-	—	—
tear	T59.3x1-	T59.3x2-	T59.3x3-	T59.3x4-	—	—
therapeutic	T41.5x1-	T41.5x2-	T41.5x3-	T41.5x4-	T41.5x5-	T41.5x6-

DRUGS & CHEMICALS

Table of Drugs & Chemicals	Accidental (Unintentional)	Self-Harm (Intentional)	Assault	Undetermined	Adverse Effect	Underdosing
Gas - continued	T59.91x-	T59.92x-	T59.93x-	T59.94x-	—	—
utility (for cooking, heating, or lighting) (piped) NEC	T59.891-	T59.892-	T59.893-	T59.894-	—	—
incomplete combustion of — see Carbon, monoxide, fuel, utilty						
in mobile container	T59.891-	T59.892-	T59.893-	T59.894-	—	—
piped (natural)	T59.891-	T59.892-	T59.893-	T59.894-	—	—
water	T58.11x-	T58.12x-	T58.13x-	T58.14x-	—	—
incomplete combustion of — see Carbon, monoxide, fuel, utility						
Gaseous substance — see Gas						
Gasoline	T52.0x1-	T52.0x2-	T52.0x3-	T52.0x4-	—	—
vapor	T52.0x1-	T52.0x2-	T52.0x3-	T52.0x4-	—	—
Gastric enzymes	T47.5x1-	T47.5x2-	T47.5x3-	T47.5x4-	T47.5x5-	T47.5x6-
Gastrografin	T50.8x1-	T50.8x2-	T50.8x3-	T50.8x4-	T50.8x5-	T50.8x6-
Gastrointestinal drug	T47.91x-	T47.92x-	T47.93x-	T47.94x-	T47.95x-	T47.96x-
biological	T47.8x1-	T47.8x2-	T47.8x3-	T47.8x4-	T47.8x5-	T47.8x6-
specified NEC	T47.8x1-	T47.8x2-	T47.8x3-	T47.8x4-	T47.8x5-	T47.8x6-
Gaultheria procumbens	T62.2x1-	T62.2x2-	T62.2x3-	T62.2x4-	—	—
Gefarnate	T44.3x1-	T44.3x2-	T44.3x3-	T44.3x4-	T44.3x5-	T44.3x6-
Gelatin (intravenous)	T45.8x1-	T45.8x2-	T45.8x3-	T45.8x4-	T45.8x5-	T45.8x6-
absorbable (sponge)	T45.7x1-	T45.7x2-	T45.7x3-	T45.7x4-	T45.7x5-	T45.7x6-
Gelfilm	T49.8x1-	T49.8x2-	T49.8x3-	T49.8x4-	T49.8x5-	T49.8x6-
Gelfoam	T45.7x1-	T45.7x2-	T45.7x3-	T45.7x4-	T45.7x5-	T45.7x6-
Gelsemine	T50.991-	T50.992-	T50.993-	T50.994-	T50.995-	T50.996-
Gelsemium (sempervirens)	T62.2x1-	T62.2x2-	T62.2x3-	T62.2x4-	—	—
Gemeprost	T48.0x1-	T48.0x2-	T48.0x3-	T48.0x4-	T48.0x5-	T48.0x6-
Gemfibrozil	T46.6x1-	T46.6x2-	T46.6x3-	T46.6x4-	T46.6x5-	T46.6x6-
Gemonil	T42.3x1-	T42.3x2-	T42.3x3-	T42.3x4-	T42.3x5-	T42.3x6-
Gentamicin	T36.5x1-	T36.5x2-	T36.5x3-	T36.5x4-	T36.5x5-	T36.5x6-
ophthalmic preparation	T49.5x1-	T49.5x2-	T49.5x3-	T49.5x4-	T49.5x5-	T49.5x6-
topical NEC	T49.0x1-	T49.0x2-	T49.0x3-	T49.0x4-	T49.0x5-	T49.0x6-
Gentian	T47.5x1-	T47.5x2-	T47.5x3-	T47.5x4-	T47.5x5-	T47.5x6-
violet	T49.0x1-	T49.0x2-	T49.0x3-	T49.0x4-	T49.0x5-	T49.0x6-
Gepefrine	T44.4x1-	T44.4x2-	T44.4x3-	T44.4x4-	T44.4x5-	T44.4x6-
Gestonorone caproate	T38.5x1-	T38.5x2-	T38.5x3-	T38.5x4-	T38.5x5-	T38.5x6-
Gexane	T49.0x1-	T49.0x2-	T49.0x3-	T49.0x4-	T49.0x5-	T49.0x6-
Gila monster (venom)	T63.111-	T63.112-	T63.113-	T63.114-	—	—
Ginger	T47.5x1-	T47.5x2-	T47.5x3-	T47.5x4-	T47.5x5-	T47.5x6-
Jamaica — see Jamaica, ginger						
Gitalin	T46.0x1-	T46.0x2-	T46.0x3-	T46.0x4-	T46.0x5-	T46.0x6-
amorphous	T46.0x1-	T46.0x2-	T46.0x3-	T46.0x4-	T46.0x5-	T46.0x6-
Gitaloxin	T46.0x1-	T46.0x2-	T46.0x3-	T46.0x4-	T46.0x5-	T46.0x6-
Gitoxin	T46.0x1-	T46.0x2-	T46.0x3-	T46.0x4-	T46.0x5-	T46.0x6-
Glafenine	T39.8x1-	T39.8x2-	T39.8x3-	T39.8x4-	T39.8x5-	T39.8x6-
Glandular extract (medicinal) NEC	T50.Z91-	T50.Z92-	T50.Z93-	T50.Z94-	T50.Z95-	T50.Z96-
Glaucarubin	T37.3x1-	T37.3x2-	T37.3x3-	T37.3x4-	T37.3x5-	T37.3x6-
Glibenclamide	T38.3x1-	T38.3x2-	T38.3x3-	T38.3x4-	T38.3x5-	T38.3x6-
Glibornuride	T38.3x1-	T38.3x2-	T38.3x3-	T38.3x4-	T38.3x5-	T38.3x6-
Gliclazide	T38.3x1-	T38.3x2-	T38.3x3-	T38.3x4-	T38.3x5-	T38.3x6-
Glimidine	T38.3x1-	T38.3x2-	T38.3x3-	T38.3x4-	T38.3x5-	T38.3x6-
Glipizide	T38.3x1-	T38.3x2-	T38.3x3-	T38.3x4-	T38.3x5-	T38.3x6-
Gliquidone	T38.3x1-	T38.3x2-	T38.3x3-	T38.3x4-	T38.3x5-	T38.3x6-
Glisolamide	T38.3x1-	T38.3x2-	T38.3x3-	T38.3x4-	T38.3x5-	T38.3x6-
Glisoxepide	T38.3x1-	T38.3x2-	T38.3x3-	T38.3x4-	T38.3x5-	T38.3x6-

Table of Drugs & Chemicals	Accidental (Unintentional)	Self-Harm (Intentional)	Assault	Undetermined	Adverse Effect	Underdosing
Globin zinc insulin	T38.3x1-	T38.3x2-	T38.3x3-	T38.3x4-	T38.3x5-	T38.3x6-
Globulin						
antilymphocytic	T50.Z11-	T50.Z12-	T50.Z13-	T50.Z14-	T50.Z15-	T50.Z16-
antirhesus	T50.Z11-	T50.Z12-	T50.Z13-	T50.Z14-	T50.Z15-	T50.Z16-
antivenin	T50.Z11-	T50.Z12-	T50.Z13-	T50.Z14-	T50.Z15-	T50.Z16-
antiviral	T50.Z11-	T50.Z12-	T50.Z13-	T50.Z14-	T50.Z15-	T50.Z16-
Glucagon	T38.3x1-	T38.3x2-	T38.3x3-	T38.3x4-	T38.3x5-	T38.3x6-
Glucocorticoids	T38.0x1-	T38.0x2-	T38.0x3-	T38.0x4-	T38.0x5-	T38.0x6-
Glucocorticosteroid	T38.0x1-	T38.0x2-	T38.0x3-	T38.0x4-	T38.0x5-	T38.0x6-
Gluconic acid	T50.991-	T50.992-	T50.993-	T50.994-	T50.995-	T50.996-
Glucosamine sulfate	T39.4x1-	T39.4x2-	T39.4x3-	T39.4x4-	T39.4x5-	T39.4x6-
Glucose	T50.3x1-	T50.3x2-	T50.3x3-	T50.3x4-	T50.3x5-	T50.3x6-
with sodium chloride	T50.3x1-	T50.3x2-	T50.3x3-	T50.3x4-	T50.3x5-	T50.3x6-
Glucosulfone sodium	T37.1x1-	T37.1x2-	T37.1x3-	T37.1x4-	T37.1x5-	T37.1x6-
Glucurolactone	T47.8x1-	T47.8x2-	T47.8x3-	T47.8x4-	T47.8x5-	T47.8x6-
Glue NEC	T52.8x1-	T52.8x2-	T52.8x3-	T52.8x4-	—	—
Glutamic acid	T47.5x1-	T47.5x2-	T47.5x3-	T47.5x4-	T47.5x5-	T47.5x6-
Glutaral (medicinal)	T49.0x1-	T49.0x2-	T49.0x3-	T49.0x4-	T49.0x5-	T49.0x6-
nonmedicinal	T65.891-	T65.892-	T65.893-	T65.894-	—	—
Glutaraldehyde (nonmedicinal)	T65.891-	T65.892-	T65.893-	T65.894-	—	—
medicinal	T49.0x1-	T49.0x2-	T49.0x3-	T49.0x4-	T49.0x5-	T49.0x6-
Glutathione	T50.6x1-	T50.6x2-	T50.6x3-	T50.6x4-	T50.6x5-	T50.6x6-
Glutethimide	T42.6x1-	T42.6x2-	T42.6x3-	T42.6x4-	T42.6x5-	T42.6x6-
Glyburide	T38.3x1-	T38.3x2-	T38.3x3-	T38.3x4-	T38.3x5-	T38.3x6-
Glycerin	T47.4x1-	T47.4x2-	T47.4x3-	T47.4x4-	T47.4x5-	T47.4x6-
Glycerol	T47.4x1-	T47.4x2-	T47.4x3-	T47.4x4-	T47.4x5-	T47.4x6-
borax	T49.6x1-	T49.6x2-	T49.6x3-	T49.6x4-	T49.6x5-	T49.6x6-
intravenous	T50.3x1-	T50.3x2-	T50.3x3-	T50.3x4-	T50.3x5-	T50.3x6-
iodinated	T48.4x1-	T48.4x2-	T48.4x3-	T48.4x4-	T48.4x5-	T48.4x6-
Glycerophosphate	T50.991-	T50.992-	T50.993-	T50.994-	T50.995-	T50.996-
Glyceryl						
gualacolate	T48.4x1-	T48.4x2-	T48.4x3-	T48.4x4-	T48.4x5-	T48.4x6-
nitrate	T46.3x1-	T46.3x2-	T46.3x3-	T46.3x4-	T46.3x5-	T46.3x6-
triacetate (topical)	T49.0x1-	T49.0x2-	T49.0x3-	T49.0x4-	T49.0x5-	T49.0x6-
trinitrate	T46.3x1-	T46.3x2-	T46.3x3-	T46.3x4-	T46.3x5-	T46.3x6-
Glycine	T50.3x1-	T50.3x2-	T50.3x3-	T50.3x4-	T50.3x5-	T50.3x6-
Glyclopyramide	T38.3x1-	T38.3x2-	T38.3x3-	T38.3x4-	T38.3x5-	T38.3x6-
Glycobiarsol	T37.3x1-	T37.3x2-	T37.3x3-	T37.3x4-	T37.3x5-	T37.3x6-
Glycols (ether)	T52.3x1-	T52.3x2-	T52.3x3-	T52.3x4-	—	—
Glyconiazide	T37.1x1-	T37.1x2-	T37.1x3-	T37.1x4-	T37.1x5-	T37.1x6-
Glycopyrrolate	T44.3x1-	T44.3x2-	T44.3x3-	T44.3x4-	T44.3x5-	T44.3x6-
Glycopyrronium	T44.3x1-	T44.3x2-	T44.3x3-	T44.3x4-	T44.3x5-	T44.3x6-
bromide	T44.3x1-	T44.3x2-	T44.3x3-	T44.3x4-	T44.3x5-	T44.3x6-
Glycoside, cardiac (stimulant)	T46.0x1-	T46.0x2-	T46.0x3-	T46.0x4-	T46.0x5-	T46.0x6-
Glycyclamide	T38.3x1-	T38.3x2-	T38.3x3-	T38.3x4-	T38.3x5-	T38.3x6-
Glycyrrhiza extract	T48.4x1-	T48.4x2-	T48.4x3-	T48.4x4-	T48.4x5-	T48.4x6-
Glycyrrhizic acid	T48.4x1-	T48.4x2-	T48.4x3-	T48.4x4-	T48.4x5-	T48.4x6-
Glycyrrhizinate potassium	T48.4x1-	T48.4x2-	T48.4x3-	T48.4x4-	T48.4x5-	T48.4x6-
Glymidine sodium	T38.3x1-	T38.3x2-	T38.3x3-	T38.3x4-	T38.3x5-	T38.3x6-
Glyphosate	T60.3x1-	T60.3x2-	T60.3x3-	T60.3x4-	—	—
Glyphylline	T48.6x1-	T48.6x2-	T48.6x3-	T48.6x4-	T48.6x5-	T48.6x6-
Gold						
colloidal (I98Au)	T45.1x1-	T45.1x2-	T45.1x3-	T45.1x4-	T45.1x5-	T45.1x6-
salts	T39.4x1-	T39.4x2-	T39.4x3-	T39.4x4-	T39.4x5-	T39.4x6-
Golden sulfide of antimony	T56.891-	T56.892-	T56.893-	T56.894-	—	—
Goldylocks	T62.2x1-	T62.2x2-	T62.2x3-	T62.2x4-	—	—
Gonadal tissue extract	T38.901-	T38.902-	T38.903-	T38.904-	T38.905-	T38.906-
female	T38.5x1-	T38.5x2-	T38.5x3-	T38.5x4-	T38.5x5-	T38.5x6-
male	T38.7x1-	T38.7x2-	T38.7x3-	T38.7x4-	T38.7x5-	T38.7x6-
Gonadorelin	T38.891-	T38.892-	T38.893-	T38.894-	T38.895-	T38.896-

DRUGS & CHEMICALS

Table of Drugs & Chemicals	POISONING Accidental (Unintentional)	POISONING Self-Harm (Intentional)	POISONING Assault	POISONING Undetermined	Adverse Effect	Underdosing
Gonadotropin	T38.891-	T38.892-	T38.893-	T38.894-	T38.895-	T38.896-
chorionic	T38.891-	T38.892-	T38.893-	T38.894-	T38.895-	T38.896-
pituitary	T38.811-	T38.812-	T38.813-	T38.814-	T38.815-	T38.816-
Goserelin	T45.1x1-	T45.1x2-	T45.1x3-	T45.1x4-	T45.1x5-	T45.1x6-
Grain alcohol	T51.0x1-	T51.0x2-	T51.0x3-	T51.0x4-	—	—
Gramicidin	T49.0x1-	T49.0x2-	T49.0x3-	T49.0x4-	T49.0x5-	T49.0x6-
Granisetron	T45.0x1-	T45.0x2-	T45.0x3-	T45.0x4-	T45.0x5-	T45.0x6-
Gratiola officinalis	T62.2x1-	T62.2x2-	T62.2x3-	T62.2x4-	—	—
Grease	T65.891-	T65.892-	T65.893-	T65.894-	—	—
Green hellebore	T62.2x1-	T62.2x2-	T62.2x3-	T62.2x4-	—	—
Green soap	T49.2x1-	T49.2x2-	T49.2x3-	T49.2x4-	T49.2x5-	T49.2x6-
Grifulvin	T36.7x1-	T36.7x2-	T36.7x3-	T36.7x4-	T36.7x5-	T36.7x6-
Griseofulvin	T36.7x1-	T36.7x2-	T36.7x3-	T36.7x4-	T36.7x5-	T36.7x6-
Growth hormone	T38.811-	T38.812-	T38.813-	T38.814-	T38.815-	T38.816-
Guaiac reagent	T50.991-	T50.992-	T50.993-	T50.994-	T50.995-	T50.996-
Guaiacol derivatives	T48.4x1-	T48.4x2-	T48.4x3-	T48.4x4-	T48.4x5-	T48.4x6-
Guaifenesin	T48.4x1-	T48.4x2-	T48.4x3-	T48.4x4-	T48.4x5-	T48.4x6-
Guaimesal	T48.4x1-	T48.4x2-	T48.4x3-	T48.4x4-	T48.4x5-	T48.4x6-
Guaiphenesin	T48.4x1-	T48.4x2-	T48.4x3-	T48.4x4-	T48.4x5-	T48.4x6-
Guamecycline	T36.4x1-	T36.4x2-	T36.4x3-	T36.4x4-	T36.4x5-	T36.4x6-
Guanabenz	T46.5x1-	T46.5x2-	T46.5x3-	T46.5x4-	T46.5x5-	T46.5x6-
Guanacline	T46.5x1-	T46.5x2-	T46.5x3-	T46.5x4-	T46.5x5-	T46.5x6-
Guanadrel	T46.5x1-	T46.5x2-	T46.5x3-	T46.5x4-	T46.5x5-	T46.5x6-
Guanatol	T37.2x1-	T37.2x2-	T37.2x3-	T37.2x4-	T37.2x5-	T37.2x6-
Guanethidine	T46.5x1-	T46.5x2-	T46.5x3-	T46.5x4-	T46.5x5-	T46.5x6-
Guanfacine	T46.5x1-	T46.5x2-	T46.5x3-	T46.5x4-	T46.5x5-	T46.5x6-
Guano	T65.891-	T65.892-	T65.893-	T65.894-	—	—
Guanochlor	T46.5x1-	T46.5x2-	T46.5x3-	T46.5x4-	T46.5x5-	T46.5x6-
Guanoclor	T46.5x1-	T46.5x2-	T46.5x3-	T46.5x4-	T46.5x5-	T46.5x6-
Guanoctine	T46.5x1-	T46.5x2-	T46.5x3-	T46.5x4-	T46.5x5-	T46.5x6-
Guanoxabenz	T46.5x1-	T46.5x2-	T46.5x3-	T46.5x4-	T46.5x5-	T46.5x6-
Guanoxan	T46.5x1-	T46.5x2-	T46.5x3-	T46.5x4-	T46.5x5-	T46.5x6-
Guar gum (medicinal)	T46.6x1-	T46.6x2-	T46.6x3-	T46.6x4-	T46.6x5-	T46.6x6-
Hachimycin	T36.7x1-	T36.7x2-	T36.7x3-	T36.7x4-	T36.7x5-	T36.7x6-
Hair						
dye	T49.4x1-	T49.4x2-	T49.4x3-	T49.4x4-	T49.4x5-	T49.4x6-
preparation NEC	T49.4x1-	T49.4x2-	T49.4x3-	T49.4x4-	T49.4x5-	T49.4x6-
Halazepam	T42.4x1-	T42.4x2-	T42.4x3-	T42.4x4-	T42.4x5-	T42.4x6-
Halcinolone	T49.0x1-	T49.0x2-	T49.0x3-	T49.0x4-	T49.0x5-	T49.0x6-
Halcinonide	T49.0x1-	T49.0x2-	T49.0x3-	T49.0x4-	T49.0x5-	T49.0x6-
Halethazole	T49.0x1-	T49.0x2-	T49.0x3-	T49.0x4-	T49.0x5-	T49.0x6-
Hallucinogen NEC	T40.901-	T40.902-	T40.903-	T40.904-	T40.905-	T40.906-
Halofantrine	T37.2x1-	T37.2x2-	T37.2x3-	T37.2x4-	T37.2x5-	T37.2x6-
Halofenate	T46.6x1-	T46.6x2-	T46.6x3-	T46.6x4-	T46.6x5-	T46.6x6-
Halometasone	T49.0x1-	T49.0x2-	T49.0x3-	T49.0x4-	T49.0x5-	T49.0x6-
Haloperidol	T43.4x1-	T43.4x2-	T43.4x3-	T43.4x4-	T43.4x5-	T43.4x6-
Haloprogin	T49.0x1-	T49.0x2-	T49.0x3-	T49.0x4-	T49.0x5-	T49.0x6-
Halotex	T49.0x1-	T49.0x2-	T49.0x3-	T49.0x4-	T49.0x5-	T49.0x6-
Halothane	T41.0x1-	T41.0x2-	T41.0x3-	T41.0x4-	T41.0x5-	T41.0x6-
Haloxazolam	T42.4x1-	T42.4x2-	T42.4x3-	T42.4x4-	T42.4x5-	T42.4x6-
Halquinols	T49.0x1-	T49.0x2-	T49.0x3-	T49.0x4-	T49.0x5-	T49.0x6-
Hamamelis	T49.2x1-	T49.2x2-	T49.2x3-	T49.2x4-	T49.2x5-	T49.2x6-
Haptendextran	T45.8x1-	T45.8x2-	T45.8x3-	T45.8x4-	T45.8x5-	T45.8x6-
Harmonyl	T46.5x1-	T46.5x2-	T46.5x3-	T46.5x4-	T46.5x5-	T46.5x6-
Hartmann's solution	T50.3x1-	T50.3x2-	T50.3x3-	T50.3x4-	T50.3x5-	T50.3x6-
Hashish	T40.7x1-	T40.7x2-	T40.7x3-	T40.7x4-	T40.7x5-	T40.7x6-
Hawaiian Woodrose seeds	T40.991-	T40.992-	T40.993-	T40.994-	—	—
HCB	T60.3x1-	T60.3x2-	T60.3x3-	T60.3x4-	—	—
HCH	T53.6x1-	T53.6x2-	T53.6x3-	T53.6x4-	—	—
medicinal	T49.0x1-	T49.0x2-	T49.0x3-	T49.0x4-	T49.0x5-	T49.0x6-
HCN	T57.3x1-	T57.3x2-	T57.3x3-	T57.3x4-	—	—
Headache cures, drugs, powders NEC	T50.901-	T50.902-	T50.903-	T50.904-	T50.905-	T50.906-
Heavenly Blue (morning glory)	T40.991-	T40.992-	T40.993-	T40.994-	—	—

Table of Drugs & Chemicals	POISONING Accidental (Unintentional)	POISONING Self-Harm (Intentional)	POISONING Assault	POISONING Undetermined	Adverse Effect	Underdosing
Heavy metal antidote	T45.8x1-	T45.8x2-	T45.8x3-	T45.8x4-	T45.8x5-	T45.8x6-
Hedaquinium	T49.0x1-	T49.0x2-	T49.0x3-	T49.0x4-	T49.0x5-	T49.0x6-
Hedge hyssop	T62.2x1-	T62.2x2-	T62.2x3-	T62.2x4-	—	—
Heet	T49.8x1-	T49.8x2-	T49.8x3-	T49.8x4-	T49.8x5-	T49.8x6-
Helenin	T37.4x1-	T37.4x2-	T37.4x3-	T37.4x4-	T37.4x5-	T37.4x6-
Helium (nonmedicinal) NEC	T59.891-	T59.892-	T59.893-	T59.894-	—	—
medicinal	T48.991-	T48.992-	T48.993-	T48.994-	T48.995-	T48.996-
Hellebore (black) (green) (white)	T62.2x1-	T62.2x2-	T62.2x3-	T62.2x4-	—	—
Hematin	T45.8x1-	T45.8x2-	T45.8x3-	T45.8x4-	T45.8x5-	T45.8x6-
Hematinic preparation	T45.8x1-	T45.8x2-	T45.8x3-	T45.8x4-	T45.8x5-	T45.8x6-
Hematological agent	T45.91x-	T45.92x-	T45.93x-	T45.94x-	T45.95x-	T45.96x-
specified NEC	T45.8x1-	T45.8x2-	T45.8x3-	T45.8x4-	T45.8x5-	T45.8x6-
Hemlock	T62.2x1-	T62.2x2-	T62.2x3-	T62.2x4-	—	—
Hemostatic	T45.621-	T45.622-	T45.623-	T45.624-	T45.625-	T45.626-
drug, systemic	T45.621-	T45.622-	T45.623-	T45.624-	T45.625-	T45.626-
Hemostyptic	T49.4x1-	T49.4x2-	T49.4x3-	T49.4x4-	T49.4x5-	T49.4x6-
Henbane	T62.2x1-	T62.2x2-	T62.2x3-	T62.2x4-	—	—
Heparin (sodium)	T45.511-	T45.512-	T45.513-	T45.514-	T45.515-	T45.516-
action reverser	T45.7x1-	T45.7x2-	T45.7x3-	T45.7x4-	T45.7x5-	T45.7x6-
Heparin-fraction	T45.511-	T45.512-	T45.513-	T45.514-	T45.515-	T45.516-
Heparinoid (systemic)	T45.511-	T45.512-	T45.513-	T45.514-	T45.515-	T45.516-
Hepatic secretion stimulant	T47.8x1-	T47.8x2-	T47.8x3-	T47.8x4-	T47.8x5-	T47.8x6-
Hepatitis B						
immune globulin	T50.Z11-	T50.Z12-	T50.Z13-	T50.Z14-	T50.Z15-	T50.Z16-
vaccine	T50.B91-	T50.B92-	T50.B93-	T50.B94-	T50.B95-	T50.B96-
Hepronicate	T46.7x1-	T46.7x2-	T46.7x3-	T46.7x4-	T46.7x5-	T46.7x6-
Heptabarb	T42.3x1-	T42.3x2-	T42.3x3-	T42.3x4-	T42.3x5-	T42.3x6-
Heptabarbital	T42.3x1-	T42.3x2-	T42.3x3-	T42.3x4-	T42.3x5-	T42.3x6-
Heptabarbitone	T42.3x1-	T42.3x2-	T42.3x3-	T42.3x4-	T42.3x5-	T42.3x6-
Heptachlor	T60.1x1-	T60.1x2-	T60.1x3-	T60.1x4-	—	—
Heptalgin	T40.2x1-	T40.2x2-	T40.2x3-	T40.2x4-	T40.2x5-	T40.2x6-
Heptaminol	T46.3x1-	T46.3x2-	T46.3x3-	T46.3x4-	T46.3x5-	T46.3x6-
Herbicide NEC	T60.3x1-	T60.3x2-	T60.3x3-	T60.3x4-	—	—
Heroin	T40.1x1-	T40.1x2-	T40.1x3-	T40.1x4-	—	—
Herplex	T49.5x1-	T49.5x2-	T49.5x3-	T49.5x4-	T49.5x5-	T49.5x6-
HES	T45.8x1-	T45.8x2-	T45.8x3-	T45.8x4-	T45.8x5-	T45.8x6-
Hesperidin	T46.991-	T46.992-	T46.993-	T46.994-	T46.995-	T46.996-
Hetacillin	T36.0x1-	T36.0x2-	T36.0x3-	T36.0x4-	T36.0x5-	T36.0x6-
Hetastarch	T45.8x1-	T45.8x2-	T45.8x3-	T45.8x4-	T45.8x5-	T45.8x6-
HETP	T60.0x1-	T60.0x2-	T60.0x3-	T60.0x4-	—	—
Hexachlorobenzene (vapor)	T60.3x1-	T60.3x2-	T60.3x3-	T60.3x4-	—	—
Hexachlorocyclohexane	T53.6x1-	T53.6x2-	T53.6x3-	T53.6x4-	—	—
Hexachlorophene	T49.0x1-	T49.0x2-	T49.0x3-	T49.0x4-	T49.0x5-	T49.0x6-
Hexadiline	T46.3x1-	T46.3x2-	T46.3x3-	T46.3x4-	T46.3x5-	T46.3x6-
Hexadimethrine (bromide)	T45.7x1-	T45.7x2-	T45.7x3-	T45.7x4-	T45.7x5-	T45.7x6-
Hexadylamine	T46.3x1-	T46.3x2-	T46.3x3-	T46.3x4-	T46.3x5-	T46.3x6-
Hexaethyl tetraphos-phate	T60.0x1-	T60.0x2-	T60.0x3-	T60.0x4-	—	—
Hexafluorenium bromide	T48.1x1-	T48.1x2-	T48.1x3-	T48.1x4-	T48.1x5-	T48.1x6-
Hexafluronium (bromide)	T48.1x1-	T48.1x2-	T48.1x3-	T48.1x4-	T48.1x5-	T48.1x6-
Hexa-germ	T49.2x1-	T49.2x2-	T49.2x3-	T49.2x4-	T49.2x5-	T49.2x6-
Hexahydrobenzol	T52.8x1-	T52.8x2-	T52.8x3-	T52.8x4-	—	—
Hexahydrocresol(s)	T51.8x1-	T51.8x2-	T51.8x3-	T51.8x4-	—	—
arsenide	T57.0x1-	T57.0x2-	T57.0x3-	T57.0x4-	—	—
arseniurated	T57.0x1-	T57.0x2-	T57.0x3-	T57.0x4-	—	—
cyanide	T57.3x1-	T57.3x2-	T57.3x3-	T57.3x4-	—	—
gas	T59.891-	T59.892-	T59.893-	T59.894-	—	—
fluoride (liquid)	T57.8x1-	T57.8x2-	T57.8x3-	T57.8x4-	—	—
vapor	T59.891-	T59.892-	T59.893-	T59.894-	—	—
phophorated	T60.0x1-	T60.0x2-	T60.0x3-	T60.0x4-	—	—
sulfate	T57.8x1-	T57.8x2-	T57.8x3-	T57.8x4-	—	—
sulfide (gas)	T59.6x1-	T59.6x2-	T59.6x3-	T59.6x4-	—	—
arseniurated	T57.0x1-	T57.0x2-	T57.0x3-	T57.0x4-	—	—
sulfurated	T57.8x1-	T57.8x2-	T57.8x3-	T57.8x4-	—	—
Hexahydrophenol	T51.8x1-	T51.8x2-	T51.8x3-	T51.8x4-	—	—

Table of Drugs & Chemicals	Accidental (Unintentional)	Self-Harm (Intentional)	Assault	Undetermined	Adverse Effect	Underdosing
Hexalen	T51.8x1-	T51.8x2-	T51.8x3-	T51.8x4-	—	—
Hexamethonium bromide	T44.2x1-	T44.2x2-	T44.2x3-	T44.2x4-	T44.2x5-	T44.2x6-
Hexamethylene	T52.8x1-	T52.8x2-	T52.8x3-	T52.8x4-	—	—
Hexamethylmelamine	T45.1x1-	T45.1x2-	T45.1x3-	T45.1x4-	T45.1x5-	T45.1x6-
Hexamidine	T49.0x1-	T49.0x2-	T49.0x3-	T49.0x4-	T49.0x5-	T49.0x6-
Hexamine (mandelate)	T37.8x1-	T37.8x2-	T37.8x3-	T37.8x4-	T37.8x5-	T37.8x6-
Hexanone, 2-hexanone	T52.4x1-	T52.4x2-	T52.4x3-	T52.4x4-	—	—
Hexanuorenium	T48.1x1-	T48.1x2-	T48.1x3-	T48.1x4-	T48.1x5-	T48.1x6-
Hexapropymate	T42.6x1-	T42.6x2-	T42.6x3-	T42.6x4-	T42.6x5-	T42.6x6-
Hexasonium iodide	T44.3x1-	T44.3x2-	T44.3x3-	T44.3x4-	T44.3x5-	T44.3x6-
Hexcarbacholine bromide	T48.1x1-	T48.1x2-	T48.1x3-	T48.1x4-	T48.1x5-	T48.1x6-
Hexemal	T42.3x1-	T42.3x2-	T42.3x3-	T42.3x4-	T42.3x5-	T42.3x6-
Hexestrol	T38.5x1-	T38.5x2-	T38.5x3-	T38.5x4-	T38.5x5-	T38.5x6-
Hexethal (sodium)	T42.3x1-	T42.3x2-	T42.3x3-	T42.3x4-	T42.3x5-	T42.3x6-
Hexetidine	T37.8x1-	T37.8x2-	T37.8x3-	T37.8x4-	T37.8x5-	T37.8x6-
Hexobarbital	T42.3x1-	T42.3x2-	T42.3x3-	T42.3x4-	T42.3x5-	T42.3x6-
rectal	T41.291-	T41.292-	T41.293-	T41.294-	T41.295-	T41.296-
sodium	T41.1x1-	T41.1x2-	T41.1x3-	T41.1x4-	T41.1x5-	T41.1x6-
Hexobendine	T46.3x1-	T46.3x2-	T46.3x3-	T46.3x4-	T46.3x5-	T46.3x6-
Hexocyclium	T44.3x1-	T44.3x2-	T44.3x3-	T44.3x4-	T44.3x5-	T44.3x6-
metilsulfate	T44.3x1-	T44.3x2-	T44.3x3-	T44.3x4-	T44.3x5-	T44.3x6-
Hexoestrol	T38.5x1-	T38.5x2-	T38.5x3-	T38.5x4-	T38.5x5-	T38.5x6-
Hexone	T52.4x1-	T52.4x2-	T52.4x3-	T52.4x4-	—	—
Hexoprenaline	T48.6x1-	T48.6x2-	T48.6x3-	T48.6x4-	T48.6x5-	T48.6x6-
Hexylcaine	T41.3x1-	T41.3x2-	T41.3x3-	T41.3x4-	T41.3x5-	T41.3x6-
Hexylresorcinol	T52.2x1-	T52.2x2-	T52.2x3-	T52.2x4-	—	—
HGH (human growth hormone)	T38.811-	T38.812-	T38.813-	T38.814-	T38.815-	T38.816-
Hinkle's pills	T47.2x1-	T47.2x2-	T47.2x3-	T47.2x4-	T47.2x5-	T47.2x6-
Histalog	T50.8x1-	T50.8x2-	T50.8x3-	T50.8x4-	T50.8x5-	T50.8x6-
Histamine (phosphate)	T50.8x1-	T50.8x2-	T50.8x3-	T50.8x4-	T50.8x5-	T50.8x6-
Histoplasmin	T50.8x1-	T50.8x2-	T50.8x3-	T50.8x4-	T50.8x5-	T50.8x6-
Holly berries	T62.2x1-	T62.2x2-	T62.2x3-	T62.2x4-	—	—
Homatropine	T44.3x1-	T44.3x2-	T44.3x3-	T44.3x4-	T44.3x5-	T44.3x6-
methylbromide	T44.3x1-	T44.3x2-	T44.3x3-	T44.3x4-	T44.3x5-	T44.3x6-
Homochlorcyclizine	T45.0x1-	T45.0x2-	T45.0x3-	T45.0x4-	T45.0x5-	T45.0x6-
Homosalate	T49.3x1-	T49.3x2-	T49.3x3-	T49.3x4-	T49.3x5-	T49.3x6-
Homo-tet	T50.Z11-	T50.Z12-	T50.Z13-	T50.Z14-	T50.Z15-	T50.Z16-
Hormone	T38.801-	T38.802-	T38.803-	T38.804-	T38.805-	T38.806-
adrenal cortical steroids	T38.0x1-	T38.0x2-	T38.0x3-	T38.0x4-	T38.0x5-	T38.0x6-
androgenic	T38.7x1-	T38.7x2-	T38.7x3-	T38.7x4-	T38.7x5-	T38.7x6-
anterior pituitary NEC	T38.811-	T38.812-	T38.813-	T38.814-	T38.815-	T38.816-
antidiabetic agents	T38.3x1-	T38.3x2-	T38.3x3-	T38.3x4-	T38.3x5-	T38.3x6-
antidiuretic	T38.891-	T38.892-	T38.893-	T38.894-	T38.895-	T38.896-
cancer therapy	T45.1x1-	T45.1x2-	T45.1x3-	T45.1x4-	T45.1x5-	T45.1x6-
follicle stimulating	T38.811-	T38.812-	T38.813-	T38.814-	T38.815-	T38.816-
gonadotropic	T38.891-	T38.892-	T38.893-	T38.894-	T38.895-	T38.896-
pituitary	T38.811-	T38.812-	T38.813-	T38.814-	T38.815-	T38.816-
growth	T38.811-	T38.812-	T38.813-	T38.814-	T38.815-	T38.816-
luteinizing	T38.811-	T38.812-	T38.813-	T38.814-	T38.815-	T38.816-
ovarian	T38.5x1-	T38.5x2-	T38.5x3-	T38.5x4-	T38.5x5-	T38.5x6-
oxytocic	T48.0x1-	T48.0x2-	T48.0x3-	T48.0x4-	T48.0x5-	T48.0x6-
parathyroid (derivatives)	T50.991-	T50.992-	T50.993-	T50.994-	T50.995-	T50.996-
pituitary (posterior) NEC	T38.891-	T38.892-	T38.893-	T38.894-	T38.895-	T38.896-
anterior	T38.811-	T38.812-	T38.813-	T38.814-	T38.815-	T38.816-
specified, NEC	T38.891-	T38.892-	T38.893-	T38.894-	T38.895-	T38.896-
thyroid	T38.1x1-	T38.1x2-	T38.1x3-	T38.1x4-	T38.1x5-	T38.1x6-
Hornet (sting)	T63.451-	T63.452-	T63.453-	T63.454-	—	—
Horse anti-human lymphocytic serum	T50.Z11-	T50.Z12-	T50.Z13-	T50.Z14-	T50.Z15-	T50.Z16-
Horticulture agent NEC	T65.91x-	T65.92x-	T65.93x-	T65.94x-	—	—
with pesticide	T60.91x-	T60.92x-	T60.93x-	T60.94x-	—	—

Table of Drugs & Chemicals	Accidental (Unintentional)	Self-Harm (Intentional)	Assault	Undetermined	Adverse Effect	Underdosing
Human						
albumin	T45.8x1-	T45.8x2-	T45.8x3-	T45.8x4-	T45.8x5-	T45.8x6-
growth hormone (HGH)	T38.811-	T38.812-	T38.813-	T38.814-	T38.815-	T38.816-
immune serum	T50.Z11-	T50.Z12-	T50.Z13-	T50.Z14-	T50.Z15-	T50.Z16-
Hyaluronidase	T45.3x1-	T45.3x2-	T45.3x3-	T45.3x4-	T45.3x5-	T45.3x6-
Hyazyme	T45.3x1-	T45.3x2-	T45.3x3-	T45.3x4-	T45.3x5-	T45.3x6-
Hycodan	T40.2x1-	T40.2x2-	T40.2x3-	T40.2x4-	T40.2x5-	T40.2x6-
Hydantoin derivative NEC	T42.0x1-	T42.0x2-	T42.0x3-	T42.0x4-	T42.0x5-	T42.0x6-
Hydeltra	T38.0x1-	T38.0x2-	T38.0x3-	T38.0x4-	T38.0x5-	T38.0x6-
Hydergine	T44.6x1-	T44.6x2-	T44.6x3-	T44.6x4-	T44.6x5-	T44.6x6-
Hydrabamine penicillin	T36.0x1-	T36.0x2-	T36.0x3-	T36.0x4-	T36.0x5-	T36.0x6-
Hydralazine	T46.5x1-	T46.5x2-	T46.5x3-	T46.5x4-	T46.5x5-	T46.5x6-
Hydrargaphen	T49.0x1-	T49.0x2-	T49.0x3-	T49.0x4-	T49.0x5-	T49.0x6-
Hydrargyri amino-chloridum	T49.0x1-	T49.0x2-	T49.0x3-	T49.0x4-	T49.0x5-	T49.0x6-
Hydrastine	T48.291-	T48.292-	T48.293-	T48.294-	T48.295-	T48.296-
Hydrazine	T54.1x1-	T54.1x2-	T54.1x3-	T54.1x4-	—	—
monoamine oxidase inhibitors	T43.1x1-	T43.1x2-	T43.1x3-	T43.1x4-	T43.1x5-	T43.1x6-
Hydrazoic acid, azides	T54.2x1-	T54.2x2-	T54.2x3-	T54.2x4-	—	—
Hydriodic acid	T48.4x1-	T48.4x2-	T48.4x3-	T48.4x4-	—	T48.4x6-
Hydrocarbon gas	T59.891-	T59.892-	T59.893-	T59.894-	—	—
incomplete combustion of — see Carbon, monoxide, fuel, utility						
liquefied (mobile container)	T59.891-	T59.892-	T59.893-	T59.894-	—	—
piped (natural)	T59.891-	T59.892-	T59.893-	T59.894-	—	—
Hydrochloric acid (liquid)	T54.2x1-	T54.2x2-	T54.2x3-	T54.2x4-	—	—
medicinal (digestant)	T47.5x1-	T47.5x2-	T47.5x3-	T47.5x4-	T47.5x5-	T47.5x6-
vapor	T59.891-	T59.892-	T59.893-	T59.894-	—	—
Hydrochlorothiazide	T50.2x1-	T50.2x2-	T50.2x3-	T50.2x4-	T50.2x5-	T50.2x6-
Hydrocodone	T40.2x1-	T40.2x2-	T40.2x3-	T40.2x4-	T40.2x5-	T40.2x6-
Hydrocortisone (derivatives)	T38.0x1-	T38.0x2-	T38.0x3-	T38.0x4-	T38.0x5-	T38.0x6-
aceponate	T49.0x1-	T49.0x2-	T49.0x3-	T49.0x4-	T49.0x5-	T49.0x6-
ENT agent	T49.6x1-	T49.6x2-	T49.6x3-	T49.6x4-	T49.6x5-	T49.6x6-
ophthalmic preparation	T49.5x1-	T49.5x2-	T49.5x3-	T49.5x4-	T49.5x5-	T49.5x6-
topical NEC	T49.0x1-	T49.0x2-	T49.0x3-	T49.0x4-	T49.0x5-	T49.0x6-
Hydrocortone	T38.0x1-	T38.0x2-	T38.0x3-	T38.0x4-	T38.0x5-	T38.0x6-
ENT agent	T49.6x1-	T49.6x2-	T49.6x3-	T49.6x4-	T49.6x5-	T49.6x6-
ophthalmic preparation	T49.5x1-	T49.5x2-	T49.5x3-	T49.5x4-	T49.5x5-	T49.5x6-
topical NEC	T49.0x1-	T49.0x2-	T49.0x3-	T49.0x4-	T49.0x5-	T49.0x6-
Hydrocyanic acid (liquid)	T57.3x1-	T57.3x2-	T57.3x3-	T57.3x4-	—	—
gas	T65.0x1-	T65.0x2-	T65.0x3-	T65.0x4-	—	—
Hydroflumethiazide	T50.2x1-	T50.2x2-	T50.2x3-	T50.2x4-	T50.2x5-	T50.2x6-
Hydrofluoric acid (liquid)	T54.2x1-	T54.2x2-	T54.2x3-	T54.2x4-	—	—
vapor	T59.891-	T59.892-	T59.893-	T59.894-	—	—
Hydrogen	T59.891-	T59.892-	T59.893-	T59.894-	—	—
arsenide	T57.0x1-	T57.0x2-	T57.0x3-	T57.0x4-	—	—
arseniureted	T57.0x1-	T57.0x2-	T57.0x3-	T57.0x4-	—	—
chloride	T57.8x1-	T57.8x2-	T57.8x3-	T57.8x4-	—	—
cyanide (salts)	T57.3x1-	T57.3x2-	T57.3x3-	T57.3x4-	—	—
gas	T57.3x1-	T57.3x2-	T57.3x3-	T57.3x4-	—	—
fluoride	T59.5x1-	T59.5x2-	T59.5x3-	T59.5x4-	—	—
vapor	T59.5x1-	T59.5x2-	T59.5x3-	T59.5x4-	—	—
peroxide	T49.0x1-	T49.0x2-	T49.0x3-	T49.0x4-	T49.0x5-	T49.0x6-
phosphureted	T57.1x1-	T57.1x2-	T57.1x3-	T57.1x4-	—	—
sulfide	T59.6x1-	T59.6x2-	T59.6x3-	T59.6x4-	—	—
arseniureted	T57.0x1-	T57.0x2-	T57.0x3-	T57.0x4-	—	—
sulfureted	T59.6x1-	T59.6x2-	T59.6x3-	T59.6x4-	—	—

DRUGS & CHEMICALS

Table of Drugs & Chemicals	POISONING Accidental (Unintentional)	POISONING Self-Harm (Intentional)	POISONING Assault	POISONING Undetermined	Adverse Effect	Underdosing
Hydromethylpyridine	T46.7x1-	T46.7x2-	T46.7x3-	T46.7x4-	T46.7x5-	T46.7x6-
Hydromorphinol	T40.2x1-	T40.2x2-	T40.2x3-	T40.2x4-	—	—
Hydromorphinone	T40.2x1-	T40.2x2-	T40.2x3-	T40.2x4-	T40.2x5-	T40.2x6-
Hydromorphone	T40.2x1-	T40.2x2-	T40.2x3-	T40.2x4-	T40.2x5-	T40.2x6-
Hydromox	T50.2x1-	T50.2x2-	T50.2x3-	T50.2x4-	T50.2x5-	T50.2x6-
Hydrophilic lotion	T49.3x1-	T49.3x2-	T49.3x3-	T49.3x4-	T49.3x5-	T49.3x6-
Hydroquinidine	T46.2x1-	T46.2x2-	T46.2x3-	T46.2x4-	T46.2x5-	T46.2x6-
Hydroquinone	T52.2x1-	T52.2x2-	T52.2x3-	T52.2x4-	—	—
vapor	T59.891-	T59.892-	T59.893-	T59.894-		
Hydrosulfuric acid (gas)	T59.6x1-	T59.6x2-	T59.6x3-	T59.6x4-	—	—
Hydrotalcite	T47.1x1-	T47.1x2-	T47.1x3-	T47.1x4-	T47.1x5-	T47.1x6-
Hydrous wool fat	T49.3x1-	T49.3x2-	T49.3x3-	T49.3x4-	T49.3x5-	T49.3x6-
Hydroxide, caustic	T54.3x1-	T54.3x2-	T54.3x3-	T54.3x4-	—	—
Hydroxocobalamin	T45.8x1-	T45.8x2-	T45.8x3-	T45.8x4-	T45.8x5-	T45.8x6-
Hydroxyamphetamine	T49.5x1-	T49.5x2-	T49.5x3-	T49.5x4-	T49.5x5-	T49.5x6-
Hydroxycarbamide	T45.1x1-	T45.1x2-	T45.1x3-	T45.1x4-	T45.1x5-	T45.1x6-
Hydroxychloroquine	T37.8x1-	T37.8x2-	T37.8x3-	T37.8x4-	T37.8x5-	T37.8x6-
Hydroxydihydrocodeinone	T40.2x1-	T40.2x2-	T40.2x3-	T40.2x4-	T40.2x5-	T40.2x6-
Hydroxyestrone	T38.5x1-	T38.5x2-	T38.5x3-	T38.5x4-	T38.5x5-	T38.5x6-
Hydroxyethyl starch	T45.8x1-	T45.8x2-	T45.8x3-	T45.8x4-	T45.8x5-	T45.8x6-
Hydroxymethylpenta-none..	T52.4x1-	T52.4x2-	T52.4x3-	T52.4x4-		
Hydroxyphenamate	T43.591-	T43.592-	T43.593-	T43.594-	T43.595-	T43.596-
Hydroxyphenylbutazone	T39.2x1-	T39.2x2-	T39.2x3-	T39.2x4-	T39.2x5-	T39.2x6-
Hydroxyprogesterone	T38.5x1-	T38.5x2-	T38.5x3-	T38.5x4-	T38.5x5-	T38.5x6-
caproate	T38.5x1-	T38.5x2-	T38.5x3-	T38.5x4-	T38.5x5-	T38.5x6-
Hydroxyquinoline (derivatives) NEC	T37.8x1-	T37.8x2-	T37.8x3-	T37.8x4-	T37.8x5-	T37.8x6-
Hydroxystilbamidine	T37.3x1-	T37.3x2-	T37.3x3-	T37.3x4-	T37.3x5-	T37.3x6-
Hydroxytoluene (nonmedicinal)	T54.0x1-	T54.0x2-	T54.0x3-	T54.0x4-	—	—
medicinal	T49.0x1-	T49.0x2-	T49.0x3-	T49.0x4-	T49.0x5-	T49.0x6-
Hydroxyurea	T45.1x1-	T45.1x2-	T45.1x3-	T45.1x4-	T45.1x5-	T45.1x6-
Hydroxyzine	T43.591-	T43.592-	T43.593-	T43.594-	T43.595-	T43.596-
Hyoscine	T44.3x1-	T44.3x2-	T44.3x3-	T44.3x4-	T44.3x5-	T44.3x6-
Hyoscyamine	T44.3x1-	T44.3x2-	T44.3x3-	T44.3x4-	T44.3x5-	T44.3x6-
Hyoscyamus	T44.3x1-	T44.3x2-	T44.3x3-	T44.3x4-	T44.3x5-	T44.3x6-
dry extract	T44.3x1-	T44.3x2-	T44.3x3-	T44.3x4-	T44.3x5-	T44.3x6-
Hypaque	T50.8x1-	T50.8x2-	T50.8x3-	T50.8x4-	T50.8x5-	T50.8x6-
Hypertussis	T50.Z11-	T50.Z12-	T50.Z13-	T50.Z14-	T50.Z15-	T50.Z16-
Hypnotic	T42.71x-	T42.72x-	T42.73x-	T42.74x-	T42.75x-	T42.76x-
anticonvulsant	T42.71x-	T42.72x-	T42.73x-	T42.74x-	T42.75x-	T42.76x-
specified NEC	T42.6x1-	T42.6x2-	T42.6x3-	T42.6x4-	T42.6x5-	T42.6x6-
Hypochlorite	T49.0x1-	T49.0x2-	T49.0x3-	T49.0x4-	T49.0x5-	T49.0x6-
Hypophysis, posterior	T38.891-	T38.892-	T38.893-	T38.894-	T38.895-	T38.896-
Hypotensive NEC	T46.5x1-	T46.5x2-	T46.5x3-	T46.5x4-	T46.5x5-	T46.5x6-
Hypromellose	T49.5x1-	T49.5x2-	T49.5x3-	T49.5x4-	T49.5x5-	T49.5x6-
Ibacitabine	T37.5x1-	T37.5x2-	T37.5x3-	T37.5x4-	T37.5x5-	T37.5x6-
Ibopamine	T44.991-	T44.992-	T44.993-	T44.994-	T44.995-	T44.996-
Ibufenac	T39.311-	T39.312-	T39.313-	T39.314-	T39.315-	T39.316-
Ibuprofen	T39.311-	T39.312-	T39.313-	T39.314-	T39.315-	T39.316-
Ibuproxam	T39.311-	T39.312-	T39.313-	T39.314-	T39.315-	T39.316-
Ibuterol	T48.6x1-	T48.6x2-	T48.6x3-	T48.6x4-	T48.6x5-	T48.6x6-
Ichthammol	T49.0x1-	T49.0x2-	T49.0x3-	T49.0x4-	T49.0x5-	T49.0x6-
Ichthyol	T49.4x1-	T49.4x2-	T49.4x3-	T49.4x4-	T49.4x5-	T49.4x6-
Idarubicin	T45.1x1-	T45.1x2-	T45.1x3-	T45.1x4-	T45.1x5-	T45.1x6-
Idrocilamide	T42.8x1-	T42.8x2-	T42.8x3-	T42.8x4-	T42.8x5-	T42.8x6-
Ifenprodil	T46.7x1-	T46.7x2-	T46.7x3-	T46.7x4-	T46.7x5-	T46.7x6-
Ifosfamide	T45.1x1-	T45.1x2-	T45.1x3-	T45.1x4-	T45.1x5-	T45.1x6-
Iletin	T38.3x1-	T38.3x2-	T38.3x3-	T38.3x4-	T38.3x5-	T38.3x6-
Ilex	T62.2x1-	T62.2x2-	T62.2x3-	T62.2x4-	—	—
Illuminating gas (after combustion)	T58.11x-	T58.12x-	T58.13x-	T58.14x-	—	—
prior to combustion	T59.891-	T59.892-	T59.893-	T59.894-	—	—

Table of Drugs & Chemicals	POISONING Accidental (Unintentional)	POISONING Self-Harm (Intentional)	POISONING Assault	POISONING Undetermined	Adverse Effect	Underdosing
Ilopan	T45.2x1-	T45.2x2-	T45.2x3-	T45.2x4-	T45.2x5-	T45.2x6-
Iloprost	T46.7x1-	T46.7x2-	T46.7x3-	T46.7x4-	T46.7x5-	T46.7x6-
Ilotycin	T36.3x1-	T36.3x2-	T36.3x3-	T36.3x4-	T36.3x5-	T36.3x6-
ophthalmic preparation	T49.5x1-	T49.5x2-	T49.5x3-	T49.5x4-	T49.5x5-	T49.5x6-
topical NEC	T49.0x1-	T49.0x2-	T49.0x3-	T49.0x4-	T49.0x5-	T49.0x6-
Imidazole-4-carboxamide	T45.1x1-	T45.1x2-	T45.1x3-	T45.1x4-	T45.1x5-	T45.1x6-
Iminostilbene	T42.1x1-	T42.1x2-	T42.1x3-	T42.1x4-	T42.1x5-	T42.1x6-
Imipenem	T36.0x1-	T36.0x2-	T36.0x3-	T36.0x4-	T36.0x5-	T36.0x6-
Imipramine	T43.011-	T43.012-	T43.013-	T43.014-	T43.015-	T43.016-
Immu-G	T50.Z11-	T50.Z12-	T50.Z13-	T50.Z14-	T50.Z15-	T50.Z16-
Immuglobin	T50.Z11-	T50.Z12-	T50.Z13-	T50.Z14-	T50.Z15-	T50.Z16-
Immune globulin	T50.Z11-	T50.Z12-	T50.Z13-	T50.Z14-	T50.Z15-	T50.Z16-
serum globulin	T50.Z11-	T50.Z12-	T50.Z13-	T50.Z14-	T50.Z15-	T50.Z16-
Immunoglobin human (intravenous) (normal)	T50.Z11-	T50.Z12-	T50.Z13-	T50.Z14-	T50.Z15-	T50.Z16-
unmodified	T45.1x1-	T45.1x2-	T45.1x3-	T45.1x4-	T45.1x5-	T45.1x6-
Immunosuppressive drug	T50.Z11-	T50.Z12-	T50.Z13-	T50.Z14-	T50.Z15-	T50.Z16-
Immu-tetanus	T50.Z11-	T50.Z12-	T50.Z13-	T50.Z14-	T50.Z15-	T50.Z16-
Indalpine	T43.221-	T43.222-	T43.223-	T43.224-	T43.225-	T43.226-
Indanazoline	T48.5x1-	T48.5x2-	T48.5x3-	T48.5x4-	T48.5x5-	T48.5x6-
Indandione (derivatives)	T45.511-	T45.512-	T45.513-	T45.514-	T45.515-	T45.516-
Indapamide	T46.5x1-	T46.5x2-	T46.5x3-	T46.5x4-	T46.5x5-	T46.5x6-
Indendione (derivatives)	T45.511-	T45.512-	T45.513-	T45.514-	T45.515-	T45.516-
Indenolol	T44.7x1-	T44.7x2-	T44.7x3-	T44.7x4-	T44.7x5-	T44.7x6-
Inderal	T44.7x1-	T44.7x2-	T44.7x3-	T44.7x4-	T44.7x5-	T44.7x6-
Indian hemp	T40.7x1-	T40.7x2-	T40.7x3-	T40.7x4-	T40.7x5-	T40.7x6-
tobacco	T62.2x1-	T62.2x2-	T62.2x3-	T62.2x4-	—	—
Indigo carmine	T50.8x1-	T50.8x2-	T50.8x3-	T50.8x4-	T50.8x5-	T50.8x6-
Indobufen	T45.521-	T45.522-	T45.523-	T45.524-	T45.525-	T45.526-
Indocin	T39.2x1-	T39.2x2-	T39.2x3-	T39.2x4-	T39.2x5-	T39.2x6-
Indocyanine green	T50.8x1-	T50.8x2-	T50.8x3-	T50.8x4-	T50.8x5-	T50.8x6-
Indometacin	T39.391-	T39.392-	T39.393-	T39.394-	T39.395-	T39.396-
Indomethacin	T39.391-	T39.392-	T39.393-	T39.394-	T39.395-	T39.396-
farnesil	T39.4x1-	T39.4x2-	T39.4x3-	T39.4x4-	T39.4x5-	T39.4x6-
Indoramin	T44.6x1-	T44.6x2-	T44.6x3-	T44.6x4-	T44.6x5-	T44.6x6-
Industrial alcohol	T51.0x1-	T51.0x2-	T51.0x3-	T51.0x4-	—	—
fumes	T59.891-	T59.892-	T59.893-	T59.894-	—	—
solvents (fumes) (vapors)	T52.91x-	T52.92x-	T52.93x-	T52.94x-	—	—
Influenza vaccine	T50.B91-	T50.B92-	T50.B93-	T50.B94-	T50.B95-	T50.B96-
Ingested substance NEC	T65.91x-	T65.92x-	T65.93x-	T65.94x-		
INH	T37.1x1-	T37.1x2-	T37.1x3-	T37.1x4-	T37.1x5-	T37.1x6-
Inhalation, gas (noxious) — see Gas						
Inhibitor angiotensin-converting enzyme	T46.4x1-	T46.4x2-	T46.4x3-	T46.4x4-	T46.4x5-	T46.4x6-
carbonic anhydrase	T50.2x1-	T50.2x2-	T50.2x3-	T50.2x4-	T50.2x5-	T50.2x6-
fibrinolysis	T45.621-	T45.622-	T45.623-	T45.624-	T45.625-	T45.626-
monoamine oxidase NEC	T43.1x1-	T43.1x2-	T43.1x3-	T43.1x4-	T43.1x5-	T43.1x6-
hydrazine	T43.1x1-	T43.1x2-	T43.1x3-	T43.1x4-	T43.1x5-	T43.1x6-
postsynaptic	T43.8x1-	T43.8x2-	T43.8x3-	T43.8x4-	T43.8x5-	T43.8x6-
prothrombin synthesis	T45.511-	T45.512-	T45.513-	T45.514-	T45.515-	T45.516-
Ink	T65.891-	T65.892-	T65.893-	T65.894-	—	—
Inorganic substance	T57.91x-	T57.92x-	T57.93x-	T57.94x-	—	—
Inosine pranobex	T37.5x1-	T37.5x2-	T37.5x3-	T37.5x4-	T37.5x5-	T37.5x6-
Inositol	T50.991-	T50.992-	T50.993-	T50.994-	T50.995-	T50.996-
nicotinate	T46.7x1-	T46.7x2-	T46.7x3-	T46.7x4-	T46.7x5-	T46.7x6-
Inproquone	T45.1x1-	T45.1x2-	T45.1x3-	T45.1x4-	T45.1x5-	T45.1x6-

DRUGS & CHEMICALS

Table of Drugs & Chemicals	POISONING Accidental (Unintentional)	Self-Harm (Intentional)	Assault	Undetermined	Adverse Effect	Underdosing
Insect (sting), venomous	T63.481-	T63.482-	T63.483-	T63.484-	—	—
ant	T63.421-	T63.422-	T63.423-	T63.424-	—	—
bee	T63.441-	T63.442-	T63.443-	T63.444-	—	—
caterpillar	T63.431-	T63.432-	T63.433-	T63.434-	—	—
hornet	T63.451-	T63.452-	T63.453-	T63.454-	—	—
wasp	T63.461-	T63.462-	T63.463-	T63.464-	—	—
Insecticide NEC	T60.91x-	T60.92x-	T60.93x-	T60.94x-	—	—
carbamate	T60.0x1-	T60.0x2-	T60.0x3-	T60.0x4-	—	—
chlorinated	T60.1x1-	T60.1x2-	T60.1x3-	T60.1x4-	—	—
mixed	T60.91x-	T60.92x-	T60.93x-	T60.94x-	—	—
organochlorine	T60.1x1-	T60.1x2-	T60.1x3-	T60.1x4-	—	—
organophosphorus	T60.0x1-	T60.0x2-	T60.0x3-	T60.0x4-	—	—
Insular tissue extract	T38.3x1-	T38.3x2-	T38.3x3-	T38.3x4-	T38.3x5-	T38.3x6-
Insulin (amorphous) (globin) (isophane) (Lente) (NPH) (Semilente) (Ultralente) (zinc)	T38.3x1-	T38.3x2-	T38.3x3-	T38.3x4-	T38.3x5-	T38.3x6-
defalan	T38.3x1-	T38.3x2-	T38.3x3-	T38.3x4-	T38.3x5-	T38.3x6-
human	T38.3x1-	T38.3x2-	T38.3x3-	T38.3x4-	T38.3x5-	T38.3x6-
injection, soluble	T38.3x1-	T38.3x2-	T38.3x3-	T38.3x4-	T38.3x5-	T38.3x6-
biphasic	T38.3x1-	T38.3x2-	T38.3x3-	T38.3x4-	T38.3x5-	T38.3x6-
intermediate acting	T38.3x1-	T38.3x2-	T38.3x3-	T38.3x4-	T38.3x5-	T38.3x6-
protamine zinc	T38.3x1-	T38.3x2-	T38.3x3-	T38.3x4-	T38.3x5-	T38.3x6-
slow acting	T38.3x1-	T38.3x2-	T38.3x3-	T38.3x4-	T38.3x5-	T38.3x6-
zinc protamine injection	T38.3x1-	T38.3x2-	T38.3x3-	T38.3x4-	T38.3x5-	T38.3x6-
suspension (amorphous) (crystalline)	T38.3x1-	T38.3x2-	T38.3x3-	T38.3x4-	T38.3x5-	T38.3x6-
Interferon (alpha) (beta) (gamma)	T37.5x1-	T37.5x2-	T37.5x3-	T37.5x4-	T37.5x5-	T37.5x6-
Intestinal motility control drug	T47.6x1-	T47.6x2-	T47.6x3-	T47.6x4-	T47.6x5-	T47.6x6-
biological	T47.8x1-	T47.8x2-	T47.8x3-	T47.8x4-	T47.8x5-	T47.8x6-
Intranarcon	T41.1x1-	T41.1x2-	T41.1x3-	T41.1x4-	T41.1x5-	T41.1x6-
Intravenous amino acids	T50.991-	T50.992-	T50.993-	T50.994-	T50.995-	T50.996-
fat suspension	T50.991-	T50.992-	T50.993-	T50.994-	T50.995-	T50.996-
Inulin	T50.8x1-	T50.8x2-	T50.8x3-	T50.8x4-	T50.8x5-	T50.8x6-
Invert sugar	T50.3x1-	T50.3x2-	T50.3x3-	T50.3x4-	T50.3x5-	T50.3x6-
Inza — see Naproxen						
Iobenzamic acid	T50.8x1-	T50.8x2-	T50.8x3-	T50.8x4-	T50.8x5-	T50.8x6-
Iocarmic acid	T50.8x1-	T50.8x2-	T50.8x3-	T50.8x4-	T50.8x5-	T50.8x6-
Iocetamic acid	T50.8x1-	T50.8x2-	T50.8x3-	T50.8x4-	T50.8x5-	T50.8x6-
Iodamide	T50.8x1-	T50.8x2-	T50.8x3-	T50.8x4-	T50.8x5-	T50.8x6-
Iodide NEC — see also Iodine	T49.0x1-	T49.0x2-	T49.0x3-	T49.0x4-	T49.0x5-	T49.0x6-
mercury (ointment)	T49.0x1-	T49.0x2-	T49.0x3-	T49.0x4-	T49.0x5-	T49.0x6-
methylate	T49.0x1-	T49.0x2-	T49.0x3-	T49.0x4-	T49.0x5-	T49.0x6-
potassium (expectorant) NEC	T48.4x1-	T48.4x2-	T48.4x3-	T48.4x4-	T48.4x5-	T48.4x6-
Iodinated contrast medium	T50.8x1-	T50.8x2-	T50.8x3-	T50.8x4-	T50.8x5-	T50.8x6-
glycerol	T48.4x1-	T48.4x2-	T48.4x3-	T48.4x4-	T48.4x5-	T48.4x6-
human serum albumin (131I)	T50.8x1-	T50.8x2-	T50.8x3-	T50.8x4-	T50.8x5-	T50.8x6-
Iodine (antiseptic, external) (tincture) NEC	T49.0x1-	T49.0x2-	T49.0x3-	T49.0x4-	T49.0x5-	T49.0x6-
125 — see also Radiation sickness, and Exposure to radioactivce isotopes	T50.8x1-	T50.8x2-	T50.8x3-	T50.8x4-	T50.8x5-	T50.8x6-
therapeutic	T50.991-	T50.992-	T50.993-	T50.994-	T50.995-	T50.996-
131 — see also Radiation sickness, and Exposure to radioactivce isotopes	T50.8x1-	T50.8x2-	T50.8x3-	T50.8x4-	T50.8x5-	T50.8x6-
therapeutic	T38.2x1-	T38.2x2-	T38.2x3-	T38.2x4-	T38.2x5-	T38.2x6-
diagnostic	T50.8x1-	T50.8x2-	T50.8x3-	T50.8x4-	T50.8x5-	T50.8x6-
for thyroid conditions (antithyroid)	T38.2x1-	T38.2x2-	T38.2x3-	T38.2x4-	T38.2x5-	T38.2x6-
solution	T49.0x1-	T49.0x2-	T49.0x3-	T49.0x4-	T49.0x5-	T49.0x6-
vapor	T59.891-	T59.892-	T59.893-	T59.894-	—	—
Iodipamide	T50.8x1-	T50.8x2-	T50.8x3-	T50.8x4-	T50.8x5-	T50.8x6-
Iodized (poppy seed) oil	T50.8x1-	T50.8x2-	T50.8x3-	T50.8x4-	T50.8x5-	T50.8x6-
Iodobismitol	T37.8x1-	T37.8x2-	T37.8x3-	T37.8x4-	T37.8x5-	T37.8x6-
Iodochlorhydroxyquin	T37.8x1-	T37.8x2-	T37.8x3-	T37.8x4-	T37.8x5-	T37.8x6-
topical	T49.0x1-	T49.0x2-	T49.0x3-	T49.0x4-	T49.0x5-	T49.0x6-
Iodochlorhydroxyquinoline	T37.8x1-	T37.8x2-	T37.8x3-	T37.8x4-	T37.8x5-	T37.8x6-
Iodocholesterol (131I)	T50.8x1-	T50.8x2-	T50.8x3-	T50.8x4-	T50.8x5-	T50.8x6-
Iodoform	T49.0x1-	T49.0x2-	T49.0x3-	T49.0x4-	T49.0x5-	T49.0x6-
Iodohippuric acid	T50.8x1-	T50.8x2-	T50.8x3-	T50.8x4-	T50.8x5-	T50.8x6-
Iodopanoic acid	T50.8x1-	T50.8x2-	T50.8x3-	T50.8x4-	T50.8x5-	T50.8x6-
Iodophthalein (sodium)	T50.8x1-	T50.8x2-	T50.8x3-	T50.8x4-	T50.8x5-	T50.8x6-
Iodopyracet	T50.8x1-	T50.8x2-	T50.8x3-	T50.8x4-	T50.8x5-	T50.8x6-
Iodoquinol	T37.8x1-	T37.8x2-	T37.8x3-	T37.8x4-	T37.8x5-	T37.8x6-
Iodoxamic acid	T50.8x1-	T50.8x2-	T50.8x3-	T50.8x4-	T50.8x5-	T50.8x6-
Iofendylate	T50.8x1-	T50.8x2-	T50.8x3-	T50.8x4-	T50.8x5-	T50.8x6-
Ioglycamic acid	T50.8x1-	T50.8x2-	T50.8x3-	T50.8x4-	T50.8x5-	T50.8x6-
Iohexol	T50.8x1-	T50.8x2-	T50.8x3-	T50.8x4-	T50.8x5-	T50.8x6-
Ion exchange resin anion	T47.8x1-	T47.8x2-	T47.8x3-	T47.8x4-	T47.8x5-	T47.8x6-
cation	T50.3x1-	T50.3x2-	T50.3x3-	T50.3x4-	T50.3x5-	T50.3x6-
cholestyramine	T46.6x1-	T46.6x2-	T46.6x3-	T46.6x4-	T46.6x5-	T46.6x6-
intestinal	T47.8x1-	T47.8x2-	T47.8x3-	T47.8x4-	T47.8x5-	T47.8x6-
Iopamidol	T50.8x1-	T50.8x2-	T50.8x3-	T50.8x4-	T50.8x5-	T50.8x6-
Iopanoic acid	T50.8x1-	T50.8x2-	T50.8x3-	T50.8x4-	T50.8x5-	T50.8x6-
Iophenoic acid	T50.8x1-	T50.8x2-	T50.8x3-	T50.8x4-	T50.8x5-	T50.8x6-
Iopodate, sodium	T50.8x1-	T50.8x2-	T50.8x3-	T50.8x4-	T50.8x5-	T50.8x6-
Iopodic acid	T50.8x1-	T50.8x2-	T50.8x3-	T50.8x4-	T50.8x5-	T50.8x6-
Iopromide	T50.8x1-	T50.8x2-	T50.8x3-	T50.8x4-	T50.8x5-	T50.8x6-
Iopydol	T50.8x1-	T50.8x2-	T50.8x3-	T50.8x4-	T50.8x5-	T50.8x6-
Iotalamic acid	T50.8x1-	T50.8x2-	T50.8x3-	T50.8x4-	T50.8x5-	T50.8x6-
Iothalamate	T50.8x1-	T50.8x2-	T50.8x3-	T50.8x4-	T50.8x5-	T50.8x6-
Iothiouracil	T38.2x1-	T38.2x2-	T38.2x3-	T38.2x4-	T38.2x5-	T38.2x6-
Iotrol	T50.8x1-	T50.8x2-	T50.8x3-	T50.8x4-	T50.8x5-	T50.8x6-
Iotrolan	T50.8x1-	T50.8x2-	T50.8x3-	T50.8x4-	T50.8x5-	T50.8x6-
Iotroxate	T50.8x1-	T50.8x2-	T50.8x3-	T50.8x4-	T50.8x5-	T50.8x6-
Iotroxic acid	T50.8x1-	T50.8x2-	T50.8x3-	T50.8x4-	T50.8x5-	T50.8x6-
Ioversol	T50.8x1-	T50.8x2-	T50.8x3-	T50.8x4-	T50.8x5-	T50.8x6-
Ioxaglate	T50.8x1-	T50.8x2-	T50.8x3-	T50.8x4-	T50.8x5-	T50.8x6-
Ioxaglic acid	T50.8x1-	T50.8x2-	T50.8x3-	T50.8x4-	T50.8x5-	T50.8x6-
Ioxitalamic acid	T50.8x1-	T50.8x2-	T50.8x3-	T50.8x4-	T50.8x5-	T50.8x6-
Ipecac	T47.7x1-	T47.7x2-	T47.7x3-	T47.7x4-	T47.7x5-	T47.7x6-
Ipecacuanha	T48.4x1-	T48.4x2-	T48.4x3-	T48.4x4-	T48.4x5-	T48.4x6-
Ipodate, calcium	T50.8x1-	T50.8x2-	T50.8x3-	T50.8x4-	T50.8x5-	T50.8x6-
Ipral	T42.3x1-	T42.3x2-	T42.3x3-	T42.3x4-	T42.3x5-	T42.3x6-
Ipratropium (bromide)	T48.6x1-	T48.6x2-	T48.6x3-	T48.6x4-	T48.6x5-	T48.6x6-

DRUGS & CHEMICALS

Table of Drugs & Chemicals	POISONING Accidental (Unintentional)	Self-Harm (Intentional)	Assault	Undetermined	Adverse Effect	Underdosing
Ipriflavone	T46.3x1-	T46.3x2-	T46.3x3-	T46.3x4-	T46.3x5-	T46.3x6-
Iprindole	T43.011-	T43.012-	T43.013-	T43.014-	T43.015-	T43.016-
Iproclozide	T43.1x1-	T43.1x2-	T43.1x3-	T43.1x4-	T43.1x5-	T43.1x6-
Iprofenin	T50.8x1-	T50.8x2-	T50.8x3-	T50.8x4-	T50.8x5-	T50.8x6-
Iproheptine	T49.2x1-	T49.2x2-	T49.2x3-	T49.2x4-	T49.2x5-	T49.2x6-
Iproniazid	T43.1x1-	T43.1x2-	T43.1x3-	T43.1x4-	T43.1x5-	T43.1x6-
Iproplatin	T45.1x1-	T45.1x2-	T45.1x3-	T45.1x4-	T45.1x5-	T45.1x6-
Iproveratril	T46.1x1-	T46.1x2-	T46.1x3-	T46.1x4-	T46.1x5-	T46.1x6-
Iron (compounds)						
(medicinal) NEC	T45.4x1-	T45.4x2-	T45.4x3-	T45.4x4-	T45.4x5-	T45.4x6-
ammonium	T45.4x1-	T45.4x2-	T45.4x3-	T45.4x4-	T45.4x5-	T45.4x6-
dextran injection	T45.4x1-	T45.4x2-	T45.4x3-	T45.4x4-	T45.4x5-	T45.4x6-
nonmedicinal	T56.891-	T56.892-	T56.893-	T56.894-	—	—
salts	T45.4x1-	T45.4x2-	T45.4x3-	T45.4x4-	T45.4x5-	T45.4x6-
sorbitex	T45.4x1-	T45.4x2-	T45.4x3-	T45.4x4-	T45.4x5-	T45.4x6-
sorbitol citric acid complex	T45.4x1-	T45.4x2-	T45.4x3-	T45.4x4-	T45.4x5-	T45.4x6-
Irrigating fluid (vaginal)	T49.8x1-	T49.8x2-	T49.8x3-	T49.8x4-	T49.8x5-	T49.8x6-
eye	T49.5x1-	T49.5x2-	T49.5x3-	T49.5x4-	T49.5x5-	T49.5x6-
Isepamicin	T36.5x1-	T36.5x2-	T36.5x3-	T36.5x4-	T36.5x5-	T36.5x6-
Isoaminile (citrate)	T48.3x1-	T48.3x2-	T48.3x3-	T48.3x4-	T48.3x5-	T48.3x6-
Isoamyl nitrite	T46.3x1-	T46.3x2-	T46.3x3-	T46.3x4-	T46.3x5-	T46.3x6-
Isobenzan	T60.1x1-	T60.1x2-	T60.1x3-	T60.1x4-	—	—
Isobutyl acetate	T52.8x1-	T52.8x2-	T52.8x3-	T52.8x4-	—	—
Isocarboxazid	T43.1x1-	T43.1x2-	T43.1x3-	T43.1x4-	T43.1x5-	T43.1x6-
Isoconazole	T49.0x1-	T49.0x2-	T49.0x3-	T49.0x4-	T49.0x5-	T49.0x6-
Isocyanate	T65.0x1-	T65.0x2-	T65.0x3-	T65.0x4-	—	—
Isoephedrine	T44.991-	T44.992-	T44.993-	T44.994-	T44.995-	T44.996-
Isoetarine	T48.6x1-	T48.6x2-	T48.6x3-	T48.6x4-	T48.6x5-	T48.6x6-
Isoethadione	T42.2x1-	T42.2x2-	T42.2x3-	T42.2x4-	T42.2x5-	T42.2x6-
Isoetharine	T44.5x1-	T44.5x2-	T44.5x3-	T44.5x4-	T44.5x5-	T44.5x6-
Isoflurane	T41.0x1-	T41.0x2-	T41.0x3-	T41.0x4-	T41.0x5-	T41.0x6-
Isoflurophate	T44.0x1-	T44.0x2-	T44.0x3-	T44.0x4-	T44.0x5-	T44.0x6-
Isomaltose, ferric complex	T45.4x1-	T45.4x2-	T45.4x3-	T45.4x4-	T45.4x5-	T45.4x6-
Isometheptene	T44.3x1-	T44.3x2-	T44.3x3-	T44.3x4-	T44.3x5-	T44.3x6-
Isoniazid	T37.1x1-	T37.1x2-	T37.1x3-	T37.1x4-	T37.1x5-	T37.1x6-
with						
rifampicin	T36.6x1-	T36.6x2-	T36.6x3-	T36.6x4-	T36.6x5-	T36.6x6-
thioacetazone	T37.1x1-	T37.1x2-	T37.1x3-	T37.1x4-	T37.1x5-	T37.1x6-
Isonicotinic acid hydrazide	T37.1x1-	T37.1x2-	T37.1x3-	T37.1x4-	T37.1x5-	T37.1x6-
Isonipecaine	T40.4x1-	T40.4x2-	T40.4x3-	T40.4x4-	T40.4x5-	T40.4x6-
Isopentaquine	T37.2x1-	T37.2x2-	T37.2x3-	T37.2x4-	T37.2x5-	T37.2x6-
Isophane insulin	T38.3x1-	T38.3x2-	T38.3x3-	T38.3x4-	T38.3x5-	T38.3x6-
Isophorone	T65.891-	T65.892-	T65.893-	T65.894-	—	—
Isophosphamide	T45.1x1-	T45.1x2-	T45.1x3-	T45.1x4-	T45.1x5-	T45.1x6-
Isopregnenone	T38.5x1-	T38.5x2-	T38.5x3-	T38.5x4-	T38.5x5-	T38.5x6-
Isoprenaline	T48.6x1-	T48.6x2-	T48.6x3-	T48.6x4-	T48.6x5-	T48.6x6-
Isopromethazine	T43.3x1-	T43.3x2-	T43.3x3-	T43.3x4-	T43.3x5-	T43.3x6-
Isopropamide	T44.3x1-	T44.3x2-	T44.3x3-	T44.3x4-	T44.3x5-	T44.3x6-
iodide	T44.3x1-	T44.3x2-	T44.3x3-	T44.3x4-	T44.3x5-	T44.3x6-
Isopropanol	T51.2x1-	T51.2x2-	T51.2x3-	T51.2x4-	—	—
Isopropyl						
acetate	T52.8x1-	T52.8x2-	T52.8x3-	T52.8x4-	—	—
alcohol	T51.2x1-	T51.2x2-	T51.2x3-	T51.2x4-	—	—
medicinal	T49.4x1-	T49.4x2-	T49.4x3-	T49.4x4-	T49.4x5-	T49.4x6-
ether	T52.8x1-	T52.8x2-	T52.8x3-	T52.8x4-	—	—
Isopropylaminophenazone	T39.2x1-	T39.2x2-	T39.2x3-	T39.2x4-	T39.2x5-	T39.2x6-
Isoproterenol	T48.6x1-	T48.6x2-	T48.6x3-	T48.6x4-	T48.6x5-	T48.6x6-
Isosorbide dinitrate	T46.3x1-	T46.3x2-	T46.3x3-	T46.3x4-	T46.3x5-	T46.3x6-
Isothipendyl	T45.0x1-	T45.0x2-	T45.0x3-	T45.0x4-	T45.0x5-	T45.0x6-
Isotretinoin	T50.991-	T50.992-	T50.993-	T50.994-	T50.995-	T50.996-
Isoxazolyl penicillin	T36.0x1-	T36.0x2-	T36.0x3-	T36.0x4-	T36.0x5-	T36.0x6-
Isoxicam	T39.391-	T39.392-	T39.393-	T39.394-	T39.395-	T39.396-
Isoxsuprine	T46.7x1-	T46.7x2-	T46.7x3-	T46.7x4-	T46.7x5-	T46.7x6-

Table of Drugs & Chemicals	POISONING Accidental (Unintentional)	Self-Harm (Intentional)	Assault	Undetermined	Adverse Effect	Underdosing
Ispagula	T47.4x1-	T47.4x2-	T47.4x3-	T47.4x4-	T47.4x5-	T47.4x6-
husk	T47.4x1-	T47.4x2-	T47.4x3-	T47.4x4-	T47.4x5-	T47.4x6-
Isradipine	T46.1x1-	T46.1x2-	T46.1x3-	T46.1x4-	T46.1x5-	T46.1x6-
I-thyroxine sodium	T38.1x1-	T38.1x2-	T38.1x3-	T38.1x4-	T38.1x5-	T38.1x6-
Itraconazole	T37.8x1-	T37.8x2-	T37.8x3-	T37.8x4-	T37.8x5-	T37.8x6-
Itramin tosilate	T46.3x1-	T46.3x2-	T46.3x3-	T46.3x4-	T46.3x5-	T46.3x6-
Ivermectin	T37.4x1-	T37.4x2-	T37.4x3-	T37.4x4-	T37.4x5-	T37.4x6-
Izoniazid	T37.1x1-	T37.1x2-	T37.1x3-	T37.1x4-	T37.1x5-	T37.1x6-
with thioacetazone	T37.1x1-	T37.1x2-	T37.1x3-	T37.1x4-	T37.1x5-	T37.1x6-
Jalap	T47.2x1-	T47.2x2-	T47.2x3-	T47.2x4-	T47.2x5-	T47.2x6-
Jamaica						
dogwood (bark)	T39.8x1-	T39.8x2-	T39.8x3-	T39.8x4-	T39.8x5-	T39.8x6-
ginger	T65.891-	T65.892-	T65.893-	T65.894-	—	—
root	T62.2x1-	T62.2x2-	T62.2x3-	T62.2x4-	—	—
Jatropha	T62.2x1-	T62.2x2-	T62.2x3-	T62.2x4-	—	—
curcas	T62.2x1-	T62.2x2-	T62.2x3-	T62.2x4-	—	—
Jectofer	T45.4x1-	T45.4x2-	T45.4x3-	T45.4x4-	T45.4x5-	T45.4x6-
Jellyfish (sting)	T63.621-	T63.622-	T63.623-	T63.624-	—	—
Jequirity (bean)	T62.2x1-	T62.2x2-	T62.2x3-	T62.2x4-	—	—
Jimson weed (stramonium)	T62.2x1-	T62.2x2-	T62.2x3-	T62.2x4-	—	—
seeds	T62.2x1-	T62.2x2-	T62.2x3-	T62.2x4-	—	—
Josamycin	T36.3x1-	T36.3x2-	T36.3x3-	T36.3x4-	T36.3x5-	T36.3x6-
Juniper tar	T49.1x1-	T49.1x2-	T49.1x3-	T49.1x4-	T49.1x5-	T49.1x6-
Kallidinogenase	T46.7x1-	T46.7x2-	T46.7x3-	T46.7x4-	T46.7x5-	T46.7x6-
Kallikrein	T46.7x1-	T46.7x2-	T46.7x3-	T46.7x4-	T46.7x5-	T46.7x6-
Kanamycin	T36.5x1-	T36.5x2-	T36.5x3-	T36.5x4-	T36.5x5-	T36.5x6-
Kantrex	T36.5x1-	T36.5x2-	T36.5x3-	T36.5x4-	T36.5x5-	T36.5x6-
Kaolin	T47.6x1-	T47.6x2-	T47.6x3-	T47.6x4-	T47.6x5-	T47.6x6-
light	T47.6x1-	T47.6x2-	T47.6x3-	T47.6x4-	T47.6x5-	T47.6x6-
Karaya (gum)	T47.4x1-	T47.4x2-	T47.4x3-	T47.4x4-	T47.4x5-	T47.4x6-
Kebuzone	T39.2x1-	T39.2x2-	T39.2x3-	T39.2x4-	T39.2x5-	T39.2x6-
Kelevan	T60.1x1-	T60.1x2-	T60.1x3-	T60.1x4-	—	—
Kemithal	T41.1x1-	T41.1x2-	T41.1x3-	T41.1x4-	T41.1x5-	T41.1x6-
Kenacort	T38.0x1-	T38.0x2-	T38.0x3-	T38.0x4-	T38.0x5-	T38.0x6-
Keratolytic drug NEC	T49.4x1-	T49.4x2-	T49.4x3-	T49.4x4-	T49.4x5-	T49.4x6-
anthracene	T49.4x1-	T49.4x2-	T49.4x3-	T49.4x4-	T49.4x5-	T49.4x6-
Keratoplastic NEC	T49.4x1-	T49.4x2-	T49.4x3-	T49.4x4-	T49.4x5-	T49.4x6-
Kerosene, kerosine (fuel)						
(solvent) NEC	T52.0x1-	T52.0x2-	T52.0x3-	T52.0x4-	—	—
insecticide	T52.0x1-	T52.0x2-	T52.0x3-	T52.0x4-	—	—
vapor	T52.0x1-	T52.0x2-	T52.0x3-	T52.0x4-	—	—
Ketamine	T41.291-	T41.292-	T41.293-	T41.294-	T41.295-	T41.296-
Ketazolam	T42.4x1-	T42.4x2-	T42.4x3-	T42.4x4-	T42.4x5-	T42.4x6-
Ketazon	T39.2x1-	T39.2x2-	T39.2x3-	T39.2x4-	T39.2x5-	T39.2x6-
Ketobemidone	T40.4x1-	T40.4x2-	T40.4x3-	T40.4x4-	—	—
Ketoconazole	T49.0x1-	T49.0x2-	T49.0x3-	T49.0x4-	T49.0x5-	T49.0x6-
Ketols	T52.4x1-	T52.4x2-	T52.4x3-	T52.4x4-	—	—
Ketone oils	T52.4x1-	T52.4x2-	T52.4x3-	T52.4x4-	—	—
Ketoprofen	T39.311-	T39.312-	T39.313-	T39.314-	T39.315-	T39.316-
Ketorolac	T39.8x1-	T39.8x2-	T39.8x3-	T39.8x4-	T39.8x5-	T39.8x6-
Ketotifen	T45.0x1-	T45.0x2-	T45.0x3-	T45.0x4-	T45.0x5-	T45.0x6-
Khat	T43.691-	T43.692-	T43.693-	T43.694-	—	—
Khellin	T46.3x1-	T46.3x2-	T46.3x3-	T46.3x4-	T46.3x5-	T46.3x6-
Khelloside	T46.3x1-	T46.3x2-	T46.3x3-	T46.3x4-	T46.3x5-	T46.3x6-
Kiln gas or vapor (carbon monoxide)	T58.8x1-	T58.8x2-	T58.8x3-	T58.8x4-	—	—
Kitasamycin	T36.3x1-	T36.3x2-	T36.3x3-	T36.3x4-	T36.3x5-	T36.3x6-
Konsyl	T47.4x1-	T47.4x2-	T47.4x3-	T47.4x4-	T47.4x5-	T47.4x6-
Kosam seed	T62.2x1-	T62.2x2-	T62.2x3-	T62.2x4-	—	—
Krait (venom)	T63.091-	T63.092-	T63.093-	T63.094-	—	—
Kwell (insecticide)	T60.1x1-	T60.1x2-	T60.1x3-	T60.1x4-	—	—
anti-infective (topical)	T49.0x1-	T49.0x2-	T49.0x3-	T49.0x4-	T49.0x5-	T49.0x6-

DRUGS & CHEMICALS

Table of Drugs & Chemicals	Accidental (Unintentional)	Self-Harm (Intentional)	Assault	Undetermined	Adverse Effect	Underdosing
Labetalol	T44.8x1-	T44.8x2-	T44.8x3-	T44.8x4-	T44.8x5-	T44.8x6-
Laburnum (seeds)	T62.2x1-	T62.2x2-	T62.2x3-	T62.2x4-	—	—
leaves	T62.2x1-	T62.2x2-	T62.2x3-	T62.2x4-	—	—
Lachesine	T49.5x1-	T49.5x2-	T49.5x3-	T49.5x4-	T49.5x5-	T49.5x6-
Lacidipine	T46.5x1-	T46.5x2-	T46.5x3-	T46.5x4-	T46.5x5-	T46.5x6-
Lacquer	T65.6x1-	T65.6x2-	T65.6x3-	T65.6x4-	—	—
Lacrimogenic gas	T59.3x1-	T59.3x2-	T59.3x3-	T59.3x4-	—	—
Lactated potassic saline	T50.3x1-	T50.3x2-	T50.3x3-	T50.3x4-	T50.3x5-	T50.3x6-
Lactic acid	T49.8x1-	T49.8x2-	T49.8x3-	T49.8x4-	T49.8x5-	T49.8x6-
Lactobacillus						
acidophilus	T47.6x1-	T47.6x2-	T47.6x3-	T47.6x4-	T47.6x5-	T47.6x6-
compound	T47.6x1-	T47.6x2-	T47.6x3-	T47.6x4-	T47.6x5-	T47.6x6-
bifidus, lyophilized	T47.6x1-	T47.6x2-	T47.6x3-	T47.6x4-	T47.6x5-	T47.6x6-
bulgaricus	T47.6x1-	T47.6x2-	T47.6x3-	T47.6x4-	T47.6x5-	T47.6x6-
sporogenes	T47.6x1-	T47.6x2-	T47.6x3-	T47.6x4-	T47.6x5-	T47.6x6-
Lactoflavin	T45.2x1-	T45.2x2-	T45.2x3-	T45.2x4-	T45.2x5-	T45.2x6-
Lactose (as excipient)	T50.901-	T50.902-	T50.903-	T50.904-	T50.905-	T50.906-
Lactuca (virosa) (extract)	T42.6x1-	T42.6x2-	T42.6x3-	T42.6x4-	T42.6x5-	T42.6x6-
Lactucarium	T42.6x1-	T42.6x2-	T42.6x3-	T42.6x4-	T42.6x5-	T42.6x6-
Lactulose	T47.3x1-	T47.3x2-	T47.3x3-	T47.3x4-	T47.3x5-	T47.3x6-
Laevo — see Levo-						
Lanatosides	T46.0x1-	T46.0x2-	T46.0x3-	T46.0x4-	T46.0x5-	T46.0x6-
Lanolin	T49.3x1-	T49.3x2-	T49.3x3-	T49.3x4-	T49.3x5-	T49.3x6-
Largactil	T43.3x1-	T43.3x2-	T43.3x3-	T43.3x4-	T43.3x5-	T43.3x6-
Larkspur	T62.2x1-	T62.2x2-	T62.2x3-	T62.2x4-	—	—
Laroxyl	T43.011-	T43.012-	T43.013-	T43.014-	T43.015-	T43.016-
Lasix	T50.1x1-	T50.1x2-	T50.1x3-	T50.1x4-	T50.1x5-	T50.1x6-
Lassar's paste	T49.4x1-	T49.4x2-	T49.4x3-	T49.4x4-	T49.4x5-	T49.4x6-
Latamoxef	T36.1x1-	T36.1x2-	T36.1x3-	T36.1x4-	T36.1x5-	T36.1x6-
Latex	T65.811-	T65.812-	T65.813-	T65.814-	—	—
Lathyrus (seed)	T62.2x1-	T62.2x2-	T62.2x3-	T62.2x4-	—	—
Laudanum	T40.0x1-	T40.0x2-	T40.0x3-	T40.0x4-	T40.0x5-	T40.0x6-
Laudexium	T48.1x1-	T48.1x2-	T48.1x3-	T48.1x4-	T48.1x5-	T48.1x6-
Laughing gas	T41.0x1-	T41.0x2-	T41.0x3-	T41.0x4-	T41.0x5-	T41.0x6-
Laurel, black or cherry	T62.2x1-	T62.2x2-	T62.2x3-	T62.2x4-	—	—
Laurolinium	T49.0x1-	T49.0x2-	T49.0x3-	T49.0x4-	T49.0x5-	T49.0x6-
Lauryl sulfoacetate	T49.2x1-	T49.2x2-	T49.2x3-	T49.2x4-	T49.2x5-	T49.2x6-
Laxative NEC	T47.4x1-	T47.4x2-	T47.4x3-	T47.4x4-	T47.4x5-	T47.4x6-
osmotic	T47.3x1-	T47.3x2-	T47.3x3-	T47.3x4-	T47.3x5-	T47.3x6-
saline	T47.3x1-	T47.3x2-	T47.3x3-	T47.3x4-	T47.3x5-	T47.3x6-
stimulant	T47.2x1-	T47.2x2-	T47.2x3-	T47.2x4-	T47.2x5-	T47.2x6-
L-dopa	T42.8x1-	T42.8x2-	T42.8x3-	T42.8x4-	T42.8x5-	T42.8x6-
Lead (dust) (fumes) (vapor) NEC	T56.0x1-	T56.0x2-	T56.0x3-	T56.0x4-	—	—
acetate	T49.2x1-	T49.2x2-	T49.2x3-	T49.2x4-	T49.2x5-	T49.2x6-
alkyl (fuel additive)	T56.0x1-	T56.0x2-	T56.0x3-	T56.0x4-	—	—
anti-infectives	T37.8x1-	T37.8x2-	T37.8x3-	T37.8x4-	T37.8x5-	T37.8x6-
antiknock compound (tetraethyl)	T56.0x1-	T56.0x2-	T56.0x3-	T56.0x4-	—	—
arsenate, arsenite (dust) (herbicide) (insecticide) (vapor)	T57.0x1-	T57.0x2-	T57.0x3-	T57.0x4-	—	—
carbonate	T56.0x1-	T56.0x2-	T56.0x3-	T56.0x4-	—	—
paint	T56.0x1-	T56.0x2-	T56.0x3-	T56.0x4-	—	—
chromate	T56.0x1-	T56.0x2-	T56.0x3-	T56.0x4-	—	—
paint	T56.0x1-	T56.0x2-	T56.0x3-	T56.0x4-	—	—
dioxide	T56.0x1-	T56.0x2-	T56.0x3-	T56.0x4-	—	—
inorganic	T56.0x1-	T56.0x2-	T56.0x3-	T56.0x4-	—	—
iodide	T56.0x1-	T56.0x2-	T56.0x3-	T56.0x4-	—	—
pigment (paint)	T56.0x1-	T56.0x2-	T56.0x3-	T56.0x4-	—	—
monoxide (dust)	T56.0x1-	T56.0x2-	T56.0x3-	T56.0x4-	—	—
paint	T56.0x1-	T56.0x2-	T56.0x3-	T56.0x4-	—	—
organic	T56.0x1-	T56.0x2-	T56.0x3-	T56.0x4-	—	—
oxide	T56.0x1-	T56.0x2-	T56.0x3-	T56.0x4-	—	—
paint	T56.0x1-	T56.0x2-	T56.0x3-	T56.0x4-	—	—
Lead (dust) (fumes) (vapor) NEC - *continued*	T56.0x1-	T56.0x2-	T56.0x3-	T56.0x4-	—	—
paint	T56.0x1-	T56.0x2-	T56.0x3-	T56.0x4-	—	—
salts	T56.0x1-	T56.0x2-	T56.0x3-	T56.0x4-	—	—
specified compound NEC	T56.0x1-	T56.0x2-	T56.0x3-	T56.0x4-	—	—
tetra-ethyl	T56.0x1-	T56.0x2-	T56.0x3-	T56.0x4-	—	—
Lebanese red	T40.7x1-	T40.7x2-	T40.7x3-	T40.7x4-	T40.7x5-	T40.7x6-
Lefetamine	T39.8x1-	T39.8x2-	T39.8x3-	T39.8x4-	T39.8x5-	T39.8x6-
Lenperone	T43.4x1-	T43.4x2-	T43.4x3-	T43.4x4-	T43.4x5-	T43.4x6-
Lente lietin (insulin)	T38.3x1-	T38.3x2-	T38.3x3-	T38.3x4-	T38.3x5-	T38.3x6-
Leptazol	T50.7x1-	T50.7x2-	T50.7x3-	T50.7x4-	T50.7x5-	T50.7x6-
Leptophos	T60.0x1-	T60.0x2-	T60.0x3-	T60.0x4-	—	—
Leritine	T40.2x1-	T40.2x2-	T40.2x3-	T40.2x4-	T40.2x5-	T40.2x6-
Letosteine	T48.4x1-	T48.4x2-	T48.4x3-	T48.4x4-	T48.4x5-	T48.4x6-
Letter	T38.1x1-	T38.1x2-	T38.1x3-	T38.1x4-	T38.1x5-	T38.1x6-
Lettuce opium	T42.6x1-	T42.6x2-	T42.6x3-	T42.6x4-	T42.6x5-	T42.6x6-
Leucinocaine	T41.3x1-	T41.3x2-	T41.3x3-	T41.3x4-	T41.3x5-	T41.3x6-
Leucocianidol	T46.991-	T46.992-	T46.993-	T46.994-	T46.995-	T46.996-
Leucovorin (factor)	T45.8x1-	T45.8x2-	T45.8x3-	T45.8x4-	T45.8x5-	T45.8x6-
Leukeran	T45.1x1-	T45.1x2-	T45.1x3-	T45.1x4-	T45.1x5-	T45.1x6-
Leuprolide	T38.891-	T38.892-	T38.893-	T38.894-	T38.895-	T38.896-
Levalbuterol	T48.6x1-	T48.6x2-	T48.6x3-	T48.6x4-	T48.6x5-	T48.6x6-
Levallorphan	T50.7x1-	T50.7x2-	T50.7x3-	T50.7x4-	T50.7x5-	T50.7x6-
Levamisole	T37.4x1-	T37.4x2-	T37.4x3-	T37.4x4-	T37.4x5-	T37.4x6-
Levanil	T42.6x1-	T42.6x2-	T42.6x3-	T42.6x4-	T42.6x5-	T42.6x6-
Levarterenol	T44.4x1-	T44.4x2-	T44.4x3-	T44.4x4-	T44.4x5-	T44.4x6-
Levdropropizine	T48.3x1-	T48.3x2-	T48.3x3-	T48.3x4-	T48.3x5-	T48.3x6-
Levobunolol	T49.5x1-	T49.5x2-	T49.5x3-	T49.5x4-	T49.5x5-	T49.5x6-
Levocabastine (hydrochloride)	T45.0x1-	T45.0x2-	T45.0x3-	T45.0x4-	T45.0x5-	T45.0x6-
Levocarnitine	T50.991-	T50.992-	T50.993-	T50.994-	T50.995-	T50.996-
Levodopa	T42.8x1-	T42.8x2-	T42.8x3-	T42.8x4-	T42.8x5-	T42.8x6-
with carbidopa	T42.8x1-	T42.8x2-	T42.8x3-	T42.8x4-	T42.8x5-	T42.8x6-
Levo-dromoran	T40.2x1-	T40.2x2-	T40.2x3-	T40.2x4-	T40.2x5-	T40.2x6-
Levoglutamide	T50.991-	T50.992-	T50.993-	T50.994-	T50.995-	T50.996-
Levoid	T38.1x1-	T38.1x2-	T38.1x3-	T38.1x4-	T38.1x5-	T38.1x6-
Levo-iso-methadone	T40.3x1-	T40.3x2-	T40.3x3-	T40.3x4-	T40.3x5-	T40.3x6-
Levomepromazine	T43.3x1-	T43.3x2-	T43.3x3-	T43.3x4-	T43.3x5-	T43.3x6-
Levonordefrin	T49.6x1-	T49.6x2-	T49.6x3-	T49.6x4-	T49.6x5-	T49.6x6-
Levonorgestrel	T38.4x1-	T38.4x2-	T38.4x3-	T38.4x4-	T38.4x5-	T38.4x6-
with ethinylestradiol	T38.5x1-	T38.5x2-	T38.5x3-	T38.5x4-	T38.5x5-	T38.5x6-
Levopromazine	T43.3x1-	T43.3x2-	T43.3x3-	T43.3x4-	T43.3x5-	T43.3x6-
Levoprome	T42.6x1-	T42.6x2-	T42.6x3-	T42.6x4-	T42.6x5-	T42.6x6-
Levopropoxyphene	T40.4x1-	T40.4x2-	T40.4x3-	T40.4x4-	T40.4x5-	T40.4x6-
Levopropylhexedrine	T50.5x1-	T50.5x2-	T50.5x3-	T50.5x4-	T50.5x5-	T50.5x6-
Levoproxyphylline	T48.6x1-	T48.6x2-	T48.6x3-	T48.6x4-	T48.6x5-	T48.6x6-
Levorphanol	T40.4x1-	T40.4x2-	T40.4x3-	T40.4x4-	T40.4x5-	T40.4x6-
Levothyroxine	T38.1x1-	T38.1x2-	T38.1x3-	T38.1x4-	T38.1x5-	T38.1x6-
sodium	T38.1x1-	T38.1x2-	T38.1x3-	T38.1x4-	T38.1x5-	T38.1x6-
Levsin	T44.3x1-	T44.3x2-	T44.3x3-	T44.3x4-	T44.3x5-	T44.3x6-
Levulose	T50.3x1-	T50.3x2-	T50.3x3-	T50.3x4-	T50.3x5-	T50.3x6-
Lewisite (gas), not in war	T57.0x1-	T57.0x2-	T57.0x3-	T57.0x4-	—	—
Librium	T42.4x1-	T42.4x2-	T42.4x3-	T42.4x4-	T42.4x5-	T42.4x6-
Lidex	T49.0x1-	T49.0x2-	T49.0x3-	T49.0x4-	T49.0x5-	T49.0x6-
Lidocaine	T41.3x1-	T41.3x2-	T41.3x3-	T41.3x4-	T41.3x5-	T41.3x6-
regional	T41.3x1-	T41.3x2-	T41.3x3-	T41.3x4-	T41.3x5-	T41.3x6-
spinal	T41.3x1-	T41.3x2-	T41.3x3-	T41.3x4-	T41.3x5-	T41.3x6-
Lidofenin	T50.8x1-	T50.8x2-	T50.8x3-	T50.8x4-	T50.8x5-	T50.8x6-
Lidoflazine	T46.1x1-	T46.1x2-	T46.1x3-	T46.1x4-	T46.1x5-	T46.1x6-
Lighter fluid	T52.0x1-	T52.0x2-	T52.0x3-	T52.0x4-	—	—
Lignin hemicellulose	T47.6x1-	T47.6x2-	T47.6x3-	T47.6x4-	T47.6x5-	T47.6x6-

DRUGS & CHEMICALS

Table of Drugs & Chemicals	Accidental (Unintentional)	Self-Harm (Intentional)	Assault	Undetermined	Adverse Effect	Underdosing
Lignocaine	T41.3x1-	T41.3x2-	T41.3x3-	T41.3x4-	T41.3x5-	T41.3x6-
regional	T41.3x1-	T41.3x2-	T41.3x3-	T41.3x4-	T41.3x5-	T41.3x6-
spinal	T41.3x1-	T41.3x2-	T41.3x3-	T41.3x4-	T41.3x5-	T41.3x6-
Ligroin(e) (solvent)	T52.0x1-	T52.0x2-	T52.0x3-	T52.0x4-	—	—
vapor	T59.891-	T59.892-	T59.893-	T59.894-	—	—
Ligustrum vulgare	T62.2x1-	T62.2x2-	T62.2x3-	T62.2x4-	—	—
Lily of the valley	T62.2x1-	T62.2x2-	T62.2x3-	T62.2x4-	—	—
Lime (chloride)	T54.3x1-	T54.3x2-	T54.3x3-	T54.3x4-	—	—
Limonene	T52.8x1-	T52.8x2-	T52.8x3-	T52.8x4-	—	—
Lincomycin	T36.8x1-	T36.8x2-	T36.8x3-	T36.8x4-	T36.8x5-	T36.8x6-
Lindane (insecticide) (nonmedicinal) (vapor)	T53.6x1-	T53.6x2-	T53.6x3-	T53.6x4-	—	—
medicinal	T49.0x1-	T49.0x2-	T49.0x3-	T49.0x4-	T49.0x5-	T49.0x6-
Liniments NEC	T49.91x-	T49.92x-	T49.93x-	T49.94x-	T49.95x-	T49.96x-
Linoleic acid	T46.6x1-	T46.6x2-	T46.6x3-	T46.6x4-	T46.6x5-	T46.6x6-
Linolenic acid	T46.6x1-	T46.6x2-	T46.6x3-	T46.6x4-	T46.6x5-	T46.6x6-
Linseed	T47.4x1-	T47.4x2-	T47.4x3-	T47.4x4-	T47.4x5-	T47.4x6-
Liothyronine	T38.1x1-	T38.1x2-	T38.1x3-	T38.1x4-	T38.1x5-	T38.1x6-
Liotrix	T38.1x1-	T38.1x2-	T38.1x3-	T38.1x4-	T38.1x5-	T38.1x6-
Lipancreatin	T47.5x1-	T47.5x2-	T47.5x3-	T47.5x4-	T47.5x5-	T47.5x6-
Lipo-alprostadil	T46.7x1-	T46.7x2-	T46.7x3-	T46.7x4-	T46.7x5-	T46.7x6-
Lipo-Lutin	T38.5x1-	T38.5x2-	T38.5x3-	T38.5x4-	T38.5x5-	T38.5x6-
Lipotropic drug NEC	T50.901-	T50.902-	T50.903-	T50.904-	T50.905-	T50.906-
Liquefied petroleum gases	T59.891-	T59.892-	T59.893-	T59.894-	—	—
piped (pure or mixed with air)	T59.891-	T59.892-	T59.893-	T59.894-	—	—
Liquid						
paraffin	T47.4x1-	T47.4x2-	T47.4x3-	T47.4x4-	T47.4x5-	T47.4x6-
petrolatum	T47.4x1-	T47.4x2-	T47.4x3-	T47.4x4-	T47.4x5-	T47.4x6-
topical	T49.3x1-	T49.3x2-	T49.3x3-	T49.3x4-	T49.3x5-	T49.3x6-
specified NEC	T65.891-	T65.892-	T65.893-	T65.894-	—	—
substance	T65.91x-	T65.92x-	T65.93x-	T65.94x-	—	—
Liquor creosolis compositus	T65.891-	T65.892-	T65.893-	T65.894-	—	—
Liquorice	T48.4x1-	T48.4x2-	T48.4x3-	T48.4x4-	T48.4x5-	T48.4x6-
extract	T47.8x1-	T47.8x2-	T47.8x3-	T47.8x4-	T47.8x5-	T47.8x6-
Lisinopril	T46.4x1-	T46.4x2-	T46.4x3-	T46.4x4-	T46.4x5-	T46.4x6-
Lisuride	T42.8x1-	T42.8x2-	T42.8x3-	T42.8x4-	T42.8x5-	T42.8x6-
Lithane	T43.8x1-	T43.8x2-	T43.8x3-	T43.8x4-	T43.8x5-	T43.8x6-
Lithium	T56.891-	T56.892-	T56.893-	T56.894-	—	—
gluconate	T43.591-	T43.592-	T43.593-	T43.594-	T43.595-	T43.596-
salts (carbonate)	T43.591-	T43.592-	T43.593-	T43.594-	T43.595-	T43.596-
Lithonate	T43.8x1-	T43.8x2-	T43.8x3-	T43.8x4-	T43.8x5-	T43.8x6-
Liver						
extract	T45.8x1-	T45.8x2-	T45.8x3-	T45.8x4-	T45.8x5-	T45.8x6-
for parenteral use	T45.8x1-	T45.8x2-	T45.8x3-	T45.8x4-	T45.8x5-	T45.8x6-
fraction 1	T45.8x1-	T45.8x2-	T45.8x3-	T45.8x4-	T45.8x5-	T45.8x6-
hydrolysate	T45.8x1-	T45.8x2-	T45.8x3-	T45.8x4-	T45.8x5-	T45.8x6-
Lizard (bite) (venom)	T63.121-	T63.122-	T63.123-	T63.124-	—	—
LMD	T45.8x1-	T45.8x2-	T45.8x3-	T45.8x4-	T45.8x5-	T45.8x6-
Lobelia	T62.2x1-	T62.2x2-	T62.2x3-	T62.2x4-	—	—
Lobeline	T50.7x1-	T50.7x2-	T50.7x3-	T50.7x4-	T50.7x5-	T50.7x6-
Local action drug NEC	T49.8x1-	T49.8x2-	T49.8x3-	T49.8x4-	T49.8x5-	T49.8x6-
Locorten	T49.0x1-	T49.0x2-	T49.0x3-	T49.0x4-	T49.0x5-	T49.0x6-
Lofepramine	T43.011-	T43.012-	T43.013-	T43.014-	T43.015-	T43.016-
Lolium temulentum	T62.2x1-	T62.2x2-	T62.2x3-	T62.2x4-	—	—
Lomotil	T47.6x1-	T47.6x2-	T47.6x3-	T47.6x4-	T47.6x5-	T47.6x6-
Lomustine	T45.1x1-	T45.1x2-	T45.1x3-	T45.1x4-	T45.1x5-	T45.1x6-
Lonidamine	T45.1x1-	T45.1x2-	T45.1x3-	T45.1x4-	T45.1x5-	T45.1x6-
Loperamide	T47.6x1-	T47.6x2-	T47.6x3-	T47.6x4-	T47.6x5-	T47.6x6-
Loprazolam	T42.4x1-	T42.4x2-	T42.4x3-	T42.4x4-	T42.4x5-	T42.4x6-
Lorajmine	T46.2x1-	T46.2x2-	T46.2x3-	T46.2x4-	T46.2x5-	T46.2x6-
Loratidine	T45.0x1-	T45.0x2-	T45.0x3-	T45.0x4-	T45.0x5-	T45.0x6-

Table of Drugs & Chemicals	Accidental (Unintentional)	Self-Harm (Intentional)	Assault	Undetermined	Adverse Effect	Underdosing
Lorazepam	T42.4x1-	T42.4x2-	T42.4x3-	T42.4x4-	T42.4x5-	T42.4x6-
Lorcainide	T46.2x1-	T46.2x2-	T46.2x3-	T46.2x4-	T46.2x5-	T46.2x6-
Lormetazepam	T42.4x1-	T42.4x2-	T42.4x3-	T42.4x4-	T42.4x5-	T42.4x6-
Lotions NEC	T49.91x-	T49.92x-	T49.93x-	T49.94x-	T49.95x-	T49.96x-
Lotusate	T42.3x1-	T42.3x2-	T42.3x3-	T42.3x4-	T42.3x5-	T42.3x6-
Lovastatin	T46.6x1-	T46.6x2-	T46.6x3-	T46.6x4-	T46.6x5-	T46.6x6-
Lowila	T49.2x1-	T49.2x2-	T49.2x3-	T49.2x4-	T49.2x5-	T49.2x6-
Loxapine	T43.591-	T43.592-	T43.593-	T43.594-	T43.595-	T43.596-
Lozenges (throat)	T49.6x1-	T49.6x2-	T49.6x3-	T49.6x4-	T49.6x5-	T49.6x6-
LSD	T40.8x1-	T40.8x2-	T40.8x3-	T40.8x4-	—	—
L-Tryptophan — *see* Amino acid						
Lubricant, eye	T49.5x1-	T49.5x2-	T49.5x3-	T49.5x4-	T49.5x5-	T49.5x6-
Lubricating oil NEC	T52.0x1-	T52.0x2-	T52.0x3-	T52.0x4-	—	—
Lucanthone	T37.4x1-	T37.4x2-	T37.4x3-	T37.4x4-	T37.4x5-	T37.4x6-
Luminal	T42.3x1-	T42.3x2-	T42.3x3-	T42.3x4-	T42.3x5-	T42.3x6-
Lung irritant (gas) NEC	T59.91x-	T59.92x-	T59.93x-	T59.94x-	—	—
Luteinizing hormone	T38.811-	T38.812-	T38.813-	T38.814-	T38.815-	T38.816-
Lutocylol	T38.5x1-	T38.5x2-	T38.5x3-	T38.5x4-	T38.5x5-	T38.5x6-
Lutromone	T38.5x1-	T38.5x2-	T38.5x3-	T38.5x4-	T38.5x5-	T38.5x6-
Lututrin	T48.291-	T48.292-	T48.293-	T48.294-	T48.295-	T48.296-
Lye (concentrated)	T54.3x1-	T54.3x2-	T54.3x3-	T54.3x4-	—	—
Lygranum (skin test)	T50.8x1-	T50.8x2-	T50.8x3-	T50.8x4-	T50.8x5-	T50.8x6-
Lymecycline	T36.4x1-	T36.4x2-	T36.4x3-	T36.4x4-	T36.4x5-	T36.4x6-
Lymphogranuloma venereum antigen	T50.8x1-	T50.8x2-	T50.8x3-	T50.8x4-	T50.8x5-	T50.8x6-
Lynestrenol	T38.4x1-	T38.4x2-	T38.4x3-	T38.4x4-	T38.4x5-	T38.4x6-
Lyovac Sodium Edecrin	T50.1x1-	T50.1x2-	T50.1x3-	T50.1x4-	T50.1x5-	T50.1x6-
Lypressin	T38.891-	T38.892-	T38.893-	T38.894-	T38.895-	T38.896-
Lysergic acid diethylamide	T40.8x1-	T40.8x2-	T40.8x3-	T40.8x4-	—	—
Lysergide	T40.8x1-	T40.8x2-	T40.8x3-	T40.8x4-	—	—
Lysine vasopressin	T38.891-	T38.892-	T38.893-	T38.894-	T38.895-	T38.896-
Lysol	T54.1x1-	T54.1x2-	T54.1x3-	T54.1x4-	—	—
Lysozyme	T49.0x1-	T49.0x2-	T49.0x3-	T49.0x4-	T49.0x5-	T49.0x6-
Lytta (vitatta)	T49.8x1-	T49.8x2-	T49.8x3-	T49.8x4-	T49.8x5-	T49.8x6-
Mace	T59.3x1-	T59.3x2-	T59.3x3-	T59.3x4-	—	—
Macrogol	T50.991-	T50.992-	T50.993-	T50.994-	T50.995-	T50.996-
Macrolide						
anabolic drug	T38.7x1-	T38.7x2-	T38.7x3-	T38.7x4-	T38.7x5-	T38.7x6-
antibiotic	T36.3x1-	T36.3x2-	T36.3x3-	T36.3x4-	T36.3x5-	T36.3x6-
Mafenide	T49.0x1-	T49.0x2-	T49.0x3-	T49.0x4-	T49.0x5-	T49.0x6-
Magaldrate	T47.1x1-	T47.1x2-	T47.1x3-	T47.1x4-	T47.1x5-	T47.1x6-
Magic mushroom	T40.991-	T40.992-	T40.993-	T40.994-	—	—
Magnamycin	T36.8x1-	T36.8x2-	T36.8x3-	T36.8x4-	T36.8x5-	T36.8x6-
Magnesia magma	T47.1x1-	T47.1x2-	T47.1x3-	T47.1x4-	T47.1x5-	T47.1x6-
Magnesium NEC	T56.891-	T56.892-	T56.893-	T56.894-	—	—
carbonate	T47.1x1-	T47.1x2-	T47.1x3-	T47.1x4-	T47.1x5-	T47.1x6-
citrate	T47.4x1-	T47.4x2-	T47.4x3-	T47.4x4-	T47.4x5-	T47.4x6-
hydroxide	T47.1x1-	T47.1x2-	T47.1x3-	T47.1x4-	T47.1x5-	T47.1x6-
oxide	T47.1x1-	T47.1x2-	T47.1x3-	T47.1x4-	T47.1x5-	T47.1x6-
peroxide	T49.0x1-	T49.0x2-	T49.0x3-	T49.0x4-	T49.0x5-	T49.0x6-
salicylate	T39.091-	T39.092-	T39.093-	T39.094-	T39.095-	T39.096-
silicofluoride	T50.3x1-	T50.3x2-	T50.3x3-	T50.3x4-	T50.3x5-	T50.3x6-
sulfate	T47.4x1-	T47.4x2-	T47.4x3-	T47.4x4-	T47.4x5-	T47.4x6-
thiosulfate	T45.0x1-	T45.0x2-	T45.0x3-	T45.0x4-	T45.0x5-	T45.0x6-
trisilicate	T47.1x1-	T47.1x2-	T47.1x3-	T47.1x4-	T47.1x5-	T47.1x6-
Malathion (medicinal)	T49.0x1-	T49.0x2-	T49.0x3-	T49.0x4-	T49.0x5-	T49.0x6-
insecticide	T60.0x1-	T60.0x2-	T60.0x3-	T60.0x4-	—	—
Male fern extract	T37.4x1-	T37.4x2-	T37.4x3-	T37.4x4-	T37.4x5-	T37.4x6-
M-AMSA	T45.1x1-	T45.1x2-	T45.1x3-	T45.1x4-	T45.1x5-	T45.1x6-
Mandelic acid	T37.8x1-	T37.8x2-	T37.8x3-	T37.8x4-	T37.8x5-	T37.8x6-
Manganese (dioxide) (salts)	T57.2x1-	T57.2x2-	T57.2x3-	T57.2x4-	—	—
medicinal	T50.991-	T50.992-	T50.993-	T50.994-	T50.995-	T50.996-

DRUGS & CHEMICALS

Table of Drugs & Chemicals	POISONING Accidental (Unintentional)	Self-Harm (Intentional)	Assault	Undetermined	Adverse Effect	Underdosing
Mannitol	T47.3x1-	T47.3x2-	T47.3x3-	T47.3x4-	T47.3x5-	T47.3x6-
hexanitrate	T46.3x1-	T46.3x2-	T46.3x3-	T46.3x4-	T46.3x5-	T46.3x6-
Mannomustine	T45.1x1-	T45.1x2-	T45.1x3-	T45.1x4-	T45.1x5-	T45.1x6-
MAO inhibitors	T43.1x1-	T43.1x2-	T43.1x3-	T43.1x4-	T43.1x5-	T43.1x6-
Mapharsen	T37.8x1-	T37.8x2-	T37.8x3-	T37.8x4-	T37.8x5-	T37.8x6-
Maphenide	T49.0x1-	T49.0x2-	T49.0x3-	T49.0x4-	T49.0x5-	T49.0x6-
Maprotiline	T43.021-	T43.022-	T43.023-	T43.024-	T43.025-	T43.026-
Marcaine	T41.3x1-	T41.3x2-	T41.3x3-	T41.3x4-	T41.3x5-	T41.3x6-
infiltration (subcutaneous)	T41.3x1-	T41.3x2-	T41.3x3-	T41.3x4-	T41.3x5-	T41.3x6-
nerve block (peripheral) (plexus)	T41.3x1-	T41.3x2-	T41.3x3-	T41.3x4-	T41.3x5-	T41.3x6-
Marezine	T45.0x1-	T45.0x2-	T45.0x3-	T45.0x4-	T45.0x5-	T45.0x6-
Marihuana	T40.7x1-	T40.7x2-	T40.7x3-	T40.7x4-	T40.7x5-	T40.7x6-
Marijuana	T40.7x1-	T40.7x2-	T40.7x3-	T40.7x4-	T40.7x5-	T40.7x6-
Marine (sting)	T63.691-	T63.692-	T63.693-	T63.694-	—	—
animals (sting)	T63.691-	T63.692-	T63.693-	T63.694-	—	—
plants (sting)	T63.711-	T63.712-	T63.713-	T63.714-	—	—
Marplan	T43.1x1-	T43.1x2-	T43.1x3-	T43.1x4-	T43.1x5-	T43.1x6-
Marsh gas	T59.891-	T59.892-	T59.893-	T59.894-		
Marsilid	T43.1x1-	T43.1x2-	T43.1x3-	T43.1x4-	T43.1x5-	T43.1x6-
Matulane	T45.1x1-	T45.1x2-	T45.1x3-	T45.1x4-	T45.1x5-	T45.1x6-
Mazindol	T50.5x1-	T50.5x2-	T50.5x3-	T50.5x4-	T50.5x5-	T50.5x6-
MCPA	T60.3x1-	T60.3x2-	T60.3x3-	T60.3x4-	—	—
MDMA	T43.621-	T43.622-	T43.623-	T43.624-	T43.625-	T43.626-
Meadow saffron	T62.2x1-	T62.2x2-	T62.2x3-	T62.2x4-	—	—
Measles virus vaccine (attenuated)	T50.B91-	T50.B92-	T50.B93-	T50.B94-	T50.B95-	T50.B96-
Meat, noxious	T62.8x1-	T62.8x2-	T62.8x3-	T62.8x4-	—	—
Meballymal	T42.3x1-	T42.3x2-	T42.3x3-	T42.3x4-	T42.3x5-	T42.3x6-
Mebanazine	T43.1x1-	T43.1x2-	T43.1x3-	T43.1x4-	T43.1x5-	T43.1x6-
Mebaral	T42.3x1-	T42.3x2-	T42.3x3-	T42.3x4-	T42.3x5-	T42.3x6-
Mebendazole	T37.4x1-	T37.4x2-	T37.4x3-	T37.4x4-	T37.4x5-	T37.4x6-
Mebeverine	T44.3x1-	T44.3x2-	T44.3x3-	T44.3x4-	T44.3x5-	T44.3x6-
Mebhydrolin	T45.0x1-	T45.0x2-	T45.0x3-	T45.0x4-	T45.0x5-	T45.0x6-
Mebumal	T42.3x1-	T42.3x2-	T42.3x3-	T42.3x4-	T42.3x5-	T42.3x6-
Mebutamate	T43.591-	T43.592-	T43.593-	T43.594-	T43.595-	T43.596-
Mecamylamine	T44.2x1-	T44.2x2-	T44.2x3-	T44.2x4-	T44.2x5-	T44.2x6-
Mechlorethamine	T45.1x1-	T45.1x2-	T45.1x3-	T45.1x4-	T45.1x5-	T45.1x6-
Mecillinam	T36.0x1-	T36.0x2-	T36.0x3-	T36.0x4-	T36.0x5-	T36.0x6-
Meclizine (hydrochloride)	T45.0x1-	T45.0x2-	T45.0x3-	T45.0x4-	T45.0x5-	T45.0x6-
Meclocycline	T36.4x1-	T36.4x2-	T36.4x3-	T36.4x4-	T36.4x5-	T36.4x6-
Meclofenamate	T39.391-	T39.392-	T39.393-	T39.394-	T39.395-	T39.396-
Meclofenamic acid	T39.391-	T39.392-	T39.393-	T39.394-	T39.395-	T39.396-
Meclofenoxate	T43.691-	T43.692-	T43.693-	T43.694-	T43.695-	T43.696-
Meclozine	T45.0x1-	T45.0x2-	T45.0x3-	T45.0x4-	T45.0x5-	T45.0x6-
Mecobalamin	T45.8x1-	T45.8x2-	T45.8x3-	T45.8x4-	T45.8x5-	T45.8x6-
Mecoprop	T60.3x1-	T60.3x2-	T60.3x3-	T60.3x4-	—	—
Mecrilate	T49.3x1-	T49.3x2-	T49.3x3-	T49.3x4-	T49.3x5-	T49.3x6-
Mecysteine	T48.4x1-	T48.4x2-	T48.4x3-	T48.4x4-	T48.4x5-	T48.4x6-
Medazepam	T42.4x1-	T42.4x2-	T42.4x3-	T42.4x4-	T42.4x5-	T42.4x6-
Medicament NEC	T50.901-	T50.902-	T50.903-	T50.904-	T50.905-	T50.906-
Medinal	T42.3x1-	T42.3x2-	T42.3x3-	T42.3x4-	T42.3x5-	T42.3x6-
Medomin	T42.3x1-	T42.3x2-	T42.3x3-	T42.3x4-	T42.3x5-	T42.3x6-
Medrogestone	T38.5x1-	T38.5x2-	T38.5x3-	T38.5x4-	T38.5x5-	T38.5x6-
Medroxalol	T44.8x1-	T44.8x2-	T44.8x3-	T44.8x4-	T44.8x5-	T44.8x6-
Medroxyprogesterone acetate (depot)	T38.5x1-	T38.5x2-	T38.5x3-	T38.5x4-	T38.5x5-	T38.5x6-
Medrysone	T49.0x1-	T49.0x2-	T49.0x3-	T49.0x4-	T49.0x5-	T49.0x6-
Mefenamic acid	T39.391-	T39.392-	T39.393-	T39.394-	T39.395-	T39.396-
Mefenorex	T50.5x1-	T50.5x2-	T50.5x3-	T50.5x4-	T50.5x5-	T50.5x6-
Mefloquine	T37.2x1-	T37.2x2-	T37.2x3-	T37.2x4-	T37.2x5-	T37.2x6-

Table of Drugs & Chemicals	POISONING Accidental (Unintentional)	Self-Harm (Intentional)	Assault	Undetermined	Adverse Effect	Underdosing
Mefruside	T50.2x1-	T50.2x2-	T50.2x3-	T50.2x4-	T50.2x5-	T50.2x6-
Megahallucinogen	T40.901-	T40.902-	T40.903-	T40.904-	T40.905-	T40.906-
Megestrol	T38.5x1-	T38.5x2-	T38.5x3-	T38.5x4-	T38.5x5-	T38.5x6-
Meglumine						
antimoniate	T37.8x1-	T37.8x2-	T37.8x3-	T37.8x4-	T37.8x5-	T37.8x6-
diatrizoate	T50.8x1-	T50.8x2-	T50.8x3-	T50.8x4-	T50.8x5-	T50.8x6-
iodipamide	T50.8x1-	T50.8x2-	T50.8x3-	T50.8x4-	T50.8x5-	T50.8x6-
iotroxate	T50.8x1-	T50.8x2-	T50.8x3-	T50.8x4-	T50.8x5-	T50.8x6-
MEK (methyl ethyl ketone)	T52.4x1-	T52.4x2-	T52.4x3-	T52.4x4-	—	—
Meladinin	T49.3x1-	T49.3x2-	T49.3x3-	T49.3x4-	T49.3x5-	T49.3x6-
Meladrazine	T44.3x1-	T44.3x2-	T44.3x3-	T44.3x4-	T44.3x5-	T44.3x6-
Melaleuca alternifolia oil	T49.0x1-	T49.0x2-	T49.0x3-	T49.0x4-	T49.0x5-	T49.0x6-
Melanizing agents	T49.3x1-	T49.3x2-	T49.3x3-	T49.3x4-	T49.3x5-	T49.3x6-
Melanocyte-stimulating hormone	T38.891-	T38.892-	T38.893-	T38.894-	T38.895-	T38.896-
Melarsonyl potassium	T37.3x1-	T37.3x2-	T37.3x3-	T37.3x4-	T37.3x5-	T37.3x6-
Melarsoprol	T37.3x1-	T37.3x2-	T37.3x3-	T37.3x4-	T37.3x5-	T37.3x6-
Melia azedarach	T62.2x1-	T62.2x2-	T62.2x3-	T62.2x4-	—	—
Melitracen	T43.011-	T43.012-	T43.013-	T43.014-	T43.015-	T43.016-
Mellaril	T43.3x1-	T43.3x2-	T43.3x3-	T43.3x4-	T43.3x5-	T43.3x6-
Meloxine	T49.3x1-	T49.3x2-	T49.3x3-	T49.3x4-	T49.3x5-	T49.3x6-
Melperone	T43.4x1-	T43.4x2-	T43.4x3-	T43.4x4-	T43.4x5-	T43.4x6-
Melphalan	T45.1x1-	T45.1x2-	T45.1x3-	T45.1x4-	T45.1x5-	T45.1x6-
Memantine	T43.8x1-	T43.8x2-	T43.8x3-	T43.8x4-	T43.8x5-	T43.8x6-
Menadiol	T45.7x1-	T45.7x2-	T45.7x3-	T45.7x4-	T45.7x5-	T45.7x6-
sodium sulfate	T45.7x1-	T45.7x2-	T45.7x3-	T45.7x4-	T45.7x5-	T45.7x6-
Menadione	T45.7x1-	T45.7x2-	T45.7x3-	T45.7x4-	T45.7x5-	T45.7x6-
sodium bisulfite	T45.7x1-	T45.7x2-	T45.7x3-	T45.7x4-	T45.7x5-	T45.7x6-
Menaphthone	T45.7x1-	T45.7x2-	T45.7x3-	T45.7x4-	T45.7x5-	T45.7x6-
Menaquinone	T45.7x1-	T45.7x2-	T45.7x3-	T45.7x4-	T45.7x5-	T45.7x6-
Menatetrenone	T45.7x1-	T45.7x2-	T45.7x3-	T45.7x4-	T45.7x5-	T45.7x6-
Meningococcal vaccine	T50.A91-	T50.A92-	T50.A93-	T50.A94-	T50.A95-	T50.A96-
Menningovax (-AC) (-C)	T50.A91-	T50.A92-	T50.A93-	T50.A94-	T50.A95-	T50.A96-
Menotropins	T38.811-	T38.812-	T38.813-	T38.814-	T38.815-	T38.816-
Menthol	T48.5x1-	T48.5x2-	T48.5x3-	T48.5x4-	T48.5x5-	T48.5x6-
Mepacrine	T37.2x1-	T37.2x2-	T37.2x3-	T37.2x4-	T37.2x5-	T37.2x6-
Meparfynol	T42.6x1-	T42.6x2-	T42.6x3-	T42.6x4-	T42.6x5-	T42.6x6-
Mepartricin	T36.7x1-	T36.7x2-	T36.7x3-	T36.7x4-	T36.7x5-	T36.7x6-
Mepazine	T43.3x1-	T43.3x2-	T43.3x3-	T43.3x4-	T43.3x5-	T43.3x6-
Mepenzolate	T44.3x1-	T44.3x2-	T44.3x3-	T44.3x4-	T44.3x5-	T44.3x6-
bromide	T44.3x1-	T44.3x2-	T44.3x3-	T44.3x4-	T44.3x5-	T44.3x6-
Meperidine	T40.4x1-	T40.4x2-	T40.4x3-	T40.4x4-	T40.4x5-	T40.4x6-
Mephebarbital	T42.3x1-	T42.3x2-	T42.3x3-	T42.3x4-	T42.3x5-	T42.3x6-
Mephenamin(e)	T42.8x1-	T42.8x2-	T42.8x3-	T42.8x4-	T42.8x5-	T42.8x6-
Mephenesin	T42.8x1-	T42.8x2-	T42.8x3-	T42.8x4-	T42.8x5-	T42.8x6-
Mephenhydramine	T45.0x1-	T45.0x2-	T45.0x3-	T45.0x4-	T45.0x5-	T45.0x6-
Mephenoxalone	T42.8x1-	T42.8x2-	T42.8x3-	T42.8x4-	T42.8x5-	T42.8x6-
Mephentermine	T44.991-	T44.992-	T44.993-	T44.994-	T44.995-	T44.996-
Mephenytoin	T42.0x1-	T42.0x2-	T42.0x3-	T42.0x4-	T42.0x5-	T42.0x6-
with phenobarbital	T42.3x1-	T42.3x2-	T42.3x3-	T42.3x4-	T42.3x5-	T42.3x6-
Mephobarbital	T42.3x1-	T42.3x2-	T42.3x3-	T42.3x4-	T42.3x5-	T42.3x6-
Mephosfolan	T60.0x1-	T60.0x2-	T60.0x3-	T60.0x4-	—	—
Mepindolol	T44.7x1-	T44.7x2-	T44.7x3-	T44.7x4-	T44.7x5-	T44.7x6-
Mepiperphenidol	T44.3x1-	T44.3x2-	T44.3x3-	T44.3x4-	T44.3x5-	T44.3x6-
Mepitiostane	T38.7x1-	T38.7x2-	T38.7x3-	T38.7x4-	T38.7x5-	T38.7x6-
Mepivacaine	T41.3x1-	T41.3x2-	T41.3x3-	T41.3x4-	T41.3x5-	T41.3x6-
epidural	T41.3x1-	T41.3x2-	T41.3x3-	T41.3x4-	T41.3x5-	T41.3x6-
Meprednisone	T38.0x1-	T38.0x2-	T38.0x3-	T38.0x4-	T38.0x5-	T38.0x6-
Meprobam	T43.591-	T43.592-	T43.593-	T43.594-	T43.595-	T43.596-
Meprobamate	T43.591-	T43.592-	T43.593-	T43.594-	T43.595-	T43.596-
Meproscillarin	T46.0x1-	T46.0x2-	T46.0x3-	T46.0x4-	T46.0x5-	T46.0x6-

DRUGS & CHEMICALS

Table of Drugs & Chemicals	POISONING Accidental (Unintentional)	Self-Harm (Intentional)	Assault	Undetermined	Adverse Effect	Underdosing
Meprylcaine	T41.3x1-	T41.3x2-	T41.3x3-	T41.3x4-	T41.3x5-	T41.3x6-
Meptazinol	T39.8x1-	T39.8x2-	T39.8x3-	T39.8x4-	T39.8x5-	T39.8x6-
Mepyramine	T45.0x1-	T45.0x2-	T45.0x3-	T45.0x4-	T45.0x5-	T45.0x6-
Mequitazine	T43.3x1-	T43.3x2-	T43.3x3-	T43.3x4-	T43.3x5-	T43.3x6-
Meralluride	T50.2x1-	T50.2x2-	T50.2x3-	T50.2x4-	T50.2x5-	T50.2x6-
Merbaphen	T50.2x1-	T50.2x2-	T50.2x3-	T50.2x4-	T50.2x5-	T50.2x6-
Merbromin	T49.0x1-	T49.0x2-	T49.0x3-	T49.0x4-	T49.0x5-	T49.0x6-
Mercaptobenzothiazole salts	T49.0x1-	T49.0x2-	T49.0x3-	T49.0x4-	T49.0x5-	T49.0x6-
Mercaptomerin	T50.2x1-	T50.2x2-	T50.2x3-	T50.2x4-	T50.2x5-	T50.2x6-
Mercaptopurine	T45.1x1-	T45.1x2-	T45.1x3-	T45.1x4-	T45.1x5-	T45.1x6-
Mercumatilin	T50.2x1-	T50.2x2-	T50.2x3-	T50.2x4-	T50.2x5-	T50.2x6-
Mercuramide	T50.2x1-	T50.2x2-	T50.2x3-	T50.2x4-	T50.2x5-	T50.2x6-
Mercurochrome	T49.0x1-	T49.0x2-	T49.0x3-	T49.0x4-	T49.0x5-	T49.0x6-
Mercurophylline	T50.2x1-	T50.2x2-	T50.2x3-	T50.2x4-	T50.2x5-	T50.2x6-
Mercury, mercurial, mercuric, mercurous (compounds) (cyanide) (fumes) (nonmedicinal) (vapor) NEC	T56.1x1-	T56.1x2-	T56.1x3-	T56.1x4-	—	—
ammoniated	T49.0x1-	T49.0x2-	T49.0x3-	T49.0x4-	T49.0x5-	T49.0x6-
anti-infective						
local	T49.0x1-	T49.0x2-	T49.0x3-	T49.0x4-	T49.0x5-	T49.0x6-
systemic	T37.8x1-	T37.8x2-	T37.8x3-	T37.8x4-	T37.8x5-	T37.8x6-
topical	T49.0x1-	T49.0x2-	T49.0x3-	T49.0x4-	T49.0x5-	T49.0x6-
chloride (ammoniated)	T49.0x1-	T49.0x2-	T49.0x3-	T49.0x4-	T49.0x5-	T49.0x6-
fungicide	T56.1x1-	T56.1x2-	T56.1x3-	T56.1x4-	—	—
diuretic NEC	T50.2x1-	T50.2x2-	T50.2x3-	T50.2x4-	T50.2x5-	T50.2x6-
fungicide	T56.1x1-	T56.1x2-	T56.1x3-	T56.1x4-	—	—
organic (fungicide)	T56.1x1-	T56.1x2-	T56.1x3-	T56.1x4-	—	—
oxide, yellow	T49.0x1-	T49.0x2-	T49.0x3-	T49.0x4-	T49.0x5-	T49.0x6-
Mersalyl	T50.2x1-	T50.2x2-	T50.2x3-	T50.2x4-	T50.2x5-	T50.2x6-
Merthiolate	T49.0x1-	T49.0x2-	T49.0x3-	T49.0x4-	T49.0x5-	T49.0x6-
ophthalmic preparation	T49.5x1-	T49.5x2-	T49.5x3-	T49.5x4-	T49.5x5-	T49.5x6-
Meruvax	T50.B91-	T50.B92-	T50.B93-	T50.B94-	T50.B95-	T50.B96-
Mesalazine	T47.8x1-	T47.8x2-	T47.8x3-	T47.8x4-	T47.8x5-	T47.8x6-
Mescal buttons	T40.991-	T40.992-	T40.993-	T40.994-	—	—
Mescaline	T40.991-	T40.992-	T40.993-	T40.994-	—	—
Mesna	T48.4x1-	T48.4x2-	T48.4x3-	T48.4x4-	T48.4x5-	T48.4x6-
Mesoglycan	T46.6x1-	T46.6x2-	T46.6x3-	T46.6x4-	T46.6x5-	T46.6x6-
Mesoridazine	T43.3x1-	T43.3x2-	T43.3x3-	T43.3x4-	T43.3x5-	T43.3x6-
Mestanolone	T38.7x1-	T38.7x2-	T38.7x3-	T38.7x4-	T38.7x5-	T38.7x6-
Mesterolone	T38.7x1-	T38.7x2-	T38.7x3-	T38.7x4-	T38.7x5-	T38.7x6-
Mestranol	T38.5x1-	T38.5x2-	T38.5x3-	T38.5x4-	T38.5x5-	T38.5x6-
Mesulergine	T42.8x1-	T42.8x2-	T42.8x3-	T42.8x4-	T42.8x5-	T42.8x6-
Mesulfen	T49.0x1-	T49.0x2-	T49.0x3-	T49.0x4-	T49.0x5-	T49.0x6-
Mesuximide	T42.2x1-	T42.2x2-	T42.2x3-	T42.2x4-	T42.2x5-	T42.2x6-
Metabutethamine	T41.3x1-	T41.3x2-	T41.3x3-	T41.3x4-	T41.3x5-	T41.3x6-
Metactesylacetate	T49.0x1-	T49.0x2-	T49.0x3-	T49.0x4-	T49.0x5-	T49.0x6-
Metacycline	T36.4x1-	T36.4x2-	T36.4x3-	T36.4x4-	T36.4x5-	T36.4x6-
Metaldehyde (snail killer) NEC	T60.8x1-	T60.8x2-	T60.8x3-	T60.8x4-	—	—
Metals (heavy) (nonmedicinal)	T56.91x-	T56.92x-	T56.93x-	T56.94x-	—	—
dust, fumes, or vapor NEC	T56.91x-	T56.92x-	T56.93x-	T56.94x-	—	—
light NEC	T56.91x-	T56.92x-	T56.93x-	T56.94x-	—	—
dust, fumes, or vapor NEC	T56.91x-	T56.92x-	T56.93x-	T56.94x-	—	—
specified NEC	T56.891-	T56.892-	T56.893-	T56.894-	—	—
thallium	T56.811-	T56.812-	T56.813-	T56.814-	—	—
Metamfetamine	T43.621-	T43.622-	T43.623-	T43.624-	T43.625-	T43.626-
Metamizole sodium	T39.2x1-	T39.2x2-	T39.2x3-	T39.2x4-	T39.2x5-	T39.2x6-
Metampicillin	T36.0x1-	T36.0x2-	T36.0x3-	T36.0x4-	T36.0x5-	T36.0x6-
Metamucil	T47.4x1-	T47.4x2-	T47.4x3-	T47.4x4-	T47.4x5-	T47.4x6-

Table of Drugs & Chemicals	POISONING Accidental (Unintentional)	Self-Harm (Intentional)	Assault	Undetermined	Adverse Effect	Underdosing
Metandienone	T38.7x1-	T38.7x2-	T38.7x3-	T38.7x4-	T38.7x5-	T38.7x6-
Metandrostenolone	T38.7x1-	T38.7x2-	T38.7x3-	T38.7x4-	T38.7x5-	T38.7x6-
Metaphen	T49.0x1-	T49.0x2-	T49.0x3-	T49.0x4-	T49.0x5-	T49.0x6-
Metaphos	T60.0x1-	T60.0x2-	T60.0x3-	T60.0x4-	—	—
Metapramine	T43.011-	T43.012-	T43.013-	T43.014-	T43.015-	T43.016-
Metaproterenol	T48.291-	T48.292-	T48.293-	T48.294-	T48.295-	T48.296-
Metaraminol	T44.4x1-	T44.4x2-	T44.4x3-	T44.4x4-	T44.4x5-	T44.4x6-
Metaxalone	T42.8x1-	T42.8x2-	T42.8x3-	T42.8x4-	T42.8x5-	T42.8x6-
Metenolone	T38.7x1-	T38.7x2-	T38.7x3-	T38.7x4-	T38.7x5-	T38.7x6-
Metergoline	T42.8x1-	T42.8x2-	T42.8x3-	T42.8x4-	T42.8x5-	T42.8x6-
Metescufylline	T46.991-	T46.992-	T46.993-	T46.994-	T46.995-	T46.996-
Metetoin	T42.0x1-	T42.0x2-	T42.0x3-	T42.0x4-	T42.0x5-	T42.0x6-
Metformin	T38.3x1-	T38.3x2-	T38.3x3-	T38.3x4-	T38.3x5-	T38.3x6-
Methacholine	T44.1x1-	T44.1x2-	T44.1x3-	T44.1x4-	T44.1x5-	T44.1x6-
Methacycline	T36.4x1-	T36.4x2-	T36.4x3-	T36.4x4-	T36.4x5-	T36.4x6-
Methadone	T40.3x1-	T40.3x2-	T40.3x3-	T40.3x4-	T40.3x5-	T40.3x6-
Methallenestril	T38.5x1-	T38.5x2-	T38.5x3-	T38.5x4-	T38.5x5-	T38.5x6-
Methallenoestril	T38.5x1-	T38.5x2-	T38.5x3-	T38.5x4-	T38.5x5-	T38.5x6-
Methamphetamine	T43.621-	T43.622-	T43.623-	T43.624-	T43.625-	T43.626-
Methampyrone	T39.2x1-	T39.2x2-	T39.2x3-	T39.2x4-	T39.2x5-	T39.2x6-
Methandienone	T38.7x1-	T38.7x2-	T38.7x3-	T38.7x4-	T38.7x5-	T38.7x6-
Methandriol	T38.7x1-	T38.7x2-	T38.7x3-	T38.7x4-	T38.7x5-	T38.7x6-
Methandrostenolone	T38.7x1-	T38.7x2-	T38.7x3-	T38.7x4-	T38.7x5-	T38.7x6-
Methane	T59.891-	T59.892-	T59.893-	T59.894-		
Methanethiol	T59.891-	T59.892-	T59.893-	T59.894-		
Methaniazide	T37.1x1-	T37.1x2-	T37.1x3-	T37.1x4-	T37.1x5-	T37.1x6-
Methanol (vapor)	T51.1x1-	T51.1x2-	T51.1x3-	T51.1x4-		
Methantheline	T44.3x1-	T44.3x2-	T44.3x3-	T44.3x4-	T44.3x5-	T44.3x6-
Methanthelinium bromide	T44.3x1-	T44.3x2-	T44.3x3-	T44.3x4-	T44.3x5-	T44.3x6-
Methaphenilene	T45.0x1-	T45.0x2-	T45.0x3-	T45.0x4-	T45.0x5-	T45.0x6-
Methapyrilene	T45.0x1-	T45.0x2-	T45.0x3-	T45.0x4-	T45.0x5-	T45.0x6-
Methaqualone (compound)	T42.6x1-	T42.6x2-	T42.6x3-	T42.6x4-	T42.6x5-	T42.6x6-
Metharbital	T42.3x1-	T42.3x2-	T42.3x3-	T42.3x4-	T42.3x5-	T42.3x6-
Methazolamide	T50.2x1-	T50.2x2-	T50.2x3-	T50.2x4-	T50.2x5-	T50.2x6-
Methdilazine	T43.3x1-	T43.3x2-	T43.3x3-	T43.3x4-	T43.3x5-	T43.3x6-
Methedrine	T43.621-	T43.622-	T43.623-	T43.624-	T43.625-	T43.626-
Methenamine (mandelate)	T37.8x1-	T37.8x2-	T37.8x3-	T37.8x4-	T37.8x5-	T37.8x6-
Methenolone	T38.7x1-	T38.7x2-	T38.7x3-	T38.7x4-	T38.7x5-	T38.7x6-
Methergine	T48.0x1-	T48.0x2-	T48.0x3-	T48.0x4-	T48.0x5-	T48.0x6-
Methetoin	T42.0x1-	T42.0x2-	T42.0x3-	T42.0x4-	T42.0x5-	T42.0x6-
Methiacil	T38.2x1-	T38.2x2-	T38.2x3-	T38.2x4-	T38.2x5-	T38.2x6-
Methicillin	T36.0x1-	T36.0x2-	T36.0x3-	T36.0x4-	T36.0x5-	T36.0x6-
Methimazole	T38.2x1-	T38.2x2-	T38.2x3-	T38.2x4-	T38.2x5-	T38.2x6-
Methiodal sodium	T50.8x1-	T50.8x2-	T50.8x3-	T50.8x4-	T50.8x5-	T50.8x6-
Methionine	T50.991-	T50.992-	T50.993-	T50.994-	T50.995-	T50.996-
Methisazone	T37.5x1-	T37.5x2-	T37.5x3-	T37.5x4-	T37.5x5-	T37.5x6-
Methisoprinol	T37.5x1-	T37.5x2-	T37.5x3-	T37.5x4-	T37.5x5-	T37.5x6-
Methitural	T42.3x1-	T42.3x2-	T42.3x3-	T42.3x4-	T42.3x5-	T42.3x6-
Methixene	T44.3x1-	T44.3x2-	T44.3x3-	T44.3x4-	T44.3x5-	T44.3x6-
Methobarbital, methobarbitone	T42.3x1-	T42.3x2-	T42.3x3-	T42.3x4-	T42.3x5-	T42.3x6-
Methocarbamol	T42.8x1-	T42.8x2-	T42.8x3-	T42.8x4-	T42.8x5-	T42.8x6-
skeletal muscle relaxant	T48.1x1-	T48.1x2-	T48.1x3-	T48.1x4-	T48.1x5-	T48.1x6-
Methohexital	T41.1x1-	T41.1x2-	T41.1x3-	T41.1x4-	T41.1x5-	T41.1x6-
Methohexitone	T41.1x1-	T41.1x2-	T41.1x3-	T41.1x4-	T41.1x5-	T41.1x6-
Methoin	T42.0x1-	T42.0x2-	T42.0x3-	T42.0x4-	T42.0x5-	T42.0x6-
Methopholine	T39.8x1-	T39.8x2-	T39.8x3-	T39.8x4-	T39.8x5-	T39.8x6-
Methopromazine	T43.3x1-	T43.3x2-	T43.3x3-	T43.3x4-	T43.3x5-	T43.3x6-
Methorate	T48.3x1-	T48.3x2-	T48.3x3-	T48.3x4-	T48.3x5-	T48.3x6-
Methoserpidine	T46.5x1-	T46.5x2-	T46.5x3-	T46.5x4-	T46.5x5-	T46.5x6-
Methotrexate	T45.1x1-	T45.1x2-	T45.1x3-	T45.1x4-	T45.1x5-	T45.1x6-
Methotrimeprazine	T43.3x1-	T43.3x2-	T43.3x3-	T43.3x4-	T43.3x5-	T43.3x6-
Methoxa-Dome	T49.3x1-	T49.3x2-	T49.3x3-	T49.3x4-	T49.3x5-	T49.3x6-

DRUGS & CHEMICALS

Table of Drugs & Chemicals	POISONING Accidental (Unintentional)	Self-Harm (Intentional)	Assault	Undetermined	Adverse Effect	Underdosing
Methoxamine	T44.4x1-	T44.4x2-	T44.4x3-	T44.4x4-	T44.4x5-	T44.4x6-
Methoxsalen	T50.991-	T50.992-	T50.993-	T50.994-	T50.995-	T50.996-
Methoxyaniline	T65.3x1-	T65.3x2-	T65.3x3-	T65.3x4-	—	—
Methoxybenzyl penicillin	T36.0x1-	T36.0x2-	T36.0x3-	T36.0x4-	T36.0x5-	T36.0x6-
Methoxychlor	T53.7x1-	T53.7x2-	T53.7x3-	T53.7x4-	—	—
Methoxy-DDT	T53.7x1-	T53.7x2-	T53.7x3-	T53.7x4-	—	—
2-Methoxyethanol	T52.3x1-	T52.3x2-	T52.3x3-	T52.3x4-	—	—
Methoxyflurane	T41.0x1-	T41.0x2-	T41.0x3-	T41.0x4-	T41.0x5-	T41.0x6-
Methoxyphenamine	T48.6x1-	T48.6x2-	T48.6x3-	T48.6x4-	T48.6x5-	T48.6x6-
Methoxypromazine	T43.3x1-	T43.3x2-	T43.3x3-	T43.3x4-	T43.3x5-	T43.3x6-
5-Methoxypsoralen (5-MOP)	T50.991-	T50.992-	T50.993-	T50.994-	T50.995-	T50.996-
8-Methoxypsoralen (8-MOP)	T50.991-	T50.992-	T50.993-	T50.994-	T50.995-	T50.996-
Methscopolamine bromide	T44.3x1-	T44.3x2-	T44.3x3-	T44.3x4-	T44.3x5-	T44.3x6-
Methsuximide	T42.2x1-	T42.2x2-	T42.2x3-	T42.2x4-	T42.2x5-	T42.2x6-
Methyclothiazide	T50.2x1-	T50.2x2-	T50.2x3-	T50.2x4-	T50.2x5-	T50.2x6-
Methyl						
acetate	T52.4x1-	T52.4x2-	T52.4x3-	T52.4x4-	—	—
acetone	T52.4x1-	T52.4x2-	T52.4x3-	T52.4x4-	—	—
acrylate	T65.891-	T65.892-	T65.893-	T65.894-	—	—
alcohol	T51.1x1-	T51.1x2-	T51.1x3-	T51.1x4-	—	—
aminophenol	T65.3x1-	T65.3x2-	T65.3x3-	T65.3x4-	—	—
amphetamine	T43.621-	T43.622-	T43.623-	T43.624-	T43.625-	T43.626-
androstanolone	T38.7x1-	T38.7x2-	T38.7x3-	T38.7x4-	T38.7x5-	T38.7x6-
atropine	T44.3x1-	T44.3x2-	T44.3x3-	T44.3x4-	T44.3x5-	T44.3x6-
benzene	T52.2x1-	T52.2x2-	T52.2x3-	T52.2x4-	—	—
benzoate	T52.8x1-	T52.8x2-	T52.8x3-	T52.8x4-	—	—
benzol	T52.2x1-	T52.2x2-	T52.2x3-	T52.2x4-	—	—
bromide (gas)	T59.891-	T59.892-	T59.893-	T59.894-	—	—
fumigant	T60.8x1-	T60.8x2-	T60.8x3-	T60.8x4-	—	—
butanol	T51.3x1-	T51.3x2-	T51.3x3-	T51.3x4-	—	—
carbonate	T52.8x1-	T52.8x2-	T52.8x3-	T52.8x4-	—	—
carbinol	T51.1x1-	T51.1x2-	T51.1x3-	T51.1x4-	—	—
CCNU	T45.1x1-	T45.1x2-	T45.1x3-	T45.1x4-	T45.1x5-	T45.1x6-
cellosolve	T52.91x-	T52.92x-	T52.93x-	T52.94x-	—	—
cellulose	T47.4x1-	T47.4x2-	T47.4x3-	T47.4x4-	T47.4x5-	T47.4x6-
chloride (gas)	T59.891-	T59.892-	T59.893-	T59.894-	—	—
chloroformate	T59.3x1-	T59.3x2-	T59.3x3-	T59.3x4-	—	—
cyclohexane	T52.8x1-	T52.8x2-	T52.8x3-	T52.8x4-	—	—
cyclohexanol	T51.8x1-	T51.8x2-	T51.8x3-	T51.8x4-	—	—
cyclohexanone	T52.8x1-	T52.8x2-	T52.8x3-	T52.8x4-	—	—
cyclohexyl acetate	T52.8x1-	T52.8x2-	T52.8x3-	T52.8x4-	—	—
demeton	T60.0x1-	T60.0x2-	T60.0x3-	T60.0x4-	—	—
dihydromorphinone	T40.2x1-	T40.2x2-	T40.2x3-	T40.2x4-	T40.2x5-	T40.2x6-
ergometrine	T48.0x1-	T48.0x2-	T48.0x3-	T48.0x4-	T48.0x5-	T48.0x6-
ergonovine	T48.0x1-	T48.0x2-	T48.0x3-	T48.0x4-	T48.0x5-	T48.0x6-
ethyl ketone	T52.4x1-	T52.4x2-	T52.4x3-	T52.4x4-	—	—
glucamine antimonate	T37.8x1-	T37.8x2-	T37.8x3-	T37.8x4-	T37.8x5-	T37.8x6-
hydrazine	T65.891-	T65.892-	T65.893-	T65.894-	—	—
iodide	T65.891-	T65.892-	T65.893-	T65.894-	—	—
isobutyl ketone	T52.4x1-	T52.4x2-	T52.4x3-	T52.4x4-	—	—
isothiocyanate	T60.3x1-	T60.3x2-	T60.3x3-	T60.3x4-	—	—
mercaptan	T59.891-	T59.892-	T59.893-	T59.894-	—	—
morphine NEC	T40.2x1-	T40.2x2-	T40.2x3-	T40.2x4-	T40.2x5-	T40.2x6-
nicotinate	T49.4x1-	T49.4x2-	T49.4x3-	T49.4x4-	T49.4x5-	T49.4x6-
paraben	T49.0x1-	T49.0x2-	T49.0x3-	T49.0x4-	T49.0x5-	T49.0x6-
parafynol	T42.6x1-	T42.6x2-	T42.6x3-	T42.6x4-	T42.6x5-	T42.6x6-
parathion	T60.0x1-	T60.0x2-	T60.0x3-	T60.0x4-	—	—
propylcarbinol	T51.3x1-	T51.3x2-	T51.3x3-	T51.3x4-	—	—
peridol	T43.4x1-	T43.4x2-	T43.4x3-	T43.4x4-	T43.4x5-	T43.4x6-
phenidate	T43.631-	T43.632-	T43.633-	T43.634-	T43.635-	T43.636-
prednisolone	T38.0x1-	T38.0x2-	T38.0x3-	T38.0x4-	T38.0x5-	T38.0x6-
ENT agent	T49.6x1-	T49.6x2-	T49.6x3-	T49.6x4-	T49.6x5-	T49.6x6-
ophthalmic preparation	T49.5x1-	T49.5x2-	T49.5x3-	T49.5x4-	T49.5x5-	T49.5x6-
topical NEC	T49.0x1-	T49.0x2-	T49.0x3-	T49.0x4-	T49.0x5-	T49.0x6-

Table of Drugs & Chemicals	POISONING Accidental (Unintentional)	Self-Harm (Intentional)	Assault	Undetermined	Adverse Effect	Underdosing
Methyl - continued						
rosaniline NEC	T49.0x1-	T49.0x2-	T49.0x3-	T49.0x4-	T49.0x5-	T49.0x6-
salicylate	T49.2x1-	T49.2x2-	T49.2x3-	T49.2x4-	T49.2x5-	T49.2x6-
sulfate (fumes)	T59.891-	T59.892-	T59.893-	T59.894-	—	—
liquid	T52.8x1-	T52.8x2-	T52.8x3-	T52.8x4-	—	—
sulfonal	T42.6x1-	T42.6x2-	T42.6x3-	T42.6x4-	T42.6x5-	T42.6x6-
testosterone	T38.7x1-	T38.7x2-	T38.7x3-	T38.7x4-	T38.7x5-	T38.7x6-
thiouracil	T38.2x1-	T38.2x2-	T38.2x3-	T38.2x4-	T38.2x5-	T38.2x6-
Methylamphetamine	T43.621-	T43.622-	T43.623-	T43.624-	T43.625-	T43.626-
Methylated spirit	T51.1x1-	T51.1x2-	T51.1x3-	T51.1x4-	—	—
Methylatropine nitrate	T44.3x1-	T44.3x2-	T44.3x3-	T44.3x4-	T44.3x5-	T44.3x6-
Methylbenactyzium bromide	T44.3x1-	T44.3x2-	T44.3x3-	T44.3x4-	T44.3x5-	T44.3x6-
Methylbenzethonium chloride	T49.0x1-	T49.0x2-	T49.0x3-	T49.0x4-	T49.0x5-	T49.0x6-
Methylcellulose	T47.4x1-	T47.4x2-	T47.4x3-	T47.4x4-	T47.4x5-	T47.4x6-
laxative	T47.4x1-	T47.4x2-	T47.4x3-	T47.4x4-	T47.4x5-	T47.4x6-
Methylchlorophenoxy-acetic acid	T60.3x1-	T60.3x2-	T60.3x3-	T60.3x4-	—	—
Methyldopa	T46.5x1-	T46.5x2-	T46.5x3-	T46.5x4-	T46.5x5-	T46.5x6-
Methyldopate	T46.5x1-	T46.5x2-	T46.5x3-	T46.5x4-	T46.5x5-	T46.5x6-
Methylene						
blue	T50.6x1-	T50.6x2-	T50.6x3-	T50.6x4-	T50.6x5-	T50.6x6-
chloride or dichloride (solvent) NEC	T53.4x1-	T53.4x2-	T53.4x3-	T53.4x4-	—	—
Methylenedioxyamphetamine	T43.621-	T43.622-	T43.623-	T43.624-	T43.625-	T43.626-
Methylenedioxymethamphetamine	T43.621-	T43.622-	T43.623-	T43.624-	T43.625-	T43.626-
Methylergometrine	T48.0x1-	T48.0x2-	T48.0x3-	T48.0x4-	T48.0x5-	T48.0x6-
Methylergonovine	T48.0x1-	T48.0x2-	T48.0x3-	T48.0x4-	T48.0x5-	T48.0x6-
Methylestrenolone	T38.5x1-	T38.5x2-	T38.5x3-	T38.5x4-	T38.5x5-	T38.5x6-
Methylethyl cellulose	T50.991-	T50.992-	T50.993-	T50.994-	T50.995-	T50.996-
Methylhexabital	T42.3x1-	T42.3x2-	T42.3x3-	T42.3x4-	T42.3x5-	T42.3x6-
Methylmorphine	T40.2x1-	T40.2x2-	T40.2x3-	T40.2x4-	T40.2x5-	T40.2x6-
Methylparaben (ophthalmic)	T49.5x1-	T49.5x2-	T49.5x3-	T49.5x4-	T49.5x5-	T49.5x6-
Methylparafynol	T42.6x1-	T42.6x2-	T42.6x3-	T42.6x4-	T42.6x5-	T42.6x6-
Methylpentynol, methylpenthynol	T42.6x1-	T42.6x2-	T42.6x3-	T42.6x4-	T42.6x5-	T42.6x6-
Methylphenidate	T43.631-	T43.632-	T43.633-	T43.634-	T43.635-	T43.636-
Methylphenobarbital	T42.3x1-	T42.3x2-	T42.3x3-	T42.3x4-	T42.3x5-	T42.3x6-
Methylpolysiloxane	T47.1x1-	T47.1x2-	T47.1x3-	T47.1x4-	T47.1x5-	T47.1x6-
Methylprednisolone — see Methyl, prednisolone						
Methylrosaniline	T49.0x1-	T49.0x2-	T49.0x3-	T49.0x4-	T49.0x5-	T49.0x6-
Methylrosanilinium chloride	T49.0x1-	T49.0x2-	T49.0x3-	T49.0x4-	T49.0x5-	T49.0x6-
Methyltestosterone	T38.7x1-	T38.7x2-	T38.7x3-	T38.7x4-	T38.7x5-	T38.7x6-
Methylthionine chloride	T50.6x1-	T50.6x2-	T50.6x3-	T50.6x4-	T50.6x5-	T50.6x6-
Methylthioninium chloride	T50.6x1-	T50.6x2-	T50.6x3-	T50.6x4-	T50.6x5-	T50.6x6-
Methylthiouracil	T38.2x1-	T38.2x2-	T38.2x3-	T38.2x4-	T38.2x5-	T38.2x6-
Methyprylon	T42.6x1-	T42.6x2-	T42.6x3-	T42.6x4-	T42.6x5-	T42.6x6-
Methysergide	T46.5x1-	T46.5x2-	T46.5x3-	T46.5x4-	T46.5x5-	T46.5x6-
Metiamide	T47.1x1-	T47.1x2-	T47.1x3-	T47.1x4-	T47.1x5-	T47.1x6-
Meticillin	T36.0x1-	T36.0x2-	T36.0x3-	T36.0x4-	T36.0x5-	T36.0x6-
Meticrane	T50.2x1-	T50.2x2-	T50.2x3-	T50.2x4-	T50.2x5-	T50.2x6-
Metildigoxin	T46.0x1-	T46.0x2-	T46.0x3-	T46.0x4-	T46.0x5-	T46.0x6-
Metipranolol	T49.5x1-	T49.5x2-	T49.5x3-	T49.5x4-	T49.5x5-	T49.5x6-
Metirosine	T46.5x1-	T46.5x2-	T46.5x3-	T46.5x4-	T46.5x5-	T46.5x6-
Metisazone	T37.5x1-	T37.5x2-	T37.5x3-	T37.5x4-	T37.5x5-	T37.5x6-
Metixene	T44.3x1-	T44.3x2-	T44.3x3-	T44.3x4-	T44.3x5-	T44.3x6-
Metizoline	T48.5x1-	T48.5x2-	T48.5x3-	T48.5x4-	T48.5x5-	T48.5x6-
Metoclopramide	T45.0x1-	T45.0x2-	T45.0x3-	T45.0x4-	T45.0x5-	T45.0x6-
Metofenazate	T43.3x1-	T43.3x2-	T43.3x3-	T43.3x4-	T43.3x5-	T43.3x6-

Table of Drugs & Chemicals	POISONING				Adverse Effect	Underdosing
	Accidental (Unintentional)	Self-Harm (Intentional)	Assault	Undetermined		
Metofoline	T39.8x1-	T39.8x2-	T39.8x3-	T39.8x4-	T39.8x5-	T39.8x6-
Metolazone	T50.2x1-	T50.2x2-	T50.2x3-	T50.2x4-	T50.2x5-	T50.2x6-
Metopon	T40.2x1-	T40.2x2-	T40.2x3-	T40.2x4-	T40.2x5-	T40.2x6-
Metoprine	T45.1x1-	T45.1x2-	T45.1x3-	T45.1x4-	T45.1x5-	T45.1x6-
Metoprolol	T44.7x1-	T44.7x2-	T44.7x3-	T44.7x4-	T44.7x5-	T44.7x6-
Metrifonate	T60.0x1-	T60.0x2-	T60.0x3-	T60.0x4-	—	—
Metrizamide	T50.8x1-	T50.8x2-	T50.8x3-	T50.8x4-	T50.8x5-	T50.8x6-
Metrizoic acid	T50.8x1-	T50.8x2-	T50.8x3-	T50.8x4-	T50.8x5-	T50.8x6-
Metronidazole	T37.8x1-	T37.8x2-	T37.8x3-	T37.8x4-	T37.8x5-	T37.8x6-
Metycaine	T41.3x1-	T41.3x2-	T41.3x3-	T41.3x4-	T41.3x5-	T41.3x6-
infiltration (subcutaneous)	T41.3x1-	T41.3x2-	T41.3x3-	T41.3x4-	T41.3x5-	T41.3x6-
nerve block (peripheral) (plexus)	T41.3x1-	T41.3x2-	T41.3x3-	T41.3x4-	T41.3x5-	T41.3x6-
topical (surface)	T41.3x1-	T41.3x2-	T41.3x3-	T41.3x4-	T41.3x5-	T41.3x6-
Metyrapone	T50.8x1-	T50.8x2-	T50.8x3-	T50.8x4-	T50.8x5-	T50.8x6-
Mevinphos	T60.0x1-	T60.0x2-	T60.0x3-	T60.0x4-	—	—
Mexazolam	T42.4x1-	T42.4x2-	T42.4x3-	T42.4x4-	T42.4x5-	T42.4x6-
Mexenone	T49.3x1-	T49.3x2-	T49.3x3-	T49.3x4-	T49.3x5-	T49.3x6-
Mexiletine	T46.2x1-	T46.2x2-	T46.2x3-	T46.2x4-	T46.2x5-	T46.2x6-
Mezereon	T62.2x1-	T62.2x2-	T62.2x3-	T62.2x4-	—	—
berries	T62.1x1-	T62.1x2-	T62.1x3-	T62.1x4-	—	—
Mezlocillin	T36.0x1-	T36.0x2-	T36.0x3-	T36.0x4-	T36.0x5-	T36.0x6-
Mianserin	T43.021-	T43.022-	T43.023-	T43.024-	T43.025-	T43.026-
Micatin	T49.0x1-	T49.0x2-	T49.0x3-	T49.0x4-	T49.0x5-	T49.0x6-
Miconazole	T49.0x1-	T49.0x2-	T49.0x3-	T49.0x4-	T49.0x5-	T49.0x6-
Micronomicin	T36.5x1-	T36.5x2-	T36.5x3-	T36.5x4-	T36.5x5-	T36.5x6-
Midazolam	T42.4x1-	T42.4x2-	T42.4x3-	T42.4x4-	T42.4x5-	T42.4x6-
Midecamycin	T36.3x1-	T36.3x2-	T36.3x3-	T36.3x4-	T36.3x5-	T36.3x6-
Mifepristone	T38.6x1-	T38.6x2-	T38.6x3-	T38.6x4-	T38.6x5-	T38.6x6-
Milk of magnesia	T47.1x1-	T47.1x2-	T47.1x3-	T47.1x4-	T47.1x5-	T47.1x6-
Millipede (tropical) (venomous)	T63.411-	T63.412-	T63.413-	T63.414-	—	—
Miltown	T43.591-	T43.592-	T43.593-	T43.594-	T43.595-	T43.596-
Milverine	T44.3x1-	T44.3x2-	T44.3x3-	T44.3x4-	T44.3x5-	T44.3x6-
Minaprine	T43.291-	T43.292-	T43.293-	T43.294-	T43.295-	T43.296-
Minaxolone	T41.291-	T41.292-	T41.293-	T41.294-	T41.295-	T41.296-
Mineral						
acids	T54.2x1-	T54.2x2-	T54.2x3-	T54.2x4-	—	—
oil (laxative) (medicinal)	T47.4x1-	T47.4x2-	T47.4x3-	T47.4x4-	T47.4x5-	T47.4x6-
emulsion	T47.2x1-	T47.2x2-	T47.2x3-	T47.2x4-	T47.2x5-	T47.2x6-
nonmedicinal	T52.0x1-	T52.0x2-	T52.0x3-	T52.0x4-	—	—
topical	T49.3x1-	T49.3x2-	T49.3x3-	T49.3x4-	T49.3x5-	T49.3x6-
salt NEC	T50.3x1-	T50.3x2-	T50.3x3-	T50.3x4-	T50.3x5-	T50.3x6-
spirits	T52.0x1-	T52.0x2-	T52.0x3-	T52.0x4-	—	—
Mineralocorticosteroid	T50.0x1-	T50.0x2-	T50.0x3-	T50.0x4-	T50.0x5-	T50.0x6-
Minocycline	T36.4x1-	T36.4x2-	T36.4x3-	T36.4x4-	T36.4x5-	T36.4x6-
Minoxidil	T46.7x1-	T46.7x2-	T46.7x3-	T46.7x4-	T46.7x5-	T46.7x6-
Miokamycin	T36.3x1-	T36.3x2-	T36.3x3-	T36.3x4-	T36.3x5-	T36.3x6-
Miotic drug	T49.5x1-	T49.5x2-	T49.5x3-	T49.5x4-	T49.5x5-	T49.5x6-
Mipafox	T60.0x1-	T60.0x2-	T60.0x3-	T60.0x4-	—	—
Mirex	T60.1x1-	T60.1x2-	T60.1x3-	T60.1x4-	—	—
Mirtazapine	T43.021-	T43.022-	T43.023-	T43.024-	T43.025-	T43.026-
Misonidazole	T37.3x1-	T37.3x2-	T37.3x3-	T37.3x4-	T37.3x5-	T37.3x6-
Misoprostol	T47.1x1-	T47.1x2-	T47.1x3-	T47.1x4-	T47.1x5-	T47.1x6-
Mithramycin	T45.1x1-	T45.1x2-	T45.1x3-	T45.1x4-	T45.1x5-	T45.1x6-
Mitobronitol	T45.1x1-	T45.1x2-	T45.1x3-	T45.1x4-	T45.1x5-	T45.1x6-
Mitoguazone	T45.1x1-	T45.1x2-	T45.1x3-	T45.1x4-	T45.1x5-	T45.1x6-
Mitolactol	T45.1x1-	T45.1x2-	T45.1x3-	T45.1x4-	T45.1x5-	T45.1x6-
Mitomycin	T45.1x1-	T45.1x2-	T45.1x3-	T45.1x4-	T45.1x5-	T45.1x6-
Mitopodozide	T45.1x1-	T45.1x2-	T45.1x3-	T45.1x4-	T45.1x5-	T45.1x6-

Table of Drugs & Chemicals	POISONING				Adverse Effect	Underdosing
	Accidental (Unintentional)	Self-Harm (Intentional)	Assault	Undetermined		
Mitotane	T45.1x1-	T45.1x2-	T45.1x3-	T45.1x4-	T45.1x5-	T45.1x6-
Mitoxantrone	T45.1x1-	T45.1x2-	T45.1x3-	T45.1x4-	T45.1x5-	T45.1x6-
Mivacurium chloride	T48.1x1-	T48.1x2-	T48.1x3-	T48.1x4-	T48.1x5-	T48.1x6-
Miyari bacteria	T47.6x1-	T47.6x2-	T47.6x3-	T47.6x4-	T47.6x5-	T47.6x6-
Moclobemide	T43.1x1-	T43.1x2-	T43.1x3-	T43.1x4-	T43.1x5-	T43.1x6-
Moderil	T46.5x1-	T46.5x2-	T46.5x3-	T46.5x4-	T46.5x5-	T46.5x6-
Mofebutazone	T39.2x1-	T39.2x2-	T39.2x3-	T39.2x4-	T39.2x5-	T39.2x6-
Mogadon — *see* Nitrazepam						
Molindone	T43.591-	T43.592-	T43.593-	T43.594-	T43.595-	T43.596-
Molsidomine	T46.3x1-	T46.3x2-	T46.3x3-	T46.3x4-	T46.3x5-	T46.3x6-
Mometasone	T49.0x1-	T49.0x2-	T49.0x3-	T49.0x4-	T49.0x5-	T49.0x6-
Monistat	T49.0x1-	T49.0x2-	T49.0x3-	T49.0x4-	T49.0x5-	T49.0x6-
Monkshood	T62.2x1-	T62.2x2-	T62.2x3-	T62.2x4-	—	—
Monoamine oxidase inhibitor NEC	T43.1x1-	T43.1x2-	T43.1x3-	T43.1x4-	T43.1x5-	T43.1x6-
hydrazine	T43.1x1-	T43.1x2-	T43.1x3-	T43.1x4-	T43.1x5-	T43.1x6-
Monobenzone	T49.4x1-	T49.4x2-	T49.4x3-	T49.4x4-	T49.4x5-	T49.4x6-
Monochloroacetic acid	T60.3x1-	T60.3x2-	T60.3x3-	T60.3x4-	—	—
Monochlorobenzene	T53.7x1-	T53.7x2-	T53.7x3-	T53.7x4-	—	—
Monoethanolamine	T46.8x1-	T46.8x2-	T46.8x3-	T46.8x4-	T46.8x5-	T46.8x6-
oleate	T46.8x1-	T46.8x2-	T46.8x3-	T46.8x4-	T46.8x5-	T46.8x6-
Monooctanoin	T50.991-	T50.992-	T50.993-	T50.994-	T50.995-	T50.996-
Monophenylbutazone	T39.2x1-	T39.2x2-	T39.2x3-	T39.2x4-	T39.2x5-	T39.2x6-
Monosodium glutamate	T65.891-	T65.892-	T65.893-	T65.894-	—	—
Monosulfiram	T49.0x1-	T49.0x2-	T49.0x3-	T49.0x4-	T49.0x5-	T49.0x6-
Monoxide, carbon — *see* Carbon, monoxide						
Monoxidine hydrochloride	T46.1x1-	T46.1x2-	T46.1x3-	T46.1x4-	T46.1x5-	T46.1x6-
Monuron	T60.3x1-	T60.3x2-	T60.3x3-	T60.3x4-	—	—
Moperone	T43.4x1-	T43.4x2-	T43.4x3-	T43.4x4-	T43.4x5-	T43.4x6-
Mopidamol	T45.1x1-	T45.1x2-	T45.1x3-	T45.1x4-	T45.1x5-	T45.1x6-
MOPP (mechlorethamine + vincristine + prednisone + procarba-zine)	T45.1x1-	T45.1x2-	T45.1x3-	T45.1x4-	T45.1x5-	T45.1x6-
Morfin	T40.2x1-	T40.2x2-	T40.2x3-	T40.2x4-	T40.2x5-	T40.2x6-
Morinamide	T37.1x1-	T37.1x2-	T37.1x3-	T37.1x4-	T37.1x5-	T37.1x6-
Morning glory seeds	T40.991-	T40.992-	T40.993-	T40.994-	—	—
Moroxydine	T37.5x1-	T37.5x2-	T37.5x3-	T37.5x4-	T37.5x5-	T37.5x6-
Morphazinamide	T37.1x1-	T37.1x2-	T37.1x3-	T37.1x4-	T37.1x5-	T37.1x6-
Morphine	T40.2x1-	T40.2x2-	T40.2x3-	T40.2x4-	T40.2x5-	T40.2x6-
antagonist	T50.7x1-	T50.7x2-	T50.7x3-	T50.7x4-	T50.7x5-	T50.7x6-
Morpholinylethylmorphine	T40.2x1-	T40.2x2-	T40.2x3-	T40.2x4-	—	—
Morsuximide	T42.2x1-	T42.2x2-	T42.2x3-	T42.2x4-	T42.2x5-	T42.2x6-
Mosapramine	T43.591-	T43.592-	T43.593-	T43.594-	T43.595-	T43.596-
Moth balls — *see also* Pesticides	T60.2x1-	T60.2x2-	T60.2x3-	T60.2x4-	—	—
naphthalene	T60.2x1-	T60.2x2-	T60.2x3-	T60.2x4-	—	—
paradichlorobenzene	T60.1x1-	T60.1x2-	T60.1x3-	T60.1x4-	—	—
Motor exhaust gas	T58.01x-	T58.02x-	T58.03x-	T58.04x-	—	—
Mouthwash (antiseptic) (zinc chloride)	T49.6x1-	T49.6x2-	T49.6x3-	T49.6x4-	T49.6x5-	T49.6x6-
Moxastine	T45.0x1-	T45.0x2-	T45.0x3-	T45.0x4-	T45.0x5-	T45.0x6-
Moxaverine	T44.3x1-	T44.3x2-	T44.3x3-	T44.3x4-	T44.3x5-	T44.3x6-
Moxisylyte	T46.7x1-	T46.7x2-	T46.7x3-	T46.7x4-	T46.7x5-	T46.7x6-
Mucilage, plant	T47.4x1-	T47.4x2-	T47.4x3-	T47.4x4-	T47.4x5-	T47.4x6-
Mucolytic drug	T48.4x1-	T48.4x2-	T48.4x3-	T48.4x4-	T48.4x5-	T48.4x6-
Mucomyst	T48.4x1-	T48.4x2-	T48.4x3-	T48.4x4-	T48.4x5-	T48.4x6-
Mucous membrane agents (external)	T49.91x-	T49.92x-	T49.93x-	T49.94x-	T49.95x-	T49.96x-
specified NEC	T49.8x1-	T49.8x2-	T49.8x3-	T49.8x4-	T49.8x5-	T49.8x6-

DRUGS & CHEMICALS

Table of Drugs & Chemicals	Poisoning Accidental (Unintentional)	Poisoning Self-Harm (Intentional)	Poisoning Assault	Poisoning Undetermined	Adverse Effect	Underdosing
Mumps						
immune globulin (human)	T50.Z11-	T50.Z12-	T50.Z13-	T50.Z14-	T50.Z15-	T50.Z16-
skin test antigen	T50.8x1-	T50.8x2-	T50.8x3-	T50.8x4-	T50.8x5-	T50.8x6-
vaccine	T50.B91-	T50.B92-	T50.B93-	T50.B94-	T50.B95-	T50.B96-
Mumpsvax	T50.B91-	T50.B92-	T50.B93-	T50.B94-	T50.B95-	T50.B96-
Mupirocin	T49.0x1-	T49.0x2-	T49.0x3-	T49.0x4-	T49.0x5-	T49.0x6-
Muriatic acid — see Hydrochloric acid						
Muromonab-CD3	T45.1x1-	T45.1x2-	T45.1x3-	T45.1x4-	T45.1x5-	T45.1x6-
Muscle affecting agents NEC	T48.201-	T48.202-	T48.203-	T48.204-	T48.205-	T48.206-
oxytocic	T48.0x1-	T48.0x2-	T48.0x3-	T48.0x4-	T48.0x5-	T48.0x6-
relaxants	T48.201-	T48.202-	T48.203-	T48.204-	T48.205-	T48.206-
central nervous system	T42.8x1-	T42.8x2-	T42.8x3-	T42.8x4-	T42.8x5-	T42.8x6-
skeletal	T48.1x1-	T48.1x2-	T48.1x3-	T48.1x4-	T48.1x5-	T48.1x6-
smooth	T44.3x1-	T44.3x2-	T44.3x3-	T44.3x4-	T44.3x5-	T44.3x6-
Muscle relaxant — see Relaxant, muscle						
Muscle-action drug NEC	T48.201-	T48.202-	T48.203-	T48.204-	T48.205-	T48.206-
Muscle-tone depressant, central NEC	T42.8x1-	T42.8x2-	T42.8x3-	T42.8x4-	T42.8x5-	T42.8x6-
specified NEC	T42.8x1-	T42.8x2-	T42.8x3-	T42.8x4-	T42.8x5-	T42.8x6-
Mushroom, noxious	T62.0x1-	T62.0x2-	T62.0x3-	T62.0x4-	—	—
Mussel, noxious	T61.781-	T61.782-	T61.783-	T61.784-		
Mustard (emetic)	T47.7x1-	T47.7x2-	T47.7x3-	T47.7x4-	T47.7x5-	T47.7x6-
black	T47.7x1-	T47.7x2-	T47.7x3-	T47.7x4-	T47.7x5-	T47.7x6-
gas, not in war	T59.91x-	T59.92x-	T59.93x-	T59.94x-	—	—
nitrogen	T45.1x1-	T45.1x2-	T45.1x3-	T45.1x4-	T45.1x5-	T45.1x6-
Mustine	T45.1x1-	T45.1x2-	T45.1x3-	T45.1x4-	T45.1x5-	T45.1x6-
M-vac	T45.1x1-	T45.1x2-	T45.1x3-	T45.1x4-	T45.1x5-	T45.1x6-
Mycifradin	T36.5x1-	T36.5x2-	T36.5x3-	T36.5x4-	T36.5x5-	T36.5x6-
topical	T49.0x1-	T49.0x2-	T49.0x3-	T49.0x4-	T49.0x5-	T49.0x6-
Mycitracin	T36.8x1-	T36.8x2-	T36.8x3-	T36.8x4-	T36.8x5-	T36.8x6-
ophthalmic preparation	T49.5x1-	T49.5x2-	T49.5x3-	T49.5x4-	T49.5x5-	T49.5x6-
Mycostatin	T36.7x1-	T36.7x2-	T36.7x3-	T36.7x4-	T36.7x5-	T36.7x6-
topical	T49.0x1-	T49.0x2-	T49.0x3-	T49.0x4-	T49.0x5-	T49.0x6-
Mycotoxins	T64.81x-	T64.82x-	T64.83x-	T64.84x-	—	—
aflatoxin	T64.01x-	T64.02x-	T64.03x-	T64.04x-	—	—
specified NEC	T64.81x-	T64.82x-	T64.83x-	T64.84x-	—	—
Mydriacyl	T44.3x1-	T44.3x2-	T44.3x3-	T44.3x4-	T44.3x5-	T44.3x6-
Mydriatic drug	T49.5x1-	T49.5x2-	T49.5x3-	T49.5x4-	T49.5x5-	T49.5x6-
Myelobromal	T45.1x1-	T45.1x2-	T45.1x3-	T45.1x4-	T45.1x5-	T45.1x6-
Myleran	T45.1x1-	T45.1x2-	T45.1x3-	T45.1x4-	T45.1x5-	T45.1x6-
Myochrysin(e)	T39.2x1-	T39.2x2-	T39.2x3-	T39.2x4-	T39.2x5-	T39.2x6-
Myoneural blocking agents	T48.1x1-	T48.1x2-	T48.1x3-	T48.1x4-	T48.1x5-	T48.1x6-
Myralact	T49.0x1-	T49.0x2-	T49.0x3-	T49.0x4-	T49.0x5-	T49.0x6-
Myristica fragrans	T62.2x1-	T62.2x2-	T62.2x3-	T62.2x4-	—	—
Myristicin	T65.891-	T65.892-	T65.893-	T65.894-		
Mysoline	T42.3x1-	T42.3x2-	T42.3x3-	T42.3x4-	T42.3x5-	T42.3x6-
Nabilone	T40.7x1-	T40.7x2-	T40.7x3-	T40.7x4-	T40.7x5-	T40.7x6-
Nabumetone	T39.391-	T39.392-	T39.393-	T39.394-	T39.395-	T39.396-
Nadolol	T44.7x1-	T44.7x2-	T44.7x3-	T44.7x4-	T44.7x5-	T44.7x6-
Nafcillin	T36.0x1-	T36.0x2-	T36.0x3-	T36.0x4-	T36.0x5-	T36.0x6-
Nafoxidine	T38.6x1-	T38.6x2-	T38.6x3-	T38.6x4-	T38.6x5-	T38.6x6-
Naftazone	T46.991-	T46.992-	T46.993-	T46.994-	T46.995-	T46.996-
Naftidrofuryl (oxalate)	T46.7x1-	T46.7x2-	T46.7x3-	T46.7x4-	T46.7x5-	T46.7x6-
Naftifine	T49.0x1-	T49.0x2-	T49.0x3-	T49.0x4-	T49.0x5-	T49.0x6-
Nail polish remover	T52.91x-	T52.92x-	T52.93x-	T52.94x-	—	—
Nalbuphine	T40.4x1-	T40.4x2-	T40.4x3-	T40.4x4-	T40.4x5-	T40.4x6-
Naled	T60.0x1-	T60.0x2-	T60.0x3-	T60.0x4-	—	—
Nalidixic acid	T37.8x1-	T37.8x2-	T37.8x3-	T37.8x4-	T37.8x5-	T37.8x6-
Nalorphine	T50.7x1-	T50.7x2-	T50.7x3-	T50.7x4-	T50.7x5-	T50.7x6-
Naloxone	T50.7x1-	T50.7x2-	T50.7x3-	T50.7x4-	T50.7x5-	T50.7x6-
Naltrexone	T50.7x1-	T50.7x2-	T50.7x3-	T50.7x4-	T50.7x5-	T50.7x6-
Namenda	T43.8x1-	T43.8x2-	T43.8x3-	T43.8x4-	T43.8x5-	T43.8x6-
Nandrolone	T38.7x1-	T38.7x2-	T38.7x3-	T38.7x4-	T38.7x5-	T38.7x6-
Naphazoline	T48.5x1-	T48.5x2-	T48.5x3-	T48.5x4-	T48.5x5-	T48.5x6-
Naphtha (painters') (petroleum)	T52.0x1-	T52.0x2-	T52.0x3-	T52.0x4-	—	—
solvent	T52.0x1-	T52.0x2-	T52.0x3-	T52.0x4-	—	—
vapor	T52.0x1-	T52.0x2-	T52.0x3-	T52.0x4-	—	—
Naphthalene (non-chlorinated)	T60.2x1-	T60.2x2-	T60.2x3-	T60.2x4-	—	—
chlorinated	T60.1x1-	T60.1x2-	T60.1x3-	T60.1x4-	—	—
vapor	T60.1x1-	T60.1x2-	T60.1x3-	T60.1x4-	—	—
insecticide or moth repellent	T60.2x1-	T60.2x2-	T60.2x3-	T60.2x4-	—	—
chlorinated	T60.1x1-	T60.1x2-	T60.1x3-	T60.1x4-	—	—
vapor	T60.2x1-	T60.2x2-	T60.2x3-	T60.2x4-	—	—
chlorinated	T60.1x1-	T60.1x2-	T60.1x3-	T60.1x4-	—	—
Naphthol	T65.891-	T65.892-	T65.893-	T65.894-		
Naphthylamine	T65.891-	T65.892-	T65.893-	T65.894-		
Naphthylthiourea (ANTU)	T60.4x1-	T60.4x2-	T60.4x3-	T60.4x4-		
Naprosyn — see Naproxen						
Naproxen	T39.311-	T39.312-	T39.313-	T39.314-	T39.315-	T39.316-
Narcotic (drug)	T40.601-	T40.602-	T40.603-	T40.604-	T40.605-	T40.606-
analgesic NEC	T40.601-	T40.602-	T40.603-	T40.604-	T40.605-	T40.606-
antagonist	T50.7x1-	T50.7x2-	T50.7x3-	T50.7x4-	T50.7x5-	T50.7x6-
specified NEC	T40.691-	T40.692-	T40.693-	T40.694-	T40.695-	T40.696-
synthetic	T40.4x1-	T40.4x2-	T40.4x3-	T40.4x4-	T40.4x5-	T40.4x6-
Narcotine	T48.3x1-	T48.3x2-	T48.3x3-	T48.3x4-	T48.3x5-	T48.3x6-
Nardil	T43.1x1-	T43.1x2-	T43.1x3-	T43.1x4-	T43.1x5-	T43.1x6-
Nasal drug NEC	T49.6x1-	T49.6x2-	T49.6x3-	T49.6x4-	T49.6x5-	T49.6x6-
Natamycin	T49.0x1-	T49.0x2-	T49.0x3-	T49.0x4-	T49.0x5-	T49.0x6-
Natrium cyanide — see Cyanide(s)						
Natural						
blood (product)	T45.8x1-	T45.8x2-	T45.8x3-	T45.8x4-	T45.8x5-	T45.8x6-
gas (piped)	T59.891-	T59.892-	T59.893-	T59.894-	—	—
incomplete combustion	T58.11x-	T58.12x-	T58.13x-	T58.14x-	—	—
Nealbarbital	T42.3x1-	T42.3x2-	T42.3x3-	T42.3x4-	T42.3x5-	T42.3x6-
Nectadon	T48.3x1-	T48.3x2-	T48.3x3-	T48.3x4-	T48.3x5-	T48.3x6-
Nedocromil	T48.6x1-	T48.6x2-	T48.6x3-	T48.6x4-	T48.6x5-	T48.6x6-
Nefopam	T39.8x1-	T39.8x2-	T39.8x3-	T39.8x4-	T39.8x5-	T39.8x6-
Nematocyst (sting)	T63.691-	T63.692-	T63.693-	T63.694-	—	—
Nembutal	T42.3x1-	T42.3x2-	T42.3x3-	T42.3x4-	T42.3x5-	T42.3x6-
Nemonapride	T43.591-	T43.592-	T43.593-	T43.594-	T43.595-	T43.596-
Neoarsphenamine	T37.8x1-	T37.8x2-	T37.8x3-	T37.8x4-	T37.8x5-	T37.8x6-
Neocinchophen	T50.4x1-	T50.4x2-	T50.4x3-	T50.4x4-	T50.4x5-	T50.4x6-
Neomycin (derivatives)	T36.5x1-	T36.5x2-	T36.5x3-	T36.5x4-	T36.5x5-	T36.5x6-
with bacitracin	T49.0x1-	T49.0x2-	T49.0x3-	T49.0x4-	T49.0x5-	T49.0x6-
neostigmine	T44.0x1-	T44.0x2-	T44.0x3-	T44.0x4-	T44.0x5-	T44.0x6-
ENT agent	T49.6x1-	T49.6x2-	T49.6x3-	T49.6x4-	T49.6x5-	T49.6x6-
ophthalmic preparation	T49.5x1-	T49.5x2-	T49.5x3-	T49.5x4-	T49.5x5-	T49.5x6-
topical NEC	T49.0x1-	T49.0x2-	T49.0x3-	T49.0x4-	T49.0x5-	T49.0x6-
Neonal	T42.3x1-	T42.3x2-	T42.3x3-	T42.3x4-	T42.3x5-	T42.3x6-
Neoprontosil	T37.0x1-	T37.0x2-	T37.0x3-	T37.0x4-	T37.0x5-	T37.0x6-
Neosalvarsan	T37.8x1-	T37.8x2-	T37.8x3-	T37.8x4-	T37.8x5-	T37.8x6-
Neosilversalvarsan	T37.8x1-	T37.8x2-	T37.8x3-	T37.8x4-	T37.8x5-	T37.8x6-
Neosporin	T36.8x1-	T36.8x2-	T36.8x3-	T36.8x4-	T36.8x5-	T36.8x6-
ENT agent	T49.6x1-	T49.6x2-	T49.6x3-	T49.6x4-	T49.6x5-	T49.6x6-
ophthalmic preparation	T49.5x1-	T49.5x2-	T49.5x3-	T49.5x4-	T49.5x5-	T49.5x6-
topical NEC	T49.0x1-	T49.0x2-	T49.0x3-	T49.0x4-	T49.0x5-	T49.0x6-

Table of Drugs & Chemicals	P O I S O N I N G				Adverse Effect	Underdosing
	Accidental (Unintentional)	Self-Harm (Intentional)	Assault	Undetermined		
Neostigmine bromide	T44.0x1-	T44.0x2-	T44.0x3-	T44.0x4-	T44.0x5-	T44.0x6-
Neraval	T42.3x1-	T42.3x2-	T42.3x3-	T42.3x4-	T42.3x5-	T42.3x6-
Neravan	T42.3x1-	T42.3x2-	T42.3x3-	T42.3x4-	T42.3x5-	T42.3x6-
Nerium oleander	T62.2x1-	T62.2x2-	T62.2x3-	T62.2x4-	—	—
Nerve gas, not in war	T59.91x-	T59.92x-	T59.93x-	T59.94x-	—	—
Nesacaine	T41.3x1-	T41.3x2-	T41.3x3-	T41.3x4-	T41.3x5-	T41.3x6-
infiltration						
(subcutaneous)	T41.3x1-	T41.3x2-	T41.3x3-	T41.3x4-	T41.3x5-	T41.3x6-
nerve block (peripheral)						
(plexus)	T41.3x1-	T41.3x2-	T41.3x3-	T41.3x4-	T41.3x5-	T41.3x6-
Netilmicin	T36.5x1-	T36.5x2-	T36.5x3-	T36.5x4-	T36.5x5-	T36.5x6-
Neurobarb	T42.3x1-	T42.3x2-	T42.3x3-	T42.3x4-	T42.3x5-	T42.3x6-
Neuroleptic drug NEC	T43.501-	T43.502-	T43.503-	T43.504-	T43.505-	T43.506-
Neuromuscular blocking drug	T48.1x1-	T48.1x2-	T48.1x3-	T48.1x4-	T48.1x5-	T48.1x6-
Neutral insulin injection	T38.3x1-	T38.3x2-	T38.3x3-	T38.3x4-	T38.3x5-	T38.3x6-
Neutral spirits	T51.0x1-	T51.0x2-	T51.0x3-	T51.0x4-	—	—
beverage	T51.0x1-	T51.0x2-	T51.0x3-	T51.0x4-	—	—
Niacin	T46.7x1-	T46.7x2-	T46.7x3-	T46.7x4-	T46.7x5-	T46.7x6-
Niacinamide	T45.2x1-	T45.2x2-	T45.2x3-	T45.2x4-	T45.2x5-	T45.2x6-
Nialamide	T43.1x1-	T43.1x2-	T43.1x3-	T43.1x4-	T43.1x5-	T43.1x6-
Niaprazine	T42.6x1-	T42.6x2-	T42.6x3-	T42.6x4-	T42.6x5-	T42.6x6-
Nicametate	T46.7x1-	T46.7x2-	T46.7x3-	T46.7x4-	T46.7x5-	T46.7x6-
Nicardipine	T46.1x1-	T46.1x2-	T46.1x3-	T46.1x4-	T46.1x5-	T46.1x6-
Nicergoline	T46.7x1-	T46.7x2-	T46.7x3-	T46.7x4-	T46.7x5-	T46.7x6-
Nickel (carbonyl) (tetra-carbonyl) (fumes) (vapor)	T56.891-	T56.892-	T56.893-	T56.894-	—	—
Nickelocene	T56.891-	T56.892-	T56.893-	T56.894-	—	—
Niclosamide	T37.4x1-	T37.4x2-	T37.4x3-	T37.4x4-	T37.4x5-	T37.4x6-
Nicofuranose	T46.7x1-	T46.7x2-	T46.7x3-	T46.7x4-	T46.7x5-	T46.7x6-
Nicomorphine	T40.2x1-	T40.2x2-	T40.2x3-	T40.2x4-	—	—
Nicorandil	T46.3x1-	T46.3x2-	T46.3x3-	T46.3x4-	T46.3x5-	T46.3x6-
Nicotiana (plant)	T62.2x1-	T62.2x2-	T62.2x3-	T62.2x4-	—	—
Nicotinamide	T45.2x1-	T45.2x2-	T45.2x3-	T45.2x4-	T45.2x5-	T45.2x6-
Nicotine (insecticide) (spray) (sulfate) NEC	T60.2x1-	T60.2x2-	T60.2x3-	T60.2x4-	—	—
from tobacco	T65.291-	T65.292-	T65.293-	T65.294-	—	—
cigarettes	T65.221-	T65.222-	T65.223-	T65.224-	—	—
not insecticide	T65.291-	T65.292-	T65.293-	T65.294-	—	—
Nicotinic acid	T46.7x1-	T46.7x2-	T46.7x3-	T46.7x4-	T46.7x5-	T46.7x6-
Nicotinyl alcohol	T46.7x1-	T46.7x2-	T46.7x3-	T46.7x4-	T46.7x5-	T46.7x6-
Nicoumalone	T45.511-	T45.512-	T45.513-	T45.514-	T45.515-	T45.516-
Nifedipine	T46.1x1-	T46.1x2-	T46.1x3-	T46.1x4-	T46.1x5-	T46.1x6-
Nifenazone	T39.2x1-	T39.2x2-	T39.2x3-	T39.2x4-	T39.2x5-	T39.2x6-
Nifuraldezone	T37.91x-	T37.92x-	T37.93x-	T37.94x-	T37.95x-	T37.96x-
Nifuratel	T37.8x1-	T37.8x2-	T37.8x3-	T37.8x4-	T37.8x5-	T37.8x6-
Nifurtimox	T37.3x1-	T37.3x2-	T37.3x3-	T37.3x4-	T37.3x5-	T37.3x6-
Nifurtoinol	T37.8x1-	T37.8x2-	T37.8x3-	T37.8x4-	T37.8x5-	T37.8x6-
Nightshade, deadly (solanum) — see also Belladonna	T62.2x1-	T62.2x2-	T62.2x3-	T62.2x4-	—	—
berry	T62.1x1-	T62.1x2-	T62.1x3-	T62.1x4-	—	—
Nikethamide	T50.7x1-	T50.7x2-	T50.7x3-	T50.7x4-	T50.7x5-	T50.7x6-
Nilstat	T36.7x1-	T36.7x2-	T36.7x3-	T36.7x4-	T36.7x5-	T36.7x6-
topical	T49.0x1-	T49.0x2-	T49.0x3-	T49.0x4-	T49.0x5-	T49.0x6-
Nilutamide	T38.6x1-	T38.6x2-	T38.6x3-	T38.6x4-	T38.6x5-	T38.6x6-
Nimesulide	T39.391-	T39.392-	T39.393-	T39.394-	T39.395-	T39.396-
Nimetazepam	T42.4x1-	T42.4x2-	T42.4x3-	T42.4x4-	T42.4x5-	T42.4x6-
Nimodipine	T46.1x1-	T46.1x2-	T46.1x3-	T46.1x4-	T46.1x5-	T46.1x6-
Nimorazole	T37.3x1-	T37.3x2-	T37.3x3-	T37.3x4-	T37.3x5-	T37.3x6-
Nimustine	T45.1x1-	T45.1x2-	T45.1x3-	T45.1x4-	T45.1x5-	T45.1x6-

Table of Drugs & Chemicals	P O I S O N I N G				Adverse Effect	Underdosing
	Accidental (Unintentional)	Self-Harm (Intentional)	Assault	Undetermined		
Niridazole	T37.4x1-	T37.4x2-	T37.4x3-	T37.4x4-	T37.4x5-	T37.4x6-
Nisentil	T40.2x1-	T40.2x2-	T40.2x3-	T40.2x4-	T40.2x5-	T40.2x6-
Nisoldipine	T46.1x1-	T46.1x2-	T46.1x3-	T46.1x4-	T46.1x5-	T46.1x6-
Nitramine	T65.3x1-	T65.3x2-	T65.3x3-	T65.3x4-	—	—
Nitrate, organic	T46.3x1-	T46.3x2-	T46.3x3-	T46.3x4-	T46.3x5-	T46.3x6-
Nitrazepam	T42.4x1-	T42.4x2-	T42.4x3-	T42.4x4-	T42.4x5-	T42.4x6-
Nitrefazole	T50.6x1-	T50.6x2-	T50.6x3-	T50.6x4-	T50.6x5-	T50.6x6-
Nitrendipine	T46.1x1-	T46.1x2-	T46.1x3-	T46.1x4-	T46.1x5-	T46.1x6-
Nitric						
acid (liquid)	T54.2x1-	T54.2x2-	T54.2x3-	T54.2x4-	—	—
vapor	T59.891-	T59.892-	T59.893-	T59.894-	—	—
oxide (gas)	T59.0x1-	T59.0x2-	T59.0x3-	T59.0x4-	—	—
Nitrimidazine	T37.3x1-	T37.3x2-	T37.3x3-	T37.3x4-	T37.3x5-	T37.3x6-
Nitrite, amyl (medicinal) (vapor)	T46.3x1-	T46.3x2-	T46.3x3-	T46.3x4-	T46.3x5-	T46.3x6-
Nitroaniline	T65.3x1-	T65.3x2-	T65.3x3-	T65.3x4-	—	—
vapor	T59.891-	T59.892-	T59.893-	T59.894-	—	—
Nitrobenzene, nitrobenzol	T65.3x1-	T65.3x2-	T65.3x3-	T65.3x4-	—	—
vapor	T65.3x1-	T65.3x2-	T65.3x3-	T65.3x4-	—	—
Nitrocellulose	T65.891-	T65.892-	T65.893-	T65.894-	—	—
lacquer	T65.891-	T65.892-	T65.893-	T65.894-	—	—
Nitrodiphenyl	T65.3x1-	T65.3x2-	T65.3x3-	T65.3x4-	—	—
Nitrofural	T49.0x1-	T49.0x2-	T49.0x3-	T49.0x4-	T49.0x5-	T49.0x6-
Nitrofurantoin	T37.8x1-	T37.8x2-	T37.8x3-	T37.8x4-	T37.8x5-	T37.8x6-
Nitrofurazone	T49.0x1-	T49.0x2-	T49.0x3-	T49.0x4-	T49.0x5-	T49.0x6-
Nitrogen	T59.0x1-	T59.0x2-	T59.0x3-	T59.0x4-	—	—
mustard	T45.1x1-	T45.1x2-	T45.1x3-	T45.1x4-	T45.1x5-	T45.1x6-
Nitroglycerin, nitro-glycerol (medicinal)	T46.3x1-	T46.3x2-	T46.3x3-	T46.3x4-	T46.3x5-	T46.3x6-
nonmedicinal	T65.5x1-	T65.5x2-	T65.5x3-	T65.5x4-	—	—
fumes	T65.5x1-	T65.5x2-	T65.5x3-	T65.5x4-	—	—
Nitroglycol	T52.3x1-	T52.3x2-	T52.3x3-	T52.3x4-	—	—
Nitrohydrochloric acid	T54.2x1-	T54.2x2-	T54.2x3-	T54.2x4-	—	—
Nitromersol	T49.0x1-	T49.0x2-	T49.0x3-	T49.0x4-	T49.0x5-	T49.0x6-
Nitronaphthalene	T65.891-	T65.892-	T65.893-	T65.894-	—	—
Nitrophenol	T54.0x1-	T54.0x2-	T54.0x3-	T54.0x4-	—	—
Nitropropane	T52.8x1-	T52.8x2-	T52.8x3-	T52.8x4-	—	—
Nitroprusside	T46.5x1-	T46.5x2-	T46.5x3-	T46.5x4-	T46.5x5-	T46.5x6-
Nitrosodimethylamine	T65.3x1-	T65.3x2-	T65.3x3-	T65.3x4-	—	—
Nitrothiazol	T37.4x1-	T37.4x2-	T37.4x3-	T37.4x4-	T37.4x5-	T37.4x6-
Nitrotoluene, nitrotoluol	T65.3x1-	T65.3x2-	T65.3x3-	T65.3x4-	—	—
vapor	T65.3x1-	T65.3x2-	T65.3x3-	T65.3x4-	—	—
Nitrous						
acid (liquid)	T54.2x1-	T54.2x2-	T54.2x3-	T54.2x4-	—	—
fumes	T59.891-	T59.892-	T59.893-	T59.894-	—	—
ether spirit	T46.3x1-	T46.3x2-	T46.3x3-	T46.3x4-	T46.3x5-	T46.3x6-
oxide	T41.0x1-	T41.0x2-	T41.0x3-	T41.0x4-	T41.0x5-	T41.0x6-
Nitroxoline	T37.8x1-	T37.8x2-	T37.8x3-	T37.8x4-	T37.8x5-	T37.8x6-
Nitrozone	T49.0x1-	T49.0x2-	T49.0x3-	T49.0x4-	T49.0x5-	T49.0x6-
Nizatidine	T47.0x1-	T47.0x2-	T47.0x3-	T47.0x4-	T47.0x5-	T47.0x6-
Nizofenone	T43.8x1-	T43.8x2-	T43.8x3-	T43.8x4-	T43.8x5-	T43.8x6-
Noctec	T42.6x1-	T42.6x2-	T42.6x3-	T42.6x4-	T42.6x5-	T42.6x6-
Noludar	T42.6x1-	T42.6x2-	T42.6x3-	T42.6x4-	T42.6x5-	T42.6x6-
Nomegestrol	T38.5x1-	T38.5x2-	T38.5x3-	T38.5x4-	T38.5x5-	T38.5x6-
Nomifensine	T43.291-	T43.292-	T43.293-	T43.294-	T43.295-	T43.296-
Nonoxinol	T49.8x1-	T49.8x2-	T49.8x3-	T49.8x4-	T49.8x5-	T49.8x6-
Nonylphenoxy (polyethoxy-ethanol)	T49.8x1-	T49.8x2-	T49.8x3-	T49.8x4-	T49.8x5-	T49.8x6-
Noptil	T42.3x1-	T42.3x2-	T42.3x3-	T42.3x4-	T42.3x5-	T42.3x6-
Noradrenaline	T44.4x1-	T44.4x2-	T44.4x3-	T44.4x4-	T44.4x5-	T44.4x6-
Noramidopyrine	T39.2x1-	T39.2x2-	T39.2x3-	T39.2x4-	T39.2x5-	T39.2x6-
methanesulfonate sodium	T39.2x1-	T39.2x2-	T39.2x3-	T39.2x4-	T39.2x5-	T39.2x6-

Table of Drugs & Chemicals	POISONING				Adverse Effect	Underdosing
	Accidental (Unintentional)	Self-Harm (Intentional)	Assault	Undetermined		
Norbormide	T60.4x1-	T60.4x2-	T60.4x3-	T60.4x4-	—	—
Nordazepam	T42.4x1-	T42.4x2-	T42.4x3-	T42.4x4-	T42.4x5-	T42.4x6-
Norepinephrine	T44.4x1-	T44.4x2-	T44.4x3-	T44.4x4-	T44.4x5-	T44.4x6-
Norethandrolone	T38.7x1-	T38.7x2-	T38.7x3-	T38.7x4-	T38.7x5-	T38.7x6-
Norethindrone	T38.4x1-	T38.4x2-	T38.4x3-	T38.4x4-	T38.4x5-	T38.4x6-
Norethisterone (acetate) (enantate)	T38.4x1-	T38.4x2-	T38.4x3-	T38.4x4-	T38.4x5-	T38.4x6-
with ethinylestradiol	T38.5x1-	T38.5x2-	T38.5x3-	T38.5x4-	T38.5x5-	T38.5x6-
Noretynodrel	T38.5x1-	T38.5x2-	T38.5x3-	T38.5x4-	T38.5x5-	T38.5x6-
Norfenefrine	T44.4x1-	T44.4x2-	T44.4x3-	T44.4x4-	T44.4x5-	T44.4x6-
Norfloxacin	T36.8x1-	T36.8x2-	T36.8x3-	T36.8x4-	T36.8x5-	T36.8x6-
Norgestrel	T38.4x1-	T38.4x2-	T38.4x3-	T38.4x4-	T38.4x5-	T38.4x6-
Norgestrienone	T38.4x1-	T38.4x2-	T38.4x3-	T38.4x4-	T38.4x5-	T38.4x6-
Norlestrin	T38.4x1-	T38.4x2-	T38.4x3-	T38.4x4-	T38.4x5-	T38.4x6-
Norlutin	T38.4x1-	T38.4x2-	T38.4x3-	T38.4x4-	T38.4x5-	T38.4x6-
Normal serum albumin (human), salt-poor	T45.8x1-	T45.8x2-	T45.8x3-	T45.8x4-	T45.8x5-	T45.8x6-
Normethandrone	T38.5x1-	T38.5x2-	T38.5x3-	T38.5x4-	T38.5x5-	T38.5x6-
Normison — see Benzodiazepines						
Normorphine	T40.2x1-	T40.2x2-	T40.2x3-	T40.2x4-	—	—
Norpseudoephedrine	T50.5x1-	T50.5x2-	T50.5x3-	T50.5x4-	T50.5x5-	T50.5x6-
Nortestosterone (furanpropionate)	T38.7x1-	T38.7x2-	T38.7x3-	T38.7x4-	T38.7x5-	T38.7x6-
Nortriptyline	T43.011-	T43.012-	T43.013-	T43.014-	T43.015-	T43.016-
Noscapine	T48.3x1-	T48.3x2-	T48.3x3-	T48.3x4-	T48.3x5-	T48.3x6-
Nose preparations	T49.6x1-	T49.6x2-	T49.6x3-	T49.6x4-	T49.6x5-	T49.6x6-
Novobiocin	T36.5x1-	T36.5x2-	T36.5x3-	T36.5x4-	T36.5x5-	T36.5x6-
Novocain (infiltration) (topical)	T41.3x1-	T41.3x2-	T41.3x3-	T41.3x4-	T41.3x5-	T41.3x6-
nerve block (peripheral) (plexus)	T41.3x1-	T41.3x2-	T41.3x3-	T41.3x4-	T41.3x5-	T41.3x6-
spinal	T41.3x1-	T41.3x2-	T41.3x3-	T41.3x4-	T41.3x5-	T41.3x6-
Noxious foodstuff	T62.91x-	T62.92x-	T62.93x-	T62.94x-	—	—
specified NEC	T62.8x1-	T62.8x2-	T62.8x3-	T62.8x4-	—	—
Noxiptiline	T43.011-	T43.012-	T43.013-	T43.014-	T43.015-	T43.016-
Noxytiolin	T49.0x1-	T49.0x2-	T49.0x3-	T49.0x4-	T49.0x5-	T49.0x6-
NPH lletin (insulin)	T38.3x1-	T38.3x2-	T38.3x3-	T38.3x4-	T38.3x5-	T38.3x6-
Numorphan	T40.2x1-	T40.2x2-	T40.2x3-	T40.2x4-	T40.2x5-	T40.2x6-
Nunol	T42.3x1-	T42.3x2-	T42.3x3-	T42.3x4-	T42.3x5-	T42.3x6-
Nupercaine (spinal anesthetic)	T41.3x1-	T41.3x2-	T41.3x3-	T41.3x4-	T41.3x5-	T41.3x6-
topical (surface)	T41.3x1-	T41.3x2-	T41.3x3-	T41.3x4-	T41.3x5-	T41.3x6-
Nutmeg oil (liniment)	T49.3x1-	T49.3x2-	T49.3x3-	T49.3x4-	T49.3x5-	T49.3x6-
Nutritional supplement	T50.901-	T50.902-	T50.903-	T50.904-	T50.905-	T50.906-
Nux vomica	T65.1x1-	T65.1x2-	T65.1x3-	T65.1x4-	—	—
Nydrazid	T37.1x1-	T37.1x2-	T37.1x3-	T37.1x4-	T37.1x5-	T37.1x6-
Nylidrin	T46.7x1-	T46.7x2-	T46.7x3-	T46.7x4-	T46.7x5-	T46.7x6-
Nystatin	T36.7x1-	T36.7x2-	T36.7x3-	T36.7x4-	T36.7x5-	T36.7x6-
topical	T49.0x1-	T49.0x2-	T49.0x3-	T49.0x4-	T49.0x5-	T49.0x6-
Nytol	T45.0x1-	T45.0x2-	T45.0x3-	T45.0x4-	T45.0x5-	T45.0x6-
Obidoxime chloride	T50.6x1-	T50.6x2-	T50.6x3-	T50.6x4-	T50.6x5-	T50.6x6-
Octafonium (chloride)	T49.3x1-	T49.3x2-	T49.3x3-	T49.3x4-	T49.3x5-	T49.3x6-
Octamethyl pyrophosphoramide	T60.0x1-	T60.0x2-	T60.0x3-	T60.0x4-	—	—
Octanoin	T50.991-	T50.992-	T50.993-	T50.994-	T50.995-	T50.996-
Octatropine methyl bromide	T44.3x1-	T44.3x2-	T44.3x3-	T44.3x4-	T44.3x5-	T44.3x6-
Octotiamine	T45.2x1-	T45.2x2-	T45.2x3-	T45.2x4-	T45.2x5-	T45.2x6-
Octoxinol (9)	T49.8x1-	T49.8x2-	T49.8x3-	T49.8x4-	T49.8x5-	T49.8x6-
Octreotide	T38.991-	T38.992-	T38.993-	T38.994-	T38.995-	T38.996-
Octyl nitrite	T46.3x1-	T46.3x2-	T46.3x3-	T46.3x4-	T46.3x5-	T46.3x6-
Oestradiol	T38.5x1-	T38.5x2-	T38.5x3-	T38.5x4-	T38.5x5-	T38.5x6-
Oestriol	T38.5x1-	T38.5x2-	T38.5x3-	T38.5x4-	T38.5x5-	T38.5x6-
Oestrogen	T38.5x1-	T38.5x2-	T38.5x3-	T38.5x4-	T38.5x5-	T38.5x6-
Oestrone	T38.5x1-	T38.5x2-	T38.5x3-	T38.5x4-	T38.5x5-	T38.5x6-
Ofloxacin	T36.8x1-	T36.8x2-	T36.8x3-	T36.8x4-	T36.8x5-	T36.8x6-
Oil (of)	T65.891-	T65.892-	T65.893-	T65.894-	—	—
bitter almond	T62.8x1-	T62.8x2-	T62.8x3-	T62.8x4-	—	—
cloves	T49.7x1-	T49.7x2-	T49.7x3-	T49.7x4-	T49.7x5-	T49.7x6-
colors	T65.6x1-	T65.6x2-	T65.6x3-	T65.6x4-	—	—
fumes	T59.891-	T59.892-	T59.893-	T59.894-	—	—
lubricating	T52.0x1-	T52.0x2-	T52.0x3-	T52.0x4-	—	—
Niobe	T52.8x1-	T52.8x2-	T52.8x3-	T52.8x4-	—	—
vitriol (liquid)	T54.2x1-	T54.2x2-	T54.2x3-	T54.2x4-	—	—
fumes	T54.2x1-	T54.2x2-	T54.2x3-	T54.2x4-	—	—
wintergreen (bitter) NEC	T49.3x1-	T49.3x2-	T49.3x3-	T49.3x4-	T49.3x5-	T49.3x6-
Oily preparation (for skin)	T49.3x1-	T49.3x2-	T49.3x3-	T49.3x4-	T49.3x5-	T49.3x6-
Ointment NEC	T49.3x1-	T49.3x2-	T49.3x3-	T49.3x4-	T49.3x5-	T49.3x6-
Olanzapine	T43.591-	T43.592-	T43.593-	T43.594-	T43.595-	T43.596-
Oleander	T62.2x1-	T62.2x2-	T62.2x3-	T62.2x4-	—	—
Oleandomycin	T36.3x1-	T36.3x2-	T36.3x3-	T36.3x4-	T36.3x5-	T36.3x6-
Oleandrin	T46.0x1-	T46.0x2-	T46.0x3-	T46.0x4-	T46.0x5-	T46.0x6-
Oleic acid	T46.6x1-	T46.6x2-	T46.6x3-	T46.6x4-	T46.6x5-	T46.6x6-
Oleovitamin A	T45.2x1-	T45.2x2-	T45.2x3-	T45.2x4-	T45.2x5-	T45.2x6-
Oleum ricini	T47.2x1-	T47.2x2-	T47.2x3-	T47.2x4-	T47.2x5-	T47.2x6-
Olive oil (medicinal) NEC	T47.4x1-	T47.4x2-	T47.4x3-	T47.4x4-	T47.4x5-	T47.4x6-
Olivomycin	T45.1x1-	T45.1x2-	T45.1x3-	T45.1x4-	T45.1x5-	T45.1x6-
Olsalazine	T47.8x1-	T47.8x2-	T47.8x3-	T47.8x4-	T47.8x5-	T47.8x6-
Omeprazole	T47.1x1-	T47.1x2-	T47.1x3-	T47.1x4-	T47.1x5-	T47.1x6-
OMPA	T60.0x1-	T60.0x2-	T60.0x3-	T60.0x4-	—	—
Oncovin	T45.1x1-	T45.1x2-	T45.1x3-	T45.1x4-	T45.1x5-	T45.1x6-
Ondansetron	T45.0x1-	T45.0x2-	T45.0x3-	T45.0x4-	T45.0x5-	T45.0x6-
Ophthaine	T41.3x1-	T41.3x2-	T41.3x3-	T41.3x4-	T41.3x5-	T41.3x6-
Ophthetic	T41.3x1-	T41.3x2-	T41.3x3-	T41.3x4-	T41.3x5-	T41.3x6-
Opiate NEC	T40.601-	T40.602-	T40.603-	T40.604-	T40.605-	T40.606-
antagonists	T50.7x1-	T50.7x2-	T50.7x3-	T50.7x4-	T50.7x5-	T50.7x6-
Opioid NEC	T40.2x1-	T40.2x2-	T40.2x3-	T40.2x4-	T40.2x5-	T40.2x6-
Opipramol	T43.011-	T43.012-	T43.013-	T43.014-	T43.015-	T43.016-
Opium alkaloids (total)	T40.0x1-	T40.0x2-	T40.0x3-	T40.0x4-	T40.0x5-	T40.0x6-
standardized powdered	T40.0x1-	T40.0x2-	T40.0x3-	T40.0x4-	T40.0x5-	T40.0x6-
tincture (camphorated)	T40.0x1-	T40.0x2-	T40.0x3-	T40.0x4-	T40.0x5-	T40.0x6-
Oracon	T38.4x1-	T38.4x2-	T38.4x3-	T38.4x4-	T38.4x5-	T38.4x6-
Oragrafin	T50.8x1-	T50.8x2-	T50.8x3-	T50.8x4-	T50.8x5-	T50.8x6-
Oral contraceptives	T38.4x1-	T38.4x2-	T38.4x3-	T38.4x4-	T38.4x5-	T38.4x6-
Oral rehydration salts	T50.3x1-	T50.3x2-	T50.3x3-	T50.3x4-	T50.3x5-	T50.3x6-
Orazamide	T50.991-	T50.992-	T50.993-	T50.994-	T50.995-	T50.996-
Orciprenaline	T48.291-	T48.292-	T48.293-	T48.294-	T48.295-	T48.296-
Organidin	T48.4x1-	T48.4x2-	T48.4x3-	T48.4x4-	T48.4x5-	T48.4x6-
Organonitrate NEC	T46.3x1-	T46.3x2-	T46.3x3-	T46.3x4-	T46.3x5-	T46.3x6-
Organophosphates	T60.0x1-	T60.0x2-	T60.0x3-	T60.0x4-	—	—
Orimune	T50.B91-	T50.B92-	T50.B93-	T50.B94-	T50.B95-	T50.B96-
Orinase	T38.3x1-	T38.3x2-	T38.3x3-	T38.3x4-	T38.3x5-	T38.3x6-
Ormeloxifene	T38.6x1-	T38.6x2-	T38.6x3-	T38.6x4-	T38.6x5-	T38.6x6-
Ornidazole	T37.3x1-	T37.3x2-	T37.3x3-	T37.3x4-	T37.3x5-	T37.3x6-
Ornithine aspartate	T50.991-	T50.992-	T50.993-	T50.994-	T50.995-	T50.996-
Ornoprostil	T47.1x1-	T47.1x2-	T47.1x3-	T47.1x4-	T47.1x5-	T47.1x6-
Orphenadrine (hydrochloride)	T42.8x1-	T42.8x2-	T42.8x3-	T42.8x4-	T42.8x5-	T42.8x6-
Ortal (sodium)	T42.3x1-	T42.3x2-	T42.3x3-	T42.3x4-	T42.3x5-	T42.3x6-
Orthoboric acid	T49.0x1-	T49.0x2-	T49.0x3-	T49.0x4-	T49.0x5-	T49.0x6-
ENT agent	T49.6x1-	T49.6x2-	T49.6x3-	T49.6x4-	T49.6x5-	T49.6x6-
ophthalmic preparation	T49.5x1-	T49.5x2-	T49.5x3-	T49.5x4-	T49.5x5-	T49.5x6-
Orthocaine	T41.3x1-	T41.3x2-	T41.3x3-	T41.3x4-	T41.3x5-	T41.3x6-
Orthodichlorobenzene	T53.7x1-	T53.7x2-	T53.7x3-	T53.7x4-	—	—

DRUGS & CHEMICALS

Table of Drugs & Chemicals	POISONING Accidental (Unintentional)	Self-Harm (Intentional)	Assault	Undetermined	Adverse Effect	Underdosing
Ortho-Novum	T38.4x1-	T38.4x2-	T38.4x3-	T38.4x4-	T38.4x5-	T38.4x6-
Orthotolidine (reagent)	T54.2x1-	T54.2x2-	T54.2x3-	T54.2x4-	—	—
Osmic acid (liquid)	T54.2x1-	T54.2x2-	T54.2x3-	T54.2x4-	—	—
fumes	T54.2x1-	T54.2x2-	T54.2x3-	T54.2x4-	—	—
Osmotic diuretics	T50.2x1-	T50.2x2-	T50.2x3-	T50.2x4-	T50.2x5-	T50.2x6-
Otilonium bromide	T44.3x1-	T44.3x2-	T44.3x3-	T44.3x4-	T44.3x5-	T44.3x6-
Otorhinolaryngological drug NEC	T49.6x1-	T49.6x2-	T49.6x3-	T49.6x4-	T49.6x5-	T49.6x6-
Ouabain(e)	T46.0x1-	T46.0x2-	T46.0x3-	T46.0x4-	T46.0x5-	T46.0x6-
Ovarian hormone	T38.5x1-	T38.5x2-	T38.5x3-	T38.5x4-	T38.5x5-	T38.5x6-
stimulant	T38.5x1-	T38.5x2-	T38.5x3-	T38.5x4-	T38.5x5-	T38.5x6-
Ovral	T38.4x1-	T38.4x2-	T38.4x3-	T38.4x4-	T38.4x5-	T38.4x6-
Ovulen	T38.4x1-	T38.4x2-	T38.4x3-	T38.4x4-	T38.4x5-	T38.4x6-
Ox bile extract	T47.5x1-	T47.5x2-	T47.5x3-	T47.5x4-	T47.5x5-	T47.5x6-
Oxacillin	T36.0x1-	T36.0x2-	T36.0x3-	T36.0x4-	T36.0x5-	T36.0x6-
Oxalic acid	T54.2x1-	T54.2x2-	T54.2x3-	T54.2x4-	—	—
ammonium salt	T50.991-	T50.992-	T50.993-	T50.994-	T50.995-	T50.996-
Oxamniquine	T37.4x1-	T37.4x2-	T37.4x3-	T37.4x4-	T37.4x5-	T37.4x6-
Oxanamide	T43.591-	T43.592-	T43.593-	T43.594-	T43.595-	T43.596-
Oxandrolone	T38.7x1-	T38.7x2-	T38.7x3-	T38.7x4-	T38.7x5-	T38.7x6-
Oxantel	T37.4x1-	T37.4x2-	T37.4x3-	T37.4x4-	T37.4x5-	T37.4x6-
Oxapium iodide	T44.3x1-	T44.3x2-	T44.3x3-	T44.3x4-	T44.3x5-	T44.3x6-
Oxaprotiline	T43.021-	T43.022-	T43.023-	T43.024-	T43.025-	T43.026-
Oxaprozin	T39.311-	T39.312-	T39.313-	T39.314-	T39.315-	T39.316-
Oxatomide	T45.0x1-	T45.0x2-	T45.0x3-	T45.0x4-	T45.0x5-	T45.0x6-
Oxazepam	T42.4x1-	T42.4x2-	T42.4x3-	T42.4x4-	T42.4x5-	T42.4x6-
Oxazimedrine	T50.5x1-	T50.5x2-	T50.5x3-	T50.5x4-	T50.5x5-	T50.5x6-
Oxazolam	T42.4x1-	T42.4x2-	T42.4x3-	T42.4x4-	T42.4x5-	T42.4x6-
Oxazolidine derivatives	T42.2x1-	T42.2x2-	T42.2x3-	T42.2x4-	T42.2x5-	T42.2x6-
Oxazolidinedione (derivative)	T42.2x1-	T42.2x2-	T42.2x3-	T42.2x4-	T42.2x5-	T42.2x6-
Oxcarbazepine	T42.1x1-	T42.1x2-	T42.1x3-	T42.1x4-	T42.1x5-	T42.1x6-
Oxedrine	T44.4x1-	T44.4x2-	T44.4x3-	T44.4x4-	T44.4x5-	T44.4x6-
Oxeladin (citrate)	T48.3x1-	T48.3x2-	T48.3x3-	T48.3x4-	T48.3x5-	T48.3x6-
Oxendolone	T38.5x1-	T38.5x2-	T38.5x3-	T38.5x4-	T38.5x5-	T38.5x6-
Oxetacaine	T41.3x1-	T41.3x2-	T41.3x3-	T41.3x4-	T41.3x5-	T41.3x6-
Oxethazine	T41.3x1-	T41.3x2-	T41.3x3-	T41.3x4-	T41.3x5-	T41.3x6-
Oxetorone	T39.8x1-	T39.8x2-	T39.8x3-	T39.8x4-	T39.8x5-	T39.8x6-
Oxiconazole	T49.0x1-	T49.0x2-	T49.0x3-	T49.0x4-	T49.0x5-	T49.0x6-
Oxidizing agent NEC	T54.91x-	T54.92x-	T54.93x-	T54.94x-	—	—
Oxipurinol	T50.4x1-	T50.4x2-	T50.4x3-	T50.4x4-	T50.4x5-	T50.4x6-
Oxitriptan	T43.291-	T43.292-	T43.293-	T43.294-	T43.295-	T43.296-
Oxitropium bromide	T48.6x1-	T48.6x2-	T48.6x3-	T48.6x4-	T48.6x5-	T48.6x6-
Oxodipine	T46.1x1-	T46.1x2-	T46.1x3-	T46.1x4-	T46.1x5-	T46.1x6-
Oxolamine	T48.3x1-	T48.3x2-	T48.3x3-	T48.3x4-	T48.3x5-	T48.3x6-
Oxolinic acid	T37.8x1-	T37.8x2-	T37.8x3-	T37.8x4-	T37.8x5-	T37.8x6-
Oxomemazine	T43.3x1-	T43.3x2-	T43.3x3-	T43.3x4-	T43.3x5-	T43.3x6-
Oxophenarsine	T37.3x1-	T37.3x2-	T37.3x3-	T37.3x4-	T37.3x5-	T37.3x6-
Oxprenolol	T44.7x1-	T44.7x2-	T44.7x3-	T44.7x4-	T44.7x5-	T44.7x6-
Oxsoralen	T49.3x1-	T49.3x2-	T49.3x3-	T49.3x4-	T49.3x5-	T49.3x6-
Oxtriphylline	T48.6x1-	T48.6x2-	T48.6x3-	T48.6x4-	T48.6x5-	T48.6x6-
Oxybate sodium	T41.291-	T41.292-	T41.293-	T41.294-	T41.295-	T41.296-
Oxybuprocaine	T41.3x1-	T41.3x2-	T41.3x3-	T41.3x4-	T41.3x5-	T41.3x6-
Oxybutynin	T44.3x1-	T44.3x2-	T44.3x3-	T44.3x4-	T44.3x5-	T44.3x6-
Oxychlorosene	T49.0x1-	T49.0x2-	T49.0x3-	T49.0x4-	T49.0x5-	T49.0x6-
Oxycodone	T40.2x1-	T40.2x2-	T40.2x3-	T40.2x4-	T40.2x5-	T40.2x6-
Oxyfedrine	T46.3x1-	T46.3x2-	T46.3x3-	T46.3x4-	T46.3x5-	T46.3x6-
Oxygen	T41.5x1-	T41.5x2-	T41.5x3-	T41.5x4-	T41.5x5-	T41.5x6-
Oxylone	T49.0x1-	T49.0x2-	T49.0x3-	T49.0x4-	T49.0x5-	T49.0x6-
ophthalmic preparation	T49.5x1-	T49.5x2-	T49.5x3-	T49.5x4-	T49.5x5-	T49.5x6-
Oxymesterone	T38.7x1-	T38.7x2-	T38.7x3-	T38.7x4-	T38.7x5-	T38.7x6-
Oxymetazoline	T48.5x1-	T48.5x2-	T48.5x3-	T48.5x4-	T48.5x5-	T48.5x6-
Oxymetholone	T38.7x1-	T38.7x2-	T38.7x3-	T38.7x4-	T38.7x5-	T38.7x6-
Oxymorphone	T40.2x1-	T40.2x2-	T40.2x3-	T40.2x4-	T40.2x5-	T40.2x6-
Oxypertine	T43.591-	T43.592-	T43.593-	T43.594-	T43.595-	T43.596-
Oxyphenbutazone	T39.2x1-	T39.2x2-	T39.2x3-	T39.2x4-	T39.2x5-	T39.2x6-
Oxyphencyclimine	T44.3x1-	T44.3x2-	T44.3x3-	T44.3x4-	T44.3x5-	T44.3x6-
Oxyphenisatine	T47.2x1-	T47.2x2-	T47.2x3-	T47.2x4-	T47.2x5-	T47.2x6-
Oxyphenonium bromide	T44.3x1-	T44.3x2-	T44.3x3-	T44.3x4-	T44.3x5-	T44.3x6-
Oxypolygelatin	T45.8x1-	T45.8x2-	T45.8x3-	T45.8x4-	T45.8x5-	T45.8x6-
Oxyquinoline (derivatives)	T37.8x1-	T37.8x2-	T37.8x3-	T37.8x4-	T37.8x5-	T37.8x6-
Oxytetracycline	T36.4x1-	T36.4x2-	T36.4x3-	T36.4x4-	T36.4x5-	T36.4x6-
Oxytocic drug NEC	T48.0x1-	T48.0x2-	T48.0x3-	T48.0x4-	T48.0x5-	T48.0x6-
Oxytocin (synthetic)	T48.0x1-	T48.0x2-	T48.0x3-	T48.0x4-	T48.0x5-	T48.0x6-
Ozone	T59.891-	T59.892-	T59.893-	T59.894-	—	—
PABA	T49.3x1-	T49.3x2-	T49.3x3-	T49.3x4-	T49.3x5-	T49.3x6-
Packed red cells	T45.8x1-	T45.8x2-	T45.8x3-	T45.8x4-	T45.8x5-	T45.8x6-
Padimate	T49.3x1-	T49.3x2-	T49.3x3-	T49.3x4-	T49.3x5-	T49.3x6-
Paint NEC	T65.6x1-	T65.6x2-	T65.6x3-	T65.6x4-	—	—
cleaner	T52.91x-	T52.92x-	T52.93x-	T52.94x-	—	—
fumes NEC	T59.891-	T59.892-	T59.893-	T59.894-	—	—
lead (fumes)	T56.0x1-	T56.0x2-	T56.0x3-	T56.0x4-	—	—
solvent NEC	T52.8x1-	T52.8x2-	T52.8x3-	T52.8x4-	—	—
stripper	T52.8x1-	T52.8x2-	T52.8x3-	T52.8x4-	—	—
Palfium	T40.2x1-	T40.2x2-	T40.2x3-	T40.2x4-	—	—
Palm kernel oil	T50.991-	T50.992-	T50.993-	T50.994-	T50.995-	T50.996-
Paludrine	T37.2x1-	T37.2x2-	T37.2x3-	T37.2x4-	T37.2x5-	T37.2x6-
PAM (pralidoxime)	T50.6x1-	T50.6x2-	T50.6x3-	T50.6x4-	T50.6x5-	T50.6x6-
Pamaquine (naphthoute)	T37.2x1-	T37.2x2-	T37.2x3-	T37.2x4-	T37.2x5-	T37.2x6-
Panadol	T39.1x1-	T39.1x2-	T39.1x3-	T39.1x4-	T39.1x5-	T39.1x6-
Pancreatic digestive secretion stimulant	T47.8x1-	T47.8x2-	T47.8x3-	T47.8x4-	T47.8x5-	T47.8x6-
dornase	T45.3x1-	T45.3x2-	T45.3x3-	T45.3x4-	T45.3x5-	T45.3x6-
Pancreatin	T47.5x1-	T47.5x2-	T47.5x3-	T47.5x4-	T47.5x5-	T47.5x6-
Pancrelipase	T47.5x1-	T47.5x2-	T47.5x3-	T47.5x4-	T47.5x5-	T47.5x6-
Pancuronium (bromide)	T48.1x1-	T48.1x2-	T48.1x3-	T48.1x4-	T48.1x5-	T48.1x6-
Pangamic acid	T45.2x1-	T45.2x2-	T45.2x3-	T45.2x4-	T45.2x5-	T45.2x6-
Panthenol	T45.2x1-	T45.2x2-	T45.2x3-	T45.2x4-	T45.2x5-	T45.2x6-
topical	T49.8x1-	T49.8x2-	T49.8x3-	T49.8x4-	T49.8x5-	T49.8x6-
Pantopon	T40.0x1-	T40.0x2-	T40.0x3-	T40.0x4-	T40.0x5-	T40.0x6-
Pantothenic acid	T45.2x1-	T45.2x2-	T45.2x3-	T45.2x4-	T45.2x5-	T45.2x6-
Panwarfin	T45.511-	T45.512-	T45.513-	T45.514-	T45.515-	T45.516-
Papain	T47.5x1-	T47.5x2-	T47.5x3-	T47.5x4-	T47.5x5-	T47.5x6-
digestant	T47.5x1-	T47.5x2-	T47.5x3-	T47.5x4-	T47.5x5-	T47.5x6-
Papaveretum	T40.0x1-	T40.0x2-	T40.0x3-	T40.0x4-	T40.0x5-	T40.0x6-
Papaverine	T44.3x1-	T44.3x2-	T44.3x3-	T44.3x4-	T44.3x5-	T44.3x6-
Para-acetamidophenol	T39.1x1-	T39.1x2-	T39.1x3-	T39.1x4-	T39.1x5-	T39.1x6-
Para-aminobenzoic acid	T49.3x1-	T49.3x2-	T49.3x3-	T49.3x4-	T49.3x5-	T49.3x6-
Para-aminophenol derivatives	T39.1x1-	T39.1x2-	T39.1x3-	T39.1x4-	T39.1x5-	T39.1x6-
Para-aminosalicylic acid	T37.1x1-	T37.1x2-	T37.1x3-	T37.1x4-	T37.1x5-	T37.1x6-
Paracetaldehyde	T42.6x1-	T42.6x2-	T42.6x3-	T42.6x4-	T42.6x5-	T42.6x6-
Paracetamol	T39.1x1-	T39.1x2-	T39.1x3-	T39.1x4-	T39.1x5-	T39.1x6-
Parachlorophenol (camphorated)	T49.0x1-	T49.0x2-	T49.0x3-	T49.0x4-	T49.0x5-	T49.0x6-
Paracodin	T40.2x1-	T40.2x2-	T40.2x3-	T40.2x4-	T40.2x5-	T40.2x6-
Paradione	T42.2x1-	T42.2x2-	T42.2x3-	T42.2x4-	T42.2x5-	T42.2x6-
Paraffin(s) (wax)	T52.0x1-	T52.0x2-	T52.0x3-	T52.0x4-	—	—
liquid (medicinal)	T47.4x1-	T47.4x2-	T47.4x3-	T47.4x4-	T47.4x5-	T47.4x6-
nonmedicinal	T52.0x1-	T52.0x2-	T52.0x3-	T52.0x4-	—	—

Table of Drugs & Chemicals	Poisoning, Accidental (Unintentional)	Poisoning, Self-Harm (Intentional)	Poisoning, Assault	Poisoning, Undetermined	Adverse Effect	Underdosing
Paraformaldehyde	T60.3x1-	T60.3x2-	T60.3x3-	T60.3x4-	—	—
Paraldehyde	T42.6x1-	T42.6x2-	T42.6x3-	T42.6x4-	T42.6x5-	T42.6x6-
Paramethadione	T42.2x1-	T42.2x2-	T42.2x3-	T42.2x4-	T42.2x5-	T42.2x6-
Paramethasone	T38.0x1-	T38.0x2-	T38.0x3-	T38.0x4-	T38.0x5-	T38.0x6-
acetate	T49.0x1-	T49.0x2-	T49.0x3-	T49.0x4-	T49.0x5-	T49.0x6-
Paraoxon	T60.0x1-	T60.0x2-	T60.0x3-	T60.0x4-	—	—
Paraquat	T60.3x1-	T60.3x2-	T60.3x3-	T60.3x4-	—	—
Parasympatholytic NEC	T44.3x1-	T44.3x2-	T44.3x3-	T44.3x4-	T44.3x5-	T44.3x6-
Parasympathomimetic drug NEC	T44.1x1-	T44.1x2-	T44.1x3-	T44.1x4-	T44.1x5-	T44.1x6-
Parathion	T60.0x1-	T60.0x2-	T60.0x3-	T60.0x4-	—	—
Parathormone	T50.991-	T50.992-	T50.993-	T50.994-	T50.995-	T50.996-
Parathyroid extract	T50.991-	T50.992-	T50.993-	T50.994-	T50.995-	T50.996-
Paratyphoid vaccine	T50.A91-	T50.A92-	T50.A93-	T50.A94-	T50.A95-	T50.A96-
Paredrine	T44.4x1-	T44.4x2-	T44.4x3-	T44.4x4-	T44.4x5-	T44.4x6-
Paregoric	T40.0x1-	T40.0x2-	T40.0x3-	T40.0x4-	T40.0x5-	T40.0x6-
Pargyline	T46.5x1-	T46.5x2-	T46.5x3-	T46.5x4-	T46.5x5-	T46.5x6-
Paris green	T57.0x1-	T57.0x2-	T57.0x3-	T57.0x4-	—	—
insecticide	T57.0x1-	T57.0x2-	T57.0x3-	T57.0x4-		
Parnate	T43.1x1-	T43.1x2-	T43.1x3-	T43.1x4-	T43.1x5-	T43.1x6-
Paromomycin	T36.5x1-	T36.5x2-	T36.5x3-	T36.5x4-	T36.5x5-	T36.5x6-
Paroxypropione	T45.1x1-	T45.1x2-	T45.1x3-	T45.1x4-	T45.1x5-	T45.1x6-
Parzone	T40.2x1-	T40.2x2-	T40.2x3-	T40.2x4-	T40.2x5-	T40.2x6-
PAS	T37.1x1-	T37.1x2-	T37.1x3-	T37.1x4-	T37.1x5-	T37.1x6-
Pasiniazid	T37.1x1-	T37.1x2-	T37.1x3-	T37.1x4	T37.1x5-	T37.1x6-
PBB (polybrominated biphenyls)	T65.891-	T65.892-	T65.893-	T65.894-	—	—
PCB	T65.891-	T65.892-	T65.893-	T65.894-	—	—
PCP						
meaning pentachlorophenol	T60.1x1-	T60.1x2-	T60.1x3-	T60.1x4-	—	—
fungicide	T60.3x1-	T60.3x2-	T60.3x3-	T60.3x4-	—	—
herbicide	T60.3x1-	T60.3x2-	T60.3x3-	T60.3x4-	—	—
insecticide	T60.1x1-	T60.1x2-	T60.1x3-	T60.1x4-	—	—
meaning phencyclidine	T40.991-	T40.992-	T40.993-	T40.994-	—	—
Peach kernel oil (emulsion)	T47.4x1-	T47.4x2-	T47.4x3-	T47.4x4-	T47.4x5-	T47.4x6-
Peanut oil (emulsion) NEC	T47.4x1-	T47.4x2-	T47.4x3-	T47.4x4-	T47.4x5-	T47.4x6-
topical	T49.3x1-	T49.3x2-	T49.3x3-	T49.3x4-	T49.3x5-	T49.3x6-
Pearly Gates (morning glory seeds)	T40.991-	T40.992-	T40.993-	T40.994-		—
Pecazine	T43.3x1-	T43.3x2-	T43.3x3-	T43.3x4-	T43.3x5-	T43.3x6-
Pectin	T47.6x1-	T47.6x2-	T47.6x3-	T47.6x4-	T47.6x5-	T47.6x6-
Pefloxacin	T37.8x1-	T37.8x2-	T37.8x3-	T37.8x4-	T37.8x5-	T37.8x6-
Pegademase, bovine	T50.Z91-	T50.Z92-	T50.Z93-	T50.Z94-	T50.Z95-	T50.Z96-
Pelletierine tannate	T37.4x1-	T37.4x2-	T37.4x3-	T37.4x4-	T37.4x5-	T37.4x6-
Pemirolast (potassium)	T48.6x1-	T48.6x2-	T48.6x3-	T48.6x4-	T48.6x5-	T48.6x6-
Pemoline	T50.7x1-	T50.7x2-	T50.7x3-	T50.7x4-	T50.7x5-	T50.7x6-
Pempidine	T44.2x1-	T44.2x2-	T44.2x3-	T44.2x4-	T44.2x5-	T44.2x6-
Penamecillin	T36.0x1-	T36.0x2-	T36.0x3-	T36.0x4-	T36.0x5-	T36.0x6-
Penbutolol	T44.7x1-	T44.7x2-	T44.7x3-	T44.7x4-	T44.7x5-	T44.7x6-
Penethamate	T36.0x1-	T36.0x2-	T36.0x3-	T36.0x4-	T36.0x5-	T36.0x6-
Penfluridol	T43.591-	T43.592-	T43.593-	T43.594-	T43.595-	T43.596-
Penflutizide	T50.2x1-	T50.2x2-	T50.2x3-	T50.2x4-	T50.2x5-	T50.2x6-
Pengitoxin	T46.0x1-	T46.0x2-	T46.0x3-	T46.0x4-	T46.0x5-	T46.0x6-
Penicillamine	T50.6x1-	T50.6x2-	T50.6x3-	T50.6x4-	T50.6x5-	T50.6x6-
Penicillin (any)	T36.0x1-	T36.0x2-	T36.0x3-	T36.0x4-	T36.0x5-	T36.0x6-
Penicillinase	T45.3x1-	T45.3x2-	T45.3x3-	T45.3x4-	T45.3x5-	T45.3x6-
Penicilloyl polylysine	T50.8x1-	T50.8x2-	T50.8x3-	T50.8x4-	T50.8x5-	T50.8x6-
Penimepicycline	T36.4x1-	T36.4x2-	T36.4x3-	T36.4x4-	T36.4x5-	T36.4x6-
Pentachloroethane	T53.6x1-	T53.6x2-	T53.6x3-	T53.6x4-	—	—
Pentachloronaphthalene	T53.7x1-	T53.7x2-	T53.7x3-	T53.7x4-	—	—
Pentachlorophenol (pesticide)	T60.1x1-	T60.1x2-	T60.1x3-	T60.1x4-	—	—
fungicide	T60.3x1-	T60.3x2-	T60.3x3-	T60.3x4-	—	—
herbicide	T60.3x1-	T60.3x2-	T60.3x3-	T60.3x4-	—	—
insecticide	T60.1x1-	T60.1x2-	T60.1x3-	T60.1x4-	—	—
Pentaerythritol	T46.3x1-	T46.3x2-	T46.3x3-	T46.3x4-	T46.3x5-	T46.3x6-
chloral	T42.6x1-	T42.6x2-	T42.6x3-	T42.6x4-	T42.6x5-	T42.6x6-
tetranitrate NEC	T46.3x1-	T46.3x2-	T46.3x3-	T46.3x4-	T46.3x5-	T46.3x6-
Pentaerythrityl tetranitrate	T46.3x1-	T46.3x2-	T46.3x3-	T46.3x4-	T46.3x5-	T46.3x6-
Pentagastrin	T50.8x1-	T50.8x2-	T50.8x3-	T50.8x4-	T50.8x5-	T50.8x6-
Pentalin	T53.6x1-	T53.6x2-	T53.6x3-	T53.6x4-	—	—
Pentamethonium bromide	T44.2x1-	T44.2x2-	T44.2x3-	T44.2x4-	T44.2x5-	T44.2x6-
Pentamidine	T37.3x1-	T37.3x2-	T37.3x3-	T37.3x4-	T37.3x5-	T37.3x6-
Pentanol	T51.3x1-	T51.3x2-	T51.3x3-	T51.3x4-	—	—
Pentapyrrolinium (bitartrate)	T44.2x1-	T44.2x2-	T44.2x3-	T44.2x4-	T44.2x5-	T44.2x6-
Pentaquine	T37.2x1-	T37.2x2-	T37.2x3-	T37.2x4-	T37.2x5-	T37.2x6-
Pentazocine	T40.4x1-	T40.4x2-	T40.4x3-	T40.4x4-	T40.4x5-	T40.4x6-
Pentetrazole	T50.7x1-	T50.7x2-	T50.7x3-	T50.7x4-	T50.7x5-	T50.7x6-
Penthienate bromide	T44.3x1-	T44.3x2-	T44.3x3-	T44.3x4-	T44.3x5-	T44.3x6-
Pentifylline	T46.7x1-	T46.7x2-	T46.7x3-	T46.7x4-	T46.7x5-	T46.7x6-
Pentobarbital	T42.3x1-	T42.3x2-	T42.3x3-	T42.3x4-	T42.3x5-	T42.3x6-
sodium	T42.3x1-	T42.3x2-	T42.3x3-	T42.3x4-	T42.3x5-	T42.3x6-
Pentobarbitone	T42.3x1-	T42.3x2-	T42.3x3-	T42.3x4-	T42.3x5-	T42.3x6-
Pentolonium tartrate	T44.2x1-	T44.2x2-	T44.2x3-	T44.2x4-	T44.2x5-	T44.2x6-
Pentosan polysulfate (sodium)	T39.8x1-	T39.8x2-	T39.8x3-	T39.8x4-	T39.8x5-	T39.8x6-
Pentostatin	T45.1x1-	T45.1x2-	T45.1x3-	T45.1x4-	T45.1x5-	T45.1x6-
Pentothal	T41.1x1-	T41.1x2-	T41.1x3-	T41.1x4-	T41.1x5-	T41.1x6-
Pentoxifylline	T46.7x1-	T46.7x2-	T46.7x3-	T46.7x4-	T46.7x5-	T46.7x6-
Pentoxyverine	T48.3x1-	T48.3x2-	T48.3x3-	T48.3x4-	T48.3x5-	T48.3x6-
Pentrinat	T46.3x1-	T46.3x2-	T46.3x3-	T46.3x4-	T46.3x5-	T46.3x6-
Pentylenetetrazole	T50.7x1-	T50.7x2-	T50.7x3-	T50.7x4-	T50.7x5-	T50.7x6-
Pentylsalicylamide	T37.1x1-	T37.1x2-	T37.1x3-	T37.1x4-	T37.1x5-	T37.1x6-
Pentymal	T42.3x1-	T42.3x2-	T42.3x3-	T42.3x4-	T42.3x5-	T42.3x6-
Peplomycin	T45.1x1-	T45.1x2-	T45.1x3-	T45.1x4-	T45.1x5-	T45.1x6-
Peppermint (oil)	T47.5x1-	T47.5x2-	T47.5x3-	T47.5x4-	T47.5x5-	T47.5x6-
Pepsin	T47.5x1-	T47.5x2-	T47.5x3-	T47.5x4-	T47.5x5-	T47.5x6-
digestant	T47.5x1-	T47.5x2-	T47.5x3-	T47.5x4-	T47.5x5-	T47.5x6-
Pepstatin	T47.1x1-	T47.1x2-	T47.1x3-	T47.1x4-	T47.1x5-	T47.1x6-
Peptavlon	T50.8x1-	T50.8x2-	T50.8x3-	T50.8x4-	T50.8x5-	T50.8x6-
Perazine	T43.3x1-	T43.3x2-	T43.3x3-	T43.3x4-	T43.3x5-	T43.3x6-
Percaine (spinal)	T41.3x1-	T41.3x2-	T41.3x3-	T41.3x4-	T41.3x5-	T41.3x6-
topical (surface)	T41.3x1-	T41.3x2-	T41.3x3-	T41.3x4-	T41.3x5-	T41.3x6-
Perchloroethylene	T53.3x1-	T53.3x2-	T53.3x3-	T53.3x4-	—	—
vapor	T53.3x1-	T53.3x2-	T53.3x3-	T53.3x4-	—	—
medicinal	T37.4x1-	T37.4x2-	T37.4x3-	T37.4x4-	T37.4x5-	T37.4x6-
Percodan	T40.2x1-	T40.2x2-	T40.2x3-	T40.2x4-	T40.2x5-	T40.2x6-
Percogesic — see also Acetaminophen	T45.0x1-	T45.0x2-	T45.0x3-	T45.0x4-	T45.0x5-	T45.0x6-
Percorten	T38.0x1-	T38.0x2-	T38.0x3-	T38.0x4-	T38.0x5-	T38.0x6-
Pergolide	T42.8x1-	T42.8x2-	T42.8x3-	T42.8x4-	T42.8x5-	T42.8x6-
Pergonal	T38.811-	T38.812-	T38.813-	T38.814-	T38.815-	T38.816-
Perhexilene	T46.3x1-	T46.3x2-	T46.3x3-	T46.3x4-	T46.3x5-	T46.3x6-
Perhexiline (maleate)	T46.3x1-	T46.3x2-	T46.3x3-	T46.3x4-	T46.3x5-	T46.3x6-
Periactin	T45.0x1-	T45.0x2-	T45.0x3-	T45.0x4-	T45.0x5-	T45.0x6-
Periciazine	T43.3x1-	T43.3x2-	T43.3x3-	T43.3x4-	T43.3x5-	T43.3x6-
Periclor	T42.6x1-	T42.6x2-	T42.6x3-	T42.6x4-	T42.6x5-	T42.6x6-
Perindopril	T46.4x1-	T46.4x2-	T46.4x3-	T46.4x4-	T46.4x5-	T46.4x6-
Perisoxal	T39.8x1-	T39.8x2-	T39.8x3-	T39.8x4-	T39.8x5-	T39.8x6-

DRUGS & CHEMICALS

Table of Drugs & Chemicals	POISONING Accidental (Unintentional)	Self-Harm (Intentional)	Assault	Undetermined	Adverse Effect	Underdosing
Peritoneal dialysis solution	T50.3x1-	T50.3x2-	T50.3x3-	T50.3x4-	T50.3x5-	T50.3x6-
Peritrate	T46.3x1-	T46.3x2-	T46.3x3-	T46.3x4-	T46.3x5-	T46.3x6-
Perlapine	T42.4x1-	T42.4x2-	T42.4x3-	T42.4x4-	T42.4x5-	T42.4x6-
Permanganate	T65.891-	T65.892-	T65.893-	T65.894-	—	—
Permethrin	T60.1x1-	T60.1x2-	T60.1x3-	T60.1x4-	—	—
Pernocton	T42.3x1-	T42.3x2-	T42.3x3-	T42.3x4-	T42.3x5-	T42.3x6-
Pernoston	T42.3x1-	T42.3x2-	T42.3x3-	T42.3x4-	T42.3x5-	T42.3x6-
Peronine	T40.2x1-	T40.2x2-	T40.2x3-	T40.2x4-	—	—
Perphenazine	T43.3x1-	T43.3x2-	T43.3x3-	T43.3x4-	T43.3x5-	T43.3x6-
Pertofrane	T43.011-	T43.012-	T43.013-	T43.014-	T43.015-	T43.016-
Pertussis immune serum (human)	T50.Z11-	T50.Z12-	T50.Z13-	T50.Z14-	T50.Z15-	T50.Z16-
vaccine (with diphtheria toxoid) (with tetanus toxoid)	T50.A11-	T50.A12-	T50.A13-	T50.A14-	T50.A15-	T50.A16-
Peruvian balsam	T49.0x1-	T49.0x2-	T49.0x3-	T49.0x4-	T49.0x5-	T49.0x6-
Peruvoside	T46.0x1-	T46.0x2-	T46.0x3-	T46.0x4-	T46.0x5-	T46.0x6-
Pesticide (dust) (fumes) (vapor) NEC	T60.91x-	T60.92x-	T60.93x-	T60.94x-	—	—
arsenic	T57.0x1-	T57.0x2-	T57.0x3-	T57.0x4-	—	—
chlorinated	T60.1x1-	T60.1x2-	T60.1x3-	T60.1x4-	—	—
cyanide	T65.0x1-	T65.0x2-	T65.0x3-	T65.0x4-	—	—
kerosene	T52.0x1-	T52.0x2-	T52.0x3-	T52.0x4-	—	—
mixture (of compounds)	T60.91x-	T60.92x-	T60.93x-	T60.94x-	—	—
naphthalene	T60.2x1-	T60.2x2-	T60.2x3-	T60.2x4-	—	—
organochlorine (compounds)	T60.1x1-	T60.1x2-	T60.1x3-	T60.1x4-	—	—
petroleum (distillate) (products) NEC	T60.8x1-	T60.8x2-	T60.8x3-	T60.8x4-	—	—
specified ingredient NEC	T60.8x1-	T60.8x2-	T60.8x3-	T60.8x4-	—	—
strychnine	T65.1x1-	T65.1x2-	T65.1x3-	T65.1x4-	—	—
thallium	T60.4x1-	T60.4x2-	T60.4x3-	T60.4x4-	—	—
Pethidine	T40.4x1-	T40.4x2-	T40.4x3-	T40.4x4-	T40.4x5-	T40.4x6-
Petrichloral	T42.6x1-	T42.6x2-	T42.6x3-	T42.6x4-	T42.6x5-	T42.6x6-
Petrol	T52.0x1-	T52.0x2-	T52.0x3-	T52.0x4-	—	—
vapor	T52.0x1-	T52.0x2-	T52.0x3-	T52.0x4-	—	—
Petrolatum	T49.3x1-	T49.3x2-	T49.3x3-	T49.3x4-	T49.3x5-	T49.3x6-
hydrophilic	T49.3x1-	T49.3x2-	T49.3x3-	T49.3x4-	T49.3x5-	T49.3x6-
liquid	T47.4x1-	T47.4x2-	T47.4x3-	T47.4x4-	T47.4x5-	T47.4x6-
topical	T49.3x1-	T49.3x2-	T49.3x3-	T49.3x4-	T49.3x5-	T49.3x6-
nonmedicinal	T52.0x1-	T52.0x2-	T52.0x3-	T52.0x4-	—	—
red veterinary	T49.3x1-	T49.3x2-	T49.3x3-	T49.3x4-	T49.3x5-	T49.3x6-
white	T49.3x1-	T49.3x2-	T49.3x3-	T49.3x4-	T49.3x5-	T49.3x6-
Petroleum (products) NEC	T52.0x1-	T52.0x2-	T52.0x3-	T52.0x4-	—	—
benzine (s) — see Ligroin						
ether — see Ligroin						
jelly — see Petrolatum						
naphtha — see Ligroin						
pesticide	T60.8x1-	T60.8x2-	T60.8x3-	T60.8x4-	—	—
solids	T52.0x1-	T52.0x2-	T52.0x3-	T52.0x4-	—	—
solvents	T52.0x1-	T52.0x2-	T52.0x3-	T52.0x4-	—	—
vapor	T52.0x1-	T52.0x2-	T52.0x3-	T52.0x4-	—	—
Peyote	T40.991-	T40.992-	T40.993-	T40.994-	—	—
Phanodorm, phanodorn	T42.3x1-	T42.3x2-	T42.3x3-	T42.3x4-	T42.3x5-	T42.3x6-
Phanquinone	T37.3x1-	T37.3x2-	T37.3x3-	T37.3x4-	T37.3x5-	T37.3x6-
Phanquone	T37.3x1-	T37.3x2-	T37.3x3-	T37.3x4-	T37.3x5-	T37.3x6-
Pharmaceutical adjunct NEC	T50.901-	T50.902-	T50.903-	T50.904-	T50.905-	T50.906-
excipient NEC	T50.901-	T50.902-	T50.903-	T50.904-	T50.905-	T50.906-
sweetener	T50.901-	T50.902-	T50.903-	T50.904-	T50.905-	T50.906-
viscous agent	T50.901-	T50.902-	T50.903-	T50.904-	T50.905-	T50.906-
Phemitone	T42.3x1-	T42.3x2-	T42.3x3-	T42.3x4-	T42.3x5-	T42.3x6-
Phenacaine	T41.3x1-	T41.3x2-	T41.3x3-	T41.3x4-	T41.3x5-	T41.3x6-
Phenacemide	T42.6x1-	T42.6x2-	T42.6x3-	T42.6x4-	T42.6x5-	T42.6x6-
Phenacetin	T39.1x1-	T39.1x2-	T39.1x3-	T39.1x4-	T39.1x5-	T39.1x6-
Phenadoxone	T40.2x1-	T40.2x2-	T40.2x3-	T40.2x4-	—	—
Phenaglycodol	T43.591-	T43.592-	T43.593-	T43.594-	T43.595-	T43.596-
Phenantoin	T42.0x1-	T42.0x2-	T42.0x3-	T42.0x4-	T42.0x5-	T42.0x6-
Phenaphthazine reagent	T50.991-	T50.992-	T50.993-	T50.994-	T50.995-	T50.996-
Phenazocine	T40.4x1-	T40.4x2-	T40.4x3-	T40.4x4-	T40.4x5-	T40.4x6-
Phenazone	T39.2x1-	T39.2x2-	T39.2x3-	T39.2x4-	T39.2x5-	T39.2x6-
Phenazopyridine	T39.8x1-	T39.8x2-	T39.8x3-	T39.8x4-	T39.8x5-	T39.8x6-
Phenbenicillin	T36.0x1-	T36.0x2-	T36.0x3-	T36.0x4-	T36.0x5-	T36.0x6-
Phenbutrazate	T50.5x1-	T50.5x2-	T50.5x3-	T50.5x4-	T50.5x5-	T50.5x6-
Phencyclidine	T40.991-	T40.992-	T40.993-	T40.994-	T40.995-	T40.996-
Phendimetrazine	T50.5x1-	T50.5x2-	T50.5x3-	T50.5x4-	T50.5x5-	T50.5x6-
Phenelzine	T43.1x1-	T43.1x2-	T43.1x3-	T43.1x4-	T43.1x5-	T43.1x6-
Phenemal	T42.3x1-	T42.3x2-	T42.3x3-	T42.3x4-	T42.3x5-	T42.3x6-
Phenergan	T42.6x1-	T42.6x2-	T42.6x3-	T42.6x4-	T42.6x5-	T42.6x6-
Pheneticillin	T36.0x1-	T36.0x2-	T36.0x3-	T36.0x4-	T36.0x5-	T36.0x6-
Pheneturide	T42.6x1-	T42.6x2-	T42.6x3-	T42.6x4-	T42.6x5-	T42.6x6-
Phenformin	T38.3x1-	T38.3x2-	T38.3x3-	T38.3x4-	T38.3x5-	T38.3x6-
Phenglutarimide	T44.3x1-	T44.3x2-	T44.3x3-	T44.3x4-	T44.3x5-	T44.3x6-
Phenicarbazide	T39.8x1-	T39.8x2-	T39.8x3-	T39.8x4-	T39.8x5-	T39.8x6-
Phenindamine	T45.0x1-	T45.0x2-	T45.0x3-	T45.0x4-	T45.0x5-	T45.0x6-
Phenindione	T45.511-	T45.512-	T45.513-	T45.514-	T45.515-	T45.516-
Pheniprazine	T43.1x1-	T43.1x2-	T43.1x3-	T43.1x4-	T43.1x5-	T43.1x6-
Pheniramine	T45.0x1-	T45.0x2-	T45.0x3-	T45.0x4-	T45.0x5-	T45.0x6-
Phenisatin	T47.2x1-	T47.2x2-	T47.2x3-	T47.2x4-	T47.2x5-	T47.2x6-
Phenmetrazine	T50.5x1-	T50.5x2-	T50.5x3-	T50.5x4-	T50.5x5-	T50.5x6-
Phenobal	T42.3x1-	T42.3x2-	T42.3x3-	T42.3x4-	T42.3x5-	T42.3x6-
Phenobarbital	T42.3x1-	T42.3x2-	T42.3x3-	T42.3x4-	T42.3x5-	T42.3x6-
with mephenytoin	T42.3x1-	T42.3x2-	T42.3x3-	T42.3x4-	T42.3x5-	T42.3x6-
phenytoin	T42.3x1-	T42.3x2-	T42.3x3-	T42.3x4-	T42.3x5-	T42.3x6-
sodium	T42.3x1-	T42.3x2-	T42.3x3-	T42.3x4-	T42.3x5-	T42.3x6-
Phenobarbitone	T42.3x1-	T42.3x2-	T42.3x3-	T42.3x4-	T42.3x5-	T42.3x6-
Phenobutiodil	T50.8x1-	T50.8x2-	T50.8x3-	T50.8x4-	T50.8x5-	T50.8x6-
Phenoctide	T49.0x1-	T49.0x2-	T49.0x3-	T49.0x4-	T49.0x5-	T49.0x6-
Phenol	T49.0x1-	T49.0x2-	T49.0x3-	T49.0x4-	T49.0x5-	T49.0x6-
disinfectant	T54.0x1-	T54.0x2-	T54.0x3-	T54.0x4-	—	—
in oil injection	T46.8x1-	T46.8x2-	T46.8x3-	T46.8x4-	T46.8x5-	T46.8x6-
medicinal	T49.1x1-	T49.1x2-	T49.1x3-	T49.1x4-	T49.1x5-	T49.1x6-
nonmedicinal NEC	T54.0x1-	T54.0x2-	T54.0x3-	T54.0x4-	—	—
pesticide	T60.8x1-	T60.8x2-	T60.8x3-	T60.8x4-	—	—
red	T50.8x1-	T50.8x2-	T50.8x3-	T50.8x4-	T50.8x5-	T50.8x6-
Phenolic preparation	T49.1x1-	T49.1x2-	T49.1x3-	T49.1x4-	T49.1x5-	T49.1x6-
Phenolphthalein	T47.2x1-	T47.2x2-	T47.2x3-	T47.2x4-	T47.2x5-	T47.2x6-
Phenolsulfonphthalein	T50.8x1-	T50.8x2-	T50.8x3-	T50.8x4-	T50.8x5-	T50.8x6-
Phenomorphan	T40.2x1-	T40.2x2-	T40.2x3-	T40.2x4-	—	—
Phenonyl	T42.3x1-	T42.3x2-	T42.3x3-	T42.3x4-	T42.3x5-	T42.3x6-
Phenoperidine	T40.4x1-	T40.4x2-	T40.4x3-	T40.4x4-	—	—
Phenopyrazone	T46.991-	T46.992-	T46.993-	T46.994-	T46.995-	T46.996-
Phenoquin	T50.4x1-	T50.4x2-	T50.4x3-	T50.4x4-	T50.4x5-	T50.4x6-
Phenothiazine (psychotropic) NEC	T43.3x1-	T43.3x2-	T43.3x3-	T43.3x4-	T43.3x5-	T43.3x6-
insecticide	T60.2x1-	T60.2x2-	T60.2x3-	T60.2x4-	—	—
Phenothrin	T49.0x1-	T49.0x2-	T49.0x3-	T49.0x4-	T49.0x5-	T49.0x6-
Phenoxybenzamine	T46.7x1-	T46.7x2-	T46.7x3-	T46.7x4-	T46.7x5-	T46.7x6-
Phenoxyethanol	T49.0x1-	T49.0x2-	T49.0x3-	T49.0x4-	T49.0x5-	T49.0x6-
Phenoxymethyl penicillin	T36.0x1-	T36.0x2-	T36.0x3-	T36.0x4-	T36.0x5-	T36.0x6-
Phenprobamate	T42.8x1-	T42.8x2-	T42.8x3-	T42.8x4-	T42.8x5-	T42.8x6-

DRUGS & CHEMICALS

Table of Drugs & Chemicals	POISONING Accidental (Unintentional)	Self-Harm (Intentional)	Assault	Undetermined	Adverse Effect	Underdosing
Phenprocoumon	T45.511-	T45.512-	T45.513-	T45.514-	T45.515-	T45.516-
Phensuximide	T42.2x1-	T42.2x2-	T42.2x3-	T42.2x4-	T42.2x5-	T42.2x6-
Phentermine	T50.5x1-	T50.5x2-	T50.5x3-	T50.5x4-	T50.5x5-	T50.5x6-
Phenthicillin	T36.0x1-	T36.0x2-	T36.0x3-	T36.0x4-	T36.0x5-	T36.0x6-
Phentolamine	T46.7x1-	T46.7x2-	T46.7x3-	T46.7x4-	T46.7x5-	T46.7x6-
Phenyl						
butazone	T39.2x1-	T39.2x2-	T39.2x3-	T39.2x4-	T39.2x5-	T39.2x6-
enediamine	T65.3x1-	T65.3x2-	T65.3x3-	T65.3x4-	—	—
hydrazine	T65.3x1-	T65.3x2-	T65.3x3-	T65.3x4-	—	—
antineoplastic	T45.1x1-	T45.1x2-	T45.1x3-	T45.1x4-	T45.1x5-	T45.1x6-
mercuric compounds — see Mercury						
salicylate	T49.3x1-	T49.3x2-	T49.3x3-	T49.3x4-	T49.3x5-	T49.3x6-
Phenylalanine mustard	T45.1x1-	T45.1x2-	T45.1x3-	T45.1x4-	T45.1x5-	T45.1x6-
Phenylbutazone	T39.2x1-	T39.2x2-	T39.2x3-	T39.2x4-	T39.2x5-	T39.2x6-
Phenylenediamine	T65.3x1-	T65.3x2-	T65.3x3-	T65.3x4-	—	—
Phenylephrine	T44.4x1-	T44.4x2-	T44.4x3-	T44.4x4-	T44.4x5-	T44.4x6-
Phenylethylbiguanide	T38.3x1-	T38.3x2-	T38.3x3-	T38.3x4-	T38.3x5-	T38.3x6-
Phenylmercuric						
acetate	T49.0x1-	T49.0x2-	T49.0x3-	T49.0x4-	T49.0x5-	T49.0x6-
borate	T49.0x1-	T49.0x2-	T49.0x3-	T49.0x4-	T49.0x5-	T49.0x6-
nitrate	T49.0x1-	T49.0x2-	T49.0x3-	T49.0x4-	T49.0x5-	T49.0x6-
Phenylmethylbarbitone	T42.3x1-	T42.3x2-	T42.3x3-	T42.3x4-	T42.3x5-	T42.3x6-
Phenylpropanol	T47.5x1-	T47.5x2-	T47.5x3-	T47.5x4-	T47.5x5-	T47.5x6-
Phenylpropanolamine	T44.991-	T44.992-	T44.993-	T44.994-	T44.995-	T44.996-
Phenylsulfthion	T60.0x1-	T60.0x2-	T60.0x3-	T60.0x4-	—	—
Phenyltoloxamine	T45.0x1-	T45.0x2-	T45.0x3-	T45.0x4-	T45.0x5-	T45.0x6-
Phenyramidol, phenyramidon	T39.8x1-	T39.8x2-	T39.8x3-	T39.8x4-	T39.8x5-	T39.8x6-
Phenytoin	T42.0x1-	T42.0x2-	T42.0x3-	T42.0x4-	T42.0x5-	T42.0x6-
with phenobarbital	T42.3x1-	T42.3x2-	T42.3x3-	T42.3x4-	T42.3x5-	T42.3x6-
pHisoHex	T49.2x1-	T49.2x2-	T49.2x3-	T49.2x4-	T49.2x5-	T49.2x6-
Pholcodine	T48.3x1-	T48.3x2-	T48.3x3-	T48.3x4-	T48.3x5-	T48.3x6-
Pholedrine	T46.991-	T46.992-	T46.993-	T46.994-	T46.995-	T46.996-
Phorate	T60.0x1-	T60.0x2-	T60.0x3-	T60.0x4-	—	—
Phosdrin	T60.0x1-	T60.0x2-	T60.0x3-	T60.0x4-	—	—
Phosfolan	T60.0x1-	T60.0x2-	T60.0x3-	T60.0x4-	—	—
Phosgene (gas)	T59.891-	T59.892-	T59.893-	T59.894-	—	—
Phosphamidon	T60.0x1-	T60.0x2-	T60.0x3-	T60.0x4-	—	—
Phosphate	T65.891-	T65.892-	T65.893-	T65.894-	—	—
laxative	T47.4x1-	T47.4x2-	T47.4x3-	T47.4x4-	T47.4x5-	T47.4x6-
organic	T60.0x1-	T60.0x2-	T60.0x3-	T60.0x4-	—	—
solvent	T52.91x-	T52.92x-	T52.93x-	T52.94x-	—	—
tricresyl	T65.891-	T65.892-	T65.893-	T65.894-	—	—
Phosphine	T57.1x1-	T57.1x2-	T57.1x3-	T57.1x4-	—	—
fumigant	T57.1x1-	T57.1x2-	T57.1x3-	T57.1x4-	—	—
Phospholine	T49.5x1-	T49.5x2-	T49.5x3-	T49.5x4-	T49.5x5-	T49.5x6-
Phosphoric acid	T54.2x1-	T54.2x2-	T54.2x3-	T54.2x4-	—	—
Phosphorus (compound) NEC	T57.1x1-	T57.1x2-	T57.1x3-	T57.1x4-	—	—
pesticide	T60.0x1-	T60.0x2-	T60.0x3-	T60.0x4-	—	—
Phthalates	T65.891-	T65.892-	T65.893-	T65.894-	—	—
Phthalic anhydride	T65.891-	T65.892-	T65.893-	T65.894-	—	—
Phthalimidoglutarimide	T42.6x1-	T42.6x2-	T42.6x3-	T42.6x4-	T42.6x5-	T42.6x6-
Phthalylsulfathiazole	T37.0x1-	T37.0x2-	T37.0x3-	T37.0x4-	T37.0x5-	T37.0x6-
Phylloquinone	T45.7x1-	T45.7x2-	T45.7x3-	T45.7x4-	T45.7x5-	T45.7x6-
Physeptone	T40.3x1-	T40.3x2-	T40.3x3-	T40.3x4-	T40.3x5-	T40.3x6-
Physostigma venenosum	T62.2x1-	T62.2x2-	T62.2x3-	T62.2x4-	—	—
Physostigmine	T49.5x1-	T49.5x2-	T49.5x3-	T49.5x4-	T49.5x5-	T49.5x6-
Phytolacca decandra	T62.2x1-	T62.2x2-	T62.2x3-	T62.2x4-	—	—
berries	T62.1x1-	T62.1x2-	T62.1x3-	T62.1x4-	—	—

Table of Drugs & Chemicals	POISONING Accidental (Unintentional)	Self-Harm (Intentional)	Assault	Undetermined	Adverse Effect	Underdosing
Phytomenadione	T45.7x1-	T45.7x2-	T45.7x3-	T45.7x4-	T45.7x5-	T45.7x6-
Phytonadione	T45.7x1-	T45.7x2-	T45.7x3-	T45.7x4-	T45.7x5-	T45.7x6-
Picoperine	T48.3x1-	T48.3x2-	T48.3x3-	T48.3x4-	T48.3x5-	T48.3x6-
Picosulfate (sodium)	T47.2x1-	T47.2x2-	T47.2x3-	T47.2x4-	T47.2x5-	T47.2x6-
Picric (acid)	T54.2x1-	T54.2x2-	T54.2x3-	T54.2x4-	—	—
Picrotoxin	T50.7x1-	T50.7x2-	T50.7x3-	T50.7x4-	T50.7x5-	T50.7x6-
Piketoprofen	T49.0x1-	T49.0x2-	T49.0x3-	T49.0x4-	T49.0x5-	T49.0x6-
Pilocarpine	T44.1x1-	T44.1x2-	T44.1x3-	T44.1x4-	T44.1x5-	T44.1x6-
Pilocarpus (jaborandi) extract	T44.1x1-	T44.1x2-	T44.1x3-	T44.1x4-	T44.1x5-	T44.1x6-
Pilsicainide (hydrochloride)	T46.2x1-	T46.2x2-	T46.2x3-	T46.2x4-	T46.2x5-	T46.2x6-
Pimaricin	T36.7x1-	T36.7x2-	T36.7x3-	T36.7x4-	T36.7x5-	T36.7x6-
Pimeclone	T50.7x1-	T50.7x2-	T50.7x3-	T50.7x4-	T50.7x5-	T50.7x6-
Pimelic ketone	T52.8x1-	T52.8x2-	T52.8x3-	T52.8x4-	—	—
Pimethixene	T45.0x1-	T45.0x2-	T45.0x3-	T45.0x4-	T45.0x5-	T45.0x6-
Piminodine	T40.2x1-	T40.2x2-	T40.2x3-	T40.2x4-	T40.2x5-	T40.2x6-
Pimozide	T43.591-	T43.592-	T43.593-	T43.594-	T43.595-	T43.596-
Pinacidil	T46.5x1-	T46.5x2-	T46.5x3-	T46.5x4-	T46.5x5-	T46.5x6-
Pinaverium bromide	T44.3x1-	T44.3x2-	T44.3x3-	T44.3x4-	T44.3x5-	T44.3x6-
Pinazepam	T42.4x1-	T42.4x2-	T42.4x3-	T42.4x4-	T42.4x5-	T42.4x6-
Pindolol	T44.7x1-	T44.7x2-	T44.7x3-	T44.7x4-	T44.7x5-	T44.7x6-
Pindone	T60.4x1-	T60.4x2-	T60.4x3-	T60.4x4-	—	—
Pine oil (disinfectant)	T65.891-	T65.892-	T65.893-	T65.894-	—	—
Pinkroot	T37.4x1-	T37.4x2-	T37.4x3-	T37.4x4-	T37.4x5-	T37.4x6-
Pipadone	T40.2x1-	T40.2x2-	T40.2x3-	T40.2x4-	—	—
Pipamazine	T45.0x1-	T45.0x2-	T45.0x3-	T45.0x4-	T45.0x5-	T45.0x6-
Pipamperone	T43.4x1-	T43.4x2-	T43.4x3-	T43.4x4-	T43.4x5-	T43.4x6-
Pipazetate	T48.3x1-	T48.3x2-	T48.3x3-	T48.3x4-	T48.3x5-	T48.3x6-
Pipemidic acid	T37.8x1-	T37.8x2-	T37.8x3-	T37.8x4-	T37.8x5-	T37.8x6-
Pipenzolate bromide	T44.3x1-	T44.3x2-	T44.3x3-	T44.3x4-	T44.3x5-	T44.3x6-
Piper cubeba	T62.2x1-	T62.2x2-	T62.2x3-	T62.2x4-	—	—
Piperacetazine	T43.3x1-	T43.3x2-	T43.3x3-	T43.3x4-	T43.3x5-	T43.3x6-
Piperacillin	T36.0x1-	T36.0x2-	T36.0x3-	T36.0x4-	T36.0x5-	T36.0x6-
Piperazine	T37.4x1-	T37.4x2-	T37.4x3-	T37.4x4-	T37.4x5-	T37.4x6-
estrone sulfate	T38.5x1-	T38.5x2-	T38.5x3-	T38.5x4-	T38.5x5-	T38.5x6-
Piperidione	T48.3x1-	T48.3x2-	T48.3x3-	T48.3x4-	T48.3x5-	T48.3x6-
Piperidolate	T44.3x1-	T44.3x2-	T44.3x3-	T44.3x4-	T44.3x5-	T44.3x6-
Piperocaine	T41.3x1-	T41.3x2-	T41.3x3-	T41.3x4-	T41.3x5-	T41.3x6-
infiltration (subcutaneous)	T41.3x1-	T41.3x2-	T41.3x3-	T41.3x4-	T41.3x5-	T41.3x6-
nerve block (peripheral) (plexus)	T41.3x1-	T41.3x2-	T41.3x3-	T41.3x4-	T41.3x5-	T41.3x6-
topical (surface)	T41.3x1-	T41.3x2-	T41.3x3-	T41.3x4-	T41.3x5-	T41.3x6-
Piperonyl butoxide	T60.8x1-	T60.8x2-	T60.8x3-	T60.8x4-	—	—
Pipethanate	T44.3x1-	T44.3x2-	T44.3x3-	T44.3x4-	T44.3x5-	T44.3x6-
Pipobroman	T45.1x1-	T45.1x2-	T45.1x3-	T45.1x4-	T45.1x5-	T45.1x6-
Pipotiazine	T43.3x1-	T43.3x2-	T43.3x3-	T43.3x4-	T43.3x5-	T43.3x6-
Pipoxizine	T45.0x1-	T45.0x2-	T45.0x3-	T45.0x4-	T45.0x5-	T45.0x6-
Pipradrol	T43.691-	T43.692-	T43.693-	T43.694-	T43.695-	T43.696-
Piprinhydrinate	T45.0x1-	T45.0x2-	T45.0x3-	T45.0x4-	T45.0x5-	T45.0x6-
Pirarubicin	T45.1x1-	T45.1x2-	T45.1x3-	T45.1x4-	T45.1x5-	T45.1x6-
Pirazinamide	T37.1x1-	T37.1x2-	T37.1x3-	T37.1x4-	T37.1x5-	T37.1x6-
Pirbuterol	T48.6x1-	T48.6x2-	T48.6x3-	T48.6x4-	T48.6x5-	T48.6x6-
Pirenzepine	T47.1x1-	T47.1x2-	T47.1x3-	T47.1x4-	T47.1x5-	T47.1x6-
Piretanide	T50.1x1-	T50.1x2-	T50.1x3-	T50.1x4-	T50.1x5-	T50.1x6-
Piribedil	T42.8x1-	T42.8x2-	T42.8x3-	T42.8x4-	T42.8x5-	T42.8x6-
Piridoxilate	T46.3x1-	T46.3x2-	T46.3x3-	T46.3x4-	T46.3x5-	T46.3x6-
Piritramide	T40.4x1-	T40.4x2-	T40.4x3-	T40.4x4-	—	—
Piromidic acid	T37.8x1-	T37.8x2-	T37.8x3-	T37.8x4-	T37.8x5-	T37.8x6-
Piroxicam	T39.391-	T39.392-	T39.393-	T39.394-	T39.395-	T39.396-
beta-cyclodextrin complex	T39.8x1-	T39.8x2-	T39.8x3-	T39.8x4-	T39.8x5-	T39.8x6-

DRUGS & CHEMICALS

Table of Drugs & Chemicals	Accidental (Unintentional)	Self-Harm (Intentional)	Assault	Undetermined	Adverse Effect	Underdosing
Pirozadil	T46.6x1-	T46.6x2-	T46.6x3-	T46.6x4-	T46.6x5-	T46.6x6-
Piscidia (bark) (erythrina)	T39.8x1-	T39.8x2-	T39.8x3-	T39.8x4-	T39.8x5-	T39.8x6-
Pitch	T65.891-	T65.892-	T65.893-	T65.894-	—	—
Pitkin's solution	T41.3x1-	T41.3x2-	T41.3x3-	T41.3x4-	T41.3x5-	T41.3x6-
Pitocin	T48.0x1-	T48.0x2-	T48.0x3-	T48.0x4-	T48.0x5-	T48.0x6-
Pitressin (tannate)	T38.891-	T38.892-	T38.893-	T38.894-	T38.895-	T38.896-
Pituitary extracts (posterior)	T38.891-	T38.892-	T38.893-	T38.894-	T38.895-	T38.896-
anterior	T38.811-	T38.812-	T38.813-	T38.814-	T38.815-	T38.816-
Pituitrin	T38.891-	T38.892-	T38.893-	T38.894-	T38.895-	T38.896-
Pivampicillin	T36.0x1-	T36.0x2-	T36.0x3-	T36.0x4-	T36.0x5-	T36.0x6-
Pivmecillinam	T36.0x1-	T36.0x2-	T36.0x3-	T36.0x4-	T36.0x5-	T36.0x6-
Placental hormone	T38.891-	T38.892-	T38.893-	T38.894-	T38.895-	T38.896-
Placidyl	T42.6x1-	T42.6x2-	T42.6x3-	T42.6x4-	T42.6x5-	T42.6x6-
Plague vaccine	T50.A91-	T50.A92-	T50.A93-	T50.A94-	T50.A95-	T50.A96-
Plant						
food or fertilizer NEC	T65.891-	T65.892-	T65.893-	T65.894-	—	—
containing herbicide	T60.3x1-	T60.3x2-	T60.3x3-	T60.3x4-	—	—
noxious, used as food	T62.2x1-	T62.2x2-	T62.2x3-	T62.2x4-	—	—
berries	T62.1x1-	T62.1x2-	T62.1x3-	T62.1x4-	—	—
seeds	T62.2x1-	T62.2x2-	T62.2x3-	T62.2x4-	—	—
specified type NEC	T62.2x1-	T62.2x2-	T62.2x3-	T62.2x4-	—	—
Plasma	T45.8x1-	T45.8x2-	T45.8x3-	T45.8x4-	T45.8x5-	T45.8x6-
expander NEC	T45.8x1-	T45.8x2-	T45.8x3-	T45.8x4-	T45.8x5-	T45.8x6-
protein fraction (human)	T45.8x1-	T45.8x2-	T45.8x3-	T45.8x4-	T45.8x5-	T45.8x6-
Plasmanate	T45.8x1-	T45.8x2-	T45.8x3-	T45.8x4-	T45.8x5-	T45.8x6-
Plasminogen (tissue) activator	T45.611-	T45.612-	T45.613-	T45.614-	T45.615-	T45.616-
Plaster dressing	T49.3x1-	T49.3x2-	T49.3x3-	T49.3x4-	T49.3x5-	T49.3x6-
Plastic dressing	T49.3x1-	T49.3x2-	T49.3x3-	T49.3x4-	T49.3x5-	T49.3x6-
Plegicil	T43.3x1-	T43.3x2-	T43.3x3-	T43.3x4-	T43.3x5-	T43.3x6-
Plicamycin	T45.1x1-	T45.1x2-	T45.1x3-	T45.1x4-	T45.1x5-	T45.1x6-
Podophyllotoxin	T49.8x1-	T49.8x2-	T49.8x3-	T49.8x4-	T49.8x5-	T49.8x6-
Podophyllum (resin)	T49.4x1-	T49.4x2-	T49.4x3-	T49.4x4-	T49.4x5-	T49.4x6-
Poison NEC	T65.91x-	T65.92x-	T65.93x-	T65.94x-	—	—
Poisonous berries	T62.1x1-	T62.1x2-	T62.1x3-	T62.1x4-	—	—
Pokeweed (any part)	T62.2x1-	T62.2x2-	T62.2x3-	T62.2x4-	—	—
Poldine metilsulfate	T44.3x1-	T44.3x2-	T44.3x3-	T44.3x4-	T44.3x5-	T44.3x6-
Polidexide (sulfate)	T46.6x1-	T46.6x2-	T46.6x3-	T46.6x4-	T46.6x5-	T46.6x6-
Polidocanol	T46.8x1-	T46.8x2-	T46.8x3-	T46.8x4-	T46.8x5-	T46.8x6-
Poliomyelitis vaccine	T50.B91-	T50.B92-	T50.B93-	T50.B94-	T50.B95-	T50.B96-
Polish (car) (floor) (furniture) (metal) (porcelain) (silver)	T65.891-	T65.892-	T65.893-	T65.894-	—	—
abrasive	T65.891-	T65.892-	T65.893-	T65.894-	—	—
porcelain	T65.891-	T65.892-	T65.893-	T65.894-	—	—
Poloxalkol	T47.4x1-	T47.4x2-	T47.4x3-	T47.4x4-	T47.4x5-	T47.4x6-
Poloxamer	T47.4x1-	T47.4x2-	T47.4x3-	T47.4x4-	T47.4x5-	T47.4x6-
Polyaminostyrene resins	T50.3x1-	T50.3x2-	T50.3x3-	T50.3x4-	T50.3x5-	T50.3x6-
Polycarbophil	T47.4x1-	T47.4x2-	T47.4x3-	T47.4x4-	T47.4x5-	T47.4x6-
Polychlorinated biphenyl	T65.891-	T65.892-	T65.893-	T65.894-	—	—
Polycycline	T36.4x1-	T36.4x2-	T36.4x3-	T36.4x4-	T36.4x5-	T36.4x6-
Polyester fumes	T59.891-	T59.892-	T59.893-	T59.894-	—	—
Polyester resin hardener	T52.91x-	T52.92x-	T52.93x-	T52.94x-	—	—
fumes	T59.891-	T59.892-	T59.893-	T59.894-	—	—
Polyestradiol phosphate	T38.5x1-	T38.5x2-	T38.5x3-	T38.5x4-	T38.5x5-	T38.5x6-
Polyethanolamine alkyl sulfate	T49.2x1-	T49.2x2-	T49.2x3-	T49.2x4-	T49.2x5-	T49.2x6-
Polyethylene adhesive	T49.3x1-	T49.3x2-	T49.3x3-	T49.3x4-	T49.3x5-	T49.3x6-
Polyferose	T45.4x1-	T45.4x2-	T45.4x3-	T45.4x4-	T45.4x5-	T45.4x6-
Polygeline	T45.8x1-	T45.8x2-	T45.8x3-	T45.8x4-	T45.8x5-	T45.8x6-

Table of Drugs & Chemicals	Accidental (Unintentional)	Self-Harm (Intentional)	Assault	Undetermined	Adverse Effect	Underdosing
Polymyxin	T36.8x1-	T36.8x2-	T36.8x3-	T36.8x4-	T36.8x5-	T36.8x6-
B	T36.8x1-	T36.8x2-	T36.8x3-	T36.8x4-	T36.8x5-	T36.8x6-
ENT agent	T49.6x1-	T49.6x2-	T49.6x3-	T49.6x4-	T49.6x5-	T49.6x6-
ophthalmic preparation	T49.5x1-	T49.5x2-	T49.5x3-	T49.5x4-	T49.5x5-	T49.5x6-
topical NEC	T49.0x1-	T49.0x2-	T49.0x3-	T49.0x4-	T49.0x5-	T49.0x6-
E sulfate (eye preparation)	T49.5x1-	T49.5x2-	T49.5x3-	T49.5x4-	T49.5x5-	T49.5x6-
Polynoxylin	T49.0x1-	T49.0x2-	T49.0x3-	T49.0x4-	T49.0x5-	T49.0x6-
Polyoestradiol phosphate	T38.5x1-	T38.5x2-	T38.5x3-	T38.5x4-	T38.5x5-	T38.5x6-
Polyoxymethyleneurea	T49.0x1-	T49.0x2-	T49.0x3-	T49.0x4-	T49.0x5-	T49.0x6-
Polysilane	T47.8x1-	T47.8x2-	T47.8x3-	T47.8x4-	T47.8x5-	T47.8x6-
Polytetrafluoroethylene (inhaled)	T59.891-	T59.892-	T59.893-	T59.894-	—	—
Polythiazide	T50.2x1-	T50.2x2-	T50.2x3-	T50.2x4-	T50.2x5-	T50.2x6-
Polyvidone	T45.8x1-	T45.8x2-	T45.8x3-	T45.8x4-	T45.8x5-	T45.8x6-
Polyvinylpyrrolidone	T45.8x1-	T45.8x2-	T45.8x3-	T45.8x4-	T45.8x5-	T45.8x6-
Pontocaine (hydrochloride) (infiltration) (topical)	T41.3x1-	T41.3x2-	T41.3x3-	T41.3x4-	T41.3x5-	T41.3x6-
nerve block (peripheral) (plexus)	T41.3x1-	T41.3x2-	T41.3x3-	T41.3x4-	T41.3x5-	T41.3x6-
spinal	T41.3x1-	T41.3x2-	T41.3x3-	T41.3x4-	T41.3x5-	T41.3x6-
Porfiromycin	T45.1x1-	T45.1x2-	T45.1x3-	T45.1x4-	T45.1x5-	T45.1x6-
Posterior pituitary hormone NEC	T38.891-	T38.892-	T38.893-	T38.894-	T38.895-	T38.896-
Pot	T40.7x1-	T40.7x2-	T40.7x3-	T40.7x4-	T40.7x5-	T40.7x6-
Potash (caustic)	T54.3x1-	T54.3x2-	T54.3x3-	T54.3x4-	—	—
Potassic saline injection (lactated)	T50.3x1-	T50.3x2-	T50.3x3-	T50.3x4-	T50.3x5-	T50.3x6-
Potassium (salts) NEC	T50.3x1-	T50.3x2-	T50.3x3-	T50.3x4-	T50.3x5-	T50.3x6-
aminobenzoate	T45.8x1-	T45.8x2-	T45.8x3-	T45.8x4-	T45.8x5-	T45.8x6-
aminosalicylate	T37.1x1-	T37.1x2-	T37.1x3-	T37.1x4-	T37.1x5-	T37.1x6-
antimony 'tartrate'	T37.8x1-	T37.8x2-	T37.8x3-	T37.8x4-	T37.8x5-	T37.8x6-
arsenite (solution)	T57.0x1-	T57.0x2-	T57.0x3-	T57.0x4-	—	—
bichromate	T56.2x1-	T56.2x2-	T56.2x3-	T56.2x4-	—	—
bisulfate	T47.3x1-	T47.3x2-	T47.3x3-	T47.3x4-	T47.3x5-	T47.3x6-
bromide	T42.6x1-	T42.6x2-	T42.6x3-	T42.6x4-	T42.6x5-	T42.6x6-
canrenoate	T50.0x1-	T50.0x2-	T50.0x3-	T50.0x4-	T50.0x5-	T50.0x6-
carbonate	T54.3x1-	T54.3x2-	T54.3x3-	T54.3x4-	—	—
chlorate NEC	T65.891-	T65.892-	T65.893-	T65.894-	—	—
chloride	T50.3x1-	T50.3x2-	T50.3x3-	T50.3x4-	T50.3x5-	T50.3x6-
citrate	T50.991-	T50.992-	T50.993-	T50.994-	T50.995-	T50.996-
cyanide	T65.0x1-	T65.0x2-	T65.0x3-	T65.0x4-	—	—
ferric hexacyanoferrate (medicinal)	T50.6x1-	T50.6x2-	T50.6x3-	T50.6x4-	T50.6x5-	T50.6x6-
nonmedicinal	T65.891-	T65.892-	T65.893-	T65.894-	—	—
fluoride	T57.8x1-	T57.8x2-	T57.8x3-	T57.8x4-	—	—
glucaldrate	T47.1x1-	T47.1x2-	T47.1x3-	T47.1x4-	T47.1x5-	T47.1x6-
hydroxide	T54.3x1-	T54.3x2-	T54.3x3-	T54.3x4-	—	—
iodate	T49.0x1-	T49.0x2-	T49.0x3-	T49.0x4-	T49.0x5-	T49.0x6-
iodide	T48.4x1-	T48.4x2-	T48.4x3-	T48.4x4-	T48.4x5-	T48.4x6-
nitrate	T57.8x1-	T57.8x2-	T57.8x3-	T57.8x4-	—	—
oxalate	T65.891-	T65.892-	T65.893-	T65.894-	—	—
perchlorate						
(nonmedicinal) NEC	T65.891-	T65.892-	T65.893-	T65.894-	—	—
antithyroid	T38.2x1-	T38.2x2-	T38.2x3-	T38.2x4-	T38.2x5-	T38.2x6-
medicinal	T38.2x1-	T38.2x2-	T38.2x3-	T38.2x4-	T38.2x5-	T38.2x6-
permanganate						
(nonmedicinal)	T65.891-	T65.892-	T65.893-	T65.894-	—	—
medicinal	T49.0x1-	T49.0x2-	T49.0x3-	T49.0x4-	T49.0x5-	T49.0x6-
sulfate	T47.2x1-	T47.2x2-	T47.2x3-	T47.2x4-	T47.2x5-	T47.2x6-

DRUGS & CHEMICALS

Table of Drugs & Chemicals	POISONING Accidental (Unintentional)	Self-Harm (Intentional)	Assault	Undetermined	Adverse Effect	Underdosing
Potassium-removing resin ..	T50.3x1-	T50.3x2-	T50.3x3-	T50.3x4-	T50.3x5-	T50.3x6-
Potassium-retaining drug ..	T50.3x1-	T50.3x2-	T50.3x3-	T50.3x4-	T50.3x5-	T50.3x6-
Povidone	T45.8x1-	T45.8x2-	T45.8x3-	T45.8x4-	T45.8x5-	T45.8x6-
iodine	T49.0x1-	T49.0x2-	T49.0x3-	T49.0x4-	T49.0x5-	T49.0x6-
Practolol	T44.7x1-	T44.7x2-	T44.7x3-	T44.7x4-	T44.7x5-	T44.7x6-
Prajmalium bitartrate	T46.2x1-	T46.2x2-	T46.2x3-	T46.2x4-	T46.2x5-	T46.2x6-
Pralidoxime (iodide)	T50.6x1-	T50.6x2-	T50.6x3-	T50.6x4-	T50.6x5-	T50.6x6-
chloride	T50.6x1-	T50.6x2-	T50.6x3-	T50.6x4-	T50.6x5-	T50.6x6-
Pramiverine	T44.3x1-	T44.3x2-	T44.3x3-	T44.3x4-	T44.3x5-	T44.3x6-
Pramocaine	T49.1x1-	T49.1x2-	T49.1x3-	T49.1x4-	T49.1x5-	T49.1x6-
Pramoxine	T49.1x1-	T49.1x2-	T49.1x3-	T49.1x4-	T49.1x5-	T49.1x6-
Prasterone	T38.7x1-	T38.7x2-	T38.7x3-	T38.7x4-	T38.7x5-	T38.7x6-
Pravastatin	T46.6x1-	T46.6x2-	T46.6x3-	T46.6x4-	T46.6x5-	T46.6x6-
Prazepam	T42.4x1-	T42.4x2-	T42.4x3-	T42.4x4-	T42.4x5-	T42.4x6-
Praziquantel	T37.4x1-	T37.4x2-	T37.4x3-	T37.4x4-	T37.4x5-	T37.4x6-
Prazitone	T43.291-	T43.292-	T43.293-	T43.294-	T43.295-	T43.296-
Prazosin	T44.6x1-	T44.6x2-	T44.6x3-	T44.6x4-	T44.6x5-	T44.6x6-
Prednicarbate	T49.0x1-	T49.0x2-	T49.0x3-	T49.0x4-	T49.0x5-	T49.0x6-
Prednimustine	T45.1x1-	T45.1x2-	T45.1x3-	T45.1x4-	T45.1x5-	T45.1x6-
Prednisolone	T38.0x1-	T38.0x2-	T38.0x3-	T38.0x4-	T38.0x5-	T38.0x6-
ENT agent	T49.6x1-	T49.6x2-	T49.6x3-	T49.6x4-	T49.6x5-	T49.6x6-
ophthalmic preparation ..	T49.5x1-	T49.5x2-	T49.5x3-	T49.5x4-	T49.5x5-	T49.5x6-
steaglate	T49.0x1-	T49.0x2-	T49.0x3-	T49.0x4-	T49.0x5-	T49.0x6-
topical NEC	T49.0x1-	T49.0x2-	T49.0x3-	T49.0x4-	T49.0x5-	T49.0x6-
Prednisone	T38.0x1-	T38.0x2-	T38.0x3-	T38.0x4-	T38.0x5-	T38.0x6-
Prednylidene	T38.0x1-	T38.0x2-	T38.0x3-	T38.0x4-	T38.0x5-	T38.0x6-
Pregnandiol	T38.5x1-	T38.5x2-	T38.5x3-	T38.5x4-	T38.5x5-	T38.5x6-
Pregneninolone	T38.5x1-	T38.5x2-	T38.5x3-	T38.5x4-	T38.5x5-	T38.5x6-
Preludin	T43.691-	T43.692-	T43.693-	T43.694-	T43.695-	T43.696-
Premarin	T38.5x1-	T38.5x2-	T38.5x3-	T38.5x4-	T38.5x5-	T38.5x6-
Premedication anesthetic	T41.201-	T41.202-	T41.203-	T41.204-	T41.205-	T41.206-
Prenalterol	T44.5x1-	T44.5x2-	T44.5x3-	T44.5x4-	T44.5x5-	T44.5x6-
Prenoxdiazine	T48.3x1-	T48.3x2-	T48.3x3-	T48.3x4-	T48.3x5-	T48.3x6-
Prenylamine	T46.3x1-	T46.3x2-	T46.3x3-	T46.3x4-	T46.3x5-	T46.3x6-
Preparation, local	T49.4x1-	T49.4x2-	T49.4x3-	T49.4x4-	T49.4x5-	T49.4x6-
Preparation H	T49.8x1-	T49.8x2-	T49.8x3-	T49.8x4-	T49.8x5-	T49.8x6-
Preservative (nonmedicinal)	T65.891-	T65.892-	T65.893-	T65.894-	—	—
medicinal	T50.901-	T50.902-	T50.903-	T50.904-	T50.905-	T50.906-
wood	T60.91x-	T60.92x-	T60.93x-	T60.94x-	—	—
Prethcamide	T50.7x1-	T50.7x2-	T50.7x3-	T50.7x4-	T50.7x5-	T50.7x6-
Pride of China	T62.2x1-	T62.2x2-	T62.2x3-	T62.2x4-	—	—
Pridinol	T44.3x1-	T44.3x2-	T44.3x3-	T44.3x4-	T44.3x5-	T44.3x6-
Prifinium bromide	T44.3x1-	T44.3x2-	T44.3x3-	T44.3x4-	T44.3x5-	T44.3x6-
Prilocaine	T41.3x1-	T41.3x2-	T41.3x3-	T41.3x4-	T41.3x5-	T41.3x6-
infiltration (subcutaneous)	T41.3x1-	T41.3x2-	T41.3x3-	T41.3x4-	T41.3x5-	T41.3x6-
nerve block (peripheral) (plexus)	T41.3x1-	T41.3x2-	T41.3x3-	T41.3x4-	T41.3x5-	T41.3x6-
regional	T41.3x1-	T41.3x2-	T41.3x3-	T41.3x4-	T41.3x5-	T41.3x6-
Primaquine	T37.2x1-	T37.2x2-	T37.2x3-	T37.2x4-	T37.2x5-	T37.2x6-
Primidone	T42.6x1-	T42.6x2-	T42.6x3-	T42.6x4-	T42.6x5-	T42.6x6-
Primula (veris)	T62.2x1-	T62.2x2-	T62.2x3-	T62.2x4-	—	—
Prinadol	T40.2x1-	T40.2x2-	T40.2x3-	T40.2x4-	T40.2x5-	T40.2x6-
Priscol, Priscoline	T44.6x1-	T44.6x2-	T44.6x3-	T44.6x4-	T44.6x5-	T44.6x6-
Pristinamycin	T36.3x1-	T36.3x2-	T36.3x3-	T36.3x4-	T36.3x5-	T36.3x6-
Privet	T62.2x1-	T62.2x2-	T62.2x3-	T62.2x4-	—	—
berries	T62.1x1-	T62.1x2-	T62.1x3-	T62.1x4-	—	—
Privine	T44.4x1-	T44.4x2-	T44.4x3-	T44.4x4-	T44.4x5-	T44.4x6-
Pro-Banthine	T44.3x1-	T44.3x2-	T44.3x3-	T44.3x4-	T44.3x5-	T44.3x6-
Probarbital	T42.3x1-	T42.3x2-	T42.3x3-	T42.3x4-	T42.3x5-	T42.3x6-
Probenecid	T50.4x1-	T50.4x2-	T50.4x3-	T50.4x4-	T50.4x5-	T50.4x6-

Table of Drugs & Chemicals	POISONING Accidental (Unintentional)	Self-Harm (Intentional)	Assault	Undetermined	Adverse Effect	Underdosing
Probucol	T46.6x1-	T46.6x2-	T46.6x3-	T46.6x4-	T46.6x5-	T46.6x6-
Procainamide	T46.2x1-	T46.2x2-	T46.2x3-	T46.2x4-	T46.2x5-	T46.2x6-
Procaine	T41.3x1-	T41.3x2-	T41.3x3-	T41.3x4-	T41.3x5-	T41.3x6-
benzylpenicillin	T36.0x1-	T36.0x2-	T36.0x3-	T36.0x4-	T36.0x5-	T36.0x6-
nerve block (periphreal) (plexus)	T41.3x1-	T41.3x2-	T41.3x3-	T41.3x4-	T41.3x5-	T41.3x6-
penicillin G	T36.0x1-	T36.0x2-	T36.0x3-	T36.0x4-	T36.0x5-	T36.0x6-
regional	T41.3x1-	T41.3x2-	T41.3x3-	T41.3x4-	T41.3x5-	T41.3x6-
spinal	T41.3x1-	T41.3x2-	T41.3x3-	T41.3x4-	T41.3x5-	T41.3x6-
Procalmidol	T43.591-	T43.592-	T43.593-	T43.594-	T43.595-	T43.596-
Procarbazine	T45.1x1-	T45.1x2-	T45.1x3-	T45.1x4-	T45.1x5-	T45.1x6-
Procaterol	T44.5x1-	T44.5x2-	T44.5x3-	T44.5x4-	T44.5x5-	T44.5x6-
Prochlorperazine	T43.3x1-	T43.3x2-	T43.3x3-	T43.3x4-	T43.3x5-	T43.3x6-
Procyclidine	T44.3x1-	T44.3x2-	T44.3x3-	T44.3x4-	T44.3x5-	T44.3x6-
Producer gas	T58.8x1-	T58.8x2-	T58.8x3-	T58.8x4-	—	—
Profadol	T40.4x1-	T40.4x2-	T40.4x3-	T40.4x4-	T40.4x5-	T40.4x6-
Profenamine	T44.3x1-	T44.3x2-	T44.3x3-	T44.3x4-	T44.3x5-	T44.3x6-
Profenil	T44.3x1-	T44.3x2-	T44.3x3-	T44.3x4-	T44.3x5-	T44.3x6-
Proflavine	T49.0x1-	T49.0x2-	T49.0x3-	T49.0x4-	T49.0x5-	T49.0x6-
Progabide	T42.6x1-	T42.6x2-	T42.6x3-	T42.6x4-	T42.6x5-	T42.6x6-
Progesterone	T38.5x1-	T38.5x2-	T38.5x3-	T38.5x4-	T38.5x5-	T38.5x6-
Progestin	T38.5x1-	T38.5x2-	T38.5x3-	T38.5x4-	T38.5x5-	T38.5x6-
oral contraceptive	T38.4x1-	T38.4x2-	T38.4x3-	T38.4x4-	T38.4x5-	T38.4x6-
Progestogen NEC	T38.5x1-	T38.5x2-	T38.5x3-	T38.5x4-	T38.5x5-	T38.5x6-
Progestone	T38.5x1-	T38.5x2-	T38.5x3-	T38.5x4-	T38.5x5-	T38.5x6-
Proglumide	T47.1x1-	T47.1x2-	T47.1x3-	T47.1x4-	T47.1x5-	T47.1x6-
Proguanil	T37.2x1-	T37.2x2-	T37.2x3-	T37.2x4-	T37.2x5-	T37.2x6-
Prolactin	T38.811-	T38.812-	T38.813-	T38.814-	T38.815-	T38.816-
Prolintane	T43.691-	T43.692-	T43.693-	T43.694-	T43.695-	T43.696-
Proloid	T38.1x1-	T38.1x2-	T38.1x3-	T38.1x4-	T38.1x5-	T38.1x6-
Proluton	T38.5x1-	T38.5x2-	T38.5x3-	T38.5x4-	T38.5x5-	T38.5x6-
Promacetin	T37.1x1-	T37.1x2-	T37.1x3-	T37.1x4-	T37.1x5-	T37.1x6-
Promazine	T43.3x1-	T43.3x2-	T43.3x3-	T43.3x4-	T43.3x5-	T43.3x6-
Promedol	T40.2x1-	T40.2x2-	T40.2x3-	T40.2x4-	—	—
Promegestone	T38.5x1-	T38.5x2-	T38.5x3-	T38.5x4-	T38.5x5-	T38.5x6-
Promethazine (teoclate)	T43.3x1-	T43.3x2-	T43.3x3-	T43.3x4-	T43.3x5-	T43.3x6-
Promin	T37.1x1-	T37.1x2-	T37.1x3-	T37.1x4-	T37.1x5-	T37.1x6-
Pronase	T45.3x1-	T45.3x2-	T45.3x3-	T45.3x4-	T45.3x5-	T45.3x6-
Pronestyl (hydrochloride) ..	T46.2x1-	T46.2x2-	T46.2x3-	T46.2x4-	T46.2x5-	T46.2x6-
Pronetalol	T44.7x1-	T44.7x2-	T44.7x3-	T44.7x4-	T44.7x5-	T44.7x6-
Prontosil	T37.0x1-	T37.0x2-	T37.0x3-	T37.0x4-	T37.0x5-	T37.0x6-
Propachlor	T60.3x1-	T60.3x2-	T60.3x3-	T60.3x4-	—	—
Propafenone	T46.2x1-	T46.2x2-	T46.2x3-	T46.2x4-	T46.2x5-	T46.2x6-
Propallylonal	T42.3x1-	T42.3x2-	T42.3x3-	T42.3x4-	T42.3x5-	T42.3x6-
Propamidine	T49.0x1-	T49.0x2-	T49.0x3-	T49.0x4-	T49.0x5-	T49.0x6-
Propane (distributed in mobile container)	T59.891-	T59.892-	T59.893-	T59.894-	—	—
distributed through pipes	T59.891-	T59.892-	T59.893-	T59.894-	—	—
incomplete combustion ..	T58.11x-	T58.12x-	T58.13x-	T58.14x-	—	—
Propanidid	T41.291-	T41.292-	T41.293-	T41.294-	T41.295-	T41.296-
Propanil	T60.3x1-	T60.3x2-	T60.3x3-	T60.3x4-	—	—
1-Propanol	T51.3x1-	T51.3x2-	T51.3x3-	T51.3x4-	—	—
2-Propanol	T51.2x1-	T51.2x2-	T51.2x3-	T51.2x4-	—	—
Propantheline	T44.3x1-	T44.3x2-	T44.3x3-	T44.3x4-	T44.3x5-	T44.3x6-
bromide	T44.3x1-	T44.3x2-	T44.3x3-	T44.3x4-	T44.3x5-	T44.3x6-
Proparacaine	T41.3x1-	T41.3x2-	T41.3x3-	T41.3x4-	T41.3x5-	T41.3x6-
Propatylnitrate	T46.3x1-	T46.3x2-	T46.3x3-	T46.3x4-	T46.3x5-	T46.3x6-
Propicillin	T36.0x1-	T36.0x2-	T36.0x3-	T36.0x4-	T36.0x5-	T36.0x6-
Propiolactone	T49.0x1-	T49.0x2-	T49.0x3-	T49.0x4-	T49.0x5-	T49.0x6-
Propiomazine	T45.0x1-	T45.0x2-	T45.0x3-	T45.0x4-	T45.0x5-	T45.0x6-
Propion gel	T49.0x1-	T49.0x2-	T49.0x3-	T49.0x4-	T49.0x5-	T49.0x6-

Table of Drugs & Chemicals	POISONING Accidental (Unintentional)	Self-Harm (Intentional)	Assault	Undetermined	Adverse Effect	Underdosing
Propionaldehyde (medicinal)	T42.6x1-	T42.6x2-	T42.6x3-	T42.6x4-	T42.6x5-	T42.6x6-
Propionate (calcium) (sodium)	T49.0x1-	T49.0x2-	T49.0x3-	T49.0x4-	T49.0x5-	T49.0x6-
Propitocaine	T41.3x1-	T41.3x2-	T41.3x3-	T41.3x4-	T41.3x5-	T41.3x6-
infiltration (subcutaneous)	T41.3x1-	T41.3x2-	T41.3x3-	T41.3x4-	T41.3x5-	T41.3x6-
nerve block (peripheral) (plexus)	T41.3x1-	T41.3x2-	T41.3x3-	T41.3x4-	T41.3x5-	T41.3x6-
Propofol	T41.291-	T41.292-	T41.293-	T41.294-	T41.295-	T41.296-
Propoxur	T60.0x1-	T60.0x2-	T60.0x3-	T60.0x4-	—	—
Propoxycaine	T41.3x1-	T41.3x2-	T41.3x3-	T41.3x4-	T41.3x5-	T41.3x6-
infiltration (subcutaneous)	T41.3x1-	T41.3x2-	T41.3x3-	T41.3x4-	T41.3x5-	T41.3x6-
nerve block (peripheral) (plexus)	T41.3x1-	T41.3x2-	T41.3x3-	T41.3x4-	T41.3x5-	T41.3x6-
topical (surface)	T41.3x1-	T41.3x2-	T41.3x3-	T41.3x4-	T41.3x5-	T41.3x6-
Propoxyphene	T40.4x1-	T40.4x2-	T40.4x3-	T40.4x4-	T40.4x5-	T40.4x6-
Propranolol	T44.7x1-	T44.7x2-	T44.7x3-	T44.7x4-	T44.7x5-	T44.7x6-
Propyl						
alcohol	T51.3x1-	T51.3x2-	T51.3x3-	T51.3x4-	—	—
carbinol	T51.3x1-	T51.3x2-	T51.3x3-	T51.3x4-	—	—
hexadrine	T44.4x1-	T44.4x2-	T44.4x3-	T44.4x4-	T44.4x5-	T44.4x6-
iodone	T50.8x1-	T50.8x2-	T50.8x3-	T50.8x4-	T50.8x5-	T50.8x6-
thiouracil	T38.2x1-	T38.2x2-	T38.2x3-	T38.2x4-	T38.2x5-	T38.2x6-
Propylaminophenothiazine	T43.3x1-	T43.3x2-	T43.3x3-	T43.3x4-	T43.3x5-	T43.3x6-
Propylene	T59.891-	T59.892-	T59.893-	T59.894-	—	—
Propylhexedrine	T48.5x1-	T48.5x2-	T48.5x3-	T48.5x4-	T48.5x5-	T48.5x6-
Propyliodone	T50.8x1-	T50.8x2-	T50.8x3-	T50.8x4-	T50.8x5-	T50.8x6-
Propylparaben (ophthalmic)	T49.5x1-	T49.5x2-	T49.5x3-	T49.5x4-	T49.5x5-	T49.5x6-
Propylthiouracil	T38.2x1-	T38.2x2-	T38.2x3-	T38.2x4-	T38.2x5-	T38.2x6-
Propyphenazone	T39.2x1-	T39.2x2-	T39.2x3-	T39.2x4-	T39.2x5-	T39.2x6-
Proquazone	T39.391-	T39.392-	T39.393-	T39.394-	T39.395-	T39.396-
Proscillaridin	T46.0x1-	T46.0x2-	T46.0x3-	T46.0x4-	T46.0x5-	T46.0x6-
Prostacyclin	T45.521-	T45.522-	T45.523-	T45.524-	T45.525-	T45.526-
Prostaglandin (I2)	T45.521-	T45.522-	T45.523-	T45.524-	T45.525-	T45.526-
E1	T46.7x1-	T46.7x2-	T46.7x3-	T46.7x4-	T46.7x5-	T46.7x6-
E2	T48.0x1-	T48.0x2-	T48.0x3-	T48.0x4-	T48.0x5-	T48.0x6-
F2 alpha	T48.0x1-	T48.0x2-	T48.0x3-	T48.0x4-	T48.0x5-	T48.0x6-
Prostigmin	T44.0x1-	T44.0x2-	T44.0x3-	T44.0x4-	T44.0x5-	T44.0x6-
Prosultiamine	T45.2x1-	T45.2x2-	T45.2x3-	T45.2x4-	T45.2x5-	T45.2x6-
Protamine sulfate	T45.7x1-	T45.7x2-	T45.7x3-	T45.7x4-	T45.7x5-	T45.7x6-
zinc insulin	T38.3x1-	T38.3x2-	T38.3x3-	T38.3x4-	T38.3x5-	T38.3x6-
Protease	T47.5x1-	T47.5x2-	T47.5x3-	T47.5x4-	T47.5x5-	T47.5x6-
Protectant, skin NEC	T49.3x1-	T49.3x2-	T49.3x3-	T49.3x4-	T49.3x5-	T49.3x6-
Protein hydrolysate	T50.991-	T50.992-	T50.993-	T50.994-	T50.995-	T50.996-
Prothiaden — see Dothiepin hydrochloride						
Prothionamide	T37.1x1-	T37.1x2-	T37.1x3-	T37.1x4-	T37.1x5-	T37.1x6-
Prothipendyl	T43.591-	T43.592-	T43.593-	T43.594-	T43.595-	T43.596-
Prothoate	T60.0x1-	T60.0x2-	T60.0x3-	T60.0x4-	—	—
Prothrombin						
activator	T45.7x1-	T45.7x2-	T45.7x3-	T45.7x4-	T45.7x5-	T45.7x6-
synthesis inhibitor	T45.511-	T45.512-	T45.513-	T45.514-	T45.515-	T45.516-
Protionamide	T37.1x1-	T37.1x2-	T37.1x3-	T37.1x4-	T37.1x5-	T37.1x6-
Protirelin	T38.891-	T38.892-	T38.893-	T38.894-	T38.895-	T38.896-
Protokylol	T48.6x1-	T48.6x2-	T48.6x3-	T48.6x4-	T48.6x5-	T48.6x6-
Protopam	T50.6x1-	T50.6x2-	T50.6x3-	T50.6x4-	T50.6x5-	T50.6x6-
Protoveratrine(s) (A) (B)	T46.5x1-	T46.5x2-	T46.5x3-	T46.5x4-	T46.5x5-	T46.5x6-
Protriptyline	T43.011-	T43.012-	T43.013-	T43.014-	T43.015-	T43.016-
Provera	T38.5x1-	T38.5x2-	T38.5x3-	T38.5x4-	T38.5x5-	T38.5x6-
Provitamin A	T45.2x1-	T45.2x2-	T45.2x3-	T45.2x4-	T45.2x5-	T45.2x6-
Proxibarbal	T42.3x1-	T42.3x2-	T42.3x3-	T42.3x4-	T42.3x5-	T42.3x6-
Proxymetacaine	T41.3x1-	T41.3x2-	T41.3x3-	T41.3x4-	T41.3x5-	T41.3x6-
Proxyphylline	T48.6x1-	T48.6x2-	T48.6x3-	T48.6x4-	T48.6x5-	T48.6x6-
Prozac — see Fluoxetine hydrochloride						
Prunus						
laurocerasus	T62.2x1-	T62.2x2-	T62.2x3-	T62.2x4-	—	—
virginiana	T62.2x1-	T62.2x2-	T62.2x3-	T62.2x4-	—	—
Prussian blue						
commercial	T65.891-	T65.892-	T65.893-	T65.894-	—	—
therapeutic	T50.6x1-	T50.6x2-	T50.6x3-	T50.6x4-	T50.6x5-	T50.6x6-
Prussic acid	T65.0x1-	T65.0x2-	T65.0x3-	T65.0x4-	—	—
vapor	T57.3x1-	T57.3x2-	T57.3x3-	T57.3x4-	—	—
Pseudoephedrine	T44.991-	T44.992-	T44.993-	T44.994-	T44.995-	T44.996-
Psilocin	T40.991-	T40.992-	T40.993-	T40.994-	—	—
Psilocybin	T40.991-	T40.992-	T40.993-	T40.994-	—	—
Psilocybine	T40.991-	T40.992-	T40.993-	T40.994-	—	—
Psoralene (nonmedicinal)	T65.891-	T65.892-	T65.893-	T65.894-	—	—
Psoralens (medicinal)	T50.991-	T50.992-	T50.993-	T50.994-	T50.995-	T50.996-
PSP (phenolsulfon-phthalein)	T50.8x1-	T50.8x2-	T50.8x3-	T50.8x4-	T50.8x5-	T50.8x6-
Psychodysleptic drug NEC	T40.901-	T40.902-	T40.903-	T40.904-	T40.905-	T40.906-
Psychostimulant	T43.601-	T43.602-	T43.603-	T43.604-	T43.605-	T43.606-
amphetamine	T43.621-	T43.622-	T43.623-	T43.624-	T43.625-	T43.626-
caffeine	T43.611-	T43.612-	T43.613-	T43.614-	T43.615-	T43.616-
methylphenidate	T43.631-	T43.632-	T43.633-	T43.634-	T43.635-	T43.636-
specified NEC	T43.691-	T43.692-	T43.693-	T43.694-	T43.695-	T43.696-
Psychotherapeutic drug NEC	T43.91x-	T43.92x-	T43.93x-	T43.94x-	T43.95x-	T43.96x-
antidepressants — see also Antidepressant						
specified NEC	T43.8x1-	T43.8x2-	T43.8x3-	T43.8x4-	T43.8x5-	T43.8x6-
tranquilizers NEC	T43.501-	T43.502-	T43.503-	T43.504-	T43.505-	T43.506-
Psychotomimetic agents	T40.901-	T40.902-	T40.903-	T40.904-	T40.905-	T40.906-
Psychotropic drug NEC	T43.91x-	T43.92x-	T43.93x-	T43.94x-	T43.95x-	T43.96x-
specified NEC	T43.8x1-	T43.8x2-	T43.8x3-	T43.8x4-	T43.8x5-	T43.8x6-
Psyllium hydrophilic mucilloid	T47.4x1-	T47.4x2-	T47.4x3-	T47.4x4-	T47.4x5-	T47.4x6-
Pteroylglutamic acid	T45.8x1-	T45.8x2-	T45.8x3-	T45.8x4-	T45.8x5-	T45.8x6-
Pteroyltriglutamate	T45.1x1-	T45.1x2-	T45.1x3-	T45.1x4-	T45.1x5-	T45.1x6-
PTFE — see Polytetrafluoroethylene						
Pulp						
devitalizing paste	T49.7x1-	T49.7x2-	T49.7x3-	T49.7x4-	T49.7x5-	T49.7x6-
dressing	T49.7x1-	T49.7x2-	T49.7x3-	T49.7x4-	T49.7x5-	T49.7x6-
Pulsatilla	T62.2x1-	T62.2x2-	T62.2x3-	T62.2x4-	—	—
Pumpkin seed extract	T37.4x1-	T37.4x2-	T37.4x3-	T37.4x4-	T37.4x5-	T37.4x6-
Purex (bleach)	T54.91x-	T54.92x-	T54.93x-	T54.94x-	—	—
Purgative NEC — see also Cathartic	T47.4x1-	T47.4x2-	T47.4x3-	T47.4x4-	T47.4x5-	T47.4x6-
Purine analogue (antineoplastic)	T45.1x1-	T45.1x2-	T45.1x3-	T45.1x4-	T45.1x5-	T45.1x6-
Purine diuretics	T50.2x1-	T50.2x2-	T50.2x3-	T50.2x4-	T50.2x5-	T50.2x6-
Purinethol	T45.1x1-	T45.1x2-	T45.1x3-	T45.1x4-	T45.1x5-	T45.1x6-
PVP	T45.8x1-	T45.8x2-	T45.8x3-	T45.8x4-	T45.8x5-	T45.8x6-
Pyrabital	T39.8x1-	T39.8x2-	T39.8x3-	T39.8x4-	T39.8x5-	T39.8x6-
Pyramidon	T39.2x1-	T39.2x2-	T39.2x3-	T39.2x4-	T39.2x5-	T39.2x6-
Pyrantel	T37.4x1-	T37.4x2-	T37.4x3-	T37.4x4-	T37.4x5-	T37.4x6-
Pyrathiazine	T45.0x1-	T45.0x2-	T45.0x3-	T45.0x4-	T45.0x5-	T45.0x6-
Pyrazinamide	T37.1x1-	T37.1x2-	T37.1x3-	T37.1x4-	T37.1x5-	T37.1x6-
Pyrazinoic acid (amide)	T37.1x1-	T37.1x2-	T37.1x3-	T37.1x4-	T37.1x5-	T37.1x6-
Pyrazole (derivatives)	T39.2x1-	T39.2x2-	T39.2x3-	T39.2x4-	T39.2x5-	T39.2x6-
Pyrazolone analgesic NEC	T39.2x1-	T39.2x2-	T39.2x3-	T39.2x4-	T39.2x5-	T39.2x6-

DRUGS & CHEMICALS

DRUGS & CHEMICALS

Table of Drugs & Chemicals	Accidental (Unintentional)	Self-Harm (Intentional)	Assault	Undetermined	Adverse Effect	Underdosing
Pyrethrin, pyrethrum (nonmedicinal)	T60.2x1-	T60.2x2-	T60.2x3-	T60.2x4-	—	—
Pyrethrum extract	T49.0x1-	T49.0x2-	T49.0x3-	T49.0x4-	T49.0x5-	T49.0x6-
Pyribenzamine	T45.0x1-	T45.0x2-	T45.0x3-	T45.0x4-	T45.0x5-	T45.0x6-
Pyridine	T52.8x1-	T52.8x2-	T52.8x3-	T52.8x4-	—	—
aldoxime methiodide	T50.6x1-	T50.6x2-	T50.6x3-	T50.6x4-	T50.6x5-	T50.6x6-
aldoxime methyl chloride	T50.6x1-	T50.6x2-	T50.6x3-	T50.6x4-	T50.6x5-	T50.6x6-
vapor	T59.891-	T59.892-	T59.893-	T59.894-		
Pyridium	T39.8x1-	T39.8x2-	T39.8x3-	T39.8x4-	T39.8x5-	T39.8x6-
Pyridostigmine bromide	T44.0x1-	T44.0x2-	T44.0x3-	T44.0x4-	T44.0x5-	T44.0x6-
Pyridoxal phosphate	T45.2x1-	T45.2x2-	T45.2x3-	T45.2x4-	T45.2x5-	T45.2x6-
Pyridoxine	T45.2x1-	T45.2x2-	T45.2x3-	T45.2x4-	T45.2x5-	T45.2x6-
Pyrilamine	T45.0x1-	T45.0x2-	T45.0x3-	T45.0x4-	T45.0x5-	T45.0x6-
Pyrimethamine	T37.2x1-	T37.2x2-	T37.2x3-	T37.2x4-	T37.2x5-	T37.2x6-
with sulfadoxine	T37.2x1-	T37.2x2-	T37.2x3-	T37.2x4-	T37.2x5-	T37.2x6-
Pyrimidine antagonist	T45.1x1-	T45.1x2-	T45.1x3-	T45.1x4-	T45.1x5-	T45.1x6-
Pyriminil	T60.4x1-	T60.4x2-	T60.4x3-	T60.4x4-	—	—
Pyrithione zinc	T49.4x1-	T49.4x2-	T49.4x3-	T49.4x4-	T49.4x5-	T49.4x6-
Pyrithyldione	T42.6x1-	T42.6x2-	T42.6x3-	T42.6x4-	T42.6x5-	T42.6x6-
Pyrogallic acid	T49.0x1-	T49.0x2-	T49.0x3-	T49.0x4-	T49.0x5-	T49.0x6-
Pyrogallol	T49.0x1-	T49.0x2-	T49.0x3-	T49.0x4-	T49.0x5-	T49.0x6-
Pyroxylin	T49.3x1-	T49.3x2-	T49.3x3-	T49.3x4-	T49.3x5-	T49.3x6-
Pyrrobutamine	T45.0x1-	T45.0x2-	T45.0x3-	T45.0x4-	T45.0x5-	T45.0x6-
Pyrrolizidine alkaloids	T62.8x1-	T62.8x2-	T62.8x3-	T62.8x4-	—	—
Pyrvinium chloride	T37.4x1-	T37.4x2-	T37.4x3-	T37.4x4-	T37.4x5-	T37.4x6-
PZI	T38.3x1-	T38.3x2-	T38.3x3-	T38.3x4-	T38.3x5-	T38.3x6-
Quaalude	T42.6x1-	T42.6x2-	T42.6x3-	T42.6x4-	T42.6x5-	T42.6x6-
Quarternary ammonium anti-infective	T49.0x1-	T49.0x2-	T49.0x3-	T49.0x4-	T49.0x5-	T49.0x6-
ganglion blocking	T44.2x1-	T44.2x2-	T44.2x3-	T44.2x4-	T44.2x5-	T44.2x6-
parasympatholytic	T44.3x1-	T44.3x2-	T44.3x3-	T44.3x4-	T44.3x5-	T44.3x6-
Quazepam	T42.4x1-	T42.4x2-	T42.4x3-	T42.4x4-	T42.4x5-	T42.4x6-
Quicklime	T54.3x1-	T54.3x2-	T54.3x3-	T54.3x4-	—	—
Quillaja extract	T48.4x1-	T48.4x2-	T48.4x3-	T48.4x4-	T48.4x5-	T48.4x6-
Quinacrine	T37.2x1-	T37.2x2-	T37.2x3-	T37.2x4-	T37.2x5-	T37.2x6-
Quinaglute	T46.2x1-	T46.2x2-	T46.2x3-	T46.2x4-	T46.2x5-	T46.2x6-
Quinalbarbital	T42.3x1-	T42.3x2-	T42.3x3-	T42.3x4-	T42.3x5-	T42.3x6-
Quinalbarbitone sodium	T42.3x1-	T42.3x2-	T42.3x3-	T42.3x4-	T42.3x5-	T42.3x6-
Quinalphos	T60.0x1-	T60.0x2-	T60.0x3-	T60.0x4-	—	—
Quinapril	T46.4x1-	T46.4x2-	T46.4x3-	T46.4x4-	T46.4x5-	T46.4x6-
Quinestradiol	T38.5x1-	T38.5x2-	T38.5x3-	T38.5x4-	T38.5x5-	T38.5x6-
Quinestradol	T38.5x1-	T38.5x2-	T38.5x3-	T38.5x4-	T38.5x5-	T38.5x6-
Quinestrol	T38.5x1-	T38.5x2-	T38.5x3-	T38.5x4-	T38.5x5-	T38.5x6-
Quinethazone	T50.2x1-	T50.2x2-	T50.2x3-	T50.2x4-	T50.2x5-	T50.2x6-
Quingestanol	T38.4x1-	T38.4x2-	T38.4x3-	T38.4x4-	T38.4x5-	T38.4x6-
Quinidine	T46.2x1-	T46.2x2-	T46.2x3-	T46.2x4-	T46.2x5-	T46.2x6-
Quinine	T37.2x1-	T37.2x2-	T37.2x3-	T37.2x4-	T37.2x5-	T37.2x6-
Quiniobine	T37.8x1-	T37.8x2-	T37.8x3-	T37.8x4-	T37.8x5-	T37.8x6-
Quinisocaine	T49.1x1-	T49.1x2-	T49.1x3-	T49.1x4-	T49.1x5-	T49.1x6-
Quinocide	T37.2x1-	T37.2x2-	T37.2x3-	T37.2x4-	T37.2x5-	T37.2x6-
Quinoline (derivatives) NEC	T37.8x1-	T37.8x2-	T37.8x3-	T37.8x4-	T37.8x5-	T37.8x6-
Quinupramine	T43.011-	T43.012-	T43.013-	T43.014-	T43.015-	T43.016-
Quotane	T41.3x1-	T41.3x2-	T41.3x3-	T41.3x4-	T41.3x5-	T41.3x6-
Rabies immune globulin (human)	T50.Z11-	T50.Z12-	T50.Z13-	T50.Z14-	T50.Z15-	T50.Z16-
vaccine	T50.B91-	T50.B92-	T50.B93-	T50.B94-	T50.B95-	T50.B96-
Racemoramide	T40.2x1-	T40.2x2-	T40.2x3-	T40.2x4-	—	—
Racemorphan	T40.2x1-	T40.2x2-	T40.2x3-	T40.2x4-	T40.2x5-	T40.2x6-
Racepinefrin	T44.5x1-	T44.5x2-	T44.5x3-	T44.5x4-	T44.5x5-	T44.5x6-
Raclopride	T43.591-	T43.592-	T43.593-	T43.594-	T43.595-	T43.596-
Radiator alcohol	T51.1x1-	T51.1x2-	T51.1x3-	T51.1x4-		
Radioactive drug NEC	T50.8x1-	T50.8x2-	T50.8x3-	T50.8x4-	T50.8x5-	T50.8x6-
Radio-opaque (drugs) (materials)	T50.8x1-	T50.8x2-	T50.8x3-	T50.8x4-	T50.8x5-	T50.8x6-
Ramifenazone	T39.2x1-	T39.2x2-	T39.2x3-	T39.2x4-	T39.2x5-	T39.2x6-
Ramipril	T46.4x1-	T46.4x2-	T46.4x3-	T46.4x4-	T46.4x5-	T46.4x6-
Ranitidine	T47.0x1-	T47.0x2-	T47.0x3-	T47.0x4-	T47.0x5-	T47.0x6-
Ranunculus	T62.2x1-	T62.2x2-	T62.2x3-	T62.2x4-	—	—
Rat poison NEC	T60.4x1-	T60.4x2-	T60.4x3-	T60.4x4-		
Rattlesnake (venom)	T63.011-	T63.012-	T63.013-	T63.014-		
Raubasine	T46.7x1-	T46.7x2-	T46.7x3-	T46.7x4-	T46.7x5-	T46.7x6-
Raudixin	T46.5x1-	T46.5x2-	T46.5x3-	T46.5x4-	T46.5x5-	T46.5x6-
Rautensin	T46.5x1-	T46.5x2-	T46.5x3-	T46.5x4-	T46.5x5-	T46.5x6-
Rautina	T46.5x1-	T46.5x2-	T46.5x3-	T46.5x4-	T46.5x5-	T46.5x6-
Rautotal	T46.5x1-	T46.5x2-	T46.5x3-	T46.5x4-	T46.5x5-	T46.5x6-
Rauwiloid	T46.5x1-	T46.5x2-	T46.5x3-	T46.5x4-	T46.5x5-	T46.5x6-
Rauwoldin	T46.5x1-	T46.5x2-	T46.5x3-	T46.5x4-	T46.5x5-	T46.5x6-
Rauwolfia (alkaloids)	T46.5x1-	T46.5x2-	T46.5x3-	T46.5x4-	T46.5x5-	T46.5x6-
Razoxane	T45.1x1-	T45.1x2-	T45.1x3-	T45.1x4-	T45.1x5-	T45.1x6-
Realgar	T57.0x1-	T57.0x2-	T57.0x3-	T57.0x4-	—	—
Recombinant (R) — see specific protein						
Red blood cells, packed	T45.8x1-	T45.8x2-	T45.8x3-	T45.8x4-	T45.8x5-	T45.8x6-
Red squill (scilliroside)	T60.4x1-	T60.4x2-	T60.4x3-	T60.4x4-	—	—
Reducing agent, industrial NEC	T65.891-	T65.892-	T65.893-	T65.894-	—	—
Refrigerant gas (chlorofluoro-carbon)	T53.5x1-	T53.5x2-	T53.5x3-	T53.5x4-	—	—
not chlorofluoro-carbon	T59.891-	T59.892-	T59.893-	T59.894-	—	—
Regroton	T50.2x1-	T50.2x2-	T50.2x3-	T50.2x4-	T50.2x5-	T50.2x6-
Rehydration salts (oral)	T50.3x1-	T50.3x2-	T50.3x3-	T50.3x4-	T50.3x5-	T50.3x6-
Rela	T42.8x1-	T42.8x2-	T42.8x3-	T42.8x4-	T42.8x5-	T42.8x6-
Relaxant, muscle anesthetic	T48.1x1-	T48.1x2-	T48.1x3-	T48.1x4-	T48.1x5-	T48.1x6-
central nervous system	T42.8x1-	T42.8x2-	T42.8x3-	T42.8x4-	T42.8x5-	T42.8x6-
skeletal NEC	T48.1x1-	T48.1x2-	T48.1x3-	T48.1x4-	T48.1x5-	T48.1x6-
smooth NEC	T44.3x1-	T44.3x2-	T44.3x3-	T44.3x4-	T44.3x5-	T44.3x6-
Remoxipride	T43.591-	T43.592-	T43.593-	T43.594-	T43.595-	T43.596-
Renese	T50.2x1-	T50.2x2-	T50.2x3-	T50.2x4-	T50.2x5-	T50.2x6-
Renografin	T50.8x1-	T50.8x2-	T50.8x3-	T50.8x4-	T50.8x5-	T50.8x6-
Replacement solution	T50.3x1-	T50.3x2-	T50.3x3-	T50.3x4-	T50.3x5-	T50.3x6-
Reproterol	T48.6x1-	T48.6x2-	T48.6x3-	T48.6x4-	T48.6x5-	T48.6x6-
Rescinnamine	T46.5x1-	T46.5x2-	T46.5x3-	T46.5x4-	T46.5x5-	T46.5x6-
Reserpin(e)	T46.5x1-	T46.5x2-	T46.5x3-	T46.5x4-	T46.5x5-	T46.5x6-
Resorcin, resorcinol (nonmedicinal)	T65.891-	T65.892-	T65.893-	T65.894-	—	—
medicinal	T49.4x1-	T49.4x2-	T49.4x3-	T49.4x4-	T49.4x5-	T49.4x6-
Respaire	T48.4x1-	T48.4x2-	T48.4x3-	T48.4x4-	T48.4x5-	T48.4x6-
Respiratory drug NEC	T48.901-	T48.902-	T48.903-	T48.904-	T48.905-	T48.906-
antiasthmatic NEC	T48.6x1-	T48.6x2-	T48.6x3-	T48.6x4-	T48.6x5-	T48.6x6-
anti-common-cold NEC	T48.5x1-	T48.5x2-	T48.5x3-	T48.5x4-	T48.5x5-	T48.5x6-
expectorant NEC	T48.4x1-	T48.4x2-	T48.4x3-	T48.4x4-	T48.4x5-	T48.4x6-
stimulant	T48.901-	T48.902-	T48.903-	T48.904-	T48.905-	T48.906-
Retinoic acid	T49.0x1-	T49.0x2-	T49.0x3-	T49.0x4-	T49.0x5-	T49.0x6-
Retinol	T45.2x1-	T45.2x2-	T45.2x3-	T45.2x4-	T45.2x5-	T45.2x6-
Rh (D) immune globulin (human)	T50.Z11-	T50.Z12-	T50.Z13-	T50.Z14-	T50.Z15-	T50.Z16-
Rhodine	T39.011-	T39.012-	T39.013-	T39.014-	T39.015-	T39.016-
RhoGAM	T50.Z11-	T50.Z12-	T50.Z13-	T50.Z14-	T50.Z15-	T50.Z16-
Rhubarb dry extract	T47.2x1-	T47.2x2-	T47.2x3-	T47.2x4-	T47.2x5-	T47.2x6-
tincture, compound	T47.2x1-	T47.2x2-	T47.2x3-	T47.2x4-	T47.2x5-	T47.2x6-

DRUGS & CHEMICALS

Table of Drugs & Chemicals	POISONING Accidental (Unintentional)	Self-Harm (Intentional)	Assault	Undetermined	Adverse Effect	Underdosing
Ribavirin	T37.5x1-	T37.5x2-	T37.5x3-	T37.5x4-	T37.5x5-	T37.5x6-
Riboflavin	T45.2x1-	T45.2x2-	T45.2x3-	T45.2x4-	T45.2x5-	T45.2x6-
Ribostamycin	T36.5x1-	T36.5x2-	T36.5x3-	T36.5x4-	T36.5x5-	T36.5x6-
Ricin	T62.2x1-	T62.2x2-	T62.2x3-	T62.2x4-	—	—
Ricinus communis	T62.2x1-	T62.2x2-	T62.2x3-	T62.2x4-	—	—
Rickettsial vaccine NEC	T50.A91-	T50.A92-	T50.A93-	T50.A94-	T50.A95-	T50.A96-
Rifabutin	T36.6x1-	T36.6x2-	T36.6x3-	T36.6x4-	T36.6x5-	T36.6x6-
Rifamide	T36.6x1-	T36.6x2-	T36.6x3-	T36.6x4-	T36.6x5-	T36.6x6-
Rifampicin	T36.6x1-	T36.6x2-	T36.6x3-	T36.6x4-	T36.6x5-	T36.6x6-
with isoniazid	T37.1x1-	T37.1x2-	T37.1x3-	T37.1x4-	T37.1x5-	T37.1x6-
Rifampin	T36.6x1-	T36.6x2-	T36.6x3-	T36.6x4-	T36.6x5-	T36.6x6-
Rifamycin	T36.6x1-	T36.6x2-	T36.6x3-	T36.6x4-	T36.6x5-	T36.6x6-
Rifaximin	T36.6x1-	T36.6x2-	T36.6x3-	T36.6x4-	T36.6x5-	T36.6x6-
Rimantadine	T37.5x1-	T37.5x2-	T37.5x3-	T37.5x4-	T37.5x5-	T37.5x6-
Rimazolium metilsulfate	T39.8x1-	T39.8x2-	T39.8x3-	T39.8x4-	T39.8x5-	T39.8x6-
Rimifon	T37.1x1-	T37.1x2-	T37.1x3-	T37.1x4-	T37.1x5-	T37.1x6-
Rimiterol	T48.6x1-	T48.6x2-	T48.6x3-	T48.6x4-	T48.6x5-	T48.6x6-
Ringer (lactate) solution	T50.3x1-	T50.3x2-	T50.3x3-	T50.3x4-	T50.3x5-	T50.3x6-
Ristocetin	T36.8x1-	T36.8x2-	T36.8x3-	T36.8x4-	T36.8x5-	T36.8x6-
Ritalin	T43.631-	T43.632-	T43.633-	T43.634-	T43.635-	T43.636-
Ritodrine	T44.5x1-	T44.5x2-	T44.5x3-	T44.5x4-	T44.5x5-	T44.5x6-
Roach killer — see Insecticide						
Rociverine	T44.3x1-	T44.3x2-	T44.3x3-	T44.3x4-	T44.3x5-	T44.3x6-
Rocky Mountain spotted fever vaccine	T50.A91-	T50.A92-	T50.A93-	T50.A94-	T50.A95-	T50.A96-
Rodenticide NEC	T60.4x1-	T60.4x2-	T60.4x3-	T60.4x4-	—	—
Rohypnol	T42.4x1-	T42.4x2-	T42.4x3-	T42.4x4-	T42.4x5-	T42.4x6-
Rokitamycin	T36.3x1-	T36.3x2-	T36.3x3-	T36.3x4-	T36.3x5-	T36.3x6-
Rolaids	T47.1x1-	T47.1x2-	T47.1x3-	T47.1x4-	T47.1x5-	T47.1x6-
Rolitetracycline	T36.4x1-	T36.4x2-	T36.4x3-	T36.4x4-	T36.4x5-	T36.4x6-
Romilar	T48.3x1-	T48.3x2-	T48.3x3-	T48.3x4-	T48.3x5-	T48.3x6-
Ronifibrate	T46.6x1-	T46.6x2-	T46.6x3-	T46.6x4-	T46.6x5-	T46.6x6-
Rosaprostol	T47.1x1-	T47.1x2-	T47.1x3-	T47.1x4-	T47.1x5-	T47.1x6-
Rose bengal sodium (131I)	T50.8x1-	T50.8x2-	T50.8x3-	T50.8x4-	T50.8x5-	T50.8x6-
Rose water ointment	T49.3x1-	T49.3x2-	T49.3x3-	T49.3x4-	T49.3x5-	T49.3x6-
Rosoxacin	T37.8x1-	T37.8x2-	T37.8x3-	T37.8x4-	T37.8x5-	T37.8x6-
Rotenone	T60.2x1-	T60.2x2-	T60.2x3-	T60.2x4-	—	—
Rotoxamine	T45.0x1-	T45.0x2-	T45.0x3-	T45.0x4-	T45.0x5-	T45.0x6-
Rough-on-rats	T60.4x1-	T60.4x2-	T60.4x3-	T60.4x4-	—	—
Roxatidine	T47.0x1-	T47.0x2-	T47.0x3-	T47.0x4-	T47.0x5-	T47.0x6-
Roxithromycin	T36.3x1-	T36.3x2-	T36.3x3-	T36.3x4-	T36.3x5-	T36.3x6-
Rt-PA	T45.611-	T45.612-	T45.613-	T45.614-	T45.615-	T45.616-
Rubbing alcohol	T51.2x1-	T51.2x2-	T51.2x3-	T51.2x4-	—	—
Rubefacient	T49.4x1-	T49.4x2-	T49.4x3-	T49.4x4-	T49.4x5-	T49.4x6-
Rubella vaccine	T50.B91-	T50.B92-	T50.B93-	T50.B94-	T50.B95-	T50.B96-
Rubeola vaccine	T50.B91-	T50.B92-	T50.B93-	T50.B94-	T50.B95-	T50.B96-
Rubidium chloride Rb82	T50.8x1-	T50.8x2-	T50.8x3-	T50.8x4-	T50.8x5-	T50.8x6-
Rubidomycin	T45.1x1-	T45.1x2-	T45.1x3-	T45.1x4-	T45.1x5-	T45.1x6-
Rue	T62.2x1-	T62.2x2-	T62.2x3-	T62.2x4-	—	—
Rufocromomycin	T45.1x1-	T45.1x2-	T45.1x3-	T45.1x4-	T45.1x5-	T45.1x6-
Russel's viper venin	T45.7x1-	T45.7x2-	T45.7x3-	T45.7x4-	T45.7x5-	T45.7x6-
Ruta (graveolens)	T62.2x1-	T62.2x2-	T62.2x3-	T62.2x4-	—	—
Rutinum	T46.991-	T46.992-	T46.993-	T46.994-	T46.995-	T46.996-
Rutoside	T46.991-	T46.992-	T46.993-	T46.994-	T46.995-	T46.996-
Sabadilla (plant)	T62.2x1-	T62.2x2-	T62.2x3-	T62.2x4-	—	—
pesticide	T60.2x1-	T60.2x2-	T60.2x3-	T60.2x4-	—	—
Saccharated iron oxide	T45.8x1-	T45.8x2-	T45.8x3-	T45.8x4-	T45.8x5-	T45.8x6-
Saccharin	T50.901-	T50.902-	T50.903-	T50.904-	T50.905-	T50.906-
Saccharomyces boulardii	T47.6x1-	T47.6x2-	T47.6x3-	T47.6x4-	T47.6x5-	T47.6x6-
Safflower oil	T46.6x1-	T46.6x2-	T46.6x3-	T46.6x4-	T46.6x5-	T46.6x6-
Safrazine	T43.1x1-	T43.1x2-	T43.1x3-	T43.1x4-	T43.1x5-	T43.1x6-
Salazosulfapyridine	T37.0x1-	T37.0x2-	T37.0x3-	T37.0x4-	T37.0x5-	T37.0x6-
Salbutamol	T48.6x1-	T48.6x2-	T48.6x3-	T48.6x4-	T48.6x5-	T48.6x6-
Salicylamide	T39.091-	T39.092-	T39.093-	T39.094-	T39.095-	T39.096-
Salicylate NEC	T39.091-	T39.092-	T39.093-	T39.094-	T39.095-	T39.096-
methyl	T49.3x1-	T49.3x2-	T49.3x3-	T49.3x4-	T49.3x5-	T49.3x6-
theobromine calcium	T50.2x1-	T50.2x2-	T50.2x3-	T50.2x4-	T50.2x5-	T50.2x6-
Salicylazosulfapyridine	T37.0x1-	T37.0x2-	T37.0x3-	T37.0x4-	T37.0x5-	T37.0x6-
Salicylhydroxamic acid	T49.0x1-	T49.0x2-	T49.0x3-	T49.0x4-	T49.0x5-	T49.0x6-
Salicylic acid	T49.4x1-	T49.4x2-	T49.4x3-	T49.4x4-	T49.4x5-	T49.4x6-
with benzoic acid	T49.4x1-	T49.4x2-	T49.4x3-	T49.4x4-	T49.4x5-	T49.4x6-
congeners	T39.091-	T39.092-	T39.093-	T39.094-	T39.095-	T39.096-
derivative	T39.091-	T39.092-	T39.093-	T39.094-	T39.095-	T39.096-
salts	T39.091-	T39.092-	T39.093-	T39.094-	T39.095-	T39.096-
Salinazid	T37.1x1-	T37.1x2-	T37.1x3-	T37.1x4-	T37.1x5-	T37.1x6-
Salmeterol	T48.6x1-	T48.6x2-	T48.6x3-	T48.6x4-	T48.6x5-	T48.6x6-
Salol	T49.3x1-	T49.3x2-	T49.3x3-	T49.3x4-	T49.3x5-	T49.3x6-
Salsalate	T39.091-	T39.092-	T39.093-	T39.094-	T39.095-	T39.096-
Salt substitute	T50.901-	T50.902-	T50.903-	T50.904-	T50.905-	T50.906-
Salt-replacing drug	T50.901-	T50.902-	T50.903-	T50.904-	T50.905-	T50.906-
Salt-retaining mineralocorticoid	T50.0x1-	T50.0x2-	T50.0x3-	T50.0x4-	T50.0x5-	T50.0x6-
Saluretic NEC	T50.2x1-	T50.2x2-	T50.2x3-	T50.2x4-	T50.2x5-	T50.2x6-
Saluron	T50.2x1-	T50.2x2-	T50.2x3-	T50.2x4-	T50.2x5-	T50.2x6-
Salvarsan 606 (neosilver) (silver)	T37.8x1-	T37.8x2-	T37.8x3-	T37.8x4-	T37.8x5-	T37.8x6-
Sambucus canadensis	T62.2x1-	T62.2x2-	T62.2x3-	T62.2x4-	—	—
berry	T62.1x1-	T62.1x2-	T62.1x3-	T62.1x4-	—	—
Sandril	T46.5x1-	T46.5x2-	T46.5x3-	T46.5x4-	T46.5x5-	T46.5x6-
Sanguinaria canadensis	T62.2x1-	T62.2x2-	T62.2x3-	T62.2x4-	—	—
Saniflush (cleaner)	T54.2x1-	T54.2x2-	T54.2x3-	T54.2x4-	—	—
Santonin	T37.4x1-	T37.4x2-	T37.4x3-	T37.4x4-	T37.4x5-	T37.4x6-
Santyl	T49.8x1-	T49.8x2-	T49.8x3-	T49.8x4-	T49.8x5-	T49.8x6-
Saralasin	T46.5x1-	T46.5x2-	T46.5x3-	T46.5x4-	T46.5x5-	T46.5x6-
Sarcolysin	T45.1x1-	T45.1x2-	T45.1x3-	T45.1x4-	T45.1x5-	T45.1x6-
Sarkomycin	T45.1x1-	T45.1x2-	T45.1x3-	T45.1x4-	T45.1x5-	T45.1x6-
Saroten	T43.011-	T43.012-	T43.013-	T43.014-	T43.015-	T43.016-
Saturnine — see Lead						
Savin (oil)	T49.4x1-	T49.4x2-	T49.4x3-	T49.4x4-	T49.4x5-	T49.4x6-
Scammony	T47.2x1-	T47.2x2-	T47.2x3-	T47.2x4-	T47.2x5-	T47.2x6-
Scarlet red	T49.8x1-	T49.8x2-	T49.8x3-	T49.8x4-	T49.8x5-	T49.8x6-
Scheele's green	T57.0x1-	T57.0x2-	T57.0x3-	T57.0x4-	—	—
insecticide	T57.0x1-	T57.0x2-	T57.0x3-	T57.0x4-	—	—
Schizontozide (blood) (tissue)	T37.2x1-	T37.2x2-	T37.2x3-	T37.2x4-	T37.2x5-	T37.2x6-
Schradan	T60.0x1-	T60.0x2-	T60.0x3-	T60.0x4-	—	—
Schweinfurth green	T57.0x1-	T57.0x2-	T57.0x3-	T57.0x4-	—	—
insecticide	T57.0x1-	T57.0x2-	T57.0x3-	T57.0x4-	—	—
Scilla, rat poison	T60.4x1-	T60.4x2-	T60.4x3-	T60.4x4-	—	—
Scillaren	T60.4x1-	T60.4x2-	T60.4x3-	T60.4x4-	—	—
Sclerosing agent	T46.8x1-	T46.8x2-	T46.8x3-	T46.8x4-	T46.8x5-	T46.8x6-
Scombrotoxin	T61.11x-	T61.12x-	T61.13x-	T61.14x-	—	—
Scopolamine	T44.3x1-	T44.3x2-	T44.3x3-	T44.3x4-	T44.3x5-	T44.3x6-
Scopolia extract	T44.3x1-	T44.3x2-	T44.3x3-	T44.3x4-	T44.3x5-	T44.3x6-
Scouring powder	T65.891-	T65.892-	T65.893-	T65.894-	—	—
Sea						
anemone (sting)	T63.631-	T63.632-	T63.633-	T63.634-	—	—
cucumber (sting)	T63.691-	T63.692-	T63.693-	T63.694-	—	—
snake (bite) (venom)	T63.091-	T63.092-	T63.093-	T63.094-	—	—
urchin spine (puncture)	T63.691-	T63.692-	T63.693-	T63.694-	—	—

DRUGS & CHEMICALS

Table of Drugs & Chemicals	POISONING Accidental (Unintentional)	Self-Harm (Intentional)	Assault	Undetermined	Adverse Effect	Underdosing
Seafood	T61.91x-	T61.92x-	T61.93x-	T61.94x-	—	—
specified NEC	T61.8x1-	T61.8x2-	T61.8x3-	T61.8x4-	—	—
Secbutabarbital	T42.3x1-	T42.3x2-	T42.3x3-	T42.3x4-	T42.3x5-	T42.3x6-
Secbutabarbitone	T42.3x1-	T42.3x2-	T42.3x3-	T42.3x4-	T42.3x5-	T42.3x6-
Secnidazole	T37.3x1-	T37.3x2-	T37.3x3-	T37.3x4-	T37.3x5-	T37.3x6-
Secobarbital	T42.3x1-	T42.3x2-	T42.3x3-	T42.3x4-	T42.3x5-	T42.3x6-
Seconal	T42.3x1-	T42.3x2-	T42.3x3-	T42.3x4-	T42.3x5-	T42.3x6-
Secretin	T50.8x1-	T50.8x2-	T50.8x3-	T50.8x4-	T50.8x5-	T50.8x6-
Sedative NEC	T42.71x-	T42.72x-	T42.73x-	T42.74x-	T42.75x-	T42.76x-
mixed NEC	T42.6x1-	T42.6x2-	T42.6x3-	T42.6x4-	T42.6x5-	T42.6x6-
Sedormid	T42.6x1-	T42.6x2-	T42.6x3-	T42.6x4-	T42.6x5-	T42.6x6-
Seed disinfectant or dressing	T60.8x1-	T60.8x2-	T60.8x3-	T60.8x4-	—	—
Seeds (poisonous)	T62.2x1-	T62.2x2-	T62.2x3-	T62.2x4-	—	—
Selegiline	T42.8x1-	T42.8x2-	T42.8x3-	T42.8x4-	T42.8x5-	T42.8x6-
Selenium NEC	T56.891-	T56.892-	T56.893-	T56.894-	—	—
disulfide or sulfide	T49.4x1-	T49.4x2-	T49.4x3-	T49.4x4-	T49.4x5-	T49.4x6-
fumes	T59.891-	T59.892-	T59.893-	T59.894-	—	—
sulfide	T49.4x1-	T49.4x2-	T49.4x3-	T49.4x4-	T49.4x5-	T49.4x6-
Selenomethionine (75Se)	T50.8x1-	T50.8x2-	T50.8x3-	T50.8x4-	T50.8x5-	T50.8x6-
Selsun	T49.4x1-	T49.4x2-	T49.4x3-	T49.4x4-	T49.4x5-	T49.4x6-
Semustine	T45.1x1-	T45.1x2-	T45.1x3-	T45.1x4-	T45.1x5-	T45.1x6-
Senega syrup	T48.4x1-	T48.4x2-	T48.4x3-	T48.4x4-	T48.4x5-	T48.4x6-
Senna	T47.2x1-	T47.2x2-	T47.2x3-	T47.2x4-	T47.2x5-	T47.2x6-
Sennoside A+B	T47.2x1-	T47.2x2-	T47.2x3-	T47.2x4-	T47.2x5-	T47.2x6-
Septisol	T49.2x1-	T49.2x2-	T49.2x3-	T49.2x4-	T49.2x5-	T49.2x6-
Seractide	T38.811-	T38.812-	T38.813-	T38.814-	T38.815-	T38.816-
Serax	T42.4x1-	T42.4x2-	T42.4x3-	T42.4x4-	T42.4x5-	T42.4x6-
Serenesil	T42.6x1-	T42.6x2-	T42.6x3-	T42.6x4-	T42.6x5-	T42.6x6-
Serenium (hydrochloride)	T37.91x-	T37.92x-	T37.93x-	T37.94x-	T37.95x-	T37.96x-
Serepax — see Oxazepam						
Sermorelin	T38.891-	T38.892-	T38.893-	T38.894-	T38.895-	T38.896-
Sernyl	T41.1x1-	T41.1x2-	T41.1x3-	T41.1x4-	T41.1x5-	T41.1x6-
Serotonin	T50.991-	T50.992-	T50.993-	T50.994-	T50.995-	T50.996-
Serpasil	T46.5x1-	T46.5x2-	T46.5x3-	T46.5x4-	T46.5x5-	T46.5x6-
Serrapeptase	T45.3x1-	T45.3x2-	T45.3x3-	T45.3x4-	T45.3x5-	T45.3x6-
Serum						
antibotulinus	T50.Z11-	T50.Z12-	T50.Z13-	T50.Z14-	T50.Z15-	T50.Z16-
anticytotoxic	T50.Z11-	T50.Z12-	T50.Z13-	T50.Z14-	T50.Z15-	T50.Z16-
antidiphtheria	T50.Z11-	T50.Z12-	T50.Z13-	T50.Z14-	T50.Z15-	T50.Z16-
antimeningococcus	T50.Z11-	T50.Z12-	T50.Z13-	T50.Z14-	T50.Z15-	T50.Z16-
anti-Rh	T50.Z11-	T50.Z12-	T50.Z13-	T50.Z14-	T50.Z15-	T50.Z16-
anti-snake-bite	T50.Z11-	T50.Z12-	T50.Z13-	T50.Z14-	T50.Z15-	T50.Z16-
antitetanic	T50.Z11-	T50.Z12-	T50.Z13-	T50.Z14-	T50.Z15-	T50.Z16-
antitoxic	T50.Z11-	T50.Z12-	T50.Z13-	T50.Z14-	T50.Z15-	T50.Z16-
complement (inhibitor)	T45.8x1-	T45.8x2-	T45.8x3-	T45.8x4-	T45.8x5-	T45.8x6-
convalescent	T50.Z11-	T50.Z12-	T50.Z13-	T50.Z14-	T50.Z15-	T50.Z16-
hemolytic complement	T45.8x1-	T45.8x2-	T45.8x3-	T45.8x4-	T45.8x5-	T45.8x6-
immune (human)	T50.Z11-	T50.Z12-	T50.Z13-	T50.Z14-	T50.Z15-	T50.Z16-
protective NEC	T50.Z11-	T50.Z12-	T50.Z13-	T50.Z14-	T50.Z15-	T50.Z16-
Setastine	T45.0x1-	T45.0x2-	T45.0x3-	T45.0x4-	T45.0x5-	T45.0x6-
Setoperone	T43.591-	T43.592-	T43.593-	T43.594-	T43.595-	T43.596-
Sewer gas	T59.91x-	T59.92x-	T59.93x-	T59.94x-	—	—
Shampoo	T55.0x1-	T55.0x2-	T55.0x3-	T55.0x4-	—	—
Shellfish, noxious, nonbacterial	T61.781-	T61.782-	T61.783-	T61.784-	—	—
Sildenafil	T46.7x1-	T46.7x2-	T46.7x3-	T46.7x4-	T46.7x5-	T46.7x6-
Silibinin	T50.991-	T50.992-	T50.993-	T50.994-	T50.995-	T50.996-
Silicone NEC	T65.891-	T65.892-	T65.893-	T65.894-	—	—
medicinal	T49.3x1-	T49.3x2-	T49.3x3-	T49.3x4-	T49.3x5-	T49.3x6-
Silvadene	T49.0x1-	T49.0x2-	T49.0x3-	T49.0x4-	T49.0x5-	T49.0x6-
Silver	T49.0x1-	T49.0x2-	T49.0x3-	T49.0x4-	T49.0x5-	T49.0x6-
anti-infectives	T49.0x1-	T49.0x2-	T49.0x3-	T49.0x4-	T49.0x5-	T49.0x6-
arsphenamine	T37.8x1-	T37.8x2-	T37.8x3-	T37.8x4-	T37.8x5-	T37.8x6-
colloidal	T49.0x1-	T49.0x2-	T49.0x3-	T49.0x4-	T49.0x5-	T49.0x6-
nitrate	T49.0x1-	T49.0x2-	T49.0x3-	T49.0x4-	T49.0x5-	T49.0x6-
ophthalmic preparation	T49.5x1-	T49.5x2-	T49.5x3-	T49.5x4-	T49.5x5-	T49.5x6-
toughened (keratolytic)	T49.4x1-	T49.4x2-	T49.4x3-	T49.4x4-	T49.4x5-	T49.4x6-
nonmedicinal (dust)	T56.891-	T56.892-	T56.893-	T56.894-	—	—
protein	T49.5x1-	T49.5x2-	T49.5x3-	T49.5x4-	T49.5x5-	T49.5x6-
salvarsan	T37.8x1-	T37.8x2-	T37.8x3-	T37.8x4-	T37.8x5-	T37.8x6-
sulfadiazine	T49.4x1-	T49.4x2-	T49.4x3-	T49.4x4-	T49.4x5-	T49.4x6-
Silymarin	T50.991-	T50.992-	T50.993-	T50.994-	T50.995-	T50.996-
Simaldrate	T47.1x1-	T47.1x2-	T47.1x3-	T47.1x4-	T47.1x5-	T47.1x6-
Simazine	T60.3x1-	T60.3x2-	T60.3x3-	T60.3x4-	—	—
Simethicone	T47.1x1-	T47.1x2-	T47.1x3-	T47.1x4-	T47.1x5-	T47.1x6-
Simfibrate	T46.6x1-	T46.6x2-	T46.6x3-	T46.6x4-	T46.6x5-	T46.6x6-
Simvastatin	T46.6x1-	T46.6x2-	T46.6x3-	T46.6x4-	T46.6x5-	T46.6x6-
Sincalide	T50.8x1-	T50.8x2-	T50.8x3-	T50.8x4-	T50.8x5-	T50.8x6-
Sinequan	T43.011-	T43.012-	T43.013-	T43.014-	T43.015-	T43.016-
Singoserp	T46.5x1-	T46.5x2-	T46.5x3-	T46.5x4-	T46.5x5-	T46.5x6-
Sintrom	T45.511-	T45.512-	T45.513-	T45.514-	T45.515-	T45.516-
Sisomicin	T36.5x1-	T36.5x2-	T36.5x3-	T36.5x4-	T36.5x5-	T36.5x6-
Sitosterols	T46.6x1-	T46.6x2-	T46.6x3-	T46.6x4-	T46.6x5-	T46.6x6-
Skeletal muscle relaxants	T48.1x1-	T48.1x2-	T48.1x3-	T48.1x4-	T48.1x5-	T48.1x6-
Skin						
agents (external)	T49.91x-	T49.92x-	T49.93x-	T49.94x-	T49.95x-	T49.96x-
specified NEC	T49.8x1-	T49.8x2-	T49.8x3-	T49.8x4-	T49.8x5-	T49.8x6-
test antigen	T50.8x1-	T50.8x2-	T50.8x3-	T50.8x4-	T50.8x5-	T50.8x6-
Sleep-eze	T45.0x1-	T45.0x2-	T45.0x3-	T45.0x4-	T45.0x5-	T45.0x6-
Sleeping draught, pill	T42.71x-	T42.72x-	T42.73x-	T42.74x-	T42.75x-	T42.76x-
Smallpox vaccine	T50.B11-	T50.B12-	T50.B13-	T50.B14-	T50.B15-	T50.B16-
Smelter fumes NEC	T56.91x-	T56.92x-	T56.93x-	T56.94x-	—	—
Smog	T59.1x1-	T59.1x2-	T59.1x3-	T59.1x4-	—	—
Smoke NEC	T59.811-	T59.812-	T59.813-	T59.814-	—	—
Smooth muscle relaxant	T44.3x1-	T44.3x2-	T44.3x3-	T44.3x4-	T44.3x5-	T44.3x6-
Snail killer NEC	T60.8x1-	T60.8x2-	T60.8x3-	T60.8x4-	—	—
Snake venom or bite	T63.001-	T63.002-	T63.003-	T63.004-	—	—
hemocoagulase	T45.7x1-	T45.7x2-	T45.7x3-	T45.7x4-	T45.7x5-	T45.7x6-
Snuff	T65.211-	T65.212-	T65.213-	T65.214-	—	—
Soap (powder) (product)	T55.0x1-	T55.0x2-	T55.0x3-	T55.0x4-	—	—
enema	T47.4x1-	T47.4x2-	T47.4x3-	T47.4x4-	T47.4x5-	T47.4x6-
medicinal, soft	T49.2x1-	T49.2x2-	T49.2x3-	T49.2x4-	T49.2x5-	T49.2x6-
superfatted	T49.2x1-	T49.2x2-	T49.2x3-	T49.2x4-	T49.2x5-	T49.2x6-
Sobrerol	T48.4x1-	T48.4x2-	T48.4x3-	T48.4x4-	T48.4x5-	T48.4x6-
Soda (caustic)	T54.3x1-	T54.3x2-	T54.3x3-	T54.3x4-	—	—
bicarb	T47.1x1-	T47.1x2-	T47.1x3-	T47.1x4-	T47.1x5-	T47.1x6-
chlorinated — see Sodium, hypochlorite						
Sodium						
l-triiodothyronine	T38.1x1-	T38.1x2-	T38.1x3-	T38.1x4-	T38.1x5-	T38.1x6-
acetosulfone	T37.1x1-	T37.1x2-	T37.1x3-	T37.1x4-	T37.1x5-	T37.1x6-
acetrizoate	T50.8x1-	T50.8x2-	T50.8x3-	T50.8x4-	T50.8x5-	T50.8x6-
acid phosphate	T50.3x1-	T50.3x2-	T50.3x3-	T50.3x4-	T50.3x5-	T50.3x6-
alginate	T47.8x1-	T47.8x2-	T47.8x3-	T47.8x4-	T47.8x5-	T47.8x6-
amidotrizoate	T50.8x1-	T50.8x2-	T50.8x3-	T50.8x4-	T50.8x5-	T50.8x6-
aminopterin	T45.1x1-	T45.1x2-	T45.1x3-	T45.1x4-	T45.1x5-	T45.1x6-
amylosulfate	T47.8x1-	T47.8x2-	T47.8x3-	T47.8x4-	T47.8x5-	T47.8x6-
amytal	T42.3x1-	T42.3x2-	T42.3x3-	T42.3x4-	T42.3x5-	T42.3x6-
antimony gluconate	T37.3x1-	T37.3x2-	T37.3x3-	T37.3x4-	T37.3x5-	T37.3x6-
arsenate	T57.0x1-	T57.0x2-	T57.0x3-	T57.0x4-	—	—
aurothiomalate	T39.4x1-	T39.4x2-	T39.4x3-	T39.4x4-	T39.4x5-	T39.4x6-
aurothiosulfate	T39.4x1-	T39.4x2-	T39.4x3-	T39.4x4-	T39.4x5-	T39.4x6-
barbiturate	T42.3x1-	T42.3x2-	T42.3x3-	T42.3x4-	T42.3x5-	T42.3x6-
basic phosphate	T47.4x1-	T47.4x2-	T47.4x3-	T47.4x4-	T47.4x5-	T47.4x6-
bicarbonate	T47.1x1-	T47.1x2-	T47.1x3-	T47.1x4-	T47.1x5-	T47.1x6-

Table of Drugs & Chemicals	POISONING Accidental (Unintentional)	POISONING Self-Harm (Intentional)	POISONING Assault	POISONING Undetermined	Adverse Effect	Underdosing
Sodium - continued						
bichromate	T57.8x1-	T57.8x2-	T57.8x3-	T57.8x4-	—	—
biphosphate	T50.3x1-	T50.3x2-	T50.3x3-	T50.3x4-	T50.3x5-	T50.3x6-
bisulfate	T65.891-	T65.892-	T65.893-	T65.894-	—	—
borate						
cleanser	T57.8x1-	T57.8x2-	T57.8x3-	T57.8x4-	—	—
eye	T49.5x1-	T49.5x2-	T49.5x3-	T49.5x4-	T49.5x5-	T49.5x6-
therapeutic	T49.8x1-	T49.8x2-	T49.8x3-	T49.8x4-	T49.8x5-	T49.8x6-
bromide	T42.6x1-	T42.6x2-	T42.6x3-	T42.6x4-	T42.6x5-	T42.6x6-
cacodylate (nonmedicinal)						
NEC	T50.8x1-	T50.8x2-	T50.8x3-	T50.8x4-	T50.8x5-	T50.8x6-
anti-infective	T37.8x1-	T37.8x2-	T37.8x3-	T37.8x4-	T37.8x5-	T37.8x6-
herbicide	T60.3x1-	T60.3x2-	T60.3x3-	T60.3x4-	—	—
calcium edetate	T45.8x1-	T45.8x2-	T45.8x3-	T45.8x4-	T45.8x5-	T45.8x6-
carbonate NEC	T54.3x1-	T54.3x2-	T54.3x3-	T54.3x4-	—	—
chlorate NEC	T65.891-	T65.892-	T65.893-	T65.894-	—	—
herbicide	T54.91x-	T54.92x-	T54.93x-	T54.94x-	—	—
chloride	T50.3x1-	T50.3x2-	T50.3x3-	T50.3x4-	T50.3x5-	T50.3x6-
with glucose	T50.3x1-	T50.3x2-	T50.3x3-	T50.3x4-	T50.3x5-	T50.3x6-
chromate	T65.891-	T65.892-	T65.893-	T65.894-	—	—
citrate	T50.991-	T50.992-	T50.993-	T50.994-	T50.995-	T50.996-
cromoglicate	T48.6x1-	T48.6x2-	T48.6x3-	T48.6x4-	T48.6x5-	T48.6x6-
cyanide	T65.0x1-	T65.0x2-	T65.0x3-	T65.0x4-	—	—
cyclamate	T50.3x1-	T50.3x2-	T50.3x3-	T50.3x4-	T50.3x5-	T50.3x6-
dehydrocholate	T45.8x1-	T45.8x2-	T45.8x3-	T45.8x4-	T45.8x5-	T45.8x6-
diatrizoate	T50.8x1-	T50.8x2-	T50.8x3-	T50.8x4-	T50.8x5-	T50.8x6-
dibunate	T48.4x1-	T48.4x2-	T48.4x3-	T48.4x4-	T48.4x5-	T48.4x6-
dioctyl sulfosuccinate	T47.4x1-	T47.4x2-	T47.4x3-	T47.4x4-	T47.4x5-	T47.4x6-
dipantoyl ferrate	T45.8x1-	T45.8x2-	T45.8x3-	T45.8x4-	T45.8x5-	T45.8x6-
edetate	T45.8x1-	T45.8x2-	T45.8x3-	T45.8x4-	T45.8x5-	T45.8x6-
ethacrynate	T50.1x1-	T50.1x2-	T50.1x3-	T50.1x4-	T50.1x5-	T50.1x6-
feredetate	T45.8x1-	T45.8x2-	T45.8x3-	T45.8x4-	T45.8x5-	T45.8x6-
fluoride — see Fluoride						
fluoroacetate (dust)						
(pesticide)	T60.4x1-	T60.4x2-	T60.4x3-	T60.4x4-	—	—
free salt	T50.3x1-	T50.3x2-	T50.3x3-	T50.3x4-	T50.3x5-	T50.3x6-
fusidate	T36.8x1-	T36.8x2-	T36.8x3-	T36.8x4-	T36.8x5-	T36.8x6-
glucaldrate	T47.1x1-	T47.1x2-	T47.1x3-	T47.1x4-	T47.1x5-	T47.1x6-
glucosulfone	T37.1x1-	T37.1x2-	T37.1x3-	T37.1x4-	T37.1x5-	T37.1x6-
glutamate	T45.8x1-	T45.8x2-	T45.8x3-	T45.8x4-	T45.8x5-	T45.8x6-
hydrogen carbonate	T50.3x1-	T50.3x2-	T50.3x3-	T50.3x4-	T50.3x5-	T50.3x6-
hydroxide	T54.3x1-	T54.3x2-	T54.3x3-	T54.3x4-	—	—
hypochlorite (bleach) NEC	T54.3x1-	T54.3x2-	T54.3x3-	T54.3x4-	—	—
disinfectant	T54.3x1-	T54.3x2-	T54.3x3-	T54.3x4-	—	—
medicinal (anti-infective) (external)	T49.0x1-	T49.0x2-	T49.0x3-	T49.0x4-	T49.0x5-	T49.0x6-
vapor	T54.3x1-	T54.3x2-	T54.3x3-	T54.3x4-	—	—
hyposulfite	T49.0x1-	T49.0x2-	T49.0x3-	T49.0x4-	T49.0x5-	T49.0x6-
indigotin disulfonate	T50.8x1-	T50.8x2-	T50.8x3-	T50.8x4-	T50.8x5-	T50.8x6-
iodide	T50.991-	T50.992-	T50.993-	T50.994-	T50.995-	T50.996-
I-131	T50.8x1-	T50.8x2-	T50.8x3-	T50.8x4-	T50.8x5-	T50.8x6-
therapeutic	T38.2x1-	T38.2x2-	T38.2x3-	T38.2x4-	T38.2x5-	T38.2x6-
iodohippurate (131I)	T50.8x1-	T50.8x2-	T50.8x3-	T50.8x4-	T50.8x5-	T50.8x6-
iopodate	T50.8x1-	T50.8x2-	T50.8x3-	T50.8x4-	T50.8x5-	T50.8x6-
iothalamate	T50.8x1-	T50.8x2-	T50.8x3-	T50.8x4-	T50.8x5-	T50.8x6-
iron edetate	T45.4x1-	T45.4x2-	T45.4x3-	T45.4x4-	T45.4x5-	T45.4x6-
lactate (compound solution)	T45.8x1-	T45.8x2-	T45.8x3-	T45.8x4-	T45.8x5-	T45.8x6-
lauryl (sulfate)	T49.2x1-	T49.2x2-	T49.2x3-	T49.2x4-	T49.2x5-	T49.2x6-
(L)-triiodothyronine	T38.1x1-	T38.1x2-	T38.1x3-	T38.1x4-	T38.1x5-	T38.1x6-

Table of Drugs & Chemicals	POISONING Accidental (Unintentional)	POISONING Self-Harm (Intentional)	POISONING Assault	POISONING Undetermined	Adverse Effect	Underdosing
Sodium - continued						
magnesium citrate	T50.991-	T50.992-	T50.993-	T50.994-	T50.995-	T50.996-
mersalate	T50.2x1-	T50.2x2-	T50.2x3-	T50.2x4-	T50.2x5-	T50.2x6-
metasilicate	T65.891-	T65.892-	T65.893-	T65.894-	—	—
metrizoate	T50.8x1-	T50.8x2-	T50.8x3-	T50.8x4-	T50.8x5-	T50.8x6-
monofluoroacetate (pesticide)	T60.1x1-	T60.1x2-	T60.1x3-	T60.1x4-	—	—
morrhuate	T46.8x1-	T46.8x2-	T46.8x3-	T46.8x4-	T46.8x5-	T46.8x6-
nafcillin	T36.0x1-	T36.0x2-	T36.0x3-	T36.0x4-	T36.0x5-	T36.0x6-
nitrate (oxidizing agent)	T65.891-	T65.892-	T65.893-	T65.894-	—	—
nitrite	T50.6x1-	T50.6x2-	T50.6x3-	T50.6x4-	T50.6x5-	T50.6x6-
nitroferricyanide	T46.5x1-	T46.5x2-	T46.5x3-	T46.5x4-	T46.5x5-	T46.5x6-
nitroprusside	T46.5x1-	T46.5x2-	T46.5x3-	T46.5x4-	T46.5x5-	T46.5x6-
oxalate	T65.891-	T65.892-	T65.893-	T65.894-	—	—
oxide/peroxide	T65.891-	T65.892-	T65.893-	T65.894-	—	—
oxybate	T41.291-	T41.292-	T41.293-	T41.294-	T41.295-	T41.296-
para-aminohippurate	T50.8x1-	T50.8x2-	T50.8x3-	T50.8x4-	T50.8x5-	T50.8x6-
perborate (nonmedicinal)						
NEC	T65.891-	T65.892-	T65.893-	T65.894-	—	—
medicinal	T49.0x1-	T49.0x2-	T49.0x3-	T49.0x4-	T49.0x5-	T49.0x6-
soap	T55.0x1-	T55.0x2-	T55.0x3-	T55.0x4-	—	—
percarbonate — see Sodium, perborate						
pertechnetate Tc99m	T50.8x1-	T50.8x2-	T50.8x3-	T50.8x4-	T50.8x5-	T50.8x6-
phosphate						
cellulose	T45.8x1-	T45.8x2-	T45.8x3-	T45.8x4-	T45.8x5-	T45.8x6-
dibasic	T47.2x1-	T47.2x2-	T47.2x3-	T47.2x4-	T47.2x5-	T47.2x6-
monobasic	T47.2x1-	T47.2x2-	T47.2x3-	T47.2x4-	T47.2x5-	T47.2x6-
phytate	T50.6x1-	T50.6x2-	T50.6x3-	T50.6x4-	T50.6x5-	T50.6x6-
picosulfate	T47.2x1-	T47.2x2-	T47.2x3-	T47.2x4-	T47.2x5-	T47.2x6-
polyhydroxyaluminium monocarbonate	T47.1x1-	T47.1x2-	T47.1x3-	T47.1x4-	T47.1x5-	T47.1x6-
polystyrene sulfonate	T50.3x1-	T50.3x2-	T50.3x3-	T50.3x4-	T50.3x5-	T50.3x6-
propionate	T49.0x1-	T49.0x2-	T49.0x3-	T49.0x4-	T49.0x5-	T49.0x6-
propyl hydroxybenzoate	T50.991-	T50.992-	T50.993-	T50.994-	T50.995-	T50.996-
psylliate	T46.8x1-	T46.8x2-	T46.8x3-	T46.8x4-	T46.8x5-	T46.8x6-
removing resins	T50.3x1-	T50.3x2-	T50.3x3-	T50.3x4-	T50.3x5-	T50.3x6-
salicylate	T39.091-	T39.092-	T39.093-	T39.094-	T39.095-	T39.096-
salt NEC	T50.3x1-	T50.3x2-	T50.3x3-	T50.3x4-	T50.3x5-	T50.3x6-
selenate	T60.2x1-	T60.2x2-	T60.2x3-	T60.2x4-	—	—
stibogluconate	T37.3x1-	T37.3x2-	T37.3x3-	T37.3x4-	T37.3x5-	T37.3x6-
sulfate	T47.4x1-	T47.4x2-	T47.4x3-	T47.4x4-	T47.4x5-	T47.4x6-
sulfoxone	T37.1x1-	T37.1x2-	T37.1x3-	T37.1x4-	T37.1x5-	T37.1x6-
tetradecyl sulfate	T46.8x1-	T46.8x2-	T46.8x3-	T46.8x4-	T46.8x5-	T46.8x6-
thiopental	T41.1x1-	T41.1x2-	T41.1x3-	T41.1x4-	T41.1x5-	T41.1x6-
thiosalicylate	T39.091-	T39.092-	T39.093-	T39.094-	T39.095-	T39.096-
thiosulfate	T50.6x1-	T50.6x2-	T50.6x3-	T50.6x4-	T50.6x5-	T50.6x6-
tolbutamide	T38.3x1-	T38.3x2-	T38.3x3-	T38.3x4-	T38.3x5-	T38.3x6-
tyropanoate	T50.8x1-	T50.8x2-	T50.8x3-	T50.8x4-	T50.8x5-	T50.8x6-
valproate	T42.6x1-	T42.6x2-	T42.6x3-	T42.6x4-	T42.6x5-	T42.6x6-
versenate	T50.6x1-	T50.6x2-	T50.6x3-	T50.6x4-	T50.6x5-	T50.6x6-
Sodium-free salt	T50.901-	T50.902-	T50.903-	T50.904-	T50.905-	T50.906-
Sodium-removing resin	T50.3x1-	T50.3x2-	T50.3x3-	T50.3x4-	T50.3x5-	T50.3x6-
Soft soap	T55.0x1-	T55.0x2-	T55.0x3-	T55.0x4-	—	—
Solanine	T62.2x1-	T62.2x2-	T62.2x3-	T62.2x4-	—	—
berries	T62.1x1-	T62.1x2-	T62.1x3-	T62.1x4-	—	—
Solanum dulcamara	T62.2x1-	T62.2x2-	T62.2x3-	T62.2x4-	—	—
berries	T62.1x1-	T62.1x2-	T62.1x3-	T62.1x4-	—	—
Solapsone	T37.1x1-	T37.1x2-	T37.1x3-	T37.1x4-	T37.1x5-	T37.1x6-
Solar lotion	T49.3x1-	T49.3x2-	T49.3x3-	T49.3x4-	T49.3x5-	T49.3x6-
Solasulfone	T37.1x1-	T37.1x2-	T37.1x3-	T37.1x4-	T37.1x5-	T37.1x6-

DRUGS & CHEMICALS

DRUGS & CHEMICALS

Table of Drugs & Chemicals	POISONING Accidental (Unintentional)	Self-Harm (Intentional)	Assault	Undetermined	Adverse Effect	Underdosing
Soldering fluid	T65.891-	T65.892-	T65.893-	T65.894-	—	—
Solid substance	T65.91x-	T65.92x-	T65.93x-	T65.94x-	—	—
specified NEC	T65.891-	T65.892-	T65.893-	T65.894-	—	—
Solvent, industrial NEC	T52.91x-	T52.92x-	T52.93x-	T52.94x-	—	—
naphtha	T52.0x1-	T52.0x2-	T52.0x3-	T52.0x4-	—	—
petroleum	T52.0x1-	T52.0x2-	T52.0x3-	T52.0x4-	—	—
specified NEC	T52.8x1-	T52.8x2-	T52.8x3-	T52.8x4-	—	—
Soma	T42.8x1-	T42.8x2-	T42.8x3-	T42.8x4-	T42.8x5-	T42.8x6-
Somatorelin	T38.891-	T38.892-	T38.893-	T38.894-	T38.895-	T38.896-
Somatostatin	T38.991-	T38.992-	T38.993-	T38.994-	T38.995-	T38.996-
Somatotropin	T38.811-	T38.812-	T38.813-	T38.814-	T38.815-	T38.816-
Somatrem	T38.811-	T38.812-	T38.813-	T38.814-	T38.815-	T38.816-
Somatropin	T38.811-	T38.812-	T38.813-	T38.814-	T38.815-	T38.816-
Sominex	T45.0x1-	T45.0x2-	T45.0x3-	T45.0x4-	T45.0x5-	T45.0x6-
Somnos	T42.6x1-	T42.6x2-	T42.6x3-	T42.6x4-	T42.6x5-	T42.6x6-
Somonal	T42.3x1-	T42.3x2-	T42.3x3-	T42.3x4-	T42.3x5-	T42.3x6-
Soneryl	T42.3x1-	T42.3x2-	T42.3x3-	T42.3x4-	T42.3x5-	T42.3x6-
Soothing syrup	T50.901-	T50.902-	T50.903-	T50.904-	T50.905-	T50.906-
Sopor	T42.6x1-	T42.6x2-	T42.6x3-	T42.6x4-	T42.6x5-	T42.6x6-
Soporific	T42.71x-	T42.72x-	T42.73x-	T42.74x-	T42.75x-	T42.76x-
Soporific drug	T42.71x-	T42.72x-	T42.73x-	T42.74x-	T42.75x-	T42.76x-
specified type NEC	T42.6x1-	T42.6x2-	T42.6x3-	T42.6x4-	T42.6x5-	T42.6x6-
Sorbide nitrate	T46.3x1-	T46.3x2-	T46.3x3-	T46.3x4-	T46.3x5-	T46.3x6-
Sorbitol	T47.4x1-	T47.4x2-	T47.4x3-	T47.4x4-	T47.4x5-	T47.4x6-
Sotalol	T44.7x1-	T44.7x2-	T44.7x3-	T44.7x4-	T44.7x5-	T44.7x6-
Sotradecol	T46.8x1-	T46.8x2-	T46.8x3-	T46.8x4-	T46.8x5-	T46.8x6-
Soysterol	T46.6x1-	T46.6x2-	T46.6x3-	T46.6x4-	T46.6x5-	T46.6x6-
Spacoline	T44.3x1-	T44.3x2-	T44.3x3-	T44.3x4-	T44.3x5-	T44.3x6-
Spanish fly	T49.8x1-	T49.8x2-	T49.8x3-	T49.8x4-	T49.8x5-	T49.8x6-
Sparine	T43.3x1-	T43.3x2-	T43.3x3-	T43.3x4-	T43.3x5-	T43.3x6-
Sparteine	T48.0x1-	T48.0x2-	T48.0x3-	T48.0x4-	T48.0x5-	T48.0x6-
Spasmolytic						
anticholinergics	T44.3x1-	T44.3x2-	T44.3x3-	T44.3x4-	T44.3x5-	T44.3x6-
autonomic	T44.3x1-	T44.3x2-	T44.3x3-	T44.3x4-	T44.3x5-	T44.3x6-
bronchial NEC	T48.6x1-	T48.6x2-	T48.6x3-	T48.6x4-	T48.6x5-	T48.6x6-
quaternary ammonium	T44.3x1-	T44.3x2-	T44.3x3-	T44.3x4-	T44.3x5-	T44.3x6-
skeletal muscle NEC	T48.1x1-	T48.1x2-	T48.1x3-	T48.1x4-	T48.1x5-	T48.1x6-
Spectinomycin	T36.5x1-	T36.5x2-	T36.5x3-	T36.5x4-	T36.5x5-	T36.5x6-
Speed	T43.621-	T43.622-	T43.623-	T43.624-	T43.625-	T43.626-
Spermicide	T49.8x1-	T49.8x2-	T49.8x3-	T49.8x4-	T49.8x5-	T49.8x6-
Spider (bite) (venom)	T63.391-	T63.392-	T63.393-	T63.394-	—	—
antivenin	T50.Z11-	T50.Z12-	T50.Z13-	T50.Z14-	T50.Z15-	T50.Z16-
Spigelia (root)	T37.4x1-	T37.4x2-	T37.4x3-	T37.4x4-	T37.4x5-	T37.4x6-
Spindle inactivator	T50.4x1-	T50.4x2-	T50.4x3-	T50.4x4-	T50.4x5-	T50.4x6-
Spiperone	T43.4x1-	T43.4x2-	T43.4x3-	T43.4x4-	T43.4x5-	T43.4x6-
Spiramycin	T36.3x1-	T36.3x2-	T36.3x3-	T36.3x4-	T36.3x5-	T36.3x6-
Spirapril	T46.4x1-	T46.4x2-	T46.4x3-	T46.4x4-	T46.4x5-	T46.4x6-
Spirilene	T43.591-	T43.592-	T43.593-	T43.594-	T43.595-	T43.596-
Spirit (s) (neutral) NEC	T51.0x1-	T51.0x2-	T51.0x3-	T51.0x4-	—	—
beverage	T51.0x1-	T51.0x2-	T51.0x3-	T51.0x4-	—	—
industrial	T51.0x1-	T51.0x2-	T51.0x3-	T51.0x4-	—	—
mineral	T52.0x1-	T52.0x2-	T52.0x3-	T52.0x4-	—	—
of salt — see Hydrochloric acid						
surgical	T51.0x1-	T51.0x2-	T51.0x3-	T51.0x4-	—	—
Spironolactone	T50.0x1-	T50.0x2-	T50.0x3-	T50.0x4-	T50.0x5-	T50.0x6-
Spiroperidol	T43.4x1-	T43.4x2-	T43.4x3-	T43.4x4-	T43.4x5-	T43.4x6-
Sponge, absorbable (gelatin)	T45.7x1-	T45.7x2-	T45.7x3-	T45.7x4-	T45.7x5-	T45.7x6-
Sporostacin	T49.0x1-	T49.0x2-	T49.0x3-	T49.0x4-	T49.0x5-	T49.0x6-
Spray (aerosol)	T65.91x-	T65.92x-	T65.93x-	T65.94x-	—	—
cosmetic	T65.891-	T65.892-	T65.893-	T65.894-	—	—
medicinal NEC	T50.901-	T50.902-	T50.903-	T50.904-	T50.905-	T50.906-
pesticides — see Pesticides						
specified content — see specific substance						
Spurge flax	T62.2x1-	T62.2x2-	T62.2x3-	T62.2x4-	—	—
Spurges	T62.2x1-	T62.2x2-	T62.2x3-	T62.2x4-	—	—
Sputum viscosity-lowering drug	T48.4x1-	T48.4x2-	T48.4x3-	T48.4x4-	T48.4x5-	T48.4x6-
Squill	T46.0x1-	T46.0x2-	T46.0x3-	T46.0x4-	T46.0x5-	T46.0x6-
rat poison	T60.4x1-	T60.4x2-	T60.4x3-	T60.4x4-	—	—
Squirting cucumber (cathartic)	T47.2x1-	T47.2x2-	T47.2x3-	T47.2x4-	T47.2x5-	T47.2x6-
Stains	T65.6x1-	T65.6x2-	T65.6x3-	T65.6x4-	—	—
Stannous fluoride	T49.7x1-	T49.7x2-	T49.7x3-	T49.7x4-	T49.7x5-	T49.7x6-
Stanolone	T38.7x1-	T38.7x2-	T38.7x3-	T38.7x4-	T38.7x5-	T38.7x6-
Stanozolol	T38.7x1-	T38.7x2-	T38.7x3-	T38.7x4-	T38.7x5-	T38.7x6-
Staphisagria or stavesacre (pediculicide)	T49.0x1-	T49.0x2-	T49.0x3-	T49.0x4-	T49.0x5-	T49.0x6-
Starch	T50.901-	T50.902-	T50.903-	T50.904-	T50.905-	T50.906-
Stelazine	T43.3x1-	T43.3x2-	T43.3x3-	T43.3x4-	T43.3x5-	T43.3x6-
Stemetil	T43.3x1-	T43.3x2-	T43.3x3-	T43.3x4-	T43.3x5-	T43.3x6-
Stepronin	T48.4x1-	T48.4x2-	T48.4x3-	T48.4x4-	T48.4x5-	T48.4x6-
Sterculia	T47.4x1-	T47.4x2-	T47.4x3-	T47.4x4-	T47.4x5-	T47.4x6-
Sternutator gas	T59.891-	T59.892-	T59.893-	T59.894-	—	—
Steroid	T38.0x1-	T38.0x2-	T38.0x3-	T38.0x4-	T38.0x5-	T38.0x6-
anabolic	T38.7x1-	T38.7x2-	T38.7x3-	T38.7x4-	T38.7x5-	T38.7x6-
androgenic	T38.7x1-	T38.7x2-	T38.7x3-	T38.7x4-	T38.7x5-	T38.7x6-
antineoplastic, hormone	T38.7x1-	T38.7x2-	T38.7x3-	T38.7x4-	T38.7x5-	T38.7x6-
estrogen	T38.5x1-	T38.5x2-	T38.5x3-	T38.5x4-	T38.5x5-	T38.5x6-
ENT agent	T49.6x1-	T49.6x2-	T49.6x3-	T49.6x4-	T49.6x5-	T49.6x6-
ophthalmic preparation	T49.5x1-	T49.5x2-	T49.5x3-	T49.5x4-	T49.5x5-	T49.5x6-
topical NEC	T49.0x1-	T49.0x2-	T49.0x3-	T49.0x4-	T49.0x5-	T49.0x6-
Stibine	T56.891-	T56.892-	T56.893-	T56.894-	—	—
Stibogluconate	T37.3x1-	T37.3x2-	T37.3x3-	T37.3x4-	T37.3x5-	T37.3x6-
Stibophen	T37.4x1-	T37.4x2-	T37.4x3-	T37.4x4-	T37.4x5-	T37.4x6-
Stilbamidine (isetionate)	T37.3x1-	T37.3x2-	T37.3x3-	T37.3x4-	T37.3x5-	T37.3x6-
Stilbestrol	T38.5x1-	T38.5x2-	T38.5x3-	T38.5x4-	T38.5x5-	T38.5x6-
Stilboestrol	T38.5x1-	T38.5x2-	T38.5x3-	T38.5x4-	T38.5x5-	T38.5x6-
Stimulant						
central nervous system — see also Psychostimulant	T43.601-	T43.602-	T43.603-	T43.604-	T43.605-	T43.606-
analeptics	T50.7x1-	T50.7x2-	T50.7x3-	T50.7x4-	T50.7x5-	T50.7x6-
opiate antagonist	T50.7x1-	T50.7x2-	T50.7x3-	T50.7x4-	T50.7x5-	
psychotherapeutic NEC — see also Psychotherapeutic drug	T43.601-	T43.602-	T43.603-	T43.604-	T43.605-	T43.606-
specified NEC	T43.691-	T43.692-	T43.693-	T43.694-	T43.695-	T43.696-
respiratory	T48.901-	T48.902-	T48.903-	T48.904-	T48.905-	T48.906-
Stone-dissolving drug	T50.901-	T50.902-	T50.903-	T50.904-	T50.905-	T50.906-
Storage battery (cells) (acid)	T54.2x1-	T54.2x2-	T54.2x3-	T54.2x4-	—	—
Stovaine	T41.3x1-	T41.3x2-	T41.3x3-	T41.3x4-	T41.3x5-	T41.3x6-
infiltration (subcutaneous)	T41.3x1-	T41.3x2-	T41.3x3-	T41.3x4-	T41.3x5-	T41.3x6-
nerve block (peripheral) (plexus)	T41.3x1-	T41.3x2-	T41.3x3-	T41.3x4-	T41.3x5-	T41.3x6-
spinal	T41.3x1-	T41.3x2-	T41.3x3-	T41.3x4-	T41.3x5-	T41.3x6-
topical (surface)	T41.3x1-	T41.3x2-	T41.3x3-	T41.3x4-	T41.3x5-	T41.3x6-

Table of Drugs & Chemicals	Accidental (Unintentional)	Self-Harm (Intentional)	Assault	Undetermined	Adverse Effect	Underdosing
Stovarsal	T37.8x1-	T37.8x2-	T37.8x3-	T37.8x4-	T37.8x5-	T37.8x6-
Stove gas — see Gas, stove						
Stoxil	T49.5x1-	T49.5x2-	T49.5x3-	T49.5x4-	T49.5x5-	T49.5x6-
Stramonium	T48.6x1-	T48.6x2-	T48.6x3-	T48.6x4-	T48.6x5-	T48.6x6-
natural state	T62.2x1-	T62.2x2-	T62.2x3-	T62.2x4-	—	—
Streptodornase	T45.3x1-	T45.3x2-	T45.3x3-	T45.3x4-	T45.3x5-	T45.3x6-
Streptoduocin	T36.5x1-	T36.5x2-	T36.5x3-	T36.5x4-	T36.5x5-	T36.5x6-
Streptokinase	T45.611-	T45.612-	T45.613-	T45.614-	T45.615-	T45.616-
Streptomycin (derivative)	T36.5x1-	T36.5x2-	T36.5x3-	T36.5x4-	T36.5x5-	T36.5x6-
Streptonivicin	T36.5x1-	T36.5x2-	T36.5x3-	T36.5x4-	T36.5x5-	T36.5x6-
Streptovarycin	T36.5x1-	T36.5x2-	T36.5x3-	T36.5x4-	T36.5x5-	T36.5x6-
Streptozocin	T45.1x1-	T45.1x2-	T45.1x3-	T45.1x4-	T45.1x5-	T45.1x6-
Streptozotocin	T45.1x1-	T45.1x2-	T45.1x3-	T45.1x4-	T45.1x5-	T45.1x6-
Stripper (paint) (solvent)	T52.8x1-	T52.8x2-	T52.8x3-	T52.8x4-	—	—
Strobane	T60.1x1-	T60.1x2-	T60.1x3-	T60.1x4-	—	—
Strofantina	T46.0x1-	T46.0x2-	T46.0x3-	T46.0x4-	T46.0x5-	T46.0x6-
Strophanthin (g) (k)	T46.0x1-	T46.0x2-	T46.0x3-	T46.0x4-	T46.0x5-	T46.0x6-
Strophanthus	T46.0x1-	T46.0x2-	T46.0x3-	T46.0x4-	T46.0x5-	T46.0x6-
Strophantin	T46.0x1-	T46.0x2-	T46.0x3-	T46.0x4-	T46.0x5-	T46.0x6-
Strophantin-g	T46.0x1-	T46.0x2-	T46.0x3-	T46.0x4-	T46.0x5-	T46.0x6-
Strychnine (nonmedicinal) (pesticide) (salts)	T65.1x1-	T65.1x2-	T65.1x3-	T65.1x4-	—	—
medicinal	T48.291-	T48.292-	T48.293-	T48.294-	T48.295-	T48.296-
Strychnos (ignatii) — see Strychnine						
Styramate	T42.8x1-	T42.8x2-	T42.8x3-	T42.8x4-	T42.8x5-	T42.8x6-
Styrene	T65.891-	T65.892-	T65.893-	T65.894-	—	—
Succinimide, antiepileptic or anticonvulsant	T42.2x1-	T42.2x2-	T42.2x3-	T42.2x4-	T42.2x5-	T42.2x6-
mercuric — see Mercury						
Succinylcholine	T48.1x1-	T48.1x2-	T48.1x3-	T48.1x4-	T48.1x5-	T48.1x6-
Succinylsulfathiazole	T37.0x1-	T37.0x2-	T37.0x3-	T37.0x4-	T37.0x5-	T37.0x6-
Sucralfate	T47.1x1-	T47.1x2-	T47.1x3-	T47.1x4-	T47.1x5-	T47.1x6-
Sucrose	T50.3x1-	T50.3x2-	T50.3x3-	T50.3x4-	T50.3x5-	T50.3x6-
Sufentanil	T40.4x1-	T40.4x2-	T40.4x3-	T40.4x4-	T40.4x5-	T40.4x6-
Sulbactam	T36.0x1-	T36.0x2-	T36.0x3-	T36.0x4-	T36.0x5-	T36.0x6-
Sulbenicillin	T36.0x1-	T36.0x2-	T36.0x3-	T36.0x4-	T36.0x5-	T36.0x6-
Sulbentine	T49.0x1-	T49.0x2-	T49.0x3-	T49.0x4-	T49.0x5-	T49.0x6-
Sulfacetamide	T49.0x1-	T49.0x2-	T49.0x3-	T49.0x4-	T49.0x5-	T49.0x6-
ophthalmic preparation	T49.5x1-	T49.5x2-	T49.5x3-	T49.5x4-	T49.5x5-	T49.5x6-
Sulfachlorpyridazine	T37.0x1-	T37.0x2-	T37.0x3-	T37.0x4-	T37.0x5-	T37.0x6-
Sulfacitine	T37.0x1-	T37.0x2-	T37.0x3-	T37.0x4-	T37.0x5-	T37.0x6-
Sulfadiasulfone sodium	T37.0x1-	T37.0x2-	T37.0x3-	T37.0x4-	T37.0x5-	T37.0x6-
Sulfadiazine	T37.0x1-	T37.0x2-	T37.0x3-	T37.0x4-	T37.0x5-	T37.0x6-
silver (topical)	T49.0x1-	T49.0x2-	T49.0x3-	T49.0x4-	T49.0x5-	T49.0x6-
Sulfadimethoxine	T37.0x1-	T37.0x2-	T37.0x3-	T37.0x4-	T37.0x5-	T37.0x6-
Sulfadimidine	T37.0x1-	T37.0x2-	T37.0x3-	T37.0x4-	T37.0x5-	T37.0x6-
Sulfadoxine	T37.0x1-	T37.0x2-	T37.0x3-	T37.0x4-	T37.0x5-	T37.0x6-
with pyrimethamine	T37.2x1-	T37.2x2-	T37.2x3-	T37.2x4-	T37.2x5-	T37.2x6-
Sulfaethidole	T37.0x1-	T37.0x2-	T37.0x3-	T37.0x4-	T37.0x5-	T37.0x6-
Sulfafurazole	T37.0x1-	T37.0x2-	T37.0x3-	T37.0x4-	T37.0x5-	T37.0x6-
Sulfaguanidine	T37.0x1-	T37.0x2-	T37.0x3-	T37.0x4-	T37.0x5-	T37.0x6-
Sulfalene	T37.0x1-	T37.0x2-	T37.0x3-	T37.0x4-	T37.0x5-	T37.0x6-
Sulfaloxate	T37.0x1-	T37.0x2-	T37.0x3-	T37.0x4-	T37.0x5-	T37.0x6-
Sulfaloxic acid	T37.0x1-	T37.0x2-	T37.0x3-	T37.0x4-	T37.0x5-	T37.0x6-
Sulfamazone	T39.2x1-	T39.2x2-	T39.2x3-	T39.2x4-	T39.2x5-	T39.2x6-
Sulfamerazine	T37.0x1-	T37.0x2-	T37.0x3-	T37.0x4-	T37.0x5-	T37.0x6-
Sulfameter	T37.0x1-	T37.0x2-	T37.0x3-	T37.0x4-	T37.0x5-	T37.0x6-
Sulfamethazine	T37.0x1-	T37.0x2-	T37.0x3-	T37.0x4-	T37.0x5-	T37.0x6-
Sulfamethizole	T37.0x1-	T37.0x2-	T37.0x3-	T37.0x4-	T37.0x5-	T37.0x6-
Sulfamethoxazole	T37.0x1-	T37.0x2-	T37.0x3-	T37.0x4-	T37.0x5-	T37.0x6-
with trimethoprim	T36.8x1-	T36.8x2-	T36.8x3-	T36.8x4-	T36.8x5-	T36.8x6-
Sulfamethoxydiazine	T37.0x1-	T37.0x2-	T37.0x3-	T37.0x4-	T37.0x5-	T37.0x6-
Sulfamethoxypyridazine	T37.0x1-	T37.0x2-	T37.0x3-	T37.0x4-	T37.0x5-	T37.0x6-
Sulfamethylthiazole	T37.0x1-	T37.0x2-	T37.0x3-	T37.0x4-	T37.0x5-	T37.0x6-
Sulfametoxydiazine	T37.0x1-	T37.0x2-	T37.0x3-	T37.0x4-	T37.0x5-	T37.0x6-
Sulfamidopyrine	T39.2x1-	T39.2x2-	T39.2x3-	T39.2x4-	T39.2x5-	T39.2x6-
Sulfamonomethoxine	T37.0x1-	T37.0x2-	T37.0x3-	T37.0x4-	T37.0x5-	T37.0x6-
Sulfamoxole	T37.0x1-	T37.0x2-	T37.0x3-	T37.0x4-	T37.0x5-	T37.0x6-
Sulfamylon	T49.0x1-	T49.0x2-	T49.0x3-	T49.0x4-	T49.0x5-	T49.0x6-
Sulfan blue (diagnostic dye)	T50.8x1-	T50.8x2-	T50.8x3-	T50.8x4-	T50.8x5-	T50.8x6-
Sulfanilamide	T37.0x1-	T37.0x2-	T37.0x3-	T37.0x4-	T37.0x5-	T37.0x6-
Sulfanilylguanidine	T37.0x1-	T37.0x2-	T37.0x3-	T37.0x4-	T37.0x5-	T37.0x6-
Sulfaperin	T37.0x1-	T37.0x2-	T37.0x3-	T37.0x4-	T37.0x5-	T37.0x6-
Sulfaphenazole	T37.0x1-	T37.0x2-	T37.0x3-	T37.0x4-	T37.0x5-	T37.0x6-
Sulfaphenylthiazole	T37.0x1-	T37.0x2-	T37.0x3-	T37.0x4-	T37.0x5-	T37.0x6-
Sulfaproxyline	T37.0x1-	T37.0x2-	T37.0x3-	T37.0x4-	T37.0x5-	T37.0x6-
Sulfapyridine	T37.0x1-	T37.0x2-	T37.0x3-	T37.0x4-	T37.0x5-	T37.0x6-
Sulfapyrimidine	T37.0x1-	T37.0x2-	T37.0x3-	T37.0x4-	T37.0x5-	T37.0x6-
Sulfarsphenamine	T37.8x1-	T37.8x2-	T37.8x3-	T37.8x4-	T37.8x5-	T37.8x6-
Sulfasalazine	T37.0x1-	T37.0x2-	T37.0x3-	T37.0x4-	T37.0x5-	T37.0x6-
Sulfasuxidine	T37.0x1-	T37.0x2-	T37.0x3-	T37.0x4-	T37.0x5-	T37.0x6-
Sulfasymazine	T37.0x1-	T37.0x2-	T37.0x3-	T37.0x4-	T37.0x5-	T37.0x6-
Sulfated amylopectin	T47.8x1-	T47.8x2-	T47.8x3-	T47.8x4-	T47.8x5-	T47.8x6-
Sulfathiazole	T37.0x1-	T37.0x2-	T37.0x3-	T37.0x4-	T37.0x5-	T37.0x6-
Sulfatostearate	T49.2x1-	T49.2x2-	T49.2x3-	T49.2x4-	T49.2x5-	T49.2x6-
Sulfinpyrazone	T50.4x1-	T50.4x2-	T50.4x3-	T50.4x4-	T50.4x5-	T50.4x6-
Sulfiram	T49.0x1-	T49.0x2-	T49.0x3-	T49.0x4-	T49.0x5-	T49.0x6-
Sulfisomidine	T37.0x1-	T37.0x2-	T37.0x3-	T37.0x4-	T37.0x5-	T37.0x6-
Sulfisoxazole	T37.0x1-	T37.0x2-	T37.0x3-	T37.0x4-	T37.0x5-	T37.0x6-
ophthalmic preparation	T49.5x1-	T49.5x2-	T49.5x3-	T49.5x4-	T49.5x5-	T49.5x6-
Sulfobromophthalein (sodium)	T50.8x1-	T50.8x2-	T50.8x3-	T50.8x4-	T50.8x5-	T50.8x6-
Sulfobromphthalein	T50.8x1-	T50.8x2-	T50.8x3-	T50.8x4-	T50.8x5-	T50.8x6-
Sulfogaiacol	T48.4x1-	T48.4x2-	T48.4x3-	T48.4x4-	T48.4x5-	T48.4x6-
Sulfomyxin	T36.8x1-	T36.8x2-	T36.8x3-	T36.8x4-	T36.8x5-	T36.8x6-
Sulfonal	T42.6x1-	T42.6x2-	T42.6x3-	T42.6x4-	T42.6x5-	T42.6x6-
Sulfonamide NEC	T37.0x1-	T37.0x2-	T37.0x3-	T37.0x4-	T37.0x5-	T37.0x6-
eye	T49.5x1-	T49.5x2-	T49.5x3-	T49.5x4-	T49.5x5-	T49.5x6-
Sulfonazide	T37.1x1-	T37.1x2-	T37.1x3-	T37.1x4-	T37.1x5-	T37.1x6-
Sulfones	T37.1x1-	T37.1x2-	T37.1x3-	T37.1x4-	T37.1x5-	T37.1x6-
Sulfonethylmethane	T42.6x1-	T42.6x2-	T42.6x3-	T42.6x4-	T42.6x5-	T42.6x6-
Sulfonmethane	T42.6x1-	T42.6x2-	T42.6x3-	T42.6x4-	T42.6x5-	T42.6x6-
Sulfonphthal, sulfonphthol	T50.8x1-	T50.8x2-	T50.8x3-	T50.8x4-	T50.8x5-	T50.8x6-
Sulfonylurea derivatives, oral	T38.3x1-	T38.3x2-	T38.3x3-	T38.3x4-	T38.3x5-	T38.3x6-
Sulforidazine	T43.3x1-	T43.3x2-	T43.3x3-	T43.3x4-	T43.3x5-	T43.3x6-
Sulfoxone	T37.1x1-	T37.1x2-	T37.1x3-	T37.1x4-	T37.1x5-	T37.1x6-
Sulfur, sulfurated, sulfuric, sulfurous, sulfuryl (compounds NEC) (medicinal)	T49.4x1-	T49.4x2-	T49.4x3-	T49.4x4-	T49.4x5-	T49.4x6-
acid	T54.2x1-	T54.2x2-	T54.2x3-	T54.2x4-	—	—
dioxide (gas)	T59.1x1-	T59.1x2-	T59.1x3-	T59.1x4-	—	—
ether — see Ether(s)						
hydrogen	T59.6x1-	T59.6x2-	T59.6x3-	T59.6x4-	—	—
medicinal (keratolytic) (ointment) NEC	T49.4x1-	T49.4x2-	T49.4x3-	T49.4x4-	T49.4x5-	T49.4x6-
ointment	T49.0x1-	T49.0x2-	T49.0x3-	T49.0x4-	T49.0x5-	T49.0x6-
pesticide (vapor)	T60.91x-	T60.92x-	T60.93x-	T60.94x-	—	—
vapor NEC	T59.891-	T59.892-	T59.893-	T59.894-	—	—

DRUGS & CHEMICALS

© 2016 Channel Publishing, Ltd.

DRUGS & CHEMICALS

Table of Drugs & Chemicals	Poisoning Accidental (Unintentional)	Poisoning Self-Harm (Intentional)	Poisoning Assault	Poisoning Undetermined	Adverse Effect	Underdosing
Sulfuric acid	T54.2x1-	T54.2x2-	T54.2x3-	T54.2x4-	—	—
Sulglicotide	T47.1x1-	T47.1x2-	T47.1x3-	T47.1x4-	T47.1x5-	T47.1x6-
Sulindac	T39.391-	T39.392-	T39.393-	T39.394-	T39.395-	T39.396-
Sulisatin	T47.2x1-	T47.2x2-	T47.2x3-	T47.2x4-	T47.2x5-	T47.2x6-
Sulisobenzone	T49.3x1-	T49.3x2-	T49.3x3-	T49.3x4-	T49.3x5-	T49.3x6-
Sulkowitch's reagent	T50.8x1-	T50.8x2-	T50.8x3-	T50.8x4-	T50.8x5-	T50.8x6-
Sulmetozine	T44.3x1-	T44.3x2-	T44.3x3-	T44.3x4-	T44.3x5-	T44.3x6-
Suloctidil	T46.7x1-	T46.7x2-	T46.7x3-	T46.7x4-	T46.7x5-	T46.7x6-
Sulph- — see also Sulf-						
Sulphadiazine	T37.0x1-	T37.0x2-	T37.0x3-	T37.0x4-	T37.0x5-	T37.0x6-
Sulphadimethoxine	T37.0x1-	T37.0x2-	T37.0x3-	T37.0x4-	T37.0x5-	T37.0x6-
Sulphadimidine	T37.0x1-	T37.0x2-	T37.0x3-	T37.0x4-	T37.0x5-	T37.0x6-
Sulphadione	T37.1x1-	T37.1x2-	T37.1x3-	T37.1x4-	T37.1x5-	T37.1x6-
Sulphafurazole	T37.0x1-	T37.0x2-	T37.0x3-	T37.0x4-	T37.0x5-	T37.0x6-
Sulphamethizole	T37.0x1-	T37.0x2-	T37.0x3-	T37.0x4-	T37.0x5-	T37.0x6-
Sulphamethoxazole	T37.0x1-	T37.0x2-	T37.0x3-	T37.0x4-	T37.0x5-	T37.0x6-
Sulphan blue	T50.8x1-	T50.8x2-	T50.8x3-	T50.8x4-	T50.8x5-	T50.8x6-
Sulphaphenazole	T37.0x1-	T37.0x2-	T37.0x3-	T37.0x4-	T37.0x5-	T37.0x6-
Sulphapyridine	T37.0x1-	T37.0x2-	T37.0x3-	T37.0x4-	T37.0x5-	T37.0x6-
Sulphasalazine	T37.0x1-	T37.0x2-	T37.0x3-	T37.0x4-	T37.0x5-	T37.0x6-
Sulphinpyrazone	T50.4x1-	T50.4x2-	T50.4x3-	T50.4x4-	T50.4x5-	T50.4x6-
Sulpiride	T43.591-	T43.592-	T43.593-	T43.594-	T43.595-	T43.596-
Sulprostone	T48.0x1-	T48.0x2-	T48.0x3-	T48.0x4-	T48.0x5-	T48.0x6-
Sulpyrine	T39.2x1-	T39.2x2-	T39.2x3-	T39.2x4-	T39.2x5-	T39.2x6-
Sultamicillin	T36.0x1-	T36.0x2-	T36.0x3-	T36.0x4-	T36.0x5-	T36.0x6-
Sulthiame	T42.6x1-	T42.6x2-	T42.6x3-	T42.6x4-	T42.6x5-	T42.6x6-
Sultiame	T42.6x1-	T42.6x2-	T42.6x3-	T42.6x4-	T42.6x5-	T42.6x6-
Sultopride	T43.591-	T43.592-	T43.593-	T43.594-	T43.595-	T43.596-
Sumatriptan	T39.8x1-	T39.8x2-	T39.8x3-	T39.8x4-	T39.8x5-	T39.8x6-
Sunflower seed oil	T46.6x1-	T46.6x2-	T46.6x3-	T46.6x4-	T46.6x5-	T46.6x6-
Superinone	T48.4x1-	T48.4x2-	T48.4x3-	T48.4x4-	T48.4x5-	T48.4x6-
Suprofen	T39.311-	T39.312-	T39.313-	T39.314-	T39.315-	T39.316-
Suramin (sodium)	T37.4x1-	T37.4x2-	T37.4x3-	T37.4x4-	T37.4x5-	T37.4x6-
Surfacaine	T41.3x1-	T41.3x2-	T41.3x3-	T41.3x4-	T41.3x5-	T41.3x6-
Surital	T41.1x1-	T41.1x2-	T41.1x3-	T41.1x4-	T41.1x5-	T41.1x6-
Sutilains	T45.3x1-	T45.3x2-	T45.3x3-	T45.3x4-	T45.3x5-	T45.3x6-
Suxamethonium (chloride)	T48.1x1-	T48.1x2-	T48.1x3-	T48.1x4-	T48.1x5-	T48.1x6-
Suxethonium (chloride)	T48.1x1-	T48.1x2-	T48.1x3-	T48.1x4-	T48.1x5-	T48.1x6-
Suxibuzone	T39.2x1-	T39.2x2-	T39.2x3-	T39.2x4-	T39.2x5-	T39.2x6-
Sweet niter spirit	T46.3x1-	T46.3x2-	T46.3x3-	T46.3x4-	T46.3x5-	T46.3x6-
Sweet oil (birch)	T49.3x1-	T49.3x2-	T49.3x3-	T49.3x4-	T49.3x5-	T49.3x6-
Sweetener	T50.901-	T50.902-	T50.903-	T50.904-	T50.905-	T50.906-
Sym-dichloroethyl ether	T53.6x1-	T53.6x2-	T53.6x3-	T53.6x4-	—	—
Sympatholytic NEC	T44.8x1-	T44.8x2-	T44.8x3-	T44.8x4-	T44.8x5-	T44.8x6-
haloalkylamine	T44.8x1-	T44.8x2-	T44.8x3-	T44.8x4-	T44.8x5-	T44.8x6-
Sympathomimetic NEC	T44.901-	T44.902-	T44.903-	T44.904-	T44.905-	T44.906-
anti-common-cold	T48.5x1-	T48.5x2-	T48.5x3-	T48.5x4-	T48.5x5-	T48.5x6-
bronchodilator	T48.6x1-	T48.6x2-	T48.6x3-	T48.6x4-	T48.6x5-	T48.6x6-
specified NEC	T44.991-	T44.992-	T44.993-	T44.994-	T44.995-	T44.996-
Synagis	T50.B91-	T50.B92-	T50.B93-	T50.B94-	T50.B95-	T50.B96-
Synalar	T49.0x1-	T49.0x2-	T49.0x3-	T49.0x4-	T49.0x5-	T49.0x6-
Synthroid	T38.1x1-	T38.1x2-	T38.1x3-	T38.1x4-	T38.1x5-	T38.1x6-
Syntocinon	T48.0x1-	T48.0x2-	T48.0x3-	T48.0x4-	T48.0x5-	T48.0x6-
Syrosingopine	T46.5x1-	T46.5x2-	T46.5x3-	T46.5x4-	T46.5x5-	T46.5x6-
Systemic drug	T45.91x-	T45.92x-	T45.93x-	T45.94x-	T45.95x-	T45.96x-
specified NEC	T45.8x1-	T45.8x2-	T45.8x3-	T45.8x4-	T45.8x5-	T45.8x6-

Table of Drugs & Chemicals	Poisoning Accidental (Unintentional)	Poisoning Self-Harm (Intentional)	Poisoning Assault	Poisoning Undetermined	Adverse Effect	Underdosing
2,4,5-T	T60.3x1-	T60.3x2-	T60.3x3-	T60.3x4-	—	—
Tablets — see also specified substance	T50.901-	T50.902-	T50.903-	T50.904-	T50.905-	T50.906-
Tace	T38.5x1-	T38.5x2-	T38.5x3-	T38.5x4-	T38.5x5-	T38.5x6-
Tacrine	T44.0x1-	T44.0x2-	T44.0x3-	T44.0x4-	T44.0x5-	T44.0x6-
Tadalafil	T46.7x1-	T46.7x2-	T46.7x3-	T46.7x4-	T46.7x5-	T46.7x6-
Talampicillin	T36.0x1-	T36.0x2-	T36.0x3-	T36.0x4-	T36.0x5-	T36.0x6-
Talbutal	T42.3x1-	T42.3x2-	T42.3x3-	T42.3x4-	T42.3x5-	T42.3x6-
Talc powder	T49.3x1-	T49.3x2-	T49.3x3-	T49.3x4-	T49.3x5-	T49.3x6-
Talcum	T49.3x1-	T49.3x2-	T49.3x3-	T49.3x4-	T49.3x5-	T49.3x6-
Taleranol	T38.6x1-	T38.6x2-	T38.6x3-	T38.6x4-	T38.6x5-	T38.6x6-
Tamoxifen	T38.6x1-	T38.6x2-	T38.6x3-	T38.6x4-	T38.6x5-	T38.6x6-
Tamsulosin	T44.6x1-	T44.6x2-	T44.6x3-	T44.6x4-	T44.6x5-	T44.6x6-
Tandearil, tanderil	T39.2x1-	T39.2x2-	T39.2x3-	T39.2x4-	T39.2x5-	T39.2x6-
Tannic acid	T49.2x1-	T49.2x2-	T49.2x3-	T49.2x4-	T49.2x5-	T49.2x6-
medicinal (astringent)	T49.2x1-	T49.2x2-	T49.2x3-	T49.2x4-	T49.2x5-	T49.2x6-
Tannin — see Tannic acid						
Tansy	T62.2x1-	T62.2x2-	T62.2x3-	T62.2x4-	—	—
TAO	T36.3x1-	T36.3x2-	T36.3x3-	T36.3x4-	T36.3x5-	T36.3x6-
Tapazole	T38.2x1-	T38.2x2-	T38.2x3-	T38.2x4-	T38.2x5-	T38.2x6-
Tar NEC	T52.0x1-	T52.0x2-	T52.0x3-	T52.0x4-	—	—
camphor	T60.1x1-	T60.1x2-	T60.1x3-	T60.1x4-	—	—
distillate	T49.1x1-	T49.1x2-	T49.1x3-	T49.1x4-	T49.1x5-	T49.1x6-
fumes	T59.891-	T59.892-	T59.893-	T59.894-	—	—
medicinal	T49.1x1-	T49.1x2-	T49.1x3-	T49.1x4-	T49.1x5-	T49.1x6-
ointment	T49.1x1-	T49.1x2-	T49.1x3-	T49.1x4-	T49.1x5-	T49.1x6-
Taractan	T43.591-	T43.592-	T43.593-	T43.594-	T43.595-	T43.596-
Tarantula (venomous)	T63.321-	T63.322-	T63.323-	T63.324-		
Tartar emetic	T37.8x1-	T37.8x2-	T37.8x3-	T37.8x4-	T37.8x5-	T37.8x6-
Tartaric acid	T65.891-	T65.892-	T65.893-	T65.894-		
Tartrate, laxative	T47.4x1-	T47.4x2-	T47.4x3-	T47.4x4-	T47.4x5-	T47.4x6-
Tartrated antimony (anti-infective)	T37.8x1-	T37.8x2-	T37.8x3-	T37.8x4-	T37.8x5-	T37.8x6-
Tauromustine	T45.1x1-	T45.1x2-	T45.1x3-	T45.1x4-	T45.1x5-	T45.1x6-
TCA — see Trichloroacetic acid						
TCDD	T53.7x1-	T53.7x2-	T53.7x3-	T53.7x4-	—	—
TDI (vapor)	T65.0x1-	T65.0x2-	T65.0x3-	T65.0x4-	—	—
Tear						
gas	T59.3x1-	T59.3x2-	T59.3x3-	T59.3x4-	—	—
solution	T49.5x1-	T49.5x2-	T49.5x3-	T49.5x4-	T49.5x5-	T49.5x6-
Teclothiazide	T50.2x1-	T50.2x2-	T50.2x3-	T50.2x4-	T50.2x5-	T50.2x6-
Teclozan	T37.3x1-	T37.3x2-	T37.3x3-	T37.3x4-	T37.3x5-	T37.3x6-
Tegafur	T45.1x1-	T45.1x2-	T45.1x3-	T45.1x4-	T45.1x5-	T45.1x6-
Tegretol	T42.1x1-	T42.1x2-	T42.1x3-	T42.1x4-	T42.1x5-	T42.1x6-
Teicoplanin	T36.8x1-	T36.8x2-	T36.8x3-	T36.8x4-	T36.8x5-	T36.8x6-
Telepaque	T50.8x1-	T50.8x2-	T50.8x3-	T50.8x4-	T50.8x5-	T50.8x6-
Tellurium	T56.891-	T56.892-	T56.893-	T56.894-	—	—
fumes	T56.891-	T56.892-	T56.893-	T56.894-	—	—
TEM	T45.1x1-	T45.1x2-	T45.1x3-	T45.1x4-	T45.1x5-	T45.1x6-
Temazepam	T42.4x1-	T42.4x2-	T42.4x3-	T42.4x4-	T42.4x5-	T42.4x6-
Temocillin	T36.0x1-	T36.0x2-	T36.0x3-	T36.0x4-	T36.0x5-	T36.0x6-
Tenamfetamine	T43.621-	T43.622-	T43.623-	T43.624-	T43.625-	T43.626-
Teniposide	T45.1x1-	T45.1x2-	T45.1x3-	T45.1x4-	T45.1x5-	T45.1x6-
Tenitramine	T46.3x1-	T46.3x2-	T46.3x3-	T46.3x4-	T46.3x5-	T46.3x6-
Tenoglicin	T48.4x1-	T48.4x2-	T48.4x3-	T48.4x4-	T48.4x5-	T48.4x6-
Tenonitrozole	T37.3x1-	T37.3x2-	T37.3x3-	T37.3x4-	T37.3x5-	T37.3x6-
Tenoxicam	T39.391-	T39.392-	T39.393-	T39.394-	T39.395-	T39.396-
TEPA	T45.1x1-	T45.1x2-	T45.1x3-	T45.1x4-	T45.1x5-	T45.1x6-
TEPP	T60.0x1-	T60.0x2-	T60.0x3-	T60.0x4-		

DRUGS & CHEMICALS

Table of Drugs & Chemicals	POISONING Accidental (Unintentional)	Self-Harm (Intentional)	Assault	Undetermined	Adverse Effect	Underdosing
Teprotide	T46.5x1-	T46.5x2-	T46.5x3-	T46.5x4-	T46.5x5-	T46.5x6-
Terazosin	T44.6x1-	T44.6x2-	T44.6x3-	T44.6x4-	T44.6x5-	T44.6x6-
Terbufos	T60.0x1-	T60.0x2-	T60.0x3-	T60.0x4-		
Terbutaline	T48.6x1-	T48.6x2-	T48.6x3-	T48.6x4-	T48.6x5-	T48.6x6-
Terconazole	T49.0x1-	T49.0x2-	T49.0x3-	T49.0x4-	T49.0x5-	T49.0x6-
Terfenadine	T45.0x1-	T45.0x2-	T45.0x3-	T45.0x4-	T45.0x5-	T45.0x6-
Teriparatide (acetate)	T50.991-	T50.992-	T50.993-	T50.994-	T50.995-	T50.996-
Terizidone	T37.1x1-	T37.1x2-	T37.1x3-	T37.1x4-	T37.1x5-	T37.1x6-
Terlipressin	T38.891-	T38.892-	T38.893-	T38.894-	T38.895-	T38.896-
Terodiline	T46.3x1-	T46.3x2-	T46.3x3-	T46.3x4-	T46.3x5-	T46.3x6-
Teroxalene	T37.4x1-	T37.4x2-	T37.4x3-	T37.4x4-	T37.4x5-	T37.4x6-
Terpin (cis) hydrate	T48.4x1-	T48.4x2-	T48.4x3-	T48.4x4-	T48.4x5-	T48.4x6-
Terramycin	T36.4x1-	T36.4x2-	T36.4x3-	T36.4x4-	T36.4x5-	T36.4x6-
Tertatolol	T44.7x1-	T44.7x2-	T44.7x3-	T44.7x4-	T44.7x5-	T44.7x6-
Tessalon	T48.3x1-	T48.3x2-	T48.3x3-	T48.3x4-	T48.3x5-	T48.3x6-
Testolactone	T38.7x1-	T38.7x2-	T38.7x3-	T38.7x4-	T38.7x5-	T38.7x6-
Testosterone	T38.7x1-	T38.7x2-	T38.7x3-	T38.7x4-	T38.7x5-	T38.7x6-
Tetanus toxoid or vaccine	T50.A91-	T50.A92-	T50.A93-	T50.A94-	T50.A95-	T50.A96-
antitoxin	T50.Z11-	T50.Z12-	T50.Z13-	T50.Z14-	T50.Z15-	T50.Z16-
immune globulin (human)	T50.Z11-	T50.Z12-	T50.Z13-	T50.Z14-	T50.Z15-	T50.Z16-
toxoid	T50.A91-	T50.A92-	T50.A93-	T50.A94-	T50.A95-	T50.A96-
with diphtheria toxoid	T50.A21-	T50.A22-	T50.A23-	T50.A24-	T50.A25-	T50.A26-
with pertussis	T50.A11-	T50.A12-	T50.A13-	T50.A14-	T50.A15-	T50.A16-
Tetrabenazine	T43.591-	T43.592-	T43.593-	T43.594-	T43.595-	T43.596-
Tetracaine	T41.3x1-	T41.3x2-	T41.3x3-	T41.3x4-	T41.3x5-	T41.3x6-
nerve block (peripheral) (plexus)	T41.3x1-	T41.3x2-	T41.3x3-	T41.3x4-	T41.3x5-	T41.3x6-
regional	T41.3x1-	T41.3x2-	T41.3x3-	T41.3x4-	T41.3x5-	T41.3x6-
spinal	T41.3x1-	T41.3x2-	T41.3x3-	T41.3x4-	T41.3x5-	T41.3x6-
Tetrachlorethylene — see Tetrachloroethylene						
Tetrachlormethiazide	T50.2x1-	T50.2x2-	T50.2x3-	T50.2x4-	T50.2x5-	T50.2x6-
2,3,7,8-Tetrachlorodibenzo-p-dioxin	T53.7x1-	T53.7x2-	T53.7x3-	T53.7x4-	—	—
Tetrachloroethane	T53.6x1-	T53.6x2-	T53.6x3-	T53.6x4-	—	—
vapor	T53.6x1-	T53.6x2-	T53.6x3-	T53.6x4-	—	—
paint or varnish	T53.6x1-	T53.6x2-	T53.6x3-	T53.6x4-	—	—
Tetrachloroethylene (liquid)	T53.3x1-	T53.3x2-	T53.3x3-	T53.3x4-	—	—
medicinal	T37.4x1-	T37.4x2-	T37.4x3-	T37.4x4-	T37.4x5-	T37.4x6-
vapor	T53.3x1-	T53.3x2-	T53.3x3-	T53.3x4-	—	—
Tetrachloromethane — see Carbon tetrachloride						
Tetracosactide	T38.811-	T38.812-	T38.813-	T38.814-	T38.815-	T38.816-
Tetracosactrin	T38.811-	T38.812-	T38.813-	T38.814-	T38.815-	T38.816-
Tetracycline	T36.4x1-	T36.4x2-	T36.4x3-	T36.4x4-	T36.4x5-	T36.4x6-
ophthalmic preparation	T49.5x1-	T49.5x2-	T49.5x3-	T49.5x4-	T49.5x5-	T49.5x6-
topical NEC	T49.0x1-	T49.0x2-	T49.0x3-	T49.0x4-	T49.0x5-	T49.0x6-
Tetradifon	T60.8x1-	T60.8x2-	T60.8x3-	T60.8x4-	—	—
Tetradotoxin	T61.771-	T61.772-	T61.773-	T61.774-		
Tetraethyl lead	T56.0x1-	T56.0x2-	T56.0x3-	T56.0x4-	—	—
pyrophosphate	T60.0x1-	T60.0x2-	T60.0x3-	T60.0x4-	—	—
Tetraethylammonium chloride	T44.2x1-	T44.2x2-	T44.2x3-	T44.2x4-	T44.2x5-	T44.2x6-
Tetraethylthiuram disulfide	T50.6x1-	T50.6x2-	T50.6x3-	T50.6x4-	T50.6x5-	T50.6x6-
Tetrahydroaminoacridine	T44.0x1-	T44.0x2-	T44.0x3-	T44.0x4-	T44.0x5-	T44.0x6-
Tetrahydrocannabinol	T40.7x1-	T40.7x2-	T40.7x3-	T40.7x4-	T40.7x5-	T40.7x6-
Tetrahydrofuran	T52.8x1-	T52.8x2-	T52.8x3-	T52.8x4-	—	—
Tetrahydronaphthalene	T52.8x1-	T52.8x2-	T52.8x3-	T52.8x4-	—	—
Tetrahydrozoline	T49.5x1-	T49.5x2-	T49.5x3-	T49.5x4-	T49.5x5-	T49.5x6-
Tetralin	T52.8x1-	T52.8x2-	T52.8x3-	T52.8x4-	—	—
Tetramethrin	T60.2x1-	T60.2x2-	T60.2x3-	T60.2x4-	—	—
Tetramethylthiuram (disulfide) NEC	T60.3x1-	T60.3x2-	T60.3x3-	T60.3x4-	—	—
medicinal	T49.0x1-	T49.0x2-	T49.0x3-	T49.0x4-	T49.0x5-	T49.0x6-
Tetramisole	T37.4x1-	T37.4x2-	T37.4x3-	T37.4x4-	T37.4x5-	T37.4x6-
Tetranicotinoyl fructose	T46.7x1-	T46.7x2-	T46.7x3-	T46.7x4-	T46.7x5-	T46.7x6-
Tetrazepam	T42.4x1-	T42.4x2-	T42.4x3-	T42.4x4-	T42.4x5-	T42.4x6-
Tetronal	T42.6x1-	T42.6x2-	T42.6x3-	T42.6x4-	T42.6x5-	T42.6x6-
Tetryl	T65.3x1-	T65.3x2-	T65.3x3-	T65.3x4-	—	—
Tetrylammonium chloride	T44.2x1-	T44.2x2-	T44.2x3-	T44.2x4-	T44.2x5-	T44.2x6-
Tetryzoline	T49.5x1-	T49.5x2-	T49.5x3-	T49.5x4-	T49.5x5-	T49.5x6-
Thalidomide	T45.1x1-	T45.1x2-	T45.1x3-	T45.1x4-	T45.1x5-	T45.1x6-
Thallium (compounds) (dust) NEC	T56.811-	T56.812-	T56.813-	T56.814-	—	—
pesticide	T60.4x1-	T60.4x2-	T60.4x3-	T60.4x4-	—	—
THC	T40.7x1-	T40.7x2-	T40.7x3-	T40.7x4-	T40.7x5-	T40.7x6-
Thebacon	T48.3x1-	T48.3x2-	T48.3x3-	T48.3x4-	T48.3x5-	T48.3x6-
Thebaine	T40.2x1-	T40.2x2-	T40.2x3-	T40.2x4-	T40.2x5-	T40.2x6-
Thenoic acid	T49.6x1-	T49.6x2-	T49.6x3-	T49.6x4-	T49.6x5-	T49.6x6-
Thenyldiamine	T45.0x1-	T45.0x2-	T45.0x3-	T45.0x4-	T45.0x5-	T45.0x6-
Theobromine (calcium salicylate)	T48.6x1-	T48.6x2-	T48.6x3-	T48.6x4-	T48.6x5-	T48.6x6-
sodium salicylate	T48.6x1-	T48.6x2-	T48.6x3-	T48.6x4-	T48.6x5-	T48.6x6-
Theophyllamine	T48.6x1-	T48.6x2-	T48.6x3-	T48.6x4-	T48.6x5-	T48.6x6-
Theophylline	T48.6x1-	T48.6x2-	T48.6x3-	T48.6x4-	T48.6x5-	T48.6x6-
aminobenzoic acid	T48.6x1-	T48.6x2-	T48.6x3-	T48.6x4-	T48.6x5-	T48.6x6-
ethylenediamine	T48.6x1-	T48.6x2-	T48.6x3-	T48.6x4-	T48.6x5-	T48.6x6-
piperazine p-amino-benzoate	T48.6x1-	T48.6x2-	T48.6x3-	T48.6x4-	T48.6x5-	T48.6x6-
Thiabendazole	T37.4x1-	T37.4x2-	T37.4x3-	T37.4x4-	T37.4x5-	T37.4x6-
Thialbarbital	T41.1x1-	T41.1x2-	T41.1x3-	T41.1x4-	T41.1x5-	T41.1x6-
Thiamazole	T38.2x1-	T38.2x2-	T38.2x3-	T38.2x4-	T38.2x5-	T38.2x6-
Thiambutosine	T37.1x1-	T37.1x2-	T37.1x3-	T37.1x4-	T37.1x5-	T37.1x6-
Thiamine	T45.2x1-	T45.2x2-	T45.2x3-	T45.2x4-	T45.2x5-	T45.2x6-
Thiamphenicol	T36.2x1-	T36.2x2-	T36.2x3-	T36.2x4-	T36.2x5-	T36.2x6-
Thiamylal	T41.1x1-	T41.1x2-	T41.1x3-	T41.1x4-	T41.1x5-	T41.1x6-
sodium	T41.1x1-	T41.1x2-	T41.1x3-	T41.1x4-	T41.1x5-	T41.1x6-
Thiazesim	T43.291-	T43.292-	T43.293-	T43.294-	T43.295-	T43.296-
Thiazides (diuretics)	T50.2x1-	T50.2x2-	T50.2x3-	T50.2x4-	T50.2x5-	T50.2x6-
Thiazinamium metilsulfate	T43.3x1-	T43.3x2-	T43.3x3-	T43.3x4-	T43.3x5-	T43.3x6-
Thiethylperazine	T43.3x1-	T43.3x2-	T43.3x3-	T43.3x4-	T43.3x5-	T43.3x6-
Thimerosal	T49.0x1-	T49.0x2-	T49.0x3-	T49.0x4-	T49.0x5-	T49.0x6-
ophthalmic preparation	T49.5x1-	T49.5x2-	T49.5x3-	T49.5x4-	T49.5x5-	T49.5x6-
Thioacetazone	T37.1x1-	T37.1x2-	T37.1x3-	T37.1x4-	T37.1x5-	T37.1x6-
with isoniazid	T37.1x1-	T37.1x2-	T37.1x3-	T37.1x4-	T37.1x5-	T37.1x6-
Thiobarbital sodium	T41.1x1-	T41.1x2-	T41.1x3-	T41.1x4-	T41.1x5-	T41.1x6-
Thiobarbiturate anesthetic	T41.1x1-	T41.1x2-	T41.1x3-	T41.1x4-	T41.1x5-	T41.1x6-
Thiobismol	T37.8x1-	T37.8x2-	T37.8x3-	T37.8x4-	T37.8x5-	T37.8x6-
Thiobutabarbital sodium	T41.1x1-	T41.1x2-	T41.1x3-	T41.1x4-	T41.1x5-	T41.1x6-
Thiocarbamate (insecticide)	T60.0x1-	T60.0x2-	T60.0x3-	T60.0x4-	—	—
Thiocarbamide	T38.2x1-	T38.2x2-	T38.2x3-	T38.2x4-	T38.2x5-	T38.2x6-
Thiocarbarsone	T37.8x1-	T37.8x2-	T37.8x3-	T37.8x4-	T37.8x5-	T37.8x6-
Thiocarlide	T37.1x1-	T37.1x2-	T37.1x3-	T37.1x4-	T37.1x5-	T37.1x6-
Thioctamide	T50.991-	T50.992-	T50.993-	T50.994-	T50.995-	T50.996-
Thioctic acid	T50.991-	T50.992-	T50.993-	T50.994-	T50.995-	T50.996-
Thiofos	T60.0x1-	T60.0x2-	T60.0x3-	T60.0x4-	—	—
Thioglycolate	T49.4x1-	T49.4x2-	T49.4x3-	T49.4x4-	T49.4x5-	T49.4x6-
Thioglycolic acid	T65.891-	T65.892-	T65.893-	T65.894-	—	—
Thioguanine	T45.1x1-	T45.1x2-	T45.1x3-	T45.1x4-	T45.1x5-	T45.1x6-
Thiomercaptomerin	T50.2x1-	T50.2x2-	T50.2x3-	T50.2x4-	T50.2x5-	T50.2x6-

DRUGS & CHEMICALS

Table of Drugs & Chemicals	POISONING Accidental (Unintentional)	Self-Harm (Intentional)	Assault	Undetermined	Adverse Effect	Underdosing
Thiomerin	T50.2x1-	T50.2x2-	T50.2x3-	T50.2x4-	T50.2x5-	T50.2x6-
Thiomersal	T49.0x1-	T49.0x2-	T49.0x3-	T49.0x4-	T49.0x5-	T49.0x6-
Thionazin	T60.0x1-	T60.0x2-	T60.0x3-	T60.0x4-	—	—
Thiopental (sodium)	T41.1x1-	T41.1x2-	T41.1x3-	T41.1x4-	T41.1x5-	T41.1x6-
Thiopentone (sodium)	T41.1x1-	T41.1x2-	T41.1x3-	T41.1x4-	T41.1x5-	T41.1x6-
Thiopropazate	T43.3x1-	T43.3x2-	T43.3x3-	T43.3x4-	T43.3x5-	T43.3x6-
Thioproperazine	T43.3x1-	T43.3x2-	T43.3x3-	T43.3x4-	T43.3x5-	T43.3x6-
Thioridazine	T43.3x1-	T43.3x2-	T43.3x3-	T43.3x4-	T43.3x5-	T43.3x6-
Thiosinamine	T49.3x1-	T49.3x2-	T49.3x3-	T49.3x4-	T49.3x5-	T49.3x6-
Thiotepa	T45.1x1-	T45.1x2-	T45.1x3-	T45.1x4-	T45.1x5-	T45.1x6-
Thiothixene	T43.4x1-	T43.4x2-	T43.4x3-	T43.4x4-	T43.4x5-	T43.4x6-
Thiouracil (benzyl) (methyl) (propyl)	T38.2x1-	T38.2x2-	T38.2x3-	T38.2x4-	T38.2x5-	T38.2x6-
Thiourea	T38.2x1-	T38.2x2-	T38.2x3-	T38.2x4-	T38.2x5-	T38.2x6-
Thiphenamil	T44.3x1-	T44.3x2-	T44.3x3-	T44.3x4-	T44.3x5-	T44.3x6-
Thiram	T60.3x1-	T60.3x2-	T60.3x3-	T60.3x4-	—	—
medicinal	T49.2x1-	T49.2x2-	T49.2x3-	T49.2x4-	T49.2x5-	T49.2x6-
Thonzylamine (systemic)	T45.0x1-	T45.0x2-	T45.0x3-	T45.0x4-	T45.0x5-	T45.0x6-
mucosal decongestant	T48.5x1-	T48.5x2-	T48.5x3-	T48.5x4-	T48.5x5-	T48.5x6-
Thorazine	T43.3x1-	T43.3x2-	T43.3x3-	T43.3x4-	T43.3x5-	T43.3x6-
Thorium dioxide suspension	T50.8x1-	T50.8x2-	T50.8x3-	T50.8x4-	T50.8x5-	T50.8x6-
Thornapple	T62.2x1-	T62.2x2-	T62.2x3-	T62.2x4-	—	—
Throat drug NEC	T49.6x1-	T49.6x2-	T49.6x3-	T49.6x4-	T49.6x5-	T49.6x6-
Thrombin	T45.7x1-	T45.7x2-	T45.7x3-	T45.7x4-	T45.7x5-	T45.7x6-
Thrombolysin	T45.611-	T45.612-	T45.613-	T45.614-	T45.615-	T45.616-
Thromboplastin	T45.7x1-	T45.7x2-	T45.7x3-	T45.7x4-	T45.7x5-	T45.7x6-
Thurfyl nicotinate	T46.7x1-	T46.7x2-	T46.7x3-	T46.7x4-	T46.7x5-	T46.7x6-
Thymol	T49.0x1-	T49.0x2-	T49.0x3-	T49.0x4-	T49.0x5-	T49.0x6-
Thymopentin	T37.5x1-	T37.5x2-	T37.5x3-	T37.5x4-	T37.5x5-	T37.5x6-
Thymoxamine	T46.7x1-	T46.7x2-	T46.7x3-	T46.7x4-	T46.7x5-	T46.7x6-
Thymus extract	T38.891-	T38.892-	T38.893-	T38.894-	T38.895-	T38.896-
Thyreotrophic hormone	T38.811-	T38.812-	T38.813-	T38.814-	T38.815-	T38.816-
Thyroglobulin	T38.1x1-	T38.1x2-	T38.1x3-	T38.1x4-	T38.1x5-	T38.1x6-
Thyroid (hormone)	T38.1x1-	T38.1x2-	T38.1x3-	T38.1x4-	T38.1x5-	T38.1x6-
Thyrolar	T38.1x1-	T38.1x2-	T38.1x3-	T38.1x4-	T38.1x5-	T38.1x6-
Thyrotrophin	T38.811-	T38.812-	T38.813-	T38.814-	T38.815-	T38.816-
Thyrotropic hormone	T38.811-	T38.812-	T38.813-	T38.814-	T38.815-	T38.816-
Thyroxine	T38.1x1-	T38.1x2-	T38.1x3-	T38.1x4-	T38.1x5-	T38.1x6-
Tiabendazole	T37.4x1-	T37.4x2-	T37.4x3-	T37.4x4-	T37.4x5-	T37.4x6-
Tiamizide	T50.2x1-	T50.2x2-	T50.2x3-	T50.2x4-	T50.2x5-	T50.2x6-
Tianeptine	T43.291-	T43.292-	T43.293-	T43.294-	T43.295-	T43.296-
Tiapamil	T46.1x1-	T46.1x2-	T46.1x3-	T46.1x4-	T46.1x5-	T46.1x6-
Tiapride	T43.591-	T43.592-	T43.593-	T43.594-	T43.595-	T43.596-
Tiaprofenic acid	T39.311-	T39.312-	T39.313-	T39.314-	T39.315-	T39.316-
Tiaramide	T39.8x1-	T39.8x2-	T39.8x3-	T39.8x4-	T39.8x5-	T39.8x6-
Ticarcillin	T36.0x1-	T36.0x2-	T36.0x3-	T36.0x4-	T36.0x5-	T36.0x6-
Ticlatone	T49.0x1-	T49.0x2-	T49.0x3-	T49.0x4-	T49.0x5-	T49.0x6-
Ticlopidine	T45.521-	T45.522-	T45.523-	T45.524-	T45.525-	T45.526-
Ticrynafen	T50.1x1-	T50.1x2-	T50.1x3-	T50.1x4-	T50.1x5-	T50.1x6-
Tidiacic	T50.991-	T50.992-	T50.993-	T50.994-	T50.995-	T50.996-
Tiemonium	T44.3x1-	T44.3x2-	T44.3x3-	T44.3x4-	T44.3x5-	T44.3x6-
iodide	T44.3x1-	T44.3x2-	T44.3x3-	T44.3x4-	T44.3x5-	T44.3x6-
Tienilic acid	T50.1x1-	T50.1x2-	T50.1x3-	T50.1x4-	T50.1x5-	T50.1x6-
Tifenamil	T44.3x1-	T44.3x2-	T44.3x3-	T44.3x4-	T44.3x5-	T44.3x6-
Tigan	T45.0x1-	T45.0x2-	T45.0x3-	T45.0x4-	T45.0x5-	T45.0x6-
Tigloidine	T44.3x1-	T44.3x2-	T44.3x3-	T44.3x4-	T44.3x5-	T44.3x6-
Tilactase	T47.5x1-	T47.5x2-	T47.5x3-	T47.5x4-	T47.5x5-	T47.5x6-
Tiletamine	T41.291-	T41.292-	T41.293-	T41.294-	T41.295-	T41.296-
Tilidine	T40.4x1-	T40.4x2-	T40.4x3-	T40.4x4-	—	—

Table of Drugs & Chemicals	POISONING Accidental (Unintentional)	Self-Harm (Intentional)	Assault	Undetermined	Adverse Effect	Underdosing
Timepidium bromide	T44.3x1-	T44.3x2-	T44.3x3-	T44.3x4-	T44.3x5-	T44.3x6-
Timiperone	T43.4x1-	T43.4x2-	T43.4x3-	T43.4x4-	T43.4x5-	T43.4x6-
Timolol	T44.7x1-	T44.7x2-	T44.7x3-	T44.7x4-	T44.7x5-	T44.7x6-
Tin (chloride) (dust) (oxide) NEC	T56.6x1-	T56.6x2-	T56.6x3-	T56.6x4-	—	—
anti-infectives	T37.8x1-	T37.8x2-	T37.8x3-	T37.8x4-	T37.8x5-	T37.8x6-
Tincture, iodine — see Iodine						
Tindal	T43.3x1-	T43.3x2-	T43.3x3-	T43.3x4-	T43.3x5-	T43.3x6-
Tinidazole	T37.3x1-	T37.3x2-	T37.3x3-	T37.3x4-	T37.3x5-	T37.3x6-
Tinoridine	T39.8x1-	T39.8x2-	T39.8x3-	T39.8x4-	T39.8x5-	T39.8x6-
Tiocarlide	T37.1x1-	T37.1x2-	T37.1x3-	T37.1x4-	T37.1x5-	T37.1x6-
Tioclomarol	T45.511-	T45.512-	T45.513-	T45.514-	T45.515-	T45.516-
Tioconazole	T49.0x1-	T49.0x2-	T49.0x3-	T49.0x4-	T49.0x5-	T49.0x6-
Tioguanine	T45.1x1-	T45.1x2-	T45.1x3-	T45.1x4-	T45.1x5-	T45.1x6-
Tiopronin	T50.991-	T50.992-	T50.993-	T50.994-	T50.995-	T50.996-
Tiotixene	T43.4x1-	T43.4x2-	T43.4x3-	T43.4x4-	T43.4x5-	T43.4x6-
Tioxolone	T49.4x1-	T49.4x2-	T49.4x3-	T49.4x4-	T49.4x5-	T49.4x6-
Tipepidine	T48.3x1-	T48.3x2-	T48.3x3-	T48.3x4-	T48.3x5-	T48.3x6-
Tiquizium bromide	T44.3x1-	T44.3x2-	T44.3x3-	T44.3x4-	T44.3x5-	T44.3x6-
Tiratricol	T38.1x1-	T38.1x2-	T38.1x3-	T38.1x4-	T38.1x5-	T38.1x6-
Tisopurine	T50.4x1-	T50.4x2-	T50.4x3-	T50.4x4-	T50.4x5-	T50.4x6-
Titanium (compounds) (vapor)	T56.891-	T56.892-	T56.893-	T56.894-	—	—
dioxide	T49.3x1-	T49.3x2-	T49.3x3-	T49.3x4-	T49.3x5-	T49.3x6-
ointment	T49.3x1-	T49.3x2-	T49.3x3-	T49.3x4-	T49.3x5-	T49.3x6-
oxide	T49.3x1-	T49.3x2-	T49.3x3-	T49.3x4-	T49.3x5-	T49.3x6-
tetrachloride	T56.891-	T56.892-	T56.893-	T56.894-	—	—
Titanocene	T56.891-	T56.892-	T56.893-	T56.894-	—	—
Titroid	T38.1x1-	T38.1x2-	T38.1x3-	T38.1x4-	T38.1x5-	T38.1x6-
Tizanidine	T42.8x1-	T42.8x2-	T42.8x3-	T42.8x4-	T42.8x5-	T42.8x6-
TMTD	T60.3x1-	T60.3x2-	T60.3x3-	T60.3x4-	—	—
TNT (fumes)	T65.3x1-	T65.3x2-	T65.3x3-	T65.3x4-	—	—
Toadstool	T62.0x1-	T62.0x2-	T62.0x3-	T62.0x4-	—	—
Tobacco NEC	T65.291-	T65.292-	T65.293-	T65.294-	—	—
cigarettes	T65.221-	T65.222-	T65.223-	T65.224-	—	—
Indian	T62.2x1-	T62.2x2-	T62.2x3-	T62.2x4-	—	—
smoke, second-hand	T65.221-	T65.222-	T65.223-	T65.224-	—	—
Tobramycin	T36.5x1-	T36.5x2-	T36.5x3-	T36.5x4-	T36.5x5-	T36.5x6-
Tocainide	T46.2x1-	T46.2x2-	T46.2x3-	T46.2x4-	T46.2x5-	T46.2x6-
Tocoferol	T45.2x1-	T45.2x2-	T45.2x3-	T45.2x4-	T45.2x5-	T45.2x6-
Tocopherol	T45.2x1-	T45.2x2-	T45.2x3-	T45.2x4-	T45.2x5-	T45.2x6-
acetate	T45.2x1-	T45.2x2-	T45.2x3-	T45.2x4-	T45.2x5-	T45.2x6-
Tocosamine	T48.0x1-	T48.0x2-	T48.0x3-	T48.0x4-	T48.0x5-	T48.0x6-
Todralazine	T46.5x1-	T46.5x2-	T46.5x3-	T46.5x4-	T46.5x5-	T46.5x6-
Tofisopam	T42.4x1-	T42.4x2-	T42.4x3-	T42.4x4-	T42.4x5-	T42.4x6-
Tofranil	T43.011-	T43.012-	T43.013-	T43.014-	T43.015-	T43.016-
Toilet deodorizer	T65.891-	T65.892-	T65.893-	T65.894-	—	—
Tolamolol	T44.7x1-	T44.7x2-	T44.7x3-	T44.7x4-	T44.7x5-	T44.7x6-
Tolazamide	T38.3x1-	T38.3x2-	T38.3x3-	T38.3x4-	T38.3x5-	T38.3x6-
Tolazoline	T46.7x1-	T46.7x2-	T46.7x3-	T46.7x4-	T46.7x5-	T46.7x6-
Tolbutamide (sodium)	T38.3x1-	T38.3x2-	T38.3x3-	T38.3x4-	T38.3x5-	T38.3x6-
Tolciclate	T49.0x1-	T49.0x2-	T49.0x3-	T49.0x4-	T49.0x5-	T49.0x6-
Tolmetin	T39.391-	T39.392-	T39.393-	T39.394-	T39.395-	T39.396-
Tolnaftate	T49.0x1-	T49.0x2-	T49.0x3-	T49.0x4-	T49.0x5-	T49.0x6-
Tolonidine	T46.5x1-	T46.5x2-	T46.5x3-	T46.5x4-	T46.5x5-	T46.5x6-
Toloxatone	T42.6x1-	T42.6x2-	T42.6x3-	T42.6x4-	T42.6x5-	T42.6x6-
Tolperisone	T44.3x1-	T44.3x2-	T44.3x3-	T44.3x4-	T44.3x5-	T44.3x6-
Tolserol	T42.8x1-	T42.8x2-	T42.8x3-	T42.8x4-	T42.8x5-	T42.8x6-

DRUGS & CHEMICALS

Table of Drugs & Chemicals	Poisoning Accidental (Unintentional)	Poisoning Self-Harm (Intentional)	Poisoning Assault	Poisoning Undetermined	Adverse Effect	Underdosing
Toluene (liquid)	T52.2x1-	T52.2x2-	T52.2x3-	T52.2x4-	—	—
diisocyanate	T65.0x1-	T65.0x2-	T65.0x3-	T65.0x4-	—	—
Toluidine	T65.891-	T65.892-	T65.893-	T65.894-	—	—
vapor	T59.891-	T59.892-	T59.893-	T59.894-	—	—
Toluol (liquid)	T52.2x1-	T52.2x2-	T52.2x3-	T52.2x4-	—	—
vapor	T52.2x1-	T52.2x2-	T52.2x3-	T52.2x4-	—	—
Toluylenediamine	T65.3x1-	T65.3x2-	T65.3x3-	T65.3x4-	—	—
Tolylene-2,4-diisocyanate	T65.0x1-	T65.0x2-	T65.0x3-	T65.0x4-	—	—
Tonic NEC	T50.901-	T50.902-	T50.903-	T50.904-	T50.905-	T50.906-
Topical action drug NEC	T49.91x-	T49.92x-	T49.93x-	T49.94x-	T49.95x-	T49.96x-
ear, nose or throat	T49.6x1-	T49.6x2-	T49.6x3-	T49.6x4-	T49.6x5-	T49.6x6-
eye	T49.5x1-	T49.5x2-	T49.5x3-	T49.5x4-	T49.5x5-	T49.5x6-
skin	T49.91x-	T49.92x-	T49.93x-	T49.94x-	T49.95x-	T49.96x-
specified NEC	T49.8x1-	T49.8x2-	T49.8x3-	T49.8x4-	T49.8x5-	T49.8x6-
Toquizine	T44.3x1-	T44.3x2-	T44.3x3-	T44.3x4-	T44.3x5-	T44.3x6-
Toremifene	T38.6x1-	T38.6x2-	T38.6x3-	T38.6x4-	T38.6x5-	T38.6x6-
Tosylchloramide sodium	T49.8x1-	T49.8x2-	T49.8x3-	T49.8x4-	T49.8x5-	T49.8x6-
Toxaphene (dust) (spray)	T60.1x1-	T60.1x2-	T60.1x3-	T60.1x4-	—	—
Toxin, diphtheria (Schick Test)	T50.8x1-	T50.8x2-	T50.8x3-	T50.8x4-	T50.8x5-	T50.8x6-
Toxoid						
combined	T50.A21-	T50.A22-	T50.A23-	T50.A24-	T50.A25-	T50.A26-
diphtheria	T50.A91-	T50.A92-	T50.A93-	T50.A94-	T50.A95-	T50.A96-
tetanus	T50.A91-	T50.A92-	T50.A93-	T50.A94-	T50.A95-	T50.A96-
Trace element NEC	T45.8x1-	T45.8x2-	T45.8x3-	T45.8x4-	T45.8x5-	T45.8x6-
Tractor fuel NEC	T52.0x1-	T52.0x2-	T52.0x3-	T52.0x4-	—	—
Tragacanth	T50.991-	T50.992-	T50.993-	T50.994-	T50.995-	T50.996-
Tramadol	T40.4x1-	T40.4x2-	T40.4x3-	T40.4x4-	T40.4x5-	T40.4x6-
Tramazoline	T48.5x1-	T48.5x2-	T48.5x3-	T48.5x4-	T48.5x5-	T48.5x6-
Tranexamic acid	T45.621-	T45.622-	T45.623-	T45.624-	T45.625-	T45.626-
Tranilast	T45.0x1-	T45.0x2-	T45.0x3-	T45.0x4-	T45.0x5-	T45.0x6-
Tranquilizer NEC	T43.501-	T43.502-	T43.503-	T43.504-	T43.505-	T43.506-
with hypnotic or sedative	T42.6x1-	T42.6x2-	T42.6x3-	T42.6x4-	T42.6x5-	T42.6x6-
benzodiazepine NEC	T42.4x1-	T42.4x2-	T42.4x3-	T42.4x4-	T42.4x5-	T42.4x6-
butyrophenone NEC	T43.4x1-	T43.4x2-	T43.4x3-	T43.4x4-	T43.4x5-	T43.4x6-
carbamate	T43.591-	T43.592-	T43.593-	T43.594-	T43.595-	T43.596-
dimethylamine	T43.3x1-	T43.3x2-	T43.3x3-	T43.3x4-	T43.3x5-	T43.3x6-
ethylamine	T43.3x1-	T43.3x2-	T43.3x3-	T43.3x4-	T43.3x5-	T43.3x6-
hydroxyzine	T43.591-	T43.592-	T43.593-	T43.594-	T43.595-	T43.596-
major NEC	T43.501-	T43.502-	T43.503-	T43.504-	T43.505-	T43.506-
penothiazine NEC	T43.3x1-	T43.3x2-	T43.3x3-	T43.3x4-	T43.3x5-	T43.3x6-
phenothiazine-based	T43.3x1-	T43.3x2-	T43.3x3-	T43.3x4-	T43.3x5-	T43.3x6-
piperazine NEC	T43.3x1-	T43.3x2-	T43.3x3-	T43.3x4-	T43.3x5-	T43.3x6-
piperidine	T43.3x1-	T43.3x2-	T43.3x3-	T43.3x4-	T43.3x5-	T43.3x6-
propylamine	T43.3x1-	T43.3x2-	T43.3x3-	T43.3x4-	T43.3x5-	T43.3x6-
specified NEC	T43.591-	T43.592-	T43.593-	T43.594-	T43.595-	T43.596-
thioxanthene NEC	T43.591-	T43.592-	T43.593-	T43.594-	T43.595-	T43.596-
Tranxene	T42.4x1-	T42.4x2-	T42.4x3-	T42.4x4-	T42.4x5-	T42.4x6-
Tranylcypromine	T43.1x1-	T43.1x2-	T43.1x3-	T43.1x4-	T43.1x5-	T43.1x6-
Trapidil	T46.3x1-	T46.3x2-	T46.3x3-	T46.3x4-	T46.3x5-	T46.3x6-
Trasentine	T44.3x1-	T44.3x2-	T44.3x3-	T44.3x4-	T44.3x5-	T44.3x6-
Travert	T50.3x1-	T50.3x2-	T50.3x3-	T50.3x4-	T50.3x5-	T50.3x6-
Trazodone	T43.211-	T43.212-	T43.213-	T43.214-	T43.215-	T43.216-
Trecator	T37.1x1-	T37.1x2-	T37.1x3-	T37.1x4-	T37.1x5-	T37.1x6-
Treosulfan	T45.1x1-	T45.1x2-	T45.1x3-	T45.1x4-	T45.1x5-	T45.1x6-
Tretamine	T45.1x1-	T45.1x2-	T45.1x3-	T45.1x4-	T45.1x5-	T45.1x6-
Tretinoin	T49.0x1-	T49.0x2-	T49.0x3-	T49.0x4-	T49.0x5-	T49.0x6-
Tretoquinol	T48.6x1-	T48.6x2-	T48.6x3-	T48.6x4-	T48.6x5-	T48.6x6-
Triacetin	T49.0x1-	T49.0x2-	T49.0x3-	T49.0x4-	T49.0x5-	T49.0x6-
Triacetoxyanthracene	T49.4x1-	T49.4x2-	T49.4x3-	T49.4x4-	T49.4x5-	T49.4x6-
Triacetyloleandomycin	T36.3x1-	T36.3x2-	T36.3x3-	T36.3x4-	T36.3x5-	T36.3x6-
Triamcinolone	T49.0x1-	T49.0x2-	T49.0x3-	T49.0x4-	T49.0x5-	T49.0x6-
ENT agent	T49.6x1-	T49.6x2-	T49.6x3-	T49.6x4-	T49.6x5-	T49.6x6-
hexacetonide	T49.0x1-	T49.0x2-	T49.0x3-	T49.0x4-	T49.0x5-	T49.0x6-
ophthalmic preparation	T49.5x1-	T49.5x2-	T49.5x3-	T49.5x4-	T49.5x5-	T49.5x6-
topical NEC	T49.0x1-	T49.0x2-	T49.0x3-	T49.0x4-	T49.0x5-	T49.0x6-
Triampyzine	T44.3x1-	T44.3x2-	T44.3x3-	T44.3x4-	T44.3x5-	T44.3x6-
Triamterene	T50.2x1-	T50.2x2-	T50.2x3-	T50.2x4-	T50.2x5-	T50.2x6-
Triazine (herbicide)	T60.3x1-	T60.3x2-	T60.3x3-	T60.3x4-	—	—
Triaziquone	T45.1x1-	T45.1x2-	T45.1x3-	T45.1x4-	T45.1x5-	T45.1x6-
Triazolam	T42.4x1-	T42.4x2-	T42.4x3-	T42.4x4-	T42.4x5-	T42.4x6-
Triazole (herbicide)	T60.3x1-	T60.3x2-	T60.3x3-	T60.3x4-	—	—
Tribenoside	T46.991-	T46.992-	T46.993-	T46.994-	T46.995-	T46.996-
Tribromacetaldehyde	T42.6x1-	T42.6x2-	T42.6x3-	T42.6x4-	T42.6x5-	T42.6x6-
Tribromoethanol, rectal	T41.291-	T41.292-	T41.293-	T41.294-	T41.295-	T41.296-
Tribromomethane	T42.6x1-	T42.6x2-	T42.6x3-	T42.6x4-	T42.6x5-	T42.6x6-
Trichlorethane	T53.2x1-	T53.2x2-	T53.2x3-	T53.2x4-	—	—
Trichlorethylene	T53.2x1-	T53.2x2-	T53.2x3-	T53.2x4-	—	—
Trichlorfon	T60.0x1-	T60.0x2-	T60.0x3-	T60.0x4-	—	—
Trichlormethiazide	T50.2x1-	T50.2x2-	T50.2x3-	T50.2x4-	T50.2x5-	T50.2x6-
Trichlormethine	T45.1x1-	T45.1x2-	T45.1x3-	T45.1x4-	T45.1x5-	T45.1x6-
Trichloroacetic acid, trichloracetic acid	T54.2x1-	T54.2x2-	T54.2x3-	T54.2x4-	—	—
medicinal	T49.4x1-	T49.4x2-	T49.4x3-	T49.4x4-	T49.4x5-	T49.4x6-
Trichloroethane	T53.2x1-	T53.2x2-	T53.2x3-	T53.2x4-	—	—
Trichloroethanol	T42.6x1-	T42.6x2-	T42.6x3-	T42.6x4-	T42.6x5-	T42.6x6-
Trichloroethyl phosphate	T42.6x1-	T42.6x2-	T42.6x3-	T42.6x4-	T42.6x5-	T42.6x6-
Trichloroethylene (liquid) (vapor)	T53.2x1-	T53.2x2-	T53.2x3-	T53.2x4-	—	—
anesthetic (gas)	T41.0x1-	T41.0x2-	T41.0x3-	T41.0x4-	T41.0x5-	T41.0x6-
vapor NEC	T53.2x1-	T53.2x2-	T53.2x3-	T53.2x4-	—	—
Trichlorofluoromethane NEC	T53.5x1-	T53.5x2-	T53.5x3-	T53.5x4-	—	—
Trichloronate	T60.0x1-	T60.0x2-	T60.0x3-	T60.0x4-	—	—
2,4,5-Trichlorophen-oxyacetic acid	T60.3x1-	T60.3x2-	T60.3x3-	T60.3x4-	—	—
Trichloropropane	T53.6x1-	T53.6x2-	T53.6x3-	T53.6x4-	—	—
Trichlorotriethylamine	T45.1x1-	T45.1x2-	T45.1x3-	T45.1x4-	T45.1x5-	T45.1x6-
Trichomonacides NEC	T37.3x1-	T37.3x2-	T37.3x3-	T37.3x4-	T37.3x5-	T37.3x6-
Trichomycin	T36.7x1-	T36.7x2-	T36.7x3-	T36.7x4-	T36.7x5-	T36.7x6-
Triclobisonium chloride	T49.0x1-	T49.0x2-	T49.0x3-	T49.0x4-	T49.0x5-	T49.0x6-
Triclocarban	T49.0x1-	T49.0x2-	T49.0x3-	T49.0x4-	T49.0x5-	T49.0x6-
Triclofos	T42.6x1-	T42.6x2-	T42.6x3-	T42.6x4-	T42.6x5-	T42.6x6-
Triclosan	T49.0x1-	T49.0x2-	T49.0x3-	T49.0x4-	T49.0x5-	T49.0x6-
Tricresyl phosphate	T65.891-	T65.892-	T65.893-	T65.894-	—	—
solvent	T52.91x-	T52.92x-	T52.93x-	T52.94x-	—	—
Tricyclamol chloride	T44.3x1-	T44.3x2-	T44.3x3-	T44.3x4-	T44.3x5-	T44.3x6-
Tridesilon	T49.0x1-	T49.0x2-	T49.0x3-	T49.0x4-	T49.0x5-	T49.0x6-
Tridihexethyl iodide	T44.3x1-	T44.3x2-	T44.3x3-	T44.3x4-	T44.3x5-	T44.3x6-
Tridione	T42.2x1-	T42.2x2-	T42.2x3-	T42.2x4-	T42.2x5-	T42.2x6-
Trientine	T45.8x1-	T45.8x2-	T45.8x3-	T45.8x4-	T45.8x5-	T45.8x6-
Triethanolamine NEC	T54.3x1-	T54.3x2-	T54.3x3-	T54.3x4-	—	—
detergent	T54.3x1-	T54.3x2-	T54.3x3-	T54.3x4-	—	—
trinitrate (biphosphate)	T46.3x1-	T46.3x2-	T46.3x3-	T46.3x4-	T46.3x5-	T46.3x6-
Triethanomelamine	T45.1x1-	T45.1x2-	T45.1x3-	T45.1x4-	T45.1x5-	T45.1x6-
Triethylenemelamine	T45.1x1-	T45.1x2-	T45.1x3-	T45.1x4-	T45.1x5-	T45.1x6-
Triethylenephosphoramide	T45.1x1-	T45.1x2-	T45.1x3-	T45.1x4-	T45.1x5-	T45.1x6-
Triethylenethiophospho-ramide	T45.1x1-	T45.1x2-	T45.1x3-	T45.1x4-	T45.1x5-	T45.1x6-
Trifluoperazine	T43.3x1-	T43.3x2-	T43.3x3-	T43.3x4-	T43.3x5-	T43.3x6-
Trifluoroethyl vinyl ether	T41.0x1-	T41.0x2-	T41.0x3-	T41.0x4-	T41.0x5-	T41.0x6-
Trifluperidol	T43.4x1-	T43.4x2-	T43.4x3-	T43.4x4-	T43.4x5-	T43.4x6-
Triflupromazine	T43.3x1-	T43.3x2-	T43.3x3-	T43.3x4-	T43.3x5-	T43.3x6-

DRUGS & CHEMICALS

Table of Drugs & Chemicals	Accidental (Unintentional)	Self-Harm (Intentional)	Assault	Undetermined	Adverse Effect	Underdosing
Trifluridine	T37.5x1-	T37.5x2-	T37.5x3-	T37.5x4-	T37.5x5-	T37.5x6-
Triflusal	T45.521-	T45.522-	T45.523-	T45.524-	T45.525-	T45.526-
Trihexyphenidyl	T44.3x1-	T44.3x2-	T44.3x3-	T44.3x4-	T44.3x5-	T44.3x6-
Triiodothyronine	T38.1x1-	T38.1x2-	T38.1x3-	T38.1x4-	T38.1x5-	T38.1x6-
Trilene	T41.0x1-	T41.0x2-	T41.0x3-	T41.0x4-	T41.0x5-	T41.0x6-
Trilostane	T38.991-	T38.992-	T38.993-	T38.994-	T38.995-	T38.996-
Trimebutine	T44.3x1-	T44.3x2-	T44.3x3-	T44.3x4-	T44.3x5-	T44.3x6-
Trimecaine	T41.3x1-	T41.3x2-	T41.3x3-	T41.3x4-	T41.3x5-	T41.3x6-
Trimeprazine (tartrate)	T44.3x1-	T44.3x2-	T44.3x3-	T44.3x4-	T44.3x5-	T44.3x6-
Trimetaphan camsilate	T44.2x1-	T44.2x2-	T44.2x3-	T44.2x4-	T44.2x5-	T44.2x6-
Trimetazidine	T46.7x1-	T46.7x2-	T46.7x3-	T46.7x4-	T46.7x5-	T46.7x6-
Trimethadione	T42.2x1-	T42.2x2-	T42.2x3-	T42.2x4-	T42.2x5-	T42.2x6-
Trimethaphan	T44.2x1-	T44.2x2-	T44.2x3-	T44.2x4-	T44.2x5-	T44.2x6-
Trimethidinium	T44.2x1-	T44.2x2-	T44.2x3-	T44.2x4-	T44.2x5-	T44.2x6-
Trimethobenzamide	T45.0x1-	T45.0x2-	T45.0x3-	T45.0x4-	T45.0x5-	T45.0x6-
Trimethoprim	T37.8x1-	T37.8x2-	T37.8x3-	T37.8x4-	T37.8x5-	T37.8x6-
with sulfamethoxazole	T36.8x1-	T36.8x2-	T36.8x3-	T36.8x4-	T36.8x5-	T36.8x6-
Trimethylcarbinol	T51.3x1-	T51.3x2-	T51.3x3-	T51.3x4-	—	—
Trimethylpsoralen	T49.3x1-	T49.3x2-	T49.3x3-	T49.3x4-	T49.3x5-	T49.3x6-
Trimeton	T45.0x1-	T45.0x2-	T45.0x3-	T45.0x4-	T45.0x5-	T45.0x6-
Trimetrexate	T45.1x1-	T45.1x2-	T45.1x3-	T45.1x4-	T45.1x5-	T45.1x6-
Trimipramine	T43.011-	T43.012-	T43.013-	T43.014-	T43.015-	T43.016-
Trimustine	T45.1x1-	T45.1x2-	T45.1x3-	T45.1x4-	T45.1x5-	T45.1x6-
Trinitrine	T46.3x1-	T46.3x2-	T46.3x3-	T46.3x4-	T46.3x5-	T46.3x6-
Trinitrobenzol	T65.3x1-	T65.3x2-	T65.3x3-	T65.3x4-	—	—
Trinitrophenol	T65.3x1-	T65.3x2-	T65.3x3-	T65.3x4-	—	—
Trinitrotoluene (fumes)	T65.3x1-	T65.3x2-	T65.3x3-	T65.3x4-	—	—
Trional	T42.6x1-	T42.6x2-	T42.6x3-	T42.6x4-	T42.6x5-	T42.6x6-
Triorthocresyl phosphate	T65.891-	T65.892-	T65.893-	T65.894-	—	—
Trioxide of arsenic	T57.0x1-	T57.0x2-	T57.0x3-	T57.0x4-	—	—
Trioxysalen	T49.4x1-	T49.4x2-	T49.4x3-	T49.4x4-	T49.4x5-	T49.4x6-
Tripamide	T50.2x1-	T50.2x2-	T50.2x3-	T50.2x4-	T50.2x5-	T50.2x6-
Triparanol	T46.6x1-	T46.6x2-	T46.6x3-	T46.6x4-	T46.6x5-	T46.6x6-
Tripelennamine	T45.0x1-	T45.0x2-	T45.0x3-	T45.0x4-	T45.0x5-	T45.0x6-
Triperiden	T44.3x1-	T44.3x2-	T44.3x3-	T44.3x4-	T44.3x5-	T44.3x6-
Triperidol	T43.4x1-	T43.4x2-	T43.4x3-	T43.4x4-	T43.4x5-	T43.4x6-
Triphenylphosphate	T65.891-	T65.892-	T65.893-	T65.894-	—	—
Triple						
bromides	T42.6x1-	T42.6x2-	T42.6x3-	T42.6x4-	T42.6x5-	T42.6x6-
carbonate	T47.1x1-	T47.1x2-	T47.1x3-	T47.1x4-	T47.1x5-	T47.1x6-
vaccine						
DPT	T50.A11-	T50.A12-	T50.A13-	T50.A14-	T50.A15-	T50.A16-
including pertussis	T50.A11-	T50.A12-	T50.A13-	T50.A14-	T50.A15-	T50.A16-
MMR	T50.B91-	T50.B92-	T50.B93-	T50.B94-	T50.B95-	T50.B96-
Triprolidine	T45.0x1-	T45.0x2-	T45.0x3-	T45.0x4-	T45.0x5-	T45.0x6-
Trisodium hydrogen edetate	T50.6x1-	T50.6x2-	T50.6x3-	T50.6x4-	T50.6x5-	T50.6x6-
Trisoralen	T49.3x1-	T49.3x2-	T49.3x3-	T49.3x4-	T49.3x5-	T49.3x6-
Trisulfapyrimidines	T37.0x1-	T37.0x2-	T37.0x3-	T37.0x4-	T37.0x5-	T37.0x6-
Trithiozine	T44.3x1-	T44.3x2-	T44.3x3-	T44.3x4-	T44.3x5-	T44.3x6-
Tritiozine	T44.3x1-	T44.3x2-	T44.3x3-	T44.3x4-	T44.3x5-	T44.3x6-
Tritoqualine	T45.0x1-	T45.0x2-	T45.0x3-	T45.0x4-	T45.0x5-	T45.0x6-
Trofosfamide	T45.1x1-	T45.1x2-	T45.1x3-	T45.1x4-	T45.1x5-	T45.1x6-
Troleandomycin	T36.3x1-	T36.3x2-	T36.3x3-	T36.3x4-	T36.3x5-	T36.3x6-
Trolnitrate (phosphate)	T46.3x1-	T46.3x2-	T46.3x3-	T46.3x4-	T46.3x5-	T46.3x6-
Tromantadine	T37.5x1-	T37.5x2-	T37.5x3-	T37.5x4-	T37.5x5-	T37.5x6-
Trometamol	T50.2x1-	T50.2x2-	T50.2x3-	T50.2x4-	T50.2x5-	T50.2x6-
Tromethamine	T50.2x1-	T50.2x2-	T50.2x3-	T50.2x4-	T50.2x5-	T50.2x6-
Tronothane	T41.3x1-	T41.3x2-	T41.3x3-	T41.3x4-	T41.3x5-	T41.3x6-
Tropacine	T44.3x1-	T44.3x2-	T44.3x3-	T44.3x4-	T44.3x5-	T44.3x6-
Tropatepine	T44.3x1-	T44.3x2-	T44.3x3-	T44.3x4-	T44.3x5-	T44.3x6-
Tropicamide	T44.3x1-	T44.3x2-	T44.3x3-	T44.3x4-	T44.3x5-	T44.3x6-
Trospium chloride	T44.3x1-	T44.3x2-	T44.3x3-	T44.3x4-	T44.3x5-	T44.3x6-
Troxerutin	T46.991-	T46.992-	T46.993-	T46.994-	T46.995-	T46.996-
Troxidone	T42.2x1-	T42.2x2-	T42.2x3-	T42.2x4-	T42.2x5-	T42.2x6-
Tryparsamide	T37.3x1-	T37.3x2-	T37.3x3-	T37.3x4-	T37.3x5-	T37.3x6-
Trypsin	T45.3x1-	T45.3x2-	T45.3x3-	T45.3x4-	T45.3x5-	T45.3x6-
Tryptizol	T43.011-	T43.012-	T43.013-	T43.014-	T43.015-	T43.016-
TSH	T38.811-	T38.812-	T38.813-	T38.814-	T38.815-	T38.816-
Tuaminoheptane	T48.5x1-	T48.5x2-	T48.5x3-	T48.5x4-	T48.5x5-	T48.5x6-
Tuberculin, purified protein derivative (PPD)	T50.8x1-	T50.8x2-	T50.8x3-	T50.8x4-	T50.8x5-	T50.8x6-
Tubocurare	T48.1x1-	T48.1x2-	T48.1x3-	T48.1x4-	T48.1x5-	T48.1x6-
Tubocurarine (chloride)	T48.1x1-	T48.1x2-	T48.1x3-	T48.1x4-	T48.1x5-	T48.1x6-
Tulobuterol	T48.6x1-	T48.6x2-	T48.6x3-	T48.6x4-	T48.6x5-	T48.6x6-
Turpentine (spirits of)	T52.8x1-	T52.8x2-	T52.8x3-	T52.8x4-	—	—
vapor	T52.8x1-	T52.8x2-	T52.8x3-	T52.8x4-	—	—
Tybamate	T43.591-	T43.592-	T43.593-	T43.594-	T43.595-	T43.596-
Tyloxapol	T48.4x1-	T48.4x2-	T48.4x3-	T48.4x4-	T48.4x5-	T48.4x6-
Tymazoline	T48.5x1-	T48.5x2-	T48.5x3-	T48.5x4-	T48.5x5-	T48.5x6-
Typhoid-paratyphoid vaccine	T50.A91-	T50.A92-	T50.A93-	T50.A94-	T50.A95-	T50.A96-
Typhus vaccine	T50.A91-	T50.A92-	T50.A93-	T50.A94-	T50.A95-	T50.A96-
Tyropanoate	T50.8x1-	T50.8x2-	T50.8x3-	T50.8x4-	T50.8x5-	T50.8x6-
Tyrothricin	T49.6x1-	T49.6x2-	T49.6x3-	T49.6x4-	T49.6x5-	T49.6x6-
ENT agent	T49.6x1-	T49.6x2-	T49.6x3-	T49.6x4-	T49.6x5-	T49.6x6-
ophthalmic preparation	T49.5x1-	T49.5x2-	T49.5x3-	T49.5x4-	T49.5x5-	T49.5x6-
Ufenamate	T39.391-	T39.392-	T39.393-	T39.394-	T39.395-	T39.396-
Ultraviolet light protectant	T49.3x1-	T49.3x2-	T49.3x3-	T49.3x4-	T49.3x5-	T49.3x6-
Undecenoic acid	T49.0x1-	T49.0x2-	T49.0x3-	T49.0x4-	T49.0x5-	T49.0x6-
Undecoylium	T49.0x1-	T49.0x2-	T49.0x3-	T49.0x4-	T49.0x5-	T49.0x6-
Undecylenic acid (derivatives)	T49.0x1-	T49.0x2-	T49.0x3-	T49.0x4-	T49.0x5-	T49.0x6-
Unna's boot	T49.3x1-	T49.3x2-	T49.3x3-	T49.3x4-	T49.3x5-	T49.3x6-
Unsaturated fatty acid	T46.6x1-	T46.6x2-	T46.6x3-	T46.6x4-	T46.6x5-	T46.6x6-
Uracil mustard	T45.1x1-	T45.1x2-	T45.1x3-	T45.1x4-	T45.1x5-	T45.1x6-
Uramustine	T45.1x1-	T45.1x2-	T45.1x3-	T45.1x4-	T45.1x5-	T45.1x6-
Urapidil	T46.5x1-	T46.5x2-	T46.5x3-	T46.5x4-	T46.5x5-	T46.5x6-
Urari	T48.1x1-	T48.1x2-	T48.1x3-	T48.1x4-	T48.1x5-	T48.1x6-
Urate oxidase	T50.4x1-	T50.4x2-	T50.4x3-	T50.4x4-	T50.4x5-	T50.4x6-
Urea	T47.3x1-	T47.3x2-	T47.3x3-	T47.3x4-	T47.3x5-	T47.3x6-
peroxide	T49.0x1-	T49.0x2-	T49.0x3-	T49.0x4-	T49.0x5-	T49.0x6-
stibamine	T37.4x1-	T37.4x2-	T37.4x3-	T37.4x4-	T37.4x5-	T37.4x6-
topical	T49.8x1-	T49.8x2-	T49.8x3-	T49.8x4-	T49.8x5-	T49.8x6-
Urethane	T45.1x1-	T45.1x2-	T45.1x3-	T45.1x4-	T45.1x5-	T45.1x6-
Urginea (maritima) (scilla) — see Squill						
Uric acid metabolism drug NEC	T50.4x1-	T50.4x2-	T50.4x3-	T50.4x4-	T50.4x5-	T50.4x6-
Uricosuric agent	T50.4x1-	T50.4x2-	T50.4x3-	T50.4x4-	T50.4x5-	T50.4x6-
Urinary anti-infective	T37.8x1-	T37.8x2-	T37.8x3-	T37.8x4-	T37.8x5-	T37.8x6-
Urofollitropin	T38.811-	T38.812-	T38.813-	T38.814-	T38.815-	T38.816-
Urokinase	T45.611-	T45.612-	T45.613-	T45.614-	T45.615-	T45.616-
Urokon	T50.8x1-	T50.8x2-	T50.8x3-	T50.8x4-	T50.8x5-	T50.8x6-
Ursodeoxycholic acid	T50.991-	T50.992-	T50.993-	T50.994-	T50.995-	T50.996-
Ursodiol	T50.991-	T50.992-	T50.993-	T50.994-	T50.995-	T50.996-
Urtica	T62.2x1-	T62.2x2-	T62.2x3-	T62.2x4-	—	—
Utility gas — see Gas, utility						

DRUGS & CHEMICALS

Table of Drugs & Chemicals	POISONING				Adverse Effect	Underdosing
	Accidental (Unintentional)	Self-Harm (Intentional)	Assault	Undetermined		
Vaccine NEC	T50.Z91-	T50.Z92-	T50.Z93-	T50.Z94-	T50.Z95-	T50.Z96-
antineoplastic	T50.Z91-	T50.Z92-	T50.Z93-	T50.Z94-	T50.Z95-	T50.Z96-
bacterial NEC	T50.A91-	T50.A92-	T50.A93-	T50.A94-	T50.A95-	T50.A96-
with other bacterial component	T50.A21-	T50.A22-	T50.A23-	T50.A24-	T50.A25-	T50.A26-
pertussis component	T50.A11-	T50.A12-	T50.A13-	T50.A14-	T50.A15-	T50.A16-
viral-rickettsial component	T50.A21-	T50.A22-	T50.A23-	T50.A24-	T50.A25-	T50.A26-
mixed NEC	T50.A21-	T50.A22-	T50.A23-	T50.A24-	T50.A25-	T50.A26-
BCG	T50.A91-	T50.A92-	T50.A93-	T50.A94-	T50.A95-	T50.A96-
cholera	T50.A91-	T50.A92-	T50.A93-	T50.A94-	T50.A95-	T50.A96-
diphtheria	T50.A91-	T50.A92-	T50.A93-	T50.A94-	T50.A95-	T50.A96-
with tetanus	T50.A21-	T50.A22-	T50.A23-	T50.A24-	T50.A25-	T50.A26-
and pertussis	T50.A11-	T50.A12-	T50.A13-	T50.A14-	T50.A15-	T50.A16-
influenza	T50.B91-	T50.B92-	T50.B93-	T50.B94-	T50.B95-	T50.B96-
measles	T50.B91-	T50.B92-	T50.B93-	T50.B94-	T50.B95-	T50.B96-
with mumps and rubella	T50.B91-	T50.B92-	T50.B93-	T50.B94-	T50.B95-	T50.B96-
meningococcal	T50.A91-	T50.A92-	T50.A93-	T50.A94-	T50.A95-	T50.A96-
mumps	T50.B91-	T50.B92-	T50.B93-	T50.B94-	T50.B95-	T50.B96-
paratyphoid	T50.A91-	T50.A92-	T50.A93-	T50.A94-	T50.A95-	T50.A96-
pertussis	T50.A11-	T50.A12-	T50.A13-	T50.A14-	T50.A15-	T50.A16-
with diphtheria	T50.A11-	T50.A12-	T50.A13-	T50.A14-	T50.A15-	T50.A16-
and tetanus	T50.A11-	T50.A12-	T50.A13-	T50.A14-	T50.A15-	T50.A16-
with other component	T50.A11-	T50.A12-	T50.A13-	T50.A14-	T50.A15-	T50.A16-
plague	T50.A91-	T50.A92-	T50.A93-	T50.A94-	T50.A95-	T50.A96-
poliomyelitis	T50.B91-	T50.B92-	T50.B93-	T50.B94-	T50.B95-	T50.B96-
poliovirus	T50.B91-	T50.B92-	T50.B93-	T50.B94-	T50.B95-	T50.B96-
rabies	T50.B91-	T50.B92-	T50.B93-	T50.B94-	T50.B95-	T50.B96-
respiratory syncytial virus	T50.B91-	T50.B92-	T50.B93-	T50.B94-	T50.B95-	T50.B96-
rickettsial NEC	T50.A91-	T50.A92-	T50.A93-	T50.A94-	T50.A95-	T50.A96-
with bacterial component	T50.A21-	T50.A22-	T50.A23-	T50.A24-	T50.A25-	T50.A26-
Rocky Mountain spotted fever	T50.A91-	T50.A92-	T50.A93-	T50.A94-	T50.A95-	T50.A96-
rubella	T50.B91-	T50.B92-	T50.B93-	T50.B94-	T50.B95-	T50.B96-
sabin oral	T50.B91-	T50.B92-	T50.B93-	T50.B94-	T50.B95-	T50.B96-
smallpox	T50.B11-	T50.B12-	T50.B13-	T50.B14-	T50.B15-	T50.B16-
TAB	T50.A91-	T50.A92-	T50.A93-	T50.A94-	T50.A95-	T50.A96-
tetanus	T50.A91-	T50.A92-	T50.A93-	T50.A94-	T50.A95-	T50.A96-
typhoid	T50.A91-	T50.A92-	T50.A93-	T50.A94-	T50.A95-	T50.A96-
typhus	T50.A91-	T50.A92-	T50.A93-	T50.A94-	T50.A95-	T50.A96-
viral NEC	T50.B91-	T50.B92-	T50.B93-	T50.B94-	T50.B95-	T50.B96-
yellow fever	T50.B91-	T50.B92-	T50.B93-	T50.B94-	T50.B95-	T50.B96-
Vaccinia immune globulin	T50.Z11-	T50.Z12-	T50.Z13-	T50.Z14-	T50.Z15-	T50.Z16-
Vaginal contraceptives	T49.8x1-	T49.8x2-	T49.8x3-	T49.8x4-	T49.8x5-	T49.8x6-
Valerian						
root	T42.6x1-	T42.6x2-	T42.6x3-	T42.6x4-	T42.6x5-	T42.6x6-
tincture	T42.6x1-	T42.6x2-	T42.6x3-	T42.6x4-	T42.6x5-	T42.6x6-
Valethamate bromide	T44.3x1-	T44.3x2-	T44.3x3-	T44.3x4-	T44.3x5-	T44.3x6-
Valisone	T49.0x1-	T49.0x2-	T49.0x3-	T49.0x4-	T49.0x5-	T49.0x6-
Valium	T42.4x1-	T42.4x2-	T42.4x3-	T42.4x4-	T42.4x5-	T42.4x6-
Valmid	T42.6x1-	T42.6x2-	T42.6x3-	T42.6x4-	T42.6x5-	T42.6x6-
Valnoctamide	T42.6x1-	T42.6x2-	T42.6x3-	T42.6x4-	T42.6x5-	T42.6x6-
Valproate (sodium)	T42.6x1-	T42.6x2-	T42.6x3-	T42.6x4-	T42.6x5-	T42.6x6-
Valproic acid	T42.6x1-	T42.6x2-	T42.6x3-	T42.6x4-	T42.6x5-	T42.6x6-
Valpromide	T42.6x1-	T42.6x2-	T42.6x3-	T42.6x4-	T42.6x5-	T42.6x6-
Vanadium	T56.891-	T56.892-	T56.893-	T56.894-	—	—
Vancomycin	T36.8x1-	T36.8x2-	T36.8x3-	T36.8x4-	T36.8x5-	T36.8x6-
Vapor — see also Gas	T59.91x-	T59.92x-	T59.93x-	T59.94x-	—	—
kiln (carbon monoxide)	T58.8x1-	T58.8x2-	T58.8x3-	T58.8x4-	—	—
lead — see Lead						
specified source NEC	T59.891-	T59.892-	T59.893-	T59.894-	—	—
Vardenafil	T46.7x1-	T46.7x2-	T46.7x3-	T46.7x4-	T46.7x5-	T46.7x6-

Table of Drugs & Chemicals	POISONING				Adverse Effect	Underdosing
	Accidental (Unintentional)	Self-Harm (Intentional)	Assault	Undetermined		
Varicose reduction drug	T46.8x1-	T46.8x2-	T46.8x3-	T46.8x4-	T46.8x5-	T46.8x6-
Varnish	T65.4x1-	T65.4x2-	T65.4x3-	T65.4x4-	—	—
cleaner	T52.91x-	T52.92x-	T52.93x-	T52.94x-	—	—
Vaseline	T49.3x1-	T49.3x2-	T49.3x3-	T49.3x4-	T49.3x5-	T49.3x6-
Vasodilan	T46.7x1-	T46.7x2-	T46.7x3-	T46.7x4-	T46.7x5-	T46.7x6-
Vasodilator						
coronary NEC	T46.3x1-	T46.3x2-	T46.3x3-	T46.3x4-	T46.3x5-	T46.3x6-
peripheral NEC	T46.7x1-	T46.7x2-	T46.7x3-	T46.7x4-	T46.7x5-	T46.7x6-
Vasopressin	T38.891-	T38.892-	T38.893-	T38.894-	T38.895-	T38.896-
Vasopressor drugs	T38.891-	T38.892-	T38.893-	T38.894-	T38.895-	T38.896-
Vecuronium bromide	T48.1x1-	T48.1x2-	T48.1x3-	T48.1x4-	T48.1x5-	T48.1x6-
Vegetable extract, astringent	T49.2x1-	T49.2x2-	T49.2x3-	T49.2x4-	T49.2x5-	T49.2x6-
Venlafaxine	T43.211-	T43.212-	T43.213-	T43.214-	T43.215-	T43.216-
Venom, venomous (bite) (sting)	T63.91x-	T63.92x-	T63.93x-	T63.94x-	—	—
ant	T63.421-	T63.422-	T63.423-	T63.424-	—	—
amphibian NEC	T63.831-	T63.832-	T63.833-	T63.834-	—	—
animal NEC	T63.891-	T63.892-	T63.893-	T63.894-	—	—
arthropod NEC	T63.481-	T63.482-	T63.483-	T63.484-	—	—
bee	T63.441-	T63.442-	T63.443-	T63.444-	—	—
centipede	T63.411-	T63.412-	T63.413-	T63.414-	—	—
fish	T63.591-	T63.592-	T63.593-	T63.594-	—	—
frog	T63.811-	T63.812-	T63.813-	T63.814-	—	—
hornet	T63.451-	T63.452-	T63.453-	T63.454-	—	—
insect NEC	T63.481-	T63.482-	T63.483-	T63.484-	—	—
lizard	T63.121-	T63.122-	T63.123-	T63.124-	—	—
marine						
animals	T63.691-	T63.692-	T63.693-	T63.694-	—	—
bluebottle	T63.611-	T63.612-	T63.613-	T63.614-	—	—
jellyfish NEC	T63.621-	T63.622-	T63.623-	T63.624-	—	—
Portugese Man-o-war	T63.611-	T63.612-	T63.613-	T63.614-	—	—
sea anemone	T63.631-	T63.632-	T63.633-	T63.634-	—	—
specified NEC	T63.691-	T63.692-	T63.693-	T63.694-	—	—
fish	T63.591-	T63.592-	T63.593-	T63.594-	—	—
sting ray	T63.511-	T63.512-	T63.513-	T63.514-	—	—
plants	T63.711-	T63.712-	T63.713-	T63.714-	—	—
millipede (tropical)	T63.411-	T63.412-	T63.413-	T63.414-	—	—
plant NEC	T63.791-	T63.792-	T63.793-	T63.794-	—	—
marine	T63.711-	T63.712-	T63.713-	T63.714-	—	—
reptile	T63.191-	T63.192-	T63.193-	T63.194-	—	—
gila monster	T63.111-	T63.112-	T63.113-	T63.114-	—	—
lizard NEC	T63.121-	T63.122-	T63.123-	T63.124-	—	—
scorpion	T63.2x1-	T63.2x2-	T63.2x3-	T63.2x4-	—	—
snake	T63.001-	T63.002-	T63.003-	T63.004-	—	—
African NEC	T63.081-	T63.082-	T63.083-	T63.084-	—	—
American (North) (South) NEC	T63.061-	T63.062-	T63.063-	T63.064-	—	—
Asian	T63.081-	T63.082-	T63.083-	T63.084-	—	—
Australian	T63.071-	T63.072-	T63.073-	T63.074-	—	—
cobra	T63.041-	T63.042-	T63.043-	T63.044-	—	—
coral snake	T63.021-	T63.022-	T63.023-	T63.024-	—	—
rattlesnake	T63.011-	T63.012-	T63.013-	T63.014-	—	—
specified NEC	T63.091-	T63.092-	T63.093-	T63.094-	—	—
taipan	T63.031-	T63.032-	T63.033-	T63.034-	—	—
specified NEC	T63.891-	T63.892-	T63.893-	T63.894-	—	—
spider	T63.301-	T63.302-	T63.303-	T63.304-	—	—
black widow	T63.311-	T63.312-	T63.313-	T63.314-	—	—
brown recluse	T63.331-	T63.332-	T63.333-	T63.334-	—	—
specified NEC	T63.391-	T63.392-	T63.393-	T63.394-	—	—
tarantula	T63.321-	T63.322-	T63.323-	T63.324-	—	—
sting ray	T63.511-	T63.512-	T63.513-	T63.514-	—	—
toad	T63.821-	T63.822-	T63.823-	T63.824-	—	—
wasp	T63.461-	T63.462-	T63.463-	T63.464-	—	—

Table of Drugs & Chemicals	POISONING				Adverse Effect	Underdosing
	Accidental (Unintentional)	Self-Harm (Intentional)	Assault	Undetermined		
Venous sclerosing drug NEC	T46.8x1-	T46.8x2-	T46.8x3-	T46.8x4-	T46.8x5-	T46.8x6-
Ventolin — see Albuterol						
Veramon	T42.3x1-	T42.3x2-	T42.3x3-	T42.3x4-	T42.3x5-	T42.3x6-
Verapamil	T46.1x1-	T46.1x2-	T46.1x3-	T46.1x4-	T46.1x5-	T46.1x6-
Veratrine	T46.5x1-	T46.5x2-	T46.5x3-	T46.5x4-	T46.5x5-	T46.5x6-
Veratrum						
album	T62.2x1-	T62.2x2-	T62.2x3-	T62.2x4-	—	—
alkaloids	T46.5x1-	T46.5x2-	T46.5x3-	T46.5x4-	T46.5x5-	T46.5x6-
viride	T62.2x1-	T62.2x2-	T62.2x3-	T62.2x4-	—	—
Verdigris	T60.3x1-	T60.3x2-	T60.3x3-	T60.3x4-	—	—
Veronal	T42.3x1-	T42.3x2-	T42.3x3-	T42.3x4-	T42.3x5-	T42.3x6-
Veroxil	T37.4x1-	T37.4x2-	T37.4x3-	T37.4x4-	T37.4x5-	T37.4x6-
Versenate	T50.6x1-	T50.6x2-	T50.6x3-	T50.6x4-	T50.6x5-	T50.6x6-
Versidyne	T39.8x1-	T39.8x2-	T39.8x3-	T39.8x4-	T39.8x5-	T39.8x6-
Vetrabutine	T48.0x1-	T48.0x2-	T48.0x3-	T48.0x4-	T48.0x5-	T48.0x6-
Vidarabine	T37.5x1-	T37.5x2-	T37.5x3-	T37.5x4-	T37.5x5-	T37.5x6-
Vienna						
green	T57.0x1-	T57.0x2-	T57.0x3-	T57.0x4-	—	—
insecticide	T60.2x1-	T60.2x2-	T60.2x3-	T60.2x4-	—	—
red	T57.0x1-	T57.0x2-	T57.0x3-	T57.0x4-	—	—
pharmaceutical dye	T50.991-	T50.992-	T50.993-	T50.994-	T50.995-	T50.996-
Vigabatrin	T42.6x1-	T42.6x2-	T42.6x3-	T42.6x4-	T42.6x5-	T42.6x6-
Viloxazine	T43.291-	T43.292-	T43.293-	T43.294-	T43.295-	T43.296-
Viminol	T39.8x1-	T39.8x2-	T39.8x3-	T39.8x4-	T39.8x5-	T39.8x6-
Vinbarbital, vinbarbitone	T42.3x1-	T42.3x2-	T42.3x3-	T42.3x4-	T42.3x5-	T42.3x6-
Vinblastine	T45.1x1-	T45.1x2-	T45.1x3-	T45.1x4-	T45.1x5-	T45.1x6-
Vinburnine	T46.7x1-	T46.7x2-	T46.7x3-	T46.7x4-	T46.7x5-	T46.7x6-
Vincamine	T45.1x1-	T45.1x2-	T45.1x3-	T45.1x4-	T45.1x5-	T45.1x6-
Vincristine	T45.1x1-	T45.1x2-	T45.1x3-	T45.1x4-	T45.1x5-	T45.1x6-
Vindesine	T45.1x1-	T45.1x2-	T45.1x3-	T45.1x4-	T45.1x5-	T45.1x6-
Vinesthene, vinethene	T41.0x1-	T41.0x2-	T41.0x3-	T41.0x4-	T41.0x5-	T41.0x6-
Vinorelbine tartrate	T45.1x1-	T45.1x2-	T45.1x3-	T45.1x4-	T45.1x5-	T45.1x6-
Vinpocetine	T46.7x1-	T46.7x2-	T46.7x3-	T46.7x4-	T46.7x5-	T46.7x6-
Vinyl						
acetate	T65.891-	T65.892-	T65.893-	T65.894-	—	—
bital	T42.3x1-	T42.3x2-	T42.3x3-	T42.3x4-	T42.3x5-	T42.3x6-
bromide	T65.891-	T65.892-	T65.893-	T65.894-	—	—
chloride	T59.891-	T59.892-	T59.893-	T59.894-	—	—
ether	T41.0x1-	T41.0x2-	T41.0x3-	T41.0x4-	T41.0x5-	T41.0x6-
Vinylbital	T42.3x1-	T42.3x2-	T42.3x3-	T42.3x4-	T42.3x5-	T42.3x6-
Vinylidene chloride	T65.891-	T65.892-	T65.893-	T65.894-	—	—
Vioform	T37.8x1-	T37.8x2-	T37.8x3-	T37.8x4-	T37.8x5-	T37.8x6-
topical	T49.0x1-	T49.0x2-	T49.0x3-	T49.0x4-	T49.0x5-	T49.0x6-
Viomycin	T36.8x1-	T36.8x2-	T36.8x3-	T36.8x4-	T36.8x5-	T36.8x6-
Viosterol	T45.2x1-	T45.2x2-	T45.2x3-	T45.2x4-	T45.2x5-	T45.2x6-
Viper (venom)	T63.091-	T63.092-	T63.093-	T63.094-	—	—
Viprynium	T37.4x1-	T37.4x2-	T37.4x3-	T37.4x4-	T37.4x5-	T37.4x6-
Viquidil	T46.7x1-	T46.7x2-	T46.7x3-	T46.7x4-	T46.7x5-	T46.7x6-
Viral vaccine NEC	T50.B91-	T50.B92-	T50.B93-	T50.B94-	T50.B95-	T50.B96-
Virginiamycin	T36.8x1-	T36.8x2-	T36.8x3-	T36.8x4-	T36.8x5-	T36.8x6-
Virugon	T37.5x1-	T37.5x2-	T37.5x3-	T37.5x4-	T37.5x5-	T37.5x6-
Viscous agent	T50.901-	T50.902-	T50.903-	T50.904-	T50.905-	T50.906-
Visine	T49.5x1-	T49.5x2-	T49.5x3-	T49.5x4-	T49.5x5-	T49.5x6-
Visnadine	T46.3x1-	T46.3x2-	T46.3x3-	T46.3x4-	T46.3x5-	T46.3x6-

Table of Drugs & Chemicals	POISONING				Adverse Effect	Underdosing
	Accidental (Unintentional)	Self-Harm (Intentional)	Assault	Undetermined		
Vitamin NEC	T45.2x1-	T45.2x2-	T45.2x3-	T45.2x4-	T45.2x5-	T45.2x6-
A	T45.2x1-	T45.2x2-	T45.2x3-	T45.2x4-	T45.2x5-	T45.2x6-
B NEC	T45.2x1-	T45.2x2-	T45.2x3-	T45.2x4-	T45.2x5-	T45.2x6-
nicotinic acid	T46.7x1-	T46.7x2-	T46.7x3-	T46.7x4-	T46.7x5-	T46.7x6-
B1	T45.2x1-	T45.2x2-	T45.2x3-	T45.2x4-	T45.2x5-	T45.2x6-
B2	T45.2x1-	T45.2x2-	T45.2x3-	T45.2x4-	T45.2x5-	T45.2x6-
B6	T45.2x1-	T45.2x2-	T45.2x3-	T45.2x4-	T45.2x5-	T45.2x6-
B12	T45.2x1-	T45.2x2-	T45.2x3-	T45.2x4-	T45.2x5-	T45.2x6-
B15	T45.2x1-	T45.2x2-	T45.2x3-	T45.2x4-	T45.2x5-	T45.2x6-
C	T45.2x1-	T45.2x2-	T45.2x3-	T45.2x4-	T45.2x5-	T45.2x6-
D	T45.2x1-	T45.2x2-	T45.2x3-	T45.2x4-	T45.2x5-	T45.2x6-
D2	T45.2x1-	T45.2x2-	T45.2x3-	T45.2x4-	T45.2x5-	T45.2x6-
D3	T45.2x1-	T45.2x2-	T45.2x3-	T45.2x4-	T45.2x5-	T45.2x6-
E	T45.2x1-	T45.2x2-	T45.2x3-	T45.2x4-	T45.2x5-	T45.2x6-
E acetate	T45.2x1-	T45.2x2-	T45.2x3-	T45.2x4-	T45.2x5-	T45.2x6-
hematopoietic	T45.8x1-	T45.8x2-	T45.8x3-	T45.8x4-	T45.8x5-	T45.8x6-
K NEC	T45.7x1-	T45.7x2-	T45.7x3-	T45.7x4-	T45.7x5-	T45.7x6-
K1	T45.7x1-	T45.7x2-	T45.7x3-	T45.7x4-	T45.7x5-	T45.7x6-
K2	T45.7x1-	T45.7x2-	T45.7x3-	T45.7x4-	T45.7x5-	T45.7x6-
PP	T45.2x1-	T45.2x2-	T45.2x3-	T45.2x4-	T45.2x5-	T45.2x6-
ulceroprotectant	T47.1x1-	T47.1x2-	T47.1x3-	T47.1x4-	T47.1x5-	T47.1x6-
Vleminckx's solution	T49.4x1-	T49.4x2-	T49.4x3-	T49.4x4-	T49.4x5-	T49.4x6-
Voltaren — see Diclofenac sodium						
Warfarin	T45.511-	T45.512-	T45.513-	T45.514-	T45.515-	T45.516-
rodenticide	T60.4x1-	T60.4x2-	T60.4x3-	T60.4x4-	—	—
sodium	T60.4x1-	T60.4x2-	T60.4x3-	T60.4x4-	—	—
Wasp (sting)	T63.461-	T63.462-	T63.463-	T63.464-	—	—
Water						
balance drug	T50.3x1-	T50.3x2-	T50.3x3-	T50.3x4-	T50.3x5-	T50.3x6-
distilled	T50.3x1-	T50.3x2-	T50.3x3-	T50.3x4-	T50.3x5-	T50.3x6-
gas — see Gas, water						
incomplete combustion of — see Carbon, monoxide, fuel, utility						
hemlock	T62.2x1-	T62.2x2-	T62.2x3-	T62.2x4-	—	—
moccasin (venom)	T63.061-	T63.062-	T63.063-	T63.064-	—	—
purified	T50.3x1-	T50.3x2-	T50.3x3-	T50.3x4-	T50.3x5-	T50.3x6-
Wax (paraffin) (petroleum)	T52.0x1-	T52.0x2-	T52.0x3-	T52.0x4-	—	—
automobile	T65.891-	T65.892-	T65.893-	T65.894-	—	—
floor	T52.0x1-	T52.0x2-	T52.0x3-	T52.0x4-	—	—
Weed killers NEC	T60.3x1-	T60.3x2-	T60.3x3-	T60.3x4-	—	—
Welldorm	T42.6x1-	T42.6x2-	T42.6x3-	T42.6x4-	T42.6x5-	T42.6x6-
White						
arsenic	T57.0x1-	T57.0x2-	T57.0x3-	T57.0x4-	—	—
hellebore	T62.2x1-	T62.2x2-	T62.2x3-	T62.2x4-	—	—
lotion (keratolytic)	T49.4x1-	T49.4x2-	T49.4x3-	T49.4x4-	T49.4x5-	T49.4x6-
spirit	T52.0x1-	T52.0x2-	T52.0x3-	T52.0x4-	—	—
Whitewash	T65.891-	T65.892-	T65.893-	T65.894-	—	—
Whole blood (human)	T45.8x1-	T45.8x2-	T45.8x3-	T45.8x4-	T45.8x5-	T45.8x6-
Wild						
black cherry	T62.2x1-	T62.2x2-	T62.2x3-	T62.2x4-	—	—
poisonous plants NEC	T62.2x1-	T62.2x2-	T62.2x3-	T62.2x4-	—	—
Window cleaning fluid	T65.891-	T65.892-	T65.893-	T65.894-	—	—
Wintergreen (oil)	T49.3x1-	T49.3x2-	T49.3x3-	T49.3x4-	T49.3x5-	T49.3x6-
Wisterine	T62.2x1-	T62.2x2-	T62.2x3-	T62.2x4-	—	—
Witch hazel	T49.2x1-	T49.2x2-	T49.2x3-	T49.2x4-	T49.2x5-	T49.2x6-
Wood alcohol or spirit	T51.1x1-	T51.1x2-	T51.1x3-	T51.1x4-	—	—
Wool fat (hydrous)	T49.3x1-	T49.3x2-	T49.3x3-	T49.3x4-	T49.3x5-	T49.3x6-
Woorali	T48.1x1-	T48.1x2-	T48.1x3-	T48.1x4-	T48.1x5-	T48.1x6-
Wormseed, American	T37.4x1-	T37.4x2-	T37.4x3-	T37.4x4-	T37.4x5-	T37.4x6-

Table of Drugs & Chemicals	POISONING Accidental (Unintentional)	Self-Harm (Intentional)	Assault	Undetermined	Adverse Effect	Underdosing	Table of Drugs & Chemicals	POISONING Accidental (Unintentional)	Self-Harm (Intentional)	Assault	Undetermined	Adverse Effect	Underdosing
Xamoterol	T44.5x1-	T44.5x2-	T44.5x3-	T44.5x4-	T44.5x5-	T44.5x6-	Zopiclone	T42.6x1-	T42.6x2-	T42.6x3-	T42.6x4-	T42.6x5-	T42.6x6-
Xanthine diuretics	T50.2x1-	T50.2x2-	T50.2x3-	T50.2x4-	T50.2x5-	T50.2x6-	Zorubicin	T45.1x1-	T45.1x2-	T45.1x3-	T45.1x4-	T45.1x5-	T45.1x6-
Xanthinol nicotinate	T46.7x1-	T46.7x2-	T46.7x3-	T46.7x4-	T46.7x5-	T46.7x6-	Zotepine	T43.591-	T43.592-	T43.593-	T43.594-	T43.595-	T43.596-
Xanthotoxin	T49.3x1-	T49.3x2-	T49.3x3-	T49.3x4-	T49.3x5-	T49.3x6-	Zovant	T45.511-	T45.512-	T45.513-	T45.514-	T45.515-	T45.516-
Xantinol nicotinate	T46.7x1-	T46.7x2-	T46.7x3-	T46.7x4-	T46.7x5-	T46.7x6-	Zoxazolamine	T42.8x1-	T42.8x2-	T42.8x3-	T42.8x4-	T42.8x5-	T42.8x6-
Xantocillin	T36.0x1-	T36.0x2-	T36.0x3-	T36.0x4-	T36.0x5-	T36.0x6-	Zuclopenthixol	T43.4x1-	T43.4x2-	T43.4x3-	T43.4x4-	T43.4x5-	T43.4x6-
Xenon (127Xe) (133Xe)	T50.8x1-	T50.8x2-	T50.8x3-	T50.8x4-	T50.8x5-	T50.8x6-	Zygadenus (venenosus)	T62.2x1-	T62.2x2-	T62.2x3-	T62.2x4-	—	—
Xenysalate	T49.4x1-	T49.4x2-	T49.4x3-	T49.4x4-	T49.4x5-	T49.4x6-	Zyprexa	T43.591-	T43.592-	T43.593-	T43.594-	T43.595-	T43.596-
Xibornol	T37.8x1-	T37.8x2-	T37.8x3-	T37.8x4-	T37.8x5-	T37.8x6-							
Xigris	T45.511-	T45.512-	T45.513-	T45.514-	T45.515-	T45.516-							
Xipamide	T50.2x1-	T50.2x2-	T50.2x3-	T50.2x4-	T50.2x5-	T50.2x6-							
Xylene (vapor)	T52.2x1-	T52.2x2-	T52.2x3-	T52.2x4-	—	—							
Xylocaine (infiltration) (topical)	T41.3x1-	T41.3x2-	T41.3x3-	T41.3x4-	T41.3x5-	T41.3x6-							
nerve block (peripheral) (plexus)	T41.3x1-	T41.3x2-	T41.3x3-	T41.3x4-	T41.3x5-	T41.3x6-							
spinal	T41.3x1-	T41.3x2-	T41.3x3-	T41.3x4-	T41.3x5-	T41.3x6-							
Xylol (vapor)	T52.2x1-	T52.2x2-	T52.2x3-	T52.2x4-	—	—							
Xylometazoline	T48.5x1-	T48.5x2-	T48.5x3-	T48.5x4-	T48.5x5-	T48.5x6-							
Yeast	T45.2x1-	T45.2x2-	T45.2x3-	T45.2x4-	T45.2x5-	T45.2x6-							
dried	T45.2x1-	T45.2x2-	T45.2x3-	T45.2x4-	T45.2x5-	T45.2x6-							
Yellow fever vaccine	T50.B91-	T50.B92-	T50.B93-	T50.B94-	T50.B95-	T50.B96-							
jasmine	T62.2x1-	T62.2x2-	T62.2x3-	T62.2x4-	—	—							
phenolphthalein	T47.2x1-	T47.2x2-	T47.2x3-	T47.2x4-	T47.2x5-	T47.2x6-							
Yew	T62.2x1-	T62.2x2-	T62.2x3-	T62.2x4-	—	—							
Yohimbic acid	T40.991-	T40.992-	T40.993-	T40.994-	T40.995-	T40.996-							
Zactane	T39.8x1-	T39.8x2-	T39.8x3-	T39.8x4-	T39.8x5-	T39.8x6-							
Zalcitabine	T37.5x1-	T37.5x2-	T37.5x3-	T37.5x4-	T37.5x5-	T37.5x6-							
Zaroxolyn	T50.2x1-	T50.2x2-	T50.2x3-	T50.2x4-	T50.2x5-	T50.2x6-							
Zephiran (topical)	T49.0x1-	T49.0x2-	T49.0x3-	T49.0x4-	T49.0x5-	T49.0x6-							
ophthalmic preparation	T49.5x1-	T49.5x2-	T49.5x3-	T49.5x4-	T49.5x5-	T49.5x6-							
Zeranol	T38.7x1-	T38.7x2-	T38.7x3-	T38.7x4-	T38.7x5-	T38.7x6-							
Zerone	T51.1x1-	T51.1x2-	T51.1x3-	T51.1x4-	—	—							
Zidovudine	T37.5x1-	T37.5x2-	T37.5x3-	T37.5x4-	T37.5x5-	T37.5x6-							
Zimeldine	T43.221-	T43.222-	T43.223-	T43.224-	T43.225-	T43.226-							
Zinc (compounds) (fumes) (vapor) NEC	T56.5x1-	T56.5x2-	T56.5x3-	T56.5x4-	—	—							
anti-infectives	T49.0x1-	T49.0x2-	T49.0x3-	T49.0x4-	T49.0x5-	T49.0x6-							
antivaricose	T46.8x1-	T46.8x2-	T46.8x3-	T46.8x4-	T46.8x5-	T46.8x6-							
bacitracin	T49.0x1-	T49.0x2-	T49.0x3-	T49.0x4-	T49.0x5-	T49.0x6-							
chloride (mouthwash)	T49.6x1-	T49.6x2-	T49.6x3-	T49.6x4-	T49.6x5-	T49.6x6-							
chromate	T56.5x1-	T56.5x2-	T56.5x3-	T56.5x4-	—	—							
gelatin	T49.3x1-	T49.3x2-	T49.3x3-	T49.3x4-	T49.3x5-	T49.3x6-							
oxide	T49.3x1-	T49.3x2-	T49.3x3-	T49.3x4-	T49.3x5-	T49.3x6-							
plaster	T49.3x1-	T49.3x2-	T49.3x3-	T49.3x4-	T49.3x5-	T49.3x6-							
peroxide	T49.0x1-	T49.0x2-	T49.0x3-	T49.0x4-	T49.0x5-	—							
pesticides	T56.5x1-	T56.5x2-	T56.5x3-	T56.5x4-	—	—							
phosphide	T60.4x1-	T60.4x2-	T60.4x3-	T60.4x4-	—	—							
pyrithionate	T49.4x1-	T49.4x2-	T49.4x3-	T49.4x4-	T49.4x5-	T49.4x6-							
stearate	T49.3x1-	T49.3x2-	T49.3x3-	T49.3x4-	T49.3x5-	T49.3x6-							
sulfate	T49.5x1-	T49.5x2-	T49.5x3-	T49.5x4-	T49.5x5-	T49.5x6-							
ENT agent	T49.6x1-	T49.6x2-	T49.6x3-	T49.6x4-	T49.6x5-	T49.6x6-							
ophthalmic solution	T49.5x1-	T49.5x2-	T49.5x3-	T49.5x4-	T49.5x5-	T49.5x6-							
topical NEC	T49.0x1-	T49.0x2-	T49.0x3-	T49.0x4-	T49.0x5-	T49.0x6-							
undecylenate	T49.0x1-	T49.0x2-	T49.0x3-	T49.0x4-	T49.0x5-	T49.0x6-							
Zineb	T60.0x1-	T60.0x2-	T60.0x3-	T60.0x4-	—	—							
Zinostatin	T45.1x1-	T45.1x2-	T45.1x3-	T45.1x4-	T45.1x5-	T45.1x6-							
Zipeprol	T48.3x1-	T48.3x2-	T48.3x3-	T48.3x4-	T48.3x5-	T48.3x6-							
Zofenopril	T46.4x1-	T46.4x2-	T46.4x3-	T46.4x4-	T46.4x5-	T46.4x6-							
Zolpidem	T42.6x1-	T42.6x2-	T42.6x3-	T42.6x4-	T42.6x5-	T42.6x6-							
Zomepirac	T39.391-	T39.392-	T39.393-	T39.394-	T39.395-	T39.396-							

DRUGS & CHEMICALS

Table of Drugs & Chemicals	POISONING				Adverse Effect	Underdosing	Table of Drugs & Chemicals	POISONING				Adverse Effect	Underdosing
	Accidental (Unintentional)	Self-Harm (Intentional)	Assault	Undetermined				Accidental (Unintentional)	Self-Harm (Intentional)	Assault	Undetermined		

A

Abandonment (causing exposure to weather conditions) (with intent to injure or kill) NEC X58

Abuse (adult) (child) (mental) (physical) (sexual) X58

Accident (to) X58
  aircraft (in transit) (powered) — *see also* Accident, transport, aircraft
    due to, caused by cataclysm — *see* Forces of nature, by type
  animal-drawn vehicle — *see* Accident, transport, animal-drawn vehicle occupant
  animal-rider — *see* Accident, transport, animal-rider
  automobile — *see* Accident, transport, car occupant
  bare foot water skier V94.4
  boat, boating — *see also* Accident, watercraft
    striking swimmer
      powered V94.11
      unpowered V94.12
  bus — *see* Accident, transport, bus occupant
  cable car, not on rails V98.0
    on rails — *see* Accident, transport, streetcar occupant
  car — *see* Accident, transport, car occupant
  caused by, due to
    animal NEC W64
    chain hoist W24.0
    cold (excessive) — *see* Exposure, cold
    corrosive liquid, substance — *see* Table of Drugs and Chemicals
    cutting or piercing instrument — *see* Contact, with, by type of instrument
    drive belt W24.0
    electric
      current — *see* Exposure, electric current
      motor (*see also* Contact, with, by type of machine) W31.3
        current (of) W86.8
    environmental factor NEC X58
    explosive material — *see* Explosion
    fire, flames — *see* Exposure, fire
    firearm missile — *see* Discharge, firearm by type
    heat (excessive) — *see* Heat
    hot — *see* Contact, with, hot
    ignition — *see* Ignition
    lifting device W24.0
    lightning — *see* subcategory T75.0
      causing fire — *see* Exposure, fire
    machine, machinery — *see* Contact, with, by type of machine
    natural factor NEC X58
    pulley (block) W24.0
    radiation — *see* Radiation
    steam X13.1
      inhalation X13.0
      pipe X16
    thunderbolt — *see* subcategory T75.0
      causing fire — *see* Exposure, fire
    transmission device W24.1
  coach — *see* Accident, transport, bus occupant
  coal car — *see* Accident, transport, industrial vehicle occupant
  diving — *see also* Fall, into, water
    with
      drowning or submersion — *see* Drowning
  forklift — *see* Accident, transport, industrial vehicle occupant
  heavy transport vehicle NOS — *see* Accident, transport, truck occupant
  ice yacht V98.2

Accident (to) X58 — *continued*
  in
    medical, surgical procedure
      as, or due to misadventure — *see* Misadventure
      causing an abnormal reaction or later complication without mention of misadventure (*see also* Complication of or following, by type of procedure) Y84.9
  land yacht V98.1
  late effect of — *see* W00-X58 with 7th character S
  logging car — *see* Accident, transport, industrial vehicle occupant
  machine, machinery — *see also* Contact, with, by type of machine
    on board watercraft V93.69
      explosion — *see* Explosion, in, watercraft
      fire — *see* Burn, on board watercraft
      powered craft V93.63
        ferry boat V93.61
        fishing boat V93.62
        jetskis V93.63
        liner V93.61
        merchant ship V93.60
        passenger ship V93.61
        sailboat V93.64
  mine tram — *see* Accident, transport, industrial vehicle occupant
  mobility scooter (motorized) — *see* Accident, transport, pedestrian, conveyance, specified type NEC
  motor scooter — *see* Accident, transport, motorcyclist
  motor vehicle NOS (traffic) (*see also* Accident, transport) V89.2
    nontraffic V89.0
    three-wheeled NOS — *see* Accident, transport, three-wheeled motor vehicle occupant
  motorcycle NOS — *see* Accident, transport, motorcyclist
  nonmotor vehicle NOS (nontraffic) (*see also* Accident, transport) V89.1
    traffic NOS V89.3
  nontraffic (victim's mode of transport NOS) V88.9
    collision (between) V88.7
      bus and truck V88.5
      car and:
        bus V88.3
        pickup V88.2
        three-wheeled motor vehicle V88.0
        train V88.6
        truck V88.4
        two-wheeled motor vehicle V88.0
        van V88.2
      specified vehicle NEC and:
        three-wheeled motor vehicle V88.1
        two-wheeled motor vehicle V88.1
    known mode of transport — *see* Accident, transport, by type of vehicle
    noncollision V88.8

Accident (to) X58 — *continued*
  on board watercraft V93.89
    powered craft V93.83
      ferry boat V93.81
      fishing boat V93.82
      jetskis V93.83
      liner V93.81
      merchant ship V93.80
      passenger ship V93.81
    unpowered craft V93.88
      canoe V93.85
      inflatable V93.86
        in tow
          recreational V94.31
          specified NEC V94.32
      kayak V93.85
      sailboat V93.84
      surfboard V93.88
      water skis V93.87
      windsurfer V93.88
  parachutist V97.29
    entangled in object V97.21
    injured on landing V97.22
  pedal cycle — *see* Accident, transport, pedal cyclist
  pedestrian (on foot)
    with
      another pedestrian W51
        with fall W03
          due to ice or snow W00.0
      on pedestrian conveyance NEC V00.09
        roller skater (in-line) V00.01
        skate boarder V00.02
      transport vehicle — *see* Accident, transport
    on pedestrian conveyance — *see* Accident, transport, pedestrian, conveyance
  pickup truck or van — *see* Accident, transport, pickup truck occupant
  quarry truck — *see* Accident, transport, industrial vehicle occupant
  railway vehicle (any) (in motion) — *see* Accident, transport, railway vehicle occupant
    due to cataclysm — *see* Forces of nature, by type
  scooter (non-motorized) — *see* Accident, transport, pedestrian, conveyance, scooter
  sequelae of — *see* W00-X58 with 7th character S
  skateboard — *see* Accident, transport, pedestrian, conveyance, skateboard
  ski(ing) — *see* Accident, transport, pedestrian, conveyance
    lift V98.3
  specified cause NEC X58
  streetcar — *see* Accident, transport, streetcar occupant
  traffic (victim's mode of transport NOS) V87.9
    collision (between) V87.7
      bus and truck V87.5
      car and:
        bus V87.3
        pickup V87.2
        three-wheeled motor vehicle V87.0
        train V87.6
        truck V87.4
        two-wheeled motor vehicle V87.0
        van V87.2
      specified vehicle NEC and:
        three-wheeled motor vehicle V87.1
        two-wheeled motor vehicle V87.1
    known mode of transport — *see* Accident, transport, by type of vehicle
    noncollision V87.8

EXTERNAL CAUSES

Accident (to) X58 — *continued*
transport (involving injury to) V99
 18 wheeler — *see* Accident, transport, truck
  occupant
 agricultural vehicle occupant (nontraffic)
  V84.9
  driver V84.5
  hanger-on V84.7
  passenger V84.6
  traffic V84.3
   driver V84.0
   hanger-on V84.2
   passenger V84.1
  while boarding or alighting V84.4
 aircraft NEC V97.89
  military NEC V97.818
   with civlian aircraft V97.810
   civilian injured by V97.811
  occupant injured (in)
   nonpowered craft accident V96.9
    balloon V96.00
     collision V96.03
     crash V96.01
     explosion V96.05
     fire V96.04
     forced landing V96.02
     specified type NEC V96.09
    glider V96.20
     collision V96.23
     crash V96.21
     explosion V96.25
     fire V96.24
     forced landing V96.22
     specified type NEC V96.29
    hang glider V96.10
     collision V96.13
     crash V96.11
     explosion V96.15
     fire V96.14
     forced landing V96.12
     specified type NEC V96.19
    specified craft NEC V96.8
   powered craft accident V95.9
    fixed wing NEC
     commercial V95.30
      collision V95.33
      crash V95.31
      explosion V95.35
      fire V95.34
      forced landing V95.32
      specified type NEC V95.39
     private V95.20
      collision V95.23
      crash V95.21
      explosion V95.25
      fire V95.24
      forced landing V95.22
      specified type NEC V95.29
    glider V95.10
     collision V95.13
     crash V95.11
     explosion V95.15
     fire V95.14
     forced landing V95.12
     specified type NEC V95.19
    helicopter V95.00
     collision V95.03
     crash V95.01
     explosion V95.05
     fire V95.04
     forced landing V95.02
     specified type NEC V95.09

Accident (to) X58 — *continued*
transport (involving injury to) V99—*continued*
 aircraft NEC V97.89 — *continued*
  occupant injured (in) — *continued*
   powered craft accident V95.9 —
    continued
    spacecraft V95.40
     collision V95.43
     crash V95.41
     explosion V95.45
     fire V95.44
     forced landing V95.42
     specified type NEC V95.49
    specified craft NEC V95.8
    ultralight V95.10
     collision V95.13
     crash V95.11
     explosion V95.15
     fire V95.14
     forced landing V95.12
     specified type NEC V95.19
   specified accident NEC V97.0
   while boarding or alighting V97.1
  person (injured by)
   falling from, in or on aircraft V97.0
   machinery on aircraft V97.89
   on ground with aircraft involvement
    V97.39
   rotating propeller V97.32
   struck by object falling from aircraft
    V97.31
   sucked into aircraft jet V97.33
   while boarding or alighting aircraft
    V97.1
 airport (battery-powered) passenger vehicle
  — *see* Accident, transport, industrial
  vehicle occupant
 all-terrain vehicle occupant (nontraffic)
  V86.99
  driver V86.59
  dune buggy — *see* Accident, transport,
   dune buggy occupant
  hanger-on V86.79
  passenger V86.69
  snowmobile — *see* Accident, transport,
   snowmobile occupant
  traffic V86.39
   driver V86.09
   hanger-on V86.29
   passenger V86.19
  while boarding or alighting V86.49
 ambulance occupant (traffic) V86.31
  driver V86.01
  hanger-on V86.21
  nontraffic V86.91
   driver V86.51
  passenger V86.11
  while boarding or alighting V86.41

Accident (to) X58 — *continued*
transport (involving injury to) V99—*continued*
 animal-drawn vehicle occupant (in) V80.929
  collision (with)
   animal V80.12
    being ridden V80.711
   animal-drawn vehicle V80.721
   bus V80.42
   car V80.42
   fixed or stationary object V80.82
   military vehicle V80.920
   nonmotor vehicle V80.791
   pedal cycle V80.22
   pedestrian V80.12
   pickup V80.42
   railway train or vehicle V80.62
   specified motor vehicle NEC V80.52
   streetcar V80.731
   truck V80.42
   two-or three-wheeled motor vehicle
    V80.32
   van V80.42
  noncollision V80.02
  specified circumstance NEC V80.928
 animal-rider V80.919
  collision (with)
   animal V80.11
    being ridden V80.710
   animal-drawn vehicle V80.720
   bus V80.41
   car V80.41
   fixed or stationary object V80.81
   military vehicle V80.910
   nonmotor vehicle V80.790
   pedal cycle V80.21
   pedestrian V80.11
   pickup V80.41
   railway train or vehicle V80.61
   specified motor vehicle NEC V80.51
   streetcar V80.730
   truck V80.41
   two-or three-wheeled motor vehicle
    V80.31
   van V80.41
  noncollision V80.018
   specified as horse rider V80.010
  specified circumstance NEC V80.918
 armored car — *see* Accident, transport, truck
  occupant
 battery-powered truck (baggage) (mail) —
  see Accident, transport, industrial vehicle
  occupant

Accident (to) X58 — *continued*
  transport (involving injury to) V99—*continued*
    bus occupant V79.9
      collision (with)
        animal (traffic) V70.9
          being ridden (traffic) V76.9
            nontraffic V76.3
              while boarding or alighting V76.4
          nontraffic V70.3
            while boarding or alighting V70.4
        animal-drawn vehicle (traffic) V76.9
          nontraffic V76.3
            while boarding or alighting V76.4
        bus (traffic) V74.9
          nontraffic V74.3
            while boarding or alighting V74.4
        car (traffic) V73.9
          nontraffic V73.3
            while boarding or alighting V73.4
        motor vehicle NOS (traffic) V79.60
          nontraffic V79.20
          specified type NEC (traffic) V79.69
            nontraffic V79.29
        pedal cycle (traffic) V71.9
          nontraffic V71.3
            while boarding or alighting V71.4
        pickup truck (traffic) V73.9
          nontraffic V73.3
            while boarding or alighting V73.4
        railway vehicle (traffic) V75.9
          nontraffic V75.3
            while boarding or alighting V75.4
        specified vehicle NEC (traffic) V76.9
          nontraffic V76.3
            while boarding or alighting V76.4
        stationary object (traffic) V77.9
          nontraffic V77.3
            while boarding or alighting V77.4
        streetcar (traffic) V76.9
          nontraffic V76.3
            while boarding or alighting V76.4
        three wheeled motor vehicle (traffic) V72.9
          nontraffic V72.3
            while boarding or alighting V72.4
        truck (traffic) V74.9
          nontraffic V74.3
            while boarding or alighting V74.4
        two wheeled motor vehicle (traffic) V72.9
          nontraffic V72.3
            while boarding or alighting V72.4
        van (traffic) V73.9
          nontraffic V73.3
            while boarding or alighting V73.4
      driver
        collision (with)
          animal (traffic) V70.5
            being ridden (traffic) V76.5
              nontraffic V76.0
            nontraffic V70.0
          animal-drawn vehicle (traffic) V76.5
            nontraffic V76.0
          bus (traffic) V74.5
            nontraffic V74.0
          car (traffic) V73.5
            nontraffic V73.0
          motor vehicle NOS (traffic) V79.40
            nontraffic V79.00
            specified type NEC (traffic) V79.49
              nontraffic V79.09
          pedal cycle (traffic) V71.5
            nontraffic V71.0
          pickup truck (traffic) V73.5
            nontraffic V73.0
          railway vehicle (traffic) V75.5
            nontraffic V75.0

Accident (to) X58 — *continued*
  transport (involving injury to) V99—*continued*
    bus occupant V79.9 — *continued*
      driver — *continued*
        collision (with) — *continued*
          specified vehicle NEC (traffic) V76.5
            nontraffic V76.0
          stationary object (traffic) V77.5
            nontraffic V77.0
          streetcar (traffic) V76.5
            nontraffic V76.0
          three wheeled motor vehicle (traffic) V72.5
            nontraffic V72.0
          truck (traffic) V74.5
            nontraffic V74.0
          two wheeled motor vehicle (traffic) V72.5
            nontraffic V72.0
          van (traffic) V73.5
            nontraffic V73.0
        noncollision accident (traffic) V78.5
          nontraffic V78.0
      hanger-on
        collision (with)
          animal (traffic) V70.7
            being ridden (traffic) V76.7
              nontraffic V76.2
            nontraffic V70.2
          animal-drawn vehicle (traffic) V76.7
            nontraffic V76.2
          bus (traffic) V74.7
            nontraffic V74.2
          car (traffic) V73.7
            nontraffic V73.2
          pedal cycle (traffic) V71.7
            nontraffic V71.2
          pickup truck (traffic) V73.7
            nontraffic V73.2
          railway vehicle (traffic) V75.7
            nontraffic V75.2
          specified vehicle NEC (traffic) V76.7
            nontraffic V76.2
          stationary object (traffic) V77.7
            nontraffic V77.2
          streetcar (traffic) V76.7
            nontraffic V76.2
          three wheeled motor vehicle (traffic) V72.7
            nontraffic V72.2
          truck (traffic) V74.7
            nontraffic V74.2
          two wheeled motor vehicle (traffic) V72.7
            nontraffic V72.2
          van (traffic) V73.7
            nontraffic V73.2
        noncollision accident (traffic) V78.7
          nontraffic V78.2
        noncollision accident (traffic) V78.9
          nontraffic V78.3
          while boarding or alighting V78.4
      nontraffic V79.3

Accident (to) X58 — *continued*
  transport (involving injury to) V99—*continued*
    bus occupant V79.9 — *continued*
      passenger
        collision (with)
          animal (traffic) V70.6
            being ridden (traffic) V76.6
              nontraffic V76.1
            nontraffic V70.1
          animal-drawn vehicle (traffic) V76.6
            nontraffic V76.1
          bus (traffic) V74.6
            nontraffic V74.1
          car (traffic) V73.6
            nontraffic V73.1
          motor vehicle NOS (traffic) V79.50
            nontraffic V79.10
            specified type NEC (traffic) V79.59
              nontraffic V79.19
          pedal cycle (traffic) V71.6
            nontraffic V71.1
          pickup truck (traffic) V73.6
            nontraffic V73.1
          railway vehicle (traffic) V75.6
            nontraffic V75.1
          specified vehicle NEC (traffic) V76.6
            nontraffic V76.1
          stationary object (traffic) V77.6
            nontraffic V77.1
          streetcar (traffic) V76.6
            nontraffic V76.1
          three wheeled motor vehicle (traffic) V72.6
            nontraffic V72.1
          truck (traffic) V74.6
            nontraffic V74.1
          two wheeled motor vehicle (traffic) V72.6
            nontraffic V72.1
          van (traffic) V73.6
            nontraffic V73.1
        noncollision accident (traffic) V78.6
          nontraffic V78.1
      specified type NEC V79.88
      military vehicle V79.81

Accident (to) X58 — *continued*
transport (involving injury to) V99—*continued*
  cable car, not on rails V98.0
    on rails — *see* Accident, transport, streetcar occupant
  car occupant V49.9
    ambulance occupant — *see* Accident, transport, ambulance occupant
    collision (with)
      animal (traffic) V40.9
        being ridden (traffic) V46.9
          nontraffic V46.3
          while boarding or alighting V46.4
        nontraffic V40.3
        while boarding or alighting V40.4
      animal-drawn vehicle (traffic) V46.9
        nontraffic V46.3
        while boarding or alighting V46.4
      bus (traffic) V44.9
        nontraffic V44.3
        while boarding or alighting V44.4
      car (traffic) V43.92
        nontraffic V43.32
        while boarding or alighting V43.42
      motor vehicle NOS (traffic) V49.60
        nontraffic V49.20
        specified type NEC (traffic) V49.69
          nontraffic V49.29
      pedal cycle (traffic) V41.9
        nontraffic V41.3
        while boarding or alighting V41.4
      pickup truck (traffic) V43.93
        nontraffic V43.33
        while boarding or alighting V43.43
      railway vehicle (traffic) V45.9
        nontraffic V45.3
        while boarding or alighting V45.4
      specified vehicle NEC (traffic) V46.9
        nontraffic V46.3
        while boarding or alighting V46.4
      sport utility vehicle (traffic) V43.91
        nontraffic V43.31
        while boarding or alighting V43.41
      stationary object (traffic) V47.92
        nontraffic V47.32
        while boarding or alighting V47.4
      streetcar (traffic) V46.9
        nontraffic V46.3
        while boarding or alighting V46.4
      three wheeled motor vehicle (traffic) V42.9
        nontraffic V42.3
        while boarding or alighting V42.4
      truck (traffic) V44.9
        nontraffic V44.3
        while boarding or alighting V44.4
      two wheeled motor vehicle (traffic) V42.9
        nontraffic V42.3
        while boarding or alighting V42.4
      van (traffic) V43.94
        nontraffic V43.34
        while boarding or alighting V43.44

Accident (to) X58 — *continued*
transport (involving injury to) V99—*continued*
  car occupant V49.9 — *continued*
    driver
      collision (with)
        animal (traffic) V40.5
          being ridden (traffic) V46.5
          nontraffic V46.0
          nontraffic V40.0
        animal-drawn vehicle (traffic) V46.5
          nontraffic V46.0
        bus (traffic) V44.5
          nontraffic V44.0
        car (traffic) V43.52
          nontraffic V43.02
        motor vehicle NOS (traffic) V49.40
          nontraffic V49.00
          specified type NEC (traffic) V49.49
            nontraffic V49.09
        pedal cycle (traffic) V41.5
          nontraffic V41.0
        pickup truck (traffic) V43.53
          nontraffic V43.03
        railway vehicle (traffic) V45.5
          nontraffic V45.0
        specified vehicle NEC (traffic) V46.5
          nontraffic V46.0
        sport utility vehicle (traffic) V43.51
          nontraffic V43.01
        stationary object (traffic) V47.52
          nontraffic V47.02
        streetcar (traffic) V46.5
          nontraffic V46.0
        three wheeled motor vehicle (traffic) V42.5
          nontraffic V42.0
        truck (traffic) V44.5
          nontraffic V44.0
        two wheeled motor vehicle (traffic) V42.5
          nontraffic V42.0
        van (traffic) V43.54
          nontraffic V43.04
      noncollision accident (traffic) V48.5
        nontraffic V48.0

Accident (to) X58 — *continued*
transport (involving injury to) V99—*continued*
  car occupant V49.9 — *continued*
    hanger-on
      collision (with)
        animal (traffic) V40.7
          being ridden (traffic) V46.7
          nontraffic V46.2
          nontraffic V40.2
        animal-drawn vehicle (traffic) V46.7
          nontraffic V46.2
        bus (traffic) V44.7
          nontraffic V44.2
        car (traffic) V43.72
          nontraffic V43.22
        pedal cycle (traffic) V41.7
          nontraffic V41.2
        pickup truck (traffic) V43.73
          nontraffic V43.23
        railway vehicle (traffic) V45.7
          nontraffic V45.2
        specified vehicle NEC (traffic) V46.7
          nontraffic V46.2
        sport utility vehicle (traffic) V43.71
          nontraffic V43.21
        stationary object (traffic) V47.7
          nontraffic V47.2
        streetcar (traffic) V46.7
          nontraffic V46.2
        three wheeled motor vehicle (traffic) V42.7
          nontraffic V42.2
        truck (traffic) V44.7
          nontraffic V44.2
        two wheeled motor vehicle (traffic) V42.7
          nontraffic V42.2
        van (traffic) V43.74
          nontraffic V43.24
      noncollision accident (traffic) V48.7
        nontraffic V48.2
    noncollision accident (traffic) V48.9
      nontraffic V48.3
      while boarding or alighting V48.4
    nontraffic V49.3

Accident (to) X58 — *continued*
  transport (involving injury to) V99—*continued*
    car occupant V49.9 — *continued*
      passenger
        collision (with)
          animal (traffic) V40.6
            being ridden (traffic) V46.6
              nontraffic V46.1
            nontraffic V40.1
          animal-drawn vehicle (traffic) V46.6
            nontraffic V46.1
          bus (traffic) V44.6
            nontraffic V44.1
          car (traffic) V43.62
            nontraffic V43.12
          motor vehicle NOS (traffic) V49.50
            nontraffic V49.10
            specified type NEC (traffic) V49.59
              nontraffic V49.19
          pedal cycle (traffic) V41.6
            nontraffic V41.1
          pickup truck (traffic) V43.63
            nontraffic V43.13
          railway vehicle (traffic) V45.6
            nontraffic V45.1
          specified vehicle NEC (traffic) V46.6
            nontraffic V46.1
          sport utility vehicle (traffic) V43.61
            nontraffic V43.11
          stationary object (traffic) V47.62
            nontraffic V47.12
          streetcar (traffic) V46.6
            nontraffic V46.1
          three wheeled motor vehicle (traffic) V42.6
            nontraffic V42.1
          truck (traffic) V44.6
            nontraffic V44.1
          two wheeled motor vehicle (traffic) V42.6
            nontraffic V42.1
          van (traffic) V43.64
            nontraffic V43.14
         noncollision accident (traffic) V48.6
          nontraffic V48.1
        specified type NEC V49.88
        military vehicle V49.81

Accident (to) X58 — *continued*
  transport (involving injury to) V99—*continued*
    coal car — *see* Accident, transport, industrial vehicle occupant
    construction vehicle occupant (nontraffic) V85.9
      driver V85.5
      hanger-on V85.7
      passenger V85.6
      traffic V85.3
        driver V85.0
        hanger-on V85.2
        passenger V85.1
      while boarding or alighting V85.4
    dirt bike rider — *see* Accident, transport, all-terrain vehicle occupant
    due to cataclysm — *see* Forces of nature, by type
    dune buggy occupant (nontraffic) V86.93
      driver V86.53
      hanger-on V86.73
      passenger V86.63
      traffic V86.33
        driver V86.03
        hanger-on V86.23
        passenger V86.13
      while boarding or alighting V86.43
    forklift — *see* Accident, transport, industrial vehicle occupant
    go cart — *see* Accident, transport, all-terrain vehicle occupant
    golf cart — *see* Accident, transport, all-terrain vehicle occupant
    heavy transport vehicle occupant — *see* Accident, transport, truck occupant
    ice yacht V98.2
    industrial vehicle occupant (nontraffic) V83.9
      driver V83.5
      hanger-on V83.7
      passenger V83.6
      traffic V83.3
        driver V83.0
        hanger-on V83.2
        passenger V83.1
      while boarding or alighting V83.4
    interurban electric car — *see* Accident, transport, streetcar
    land yacht V98.1
    logging car — *see* Accident, transport, industrial vehicle occupant
    military vehicle occupant (traffic) V86.34
      driver V86.04
      hanger-on V86.24
      nontraffic V86.94
        driver V86.54
        hanger-on V86.74
        passenger V86.64
      passenger V86.14
      while boarding or alighting V86.44
    mine tram — *see* Accident, transport, industrial vehicle occupant
    motor vehicle NEC occupant (traffic) V89.2
    motorcoach — *see* Accident, transport, bus occupant

Accident (to) X58 — *continued*
  transport (involving injury to) V99—*continued*
    motorcyclist V29.9
      collision (with)
        animal (traffic) V20.9
          being ridden (traffic) V26.9
            nontraffic V26.2
            while boarding or alighting V26.3
          nontraffic V20.2
          while boarding or alighting V20.3
        animal-drawn vehicle (traffic) V26.9
          nontraffic V26.2
          while boarding or alighting V26.3
        bus (traffic) V24.9
          nontraffic V24.2
          while boarding or alighting V24.3
        car (traffic) V23.9
          nontraffic V23.2
          while boarding or alighting V23.3
        motor vehicle NOS (traffic) V29.60
          nontraffic V29.20
          specified type NEC (traffic) V29.69
            nontraffic V29.29
        pedal cycle (traffic) V21.9
          nontraffic V21.2
          while boarding or alighting V21.3
        pickup truck (traffic) V23.9
          nontraffic V23.2
          while boarding or alighting V23.3
        railway vehicle (traffic) V25.9
          nontraffic V25.2
          while boarding or alighting V25.3
        specified vehicle NEC (traffic) V26.9
          nontraffic V26.2
          while boarding or alighting V26.3
        stationary object (traffic) V27.9
          nontraffic V27.2
          while boarding or alighting V27.3
        streetcar (traffic) V26.9
          nontraffic V26.2
          while boarding or alighting V26.3
        three wheeled motor vehicle (traffic) V22.9
          nontraffic V22.2
          while boarding or alighting V22.3
        truck (traffic) V24.9
          nontraffic V24.2
          while boarding or alighting V24.3
        two wheeled motor vehicle (traffic) V22.9
          nontraffic V22.2
          while boarding or alighting V22.3
        van (traffic) V23.9
          nontraffic V23.2
          while boarding or alighting V23.3

Accident (to) X58 — *continued*
  transport (involving injury to) V99—*continued*
    motorcyclist V29.9 — *continued*
      driver
        collision (with)
          animal (traffic) V20.4
            being ridden (traffic) V26.4
              nontraffic V26.0
            nontraffic V20.0
          animal-drawn vehicle (traffic) V26.4
            nontraffic V26.0
          bus (traffic) V24.4
            nontraffic V24.0
          car (traffic) V23.4
            nontraffic V23.0
          motor vehicle NOS (traffic) V29.40
            nontraffic V29.00
            specified type NEC (traffic) V29.49
              nontraffic V29.09
          pedal cycle (traffic) V21.4
            nontraffic V21.0
          pickup truck (traffic) V23.4
            nontraffic V23.0
          railway vehicle (traffic) V25.4
            nontraffic V25.0
          specified vehicle NEC (traffic) V26.4
            nontraffic V26.0
          stationary object (traffic) V27.4
            nontraffic V27.0
          streetcar (traffic) V26.4
            nontraffic V26.0
          three wheeled motor vehicle (traffic)
            V22.4
            nontraffic V22.0
          truck (traffic) V24.4
            nontraffic V24.0
          two wheeled motor vehicle (traffic)
            V22.4
            nontraffic V22.0
          van (traffic) V23.4
            nontraffic V23.0
        noncollision accident (traffic) V28.4
          nontraffic V28.0
      noncollision accident (traffic) V28.9
        nontraffic V28.2
        while boarding or alighting V28.3
      nontraffic V29.3

Accident (to) X58 — *continued*
  transport (involving injury to) V99—*continued*
    motorcyclist V29.9 — *continued*
      passenger
        collision (with)
          animal (traffic) V20.5
            being ridden (traffic) V26.5
              nontraffic V26.1
            nontraffic V20.1
          animal-drawn vehicle (traffic) V26.5
            nontraffic V26.1
          bus (traffic) V24.5
            nontraffic V24.1
          car (traffic) V23.5
            nontraffic V23.1
          motor vehicle NOS (traffic) V29.50
            nontraffic V29.10
            specified type NEC (traffic) V29.59
              nontraffic V29.19
          pedal cycle (traffic) V21.5
            nontraffic V21.1
          pickup truck (traffic) V23.5
            nontraffic V23.1
          railway vehicle (traffic) V25.5
            nontraffic V25.1
          specified vehicle NEC (traffic) V26.5
            nontraffic V26.1
          stationary object (traffic) V27.5
            nontraffic V27.1
          streetcar (traffic) V26.5
            nontraffic V26.1
          three wheeled motor vehicle (traffic)
            V22.5
            nontraffic V22.1
          truck (traffic) V24.5
            nontraffic V24.1
          two wheeled motor vehicle (traffic)
            V22.5
            nontraffic V22.1
          van (traffic) V23.5
            nontraffic V23.1
        noncollision accident (traffic) V28.5
          nontraffic V28.1
      specified type NEC V29.88
        military vehicle V29.81

Accident (to) X58 — *continued*
  transport (involving injury to) V99—*continued*
    occupant (of)
      aircraft (powered) V95.9
        fixed wing
          commercial — *see* Accident, transport,
            aircraft, occupant, powered, fixed
            wing, commercial
          private — *see* Accident, transport,
            aircraft, occupant, powered, fixed
            wing, private
        nonpowered V96.9
        specified NEC V95.8
      airport battery-powered vehicle — *see*
        Accident, transport, industrial vehicle
        occupant
      all-terrain vehicle (ATV) — *see* Accident,
        transport, all-terrain vehicle occupant
      animal-drawn vehicle — *see* Accident,
        transport, animal-drawn vehicle
        occupant
      automobile — *see* Accident, transport, car
        occupant
      balloon V96.00
      battery-powered vehicle — *see* Accident,
        transport, industrial vehicle occupant
      bicycle — *see* Accident, transport, pedal
        cyclist
        motorized — *see* Accident, transport,
          motorcycle rider
      boat NEC — *see* Accident, watercraft
      bulldozer — *see* Accident, transport,
        construction vehicle occupant
      bus — *see* Accident, transport, bus
        occupant
      cable car (on rails) — *see also* Accident,
        transport, streetcar occupant
        not on rails V98.0
      car — *see also* Accident, transport, car
        occupant
        cable (on rails) — *see also* Accident,
          transport, streetcar occupant
          not on rails V98.0
      coach — *see* Accident, transport, bus
        occupant
      coal-car — *see* Accident, transport,
        industrial vehicle occupant
      digger — *see* Accident, transport,
        construction vehicle occupant
      dump truck — *see* Accident, transport,
        construction vehicle occupant
      earth-leveler — *see* Accident, transport,
        construction vehicle occupant
      farm machinery (self-propelled) — *see*
        Accident, transport, agricultural
        vehicle occupant
      forklift — *see* Accident, transport,
        industrial vehicle occupant
      glider (unpowered) V96.20
        hang V96.10
        powered (microlight) (ultralight) — *see*
          Accident, transport, aircraft,
          occupant, powered, glider
      glider (unpowered) NEC V96.20
      hang-glider V96.10
      harvester — *see* Accident, transport,
        agricultural vehicle occupant
      heavy (transport) vehicle — *see* Accident,
        transport, truck occupant
      helicopter — *see* Accident, transport,
        aircraft, occupant, helicopter
      ice-yacht V98.2
      kite (carrying person) V96.8
      land-yacht V98.1
      logging car — *see* Accident, transport,
        industrial vehicle occupant

Accident (to) X58 — *continued*
transport (involving injury to) V99—*continued*
occupant (of) — *continued*
mechanical shovel — *see* Accident, transport, construction vehicle occupant
microlight — *see* Accident, transport, aircraft, occupant, powered, glider
minibus — *see* Accident, transport, pickup truck occupant
minivan — *see* Accident, transport, pickup truck occupant
moped — *see* Accident, transport, motorcycle
motor scooter — *see* Accident, transport, motorcycle
motorcycle (with sidecar) — *see* Accident, transport, motorcycle
pedal cycle — *see also* Accident, transport, pedal cyclist
pickup (truck) — *see* Accident, transport, pickup truck occupant
railway (train) (vehicle) (subterranean) (elevated) — *see* Accident, transport, railway vehicle occupant
rickshaw — *see* Accident, transport, pedal cycle
motorized — *see* Accident, transport, three-wheeled motor vehicle
pedal driven — *see* Accident, transport, pedal cyclist
road-roller — *see* Accident, transport, construction vehicle occupant
ship NOS V94.9
ski-lift (chair) (gondola) V98.3
snowmobile — *see* Accident, transport, snowmobile occupant
spacecraft, spaceship — *see* Accident, transport, aircraft, occupant, spacecraft
sport utility vehicle — *see* Accident, transport, pickup truck occupant
streetcar (interurban) (operating on public street or highway) — *see* Accident, transport, streetcar occupant
SUV — *see* Accident, transport, pickup truck occupant
téléférique V98.0
three-wheeled vehicle (motorized) — *see also* Accident, transport, three-wheeled motor vehicle occupant
nonmotorized — *see* Accident, transport, pedal cycle
tractor (farm) (and trailer) — *see* Accident, transport, agricultural vehicle occupant
train — *see* Accident, transport, railway vehicle occupant
tram — *see* Accident, transport, streetcar occupant
in mine or quarry — *see* Accident, transport, industrial vehicle occupant
tricycle — *see* Accident, transport, pedal cycle
motorized — *see* Accident, transport, three-wheeled motor vehicle
trolley — *see* Accident, transport, streetcar occupant
in mine or quarry — *see* Accident, transport, industrial vehicle occupant
tub, in mine or quarry — *see* Accident, transport, industrial vehicle occupant
ultralight — *see* Accident, transport, aircraft, occupant, powered, glider
van — *see* Accident, transport, van occupant

Accident (to) X58 — *continued*
transport (involving injury to) V99—*continued*
occupant (of) — *continued*
vehicle NEC V89.9
heavy transport — *see* Accident, transport, truck occupant
motor (traffic) NEC V89.2
nontraffic NEC V89.0
watercraft NOS V94.9
causing drowning — *see* Drowning, resulting from accident to boat
parachutist V97.29
after accident to aircraft — *see* Accident, transport, aircraft
entangled in object V97.21
injured on landing V97.22
pedal cyclist V19.9
collision (with)
animal (traffic) V10.9
being ridden (traffic) V16.9
nontraffic V16.2
while boarding or alighting V16.3
nontraffic V10.2
while boarding or alighting V10.3
animal-drawn vehicle (traffic) V16.9
nontraffic V16.2
while boarding or alighting V16.3
bus (traffic) V14.9
nontraffic V14.2
while boarding or alighting V14.3
car (traffic) V13.9
nontraffic V13.2
while boarding or alighting V13.3
motor vehicle NOS (traffic) V19.60
nontraffic V19.20
specified type NEC (traffic) V19.69
nontraffic V19.29
pedal cycle (traffic) V11.9
nontraffic V11.2
while boarding or alighting V11.3
pickup truck (traffic) V13.9
nontraffic V13.2
while boarding or alighting V13.3
railway vehicle (traffic) V15.9
nontraffic V15.2
while boarding or alighting V15.3
specified vehicle NEC (traffic) V16.9
nontraffic V16.2
while boarding or alighting V16.3
stationary object (traffic) V17.9
nontraffic V17.2
while boarding or alighting V17.3
streetcar (traffic) V16.9
nontraffic V16.2
while boarding or alighting V16.3
three wheeled motor vehicle (traffic) V12.9
nontraffic V12.2
while boarding or alighting V12.3
truck (traffic) V14.9
nontraffic V14.2
while boarding or alighting V14.3
two wheeled motor vehicle (traffic) V12.9
nontraffic V12.2
while boarding or alighting V12.3
van (traffic) V13.9
nontraffic V13.2
while boarding or alighting V13.3

Accident (to) X58 — *continued*
transport (involving injury to) V99—*continued*
pedal cyclist V19.9 — *continued*
driver
collision (with)
animal (traffic) V10.4
being ridden (traffic) V16.4
nontraffic V16.0
nontraffic V10.0
animal-drawn vehicle (traffic) V16.4
nontraffic V16.0
bus (traffic) V14.4
nontraffic V14.0
car (traffic) V13.4
nontraffic V13.0
motor vehicle NOS (traffic) V19.40
nontraffic V19.00
specified type NEC (traffic) V19.49
nontraffic V19.09
pedal cycle (traffic) V11.4
nontraffic V11.0
pickup truck (traffic) V13.4
nontraffic V13.0
railway vehicle (traffic) V15.4
nontraffic V15.0
specified vehicle NEC (traffic) V16.4
nontraffic V16.0
stationary object (traffic) V17.4
nontraffic V17.0
streetcar (traffic) V16.4
nontraffic V16.0
three wheeled motor vehicle (traffic) V12.4
nontraffic V12.0
truck (traffic) V14.4
nontraffic V14.0
two wheeled motor vehicle (traffic) V12.4
nontraffic V12.0
van (traffic) V13.4
nontraffic V13.0
noncollision accident (traffic) V18.4
nontraffic V18.0
noncollision accident (traffic) V18.9
nontraffic V18.2
while boarding or alighting V18.3
nontraffic V19.3

EXTERNAL CAUSES

Accident (to) X58 — *continued*
  transport (involving injury to) V99—*continued*
    pedal cyclist V19.9 — *continued*
      passenger
        collision (with)
          animal (traffic) V10.5
            being ridden (traffic) V16.5
              nontraffic V16.1
            nontraffic V10.1
          animal-drawn vehicle (traffic) V16.5
            nontraffic V16.1
          bus (traffic) V14.5
            nontraffic V14.1
          car (traffic) V13.5
            nontraffic V13.1
          motor vehicle NOS (traffic) V19.50
            nontraffic V19.10
            specified type NEC (traffic) V19.59
              nontraffic V19.19
          pedal cycle (traffic) V11.5
            nontraffic V11.1
          pickup truck (traffic) V13.5
            nontraffic V13.1
          railway vehicle (traffic) V15.5
            nontraffic V15.1
          specified vehicle NEC (traffic) V16.5
            nontraffic V16.1
          stationary object (traffic) V17.5
            nontraffic V17.1
          streetcar (traffic) V16.5
            nontraffic V16.1
          three wheeled motor vehicle (traffic)
            V12.5
            nontraffic V12.1
          truck (traffic) V14.5
            nontraffic V14.1
          two wheeled motor vehicle (traffic)
            V12.5
            nontraffic V12.1
          van (traffic) V13.5
            nontraffic V13.1
         noncollision accident (traffic) V18.5
          nontraffic V18.1
      specified type NEC V19.88
        military vehicle V19.81

Accident (to) X58 — *continued*
  transport (involving injury to) V99—*continued*
    pedestrian
      conveyance (occupant) V09.9
        babystroller V00.828
          collision (with) V09.9
            animal being ridden or animal
              drawn vehicle V06.99
              nontraffic V06.09
              traffic V06.19
            bus or heavy transport V04.99
              nontraffic V04.09
              traffic V04.19
            car V03.99
              nontraffic V03.09
              traffic V03.19
            pedal cycle V01.99
              nontraffic V01.09
              traffic V01.19
            pickup truck or van V03.99
              nontraffic V03.09
              traffic V03.19
            railway (train) (vehicle) V05.99
              nontraffic V05.09
              traffic V05.19
            stationary object V00.822
            streetcar V06.99
              nontraffic V06.09
              traffic V06.19
            two-or three-wheeled motor vehicle
              V02.99
              nontraffic V02.09
              traffic V02.19
            vehicle V09.9
              animal-drawn V06.99
                nontraffic V06.09
                traffic V06.19
              motor
                nontraffic V09.00
                traffic V09.20
        fall V00.821
        nontraffic V09.1
          involving motor vehicle NEC
            V09.00
        traffic V09.3
          involving motor vehicle NEC
            V09.20

Accident (to) X58 — *continued*
  transport (involving injury to) V99—*continued*
    pedestrian — *continued*
      conveyance (occupant) V09.9 —
        continued
        flat-bottomed NEC V00.388
        collision (with) V09.9
          animal being ridden or animal
            drawn vehicle V06.99
            nontraffic V06.09
            traffic V06.19
          bus or heavy transport V04.99
            nontraffic V04.09
            traffic V04.19
          car V03.99
            nontraffic V03.09
            traffic V03.19
          pedal cycle V01.99
            nontraffic V01.09
            traffic V01.19
          pickup truck or van V03.99
            nontraffic V03.09
            traffic V03.19
          railway (train) (vehicle) V05.99
            nontraffic V05.09
            traffic V05.19
          stationary object V00.382
          streetcar V06.99
            nontraffic V06.09
            traffic V06.19
          two-or three-wheeled motor vehicle
            V02.99
            nontraffic V02.09
            traffic V02.19
          vehicle V09.9
            animal-drawn V06.99
             nontraffic V06.09
             traffic V06.19
            motor
             nontraffic V09.00
             traffic V09.20
        fall V00.381
        nontraffic V09.1
          involving motor vehicle NEC
            V09.00
      snow
        board — *see* Accident, transport,
          pedestrian, conveyance, snow
          board
        ski — *see* Accident, transport,
          pedestrian, conveyance, skis
          (snow)
      traffic V09.3
        involving motor vehicle NEC
          V09.20

Accident (to) X58 — *continued*
transport (involving injury to) V99—*continued*
pedestrian — *continued*
conveyance (occupant) V09.9 —
continued
gliding type NEC V00.288
collision (with) V09.9
animal being ridden or animal
drawn vehicle V06.99
nontraffic V06.09
traffic V06.19
bus or heavy transport V04.99
nontraffic V04.09
traffic V04.19
car V03.99
nontraffic V03.09
traffic V03.19
pedal cycle V01.99
nontraffic V01.09
traffic V01.19
pick-up truck or van V03.99
nontraffic V03.09
traffic V03.19
railway (train) (vehicle) V05.99
nontraffic V05.09
traffic V05.19
stationary object V00.282
streetcar V06.99
nontraffic V06.09
traffic V06.19
two-or three-wheeled motor vehicle
V02.99
nontraffic V02.09
traffic V02.19
vehicle V09.9
animal-drawn V06.99
nontraffic V06.09
traffic V06.19
motor
nontraffic V09.00
traffic V09.20
fall V00.281
heelies — *see* Accident, transport,
pedestrian, conveyance, heelies
ice skate — *see* Accident, transport,
pedestrian, conveyance, ice skate
nontraffic V09.1
involving motor vehicle NEC
V09.00
sled — *see* Accident, transport,
pedestrian, conveyance, sled
traffic V09.3
involving motor vehicle NEC
V09.20
wheelies — *see* Accident, transport,
pedestrian, conveyance, heelies

Accident (to) X58 — *continued*
transport (involving injury to) V99—*continued*
pedestrian — *continued*
conveyance (occupant) V09.9 —
continued
heelies V00.158
colliding with stationary object
V00.152
fall V00.151
ice skates V00.218
collision (with) V09.9
animal being ridden or animal
drawn vehicle V06.99
nontraffic V06.09
traffic V06.19
bus or heavy transport V04.99
nontraffic V04.09
traffic V04.19
car V03.99
nontraffic V03.09
traffic V03.19
pedal cycle V01.99
nontraffic V01.09
traffic V01.19
pick-up truck or van V03.99
nontraffic V03.09
traffic V03.19
railway (train) (vehicle) V05.99
nontraffic V05.09
traffic V05.19
stationary object V00.212
streetcar V06.99
nontraffic V06.09
traffic V06.19
two-or three-wheeled motor vehicle
V02.99
nontraffic V02.09
traffic V02.19
vehicle V09.9
animal-drawn V06.99
nontraffic V06.09
traffic V06.19
motor
nontraffic V09.00
traffic V09.20
fall V00.211
nontraffic V09.1
involving motor vehicle NEC
V09.00
traffic V09.3
involving motor vehicle NEC
V09.20

Accident (to) X58 — *continued*
transport (involving injury to) V99—*continued*
pedestrian — *continued*
conveyance (occupant) V09.9 —
continued
motorized mobility scooter V00.838
collision with stationary object
V00.832
fall from V00.831
nontraffic V09.1
involving motor vehicle V09.00
military V09.01
specified type NEC V09.09
roller skates (non in-line) V00.128
collision (with) V09.9
animal being ridden or animal
drawn vehicle V06.91
nontraffic V06.01
traffic V06.11
bus or heavy transport V04.91
nontraffic V04.01
traffic V04.11
car V03.91
nontraffic V03.01
traffic V03.11
pedal cycle V01.91
nontraffic V01.01
traffic V01.11
pickup truck or van V03.91
nontraffic V03.01
traffic V03.11
railway (train) (vehicle) V05.91
nontraffic V05.01
traffic V05.11
stationary object V00.122
streetcar V06.91
nontraffic V06.01
traffic V06.11
two-or three-wheeled motor vehicle
V02.91
nontraffic V02.01
traffic V02.11
vehicle V09.9
animal-drawn V06.91
nontraffic V06.01
traffic V06.11
motor
nontraffic V09.00
traffic V09.20
fall V00.121
in-line V00.118
collision — *see also* Accident,
transport, pedestrian,
conveyance occupant, roller
skates, collision
with stationary object V00.112
fall V00.111
nontraffic V09.1
involving motor vehicle NEC
V09.00
traffic V09.3
involving motor vehicle NEC
V09.20

Accident (to) X58 — *continued*
transport (involving injury to) V99—*continued*
pedestrian — *continued*
conveyance (occupant) V09.9 —
continued
rolling shoes V00.158
colliding with stationary object
V00.152
fall V00.151
rolling type NEC V00.188
collision (with) V09.9
animal being ridden or animal
drawn vehicle V06.99
nontraffic V06.09
traffic V06.19
bus or heavy transport V04.99
nontraffic V04.09
traffic V04.19
car V03.99
nontraffic V03.09
traffic V03.19
pedal cycle V01.99
nontraffic V01.09
traffic V01.19
pickup truck or van V03.99
nontraffic V03.09
traffic V03.19
railway (train) (vehicle) V05.99
nontraffic V05.09
traffic V05.19
stationary object V00.182
streetcar V06.99
nontraffic V06.09
traffic V06.19
two-or three-wheeled motor vehicle
V02.99
nontraffic V02.09
traffic V02.19
vehicle V09.9
animal-drawn V06.99
nontraffic V06.09
traffic V06.19
motor
nontraffic V09.00
traffic V09.20
fall V00.181
in-line roller skate — *see* Accident,
transport, pedestrian,
conveyance, roller skate, in-line
nontraffic V09.1
involving motor vehicle NEC
V09.00
roller skate — *see* Accident, transport,
pedestrian, conveyance, roller
skate
scooter (non-motorized) — *see*
Accident, transport, pedestrian,
conveyance, scooter
skateboard — *see* Accident, transport,
pedestrian, conveyance,
skateboard
traffic V09.3
involving motor vehicle NEC
V09.20

Accident (to) X58 — *continued*
transport (involving injury to) V99—*continued*
pedestrian — *continued*
conveyance (occupant) V09.9 —
continued
scooter (non-motorized) V00.148
collision (with) V09.9
animal being ridden or animal
drawn vehicle V06.99
nontraffic V06.09
traffic V06.19
bus or heavy transport V04.99
nontraffic V04.09
traffic V04.19
car V03.99
nontraffic V03.09
traffic V03.19
pedal cycle V01.99
nontraffic V01.09
traffic V01.19
pickup truck or van V03.99
nontraffic V03.09
traffic V03.19
railway (train) (vehicle) V05.99
nontraffic V05.09
traffic V05.19
stationary object V00.142
streetcar V06.99
nontraffic V06.09
traffic V06.19
two-or three-wheeled motor vehicle
V02.99
nontraffic V02.09
traffic V02.19
vehicle V09.9
animal-drawn V06.99
nontraffic V06.09
traffic V06.19
motor
nontraffic V09.00
traffic V09.20
fall V00.141
nontraffic V09.1
involving motor vehicle NEC
V09.00
traffic V09.3
involving motor vehicle NEC
V09.20

Accident (to) X58 — *continued*
transport (involving injury to) V99—*continued*
pedestrian — *continued*
conveyance (occupant) V09.9 —
continued
skate board V00.138
collision (with) V09.9
animal being ridden or animal
drawn vehicle V06.92
nontraffic V06.02
traffic V06.12
bus or heavy transport V04.92
nontraffic V04.02
traffic V04.12
car V03.92
nontraffic V03.02
traffic V03.12
pedal cycle V01.92
nontraffic V01.02
traffic V01.12
pickup truck or van V03.92
nontraffic V03.02
traffic V03.12
railway (train) (vehicle) V05.92
nontraffic V05.02
traffic V05.12
stationary object V00.132
streetcar V06.92
nontraffic V06.02
traffic V06.12
two-or three-wheeled motor vehicle
V02.92
nontraffic V02.02
traffic V02.12
vehicle V09.9
animal-drawn V06.92
nontraffic V06.02
traffic V06.12
motor
nontraffic V09.00
traffic V09.20
fall V00.131
nontraffic V09.1
involving motor vehicle NEC
V09.00
traffic V09.3
involving motor vehicle NEC
V09.20

Accident (to) X58 — *continued*
  transport (involving injury to) V99—*continued*
    pedestrian — *continued*
      conveyance (occupant) V09.9 —
        continued
        skis (snow) V00.328
          collision (with) V09.9
            animal being ridden or animal
              drawn vehicle V06.99
              nontraffic V06.09
              traffic V06.19
            bus or heavy transport V04.99
              nontraffic V04.09
              traffic V04.19
            car V03.99
              nontraffic V03.09
              traffic V03.19
            pedal cycle V01.99
              nontraffic V01.09
              traffic V01.19
            pickup truck or van V03.99
              nontraffic V03.09
              traffic V03.19
            railway (train) (vehicle) V05.99
              nontraffic V05.09
              traffic V05.19
            stationary object V00.322
            streetcar V06.99
              nontraffic V06.09
              traffic V06.19
            two-or three-wheeled motor vehicle
              V02.99
              nontraffic V02.09
              traffic V02.19
            vehicle V09.9
              animal-drawn V06.99
                nontraffic V06.09
                traffic V06.19
              motor
                nontraffic V09.00
                traffic V09.20
        fall V00.321
        nontraffic V09.1
          involving motor vehicle NEC
            V09.00
        traffic V09.3
          involving motor vehicle NEC
            V09.20

Accident (to) X58 — *continued*
  transport (involving injury to) V99—*continued*
    pedestrian — *continued*
      conveyance (occupant) V09.9 —
        continued
        sled V00.228
          collision (with) V09.9
            animal being ridden or animal
              drawn vehicle V06.99
              nontraffic V06.09
              traffic V06.19
            bus or heavy transport V04.99
              nontraffic V04.09
              traffic V04.19
            car V03.99
              nontraffic V03.09
              traffic V03.19
            pedal cycle V01.99
              nontraffic V01.09
              traffic V01.19
            pickup truck or van V03.99
              nontraffic V03.09
              traffic V03.19
            railway (train) (vehicle) V05.99
              nontraffic V05.09
              traffic V05.19
            stationary object V00.222
            streetcar V06.99
              nontraffic V06.09
            traffic V06.19
            two-or three-wheeled motor vehicle
              V02.99
              nontraffic V02.09
              traffic V02.19
            vehicle V09.9
              animal-drawn V06.99
                nontraffic V06.09
                traffic V06.19
              motor
                nontraffic V09.00
                traffic V09.20
        fall V00.221
        nontraffic V09.1
          involving motor vehicle NEC
            V09.00
        traffic V09.3
          involving motor vehicle NEC
            V09.20

Accident (to) X58 — *continued*
  transport (involving injury to) V99—*continued*
    pedestrian — *continued*
      conveyance (occupant) V09.9 —
        continued
        snow board V00.318
          collision (with) V09.9
            animal being ridden or animal
              drawn vehicle V06.99
              nontraffic V06.09
              traffic V06.19
            bus or heavy transport V04.99
              nontraffic V04.09
              traffic V04.19
            car V03.99
              nontraffic V03.09
              traffic V03.19
            pedal cycle V01.99
              nontraffic V01.09
              traffic V01.19
            pickup truck or van V03.99
              nontraffic V03.09
              traffic V03.19
            railway (train) (vehicle) V05.99
              nontraffic V05.09
              traffic V05.19
            stationary object V00.312
            streetcar V06.99
              nontraffic V06.09
              traffic V06.19
            two-or three-wheeled motor vehicle
              V02.99
              nontraffic V02.09
              traffic V02.19
            vehicle V09.9
              animal-drawn V06.99
                nontraffic V06.09
                traffic V06.19
              motor
                nontraffic V09.00
                traffic V09.20
        fall V00.311
        nontraffic V09.1
          involving motor vehicle NEC
            V09.00
        traffic V09.3
          involving motor vehicle NEC
            V09.20

Accident (to) X58 — *continued*
  transport (involving injury to) V99—*continued*
   pedestrian — *continued*
    conveyance (occupant) V09.9 —
     continued
     specified type NEC V00.898
      collision (with) V09.9
       animal being ridden or animal
        drawn vehicle V06.99
        nontraffic V06.09
        traffic V06.19
       bus or heavy transport V04.99
        nontraffic V04.09
        traffic V04.19
       car V03.99
        nontraffic V03.09
        traffic V03.19
       pedal cycle V01.99
        nontraffic V01.09
        traffic V01.19
       pickup truck or van V03.99
        nontraffic V03.09
        traffic V03.19
       railway (train) (vehicle) V05.99
        nontraffic V05.09
        traffic V05.19
       stationary object V00.892
       streetcar V06.99
        nontraffic V06.09
        traffic V06.19
       two-or three-wheeled motor vehicle
        V02.99
        nontraffic V02.09
        traffic V02.19
       vehicle V09.9
        animal-drawn V06.99
         nontraffic V06.09
         traffic V06.19
        motor
         nontraffic V09.00
         traffic V09.20
     fall V00.891
     nontraffic V09.1
      involving motor vehicle NEC
       V09.00
     traffic V09.3
      involving motor vehicle NEC
       V09.20

Accident (to) X58 — *continued*
  transport (involving injury to) V99—*continued*
   pedestrian — *continued*
    conveyance (occupant) V09.9 —
     continued
     traffic V09.3
      involving motor vehicle V09.20
       military V09.21
       specified type NEC V09.29
    wheelchair (powered) V00.818
     collision (with) V09.9
      animal being ridden or animal
       drawn vehicle V06.99
       nontraffic V06.09
       traffic V06.19
      bus or heavy transport V04.99
       nontraffic V04.09
       traffic V04.19
      car V03.99
       nontraffic V03.09
       traffic V03.19
      pedal cycle V01.99
       nontraffic V01.09
       traffic V01.19
      pickup truck or van V03.99
       nontraffic V03.09
       traffic V03.19
      railway (train) (vehicle) V05.99
       nontraffic V05.09
       traffic V05.19
      stationary object V00.812
      streetcar V06.99
       nontraffic V06.09
       traffic V06.19
      two-or three-wheeled motor vehicle
       V02.99
       nontraffic V02.09
       traffic V02.19
      vehicle V09.9
       animal-drawn V06.99
        nontraffic V06.09
        traffic V06.19
       motor
        nontraffic V09.00
        traffic V09.20
    fall V00.811
    nontraffic V09.1
     involving motor vehicle NEC
      V09.00
    traffic V09.3
     involving motor vehicle NEC
      V09.20
    wheeled shoe V00.158
     colliding with stationary object
      V00.152
     fall V00.151

Accident (to) X58 — *continued*
  transport (involving injury to) V99—*continued*
   pedestrian — *continued*
    on foot — *see also* Accident, pedestrian
     collision (with)
      animal being ridden or animal drawn
       vehicle V06.90
       nontraffic V06.00
       traffic V06.10
      bus or heavy transport V04.90
       nontraffic V04.00
       traffic V04.10
      car V03.90
       nontraffic V03.00
       traffic V03.10
      pedal cycle V01.90
       nontraffic V01.00
       traffic V01.10
      pickup truck or van V03.90
       nontraffic V03.00
       traffic V03.10
      railway (train) (vehicle) V05.90
       nontraffic V05.00
       traffic V05.10
      streetcar V06.90
       nontraffic V06.00
       traffic V06.10
      two-or three-wheeled motor vehicle
       V02.90
       nontraffic V02.00
       traffic V02.10
      vehicle V09.9
       animal-drawn V06.90
        nontraffic V06.00
        traffic V06.10
       motor
        nontraffic V09.00
        traffic V09.20
   nontraffic V09.1
    involving motor vehicle V09.00
     military V09.01
     specified type NEC V09.09
   traffic V09.3
    involving motor vehicle V09.20
     military V09.21
     specified type NEC V09.29

Accident (to) X58 — *continued*
  transport (involving injury to) V99—*continued*
    person NEC (unknown way or
      transportation) V99
      collision (between)
        bus (with)
          heavy transport vehicle (traffic) V87.5
            nontraffic V88.5
        car (with)
          bus (traffic) V87.3
            nontraffic V88.3
          heavy transport vehicle (traffic) V87.4
            nontraffic V88.4
          nontraffic V88.5
          pickup truck or van (traffic) V87.2
            nontraffic V88.2
          train or railway vehicle (traffic) V87.6
            nontraffic V88.6
          two-or three-wheeled motor vehicle
            (traffic) V87.0
            nontraffic V88.0
        motor vehicle (traffic) NEC V87.7
          nontraffic V88.7
        two-or three-wheeled vehicle (with)
          (traffic)
          motor vehicle NEC V87.1
            nontraffic V88.1
        nonmotor vehicle (collision) (noncollision)
          (traffic) V87.9
          nontraffic V88.9

Accident (to) X58 — *continued*
  transport (involving injury to) V99—*continued*
    pickup truck occupant V59.9
      collision (with)
        animal (traffic) V50.9
          being ridden (traffic) V56.9
            nontraffic V56.3
            while boarding or alighting V56.4
          nontraffic V50.3
          while boarding or alighting V50.4
        animal-drawn vehicle (traffic) V56.9
          nontraffic V56.3
          while boarding or alighting V56.4
        bus (traffic) V54.9
          nontraffic V54.3
          while boarding or alighting V54.4
        car (traffic) V53.9
          nontraffic V53.3
          while boarding or alighting V53.4
        motor vehicle NOS (traffic) V59.60
          nontraffic V59.20
          specified type NEC (traffic) V59.69
            nontraffic V59.29
        pedal cycle (traffic) V51.9
          nontraffic V51.3
          while boarding or alighting V51.4
        pickup truck (traffic) V53.9
          nontraffic V53.3
          while boarding or alighting V53.4
        railway vehicle (traffic) V55.9
          nontraffic V55.3
          while boarding or alighting V55.4
        specified vehicle NEC (traffic) V56.9
          nontraffic V56.3
          while boarding or alighting V56.4
        stationary object (traffic) V57.9
          nontraffic V57.3
          while boarding or alighting V57.4
        streetcar (traffic) V56.9
          nontraffic V56.3
          while boarding or alighting V56.4
        three wheeled motor vehicle (traffic)
          V52.9
          nontraffic V52.3
          while boarding or alighting V52.4
        truck (traffic) V54.9
          nontraffic V54.3
          while boarding or alighting V54.4
        two wheeled motor vehicle (traffic)
          V52.9
          nontraffic V52.3
          while boarding or alighting V52.4
        van (traffic) V53.9
          nontraffic V53.3
          while boarding or alighting V53.4

Accident (to) X58 — *continued*
  transport (involving injury to) V99—*continued*
    pickup truck occupant V59.9 — *continued*
      driver
        collision (with)
          animal (traffic) V50.5
            being ridden (traffic) V56.5
              nontraffic V56.0
            nontraffic V50.0
          animal-drawn vehicle (traffic) V56.5
            nontraffic V56.0
          bus (traffic) V54.5
            nontraffic V54.0
          car (traffic) V53.5
            nontraffic V53.0
          motor vehicle NOS (traffic) V59.40
            nontraffic V59.00
            specified type NEC (traffic) V59.49
              nontraffic V59.09
          pedal cycle (traffic) V51.5
            nontraffic V51.0
          pickup truck (traffic) V53.5
            nontraffic V53.0
          railway vehicle (traffic) V55.5
            nontraffic V55.0
          specified vehicle NEC (traffic) V56.5
            nontraffic V56.0
          stationary object (traffic) V57.5
            nontraffic V57.0
          streetcar (traffic) V56.5
            nontraffic V56.0
          three wheeled motor vehicle (traffic)
            V52.5
            nontraffic V52.0
          truck (traffic) V54.5
            nontraffic V54.0
          two wheeled motor vehicle (traffic)
            V52.5
            nontraffic V52.0
          van (traffic) V53.5
            nontraffic V53.0
        noncollision accident (traffic) V58.5
          nontraffic V58.0

Accident (to) X58 — *continued*
  transport (involving injury to) V99—*continued*
    streetcar occupant V82.9
      collision (with) V82.3
        motor vehicle (traffic) V82.1
        nontraffic V82.0
        rolling stock V82.2
      during derailment V82.7
        with antecedent collision — *see*
          Accident, transport, streetcar
          occupant, collision
      fall (in streetcar) V82.5
        during derailment V82.7
          with antecedent collision — *see*
            Accident, transport, streetcar
            occupant, collision
      from streetcar V82.6
        during derailment V82.7
          with antecedent collision — *see*
            Accident, transport, streetcar
            occupant, collision
        while boarding or alighting V82.4
      while boarding or alighting V82.4
      specified type NEC V82.8
      while boarding or alighting V82.4

Accident (to) X58 — *continued*
  transport (involving injury to) V99—*continued*
    three-wheeled motor vehicle occupant V39.9
      collision (with)
        animal (traffic) V30.9
          being ridden (traffic) V36.9
            nontraffic V36.3
            while boarding or alighting V36.4
          nontraffic V30.3
          while boarding or alighting V30.4
        animal-drawn vehicle (traffic) V36.9
          nontraffic V36.3
          while boarding or alighting V36.4
        bus (traffic) V34.9
          nontraffic V34.3
          while boarding or alighting V34.4
        car (traffic) V33.9
          nontraffic V33.3
          while boarding or alighting V33.4
        motor vehicle NOS (traffic) V39.60
          nontraffic V39.20
          specified type NEC (traffic) V39.69
            nontraffic V39.29
        pedal cycle (traffic) V31.9
          nontraffic V31.3
          while boarding or alighting V31.4
        pickup truck (traffic) V33.9
          nontraffic V33.3
          while boarding or alighting V33.4
        railway vehicle (traffic) V35.9
          nontraffic V35.3
          while boarding or alighting V35.4
        specified vehicle NEC (traffic) V36.9
          nontraffic V36.3
          while boarding or alighting V36.4
        stationary object (traffic) V37.9
          nontraffic V37.3
          while boarding or alighting V37.4
        streetcar (traffic) V36.9
          nontraffic V36.3
          while boarding or alighting V36.4
        three wheeled motor vehicle (traffic)
          V32.9
          nontraffic V32.3
          while boarding or alighting V32.4
        truck (traffic) V34.9
          nontraffic V34.3
          while boarding or alighting V34.4
        two wheeled motor vehicle (traffic)
          V32.9
          nontraffic V32.3
          while boarding or alighting V32.4
        van (traffic) V33.9
          nontraffic V33.3
          while boarding or alighting V33.4

Accident (to) X58 — *continued*
  transport (involving injury to) V99—*continued*
    three-wheeled motor vehicle occupant
      V39.9 — *continued*
      driver
        collision (with)
          animal (traffic) V30.5
            being ridden (traffic) V36.5
              nontraffic V36.0
            nontraffic V30.0
          animal-drawn vehicle (traffic) V36.5
            nontraffic V36.0
          bus (traffic) V34.5
            nontraffic V34.0
          car (traffic) V33.5
            nontraffic V33.0
          motor vehicle NOS (traffic) V39.40
          nontraffic V39.00
            specified type NEC (traffic) V39.49
              nontraffic V39.09
          pedal cycle (traffic) V31.5
            nontraffic V31.0
          pickup truck (traffic) V33.5
            nontraffic V33.0
          railway vehicle (traffic) V35.5
            nontraffic V35.0
          specified vehicle NEC (traffic) V36.5
            nontraffic V36.0
          stationary object (traffic) V37.5
            nontraffic V37.0
          streetcar (traffic) V36.5
            nontraffic V36.0
          three wheeled motor vehicle (traffic)
            V32.5
            nontraffic V32.0
          truck (traffic) V34.5
            nontraffic V34.0
          two wheeled motor vehicle (traffic)
            V32.5
            nontraffic V32.0
          van (traffic) V33.5
            nontraffic V33.0
        noncollision accident (traffic) V38.5
          nontraffic V38.0

EXTERNAL CAUSES

Accident (to) X58 — *continued*
  transport (involving injury to) V99—*continued*
    three-wheeled motor vehicle occupant
      V39.9 — *continued*
      hanger-on
        collision (with)
          animal (traffic) V30.7
            being ridden (traffic) V36.7
              nontraffic V36.2
            nontraffic V30.2
          animal-drawn vehicle (traffic) V36.7
            nontraffic V36.2
          bus (traffic) V34.7
            nontraffic V34.2
          car (traffic) V33.7
            nontraffic V33.2
          pedal cycle (traffic) V31.7
            nontraffic V31.2
          pickup truck (traffic) V33.7
            nontraffic V33.2
          railway vehicle (traffic) V35.7
            nontraffic V35.2
          specified vehicle NEC (traffic) V36.7
            nontraffic V36.2
          stationary object (traffic) V37.7
            nontraffic V37.2
          streetcar (traffic) V36.7
            nontraffic V36.2
          three wheeled motor vehicle (traffic)
            V32.7
            nontraffic V32.2
          truck (traffic) V34.7
            nontraffic V34.2
          two wheeled motor vehicle (traffic)
            V32.7
            nontraffic V32.2
          van (traffic) V33.7
            nontraffic V33.2
        noncollision accident (traffic) V38.7
          nontraffic V38.2

Accident (to) X58 — *continued*
  transport (involving injury to) V99—*continued*
    three-wheeled motor vehicle occupant
      V39.9 — *continued*
      noncollision accident (traffic) V38.9
        nontraffic V38.3
        while boarding or alighting V38.4
    nontraffic V39.3
    passenger
      collision (with)
        animal (traffic) V30.6
          being ridden (traffic) V36.6
            nontraffic V36.1
          nontraffic V30.1
        animal-drawn vehicle (traffic) V36.6
          nontraffic V36.1
        bus (traffic) V34.6
          nontraffic V34.1
        car (traffic) V33.6
          nontraffic V33.1
        motor vehicle NOS (traffic) V39.50
          nontraffic V39.10
          specified type NEC (traffic) V39.59
            nontraffic V39.19
        pedal cycle (traffic) V31.6
          nontraffic V31.1
        pickup truck (traffic) V33.6
          nontraffic V33.1
        railway vehicle (traffic) V35.6
          nontraffic V35.1
        specified vehicle NEC (traffic) V36.6
          nontraffic V36.1
        stationary object (traffic) V37.6
          nontraffic V37.1
        streetcar (traffic) V36.6
          nontraffic V36.1
        three wheeled motor vehicle (traffic)
          V32.6
          nontraffic V32.1
        truck (traffic) V34.6
          nontraffic V34.1
        two wheeled motor vehicle (traffic)
          V32.6
          nontraffic V32.1
        van (traffic) V33.6
          nontraffic V33.1
      noncollision accident (traffic) V38.6
        nontraffic V38.1
    specified type NEC V39.89
      military vehicle V39.81

Accident (to) X58 — *continued*
  transport (involving injury to) V99—*continued*
    tractor (farm) (and trailer) — *see* Accident,
      transport, agricultural vehicle occupant
    tram — *see* Accident, transport, streetcar
      in mine or quarry — *see* Accident,
        transport, industrial vehicle occupant
    trolley — *see* Accident, transport, streetcar
      in mine or quarry — *see* Accident,
        transport, industrial vehicle occupant
    truck (heavy) occupant V69.9
      collision (with)
        animal (traffic) V60.9
          being ridden (traffic) V66.9
            nontraffic V66.3
            while boarding or alighting V66.4
          nontraffic V60.3
          while boarding or alighting V60.4
        animal-drawn vehicle (traffic) V66.9
          nontraffic V66.3
          while boarding or alighting V66.4
        bus (traffic) V64.9
          nontraffic V64.3
          while boarding or alighting V64.4
        car (traffic) V63.9
          nontraffic V63.3
          while boarding or alighting V63.4
        motor vehicle NOS (traffic) V69.60
          nontraffic V69.20
          specified type NEC (traffic) V69.69
            nontraffic V69.29
        pedal cycle (traffic) V61.9
          nontraffic V61.3
          while boarding or alighting V61.4
        pickup truck (traffic) V63.9
          nontraffic V63.3
          while boarding or alighting V63.4
        railway vehicle (traffic) V65.9
          nontraffic V65.3
          while boarding or alighting V65.4
        specified vehicle NEC (traffic) V66.9
          nontraffic V66.3
          while boarding or alighting V66.4
        stationary object (traffic) V67.9
          nontraffic V67.3
          while boarding or alighting V67.4
        streetcar (traffic) V66.9
          nontraffic V66.3
          while boarding or alighting V66.4
        three wheeled motor vehicle (traffic)
          V62.9
          nontraffic V62.3
          while boarding or alighting V62.4
        truck (traffic) V64.9
          nontraffic V64.3
          while boarding or alighting V64.4
        two wheeled motor vehicle (traffic)
          V62.9
          nontraffic V62.3
          while boarding or alighting V62.4
        van (traffic) V63.9
          nontraffic V63.3
          while boarding or alighting V63.4

© 2016 Channel Publishing Ltd

Accident (to) X58 — *continued*
  transport (involving injury to) V99—*continued*
    truck (heavy) occupant V69.9 — *continued*
      driver
        collision (with)
          animal (traffic) V60.5
            being ridden (traffic) V66.5
              nontraffic V66.0
            nontraffic V60.0
          animal-drawn vehicle (traffic) V66.5
            nontraffic V66.0
          bus (traffic) V64.5
            nontraffic V64.0
          car (traffic) V63.5
            nontraffic V63.0
          motor vehicle NOS (traffic) V69.40
            nontraffic V69.00
            specified type NEC (traffic) V69.49
              nontraffic V69.09
          pedal cycle (traffic) V61.5
            nontraffic V61.0
          pickup truck (traffic) V63.5
            nontraffic V63.0
          railway vehicle (traffic) V65.5
            nontraffic V65.0
          specified vehicle NEC (traffic) V66.5
            nontraffic V66.0
          stationary object (traffic) V67.5
            nontraffic V67.0
          streetcar (traffic) V66.5
            nontraffic V66.0
          three wheeled motor vehicle (traffic)
            V62.5
            nontraffic V62.0
          truck (traffic) V64.5
            nontraffic V64.0
          two wheeled motor vehicle (traffic)
            V62.5
            nontraffic V62.0
          van (traffic) V63.5
            nontraffic V63.0
        noncollision accident (traffic) V68.5
          nontraffic V68.0

Accident (to) X58 — *continued*
  transport (involving injury to) V99—*continued*
    truck (heavy) occupant V69.9 — *continued*
      dump — *see* Accident, transport,
        construction vehicle occupant
      hanger-on
        collision (with)
          animal (traffic) V60.7
            being ridden (traffic) V66.7
              nontraffic V66.2
            nontraffic V60.2
          animal-drawn vehicle (traffic) V66.7
            nontraffic V66.2
          bus (traffic) V64.7
            nontraffic V64.2
          car (traffic) V63.7
            nontraffic V63.2
          pedal cycle (traffic) V61.7
            nontraffic V61.2
          pickup truck (traffic) V63.7
            nontraffic V63.2
          railway vehicle (traffic) V65.7
            nontraffic V65.2
          specified vehicle NEC (traffic) V66.7
            nontraffic V66.2
          stationary object (traffic) V67.7
            nontraffic V67.2
          streetcar (traffic) V66.7
            nontraffic V66.2
          three wheeled motor vehicle (traffic)
            V62.7
            nontraffic V62.2
          truck (traffic) V64.7
            nontraffic V64.2
          two wheeled motor vehicle (traffic)
            V62.7
            nontraffic V62.2
          van (traffic) V63.7
            nontraffic V63.2
        noncollision accident (traffic) V68.7
          nontraffic V68.2

Accident (to) X58 — *continued*
  transport (involving injury to) V99—*continued*
    truck (heavy) occupant V69.9 — *continued*
      noncollision accident (traffic) V68.9
        nontraffic V68.3
        while boarding or alighting V68.4
      nontraffic V69.3
      passenger
        collision (with)
          animal (traffic) V60.6
            being ridden (traffic) V66.6
              nontraffic V66.1
            nontraffic V60.1
          animal-drawn vehicle (traffic) V66.6
            nontraffic V66.1
          bus (traffic) V64.6
            nontraffic V64.1
          car (traffic) V63.6
            nontraffic V63.1
          motor vehicle NOS (traffic) V69.50
            nontraffic V69.10
            specified type NEC (traffic) V69.59
              nontraffic V69.19
          pedal cycle (traffic) V61.6
            nontraffic V61.1
          pickup truck (traffic) V63.6
            nontraffic V63.1
          railway vehicle (traffic) V65.6
            nontraffic V65.1
          specified vehicle NEC (traffic) V66.6
            nontraffic V66.1
          stationary object (traffic) V67.6
            nontraffic V67.1
          streetcar (traffic) V66.6
            nontraffic V66.1
          three wheeled motor vehicle (traffic)
            V62.6
            nontraffic V62.1
          truck (traffic) V64.6
            nontraffic V64.1
          two wheeled motor vehicle (traffic)
            V62.6
            nontraffic V62.1
          van (traffic) V63.6
            nontraffic V63.1
        noncollision accident (traffic) V68.6
          nontraffic V68.1
      pickup — *see* Accident, transport, pickup
        truck occupant
      specified type NEC V69.88
        military vehicle V69.81

EXTERNAL CAUSES

Accident (to) X58 — *continued*
transport (involving injury to) V99—*continued*
van occupant V59.9
collision (with)
animal (traffic) V50.9
being ridden (traffic) V56.9
nontraffic V56.3
while boarding or alighting V56.4
nontraffic V50.3
while boarding or alighting V50.4
animal-drawn vehicle (traffic) V56.9
nontraffic V56.3
while boarding or alighting V56.4
bus (traffic) V54.9
nontraffic V54.3
while boarding or alighting V54.4
car (traffic) V53.9
nontraffic V53.3
while boarding or alighting V53.4
motor vehicle NOS (traffic) V59.60
nontraffic V59.20
specified type NEC (traffic) V59.69
nontraffic V59.29
pedal cycle (traffic) V51.9
nontraffic V51.3
while boarding or alighting V51.4
pickup truck (traffic) V53.9
nontraffic V53.3
while boarding or alighting V53.4
railway vehicle (traffic) V55.9
nontraffic V55.3
while boarding or alighting V55.4
specified vehicle NEC (traffic) V56.9
nontraffic V56.3
while boarding or alighting V56.4
stationary object (traffic) V57.9
nontraffic V57.3
while boarding or alighting V57.4
streetcar (traffic) V56.9
nontraffic V56.3
while boarding or alighting V56.4
three wheeled motor vehicle (traffic)
V52.9
nontraffic V52.3
while boarding or alighting V52.4
truck (traffic) V54.9
nontraffic V54.3
while boarding or alighting V54.4
two wheeled motor vehicle (traffic)
V52.9
nontraffic V52.3
while boarding or alighting V52.4
van (traffic) V53.9
nontraffic V53.3
while boarding or alighting V53.4

Accident (to) X58 — *continued*
transport (involving injury to) V99—*continued*
van occupant V59.9 — *continued*
driver
collision (with)
animal (traffic) V50.5
being ridden (traffic) V56.5
nontraffic V56.0
nontraffic V50.0
animal-drawn vehicle (traffic) V56.5
nontraffic V56.0
bus (traffic) V54.5
nontraffic V54.0
car (traffic) V53.5
nontraffic V53.0
motor vehicle NOS (traffic) V59.40
nontraffic V59.00
specified type NEC (traffic) V59.49
nontraffic V59.09
pedal cycle (traffic) V51.5
nontraffic V51.0
pickup truck (traffic) V53.5
nontraffic V53.0
railway vehicle (traffic) V55.5
nontraffic V55.0
specified vehicle NEC (traffic) V56.5
nontraffic V56.0
stationary object (traffic) V57.5
nontraffic V57.0
streetcar (traffic) V56.5
nontraffic V56.0
three wheeled motor vehicle (traffic)
V52.5
nontraffic V52.0
truck (traffic) V54.5
nontraffic V54.0
two wheeled motor vehicle (traffic)
V52.5
nontraffic V52.0
van (traffic) V53.5
nontraffic V53.0
noncollision accident (traffic) V58.5
nontraffic V58.0

Accident (to) X58 — *continued*
transport (involving injury to) V99—*continued*
van occupant V59.9 — *continued*
hanger-on
collision (with)
animal (traffic) V50.7
being ridden (traffic) V56.7
nontraffic V56.2
nontraffic V50.2
animal-drawn vehicle (traffic) V56.7
nontraffic V56.2
bus (traffic) V54.7
nontraffic V54.2
car (traffic) V53.7
nontraffic V53.2
pedal cycle (traffic) V51.7
nontraffic V51.2
pickup truck (traffic) V53.7
nontraffic V53.2
railway vehicle (traffic) V55.7
nontraffic V55.2
specified vehicle NEC (traffic) V56.7
nontraffic V56.2
stationary object (traffic) V57.7
nontraffic V57.2
streetcar (traffic) V56.7
nontraffic V56.2
three wheeled motor vehicle (traffic)
V52.7
nontraffic V52.2
truck (traffic) V54.7
nontraffic V54.2
two wheeled motor vehicle (traffic)
V52.7
nontraffic V52.2
van (traffic) V53.7
nontraffic V53.2
noncollision accident (traffic) V58.7
nontraffic V58.2

Accident (to) X58 — *continued*
  transport (involving injury to) V99—*continued*
    van occupant V59.9 — *continued*
      noncollision accident (traffic) V58.9
        nontraffic V58.3
        while boarding or alighting V58.4
      nontraffic V59.3
      passenger
        collision (with)
          animal (traffic) V50.6
            being ridden (traffic) V56.6
              nontraffic V56.1
            nontraffic V50.1
          animal-drawn vehicle (traffic) V56.6
            nontraffic V56.1
          bus (traffic) V54.6
            nontraffic V54.1
          car (traffic) V53.6
            nontraffic V53.1
          motor vehicle NOS (traffic) V59.50
            nontraffic V59.10
            specified type NEC (traffic) V59.59
              nontraffic V59.19
          pedal cycle (traffic) V51.6
            nontraffic V51.1
          pickup truck (traffic) V53.6
            nontraffic V53.1
          railway vehicle (traffic) V55.6
            nontraffic V55.1
          specified vehicle NEC (traffic) V56.6
            nontraffic V56.1
          stationary object (traffic) V57.6
            nontraffic V57.1
          streetcar (traffic) V56.6
            nontraffic V56.1
          three wheeled motor vehicle (traffic)
            V52.6
            nontraffic V52.1
          truck (traffic) V54.6
            nontraffic V54.1
          two wheeled motor vehicle (traffic)
            V52.6
            nontraffic V52.1
          van (traffic) V53.6
            nontraffic V53.1
      noncollision accident (traffic) V58.6
        nontraffic V58.1
      specified type NEC V59.88
      military vehicle V59.81

Accident (to) X58 — *continued*
  transport (involving injury to) V99—*continued*
    watercraft occupant — *see* Accident,
      watercraft
    vehicle NEC V89.9
      animal-drawn NEC — *see* Accident,
        transport, animal-drawn vehicle
        occupant
    special
      agricultural — *see* Accident, transport,
        agricultural vehicle occupant
      construction — *see* Accident, transport,
        construction vehicle occupant
      industrial — *see* Accident, transport,
        industrial vehicle occupant
      three-wheeled NEC (motorized) — *see*
        Accident, transport, three-wheeled
        motor vehicle occupant
  watercraft V94.9
    causing
      drowning — *see* Drowning, due to,
        accident to, watercraft
      injury NEC V91.89
        crushed between craft and object
          V91.19
          powered craft V91.13
            ferry boat V91.11
            fishing boat V91.12
            jetskis V91.13
            liner V91.11
            merchant ship V91.10
            passenger ship V91.11
          unpowered craft V91.18
            canoe V91.15
            inflatable V91.16
            kayak V91.15
            sailboat V91.14
            surfboard V91.18
            windsurfer V91.18
        fall on board V91.29
          powered craft V91.23
            ferry boat V91.21
            fishing boat V91.22
            jetskis V91.23
            liner V91.21
            merchant ship V91.20
            passenger ship V91.21
          unpowered craft
            canoe V91.25
            inflatable V91.26
            kayak V91.25
            sailboat V91.24
        fire on board causing burn V91.09
          powered craft V91.03
            ferry boat V91.01
            fishing boat V91.02
            jetskis V91.03
            liner V91.01
            merchant ship V91.00
            passenger ship V91.01
          unpowered craft V91.08
            canoe V91.05
            inflatable V91.06
            kayak V91.05
            sailboat V91.04
            surfboard V91.08
            water skis V91.07
            windsurfer V91.08

Accident (to) X58 — *continued*
  watercraft V94.9 — *continued*
    causing — *continued*
      injury NEC V91.89 — *continued*
        hit by falling object V91.39
          powered craft V91.33
            ferry boat V91.31
            fishing boat V91.32
            jetskis V91.33
            liner V91.31
            merchant ship V91.30
            passenger ship V91.31
          unpowered craft V91.38
            canoe V91.35
            inflatable V91.36
            kayak V91.35
            sailboat V91.34
            surfboard V91.38
            water skis V91.37
            windsurfer V91.38
        specified type NEC V91.89
          powered craft V91.83
            ferry boat V91.81
            fishing boat V91.82
            jetskis V91.83
            liner V91.81
            merchant ship V91.80
            passenger ship V91.81
          unpowered craft V91.88
            canoe V91.85
            inflatable V91.86
            kayak V91.85
            sailboat V91.84
            surfboard V91.88
            water skis V91.87
            windsurfer V91.88
    due to, caused by cataclysm — *see* Forces of
      nature, by type
    military NEC V94.818
      with civilian watercraft V94.810
      civilian in water injured by V94.811
    nonpowered, struck by
      nonpowered vessel V94.22
      powered vessel V94.21
    specified type NEC V94.89
    striking swimmer
      powered V94.11
      unpowered V94.12

EXTERNAL CAUSES

Acid throwing (assault) Y08.89

Activity (involving) (of victim at time of event) Y93.9
  aerobic and step exercise (class) Y93.A3
  alpine skiing Y93.23
  animal care NEC Y93.K9
  arts and handcrafts NEC Y93.D9
  athletics NEC Y93.79
  athletics played as a team or group NEC Y93.69
  athletics played individually NEC Y93.59
  baking Y93.G3
  ballet Y93.41
  barbells Y93.B3
  BASE (Building, Antenna, Span, Earth) jumping Y93.33
  baseball Y93.64
  basketball Y93.67
  bathing (personal) Y93.E1
  beach volleyball Y93.68
  bike riding Y93.55
  blackout game Y93.85
  boogie boarding Y93.18
  bowling Y93.54
  boxing Y93.71
  brass instrument playing Y93.J4
  building construction Y93.H3
  bungee jumping Y93.34
  calisthenics Y93.A2
  canoeing (in calm and turbulent water) Y93.16
  capture the flag Y93.6A
  cardiorespiratory exercise NEC Y93.A9
  caregiving (providing) NEC Y93.F9
    bathing Y93.F1
    lifting Y93.F2
  cellular
    communication device Y93.C2
    telephone Y93.C2
  challenge course Y93.A5
  cheerleading Y93.45
  choking game Y93.85
  circuit training Y93.A4
  cleaning
    floor Y93.E5
  climbing NEC Y93.39
    mountain Y93.31
    rock Y93.31
    wall Y93.31
  clothing care and maintenance NEC Y93.E9
  combatives Y93.75
  computer
    keyboarding Y93.C1
    technology NEC Y93.C9
  confidence course Y93.A5
  construction (building) Y93.H3
  cooking and baking Y93.G3
  cool down exercises Y93.A2
  cricket Y93.69
  crocheting Y93.D1
  cross country skiing Y93.24
  dancing (all types) Y93.41
  digging
    dirt Y93.H1
  dirt digging Y93.H1
  dishwashing Y93.G1
  diving (platform) (springboard) Y93.12
    underwater Y93.15
  dodge ball Y93.6A
  downhill skiing Y93.23
  drum playing Y93.J2
  dumbbells Y93.B3
  electronic
    devices NEC Y93.C9
      hand held interactive Y93.C2
    game playing (using) (with)
      interactive device Y93.C2
      keyboard or other stationary device Y93.C1
  elliptical machine Y93.A1

Activity (involving) (of victim at time of event) Y93.9 — *continued*
  exercise(s)
    machines ((primarily) for)
      cardiorespiratory conditioning Y93.A1
      muscle strengthening Y93.B1
    muscle strengthening (non-machine) NEC Y93.B9
  external motion NEC Y93.I9
    rollercoaster Y93.I1
  fainting game Y93.85
  field hockey Y93.65
  figure skating (pairs) (singles) Y93.21
  flag football Y93.62
  floor mopping and cleaning Y93.E5
  food preparation and clean up Y93.G1
  football (American) NOS Y93.61
    flag Y93.62
    tackle Y93.61
    touch Y93.62
  four square Y93.6A
  free weights Y93.B3
  frisbee (ultimate) Y93.74
  furniture
    building Y93.D3
    finishing Y93.D3
    repair Y93.D3
  game playing (electronic)
    using interactive device Y93.C2
    using keyboard or other stationary device Y93.C1
  gardening Y93.H2
  golf Y93.53
  grass drills Y93.A6
  grilling and smoking food Y93.G2
  grooming and shearing an animal Y93.K3
  guerilla drills Y93.A6
  gymnastics (rhythmic) Y93.43
  hand held interactive electronic device Y93.C2
  handball Y93.73
  handcrafts NEC Y93.D9
  hang gliding Y93.35
  hiking (on level or elevated terrain) Y93.01
  hockey (ice) Y93.22
    field Y93.65
  horseback riding Y93.52
  household (interior) maintenance NEC Y93.E9
  ice NEC Y93.29
    dancing Y93.21
    hockey Y93.22
    skating Y93.21
  inline roller skating Y93.51
  ironing Y93.E4
  judo Y93.75
  jumping (off) NEC Y93.39
    BASE (Building, Antenna, Span, Earth) Y93.33
    bungee Y93.34
    jacks Y93.A2
    rope Y93.56
  jumping jacks Y93.A2
  jumping rope Y93.56
  karate Y93.75
  kayaking (in calm and turbulent water) Y93.16
  keyboarding (computer) Y93.C1
  kickball Y93.6A
  knitting Y93.D1
  lacrosse Y93.65
  land maintenance NEC Y93.H9
  landscaping Y93.H2
  laundry Y93.E2
  machines (exercise)
    primarily for cardiorespiratory conditioning Y93.A1
    primarily for muscle strengthening Y93.B1

Activity (involving) (of victim at time of event) Y93.9 — *continued*
  maintenance
    exterior building NEC Y93.H9
    household (interior) NEC Y93.E9
    land Y93.H9
    property Y93.H9
  marching (on level or elevated terrain) Y93.01
  martial arts Y93.75
  microwave oven Y93.G3
  milking an animal Y93.K2
  mopping (floor) Y93.E5
  mountain climbing Y93.31
  muscle strengthening
    exercises (non-machine) NEC Y93.B9
    machines Y93.B1
  musical keyboard (electronic) playing Y93.J1
  nordic skiing Y93.24
  obstacle course Y93.A5
  oven (microwave) Y93.G3
  packing up and unpacking in moving to a new residence Y93.E6
  parasailing Y93.19
  pass out game Y93.85
  percussion instrument playing NEC Y93.J2
  personal
    bathing and showering Y93.E1
    hygiene NEC Y93.E8
    showering Y93.E1
  physical games generally associated with school recess, summer camp and children Y93.6A
  physical training NEC Y93.A9
  piano playing Y93.J1
  pilates Y93.B4
  platform diving Y93.12
  playing musical instrument
    brass instrument Y93.J4
    drum Y93.J2
    musical keyboard (electronic) Y93.J1
    percussion instrument NEC Y93.J2
    piano Y93.J1
    string instrument Y93.J3
    winds instrument Y93.J4
  property maintenance
    exterior NEC Y93.H9
    interior NEC Y93.E9
  pruning (garden and lawn) Y93.H2
  pull-ups Y93.B2
  push-ups Y93.B2
  racquetball Y93.73
  rafting (in calm and turbulent water) Y93.16
  raking (leaves) Y93.H1
  rappelling Y93.32
  refereeing a sports activity Y93.81
  residential relocation Y93.E6
  rhythmic gymnastics Y93.43
  rhythmic movement NEC Y93.49
  riding
    horseback Y93.52
    rollercoaster Y93.I1
  rock climbing Y93.31
  roller skating (inline) Y93.51
  rollercoaster riding Y93.I1
  rough housing and horseplay Y93.83
  rowing (in calm and turbulent water) Y93.16
  rugby Y93.63
  running Y93.02
  SCUBA diving Y93.15
  sewing Y93.D2
  shoveling Y93.H1
    dirt Y93.H1
    snow Y93.H1
  showering (personal) Y93.E1
  sit-ups Y93.B2
  skateboarding Y93.51
  skating (ice) Y93.21
    roller Y93.51

Activity (involving) (of victim at time of event)
Y93.9 — *continued*
skiing (alpine) (downhill) Y93.23
cross country Y93.24
nordic Y93.24
water Y93.17
sledding (snow) Y93.23
sleeping (sleep) Y93.84
smoking and grilling food Y93.G2
snorkeling Y93.15
snow NEC Y93.29
boarding Y93.23
shoveling Y93.H1
sledding Y93.23
tubing Y93.23
soccer Y93.66
softball Y93.64
specified NEC Y93.89
spectator at an event Y93.82
sports NEC Y93.79
sports played as a team or group NEC Y93.69
sports played individually NEC Y93.59
springboard diving Y93.12
squash Y93.73
stationary bike Y93.A1
step (stepping) exercise (class) Y93.A3
stepper machine Y93.A1
stove Y93.G3
string instrument playing Y93.J3
surfing Y93.18
wind Y93.18
swimming Y93.11
tackle football Y93.61
tap dancing Y93.41
tennis Y93.73
tobogganing Y93.23
touch football Y93.62
track and field events (non-running) Y93.57
running Y93.02
trampoline Y93.44
treadmill Y93.A1
trimming shrubs Y93.H2
tubing (in calm and turbulent water) Y93.16
snow Y93.23
ultimate frisbee Y93.74
underwater diving Y93.15
unpacking in moving to a new residence Y93.E6
use of stove, oven and microwave oven Y93.G3
vacuuming Y93.E3
volleyball (beach) (court) Y93.68
wake boarding Y93.17
walking (on level or elevated terrain) Y93.01
an animal Y93.K1
walking an animal Y93.K1
wall climbing Y93.31
warm up and cool down exercises Y93.A2
water NEC Y93.19
aerobics Y93.14
craft NEC Y93.19
exercise Y93.14
polo Y93.13
skiing Y93.17
sliding Y93.18
survival training and testing Y93.19
weeding (garden and lawn) Y93.H2
wind instrument playing Y93.J4
windsurfing Y93.18
wrestling Y93.72
yoga Y93.42
Adverse effect of drugs — *see* Table of Drugs and Chemicals
Aerosinusitis — *see* Air, pressure
After-effect, late — *see* Sequelae

Air
blast in war operations — *see* War operations, air blast
pressure
change, rapid
during
ascent W94.29
while (in) (surfacing from)
aircraft W94.23
deep water diving W94.21
underground W94.22
descent W94.39
in
aircraft W94.31
water W94.32
high, prolonged W94.0
low, prolonged W94.12
due to residence or long visit at high altitude W94.11
Alpine sickness W94.11
Altitude sickness W94.11
Anaphylactic shock, anaphylaxis — *see* Table of Drugs and Chemicals
Andes disease W94.11
Arachnidism, arachnoidism X58
Arson (with intent to injure or kill) X97
Asphyxia, asphyxiation
by
food (bone) (seed) — *see* categories T17 and T18
gas — *see also* Table of Drugs and Chemicals
legal
execution — *see* Legal, intervention, gas
intervention — *see* Legal, intervention, gas
from
fire — *see also* Exposure, fire
in war operations — *see* War operations, fire
ignition — *see* Ignition
vomitus T17.81
in war operations — *see* War operations, restriction of airway
Aspiration
food (any type) (into respiratory tract) (with asphyxia, obstruction respiratory tract, suffocation) — *see* categories T17 and T18
foreign body — *see* Foreign body, aspiration
vomitus (with asphyxia, obstruction respiratory tract, suffocation) T17.81-
Assassination (attempt) — *see* Assault
Assault (homicidal) (by) (in) Y09
arson X97
bite (of human being) Y04.1
bodily force Y04.8
bite Y04.1
bumping into Y04.2
sexual — *see* subcategories T74.0, T76.0
unarmed fight Y04.0
bomb X96.9
antipersonnel X96.0
fertilizer X96.3
gasoline X96.1
letter X96.2
petrol X96.1
pipe X96.3
specified NEC X96.8
brawl (hand) (fists) (foot) (unarmed) Y04.0
burning, burns (by fire) NEC X97
acid Y08.89
caustic, corrosive substance Y08.89
chemical from swallowing caustic, corrosive substance — *see* Table of Drugs and Chemicals
cigarette(s) X97

Assault (homicidal) (by) (in) Y09 — *continued*
burning, burns (by fire) NEC X97 — *continued*
hot object X98.9
fluid NEC X98.2
household appliance X98.3
specified NEC X98.8
steam X98.0
tap water X98.1
vapors X98.0
scalding — *see* Assault, burning
steam X98.0
vitriol Y08.89
caustic, corrosive substance (gas) Y08.89
crashing of
aircraft Y08.81
motor vehicle Y03.8
pushed in front of Y02.0
run over Y03.0
specified NEC Y03.8
cutting or piercing instrument X99.9
dagger X99.2
glass X99.0
knife X99.1
specified NEC X99.8
sword X99.2
dagger X99.2
drowning (in) X92.9
bathtub X92.0
natural water X92.3
specified NEC X92.8
swimming pool X92.1
following fall X92.2
dynamite X96.8
explosive(s) (material) X96.9
fight (hand) (fists) (foot) (unarmed) Y04.0
with weapon — *see* Assault, by type of weapon
fire X97
firearm X95.9
airgun X95.01
handgun X93
hunting rifle X94.1
larger X94.9
specified NEC X94.8
machine gun X94.2
shotgun X94.0
specified NEC X95.8
from high place Y01
gunshot (wound) NEC — *see* Assault, firearm, by type
incendiary device X97
injury Y09
to child due to criminal abortion attempt NEC Y08.89
knife X99.1
late effect of — *see* X92-Y08 with 7th character S
placing before moving object NEC Y02.8
motor vehicle Y02.0
poisoning — *see* categories T36-T65 with 7th character S
puncture, any part of body — *see* Assault, cutting or piercing instrument
pushing
before moving object NEC Y02.8
motor vehicle Y02.0
subway train Y02.1
train Y02.1
rape T74.2-
scalding — *see* Assault, burning
sequelae of — *see* X92-Y08 with 7th character S
sexual (by bodily force) T74.2-
shooting — *see* Assault, firearm
specified means NEC Y08.89
stab, any part of body — *see* Assault, cutting or piercing instrument
steam X98.0

EXTERNAL CAUSES

Assault (homicidal) (by) (in) Y09 — *continued*
　striking against
　　other person Y04.2
　　sports equipment Y08.09
　　　baseball bat Y08.02
　　　hockey stick Y08.01
　struck by
　　sports equipment Y08.09
　　　baseball bat Y08.02
　　　hockey stick Y08.01
　submersion — *see* Assault, drowning
　violence Y09
　weapon Y09
　　blunt Y00
　　cutting or piercing — *see* Assault, cutting or
　　　piercing instrument
　　firearm — *see* Assault, firearm
　wound Y09
　　cutting — *see* Assault, cutting or piercing
　　　instrument
　　gunshot — *see* Assault, firearm
　　knife X99.1
　　piercing — *see* Assault, cutting or piercing
　　　instrument
　　puncture — *see* Assault, cutting or piercing
　　　instrument
　　stab — *see* Assault, cutting or piercing
　　　instrument
Attack by mammals NEC W55.89
Avalanche — *see* Landslide
Aviator's disease — *see* Air, pressure

B

Barotitis, barodontalgia, barosinusitis, barotrauma (otitic) (sinus) — *see* Air, pressure
Battered (baby) (child) (person) (syndrome) X58
Bayonet wound W26.1
　in
　　legal intervention — *see* Legal, intervention, sharp object, bayonet
　　war operations — *see* War operations, combat
　stated as undetermined whether accidental or intentional Y28.8
　suicide (attempt) X78.2
Bean in nose — *see* categories T17 and T18
Bed set on fire NEC — *see* Exposure, fire, uncontrolled, building, bed
Beheading (by guillotine)
　homicide X99.9
　legal execution — *see* Legal, intervention
Bending, injury in (prolonged) (static) X50.1
Bends — *see* Air, pressure, change
Bite, bitten by
　alligator W58.01
　arthropod (nonvenomous) NEC W57
　bull W55.21
　cat W55.01
　cow W55.21
　crocodile W58.11
　dog W54.0
　goat W55.31
　hoof stock NEC W55.31
　horse W55.11
　human being (accidentally) W50.3
　　with intent to injure or kill Y04.1
　　as, or caused by, a crowd or human stampede (with fall) W52
　　assault Y04.1
　　homicide (attempt) Y04.1
　　in
　　　fight Y04.1
　insect (nonvenomous) W57
　lizard (nonvenomous) W59.01
　mammal NEC W55.81
　　marine W56.31
　marine animal (nonvenomous) W56.81
　millipede W57
　moray eel W56.51
　mouse W53.01
　person(s) (accidentally) W50.3
　　with intent to injure or kill Y04.1
　　as, or caused by, a crowd or human stampede (with fall) W52
　　assault Y04.1
　　homicide (attempt) Y04.1
　　in
　　　fight Y04.1
　pig W55.41
　raccoon W55.51
　rat W53.11
　reptile W59.81
　　lizard W59.01
　　snake W59.11
　　turtle W59.21
　　　terrestrial W59.81
　rodent W53.81
　　mouse W53.01
　　rat W53.11
　　specified NEC W53.81
　　squirrel W53.21
　shark W56.41
　sheep W55.31
　snake (nonvenomous) W59.11
　spider (nonvenomous) W57
　squirrel W53.21

Blast (air) in war operations — *see* War operations, blast
Blizzard X37.2
Blood alcohol level Y90.9
　100-119mg/100ml Y90.5
　120-199mg/100ml Y90.6
　20-39mg/100ml Y90.1
　200-239mg/100ml Y90.7
　40-59mg/100ml Y90.2
　60-79mg/100ml Y90.3
　80-99mg/100ml Y90.4
　less than 20mg/100ml Y90.0
　presence in blood, level not specified Y90.9
Blow X58
　by law-enforcing agent, police (on duty) — *see* Legal, intervention, manhandling
　　blunt object — *see* Legal, intervention, blunt object
Blowing up — *see* Explosion
Brawl (hand) (fists) (foot) Y04.0
Breakage (accidental) (part of)
　ladder (causing fall) W11
　scaffolding (causing fall) W12
Broken
　glass, contact with — *see* Contact, with, glass
　power line (causing electric shock) W85
Bumping against, into (accidentally)
　object NEC W22.8
　　with fall — *see* Fall, due to, bumping against, object
　　caused by crowd or human stampede (with fall) W52
　　sports equipment W21.9
　person(s) W51
　　with fall W03
　　　due to ice or snow W00.0
　　assault Y04.2
　　caused by, a crowd or human stampede (with fall) W52
　　homicide (attempt) Y04.2
　sports equipment W21.9
Burn, burned, burning (accidental) (by) (from) (on)
　acid NEC — *see* Table of Drugs and Chemicals
　bed linen — *see* Exposure, fire, uncontrolled, in building, bed
　blowtorch X08.8
　　with ignition of clothing NEC X06.2
　　　nightwear X05
　bonfire, campfire (controlled) — *see also* Exposure, fire, controlled, not in building
　　uncontrolled — *see* Exposure, fire, uncontrolled, not in building
　candle X08.8
　　with ignition of clothing NEC X06.2
　　　nightwear X05
　caustic liquid, substance (external) (internal) NEC — *see* Table of Drugs and Chemicals
　chemical (external) (internal) — *see also* Table of Drugs and Chemicals
　　in war operations — *see* War operations. fire
　cigar(s) or cigarette(s) X08.8
　　with ignition of clothing NEC X06.2
　　　nightwear X05
　clothes, clothing NEC (from controlled fire) X06.2
　　with conflagration — *see* Exposure, fire, uncontrolled, building
　　not in building or structure — *see* Exposure, fire, uncontrolled, not in building
　cooker (hot) X15.8
　　stated as undetermined whether accidental or intentional Y27.3
　　suicide (attempt) X77.3
　electric blanket X16
　engine (hot) X17

Burn, burned, burning (accidental) (by) (from) (on) — *continued*
  fire, flames — *see* Exposure, fire
  flare, Very pistol — *see* Discharge, firearm NEC
  heat
    from appliance (electrical) (household) X15.8
      cooker X15.8
      hotplate X15.2
      kettle X15.8
      light bulb X15.8
      saucepan X15.3
      skillet X15.3
      stated as undetermined whether accidental or intentional Y27.3
      stove X15.0
      suicide (attempt) X77.3
      toaster X15.1
    in local application or packing during medical or surgical procedure Y63.5
  heating
    appliance, radiator or pipe X16
  homicide (attempt) — *see* Assault, burning
  hot
    air X14.1
    cooker X15.8
    drink X10.0
    engine X17
    fat X10.2
    fluid NEC X12
    food X10.1
    gases X14.1
    heating appliance X16
    household appliance NEC X15.8
    kettle X15.8
    liquid NEC X12
    machinery X17
    metal (molten) (liquid) NEC X18
    object (not producing fire or flames) NEC X19
    oil (cooking) X10.2
    pipe(s) X16
    radiator X16
    saucepan (glass) (metal) X15.3
    stove (kitchen) X15.0
    substance NEC X19
      caustic or corrosive NEC — *see* Table of Drugs and Chemicals
    toaster X15.1
    tool X17
    vapor X13.1
    water (tap) — *see* Contact, with, hot, tap water
  hotplate X15.2
    suicide (attempt) X77.3
  ignition — *see* Ignition
  in war operations — *see* War operations, fire
  inflicted by other person X97
    by hot objects, hot vapor, and steam — *see* Assault, burning, hot object
  internal, from swallowed caustic, corrosive liquid, substance — *see* Table of Drugs and Chemicals
  iron (hot) X15.8
    stated as undetermined whether accidental or intentional Y27.3
    suicide (attempt) X77.3
  kettle (hot) X15.8
    stated as undetermined whether accidental or intentional Y27.3
    suicide (attempt) X77.3
  lamp (flame) X08.8
    with ignition of clothing NEC X06.2
      nightwear X05
  lighter (cigar) (cigarette) X08.8
    with ignition of clothing NEC X06.2
      nightwear X05

Burn, burned, burning (accidental) (by) (from) (on) — *continued*
  lightning — *see* subcategory T75.0
    causing fire — *see* Exposure, fire
  liquid (boiling) (hot) NEC X12
    stated as undetermined whether accidental or intentional Y27.2
    suicide (attempt) X77.2
  local application of externally applied substance in medical or surgical care Y63.5
  machinery (hot) X17
  matches X08.8
    with ignition of clothing NEC X06.2
      nightwear X05
  mattress — *see* Exposure, fire, uncontrolled, building, bed
  medicament, externally applied Y63.5
  metal (hot) (liquid) (molten) NEC X18
  nightwear (nightclothes, nightdress, gown, pajamas, robe) X05
  object (hot) NEC X19
  on board watercraft
    due to
      accident to watercraft V91.09
        powered craft V91.03
          ferry boat V91.01
          fishing boat V91.02
          jetskis V91.03
          liner V91.01
          merchant ship V91.00
          passenger ship V91.01
        unpowered craft V91.08
          canoe V91.05
          inflatable V91.06
          kayak V91.05
          sailboat V91.04
          surfboard V91.08
          water skis V91.07
          windsurfer V91.08
      fire on board V93.09
        ferry boat V93.01
        fishing boat V93.02
        jetskis V93.03
        liner V93.01
        merchant ship V93.00
        passenger ship V93.01
        powered craft NEC V93.03
        sailboat V93.04
      specified heat source NEC on board V93.19
        ferry boat V93.11
        fishing boat V93.12
        jetskis V93.13
        liner V93.11
        merchant ship V93.10
        passenger ship V93.11
        powered craft NEC V93.13
        sailboat V93.14
  pipe (hot) X16
    smoking X08.8
    with ignition of clothing NEC X06.2
      nightwear X05
  powder — *see* Powder burn
  radiator (hot) X16
  saucepan (hot) (glass) (metal) X15.3
    stated as undetermined whether accidental or intentional Y27.3
    suicide (attempt) X77.3
  self-inflicted X76
    stated as undetermined whether accidental or intentional Y26
  stated as undetermined whether accidental or intentional Y27.0

Burn, burned, burning (accidental) (by) (from) (on) — *continued*
  steam X13.1
    pipe X16
    stated as undetermined whether accidental or intentional Y27.8
    stated as undetermined whether accidental or intentional Y27.0
    suicide (attempt) X77.0
  stove (hot) (kitchen) X15.0
    stated as undetermined whether accidental or intentional Y27.3
    suicide (attempt) X77.3
  substance (hot) NEC X19
    boiling X12
      stated as undetermined whether accidental or intentional Y27.2
      suicide (attempt) X77.2
    molten (metal) X18
    suicide (attempt) NEC X76
    hot
      household appliance X77.3
      object X77.9
  therapeutic misadventure
    heat in local application or packing during medical or surgical procedure Y63.5
    overdose of radiation Y63.2
  toaster (hot) X15.1
    stated as undetermined whether accidental or intentional Y27.3
    suicide (attempt) X77.3
  tool (hot) X17
  torch, welding X08.8
    with ignition of clothing NEC X06.2
      nightwear X05
  trash fire (controlled) — *see* Exposure, fire, controlled, not in building
    uncontrolled — *see* Exposure, fire, uncontrolled, not in building
  vapor (hot) X13.1
    stated as undetermined whether accidental or intentional Y27.0
    suicide (attempt) X77.0
  Very pistol — *see* Discharge, firearm NEC

Butted by animal W55.82
  bull W55.22
  cow W55.22
  goat W55.32
  horse W55.12
  pig W55.42
  sheep W55.32

C

Caisson disease — *see* Air, pressure, change
Campfire (exposure to) (controlled) — *see also* Exposure, fire, controlled, not in building
  uncontrolled — *see* Exposure, fire, uncontrolled, not in building
Capital punishment (any means) — *see* Legal, intervention
Car sickness T75.3
Casualty (not due to war) NEC X58
  war — *see* War operations
Cat
  bite W55.01
  scratch W55.03
Cataclysm, cataclysmic (any injury) NEC — *see* Forces of nature
Catching fire — *see* Exposure, fire
Caught
  between
    folding object W23.0
    objects (moving) (stationary and moving) W23.0
      and machinery — *see* Contact, with, by type of machine
      stationary W23.1
    sliding door and door frame W23.0
  by, in
    machinery (moving parts of) — *see* Contact, with, by type of machine
    washing-machine wringer W23.0
  under packing crate (due to losing grip) W23.1
Cave-in caused by cataclysmic earth surface movement or eruption — *see* Landslide
Change(s) in air pressure — *see* Air, pressure, change
Choked, choking (on) (any object except food or vomitus)
  food (bone) (seed) — *see* categories T17 and T18
  vomitus T17.81-
Civil insurrection — *see* War operations
Cloudburst (any injury) X37.8
Cold, exposure to (accidental) (excessive) (extreme) (natural) (place) NEC — *see* Exposure, cold
Collapse
  building W20.1
    burning (uncontrolled fire) X00.2
  dam or man-made structure (causing earth movement) X36.0
  machinery — *see* Contact, with, by type of machine
  structure W20.1
    burning (uncontrolled fire) X00.2
Collision (accidental) NEC (*see also* Accident, transport) V89.9
  pedestrian W51
    with fall W03
      due to ice or snow W00.0
      involving pedestrian conveyance — *see* Accident, transport, pedestrian, conveyance
    and
      crowd or human stampede (with fall) W52
      object W22.8
        with fall — *see* Fall, due to, bumping against, object
    person(s) — *see* Collision, pedestrian

Collision (accidental) NEC (*see also* Accident, transport) V89.9 — *continued*
  transport vehicle NEC V89.9
    and
      avalanche, fallen or not moving — *see* Accident, transport
        falling or moving — *see* Landslide
      landslide, fallen or not moving — *see* Accident, transport
        falling or moving — *see* Landslide
      due to cataclysm — *see* Forces of nature, by type
      intentional, purposeful suicide (attempt) — *see* Suicide, collision
Combustion, spontaneous — *see* Ignition
Complication (delayed) of or following (medical or surgical procedure) Y84.9
  with misadventure — *see* Misadventure
  amputation of limb(s) Y83.5
  anastomosis (arteriovenous) (blood vessel) (gastrojejunal) (tendon) (natural or artificial material) Y83.2
  aspiration (of fluid) Y84.4
    tissue Y84.8
  biopsy Y84.8
  blood
    sampling Y84.7
    transfusion
      procedure Y84.8
  bypass Y83.2
  catheterization (urinary) Y84.6
    cardiac Y84.0
  colostomy Y83.3
  cystostomy Y83.3
  dialysis (kidney) Y84.1
  drug — *see* Table of Drugs and Chemicals
  due to misadventure — *see* Misadventure
  duodenostomy Y83.3
  electroshock therapy Y84.3
  external stoma, creation of Y83.3
  formation of external stoma Y83.3
  gastrostomy Y83.3
  graft Y83.2
  hypothermia (medically-induced) Y84.8
  implant, implantation (of)
    artificial
      internal device (cardiac pacemaker) (electrodes in brain) (heart valve prosthesis) (orthopedic) Y83.1
      material or tissue (for anastomosis or bypass) Y83.2
        with creation of external stoma Y83.3
      natural tissues (for anastomosis or bypass) Y83.2
        with creation of external stoma Y83.3
  infusion
    procedure Y84.8
  injection — *see* Table of Drugs and Chemicals
    procedure Y84.8
  insertion of gastric or duodenal sound Y84.5
  insulin-shock therapy Y84.3
  paracentesis (abdominal) (thoracic) (aspirative) Y84.4
  procedures other than surgical operation — *see* Complication of or following, by type of procedure
  radiological procedure or therapy Y84.2
  removal of organ (partial) (total) NEC Y83.6
  sampling
    blood Y84.7
    fluid NEC Y84.4
    tissue Y84.8
  shock therapy Y84.3

Complication (delayed) of or following (medical or surgical procedure) Y84.9 — *continued*
  surgical operation NEC (*see also* Complication of or following, by type of operation) Y83.9
    reconstructive NEC Y83.4
      with
        anastomosis, bypass or graft Y83.2
        formation of external stoma Y83.3
      specified NEC Y83.8
  transfusion — *see also* Table of Drugs and Chemicals
    procedure Y84.8
  transplant, transplantation (heart) (kidney) (liver) (whole organ, any) Y83.0
    partial organ Y83.4
  ureterostomy Y83.3
  vaccination — *see also* Table of Drugs and Chemicals
    procedure Y84.8
Compression
  divers' squeeze — *see* Air, pressure, change
  trachea by
    food (lodged in esophagus) — *see* categories T17 and T18
    vomitus (lodged in esophagus) T17.81-
Conflagration — *see* Exposure, fire, uncontrolled
Constriction (external)
  hair W49.01
  jewelry W49.04
  ring W49.04
  rubber band W49.03
  specified item NEC W49.09
  string W49.02
  thread W49.02
Contact (accidental)
  with
    abrasive wheel (metalworking) W31.1
    alligator W58.09
      bite W58.01
      crushing W58.03
      strike W58.02
    amphibian W62.9
      frog W62.0
      toad W62.1
    animal (nonvenomous) NEC W64
      marine W56.89
        bite W56.81
        dolphin — *see* Contact, with, dolphin
        fish NEC — *see* Contact, with, fish
        mammal — *see* Contact, with, mammal, marine
        orca — *see* Contact, with, orca
        sea lion — *see* Contact, with, sea lion
        shark — *see* Contact, with, shark
        strike W56.82
    animate mechanical force NEC W64
    arrow W21.89
      not thrown, projected or falling W45.8
    arthropods (nonvenomous) W57
    axe W27.0
    band-saw (industrial) W31.2
    bayonet — *see* Bayonet wound
    bee(s) X58
    bench-saw (industrial) W31.2
    bird W61.99
      bite W61.91
      chicken — *see* Contact, with, chicken
      duck — *see* Contact, with, duck
      goose — *see* Contact, with, goose
      macaw — *see* Contact, with, macaw
      parrot — *see* Contact, with, parrot
      psittacine — *see* Contact, with, psittacine
      strike W61.92
      turkey — *see* Contact, with, turkey
    blender W29.0

EXTERNAL CAUSES

Contact (accidental) — *continued*
　with — *continued*
　　boiling water X12
　　　stated as undetermined whether accidental
　　　　or intentional Y27.2
　　　suicide (attempt) X77.2
　　bore, earth-drilling or mining (land)
　　　(seabed) W31.0
　　buffalo — *see* Contact, with, hoof stock NEC
　　bull W55.29
　　　bite W55.21
　　　gored W55.22
　　　strike W55.22
　　bumper cars W31.81
　　camel — *see* Contact, with, hoof stock NEC
　　can
　　　lid W26.8
　　　opener W27.4
　　　　powered W29.0
　　cat W55.09
　　　bite W55.01
　　　scratch W55.03
　　caterpillar (venomous) X58
　　centipede (venomous) X58
　　chain
　　　hoist W24.0
　　　　agricultural operations W30.89
　　　saw W29.3
　　chicken W61.39
　　　peck W61.33
　　　strike W61.32
　　chisel W27.0
　　circular saw W31.2
　　cobra X58
　　combine (harvester) W30.0
　　conveyer belt W24.1
　　cooker (hot) X15.8
　　　stated as undetermined whether accidental
　　　　or intentional Y27.3
　　　suicide (attempt) X77.3
　　coral X58
　　cotton gin W31.82
　　cow W55.29
　　　bite W55.21
　　　strike W55.22
　　crane W24.0
　　　agricultural operations W30.89
　　crocodile W58.19
　　　bite W58.11
　　　crushing W58.13
　　　strike W58.12
　　dagger W26.1
　　　stated as undetermined whether accidental
　　　　or intentional Y28.2
　　　suicide (attempt) X78.2
　　dairy equipment W31.82
　　dart W21.89
　　　not thrown, projected or falling W45.8
　　deer — *see* Contact, with, hoof stock NEC
　　derrick W24.0
　　　agricultural operations W30.89
　　　　hay W30.2
　　dog W54.8
　　　bite W54.0
　　　strike W54.1
　　dolphin W56.09
　　　bite W56.01
　　　strike W56.02
　　donkey — *see* Contact, with, hoof stock NEC
　　drill (powered) W29.8
　　　earth (land) (seabed) W31.0
　　　nonpowered W27.8
　　drive belt W24.0
　　　agricultural operations W30.89
　　dry ice — *see* Exposure, cold, man-made
　　dryer (clothes) (powered) (spin) W29.2

Contact (accidental) — *continued*
　with — *continued*
　　duck W61.69
　　　bite W61.61
　　　strike W61.62
　　earth(-)
　　　drilling machine (industrial) W31.0
　　　scraping machine in stationary use
　　　　W31.83
　　edge of stiff paper W26.2
　　electric
　　　beater W29.0
　　　blanket X16
　　　fan W29.2
　　　　commercial W31.82
　　　knife W29.1
　　　mixer W29.0
　　elevator (building) W24.0
　　　agricultural operations W30.89
　　　　grain W30.3
　　engine(s), hot NEC X17
　　excavating machine W31.0
　　farm machine W30.9
　　feces — *see* Contact, with, by type of animal
　　fer de lance X58
　　fish W56.59
　　　bite W56.51
　　　shark — *see* Contact, with, shark
　　　strike W56.52
　　flying horses W31.81
　　forging (metalworking) machine W31.1
　　fork W27.4
　　forklift (truck) W24.0
　　　agricultural operations W30.89
　　frog W62.0
　　garden
　　　cultivator (powered) W29.3
　　　　riding W30.89
　　　fork W27.1
　　gas turbine W31.3
　　Gila monster X58
　　giraffe — *see* Contact, with, hoof stock NEC
　　glass (sharp) (broken) W25
　　　with subsequent fall W18.02
　　　assault X99.0
　　　due to fall — *see* Fall, by type
　　　stated as undetermined whether accidental
　　　　or intentional Y28.0
　　　suicide (attempt) X78.0
　　goat W55.39
　　　bite W55.31
　　　strike W55.32
　　goose W61.59
　　　bite W61.51
　　　strike W61.52
　　hand
　　　saw W27.0
　　　tool (not powered) NEC W27.8
　　　　powered W29.8
　　harvester W30.0
　　hay-derrick W30.2
　　heat NEC X19
　　　from appliance (electrical) (household) —
　　　　see Contact, with, hot, household
　　　　appliance
　　　heating appliance X16
　　heating
　　　appliance (hot) X16
　　　pad (electric) X16
　　hedge-trimmer (powered) W29.3
　　hoe W27.1
　　hoist (chain) (shaft) NEC W24.0
　　　agricultural W30.89
　　hoof stock NEC W55.39
　　　bite W55.31
　　　strike W55.32
　　hornet(s) X58

Contact (accidental) — *continued*
　with — *continued*
　　horse W55.19
　　　bite W55.11
　　　strike W55.12
　　hot
　　　air X14.1
　　　　inhalation X14.0
　　　cooker X15.8
　　　drinks X10.0
　　　engine X17
　　　fats X10.2
　　　fluids NEC X12
　　　　assault X98.2
　　　　suicide (attempt) X77.2
　　　　undetermined whether accidental or
　　　　　intentional Y27.2
　　　food X10.1
　　　gases X14.1
　　　　inhalation X14.0
　　　heating appliance X16
　　　household appliance X15.8
　　　　assault X98.3
　　　　cooker X15.8
　　　　hotplate X15.2
　　　　kettle X15.8
　　　　light bulb X15.8
　　　　object NEC X19
　　　　　assault X98.8
　　　　　stated as undetermined whether
　　　　　　accidental or intentional Y27.9
　　　　　suicide (attempt) X77.8
　　　　saucepan X15.3
　　　　skillet X15.3
　　　　stated as undetermined whether
　　　　　accidental or intentional Y27.3
　　　　stove X15.0
　　　　suicide (attempt) X77.3
　　　　toaster X15.1
　　　kettle X15.8
　　　light bulb X15.8
　　　liquid NEC (*see also* Burn) X12
　　　　drinks X10.0
　　　　stated as undetermined whether
　　　　　accidental or intentional Y27.2
　　　　suicide (attempt) X77.2
　　　　tap water X11.8
　　　　　stated as undetermined whether
　　　　　　accidental or intentional Y27.1
　　　　　suicide (attempt) X77.1
　　　machinery X17
　　　metal (molten) (liquid) NEC X18
　　　object (not producing fire or flames) NEC
　　　　X19
　　　oil (cooking) X10.2
　　　pipe X16
　　　plate X15.2
　　　radiator X16
　　　saucepan (glass) (metal) X15.3
　　　skillet X15.3
　　　stove (kitchen) X15.0
　　　substance NEC X19
　　　tap-water X11.8
　　　　assault X98.1
　　　　heated on stove X12
　　　　　stated as undetermined whether
　　　　　　accidental or intentional Y27.2
　　　　　suicide (attempt) X77.2
　　　　in bathtub X11.0
　　　　running X11.1
　　　　stated as undetermined whether
　　　　　accidental or intentional Y27.1
　　　　suicide (attempt) X77.1
　　　toaster X15.1
　　　tool X17
　　　vapors X13.1
　　　　inhalation X13.0

Contact (accidental) — *continued*
  with — *continued*
    hot — *continued*
      water (tap) X11.8
        boiling X12
          stated as undetermined whether
            accidental or intentional Y27.2
          suicide (attempt) X77.2
        heated on stove X12
          stated as undetermined whether
            accidental or intentional Y27.2
          suicide (attempt) X77.2
        in bathtub X11.0
        running X11.1
        stated as undetermined whether
          accidental or intentional Y27.1
        suicide (attempt) X77.1
    hotplate X15.2
    ice-pick W27.4
    insect (nonvenomous) NEC W57
    kettle (hot) X15.8
    knife W26.0
      assault X99.1
      electric W29.1
      stated as undetermined whether accidental
        or intentional Y28.1
      suicide (attempt) X78.1
    lathe (metalworking) W31.1
      turnings W45.8
      woodworking W31.2
    lawnmower (powered) (ridden) W28
      causing electrocution W86.8
        suicide (attempt) X83.1
      unpowered W27.1
    lift, lifting (devices) W24.0
      agricultural operations W30.89
      shaft W24.0
    liquefied gas — *see* Exposure, cold, man-
      made
    liquid air, hydrogen, nitrogen — *see*
      Exposure, cold, man-made
    lizard (nonvenomous) W59.09
      bite W59.01
      strike W59.02
    llama — *see* Contact, with, hoof stock NEC
    macaw W61.19
      bite W61.11
      strike W61.12
    machine, machinery W31.9
      abrasive wheel W31.1
      agricultural including animal-powered
        W30.9
        combine harvester W30.0
        grain storage elevator W30.3
        hay derrick W30.2
        power take-off device W30.1
        reaper W30.0
        specified NEC W30.89
        thresher W30.0
        transport vehicle, stationary W30.81
      band saw W31.2
      bench saw W31.2
      circular saw W31.2
      commercial NEC W31.82
      drilling, metal (industrial) W31.1
      earth-drilling W31.0
      earthmoving or scraping W31.89
      excavating W31.89
      forging machine W31.1
      gas turbine W31.3
      hot X17
      internal combustion engine W31.3
      land drill W31.0
      lathe W31.1
      lifting (devices) W24.0
      metal drill W31.1
      metalworking (industrial) W31.1
      milling, metal W31.1

Contact (accidental) — *continued*
  with — *continued*
    machine, machinery W31.9 — *continued*
      mining W31.0
      molding W31.2
      overhead plane W31.2
      power press, metal W31.1
      prime mover W31.3
      printing W31.89
      radial saw W31.2
      recreational W31.81
      roller-coaster W31.81
      rolling mill, metal W31.1
      sander W31.2
      seabed drill W31.0
      shaft
        hoist W31.0
        lift W31.0
      specified NEC W31.89
      spinning W31.89
      steam engine W31.3
      transmission W24.1
      undercutter W31.0
      water driven turbine W31.3
      weaving W31.89
      woodworking or forming (industrial)
        W31.2
    mammal (feces) (urine) W55.89
      bull — *see* Contact, with, bull
      cat — *see* Contact, with, cat
      cow — *see* Contact, with, cow
      goat — *see* Contact, with, goat
      hoof stock — *see* Contact, with, hoof stock
      horse — *see* Contact, with, horse
      marine W56.39
        dolphin — *see* Contact, with, dolphin
        orca — *see* Contact, with, orca
        sea lion — *see* Contact, with, sea lion
        specified NEC W56.39
          bite W56.31
          strike W56.32
      pig — *see* Contact, with, pig
      raccoon — *see* Contact, with, raccoon
      rodent — *see* Contact, with, rodent
      sheep — *see* Contact, with, sheep
      specified NEC W55.89
        bite W55.81
        strike W55.82
    marine
      animal W56.89
        bite W56.81
        dolphin — *see* Contact, with, dolphin
        fish NEC — *see* Contact, with, fish
        mammal — *see* Contact, with, mammal,
          marine
        orca — *see* Contact, with, orca
        sea lion — *see* Contact, with, sea lion
        shark — *see* Contact, with, shark
        strike W56.82
    meat
      grinder (domestic) W29.0
        industrial W31.82
        nonpowered W27.4
      slicer (domestic) W29.0
        industrial W31.82
    merry go round W31.81
    metal, hot (liquid) (molten) NEC X18
    millipede W57
    nail W45.0
      gun W29.4
    needle (sewing) W27.3
      hypodermic W46.0
        contaminated W46.1

Contact (accidental) — *continued*
  with — *continued*
    object (blunt) NEC
      hot NEC X19
      legal intervention — *see* Legal,
        intervention, blunt object
      sharp NEC W45.8
        inflicted by other person NEC W45.8
          stated as
            intentional homicide (attempt) — *see*
              Assault, cutting or piercing
              instrument
          legal intervention — *see* Legal,
            intervention, sharp object
          self-inflicted X78.9
    orca W56.29
      bite W56.21
      strike W56.22
    overhead plane W31.2
    paper (as sharp object) W26.2
    paper-cutter W27.5
    parrot W61.09
      bite W61.01
      strike W61.02
    pig W55.49
      bite W55.41
      strike W55.42
    pipe, hot X16
    pitchfork W27.1
    plane (metal) (wood) W27.0
      overhead W31.2
    plant thorns, spines, sharp leaves or other
      mechanisms W60
    powered
      garden cultivator W29.3
      household appliance, implement, or
        machine W29.8
      saw (industrial) W31.2
        hand W29.8
    printing machine W31.89
    psittacine bird W61.29
      bite W61.21
      macaw — *see* Contact, with, macaw
      parrot — *see* Contact, with, parrot
      strike W61.22
    pulley (block) (transmission) W24.0
      agricultural operations W30.89
    raccoon W55.59
      bite W55.51
      strike W55.52
    radial-saw (industrial) W31.2
    radiator (hot) X16
    rake W27.1
    rattlesnake X58
    reaper W30.0
    reptile W59.89
      lizard — *see* Contact, with, lizard
      snake — *see* Contact, with, snake
      specified NEC W59.89
        bite W59.81
        crushing W59.83
        strike W59.82
      turtle — *see* Contact, with, turtle
    rivet gun (powered) W29.4
    road scraper — *see* Accident, transport,
      construction vehicle
    rodent (feces) (urine) W53.89
      bite W53.81
      mouse W53.09
        bite W53.01
      rat W53.19
        bite W53.11
      specified NEC W53.89
        bite W53.81
      squirrel W53.29
        bite W53.21
    roller coaster W31.81

EXTERNAL CAUSES

Contact (accidental) — *continued*
  with — *continued*
    rope NEC W24.0
      agricultural operations W30.89
    saliva — *see* Contact, with, by type of
        animal
    sander W29.8
      industrial W31.2
    saucepan (hot) (glass) (metal) X15.3
    saw W27.0
      band (industrial) W31.2
      bench (industrial) W31.2
      chain W29.3
      hand W27.0
    sawing machine, metal W31.1
    scissors W27.2
    scorpion X58
    screwdriver W27.0
      powered W29.8
    sea
      anemone, cucumber or urchin (spine) X58
      lion W56.19
        bite W56.11
        strike W56.12
    serpent — *see* Contact, with, snake, by type
    sewing-machine (electric) (powered) W29.2
      not powered W27.8
    shaft (hoist) (lift) (transmission) NEC W24.0
      agricultural W30.89
    shark W56.49
      bite W56.41
      strike W56.42
    sharp object(s) W26.9
      specified NEC W26.8
    shears (hand) W27.2
      powered (industrial) W31.1
        domestic W29.2
    sheep W55.39
      bite W55.31
      strike W55.32
    shovel W27.8
      steam — *see* Accident, transport,
          construction vehicle
    snake (nonvenomous) W59.19
      bite W59.11
      crushing W59.13
      strike W59.12
    spade W27.1
    spider (venomous) X58
    spin-drier W29.2
    spinning machine W31.89
    splinter W45.8
    sports equipment W21.9
    staple gun (powered) W29.8
    steam X13.1
      engine W31.3
      inhalation X13.0
      pipe X16
      shovel W31.89
    stove (hot) (kitchen) X15.0
    substance, hot NEC X19
      molten (metal) X18
    sword W26.1
      assault X99.2
      stated as undetermined whether accidental
          or intentional Y28.2
      suicide (attempt) X78.2
    tarantula X58
    thresher W30.0
    tin can lid W26.8
    toad W62.1
    toaster (hot) X15.1

Contact (accidental) — *continued*
  with — *continued*
    tool W27.8
      hand (not powered) W27.8
        auger W27.0
        axe W27.0
        can opener W27.4
        chisel W27.0
        fork W27.4
        garden W27.1
        handsaw W27.0
        hoe W27.1
        ice-pick W27.4
        kitchen utensil W27.4
        manual
          lawn mower W27.1
          sewing machine W27.8
        meat grinder W27.4
        needle (sewing) W27.3
          hypodermic W46.0
            contaminated W46.1
        paper cutter W27.5
        pitchfork W27.1
        rake W27.1
        scissors W27.2
        screwdriver W27.0
        specified NEC W27.8
        workbench W27.0
      hot X17
      powered W29.8
        blender W29.0
          commercial W31.82
        can opener W29.0
          commercial W31.82
        chainsaw W29.3
        clothes dryer W29.2
          commercial W31.82
        dishwasher W29.2
          commercial W31.82
        edger W29.3
        electric fan W29.2
          commercial W31.82
        electric knife W29.1
        food processor W29.0
          commercial W31.82
        garbage disposal W29.0
          commercial W31.82
        garden tool W29.3
        hedge trimmer W29.3
        ice maker W29.0
          commercial W31.82
        kitchen appliance W29.0
          commercial W31.82
        lawn mower W28
        meat grinder W29.0
          commercial W31.82
        mixer W29.0
          commercial W31.82
        rototiller W29.3
        sewing machine W29.2
          commercial W31.82
        washing machine W29.2
          commercial W31.82
    transmission device (belt, cable, chain, gear,
        pinion, shaft) W24.1
      agricultural operations W30.89
    turbine (gas) (water-driven) W31.3
    turkey W61.49
      peck W61.43
      strike W61.42
    turtle (nonvenomous) W59.29
      bite W59.21
      strike W59.22
      terrestrial W59.89
        bite W59.81
        crushing W59.83
        strike W59.82

Contact (accidental) — *continued*
  with — *continued*
    under-cutter W31.0
    urine — *see* Contact, with, by type of animal
    vehicle
      agricultural use (transport) — *see*
          Accident, transport, agricultural
          vehicle
        not on public highway W30.81
      industrial use (transport) — *see* Accident,
          transport, industrial vehicle
        not on public highway W31.83
      off-road use (transport) — *see* Accident,
          transport, all-terrain or off-road
          vehicle
        not on public highway W31.83
      special construction use (transport) — *see*
          Accident, transport, construction
          vehicle
        not on public highway W31.83
    venomous
      animal X58
      arthropods X58
      lizard X58
      marine animal NEC X58
      marine plant NEC X58
      millipedes (tropical) X58
      plant(s) X58
      snake X58
      spider X58
      viper X58
    washing-machine (powered) W29.2
    wasp X58
    weaving-machine W31.89
    winch W24.0
      agricultural operations W30.89
    wire NEC W24.0
      agricultural operations W30.89
    wood slivers W45.8
    yellow jacket X58
    zebra — *see* Contact, with, hoof stock NEC
  pressure X50.9
  stress X50.9
Coup de soleil X32
Crash
  aircraft (in transit) (powered) V95.9
    balloon V96.01
    fixed wing NEC (private) V95.21
      commercial V95.31
    glider V96.21
      hang V96.11
      powered V95.11
    helicopter V95.01
    in war operations — *see* War operations,
        destruction of aircraft
    microlight V95.11
    nonpowered V96.9
      specified NEC V96.8
    powered NEC V95.8
    stated as
      homicide (attempt) Y08.81
      suicide (attempt) X83.0
    ultralight V95.11
  spacecraft V95.41
  transport vehicle NEC (*see also* Accident,
      transport) V89.9
    homicide (attempt) Y03.8
    motor NEC (traffic) V89.2
      homicide (attempt) Y03.8
      suicide (attempt) — *see* Suicide, collision
Cruelty (mental) (physical) (sexual) X58

EXTERNAL CAUSES

Crushed (accidentally) X58
  between objects (moving) (stationary and
    moving) W23.0
    stationary W23.1
  by
    alligator W58.03
    avalanche NEC — *see* Landslide
    cave-in W20.0
      caused by cataclysmic earth surface
        movement — *see* Landslide
    crocodile W58.13
    crowd or human stampede W52
    falling
      aircraft V97.39
        in war operations — *see* War
          operations, destruction of aircraft
      earth, material W20.0
        caused by cataclysmic earth surface
          movement — *see* Landslide
      object NEC W20.8
    landslide NEC — *see* Landslide
    lizard (nonvenomous) W59.09
    machinery — *see* Contact, with, by type of
      machine
    reptile NEC W59.89
    snake (nonvenomous) W59.13
  in
    machinery — *see* Contact, with, by type of
      machine
Cut, cutting (any part of body) (accidental) —
  see also Contact, with, by object or machine
  during medical or surgical treatment as
    misadventure — *see* Index to Diseases and
    Injuries, Complications
  homicide (attempt) — *see* Assault, cutting or
    piercing instrument
  inflicted by other person — *see* Assault, cutting
    or piercing instrument
  legal
    execution — *see* Legal, intervention
    intervention — *see* Legal, intervention, sharp
      object
  machine NEC (*see also* Contact, with, by type
    of machine) W31.9
  self-inflicted — *see* Suicide, cutting or piercing
    instrument
  suicide (attempt) — *see* Suicide, cutting or
    piercing instrument
Cyclone (any injury) X37.1

D

Decapitation (accidental circumstances) NEC
  X58
  homicide X99.9
  legal execution — *see* Legal, intervention
Dehydration from lack of water X58
Deprivation X58
Derailment (accidental)
  railway (rolling stock) (train) (vehicle) (without
    antecedent collision) V81.7
    with antecedent collision — *see* Accident,
      transport, railway vehicle occupant
  streetcar (without antecedent collision) V82.7
    with antecedent collision — *see* Accident,
      transport, streetcar occupant
Descent
  parachute (voluntary) (without accident to
    aircraft) V97.29
    due to accident to aircraft — *see* Accident,
      transport, aircraft
Desertion X58
Destitution X58
Disability, late effect or sequela of injury
  — *see* Sequelae
Discharge (accidental)
  airgun W34.010
    assault X95.01
    homicide (attempt) X95.01
    stated as undetermined whether accidental
      or intentional Y24.0
    suicide (attempt) X74.01
  BB gun — *see* Discharge, airgun
  firearm (accidental) W34.00
    assault X95.9
    handgun (pistol) (revolver) W32.0
      assault X93
      homicide (attempt) X93
      legal intervention — *see* Legal,
        intervention, firearm, handgun
      stated as undetermined whether accidental
        or intentional Y22
      suicide (attempt) X72
    homicide (attempt) X95.9
    hunting rifle W33.02
      assault X94.1
      homicide (attempt) X94.1
      legal intervention
        injuring
          bystander Y35.032
          law enforcement personnel Y35.031
          suspect Y35.033
      stated as undetermined whether accidental
        or intentional Y23.1
      suicide (attempt) X73.1
    larger W33.00
      assault X94.9
      homicide (attempt) X94.9
      hunting rifle — *see* Discharge, firearm,
        hunting rifle
      legal intervention — *see* Legal,
        intervention, firearm by type of
        firearm
      machine gun — *see* Discharge, firearm,
        machine gun
      shotgun — *see* Discharge, firearm, shotgun
      specified NEC W33.09
        assault X94.8
        homicide (attempt) X94.8
        legal intervention
          injuring
            bystander Y35.092
            law enforcement personnel Y35.091
            suspect Y35.093
        stated as undetermined whether
          accidental or intentional Y23.8

Discharge (accidental) — *continued*
  firearm (accidental) W34.00 — *continued*
    larger W33.00 — *continued*
      specified NEC W33.09 — *continued*
        suicide (attempt) X73.8
      stated as undetermined whether accidental
        or intentional Y23.9
      suicide (attempt) X73.9
    legal intervention
      injuring
        bystander Y35.002
        law enforcement personnel Y35.001
        suspect Y35.03
      using rubber bullet
        injuring
          bystander Y35.042
          law enforcement personnel Y35.041
          suspect Y35.043
    machine gun W33.03
      assault X94.2
      homicide (attempt) X94.2
      legal intervention — *see* Legal,
        intervention, firearm, machine gun
      stated as undetermined whether accidental
        or intentional Y23.3
      suicide (attempt) X73.2
    pellet gun — *see* Discharge, airgun
    shotgun W33.01
      assault X94.0
      homicide (attempt) X94.0
      legal intervention — *see* Legal,
        intervention, firearm, specified NEC
      stated as undetermined whether accidental
        or intentional Y23.0
      suicide (attempt) X73.0
    specified NEC W34.09
      assault X95.8
      homicide (attempt) X95.8
      legal intervention — *see* Legal,
        intervention, firearm, specified NEC
      stated as undetermined whether accidental
        or intentional Y24.8
      suicide (attempt) X74.8
    stated as undetermined whether accidental
      or intentional Y24.9
    suicide (attempt) X74.9
    Very pistol W34.09
      assault X95.8
      homicide (attempt) X95.8
      stated as undetermined whether accidental
        or intentional Y24.8
      suicide (attempt) X74.8
  firework(s) W39
    stated as undetermined whether accidental
      or intentional Y25
  gas-operated gun NEC W34.018
    airgun — *see* Discharge, airgun
    assault X95.09
    homicide (attempt) X95.09
    paintball gun — *see* Discharge, paintball
      gun
    stated as undetermined whether accidental
      or intentional Y24.8
    suicide (attempt) X74.09
  gun NEC — *see also* Discharge, firearm NEC
    air — *see* Discharge, airgun
    BB — *see* Discharge, airgun
    for single hand use — *see* Discharge,
      firearm, handgun
    hand — *see* Discharge, firearm, handgun
    machine — *see* Discharge, firearm, machine
      gun
    other specified — *see* Discharge, firearm
      NEC
    paintball — *see* Discharge, paintball gun
    pellet — *see* Discharge, airgun
  handgun — *see* Discharge, firearm, handgun

Discharge (accidental) — *continued*
  machine gun — *see* Discharge, firearm,
    machine gun
  paintball gun W34.011
    assault X95.02
    homicide (attempt) X95.02
    stated as undetermined whether accidental
      or intentional Y24.8
    suicide (attempt) X74.02
  pistol — *see* Discharge, firearm, handgun
    flare — *see* Discharge, firearm, Very pistol
    pellet — *see* Discharge, airgun
    Very — *see* Discharge, firearm, Very pistol
  revolver — *see* Discharge, firearm, handgun
  rifle (hunting) — *see* Discharge, firearm,
    hunting rifle
  shotgun — *see* Discharge, firearm, shotgun
  spring-operated gun NEC W34.018
    assault X95.09
    homicide (attempt) X95.09
    stated as undetermined whether accidental
      or intentional Y24.8
    suicide (attempt) X74.09
Disease
  Andes W94.11
  aviator's — *see* Air, pressure
  range W94.11
**Diver's disease, palsy, paralysis,
  squeeze** — *see* Air, pressure
Diving (into water) — *see* Accident, diving
Dog bite W54.0
Dragged by transport vehicle NEC (*see also*
  Accident, transport) V09.9
Drinking poison (accidental) — *see* Table of
  Drugs and Chemicals
**Dropped (accidentally) while being
  carried or supported by other person**
  W04

Drowning (accidental) W74
  assault X92.9
  due to
    accident (to)
      machinery — *see* Contact, with, by type of
        machine
      watercraft V90.89
        burning V90.29
          powered V90.23
            fishing boat V90.22
            jetskis V90.23
            merchant ship V90.20
            passenger ship V90.21
          unpowered V90.28
            canoe V90.25
            inflatable V90.26
            kayak V90.25
            sailboat V90.24
            water skis V90.27
        crushed V90.39
          powered V90.33
            fishing boat V90.32
            jetskis V90.33
            merchant ship V90.30
            passenger ship V90.31
          unpowered V90.38
            canoe V90.35
            inflatable V90.36
            kayak V90.35
            sailboat V90.34
            water skis V90.37
        overturning V90.09
          powered V90.03
            fishing boat V90.02
            jetskis V90.03
            merchant ship V90.00
            passenger ship V90.01
          unpowered V90.08
            canoe V90.05
            inflatable V90.06
            kayak V90.05
            sailboat V90.04
        sinking V90.19
          powered V90.13
            fishing boat V90.12
            jetskis V90.13
            merchant ship V90.10
            passenger ship V90.11
          unpowered V90.18
            canoe V90.15
            inflatable V90.16
            kayak V90.15
            sailboat V90.14
        specified type NEC V90.89
          powered V90.83
            fishing boat V90.82
            jetskis V90.83
            merchant ship V90.80
            passenger ship V90.81
          unpowered V90.88
            canoe V90.85
            inflatable V90.86
            kayak V90.85
            sailboat V90.84
            water skis V90.87

Drowning (accidental) W74 — *continued*
  due to — *continued*
    avalanche — *see* Landslide
    cataclysmic
      earth surface movement NEC — *see* Forces
        of nature, earth movement
      storm — *see* Forces of nature, cataclysmic
        storm
    cloudburst X37.8
    cyclone X37.1
    fall overboard (from) V92.09
      powered craft V92.03
        ferry boat V92.01
        fishing boat V92.02
        jetskis V92.03
        liner V92.01
        merchant ship V92.00
        passenger ship V92.01
    resulting from
      accident to watercraft — *see* Drowning,
        due to, accident to, watercraft
      being washed overboard (from) V92.29
        powered craft V92.23
          ferry boat V92.21
          fishing boat V92.22
          jetskis V92.23
          liner V92.21
          merchant ship V92.20
          passenger ship V92.21
        unpowered craft V92.28
          canoe V92.25
          inflatable V92.26
          kayak V92.25
          sailboat V92.24
          surfboard V92.28
          water skis V92.27
          windsurfer V92.28
      motion of watercraft V92.19
        powered craft V92.13
          ferry boat V92.11
          fishing boat V92.12
          jetskis V92.13
          liner V92.11
          merchant ship V92.10
          passenger ship V92.11
        unpowered craft
          canoe V92.15
          inflatable V92.16
          kayak V92.15
          sailboat V92.14
      unpowered craft V92.08
        canoe V92.05
        inflatable V92.06
        kayak V92.05
        sailboat V92.04
        surfboard V92.08
        water skis V92.07
        windsurfer V92.08
    hurricane X37.0
    jumping into water from watercraft (involved
      in accident) — *see also* Drowning, due
      to, accident to, watercraft
      without accident to or on watercraft
        W16.711
    tidal wave NEC — *see* Forces of nature, tidal
      wave
    torrential rain X37.8

EXTERNAL CAUSES

Drowning (accidental) W74 — *continued*
following
  fall
    into
      bathtub W16.211
      bucket W16.221
      fountain — *see* Drowning, following,
        fall, into, water, specified NEC
      quarry — *see* Drowning, following, fall,
        into, water, specified NEC
      reservoir — *see* Drowning, following,
        fall, into, water, specified NEC
      swimming pool W16.011
        stated as undetermined whether
          accidental or intentional Y21.3
        striking
          bottom W16.021
          wall W16.031
        suicide (attempt) X71.2
      water NOS W16.41
        natural (lake) (open sea) (pond) (river)
          (stream) W16.111
          striking
            bottom W16.121
            side W16.131
        specified NEC W16.311
          striking
            bottom W16.321
            wall W16.331
  overboard NEC — *see* Drowning, due to,
    fall overboard
jump or dive
  from boat W16.711
    striking bottom W16.721
  into
    fountain — *see* Drowning, following,
      jump or dive, into, water, specified
      NEC
    quarry — *see* Drowning, following, jump
      or dive, into, water, specified NEC
    reservoir — *see* Drowning, following,
      jump or dive, into, water, specified
      NEC
    swimming pool W16.511
      striking
        bottom W16.521
        wall W16.531
      suicide (attempt) X71.2
    water NOS W16.91
      natural (lake) (open sea) (pond) (river)
        (stream) W16.611
      specified NEC W16.811
        striking
          bottom W16.821
          wall W16.831
      striking bottom W16.621

Drowning (accidental) W74 — *continued*
homicide (attempt) X92.9
in
  bathtub (accidental) W65
    assault X92.0
    following fall W16.211
      stated as undetermined whether
        accidental or intentional Y21.1
    stated as undetermined whether accidental
      or intentional Y21.0
    suicide (attempt) X71.0
  lake — *see* Drowning, in, natural water
  natural water (lake) (open sea) (pond) (river)
    (stream) W69
    assault X92.3
    following
      dive or jump W16.611
        striking bottom W16.621
      fall W16.111
        striking
          bottom W16.121
          side W16.131
    stated as undetermined whether accidental
      or intentional Y21.4
    suicide (attempt) X71.3
  quarry — *see* Drowning, in, specified place
    NEC
  quenching tank — *see* Drowning, in,
    specified place NEC
  reservoir — *see* Drowning, in, specified
    place NEC
  river — *see* Drowning, in, natural water
  sea — *see* Drowning, in, natural water
  specified place NEC W73
    assault X92.8
    following
      dive or jump W16.811
        striking
          bottom W16.821
          wall W16.831
      fall W16.311
        striking
          bottom W16.321
          wall W16.331
    stated as undetermined whether accidental
      or intentional Y21.8
    suicide (attempt) X71.8
  stream — *see* Drowning, in, natural water
  swimming pool W67
    assault X92.1
    following fall X92.2
    following
      dive or jump W16.511
        striking
          bottom W16.521
          wall W16.531
      fall W16.011
        striking
          bottom W16.021
          wall W16.031
    stated as undetermined whether accidental
      or intentional Y21.2
    following fall Y21.3
    suicide (attempt) X71.1
    following fall X71.2
  war operations — *see* War operations,
    restriction of airway
resulting from accident to watercraft — *see*
  Drowning, due to, accident, watercraft
self-inflicted X71.9
stated as undetermined whether accidental or
  intentional Y21.9
suicide (attempt) X71.9

E

Earth falling (on) W20.0
  caused by cataclysmic earth surface movement
    or eruption — *see* Landslide
Earth (surface) movement NEC — *see*
  Forces of nature, earth movement
Earthquake (any injury) X34
Effect(s) (adverse) of
  air pressure (any) — *see* Air, pressure
  cold, excessive (exposure to) — *see* Exposure,
    cold
  heat (excessive) — *see* Heat
  hot place (weather) — *see* Heat
  insolation X30
  late — *see* Sequelae
  motion — *see* Motion
  nuclear explosion or weapon in war
    operations — *see* War operations, nuclear
    weapon
  radiation — *see* Radiation
  travel — *see* Travel
Electric shock (accidental) (by) (in) — *see*
  Exposure, electric current
Electrocution (accidental) — *see* Exposure,
  electric current
Endotracheal tube wrongly placed
  during anesthetic procedure
Entanglement
  in
    bed linen, causing suffocation — *see*
      category T71
    wheel of pedal cycle V19.88
Entry of foreign body or material — *see*
  Foreign body
Environmental pollution related
  condition — *see* Z57
Execution, legal (any method) — *see* Legal,
  intervention
Exhaustion
  cold — *see* Exposure, cold
  due to excessive exertion (*see also*
    Overexertion) X50.9
  heat — *see* Heat
Explosion (accidental) (of) (with secondary fire)
  W40.9
  acetylene W40.1
  aerosol can W36.1
  air tank (compressed) (in machinery) W36.2
  aircraft (in transit) (powered) NEC V95.9
    balloon V96.05
    fixed wing NEC (private) V95.25
      commercial V95.35
    glider V96.25
      hang V96.15
      powered V95.15
    helicopter V95.05
    in war operations — *see* War operations,
      destruction of aircraft
    microlight V95.15
    nonpowered V96.9
      specified NEC V96.8
    powered NEC V95.8
    stated as
      homicide (attempt) Y03.8
      suicide (attempt) X83.0
    ultralight V95.15
  anesthetic gas in operating room W40.1
  antipersonnel bomb W40.8
    assault X96.0
    homicide (attempt) X96.0
    suicide (attempt) X75
  assault X96.9
  bicycle tire W37.0
  blasting (cap) (materials) W40.0
  boiler (machinery), not on transport vehicle
    W35
    on watercraft — *see* Explosion, in, watercraft

Explosion (accidental) (of) (with secondary fire)
W40.9 — *continued*
butane W40.1
caused by other person X96.9
coal gas W40.1
detonator W40.0
dump (munitions) W40.8
dynamite W40.0
  in
    assault X96.8
    homicide (attempt) X96.8
    legal intervention
      injuring
        bystander Y35.112
        law enforcement personnel Y35.111
        suspect Y35.113
    suicide (attempt) X75
explosive (material) W40.9
  gas W40.1
  in blasting operation W40.0
  specified NEC W40.8
    in
      assault X96.8
      homicide (attempt) X96.8
      legal intervention
        injuring
          bystander Y35.192
          law enforcement personnel Y35.191
          suspect Y35.193
      suicide (attempt) X75
factory (munitions) W40.8
fertilizer bomb W40.8
  assault X96.3
  homicide (attempt) X96.3
  suicide (attempt) X75
fire-damp W40.1
firearm (parts) NEC W34.19
  airgun W34.110
  BB gun W34.110
  gas, air or spring-operated gun NEC W34.118
  hangun W32.1
  hunting rifle W33.12
  larger firearm W33.10
    specified NEC W33.19
  machine gun W33.13
  paintball gun W34.111
  pellet gun W34.110
  shotgun W33.11
  Very pistol [flare] W34.19
fireworks W39
gas (coal) (explosive) W40.1
  cylinder W36.9
    aerosol can W36.1
    air tank W36.2
    pressurized W36.3
    specified NEC W36.8
gasoline (fumes) (tank) not in moving motor vehicle W40.1
  bomb W40.8
    assault X96.1
    homicide (attempt) X96.1
    suicide (attempt) X75
  in motor vehicle — *see* Accident, transport, by type of vehicle
grain store W40.8
grenade W40.8
  in
    assault X96.8
    homicide (attempt) X96.8
    legal intervention
      injuring
        bystander Y35.192
        law enforcement personnel Y35.191
        suspect Y35.193
    suicide (attempt) X75
handgun (parts) — *see* Explosion, firearm, hangun (parts)

Explosion (accidental) (of) (with secondary fire)
W40.9 — *continued*
homicide (attempt) X96.9
  antipersonnel bomb — *see* Explosion, antipersonnel bomb
  fertilizer bomb — *see* Explosion, fertilizer bomb
  gasoline bomb — *see* Explosion, gasoline bomb
  letter bomb — *see* Explosion, letter bomb
  pipe bomb — *see* Explosion, pipe bomb
  specified NEC X96.8
hose, pressurized W37.8
hot water heater, tank (in machinery) W35
  on watercraft — *see* Explosion, in, watercraft
in, on
  dump W40.8
  factory W40.8
  mine (of explosive gases) NEC W40.1
  watercraft V93.59
    powered craft V93.53
      ferry boat V93.51
      fishing boat V93.52
      jetskis V93.53
      liner V93.51
      merchant ship V93.50
      passenger ship V93.51
      sailboat V93.54
letter bomb W40.8
  assault X96.2
  homicide (attempt) X96.2
  suicide (attempt) X75
machinery — *see also* Contact, with, by type of machine
  on board watercraft — *see* Explosion, in, watercraft
  pressure vessel — *see* Explosion, by type of vessel
methane W40.1
mine W40.1
missile NEC W40.8
mortar bomb W40.8
  in
    assault X96.8
    homicide (attempt) X96.8
    legal intervention
      injuring
        bystander Y35.192
        law enforcement personnel Y35.191
        suspect Y35.193
    suicide (attempt) X75
munitions (dump) (factory) W40.8
pipe, pressurized W37.8
  bomb W40.8
    assault X96.4
    homicide (attempt) X96.4
    suicide (attempt) X75
pressure, pressurized
  cooker W38
  gas tank (in machinery) W36.3
  hose W37.8
  pipe W37.8
  specified device NEC W38
  tire W37.8
    bicycle W37.0
  vessel (in machinery) W38
propane W40.1
self-inflicted X75
shell (artillery) NEC W40.8
  during war operations — *see* War operations, explosion
  in
    legal intervention
      injuring
        bystander Y35.122
        law enforcement personnel Y35.121
        suspect Y35.123
  war — *see* War operations, explosion

Explosion (accidental) (of) (with secondary fire)
W40.9 — *continued*
spacecraft V95.45
stated as undetermined whether accidental or intentional Y25
steam or water lines (in machinery) W37.8
stove W40.9
suicide (attempt) X75
tire, pressurized W37.8
  bicycle W37.0
undetermined whether accidental or intentional Y25
vehicle tire NEC W37.8
  bicycle W37.0
war operations — *see* War operations, explosion

Exposure (to) X58
air pressure change — *see* Air, pressure
cold (accidental) (excessive) (extreme) (natural) (place) X31
  assault Y08.89
  due to
    man-made conditions W93.8
      dry ice (contact) W93.01
        inhalation W93.02
      liquid air (contact) (hydrogen) (nitrogen) W93.11
        inhalation W93.12
      refrigeration unit (deep freeze) W93.2
    suicide (attempt) X83.2
    weather (conditions) X31
  homicide (attempt) Y08.89
  self-inflicted X83.2
due to abandonment or neglect X58
electric current W86.8
  appliance (faulty) W86.8
    domestic W86.0
  caused by other person Y08.89
  conductor (faulty) W86.1
  control apparatus (faulty) W86.1
  electric power generating plant, distribution station W86.1
  electroshock gun — *see* Exposure, electric current, taser
  high-voltage cable W85
  homicide (attempt) Y08.89
  legal execution — *see* Legal, intervention, specified means NEC
  lightning — *see* subcategory T75.0
  live rail W86.8
  misadventure in medical or surgical procedure in electroshock therapy Y63.4
  motor (electric) (faulty) W86.8
    domestic W86.0
    self-inflicted X83.1
  specified NEC W86.8
    domestic W86.0
  stun gun — *see* Exposure, electric current, taser
  suicide (attempt) X83.1
  taser W86.8
    assault Y08.89
    legal intervention — *see* category Y35
    self-harm (intentional) X83.8
    undetermined intent Y33
  third rail W86.8
  transformer (faulty) W86.1
  transmission lines W85
environmental tobacco smoke X58
excessive
  cold — *see* Exposure, cold
  heat (natural) NEC X30
    man-made W92
factor(s) NOS X58
  environmental NEC X58
    man-made NEC W99
    natural NEC — *see* Forces of nature
  specified NEC X58

EXTERNAL CAUSES

EXTERNAL CAUSES

Exposure (to) X58— *continued*
fire, flames (accidental) X08.8
  assault X97
  campfire — *see* Exposure, fire, controlled,
    not in building
  controlled (in)
    with ignition (of) clothing (*see also* Ignition,
      clothes) X06.2
      nightwear X05
    bonfire — *see* Exposure, fire, controlled,
      not in building
    brazier (in building or structure) — *see also*
      Exposure, fire, controlled, building
      not in building or structure — *see*
        Exposure, fire, controlled, not in
        building
    building or structure X02.0
      with
        fall from building X02.3
        from building X02.5
        injury due to building collapse X02.2
        smoke inhalation X02.1
      hit by object from building X02.4
      specified mode of injury NEC X02.8
    fireplace, furnace or stove — *see*
      Exposure, fire, controlled, building
    not in building or structure X03.0
      with
        fall X03.3
        smoke inhalation X03.1
      hit by object X03.4
      specified mode of injury NEC X03.8
    trash — *see* Exposure, fire, controlled, not
      in building
  fireplace — *see* Exposure, fire, controlled,
    building
  fittings or furniture (in building or structure)
    (uncontrolled) — *see* Exposure, fire,
    uncontrolled, building
  forest (uncontrolled) — *see* Exposure, fire,
    uncontrolled, not in building
  grass (uncontrolled) — *see* Exposure, fire,
    uncontrolled, not in building
  hay (uncontrolled) — *see* Exposure, fire,
    uncontrolled, not in building
  homicide (attempt) X97
  ignition of highly flammable material X04
  in, of, on, starting in
    machinery — *see* Contact, with, by type of
      machine
    motor vehicle (in motion) (*see also*
      Accident, transport, occupant by type
      of vehicle) V87.8
      with collision — *see* Collision
    railway rolling stock, train, vehicle V81.81
      with collision — *see* Accident, transport,
        railway vehicle occupant
    street car (in motion) V82.8
      with collision — *see* Accident, transport,
        streetcar occupant
    transport vehicle NEC — *see also* Accident,
      transport
      with collision — *see* Collision
    war operations — *see also* War operations,
      fire
      from nuclear explosion — *see* War
        operations, nuclear weapons

Exposure (to) X58— *continued*
fire, flames (accidental) X08.8 — *continued*
  in, of, on, starting in — *continued*
    watercraft (in transit) (not in transit)
      V91.09
      localized — *see* Burn, on board
        watercraft, due to, fire on board
      powered craft V91.03
        ferry boat V91.01
        fishing boat V91.02
        jet skis V91.03
        liner V91.01
        merchant ship V91.00
        passenger ship V91.01
      unpowered craft V91.08
        canoe V91.05
        inflatable V91.06
        kayak V91.05
        sailboat V91.04
        surfboard V91.08
        waterskis V91.07
        windsurfer V91.08
  lumber (uncontrolled) — *see* Exposure, fire,
    uncontrolled, not in building
  mine (uncontrolled) — *see* Exposure, fire,
    uncontrolled, not in building
  prairie (uncontrolled) — *see* Exposure, fire,
    uncontrolled, not in building
  resulting from
    explosion — *see* Explosion
    lightning X08.8
  self-inflicted X76
  specified NEC X08.8
  started by other person X97
  stated as undetermined whether accidental
    or intentional Y26
  stove — *see* Exposure, fire, controlled,
    building
  suicide (attempt) X76
  tunnel (uncontrolled) — *see* Exposure, fire,
    uncontrolled, not in building
  uncontrolled
    in building or structure X00.0
      with
        fall from building X00.3
        injury due to building collapse X00.2
        jump from building X00.5
        smoke inhalation X00.1
      bed X08.00
        due to
          cigarette X08.01
          specified material NEC X08.09
      furniture NEC X08.20
        due to
          cigarette X08.21
          specified material NEC X08.29
      hit by object from building X00.4
      sofa X08.10
        due to
          cigarette X08.11
          specified material NEC X08.19
      specified mode of injury NEC X00.8
    not in building or structure (any) X01.0
      with
        fall X01.3
        smoke inhalation X01.1
      hit by object X01.4
      specified mode of injury NEC X01.8
  undetermined whether accidental or
    intentional Y26
forces of nature NEC — *see* Forces of nature
G-forces (abnormal) W49.9
gravitational forces (abnormal) W49.9
heat (natural) NEC — *see* Heat
high-pressure jet (hydraulic) (pneumatic)
  W49.9
hydraulic jet W49.9
inanimate mechanical force W49.9

Exposure (to) X58— *continued*
jet, high-pressure (hydraulic) (pneumatic)
  W49.9
lightning — *see* subcategory T75.0
  causing fire — *see* Exposure, fire
mechanical forces NEC W49.9
  animate NEC W64
  inanimate NEC W49.9
noise W42.9
  supersonic W42.0
noxious substance — *see* Table of Drugs and
  Chemicals
pneumatic jet W49.9
prolonged in deep-freeze unit or refrigerator
  W93.2
radiation — *see* Radiation
smoke — *see also* Exposure, fire
  tobacco, second hand Z77.22
specified factors NEC X58
sunlight X32
  man-made (sun lamp) W89.8
    tanning bed W89.1
supersonic waves W42.0
transmission line(s), electric W85
vibration W49.9
waves
  infrasound W49.9
  sound W42.9
  supersonic W42.0
weather NEC — *see* Forces of nature
External cause status Y99.9
child assisting in compensated work for family
  Y99.8
civilian activity done for financial or other
  compensation Y99.0
civilian activity done for income or pay Y99.0
family member assisting in compensated work
  for other family member Y99.8
hobby not done for income Y99.8
leisure activity Y99.8
military activity Y99.1
off-duty activity of military personnel Y99.8
recreation or sport not for income or while a
  student Y99.8
specified NEC Y99.8
student activity Y99.8
volunteer activity Y99.2

F

Factors, supplemental
  alcohol
    blood level
      100-119mg/100ml Y90.5
      120-199mg/100ml Y90.6
      20-39mg/100ml Y90.1
      200-239mg/100ml Y90.7
      240mg/100ml or more Y90.8
      40-59mg/100ml Y90.2
      60-79mg/100ml Y90.3
      80-99mg/100ml Y90.4
      less than 20mg/100ml Y90.0
      presence in blood, level not specified
        Y90.9
      presence in blood, but level not specified
        Y90.9
    environmental-pollution-related condition —
      see Z57
    nosocomial condition Y95
    work-related condition Y99.0
Failure
  in suture or ligature during surgical procedure
    Y65.2
  mechanical, of instrument or apparatus (any)
    (during any medical or surgical
    procedure) Y65.8
  sterile precautions (during medical and
    surgical care) — see Misadventure, failure,
    sterile precautions, by type ofprocedure
  to
    introduce tube or instrument Y65.4
      endotracheal tube during anesthesia
        Y65.3
    make curve (transport vehicle) NEC —
      Accident, transport
    remove tube or instrument Y65.4
Fall, falling (accidental) W19
  building W20.1
    burning (uncontrolled fire) X00.3
  down
    embankment W17.81
    escalator W10.0
    hill W17.81
    ladder W11
    ramp W10.2
    stairs, steps W10.9
  due to
    bumping against
      object W18.00
        sharp glass W18.02
        specified NEC W18.09
        sports equipment W18.01
      person W03
        due to ice or snow W00.0
        on pedestrian conveyance — see
          Accident, transport, pedestrian,
          conveyance
    collision with another person W03
      due to ice or snow W00.0
      involving pedestrian conveyance — see
        Accident, transport, pedestrian,
        conveyance
    grocery cart tipping over W17.82
    ice or snow W00.9
      from one level to another W00.2
      on stairs or steps W00.1
      involving pedestrian conveyance — see
        Accident, transport, pedestrian,
        conveyance
      on same level W00.0

Fall, falling (accidental) W19 — continued
  due to — continued
    slipping (on moving sidewalk) W01.0
      with subsequent striking against object
        W01.10
        furniture W01.190
        sharp object W01.119
          glass W01.110
          power tool or machine W01.111
          specified NEC W01.118
        specified NEC W01.198
    striking against
      object W18.00
        sharp glass W18.02
        specified NEC W18.09
        sports equipment W18.01
      person W03
        due to ice or snow W00.0
        on pedestrian conveyance — see
          Accident, transport, pedestrian,
          conveyance
  earth (with asphyxia or suffocation (by
    pressure)) — see Earth, falling
  from, off, out of
    aircraft NEC (with accident to aircraft NEC)
      V97.0
      while boarding or alighting V97.1
    balcony W13.0
    bed W06
    boat, ship, watercraft NEC (with drowning
      or submersion) — see Drowning, due to,
      fall overboard
      with hitting bottom or object V94.0
    bridge W13.1
    building W13.9
      burning (uncontrolled fire) X00.3
    cavity W17.2
    chair W07
    cherry picker W17.89
    cliff W15
    dock W17.4
    embankment W17.81
    escalator W10.0
    flagpole W13.8
    furniture NEC W08
    grocery cart W17.82
    haystack W17.89
    high place NEC W17.89
      stated as undetermined whether accidental
        or intentional Y30
    hole W17.2
    incline W10.2
    ladder W11
    lifting device W17.89
    machine, machinery — see also Contact,
      with, by type of machine
      not in operation W17.89
    manhole W17.1
    mobile elevated work platform [MEWP]
      W17.89
    motorized mobility scooter W05.2
    one level to another NEC W17.89
      intentional, purposeful, suicide (attempt)
        X80
      stated as undetermined whether accidental
        or intentional Y30
    pit W17.2
    playground equipment W09.8
      jungle gym W09.2
      slide W09.0
      swing W09.1
    quarry W17.89
    railing W13.9
    ramp W10.2
    roof W13.2
    scaffolding W12
    scooter (nonmotorized) W05.1
      motorized mobility W05.2

Fall, falling (accidental) W19 — continued
  from, off, out of — continued
    sky lift W17.89
    stairs, steps W10.9
      curb W10.1
      due to ice or snow W00.1
      escalator W10.0
      incline W10.2
      ramp W10.2
      sidewalk curb W10.1
      specified NEC W10.8
    stepladder W11
    storm drain W17.1
    streetcar NEC V82.6
      with antecedent collision — see Accident,
        transport, streetcar occupant
      while boarding or alighting V82.4
    structure NEC W13.8
      burning (uncontrolled fire) X00.3
    table W08
    toilet W18.11
      with subsequent striking against object
        W18.12
    train NEC V81.6
      during derailment (without antecedent
        collision) V81.7
      with antecedent collision — see
        Accident, transport, railway vehicle
        occupant
      while boarding or alighting V81.4
    transport vehicle after collision — see
      Accident, transport, by type of vehicle,
      collision
    tree W14
    vehicle (in motion) NEC (see also Accident,
      transport) V89.9
      motor NEC (see also Accident, transport,
        occupant, by type of vehicle) V87.8
      stationary W17.89
        while boarding or alighting — see
          Accident, transport, by type of
          vehicle, while boarding or alighting
    viaduct W13.8
    wall W13.8
    watercraft — see also Drowning, due to, fall
      overboard
      with hitting bottom or object V94.0
    well W17.0
    wheelchair, non-moving W05.0
      powered — see Accident, transport,
        pedestrian, conveyance occupant,
        specified type NEC
    window W13.4
  in, on
    aircraft NEC V97.0
      with accident to aircraft V97.0
      while boarding or alighting V97.1
    bathtub (empty) W18.2
      filled W16.212
        causing drowning W16.211
    escalator W10.0
    incline W10.2
    ladder W11
    machine, machinery — see Contact, with, by
      type of machine
    object, edged, pointed or sharp (with cut) —
      see Fall, by type
    playground equipment W09.8
      jungle gym W09.2
      slide W09.0
      swing W09.1
    ramp W10.2
    scaffolding W12
    shower W18.2
      causing drowning W16.211

EXTERNAL CAUSES

Fall, falling (accidental) W19 — *continued*
  in, on — *continued*
    staircase, stairs, steps W10.9
      curb W10.1
      due to ice or snow W00.1
      escalator W10.0
      incline W10.2
      specified NEC W10.8
    streetcar (without antecedent collision) V82.5
      with antecedent collision — *see* Accident,
        transport, streetcar occupant
      while boarding or alighting V82.4
    train (without antecedent collision) V81.5
      with antecedent collision — *see* Accident,
        transport, railway vehicle occupant
      during derailment (without antecedent
        collision) V81.7
        with antecedent collision — *see*
          Accident, transport, railway vehicle
          occupant
      while boarding or alighting V81.4
    transport vehicle after collision — *see*
      Accident, transport, by type of vehicle,
      collision
    watercraft V93.39
      due to
        accident to craft V91.29
          powered craft V91.23
            ferry boat V91.21
            fishing boat V91.22
            jetskis V91.23
            liner V91.21
            merchant ship V91.20
            passenger ship V91.21
          unpowered craft
            canoe V91.25
            inflatable V91.26
            kayak V91.25
            sailboat V91.24
        powered craft V93.33
          ferry boat V93.31
          fishing boat V93.32
          jetskis V93.33
          liner V93.31
          merchant ship V93.30
          passenger ship V93.31
        unpowered craft V93.38
          canoe V93.35
          inflatable V93.36
          kayak V93.35
          sailboat V93.34
          surfboard V93.38
          windsurfer V93.38
  into
    cavity W17.2
    dock W17.4
    fire — *see* Exposure, fire, by type
    haystack W17.89
    hole W17.2
    lake — *see* Fall, into, water
    manhole W17.1
    moving part of machinery — *see* Contact,
      with, by type of machine
    ocean — *see* Fall, into, water
    opening in surface NEC W17.89
    pit W17.2
    pond — *see* Fall, into, water
    quarry W17.89
    river — *see* Fall, into, water
    shaft W17.89
    storm drain W17.1
    stream — *see* Fall, into, water
    swimming pool — *see also* Fall, into, water,
      in, swimming pool
      empty W17.3
    tank W17.89

Fall, falling (accidental) W19 — *continued*
  into — *continued*
    water W16.42
      causing drowning W16.41
      from watercraft — *see* Drowning, due to,
        fall overboard
      hitting diving board W21.4
      in
        bathtub W16.212
          causing drowning W16.211
        bucket W16.222
          causing drowning W16.221
        natural body of water W16.112
          causing drowning W16.111
          striking
            bottom W16.122
              causing drowning W16.121
            side W16.132
              causing drowning W16.131
        specified water NEC W16.312
          causing drowning W16.311
          striking
            bottom W16.322
              causing drowning W16.321
            wall W16.332
              causing drowning W16.331
        swimming pool W16.012
          causing drowning W16.011
          striking
            bottom W16.022
              causing drowning W16.021
            wall W16.032
              causing drowning W16.031
        utility bucket W16.222
          causing drowning W16.221
      well W17.0
  involving
    bed W06
    chair W07
    furniture NEC W08
    glass — *see* Fall, by type
    playground equipment W09.8
      jungle gym W09.2
      slide W09.0
      swing W09.1
    roller blades — *see* Accident, transport,
      pedestrian, conveyance
    skateboard(s) — *see* Accident, transport,
      pedestrian, conveyance
    skates (ice) (in line) (roller) — *see* Accident,
      transport, pedestrian, conveyance
    skis — *see* Accident, transport, pedestrian,
      conveyance
    table W08
    wheelchair, non-moving W05.0
      powered — *see* Accident, transport,
        pedestrian, conveyance, specified type
        NEC
  object — *see* Struck by, object, falling
  off
    toilet W18.11
      with subsequent striking against object
        W18.12
  on same level W18.30
    due to
      specified NEC W18.39
      stepping on an object W18.31
  out of
    bed W06
    building NEC W13.8
    chair W07
    furniture NEC W08
    wheelchair, non-moving W05.0
      powered — *see* Accident, transport,
        pedestrian, conveyance, specified type
        NEC
    window W13.4

Fall, falling (accidental) W19 — *continued*
  over
    animal W01.0
    cliff W15
    embankment W17.81
    small object W01.0
    rock W20.8
    same level W18.30
      from
        being crushed, pushed, or stepped on by
          a crowd or human stampede W52
        collision, pushing, shoving, by or with
          other person W03
        slipping, stumbling, tripping W01.0
      involving ice or snow W00.0
      involving skates (ice) (roller), skateboard,
        skis — *see* Accident, transport,
        pedestrian, conveyance
    snowslide (avalanche) — *see* Landslide
    stone W20.8
    structure W20.1
      burning (uncontrolled fire) X00.3
    through
      bridge W13.1
      floor W13.3
      roof W13.2
      wall W13.8
      window W13.4
    timber W20.8
    tree (caused by lightning) W20.8
    while being carried or supported by other
      person(s) W04
Fallen on by
  animal (not being ridden) NEC W55.89
Felo-de-se — *see* Suicide
Fight (hand) (fists) (foot) — *see* Assault, fight
Fire (accidental) — *see* Exposure, fire
Firearm discharge — *see* Discharge, firearm
**Fireball effects from nuclear explosion in
    war operations** — *see* War operations,
    nuclear weapons
Fireworks (explosion) W39
Flash burns from explosion — *see* Explosion
Flood (any injury) (caused by) X38
  collapse of man-made structure causing earth
    movement X36.0
  tidal wave — *see* Forces of nature, tidal wave
Food (any type) in
  air passages (with asphyxia, obstruction, or
    suffocation) — *see* categories T17 and T18
  alimentary tract causing asphyxia (due to
    compression of trachea) — *see* categories
    T17 and T18
Forces of nature X39.8
  avalanche X36.1
    causing transport accident — *see* Accident,
      transport, by type of vehicle
  blizzard X37.2
  cataclysmic storm X37.9
    with flood X38
    blizzard X37.2
    cloudburst X37.8
    cyclone X37.1
    dust storm X37.3
    hurricane X37.0
    specified storm NEC X37.8
    storm surge X37.0
    tornado X37.1
    twister X37.1
    typhoon X37.0
  cloudburst X37.8
  cold (natural) X31
  cyclone X37.1
  dam collapse causing earth movement X36.0
  dust storm X37.3
  earth movement X36.1
    caused by dam or structure collapse X36.0
    earthquake X34

EXTERNAL CAUSES

Forces of nature X39.8 — *continued*
 earthquake X34
 flood (caused by) X38
  dam collapse X36.0
  tidal wave — *see* Forces of nature, tidal
   wave
 heat (natural) X30
 hurricane X37.0
 landslide X36.1
  causing transport accident — *see* Accident,
   transport, by type of vehicle
 lightning — *see* subcategory T75.0
  causing fire — *see* Exposure, fire
 mudslide X36.1
  causing transport accident — *see* Accident,
   transport, by type of vehicle
 radiation (natural) X39.08
  radon X39.01
 radon X39.01
 specified force NEC X39.8
 storm surge X37.0
 structure collapse causing earth movement
   X36.0
 sunlight X32
 tidal wave X37.41
  due to
   earthquake X37.41
   landslide X37.43
   storm X37.42
   volcanic eruption X37.41
 tornado X37.1
 tsunami X37.41
 twister X37.1
 typhoon X37.0
 volcanic eruption X35
Foreign body
 aspiration — *see* Index to Diseases and
  Injuries, Foreign body, respiratory tract
 embedded in skin W45
 entering through skin W45.8
  can lid W26.8
  nail W45.0
  paper W26.2
  specified NEC W45.8
  splinter W45.8
Forest fire (exposure to) — *see* Exposure, fire,
  uncontrolled, not in building
Found injured X58
 from exposure (to) — *see* Exposure
 on
  highway, road(way), street V89.9
  railway right of way V81.9
Fracture (circumstances unknown or
  unspecified) X58
 due to specified cause NEC X58
Freezing — *see* Exposure, cold
Frostbite X31
 due to man-made conditions — *see* Exposure,
  cold, man-made
Frozen — *see* Exposure, cold

G

Gored by bull W55.22
Gunshot wound W34.00

H

Hailstones, injured by X39.8
Hanged herself or himself — *see* Hanging,
 self-inflicted
Hanging (accidental) (*see also* category) T71
 legal execution — *see* Legal, intervention,
  specified means NEC
Heat (effects of) (excessive) X30
 due to
  man-made conditions W92
   on board watercraft V93.29
    fishing boat V93.22
    merchant ship V93.20
    passenger ship V93.21
    sailboat V93.24
    specified powered craft NEC V93.23
  weather (conditions) X30
 from
  electric heating apparatus causing burning
   X16
  nuclear explosion in war operations — *see*
   War operations, nuclear weapons
  inappropriate in local application or packing
   in medical or surgical procedure Y63.5
Hemorrhage
 delayed following medical or surgical
  treatment without mention of misadventure
  — *see* Index to Diseases and Injuries,
  Complication(s)
 during medical or surgical treatment as
  misadventure — *see* Index to Diseases and
  Injuries, Complication(s)
High
 altitude (effects) — *see* Air, pressure, low
 level of radioactivity, effects — *see* Radiation
 pressure (effects) — *see* Air, pressure, high
 temperature, effects — *see* Heat
Hit, hitting (accidental) by — *see* Struck by
Hitting against — *see* Striking against
Homicide (attempt) (justifiable) — *see* Assault
Hot
 place, effects — *see also* Heat
 weather, effects X30
House fire (uncontrolled) — *see* Exposure, fire,
  uncontrolled, building
Humidity, causing problem X39.8
Hunger X58
Hurricane (any injury) X37.0
Hypobarism, hypobaropathy — *see* Air,
  pressure, low

I

EXTERNAL CAUSES

Ictus
caloris — *see also* Heat
solaris X30

Ignition (accidental) (*see also* Exposure, fire)
X08.8
anesthetic gas in operating room W40.1
apparel X06.2
from highly flammable material X04
nightwear X05
bed linen (sheets) (spreads) (pillows) (mattress)
— *see* Exposure, fire, uncontrolled,
building, bed
benzine X04
clothes, clothing NEC (from controlled fire)
X06.2
from
highly flammable material X04
ether X04
in operating room W40.1
explosive material — *see* Explosion
gasoline X04
jewelry (plastic) (any) X06.0
kerosene X04
material
explosive — *see* Explosion
highly flammable with secondary explosion
X04
nightwear X05
paraffin X04
petrol X04
Immersion (accidental) — *see also* Drowning
hand or foot due to cold (excessive) X31
Implantation of quills of porcupine
W55.89
Inanition (from) (hunger) X58
thirst X58
Inappropriate operation performed
correct operation on wrong side or body part
(wrong side) (wrong site) Y65.53
operation intended for another patient done
on wrong patient Y65.52
wrong operation performed on correct patient
Y65.51
Inattention after, at birth (homicidal intent)
(infanticidal intent) X58
Incident, adverse
device
anesthesiology Y70.8
accessory Y70.2
diagnostic Y70.0
miscellaneous Y70.8
monitoring Y70.0
prosthetic Y70.2
rehabilitative Y70.1
surgical Y70.3
therapeutic Y70.1
cardiovascular Y71.8
accessory Y71.2
diagnostic Y71.0
miscellaneous Y71.8
monitoring Y71.0
prosthetic Y71.2
rehabilitative Y71.1
surgical Y71.3
therapeutic Y71.1
gastroenterology Y73.8
accessory Y73.2
diagnostic Y73.0
miscellaneous Y73.8
monitoring Y73.0
prosthetic Y73.2
rehabilitative Y73.1
surgical Y73.3
therapeutic Y73.1

Incident, adverse — *continued*
device — *continued*
general
hospital Y74.8
accessory Y74.2
diagnostic Y74.0
miscellaneous Y74.8
monitoring Y74.0
prosthetic Y74.2
rehabilitative Y74.1
surgical Y74.3
therapeutic Y74.1
surgical Y81.8
accessory Y81.2
diagnostic Y81.0
miscellaneous Y81.8
monitoring Y81.0
prosthetic Y81.2
rehabilitative Y81.1
surgical Y81.3
therapeutic Y81.1
gynecological Y76.8
accessory Y76.2
diagnostic Y76.0
miscellaneous Y76.8
monitoring Y76.0
prosthetic Y76.2
rehabilitative Y76.1
surgical Y76.3
therapeutic Y76.1
medical Y82.9
specified type NEC Y82.8
neurological Y75.8
accessory Y75.2
diagnostic Y75.0
miscellaneous Y75.8
monitoring Y75.0
prosthetic Y75.2
rehabilitative Y75.1
surgical Y75.3
therapeutic Y75.1
obstetrical Y76.8
accessory Y76.2
diagnostic Y76.0
miscellaneous Y76.8
monitoring Y76.0
prosthetic Y76.2
rehabilitative Y76.1
surgical Y76.3
therapeutic Y76.1
ophthalmic Y77.8
accessory Y77.2
diagnostic Y77.0
miscellaneous Y77.8
monitoring Y77.0
prosthetic Y77.2
rehabilitative Y77.1
surgical Y77.3
therapeutic Y77.1
orthopedic Y79.8
accessory Y79.2
diagnostic Y79.0
miscellaneous Y79.8
monitoring Y79.0
prosthetic Y79.2
rehabilitative Y79.1
surgical Y79.3
therapeutic Y79.1
otorhinolaryngological Y72.8
accessory Y72.2
diagnostic Y72.0
miscellaneous Y72.8
monitoring Y72.0
prosthetic Y72.2
rehabilitative Y72.1
surgical Y72.3
therapeutic Y72.1

Incident, adverse — *continued*
device — *continued*
personal use Y74.8
accessory Y74.2
diagnostic Y74.0
miscellaneous Y74.8
monitoring Y74.0
prosthetic Y74.2
rehabilitative Y74.1
surgical Y74.3
therapeutic Y74.1
physical medicine Y80.8
accessory Y80.2
diagnostic Y80.0
miscellaneous Y80.8
monitoring Y80.0
prosthetic Y80.2
rehabilitative Y80.1
surgical Y80.3
therapeutic Y80.1
plastic surgical Y81.8
accessory Y81.2
diagnostic Y81.0
miscellaneous Y81.8
monitoring Y81.0
prosthetic Y81.2
rehabilitative Y81.1
surgical Y81.3
therapeutic Y81.1
radiological Y78.8
accessory Y78.2
diagnostic Y78.0
miscellaneous Y78.8
monitoring Y78.0
prosthetic Y78.2
rehabilitative Y78.1
surgical Y78.3
therapeutic Y78.1
urology Y73.8
accessory Y73.2
diagnostic Y73.0
miscellaneous Y73.8
monitoring Y73.0
prosthetic Y73.2
rehabilitative Y73.1
surgical Y73.3
therapeutic Y73.1
Incineration (accidental) — *see* Exposure, fire
Infanticide — *see* Assault
Infrasound waves (causing injury) W49.9
Ingestion
foreign body (causing injury) (with obstruction)
— *see* Foreign body, alimentary canal
poisonous
plant(s) X58
substance NEC — *see* Table of Drugs and
Chemicals
Inhalation
excessively cold substance, man-made — *see*
Exposure, cold, man-made
food (any type) (into respiratory tract) (with
asphyxia, obstruction respiratory tract,
suffocation) — *see* categories T17 and T18
foreign body — *see* Foreign body, aspiration
gastric contents (with asphyxia, obstruction
respiratory passage, suffocation) T17.81-
hot air or gases X14.0
liquid air, hydrogen, nitrogen W93.12
suicide (attempt) X83.2
steam X13.0
assault X98.0
stated as undetermined whether accidental
or intentional Y27.0
suicide (attempt) X77.0
toxic gas — *see* Table of Drugs and Chemicals
vomitus (with asphyxia, obstruction respiratory
passage, suffocation) T17.81-

Injury, injured (accidental(ly)) NOS X58
  by, caused by, from
    assault — *see* Assault
    law-enforcing agent, police, in course of
      legal intervention — *see* Legal
      intervention
    suicide (attempt) X83.8
  due to, in
    civil insurrection — *see* War operations
    fight (*see also* Assault, fight) Y04.0
    war operations — *see* War operations
  homicide (*see also* Assault) Y09
  inflicted (by)
    in course of arrest (attempted), suppression
      of disturbance, maintenance of order, by
      law-enforcing agents — *see* Legal
      intervention
    other person
      stated as
        accidental X58
        intentional, homicide (attempt) — *see*
          Assault
        undetermined whether accidental or
          intentional Y33
    purposely (inflicted) by other person(s) — *see*
      Assault
    self-inflicted X83.8
      stated as accidental X58
    specified cause NEC X58
    undetermined whether accidental or intentional
      Y33
Insolation, effects X30
Insufficient nourishment X58
Interruption of respiration (by)
  food (lodged in esophagus) — *see* categories
    T17 and T18
  vomitus (lodged in esophagus) T17.81-
Intervention, legal — *see* Legal intervention
Intoxication
  drug — *see* Table of Drugs and Chemicals
  poison — *see* Table of Drugs and Chemicals

J

Jammed (accidentally)
  between objects (moving) (stationary and
    moving) W23.0
  stationary W23.1
Jumped, jumping
  before moving object NEC X81.8
    motor vehicle X81.0
    subway train X81.1
    train X81.1
    undetermined whether accidental or
      intentional Y31
  from
    boat (into water) voluntarily, without
      accident (to or on boat) W16.712
      with
        accident to or on boat — *see* Accident,
          watercraft
        drowning or submersion W16.711
          suicide (attempt) X71.3
        striking bottom W16.722
          causing drowning W16.721
    building (*see also* Jumped, from, high place)
      W13.9
      burning (uncontrolled fire) X00.5
    high place NEC W17.89
      suicide (attempt) X80
      undetermined whether accidental or
        intentional Y30
    structure (*see also* Jumped, from, high place)
      W13.9
      burning (uncontrolled fire) X00.5
  into water W16.92
    causing drowning W16.91
    from, off watercraft — *see* Jumped, from,
      boat
    in
      natural body W16.612
        causing drowning W16.611
        striking bottom W16.622
          causing drowning W16.621
      specified place NEC W16.812
        causing drowning W16.811
        striking
          bottom W16.822
            causing drowning W16.821
          wall W16.832
            causing drowning W16.831
      swimming pool W16.512
        causing drowning W16.511
        striking
          bottom W16.522
            causing drowning W16.521
          wall W16.532
            causing drowning W16.531
  suicide (attempt) X71.3

K

Kicked by
  animal NEC W55.82
  person(s) (accidentally) W50.1
    with intent to injure or kill Y04.0
    as, or caused by, a crowd or human
      stampede (with fall) W52
    assault Y04.0
    homicide (attempt) Y04.0
    in
      fight Y04.0
      legal intervention
        injuring
          bystander Y35.812
          law enforcement personnel Y35.811
          suspect Y35.813
Kicking
  against
    object W22.8
      sports equipment W21.9
    stationary W22.09
      sports equipment W21.89
    person — *see* Striking against, person
    sports equipment W21.9
  carpet stretcher with knee X50.3
Killed, killing (accidentally) NOS (*see also*
  Injury) X58
  in
    action — *see* War operations
    brawl, fight (hand) (fists) (foot) Y04.0
      by weapon — *see also* Assault
        cutting, piercing — *see* Assault, cutting
          or piercing instrument
        firearm — *see* Discharge, firearm, by
          type, homicide
  self
    stated as
      accident NOS X58
      suicide — *see* Suicide
      undetermined whether accidental or
        intentional Y33
Kneeling (prolonged) (static) X50.1
Knocked down (accidentally) (by) NOS X58
  animal (not being ridden) NEC — *see also*
    Struck by, by type of animal
  crowd or human stampede W52
  person W51
    in brawl, fight Y04.0
  transport vehicle NEC (*see also* Accident,
    transport) V09.9

L

Laceration NEC — *see* Injury
Lack of
  care (helpless person) (infant) (newborn) X58
  food except as result of abandonment or neglect X58
    due to abandonment or neglect X58
  water except as result of transport accident X58
    due to transport accident — *see* Accident, transport, by type
  helpless person, infant, newborn X58
Landslide (falling on transport vehicle) X36.1
  caused by collapse of man-made structure X36.0
Late effect — *see* Sequelae
Legal
  execution (any method) — *see* Legal, intervention
  intervention (by)
    baton — *see* Legal, intervention, blunt object, baton
    bayonet — *see* Legal, intervention, sharp object, bayonet
    blow — *see* Legal, intervention, manhandling
    blunt object
      baton
        injuring
          bystander Y35.312
          law enforcement personnel Y35.311
          suspect Y35.313
      injuring
        bystander Y35.302
        law enforcement personnel Y35.301
        suspect Y35.303
      specified NEC
        injuring
          bystander Y35.392
          law enforcement personnel Y35.391
          suspect Y35.393
      stave
        injuring
          bystander Y35.392
          law enforcement personnel Y35.391
          suspect Y35.393
    bomb — *see* Legal, intervention, explosive
    cutting or piercing instrument — *see* Legal, intervention, sharp object
    dynamite — *see* Legal, intervention, explosive, dynamite
    explosive(s)
      dynamite
        injuring
          bystander Y35.112
          law enforcement personnel Y35.111
          suspect Y35.113
      grenade
        injuring
          bystander Y35.192
          law enforcement personnel Y35.191
          suspect Y35.193
      injuring
        bystander Y35.102
        law enforcement personnel Y35.101
        suspect Y35.103
      mortar bomb
        injuring
          bystander Y35.192
          law enforcement personnel Y35.191
          suspect Y35.193
      shell
        injuring
          bystander Y35.122
          law enforcement personnel Y35.121
          suspect Y35.123

Legal — *continued*
  intervention (by) — *continued*
    explosive(s) — *continued*
      specified NEC
        injuring
          bystander Y35.192
          law enforcement personnel Y35.191
          suspect Y35.193
    firearm(s) (discharge)
      handgun
        injuring
          bystander Y35.022
          law enforcement personnel Y35.021
          suspect Y35.023
      injuring
        bystander Y35.002
        law enforcement personnel Y35.001
        suspect Y35.003
      machine gun
        injuring
          bystander Y35.012
          law enforcement personnel Y35.011
          suspect Y35.013
      rifle pellet
        injuring
          bystander Y35.032
          law enforcement personnel Y35.031
          suspect Y35.033
      rubber bullet
        injuring
          bystander Y35.042
          law enforcement personnel Y35.041
          suspect Y35.043
      shotgun — *see* Legal, intervention, firearm, specified NEC
      specified NEC
        injuring
          bystander Y35.092
          law enforcement personnel Y35.091
          suspect Y35.093
    gas (asphyxiation) (poisoning)
      injuring
        bystander Y35.202
        law enforcement personnel Y35.201
        suspect Y35.203
      specified NEC
        injuring
          bystander Y35.292
          law enforcement personnel Y35.291
          suspect Y35.293
      tear gas
        injuring
          bystander Y35.212
          law enforcement personnel Y35.211
          suspect Y35.213
    grenade — *see* Legal, intervention, explosive, grenade
    injuring
      bystander Y35.92
      law enforcement personnel Y35.91
      suspect Y35.93
    late effect (of) — *see* with 7th character S Y35
    manhandling
      injuring
        bystander Y35.812
        law enforcement personnel Y35.811
        suspect Y35.813
    sequelae (of) — *see* with 7th character S Y35
    sharp objects
      bayonet
        injuring
          bystander Y35.412
          law enforcement personnel Y35.411
          suspect Y35.413

Legal — *continued*
  intervention (by) — *continued*
    sharp objects — *continued*
      injuring
        bystander Y35.402
        law enforcement personnel Y35.401
        suspect Y35.403
      specified NEC
        injuring
          bystander Y35.492
          law enforcement personnel Y35.491
          suspect Y35.493
    specified means NEC
      injuring
        bystander Y35.892
        law enforcement personnel Y35.891
        suspect Y35.893
    stabbing — *see* Legal, intervention, sharp object
    stave — *see* Legal, intervention, blunt object, stave
    tear gas — *see* Legal, intervention, gas, tear gas
    truncheon — *see* Legal, intervention, blunt object, stave
Lifting — *see* Overexertion
  heavy objects X50.0
  weights X50.0
Lightning (shock) (stroke) (struck by) — *see* subcategory T75.0
  causing fire — *see* Exposure, fire
Loss of control (transport vehicle) NEC — *see* Accident, transport
Lost at sea NOS — *see* Drowning, due to, fall overboard
Low
  pressure (effects) — seeAir, pressure, low
  temperature (effects) — *see* Exposure, cold
Lying before train, vehicle or other moving object X81.8
  subway train X81.1
  train X81.1
  undetermined whether accidental or intentional Y31
Lynching — *see* Assault

M

Malfunction (mechanism or component) (of)
 firearm W34.10
  airgun W34.110
  BB gun W34.110
  gas, air or spring-operated gun NEC
   W34.118
  handgun W32.1
  hunting rifle W33.12
  larger firearm W33.10
   specified NEC W33.19
  machine gun W33.13
  paintball gun W34.111
  pellet gun W34.110
  shotgun W33.11
  specified NEC W34.19
  Very pistol [flare] W34.19
 handgun — *see* Malfunction, firearm, handgun
Maltreatment — *see* Perpetrator
Mangled (accidentally) NOS X58
Manhandling (in brawl, fight) Y04.0
 legal intervention — *see* Legal, intervention,
  manhandling
Manslaughter (nonaccidental) — *see* Assault
Mauled by animal NEC W55.89
Medical procedure, complication of
 (delayed or as an abnormal reaction without
  mention of misadventure) — *see* Complication
  of or following, by specified type of
  procedure
 due to or as a result of misadventure — *see*
  Misadventure
Melting (due to fire) — *see also* Exposure, fire
 apparel NEC X06.3
 clothes, clothing NEC X06.3
  nightwear X05
 fittings or furniture (burning building)
  (uncontrolled fire) X00.8
 nightwear X05
 plastic jewelry X06.1
Mental cruelty X58
Military operations (injuries to military and
 civilians occuring during peacetime on
 military property and during routine military
 exercises and operations) (by) (from)
 (involving) Y37.90-
 air blast Y37.20-
 aircraft
  destruction — *see* Military operations,
   destruction of aircraft
  airway restriction — *see* Military operations,
   restriction of airways
  asphyxiation — *see* Military operations,
   restriction of airways
 biological weapons Y37.6x-
 blast Y37.20-
 blast fragments Y37.20-
 blast wave Y37.20-
 blast wind Y37.20-
 bomb Y37.20-
  dirty Y37.50-
  gasoline Y37.31-
  incendiary Y37.31-
  petrol Y37.31-
 bullet Y37.43-
  incendiary Y37.32-
  rubber Y37.41-
 chemical weapons Y37.7x-
 combat
  hand to hand (unarmed) combat Y37.44-
  using blunt or piercing object Y37.45-
 conflagration — *see* Military operations, fire
 conventional warfare NEC Y37.49-
 depth-charge Y37.01-

Military operations (injuries to military and
 civilians occuring during peacetime on
 military property and during routine military
 exercises and operations) (by) (from)
 (involving) Y37.90- — *continued*
 destruction of aircraft Y37.10-
  due to
   air to air missile Y37.11-
   collision with other aircraft Y37.12-
   detonation (accidental) of onboard
    munitions and explosives Y37.14-
   enemy fire or explosives Y37.11-
   explosive placed on aircraft Y37.11-
   onboard fire Y37.13-
   rocket propelled grenade [RPG] Y37.11-
   small arms fire Y37.11-
   surface to air missile Y37.11-
  specified NEC Y37.19-
 detonation (accidental) of
  onboard marine weapons Y37.05-
  own munitions or munitions launch device
   Y37.24-
 dirty bomb Y37.50-
 explosion (of) Y37.20-
  aerial bomb Y37.21-
  bomb NOS (*see also* Military operations,
   bomb(s)) Y37.20-
  fragments Y37.20-
  grenade Y37.29-
  guided missile Y37.22-
  improvised explosive device [IED] (person-
   borne) (roadside) (vehicle-borne)
   Y37.23-
  land mine Y37.29-
  marine mine (at sea) (in harbor) Y37.02-
  marine weapon Y37.00-
   specified NEC Y37.09-
  own munitions or munitions launch device
   (accidental) Y37.24-
  sea-based artillery shell Y37.03-
  specified NEC Y37.29-
  torpedo Y37.04-
 fire Y37.30-
  specified NEC Y37.39-
 firearms
  discharge Y37.43-
  pellets Y37.42-
 flamethrower Y37.33-
 fragments (from) (of)
  improvised explosive device [IED] (person-
   borne) (roadside) (vehicle-borne)
   Y37.26-
  munitions Y37.25-
  specified NEC Y37.29-
  weapons Y37.27-
 friendly fire Y37.92-
 hand to hand (unarmed) combat Y37.44-
 hot substances — *see* Military operations, fire
 incendiary bullet Y37.32-
 nuclear weapon (effects of) Y37.50-
  acute radiation exposure Y37.54-
  blast pressure Y37.51-
  direct blast Y37.51-
  direct heat Y37.53-
  fallout exposure Y37.54-
  fireball Y37.53-
  indirect blast (struck or crushed by blast
   debris) (being thrown by blast) Y37.52-
  ionizing radiation (immediate exposure)
   Y37.54-
  nuclear radiation Y37.54-
  radiation
   ionizing (immediate exposure) Y37.54-
   nuclear Y37.54-
   thermal Y37.53-
  secondary effects Y37.54-
  specified NEC Y37.59-
  thermal radiation Y37.53-

Military operations (injuries to military and
 civilians occuring during peacetime on
 military property and during routine military
 exercises and operations) (by) (from)
 (involving) Y37.90- — *continued*
 restriction of air (airway)
  intentional Y37.46-
  unintentional Y37.47-
 rubber bullets Y37.41-
 shrapnel NOS Y37.29-
 suffocation — *see* Military operations,
  restriction of airways
 unconventional warfare NEC Y37.7x-
 underwater blast NOS Y37.00-
 warfare
  conventional NEC Y37.49-
  unconventional NEC Y37.7x-
 weapon of mass destruction [WMD] Y37.91-
 weapons
  biological weapons Y37.6x-
  chemical Y37.7x-
  nuclear (effects of) Y37.50-
   acute radiation exposure Y37.54-
   blast pressure Y37.51-
   direct blast Y37.51-
   direct heat Y37.53-
   fallout exposure Y37.54-
   fireball Y37.53-
   indirect blast (struck or crushed by blast
    debris) (being thrown by blast)
    Y37.52-
   radiation
    ionizing (immediate exposure) Y37.54-
    nuclear Y37.54-
    thermal Y37.53-
   secondary effects Y37.54-
   specified NEC Y37.59-
 of mass destruction [WMD] Y37.91-
**Misadventure(s) to patient(s) during
 surgical or medical care** Y69
 contaminated medical or biological substance
  (blood, drug, fluid) Y64.9
  administered (by) NEC Y64.9
   immunization Y64.1
   infusion Y64.0
   injection Y64.1
   specified means NEC Y64.8
   transfusion Y64.0
   vaccination Y64.1
 excessive amount of blood or other fluid
  during transfusion or infusion Y63.0
 failure
  in dosage Y63.9
   electroshock therapy Y63.4
   inappropriate temperature (too hot or too
    cold) in local application and packing
    Y63.5
   infusion
    excessive amount of fluid Y63.0
    incorrect dilution of fluid Y63.1
   insulin-shock therapy Y63.4
   nonadministration of necessary drug or
    biological substance Y63.6
   overdose — *see* Table of Drugs and
    Chemicals
    radiation, in therapy Y63.2
   radiation
    overdose Y63.2
   specified procedure NEC Y63.8
   transfusion
    excessive amount of blood Y63.0
  mechanical, of instrument or apparatus (any)
   (during any procedure) Y65.8
  sterile precautions (during procedure) Y62.9
   aspiration of fluid or tissue (by puncture or
    catheterization, except heart) Y62.6
   biopsy (except needle aspiration) Y62.8
    needle (aspirating) Y62.6
   blood sampling Y62.6

Misadventure(s) to patient(s) during surgical or medical care Y69 — *continued*
  failure — *continued*
    sterile precautions (during procedure) Y62.9 — *continued*
      catheterization Y62.6
        heart Y62.5
      dialysis (kidney) Y62.2
      endoscopic examination Y62.4
      enema Y62.8
      immunization Y62.3
      infusion Y62.1
      injection Y62.3
      needle biopsy Y62.6
      paracentesis (abdominal) (thoracic) Y62.6
      perfusion Y62.2
      puncture (lumbar) Y62.6
      removal of catheter or packing Y62.8
      specified procedure NEC Y62.8
      surgical operation Y62.0
      transfusion Y62.1
      vaccination Y62.3
    suture or ligature during surgical procedure Y65.2
    to introduce or to remove tube or instrument — *see* Failure, to
  hemorrhage — *see* Index to Diseases and Injuries, Complication(s)
  inadvertent exposure of patient to radiation Y63.3
  inappropriate
    operation performed — *see* Inappropriate operation performed
    temperature (too hot or too cold) in local application or packing Y63.5
  infusion (*see also* Misadventure, by type, infusion) Y69
    excessive amount of fluid Y63.0
    incorrect dilution of fluid Y63.1
    wrong fluid Y65.1
  mismatched blood in transfusion Y65.0
  nonadministration of necessary drug or biological substance Y63.6
  overdose — *see* Table of Drugs and Chemicals
  radiation (in therapy)
  perforation — *see* Index to Diseases and Injuries, Complication(s)
  performance of inappropriate operation — *see* Inappropriate operation performed
  puncture — *see* Index to Diseases and Injuries, Complication(s)
  specified type NEC Y65.8
    failure
      suture or ligature during surgical operation Y65.2
      to introduce or to remove tube or instrument — *see* Failure, to
    infusion of wrong fluid Y65.1
    performance of inappropriate operation — *see* Inappropriate operation performed
    transfusion of mismatched blood Y65.0
    wrong
      fluid in infusion Y65.1
      placement of endotracheal tube during anesthetic procedure Y65.3
  transfusion — *see* Misadventure, by type, transfusion
    excessive amount of blood Y63.0
    mismatched blood Y65.0
  wrong
    drug given in error — *see* Table of Drugs and Chemicals
    fluid in infusion Y65.1
    placement of endotracheal tube during anesthetic procedure Y65.3
Mismatched blood in transfusion Y65.0
Motion sickness T75.3
Mountain sickness W94.11
Mudslide (of cataclysmic nature) — *see* Landslide

Murder (attempt) — *see* Assault

N

Nail
  contact with W45.0
    gun W29.4
  embedded in skin W45.0
Neglect (criminal) (homicidal intent) X58
Noise (causing injury) (pollution) W42.9
  supersonic W42.0
Nonadministration (of)
  drug or biological substance (necessary) Y63.6
  surgical and medical care Y66
Nosocomial condition Y95

O

Object
  falling
    from, in, on, hitting
      machinery — *see* Contact, with, by type of machine
    set in motion by
      accidental explosion or rupture of pressure vessel W38
      firearm — *see* Discharge, firearm, by type
      machine(ry) — *see* Contact, with, by type of machine
Overdose (drug) — *see* Table of Drugs and Chemicals
  radiation Y63.2
Overexertion X50.9
  from
    prolonged static or awkward postures X50.1
    repetitive movements X50.3
    specified strenuous movements or postures NEC X50.9
    strenuous movement or load X50.0
Overexposure (accidental) (to)
  cold (*see also* Exposure, cold) X31
    due to man-made conditions — *see* Exposure, cold, man-made
  heat (*see also* Heat) X30
  radiation — *see* Radiation
  radioactivity W88.0
  sun (sunburn) X32
  weather NEC — *see* Forces of nature
  wind NEC — *see* Forces of nature
Overheated — *see* Heat
Overturning (accidental)
  machinery — *see* Contact, with, by type of machine
  transport vehicle NEC (*see also* Accident, transport) V89.9
  watercraft (causing drowning, submersion) — *see also* Drowning, due to, accident to, watercraft, overturning
    causing injury except drowning or submersion — *see* Accident, watercraft, causing, injury NEC

P

Parachute descent (voluntary) (without accident to aircraft) V97.29
  due to accident to aircraft — *see* Accident, transport, aircraft
Pecked by bird W61.99
Perforation during medical or surgical treatment as misadventure — *see* Index to Diseases and Injuries, Complication(s)
Perpetrator, perpetration, of assault, maltreatment and neglect (by) Y07.9
  boyfriend Y07.03
  brother Y07.410
    stepbrother Y07.435
  coach Y07.53
  cousin
    female Y07.491
    male Y07.490
  daycare provider Y07.519
    at-home
      adult care Y07.512
      childcare Y07.510
    care center
      adult care Y07.513
      childcare Y07.511
  family member NEC Y07.499
  father Y07.11
    adoptive Y07.13
    foster Y07.420
    stepfather Y07.430
  foster father Y07.420
  foster mother Y07.421
  girl friend Y07.04
  healthcare provider Y07.529
    mental health Y07.521
    specified NEC Y07.528
  husband Y07.01
  instructor Y07.53
  mother Y07.12
    adoptive Y07.14
    foster Y07.421
    stepmother Y07.433
  nonfamily member Y07.50
    specified NEC Y07.59
  nurse Y07.528
  occupational therapist Y07.528
  partner of parent
    female Y07.434
    male Y07.432
  physical therapist Y07.528
  sister Y07.411
  speech therapist Y07.528
  stepbrother Y07.435
  stepfather Y07.430
  stepmother Y07.433
  stepsister Y07.436
  teacher Y07.53
  wife Y07.02
Piercing — *see* Contact, with, by type of object or machine
Pinched
  between objects (moving) (stationary and moving) W23.0
    stationary W23.1
Pinned under machine(ry) — *see* Contact, with, by type of machine
Place of occurrence Y92.9
  abandoned house Y92.89
  airplane Y92.813
  airport Y92.520
  ambulatory health services establishment NEC Y92.538
  ambulatory surgery center Y92.530
  amusement park Y92.831

Place of occurrence Y92.9 — *continued*
  apartment (co-op) — *see* Place of occurrence, residence, apartment
  assembly hall Y92.29
  bank Y92.510
  barn Y92.71
  baseball field Y92.320
  basketball court Y92.310
  beach Y92.832
  boarding house — *see* Place of occurrence, residence, boarding house
  boat Y92.814
  bowling alley Y92.39
  bridge Y92.89
  building under construction Y92.61
  bus Y92.811
    station Y92.521
  cafe Y92.511
  campsite Y92.833
  campus — *see* Place of occurrence, school
  canal Y92.89
  car Y92.810
  casino Y92.59
  children's home — *see* Place of occurrence, residence, institutional, orphanage
  church Y92.22
  cinema Y92.26
  clubhouse Y92.29
  coal pit Y92.64
  college (community) Y92.214
  condominium — *see* Place of occurrence, residence, apartment
  construction area — *see* Place of occurrence, industrial and construction area
  convalescent home — *see* Place of occurrence, residence, institutional, nursing home
  court-house Y92.240
  cricket ground Y92.328
  cultural building Y92.258
    art gallery Y92.250
    museum Y92.251
    music hall Y92.252
    opera house Y92.253
    specified NEC Y92.258
    theater Y92.254
  dancehall Y92.252
  day nursery Y92.210
  dentist office Y92.531
  derelict house Y92.89
  desert Y92.820
  dock NOS Y92.89
  dockyard Y92.62
  doctor's office Y92.531
  dormitory — *see* Place of occurrence, residence, institutional, school dormitory
  dry dock Y92.62
  factory (building) (premises) Y92.63
  farm (land under cultivation) (outbuildings) Y92.79
    barn Y92.71
    chicken coop Y92.72
    field Y92.73
    hen house Y92.72
    house — *see* Place of occurrence, residence, house
    orchard Y92.74
    specified NEC Y92.79
  football field Y92.321
  forest Y92.821
  freeway Y92.411
  gallery Y92.250
  garage (commercial) Y92.59
    boarding house Y92.044
    military base Y92.135
    mobile home Y92.025
    nursing home Y92.124
    orphanage Y92.114
    private house Y92.015

Place of occurrence Y92.9 — *continued*
  garage (commercial) Y92.59 — *continued*
    reform school Y92.155
  gas station Y92.524
  gasworks Y92.69
  golf course Y92.39
  gravel pit Y92.64
  grocery Y92.512
  gymnasium Y92.39
  handball court Y92.318
  harbor Y92.89
  harness racing course Y92.39
  healthcare provider office Y92.531
  highway (interstate) Y92.411
  hill Y92.828
  hockey rink Y92.330
  home — *see* Place of occurrence, residence
  hospice — *see* Place of occurrence, residence, institutional, nursing home
  hospital Y92.239
    cafeteria Y92.233
    corridor Y92.232
    operating room Y92.234
    patient
      bathroom Y92.231
      room Y92.230
    specified NEC Y92.238
  hotel Y92.59
  house — *see also* Place of occurrence, residence
    abandoned Y92.89
    under construction Y92.61
  industrial and construction area (yard) Y92.69
    building under construction Y92.61
    dock Y92.62
    dry dock Y92.62
    factory Y92.63
    gasworks Y92.69
    mine Y92.64
    oil rig Y92.65
    pit Y92.64
    power station Y92.69
    shipyard Y92.62
    specified NEC Y92.69
    tunnel under construction Y92.69
    workshop Y92.69
  kindergarten Y92.211
  lacrosse field Y92.328
  lake Y92.828
  library Y92.241
  mall Y92.59
  market Y92.512
  marsh Y92.828
  military
    base — *see* Place of occurrence, residence, institutional, military base
    training ground Y92.84
  mine Y92.64
  mosque Y92.22
  motel Y92.59
  motorway (interstate) Y92.411
  mountain Y92.828
  movie-house Y92.26
  museum Y92.251
  music-hall Y92.252
  not applicable Y92.9
  nuclear power station Y92.69
  nursing home — *see* Place of occurrence, residence, institutional, nursing home
  office building Y92.59
  offshore installation Y92.65
  oil rig Y92.65
  old people's home — *see* Place of occurrence, residence, institutional, specified NEC
  opera-house Y92.253
  orphanage — *see* Place of occurrence, residence, institutional, orphanage
  outpatient surgery center Y92.530

EXTERNAL CAUSES

Place of occurrence Y92.9 — *continued*
store Y92.512
stream Y92.828
street and highway Y92.410
  bike path Y92.482
  freeway Y92.411
  highway ramp Y92.415
  interstate highway Y92.411
  local residential or business street Y92.414
  motorway Y92.411
  parking lot Y92.481
  parkway Y92.412
  sidewalk Y92.480
  specified NEC Y92.488
  state road Y92.413
subway car Y92.816
supermarket Y92.512
swamp Y92.828
swimming pool (public) Y92.34
  private (at) Y92.095
    boarding house Y92.045
    military base Y92.136
    mobile home Y92.026
    nursing home Y92.125
    orphanage Y92.115
    prison Y92.146
    reform school Y92.156
    single family residence Y92.016
synagogue Y92.22
television station Y92.59
tennis court Y92.312
theater Y92.254
trade area Y92.59
  bank Y92.510
  cafe Y92.511
  casino Y92.59
  garage Y92.59
  hotel Y92.59
  market Y92.512
  office building Y92.59
  radio station Y92.59
  restaurant Y92.511
  shop Y92.513
  shopping mall Y92.59
  store Y92.512
  supermarket Y92.512
  television station Y92.59
  warehouse Y92.59
trailer park, residential — *see* Place of occurrence, residence, mobile home
trailer site NOS Y92.89
train Y92.815
  station Y92.522
truck Y92.812
tunnel under construction Y92.69
university Y92.214
urgent (health) care center Y92.532
vehicle (transport) Y92.818
  airplane Y92.813
  boat Y92.814
  bus Y92.811
  car Y92.810
  specified NEC Y92.818
  subway car Y92.816
  train Y92.815
  truck Y92.812
warehouse Y92.59
water reservoir Y92.89
wilderness area Y92.828
  desert Y92.820
  forest Y92.821
  marsh Y92.828
  mountain Y92.828
  prairie Y92.828
  specified NEC Y92.828
  swamp Y92.828
workshop Y92.69

Place of occurrence Y92.9 — *continued*
yard, private Y92.096
  boarding house Y92.046
  mobile home Y92.027
  single family house Y92.017
youth center Y92.29
zoo (zoological garden) Y92.834
Plumbism — *see* Table of Drugs and Chemicals, lead
Poisoning (accidental) (by) — *see also* Table of Drugs and Chemicals
by plant, thorns, spines, sharp leaves or other mechanisms NEC X58
carbon monoxide
  generated by
    motor vehicle — *see* Accident, transport
    watercraft (in transit) (not in transit) V93.89
      ferry boat V93.81
      fishing boat V93.82
      jet skis V93.83
      liner V93.81
      merchant ship V93.80
      passenger ship V93.81
      powered craft NEC V93.83
caused by injection of poisons into skin by plant thorns, spines, sharp leaves X58
marine or sea plants (venomous) X58
exhaust gas
  generated by
    motor vehicle — *see* Accident, transport
    watercraft (in transit) (not in transit) V93.89
      ferry boat V93.81
      fishing boat V93.82
      jet skis V93.83
      liner V93.81
      merchant ship V93.80
      passenger ship V93.81
      powered craft NEC V93.83
fumes or smoke due to
  explosion (*see also* Explosion) W40.9
  fire — *see* Exposure, fire
  ignition — *see* Ignition
gas
  in legal intervention — *see* Legal, intervention, gas
  legal execution — *see* Legal, intervention, gas
in war operations — *see* War operations
legal execution — *see* Legal, intervention
intervention
  by gas — *see* Legal, intervention, gas
  by other specified means — *see* Legal, intervention, specified means NEC
Powder burn (by) (from)
airgun W34.110
BB gun W34.110
firearm NEC W34.19
gas, air or spring-operated gun NEC W34.118
handgun W32.1
hunting rifle W33.12
larger firearm W33.10
  specified NEC W33.19
machine gun W33.13
paintball gun W34.111
pellet gun W34.110
shotgun W33.11
Very pistol [flare] W34.19
Premature cessation (of) surgical and medical care Y66
Privation (food) (water) X58

Procedure (operation)
correct, on wrong side or body part (wrong side) (wrong site) Y65.53
intended for another patient done on wrong patient Y65.52
performed on patient not scheduled for surgery Y65.52
performed on wrong patient Y65.52
wrong, performed on correct patient Y65.51
Prolonged
sitting in transport vehicle — *see* Travel, by type of vehicle
stay in
  high altitude as cause of anoxia, barodontalgia, barotitis or hypoxia W94.11
  weightless environment X52
Pulling, excessive (*see also* Overexertion) X50.9
Puncture, puncturing — *see also* Contact, with, by type of object or machine
by
  plant thorns, spines, sharp leaves or other mechanisms NEC W60
during medical or surgical treatment as misadventure — *see* Index to Diseases and Injuries, Complication(s)
Pushed, pushing (accidental) (injury in)
by other person(s) (accidental) W51
  with fall W03
    due to ice or snow W00.0
  as, or caused by, a crowd or human stampede (with fall) W52
before moving object NEC Y02.8
  motor vehicle Y02.0
  subway train Y02.1
  train Y02.1
from
  high place NEC
    in accidental circumstances W17.89
    stated as
      intentional, homicide (attempt) Y01
      undetermined whether accidental or intentional Y30
  transport vehicle NEC (*see also* Accident, transport) V89.9
    stated as
      intentional, homicide (attempt) Y08.89
overexertion X50.9

EXTERNAL CAUSES

Q

R

Radiation (exposure to)
arc lamps W89.0
atomic power plant (malfunction) NEC W88.1
complication of or abnormal reaction to
    medical radiotherapy Y84.2
electromagnetic, ionizing W88.0
gamma rays W88.1
in
    war operations (from or following nuclear
        explosion) — see War operations
inadvertent exposure of patient (receiving test
    or therapy) Y63.3
infrared (heaters and lamps) W90.1
    excessive heat from W92
ionized, ionizing (particles, artificially
    accelerated)
    radioisotopes W88.1
    specified NEC W88.8
    x-rays W88.0
isotopes, radioactive — see Radiation,
    radioactive isotopes
laser(s) W90.2
    in war operations — see War operations
    misadventure in medical care Y63.2
light sources (man-made visible and ultraviolet)
    W89.9
    natural X32
    specified NEC W89.8
    tanning bed W89.1
    welding light W89.0
man-made visible light W89.9
    specified NEC W89.8
    tanning bed W89.1
    welding light W89.0
microwave W90.8
misadventure in medical or surgical procedure
    Y63.2
natural NEC X39.08
    radon X39.01
overdose (in medical or surgical procedure)
    Y63.2
radar W90.0
radioactive isotopes (any) W88.1
    atomic power plant malfunction W88.1
    misadventure in medical or surgical
        treatment Y63.2
radiofrequency W90.0
radium NEC W88.1
sun X32
ultraviolet (light) (man-made) W89.9
    natural X32
    specified NEC W89.8
    tanning bed W89.1
    welding light W89.0
welding arc, torch, or light W89.0
    excessive heat from W92
x-rays (hard) (soft) W88.0
Range disease W94.11
Rape (attempted) T74.2-
Rat bite W53.11
Reaching (prolonged) (static) X50.1
**Reaction, abnormal to medical
    procedure** (see also Complication of or
    following, by type of procedure) Y84.9
with misadventure — see Misadventure
biologicals — see Table of Drugs and
    Chemicals
drugs — see Table of Drugs and Chemicals
vaccine — see Table of Drugs and Chemicals

Recoil
airgun W34.110
BB gun W34.110
firearm NEC W34.19
gas, air or spring-operated gun NEC
    W34.118
handgun W32.1
hunting rifle W33.12
larger firearm W33.10
    specified NEC W33.19
machine gun W33.13
paintball gun W34.111
pellet W34.110
shotgun W33.11
Very pistol [flare] W34.19
Reduction in
atmospheric pressure — see Air, pressure,
    change
Rock falling on or hitting (accidentally)
    (person) W20.8
    in cave-in W20.0
Run over (accidentally) (by)
animal (not being ridden) NEC W55.89
machinery — see Contact, with, by specified
    type of machine
transport vehicle NEC (see also Accident,
    transport) V09.9
    intentional homicide (attempt) Y03.0
    motor NEC V09.20
        intentional homicide (attempt) Y03.0
Running
before moving object X81.8
    motor vehicle X81.0
Running off, away
animal (being ridden) (see also Accident,
    transport) V80.918
    not being ridden W55.89
animal-drawn vehicle NEC (see also Accident,
    transport) V80.928
highway, road(way), street
    transport vehicle NEC (see also Accident,
        transport) V89.9
Rupture pressurized devices — see
    Explosion, by type of device

S

Saturnism — see Table of Drugs and
    Chemicals, lead
Scald, scalding (accidental) (by) (from) (in)
    X19
air (hot) X14.1
gases (hot) X14.1
homicide (attempt) — see Assault, burning, hot
    object
inflicted by other person
    stated as intentional, homicide (attempt) —
        see Assault, burning, hot object
liquid (boiling) (hot) NEC X12
    stated as undetermined whether accidental
        or intentional Y27.2
    suicide (attempt) X77.2
local application of externally applied
    substance in medical or surgical care
    Y63.5
metal (molten) (liquid) (hot) NEC X18
self-inflicted X77.9
stated as undetermined whether accidental or
    intentional Y27.8
steam X13.1
    assault X98.0
    stated as undetermined whether accidental
        or intentional Y27.0
    suicide (attempt) X77.0
suicide (attempt) X77.9
vapor (hot) X13.1
    assault X98.0
    stated as undetermined whether accidental
        or intentional Y27.0
    suicide (attempt) X77.0
Scratched by
cat W55.03
person(s) (accidentally) W50.4
    with intent to injure or kill Y04.0
    as, or caused by, a crowd or human
        stampede (with fall) W52
    assault Y04.0
    homicide (attempt) Y04.0
    in
        fight Y04.0
        legal intervention
            injuring
                bystander Y35.892
                law enforcement personnel Y35.891
                suspect Y35.893
Seasickness T75.3
Self-harm NEC — see also External cause by
    type, undetermined whether accidental or
    intentional
intentional — see Suicide
poisoning NEC — see Table of Drugs and
    Chemicals, accident
Self-inflicted (injury) NEC — see also External
    cause by type, undetermined whether
    accidental or intentional
intentional — see Suicide
poisoning NEC — see Table of Drugs and
    Chemicals, accident
Sequelae (of)
accident NEC — see W00-X58 with 7th
    character S
assault (homicidal) (any means) — see X92-
    Y08 with 7th character S
homicide, attempt (any means) — see X92-Y08
    with 7th character S
injury undetermined whether accidentally or
    purposely inflicted — see Y21-Y33 with
    7th character S
intentional self-harm (classifiable to X71-X83)
    — see X71-X83 with 7th character S
legal intervention — see with 7th character S
    Y35

Sequelae (of) — continued
  motor vehicle accident — see V00-V99 with 7th character S
  suicide, attempt (any means) — see X71-X83 with 7th character S
  transport accident — see V00-V99 with 7th character S
  war operations — see War operations
Shock
  electric — see Exposure, electric current
  from electric appliance (any) (faulty) W86.8
    domestic W86.0
    suicide (attempt) X83.1
Shooting, shot (accidental(ly)) — see also Discharge, firearm, by type
  herself or himself — see Discharge, firearm by type, self-inflicted
  homicide (attempt) — see Discharge, firearm by type, homicide
  in war operations — see War operations
  inflicted by other person — see Discharge, firearm by type, homicide
    accidental — see Discharge, firearm, by type of firearm
  legal
    execution — see Legal, intervention, firearm
    intervention — see Legal, intervention, firearm
  self-inflicted — see Discharge, firearm by type, suicide
    accidental — see Discharge, firearm, by type of firearm
  suicide (attempt) — see Discharge, firearm by type, suicide
Shoving (accidentally) by other person — see Pushed, by other person
Sickness
  alpine W94.11
  motion — see Motion
  mountain W94.11
Sinking (accidental)
  watercraft (causing drowning, submersion) — see also Drowning, due to, accident to, watercraft, sinking
    causing injury except drowning or submersion — see Accident, watercraft, causing, injury NEC
Siriasis X32
Sitting (prolonged) (static) X50.1
Slashed wrists — see Cut, self-inflicted
Slipping (accidental) (on same level) (with fall) W01.0
  on
    ice W00.0
      with skates — see Accident, transport, pedestrian, conveyance
    mud W01.0
    oil W01.0
    snow W00.0
      with skis — see Accident, transport, pedestrian, conveyance
    surface (slippery) (wet) NEC W01.0
  without fall W18.40
    due to
      specified NEC W18.49
      stepping from one level to another W18.43
      stepping in hole or opening W18.42
      stepping on object W18.41
Sliver, wood, contact with W45.8
Smoldering (due to fire) — see Exposure, fire
Sodomy (attempted) by force T74.2-
Sound waves (causing injury) W42.9
  supersonic W42.0
Splinter, contact with W45.8
Stab, stabbing — see Cut
Standing (prolonged) (static) X50.1
Starvation X58

Status of external cause Y99.9
  child assisting in compensated work for family Y99.8
  civilian activity done for financial or other compensation Y99.0
  civilian activity done for income or pay Y99.0
  family member assisting in compensated work for other family member Y99.8
  hobby not done for income Y99.8
  leisure activity Y99.8
  military activity Y99.1
  off-duty activity of military personnel Y99.8
  recreation or sport not for income or while a student Y99.8
  specified NEC Y99.8
  student activity Y99.8
  volunteer activity Y99.2
Stepped on
  by
    animal (not being ridden) NEC W55.89
    crowd or human stampede W52
    person W50.0
Stepping on
  object W22.8
    with fall W18.31
    sports equipment W21.9
    stationary W22.09
      sports equipment W21.89
  person W51
    by crowd or human stampede W52
  sports equipment W21.9
Sting
  arthropod, nonvenomous W57
  insect, nonvenomous W57
Storm (cataclysmic) — see Forces of nature, cataclysmic storm
Straining, excessive (see also Overexertion) X50.9
Strangling — see Strangulation
Strangulation (accidental) — see category T71
Strenuous movements (see also Overexertion) X50.9
Striking against
  airbag (automobile) W22.10
    driver side W22.11
    front passenger side W22.12
    specified NEC W22.19
  bottom when
    diving or jumping into water (in) W16.822
      causing drowning W16.821
      from boat W16.722
        causing drowning W16.721
      natural body W16.622
        causing drowning W16.821
      swimming pool W16.522
        causing drowning W16.521
    falling into water (in) W16.322
      causing drowning W16.321
    fountain — see Striking against, bottom when, falling into water, specified NEC
    natural body W16.122
      causing drowning W16.121
    reservoir — see Striking against, bottom when, falling into water, specified NEC
    specified NEC W16.322
      causing drowning W16.321
    swimming pool W16.022
      causing drowning W16.021
  diving board (swimming pool) W21.4
  object W22.8
    with
      drowning or submersion — see Drowning
      fall — see Fall, due to, bumping against, object
    caused by crowd or human stampede (with fall) W52
    furniture W22.03

Striking against — continued
  object W22.8 — continued
    lamppost W22.02
    sports equipment W21.9
    stationary W22.09
      sports equipment W21.89
    wall W22.01
  person(s) W51
    with fall W03
      due to ice or snow W00.0
    as, or caused by, a crowd or human stampede (with fall) W52
    assault Y04.2
    homicide (attempt) Y04.2
  sports equipment W21.9
  wall (when) W22.01
    diving or jumping into water (in) W16.832
      causing drowning W16.831
      swimming pool W16.532
        causing drowning W16.531
    falling into water (in) W16.332
      causing drowning W16.331
    fountain — see Striking against, wall when, falling into water, specified NEC
    natural body W16.132
      causing drowning W16.131
    reservoir — see Striking against, wall when, falling into water, specified NEC
    specified NEC W16.332
      causing drowning W16.331
    swimming pool W16.032
      causing drowning W16.031
  swimming pool (when) W22.042
    causing drowning W22.041
    diving or jumping into water W16.532
      causing drowning W16.531
    falling into water W16.032
      causing drowning W16.031
Struck (accidentally) by
  airbag (automobile) W22.10
    driver side W22.11
    front passenger side W22.12
    specified NEC W22.19
  alligator W58.02
  animal (not being ridden) NEC W55.89
  avalanche — see Landslide
  ball (hit) (thrown) W21.00
    assault Y08.09
    baseball W21.03
    basketball W21.05
    football W21.01
    golf ball W21.04
    soccer W21.02
    softball W21.07
    specified NEC W21.09
    volleyball W21.06
  bat or racquet
    baseball bat W21.11
      assault Y08.02
    golf club W21.13
      assault Y08.09
    specified NEC W21.19
      assault Y08.09
    tennis racquet W21.12
      assault Y08.09
  bullet — see also Discharge, firearm by type
    in war operations — see War operations
  crocodile W58.12
  dog W54.1
  flare, Very pistol — see Discharge, firearm NEC
  hailstones X39.8

Struck (accidentally) by — *continued*
  hockey (ice)
    field
      puck W21.221
      stick W21.211
    puck W21.220
    stick W21.210
    assault Y08.01
  landslide — *see* Landslide
  law-enforcement agent (on duty) — *see* Legal, intervention, manhandling
    with blunt object — *see* Legal, intervention, blunt object
  lightning — *see* subcategory T75.0
    causing fire — *see* Exposure, fire
  machine — *see* Contact, with, by type of machine
  mammal NEC W55.89
    marine W56.32
  marine animal W56.82
  missile
    firearm — *see* Discharge, firearm by type
    in war operations — *see* War operations, missile
  object W22.8
    blunt W22.8
      assault Y00
      suicide (attempt) X79
      undetermined whether accidental or intentional Y29
    falling W20.8
      from, in, on
        building W20.1
          burning (uncontrolled fire) X00.4
        cataclysmic
          earth surface movement NEC — *see* Landslide
          storm — *see* Forces of nature, cataclysmic storm
        cave-in W20.0
        earthquake X34
        machine (in operation) — *see* Contact, with, by type of machine
        structure W20.1
          burning X00.4
        transport vehicle (in motion) — *see* Accident, transport, by type of vehicle
        watercraft W93.49
          due to
            accident to craft V91.39
              powered craft V91.33
                ferry boat V91.31
                fishing boat V91.32
                jetskis V91.33
                liner V91.31
                merchant ship V91.30
                passenger ship V91.31
              unpowered craft V91.38
                canoe V91.35
                inflatable V91.36
                kayak V91.35
                sailboat V91.34
                surfboard V91.38
                windsurfer V91.38
            powered craft V93.43
              ferry boat V93.41
              fishing boat V93.42
              jetskis V93.43
              liner V93.41
              merchant ship V93.40
              passenger ship V93.41
            unpowered craft V93.48
              sailboat V93.44
              surfboard V93.48
              windsurfer V93.48

Struck (accidentally) by — *continued*
  object W22.8 — *continued*
    moving NEC W20.8
    projected W20.8
      assault Y00
      in sports W21.9
      assault Y08.09
      ball W21.00
        baseball W21.03
        basketball W21.05
        football W21.01
        golf ball W21.04
        soccer W21.02
        softball W21.07
        specified NEC W21.09
        volleyball W21.06
      bat or racquet
        baseball bat W21.11
          assault Y08.02
        golf club W21.13
          assault Y08.09
        specified NEC W21.19
          assault Y08.09
        tennis racquet W21.12
          assault Y08.09
      hockey (ice)
        field
          puck W21.221
          stick W21.211
        puck W21.220
        stick W21.210
        assault Y08.01
      specified NEC W21.89
    set in motion by explosion — *see* Explosion
    thrown W20.8
      assault Y00
      in sports W21.9
      assault Y08.09
      ball W21.00
        baseball W21.03
        basketball W21.05
        football W21.01
        golf ball W21.04
        soccer W21.02
        soft ball W21.07
        specified NEC W21.09
        volleyball W21.06
      bat or racquet
        baseball bat W21.11
          assault Y08.02
        golf club W21.13
          assault Y08.09
        specified NEC W21.19
          assault Y08.09
        tennis racquet W21.12
          assault Y08.09
      hockey (ice)
        field
          puck W21.221
          stick W21.211
        puck W21.220
        stick W21.210
        assault Y08.01
      specified NEC W21.89
  other person(s) W50.0
    with
      blunt object W22.8
        intentional, homicide (attempt) Y00
        sports equipment W21.9
        undetermined whether accidental or intentional Y29
      fall W03
        due to ice or snow W00.0
    as, or caused by, a crowd or human stampede (with fall) W52
    assault Y04.2
    homicide (attempt) Y04.2

Struck (accidentally) by — *continued*
  other person(s) W50.0 — *continued*
    in legal intervention
      injuring
        bystander Y35.812
        law enforcement personnel Y35.811
        suspect Y35.813
    sports equipment W21.9
  police (on duty) — *see* Legal, intervention, manhandling
    with blunt object — *see* Legal, intervention, blunt object
  sports equipment W21.9
    assault Y08.09
    ball W21.00
      baseball W21.03
      basketball W21.05
      football W21.01
      golf ball W21.04
      soccer W21.02
      soft ball W21.07
      specified NEC W21.09
      volleyball W21.06
    bat or racquet
      baseball bat W21.11
        assault Y08.02
      golf club W21.13
        assault Y08.09
      specified NEC W21.19
      tennis racquet W21.12
        assault Y08.09
    cleats (shoe) W21.31
    foot wear NEC W21.39
    football helmet W21.81
    hockey (ice)
      field
        puck W21.221
        stick W21.211
      puck W21.220
      stick W21.210
      assault Y08.01
    skate blades W21.32
    specified NEC W21.89
      assault Y08.09
  thunderbolt — *see* subcategory T75.0
    causing fire — *see* Exposure, fire
  transport vehicle NEC (*see also* Accident, transport) V09.9
    intentional, homicide (attempt) Y03.0
    motor NEC (*see also* Accident, transport) V09.20
      homicide Y03.0
  vehicle (transport) NEC — *see* Accident, transport, by type of vehicle
    stationary (falling from jack, hydraulic lift, ramp) W20.8

Stumbling
  over
    animal NEC W01.0
      with fall W18.09
    carpet, rug or (small) object W22.8
      with fall W18.09
    person W51
      with fall W03
        due to ice or snow W00.0
  without fall W18.40
    due to
      specified NEC W18.49
      stepping from one level to another W18.43
      stepping into hole or opening W18.42
      stepping on object W18.41
Submersion (accidental) — *see* Drowning

Suffocation (accidental) (by external means)
(by pressure) (mechanical) (*see also* category)
T71
  due to, by
    avalanche — *see* Landslide
    explosion — *see* Explosion
    fire — *see* Exposure, fire
    food, any type (aspiration) (ingestion)
      (inhalation) — *see* categories T17 and
      T18
    ignition — *see* Ignition
    landslide — *see* Landslide
    machine(ry) — *see* Contact, with, by type of
      machine
    vomitus (aspiration) (inhalation) T17.81-
  in
    burning building X00.8
Suicide, suicidal (attempted) (by) X83.8
  blunt object X79
  burning, burns X76
    hot object X77.9
      fluid NEC X77.2
      household appliance X77.3
      specified NEC X77.8
      steam X77.0
      tap water X77.1
      vapors X77.0
  caustic substance — *see* Table of Drugs and
    Chemicals
  cold, extreme X83.2
  collision of motor vehicle with
    motor vehicle X82.0
    specified NEC X82.8
    train X82.1
    tree X82.2
  crashing of aircraft X83.0
  cut (any part of body) X78.9
  cutting or piercing instrument X78.9
    dagger X78.2
    glass X78.0
    knife X78.1
    specified NEC X78.8
    sword X78.2
  drowning (in) X71.9
    bathtub X71.0
    natural water X71.3
    specified NEC X71.8
    swimming pool X71.1
      following fall X71.2
  electrocution X83.1
  explosive(s) (material) X75
  fire, flames X76
  firearm X74.9
    airgun X74.01
    handgun X72
    hunting rifle X73.1
    larger X73.9
      specified NEC X73.8
    machine gun X73.2
    shotgun X73.0
    specified NEC X74.8
  hanging X83.8
  hot object — *see* Suicide, burning, hot object
  jumping
    before moving object X81.8
      motor vehicle X81.0
      subway train X81.1
      train X81.1
    from high place X80
  late effect of attempt — *see* X71-X83 with 7th
    character S
  lying before moving object, train, vehicle
    X81.8
  poisoning — *see* Table of Drugs and Chemicals
  puncture (any part of body) — *see* Suicide,
    cutting or piercing instrument
  scald — *see* Suicide, burning, hot object

Suicide, suicidal (attempted) (by) X83.8 —
  continued
  sequelae of attempt — *see* X71-X83 with 7th
    character S
  sharp object (any) — *see* Suicide, cutting or
    piercing instrument
  shooting — *see* Suicide, firearm
  specified means NEC X83.8
  stab (any part of body) — *see* Suicide, cutting
    or piercing instrument
  steam, hot vapors X77.0
  strangulation X83.8
  submersion — *see* Suicide, drowning
  suffocation X83.8
  wound NEC X83.8
Sunstroke X32
Supersonic waves (causing injury) W42.0
Surgical procedure, complication of
    (delayed or as an abnormal reaction without
    mention of misadventure) — *see also*
    Complication of or following, by type of
    procedure
  due to or as a result of misadventure — *see*
    Misadventure
Swallowed, swallowing
  foreign body — *see* Foreign body, alimentary
    canal
  poison — *see* Table of Drugs and Chemicals
  substance
    caustic or corrosive — *see* Table of Drugs
      and Chemicals
    poisonous — *see* Table of Drugs and
      Chemicals

T

Tackle in sport W03
Terrorism (involving) Y38.80
  biological weapons Y38.6x-
  chemical weapons Y38.7x-
  conflagration Y38.3x-
  drowning and submersion Y38.89-
  explosion Y38.2x-
    destruction of aircraft Y38.1x-
    marine weapons Y38.0x-
  fire Y38.3x-
  firearms Y38.4x-
  hot substances Y38.3x-
  lasers Y38.89-
  nuclear weapons Y38.5x-
  piercing or stabbing instruments Y38.89-
  secondary effects Y38.9x-
  specified method NEC Y38.89-
  suicide bomber Y38.81-
Thirst X58
Threat to breathing
  aspiration — *see* Aspiration
  due to cave-in, falling earth or substance NEC
    — *see* category T71
Thrown (accidentally)
  against part (any) of or object in transport
    vehicle (in motion) NEC — *see also*
    Accident, transport
  from
    high place, homicide (attempt) Y01
    machinery — *see* Contact, with, by type of
      machine
    transport vehicle NEC (*see also* Accident,
      transport) V89.9
  off — *see* Thrown, from
Thunderbolt — *see* subcategory T75.0
  causing fire — *see* Exposure, fire
Tidal wave (any injury) NEC — *see* Forces of
  nature, tidal wave
Took
  overdose (drug) — *see* Table of Drugs and
    Chemicals
  poison — *see* Table of Drugs and Chemicals
Tornado (any injury) X37.1
Torrential rain (any injury) X37.8
Torture X58
Trampled by animal NEC W55.89
Trapped (accidentally)
  between objects (moving) (stationary and
    moving) — *see* Caught
  by part (any) of
    motorcycle V29.88
    pedal cycle V19.88
    transport vehicle NEC (*see also* Accident,
      transport) V89.9
Travel (effects) (sickness) T75.3
Tree falling on or hitting (accidentally)
  (person) W20.8
Tripping
  over
    animal W01.0
      with fall W01.0
    carpet, rug or (small) object W22.8
      with fall W18.09
    person W51
      with fall W03
        due to ice or snow W00.0
  without fall W18.40
    due to
      specified NEC W18.49
      stepping from one level to another
        W18.43
      stepping into hole or opening W18.42
      stepping on object W18.41

EXTERNAL CAUSES

Twisted by person(s) (accidentally) W50.2
  with intent to injure or kill Y04.0
  as, or caused by, a crowd or human stampede
    (with fall) W52
  assault Y04.0
  homicide (attempt) Y04.0
  in
    fight Y04.0
    legal intervention — *see* Legal, intervention,
      manhandling
Twisting (prolonged) (static) X50.1

U

**Underdosing of necessary drugs,
  medicaments or biological
  substances** Y63.6
Undetermined intent (contact) (exposure)
  automobile collision Y32
  blunt object Y29
  drowning (submersion) (in) Y21.9
    bathtub Y21.0
      after fall Y21.1
    natural water (lake) (ocean) (pond) (river)
      (stream) Y21.4
    specified place NEC Y21.8
    swimming pool Y21.2
      after fall Y21.3
  explosive material Y25
  fall, jump or push from high place Y30
  falling, lying or running before moving object
    Y31
  fire Y26
  firearm discharge Y24.9
    airgun (BB) (pellet) Y24.0
    handgun (pistol) (revolver) Y22
    hunting rifle Y23.1
    larger Y23.9
      hunting rifle Y23.1
      machine gun Y23.3
      military Y23.2
      shotgun Y23.0
      specified type NEC Y23.8
    machine gun Y23.3
    military Y23.2
    shotgun Y23.0
    specified type NEC Y24.8
    Very pistol Y24.8
  hot object Y27.9
    fluid NEC Y27.2
    household appliance Y27.3
    specified object NEC Y27.8
    steam Y27.0
    tap water Y27.1
    vapor Y27.0
  jump, fall or push from high place Y30
  lying, falling or running before moving object
    Y31
  motor vehicle crash Y32
  push, fall or jump from high place Y30
  running, falling or lying before moving object
    Y31
  sharp object Y28.9
    dagger Y28.2
    glass Y28.0
    knife Y28.1
    specified object NEC Y28.8
    sword Y28.2
  smoke Y26
  specified event NEC Y33
Use of hand as hammer X50.3

V

Vibration (causing injury) W49.9
Victim (of)
  avalanche — *see* Landslide
  earth movements NEC — *see* Forces of nature,
    earth movement
  earthquake X34
  flood — *see* Flood
  landslide — *see* Landslide
  lightning — *see* subcategory T75.0
    causing fire — *see* Exposure, fire
  storm (cataclysmic) NEC — *see* Forces of
    nature, cataclysmic storm
  volcanic eruption X35
Volcanic eruption (any injury) X35
Vomitus, gastric contents in air passages
  (with asphyxia, obstruction or suffocation)
  T17.81-

W

Walked into stationary object (any)
W22.09
furniture W22.03
lamppost W22.02
wall W22.01
War operations (injuries to military personnel
and civilians during war, civil insurrection
and peacekeeping missions) (by) (from)
(involving) Y36.90
after cessation of hostilities Y36.89-
explosion (of)
bomb placed during war operations
Y36.82-
mine placed during war operations
Y36.81-
specified NEC Y36.88-
air blast Y36.20-
aircraft
destruction — *see* War operations,
destruction of aircraft
airway restriction — *see* War operations,
restriction of airways
asphyxiation — *see* War operations, restriction
of airways
biological weapons Y36.6x-
blast Y36.20-
blast fragments Y36.20-
blast wave Y36.20-
blast wind Y36.20-
bomb Y36.20-
dirty Y36.50-
gasoline Y36.31-
incendiary Y36.31-
petrol Y36.31-
bullet Y36.43-
incendiary Y36.32-
rubber Y36.41-
chemical weapons Y36.7x-
combat
hand to hand (unarmed) combat Y36.44-
using blunt or piercing object Y36.45-
conflagration — *see* War operations, fire
conventional warfare NEC Y36.49-
depth-charge Y36.01-
destruction of aircraft Y36.10-
due to
air to air missile Y36.11-
collision with other aircraft Y36.12-
detonation (accidental) of onboard
munitions and explosives Y36.14-
enemy fire or explosives Y36.11-
explosive placed on aircraft Y36.11-
onboard fire Y36.13-
rocket propelled grenade [RPG] Y36.11-
small arms fire Y36.11-
surface to air missile Y36.11-
specified NEC Y36.19-
detonation (accidental) of
onboard marine weapons Y36.05-
own munitions or munitions launch device
Y36.24-
dirty bomb Y36.50-

War operations (injuries to military personnel
and civilians during war, civil insurrection
and peacekeeping missions) (by) (from)
(involving) Y36.90 — *continued*
explosion (of) Y36.20-
aerial bomb Y36.21-
after cessation of hostilities
bomb placed during war operations
Y36.82-
mine placed during war operations
Y36.81-
bomb NOS (*see also* War operations,
bomb(s)) Y36.20-
fragments Y36.20-
grenade Y36.29-
guided missile Y36.22-
improvised explosive device [IED] (person-
borne) (roadside) (vehicle-borne)
Y36.23-
land mine Y36.29-
marine mine (at sea) (in harbor) Y36.02-
marine weapon Y36.00-
specified NEC Y36.09-
own munitions or munitions launch device
(accidental) Y36.24-
sea-based artillery shell Y36.03-
specified NEC Y36.29-
torpedo Y36.04-
fire Y36.30-
specified NEC Y36.39-
firearms
discharge Y36.43-
pellets Y36.42-
flamethrower Y36.33-
fragments (from) (of)
improvised explosive device [IED] (person-
borne) (roadside) (vehicle-borne)
Y36.26-
munitions Y36.25-
specified NEC Y36.29-
weapons Y36.27-
friendly fire Y36.92
hand to hand (unarmed) combat Y36.44-
hot substances — *see* War operations, fire
incendiary bullet Y36.32-
nuclear weapon (effects of) Y36.50-
acute radiation exposure Y36.54-
blast pressure Y36.51-
direct blast Y36.51-
direct heat Y36.53-
fallout exposure Y36.54-
fireball Y36.53-
indirect blast (struck or crushed by blast
debris) (being thrown by blast) Y36.52-
ionizing radiation (immediate exposure)
Y36.54-
nuclear radiation Y36.54-
radiation
ionizing (immediate exposure) Y36.54-
nuclear Y36.54-
thermal Y36.53-
secondary effects Y36.54-
specified NEC Y36.59-
thermal radiation Y36.53-
restriction of air (airway)
intentional Y36.46-
unintentional Y36.47-
rubber bullets Y36.41-
shrapnel NOS Y36.29-
suffocation — *see* War operations, restriction
of airways
unconventional warfare NEC Y36.7x-
underwater blast NOS Y36.00-
warfare
conventional NEC Y36.49-
unconventional NEC Y36.7x-

War operations (injuries to military personnel
and civilians during war, civil insurrection
and peacekeeping missions) (by) (from)
(involving) Y36.90 — *continued*
weapon of mass destruction [WMD] Y36.91
weapons
biological weapons Y36.6x-
chemical Y36.7x-
nuclear (effects of) Y36.50-
acute radiation exposure Y36.54-
blast pressure Y36.51-
direct blast Y36.51-
direct heat Y36.53-
fallout exposure Y36.54-
fireball Y36.53-
radiation
ionizing (immediate exposure) Y36.54-
nuclear Y36.54-
thermal Y36.53-
secondary effects Y36.54-
specified NEC Y36.59-
of mass destruction [WMD] Y36.91
Washed
away by flood — *see* Flood
off road by storm (transport vehicle) — *see*
Forces of nature, cataclysmic storm
Weather exposure NEC — *see* Forces of
nature
Weightlessness (causing injury) (effects of) (in
spacecraft, real or simulated) X52
Work related condition Y99.0
Wound (accidental) NEC (*see also* Injury) X58
battle (*see also* War operations) Y36.90
gunshot — *see* Discharge, firearm by type
Wreck transport vehicle NEC (*see also*
Accident, transport) V89.9
Wrong
device implanted into correct surgical site
Y65.51
fluid in infusion Y65.1
patient, procedure performed on Y65.52
procedure (operation) on correct patient
Y65.51

X

Y

Z

Chapter 1 – Certain infectious and parasitic diseases (A00-B99)

Includes: Diseases generally recognized as communicable or transmissible

Use additional code to identify resistance to antimicrobial drugs (Z16.-)

Excludes 1: certain localized infections — see body system, related chapters

Excludes ❷: carrier or suspected carrier of infectious disease (Z22.-)
infectious and parasitic diseases complicating pregnancy, childbirth and the puerperium (O98.-)
infectious and parasitic diseases specific to the perinatal period (P35-P39)
influenza and other acute respiratory infections (J00-J22)

This chapter contains the following blocks:

A00-A09	Intestinal infectious diseases
A15-A19	Tuberculosis
A20-A28	Certain zoonotic bacterial diseases
A30-A49	Other bacterial diseases
A50-A64	Infections with a predominantly sexual mode of transmission
A65-A69	Other spirochetal diseases
A70-A74	Other diseases caused by chlamydiae
A75-A79	Rickettsioses
A80-A89	Viral and prion infections of the central nervous system
A90-A99	Arthropod-borne viral fevers and viral hemorrhagic fevers
B00-B09	Viral infections characterized by skin and mucous membrane lesions
B10	Other human herpesviruses
B15-B19	Viral hepatitis
B20	Human immunodeficiency virus [HIV] disease
B25-B34	Other viral diseases
B35-B49	Mycoses
B50-B64	Protozoal diseases
B65-B83	Helminthiases
B85-B89	Pediculosis, acariasis and other infestations
B90-B94	Sequelae of infectious and parasitic diseases
B95-B97	Bacterial and viral infectious agents
B99	Other infectious diseases

Chapter-Specific Coding Guidelines

C. Chapter-Specific Coding Guidelines
In addition to general coding guidelines, there are guidelines for specific diagnoses and/or conditions in the classification. Unless otherwise indicated, these guidelines apply to all health care settings. Please refer to Section II for guidelines on the selection of principal diagnosis.

1. Chapter 1: Certain Infectious and Parasitic Diseases (A00-B99)

a. Human Immunodeficiency Virus (HIV) Infections

1) Code only confirmed cases
Code only confirmed cases of HIV infection/illness. This is an exception to the hospital inpatient guideline Section II, H.

In this context, "confirmation" does not require documentation of positive serology or culture for HIV; the provider's diagnostic statement that the patient is HIV positive, or has an HIV-related illness is sufficient.

2) Selection and sequencing of HIV codes

(a) Patient admitted for HIV-related condition
If a patient is admitted for an HIV-related condition, the principal diagnosis should be B20, Human immunodeficiency virus [HIV] disease followed by additional diagnosis codes for all reported HIV-related conditions.

(b) Patient with HIV disease admitted for unrelated condition
If a patient with HIV disease is admitted for an unrelated condition (such as a traumatic injury), the code for the unrelated condition (e.g., the nature of injury code) should be the principal diagnosis. Other diagnoses would be B20 followed by additional diagnosis codes for all reported HIV-related conditions.

(c) Whether the patient is newly diagnosed
Whether the patient is newly diagnosed or has had previous admissions/encounters for HIV conditions is irrelevant to the sequencing decision.

(d) Asymptomatic human immunodeficiency virus
Z21, Asymptomatic human immunodeficiency virus [HIV] infection status, is to be applied when the patient without any documentation of symptoms is listed as being "HIV positive," "known HIV," "HIV test positive," or similar terminology. Do not use this code if the term "AIDS" is used or if the patient is treated for any HIV-related illness or is described as having any condition(s) resulting from his/her HIV positive status; use B20 in these cases.

(e) Patients with inconclusive HIV serology
Patients with inconclusive HIV serology, but no definitive diagnosis or manifestations of the illness, may be assigned code R75, Inconclusive laboratory evidence of human immunodeficiency virus [HIV].

(f) Previously diagnosed HIV-related illness
Patients with any known prior diagnosis of an HIV-related illness should be coded to B20. Once a patient has developed an HIV-related illness, the patient should always be assigned code B20 on every subsequent admission/encounter. Patients previously diagnosed with any HIV illness (B20) should never be assigned to R75 or Z21, Asymptomatic human immunodeficiency virus [HIV] infection status.

(g) HIV Infection in Pregnancy, Childbirth and the Puerperium
During pregnancy, childbirth or the puerperium, a patient admitted (or presenting for a health care encounter) because of an HIV-related illness should receive a principal diagnosis code of O98.7-, Human immunodeficiency [HIV] disease complicating pregnancy, childbirth and the puerperium, followed by B20 and the code(s) for the HIV-related illness(es). Codes from Chapter 15 always take sequencing priority.

Patients with asymptomatic HIV infection status admitted (or presenting for a health care encounter) during pregnancy, childbirth, or the puerperium should receive codes of O98.7- and Z21.

(h) Encounters for testing for HIV
If a patient is being seen to determine his/her HIV status, use code Z11.4, Encounter for screening for human immunodeficiency virus [HIV]. Use additional codes for any associated high risk behavior.

If a patient with signs or symptoms is being seen for HIV testing, code the signs and symptoms. An additional counseling code Z71.7, Human immunodeficiency virus [HIV] counseling, may be used if counseling is provided during the encounter for the test.

When a patient returns to be informed of his/her HIV test results and the test result is negative, use code Z71.7, Human immunodeficiency virus [HIV] counseling.

If the results are positive, see previous guidelines and assign codes as appropriate.

b. Infectious agents as the cause of diseases classified to other chapters
Certain infections are classified in chapters other than Chapter 1 and no organism is identified as part of the infection code. In these instances, it is necessary to use an additional code from Chapter 1 to identify the organism. A code from category B95, Streptococcus, Staphylococcus, and Enterococcus as the cause of diseases classified to other chapters, B96, Other bacterial agents as the cause of diseases classified to other chapters, or B97, Viral agents as the cause of diseases classified to other chapters, is to be used as an additional code to identify the organism. An instructional note will be found at the infection code advising that an additional organism code is required.

c. Infections resistant to antibiotics
Many bacterial infections are resistant to current antibiotics. It is necessary to identify all infections documented as antibiotic resistant. Assign a code from category Z16, Resistance to antimicrobial drugs, following the infection code only if the infection code does not identify drug resistance.

d. Sepsis, Severe Sepsis, and Septic Shock

1) Coding of Sepsis and Severe Sepsis

(a) Sepsis
For a diagnosis of sepsis, assign the appropriate code for the underlying systemic infection. If the type of infection or causal organism is not further specified, assign code A41.9, Sepsis, unspecified organism.

A code from subcategory R65.2, Severe sepsis, should not be assigned unless severe sepsis or an associated acute organ dysfunction is documented.

(i) Negative or inconclusive blood cultures and sepsis
Negative or inconclusive blood cultures do not preclude a diagnosis of sepsis in patients with clinical evidence of the condition, however, the provider should be queried.

(ii) Urosepsis
The term urosepsis is a nonspecific term. It is not to be considered synonymous with sepsis. It has no default code in the Alphabetic Index. Should a provider use this term, he/she must be queried for clarification.

Excludes 1: = NOT CODED HERE! (Do not code both)   *Excludes ❷:* = Not Included Here

(iii) Sepsis with organ dysfunction

If a patient has sepsis and associated acute organ dysfunction or multiple organ dysfunction (MOD), follow the instructions for coding severe sepsis.

(iv) Acute organ dysfunction that is not clearly associated with the sepsis

If a patient has sepsis and an acute organ dysfunction, but the medical record documentation indicates that the acute organ dysfunction is related to a medical condition other than the sepsis, do not assign a code from subcategory R65.2, Severe sepsis. An acute organ dysfunction must be associated with the sepsis in order to assign the severe sepsis code. If the documentation is not clear as to whether an acute organ dysfunction is related to the sepsis or another medical condition, query the provider.

(b) Severe sepsis

The coding of severe sepsis requires a minimum of 2 codes: first a code for the underlying systemic infection, followed by a code from subcategory R65.2, Severe sepsis. If the causal organism is not documented, assign code A41.9, Sepsis, unspecified organism, for the infection. Additional code(s) for the associated acute organ dysfunction are also required.

Due to the complex nature of severe sepsis, some cases may require querying the provider prior to assignment of the codes.

2) Septic shock

(a) Septic shock

Septic shock generally refers to circulatory failure associated with severe sepsis, and therefore, it represents a type of acute organ dysfunction.

For cases of septic shock, the code for the systemic infection should be sequenced first, followed by code R65.21, Severe sepsis with septic shock or code T81.12, Postprocedural septic shock. Any additional codes for the other acute organ dysfunctions should also be assigned. As noted in the sequencing instructions in the Tabular List, the code for septic shock cannot be assigned as a principal diagnosis.

3) Sequencing of severe sepsis

If severe sepsis is present on admission, and meets the definition of principal diagnosis, the underlying systemic infection should be assigned as principal diagnosis followed by the appropriate code from subcategory R65.2 as required by the sequencing rules in the Tabular List. A code from subcategory R65.2 can never be assigned as a principal diagnosis.

When severe sepsis develops during an encounter (it was not present on admission) the underlying systemic infection and the appropriate code from subcategory R65.2 should be assigned as secondary diagnoses.

Severe sepsis may be present on admission but the diagnosis may not be confirmed until sometime after admission. If the documentation is not clear whether severe sepsis was present on admission, the provider should be queried.

4) Sepsis and severe sepsis with a localized infection

If the reason for admission is both sepsis or severe sepsis and a localized infection, such as pneumonia or cellulitis, a code(s) for the underlying systemic infection should be assigned first and the code for the localized infection should be assigned as a secondary diagnosis. If the patient has severe sepsis, a code from subcategory R65.2 should also be assigned as a secondary diagnosis. If the patient is admitted with a localized infection, such as pneumonia, and sepsis/severe sepsis doesn't develop until after admission, the localized infection should be assigned first, followed by the appropriate sepsis/severe sepsis codes.

5) Sepsis due to a postprocedural infection

(a) Documentation of causal relationship

As with all postprocedural complications, code assignment is based on the provider's documentation of the relationship between the infection and the procedure.

(b) Sepsis due to a postprocedural infection

For such cases, the postprocedural infection code, such as, T80.2, Infections following infusion, transfusion, and therapeutic injection, T81.4, Infection following a procedure, T88.0, Infection following immunization, or O86.0, Infection of obstetric surgical wound, should be coded first, followed by the code for the specific infection. If the patient has severe sepsis the appropriate code from subcategory R65.2 should also be assigned with the additional code(s) for any acute organ dysfunction.

(c) Postprocedural infection and postprocedural septic shock

In cases where a postprocedural infection has occurred and has resulted in severe sepsis the code for the precipitating complication such as code T81.4, Infection following a procedure, or O86.0, Infection of obstetrical surgical wound should be coded first followed by code R65.20, Severe sepsis without septic shock and a code for the systemic infection. A code for the systemic infection should also be assigned.

If a postprocedural infection has resulted in postprocedural septic shock, the code for the precipitating complication such as T81.4, Infection following a procedure, or O86.0, Infection of obstetrical surgical wound should be coded first followed by code T81.12-, Postprocedural septic shock. A code for the systemic infection should also be assigned.

6) Sepsis and severe sepsis associated with a noninfectious process (condition)

In some cases a noninfectious process (condition), such as trauma, may lead to an infection which can result in sepsis or severe sepsis. If sepsis or severe sepsis is documented as associated with a noninfectious condition, such as a burn or serious injury, and this condition meets the definition for principal diagnosis, the code for the noninfectious condition should be sequenced first, followed by the code for the resulting infection. If severe sepsis, is present a code from subcategory R65.2 should also be assigned with any associated organ dysfunction(s) codes. It is not necessary to assign a code from subcategory R65.1, Systemic inflammatory response syndrome (SIRS) of non-infectious origin, for these cases.

If the infection meets the definition of principal diagnosis it should be sequenced before the non-infectious condition. When both the associated non-infectious condition and the infection meet the definition of principal diagnosis either may be assigned as principal diagnosis.

Only one code from category R65, Symptoms and signs specifically associated with systemic inflammation and infection, should be assigned. Therefore, when a non-infectious condition leads to an infection resulting in severe sepsis, assign the appropriate code from subcategory R65.2, Severe sepsis. Do not additionally assign a code from subcategory R65.1, Systemic inflammatory response syndrome (SIRS) of non-infectious origin.

See Section I.C.18. SIRS due to non-infectious process.

7) Sepsis and septic shock complicating abortion, pregnancy, childbirth, and the puerperium

See Section I.C.15. Sepsis and septic shock complicating abortion, pregnancy, childbirth and the puerperium.

8) Newborn sepsis

See Section I.C.16.f. Bacterial sepsis of Newborn.

e. Methicillin Resistant *Staphylococcus aureus* (MRSA) Conditions

1) Selection and sequencing of MRSA codes

(a) Combination codes for MRSA infection

When a patient is diagnosed with an infection that is due to methicillin resistant *Staphylococcus aureus* (MRSA), and that infection that has a combination code that includes the causal organism (e.g., sepsis, pneumonia) assign the appropriate combination code for the condition (e.g., code A41.02, Sepsis due to methicillin resistant Staphylococcus aureus or code J15.212, Pneumonia due to methicillin resistant Staphylococcus aureus). Do not assign code B95.62, Methicillin resistant Staphylococcus aureus infection as the cause of the diseases classified elsewhere, as an additional code because the combination code includes the type of infection and the MRSA organism. Do not assign a code from subcategory Z16.11, Resistance to penicillins, as an additional diagnosis.

See Section C.1. for instructions on coding and sequencing of sepsis and severe sepsis.

(b) Other codes for MRSA infection

When there is documentation of a current infection (e.g., wound infection, stitch abscess, urinary tract infection) due to MRSA, and that infection does not have a combination code that includes the causal organism, assign the appropriate code to identify the condition along with code B95.62, Methicillin resistant Staphylococcus aureus infection as the cause of diseases classified elsewhere for the MRSA infection. Do not assign a code from subcategory Z16.11, Resistance to penicillins.

(c)   Methicillin susceptible Staphylococcus aureus (MSSA) and MRSA colonization

The condition or state of being colonized or carrying MSSA or MRSA is called colonization or carriage, while an individual person is described as being colonized or being a carrier. Colonization means that MSSA and MSRA is present on or in the body without necessarily causing illness. A positive MRSA colonization test might be documented by the provider as "MRSA screen positive" or "MRSA nasal swab positive".

Assign code Z22.322, Carrier or suspected carrier of methicillin resistant Staphylococcus aureus, for patients documented as having MRSA colonization. Assign code Z22.321, Carrier or suspected carrier of methicillin susceptible Staphylococcus aureus, for patient documented as having MSSA colonization. Colonization is not necessarily indicative of a disease process or as the cause of a specific condition the patient may have unless documented as such by the provider.

(d)   MRSA colonization and infection

If a patient is documented as having both MRSA colonization and infection during a hospital admission, code Z22.322, Carrier or suspected carrier of methicillin resistant Staphylococcus aureus, and a code for the MRSA infection may both be assigned.

f.   Zika virus infections

1)   Code only confirmed cases

Code only a confirmed diagnosis of Zika virus (A92.5, Zika virus disease) as documented by the provider. This is an exception to the hospital inpatient guideline Section II, H. In this context, "confirmation" does not require documentation of the type of test performed; the physician's diagnostic statement that the condition is confirmed is sufficient. This code should be assigned regardless of the stated mode of transmission.

If the provider documents "suspected", "possible" or "probable" Zika, do not assign code A92.5. Assign a code(s) explaining the reason for the encounter (such as fever, rash, or joint pain) or Z20.828, Contact with and (suspected) exposure to other viral communicable diseases.

Intestinal infectious diseases (A00-A09)

A00- <u>Cholera</u> — An acute infectious disease caused by Vibrio cholerae manifested by diarrhea and severe dehydration.

cc**A00.0** Cholera due to Vibrio cholerae 01, biovar <u>cholerae</u>
Classical cholera

cc**A00.1** Cholera due to Vibrio cholerae 01, biovar <u>el tor</u>
Cholera el tor

cc**A00.9** Cholera, unspecified

A01- **Typhoid and paratyphoid fevers** — An acute infectious disease caused by a Salmonella organism and characterized by acute fever and Peyer's patches in the intestines.

A01.0- <u>Typhoid</u> fever — A form due to infection with Salmonella typhi.
Infection due to Salmonella typhi

cc**A01.00** Typhoid fever, unspecified

cc**A01.01** Typhoid <u>meningitis</u>

cc**A01.02** Typhoid fever with <u>heart</u> involvement
Typhoid endocarditis
Typhoid myocarditis

cc**A01.03** Typhoid <u>pneumonia</u>

cc**A01.04** Typhoid <u>arthritis</u>

cc**A01.05** Typhoid <u>osteomyelitis</u>

cc**A01.09** Typhoid fever with other complications

cc**A01.1** <u>Paratyphoid</u> fever <u>A</u> — A form due to infection with Salmonella enteritidis paratyphi A.

cc**A01.2** <u>Paratyphoid</u> fever <u>B</u> — A form due to infection with Salmonella enteritidis paratyphi B.

cc**A01.3** <u>Paratyphoid</u> fever <u>C</u> — A form due to infection with Salmonella enteritidis paratyphi C.

cc**A01.4** <u>Paratyphoid</u> fever, unspecified
Infection due to Salmonella paratyphi NOS

A02- <u>Other salmonella</u> infections — Cellular injury due to competitive metabolism after invasion and multiplication of Salmonella organisms.
Includes: Infection or foodborne intoxication due to any Salmonella species other than S. typhi and S. paratyphi

cc**A02.0** Salmonella <u>enteritis</u> — Infection of the gastrointestinal tract by Salmonella.
Salmonellosis

mcc**A02.1** Salmonella <u>sepsis</u> — A systemic disease caused by persistence of Salmonella and/or their toxins in the blood.

A02.2- <u>Localized</u> salmonella infections

A02.20 Localized salmonella infection, unspecified

mcc**A02.21** Salmonella <u>meningitis</u>

mcc**A02.22** Salmonella <u>pneumonia</u>

cc**A02.23** Salmonella <u>arthritis</u>

cc**A02.24** Salmonella <u>osteomyelitis</u>

cc**A02.25** Salmonella <u>pyelonephritis</u>
Salmonella tubulo-interstitial nephropathy

cc**A02.29** Salmonella with other localized infection

cc**A02.8** Other specified salmonella infections

cc**A02.9** Salmonella infection, unspecified

A03- <u>Shigellosis</u> — An acute infectious disease due to the genus shigella, tribe Salmonelleae, which causes dysentery.

cc**A03.0** Shigellosis due to Shigella dysenteriae
Group A shigellosis [Shiga-Kruse dysentery]

A03.1 Shigellosis due to Shigella flexneri
Group B shigellosis

A03.2 Shigellosis due to Shigella boydii
Group C shigellosis

A03.3 Shigellosis due to Shigella sonnei
Group D shigellosis

A03.8 Other shigellosis

A03.9 Shigellosis, unspecified
Bacillary dysentery NOS

A04- <u>Other bacterial intestinal</u> infections — Escherichia coli – Intestinal infection due to the species Escherichia coli in massive numbers, although common in man's intestinal flora.
Excludes 1: *bacterial foodborne intoxications, NEC (A05.-)*
tuberculous enteritis (A18.32)

cc**A04.0** Enteropathogenic <u>Escherichia coli</u> infection

cc**A04.1** Enterotoxigenic <u>Escherichia coli</u> infection

cc**A04.2** Enteroinvasive <u>Escherichia coli</u> infection

cc**A04.3** Enterohemorrhagic <u>Escherichia coli</u> infection

cc**A04.4** Other intestinal <u>Escherichia coli</u> infections
Escherichia coli enteritis NOS

cc**A04.5** Campylobacter enteritis

cc**A04.6** Enteritis due to Yersinia enterocolitica
Excludes 1: *extraintestinal yersiniosis (A28.2)*

cc**A04.7** Enterocolitis due to Clostridium difficile
Foodborne intoxication by Clostridium difficile
Pseudomembraneous colitis

cc**A04.8** Other specified bacterial intestinal infections

cc**A04.9** Bacterial intestinal infection, unspecified
Bacterial enteritis NOS

A05- Other bacterial <u>foodborne</u> intoxications, not elsewhere classified
Excludes 1: *Clostridium difficile foodborne intoxication and infection (A04.7)*
Escherichia coli infection (A04.0-A04.4)
listeriosis (A32.-)
salmonella foodborne intoxication and infection (A02.-)
toxic effect of noxious foodstuffs (T61-T62)

cc**A05.0** Foodborne staphylococcal intoxication

cc**A05.1** Botulism food poisoning — A form caused by the neurotoxin (Botulin) produced by the growth of Clostridium botulinum in improperly canned or preserved foods.
Botulism NOS
Classical foodborne intoxication due to Clostridium botulinum
Excludes 1: *infant botulism (A48.51)*
wound botulism (A48.52)

cc**A05.2** Foodborne Clostridium perfringens [Clostridium welchii] intoxication
Enteritis necroticans
Pig-bel

cc**A05.3** Foodborne Vibrio parahaemolyticus intoxication

cc**A05.4** Foodborne Bacillus cereus intoxication

cc**A05.5** Foodborne Vibrio vulnificus intoxication

cc**A05.8** Other specified bacterial foodborne intoxications

A05.9 Bacterial foodborne intoxication, unspecified

A06- <u>Amebiasis</u> — The state of being infected with Entamoeba histolytica.
Includes: Infection due to Entamoeba histolytica
Excludes 1: *other protozoal intestinal diseases (A07.-)*
Excludes ❷: *acanthamebiasis (B60.1-)*
Naegleriasis (B60.2)

cc**A06.0** Acute amebic dysentery
Acute amebiasis
Intestinal amebiasis NOS

cc**A06.1** Chronic intestinal amebiasis

cc**A06.2** Amebic nondysenteric colitis

cc**A06.3** Ameboma of intestine
Ameboma NOS

mcc**A06.4** Amebic liver abscess
Hepatic amebiasis

mcc**A06.5** Amebic lung abscess
Amebic abscess of lung (and liver)

mcc**A06.6** Amebic brain abscess
Amebic abscess of brain (and liver) (and lung)

A06.7 Cutaneous amebiasis

A06.8- Amebic infection of other sites

cc**A06.81** Amebic cystitis

cc**A06.82** Other amebic genitourinary infections
Amebic balanitis
Amebic vesiculitis
Amebic vulvovaginitis

A00-A06

cc **A06.89** **Other amebic infections**
    Amebic appendicitis
    Amebic splenic abscess

A06.9 **Amebiasis, unspecified**

A07- **Other protozoal intestinal diseases**

A07.0 **Balantidiasis** — Infection of the colon by the protozoa Balantidium coli.
    Balantidial dysentery

cc **A07.1** **Giardiasis [lambliasis]** — Infection of the small intestine by the species Giardia lamblia.

cc **A07.2** **Cryptosporidiosis** — Intestinal infection caused by Cryptosporidium parvum.

cc **A07.3** **Isosporiasis**
    Infection due to Isospora belli and Isospora hominis
    Intestinal coccidiosis
    Isosporosis

cc **A07.4** **Cyclosporiasis** — Intestinal infection, with severe diarrhea, caused by Cyclospora cayetanensis, associated with eating contaminated raspberries.

cc **A07.8** **Other specified protozoal intestinal diseases**
    Intestinal microsporidiosis
    Intestinal trichomoniasis
    Sarcocystosis
    Sarcosporidiosis

cc **A07.9** **Protozoal intestinal disease, unspecified**
    Flagellate diarrhea
    Protozoal colitis
    Protozoal diarrhea
    Protozoal dysentery

A08- **Viral and other specified intestinal infections**
    Excludes 1: *influenza with involvement of gastrointestinal tract (J09.x3, J10.2, J11.2)*

cc **A08.0** **Rotaviral enteritis** — Inflammation of the intestine, primarily the small intestine, caused by a group of RNA viruses and often seen in children.

A08.1- **Acute gastroenteropathy due to Norwalk agent and other small round viruses**

cc **A08.11** **Acute gastroenteropathy due to Norwalk agent** — Inflammation of the intestine, primarily the small intestine, caused by the adenovirus group of disease-causing viruses.
    Acute gastroenteropathy due to Norovirus
    Acute gastroenteropathy due to Norwalk-like agent

cc **A08.19** **Acute gastroenteropathy due to other small round viruses**
    Acute gastroenteropathy due to small round virus [SRV] NOS

cc **A08.2** **Adenoviral enteritis**

A08.3- **Other viral enteritis**

cc **A08.31** **Calicivirus enteritis** — Inflammation of the intestine, primarily the small intestine, caused by a subgroup of Picornaviruses.

cc **A08.32** **Astrovirus enteritis** — Inflammation of the intestine, primarily the small intestine, caused by the Astrovirus.

cc **A08.39** **Other viral enteritis**
    Coxsackie virus enteritis — Inflammation of the intestine, primarily the small intestine, caused by the Coxsackie virus from the enterovirus group.
    Echovirus enteritis — Inflammation of the intestine, primarily the small intestine, caused by the Echovirus from the enterovirus group.
    Enterovirus enteritis NEC
    Torovirus enteritis

A08.4 **Viral intestinal infection, unspecified**
    Viral enteritis NOS
    Viral gastroenteritis NOS
    Viral gastroenteropathy NOS

A08.8 **Other specified intestinal infections**

A09 **Infectious gastroenteritis and colitis, unspecified** — Inflammation of the
cc colon, small intestine, and stomach of an infectious origin.
    Infectious colitis NOS
    Infectious enteritis NOS
    Infectious gastroenteritis NOS
    Excludes 1: *colitis NOS (K52.9)*
        diarrhea NOS (R19.7)
        enteritis NOS (K52.9)
        gastroenteritis NOS (K52.9)
        noninfective gastroenteritis and colitis, unspecified (K52.9)

Tuberculosis (A15-A19)

Includes: Infections due to Mycobacterium tuberculosis and Mycobacterium bovis

Excludes 1: *congenital tuberculosis (P37.0)*
    nonspecific reaction to test for tuberculosis without active tuberculosis (R76.1-)
    pneumoconiosis associated with tuberculosis, any type in A15 (J65)
    positive PPD (R76.11)
    positive tuberculin skin test without active tuberculosis (R76.11)
    sequelae of tuberculosis (B90.-)
    silicotuberculosis (J65)

A15- **Respiratory tuberculosis** — An infectious disease caused by Mycobacterium tuberculosis or Mycobacterium bovis and characterized by involvement of respiratory tissues.

cc **A15.0** **Tuberculosis of lung**
    Tuberculous bronchiectasis
    Tuberculous fibrosis of lung
    Tuberculous pneumonia
    Tuberculous pneumothorax

cc **A15.4** **Tuberculosis of intrathoracic lymph nodes**
    Tuberculosis of hilar lymph nodes
    Tuberculosis of mediastinal lymph nodes
    Tuberculosis of tracheobronchial lymph nodes
    Excludes 1: *tuberculosis specified as primary (A15.7)*

cc **A15.5** **Tuberculosis of larynx, trachea and bronchus**
    Tuberculosis of bronchus
    Tuberculosis of glottis
    Tuberculosis of larynx
    Tuberculosis of trachea

cc **A15.6** **Tuberculous pleurisy**
    Tuberculosis of pleura
    Tuberculous empyema
    Excludes 1: *primary respiratory tuberculosis (A15.7)*

cc **A15.7** **Primary respiratory tuberculosis**

cc **A15.8** **Other respiratory tuberculosis**
    Mediastinal tuberculosis
    Nasopharyngeal tuberculosis
    Tuberculosis of nose
    Tuberculosis of sinus [any nasal]

cc **A15.9** **Respiratory tuberculosis unspecified**

A17- **Tuberculosis of nervous system** — An infectious disease caused by Mycobacterium tuberculosis or Mycobacterium bovis and characterized by involvement of meninges and the nervous system.

MCC **A17.0** **Tuberculous meningitis**
    Tuberculosis of meninges (cerebral) (spinal)
    Tuberculous leptomeningitis
    Excludes 1: *tuberculous meningoencephalitis (A17.82)*

MCC **A17.1** **Meningeal tuberculoma**
    Tuberculoma of meninges (cerebral) (spinal)
    Excludes ❷: *tuberculoma of brain and spinal cord (A17.81)*

A17.8- **Other tuberculosis of nervous system**

MCC **A17.81** **Tuberculoma of brain and spinal cord**
    Tuberculous abscess of brain and spinal cord

MCC **A17.82** **Tuberculous meningoencephalitis**
    Tuberculous myelitis

MCC **A17.83** **Tuberculous neuritis**
    Tuberculous mononeuropathy

MCC **A17.89** **Other tuberculosis of nervous system**
    Tuberculous polyneuropathy

cc **A17.9** **Tuberculosis of nervous system, unspecified**

A18- **Tuberculosis of other organs**

A18.0- **Tuberculosis of bones and joints**

cc **A18.01** **Tuberculosis of spine**
    Pott's disease or curvature of spine
    Tuberculous arthritis
    Tuberculous osteomyelitis of spine
    Tuberculous spondylitis

cc **A18.02** **Tuberculous arthritis of other joints**
    Tuberculosis of hip (joint)
    Tuberculosis of knee (joint)

cc **A18.03** **Tuberculosis of other bones**
    Tuberculous mastoiditis
    Tuberculous osteomyelitis

A06 - A18

cc **A18.09** **Other musculoskeletal tuberculosis**
  Tuberculous myositis
  Tuberculous synovitis
  Tuberculous tenosynovitis

A18.1- **Tuberculosis of** <u>genitourinary</u> **system** — An infectious disease caused by Mycobacterium tuberculosis or Mycobacterium bovis and characterized by involvement of the genitourinary system.

cc **A18.10** **Tuberculosis of genitourinary system, unspecified**

cc **A18.11** **Tuberculosis of kidney and ureter**

cc **A18.12** **Tuberculosis of bladder**

cc **A18.13** **Tuberculosis of other urinary organs**
  Tuberculous urethritis

cc **A18.14** **Tuberculosis of prostate** — [♂, Age/15-124]

cc **A18.15** **Tuberculosis of other male genital organs** — [♂]

cc **A18.16** **Tuberculosis of cervix** — [♀]

cc **A18.17** **Tuberculous female pelvic inflammatory disease** — [♀]
  Tuberculous endometritis
  Tuberculous oophoritis and salpingitis

cc **A18.18** **Tuberculosis of other female genital organs** — [♀]
  Tuberculous ulceration of vulva

cc **A18.2** **Tuberculous peripheral** <u>lymphadenopathy</u>
  Tuberculous adenitis
  Excludes ❷: *tuberculosis of bronchial and mediastinal lymph nodes (A15.4)*
        tuberculosis of mesenteric and retroperitoneal lymph nodes (A18.39)
        tuberculous tracheobronchial adenopathy (A15.4)

A18.3- **Tuberculosis of** <u>intestines</u>, **peritoneum and mesenteric glands**

MCC **A18.31** **Tuberculous peritonitis**
  Tuberculous ascites

cc **A18.32** **Tuberculous enteritis**
  Tuberculosis of anus and rectum
  Tuberculosis of intestine (large) (small)

cc **A18.39** **Retroperitoneal tuberculosis**
  Tuberculosis of mesenteric glands
  Tuberculosis of retroperitoneal (lymph glands)

cc **A18.4** **Tuberculosis of** <u>skin</u> **and subcutaneous tissue**
  Erythema induratum, tuberculous
  Lupus excedens
  Lupus vulgaris NOS
  Lupus vulgaris of eyelid
  Scrofuloderma
  Tuberculosis of external ear
  Excludes ❷: *lupus erythematosus (L93.-)*
        lupus NOS (M32.9)
        systemic (M32.-)

A18.5- **Tuberculosis of** <u>eye</u>
  Excludes ❷: *lupus vulgaris of eyelid (A18.4)*

cc **A18.50** **Tuberculosis of eye, unspecified**

cc **A18.51** **Tuberculous episcleritis**

cc **A18.52** **Tuberculous keratitis**
  Tuberculous interstitial keratitis
  Tuberculous keratoconjunctivitis (interstitial) (phlyctenular)

cc **A18.53** **Tuberculous chorioretinitis**

cc **A18.54** **Tuberculous iridocyclitis**

cc **A18.59** **Other tuberculosis of eye**
  Tuberculous conjunctivitis

cc **A18.6** **Tuberculosis of (inner) (middle)** <u>ear</u>
  Tuberculous otitis media
  Excludes ❷: *tuberculosis of external ear (A18.4)*
        tuberculous mastoiditis (A18.03)

cc **A18.7** **Tuberculosis of** <u>adrenal</u> **glands**
  Tuberculous Addison's disease

A18.8- **Tuberculosis of** <u>other specified</u> **organs**

cc **A18.81** **Tuberculosis of thyroid gland**

cc **A18.82** **Tuberculosis of other endocrine glands**
  Tuberculosis of pituitary gland
  Tuberculosis of thymus gland

cc **A18.83** **Tuberculosis of digestive tract organs, not elsewhere classified**
  Excludes 1: *tuberculosis of intestine (A18.32)*

cc **A18.84** **Tuberculosis of heart**
  Tuberculous cardiomyopathy
  Tuberculous endocarditis
  Tuberculous myocarditis
  Tuberculous pericarditis

cc **A18.85** **Tuberculosis of spleen**

cc **A18.89** **Tuberculosis of other sites**
  Tuberculosis of muscle
  Tuberculous cerebral arteritis

A19- <u>Miliary</u> **tuberculosis** — An infectious disease caused by Mycobacterium tuberculosis or Mycobacterium bovis and characterized by dissemination of viable tubercle bacilli into the bloodstream with infection throughout the body.
  Includes: Disseminated tuberculosis
        Generalized tuberculosis
        Tuberculous polyserositis

MCC **A19.0** **Acute miliary tuberculosis of a single specified site**

MCC **A19.1** **Acute miliary tuberculosis of multiple sites**

MCC **A19.2** **Acute miliary tuberculosis, unspecified**

MCC **A19.8** **Other miliary tuberculosis**

MCC **A19.9** **Miliary tuberculosis, unspecified**

Certain zoonotic bacterial diseases (A20-A28)

A20- <u>Plague</u> — A febrile infectious disease caused by Yersinia pestis, characterized by acute fever and chills followed by prostration and commonly marked with delirium, headache, vomiting, and diarrhea. Primarily a disease of rodents, it is transmitted to man by the bite of infected fleas and communicated from patient to patient.
  Includes: Infection due to Yersinia pestis

MCC **A20.0** **Bubonic plague**

MCC **A20.1** **Cellulocutaneous plague**

MCC **A20.2** **Pneumonic plague**

MCC **A20.3** **Plague meningitis**

MCC **A20.7** **Septicemic plague**

MCC **A20.8** **Other forms of plague**
  Abortive plague
  Asymptomatic plague
  Pestis minor

MCC **A20.9** **Plague, unspecified**

A21- <u>Tularemia</u> — A febrile infectious disease (resembling plague) caused by Francisella tularensis, and characterized by fever, chills, headache, and myalgia. It is transmitted to man by bites from infected flies, fleas, ticks, and lice.
  Includes: Deer-fly fever
        Infection due to Francisella tularensis
        Rabbit fever

cc **A21.0** **Ulceroglandular tularemia**

cc **A21.1** **Oculoglandular tularemia**
  Ophthalmic tularemia

cc **A21.2** **Pulmonary tularemia**

cc **A21.3** **Gastrointestinal tularemia**
  Abdominal tularemia

cc **A21.7** **Generalized tularemia**

cc **A21.8** **Other forms of tularemia**

cc **A21.9** **Tularemia, unspecified**

A22- <u>Anthrax</u> — An infectious disease caused by Bacillus anthracis and characterized by ulcerated papules which form black eschars with following necrosis. It is transmitted to man by direct and indirect contact with infected animals and their commerical products.
  Includes: Infection due to Bacillus anthracis

cc **A22.0** **Cutaneous anthrax**
  Malignant carbuncle
  Malignant pustule

MCC **A22.1** **Pulmonary anthrax**
  Inhalation anthrax
  Ragpicker's disease
  Woolsorter's disease

cc **A22.2** **Gastrointestinal anthrax**

MCC **A22.7** **Anthrax sepsis**

cc **A22.8** **Other forms of anthrax**
  Anthrax meningitis

cc **A22.9** **Anthrax, unspecified**

Excludes 1: = NOT CODED HERE! (Do not code both)   **Excludes ❷:** = Not Included Here

A23- **Brucellosis** — An infectious disease caused by Brucella bacterial species, characterized by fever, chills, headache, aches and pains, and weakness.
  Includes: Malta fever
              Mediterranean fever
              Undulant fever
  A23.0   **Brucellosis due to Brucella melitensis**
  A23.1   **Brucellosis due to Brucella abortus**
  A23.2   **Brucellosis due to Brucella suis**
  A23.3   **Brucellosis due to Brucella canis**
cc **A23.8**   **Other brucellosis**
cc **A23.9**   **Brucellosis, unspecified**

A24- **Glanders and melioidosis**
cc **A24.0**   **Glanders** — An infectious disease caused by Pseudomonas mallei and characterized by inflammation of mucous membranes and development of nodules of the skin which break down to ulcers. It is transmitted to man by infected horses.
              Infection due to Pseudomonas mallei
              Malleus
cc **A24.1**   **Acute and fulminating melioidosis**
              Melioidosis pneumonia
              Melioidosis sepsis
cc **A24.2**   **Subacute and chronic melioidosis**
cc **A24.3**   **Other melioidosis**
cc **A24.9**   **Melioidosis, unspecified** — An infectious disease caused by Pseudomonas pseudomallei, variously marked by fever, chills, bloodstained sputum, diarrhea, abdominal pain, and in less acute cases granulomatous pneumonia and multiple skin abscess formations.
              Infection due to Pseudomonas pseudomallei NOS
              Whitmore's disease

A25- **Rat-bite fevers**
cc **A25.0**   **Spirillosis** — An infectious disease caused by Spirillum minor and characterized by local inflammation at the site of the rat bite, regional lymphadenopathy, macular red-brown rash, and fever of sudden onset.
              Sodoku
cc **A25.1**   **Streptobacillosis** — An infectious disease caused by Streptobacillus moniliformis and characterized by sudden onset of fever, erythematous eruption, polyarthritis, adenitis, headache, and vomiting.
              Epidemic arthritic erythema
              Haverhill fever
              Streptobacillary rat-bite fever
cc **A25.9**   **Rat-bite fever, unspecified**

A26- **Erysipeloid** — An infectious disease caused by Erysipelothrix insidiosa or Erysipelothrix rhusiopathiae and characterized by local inflammation at an abrasion site after contact with infected meat.
  A26.0   **Cutaneous erysipeloid**
              Erythema migrans
MCC **A26.7**   **Erysipelothrix sepsis**
  A26.8   **Other forms of erysipeloid**
  A26.9   **Erysipeloid, unspecified**

A27- **Leptospirosis** — An infectious bacterial disease caused by the genus Leptospira and generally characterized by fever, chills, headache, malaise, and occasionally meningitis, uveitis, hepatitis, and nephritis.
cc **A27.0**   **Leptospirosis icterohemorrhagica** — A form caused by Leptospira icterhaemorrhagiae and characterized by fever, jaundice, myalgia, hemorrhage, anemia, and sometimes vascular collapse.
              Leptospiral or spirochetal jaundice (hemorrhagic)
              Weil's disease
  A27.8- **Other forms of leptospirosis**
MCC **A27.81** **Aseptic meningitis in leptospirosis**
cc **A27.89** **Other forms of leptospirosis**
cc **A27.9**   **Leptospirosis, unspecified**

A28- **Other zoonotic bacterial diseases, not elsewhere classified**
cc **A28.0**   **Pasteurellosis** — An infectious disease caused by Pasteurella multocida and variously characterized by local infections, respiratory infections, or systemic infections such as meningitis and bacteremia.
cc **A28.1**   **Cat-scratch disease** — An infectious disease caused by Bartonella henselae and characterized by regional lymphadenitis, granulomatous skin reaction at the site of injury from a cat, and mild fever.
              Cat-scratch fever
cc **A28.2**   **Extraintestinal yersiniosis**
  Excludes 1:   enteritis due to Yersinia enterocolitica (A04.6)
              plague (A20.-)

cc **A28.8**   **Other specified zoonotic bacterial diseases, not elsewhere classified**
cc **A28.9**   **Zoonotic bacterial disease, unspecified**

Other bacterial diseases (A30-A49)

A30- **Leprosy [Hansen's disease]** — A chronic infectious disease caused by Mycobacterium leprae and primarily characterized by granulomatous lesions of the skin, peripheral nerves, and mucous membranes.
  Includes: Infection due to Mycobacterium leprae
  Excludes 1:   sequelae of leprosy (B92)
cc **A30.0**   **Indeterminate leprosy**
              I leprosy
cc **A30.1**   **Tuberculoid leprosy**
              TT leprosy
cc **A30.2**   **Borderline tuberculoid leprosy**
              BT leprosy
cc **A30.3**   **Borderline leprosy**
              BB leprosy
cc **A30.4**   **Borderline lepromatous leprosy**
              BL leprosy
cc **A30.5**   **Lepromatous leprosy**
              LL leprosy
cc **A30.8**   **Other forms of leprosy**
cc **A30.9**   **Leprosy, unspecified**

A31- **Infection due to other mycobacteria**
  Excludes ❷: leprosy (A30.-)
              tuberculosis (A15-A19)
cc **A31.0**   **Pulmonary mycobacterial infection**
              Infection due to Mycobacterium avium
              Infection due to Mycobacterium intracellulare [Battey bacillus]
              Infection due to Mycobacterium kansasii
cc **A31.1**   **Cutaneous mycobacterial infection**
              Buruli ulcer
              Infection due to Mycobacterium marinum
              Infection due to Mycobacterium ulcerans
cc **A31.2**   **Disseminated mycobacterium avium-intracellulare complex (DMAC)**
              MAC sepsis
cc **A31.8**   **Other mycobacterial infections**
cc **A31.9**   **Mycobacterial infection, unspecified**
              Atypical mycobacterial infection NOS
              Mycobacteriosis NOS

A32- **Listeriosis** — An infectious disease caused by Listeria monocytogenes and characterized by sore throat with glandular swelling, monocytosis, septicemia, conjunctivitis, involvement of the liver, and localized purulent mucous membrane inflammations.
  Includes: Listerial foodborne infection
  Excludes 1:   neonatal (disseminated) listeriosis (P37.2)
cc **A32.0**   **Cutaneous listeriosis**
  A32.1- **Listerial meningitis and meningoencephalitis**
cc **A32.11** **Listerial meningitis**
cc **A32.12** **Listerial meningoencephalitis**
MCC **A32.7**   **Listerial sepsis**
  A32.8- **Other forms of listeriosis**
cc **A32.81** **Oculoglandular listeriosis**
cc **A32.82** **Listerial endocarditis**
cc **A32.89** **Other forms of listeriosis**
              Listerial cerebral arteritis
cc **A32.9**   **Listeriosis, unspecified**

A33 **Tetanus neonatorum** — [Age/0]
MCC

A34 **Obstetrical tetanus** — [♀, Age/12-55]
CC

A35 **Other tetanus** — An infectious disease complication of wounds caused by the toxin
MCC produced by Clostridium tetani and characterized by tonic spasms of the voluntary muscles, hyperreflexia resulting in trismus (lockjaw), severe cases developing generalized convulsions and respiratory distress.
  Tetanus NOS
  Excludes 1:   obstetrical tetanus (A34)
              tetanus neonatorum (A33)

Excludes 1: = NOT CODED HERE! (Do not code both)   **531**   *Excludes ❷:* = Not Included Here

A36- <u>Diphtheria</u> — An infectious disease caused by Corynebacterium diphtheriae, and characterized by a membrane in the pharynx, sore throat, fever, nausea, vomiting, headache, and chills.

cc **A36.0** **Pharyngeal diphtheria**
Diphtheritic membranous angina
Tonsillar diphtheria

cc **A36.1** **Nasopharyngeal diphtheria**

cc **A36.2** **Laryngeal diphtheria**
Diphtheritic laryngotracheitis

cc **A36.3** **Cutaneous diphtheria**
Excludes ❷: erythrasma (L08.1)

A36.8- **Other diphtheria**

cc **A36.81** **Diphtheritic cardiomyopathy**
Diphtheritic myocarditis

cc **A36.82** **Diphtheritic radiculomyelitis**

cc **A36.83** **Diphtheritic polyneuritis**

cc **A36.84** **Diphtheritic tubulo-interstitial nephropathy**

cc **A36.85** **Diphtheritic cystitis**

cc **A36.86** **Diphtheritic conjunctivitis**

cc **A36.89** **Other diphtheritic complications**
Diphtheritic peritonitis

cc **A36.9** **Diphtheria, unspecified**

A37- <u>Whooping cough</u> — An infectious disease caused by Bordetella pertussis and characterized by progressive and repetitive paroxysmal coughing, mild systemic complaints, lymphocytosis, and inspiratory whoop.

A37.0- **Whooping cough due to Bordetella pertussis**

cc **A37.00** **Whooping cough due to Bordetella pertussis without pneumonia**

mcc **A37.01** **Whooping cough due to Bordetella pertussis with pneumonia**

A37.1- **Whooping cough due to Bordetella parapertussis**

cc **A37.10** **Whooping cough due to Bordetella parapertussis without pneumonia**

mcc **A37.11** **Whooping cough due to Bordetella parapertussis with pneumonia**

A37.8- **Whooping cough due to other Bordetella species**

cc **A37.80** **Whooping cough due to other Bordetella species without pneumonia**

mcc **A37.81** **Whooping cough due to other Bordetella species with pneumonia**

A37.9- **Whooping cough, unspecified species**

cc **A37.90** **Whooping cough, unspecified species without pneumonia**

mcc **A37.91** **Whooping cough, unspecified species with pneumonia**

A38- <u>Scarlet fever</u> — An acute febrile infectious disease caused by Group A Streptococcus and characterized by high fever, sore throat, and skin rash.
Includes: scarlatina
Excludes ❷: streptococcal sore throat (J02.0)

cc **A38.0** **Scarlet fever with otitis media**

cc **A38.1** **Scarlet fever with myocarditis**

cc **A38.8** **Scarlet fever with other complications**

cc **A38.9** **Scarlet fever, uncomplicated**
Scarlet fever, NOS

A39- <u>Meningococcal</u> **infection** — Infectious diseases caused by Neisseria meningitidis.

mcc **A39.0** **Meningococcal meningitis** — A form characterized by inflammation of the cerebral and spinal meninges.

mcc **A39.1** **Waterhouse-Friderichsen syndrome** — The fulminating form characterized by abrupt sudden high fever, chills, myalgias, nausea, vomiting, headache, widespread ecchymotic rash, and buccal mucosa and conjunctival hemorrhages, with cyanosis, hypotension, profound shock, and bilateral adrenal hemorrhages.
Meningococcal hemorrhagic adrenalitis
Meningococcic adrenal syndrome

mcc **A39.2** **Acute meningococcemia**

mcc **A39.3** **Chronic meningococcemia**

mcc **A39.4** **Meningococcemia, unspecified**

A39.5- **Meningococcal heart disease**

mcc **A39.50** **Meningococcal carditis, unspecified**

mcc **A39.51** **Meningococcal endocarditis**

mcc **A39.52** **Meningococcal myocarditis**

mcc **A39.53** **Meningococcal pericarditis**

A39.8- **Other meningococcal infections**

mcc **A39.81** **Meningococcal encephalitis**

cc **A39.82** **Meningococcal retrobulbar neuritis**

cc **A39.83** **Meningococcal arthritis**

cc **A39.84** **Postmeningococcal arthritis**

cc **A39.89** **Other meningococcal infections**
Meningococcal conjunctivitis

cc **A39.9** **Meningococcal infection, unspecified**
Meningococcal disease NOS

A40- <u>Streptococcal sepsis</u> — Streptococcal bacteria in the bloodstream marked by high fever, shaking, chills, prostration, and if untreated, hypotension, shock, and death.
Code first: Postprocedural streptococcal sepsis (T81.4-)
Streptococcal sepsis during labor (O75.3)
Streptococcal sepsis following abortion or ectopic or molar pregnancy (O03-O07, O08.0)
Streptococcal sepsis following immunization (T88.0)
Streptococcal sepsis following infusion, transfusion or therapeutic injection (T80.2-)
Excludes 1: neonatal (P36.0-P36.1)
puerperal sepsis (O85)
sepsis due to Streptococcus, group D (A41.81)

mcc **A40.0** **Sepsis due to streptococcus, group A**

mcc **A40.1** **Sepsis due to streptococcus, group B**

mcc **A40.3** **Sepsis due to Streptococcus pneumoniae**
Pneumococcal sepsis

mcc **A40.8** **Other streptococcal sepsis**

mcc **A40.9** **Streptococcal sepsis, unspecified**

A41-   <u>Other sepsis</u>
    AHA 16:1Q:p32 – Resolving sepsis
    Code first: Postprocedural sepsis (T81.4-)
              Sepsis during labor (O75.3)
              Sepsis following abortion, ectopic or molar pregnancy
                (O03-O07, O08.0)
              Sepsis following immunization (T88.0)
              Sepsis following infusion, transfusion or therapeutic injection
                (T80.2-)
    Excludes 1: *bacteremia NOS (R78.81)*
                neonatal (P36.-)
                puerperal sepsis (O85)
                streptococcal sepsis (A40.-)
    Excludes ❷: *sepsis (due to) (in) actinomycotic (A42.7)*
                sepsis (due to) (in) anthrax (A22.7)
                sepsis (due to) (in) candidal (B37.7)
                sepsis (due to) (in) Erysipelothrix (A26.7)
                sepsis (due to) (in) extraintestinal yersiniosis (A28.2)
                sepsis (due to) (in) gonococcal (A54.86)
                sepsis (due to) (in) herpesviral (B00.7)
                sepsis (due to) (in) listerial (A32.7)
                sepsis (due to) (in) melioidosis (A24.1)
                sepsis (due to) (in) meningococcal (A39.2-A39.4)
                sepsis (due to) (in) plague (A20.7)
                sepsis (due to) (in) tularemia (A21.7)
                toxic shock syndrome (A48.3)

A41.0-   **Sepsis due to <u>Staphylococcus aureus</u>** — Staphylococcus aureus bacteria in the bloodstream marked by high fever, shaking, chills, prostration, and if untreated, hypotension, shock, and death.

  ᴹᶜᶜ**A41.01**   <u>Sepsis due to methicillin **susceptible** Staphylococcus aureus</u> — A form caused by a form of the bacterium Staphylococcus aureus that is susceptible to antibiotic treatment.
        MSSA sepsis
        Staphylococcus aureus sepsis NOS

  ᴹᶜᶜ**A41.02**   <u>Sepsis due to methicillin **resistant** Staphylococcus aureus</u> — A form caused by a form of the bacterium Staphylococcus aureus that is resistant to treatment from beta-lactam class antibiotics.

ᴹᶜᶜ**A41.1**   **Sepsis due to other specified staphylococcus**
      Coagulase negative staphylococcus sepsis

ᴹᶜᶜ**A41.2**   **Sepsis due to unspecified staphylococcus**

ᴹᶜᶜ**A41.3**   **Sepsis due to <u>Hemophilus influenzae</u>**

ᴹᶜᶜ**A41.4**   **Sepsis due to anaerobes**
    Excludes 1: *gas gangrene (A48.0)*

A41.5-   **Sepsis due to other Gram-negative organisms**

  ᴹᶜᶜ**A41.50**   **Gram-negative sepsis, unspecified**
        Gram-negative sepsis NOS

  ᴹᶜᶜ**A41.51**   **Sepsis due to <u>Escherichia coli [E. coli]</u>**

  ᴹᶜᶜ**A41.52**   **Sepsis due to <u>Pseudomonas</u>**
        Pseudomonas aeroginosa

  ᴹᶜᶜ**A41.53**   **Sepsis due to <u>Serratia</u>**

  ᴹᶜᶜ**A41.59**   **Other Gram-negative sepsis**

A41.8-   **Other specified sepsis**

  ᴹᶜᶜ**A41.81**   **Sepsis due to <u>Enterococcus</u>**

  ᴹᶜᶜ**A41.89**   **Other specified sepsis**

ᴹᶜᶜ**A41.9**   **Sepsis, unspecified organism**
      Septicemia NOS

A42-   <u>Actinomycosis</u> — A group of gram-positive infectious diseases classified to the bacterial families Actinomycetaceae and Propionibacteriaceae, often by Actinomyces israelii.
    Excludes 1: *actinomycetoma (B47.1)*

ᶜᶜ**A42.0**   **Pulmonary actinomycosis**

ᶜᶜ**A42.1**   **Abdominal actinomycosis**

ᶜᶜ**A42.2**   **Cervicofacial actinomycosis**

ᴹᶜᶜ**A42.7**   **Actinomycotic sepsis**

A42.8-   **Other forms of actinomycosis**

  ᶜᶜ**A42.81**   **Actinomycotic meningitis**

  ᶜᶜ**A42.82**   **Actinomycotic encephalitis**

  ᶜᶜ**A42.89**   **Other forms of actinomycosis**

ᶜᶜ**A42.9**   **Actinomycosis, unspecified**

A43-   <u>Nocardiosis</u> — Infection by bacterium of the genus Nocardia, most commonly Nocardia asteroides or Nocardia brasiliensis.

ᶜᶜ**A43.0**   **Pulmonary nocardiosis**

ᶜᶜ**A43.1**   **Cutaneous nocardiosis**

ᶜᶜ**A43.8**   **Other forms of nocardiosis**

ᶜᶜ**A43.9**   **Nocardiosis, unspecified**

A44-   <u>Bartonellosis</u> — An infectious bacterial disease caused by Bartonella bacilliformis, and characterized by acute febrile hemolytic anemia, and hemangioma-like nodules on the skin.

ᶜᶜ**A44.0**   **Systemic bartonellosis**
      Oroya fever

ᶜᶜ**A44.1**   **Cutaneous and mucocutaneous bartonellosis**
      Verruga peruana

ᶜᶜ**A44.8**   **Other forms of bartonellosis**

ᶜᶜ**A44.9**   **Bartonellosis, unspecified**

A46   <u>Erysipelas</u> — An infectious contagious disease of the skin and subcutaneous tissue caused by Group A Beta-hemolytic Streptococcus, and characterized by obstructed lymphatics, redness and swelling of the affected areas, and sometimes large tension bullae.
    Excludes 1: *postpartum or puerperal erysipelas (O86.89)*

A48-   **Other bacterial diseases, not elsewhere classified**
    Excludes 1: *actinomycetoma (B47.1)*

ᴹᶜᶜ**A48.0**   **Gas gangrene** — An acute infectious disease caused by the genus Clostridium, and characterized by severe, painful histotoxic infection of muscles and subcutaneous tissues which fill with gas and a serosanguineous exudate.
      Clostridial cellulitis
      Clostridial myonecrosis

ᴹᶜᶜ**A48.1**   **Legionnaires' disease** — An infectious disease caused by the genus Legionella, usually by Legionella pneumophila and characterized by infection of the respiratory sytem, fever, chills, and cough.

A48.2   **Nonpneumonic Legionnaires' disease [Pontiac fever]** — A milder form resembling the flu.

ᴹᶜᶜ**A48.3**   **Toxic shock syndrome** — An acute infectious bacterial disease caused by Staphylococcus aureus or Group A Streptococcus bacteria, characterized by abrupt onset of high fever, vomiting, diarrhea, sunburn-like rash, and myalgia, followed by hypotension and in severe cases, shock and multi-organ failure.
      Use additional code to identify the organism (B95, B96)
    Excludes 1: *endotoxic shock NOS (R57.8)*
                sepsis NOS (A41.9)

A48.4   **Brazilian purpuric fever**
      Systemic Hemophilus aegyptius infection

A48.5-   **Other specified botulism**
      Non-foodborne intoxication due to toxins of Clostridium botulinum [C. botulinum]
    Excludes 1: *food poisoning due to toxins of Clostridium botulinum (A05.1)*

  ᶜᶜ**A48.51**   **Infant botulism** — [Age/0-17]

  ᶜᶜ**A48.52**   **Wound botulism**
        Non-foodborne botulism NOS
        Use additional code for associated wound

A48.8   **Other specified bacterial diseases**

A49-   **Bacterial <u>infection</u> of <u>unspecified site</u>**
    Excludes 1: *bacterial agents as the cause of diseases classified elsewhere (B95-B96)*
                chlamydial infection NOS (A74.9)
                meningococcal infection NOS (A39.9)
                rickettsial infection NOS (A79.9)
                spirochetal infection NOS (A69.9)

A49.0-   **Staphylococcal infection, unspecified site**

  A49.01   **Methicillin <u>susceptible</u> Staphylococcus aureus <u>infection</u>, unspecified site** — An infection caused by a form of the bacterium Staphylococcus aureus that is susceptible to antibiotic treatment.
        Methicillin susceptible Staphylococcus aureus (MSSA) infection
        Staphylococcus aureus infection NOS

  A49.02   **Methicillin <u>resistant</u> Staphylococcus aureus <u>infection</u>, unspecified site** — An infection caused by a form of the bacterium Staphylococcus aureus that is resistant to treatment from beta-lactam class antibiotics.
        Methicillin resistant Staphylococcus aureus (MRSA) infection

A49.1   **Streptococcal infection, unspecified site**

A49.2   **Hemophilus influenzae infection, unspecified site**

A49.3   **Mycoplasma infection, unspecified site**

A49.8   **Other bacterial infections of unspecified site**

A49.9   **Bacterial infection, unspecified**
    Excludes 1: *bacteremia NOS (R78.81)*

A41–A49

Infections with a <u>predominantly sexual mode</u> of transmission (A50-A64)

> **Excludes 1:** human immunodeficiency virus [HIV] disease (B20)
> nonspecific and nongonococcal urethritis (N34.1)
> Reiter's disease (M02.3-)

A50- <u>Congenital</u> syphilis — An infectious bacterial disease caused by Treponema pallidum, which is transmitted transplacentally to the fetus from an infected pregnant woman.

- **A50.0-** **Early congenital syphilis, symptomatic** — A form characterized by an enlarged liver and spleen, periostitis and osteochondritis, purulent nasal discharge, and skin lesions and patches on mucous membranes.
  > Any congenital syphilitic condition specified as early or manifest less than two years after birth.

  - cc **A50.01** **Early congenital syphilitic oculopathy**
  - cc **A50.02** **Early congenital syphilitic osteochondropathy**
  - cc **A50.03** **Early congenital syphilitic pharyngitis**
    Early congenital syphilitic laryngitis
  - cc **A50.04** **Early congenital syphilitic pneumonia**
  - cc **A50.05** **Early congenital syphilitic rhinitis**
  - cc **A50.06** **Early cutaneous congenital syphilis**
  - cc **A50.07** **Early mucocutaneous congenital syphilis**
  - cc **A50.08** **Early visceral congenital syphilis**
  - cc **A50.09** **Other early congenital syphilis, symptomatic**

- **A50.1** **Early congenital syphilis, latent**
  > Congenital syphilis without clinical manifestations, with positive serological reaction and negative spinal fluid test, less than two years after birth

- cc **A50.2** **Early congenital syphilis, unspecified**
  > Congenital syphilis NOS less than two years after birth

- **A50.3-** **Late congenital syphilitic oculopathy**
  > **Excludes 1:** Hutchinson's triad (A50.53)

  - cc **A50.30** **Late congenital syphilitic oculopathy, unspecified**
  - cc **A50.31** **Late congenital syphilitic interstitial keratitis**
  - cc **A50.32** **Late congenital syphilitic chorioretinitis**
  - cc **A50.39** **Other late congenital syphilitic oculopathy**

- **A50.4-** **Late congenital neurosyphilis [juvenile neurosyphilis]**
  > Use additional code to identify any associated mental disorder
  > **Excludes 1:** Hutchinson's triad (A50.53)

  - cc **A50.40** **Late congenital neurosyphilis, unspecified**
    Juvenile neurosyphilis NOS
  - mcc **A50.41** **Late congenital syphilitic meningitis**
  - mcc **A50.42** **Late congenital syphilitic encephalitis**
  - cc **A50.43** **Late congenital syphilitic polyneuropathy**
  - cc **A50.44** **Late congenital syphilitic optic nerve atrophy**
  - cc **A50.45** **Juvenile general paresis**
    Dementia paralytica juvenilis
    Juvenile tabetoparetic neurosyphilis
  - cc **A50.49** **Other late congenital neurosyphilis**
    Juvenile tabes dorsalis

- **A50.5-** **Other late congenital syphilis, symptomatic**
  > Any congenital syphilitic condition specified as late or manifest two years or more after birth

  - cc **A50.51** **Clutton's joints**
  - cc **A50.52** **Hutchinson's teeth**
  - cc **A50.53** **Hutchinson's triad**
  - cc **A50.54** **Late congenital cardiovascular syphilis**
  - cc **A50.55** **Late congenital syphilitic arthropathy**
  - cc **A50.56** **Late congenital syphilitic osteochondropathy**
  - cc **A50.57** **Syphilitic saddle nose**
  - cc **A50.59** **Other late congenital syphilis, symptomatic**

- **A50.6** **Late congenital syphilis, latent**
  > Congenital syphilis without clinical manifestations, with positive serological reaction and negative spinal fluid test, two years or more after birth

- **A50.7** **Late congenital syphilis, unspecified**
  > Congenital syphilis NOS two years or more after birth

- **A50.9** **Congenital syphilis, unspecified**

A51- <u>Early</u> **syphilis** — The acquired infectious bacterial disease caused by Treponema pallidum.

- **A51.0** **Primary genital syphilis** — A first stage form characterized by a small, painless open sore or ulcer (called a chancre) on the genitals that heals by itself in 3 to 6 weeks.
  > Syphilitic chancre NOS

- **A51.1** **Primary anal syphilis** — A first stage form characterized by a small, painless open sore or ulcer (called a chancre) on the anus or rectum that heals by itself in 3 to 6 weeks.

- **A51.2** **Primary syphilis of other sites** — A first stage form characterized by a small, painless open sore or ulcer (called a chancre) on the mouth, skin, or other areas that heals by itself in 3 to 6 weeks.

- **A51.3-** **Secondary syphilis of skin and mucous membranes** — The second stage of the acquired infectious bacterial disease caused by Treponema pallidum.

  - cc **A51.31** **Condyloma latum**
  - cc **A51.32** **Syphilitic alopecia**
  - cc **A51.39** **Other secondary syphilis of skin**
    Syphilitic leukoderma
    Syphilitic mucous patch
    > **Excludes 1:** late syphilitic leukoderma (A52.79)

- **A51.4-** **Other secondary syphilis** — The second stage of the acquired infectious bacterial disease caused by Treponema pallidum.

  - mcc **A51.41** **Secondary syphilitic meningitis**
  - cc **A51.42** **Secondary syphilitic female pelvic disease** — [♀]
  - cc **A51.43** **Secondary syphilitic oculopathy**
    Secondary syphilitic chorioretinitis
    Secondary syphilitic iridocyclitis, iritis
    Secondary syphilitic uveitis
  - cc **A51.44** **Secondary syphilitic nephritis**
  - cc **A51.45** **Secondary syphilltic hepatitis**
  - cc **A51.46** **Secondary syphilitic osteopathy**
  - cc **A51.49** **Other secondary syphilitic conditions**
    Secondary syphilitic lymphadenopathy
    Secondary syphilitic myositis

- **A51.5** **Early syphilis, latent**
  > Syphilis (acquired) without clinical manifestations, with positive serological reaction and negative spinal fluid test, less than two years after infection

- **A51.9** **Early syphilis, unspecified**

A52- <u>Late</u> **syphilis** — The third stage of the acquired infectious bacterial disease caused by Treponema pallidum.

- **A52.0-** **Cardiovascular and cerebrovascular syphilis**

  - cc **A52.00** **Cardiovascular syphilis, unspecified**
  - cc **A52.01** **Syphilitic aneurysm of aorta**
  - cc **A52.02** **Syphilitic aortitis**
  - cc **A52.03** **Syphilitic endocarditis**
    Syphilitic aortic valve incompetence or stenosis
    Syphilitic mitral valve stenosis
    Syphilitic pulmonary valve regurgitation
  - cc **A52.04** **Syphilitic cerebral arteritis**
  - cc **A52.05** **Other cerebrovascular syphilis**
    Syphilitic cerebral aneurysm (ruptured) (non-ruptured)
    Syphilitic cerebral thrombosis
  - cc **A52.06** **Other syphilitic heart involvement**
    Syphilitic coronary artery disease
    Syphilitic myocarditis
    Syphilitic pericarditis
  - cc **A52.09** **Other cardiovascular syphilis**

- **A52.1-** **Symptomatic neurosyphilis**

  - cc **A52.10** **Symptomatic neurosyphilis, unspecified**
  - cc **A52.11** **Tabes dorsalis**
    Locomotor ataxia (progressive)
    Tabetic neurosyphilis
  - cc **A52.12** **Other cerebrospinal syphilis**
  - mcc **A52.13** **Late syphilitic meningitis**
  - mcc **A52.14** **Late syphilitic encephalitis**
  - cc **A52.15** **Late syphilitic neuropathy**
    Late syphilitic acoustic neuritis
    Late syphilitic optic (nerve) atrophy
    Late syphilitic polyneuropathy
    Late syphilitic retrobulbar neuritis
  - cc **A52.16** **Charcot's arthropathy (tabetic)**

A 5 0 – A 5 2

cc **A52.17** **General paresis**
Dementia paralytica

cc **A52.19** **Other symptomatic neurosyphilis**
Syphilitic parkinsonism

cc **A52.2** **Asymptomatic neurosyphilis**

cc **A52.3** **Neurosyphilis, unspecified**
Gumma (syphilitic)
Syphilis (late)
Syphiloma

A52.7- **Other symptomatic late syphilis**

cc **A52.71** **Late syphilitic oculopathy**
Late syphilitic chorioretinitis
Late syphilitic episcleritis

cc **A52.72** **Syphilis of lung and bronchus**

cc **A52.73** **Symptomatic late syphilis of other respiratory organs**

cc **A52.74** **Syphilis of liver and other viscera**
Late syphilitic peritonitis

cc **A52.75** **Syphilis of kidney and ureter**
Syphilitic glomerular disease

cc **A52.76** **Other genitourinary symptomatic late syphilis**
Late syphilitic female pelvic inflammatory disease

cc **A52.77** **Syphilis of bone and joint**

cc **A52.78** **Syphilis of other musculoskeletal tissue**
Late syphilitic bursitis
Syphilis [stage unspecified] of bursa
Syphilis [stage unspecified] of muscle
Syphilis [stage unspecified] of synovium
Syphilis [stage unspecified] of tendon

cc **A52.79** **Other symptomatic late syphilis**
Late syphilitic leukoderma
Syphilis of adrenal gland
Syphilis of pituitary gland
Syphilis of thyroid gland
Syphilitic splenomegaly
Excludes 1: *syphilitic leukoderma (secondary) (A51.39)*

A52.8 **Late syphilis, latent**
Syphilis (acquired) without clinical manifestations, with positive serological reaction and negative spinal fluid test, two years or more after infection

A52.9 **Late syphilis, unspecified**

A53- **Other and unspecified syphilis**

A53.0 **Latent syphilis, unspecified as early or late**
Latent syphilis NOS
Positive serological reaction for syphilis

A53.9 **Syphilis, unspecified**
Infection due to Treponema pallidum NOS
Syphilis (acquired) NOS
Excludes 1: *syphilis NOS under two years of age (A50.2)*

A54- **Gonococcal infection** — An infectious bacterial disease caused by Neisseria gonorrhoeae and characterized by a purulent, sexually transmitted infection most commonly affecting the urethra and genital organs.

A54.0- **Gonococcal infection of lower genitourinary tract <u>without</u> periurethral or accessory gland abscess**
Excludes 1: *gonococcal infection with genitourinary gland abscess (A54.1)*
gonococcal infection with periurethral abscess (A54.1)

cc **A54.00** **Gonococcal infection of lower genitourinary tract, unspecified**

cc **A54.01** **Gonococcal cystitis and urethritis, unspecified**

cc **A54.02** **Gonococcal vulvovaginitis, unspecified —[♀]**

cc **A54.03** **Gonococcal cervicitis, unspecified —[♀]**

cc **A54.09** **Other gonococcal infection of lower genitourinary tract**

cc **A54.1** **Gonococcal infection of lower genitourinary tract <u>with</u> periurethral and accessory gland abscess**
Gonococcal Bartholin's gland abscess

A54.2- **Gonococcal pelviperitonitis and other gonococcal genitourinary infection**

cc **A54.21** **Gonococcal infection of kidney and ureter**

cc **A54.22** **Gonococcal prostatitis —[♂]**

cc **A54.23** **Gonococcal infection of other male genital organs —[♂]**
Gonococcal epididymitis
Gonococcal orchitis

cc **A54.24** **Gonococcal female pelvic inflammatory disease —[♀]**
Gonococcal pelviperitonitis
Excludes 1: *gonococcal peritonitis (A54.85)*

cc **A54.29** **Other gonococcal genitourinary infections**

A54.3- **Gonococcal infection of eye**

cc **A54.30** **Gonococcal infection of eye, unspecified**

cc **A54.31** **Gonococcal conjunctivitis**
Ophthalmia neonatorum due to gonococcus

cc **A54.32** **Gonococcal iridocyclitis**

cc **A54.33** **Gonococcal keratitis**

cc **A54.39** **Other gonococcal eye infection**
Gonococcal endophthalmia

A54.4- **Gonococcal infection of musculoskeletal system**

cc **A54.40** **Gonococcal infection of musculoskeletal system, unspecified**

cc **A54.41** **Gonococcal spondylopathy**

cc **A54.42** **Gonococcal arthritis**
Excludes ❷: *gonococcal infection of spine (A54.41)*

cc **A54.43** **Gonococcal osteomyelitis**
Excludes ❷: *gonococcal infection of spine (A54.41)*

cc **A54.49** **Gonococcal infection of other musculoskeletal tissue**
Gonococcal bursitis
Gonococcal myositis
Gonococcal synovitis
Gonococcal tenosynovitis

A54.5 **Gonococcal pharyngitis**

A54.6 **Gonococcal infection of anus and rectum**

A54.8- **Other gonococcal infections**

mcc **A54.81** **Gonococcal meningitis**

cc **A54.82** **Gonococcal brain abscess**

cc **A54.83** **Gonococcal heart infection**
Gonococcal endocarditis
Gonococcal myocarditis
Gonococcal pericarditis

cc **A54.84** **Gonococcal pneumonia**

cc **A54.85** **Gonococcal peritonitis**
Excludes 1: *gonococcal pelviperitonitis (A54.24)*

mcc **A54.86** **Gonococcal sepsis**

cc **A54.89** **Other gonococcal infections**
Gonococcal keratoderma
Gonococcal lymphadenitis

cc **A54.9** **Gonococcal infection, unspecified**

A55 **Chlamydial lymphogranuloma (venereum)** — An infectious bacterial disease caused by Chlamydia trachomatis and characterized by a painless primary urethral lesion and regional lymphadenopathy which is transmitted sexually.
Climatic or tropical bubo
Durand-Nicolas-Favre disease
Esthiomene
Lymphogranuloma inguinale

A56- **Other sexually transmitted chlamydial diseases**
Includes: Sexually transmitted diseases due to Chlamydia Trachomatis
Excludes 1: *neonatal chlamydial conjunctivitis (P39.1)*
neonatal chlamydial pneumonia (P23.1)
Excludes ❷: *chlamydial lymphogranuloma (A55)*
conditions classified to A74.-

A56.0- **Chlamydial infection of lower genitourinary tract** — An infectious bacterial disease caused by Chlamydia trachomatis affecting the lower genitourinary tract.

A56.00 **Chlamydial infection of lower genitourinary tract, unspecified**

A56.01 **Chlamydial cystitis and urethritis**

A56.02 **Chlamydial vulvovaginitis —[♀]**

A56.09 **Other chlamydial infection of lower genitourinary tract**
Chlamydial cervicitis

A56.1- **Chlamydial infection of pelviperitoneum and other genitourinary organs**

A56.11 **Chlamydial female pelvic inflammatory disease —[♀]**

A56.19 **Other chlamydial genitourinary infection**
Chlamydial epididymitis
Chlamydial orchitis

A56.2 **Chlamydial infection of genitourinary tract, unspecified**

A
5
2
-
A
5
6

A56.3   **Chlamydial infection of anus and rectum**

A56.4   **Chlamydial infection of pharynx**

A56.8   **Sexually transmitted chlamydial infection of other sites**

A57   <u>**Chancroid**</u> — An infectious, bacterial disease caused by Haemophilus ducreyi and characterized by a painful genital ulceration and diffuse inguinal lymphadenitis that is transmitted sexually.
     Ulcus molle

A58   <u>**Granuloma inguinale**</u> — An infectious bacterial disease caused by Calymmatobacterium granulomatis and characterized by a mildly painful cutaneous or mucocutaneous genital lesion that is transmitted sexually.
     Donovanosis

A59-   <u>**Trichomoniasis**</u> — A parasitic disease caused by Trichomonas vaginalis and principally affecting the lower genitourinary tract that is transmitted sexually.
     Excludes ❷: intestinal trichomoniasis (A07.8)

   A59.0-   **Urogenital trichomoniasis**

     A59.00   **Urogenital trichomoniasis, unspecified**
         Fluor (vaginalis) due to Trichomonas
         Leukorrhea (vaginalis) due to Trichomonas

     A59.01   **Trichomonal vulvovaginitis** —[♀]

     A59.02   **Trichomonal prostatitis** —[♂]

     A59.03   **Trichomonal cystitis and urethritis**

     A59.09   **Other urogenital trichomoniasis**
         Trichomonas cervicitis

   A59.8   **Trichomoniasis of other sites**

   A59.9   **Trichomoniasis, unspecified**

A60-   <u>**Anogenital herpesviral [herpes simplex] infections**</u> — Viral infections of the genitourinary tract caused by herpes simplex virus, Type 2, and characterized by herpetic vesicles that is transmitted sexually and may be accompanied by fever, headache, and malaise.

   A60.0-   **Herpesviral infection of genitalia and urogenital tract**

     A60.00   **Herpesviral infection of urogenital system, unspecified**

     A60.01   **Herpesviral infection of penis** —[♂]

     A60.02   **Herpesviral infection of other male genital organs** —[♂]

     A60.03   **Herpesviral cervicitis** —[♀]

     A60.04   **Herpesviral vulvovaginitis** —[♀]
         Herpesviral [herpes simplex] ulceration
         Herpesviral [herpes simplex] vaginitis
         Herpesviral [herpes simplex] vulvitis

     A60.09   **Herpesviral infection of other urogenital tract**

   A60.1   **Herpesviral infection of perianal skin and rectum**

   A60.9   **Anogenital herpesviral infection, unspecified**

A63-   **Other predominantly sexually transmitted diseases, not elsewhere classified**
     Excludes ❷: molluscum contagiosum (B08.1)
           papilloma of cervix (D26.0)

   A63.0   **Anogenital (venereal) warts** — An epidermal infectious viral disease caused by a human papillomavirus and characterized by cauliflower-like growths on the external genitals and transmitted mainly through infected genital contact.
     Anogenital warts due to (human) papillomavirus [HPV]
     Condyloma acuminatum

   A63.8   **Other specified predominantly sexually transmitted diseases**

A64   **Unspecified sexually transmitted disease**

Other spirochetal diseases (A65-A69)

Excludes ❷: leptospirosis (A27.-)
          syphilis (A50-A53)

A65   <u>**Nonvenereal syphilis**</u> — An infectious bacterial disease caused by species of Spirochaeta that are very similar to, but different from, syphilis.
     Bejel — An infectious bacterial disease caused by Treponema pallidum and characterized by a primary oral lesion, rashes, papillomas, and occasionally by laryngitis, pharyngitis, periostitis, generalized lymphadenopathy, and nodular ulcerations.
     Endemic syphilis
     Njovera

A66-   <u>**Yaws**</u> — An infectious bacterial disease caused by Treponema pertenue and characterized by a primary granulomatous lesion, later crops of granulomatous papules, and ulcerative necrosis of the lesions.
   Includes: **Bouba**
          Frambesia (tropica)
          Pian

   A66.0   **Initial lesions of yaws**
     Chancre of yaws
     Frambesia, initial or primary
     Initial frambesial ulcer
     Mother yaw

   A66.1   **Multiple papillomata and wet crab yaws**
     Frambesioma
     Pianoma
     Plantar or palmar papilloma of yaws

   A66.2   **Other early skin lesions of yaws**
     Cutaneous yaws, less than five years after infection
     Early yaws (cutaneous) (macular) (maculopapular) (micropapular)
       (papular)
     Frambeside of early yaws

   A66.3   **Hyperkeratosis of yaws**
     Ghoul hand
     Hyperkeratosis, palmar or plantar (early) (late) due to yaws
     Worm-eaten soles

   A66.4   **Gummata and ulcers of yaws**
     Gummatous frambeside
     Nodular late yaws (ulcerated)

   A66.5   **Gangosa**
     Rhinopharyngitis mutilans

   A66.6   **Bone and joint lesions of yaws**
     Yaws ganglion
     Yaws goundou
     Yaws gumma, bone
     Yaws gummatous osteitis or periostitis
     Yaws hydrarthrosis
     Yaws osteitis
     Yaws periostitis (hypertrophic)

   A66.7   **Other manifestations of yaws**
     Juxta-articular nodules of yaws
     Mucosal yaws

   A66.8   **Latent yaws**
     Yaws without clinical manifestations, with positive serology

   A66.9   **Yaws, unspecified**

A67-   <u>**Pinta [carate]**</u> — An infectious bacterial disease caused by Treponema carateum and characterized by chronic dermatosis with depigmentation.

   A67.0   **Primary lesions of pinta**
     Chancre (primary) of pinta
     Papule (primary) of pinta

   A67.1   **Intermediate lesions of pinta**
     Erythematous plaques of pinta
     Hyperchromic lesions of pinta
     Hyperkeratosis of pinta
     Pintids

   A67.2   **Late lesions of pinta**
     Achromic skin lesions of pinta
     Cicatricial skin lesions of pinta
     Dyschromic skin lesions of pinta

   A67.3   **Mixed lesions of pinta**
     Achromic with hyperchromic skin lesions of pinta [carate]

   A67.9   **Pinta, unspecified**

Excludes 1: = NOT CODED HERE! (Do not code both)

Excludes ❷: = Not Included Here

A68- **Relapsing fevers** — An infectious bacterial disease caused by the genus Borrelia that is characterized by febrile episodes with interim afebrile periods.

Includes: Recurrent fever

Excludes ❷: *Lyme disease (A69.2-)*

cc **A68.0** **Louse-borne relapsing fever** — A form transmitted to man by the human body louse that is caused by Borrelia recurrentis.

Relapsing fever due to Borrelia recurrentis

cc **A68.1** **Tick-borne relapsing fever** — A form transmitted to man by ticks.

Relapsing fever due to any Borrelia species other than Borrelia recurrentis

cc **A68.9** **Relapsing fever, unspecified**

A69- **Other spirochetal infections**

A69.0 **Necrotizing ulcerative stomatitis** — An inflammatory bacterial disease characterized by ulcerative oral lesions with severe pain.

Cancrum oris
Fusospirochetal gangrene
Noma
Stomatitis gangrenosa

cc **A69.1** **Other Vincent's infections**

Fusospirochetal pharyngitis
Necrotizing ulcerative (acute) gingivitis
Necrotizing ulcerative (acute) gingivostomatitis
Spirochetal stomatitis
Trench mouth
Vincent's angina
Vincent's gingivitis

A69.2- **Lyme disease** — An infectious bacterial disease that is transmitted by ticks, caused by Borella burgdorferi and characterized by erythematous lesions, arthritis, myalgia, malaise, and other multiple systemic manifestations.

Erythema chronicum migrans due to Borrelia burgdorferi

cc **A69.20** **Lyme disease, unspecified**

cc **A69.21** **Meningitis due to Lyme disease**

cc **A69.22** **Other neurologic disorders in Lyme disease**

Cranial neuritis
Meningoencephalitis
Polyneuropathy

cc **A69.23** **Arthritis due to Lyme disease**

cc **A69.29** **Other conditions associated with Lyme disease**

Myopericarditis due to Lyme disease

A69.8 **Other specified spirochetal infections**

A69.9 **Spirochetal infection, unspecified**

Other diseases caused by chlamydiae (A70-A74)

Excludes 1: *sexually transmitted chlamydial diseases (A55-A56)*

A70 **Chlamydia psittaci infections** — An infectious bacterial disease caused by
cc   Chlamydia psittaci and characterized by sore throat, myalgia, cough, confusion, weakness, fever, hepatosplenomegaly, and headache.

Ornithosis
Parrot fever
Psittacosis

A71- **Trachoma** — An infectious bacterial disease caused by Chlamydia trachomatis and characterized by acute inflammation of the conjunctiva.

Excludes 1: *sequelae of trachoma (B94.0)*

A71.0 **Initial stage of trachoma**

Trachoma dubium

A71.1 **Active stage of trachoma**

Granular conjunctivitis (trachomatous)
Trachomatous follicular conjunctivitis
Trachomatous pannus

A71.9 **Trachoma, unspecified**

A74- **Other diseases caused by chlamydiae**

Excludes 1: *neonatal chlamydial conjunctivitis (P39.1)*
neonatal chlamydial pneumonia (P23.1)
Reiter's disease (M02.3-)
sexually transmitted chlamydial diseases (A55-A56)

Excludes ❷: *chlamydial pneumonia (J16.0)*

A74.0 **Chlamydial conjunctivitis** — An infectious bacterial disease caused by Chlamydia trachomatis affecting the conjunctiva.

Paratrachoma

A74.8- **Other chlamydial diseases**

A74.81 **Chlamydial peritonitis**

A74.89 **Other chlamydial diseases**

A74.9 **Chlamydial infection, unspecified**

Chlamydiosis NOS

Rickettsioses (A75-A79)

A75- **Typhus fever**

Excludes 1: *rickettsiosis due to Ehrlichia sennetsu (A79.81)*

cc **A75.0** **Epidemic louse-borne typhus fever due to Rickettsia prowazekii** — An infectious bacterial disease caused by Rickettsia prowazekii and characterized by high fever, severe inflammation of the brain, and maculopapular rash, transmitted to man by lice.

Classical typhus (fever)
Epidemic (louse-borne) typhus

cc **A75.1** **Recrudescent typhus [Brill's disease]** — A recrudescence of louse-borne (epidemic) typhus occurs when latent infection reactivates with the same symptoms but of lower intensity.

Brill-Zinsser disease

cc **A75.2** **Typhus fever due to Rickettsia typhi** — An infectious bacterial disease caused by Rickettsia typhi and characterized by fever and a maculopapular rash, transmitted to man by fleas.

Murine (flea-borne) typhus

cc **A75.3** **Typhus fever due to Rickettsia tsutsugamushi** — An infectious bacterial disease caused by Orientia tsutsugamushi and characterized by fever and a maculopapular rash, transmitted to man by mites.

Scrub (mite-borne) typhus
Tsutsugamushi fever

cc **A75.9** **Typhus fever, unspecified**

Typhus (fever) NOS

A77- **Spotted fever [tick-borne rickettsioses]**

cc **A77.0** **Spotted fever due to Rickettsia rickettsii** — An infectious bacterial disease caused by Rickettsia rickettsii and characterized by fever, skin rash, myalgias, intense headache, and prostration, transmitted to man by ticks.

Rocky Mountain spotted fever
Sao Paulo fever

cc **A77.1** **Spotted fever due to Rickettsia conorii** — An infectious bacterial disease caused by Rickettsia conorii and characterized by a primary lesion at the site of tick attachment, a maculopapular exanthem, headache, photophobia, arthralgia, and diffuse myalgia, transmitted to man by ticks.

African tick typhus
Boutonneuse fever
India tick typhus
Kenya tick typhus
Marseilles fever
Mediterranean tick fever

cc **A77.2** **Spotted fever due to Rickettsia siberica**

North Asian tick fever
Siberian tick typhus

cc **A77.3** **Spotted fever due to Rickettsia australis**

Queensland tick typhus

A77.4- **Ehrlichiosis** — An infectious bacterial disease caused by the genus Ehrlichia and characterized by symptoms that may include fever, headache, myalgia, thrombocytopenia, and leukopenia, transmitted to man by ticks.

Excludes 1: *Rickettsiosis due to Ehrlichia sennetsu (A79.81)*

cc **A77.40** **Ehrlichiosis, unspecified**

cc **A77.41** **Ehrlichiosis chafeensis [E. chafeensis]**

cc **A77.49** **Other ehrlichiosis**

cc **A77.8** **Other spotted fevers**

cc **A77.9** **Spotted fever, unspecified**

Tick-borne typhus NOS

A78 **Q fever** — An infectious bacterial disease caused by Coxiella burnetii and characterized
cc   by severe headache, sweating, fever, and pneumonia.

Infection due to Coxiella burnetii
Nine Mile fever
Quadrilateral fever

A79- **Other rickettsioses**

cc **A79.0** **Trench fever** — An infectious bacterial disease caused by Rochalimaea quintana and characterized by recurrent febrile episodes, severe headache, profuse sweating, myalgias, a macular rash on the chest and abdomen, and splenomegaly, transmitted to man by lice.

Quintan fever
Wolhynian fever

cc **A79.1** **Rickettsialpox due to Rickettsia akari**

Kew Garden fever
Vesicular rickettsiosis

A79.8- **Other specified rickettsioses**

cc **A79.81** **Rickettsiosis due to Ehrlichia sennetsu**

cc **A79.89** **Other specified rickettsioses**

cc **A79.9** **Rickettsiosis, unspecified**

Rickettsial infection NOS

A
6
8
|
A
7
9

Viral and prion infections of the central nervous system (A80-A89)

Excludes 1:   postpolio syndrome (G14)
               sequelae of poliomyelitis (B91)
               sequelae of viral encephalitis (B94.1)

A80-   Acute poliomyelitis — A viral infectious disease caused by the poliovirus, a human enterovirus, and characterized by fever, muscular pain, spasm, and paralysis which may affect the central nervous system and cause permanent muscular deformity.

MCC **A80.0   Acute paralytic poliomyelitis, vaccine-associated**

MCC **A80.1   Acute paralytic poliomyelitis, wild virus, imported**

MCC **A80.2   Acute paralytic poliomyelitis, wild virus, indigenous**

A80.3-   Acute paralytic poliomyelitis, other and unspecified

MCC **A80.30   Acute paralytic poliomyelitis, unspecified**

MCC **A80.39   Other acute paralytic poliomyelitis**

A80.4   Acute nonparalytic poliomyelitis

A80.9   Acute poliomyelitis, unspecified

A81-   Atypical virus infections of central nervous system
   Includes: Diseases of the central nervous system caused by prions
   Use additional code to identify:
      Dementia with behavioral disturbance (F02.81)
      Dementia without behavioral disturbance (F02.80)

A81.0-   Creutzfeldt-Jakob disease

CC **A81.00   Creutzfeldt-Jakob disease, unspecified**
         Jakob-Creutzfeldt disease, unspecified

CC **A81.01   Variant Creutzfeldt-Jakob disease** — A transmissible spongiform encephalopathy (TSE) causing prominent psychiatric/behavioral symptoms with delayed neurologic signs that results in death and is related to "mad cow disease" (bovine spongiform encephalopathy).
         vCJD

CC **A81.09   Other Creutzfeldt-Jakob disease** — A transmissible spongiform encephalopathy (TSE) causing progressive presenile dementia, encephalopathy, and a downhill course resulting in death.
         CJD
         Familial Creutzfeldt-Jakob disease
         Iatrogenic Creutzfeldt-Jakob disease
         Sporadic Creutzfeldt-Jakob disease
         Subacute spongiform encephalopathy (with dementia)

CC **A81.1   Subacute sclerosing panencephalitis** — A rare viral infectious disease affecting the brain and causing progressive mental deterioration with blindness, profound dementia, and hypothalmic dysfunction in the terminal phase.
         Dawson's inclusion body encephalitis
         Van Bogaert's sclerosing leukoencephalopathy

CC **A81.2   Progressive multifocal leukoencephalopathy** — A viral infectious disease characterized by demyelination of the cerebral cortex in immunologically compromised patients with symptoms of confusion, disorientation, poor memory, speech and visual disturbances, weakness, and paralysis.
         Multifocal leukoencephalopathy NOS

A81.8-   Other atypical virus infections of central nervous system

CC **A81.81   Kuru** — A transmissible spongiform encephalopathy (TSE) affecting the central nervous system causing tremors, flaccid paralysis, and death; found in the Fore and neighboring peoples of the mountainous regions of Papua New Guinea who practice ritualistic cannibalism.

CC **A81.82   Gerstmann-Sträussler-Scheinker syndrome** — A prion disease caused by the inheritance of a PrP gene with mutations and characterized by difficulty speaking, unsteadiness, and amyloid plaques.
         GSS syndrome

CC **A81.83   Fatal familial insomnia** — A prion disease caused by the inheritance of a PrP gene with mutations and characterized by complete sleeplessness and pathological lesions in the thalamus.
         FFI

CC **A81.89   Other atypical virus infections of central nervous system**

CC **A81.9   Atypical virus infection of central nervous system, unspecified**
         Prion diseases of the central nervous system NOS

A82-   Rabies — An infectious viral disease caused by the rabies virus and characterized by infection of the central nervous system with fever, excitation, convulsions, lacrimation, salivation, paralysis, pharyngeal spasms, coma, and usually death.

CC **A82.0   Sylvatic rabies**

CC **A82.1   Urban rabies**

CC **A82.9   Rabies, unspecified**

A83-   Mosquito-borne viral encephalitis — A group of infectious viral diseases characterized by inflammation of the brain and transmitted to man by mosquitoes.
   Includes: Mosquito-borne viral meningoencephalitis
   Excludes ❷: Venezuelan equine encephalitis (A92.2)
               West Nile fever (A92.3-)
               West Nile virus (A92.3-)

MCC **A83.0   Japanese encephalitis**

MCC **A83.1   Western equine encephalitis**

MCC **A83.2   Eastern equine encephalitis**

MCC **A83.3   St. Louis encephalitis**

MCC **A83.4   Australian encephalitis**
         Kunjin virus disease

MCC **A83.5   California encephalitis**
         California meningoencephalitis
         La Crosse encephalitis

MCC **A83.6   Rocio virus disease**

MCC **A83.8   Other mosquito-borne viral encephalitis**

MCC **A83.9   Mosquito-borne viral encephalitis, unspecified**

A84-   Tick-borne viral encephalitis — A group of infectious viral diseases (arbovirus) caused by the genus Flavivirus, and characterized by convulsions, fever, nuchal rigidity, nausea, vomiting, and paralysis in its severe form, and transmitted to man by ticks.
   Includes: Tick-borne viral meningoencephalitis

MCC **A84.0   Far Eastern tick-borne encephalitis [Russian spring-summer encephalitis]**

MCC **A84.1   Central European tick-borne encephalitis**

MCC **A84.8   Other tick-borne viral encephalitis**
         Louping ill
         Powassan virus disease

MCC **A84.9   Tick-borne viral encephalitis, unspecified**

A85-   Other viral encephalitis, not elsewhere classified
   Includes: Specified viral encephalomyelitis NEC
               Specified viral meningoencephalitis NEC
   Excludes 1:   benign myalgic encephalomyelitis (G93.3)
               encephalitis due to cytomegalovirus (B25.8)
               encephalitis due to herpesvirus NEC (B10.0-)
               encephalitis due to herpesvirus [herpes simplex] (B00.4)
               encephalitis due to measles virus (B05.0)
               encephalitis due to mumps virus (B26.2)
               encephalitis due to poliomyelitis virus (A80.-)
               encephalitis due to zoster (B02.0)
               lymphocytic choriomeningitis (A87.2)

CC **A85.0   Enteroviral encephalitis**
         Enteroviral encephalomyelitis

CC **A85.1   Adenoviral encephalitis**
         Adenoviral meningoencephalitis

MCC **A85.2   Arthropod-borne viral encephalitis, unspecified**
   Excludes 1:   West Nile virus with encephalitis (A92.31)

CC **A85.8   Other specified viral encephalitis**
         Encephalitis lethargica
         Von Economo-Cruchet disease

A86   Unspecified viral encephalitis
CC   Viral encephalomyelitis NOS
         Viral meningoencephalitis NOS

A87-   Viral meningitis — A viral infectious inflammation of the meninges caused by Enteroviruses and characterized by malaise, fever, headache, stiff neck, and a relatively shorter benign course than bacterial meningitis.
   Excludes 1:   meningitis due to herpesvirus [herpes simplex] (B00.3)
               meningitis due to measles virus (B05.1)
               meningitis due to mumps virus (B26.1)
               meningitis due to poliomyelitis virus (A80.-)
               meningitis due to zoster (B02.1)

CC **A87.0   Enteroviral meningitis**
         Coxsackievirus meningitis
         Echovirus meningitis

CC **A87.1   Adenoviral meningitis**

CC **A87.2   Lymphocytic choriomeningitis**
         Lymphocytic meningoencephalitis

CC **A87.8   Other viral meningitis**

CC **A87.9   Viral meningitis, unspecified**

A88- **Other viral infections of central nervous system, not elsewhere classified**

   Excludes 1:   *viral encephalitis NOS (A86)*
                        viral meningitis NOS (A87.9)

cc **A88.0** **Enteroviral exanthematous fever [Boston exanthem]** — A viral infectious inflammation of the central nervous system caused by Enteroviruses.

   A88.1 **Epidemic vertigo**

cc **A88.8** **Other specified viral infections of central nervous system**

A89 **Unspecified viral infection of central nervous system**
cc

Arthropod-borne viral fevers and viral hemorrhagic fevers (A90-A99)

A90 **Dengue fever [classical dengue]** — A mosquito-borne viral disease caused by
cc the dengue virus that is characterized by fever, headache, severe myalgias, and characteristic rash.

   Excludes 1:   *dengue hemorrhagic fever (A91)*

A91 **Dengue hemorrhagic fever** — A mosquito-borne viral disease caused by
cc the dengue virus that is characterized by fever, headache, severe myalgias, and characteristic rash that then develops bleeding, low platelet count, and dangerously low blood pressure.

A92- **Other mosquito-borne viral fevers** — Infectious febrile viral diseases transmitted by mosquitoes.

   Excludes 1:   *Ross River disease (B33.1)*

cc **A92.0** **Chikungunya virus disease**
        Chikungunya (hemorrhagic) fever

cc **A92.1** **O'nyong-nyong fever**

cc **A92.2** **Venezuelan equine fever**
        Venezuelan equine encephalitis
        Venezuelan equine encephalomyelitis virus disease

   A92.3- **West Nile virus infection** — An infectious disease caused by the genus Flavivirus and characterized by a mild fever and flu-like symptoms and in severe cases, encephalitis. It originated in Africa and was first identified in the United States in 1999.
        West Nile fever

mcc **A92.30** **West Nile virus infection, unspecified**
        West Nile fever NOS
        West Nile fever without complications
        West Nile virus NOS

mcc **A92.31** **West Nile virus infection with encephalitis**
        West Nile encephalitis
        West Nile encephalomyelitis

mcc **A92.32** **West Nile virus infection with other neurologic manifestation**
        Use additional code to specify the neurologic manifestation

mcc **A92.39** **West Nile virus infection with other complications**
        Use additional code to specify the other conditions

cc **A92.4** **Rift Valley fever**

cc **A92.5** **Zika virus disease** — An infectious disease caused by the Zika virus that is characterized by fever, maculopapular rash, joint pain, and conjunctivitis, and infection during pregnancy can cause fetal microcephaly or other birth defects.
        Zika virus fever
        Zika virus infection
        Zika NOS

cc **A92.8** **Other specified mosquito-borne viral fevers**

cc **A92.9** **Mosquito-borne viral fever, unspecified**

A93- **Other arthropod-borne viral fevers, not elsewhere classified**

cc **A93.0** **Oropouche virus disease**
        Oropouche fever

cc **A93.1** **Sandfly fever**
        Pappataci fever
        Phlebotomus fever

cc **A93.2** **Colorado tick fever**

cc **A93.8** **Other specified arthropod-borne viral fevers**
        Piry virus disease
        Vesicular stomatitis virus disease [Indiana fever]

A94 **Unspecified arthropod-borne viral fever**
cc   Arboviral fever NOS
        Arbovirus infection NOS

A95- **Yellow fever** — A mosquito-borne viral disease caused by the genus Flavivirus that is characterized by fever, chills, jaundice, albuminuria, hemorrhage, and renal damage.

cc **A95.0** **Sylvatic yellow fever**
        Jungle yellow fever

cc **A95.1** **Urban yellow fever**

cc **A95.9** **Yellow fever, unspecified**

A96- **Arenaviral hemorrhagic fever** — Hemorrhagic fevers caused by Arenaviruses.

cc **A96.0** **Junin hemorrhagic fever**
        Argentinian hemorrhagic fever

cc **A96.1** **Machupo hemorrhagic fever**
        Bolivian hemorrhagic fever

   A96.2 **Lassa fever**

cc **A96.8** **Other arenaviral hemorrhagic fevers**

cc **A96.9** **Arenaviral hemorrhagic fever, unspecified**

A98- **Other viral hemorrhagic fevers, not elsewhere classified**

   Excludes 1:   *chikungunya hemorrhagic fever (A92.0)*
                        dengue hemorrhagic fever (A91)

cc **A98.0** **Crimean-Congo hemorrhagic fever**
        Central Asian hemorrhagic fever

cc **A98.1** **Omsk hemorrhagic fever**

cc **A98.2** **Kyasanur Forest disease**

   A98.3 **Marburg virus disease**

   A98.4 **Ebola virus disease**

cc **A98.5** **Hemorrhagic fever with renal syndrome**
        Epidemic hemorrhagic fever
        Korean hemorrhagic fever
        Russian hemorrhagic fever
        Hantaan virus disease
        Hantavirus disease with renal manifestations
        Nephropathia epidemica
        Songo fever

     Excludes 1:   *hantavirus (cardio)-pulmonary syndrome (B33.4)*

cc **A98.8** **Other specified viral hemorrhagic fevers**

A99 **Unspecified viral hemorrhagic fever**
cc

Viral infections characterized by skin and mucous membrane lesions (B00-B09)

B00- **Herpesviral [herpes simplex] infections** — A viral infectious disease affecting the skin and mucous membranes caused by the herpes simplex virus, usually Type 1.

   Excludes 1:   *congenital herpesviral infections (P35.2)*
   Excludes ❷: *anogenital herpesviral infection (A60.-)*
                      gammaherpesviral mononucleosis (B27.0-)
                      herpangina (B08.5)

   B00.0 **Eczema herpeticum**
        Kaposi's varicelliform eruption

   B00.1 **Herpesviral vesicular dermatitis**
        Herpes simplex facialis
        Herpes simplex labialis
        Herpes simplex otitis externa
        Vesicular dermatitis of ear
        Vesicular dermatitis of lip

cc **B00.2** **Herpesviral gingivostomatitis and pharyngotonsillitis**
        Herpesviral pharyngitis

mcc **B00.3** **Herpesviral meningitis**

mcc **B00.4** **Herpesviral encephalitis**
        Herpesviral meningoencephalitis
        Simian B disease

     Excludes 1:   *herpesviral encephalitis due to herpesvirus 6 and 7 (B10.01, B10.09)*
                        non-simplex herpesviral encephalitis (B10.0-)

   B00.5- **Herpesviral ocular disease**

cc **B00.50** **Herpesviral ocular disease, unspecified**

cc **B00.51** **Herpesviral iridocyclitis**
        Herpesviral iritis
        Herpesviral uveitis, anterior

cc **B00.52** **Herpesviral keratitis**
        Herpesviral keratoconjunctivitis

cc **B00.53** **Herpesviral conjunctivitis**

cc **B00.59** **Other herpesviral disease of eye**
        Herpesviral dermatitis of eyelid

A88 - B00

Excludes 1: = NOT CODED HERE! (Do not code both)   **539**   *Excludes ❷: =* Not Included Here

MCC **B00.7** <u>Disseminated</u> herpesviral disease
Herpesviral sepsis

B00.8- Other forms of herpesviral infections

CC **B00.81** Herpesviral <u>hepatitis</u>

MCC **B00.82** Herpes simplex <u>myelitis</u>

CC **B00.89** Other herpesviral infection
Herpesviral whitlow

B00.9 Herpesviral infection, unspecified
Herpes simplex infection NOS

B01- <u>Varicella</u> [chickenpox] — A highly contagious viral disease caused by Varicella-zoster virus, (the same virus which causes herpes zoster) that is characterized by fever and a rash which progresses rapidly from macules to papules to vesicles to pustules to crusts.

CC **B01.0** Varicella meningitis

B01.1- Varicella encephalitis, myelitis and encephalomyelitis
Postchickenpox encephalitis, myelitis and encephalomyelitis

MCC **B01.11** Varicella encephalitis and encephalomyelitis
Postchickenpox encephalitis and encephalomyelitis

MCC **B01.12** Varicella myelitis
Postchickenpox myelitis

MCC **B01.2** Varicella pneumonia

B01.8- Varicella with other complications

CC **B01.81** Varicella keratitis

CC **B01.89** Other varicella complications

CC **B01.9** Varicella without complication
Varicella NOS

B02- Zoster [herpes zoster] — A viral infectious disease caused by Varicella-zoster virus, (the same virus which causes chickenpox) that is characterized by unilateral radicular pain and a vesicular eruption to the surface area of an infected spinal or cerebral sensory ganglion.
Includes: Shingles
Zona

CC **B02.0** Zoster <u>encephalitis</u>
Zoster meningoencephalitis

MCC **B02.1** Zoster <u>meningitis</u>

B02.2- Zoster with <u>other nervous</u> system involvement

CC **B02.21** Postherpetic geniculate ganglionitis

CC **B02.22** Postherpetic trigeminal neuralgia

CC **B02.23** Postherpetic polyneuropathy

MCC **B02.24** Postherpetic myelitis
Herpes zoster myelitis

CC **B02.29** Other postherpetic nervous system involvement
Postherpetic radiculopathy

B02.3- Zoster <u>ocular</u> disease

CC **B02.30** Zoster ocular disease, unspecified

CC **B02.31** Zoster conjunctivitis

CC **B02.32** Zoster iridocyclitis

CC **B02.33** Zoster keratitis
Herpes zoster keratoconjunctivitis

CC **B02.34** Zoster scleritis

CC **B02.39** Other herpes zoster eye disease
Zoster blepharitis

CC **B02.7** <u>Disseminated</u> zoster

CC **B02.8** Zoster with other complications
Herpes zoster otitis externa

B02.9 Zoster without complications
Zoster NOS

B03 Smallpox
CC Note: In 1980 the 33rd World Health Assembly declared that smallpox had been eradicated. The classification is maintained for surveillance purposes.

B04 Monkeypox — An infectious viral disease caused by the Monkeypox virus that is
CC characterized by fever, rash, respiratory symptoms, and lymphadenopathy.

B05- <u>Measles</u> — A contagious viral infection caused by the measles virus, and characterized by fever, conjunctivitis, and a generalized maculopapular eruption.
Includes: Morbilli
Excludes 1:   *subacute sclerosing panencephalitis (A81.1)*

MCC **B05.0** Measles complicated by encephalitis
Postmeasles encephalitis

CC **B05.1** Measles complicated by meningitis
Postmeasles meningitis

MCC **B05.2** Measles complicated by pneumonia
Postmeasles pneumonia

B05.3 Measles complicated by otitis media
Postmeasles otitis media

CC **B05.4** Measles with intestinal complications

B05.8- Measles with other complications

CC **B05.81** Measles keratitis and keratoconjunctivitis

CC **B05.89** Other measles complications

B05.9 Measles without complication
Measles NOS

B06- <u>Rubella</u> [German measles] — A contagious viral infection caused by the rubella virus, and characterized by a three-day generalized maculopapular rash.
Excludes 1:   *congenital rubella (P35.0)*

B06.0- Rubella with neurological complications

CC **B06.00** Rubella with neurological complication, unspecified

MCC **B06.01** Rubella encephalitis
Rubella meningoencephalitis

CC **B06.02** Rubella meningitis

CC **B06.09** Other neurological complications of rubella

B06.8- Rubella with other complications

CC **B06.81** Rubella pneumonia

CC **B06.82** Rubella arthritis

CC **B06.89** Other rubella complications

B06.9 Rubella without complication
Rubella NOS

B07- <u>Viral warts</u> — An epidermal infectious viral disease caused by a human papillomavirus, that is characterized by a raised, round papillomatous growth with a horny surface that is most often located on the dorsal aspect of the hands and fingers.
Includes: Verruca simplex
Verruca vulgaris
Viral warts due to human papillomavirus
Excludes ❷: *anogenital (venereal) warts (A63.0)*
papilloma of bladder (D41.4)
papilloma of cervix (D26.0)
papilloma larynx (D14.1)

B07.0 Plantar wart — A form characterized by location on the soles of the feet, and lying deep within the epidermis.
Verruca plantaris

B07.8 Other viral warts
Common wart
Flat wart
Verruca plana

B07.9 Viral wart, unspecified

B08- Other viral infections characterized by skin and mucous membrane lesions, not elsewhere classified
Excludes 1:   *vesicular stomatitis virus disease (A93.8)*

B08.0- Other orthopoxvirus infections
Excludes ❷: *monkeypox (B04)*

B08.01- Cowpox and vaccinia not from vaccine

B08.010 Cowpox — A viral infectious disease of cattle that is caused by the Cowpox virus, which infects man through skin contact and is characterized by vesicopustular lesions on the hands, face, and/or other cutaneous sites.

B08.011 Vaccinia not from vaccine — An infection that results from the accidentally induced vaccinia virus and is not from an intentional medical care vaccination.
Excludes 1:   *vaccinia (from vaccination) (generalized) (T88.1)*

B08.02 Orf virus disease
Contagious pustular dermatitis
Ecthyma contagiosum

B08.03 Pseudocowpox [milker's node] — A viral disease characterized by circumscribed nodules on the hands of workers who milk cows infected with cowpox.

Excludes 1: = NOT CODED HERE! (Do not code both)   **540**   *Excludes ❷:* = Not Included Here

B08.04 **Paravaccinia, unspecified**

B08.09 **Other orthopoxvirus infections**
Orthopoxvirus infection NOS

B08.1 **Molluscum contagiosum** — An infectious viral disease caused by a Poxvirus, and characterized by discrete pearly skin papules containing caseous matter.

B08.2- **Exanthema subitum [sixth disease]** — A sudden, mild viral illness caused by the human herpesvirus that is characterized by a few days of fever, followed by a faint pink rash, usually seen on the trunk.
Roseola infantum

B08.20 **Exanthema subitum [sixth disease], unspecified** — [Age/0-17]
Roseola infantum, unspecified

B08.21 **Exanthema subitum [sixth disease] due to human herpesvirus 6** — [Age/0-17]
Roseola infantum due to human herpesvirus 6

B08.22 **Exanthema subitum [sixth disease] due to human herpesvirus 7** — [Age/0-17]
Roseola infantum due to human herpesvirus 7

cc B08.3 **Erythema infectiosum [fifth disease]** — A contagious viral infectious disease that is caused by Parvovirus B19 and is characterized by a rose-colored macular rash, occurring mainly in children.

B08.4 **Enteroviral vesicular stomatitis with exanthem** — An infectious viral disease caused by Coxsackie A virus, and characterized by vesicular eruption of hands, feet, and mouth. NOTE: Foot and mouth disease (B08.8) is a separate and different infection.
Hand, foot and mouth disease

B08.5 **Enteroviral vesicular pharyngitis**
Herpangina

B08.6- **Parapoxvirus infections**

B08.60 **Parapoxvirus infection, unspecified**

B08.61 **Bovine stomatitis** — A cutaneous infection in humans caused by contact with cattle infected with bovine papular stomatitis.

B08.62 **Sealpox** — A cutaneous infection in humans caused by contact with seals and sea lions infected with the sealpox virus.

B08.69 **Other parapoxvirus infections**

B08.7- **Yatapoxvirus infections**

B08.70 **Yatapoxvirus infection, unspecified**

cc B08.71 **Tanapox virus disease** — A viral infection caused by the Tanapox virus that is characterized by fever, headaches, and often itching at the cutaneous lesion sites.

B08.72 **Yaba pox virus disease** — A viral infection caused by the Yaba monkey tumor virus that is characterized by a tumor or nodule containing histiocytes.
Yaba monkey tumor disease

B08.79 **Other yatapoxvirus infections**

B08.8 **Other specified viral infections characterized by skin and mucous membrane lesions**
Enteroviral lymphonodular pharyngitis
Foot-and-mouth disease — An infectious viral disease caused by picornavirus affecting cattle and rarely humans.
Poxvirus NEC

B09 **Unspecified viral infection characterized by skin and mucous membrane lesions**
Viral enanthema NOS
Viral exanthema NOS

Other human herpesviruses (B10)

B10- **Other human herpesviruses**
Excludes ❷: cytomegalovirus (B25.9)
Epstein-Barr virus (B27.0-)
herpes NOS (B00.9)
herpes simplex (B00-)
herpes zoster (B02-)
human herpesvirus NOS (B00-)
human herpesvirus 1 and 2 (B00-)
human herpesvirus 3 (B01.-, B02.-)
human herpesvirus 4 (B27.0-)
human herpesvirus 5 (B25-)
varicella (B01-)
zoster (B02-)

B10.0- **Other human herpesvirus encephalitis** — Inflammation of the brain caused by a human herpesvirus infection.
Excludes ❷: herpes encephalitis NOS (B00.4)
herpes simplex encephalitis (B00.4)
human herpesvirus encephalitis (B00.4)
simian B herpes virus encephalitis (B00.4)

MCC B10.01 **Human herpesvirus 6 encephalitis**

MCC B10.09 **Other human herpesvirus encephalitis**
Human herpesvirus 7 encephalitis

B10.8- **Other human herpesvirus infection**

B10.81 **Human herpesvirus 6 infection**

B10.82 **Human herpesvirus 7 infection**

B10.89 **Other human herpesvirus infection**
Human herpesvirus 8 infection
Kaposi's sarcoma-associated herpesvirus infection

Viral hepatitis (B15-B19)

Excludes 1: sequelae of viral hepatitis (B94.2)
Excludes ❷: cytomegaloviral hepatitis (B25.1)
herpesviral [herpes simplex] hepatitis (B00.81)

B15- **Acute hepatitis A** — The initial/first stage (within the first 6 months after someone is exposed) of an infection and inflammation of the liver caused by the hepatitis A virus, that is characterized by jaundice, anorexia, nausea, dark urine, pale stool, and vomiting.

MCC B15.0 **Hepatitis A with hepatic coma**

cc B15.9 **Hepatitis A without hepatic coma**
Hepatitis A (acute) (viral) NOS

B16- **Acute hepatitis B** — The initial/first stage (within the first 6 months after someone is exposed) of an infection and inflammation of the liver caused by the hepatitis B virus, that Is characterized by jaundice, urticarial skin lesions, and arthritis.

MCC B16.0 **Acute hepatitis B with delta-agent with hepatic coma**

cc B16.1 **Acute hepatitis B with delta-agent without hepatic coma**

MCC B16.2 **Acute hepatitis B without delta-agent with hepatic coma**

cc B16.9 **Acute hepatitis B without delta-agent and without hepatic coma**
Hepatitis B (acute) (viral) NOS

B17- **Other acute viral hepatitis** — The initial/first stage (within the first 6 months after someone is exposed) of an infection and inflammation of the liver caused by a hepatitis virus.

cc B17.0 **Acute delta-(super) infection of hepatitis B carrier**

B17.1- **Acute hepatitis C**

cc B17.10 **Acute hepatitis C without hepatic coma**
Acute hepatitis C NOS

MCC B17.11 **Acute hepatitis C with hepatic coma**

cc B17.2 **Acute hepatitis E**

cc B17.8 **Other specified acute viral hepatitis**
Hepatitis non-A non-B (acute) (viral) NEC

cc B17.9 **Acute viral hepatitis, unspecified**
Acute hepatitis NOS
Acute infectious hepatitis NOS

B08
|
B17

B18- <u>Chronic</u> **viral hepatitis** — The second, long-term illness stage of an infection and inflammation of the liver caused by a hepatitis virus.
  Includes: Carrier of viral hepatitis
  cc **B18.0** **Chronic viral hepatitis B with delta-agent**
  cc **B18.1** **Chronic viral hepatitis B without delta-agent**
    Carrier of viral hepatitis B
    Chronic (viral) hepatitis B
  B18.2 **Chronic viral hepatitis C**
    Carrier of viral hepatitis C
  cc **B18.8** **Other chronic viral hepatitis**
    Carrier of other viral hepatitis
  cc **B18.9** **Chronic viral hepatitis, unspecified**
    Carrier of unspecified viral hepatitis

B19- <u>Unspecified</u> **viral hepatitis**
  mcc **B19.0** **Unspecified viral hepatitis with hepatic coma**
  B19.1- **Unspecified viral hepatitis B**
    cc **B19.10** **Unspecified viral hepatitis B without hepatic coma**
      Unspecified viral hepatitis B NOS
    mcc **B19.11** **Unspecified viral hepatitis B with hepatic coma**
  B19.2- **Unspecified viral hepatitis C**
    B19.20 **Unspecified viral hepatitis C without hepatic coma**
      Viral hepatitis C NOS
    mcc **B19.21** **Unspecified viral hepatitis C with hepatic coma**
  cc **B19.9** **Unspecified viral hepatitis without hepatic coma**
    Viral hepatitis NOS

Human immunodeficiency virus [HIV] disease (B20)

B20 **Human immunodeficiency virus [HIV] disease** — A viral infectious disease
mcc caused by the human immunodeficiency virus that attacks the immune system causing the body to have trouble fighting off disease.
  Includes: Acquired immune deficiency syndrome [AIDS]
    AIDS-related complex [ARC]
    HIV infection, symptomatic
  Code first Human immunodeficiency virus [HIV] disease complicating pregnancy, childbirth and the puerperium, if applicable (O98.7-)
  Use additional code(s) to identify all manifestations of HIV infection
  Excludes 1: *asymptomatic human immunodeficiency virus [HIV] infection status (Z21)*
    exposure to HIV virus (Z20.6)
    inconclusive serologic evidence of HIV (R75)

Other viral diseases (B25-B34)

B25- <u>Cytomegaloviral disease</u> — An infectious viral disease caused by the Cytomegalovirus that is characterized by fever and swollen glands.
  Excludes 1: *congenital cytomegalovirus infection (P35.1)*
    cytomegaloviral mononucleosis (B27.1-)
  mcc **B25.0** **Cytomegaloviral pneumonitis**
  cc **B25.1** **Cytomegaloviral hepatitis**
  mcc **B25.2** **Cytomegaloviral pancreatitis**
  cc **B25.8** **Other cytomegaloviral diseases**
    Cytomegaloviral encephalitis
  cc **B25.9** **Cytomegaloviral disease, unspecified**

B26- <u>Mumps</u> — An infectious viral disease of the paramyxovirus group, and marked most commonly by inflammation of parotid glands.
  Includes: Epidemic parotitis
    Infectious parotitis
  cc **B26.0** **Mumps orchitis** — [♂]
  mcc **B26.1** **Mumps meningitis**
  mcc **B26.2** **Mumps encephalitis**
  cc **B26.3** **Mumps pancreatitis**
  B26.8- **Mumps with other complications**
    cc **B26.81** **Mumps hepatitis**
    cc **B26.82** **Mumps myocarditis**
    cc **B26.83** **Mumps nephritis**
    cc **B26.84** **Mumps polyneuropathy**
    cc **B26.85** **Mumps arthritis**
    cc **B26.89** **Other mumps complications**
  B26.9 **Mumps without complication**
    Mumps NOS
    Mumps parotitis NOS

B27- <u>Infectious mononucleosis</u>
  Includes: Glandular fever
    Monocytic angina
    Pfeiffer's disease
  B27.0- **Gammaherpesviral mononucleosis** — An infectious viral disease caused by Epstein-Barr virus, that is characterized by inflammation of the pharynx, fever, malaise, lymphadenopathy, and hepatosplenomegaly.
    Mononucleosis due to Epstein-Barr virus
    B27.00 **Gammaherpesviral mononucleosis without complication**
    B27.01 **Gammaherpesviral mononucleosis with polyneuropathy**
    B27.02 **Gammaherpesviral mononucleosis with meningitis**
    B27.09 **Gammaherpesviral mononucleosis with other complications**
      Hepatomegaly in gammaherpesviral mononucleosis
  B27.1- **Cytomegaloviral mononucleosis** — An infectious viral disease caused by cytomegalovirus that is characterized by inflammation of the pharynx, fever, malaise, lymphadenopathy, and hepatosplenomegaly.
    B27.10 **Cytomegaloviral mononucleosis without complications**
    B27.11 **Cytomegaloviral mononucleosis with polyneuropathy**
    B27.12 **Cytomegaloviral mononucleosis with meningitis**
    B27.19 **Cytomegaloviral mononucleosis with other complication**
      Hepatomegaly in cytomegaloviral mononucleosis
  B27.8- **Other infectious mononucleosis**
    B27.80 **Other infectious mononucleosis without complication**
    B27.81 **Other infectious mononucleosis with polyneuropathy**
    B27.82 **Other infectious mononucleosis with meningitis**
    B27.89 **Other infectious mononucleosis with other complication**
      Hepatomegaly in other infectious mononucleosis
  B27.9- **Infectious mononucleosis, unspecified**
    B27.90 **Infectious mononucleosis, unspecified without complication**
    B27.91 **Infectious mononucleosis, unspecified with polyneuropathy**
    B27.92 **Infectious mononucleosis, unspecified with meningitis**
    B27.99 **Infectious mononucleosis, unspecified with other complication**
      Hepatomegaly in unspecified infectious mononucleosis

B30- <u>Viral conjunctivitis</u> — An infectious viral disease usually caused by an Adenovirus that is characterized by inflammation of the conjunctiva.
  Excludes 1: *herpesviral [herpes simplex] ocular disease (B00.5)*
    ocular zoster (B02.3)
  B30.0 **Keratoconjunctivitis due to adenovirus**
    Epidemic keratoconjunctivitis
    Shipyard eye
  B30.1 **Conjunctivitis due to adenovirus**
    Acute adenoviral follicular conjunctivitis
    Swimming-pool conjunctivitis
  B30.2 **Viral pharyngoconjunctivitis**
  B30.3 **Acute epidemic hemorrhagic conjunctivitis (enteroviral)**
    Conjunctivitis due to coxsackievirus 24
    Conjunctivitis due to enterovirus 70
    Hemorrhagic conjunctivitis (acute) (epidemic)
  B30.8 **Other viral conjunctivitis**
    Newcastle conjunctivitis
  B30.9 **Viral conjunctivitis, unspecified**

B33- **Other viral diseases, not elsewhere classified**
  B33.0 **Epidemic myalgia** — An infectious viral disease caused by Coxsackie B virus, and characterized by sudden, sharp, paroxysmal chest pain, headache, myalgia, and fever of brief duration.
    Bornholm disease
  cc **B33.1** **Ross River disease**
    Epidemic polyarthritis and exanthema
    Ross River fever
  B33.2- **Viral carditis** — An infectious viral disease of the heart caused by the Coxsackie virus.
    Coxsackie (virus) carditis
    cc **B33.20** **Viral carditis, unspecified**
    cc **B33.21** **Viral endocarditis**
    cc **B33.22** **Viral myocarditis**
    cc **B33.23** **Viral pericarditis**
    B33.24 **Viral cardiomyopathy**

B18-B33

Excludes 1: = NOT CODED HERE! (Do not code both)   *Excludes ❷:* = Not Included Here

B33.3   Retrovirus infections, not elsewhere classified
　　　　Retrovirus infection NOS

cc **B33.4   Hantavirus (cardio)-pulmonary syndrome [HPS] [HCPS]** — An infectious viral disease caused by an RNA virus, that is characterized by fever, cough, muscle aches, headache, lethargy, and shortness-of-breath, which can rapidly deteriorate into acute respiratory failure.
　　　　Hantavirus disease with pulmonary manifestations
　　　　Sin nombre virus disease
　　　　Use additional code to identify any associated acute kidney failure
　　　　　(N17.9)
　　　　Excludes 1:　hantavirus disease with renal manifestations (A98.5)
　　　　　　　　　　hemorrhagic fever with renal manifestations (A98.5)

B33.8   Other specified viral diseases
　　　　Excludes 1:　anogenital human papillomavirus infection (A63.0)
　　　　　　　　　　viral warts due to human papillomavirus infection (B07)

B34-   Viral infection of unspecified site
　　　　Excludes 1:　anogenital human papillomavirus infection (A63.0)
　　　　　　　　　　cytomegaloviral disease NOS (B25.9)
　　　　　　　　　　herpesvirus [herpes simplex] infection NOS (B00.9)
　　　　　　　　　　retrovirus infection NOS (B33.3)
　　　　　　　　　　viral agents as the cause of diseases classified elsewhere
　　　　　　　　　　　(B97-)
　　　　　　　　　　viral warts due to human papillomavirus infection (B07)

B34.0   Adenovirus infection, unspecified

B34.1   Enterovirus infection, unspecified
　　　　Coxsackievirus infection NOS
　　　　Echovirus infection NOS

B34.2   Coronavirus infection, unspecified
　　　　Excludes 1:　pneumonia due to SARS-associated coronavirus
　　　　　　　　　　(J12.81)

cc **B34.3   Parvovirus infection, unspecified**

B34.4   Papovavirus infection, unspecified

B34.8   Other viral infections of unspecified site

B34.9   Viral infection, unspecified
　　　　Viremia NOS

Mycoses (B35-B49)

Excludes ❷:　hypersensitivity pneumonitis due to organic dust (J67.-)
　　　　　　mycosis fungoides (C84.0-)

B35-   Dermatophytosis — A group of infectious superficial fungal skin diseases caused by a dermatophyte.
　　　　Includes:　Favus
　　　　　　　　Infections due to species of Epidermophyton, Micro-sporum and
　　　　　　　　　Trichophyton
　　　　　　　　Tinea, any type except those in B36.-

B35.0   Tinea barbae and tinea capitis
　　　　Beard ringworm
　　　　Kerion
　　　　Scalp ringworm
　　　　Sycosis, mycotic

B35.1   Tinea unguium
　　　　Dermatophytic onychia
　　　　Dermatophytosis of nail
　　　　Onychomycosis
　　　　Ringworm of nails

B35.2   Tinea manuum
　　　　Dermatophytosis of hand
　　　　Hand ringworm

B35.3   Tinea pedis
　　　　Athlete's foot
　　　　Dermatophytosis of foot
　　　　Foot ringworm

B35.4   Tinea corporis
　　　　Ringworm of the body

B35.5   Tinea imbricata
　　　　Tokelau

B35.6   Tinea cruris
　　　　Dhobi itch
　　　　Groin ringworm
　　　　Jock itch

B35.8   Other dermatophytoses
　　　　Disseminated dermatophytosis
　　　　Granulomatous dermatophytosis

B35.9   Dermatophytosis, unspecified
　　　　Ringworm NOS

B36-   Other superficial mycoses

B36.0   Pityriasis versicolor — A superficial fungal skin disease characterized by discolored, hyperpigmented spots or plaques on the chest and back with a slight scale formation.
　　　　Tinea flava
　　　　Tinea versicolor

B36.1   Tinea nigra — A superficial fungal skin disease characterized by black discoloration of the skin and caused by Cladosporium Wernecki.
　　　　Keratomycosis nigricans palmaris
　　　　Microsporosis nigra
　　　　Pityriasis nigra

B36.2   White piedra — A superficial fungal skin disease characterized by white fungal masses on the hair shafts, which may occasionally cause a systemic infection in debilitated patients.
　　　　Tinea blanca

B36.3   Black piedra — A superficial fungal skin disease characterized by black nodular masses of fungi on the hair shafts.

B36.8   Other specified superficial mycoses

B36.9   Superficial mycosis, unspecified

B37-   Candidiasis — Infectious fungal diseases caused by the genus Candida, and characterized by stubborn infection of the moist areas of the body.
　　　　Includes:　Candidosis
　　　　　　　　Moniliasis
　　　　Excludes 1:　neonatal candidiasis (P37.5)

cc **B37.0   Candidal stomatitis** — A form characterized by whitish spots in the mouth, caused by Candida albicans.
　　　　Oral thrush

mcc **B37.1   Pulmonary candidiasis** — A form characterized by infection of the lung tissues that can develop into pneumonia.
　　　　Candidal bronchitis
　　　　Candidal pneumonia

B37.2   Candidiasis of skin and nail
　　　　Candidal onychia
　　　　Candidal paronychia
　　　　Excludes ❷:　diaper dermatitis (L22)

B37.3   Candidiasis of vulva and vagina — [♀]
　　　　Candidal vulvovaginitis
　　　　Monilial vulvovaginitis
　　　　Vaginal thrush

B37.4-   Candidiasis of other urogenital sites

　cc **B37.41   Candidal cystitis and urethritis**

　　B37.42   Candidal balanitis

　cc **B37.49   Other urogenital candidiasis**
　　　　Candidal pyelonephritis

mcc **B37.5   Candidal meningitis**

mcc **B37.6   Candidal endocarditis**

mcc **B37.7   Candidal sepsis**
　　　　AHA 14:2Q:p13 – Sepsis due to non-Candida Albicans
　　　　AHA 14:4Q:p46 – Sepsis due to non-Candida Albicans, clarification
　　　　Disseminated candidiasis
　　　　Systemic candidiasis

B37.8-   Candidiasis of other sites

　cc **B37.81   Candidal esophagitis**

　cc **B37.82   Candidal enteritis**
　　　　Candidal proctitis

　cc **B37.83   Candidal cheilitis**

　cc **B37.84   Candidal otitis externa**

　cc **B37.89   Other sites of candidiasis**
　　　　Candidal osteomyelitis

B37.9   Candidiasis, unspecified
　　　　Thrush NOS

B
3
3
I
B
3
7

B38- **Coccidioidomycosis** — Infectious fungal diseases caused by Coccidioides immitis, and characterized by respiratory origin of pulmonary disease, and dissemination.

cc **B38.0** **Acute pulmonary coccidioidomycosis**

cc **B38.1** **Chronic pulmonary coccidioidomycosis**

cc **B38.2** **Pulmonary coccidioidomycosis, unspecified**

cc **B38.3** **Cutaneous coccidioidomycosis**

mcc **B38.4** **Coccidioidomycosis meningitis**

cc **B38.7** **Disseminated coccidioidomycosis**
Generalized coccidioidomycosis

B38.8- **Other forms of coccidioidomycosis**

cc **B38.81** Prostatic coccidioidomycosis — [♂]

cc **B38.89** Other forms of coccidioidomycosis

cc **B38.9** **Coccidioidomycosis, unspecified**

B39- **Histoplasmosis** — Infectious fungal diseases caused by the genus Histoplasma.
Code first associated AIDS (B20)
Use additional code for any associated manifestations, such as:
Eendocarditis (I39)
Meningitis (G02)
Pericarditis (I32)
Retinitits (H32)

mcc **B39.0** **Acute pulmonary histoplasmosis capsulati**

mcc **B39.1** **Chronic pulmonary histoplasmosis capsulati**

mcc **B39.2** **Pulmonary histoplasmosis capsulati, unspecified**

cc **B39.3** **Disseminated histoplasmosis capsulati**
Generalized histoplasmosis capsulati

B39.4 **Histoplasmosis capsulati, unspecified**
American histoplasmosis

B39.5 **Histoplasmosis duboisii**
African histoplasmosis

B39.9 **Histoplasmosis, unspecified**

B40- **Blastomycosis** — An infectious fungal disease caused by Blastomyces dermatitidis, and characterized by involvement of the skin, lungs, and other viscera, occurring primarily in North America.
Excludes 1: *Brazilian blastomycosis (B41.-)*
keloidal blastomycosis (B48.0)

cc **B40.0** **Acute pulmonary blastomycosis**

cc **B40.1** **Chronic pulmonary blastomycosis**

cc **B40.2** **Pulmonary blastomycosis, unspecified**

cc **B40.3** **Cutaneous blastomycosis**

cc **B40.7** **Disseminated blastomycosis**
Generalized blastomycosis

B40.8- **Other forms of blastomycosis**

cc **B40.81** **Blastomycotic meningoencephalitis**
Meningomyelitis due to blastomycosis

cc **B40.89** **Other forms of blastomycosis**

cc **B40.9** **Blastomycosis, unspecified**

B41- **Paracoccidioidomycosis** — An infectious fungal disease caused by Paracoccidioides brasiliensis, and characterized by systemic infection which may affect a few organs to almost all organs.
Includes: Brazilian blastomycosis
Lutz' disease

cc **B41.0** **Pulmonary paracoccidioidomycosis**

cc **B41.7** **Disseminated paracoccidioidomycosis**
Generalized paracoccidioidomycosis

cc **B41.8** **Other forms of paracoccidioidomycosis**

cc **B41.9** **Paracoccidioidomycosis, unspecified**

B42- **Sporotrichosis** — An infectious fungal disease caused by Sporothrix schenckii, and characterized primarily by suppurating nodules along the lymphatics of the skin and subcutaneous tissue, and occasionally developing into other tissues and organs.

B42.0 **Pulmonary sporotrichosis**

B42.1 **Lymphocutaneous sporotrichosis**

B42.7 **Disseminated sporotrichosis**
Generalized sporotrichosis

B42.8- **Other forms of sporotrichosis**

B42.81 **Cerebral sporotrichosis**
Meningitis due to sporotrichosis

B42.82 **Sporotrichosis arthritis**

B42.89 **Other forms of sporotrichosis**

B42.9 **Sporotrichosis, unspecified**

B43- **Chromomycosis** and **pheomycotic abscess** — An infectious fungal disease caused by closely related fungal organisms Cladosporium carrionii, Fonsecaea pedrosoi, Fonsecaea compactum, and Phialophora verrucosa, and characterized by chronic granulomatous nodules in the skin and subcutaneous tissue and occasionally multiple subcutaneous pheomycotic cysts and abscesses.

B43.0 **Cutaneous chromomycosis**
Dermatitis verrucosa

B43.1 **Pheomycotic brain abscess**
Cerebral chromomycosis

B43.2 **Subcutaneous pheomycotic abscess and cyst**

B43.8 **Other forms of chromomycosis**

B43.9 **Chromomycosis, unspecified**

B44- **Aspergillosis** — An infectious fungal disease caused by the genus Aspergillus, and characterized by inflammatory granulomatous lesions in the skin, ear, orbit, nasal sinuses, lungs, and occasionally in the bones and meninges.
Includes: Aspergilloma

mcc **B44.0** **Invasive pulmonary aspergillosis**

cc **B44.1** **Other pulmonary aspergillosis**

cc **B44.2** **Tonsillar aspergillosis**

cc **B44.7** **Disseminated aspergillosis**
Generalized aspergillosis

B44.8- **Other forms of aspergillosis**

cc **B44.81** **Allergic bronchopulmonary aspergillosis**

cc **B44.89** **Other forms of aspergillosis**

cc **B44.9** **Aspergillosis, unspecified**

B45- **Cryptococcosis** — An infectious fungal disease caused by Cryptococcus neoformans, and characterized by involving the lungs, skin, brain, and meninges.

cc **B45.0** **Pulmonary cryptococcosis**

mcc **B45.1** **Cerebral cryptococcosis**
Cryptococcal meningitis
Cryptococcosis meningocerebralis

cc **B45.2** **Cutaneous cryptococcosis**

cc **B45.3** **Osseous cryptococcosis**

cc **B45.7** **Disseminated cryptococcosis**
Generalized cryptococcosis

cc **B45.8** **Other forms of cryptococcosis**

cc **B45.9** **Cryptococcosis, unspecified**

B46- **Zygomycosis** — A group of infectious fungal (Zygomycetes) diseases marked by a variety of manifestations depending upon which organism is the infective agent and the body part(s) infected.

mcc **B46.0** **Pulmonary mucormycosis**

mcc **B46.1** **Rhinocerebral mucormycosis**

mcc **B46.2** **Gastrointestinal mucormycosis**

mcc **B46.3** **Cutaneous mucormycosis**
Subcutaneous mucormycosis

mcc **B46.4** **Disseminated mucormycosis**
Generalized mucormycosis

mcc **B46.5** **Mucormycosis, unspecified**

mcc **B46.8** **Other zygomycoses**
Entomophthoromycosis

mcc **B46.9** **Zygomycosis, unspecified**
Phycomycosis NOS

B47- **Mycetoma**

cc **B47.0** **Eumycetoma** — A fungal disease (Eumycetes) that is characterized by chronic, suppurative, granulomatous subcutaneous tissues and bones with sinus formation.
Madura foot, mycotic
Maduromycosis

cc **B47.1** **Actinomycetoma** — An infectious disease caused by actinomycetes that is characterized by chronic, suppurative, granulomatous subcutaneous tissues and bones with sinus formation.

cc **B47.9** **Mycetoma, unspecified**
Madura foot NOS

B48-   <u>Other mycoses</u>, not elsewhere classified

B48.0   **Lobomycosis** — An infectious fungal disease caused by Loboa loboi that is characterized by slow-growing keloid-like skin tumors.
> Keloidal blastomycosis
> Lobo's disease

B48.1   **Rhinosporidiosis** — An infectious fungal disease caused by Rhinosporidium seeberi that is characterized by small tumor-like masses usually in the nose and nasopharynx.

cc **B48.2**   **Allescheriasis** — An infectious fungal disease caused by Allescheria [Petriellidium] boydii that is characterized by suppurative, granulomatous skin and subcutaneous lesions.
> Infection due to Pseudallescheria boydii

> *Excludes 1:*   eumycetoma (B47.0)

cc **B48.3**   **Geotrichosis** — A fungal infection caused by Geotrichum candidum that affects the oral cavity and sometimes the lungs.
> Geotrichum stomatitis

cc **B48.4**   **Penicillosis** — A fungal infection caused by Penicillium marneffei that affects immunocompromised patients that is characterized by fever, skin lesions, and lymphandenopathy.

cc **B48.8**   **Other specified mycoses**
> AHA 14:2Q:p13 – Sepsis due to non-Candida Albicans
> AHA 14:4Q:p46 – Sepsis due to non-Candida Albicans, clarification
> Adiaspiromycosis
> Infection of tissue and organs by Alternaria
> Infection of tissue and organs by Drechslera
> Infection of tissue and organs by Fusarium
> Infection of tissue and organs by saprophytic fungi NEC

B49   **Unspecified mycosis**
cc
> Fungemia NOS

Protozoal diseases (B50-B64)

> *Excludes 1:*   amebiasis (A06.-)
>   other protozoal intestinal diseases (A07.-)

B50-   **Plasmodium <u>falciparum malaria</u>** — A mosquito-borne parasitic disease caused by Plasmodium falciparum that is characterized by respiratory distress, severe anemia, pulmonary edema, circulatory shock, and organ failure.
> Includes: Mixed infections of Plasmodium falciparum with any other Plasmodium species

cc **B50.0**   **Plasmodium falciparum malaria with cerebral complications**
> Cerebral malaria NOS

cc **B50.8**   **Other severe and complicated Plasmodium falciparum malaria**
> Severe or complicated Plasmodium falciparum malaria NOS

mcc **B50.9**   **Plasmodium falciparum malaria, unspecified**

B51-   **Plasmodium <u>vivax malaria</u>** — A mosquito-borne parasitic disease caused by Plasmodium vivax that is characterized by fever, headache, chills and vomiting, respiratory distress, anemia, and weakness. Clinical relapses may occur weeks to months after the first infection.
> Includes: Mixed infections of Plasmodium vivax with other Plasmodium species, except Plasmodium falciparum

> *Excludes 1:*   *Plasmodium vivav with Plasmodium falciparum (B50.-)*

cc **B51.0**   **Plasmodium vivax malaria with rupture of spleen**

cc **B51.8**   **Plasmodium vivax malaria with other complications**

cc **B51.9**   **Plasmodium vivax malaria without complication**
> Plasmodium vivax malaria NOS

B52-   **Plasmodium malariae malaria** — A mosquito-borne parasitic disease caused by Plasmodium malariae that is characterized by fever, headache, chills and vomiting, respiratory distress, anemia, and weakness.
> Includes: Mixed infections of Plasmodium malariae with other Plasmodium species, except Plasmodium falciparum and Plasmodium vivax

> *Excludes 1:*   *Plasmodium falciparum (B50.-)*
>   *Plasmodium vivax (B51.-)*

cc **B52.0**   **Plasmodium malariae malaria with nephropathy**

cc **B52.8**   **Plasmodium malariae malaria with other complications**

cc **B52.9**   **Plasmodium malariae malaria without complication**
> Plasmodium malariae malaria NOS

B53-   **Other specified malaria**

cc **B53.0**   **Plasmodium <u>ovale malaria</u>** — A mosquito-borne parasitic disease caused by Plasmodium ovale that is characterized by fever, headache, chills and vomiting, respiratory distress, anemia, and weakness. Clinical relapses may occur weeks to months after the first infection.
> *Excludes 1:*   *Plasmodium ovale with Plasmodium falciparum (B50.-)*
>   *Plasmodium ovale with Plasmodium malariae (B52.-)*
>   *Plasmodium ovale with Plasmodium vivax (B51.-)*

cc **B53.1**   **Malaria due to <u>simian plasmodia</u>** — A mosquito-borne parasitic disease caused by Plasmodium knowlesi that is characterized by fever, headache, chills and vomiting, respiratory distress, anemia, and weakness.
> *Excludes 1:*   *malaria due to simian plasmodia with Plasmodium falciparum (B50.-)*
>   *malaria due to simian plasmodia with Plasmodium malariae (B52.-)*
>   *malaria due to simian plasmodia with Plasmodium ovale (B53.0)*
>   *malaria due to simian plasmodia with Plasmodium vivax (B51.-)*

cc **B53.8**   **Other malaria, not elsewhere classified**

B54   <u>Unspecified malaria</u>
cc

B55-   <u>Leishmaniasis</u> — Parasitic diseases caused by the protozoan genus Leishmaniasis through the bite of sandflies.

cc **B55.0**   **Visceral leishmaniasis** — Leishmaniasis that is characterized by fever, chills, weight loss, splenomegaly, leukopenia, anemia, and potentially fatal if untreated.
> Kala-azar
> Post-kala-azar dermal leishmaniasis

cc **B55.1**   **Cutaneous leishmaniasis** — Leishmaniasis that is characterized by ulcerated sores with small papules on the edge of the sore.

cc **B55.2**   **Mucocutaneous leishmaniasis** — Leishmaniasis that is characterized by ulceration of the skin and mucous membranes of the throat and nose.

cc **B55.9**   **Leishmaniasis, unspecified**

B56-   **African trypanosomiasis**

cc **B56.0**   **Gambiense trypanosomiasis** — A parasitic disease caused by Trypanosoma brucei gambiense, and characterized by a primary lesion at the tsetse fly bite, fever, lymphadenopathy (especially of posterior neck), and invasion of the central nervous system with somnolence and coma which develops slower than the Rhodesian form.
> Infection due to Trypanosoma brucei gambiense
> West African sleeping sickness

cc **B56.1**   **Rhodesiense trypanosomiasis** — A parasitic disease caused by Trypanosoma brucei rhodesiense that is characterized by a primary lesion at the tsetse fly bite, fever, lymphadenopathy (especially of posterior neck), and invasion of the central nervous system with somnolence and coma which develops more rapidly than the Gambian form.
> East African sleeping sickness
> Infection due to Trypanosoma brucei rhodesiense

cc **B56.9**   **African trypanosomiasis, unspecified**
> Sleeping sickness NOS

B57-   <u>Chagas'</u> **disease** — A parasitic disease caused by Trypanosoma cruzi that is characterized by primary lesion at the site of entry (skin, conjunctiva), fever, headache, swollen lymph glands, facial and generalized edema, and can progress to involve various organs.
> Includes: American trypanosomiasis
>   Infection due to Trypanosoma cruzi

cc **B57.0**   **Acute Chagas' disease with heart involvement**
> Acute Chagas' disease with myocarditis

cc **B57.1**   **Acute Chagas' disease without heart involvement**
> Acute Chagas' disease NOS

cc **B57.2**   **Chagas' disease (chronic) with heart involvement**
> American trypanosomiasis NOS
> Chagas' disease (chronic) NOS
> Chagas' disease (chronic) with myocarditis
> Trypanosomiasis NOS

B57.3-   **Chagas' disease (chronic) with digestive system involvement**

cc **B57.30**   **Chagas' disease with digestive system involvement, unspecified**

cc **B57.31**   **Megaesophagus in Chagas' disease**

cc **B57.32**   **Megacolon in Chagas' disease**

cc **B57.39**   **Other digestive system involvement in Chagas' disease**

B 4 8 – B 5 7

B57.4- Chagas' disease (chronic) with nervous system involvement

cc **B57.40** Chagas' disease with nervous system involvement, unspecified

cc **B57.41** Meningitis in Chagas' disease

cc **B57.42** Meningoencephalitis in Chagas' disease

cc **B57.49** Other nervous system involvement in Chagas' disease

cc **B57.5** Chagas' disease (chronic) with other organ involvement

B58- Toxoplasmosis — *A parasitic disease caused by Toxoplasma gondii, and characterized by involvement of various organs.*
   Includes: Infection due to Toxoplasma gondii
   Excludes 1:   *congenital toxoplasmosis (P37.1)*

B58.0- Toxoplasma oculopathy

cc **B58.00** Toxoplasma oculopathy, unspecified

cc **B58.01** Toxoplasma chorioretinitis

cc **B58.09** Other toxoplasma oculopathy
      Toxoplasma uveitis

cc **B58.1** Toxoplasma hepatitis

MCC **B58.2** Toxoplasma meningoencephalitis

MCC **B58.3** Pulmonary toxoplasmosis

B58.8- Toxoplasmosis with other organ involvement

MCC **B58.81** Toxoplasma myocarditis

cc **B58.82** Toxoplasma myositis

cc **B58.83** Toxoplasma tubulo-interstitial nephropathy
      Toxoplasma pyelonephritis

cc **B58.89** Toxoplasmosis with other organ involvement

cc **B58.9** Toxoplasmosis, unspecified

B59 Pneumocystosis — *A highly contagious interstitial plasma cell pneumonia caused by*
MCC *Pneumocystis carinii and Pneumocystis jiroveci that is usually seen in immunocompromised patients.*
      Pneumonia due to Pneumocystis carinii
      Pneumonia due to Pneumocystis jiroveci

B60- Other protozoal diseases, not elsewhere classified
   Excludes 1:   *cryptosporidiosis (A07.2)*
      intestinal microsporidiosis (A07.8)
      isosporiasis (A07.3)

cc **B60.0** Babesiosis — *An infectious parasitic (tick-borne) disease caused by the genus Babesia, and characterized by a malaria-like fever, myalgia, hemolytic anemia, and splenomegaly.*
      Piroplasmosis

B60.1- Acanthamebiasis — *An infectious parasitic disease caused by the free-living soil and water ameoba Acanthameoba that is characterized by skin ulcers and granulomas, and can progress to infect the meninges.*

cc **B60.10** Acanthamebiasis, unspecified

B60.11 Meningoencephalitis due to Acanthamoeba (culbertsoni)

B60.12 Conjunctivitis due to Acanthamoeba

B60.13 Keratoconjunctivitis due to Acanthamoeba —
      [Unacceptable PDX]

cc **B60.19** Other acanthamebic disease

cc **B60.2** Naegleriasis — *An infectious parasitic disease caused by the free-living soil and warm water ameoba Naegleria fowleri that is characterized by infection of the nervous system and brain.*
      Primary amebic meningoencephalitis

B60.8 Other specified protozoal diseases
      Microsporidiosis

B64 Unspecified protozoal disease

Helminthiases (B65-B83)

B65- Schistosomiasis [bilharziasis] — *A parasitic disease caused by the genus Schistosoma (caused by schistosomes worms) that is characterized by abdominal pain and infection of the gastrointestinal and urinary tracts.*
   Includes: Snail fever

cc **B65.0** Schistosomiasis due to Schistosoma haematobium [urinary schistosomiasis]

cc **B65.1** Schistosomiasis due to Schistosoma mansoni [intestinal schistosomiasis]

cc **B65.2** Schistosomiasis due to Schistosoma japonicum
      Asiatic schistosomiasis

cc **B65.3** Cercarial dermatitis
      Swimmer's itch

cc **B65.8** Other schistosomiasis
      Infection due to Schistosoma intercalatum
      Infection due to Schistosoma mattheei
      Infection due to Schistosoma mekongi

cc **B65.9** Schistosomiasis, unspecified

B66- Other fluke infections

cc **B66.0** Opisthorchiasis — *A parasitic disease caused by Opisthorchis felineus and viverrini that is characterized by liver infestation which, in its severe form, presents hepatomegaly, jaundice, liver abscess, and pancreatitis.*
      Infection due to cat liver fluke
      Infection due to Opisthorchis (felineus) (viverrini)

cc **B66.1** Clonorchiasis — *A parasitic disease caused by Clonorchis (Oristhorchis) sinensis that is characterized by infestation and inflammation of the gallbladder, bile ducts, and liver.*
      Chinese liver fluke disease
      Infection due to Clonorchis sinensis
      Oriental liver fluke disease

cc **B66.2** Dicroceliasis — *A parasitic disease caused by Dicrocoelium dendriticum that is characterized by infection of the bile ducts.*
      Infection due to Dicrocoelium dendriticum
      Lancet fluke infection

cc **B66.3** Fascioliasis — *A parasitic disease caused by the genus Fasciola with symptoms characterized by fever, malaise, urticaria, and nonproductive cough, with large flukes obstructing the biliary tract where they live.*
      Infection due to Fasciola gigantica
      Infection due to Fasciola hepatica
      Infection due to Fasciola indica
      Sheep liver fluke disease

cc **B66.4** Paragonimiasis — *A parasitic disease caused by the genus Paragonimus that is characterized by lung infestation with resulting hemoptysis, fever, and occasionally by pleural conditions, and right heart failure.*
      Infection due to Paragonimus species
      Lung fluke disease
      Pulmonary distomiasis

cc **B66.5** Fasciolopsiasis — *A parasitic disease caused by Fasciolopsis buski that is characterized by abdominal pain, intermittent diarrhea, flatus, and excessive appetite or anorexia.*
      Infection due to Fasciolopsis buski
      Intestinal distomiasis

cc **B66.8** Other specified fluke infections
      Echinostomiasis
      Heterophyiasis
      Metagonimiasis
      Nanophyetiasis
      Watsoniasis

B66.9 Fluke infection, unspecified

B67- Echinococcosis — *A parasitic disease caused by Echinococcus granulosus that is characterized by chronic space-occupying lesions of various organs.*
   Includes: Hydatidosis

cc **B67.0** Echinococcus granulosus infection of liver

cc **B67.1** Echinococcus granulosus infection of lung

cc **B67.2** Echinococcus granulosus infection of bone

B67.3- Echinococcus granulosus infection, other and multiple sites

cc **B67.31** Echinococcus granulosus infection, thyroid gland

cc **B67.32** Echinococcus granulosus infection, multiple sites

cc **B67.39** Echinococcus granulosus infection, other sites

cc **B67.4** Echinococcus granulosus infection, unspecified
      Dog tapeworm (infection)

cc **B67.5** Echinococcus multilocularis infection of liver

B67.6- Echinococcus multilocularis infection, other and multiple sites

cc **B67.61** Echinococcus multilocularis infection, multiple sites

cc **B67.69** Echinococcus multilocularis infection, other sites

cc **B67.7** Echinococcus multilocularis infection, unspecified

cc **B67.8** Echinococcosis, unspecified, of liver

B67.9- Echinococcosis, other and unspecified

cc **B67.90** Echinococcosis, unspecified
      Echinococcosis NOS

cc **B67.99** Other echinococcosis

B
5
7
–
B
6
7

B68- Taeniasis — A parasitic disease caused by adult intestinal tapeworms growing to 3 to 25 feet (1 to 7.5 m) in length.
> *Excludes 1: cysticercosis (B69.-)*

cc **B68.0 Taenia solium taeniasis**
> Pork tapeworm (infection)

cc **B68.1 Taenia saginata taeniasis**
> Beef tapeworm (infection)
> Infection due to adult tapeworm Taenia saginata

cc **B68.9 Taeniasis, unspecified**

B69- Cysticercosis — A parasitic disease caused by the larvae of Taenia solium and characterized by mechanical injury at the larval site which may infest the muscle and often the brain and meninges.
> Includes: Cysticerciasis infection due to larval form of Taenia solium

cc **B69.0 Cysticercosis of central nervous system**

cc **B69.1 Cysticercosis of eye**

B69.8- Cysticercosis of other sites

cc **B69.81 Myositis in cysticercosis**

cc **B69.89 Cysticercosis of other sites**

cc **B69.9 Cysticercosis, unspecified**

B70- Diphyllobothriasis and sparganosis

cc **B70.0 Diphyllobothriasis** — A parasitic disease caused by Diphyllobothrium latum, characterized by a small intestinal tapeworm of up to 30 feet (9 m) in length, and acquired from eating infected raw or undercooked freshwater fish.
> Diphyllobothrium (adult) (latum) (pacificum) infection
> Fish tapeworm (infection)
> *Excludes ❷: larval diphyllobothriasis (B70.1)*

cc **B70.1 Sparganosis** — A parasitic disease caused by the larvae identified below and characterized by invasion of subcutaneous tissue, causing inflammation and fibrosis.
> Infection due to Sparganum (mansoni) (proliferum)
> Infection due to Spirometra larva
> Larval diphyllobothriasis
> Spirometrosis

B71- Other cestode infections

cc **B71.0 Hymenolepiasis** — A parasitic disease caused by Hymenolepis nana and characterized by a 1.6 inch (4 cm) ileal tapeworm which has a lifespan of a few weeks.
> Dwarf tapeworm infection
> Rat tapeworm (infection)

cc **B71.1 Dipylidiasis**

cc **B71.8 Other specified cestode infections**
> Coenurosis

B71.9 Cestode infection, unspecified
> Tapeworm (infection) NOS

B72 Dracunculiasis — A parasitic disease caused by the guinea worm that is characterized
cc by development of a worm under the skin causing burning pain at the site.
> Includes: Guinea worm infection
> Infection due to Dracunculus medinensis

B73- Onchocerciasis — A parasitic disease caused by Onchocerca volvulus that is characterized by skin nodules, eye lesions, and dermatitis with lymphatic symptoms.
> Includes: Onchocerca volvulus infection
> Onchocercosis
> River blindness

B73.0- Onchocerciasis with eye disease

cc **B73.00 Onchocerciasis with eye involvement, unspecified**

cc **B73.01 Onchocerciasis with endophthalmitis**

cc **B73.02 Onchocerciasis with glaucoma**

cc **B73.09 Onchocerciasis with other eye involvement**
> Infestation of eyelid due to onchocerciasis

cc **B73.1 Onchocerciasis without eye disease**

B74- Filariasis
> *Excludes ❷: onchocerciasis (B73)*
> *tropical (pulmonary) eosinophilia NOS (J82)*

cc **B74.0 Filariasis due to Wuchereria bancrofti** — A parasitic disease caused by Wuchereria bancrofti that is characterized by frequent attacks of fever, lymphangitis, lymphadenitis, and in the most severe cases elephantiasis.
> Bancroftian elephantiasis
> Bancroftian filariasis

cc **B74.1 Filariasis due to Brugia malayi** — A parasitic disease caused by Brugia malayi and characterized usually by more acute symptoms than bancroftian filariasis, and in which elephantiasis is more common, but spares the bladder and genitalia.

cc **B74.2 Filariasis due to Brugia timori** — A parasitic disease caused by Brugia malayi.

cc **B74.3 Loiasis** — A parasitic disease caused by Loa loa, and characterized by worms 1 to 2 inches (2.5 to 5 cm) in length which move freely in connective tissue giving rise to edematous swelling (Calabar swellings), and frequently infest the conjunctiva with occasional serious complications such as encephalitis.
> Calabar swelling
> Eyeworm disease of Africa
> Loa loa infection

cc **B74.4 Mansonelliasis** — A parasitic disease caused by Mansonella ozzardi that is characterized by adult worms inhabiting the visceral adipose tissue, and are usually asymptomatic.
> Infection due to Mansonella ozzardi
> Infection due to Mansonella perstans
> Infection due to Mansonella streptocerca

cc **B74.8 Other filariases**
> Dirofilariasis

cc **B74.9 Filariasis, unspecified**

B75 Trichinellosis — A parasitic disease caused by Trichinella spiralis, and characterized in
cc the early stages by diarrhea, nausea, colic, and fever, and in the later stages characterized by stiffness, pain, swelling of the muscles, splinter hemorrhages, sweating, and insomnia.
> Includes: Infection due to Trichinella species
> Trichiniasis

B76- Hookworm diseases
> Includes: Uncinariasis

cc **B76.0 Ancylostomiasis** — A parasitic disease caused by genus Ancylostoma that is characterized by adult worms in the small intestine, causing abdominal pain, diarrhea, malnutrition, and in severe cases anemia.
> Infection due to Ancylostoma species

cc **B76.1 Necatoriasis** — A parasitic disease caused by Necator americanus that is characterized by adult worms in the small intestine causing abdominal pain, diarrhea, and malnutrition.
> Infection due to Necator americanus

cc **B76.8 Other hookworm diseases**

cc **B76.9 Hookworm disease, unspecified**
> Cutaneous larva migrans NOS

B77- Ascariasis — A parasitic disease caused by Ascaris lumbricoides that is characterized by giant intestinal worms and in severe cases by pneumonitis and intestinal blockage.
> Includes: Ascaridiasis
> Roundworm infection

cc **B77.0 Ascariasis with intestinal complications**

B77.8- Ascariasis with other complications

mcc **B77.81 Ascariasis pneumonia**

cc **B77.89 Ascariasis with other complications**

cc **B77.9 Ascariasis, unspecified**

B78- Strongyloidiasis — A parasitic disease caused by Strongyloides stercoralis and characterized by roundworm infestation of the small intestine with watery, mucus diarrhea, and migratory larvae infestation of the lungs, rupturing the alveoli.
> *Excludes 1: trichostrongyliasis (B81.2)*

cc **B78.0 Intestinal strongyloidiasis**

B78.1 Cutaneous strongyloidiasis

cc **B78.7 Disseminated strongyloidiasis**

cc **B78.9 Strongyloidiasis, unspecified**

B79 Trichuriasis — A parasitic disease caused by Trichuris trichiura, and characterized by
cc whipworm infestation of the large intestine and rectum causing chronic diarrhea, mucus stools, and rectal prolapse.
> Includes: Trichocephaliasis
> Whipworm (disease) (infection)

B80 Enterobiasis — A parasitic disease caused by Enterobius vermicularis that is
cc characterized by pinworm infestation of the large intestine causing intense perineal itching in symptomatic patients.
> Includes: Oxyuriasis
> Pinworm infection
> Threadworm infection

B81- Other intestinal helminthiases, not elsewhere classified
> *Excludes 1: angiostrongyliasis due to Parastrongylus cantonensis (B83.2)*

cc **B81.0 Anisakiasis** — A parasitic disease caused by Ascaris lumbricoides and characterized by giant intestinal worms and in severe cases by pneumonitis and intestinal blockage.
> Infection due to Anisakis larva

cc **B81.1 Intestinal capillariasis** — A parasitic disease caused by Capillaria philippinensis, and characterized by adult worms infesting the small intestine causing rampant diarrhea, malabsorption, electrolyte imbalance, and in severe cases lead to death.
> Capillariasis NOS
> Infection due to Capillaria philippinensis
> *Excludes ❷: hepatic capillariasis (B83.8)*

B 6 8 – B 8 1

B81 – B89

cc **B81.2** **Trichostrongyliasis** — A parasitic disease caused by the genus Trichostrongylus, and characterized by worms infesting the intestines causing anemia in some patients, but patients usually are infected with other intestinal parasites making symptom differentiation difficult.

cc **B81.3** **Intestinal angiostrongyliasis**
Angiostrongyliasis due to Parastrongylus costaricensis

cc **B81.4** **Mixed intestinal helminthiases**
Infection due to intestinal helminths classified to more than one of the categories B65.0-B81.3 and B81.8
Mixed helminthiasis NOS

cc **B81.8** **Other specified intestinal helminthiases**
Infection due to Oesophagostomum species [esophagostomiasis]
Infection due to Ternidens diminutus [ternidensiasis]

B82- **Unspecified intestinal parasitism**

cc **B82.0** **Intestinal helminthiasis, unspecified**

B82.9 **Intestinal parasitism, unspecified**

B83- **Other helminthiases**
Excludes 1: *capillariasis NOS (B81.1)*
Excludes ❷: *intestinal capillariasis (B81.1)*

B83.0 **Visceral larva migrans** — A parasitic disease caused by the larva of genus Toxocara, and characterized by migrating larvae causing eosinophilia, visceral involvement, and fever.
Toxocariasis

B83.1 **Gnathostomiasis** — A parasitic disease caused by Gnathostoma spinigerum, and characterized by worm infestation causing subcutaneous abscesses.
Wandering swelling

B83.2 **Angiostrongyliasis due to Parastrongylus cantonensis** — A parasitic disease of larval infestation characterized by larval migration to the central nervous system resulting in eosinophilic meningoencephalitis.
Eosinophilic meningoencephalitis due to Parastrongylus cantonensis
Excludes ❷: *intestinal angiostrongyliasis (B81.3)*

B83.3 **Syngamiasis** — A parasitic disease caused by Syngamus trachea (gapeworm) in humans that is characterized by worm infestation in the trachea, usually found in birds.
Syngamosis

B83.4 **Internal hirudiniasis** — A parasitic infestation of leeches to the mouth, pharynx, or larynx.
Excludes ❷: *external hirudiniasis (B88.3)*

B83.8 **Other specified helminthiases**
Acanthocephaliasis
Gongylonemiasis
Hepatic capillariasis
Metastrongyliasis
Thelaziasis

B83.9 **Helminthiasis, unspecified**
Worms NOS
Excludes 1: *intestinal helminthiasis NOS (B82.0)*

Pediculosis, acariasis and other infestations (B85-B89)

B85- **Pediculosis** and **phthiriasis** — Parasitic diseases caused by lice, and marked by intense itching.

B85.0 **Pediculosis due to Pediculus humanus capitis**
Head-louse infestation

B85.1 **Pediculosis due to Pediculus humanus corporis**
Body-louse infestation

B85.2 **Pediculosis, unspecified**

B85.3 **Phthiriasis**
Infestation by crab-louse
Infestation by Phthirus pubis

B85.4 **Mixed pediculosis and phthiriasis**
Infestation classifiable to more than one of the categories B85.0-B85.3

B86 **Scabies** — A parasitic infestation of the skin by Sarcoptes scabiei, and characterized by nocturnal itching and rash, due to the burrowing under the skin by mites.
Sarcoptic itch

B87- **Myiasis** — A parasitic infestation of the body by fly maggots.
Includes: Infestation by larva of flies

B87.0 **Cutaneous myiasis**
Creeping myiasis

B87.1 **Wound myiasis**
Traumatic myiasis

B87.2 **Ocular myiasis**

B87.3 **Nasopharyngeal myiasis**
Laryngeal myiasis

B87.4 **Aural myiasis**

B87.8- **Myiasis of other sites**

B87.81 **Genitourinary myiasis**

B87.82 **Intestinal myiasis**

B87.89 **Myiasis of other sites**

B87.9 **Myiasis, unspecified**

B88- **Other infestations**

B88.0 **Other acariasis** — Parasitic infestations of mites.
Acarine dermatitis
Dermatitis due to Demodex species
Dermatitis due to Dermanyssus gallinae
Dermatitis due to Liponyssoides sanguineus
Trombiculosis
Excludes ❷: *scabies (B86)*

B88.1 **Tungiasis [sandflea infestation]** — A skin-burrowing flea which causes intense irritation and, in severe cases, ulceration.

B88.2 **Other arthropod infestations**
Scarabiasis

B88.3 **External hirudiniasis** — A parasitic infestation of leeches to the skin.
Leech infestation NOS
Excludes ❷: *internal hirudiniasis (B83.4)*

B88.8 **Other specified infestations**
Ichthyoparasitism due to Vandellia cirrhosa
Linguatulosis
Porocephaliasis

B88.9 **Infestation, unspecified**
Infestation (skin) NOS
Infestation by mites NOS
Skin parasites NOS

B89 **Unspecified parasitic disease**

Sequelae of infectious and parasitic diseases (B90-B94)

Note: Categories B90-B94 are to be used to indicate conditions in categories A00-B89 as the cause of sequelae, which are themselves classified elsewhere. The "sequelae" include conditions specified as such; they also include residuals of diseases classifiable to the above categories if there is evidence that the disease itself is no longer present. Codes from these categories are not to be used for chronic infections. Code chronic current infections to active infectious disease as appropriate.

Code first condition resulting from (sequela) the infectious or parasitic disease

B90- <u>Sequelae</u> of tuberculosis

   B90.0 Sequelae of central nervous system tuberculosis

   B90.1 Sequelae of genitourinary tuberculosis

   B90.2 Sequelae of tuberculosis of bones and joints

   B90.8 Sequelae of tuberculosis of other organs
   Excludes ❷: sequelae of respiratory tuberculosis (B90.9)

   B90.9 Sequelae of respiratory and unspecified tuberculosis
   Sequelae of tuberculosis NOS

B91 <u>Sequelae</u> of poliomyelitis
   Excludes 1: postpolio syndrome (G14)

B92 <u>Sequelae</u> of leprosy

B94- <u>Sequelae</u> of other and unspecified infectious and parasitic diseases

   B94.0 Sequelae of trachoma

   B94.1 Sequelae of viral encephalitis

   B94.2 Sequelae of viral hepatitis

   B94.8 Sequelae of other specified infectious and parasitic diseases

   B94.9 Sequelae of unspecified infectious and parasitic disease

Bacterial and viral infectious agents (B95-B97)

Note: These categories are provided for use as supplementary or additional codes to identify the infectious agent(s) in diseases classified elsewhere.

B95- <u>Streptococcus, Staphylococcus, and Enterococcus</u> as the cause of diseases classified elsewhere

   B95.0 Streptococcus, group A, as the cause of diseases classified elsewhere

   B95.1 Streptococcus, group B, as the cause of diseases classified elsewhere

   B95.2 Enterococcus as the cause of diseases classified elsewhere

   B95.3 Streptococcus pneumoniae as the cause of diseases classified elsewhere

   B95.4 Other streptococcus as the cause of diseases classified elsewhere

   B95.5 Unspecified streptococcus as the cause of diseases classified elsewhere

   B95.6- Staphylococcus aureus as the cause of diseases classified elsewhere

      B95.61 <u>Methicillin susceptible</u> Staphylococcus aureus infection as the cause of diseases classified elsewhere
      Methicillin susceptible Staphylococcus aureus (MSSA) infection as the cause of diseases classified elsewhere
      Staphylococcus aureus infection NOS as the cause of diseases classified elsewhere

      B95.62 <u>Methicillin resistant</u> Staphylococcus aureus infection as the cause of diseases classified elsewhere
      Methicillin resistant Staphylococcus aureus (MRSA) infection as the cause of diseases classified elsewhere

   B95.7 Other staphylococcus as the cause of diseases classified elsewhere

   B95.8 Unspecified staphylococcus as the cause of diseases classified elsewhere

B96- <u>Other bacterial agents</u> as the cause of diseases classified elsewhere

   B96.0 Mycoplasma pneumoniae [M. pneumoniae] as the cause of diseases classified elsewhere
   Pleuro-pneumonia-like-organism [PPLO]

   B96.1 Klebsiella pneumoniae [K. pneumoniae] as the cause of diseases classified elsewhere

   B96.2- Escherichia coli [E. coli] as the cause of diseases classified elsewhere

      B96.20 Unspecified Escherichia coli [E. coli] as the cause of diseases classified elsewhere
      Escherichia coli [E. coli] NOS

      B96.21 Shiga toxin-producing Escherichia coli [E. coli] (STEC) O157 as the cause of diseases classified elsewhere
      E. coli O157:H- (nonmotile) with confirmation of Shiga toxin
      E. coli O157 with confirmation of Shiga toxin when H antigen is unknown, or is not H7
      O157:H7 Escherichia coli [E. coli] with or without confirmation of Shiga toxin-production
      Shiga toxin-producing Escherichia coli [E. coli] O157:H7 with or without confirmation of Shiga toxin-production
      STEC O157:H7 with or without confirmation of Shiga toxin-production

      B96.22 Other specified Shiga toxin-producing Escherichia coli [E. coli] (STEC) as the cause of diseases classified elsewhere
      Non-O157 Shiga toxin-producing Escherichia coli [E. coli]
      Non-O157 Shiga toxin-producing Escherichia coli [E. coli] with known O group

      B96.23 Unspecified Shiga toxin-producing Escherichia coli [E. coli] (STEC) as the cause of diseases classified elsewhere
      Shiga toxin-producing Escherichia coli [E. coli] with specified O group
      STEC NOS

      B96.29 Other Escherichia coli [E. coli] as the cause of diseases classified elsewhere
      Non-Shiga toxin-producing [E. coli]

   B96.3 Hemophilus influenzae [H. influenzae] as the cause of diseases classified elsewhere

   B96.4 Proteus (mirabilis) (morganii) as the cause of diseases classified elsewhere

   B96.5 Pseudomonas (aeruginosa) (mallei) (pseudomallei) as the cause of diseases classified elsewhere
   AHA 15:1Q:p18 – Auricular chondritis due to Pseudomonas aeruginosa

   B96.6 Bacteroides fragilis [B. fragilis] as the cause of diseases classified elsewhere

   B96.7 Clostridium perfringens [C. perfringens] as the cause of diseases classified elsewhere

   B96.8- Other specified bacterial agents as the cause of diseases classified elsewhere

      B96.81 Helicobacter pylori [H. pylori] as the cause of diseases classified elsewhere

      B96.82 Vibrio vulnificus as the cause of diseases classified elsewhere

      B96.89 Other specified bacterial agents as the cause of diseases classified elsewhere

B97- <u>Viral</u> agents as the cause of diseases classified elsewhere

   B97.0 Adenovirus as the cause of diseases classified elsewhere

   B97.1- Enterovirus as the cause of diseases classified elsewhere

      B97.10 Unspecified enterovirus as the cause of diseases classified elsewhere

      B97.11 Coxsackievirus as the cause of diseases classified elsewhere

      B97.12 Echovirus as the cause of diseases classified elsewhere

      B97.19 Other enterovirus as the cause of diseases classified elsewhere

B90 – B97

B97.2-   Coronavirus as the cause of diseases classified elsewhere

cc B97.21   SARS-associated coronavirus as the cause of diseases classified elsewhere
> *Excludes 1:   pneumonia due to SARS-associated coronavirus (J12.81)*

B97.29   Other coronavirus as the cause of diseases classified elsewhere

B97.3-   Retrovirus as the cause of diseases classified elsewhere
> *Excludes 1:   Human immunodeficiency virus [HIV] disease (B20)*

B97.30   Unspecified retrovirus as the cause of diseases classified elsewhere

B97.31   Lentivirus as the cause of diseases classified elsewhere

B97.32   Oncovirus as the cause of diseases classified elsewhere

cc B97.33   Human T-cell lymphotrophic virus, type I [HTLV-I] as the cause of diseases classified elsewhere

cc B97.34   Human T-cell lymphotrophic virus, type II [HTLV-II] as the cause of diseases classified elsewhere

cc B97.35   Human immunodeficiency virus, type 2 [HIV 2] as the cause of diseases classified elsewhere

B97.39   Other retrovirus as the cause of diseases classified elsewhere

B97.4   Respiratory syncytial virus as the cause of diseases classified elsewhere

B97.5   Reovirus as the cause of diseases classified elsewhere

B97.6   Parvovirus as the cause of diseases classified elsewhere

B97.7   Papillomavirus as the cause of diseases classified elsewhere

B97.8-   Other viral agents as the cause of diseases classified elsewhere

B97.81   Human metapneumovirus as the cause of diseases classified elsewhere

B97.89   Other viral agents as the cause of diseases classified elsewhere

Other infectious diseases (B99)

B99-   <u>Other and unspecified infectious diseases</u>

B99.8   Other infectious disease

B99.9   Unspecified infectious disease

Chapter 2 – Neoplasms (C00-D49)

Note: Functional activity
All neoplasms are classified in this chapter, whether they are functionally active or not. An additional code from Chapter 4 may be used, to identify functional activity associated with any neoplasm.
Morphology [Histology]
Chapter 2 classifies neoplasms primarily by site (topography), with broad groupings for behavior, malignant, in situ, benign, etc. The Table of Neoplasms should be used to identify the correct topography code. In a few cases, such as for malignant melanoma and certain neuroendocrine tumors, the morphology (histologic type) is included in the category and codes.
Primary malignant neoplasms overlapping site boundaries
A primary malignant neoplasm that overlaps two or more contiguous (next to each other) sites should be classified to the subcategory/code .8 ("overlapping lesion"), unless the combination is specifically indexed elsewhere. For multiple neoplasms of the same site that are not contiguous, such as tumors in different quadrants of the same breast, codes for each site should be assigned.
Malignant neoplasm of ectopic tissue
Malignant neoplasms of ectopic tissue are to be coded to the site mentioned, e.g., ectopic pancreatic malignant neoplasms are coded to pancreas, unspecified (C25.9).

This chapter contains the following blocks:

C00-C14	**Malignant neoplasm of lip, oral cavity and pharynx**
C15-C26	**Malignant neoplasm of digestive organs**
C30-C39	**Malignant neoplasm of respiratory and intrathoracic organs**
C40-C41	**Malignant neoplasm of bone and articular cartilage**
C43-C44	**Melanoma and other malignant neoplasms of skin**
C45-C49	**Malignant neoplasms of mesothelial and soft tissue**
C50	**Malignant neoplasm of breast**
C51-C58	**Malignant neoplasm of female genital organs**
C60-C63	**Malignant neoplasms of male genital organs**
C64-C68	**Malignant neoplasm of urinary tract**
C69-C72	**Malignant neoplasms of eye, brain and other parts of central nervous system**
C73-C75	**Malignant neoplasm of thyroid and other endocrine glands**
C7A	**Malignant neuroendocrine tumors**
C7B	**Secondary neuroendocrine tumors**
C76-C80	**Malignant neoplasms of ill-defined, other secondary and unspecified sites**
C81-C96	**Malignant neoplasms of lymphoid, hematopoietic and related tissue**
D00-D09	**In situ neoplasms**
D10-D36	**Benign neoplasms, except benign neuroendocrine tumors**
D3A	**Benign neuroendocrine tumors**
D37-D48	**Neoplasms of uncertain behavior, polycythemia vera and myelodysplastic syndromes**
D49	**Neoplasms of unspecified behavior**

Chapter-Specific Coding Guidelines

C. Chapter-Specific Coding Guidelines
In addition to general coding guidelines, there are guidelines for specific diagnoses and/or conditions in the classification. Unless otherwise indicated, these guidelines apply to all health care settings. Please refer to Section II for guidelines on the selection of principal diagnosis.

2. Chapter 2: Neoplasms (C00-D49)

General guidelines

Chapter 2 of the ICD-10-CM contains the codes for most benign and all malignant neoplasms. Certain benign neoplasms, such as prostatic adenomas, may be found in the specific body system chapters. To properly code a neoplasm it is necessary to determine from the record if the neoplasm is benign, in-situ, malignant, or of uncertain histologic behavior. If malignant, any secondary (metastatic) sites should also be determined.

Primary malignant neoplasms overlapping site boundaries

A primary malignant neoplasm that overlaps two or more contiguous (next to each other) sites should be classified to the subcategory/code .8 ('overlapping lesion'), unless the combination is specifically indexed elsewhere. For multiple neoplasms of the same site that are not contiguous such as tumors in different quadrants of the same breast, codes for each site should be assigned.

Malignant neoplasm of ectopic tissue

Malignant neoplasms of ectopic tissue are to be coded to the site of origin mentioned, e.g., ectopic pancreatic malignant neoplasms involving the stomach are coded to pancreas, unspecified (C25.9).

The neoplasm table in the Alphabetic Index should be referenced first. However, if the histological term is documented, that term should be referenced first, rather than going immediately to the Neoplasm Table, in order to determine which column in the Neoplasm Table is appropriate. For example, if the documentation indicates "adenoma," refer to the term in the Alphabetic Index to review the entries under this term and the instructional note to "see also neoplasm, by site, benign." The table provides the proper code based on the type of neoplasm and the site. It is important to select the proper column in the table that corresponds to the type of neoplasm. The Tabular List should then be referenced to verify that the correct code has been selected from the table and that a more specific site code does not exist.

See Section I.C.21. Factors influencing health status and contact with health services, Status, for information regarding Z15.0, codes for genetic susceptibility to cancer.

a. Treatment directed at the malignancy
If the treatment is directed at the malignancy, designate the malignancy as the principal diagnosis.

The only exception to this guideline is if a patient admission/encounter is solely for the administration of chemotherapy, immunotherapy or radiation therapy, assign the appropriate Z51.– code as the first-listed or principal diagnosis, and the diagnosis or problem for which the service is being performed as a secondary diagnosis.

b. Treatment of secondary site
When a patient is admitted because of a primary neoplasm with metastasis and treatment is directed toward the secondary site only, the secondary neoplasm is designated as the principal diagnosis even though the primary malignancy is still present.

c. Coding and sequencing of complications
Coding and sequencing of complications associated with the malignancies or with the therapy thereof are subject to the following guidelines:

1) Anemia associated with malignancy
When admission/encounter is for management of an anemia associated with the malignancy, and the treatment is only for anemia, the appropriate code for the malignancy is sequenced as the principal or first-listed diagnosis followed by the appropriate code for the anemia (such as code D63.0, Anemia in neoplastic disease).

2) Anemia associated with chemotherapy, immunotherapy and radiation therapy
When the admission/encounter is for management of an anemia associated with an adverse effect of the administration of chemotherapy or immunotherapy and the only treatment is for the anemia, the anemia code is sequenced first followed by the appropriate codes for the neoplasm and the adverse effect (T45.1X5, Adverse effect of antineoplastic and immunosuppressive drugs).

When the admission/encounter is for management of an anemia associated with an adverse effect of radiotherapy, the anemia code should be sequenced first, followed by the appropriate neoplasm code and code Y84.2, Radiological procedure and radiotherapy as the cause of abnormal reaction of the patient, or of later complication, without mention of misadventure at the time of the procedure.

3) Management of dehydration due to the malignancy
When the admission/encounter is for management of dehydration due to the malignancy and only the dehydration is being treated (intravenous rehydration), the dehydration is sequenced first, followed by the code(s) for the malignancy.

4) Treatment of a complication resulting from a surgical procedure
When the admission/encounter is for treatment of a complication resulting from a surgical procedure, designate the complication as the principal or first-listed diagnosis if treatment is directed at resolving the complication.

d. Primary malignancy previously excised
When a primary malignancy has been previously excised or eradicated from its site and there is no further treatment directed to that site and there is no evidence of any existing primary malignancy, a code from category Z85, Personal history of malignant neoplasm, should be used to indicate the former site of the malignancy. Any mention of extension, invasion, or metastasis to another site is coded as a secondary malignant neoplasm to that site. The secondary site may be the principal or first-listed with the Z85 code used as a secondary code.

e. Admissions/Encounters involving chemotherapy, immunotherapy and radiation therapy

1) Episode of care involves surgical removal of neoplasm
When an episode of care involves the surgical removal of a neoplasm, primary or secondary site, followed by adjunct chemotherapy or radiation treatment during the same episode of care, the code for the neoplasm should be assigned as principal or first-listed diagnosis.

2) Patient admission/encounter solely for administration of chemotherapy, immunotherapy and radiation therapy

If a patient admission/encounter is solely for the administration of chemotherapy, immunotherapy or radiation therapy assign code Z51.0, Encounter for antineoplastic radiation therapy, or Z51.11, Encounter for antineoplastic chemotherapy, or Z51.12, Encounter for antineoplastic immunotherapy as the first-listed or principal diagnosis. If a patient receives more than one of these therapies during the same admission more than one of these codes may be assigned, in any sequence.

The malignancy for which the therapy is being administered should be assigned as a secondary diagnosis.

3) Patient admitted for radiation therapy, chemotherapy or immunotherapy and develops complications

When a patient is admitted for the purpose of radiotherapy, immunotherapy or chemotherapy and develops complications such as uncontrolled nausea and vomiting or dehydration, the principal or first-listed diagnosis is Z51.0, Encounter for antineoplastic radiation therapy, or Z51.11, Encounter for antineoplastic chemotherapy, or Z51.12, Encounter for antineoplastic immunotherapy followed by any codes for the complications.

f. Admission/encounter to determine extent of malignancy

When the reason for admission/encounter is to determine the extent of the malignancy, or for a procedure such as paracentesis or thoracentesis, the primary malignancy or appropriate metastatic site is designated as the principal or first-listed diagnosis, even though chemotherapy or radiotherapy is administered.

g. Symptoms, signs, and abnormal findings listed in Chapter 18 associated with neoplasms

Symptoms, signs, and ill-defined conditions listed in Chapter 18 characteristic of, or associated with, an existing primary or secondary site malignancy cannot be used to replace the malignancy as principal or first-listed diagnosis, regardless of the number of admissions or encounters for treatment and care of the neoplasm.

See section I.C.21. Factors influencing health status and contact with health services, Encounter for prophylactic organ removal.

h. Admission/encounter for pain control/management

See Section I.C.6. for information on coding admission/encounter for pain control/management.

i. Malignancy in two or more noncontiguous sites

A patient may have more than one malignant tumor in the same organ. These tumors may represent different primaries or metastatic disease, depending on the site. Should the documentation be unclear, the provider should be queried as to the status of each tumor so that the correct codes can be assigned.

j. Disseminated malignant neoplasm, unspecified

Code C80.0, Disseminated malignant neoplasm, unspecified, is for use only in those cases where the patient has advanced metastatic disease and no known primary or secondary sites are specified. It should not be used in place of assigning codes for the primary site and all known secondary sites.

k. Malignant neoplasm without specification of site

Code C80.1, Malignant (primary) neoplasm, unspecified, equates to Cancer, unspecified. This code should only be used when no determination can be made as to the primary site of a malignancy. This code should rarely be used in the inpatient setting.

l. Sequencing of neoplasm codes

1) Encounter for treatment of primary malignancy

If the reason for the encounter is for treatment of a primary malignancy, assign the malignancy as the principal/first-listed diagnosis. The primary site is to be sequenced first, followed by any metastatic sites.

2) Encounter for treatment of secondary malignancy

When an encounter is for a primary malignancy with metastasis and treatment is directed toward the metastatic (secondary) site(s) only, the metastatic site(s) is designated as the principal/first-listed diagnosis. The primary malignancy is coded as an additional code.

3) Malignant neoplasm in a pregnant patient

When a pregnant woman has a malignant neoplasm, a code from subcategory O9A.1-, Malignant neoplasm complicating pregnancy, childbirth, and the puerperium, should be sequenced first, followed by the appropriate code from Chapter 2 to indicate the type of neoplasm.

4) Encounter for complication associated with a neoplasm

When an encounter is for management of a complication associated with a neoplasm, such as dehydration, and the treatment is only for the complication, the complication is coded first, followed by the appropriate code(s) for the neoplasm.

The exception to this guideline is anemia. When the admission/encounter is for management of an anemia associated with the malignancy, and the treatment is only for anemia, the appropriate code for the malignancy is sequenced as the principal or first-listed diagnosis followed by code D63.0, Anemia in neoplastic disease.

5) Complication from surgical procedure for treatment of a neoplasm

When an encounter is for treatment of a complication resulting from a surgical procedure performed for the treatment of the neoplasm, designate the complication as the principal/first-listed diagnosis. See guideline regarding the coding of a current malignancy versus personal history to determine if the code for the neoplasm should also be assigned.

6) Pathologic fracture due to a neoplasm

When an encounter is for a pathological fracture due to a neoplasm, and the focus of treatment is the fracture, a code from subcategory M84.5, Pathological fracture in neoplastic disease, should be sequenced first, followed by the code for the neoplasm.

If the focus of treatment is the neoplasm with an associated pathological fracture, the neoplasm code should be sequenced first, followed by a code from M84.5 for the pathological fracture.

m. Current malignancy versus personal history of malignancy

When a primary malignancy has been excised but further treatment, such as an additional surgery for the malignancy, radiation therapy or chemotherapy is directed to that site, the primary malignancy code should be used until treatment is completed.

When a primary malignancy has been previously excised or eradicated from its site, there is no further treatment (of the malignancy) directed to that site, and there is no evidence of any existing primary malignancy, a code from category Z85, Personal history of malignant neoplasm, should be used to indicate the former site of the malignancy.

See Section I.C.21. Factors influencing health status and contact with health services, History (of).

n. Leukemia, Multiple Myeloma, and Malignant Plasma Cell Neoplasms in remission versus personal history

The categories for leukemia, and category C90, Multiple myeloma and malignant plasma cell neoplasms, have codes indicating whether or not the leukemia has achieved remission. There are also codes Z85.6, Personal history of leukemia, and Z85.79, Personal history of other malignant neoplasms of lymphoid, hematopoietic and related tissues. If the documentation is unclear, as to whether the leukemia has achieved remission, the provider should be queried.

See Section I.C.21. Factors influencing health status and contact with health services, History (of).

o. Aftercare following surgery for neoplasm

See Section I.C.21. Factors influencing health status and contact with health services, Aftercare.

p. Follow-up care for completed treatment of a malignancy

See Section I.C.21. Factors influencing health status and contact with health services, Follow-up.

q. Prophylactic organ removal for prevention of malignancy

See Section I.C.21. Factors influencing health status and contact with health services, Prophylactic organ removal.

r. Malignant neoplasm associated with transplanted organ

A malignant neoplasm of a transplanted organ should be coded as a transplant complication. Assign first the appropriate code from category T86.-, Complications of transplanted organs and tissue, followed by code C80.2, Malignant neoplasm associated with transplanted organ. Use an additional code for the specific malignancy.

Excludes 1: = NOT CODED HERE! (Do not code both)

Excludes ❷: = Not Included Here

Malignant neoplasms (C00-C96)

Malignant neoplasms, stated or presumed to be primary (of specified sites), and certain specified histologies, except neuroendocrine, and of lymphoid, hematopoietic and related tissue (C00-C75)

Malignant neoplasms of lip, oral cavity and pharynx (C00-C14)

C00- **Malignant neoplasm of lip** — Any new and abnormal growth of the lips in which tissue growth is uncontrolled and has the properties of anaplasia, invasion, and metastases.
  Use additional code to identify:
    Alcohol abuse and dependence (F10.-)
    History of tobacco dependence (Z87.891)
    Tobacco dependence (F17.-)
    Tobacco use (Z72.0)
  Excludes 1: *malignant melanoma of lip (C43.0)*
            Merkel cell carcinoma of lip (C4A.0)
            other and unspecified malignant neoplasm of skin of lip (C44.0-)
  ANATOMY OF THE LIPS — The lips are the highly mobile upper and lower skeletal muscle margins of the anterior wall of the oral cavity.
  PHYSIOLOGY OF THE LIPS — The lips have a variety of sensory receptors that are useful in judging the temperature and texture of foods. Their normal reddish color is due to an abundance of blood vessels near their surfaces.

C00.0 **Malignant neoplasm of <u>external</u> <u>upper</u> lip**
    Malignant neoplasm of lipstick area of upper lip
    Malignant neoplasm of upper lip NOS
    Malignant neoplasm of vermilion border of upper lip

C00.1 **Malignant neoplasm of <u>external</u> <u>lower</u> lip**
    Malignant neoplasm of lower lip NOS
    Malignant neoplasm of lipstick area of lower lip
    Malignant neoplasm of vermilion border of lower lip

C00.2 **Malignant neoplasm of external lip, unspecified**
    Malignant neoplasm of vermilion border of lip NOS

C00.3 **Malignant neoplasm of <u>upper</u> lip, <u>inner</u> aspect**
    Malignant neoplasm of buccal aspect of upper lip
    Malignant neoplasm of frenulum of upper lip
    Malignant neoplasm of mucosa of upper lip
    Malignant neoplasm of oral aspect of upper lip

C00.4 **Malignant neoplasm of <u>lower</u> lip, <u>inner</u> aspect**
    Malignant neoplasm of buccal aspect of lower lip
    Malignant neoplasm of frenulum of lower lip
    Malignant neoplasm of mucosa of lower lip
    Malignant neoplasm of oral aspect of lower lip

C00.5 **Malignant neoplasm of lip, unspecified, inner aspect**
    Malignant neoplasm of buccal aspect of lip, unspecified
    Malignant neoplasm of frenulum of lip, unspecified
    Malignant neoplasm of mucosa of lip, unspecified
    Malignant neoplasm of oral aspect of lip, unspecified

C00.6 **Malignant neoplasm of <u>commissure</u> of lip, unspecified**

C00.8 **Malignant neoplasm of <u>overlapping</u> sites of lip**

C00.9 **Malignant neoplasm of lip, unspecified**

C01 **Malignant neoplasm of <u>base of tongue</u>** — Any new and abnormal growth of the base of the tongue (the posterior third of the tongue which is attached to the floor of the mouth) in which tissue growth is uncontrolled and has the properties of anaplasia, invasion, and metastases.
    Malignant neoplasm of dorsal surface of base of tongue
    Malignant neoplasm of fixed part of tongue NOS
    Malignant neoplasm of posterior third of tongue
  Use additional code to identify:
    Alcohol abuse and dependence (F10.-)
    History of tobacco dependence (Z87.891)
    Tobacco dependence (F17.-)
    Tobacco use (Z72.0)

C02- **Malignant neoplasm of other and unspecified parts of tongue** — Any new and abnormal growth of the tongue (other than the base) in which tissue growth is uncontrolled and has the properties of anaplasia, invasion, and metastases.
  Use additional code to identify:
    Alcohol abuse and dependence (F10.-)
    History of tobacco dependence (Z87.891)
    Tobacco dependence (F17.-)
    Tobacco use (Z72.0)
  ANATOMY OF THE TONGUE —The tongue is the movable, muscular organ on the floor of the mouth. The lingual tonsils are a mass of lymphoid tissue at the root, and the frenulum is the mucous membrane fold which attaches the undersurface of the tongue to the floor of the mouth.
  PHYSIOLOGY OF THE TONGUE — The tongue functions primarily as the organ for sense of taste, as well as aiding in the chewing and swallowing of food, and the articulation of sound. The lingual tonsils aid in the elimination of bacteria entering the oral cavity. The frenulum somewhat restricts the movement of the tongue.

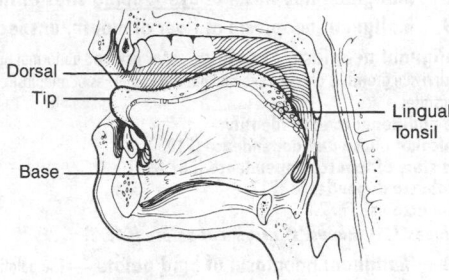

Dorsal
Tip
Lingual Tonsil
Base

TONGUE — SAGITTAL VIEW

C02.0 **Malignant neoplasm of <u>dorsal surface</u> of tongue**
    Malignant neoplasm of anterior two-thirds of tongue, dorsal surface
  Excludes ❷: *malignant neoplasm of dorsal surface of base of tongue (C01)*

C02.1 **Malignant neoplasm of <u>border</u> of tongue**
    Malignant neoplasm of tip of tongue

C02.2 **Malignant neoplasm of <u>ventral</u> surface of tongue**
    Malignant neoplasm of anterior two-thirds of tongue, ventral surface
    Malignant neoplasm of frenulum linguae

C02.3 **Malignant neoplasm of <u>anterior two-thirds</u> of tongue, part unspecified**
    Malignant neoplasm of middle third of tongue NOS
    Malignant neoplasm of mobile part of tongue NOS

C02.4 **Malignant neoplasm of <u>lingual</u> tonsil** — A mass of lymphoid tissue at the root of the tongue.
  Excludes ❷: *malignant neoplasm of tonsil NOS (C09.9)*

C02.8 **Malignant neoplasm of <u>overlapping</u> sites of tongue**
    Malignant neoplasm of two or more contiguous sites of tongue

C02.9 **Malignant neoplasm of tongue, unspecified**

C03- **Malignant neoplasm of <u>gum</u>** — Any new and abnormal growth of the gums in which tissue growth is uncontrolled and has the properties of anaplasia, invasion, and metastases.
  Includes: Malignant neoplasm of alveolar (ridge) mucosa
            Malignant neoplasm of gingiva
  Use additional code to identify:
    Alcohol abuse and dependence (F10.-)
    History of tobacco dependence (Z87.891)
    Tobacco dependence (F17.-)
    Tobacco use (Z72.0)
  Excludes ❷: *malignant odontogenic neoplasms (C41.0-C41.1)*
  ANATOMY OF THE GUMS — The gums (gingiva) are fibrous and mucous membrane tissues which surround the roots of erupted teeth and the crowns of unerupted teeth, and cover the alveolar process of the maxilla and mandible.
  PHYSIOLOGY OF THE GUMS — The gums (gingiva) function to help protect and support the roots of the teeth.

C03.0 **Malignant neoplasm of <u>upper</u> gum**

C03.1 **Malignant neoplasm of <u>lower</u> gum**

C03.9 **Malignant neoplasm of gum, unspecified**

C
0
0
I
C
0
3

Excludes 1: = NOT CODED HERE! (Do not code both)   *Excludes ❷:* = Not Included Here

C04-   **Malignant neoplasm of <u>floor of mouth</u>** — Any new and abnormal growth of the floor of the mouth in which tissue growth is uncontrolled and has the properties of anaplasia, invasion, and metastases.
    Use additional code to identify:
      Alcohol abuse and dependence (F10.-)
      History of tobacco dependence (Z87.891)
      Tobacco dependence (F17.-)
      Tobacco use (Z72.0)
    ANATOMY OF THE FLOOR OF MOUTH — The floor of mouth is the musculomembranous tissue which forms the inferior wall of the oral cavity.
    PHYSIOLOGY OF THE FLOOR OF MOUTH — The floor of mouth functions to enclose the inferior floor of the oral cavity between the mandibular bodies.

    C04.0   **Malignant neoplasm of <u>anterior</u> floor of mouth**
        Malignant neoplasm of anterior to the premolar-canine junction

    C04.1   **Malignant neoplasm of <u>lateral</u> floor of mouth**

    C04.8   **Malignant neoplasm of <u>overlapping</u> sites of floor of mouth**

    C04.9   **Malignant neoplasm of floor of mouth, unspecified**

C05-   **Malignant neoplasm of <u>palate</u>** — Any new and abnormal growth of the palate in which tissue growth is uncontrolled and has the properties of anaplasia, invasion, and metastases.
    Use additional code to identify:
      Alcohol abuse and dependence (F10.-)
      History of tobacco dependence (Z87.891)
      Tobacco dependence (F17.-)
      Tobacco use (Z72.0)
    Excludes 1:   *Kaposi's sarcoma of palate (C46.2)*

    C05.0   **Malignant neoplasm of <u>hard</u> palate** — The palatine process of the maxilla that separates the nasal and oral cavities.

    C05.1   **Malignant neoplasm of <u>soft</u> palate** — The muscular extension of the hard palate in the superior-posterior portion of the oral cavity.
        Excludes ❷: *malignant neoplasm of nasopharyngeal surface of soft palate (C11.3)*

    C05.2   **Malignant neoplasm of <u>uvula</u>** — The cone-shaped projection of the soft palate which hangs over the area of the root of the tongue.

    C05.8   **Malignant neoplasm of <u>overlapping</u> sites of palate**

    C05.9   **Malignant neoplasm of palate, unspecified**
        Malignant neoplasm of roof of mouth

C06-   **Malignant neoplasm of other and unspecified parts of mouth** — Any new and abnormal growth of the other and unspecified parts of the mouth in which tissue growth is uncontrolled, and has the properties of anaplasia, invasion and metastases.
    Use additional code to identify:
      Alcohol abuse and dependence (F10.-)
      History of tobacco dependence (Z87.891)
      Tobacco dependence (F17.-)
      Tobacco use (Z72.0)
    ANATOMY OF OTHER PARTS OF THE MOUTH — The cheeks are the layers of skin, subcutaneous tissue, and certain muscles which form the lateral walls of the oral cavity. The vestibule is the space which lies between the cheeks or lips and the gingiva and teeth. The hard palate is the superior wall of the oral cavity formed by the palatine processes of the maxilla. The soft palate is the muscular extension of the hard palate in the superior-posterior oral cavity. The uvula is the cone-shaped projection of the soft palate. The retromolar area is the nonspecific area of tissue located behind the third molar teeth.
    PHYSIOLOGY OF OTHER PARTS OF THE MOUTH — The cheeks have certain muscles which are associated with chewing and facial expression. The soft palate contracts to allow swallowing, and prevents food from entering the nasal cavity.

    C06.0   **Malignant neoplasm of <u>cheek mucosa</u>** — The mucous membrane of the cheeks.
        Malignant neoplasm of buccal mucosa NOS
        Malignant neoplasm of internal cheek

    C06.1   **Malignant neoplasm of <u>vestibule</u> of mouth** — The lining between the cheeks and lips, and the gingiva and teeth.
        Malignant neoplasm of buccal sulcus (upper) (lower)
        Malignant neoplasm of labial sulcus (upper) (lower)

    C06.2   **Malignant neoplasm of <u>retromolar area</u>** — The nonspecific area of tissue located behind the third molar.

    C06.8-   **Malignant neoplasm of overlapping sites of other and unspecified parts of mouth**

      C06.80   **Malignant neoplasm of overlapping sites of unspecified parts of mouth**

      C06.89   **Malignant neoplasm of overlapping sites of other parts of mouth**
          "Book leaf" neoplasm [ventral surface of tongue and floor of mouth]

    C06.9   **Malignant neoplasm of mouth, unspecified**
        Malignant neoplasm of minor salivary gland, unspecified site
        Malignant neoplasm of oral cavity NOS

C07   **Malignant neoplasm of <u>parotid gland</u>** — Any new and abnormal growth of the parotid gland in which tissue growth is uncontrolled and has the properties of anaplasia, invasion, and metastases.
    Use additional code to identify:
      Alcohol abuse and dependence (F10.-)
      Exposure to environmental tobacco smoke (Z77.22)
      Exposure to tobacco smoke in the perinatal period (P96.81)
      History of tobacco dependence (Z87.891)
      Occupational exposure to environmental tobacco smoke (Z57.31)
      Tobacco dependence (F17.-)
      Tobacco use (Z72.0)

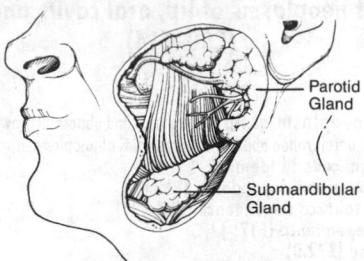

Parotid Gland

Submandibular Gland

PAROTID GLAND

C08-   **Malignant neoplasm of other and unspecified major salivary glands**
    Includes: malignant neoplasm of salivary ducts
    Use additional code to identify:
      Alcohol abuse and dependence (F10.-)
      Exposure to environmental tobacco smoke (Z77.22)
      Exposure to tobacco smoke in the perinatal period (P96.81)
      History of tobacco dependence (Z87.891)
      Occupational exposure to environmental tobacco smoke (Z57.31)
      Tobacco dependence (F17.-)
      Tobacco use (Z72.0)
    Excludes 1:   *malignant neoplasms of specified minor salivary glands which are classified according to their anatomical location*
    Excludes ❷: *malignant neoplasms of minor salivary glands NOS (C06.9)*
                 malignant neoplasm of parotid gland (C07)
    ANATOMY OF THE MAJOR SALIVARY GLANDS — There are three pairs of major salivary glands. The two parotid glands lie above the mouth, and below and in front of the ears with ducts (Stenson's ducts) which run down through the cheeks and empty into the roof of the mouth opposite of the second molar. The two submandibular (submaxillary) glands lie in the floor of the mouth on the inside surface of the mandible, with ducts (Wharton's ducts) opening beneath the tongue, and with other ducts opening near the frenulum of the tongue. The two sublingual glands lie beneath the tongue, with ducts opening near the frenulum of the tongue. Both sympathetic and parasympathetic nerves stimulate the major salivary glands.
    PHYSIOLOGY OF THE MAJOR SALIVARY GLANDS — The major salivary glands function to secrete saliva which moistens food particles, helps to bind them together, and begins digestion of carbohydrates. Saliva also dissolves various food chemicals so they can be tasted. There are two types of secretory cells. Serous cells produce a watery fluid which contains a digestive enzyme, called amylase. Mucous cells produce a thick stringy liquid that binds food together and acts as a lubricant during swallowing. Sympathetic nerves stimulate the glands to secrete a small quantity of saliva to keep the mouth moist. Parasympathetic nerves stimulate the glands reflexly when the person sees, smells, or even thinks about pleasant food.

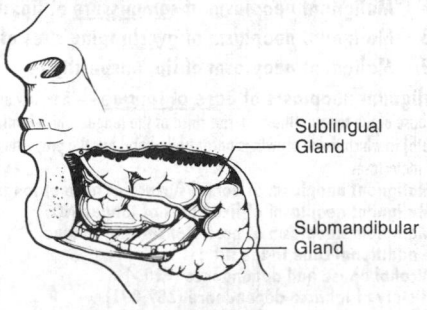

Sublingual Gland

Submandibular Gland

SALIVARY GLANDS

    C08.0   **Malignant neoplasm of <u>submandibular gland</u>** — Any new and abnormal growth of the submandibular (submaxillary) glands in which tissue growth is uncontrolled and has the properties of anaplasia, invasion, and metastases.
        Malignant neoplasm of submaxillary gland

    C08.1   **Malignant neoplasm of <u>sublingual gland</u>** — Any new and abnormal growth of the sublingual glands in which tissue growth is uncontrolled and has the properties of anaplasia, invasion, and metastases.

(Left margin tab) **C04-C08**

(Right margin, vertical) © 2016 Channel Publishing, Ltd

C08.9 **Malignant neoplasm of major salivary gland, unspecified**
Malignant neoplasm of salivary gland (major) NOS

C09- **Malignant neoplasm of <u>tonsil</u>** — Any new and abnormal growth of the tonsils (the small, almond-shaped masses of lymphatic tissue on either side of the tongue in the posterior oral cavity) in which tissue growth is uncontrolled and has the properties of anaplasia, invasion, and metastases.
Use additional code to identify:
Alcohol abuse and dependence (F10.-)
Exposure to environmental tobacco smoke (Z77.22)
Exposure to tobacco smoke in the perinatal period (P96.81)
History of tobacco dependence (Z87.891)
Occupational exposure to environmental tobacco smoke (Z57.31)
Tobacco dependence (F17.-)
Tobacco use (Z72.0)
Excludes ❷: *malignant neoplasm of lingual tonsil (C02.4)*
malignant neoplasm of pharyngeal tonsil (C11.1)

C09.0 **Malignant neoplasm of tonsillar <u>fossa</u>** — The depression in which the tonsils are located.

C09.1 **Malignant neoplasm of tonsillar <u>pillar</u> (anterior) (posterior)** — The mucous membrane folds attached to the soft palate.

C09.8 **Malignant neoplasm of <u>overlapping</u> sites of tonsil**

C09.9 **Malignant neoplasm of tonsil, unspecified**
Malignant neoplasm of tonsil NOS
Malignant neoplasm of faucial tonsils
Malignant neoplasm of palatine tonsils

C10- **Malignant neoplasm of <u>oropharynx</u>** — Any new and abnormal growth of the oropharynx in which tissue growth is uncontrolled and has the properties of anaplasia, invasion, and metastases.
Use additional code to identify:
Alcohol abuse and dependence (F10.-)
Exposure to environmental tobacco smoke (Z77.22)
Exposure to tobacco smoke in the perinatal period (P96.81)
History of tobacco dependence (Z87.891)
Occupational exposure to environmental tobacco smoke (Z57.31)
Tobacco dependence (F17.-)
Tobacco use (Z72.0)
Excludes ❷: *malignant neoplasm of tonsil (C09.-)*
ANATOMY OF THE OROPHARYNX — The tonsils are masses of lymphatic tissue located on either side of the tongue in the posterior oral cavity. The tonsillar fossa is the depression in which the tonsils are located. The tonsillar pillars are the mucous membrane folds attached to the soft palate. The vallecula is the anterior and medial surface of the pharyngoepiglottic fold.
PHYSIOLOGY OF THE OROPHARYNX — The tonsils function to help fight off bacteria by releasing bacteria-consuming phagocytes.

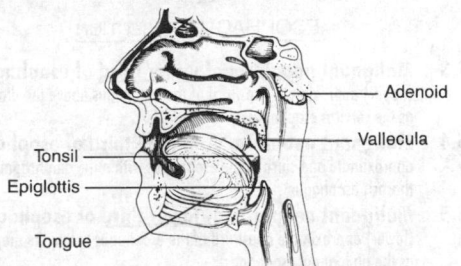

OROPHARYNX

C10.0 **Malignant neoplasm of <u>vallecula</u>** — The depression between the lateral and median glossoepiglottic folds on each side.

C10.1 **Malignant neoplasm of anterior surface of <u>epiglottis</u>** — That portion of the lip-like structure covering the larynx which faces the oral cavity.
Malignant neoplasm of epiglottis, free border [margin]
Malignant neoplasm of glossoepiglottic fold(s)
Excludes ❷: *malignant neoplasm of epiglottis (suprahyoid portion) NOS (C32.1)*

C10.2 **Malignant neoplasm of <u>lateral wall</u> of oropharynx**

C10.3 **Malignant neoplasm of <u>posterior wall</u> of oropharynx**

C10.4 **Malignant neoplasm of <u>branchial cleft</u>** — An area of the lateral part of the neck that is present from the failure of obliteration of the second branchial cleft in embryonic development.
Malignant neoplasm of branchial cyst [site of neoplasm]

C10.8 **Malignant neoplasm of <u>overlapping</u> sites of oropharynx**
Malignant neoplasm of junctional region of oropharynx

C10.9 **Malignant neoplasm of oropharynx, unspecified**

C11- **Malignant neoplasm of <u>nasopharynx</u>** — Any new and abnormal growth of the nasopharynx in which tissue growth is uncontrolled and has the properties of anaplasia, invasion, and metastases.
Use additional code to identify:
Exposure to environmental tobacco smoke (Z77.22)
Exposure to tobacco smoke in the perinatal period (P96.81)
History of tobacco dependence (Z87.891)
Occupational exposure to environmental tobacco smoke (Z57.31)
Tobacco dependence (F17.-)
Tobacco use (Z72.0)
ANATOMY OF THE NASOPHARYNX — The nasopharynx is the upper portion of the pharynx which lies above the soft palate. The adenoids are the masses of lymphatic tissue in the posterior wall of the nasopharynx.
PHYSIOLOGY OF THE NASOPHARYNX — The nasopharynx functions to connect the nasal cavity with the back of the oral cavity to allow nasal breathing and sinus drainage. The adenoids help in the prevention of bacteria entering the body.

C11.0 **Malignant neoplasm of <u>superior wall</u> of nasopharynx**

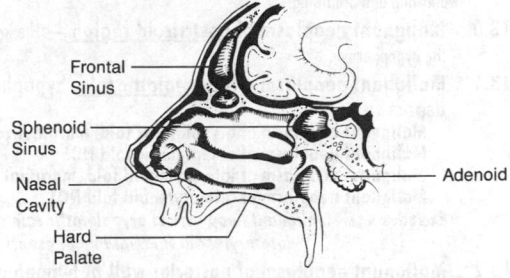

NASOPHARYNX

Malignant neoplasm of roof of nasopharynx — The upper limit of the nasopharynx.

C11.1 **Malignant neoplasm of <u>posterior wall</u> of nasopharynx**
Malignant neoplasm of adenoid — A mass of lymphatic tissue in the posterior wall.
Malignant neoplasm of pharyngeal tonsil — Synonym for Adenoid.

C11.2 **Malignant neoplasm of <u>lateral wall</u> of nasopharynx**
Malignant neoplasm of fossa of Rosenmüller — Synonym for Pharyngeal Recess.
Malignant neoplasm of opening of auditory tube — The area where the auditory (Eustachian) tube enters the nasopharynx from the middle ear.
Malignant neoplasm of pharyngeal recess — Slit-like lateral extension in the nasopharyngeal wall.

C11.3 **Malignant neoplasm of <u>anterior wall</u> of nasopharynx**
Malignant neoplasm of floor of nasopharynx
Malignant neoplasm of nasopharyngeal (anterior) (posterior) surface of soft palate
Malignant neoplasm of posterior margin of nasal choana
Malignant neoplasm of posterior margin of nasal septum

C11.8 **Malignant neoplasm of <u>overlapping</u> sites of nasopharynx**

C11.9 **Malignant neoplasm of nasopharynx, unspecified**
Malignant neoplasm of nasopharyngeal wall NOS

C12 **Malignant neoplasm of <u>pyriform sinus</u>** — Any new and abnormal growth of the pyriform sinus (the elongated depression of the hypopharynx lying between the laryngeal opening and the outer wall of the hypopharynx) in which tissue growth is uncontrolled and has the properties of anaplasia, invasion, and metastases.
Malignant neoplasm of pyriform fossa
Use additional code to identify:
Exposure to environmental tobacco smoke (Z77.22)
Exposure to tobacco smoke in the perinatal period (P96.81)
History of tobacco dependence (Z87.891)
Occupational exposure to environmental tobacco smoke (Z57.31)
Tobacco dependence (F17.-)
Tobacco use (Z72.0)

C08 - C12

C13-   **Malignant neoplasm of <u>hypopharynx</u>** — Any new and abnormal growth of the hypopharynx in which tissue growth is uncontrolled and has the properties of anaplasia, invasion, and metastases.

Use additional code to identify:
Exposure to environmental tobacco smoke (Z77.22)
Exposure to tobacco smoke in the perinatal period (P96.81)
History of tobacco dependence (Z87.891)
Occupational exposure to environmental tobacco smoke (Z57.31)
Tobacco dependence (F17.-)
Tobacco use (Z72.0)

Excludes ❷: *malignant neoplasm of pyriform sinus (C12)*

ANATOMY OF THE HYPOPHARYNX — The hypopharynx is the cavity which lies from the upper border of the epiglottis to the opening of the larynx and esophagus. The pyriform sinus is the elongated depression of the hypopharynx lying between the laryngeal opening and the outer wall of the hypopharynx. The aryepiglottic fold is the mucous membrane fold on each side of the epiglottis.

PHYSIOLOGY OF THE HYPOPHARYNX — The hypopharynx functions to help in swallowing and breathing.

C13.0   **Malignant neoplasm of <u>postcricoid region</u>** — The lower portion of the hypopharnyx.

C13.1   **Malignant neoplasm of <u>aryepiglottic fold</u>, hypopharyngeal aspect**
Malignant neoplasm of aryepiglottic fold, marginal zone
Malignant neoplasm of aryepiglottic fold NOS
Malignant neoplasm of interarytenoid fold, marginal zone
Malignant neoplasm of interarytenoid fold NOS
Excludes ❷: *malignant neoplasm of aryepiglottic fold or interarytenoid fold, laryngeal aspect (C32.1)*

C13.2   **Malignant neoplasm of <u>posterior wall</u> of hypopharynx**

C13.8   **Malignant neoplasm of <u>overlapping</u> sites of hypopharynx**

C13.9   **Malignant neoplasm of hypopharynx, unspecified**
Malignant neoplasm of hypopharyngeal wall NOS

C14-   **Malignant neoplasm of other and ill-defined sites in the lip, oral cavity and pharynx**

Use additional code to identify:
Alcohol abuse and dependence (F10.-)
Exposure to environmental tobacco smoke (Z77.22)
Exposure to tobacco smoke in the perinatal period (P96.81)
History of tobacco dependence (Z87.891)
Occupational exposure to environmental tobacco smoke (Z57.31)
Tobacco dependence (F17.-)
Tobacco use (Z72.0)

Excludes 1:   *malignant neoplasm of oral cavity NOS (C06.9)*

C14.0   **Malignant neoplasm of pharynx, unspecified**

C14.2   **Malignant neoplasm of Waldeyer's ring** — Any new and abnormal growth of Waldeyer's ring (the ring of lymphoid tissue located in the nasopharynx and oropharynx) in which tissue growth is uncontrolled and has the properties of anaplasia, invasion, and metastases.

C14.8   **Malignant neoplasm of overlapping sites of lip, oral cavity and pharynx**
Primary malignant neoplasm of two or more contiguous sites of lip, oral cavity and pharynx
Excludes 1:   *"book leaf" neoplasm [ventral surface of tongue and floor of mouth] (C06.89)*

Malignant neoplasms of digestive organs (C15-C26)

Excludes 1:   **Kaposi's sarcoma of gastrointestinal sites (C46.4)**
Excludes ❷: **gastrointestinal stromal tumors (C49.A-)**

C15-   **Malignant neoplasm of <u>esophagus</u>** — Any new and abnormal growth of the esophagus in which tissue growth is uncontrolled and has the properties of anaplasia, invasion, and metastases.

Use additional code to identify:
Alcohol abuse and dependence (F10.-)

ANATOMY OF THE ESOPHAGUS — The esophagus, located between the pharynx and stomach, is a collapsible musculomembranous alimentary tract tube about 10 inches (25 cm) long. The esophagus is lined with mucous glands.

PHYSIOLOGY OF THE ESOPHAGUS — The esophagus is the passageway for food from the mouth to the stomach. The mucous glands moisten and lubricate the inner lining to facilitate the passage of food. Situated just above the stomach opening lies the contracted circular muscles which prevent regurgitation.

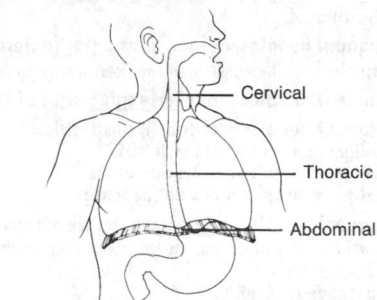

ESOPHAGUS — ANTERIOR VIEW

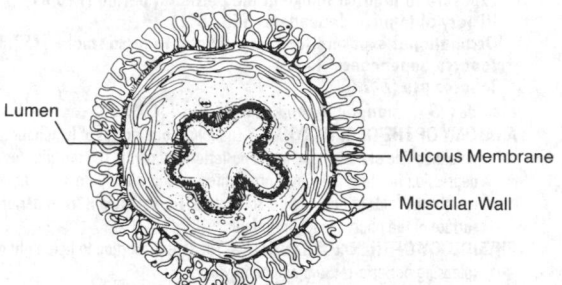

ESOPHAGUS — SECTION

cc **C15.3**   **Malignant neoplasm of <u>upper third</u> of esophagus** — The proximal (upper) approximate one-third of the esophagus above the diaphragm (also known as the cervical esophagus).

cc **C15.4**   **Malignant neoplasm of <u>middle third</u> of esophagus** — The middle approximate one-third of the esophagus within the diaphragm (also known as the thoracic esophagus).

cc **C15.5**   **Malignant neoplasm of <u>lower third</u> of esophagus** — The distal (lower) approximate one-third of the esophagus below the diaphragm (also known as the abdominal esophagus).
Excludes 1:   *malignant neoplasm of cardio-esophageal junction (C16.0)*

cc **C15.8**   **Malignant neoplasm of <u>overlapping</u> sites of esophagus**

cc **C15.9**   **Malignant neoplasm of esophagus, unspecified**

C16-   Malignant neoplasm of <u>stomach</u> — Any new and abnormal growth of the stomach in which tissue growth is uncontrolled and has the properties of anaplasia, invasion, and metastases.
   Use additional code to identify:
      Alcohol abuse and dependence (F10.-)
   Excludes ❷: malignant carcinoid tumor of the stomach (C7A.092)
   ANATOMY OF THE STOMACH — The stomach, located in the upper abdomen, is a pouch-like organ of the alimentary tract connecting with the esophagus in the proximal (upper) portion and the duodenum in the distal (lower) portion and is about 10 to 12 inches (25 to 30 cm) long. The cardia lies at the opening of the esophagus at the fundus of the stomach. The fundus is the upper ballooned area of the stomach. The body is the main part of the stomach and is located between the fundus and the pyloric antrum and the duodenum. When empty, the mucous membrane on the interior surface forms longitudinal folds, called rugae. There are three mucosal glands which secrete digestive juices and mucus. These are the gastric glands, which are located throughout the body of the stomach; the cardiac glands, which are found near the esophageal opening; and the pyloric glands, which are located in the pyloric (distal) region. There are three layers of smooth muscle, and a serosal covering of visceral peritoneum. The vagus nerve stimulates the gastric glands. The stomach has a rich arterial blood supply through the celiac artery. The venous blood is drained into the hepatic portal system.
   PHYSIOLOGY OF THE STOMACH — The stomach functions to receive food from the esophagus, mixes it with the gastric juice, initiates the digestion of proteins with pepsin, carries on a limited amount of absorption, and moves food into the small intestine by peristaltic muscle action. The gastric glands produce mucous, digestive enzymes (pepsin), hydrochloric acid, and an intrinsic factor, forming the gastric juice. The mucous is thought to help prevent the pepsin and hydrochloric acid from digesting the stomach surface. The stomach may absorb small quantities of water, glucose, certain salts, and alcohol. The parasympathetic vagus nerve stimulates the gastric glands to secrete large amounts of gastric juice which, in turn, releases gastrin, a hormone that causes the gastric glands to increase their secretory activity.

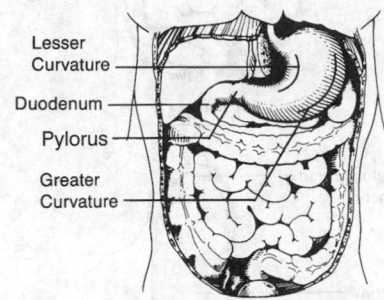

STOMACH

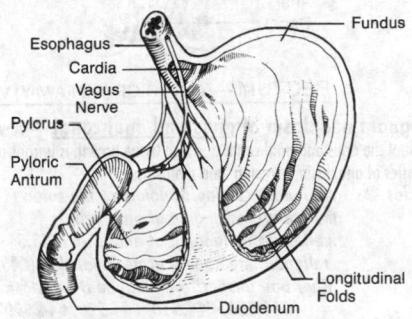

STOMACH — ANTERIOR (CUT-AWAY) VIEW

cc **C16.0   Malignant neoplasm of <u>cardia</u>** — The opening and junction of the stomach from the esophagus.
      Malignant neoplasm of cardiac orifice
      Malignant neoplasm of cardio-esophageal junction
      Malignant neoplasm of esophagus and stomach
      Malignant neoplasm of gastro-esophageal junction

cc **C16.1   Malignant neoplasm of <u>fundus</u> of stomach** — The ballooned upper end of the stomach lying above a transverse line drawn from the cardia.

cc **C16.2   Malignant neoplasm of <u>body</u> of stomach** — The main pouch-like portion.

cc **C16.3   Malignant neoplasm of <u>pyloric antrum</u>** — That portion between the body and the pylorus.
      Malignant neoplasm of gastric antrum

cc **C16.4   Malignant neoplasm of <u>pylorus</u>** — The opening between the pyloric antrum and the duodenum.
      Malignant neoplasm of prepylorus
      Malignant neoplasm of pyloric canal

cc **C16.5   Malignant neoplasm of lesser curvature of stomach, unspecified** — The smaller, innermost curved vertical portion from the esophagus to the duodenum.
      Malignant neoplasm of lesser curvature of stomach, not classifiable to C16.1-C16.4

cc **C16.6   Malignant neoplasm of greater curvature of stomach, unspecified** — The larger, outermost curved vertical portion from the esophagus to the duodenum.
      Malignant neoplasm of greater curvature of stomach, not classifiable to C16.0-C16.4

cc **C16.8   Malignant neoplasm of <u>overlapping</u> sites of stomach**

cc **C16.9   Malignant neoplasm of stomach, unspecified**
      Gastric cancer NOS

C17-   Malignant neoplasm of <u>small intestine</u> — Any new and abnormal growth of the small intestine, including duodenum, in which tissue growth is uncontrolled and has the properties of anaplasia, invasion, and metastases.
   Excludes 1:   malignant carcinoid tumors of the small intestine (C7A.01)
   ANATOMY OF THE SMALL INTESTINE — The small intestine is the tubular organ of the alimentary tract between the stomach and large intestine and is about 16 to 20 feet (5 to 6 m) long, and has 3 parts: Duodenum, jejunum, and ileum. The duodenum is the first portion about 10 inches (25 cm) long connected at its proximal end to the stomach. The jejunum is the middle, approximately two-fifths, portion. The ileum is the distal portion which connects with the large intestine. Both the jejunum and ileum are suspended from the posterior abdominal wall by the mesentery.
   PHYSIOLOGY OF THE SMALL INTESTINE — The small intestine functions to absorb water and the nutrients produced through digestion. The food is passed through the small intestine by the contraction of its circular smooth muscle layer, called peristalsis. The duodenum releases several enzymes and mixes the pancreatic and bile juices with food from the stomach. The jejunum and ileum continue mixing and absorbing until the remaining substances pass into the large intestine.

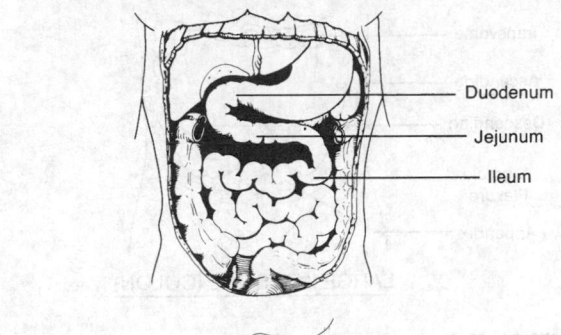

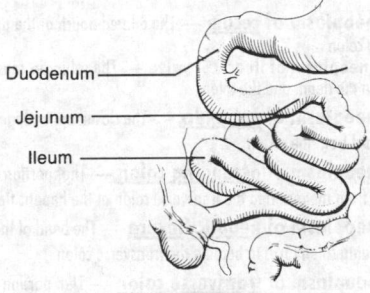

SMALL INTESTINE

cc **C17.0   Malignant neoplasm of <u>duodenum</u>** — The most proximal portion connected with the stomach.

cc **C17.1   Malignant neoplasm of <u>jejunum</u>** — The middle portion which is larger in diameter than the ileum.

cc **C17.2   Malignant neoplasm of <u>ileum</u>** — The distal portion connecting with the cecum.
   Excludes 1:   malignant neoplasm of ileocecal valve (C18.0)

cc **C17.3   <u>Meckel's</u> diverticulum, malignant** — A sacculation or appendage of the ileum, specified as malignant.
   Excludes 1:   Meckel's diverticulum, congenital (Q43.0)

cc **C17.8   Malignant neoplasm of <u>overlapping</u> sites of small intestine**

cc **C17.9   Malignant neoplasm of small intestine, unspecified**

C 1 6 - C 1 7

Excludes 1: = NOT CODED HERE! (Do not code both)   **557**   *Excludes ❷: = Not Included Here*

C18- **Malignant neoplasm of <u>colon</u>** — Any new and abnormal growth of the large intestine in which tissue growth is uncontrolled and has the properties of anaplasia, invasion, and metastases.

  Excludes 1:   *malignant carcinoid tumors of the colon (C7A.02-)*

  ANATOMY OF THE COLON — The colon (large intestine) is the tubular organ of the alimentary tract between the small intestine and the rectum, and is about 5 feet (1.5 m) long. The colon has four main segments: Ascending, transverse, descending, and sigmoid. The ascending colon arises from the cecum, the pouch-like structure, and continues upwards where it turns (hepatic flexure) and connects to the transverse colon. The transverse colon extends horizontally and turns (splenic flexure) downward connecting to the descending colon. The descending colon extends downward to the rectum, and is called the sigmoid (flexure) colon where it makes an S-shaped curve over the pelvic brim. The appendix projects downward from the cecum.

  PHYSIOLOGY OF THE COLON — The colon (large intestine) functions in a minor capacity to absorb water and electrolytes, and to move by peristalsis, nonabsorbed substances to the rectum for defecation. Many bacteria normally inhabit the colon and serve to further break down substances for colonic absorption.

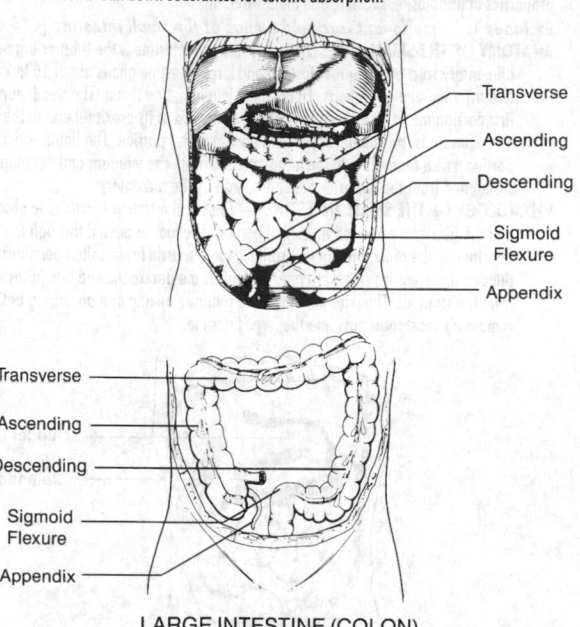

LARGE INTESTINE (COLON)

cc C18.0 **Malignant neoplasm of <u>cecum</u>** — The dilated pouch at the proximal end of the ascending colon.

  Malignant neoplasm of ileocecal valve — The sphincter muscle valve between the ileum and the colon.

cc C18.1 **Malignant neoplasm of <u>appendix</u>** — The closed appendage which projects downward from the cecum.

cc C18.2 **Malignant neoplasm of <u>ascending colon</u>** — That portion which extends upward from the cecum to the transverse colon at the hepatic flexure.

cc C18.3 **Malignant neoplasm of <u>hepatic flexure</u>** — The bend of the colon where the ascending colon turns to become the transverse colon.

cc C18.4 **Malignant neoplasm of <u>transverse colon</u>** — That portion which lies horizontally between ascending colon at the hepatic flexure and the descending colon at the splenic flexure.

cc C18.5 **Malignant neoplasm of <u>splenic flexure</u>** — The bend of the colon where the transverse colon turns downward to become the descending colon.

cc C18.6 **Malignant neoplasm of <u>descending colon</u>** — That portion which extends downward from the transeverse colon at the splenic flexure to the sigmoid colon.

cc C18.7 **Malignant neoplasm of <u>sigmoid colon</u>** — That portion of the colon from the descending colon to the rectum, which forms an S-shaped curve over the pelvic brim.

  Malignant neoplasm of sigmoid (flexure)

  Excludes 1:   *malignant neoplasm of rectosigmoid junction (C19)*

cc C18.8 **Malignant neoplasm of <u>overlapping</u> sites of colon**

cc C18.9 **Malignant neoplasm of colon, unspecified**

  Malignant neoplasm of large intestine NOS

C19 **Malignant neoplasm of <u>rectosigmoid junction</u>** — Any new and abnormal
cc growth of the rectosigmoid junction in which tissue growth is uncontrolled and has the properties of anaplasia, invasion, and metastases.

  Malignant neoplasm of colon with rectum

  Malignant neoplasm of rectosigmoid (colon)

  Excludes 1:   *malignant carcinoid tumors of the colon (C7A.02-)*

C20 **Malignant neoplasm of <u>rectum</u>** — Any new and abnormal growth of the rectum
cc in which tissue growth is uncontrolled and has the properties of anaplasia, invasion, and metastases.

  Malignant neoplasm of rectal ampulla — The dilated portion just proximal to the anus.

  Excludes 1:   *malignant carcinoid tumor of the rectum (C7A.026)*

  ANATOMY OF THE RECTUM AND ANUS — The rectum is the musculomembranous portion of the alimentary tract between the colon and anus, approximately 5 inches (13 cm) long. The anus is the internal canal from the rectum which ends the alimentary tract at the anal opening. The rectosigmoid junction is that portion of the alimentary tract between the distal end of the sigmoid colon and the proximal end of the rectum.

  PHYSIOLOGY OF THE RECTUM AND ANUS — The rectum and anus function to eliminate feces from the alimentary tract. A reflex signal is sent when the rectum fills and urgency to defecate is perceived. The external voluntary muscle is voluntarily relaxed to defecate.

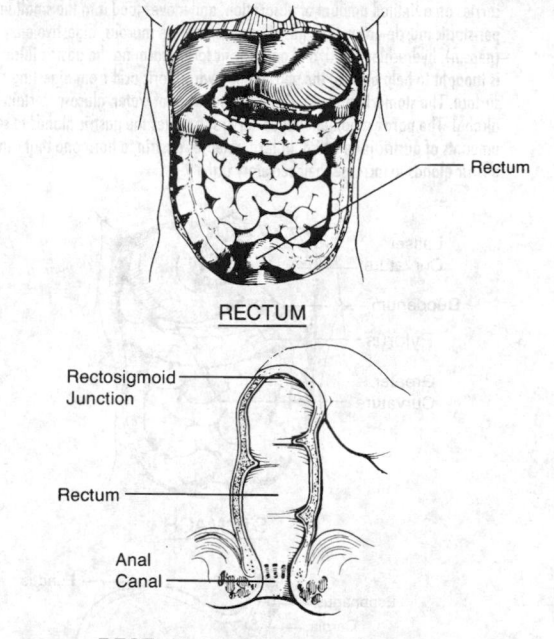

RECTUM

RECTUM — ANTERIOR (CUT-AWAY) VIEW

C21- **Malignant neoplasm of <u>anus and anal canal</u>** — Any new and abnormal growth of the anus and anal canal in which tissue growth is uncontrolled and has the properties of anaplasia, invasion, and metastases.

  Excludes ❷: *malignant carcinoid tumors of the colon (C7A.02-)*
        malignant melanoma of anal margin (C43.51)
        malignant melanoma of anal skin (C43.51)
        malignant melanoma of perianal skin (C43.51)
        other and unspecified malignant neoplasm of anal margin (C44.500, C44.510, C44.520, C44.590)
        other and unspecified malignant neoplasm of anal skin (C44.500, C44.510, C44.520, C44.590)
        other and unspecified malignant neoplasm of perianal skin (C44.500, C44.510, C44.520, C44.590)

cc C21.0 **Malignant neoplasm of anus, unspecified**

cc C21.1 **Malignant neoplasm of <u>anal canal</u>** — That portion of the alimentary tract between the sigmoid colon and the external opening of the anus.

  Malignant neoplasm of anal sphincter

cc C21.2 **Malignant neoplasm of <u>cloacogenic zone</u>** — The anorectal region originating from a persistant remnant of the cloacal membrane of the embryo.

cc C21.8 **Malignant neoplasm of <u>overlapping</u> sites of rectum, anus and anal canal**

  Malignant neoplasm of anorectal junction

  Malignant neoplasm of anorectum

  Primary malignant neoplasm of two or more contiguous sites of rectum, anus and anal canal

---

Excludes 1: = NOT CODED HERE! (Do not code both)

Excludes ❷: = Not Included Here

C22- Malignant neoplasm of <u>liver</u> and intrahepatic bile ducts — Any new and abnormal growth of the liver and intrahepatic ducts in which the tissue growth is uncontrolled, and has the properties of anaplasia, invasion and metastases.

Use additional code to identify:
   Alcohol abuse and dependence (F10.-)
   Hepatitis B (B16.-, B18.0-B18.1)
   Hepatitis C (B17.1-, B18.2)
   Excludes 1:   *malignant neoplasm of biliary tract NOS (C24.9)*
                    secondary malignant neoplasm of liver and intrahepatic bile duct (C78.7)

ANATOMY OF THE LIVER — The liver is the largest organ in the body, weighing about 3 pounds (1 kg) in the adult. Located in the upper right quadrant of the abdominal cavity, its superior surface lies under the dome of the diaphragm. There are 4 lobes of the liver. The common bile duct is formed by the joining of the hepatic duct, which carries bile from the liver, and the cystic duct, which carries bile from the gallbladder. The common duct then carries the bile into the duodenum through an opening on the duodenal papilla. The hepatic artery furnishes arterial blood for the nourishment of the liver cells. The portal vein carries blood containing products of digestion from the intestinal tract into the liver. Internally, the liver lobules are the functional units of liver substance. Bile is secreted by the liver cells into tiny canals, or canaliculi, and then is emptied into a bile duct.

PHYSIOLOGY OF THE LIVER — One of the regulatory functions of the liver is that of controlling the blood sugar level. The liver is able to both absorb excess sugar and dispense it into the blood. The liver also stores and secretes other essential nutrients. It chemically processes these materials and detoxifies many substances that could be harmful if allowed to accumulate in the body. Its bile salts are necessary for the absorption of vitamin K from the gastrointestinal tract, which in turn, is needed for the production of prothrombin. Another important liver function is that of producing bile. A brownish-yellow fluid, it is secreted continuously by the liver in amounts averaging about 20 fluid ounces (600 ml). per day. Bile contains the bile salts which are very important in the digestion of fat.

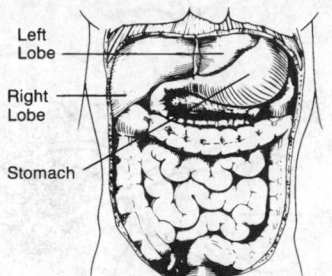

LIVER — ANTERIOR VIEW

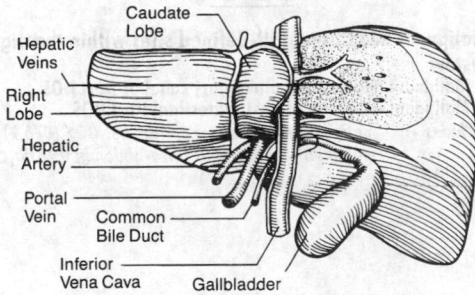

LIVER — POSTERIOR VIEW

cc **C22.0**   <u>Liver cell</u> carcinoma — A form originating in the liver cells.
         Hepatocellular carcinoma
         Hepatoma

cc **C22.1**   <u>Intrahepatic bile duct</u> carcinoma — The small channels between the hepatic lobules, which drain into the bile ductules.
         Cholangiocarcinoma
         Excludes 1:   *malignant neoplasm of hepatic duct (C24.0)*

cc **C22.2**   <u>Hepatoblastoma</u> — A malignant intrahepatic tumor occurring in infants and young children and consisting chiefly of embryonic hepatic tissue.

cc **C22.3**   <u>Angiosarcoma</u> of liver
         Kupffer cell sarcoma

cc **C22.4**   **Other sarcomas of liver**

cc **C22.7**   **Other specified carcinomas of liver**

cc **C22.8**   **Malignant neoplasm of liver, primary, unspecified as to type**

cc **C22.9**   **Malignant neoplasm of liver, not specified as primary or secondary**

C23 Malignant neoplasm of <u>gallbladder</u> — Any new and abnormal
cc   growth of the gallbladder in which tissue growth is uncontrolled and has the properties of anaplasia, invasion, and metastases.

ANATOMY OF THE GALLBLADDER — The gallbladder is the musculomembranous, pear-shaped bile reservoir located on the undersurface of the liver. The cystic duct is the tubular drain of the gallbladder which merges with the hepatic duct to form the common bile duct. The common bile duct merges with the pancreatic duct in the dilatated area known as the ampulla of Vater. The sphincter of Oddi is the muscle which encircles the bile duct where it enters the duodenum.

PHYSIOLOGY OF THE GALLBLADDER — The gallbladder functions to store and concentrate the bile and release the bile on demand to the small intestine for the digestion of fats. The cystic duct, hepatic duct, and common bile duct convey the bile into the duodenum. The sphincter of Oddi contracts to prevent reflux of intestinal contents back into the bile ducts.

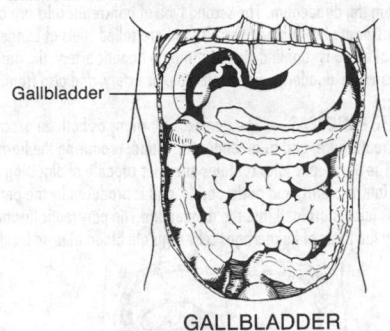

GALLBLADDER

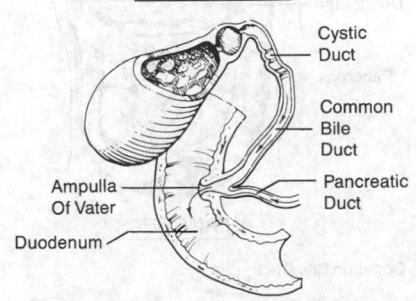

GALLBLADDER — ANTERIOR (CUT-AWAY) VIEW

C24- Malignant neoplasm of other and unspecified parts of biliary tract
      Excludes 1:   *malignant neoplasm of intrahepatic bile duct (C22.1)*

cc **C24.0**   **Malignant neoplasm of <u>extrahepatic bile duct</u>** — Any new and abnormal growth in an extrahepatic bile duct (bile ducts which are not within the liver capsule) in which tissue growth is uncontrolled and has the properties of anaplasia, invasion, and metastases.
         Malignant neoplasm of biliary duct or passage NOS
         Malignant neoplasm of common bile duct
         Malignant neoplasm of cystic duct
         Malignant neoplasm of hepatic duct

cc **C24.1**   **Malignant neoplasm of <u>ampulla of Vater</u>** — Any new and abnormal growth of the ampulla of Vater (the dilatation formed by the merger of the pancreatic and common bile ducts just proximal to opening into the duodenum) in which tissue growth is uncontrolled and has the properties of anaplasia, invasion, and metastases.

cc **C24.8**   **Malignant neoplasm of <u>overlapping</u> sites of biliary tract**
         Malignant neoplasm involving both intrahepatic and extrahepatic bile ducts
         Primary malignant neoplasm of two or more contiguous sites of biliary tract

cc **C24.9**   **Malignant neoplasm of biliary tract, unspecified**

C 2 2 - C 2 4

C25- **Malignant neoplasm of** <u>pancreas</u> — Any new and abnormal growth of the pancreas and pancreatic ducts in which the tissue growth is uncontrolled and has the properties of anaplasia, invasion, and metastases.

Code also exocrine pancreatic insufficiency (K86.81)
Use additional code to identify:
   Alcohol abuse and dependence (F10.-)

ANATOMY OF THE PANCREAS — The pancreas is a slender organ about 6 to 9 inches (15 to 23 cm) long lying horizontally and located in the abdomen behind and under the stomach. The pancreas is divided into 3 areas. The head, lying in the curve formed by the duodenum; the body, the main portion, lying between the head and tail; and the tail, the most lateral portion blunting up against the spleen. The cells that produce pancreatic juice are called pancreatic acinar cells, and they make up the bulk of the pancreas. These cells are clustered around tiny tubes which drain into the pancreatic duct (duct of Wirsung). This duct connects with the duodenum at the same place where the bile ducts join the duodenum. The second type of pancreatic cells are arranged in groups closely associated with blood vessels, and are called islets of Langerhans. The pancreas arterial blood is supplied via the common hepatic artery, the gastroduodenal artery, the pancreatico-duodenal arches, the splenic artery, and also from the superior mesenteric artery.

PHYSIOLOGY OF THE PANCREAS — The pancreas functions as both an exocrine gland, producing pancreatic juice, and as an endocrine gland, producing the hormones insulin and glucagon. The pancreatic juice contains enzymes capable of digesting carbohydrates, fats, proteins, and nucleic acids, and is produced by the pancreatic acinar cells. This juice is drained into the duodenum. The pancreatic hormones which are produced by the islets of Langerhans cells regulate blood glucose level.

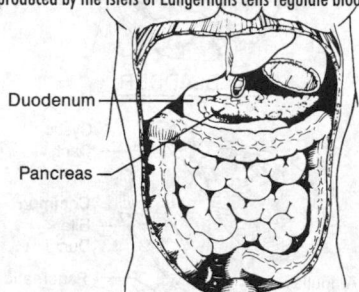

Duodenum
Pancreas

PANCREAS

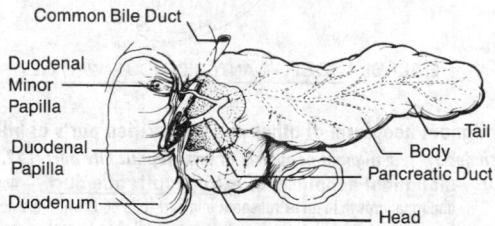

Common Bile Duct
Duodenal Minor Papilla
Duodenal Papilla
Duodenum
Tail
Body
Pancreatic Duct
Head

PANCREAS — ANTERIOR VIEW

CC **C25.0** **Malignant neoplasm of** <u>head</u> **of pancreas** — The medial portion lying in the duodenal curve.

CC **C25.1** **Malignant neoplasm of** <u>body</u> **of pancreas** — The main portion lying horizontally between the head and tail.

CC **C25.2** **Malignant neoplasm of** <u>tail</u> **of pancreas** — The most lateral portion blunting up against the spleen.

CC **C25.3** **Malignant neoplasm of** <u>pancreatic duct</u> — The duct that runs the length of the pancreas emptying the pancreatic juice into the duodenum.

CC **C25.4** **Malignant neoplasm of** <u>endocrine</u> **pancreas** — The cells within the pancreas that produce hormones.
   Malignant neoplasm of islets of Langerhans
   Use additional code to identify any functional activity

CC **C25.7** **Malignant neoplasm of other parts of pancreas**
   Malignant neoplasm of neck of pancreas

CC **C25.8** **Malignant neoplasm of** <u>overlapping</u> **sites of pancreas**

CC **C25.9** **Malignant neoplasm of pancreas, unspecified**

C26- **Malignant neoplasm of other and ill-defined digestive organs**
   Excludes 1: *malignant neoplasm of peritoneum and retroperitoneum (C48.-)*

C26.0 **Malignant neoplasm of intestinal tract, part unspecified**
   Malignant neoplasm of intestine NOS

C26.1 **Malignant neoplasm of** <u>spleen</u> — Any new and abnormal growth of the spleen in which the tissue growth is uncontrolled and has the properties of anaplasia, invasion, and metastases.
   Excludes 1: *Hodgkin lymphoma (C81.-)*
          non-Hodgkin lymphoma (C82-C85)

ANATOMY OF THE SPLEEN —The spleen is a gland-like organ, located in the upper abdomen behind the stomach and at the tail of the pancreas, and is about 5 inches (13 cm) in length. The spleen contains both white pulp and red pulp.

PHYSIOLOGY OF THE SPLEEN — The spleen functions as both a large lymph node (white pulp) that filters the blood and produces lymphocytes and monocytes, and as a red blood cell reservoir (red pulp) and disintegrator of worn-out red blood cells. It also plays a role in producing antibodies. Although important, the spleen is not essential to life.

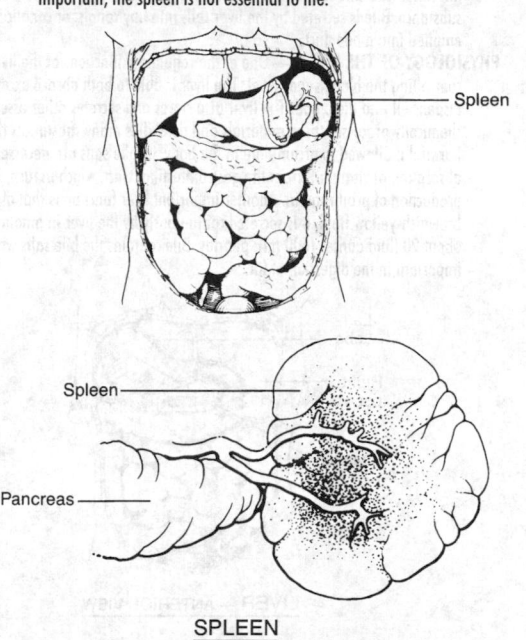

Spleen
Spleen
Pancreas

SPLEEN

C26.9 **Malignant neoplasm of ill-defined sites within the digestive system**
   Malignant neoplasm of alimentary canal or tract NOS
   Malignant neoplasm of gastrointestinal tract NOS
   Excludes 1: *malignant neoplasm of abdominal NOS (C76.2)*
          malignant neoplasm of intra-abdominal NOS (C76.2)

Excludes 1: = NOT CODED HERE! (Do not code both)   **560**   *Excludes ❷:* = Not Included Here

Malignant neoplasms of respiratory and intrathoracic organs (C30-C39)

    Includes: Malignant neoplasm of middle ear
    Excludes 1:   mesothelioma (C45.-)

C30- **Malignant neoplasm of nasal cavity and middle ear**

    C30.0 **Malignant neoplasm of <u>nasal cavity</u>** — Any new and abnormal growth of the nasal cavity in which the tissue growth is uncontrolled and has the properties of anaplasia, invasion, and metastases.

        Malignant neoplasm of cartilage of nose
        Malignant neoplasm of nasal concha
        Malignant neoplasm of internal nose
        Malignant neoplasm of septum of nose
        Malignant neoplasm of vestibule of nose

      Excludes 1:   *malignant melanoma of skin of nose (C43.31)*
                 malignant neoplasm of nasal bone (C41.0)
                 malignant neoplasm of nose NOS (C76.0)
                 malignant neoplasm of olfactory bulb (C72.2-)
                 malignant neoplasm of posterior margin of nasal septum and choana (C11.3)
                 malignant neoplasm of turbinates (C41.0)
                 other and unspecified malignant neoplasm of skin of nose (C44.301, C44.311, C44.321, C44.391)

      ANATOMY OF THE NASAL CAVITIES — The nasal cavity is located between the external nose and the nasopharynx with the nasal bones, and parts of the ethmoid, frontal, sphenoid, vomer, and palatine bones forming the roof, and the maxilla and palatine bones forming the floor.

      PHYSIOLOGY OF THE NASAL CAVITIES — The nasal cavity functions to moisten, filter, and warm air as it passes to the lungs. It also contains the sense of smell organ, and helps with speech.

    C30.1 **Malignant neoplasm of <u>middle ear</u>** — Any new and abnormal growth of the middle ear in which the tissue growth is uncontrolled and has the properties of anaplasia, invasion, and metastases.

        Malignant neoplasm of antrum tympanicum
        Malignant neoplasm of auditory tube
        Malignant neoplasm of eustachian tube
        Malignant neoplasm of inner ear
        Malignant neoplasm of mastoid air cells
        Malignant neoplasm of tympanic cavity

      Excludes 1:   *malignant melanoma of skin of (external) ear (C43.2-)*
                 malignant neoplasm of auricular canal (external) (C43.2-,C44.2-)
                 malignant neoplasm of bone of ear (meatus) (C41.0)
                 malignant neoplasm of cartilage of ear (C49.0)
                 other and unspecified malignant neoplasm of skin of (external) ear (C44.2-)

      ANATOMY OF THE MIDDLE EAR — The middle ear is the air-filled space behind the tympanic membrane of the external ear which connects the inner ear, mastoid cells, ossicles, and auditory tube. The auditory tube (Eustachian tube) passes between the middle ear and the nasopharynx.

      PHYSIOLOGY OF THE MIDDLE EAR — The middle ear transfers, modulates, and amplifies the sound to the inner ear. The auditory tube functions to equalize air pressure within the middle ear to the outside air pressure, and to drain any fluid that may unnaturally accumulate in the middle ear.

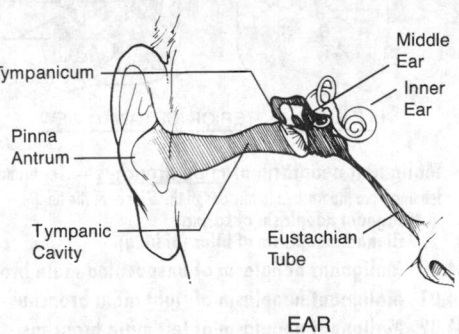

EAR

C31- **Malignant neoplasm of accessory <u>sinuses</u>** — Any new and abnormal growth of the accessory sinuses in which the tissue growth is uncontrolled and has the properties of anaplasia, invasion, and metastases.

  ANATOMY OF THE ACCESSORY SINUSES — The paired paranasal sinuses (maxillary, ethmoidal, frontal, and sphenoidal) are the bony cavities lined with mucous membranes which communicate with the nasal cavity.

  PHYSIOLOGY OF THE ACCESSORY SINUSES — The paranasal cavities function to lighten the bones of the skull, warm air, and give resonance to the voice.

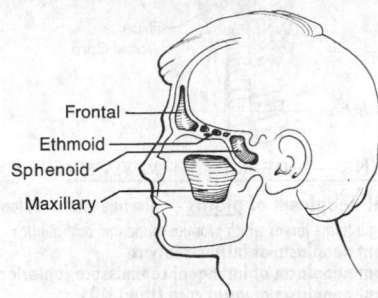

ACCESSORY SINUSES

    C31.0 **Malignant neoplasm of <u>maxillary</u> sinus** — The largest of the one of the four paired, air-filled paranasal sinuses located under the eye in the maxillary bone.

        Malignant neoplasm of antrum (Highmore) (maxillary)

    C31.1 **Malignant neoplasm of <u>ethmoidal</u> sinus** — One of the four paired, air-filled paranasal sinuses located within the ethmoid bone cavities that lies between the nose and the eyes.

    C31.2 **Malignant neoplasm of <u>frontal</u> sinus** — One of the four paired, air-filled paranasal sinuses located above the eye in the frontal bone.

    C31.3 **Malignant neoplasm of <u>sphenoid</u> sinus** — One of the four paired, air-filled paranasal sinuses located behind the eyes and nose in the sphenoid bone.

    C31.8 **Malignant neoplasm of <u>overlapping</u> sites of accessory sinuses**

    C31.9 **Malignant neoplasm of accessory sinus, unspecified**

C32- **Malignant neoplasm of <u>larynx</u>** — Any new and abnormal growth of the larynx in which tissue growth is uncontrolled and has the properties of anaplasia, invasion, and metastases.

  Use additional code to identify:
    Alcohol abuse and dependence (F10.-)
    Exposure to environmental tobacco smoke (Z77.22)
    Exposure to tobacco smoke in the perinatal period (P96.81)
    History of tobacco dependence (Z87.891)
    Occupational exposure to environmental tobacco smoke (Z57.31)
    Tobacco dependence (F17.-)
    Tobacco use (Z72.0)

  ANATOMY OF THE LARYNX — The larynx is the musculocartilaginous structure, lined with mucous membrane located between the root of the tongue and the trachea. The glottis is the slit-like opening of the larynx formed by the true vocal cords. The supraglottis is that portion of the larynx situated above the glottis. There are nine laryngeal cartilages, three paired and three single.

  PHYSIOLOGY OF THE LARYNX — The larynx functions to guard the entrance of the trachea from food and liquids, to control the expulsion of air, and to produce sound. The glottis produces sound, controls pitch, and when closed prevents food from entering the trachea. The supraglottis is an area of the larynx which helps to prevent food and liquid from entering the trachea. The laryngeal cartilages frame and support the larynx and its muscles.

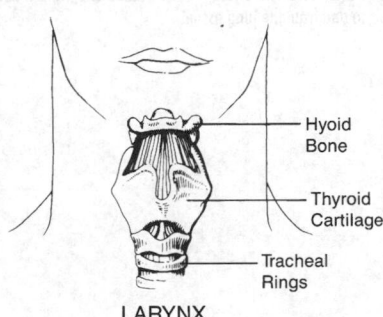

LARYNX

Continued on next page

Continued from previous page

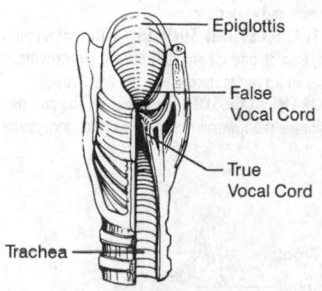

LARYNX — ANTERIOR (CUT-AWAY) VIEW

C32.0 **Malignant neoplasm of glottis** — The true vocal cords formed by the two folds opening into the larynx which produce sound and control pitch.
    Malignant neoplasm of intrinsic larynx
    Malignant neoplasm of laryngeal commissure (anterior) (posterior)
    Malignant neoplasm of vocal cord (true) NOS

C32.1 **Malignant neoplasm of supraglottis** — That portion of the larynx situated above the glottis.
    Malignant neoplasm of aryepiglottic fold or interarytenoid fold, laryngeal aspect
    Malignant neoplasm of epiglottis (suprahyoid portion) NOS
    Malignant neoplasm of extrinsic larynx
    Malignant neoplasm of false vocal cord
    Malignant neoplasm of posterior (laryngeal) surface of epiglottis
    Malignant neoplasm of ventricular bands
    Excludes ❷: *malignant neoplasm of anterior surface of epiglottis (C10.1)*
        malignant neoplasm of aryepiglottic fold or interarytenoid fold, hypopharyngeal aspect (C13.1)
        malignant neoplasm of aryepiglottic fold or interarytenoid fold, marginal zone (C13.1)
        malignant neoplasm of aryepiglottic fold or interarytenoid fold NOS (C13.1)

C32.2 **Malignant neoplasm of subglottis** — That portion of the larynx just below the true vocal cords and above the trachea.

C32.3 **Malignant neoplasm of laryngeal cartilage** — The 9 fibrous connective tissue structures which frame and support the larynx and its muscles.

C32.8 **Malignant neoplasm of overlapping sites of larynx**

C32.9 **Malignant neoplasm of larynx, unspecified**

C33 **Malignant neoplasm of trachea** — Any new and abnormal growth of the trachea
cc   in which tissue growth is uncontrolled and has the properties of anaplasia, invasion, and metastases.
    Use additional code to identify:
    Exposure to environmental tobacco smoke (Z77.22)
    Exposure to tobacco smoke in the perinatal period (P96.81)
    History of tobacco dependence (Z87.891)
    Occupational exposure to environmental tobacco smoke (Z57.31)
    Tobacco dependence (F17.-)
    Tobacco use (Z72.0)
ANATOMY OF THE TRACHEA — The trachea is a cylindrical tube about 1 inch (2.5 cm) in length. It extends downward in front of the esophagus and into the thoracic cavity, where it splits into the right and left bronchi.
PHYSIOLOGY OF THE TRACHEA — The trachea and bronchi allow for the rapid transport of air to and from the lung tissue.

C34- **Malignant neoplasm of bronchus and lung** — Any new and abnormal growth of the bronchus and lungs in which the tissue growth is uncontrolled and has the properties of anaplasia, invasion, and metastases.
    Use additional code to identify:
    Exposure to environmental tobacco smoke (Z77.22)
    Exposure to tobacco smoke in the perinatal period (P96.81)
    History of tobacco dependence (Z87.891)
    Occupational exposure to environmental tobacco smoke (Z57.31)
    Tobacco dependence (F17.-)
    Tobacco use (Z72.0)
    Excludes 1:   *Kaposi's sarcoma of lung (C46.5-)*
        malignant carcinoid tumor of the bronchus and lung (C7A.090)
ANATOMY OF THE BRONCHUS AND LUNGS — The bronchial tree consists of branched airways leading from the trachea to the microscopic air sacs. The 2 main branches, the right and left bronchi, subdivide into secondary or lobar bronchi which, in turn, branch into finer tubes down to the bronchioles. The lungs are soft, spongy, cone-shaped organs located in the thoracic cavity. The right and left lungs are separated medially by the heart and the mediastinum, and they are enclosed by the diaphragm and the thoracic cage. The right lung is divided into 3 lobes called the upper (superior), middle, and lower (inferior). The left lung is divided into 2 lobes, the upper and lower. The lobes are subdivided into lobules which are composed of bronchioles, alveolar sacs, alveoli, nerves, and associated blood and lymphatic vessels. The alveoli are thin-walled, microscopic air sacs that open only on the side communicating with the inhaled air. Venous blood is pumped from the right ventricle of the heart to the lungs by the right and left pulmonary arteries. (NOTE: Pulmonary arteries carry venous blood, the opposite of the rest of the arteries.) The arterialized blood returns to the left atrium of the heart via the pulmonary veins. (NOTE: Blood vessels with blood flow going to the heart are termed veins.)
PHYSIOLOGY OF THE BRONCHUS AND LUNGS — The lungs are organs that perform pulmonary ventilation. The alveoli are the microscopic structures responsible for the exchange of oxygen into the blood and carbon dioxide out of the body. Inspiration (inhalation) and expiration (exhalation) are complex central nervous system functions. Two groups of nerve cell bodies in the medulla of the brain compose the inspiratory center and the expiratory center. These 2 centers act reciprocally; that is, when one is stimulated and discharging, the other is inhibited. Both centers discharge nerve impulses to the intercostal muscles. When the inspiration center discharges nerve impulses, the diaphragm moves down and the external intercostal muscles contract, causing inflation. Inflation of the lungs causes stimulation of stretch receptors, which send impulses to the medulla, which in turn stimulates the expiratory center. Two other respiratory centers are contained in the pons which modify and control the medullary centers' activities, and are called the apneustic center and the pneumotaxic center. In addition to the above centers, there is also a chemical reaction which helps to control pulmonary ventilation. The carbon dioxide level in the blood is directly measured by the medulla, and respiration is adjusted accordingly. A decrease in the oxygen level, sensed by nerve endings in the common carotid artery and the aortic arch, will also stimulate a respiratory adjustment, but it does not play a noticeable difference in pulmonary ventilation.

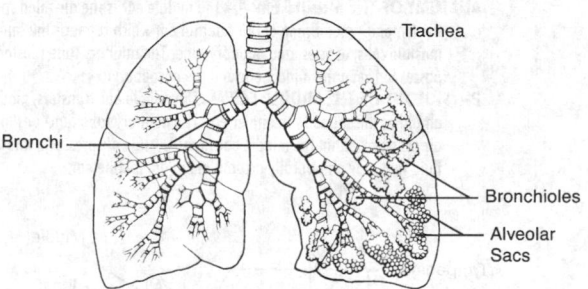

LUNGS — ANTERIOR (CUT-AWAY) VIEW

C34.0- **Malignant neoplasm of main bronchus** — The branched airways leading from the trachea to any one of the 5 lobes of the lung.
    Malignant neoplasm of carina
    Malignant neoplasm of hilus (of lung)

cc C34.00 **Malignant neoplasm of unspecified main bronchus**

cc C34.01 **Malignant neoplasm of right main bronchus**

cc C34.02 **Malignant neoplasm of left main bronchus**

C34.1- **Malignant neoplasm of upper lobe, bronchus or lung** — The two uppermost cone-shaped organs of respiration.

cc C34.10 **Malignant neoplasm of upper lobe, unspecified bronchus or lung**

cc C34.11 **Malignant neoplasm of upper lobe, right bronchus or lung**

cc C34.12 **Malignant neoplasm of upper lobe, left bronchus or lung**

cc **C34.2   Malignant neoplasm of <u>middle lobe, bronchus or lung</u>** — The single cone-shaped organ of respiration located between the upper and lower lobes of the right side.

C34.3-   Malignant neoplasm of <u>lower lobe, bronchus or lung</u> — The two lowermost cone-shaped organs of respiration.

cc **C34.30   Malignant neoplasm of lower lobe, unspecified bronchus or lung**

cc **C34.31   Malignant neoplasm of lower lobe, <u>right</u> bronchus or lung**

cc **C34.32   Malignant neoplasm of lower lobe, <u>left</u> bronchus or lung**

C34.8-   Malignant neoplasm of <u>overlapping sites</u> of bronchus and lung

cc **C34.80   Malignant neoplasm of overlapping sites of unspecified bronchus and lung**

cc **C34.81   Malignant neoplasm of overlapping sites of <u>right</u> bronchus and lung**

cc **C34.82   Malignant neoplasm of overlapping sites of <u>left</u> bronchus and lung**

C34.9-   Malignant neoplasm of <u>unspecified part</u> of bronchus or lung

cc **C34.90   Malignant neoplasm of unspecified part of unspecified bronchus or lung**
Lung cancer NOS

cc **C34.91   Malignant neoplasm of unspecified part of <u>right</u> bronchus or lung**

cc **C34.92   Malignant neoplasm of unspecified part of <u>left</u> bronchus or lung**

C37   Malignant neoplasm of <u>thymus</u> — Any new and abnormal growth of the thymus
cc   (the flat bi-lobed organ lying behind the sternum which is large during childhood but shrinks dramatically in the adult, and is composed of lymphoid material, and possibly some hormonal endocrine tissue) in which tissue growth is uncontrolled and has the properties of anaplasia, invasion, and metastases.
ANATOMY OF THE THYMUS — The thymus is the small, flat bi-lobed organ lying behind the sternum, and composed of lymphoid material.
PHYSIOLOGY OF THE THYMUS — The thymus functions during childhood by producing lymphocytes and aids in the development of the individual's immunity.
Excludes 1:   malignant carcinoid tumor of the thymus (C7A.091)

C38-   Malignant neoplasm of heart, mediastinum and pleura — Any new and abnormal growth of the heart, mediastinum, and pleura in which the tissue growth is uncontrolled and has the properties of anaplasia, invasion, and metastases.
Excludes 1:   mesothelioma (C45.-)
ANATOMY OF THE HEART, MEDIASTINUM, AND PLEURA — The heart is the 4 chambered, muscular, blood pumping organ behind the mediastinum in the thorax, and is approximately 5.5 inches (14 cm) long and 3.5 inches (9 cm) wide. The heart has 3 layers: The endocardium, myocardium, and pericardium. The endocardium is the interior lining of endothelium. The myocardium is the thick muscular layer. The pericardium is the double-layered serous membrane protecting the heart from friction as it beats. The heart has 4 valves and 4 chambers: The tricuspid valve, mitral valve, aortic valve, the pulmonary valve, right and left atria and right and left ventricles. The mediastinum is the mass of tissue between the sternum and vertebral column which divides the thoracic cavity. The pleura are closed double-layered serous membranous sacs surrounding the lungs. The parietal pleura is the layer which lines the thoracic walls opposite to the visceral pleura. The visceral pleura is the layer which adheres to the lungs and together with the parietal, forms the pleural cavity.
PHYSIOLOGY OF THE HEART, MEDIASTINUM, AND PLEURA — The heart functions to pump and maintain sufficient pressure of the blood to constantly meet the needs of the body cells. The venous blood is returned from the body via the inferior and superior vena cava to the right atrium where it is pooled momentarily before the tricuspid valve opens and allows the venous blood to enter the right ventricle. The right ventricle then contracts forcing the blood through the pulmonary valve to the lungs. The lungs return the reoxygenated blood to the left atrium where it is pooled momentarily before the mitral valve opens and allows the venous blood to enter the left ventricle. The left ventricle then contracts, forcing the blood through the aortic valve to all the tissues of the body. The pleura functions to prevent friction of the lungs against the thoracic wall during respiration. There is a small amount of serous fluid in the pleural cavity which lubricates the facing membranes.

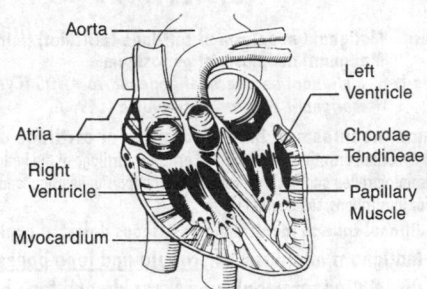

HEART — ANTERIOR (CUT-AWAY) VIEW

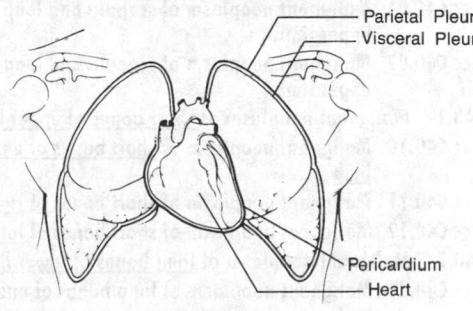

PLEURA

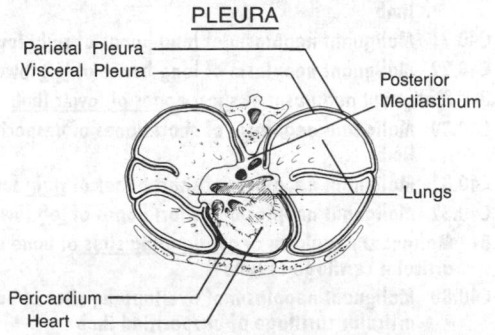

PLEURA — TRANSVERSE SECTION

cc **C38.0   Malignant neoplasm of <u>heart</u>** — The hollow, 4 chambered muscular organ which pumps the blood and maintains circulation.
Malignant neoplasm of pericardium
Excludes 1:   malignant neoplasm of great vessels (C49.3)

cc **C38.1   Malignant neoplasm of <u>anterior mediastinum</u>** — That portion of the cavity which lies in front, near the chest that contains the heart.

C34 - C38

cc **C38.2** **Malignant neoplasm of** <u>posterior mediastinum</u> — That portion of the cavity which lies behind the heart and contains the descending aorta, thoracic duct, the esophagus, and the vagus nerve.

cc **C38.3** **Malignant neoplasm of mediastinum, part unspecified**

cc **C38.4** **Malignant neoplasm of** <u>pleura</u> — The pleura are closed double-layered serous membranous sacs surrounding the lungs.

cc **C38.8** **Malignant neoplasm of** <u>overlapping sites</u> **of heart, mediastinum and pleura**

C39- **Malignant neoplasm of other and ill-defined sites in the respiratory system and intrathoracic organs**
Use additional code to identify:
Exposure to environmental tobacco smoke (Z77.22)
Exposure to tobacco smoke in the perinatal period (P96.81)
History of tobacco dependence (Z87.891)
Occupational exposure to environmental tobacco smoke (Z57.31)
Tobacco dependence (F17.-)
Tobacco use (Z72.0)
Excludes 1: *intrathoracic malignant neoplasm NOS (C76.1)*
thoracic malignant neoplasm NOS (C76.1)

C39.0 **Malignant neoplasm of upper respiratory tract, part unspecified**

C39.9 **Malignant neoplasm of lower respiratory tract, part unspecified**
Malignant neoplasm of respiratory tract NOS

Malignant neoplasms of bone and articular cartilage (C40-C41)

Includes: Malignant neoplasm of cartilage (articular) (joint)
Malignant neoplasm of periosteum
Excludes 1: *malignant neoplasm of bone marrow NOS (C96.9)*
malignant neoplasm of synovia (C49.-)

C40- **Malignant neoplasm of bone and articular cartilage of limbs** — Any new and abnormal growth of the bone and articular cartilage of the limbs in which tissue growth is uncontrolled and has the properties of anaplasia, invasion, and metastases. NOTE: For illustrations, see Chapter19.
Use additional code to identify major osseous defect, if applicable (M89.7-)

C40.0- **Malignant neoplasm of** <u>scapula and long bones of upper limb</u>

cc **C40.00** **Malignant neoplasm of scapula and long bones of unspecified upper limb**

cc **C40.01** **Malignant neoplasm of scapula and long bones of** <u>right</u> **upper limb**

cc **C40.02** **Malignant neoplasm of scapula and long bones of** <u>left</u> **upper limb**

C40.1- **Malignant neoplasm of** <u>short bones of upper limb</u>

cc **C40.10** **Malignant neoplasm of** <u>short bones of unspecified upper limb</u>

cc **C40.11** **Malignant neoplasm of short bones of** <u>right</u> **upper limb**

cc **C40.12** **Malignant neoplasm of short bones of** <u>left</u> **upper limb**

C40.2- **Malignant neoplasm of** <u>long bones of lower limb</u>

cc **C40.20** **Malignant neoplasm of long bones of unspecified lower limb**

cc **C40.21** **Malignant neoplasm of long bones of** <u>right</u> **lower limb**

cc **C40.22** **Malignant neoplasm of long bones of** <u>left</u> **lower limb**

C40.3- **Malignant neoplasm of** <u>short bones of lower limb</u>

cc **C40.30** **Malignant neoplasm of short bones of unspecified lower limb**

cc **C40.31** **Malignant neoplasm of short bones of** <u>right</u> **lower limb**

cc **C40.32** **Malignant neoplasm of short bones of** <u>left</u> **lower limb**

C40.8- **Malignant neoplasm of** <u>overlapping sites</u> **of bone and articular cartilage of limb**

cc **C40.80** **Malignant neoplasm of overlapping sites of bone and articular cartilage of unspecified limb**

cc **C40.81** **Malignant neoplasm of overlapping sites of bone and articular cartilage of** <u>right</u> **limb**

cc **C40.82** **Malignant neoplasm of overlapping sites of bone and articular cartilage of** <u>left</u> **limb**

C40.9- **Malignant neoplasm of unspecified bones and articular cartilage of limb**

cc **C40.90** **Malignant neoplasm of unspecified bones and articular cartilage of unspecified limb**

cc **C40.91** **Malignant neoplasm of unspecified bones and articular cartilage of** <u>right</u> **limb**

cc **C40.92** **Malignant neoplasm of unspecified bones and articular cartilage of** <u>left</u> **limb**

C41- **Malignant neoplasm of bone and articular cartilage of other and unspecified sites** — Any new and abnormal growth of the bone and articular cartilage other than the limbs in which tissue growth is uncontrolled and has the properties of anaplasia, invasion, and metastases. NOTE: For illustrations, see Chapter19.
Excludes 1: *malignant neoplasm of bones of limbs (C40.-)*
malignant neoplasm of cartilage of ear (C49.0)
malignant neoplasm of cartilage of eyelid (C49.0)
malignant neoplasm of cartilage of larynx (C32.3)
malignant neoplasm of cartilage of limbs (C40.-)
malignant neoplasm of cartilage of nose (C30.0)

cc **C41.0** **Malignant neoplasm of** <u>bones of skull and face</u>
Malignant neoplasm of maxilla (superior)
Malignant neoplasm of orbital bone
Excludes ❷: *carcinoma, any type except intraosseous or odontogenic of:*
maxillary sinus (C31.0)
upper jaw (C03.0)
malignant neoplasm of jaw bone (lower) (C41.1)

cc **C41.1** **Malignant neoplasm of** <u>mandible</u>
Malignant neoplasm of inferior maxilla
Malignant neoplasm of lower jaw bone
Excludes ❷: *carcinoma, any type except intraosseous or odontogenic of:*
jaw NOS (C03.9)
lower (C03.1)
malignant neoplasm of upper jaw bone (C41.0)

cc **C41.2** **Malignant neoplasm of** <u>vertebral column</u>
Excludes 1: *malignant neoplasm of sacrum and coccyx (C41.4)*

cc **C41.3** **Malignant neoplasm of** <u>ribs, sternum and clavicle</u>

cc **C41.4** **Malignant neoplasm of** <u>pelvic bones, sacrum and coccyx</u>

cc **C41.9** **Malignant neoplasm of bone and articular cartilage, unspecified**

Melanoma and other malignant neoplasms of skin (C43-C44)

C43- **Malignant** <u>melanoma</u> **of skin** — Any new and abnormal growth of the melanin-pigmented cells in which tissue growth is uncontrolled and has the properties of anaplasia, invasion, and metastases; usually developing from a nevus.
Excludes 1: *melanoma in situ (D03.-)*
Excludes ❷: *malignant melanoma of skin of genital organs (C51-C52, C60.-, C63.-)*
Merkel cell carcinoma (C4A.-)
sites other than skin — code to malignant neoplasm of the site

C43.0 **Malignant melanoma of** <u>lip</u>
Excludes 1: *malignant neoplasm of vermilion border of lip (C00.0-C00.2)*

C43.1- **Malignant melanoma of** <u>eyelid, including canthus</u>

C43.10 **Malignant melanoma of unspecified eyelid, including canthus**

C43.11 **Malignant melanoma of** <u>right</u> **eyelid, including canthus**

C43.12 **Malignant melanoma of** <u>left</u> **eyelid, including canthus**

C43.2- **Malignant melanoma of** <u>ear and external auricular canal</u>

C43.20 **Malignant melanoma of unspecified ear and external auricular canal**

C43.21 **Malignant melanoma of** <u>right</u> **ear and external auricular canal**

C43.22 **Malignant melanoma of** <u>left</u> **ear and external auricular canal**

C43.3- **Malignant melanoma of other and unspecified parts of face**

C43.30 **Malignant melanoma of unspecified part of face**

C43.31 **Malignant melanoma of** <u>nose</u>

C43.39 **Malignant melanoma of other parts of face**

C43.4 **Malignant melanoma of** <u>scalp and neck</u>

C 3 8 - C 4 3

C43.5- Malignant melanoma of <u>trunk</u>
 Excludes ❷*: malignant neoplasm of anus NOS (C21.0)*
 malignant neoplasm of scrotum (C63.2)

 C43.51 Malignant melanoma of <u>anal skin</u>
  Malignant melanoma of anal margin
  Malignant melanoma of perianal skin

 C43.52 Malignant melanoma of <u>skin of breast</u>

 C43.59 Malignant melanoma of other part of <u>trunk</u>

C43.6- Malignant melanoma of <u>upper limb</u>, including shoulder

 C43.60 Malignant melanoma of unspecified upper limb, including shoulder

 C43.61 Malignant melanoma of <u>right</u> upper limb, including shoulder

 C43.62 Malignant melanoma of <u>left</u> upper limb, including shoulder

C43.7- Malignant melanoma of <u>lower limb</u>, including hip

 C43.70 Malignant melanoma of unspecified lower limb, including hip

 C43.71 Malignant melanoma of <u>right</u> lower limb, including hip

 C43.72 Malignant melanoma of <u>left</u> lower limb, including hip

C43.8 Malignant melanoma of <u>overlapping sites</u> of skin

C43.9 Malignant melanoma of skin, unspecified
  Malignant melanoma of unspecified site of skin
  Melanoma (malignant) NOS

C4A- <u>Merkel cell</u> carcinoma — An aggressive neuroendocrine skin cancer that arises from Merkel cells in the epidermis and is often associated with the Merkel cell polyomavirus (MCV).

C4A.0 Merkel cell carcinoma of <u>lip</u>
 Excludes 1: malignant neoplasm of vermilion border of lip (C00.0-C00.2)

C4A.1- Merkel cell carcinoma of <u>eyelid, including canthus</u>

 C4A.10 Merkel cell carcinoma of unspecified eyelid, including canthus

 C4A.11 Merkel cell carcinoma of <u>right</u> eyelid, including canthus

 C4A.12 Merkel cell carcinoma of <u>left</u> eyelid, including canthus

C4A.2- Merkel cell carcinoma of <u>ear and external auricular canal</u>

 C4A.20 Merkel cell carcinoma of unspecified ear and external auricular canal

 C4A.21 Merkel cell carcinoma of <u>right</u> ear and external auricular canal

 C4A.22 Merkel cell carcinoma of <u>left</u> ear and external auricular canal

C4A.3- Merkel cell carcinoma of other and unspecified parts of face

 C4A.30 Merkel cell carcinoma of unspecified part of face

 C4A.31 Merkel cell carcinoma of <u>nose</u>

 C4A.39 Merkel cell carcinoma of other parts of face

C4A.4 Merkel cell carcinoma of <u>scalp and neck</u>

C4A.5- Merkel cell carcinoma of trunk
 Excludes ❷*: malignant neoplasm of anus NOS (C21.0)*
 malignant neoplasm of scrotum (C63.2)

 C4A.51 Merkel cell carcinoma of <u>anal skin</u>
  Merkel cell carcinoma of anal margin
  Merkel cell carcinoma of perianal skin

 C4A.52 Merkel cell carcinoma of <u>skin of breast</u>

 C4A.59 Merkel cell carcinoma of other part of trunk

C4A.6- Merkel cell carcinoma of <u>upper limb</u>, including shoulder

 C4A.60 Merkel cell carcinoma of unspecified upper limb, including shoulder

 C4A.61 Merkel cell carcinoma of <u>right</u> upper limb, including shoulder

 C4A.62 Merkel cell carcinoma of <u>left</u> upper limb, including shoulder

C4A.7- Merkel cell carcinoma of <u>lower limb</u>, including hip

 C4A.70 Merkel cell carcinoma of unspecified lower limb, including hip

 C4A.71 Merkel cell carcinoma of <u>right</u> lower limb, including hip

 C4A.72 Merkel cell carcinoma of <u>left</u> lower limb, including hip

C4A.8 Merkel cell carcinoma of <u>overlapping sites</u>

C4A.9 Merkel cell carcinoma, unspecified
  Merkel cell carcinoma of unspecified site
  Merkel cell carcinoma NOS

C44- <u>Other and unspecified malignant</u> neoplasm of <u>skin</u> — Any new and abnormal growth of the skin (basal cell carcinoma arises in the skin's basal cells) (squamous cell carcinoma arises in the skin's squamous cells) that is not classified elsewhere in which tissue growth is uncontrolled and has the properties of anaplasia, invasion, and metastases.
 Includes: **Malignant neoplasm of sebaceous glands** — The holocrine glands which secrete a mixture of fatty material and cellular debris onto the hairs and help to keep the skin soft, pliable, and relatively waterproof.
  Malignant neoplasm of sweat glands — The sweat glands of two types; the large apocrine glands of the axilla and perianal tissues that when stimulated by emotion produce sweat with an odor, and the smaller eccrine glands which produce the watery sweat for body cooling after stimulation from a rise in body temperature.
 Excludes 1: *Kaposi's sarcoma of skin (C46.0)*
 malignant melanoma of skin (C43.-)
 malignant neoplasm of skin of genital organs (C51-C52, C60.-, C63.2)
 Merkel cell carcinoma (C4A.-)
 ANATOMY OF THE SKIN — The skin is the outer covering of the body, consisting of the epidermis and dermis, and which rests upon the subcutaneous tissue. The epidermis is the outermost layer of the skin which develops keratin, a tough, fibrous waterproof protein, and lacks blood vessels. The dermis is the tough, elastic vascular connective tissue layer of the skin which contains the sebaceous and sweat glands.
 PHYSIOLOGY OF THE SKIN — The skin functions to protect the body from invading microorganisms, limits the loss of water from deep tissues, assists in homeostasis, aids in the regulation of body temperature, acts as the sense organ for the cutaneous senses, and is a source of vitamin D when it is exposed to light.

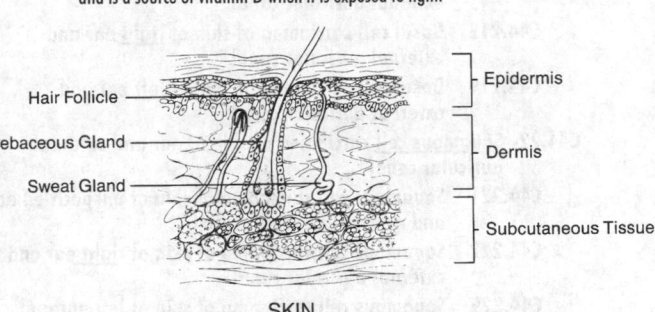

Hair Follicle — Epidermis
Sebaceous Gland — Dermis
Sweat Gland — Subcutaneous Tissue

SKIN

C44.0- Other and unspecified malignant neoplasm of skin of <u>lip</u>
 Excludes 1: malignant neoplasm of lip (C00.-)

 C44.00 <u>Unspecified</u> malignant neoplasm of skin of lip

 C44.01 <u>Basal cell</u> carcinoma of skin of lip

 C44.02 <u>Squamous cell</u> carcinoma of skin of lip

 C44.09 <u>Other specified</u> malignant neoplasm of skin of lip

C44.1- Other and unspecified malignant neoplasm of skin of <u>eyelid, including canthus</u>
 Excludes 1: connective tissue of eyelid (C49.0)

 C44.10- <u>Unspecified</u> malignant neoplasm of skin of eyelid, including canthus

  C44.101 Unspecified malignant neoplasm of skin of unspecified eyelid, including canthus

  C44.102 Unspecified malignant neoplasm of skin of <u>right</u> eyelid, including canthus

  C44.109 Unspecified malignant neoplasm of skin of <u>left</u> eyelid, including canthus

 C44.11- <u>Basal cell</u> carcinoma of skin of eyelid, including canthus

  C44.111 Basal cell carcinoma of skin of unspecified eyelid, including canthus

  C44.112 Basal cell carcinoma of skin of <u>right</u> eyelid, including canthus

  C44.119 Basal cell carcinoma of skin of <u>left</u> eyelid, including canthus

 C44.12- <u>Squamous cell</u> carcinoma of skin of eyelid, including canthus

  C44.121 Squamous cell carcinoma of skin of unspecified eyelid, including canthus

  C44.122 Squamous cell carcinoma of skin of <u>right</u> eyelid, including canthus

C44.129   Squamous cell carcinoma of skin of <u>left</u> eyelid, including canthus

C44.19-   <u>Other specified</u> malignant neoplasm of skin of eyelid, including canthus

     C44.191   Other specified malignant neoplasm of skin of unspecified eyelid, including canthus

     C44.192   Other specified malignant neoplasm of skin of <u>right</u> eyelid, including canthus

     C44.199   Other specified malignant neoplasm of skin of <u>left</u> eyelid, including canthus

C44.2-   Other and unspecified malignant neoplasm of skin of <u>ear and external auricular canal</u>

     Excludes 1:   connective tissue of ear (C49.0)

C44.20-   <u>Unspecified</u> malignant neoplasm of skin of ear and external auricular canal

     C44.201   Unspecified malignant neoplasm of skin of unspecified ear and external auricular canal

     C44.202   Unspecified malignant neoplasm of skin of <u>right</u> ear and external auricular canal

     C44.209   Unspecified malignant neoplasm of skin of <u>left</u> ear and external auricular canal

C44.21-   <u>Basal cell</u> carcinoma of skin of ear and external auricular canal

     C44.211   Basal cell carcinoma of skin of unspecified ear and external auricular canal

     C44.212   Basal cell carcinoma of skin of <u>right</u> ear and external auricular canal

     C44.219   Basal cell carcinoma of skin of <u>left</u> ear and external auricular canal

C44.22-   <u>Squamous cell</u> carcinoma of skin of ear and external auricular canal

     C44.221   Squamous cell carcinoma of skin of unspecified ear and external auricular canal

     C44.222   Squamous cell carcinoma of skin of <u>right</u> ear and external auricular canal

     C44.229   Squamous cell carcinoma of skin of <u>left</u> ear and external auricular canal

C44.29-   <u>Other specified</u> malignant neoplasm of skin of ear and external auricular canal

     C44.291   Other specified malignant neoplasm of skin of unspecified ear and external auricular canal

     C44.292   Other specified malignant neoplasm of skin of <u>right</u> ear and external auricular canal

     C44.299   Other specified malignant neoplasm of skin of <u>left</u> ear and external auricular canal

C44.3-   Other and unspecified malignant neoplasm of skin of <u>other and unspecified parts of face</u>

C44.30-   <u>Unspecified</u> malignant neoplasm of skin of other and unspecified parts of face

     C44.300   Unspecified malignant neoplasm of skin of unspecified part of face

     C44.301   Unspecified malignant neoplasm of skin of <u>nose</u>

     C44.309   Unspecified malignant neoplasm of skin of <u>other parts</u> of face

C44.31-   <u>Basal cell</u> carcinoma of skin of other and unspecified parts of face

     C44.310   Basal cell carcinoma of skin of unspecified parts of face

     C44.311   Basal cell carcinoma of skin of <u>nose</u>

     C44.319   Basal cell carcinoma of skin of <u>other parts</u> of face

C44.32-   <u>Squamous cell</u> carcinoma of skin of other and unspecified parts of face

     C44.320   Squamous cell carcinoma of skin of unspecified parts of face

     C44.321   Squamous cell carcinoma of skin of <u>nose</u>

     C44.329   Squamous cell carcinoma of skin of <u>other parts</u> of face

C44.39-   <u>Other specified</u> malignant neoplasm of skin of other and unspecified parts of face

     C44.390   Other specified malignant neoplasm of skin of unspecified parts of face

     C44.391   Other specified malignant neoplasm of skin of <u>nose</u>

     C44.399   Other specified malignant neoplasm of skin of <u>other parts</u> of face

C44.4-   Other and unspecified malignant neoplasm of skin of <u>scalp and neck</u>

C44.40   <u>Unspecified</u> malignant neoplasm of skin of scalp and neck

C44.41   <u>Basal cell</u> carcinoma of skin of scalp and neck

C44.42   <u>Squamous cell</u> carcinoma of skin of scalp and neck

C44.49   <u>Other specified</u> malignant neoplasm of skin of scalp and neck

C44.5-   Other and unspecified malignant neoplasm of skin of <u>trunk</u>

     Excludes 1:   anus NOS (C21.0)
                 scrotum (C63.2)

C44.50-   <u>Unspecified</u> malignant neoplasm of skin of trunk

     C44.500   Unspecified malignant neoplasm of <u>anal skin</u>
                 Unspecified malignant neoplasm of anal margin
                 Unspecified malignant neoplasm of perianal skin

     C44.501   Unspecified malignant neoplasm of skin of <u>breast</u>

     C44.509   Unspecified malignant neoplasm of skin of other part of trunk

C44.51-   <u>Basal cell</u> carcinoma of skin of trunk

     C44.510   Basal cell carcinoma of <u>anal skin</u>
                 Basal cell carcinoma of anal margin
                 Basal cell carcinoma of perianal skin

     C44.511   Basal cell carcinoma of skin of <u>breast</u>

     C44.519   Basal cell carcinoma of skin of other part of trunk

C44.52-   <u>Squamous cell</u> carcinoma of skin of trunk

     C44.520   Squamous cell carcinoma of <u>anal skin</u>
                 Squamous cell carcinoma of anal margin
                 Squamous cell carcinoma of perianal skin

     C44.521   Squamous cell carcinoma of skin of <u>breast</u>

     C44.529   Squamous cell carcinoma of skin of other part of trunk

C44.59-   <u>Other specified</u> malignant neoplasm of skin of trunk

     C44.590   Other specified malignant neoplasm of <u>anal skin</u>
                 Other specified malignant neoplasm of anal margin
                 Other specified malignant neoplasm of perianal skin

     C44.591   Other specified malignant neoplasm of skin of <u>breast</u>

     C44.599   Other specified malignant neoplasm of skin of other part of trunk

C44.6-   Other and unspecified malignant neoplasm of skin of <u>upper limb</u>, including shoulder

C44.60-   <u>Unspecified</u> malignant neoplasm of skin of upper limb, including shoulder

     C44.601   Unspecified malignant neoplasm of skin of unspecified upper limb, including shoulder

     C44.602   Unspecified malignant neoplasm of skin of <u>right</u> upper limb, including shoulder

     C44.609   Unspecified malignant neoplasm of skin of <u>left</u> upper limb, including shoulder

C44.61-   <u>Basal cell</u> carcinoma of skin of upper limb, including shoulder

     C44.611   Basal cell carcinoma of skin of unspecified upper limb, including shoulder

     C44.612   Basal cell carcinoma of skin of <u>right</u> upper limb, including shoulder

     C44.619   Basal cell carcinoma of skin of <u>left</u> upper limb, including shoulder

C44.62- <u>Squamous cell</u> carcinoma of skin of upper limb, including shoulder

    C44.621 Squamous cell carcinoma of skin of unspecified upper limb, including shoulder

    C44.622 Squamous cell carcinoma of skin of <u>right</u> upper limb, including shoulder

    C44.629 Squamous cell carcinoma of skin of <u>left</u> upper limb, including shoulder

C44.69- <u>Other specified</u> malignant neoplasm of skin of upper limb, including shoulder

    C44.691 Other specified malignant neoplasm of skin of unspecified upper limb, including shoulder

    C44.692 Other specified malignant neoplasm of skin of <u>right</u> upper limb, including shoulder

    C44.699 Other specified malignant neoplasm of skin of <u>left</u> upper limb, including shoulder

C44.7- Other and unspecified malignant neoplasm of skin of <u>lower limb</u>, including hip

C44.70- <u>Unspecified</u> malignant neoplasm of skin of lower limb, including hip

    C44.701 Unspecified malignant neoplasm of skin of unspecified lower limb, including hip

    C44.702 Unspecified malignant neoplasm of skin of <u>right</u> lower limb, including hip

    C44.709 Unspecified malignant neoplasm of skin of <u>left</u> lower limb, including hip

C44.71- <u>Basal cell</u> carcinoma of skin of lower limb, including hip

    C44.711 Basal cell carcinoma of skin of unspecified lower limb, including hip

    C44.712 Basal cell carcinoma of skin of <u>right</u> lower limb, including hip

    C44.719 Basal cell carcinoma of skin of <u>left</u> lower limb, including hip

C44.72- <u>Squamous cell</u> carcinoma of skin of lower limb, including hip

    C44.721 Squamous cell carcinoma of skin of unspecified lower limb, including hip

    C44.722 Squamous cell carcinoma of skin of <u>right</u> lower limb, including hip

    C44.729 Squamous cell carcinoma of skin of <u>left</u> lower limb, including hip

C44.79- <u>Other specified</u> malignant neoplasm of skin of lower limb, including hip

    C44.791 Other specified malignant neoplasm of skin of unspecified lower limb, including hip

    C44.792 Other specified malignant neoplasm of skin of <u>right</u> lower limb, including hip

    C44.799 Other specified malignant neoplasm of skin of <u>left</u> lower limb, including hip

C44.8- Other and unspecified malignant neoplasm of <u>overlapping sites</u> of skin

    C44.80 <u>Unspecified</u> malignant neoplasm of overlapping sites of skin

    C44.81 <u>Basal cell</u> carcinoma of overlapping sites of skin

    C44.82 <u>Squamous cell</u> carcinoma of overlapping sites of skin

    C44.89 <u>Other specified</u> malignant neoplasm of overlapping sites of skin

C44.9- Other and unspecified malignant neoplasm of skin, unspecified

    C44.90 <u>Unspecified</u> malignant neoplasm of skin, unspecified
        Malignant neoplasm of unspecified site of skin

    C44.91 <u>Basal cell</u> carcinoma of skin, unspecified

    C44.92 <u>Squamous cell</u> carcinoma of skin, unspecified

    C44.99 <u>Other specified</u> malignant neoplasm of skin, unspecified

Malignant neoplasms of mesothelial and soft tissue (C45-C49)

C45- <u>Mesothelioma</u> — Any new and abnormal growth of the tissue that lines most of the internal organs (mesothelium) in which tissue growth is uncontrolled and has the properties of anaplasia, invasion, and metastases and is most often associated with asbestos exposure.

cc **C45.0** Mesothelioma of <u>pleura</u>
    Excludes 1:   *other malignant neoplasm of pleura (C38.4)*

cc **C45.1** Mesothelioma of <u>peritoneum</u>
    Mesothelioma of cul-de-sac
    Mesothelioma of mesentery
    Mesothelioma of mesocolon
    Mesothelioma of omentum
    Mesothelioma of peritoneum (parietal) (pelvic)
    Excludes 1:   *other malignant neoplasm of soft tissue of peritoneum (C48.-)*

cc **C45.2** Mesothelioma of <u>pericardium</u>
    Excludes 1:   *other malignant neoplasm of pericardium (C38.0)*

    C45.7 Mesothelioma of other sites

    C45.9 Mesothelioma, unspecified

C46- <u>Kaposi's sarcoma</u> — Any new and abnormal growth of cells that line the lymph and blood vessels (endothelium) in which tissue growth is uncontrolled and has the properties of anaplasia and invasion and is often seen in HIV disease and other immunocompromised conditions.
    Code first any human immunodeficiency virus [HIV] disease (B20)

cc **C46.0** Kaposi's sarcoma of <u>skin</u>

cc **C46.1** Kaposi's sarcoma of <u>soft tissue</u>
    Kaposi's sarcoma of blood vessel
    Kaposi's sarcoma of connective tissue
    Kaposi's sarcoma of fascia
    Kaposi's sarcoma of ligament
    Kaposi's sarcoma of lymphatic(s) NEC
    Kaposi's sarcoma of muscle
    Excludes ❷: *Kaposi's sarcoma of lymph glands and nodes (C46.3)*

cc **C46.2** Kaposi's sarcoma of <u>palate</u>

cc **C46.3** Kaposi's sarcoma of <u>lymph nodes</u>

cc **C46.4** Kaposi's sarcoma of <u>gastrointestinal</u> sites

    C46.5- Kaposi's sarcoma of <u>lung</u>

cc **C46.50** Kaposi's sarcoma of unspecified lung

cc **C46.51** Kaposi's sarcoma of <u>right</u> lung

cc **C46.52** Kaposi's sarcoma of <u>left</u> lung

cc **C46.7** Kaposi's sarcoma of other sites

cc **C46.9** Kaposi's sarcoma, unspecified
    Kaposi's sarcoma of unspecified site

C47- Malignant neoplasm of <u>peripheral nerves</u> and <u>autonomic nervous system</u> — Any new and abnormal growth of the peripheral and autonomic nervous system in which tissue growth is uncontrolled and has the properties of anaplasia, invasion, and metastases.
    Includes: Malignant neoplasm of sympathetic and parasympathetic nerves and ganglia
    Excludes 1:   *Kaposi's sarcoma of soft tissue (C46.1)*

cc **C47.0** Malignant neoplasm of peripheral nerves of head, face and neck
    Excludes 1:   *malignant neoplasm of peripheral nerves of orbit (C69.6-)*

    C47.1- Malignant neoplasm of peripheral nerves of <u>upper limb</u>, including shoulder

cc **C47.10** Malignant neoplasm of peripheral nerves of unspecified upper limb, including shoulder

cc **C47.11** Malignant neoplasm of peripheral nerves of <u>right</u> upper limb, including shoulder

cc **C47.12** Malignant neoplasm of peripheral nerves of <u>left</u> upper limb, including shoulder

    C47.2- Malignant neoplasm of peripheral nerves of <u>lower limb</u>, including hip

cc **C47.20** Malignant neoplasm of peripheral nerves of unspecified lower limb, including hip

cc **C47.21** Malignant neoplasm of peripheral nerves of <u>right</u> lower limb, including hip

cc **C47.22** Malignant neoplasm of peripheral nerves of <u>left</u> lower limb, including hip

C 4 4 - C 4 7

Excludes 1: = NOT CODED HERE! (Do not code both)   567   *Excludes ❷:* = Not Included Here

CC **C47.3** **Malignant neoplasm of peripheral nerves of <u>thorax</u>**

CC **C47.4** **Malignant neoplasm of peripheral nerves of <u>abdomen</u>**

CC **C47.5** **Malignant neoplasm of peripheral nerves of <u>pelvis</u>**

CC **C47.6** **Malignant neoplasm of peripheral nerves of trunk, unspecified**
> Malignant neoplasm of peripheral nerves of unspecified part of trunk

CC **C47.8** **Malignant neoplasm of <u>overlapping sites</u> of peripheral nerves and autonomic nervous system**

CC **C47.9** **Malignant neoplasm of peripheral nerves and autonomic nervous system, unspecified**
> Malignant neoplasm of unspecified site of peripheral nerves and autonomic nervous system

C48- **Malignant neoplasm of retroperitoneum and peritoneum** — Any new and abnormal growth of the retroperitoneum and peritoneum in which tissue growth is uncontrolled and has the properties of anaplasia, invasion, and metastases.
> *Excludes 1:* *Kaposi's sarcoma of connective tissue (C46.1)*
> *mesothelioma (C45.-)*

ANATOMY OF THE RETROPERITONEUM AND PERITONEUM — The retroperitoneum is the space behind the peritoneum and borders the deep muscles of the back which contain the kidneys, adrenals, most of the duodenum, ascending and descending colon, and the pancreas. The peritoneum is the serous membrane which contains most of the abdominal contents, and where it is doubled upon itself it forms supporting structures called ligaments.

PHYSIOLOGY OF THE RETROPERITONEUM AND PERITONEUM —The peritoneum encapsules and protects the abdominal visceral organs allowing them to move slightly without damaging function.

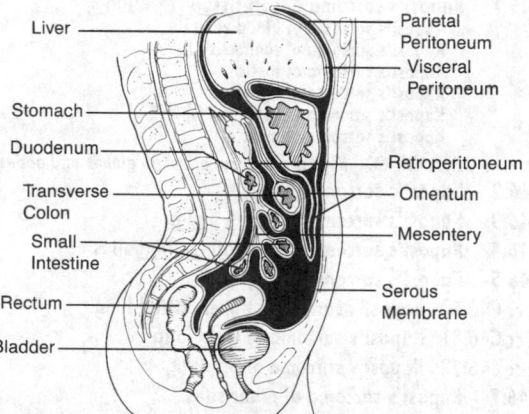

PERITONEUM — (FEMALE) SAGITTAL VIEW

CC **C48.0** **Malignant neoplasm of <u>retroperitoneum</u>** — The space which is behind the peritoneum and borders the deep muscles of the back.

CC **C48.1** **Malignant neoplasm of specified parts of <u>peritoneum</u>**
> **Malignant neoplasm of cul-de-sac** — The area formed by the peritoneal fold behind the uterus and between the rectum and uterus.
> **Malignant neoplasm of mesentery** — The peritoneal fold encircling most of the small bowel and attached to the posterior abdominal wall.
> **Malignant neoplasm of mesocolon** — The peritoneal fold attaching the colon to the posterior abdominal wall.
> **Malignant neoplasm of omentum** — The peritoneal fold attached to the stomach and extending down over the abdominal cavity.
> **Malignant neoplasm of parietal peritoneum** — The serous membrane that lines the abdominal walls and the undersurface of the diaphragm.
> **Malignant neoplasm of pelvic peritoneum** — The serous membrane that lines the pelvic cavity which is continuous with the parietal peritoneum.

CC **C48.2** **Malignant neoplasm of peritoneum, unspecified**

CC **C48.8** **Malignant neoplasm of <u>overlapping sites</u> of retroperitoneum and peritoneum**

C49- **Malignant neoplasm of <u>other connective and soft tissue</u>** — Any new and abnormal growth of the connective and other soft tissue in which tissue growth is uncontrolled and has the properties of anaplasia, invasion invasion, and metastases.
> **Includes:** **Malignant neoplasm of blood vessel** — The musculomembranous tubes of the cardiovascular system that carry blood from the heart to the body cells and back again.
> **Malignant neoplasm of bursa** — A pad-like sac or cavity of connective tissue lined with a synovial membrane which contains a viscid fluid and serves to prevent friction between structures where friction is likely to occur.
> **Malignant neoplasm of cartilage** — The tough but flexible tissue that covers the ends of the bones at a joint and gives shape and support to other body parts.
> **Malignant neoplasm of fascia** — A fibrous membrane which covers, supports, and separates muscles, and lies between the skin and underlying tissue.
> **Malignant neoplasm of fat** — A soft mass of adipose tissue which creates pads between various organs, and serves as an energy reserve for the body.
> **Malignant neoplasm of ligament, except uterine** — A band of fibrous connective tissue that connects bones and cartilages, serving to support and strengthen joints.
> **Malignant neoplasm of lymphatic vessel** — The musculomembranous tubes of the lymphatic system that carry lymph fluid.
> **Malignant neoplasm of muscle** — Groups of tissue made up of cells that contract together to produce movement.
> **Malignant neoplasm of synovia** — The transparent alkaline fluid (synovial fluid) secreted by the synovial membranes into the joints, bursa, and tendons.
> **Malignant neoplasm of tendon (sheath)** — The fibrous connective tissue cords which attach the muscles to bones and other structures.

> *Excludes 1:* *malignant neoplasm of cartilage (of):*
> *articular (C40-C41)*
> *larynx (C32.3)*
> *nose (C30.0)*
> *malignant neoplasm of connective tissue of breast (C50.-)*

> *Excludes ❷:* *Kaposi's sarcoma of soft tissue (C46.1)*
> *malignant neoplasm of heart (C38.0)*
> *malignant neoplasm of peripheral nerves and autonomic nervous system (C47.-)*
> *malignant neoplasm of peritoneum (C48.2)*
> *malignant neoplasm of retroperitoneum (C48.0)*
> *malignant neoplasm of uterine ligament (C57.3)*
> *mesothelioma (C45.-)*

CC **C49.0** **Malignant neoplasm of connective and soft tissue of <u>head, face and neck</u>**
> Malignant neoplasm of connective tissue of ear
> Malignant neoplasm of connective tissue of eyelid
> *Excludes 1:* *connective tissue of orbit (C69.6-)*

C49.1- **Malignant neoplasm of connective and soft tissue of <u>upper limb</u>, including shoulder**

CC **C49.10** **Malignant neoplasm of connective and soft tissue of unspecified upper limb, including shoulder**

CC **C49.11** **Malignant neoplasm of connective and soft tissue of <u>right</u> upper limb, including shoulder**

CC **C49.12** **Malignant neoplasm of connective and soft tissue of <u>left</u> upper limb, including shoulder**

C49.2- **Malignant neoplasm of connective and soft tissue of <u>lower limb</u>, including hip**

CC **C49.20** **Malignant neoplasm of connective and soft tissue of unspecified lower limb, including hip**

CC **C49.21** **Malignant neoplasm of connective and soft tissue of <u>right</u> lower limb, including hip**

CC **C49.22** **Malignant neoplasm of connective and soft tissue of <u>left</u> lower limb, including hip**

CC **C49.3** **Malignant neoplasm of connective and soft tissue of <u>thorax</u>**
> AHA 15:3Q:p19 – Synovial sarcoma, chest
> Malignant neoplasm of axilla
> Malignant neoplasm of diaphragm
> Malignant neoplasm of great vessels
> *Excludes 1:* *malignant neoplasm of breast (C50.-)*
> *malignant neoplasm of heart (C38.0)*
> *malignant neoplasm of mediastinum (C38.1-C38.3)*
> *malignant neoplasm of thymus (C37)*

CC **C49.4** **Malignant neoplasm of connective and soft tissue of <u>abdomen</u>**
> Malignant neoplasm of abdominal wall
> Malignant neoplasm of hypochondrium

C47-C49

cc **C49.5** **Malignant neoplasm of connective and soft tissue of <u>pelvis</u>**
Malignant neoplasm of buttock
Malignant neoplasm of groin
Malignant neoplasm of perineum

cc **C49.6** **Malignant neoplasm of connective and soft tissue of trunk, unspecified**
Malignant neoplasm of back NOS

cc **C49.8** **Malignant neoplasm of <u>overlapping sites</u> of connective and soft tissue**
Primary malignant neoplasm of two or more contiguous sites of connective and soft tissue

cc **C49.9** **Malignant neoplasm of connective and soft tissue, unspecified**

C49.A- **Gastrointestinal stromal tumor** — A soft tissue sarcoma of the gastrointestinal tract (GIST) originating from interstitial cells of Cajal.

cc **C49.A0** **Gastrointestinal stromal tumor, unspecified site**

cc **C49.A1** **Gastrointestinal stromal tumor of esophagus**

cc **C49.A2** **Gastrointestinal stromal tumor of stomach**

cc **C49.A3** **Gastrointestinal stromal tumor of small intestine**

cc **C49.A4** **Gastrointestinal stromal tumor of large intestine**

cc **C49.A5** **Gastrointestinal stromal tumor of rectum**

cc **C49.A9** **Gastrointestinal stromal tumor of other sites**

Malignant neoplasms of breast (C50)

C50- **Malignant neoplasm of <u>breast</u>** — Any new and abnormal growth of the breast in which tissue growth is uncontrolled and has the properties of anaplasia, invasion, and metastases.
Includes: Connective tissue of breast
Paget's disease of breast
Paget's disease of nipple
Use additional code to identify estrogen receptor status (Z17.0, Z17.1)
Excludes 1:   skin of breast (C44.501, C44.511, C44.521, C44.591)
ANATOMY OF THE FEMALE BREAST — The female breast is the modified cutaneous glandular prominence overlying the pectoral muscle on the anterior chest, and contains the milk-producing mammary glands. The areola is the circular pigmented area around the nipple. The nipple is the pigmented projection and contains the ends of the mammary ducts.
PHYSIOLOGY OF THE FEMALE BREAST — The female breast functions to secrete nourishing milk for the newborn. During pregnancy, hormones increase the size of the mammary glands, and following delivery, the pituitary gland secretes prolactin, which stimulates the mammary glands to produce milk. The mammary ducts convey the milk to the nipple.

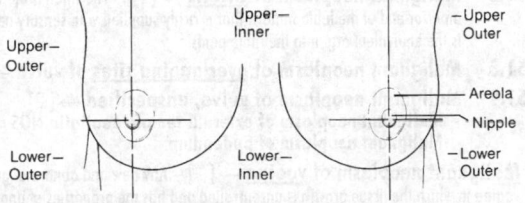

FEMALE BREASTS — ANTERIOR VIEW (QUADRANTS)

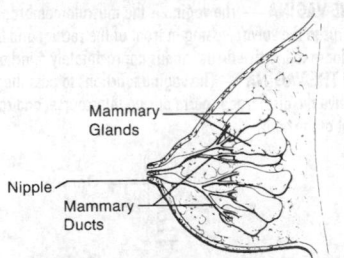

FEMALE BREAST — SAGITTAL VIEW

C50.0- **Malignant neoplasm of <u>nipple and areola</u>** — Nipple – The projection arising from the approximate center of the areola that contains the ends of the mammary ducts. Areola – The pigmented circular or elliptical area of the approximate center of the breast with the nipple projecting.

C50.01- **Malignant neoplasm of nipple and areola, <u>female</u>**

C50.011 **Malignant neoplasm of nipple and areola, <u>right</u> female breast** — [♀]

C50.012 **Malignant neoplasm of nipple and areola, <u>left</u> female breast** — [♀]

C50.019 **Malignant neoplasm of nipple and areola, unspecified female breast** — [♀]

C50.02- **Malignant neoplasm of nipple and areola, <u>male</u>**

C50.021 **Malignant neoplasm of nipple and areola, <u>right</u> male breast** — [♂]

C50.022 **Malignant neoplasm of nipple and areola, <u>left</u> male breast** — [♂]

C50.029 **Malignant neoplasm of nipple and areola, unspecified male breast** — [♂]

C50.1- **Malignant neoplasm of <u>central portion</u> of breast** — The general area that is located behind the areola in the center of breast mass.

C50.11- **Malignant neoplasm of central portion of breast, <u>female</u>**

C50.111 **Malignant neoplasm of central portion of <u>right</u> female breast** — [♀]

C50.112 **Malignant neoplasm of central portion of <u>left</u> female breast** — [♀]

C50.119 **Malignant neoplasm of central portion of unspecified female breast** — [♀]

C50.12- **Malignant neoplasm of central portion of breast, <u>male</u>**

C50.121 **Malignant neoplasm of central portion of <u>right</u> male breast** — [♂]

C50.122 **Malignant neoplasm of central portion of <u>left</u> male breast** — [♂]

C50.129 **Malignant neoplasm of central portion of unspecified male breast** — [♂]

C50.2- **Malignant neoplasm of <u>upper-inner quadrant</u> of breast** — That area above the nipple and towards the other breast.

C50.21- **Malignant neoplasm of upper-inner quadrant of breast, <u>female</u>**

C50.211 **Malignant neoplasm of upper-inner quadrant of <u>right</u> female breast** — [♀]

C50.212 **Malignant neoplasm of upper-inner quadrant of <u>left</u> female breast** — [♀]

C50.219 **Malignant neoplasm of upper-inner quadrant of unspecified female breast** — [♀]

C50.22- **Malignant neoplasm of upper-inner quadrant of breast, <u>male</u>**

C50.221 **Malignant neoplasm of upper-inner quadrant of <u>right</u> male breast** — [♂]

C50.222 **Malignant neoplasm of upper-inner quadrant of <u>left</u> male breast** — [♂]

C50.229 **Malignant neoplasm of upper-inner quadrant of unspecified male breast** — [♂]

C50.3- **Malignant neoplasm of <u>lower-inner quadrant</u> of breast** — That area below the nipple and towards the other breast.

C50.31- **Malignant neoplasm of lower-inner quadrant of breast, <u>female</u>**

C50.311 **Malignant neoplasm of lower-inner quadrant of <u>right</u> female breast** — [♀]

C50.312 **Malignant neoplasm of lower-inner quadrant of <u>left</u> female breast** — [♀]

C50.319 **Malignant neoplasm of lower-inner quadrant of unspecified female breast** — [♀]

C50.32- **Malignant neoplasm of lower-inner quadrant of breast, <u>male</u>**

C50.321 **Malignant neoplasm of lower-inner quadrant of <u>right</u> male breast** — [♂]

C50.322 **Malignant neoplasm of lower-inner quadrant of <u>left</u> male breast** — [♂]

C50.329 **Malignant neoplasm of lower-inner quadrant of unspecified male breast** — [♂]

C50.4- **Malignant neoplasm of <u>upper-outer quadrant</u> of breast** — That area above the nipple and to the side of the body.

C50.41- **Malignant neoplasm of upper-outer quadrant of breast, <u>female</u>**

C50.411 **Malignant neoplasm of upper-outer quadrant of <u>right</u> female breast** — [♀]

C50.412 **Malignant neoplasm of upper-outer quadrant of <u>left</u> female breast** — [♀]

C49 – C50

Excludes 1: = NOT CODED HERE! (Do not code both)

Excludes ❷: = Not Included Here

C50.419 Malignant neoplasm of upper-outer quadrant of unspecified female breast — [♀]

C50.42- Malignant neoplasm of upper-outer quadrant of breast, male

   C50.421 Malignant neoplasm of upper-outer quadrant of right male breast — [♂]

   C50.422 Malignant neoplasm of upper-outer quadrant of left male breast — [♂]

   C50.429 Malignant neoplasm of upper-outer quadrant of unspecified male breast — [♂]

C50.5- Malignant neoplasm of <u>lower-outer quadrant</u> of breast — That area below the nipple and to the side of the body.

C50.51- Malignant neoplasm of lower-outer quadrant of breast, <u>female</u>

   C50.511 Malignant neoplasm of lower-outer quadrant of <u>right</u> female breast — [♀]

   C50.512 Malignant neoplasm of lower-outer quadrant of <u>left</u> female breast — [♀]

   C50.519 Malignant neoplasm of lower-outer quadrant of unspecified female breast — [♀]

C50.52- Malignant neoplasm of lower-outer quadrant of breast, <u>male</u>

   C50.521 Malignant neoplasm of lower-outer quadrant of <u>right</u> male breast — [♂]

   C50.522 Malignant neoplasm of lower-outer quadrant of <u>left</u> male breast — [♂]

   C50.529 Malignant neoplasm of lower-outer quadrant of unspecified male breast — [♂]

C50.6- Malignant neoplasm of <u>axillary tail</u> of breast — That area which tapers away from the breast towards the axilla.

C50.61- Malignant neoplasm of axillary tail of breast, <u>female</u>

   C50.611 Malignant neoplasm of axillary tail of <u>right</u> female breast — [♀]

   C50.612 Malignant neoplasm of axillary tail of <u>left</u> female breast — [♀]

   C50.619 Malignant neoplasm of axillary tail of unspecified female breast — [♀]

C50.62- Malignant neoplasm of axillary tail of breast, <u>male</u>

   C50.621 Malignant neoplasm of axillary tail of <u>right</u> male breast — [♂]

   C50.622 Malignant neoplasm of axillary tail of <u>left</u> male breast — [♂]

   C50.629 Malignant neoplasm of axillary tail of unspecified male breast — [♂]

C50.8- Malignant neoplasm of <u>overlapping sites</u> of breast

C50.81- Malignant neoplasm of overlapping sites of breast, <u>female</u>

   C50.811 Malignant neoplasm of overlapping sites of <u>right</u> female breast — [♀]

   C50.812 Malignant neoplasm of overlapping sites of <u>left</u> female breast — [♀]

   C50.819 Malignant neoplasm of overlapping sites of unspecified female breast — [♀]

C50.82- Malignant neoplasm of overlapping sites of breast, <u>male</u>

   C50.821 Malignant neoplasm of overlapping sites of <u>right</u> male breast — [♂]

   C50.822 Malignant neoplasm of overlapping sites of <u>left</u> male breast — [♂]

   C50.829 Malignant neoplasm of overlapping sites of unspecified male breast — [♂]

C50.9- Malignant neoplasm of breast of unspecified site

C50.91- Malignant neoplasm of breast of unspecified site, <u>female</u>

   C50.911 Malignant neoplasm of unspecified site of <u>right</u> female breast — [♀]

   C50.912 Malignant neoplasm of unspecified site of <u>left</u> female breast — [♀]

   C50.919 Malignant neoplasm of unspecified site of unspecified female breast — [♀]

C50.92- Malignant neoplasm of breast of unspecified site, <u>male</u>

   C50.921 Malignant neoplasm of unspecified site of <u>right</u> male breast — [♂]

   C50.922 Malignant neoplasm of unspecified site of <u>left</u> male breast — [♂]

   C50.929 Malignant neoplasm of unspecified site of unspecified male breast — [♂]

Malignant neoplasms of female genital organs (C51-C58)

Includes: Malignant neoplasm of skin of female genital organs

C51- Malignant neoplasm of <u>vulva</u> — Any new and abnormal growth of the vulva in which the tissue growth is uncontrolled and has the properties of anaplasia, invasion, and metastases.

Excludes 1: carcinoma in situ of vulva (D07.1)

ANATOMY OF THE VULVA — The vulva is the group of external female genital organs comprising the labia majora, labia minora, clitoris, and vestibular glands.

PHYSIOLOGY OF THE VULVA — The vulva functions to protect the genital organs at the entrance of the vagina, and aid in sexual stimulation and lubrication during intercourse.

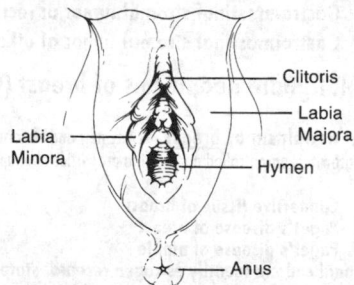

EXTERNAL FEMALE GENITALS

C51.0 Malignant neoplasm of <u>labium majus</u> — [♀] — The longitudinal cutaneous folds of skin covering adipose tissue which enclose and protect the other female reproductive organs.

   Malignant neoplasm of Bartholin's [greater vestibular] gland — The mucous-secreting glands on each side of the vaginal orifice.

C51.1 Malignant neoplasm of <u>labium minus</u> — [♀] — The longitudinal flaps of skin on both sides of the vaginal opening and located within the labia majora that merge to form a hood-like covering around the clitoris.

C51.2 Malignant neoplasm of <u>clitoris</u> — [♀] — The small projection at the anterior end of the labia minora that is richly supplied with sensory nerve fibers and is the equivalent organ to the male penis.

C51.8 Malignant neoplasm of <u>overlapping sites</u> of vulva — [♀]

C51.9 Malignant neoplasm of vulva, unspecified — [♀]
   Malignant neoplasm of external female genitalia NOS
   Malignant neoplasm of pudendum

C52 Malignant neoplasm of <u>vagina</u> — [♀] — Any new and abnormal growth of the vagina in which the tissue growth is uncontrolled and has the properties of anaplasia, invasion, and metastases.

Excludes 1: carcinoma in situ of vagina (D07.2)

ANATOMY OF THE VAGINA — The vagina is the musculomembranous tube extending from the uterus to the vulva, passing in front of the rectum and behind the bladder, and attached by loose connective tissue, and is approximately 4 inches (10 cm) in length.

PHYSIOLOGY OF THE VAGINA — The vagina functions to pass the fetus to birth during delivery, receive the discharged sperm during intercourse, and convey the menstrual discharge out of the body.

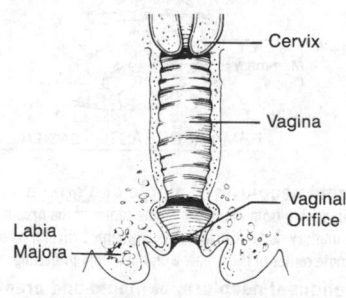

VAGINA — CUT-AWAY VIEW

Excludes 1: = NOT CODED HERE! (Do not code both)

Excludes ❷: = Not Included Here

C53- **Malignant neoplasm of <u>cervix</u> uteri** — The lower neck of the uterus which extends downward into the upper portion of the vagina.

    Excludes 1:   *carcinoma in situ of cervix uteri (D06.-)*

  C53.0   **Malignant neoplasm of <u>endo</u>cervix** — [♀] – The mucous membrane lining of the cervix.

  C53.1   **Malignant neoplasm of <u>exo</u>cervix** — [♀] – That part of the cervix lined with squamous epithelium extending onto the lip of the cervix.

  C53.8   **Malignant neoplasm of <u>overlapping sites</u> of cervix uteri** — [♀]

  C53.9   **Malignant neoplasm of cervix uteri, unspecified** — [♀]

C54- **Malignant neoplasm of <u>corpus</u> uteri** — Any new and abnormal growth of the

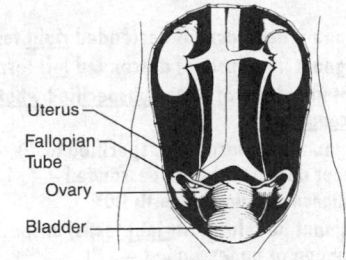

Uterus
Fallopian Tube
Ovary
Bladder

UTERUS AND ADNEXA

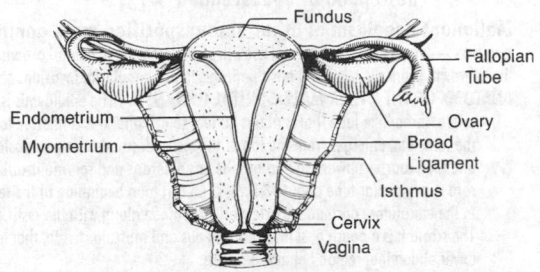

Fundus
Fallopian Tube
Ovary
Broad Ligament
Isthmus
Cervix
Vagina
Endometrium
Myometrium

UTERUS AND ADNEXA — CUT-AWAY

body of the uterus in which tissue growth is uncontrolled and has the properties of anaplasia, invasion, and metastases.

ANATOMY OF THE UTERUS — The uterus is the hollow, muscular organ which receives the embryo and is about 2.8 inches (7 cm) in length, and up to 2 Inches (5 cm) in width. The cervix is the lower third of the uterus which extends downward into the upper portion of the vagina. The isthmus is the narrowed lower end of the body of the uterus. The body is the bulky upper portion with the dome above the fallopian tube orifices, called the fundus. The endometrium is the mucous membrane interior lining upon the thick muscular myometrium of the body.

PHYSIOLOGY OF THE UTERUS — The uterus functions to receive the embryo, serves as attachment for the placenta, enlarges to allow for the fetus to grow, and rhythmically contracts for delivery of the fetus.

  C54.0   **Malignant neoplasm of <u>isthmus</u> uteri** — [♀] – The narrowed part between the body and the cervix.

      Malignant neoplasm of lower uterine segment

  C54.1   **Malignant neoplasm of <u>endometrium</u>** — [♀] – The endometrium is the mucous membrane interior lining upon the thick muscular myometrium of the body.

  C54.2   **Malignant neoplasm of <u>myometrium</u>** — [♀] – The thick, smooth muscle layer of the uterine walls which is interlaced with connective tissue.

  C54.3   **Malignant neoplasm of <u>fundus</u> uteri** — [♀] – The dome-shaped portion above the orifices of the fallopian tubes.

  C54.8   **Malignant neoplasm of <u>overlapping sites</u> of corpus uteri** — [♀]

  C54.9   **Malignant neoplasm of corpus uteri, unspecified** — [♀]

C55   **Malignant neoplasm of uterus, part unspecified** — [♀]

C56- **Malignant neoplasm of <u>ovary</u>** — Any new and abnormal growth of the ovary (the flat, ovoid paired sexual glands in the female which produce the human reproductive cell, the ova) in which tissue growth is uncontrolled and has the properties of anaplasia, invasion, and metastases.

  Use additional code to identify any functional activity

  ANATOMY OF THE OVARIES — The ovaries are the paired, flat, ovoid female sexual glands located on each side of the uterus and attached to the broad ligament, and are approximately 1.4 inches (3.5 cm) in length and 0.8 inches (2 cm) in width.

  PHYSIOLOGY OF THE OVARIES — The ovaries function to produce the human reproductive cell, and produce sexual hormones.

cc **C56.1**   **Malignant neoplasm of <u>right</u> ovary** — [♀]

cc **C56.2**   **Malignant neoplasm of <u>left</u> ovary** — [♀]

cc **C56.9**   **Malignant neoplasm of unspecified ovary** — [♀]

C57- **Malignant neoplasm of other and unspecified female genital organs** — Any new and abnormal growth of the other uterine adnexa in which tissue growth is uncontrolled and has the properties of anaplasia, invasion, and metastases.

  C57.0-   **Malignant neoplasm of <u>fallopian tube</u>** — The long, slender tube that extends from the uterus to the area next to the ovary which transfers the ova to the uterus for implantation.

      Malignant neoplasm of oviduct

      Malignant neoplasm of uterine tube

  C57.00   **Malignant neoplasm of unspecified fallopian tube** — [♀]

  C57.01   **Malignant neoplasm of <u>right</u> fallopian tube** — [♀]

  C57.02   **Malignant neoplasm of <u>left</u> fallopian tube** — [♀]

  C57.1-   **Malignant neoplasm of <u>broad ligament</u>** — The peritoneal fold that supports the uterus on each side.

  C57.10   **Malignant neoplasm of unspecified broad ligament** — [♀]

  C57.11   **Malignant neoplasm of <u>right</u> broad ligament** — [♀]

  C57.12   **Malignant neoplasm of <u>left</u> broad ligament** — [♀]

  C57.2-   **Malignant neoplasm of <u>round ligament</u>** — The fibromuscular band attached to the uterus, just below the fallopian tube entrance, and to the pelvic wall.

  C57.20   **Malignant neoplasm of unspecified round ligament** — [♀]

  C57.21   **Malignant neoplasm of <u>right</u> round ligament** — [♀]

  C57.22   **Malignant neoplasm of <u>left</u> round ligament** — [♀]

  C57.3   **Malignant neoplasm of <u>parametrium</u>** — [♀] – The loose connective tissue between the serous layers of the broad ligaments.

      Malignant neoplasm of uterine ligament NOS

  C57.4   **Malignant neoplasm of uterine adnexa, unspecified** — [♀]

  C57.7   **Malignant neoplasm of other specified female genital organs** — [♀]

      Malignant neoplasm of wolffian body or duct

  C57.8   **Malignant neoplasm of <u>overlapping sites</u> of female genital organs** — [♀]

      Primary malignant neoplasm of two or more contiguous sites of the female genital organs whose point of origin cannot be determined

      Primary tubo-ovarian malignant neoplasm whose point of origin cannot be determined

      Primary utero-ovarian malignant neoplasm whose point of origin cannot be determined

  C57.9   **Malignant neoplasm of female genital organ, unspecified** — [♀]

      Malignant neoplasm of female genitourinary tract NOS

C58   **Malignant neoplasm of <u>placenta</u>** — [♀, Age/12-55] – Any new and abnormal growth of the placenta in which tissue growth is uncontrolled and has the properties of anaplasia, invasion, and metastases.

  Includes: **Choriocarcinoma NOS**

             Chorionepithelioma NOS

  Excludes 1:   *chorioadenoma (destruens) (D39.2)*

             hydatidiform mole NOS (O01.9)

             invasive hydatidiform mole (D39.2)

             male choriocarcinoma NOS (C62.9-)

             malignant hydatidiform mole (D39.2)

ANATOMY OF THE PLACENTA — The placenta is the highly vascular disc-shaped organ within the pregnant uterus which connects with the fetus through the umbilical cord.

PHYSIOLOGY OF THE PLACENTA — The placenta functions to provide the fetus with nourishment, to filter the maternal blood, and, as an endocrine gland, to produce chorionic gonadotrophins, estrogen, and progesterone.

C 5 3 – C 5 8

Excludes 1: = NOT CODED HERE! (Do not code both)   **571**   ***Excludes ❷:*** = Not Included Here

Malignant neoplasms of male genital organs (C60-C63)

Includes: Malignant neoplasm of skin of male genital organs

C60- **Malignant neoplasm of <u>penis</u>** — Any new and abnormal growth of the penis in which the tissue growth is uncontrolled and has the properties of anaplasia, invasion, and metastases.

ANATOMY OF THE PENIS — The penis is a cylindrical organ which contains the urethra, located at the base of the male perineum. The body (shaft) is composed of 3 columns of erectile tissue, including a pair of dorsally located corpora cavernosa and a single corpus spongiosum below. The corpus spongiosum, through which the urethra extends, is enlarged at its distal end to form a sensitive, cone-shaped glans penis. A loose fold of skin, called the prepuce (foreskin) covers the glans penis, unless removed by circumcision.

PHYSIOLOGY OF THE PENIS — The penis functions as the specialized organ in the male that when erect is inserted into the female vagina for sexual intercourse. It also functions to convey urine and seminal fluid through the urethra to the outside. Erection is obtained by sexual excitement, stimulating parasympathetic nerve impulses causing blood engorgement of the corpora cavernosa and corpus spongiosum.

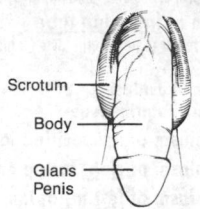

Scrotum
Body
Glans Penis

PENIS — FRONTAL VIEW

C60.0 **Malignant neoplasm of <u>prepuce</u>** — [♂] – The foreskin which covers the glans penis, unless circumcision has been performed.
Malignant neoplasm of foreskin

C60.1 **Malignant neoplasm of <u>glans</u> penis** — [♂] – The cone-shaped distal end of the penis that contains numerous sensory nerve fibers.

C60.2 **Malignant neoplasm of <u>body</u> of penis** — [♂] – The shaft of the penis composed of 3 columns of erectile tissue.
Malignant neoplasm of corpus cavernosum — The pair of dorsally located erectile tissue columns running the length of the penis.

C60.8 **Malignant neoplasm of <u>overlapping sites</u> of penis** — [♂]

C60.9 **Malignant neoplasm of penis, unspecified** — [♂]
Malignant neoplasm of skin of penis NOS

C61 **Malignant neoplasm of <u>prostate</u>** — [♂] – Any new and abnormal growth of the prostate in which tissue growth is uncontrolled and has the properties of anaplasia, invasion, and metastases.
Use additional code to identify:
Hormone sensitivity status (Z19.1-Z19.2)
Rising PSA following treatment for malignant neoplasm of prostate (R97.21)
Excludes 1: *malignant neoplasm of seminal vesicle (C63.7)*
ANATOMY OF THE PROSTATE — The prostate is a walnut-shaped gland which surrounds the bladder neck, and is contracted by smooth muscle with ducts opening into the urethra, and is 1.6 inches (4 cm) across and 1.2 inches (3 cm) thick.
PHYSIOLOGY OF THE PROSTATE — The prostate secretes a thin, milky fluid with an alkaline pH which enhances the motility of sperm cells and neutralizes the acidic pH of the vagina.

C62- **Malignant neoplasm of <u>testis</u>** — Any new and abnormal growth of the testis in which tissue growth is uncontrolled and has the properties of anaplasia, invasion, and metastases.
Use additional code to identify any functional activity
ANATOMY OF THE TESTES — The testes are the ovoid structures in the scrotum, suspended by a spermatic cord, and approximately 2 inches (5 cm) in length and 1.2 inches (3 cm) in diameter. Each testis is enclosed by a tough, white fibrous capsule called the tunica albuginea.
PHYSIOLOGY OF THE TESTES — The testes function to produce sperm cells for human reproduction, and secrete male hormones.

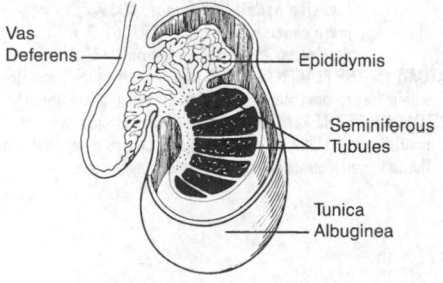

Vas Deferens
Epididymis
Seminiferous Tubules
Tunica Albuginea

TESTIS — CUT-AWAY

C62.0- **Malignant neoplasm of <u>undescended</u> testis** — A testis which has failed to descend into the scrotum and remains in the inguinal canal.
Malignant neoplasm of ectopic testis
Malignant neoplasm of retained testis

C62.00 **Malignant neoplasm of unspecified undescended testis** — [♂]

C62.01 **Malignant neoplasm of undescended <u>right</u> testis** — [♂]

C62.02 **Malignant neoplasm of undescended <u>left</u> testis** — [♂]

C62.1- **Malignant neoplasm of <u>descended</u> testis** — The normal position of the testis in the scrotum.
Malignant neoplasm of scrotal testis

C62.10 **Malignant neoplasm of unspecified descended testis** — [♂]

C62.11 **Malignant neoplasm of descended <u>right</u> testis** — [♂]

C62.12 **Malignant neoplasm of descended <u>left</u> testis** — [♂]

C62.9- **Malignant neoplasm of testis, <u>unspecified whether descended or undescended</u>**

C62.90 **Malignant neoplasm of unspecified testis, unspecified whether descended or undescended** — [♂]
Malignant neoplasm of testis NOS

C62.91 **Malignant neoplasm of <u>right</u> testis, unspecified whether descended or undescended** — [♂]

C62.92 **Malignant neoplasm of <u>left</u> testis, unspecified whether descended or undescended** — [♂]

C63- **Malignant neoplasm of other and unspecified male genital organs** — Any new and abnormal growth of the other male genital organs in which the tissue growth is uncontrolled and has the properties of anaplasia, invasion, and metastases.
ANATOMY OF THE OTHER MALE GENITAL ORGANS — The epididymis is a tightly coiled, threadlike tube that is about 20 feet (6 m) long. It is connected to ducts within the testis and emerges from the top of the testis, descends along its posterior surface, and then courses upward to become the vas deferans and spermatic cord. The spermatic cord is a muscular tube about 18 inches (45 cm) long beginning at the testis and ending in the ejaculatory duct, and is externally contained along with the testis, in the scrotum. The scrotum is a pouch of skin, subcutaneous and muscular tissue, that hangs from the lower abdominal region behind the penis.
PHYSIOLOGY OF THE OTHER MALE GENITAL ORGANS — The epididymis functions to store and mature sperm cells, and to transport the sperm from the testicular ducts to the spermatic cord. The spermatic cord transports the sperm to the ejaculatory duct. The scrotum protects the testis and spermatic cord by contracting and relaxing the dartos muscle.

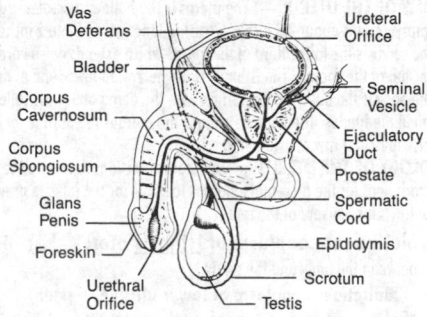

Vas Deferans
Bladder
Corpus Cavernosum
Corpus Spongiosum
Glans Penis
Foreskin
Urethral Orifice
Ureteral Orifice
Seminal Vesicle
Ejaculatory Duct
Prostate
Spermatic Cord
Epididymis
Scrotum
Testis

MALE GENITAL ORGANS — SAGITTAL VIEW

C63.0- **Malignant neoplasm of <u>epididymis</u>** — The tightly coiled tube attached to each testis where sperm cells mature and are stored.

C63.00 **Malignant neoplasm of unspecified epididymis** — [♂]

C63.01 **Malignant neoplasm of <u>right</u> epididymis** — [♂]

C63.02 **Malignant neoplasm of <u>left</u> epididymis** — [♂]

C63.1- **Malignant neoplasm of <u>spermatic cord</u>** — The muscular tube which transports the sperm from the epididymis to the ejaculatory duct.

C63.10 **Malignant neoplasm of unspecified spermatic cord** — [♂]

C63.11 **Malignant neoplasm of <u>right</u> spermatic cord** — [♂]

C63.12 **Malignant neoplasm of <u>left</u> spermatic cord** — [♂]

C63.2 **Malignant neoplasm of <u>scrotum</u>** — [♂] – The pouch of skin, subcutaneous, and muscular tissue that encloses and protects the testes, and hangs from the trunk behind the penis.
Malignant neoplasm of skin of scrotum — The protective dermal covering of the scrotum.

Excludes 1: = NOT CODED HERE! (Do not code both)

Excludes ❷: = Not Included Here

C60 - C63

C63.7 **Malignant neoplasm of other specified male genital organs** — [♂]

    Malignant neoplasm of seminal vesicle — The tube-like glands attached to the vas deferens near the base of the bladder which secrete a slightly alkaline fluid rich in nutrients and prostaglandins.

    Malignant neoplasm of tunica vaginalis — The serous membrane covering the front and sides of the testis and epididymis.

C63.8 **Malignant neoplasm of overlapping sites of male genital organs** — [♂]

    Primary malignant neoplasm of two or more contiguous sites of male genital organs whose point of origin cannot be determined

C63.9 **Malignant neoplasm of male genital organ, unspecified** — [♂]

    Malignant neoplasm of male genitourinary tract NOS

Malignant neoplasms of urinary tract (C64-C68)

C64- **Malignant neoplasm of kidney, except renal pelvis** — Any new and abnormal growth of the kidney in which the tissue growth is uncontrolled and has the properties of anaplasia, invasion, and metastases.

    Excludes 1:   *malignant carcinoid tumor of the kidney (C7A.093)*
                malignant neoplasm of renal calyces (C65.-)
                malignant neoplasm of renal pelvis (C65.-)

    ANATOMY OF THE KIDNEYS — The kidneys are reddish-brown, bean-shaped organs about 4.7 inches (12 cm) long, 2.3 inches (6 cm) wide, and 1.2 inches (3 cm) thick, and are located on either side of the vertebral column in the retroperitoneal space. The kidneys are supplied with arterial blood from the renal arteries which branch off from the aorta, and are drained by the renal veins which connect with the inferior vena cava. The renal pelvis is the funnel-shaped urinary collecting system of the kidney at the upper end of a ureter.

    PHYSIOLOGY OF THE KIDNEYS — The kidneys function to remove metabolic wastes from the blood by transferring them into the urine. They also regulate red blood cell production, blood pressure, calcium absorption, and the pH level of the blood.

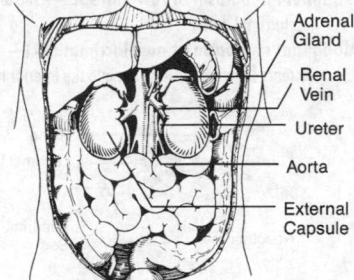

KIDNEY — ANTERIOR VIEW

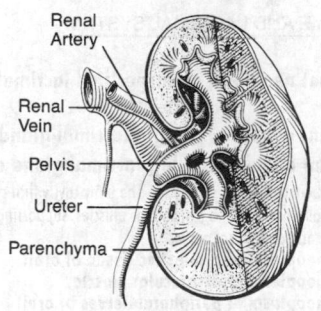

KIDNEY — (CUT AWAY VIEW)

cc **C64.1** **Malignant neoplasm of right kidney, except renal pelvis**

cc **C64.2** **Malignant neoplasm of left kidney, except renal pelvis**

cc **C64.9** **Malignant neoplasm of unspecified kidney, except renal pelvis**

C65- **Malignant neoplasm of renal pelvis** — Any new and abnormal growth of the kidney pelvis in which the tissue growth is uncontrolled and has the properties of anaplasia, invasion, and metastases.

    Includes: **Malignant neoplasm of pelviureteric junction** — The funnel-shaped urine collecting system of the kidneys.

              Malignant neoplasm of renal calyces — The minor subdivisions of the renal pelvis.

cc **C65.1** **Malignant neoplasm of right renal pelvis**

cc **C65.2** **Malignant neoplasm of left renal pelvis**

cc **C65.9** **Malignant neoplasm of unspecified renal pelvis**

C66- **Malignant neoplasm of ureter** — Any new and abnormal growth of the ureter (the musculomembranous tubes which convey urine from the kidneys to the bladder) in which the tissue growth is uncontrolled and has the properties of anaplasia, invasion, and metastases.

    Excludes 1:   *malignant neoplasm of ureteric orifice of bladder (C67.6)*

cc **C66.1** **Malignant neoplasm of right ureter**

cc **C66.2** **Malignant neoplasm of left ureter**

cc **C66.9** **Malignant neoplasm of unspecified ureter**

C67- **Malignant neoplasm of bladder** — Any new and abnormal growth of the bladder in which the tissue growth is uncontrolled and has the properties of anaplasia, invasion, and metastases.

    AHA 16:1Q:p19 – Malignant neoplasm of neobladder

    ANATOMY OF THE BLADDER — The urinary bladder is a hollow, collapsible musculomembranous organ, and is located within the pelvic cavity, behind the symphysis pubis. In the male, it lies against the rectum, and in the female it lies against the vagina and uterus. When filled it may contain 17 fluid ounces (500 ml) of urine and pushes upward indenting the abdominal cavity. The trigone area is the floor of the bladder formed by three points, the two ureteral orifices and the urethral orifice. The dome is the expandable superior surface of the bladder. The bladder neck is that area surrounding the urethral orifice. The ureteric orifice is that area surrounding the ureteral openings. The urachus in the adult forms the middle umbilical ligament of the bladder.

    PHYSIOLOGY OF THE BLADDER — The urinary bladder functions as a reservoir for the urine produced by the kidneys until the individual expels the urine (micturition). Micturition occurs when the bladder becomes distended with urine and stretch receptor nerves signal the micturition center in the sacral spinal cord. Parasympathetic nerve impulses start rhythmically contracting the bladder and the individual senses an urgency to urinate. Following the midbrain decision to urinate, the external urethral

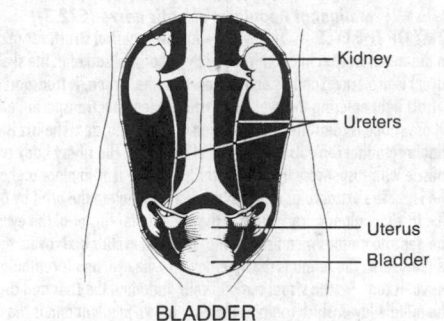

BLADDER

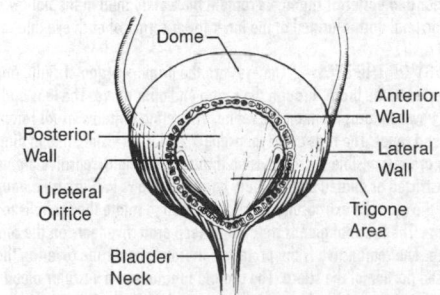

BLADDER — ANTERIOR (CUT-AWAY) VIEW

sphincter is relaxed, and urination begins as the bladder muscle contracts.

C67.0 **Malignant neoplasm of trigone of bladder** — The area of the bladder floor formed by the ureteral orifices and the urethral orifice.

C67.1 **Malignant neoplasm of dome of bladder** — The expandable superior surface of the bladder.

C67.2 **Malignant neoplasm of lateral wall of bladder**

C67.3 **Malignant neoplasm of anterior wall of bladder**

C67.4 **Malignant neoplasm of posterior wall of bladder**

C67.5 **Malignant neoplasm of bladder neck** — The outlet area of bladder surrounding the urethral orifice.

    Malignant neoplasm of internal urethral orifice

C67.6 **Malignant neoplasm of ureteric orifice** — The opening of a ureter into the bladder.

C67.7 **Malignant neoplasm of urachus** — The fetal urinary tract that in the adult forms the middle umbilical ligament of the bladder.

C67.8 **Malignant neoplasm of overlapping sites of bladder**

C67.9 **Malignant neoplasm of bladder, unspecified**

C63 - C67

Excludes 1: = NOT CODED HERE! (Do not code both)   **573**   *Excludes ❷:* = Not Included Here

C68- Malignant neoplasm of other and unspecified urinary organs

    Excludes 1:   *malignant neoplasm of female genitourinary tract NOS (C57.9)*
                 malignant neoplasm of male genitourinary tract NOS (C63.9)

cc **C68.0 Malignant neoplasm of <u>urethra</u>** — Any new and abnormal growth of the urethra (the musculomembranous tube which conveys urine from the bladder to the outside at the urethral orifice) in which the tissue growth is uncontrolled and has the properties of anaplasia, invasion, and metastases.

    Excludes 1:   *malignant neoplasm of urethral orifice of bladder (C67.5)*

cc **C68.1 Malignant neoplasm of <u>paraurethral glands</u>** — Any new and abnormal growth of the paraurethral glands (the small rudimentary glands that open on either side of the posterior portion of the urethral orifice) in which the tissue growth is uncontrolled and has the properties of anaplasia, invasion, and metastases.

cc **C68.8 Malignant neoplasm of overlapping sites of urinary organs**
        Primary malignant neoplasm of two or more contiguous sites of urinary organs whose point of origin cannot be determined

cc **C68.9 Malignant neoplasm of urinary organ, unspecified**
        Malignant neoplasm of urinary system NOS

Malignant neoplasms of eye, brain and other parts of central nervous system (C69-C72)

C69- Malignant neoplasm of <u>eye and adnexa</u> — Any new and abnormal growth of the eye and adnexa in which the tissue growth is uncontrolled and has the properties of anaplasia, invasion, and metastases.

    Excludes 1:   *malignant neoplasm of connective tissue of eyelid (C49.0)*
                 malignant neoplasm of eyelid (skin) (C43.1-, C44.1-)
                 malignant neoplasm of optic nerve (C72.3-)

ANATOMY OF THE EYES — The eyes are hollow spherical structures about 1 inch (2.5 cm) in diameter, located in and protected by the orbital socket in the skull. The sclera (outer layer) is protective, and its anterior portion, the cornea, is transparent so that it can refract light entering the eye. The crystalline lens is a transparent elastic structure whose shape is controlled by the action of ciliary muscles. The iris is a muscular diaphragm that controls the dilation of the pupil. The ciliary body consists of smooth muscle with suspensory ligaments which hold the lens in place and adjust the focus of the lens. The extraocular muscles attach the eyeball to the orbit by 6 different muscles. The lacrimal glands are located in the upper outer corner of the eyes. The conjunctiva is the delicate mucous membrane which lines the eyelids and covers the exposed surface of the sclera. The retina is the inner layer of the eye, and is continuous with the optic nerve. It contains the visual receptor cells, including the rods and cones. The choroid is the middle layer which contains the dark brown pigment and is the vascular layer. The anterior and posterior chambers contain the watery fluid in the hollow bulk of the eye. The lacrimal duct is located at the inner lower corner of each eye and connects with the nasal cavity.

PHYSIOLOGY OF THE EYES — The eyes are the primary organ of sight, and are directly connected to the brain through the retina and optic nerve. The lens and cornea refract light waves to focus them on the retina. The retina contains visual receptor cells, called rods and cones. The rods are responsible for colorless vision, like in dim light, and the cones are responsible for color vision through their light-sensitive pigment sets. The iris is constricted or dilated by the ciliary body and allows for varying amounts of light to enter the eye. The extraocular muscles function to rotate the eyeballs to look at desired objects . The lacrimal glands function to keep protective tears on the conjunctiva and cornea. The conjunctiva is the protective mucous membrane covering the eyelids and exposed portion of the sclera. The choroid functions as a vascular blood supply to most eye structures and absorbs excess light through its dark pigment. The lacrimal duct drains the tears from the eyes into the nasal cavities.

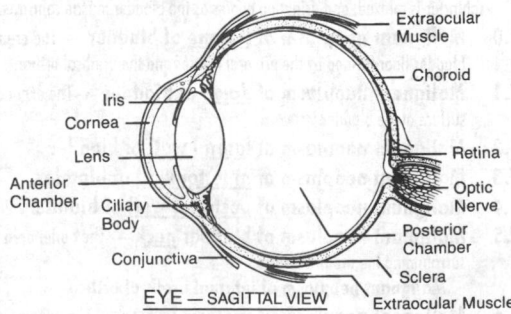

EYE — SAGITTAL VIEW

C69.0- Malignant neoplasm of <u>conjunctiva</u> — The delicate mucous membrane that lines the eyelids and exposed surface of the sclera.

    C69.00 Malignant neoplasm of unspecified conjunctiva

    C69.01 Malignant neoplasm of <u>right</u> conjunctiva

    C69.02 Malignant neoplasm of <u>left</u> conjunctiva

C69.1- Malignant neoplasm of <u>cornea</u> — The clear, transparent fibrous outer tissue layer of the anterior eyeball including the iris, pupil, and anterior chamber that is continuous with the sclera.

    C69.10 Malignant neoplasm of unspecified cornea

    C69.11 Malignant neoplasm of <u>right</u> cornea

    C69.12 Malignant neoplasm of <u>left</u> cornea

C69.2- Malignant neoplasm of <u>retina</u> — The innermost layer of the eyeball, consisting of an outer pigmented layer and an inner nervous layer which includes the rods and cones and is continuous with the optic nerve.

    Excludes 1:   *dark area on retina (D49.81)*
                 neoplasm of unspecified behavior of retina and choroid (D49.81)
                 retinal freckle (D49.81)

    C69.20 Malignant neoplasm of unspecified retina

    C69.21 Malignant neoplasm of <u>right</u> retina

    C69.22 Malignant neoplasm of <u>left</u> retina

C69.3- Malignant neoplasm of <u>choroid</u> — The thin, dark brown pigmented vascular layer between the retina and the sclera that covers the eyeball, except for the anterior light-entering portion.

    C69.30 Malignant neoplasm of unspecified choroid

    C69.31 Malignant neoplasm of <u>right</u> choroid

    C69.32 Malignant neoplasm of <u>left</u> choroid

C69.4- Malignant neoplasm of <u>ciliary body</u> — The smooth muscle layer which adjusts the iris and lens.

    C69.40 Malignant neoplasm of unspecified ciliary body

    C69.41 Malignant neoplasm of <u>right</u> ciliary body

    C69.42 Malignant neoplasm of <u>left</u> ciliary body

C69.5- Malignant neoplasm of <u>lacrimal gland and duct</u> — The tear-secreting glands and their ducts that lie at the upper-outer angle of the orbit.

    Malignant neoplasm of lacrimal sac — The dilated upper end of the nasolacrimal duct.

    Malignant neoplasm of nasolacrimal duct — The passage which conveys the tears from the lacrimal sac into the interior nasal meatus.

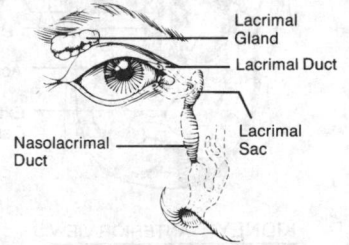

EYE AND LACRIMAL SYSTEM

    C69.50 Malignant neoplasm of unspecified lacrimal gland and duct

    C69.51 Malignant neoplasm of <u>right</u> lacrimal gland and duct

    C69.52 Malignant neoplasm of <u>left</u> lacrimal gland and duct

C69.6- Malignant neoplasm of <u>orbit</u> — The bony cavity that contains and protects the eyeball, including the extraocular muscles, supporting and connecting connective tissue, and peripheral nerves.

    Malignant neoplasm of connective tissue of orbit
    Malignant neoplasm of extraocular muscle
    Malignant neoplasm of peripheral nerves of orbit
    Malignant neoplasm of retrobulbar tissue
    Malignant neoplasm of retro-ocular tissue

    Excludes 1:   *malignant neoplasm of orbital bone (C41.0)*

    C69.60 Malignant neoplasm of unspecified orbit

    C69.61 Malignant neoplasm of <u>right</u> orbit

    C69.62 Malignant neoplasm of <u>left</u> orbit

C69.8- Malignant neoplasm of <u>overlapping sites</u> of eye and adnexa

    C69.80 Malignant neoplasm of overlapping sites of unspecified eye and adnexa

    C69.81 Malignant neoplasm of overlapping sites of <u>right</u> eye and adnexa

    C69.82 Malignant neoplasm of overlapping sites of <u>left</u> eye and adnexa

C69.9- Malignant neoplasm of unspecified site of eye
Malignant neoplasm of eyeball

C69.90 Malignant neoplasm of unspecified site of unspecified eye

C69.91 Malignant neoplasm of unspecified site of <u>right</u> eye

C69.92 Malignant neoplasm of unspecified site of <u>left</u> eye

C70- **Malignant neoplasm of <u>meninges</u>** — Any new and abnormal growth of the meninges in which tissue growth is uncontrolled and has the properties of anaplasia, invasion, and metastases.

CC **C70.0** **Malignant neoplasm of <u>cerebral</u> meninges** — The three protective covering membranes of the brain, consisting of the dura mater (outermost), the arachnoid (middle), and the pia mater (innermost) that are continuous with the spinal meninges.

CC **C70.1** **Malignant neoplasm of <u>spinal</u> meninges** — The three protective covering membranes of the spinal cord which are continuous with the cerebral meninges.

CC **C70.9** **Malignant neoplasm of meninges, unspecified**

C71- **Malignant neoplasm of <u>brain</u>** — Any new and abnormal growth of the brain in which tissue growth is uncontrolled and has the properties of anaplasia, invasion, and metastases.

AHA 14:3Q:p3 – Astrocytoma

Excludes 1: *malignant neoplasm of cranial nerves (C72.2-C72.5)*
retrobulbar malignant neoplasm (C69.6-)

ANATOMY OF THE BRAIN — The brain is the largest and most complex part of the nervous system, and is located in the cranial cavity. The cerebrum is the largest part of the brain, and is divided sagittally (front and back through the center) into 2 hemispheres. The corpus callosum lies below and connects the 2 hemispheres. The thalamus lies below the corpus callosum on either side of the third ventricle. The hypothalamus lies above the brain stem and forms the floor of the third ventricle. The basal ganglia are masses of gray matter located deep within the cerebral hemispheres, including the globus pallidus. The corpus striatum consists of 2 of the basal ganglia, the caudate and lentiform nuclei. The frontal lobe forms the anterior portion of each cerebral hemisphere. The temporal lobes lie below the frontal lobe on the lateral side of each cerebral hemisphere. The parietal lobe forms the superior portion of the cerebrum, lying posterior to the frontal lobe. The occipital lobe forms the posterior portion of each cerebral hemisphere. The ventricles are a series of interconnected cavities of the brain and are continuous with the central canal of the spinal cord, which are filled with the cerebrospinal fluid. The cerebellum is the second largest portion of the brain, located below the occipital lobe and behind the brain stem. The brain stem connects the upper end of the spinal cord with the cerebrum. It contains the pons, cerebral peduncle, medulla oblongata, and midbrain. The tapetum is a layer of fibers from the corpus callosum forming the roof and lateral walls of the lateral ventricles.

PHYSIOLOGY OF THE BRAIN — The cerebrum, including its lobes and cerebral cortex, is concerned with the higher brain functions, such as memory, thought, reasoning, and voluntary muscle control. The basal ganglia function as relay stations for motor impulses. The thalamus functions as a central relay station for sensory impulses. The hypothalamus functions to control homeostasis by regulation of the heart rate, arterial blood pressure, body temperature, body weight, and sleep. The ventricles are filled by continuously replaced cerebrospinal fluid which serves to protect the brain by absorbing shocks and removing any waste substances. It also provides a stable ionic concentration in the central nervous system, which is important for maximum nerve impulse transfers. The cerebellum functions primarily as a reflex center in the coordination of skeletal muscle movements and the maintenance of equilibrium. The pons transmits impulses between the cerebrum and other parts of the nervous system and contains centers that help to regulate the rate and depth of breathing. The medulla oblongata transmits all ascending and descending impulses, and contains several vital and nonvital reflex centers. The midbrain contains reflex centers associated with eye and head movements.

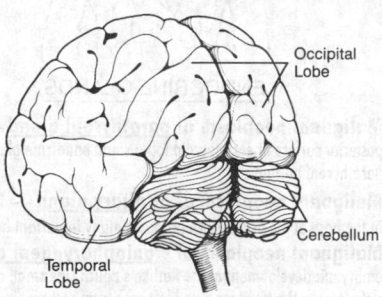

BRAIN — POSTERIOR VIEW

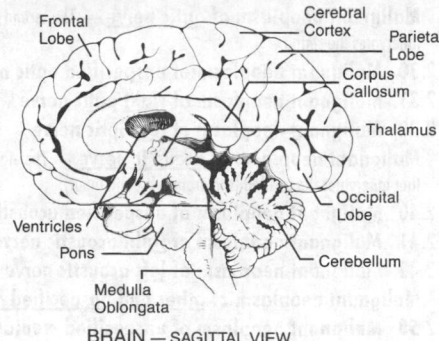

BRAIN — SAGITTAL VIEW

CC **C71.0** **Malignant neoplasm of <u>cerebrum</u>, except lobes and ventricles**
Malignant neoplasm of supratentorial NOS

CC **C71.1** **Malignant neoplasm of <u>frontal lobe</u>** — The anterior portion of the cerebral hemispheres.

CC **C71.2** **Malignant neoplasm of <u>temporal lobe</u>** — The lower lateral portion of the cerebral hemispheres.

CC **C71.3** **Malignant neoplasm of <u>parietal lobe</u>** — The upper central portion of the cerebral hemispheres.

CC **C71.4** **Malignant neoplasm of <u>occipital lobe</u>** — The posterior portion of the cerebral hemispheres.

CC **C71.5** **Malignant neoplasm of <u>cerebral ventricle</u>** — The three cavities within the brain that are filled with cerebrospinal fluid, including the two lateral ventricles and the third ventricle.

Excludes 1: *malignant neoplasm of fourth cerebral ventricle (C71.7)*

CC **C71.6** **Malignant neoplasm of <u>cerebellum</u>** — That part of the brain, below the occipital lobe of the cerebrum and posterior to the brain stem, that functions to control the voluntary muscles and coordination.

CC **C71.7** **Malignant neoplasm of <u>brain stem</u>** — The stem-like portion of the brain connecting the cerebrum with the spinal cord.

Malignant neoplasm of fourth cerebral ventricle — The cavity within the brain that is filled with cerebrospinal fluid and located at the base of the brain surrounding the pons.

Infratentorial malignant neoplasm NOS

CC **C71.8** **Malignant neoplasm of <u>overlapping sites</u> of brain**

CC **C71.9** **Malignant neoplasm of brain, unspecified**

C72- **Malignant neoplasm of spinal cord, cranial nerves and other parts of central nervous system** — Any new and abnormal growth of the spinal cord, cranial nerves, and other parts of the central nervous system in which tissue growth is uncontrolled and has the properties of anaplasia, invasion, and metastases.

Excludes 1: *malignant neoplasm of meninges (C70.-)*
malignant neoplasm of peripheral nerves and autonomic nervous system (C47.-)

ANATOMY OF THE NERVOUS SYSTEM, OTHER THAN THE BRAIN — The cranial nerves are the 12 pairs of nerves arising from the brain stem and cerebrum and serving the various organs of the head. The meninges, both cerebral and spinal are the 3 membranes which completely enclose the brain and spinal cord, and contain the cerebrospinal fluid. The spinal cord is the vertebral canal extension of the central nervous system with most of the body's nerves leaving and entering along its length.

PHYSIOLOGY OF THE NERVOUS SYSTEM, OTHER THAN THE BRAIN — The cranial nerves serve the various specific organs of the head, with some being sensory only (olfactory, optic), others are mostly motor (abducens), while most are of mixed sensory and motor nerves. The meninges function to protect the brain and spinal cord from injury and infection, and contain the cerebrospinal fluid. The spinal cord functions to supply the body with 31 pairs of nerves that branch out to serve all the parts of the body below the neck.

CC **C72.0** **Malignant neoplasm of <u>spinal cord</u>** — That part of the central nervous system found in the vertebral column canal which is continuous with the medulla oblongata.

CC **C72.1** **Malignant neoplasm of <u>cauda equina</u>** — The group of spinal nerve roots that extend from the lower part of the spinal cord.

C72.2- **Malignant neoplasm of <u>olfactory nerve</u>** — The first cranial nerve that receives sensory impulses of smell from the nasal cavity.

Malignant neoplasm of olfactory bulb

CC **C72.20** **Malignant neoplasm of unspecified olfactory nerve**

CC **C72.21** **Malignant neoplasm of <u>right</u> olfactory nerve**

CC **C72.22** **Malignant neoplasm of <u>left</u> olfactory nerve**

C
6
9
-
C
7
2

Excludes 1: = NOT CODED HERE! (Do not code both)   *Excludes ❷:* = Not Included Here

C72.3- Malignant neoplasm of <u>optic nerve</u> — The second cranial nerve that innervates the retina.

cc **C72.30** Malignant neoplasm of unspecified optic nerve

cc **C72.31** Malignant neoplasm of <u>right</u> optic nerve

cc **C72.32** Malignant neoplasm of <u>left</u> optic nerve

C72.4- Malignant neoplasm of <u>acoustic nerve</u> — The eighth cranial nerve that innervates the cochlea (the organ of sound input).

cc **C72.40** Malignant neoplasm of unspecified acoustic nerve

cc **C72.41** Malignant neoplasm of <u>right</u> acoustic nerve

cc **C72.42** Malignant neoplasm of <u>left</u> acoustic nerve

C72.5- Malignant neoplasm of <u>other and unspecified cranial nerves</u>

cc **C72.50** Malignant neoplasm of unspecified cranial nerve
   Malignant neoplasm of cranial nerve NOS

cc **C72.59** Malignant neoplasm of other cranial nerves

cc **C72.9-** Malignant neoplasm of central nervous system, unspecified
   Malignant neoplasm of unspecified site of central nervous system
   Malignant neoplasm of nervous system NOS

Malignant neoplasms of thyroid and other endocrine glands (C73-C75)

C73 Malignant neoplasm of <u>thyroid</u> gland — Any new and abnormal growth of the thyroid gland in which tissue growth is uncontrolled and has the properties of anaplasia, invasion, and metastases.

Use additional code to identify any functional activity

ANATOMY OF THE THYROID — The thyroid gland is the bi-lobed endocrine gland of the front of the neck and joined by a narrow isthmus.

PHYSIOLOGY OF THE THYROID — The thyroid gland produces the hormones (thyroxine and triiodothyronine) which help to regulate the metabolic rate of the body.

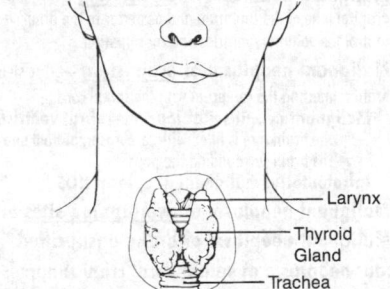

— Larynx
— Thyroid Gland
— Trachea

THYROID GLAND

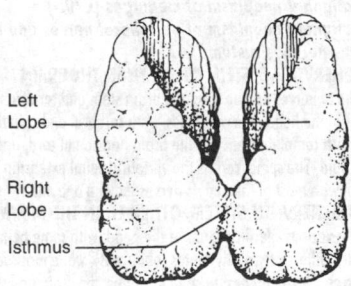

Left Lobe
Right Lobe
Isthmus

THYROID GLAND — ANTERIOR (DETAIL) VIEW

C74- Malignant neoplasm of <u>adrenal</u> gland — Any new and abnormal growth of the adrenal gland in which tissue growth is uncontrolled and has the properties of anaplasia, invasion, and metastases.

ANATOMY OF THE ADRENAL GLAND — The adrenal gland is the pyramid-shaped endocrine gland which sits upon the top of each kidney, and is highly vascular.

PHYSIOLOGY OF THE ADRENAL GLAND — The adrenal gland produces several important hormones, among them: Adrenalin, noradrenalin, aldosterone, cortisol, and some sex hormones.

C74.0- Malignant neoplasm of <u>cortex</u> of adrenal gland — The bulk of the gland covering the medulla that contains the steroid-producing cells.

cc **C74.00** Malignant neoplasm of cortex of unspecified adrenal gland

cc **C74.01** Malignant neoplasm of cortex of <u>right</u> adrenal gland

cc **C74.02** Malignant neoplasm of cortex of <u>left</u> adrenal gland

C74.1- Malignant neoplasm of <u>medulla</u> of adrenal gland — The inner portion of the gland that contains the epinephrine- (adrenaline) and norepinephrine- (noradrenaline) producing cells.

cc **C74.10** Malignant neoplasm of medulla of unspecified adrenal gland

cc **C74.11** Malignant neoplasm of medulla of <u>right</u> adrenal gland

cc **C74.12** Malignant neoplasm of medulla of <u>left</u> adrenal gland

C74.9- Malignant neoplasm of unspecified part of adrenal gland

cc **C74.90** Malignant neoplasm of unspecified part of unspecified adrenal gland

cc **C74.91** Malignant neoplasm of unspecified part of <u>right</u> adrenal gland

cc **C74.92** Malignant neoplasm of unspecified part of <u>left</u> adrenal gland

C75- Malignant neoplasms of other <u>endocrine glands</u> and related structures — Any new and abnormal growth of the other endocrine glands and related structures in which tissue growth is uncontrolled and has the properties of anaplasia, invasion, and metastases.

Excludes 1: malignant carcinoid tumors (C7A.0-)
   malignant neoplasm of adrenal gland (C74.-)
   malignant neoplasm of endocrine pancreas (C25.4)
   malignant neoplasm of islets of Langerhans (C25.4)
   malignant neoplasm of ovary (C56.-)
   malignant neoplasm of testis (C62.-)
   malignant neoplasm of thymus (C37)
   malignant neoplasm of thyroid gland (C73)
   malignant neuroendocrine tumors (C7A.-)

ANATOMY OF THE PARATHYROID GLANDS, PITUITARY GLAND, PINEAL GLAND, AND THE CAROTID AND AORTIC BODIES — The parathyroid glands are 4 small glands, 2 on the posterior surface of the thyroid lobes. The pituitary gland is the small endocrine gland located in the sella turcica of the sphenoid bone at the base of the cerebrum, and is about 0.4 inches (1 cm) in diameter. The pineal gland is the small endocrine gland located below the posterior base of the corpus callosum, and attached to the upper portion of the thalamus. The carotid bodies are small neurovascular structures at the carotid bifurcation. The aortic body is the small neurovascular structure located at the aortic arch.

PHYSIOLOGY OF THE PARATHYROID GLANDS, PITUITARY GLAND, PINEAL GLAND, AND THE CAROTID AND AORTIC BODIES — The parathyroid glands secretes one hormone, the parathyroid hormone which causes an increase in the blood calcium level and a decrease in the blood phosphate level. The pituitary gland functions as the central endocrine gland by producing hormones which stimulate many of the other endocrine glands, and has 2 lobes. The anterior lobe (adenohypophysis) produces the growth hormone, prolactin, thyroid-stimulating hormone, follicle-stimulating and luteinizing hormones, and adrenocorticotropic hormone. The posterior lobe (neurohypophysis) secretes the antidiuretic hormone, and oxytocin. The pineal gland produces the hormone melatonin. The aortic body monitors and regulates the reflex respiration.

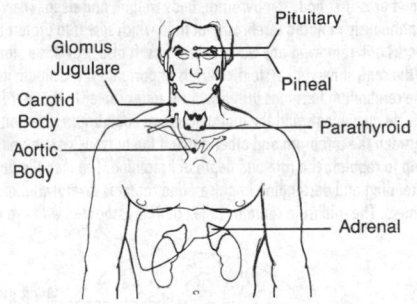

Pituitary
Glomus Jugulare
Carotid Body
Aortic Body
Pineal
Parathyroid
Adrenal

ENDOCRINE GLANDS

cc **C75.0** Malignant neoplasm of <u>parathyroid gland</u> — The four (two on the posterior surface of each thyroid lobe) small endocrine glands which secrete the parathyroid hormone.

cc **C75.1** Malignant neoplasm of <u>pituitary gland</u> — The small endocrine gland at the base of the brain which produces many important hormones.

cc **C75.2** Malignant neoplasm of <u>craniopharyngeal duct</u> — The duct of embryonic development of the Rathke's pouch (the small colloid-filled cysts and clefts next to the pituitary gland left over from embryonic development).

cc **C75.3** Malignant neoplasm of <u>pineal gland</u> — The small endocrine gland below the posterior base of the corpus callosum, which produces the hormone melatonin.

cc **C75.4** Malignant neoplasm of <u>carotid body</u> — The small neurovascular structures at the bifurcation of the carotid arteries which monitor the oxygen content of the blood.

Excludes 1: = NOT CODED HERE! (Do not code both)

Excludes ❷: = Not Included Here

C72-C75

cc **C75.5** Malignant neoplasm of <u>aortic body</u> and other paraganglia —
The aortic body is the small neurovascular structure at the aortic arch which monitors and regulates reflex respiration.

cc **C75.8** Malignant neoplasm with <u>pluriglandular involvement</u>, unspecified

cc **C75.9** Malignant neoplasm of endocrine gland, unspecified

Malignant neuroendocrine tumors (C7A)

C7A- Malignant <u>neuroendocrine tumors</u> — Any new and abnormal growth that arises from endocrine or neuroendocrine cells rather than from where the tumor is located in which the tissue growth is uncontrolled and has the properties of anaplasia, invasion, and metastases (also known as carcinoid tumors, especially when arising in the gastrointestinal tract).
Code also any associated multiple endocrine neoplasia [MEN] syndromes (E31.2-)
Use additional code to identify any associated endocrine syndrome, such as:
Carcinoid syndrome (E34.0)
Excludes ❷: *malignant pancreatic islet cell tumors (C25.4)*
Merkel cell carcinoma (C4A.-)

C7A.0- Malignant <u>carcinoid</u> tumors

cc **C7A.00** Malignant carcinoid tumor of unspecified site

C7A.01- Malignant carcinoid tumors of the <u>small intestine</u>

cc **C7A.010** Malignant carcinoid tumor of the <u>duodenum</u>

cc **C7A.011** Malignant carcinoid tumor of the <u>jejunum</u>

cc **C7A.012** Malignant carcinoid tumor of the <u>ileum</u>

cc **C7A.019** Malignant carcinoid tumor of the small intestine, unspecified portion

C7A.02- Malignant carcinoid tumors of the <u>appendix, large intestine, and rectum</u>

cc **C7A.020** Malignant carcinoid tumor of the <u>appendix</u>

cc **C7A.021** Malignant carcinoid tumor of the <u>cecum</u>

cc **C7A.022** Malignant carcinoid tumor of the <u>ascending colon</u>

cc **C7A.023** Malignant carcinoid tumor of the <u>transverse colon</u>

cc **C7A.024** Malignant carcinoid tumor of the <u>descending colon</u>

cc **C7A.025** Malignant carcinoid tumor of the <u>sigmoid colon</u>

cc **C7A.026** Malignant carcinoid tumor of the <u>rectum</u>

cc **C7A.029** Malignant carcinoid tumor of the large intestine, unspecified portion
Malignant carcinoid tumor of the colon NOS

C7A.09- Malignant <u>carcinoid</u> tumors of other sites

cc **C7A.090** Malignant carcinoid tumor of the <u>bronchus and lung</u>

cc **C7A.091** Malignant carcinoid tumor of the <u>thymus</u>

cc **C7A.092** Malignant carcinoid tumor of the <u>stomach</u>

cc **C7A.093** Malignant carcinoid tumor of the <u>kidney</u>

cc **C7A.094** Malignant carcinoid tumor of the foregut, unspecified

cc **C7A.095** Malignant carcinoid tumor of the midgut, unspecified

cc **C7A.096** Malignant carcinoid tumor of the hindgut, unspecified

cc **C7A.098** Malignant carcinoid tumors of other sites

cc **C7A.1** Malignant <u>poorly differentiated</u> neuroendocrine tumors
High grade neuroendocrine carcinoma, any site
Malignant poorly differentiated neuroendocrine carcinoma, any site
Malignant poorly differentiated neuroendocrine tumor NOS

cc **C7A.8** Other malignant neuroendocrine tumors

Secondary neuroendocrine tumors (C7B)

C7B- <u>Secondary neuroendocrine tumors</u> — The migration of malignant neuroendocrine cells from an original (primary) site to other sites in the body.
Use additional code to identify any functional activity

C7B.0- <u>Secondary carcinoid</u> tumors

C7B.00 Secondary carcinoid tumors, unspecified site

cc **C7B.01** Secondary carcinoid tumors of <u>distant lymph nodes</u>

cc **C7B.02** Secondary carcinoid tumors of <u>liver</u>

cc **C7B.03** Secondary carcinoid tumors of <u>bone</u>

cc **C7B.04** Secondary carcinoid tumors of <u>peritoneum</u>
Mesentary metastasis of carcinoid tumor

cc **C7B.09** Secondary carcinoid tumors of other sites

C7B.1 <u>Secondary Merkel cell</u> carcinoma — The migration of malignant Merkel cell carcinoma cells from an original (primary) site to other sites in the body.
Merkel cell carcinoma nodal presentation
Merkel cell carcinoma visceral metastatic presentation

cc **C7B.8** Other secondary neuroendocrine tumors

Malignant neoplasms of ill-defined, other secondary and unspecified sites (C76-C80)

C76- Malignant neoplasm of other and ill-defined sites — Any new and abnormal growth of the other and ill-defined sites in which tissue growth is uncontrolled and has the properties of anaplasia, invasion, and metastases.
Excludes 1: *malignant neoplasm of female genitourinary tract NOS (C57.9)*
malignant neoplasm of male genitourinary tract NOS (C63.9)
malignant neoplasm of lymphoid, hematopoietic and related tissue (C81-C96)
malignant neoplasm of skin (C44.-)
malignant neoplasm of unspecified site NOS (C80.1)

C76.0 Malignant neoplasm of head, face and neck
Malignant neoplasm of cheek NOS
Malignant neoplasm of nose NOS

C76.1 Malignant neoplasm of thorax
Intrathoracic malignant neoplasm NOS
Malignant neoplasm of axilla NOS
Thoracic malignant neoplasm NOS

C76.2 Malignant neoplasm of abdomen

C76.3 Malignant neoplasm of pelvis
Malignant neoplasm of groin NOS
Malignant neoplasm of sites overlapping systems within the pelvis
Rectovaginal (septum) malignant neoplasm
Rectovesical (septum) malignant neoplasm

C76.4- Malignant neoplasm of <u>upper limb</u>

C76.40 Malignant neoplasm of unspecified upper limb

C76.41 Malignant neoplasm of <u>right</u> upper limb

C76.42 Malignant neoplasm of <u>left</u> upper limb

C76.5- Malignant neoplasm of <u>lower limb</u>

C76.50 Malignant neoplasm of unspecified lower limb

C76.51 Malignant neoplasm of <u>right</u> lower limb

C76.52 Malignant neoplasm of <u>left</u> lower limb

C76.8 Malignant neoplasm of other specified ill-defined sites
Malignant neoplasm of overlapping ill-defined sites

C 7 5 - C 7 6

C77- Secondary and unspecified malignant neoplasm of lymph nodes — The migration of malignant cells from an original (primary) site to any of the lymph nodes.

> Excludes 1:   malignant neoplasm of lymph nodes, specified as primary (C81-C86, C88, C96.-)
> mesentary metastasis of carcinoid tumor (C7B.04)
> secondary carcinoid tumors of distant lymph nodes (C7B.01)

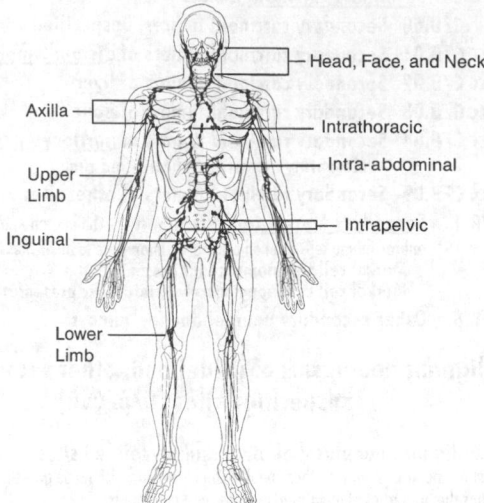

Head, Face, and Neck
Axilla
Intrathoracic
Intra-abdominal
Upper Limb
Intrapelvic
Inguinal
Lower Limb

LYMPH NODES

cc **C77.0** Secondary and unspecified malignant neoplasm of lymph nodes of head, face and neck
Secondary and unspecified malignant neoplasm of supraclavicular lymph nodes

cc **C77.1** Secondary and unspecified malignant neoplasm of intrathoracic lymph nodes

cc **C77.2** Secondary and unspecified malignant neoplasm of intra-abdominal lymph nodes

cc **C77.3** Secondary and unspecified malignant neoplasm of axilla and upper limb lymph nodes
Secondary and unspecified malignant neoplasm of pectoral lymph nodes

cc **C77.4** Secondary and unspecified malignant neoplasm of inguinal and lower limb lymph nodes

cc **C77.5** Secondary and unspecified malignant neoplasm of intrapelvic lymph nodes

cc **C77.8** Secondary and unspecified malignant neoplasm of lymph nodes of multiple regions

cc **C77.9** Secondary and unspecified malignant neoplasm of lymph node, unspecified

C78- Secondary malignant neoplasm of respiratory and digestive organs — The migration of malignant cells from an original (primary) site to the tissues of the respiratory and digestive organs.

> Excludes 1:   secondary carcinoid tumors of liver (C7B.02)
> secondary carcinoid tumors of peritoneum (C7B.04)
> Excludes ❷: lymph node metastases (C77.0)

C78.0- Secondary malignant neoplasm of lung

cc **C78.00** Secondary malignant neoplasm of unspecified lung

cc **C78.01** Secondary malignant neoplasm of right lung

cc **C78.02** Secondary malignant neoplasm of left lung

cc **C78.1** Secondary malignant neoplasm of mediastinum

cc **C78.2** Secondary malignant neoplasm of pleura

C78.3- Secondary malignant neoplasm of other and unspecified respiratory organs

cc **C78.30** Secondary malignant neoplasm of unspecified respiratory organ

cc **C78.39** Secondary malignant neoplasm of other respiratory organs

cc **C78.4** Secondary malignant neoplasm of small intestine

cc **C78.5** Secondary malignant neoplasm of large intestine and rectum

cc **C78.6** Secondary malignant neoplasm of retroperitoneum and peritoneum

cc **C78.7** Secondary malignant neoplasm of liver and intrahepatic bile duct

C78.8- Secondary malignant neoplasm of other and unspecified digestive organs

cc **C78.80** Secondary malignant neoplasm of unspecified digestive organ

cc **C78.89** Secondary malignant neoplasm of other digestive organs
Code also exocrine pancreatic insufficiency (K86.81)

C79- Secondary malignant neoplasm of other and unspecified sites — The migration of malignant cells from an original (primary) site to other tissues.

> Excludes 1:   secondary carcinoid tumors (C7B.-)
> secondary neuroendocrine tumors (C7B.-)
> Excludes ❷: lymph node metastases (C77.0)

C79.0- Secondary malignant neoplasm of kidney and renal pelvis

cc **C79.00** Secondary malignant neoplasm of unspecified kidney and renal pelvis

cc **C79.01** Secondary malignant neoplasm of right kidney and renal pelvis

cc **C79.02** Secondary malignant neoplasm of left kidney and renal pelvis

C79.1- Secondary malignant neoplasm of bladder and other and unspecified urinary organs

cc **C79.10** Secondary malignant neoplasm of unspecified urinary organs

cc **C79.11** Secondary malignant neoplasm of bladder

cc **C79.19** Secondary malignant neoplasm of other urinary organs

cc **C79.2** Secondary malignant neoplasm of skin
> Excludes 1:   secondary Merkel cell carcinoma (C7B.1)

C79.3- Secondary malignant neoplasm of brain and cerebral meninges

cc **C79.31** Secondary malignant neoplasm of brain

cc **C79.32** Secondary malignant neoplasm of cerebral meninges

C79.4- Secondary malignant neoplasm of other and unspecified parts of nervous system

cc **C79.40** Secondary malignant neoplasm of unspecified part of nervous system

cc **C79.49** Secondary malignant neoplasm of other parts of nervous system

C79.5- Secondary malignant neoplasm of bone and bone marrow
> Excludes 1:   secondary carcinoid tumors of bone (C7B.03)

cc **C79.51** Secondary malignant neoplasm of bone

cc **C79.52** Secondary malignant neoplasm of bone marrow

C79.6- Secondary malignant neoplasm of ovary

cc **C79.60** Secondary malignant neoplasm of unspecified ovary — [♀]

cc **C79.61** Secondary malignant neoplasm of right ovary — [♀]

cc **C79.62** Secondary malignant neoplasm of left ovary — [♀]

C79.7- Secondary malignant neoplasm of adrenal gland

cc **C79.70** Secondary malignant neoplasm of unspecified adrenal gland

cc **C79.71** Secondary malignant neoplasm of right adrenal gland

cc **C79.72** Secondary malignant neoplasm of left adrenal gland

C79.8- Secondary malignant neoplasm of other specified sites

cc **C79.81** Secondary malignant neoplasm of breast

cc **C79.82** Secondary malignant neoplasm of genital organs

cc **C79.89** Secondary malignant neoplasm of other specified sites

cc **C79.9** Secondary malignant neoplasm of unspecified site
Metastatic cancer NOS
Metastatic disease NOS
> Excludes 1:   carcinomatosis NOS (C80.0)
> generalized cancer NOS (C80.0)
> malignant (primary) neoplasm of unspecified site (C80.1)

Excludes 1: = NOT CODED HERE! (Do not code both)

Excludes ❷: = Not Included Here

C80- **Malignant neoplasm <u>without specification of site</u>** — Any new and abnormal growth of an unspecified site in which the tissue growth has the properties of anaplasia, invasion, and metastases.
    Excludes 1:   *malignant carcinoid tumor of unspecified site (C7A.00)*
               malignant neoplasm of specified multiple sites — code to each site

cc **C80.0** **<u>Disseminated</u> malignant neoplasm, unspecified**
    Carcinomatosis NOS
    Generalized cancer, unspecified site (primary) (secondary)
    Generalized malignancy, unspecified site (primary) (secondary)

C80.1 **Malignant (primary) neoplasm, unspecified**
    Cancer NOS
    Cancer unspecified site (primary)
    Carcinoma unspecified site (primary)
    Malignancy unspecified site (primary)
    Excludes 1:   *secondary malignant neoplasm of unspecified site (C79.9)*

cc **C80.2** **Malignant neoplasm associated with <u>transplanted organ</u>** —
    [Unacceptable PDX]
    Code first complication of transplanted organ (T86.-)
    Use additional code to identify the specific malignancy

Malignant neoplasms of lymphoid, hematopoietic and related tissue (C81-C96)

    Excludes ❷: *Kaposi's sarcoma of lymph nodes (C46.3)*
                  secondary and unspecified neoplasm of lymph nodes (C77.-)
                  secondary neoplasm of bone marrow (C79.52)
                  secondary neoplasm of spleen (C78.89)

C81- **<u>Hodgkin lymphoma</u>** — A malignant lymphoma (a malignancy that starts in the white blood cells called lymphocytes) of the lymphatic system (lymph, lymph nodes, lymph vessels) characterized by the histologic identification of Reed-Stemberg cells.
    Excludes 1:   *personal history of Hodgkin lymphoma (Z85.71)*

C81.0- **<u>Nodular lymphocyte predominant</u> Hodgkin lymphoma** — A form marked by large cell variants of Reed-Stemberg cells called popcorn cells.

cc **C81.00** **Nodular lymphocyte predominant Hodgkin lymphoma, unspecified site**

cc **C81.01** **Nodular lymphocyte predominant Hodgkin lymphoma, lymph nodes of <u>head, face, and neck</u>**

cc **C81.02** **Nodular lymphocyte predominant Hodgkin lymphoma, <u>intrathoracic</u> lymph nodes**

cc **C81.03** **Nodular lymphocyte predominant Hodgkin lymphoma, <u>intra-abdominal</u> lymph nodes**

cc **C81.04** **Nodular lymphocyte predominant Hodgkin lymphoma, lymph nodes of <u>axilla and upper limb</u>**

cc **C81.05** **Nodular lymphocyte predominant Hodgkin lymphoma, lymph nodes of <u>inguinal region and lower limb</u>**

cc **C81.06** **Nodular lymphocyte predominant Hodgkin lymphoma, <u>intrapelvic</u> lymph nodes**

cc **C81.07** **Nodular lymphocyte predominant Hodgkin lymphoma, <u>spleen</u>**

cc **C81.08** **Nodular lymphocyte predominant Hodgkin lymphoma, lymph nodes of <u>multiple sites</u>**

cc **C81.09** **Nodular lymphocyte predominant Hodgkin lymphoma, <u>extranodal and solid organ sites</u>**

C81.1- **<u>Nodular sclerosis</u> Hodgkin lymphoma** — A form marked by large tumor nodules with extensive scar tissue and lacunar cells.
    Nodular sclerosis classical Hodgkin lymphoma

cc **C81.10** **Nodular sclerosis Hodgkin lymphoma, unspecified site**

cc **C81.11** **Nodular sclerosis Hodgkin lymphoma, lymph nodes of <u>head, face, and neck</u>**

cc **C81.12** **Nodular sclerosis Hodgkin lymphoma, <u>intrathoracic</u> lymph nodes**

cc **C81.13** **Nodular sclerosis Hodgkin lymphoma, <u>intra-abdominal</u> lymph nodes**

cc **C81.14** **Nodular sclerosis Hodgkin lymphoma, lymph nodes of <u>axilla and upper limb</u>**

cc **C81.15** **Nodular sclerosis Hodgkin lymphoma, lymph nodes of <u>inguinal region and lower limb</u>**

cc **C81.16** **Nodular sclerosis Hodgkin lymphoma, <u>intrapelvic</u> lymph nodes**

cc **C81.17** **Nodular sclerosis Hodgkin lymphoma, <u>spleen</u>**

cc **C81.18** **Nodular sclerosis Hodgkin lymphoma, lymph nodes of <u>multiple sites</u>**

cc **C81.19** **Nodular sclerosis Hodgkin lymphoma, <u>extranodal and solid organ sites</u>**

C81.2- **<u>Mixed cellularity</u> Hodgkin lymphoma** — A form marked by many Reed-Stemberg cells and the presence of several other types of cells.
    Mixed cellularity classical Hodgkin lymphoma

cc **C81.20** **Mixed cellularity Hodgkin lymphoma, unspecified site**

cc **C81.21** **Mixed cellularity Hodgkin lymphoma, lymph nodes of <u>head, face, and neck</u>**

cc **C81.22** **Mixed cellularity Hodgkin lymphoma, <u>intrathoracic</u> lymph nodes**

cc **C81.23** **Mixed cellularity Hodgkin lymphoma, <u>intra-abdominal</u> lymph nodes**

cc **C81.24** **Mixed cellularity Hodgkin lymphoma, lymph nodes of <u>axilla and upper limb</u>**

cc **C81.25** **Mixed cellularity Hodgkin lymphoma, lymph nodes of <u>inguinal region and lower limb</u>**

cc **C81.26** **Mixed cellularity Hodgkin lymphoma, <u>intrapelvic</u> lymph nodes**

cc **C81.27** **Mixed cellularity Hodgkin lymphoma, <u>spleen</u>**

cc **C81.28** **Mixed cellularity Hodgkin lymphoma, lymph nodes of <u>multiple sites</u>**

cc **C81.29** **Mixed cellularity Hodgkin lymphoma, <u>extranodal and solid organ sites</u>**

C81.3- **<u>Lymphocyte depleted</u> Hodgkin lymphoma** — A form marked by an abundance of Reed-Stemberg cells and few normal cells.
    Lymphocyte depleted classical Hodgkin lymphoma

cc **C81.30** **Lymphocyte depleted Hodgkin lymphoma, unspecified site**

cc **C81.31** **Lymphocyte depleted Hodgkin lymphoma, lymph nodes of <u>head, face, and neck</u>**

cc **C81.32** **Lymphocyte depleted Hodgkin lymphoma, <u>intrathoracic</u> lymph nodes**

cc **C81.33** **Lymphocyte depleted Hodgkin lymphoma, <u>intra-abdominal</u> lymph nodes**

cc **C81.34** **Lymphocyte depleted Hodgkin lymphoma, lymph nodes of <u>axilla and upper limb</u>**

cc **C81.35** **Lymphocyte depleted Hodgkin lymphoma, lymph nodes of <u>inguinal region and lower limb</u>**

cc **C81.36** **Lymphocyte depleted Hodgkin lymphoma, <u>Intrapelvic</u> lymph nodes**

cc **C81.37** **Lymphocyte depleted Hodgkin lymphoma, <u>spleen</u>**

cc **C81.38** **Lymphocyte depleted Hodgkin lymphoma, lymph nodes of <u>multiple sites</u>**

cc **C81.39** **Lymphocyte depleted Hodgkin lymphoma, <u>extranodal and solid organ sites</u>**

C81.4- **<u>Lymphocyte-rich</u> Hodgkin lymphoma** — A form marked by an abundance of normal-appearing lymphocytes and classic Reed-Stemberg cells.
    Excludes 1:   *nodular lymphocyte predominant Hodgkin lymphoma (C81.0-)*
    Lymphocyte-rich classical Hodgkin lymphoma

cc **C81.40** **Lymphocyte-rich Hodgkin lymphoma, unspecified site**

cc **C81.41** **Lymphocyte-rich Hodgkin lymphoma, lymph nodes of <u>head, face, and neck</u>**

cc **C81.42** **Lymphocyte-rich Hodgkin lymphoma, <u>intrathoracic</u> lymph nodes**

cc **C81.43** **Lymphocyte-rich Hodgkin lymphoma, <u>intra-abdominal</u> lymph nodes**

cc **C81.44** **Lymphocyte-rich Hodgkin lymphoma, lymph nodes of <u>axilla and upper limb</u>**

cc **C81.45** **Lymphocyte-rich Hodgkin lymphoma, lymph nodes of <u>inguinal region and lower limb</u>**

cc **C81.46** **Lymphocyte-rich Hodgkin lymphoma, <u>intrapelvic</u> lymph nodes**

cc **C81.47** **Lymphocyte-rich Hodgkin lymphoma, <u>spleen</u>**

cc **C81.48** **Lymphocyte-rich Hodgkin lymphoma, lymph nodes of <u>multiple sites</u>**

cc **C81.49** **Lymphocyte-rich Hodgkin lymphoma, <u>extranodal and solid organ sites</u>**

C80 - C81

C81.7- <u>Other</u> Hodgkin lymphoma
  Classical Hodgkin lymphoma NOS
  Other classical Hodgkin lymphoma
  cc **C81.70** Other Hodgkin lymphoma, unspecified site
  cc **C81.71** Other Hodgkin lymphoma, lymph nodes of <u>head, face, and neck</u>
  cc **C81.72** Other Hodgkin lymphoma, <u>intrathoracic</u> lymph nodes
  cc **C81.73** Other Hodgkin lymphoma, <u>intra-abdominal</u> lymph nodes
  cc **C81.74** Other Hodgkin lymphoma, lymph nodes of <u>axilla and upper limb</u>
  cc **C81.75** Other Hodgkin lymphoma, lymph nodes of <u>inguinal region and lower limb</u>
  cc **C81.76** Other Hodgkin lymphoma, <u>intrapelvic</u> lymph nodes
  cc **C81.77** Other Hodgkin lymphoma, <u>spleen</u>
  cc **C81.78** Other Hodgkin lymphoma, lymph nodes of <u>multiple sites</u>
  cc **C81.79** Other Hodgkin lymphoma, <u>extranodal and solid organ sites</u>

C81.9- Hodgkin lymphoma, <u>unspecified</u>
  cc **C81.90** Hodgkin lymphoma, unspecified, unspecified site
  cc **C81.91** Hodgkin lymphoma, unspecified, lymph nodes of <u>head, face, and neck</u>
  cc **C81.92** Hodgkin lymphoma, unspecified, <u>intrathoracic</u> lymph nodes
  cc **C81.93** Hodgkin lymphoma, unspecified, <u>intra-abdominal</u> lymph nodes
  cc **C81.94** Hodgkin lymphoma, unspecified, lymph nodes of <u>axilla and upper limb</u>
  cc **C81.95** Hodgkin lymphoma, unspecified, lymph nodes of <u>inguinal region and lower limb</u>
  cc **C81.96** Hodgkin lymphoma, unspecified, <u>intrapelvic</u> lymph nodes
  cc **C81.97** Hodgkin lymphoma, unspecified, <u>spleen</u>
  cc **C81.98** Hodgkin lymphoma, unspecified, lymph nodes of <u>multiple sites</u>
  cc **C81.99** Hodgkin lymphoma, unspecified, <u>extranodal and solid organ sites</u>

C82- <u>Follicular</u> lymphoma — A (non-Hodgkin lymphoma) lymphoma characterized by the histologic identification of certain follicle center B-cell lymphocytes, called centrocytes (small cells) and centroblasts (large cells). Grading of follicular lymphoma is based on various morphological criteria, most commonly by the number of abnormal cells detected under a high-power field microscope.
  Includes: Follicular lymphoma with or without diffuse areas
  Excludes 1: *mature T/NK-cell lymphomas (C84.-)*
      personal history of non-Hodgkin lymphoma (Z85.72)

C82.0- Follicular lymphoma <u>grade I</u>
  cc **C82.00** Follicular lymphoma grade I, unspecified site
  cc **C82.01** Follicular lymphoma grade I, lymph nodes of <u>head, face, and neck</u>
  cc **C82.02** Follicular lymphoma grade I, <u>intrathoracic</u> lymph nodes
  cc **C82.03** Follicular lymphoma grade I, <u>intra-abdominal</u> lymph nodes
  cc **C82.04** Follicular lymphoma grade I, lymph nodes of <u>axilla and upper limb</u>
  cc **C82.05** Follicular lymphoma grade I, lymph nodes of <u>inguinal region and lower limb</u>
  cc **C82.06** Follicular lymphoma grade I, <u>intrapelvic</u> lymph nodes
  cc **C82.07** Follicular lymphoma grade I, <u>spleen</u>
  cc **C82.08** Follicular lymphoma grade I, lymph nodes of <u>multiple sites</u>
  cc **C82.09** Follicular lymphoma grade I, <u>extranodal and solid organ sites</u>

C82.1- Follicular lymphoma <u>grade II</u>
  cc **C82.10** Follicular lymphoma grade II, unspecified site
  cc **C82.11** Follicular lymphoma grade II, lymph nodes of <u>head, face, and neck</u>
  cc **C82.12** Follicular lymphoma grade II, <u>intrathoracic</u> lymph nodes
  cc **C82.13** Follicular lymphoma grade II, <u>intra-abdominal</u> lymph nodes
  cc **C82.14** Follicular lymphoma grade II, lymph nodes of <u>axilla and upper limb</u>

cc **C82.15** Follicular lymphoma grade II, lymph nodes of <u>inguinal region and lower limb</u>
cc **C82.16** Follicular lymphoma grade II, <u>intrapelvic</u> lymph nodes
cc **C82.17** Follicular lymphoma grade II, <u>spleen</u>
cc **C82.18** Follicular lymphoma grade II, lymph nodes of <u>multiple sites</u>
cc **C82.19** Follicular lymphoma grade II, <u>extranodal and solid organ sites</u>

C82.2- Follicular lymphoma <u>grade III, unspecified</u>
  cc **C82.20** Follicular lymphoma grade III, unspecified, unspecified site
  cc **C82.21** Follicular lymphoma grade III, unspecified, lymph nodes of <u>head, face, and neck</u>
  cc **C82.22** Follicular lymphoma grade III, unspecified, <u>intrathoracic</u> lymph nodes
  cc **C82.23** Follicular lymphoma grade III, unspecified, <u>intra-abdominal</u> lymph nodes
  cc **C82.24** Follicular lymphoma grade III, unspecified, lymph nodes of <u>axilla and upper limb</u>
  cc **C82.25** Follicular lymphoma grade III, unspecified, lymph nodes of <u>inguinal region and lower limb</u>
  cc **C82.26** Follicular lymphoma grade III, unspecified, <u>intrapelvic</u> lymph nodes
  cc **C82.27** Follicular lymphoma grade III, unspecified, <u>spleen</u>
  cc **C82.28** Follicular lymphoma grade III, unspecified, lymph nodes of <u>multiple sites</u>
  cc **C82.29** Follicular lymphoma grade III, unspecified, <u>extranodal and solid organ sites</u>

C82.3- Follicular lymphoma <u>grade IIIa</u>
  cc **C82.30** Follicular lymphoma grade IIIa, unspecified site
  cc **C82.31** Follicular lymphoma grade IIIa, lymph nodes of <u>head, face, and neck</u>
  cc **C82.32** Follicular lymphoma grade IIIa, <u>intrathoracic</u> lymph nodes
  cc **C82.33** Follicular lymphoma grade IIIa, <u>intra-abdominal</u> lymph nodes
  cc **C82.34** Follicular lymphoma grade IIIa, lymph nodes of <u>axilla and upper limb</u>
  cc **C82.35** Follicular lymphoma grade IIIa, lymph nodes of <u>inguinal region and lower limb</u>
  cc **C82.36** Follicular lymphoma grade IIIa, <u>intrapelvic</u> lymph nodes
  cc **C82.37** Follicular lymphoma grade IIIa, <u>spleen</u>
  cc **C82.38** Follicular lymphoma grade IIIa, lymph nodes of <u>multiple sites</u>
  cc **C82.39** Follicular lymphoma grade IIIa, <u>extranodal and solid organ sites</u>

C82.4- Follicular lymphoma <u>grade IIIb</u>
  cc **C82.40** Follicular lymphoma grade IIIb, unspecified site
  cc **C82.41** Follicular lymphoma grade IIIb, lymph nodes of <u>head, face, and neck</u>
  cc **C82.42** Follicular lymphoma grade IIIb, <u>intrathoracic</u> lymph nodes
  cc **C82.43** Follicular lymphoma grade IIIb, <u>intra-abdominal</u> lymph nodes
  cc **C82.44** Follicular lymphoma grade IIIb, lymph nodes of <u>axilla and upper limb</u>
  cc **C82.45** Follicular lymphoma grade IIIb, lymph nodes of <u>inguinal region and lower limb</u>
  cc **C82.46** Follicular lymphoma grade IIIb, <u>intrapelvic</u> lymph nodes
  cc **C82.47** Follicular lymphoma grade IIIb, <u>spleen</u>
  cc **C82.48** Follicular lymphoma grade IIIb, lymph nodes of <u>multiple sites</u>
  cc **C82.49** Follicular lymphoma grade IIIb, <u>extranodal and solid organ sites</u>

C82.5- <u>Diffuse follicle center</u> lymphoma
  cc **C82.50** Diffuse follicle center lymphoma, unspecified site
  cc **C82.51** Diffuse follicle center lymphoma, lymph nodes of <u>head, face, and neck</u>

cc **C82.52** Diffuse follicle center lymphoma, <u>intrathoracic</u> lymph nodes

cc **C82.53** Diffuse follicle center lymphoma, <u>intra-abdominal</u> lymph nodes

cc **C82.54** Diffuse follicle center lymphoma, lymph nodes of <u>axilla and upper limb</u>

cc **C82.55** Diffuse follicle center lymphoma, lymph nodes of <u>inguinal region and lower limb</u>

cc **C82.56** Diffuse follicle center lymphoma, <u>intrapelvic</u> lymph nodes

cc **C82.57** Diffuse follicle center lymphoma, <u>spleen</u>

cc **C82.58** Diffuse follicle center lymphoma, lymph nodes of <u>multiple sites</u>

cc **C82.59** Diffuse follicle center lymphoma, <u>extranodal and solid organ sites</u>

C82.6- <u>Cutaneous follicle center</u> lymphoma

cc **C82.60** Cutaneous follicle center lymphoma, unspecified site

cc **C82.61** Cutaneous follicle center lymphoma, lymph nodes of <u>head, face, and neck</u>

cc **C82.62** Cutaneous follicle center lymphoma, <u>intrathoracic</u> lymph nodes

cc **C82.63** Cutaneous follicle center lymphoma, <u>intra-abdominal</u> lymph nodes

cc **C82.64** Cutaneous follicle center lymphoma, lymph nodes of <u>axilla and upper limb</u>

cc **C82.65** Cutaneous follicle center lymphoma, lymph nodes of <u>inguinal region and lower limb</u>

cc **C82.66** Cutaneous follicle center lymphoma, intrapelvic lymph nodes

cc **C82.67** Cutaneous follicle center lymphoma, <u>spleen</u>

cc **C82.68** Cutaneous follicle center lymphoma, lymph nodes of <u>multiple sites</u>

cc **C82.69** Cutaneous follicle center lymphoma, <u>extranodal and solid organ sites</u>

C82.8- <u>Other types</u> of follicular lymphoma

cc **C82.80** Other types of follicular lymphoma, unspecified site

cc **C82.81** Other types of follicular lymphoma, lymph nodes of <u>head, face, and neck</u>

cc **C82.82** Other types of follicular lymphoma, <u>intrathoracic</u> lymph nodes

cc **C82.83** Other types of follicular lymphoma, <u>intra-abdominal</u> lymph nodes

cc **C82.84** Other types of follicular lymphoma, lymph nodes of <u>axilla and upper limb</u>

cc **C82.85** Other types of follicular lymphoma, lymph nodes of <u>inguinal region and lower limb</u>

cc **C82.86** Other types of follicular lymphoma, <u>intrapelvic</u> lymph nodes

cc **C82.87** Other types of follicular lymphoma, <u>spleen</u>

cc **C82.88** Other types of follicular lymphoma, lymph nodes of <u>multiple sites</u>

cc **C82.89** Other types of follicular lymphoma, <u>extranodal and solid organ sites</u>

C82.9- Follicular lymphoma, <u>unspecified</u>

cc **C82.90** Follicular lymphoma, unspecified, unspecified site

cc **C82.91** Follicular lymphoma, unspecified, lymph nodes of <u>head, face, and neck</u>

cc **C82.92** Follicular lymphoma, unspecified, <u>intrathoracic</u> lymph nodes

cc **C82.93** Follicular lymphoma, unspecified, <u>intra-abdominal</u> lymph nodes

cc **C82.94** Follicular lymphoma, unspecified, lymph nodes of <u>axilla and upper limb</u>

cc **C82.95** Follicular lymphoma, unspecified, lymph nodes of <u>inguinal region and lower limb</u>

cc **C82.96** Follicular lymphoma, unspecified, <u>intrapelvic</u> lymph nodes

cc **C82.97** Follicular lymphoma, unspecified, <u>spleen</u>

cc **C82.98** Follicular lymphoma, unspecified, lymph nodes of <u>multiple sites</u>

cc **C82.99** Follicular lymphoma, unspecified, <u>extranodal and solid organ sites</u>

C83- <u>Non-follicular</u> lymphoma — A (non-Hodgkin lymphoma) lymphoma characterized by the histologic identification of malignant B-cell lymphocytes.

    Excludes 1:   *personal history of non-Hodgkin lymphoma (Z85.72)*

  C83.0- <u>Small cell</u> B-cell lymphoma
     Lymphoplasmacytic lymphoma
     Nodal marginal zone lymphoma
     Non-leukemic variant of B-CLL
     Splenic marginal zone lymphoma
    Excludes 1:   *chronic lymphocytic leukemia (C91.1)*
                mature T/NK-cell lymphomas (C84.-)
                Waldenström macroglobulinemia (C88.0)

cc **C83.00** Small cell B-cell lymphoma, unspecified site

cc **C83.01** Small cell B-cell lymphoma, lymph nodes of <u>head, face, and neck</u>

cc **C83.02** Small cell B-cell lymphoma, <u>intrathoracic</u> lymph nodes

cc **C83.03** Small cell B-cell lymphoma, <u>intra-abdominal</u> lymph nodes

cc **C83.04** Small cell B-cell lymphoma, lymph nodes of <u>axilla and upper limb</u>

cc **C83.05** Small cell B-cell lymphoma, lymph nodes of <u>inguinal region and lower limb</u>

cc **C83.06** Small cell B-cell lymphoma, intrapelvic lymph nodes

cc **C83.07** Small cell B-cell lymphoma, <u>spleen</u>

cc **C83.08** Small cell B-cell lymphoma, lymph nodes of <u>multiple sites</u>

cc **C83.09** Small cell B-cell lymphoma, <u>extranodal and solid organ sites</u>

  C83.1- <u>Mantle cell</u> lymphoma
     Centrocytic lymphoma
     Malignant lymphomatous polyposis

cc **C83.10** Mantle cell lymphoma, unspecified site

cc **C83.11** Mantle cell lymphoma, lymph nodes of <u>head, face, and neck</u>

cc **C83.12** Mantle cell lymphoma, <u>intrathoracic</u> lymph nodes

cc **C83.13** Mantle cell lymphoma, <u>intra-abdominal</u> lymph nodes

cc **C83.14** Mantle cell lymphoma, lymph nodes of <u>axilla and upper limb</u>

cc **C83.15** Mantle cell lymphoma, lymph nodes of <u>inguinal region and lower limb</u>

cc **C83.16** Mantle cell lymphoma, <u>intrapelvic</u> lymph nodes

cc **C83.17** Mantle cell lymphoma, <u>spleen</u>

cc **C83.18** Mantle cell lymphoma, lymph nodes of <u>multiple sites</u>

cc **C83.19** Mantle cell lymphoma, <u>extranodal and solid organ sites</u>

  C83.3- <u>Diffuse large</u> B-cell lymphoma
     Anaplastic diffuse large B-cell lymphoma
     CD30-positive diffuse large B-cell lymphoma
     Centroblastic diffuse large B-cell lymphoma
     Diffuse large B-cell lymphoma, subtype not specified
     Immunoblastic diffuse large B-cell lymphoma
     Plasmablastic diffuse large B-cell lymphoma
     T-cell rich diffuse large B-cell lymphoma
    Excludes 1:   *mediastinal (thymic) large B-cell lymphoma (C85.2-)*
                mature T/NK-cell lymphomas (C84.-)

cc **C83.30** Diffuse large B-cell lymphoma, unspecified site

cc **C83.31** Diffuse large B-cell lymphoma, lymph nodes of <u>head, face, and neck</u>

cc **C83.32** Diffuse large B-cell lymphoma, <u>intrathoracic</u> lymph nodes

cc **C83.33** Diffuse large B-cell lymphoma, <u>intra-abdominal</u> lymph nodes

cc **C83.34** Diffuse large B-cell lymphoma, lymph nodes of <u>axilla and upper limb</u>

cc **C83.35** Diffuse large B-cell lymphoma, lymph nodes of <u>inguinal region and lower limb</u>

cc **C83.36** Diffuse large B-cell lymphoma, <u>intrapelvic</u> lymph nodes

cc **C83.37** Diffuse large B-cell lymphoma, <u>spleen</u>

cc **C83.38** Diffuse large B-cell lymphoma, lymph nodes of <u>multiple sites</u>

C 8 2 - C 8 3

Excludes 1: = NOT CODED HERE! (Do not code both)   **581**   *Excludes ❷:* = Not Included Here

cc **C83.39** Diffuse large B-cell lymphoma, <u>extranodal and solid organ sites</u>

C83.5- <u>Lymphoblastic</u> (diffuse) lymphoma
B-precursor lymphoma
Lymphoblastic B-cell lymphoma
Lymphoblastic lymphoma NOS
Lymphoblastic T-cell lymphoma
T-precursor lymphoma

cc **C83.50** Lymphoblastic (diffuse) lymphoma, unspecified site

cc **C83.51** Lymphoblastic (diffuse) lymphoma, lymph nodes of <u>head, face, and neck</u>

cc **C83.52** Lymphoblastic (diffuse) lymphoma, <u>intrathoracic</u> lymph nodes

cc **C83.53** Lymphoblastic (diffuse) lymphoma, <u>intra-abdominal</u> lymph nodes

cc **C83.54** Lymphoblastic (diffuse) lymphoma, lymph nodes of <u>axilla and upper limb</u>

cc **C83.55** Lymphoblastic (diffuse) lymphoma, lymph nodes of <u>inguinal region and lower limb</u>

cc **C83.56** Lymphoblastic (diffuse) lymphoma, <u>intrapelvic</u> lymph nodes

cc **C83.57** Lymphoblastic (diffuse) lymphoma, <u>spleen</u>

cc **C83.58** Lymphoblastic (diffuse) lymphoma, lymph nodes of <u>multiple sites</u>

cc **C83.59** Lymphoblastic (diffuse) lymphoma, <u>extranodal and solid organ sites</u>

C83.7- <u>Burkitt</u> lymphoma
Atypical Burkitt lymphoma
Burkitt-like lymphoma
Excludes 1:   mature B-cell leukemia Burkitt type (C91.A-)

cc **C83.70** Burkitt lymphoma, unspecified site

cc **C83.71** Burkitt lymphoma, lymph nodes of <u>head, face, and neck</u>

cc **C83.72** Burkitt lymphoma, <u>intrathoracic</u> lymph nodes

cc **C83.73** Burkitt lymphoma, <u>intra-abdominal</u> lymph nodes

cc **C83.74** Burkitt lymphoma, lymph nodes of <u>axilla and upper limb</u>

cc **C83.75** Burkitt lymphoma, lymph nodes of <u>inguinal region and lower limb</u>

cc **C83.76** Burkitt lymphoma, <u>intrapelvic</u> lymph nodes

cc **C83.77** Burkitt lymphoma, <u>spleen</u>

cc **C83.78** Burkitt lymphoma, lymph nodes of <u>multiple sites</u>

cc **C83.79** Burkitt lymphoma, <u>extranodal and solid organ sites</u>

C83.8- <u>Other non-follicular</u> lymphoma
Intravascular large B-cell lymphoma
Lymphoid granulomatosis
Primary effusion B-cell lymphoma
Excludes 1:   mediastinal (thymic) large B-cell lymphoma (C85.2-)
T-cell rich B-cell lymphoma (C83.3-)

cc **C83.80** Other non-follicular lymphoma, unspecified site

cc **C83.81** Other non-follicular lymphoma, lymph nodes of <u>head, face, and neck</u>

cc **C83.82** Other non-follicular lymphoma, <u>intrathoracic</u> lymph nodes

cc **C83.83** Other non-follicular lymphoma, <u>intra-abdominal</u> lymph nodes

cc **C83.84** Other non-follicular lymphoma, lymph nodes of <u>axilla and upper limb</u>

cc **C83.85** Other non-follicular lymphoma, lymph nodes of <u>inguinal region and lower limb</u>

cc **C83.86** Other non-follicular lymphoma, <u>intrapelvic</u> lymph nodes

cc **C83.87** Other non-follicular lymphoma, <u>spleen</u>

cc **C83.88** Other non-follicular lymphoma, lymph nodes of <u>multiple sites</u>

cc **C83.89** Other non-follicular lymphoma, <u>extranodal and solid organ sites</u>

C83.9- Non-follicular (diffuse) lymphoma, <u>unspecified</u>

cc **C83.90** Non-follicular (diffuse) lymphoma, unspecified, unspecified site

cc **C83.91** Non-follicular (diffuse) lymphoma, unspecified, lymph nodes of <u>head, face, and neck</u>

cc **C83.92** Non-follicular (diffuse) lymphoma, unspecified, <u>intrathoracic</u> lymph nodes

cc **C83.93** Non-follicular (diffuse) lymphoma, unspecified, <u>intra-abdominal</u> lymph nodes

cc **C83.94** Non-follicular (diffuse) lymphoma, unspecified, lymph nodes of <u>axilla and upper limb</u>

cc **C83.95** Non-follicular (diffuse) lymphoma, unspecified, lymph nodes of <u>inguinal region and lower limb</u>

cc **C83.96** Non-follicular (diffuse) lymphoma, unspecified, <u>intrapelvic</u> lymph nodes

cc **C83.97** Non-follicular (diffuse) lymphoma, unspecified, <u>spleen</u>

cc **C83.98** Non-follicular (diffuse) lymphoma, unspecified, lymph nodes of <u>multiple sites</u>

cc **C83.99** Non-follicular (diffuse) lymphoma, unspecified, <u>extranodal and solid organ sites</u>

C84- <u>Mature T/NK-cell</u> lymphomas — A (non-Hodgkin lymphoma) lymphoma characterized by the histologic identification of malignant T- and NK-cell lymphocytes.
Excludes 1:   personal history of non-Hodgkin lymphoma (Z85.72)

C84.0- <u>Mycosis fungoides</u>
Excludes 1:   peripheral T-cell lymphoma, not classified (C84.4-)

cc **C84.00** Mycosis fungoides, unspecified site

cc **C84.01** Mycosis fungoides, lymph nodes of <u>head, face, and neck</u>

cc **C84.02** Mycosis fungoides, <u>intrathoracic</u> lymph nodes

cc **C84.03** Mycosis fungoides, <u>intra-abdominal</u> lymph nodes

cc **C84.04** Mycosis fungoides, lymph nodes of <u>axilla and upper limb</u>

cc **C84.05** Mycosis fungoides, lymph nodes of <u>inguinal region and lower limb</u>

cc **C84.06** Mycosis fungoides, <u>intrapelvic</u> lymph nodes

cc **C84.07** Mycosis fungoides, <u>spleen</u>

cc **C84.08** Mycosis fungoides, lymph nodes of <u>multiple sites</u>

cc **C84.09** Mycosis fungoides, <u>extranodal and solid organ sites</u>

C84.1- <u>Sézary disease</u>

cc **C84.10** Sézary disease, unspecified site

cc **C84.11** Sézary disease, lymph nodes of <u>head, face, and neck</u>

cc **C84.12** Sézary disease, <u>intrathoracic</u> lymph nodes

cc **C84.13** Sézary disease, <u>intra-abdominal</u> lymph nodes

cc **C84.14** Sézary disease, lymph nodes of <u>axilla and upper limb</u>

cc **C84.15** Sézary disease, lymph nodes of <u>inguinal region and lower limb</u>

cc **C84.16** Sézary disease, <u>intrapelvic</u> lymph nodes

cc **C84.17** Sézary disease, <u>spleen</u>

cc **C84.18** Sézary disease, lymph nodes of <u>multiple sites</u>

cc **C84.19** Sézary disease, <u>extranodal and solid organ sites</u>

C84.4- <u>Peripheral T-cell</u> lymphoma, not classified
Lennert's lymphoma
Lymphoepithelioid lymphoma
Mature T-cell lymphoma, not elsewhere classified

cc **C84.40** Peripheral T-cell lymphoma, not classified, unspecified site

cc **C84.41** Peripheral T-cell lymphoma, not classified, lymph nodes of <u>head, face, and neck</u>

cc **C84.42** Peripheral T-cell lymphoma, not classified, <u>intrathoracic</u> lymph nodes

cc **C84.43** Peripheral T-cell lymphoma, not classified, <u>intra-abdominal</u> lymph nodes

cc **C84.44** Peripheral T-cell lymphoma, not classified, lymph nodes of <u>axilla and upper limb</u>

cc **C84.45** Peripheral T-cell lymphoma, not classified, lymph nodes of <u>inguinal region and lower limb</u>

cc **C84.46** Peripheral T-cell lymphoma, not classified, <u>intrapelvic</u> lymph nodes

cc **C84.47** Peripheral T-cell lymphoma, not classified, <u>spleen</u>

cc **C84.48** Peripheral T-cell lymphoma, not classified, lymph nodes of <u>multiple sites</u>

cc **C84.49** Peripheral T-cell lymphoma, not classified, <u>extranodal and solid organ sites</u>

C83 - C84

C84.6- **Anaplastic large cell** lymphoma, ALK-**positive**
    Anaplastic large cell lymphoma, CD30-positive

cc **C84.60** Anaplastic large cell lymphoma, ALK-positive, unspecified site

cc **C84.61** Anaplastic large cell lymphoma, ALK-positive, lymph nodes of <u>head, face, and neck</u>

cc **C84.62** Anaplastic large cell lymphoma, ALK-positive, <u>intrathoracic</u> lymph nodes

cc **C84.63** Anaplastic large cell lymphoma, ALK-positive, <u>intra-abdominal</u> lymph nodes

cc **C84.64** Anaplastic large cell lymphoma, ALK-positive, lymph nodes of <u>axilla and upper limb</u>

cc **C84.65** Anaplastic large cell lymphoma, ALK-positive, lymph nodes of <u>inguinal region and lower limb</u>

cc **C84.66** Anaplastic large cell lymphoma, ALK-positive, <u>intrapelvic</u> lymph nodes

cc **C84.67** Anaplastic large cell lymphoma, ALK-positive, <u>spleen</u>

cc **C84.68** Anaplastic large cell lymphoma, ALK-positive, lymph nodes of <u>multiple sites</u>

cc **C84.69** Anaplastic large cell lymphoma, ALK-positive, <u>extranodal and solid organ sites</u>

C84.7- **Anaplastic large cell** lymphoma, ALK-**negative**
    Excludes 1:   *primary cutaneous CD30-positive T-cell proliferations (C86.6-)*

cc **C84.70** Anaplastic large cell lymphoma, ALK-negative, unspecified site

cc **C84.71** Anaplastic large cell lymphoma, ALK-negative, lymph nodes of <u>head, face, and neck</u>

cc **C84.72** Anaplastic large cell lymphoma, ALK-negative, <u>intrathoracic</u> lymph nodes

cc **C84.73** Anaplastic large cell lymphoma, ALK-negative, <u>intra-abdominal</u> lymph nodes

cc **C84.74** Anaplastic large cell lymphoma, ALK-negative, lymph nodes of <u>axilla and upper limb</u>

cc **C84.75** Anaplastic large cell lymphoma, ALK-negative, lymph nodes of <u>inguinal region and lower limb</u>

cc **C84.76** Anaplastic large cell lymphoma, ALK-negative, <u>intrapelvic</u> lymph nodes

cc **C84.77** Anaplastic large cell lymphoma, ALK-negative, <u>spleen</u>

cc **C84.78** Anaplastic large cell lymphoma, ALK-negative, lymph nodes of <u>multiple sites</u>

cc **C84.79** Anaplastic large cell lymphoma, ALK-negative, <u>extranodal and solid organ sites</u>

C84.A- **Cutaneous T-cell** lymphoma, unspecified

cc **C84.A0** Cutaneous T-cell lymphoma, unspecified, unspecified site

cc **C84.A1** Cutaneous T-cell lymphoma, unspecified lymph nodes of <u>head, face, and neck</u>

cc **C84.A2** Cutaneous T-cell lymphoma, unspecified, <u>intrathoracic</u> lymph nodes

cc **C84.A3** Cutaneous T-cell lymphoma, unspecified, <u>intra-abdominal</u> lymph nodes

cc **C84.A4** Cutaneous T-cell lymphoma, unspecified, lymph nodes of <u>axilla and upper limb</u>

cc **C84.A5** Cutaneous T-cell lymphoma, unspecified, lymph nodes of <u>inguinal region and lower limb</u>

cc **C84.A6** Cutaneous T-cell lymphoma, unspecified, <u>intrapelvic</u> lymph nodes

cc **C84.A7** Cutaneous T-cell lymphoma, unspecified, <u>spleen</u>

cc **C84.A8** Cutaneous T-cell lymphoma, unspecified, lymph nodes of <u>multiple sites</u>

cc **C84.A9** Cutaneous T-cell lymphoma, unspecified, <u>extranodal and solid organ sites</u>

C84.Z- **Other mature T/NK-cell** lymphomas
    Note: If T-cell lineage or involvement is mentioned in conjunction with a specific lymphoma, code to the more specific description.
    Excludes 1:   *angioimmunoblastic T-cell lymphoma (C86.5)*
                  blastic NK-cell lymphoma (C86.4)
                  enteropathy-type T-cell lymphoma (C86.2)
                  extranodal NK-cell lymphoma, nasal type (C86.0)
                  hepatosplenic T-cell lymphoma (C86.1)
                  primary cutaneous CD30-positive T-cell proliferations (C86.6)
                  subcutaneous panniculitis-like T-cell lymphoma (C86.3)
                  T-cell leukemia (C91.1-)

cc **C84.Z0** Other mature T/NK-cell lymphomas, unspecified site

cc **C84.Z1** Other mature T/NK-cell lymphomas, lymph nodes of <u>head, face, and neck</u>

cc **C84.Z2** Other mature T/NK-cell lymphomas, <u>intrathoracic</u> lymph nodes

cc **C84.Z3** Other mature T/NK-cell lymphomas, <u>intra-abdominal</u> lymph nodes

cc **C84.Z4** Other mature T/NK-cell lymphomas, lymph nodes of <u>axilla and upper limb</u>

cc **C84.Z5** Other mature T/NK-cell lymphomas, lymph nodes of <u>inguinal region and lower limb</u>

cc **C84.Z6** Other mature T/NK-cell lymphomas, <u>intrapelvic</u> lymph nodes

cc **C84.Z7** Other mature T/NK-cell lymphomas, <u>spleen</u>

cc **C84.Z8** Other mature T/NK-cell lymphomas, lymph nodes of <u>multiple sites</u>

cc **C84.Z9** Other mature T/NK-cell lymphomas, <u>extranodal and solid organ sites</u>

C84.9- **Mature T/NK-cell lymphomas, <u>unspecified</u>**
    NK/T cell lymphoma NOS
    Excludes 1:   *mature T-cell lymphoma, not elsewhere classified (C84.4-)*

cc **C84.90** Mature T/NK-cell lymphomas, unspecified, unspecified site

cc **C84.91** Mature T/NK-cell lymphomas, unspecified, lymph nodes of <u>head, face, and neck</u>

cc **C84.92** Mature T/NK-cell lymphomas, unspecified, <u>intrathoracic</u> lymph nodes

cc **C84.93** Mature T/NK-cell lymphomas, unspecified, <u>intra-abdominal</u> lymph nodes

cc **C84.94** Mature T/NK-cell lymphomas, unspecified, lymph nodes of <u>axilla and upper limb</u>

cc **C84.95** Mature T/NK-cell lymphomas, unspecified, lymph nodes of <u>inguinal region and lower limb</u>

cc **C84.96** Mature T/NK-cell lymphomas, unspecified, <u>intrapelvic</u> lymph nodes

cc **C84.97** Mature T/NK-cell lymphomas, unspecified, <u>spleen</u>

cc **C84.98** Mature T/NK-cell lymphomas, unspecified, lymph nodes of <u>multiple sites</u>

cc **C84.99** Mature T/NK-cell lymphomas, unspecified, <u>extranodal and solid organ sites</u>

C85- **Other specified and unspecified types of non-Hodgkin** lymphoma
    Excludes 1:   *other specified types of T/NK-cell lymphoma (C86.-)*
                  personal history of non-Hodgkin lymphoma (Z85.72)

C85.1- **Unspecified B-cell** lymphoma
    Note: If B-cell lineage or involvement is mentioned in conjunction with a specific lymphoma, code to the more specific description.

cc **C85.10** Unspecified B-cell lymphoma, unspecified site

cc **C85.11** Unspecified B-cell lymphoma, lymph nodes of <u>head, face, and neck</u>

cc **C85.12** Unspecified B-cell lymphoma, <u>intrathoracic</u> lymph nodes

cc **C85.13** Unspecified B-cell lymphoma, <u>intra-abdominal</u> lymph nodes

cc **C85.14** Unspecified B-cell lymphoma, lymph nodes of <u>axilla and upper limb</u>

cc **C85.15** Unspecified B-cell lymphoma, lymph nodes of <u>inguinal region and lower limb</u>

C84 – C85

Excludes 1: = NOT CODED HERE! (Do not code both)

Excludes ❷: = Not Included Here

cc **C85.16** Unspecified B-cell lymphoma, <u>intrapelvic</u> lymph nodes

cc **C85.17** Unspecified B-cell lymphoma, <u>spleen</u>

cc **C85.18** Unspecified B-cell lymphoma, lymph nodes of <u>multiple sites</u>

cc **C85.19** Unspecified B-cell lymphoma, <u>extranodal and solid organ sites</u>

C85.2- <u>Mediastinal (thymic) large B-cell</u> lymphoma

cc **C85.20** Mediastinal (thymic) large B-cell lymphoma, unspecified site

cc **C85.21** Mediastinal (thymic) large B-cell lymphoma, lymph nodes of <u>head, face, and neck</u>

cc **C85.22** Mediastinal (thymic) large B-cell lymphoma, <u>intrathoracic</u> lymph nodes

cc **C85.23** Mediastinal (thymic) large B-cell lymphoma, <u>intra-abdominal</u> lymph nodes

cc **C85.24** Mediastinal (thymic) large B-cell lymphoma, lymph nodes of <u>axilla and upper limb</u>

cc **C85.25** Mediastinal (thymic) large B-cell lymphoma, lymph nodes of <u>inguinal region and lower limb</u>

cc **C85.26** Mediastinal (thymic) large B-cell lymphoma, <u>intrapelvic</u> lymph nodes

cc **C85.27** Mediastinal (thymic) large B-cell lymphoma, <u>spleen</u>

cc **C85.28** Mediastinal (thymic) large B-cell lymphoma, lymph nodes of <u>multiple sites</u>

cc **C85.29** Mediastinal (thymic) large B-cell lymphoma, <u>extranodal and solid organ sites</u>

C85.8- <u>Other specified types of non-Hodgkin</u> lymphoma

cc **C85.80** Other specified types of non-Hodgkin lymphoma, unspecified site

cc **C85.81** Other specified types of non-Hodgkin lymphoma, lymph nodes of <u>head, face, and neck</u>

cc **C85.82** Other specified types of non-Hodgkin lymphoma, <u>intrathoracic</u> lymph nodes

cc **C85.83** Other specified types of non-Hodgkin lymphoma, <u>intra-abdominal</u> lymph nodes

cc **C85.84** Other specified types of non-Hodgkin lymphoma, lymph nodes of <u>axilla and upper limb</u>

cc **C85.85** Other specified types of non-Hodgkin lymphoma, lymph nodes of <u>inguinal region and lower limb</u>

cc **C85.86** Other specified types of non-Hodgkin lymphoma, <u>intrapelvic</u> lymph nodes

cc **C85.87** Other specified types of non-Hodgkin lymphoma, <u>spleen</u>

cc **C85.88** Other specified types of non-Hodgkin lymphoma, lymph nodes of <u>multiple sites</u>

cc **C85.89** Other specified types of non-Hodgkin lymphoma, <u>extranodal and solid organ sites</u>

C85.9- Non-Hodgkin lymphoma, <u>unspecified</u>
Lymphoma NOS
Malignant lymphoma NOS
Non-Hodgkin lymphoma NOS

cc **C85.90** Non-Hodgkin lymphoma, unspecified, unspecified site

cc **C85.91** Non-Hodgkin lymphoma, unspecified, lymph nodes of <u>head, face, and neck</u>

cc **C85.92** Non-Hodgkin lymphoma, unspecified, <u>intrathoracic</u> lymph nodes

cc **C85.93** Non-Hodgkin lymphoma, unspecified, <u>intra-abdominal</u> lymph nodes

cc **C85.94** Non-Hodgkin lymphoma, unspecified, lymph nodes of <u>axilla and upper limb</u>

cc **C85.95** Non-Hodgkin lymphoma, unspecified, lymph nodes of <u>inguinal region and lower limb</u>

cc **C85.96** Non-Hodgkin lymphoma, unspecified, <u>intrapelvic</u> lymph nodes

cc **C85.97** Non-Hodgkin lymphoma, unspecified, <u>spleen</u>

cc **C85.98** Non-Hodgkin lymphoma, unspecified, lymph nodes of <u>multiple sites</u>

cc **C85.99** Non-Hodgkin lymphoma, unspecified, <u>extranodal and solid organ sites</u>

C86- <u>Other specified types of T/NK-cell</u> lymphoma
Excludes 1: *anaplastic large cell lymphoma, ALK negative (C84.7-)*
anaplastic large cell lymphoma, ALK positive (C84.6-)
mature T/NK-cell lymphomas (C84.-)
other specified types of non-Hodgkin lymphoma (C85.8-)

cc **C86.0** <u>Extranodal NK/T-cell</u> lymphoma, nasal type

cc **C86.1** <u>Hepatosplenic</u> T-cell lymphoma
Alpha-beta and gamma delta types

cc **C86.2** <u>Enteropathy-type</u> (intestinal) T-cell lymphoma
Enteropathy associated T-cell lymphoma

cc **C86.3** <u>Subcutaneous panniculitis-like</u> T-cell lymphoma

cc **C86.4** <u>Blastic NK-cell</u> lymphoma

cc **C86.5** <u>Angioimmunoblastic</u> T-cell lymphoma
Angioimmunoblastic lymphadenopathy with dysproteinemia (AILD)

cc **C86.6** <u>Primary cutaneous CD30-positive</u> T-cell proliferations
Lymphomatoid papulosis
Primary cutaneous anaplastic large cell lymphoma
Primary cutaneous CD30-positive large T-cell lymphoma

C88- <u>Malignant immunoproliferative diseases and certain other B-cell lymphomas</u>
Excludes 1: *B-cell lymphoma, unspecified (C85.1-)*
personal history of other malignant neoplasms of lymphoid, hematopoietic and related tissues (Z85.79)

C88.0 Waldenström macroglobulinemia
Lymphoplasmacytic lymphoma with IgM-production
Macroglobulinemia (idiopathic) (primary)
Excludes 1: *small cell B-cell lymphoma (C83.0)*

cc **C88.2** Heavy chain disease
Franklin disease
Gamma heavy chain disease
Mu heavy chain disease

cc **C88.3** Immunoproliferative small intestinal disease
Alpha heavy chain disease
Mediterranean lymphoma

cc **C88.4** Extranodal marginal zone B-cell lymphoma of mucosa-associated lymphoid tissue [MALT-lymphoma]
Lymphoma of skin-associated lymphoid tissue [SALT-lymphoma]
Lymphoma of bronchial-associated lymphoid tissue [BALT-lymphoma]
Excludes 1: *high malignant (diffuse large B-cell) lymphoma (C83.3-)*

cc **C88.8** Other malignant immunoproliferative diseases

cc **C88.9** Malignant immunoproliferative disease, unspecified
Immunoproliferative disease NOS

C90- <u>Multiple myeloma and malignant plasma cell neoplasms</u>
Excludes 1: *personal history of other malignant neoplasms of lymphoid, hematopoietic and related tissues (Z85.79)*

C90.0- <u>Multiple myeloma</u> — A malignancy affecting plasma cells (a type of white blood cell).
Kahler's disease
Medullary plasmacytoma
Myelomatosis
Plasma cell myeloma
Excludes 1: *solitary myeloma (C90.3-)*
solitary plasmactyoma (C90.3-)

cc **C90.00** Multiple myeloma <u>not</u> having achieved remission
Multiple myeloma with failed remission
Multiple myeloma NOS

cc **C90.01** Multiple myeloma <u>in remission</u>

cc **C90.02** Multiple myeloma <u>in relapse</u>

C90.1- <u>Plasma cell leukemia</u> — A very aggressive malignancy affecting plasma cells (a type of white blood cell), often evolving from multiple myeloma.
Plasmacytic leukemia

cc **C90.10** Plasma cell leukemia <u>not</u> having achieved remission
Plasma cell leukemia with failed remission
Plasma cell leukemia NOS

cc **C90.11** Plasma cell leukemia <u>in remission</u>

cc **C90.12** Plasma cell leukemia <u>in relapse</u>

C90.2- **Extramedullary plasmacytoma** — A malignant plasma cell tumor forming a solid mass affecting the soft tissues.

cc **C90.20** **Extramedullary plasmacytoma not having achieved remission**
Extramedullary plasmacytoma with failed remission
Extramedullary plasmacytoma NOS

cc **C90.21** **Extramedullary plasmacytoma in remission**

cc **C90.22** **Extramedullary plasmacytoma in relapse**

C90.3- **Solitary plasmacytoma** — A malignant plasma cell tumor forming a solid mass affecting the bones.
Localized malignant plasma cell tumor NOS
Plasmacytoma NOS
Solitary myeloma

cc **C90.30** **Solitary plasmacytoma not having achieved remission**
Solitary plasmacytoma with failed remission
Solitary plasmacytoma NOS

cc **C90.31** **Solitary plasmacytoma in remission**

cc **C90.32** **Solitary plasmacytoma in relapse**

C91- **Lymphoid leukemia** — A malignancy affecting circulating lymphocytes, a type of white blood cell, that originates in the bone marrow.
Excludes 1:   personal history of leukemia (Z85.6)

C91.0- **Acute lymphoblastic leukemia [ALL]**
Note: Code C91.0 should only be used for T-cell and B-cell precursor leukemia

cc **C91.00** **Acute lymphoblastic leukemia not having achieved remission**
Acute lymphoblastic leukemia with failed remission
Acute lymphoblastic leukemia NOS

cc **C91.01** **Acute lymphoblastic leukemia, in remission**

cc **C91.02** **Acute lymphoblastic leukemia, in relapse**

C91.1- **Chronic lymphocytic leukemia of B-cell type**
Lymphoplasmacytic leukemia
Richter syndrome
Excludes 1:   lymphoplasmacytic lymphoma (C83.0-)

cc **C91.10** **Chronic lymphocytic leukemia of B-cell type not having achieved remission**
Chronic lymphocytic leukemia of B-cell type with failed remission
Chronic lymphocytic leukemia of B-cell type NOS

cc **C91.11** **Chronic lymphocytic leukemia of B-cell type in remission**

cc **C91.12** **Chronic lymphocytic leukemia of B-cell type in relapse**

C91.3- **Prolymphocytic leukemia of B-cell type**

cc **C91.30** **Prolymphocytic leukemia of B-cell type not having achieved remission**
Prolymphocytic leukemia of B-cell type with failed remission
Prolymphocytic leukemia of B-cell type NOS

cc **C91.31** **Prolymphocytic leukemia of B-cell type, in remission**

cc **C91.32** **Prolymphocytic leukemia of B-cell type, in relapse**

C91.4- **Hairy cell leukemia**
Leukemic reticuloendotheliosis

cc **C91.40** **Hairy cell leukemia not having achieved remission**
Hairy cell leukemia with failed remission
Hairy cell leukemia NOS

cc **C91.41** **Hairy cell leukemia, in remission**

cc **C91.42** **Hairy cell leukemia, in relapse**

C91.5- **Adult T-cell lymphoma/leukemia (HTLV-1-associated)**
Acute variant of adult T-cell lymphoma/leukemia (HTLV-1-associated)
Chronic variant of adult T-cell lymphoma/leukemia (HTLV-1-associated)
Lymphomatoid variant of adult T-cell lymphoma/leukemia (HTLV-1-associated)
Smouldering variant of adult T-cell lymphoma/leukemia (HTLV-1-associated)

cc **C91.50** **Adult T-cell lymphoma/leukemia (HTLV-1-associated) not having achieved remission** — [Age/15-124]
Adult T-cell lymphoma/leukemia (HTLV-1-associated) with failed remission
Adult T-cell lymphoma/leukemia (HTLV-1-associated) NOS

cc **C91.51** **Adult T-cell lymphoma/leukemia (HTLV-1-associated), in remission** — [Age/15-124]

cc **C91.52** **Adult T-cell lymphoma/leukemia (HTLV-1-associated), in relapse** — [Age/15-124]

C91.6- **Prolymphocytic leukemia of T-cell type**

cc **C91.60** **Prolymphocytic leukemia of T-cell type not having achieved remission**
Prolymphocytic leukemia of T-cell type with failed remission
Prolymphocytic leukemia of T-cell type NOS

cc **C91.61** **Prolymphocytic leukemia of T-cell type, in remission**

cc **C91.62** **Prolymphocytic leukemia of T-cell type, in relapse**

C91.A- **Mature B-cell leukemia Burkitt-type**
Excludes 1:   Burkitt lymphoma (C83.7-)

cc **C91.A0** **Mature B-cell leukemia Burkitt-type not having achieved remission**
Mature B-cell leukemia Burkitt-type with failed remission
Mature B-cell leukemia Burkitt-type NOS

cc **C91.A1** **Mature B-cell leukemia Burkitt-type, in remission**

cc **C91.A2** **Mature B-cell leukemia Burkitt-type, in relapse**

C91.Z- **Other lymphoid leukemia**
T-cell large granular lymphocytic leukemia (associated with rheumatoid arthritis)

cc **C91.Z0** **Other lymphoid leukemia not having achieved remission**
Other lymphoid leukemia with failed remission
Other lymphoid leukemia NOS

cc **C91.Z1** **Other lymphoid leukemia, in remission**

cc **C91.Z2** **Other lymphoid leukemia, in relapse**

C91.9- **Lymphoid leukemia, unspecified**

cc **C91.90** **Lymphoid leukemia, unspecified not having achieved remission**
Lymphoid leukemia with failed remission
Lymphoid leukemia NOS

cc **C91.91** **Lymphoid leukemia, unspecified, in remission**

cc **C91.92** **Lymphoid leukemia, unspecified, in relapse**

C92 **Myeloid leukemia** — A malignancy affecting white blood cell development in which the bone marrow makes abnormal myeloblasts, red blood cells, and platelets.
Includes: Granulocytic leukemia
Myelogenous leukemia
Excludes 1:   personal history of leukemia (Z85.6)

C92.0- **Acute myeloblastic leukemia**
Acute myeloblastic leukemia, minimal differentiation
Acute myeloblastic leukemia (with maturation)
Acute myeloblastic leukemia 1/ETO
Acute myeloblastic leukemia M0
Acute myeloblastic leukemia M1
Acute myeloblastic leukemia M2
Acute myeloblastic leukemia with t(8;21)
Acute myeloblastic leukemia (without a FAB classification) NOS
Refractory anemia with excess blasts in transformation [RAEB T]
Excludes 1:   acute exacerbation of chronic myeloid leukemia (C92.10)
refractory anemia with excess of blasts not in transformation (D46.2-)

cc **C92.00** **Acute myeloblastic leukemia, not having achieved remission**
Acute myeloblastic leukemia with failed remission
Acute myeloblastic leukemia NOS

cc **C92.01** **Acute myeloblastic leukemia, in remission**

cc **C92.02** **Acute myeloblastic leukemia, in relapse**

C92.1- **Chronic myeloid leukemia, BCR/ABL-positive**
Chronic myelogenous leukemia, Philadelphia chromosome (Ph1) positive
Chronic myelogenous leukemia, t(9;22) (q34;q11)
Chronic myelogenous leukemia with crisis of blast cells
Excludes 1:   atypical chronic myeloid leukemia BCR/ABL-negative (C92.2-)
chronic myelomonocytic leukemia (C93.1-)
chronic myeloproliferative disease (D47.1)

cc **C92.10** **Chronic myeloid leukemia, BCR/ABL-positive, not having achieved remission**
Chronic myeloid leukemia, BCR/ABL-positive with failed remission
Chronic myeloid leukemia, BCR/ABL-positive NOS

cc **C92.11** **Chronic myeloid leukemia, BCR/ABL-positive, in remission**

cc **C92.12** **Chronic myeloid leukemia, BCR/ABL-positive, in relapse**

C90 - C92

C92.2- **Atypical chronic** myeloid leukemia, **BCR/ABL-negative**

cc **C92.20** Atypical chronic myeloid leukemia, BCR/ABL-negative, **not** having achieved remission
Atypical chronic myeloid leukemia, BCR/ABL-negative with failed remission
Atypical chronic myeloid leukemia, BCR/ABL-negative NOS

cc **C92.21** Atypical chronic myeloid leukemia, BCR/ABL-negative, **in remission**

cc **C92.22** Atypical chronic myeloid leukemia, BCR/ABL-negative, **in relapse**

C92.3- Myeloid **sarcoma**
A malignant tumor of immature myeloid cells
Chloroma
Granulocytic sarcoma

cc **C92.30** Myeloid sarcoma, **not having achieved remission**
Myeloid sarcoma with failed remission
Myeloid sarcoma NOS

cc **C92.31** Myeloid sarcoma, **in remission**

cc **C92.32** Myeloid sarcoma, **in relapse**

C92.4- **Acute promyelocytic** leukemia
AML M3
AML Me with t(15;17) and variants

cc **C92.40** Acute promyelocytic leukemia, **not** having achieved remission
Acute promyelocytic leukemia with failed remission
Acute promyelocytic leukemia NOS

cc **C92.41** Acute promyelocytic leukemia, **in remission**

cc **C92.42** Acute promyelocytic leukemia, **in relapse**

C92.5- **Acute myelomonocytic** leukemia
AML M4
AML M4 Eo with inv(16) or t(16;16)

cc **C92.50** Acute myelomonocytic leukemia, **not** having achieved remission
Acute myelomonocytic leukemia with failed remission
Acute myelomonocytic leukemia NOS

cc **C92.51** Acute myelomonocytic leukemia, **in remission**

cc **C92.52** Acute myelomonocytic leukemia, **in relapse**

C92.6- **Acute myeloid** leukemia **with 11q23-abnormality**
Acute myeloid leukemia with variation of MLL-gene

cc **C92.60** Acute myeloid leukemia with 11q23-abnormality **not** having achieved remission
Acute myeloid leukemia with 11q23-abnormality with failed remission
Acute myeloid leukemia with 11q23-abnormality NOS

cc **C92.61** Acute myeloid leukemia with 11q23-abnormality **in remission**

cc **C92.62** Acute myeloid leukemia with 11q23-abnormality **in relapse**

C92.A- **Acute myeloid** leukemia **with multilineage dysplasia**
Acute myeloid leukemia with dysplasia of remaining hematopoesis and/or myelodysplastic disease in its history

cc **C92.A0** Acute myeloid leukemia with multilineage dysplasia, **not** having achieved remission
Acute myeloid leukemia with multilineage dysplasia with failed remission
Acute myeloid leukemia with multilineage dysplasia NOS

cc **C92.A1** Acute myeloid leukemia with multilineage dysplasia, **in remission**

cc **C92.A2** Acute myeloid leukemia with multilineage dysplasia, **in relapse**

C92.Z- **Other** myeloid leukemia

cc **C92.Z0** Other myeloid leukemia **not having achieved remission**
Myeloid leukemia NEC with failed remission
Myeloid leukemia NEC

cc **C92.Z1** Other myeloid leukemia, **in remission**

cc **C92.Z2** Other myeloid leukemia, **in relapse**

C92.9- Myeloid leukemia, **unspecified**

cc **C92.90** Myeloid leukemia, unspecified, **not** having achieved remission
Myeloid leukemia, unspecified with failed remission
Myeloid leukemia, unspecified NOS

cc **C92.91** Myeloid leukemia, unspecified **in remission**

cc **C92.92** Myeloid leukemia, unspecified **in relapse**

C93- **Monocytic** leukemia — A malignancy affecting white blood cell development in which the bone marrow makes an excessive number of monocytes.

Includes: Monocytoid leukemia

Excludes 1:   *personal history of leukemia (Z85.6)*

C93.0- **Acute monoblastic/monocytic** leukemia
AML M5
AML M5a
AML M5b

cc **C93.00** Acute monoblastic/monocytic leukemia, **not** having achieved remission
Acute monoblastic/monocytic leukemia with failed remission
Acute monoblastic/monocytic leukemia NOS

cc **C93.01** Acute monoblastic/monocytic leukemia, **in remission**

cc **C93.02** Acute monoblastic/monocytic leukemia, **in relapse**

C93.1- **Chronic myelomonocytic** leukemia
Chronic monocytic leukemia
CMML-1
CMML-2
CMML with eosinophilia

cc **C93.10** Chronic myelomonocytic leukemia **not having achieved remission**
Chronic myelomonocytic leukemia with failed remission
Chronic myelomonocytic leukemia NOS

cc **C93.11** Chronic myelomonocytic leukemia, **in remission**

cc **C93.12** Chronic myelomonocytic leukemia, **in relapse**

C93.3- **Juvenile myelomonocytic** leukemia

cc **C93.30** Juvenile myelomonocytic leukemia, **not** having achieved remission — [Age/0-17]
Juvenile myelomonocytic leukemia with failed remission
Juvenile myelomonocytic leukemia NOS

cc **C93.31** Juvenile myelomonocytic leukemia, **in remission** — [Age/0-17]

cc **C93.32** Juvenile myelomonocytic leukemia, **in relapse** — [Age/0-17]

C93.Z- **Other monocytic** leukemia

cc **C93.Z0** Other monocytic leukemia, **not having achieved remission**
Other monocytic leukemia NOS

cc **C93.Z1** Other monocytic leukemia, **in remission**

cc **C93.Z2** Other monocytic leukemia, **in relapse**

C93.9- **Monocytic** leukemia, **unspecified**

cc **C93.90** Monocytic leukemia, unspecified, **not** having achieved remission
Monocytic leukemia, unspecified with failed remission
Monocytic leukemia, unspecified NOS

cc **C93.91** Monocytic leukemia, unspecified **in remission**

cc **C93.92** Monocytic leukemia, unspecified **in relapse**

C94- Other leukemias of specified cell type
Excludes 1:   *leukemic reticuloendotheliosis (C91.4-)*
myelodysplastic syndromes (D46.-)
personal history of leukemia (Z85.6)
plasma cell leukemia (C90.1-)

C94.0- **Acute erythroid** leukemia
Acute myeloid leukemia M6(a)(b)
Erythroleukemia

cc **C94.00** Acute erythroid leukemia, **not having achieved remission**
Acute erythroid leukemia with failed remission
Acute erythroid leukemia NOS

cc **C94.01** Acute erythroid leukemia, **in remission**

cc **C94.02** Acute erythroid leukemia, **in relapse**

C94.2- **Acute megakaryoblastic** leukemia
Acute myeloid leukemia M7
Acute megakaryocytic leukemia

cc **C94.20** Acute megakaryoblastic leukemia **not** having achieved remission
Acute megakaryoblastic leukemia with failed remission
Acute megakaryoblastic leukemia NOS

cc **C94.21** Acute megakaryoblastic leukemia, **in remission**

cc **C94.22** Acute megakaryoblastic leukemia, **in relapse**

C94.3- **Mast cell** leukemia

cc **C94.30** Mast cell leukemia **not having achieved remission**
Mast cell leukemia with failed remission
Mast cell leukemia NOS

cc **C94.31** Mast cell leukemia, **in remission**

cc **C94.32** Mast cell leukemia, **in relapse**

Excludes 1: = NOT CODED HERE! (Do not code both)   **586**   *Excludes ❷:* = Not Included Here

C 9 2 - C 9 4

C94.4- <u>Acute panmyelosis</u> with myelofibrosis
　　Acute myelofibrosis
　　Excludes 1:   myelofibrosis NOS (D75.81)
　　　　　　　secondary myelofibrosis NOS (D75.81)

cc **C94.40** Acute panmyelosis with myelofibrosis <u>not</u> having achieved remission
　　Acute myelofibrosis NOS
　　Acute panmyelosis with myelofibrosis with failed remission
　　Acute panmyelosis NOS

cc **C94.41** Acute panmyelosis with myelofibrosis, <u>in remission</u>

cc **C94.42** Acute panmyelosis with myelofibrosis, <u>in relapse</u>

cc **C94.6** Myelodysplastic disease, not classified
　　Myeloproliferative disease, not classified

C94.8- <u>Other specified</u> leukemias
　　Aggressive NK-cell leukemia
　　Acute basophilic leukemia

cc **C94.80** Other specified leukemias <u>not</u> having achieved remission
　　Other specified leukemia with failed remission
　　Other specified leukemias NOS

cc **C94.81** Other specified leukemias, <u>in remission</u>

cc **C94.82** Other specified leukemias, <u>in relapse</u>

C95- Leukemia of <u>unspecified cell type</u>
　　Excludes 1:   personal history of leukemia (Z85.6)

C95.0- <u>Acute</u> leukemia of unspecified cell type
　　Acute bilineal leukemia
　　Acute mixed lineage leukemia
　　Biphenotypic acute leukemia
　　Stem cell leukemia of unclear lineage
　　Excludes 1:   acute exacerbation of unspecified chronic leukemia (C95.10)

cc **C95.00** Acute leukemia of unspecified cell type <u>not</u> having achieved remission
　　Acute leukemia of unspecified cell type with failed remission
　　Acute leukemia NOS

cc **C95.01** Acute leukemia of unspecified cell type, <u>in remission</u>

cc **C95.02** Acute leukemia of unspecified cell type, <u>in relapse</u>

C95.1- <u>Chronic</u> leukemia of unspecified cell type

cc **C95.10** Chronic leukemia of unspecified cell type <u>not</u> having achieved remission
　　Chronic leukemia of unspecified cell type with failed remission
　　Chronic leukemia NOS

cc **C95.11** Chronic leukemia of unspecified cell type, <u>in remission</u>

cc **C95.12** Chronic leukemia of unspecified cell type, <u>in relapse</u>

C95.9- Leukemia, <u>unspecified</u>

cc **C95.90** Leukemia, unspecified <u>not</u> having achieved remission
　　Leukemia unspecified with failed remission
　　Leukemia NOS

cc **C95.91** Leukemia, unspecified, <u>in remission</u>

cc **C95.92** Leukemia, unspecified, <u>in relapse</u>

C96- Other and unspecified malignant neoplasms of lymphoid, hematopoietic and related tissue
　　Excludes 1:   personal history of other malignant neoplasms of lymphoid, hematopoietic and related tissues (Z85.79)

cc **C96.0** Multifocal and <u>multisystemic</u> (disseminated) Langerhans-cell histiocytosis
　　Histiocytosis X, multisystemic
　　Letterer-Siwe disease
　　Excludes 1:   adult pulmonary Langerhans-cell histiocytosis (J84.82)
　　　　　　multifocal and unisystemic Langerhans-cell histiocytosis (C96.5)
　　　　　　unifocal Langerhans-cell histiocytosis (C96.6)

cc **C96.2** Malignant <u>mast cell</u> tumor
　　Aggressive systemic mastocytosis
　　Mast cell sarcoma
　　Excludes 1:   indolent mastocytosis (D47.0)
　　　　　　mast cell leukemia (C94.30)
　　　　　　mastocytosis (congenital) (cutaneous) (Q82.2)

cc **C96.4** Sarcoma of <u>dendritic cells</u> (accessory cells)
　　Follicular dendritic cell sarcoma
　　Interdigitating dendritic cell sarcoma
　　Langerhans cell sarcoma

cc **C96.5** Multifocal and <u>unisystemic</u> Langerhans-cell histiocytosis
　　Hand-Schüller-Christian disease
　　Histiocytosis X, multifocal
　　Excludes 1:   multifocal and multisystemic (disseminated) Langerhans-cell histiocytosis (C96.0)
　　　　　　unifocal Langerhans-cell histiocytosis (C96.6)

cc **C96.6** <u>Unifocal Langerhans-cell histiocytosis</u>
　　Eosinophilic granuloma
　　Histiocytosis X, unifocal
　　Histiocytosis X NOS
　　Langerhans-cell histiocytosis NOS
　　Excludes 1:   multifocal and multisysemic (disseminated) Langerhans-cell histiocytosis (C96.0)
　　　　　　multifocal and unisystemic Langerhans-cell histiocytosis (C96.5)

cc **C96.A** Histiocytic sarcoma
　　Malignant histiocytosis

cc **C96.Z** Other specified malignant neoplasms of lymphoid, hematopoietic and related tissue

cc **C96.9** Malignant neoplasm of lymphoid, hematopoietic and related tissue, unspecified

In situ neoplasms (D00-D09)

Includes:　Bowen's disease
　　　　Erythroplasia
　　　　Grade III intraepithelial neoplasia
　　　　Queyrat's erythroplasia

D00- <u>Carcinoma in situ</u> of oral cavity, esophagus and stomach — Malignant neoplastic tumor cells that still remain within the epithelium without invasion of the basement membrane.
　　Excludes 1:   melanoma in situ (D03.-)

D00.0- Carcinoma in situ of <u>lip, oral cavity and pharynx</u>
　　Use additional code to identify:
　　Exposure to environmental tobacco smoke (Z77.22)
　　Exposure to tobacco smoke in the perinatal period (P96.81)
　　History of tobacco dependence (Z87.891)
　　Occupational exposure to environmental tobacco smoke (Z57.31)
　　Tobacco dependence (F17.-)
　　Tobacco use (Z72.0)
　　Excludes 1:   carcinoma in situ of aryepiglottic fold or interarytenoid fold, laryngeal aspect (D02.0)
　　　　　　carcinoma in situ of epiglottis NOS (D02.0)
　　　　　　carcinoma in situ of epiglottis suprahyoid portion (D02.0)
　　　　　　carcinoma in situ of skin of lip (D03.0, D04.0)

D00.00 Carcinoma in situ of oral cavity, unspecified site

D00.01 Carcinoma in situ of <u>labial mucosa and vermilion border</u>

D00.02 Carcinoma in situ of <u>buccal</u> mucosa

D00.03 Carcinoma in situ of <u>gingiva</u> and edentulous alveolar ridge

D00.04 Carcinoma in situ of <u>soft</u> palate

D00.05 Carcinoma in situ of <u>hard</u> palate

D00.06 Carcinoma in situ of <u>floor</u> of mouth

D00.07 Carcinoma in situ of <u>tongue</u>

D00.08 Carcinoma in situ of <u>pharynx</u>
　　Carcinoma in situ of aryepiglottic fold NOS
　　Carcinoma in situ of hypopharyngeal aspect of aryepiglottic fold
　　Carcinoma in situ of marginal zone of aryepiglottic fold

D00.1 Carcinoma in situ of <u>esophagus</u>

D00.2 Carcinoma in situ of <u>stomach</u>

D01- <u>Carcinoma in situ</u> of other and unspecified digestive organs
　　Excludes 1:   melanoma in situ (D03.-)

D01.0 Carcinoma in situ of <u>colon</u>
　　Excludes 1:   carcinoma in situ of rectosigmoid junction (D01.1)

D01.1 Carcinoma in situ of <u>rectosigmoid</u> junction

D01.2 Carcinoma in situ of <u>rectum</u>

D01.3 Carcinoma in situ of <u>anus and anal canal</u>
　　Anal intraepithelial neoplasia III [AIN III]
　　Severe dysplasia of anus
　　Excludes 1:   anal intraepithelial neoplasia I and II [AIN I and AIN II] (K62.82)
　　　　　　carcinoma in situ of anal margin (D04.5)
　　　　　　carcinoma in situ of anal skin (D04.5)
　　　　　　carcinoma in situ of perianal skin (D04.5)

C94 - D01

Excludes 1: = NOT CODED HERE! (Do not code both)　　　**587**　　　*Excludes ❷:* = Not Included Here

D01.4- Carcinoma in situ of other and unspecified parts of intestine
> *Excludes 1:* *carcinoma in situ of ampulla of Vater (D01.5)*

D01.40 Carcinoma in situ of unspecified part of intestine

D01.49 Carcinoma in situ of other parts of intestine

D01.5 Carcinoma in situ of <u>liver, gallbladder and bile ducts</u>
Carcinoma in situ of ampulla of Vater

D01.7 Carcinoma in situ of other specified digestive organs
Carcinoma in situ of pancreas

D01.9 Carcinoma in situ of digestive organ, unspecified

D02- <u>Carcinoma in situ</u> of middle ear and respiratory system — Malignant neoplastic tumor cells that still remain within the epithelium without invasion of the basement membrane.
Use additional code to identify:
Exposure to environmental tobacco smoke (Z77.22)
Exposure to tobacco smoke in the perinatal period (P96.81)
History of tobacco dependence (Z87.891)
Occupational exposure to environmental tobacco smoke (Z57.31)
Tobacco dependence (F17.-)
Tobacco use (Z72.0)
> *Excludes 1:* *melanoma in situ (D03.-)*

D02.0 Carcinoma in situ of <u>larynx</u>
Carcinoma in situ of aryepiglottic fold or interarytenoid fold, laryngeal aspect
Carcinoma in situ of epiglottis (suprahyoid portion)
> *Excludes 1:* *carcinoma in situ of aryepiglottic fold or interarytenoid fold NOS (D00.08)*
> *carcinoma in situ of hypopharyngeal aspect (D00.08)*
> *carcinoma in situ of marginal zone (D00.08)*

D02.1 Carcinoma in situ of <u>trachea</u>

D02.2- Carcinoma in situ of <u>bronchus and lung</u>

D02.20 Carcinoma in situ of unspecified bronchus and lung

D02.21 Carcinoma in situ of <u>right</u> bronchus and lung

D02.22 Carcinoma in situ of <u>left</u> bronchus and lung

D02.3 Carcinoma in situ of other parts of respiratory system
Carcinoma in situ of accessory sinuses
Carcinoma in situ of middle ear
Carcinoma in situ of nasal cavities
> *Excludes 1:* *carcinoma in situ of ear (external) (skin) (D04.2-)*
> *carcinoma in situ of nose NOS (D09.8)*
> *carcinoma in situ of skin of nose (D04.3)*

D02.4 Carcinoma in situ of respiratory system, unspecified

D03- <u>Melanoma in situ</u> — Malignant melanoma tumor cells that still remain within the epidermis (the outermost layer of skin) without invasion of the deeper tissue layers.

D03.0 Melanoma in situ of <u>lip</u>

D03.1- Melanoma in situ of <u>eyelid, including canthus</u>

D03.10 Melanoma in situ of unspecified eyelid, including canthus

D03.11 Melanoma in situ of <u>right</u> eyelid, including canthus

D03.12 Melanoma in situ of <u>left</u> eyelid, including canthus

D03.2- Melanoma in situ of ear and external auricular canal

D03.20 Melanoma in situ of unspecified <u>ear and external auricular canal</u>

D03.21 Melanoma in situ of <u>right</u> ear and external auricular canal

D03.22 Melanoma in situ of <u>left</u> ear and external auricular canal

D03.3- Melanoma in situ of other and unspecified parts of face

D03.30 Melanoma in situ of unspecified part of face

D03.39 Melanoma in situ of other parts of face

D03.4 Melanoma in situ of <u>scalp and neck</u>

D03.5- Melanoma in situ of trunk

D03.51 Melanoma in situ of <u>anal skin</u>
Melanoma in situ of anal margin
Melanoma in situ of perianal skin

D03.52 Melanoma in situ of <u>breast</u> (skin) (soft tissue)

D03.59 Melanoma in situ of other part of trunk

D03.6- Melanoma in situ of <u>upper limb</u>, including shoulder

D03.60 Melanoma in situ of unspecified upper limb, including shoulder

D03.61 Melanoma in situ of <u>right</u> upper limb, including shoulder

D03.62 Melanoma in situ of <u>left</u> upper limb, including shoulder

D03.7- Melanoma in situ of <u>lower limb</u>, including hip

D03.70 Melanoma in situ of unspecified lower limb, including hip

D03.71 Melanoma in situ of <u>right</u> lower limb, including hip

D03.72 Melanoma in situ of <u>left</u> lower limb, including hip

D03.8 Melanoma in situ of other sites
Melanoma in situ of scrotum
> *Excludes 1:* *carcinoma in situ of scrotum (D07.61)*

D03.9 Melanoma in situ, unspecified

D04- <u>Carcinoma in situ</u> of <u>skin</u> — Malignant neoplastic (non-melanoma) tumor cells that still remain within the epidermis (the outermost layer of skin) without invasion of the deeper tissue layers.
> *Excludes 1:* *erythroplasia of Queyrat (penis) NOS (D07.4)*
> *melanoma in situ (D03.-)*

D04.0 Carcinoma in situ of <u>skin</u> of lip
> *Excludes 1:* *carcinoma in situ of vermilion border of lip (D00.01)*

D04.1- Carcinoma in situ of <u>skin</u> of <u>eyelid, including canthus</u>

D04.10 Carcinoma in situ of skin of unspecified eyelid, including canthus

D04.11 Carcinoma in situ of skin of <u>right</u> eyelid, including canthus

D04.12 Carcinoma in situ of skin of <u>left</u> eyelid, including canthus

D04.2- Carcinoma in situ of <u>skin</u> of <u>ear and external auricular canal</u>

D04.20 Carcinoma in situ of skin of unspecified ear and external auricular canal

D04.21 Carcinoma in situ of skin of <u>right</u> ear and external auricular canal

D04.22 Carcinoma in situ of skin of <u>left</u> ear and external auricular canal

D04.3- Carcinoma in situ of <u>skin</u> of other and unspecified parts of face

D04.30 Carcinoma in situ of skin of unspecified part of face

D04.39 Carcinoma in situ of skin of other parts of face

D04.4 Carcinoma in situ of <u>skin</u> of <u>scalp and neck</u>

D04.5 Carcinoma in situ of <u>skin</u> of <u>trunk</u>
Carcinoma in situ of anal margin
Carcinoma in situ of anal skin
Carcinoma in situ of perianal skin
Carcinoma in situ of skin of breast
> *Excludes 1:* *carcinoma in situ of anus NOS (D01.3)*
> *carcinoma in situ of scrotum (D07.61)*
> *carcinoma in situ of skin of genital organs (D07.-)*

D04.6- Carcinoma in situ of <u>skin</u> of <u>upper limb</u>, including shoulder

D04.60 Carcinoma in situ of skin of unspecified upper limb, including shoulder

D04.61 Carcinoma in situ of skin of <u>right</u> upper limb, including shoulder

D04.62 Carcinoma in situ of skin of <u>left</u> upper limb, including shoulder

D04.7- Carcinoma in situ of <u>skin</u> of <u>lower limb</u>, including hip

D04.70 Carcinoma in situ of skin of unspecified lower limb, including hip

D04.71 Carcinoma in situ of skin of <u>right</u> lower limb, including hip

D04.72 Carcinoma in situ of skin of <u>left</u> lower limb, including hip

D04.8 Carcinoma in situ of <u>skin</u> of other sites

D04.9 Carcinoma in situ of <u>skin</u>, unspecified

D05- <u>Carcinoma in situ</u> of breast — Malignant neoplastic tumor cells that still remain within the epithelium without invasion of the basement membrane.
> *Excludes 1:* *carcinoma in situ of skin of breast (D04.5)*
> *melanoma in situ of breast (skin) (D03.5)*
> *Paget's disease of breast or nipple (C50.-)*

D05.0- <u>Lobular</u> carcinoma in situ of breast

D05.00 Lobular carcinoma in situ of unspecified breast

D05.01 Lobular carcinoma in situ of <u>right</u> breast

D05.02 Lobular carcinoma in situ of <u>left</u> breast

D05.1- <u>Intraductal</u> carcinoma in situ of breast

D05.10 Intraductal carcinoma in situ of unspecified breast

D05.11 Intraductal carcinoma in situ of <u>right</u> breast

D05.12 Intraductal carcinoma in situ of <u>left</u> breast

D
0
1
-
D
0
5

D05.8- <u>Other specified type</u> of carcinoma in situ of breast

D05.80 Other specified type of carcinoma in situ of unspecified breast

D05.81 Other specified type of carcinoma in situ of <u>right</u> breast

D05.82 Other specified type of carcinoma in situ of <u>left</u> breast

D05.9- <u>Unspecified</u> type of carcinoma in situ of breast

D05.90 Unspecified type of carcinoma in situ of unspecified breast

D05.91 Unspecified type of carcinoma in situ of <u>right</u> breast

D05.92 Unspecified type of carcinoma in situ of <u>left</u> breast

D06- <u>Carcinoma in situ</u> of cervix uteri — Malignant neoplastic tumor cells that still remain within the surface layer of the cervix without invasion of the basement membrane.

Includes: Cervical adenocarcinoma in situ
Cervical intraepithelial glandular neoplasia
Cervical intraepithelial neoplasia III [CIN III]
Severe dysplasia of cervix uteri

Excludes 1: *cervical intraepithelial neoplasia II [CIN II] (N87.1)*
cytologic evidence of malignancy of cervix without histologic confirmation (R87.614)
high grade squamous intraepithelial lesion (HGSIL) of cervix (R87.613)
melanoma in situ of cervix (D03.5)
moderate cervical dysplasia (N87.1)

D06.0 Carcinoma in situ of <u>endocervix</u> — [♀]

D06.1 Carcinoma in situ of <u>exocervix</u> — [♀]

D06.7 Carcinoma in situ of other parts of cervix — [♀]

D06.9 Carcinoma in situ of cervix, unspecified — [♀]

D07- <u>Carcinoma in situ</u> of other and unspecified genital organs — Malignant neoplastic tumor cells that still remain within the surface layer without invasion of the basement membrane.

Excludes 1: *melanoma in situ of trunk (D03.5)*

D07.0 Carcinoma in situ of <u>endometrium</u> — [♀]

D07.1 Carcinoma in situ of <u>vulva</u> — [♀]
Severe dysplasia of vulva
Vulvar intraepithelial neoplasia III [VIN III]

Excludes 1: *moderate dysplasia of vulva (N90.1)*
vulvar intraepithelial neoplasia II [VIN II] (N90.1)

D07.2 Carcinoma in situ of <u>vagina</u> — [♀]
Severe dysplasia of vagina
Vaginal intraepithelial neoplasia III [VAIN III]

Excludes 1: *moderate dysplasia of vagina (N89.1)*
vaginal intraepithelial neoplasia II [VIN II] (N89.1)

D07.3- Carcinoma in situ of other and unspecified female genital organs

D07.30 Carcinoma in situ of unspecified female genital organs — [♀]

D07.39 Carcinoma in situ of other female genital organs — [♀]

D07.4 Carcinoma in situ of <u>penis</u> — [♂]
Erythroplasia of Queyrat NOS

D07.5 Carcinoma in situ of <u>prostate</u> — [♂]
Prostatic intraepithelial neoplasia III (PIN III)
Severe dysplasia of prostate

Excludes 1: *dysplasia (mild) (moderate) of prostate (N42.3-)*
prostatic intraepithelial neoplasia II [PIN II] (N42.3-)

D07.6- Carcinoma in situ of other and unspecified male genital organs

D07.60 Carcinoma in situ of unspecified male genital organs — [♂]

D07.61 Carcinoma in situ of <u>scrotum</u> — [♂]

D07.69 Carcinoma in situ of other male genital organs — [♂]

D09- <u>Carcinoma in situ</u> of other and unspecified sites — Malignant neoplastic tumor cells that still remain within the surface layer without invasion of the basement membrane.

Excludes 1: *melanoma in situ (D03.-)*

D09.0 Carcinoma in situ of <u>bladder</u>

D09.1- Carcinoma in situ of other and unspecified urinary organs

D09.10 Carcinoma in situ of unspecified urinary organ

D09.19 Carcinoma in situ of other urinary organs

D09.2- Carcinoma in situ of <u>eye</u>

Excludes 1: *carcinoma in situ of skin of eyelid (D04.1-)*

D09.20 Carcinoma in situ of unspecified eye

D09.21 Carcinoma in situ of <u>right</u> eye

D09.22 Carcinoma in situ of <u>left</u> eye

D09.3 Carcinoma in situ of <u>thyroid</u> and other endocrine glands

Excludes 1: *carcinoma in situ of endocrine pancreas (D01.7)*
carcinoma in situ of ovary (D07.39)
carcinoma in situ of testis (D07.69)

D09.8 Carcinoma in situ of other specified sites

D09.9 Carcinoma in situ, unspecified

Benign neoplasms, except benign neuroendocrine tumors (D10-D36)

D10- <u>Benign neoplasm</u> of mouth and pharynx — Any new and abnormal growth in which tumor cells progressively multiply, but lack the properties of invasion and metastases (see Malignant Neoplasm code catgories, by site, for anatomical description).

D10.0 Benign neoplasm of <u>lip</u>
Benign neoplasm of lip (frenulum) (inner aspect) (mucosa) (vermilion border)

Excludes 1: *benign neoplasm of skin of lip (D22.0, D23.0)*

D10.1 Benign neoplasm of <u>tongue</u>
Benign neoplasm of lingual tonsil

D10.2 Benign neoplasm of <u>floor</u> of mouth

D10.3- Benign neoplasm of other and unspecified parts of mouth

D10.30 Benign neoplasm of unspecified part of mouth

D10.39 Benign neoplasm of other parts of mouth
Benign neoplasm of minor salivary gland NOS

Excludes 1: *benign odontogenic neoplasms (D16.4-D16.5)*
benign neoplasm of mucosa of lip (D10.0)
benign neoplasm of nasopharyngeal surface of soft palate (D10.6)

D10.4 Benign neoplasm of <u>tonsil</u>
Benign neoplasm of tonsil (faucial) (palatine)

Excludes 1: *benign neoplasm of lingual tonsil (D10.1)*
benign neoplasm of pharyngeal tonsil (D10.6)
benign neoplasm of tonsillar fossa (D10.5)
benign neoplasm of tonsillar pillars (D10.5)

D10.5 Benign neoplasm of other parts of oropharynx
Benign neoplasm of epiglottis, anterior aspect
Benign neoplasm of tonsillar fossa
Benign neoplasm of tonsillar pillars
Benign neoplasm of vallecula

Excludes 1: *benign neoplasm of epiglottis NOS (D14.1)*
benign neoplasm of epiglottis, suprahyoid portion (D14.1)

D10.6 Benign neoplasm of <u>nasopharynx</u>
Benign neoplasm of pharyngeal tonsil
Benign neoplasm of posterior margin of septum and choanae

D10.7 Benign neoplasm of <u>hypopharynx</u>

D10.9 Benign neoplasm of pharynx, unspecified

D11- <u>Benign neoplasm</u> of major salivary glands — Any new and abnormal growth in which tumor cells progressively multiply, but lack the properties of invasion and metastases (see Malignant Neoplasm code catgories, by site, for anatomical description).

Excludes 1: *benign neoplasms of specified minor salivary glands which are classified according to their anatomic allocation*
benign neoplasms of minor salivary glands NOS (D10.39)

D11.0 Benign neoplasm of <u>parotid</u> gland

D11.7 Benign neoplasm of other major salivary glands
Benign neoplasm of sublingual salivary gland
Benign neoplasm of submandibular salivary gland

D11.9 Benign neoplasm of major salivary gland, unspecified

D12- <u>Benign neoplasm</u> of colon, rectum, anus and anal canal — Any new and abnormal growth in which tumor cells progressively multiply, but lack the properties of invasion and metastases (see Malignant Neoplasm code catgories, by site, for anatomical description).

Excludes 1: *benign carcinoid tumors of the large intestine, and rectum (D3A.02-)*

D12.0 Benign neoplasm of <u>cecum</u>
Benign neoplasm of ileocecal valve

D12.1 Benign neoplasm of <u>appendix</u>

Excludes 1: *benign carcinoid tumor of the appendix (D3A.020)*

D12.2 Benign neoplasm of <u>ascending colon</u>

D12.3 Benign neoplasm of <u>transverse colon</u>
Benign neoplasm of hepatic flexure
Benign neoplasm of splenic flexure

D12.4 Benign neoplasm of <u>descending colon</u>

D05 - D12

Excludes 1: = NOT CODED HERE! (Do not code both)

Excludes ❷: = Not Included Here

D12.5 Benign neoplasm of <u>sigmoid colon</u>

D12.6 Benign neoplasm of colon, unspecified
Adenomatosis of colon
Benign neoplasm of large intestine NOS
Polyposis (hereditary) of colon
Excludes 1: inflammatory polyp of colon (K51.4-)
polyp of colon NOS (K63.5)

D12.7 Benign neoplasm of <u>rectosigmoid</u> junction

D12.8 Benign neoplasm of <u>rectum</u>
Excludes 1: benign carcinoid tumor of the rectum (D3A.026)

D12.9 Benign neoplasm of <u>anus and anal canal</u>
Benign neoplasm of anus NOS
Excludes 1: benign neoplasm of anal margin (D22.5, D23.5)
benign neoplasm of anal skin (D22.5, D23.5)
benign neoplasm of perianal skin (D22.5, D23.5)

D13- <u>Benign neoplasm</u> of other and ill-defined parts of digestive
system — Any new and abnormal growth in which tumor cells progressively multiply, but
lack the properties of invasion and metastases (see Malignant Neoplasm code catgories, by
site, for anatomical description).
Excludes 1: benign stromal tumors of digestive system (D21.4)

D13.0 Benign neoplasm of <u>esophagus</u>

D13.1 Benign neoplasm of <u>stomach</u>
Excludes 1: benign carcinoid tumor of the stomach (D3A.092)

D13.2 Benign neoplasm of <u>duodenum</u>
Excludes 1: benign carcinoid tumor of the duodenum (D3A.010)

D13.3- Benign neoplasm of other and unspecified parts of small
intestine
Excludes 1: benign carcinoid tumors of the small intestine(D3A.01-)
benign neoplasm of ileocecal valve (D12.0)

  D13.30 Benign neoplasm of unspecified part of small intestine

  D13.39 Benign neoplasm of other parts of small intestine

D13.4 Benign neoplasm of <u>liver</u>
Benign neoplasm of intrahepatic bile ducts

D13.5 Benign neoplasm of <u>extrahepatic bile ducts</u>

D13.6 Benign neoplasm of <u>pancreas</u>
Excludes 1: benign neoplasm of endocrine pancreas (D13.7)

D13.7 Benign neoplasm of <u>endocrine pancreas</u>
Islet cell tumor
Benign neoplasm of islets of Langerhans
Use additional code to identify any functional activity.

D13.9 Benign neoplasm of ill-defined sites within the digestive
system
Benign neoplasm of digestive system NOS
Benign neoplasm of intestine NOS
Benign neoplasm of spleen

D14- <u>Benign neoplasm</u> of middle ear and respiratory system — Any new and
abnormal growth in which tumor cells progressively multiply, but lack the properties of
invasion and metastases (see Malignant Neoplasm code catgories, by site, for anatomical
description).

D14.0 Benign neoplasm of middle ear, nasal cavity and accessory
sinuses
Benign neoplasm of cartilage of nose
Excludes 1: benign neoplasm of auricular canal (external) (D22.2-,
D23.2-)
benign neoplasm of bone of ear (D16.4)
benign neoplasm of bone of nose (D16.4)
benign neoplasm of cartilage of ear (D21.0)
benign neoplasm of ear (external) (skin) (D22.2-,
D23.2-)
benign neoplasm of nose NOS (D36.7)
benign neoplasm of skin of nose (D22.39, D23.39)
benign neoplasm of olfactory bulb (D33.3)
benign neoplasm of posterior margin of septum and
choanae (D10.6)
polyp of accessory sinus (J33.8)
polyp of ear (middle) (H74.4)
polyp of nasal (cavity) (J33.-)

D14.1 Benign neoplasm of <u>larynx</u>
Adenomatous polyp of larynx
Benign neoplasm of epiglottis (suprahyoid portion)
Excludes 1: benign neoplasm of epiglottis, anterior aspect (D10.5)
polyp (nonadenomatous) of vocal cord or larynx (J38.1)

D14.2 Benign neoplasm of <u>trachea</u>

D14.3- Benign neoplasm of <u>bronchus and lung</u>
Excludes 1: benign carcinoid tumor of the bronchus and lung
(D3A.090)

  D14.30 Benign neoplasm of unspecified bronchus and lung

  D14.31 Benign neoplasm of <u>right</u> bronchus and lung

  D14.32 Benign neoplasm of <u>left</u> bronchus and lung

D14.4 Benign neoplasm of respiratory system, unspecified

D15- <u>Benign neoplasm</u> of other and unspecified intrathoracic organs —
Any new and abnormal growth in which tumor cells progressively multiply, but lack the
properties of invasion and metastases (see Malignant Neoplasm code catgories, by site, for
anatomical description).
Excludes 1: benign neoplasm of mesothelial tissue (D19.-)

D15.0 Benign neoplasm of <u>thymus</u>
Excludes 1: benign carcinoid tumor of the thymus (D3A.091)

D15.1 Benign neoplasm of <u>heart</u>
Excludes 1: benign neoplasm of great vessels (D21.3)

D15.2 Benign neoplasm of <u>mediastinum</u>

D15.7 Benign neoplasm of other specified intrathoracic organs

D15.9 Benign neoplasm of intrathoracic organ, unspecified

D16- <u>Benign neoplasm</u> of bone and articular cartilage — Any new and
abnormal growth of in which tumor cells progressively multiply, but lack the properties of
invasion and metastases (see Malignant Neoplasm code catgories, by site, for anatomical
description).
Excludes 1: benign neoplasm of connective tissue of ear (D21.0)
benign neoplasm of connective tissue of eyelid (D21.0)
benign neoplasm of connective tissue of larynx (D14.1)
benign neoplasm of connective tissue of nose (D14.0)
benign neoplasm of synovia (D21.-)

D16.0- Benign neoplasm of <u>scapula and long bones of upper limb</u>

  D16.00 Benign neoplasm of scapula and long bones of
unspecified upper limb

  D16.01 Benign neoplasm of scapula and long bones of <u>right</u>
upper limb

  D16.02 Benign neoplasm of scapula and long bones of <u>left</u> upper
limb

D16.1- Benign neoplasm of <u>short bones of upper limb</u>

  D16.10 Benign neoplasm of short bones of unspecified upper
limb

  D16.11 Benign neoplasm of short bones of <u>right</u> upper limb

  D16.12 Benign neoplasm of short bones of <u>left</u> upper limb

D16.2- Benign neoplasm of <u>long bones of lower limb</u>

  D16.20 Benign neoplasm of long bones of unspecified lower limb

  D16.21 Benign neoplasm of long bones of <u>right</u> lower limb

  D16.22 Benign neoplasm of long bones of <u>left</u> lower limb

D16.3- Benign neoplasm of <u>short bones of lower limb</u>

  D16.30 Benign neoplasm of short bones of unspecified lower
limb

  D16.31 Benign neoplasm of short bones of <u>right</u> lower limb

  D16.32 Benign neoplasm of short bones of <u>left</u> lower limb

D16.4 Benign neoplasm of <u>bones of skull and face</u>
Benign neoplasm of maxilla (superior)
Benign neoplasm of orbital bone
Keratocyst of maxilla
Keratocystic odontogenic tumor of maxilla
Excludes ❷: benign neoplasm of lower jaw bone (D16.5)

D16.5 Benign neoplasm of <u>lower jaw</u> bone
Keratocyst of mandible
Keratocystic odontogenic tumor of mandible

D16.6 Benign neoplasm of <u>vertebral</u> column
Excludes 1: benign neoplasm of sacrum and coccyx (D16.8)

D16.7 Benign neoplasm of <u>ribs, sternum and clavicle</u>

D16.8 Benign neoplasm of <u>pelvic bones, sacrum and coccyx</u>

D16.9 Benign neoplasm of bone and articular cartilage, unspecified

D17- <u>Benign lipomatous</u> neoplasm — Any new and abnormal growth of adipose cells
(fat) in which tumor cells progressively multiply, but lack the properties of invasion and
metastases (see Malignant Neoplasm code catgories, by site, for anatomical description).

D17.0 Benign lipomatous neoplasm of <u>skin</u> and subcutaneous tissue
of <u>head, face and neck</u>

D17.1 Benign lipomatous neoplasm of <u>skin</u> and subcutaneous tissue
of <u>trunk</u>

D12-D17

D17.2- Benign lipomatous neoplasm of <u>skin</u> and subcutaneous tissue of <u>limb</u>

  D17.20 Benign lipomatous neoplasm of skin and subcutaneous tissue of unspecified limb

  D17.21 Benign lipomatous neoplasm of skin and subcutaneous tissue of <u>right</u> arm

  D17.22 Benign lipomatous neoplasm of skin and subcutaneous tissue of <u>left</u> arm

  D17.23 Benign lipomatous neoplasm of skin and subcutaneous tissue of <u>right</u> leg

  D17.24 Benign lipomatous neoplasm of skin and subcutaneous tissue of <u>left</u> leg

D17.3- Benign lipomatous neoplasm of <u>skin</u> and subcutaneous tissue of other and unspecified sites

  D17.30 Benign lipomatous neoplasm of skin and subcutaneous tissue of unspecified sites

  D17.39 Benign lipomatous neoplasm of skin and subcutaneous tissue of other sites

D17.4 Benign lipomatous neoplasm of <u>intrathoracic organs</u>

D17.5 Benign lipomatous neoplasm of <u>intra-abdominal organs</u>
  Excludes 1: *benign lipomatous neoplasm of peritoneum and retroperitoneum (D17.79)*

D17.6 Benign lipomatous neoplasm of <u>spermatic cord</u> — [♂]

D17.7- Benign lipomatous neoplasm of other sites

  D17.71 Benign lipomatous neoplasm of <u>kidney</u>

  D17.72 Benign lipomatous neoplasm of <u>other genitourinary organ</u>

  D17.79 Benign lipomatous neoplasm of <u>other sites</u>
    Benign lipomatous neoplasm of peritoneum
    Benign lipomatous neoplasm of retroperitoneum

D17.9 Benign lipomatous neoplasm, unspecified
    Lipoma NOS

D18- Hemangioma and lymphangioma, any site
  Excludes 1: *benign neoplasm of glomus jugulare (D35.6)*
          blue or pigmented nevus (D22.-)
          nevus NOS (D22.-)
          vascular nevus (Q82.5)

D18.0- <u>Hemangioma</u> — Any new and abnormal growth of in which tumor cells of newly formed blood vessels progressively multiply, but lack the properties of invasion and metastases.
    Angioma NOS
    Cavernous nevus

  D18.00 Hemangioma unspecified site

  D18.01 Hemangioma of <u>skin</u> and subcutaneous tissue

  D18.02 Hemangioma of <u>intracranial</u> structures

  D18.03 Hemangioma of <u>intra-abdominal</u> structures

  D18.09 Hemangioma of other sites

D18.1 <u>Lymphangioma</u>, any site — Any new and abnormal growth in which tumor cells of newly formed lymph spaces and channels progressively multiply, but lack the properties of invasion and metastases.

D19- <u>Benign neoplasm</u> of <u>mesothelial tissue</u> — Any new and abnormal growth of the tissue that lines most of the internal organs (mesothelium) in which tumor cells progressively multiply, but lack the properties of invasion and metastases (see Malignant Neoplasm code catgories, by site, for anatomical description).

D19.0 Benign neoplasm of mesothelial tissue of <u>pleura</u>

D19.1 Benign neoplasm of mesothelial tissue of <u>peritoneum</u>

D19.7 Benign neoplasm of mesothelial tissue of other sites

D19.9 Benign neoplasm of mesothelial tissue, unspecified
    Benign mesothelioma NOS

D20- <u>Benign neoplasm</u> of <u>soft tissue</u> of retroperitoneum and peritoneum — Any new and abnormal growth in which tumor cells progressively multiply, but lack the properties of invasion and metastases (see Malignant Neoplasm code catgories, by site, for anatomical description).
  Excludes 1: *benign lipomatous neoplasm of peritoneum and retroperitoneum (D17.79)*
          benign neoplasm of mesothelial tissue (D19.-)

D20.0 Benign neoplasm of soft tissue of <u>retroperitoneum</u>

D20.1 Benign neoplasm of soft tissue of <u>peritoneum</u>

D21- <u>Other benign neoplasms</u> of <u>connective</u> and other soft tissue — Any new and abnormal growth in which tumor cells progressively multiply, but lack the properties of invasion and metastases (see Malignant Neoplasm code catgories, by site, for anatomical description).
  Includes: Benign neoplasm of blood vessel
             Benign neoplasm of bursa
             Benign neoplasm of cartilage
             Benign neoplasm of fascia
             Benign neoplasm of fat
             Benign neoplasm of ligament, except uterine
             Benign neoplasm of lymphatic channel
             Benign neoplasm of muscle
             Benign neoplasm of synovia
             Benign neoplasm of tendon (sheath)
             Benign stromal tumors
  Excludes 1: *benign neoplasm of articular cartilage (D16.-)*
          benign neoplasm of cartilage of larynx (D14.1)
          benign neoplasm of cartilage of nose (D14.0)
          benign neoplasm of connective tissue of breast (D24.-)
          benign neoplasm of peripheral nerves and autonomic nervous system (D36.1-)
          benign neoplasm of peritoneum (D20.1)
          benign neoplasm of retroperitoneum (D20.0)
          benign neoplasm of uterine ligament, any (D28.2)
          benign neoplasm of vascular tissue (D18.-)
          hemangioma (D18.0-)
          lipomatous neoplasm (D17.-)
          lymphangioma (D18.1)
          uterine leiomyoma (D25.-)

D21.0 Benign neoplasm of connective and other soft tissue of <u>head, face and neck</u>
    Benign neoplasm of connective tissue of ear
    Benign neoplasm of connective tissue of eyelid
  Excludes 1: *benign neoplasm of connective tissue of orbit (D31.6-)*

D21.1- Benign neoplasm of connective and other soft tissue of <u>upper limb</u>, including shoulder

  D21.10 Benign neoplasm of connective and other soft tissue of unspecified upper limb, including shoulder

  D21.11 Benign neoplasm of connective and other soft tissue of <u>right</u> upper limb, including shoulder

  D21.12 Benign neoplasm of connective and other soft tissue of <u>left</u> upper limb, including shoulder

D21.2- Benign neoplasm of connective and other soft tissue of <u>lower limb</u>, including hip

  D21.20 Benign neoplasm of connective and other soft tissue of unspecified lower limb, including hip

  D21.21 Benign neoplasm of connective and other soft tissue of <u>right</u> lower limb, including hip

  D21.22 Benign neoplasm of connective and other soft tissue of <u>left</u> lower limb, including hip

D21.3 Benign neoplasm of connective and other soft tissue of <u>thorax</u>
    Benign neoplasm of axilla
    Benign neoplasm of diaphragm
    Benign neoplasm of great vessels
  Excludes 1: *benign neoplasm of heart (D15.1)*
          benign neoplasm of mediastinum (D15.2)
          benign neoplasm of thymus (D15.0)

D21.4 Benign neoplasm of connective and other soft tissue of <u>abdomen</u>
    Benign stromal tumors of abdomen

D21.5 Benign neoplasm of connective and other soft tissue of <u>pelvis</u>
  Excludes 1: *benign neoplasm of any uterine ligament (D28.2)*
          uterine leiomyoma (D25.-)

D21.6 Benign neoplasm of connective and other soft tissue of trunk, unspecified
    Benign neoplasm of back NOS

D21.9 Benign neoplasm of connective and other soft tissue, unspecified

---

Excludes 1: = NOT CODED HERE! (Do not code both)   **591**   *Excludes ❷:* = Not Included Here

D22- **Melanocytic nevi** — Any new and abnormal growth in which pigment-producing cells (a type of melanocyte) progressively multiply, but lack the properties of invasion and metastases (see Malignant Neoplasm code catgories, by site, for anatomical description).
    Includes: Atypical nevus
                 Blue hairy pigmented nevus
                 Nevus NOS

D22.0 **Melanocytic nevi of** <u>lip</u>

D22.1- **Melanocytic nevi of** <u>eyelid, including canthus</u>

    D22.10 Melanocytic nevi of unspecified eyelid, including canthus

    D22.11 Melanocytic nevi of <u>right</u> eyelid, including canthus

    D22.12 Melanocytic nevi of <u>left</u> eyelid, including canthus

D22.2- **Melanocytic nevi of** <u>ear and external auricular canal</u>

    D22.20 Melanocytic nevi of unspecified ear and external auricular canal

    D22.21 Melanocytic nevi of <u>right</u> ear and external auricular canal

    D22.22 Melanocytic nevi of <u>left</u> ear and external auricular canal

D22.3- **Melanocytic nevi of other and unspecified parts of face**

    D22.30 Melanocytic nevi of unspecified part of face

    D22.39 Melanocytic nevi of other parts of face

D22.4 **Melanocytic nevi of** <u>scalp and neck</u>

D22.5 **Melanocytic nevi of** <u>trunk</u>
        Melanocytic nevi of anal margin
        Melanocytic nevi of anal skin
        Melanocytic nevi of perianal skin
        Melanocytic nevi of skin of breast

D22.6- **Melanocytic nevi of** <u>upper limb</u>, including shoulder

    D22.60 Melanocytic nevi of unspecified upper limb, including shoulder

    D22.61 Melanocytic nevi of <u>right</u> upper limb, including shoulder

    D22.62 Melanocytic nevi of <u>left</u> upper limb, including shoulder

D22.7- **Melanocytic nevi of** <u>lower limb</u>, including hip

    D22.70 Melanocytic nevi of unspecified lower limb, including hip

    D22.71 Melanocytic nevi of <u>right</u> lower limb, including hip

    D22.72 Melanocytic nevi of <u>left</u> lower limb, including hip

D22.9 **Melanocytic nevi, unspecified**

D23- **Other benign neoplasms** of <u>skin</u> — Any new and abnormal growth in which skin cells progressively multiply, but lack the properties of invasion and metastases (see Malignant Neoplasm code catgories, by site, for anatomical description).
    Includes: Benign neoplasm of hair follicles
                 Benign neoplasm of sebaceous glands
                 Benign neoplasm of sweat glands
    Excludes 1:   *benign lipomatous neoplasms of skin (D17.0-D17.3)*
                    melanocytic nevi (D22.-)

D23.0 <u>Other</u> benign neoplasm of <u>skin</u> of <u>lip</u>
    Excludes 1:   *benign neoplasm of vermilion border of lip (D10.0)*

D23.1- <u>Other</u> benign neoplasm of <u>skin</u> of <u>eyelid, including canthus</u>

    D23.10 Other benign neoplasm of skin of unspecified eyelid, including canthus

    D23.11 Other benign neoplasm of skin of <u>right</u> eyelid, including canthus

    D23.12 Other benign neoplasm of skin of <u>left</u> eyelid, including canthus

D23.2- <u>Other</u> benign neoplasm of <u>skin</u> of <u>ear and external auricular canal</u>

    D23.20 Other benign neoplasm of skin of unspecified ear and external auricular canal

    D23.21 Other benign neoplasm of skin of <u>right</u> ear and external auricular canal

    D23.22 Other benign neoplasm of skin of <u>left</u> ear and external auricular canal

D23.3- <u>Other</u> benign neoplasm of <u>skin</u> of other and unspecified parts of face

    D23.30 Other benign neoplasm of skin of unspecified part of face

    D23.39 Other benign neoplasm of skin of other parts of face

D23.4 <u>Other</u> benign neoplasm of <u>skin</u> of <u>scalp and neck</u>

D23.5 <u>Other</u> benign neoplasm of <u>skin</u> of <u>trunk</u>
        Other benign neoplasm of anal margin
        Other benign neoplasm of anal skin
        Other benign neoplasm of perianal skin
        Other benign neoplasm of skin of breast
    Excludes 1:   *benign neoplasm of anus NOS (D12.9)*

D23.6- <u>Other</u> benign neoplasm of <u>skin</u> of <u>upper limb</u>, including shoulder

    D23.60 Other benign neoplasm of skin of unspecified upper limb, including shoulder

    D23.61 Other benign neoplasm of skin of <u>right</u> upper limb, including shoulder

    D23.62 Other benign neoplasm of skin of <u>left</u> upper limb, including shoulder

D23.7- <u>Other</u> benign neoplasm of <u>skin</u> of <u>lower limb</u>, including hip

    D23.70 Other benign neoplasm of skin of unspecified lower limb, including hip

    D23.71 Other benign neoplasm of skin of <u>right</u> lower limb, including hip

    D23.72 Other benign neoplasm of skin of <u>left</u> lower limb, including hip

D23.9 <u>Other</u> benign neoplasm of <u>skin</u>, unspecified

D24- **Benign neoplasm** of breast — Any new and abnormal growth in which tumor cells progressively multiply, but lack the properties of invasion and metastases (see Malignant Neoplasm code catgories, by site, for anatomical description).
    Includes: Benign neoplasm of connective tissue of breast
                 Benign neoplasm of soft parts of breast
                 Fibroadenoma of breast
    Excludes ❷: *adenofibrosis of breast (N60.2)*
                    benign cyst of breast (N60.-)
                    benign mammary dysplasia (N60.-)
                    benign neoplasm of skin of breast (D22.5, D23.5)
                    fibrocystic disease of breast (N60.-)

D24.1 **Benign neoplasm of** <u>right</u> breast

D24.2 **Benign neoplasm of** <u>left</u> breast

D24.9 **Benign neoplasm of unspecified breast**

D25- **Leiomyoma** of uterus — Any new and abnormal growth in which tumor cells progressively multiply, but lack the properties of invasion and metastases (see Malignant Neoplasm code catgories, by site, for anatomical description).
    Includes: Uterine fibroid
                 Uterine fibromyoma
                 Uterine myoma

D25.0 <u>Submucous</u> leiomyoma of uterus — [♀]

D25.1 <u>Intramural</u> leiomyoma of uterus — [♀]
        Interstitial leiomyoma of uterus

D25.2 <u>Subserosal</u> leiomyoma of uterus — [♀]
        Subperitoneal leiomyoma of uterus

D25.9 **Leiomyoma of uterus, unspecified** — [♀]

D26- **Other** benign neoplasms of <u>uterus</u> — Any new and abnormal growth in which tumor cells progressively multiply, but lack the properties of invasion and metastases (see Malignant Neoplasm code catgories, by site, for anatomical description).

D26.0 **Other benign neoplasm of** <u>cervix uteri</u> — [♀]

D26.1 **Other benign neoplasm of** <u>corpus uteri</u> — [♀]

D26.7 **Other benign neoplasm of other parts of uterus** — [♀]

D26.9 **Other benign neoplasm of uterus, unspecified** — [♀]

D27- **Benign neoplasm** of ovary — Any new and abnormal growth in which tumor cells progressively multiply, but lack the properties of invasion and metastases (see Malignant Neoplasm code catgories, by site, for anatomical description).
    Use additional code to identify any functional activity.
    Excludes ❷: *corpus albicans cyst (N83.2-)*
                    corpus luteum cyst (N83.1-)
                    endometrial cyst (N80.1)
                    follicular (atretic) cyst (N83.0-)
                    graafian follicle cyst (N83.0-)
                    ovarian cyst NEC (N83.2-)
                    ovarian retention cyst (N83.2-)

D27.0 **Benign neoplasm of** <u>right</u> ovary — [♀]

D27.1 **Benign neoplasm of** <u>left</u> ovary — [♀]

D27.9 **Benign neoplasm of unspecified ovary** — [♀]

D22-D27

D28- **Benign neoplasm** of other and unspecified female genital organs — Any new and abnormal growth in which tumor cells progressively multiply, but lack the properties of invasion and metastases (see Malignant Neoplasm code catgories, by site, for anatomical description).

    Includes: Adenomatous polyp
                Benign neoplasm of skin of female genital organs
                Benign teratoma
    Excludes 1:   *epoophoron cyst (Q50.5)*
                fimbrial cyst (Q50.4)
                Gartner's duct cyst (Q52.4)
                parovarian cyst (Q50.5)

   D28.0 Benign neoplasm of **vulva** — [♀]

   D28.1 Benign neoplasm of **vagina** — [♀]

   D28.2 Benign neoplasm of **uterine tubes and ligaments** — [♀]
          Benign neoplasm of fallopian tube
          Benign neoplasm of uterine ligament (broad) (round)

   D28.7 Benign neoplasm of other specified female genital organs — [♀]

   D28.9 Benign neoplasm of female genital organ, unspecified — [♀]

D29- **Benign neoplasm** of male genital organs — Any new and abnormal growth in which tumor cells progressively multiply, but lack the properties of invasion and metastases (see Malignant Neoplasm code catgories, by site, for anatomical description).

    Includes: Benign neoplasm of skin of male genital organs

   D29.0 Benign neoplasm of **penis** — [♂]

   D29.1 Benign neoplasm of **prostate** — [♂]
       Excludes 1:   *enlarged prostate (N40.-)*

   D29.2- Benign neoplasm of **testis**
       Use additional code to identify any functional activity.

      D29.20 Benign neoplasm of unspecified testis — [♂]

      D29.21 Benign neoplasm of **right** testis — [♂]

      D29.22 Benign neoplasm of **left** testis — [♂]

   D29.3- Benign neoplasm of **epididymis**

      D29.30 Benign neoplasm of unspecified epididymis — [♂]

      D29.31 Benign neoplasm of **right** epididymis — [♂]

      D29.32 Benign neoplasm of **left** epididymis — [♂]

   D29.4 Benign neoplasm of **scrotum** — [♂]
         Benign neoplasm of skin of scrotum

   D29.8 Benign neoplasm of other specified male genital organs — [♂]
         Benign neoplasm of seminal vesicle
         Benign neoplasm of spermatic cord
         Benign neoplasm of tunica vaginalis

   D29.9 Benign neoplasm of male genital organ, unspecified — [♂]

D30- **Benign neoplasm** of urinary organs — Any new and abnormal growth in which tumor cells progressively multiply, but lack the properties of invasion and metastases (see Malignant Neoplasm code catgories, by site, for anatomical description).

   D30.0- Benign neoplasm of **kidney**
       Excludes 1:   *benign carcinoid tumor of the kidney (D3A.093)*
                 benign neoplasm of renal calyces (D30.1-)
                 benign neoplasm of renal pelvis (D30.1-)

      D30.00 Benign neoplasm of unspecified kidney

      D30.01 Benign neoplasm of **right** kidney

      D30.02 Benign neoplasm of **left** kidney

   D30.1- Benign neoplasm of **renal pelvis**

      D30.10 Benign neoplasm of unspecified renal pelvis

      D30.11 Benign neoplasm of **right** renal pelvis

      D30.12 Benign neoplasm of **left** renal pelvis

   D30.2- Benign neoplasm of **ureter**
       Excludes 1:   *benign neoplasm of ureteric orifice of bladder (D30.3)*

      D30.20 Benign neoplasm of unspecified ureter

      D30.21 Benign neoplasm of **right** ureter

      D30.22 Benign neoplasm of **left** ureter

   D30.3 Benign neoplasm of **bladder**
         Benign neoplasm of ureteric orifice of bladder
         Benign neoplasm of urethral orifice of bladder

   D30.4 Benign neoplasm of **urethra**
       Excludes 1:   *benign neoplasm of urethral orifice of bladder (D30.3)*

   D30.8 Benign neoplasm of other specified urinary organs
         Benign neoplasm of paraurethral glands

   D30.9 Benign neoplasm of urinary organ, unspecified
         Benign neoplasm of urinary system NOS

D31- **Benign neoplasm** of eye and adnexa — Any new and abnormal growth in which tumor cells progressively multiply, but lack the properties of invasion and metastases (see Malignant Neoplasm code catgories, by site, for anatomical description).
    Excludes 1:   *benign neoplasm of connective tissue of eyelid (D21.0)*
                benign neoplasm of optic nerve (D33.3)
                benign neoplasm of skin of eyelid (D22.1-, D23.1-)

   D31.0- Benign neoplasm of **conjunctiva**

      D31.00 Benign neoplasm of unspecified conjunctiva

      D31.01 Benign neoplasm of **right** conjunctiva

      D31.02 Benign neoplasm of **left** conjunctiva

   D31.1- Benign neoplasm of **cornea**

      D31.10 Benign neoplasm of unspecified cornea

      D31.11 Benign neoplasm of **right** cornea

      D31.12 Benign neoplasm of **left** cornea

   D31.2- Benign neoplasm of **retina**
       Excludes 1:   *dark area on retina (D49.81)*
                 hemangioma of retina (D49.81)
                 neoplasm of unspecified behavior of retina and choroid (D49.81)
                 retinal freckle (D49.81)

      D31.20 Benign neoplasm of unspecified retina

      D31.21 Benign neoplasm of **right** retina

      D31.22 Benign neoplasm of **left** retina

   D31.3- Benign neoplasm of **choroid**

      D31.30 Benign neoplasm of unspecified choroid

      D31.31 Benign neoplasm of **right** choroid

      D31.32 Benign neoplasm of **left** choroid

   D31.4- Benign neoplasm of **ciliary body**

      D31.40 Benign neoplasm of unspecified ciliary body

      D31.41 Benign neoplasm of **right** ciliary body

      D31.42 Benign neoplasm of **left** ciliary body

   D31.5- Benign neoplasm of **lacrimal gland and duct**
         Benign neoplasm of lacrimal sac
         Benign neoplasm of nasolacrimal duct

      D31.50 Benign neoplasm of unspecified lacrimal gland and duct

      D31.51 Benign neoplasm of **right** lacrimal gland and duct

      D31.52 Benign neoplasm of **left** lacrimal gland and duct

   D31.6- Benign neoplasm of unspecified site of orbit
         Benign neoplasm of connective tissue of orbit
         Benign neoplasm of extraocular muscle
         Benign neoplasm of peripheral nerves of orbit
         Benign neoplasm of retrobulbar tissue
         Benign neoplasm of retro-ocular tissue
       Excludes 1:   *benign neoplasm of orbital bone (D16.4)*

      D31.60 Benign neoplasm of unspecified site of unspecified orbit

      D31.61 Benign neoplasm of unspecified site of **right** orbit

      D31.62 Benign neoplasm of unspecified site of **left** orbit

   D31.9- Benign neoplasm of unspecified part of eye
         Benign neoplasm of eyeball

      D31.90 Benign neoplasm of unspecified part of unspecified eye

      D31.91 Benign neoplasm of unspecified part of **right** eye

      D31.92 Benign neoplasm of unspecified part of **left** eye

D32- **Benign neoplasm** of meninges — Any new and abnormal growth in which tumor cells progressively multiply, but lack the properties of invasion and metastases (see Malignant Neoplasm code catgories, by site, for anatomical description).

   D32.0 Benign neoplasm of **cerebral meninges**

   D32.1 Benign neoplasm of **spinal meninges**

   D32.9 Benign neoplasm of meninges, unspecified
         Meningioma NOS

Excludes 1: = NOT CODED HERE! (Do not code both)   **593**   *Excludes ❷:* = Not Included Here

D33- **Benign neoplasm** of brain and other parts of central nervous system — Any new and abnormal growth in which tumor cells progressively multiply, but lack the properties of invasion and metastases (see Malignant Neoplasm code catgories, by site, for anatomical description).
Excludes 1: angioma (D18.0-)
benign neoplasm of meninges (D32.-)
benign neoplasm of peripheral nerves and autonomic nervous system (D36.1-)
hemangioma (D18.0-)
neurofibromatosis (Q85.0-)
retro-ocular benign neoplasm (D31.6-)

D33.0 Benign neoplasm of brain, supratentorial
Benign neoplasm of cerebral ventricle
Benign neoplasm of cerebrum
Benign neoplasm of frontal lobe
Benign neoplasm of occipital lobe
Benign neoplasm of parietal lobe
Benign neoplasm of temporal lobe
Excludes 1: benign neoplasm of fourth ventricle (D33.1)

D33.1 Benign neoplasm of brain, infratentorial
Benign neoplasm of brain stem
Benign neoplasm of cerebellum
Benign neoplasm of fourth ventricle

D33.2 Benign neoplasm of brain, unspecified

D33.3 Benign neoplasm of cranial nerves
Benign neoplasm of olfactory bulb

D33.4 Benign neoplasm of spinal cord

D33.7 Benign neoplasm of other specified parts of central nervous system

D33.9 Benign neoplasm of central nervous system, unspecified
Benign neoplasm of nervous system (central) NOS

D34 **Benign neoplasm** of thyroid gland — Any new and abnormal growth in which tumor cells progressively multiply, but lack the properties of invasion and metastases (see Malignant Neoplasm code catgories, by site, for anatomical description).
Use additional code to identify any functional activity

D35- **Benign neoplasm** of other and unspecified endocrine glands — Any new and abnormal growth in which tumor cells progressively multiply, but lack the properties of invasion and metastases (see Malignant Neoplasm code catgories, by site, for anatomical description).
Use additional code to identify any functional activity
Excludes 1: benign neoplasm of endocrine pancreas (D13.7)
benign neoplasm of ovary (D27.-)
benign neoplasm of testis (D29.2.-)
benign neoplasm of thymus (D15.0)

D35.0- Benign neoplasm of adrenal gland
D35.00 Benign neoplasm of unspecified adrenal gland
D35.01 Benign neoplasm of right adrenal gland
D35.02 Benign neoplasm of left adrenal gland

D35.1 Benign neoplasm of parathyroid gland

D35.2 Benign neoplasm of pituitary gland
AHA 14:3Q:p22 – Pituitary macroadenoma

D35.3 Benign neoplasm of craniopharyngeal duct

D35.4 Benign neoplasm of pineal gland

D35.5 Benign neoplasm of carotid body

D35.6 Benign neoplasm of aortic body and other paraganglia
Benign tumor of glomus jugulare

D35.7 Benign neoplasm of other specified endocrine glands

D35.9 Benign neoplasm of endocrine gland, unspecified
Benign neoplasm of unspecified endocrine gland

D36- **Benign neoplasm** of other and unspecified sites — Any new and abnormal growth in which tumor cells progressively multiply, but lack the properties of invasion and metastases (see Malignant Neoplasm code catgories, by site, for anatomical description).

D36.0 Benign neoplasm of lymph nodes
Excludes 1: lymphangioma (D18.1)

D36.1- Benign neoplasm of peripheral nerves and autonomic nervous system
Excludes 1: benign neoplasm of peripheral nerves of orbit (D31.6-)
neurofibromatosis (Q85.0-)

D36.10 Benign neoplasm of peripheral nerves and autonomic nervous system, unspecified

D36.11 Benign neoplasm of peripheral nerves and autonomic nervous system of face, head, and neck

D36.12 Benign neoplasm of peripheral nerves and autonomic nervous system, upper limb, including shoulder

D36.13 Benign neoplasm of peripheral nerves and autonomic nervous system of lower limb, including hip

D36.14 Benign neoplasm of peripheral nerves and autonomic nervous system of thorax

D36.15 Benign neoplasm of peripheral nerves and autonomic nervous system of abdomen

D36.16 Benign neoplasm of peripheral nerves and autonomic nervous system of pelvis

D36.17 Benign neoplasm of peripheral nerves and autonomic nervous system of trunk, unspecified

D36.7 Benign neoplasm of other specified sites
Benign neoplasm of nose NOS

D36.9 Benign neoplasm, unspecified site

Benign neuroendocrine tumors (D3A)

D3A- **Benign neuroendocrine tumors** — Any new and abnormal growth that arises from endocrine or neuroendocrine cells rather than from where the tumor is located in which tumor cells progressively multiply, but lack the properties of invasion and metastases (see Malignant Neoplasm code catgories, by site, for anatomical description).
Use additional code to identify any associated endocrine syndrome, such as:
Carcinoid syndrome (E34.0)
Excludes ❷: benign pancreatic islet cell tumors (D13.7)
Code also any associated multiple endocrine neoplasia [MEN] syndromes (E31.2-)

D3A.0- Benign carcinoid tumors
D3A.00 Benign carcinoid tumor of unspecified site
Carcinoid tumor NOS

D3A.01- Benign carcinoid tumors of the small intestine
D3A.010 Benign carcinoid tumor of the duodenum
D3A.011 Benign carcinoid tumor of the jejunum
D3A.012 Benign carcinoid tumor of the ileum
D3A.019 Benign carcinoid tumor of the small intestine, unspecified portion

D3A.02- Benign carcinoid tumors of the appendix, large intestine, and rectum
D3A.020 Benign carcinoid tumor of the appendix
D3A.021 Benign carcinoid tumor of the cecum
D3A.022 Benign carcinoid tumor of the ascending colon
D3A.023 Benign carcinoid tumor of the transverse colon
D3A.024 Benign carcinoid tumor of the descending colon
D3A.025 Benign carcinoid tumor of the sigmoid colon
D3A.026 Benign carcinoid tumor of the rectum
D3A.029 Benign carcinoid tumor of the large intestine, unspecified portion
Benign carcinoid tumor of the colon NOS

D3A.09- Benign carcinoid tumors of other sites
D3A.090 Benign carcinoid tumor of the bronchus and lung
D3A.091 Benign carcinoid tumor of the thymus
D3A.092 Benign carcinoid tumor of the stomach
D3A.093 Benign carcinoid tumor of the kidney
D3A.094 Benign carcinoid tumor of the foregut, unspecified
D3A.095 Benign carcinoid tumor of the midgut, unspecified
D3A.096 Benign carcinoid tumor of the hindgut, unspecified
D3A.098 Benign carcinoid tumors of other sites

D3A.8 Other benign neuroendocrine tumors
Neuroendocrine tumor NOS

Neoplasms of uncertain behavior, polycythemia vera and myelodysplastic syndromes (D37-D48)

Note: Categories D37-D44, and D48 classify by site neoplasms of uncertain behavior, i.e., histologic confirmation whether the neoplasm is malignant or benign cannot be made.
Excludes 1:   neoplasms of unspecified behavior (D49.-)

D37- Neoplasm of <u>uncertain behavior</u> of oral cavity and digestive organs — See Note and Excludes 1 at code block D37-D48.
Excludes 1:   stromal tumors of uncertain behavior of digestive system (D48.1)

D37.0- Neoplasm of uncertain behavior of lip, oral cavity and pharynx
Excludes 1:   neoplasm of uncertain behavior of aryepiglottic fold or interarytenoid fold, laryngeal aspect (D38.0)
neoplasm of uncertain behavior of epiglottis NOS (D38.0)
neoplasm of uncertain behavior of skin of lip (D48.5)
neoplasm of uncertain behavior of suprahyoid portion of epiglottis (D38.0)

D37.01 Neoplasm of uncertain behavior of <u>lip</u>
Neoplasm of uncertain behavior of vermilion border of lip

D37.02 Neoplasm of uncertain behavior of <u>tongue</u>

D37.03- Neoplasm of uncertain behavior of the <u>major</u> salivary glands

D37.030 Neoplasm of uncertain behavior of the <u>parotid</u> salivary glands

D37.031 Neoplasm of uncertain behavior of the <u>sublingual</u> salivary glands

D37.032 Neoplasm of uncertain behavior of the <u>submandibular</u> salivary glands

D37.039 Neoplasm of uncertain behavior of the major salivary glands, unspecified

D37.04 Neoplasm of uncertain behavior of the <u>minor</u> salivary glands
Neoplasm of uncertain behavior of submucosal salivary glands of lip
Neoplasm of uncertain behavior of submucosal salivary glands of cheek
Neoplasm of uncertain behavior of submucosal salivary glands of hard palate
Neoplasm of uncertain behavior of submucosal salivary glands of soft palate

D37.05 Neoplasm of uncertain behavior of <u>pharynx</u>
Neoplasm of uncertain behavior of aryepiglottic fold of pharynx NOS
Neoplasm of uncertain behavior of hypopharyngeal aspect of aryepiglottic fold of pharynx
Neoplasm of uncertain behavior of marginal zone of aryepiglottic fold of pharynx

D37.09 Neoplasm of uncertain behavior of other specified sites of the oral cavity

D37.1 Neoplasm of uncertain behavior of <u>stomach</u>

D37.2 Neoplasm of uncertain behavior of <u>small intestine</u>

D37.3 Neoplasm of uncertain behavior of <u>appendix</u>

D37.4 Neoplasm of uncertain behavior of <u>colon</u>

D37.5 Neoplasm of uncertain behavior of <u>rectum</u>
Neoplasm of uncertain behavior of rectosigmoid junction

D37.6 Neoplasm of uncertain behavior of <u>liver, gallbladder and bile ducts</u>
Neoplasm of uncertain behavior of ampulla of Vater

D37.8 Neoplasm of uncertain behavior of other specified digestive organs
Neoplasm of uncertain behavior of anal canal
Neoplasm of uncertain behavior of anal sphincter
Neoplasm of uncertain behavior of anus NOS
Neoplasm of uncertain behavior of esophagus
Neoplasm of uncertain behavior of intestine NOS
Neoplasm of uncertain behavior of pancreas
Excludes 1:   neoplasm of uncertain behavior of anal margin (D48.5)
neoplasm of uncertain behavior of anal skin (D48.5)
neoplasm of uncertain behavior of perianal skin (D48.5)

D37.9 Neoplasm of uncertain behavior of digestive organ, unspecified

D38- Neoplasm of <u>uncertain behavior</u> of middle ear and respiratory and intrathoracic organs — See Note and Excludes 1 at code block D37-D48.
Excludes 1:   neoplasm of uncertain behavior of heart (D48.7)

D38.0 Neoplasm of uncertain behavior of <u>larynx</u>
Neoplasm of uncertain behavior of aryepiglottic fold or interarytenoid fold, laryngeal aspect
Neoplasm of uncertain behavior of epiglottis (suprahyoid portion)
Excludes 1:   neoplasm of uncertain behavior of aryepiglottic fold or interarytenoid fold NOS (D37.05)
neoplasm of uncertain behavior of hypopharyngeal aspect of aryepiglottic fold (D37.05)
neoplasm of uncertain behavior of marginal zone of aryepiglottic fold (D37.05)

D38.1 Neoplasm of uncertain behavior of <u>trachea, bronchus and lung</u>

D38.2 Neoplasm of uncertain behavior of <u>pleura</u>

D38.3 Neoplasm of uncertain behavior of <u>mediastinum</u>

D38.4 Neoplasm of uncertain behavior of <u>thymus</u>

D38.5 Neoplasm of uncertain behavior of other respiratory organs
Neoplasm of uncertain behavior of accessory sinuses
Neoplasm of uncertain behavior of cartilage of nose
Neoplasm of uncertain behavior of middle ear
Neoplasm of uncertain behavior of nasal cavities
Excludes 1:   neoplasm of uncertain behavior of ear (external) (skin) (D48.5)
neoplasm of uncertain behavior of nose NOS (D48.7)
neoplasm of uncertain behavior of skin of nose (D48.5)

D38.6 Neoplasm of uncertain behavior of respiratory organ, unspecified

D39- Neoplasm of <u>uncertain behavior</u> of female genital organs — See Note and Excludes 1 at code block D37-D48.

D39.0 Neoplasm of uncertain behavior of <u>uterus</u> — [♀]

D39.1- Neoplasm of uncertain behavior of <u>ovary</u>
Use additional code to identify any functional activity.

D39.10 Neoplasm of uncertain behavior of unspecified ovary — [♀]

D39.11 Neoplasm of uncertain behavior of <u>right</u> ovary — [♀]

D39.12 Neoplasm of uncertain behavior of <u>left</u> ovary — [♀]

D39.2 Neoplasm of uncertain behavior of <u>placenta</u> — [♀, Age/12-55]
Chorioadenoma destruens
Invasive hydatidiform mole
Malignant hydatidiform mole
Excludes 1:   hydatidiform mole NOS (O01.9)

D39.8 Neoplasm of uncertain behavior of other specified female genital organs — [♀]
Neoplasm of uncertain behavior of skin of female genital organs

D39.9 Neoplasm of uncertain behavior of female genital organ, unspecified — [♀]

D40- Neoplasm of <u>uncertain behavior</u> of male genital organs — See Note and Excludes 1 at code block D37-D48.

D40.0 Neoplasm of uncertain behavior of <u>prostate</u> — [♂]

D40.1- Neoplasm of uncertain behavior of <u>testis</u>

D40.10 Neoplasm of uncertain behavior of unspecified testis — [♂]

D40.11 Neoplasm of uncertain behavior of <u>right</u> testis — [♂]

D40.12 Neoplasm of uncertain behavior of <u>left</u> testis — [♂]

D40.8 Neoplasm of uncertain behavior of other specified male genital organs — [♂]
Neoplasm of uncertain behavior of skin of male genital organs

D40.9 Neoplasm of uncertain behavior of male genital organ, unspecified — [♂]

D41- Neoplasm of <u>uncertain behavior</u> of urinary organs — See Note and Excludes 1 at code block D37-D48.

D41.0- Neoplasm of uncertain behavior of <u>kidney</u>
Excludes 1:   neoplasm of uncertain behavior of renal pelvis (D41.1-)

D41.00 Neoplasm of uncertain behavior of unspecified kidney

D41.01 Neoplasm of uncertain behavior of <u>right</u> kidney

D41.02 Neoplasm of uncertain behavior of <u>left</u> kidney

D37 - D41

D41.1- Neoplasm of uncertain behavior of <u>renal pelvis</u>

 D41.10 Neoplasm of uncertain behavior of unspecified renal pelvis

 D41.11 Neoplasm of uncertain behavior of <u>right</u> renal pelvis

 D41.12 Neoplasm of uncertain behavior of <u>left</u> renal pelvis

D41.2- Neoplasm of uncertain behavior of <u>ureter</u>

 D41.20 Neoplasm of uncertain behavior of unspecified ureter

 D41.21 Neoplasm of uncertain behavior of <u>right</u> ureter

 D41.22 Neoplasm of uncertain behavior of <u>left</u> ureter

D41.3 Neoplasm of uncertain behavior of <u>urethra</u>

D41.4 Neoplasm of uncertain behavior of <u>bladder</u>

D41.8 Neoplasm of uncertain behavior of other specified urinary organs

D41.9 Neoplasm of uncertain behavior of unspecified urinary organ

D42- Neoplasm of <u>uncertain behavior</u> of meninges — See Note and Excludes 1 at code block D37-D48.

D42.0 Neoplasm of uncertain behavior of <u>cerebral meninges</u>

D42.1 Neoplasm of uncertain behavior of <u>spinal meninges</u>

D42.9 Neoplasm of uncertain behavior of meninges, unspecified

D43- Neoplasm of <u>uncertain behavior</u> of brain and central nervous system — See Note and Excludes 1 at code block D37-D48.
 Excludes 1: neoplasm of uncertain behavior of peripheral nerves and autonomic nervous system (D48.2)

D43.0 Neoplasm of uncertain behavior of <u>brain, supratentorial</u>
 Neoplasm of uncertain behavior of cerebral ventricle
 Neoplasm of uncertain behavior of cerebrum
 Neoplasm of uncertain behavior of frontal lobe
 Neoplasm of uncertain behavior of occipital lobe
 Neoplasm of uncertain behavior of parietal lobe
 Neoplasm of uncertain behavior of temporal lobe
 Excludes 1: neoplasm of uncertain behavior of fourth ventricle (D43.1)

D43.1 Neoplasm of uncertain behavior of <u>brain, infratentorial</u>
 Neoplasm of uncertain behavior of brain stem
 Neoplasm of uncertain behavior of cerebellum
 Neoplasm of uncertain behavior of fourth ventricle

D43.2 Neoplasm of uncertain behavior of brain, unspecified

D43.3 Neoplasm of uncertain behavior of <u>cranial nerves</u>

D43.4 Neoplasm of uncertain behavior of <u>spinal cord</u>

D43.8 Neoplasm of uncertain behavior of other specified parts of central nervous system

D43.9 Neoplasm of uncertain behavior of central nervous system, unspecified
 Neoplasm of uncertain behavior of nervous system (central) NOS

D44- Neoplasm of <u>uncertain behavior</u> of endocrine glands — See Note and Excludes 1 at code block D37-D48.
 Excludes 1: multiple endocrine adenomatosis (E31.2-)
  multiple endocrine neoplasia (E31.2-)
  neoplasm of uncertain behavior of endocrine pancreas(D37.8)
  neoplasm of uncertain behavior of ovary (D39.1-)
  neoplasm of uncertain behavior of testis (D40.1-)
  neoplasm of uncertain behavior of thymus (D38.4)

D44.0 Neoplasm of uncertain behavior of <u>thyroid gland</u>

D44.1- Neoplasm of uncertain behavior of <u>adrenal gland</u>
 Use additional code to identify any functional activity.

 D44.10 Neoplasm of uncertain behavior of unspecified adrenal gland

 D44.11 Neoplasm of uncertain behavior of <u>right</u> adrenal gland

 D44.12 Neoplasm of uncertain behavior of <u>left</u> adrenal gland

D44.2 Neoplasm of uncertain behavior of <u>parathyroid gland</u>

D44.3 Neoplasm of uncertain behavior of <u>pituitary gland</u>
 Use additional code to identify any functional activity.

D44.4 Neoplasm of uncertain behavior of <u>craniopharyngeal duct</u>

D44.5 Neoplasm of uncertain behavior of <u>pineal gland</u>

D44.6 Neoplasm of uncertain behavior of <u>carotid body</u>

D44.7 Neoplasm of uncertain behavior of <u>aortic body</u> and other <u>paraganglia</u>

D44.9 Neoplasm of uncertain behavior of unspecified endocrine gland

D45 <u>Polycythemia vera</u> — A neoplastic proliferation disorder that is characterized by an abnormally high production and concentration of red blood cells (erythrocytes).
 Excludes 1: familial polycythemia (D75.0)
  secondary polycythemia (D75.1)

D46- <u>Myelodysplastic syndromes</u> — A neoplastic bone marrow cell production disorder in which immature cells to not develop normally into mature, healthy cells.
 Use additional code for adverse effect, if applicable, to identify drug (T36-T50 with fifth or sixth character 5)
 Excludes ❷: drug-induced aplastic anemia (D61.1)

D46.0 Refractory anemia <u>without</u> ring sideroblasts, so stated
 Refractory anemia without sideroblasts, without excess of blasts

D46.1 Refractory anemia <u>with</u> ring sideroblasts — A form producing too few red blood cells and those cells have too much iron inside the cell.
 RARS

D46.2- Refractory anemia <u>with excess of blasts</u> [RAEB] — A form producing too few red blood cells and a greater than normal number of blast cells.

 D46.20 Refractory anemia with excess of blasts, unspecified
  RAEB NOS

 D46.21 Refractory anemia with excess of <u>blasts</u> 1
  RAEB 1

 CC **D46.22** Refractory anemia with excess of <u>blasts</u> 2
  RAEB 2

D46.A Refractory cytopenia with multilineage dysplasia — A form producing too few of at least two types of blood cells (red blood cells, white blood cells, or platelets).

D46.B Refractory cytopenia with multilineage dysplasia <u>and ring sideroblasts</u> — A form producing too few of at least two types of blood cells (red blood cells, white blood cells, or platelets) and those red blood cells have too much iron inside the cell.
 RCMD RS

CC **D46.C** Myelodysplastic syndrome with isolated del(5q) chromosomal abnormality — A form producing too few red blood cells that is characterized by changes in chromosome 5.
 Myelodysplastic syndrome with 5q deletion
 5q minus syndrome NOS

D46.4 Refractory anemia, unspecified

D46.Z Other myelodysplastic syndromes
 Excludes 1: chronic myelomonocytic leukemia (C93.1-)

D46.9 Myelodysplastic syndrome, unspecified
 Myelodysplasia NOS

D47- Other neoplasms of <u>uncertain behavior</u> of lymphoid, hematopoietic and related tissue

CC **D47.0** <u>Histiocytic and mast cell tumors</u> of uncertain behavior
 Indolent systemic mastocytosis
 Mast cell tumor NOS
 Mastocytoma NOS
 Excludes 1: malignant mast cell tumor (C96.2)
  mastocytosis (congenital) (cutaneous) (Q82.2)

CC **D47.1** <u>Chronic myeloproliferative disease</u> — A neoplastic bone marrow cell production disorder in which too many blood cells (red blood cells, white blood cells, or platelets) are produced.
 Chronic neutrophilic leukemia
 Myeloproliferative disease, unspecified
 Excludes 1: atypical chronic myeloid leukemia BCR/ABL-negative (C92.2-)
  chronic myeloid leukemia BCR/ABL-positive (C92.1-)
  myelofibrosis NOS (D75.81)
  myelophthisic anemia (D61.82)
  myelophthisis (D61.82)
  secondary myelofibrosis NOS (D75.81)

D47.2 <u>Monoclonal gammopathy</u>
 Monoclonal gammopathy of undetermined significance [MGUS]

D47.3 <u>Essential (hemorrhagic) thrombocythemia</u> — A neoplastic bone marrow cell production disorder in which too many platelets are formed.
 Essential thrombocytosis
 Idiopathic hemorrhagic thrombocythemia

D47.4 <u>Osteomyelofibrosis</u>
 Chronic idiopathic myelofibrosis
 Myelofibrosis (idiopathic) (with myeloid metaplasia)
 Myelosclerosis (megakaryocytic) with myeloid metaplasia
 Secondary myelofibrosis in myeloproliferative disease
 Excludes 1: acute myelofibrosis (C94.4-)

D41-D47

D47.Z- Other specified neoplasms of uncertain behavior of lymphoid, hematopoietic and related tissue

CC **D47.Z1** Post-transplant lymphoproliferative disorder (PTLD) —
[Unacceptable PDX]
Code first complications of transplanted organs and tissue (T86.-)

CC **D47.Z2** Castleman disease — A lymphoproliferative disorder with varying clinical features that is characterized by proliferation of morphologically benign lymphocytes.
Code also if applicable human herpesvirus 8 infection (B10.89)
Excludes ❷: Kaposi's sarcoma (C46-)

CC **D47.Z9** Other specified neoplasms of uncertain behavior of lymphoid, hematopoietic and related tissue
Histiocytic tumors of uncertain behavior

CC **D47.9** Neoplasm of uncertain behavior of lymphoid, hematopoietic and related tissue, unspecified
Lymphoproliferative disease NOS

D48- Neoplasm of <u>uncertain behavior</u> of other and unspecified sites — See Note and Excludes 1 at code block D37-D48.
Excludes 1: neurofibromatosis (nonmalignant) (Q85.0-)

D48.0 Neoplasm of uncertain behavior of <u>bone and articular cartilage</u>
Excludes 1: neoplasm of uncertain behavior of cartilage of ear (D48.1)
neoplasm of uncertain behavior of cartilage of larynx (D38.0)
neoplasm of uncertain behavior of cartilage of nose (D38.5)
neoplasm of uncertain behavior of connective tissue of eyelid (D48.1)
neoplasm of uncertain behavior of synovia (D48.1)

D48.1 Neoplasm of uncertain behavior of <u>connective and other soft tissue</u>
Neoplasm of uncertain behavior of connective tissue of ear
Neoplasm of uncertain behavior of connective tissue of eyelid
Stromal tumors of uncertain behavior of digestive system
Excludes 1: neoplasm of uncertain behavior of articular cartilage (D48.0)
neoplasm of uncertain behavior of cartilage of larynx (D38.0)
neoplasm of uncertain behavior of cartilage of nose (D38.5)
neoplasm of uncertain behavior of connective tissue of breast (D48.6-)

D48.2 Neoplasm of uncertain behavior of <u>peripheral nerves and autonomic nervous system</u>
Excludes 1: neoplasm of uncertain behavior of peripheral nerves of orbit (D48.7)

D48.3 Neoplasm of uncertain behavior of <u>retroperitoneum</u>

D48.4 Neoplasm of uncertain behavior of <u>peritoneum</u>

D48.5 Neoplasm of uncertain behavior of <u>skin</u>
Neoplasm of uncertain behavior of anal margin
Neoplasm of uncertain behavior of anal skin
Neoplasm of uncertain behavior of perianal skin
Neoplasm of uncertain behavior of skin of breast
Excludes 1: neoplasm of uncertain behavior of anus NOS (D37.8)
neoplasm of uncertain behavior of skin of genital organs (D39.8, D40.8)
neoplasm of uncertain behavior of vermilion border of lip (D37.0)

D48.6- Neoplasm of uncertain behavior of <u>breast</u>
Neoplasm of uncertain behavior of connective tissue of breast
Cystosarcoma phyllodes
Excludes 1: neoplasm of uncertain behavior of skin of breast (D48.5)

D48.60 Neoplasm of uncertain behavior of unspecified breast

D48.61 Neoplasm of uncertain behavior of <u>right</u> breast

D48.62 Neoplasm of uncertain behavior of <u>left</u> breast

D48.7 Neoplasm of uncertain behavior of other specified sites
Neoplasm of uncertain behavior of eye
Neoplasm of uncertain behavior of heart
Neoplasm of uncertain behavior of peripheral nerves of orbit
Excludes 1: neoplasm of uncertain behavior of connective tissue (D48.1)
neoplasm of uncertain behavior of skin of eyelid (D48.5)

D48.9 Neoplasm of uncertain behavior, unspecified

Neoplasms of unspecified behavior (D49)

D49- Neoplasms of <u>unspecified behavior</u>
Note: Category D49 classifies by site neoplasms of unspecified morphology and behavior. The term "mass", unless otherwise stated, is not to be regarded as a neoplastic growth.
Includes: "Growth" NOS
Neoplasm NOS
New growth NOS
Tumor NOS
Excludes 1: neoplasms of uncertain behavior (D37-D44, D48)

D49.0 Neoplasm of unspecified behavior of <u>digestive system</u>
Excludes 1: neoplasm of unspecified behavior of margin of anus (D49.2)
neoplasm of unspecified behavior of perianal skin (D49.2)
neoplasm of unspecified behavior of skin of anus (D49.2)

D49.1 Neoplasm of unspecified behavior of <u>respiratory system</u>

D49.2 Neoplasm of unspecified behavior of <u>bone, soft tissue, and skin</u>
Excludes 1: neoplasm of unspecified behavior of anal canal (D49.0)
neoplasm of unspecified behavior of anus NOS (D49.0)
neoplasm of unspecified behavior of bone marrow (D49.89)
neoplasm of unspecified behavior of cartilage of larynx (D49.1)
neoplasm of unspecified behavior of cartilage of nose (D49.1)
neoplasm of unspecified behavior of connective tissue of breast (D49.3)
neoplasm of unspecified behavior of skin of genital organs (D49.59)
neoplasm of unspecified behavior of vermilion border of lip (D49.0)

D49.3 Neoplasm of unspecified behavior of <u>breast</u>
Excludes 1: neoplasm of unspecified behavior of skin of breast (D49.2)

D49.4 Neoplasm of unspecified behavior of <u>bladder</u>

D49.5- Neoplasm of unspecified behavior of <u>other genitourinary organs</u>

D49.51- Neoplasm of unspecified behavior of <u>kidney</u>

D49.511 Neoplasm of unspecified behavior of <u>right</u> kidney

D49.512 Neoplasm of unspecified behavior of <u>left</u> kidney

D49.519 Neoplasm of unspecified behavior of <u>unspecified</u> kidney

D49.59 Neoplasm of unspecified behavior of other genitourinary organ

D49.6 Neoplasm of unspecified behavior of <u>brain</u>
Excludes 1: neoplasm of unspecified behavior of cerebral meninges (D49.7)
neoplasm of unspecified behavior of cranial nerves (D49.7)

D49.7 Neoplasm of unspecified behavior of <u>endocrine glands and other parts of nervous system</u>
Excludes 1: neoplasm of unspecified behavior of peripheral, sympathetic, and parasympathetic nerves and ganglia (D49.2)

D49.8- Neoplasm of unspecified behavior of other specified sites
Excludes 1: neoplasm of unspecified behavior of eyelid (skin) (D49.2)
neoplasm of unspecified behavior of eyelid cartilage (D49.2)
neoplasm of unspecified behavior of great vessels (D49.2)
neoplasm of unspecified behavior of optic nerve (D49.7)

D49.81 Neoplasm of unspecified behavior of retina and choroid
Dark area on retina
Retinal freckle

D49.89 Neoplasm of unspecified behavior of other specified sites

D49.9 Neoplasm of unspecified behavior of unspecified site

D47 I D49

D49‑D49

Chapter 3 – Diseases of the blood and blood-forming organs and certain disorders involving the immune mechanism (D50-D89)

Excludes ❷: *autoimmune disease (systemic) NOS (M35.9)*

certain conditions originating in the perinatal period (P00-P96)

complications of pregnancy, childbirth and the puerperium (O00-O9A)

congenital malformations, deformations and chromosomal abnormalities (Q00-Q99)

endocrine, nutritional and metabolic diseases (E00-E88)

human immunodeficiency virus [HIV] disease (B20)

injury, poisoning and certain other consequences of external causes (S00-T88)

neoplasms (C00-D49)

symptoms, signs and abnormal clinical and laboratory findings, not elsewhere classified (R00-R94)

This chapter contains the following blocks:

D50-D53	Nutritional anemias
D55-D59	Hemolytic anemias
D60-D64	Aplastic and other anemias and other bone marrow failure syndromes
D65-D69	Coagulation defects, purpura and other hemorrhagic conditions
D70-D77	Other disorders of blood and blood-forming organs
D78	Intraoperative and postprocedural complications of the spleen
D80-D89	Certain disorders involving the immune mechanism

Chapter-Specific Coding Guidelines

C.   Chapter-Specific Coding Guidelines

In addition to general coding guidelines, there are guidelines for specific diagnoses and/or conditions in the classification. Unless otherwise indicated, these guidelines apply to all health care settings. Please refer to Section II for guidelines on the selection of principal diagnosis.

3.   Chapter 3: Disease of the Blood and Blood-forming Organs and Certain Disorders Involving the Immune Mechanism (D50-D89)

Reserved for future guideline expansion

Nutritional anemias (D50-D53)

D50-   <u>Iron deficiency</u> anemia — An abnormal reduction of red blood cells caused by low or absent iron stores.

     Includes: Asiderotic anemia
                 Hypochromic anemia

D50.0   Iron deficiency anemia secondary to <u>blood loss</u> (chronic)

       Posthemorrhagic anemia (chronic)

       Excludes 1:   *acute posthemorrhagic anemia (D62)*
                      congenital anemia from fetal blood loss (P61.3)

D50.1   Sideropenic dysphagia

       Kelly-Paterson syndrome

       Plummer-Vinson syndrome

D50.8   Other iron deficiency anemias

       Iron deficiency anemia due to inadequate dietary iron intake

D50.9   Iron deficiency anemia, unspecified

D51-   <u>Vitamin B12 deficiency</u> anemia — A megaloblastic anemia characterized by decreased levels of vitamin B12 absorption.

     Excludes 1:   *vitamin B12 deficiency (E53.8)*

D51.0   Vitamin B12 deficiency anemia due to <u>intrinsic factor</u> deficiency

       Addison anemia

       Biermer anemia

       Pernicious (congenital) anemia

       Congenital intrinsic factor deficiency

D51.1   Vitamin B12 deficiency anemia due to <u>selective vitamin B12</u> malabsorption with proteinuria

       Imerslund (Gräsbeck) syndrome

       Megaloblastic hereditary anemia

D51.2   <u>Transcobalamin II</u> deficiency

D51.3   Other dietary vitamin B12 deficiency anemia

       Vegan anemia

D51.8   Other vitamin B12 deficiency anemias

D51.9   Vitamin B12 deficiency anemia, unspecified

D52-   <u>Folate deficiency</u> anemia — Megaloblastic anemia caused by the lack of folic acid (one of the B vitamins) in the blood.

     Excludes 1:   *folate deficiency without anemia (E53.8)*

D52.0   <u>Dietary</u> folate deficiency anemia

       Nutritional megaloblastic anemia

D52.1   <u>Drug-induced</u> folate deficiency anemia

       Use additional code for adverse effect, if applicable, to identify drug (T36-T50 with fifth or sixth character 5)

D52.8   Other folate deficiency anemias

D52.9   Folate deficiency anemia, unspecified

       Folic acid deficiency anemia NOS

D53-   <u>Other nutritional</u> anemias

     Includes: Megaloblastic anemia unresponsive to vitamin B12 or folate therapy

D53.0   <u>Protein</u> deficiency anemia — An abnormal reduction of blood cells due to decreased protein intake.

       Amino-acid deficiency anemia

       Orotaciduric anemia

       Excludes 1:   *Lesch-Nyhan syndrome (E79.1)*

D53.1   Other megaloblastic anemias, not elsewhere classified

       Megaloblastic anemia NOS

       Excludes 1:   *Di Guglielmo's disease (C94.0)*

D53.2   <u>Scorbutic</u> anemia

       Excludes 1:   *scurvy (E54)*

D53.8   Other specified nutritional anemias

       Anemia associated with deficiency of copper

       Anemia associated with deficiency of molybdenum

       Anemia associated with deficiency of zinc

       Excludes 1:   *nutritional deficiencies without anemia, such as:*
                           copper deficiency NOS (E61.0)
                           molybdenum deficiency NOS (E61.5)
                           zinc deficiency NOS (E60)

D53.9   Nutritional anemia, unspecified

       Simple chronic anemia

       Excludes 1:   *anemia NOS (D64.9)*

Hemolytic anemias (D55-D59)

D55-   Anemia due to <u>enzyme disorders</u> — An abnormal reduction of red blood cells due to the breakdown of red blood cells caused by enzyme disorders.

     Excludes 1:   *drug-induced enzyme deficiency anemia (D59.2)*

D55.0   Anemia due to glucose-6-phosphate dehydrogenase [G6PD] deficiency — A genetic form caused by a deficiency of the enzyme glucose-6-phosphate dehydrogenase.

       Favism

       G6PD deficiency anemia

D55.1   Anemia due to other disorders of glutathione metabolism

       Anemia (due to) enzyme deficiencies, except G6PD, related to the hexose monophosphate [HMP] shunt pathway

       Anemia (due to) hemolytic nonspherocytic (hereditary), type I

D55.2   Anemia due to disorders of glycolytic enzymes — A genetic form caused by a deficiency of the glycolytic enzymes (hexokinase, pyruvate kinase, triose-phosphate isomerase).

       Hemolytic nonspherocytic (hereditary) anemia, type II

       Hexokinase deficiency anemia

       Pyruvate kinase [PK] deficiency anemia

       Triose-phosphate isomerase deficiency anemia

       Excludes 1:   *disorders of glycolysis not associated with anemia (E74.8)*

D55.3   Anemia due to disorders of nucleotide metabolism

D55.8   Other anemias due to enzyme disorders

D55.9   Anemia due to enzyme disorder, unspecified

D50 – D55

D56-   <u>Thalassemia</u> — A group of hereditary hemolytic anemias in which the body makes an abnormal form of hemoglobin that has limited capacity to carry oxygen.
> *Excludes 1:*   *sickle-cell thalassemia (D57.4-)*

D56.0   <u>Alpha</u> thalassemia — A severe form involving defective alpha hemoglobin chain genes.
> Alpha thalassemia major
> Hemoglobin H Constant Spring
> Hemoglobin H disease
> Hydrops fetalis due to alpha thalassemia
> Severe alpha thalassemia
> Triple gene defect alpha thalassemia
> Use additional code, if applicable, for hydrops fetalis due to alpha thalassemia (P56.99)
> *Excludes 1:*   *alpha thalassemia trait or minor (D56.3)*
>   *asymptomatic alpha thalassemia (D56.3)*
>   *hydrops fetalis due to isoimmunization (P56.0)*
>   *hydrops fetalis not due to immune hemolysis (P83.2)*

D56.1   <u>Beta</u> thalassemia — A severe form involving defective beta hemoglobin chain genes.
> Beta thalassemia major
> Cooley's anemia
> Homozygous beta thalassemia
> Severe beta thalassemia
> Thalassemia intermedia
> Thalassemia major
> *Excludes 1:*   *beta thalassemia minor (D56.3)*
>   *beta thalassemia trait (D56.3)*
>   *delta-beta thalassemia (D56.2)*
>   *hemoglobin E-beta thalassemia (D56.5)*
>   *sickle-cell beta thalassemia (D57.4-)*

D56.2   <u>Delta-beta</u> thalassemia — A form involving defective portions of both beta and delta hemoglobin chain genes.
> Homozygous delta-beta thalassemia
> *Excludes 1:*   *delta-beta thalassemia minor (D56.3)*
>   *delta-beta thalassemia trait (D56.3)*

D56.3   Thalassemia <u>minor</u> — A less severe form involving defective hemoglobin chain genes.
> Alpha thalassemia minor
> Alpha thalassemia silent carrier
> Alpha thalassemia trait
> Beta thalassemia minor
> Beta thalassemia trait
> Delta-beta thalassemia minor
> Delta-beta thalassemia trait
> Thalassemia trait NOS
> *Excludes 1:*   *alpha thalassemia (D56.0)*
>   *beta thalassemia (D56.1)*
>   *delta-beta thalassemia (D56.2)*
>   *hemoglobin E-beta thalassemia (D56.5)*
>   *sickle-cell trait (D57.3)*

D56.4   **Hereditary persistence of fetal hemoglobin [HPFH]**

D56.5   <u>Hemoglobin E-beta</u> thalassemia — A beta chain variant hemoglobinopathy characteized by the presence of variant hemoglobin E.
> *Excludes 1:*   *beta thalassemia (D56.1)*
>   *beta thalassemia minor (D56.3)*
>   *beta thalassemia trait (D56.3)*
>   *delta-beta thalassemia (D56.2)*
>   *delta-beta thalassemia trait (D56.3)*
>   *hemoglobin E disease (D58.2)*
>   *other hemoglobinopathies (D58.2)*
>   *sickle-cell beta thalassemia (D57.4-)*

D56.8   **Other thalassemias**
> Dominant thalassemia
> Hemoglobin C thalassemia
> Mixed thalassemia
> Thalassemia with other hemoglobinopathy
> *Excludes 1:*   *hemoglobin C disease (D58.2)*
>   *hemoglobin E disease (D58.2)*
>   *other hemoglobinopathies (D58.2)*
>   *sickle-cell anemia (D57.-)*
>   *sickle-cell thalassemia (D57.4)*

D56.9   **Thalassemia, unspecified**
> Mediterranean anemia (with other hemoglobinopathy)

D57-   <u>Sickle-cell</u> disorders — A hereditary hemolytic disease characterized by abnormal, shortened-lifespan, crescent-shaped hemoglobin resulting in decreased oxygenation of the tissues.
> **Use additional code for any associated fever (R50.81)**
> *Excludes 1:*   *other hemoglobinopathies (D58.-)*

D57.0-   <u>Hb-SS</u> disease <u>with crisis</u> — A form in which the patient has abnormal hemoglobin SS, and is experiencing the painful symptoms and conditions caused by the sickled red blood cells which block the blood flow, resulting in significant loss of oxygenation of the tissues.
> Sickle-cell disease NOS with crisis
> Hb-SS disease with vasoocclusive pain

MCC D57.00   **Hb-SS disease with crisis, unspecified**

MCC D57.01   **Hb-SS disease with acute chest syndrome**

MCC D57.02   **Hb-SS disease with splenic sequestration**

D57.1   **Sickle-cell disease <u>without</u> crisis**
> Hb-SS disease without crisis
> Sickle-cell anemia NOS
> Sickle-cell disease NOS
> Sickle-cell disorder NOS

D57.2-   **Sickle-cell/<u>Hb-C</u> disease** — A form in which the patient has abnormal hemoglobin C.
> Hb-SC disease
> Hb-S/Hb-C disease

D57.20   **Sickle-cell/Hb-C disease <u>without</u> crisis**

D57.21-   **Sickle-cell/Hb-C disease <u>with crisis</u>** — A form in which the patient is experiencing the painful symptoms and conditions caused by the sickled red blood cells which block the blood flow, resulting in significant loss of oxygenation of the tissues.

MCC D57.211   **Sickle-cell/Hb-C disease with acute chest syndrome** — A form involving the chest (lungs) with symptoms that resemble pneumonia.

MCC D57.212   **Sickle-cell/Hb-C disease with splenic sequestration** — A form resulting from the sickled cells pooling in the spleen causing pain, damage to the spleen, and sometimes life-threatening drop in hemoglobin.

MCC D57.219   **Sickle-cell/Hb-C disease with crisis, unspecified**
> Sickle-cell/Hb-C disease with crisis NOS

D57.3   **Sickle-cell <u>trait</u>** — The usually asymptomatic condition of crescent-shaped hemoglobin S inherited from one of the patient's parents.
> Hb-S trait
> Heterozygous hemoglobin S

D57.4-   **Sickle-cell <u>thalassemia</u>** — A form in which the patient has both the abnormal hemoglobin S gene and the thalassemia gene.
> Sickle-cell beta thalassemia
> Thalassemia Hb-S disease

D57.40   **Sickle-cell thalassemia <u>without</u> crisis**
> Microdrepanocytosis
> Sickle-cell thalassemia NOS

D57.41-   **Sickle-cell thalassemia <u>with crisis</u>**
> Sickle-cell thalassemia with vasoocclusive pain

MCC D57.411   **Sickle-cell thalassemia with acute chest syndrome** — A form involving the chest (lungs) with symptoms that resemble pneumonia.

MCC D57.412   **Sickle-cell thalassemia with splenic sequestration** — A form resulting from the sickled cells pooling in the spleen causing pain, damage to the spleen, and sometimes a life-threatening drop in hemoglobin.

MCC D57.419   **Sickle-cell thalassemia with crisis, unspecified**
> Sickle-cell thalassemia with crisis NOS

D57.8-   **<u>Other</u> sickle-cell disorders**
> Hb-SD disease
> Hb-SE disease

D57.80   **Other sickle-cell disorders <u>without</u> crisis**

D57.81-   **Other sickle-cell disorders <u>with crisis</u>**

MCC D57.811   **Other sickle-cell disorders with acute chest syndrome**

MCC D57.812   **Other sickle-cell disorders with splenic sequestration**

MCC D57.819   **Other sickle-cell disorders with crisis, unspecified**
> Other sickle-cell disorders with crisis NOS

D 5 6 - D 5 7

Excludes 1: = NOT CODED HERE! (Do not code both)   **600**   *Excludes ❷:* = Not Included Here

D58- <u>Other hereditary</u> **hemolytic anemias**

  Excludes 1: *hemolytic anemia of the newborn (P55.-)*

  D58.0 **Hereditary spherocytosis** — An inherited hemolytic anemia in which erythrocytes assume a spheroid shape that is characterized by hemolysis, jaundice, and splenomegaly.

    Acholuric (familial) jaundice
    Congenital (spherocytic) hemolytic icterus
    Minkowski-Chauffard syndrome

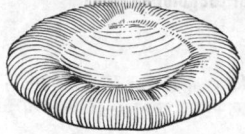 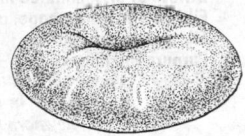

  NORMAL RED BLOOD CELL   SPHEROCYTOSIS, RED BLOOD CELL

  D58.1 **Hereditary elliptocytosis** — A hereditary disorder in which the greater proportion of [BT] erythrocytes are elliptical in shape, and which is characterized by varying degrees of increased red cell destruction and anemia.

    Elliptocytosis (congenital)
    Ovalocytosis (congenital) (hereditary)

  D58.2 **Other hemoglobinopathies**
    Abnormal hemoglobin NOS
    Congenital Heinz body anemia
    Hb-C disease
    Hb-D disease
    Hb-E disease
    Hemoglobinopathy NOS
    Unstable hemoglobin hemolytic disease

    Excludes 1: *familial polycythemia (D75.0)*
        Hb-M disease (D74.0)
        hemoglobin E-beta thalassemia (D56.5)
        hereditary persistence of fetal hemoglobin [HPFH] (D56.4)
        high-altitude polycythemia (D75.1)
        methemoglobinemia (D74.-)
        other hemoglobinopathies with thalassemia (D56.8)

  CC **D58.8** **Other specified hereditary hemolytic anemias**
    Stomatocytosis

  CC **D58.9** **Hereditary hemolytic anemia, unspecified**

D59- <u>Acquired</u> **hemolytic anemia** — An abnormal reduction of red blood cells caused by an increased rate of red blood cell destruction and inability of the bone marrow to compensate, which is due to causes other than hereditary factors.

  CC **D59.0** <u>Drug-induced</u> **autoimmune hemolytic anemia**
    Use additional code for adverse effect, if applicable, to identify drug (T36-T50 with fifth or sixth character 5)

  CC **D59.1** **Other autoimmune hemolytic anemias** — Acquired hemolytic anemia characterized by serum antibodies attacking red blood cells that is caused by the adverse chemical reaction of drugs.
    Autoimmune hemolytic disease (cold type) (warm type)
    Chronic cold hemagglutinin disease
    Cold agglutinin disease
    Cold agglutinin hemoglobinuria
    Cold type (secondary) (symptomatic) hemolytic anemia
    Warm type (secondary) (symptomatic) hemolytic anemia

    Excludes 1: *Evans syndrome (D69.41)*
        hemolytic disease of newborn (P55.-)
        paroxysmal cold hemoglobinuria (D59.6)

  CC **D59.2** <u>Drug-induced</u> **nonautoimmune hemolytic anemia**
    Drug-induced enzyme deficiency anemia
    Use additional code for adverse effect, if applicable, to identify drug (T36-T50 with fifth or sixth character 5)

  MCC **D59.3** **Hemolytic-uremic syndrome** — A syndrome characterized by microangiopathic anemia, severe thrombocytopenia, and renal failure.
    Use additional code to identify associated:
    E. coli infection (B96.2-)
    Pneumococcal pneumonia (J13)
    Shigella dysenteriae (A03.9)

  CC **D59.4** **Other nonautoimmune hemolytic anemias**
    Mechanical hemolytic anemia
    Microangiopathic hemolytic anemia
    Toxic hemolytic anemia

  D59.5 **Paroxysmal nocturnal hemoglobinuria [Marchiafava-Micheli]**
    Excludes 1: *hemoglobinuria NOS (R82.3)*

D59.6 **Hemoglobinuria due to hemolysis from other external causes**
  Hemoglobinuria from exertion
  March hemoglobinuria
  Paroxysmal cold hemoglobinuria
  Use additional code (Chapter 20) to identify external cause
  Excludes 1: *hemoglobinuria NOS (R82.3)*

D59.8 **Other acquired hemolytic anemias**

CC **D59.9** **Acquired hemolytic anemia, unspecified**
  Idiopathic hemolytic anemia, chronic

Aplastic and other anemias and other bone marrow failure syndromes (D60-D64)

D60- <u>Acquired pure red cell aplasia</u> **[erythroblastopenia]** — A bone marrow disorder characterized by decreased production of red blood cells that is often chronic and associated with underlying disorders such as thymomas and autoimmune diseases.
  Includes: **Red cell aplasia (acquired) (adult) (with thymoma)**
  Excludes 1: *congenital red cell aplasia (D61.01)*

MCC **D60.0** <u>Chronic</u> **acquired pure red cell aplasia**

MCC **D60.1** <u>Transient</u> **acquired pure red cell aplasia**

MCC **D60.8** **Other acquired pure red cell aplasias**

MCC **D60.9** **Acquired pure red cell aplasia, unspecified**

D61- <u>Other aplastic</u> **anemias and other bone marrow failure syndromes**
  Excludes 1: *neutropenia (D70.-)*

  D61.0- <u>Constitutional</u> **aplastic anemia**

    CC **D61.01** **Constitutional (pure) red blood cell aplasia** — An inherited, progressive hypoplasia of the bone marrow that is characterized by slow growth, abnormal weakness, deformities, and defects and is unaccompanied by leukopenia and thrombocytopenia.
      Blackfan-Diamond syndrome
      Congenital (pure) red cell aplasia
      Familial hypoplastic anemia
      Primary (pure) red cell aplasia
      Red cell (pure) aplasia of infants
      Excludes 1: *acquired red cell aplasia (D60.9)*

    CC **D61.09** **Other constitutional aplastic anemia**
      Fanconi's anemia — An inherited disorder that results in deficiency of all bone marrow elements including red blood cells, white blood cells, and platelets and is characterized by skin pigment changes, musculoskeletal deformities, and short stature.
      Pancytopenia with malformations

  MCC **D61.1** <u>Drug-induced</u> **aplastic anemia** — Decreased bone marrow production of red blood cells due to the chemical effects of drugs.
    Use additional code for adverse effect, if applicable, to identify drug (T36-T50 with fifth or sixth character 5)

  MCC **D61.2** **Aplastic anemia <u>due to other</u> external agents**
    Code first, if applicable, toxic effects of substances chiefly nonmedicinal as to source (T51-T65)

  MCC **D61.3** <u>Idiopathic</u> **aplastic anemia**

  D61.8- **Other specified aplastic anemias and other bone marrow failure syndromes**

    D61.81- <u>Pancytopenia</u> — A deficiency of all bone marrow elements including red and white blood cells and platelets.
      Excludes 1: *pancytopenia (due to) (with) aplastic anemia (D61.9)*
          pancytopenia (due to) (with) bone marrow infiltration (D61.82)
          pancytopenia (due to) (with) congenital (pure) red cell aplasia (D61.01)
          pancytopenia (due to) (with) hairy cell leukemia (C91.4-)
          pancytopenia (due to) (with) human immunodeficiency virus disease (B20.-)
          pancytopenia (due to) (with) leukoerythroblastic anemia (D61.82)
          pancytopenia (due to) (with) myeloproliferative disease (D47.1)
      Excludes ❷: *pancytopenia (due to) (with) myelodysplastic syndromes (D46.-)*

    MCC **D61.810** **Antineoplastic <u>chemotherapy induced</u> pancytopenia**
      Excludes ❷: *aplastic anemia due to antineoplastic chemotherapy (D61.1)*

    MCC **D61.811** **Other <u>drug-induced</u> pancytopenia**
      Excludes ❷: *aplastic anemia due to drugs (D61.1)*

    CC **D61.818** **Other pancytopenia**

Excludes 1: = NOT CODED HERE! (Do not code both)   **601**   *Excludes ❷:* = Not Included Here

CC D61.82 Myelophthisis — A condition of bone marrow failure that results from the destruction of bone marrow precursor cells.
  Leukoerythroblastic anemia
  Myelophthisic anemia
  Panmyelophthisis
  Excludes 1: *idiopathic myelofibrosis (D47.1)*
      myelofibrosis NOS (D75.81)
      myelofibrosis with myeloid metaplasia (D47.4)
      primary myelofibrosis (D47.1)
      secondary myelofibrosis (D75.81)
  Code also the underlying disorder, such as:
    Malignant neoplasm of breast (C50.-)
    Tuberculosis (A15.-)

MCC D61.89 Other specified aplastic anemias and other bone marrow failure syndromes

CC D61.9 Aplastic anemia, unspecified
  Hypoplastic anemia NOS
  Medullary hypoplasia

D62 Acute posthemorrhagic anemia — An abnormal reduction of red blood cells due
CC to the voluminous escape of blood from the body, more rapidly than the body can replace it.
  Excludes 1: *anemia due to chronic blood loss (D50.0)*
      blood loss anemia NOS (D50.0)
      congenital anemia from fetal blood loss (P61.3)

D63- Anemia in chronic diseases classified elsewhere

  D63.0 Anemia in neoplastic disease — [Not Allowed as PDX]
    Code first neoplasm (C00-D49)
    Excludes 1: *anemia due to antineoplastic chemotherapy (D64.81)*
        aplastic anemia due to antineoplastic chemotherapy (D61.1)

  D63.1 Anemia in chronic kidney disease — [Not Allowed as PDX]
    Erythropoietin resistant anemia (EPO resistant anemia)
    Code first underlying chronic kidney disease (CKD) (N18.-)

  D63.8 Anemia in other chronic diseases classified elsewhere —
    [Not Allowed as PDX]
    Code first underlying disease, such as:
      Diphyllobothriasis (B70.0)
      Hookworm disease (B76.0-B76.9)
      Hypothyroidism (E00.0-E03.9)
      Malaria (B50.0-B54)
      Symptomatic late syphilis (A52.79)
      Tuberculosis (A18.89)

D64- Other anemias
  Excludes 1: *refractory anemia (D46.-)*
      refractory anemia with excess blasts in transformation [RAEB T] (C92.0-)

  D64.0 Hereditary sideroblastic anemia — An abnormal reduction of red blood cells caused by a defect in the final stage of hemesynthesis, and which is marked by hypochromic red blood cells and elevated serum iron.
    Sex-linked hypochromic sideroblastic anemia

  D64.1 Secondary sideroblastic anemia due to disease —
    [Not Allowed as PDX]
    Code first underlying disease

  D64.2 Secondary sideroblastic anemia due to drugs and toxins
    Code first poisoning due to drug or toxin, if applicable (T36-T65 with fifth or sixth character 1-4 or 6)
    Use additional code for adverse effect, if applicable, to identify drug (T36-T50 with fifth or sixth character 5)

  D64.3 Other sideroblastic anemias
    Sideroblastic anemia NOS
    Pyridoxine-responsive sideroblastic anemia NEC

  D64.4 Congenital dyserythropoietic anemia
    Dyshematopoietic anemia (congenital)
    Excludes 1: *Blackfan-Diamond syndrome (D61.01)*
        Di Guglielmo's disease (C94.0)

  D64.8- Other specified anemias

    D64.81 Anemia due to antineoplastic chemotherapy
      AHA 14:4Q:p22 – Anemia secondary to chemotherapy
      Antineoplastic chemotherapy induced anemia
      Excludes 1: *aplastic anemia due to antineoplastic chemotherapy (D61.1)*
      Excludes ❷: *anemia in neoplastic disease (D63.0)*

    D64.89 Other specified anemias
      Infantile pseudoleukemia

  D64.9 Anemia, unspecified

Coagulation defects, purpura and other hemorrhagic conditions (D65-D69)

D65 Disseminated intravascular coagulation [defibrination syndrome] —
MCC An acquired syndrome characterized by consumption coagulopathy and fibrinolysis.
  Afibrinogenemia, acquired
  Consumption coagulopathy
  Diffuse or disseminated intravascular coagulation [DIC]
  Fibrinolytic hemorrhage, acquired
  Fibrinolytic purpura
  Purpura fulminans
  Excludes 1: *disseminated intravascular coagulation (complicating):*
      abortion or ectopic or molar pregnancy (O00-O07, O08.1)
      in newborn (P60)
      pregnancy, childbirth and the puerperium (O45.0, O46.0, O67.0, O72.3)

D66 Hereditary factor VIII deficiency — A hereditary deficiency of Factor VIII,
MCC antihemophilic factor, characterized by recurrent hemarthroses, muscular hematomas, retroperitoneal bleeding, and easy bruising.
  Classical hemophilia
  Deficiency factor VIII (with functional defect)
  Hemophilia NOS
  Hemophilia A
  Excludes 1: *factor VIII deficiency with vascular defect (D68.0)*

D67 Hereditary factor IX deficiency — A hereditary deficiency of Factor IX, plasma
MCC thromboplastin component factor, characterized by severe joint and soft tissue bleeding.
  Christmas disease
  Factor IX deficiency (with functional defect)
  Hemophilia B
  Plasma thromboplastin component [PTC] deficiency

D68- Other coagulation defects
  Excludes 1: *abnormal coagulation profile (R79.1)*
      coagulation defects complicating abortion or ectopic or molar pregnancy (O00-O07, O08.1)
      coagulation defects complicating pregnancy, childbirth and the puerperium (O45.0, O46.0, O67.0, O72.3)

CC D68.0 Von Willebrand's disease — A hereditary disease caused by abnormal blood vessels in association with Factor VIII deficiency, and is characterized by superficial skin and mucous membrane bleeding, and some mild joint bleeding.
    Angiohemophilia
    Factor VIII deficiency with vascular defect
    Vascular hemophilia
    Excludes 1: *capillary fragility (hereditary) (D69.8)*
        factor VIII deficiency NOS (D66)
        factor VIII deficiency with functional defect (D66)

CC D68.1 Hereditary factor XI deficiency — A hereditary deficiency of Factor XI, plasma thromboplastin antecedent factor, characterized by mild mucosal bleeding, bruising, and epistaxis.
    Hemophilia C
    Plasma thromboplastin antecedent [PTA] deficiency
    Rosenthal's disease

CC D68.2 Hereditary deficiency of other clotting factors
    AC globulin deficiency
    Congenital afibrinogenemia
    Deficiency of factor I [fibrinogen]
    Deficiency of factor II [prothrombin]
    Deficiency of factor V [labile]
    Deficiency of factor VII [stable]
    Deficiency of factor X [Stuart-Prower]
    Deficiency of factor XII [Hageman]
    Deficiency of factor XIII [fibrin stabilizing]
    Dysfibrinogenemia (congenital)
    Hypoproconvertinemia
    Owren's disease
    Proaccelerin deficiency

D68.3- Hemorrhagic disorder due to circulating anticoagulants
    AHA 16:1Q:p14x2 – Duodenal ulcer with hemorrhage due to Coumadin therapy

  D68.31- Hemorrhagic disorder due to intrinsic circulating anticoagulants, antibodies, or inhibitors

    CC D68.311 Acquired hemophilia — A bleeding disorder from a non-genetic origin that is caused by substances in the blood circulation that delays or prevents normal blood clotting.
        Autoimmune hemophilia
        Autoimmune inhibitors to clotting factors
        Secondary hemophilia

CC **D68.312** <u>Antiphospholipid antibody</u> with hemorrhagic disorder — A bleeding disorder that is due to the autoimmune production of antibodies against phospholipids (cell membrane component).
  Lupus anticoagulant (LAC) with hemorrhagic disorder
  Systemic lupus erythematosus [SLE] inhibitor with hemorrhagic disorder
  Excludes 1: antiphospholipid antibody finding without diagnosis (R76.0)
  antiphospholipid antibody syndrome (D68.61)
  antiphospholipid antibody with hypercoagulable state (D68.61)
  lupus anticoagulant (LAC) finding without diagnosis (R76.0)
  lupus anticoagulant (LAC) with hypercoagulable state (D68.62)
  systemic lupus erythematosus [SLE] inhibitor finding without diagnosis (R76.0)
  systemic lupus erythematosus [SLE] inhibitor with hypercoagulable state (D68.62)

CC **D68.318** **Other hemorrhagic disorder due to intrinsic circulating anticoagulants, antibodies, or inhibitors**
  Antithromboplastinemia
  Antithromboplastinogenemia
  Hemorrhagic disorder due to intrinsic increase in antithrombin
  Hemorrhagic disorder due to intrinsic increase in anti-VIIIa
  Hemorrhagic disorder due to intrinsic increase in anti-IXa
  Hemorrhagic disorder due to intrinsic increase in anti-XIa

CC **D68.32** **Hemorrhagic disorder due to <u>extrinsic</u> circulating anticoagulants**
  AHA 16:1Q:p15 – Hemorrhage due to Prasugrel (Effient®)
  Drug-induced hemorrhagic disorder
  Hemorrhagic disorder due to increase in anti-IIa
  Hemorrhagic disorder due to increase in anti-Xa
  Hyperheparinemia
  Use additional code for adverse effect, if applicable, to identify drug (T45.515-, T45.525-)

CC **D68.4** **Acquired coagulation factor deficiency** — Decreased production of coagulation factors.
  Deficiency of coagulation factor due to liver disease
  Deficiency of coagulation factor due to vitamin K deficiency
  Excludes 1: vitamin K deficiency of newborn (P53)

D68.5- <u>Primary</u> **thrombophilia** — An inherited condition of an increased tendency to form blood clots (thrombosis), potentially leading to deep vein thrombosis or pulmonary embolism.
  Primary hypercoagulable states
  Excludes 1: antiphospholipid syndrome (D68.61)
  lupus anticoagulant (D68.62)
  secondary activated protein C resistance (D68.69)
  secondary antiphospholipid antibody syndrome (D68.69)
  secondary lupus anticoagulant with hypercoagulable state (D68.69)
  secondary systemic lupus erythematosus [SLE] inhibitor with hypercoagulable state (D68.69)
  systemic lupus erythematosus [SLE] inhibitor finding without diagnosis (R76.0)
  systemic lupus erythematosus [SLE] inhibitor with hemorrhagic disorder (D68.312)
  thrombotic thrombocytopenic purpura (M31.1)

CC **D68.51** **Activated <u>protein C</u> resistance** — A form caused by the body's poor response to activated protein C that poses a major risk factor for venous thromboembolism.
  Factor V Leiden mutation

CC **D68.52** <u>Prothrombin</u> **gene mutation** — A form that impairs the prothrombin anticoagulant process.

CC **D68.59** **Other primary thrombophilia**
  Antithrombin III deficiency
  Hypercoagulable state NOS
  Primary hypercoagulable state NEC
  Primary thrombophilia NEC
  Protein C deficiency
  Protein S deficiency
  Thrombophilia NOS

D68.6- **Other thrombophilia**
  Other hypercoagulable states
  Excludes 1: diffuse or disseminated intravascular coagulation [DIC] (D65)
  heparin induced thrombocytopenia (HIT) (D75.82)
  hyperhomocysteinemia (E72.11)

CC **D68.61** **Antiphospholipid syndrome** — An increased tendency to form blood clots (thrombosis) that is due to the autoimmune production of antibodies against phospholipids (cell membrane component).
  Anticardiolipin syndrome
  Antiphospholipid antibody syndrome
  Excludes 1: antiphospholipid antibody finding without diagnosis (R76.0)
  antiphospholipid antibody with hemorrhagic disorder (D68.312)
  lupus anticoagulant syndrome (D68.62)

CC **D68.62** **Lupus anticoagulant syndrome** — An increased tendency to form blood clots (thrombosis) that is associated with systemic lupus.
  Lupus anticoagulant
  Presence of systemic lupus erythematosus [SLE] inhibitor
  Excludes 1: anticardiolipin syndrome (D68.61)
  antiphospholipid syndrome (D68.61)
  lupus anticoagulant (LAC) finding without diagnosis (R76.0)
  lupus anticoagulant (LAC) with hemorrhagic disorder (D68.312)

CC **D68.69** **Other thrombophilia**
  Hypercoagulable states NEC
  Secondary hypercoagulable state NOS

CC **D68.8** **Other specified coagulation defects**
  Excludes 1: hemorrhagic disease of newborn (P53)

CC **D68.9** **Coagulation defect, unspecified**

D69- <u>Purpura</u> **and other hemorrhagic conditions**
  Excludes 1: benign hypergammaglobulinemic purpura (D89.0)
  cryoglobulinemic purpura (D89.1)
  essential (hemorrhagic) thrombocythemia (D47.3)
  hemorrhagic thrombocythemia (D47.3)
  purpura fulminans (D65)
  thrombotic thrombocytopenic purpura (M31.1)
  Waldenström hypergammaglobulinemic purpura (D89.0)

CC **D69.0** <u>Allergic</u> **purpura** — A condition characterized by skin and mucous membrane hemorrhages that is caused by a variety of agents including bacteria, drugs, and food.
  Allergic vasculitis
  Nonthrombocytopenic hemorrhagic purpura
  Nonthrombocytopenic idiopathic purpura
  Purpura anaphylactoid
  Purpura Henoch(-Schönlein)
  Purpura rheumatica
  Vascular purpura
  Excludes 1: thrombocytopenic hemorrhagic purpura (D69.3)

D69.1 **Qualitative platelet defects** — Blood coagulation disorders caused by platelet cellular abnormalities.
  Bernard-Soulier [giant platelet] syndrome
  Glanzmann's disease
  Grey platelet syndrome
  Thromboasthenia (hemorrhagic) (hereditary)
  Thrombocytopathy
  Excludes 1: von Willebrand's disease (D68.0)

D69.2 <u>Other</u> **nonthrombocytopenic purpura**
  Purpura NOS
  Purpura simplex — Nonthrombocytopenic purpura which is not associated with vascular or intravascular abnormalities, and marked by persistent bruising.
  Senile purpura

CC **D69.3** <u>Immune</u> **thrombocytopenic purpura** — An autoimmune form characterized by development of antibodies to one's own platelets, resulting in destruction of the platelets by phagocytosis.
  Hemorrhagic (thrombocytopenic) purpura
  Idiopathic thrombocytopenic purpura
  Tidal platelet dysgenesis

D69.4- **Other <u>primary</u> thrombocytopenia**
  Excludes 1: transient neonatal thrombocytopenia (P61.0)
  Wiskott-Aldrich syndrome (D82.0)

CC **D69.41** **Evans syndrome** — An abnormally decreased platelet count with purpural hemorrhages of the skin that is marked by hemolytic anemia of an autoimmune cause.

D68
|
D69

CC **D69.42 Congenital and hereditary thrombocytopenia purpura** — An inherited abnormally decreased platelet count with purpural hemorrhages of the skin.
Congenital thrombocytopenia
Hereditary thrombocytopenia
Code first congenital or hereditary disorder, such as:
Thrombocytopenia with absent radius (TAR syndrome) (Q87.2)

D69.49 Other primary thrombocytopenia
Megakaryocytic hypoplasia
Primary thrombocytopenia NOS

D69.5- Secondary thrombocytopenia — An abnormally decreased platelet count with purpural hemorrhages of the skin resulting from an underlying disease or an external cause.
AHA 14:4Q:p22 – Secondary thrombocytopenia
Excludes 1:   heparin induced thrombocytopenia (HIT) (D75.82)
transient thrombocytopenia of newborn (P61.0)

D69.51 Posttransfusion purpura — A form resulting from blood transfusions.
Posttransfusion purpura from whole blood (fresh) or blood products
PTP

D69.59 Other secondary thrombocytopenia

D69.6 Thrombocytopenia, unspecified

D69.8 Other specified hemorrhagic conditions
Capillary fragility (hereditary)
Vascular pseudohemophilia

D69.9 Hemorrhagic condition, unspecified

Other disorders of blood and blood-forming organs (D70-D77)

D70- Neutropenia — An abnormally low number of neutrophils in the blood.
Includes: Agranulocytosis
Decreased absolute neurophile count (ANC)
Use additional code for any associated:
Fever (R50.81)
Mucositis (J34.81, K12.3-, K92.81, N76.81)
Excludes 1:   neutropenic splenomegaly (D73.81)
transient neonatal neutropenia (P61.5)

D70.0 Congenital agranulocytosis — An inherited form characterized by severe neutropenia and frequent, recurrent infections.
Congenital neutropenia
Infantile genetic agranulocytosis
Kostmann's disease

D70.1 Agranulocytosis secondary to cancer chemotherapy
AHA 14:4Q:p22 – Neutropenia secondary to chemotherapy
Use additional code for adverse effect, if applicable, to identify drug (T45.1x5-)
Code also underlying neoplasm

D70.2 Other drug-induced agranulocytosis
Use additional code for adverse effect, if applicable, to identify drug (T36-T50 with fifth or sixth character 5)

D70.3 Neutropenia due to infection

D70.4 Cyclic neutropenia — A form characterized by periodic neutropenia with subsequent infections, followed by peripheral neutrophil recovery.
Cyclic hematopoiesis
Periodic neutropenia

D70.8 Other neutropenia

D70.9 Neutropenia, unspecified

D71 Functional disorders of polymorphonuclear neutrophils — Inhibiting disorders of granular leukocytes marked by decreased survival or abnormal pooling.
Cell membrane receptor complex [CR3] defect
Chronic (childhood) granulomatous disease
Congenital dysphagocytosis
Progressive septic granulomatosis

D72- Other disorders of white blood cells
Excludes 1:   basophilia (D72.824)
immunity disorders (D80-D89)
neutropenia (D70)
preleukemia (syndrome) (D46.9)

D72.0 Genetic anomalies of leukocytes
Alder (granulation) (granulocyte) anomaly
Alder syndrome
Hereditary leukocytic hypersegmentation
Hereditary leukocytic hyposegmentation
Hereditary leukomelanopathy
May-Hegglin (granulation) (granulocyte) anomaly
May-Hegglin syndrome
Pelger-Huët (granulation) (granulocyte) anomaly
Pelger-Huët syndrome
Excludes 1:   Chédiak (-Steinbrinck)-Higashi syndrome (E70.330)

D72.1 Eosinophilia — The abnormal accumulation of eosinophil type granular leukocytes in the blood.
Allergic eosinophilia
Hereditary eosinophilia
Excludes 1:   Löffler's syndrome (J82)
pulmonary eosinophilia (J82)

D72.8- Other specified disorders of white blood cells
Excludes 1:   leukemia (C91-C95)

D72.81- Decreased white blood cell count
Excludes 1:   neutropenia (D70.-)

D72.810 Lymphocytopenia — An abnormally low number of lymphocytes in the blood.
Decreased lymphocytes

D72.818 Other decreased white blood cell count
Basophilic leukopenia
Eosinophilic leukopenia
Monocytopenia
Other decreased leukocytes
Plasmacytopenia

D72.819 Decreased white blood cell count, unspecified
Decreased leukocytes, unspecified
Leukocytopenia, unspecified
Leukopenia
Excludes 1:   malignant leukopenia (D70.9)

D72.82- Elevated white blood cell count — An abnormally high number of white blood cells.
Excludes 1:   eosinophilia (D72.1)

D72.820 Lymphocytosis (symptomatic) — An abnormal excess of lymphocytes in the blood.
Elevated lymphocytes

D72.821 Monocytosis (symptomatic) — An abnormal increase in the proportion of monocytes in the blood.
Excludes 1:   infectious mononucleosis (B27.-)

D72.822 Plasmacytosis — An abnormal increase of plasma cells in the blood.

D72.823 Leukemoid reaction — A severe form of leukocytosis that closely resembles leukemia by morphologic appearance, but is due to a physiologic response to stress, infection, or a disease process.
Basophilic leukemoid reaction
Leukemoid reaction NOS
Lymphocytic leukemoid reaction
Monocytic leukemoid reaction
Myelocytic leukemoid reaction
Neutrophilic leukemoid reaction

D72.824 Basophilia — An abnormal increase of basophils in the blood.

D72.825 Bandemia — An abnormal excess of immature white blood cells (band cells) that is not due to a confirmed infection.
Bandemia without diagnosis of specific infection
Excludes 1:   confirmed infection — code to infection
leukemia (C91.-, C92.-, C93.-, C94.-, C95.-)

D72.828 Other elevated white blood cell count

D72.829 Elevated white blood cell count, unspecified
Elevated leukocytes, unspecified
Leukocytosis, unspecified

D72.89 Other specified disorders of white blood cells
Abnormality of white blood cells NEC

D72.9 Disorder of white blood cells, unspecified
Abnormal leukocyte differential NOS

D69 - D72

D73- Diseases of spleen

D73.0 Hyposplenism — The reduced function of the spleen.
> Atrophy of spleen
>
> *Excludes 1:* *asplenia (congenital) (Q89.01)*
> *postsurgical absence of spleen (Z90.81)*

D73.1 Hypersplenism — Increased function of the spleen resulting in the removal of blood cells too early.
> *Excludes 1:* *neutropenic splenomegaly (D73.81)*
> *primary splenic neutropenia (D73.81)*
> *splenitis, splenomegaly in late syphilis (A52.79)*
> *splenitis, splenomegaly in tuberculosis (A18.85)*
> *splenomegaly NOS (R16.1)*
> *splenomegaly congenital (Q89.0)*

D73.2 Chronic congestive splenomegaly — Enlargement of the spleen often associated with portal hypertension.

D73.3 Abscess of spleen — A localized collection of pus caused by the disintegration of splenic tissue.

D73.4 Cyst of spleen — A fluid-filled sac within the spleen.

D73.5 Infarction of spleen — Ischemic tissue necrosis of the spleen.
> Splenic rupture, nontraumatic
> Torsion of spleen
>
> *Excludes 1:* *rupture of spleen due to Plasmodium vivax malaria (B51.0)*
> *traumatic rupture of spleen (S36.03-)*

D73.8- Other diseases of spleen

D73.81 Neutropenic splenomegaly — The enlargement of the spleen that results from the abnormal pooling of granular leukocytes.
> Werner-Schultz disease

D73.89 Other diseases of spleen
> Fibrosis of spleen NOS
> Perisplenitis
> Splenitis NOS

D73.9 Disease of spleen, unspecified

D74- Methemoglobinemia — The abnormal presence of methemoglobin in the blood which inhibits normal oxygen combination with iron resulting in cyanosis.

cc **D74.0 Congenital methemoglobinemia**
> Congenital NADH-methemoglobin reductase deficiency
> Hemoglobin-M [Hb-M] disease
> Methemoglobinemia, hereditary

cc **D74.8 Other methemoglobinemias**
> Acquired methemoglobinemia (with sulfhemoglobinemia)
> Toxic methemoglobinemia

cc **D74.9 Methemoglobinemia, unspecified**

D75- Other and unspecified diseases of blood and blood-forming organs
> *Excludes ❷:* *acute lymphadenitis (L04.-)*
> *chronic lymphadenitis (I88.1)*
> *enlarged lymph nodes (R59.-)*
> *hypergammaglobulinemia NOS (D89.2)*
> *lymphadenitis NOS (I88.9)*
> *mesenteric lymphadenitis (acute) (chronic) (I88.0)*

D75.0 Familial erythrocytosis — A hereditary increase in the total red blood cell mass.
> Benign polycythemia
> Familial polycythemia
>
> *Excludes 1:* *hereditary ovalocytosis (D58.1)*

D75.1 Secondary polycythemia — An abnormal increase in the total red blood cell mass caused as a consequence of a disease, or an external cause.
> Acquired polycythemia
> Emotional polycythemia
> Erythrocytosis NOS
> Hypoxemic polycythemia
> Nephrogenous polycythemia
> Polycythemia due to erythropoietin
> Polycythemia due to fall in plasma volume
> Polycythemia due to high altitude
> Polycythemia due to stress
> Polycythemia NOS
> Relative polycythemia
>
> *Excludes 1:* *polycythemia neonatorum (P61.1)*
> *polycythemia vera (D45)*

D75.8- Other specified diseases of blood and blood-forming organs

cc **D75.81 Myelofibrosis** — [Not Allowed as PDX] — Replacement of the bone marrow with fibrous tissue that is usually secondary to a disease process.
> Myelofibrosis NOS
> Secondary myelofibrosis NOS
> Code first the underlying disorder, such as:
>   Malignant neoplasm of breast (C50.-)
> Use additional code, if applicable, for associated therapy-related myelodysplastic syndrome (D46.-)
> Use additional code for adverse effect, if applicable, to identify drug (T45.1x5-)
>
> *Excludes 1:* *acute myelofibrosis (C94.4-)*
> *idiopathic myelofibrosis (D47.1)*
> *leukoerythroblastic anemia (D61.82)*
> *myelofibrosis with myeloid metaplasia (D47.4)*
> *myelophthisic anemia (D61.82)*
> *myelophthisis (D61.82)*
> *primary myelofibrosis (D47.1)*

D75.82 Heparin induced thrombocytopenia (HIT)

D75.89 Other specified diseases of blood and blood-forming organs

D75.9 Disease of blood and blood-forming organs, unspecified

D76- Other specified diseases with participation of lymphoreticular and reticulohistiocytic tissue
> *Excludes 1:* *(Abt-) Letterer-Siwe disease (C96.0)*
> *eosinophilic granuloma (C96.6)*
> *Hand-Schüller-Christian disease (C96.5)*
> *histiocytic medullary reticulosis (C96.9)*
> *histiocytic sarcoma (C96.A)*
> *histiocytosis X, multifocal (C96.5)*
> *histiocytosis X, unifocal (C96.6)*
> *Langerhans-cell histiocytosis, multifocal (C96.5)*
> *Langerhans-cell histiocytosis NOS (C96.6)*
> *Langerhans-cell histiocytosis, unifocal (C96.6)*
> *leukemic reticuloendotheliosis (C91.4-)*
> *lipomelanotic reticulosis (I89.8)*
> *malignant histiocytosis (C96.A)*
> *malignant reticulosis (C86.0)*
> *nonlipid reticuloendotheliosis (C96.0)*

cc **D76.1 Hemophagocytic lymphohistiocytosis** — The abnormal activation of lymphocytes and macrophages that destroy healthy blood cells.
> Familial hemophagocytic reticulosis
> Histiocytoses of mononuclear phagocytes

cc **D76.2 Hemophagocytic syndrome, infection-associated**
> Use additional code to identify infectious agent or disease.

cc **D76.3 Other histiocytosis syndromes**
> Reticulohistiocytoma (giant-cell)
> Sinus histiocytosis with massive lymphadenopathy
> Xanthogranuloma

D77 Other disorders of blood and blood-forming organs in diseases classified elsewhere — [Not Allowed as PDX]
> Code first underlying disease, such as:
> Amyloidosis (E85.-)
> Congenital early syphilis (A50.0)
> Echinococcosis (B67.0-B67.9)
> Malaria (B50.0-B54)
> Schistosomiasis [bilharziasis] (B65.0-B65.9)
> Vitamin C deficiency (E54)
>
> *Excludes 1:* *rupture of spleen due to Plasmodium vivax malaria (B51.0)*
> *splenitis, splenomegaly in late syphilis (A52.79)*
> *splenitis, splenomegaly in tuberculosis (A18.85)*

D73 | D77

Excludes 1: = NOT CODED HERE! (Do not code both)   **605**   *Excludes ❷:* = Not Included Here

Intraoperative and postprocedural complications of the spleen (D78)

D78- Intraoperative and postprocedural complications of the <u>spleen</u>

  D78.0- <u>Intraoperative hemorrhage</u> and hematoma of the spleen complicating a procedure

    Excludes 1: intraoperative hemorrhage and hematoma of the spleen due to accidental puncture or laceration during a procedure (D78.1-)

    cc D78.01 Intraoperative hemorrhage and hematoma of the spleen complicating a procedure on the spleen

    cc D78.02 Intraoperative hemorrhage and hematoma of the spleen complicating other procedure

  D78.1- <u>Accidental puncture</u> and laceration of the spleen during a procedure

    cc D78.11 Accidental puncture and laceration of the spleen during a procedure on the spleen

    cc D78.12 Accidental puncture and laceration of the spleen during other procedure

  D78.2- <u>Postprocedural hemorrhage</u> of the spleen following a procedure

    cc D78.21 Postprocedural <u>hemorrhage</u> of the spleen following a procedure on the spleen

    cc D78.22 Postprocedural <u>hemorrhage</u> of the spleen following other procedure

  D78.3- <u>Postprocedural hematoma and seroma</u> of the spleen following a procedure

    cc D78.31 Postprocedural <u>hematoma</u> of the spleen following a procedure on the spleen

    cc D78.32 Postprocedural <u>hematoma</u> of the spleen following other procedure

    cc D78.33 Postprocedural <u>seroma</u> of the spleen following a procedure on the spleen

    cc D78.34 Postprocedural <u>seroma</u> of the spleen following other procedure

  D78.8- Other intraoperative and postprocedural complications of the spleen

    Use additional code, if applicable, to further specify disorder

    cc D78.81 Other intraoperative complications of the spleen

    cc D78.89 Other postprocedural complications of the spleen

Certain disorders involving the immune mechanism (D80-D89)

  Includes: Defects in the complement system
      Immunodeficiency disorders, except human immunodeficiency virus [HIV] disease
      Sarcoidosis

  Excludes 1: autoimmune disease (systemic) NOS (M35.9)
      functional disorders of polymorphonuclear neutrophils (D71)
      human immunodeficiency virus [HIV] disease (B20)

D80- Immunodeficiency with predominantly antibody defects

  cc D80.0 <u>Hereditary</u> hypogammaglobulinemia — An inherited immunological deficiency state characterized by abnormally low levels of gammaglobulins.
    Autosomal recessive agammaglobulinemia (Swiss type)
    X-linked agammaglobulinemia [Bruton] (with growth hormone deficiency)

  cc D80.1 <u>Nonfamilial</u> hypogammaglobulinemia — An immunological deficiency state characterized by abnormally low levels of gammaglobulins.
    Agammaglobulinemia with immunoglobulin-bearing B-lymphocytes
    Common variable agammaglobulinemia [CVAgamma]
    Hypogammaglobulinemia NOS

  cc D80.2 <u>Selective</u> deficiency of immunoglobulin <u>A [IgA]</u> — An immunological deficiency state characterized by abnormally low levels of IgA class immunoglobins.

  cc D80.3 <u>Selective</u> deficiency of immunoglobulin <u>G [IgG] subclasses</u> — An immunological deficiency state characterized by abnormally low levels of IgG class immunoglobins.

  cc D80.4 <u>Selective</u> deficiency of immunoglobulin <u>M [IgM]</u> — An immunological deficiency state characterized by abnormally low levels of IgM class immunoglobins.

  cc D80.5 <u>Immunodeficiency</u> with increased immunoglobulin <u>M [IgM]</u> — An immunological deficiency state characterized by increased levels of IgM class immunoglobins.

  cc D80.6 <u>Antibody deficiency</u> with near-normal immunoglobulins or with hyperimmunoglobulinemia

  cc D80.7 Transient hypogammaglobulinemia of <u>infancy</u>

  cc D80.8 Other immunodeficiencies with predominantly antibody defects
    Kappa light chain deficiency

  cc D80.9 Immunodeficiency with predominantly antibody defects, unspecified

D81- <u>Combined immunodeficiencies</u> — Immunological deficiency of both humoral and cell-mediated immunity.

  Excludes 1: autosomal recessive agammaglobulinemia (Swiss type) (D80.0)

  cc D81.0 Severe combined immunodeficiency [SCID] <u>with reticular dysgenesis</u>

  cc D81.1 Severe combined immunodeficiency [SCID] <u>with low T- and B-cell numbers</u>

  cc D81.2 Severe combined immunodeficiency [SCID] <u>with low or normal B-cell numbers</u>

  cc D81.3 <u>Adenosine</u> deaminase [ADA] deficiency

  cc D81.4 <u>Nezelof's</u> syndrome

  cc D81.5 <u>Purine</u> nucleoside phosphorylase [PNP] deficiency

  cc D81.6 Major histocompatibility complex <u>class I</u> deficiency
    Bare lymphocyte syndrome

  cc D81.7 Major histocompatibility complex <u>class II</u> deficiency

  D81.8- Other combined immunodeficiencies

    D81.81- Biotin-dependent carboxylase deficiency
      Multiple carboxylase deficiency
      Excludes 1: biotin-dependent carboxylase deficiency due to dietary deficiency of biotin (E53.8)

      D81.810 Biotinidase deficiency

      D81.818 Other biotin-dependent carboxylase deficiency
        Holocarboxylase synthetase deficiency
        Other multiple carboxylase deficiency

      D81.819 Biotin-dependent carboxylase deficiency, unspecified
        Multiple carboxylase deficiency, unspecified

    cc D81.89 Other combined immunodeficiencies

  cc D81.9 Combined immunodeficiency, unspecified
    Severe combined immunodeficiency disorder [SCID] NOS

D82- <u>Immunodeficiency</u> associated with other <u>major defects</u>

  Excludes 1: ataxia telangiectasia [Louis-Bar] (G11.3)

  cc D82.0 Wiskott-Aldrich syndrome
    Immunodeficiency with thrombocytopenia and eczema

  cc D82.1 Di George's syndrome
    Pharyngeal pouch syndrome
    Thymic alymphoplasia
    Thymic aplasia or hypoplasia with immunodeficiency

  D82.2 Immunodeficiency with short-limbed stature

  D82.3 Immunodeficiency following hereditary defective response to Epstein-Barr virus
    X-linked lymphoproliferative disease

  D82.4 Hyperimmunoglobulin E [IgE] syndrome

  D82.8 Immunodeficiency associated with other specified major defects

  D82.9 Immunodeficiency associated with major defect, unspecified

D83- <u>Common variable</u> immunodeficiency

  cc D83.0 Common variable immunodeficiency with predominant abnormalities of B-cell numbers and function

  cc D83.1 Common variable immunodeficiency with predominant immunoregulatory T-cell disorders

  cc D83.2 Common variable immunodeficiency with autoantibodies to B- or T-cells

  cc D83.8 Other common variable immunodeficiencies

  cc D83.9 Common variable immunodeficiency, unspecified

Excludes 1: = NOT CODED HERE! (Do not code both)   **606**   *Excludes ❷: = Not Included Here*

D84-   <u>Other</u> **immunodeficiencies**

D84.0   **Lymphocyte function antigen-1 [LFA-1] defect**

D84.1   **Defects in the complement system**
         C1 esterase inhibitor [C1-INH] deficiency

cc **D84.8**   **Other specified immunodeficiencies**

cc **D84.9**   **Immunodeficiency, unspecified**

D86-   <u>Sarcoidosis</u> — A chronic, progressive disease of unknown etiology characterized by granulomatous cells collecting into nodule-like masses that may affect any organ or tissue, including the liver, lungs, skin, lymph nodes, spleen, and eyes.

D86.0   **Sarcoidosis of lung**

D86.1   **Sarcoidosis of lymph nodes**

D86.2   **Sarcoidosis of lung with sarcoidosis of lymph nodes**

D86.3   **Sarcoidosis of skin**

D86.8-   **Sarcoidosis of other sites**

   D86.81   **Sarcoid meningitis**

   D86.82   **Multiple cranial nerve palsies in sarcoidosis**

   D86.83   **Sarcoid iridocyclitis**

   D86.84   **Sarcoid pyelonephritis**
            Tubulo-interstitial nephropathy in sarcoidosis

   D86.85   **Sarcoid myocarditis**

   D86.86   **Sarcoid arthropathy**
            Polyarthritis in sarcoidosis

   D86.87   **Sarcoid myositis**

   D86.89   **Sarcoidosis of other sites**
            Hepatic granuloma
            Uveoparotid fever [Heerfordt]

D86.9   **Sarcoidosis, unspecified**

D89-   **Other disorders involving the immune mechanism, not elsewhere classified**
      Excludes 1:   *hyperglobulinemia NOS (R77.1)*
               monoclonal gammopathy (of undetermined significance) (D47.2)
      Excludes ❷: *transplant failure and rejection (T86.-)*

D89.0   **Polyclonal hypergammaglobulinemia** — The abnormal excess of multiple types of immunoglobulins in the blood.
         Benign hypergammaglobulinemic purpura
         Polyclonal gammopathy NOS

D89.1   **Cryoglobulinemia** — The abnormal presence of cryoglobins (certain temperature sensitive proteins) in the blood.
         Cryoglobulinemic purpura
         Cryoglobulinemic vasculitis
         Essential cryoglobulinemia
         Idiopathic cryoglobulinemia
         Mixed cryoglobulinemia
         Primary cryoglobulinemia
         Secondary cryoglobulinemia

D89.2   **Hypergammaglobulinemia, unspecified**

D89.3   **Immune reconstitution syndrome**
         Immune reconstitution inflammatory syndrome [IRIS]
         Use additional code for adverse effect, if applicable, to identify drug (T36-T50 with fifth or sixth character 5)

D89.4-   **Mast cell activation syndrome and related disorders**
      Excludes 1:   *aggressive systemic mastocytosis (C96.2)*
               cutaneous mastocytosis (Q82.2)
               indolent systemic mastocytosis (D47.0)
               malignant mastocytoma (C96.2)
               mast cell leukemia (C94.3-)
               mastocytoma (D47.0)
               systemic mastocytosis associated with a clonal hematologic non-mast cell lineage disease (SM-AHNMD) (D47.0)

   D89.40   **Mast cell activation, unspecified**
            Mast cell activation disorder, unspecified
            Mast cell activation syndrome, NOS

   D89.41   **Monoclonal mast cell activation syndrome** — A disorder involving hyperresponsive mast cells that is characterized by flushing, pruritis, urticaria, headache, gastrointestinal symptoms, and hypotension.

   D89.42   **Idiopathic mast cell activation syndrome** — A form without an underlying cause.

   D89.43   **Secondary mast cell activation** — A form occurring as an indirect result of another disease or condition.
            Secondary mast cell activation syndrome
            Code also underlying etiology, if known

D89.49   **Other mast cell activation disorder**
         Other mast cell activation syndrome

D89.8-   **Other specified disorders involving the immune mechanism, not elsewhere classified**

D89.81-   **Graft-versus-host disease** — A condition in which the donor tissue or organ (graft) contains immunogenic cells that attack the recipient's (host) tissue, most often the skin, eyes, blood, liver, and gastrointestinal tract.
         Code first underlying cause, such as:
            Complications of transplanted organs and tissue (T86.-)
            Complications of blood transfusion (T80.89)
         Use additional code to identify associated manifestations, such as:
            Desquamative dermatitis (L30.8)
            Diarrhea (R19.7)
            Elevated bilirubin (R17)
            Hair loss (L65.9)

cc **D89.810**   <u>**Acute**</u> **graft-versus-host disease** —
            [Unacceptable PDX] – A form usually appearing within two months of the transplant.

cc **D89.811**   <u>**Chronic**</u> **graft-versus-host disease** —
            [Unacceptable PDX] – A form usually appearing during the third month of the transplant or later.

cc **D89.812**   <u>**Acute on chronic**</u> **graft-versus-host disease** —
            [Unacceptable PDX]

cc **D89.813**   **Graft-versus-host disease, unspecified** —
            [Unacceptable PDX]

D89.82   **Autoimmune lymphoproliferative syndrome [ALPS]** — An inherited disorder of the immune system that is characterized by an excessive accumulation of lymphocytes in the body that often results in anemia, thrombocytopenia, and neutropenia.

D89.89   **Other specified disorders involving the immune mechanism, not elsewhere classified**
         Excludes 1:   *human immunodeficiency virus disease (B20)*

D89.9   **Disorder involving the immune mechanism, unspecified**
         AHA 15:3Q:p22 – Immunocompromised state not due to medication or underlying disease
         Immune disease NOS

D 8 4 I D 8 9

Chapter 4 – Endocrine, nutritional and metabolic diseases (E00-E89)

Note: All neoplasms, whether functionally active or not, are classified in Chapter 2. Appropriate codes in this chapter (i.e. E05.8, E07.0, E16-E31, E34.-) may be used as additional codes to indicate either functional activity by neoplasms and ectopic endocrine tissue or hyperfunction and hypofunction of endocrine glands associated with neoplasms and other conditions classified elsewhere.

Excludes 1:   *transitory endocrine and metabolic disorders specific to newborn (P70-P74)*

This chapter contains the following blocks:

E00-E07	Disorders of thyroid gland
E08-E13	Diabetes mellitus
E15-E16	Other disorders of glucose regulation and pancreatic internal secretion
E20-E35	Disorders of other endocrine glands
E36	Intraoperative complications of endocrine system
E40-E46	Malnutrition
E50-E64	Other nutritional deficiencies
E65-E68	Overweight, obesity and other hyperalimentation
E70-E88	Metabolic disorders
E89	Postprocedural endocrine and metabolic complications and disorders, not elsewhere classified

Chapter-Specific Coding Guidelines

C. Chapter-Specific Coding Guidelines

In addition to general coding guidelines, there are guidelines for specific diagnoses and/or conditions in the classification. Unless otherwise indicated, these guidelines apply to all health care settings. Please refer to Section II for guidelines on the selection of principal diagnosis.

4. Chapter 4: Endocrine, Nutritional, and Metabolic Diseases (E00-E89)

a. Diabetes mellitus

The diabetes mellitus codes are combination codes that include the type of diabetes mellitus, the body system affected, and the complications affecting that body system. As many codes within a particular category as are necessary to describe all of the complications of the disease may be used. They should be sequenced based on the reason for a particular encounter. Assign as many codes from categories E08 – E13 as needed to identify all of the associated conditions that the patient has.

1) Type of diabetes

The age of a patient is not the sole determining factor, though most type 1 diabetics develop the condition before reaching puberty. For this reason type 1 diabetes mellitus is also referred to as juvenile diabetes.

2) Type of diabetes mellitus not documented

If the type of diabetes mellitus is not documented in the medical record the default is E11.-, Type 2 diabetes mellitus.

3) Diabetes mellitus and the use of insulin *and oral hypoglycemics*

If the documentation in a medical record does not indicate the type of diabetes but does indicate that the patient uses insulin, code E11, Type 2 diabetes mellitus, should be assigned. Code Z79.4, Long-term (current) use of insulin, or Z79.84, Long term (current) use of oral hypoglycemic drugs, should also be assigned to indicate that the patient uses insulin or hypoglycemic drugs. Code Z79.4 should not be assigned if insulin is given temporarily to bring a type 2 patient's blood sugar under control during an encounter.

4) Diabetes mellitus in pregnancy and gestational diabetes

See Section I.C.15. Diabetes mellitus in pregnancy.
See Section I.C.15. Gestational (pregnancy induced) diabetes.

5) Complications due to insulin pump malfunction

(a) Underdose of insulin due to insulin pump failure

An underdose of insulin due to an insulin pump failure should be assigned to a code from subcategory T85.6, Mechanical complication of other specified internal and external prosthetic devices, implants and grafts, that specifies the type of pump malfunction, as the principal or first-listed code, followed by code T38.3x6-, Underdosing of insulin and oral hypoglycemic [antidiabetic] drugs. Additional codes for the type of diabetes mellitus and any associated complications due to the underdosing should also be assigned.

(b) Overdose of insulin due to insulin pump failure

The principal or first-listed code for an encounter due to an insulin pump malfunction resulting in an overdose of insulin, should also be T85.6-, Mechanical complication of other specified internal and external prosthetic devices, implants and grafts, followed by code T38.3x1-, Poisoning by insulin and oral hypoglycemic [antidiabetic] drugs, accidental (unintentional).

6) Secondary diabetes mellitus

Codes under categories E08, Diabetes mellitus due to underlying condition, and E09, Drug or chemical induced diabetes mellitus, and E13, Other specified diabetes mellitus, identify complications/manifestations associated with secondary diabetes mellitus. Secondary diabetes is always caused by another condition or event (e.g., cystic fibrosis, malignant neoplasm of pancreas, pancreatectomy, adverse effect of drug, or poisoning).

(a) Secondary diabetes mellitus and the use of insulin *or oral hypoglycemic drugs*

For patients who routinely use insulin or hypoglycemic drugs, code Z79.4, Long-term (current) use of insulin, or Z79.84, Long term (current) use of oral hypoglycemic drugs, should also be assigned. Code Z79.4 should not be assigned if insulin is given temporarily to bring a patient's blood sugar under control during an encounter.

(b) Assigning and sequencing secondary diabetes codes and its causes

The sequencing of the secondary diabetes codes in relationship to codes for the cause of the diabetes is based on the Tabular List instructions for categories E08, E09 and E13.

(i) Secondary diabetes mellitus due to pancreatectomy

For postpancreatectomy diabetes mellitus (lack of insulin due to the surgical removal of all or part of the pancreas), assign code E89.1, Postprocedural hypoinsulinemia. Assign a code from category E13 and a code from subcategory Z90.41-, Acquired absence of pancreas, as additional codes.

(ii) Secondary diabetes due to drugs

Secondary diabetes may be caused by an adverse effect of correctly administered medications, poisoning or sequela of poisoning.

See section I.C.19.e for coding of adverse effects and poisoning, and section I.C.20 for external cause code reporting.

Disorders of thyroid gland (E00-E07)

E00-   Congenital <u>iodine-deficiency</u> syndrome — The fetal developmental failure of the thyroid gland to secrete enough thyroid hormones to maintain the normal metabolic rate (congenital hypothyroidism) that is characterized by arrested physical and mental development, dystrophy of the bones and soft parts, and lowered basal metabolism.

Use additional code (F70-F79) to identify associated intellectual disabilities.

Excludes 1:   *subclinical iodine-deficiency hypothyroidism (E02)*

E00.0   Congenital iodine-deficiency syndrome, <u>neurological</u> type
Endemic cretinism, neurological type

E00.1   Congenital iodine-deficiency syndrome, <u>myxedematous</u> type
Endemic hypothyroid cretinism
Endemic cretinism, myxedematous type

E00.2   Congenital iodine-deficiency syndrome, <u>mixed</u> type
Endemic cretinism, mixed type

E00.9   Congenital iodine-deficiency syndrome, unspecified
Congenital iodine-deficiency hypothyroidism NOS
Endemic cretinism NOS

E01-   Iodine-deficiency related <u>thyroid disorders</u> and allied conditions
Excludes 1:   *congenital iodine-deficiency syndrome (E00.-)*
      subclinical iodine-deficiency hypothyroidism (E02)

E01.0   Iodine-deficiency related <u>diffuse</u> (endemic) goiter — An enlargement of the thyroid gland with associated swelling in the front part of the neck that is associated with dietary iodine deficiency.

E01.1   Iodine-deficiency related <u>multinodular</u> (endemic) goiter — An enlargement of the thyroid gland with associated swelling in the front part of the neck that is associated with dietary iodine deficiency and characterized by the formation of multiple nodules within the thyroid.

Iodine-deficiency related nodular goiter

E01.2   Iodine-deficiency related (endemic) goiter, unspecified
Endemic goiter NOS

E01.8   Other iodine-deficiency related thyroid disorders and allied conditions
Acquired iodine-deficiency hypothyroidism NOS

E02   <u>Subclinical</u> iodine-deficiency <u>hypothyroidism</u> — A milder form of hypothyroidism that is associated with dietary iodine deficiency.

E03-   <u>Other</u> hypothyroidism
Excludes 1:   *iodine-deficiency related hypothyroidism (E00-E02)*
      postprocedural hypothyroidism (E89.0)

E03.0   <u>Congenital</u> hypothyroidism <u>with</u> diffuse goiter — The failure of the thyroid gland to secrete enough thyroid hormones that is present at birth and causes a general inflammation of the thyroid gland.
Congenital parenchymatous goiter (nontoxic)
Congenital goiter (nontoxic) NOS
Excludes 1:   *transitory congenital goiter with normal function (P72.0)*

E00 - E03

Excludes 1: = NOT CODED HERE! (Do not code both)   *Excludes ❷:* = Not Included Here

E03.1   Congenital hypothyroidism without goiter
Aplasia of thyroid (with myxedema)
Congenital atrophy of thyroid
Congenital hypothyroidism NOS

E03.2   Hypothyroidism due to medicaments and other exogenous substances
Code first poisoning due to drug or toxin, if applicable (T36-T65 with fifth or sixth character 1-4 or 6)
Use additional code for adverse effect, if applicable, to identify drug (T36-T50 with fifth or sixth character 5)

E03.3   Postinfectious hypothyroidism

E03.4   Atrophy of thyroid (acquired)
Excludes 1:   congenital atrophy of thyroid (E03.1)

MCC **E03.5   Myxedema coma** — A life-threatening form of severe, longstanding hypothyroidism that is characterized by loss of brain function.

E03.8   Other specified hypothyroidism

E03.9   Hypothyroidism, unspecified
Myxedema NOS

E04-   Other nontoxic goiter
Excludes 1:   congenital goiter (NOS) (diffuse) (parenchymatous) (E03.0)
iodine-deficiency related goiter (E00-E02)

E04.0   Nontoxic diffuse goiter — Hypertrophy of the thyroid with a generalized enlargement of the thyroid gland.
Diffuse (colloid) nontoxic goiter
Simple nontoxic goiter

E04.1   Nontoxic single thyroid nodule — Hypertrophy of the thyroid with the presence of a single nodule.
Colloid nodule (cystic) (thyroid)
Nontoxic uninodular goiter
Thyroid (cystic) nodule NOS

E04.2   Nontoxic multinodular goiter — Hypertrophy of the thyroid with the presence of multiple nodules.
Cystic goiter NOS
Multinodular (cystic) goiter NOS

E04.8   Other specified nontoxic goiter

E04.9   Nontoxic goiter, unspecified
Goiter NOS
Nodular goiter (nontoxic) NOS

E05-   Thyrotoxicosis [hyperthyroidism] — The condition of elevated levels of circulating thyroid hormones.
Excludes 1:   chronic thyroiditis with transient thyrotoxicosis (E06.2)
neonatal thyrotoxicosis (P72.1)

E05.0-   Thyrotoxicosis with diffuse goiter — A form marked by a generalized enlargement of the thyroid gland.
Exophthalmic or toxic goiter NOS
Graves' disease
Toxic diffuse goiter

E05.00   Thyrotoxicosis with diffuse goiter without thyrotoxic crisis or storm

MCC **E05.01   Thyrotoxicosis with diffuse goiter with thyrotoxic crisis or storm** — An acute, life-threatening state of excessive release of thyroid hormones that is characterized by a rapid increase in the body's temperature, blood pressure, and heart rate.

E05.1-   Thyrotoxicosis with toxic single thyroid nodule — A form marked by the presence of a single nodule.
Thyrotoxicosis with toxic uninodular goiter

E05.10   Thyrotoxicosis with toxic single thyroid nodule without thyrotoxic crisis or storm

MCC **E05.11   Thyrotoxicosis with toxic single thyroid nodule with thyrotoxic crisis or storm** — An acute, life-threatening state of excessive release of thyroid hormones that is characterized by a rapid increase in the body's temperature, blood pressure, and heart rate.

E05.2-   Thyrotoxicosis with toxic multinodular goiter — A form marked by the presence of multiple nodules.
Toxic nodular goiter NOS

E05.20   Thyrotoxicosis with toxic multinodular goiter without thyrotoxic crisis or storm

MCC **E05.21   Thyrotoxicosis with toxic multinodular goiter with thyrotoxic crisis or storm** — An acute, life-threatening state of excessive release of thyroid hormones that is characterized by a rapid increase in the body's temperature, blood pressure, and heart rate.

E05.3-   Thyrotoxicosis from ectopic thyroid tissue — A form marked by thyroid-tissue hormones from a thyroid nodule which is not within the thyroid gland.

E05.30   Thyrotoxicosis from ectopic thyroid tissue without thyrotoxic crisis or storm

MCC **E05.31   Thyrotoxicosis from ectopic thyroid tissue with thyrotoxic crisis or storm** — An acute, life-threatening state of excessive release of thyroid hormones that is characterized by a rapid increase in the body's temperature, blood pressure, and heart rate.

E05.4-   Thyrotoxicosis factitia — A form marked by the ingestion of excessive amounts of exogenous thyroid hormone.

E05.40   Thyrotoxicosis factitia without thyrotoxic crisis or storm

MCC **E05.41   Thyrotoxicosis factitia with thyrotoxic crisis or storm** — An acute, life-threatening state of excessive release of thyroid hormones that is characterized by a rapid increase in the body's temperature, blood pressure, and heart rate.

E05.8-   Other thyrotoxicosis
Overproduction of thyroid-stimulating hormone

E05.80   Other thyrotoxicosis without thyrotoxic crisis or storm

MCC **E05.81   Other thyrotoxicosis with thyrotoxic crisis or storm** — An acute, life-threatening state of excessive release of thyroid hormones that is characterized by a rapid increase in the body's temperature, blood pressure, and heart rate.

E05.9-   Thyrotoxicosis, unspecified
Hyperthyroidism NOS

E05.90   Thyrotoxicosis, unspecified without thyrotoxic crisis or storm

MCC **E05.91   Thyrotoxicosis, unspecified with thyrotoxic crisis or storm**

E06-   Thyroiditis — Inflammation of the thyroid gland.
Excludes 1:   postpartum thyroiditis (O90.5)

CC **E06.0   Acute thyroiditis** — A sudden, severe onset of inflammation of the thyroid gland usually caused by a bacterial infection.
Abscess of thyroid
Pyogenic thyroiditis
Suppurative thyroiditis
Use additional code (B95-B97) to identify infectious agent.

E06.1   Subacute thyroiditis — Inflammation of the thyroid marked by the presence of giant cells, granulomas in the gland, and masses of colloid.
de Quervain thyroiditis
Giant-cell thyroiditis
Granulomatous thyroiditis
Nonsuppurative thyroiditis
Viral thyroiditis
Excludes 1:   autoimmune thyroiditis (E06.3)

E06.2   Chronic thyroiditis with transient thyrotoxicosis — A form with brief periods of elevated circulating thyroid hormones.
Excludes 1:   autoimmune thyroiditis (E06.3)

E06.3   Autoimmune thyroiditis — An autoimmune disease of progressive inflammation of the thyroid gland characterized by diffuse lymphocytic infiltration and fibrotic replacement of thyroid tissue.
Hashimoto's thyroiditis
Hashitoxicosis (transient)
Lymphadenoid goiter
Lymphocytic thyroiditis
Struma lymphomatosa

E06.4   Drug-induced thyroiditis
Use additional code for adverse effect, if applicable, to identify drug (T36-T50 with fifth or sixth character 5)

E06.5   Other chronic thyroiditis
Chronic fibrous thyroiditis
Chronic thyroiditis NOS
Ligneous thyroiditis
Riedel thyroiditis

E06.9   Thyroiditis, unspecified

E07-   Other disorders of thyroid

E07.0   Hypersecretion of calcitonin — A condition resulting in the body's depletion of calcium and phosphate levels caused by thyrocalcitonin (a thyroid hormone which responds to excessive calcium in the body).
C-cell hyperplasia of thyroid
Hypersecretion of thyrocalcitonin

E07.1   Dyshormogenetic goiter — Thyroid hyperplasia due to enzyme defects in thyroid-hormone synthesis.
Familial dyshormogenetic goiter
Pendred's syndrome
Excludes 1:   transitory congenital goiter with normal function (P72.0)

E07.8-   Other specified disorders of thyroid

E07.81   Sick-euthyroid syndrome — A transient alteration in thyroid hormone metabolism (low levels of serum thyroid hormones) caused by a nonthyroidal illness or condition.
Euthyroid sick-syndrome

E03 - E07

E07.89   Other specified disorders of thyroid
Abnormality of thyroid-binding globulin
Hemorrhage of thyroid
Infarction of thyroid

E07.9   Disorder of thyroid, unspecified

Diabetes mellitus (E08-E13)

E08-   Diabetes mellitus due to <u>underlying condition</u> — A complex metabolic syndrome characterized by consistently high blood sugar (glucose) levels, glycosuria, and metabolic effects caused by faulty pancreatic insulin production, thus producing insufficient amounts of insulin that is due to another medical condition.

AHA 13:3Q:p20 – Hyperglycemia together with another diabetes code
AHA 13:3Q:p20 – Uncontrolled type 1 diabetes with ketoacidosis
AHA 16:1Q:p12 – Cause-and-effect condition relationships
Code first the underlying condition, such as:
Congenital rubella (P35.0)
Cushing's syndrome (E24.-)
Cystic fibrosis (E84.-)
Malignant neoplasm (C00-C96)
Malnutrition (E40-E46)
Pancreatitis and other diseases of the pancreas (K85-, K86-)
Use additional code to identify control using:
Insulin (Z79.4)
Oral antidiabetic drugs (Z79.84)
Oral hypoglycemic drugs (Z79.84)
Excludes 1:   *drug or chemical induced diabetes mellitus (E09-)*
gestational diabetes (O24.4-)
neonatal diabetes mellitus (P70.2)
postpancreatectomy diabetes mellitus (E13-)
postprocedural diabetes mellitus (E13-)
secondary diabetes mellitus NEC (E13-)
type 1 diabetes mellitus (E10-)
type 2 diabetes mellitus (E11-)

E08.0-   Diabetes mellitus due to <u>underlying condition</u> with <u>hyperosmolarity</u> — A form with extremely high blood sugar (glucose) levels and without the presence of ketones.

MCC **E08.00   Diabetes mellitus due to underlying condition with hyperosmolarity <u>without</u> nonketotic hyperglycemic-hyperosmolar coma (NKHHC)** — [Not Allowed as PDX]

MCC **E08.01   Diabetes mellitus due to underlying condition with hyperosmolarity <u>with coma</u>** — [Not Allowed as PDX]

E08.1-   Diabetes mellitus due to <u>underlying condition</u> with <u>ketoacidosis</u> — The potentially life-threatening complication of ketone poisoning caused by very low insulin that forces the body to use fat for fuel. When the fat breaks down, its waste products (acids called ketone bodies) build up in the blood and urine.

MCC **E08.10   Diabetes mellitus due to underlying condition with ketoacidosis <u>without</u> coma** — [Not Allowed as PDX]

MCC **E08.11   Diabetes mellitus due to underlying condition with ketoacidosis <u>with coma</u>** — [Not Allowed as PDX]

E08.2-   Diabetes mellitus due to <u>underlying condition</u> with <u>kidney</u> complications

E08.21   Diabetes mellitus due to underlying condition with diabetic <u>nephropathy</u> — [Not Allowed as PDX] – A progressive kidney disease caused by damage to the blood capillaries of the kidney's glomeruli that is due to the long-term effects of diabetes.
Diabetes mellitus due to underlying condition with intercapillary glomerulosclerosis
Diabetes mellitus due to underlying condition with intracapillary glomerulonephrosis
Diabetes mellitus due to underlying condition with Kimmelstiel-Wilson disease

E08.22   Diabetes mellitus due to underlying condition with diabetic <u>chronic kidney disease</u> — [Not Allowed as PDX]
Use additional code to identify stage of chronic kidney disease (N18.1-N18.6)

E08.29   Diabetes mellitus due to underlying condition with other diabetic kidney complication — [Not Allowed as PDX]
Renal tubular degeneration in diabetes mellitus due to underlying condition

E08.3-   Diabetes mellitus due to <u>underlying condition</u> with ophthalmic complications

E08.31-   Diabetes mellitus due to underlying condition with <u>unspecified</u> diabetic retinopathy — A diabetic complication caused by damage to the blood vessels of the retina.

E08.311   Diabetes mellitus due to underlying condition with unspecified diabetic retinopathy <u>with macular edema</u> — [Not Allowed as PDX]

E08.319   Diabetes mellitus due to underlying condition with unspecified diabetic retinopathy <u>without</u> macular edema — [Not Allowed as PDX]

E08.32-   Diabetes mellitus due to underlying condition with <u>mild</u> nonproliferative diabetic retinopathy
Diabetes mellitus due to underlying condition with nonproliferative diabetic retinopathy NOS
One of the following 7th characters is to be assigned to codes in subcategory E08.32- to designate laterality of the disease:
1   Right eye
2   Left eye
3   Bilateral
9   Unspecified eye

E08.321-   Diabetes mellitus due to underlying condition with mild nonproliferative diabetic retinopathy <u>with</u> macular edema — [Not Allowed as PDX]

E08.329-   Diabetes mellitus due to underlying condition with mild nonproliferative diabetic retinopathy <u>without</u> macular edema — [Not Allowed as PDX]

E08.33-   Diabetes mellitus due to underlying condition with <u>moderate</u> <u>non</u>proliferative diabetic retinopathy
One of the following 7th characters is to be assigned to codes in subcategory E08.33- to designate laterality of the disease:
1   Right eye
2   Left eye
3   Bilateral
9   Unspecified eye

E08.331-   Diabetes mellitus due to underlying condition with moderate nonproliferative diabetic retinopathy <u>with macular edema</u> — [Not Allowed as PDX]

E08.339-   Diabetes mellitus due to underlying condition with moderate nonproliferative diabetic retinopathy <u>without</u> macular edema — [Not Allowed as PDX]

E08.34-   Diabetes mellitus due to underlying condition with <u>severe</u> <u>non</u>proliferative diabetic retinopathy
One of the following 7th characters is to be assigned to codes in subcategory E08.34- to designate laterality of the disease:
1   Right eye
2   Left eye
3   Bilateral
9   Unspecified eye

E08.341-   Diabetes mellitus due to underlying condition with severe nonproliferative diabetic retinopathy <u>with</u> macular edema — [Not Allowed as PDX]

E08.349-   Diabetes mellitus due to underlying condition with severe nonproliferative diabetic retinopathy <u>without</u> macular edema — [Not Allowed as PDX]

E08.35-   Diabetes mellitus due to underlying condition with <u>proliferative</u> diabetic retinopathy
One of the following 7th characters is to be assigned to codes in subcategory E08.35- to designate laterality of the disease:
1   Right eye
2   Left eye
3   Bilateral
9   Unspecified eye

E08.351-   Diabetes mellitus due to underlying condition with proliferative diabetic retinopathy <u>with macular edema</u> — [Not Allowed as PDX]

E07-E08

E08.352- Diabetes mellitus due to underlying condition with proliferative diabetic retinopathy <u>with traction retinal detachment involving the macula</u> — [Not Allowed as PDX]

E08.353- Diabetes mellitus due to underlying condition with proliferative diabetic retinopathy with traction retinal detachment <u>not</u> involving the macula — [Not Allowed as PDX]

E08.354- Diabetes mellitus due to underlying condition with proliferative diabetic retinopathy <u>with combined</u> traction retinal detachment and rhegmatogenous retinal detachment — [Not Allowed as PDX]

E08.355- Diabetes mellitus due to underlying condition <u>with stable</u> proliferative diabetic retinopathy — [Not Allowed as PDX]

E08.359- Diabetes mellitus due to underlying condition with proliferative diabetic retinopathy <u>without</u> macular edema — [Not Allowed as PDX]

E08.36 Diabetes mellitus due to underlying condition with diabetic <u>cataract</u> — [Not Allowed as PDX] — The diabetic complication resulting in the clouding of the ocular lens.

E08.37x- Diabetes mellitus due to underlying condition with diabetic macular edema, <u>resolved</u> following treatment — [Not Allowed as PDX]

> One of the following 7th characters is to be assigned to code E08.37x- to designate laterality of the disease:
> 1   Right eye
> 2   Left eye
> 3   Bilateral
> 9   Unspecified eye

E08.39 Diabetes mellitus due to underlying condition with other diabetic <u>ophthalmic complication</u> — [Not Allowed as PDX]
Use additional code to identify manifestation, such as:
    Diabetic glaucoma (H40-H42)

E08.4- Diabetes mellitus due to <u>underlying condition</u> with <u>neurological</u> complications

E08.40 Diabetes mellitus due to underlying condition with diabetic <u>neuropathy</u>, <u>unspecified</u> — [Not Allowed as PDX]

E08.41 Diabetes mellitus due to underlying condition with diabetic <u>mononeuropathy</u> — [Not Allowed as PDX] — The diabetic nerve damage complication caused by microvascular damage to nerves in a single location.

E08.42 Diabetes mellitus due to underlying condition with diabetic <u>polyneuropathy</u> — [Not Allowed as PDX] — The diabetic nerve damage complication caused by microvascular damage to multiple nerves in various locations.
    Diabetes mellitus due to underlying condition with diabetic neuralgia

E08.43 Diabetes mellitus due to underlying condition with diabetic <u>autonomic (poly)neuropathy</u> — [Not Allowed as PDX] — The diabetic nerve damage complication caused by microvascular damage to autonomic (internal organs) nerves in various locations.
    AHA 13:4Q:p114 – Diabetic gastroparesis
    Diabetes mellitus due to underlying condition with diabetic gastroparesis

E08.44 Diabetes mellitus due to underlying condition with diabetic <u>amyotrophy</u> — [Not Allowed as PDX] — The diabetic nerve damage complication caused by microvascular damage to the nerves of the hips, buttocks, thighs, or legs and usually on one side of the body.

E08.49 Diabetes mellitus due to underlying condition with other diabetic neurological complication — [Not Allowed as PDX]

E08.5- Diabetes mellitus due to <u>underlying condition</u> with <u>circulatory</u> complications

E08.51 Diabetes mellitus due to underlying condition with <u>diabetic peripheral angiopathy without</u> gangrene — [Not Allowed as PDX] — The diabetic complication causing decay of the lining of peripheral blood vessels.

cc E08.52 Diabetes mellitus due to underlying condition with <u>diabetic peripheral angiopathy with gangrene</u> — [Not Allowed as PDX]
    Diabetes mellitus due to underlying condition with diabetic gangrene

E08.59 Diabetes mellitus due to underlying condition with other circulatory complications — [Not Allowed as PDX]

E08.6- Diabetes mellitus due to <u>underlying condition</u> with other specified complications

E08.61- Diabetes mellitus due to underlying condition with diabetic <u>arthropathy</u>

E08.610 Diabetes mellitus due to underlying condition with diabetic <u>neuropathic</u> arthropathy — [Not Allowed as PDX] — The diabetic complication of neurovascular damage of joints resulting in loss of sensation and subsequent joint damage.
    Diabetes mellitus due to underlying condition with Charcot's joints

E08.618 Diabetes mellitus due to underlying condition with other diabetic arthropathy — [Not Allowed as PDX]

E08.62- Diabetes mellitus due to underlying condition with <u>skin</u> complications

E08.620 Diabetes mellitus due to underlying condition with diabetic <u>dermatitis</u> — [Not Allowed as PDX] — The diabetic complication of cutaneous damage resulting in various skin conditions (inflammation, infection, lesions).
    Diabetes mellitus due to underlying condition with diabetic necrobiosis lipoidica

E08.621 Diabetes mellitus due to underlying condition with <u>foot ulcer</u> — [Not Allowed as PDX]
Use additional code to identify site of ulcer (L97.4-, L97.5-)

E08.622 Diabetes mellitus due to underlying condition with <u>other skin ulcer</u> — [Not Allowed as PDX]
Use additional code to identify site of ulcer (L97.1-L97.9, L98.41-L98.49)

E08.628 Diabetes mellitus due to underlying condition with other skin complications — [Not Allowed as PDX]

E08.63- Diabetes mellitus due to underlying condition with <u>oral</u> complications

E08.630 Diabetes mellitus due to underlying condition with periodontal disease — [Not Allowed as PDX]

E08.638 Diabetes mellitus due to underlying condition with other oral complications — [Not Allowed as PDX]

E08.64- Diabetes mellitus due to underlying condition with <u>hypoglycemia</u>

MCC E08.641 Diabetes mellitus due to underlying condition with hypoglycemia <u>with coma</u> — [Not Allowed as PDX]

E08.649 Diabetes mellitus due to underlying condition with hypoglycemia <u>without</u> coma — [Not Allowed as PDX]

E08.65 Diabetes mellitus due to underlying condition with <u>hyperglycemia</u> — [Not Allowed as PDX] — The diabetic condition of having high sugar (glucose) levels in the blood and urine causing excessive thirst and frequent urination.

E08.69 Diabetes mellitus due to underlying condition with <u>other specified</u> complication — [Not Allowed as PDX]
Use additional code to identify complication

E08.8 Diabetes mellitus due to <u>underlying condition</u> with <u>unspecified</u> complications — [Not Allowed as PDX]

E08.9 Diabetes mellitus due to <u>underlying condition</u> <u>without</u> complications — [Not Allowed as PDX]

E08-E08

E09- <u>Drug or chemical induced</u> **diabetes mellitus** — A complex metabolic syndrome characterized by consistently high blood sugar (glucose) levels, glycosuria, and metabolic effects caused by faulty pancreatic insulin production, thus producing insufficient amounts of insulin that is due to effect of a drug or chemical.

AHA 13:3Q:p20 – Hyperglycemia together with another diabetes code
AHA 13:3Q:p20 – Uncontrolled type 1 diabetes with ketoacidosis
AHA 16:1Q:p12 – Cause-and-effect condition relationships
Code first poisoning due to drug or toxin, if applicable (T36-T65 with fifth or sixth character 1-4 or 6)
Use additional code for adverse effect, if applicable, to identify drug (T36-T50 with fifth or sixth character 5)
Use additional code to identify control using:
   Insulin (Z79.4)
   Oral antidiabetic drugs (Z79.84)
   Oral hypoglycemic drugs (Z79.84)
Excludes 1: *diabetes mellitus due to underlying condition (E08.-)*
     gestational diabetes (O24.4-)
     neonatal diabetes mellitus (P70.2)
     postpancreatectomy diabetes mellitus (E13.-)
     postprocedural diabetes mellitus (E13.-)
     secondary diabetes mellitus NEC (E13.-)
     type 1 diabetes mellitus (E10.-)
     type 2 diabetes mellitus (E11.-)

E09.0- <u>Drug or chemical induced</u> **diabetes mellitus with** <u>hyperosmolarity</u> — A form with extremely high blood sugar (glucose) levels and without the presence of ketones.

MCC **E09.00 Drug or chemical induced diabetes mellitus with hyperosmolarity <u>without</u> nonketotic hyperglycemic-hyperosmolar coma (NKHHC)**

MCC **E09.01 Drug or chemical induced diabetes mellitus with hyperosmolarity <u>with</u> coma**

E09.1- <u>Drug or chemical induced</u> **diabetes mellitus with** <u>ketoacidosis</u> — The potentially life-threatening complication of ketone poisoning caused by very low insulin that forces the body to use fat for fuel. When the fat breaks down, its waste products (acids called ketone bodies) build up in the blood and urine.

MCC **E09.10 Drug or chemical induced diabetes mellitus with ketoacidosis <u>without</u> coma**

MCC **E09.11 Drug or chemical induced diabetes mellitus with ketoacidosis <u>with</u> coma**

E09.2- <u>Drug or chemical induced</u> **diabetes mellitus with** <u>kidney</u> **complications**

   E09.21 Drug or chemical induced diabetes mellitus with diabetic <u>nephropathy</u> — A progressive kidney disease caused by damage to the blood capillaries of the kidney's glomeruli that is due to the long-term effects of diabetes.
     Drug or chemical induced diabetes mellitus with intercapillary glomerulosclerosis
     Drug or chemical induced diabetes mellitus with intracapillary glomerulonephrosis
     Drug or chemical induced diabetes mellitus with Kimmelstiel-Wilson disease

   E09.22 Drug or chemical induced diabetes mellitus with diabetic <u>chronic kidney disease</u>
     Use additional code to identify stage of chronic kidney disease (N18.1-N18.6)

   E09.29 Drug or chemical induced diabetes mellitus with other diabetic kidney complication
     Drug or chemical induced diabetes mellitus with renal tubular degeneration

E09.3- <u>Drug or chemical induced</u> **diabetes mellitus with ophthalmic complications**

   E09.31- Drug or chemical induced diabetes mellitus with <u>unspecified</u> **diabetic retinopathy** — A diabetic complication caused by damage to the blood vessels of the retina.

     E09.311 Drug or chemical induced diabetes mellitus with unspecified diabetic retinopathy <u>with macular edema</u>

     E09.319 Drug or chemical induced diabetes mellitus with unspecified diabetic retinopathy <u>without</u> macular edema

E09.32- Drug or chemical induced diabetes mellitus with <u>mild</u> <u>non</u>**proliferative diabetic retinopathy**
   Drug or chemical induced diabetes mellitus with nonproliferative diabetic retinopathy NOS
   One of the following 7th characters is to be assigned to codes in subcategory E09.32- to designate laterality of the disease:
    1 **Right eye**
    2 **Left eye**
    3 **Bilateral**
    9 **Unspecified eye**

   E09.321- Drug or chemical induced diabetes mellitus with mild nonproliferative diabetic retinopathy <u>with macular edema</u>

   E09.329- Drug or chemical induced diabetes mellitus with mild nonproliferative diabetic retinopathy <u>without</u> macular edema

E09.33- Drug or chemical induced diabetes mellitus with <u>moderate</u> <u>non</u>**proliferative diabetic retinopathy**
   One of the following 7th characters is to be assigned to codes in subcategory E09.33- to designate laterality of the disease:
    1 **Right eye**
    2 **Left eye**
    3 **Bilateral**
    9 **Unspecified eye**

   E09.331- Drug or chemical induced diabetes mellitus with moderate nonproliferative diabetic retinopathy <u>with macular edema</u>

   E09.339- Drug or chemical induced diabetes mellitus with moderate nonproliferative diabetic retinopathy <u>without</u> macular edema

E09.34- Drug or chemical induced diabetes mellitus with <u>severe</u> <u>non</u>**proliferative diabetic retinopathy**
   One of the following 7th characters is to be assigned to codes in subcategory E09.34- to designate laterality of the disease:
    1 **Right eye**
    2 **Left eye**
    3 **Bilateral**
    9 **Unspecified eye**

   E09.341- Drug or chemical induced diabetes mellitus with severe nonproliferative diabetic retinopathy <u>with macular edema</u>

   E09.349- Drug or chemical induced diabetes mellitus with severe nonproliferative diabetic retinopathy <u>without</u> macular edema

E09.35- Drug or chemical induced diabetes mellitus with <u>proliferative</u> **diabetic retinopathy**
   One of the following 7th characters is to be assigned to codes in subcategory E09.35- to designate laterality of the disease:
    1 **Right eye**
    2 **Left eye**
    3 **Bilateral**
    9 **Unspecified eye**

   E09.351- Drug or chemical induced diabetes mellitus with proliferative diabetic retinopathy <u>with macular edema</u>

   E09.352- Drug or chemical induced diabetes mellitus with proliferative diabetic retinopathy <u>with traction retinal detachment involving the macula</u> — [Not Allowed as PDX]

   E09.353- Drug or chemical induced diabetes mellitus with proliferative diabetic retinopathy with traction retinal detachment <u>not</u> involving the macula — [Not Allowed as PDX]

   E09.354- Drug or chemical induced diabetes mellitus with proliferative diabetic retinopathy <u>with combined</u> traction retinal detachment and rhegmatogenous retinal detachment — [Not Allowed as PDX]

E09 - E09

E 0 9 - E 0 9

E09.355- Drug or chemical induced diabetes mellitus <u>with stable</u> proliferative diabetic retinopathy —
[Not Allowed as PDX]

E09.359- Drug or chemical induced diabetes mellitus with proliferative diabetic retinopathy <u>without</u> macular edema

E09.36 Drug or chemical induced diabetes mellitus with diabetic <u>cataract</u> — The diabetic complication resulting in the clouding of the ocular lens.

E09.37x- Drug or chemical induced diabetes mellitus with diabetic macular edema, <u>resolved</u> following treatment —
[Not Allowed as PDX]

One of the following 7th characters is to be assigned to code E09.37x- to designate laterality of the disease:
1   Right eye
2   Left eye
3   Bilateral
9   Unspecified eye

E09.39 Drug or chemical induced diabetes mellitus with other diabetic <u>ophthalmic complication</u>
Use additional code to identify manifestation, such as:
Diabetic glaucoma (H40-H42)

E09.4- <u>Drug or chemical induced</u> diabetes mellitus with <u>neurological</u> complications

E09.40 Drug or chemical induced diabetes mellitus with neurological complications with diabetic <u>neuropathy, unspecified</u>

E09.41 Drug or chemical induced diabetes mellitus with neurological complications with diabetic <u>mononeuropathy</u> — The diabetic nerve damage complication caused by microvascular damage to nerves in a single location.

E09.42 Drug or chemical induced diabetes mellitus with neurological complications with diabetic <u>polyneuropathy</u> — The diabetic nerve damage complication caused by microvascular damage to multiple nerves in various locations.
Drug or chemical induced diabetes mellitus with diabetic neuralgia

E09.43 Drug or chemical induced diabetes mellitus with neurological complications with diabetic <u>autonomic (poly)neuropathy</u> — The diabetic nerve damage complication caused by microvascular damage to autonomic (internal organs) nerves in various locations.
AHA 13:4Q:p114 – Diabetic gastroparesis
Drug or chemical induced diabetes mellitus with diabetic gastroparesis

E09.44 Drug or chemical induced diabetes mellitus with neurological complications with diabetic <u>amyotrophy</u> — The diabetic nerve damage complication caused by microvascular damage to the nerves of the hips, buttocks, thighs, or legs and usually on one side of the body.

E09.49 Drug or chemical induced diabetes mellitus with neurological complications with other diabetic neurological complication

E09.5- <u>Drug or chemical induced</u> diabetes mellitus with <u>circulatory</u> complications

E09.51 Drug or chemical induced diabetes mellitus with <u>diabetic peripheral angiopathy without</u> gangrene — The diabetic complication causing decay of the lining of peripheral blood vessels.

CC E09.52 Drug or chemical induced diabetes mellitus with <u>diabetic peripheral angiopathy with gangrene</u>
Drug or chemical induced diabetes mellitus with diabetic gangrene

E09.59 Drug or chemical induced diabetes mellitus with other circulatory complications

E09.6- <u>Drug or chemical induced</u> diabetes mellitus with other specified complications

E09.61- Drug or chemical induced diabetes mellitus with diabetic <u>arthropathy</u>

E09.610 Drug or chemical induced diabetes mellitus with diabetic <u>neuropathic</u> arthropathy — The diabetic complication of neurovascular damage of joints resulting in loss of sensation and subsequent joint damage.
Drug or chemical induced diabetes mellitus with Charcot's joints

E09.618 Drug or chemical induced diabetes mellitus with other diabetic arthropathy

E09.62- Drug or chemical induced diabetes mellitus with <u>skin</u> complications

E09.620 Drug or chemical induced diabetes mellitus with diabetic <u>dermatitis</u> — The diabetic complication of cutaneous damage resulting in various skin conditions (inflammation, infection, lesions).
Drug or chemical induced diabetes mellitus with diabetic necrobiosis lipoidica

E09.621 Drug or chemical induced diabetes mellitus with <u>foot ulcer</u>
Use additional code to identify site of ulcer (L97.4-, L97.5-)

E09.622 Drug or chemical induced diabetes mellitus with <u>other skin ulcer</u>
Use additional code to identify site of ulcer (L97.1-L97.9, L98.41-L98.49)

E09.628 Drug or chemical induced diabetes mellitus with other skin complications

E09.63- Drug or chemical induced diabetes mellitus with <u>oral</u> complications

E09.630 Drug or chemical induced diabetes mellitus with periodontal disease

E09.638 Drug or chemical induced diabetes mellitus with other oral complications

E09.64- Drug or chemical induced diabetes mellitus with <u>hypoglycemia</u>

MCC E09.641 Drug or chemical induced diabetes mellitus with hypoglycemia <u>with coma</u>

E09.649 Drug or chemical induced diabetes mellitus with hypoglycemia <u>without</u> coma

E09.65 Drug or chemical induced diabetes mellitus with <u>hyperglycemia</u> — The diabetic condition of having high sugar (glucose) levels in the blood and urine causing excessive thirst and frequent urination.

E09.69 Drug or chemical induced diabetes mellitus with <u>other specified</u> complication
Use additional code to identify complication

E09.8 <u>Drug or chemical induced</u> diabetes mellitus with <u>unspecified</u> complications

E09.9 <u>Drug or chemical induced</u> diabetes mellitus <u>without</u> complications

E09-E09

E10-   Type 1 diabetes mellitus — A complex metabolic syndrome characterized by consistently high blood (glucose) sugar, glycosuria, and metabolic effects caused by severely faulty pancreatic insulin production, thus producing little or no insulin.

AHA 13:3Q:p20 – Hyperglycemia together with another diabetes code

AHA 13:3Q:p20 – Uncontrolled type 1 diabetes with ketoacidosis

AHA 16:1Q:p12 – Cause-and-effect condition relationships

Includes: Brittle diabetes (mellitus)
Diabetes (mellitus) due to autoimmune process
Diabetes (mellitus) due to immune mediated pancreatic islet beta-cell destruction
Idiopathic diabetes (mellitus)
Juvenile onset diabetes (mellitus)
Ketosis-prone diabetes (mellitus)

Excludes 1:   diabetes mellitus due to underlying condition (E08.-)
drug or chemical induced diabetes mellitus (E09.-)
gestational diabetes (O24.4-)
hyperglycemia NOS (R73.9)
neonatal diabetes mellitus (P70.2)
postpancreatectomy diabetes mellitus (E13.-)
postprocedural diabetes mellitus (E13.-)
secondary diabetes mellitus NEC (E13.-)
type 2 diabetes mellitus (E11.-)

E10.1-   Type 1 diabetes mellitus with ketoacidosis — The potentially life-threatening complication of ketone poisoning caused by very low insulin that forces the body to use fat for fuel. When the fat breaks down, its waste products (acids called ketone bodies) build up in the blood and urine.

MCC **E10.10**   Type 1 diabetes mellitus with ketoacidosis without coma

MCC **E10.11**   Type 1 diabetes mellitus with ketoacidosis with coma

E10.2-   Type 1 diabetes mellitus with kidney complications

    E10.21   Type 1 diabetes mellitus with diabetic nephropathy — A progressive kidney disease caused by damage to the blood capillaries of the kidney's glomeruli that is due to the long-term effects of diabetes.
Type 1 diabetes mellitus with intercapillary glomerulosclerosis
Type 1 diabetes mellitus with intracapillary glomerulonephrosis
Type 1 diabetes mellitus with Kimmelstiel-Wilson disease

    E10.22   Type 1 diabetes mellitus with diabetic chronic kidney disease
Use additional code to identify stage of chronic kidney disease (N18.1-N18.6)

    E10.29   Type 1 diabetes mellitus with other diabetic kidney complication
Type 1 diabetes mellitus with renal tubular degeneration

E10.3-   Type 1 diabetes mellitus with ophthalmic complications

    E10.31-   Type 1 diabetes mellitus with unspecified diabetic retinopathy — A diabetic complication caused by damage to the blood vessels of the retina.

       E10.311   Type 1 diabetes mellitus with unspecified diabetic retinopathy with macular edema

       E10.319   Type 1 diabetes mellitus with unspecified diabetic retinopathy without macular edema

    E10.32-   Type 1 diabetes mellitus with mild nonproliferative diabetic retinopathy
Type 1 diabetes mellitus with nonproliferative diabetic retinopathy NOS

One of the following 7th characters is to be assigned to codes in subcategory E10.32- to designate laterality of the disease:
1   Right eye
2   Left eye
3   Bilateral
9   Unspecified eye

       E10.321-   Type 1 diabetes mellitus with mild nonproliferative diabetic retinopathy with macular edema

       E10.329-   Type 1 diabetes mellitus with mild nonproliferative diabetic retinopathy without macular edema

E10.33-   Type 1 diabetes mellitus with moderate nonproliferative diabetic retinopathy

One of the following 7th characters is to be assigned to codes in subcategory E10.33- to designate laterality of the disease:
1   Right eye
2   Left eye
3   Bilateral
9   Unspecified eye

    E10.331-   Type 1 diabetes mellitus with moderate nonproliferative diabetic retinopathy with macular edema

    E10.339-   Type 1 diabetes mellitus with moderate nonproliferative diabetic retinopathy without macular edema

E10.34-   Type 1 diabetes mellitus with severe nonproliferative diabetic retinopathy

One of the following 7th characters is to be assigned to codes in subcategory E10.34- to designate laterality of the disease:
1   Right eye
2   Left eye
3   Bilateral
9   Unspecified eye

    E10.341-   Type 1 diabetes mellitus with severe nonproliferative diabetic retinopathy with macular edema

    E10.349-   Type 1 diabetes mellitus with severe nonproliferative diabetic retinopathy without macular edema

E10.35-   Type 1 diabetes mellitus with proliferative diabetic retinopathy

One of the following 7th characters is to be assigned to codes in subcategory E10.35- to designate laterality of the disease:
1   Right eye
2   Left eye
3   Bilateral
9   Unspecified eye

    E10.351-   Type 1 diabetes mellitus with proliferative diabetic retinopathy with macular edema

    E10.352-   Type 1 diabetes mellitus with proliferative diabetic retinopathy with traction retinal detachment involving the macula — [Not Allowed as PDX]

    E10.353-   Type 1 diabetes mellitus with proliferative diabetic retinopathy with traction retinal detachment not involving the macula — [Not Allowed as PDX]

    E10.354-   Type 1 diabetes mellitus with proliferative diabetic retinopathy with combined traction retinal detachment and rhegmatogenous retinal detachment — [Not Allowed as PDX]

    E10.355-   Type 1 diabetes mellitus with stable proliferative diabetic retinopathy — [Not Allowed as PDX]

    E10.359-   Type 1 diabetes mellitus with proliferative diabetic retinopathy without macular edema

E10.36   Type 1 diabetes mellitus with diabetic cataract — The diabetic complication resulting in the clouding of the ocular lens.

E10.37x- Type 1 diabetes mellitus with diabetic macular edema, resolved following treatment — [Not Allowed as PDX]

One of the following 7th characters is to be assigned to code E10.37x- to designate laterality of the disease:
1   Right eye
2   Left eye
3   Bilateral
9   Unspecified eye

E10.39   Type 1 diabetes mellitus with other diabetic ophthalmic complication
Use additional code to identify manifestation, such as:
Diabetic glaucoma (H40-H42)

E10 – E10

E10.4-   **Type 1** diabetes mellitus with <u>neurological</u> complications

E10.40   <u>Type 1</u> diabetes mellitus with diabetic <u>neuropathy, unspecified</u>

E10.41   <u>Type 1</u> diabetes mellitus with diabetic <u>mononeuropathy</u> — The diabetic nerve damage complication caused by microvascular damage to nerves in a single location.

E10.42   Type 1 diabetes mellitus with diabetic <u>polyneuropathy</u> — The diabetic nerve damage complication caused by microvascular damage to multiple nerves in various locations.

    Type 1 diabetes mellitus with diabetic neuralgia

E10.43   <u>Type 1</u> diabetes mellitus with diabetic <u>autonomic (poly)neuropathy</u> — The diabetic nerve damage complication caused by microvascular damage to autonomic (internal organs) nerves in various locations.

    AHA 13:4Q:p114 – Diabetic gastroparesis
    Type 1 diabetes mellitus with diabetic gastroparesis

E10.44   <u>Type 1</u> diabetes mellitus with diabetic <u>amyotrophy</u> — The diabetic nerve damage complication caused by microvascular damage to the nerves of the hips, buttocks, thighs, or legs and usually on one side of the body.

E10.49   <u>Type 1</u> diabetes mellitus with other diabetic neurological complication

E10.5-   **Type 1** diabetes mellitus with <u>circulatory</u> complications

E10.51   <u>Type 1</u> diabetes mellitus with diabetic <u>peripheral angiopathy without</u> gangrene — The diabetic complication causing decay of the lining of peripheral blood vessels.

cc E10.52   <u>Type 1</u> diabetes mellitus with diabetic <u>peripheral angiopathy with gangrene</u>

    Type 1 diabetes mellitus with diabetic gangrene

E10.59   <u>Type 1</u> diabetes mellitus with other circulatory complications

E10.6-   **Type 1** diabetes mellitus with <u>other specified</u> complications

E10.61-   <u>Type 1</u> diabetes mellitus with diabetic <u>arthropathy</u>

E10.610   <u>Type 1</u> diabetes mellitus with diabetic <u>neuropathic arthropathy</u> — The diabetic complication of neurovascular damage of joints resulting in loss of sensation and subsequent joint damage.

    Type 1 diabetes mellitus with Charcot's joints

E10.618   <u>Type 1</u> diabetes mellitus with other diabetic arthropathy

E10.62-   <u>Type 1</u> diabetes mellitus with <u>skin</u> complications

E10.620   <u>Type 1</u> diabetes mellitus with diabetic <u>dermatitis</u> — The diabetic complication of cutaneous damage resulting in various skin conditions (inflammation, infection, lesions).

    Type 1 diabetes mellitus with diabetic necrobiosis lipoidica

E10.621   <u>Type 1</u> diabetes mellitus with <u>foot ulcer</u>
    Use additional code to identify site of ulcer (L97.4-, L97.5-)

E10.622   <u>Type 1</u> diabetes mellitus with <u>other skin ulcer</u>
    Use additional code to identify site of ulcer (L97.1-L97.9, L98.41-L98.49)

E10.628   Type 1 diabetes mellitus with other skin complications

E10.63-   <u>Type 1</u> diabetes mellitus with <u>oral</u> complications

E10.630   <u>Type 1</u> diabetes mellitus with periodontal disease

E10.638   <u>Type 1</u> diabetes mellitus with other oral complications

E10.64-   <u>Type 1</u> diabetes mellitus with <u>hypoglycemia</u>

MCC E10.641   <u>Type 1</u> diabetes mellitus with hypoglycemia <u>with coma</u>

E10.649   <u>Type 1</u> diabetes mellitus with hypoglycemia <u>without</u> coma

E10.65   <u>Type 1</u> diabetes mellitus with <u>hyperglycemia</u> — The diabetic condition of having high sugar (glucose) levels in the blood and urine causing excessive thirst and frequent urination.

E10.69   <u>Type 1</u> diabetes mellitus with <u>other specified</u> complication
    Use additional code to identify complication

E10.8   <u>Type 1</u> diabetes mellitus with <u>unspecified</u> complications

E10.9   <u>Type 1</u> diabetes mellitus <u>without</u> complications

---

E11-   <u>Type 2</u> diabetes mellitus — A complex metabolic syndrome characterized by consistently high blood sugar (glucose) levels, glycosuria, and metabolic effects caused by the body's inability to properly use the insulin produced (insulin resistance) and eventually resulting in faulty pancreatic insulin production, thus producing insufficient amounts of insulin.

    AHA 13:3Q:p20 – Hyperglycemia together with another diabetes code
    AHA 13:3Q:p20 – Uncontrolled type 1 diabetes with ketoacidosis
    AHA 16:1Q:p12 – Cause-and-effect condition relationships
Includes: Diabetes (mellitus) due to insulin secretory defect
       Diabetes NOS
       Insulin resistant diabetes (mellitus)
Use additional code to identify control using:
    Insulin (Z79.4)
    Oral antidiabetic drugs (Z79.84)
    Oral hypoglycemic drugs (Z79.84)
Excludes 1:   *diabetes mellitus due to underlying condition (E08.-)*
       drug or chemical induced diabetes mellitus (E09.-)
       gestational diabetes (O24.4-)
       neonatal diabetes mellitus (P70.2)
       postpancreatectomy diabetes mellitus (E13.-)
       postprocedural diabetes mellitus (E13.-)
       secondary diabetes mellitus NEC (E13.-)
       type 1 diabetes mellitus (E10.-)

E11.0-   <u>Type 2</u> diabetes mellitus with <u>hyperosmolarity</u> — A form with extremely high blood sugar (glucose) levels and without the presence of ketones.

MCC E11.00   <u>Type 2</u> diabetes mellitus with hyperosmolarity <u>without</u> nonketotic hyperglycemic-hyperosmolar coma (NKHHC)

MCC E11.01   <u>Type 2</u> diabetes mellitus with hyperosmolarity <u>with coma</u>

E11.2-   <u>Type 2</u> diabetes mellitus with <u>kidney</u> complications

E11.21   <u>Type 2</u> diabetes mellitus with diabetic <u>nephropathy</u> — A progressive kidney disease caused by damage to the blood capillaries of the kidney's glomeruli that is due to the long-term effects of diabetes.

    Type 2 diabetes mellitus with intercapillary glomerulosclerosis
    Type 2 diabetes mellitus with intracapillary glomerulonephrosis
    Type 2 diabetes mellitus with Kimmelstiel-Wilson disease

E11.22   <u>Type 2</u> diabetes mellitus with diabetic <u>chronic kidney disease</u>
    Use additional code to identify stage of chronic kidney disease (N18.1-N18.6)

E11.29   <u>Type 2</u> diabetes mellitus with other diabetic kidney complication

    Type 2 diabetes mellitus with renal tubular degeneration

E11.3-   <u>Type 2</u> diabetes mellitus with <u>ophthalmic</u> complications

E11.31-   <u>Type 2</u> diabetes mellitus with <u>unspecified</u> diabetic retinopathy — A diabetic complication caused by damage to the blood vessels of the retina.

E11.311   <u>Type 2</u> diabetes mellitus with unspecified diabetic retinopathy <u>with macular edema</u>

E11.319   <u>Type 2</u> diabetes mellitus with unspecified diabetic retinopathy <u>without</u> macular edema

E11.32-   <u>Type 2</u> diabetes mellitus with <u>mild nonproliferative</u> diabetic retinopathy

    Type 2 diabetes mellitus with nonproliferative diabetic retinopathy NOS

One of the following 7th characters is to be assigned to codes in subcategory E11.32- to designate laterality of the disease:
    1   Right eye
    2   Left eye
    3   Bilateral
    9   Unspecified eye

E11.321-   <u>Type 2</u> diabetes mellitus with mild nonproliferative diabetic retinopathy <u>with macular edema</u>

E11.329-   <u>Type 2</u> diabetes mellitus with mild nonproliferative diabetic retinopathy <u>without</u> macular edema

E10 - E11 *(side tab)*

E11.33-   <u>Type 2</u> diabetes mellitus with <u>moderate</u> <u>non</u>proliferative diabetic retinopathy

> **One of the following 7th characters is to be assigned to codes in subcategory E11.33- to designate laterality of the disease:**
> 1   **Right eye**
> 2   **Left eye**
> 3   **Bilateral**
> 9   **Unspecified eye**

E11.331-   <u>Type 2</u> diabetes mellitus with moderate nonproliferative diabetic retinopathy <u>with macular edema</u>

E11.339-   <u>Type 2</u> diabetes mellitus with moderate nonproliferative diabetic retinopathy <u>without</u> macular edema

E11.34-   <u>Type 2</u> diabetes mellitus with <u>severe</u> <u>non</u>proliferative diabetic retinopathy

> **One of the following 7th characters is to be assigned to codes in subcategory E11.34- to designate laterality of the disease:**
> 1   **Right eye**
> 2   **Left eye**
> 3   **Bilateral**
> 9   **Unspecified eye**

E11.341-   <u>Type 2</u> diabetes mellitus with severe nonproliferative diabetic retinopathy <u>with macular edema</u>

E11.349-   <u>Type 2</u> diabetes mellitus with severe nonproliferative diabetic retinopathy <u>without</u> macular edema

E11.35-   <u>Type 2</u> diabetes mellitus with <u>proliferative</u> diabetic retinopathy

> **One of the following 7th characters is to be assigned to codes in subcategory E11.35- to designate laterality of the disease:**
> 1   **Right eye**
> 2   **Left eye**
> 3   **Bilateral**
> 9   **Unspecified eye**

E11.351-   <u>Type 2</u> diabetes mellitus with proliferative diabetic retinopathy <u>with macular edema</u>

E11.352-   <u>Type 2</u> diabetes mellitus with proliferative diabetic retinopathy <u>with traction retinal detachment involving the macula</u> — [Not Allowed as PDX]

E11.353-   <u>Type 2</u> diabetes mellitus with proliferative diabetic retinopathy with traction retinal detachment <u>not</u> involving the macula — [Not Allowed as PDX]

E11.354-   <u>Type 2</u> diabetes mellitus with proliferative diabetic retinopathy <u>with combined</u> traction retinal detachment and rhegmatogenous retinal detachment — [Not Allowed as PDX]

E11.355-   <u>Type 2</u> diabetes mellitus <u>with stable</u> proliferative diabetic retinopathy — [Not Allowed as PDX]

E11.359-   <u>Type 2</u> diabetes mellitus with proliferative diabetic retinopathy <u>without</u> macular edema

E11.36   <u>Type 2</u> diabetes mellitus with diabetic <u>cataract</u> — The diabetic complication resulting in the clouding of the ocular lens.

E11.37x- <u>Type 2</u> diabetes mellitus with diabetic macular edema, <u>resolved</u> following treatment — [Not Allowed as PDX]

> **One of the following 7th characters is to be assigned to code E11.37x- to designate laterality of the disease:**
> 1   **Right eye**
> 2   **Left eye**
> 3   **Bilateral**
> 9   **Unspecified eye**

E11.39   <u>Type 2</u> diabetes mellitus with other diabetic <u>ophthalmic</u> <u>complication</u>
Use additional code to identify manifestation, such as:
    Diabetic glaucoma (H40-H42)

E11.4-   <u>Type 2</u> diabetes mellitus with <u>neurological</u> complications

E11.40   <u>Type 2</u> diabetes mellitus with diabetic <u>neuropathy, unspecified</u>

E11.41   <u>Type 2</u> diabetes mellitus with diabetic <u>mononeuropathy</u> — The diabetic nerve damage complication caused by microvascular damage to nerves in a single location.

E11.42   <u>Type 2</u> diabetes mellitus with diabetic <u>polyneuropathy</u> — The diabetic nerve damage complication caused by microvascular damage to multiple nerves in various locations.
    Type 2 diabetes mellitus with diabetic neuralgia

E11.43   <u>Type 2</u> diabetes mellitus with diabetic <u>autonomic (poly)neuropathy</u> — The diabetic nerve damage complication caused by microvascular damage to autonomic (internal organs) nerves in various locations.
    AHA 13:4Q:p114 – Diabetic gastroparesis
    Type 2 diabetes mellitus with diabetic gastroparesis

E11.44   <u>Type 2</u> diabetes mellitus with diabetic <u>amyotrophy</u> — The diabetic nerve damage complication caused by microvascular damage to the nerves of the hips, buttocks, thighs, or legs and usually on one side of the body.

E11.49   <u>Type 2</u> diabetes mellitus with other diabetic neurological complication

E11.5-   <u>Type 2</u> diabetes mellitus with <u>circulatory</u> complications

E11.51   <u>Type 2</u> diabetes mellitus with diabetic <u>peripheral angiopathy without gangrene</u> — The diabetic complication causing decay of the lining of peripheral blood vessels.

CC **E11.52**   <u>Type 2</u> diabetes mellitus with diabetic <u>peripheral angiopathy with gangrene</u>
    Type 2 diabetes mellitus with diabetic gangrene

E11.59   <u>Type 2</u> diabetes mellitus with other circulatory complications

E11.6-   <u>Type 2</u> diabetes mellitus with <u>other specified</u> complications

E11.61-   <u>Type 2</u> diabetes mellitus with diabetic <u>arthropathy</u>

E11.610   <u>Type 2</u> diabetes mellitus with diabetic <u>neuropathic arthropathy</u> — The diabetic complication of neurovascular damage of joints resulting in loss of sensation and subsequent joint damage.
    Type 2 diabetes mellitus with Charcot's joints

E11.618   <u>Type 2</u> diabetes mellitus with other diabetic arthropathy

E11.62-   <u>Type 2</u> diabetes mellitus with <u>skin</u> complications

E11.620   <u>Type 2</u> diabetes mellitus with diabetic <u>dermatitis</u> — The diabetic complication of cutaneous damage resulting in various skin conditions (inflammation, infection, lesions).
    Type 2 diabetes mellitus with diabetic necrobiosis lipoidica

E11.621   <u>Type 2</u> diabetes mellitus with <u>foot ulcer</u>
Use additional code to identify site of ulcer (L97.4-, L97.5-)

E11.622   <u>Type 2</u> diabetes mellitus with <u>other skin ulcer</u>
Use additional code to identify site of ulcer (L97.1-L97.9, L98.41-L98.49)

E11.628   <u>Type 2</u> diabetes mellitus with other skin complications

E11.63-   <u>Type 2</u> diabetes mellitus with <u>oral</u> complications

E11.630   <u>Type 2</u> diabetes mellitus with periodontal disease

E11.638   <u>Type 2</u> diabetes mellitus with other oral complications

E11.64-   <u>Type 2</u> diabetes mellitus with <u>hypoglycemia</u>

MCC **E11.641**   <u>Type 2</u> diabetes mellitus with hypoglycemia <u>with coma</u>

E11.649   <u>Type 2</u> diabetes mellitus with hypoglycemia <u>without</u> coma
    AHA 15:3Q:p21 – Diabetes mellitus with acute encephalopathy secondary to hypoglycemia

E11.65   <u>Type 2</u> diabetes mellitus with <u>hyperglycemia</u> — The diabetic condition of having high sugar (glucose) levels in the blood and urine causing excessive thirst and frequent urination.

E11.69   <u>Type 2</u> diabetes mellitus with <u>other specified</u> complication
Use additional code to identify complication

E11.8   <u>Type 2</u> diabetes mellitus with <u>unspecified</u> complications

E11.9   <u>Type 2</u> diabetes mellitus <u>without</u> complications — [Questionable Admission]

E11 | E11 | E11

E13- <u>Other specified</u> **diabetes mellitus** — A complex metabolic syndrome characterized by consistently high blood sugar (glucose) levels, glycosuria, and metabolic effects caused by faulty pancreatic insulin production, thus producing insufficient amounts of insulin.

    AHA 13:3Q:p20 – Hyperglycemia together with another diabetes code
    AHA 13:3Q:p20 – Uncontrolled type 1 diabetes with ketoacidosis
    AHA 16:1Q:p12 – Cause-and-effect condition relationships
    Includes: **Diabetes mellitus due to genetic defects of beta-cell function**
                Diabetes mellitus due to genetic defects in insulin action
                Postpancreatectomy diabetes mellitus
                Postprocedural diabetes mellitus
                Secondary diabetes mellitus NEC
    Use additional code to identify control using:
        Insulin (Z79.4)
        Oral antidiabetic drugs (Z79.84)
        Oral hypoglycemic drugs (Z79.84)
    Excludes 1:   *diabetes (mellitus) due to autoimmune process (E10.-)*
                diabetes (mellitus) due to immune mediated pancreatic islet beta-cell destruction (E10.-)
                diabetes mellitus due to underlying condition (E08.-)
                drug or chemical induced diabetes mellitus (E09.-)
                gestational diabetes (O24.4-)
                neonatal diabetes mellitus (P70.2)
                type 1 diabetes mellitus (E10.-)
                type 2 diabetes mellitus (E11.-)

E13.0- <u>Other specified</u> **diabetes mellitus with <u>hyperosmolarity</u>** — A form with extremely high blood sugar (glucose) levels and without the presence of ketones.

MCC **E13.00** **Other specified diabetes mellitus with hyperosmolarity <u>without</u> nonketotic hyperglycemic-hyperosmolar coma (NKHHC)**

MCC **E13.01** **Other specified diabetes mellitus with hyperosmolarity <u>with coma</u>**

E13.1- <u>Other specified</u> **diabetes mellitus with <u>ketoacidosis</u>** — The potentially life-threatening complication of ketone poisoning caused by very low insulin that forces the body to use fat for fuel. When the fat breaks down, its waste products (acids called ketone bodies) build up in the blood and urine.

MCC **E13.10** **Other specified diabetes mellitus with ketoacidosis <u>without</u> coma**
    AHA 13:1Q:p26 – Type 2 diabetes mellitus with diabetic ketoacidosis
    AHA 16:2Q:p10 – Unspecified diabetes type with ketoacidosis

MCC **E13.11** **Other specified diabetes mellitus with ketoacidosis <u>with coma</u>**

E13.2- **Other specified diabetes mellitus with <u>kidney</u> complications**

  E13.21 **Other specified diabetes mellitus with diabetic <u>nephropathy</u>** — A progressive kidney disease caused by damage to the blood capillaries of the kidney's glomeruli that is due to the long-term effects of diabetes.
      Other specified diabetes mellitus with intercapillary glomerulosclerosis
      Other specified diabetes mellitus with intracapillary glomerulonephrosis
      Other specified diabetes mellitus with Kimmelstiel-Wilson disease

  E13.22 **Other specified diabetes mellitus with diabetic <u>chronic kidney disease</u>**
    Use additional code to identify stage of chronic kidney disease (N18.1-N18.6)

  E13.29 **Other specified diabetes mellitus with other diabetic kidney complication**
      Other specified diabetes mellitus with renal tubular degeneration

E13.3- <u>Other specified</u> **diabetes mellitus with ophthalmic complications**

  E13.31- **Other specified diabetes mellitus with <u>unspecified diabetic retinopathy</u>** — A diabetic complication caused by damage to the blood vessels of the retina.

    E13.311 **Other specified diabetes mellitus with unspecified diabetic retinopathy <u>with macular edema</u>**

    E13.319 **Other specified diabetes mellitus with unspecified diabetic retinopathy <u>without</u> macular edema**

E13.32- **Other specified diabetes mellitus with <u>mild nonproliferative</u> diabetic retinopathy**
    Other specified diabetes mellitus with nonproliferative diabetic retinopathy NOS
    One of the following 7th characters is to be assigned to codes in subcategory E13.32- to designate laterality of the disease:
      1   Right eye
      2   Left eye
      3   Bilateral
      9   Unspecified eye

  E13.321- **Other specified diabetes mellitus with mild nonproliferative diabetic retinopathy <u>with macular edema</u>**

  E13.329- **Other specified diabetes mellitus with mild nonproliferative diabetic retinopathy <u>without</u> macular edema**

E13.33- **Other specified diabetes mellitus with <u>moderate nonproliferative</u> diabetic retinopathy**
    One of the following 7th characters is to be assigned to codes in subcategory E13.33- to designate laterality of the disease:
      1   Right eye
      2   Left eye
      3   Bilateral
      9   Unspecified eye

  E13.331- **Other specified diabetes mellitus with moderate nonproliferative diabetic retinopathy <u>with macular edema</u>**

  E13.339- **Other specified diabetes mellitus with moderate nonproliferative diabetic retinopathy <u>without</u> macular edema**

E13.34- **Other specified diabetes mellitus with <u>severe nonproliferative</u> diabetic retinopathy**
    One of the following 7th characters is to be assigned to codes in subcategory E13.34- to designate laterality of the disease:
      1   Right eye
      2   Left eye
      3   Bilateral
      9   Unspecified eye

  E13.341- **Other specified diabetes mellitus with severe nonproliferative diabetic retinopathy <u>with macular edema</u>**

  E13.349- **Other specified diabetes mellitus with severe nonproliferative diabetic retinopathy <u>without</u> macular edema**

E13.35- **Other specified diabetes mellitus with <u>proliferative</u> diabetic retinopathy**
    One of the following 7th characters is to be assigned to codes in subcategory E13.35- to designate laterality of the disease:
      1   Right eye
      2   Left eye
      3   Bilateral
      9   Unspecified eye

  E13.351- **Other specified diabetes mellitus with proliferative diabetic retinopathy <u>with macular edema</u>**

  E13.352- **Other specified diabetes mellitus with proliferative diabetic retinopathy <u>with traction retinal detachment involving the macula</u>** — [Not Allowed as PDX]

  E13.353- **Other specified diabetes mellitus with proliferative diabetic retinopathy with traction retinal detachment <u>not</u> involving the macula** — [Not Allowed as PDX]

  E13.354- **Other specified diabetes mellitus with proliferative diabetic retinopathy <u>with combined</u> traction retinal detachment and rhegmatogenous retinal detachment** — [Not Allowed as PDX]

Excludes 1: = NOT CODED HERE! (Do not code both)   **618**   *Excludes ❷:* = Not Included Here

E 1 3 - E 13

E13.355- Other specified diabetes mellitus <u>with stable</u> proliferative diabetic retinopathy — [Not Allowed as PDX]

E13.359- Other specified diabetes mellitus with proliferative diabetic retinopathy <u>without</u> macular edema

E13.36 Other specified diabetes mellitus with diabetic <u>cataract</u> — The diabetic complication resulting in the clouding of the ocular lens.

E13.37x- Other specified diabetes mellitus with diabetic macular edema, <u>resolved</u> following treatment — [Not Allowed as PDX]

> **One of the following 7th characters is to be assigned to code E13.37x- to designate laterality of the disease:**
> 1   Right eye
> 2   Left eye
> 3   Bilateral
> 9   Unspecified eye

E13.39 Other specified diabetes mellitus with other diabetic <u>ophthalmic complication</u>
Use additional code to identify manifestation, such as:
Diabetic glaucoma (H40-H42)

E13.4- <u>Other specified</u> diabetes mellitus with <u>neurological</u> complications

E13.40 Other specified diabetes mellitus with diabetic <u>neuropathy, unspecified</u>

E13.41 Other specified diabetes mellitus with diabetic <u>mononeuropathy</u> — The diabetic nerve damage complication caused by microvascular damage to nerves in a single location.

E13.42 Other specified diabetes mellitus with diabetic <u>polyneuropathy</u> — The diabetic nerve damage complication caused by microvascular damage to multiple nerves in various locations.
> Other specified diabetes mellitus with diabetic neuralgia

E13.43 Other specified diabetes mellitus with diabetic <u>autonomic</u> (poly)neuropathy — The diabetic nerve damage complication caused by microvascular damage to autonomic (internal organs) nerves in various locations.
> AHA 13:4Q:p114 – Diabetic gastroparesis
> Other specified diabetes mellitus with diabetic gastroparesis

E13.44 Other specified diabetes mellitus with diabetic <u>amyotrophy</u> — The diabetic nerve damage complication caused by microvascular damage to the nerves of the hips, buttocks, thighs, or legs and usually on one side of the body.

E13.49 Other specified diabetes mellitus with other diabetic neurological complication

E13.5- <u>Other specified</u> diabetes mellitus with <u>circulatory</u> complications

E13.51 Other specified diabetes mellitus with diabetic <u>peripheral angiopathy without</u> gangrene — The diabetic complication causing decay of the lining of peripheral blood vessels.

CC E13.52 Other specified diabetes mellitus with diabetic <u>peripheral angiopathy with gangrene</u>
> Other specified diabetes mellitus with diabetic gangrene

E13.59 Other specified diabetes mellitus with other circulatory complications

E13.6- <u>Other specified</u> diabetes mellitus with other specified complications

E13.61- Other specified diabetes mellitus with diabetic <u>arthropathy</u>

E13.610 Other specified diabetes mellitus with diabetic <u>neuropathic</u> arthropathy — The diabetic complication of neurovascular damage of joints resulting in loss of sensation and subsequent joint damage.
> Other specified diabetes mellitus with Charcot's joints

E13.618 Other specified diabetes mellitus with other diabetic arthropathy

E13.62- Other specified diabetes mellitus with <u>skin</u> complications

E13.620 Other specified diabetes mellitus with diabetic <u>dermatitis</u> — The diabetic complication of cutaneous damage resulting in various skin conditions (inflammation, infection, lesions).
> Other specified diabetes mellitus with diabetic necrobiosis lipoidica

E13.621 Other specified diabetes mellitus with <u>foot ulcer</u>
Use additional code to identify site of ulcer (L97.4-, L97.5-)

E13.622 Other specified diabetes mellitus with <u>other skin ulcer</u>
Use additional code to identify site of ulcer (L97.1-L97.9, L98.41-L98.49)

E13.628 Other specified diabetes mellitus with other skin complications

E13.63- Other specified diabetes mellitus with <u>oral</u> complications

E13.630 Other specified diabetes mellitus with periodontal disease

E13.638 Other specified diabetes mellitus with other oral complications

E13.64- Other specified diabetes mellitus with <u>hypoglycemia</u>

MCC E13.641 Other specified diabetes mellitus with hypoglycemia <u>with coma</u>

E13.649 Other specified diabetes mellitus with hypoglycemia <u>without</u> coma

E13.65 Other specified diabetes mellitus with <u>hyperglycemia</u> — The diabetic condition of having high sugar (glucose) levels in the blood and urine causing excessive thirst and frequent urination.

E13.69 Other specified diabetes mellitus with <u>other specified complication</u>
Use additional code to identify complication

E13.8 <u>Other specified</u> diabetes mellitus with <u>unspecified</u> complications

E13.9 <u>Other specified</u> diabetes mellitus <u>without</u> complications — [Questionable Admission]

Other disorders of glucose regulation and pancreatic internal secretion (E15-E16)

E15 <u>Nondiabetic</u> hypoglycemic coma — Unarousable unconsciousness due to a decreased level of blood glucose.
CC
Includes: Drug-induced insulin coma in nondiabetic
Hyperinsulinism with hypoglycemic coma
Hypoglycemic coma NOS

E16- Other disorders of pancreatic internal secretion

E16.0 <u>Drug-induced hypoglycemia</u> without coma
Use additional code for adverse effect, if applicable, to identify drug (T36-T50 with fifth or sixth character 5)
Excludes 1:   *diabetes with hypoglycemia without coma (E09.692)*

E16.1 Other hypoglycemia
Functional hyperinsulinism
Functional nonhyperinsulinemic hypoglycemia
Hyperinsulinism NOS
Hyperplasia of pancreatic islet beta cells NOS
Excludes 1:   *diabetes with hypoglycemia (E08.649, E10.649, E11.649, E13.649)*
hypoglycemia in infant of diabetic mother (P70.1)
neonatal hypoglycemia (P70.4)

E16.2 Hypoglycemia, unspecified
Excludes 1:   *diabetes with hypoglycemia (E08.649, E10.649, E11.649, E13.649)*

E16.3 Increased secretion of glucagon
Hyperplasia of pancreatic endocrine cells with glucagon excess

E16.4 Increased secretion of gastrin
Hypergastrinemia
Hyperplasia of pancreatic endocrine cells with gastrin excess
Zollinger-Ellison syndrome — A syndrome characterized by gastrin-secreting, pancreatic tumors causing hyperacidity, and ulcers in the stomach and duodenum.

E16.8 Other specified disorders of pancreatic internal secretion
Increased secretion from endocrine pancreas of growth hormone-releasing hormone
Increased secretion from endocrine pancreas of pancreatic polypeptide
Increased secretion from endocrine pancreas of somatostatin
Increased secretion from endocrine pancreas of vasoactive-intestinal polypeptide

E16.9 Disorder of pancreatic internal secretion, unspecified
Islet-cell hyperplasia NOS
Pancreatic endocrine cell hyperplasia NOS

E 1 3 - E 1 6

Excludes 1: = NOT CODED HERE! (Do not code both)

Excludes ❷: = Not Included Here

Disorders of other endocrine glands (E20-E35)

Excludes 1: *galactorrhea (N64.3)*
gynecomastia (N62)

E20- Hypoparathyroidism — Abnormal decrease in the function of the parathyroid glands.
Excludes 1: *Di George's syndrome (D82.1)*
postprocedural hypoparathyroidism (E89.2)
tetany NOS (R29.0)
transitory neonatal hypoparathyroidism (P71.4)

E20.0 <u>Idiopathic</u> hypoparathyroidism

E20.1 <u>Pseudo</u>hypoparathyroidism

E20.8 Other hypoparathyroidism

E20.9 Hypoparathyroidism, unspecified
Parathyroid tetany

E21- Hyperparathyroidism and other disorders of parathyroid gland
Excludes 1: *adult osteomalacia (M83.-)*
ectopic hyperparathyroidism (E34.2)
familial hypocalciuric hypercalcemia (E83.52)
hungry bone syndrome (E83.81)
infantile and juvenile osteomalacia (E55.0)

E21.0 <u>Primary</u> hyperparathyroidism — Abnormally increased activity of the parathyroid glands that secrete too much parathyroid hormone occurring as a result of a parathyroid condition, most commonly an adenoma.
Hyperplasia of parathyroid
Osteitis fibrosa cystica generalisata [von Recklinghausen's disease of bone]

E21.1 <u>Secondary</u> hyperparathyroidism, not elsewhere classified
Excludes 1: *secondary hyperparathyroidism of renal origin (N25.81)*

E21.2 Other hyperparathyroidism
Tertiary hyperparathyroidism
Excludes 1: *familial hypocalciuric hypercalcemia (E83.52)*

E21.3 Hyperparathyroidism, unspecified

E21.4 Other specified disorders of parathyroid gland

E21.5 Disorder of parathyroid gland, unspecified

E22- Hyperfunction of pituitary gland
Excludes 1: *Cushing's syndrome (E24.-)*
Nelson's syndrome (E24.1)
overproduction of ACTH not associated with Cushing's disease (E27.0)
overproduction of pituitary ACTH (E24.0)
overproduction of thyroid-stimulating hormone (E05.8-)

E22.0 Acromegaly and pituitary gigantism — ACROMEGALY – A chronic disease of middle-aged persons characterized by elongation and enlargement of bones of the extremities and certain head bones caused by the hypersecretion of the pituitary growth hormone. GIGANTISM – Excessive development of the bones of the hands, feet, and face due to the overproduction of the growth hormone.
Overproduction of growth hormone
Excludes 1: *constitutional gigantism (E34.4)*
constitutional tall stature (E34.4)
increased secretion from endocrine pancreas of growth hormone-releasing hormone (E16.8)

cc **E22.1** Hyperprolactinemia
Use additional code for adverse effect, if applicable, to identify drug (T36-T50 with fifth or sixth character 5)

cc **E22.2** Syndrome of inappropriate secretion of antidiuretic hormone

cc **E22.8** Other hyperfunction of pituitary gland
Central precocious puberty

cc **E22.9** Hyperfunction of pituitary gland, unspecified

E23- Hypofunction and other disorders of the pituitary gland
Includes: The listed conditions whether the disorder is in the pituitary or the hypothalamus
Excludes 1: *postprocedural hypopituitarism (E89.3)*

cc **E23.0** Hypopituitarism — Defective or absent function of the entire pituitary gland.
Fertile eunuch syndrome
Hypogonadotropic hypogonadism
Idiopathic growth hormone deficiency
Isolated deficiency of gonadotropin
Isolated deficiency of growth hormone
Isolated deficiency of pituitary hormone
Kallmann's syndrome
Lorain-Levi short stature
Necrosis of pituitary gland (postpartum)
Panhypopituitarism
Pituitary cachexia
Pituitary insufficiency NOS
Pituitary short stature
Sheehan's syndrome
Simmonds' disease

E23.1 <u>Drug-induced</u> hypopituitarism
Use additional code for adverse effect, if applicable, to identify drug (T36-T50 with fifth or sixth character 5)

cc **E23.2** <u>Diabetes insipidus</u> — A disorder characterized by excessive water intake and output, which results from inadequate pituitary secretion of antidiuretic hormone (vasopressin).
Excludes 1: *nephrogenic diabetes insipidus (N25.1)*

E23.3 Hypothalamic dysfunction, not elsewhere classified
Excludes 1: *Prader-Willi syndrome (Q87.1)*
Russell-Silver syndrome (Q87.1)

E23.6 Other disorders of pituitary gland
Abscess of pituitary
Adiposogenital dystrophy

E23.7 Disorder of pituitary gland, unspecified

E24- Cushing's syndrome
Excludes 1: *congenital adrenal hyperplasia (E25.0)*

cc **E24.0** <u>Pituitary-dependent</u> Cushing's disease — A syndrome resulting from hypersecretion of the adrenal cortex in which there is excessive production of cortisol caused by dysfunction of the pituitary gland upon the adrenal gland that is characterized by adiposity, osteoporosis, amenorrhea, impotence, capillary fragility, edema, and bruisability.
Overproduction of pituitary ACTH
Pituitary-dependent hypercorticalism

E24.1 <u>Nelson's</u> syndrome

cc **E24.2** <u>Drug-induced</u> Cushing's syndrome — A syndrome resulting from taking too much glucosteroid medicine that is characterized by adiposity, osteoporosis, amenorrhea, impotence, capillary fragility, edema, and bruisability.
Use additional code for adverse effect, if applicable, to identify drug (T36-T50 with fifth or sixth character 5)

cc **E24.3** <u>Ectopic ACTH</u> syndrome — A form caused by the production of ACTH by tissue other than the pituitary gland, such as an oat cell carcinoma of the lung.

cc **E24.4** <u>Alcohol-induced</u> pseudo-Cushing's syndrome

cc **E24.8** Other Cushing's syndrome

cc **E24.9** Cushing's syndrome, unspecified

E25- Adrenogenital disorders — Disorders of the genital organs resulting from adrenal dysfunction.
Includes: Adrenogenital syndromes, virilizing or feminizing, whether acquired or due to adrenal hyperplasia consequent on inborn enzyme defects in hormone synthesis
Female adrenal pseudohermaphroditism
Female heterosexual precocious pseudopuberty
Male isosexual precocious pseudopuberty
Male macrogenitosomia praecox
Male sexual precocity with adrenal hyperplasia
Male virilization (female)
Excludes 1: *indeterminate sex and pseudohermaphroditism (Q56)*
chromosomal abnormalities (Q90-Q99)

E25.0 <u>Congenital</u> adrenogenital disorders associated with enzyme deficiency
Congenital adrenal hyperplasia
21-Hydroxylase deficiency
Salt-losing congenital adrenal hyperplasia

E25.8 Other adrenogenital disorders
Idiopathic adrenogenital disorder
Use additional code for adverse effect, if applicable, to identify drug (T36-T50 with fifth or sixth character 5)

E25.9 Adrenogenital disorder, unspecified
Adrenogenital syndrome NOS

E20–E25

Excludes 1: = NOT CODED HERE! (Do not code both)   620   **Excludes ❷: = Not Included Here**

E26-   Hyperaldosteronism — A disease of electrolyte metabolism caused by the excessive secretion of aldosterone, and marked by hypertension, hypocholemia, alkalosis, muscular weakness, polyuria, and polydypsia.

E26.0-   Primary hyperaldosteronism — A form caused by diseases of the adrenal glands.

E26.01   Conn's syndrome — A form due to a tumor of a single adrenal gland.
Code also adrenal adenoma (D35.0-)

E26.02   Glucocorticoid-remediable aldosteronism — An inherited form that results from the formation of a hybrid gene.
Familial aldosteronism type I

E26.09   Other primary hyperaldosteronism
Primary aldosteronism due to adrenal hyperplasia (bilateral)

E26.1   Secondary hyperaldosteronism — A form caused by non-adrenal conditions producing an effect upon the adrenal glands.

E26.8-   Other hyperaldosteronism

E26.81   Bartter's syndrome — An inherited form caused by hyperplasia of the juxtaglomerular cells of the kidney and also marked by hypokalemic alkalosis and short stature.

E26.89   Other hyperaldosteronism

E26.9   Hyperaldosteronism, unspecified
Aldosteronism NOS
Hyperaldosteronism NOS

E27-   Other disorders of adrenal gland

cc **E27.0   Other adrenocortical overactivity**
Overproduction of ACTH, not associated with Cushing's disease
Premature adrenarche
Excludes 1:   *Cushing's syndrome (E24.-)*

cc **E27.1   Primary adrenocortical insufficiency** — A condition of decreased cortisol production that results in a variety of symptoms including malaise, loss of appetite, orthostatic hypotension, weight loss, anemia, pre-renal azotemia, hyperpigmentation, and hyponatremia.
Addison's disease
Autoimmune adrenalitis
Excludes 1:   *Addison only phenotype adrenoleukodystrophy (E71.528)*
     amyloidosis (E85.-)
     tuberculous Addison's disease (A18.7)
     Waterhouse-Friderichsen syndrome (A39.1)

cc **E27.2   Addisonian crisis** — A sudden, severe decrease in adrenal cortex cortisol production causing serious exacerbation of symptoms, notably low blood pressure and dehydration.
Adrenal crisis
Adrenocortical crisis

cc **E27.3   Drug-induced adrenocortical insufficiency**
Use additional code for adverse effect, if applicable, to identify drug (T36-T50 with fifth or sixth character 5)

E27.4-   Other and unspecified adrenocortical insufficiency
Excludes 1:   *adrenoleukodystrophy [Addison-Schilder] (E71.528)*
     Waterhouse-Friderichsen syndrome (A39.1)

cc **E27.40   Unspecified adrenocortical insufficiency**
Adrenocortical insufficiency NOS
Hypoaldosteronism

cc **E27.49   Other adrenocortical insufficiency**
Adrenal hemorrhage
Adrenal infarction

cc **E27.5   Adrenomedullary hyperfunction** — A condition in which the adrenal medulla oversecretes its hormones.
Adrenomedullary hyperplasia
Catecholamine hypersecretion

E27.8   Other specified disorders of adrenal gland
Abnormality of cortisol-binding globulin

E27.9   Disorder of adrenal gland, unspecified

E28-   Ovarian dysfunction — Disturbance or impairment of the normal ovarian hormonal function.
Excludes 1:   *isolated gonadotropin deficiency (E23.0)*
     postprocedural ovarian failure (E89.4-)

E28.0   Estrogen excess — [♀]
Use additional code for adverse effect, if applicable, to identify drug (T36-T50 with fifth or sixth character 5)

E28.1   Androgen excess — [♀]
Hypersecretion of ovarian androgens
Use additional code for adverse effect, if applicable, to identify drug (T36-T50 with fifth or sixth character 5)

E28.2   Polycystic ovarian syndrome — [♀] — An endocrine system disorder involving the ovaries of uncertain origin that is characterized by menstrual disorders, ovarian cysts, infertility, increased levels of male hormones, and metabolic effects.
Sclerocystic ovary syndrome
Stein-Leventhal syndrome

E28.3-   Primary ovarian failure — Abnormal ovarian function due to a disorder within the ovaries themselves.
Excludes 1:   *pure gonadal dysgenesis (Q99.1)*
     Turner's syndrome (Q96.-)

E28.31-   Premature menopause — The earlier than normal cessation of menstruation.

E28.310   Symptomatic premature menopause — [♀, Age/15-124]
Symptoms such as flushing, sleeplessness, headache, lack of concentration, associated with premature menopause

E28.319   Asymptomatic premature menopause — [♀, Age/15-124]
Premature menopause NOS

E28.39   Other primary ovarian failure — [♀]
Decreased estrogen
Resistant ovary syndrome

E28.8   Other ovarian dysfunction — [♀]
Ovarian hyperfunction NOS
Excludes 1:   *postprocedural ovarian failure (E89.4-)*

E28.9   Ovarian dysfunction, unspecified — [♀]

E29-   Testicular dysfunction — Disturbance or impairment of the normal testicular hormonal function.
Excludes 1:   *androgen insensitivity syndrome (E34.5-)*
     azoospermia or oligospermia NOS (N46.0-N46.1)
     isolated gonadotropin deficiency (E23.0)
     Klinefelter's syndrome (Q98.0-Q98.1, Q98.4)

E29.0   Testicular hyperfunction — [♂] — An abnormal increase in the production of testicular hormones.
Hypersecretion of testicular hormones

E29.1   Testicular hypofunction — [♂] — An abnormal decrease in the production of testicular hormones.
Defective biosynthesis of testicular androgen NOS
5-delta-Reductase deficiency (with male pseudohermaphroditism)
Testicular hypogonadism NOS
Use additional code for adverse effect, if applicable, to identify drug (T36-T50 with fifth or sixth character 5)
Excludes 1:   *postprocedural testicular hypofunction (E89.5)*

E29.8   Other testicular dysfunction — [♂]

E29.9   Testicular dysfunction, unspecified — [♂]

E30-   Disorders of puberty, not elsewhere classified

E30.0   Delayed puberty — Development of secondary sexual characteristics after the average period for that development.
Constitutional delay of puberty
Delayed sexual development

E30.1   Precocious puberty — [Age/0-17] — Early development of secondary sexual characteristics.
Precocious menstruation
Excludes 1:   *Albright (-McCune) (-Sternberg) syndrome (Q78.1)*
     central precocious puberty (E22.8)
     congenital adrenal hyperplasia (E25.0)
     female heterosexual precocious pseudopuberty (E25.-)
     male isosexual precocious pseudopuberty (E25.-)

E30.8   Other disorders of puberty — [Age/0-17]
Premature thelarche

E30.9   Disorder of puberty, unspecified

E31-   Polyglandular dysfunction — A condition in which mulitple endocrine glands dysfunction sequentially or simultaneously that is due to a common cause.
Excludes 1:   *ataxia telangiectasia [Louis-Bar] (G11.3)*
     dystrophia myotonica [Steinert] (G71.11)
     pseudohypoparathyroidism (E20.1)

E31.0   Autoimmune polyglandular failure — A form due to an autoimmune disorder.
Schmidt's syndrome

E31.1   Polyglandular hyperfunction — A form in which the dysfunctioning glands produce an increased volume of hormones.
Excludes 1:   *multiple endocrine adenomatosis (E31.2-)*
     multiple endocrine neoplasia (E31.2-)

E
2
6
I
E
3
1

Excludes 1: = NOT CODED HERE! (Do not code both)   **621**   *Excludes ❷:* = Not Included Here

E31.2- **Multiple endocrine neoplasia [MEN] syndromes** — A group of genetically distinct familial diseases involving adenomatous hyperplasia and tumor formation (malignant or benign) in several endocrine glands.
    Multiple endocrine adenomatosis
    Code also any associated malignancies and other conditions associated with the syndromes

  E31.20 **Multiple endocrine neoplasia [MEN] syndrome, unspecified**
      Multiple endocrine adenomatosis NOS
      Multiple endocrine neoplasia [MEN] syndrome NOS

  E31.21 **Multiple endocrine neoplasia [MEN] type I** — A form involving tumors of the parathyroid glands, pancreatic islet cells, and pituitary gland that often results in the development of kidney stones and peptic ulcer disease.
      Wermer's syndrome

  E31.22 **Multiple endocrine neoplasia [MEN] type IIA** — A form characterized by medullary carcinoma of the thyroid gland and pheochromocytomas, which usually raises blood pressure, sometimes to severe levels, and hyperparathyroidism.
      Sipple's syndrome

  E31.23 **Multiple endocrine neoplasia [MEN] type IIB** — A form with similar features to MEN type IIA, but with the additional distinct feature of mucosal neuromas.

E31.8 **Other polyglandular dysfunction**

E31.9 **Polyglandular dysfunction, unspecified**

E32- **Diseases of thymus**
  Excludes 1:   *aplasia or hypoplasia of thymus with immunodeficiency (D82.1)*
          myasthenia gravis (G70.0)

E32.0 **Persistent hyperplasia of thymus** — A sustained, abnormal increase of thymus cells.
    Hypertrophy of thymus

cc **E32.1** **Abscess of thymus** — A localized collection of pus caused by the disintegration of thymus cells.

E32.8 **Other diseases of thymus**
  Excludes 1:   *aplasia or hypoplasia with immunodeficiency (D82.1)*
          thymoma (D15.0)

E32.9 **Disease of thymus, unspecified**

E34- **Other endocrine disorders**
  Excludes 1:   *pseudohypoparathyroidism (E20.1)*

cc **E34.0** **Carcinoid syndrome** — A symptom complex caused by catecholamine secretion from carcinoid tumors.
    Note: May be used as an additional code to identify functional activity associated with a carcinoid tumor.

E34.1 **Other hypersecretion of intestinal hormones**

E34.2 **Ectopic hormone secretion, not elsewhere classified**
  Excludes 1:   *ectopic ACTH syndrome (E24.3)*

E34.3 **Short stature due to endocrine disorder** — The condition of being abnormally small in whole body size that is due to an endocrine developmental dysfunction.
    Constitutional short stature
    Laron-type short stature
  Excludes 1:   *achondroplastic short stature (Q77.4)*
          hypochondroplastic short stature (Q77.4)
          nutritional short stature (E45)
          pituitary short stature (E23.0)
          progeria (E34.8)
          renal short stature (N25.0)
          Russell-Silver syndrome (Q87.1)
          short-limbed stature with immunodeficiency (D82.2)
          short stature in specific dysmorphic syndromes — code to syndrome – see Alphabetical Index
          short stature NOS (R62.52)

E34.4 **Constitutional tall stature** — A condition of excessive growth that is caused by over-production of growth hormone.
    Constitutional gigantism

E34.5- **Androgen insensitivity syndrome** — A condition in which an individual is chromosomally-male (testes with testicular function), but can develop a wide range of gender characteristics from typical female external genitalia to predominantly male genitalia, that is due to the inability to respond to the male hormones (androgens).

  E34.50 **Androgen insensitivity syndrome, unspecified**
      Androgen insensitivity NOS

  E34.51 **Complete androgen insensitivity syndrome** — A form in which the individual develops normal female external genitalia including a vagina (but no uterus or ovaries) and has undescended testes.
      Complete androgen insensitivity
      de Quervain syndrome
      Goldberg-Maxwell syndrome

  E34.52 **Partial androgen insensitivity syndrome** — A form in which the external genitalia development ranges between underdeveloped male external genitalia to partially-developed female genitalia.
      Partial androgen insensitivity
      Reifenstein syndrome

E34.8 **Other specified endocrine disorders**
    Pineal gland dysfunction
    Progeria
  Excludes 2:   *pseudohypoparathyroidism (E20.1)*

E34.9 **Endocrine disorder, unspecified**
    Endocrine disturbance NOS
    Hormone disturbance NOS

E35 **Disorders of endocrine glands in diseases classified elsewhere** — [Not Allowed as PDX]
  Code first underlying disease, such as:
    Late congenital syphilis of thymus gland [Dubois disease] (A50.5)
  Use additional code, if applicable, to identify:
    Sequelae of tuberculosis of other organs (B90.8)
  Excludes 1:   *Echinococcus granulosus infection of thyroid gland (B67.3)*
          meningococcal hemorrhagic adrenalitis (A39.1)
          syphilis of endocrine gland (A52.79)
          tuberculosis of adrenal gland, except calcification (A18.7)
          tuberculosis of endocrine gland NEC (A18.82)
          tuberculosis of thyroid gland (A18.81)
          Waterhouse-Friderichsen syndrome (A39.1)

Intraoperative complications of endocrine system (E36)

E36- **Intraoperative complications of endocrine system**
  Excludes 2:   *postprocedural endocrine and metabolic complications and disorders, not elsewhere classified (E89.-)*

E36.0- **Intraoperative hemorrhage and hematoma of an endocrine system organ or structure complicating a procedure**
  Excludes 1:   *intraoperative hemorrhage and hematoma of an endocrine system organ or structure due to accidental puncture or laceration during a procedure (E36.1-)*

  cc **E36.01** **Intraoperative hemorrhage and hematoma of an endocrine system organ or structure complicating an endocrine system procedure**

  cc **E36.02** **Intraoperative hemorrhage and hematoma of an endocrine system organ or structure complicating other procedure**

E36.1- **Accidental puncture and laceration of an endocrine system organ or structure during a procedure**

  cc **E36.11** **Accidental puncture and laceration of an endocrine system organ or structure during an endocrine system procedure**

  cc **E36.12** **Accidental puncture and laceration of an endocrine system organ or structure during other procedure**

E36.8 **Other intraoperative complications of endocrine system**
    Use additional code, if applicable, to further specify disorder

E3 1 – E3 6

Malnutrition (E40-E46)

Excludes 1: *intestinal malabsorption (K90.-)*
sequelae of protein-calorie malnutrition (E64.0)
Excludes ❷: *nutritional anemias (D50-D53)*
starvation (T73.0)

E40 **Kwashiorkor** — A severe, protein-deficiency type of malnutrition marked by changes in
MCC skin and hair pigment, edema, retarded growth, and pathologic changes in the liver.
  **Severe malnutrition with nutritional edema with dyspigmentation of skin
  and hair**
  Excludes 1: *marasmic kwashiorkor (E42)*

E41 **Nutritional marasmus** — A protein-calorie malnutrition due to a deficiency in calorie
MCC intake that is characterized by severe tissue wasting, loss of subcutaneous fat, and often
  dehydration.
  Severe malnutrition with marasmus
  Excludes 1: *marasmic kwashiorkor (E42)*

E42 **Marasmic kwashiorkor**
MCC **Intermediate form severe protein-calorie malnutrition**
  **Severe protein-calorie malnutrition with signs of both kwashiorkor and
  marasmus**

E43 **Unspecified severe protein-calorie malnutrition**
MCC **Starvation edema**

E44- **Protein-calorie malnutrition of moderate and mild degree**
  CC E44.0 **Moderate protein-calorie malnutrition**
  CC E44.1 **Mild protein-calorie malnutrition**

E45 **Retarded development following protein-calorie malnutrition** — An
CC abnormally undersized person resulting from malnutrition.
  Nutritional short stature
  Nutritional stunting
  Physical retardation due to malnutrition

E46 **Unspecified protein-calorie malnutrition**
CC **Malnutrition NOS**
  Protein-calorie imbalance NOS
  Excludes 1: *nutritional deficiency NOS (E63.9)*

Other nutritional deficiencies (E50-E64)

Excludes ❷: *nutritional anemias (D50-D53)*

E50- **Vitamin A deficiency** — A nutritional disorder resulting from less than the normal
  amount of vitamin A in the diet.
  Excludes 1: *sequelae of vitamin A deficiency (E64.1)*
  E50.0 **Vitamin A deficiency with conjunctival xerosis** — A form marked by
  dryness of the conjunctiva.
  E50.1 **Vitamin A deficiency with Bitot's spot and conjunctival
  xerosis** — A form marked by dryness of the conjunctiva with foamy gray,
  triangular spots on the conjunctiva.
  Bitot's spot in the young child
  E50.2 **Vitamin A deficiency with corneal xerosis** — A form marked by
  dryness of the cornea.
  E50.3 **Vitamin A deficiency with corneal ulceration and xerosis** — A
  form marked by dryness of the cornea, with local, necrotic corneal tissue defects.
  E50.4 **Vitamin A deficiency with keratomalacia** — A form marked by
  softening of the cornea.
  E50.5 **Vitamin A deficiency with night blindness** — A form marked by the
  inability to see at night.
  E50.6 **Vitamin A deficiency with xerophthalmic scars of cornea** — A
  form marked by opaque regions on the cornea.
  E50.7 **Other ocular manifestations of vitamin A deficiency**
  Xerophthalmia NOS
  E50.8 **Other manifestations of vitamin A deficiency**
  Follicular keratosis — A form marked by horny growth of the skin.
  Xeroderma — A form marked by dry, rough, discolored, and sometimes scaly
  skin.
  E50.9 **Vitamin A deficiency, unspecified**
  Hypovitaminosis A NOS

E51- **Thiamine deficiency**
  Excludes 1: *sequelae of thiamine deficiency (E64.8)*
  E51.1- **Beriberi** — A nutritional disorder resulting from less than the normal amount of
  thiamine in the diet, which is marked by peripheral neurologic, cerebral, and
  cardiovascular abnormalities.
  CC E51.11 **Dry beriberi** — A form affecting the peripheral nervous system.
  Beriberi NOS
  Beriberi with polyneuropathy
  CC E51.12 **Wet beriberi** — A form affecting the cardiovascular and circulatory
  systems.
  Beriberi with cardiovascular manifestations
  Cardiovascular beriberi
  Shoshin disease
  CC E51.2 **Wernicke's encephalopathy** — A condition marked by neurological
  symptoms caused by depletion of the vitamin B1 reserves.
  CC E51.8 **Other manifestations of thiamine deficiency**
  CC E51.9 **Thiamine deficiency, unspecified**

E52 **Niacin deficiency [pellagra]** — A nutritional disorder resulting from less than the
  normal amount of niacin in the diet.
  Niacin (-tryptophan) deficiency
  Nicotinamide deficiency
  Pellagra (alcoholic)
  Excludes 1: *sequelae of niacin deficiency (E64.8)*

E53- **Deficiency of other B group vitamins**
  Excludes 1: *sequelae of vitamin B deficiency (E64.8)*
  CC E53.0 **Riboflavin deficiency** — A nutritional disorder resulting from less than the
  normal amount of riboflavin (B2) in the diet, which is marked by stomatitis, lip
  lesions, seborrhea of the nose, and vascularization of cornea.
  Ariboflavinosis
  Vitamin B2 deficiency
  E53.1 **Pyridoxine deficiency** — A nutritional disorder resulting from less than the
  normal amount of vitamin B6 in the diet, which is marked by dermatitis around the
  eyes and mouth, neuritis, anorexia, nausea, and vomiting.
  Vitamin B6 deficiency
  Excludes 1: *pyridoxine-responsive sideroblastic anemia (D64.3)*
  E53.8 **Deficiency of other specified B group vitamins**
  Biotin deficiency
  Cyanocobalamin deficiency
  Folate deficiency
  Folic acid deficiency
  Pantothenic acid deficiency
  Vitamin B12 deficiency
  Excludes 1: *folate deficiency anemia (D52.-)*
  vitamin B12 deficiency anemia (D51.-)
  E53.9 **Vitamin B deficiency, unspecified**

E54 **Ascorbic acid deficiency** — A nutritional disorder resulting from less than the
  normal amount of vitamin C in the diet, which is marked by lowered resistance to infections,
  joint tenderness, and susceptibility to dental disorders.
  Deficiency of vitamin C
  Scurvy
  Excludes 1: *scorbutic anemia (D53.2)*
  sequelae of vitamin C deficiency (E64.2)

E55- **Vitamin D deficiency** — A nutritional disorder resulting from less than the normal
  amount of vitamin D in the diet, which is marked by bone disorders.
  Excludes 1: *adult osteomalacia (M83.-)*
  osteoporosis (M80.-)
  sequelae of rickets (E64.3)
  CC E55.0 **Rickets, active** — A form marked by inadequate deposition of lime salts in
  developing cartilage and newly formed bone causing malformation which is seen
  during childhood.
  Infantile osteomalacia
  Juvenile osteomalacia
  Excludes 1: *celiac rickets (K90.0)*
  Crohn's rickets (K50.-)
  hereditary vitamin D-dependent rickets (E83.32)
  inactive rickets (E64.3)
  renal rickets (N25.0)
  sequelae of rickets (E64.3)
  vitamin D-resistant rickets (E83.31)
  E55.9 **Vitamin D deficiency, unspecified**
  Avitaminosis D — Less than the normal amount of vitamin D in the diet.

E40 I E55

Excludes 1: = NOT CODED HERE! (Do not code both)

Excludes ❷: = Not Included Here

E56- Other vitamin deficiencies
   Excludes 1:   sequelae of other vitamin deficiencies (E64.8)

   E56.0   **Deficiency of vitamin E**
   E56.1   **Deficiency of vitamin K**
      Excludes 1:   deficiency of coagulation factor due to vitamin K deficiency (D68.4)
      vitamin K deficiency of newborn (P53)
   E56.8   **Deficiency of other vitamins**
   E56.9   **Vitamin deficiency, unspecified**

E58   Dietary calcium deficiency
   Excludes 1:   disorders of calcium metabolism (E83.5-)
   sequelae of calcium deficiency (E64.8)

E59   Dietary selenium deficiency
   Keshan disease
   Excludes 1:   sequelae of selenium deficiency (E64.8)

E60   Dietary zinc deficiency

E61- Deficiency of other nutrient elements
   Use additional code for adverse effect, if applicable, to identify drug   (T36-T50 with fifth or sixth character 5)
   Excludes 1:   disorders of mineral metabolism (E83.-)
   iodine deficiency related thyroid disorders (E00-E02)
   sequelae of malnutrition and other nutritional deficiencies (E64.-)

   E61.0   **Copper deficiency**
   E61.1   **Iron deficiency**
      Excludes 1:   iron deficiency anemia (D50.-)
   E61.2   **Magnesium deficiency**
   E61.3   **Manganese deficiency**
   E61.4   **Chromium deficiency**
   E61.5   **Molybdenum deficiency**
   E61.6   **Vanadium deficiency**
   E61.7   **Deficiency of multiple nutrient elements**
   E61.8   **Deficiency of other specified nutrient elements**
   E61.9   **Deficiency of nutrient element, unspecified**

E63- Other nutritional deficiencies
   Excludes 1:   dehydration (E86.0)
   failure to thrive, adult (R62.7)
   failure to thrive, child (R62.51)
   feeding problems in newborn (P92.-)
   sequelae of malnutrition and other nutritional deficiencies (E64.-)

   E63.0   **Essential fatty acid [EFA] deficiency**
   E63.1   **Imbalance of constituents of food intake**
   E63.8   **Other specified nutritional deficiencies**
   E63.9   **Nutritional deficiency, unspecified**

E64- Sequelae of malnutrition and other nutritional deficiencies
   Note: This category is to be used to indicate conditions in categories E43, E44, E46, E50-E63 as the cause of sequelae, which are themselves classified elsewhere. The "sequelae" include conditions specified as such; they also include the late effects of diseases classifiable to the above categories if the disease itself is no longer present
   Code first condition resulting from (sequela) of malnutrition and other nutritional deficiencies

   CC **E64.0**   **Sequelae of protein-calorie malnutrition**
      Excludes ❷: retarded development following protein-calorie malnutrition (E45)
   E64.1   **Sequelae of vitamin A deficiency**
   E64.2   **Sequelae of vitamin C deficiency**
   E64.3   **Sequelae of rickets**
   E64.8   **Sequelae of other nutritional deficiencies**
   E64.9   **Sequelae of unspecified nutritional deficiency**

Overweight, obesity and other hyperalimentation (E65-E68)

E65   Localized adiposity — An abnormal amount of fat concentrated in one part of the body.
   Fat pad — An abnormal amount of fat concentrated into a well-defined circumscribed area.

E66- Overweight and obesity — The abnormally increased body weight for height due to the excess storage of body fat.
   Code first obesity complicating pregnancy, childbirth and the puerperium, if applicable (O99.21-)
   Use additional code to identify body mass index (BMI), if known (Z68.-)
   Excludes 1:   adiposogenital dystrophy (E23.6)
   lipomatosis NOS (E88.2)
   lipomatosis dolorosa [Dercum] (E88.2)
   Prader-Willi syndrome (Q87.1)

   E66.0-   **Obesity due to excess calories** — A form caused by the excess intake of food calories that is not due to a medical, genetic, or psychiatric condition, and is not drug-induced.

      E66.01   **Morbid (severe) obesity due to excess calories** — A form usually identified and diagnosed as at least twice a person's ideal weight, 100 pounds over a person's ideal weight, or a body mass index (BMI) that is greater than 40.
         Excludes 1:   morbid (severe) obesity with alveolar hypoventilation (E66.2)
      E66.09   **Other obesity due to excess calories** — [Questionable Admission]
   E66.1   **Drug-induced obesity** — [Questionable Admission]
      Use additional code for adverse effect, if applicable, to identify drug (T36-T50 with fifth or sixth character 5)
   CC **E66.2**   **Morbid (severe) obesity with alveolar hypoventilation** — A condition of decreased oxygen levels and elevated carbon dioxide levels that is associated with obesity.
      Obesity hypoventilation syndrome (OHS)
      Pickwickian syndrome
   E66.3   **Overweight** — The first grade of the overweight/obesity continuum, followed by obesity, morbid obesity, and superobesity, or simply a person's weight (excessive bone and muscle mass) that is in greater proportion to their height.
   E66.8   **Other obesity** — [Questionable Admission]
   E66.9   **Obesity, unspecified** — [Questionable Admission]
      Obesity NOS

E67- Other hyperalimentation — The excessive ingestion or administration of nutrients into the body.
   Excludes 1:   hyperalimentation NOS (R63.2)
   sequelae of hyperalimentation (E68)

   E67.0   **Hypervitaminosis A** — A disorder caused by excessive amounts of vitamin A in the blood, marked by skin pigmentation, pruritis, and loss of hair.
   E67.1   **Hypercarotinemia** — An excessive amount of the yellow or red pigment, carotene, in the blood.
   E67.2   **Megavitamin-B6 syndrome** — A disorder caused by excessive amounts of vitamin B6 in the blood.
   E67.3   **Hypervitaminosis D** — A disorder caused by excessive amounts of vitamin D in the blood, marked by weakness, fatigue, and loss of weight.
   E67.8   **Other specified hyperalimentation**

E68   Sequelae of hyperalimentation
   Code first condition resulting from (sequela) of hyperalimentation

Metabolic disorders (E70-E88)

   Excludes 1:   androgen insensitivity syndrome (E34.5-)
   congenital adrenal hyperplasia (E25.0)
   Ehlers-Danlos syndrome (Q79.6)
   hemolytic anemias attributable to enzyme disorders (D55.-)
   Marfan's syndrome (Q87.4)
   5-alpha-reductase deficiency (E29.1)

E70- Disorders of aromatic amino-acid metabolism — Abnormalities of a group of chemically similar organic compounds that form the chief structure of proteins.

   CC **E70.0**   **Classical phenylketonuria** — An inherited disease caused by the body's failure to oxidize the amino-acid phenylalanine, resulting in tremor, spasticity, convulsions, and mental deficiency.
   CC **E70.1**   **Other hyperphenylalaninemias**
   E70.2-   **Disorders of tyrosine metabolism**
      Excludes 1:   transitory tyrosinemia of newborn (P74.5)
      CC **E70.20**   **Disorder of tyrosine metabolism, unspecified**
      CC **E70.21**   **Tyrosinemia** — The abnormal level of tyrosine in the blood.
         Hypertyrosinemia

E56 - E70

cc **E70.29   Other disorders of tyrosine metabolism**
Alkaptonuria — The abnormal presence of alkapton bodies in the urine.
Ochronosis — A disorder characterized by discoloration of certain tissues of the body caused by the deposit of alkapton bodies.

E70.3-   Albinism — A disorder characterized by absence of pigment in the skin, hair, and eyes.

cc **E70.30   Albinism, unspecified**

E70.31- Ocular albinism

cc **E70.310   X-linked ocular albinism**

cc **E70.311   Autosomal recessive ocular albinism**

cc **E70.318   Other ocular albinism**

cc **E70.319   Ocular albinism, unspecified**

E70.32- Oculocutaneous albinism
Excludes 1:   Chediak-Higashi syndrome (E70.330)
Hermansky-Pudlak syndrome (E70.331)

cc **E70.320   Tyrosinase negative oculocutaneous albinism**
Albinism I
Oculocutaneous albinism ty-neg

cc **E70.321   Tyrosinase positive oculocutaneous albinism**
Albinism II
Oculocutaneous albinism ty-pos

cc **E70.328   Other oculocutaneous albinism**
Cross syndrome

cc **E70.329   Oculocutaneous albinism, unspecified**

E70.33- Albinism with hematologic abnormality

cc **E70.330   Chediak-Higashi syndrome**

cc **E70.331   Hermansky-Pudlak syndrome**

cc **E70.338   Other albinism with hematologic abnormality**

cc **E70.339   Albinism with hematologic abnormality, unspecified**

cc **E70.39   Other specified albinism**
Piebaldism

E70.4-   Disorders of histidine metabolism — Abnormal function of the amino acid, histidine, which is essential for the optimal growth of infants, and breaks down to produce histamine.

cc **E70.40   Disorders of histidine metabolism, unspecified**

cc **E70.41   Histidinemia** — An inherited histidine metabolic defect characterized by excessive amounts of histidine in the blood and urine.

cc **E70.49   Other disorders of histidine metabolism**

cc **E70.5   Disorders of tryptophan metabolism**

cc **E70.8   Other disorders of aromatic amino-acid metabolism**

cc **E70.9   Disorder of aromatic amino-acid metabolism, unspecified**

E71- Disorders of branched-chain amino-acid metabolism and fatty-acid metabolism — Abnormal function of the amino acids essential for the optimal growth of infants.

cc **E71.0   Maple-syrup-urine disease** — An inherited enzyme defect in the metabolism of branched-chain amino acids.

E71.1- Other disorders of branched-chain amino-acid metabolism

E71.11- Branched-chain organic acidurias

cc **E71.110   Isovaleric acidemia**

cc **E71.111   3-methylglutaconic aciduria**

cc **E71.118   Other branched-chain organic acidurias**

E71.12- Disorders of propionate metabolism

cc **E71.120   Methylmalonic acidemia**

cc **E71.121   Propionic acidemia**

cc **E71.128   Other disorders of propionate metabolism**

cc **E71.19   Other disorders of branched-chain amino-acid metabolism**
Hyperleucine-isoleucinemia
Hypervalinemia

cc **E71.2   Disorder of branched-chain amino-acid metabolism, unspecified**

E71.3-   Disorders of fatty-acid metabolism — Conditions resulting from the abnormal fatty acid chemical process that may be characterized by hypoglycemia, coma, muscle weakness, cardiomyopathy, or rhabdomyalgias.
Excludes 1:   peroxisomal disorders (E71.5)
Refsum's disease (G60.1)
Schilder's disease (G37.0)
Excludes ❷: carnitine deficiency due to inborn error of metabolism (E71.42)

E71.30   Disorder of fatty-acid metabolism, unspecified

E71.31- Disorders of fatty-acid oxidation

cc **E71.310   Long chain/very long chain acyl CoA dehydrogenase deficiency**
LCAD
VLCAD

cc **E71.311   Medium chain acyl CoA dehydrogenase deficiency**
MCAD

cc **E71.312   Short chain acyl CoA dehydrogenase deficiency**
SCAD

cc **E71.313   Glutaric aciduria type II**
Glutaric aciduria type II A
Glutaric aciduria type II B
Glutaric aciduria type II C
Excludes 1:   glutaric aciduria (type 1) NOS (E72.3)

cc **E71.314   Muscle carnitine palmitoyltransferase deficiency**

cc **E71.318   Other disorders of fatty-acid oxidation**

cc **E71.32   Disorders of ketone metabolism**

cc **E71.39   Other disorders of fatty-acid metabolism**

E71.4-   Disorders of carnitine metabolism
Excludes 1:   muscle carnitine palmitoyltransferase deficiency (E71.314)

E71.40   Disorder of carnitine metabolism, unspecified

E71.41   Primary carnitine deficiency — A condition of lower than normal levels of carnitine concentration in plasma or tissues that is caused by a defect in the carnitine transporter mechanism.

E71.42   Carnitine deficiency due to inborn errors of metabolism — A form caused by metabolic disorders.
Code also associated inborn error or metabolism

E71.43   Iatrogenic carnitine deficiency — A form resulting from medical treatment.
Carnitine deficiency due to hemodialysis
Carnitine deficiency due to valproic acid therapy

E71.44- Other secondary carnitine deficiency

E71.440   Ruvalcaba-Myhre-Smith syndrome

E71.448   Other secondary carnitine deficiency

E71.5-   Peroxisomal disorders — Inherited conditions resulting from the abnormal formation or functioning of the subcellular membrane-bound organelles (peroxisomes) that contain enzymes involved in the metabolism of very long chain fatty acids.
Excludes 1:   Schilder's disease (G37.0)

cc **E71.50   Peroxisomal disorder, unspecified**

E71.51- Disorders of peroxisome biogenesis
Group 1 peroxisomal disorders
Excludes 1:   Refsum's disease (G60.1)

cc **E71.510   Zellweger syndrome** — A genetic peroxisomal leukodystrophy disorder characterized by enlarged liver, lack of muscle tone, mental retardation, and vision disturbances.

cc **E71.511   Neonatal adrenoleukodystrophy** — A form of X-linked adrenoleukodystrophy (see inclusion term below) occurring in the neonatal period.
Excludes 1:   X-linked adrenoleukodystrophy (E71.42-)

cc **E71.518   Other disorders of peroxisome biogenesis**

E71.52- X-linked adrenoleukodystrophy — A genetic peroxisomal disorder occurring in childhood that is characterized by mental retardation, spasticity, blindness, and is invariably fatal.

cc **E71.520   Childhood cerebral X-linked adrenoleukodystrophy**

cc **E71.521   Adolescent X-linked adrenoleukodystrophy**

cc **E71.522   Adrenomyeloneuropathy**

cc **E71.528   Other X-linked adrenoleukodystrophy**
Addison only phenotype adrenoleukodystrophy
Addison-Schilder adrenoleukodystrophy

cc **E71.529   X-linked adrenoleukodystrophy, unspecified type**

cc **E71.53   Other group 2 peroxisomal disorders**

E
7
0
|
E
7
1

Excludes 1: = NOT CODED HERE! (Do not code both)   625   *Excludes ❷:* = Not Included Here

E71.54- Other peroxisomal disorders

cc **E71.540 Rhizomelic chondrodysplasia punctata** — A genetic peroxisomal disorder characterized by shortening of the proximal limbs and joints, round face, high forehead, and a small, upturned nose.

> Excludes 1:   chondrodysplasia punctata NOS (Q77.3)

cc **E71.541 Zellweger-like syndrome**

cc **E71.542 Other group 3 peroxisomal disorders**

cc **E71.548 Other peroxisomal disorders**

E72- Other disorders of amino-acid metabolism

> Excludes 1:   disorders of:
> aromatic amino-acid metabolism (E70.-)
> branched-chain amino-acid metabolism (E71.0-E71.2)
> fatty-acid metabolism (E71.3)
> gout (M1A.-, M10.-)
> purine and pyrimidine metabolism (E79.-)

E72.0- Disorders of amino-acid transport — Abnormalities of a group of chemically similar organic compounds that form the chief structure of proteins.

> Excludes 1:   disorders of tryptophan metabolism (E70.5)

cc **E72.00 Disorders of amino-acid transport, unspecified**

cc **E72.01 Cystinuria** — An inherited, metabolic disorder characterized by large amounts of cystine in the urine resulting in the formation of urinary calculi.

cc **E72.02 Hartnup's disease** — A disorder of the intestinal and renal transport of amino acids, marked by amino acid in the urine, skin rash, and other biochemical abnormalities.

cc **E72.03 Lowe's syndrome**

> Use additional code for associated glaucoma (H42)

cc **E72.04 Cystinosis** — An inherited disease of cystine metabolism resulting in abnormal deposition of cystine in body tissues.

> Fanconi (-de Toni) (-Debré) syndrome with cystinosis

> Excludes 1:   Fanconi (-de Toni) (-Debré) syndrome without cystinosis (E72.09)

cc **E72.09 Other disorders of amino-acid transport**

> Fanconi (-de Toni) (-Debré) syndrome, unspecified

E72.1- Disorders of sulfur-bearing amino-acid metabolism — The abnormal function of amino acids containing sulphur compounds.

> Excludes 1:   cystinosis (E72.04)
> cystinuria (E72.01)
> transcobalamin II deficiency (D51.2)

cc **E72.10 Disorders of sulfur-bearing amino-acid metabolism, unspecified**

cc **E72.11 Homocystinuria** — The abnormal presence of large amounts of homocystine in the urine caused by an error of sulfur amino acid metabolism due to a deficiency of the liver enzyme cystathionine synthase.

> Cystathionine synthase deficiency

cc **E72.12 Methylenetetrahydrofolate reductase deficiency**

cc **E72.19 Other disorders of sulfur-bearing amino-acid metabolism**

> Cystathioninuria
> Methioninemia
> Sulfite oxidase deficiency

E72.2- Disorders of urea cycle metabolism — Abnormal function of the series of reactions that produce urea, which is important in removing ammonia from the body.

> Excludes 1:   disorders of ornithine metabolism (E72.4)

cc **E72.20 Disorder of urea cycle metabolism, unspecified**

> Hyperammonemia

> Excludes 1:   hyperammonemia-hyperornithinemia-homocitrullinemia syndrome E72.4
> transient hyperammonemia of newborn (P74.6)

cc **E72.21 Argininemia**

cc **E72.22 Arginosuccinic aciduria**

cc **E72.23 Citrullinemia**

cc **E72.29 Other disorders of urea cycle metabolism**

cc **E72.3 Disorders of lysine and hydroxylysine metabolism** — The abnormal function of lysine and hydroxylysine metabolism.

> Glutaric aciduria NOS
> Glutaric aciduria (type I)
> Hydroxylysinemia
> Hyperlysinemia

> Excludes 1:   glutaric aciduria type II (E71.313)
> Refsum's dsease (G60.1)
> Zellweger syndrome (E71.510)

cc **E72.4 Disorders of ornithine metabolism** — The abnormal function of orinthine metabolism.

> Hyperammonemia-Hyperornithinemia-Homocitrullinemia syndrome
> Ornithinemia (types I, II)
> Ornithine transcarbamylase deficiency

> Excludes 1:   hereditary choroidal dystrophy (H31.2-)

E72.5- Disorders of glycine metabolism — The abnormal function of glycine metabolism.

cc **E72.50 Disorder of glycine metabolism, unspecified**

cc **E72.51 Non-ketotic hyperglycinemia**

cc **E72.52 Trimethylaminuria**

cc **E72.53 Hyperoxaluria**

> Oxalosis
> Oxaluria

cc **E72.59 Other disorders of glycine metabolism**

> D-glycericacidemia
> Hyperhydroxyprolinemia
> Hyperprolinemia (types I, II)
> Sarcosinemia

cc **E72.8 Other specified disorders of amino-acid metabolism**

> Disorders of beta-amino-acid metabolism
> Disorders of gamma-glutamyl cycle

cc **E72.9 Disorder of amino-acid metabolism, unspecified**

E73- Lactose intolerance — Abnormal decrease or impaired digestion of lactose, a sugar found in milk.

E73.0 Congenital lactase deficiency — An inherited condition of insufficient levels of the enzyme lactase.

E73.1 Secondary lactase deficiency — A condition of insufficient levels of the enzyme lactase that is due to disease conditions, usually of the small intestine.

E73.8 Other lactose intolerance

E73.9 Lactose intolerance, unspecified

E74- Other disorders of carbohydrate metabolism

> Excludes 1:   diabetes mellitus (E08-E13)
> hypoglycemia NOS (E16.2)
> increased secretion of glucagon (E16.3)
> mucopolysaccharidosis (E76.0-E76.3)

E74.0- Glycogen storage disease — An inherited metabolic disorder of glycogen storage.

cc **E74.00 Glycogen storage disease, unspecified**

cc **E74.01 von Gierke disease**

> Type I glycogen storage disease

cc **E74.02 Pompe disease**

> Cardiac glycogenosis
> Type II glycogen storage disease

cc **E74.03 Cori disease**

> Forbes disease
> Type III glycogen storage disease

cc **E74.04 McArdle disease**

> Type V glycogen storage disease

cc **E74.09 Other glycogen storage disease**

> Andersen disease
> Hers disease
> Tauri disease
> Glycogen storage disease, types 0, IV, VI-XI
> Liver phosphorylase deficiency
> Muscle phosphofructokinase deficiency

E74.1- Disorders of fructose metabolism — A metabolic disorder of fructose metabolism.

> Excludes 1:   muscle phosphofructokinase deficiency (E74.09)

E74.10 Disorder of fructose metabolism, unspecified

E74.11 Essential fructosuria — A benign, hereditary carbohydrate metabolism disorder characterized by fructosemia and fructosuria.

> Fructokinase deficiency

E74.12 Hereditary fructose intolerance — A hereditary disorder involving deficient activity of the hepatic enzyme fructose-1-phosphate aldolase, marked by hypoglycemia in infants' diets.

> Fructosemia

E74.19 Other disorders of fructose metabolism

> Fructose-1, 6-diphosphatase deficiency

E74.2- Disorders of <u>galactose metabolism</u> — A metabolic disorder of galactose metabolism.

cc **E74.20** Disorders of galactose metabolism, unspecified

cc **E74.21** Galactosemia — An inherited disorder of galactose metabolism marked by hepatomegaly, cataracts, and mental retardation.

cc **E74.29** Other disorders of galactose metabolism
Galactokinase deficiency

E74.3- Other disorders of intestinal carbohydrate absorption
Excludes ❷: *lactose intolerance (E73.-)*

E74.31 Sucrase-isomaltase deficiency

E74.39 Other disorders of intestinal carbohydrate absorption
Disorder of intestinal carbohydrate absorption NOS
Glucose-galactose malabsorption
Sucrase deficiency

cc **E74.4** Disorders of <u>pyruvate metabolism and gluconeogenesis</u>
Deficiency of phosphoenolpyruvate carboxykinase
Deficiency of pyruvate carboxylase
Deficiency of pyruvate dehydrogenase
Excludes 1: *disorders of pyruvate metabolism and gluconeogenesis with anemia (D55.-)*
Leigh's syndrome (G31.82)

cc **E74.8** Other specified disorders of carbohydrate metabolism
Essential pentosuria
Renal glycosuria

E74.9 Disorder of carbohydrate metabolism, unspecified

E75- Disorders of <u>sphingolipid metabolism</u> and <u>other lipid storage disorders</u> — Inherited disorders characterized by abnormal cellular lipid metabolism.
Excludes 1: *mucolipidosis, types I-III (E77.0-E77.1)*
Refsum's disease (G60.1)

E75.0- GM2 gangliosidosis — An inherited abnormal accumulation of GM2 ganglioside in lysosomes.

cc **E75.00** GM2 gangliosidosis, unspecified

cc **E75.01** Sandhoff disease

cc **E75.02** Tay-Sachs disease — A form with hexosaminidase A enzyme deficiency that is characterized by neurodegeneration, difficulty swallowing, and physical developmental disabilities.

cc **E75.09** Other GM2 gangliosidosis
Adult GM2 gangliosidosis
Juvenile GM2 gangliosidosis

E75.1- Other and unspecified gangliosidosis

cc **E75.10** Unspecified gangliosidosis
Gangliosidosis NOS

cc **E75.11** Mucolipidosis IV

cc **E75.19** Other gangliosidosis
GM1 gangliosidosis
GM3 gangliosidosis

E75.2- Other sphingolipidosis — Inherited lipid storage disorders relating to sphingolipid metabolism.
Excludes 1: *adrenoleukodystrophy [Addison-Schilder] (E71.528)*

E75.21 Fabry (-Anderson) disease — A form with a-galactosidase A enzyme deficiency that is characterized by full body and/or limb pain, infarction of organs, and fatigue.

E75.22 Gaucher disease — A form with glucocerebrosidase enzyme deficiency that is characterized by bruising, fatigue, anemia, hepatosplenomegaly, and pancytopenia.

cc **E75.23** Krabbe disease — A form with galactocerebrosidase enzyme deficiency that is characterized by spasticity, neurodegeneration, blindness, and seizures.

E75.24- Niemann-Pick disease — A form with sphingomyelinase enzyme deficiency that is characterized by mental retardation, spasticity, splenomegaly, and thrombocytopenia.

E75.240 Niemann-Pick disease type A

E75.241 Niemann-Pick disease type B

E75.242 Niemann-Pick disease type C

E75.243 Niemann-Pick disease type D

E75.248 Other Niemann-Pick disease

E75.249 Niemann-Pick disease, unspecified

cc **E75.25** Metachromatic leukodystrophy

cc **E75.29** Other sphingolipidosis
Farber's syndrome
Sulfatase deficiency
Sulfatide lipidosis

E75.3 Sphingolipidosis, unspecified

cc **E75.4** Neuronal ceroid lipofuscinosis
Batten disease
Bielschowsky-Jansky disease
Kufs disease
Spielmeyer-Vogt disease

E75.5 Other lipid storage disorders
Cerebrotendinous cholesterosis [van Bogaert-Scherer-Epstein]
Wolman's disease

E75.6 Lipid storage disorder, unspecified

E76- Disorders of <u>glycosaminoglycan metabolism</u> — Inherited diseases of defective glycosaminoglycan metabolism causing abnormal accumulation in the tissues.

E76.0- Mucopolysaccharidosis, <u>type I</u>

cc **E76.01** Hurler's syndrome

cc **E76.02** Hurler-Scheie syndrome

cc **E76.03** Scheie's syndrome

cc **E76.1** Mucopolysaccharidosis, <u>type II</u>
Hunter's syndrome

E76.2- Other mucopolysaccharidoses

E76.21- Morquio mucopolysaccharidoses

cc **E76.210** Morquio A mucopolysaccharidoses
Classic Morquio syndrome
Morquio syndrome A
Mucopolysaccharidosis, type IVA

cc **E76.211** Morquio B mucopolysaccharidoses
Morquio-like mucopolysaccharidoses
Morquio-like syndrome
Morquio syndrome B
Mucopolysaccharidosis, type IVB

cc **E76.219** Morquio mucopolysaccharidoses, unspecified
Morquio syndrome
Mucopolysaccharidosis, type IV

cc **E76.22** Sanfilippo mucopolysaccharidoses
Mucopolysaccharidosis, type III (A) (B) (C) (D)
Sanfilippo A syndrome
Sanfilippo B syndrome
Sanfilippo C syndrome
Sanfilippo D syndrome

cc **E76.29** Other mucopolysaccharidoses
beta-Glucuronidase deficiency
Maroteaux-Lamy (mild) (severe) syndrome
Mucopolysaccharidosis, types VI, VII

cc **E76.3** Mucopolysaccharidosis, unspecified

cc **E76.8** Other disorders of glucosaminoglycan metabolism

cc **E76.9** Glucosaminoglycan metabolism disorder, unspecified

E77- Disorders of <u>glycoprotein metabolism</u> — Inherited diseases of defective glycoprotein metabolism causing abnormal accumulation in the tissues.

E77.0 Defects in post-translational modification of lysosomal enzymes
Mucolipidosis II [I-cell disease]
Mucolipidosis III [pseudo-Hurler polydystrophy]

E77.1 Defects in glycoprotein degradation
Aspartylglucosaminuria
Fucosidosis
Mannosidosis
Sialidosis [mucolipidosis I]

E77.8 Other disorders of glycoprotein metabolism

E77.9 Disorder of glycoprotein metabolism, unspecified

E78- Disorders of <u>lipoprotein metabolism</u> and <u>other lipidemias</u> — Inherited diseases of defective lipoprotein metabolism causing abnormal accumulation in the tissues, and disorders involving lipids in the blood.
Excludes 1: *sphingolipidosis (E75.0-E75.3)*

E78.0- Pure hypercholesterolemia — A disorder caused by an increase in beta lipoproteins and cholesterol in the plasma.

E78.00 Pure hypercholesterolemia, unspecified
Fredrickson's hyperlipoproteinemia, type IIa
Hyperbetalipoproteinemia
Low-density-lipoprotein-type [LDL] hyperlipoproteinemia

E78.01 Familial hypercholesterolemia — A form caused by genetic mutations involved in LDL-C metabolism.

E78.1 **Pure hyperglyceridemia** — A disorder caused by an increase in triglycerides or pre-beta lipoproteins in the plasma.
    Elevated fasting triglycerides
    Endogenous hyperglyceridemia
    Fredrickson's hyperlipoproteinemia, type IV
    Hyperlipidemia, group B
    Hyperprebetalipoproteinemia
    Very-low-density-lipoprotein-type [VLDL] hyperlipoproteinemia

E78.2 **Mixed hyperlipidemia** — A disorder caused by an increase of beta lipoproteins and cholesterol, and triglycerides and pre-beta lipoproteins in the plasma.
    Broad- or floating-betalipoproteinemia
    Combined hyperlipidemia NOS
    Elevated cholesterol with elevated triglycerides NEC
    Fredrickson's hyperlipoproteinemia, type IIb or III
    Hyperbetalipoproteinemia with prebetalipoproteinemia
    Hypercholesteremia with endogenous hyperglyceridemia
    Hyperlipidemia, group C
    Tubo-eruptive xanthoma
    Xanthoma tuberosum
    Excludes 1:   *cerebrotendinous cholesterosis [van Bogaert-Scherer-Epstein] (E75.5)*
         familial combined hyperlipidemia (E78.4)

E78.3 **Hyperchylomicronemia** — A disorder caused by the presence of large quantities of chylomicrons resulting from an absence or deficiency of the lipoprotein lipase.
    Chylomicron retention disease
    Fredrickson's hyperlipoproteinemia, type I or V
    Hyperlipidemia, group D
    Mixed hyperglyceridemia

E78.4 **Other hyperlipidemia**
    Familial combined hyperlipidemia

E78.5 **Hyperlipidemia, unspecified**

E78.6 **Lipoprotein deficiency** — An abnormal decrease in the blood plasma lipoprotein levels.
    Abetalipoproteinemia
    Depressed HDL cholesterol
    High-density lipoprotein deficiency
    Hypoalphalipoproteinemia
    Hypobetalipoproteinemia (familial)
    Lecithin cholesterol acyltransferase deficiency
    Tangier disease

E78.7- **Disorders of bile acid and cholesterol metabolism**
    Excludes 1:   *Niemann-Pick disease type C (E75.242)*

  E78.70 **Disorder of bile acid and cholesterol metabolism, unspecified**

cc **E78.71** **Barth syndrome**

cc **E78.72** **Smith-Lemli-Opitz syndrome**

  E78.79 **Other disorders of bile acid and cholesterol metabolism**

E78.8- **Other disorders of lipoprotein metabolism**

  E78.81 **Lipoid dermatoarthritis**

  E78.89 **Other lipoprotein metabolism disorders**

E78.9 **Disorder of lipoprotein metabolism, unspecified**

E79- **Disorders of purine and pyrimidine metabolism** — Inherited diseases of defective purine and pyrimidine metabolism causing abnormal accumulation in the tissues.
    Excludes 1:   *Ataxia-telangiectasia (Q87.1)*
         Bloom's syndrome (Q82.8)
         Cockayne's syndrome (Q87.1)
         calculus of kidney (N20.0)
         combined immunodeficiency disorders (D81.-)
         Fanconi's anemia (D61.09)
         gout (M1A.-, M10.-)
         orotaciduric anemia (D53.0)
         progeria (E34.8)
         Werner's syndrome (E34.8)
         xeroderma pigmentosum (Q82.1)

E79.0 **Hyperuricemia without signs of inflammatory arthritis and tophaceous disease**
    Asymptomatic hyperuricemia

cc **E79.1** **Lesch-Nyhan syndrome**
    HGPRT deficiency

cc **E79.2** **Myoadenylate deaminase deficiency**

cc **E79.8** **Other disorders of purine and pyrimidine metabolism**
    Hereditary xanthinuria

cc **E79.9** **Disorder of purine and pyrimidine metabolism, unspecified**

E80- **Disorders of porphyrin and bilirubin metabolism** — Inherited diseases of defective porphyrin and bilirubin metabolism causing abnormal accumulation in the tissues.
    Includes: Defects of catalase and peroxidase

cc **E80.0** **Hereditary erythropoietic porphyria**
    Congenital erythropoietic porphyria
    Erythropoietic protoporphyria

cc **E80.1** **Porphyria cutanea tarda**

  E80.2- **Other and unspecified porphyria**

cc **E80.20** **Unspecified porphyria**
    Porphyria NOS

cc **E80.21** **Acute intermittent (hepatic) porphyria**

cc **E80.29** **Other porphyria**
    Hereditary coproporphyria

cc **E80.3** **Defects of catalase and peroxidase**
    Acatalasia [Takahara]

E80.4 **Gilbert syndrome**

E80.5 **Crigler-Najjar syndrome**

E80.6 **Other disorders of bilirubin metabolism**
    Dubin-Johnson syndrome
    Rotor's syndrome

E80.7 **Disorder of bilirubin metabolism, unspecified**

E83- **Disorders of mineral metabolism** — Abnormal chemical processing of the organic, life-sustaining chemical process of the nonorganic homogenous solid substances.
    Excludes 1:   *dietary mineral deficiency (E58-E61)*
         parathyroid disorders (E20-E21)
         vitamin D deficiency (E55.-)

E83.0- **Disorders of copper metabolism** — Abnormal chemical processing of the metallic element copper, which is essential to several enzyme systems.

  E83.00 **Disorder of copper metabolism, unspecified**

  E83.01 **Wilson's disease** — A hereditary, degenerative syndrome that allows abnormal accumulation of copper in various organs (brain, liver, kidney, and cornea) due to a defect in copper metabolism.
    Code also associated Kayser Fleischer ring (H18.04-)

  E83.09 **Other disorders of copper metabolism**
    Menkes' (kinky hair) (steely hair) disease

E83.1- **Disorders of iron metabolism** — Abnormal chemical processing of the metallic element iron, which is essential in the formation of hemoglobin.
    Excludes 1:   *iron deficiency anemia (D50.-)*
         sideroblastic anemia (D64.0-D64.3)

  E83.10 **Disorder of iron metabolism, unspecified**

  E83.11- **Hemochromatosis** — A disease of iron metabolism characterized by excessive iron deposition in tissues, especially the liver, bronze-like pigmentation of the skin, and diabetes mellitus.

    E83.110 **Hereditary hemochromatosis**
        Bronzed diabetes
        Pigmentary cirrhosis (of liver)
        Primary (hereditary) hemochromatosis

    E83.111 **Hemochromatosis due to repeated red blood cell transfusions**
        Iron overload due to repeated red blood cell transfusions
        Transfusion (red blood cell) associated hemochromatosis

    E83.118 **Other hemochromatosis**

    E83.119 **Hemochromatosis, unspecified**

  E83.19 **Other disorders of iron metabolism**
    Use additional code, if applicable, for idiopathic pulmonary hemosiderosis (J84.03)

E83.2 **Disorders of zinc metabolism** — Abnormal chemical processing of the metallic element zinc, which is essential in the body's general nutrition.
    Acrodermatitis enteropathica

E83.3- **Disorders of phosphorus metabolism and phosphatases** — Abnormal chemical processing of the nonmetallic element phosphorus, which is essential in energy metabolism, bone minerlization, and for conversion of glycogen to glucose.
    Excludes 1:   *adult osteomalacia (M83.-)*
         osteoporosis (M80.-)

  E83.30 **Disorder of phosphorus metabolism, unspecified**

  E83.31 **Familial hypophosphatemia**
    Vitamin D-resistant osteomalacia
    Vitamin D-resistant rickets
    Excludes 1:   *vitamin D-deficiency rickets (E55.0)*

Excludes 1: = NOT CODED HERE! (Do not code both)   **628**   *Excludes* ❷ = Not Included Here

E83.32 **Hereditary vitamin D-dependent rickets (type 1) (type 2)**
25-hydroxyvitamin D 1-alpha-hydroxylase deficiency
Pseudovitamin D deficiency
Vitamin D receptor defect

E83.39 **Other disorders of phosphorus metabolism**
Acid phosphatase deficiency
Hypophosphatasia

E83.4- **Disorders of** <u>magnesium metabolism</u> — Abnormal chemical processing of the metallic element magnesium, which activates certain enzymes to catalyze phosphate ions.

E83.40 **Disorders of magnesium metabolism, unspecified**

E83.41 **Hypermagnesemia**

E83.42 **Hypomagnesemia**

E83.49 **Other disorders of magnesium metabolism**

E83.5- **Disorders of** <u>calcium metabolism</u> — Abnormal chemical processing of the metallic element calcium, which is essential to bone formation, blood coagulation, lactation, and for function of the nerves and muscles.
> *Excludes 1:*   *chondrocalcinosis (M11.1-M11.2)*
> *hungry bone syndrome (E83.81)*
> *hyperparathyroidism (E21.0-E21.3)*

E83.50 **Unspecified disorder of calcium metabolism**

E83.51 **Hypocalcemia** — An abnormal decrease of calcium in the blood.

E83.52 **Hypercalcemia** — An excessive amount of calcium in the blood.
Familial hypocalciuric hypercalcemia

E83.59 **Other disorders of calcium metabolism**
Idiopathic hypercalciuria

E83.8- **Other disorders of mineral metabolism**

E83.81 **Hungry bone syndrome** — A hypocalcemic condition that is characterized by the sudden removal of serum calcium from the circulation and deposition into the bones, that is most often due to parathyroidectomy for hyperparathyroidism.

E83.89 **Other disorders of mineral metabolism**

E83.9 **Disorder of mineral metabolism, unspecified**

E84- <u>Cystic fibrosis</u> — An inherited disease of infants and children of the exocrine glands, marked by chronic pulmonary disease, frequent lung infections with mucous, pancreas and gastrointestinal dysfucntion, and poor growth in children.
Includes: **Mucoviscidosis**
Code also exocrine pancreatic insufficiency (K86.81)

MCC **E84.0** **Cystic fibrosis with** <u>pulmonary</u> **manifestations** — A form affecting the respiratory system with chronic obstructive pulmonary disease, frequent lung infections, and/or respiratory failure.
Use additional code to identify any infectious organism present, such as:
Pseudomonas (B96.5)

E84.1- **Cystic fibrosis with** <u>intestinal</u> **manifestations** — A form affecting the gastrointestinal system with malabsorption, pancreatic insufficiency, and/or organ involvement.

MCC **E84.11** **Meconium ileus in cystic fibrosis** — [Age/0] — An obstruction of the ileum in the newborn due to blocking of the intestine with thick meconium.
> *Excludes 1:*   *meconium ileus not due to cystic fibrosis (P76.0)*

CC **E84.19** **Cystic fibrosis with other intestinal manifestations**
Distal intestinal obstruction syndrome

CC **E84.8** **Cystic fibrosis with other manifestations**

CC **E84.9** **Cystic fibrosis, unspecified**

E85- <u>Amyloidosis</u> — A metabolic disorder marked by the deposition of an abnormal protein (amyloid - inappropriately folded proteins) in organs and tissues in amounts sufficient to impair normal function.
> *Excludes 1:*   *Alzheimer's disease (G30.0-)*

CC **E85.0** <u>Non-</u>**neuropathic heredofamilial amyloidosis** — A hereditary form characterized by regular attacks of inflammation in the lining of the abdominal cavity, chest cavity, skin or joints, along with recurrent high fevers.
Hereditary amyloid nephropathy

CC **E85.1** <u>Neuropathic</u> **heredofamilial amyloidosis** — A hereditary form characterized by paresthesias, sharp pains, and diminished sensitivity to pain.
AHA 12:4Q:p99 – Neuropathic heredofamilial amyloidosis
Amyloid polyneuropathy (Portuguese)

CC **E85.2** **Heredofamilial amyloidosis, unspecified**

CC **E85.3** <u>Secondary</u> **systemic amyloidosis**
Hemodialysis-associated amyloidosis

CC **E85.4** **Organ-limited amyloidosis**
Localized amyloidosis

CC **E85.8** **Other amyloidosis**

CC **E85.9** **Amyloidosis, unspecified**

E86- <u>Volume depletion</u> — Abnormally decreased body fluid levels.
Use additional code(s) for any associated disorders of electrolyte and acid-base balance (E87.-)
> *Excludes 1:*   *dehydration of newborn (P74.1)*
> *hypovolemic shock NOS (R57.1)*
> *postprocedural hypovolemic shock (T81.19)*
> *traumatic hypovolemic shock (T79.4)*

E86.0 **Dehydration** — The abnormal depletion of the total body water level that is necessary for normal cellular function.
AHA 14:1Q:p7 – Dehydration with hypernatremia/hyponatremia

E86.1 **Hypovolemia** — The abnormal depletion of the blood volume, especially the volume of blood plasma.
Depletion of volume of plasma

E86.9 **Volume depletion, unspecified**

E87- <u>Other disorders of fluid, electrolyte and acid-base balance</u>
> *Excludes 1:*   *diabetes insipidus (E23.2)*
> *electrolyte imbalance associated with hyperemesis gravidarum (O21.1)*
> *electrolyte imbalance following ectopic or molar pregnancy (O08.5)*
> *familial periodic paralysis (G72.3)*

CC **E87.0** <u>Hyperosmolality and hypernatremia</u> — An abnormally increased osmolar/sodium concentration.
AHA 14:1Q:p7 – Dehydration with hypernatremia
Sodium [Na] excess — An abnormally high sodium level in the blood.
Sodium [Na] overload — An abnormally high sodium level in the blood.

CC **E87.1** <u>Hypo-osmolality and hyponatremia</u> — An abnormally decreased osmolar/sodium concentration.
AHA 14:1Q:p7 – Dehydration with hyponatremia
Sodium [Na] deficiency — An abnormally low sodium level in the blood.
> *Excludes 1:*   *syndrome of inappropriate secretion of antidiuretic hormone (E22.2)*

CC **E87.2** **Acidosis** — The condition of excessive acidity of body fluids, due to the accumulation of acids, or the reduction of base concentration.
Acidosis NOS
Lactic acidosis — A form caused by excessive lactic acid in the body fluids.
Metabolic acidosis — A form resulting from acid increase other than carbonic acid.
Respiratory acidosis — A form resulting from the excess retention of carbon dioxide in the body.
> *Excludes 1:*   *diabetic acidosis — see categories E08-E10, E13 with ketoacidosis*

CC **E87.3** **Alkalosis** — The condition of excessive alkalinity (base) of body fluids, due to the accumulation of alkalies or the reduction of acids.
Alkalosis NOS
Metabolic alkalosis — A form resulting from the loss of noncarbonic acids, often from excessive vomiting.
Respiratory alkalosis — A form resulting from the excess loss of carbon dioxide in the body, often from hyperventilation.

CC **E87.4** **Mixed disorder of acid-base balance**

E87.5 **Hyperkalemia** — The abnormally increased potassium level in the blood.
Potassium [K] excess
Potassium [K] overload

E87.6 **Hypokalemia** — The abnormally decreased potassium level in the blood.
Potassium [K] deficiency

E87.7- <u>Fluid overload</u> — Abnormally increased body fluid levels.
> *Excludes 1:*   *edema NOS (R60.9)*
> *fluid retention (R60.9)*

E87.70 **Fluid overload, unspecified**

E87.71 <u>Transfusion associated circulatory overload</u> — The condition of increased body fluid levels due to recent transfusion of blood and/or blood components that is characterized by acute respiratory distress, increased blood pressure, and a positive fluid balance.
Fluid overload due to transfusion (blood) (blood components)
TACO

E87.79 **Other fluid overload**

E87.8 **Other disorders of electrolyte and fluid balance, not elsewhere classified**
Electrolyte imbalance NOS
Hyperchloremia
Hypochloremia

E
8
3
–
E
8
7

Excludes 1: = NOT CODED HERE! (Do not code both)   *Excludes ❷* = Not Included Here

E88-   Other and unspecified metabolic disorders
Use additional codes for associated conditions
Excludes 1:   histiocytosis X (chronic) (C96.6)

E88.0-   Disorders of plasma-protein metabolism, not elsewhere classified
Excludes 1:   disorder of lipoprotein metabolism (E78.-)
monoclonal gammopathy (of undetermined significance) (D47.2)
polyclonal hypergammaglobulinemia (D89.0)
Waldenström macroglobulinemia (C88.0)

E88.01   Alpha-1-antitrypsin deficiency — An inherited plasma protein disorder resulting in liver and lung damage.
AAT deficiency

E88.09   Other disorders of plasma-protein metabolism, not elsewhere classified
Bisalbuminemia

E88.1   Lipodystrophy, not elsewhere classified
Lipodystrophy NOS
Excludes 1:   Whipple's disease (K90.81)

E88.2   Lipomatosis, not elsewhere classified
Lipomatosis NOS
Lipomatosis (Check) dolorosa [Dercum]

MCC **E88.3   Tumor lysis syndrome** — A group of metabolic conditions that are caused by the byproducts of tumor necrosis and are characterized by hyperkalemia, hyperphosphatemia, hyperuricemia, and hypocalcemia and can lead to acute renal failure.
Tumor lysis syndrome (spontaneous)
Tumor lysis syndrome following antineoplastic drug chemotherapy
Use additional code for adverse effect, if applicable, to identify drug (T45.1X5-)

E88.4-   Mitochondrial metabolism disorders — Inherited conditions resulting from the disturbances/dysfunction of mitochondrial DNA.
Excludes 1:   disorders of pyruvate metabolism (E74.4)
Kearns-Sayre syndrome (H49.81)
Leber's disease (H47.22)
Leigh's encephalopathy (G31.82)
Mitochondrial myopathy, NEC (G71.3)
Reye's syndrome (G93.7)

CC **E88.40   Mitochondrial metabolism disorder, unspecified**

CC **E88.41   MELAS syndrome** — A form characterized by migraine-like attacks, encephalopathy, myopathy, and strokes.
Mitochondrial myopathy, encephalopathy, lactic acidosis and stroke-like episodes

CC **E88.42   MERRF syndrome** — A form characterized by seizure disorder, myoclonus, progressive ataxia, and spasticity, with muscle biopsies that reveal ragged red fibers.
Myoclonic epilepsy associated with ragged-red fibers
Code also progressive myoclonic epilepsy (G40.3-)

CC **E88.49   Other mitochondrial metabolism disorders**

E88.8-   Other specified metabolic disorders

E88.81   Metabolic syndrome — A disorder of energy utilization and storage.
Dysmetabolic syndrome X
Use additional codes for associated manifestations, such as:
Obesity (E66.-)

E88.89   Other specified metabolic disorders
Launois-Bensaude adenolipomatosis
Excludes 1:   adult pulmonary Langerhans cell histiocytosis (J84.82)

E88.9   Metabolic disorder, unspecified

Postprocedural endocrine and metabolic complications and disorders, not elsewhere classified (E89)

E89-   Postprocedural endocrine and metabolic complications and disorders, not elsewhere classified
Excludes ❷: intraoperative complications of endocrine system organ or structure (E36.0-, E36.1-, E36.8)

E89.0   Postprocedural hypothyroidism
Postirradiation hypothyroidism
Postsurgical hypothyroidism

CC **E89.1   Postprocedural hypoinsulinemia**
Postpancreatectomy hyperglycemia
Postsurgical hypoinsulinemia
Use additional code, if applicable, to identify:
Acquired absence of pancreas (Z90.41-)
Diabetes mellitus (postpancreatectomy) (postprocedural) (E13.-)
Insulin use (Z79.4)
Excludes 1:   transient postprocedural hyperglycemia (R73.9)
transient postprocedural hypoglycemia (E16.2)

E89.2   Postprocedural hypoparathyroidism
Parathyroprival tetany

E89.3   Postprocedural hypopituitarism
Postirradiation hypopituitarism

E89.4-   Postprocedural ovarian failure

E89.40   Asymptomatic postprocedural ovarian failure — [♀]
Postprocedural ovarian failure NOS

E89.41   Symptomatic postprocedural ovarian failure — [♀]
Symptoms such as flushing, sleeplessness, headache, lack of concentration, associated with postprocedural menopause

E89.5   Postprocedural testicular hypofunction — [♂]

CC **E89.6   Postprocedural adrenocortical (-medullary) hypofunction**

E89.8-   Other postprocedural endocrine and metabolic complications and disorders

E89.81-   Postprocedural hemorrhage of an endocrine system organ or structure following a procedure

CC **E89.810   Postprocedural hemorrhage of an endocrine system organ or structure following an endocrine system procedure**

CC **E89.811   Postprocedural hemorrhage of an endocrine system organ or structure following other procedure**

E89.82-   Postprocedural hematoma and seroma of an endocrine system organ or structure

CC **E89.820   Postprocedural hematoma of an endocrine system organ or structure following an endocrine system procedure**

CC **E89.821   Postprocedural hematoma of an endocrine system organ or structure following other procedure**

CC **E89.822   Postprocedural seroma of an endocrine system organ or structure following an endocrine system procedure**

CC **E89.823   Postprocedural seroma of an endocrine system organ or structure following other procedure**

CC **E89.89   Other postprocedural endocrine and metabolic complications and disorders**
Use additional code, if applicable, to further specify disorder

---

Excludes 1: = NOT CODED HERE! (Do not code both)

Excludes ❷: = Not Included Here

Chapter – 5 Mental, behavioral and neurodevelopmental disorders (F01-F99)

Includes: Disorders of psychological development
Excludes ❷: symptoms, signs and abnormal clinical laboratory findings, not elsewhere classified (R00-R99)

This chapter contains the following blocks:

F01-F09	Mental disorders due to known physiological conditions
F10-F19	Mental and behavioral disorders due to psychoactive substance use
F20-F29	Schizophrenia, schizotypal, delusional, and other non-mood psychotic disorders
F30-F39	Mood [affective] disorders
F40-F48	Anxiety, dissociative, stress-related, somatoform and other nonpsychotic mental disorders
F50-F59	Behavioral syndromes associated with physiological disturbances and physical factors
F60-F69	Disorders of adult personality and behavior
F70-F79	Intellectual disabilities
F80-F89	Pervasive and specific developmental disorders
F90-F98	Behavioral and emotional disorders with onset usually occurring in childhood and adolescence
F99	Unspecified mental disorder

Chapter-Specific Coding Guidelines

C.   Chapter-Specific Coding Guidelines
In addition to general coding guidelines, there are guidelines for specific diagnoses and/or conditions in the classification. Unless otherwise indicated, these guidelines apply to all health care settings. Please refer to Section II for guidelines on the selection of principal diagnosis.

5.   Chapter 5: Mental and Behavioral Disorders (F01 – F99)

a.   Pain disorders related to psychological factors
Assign code F45.41, for pain that is exclusively related to psychological disorders. As indicated by the Excludes1 note under category G89, a code from category G89 should not be assigned with code F45.41.

Code F45.42, Pain disorders with related psychological factors, should be used should be used with a code from category G89, Pain, not elsewhere classified, if there is documentation of a psychological component for a patient with acute or chronic pain.

See Section I.C.6. Pain.

b.   Mental and behavioral disorders due to psychoactive substance use

1)   In Remission
Selection of codes for "in remission" for categories F10-F19, Mental and behavioral disorders due to psychoactive substance use (categories F10-F19 with -.21) requires the provider's clinical judgment. The appropriate codes for "in remission" are assigned only on the basis of provider documentation (as defined in the Official Guidelines for Coding and Reporting).

2)   Psychoactive Substance Use, Abuse And Dependence
When the provider documentation refers to use, abuse and dependence of the same substance (e.g. alcohol, opioid, cannabis, etc.), only one code should be assigned to identify the pattern of use based on the following hierarchy:
- If both use and abuse are documented, assign only the code for abuse
- If both abuse and dependence are documented, assign only the code for dependence
- If use, abuse and dependence are all documented, assign only the code for dependence
- If both use and dependence are documented, assign only the code for dependence

3)   Psychoactive Substance Use
As with all other diagnoses, the codes for psychoactive substance use (F10.9-, F11.9-, F12.9-, F13.9-, F14.9-, F15.9-, F16.9-) should only be assigned based on provider documentation and when they meet the definition of a reportable diagnosis (see Section III, Reporting Additional Diagnoses). The codes are to be used only when the psychoactive substance use is associated with a mental or behavioral disorder, and such a relationship is documented by the provider.

Mental disorders due to known physiological conditions (F01-F09)

Note: This block comprises a range of mental disorders grouped together on the basis of their having in common a demonstrable etiology in cerebral disease, brain injury, or other insult leading to cerebral

dysfunction. The dysfunction may be primary, as in diseases, injuries, and insults that affect the brain directly and selectively; or secondary, as in systemic diseases and disorders that attack the brain only as one of the multiple organs or systems of the body that are involved.

F01-   Vascular dementia
Vascular dementia as a result of infarction of the brain due to vascular disease, including hypertensive cerebrovascular disease
Includes: Arteriosclerotic dementia
Code first the underlying physiological condition or sequelae of cerebrovascular disease

F01.5-   Vascular dementia

F01.50   Vascular dementia without behavioral disturbance —
[Age/15-124]
Major neurocognitive disorder without behavioral disturbance

cc **F01.51   Vascular dementia with behavioral disturbance —**
[Age/15-124]
Major neurocognitive disorder due to vascular disease, with behavioral disturbance
Major neurocognitive disorder with aggressive behavior
Major neurocognitive disorder with combative behavior
Major neurocognitive disorder with violent behavior
Vascular dementia with aggressive behavior
Vascular dementia with combative behavior
Vascular dementia with violent behavior
Use additional code, if applicable, to identify wandering in vascular dementia (Z91.83)

F02-   Dementia in other diseases classified elsewhere
Includes: Major neurocognitive disorder in other diseases classified elsewhere
Code first the underlying physiological condition, such as:
Alzheimer's (G30.-)
Cerebral lipidosis (E75.4)
Creutzfeldt-Jakob disease (A81.0-)
Dementia with Lewy bodies (G31.83)
Dementia with Parkinsonism (G31.83)
Epilepsy and recurrent seizures (G40.-)
Frontotemporal dementia (G31.09)
Hepatolenticular degeneration (E83.0)
Human immunodeficiency virus [HIV] disease (B20)
Huntington's disease (G10)
Hypercalcemia (E83.52)
Hypothyroidism, acquired (E00-E03.-)
Intoxications (T36-T65)
Jakob-Creutzfeldt disease (A81.0-)
Multiple sclerosis (G35)
Neurosyphilis (A52.17)
Niacin deficiency [pellagra] (E52)
Parkinson's disease (G20)
Pick's disease (G31.01)
Polyarteritis nodosa (M30.0)
Prion disease (A81.9)
Systemic lupus erythematosus (M32.-)
Traumatic brain injury (S06.-)
Trypanosomiasis (B56.-, B57.-)
Vitamin B deficiency (E53.8)
Excludes ❷: dementia in alcohol and psychoactive substance disorders (F10-F19, with .17, .27, .97)
vascular dementia (F01.5-)

F02.8-   Dementia in other diseases classified elsewhere

F02.80   Dementia in other diseases classified elsewhere without behavioral disturbance — [Not Allowed as PDX]
Dementia in other diseases classified elsewhere NOS
Major neurocognitive disorder in other diseases classified elsewhere

cc **F02.81   Dementia in other diseases classified elsewhere with behavioral disturbance** — [Not Allowed as PDX]
Dementia in other diseases classified elsewhere with aggressive behavior
Dementia in other diseases classified elsewhere with combative behavior
Dementia in other diseases classified elsewhere with violent behavior
Major neurocognitive disorder in other diseases classified elsewhere with aggressive behavior
Major neurocognitive disorder in other diseases classified elsewhere with combative behavior
Major neurocognitive disorder in other diseases classified elsewhere with violent behavior
Use additional code, if applicable, to identify wandering in dementia in conditions classified elsewhere (Z91.83)

F 0 0 - F 0 2

Excludes 1: = NOT CODED HERE! (Do not code both)

Excludes ❷: = Not Included Here

F03- <u>Unspecified</u> <u>dementia</u>
Presenile dementia NOS
Presenile psychosis NOS
Primary degenerative dementia NOS
Senile dementia NOS
Senile dementia depressed or paranoid type
Senile psychosis NOS
Excludes 1:   *senility NOS (R41.81)*
Excludes ❷: *mild memory disturbance due to known physiological condition (F06.8)*
   senile dementia with delirium or acute confusional state (F05)

F03.9-   Unspecified dementia

F03.90   Unspecified dementia without behavioral disturbance —
[Age/15-124]
Dementia NOS

CC **F03.91**   Unspecified dementia with behavioral disturbance —
[Age/15-124]
Unspecified dementia with aggressive behavior
Unspecified dementia with combative behavior
Unspecified dementia with violent behavior
Use additional code, if applicable, to identify wandering in unspecified dementia (Z91.83)

F04   <u>Amnestic disorder due to known physiological condition</u>
Korsakov's psychosis or syndrome, nonalcoholic
Code first the underlying physiological condition
Excludes 1:   *amnesia NOS (R41.3)*
   anterograde amnesia (R41.1)
   dissociative amnesia (F44.0)
   retrograde amnesia (R41.2)
Excludes ❷: *alcohol-induced or unspecified Korsakov's syndrome (F10.26, F10.96)*
   Korsakov's syndrome induced by other psychoactive substances (F13.26, F13.96, F19.16, F19.26, F19.96)

F05   <u>Delirium due to known physiological condition</u>
CC
Acute or subacute brain syndrome
Acute or subacute confusional state (nonalcoholic)
Acute or subacute infective psychosis
Acute or subacute organic reaction
Acute or subacute psycho-organic syndrome
Delirium of mixed etiology
Delirium superimposed on dementia
Sundowning
Code first the underlying physiological condition
Excludes 1:   *delirium NOS (R41.0)*
Excludes ❷: *delirium tremens alcohol-induced or unspecified (F10.231, F10.921)*

F06-   <u>Other mental disorders due to known physiological condition</u>
Includes: Mental disorders due to endocrine disorder
   Mental disorders due to exogenous hormone
   Mental disorders due to exogenous toxic substance
   Mental disorders due to primary cerebral disease
   Mental disorders due to somatic illness
   Mental disorders due to systemic disease affecting the brain
Code first the underlying physiological condition
Excludes 1:   *unspecified dementia (F03)*
Excludes ❷: *delirium due to known physiological condition (F05)*
   dementia as classified in F01-F02
   other mental disorders associated with alcohol and other psychoactive substances (F10-F19)

CC **F06.0**   <u>Psychotic</u> disorder with <u>hallucinations</u> due to known physiological condition
CC
Organic hallucinatory state (nonalcoholic)
Excludes ❷: *hallucinations and perceptual disturbance induced by alcohol and other psychoactive substances (F10-F19 with .151, .251, .951)*
   schizophrenia (F20.-)

F06.1   <u>Catatonic</u> disorder due to known physiological condition
Catatonia associated with another mental disorder
Catatonia NOS
Excludes 1:   *catatonic stupor (R40.1)*
   stupor NOS (R40.1)
Excludes ❷: *catatonic schizophrenia (F20.2)*
   dissociative stupor (F44.2)

CC **F06.2**   <u>Psychotic</u> disorder with <u>delusions</u> due to known physiological condition
Paranoid and paranoid-hallucinatory organic states
Schizophrenia-like psychosis in epilepsy
Excludes ❷: *alcohol and drug-induced psychotic disorder (F10-F19 with .150, .250, .950)*
   brief psychotic disorder (F23)
   delusional disorder (F22)
   schizophrenia (F20.-)

F06.3-   <u>Mood</u> disorder <u>due to known physiological condition</u>
Excludes ❷: *mood disorders due to alcohol and other psychoactive substances (F10-F19 with .14, .24, .94)*
   mood disorders, not due to known physiological condition or unspecified (F30-F39)

F06.30   Mood disorder due to known physiological condition, unspecified

F06.31   Mood disorder due to known physiological condition with <u>depressive features</u>

F06.32   Mood disorder due to known physiological condition with <u>major depressive-like</u> episode

F06.33   Mood disorder due to known physiological condition with <u>manic</u> features

F06.34   Mood disorder due to known physiological condition with <u>mixed</u> features

F06.4   <u>Anxiety</u> disorder <u>due to known physiological condition</u>
Excludes ❷: *anxiety disorders due to alcohol and other psychoactive substances (F10-F19 with .180, .280, .980)*
   anxiety disorders, not due to known physiological condition or unspecified (F40.-, F41.-)

F06.8   <u>Other specified</u> mental disorders <u>due to known physiological condition</u>
Epileptic psychosis NOS
Organic dissociative disorder
Organic emotionally labile [asthenic] disorder

F07-   <u>Personality and behavioral</u> disorders <u>due to known physiological condition</u>
Code first the underlying physiological condition

F07.0   <u>Personality change</u> due to known physiological condition
Frontal lobe syndrome
Limbic epilepsy personality syndrome
Lobotomy syndrome
Organic personality disorder
Organic pseudopsychopathic personality
Organic pseudoretarded personality
Postleucotomy syndrome
Code first underlying physiological condition
Excludes 1:   *mild cognitive impairment (G31.84)*
   postconcussional syndrome (F07.81)
   postencephalitic syndrome (F07.89)
   signs and symptoms involving emotional state (R45.-)
Excludes ❷: *specific personality disorder (F60.-)*

F07.8-   Other personality and behavioral disorders due to known physiological condition

F07.81   <u>Postconcussional syndrome</u>
Postcontusional syndrome (encephalopathy)
Post-traumatic brain syndrome, nonpsychotic
Use additional code to identify associated post-traumatic headache, if applicable (G44.3-)
Excludes 1:   *current concussion (brain) (S06.0-)*
   postencephalitic syndrome (F07.89)

F07.89   Other personality and behavioral disorders due to known physiological condition
Postencephalitic syndrome
Right hemispheric organic affective disorder

F07.9   Unspecified personality and behavioral disorder due to known physiological condition
Organic psychosyndrome

F09   <u>Unspecified</u> mental disorder <u>due to known physiological condition</u>
Mental disorder NOS due to known physiological condition
Organic brain syndrome NOS
Organic mental disorder NOS
Organic psychosis NOS
Symptomatic psychosis NOS
Code first the underlying physiological condition
Excludes 1:   *psychosis NOS (F29)*

F 0 3 - F 0 9

Mental and behavioral disorders due to psychoactive substance use (F10-F19)

F10- Alcohol related disorders
Use additional code for blood alcohol level, if applicable (Y90.-)

F10.1- Alcohol abuse
Excludes 1:   alcohol dependence (F10.2-)
alcohol use, unspecified (F10.9-)

F10.10 Alcohol abuse, uncomplicated
Alcohol use disorder, mild

F10.12- Alcohol abuse with intoxication

F10.120 Alcohol abuse with intoxication, uncomplicated

cc **F10.121** Alcohol abuse with intoxication delirium

F10.129 Alcohol abuse with intoxication, unspecified

cc **F10.14** Alcohol abuse with alcohol-induced mood disorder
Alcohol use disorder, mild, with alcohol-induced bipolar or related disorder
Alcohol use disorder, mild, with alcohol-induced depressive disorder

F10.15- Alcohol abuse with alcohol-induced psychotic disorder

F10.150 Alcohol abuse with alcohol-induced psychotic disorder with delusions

cc **F10.151** Alcohol abuse with alcohol-induced psychotic disorder with hallucinations

cc **F10.159** Alcohol abuse with alcohol-induced psychotic disorder, unspecified

F10.18- Alcohol abuse with other alcohol-induced disorders

cc **F10.180** Alcohol abuse with alcohol-induced anxiety disorder

cc **F10.181** Alcohol abuse with alcohol-induced sexual dysfunction

F10.182 Alcohol abuse with alcohol-induced sleep disorder

cc **F10.188** Alcohol abuse with other alcohol-induced disorder

cc **F10.19** Alcohol abuse with unspecified alcohol-induced disorder

F10.2- Alcohol dependence
Excludes 1:   alcohol abuse (F10.1-)
alcohol use, unspecified (F10.9-)
Excludes ❷: toxic effect of alcohol (T51.0-)

F10.20 Alcohol dependence, uncomplicated
Alcohol use disorder, moderate
Alcohol use disorder, severe

F10.21 Alcohol dependence, in remission

F10.22- Alcohol dependence with intoxication
Acute drunkenness (in alcoholism)
Excludes ❷: alcohol dependence with withdrawal (F10.23-)

F10.220 Alcohol dependence with intoxication, uncomplicated

cc **F10.221** Alcohol dependence with intoxication delirium

F10.229 Alcohol dependence with intoxication, unspecified

F10.23- Alcohol dependence with withdrawal
AHA 15:2Q:p15 – Alcohol withdrawal with alcohol abuse
Excludes ❷: alcohol dependence with intoxication (F10.22-)

cc **F10.230** Alcohol dependence with withdrawal, uncomplicated

cc **F10.231** Alcohol dependence with withdrawal delirium

cc **F10.232** Alcohol dependence with withdrawal with perceptual disturbance

cc **F10.239** Alcohol dependence with withdrawal, unspecified

cc **F10.24** Alcohol dependence with alcohol-induced mood disorder
Alcohol use disorder, moderate, with alcohol-induced bipolar or related disorder
Alcohol use disorder, moderate, with alcohol-induced depressive disorder
Alcohol use disorder, severe, with alcohol-induced bipolar or related disorder
Alcohol use disorder, severe, with alcohol-induced depressive disorder

F10.25- Alcohol dependence with alcohol-induced psychotic disorder

F10.250 Alcohol dependence with alcohol-induced psychotic disorder with delusions

cc **F10.251** Alcohol dependence with alcohol-induced psychotic disorder with hallucinations

cc **F10.259** Alcohol dependence with alcohol-induced psychotic disorder, unspecified

F10.26 Alcohol dependence with alcohol-induced persisting amnestic disorder
Alcohol use disorder, moderate, with alcohol-induced major neurocognitive disorder, amnestic-confabulatory type
Alcohol use disorder, severe, with alcohol-induced major neurocognitive disorder, amnestic-confabulatory type

cc **F10.27** Alcohol dependence with alcohol-induced persisting dementia
Alcohol use disorder, moderate, with alcohol-induced major neurocognitive disorder, nonamnestic-confabulatory type
Alcohol use disorder, severe, with alcohol-induced major neurocognitive disorder, nonamnestic-confabulatory type

F10.28- Alcohol dependence with other alcohol-induced disorders

cc **F10.280** Alcohol dependence with alcohol-induced anxiety disorder

cc **F10.281** Alcohol dependence with alcohol-induced sexual dysfunction

F10.282 Alcohol dependence with alcohol-induced sleep disorder

cc **F10.288** Alcohol dependence with other alcohol-induced disorder
Alcohol use disorder, moderate, with alcohol-induced mild neurocognitive disorder
Alcohol use disorder, severe, with alcohol-induced mild neurocognitive disorder

cc **F10.29** Alcohol dependence with unspecified alcohol-induced disorder

F10.9- Alcohol use, unspecified
Excludes 1:   alcohol abuse (F10.1-)
alcohol dependence (F10.2-)

F10.92- Alcohol use, unspecified with intoxication

F10.920 Alcohol use, unspecified with intoxication, uncomplicated

cc **F10.921** Alcohol use, unspecified with intoxication delirium

F10.929 Alcohol use, unspecified with intoxication, unspecified

cc **F10.94** Alcohol use, unspecified with alcohol-induced mood disorder
Alcohol-induced bipolar or related disorder, without use disorder
Alcohol-induced depressive disorder, without use disorder

F10.95- Alcohol use, unspecified with alcohol-induced psychotic disorder

F10.950 Alcohol use, unspecified with alcohol-induced psychotic disorder with delusions

cc **F10.951** Alcohol use, unspecified with alcohol-induced psychotic disorder with hallucinations

cc **F10.959** Alcohol use, unspecified with alcohol-induced psychotic disorder, unspecified
Alcohol-induced psychotic disorder, without use disorder

F10.96 Alcohol use, unspecified with alcohol-induced persisting amnestic disorder
Alcohol-induced major neurocognitive disorder, amnestic-confabulatory type, without use disorder

F10.97 Alcohol use, unspecified with alcohol-induced persisting dementia
Alcohol-induced major neurocognitive disorder, nonamnestic-confabulatory type, without use disorder

F10.98- Alcohol use, unspecified with other alcohol-induced disorders

cc **F10.980** Alcohol use, unspecified with alcohol-induced anxiety disorder
Alcohol-induced anxiety disorder, without use disorder

cc **F10.981** Alcohol use, unspecified with alcohol-induced sexual dysfunction
Alcohol-induced sexual dysfunction, without use disorder

Excludes 1: = NOT CODED HERE! (Do not code both)   **633**   *Excludes ❷:* = Not Included Here

F10.982 Alcohol use, unspecified with alcohol-induced <u>sleep</u> disorder
Alcohol-induced sleep disorder, without use disorder

cc **F10.988 Alcohol use, unspecified with other alcohol-induced disorder**
Alcohol-induced mild neurocognitive disorder, without use disorder

cc **F10.99 Alcohol use, unspecified with unspecified alcohol-induced disorder**

F11- <u>Opioid related disorders</u>

F11.1- Opioid abuse
Excludes 1: opioid dependence (F11.2-)
opioid use, unspecified (F11.9-)

F11.10 Opioid abuse, <u>uncomplicated</u>
Opioid use disorder, mild

F11.12- Opioid abuse <u>with intoxication</u>

F11.120 Opioid abuse with intoxication, <u>uncomplicated</u>

cc **F11.121 Opioid abuse with intoxication <u>delirium</u>**

F11.122 Opioid abuse with intoxication <u>with perceptual disturbance</u>

F11.129 Opioid abuse with intoxication, <u>unspecified</u>

F11.14 Opioid abuse <u>with</u> opioid-induced <u>mood</u> disorder
Opioid use disorder, mild, with opioid-induced depressive disorder

F11.15- Opioid abuse <u>with</u> opioid-induced <u>psychotic</u> disorder

cc **F11.150 Opioid abuse with opioid-induced psychotic disorder <u>with delusions</u>**

cc **F11.151 Opioid abuse with opioid-induced psychotic disorder <u>with hallucinations</u>**

F11.159 Opioid abuse with opioid-induced psychotic disorder, unspecified

F11.18- Opioid abuse <u>with</u> <u>other</u> opioid-induced disorder

F11.181 Opioid abuse with opioid-induced <u>sexual</u> <u>dysfunction</u>

F11.182 Opioid abuse with opioid-induced <u>sleep</u> disorder

F11.188 Opioid abuse with other opioid-induced disorder

F11.19 Opioid abuse with unspecified opioid-induced disorder

F11.2- <u>Opioid dependence</u>
Excludes 1: opioid abuse (F11.1-)
opioid use, unspecified (F11.9-)
Excludes ❷: opioid poisoning (T40.0-T40.2-)

cc **F11.20 Opioid dependence, <u>uncomplicated</u>**
Opioid use disorder, moderate
Opioid use disorder, severe

F11.21 Opioid dependence, in remission

F11.22- Opioid dependence <u>with intoxication</u>
Excludes 1: opioid dependence with withdrawal (F11.23)

F11.220 Opioid dependence with intoxication, <u>uncomplicated</u>

cc **F11.221 Opioid dependence with intoxication <u>delirium</u>**

cc **F11.222 Opioid dependence with intoxication <u>with perceptual disturbance</u>**

F11.229 Opioid dependence with intoxication, <u>unspecified</u>

cc **F11.23 Opioid dependence with withdrawal**
Excludes 1: opioid dependence with intoxication (F11.22-)

F11.24 Opioid dependence <u>with</u> opioid-induced <u>mood</u> disorder
Opioid use disorder, moderate, with opioid-induced depressive disorder

F11.25- Opioid dependence <u>with</u> opioid-induced <u>psychotic</u> disorder

cc **F11.250 Opioid dependence with opioid-induced psychotic disorder <u>with delusions</u>**

cc **F11.251 Opioid dependence with opioid-induced psychotic disorder <u>with hallucinations</u>**

cc **F11.259 Opioid dependence with opioid-induced psychotic disorder, unspecified**

F11.28- Opioid dependence <u>with</u> <u>other</u> opioid-induced disorder

cc **F11.281 Opioid dependence <u>with</u> opioid-induced <u>sexual</u> <u>dysfunction</u>**

cc **F11.282 Opioid dependence with opioid-induced <u>sleep</u> disorder**

cc **F11.288 Opioid dependence with other opioid-induced disorder**

F11.29 Opioid dependence with unspecified opioid-induced disorder

F11.9- <u>Opioid use, unspecified</u>
Excludes 1: opioid abuse (F11.1-)
opioid dependence (F11.2-)

F11.90 Opioid use, unspecified, <u>uncomplicated</u>

F11.92- Opioid use, unspecified <u>with intoxication</u>
Excludes 1: opioid use, unspecified with withdrawal (F11.93)

F11.920 Opioid use, unspecified with intoxication, <u>uncomplicated</u>

cc **F11.921 Opioid use, unspecified with intoxication <u>delirium</u>**
Opioid-induced delirium

F11.922 Opioid use, unspecified with intoxication <u>with perceptual disturbance</u>

F11.929 Opioid use, unspecified with intoxication, unspecified

cc **F11.93 Opioid use, unspecified <u>with withdrawal</u>**
Excludes 1: opioid use, unspecified with intoxication (F11.92-)

F11.94 Opioid use, unspecified <u>with</u> opioid-induced <u>mood</u> disorder
Opioid-induced depressive disorder, without use disorder

F11.95- Opioid use, unspecified <u>with</u> opioid-induced <u>psychotic</u> disorder

cc **F11.950 Opioid use, unspecified with opioid-induced psychotic disorder <u>with delusions</u>**

cc **F11.951 Opioid use, unspecified with opioid-induced psychotic disorder <u>with hallucinations</u>**

F11.959 Opioid use, unspecified with opioid-induced psychotic disorder, unspecified

F11.98- Opioid use, unspecified <u>with</u> <u>other</u> specified opioid-induced disorder

F11.981 Opioid use, unspecified <u>with</u> opioid-induced <u>sexual</u> <u>dysfunction</u>
Opioid-induced sexual dysfunction, without use disorder

F11.982 Opioid use, unspecified <u>with</u> opioid-induced <u>sleep</u> disorder
Opioid-induced sleep disorder, without use disorder

F11.988 Opioid use, unspecified <u>with</u> <u>other</u> opioid-induced disorder
Opioid-induced anxiety disorder, without use disorder

F11.99 Opioid use, unspecified with unspecified opioid-induced disorder

F12- <u>Cannabis related disorders</u>
Includes: Marijuana

F12.1- Cannabis <u>abuse</u>
Excludes 1: cannabis dependence (F12.2-)
cannabis use, unspecified (F12.9-)

F12.10 Cannabis abuse, <u>uncomplicated</u>
Cannabis use disorder, mild

F12.12- Cannabis abuse <u>with intoxication</u>

F12.120 Cannabis abuse with intoxication, <u>uncomplicated</u>

cc **F12.121 Cannabis abuse with intoxication <u>delirium</u>**

F12.122 Cannabis abuse with intoxication <u>with perceptual disturbance</u>

F12.129 Cannabis abuse with intoxication, <u>unspecified</u>

F12.15- Cannabis abuse <u>with</u> <u>psychotic</u> disorder

cc **F12.150 Cannabis abuse with psychotic disorder <u>with delusions</u>**

cc **F12.151 Cannabis abuse with psychotic disorder <u>with hallucinations</u>**

F12.159 Cannabis abuse with psychotic disorder, unspecified

F12.18- Cannabis abuse <u>with</u> <u>other</u> cannabis-induced disorder

F12.180 Cannabis abuse with cannabis-induced <u>anxiety</u> disorder

F10-F12 (side tab)

F12.188   Cannabis abuse with other cannabis-induced disorder
Cannabis use disorder, mild, with cannabis-induced sleep disorder

F12.19   Cannabis abuse with unspecified cannabis-induced disorder

F12.2-   Cannabis dependence
Excludes 1:   cannabis abuse (F12.1-)
cannabis use, unspecified (F12.9-)
Excludes ❷: cannabis poisoning (T40.7-)

F12.20   Cannabis dependence, uncomplicated
Cannabis use disorder, moderate
Cannabis use disorder, severe

F12.21   Cannabis dependence, in remission

F12.22-   Cannabis dependence with intoxication

F12.220   Cannabis dependence with intoxication, uncomplicated

ccF12.221   Cannabis dependence with intoxication delirium

F12.222   Cannabis dependence with intoxication with perceptual disturbance

F12.229   Cannabis dependence with intoxication, unspecified

F12.25-   Cannabis dependence with psychotic disorder

ccF12.250   Cannabis dependence with psychotic disorder with delusions

ccF12.251   Cannabis dependence with psychotic disorder with hallucinations

F12.259   Cannabis dependence with psychotic disorder, unspecified

F12.28-   Cannabis dependence with other cannabis-induced disorder

F12.280   Cannabis dependence with cannabis-induced anxiety disorder

F12.288   Cannabis dependence with other cannabis-induced disorder
Cannabis use disorder, moderate, with cannabis-induced sleep disorder
Cannabis use disorder, severe, with cannabis-induced sleep disorder
Cannabis withdrawal

F12.29   Cannabis dependence with unspecified cannabis-induced disorder

F12.9-   Cannabis use, unspecified
Excludes 1:   cannabis abuse (F12.1-)
cannabis dependence (F12.2-)

F12.90   Cannabis use, unspecified, uncomplicated

F12.92-   Cannabis use, unspecified with intoxication

F12.920   Cannabis use, unspecified with intoxication, uncomplicated

ccF12.921   Cannabis use, unspecified with intoxication delirium

F12.922   Cannabis use, unspecified with intoxication with perceptual disturbance

F12.929   Cannabis use, unspecified with intoxication, unspecified

F12.95-   Cannabis use, unspecified with psychotic disorder

ccF12.950   Cannabis use, unspecified with psychotic disorder with delusions

ccF12.951   Cannabis use, unspecified with psychotic disorder with hallucinations

F12.959   Cannabis use, unspecified with psychotic disorder, unspecified
Cannabis-induced psychotic disorder, without use disorder

F12.98-   Cannabis use, unspecified with other cannabis-induced disorder

F12.980   Cannabis use, unspecified with anxiety disorder
Cannabis-induced anxiety disorder, without use disorder

F12.988   Cannabis use, unspecified with other cannabis-induced disorder
Cannabis-induced sleep disorder, without use disorder

F12.99   Cannabis use, unspecified with unspecified cannabis-induced disorder

F13-   Sedative, hypnotic, or anxiolytic related disorders

F13.1-   Sedative, hypnotic or anxiolytic-related abuse
Excludes 1:   sedative, hypnotic or anxiolytic-related dependence (F13.2-)
sedative, hypnotic, or anxiolytic use, unspecified (F13.9-)

F13.10   Sedative, hypnotic or anxiolytic abuse, uncomplicated
Sedative, hypnotic, or anxiolytic use disorder, mild

F13.12-   Sedative, hypnotic or anxiolytic abuse with intoxication

F13.120   Sedative, hypnotic or anxiolytic abuse with intoxication, uncomplicated

ccF13.121   Sedative, hypnotic or anxiolytic abuse with intoxication delirium

F13.129   Sedative, hypnotic or anxiolytic abuse with intoxication, unspecified

F13.14   Sedative, hypnotic or anxiolytic abuse with sedative, hypnotic or anxiolytic-induced mood disorder
Sedative, hypnotic, or anxiolytic use disorder, mild, with sedative, hypnotic, or anxiolytic-induced bipolar or related disorder
Sedative, hypnotic, or anxiolytic use disorder, mild, with sedative, hypnotic, or anxiolytic-induced depressive disorder

F13.15-   Sedative, hypnotic or anxiolytic abuse with sedative, hypnotic or anxiolytic-induced psychotic disorder

ccF13.150   Sedative, hypnotic or anxiolytic abuse with sedative, hypnotic or anxiolytic-induced psychotic disorder with delusions

ccF13.151   Sedative, hypnotic or anxiolytic abuse with sedative, hypnotic or anxiolytic-induced psychotic disorder with hallucinations

F13.159   Sedative, hypnotic or anxiolytic abuse with sedative, hypnotic or anxiolytic-induced psychotic disorder, unspecified

F13.18-   Sedative, hypnotic or anxiolytic abuse with other sedative, hypnotic or anxiolytic-induced disorders

F13.180   Sedative, hypnotic or anxiolytic abuse with sedative, hypnotic or anxiolytic-induced anxiety disorder

F13.181   Sedative, hypnotic or anxiolytic abuse with sedative, hypnotic or anxiolytic-induced sexual dysfunction

F13.182   Sedative, hypnotic or anxiolytic abuse with sedative, hypnotic or anxiolytic-induced sleep disorder

F13.188   Sedative, hypnotic or anxiolytic abuse with other sedative, hypnotic or anxiolytic-induced disorder

F13.19   Sedative, hypnotic or anxiolytic abuse with unspecified sedative, hypnotic or anxiolytic-induced disorder

F13.2-   Sedative, hypnotic or anxiolytic-related dependence
Excludes 1:   sedative, hypnotic or anxiolytic-related abuse (F13.1-)
sedative, hypnotic, or anxiolytic use, unspecified (F13.9-)
Excludes ❷: sedative, hypnotic, or anxiolytic poisoning (T42.-)

ccF13.20   Sedative, hypnotic or anxiolytic dependence, uncomplicated

F13.21   Sedative, hypnotic or anxiolytic dependence, in remission

F13.22-   Sedative, hypnotic or anxiolytic dependence with intoxication
Excludes 1:   sedative, hypnotic or anxiolytic dependence with withdrawal (F13.23-)

F13.220   Sedative, hypnotic or anxiolytic dependence with intoxication, uncomplicated

ccF13.221   Sedative, hypnotic or anxiolytic dependence with Intoxication delirium

F13.229   Sedative, hypnotic or anxiolytic dependence with intoxication, unspecified

F
1
2
-
F
1
3

F13.23- Sedative, hypnotic or anxiolytic dependence <u>with</u> <u>withdrawal</u>
Sedative, hypnotic, or anxiolytic use disorder, moderate
Sedative, hypnotic, or anxiolytic use disorder, severe
Excludes 1: sedative, hypnotic or anxiolytic dependence with intoxication (F13.22-)

cc **F13.230** Sedative, hypnotic or anxiolytic dependence with withdrawal, <u>uncomplicated</u>

cc **F13.231** Sedative, hypnotic or anxiolytic dependence <u>with</u> withdrawal <u>delirium</u>

cc **F13.232** Sedative, hypnotic or anxiolytic dependence with withdrawal <u>with perceptual disturbance</u>
Sedative, hypnotic, or anxiolytic withdrawal with perceptual disturbances

cc **F13.239** Sedative, hypnotic or anxiolytic dependence with withdrawal, unspecified
Sedative, hypnotic, or anxiolytic withdrawal without perceptual disturbances

F13.24 Sedative, hypnotic or anxiolytic dependence <u>with</u> sedative, hypnotic or anxiolytic-induced <u>mood</u> disorder
Sedative, hypnotic, or anxiolytic use disorder, moderate, with sedative, hypnotic, or anxiolytic-induced bipolar or related disorder
Sedative, hypnotic, or anxiolytic use disorder, moderate, with sedative, hypnotic, or anxiolytic-induced depressive disorder
Sedative, hypnotic, or anxiolytic use disorder, severe, with sedative, hypnotic, or anxiolytic-induced bipolar or related disorder
Sedative, hypnotic, or anxiolytic use disorder, severe, with sedative, hypnotic, or anxiolytic-induced depressive disorder

F13.25- Sedative, hypnotic or anxiolytic dependence <u>with</u> sedative, hypnotic or anxiolytic-induced <u>psychotic</u> disorder

cc **F13.250** Sedative, hypnotic or anxiolytic dependence with sedative, hypnotic or anxiolytic-induced psychotic disorder <u>with delusions</u>

cc **F13.251** Sedative, hypnotic or anxiolytic dependence with sedative, hypnotic or anxiolytic-induced psychotic disorder <u>with hallucinations</u>

cc **F13.259** Sedative, hypnotic or anxiolytic dependence with sedative, hypnotic or anxiolytic-induced psychotic disorder, <u>unspecified</u>

cc **F13.26** Sedative, hypnotic or anxiolytic dependence <u>with</u> sedative, hypnotic or anxiolytic-induced <u>persisting amnestic</u> disorder

cc **F13.27** Sedative, hypnotic or anxiolytic dependence <u>with</u> sedative, hypnotic or anxiolytic-induced <u>persisting dementia</u>
Sedative, hypnotic, or anxiolytic use disorder, moderate, with sedative, hypnotic, or anxiolytic-induced major neurocognitive disorder
Sedative, hypnotic, or anxiolytic use disorder, severe, with sedative, hypnotic, or anxiolytic-induced major neurocognitive disorder

F13.28- Sedative, hypnotic or anxiolytic dependence <u>with other</u> sedative, hypnotic or anxiolytic-induced disorders

cc **F13.280** Sedative, hypnotic or anxiolytic dependence <u>with</u> sedative, hypnotic or anxiolytic-induced <u>anxiety</u> disorder

cc **F13.281** Sedative, hypnotic or anxiolytic dependence <u>with</u> sedative, hypnotic or anxiolytic-induced <u>sexual dysfunction</u>

cc **F13.282** Sedative, hypnotic or anxiolytic dependence <u>with</u> sedative, hypnotic or anxiolytic-induced <u>sleep</u> disorder

cc **F13.288** Sedative, hypnotic or anxiolytic dependence with other sedative, hypnotic or anxiolytic-induced disorder
Sedative, hypnotic, or anxiolytic use disorder, moderate, with sedative, hypnotic, or anxiolytic-induced mild neurocognitive disorder
Sedative, hypnotic, or anxiolytic use disorder, severe, with sedative, hypnotic, or anxiolytic-induced mild neurocognitive disorder

F13.29 Sedative, hypnotic or anxiolytic dependence with unspecified sedative, hypnotic or anxiolytic-induced disorder

F13.9- <u>Sedative, hypnotic or anxiolytic-related use, unspecified</u>
Excludes 1: sedative, hypnotic or anxiolytic-related abuse (F13.1-)
sedative, hypnotic or anxiolytic-related dependence (F13.2-)

F13.90 Sedative, hypnotic, or anxiolytic use, unspecified, <u>uncomplicated</u>

F13.92- Sedative, hypnotic or anxiolytic use, unspecified <u>with intoxication</u>
Excludes 1: sedative, hypnotic or anxiolytic use, unspecified with withdrawal (F13.93-)

F13.920 Sedative, hypnotic or anxiolytic use, unspecified with intoxication, <u>uncomplicated</u>

cc **F13.921** Sedative, hypnotic or anxiolytic use, unspecified with intoxication <u>delirium</u>
Sedative, hypnotic, or anxiolytic-induced delirium

F13.929 Sedative, hypnotic or anxiolytic use, unspecified with intoxication, <u>unspecified</u>

F13.93- Sedative, hypnotic or anxiolytic use, unspecified <u>with withdrawal</u>
Excludes 1: sedative, hypnotic or anxiolytic use, unspecified with intoxication (F13.92-)

cc **F13.930** Sedative, hypnotic or anxiolytic use, unspecified with withdrawal, <u>uncomplicated</u>

cc **F13.931** Sedative, hypnotic or anxiolytic use, unspecified with withdrawal <u>delirium</u>

cc **F13.932** Sedative, hypnotic or anxiolytic use, unspecified with withdrawal <u>with perceptual disturbances</u>

cc **F13.939** Sedative, hypnotic or anxiolytic use, unspecified with withdrawal, unspecified

F13.94 Sedative, hypnotic or anxiolytic use, unspecified <u>with</u> sedative, hypnotic or anxiolytic-induced <u>mood</u> disorder
Sedative, hypnotic, or anxiolytic-induced bipolar or related disorder, without use disorder
Sedative, hypnotic, or anxiolytic-induced depressive disorder, without use disorder

F13.95- Sedative, hypnotic or anxiolytic use, unspecified <u>with</u> sedative, hypnotic or anxiolytic-induced <u>psychotic</u> disorder

cc **F13.950** Sedative, hypnotic or anxiolytic use, unspecified with sedative, hypnotic or anxiolytic-induced psychotic disorder <u>with delusions</u>

cc **F13.951** Sedative, hypnotic or anxiolytic use, unspecified with sedative, hypnotic or anxiolytic-induced psychotic disorder <u>with hallucinations</u>

F13.959 Sedative, hypnotic or anxiolytic use, unspecified with sedative, hypnotic or anxiolytic-induced psychotic disorder, unspecified
Sedative, hypnotic, or anxiolytic-induced psychotic disorder, without use disorder

F13.96 Sedative, hypnotic or anxiolytic use, unspecified <u>with</u> sedative, hypnotic or anxiolytic-induced <u>persisting amnestic</u> disorder

cc **F13.97** Sedative, hypnotic or anxiolytic use, unspecified <u>with</u> sedative, hypnotic or anxiolytic-induced <u>persisting dementia</u>
Sedative, hypnotic, or anxiolytic-induced major neurocognitive disorder, without use disorder

F13.98- Sedative, hypnotic or anxiolytic use, unspecified <u>with other</u> sedative, hypnotic or anxiolytic-induced disorders

F13.980 Sedative, hypnotic or anxiolytic use, unspecified <u>with</u> sedative, hypnotic or anxiolytic-induced <u>anxiety</u> disorder
Sedative, hypnotic, or anxiolytic-induced anxiety disorder, without use disorder

F13.981 Sedative, hypnotic or anxiolytic use, unspecified <u>with</u> sedative, hypnotic or anxiolytic-induced <u>sexual dysfunction</u>
Sedative, hypnotic, or anxiolytic-induced sexual dysfunction disorder, without use disorder

F13 - F13

F13.982 Sedative, hypnotic or anxiolytic use, unspecified **with** sedative, hypnotic or anxiolytic-induced **sleep** disorder
Sedative, hypnotic, or anxiolytic-induced sleep disorder, without use disorder

F13.988 Sedative, hypnotic or anxiolytic use, unspecified with other sedative, hypnotic or anxiolytic-induced disorder
Sedative, hypnotic, or anxiolytic-induced mild neurocognitive disorder

F13.99 Sedative, hypnotic or anxiolytic use, unspecified with unspecified sedative, hypnotic or anxiolytic-induced disorder

F14- Cocaine related disorders
Excludes ❷: other stimulant-related disorders (F15.-)

F14.1- Cocaine **abuse**
Excludes 1:   cocaine dependence (F14.2-)
cocaine use, unspecified (F14.9-)

F14.10 Cocaine abuse, **uncomplicated**
Cocaine use disorder, mild

F14.12- Cocaine abuse **with intoxication**

F14.120 Cocaine abuse with intoxication, **uncomplicated**

cc **F14.121** Cocaine abuse with intoxication **with delirium**

F14.122 Cocaine abuse with intoxication **with perceptual disturbance**

F14.129 Cocaine abuse with intoxication, **unspecified**

F14.14 Cocaine abuse **with** cocaine-induced **mood** disorder
Cocaine use disorder, mild, with cocaine-induced bipolar or related disorder
Cocaine use disorder, mild, with cocaine-induced depressive disorder

F14.15- Cocaine abuse **with** cocaine-induced **psychotic** disorder

cc **F14.150** Cocaine abuse with cocaine-induced psychotic disorder **with delusions**

cc **F14.151** Cocaine abuse with cocaine-induced psychotic disorder **with hallucinations**

F14.159 Cocaine abuse with cocaine-induced psychotic disorder, unspecified

F14.18 Cocaine abuse **with other** cocaine-induced disorder

F14.180 Cocaine abuse **with** cocaine-induced **anxiety** disorder

F14.181 Cocaine abuse with cocaine-induced **sexual dysfunction**

F14.182 Cocaine abuse **with** cocaine-induced **sleep** disorder

F14.188 Cocaine abuse with other cocaine-induced disorder
Cocaine use disorder, mild, with cocaine-induced obsessive-compulsive or related disorder

F14.19 Cocaine abuse with unspecified cocaine-induced disorder

F14.2- Cocaine **dependence**
Excludes 1:   cocaine abuse (F14.1-)
cocaine use, unspecified (F14.9-)
Excludes ❷: cocaine poisoning (T40.5-)

cc **F14.20** Cocaine dependence, **uncomplicated**
Cocaine use disorder, moderate
Cocaine use disorder, severe

F14.21 Cocaine dependence, **in remission**

F14.22- Cocaine dependence **with intoxication**
Excludes 1:   cocaine dependence with withdrawal (F14.23)

F14.220 Cocaine dependence with intoxication, **uncomplicated**

cc **F14.221** Cocaine dependence with intoxication **delirium**

cc **F14.222** Cocaine dependence with intoxication **with perceptual disturbance**

cc **F14.229** Cocaine dependence with intoxication, **unspecified**

cc **F14.23** Cocaine dependence **with withdrawal**
Excludes 1:   cocaine dependence with intoxication (F14.22-)

F14.24 Cocaine dependence **with** cocaine-induced **mood** disorder
Cocaine use disorder, moderate, with cocaine-induced bipolar or related disorder
Cocaine use disorder, moderate, with cocaine-induced depressive disorder
Cocaine use disorder, severe, with cocaine-induced bipolar or related disorder
Cocaine use disorder, severe, with cocaine-induced depressive disorder

F14.25- Cocaine dependence **with** cocaine-induced **psychotic** disorder

cc **F14.250** Cocaine dependence with cocaine-induced psychotic disorder **with delusions**

cc **F14.251** Cocaine dependence with cocaine-induced psychotic disorder **with hallucinations**

cc **F14.259** Cocaine dependence with cocaine-induced psychotic disorder, unspecified

F14.28- Cocaine dependence **with other** cocaine-induced disorder

cc **F14.280** Cocaine dependence with cocaine-induced **anxiety** disorder

cc **F14.281** Cocaine dependence with cocaine-induced **sexual dysfunction**

cc **F14.282** Cocaine dependence with cocaine-induced **sleep** disorder

cc **F14.288** Cocaine dependence with other cocaine-induced disorder
Cocaine use disorder, moderate, with cocaine-induced obsessive-compulsive or related disorder
Cocaine use disorder, severe, with cocaine-induced obsessive-compulsive or related disorder

F14.29 Cocaine dependence with unspecified cocaine-induced disorder

F14.9- Cocaine **use, unspecified**
Excludes 1:   cocaine abuse (F14.1-)
cocaine dependence (F14.2-)

F14.90 Cocaine use, unspecified, **uncomplicated**

F14.92- Cocaine use, unspecified **with intoxication**

F14.920 Cocaine use, unspecified with intoxication, **uncomplicated**

cc **F14.921** Cocaine use, unspecified with intoxication **delirium**

F14.922 Cocaine use, unspecified with intoxication **with perceptual disturbance**

F14.929 Cocaine use, unspecified with intoxication, **unspecified**

F14.94 Cocaine use, unspecified **with** cocaine-induced **mood** disorder
Cocaine-induced bipolar or related disorder, without use disorder
Cocaine-induced depressive disorder, without use disorder

F14.95- Cocaine use, unspecified **with** cocaine-induced **psychotic** disorder

cc **F14.950** Cocaine use, unspecified with cocaine-induced psychotic disorder **with delusions**

cc **F14.951** Cocaine use, unspecified with cocaine-induced psychotic disorder **with hallucinations**

F14.959 Cocaine use, unspecified with cocaine-induced psychotic disorder, unspecified
Cocaine-induced psychotic disorder, without use disorder

F14.98- Cocaine use, unspecified **with other** specified cocaine-induced disorder

F14.980 Cocaine use, unspecified with cocaine-induced **anxiety** disorder
Cocaine-induced anxiety disorder, without use disorder

F14.981 Cocaine use, unspecified with cocaine-induced **sexual dysfunction**
Cocaine-induced sexual dysfunction disorder, without use disorder

F14.982 Cocaine use, unspecified with cocaine-induced **sleep** disorder
Cocaine-induced sleep disorder, without use disorder

F13 - F14

F14.988 Cocaine use, unspecified with other cocaine-induced disorder
  Cocaine-induced obsessive compulsive or related disorder

F14.99 Cocaine use, unspecified with unspecified cocaine-induced disorder

F15- Other stimulant related disorders
  Includes: Amphetamine-related disorders
    Caffeine
  Excludes ❷: cocaine-related disorders (F14.-)

F15.1- Other stimulant abuse
  Excludes 1: other stimulant dependence (F15.2-)
    other stimulant use, unspecified (F15.9-)

F15.10 Other stimulant abuse, uncomplicated
  Amphetamine type substance use disorder, mild
  Other or unspecified stimulant use disorder, mild

F15.12- Other stimulant abuse with intoxication

  F15.120 Other stimulant abuse with intoxication, uncomplicated

CC **F15.121** Other stimulant abuse with intoxication delirium

  F15.122 Other stimulant abuse with intoxication with perceptual disturbance
  Amphetamine or other stimulant use disorder, mild, with amphetamine or other stimulant intoxication, with perceptual disturbances

  F15.129 Other stimulant abuse with intoxication, unspecified
  Amphetamine or other stimulant use disorder, mild, with amphetamine or other stimulant intoxication, without perceptual disturbances

F15.14 Other stimulant abuse with stimulant-induced mood disorder
  Amphetamine or other stimulant use disorder, mild, with amphetamine or other stimulant-induced bipolar or related disorder
  Amphetamine or other stimulant use disorder, mild, with amphetamine or other stimulant-induced depressive disorder

F15.15- Other stimulant abuse with stimulant-induced psychotic disorder

CC **F15.150** Other stimulant abuse with stimulant-induced psychotic disorder with delusions

CC **F15.151** Other stimulant abuse with stimulant-induced psychotic disorder with hallucinations

  F15.159 Other stimulant abuse with stimulant-induced psychotic disorder, unspecified

F15.18- Other stimulant abuse with other stimulant-induced disorder

  F15.180 Other stimulant abuse with stimulant-induced anxiety disorder

  F15.181 Other stimulant abuse with stimulant-induced sexual dysfunction

  F15.182 Other stimulant abuse with stimulant-induced sleep disorder

  F15.188 Other stimulant abuse with other stimulant-induced disorder
  Amphetamine or other stimulant use disorder, mild, with amphetamine or other stimulant-induced obsessive-compulsive or related disorder

F15.19 Other stimulant abuse with unspecified stimulant-induced disorder

F15.2- Other stimulant dependence
  Excludes 1: other stimulant abuse (F15.1-)
    other stimulant use, unspecified (F15.9-)

CC **F15.20** Other stimulant dependence, uncomplicated
  Amphetamine type substance use disorder, moderate
  Amphetamine type substance use disorder, severe
  Other or unspecified stimulant use disorder, moderate
  Other or unspecified stimulant use disorder, severe

F15.21 Other stimulant dependence, in remission

F15.22- Other stimulant dependence with intoxication
  Excludes 1: other stimulant dependence with withdrawal (F15.23)

  F15.220 Other stimulant dependence with intoxication, uncomplicated

CC **F15.221** Other stimulant dependence with intoxication delirium

CC **F15.222** Other stimulant dependence with intoxication with perceptual disturbance
  Amphetamine or other stimulant use disorder, moderate, with amphetamine or other stimulant intoxication, with perceptual disturbances
  Amphetamine or other stimulant use disorder, severe, with amphetamine or other stimulant intoxication, with perceptual disturbances

  F15.229 Other stimulant dependence with intoxication, unspecified
  Amphetamine or other stimulant use disorder, moderate, with amphetamine or other stimulant intoxication, without perceptual disturbances
  Amphetamine or other stimulant use disorder, severe, with amphetamine or other stimulant intoxication, without perceptual disturbances

CC **F15.23** Other stimulant dependence with withdrawal
  Amphetamine or other stimulant withdrawal
  Excludes 1: other stimulant dependence with intoxication (F15.22-)

F15.24 Other stimulant dependence with stimulant-induced mood disorder
  Amphetamine or other stimulant use disorder, moderate, with amphetamine or other stimulant-induced bipolar or related disorder
  Amphetamine or other stimulant use disorder, moderate, with amphetamine or other stimulant-induced depressive disorder
  Amphetamine or other stimulant use disorder, severe, with amphetamine or other stimulant-induced bipolar or related disorder
  Amphetamine or other stimulant use disorder, severe, with amphetamine or other stimulant-induced depressive disorder

F15.25- Other stimulant dependence with stimulant-induced psychotic disorder

CC **F15.250** Other stimulant dependence with stimulant-induced psychotic disorder with delusions

CC **F15.251** Other stimulant dependence with stimulant-induced psychotic disorder with hallucinations

CC **F15.259** Other stimulant dependence with stimulant-induced psychotic disorder, unspecified

F15.28- Other stimulant dependence with other stimulant-induced disorder

CC **F15.280** Other stimulant dependence with stimulant-induced anxiety disorder

CC **F15.281** Other stimulant dependence with stimulant-induced sexual dysfunction

CC **F15.282** Other stimulant dependence with stimulant-induced sleep disorder

CC **F15.288** Other stimulant dependence with other stimulant-induced disorder
  Amphetamine or other stimulant use disorder, moderate, with amphetamine or other stimulant-induced obsessive-compulsive or related disorder
  Amphetamine or other stimulant use disorder, severe, with amphetamine or other stimulant-induced obsessive-compulsive or related disorder

F15.29 Other stimulant dependence with unspecified stimulant-induced disorder

F15.9- Other stimulant use, unspecified
  Excludes 1: other stimulant abuse (F15.1-)
    other stimulant dependence (F15.2-)

F15.90 Other stimulant use, unspecified, uncomplicated

F14-F15

F15.92- Other stimulant use, unspecified <u>with intoxication</u>
> *Excludes 1:*   *other stimulant use, unspecified with withdrawal (F15.93)*

F15.920 Other stimulant use, unspecified with intoxication, <u>uncomplicated</u>

cc **F15.921** Other stimulant use, unspecified with intoxication <u>delirium</u>
> Amphetamine or other stimulant-induced delirium

F15.922 Other stimulant use, unspecified with intoxication <u>with perceptual disturbance</u>

F15.929 Other stimulant use, unspecified with intoxication, <u>unspecified</u>
> Caffeine intoxication

cc **F15.93** Other stimulant use, unspecified, <u>with withdrawal</u>
> Caffeine withdrawal
> *Excludes 1:*   *other stimulant use, unspecified with intoxication (F15.92-)*

F15.94 Other stimulant use, unspecified <u>with</u> stimulant-induced <u>mood</u> disorder
> Amphetamine or other stimulant-induced bipolar or related disorder, without use disorder
> Amphetamine or other stimulant-induced depressive disorder, without use disorder

F15.95- Other stimulant use, unspecified <u>with</u> stimulant-induced <u>psychotic</u> disorder

cc **F15.950** Other stimulant use, unspecified with stimulant-induced psychotic disorder <u>with delusions</u>

cc **F15.951** Other stimulant use, unspecified with stimulant-induced psychotic disorder <u>with hallucinations</u>

F15.959 Other stimulant use, unspecified with stimulant-induced psychotic disorder, unspecified
> Amphetamine or other stimulant-induced psychotic disorder, without use disorder

F15.98- Other stimulant use, unspecified <u>with other</u> stimulant-induced disorder

F15.980 Other stimulant use, unspecified with stimulant-induced <u>anxiety</u> disorder
> Amphetamine or other stimulant-induced anxiety disorder, without use disorder
> Caffeine-induced anxiety disorder, without use disorder

F15.981 Other stimulant use, unspecified with stimulant-induced <u>sexual dysfunction</u>
> Amphetamine or other stimulant-induced sexual dysfunction disorder, without use disorder

F15.982 Other stimulant use, unspecified with stimulant-induced <u>sleep</u> disorder
> Amphetamine or other stimulant-induced sleep disorder, without use disorder
> Caffeine-induced sleep disorder, without use disorder

F15.988 Other stimulant use, unspecified with other stimulant-Induced disorder
> Amphetamine or other stimulant-induced obsessive-compulsive or related disorder, without use disorder

F15.99 Other stimulant use, unspecified with unspecified stimulant-induced disorder

F16- <u>Hallucinogen related disorders</u>
> Includes: Ecstasy
>   PCP
>   Phencyclidine

F16.1- Hallucinogen <u>abuse</u>
> *Excludes 1:*   *hallucinogen dependence (F16.2-)*
>   *hallucinogen use, unspecified (F16.9-)*

F16.10 Hallucinogen abuse, <u>uncomplicated</u>
> Other hallucinogen use disorder, mild
> Phencyclidine use disorder, mild

F16.12- Hallucinogen abuse <u>with intoxication</u>

F16.120 Hallucinogen abuse with intoxication, <u>uncomplicated</u>

cc **F16.121** Hallucinogen abuse with intoxication with <u>delirium</u>

F16.122 Hallucinogen abuse with intoxication <u>with perceptual disturbance</u>

F16.129 Hallucinogen abuse with intoxication, <u>unspecified</u>

F16.14 Hallucinogen abuse <u>with</u> hallucinogen-induced <u>mood</u> disorder
> Other hallucinogen use disorder, mild, with other hallucinogen-induced bipolar or related disorder
> Other hallucinogen use disorder, mild, with other hallucinogen-induced depressive disorder
> Phencyclidine use disorder, mild, with phencyclidine-induced bipolar or related disorder
> Phencyclidine use disorder, mild, with phencyclidine-induced depressive disorder

F16.15- Hallucinogen abuse <u>with</u> hallucinogen-induced <u>psychotic</u> disorder

cc **F16.150** Hallucinogen abuse with hallucinogen-induced psychotic disorder <u>with delusions</u>

cc **F16.151** Hallucinogen abuse with hallucinogen-induced psychotic disorder <u>with hallucinations</u>

F16.159 Hallucinogen abuse with hallucinogen-induced psychotic disorder, unspecified

F16.18- Hallucinogen abuse <u>with other</u> hallucinogen-induced disorder

F16.180 Hallucinogen abuse with hallucinogen-induced <u>anxiety</u> disorder

F16.183 Hallucinogen abuse with hallucinogen <u>persisting perception disorder (flashbacks)</u>

F16.188 Hallucinogen abuse with other hallucinogen-induced disorder

F16.19 Hallucinogen abuse with unspecified hallucinogen-induced disorder

F16.2- Hallucinogen <u>dependence</u>
> *Excludes 1:*   *hallucinogen abuse (F16.1-)*
>   *hallucinogen use, unspecified (F16.9-)*

cc **F16.20** Hallucinogen dependence, <u>uncomplicated</u>
> Other hallucinogen use disorder, moderate
> Other hallucinogen use disorder, severe
> Phencyclidine use disorder, moderate
> Phencyclidine use disorder, severe

F16.21 Hallucinogen dependence, <u>in remission</u>

F16.22- Hallucinogen dependence <u>with intoxication</u>

F16.220 Hallucinogen dependence with intoxication, <u>uncomplicated</u>

cc **F16.221** Hallucinogen dependence with intoxication with <u>delirium</u>

F16.229 Hallucinogen dependence with intoxication, <u>unspecified</u>

F16.24 Hallucinogen dependence <u>with</u> hallucinogen-induced <u>mood</u> disorder
> Other hallucinogen use disorder, moderate, with other hallucinogen-induced bipolar or related disorder
> Other hallucinogen use disorder, moderate, with other hallucinogen-induced depressive disorder
> Other hallucinogen use disorder, severe, with other hallucinogen-induced bipolar or related disorder
> Other hallucinogen use disorder, severe, with other hallucinogen-induced depressive disorder
> Phencyclidine use disorder, moderate, with phencyclidine-induced bipolar or related disorder
> Phencyclidine use disorder, moderate, with phencyclidine-induced depressive disorder
> Phencyclidine use disorder, severe, with phencyclidine-induced bipolar or related disorder
> Phencyclidine use disorder, severe, with phencyclidine-induced depressive disorder

F16.25- Hallucinogen dependence <u>with</u> hallucinogen-induced <u>psychotic</u> disorder

cc **F16.250** Hallucinogen dependence with hallucinogen-induced psychotic disorder <u>with delusions</u>

cc **F16.251** Hallucinogen dependence with hallucinogen-induced psychotic disorder <u>with hallucinations</u>

cc **F16.259** Hallucinogen dependence with hallucinogen-induced psychotic disorder, unspecified

F16.28- Hallucinogen dependence <u>with other</u> hallucinogen-induced disorder

cc **F16.280** Hallucinogen dependence <u>with</u> hallucinogen-induced <u>anxiety</u> disorder

F15 - F16

© 2016 Channel Publishing, Ltd.

CC **F16.283** Hallucinogen dependence <u>with</u> hallucinogen <u>persisting perception disorder (flashbacks)</u>

CC **F16.288** Hallucinogen dependence with other hallucinogen-induced disorder

F16.29 Hallucinogen dependence with unspecified hallucinogen-induced disorder

F16.9- Hallucinogen <u>use, unspecified</u>
Excludes 1: *hallucinogen abuse (F16.1-)*
hallucinogen dependence (F16.2-)

F16.90 Hallucinogen use, unspecified, <u>uncomplicated</u>

F16.92- Hallucinogen use, unspecified <u>with intoxication</u>

F16.920 Hallucinogen use, unspecified with intoxication, <u>uncomplicated</u>

CC **F16.921** Hallucinogen use, unspecified with intoxication with <u>delirium</u>
Other hallucinogen intoxication delirium

F16.929 Hallucinogen use, unspecified with intoxication, <u>unspecified</u>

F16.94 Hallucinogen use, unspecified <u>with</u> hallucinogen-induced <u>mood</u> disorder
Other hallucinogen-induced bipolar or related disorder, without use disorder
Other hallucinogen-induced depressive disorder, without use disorder
Phencyclidine-induced bipolar or related disorder, without use disorder
Phencyclidine-induced depressive disorder, without use disorder

F16.95- Hallucinogen use, unspecified <u>with</u> hallucinogen-induced <u>psychotic</u> disorder

CC **F16.950** Hallucinogen use, unspecified with hallucinogen-induced psychotic disorder <u>with delusions</u>

CC **F16.951** Hallucinogen use, unspecified with hallucinogen-induced psychotic disorder <u>with hallucinations</u>

F16.959 Hallucinogen use, unspecified with hallucinogen-induced psychotic disorder, unspecified
Other hallucinogen-induced psychotic disorder, without use disorder
Phencyclidine-induced psychotic disorder, without use disorder

F16.98- Hallucinogen use, unspecified <u>with</u> <u>other</u> specified hallucinogen-induced disorder

F16.980 Hallucinogen use, unspecified with hallucinogen-induced <u>anxiety</u> disorder
Other hallucinogen-induced anxiety disorder, without use disorder
Phencyclidine-induced anxiety disorder, without use disorder

F16.983 Hallucinogen use, unspecified <u>with</u> hallucinogen persisting perception disorder (flashbacks)

F16.988 Hallucinogen use, unspecified with other hallucinogen-induced disorder

F16.99 Hallucinogen use, unspecified with unspecified hallucinogen-induced disorder

F17- <u>Nicotine dependence</u>
Excludes 1: *history of tobacco dependence (Z87.891)*
tobacco use NOS (Z72.0)
Excludes ❷: *tobacco use (smoking) during pregnancy, childbirth and the puerperium (O99.33-)*
toxic effect of nicotine (T65.2-)

F17.2- Nicotine <u>dependence</u>
AHA 13:4Q:p108 – Smoker
AHA 13:4Q:p108 – Nicotine dependence

F17.20- Nicotine <u>dependence, unspecified</u>

F17.200 Nicotine dependence, unspecified, <u>uncomplicated</u> — [Unacceptable PDX]
Tobacco use disorder, mild
Tobacco use disorder, moderate
Tobacco use disorder, severe

F17.201 Nicotine dependence, unspecified, in remission — [Unacceptable PDX]

CC **F17.203** Nicotine dependence unspecified, <u>with withdrawal</u>
Tobacco withdrawal

F17.208 Nicotine dependence, unspecified, with other nicotine-induced disorders

F17.209 Nicotine dependence, unspecified, with unspecified nicotine-induced disorders

F17.21- Nicotine dependence, <u>cigarettes</u>
AHA 13:4Q:p109 – Nicotine dependence and COPD

F17.210 Nicotine dependence, cigarettes, <u>uncomplicated</u> — [Unacceptable PDX]

F17.211 Nicotine dependence, cigarettes, <u>in remission</u> — [Unacceptable PDX]

CC **F17.213** Nicotine dependence, cigarettes, <u>with withdrawal</u>

F17.218 Nicotine dependence, cigarettes, with other nicotine-induced disorders

F17.219 Nicotine dependence, cigarettes, with unspecified nicotine-induced disorders

F17.22- Nicotine dependence, <u>chewing tobacco</u>

F17.220 Nicotine dependence, chewing tobacco, <u>uncomplicated</u> — [Unacceptable PDX]

F17.221 Nicotine dependence, chewing tobacco, <u>in remission</u> — [Unacceptable PDX]

CC **F17.223** Nicotine dependence, chewing tobacco, <u>with withdrawal</u>

F17.228 Nicotine dependence, chewing tobacco, with other nicotine-induced disorders

F17.229 Nicotine dependence, chewing tobacco, with unspecified nicotine-induced disorders

F17.29- Nicotine dependence, <u>other tobacco product</u>

F17.290 Nicotine dependence, other tobacco product, <u>uncomplicated</u> — [Unacceptable PDX]

F17.291 Nicotine dependence, other tobacco product, <u>in remission</u> — [Unacceptable PDX]

CC **F17.293** Nicotine dependence, other tobacco product, <u>with withdrawal</u>

F17.298 Nicotine dependence, other tobacco product, with other nicotine-induced disorders

F17.299 Nicotine dependence, other tobacco product, with unspecified nicotine-induced disorders

F18- <u>Inhalant related disorders</u>
Includes: Volatile solvents

F18.1- Inhalant <u>abuse</u>
Excludes 1: *inhalant dependence (F18.2-)*
inhalant use, unspecified (F18.9-)

F18.10 Inhalant abuse, <u>uncomplicated</u>
Inhalant use disorder, mild

F18.12- Inhalant abuse <u>with intoxication</u>

F18.120 Inhalant abuse with intoxication, <u>uncomplicated</u>

CC **F18.121** Inhalant abuse with intoxication <u>delirium</u>

F18.129 Inhalant abuse with intoxication, <u>unspecified</u>

F18.14 Inhalant abuse <u>with</u> inhalant-induced <u>mood</u> disorder
Inhalant use disorder, mild, with inhalant-induced depressive disorder

F18.15- Inhalant abuse <u>with</u> inhalant-induced <u>psychotic</u> disorder

CC **F18.150** Inhalant abuse with inhalant-induced psychotic disorder <u>with delusions</u>

CC **F18.151** Inhalant abuse with inhalant-induced psychotic disorder <u>with hallucinations</u>

F18.159 Inhalant abuse with inhalant-induced psychotic disorder, unspecified

CC **F18.17** Inhalant abuse <u>with</u> inhalant-induced <u>dementia</u>
Inhalant use disorder, mild, with inhalant-induced major neurocognitive disorder

F18.18- Inhalant abuse <u>with</u> <u>other</u> inhalant-induced disorders

F18.180 Inhalant abuse with inhalant-induced <u>anxiety</u> disorder

F18.188 Inhalant abuse with other inhalant-induced disorder
Inhalant use disorder, mild, with inhalant-induced mild neurocognitive disorder

F18.19 Inhalant abuse with unspecified inhalant-induced disorder

F18.2-   Inhalant <u>dependence</u>
> *Excludes 1:*   *inhalant abuse (F18.1-)*
> *inhalant use, unspecified (F18.9-)*

cc **F18.20   Inhalant dependence,** <u>uncomplicated</u>
> Inhalant use disorder, moderate
> Inhalant use disorder, severe

F18.21   Inhalant dependence, <u>in remission</u>

F18.22-   Inhalant dependence <u>with intoxication</u>

> **F18.220   Inhalant dependence with intoxication,** <u>uncomplicated</u>

> cc **F18.221   Inhalant dependence with intoxication** <u>delirium</u>

> **F18.229   Inhalant dependence with intoxication,** <u>unspecified</u>

F18.24   Inhalant dependence <u>with</u> inhalant-induced <u>mood</u> disorder
> Inhalant use disorder, moderate, with inhalant-induced depressive disorder
> Inhalant use disorder, severe, with inhalant-induced depressive disorder

F18.25-   Inhalant dependence <u>with</u> inhalant-induced <u>psychotic</u> disorder

> cc **F18.250   Inhalant dependence with inhalant-induced psychotic disorder** <u>with delusions</u>

> cc **F18.251   Inhalant dependence with inhalant-induced psychotic disorder** <u>with hallucinations</u>

> cc **F18.259   Inhalant dependence with inhalant-induced psychotic disorder, unspecified**

cc **F18.27   Inhalant dependence** <u>with</u> inhalant-induced <u>dementia</u>
> Inhalant use disorder, moderate, with inhalant-induced major neurocognitive disorder
> Inhalant use disorder, severe, with inhalant-induced major neurocognitive disorder

F18.28-   Inhalant dependence <u>with</u> <u>other</u> inhalant-induced disorders

> cc **F18.280   Inhalant dependence with inhalant-induced** <u>anxiety</u> disorder

> cc **F18.288   Inhalant dependence with other inhalant-induced disorder**
> > Inhalant use disorder, moderate, with inhalant-induced mild neurocognitive disorder
> > Inhalant use disorder, severe, with inhalant-induced mild neurocognitive disorder

F18.29   Inhalant dependence with unspecified inhalant-induced disorder

F18.9-   Inhalant use, <u>unspecified</u>
> *Excludes 1:*   *inhalant abuse (F18.1-)*
> *inhalant dependence (F18.2-)*

F18.90   Inhalant use, unspecified, <u>uncomplicated</u>

F18.92-   Inhalant use, unspecified <u>with intoxication</u>

> **F18.920   Inhalant use, unspecified with intoxication,** <u>uncomplicated</u>

> cc **F18.921   Inhalant use, unspecified with intoxication with** <u>delirium</u>

> **F18.929   Inhalant use, unspecified with intoxication,** <u>unspecified</u>

F18.94   Inhalant use, unspecified <u>with</u> inhalant-induced <u>mood</u> disorder
> Inhalant-induced depressive disorder

F18.95-   Inhalant use, unspecified <u>with</u> inhalant-induced <u>psychotic</u> disorder

> cc **F18.950   Inhalant use, unspecified with inhalant-induced psychotic disorder** <u>with delusions</u>

> cc **F18.951   Inhalant use, unspecified with inhalant-induced psychotic disorder** <u>with hallucinations</u>

> **F18.959   Inhalant use, unspecified with inhalant-induced psychotic disorder, unspecified**

cc **F18.97   Inhalant use, unspecified** <u>with</u> inhalant-induced <u>persisting dementia</u>
> Inhalant-induced major neurocognitive disorder

F18.98-   Inhalant use, unspecified <u>with</u> <u>other</u> inhalant-induced disorders

> **F18.980   Inhalant use, unspecified with inhalant-induced** <u>anxiety</u> disorder

F18.988   Inhalant use, unspecified with other inhalant-induced disorder
> Inhalant-induced mild neurocognitive disorder

F18.99   Inhalant use, unspecified with unspecified inhalant-induced disorder

F19-   Other psychoactive substance related disorders
> Includes: Polysubstance drug use (indiscriminate drug use)

F19.1-   Other psychoactive substance <u>abuse</u>
> *Excludes 1:*   *other psychoactive substance dependence (F19.2-)*
> *other psychoactive substance use, unspecified (F19.9-)*

F19.10   Other psychoactive substance abuse, <u>uncomplicated</u>
> Other (or unknown) substance use disorder, mild

F19.12-   Other psychoactive substance abuse <u>with intoxication</u>

> **F19.120   Other psychoactive substance abuse with intoxication,** <u>uncomplicated</u>

> cc **F19.121   Other psychoactive substance abuse with intoxication** <u>delirium</u>

> **F19.122   Other psychoactive substance abuse with intoxication** <u>with perceptual disturbances</u>

> **F19.129   Other psychoactive substance abuse with intoxication, unspecified**

F19.14   Other psychoactive substance abuse <u>with</u> psychoactive substance-induced mood disorder
> Other (or unknown) substance use disorder, mild, with other (or unknown) substance-induced bipolar or related disorder
> Other (or unknown) substance use disorder, mild, with other (or unknown) substance-induced depressive disorder

F19.15-   Other psychoactive substance abuse <u>with</u> psychoactive substance-induced <u>psychotic</u> disorder

> cc **F19.150   Other psychoactive substance abuse with psychoactive substance-induced psychotic disorder** <u>with delusions</u>

> cc **F19.151   Other psychoactive substance abuse with psychoactive substance-induced psychotic disorder** <u>with hallucinations</u>

> **F19.159   Other psychoactive substance abuse with psychoactive substance-induced psychotic disorder, unspecified**

F19.16   Other psychoactive substance abuse <u>with</u> psychoactive substance-induced <u>persisting amnestic</u> disorder

cc **F19.17   Other psychoactive substance abuse** <u>with</u> psychoactive substance-induced <u>persisting dementia</u>
> Other (or unknown) substance use disorder, mild, with other (or unknown) substance-induced major neurocognitive disorder

F19.18-   Other psychoactive substance abuse <u>with</u> <u>other</u> psychoactive substance-induced disorders

> **F19.180   Other psychoactive substance abuse with psychoactive substance-induced** <u>anxiety</u> disorder

> **F19.181   Other psychoactive substance abuse** <u>with</u> psychoactive substance-induced <u>sexual dysfunction</u>

> **F19.182   Other psychoactive substance abuse** <u>with</u> psychoactive substance-induced <u>sleep</u> disorder

> **F19.188   Other psychoactive substance abuse with other psychoactive substance-induced disorder**
> > Other (or unknown) substance use disorder, mild, with other (or unknown) substance-induced mild neurocognitive disorder
> > Other (or unknown) substance use disorder, mild, with other (or unknown) substance-induced obsessive-compulsive or related disorder

F19.19   Other psychoactive substance abuse with unspecified psychoactive substance-induced disorder

F19.2-   Other psychoactive substance <u>dependence</u>
> *Excludes 1:*   *other psychoactive substance abuse (F19.1-)*
> *other psychoactive substance use, unspecified (F19.9-)*

cc **F19.20   Other psychoactive substance dependence,** <u>uncomplicated</u>
> Other (or unknown) substance use disorder, moderate
> Other (or unknown) substance use disorder, severe

F19.21   Other psychoactive substance dependence, <u>in remission</u>

F18 - F19

Excludes 1: = NOT CODED HERE! (Do not code both)   **641**   *Excludes* ❷: = Not Included Here

F19-F19

F19.22- Other psychoactive substance dependence <u>with intoxication</u>

Excludes 1: *other psychoactive substance dependence with withdrawal (F19.23-)*

F19.220 Other psychoactive substance dependence with intoxication, <u>uncomplicated</u>

cc F19.221 Other psychoactive substance dependence with intoxication <u>delirium</u>

cc F19.222 Other psychoactive substance dependence with intoxication <u>with perceptual disturbance</u>

F19.229 Other psychoactive substance dependence with intoxication, <u>unspecified</u>

F19.23- Other psychoactive substance dependence <u>with withdrawal</u>

Excludes 1: *other psychoactive substance dependence with intoxication (F19.22-)*

cc F19.230 Other psychoactive substance dependence with withdrawal, <u>uncomplicated</u>

cc F19.231 Other psychoactive substance dependence with withdrawal <u>delirium</u>

cc F19.232 Other psychoactive substance dependence with withdrawal <u>with perceptual disturbance</u>

cc F19.239 Other psychoactive substance dependence with withdrawal, <u>unspecified</u>

F19.24 Other psychoactive substance dependence <u>with</u> psychoactive substance-induced <u>mood</u> disorder

Other (or unknown) substance use disorder, moderate, with other (or unknown) substance-induced bipolar or related disorder

Other (or unknown) substance use disorder, moderate, with other (or unknown) substance-induced depressive disorder

Other (or unknown) substance use disorder, severe, with other (or unknown) substance-induced bipolar or related disorder

Other (or unknown) substance use disorder, severe, with other (or unknown) substance-induced depressive disorder

F19.25- Other psychoactive substance dependence <u>with</u> psychoactive substance-induced <u>psychotic</u> disorder

cc F19.250 Other psychoactive substance dependence with psychoactive substance-induced psychotic disorder <u>with delusions</u>

cc F19.251 Other psychoactive substance dependence with psychoactive substance-induced psychotic disorder <u>with hallucinations</u>

cc F19.259 Other psychoactive substance dependence with psychoactive substance-induced psychotic disorder, unspecified

cc **F19.26** Other psychoactive substance dependence <u>with</u> psychoactive substance-induced <u>persisting amnestic</u> disorder

cc **F19.27** Other psychoactive substance dependence <u>with</u> psychoactive substance-induced <u>persisting dementia</u>

Other (or unknown) substance use disorder, moderate, with other (or unknown) substance-induced major neurocognitive disorder

Other (or unknown) substance use disorder, severe, with other (or unknown) substance-induced major neurocognitive disorder

F19.28- Other psychoactive substance dependence <u>with other</u> psychoactive substance-induced disorders

cc F19.280 Other psychoactive substance dependence with psychoactive substance-induced <u>anxiety</u> disorder

cc F19.281 Other psychoactive substance dependence with psychoactive substance-induced <u>sexual dysfunction</u>

cc F19.282 Other psychoactive substance dependence with psychoactive substance-induced <u>sleep</u> disorder

cc F19.288 Other psychoactive substance dependence with other psychoactive substance-induced disorder

Other (or unknown) substance use disorder, moderate, with other (or unknown) substance-induced mild neurocognitive disorder

Other (or unknown) substance use disorder, severe, with other (or unknown) substance-induced mild neurocognitive disorder

Other (or unknown) substance use disorder, moderate, with other (or unknown) substance-induced obsessive-compulsive or related disorder

Other (or unknown) substance use disorder, severe, with other (or unknown) substance-induced obsessive-compulsive or related disorder

F19.29 Other psychoactive substance dependence with unspecified psychoactive substance-induced disorder

F19.9- Other psychoactive substance <u>use, unspecified</u>

Excludes 1: *other psychoactive substance abuse (F19.1-)*
other psychoactive substance dependence (F19.2-)

F19.90 Other psychoactive substance use, unspecified, <u>uncomplicated</u>

F19.92- Other psychoactive substance use, unspecified <u>with intoxication</u>

Excludes 1: *other psychoactive substance use, unspecified with withdrawal (F19.93)*

F19.920 Other psychoactive substance use, unspecified with intoxication, <u>uncomplicated</u>

cc F19.921 Other psychoactive substance use, unspecified with intoxication <u>with delirium</u>

Other (or unknown) substance-induced delirium

F19.922 Other psychoactive substance use, unspecified with intoxication <u>with perceptual disturbance</u>

F19.929 Other psychoactive substance use, unspecified with intoxication, <u>unspecified</u>

F19.93- Other psychoactive substance use, unspecified <u>with withdrawal</u>

Excludes 1: *other psychoactive substance use, unspecified with intoxication (F19.92-)*

cc F19.930 Other psychoactive substance use, unspecified with withdrawal, <u>uncomplicated</u>

cc F19.931 Other psychoactive substance use, unspecified with withdrawal <u>delirium</u>

cc F19.932 Other psychoactive substance use, unspecified with withdrawal <u>with perceptual disturbance</u>

cc F19.939 Other psychoactive substance use, unspecified with withdrawal, <u>unspecified</u>

F19.94 Other psychoactive substance use, unspecified <u>with</u> psychoactive substance-induced <u>mood</u> disorder

Other (or unknown) substance-induced bipolar or related disorder, without use disorder

Other (or unknown) substance-induced depressive disorder, without use disorder

F19.95- Other psychoactive substance use, unspecified <u>with</u> psychoactive substance-induced <u>psychotic</u> disorder

cc F19.950 Other psychoactive substance use, unspecified with psychoactive substance-induced psychotic disorder <u>with delusions</u>

cc F19.951 Other psychoactive substance use, unspecified with psychoactive substance-induced psychotic disorder <u>with hallucinations</u>

F19.959 Other psychoactive substance use, unspecified with psychoactive substance-induced psychotic disorder, unspecified

Other (or unknown) substance-induced psychotic disorder, without use disorder

F19.96 Other psychoactive substance use, unspecified <u>with</u> psychoactive substance-induced <u>persisting amnestic</u> disorder

cc **F19.97** Other psychoactive substance use, unspecified <u>with</u> psychoactive substance-induced <u>persisting dementia</u>

Other (or unknown) substance-induced major neurocognitive disorder, without use disorder

F19.98- Other psychoactive substance use, unspecified <u>with</u> <u>other</u> psychoactive substance-induced disorders

F19.980 Other psychoactive substance use, unspecified <u>with</u> psychoactive substance-induced <u>anxiety</u> disorder
Other (or unknown) substance-induced anxiety disorder, without use disorder

F19.981 Other psychoactive substance use, unspecified <u>with</u> psychoactive substance-induced <u>sexual dysfunction</u>
Other (or unknown) substance-induced sexual dysfunction, without use disorder

F19.982 Other psychoactive substance use, unspecified <u>with</u> psychoactive substance-induced <u>sleep</u> disorder
Other (or unknown) substance-induced sleep disorder, without use disorder

F19.988 Other psychoactive substance use, unspecified with other psychoactive substance-induced disorder
Other (or unknown) substance-induced mild neurocognitive disorder, without use disorder
Other (or unknown) substance-induced obsessive-compulsive or related disorder, without use disorder

F19.99 Other psychoactive substance use, unspecified with unspecified psychoactive substance-induced disorder

Schizophrenia, schizotypal, delusional, and other non-mood psychotic disorders (F20-F29)

F20- <u>Schizophrenia</u>
Excludes 1: brief psychotic disorder (F23)
cyclic schizophrenia (F25.0)
mood [affective] disorders with psychotic symptoms (F30.2, F31.2, F31.5, F31.64, F32.3, F33.3)
schizoaffective disorder (F25.-)
schizophrenic reaction NOS (F23)
Excludes ❷: schizophrenic reaction in:
alcoholism (F10.15-, F10.25-, F10.95-)
brain disease (F06.2)
epilepsy (F06.2)
psychoactive drug use (F11-F19 with .15, .25, .95)
schizotypal disorder (F21)

CC **F20.0** Paranoid schizophrenia
Paraphrenic schizophrenia
Excludes 1: involutional paranoid state (F22)
paranoia (F22)

CC **F20.1** Disorganized schizophrenia
Hebephrenic schizophrenia
Hebephrenia

CC **F20.2** Catatonic schizophrenia
Schizophrenic catalepsy
Schizophrenic catatonia
Schizophrenic flexibilitas cerea
Excludes 1: catatonic stupor (R40.1)

F20.3 Undifferentiated schizophrenia
Atypical schizophrenia
Excludes 1: acute schizophrenia-like psychotic disorder (F23)
Excludes ❷: post-schizophrenic depression (F32.89)

CC **F20.5** Residual schizophrenia
Restzustand (schizophrenic)
Schizophrenic residual state

F20.8- Other schizophrenia

CC **F20.81** Schizophreniform disorder
Schizophreniform psychosis NOS

CC **F20.89** Other schizophrenia
Cenesthopathic schizophrenia
Simple schizophrenia

F20.9 Schizophrenia, unspecified

F21 <u>Schizotypal</u> disorder
Borderline schizophrenia
Latent schizophrenia
Latent schizophrenic reaction
Prepsychotic schizophrenia
Prodromal schizophrenia
Pseudoneurotic schizophrenia
Pseudopsychopathic schizophrenia
Schizotypal personality disorder
Excludes ❷: Asperger's syndrome (F84.5)
schizoid personality disorder (F60.1)

F22 Delusional disorders
Delusional dysmorphophobia
Involutional paranoid state
Paranoia
Paranoia querulans
Paranoid psychosis
Paranoid state
Paraphrenia (late)
Sensitiver Beziehungswahn
Excludes 1: mood [affective] disorders with psychotic symptoms (F30.2, F31.2, F31.5, F31.64, F32.3, F33.3)
paranoid schizophrenia (F20.0)
Excludes ❷: paranoid personality disorder (F60.0)
paranoid psychosis, psychogenic (F23)
paranoid reaction (F23)

F23 <u>Brief</u> psychotic disorder
CC Paranoid reaction
Psychogenic paranoid psychosis
Excludes ❷: mood [affective] disorders with psychotic symptoms (F30.2, F31.2, F31.5, F31.64, F32.3, F33.3)

F24 <u>Shared</u> psychotic disorder
Folie à deux
Induced paranoid disorder
Induced psychotic disorder

F25- <u>Schizoaffective</u> disorders
Excludes 1: mood [affective] disorders with psychotic symptoms (F30.2, F31.2, F31.5, F31.64, F32.3, F33.3)
schizophrenia (F20.-)

F25.0 Schizoaffective disorder, <u>bipolar</u> type
Cyclic schizophrenia
Schizoaffective disorder, manic type
Schizoaffective disorder, mixed type
Schizoaffective psychosis, bipolar type
Schizophreniform psychosis, manic type

F25.1 Schizoaffective disorder, <u>depressive</u> type
Schizoaffective psychosis, depressive type
Schizophreniform psychosis, depressive type

F25.8 Other schizoaffective disorders

F25.9 Schizoaffective disorder, unspecified
Schizoaffective psychosis NOS

F28 Other psychotic disorder <u>not</u> due to a substance or known physiological condition
Chronic hallucinatory psychosis

F29 Unspecified psychosis <u>not</u> due to a substance or known physiological condition
Psychosis NOS
Excludes 1: mental disorder NOS (F99)
unspecified mental disorder due to known physiological condition (F09)

Mood [affective] disorders (F30-F39)

F30- <u>Manic episode</u>
Includes: Bipolar disorder, single manic episode
Mixed affective episode
Excludes 1: bipolar disorder (F31.-)
major depressive disorder, single episode (F32.-)
major depressive disorder, recurrent (F33.-)

F30.1- Manic episode <u>without</u> psychotic symptoms

CC **F30.10** Manic episode without psychotic symptoms, unspecified

CC **F30.11** Manic episode without psychotic symptoms, <u>mild</u>

CC **F30.12** Manic episode without psychotic symptoms, <u>moderate</u>

CC **F30.13** Manic episode, severe, without psychotic symptoms

CC **F30.2** Manic episode, severe <u>with psychotic symptoms</u>
Manic stupor
Mania with mood-congruent psychotic symptoms
Mania with mood-incongruent psychotic symptoms

F30.3 Manic episode in <u>partial</u> remission

F30.4 Manic episode in <u>full</u> remission

F30.8 Other manic episodes
Hypomania

CC **F30.9** Manic episode, unspecified
Mania NOS

F
1
9
-
F
3
0

F31-   Bipolar disorder
  Includes: Manic-depressive illness
             Manic-depressive psychosis
             Manic-depressive reaction
  Excludes 1:   bipolar disorder, single manic episode (F30.-)
             major depressive disorder, single episode (F32.-)
             major depressive disorder, recurrent (F33.-)
  Excludes ❷: cyclothymia (F34.0)

cc **F31.0   Bipolar disorder, current episode hypomanic**

F31.1-   Bipolar disorder, current episode manic without psychotic features

cc **F31.10   Bipolar disorder, current episode manic without psychotic features, unspecified**

cc **F31.11   Bipolar disorder, current episode manic without psychotic features, mild**

cc **F31.12   Bipolar disorder, current episode manic without psychotic features, moderate**

cc **F31.13   Bipolar disorder, current episode manic without psychotic features, severe**

cc **F31.2   Bipolar disorder, current episode manic severe with psychotic features**
             Bipolar disorder, current episode manic with mood-congruent psychotic symptoms
             Bipolar disorder, current episode manic with mood-incongruent psychotic symptoms

F31.3-   Bipolar disorder, current episode depressed, mild or moderate severity

cc **F31.30   Bipolar disorder, current episode depressed, mild or moderate severity, unspecified**

cc **F31.31   Bipolar disorder, current episode depressed, mild**

cc **F31.32   Bipolar disorder, current episode depressed, moderate**

cc **F31.4   Bipolar disorder, current episode depressed, severe, without psychotic features**

cc **F31.5   Bipolar disorder, current episode depressed, severe, with psychotic features**
             Bipolar disorder, current episode depressed with mood-incongruent psychotic symptoms
             Bipolar disorder, current episode depressed with mood-congruent psychotic symptoms

F31.6-   Bipolar disorder, current episode mixed

cc **F31.60   Bipolar disorder, current episode mixed, unspecified**

cc **F31.61   Bipolar disorder, current episode mixed, mild**

cc **F31.62   Bipolar disorder, current episode mixed, moderate**

cc **F31.63   Bipolar disorder, current episode mixed, severe, without psychotic features**

cc **F31.64   Bipolar disorder, current episode mixed, severe, with psychotic features**
             Bipolar disorder, current episode mixed with mood-congruent psychotic symptoms
             Bipolar disorder, current episode mixed with mood-incongruent psychotic symptoms

F31.7-   Bipolar disorder, currently in remission

F31.70   Bipolar disorder, currently in remission, most recent episode unspecified

F31.71   Bipolar disorder, in partial remission, most recent episode hypomanic

F31.72   Bipolar disorder, in full remission, most recent episode hypomanic

F31.73   Bipolar disorder, in partial remission, most recent episode manic

F31.74   Bipolar disorder, in full remission, most recent episode manic

F31.75   Bipolar disorder, in partial remission, most recent episode depressed

F31.76   Bipolar disorder, in full remission, most recent episode depressed

F31.77   Bipolar disorder, in partial remission, most recent episode mixed

F31.78   Bipolar disorder, in full remission, most recent episode mixed

F31.8-   Other bipolar disorders

cc **F31.81   Bipolar II disorder**

cc **F31.89   Other bipolar disorder**
             Recurrent manic episodes NOS

F31.9   Bipolar disorder, unspecified

F32-   Major depressive disorder, single episode
  Includes: Single episode of agitated depression
             Single episode of depressive reaction
             Single episode of major depression
             Single episode of psychogenic depression
             Single episode of reactive depression
             Single episode of vital depression
  Excludes 1:   bipolar disorder (F31.-)
             manic episode (F30.-)
             recurrent depressive disorder (F33.-)
  Excludes ❷: adjustment disorder (F43.2)

cc **F32.0   Major depressive disorder, single episode, mild**

cc **F32.1   Major depressive disorder, single episode, moderate**

cc **F32.2   Major depressive disorder, single episode, severe without psychotic features**

cc **F32.3   Major depressive disorder, single episode, severe with psychotic features**
             Single episode of major depression with mood-congruent psychotic symptoms
             Single episode of major depression with mood-incongruent psychotic symptoms
             Single episode of major depression with psychotic symptoms
             Single episode of psychogenic depressive psychosis
             Single episode of psychotic depression
             Single episode of reactive depressive psychosis

F32.4   Major depressive disorder, single episode, in partial remission

F32.5   Major depressive disorder, single episode, in full remission

F32.8-   Other depressive episodes

F32.81   Premenstrual dysphoric disorder —[♀]
             Excludes 1:   premenstrual tension syndrome (N94.3)

F32.89   Other specified depressive episodes
             Atypical depression
             Post-schizophrenic depression
             Single episode of "masked" depression NOS

F32.9   Major depressive disorder, single episode, unspecified
             AHA 13:4Q:p107 – Chronic depression
             Depression NOS
             Depressive disorder NOS
             Major depression NOS

F33-   Major depressive disorder, recurrent
  Includes: Recurrent episodes of depressive reaction
             Recurrent episodes of endogenous depression
             Recurrent episodes of major depression
             Recurrent episodes of psychogenic depression
             Recurrent episodes of reactive depression
             Recurrent episodes of seasonal depressive disorder
             Recurrent episodes of vital depression
  Excludes 1:   bipolar disorder (F31.-)
             manic episode (F30.-)

cc **F33.0   Major depressive disorder, recurrent, mild**

cc **F33.1   Major depressive disorder, recurrent, moderate**

cc **F33.2   Major depressive disorder, recurrent severe without psychotic features**

cc **F33.3   Major depressive disorder, recurrent, severe with psychotic symptoms**
             Endogenous depression with psychotic symptoms
             Recurrent severe episodes of major depression with mood-congruent psychotic symptoms
             Recurrent severe episodes of major depression with mood-incongruent psychotic symptoms
             Recurrent severe episodes of major depression with psychotic symptoms
             Recurrent severe episodes of psychogenic depressive psychosis
             Recurrent severe episodes of psychotic depression
             Recurrent severe episodes of reactive depressive psychosis

F33.4-   Major depressive disorder, recurrent, in remission

cc **F33.40   Major depressive disorder, recurrent, in remission, unspecified**

F33.41   Major depressive disorder, recurrent, in partial remission

F33.42   Major depressive disorder, recurrent, in full remission

F
3
1
–
F
3
3

Excludes 1: = NOT CODED HERE! (Do not code both)   **644**   *Excludes ❷:* = Not Included Here

cc **F33.8**   **Other recurrent depressive disorders**
Recurrent brief depressive episodes

cc **F33.9**   **Major depressive disorder, recurrent, unspecified**
Monopolar depression NOS

F34-   <u>Persistent mood [affective] disorders</u>

  F34.0   **Cyclothymic disorder**
Affective personality disorder
Cycloid personality
Cyclothymia
Cyclothymic personality

  F34.1   **Dysthymic disorder**
Depressive neurosis
Depressive personality disorder
Dysthymia
Neurotic depression
Persistent anxiety depression
Persistent depressive disorder

Excludes ❷*:*   *anxiety depression (mild or not persistent) (F41.8)*

  F34.8-   **Other persistent mood [affective] disorders**

cc **F34.81**   **Disruptive mood dysregulation disorder**

cc **F34.89**   **Other specified persistent mood disorders**

cc **F34.9**   **Persistent mood [affective] disorder, unspecified**

F39   **Unspecified mood [affective] disorder**
Affective psychosis NOS

Anxiety, dissociative, stress-related, somatoform and other nonpsychotic mental disorders (F40-F48)

F40-   <u>Phobic anxiety</u> **disorders**

  F40.0-   <u>Agoraphobia</u>

    F40.00   **Agoraphobia, unspecified**

    F40.01   **Agoraphobia <u>with panic disorder</u>**
Panic disorder with agoraphobia

Excludes 1:   *panic disorder without agoraphobia (F41.0)*

    F40.02   **Agoraphobia <u>without</u> panic disorder**

  F40.1-   <u>Social phobias</u>
Anthropophobia
Social anxiety disorder of childhood
Social neurosis

    F40.10   **Social phobia, unspecified**

    F40.11   **Social phobia, generalized**

  F40.2-   <u>Specific (isolated) phobias</u>

Excludes ❷*:*   *dysmorphophobia (nondelusional) (F45.22)*
nosophobia (F45.22)

    F40.21-   <u>Animal</u> **type phobia**

      F40.210   **Arachnophobia**
Fear of spiders

      F40.218   **Other animal type phobia**

    F40.22-   <u>Natural environment</u> **type phobia**

      F40.220   **Fear of thunderstorms**

      F40.228   **Other natural environment type phobia**

    F40.23-   **Blood, injection, injury type phobia**

      F40.230   **Fear of blood**

      F40.231   **Fear of injections and transfusions**

      F40.232   **Fear of other medical care**

      F40.233   **Fear of injury**

    F40.24-   <u>Situational type</u> **phobia**

      F40.240   **Claustrophobia**

      F40.241   **Acrophobia**

      F40.242   **Fear of bridges**

      F40.243   **Fear of flying**

      F40.248   **Other situational type phobia**

    F40.29-   <u>Other specified</u> **phobia**

      F40.290   **Androphobia**
Fear of men

      F40.291   **Gynephobia**
Fear of women

      F40.298   **Other specified phobia**

  F40.8   **Other phobic anxiety disorders**
Phobic anxiety disorder of childhood

F40.9   **Phobic anxiety disorder, unspecified**
Phobia NOS
Phobic state NOS

F41-   <u>Other anxiety disorders</u>

Excludes ❷*:*   *anxiety in:*
acute stress reaction (F43.0)
transient adjustment reaction (F43.2)
neurasthenia (F48.8)
psychophysiologic disorders (F45.-)
separation anxiety (F93.0)

  F41.0   <u>Panic</u> **disorder [episodic paroxysmal anxiety] without agoraphobia**
Panic attack
Panic state

Excludes 1:   *panic disorder with agoraphobia (F40.01)*

  F41.1   <u>Generalized</u> **anxiety disorder**
Anxiety neurosis
Anxiety reaction
Anxiety state
Overanxious disorder

Excludes ❷*:*   *neurasthenia (F48.8)*

  F41.3   **Other <u>mixed</u> anxiety disorders**

  F41.8   **Other specified anxiety disorders**
Anxiety depression (mild or not persistent)
Anxiety hysteria
Mixed anxiety and depressive disorder

  F41.9   **Anxiety disorder, unspecified**
Anxiety NOS

F42-   <u>Obsessive-compulsive disorder</u>

Excludes ❷*:*   *obsessive-compulsive personality (disorder) (F60.5)*
obsessive-compulsive symptoms occurring in depression (F32-F33)
obsessive-compulsive symptoms occurring in schizophrenia (F20.-)

  F42.2   **Mixed obsessional thoughts and acts**

  F42.3   **Hoarding disorder**

  F42.4   **Excoriation (skin-picking) disorder**

Excludes 1:   *factitial dermatitis (L98.1)*
other specified behavioral and emotional disorders with onset usually occurring in early childhood and adolescence (F98.8)

  F42.8   **Other obsessive-compulsive disorder**
Anancastic neurosis
Obsessive-compulsive neurosis

  F42.9   **Obsessive-compulsive disorder, unspecified**

F43-   **Reaction to severe stress, and adjustment disorders**

  F43.0   **Acute stress reaction**
Acute crisis reaction
Acute reaction to stress
Combat and operational stress reaction
Combat fatigue
Crisis state
Psychic shock

  F43.1-   **Post-traumatic stress disorder (PTSD)**
Traumatic neurosis

    F43.10   **Post-traumatic stress disorder, unspecified**

    F43.11   **Post-traumatic stress disorder, acute**

    F43.12   **Post-traumatic stress disorder, chronic**

  F43.2-   <u>Adjustment disorders</u>
Culture shock
Grief reaction
Hospitalism in children

Excludes ❷*:*   *separation anxiety disorder of childhood (F93.0)*

    F43.20   **Adjustment disorder, unspecified**

    F43.21   **Adjustment disorder <u>with depressed mood</u>**
AHA 14:1Q:p25 – Complicated bereavement

    F43.22   **Adjustment disorder <u>with anxiety</u>**

    F43.23   **Adjustment disorder <u>with mixed anxiety and depressed mood</u>**

    F43.24   **Adjustment disorder <u>with disturbance of conduct</u>**

    F43.25   **Adjustment disorder <u>with mixed disturbance of emotions and conduct</u>**

    F43.29   **Adjustment disorder <u>with other symptoms</u>**

F33 - F43

Excludes 1: = NOT CODED HERE! (Do not code both)   **645**   *Excludes* ❷*:* = Not Included Here

F43.8 **Other reactions to severe stress**
Other specified trauma and stressor-related disorder

F43.9 **Reaction to severe stress, unspecified**
Trauma and stressor-related disorder, NOS

F44- **Dissociative and conversion disorders**
Includes: Conversion hysteria
Conversion reaction
Hysteria
Hysterical psychosis
Excludes ❷: malingering [conscious simulation] (Z76.5)

F44.0 **Dissociative amnesia**
Excludes 1: amnesia NOS (R41.3)
anterograde amnesia (R41.1)
dissociative amnesia with dissociative fugue (F44.1)
retrograde amnesia (R41.2)
Excludes ❷: alcohol-or other psychoactive substance-induced amnestic disorder (F10, F13, F19 with .26, .96)
amnestic disorder due to known physiological condition (F04)
postictal amnesia in epilepsy (G40.-)

F44.1 **Dissociative fugue**
Dissociative amnesia with dissociative fugue
Excludes ❷: postictal fugue in epilepsy (G40.-)

F44.2 **Dissociative stupor**
Excludes 1: catatonic stupor (R40.1)
stupor NOS (R40.1)
Excludes ❷: catatonic disorder due to known physiological condition (F06.1)
depressive stupor (F32, F33)
manic stupor (F30, F31)

F44.4 **Conversion disorder with motor symptom or deficit**
Dissociative motor disorders
Psychogenic aphonia
Psychogenic dysphonia

F44.5 **Conversion disorder with seizures or convulsions**
Dissociative convulsions

F44.6 **Conversion disorder with sensory symptom or deficit**
Dissociative anesthesia and sensory loss
Psychogenic deafness

F44.7 **Conversion disorder with mixed symptom presentation**

F44.8- **Other dissociative and conversion disorders**

F44.81 **Dissociative identity disorder**
Multiple personality disorder

F44.89 **Other dissociative and conversion disorders**
Ganser's syndrome
Psychogenic confusion
Psychogenic twilight state
Trance and possession disorders

F44.9 **Dissociative and conversion disorder, unspecified**
Dissociative disorder NOS

F45- **Somatoform disorders**
Excludes ❷: dissociative and conversion disorders (F44.-)
factitious disorders (F68.1-)
hair-plucking (F63.3)
lalling (F80.0)
lisping (F80.0)
malingering [conscious simulation] (Z76.5)
nail-biting (F98.8)
psychological or behavioral factors associated with disorders or diseases classified elsewhere (F54)
sexual dysfunction, not due to a substance or known physiological condition (F52.-)
thumb-sucking (F98.8)
tic disorders (in childhood and adolescence) (F95.-)
Tourette's syndrome (F95.2)
trichotillomania (F63.3)

F45.0 **Somatization disorder**
Briquet's disorder
Multiple psychosomatic disorder

F45.1 **Undifferentiated somatoform disorder**
Somatic symptom disorder
Undifferentiated psychosomatic disorder

F45.2- **Hypochondriacal disorders**
Excludes ❷: delusional dysmorphophobia (F22)
fixed delusions about bodily functions or shape (F22)

F45.20 **Hypochondriacal disorder, unspecified**

F45.21 **Hypochondriasis**
Hypochondriacal neurosis
Illness anxiety disorder

F45.22 **Body dysmorphic disorder**
Dysmorphophobia (nondelusional)
Nosophobia

F45.29 **Other hypochondriacal disorders**

F45.4- **Pain disorders related to psychological factors**
Excludes 1: pain NOS (R52)

F45.41 **Pain disorder exclusively related to psychological factors**
Somatoform pain disorder (persistent)

F45.42 **Pain disorder with related psychological factors**
Code also associated acute or chronic pain (G89.-)

F45.8 **Other somatoform disorders**
Psychogenic dysmenorrhea
Psychogenic dysphagia, including "globus hystericus"
Psychogenic pruritus
Psychogenic torticollis
Somatoform autonomic dysfunction
Teeth grinding
Excludes 1: sleep related teeth grinding (G47.63)

F45.9 **Somatoform disorder, unspecified**
Psychosomatic disorder NOS

F48- **Other nonpsychotic mental disorders**

F48.1 **Depersonalization-derealization syndrome**

F48.2 **Pseudobulbar affect**
Involuntary emotional expression disorder
Code first underlying cause, if known, such as:
Amyotrophic lateral sclerosis (G12.21)
Multiple sclerosis (G35)
Sequelae of cerebrovascular disease (I69-)
Sequelae of traumatic intracranial injury (S06-)

F48.8 **Other specified nonpsychotic mental disorders**
Dhat syndrome
Neurasthenia
Occupational neurosis, including writer's cramp
Psychasthenia
Psychasthenic neurosis
Psychogenic syncope

F48.9 **Nonpsychotic mental disorder, unspecified**
Neurosis NOS

Behavioral syndromes associated with physiological disturbances and physical factors (F50-F59)

F50- **Eating disorders**
Excludes 1: anorexia NOS (R63.0)
feeding difficulties (R63.3)
polyphagia (R63.2)
Excludes ❷: feeding disorder in infancy or childhood (F98.2-)

F50.0- **Anorexia nervosa**
Excludes 1: loss of appetite (R63.0)
psychogenic loss of appetite (F50.89)

CC **F50.00** Anorexia nervosa, unspecified

CC **F50.01** Anorexia nervosa, restricting type

CC **F50.02** Anorexia nervosa, binge eating/purging type
Excludes 1: bulimia nervosa (F50.2)

CC **F50.2** **Bulimia nervosa**
Bulimia NOS
Hyperorexia nervosa
Excludes 1: anorexia nervosa, binge eating/purging type (F50.02)

F50.8- **Other eating disorders**
Excludes ❷: pica of infancy and childhood (F98.3)

F50.81 **Binge eating disorder**

F50.89 **Other specified eating disorder**
Pica in adults
Psychogenic loss of appetite

F50.9 **Eating disorder, unspecified**
Atypical anorexia nervosa
Atypical bulimia nervosa

F43-F50

F51- Sleep disorders not due to a substance or known physiological condition

Excludes ❷: *organic sleep disorders (G47.-)*

F51.0- Insomnia not due to a substance or known physiological condition

Excludes ❷: *alcohol related insomnia (F10.182, F10.282, F10.982),*
drug-related insomnia (F11.182, F11.282, F11.982,
F13.182, F13.282, F13.982, F14.182, F14.282,
F14.982, F15.182, F15.282, F15.982, F19.182,
F19.282, F19.982)
insomnia NOS (G47.0-)
insomnia due to known physiological condition
(G47.0-)
organic insomnia (G47.0-)
sleep deprivation (Z72.820)

F51.01 Primary insomnia
Idiopathic insomnia

F51.02 Adjustment insomnia

F51.03 Paradoxical insomnia

F51.04 Psychophysiologic insomnia

F51.05 Insomnia due to other mental disorder
Code also associated mental disorder

F51.09 Other insomnia not due to a substance or known physiological condition

F51.1- Hypersomnia not due to a substance or known physiological condition

Excludes ❷: *alcohol related hypersomnia (F10.182, F10.282,*
F10.982)
drug-related hypersomnia (F11.182, F11.282, F11.982,
F13.182, F13.282, F13.982, F14.182, F14.282,
F14.982, F15.182, F15.282, F15.982, F19.182,
F19.282, F19.982)
hypersomnia NOS (G47.10)
hypersomnia due to known physiological condition
(G47.10)
idiopathic hypersomnia (G47.11, G47.12)
narcolepsy (G47.4-)

F51.11 Primary hypersomnia

F51.12 Insufficient sleep syndrome
Excludes 1: *sleep deprivation (Z72.820)*

F51.13 Hypersomnia due to other mental disorder
Code also associated mental disorder

F51.19 Other hypersomnia not due to a substance or known physiological condition

F51.3 Sleepwalking [somnambulism]

F51.4 Sleep terrors [night terrors]

F51.5 Nightmare disorder
Dream anxiety disorder

F51.8 Other sleep disorders not due to a substance or known physiological condition

F51.9 Sleep disorder not due to a substance or known physiological condition, unspecified
Emotional sleep disorder NOS

F52- Sexual dysfunction not due to a substance or known physiological condition

Excludes ❷: *Dhat syndrome (F48.8)*

F52.0 Hypoactive sexual desire disorder
Lack or loss of sexual desire
Sexual anhedonia
Excludes 1: *decreased libido (R68.82)*

F52.1 Sexual aversion disorder
Sexual aversion and lack of sexual enjoyment

F52.2- Sexual arousal disorders
Failure of genital response

F52.21 Male erectile disorder — [♂]
Psychogenic impotence
Excludes 1: *impotence of organic origin (N52.-)*
impotence NOS (N52.-)

F52.22 Female sexual arousal disorder — [♀]

F52.3- Orgasmic disorder
Inhibited orgasm
Psychogenic anorgasmy

F52.31 Female orgasmic disorder — [♀]

F52.32 Male orgasmic disorder — [♂]
Delayed ejaculation

F52.4 Premature ejaculation — [♂]

F52.5 Vaginismus not due to a substance or known physiological condition — [♀]
Psychogenic vaginismus
Excludes ❷: *vaginismus (due to a known physiological condition)*
(N94.2)

F52.6 Dyspareunia not due to a substance or known physiological condition — [♀]
Genito-pelvic pain penetration disorder
Psychogenic dyspareunia
Excludes ❷: *dyspareunia (due to a known physiological condition)*
(N94.1-)

F52.8 Other sexual dysfunction not due to a substance or known physiological condition
Excessive sexual drive
Nymphomania
Satyriasis

F52.9 Unspecified sexual dysfunction not due to a substance or known physiological condition — [Unacceptable PDX]
Sexual dysfunction NOS

F53 Puerperal psychosis — [♀, Age/12-55]
Postpartum depression
Excludes 1: *mood disorders with psychotic features (F30.2, F31.2, F31.5,*
F31.64, F32.3, F33.3)
postpartum dysphoria (O90.6)
psychosis in schizophrenia, schizotypal, delusional, and other
psychotic disorders (F20-F29)

F54 Psychological and behavioral factors associated with disorders or diseases classified elsewhere — [Not Allowed as PDX]
Psychological factors affecting physical conditions
Code first the associated physical disorder, such as:
Asthma (J45.-)
Dermatitis (L23-L25)
Gastric ulcer (K25.-)
Mucous colitis (K58.-)
Ulcerative colitis (K51.-)
Urticaria (L50.-)
Excludes ❷: *tension-type headache (G44.2)*

F55- Abuse of non-psychoactive substances
Excludes ❷: *abuse of psychoactive substances (F10-F19)*

F55.0 Abuse of antacids

F55.1 Abuse of herbal or folk remedies

F55.2 Abuse of laxatives

F55.3 Abuse of steroids or hormones

F55.4 Abuse of vitamins

F55.8 Abuse of other non-psychoactive substances

F59 Unspecified behavioral syndromes associated with physiological disturbances and physical factors
Psychogenic physiological dysfunction NOS

Disorders of adult personality and behavior (F60-F69)

F60- Specific personality disorders

F60.0 Paranoid personality disorder
Expansive paranoid personality (disorder)
Fanatic personality (disorder)
Querulant personality (disorder)
Paranoid personality (disorder)
Sensitive paranoid personality (disorder)
Excludes ❷: *paranoia (F22)*
paranoia querulans (F22)
paranoid psychosis (F22)
paranoid schizophrenia (F20.0)
paranoid state (F22)

F60.1 Schizoid personality disorder
Excludes ❷: *Asperger's syndrome (F84.5)*
delusional disorder (F22)
schizoid disorder of childhood (F84.5)
schizophrenia (F20.-)
schizotypal disorder (F21)

F 5 1 I F 6 0

Excludes 1: = NOT CODED HERE! (Do not code both)   647   Excludes ❷: = Not Included Here

F60.2 Antisocial personality disorder
Amoral personality (disorder)
Asocial personality (disorder)
Dissocial personality disorder
Psychopathic personality (disorder)
Sociopathic personality (disorder)
Excludes 1: *conduct disorders (F91.-)*
Excludes ❷: *borderline personality disorder (F60.3)*

F60.3 Borderline personality disorder
Aggressive personality (disorder)
Emotionally unstable personality disorder
Explosive personality (disorder)
Excludes ❷: *antisocial personality disorder (F60.2)*

F60.4 Histrionic personality disorder
Hysterical personality (disorder)
Psychoinfantile personality (disorder)

F60.5 Obsessive-compulsive personality disorder
Anankastic personality (disorder)
Compulsive personality (disorder)
Obsessional personality (disorder)
Excludes ❷: *obsessive-compulsive disorder (F42.-)*

F60.6 Avoidant personality disorder
Anxious personality disorder

F60.7 Dependent personality disorder
Asthenic personality (disorder)
Inadequate personality (disorder)
Passive personality (disorder)

F60.8- Other specific personality disorders
F60.81 Narcissistic personality disorder
F60.89 Other specific personality disorders
Eccentric personality disorder
"Haltlose" type personality disorder
Immature personality disorder
Passive-aggressive personality disorder
Psychoneurotic personality disorder
Self-defeating personality disorder

F60.9 Personality disorder, unspecified
Character disorder NOS
Character neurosis NOS
Pathological personality NOS

F63- Impulse disorders
Excludes ❷: *habitual excessive use of alcohol or psychoactive substances (F10-F19)*
impulse disorders involving sexual behavior (F65.-)

F63.0 Pathological gambling
Compulsive gambling
Excludes 1: *gambling and betting NOS (Z72.6)*
Excludes ❷: *excessive gambling by manic patients (F30, F31)*
gambling in antisocial personality disorder (F60.2)

F63.1 Pyromania
Pathological fire-setting
Excludes ❷: *fire-setting (by) (in):*
adult with antisocial personality disorder (F60.2)
alcohol or psychoactive substance intoxication (F10-F19)
conduct disorders (F91.-)
mental disorders due to known physiological condition (F01-F09)
schizophrenia (F20.-)

F63.2 Kleptomania
Pathological stealing
Excludes 1: *shoplifting as the reason for observation for suspected mental disorder (Z03.8)*
Excludes ❷: *depressive disorder with stealing (F31-F33)*
stealing due to underlying mental condition-code to mental condition
stealing in mental disorders due to known physiological condition (F01-F09)

F63.3 Trichotillomania
Hair plucking
Excludes ❷: *other stereotyped movement disorder (F98.4)*

F63.8- Other impulse disorders
F63.81 Intermittent explosive disorder
F63.89 Other impulse disorders

F63.9 Impulse disorder, unspecified
Impulse control disorder NOS

F64- Gender identity disorders
F64.0 Transsexualism
Gender identity disorder in adolescence and adulthood
Gender dysphoria in adolescence and adults

F64.1 Dual role transvestism
Use additional code to identify sex reassignment status (Z87.890)
Excludes 1: *gender identity disorder in childhood (F64.2)*
Excludes ❷: *fetishistic transvestism (F65.1)*

F64.2 Gender identity disorder of childhood — [Age/0-17]
Gender dysphoria in children
Excludes 1: *gender identity disorder in adolescence and adulthood (F64.0)*
Excludes ❷: *sexual maturation disorder (F66)*

F64.8 Other gender identity disorders

F64.9 Gender identity disorder, unspecified
Gender-role disorder NOS

F65- Paraphilias
F65.0 Fetishism
F65.1 Transvestic fetishism
Fetishistic transvestism
F65.2 Exhibitionism
F65.3 Voyeurism
F65.4 Pedophilia
F65.5- Sadomasochism
F65.50 Sadomasochism, unspecified
F65.51 Sexual masochism
F65.52 Sexual sadism
F65.8- Other paraphilias
F65.81 Frotteurism
F65.89 Other paraphilias
Necrophilia
F65.9 Paraphilia, unspecified
Sexual deviation NOS

F66 Other sexual disorders
Sexual maturation disorder
Sexual relationship disorder

F68- Other disorders of adult personality and behavior
F68.1- Factitious disorder
Compensation neurosis
Elaboration of physical symptoms for psychological reasons
Hospital hopper syndrome
Münchausen's syndrome
Peregrinating patient
Excludes ❷: *factitial dermatitis (L98.1)*
person feigning illness (with obvious motivation) (Z76.5)

cc **F68.10 Factitious disorder, unspecified**
F68.11 Factitious disorder with predominantly psychological signs and symptoms
cc **F68.12 Factitious disorder with predominantly physical signs and symptoms**
F68.13 Factitious disorder with combined psychological and physical signs and symptoms
F68.8 Other specified disorders of adult personality and behavior

F69 Unspecified disorder of adult personality and behavior — [Age/15-124]

Intellectual disabilities (F70-F79)

Code first any associated physical or developmental disorders
Excludes 1: *borderline intellectual functioning, IQ above 70 to 84 (R41.83)*

F70 Mild intellectual disabilities
IQ level 50-55 to approximately 70
Mild mental subnormality

F71 Moderate intellectual disabilities
IQ level 35-40 to 50-55
Moderate mental subnormality

F72 Severe intellectual disabilities
cc
IQ 20-25 to 35-40
Severe mental subnormality

F73 Profound intellectual disabilities
cc
IQ level below 20-25
Profound mental subnormality

Excludes 1: = NOT CODED HERE! (Do not code both)

Excludes ❷: = Not Included Here

F60 - F73

F78   Other intellectual disabilities

F79   Unspecified intellectual disabilities
Mental deficiency NOS
Mental subnormality NOS

Pervasive and specific developmental disorders (F80-F89)

F80-   Specific developmental disorders of speech and language

F80.0   Phonological disorder
Dyslalia
Functional speech articulation disorder
Lalling
Lisping
Phonological developmental disorder
Speech articulation developmental disorder
Speech-sound disorder
Excludes 1:   speech articulation impairment due to aphasia NOS (R47.01)
speech articulation impairment due to apraxia (R48.2)
Excludes ❷: speech articulation impairment due to hearing loss (F80.4)
speech articulation impairment due to intellectual disabilities (F70-F79)
speech articulation impairment with expressive language developmental disorder (F80.1)
speech articulation impairment with mixed receptive expressive language developmental disorder (F80.2)

F80.1   Expressive language disorder
Developmental dysphasia or aphasia, expressive type
Excludes 1:   mixed receptive-expressive language disorder (F80.2)
dysphasia and aphasia NOS (R47.-)
Excludes ❷: acquired aphasia with epilepsy [Landau-Kleffner] (G40.80-)
intellectual disabilities (F70-F79)
pervasive developmental disorders (F84.-)
selective mutism (F94.0)

F80.2   Mixed receptive-expressive language disorder
Developmental dysphasia or aphasia, receptive type
Developmental Wernicke's aphasia
Excludes 1:   central auditory processing disorder (H93.25)
dysphasia or aphasia NOS (R47.-)
expressive language disorder (F80.1)
expressive type dysphasia or aphasia (F80.1)
word deafness (H93.25)
Excludes ❷: acquired aphasia with epilepsy [Landau-Kleffner] (G40.80-)
intellectual disabilities (F70-F79)
pervasive developmental disorders (F84.-)
selective mutism (F94.0)

F80.4   Speech and language development delay due to hearing loss
Code also type of hearing loss (H90.-, H91.-)

F80.8-   Other developmental disorders of speech and language

F80.81   Childhood onset fluency disorder
Cluttering NOS
Stuttering NOS
Excludes 1:   adult onset fluency disorder (F98.5)
fluency disorder in conditions classified elsewhere (R47.82)
fluency disorder (stuttering) following cerebrovascular disease (I69. with final characters -23)

F80.82   Social pragmatic communication disorder
Excludes 1:   Asperger's syndrome (F84.5)
autistic disorder (F84.0)

F80.89   Other developmental disorders of speech and language

F80.9   Developmental disorder of speech and language, unspecified
Communication disorder NOS
Language disorder NOS

F81-   Specific developmental disorders of scholastic skills

F81.0   Specific reading disorder
"Backward reading"
Developmental dyslexia
Specific reading retardation
Excludes 1:   alexia NOS (R48.0)
dyslexia NOS (R48.0)

F81.2   Mathematics disorder
Developmental acalculia
Developmental arithmetical disorder
Developmental Gerstmann's syndrome
Excludes 1:   acalculia NOS (R48.8)
Excludes ❷: arithmetical difficulties associated with a reading disorder (F81.0)
arithmetical difficulties associated with a spelling disorder (F81.81)
arithmetical difficulties due to inadequate teaching (Z55.8)

F81.8-   Other developmental disorders of scholastic skills

F81.81   Disorder of written expression
Specific spelling disorder

F81.89   Other developmental disorders of scholastic skills

F81.9   Developmental disorder of scholastic skills, unspecified —
[Unacceptable PDX]
Knowledge acquisition disability NOS
Learning disability NOS
Learning disorder NOS

F82   Specific developmental disorder of motor function
Clumsy child syndrome
Developmental coordination disorder
Developmental dyspraxia
Excludes 1:   abnormalities of gait and mobility (R26.-)
lack of coordination (R27.-)
Excludes ❷: lack of coordination secondary to intellectual disabilities (F70-F79)

F84-   Pervasive developmental disorders
Use additional code to identify any associated medical condition and intellectual disabilities

cc **F84.0   Autistic disorder**
Autism spectrum disorder
Infantile autism
Infantile psychosis
Kanner's syndrome
Excludes 1:   Asperger's syndrome (F84.5)

cc **F84.2   Rett's syndrome**
Excludes 1:   Asperger's syndrome (F84.5)
autistic disorder (F84.0)
other childhood disintegrative disorder (F84.3)

cc **F84.3   Other childhood disintegrative disorder — [Age/0-17]**
Dementia infantilis
Disintegrative psychosis
Heller's syndrome
Symbiotic psychosis
Use additional code to identify any associated neurological condition
Excludes 1:   Asperger's syndrome (F84.5)
autistic disorder (F84.0)
Rett's syndrome (F84.2)

cc **F84.5   Asperger's syndrome**
Asperger's disorder
Autistic psychopathy
Schizoid disorder of childhood

cc **F84.8   Other pervasive developmental disorders**
Overactive disorder associated with intellectual disabilities and stereotyped movements

cc **F84.9   Pervasive developmental disorder, unspecified**
Atypical autism

F88   Other disorders of psychological development
Developmental agnosia
Global developmental delay
Other specified neurodevelopmental disorder

F89   Unspecified disorder of psychological development
Developmental disorder NOS
Neurodevelopmental disorder NOS

F78 – F89

Behavioral and emotional disorders with onset usually occurring in childhood and adolescence (F90-F98)

Note: Codes within categories F90-F98 may be used regardless of the age of a patient. These disorders generally have onset within the childhood or adolescent years, but may continue throughout life or not be diagnosed until adulthood.

F90- **Attention-deficit hyperactivity disorders**
Includes: Attention deficit disorder with hyperactivity
Attention deficit syndrome with hyperactivity
Excludes ❷: anxiety disorders (F40.-, F41.-)
mood [affective] disorders (F30-F39)
pervasive developmental disorders (F84.-)
schizophrenia (F20.-)

F90.0 Attention-deficit hyperactivity disorder, predominantly <u>inattentive</u> type

F90.1 Attention-deficit hyperactivity disorder, predominantly <u>hyperactive</u> type

F90.2 Attention-deficit hyperactivity disorder, <u>combined</u> type

F90.8 Attention-deficit hyperactivity disorder, other type

F90.9 Attention-deficit hyperactivity disorder, unspecified type
Attention-deficit hyperactivity disorder of childhood or adolescence NOS
Attention-deficit hyperactivity disorder NOS

F91- <u>Conduct disorders</u>
Excludes 1: antisocial behavior (Z72.81-)
antisocial personality disorder (F60.2)
Excludes ❷: conduct problems associated with attention-deficit
hyperactivity disorder (F90.-)
mood [affective] disorders (F30-F39)
pervasive developmental disorders (F84.-)
schizophrenia (F20.-)

F91.0 Conduct disorder <u>confined to family context</u>

F91.1 Conduct disorder, <u>childhood-onset</u> type
Unsocialized conduct disorder
Conduct disorder, solitary aggressive type
Unsocialized aggressive disorder

F91.2 Conduct disorder, <u>adolescent-onset</u> type
Socialized conduct disorder
Conduct disorder, group type

F91.3 <u>Oppositional defiant</u> disorder

F91.8 Other conduct disorders
Other specified conduct disorder
Other specified disruptive disorder

F91.9 Conduct disorder, unspecified
Behavioral disorder NOS
Conduct disorder NOS
Disruptive behavior disorder NOS
Disruptive disorder NOS

F93- **Emotional disorders with onset specific to childhood**

F93.0 Separation anxiety disorder of childhood
Excludes ❷: mood [affective] disorders (F30-F39)
nonpsychotic mental disorders (F40-F48)
phobic anxiety disorder of childhood (F40.8)
social phobia (F40.1)

F93.8 Other childhood emotional disorders
Identity disorder
Excludes ❷: gender identity disorder of childhood (F64.2)

F93.9 Childhood emotional disorder, unspecified

F94- **Disorders of social functioning with onset specific to childhood and adolescence**

F94.0 Selective mutism
Elective mutism
Excludes ❷: pervasive developmental disorders (F84.-)
schizophrenia (F20.-)
specific developmental disorders of speech and
language (F80.-)
transient mutism as part of separation anxiety in young
children (F93.0)

F94.1 Reactive attachment disorder of childhood
Use additional code to identify any associated failure to thrive or growth retardation
Excludes 1: disinhibited attachment disorder of childhood (F94.2)
normal variation in pattern of selective attachment
Excludes ❷: Asperger's syndrome (F84.5)
maltreatment syndromes (T74.-)
sexual or physical abuse in childhood, resulting in
psychosocial problems (Z62.81-)

F94.2 Disinhibited attachment disorder of childhood
Affectionless psychopathy
Institutional syndrome
Excludes 1: reactive attachment disorder of childhood (F94.1)
Excludes ❷: Asperger's syndrome (F84.5)
attention-deficit hyperactivity disorders (F90.-)
hospitalism in children (F43.2-)

F94.8 Other childhood disorders of social functioning

F94.9 Childhood disorder of social functioning, unspecified

F95- **Tic disorder**

F95.0 Transient tic disorder
Provisional tic disorder

F95.1 Chronic motor or vocal tic disorder

F95.2 Tourette's disorder
Combined vocal and multiple motor tic disorder [de la Tourette]
Tourette's syndrome

F95.8 Other tic disorders

F95.9 Tic disorder, unspecified
Tic NOS

F98- **Other behavioral and emotional disorders with onset usually occurring in childhood and adolescence**
Excludes ❷: breath-holding spells (R06.89)
gender identity disorder of childhood (F64.2)
Kleine-Levin syndrome (G47.13)
obsessive-compulsive disorder (F42.-)
sleep disorders not due to a substance or known physiological
condition (F51.-)

F98.0 Enuresis <u>not</u> due to a substance or known physiological condition
Enuresis (primary) (secondary) of nonorganic origin
Functional enuresis
Psychogenic enuresis
Urinary incontinence of nonorganic origin
Excludes 1: enuresis NOS (R32)

F98.1 Encopresis <u>not</u> due to a substance or known physiological condition
Functional encopresis
Incontinence of feces of nonorganic origin
Psychogenic encopresis
Use additional code to identify the cause of any coexisting constipation
Excludes 1: encopresis NOS (R15.-)

F98.2- Other feeding disorders of infancy and childhood
Excludes 1: feeding difficulties (R63.3)
Excludes ❷: anorexia nervosa and other eating disorders (F50.-)
feeding problems of newborn (P92.-)
pica of infancy or childhood (F98.3)

F98.21 Rumination disorder of infancy

F98.29 Other feeding disorders of infancy and early childhood

F98.3 Pica of infancy and childhood

F98.4   **Stereotyped movement disorders**
     Stereotype/habit disorder
     Excludes 1:   *abnormal involuntary movements (R25.-)*
     Excludes ❷: *compulsions in obsessive-compulsive disorder (F42.-)*
               hair plucking (F63.3)
               movement disorders of organic origin (G20-G25)
               nail-biting (F98.8)
               nose-picking (F98.8)
               stereotypies that are part of a broader psychiatric
                   condition (F01-F95)
               thumb-sucking (F98.8)
               tic disorders (F95.-)
               trichotillomania (F63.3)

F98.5   **Adult onset fluency disorder**
     Excludes 1:   *childhood onset fluency disorder (F80.81)*
               dysphasia (R47.02)
               fluency disorder in conditions classified elsewhere
                   (R47.82)
               fluency disorder (stuttering) following cerebrovascular
                   disease (I69. with final characters -23)
               tic disorders (F95.-)

F98.8   **Other specified behavioral and emotional disorders with onset usually occurring in childhood and adolescence**
     Excessive masturbation
     Nail-biting
     Nose-picking
     Thumb-sucking

F98.9   **Unspecified behavioral and emotional disorders with onset usually occurring in childhood and adolescence**

Unspecified mental disorder (F99)

F99   **Mental disorder, not otherwise specified**
     Mental illness NOS
     Excludes 1:   *unspecified mental disorder due to known physiological*
                  condition (F09)

F
9
8
–
F
9
9

Chapter 6 – Diseases of the nervous system (G00-G99)

Excludes ❷: *certain conditions originating in the perinatal period (P04-P96)*
certain infectious and parasitic diseases (A00-B99)
complications of pregnancy, childbirth and the puerperium (O00-O9A)
congenital malformations, deformations, and chromosomal abnormalities (Q00-Q99)
endocrine, nutritional and metabolic diseases (E00-E88)
injury, poisoning and certain other consequences of external causes (S00-T88)
neoplasms (C00-D49)
symptoms, signs and abnormal clinical and laboratory findings, not elsewhere classified (R00-R94)

This chapter contains the following blocks:

G00-G09	Inflammatory diseases of the central nervous system
G10-G14	Systemic atrophies primarily affecting the central nervous system
G20-G26	Extrapyramidal and movement disorders
G30-G32	Other degenerative diseases of the nervous system
G35-G37	Demyelinating diseases of the central nervous system
G40-G47	Episodic and paroxysmal disorders
G50-G59	Nerve, nerve root and plexus disorders
G60-G65	Polyneuropathies and other disorders of the peripheral nervous system
G70-G73	Diseases of myoneural junction and muscle
G80-G83	Cerebral palsy and other paralytic syndromes
G89-G99	Other disorders of the nervous system

Chapter-Specific Coding Guidelines

C. Chapter-Specific Coding Guidelines
In addition to general coding guidelines, there are guidelines for specific diagnoses and/or conditions in the classification. Unless otherwise indicated, these guidelines apply to all health care settings. Please refer to Section II for guidelines on the selection of principal diagnosis.

6. Chapter 6: Diseases of Nervous System and Sense Organs (G00-G99)

a. Dominant/nondominant side
Codes from category G81, Hemiplegia and hemiparesis, and subcategories, G83.1, Monoplegia of lower limb, G83.2, Monoplegia of upper limb, and G83.3, Monoplegia, unspecified, identify whether the dominant or nondominant side is affected. Should the affected side be documented, but not specified as dominant or nondominant, and the classification system does not indicate a default, code selection is as follows:
- For ambidextrous patients, the default should be dominant.
- If the left side is affected, the default is non-dominant.
- If the right side is affected, the default is dominant.

b. Pain - Category G89

1) General coding information
Codes in category G89, Pain, not elsewhere classified, may be used in conjunction with codes from other categories and chapters to provide more detail about acute or chronic pain and neoplasm-related pain, unless otherwise indicated below.

If the pain is not specified as acute or chronic, post-thoracotomy, postprocedural, or neoplasm-related, do not assign codes from category G89.

A code from category G89 should not be assigned if the underlying (definitive) diagnosis is known, unless the reason for the encounter is pain control/management and not management of the underlying condition.

When an admission or encounter is for a procedure aimed at treating the underlying condition (e.g., spinal fusion, kyphoplasty), a code for the underlying condition (e.g., vertebral fracture, spinal stenosis) should be assigned as the principal diagnosis. No code from category G89 should be assigned.

(a) Category G89 Codes as Principal or First-Listed Diagnosis
Category G89 codes are acceptable as principal diagnosis or the first-listed code:
- When pain control or pain management is the reason for the admission/encounter (e.g., a patient with displaced intervertebral disc, nerve impingement and severe back pain presents for injection of steroid into the spinal canal). The underlying cause of the pain should be reported as an additional diagnosis, if known.

- When a patient is admitted for the insertion of a neurostimulator for pain control, assign the appropriate pain code as the principal or first-listed diagnosis. When an admission or encounter is for a procedure aimed at treating the underlying condition and a neurostimulator is inserted for pain control during the same admission/encounter, a code for the underlying condition should be assigned as the principal diagnosis and the appropriate pain code should be assigned as a secondary diagnosis.

(b) Use of Category G89 Codes in Conjunction with Site Specific Pain Codes

(i) Assigning Category G89 and Site-Specific Pain Codes
Codes from category G89 may be used in conjunction with codes that identify the site of pain (including codes from chapter 18) if the category G89 code provides additional information. For example, if the code describes the site of the pain, but does not fully describe whether the pain is acute or chronic, then both codes should be assigned.

(ii) Sequencing of Category G89 Codes with Site-Specific Pain Codes
The sequencing of category G89 codes with site-specific pain codes (including chapter 18 codes), is dependent on the circumstances of the encounter/admission as follows:
- If the encounter is for pain control or pain management, assign the code from category G89 followed by the code identifying the specific site of pain (e.g., encounter for pain management for acute neck pain from trauma is assigned code G89.11, Acute pain due to trauma, followed by code M54.2, Cervicalgia, to identify the site of pain).

- If the encounter is for any other reason except pain control or pain management, and a related definitive diagnosis has not been established (confirmed) by the provider, assign the code for the specific site of pain first, followed by the appropriate code from category G89.

2) Pain due to devices, implants and grafts
See Section I.C.19. Pain due to medical devices.

3) Postoperative Pain
The provider's documentation should be used to guide the coding of postoperative pain, as well as *Section III. Reporting Additional Diagnoses and Section IV. Diagnostic Coding and Reporting in the Outpatient Setting.*

The default for post-thoracotomy and other postoperative pain not specified as acute or chronic is the code for the acute form.

Routine or expected postoperative pain immediately after surgery should not be coded.

(a) Postoperative pain not associated with specific postoperative complication
Postoperative pain not associated with a specific postoperative complication is assigned to the appropriate postoperative pain code in category G89.

(b) Postoperative pain associated with specific postoperative complication
Postoperative pain associated with a specific postoperative complication (such as painful wire sutures) is assigned to the appropriate code(s) found in Chapter 19, Injury, poisoning, and certain other consequences of external causes. If appropriate, use additional code(s) from category G89 to identify acute or chronic pain (G89.18 or G89.28).

4) Chronic pain
Chronic pain is classified to subcategory G89.2. There is no time frame defining when pain becomes chronic pain. The provider's documentation should be used to guide use of these codes.

5) Neoplasm Related Pain
Code G89.3 is assigned to pain documented as being related, associated or due to cancer, primary or secondary malignancy, or tumor. This code is assigned regardless of whether the pain is acute or chronic.

This code may be assigned as the principal or first-listed code when the stated reason for the admission/encounter is documented as pain control/pain management. The underlying neoplasm should be reported as an additional diagnosis.
When the reason for the admission/encounter is management of the neoplasm and the pain associated with the neoplasm is also documented, code G89.3 may be assigned as an additional diagnosis. It is not necessary to assign an additional code for the site of the pain.

See Section I.C.2 for instructions on the sequencing of neoplasms for all other stated reasons for the admission/encounter (except for pain control/pain management).

6) Chronic pain syndrome
Central pain syndrome (G89.0) and chronic pain syndrome (G89.4) are different than the term "chronic pain," and therefore codes should only be used when the provider has specifically documented this condition.
See Section I.C.5. Pain disorders related to psychological factors.

G00 - G00

Excludes 1: = NOT CODED HERE! (Do not code both)

Excludes ❷: = Not Included Here

Inflammatory diseases of the central nervous system (G00-G09)

G00- **Bacterial meningitis, <u>not elsewhere classified</u>** — Bacterial inflammation of the meninges.
Includes: **Bacterial arachnoiditis** — Bacterial inflammation of the arachnoidea, the delicate membrane between the dura mater and the pia mater.
Bacterial leptomeningitis — Bacterial inflammation of the pia mater and the arachnoid membranes.
Bacterial meningitis — Bacterial inflammation of the meninges.
Bacterial pachymeningitis — Bacterial inflammation of the dura mater.
Excludes 1: *bacterial:*
meningoencephalitis (G04.2)
meningomyelitis (G04.2)

MCC **G00.0** **Hemophilus meningitis** — A form due to hemophilus microorganisms.
Meningitis due to Hemophilus influenzae

MCC **G00.1** **Pneumococcal meningitis** — A form due to pneumococcal microorganisms.
Meningitis due to Streptococcal pneumoniae

MCC **G00.2** **Streptococcal meningitis** — A form due to streptococcal microorganisms.
Use additional code to further identify organism (B95.0-B95.5)

MCC **G00.3** **Staphylococcal meningitis** — A form due to staphylococcal microorganisms.
Use additional code to further identify organism (B95.61-B95.8)

MCC **G00.8** **Other bacterial meningitis**
Meningitis due to Escherichia coli
Meningitis due to Friedländer's bacillus
Meningitis due to Klebsiella
Use additional code to further identify organism (B96.-)

MCC **G00.9** **Bacterial meningitis, unspecified**
Meningitis due to gram-negative bacteria, unspecified
Purulent meningitis NOS
Pyogenic meningitis NOS
Suppurative meningitis NOS

G01 **<u>Meningitis in bacterial diseases classified elsewhere</u>** —
MCC **[Not Allowed as PDX]**
Code first underlying disease
Excludes 1: *meningitis (in):*
gonococcal (A54.81)
leptospirosis (A27.81)
listeriosis (A32.11)
Lyme disease (A69.21)
meningococcal (A39.0)
neurosyphilis (A52.13)
tuberculosis (A17.0)
meningoencephalitis and meningomyelitis in bacterial diseases classified elsewhere (G05)

G02 **<u>Meningitis in other infectious and parasitic diseases classified</u>**
MCC **<u>elsewhere</u>** — **[Not Allowed as PDX]**
Code first underlying disease, such as:
African trypanosomiasis (B56-)
Poliovirus infection (A80-)
Excludes 1: *candidal meningitis (B37.5)*
coccidioidomycosis meningitis (B38.4)
cryptococcal meningitis (B45.1)
herpesviral [herpes simplex] meningitis (B00.3)
infectious mononucleosis complicated by meningitis (B27- with fifth character 2)
measles complicated by meningitis (B05.1)
meningoencephalitis and meningomyelitis in other infectious and parasitic diseases classified elsewhere (G05)
mumps meningitis (B26.1)
rubella meningitis (B06.02)
varicella [chickenpox] meningitis (B01.0)
zoster meningitis (B02.1)

G03- **<u>Meningitis due to other and unspecified causes</u>**
Includes: **Arachnoiditis NOS**
Leptomeningitis NOS
Meningitis NOS
Pachymeningitis NOS
Excludes 1: *meningoencephalitis (G04.-)*
meningomyelitis (G04.-)

MCC **G03.0** **Nonpyogenic meningitis** — Inflammation of the meninges characterized by the lack of pus in the cerebrospinal fluid.
Aseptic meningitis
Nonbacterial meningitis

CC **G03.1** **Chronic meningitis**

CC **G03.2** **Benign recurrent meningitis [Mollaret]**

MCC **G03.8** **Meningitis due to other specified causes**
MCC **G03.9** **Meningitis, unspecified**
Arachnoiditis (spinal) NOS

G04- **Encephalitis, myelitis and encephalomyelitis**
Includes: **Acute ascending myelitis** — Inflammation of the spinal cord that is characterized by the progression of myelopathy toward the head.
Meningoencephalitis — Inflammation of the brain and the meninges that is not of bacterial origin.
Meningomyelitis — Inflammation of the spinal cord and its membranes that is not of bacterial origin.
Excludes 1: *encephalopathy NOS (G93.40)*
Excludes ❷: *acute transverse myelitis (G37.3-)*
alcoholic encephalopathy (G31.2)
benign myalgic encephalomyelitis (G93.3)
multiple sclerosis (G35)
subacute necrotizing myelitis (G37.4)
toxic encephalitis (G92)
toxic encephalopathy (G92)

G04.0- **<u>Acute disseminated encephalitis</u>** and encephalomyelitis (ADEM)
Excludes 1: *acute necrotizing hemorrhagic encephalopathy (G04.3-)*
other noninfectious acute disseminated encephalomyelitis (noninfectious ADEM) (G04.81)

MCC **G04.00** **Acute disseminated encephalitis and encephalomyelitis, unspecified**

MCC **G04.01** **<u>Postinfectious</u> acute disseminated encephalitis and encephalomyelitis (postinfectious ADEM)** — An inflammatory demyelinating disease of the brain and/or spinal cord following an infection.
Excludes 1: *post chickenpox encephalitis (B01.1)*
post measles encephalitis (B05.0)
post measles myelitis (B05.1)

MCC **G04.02** **<u>Postimmunization</u> acute disseminated encephalitis, myelitis and encephalomyelitis** — An inflammatory demyelinating disease of the brain and/or spinal cord following an immunization.
Encephalitis, post immunization
Encephalomyelitis, post immunization
Use additional code to identify the vaccine (T50.A-, T50.B-, T50.Z-)

CC **G04.1** **Tropical spastic paraplegia** — A chronic and progressive disease of the nervous system caused by infection with the human T-cell lymphotrophic virus (HTLV-1).

MCC **G04.2** **Bacterial meningoencephalitis and meningomyelitis, not elsewhere classified**

G04.3- **<u>Acute necrotizing hemorrhagic encephalopathy</u>**
Excludes 1: *acute disseminated encephalitis and encephalomyelitis (G04.0-)*

MCC **G04.30** **Acute necrotizing hemorrhagic encephalopathy, unspecified**

MCC **G04.31** **<u>Postinfectious</u> acute necrotizing hemorrhagic encephalopathy** — An inflammatory autoimmune demyelinating disease of the brain that destroys white matter following an infection.

MCC **G04.32** **<u>Postimmunization</u> acute necrotizing hemorrhagic encephalopathy** — An inflammatory autoimmune demyelinating disease of the brain that destroys white matter following an immunization.
Use additional code to identify the vaccine (T50.A-, T50.B-, T50.Z-)

MCC **G04.39** **Other acute necrotizing hemorrhagic encephalopathy**
Code also underlying etiology, if applicable

G04.8- **Other encephalitis, myelitis and encephalomyelitis**
Code also any associated seizure (G40.-, R56.9)

MCC **G04.81** **Other encephalitis and encephalomyelitis**
Noninfectious acute disseminated encephalomyelitis (noninfectious ADEM)

MCC **G04.89** **Other myelitis**

G04.9- **Encephalitis, myelitis and encephalomyelitis, unspecified**

MCC **G04.90** **Encephalitis and encephalomyelitis, unspecified**
Ventriculitis (cerebral) NOS

MCC **G04.91** **Myelitis, unspecified**

Excludes 1: = NOT CODED HERE! (Do not code both)   **654**   *Excludes ❷:* = Not Included Here

G00-G04

G05- Encephalitis, myelitis and encephalomyelitis _in diseases classified elsewhere_
Code first underlying disease, such as:
    Human immunodeficiency virus [HIV] disease (B20)
    Poliovirus (A80.-)
    Suppurative otitis media (H66.01-H66.4)
    Trichinellosis (B75)
Excludes 1:   _adenoviral encephalitis, myelitis and encephalomyelitis (A85.1)_
        congenital toxoplasmosis encephalitis, myelitis and encephalomyelitis (P37.1)
        cytomegaloviral encephalitis, myelitis and encephalomyelitis (B25.8)
        encephalitis, myelitis and encephalomyelitis (in) measles (B05.0)
        encephalitis, myelitis and encephalomyelitis (in) systemic lupus erythematosus (M32.19)
        enteroviral encephalitis, myelitis and encephalomyelitis (A85.0)
        eosinophilic meningoencephalitis (B83.2)
        herpesviral [herpes simplex] encephalitis, myelitis and encephalomyelitis (B00.4)
        listerial encephalitis, myelitis and encephalomyelitis (A32.12)
        meningococcal encephalitis, myelitis and encephalomyelitis (A39.81)
        mumps encephalitis, myelitis and encephalomyelitis (B26.2)
        postchickenpox encephalitis, myelitis and encephalomyelitis (B01.1-)
        rubella encephalitis, myelitis and encephalomyelitis (B06.01)
        toxoplasmosis encephalitis, myelitis and encephalomyelitis (B58.2)
        zoster encephalitis, myelitis and encephalomyelitis (B02.0)

MCC G05.3   Encephalitis and encephalomyelitis in diseases classified elsewhere — [Not Allowed as PDX]
        Meningoencephalitis in diseases classified elsewhere

MCC G05.4   Myelitis in diseases classified elsewhere — [Not Allowed as PDX]
        Meningomyelitis in diseases classified elsewhere

G06- Intracranial and intraspinal abscess and granuloma
        Use additional code (B95-B97) to identify infectious agent.

MCC G06.0   Intracranial abscess and granuloma — A localized collection of pus caused by the disintegration of tissue in the brain or its membranes that usually occurs as a secondary infection.
        Brain [any part] abscess (embolic)
        Cerebellar abscess (embolic)
        Cerebral abscess (embolic)
        Intracranial epidural abscess or granuloma
        Intracranial extradural abscess or granuloma
        Intracranial subdural abscess or granuloma
        Otogenic abscess (embolic)
        Excludes 1:   _tuberculous intracranial abscess and granuloma (A17.81)_

MCC G06.1   Intraspinal abscess and granuloma — A localized collection of pus caused by the disintegration of tissue in the spinal cord or its membranes that usually occurs as a secondary infection.
        Abscess (embolic) of spinal cord [any part]
        Intraspinal epidural abscess or granuloma
        Intraspinal extradural abscess or granuloma
        Intraspinal subdural abscess or granuloma
        Excludes 1:   _tuberculous intraspinal abscess and granuloma (A17.81)_

MCC G06.2   Extradural and subdural abscess, unspecified

G07   Intracranial and intraspinal abscess and granuloma in diseases
MCC   classified elsewhere — [Not Allowed as PDX]
        Code first underlying disease, such as:
        Schistosomiasis granuloma of brain (B65.-)
        Excludes 1:   _abscess of brain:_
            amebic (A06.6)
            chromomycotic (B43.1)
            gonococcal (A54.82)
            tuberculous (A17.81)
            tuberculoma of meninges (A17.1)

G08   Intracranial and intraspinal phlebitis and thrombophlebitis —
MCC   Inflammation, or inflammation with thrombus formation, of the large venous channels which drain the cerebrum, some diploic and meningeal veins into the neck, and from the spinal cord. NOTE: Code G08 refers to phlebitis and thrombophlebitis due to a pus producing microorganism or its poisonous products. See "of nonpyogenic origin" in excludes below.
        Septic embolism of intracranial or intraspinal venous sinuses and veins
        Septic endophlebitis of intracranial or intraspinal venous sinuses and veins
        Septic phlebitis of intracranial or intraspinal venous sinuses and veins
        Septic thrombophlebitis of intracranial or intraspinal venous sinuses and veins
        Septic thrombosis of intracranial or intraspinal venous sinuses and veins
        Excludes 1:   _intracranial phlebitis and thrombophlebitis complicating:_
            abortion, ectopic or molar pregnancy (O00-O07, O08.7)
            pregnancy, childbirth and the puerperium (O22.5, O87.3)
            nonpyogenic intracranial phlebitis and thrombophlebitis (I67.6)
        Excludes ❷: _intracranial phlebitis and thrombophlebitis complicating nonpyogenic intraspinal phlebitis and thrombophlebitis (G95.1)_

G09   Sequelae of inflammatory diseases of central nervous system
        Note: Category G09 is to be used to indicate conditions whose primary classification is to G00-G08 as the cause of sequelae, themselves classifiable elsewhere. The "sequelae" include conditions specified as residuals.
        Code first condition resulting from (sequela) of inflammatory diseases of central nervous system

Systemic atrophies primarily affecting the central nervous system (G10-G14)

G10   Huntington's disease — A hereditary, degenerative disease characterized by
CC   involuntary, abrupt, spasmodic, irregular movements of short duration involving the fingers, hands, arms, face, tongue, or head and chronic dementia.
        Huntington's chorea
        Huntington's dementia

G11- Hereditary ataxia — Inherited disorders characterized by slowly progressive incoordination of gait with poor coordination of hands, speech, and eye movements and often developing cerebellar atrophy.
        Excludes ❷: _cerebral palsy (G80.-)_
            hereditary and idiopathic neuropathy (G60.-)
            metabolic disorders (E70-E88)

CC G11.0   Congenital nonprogressive ataxia

CC G11.1   Early-onset cerebellar ataxia
        Early-onset cerebellar ataxia with essential tremor
        Early-onset cerebellar ataxia with myoclonus [Hunt's ataxia]
        Early-onset cerebellar ataxia with retained tendon reflexes
        Friedreich's ataxia (autosomal recessive)
        X-linked recessive spinocerebellar ataxia

CC G11.2   Late-onset cerebellar ataxia — [Age/15-124]

CC G11.3   Cerebellar ataxia with defective DNA repair
        Ataxia telangiectasia [Louis-Bar]
        Excludes ❷: _Cockayne's syndrome (Q87.1)_
            other disorders of purine and pyrimidine metabolism (E79.-)
            xeroderma pigmentosum (Q82.1)

CC G11.4   Hereditary spastic paraplegia — An inherited paraplegia characterized by spasticity of the muscles of the paralyzed part and increased tendon reflexes.

CC G11.8   Other hereditary ataxias

CC G11.9   Hereditary ataxia, unspecified
        Hereditary cerebellar ataxia NOS
        Hereditary cerebellar degeneration
        Hereditary cerebellar disease
        Hereditary cerebellar syndrome

G12- Spinal muscular atrophy and related syndromes — A wasting of muscle tissues caused by the progressive degeneration of the motor cells of the spinal cord.

CC G12.0   Infantile spinal muscular atrophy, type I [Werdnig-Hoffman] — A hereditary spinal muscular atrophy disease present at birth, caused by the degeneration of the anterior horn cells of the spinal cord and is marked by decreased fetal movements in utero, progressive muscular weakness, hypotonia, complete flaccid paralysis, and death.

G05 I G12

cc **G12.1 Other inherited spinal muscular atrophy**
Adult form spinal muscular atrophy
Childhood form, type II spinal muscular atrophy
Distal spinal muscular atrophy
Juvenile form, type III spinal muscular atrophy [Kugelberg-Welander] — Spinal muscular atrophy caused by the degeneration of anterior horn cells of the spinal cord beginning in adolescence and marked by wasting and weakness of the legs and pelvic girdle.
Progressive bulbar palsy of childhood [Fazio-Londe]
Scapuloperoneal form spinal muscular atrophy

G12.2- Motor neuron disease — Degeneration of the motor neurons of the brain and spinal cord.

cc **G12.20 Motor neuron disease, unspecified**

cc **G12.21 Amyotrophic lateral sclerosis** — [Age/15-124] – A progressive, degenerative disease of the motor neurons in the brain and spinal cord characterized by atrophy and weakness of the muscles innervated by them, and eventually dysphagia, dysarthria, and facial weakness (also called Lou Gehrig's disease).
Progressive spinal muscle atrophy

cc **G12.22 Progressive bulbar palsy** — A type of amyotrophic lateral sclerosis caused by degeneration of the motor neurons of the cranial nerve nuclei, and characterized by progressive weakness and wasting of the pharyngeal muscles, the tongue, the facial muscles, dysarthria, and dysphagia.

cc **G12.29 Other motor neuron disease**
Familial motor neuron disease
Primary lateral sclerosis

cc **G12.8 Other spinal muscular atrophies and related syndromes**

cc **G12.9 Spinal muscular atrophy, unspecified**

G13- Systemic atrophies primarily affecting central nervous system in diseases classified elsewhere

G13.0 Paraneoplastic neuromyopathy and neuropathy — [Not Allowed as PDX]
Carcinomatous neuromyopathy
Sensorial paraneoplastic neuropathy [Denny Brown]
Code first underlying neoplasm (C00-D49)

G13.1 Other systemic atrophy primarily affecting central nervous system in neoplastic disease — [Not Allowed as PDX]
Paraneoplastic limbic encephalopathy
Code first underlying neoplasm (C00-D49)

G13.2 Systemic atrophy primarily affecting central nervous system in myxedema — [Not Allowed as PDX]
Code first underlying disease, such as:
Hypothyroidism (E03-)
Myxedematous congenital iodine deficiency (E00.1)

G13.8 Systemic atrophy primarily affecting central nervous system in other diseases classified elsewhere — [Not Allowed as PDX]
Code first underlying disease

G14 Postpolio syndrome — A condition presenting long after the acute infection phase (often decades later) characterized by slowly progressive muscle weakness, pain, fatigue, and muscle atrophy.
Includes: Postpolio myelitic syndrome
Excludes 1: *sequelae of poliomyelitis (B91)*

Extrapyramidal and movement disorders (G20-G26)

G20 Parkinson's disease — A chronic, degenerative nervous system disease that causes the destruction of dopamine-producing cells and is characterized by a fine, slowly spreading tremor, muscular weakness and rigidity, and a peculiar gait.
Hemiparkinsonism
Idiopathic Parkinsonism or Parkinson's disease
Paralysis agitans
Parkinsonism or Parkinson's disease NOS
Primary Parkinsonism or Parkinson's disease
Excludes 1: *dementia with Parkinsonism (G31.83)*

G21- Secondary parkinsonism — A symptom complex with similar characteristics to Parkinson's disease that is caused as a consequence of other diseases or external agents.
Excludes 1: *dementia with Parkinsonism (G31.83)*
Huntington's disease (G10)
Shy-Drager syndrome (G90.3)
syphilitic Parkinsonism (A52.19)

MCC **G21.0 Malignant neuroleptic syndrome** — A condition characterized by multiple symptoms, including hyperthermia and rigidity that is caused by an adverse effect of neuroleptic (antipsychotic) drug therapy.
Use additional code for adverse effect, if applicable, to identify drug (T43.3x5, T43.4x5, T43.505, T43.595)
Excludes 1: *neuroleptic induced parkinsonism (G21.11)*

G21.1- Other drug-induced secondary parkinsonism

cc **G21.11 Neuroleptic induced parkinsonism**
Use additional code for adverse effect, if applicable, to identify drug (T43.3x5, T43.4x5, T43.505, T43.595)
Excludes 1: *malignant neuroleptic syndrome (G21.0)*

cc **G21.19 Other drug-induced secondary parkinsonism**
Use additional code for adverse effect, if applicable, to identify drug (T36-T50 with fifth or sixth character 5)

cc **G21.2 Secondary parkinsonism due to other external agents**
Code first (T51-T65) to identify external agent

cc **G21.3 Postencephalitic parkinsonism**

G21.4 Vascular parkInsonism

cc **G21.8 Other secondary parkinsonism**

cc **G21.9 Secondary parkinsonism, unspecified**

G23- Other degenerative diseases of basal ganglia — Deterioration of the masses of gray matter at the base of the cerebral hemispheres which function to relay motor impulses.
Excludes ❷: *multi-system degeneration of the autonomic nervous system (G90.3)*

cc **G23.0 Hallervorden-Spatz disease** — A hereditary degeneration of the globus pallidus marked by accumulations of iron pigment, progressive rigidity, choreoathetoid movements, dysarthria, and progressive mental deterioration.
Pigmentary pallidal degeneration

cc **G23.1 Progressive supranuclear ophthalmoplegia [Steele-Richardson-Olszewski]** — A chronic degenerative disease involving the basal ganglia characterized by early paralysis of the eye movements, parkinsonian features, generalized spasticity, progressive dysarthria, and mild dementia.
Progressive supranuclear palsy

cc **G23.2 Striatonigral degeneration** — The degeneration of the striatonigral elements of the basal ganglia characterized by gait imbalance, rigidity, progressive spasticity, and speech which becomes slow and indistinct.

cc **G23.8 Other specified degenerative diseases of basal ganglia**
Calcification of basal ganglia

cc **G23.9 Degenerative disease of basal ganglia, unspecified**

G24- Dystonia — A movement disorder characterized by involuntary muscle contractions.
Includes: Dyskinesia
Excludes ❷: *athetoid cerebral palsy (G80.3)*

G24.0- Drug-induced dystonia — A condition characterized by abnormal postures and muscle spasms that is caused by drugs.
Use additional code for adverse effect, if applicable, to identify drug (T36-T50 with fifth or sixth character 5)

G24.01 Drug-induced subacute dyskinesia
Drug-induced blepharospasm
Drug-induced orofacial dyskinesia
Neuroleptic induced tardive dyskinesia
Tardive dyskinesia

cc **G24.02 Drug-induced acute dystonia**
Acute dystonic reaction to drugs
Neuroleptic induced acute dystonia

cc **G24.09 Other drug-induced dystonia**

G24.1 Genetic torsion dystonia — A hereditary movement disorder characterized by painful contortions of the muscles of the trunk and extremities that produces twisting and repetitive movements and abnormal posture.
Dystonia deformans progressiva
Dystonia musculorum deformans
Familial torsion dystonia
Idiopathic familial dystonia
Idiopathic (torsion) dystonia NOS
(Schwalbe-) Ziehen-Oppenheim disease

cc **G24.2 Idiopathic nonfamilial dystonia** — A form of unknown cause.

G24.3 Spasmodic torticollis — A form causing the head to rotate to one side and pull down toward the chest.
Excludes 1: *congenital torticollis (Q68.0)*
hysterical torticollis (F44.4)
ocular torticollis (R29.891)
psychogenic torticollis (F45.8)
torticollis NOS (M43.6)
traumatic recurrent torticollis (S13.4)

G24.4 Idiopathic orofacial dystonia — A form affecting the jaw, lips, and/or tongue.
Orofacial dyskinesia
Excludes 1: *drug induced orofacial dyskinesia (G24.01)*

G24.5 Blepharospasm — A form affecting the eyelids which may close for extended periods of time.
Excludes 1: *drug induced blepharospasm (G24.01)*

G
1
2
-
G
2
4

cc **G24.8   Other dystonia**
　　　　Acquired torsion dystonia NOS

G24.9   Dystonia, unspecified
　　　　Dyskinesia NOS

G25- Other extrapyramidal and movement disorders — EXTRAPYRAMIDAL
DISEASE — A dysfunction of the nerve fibers which are important in maintenance of
equilibrium and muscle tone. MOVEMENT DISORDERS — Varying degrees of inability to
voluntarily control muscle action.

　　Excludes ❷: *sleep related movement disorders (G47.6-)*

G25.0   Essential tremor — A movement disorder characterized by bilateral,
symmetric, involuntary quivering which begins in the fingers and hands.
　　　　Familial tremor

　　　Excludes 1:   tremor NOS (R25.1)

G25.1   Drug-induced tremor — A tremor movement disorder caused by effects of
drugs.
　　　　**Use additional code for adverse effect, if applicable, to identify drug
　　　　(T36-T50 with fifth or sixth character 5)**

G25.2   Other specified forms of tremor
　　　　Intention tremor

G25.3   Myoclonus — The sudden, involuntary twitching contractions (jerks) of a muscle
or a group of muscles.
　　　　Drug-induced myoclonus
　　　　Palatal myoclonus
　　　　**Use additional code for adverse effect, if applicable, to identify drug
　　　　(T36-T50 with fifth or sixth character 5)**

　　　Excludes 1:   facial myokymia (G51.4)
　　　　　　　　myoclonic epilepsy (G40.-)

G25.4   Drug-induced chorea
　　　　**Use additional code for adverse effect, if applicable, to identify drug
　　　　(T36-T50 with fifth or sixth character 5)**

G25.5   Other chorea
　　　　Chorea NOS

　　　Excludes 1:   chorea NOS with heart involvement (I02.0)
　　　　　　　　Huntington's chorea (G10)
　　　　　　　　rheumatic chorea (I02.-)
　　　　　　　　Sydenham's chorea (I02.-)

G25.6- Drug-induced tics and other tics of organic origin

　　G25.61   Drug-induced tics
　　　　　**Use additional code for adverse effect, if applicable, to identify
　　　　　drug (T36-T50 with fifth or sixth character 5)**

　　G25.69   Other tics of organic origin — Repetitive, spasmodic movements or
　　　　　twitching that occur in an irregular fashion and resemble voluntary
　　　　　movements and are of nonpsychogenic origin.

　　　　Excludes 1:   habit spasm (F95.9)
　　　　　　　　　tic NOS (F95.9)
　　　　　　　　　Tourette's syndrome (F95.2)

G25.7- Other and unspecified drug induced movement disorders
　　　　**Use additional code for adverse effect, if applicable, to identify drug
　　　　(T36-T50 with fifth or sixth character 5)**

　　G25.70   Drug-induced movement disorder, unspecified

　　G25.71   Drug-induced akathisia
　　　　　Drug-induced acathisia
　　　　　Neuroleptic induced acute akathisia

　　G25.79   Other drug-induced movement disorders

G25.8- Other specified extrapyramidal and movement disorders

　　G25.81   Restless legs syndrome — Discomfort deep inside the legs that is
　　　　　relieved by keeping the legs in motion.

cc 　**G25.82   Stiff-man syndrome** — A condition characterized by progressive
　　　　　painful fluctuating rigidity of the trunk and limb muscles of an unknown
　　　　　origin.

　　G25.83   Benign shuddering attacks — A neurological phenomenon
　　　　　movement disorder that is usually seen in children and is nonepileptic in
　　　　　origin.

　　G25.89   Other specified extrapyramidal and movement disorders

cc **G25.9   Extrapyramidal and movement disorder, unspecified**

**G26   Extrapyramidal and movement disorders in diseases classified
elsewhere** — [Not Allowed as PDX]
　　Code first underlying disease

Other degenerative diseases of the nervous system (G30-G32)

G30- Alzheimer's disease — Diffuse atrophy of the cerebral cortex due to neuronal
degeneration and marked by increasing loss of memory, intellectual function, and
disturbances in speech.
Includes: Alzheimer's dementia senile and presenile forms
Use additional code to identify:
　　Delirium, if applicable (F05)
　　Dementia with behavioral disturbance (F02.81)
　　Dementia without behavioral disturbance (F02.80)

　　Excludes 1:   senile degeneration of brain NEC (G31.1)
　　　　　　　　senile dementia NOS (F03)
　　　　　　　　senility NOS (R41.81)

G30.0   Alzheimer's disease with early onset

G30.1   Alzheimer's disease with late onset — [Age/15-124]

G30.8   Other Alzheimer's disease

G30.9   Alzheimer's disease, unspecified

**G31- Other degenerative diseases of nervous system, not elsewhere
classified**
Use additional code to identify:
　　Dementia with behavioral disturbance (F02.81)
　　Dementia without behavioral disturbance (F02.80)

　　Excludes ❷: *Reye's syndrome (G93.7)*

G31.0- Frontotemporal dementia — A neurodegenerative disorder of the frontal
and anterior temporal lobes of the brain.

　　G31.01   Pick's disease — A form marked by severe atrophy of the frontal and
　　　　　temporal lobes that is characterized by symptoms similar to Alzheimer's
　　　　　disease with personality, orientation, and attention span more affected.
　　　　　Primary progressive aphasia
　　　　　Progressive isolated aphasia

　　G31.09   Other frontotemporal dementia
　　　　　Frontal dementia — A form signifying neuropsychological features
　　　　　localized to the frontal lobes.

G31.1   Senile degeneration of brain, not elsewhere classified

　　　Excludes 1:   Alzheimer's disease (G30.-)
　　　　　　　　senility NOS (R41.81)

G31.2   Degeneration of nervous system due to alcohol
　　　　Alcoholic cerebellar ataxia
　　　　Alcoholic cerebellar degeneration
　　　　Alcoholic cerebral degeneration
　　　　Alcoholic encephalopathy
　　　　Dysfunction of the autonomic nervous system due to alcohol
　　　　Code also associated alcoholism (F10-)

G31.8- Other specified degenerative diseases of nervous system

cc **G31.81   Alpers disease** — Deterioration of the nerve cells and glia in all layers of
　　　　　the cerebral cortex and marked by symptoms in early infancy of convulsions,
　　　　　dementia, blindness, deafness, and paralysis.

　　　　　Grey-matter degeneration

cc **G31.82   Leigh's disease** —Deterioration and symmetrical areas of necrosis in the
　　　　　midbrain and pons and substance of the medulla, with involvement of the
　　　　　cerebral hemispheres and cerebellum probably caused by a defect involving
　　　　　tricarboxylic acid cycle, and marked by cerebellar ataxia, hemiparesis,
　　　　　quadriplegia, and in the severe form death.

　　　　　Subacute necrotizing encephalopathy

　　G31.83   Dementia with Lewy bodies — A neurodegenerative disorder with
　　　　　Parkinsonian motor features that is characterized by unexplained falls,
　　　　　prominent visual hallucinations, delusions, and gait abnormalities.
　　　　　Dementia with Parkinsonism
　　　　　Lewy body dementia
　　　　　Lewy body disease

　　G31.84   Mild cognitive impairment, so stated — A mental-functioning
　　　　　disorder in which the patient demonstrates some degree of mental impairment
　　　　　but does not meet the criteria for dementia.

　　　　Excludes 1:   age related cognitive decline (R41.81)
　　　　　　　　　altered mental status (R41.82)
　　　　　　　　　cerebral degeneration (G31.9)
　　　　　　　　　change in mental status (R41.82)
　　　　　　　　　*cognitive deficits following (sequelae of) cerebral
　　　　　　　　　　　hemorrhage or infarction (I69.01-, I69.11-,
　　　　　　　　　　　I69.21-, I69.31-, I69.81-, I69.91-)*
　　　　　　　　　*cognitive impairment due to intracranial or head
　　　　　　　　　　　injury (S06.-)*
　　　　　　　　　dementia (F01-, F02-, F03)
　　　　　　　　　mild memory disturbance (F06.8)
　　　　　　　　　neurologic neglect syndrome (R41.4)
　　　　　　　　　personality change, nonpsychotic (F68.8)

G24 - G31

Excludes 1: = NOT CODED HERE! (Do not code both)　　　**657**　　　*Excludes* ❷: = Not Included Here

G31.85 Corticobasal degeneration

G31.89 Other specified degenerative diseases of nervous system

G31.9 Degenerative disease of nervous system, unspecified

G32- Other degenerative disorders of nervous system in diseases classified elsewhere

cc **G32.0 Subacute combined degeneration of spinal cord in diseases classified elsewhere** — [Not Allowed as PDX]
Dana-Putnam syndrome
Sclerosis of spinal cord (combined) (dorsolateral) (posterolateral)
Code first underlying disease, such as:
Anemia (D51.9)
Dietary (D51.3)
Pernicious (D51.0)
Vitamin B12 deficiency (E53.8)
Excludes 1:   syphilitic combined degeneration of spinal cord (A52.11)

G32.8- Other specified degenerative disorders of nervous system in diseases classified elsewhere
Code first underlying disease, such as:
Amyloidosis cerebral degeneration (E85.-)
Cerebral degeneration (due to) hypothyroidism (E00.0-E03.9)
Cerebral degeneration (due to) neoplasm (C00-D49)
Cerebral degeneration (due to) vitamin B deficiency, except thiamine (E52-E53-)
Excludes 1:   superior hemorrhagic polioencephalitis [Wernicke's encephalopathy] (E51.2)

cc **G32.81 Cerebellar ataxia in diseases classified elsewhere** — [Not Allowed as PDX]
Code first underlying disease, such as:
Celiac disease (with gluten ataxia) (K90.0)
Cerebellar ataxia (in) neoplastic disease (paraneoplastic cerebellar degeneration) (C00-D49)
Non-celiac gluten ataxia (M35.9)
Excludes 1:   systemic atrophy primarily affecting the central nervous system in alcoholic cerebellar ataxia (G13.2)
systemic atrophy primarily affecting the central nervous system in myxedema (G13.2)

G32.89 Other specified degenerative disorders of nervous system in diseases classified elsewhere — [Not Allowed as PDX]
Degenerative encephalopathy in diseases classified elsewhere

Demyelinating diseases of the central nervous system (G35-G37)

G35 Multiple sclerosis — A demyelinating disease of the white matter of the central nervous system of unknown etiology and characterized by paralysis or paresis of the upper or lower limbs, visual loss, paresthesia, speech disturbances, and occasionally dementia.
Disseminated multiple sclerosis
Generalized multiple sclerosis
Multiple sclerosis NOS
Multiple sclerosis of brain stem
Multiple sclerosis of cord

G36- Other acute disseminated demyelination — Destruction of the myelin sheath surrounding nerve fibers of the central nervous system.
Excludes 1:   postinfectious encephalitis and encephalomyelitis NOS (G04.01)

cc **G36.0 Neuromyelitis optica [Devic]** — A combined demyelination of the optic nerve and the spinal cord that is marked by visual loss and possibly blindness, and flaccid paralysis of the extremities.
Demyelination in optic neuritis
Excludes 1:   optic neuritis NOS (H46)

cc **G36.1 Acute and subacute hemorrhagic leukoencephalitis [Hurst]**

cc **G36.8 Other specified acute disseminated demyelination**

cc **G36.9 Acute disseminated demyelination, unspecified**

G37- Other demyelinating diseases of central nervous system

cc **G37.0 Diffuse sclerosis of central nervous system** — Myelinoclastic diffuse sclerosis characterized by mental and neurologic deterioration, intellectual deterioration, increased spasticity, blindness, and deafness.
Periaxial encephalitis
Schilder's disease
Excludes 1:   X linked adrenoleukodystrophy (E71.52-)

cc **G37.1 Central demyelination of corpus callosum** — A degeneration of the corpus callosum of unknown etiology characterized by diffuse signs of cerebral disease, mental symptoms, convulsions, tremors, and other motor disabilities.

cc **G37.2 Central pontine myelinolysis** — A disease caused by the destruction of myelin localized to the base of the pons and characterized by quadriplegia, and facial, glossal, and pharyngeal paralysis with mutism.

cc **G37.3 Acute transverse myelitis in demyelinating disease of central nervous system** — A rapidly developing inflammation of the spinal cord.
Acute transverse myelitis NOS
Acute transverse myelopathy
Excludes 1:   multiple sclerosis (G35)
neuromyelitis optica [Devic] (G36.0)

MCC **G37.4 Subacute necrotizing myelitis of central nervous system**

cc **G37.5 Concentric sclerosis [Balo] of central nervous system** — A demyelinating disease characterized by concentric areas of demyelination and without recognizable clinical symptoms.

cc **G37.8 Other specified demyelinating diseases of central nervous system**

cc **G37.9 Demyelinating disease of central nervous system, unspecified**

Episodic and paroxysmal disorders (G40-G47)

G40- Epilepsy and recurrent seizures — A neurological disorder of excessive and abnormal brain cell activity that is characterized by a sudden change in how the cells of the brain send electrical signals that causes susceptibility to recurrent seizures. STATUS EPILEPTICUS — An epileptic seizure of greater than five minutes or more than one seizure within a five-minute period without recovery between them.
Note: The following terms are to be considered equivalent to intractable: pharmacoresistant (pharmacologically resistant), treatment resistant, refractory (medically) and poorly controlled.
Excludes 1:   conversion disorder with seizures (F44.5)
convulsions NOS (R56.9)
post traumatic seizures (R56.1)
seizure (convulsive) NOS (R56.9)
seizure of newborn (P90)
Excludes ❷: hippocampal sclerosis (G93.81)
mesial temporal sclerosis (G93.81)
temporal sclerosis (G93.81)
Todd's paralysis (G83.84)

G40.0- Localization-related (focal) (partial) idiopathic epilepsy and epileptic syndromes with seizures of localized onset — A type that begins in a limited region of the brain that is characterized by a dazed or staring expression.
Benign childhood epilepsy with centrotemporal EEG spikes
Childhood epilepsy with occipital EEG paroxysms
Excludes 1:   adult onset localization-related epilepsy (G40.1-, G40.2-)

G40.00- Localization-related (focal) (partial) idiopathic epilepsy and epileptic syndromes with seizures of localized onset, **not** intractable
Localization-related (focal) (partial) idiopathic epilepsy and epileptic syndromes with seizures of localized onset without intractability

cc **G40.001 Localization-related (focal) (partial) idiopathic epilepsy and epileptic syndromes with seizures of localized onset, not intractable, with status epilepticus**

cc **G40.009 Localization-related (focal) (partial) idiopathic epilepsy and epileptic syndromes with seizures of localized onset, not intractable, without status epilepticus**
Localization-related (focal) (partial) idiopathic epilepsy and epileptic syndromes with seizures of localized onset NOS

G40.01- Localization-related (focal) (partial) idiopathic epilepsy and epileptic syndromes with seizures of localized onset, **intractable**

cc **G40.011 Localization-related (focal) (partial) idiopathic epilepsy and epileptic syndromes with seizures of localized onset, intractable, with status epilepticus**

cc **G40.019 Localization-related (focal) (partial) idiopathic epilepsy and epileptic syndromes with seizures of localized onset, intractable, without status epilepticus**

G40.1- <u>Localization-related</u> (focal) (partial) symptomatic epilepsy and epileptic syndromes <u>with simple partial seizures</u> — A type that begins in a limited region of the brain and is characterized by uncontrolled shaking, altered emotions, and sensory changes, but without loss of consciousness.
>> Attacks without alteration of consciousness
>> Epilepsia partialis continua [Kozhevnikof]
>> Simple partial seizures developing into secondarily generalized seizures

G40.10- Localization-related (focal) (partial) symptomatic epilepsy and epileptic syndromes with simple partial seizures, <u>not</u> intractable
>> Localization-related (focal) (partial) symptomatic epilepsy and epileptic syndromes with simple partial seizures without intractability

cc **G40.101** Localization-related (focal) (partial) symptomatic epilepsy and epileptic syndromes with simple partial seizures, <u>not</u> intractable, <u>with status epilepticus</u>

cc **G40.109** Localization-related (focal) (partial) symptomatic epilepsy and epileptic syndromes with simple partial seizures, <u>not</u> intractable, <u>without</u> status epilepticus
>> Localization-related (focal) (partial) symptomatic epilepsy and epileptic syndromes with simple partial seizures NOS

G40.11- Localization-related (focal) (partial) symptomatic epilepsy and epileptic syndromes with simple partial seizures, <u>intractable</u>

cc **G40.111** Localization-related (focal) (partial) symptomatic epilepsy and epileptic syndromes with simple partial seizures, intractable, <u>with status epilepticus</u>

cc **G40.119** Localization-related (focal) (partial) symptomatic epilepsy and epileptic syndromes with simple partial seizures, intractable, <u>without</u> status epilepticus

G40.2- <u>Localization-related</u> (focal) (partial) symptomatic epilepsy and epileptic syndromes <u>with complex partial seizures</u> — A type that begins in a limited region of the brain that is characterized by a dazed or staring expression, repetitious, purposeless movements, and a loss of consciousness.
>> Attacks with alteration of consciousness, often with automatisms
>> Complex partial seizures developing into secondarily generalized seizures

G40.20- Localization-related (focal) (partial) symptomatic epilepsy and epileptic syndromes with complex partial seizures, <u>not</u> intractable
>> Localization-related (focal) (partial) symptomatic epilepsy and epileptic syndromes with complex partial seizures without intractability

cc **G40.201** Localization-related (focal) (partial) symptomatic epilepsy and epileptic syndromes with complex partial seizures, <u>not</u> intractable, <u>with status epilepticus</u>

cc **G40.209** Localization-related (focal) (partial) symptomatic epilepsy and epileptic syndromes with complex partial seizures, <u>not</u> intractable, <u>without</u> status epilepticus
>> Localization-related (focal) (partial) symptomatic epilepsy and epileptic syndromes with complex partial seizures NOS

G40.21- Localization-related (focal) (partial) symptomatic epilepsy and epileptic syndromes with complex partial seizures, <u>intractable</u>

cc **G40.211** Localization-related (focal) (partial) symptomatic epilepsy and epileptic syndromes with complex partial seizures, intractable, <u>with status epilepticus</u>

cc **G40.219** Localization-related (focal) (partial) symptomatic epilepsy and epileptic syndromes with complex partial seizures, intractable, <u>without</u> status epilepticus

G40.3- <u>Generalized</u> idiopathic epilepsy and epileptic syndromes — A type characterized by the electrical discharge spread to involve all of the brain, symmetric tonic contraction of all voluntary muscles, decerebrate posturing, followed by clonic violent expiratory contractions with expulsion of saliva, possibly tongue biting, and loss of consciousness.
>> Code also MERRF syndrome, if applicable (E88.42)

G40.30- <u>Generalized</u> idiopathic epilepsy and epileptic syndromes, <u>not</u> intractable
>> Generalized idiopathic epilepsy and epileptic syndromes without intractability

MCC **G40.301** <u>Generalized</u> idiopathic epilepsy and epileptic syndromes, <u>not</u> intractable, <u>with status epilepticus</u>

G40.309 <u>Generalized</u> idiopathic epilepsy and epileptic syndromes, <u>not</u> intractable, <u>without</u> status epilepticus
>> Generalized idiopathic epilepsy and epileptic syndromes NOS

G40.31- <u>Generalized</u> idiopathic epilepsy and epileptic syndromes, <u>intractable</u>

MCC **G40.311** <u>Generalized</u> idiopathic epilepsy and epileptic syndromes, intractable, <u>with status epilepticus</u>

MCC **G40.319** <u>Generalized</u> idiopathic epilepsy and epileptic syndromes, intractable, <u>without</u> status epilepticus

G40.A- <u>Absence epileptic</u> syndrome — A type characterized by staring, brief lapses of awareness and subtle body movements, but without post-seizure confusion, contractions of convulsions, or loss of consciousness.
>> Absence epileptic syndrome NOS
>> Childhood absence epilepsy [pyknolepsy]
>> Juvenile absence epilepsy

G40.A0- Absence epileptic syndrome, <u>not</u> intractable

G40.A01 Absence epileptic syndrome, not intractable, <u>with status epilepticus</u>

G40.A09 Absence epileptic syndrome, not intractable, <u>without</u> status epilepticus

G40.A1- Absence epileptic syndrome, <u>intractable</u>

cc **G40.A11** Absence epileptic syndrome, intractable, <u>with status epilepticus</u>

cc **G40.A19** Absence epileptic syndrome, intractable, <u>without</u> status epilepticus

G40.B- <u>Juvenile myoclonic</u> epilepsy [impulsive petit mal] — A form that manifests itself usually between the ages of 12 and 18.

G40.B0- Juvenile myoclonic epilepsy, <u>not</u> intractable

cc **G40.B01** Juvenile myoclonic epilepsy, not intractable, <u>with status epilepticus</u>

cc **G40.B09** Juvenile myoclonic epilepsy, not intractable, <u>without</u> status epilepticus

G40.B1- Juvenile myoclonic epilepsy, <u>intractable</u>

cc **G40.B11** Juvenile myoclonic epilepsy, intractable, <u>with status epilepticus</u>

cc **G40.B19** Juvenile myoclonic epilepsy, intractable, <u>without</u> status epilepticus

G40.4- <u>Other generalized</u> epilepsy and epileptic syndromes
>> Epilepsy with grand mal seizures on awakening
>> Epilepsy with myoclonic absences
>> Epilepsy with myoclonic-astatic seizures
>> Grand mal seizure NOS
>> Nonspecific atonic epileptic seizures
>> Nonspecific clonic epileptic seizures
>> Nonspecific myoclonic epileptic seizures
>> Nonspecific tonic epileptic seizures
>> Nonspecific tonic-clonic epileptic seizures
>> Symptomatic early myoclonic encephalopathy

G40.40- Other <u>generalized</u> epilepsy and epileptic syndromes, <u>not</u> intractable
>> Other generalized epilepsy and epileptic syndromes without intractability
>> Other generalized epilepsy and epileptic syndromes NOS

G40.401 Other <u>generalized</u> epilepsy and epileptic syndromes, <u>not</u> intractable, <u>with status epilepticus</u>

G40.409 Other <u>generalized</u> epilepsy and epileptic syndromes, <u>not</u> intractable, <u>without</u> status epilepticus

G40 - G40

G40.41- Other <u>generalized</u> epilepsy and epileptic syndromes, <u>intractable</u>

  cc **G40.411** Other <u>generalized</u> epilepsy and epileptic syndromes, intractable, <u>with status epilepticus</u>

  cc **G40.419** Other <u>generalized</u> epilepsy and epileptic syndromes, intractable, <u>without</u> status epilepticus

G40.5- Epileptic seizures <u>related to external causes</u>
    Epileptic seizures related to alcohol
    Epileptic seizures related to drugs
    Epileptic seizures related to hormonal changes
    Epileptic seizures related to sleep deprivation
    Epileptic seizures related to stress
    Use additional code for adverse effect, if applicable, to identify drug (T36-T50 with fifth or sixth digit 5)
    Code also, if applicable, associated epilepsy and recurrent seizures (G40-)

G40.50- Epileptic seizures related to external causes, <u>not</u> intractable

  cc **G40.501** Epileptic seizures related to external causes, <u>not</u> intractable, <u>with status epilepticus</u>

  cc **G40.509** Epileptic seizures related to external causes, <u>not</u> intractable, <u>without</u> status epilepticus
      Epileptic seizures related to external causes NOS

G40.8- <u>Other epilepsy</u> and recurrent seizures
    Epilepsies and epileptic syndromes undetermined as to whether they are focal or generalized
    Landau-Kleffner syndrome

G40.80- Other epilepsy

  cc **G40.801** Other epilepsy, <u>not</u> intractable, <u>with status epilepticus</u>
      Other epilepsy without intractability with status epilepticus

  cc **G40.802** Other epilepsy, <u>not</u> intractable, <u>without</u> status epilepticus
      Other epilepsy NOS
      Other epilepsy without intractability without status epilepticus

  cc **G40.803** Other epilepsy, <u>intractable</u>, <u>with status epilepticus</u>

  cc **G40.804** Other epilepsy, <u>intractable</u>, <u>without</u> status epilepticus

G40.81- Lennox-Gastaut syndrome

  cc **G40.811** Lennox-Gastaut syndrome, <u>not</u> intractable, <u>with status epilepticus</u>

  cc **G40.812** Lennox-Gastaut syndrome, <u>not</u> intractable, <u>without</u> status epilepticus

  cc **G40.813** Lennox-Gastaut syndrome, <u>intractable</u>, <u>with status epilepticus</u>

  cc **G40.814** Lennox-Gastaut syndrome, <u>intractable</u>, <u>without</u> status epilepticus

G40.82- Epileptic spasms — A type characterized by brief, sudden spasms of the flexor muscles of the neck, trunk, and limbs manifesting during the first year of life.
    Infantile spasms
    Salaam attacks
    West's syndrome

  cc **G40.821** Epileptic spasms, <u>not</u> intractable, <u>with status epilepticus</u>

  cc **G40.822** Epileptic spasms, <u>not</u> intractable, <u>without</u> status epilepticus

  cc **G40.823** Epileptic spasms, <u>intractable</u>, <u>with status epilepticus</u>

  cc **G40.824** Epileptic spasms, <u>intractable</u>, <u>without</u> status epilepticus

  cc **G40.89** Other seizures
     Excludes 1:   post traumatic seizures (R56.1)
             recurrent seizures NOS (G40.909)
             seizure NOS (R56.9)

G40.9- <u>Epilepsy, unspecified</u>

G40.90- Epilepsy, unspecified, <u>not</u> intractable
    Epilepsy, unspecified, without intractability

    G40.901 Epilepsy, unspecified, <u>not</u> intractable, <u>with status epilepticus</u>

    G40.909 Epilepsy, unspecified, <u>not</u> intractable, <u>without</u> status epilepticus
      Epilepsy NOS
      Epileptic convulsions NOS
      Epileptic fits NOS
      Epileptic seizures NOS
      Recurrent seizures NOS
      Seizure disorder NOS

G40.91- Epilepsy, unspecified, <u>intractable</u>
    Intractable seizure disorder NOS

  cc **G40.911** Epilepsy, unspecified, intractable, <u>with status epilepticus</u>

  cc **G40.919** Epilepsy, unspecified, intractable, <u>without</u> status epilepticus

G43- <u>Migraine</u> — A neurological primary headache disorder that is characterized by episodic attacks of headache and associated symptoms.
  Note: The following terms are to be considered equivalent to intractable: pharmacoresistant (pharmacologically resistant), treatment resistant, refractory (medically) and poorly controlled.
  Use additional code for adverse effect, if applicable, to identify drug (T36-T50 with fifth or sixth character 5)
  Excludes 1:   headache NOS (R51)
            lower half migraine (G44.00)
  Excludes ❷: headache syndromes (G44.-)

G43.0- <u>Migraine without aura</u> — A form characterized by moderate to severe headaches lasting 4-72 hours with varying symptoms including nausea and/or vomiting, photophobia, and phonophobia.
    Common migraine
  Excludes 1:   chronic migraine without aura (G43.7-)

G43.00- Migraine without aura, <u>not</u> intractable
    Migraine without aura without mention of refractory migraine

    G43.001 Migraine without aura, <u>not</u> intractable, <u>with status migrainosus</u> — A form lasting more than 72 hours.

    G43.009 Migraine without aura, <u>not</u> intractable, <u>without</u> status migrainosus
      Migraine without aura NOS

G43.01- Migraine without aura, <u>intractable</u> — INTRACTABLE – Provider stated, and/or see Note at G43-.
    Migraine without aura with refractory migraine

    G43.011 Migraine without aura, intractable, <u>with status migrainosus</u> — A form lasting more than 72 hours.

    G43.019 Migraine without aura, intractable, <u>without</u> status migrainosus

G43.1- <u>Migraine with aura</u> — A form characterized by moderate to severe headaches with preceding or accompanying visual (most common), sensory, motor, and/or speech aura with the features of "migraine without aura" usually following the aura symptoms.
    Basilar migraine
    Classical migraine
    Migraine equivalents
    Migraine preceded or accompanied by transient focal neurological phenomena
    Migraine triggered seizures
    Migraine with acute-onset aura
    Migraine with aura without headache (migraine equivalents)
    Migraine with prolonged aura
    Migraine with typical aura
    Retinal migraine
  Code also any associated seizure (G40.-, R56.9)
  Excludes 1:   persistent migraine aura (G43.5-, G43.6-)

G43.10- Migraine with aura, <u>not</u> intractable
    Migraine with aura without mention of refractory migraine

    G43.101 Migraine with aura, <u>not</u> intractable, <u>with status migrainosus</u> — A form lasting more than 72 hours.

    G43.109 Migraine with aura, <u>not</u> intractable, <u>without</u> status migrainosus
      Migraine with aura NOS

G43.11- Migraine with aura, <u>intractable</u> — INTRACTABLE – Provider stated, and/or see Note at G43-.
    Migraine with aura with refractory migraine

    G43.111 Migraine with aura, intractable, <u>with status migrainosus</u> — A form lasting more than 72 hours.

    G43.119 Migraine with aura, intractable, <u>without</u> status migrainosus

---

Excludes 1: = NOT CODED HERE! (Do not code both)   **660**   *Excludes ❷:* = Not Included Here

G43.4- <u>Hemiplegic</u> migraine — A form characterized by recurrent headaches with aura and temporary, unilateral hemiparesis or hemiplegia.
- Familial migraine
- Sporadic migraine

G43.40- Hemiplegic migraine, <u>not</u> intractable
- Hemiplegic migraine without refractory migraine

G43.401 Hemiplegic migraine, <u>not</u> intractable, <u>with status migrainosus</u> — A form lasting more than 72 hours.

G43.409 Hemiplegic migraine, <u>not</u> intractable, <u>without</u> status migrainosus
- Hemiplegic migraine NOS

G43.41- Hemiplegic migraine, <u>intractable</u> — INTRACTABLE – Provider stated, and/or see Note at G43-.
- Hemiplegic migraine with refractory migraine

G43.411 Hemiplegic migraine, intractable, <u>with status migrainosus</u> — A form lasting more than 72 hours.

G43.419 Hemiplegic migraine, intractable, <u>without</u> status migrainosus

G43.5- <u>Persistent</u> migraine aura <u>without</u> cerebral infarction — A form characterized by aura symptoms that persist for more than two weeks and are without radiographic evidence of infarction.

G43.50- Persistent migraine aura without cerebral infarction, <u>not</u> intractable
- Persistent migraine aura without cerebral infarction, without refractory migraine

G43.501 Persistent migraine aura without cerebral infarction, not intractable, <u>with status migrainosus</u> — A form lasting more than 72 hours.

G43.509 Persistent migraine aura without cerebral infarction, not intractable, <u>without</u> status migrainosus
- Persistent migraine aura NOS

G43.51- Persistent migraine aura without cerebral infarction, <u>intractable</u> — INTRACTABLE – Provider stated, and/or see Note at G43-.
- Persistent migraine aura without cerebral infarction, with refractory migraine

G43.511 Persistent migraine aura without cerebral infarction, intractable, <u>with status migrainosus</u> — A form lasting more than 72 hours.

G43.519 Persistent migraine aura without cerebral infarction, intractable, <u>without</u> status migrainosus

G43.6- <u>Persistent</u> migraine aura <u>with cerebral infarction</u> — A form characterized by aura symptoms that are not reversible within seven days and/or are associated with radiographic evidence of infarction.
- Code also the type of cerebral infarction (I63.-)

G43.60- Persistent migraine aura with cerebral infarction, <u>not</u> intractable
- Persistent migraine aura with cerebral infarction, without refractory migraine

cc **G43.601** Persistent migraine aura with cerebral infarction, <u>not</u> intractable, <u>with status migrainosus</u> — A form lasting more than 72 hours.

cc **G43.609** Persistent migraine aura with cerebral infarction, <u>not</u> intractable, <u>without</u> status migrainosus

G43.61- Persistent migraine aura with cerebral infarction, <u>intractable</u> — INTRACTABLE – Provider stated, and/or see Note at G43-.
- Persistent migraine aura with cerebral infarction, with refractory migraine

cc **G43.611** Persistent migraine aura with cerebral infarction, intractable, <u>with status migrainosus</u> — A form lasting more than 72 hours.

cc **G43.619** Persistent migraine aura with cerebral infarction, intractable, <u>without</u> status migrainosus

G43.7 <u>Chronic</u> migraine <u>without aura</u> — A form marked by headache occurring 15 or more days per month for more than three months and is not the result of medication overuse.
- Transformed migraine
- *Excludes 1:*   *migraine without aura (G43.0-)*

G43.70- Chronic migraine without aura, <u>not</u> intractable
- Chronic migraine without aura, without refractory migraine

G43.701 Chronic migraine without aura, <u>not</u> intractable, <u>with status migrainosus</u> — A form lasting more than 72 hours.

G43.709 Chronic migraine without aura, <u>not</u> intractable, <u>without</u> status migrainosus
- Chronic migraine without aura NOS

G43.71- Chronic migraine without aura, <u>intractable</u> — INTRACTABLE – Provider stated, and/or see Note at G43-.
- Chronic migraine without aura, with refractory migraine

G43.711 Chronic migraine without aura, intractable, <u>with status migrainosus</u> — A form lasting more than 72 hours.

G43.719 Chronic migraine without aura, intractable, <u>without</u> status migrainosus

G43.A- <u>Cyclical vomiting</u> — A form marked by intense nausea and vomiting that lasts from one hour to days and is without headache.

G43.A0 Cyclical vomiting, <u>not</u> intractable
- Cyclical vomiting, without refractory migraine

G43.A1 Cyclical vomiting, <u>intractable</u> — INTRACTABLE – Provider stated, and/or see Note at G43-.
- Cyclical vomiting, with refractory migraine

G43.B- <u>Ophthalmoplegic</u> migraine — A form marked by severe headache and pain usually surrounding the eyeball that is often associated with eye muscle weakness.

G43.B0 Ophthalmoplegic migraine, <u>not</u> intractable
- Ophthalmoplegic migraine, without refractory migraine

G43.B1 Ophthalmoplegic migraine, <u>intractable</u> — INTRACTABLE – Provider stated, and/or see Note at G43-.
- Ophthalmoplegic migraine, with refractory migraine

G43.C- <u>Periodic headache syndromes in child or adult</u> — Other forms that affect children, adolescents, or adults with varying symptoms including abdominal pain and vertigo.

G43.C0 Periodic headache syndromes in child or adult, <u>not</u> intractable
- Periodic headache syndromes in child or adult, without refractory migraine

G43.C1 Periodic headache syndromes in child or adult, <u>intractable</u> — INTRACTABLE – Provider stated, and/or see Note at G43-.
- Periodic headache syndromes in child or adult, with refractory migraine

G43.D- <u>Abdominal migraine</u> — A form marked by abdominal pain, nausea, and vomiting that is usually seen in children.

G43.D0 Abdominal migraine, <u>not</u> intractable
- Abdominal migraine, without refractory migraine

G43.D1 Abdominal migraine, <u>intractable</u> — INTRACTABLE – Provider stated, and/or see Note at G43-.
- Abdominal migraine, with refractory migraine

G43.8- <u>Other</u> migraine

G43.80- Other migraine, <u>not</u> intractable
- Other migraine, without refractory migraine

G43.801 Other migraine, <u>not</u> intractable, <u>with status migrainosus</u> — A form lasting more than 72 hours.

G43.809 Other migraine, <u>not</u> intractable, <u>without</u> status migrainosus

G43.81- Other migraine, <u>intractable</u> — INTRACTABLE – Provider stated, and/or see Note at G43-.
- Other migraine, with refractory migraine

G43.811 Other migraine, intractable, <u>with status migrainosus</u> — A form lasting more than 72 hours.

G43.819 Other migraine, intractable, <u>without</u> status migrainosus

G43.82- Menstrual migraine, <u>not</u> intractable — A form characterized by being associated with the menstrual cycle.
- Menstrual headache, not intractable
- Menstrual migraine, without refractory migraine
- Menstrually related migraine, not intractable
- Pre-menstrual headache, not intractable
- Pre-menstrual migraine, not intractable
- Pure menstrual migraine, not intractable
- Code also associated premenstrual tension syndrome (N94.3)

G43.821 Menstrual migraine, <u>not</u> intractable, <u>with status migrainosus</u> — [♀] – A form lasting more than 72 hours.

G43.829 Menstrual migraine, <u>not</u> intractable, <u>without</u> status migrainosus — [♀]
- Menstrual migraine NOS

Excludes 1: = NOT CODED HERE! (Do not code both)   **661**   *Excludes ❷:* = Not Included Here

G43.83- **Menstrual migraine, <u>intractable</u>** — A form characterized by being associated with the menstrual cycle. INTRACTABLE – Provider stated, and/or see Note at G43-.
Menstrual headache, intractable
Menstrual migraine, with refractory migraine
Menstrually related migraine, intractable
Pre-menstrual headache, intractable
Pre-menstrual migraine, intractable
Pure menstrual migraine, intractable
Code also associated premenstrual tension syndrome (N94.3)

    G43.831 **Menstrual migraine, <u>intractable</u>, <u>with status</u> <u>migrainosus</u>** — [♀] – A form lasting more than 72 hours.

    G43.839 **Menstrual migraine, <u>intractable</u>, <u>without</u> status migrainosus** — [♀]

G43.9- **Migraine, <u>unspecified</u>**

  G43.90- **Migraine, unspecified, <u>not</u> intractable**
    Migraine, unspecified, without refractory migraine

    G43.901 **Migraine, unspecified, <u>not</u> intractable, <u>with status</u> <u>migrainosus</u>** — A form lasting more than 72 hours.
      Status migrainosus NOS

    G43.909 **Migraine, unspecified, <u>not</u> intractable, <u>without</u> status migrainosus**
      Migraine NOS

  G43.91- **Migraine, unspecified, <u>intractable</u>** — INTRACTABLE – Provider stated, and/or see Note at G43-.
    Migraine, unspecified, with refractory migraine

    G43.911 **Migraine, unspecified, intractable, <u>with status</u> <u>migrainosus</u>** — A form lasting more than 72 hours.

    G43.919 **Migraine, unspecified, intractable, <u>without</u> status migrainosus**

G44- **Other headache syndromes**
  Excludes 1:   *headache NOS (R51)*
  Excludes ❷: *atypical facial pain (G50.1)*
        headache due to lumbar puncture (G97.1)
        migraines (G43.-)
        trigeminal neuralgia (G50.0)

G44.0- **Cluster headaches and other trigeminal autonomic cephalgias (TAC)** — CLUSTER HEADACHE – A neurological primary headache disorder that is characterized by extremely painful, unilateral headaches that typically occur at the same time of day for several weeks until the "cluster" period is over. TRIGEMINAL AUTONOMIC CEPHALGIAS – A group of primary headaches that involves the activation of the trigeminal-autonomic reflex.

  G44.00- **<u>Cluster headache syndrome, unspecified</u>**
    Ciliary neuralgia
    Cluster headache NOS
    Histamine cephalgia
    Lower half migraine
    Migrainous neuralgia

    G44.001 **Cluster headache syndrome, unspecified, <u>intractable</u>** — INTRACTABLE – Provider stated (also review Note at G43-).

    G44.009 **Cluster headache syndrome, unspecified, <u>not</u> intractable**
      Cluster headache syndrome NOS

  G44.01- **<u>Episodic</u> cluster headache** — A form that is characterized by cycles of headaches (commonly one to several per day for several weeks) followed by a pain-free interval of months to years.

    G44.011 **Episodic cluster headache, <u>intractable</u>** — INTRACTABLE – Provider stated (also review Note at G43-).

    G44.019 **Episodic cluster headache, <u>not</u> intractable**
      Episodic cluster headache NOS

  G44.02- **<u>Chronic</u> cluster headache** — A form that is characterized by cycles of headaches without sustained periods of remission.

    G44.021 **Chronic cluster headache, <u>intractable</u>** — INTRACTABLE – Provider stated (also review Note at G43-).

    G44.029 **Chronic cluster headache, <u>not</u> intractable**
      Chronic cluster headache NOS

G44.03- **<u>Episodic paroxysmal hemicrania</u>** — A type of primary headache that is characterized by throbbing, claw-like, or boring pain usually on one side of the face, has a duration of minutes to less than one hour, occurs multiple times per day, and has sustained periods of remission.
    Paroxysmal hemicrania NOS

    G44.031 **Episodic paroxysmal hemicrania, <u>intractable</u>**
      INTRACTABLE – Provider stated (also review Note at G43-).

    G44.039 **Episodic paroxysmal hemicrania, <u>not</u> intractable**
      Episodic paroxysmal hemicrania NOS

G44.04- **<u>Chronic paroxysmal hemicrania</u>** — A type of primary headache that is characterized by throbbing, claw-like, or boring pain usually on one side of the face, has a duration of minutes to less than one hour, occurs multiple times per day, and does not have sustained periods of remission.

    G44.041 **Chronic paroxysmal hemicrania, <u>intractable</u>** —
      INTRACTABLE – Provider stated (also review Note at G43-).

    G44.049 **Chronic paroxysmal hemicrania, <u>not</u> intractable**
      Chronic paroxysmal hemicrania NOS

G44.05- **Short lasting unilateral <u>neuralgiform headache</u> with conjunctival injection and tearing (SUNCT)** — A type of primary headache that is characterized by a very short duration (less than a minute), occurs very frequently (many times per hour), watery eyes, and bloodshot eyes that are caused by the dilation of blood vessels.

    G44.051 **Short lasting unilateral neuralgiform headache with conjunctival injection and tearing (SUNCT), <u>intractable</u>** — INTRACTABLE – Provider stated (also review Note at G43-).

    G44.059 **Short lasting unilateral neuralgiform headache with conjunctival injection and tearing (SUNCT), <u>not</u> intractable**
      Short lasting unilateral neuralgiform headache with conjunctival injection and tearing (SUNCT) NOS

G44.09- **Other <u>trigeminal autonomic cephalgias (TAC)</u>**

    G44.091 **Other trigeminal autonomic cephalgias (TAC), <u>intractable</u>** — INTRACTABLE – Provider stated (also review Note at G43-).

    G44.099 **Other trigeminal autonomic cephalgias (TAC), <u>not</u> intractable**

G44.1 **<u>Vascular headache, not elsewhere classified</u>**
  Excludes ❷: *cluster headache (G44.0)*
        complicated headache syndromes (G44.5-)
        drug-induced headache (G44.4-)
        migraine (G43-)
        other specified headache syndromes (G44.8-)
        post-traumatic headache (G44.3-)
        tension-type headache (G44.2-)

G44.2- **<u>Tension-type</u> headache** — A common type of primary headache characterized by a mild to moderate pain, tightness in the muscles of the head, and tenderness of the head muscles and is not associated with a psychological condition.

  G44.20- **Tension-type headache, <u>unspecified</u>**

    G44.201 **Tension-type headache, unspecified, <u>intractable</u>** — INTRACTABLE – Provider stated (also review Note at G43-).

    G44.209 **Tension-type headache, unspecified, <u>not</u> intractable**
      Tension headache NOS

  G44.21- **<u>Episodic</u> tension-type headache** — A form that occurs less than several times a month (approximately 15 or less).

    G44.211 **Episodic tension-type headache, <u>intractable</u>** — INTRACTABLE – Provider stated (also review Note at G43-).

    G44.219 **Episodic tension-type headache, <u>not</u> intractable**
      Episodic tension-type headache NOS

  G44.22- **<u>Chronic</u> tension-type headache** — A form that occurs more than several times a month (approximately 15 or more).

    G44.221 **Chronic tension-type headache, <u>intractable</u>** — INTRACTABLE – Provider stated (also review Note at G43-).

    G44.229 **Chronic tension-type headache, <u>not</u> intractable**
      Chronic tension-type headache NOS

G44.3- **<u>Post-traumatic</u> headache** — A type of headache that is the result of a head injury and that usually starts within two weeks post injury.

  G44.30- **Post-traumatic headache, <u>unspecified</u>**

    G44.301 **Post-traumatic headache, unspecified, <u>intractable</u>** — INTRACTABLE – Provider stated (also review Note at G43-).

G43 - G44

© 2016 Channel Publishing, Ltd

G44.309 Post-traumatic headache, unspecified, <u>not</u> intractable
Post-traumatic headache NOS

G44.31- <u>Acute</u> post-traumatic headache — A form that goes away by the third month.

G44.311 Acute post-traumatic headache, <u>intractable</u> — INTRACTABLE – Provider stated (also review Note at G43-).

G44.319 Acute post-traumatic headache, <u>not</u> intractable
Acute post-traumatic headache NOS

G44.32- <u>Chronic</u> post-traumatic headache — A form that continues beyond the third month.

G44.321 Chronic post-traumatic headache, <u>intractable</u> — INTRACTABLE – Provider stated (also review Note at G43-).

G44.329 Chronic post-traumatic headache, <u>not</u> intractable
Chronic post-traumatic headache NOS

G44.4- <u>Drug-induced</u> headache, not elsewhere classified
Medication overuse headache — A type of headache that is the result of excessive use of medication (often medication used for headaches) which resolves after the medication is withdrawn.
Use additional code for adverse effect, if applicable, to identify drug (T36-T50 with fifth or sixth character 5)

G44.40 Drug-induced headache, not elsewhere classified, <u>not</u> intractable

G44.41 Drug-induced headache, not elsewhere classified, <u>intractable</u> — INTRACTABLE – Provider stated (also review Note at G43-).

G44.5- Complicated headache syndromes

G44.51 Hemicrania continua — A type of primary headache that is characterized by unilateral, daily, and continuous headaches that are without pain-free periods and respond to therapeutic doses of indomethacin.

G44.52 New daily persistent headache (NDPH) — A type of primary headache that is characterized by daily and unremitting pain that continues for more than three months and is bilateral in location.

G44.53 Primary thunderclap headache — A type of primary headache that is characterized by very sudden onset (usually less than one minute) and very severe pain that is not due to an underlying pathology like cerebral hemorrhage.

G44.59 Other complicated headache syndrome

G44.8- Other specified headache syndromes

G44.81 Hypnic headache — A type of primary headache that is characterized by onset during sleep ("alarm clock" headache), begins after the age of 50, and is short-lived (typically 30 minutes).

G44.82 Headache associated with sexual activity — A type of primary headache that is characterized by a dull, bilateral ache during sexual activity and increases with sexual excitement.
Orgasmic headache
Preorgasmic headache

G44.83 Primary cough headache — A type of primary headache that is characterized by onset due to coughing and usually lasts less than 30 minutes.

G44.84 Primary exertional headache — A type of primary headache that is characterized by onset due to physical exertion and may last from minutes to two days.

G44.85 Primary stabbing headache — A type of primary headache that is characterized by sharp, jabbing-like pains in the orbit, temple, and parietal areas that recurs at irregular intervals from one to many per day.

G44.89 Other headache syndrome

G45- <u>Transient cerebral ischemic attacks</u> and related syndromes — An episode of neurologic dysfunction caused by temporary decreased blood flow to the brain, spinal cord, or retina and without residual effects or infarction.
*Excludes 1:   neonatal cerebral ischemia (P91.0)
transient retinal artery occlusion (H34.0-)*

cc **G45.0 Vertebro-basilar artery syndrome** — A form originating in the vertebral and basilar arteries.

cc **G45.1 Carotid artery syndrome (hemispheric)** — A form originating in a carotid artery that usually affects one hemisphere of the brain that is often caused by anatomical compression of a carotid artery while turning the head to one side for a brief to extended period of time.

cc **G45.2 Multiple and bilateral precerebral artery syndromes**

cc **G45.3 Amaurosis fugax** — A form characterized by transient visual loss in one eye.

G45.4 Transient global amnesia — A neurologic condition characterized by an acute, temporary loss of short-term memory.
Excludes 1:   amnesia NOS (R41.3)

cc **G45.8 Other transient cerebral ischemic attacks and related syndromes**

cc **G45.9 Transient cerebral ischemic attack, unspecified**
Spasm of cerebral artery
TIA
Transient cerebral ischemia NOS

G46- <u>Vascular syndromes of brain in cerebrovascular diseases</u> — The symptomatic conditions resulting from a cerebrovascular disease (occlusion, sclerosis, etc.) to a particular artery and the part of the brain it supplies.
Code first underlying cerebrovascular disease (I60-I69)

cc **G46.0 Middle cerebral artery syndrome**

cc **G46.1 Anterior cerebral artery syndrome**

cc **G46.2 Posterior cerebral artery syndrome**

G46.3 Brain stem stroke syndrome
Benedikt syndrome
Claude syndrome
Foville syndrome
Millard-Gubler syndrome
Wallenberg syndrome
Weber syndrome

G46.4 Cerebellar stroke syndrome

G46.5 Pure motor lacunar syndrome

G46.6 Pure sensory lacunar syndrome

G46.7 Other lacunar syndromes

G46.8 Other vascular syndromes of brain in cerebrovascular diseases

G47- <u>Sleep disorders</u> — A condition that affects or disrupts the natural sleep pattern.
*Excludes ❷: nightmares (F51.5)
nonorganic sleep disorders (F51.-)
sleep terrors (F51.4)
sleepwalking (F51.3)*

G47.0- <u>Insomnia</u> — A condition that disrupts the natural sleep pattern that is characterized by poor quality sleep, difficulty falling asleep, difficulty staying asleep, waking up too early, and multiple spontaneous awakenings.
*Excludes ❷: alcohol related insomnia (F10.182, F10.282, F10.982)
drug-related insomnia F11.182, F11.282, F11.982, F13.182, F13.282, F13.982, F14.182, F14.282, F14.982, F15.182, F15.282, F15.982, F19.182, F19.282, F19.982
idiopathic insomnia (F51.01)
insomnia due to a mental disorder (F51.05)
insomnia not due to a substance or known physiological condition (F51.0-)
nonorganic insomnia (F51.0-)
primary insomnia (F51.01)
sleep apnea (G47.3-)*

G47.00 Insomnia, unspecified
Insomnia NOS

G47.01 Insomnia due to medical condition
Code also associated medical condition

G47.09 Other insomnia

G47.1- <u>Hypersomnia</u> — A condition of excessive daytime sleepiness that is not relieved by naps or prolonged sleep periods and often results in difficulty waking up, long nighttime sleeping, decreased energy, confusion, disorientation, and poor motor coordination.
*Excludes ❷: alcohol-related hypersomnia (F10.182, F10.282, F10.982)
drug-related hypersomnia F11.182, F11.282, F11.982, F13.182, F13.282, F13.982, F14.182, F14.282, F14.982, F15.182, F15.282, F15.982, F19.182, F19.282, F19.982
hypersomnia due to a mental disorder (F51.13)
hypersomnia not due to a substance or known physiological condition (F51.1-)
primary hypersomnia (F51.11)
sleep apnea (G47.3-)*

G47.10 Hypersomnia, unspecified
Hypersomnia NOS

G47.11 <u>Idiopathic</u> hypersomnia <u>with long sleep time</u>
Idiopathic hypersomnia NOS

G47.12 <u>Idiopathic</u> hypersomnia <u>without</u> long sleep time

G47.13 Recurrent hypersomnia — A form that lasts for days to weeks at a time and occurs several times a year.
Kleine-Levin syndrome
Menstrual related hypersomnia

G47.14 Hypersomnia due to medical condition
Code also associated medical condition

G47.19 Other hypersomnia

G44 - G47

G47.2- <u>Circadian rhythm</u> sleep disorders — A condition that affects or disrupts the normal 24-hour sleep-wake pattern.
　　　　Disorders of the sleep wake schedule
　　　　Inversion of nyctohemeral rhythm
　　　　Inversion of sleep rhythm

G47.20 Circadian rhythm sleep disorder, unspecified type
　　　　Sleep wake schedule disorder NOS

G47.21 Circadian rhythm sleep disorder, <u>delayed</u> sleep phase type — A form in which the patient goes to bed later than desired and rises later than desired.
　　　　Delayed sleep phase syndrome

G47.22 Circadian rhythm sleep disorder, <u>advanced</u> sleep phase type — A form in which the patient goes to bed earlier than desired and rises earlier than desired.

G47.23 Circadian rhythm sleep disorder, <u>irregular</u> sleep wake type — A form in which the patient has difficulty establishing a natural sleep-wake pattern.
　　　　Irregular sleep-wake pattern

G47.24 Circadian rhythm sleep disorder, <u>free</u> running type — A form occurring in patients who are not synchronized to the normal 24-hour day due to absence of environmental cues (e.g., blind persons).

G47.25 Circadian rhythm sleep disorder, <u>jet lag type</u> — A form characterized by difficulty adjusting to rapid travel over several time zones that results in lack of alertness and sleepiness.

G47.26 Circadian rhythm sleep disorder, <u>shift work</u> type — A form characterized by difficulty adjusting to night-shift work or varying shift-work schedules.

G47.27 Circadian rhythm sleep disorder in conditions classified elsewhere — [Not Allowed as PDX]
　　　　Code first underlying condition

G47.29 Other circadian rhythm sleep disorder

G47.3- <u>Sleep apnea</u> — The periodic cessation of breathing during sleep that is not classified elsewhere (see Excludes 1 below).
　　　Code also any associated underlying condition
　　　Excludes 1:　*apnea NOS (R06.81)*
　　　　　　　　　Cheyne-Stokes breathing (R06.3)
　　　　　　　　　pickwickian syndrome (E66.2)
　　　　　　　　　sleep apnea of newborn (P28.3)

G47.30 Sleep apnea, unspecified
　　　　Sleep apnea NOS

G47.31 <u>Primary</u> central sleep apnea — A form associated with a lack of sufficient neural impulses to the respiratory system.

G47.32 <u>High altitude</u> periodic breathing — A normal phenomenon form that occurs at higher altitudes and is characterized by brief apneic periods (3 to 10 seconds), but is not associated with altitude illness.

G47.33 <u>Obstructive</u> sleep apnea (adult) (pediatric) — A form that is due to structural abnormalities in the back of the throat that briefly collapses and blocks the airway.
　　　Excludes 1:　*obstructive sleep apnea of newborn (P28.3)*

G47.34 <u>Idiopathic</u> sleep related nonobstructive alveolar hypoventilation — A condition of insufficient ventilation during sleep that causes deficient oxygenation of the blood, but is not due to an obstructive airway condition.
　　　　Sleep related hypoxia

G47.35 <u>Congenital</u> central alveolar hypoventilation syndrome — A condition of insufficient ventilation during sleep that causes deficient oxygenation of the blood that has been determined as congenital in origin. (Note: see Excludes above)

G47.36 Sleep related hypoventilation in conditions classified elsewhere — [Not Allowed as PDX]
　　　　Sleep related hypoxemia in conditions classified elsewhere
　　　　Code first underlying condition

G47.37 Central sleep apnea <u>in conditions classified elsewhere</u> — [Not Allowed as PDX]
　　　　Code first underlying condition

G47.39 Other sleep apnea

G47.4- Narcolepsy and cataplexy

G47.41- Narcolepsy — A neurological disorder of chronic recurrent attacks of drowsiness and sleep during the daytime.

　　G47.411 Narcolepsy <u>with cataplexy</u> — A form with the sudden, brief loss of muscle control triggered by strong emotion or emotional response.

　　G47.419 Narcolepsy <u>without</u> cataplexy
　　　　　Narcolepsy NOS

G47.42- Narcolepsy in conditions classified elsewhere
　　　　Code first underlying condition

　　G47.421 Narcolepsy in conditions classified elsewhere <u>with cataplexy</u> — [Not Allowed as PDX]

　　G47.429 Narcolepsy in conditions classified elsewhere <u>without</u> cataplexy — [Not Allowed as PDX]

G47.5- <u>Parasomnia</u> — The condition of abnormal behavioral or physiological events associated with sleep and sleep stages.
　　　Excludes 1:　*alcohol induced parasomnia (F10.182, F10.282, F10.982),*
　　　　　　　　　drug induced parasomnia (F11.182, F11.282, F11.982, F13.182, F13.282, F13.982, F14.182, F14.282, F14.982, F15.182, F15.282, F15.982, F19.182, F19.282, F19.982)
　　　　　　　　　parasomnia not due to a substance or known physiological condition (F51.8)

G47.50 Parasomnia, unspecified
　　　　Parasomnia NOS

G47.51 Confusional arousals — A form that may begin with yelling or crying and violently moving around in bed, in which the sleeper seems to be alert and upset after awakening.

G47.52 REM sleep behavior disorder — A form that occurs during the rapid eye movement state of sleep, in which the sleeper acts out his or her dream.

G47.53 Recurrent isolated sleep paralysis — A form with the sensation of feeling paralyzed upon awakening.

G47.54 Parasomnia in conditions classified elsewhere — [Not Allowed as PDX]
　　　　Code first underlying condition

G47.59 Other parasomnia

G47.6- Sleep related movement disorders — The condition of involuntary movement occurring during sleep.
　　　Excludes ❷:　*restless legs syndrome (G25.81)*

G47.61 Periodic limb movement disorder — A form characterized by the repetitive, brief involuntary movement of the limbs (usually legs) during sleep that occurs between non-movement periods.
　　　　Periodic limb movement disorder

G47.62 Sleep related leg cramps — A form involving the painful contraction of the leg muscles.

G47.63 Sleep related bruxism — A form involving the grinding of the teeth during sleep.
　　　Excludes 1:　*psychogenic bruxism (F45.8)*

G47.69 Other sleep related movement disorders

G47.8 Other sleep disorders

G47.9 Sleep disorder, unspecified
　　　　Sleep disorder NOS

Nerve, nerve root and plexus disorders (G50-G59)

　Excludes 1:　*current traumatic nerve, nerve root and plexus disorders — see Injury, nerve by body region*
　　　　　　　neuralgia NOS (M79.2)
　　　　　　　neuritis NOS (M79.2)
　　　　　　　peripheral neuritis in pregnancy (O26.82-)
　　　　　　　radiculitis NOS (M54.1-)

G50- Disorders of <u>trigeminal nerve</u>
　　Includes:　Disorders of 5th cranial nerve

G50.0 Trigeminal neuralgia — A sudden, severe, excruciating episodic pain in the area supplied by the trigeminal nerve.
　　　　Syndrome of paroxysmal facial pain
　　　　Tic douloureux

G50.1 Atypical facial pain

G50.8 Other disorders of trigeminal nerve

G50.9 Disorder of trigeminal nerve, unspecified

G51- <u>Facial nerve</u> disorders
　　Includes:　Disorders of 7th cranial nerve

G51.0 Bell's palsy — Facial paralysis caused by a lesion of the facial nerve and marked by characteristic distortion of the face.
　　　　Facial palsy

G51.1 Geniculate ganglionitis — Inflammation of the geniculate ganglion characterized by severe, sharp pain occurring in the region of the external ear.
　　　Excludes 1:　*postherpetic geniculate ganglionitis (B02.21)*

Excludes 1: = NOT CODED HERE! (Do not code both)　　　　**664**　　　　*Excludes ❷:* = Not Included Here

G51.2 **Melkersson's syndrome** — A hereditary facial palsy characterized by facial swelling and occasionally fissured tongue.
  Melkersson-Rosenthal syndrome

G51.3 **Clonic hemifacial spasm**

G51.4 **Facial myokymia**

G51.8 **Other disorders of facial nerve**

G51.9 **Disorder of facial nerve, unspecified**

G52- **Disorders of other cranial nerves**
  Excludes ②: *disorders of acoustic [8th] nerve (H93.3)*
      disorders of optic [2nd] nerve (H46, H47.0)
      paralytic strabismus due to nerve palsy (H49.0-H49.2)

G52.0 **Disorders of olfactory nerve**
  Disorders of 1st cranial nerve

G52.1 **Disorders of glossopharyngeal nerve**
  Disorder of 9th cranial nerve
  Glossopharyngeal neuralgia — Pharyngeal spasms of pain in the sensory distribution of the ninth cranial nerve.

G52.2 **Disorders of vagus nerve**
  Disorders of pneumogastric [10th] nerve

G52.3 **Disorders of hypoglossal nerve**
  Disorders of 12th cranial nerve

G52.7 **Disorders of multiple cranial nerves**
  Polyneuritis cranialis — Inflammation of two or more of the cranial nerves at the same time.

G52.8 **Disorders of other specified cranial nerves**

G52.9 **Cranial nerve disorder, unspecified**

G53 **Cranial nerve disorders in diseases classified elsewhere** —
  [Not Allowed as PDX]
  Code first underlying disease, such as:
    Neoplasm (C00-D49)
  Excludes 1: *multiple cranial nerve palsy in sarcoidosis (D86.82)*
      multiple cranial nerve palsy in syphilis (A52.15)
      postherpetic geniculate ganglionitis (B02.21)
      postherpetic trigeminal neuralgia (B02.22)

G54- **Nerve root and plexus disorders**
  Excludes 1: *current traumatic nerve root and plexus disorders — see nerve injury by body region*
      intervertebral disc disorders (M50-M51)
      neuralgia or neuritis NOS (M79.2)
      neuritis or radiculitis brachial NOS (M54.13)
      neuritis or radiculitis lumbar NOS (M54.16)
      neuritis or radiculitis lumbosacral NOS (M54.17)
      neuritis or radiculitis thoracic NOS (M54.14)
      radiculitis NOS (M54.10)
      radiculopathy NOS (M54.10)
      spondylosis (M47.-)

G54.0 **Brachial plexus disorders**
  Thoracic outlet syndrome — Compression of the brachial plexus nerve trunks characterized by numbness and tingling of the hand, weakness and wasting of the small muscles of the hand, and painful paresthesias.

G54.1 **Lumbosacral plexus disorders**

G54.2 **Cervical root disorders, not elsewhere classified**

G54.3 **Thoracic root disorders, not elsewhere classified** —
  [Unacceptable PDX]

G54.4 **Lumbosacral root disorders, not elsewhere classified**

G54.5 **Neuralgic amyotrophy** — Pain across the shoulder and upper arm, with atrophy and paralysis of the muscles of the shoulder girdle.
  Parsonage-Aldren-Turner syndrome
  Shoulder-girdle neuritis
  Excludes 1: *neuralgic amyotrophy in diabetes mellitus (E08-E13 with .44)*

G54.6 **Phantom limb syndrome with pain** — The sensation that pain exists in the amputated part of the limb due to stimulation of those transsected nerve ends which normally innervate the distal part of that limb.

G54.7 **Phantom limb syndrome without pain** — The sensation that the limb exists in the amputated part of the limb.
  Phantom limb syndrome NOS

G54.8 **Other nerve root and plexus disorders**

G54.9 **Nerve root and plexus disorder, unspecified**

G55 **Nerve root and plexus compressions** in diseases classified elsewhere — [Not Allowed as PDX]
  Code first underlying disease, such as:
    Neoplasm (C00-D49)
  Excludes 1: *nerve root compression (due to) (in) ankylosing spondylitis (M45.-)*
      nerve root compression (due to) (in) dorsopathies (M53.-, M54.-)
      nerve root compression (due to) (in) intervertebral disc disorders (M50.1.-, M51.1.-)
      nerve root compression (due to) (in) spondylopathies (M46.-, M48.-)

G56- **Mononeuropathies of upper limb**
  Excludes 1: *current traumatic nerve disorder — see nerve injury by body region*

  G56.0- **Carpal tunnel syndrome** — Fluctuating numbness, paresthesias, and pain in the hand due to compression of the median nerve at the wrist.
    G56.00 **Carpal tunnel syndrome, unspecified upper limb**
    G56.01 **Carpal tunnel syndrome, right upper limb**
    G56.02 **Carpal tunnel syndrome, left upper limb**
    G56.03 **Carpal tunnel syndrome, bilateral upper limbs**

  G56.1- **Other lesions of median nerve**
    G56.10 **Other lesions of median nerve, unspecified upper limb**
    G56.11 **Other lesions of median nerve, right upper limb**
    G56.12 **Other lesions of median nerve, left upper limb**
    G56.13 **Other lesions of median nerve, bilateral upper limbs**

  G56.2- **Lesion of ulnar nerve** — Pain, numbness, and weakness of the hand and forearm caused by injury or compression of the ulnar nerve at the elbow.
    Tardy ulnar nerve palsy
    G56.20 **Lesion of ulnar nerve, unspecified upper limb**
    G56.21 **Lesion of ulnar nerve, right upper limb**
    G56.22 **Lesion of ulnar nerve, left upper limb**
    G56.23 **Lesion of ulnar nerve, bilateral upper limbs**

  G56.3- **Lesion of radial nerve** — Wrist drop, paralysis of the extension of the elbow, weakness of elbow flexion, and paralysis of the extension of the fingers, thumb, and wrist due to a lesion of the radial nerve.
    G56.30 **Lesion of radial nerve, unspecified upper limb**
    G56.31 **Lesion of radial nerve, right upper limb**
    G56.32 **Lesion of radial nerve, left upper limb**
    G56.33 **Lesion of radial nerve, bilateral upper limbs**

  G56.4- **Causalgia of upper limb** — A condition characterized by intense burning pain of the upper limb with skin sensitivity, discoloration, and increased localized temperature that is most likely due to peripheral nerve damage.
    Complex regional pain syndrome II of upper limb — A form identified as following a distinct nerve injury.
    Excludes 1: *complex regional pain syndrome I of lower limb (G90.52-)*
        complex regional pain syndrome I of upper limb (G90.51-)
        complex regional pain syndrome II of lower limb (G57.7-)
        reflex sympathetic dystrophy of lower limb (G90.52-)
        reflex sympathetic dystrophy of upper limb (G90.51-)
    G56.40 **Causalgia of unspecified upper limb**
    G56.41 **Causalgia of right upper limb**
    G56.42 **Causalgia of left upper limb**
    G56.43 **Causalgia of bilateral upper limbs**

  G56.8- **Other specified mononeuropathies of upper limb**
    Interdigital neuroma of upper limb
    G56.80 **Other specified mononeuropathies of unspecified upper limb**
    G56.81 **Other specified mononeuropathies of right upper limb**
    G56.82 **Other specified mononeuropathies of left upper limb**
    G56.83 **Other specified mononeuropathies of bilateral upper limbs**

  G56.9- **Unspecified mononeuropathy of upper limb**
    G56.90 **Unspecified mononeuropathy of unspecified upper limb**
    G56.91 **Unspecified mononeuropathy of right upper limb**
    G56.92 **Unspecified mononeuropathy of left upper limb**
    G56.93 **Unspecified mononeuropathy of bilateral upper limbs**

G51 - G56

Excludes 1: = NOT CODED HERE! (Do not code both)   **665**   *Excludes ②: = Not Included Here*

G57- **Mononeuropathies of lower limb**
    Excludes 1:   *current traumatic nerve disorder — see nerve injury by body region*

  G57.0- **Lesion of sciatic nerve**
    Excludes 1:   *sciatica NOS (M54.3-)*
    Excludes ❷: *sciatica attributed to intervertebral disc disorder (M51.1.-)*

    G57.00 Lesion of sciatic nerve, unspecified lower limb
    G57.01 Lesion of sciatic nerve, <u>right</u> lower limb
    G57.02 Lesion of sciatic nerve, <u>left</u> lower limb
    G57.03 Lesion of sciatic nerve, <u>bilateral</u> lower limbs

  G57.1- **Meralgia paresthetica** — Compression of the femoral cutaneous nerve at the inguinal ligament characterized by paresthesia, pain, and numbness of the outer surface of the thigh.
    Lateral cutaneous nerve of thigh syndrome
    G57.10 Meralgia paresthetica, unspecified lower limb
    G57.11 Meralgia paresthetica, <u>right</u> lower limb
    G57.12 Meralgia paresthetica, <u>left</u> lower limb
    G57.13 Meralgia paresthetica, <u>bilateral</u> lower limbs

  G57.2- **Lesion of femoral nerve**
    G57.20 Lesion of femoral nerve, unspecified lower limb
    G57.21 Lesion of femoral nerve, <u>right</u> lower limb
    G57.22 Lesion of femoral nerve, <u>left</u> lower limb
    G57.23 Lesion of femoral nerve, <u>bilateral</u> lower limbs

  G57.3- **Lesion of lateral popliteal nerve**
    Peroneal nerve palsy
    G57.30 Lesion of lateral popliteal nerve, unspecified lower limb
    G57.31 Lesion of lateral popliteal nerve, <u>right</u> lower limb
    G57.32 Lesion of lateral popliteal nerve, <u>left</u> lower limb
    G57.33 Lesion of lateral popliteal nerve, <u>bilateral</u> lower limbs

  G57.4- **Lesion of medial popliteal nerve**
    G57.40 Lesion of medial popliteal nerve, unspecified lower limb
    G57.41 Lesion of medial popliteal nerve, <u>right</u> lower limb
    G57.42 Lesion of medial popliteal nerve, <u>left</u> lower limb
    G57.43 Lesion of medial popliteal nerve, <u>bilateral</u> lower limbs

  G57.5- **Tarsal tunnel syndrome** — Compression of the posterior tibial nerve characterized by pain, numbness, and tingling of the sole of the foot.
    G57.50 Tarsal tunnel syndrome, unspecified lower limb
    G57.51 Tarsal tunnel syndrome, <u>right</u> lower limb
    G57.52 Tarsal tunnel syndrome, <u>left</u> lower limb
    G57.53 Tarsal tunnel syndrome, <u>bilateral</u> lower limbs

  G57.6- **Lesion of plantar nerve**
    Morton's metatarsalgia — Episodic pain, or traumatic nodular mass of nerve tissue in the region of the third and fourth metatarsals of the foot.
    G57.60 Lesion of plantar nerve, unspecified lower limb
    G57.61 Lesion of plantar nerve, <u>right</u> lower limb
    G57.62 Lesion of plantar nerve, <u>left</u> lower limb
    G57.63 Lesion of plantar nerve, <u>bilateral</u> lower limbs

  G57.7- **Causalgia of lower limb** — A condition characterized by intense burning pain of the lower limb with skin sensitivity, discoloration, and increased localized temperature that is most likely due to peripheral nerve damage.
    Complex regional pain syndrome II of lower limb
    Excludes 1:   *complex regional pain syndrome I of lower limb (G90.52-)*
          complex regional pain syndrome I of upper limb (G90.51-)
          complex regional pain syndrome II of upper limb (G56.4-)
          reflex sympathetic dystrophy of lower limb (G90.52-)
          reflex sympathetic dystrophy of upper limb (G90.51-)
    G57.70 Causalgia of unspecified lower limb
    G57.71 Causalgia of <u>right</u> lower limb
    G57.72 Causalgia of <u>left</u> lower limb
    G57.73 Causalgia of <u>bilateral</u> lower limbs

G57.8- **Other specified mononeuropathies of lower limb**
    Interdigital neuroma of lower limb
    G57.80 Other specified mononeuropathies of unspecified lower limb
    G57.81 Other specified mononeuropathies of <u>right</u> lower limb
    G57.82 Other specified mononeuropathies of <u>left</u> lower limb
    G57.83 Other specified mononeuropathies of <u>bilateral</u> lower limbs

G57.9- **Unspecified mononeuropathy of lower limb**
    G57.90 Unspecified mononeuropathy of unspecified lower limb
    G57.91 Unspecified mononeuropathy of <u>right</u> lower limb
    G57.92 Unspecified mononeuropathy of <u>left</u> lower limb
    G57.93 Unspecified mononeuropathy of <u>bilateral</u> lower limbs

G58- **Other mononeuropathies**
  G58.0 **Intercostal neuropathy**
  G58.7 **Mononeuritis multiplex**
  G58.8 **Other specified mononeuropathies**
  G58.9 **Mononeuropathy, unspecified**

G59 **Mononeuropathy in diseases classified elsewhere** — [Not Allowed as PDX]
  Code first underlying disease
    Excludes 1:   *diabetic mononeuropathy (E08-E13 with .41)*
          syphilitic nerve paralysis (A52.19)
          syphilitic neuritis (A52.15)
          tuberculous mononeuropathy (A17.83)

Polyneuropathies and other disorders of the peripheral nervous system (G60-G65)

    Excludes 1:   *neuralgia NOS (M79.2)*
          neuritis NOS (M79.2)
          peripheral neuritis in pregnancy (O26.82-)
          radiculitis NOS (M54.10)

G60- **Hereditary and idiopathic neuropathy** — A peripheral nerve disease that is genetically transmitted or is of unknown origin.
  G60.0 **Hereditary motor and sensory neuropathy** — An inherited neuropathy characterized by lightning pains, hyperkeratosis feet, painless ulcers, severe distal sensory loss, and muscle wasting.
    Charcot-Marie-Tooth disease
    Déjérine-Sottas disease
    Hereditary motor and sensory neuropathy, types I-IV
    Hypertrophic neuropathy of infancy
    Peroneal muscular atrophy (axonal type) (hypertrophic type)
    Roussy-Levy syndrome
  CC **G60.1** **Refsum's disease** — An inherited defect of acid metabolism characterized by chronic polyneuritis, retinitis pigmentosa, and mild ataxia.
    Infantile Refsum disease
  G60.2 **Neuropathy in association with hereditary ataxia**
  G60.3 **Idiopathic progressive neuropathy** — A condition of increasingly persistent disease of the peripheral nerves of undetermined origin.
  G60.8 **Other hereditary and idiopathic neuropathies**
    Dominantly inherited sensory neuropathy
    Morvan's disease
    Nelaton's syndrome
    Recessively inherited sensory neuropathy
  G60.9 **Hereditary and idiopathic neuropathy, unspecified**

G61- **Inflammatory polyneuropathy** — Disease of the nervous system caused by inflammation and cellular damage.
  CC **G61.0** **Guillain-Barre syndrome** — An acute progressive ascending motor neuron paralysis of unknown etiology (most likely autoimmune) characterized by paresthesia, flaccid paralysis, spreading from the legs towards the head, and in some cases respiratory paralysis.
    AHA 14:2Q:p4 – Acute inflammatory demyelinating polyneuropathy
    Acute (post-)infective polyneuritis
    Miller Fisher Syndrome
  G61.1 **Serum neuropathy**
    Use additional code for adverse effect, if applicable, to identify serum (T50-)
  G61.8- **Other inflammatory polyneuropathies**
  CC **G61.81** **Chronic inflammatory demyelinating polyneuritis** — A slowly progressive sensorimotor condition characterized by symmetrical weakness and paresthesias.
    G61.82 **Multifocal motor neuropathy**
      MMN

Side tab: **G 5 7 - G 6 1**

G61.89 Other inflammatory polyneuropathies

G61.9 Inflammatory polyneuropathy, unspecified

G62- Other and unspecified polyneuropathies

G62.0 Drug-induced polyneuropathy — Damage of multiple peripheral nerves due to the cellular damaging effects of drugs.
Use additional code for adverse effect, if applicable, to identify drug (T36-T50 with fifth or sixth character 5)

G62.1 Alcoholic polyneuropathy — Damage of the peripheral nerves due to the cellular destructive effects of excess alcohol.

G62.2 Polyneuropathy due to other toxic agents
Code first (T51-T65) to identify toxic agent

G62.8- Other specified polyneuropathies

cc **G62.81 Critical illness polyneuropathy** — A functional disturbance or damage of the peripheral nervous system that is associated with sepsis, multi-organ failure, and SIRS.
Acute motor neuropathy

G62.82 Radiation-induced polyneuropathy
Use additional external cause code (W88-W90, X39.0-) to identify cause

G62.89 Other specified polyneuropathies
AHA 16:2Q:p11 – Anti-MAG peripheral neuropathy

G62.9 Polyneuropathy, unspecified
Neuropathy NOS

G63 Polyneuropathy in diseases classified elsewhere — [Not Allowed as PDX]
AHA 12:4Q:p99 – Polyneuropathy
Code first underlying disease, such as:
  Amyloidosis (E85.-)
  Endocrine disease, except diabetes (E00-E07, E15-E16, E20-E34)
  Metabolic diseases (E70-E88)
  Neoplasm (C00-D49)
  Nutritional deficiency (E40-E64)
Excludes 1:   polyneuropathy (in):
                diabetes mellitus (E08-E13 with .42)
                diphtheria (A36.83)
                infectious mononucleosis (B27.0-B27.9 with 1)
                Lyme disease (A69.22)
                mumps (B26.84)
                postherpetic (B02.23)
                rheumatoid arthritis (M05.33)
                scleroderma (M34.83)
                systemic lupus erythematosus (M32.19)

G64 Other disorders of peripheral nervous system
Disorder of peripheral nervous system NOS

G65- Sequelae of inflammatory and toxic polyneuropathies
Code first condition resulting from (sequela) of inflammatory and toxic polyneuropathies

G65.0 Sequelae of Guillain-Barré syndrome

G65.1 Sequelae of other inflammatory polyneuropathy

G65.2 Sequelae of toxic polyneuropathy

Diseases of myoneural junction and muscle (G70-G73)

G70- Myasthenia gravis and other myoneural disorders
Excludes 1:   botulism (A05.1, A48.51-A48.52)
                transient neonatal myasthenia gravis (P94.0)

G70.0- Myasthenia gravis — An autoimmune condition characterized by progressive muscular weakness on exertion followed by recovery of strength after a period of rest.

G70.00 Myasthenia gravis without (acute) exacerbation
Myasthenia gravis NOS

MCC **G70.01 Myasthenia gravis with (acute) exacerbation** — A relatively sudden, severe onset of difficulty breathing caused by significant weakness of the muscles that control breathing.
Myasthenia gravis in crisis

G70.1 Toxic myoneural disorders — Disorders of the muscles and nerves caused by the cellular damaging effect of toxic substances.
Code first (T51-T65) to identify toxic agent

G70.2 Congenital and developmental myasthenia

G70.8- Other specified myoneural disorders

cc **G70.80 Lambert-Eaton syndrome, unspecified** — An autoimmune, neuromuscular junction disorder that is characterized by muscle weakness, difficulty swallowing, dry mouth, and vision changes.
Lambert-Eaton syndrome NOS

cc **G70.81 Lambert-Eaton syndrome in disease classified elsewhere** — [Not Allowed as PDX]
Code first underlying disease
Excludes 1:   Lambert-Eaton syndrome in neoplastic disease (G73.1)

G70.89 Other specified myoneural disorders

G70.9 Myoneural disorder, unspecified

G71- Primary disorders of muscles
Excludes❷: arthrogryposis multiplex congenita (Q74.3)
                metabolic disorders (E70-E88)
                myositis (M60.-)

cc **G71.0 Muscular dystrophy** — A group of inherited muscular dystrophies characterized by progressive muscular weakness and degeneration of muscle fibers.
Autosomal recessive, childhood type, muscular dystrophy resembling Duchenne or Becker muscular dystrophy
Benign [Becker] muscular dystrophy
Benign scapuloperoneal muscular dystrophy with early contractures [Emery-Dreifuss]
Congenital muscular dystrophy NOS
Congenital muscular dystrophy with specific morphological abnormalities of the muscle fiber
Distal muscular dystrophy
Facioscapulohumeral muscular dystrophy
Limb-girdle muscular dystrophy
Ocular muscular dystrophy
Oculopharyngeal muscular dystrophy
Scapuloperoneal muscular dystrophy
Severe [Duchenne] muscular dystrophy

G71.1- Myotonic disorders — Disorders characterized by sustained contraction of muscles with decreased ability of muscular relaxation.

G71.11 Myotonic muscular dystrophy — An inherited disorder of the muscles that is characterized by progressive muscular weakness and wasting, cataracts, heart conduction defects, and endocrine changes.
Dystrophia myotonica [Steinert]
Myotonia atrophica
Myotonic dystrophy
Proximal myotonic myopathy (PROMM)
Steinert disease

G71.12 Myotonia congenita — An inherited disorder of the muscles that usually begins in childhood and is characterized by very stiff muscles of the hands, legs, and eyelids and associated muscular hypertrophy.
Acetazolamide responsive myotonia congenita
Dominant myotonia congenita [Thomsen disease]
Myotonia levior
Recessive myotonia congenita [Becker disease]

G71.13 Myotonic chondrodystrophy — An inherited disorder of the muscles with onset at or soon after birth that is characterized by a more severe form of myotonia, muscular hypertrophy, and multiple skeletal deformities.
Chondrodystrophic myotonia
Congenital myotonic chondrodystrophy
Schwartz-Jampel disease

G71.14 Drug-induced myotonia
Use additional code for adverse effect, if applicable, to identify drug (T36-T50 with fifth or sixth character 5)

G71.19 Other specified myotonic disorders
Myotonia fluctuans
Myotonia permanens
Neuromyotonia [Isaacs]
Paramyotonia congenita (of von Eulenburg)
Pseudomyotonia
Symptomatic myotonia

cc **G71.2 Congenital myopathies** — An inherited group of rare disorders characterized by slowly progressive or nonprogressive myopathy.
Central core disease
Fiber-type disproportion
Minicore disease
Multicore disease
Myotubular (centronuclear) myopathy
Nemaline myopathy
Excludes 1:   arthrogryposis multiplex congenita (Q74.3)

G71.3 Mitochondrial myopathy, not elsewhere classified
Excludes 1:   Kearns-Sayre syndrome (H49.81)
                Leber's disease (H47.21)
                Leigh's encephalopathy (G31.82)
                mitochondrial metabolism disorders (E88.4.-)
                Reye's syndrome (G93.7)

G71.8 Other primary disorders of muscles

G71.9 Primary disorder of muscle, unspecified
Hereditary myopathy NOS

G61 - G71

Excludes 1: = NOT CODED HERE! (Do not code both)

Excludes ❷: = Not Included Here

G72- Other and unspecified myopathies

    Excludes 1:   arthrogryposis multiplex congenita (Q74.3)
                  dermatopolymyositis (M33.-)
                  ischemic infarction of muscle (M62.2-)
                  myositis (M60.-)
                  polymyositis (M33.2.-)

cc **G72.0 Drug-induced myopathy**
    Use additional code for adverse effect, if applicable, to identify drug (T36-T50 with fifth or sixth character 5)

cc **G72.1 Alcoholic myopathy**
    Use additional code to identify alcoholism (F10.-)

cc **G72.2 Myopathy due to other toxic agents**
    Code first (T51-T65) to identify toxic agent

G72.3 Periodic paralysis — An inherited disorder of the voluntary muscles that is characterized by sudden attacks of weakness and paralysis.
    Familial periodic paralysis
    Hyperkalemic periodic paralysis (familial)
    Hypokalemic periodic paralysis (familial)
    Myotonic periodic paralysis (familial)
    Normokalemic paralysis (familial)
    Potassium sensitive periodic paralysis

    Excludes 1:   paramyotonia congenita (of von Eulenburg) (G71.19)

G72.4- Inflammatory and immune myopathies, not elsewhere classified

    G72.41 Inclusion body myositis [IBM] — An inflammatory muscle disease that is characterized by slowly progressive weakness that leads to balance problems, impaired finger gripping, and dysphagia.

    G72.49 Other inflammatory and immune myopathies, not elsewhere classified
        Inflammatory myopathy NOS

G72.8- Other specified myopathies

cc **G72.81 Critical illness myopathy** — A functional disturbance or damage to the neuromuscular system that is associated with sepsis, multi-organ failure, and SIRS.
        Acute necrotizing myopathy
        Acute quadriplegic myopathy
        Intensive care (ICU) myopathy
        Myopathy of critical illness

    G72.89 Other specified myopathies

G72.9 Myopathy, unspecified

G73- Disorders of myoneural junction and muscle in diseases classified elsewhere

cc **G73.1 Lambert-Eaton syndrome in neoplastic disease** —
    [Unacceptable PDX] [Not Allowed as PDX]
    Code first underlying neoplasm (C00-D49)
    Excludes 1:   Lambert-Eaton syndrome not associated with neoplasm (G70.80-G70.81)

cc **G73.3 Myasthenic syndromes in other diseases classified elsewhere** — [Not Allowed as PDX]
    Code first underlying, such as:
        Neoplasm (C00-D49)
        Thyrotoxicosis (E05.-)

G73.7 Myopathy in diseases classified elsewhere — [Not Allowed as PDX]
    Code first underlying disease, such as:
        Glycogen storage disease (E74.0)
        Hyperparathyroidism (E21.0, E21.3)
        Hypoparathyroidism (E20.-)
        Lipid storage disorders (E75.-)
    Excludes 1:   myopathy in:
                rheumatoid arthritis (M05.32)
                sarcoidosis (D86.87)
                scleroderma (M34.82)
                sicca syndrome [Sjögren] (M35.03)
                systemic lupus erythematosus (M32.19)

Cerebral palsy and other paralytic syndromes (G80-G83)

G80- Cerebral palsy — A nonprogressive, brain damaging disturbance of the prenatal or perinatal period characterized by persistent, qualitative motor dysfunction, paralysis, and in severe cases mental retardation.

    Excludes 1:   hereditary spastic paraplegia (G11.4)

MCC **G80.0 Spastic quadriplegic cerebral palsy** — A form characterized by paralysis of all four limbs.
    Congenital spastic paralysis (cerebral)

cc **G80.1 Spastic diplegic cerebral palsy** — The most common form due to bilateral damage of the corticospinal tracts and characterized by lower limb paralysis showing the typical "scissor" gait and is associated with prematurity.
    Spastic cerebral palsy NOS

cc **G80.2 Spastic hemiplegic cerebral palsy** — A form resulting from damage to the sensorimotor cortex that controls one side of the body and characterized by hemiparesis, growth arrest of the affected limbs, sensory deficits, and occasionally a seizure disorder which is usually associated with head trauma and is present at birth.

cc **G80.3 Athetoid cerebral palsy** — A form damaging the basal ganglia that is characterized by uncontrolled movements of the trunk and extremities.
    Double athetosis (syndrome)
    Dyskinetic cerebral palsy
    Dystonic cerebral palsy
    Vogt disease

G80.4 Ataxic cerebral palsy — A rare form that is characterized by movements that are not smooth and appear jerky.

G80.8 Other cerebral palsy
    Mixed cerebral palsy syndromes

G80.9 Cerebral palsy, unspecified
    Cerebral palsy NOS

G81- Hemiplegia and hemiparesis — Paralysis of one side of the body.
    AHA 14:1Q:p23 – Hemiplegia
    AHA 15:1Q:p25 – Left sided (nondominant) weakness
    Note: This category is to be used only when hemiplegia (complete) (incomplete) is reported without further specification, or is stated to be old or longstanding but of unspecified cause. The category is also for use in multiple coding to identify these types of hemiplegia resulting from any cause.

    Excludes 1:   congenital cerebral palsy (G80.-)
                hemiplegia and hemiparesis due to sequela of cerebrovascular disease (I69.05-, I69.15-, I69.25-, I69.35-, I69.85-, I69.95-)

G81.0- Flaccid hemiplegia — Paralysis of one side of the body with loss of tone of the muscles of the paralyzed part and absence of tendon reflexes.

cc **G81.00 Flaccid hemiplegia affecting unspecified side**
cc **G81.01 Flaccid hemiplegia affecting right dominant side**
cc **G81.02 Flaccid hemiplegia affecting left dominant side**
cc **G81.03 Flaccid hemiplegia affecting right nondominant side**
cc **G81.04 Flaccid hemiplegia affecting left nondominant side**

G81.1- Spastic hemiplegia — Paralysis of one side of the body marked by spasticity of the muscles of the paralyzed part and increased tendon reflexes.

cc **G81.10 Spastic hemiplegia affecting unspecified side**
cc **G81.11 Spastic hemiplegia affecting right dominant side**
cc **G81.12 Spastic hemiplegia affecting left dominant side**
cc **G81.13 Spastic hemiplegia affecting right nondominant side**
cc **G81.14 Spastic hemiplegia affecting left nondominant side**

G81.9- Hemiplegia, unspecified

cc **G81.90 Hemiplegia, unspecified affecting unspecified side**
cc **G81.91 Hemiplegia, unspecified affecting right dominant side**
cc **G81.92 Hemiplegia, unspecified affecting left dominant side**
cc **G81.93 Hemiplegia, unspecified affecting right nondominant side**
cc **G81.94 Hemiplegia, unspecified affecting left nondominant side**

G72 - G81

G82- Paraplegia (paraparesis) and quadriplegia (quadriparesis)
  Note: This category is to be used only when the listed conditions are reported without further specification, or are stated to be old or longstanding but of unspecified cause. The category is also for use in multiple coding to identify these conditions resulting from any cause.
    Excludes 1: *congenital cerebral palsy (G80.-)*
        functional quadriplegia (R53.2)
        hysterical paralysis (F44.4)

  G82.2- Paraplegia — Loss or impairment of function of the legs and lower part of the body.
      Paralysis of both lower limbs NOS
      Paraparesis (lower) NOS
      Paraplegia (lower) NOS
    CC **G82.20 Paraplegia, unspecified**
    CC **G82.21 Paraplegia, complete**
    CC **G82.22 Paraplegia, incomplete**

  G82.5- Quadriplegia — Loss or impairment of motor function of all four limbs.
    MCC **G82.50 Quadriplegia, unspecified**
    MCC **G82.51 Quadriplegia, C1-C4 complete**
    MCC **G82.52 Quadriplegia, C1-C4 incomplete**
    MCC **G82.53 Quadriplegia, C5-C7 complete**
    MCC **G82.54 Quadriplegia, C5-C7 incomplete**

G83- Other paralytic syndromes
  Note: This category is to be used only when the listed conditions are reported without further specification, or are stated to be old or longstanding but of unspecified cause. The category is also for use in multiple coding to identify these conditions resulting from any cause.
  Includes: Paralysis (complete) (incomplete), except as in G80-G82

  CC **G83.0 Diplegia of upper limbs** — Loss or impairment of function of the upper limbs.
      Diplegia (upper)
      Paralysis of both upper limbs

  G83.1- Monoplegia of lower limb — Loss or impairment of function of one of the lower limbs.
      Paralysis of lower limb
    Excludes 1: *monoplegia of lower limbs due to sequela of cerebrovascular disease (I69.04-, I69.14-, I69.24-, I69.34-, I69.84-, I69.94-)*

    G83.10 Monoplegia of lower limb affecting unspecified side
    G83.11 Monoplegia of lower limb affecting right dominant side
    G83.12 Monoplegia of lower limb affecting left dominant side
    G83.13 Monoplegia of lower limb affecting right nondominant side
    G83.14 Monoplegia of lower limb affecting left nondominant side

  G83.2- Monoplegia of upper limb — Loss or impairment of function of one of the upper limbs.
      Paralysis of upper limb
    Excludes 1: *monoplegia of upper limbs due to sequela of cerebrovascular disease (I69.03-, I69.13-, I69.23-, I69.33-, I69.83-, I69.93-)*

    G83.20 Monoplegia of upper limb affecting unspecified side
    G83.21 Monoplegia of upper limb affecting right dominant side
    G83.22 Monoplegia of upper limb affecting left dominant side
    G83.23 Monoplegia of upper limb affecting right nondominant side
    G83.24 Monoplegia of upper limb affecting left nondominant side

  G83.3- Monoplegia, unspecified
    G83.30 Monoplegia, unspecified affecting unspecified side
    G83.31 Monoplegia, unspecified affecting right dominant side
    G83.32 Monoplegia, unspecified affecting left dominant side
    G83.33 Monoplegia, unspecified affecting right nondominant side
    G83.34 Monoplegia, unspecified affecting left nondominant side

  CC **G83.4 Cauda equina syndrome** — Compression of the spinal nerve roots marked by areflexic paralysis, paresthesia, and dull aching pains of the perineum, bladder, and sacrum.
      Neurogenic bladder due to cauda equina syndrome — Dysfunction of the urinary bladder due to cauda equina syndrome.
    Excludes 1: *cord bladder NOS (G95.89)*
        neurogenic bladder NOS (N31.9)

MCC **G83.5 Locked-in state** — A condition marked by a severe, nonreactive paralysis while remaining conscious.

  G83.8- Other specified paralytic syndromes
    Excludes 1: *paralytic syndromes due to current spinal cord injury-code to spinal cord injury (S14, S24, S34)*

    G83.81 Brown-Séquard syndrome
    G83.82 Anterior cord syndrome
    G83.83 Posterior cord syndrome
    G83.84 Todd's paralysis (postepileptic)
    G83.89 Other specified paralytic syndromes
  G83.9 Paralytic syndrome, unspecified

Other disorders of the nervous system (G89-G99)

G89- Pain, not elsewhere classified
  Code also related psychological factors associated with pain (F45.42)
    Excludes 1: *generalized pain NOS (R52)*
        pain disorders exclusively related to psychological factors (F45.41)
        pain NOS (R52)
    Excludes ❷: *atypical face pain (G50.1)*
        headache syndromes (G44.-)
        localized pain, unspecified type — code to pain by site, such as:
          abdomen pain (R10.-)
          back pain (M54.9)
          breast pain (N64.4)
          chest pain (R07.1-R07.9)
          ear pain (H92.0-)
          eye pain (H57.1)
          headache (R51)
          joint pain (M25.5-)
          limb pain (M79.6-)
          lumbar region pain (M54.5)
          painful urination (R30.9)
          pelvic and perineal pain (R10.2)
          shoulder pain (M25.51-)
          spine pain (M54.-)
          throat pain (R07.0)
          tongue pain (K14.6)
          tooth pain (K08.8)
        migraines (G43.-)
        myalgia (M79.1)
        pain from prosthetic devices, implants, and grafts (T82.84, T83.84, T84.84, T85.84-)
        phantom limb syndrome with pain (G54.6)
        renal colic (N23)
        vulvar vestibulitis (N94.810)
        vulvodynia (N94.81-)

  G89.0 Central pain syndrome — Pain caused by damage to the central nervous system.
      Déjérine-Roussy syndrome
      Myelopathic pain syndrome
      Thalamic pain syndrome (hyperesthetic)

  G89.1- Acute pain, not elsewhere classified
    G89.11 Acute pain due to trauma
    G89.12 Acute post-thoracotomy pain
        Post-thoracotomy pain NOS
    G89.18 Other acute postprocedural pain
        Postoperative pain NOS
        Postprocedural pain NOS

  G89.2- Chronic pain, not elsewhere classified
    Excludes 1: *causalgia, lower limb (G57.7-)*
        causalgia, upper limb (G56.4-)
        central pain syndrome (G89.0)
        chronic pain syndrome (G89.4)
        complex regional pain syndrome II, lower limb (G57.7-)
        complex regional pain syndrome II, upper limb (G56.4-)
        neoplasm related chronic pain (G89.3)
        reflex sympathetic dystrophy (G90.5-)

    G89.21 Chronic pain due to trauma
    G89.22 Chronic post-thoracotomy pain
    G89.28 Other chronic postprocedural pain
        Other chronic postoperative pain
    G89.29 Other chronic pain

G82 - G89

G89.3 <u>Neoplasm</u> related pain (acute) (chronic)
Cancer associated pain
Pain due to malignancy (primary) (secondary)
Tumor associated pain

G89.4 <u>Chronic pain syndrome</u>
Chronic pain associated with significant psychosocial dysfunction

G90- **Disorders of autonomic nervous system**
Excludes 1: *dysfunction of the autonomic nervous system due to alcohol (G31.2)*

G90.0- **Idiopathic peripheral autonomic neuropathy**

G90.01 **Carotid sinus syncope** — *A temporary loss of consciousness due to the overactivity of the carotid sinus reflex.*
Carotid sinus syndrome

G90.09 **Other idiopathic peripheral autonomic neuropathy**
Idiopathic peripheral autonomic neuropathy NOS

G90.1 **Familial dysautonomia [Riley-Day]**

G90.2 **Horner's syndrome**
Bernard(-Horner) syndrome
Cervical sympathetic dystrophy or paralysis

CC **G90.3** **Multi-system degeneration of the autonomic nervous system**
Neurogenic orthostatic hypotension [Shy-Drager]
Excludes 1: *orthostatic hypotension NOS (I95.1)*

G90.4 **Autonomic dysreflexia** — *A condition of the spinal cord sympathetic nervous system signals resulting in hypertension, vasoconstriction, bradycardia, blurred vision, and sweating.*
Use additional code to identify the cause, such as:
Fecal impaction (K56.41)
Pressure ulcer (pressure area) (L89.-)
Urinary tract infection (N39.0)

G90.5- **Complex regional pain syndrome I (CRPS I)** — *A condition most often affecting one of the limbs of the sympathetic nervous system marked by burning pain, sweating, hyperesthesia, and skin atrophy most likely caused as a result of an injury to nerves or blood vessels.*
Reflex sympathetic dystrophy
Excludes 1: *causalgia of lower limb (G57.7-)*
causalgia of upper limb (G56.4-)
complex regional pain syndrome II of lower limb (G57.7-)
complex regional pain syndrome II of upper limb (G56.4-)

CC **G90.50** **Complex regional pain syndrome I, unspecified**

G90.51- **Complex regional pain syndrome I of <u>upper</u> limb**

CC **G90.511** **Complex regional pain syndrome I of <u>right</u> upper limb**

CC **G90.512** **Complex regional pain syndrome I of <u>left</u> upper limb**

CC **G90.513** **Complex regional pain syndrome I of upper limb, <u>bilateral</u>**

CC **G90.519** **Complex regional pain syndrome I of <u>unspecified</u> upper limb**

G90.52- **Complex regional pain syndrome I of <u>lower</u> limb**

CC **G90.521** **Complex regional pain syndrome I of <u>right</u> lower limb**

CC **G90.522** **Complex regional pain syndrome I of <u>left</u> lower limb**

CC **G90.523** **Complex regional pain syndrome I of lower limb, <u>bilateral</u>**

CC **G90.529** **Complex regional pain syndrome I of <u>unspecified</u> lower limb**

CC **G90.59** **Complex regional pain syndrome I of other specified site**

G90.8 **Other disorders of autonomic nervous system**

G90.9 **Disorder of the autonomic nervous system, unspecified**

G91- <u>Hydrocephalus</u> — *An abnormal accumulation of cerebrospinal fluid.*
Includes: **Acquired hydrocephalus**
Excludes 1: *Arnold-Chiari syndrome with hydrocephalus (Q07.-)*
congenital hydrocephalus (Q03.-)
spina bifida with hydrocephalus (Q05.-)

CC **G91.0** <u>Communicating</u> hydrocephalus — *An abnormal accumulation of cerebrospinal fluid that is secondary to a disease process.*
Secondary normal pressure hydrocephalus

CC **G91.1** <u>Obstructive</u> hydrocephalus — *An abnormal accumulation of cerebrospinal fluid that develops as a result of a blockage in the normal circulation of cerebrospinal fluid within the brain.*

CC **G91.2** <u>(Idiopathic) normal pressure</u> hydrocephalus — *An abnormal accumulation of cerebrospinal fluid that is characterized by dementia, urinary incontinence, and gait disturbance and is without a known cause.*
Normal pressure hydrocephalus NOS

CC **G91.3** <u>Post-traumatic</u> hydrocephalus, unspecified

G91.4 **Hydrocephalus <u>in diseases classified elsewhere</u>** —
[Not Allowed as PDX]
AHA 14:3Q:p3 – Hydrocephalus in disease classified elsewhere
Code first underlying condition, such as:
Congenital syphilis (A50.4-)
Neoplasm (C00-D49)
Excludes 1: *hydrocephalus due to congenital toxoplasmosis (P37.1)*

CC **G91.8** **Other hydrocephalus**

CC **G91.9** **Hydrocephalus, unspecified**

G92 **Toxic encephalopathy** — *A degenerative condition of the brain caused by the toxic*
MCC *effect of certain substances.*
Toxic encephalitis
Toxic metabolic encephalopathy
Code first (T51-T65) to identify toxic agent

G93- **Other disorders of brain**

G93.0 **Cerebral cysts** — *An encapsulated fluid-filled cyst of the brain and meninges.*
Arachnoid cyst
Porencephalic cyst, acquired
Excludes 1: *acquired periventricular cysts of newborn (P91.1)*
congenital cerebral cysts (Q04.6)

CC **G93.1** **Anoxic brain damage, not elsewhere classified** — *Cellular brain tissue injury due to the absence or lack of oxygen.*
Excludes 1: *cerebral anoxia due to anesthesia during labor and delivery (O74.3)*
cerebral anoxia due to anesthesia during the puerperium (O89.2)
neonatal anoxia (P84)

G93.2 **Benign intracranial hypertension** — *Cerebral edema resulting in raised intracranial pressure with headache, nausea, vomiting, and occasional sixth nerve palsy.*
Excludes 1: *hypertensive encephalopathy (I67.4)*

G93.3 **Postviral fatigue syndrome** — *The abnormal lack or loss of strength after recovery from a viral infection.*
Benign myalgic encephalomyelitis
Excludes 1: *chronic fatigue syndrome NOS (R53.82)*

G93.4- **Other and unspecified encephalopathy**
Excludes 1: *alcoholic encephalopathy (G31.2)*
encephalopathy in diseases classified elsewhere (G94)
hypertensive encephalopathy (I67.4)
toxic (metabolic) encephalopathy (G92)

MCC **G93.40** **Encephalopathy, unspecified**

MCC **G93.41** **Metabolic encephalopathy** — *A generalized cerebral dysfunction due to metabolic disorders.*
AHA 15:3Q:p21 – Diabetes mellitus with acute encephalopathy secondary to hypoglycemia
Septic encephalopathy

MCC **G93.49** **Other encephalopathy**
Encephalopathy NEC

MCC **G93.5** **Compression of brain** — *Pressure on the brain usually due to space-occupying diseases.*
Arnold-Chiari type 1 compression of brain
Compression of brain (stem)
Herniation of brain (stem)
Excludes 1: *diffuse traumatic compression of brain (S06.2-)*
focal traumatic compression of brain (S06.3-)

MCC **G93.6** **Cerebral edema** — *An excessive accumulation of fluid in the brain substance.*
Excludes 1: *cerebral edema due to birth injury (P11.0)*
traumatic cerebral edema (S06.1-)

G89 - G93

MCC **G93.7**   **Reye's syndrome** — [Age/0-17] — An acute encephalopathy in children usually following certain infections and marked by fatty degeneration of the liver, rapid development of brain swelling, hepatomegaly, and seizures.
     Code first (T39.0-), if salicylates-induced

G93.8-   **Other specified disorders of brain**

     G93.81   **Temporal sclerosis** — The condition of loss of neurons and scarring of the temporal lobe that is usually due to brain injuries or diseases and results in seizure activity.
       Hippocampal sclerosis
       Mesial temporal sclerosis

    MCC **G93.82**   **Brain death** — The condition of complete and irreversible cessation of all brain function and activity.

     G93.89   **Other specified disorders of brain**
       Postradiation encephalopathy

G93.9   **Disorder of brain, unspecified**

G94   **Other disorders of brain in diseases classified elsewhere** —
[Not Allowed as PDX]
Code first underlying disease
Excludes 1:   encephalopathy in congenital syphilis (A50.49)
           encephalopathy in influenza (J09.X9, J10.81, J11.81)
           encephalopathy in syphilis (A52.19)
           hydrocephalus in diseases classified elsewhere (G91.4)

G95-   **Other and unspecified diseases of spinal cord**
Excludes ❷: myelitis (G04.-)

CC **G95.0**   **Syringomyelia and syringobulbia** — SYRINGOMYELIA – A destructive spinal cord condition resulting in cavity formation and characterized by weakness and wasting of the small muscles of the hand, with accompanying loss of pain sensation. SYRINGOBULBIA – A destructive cavitary disorder of the brainstem characterized by weakness and wasting of the tongue, dysphagia, dysarthria, and general loss of sensation to the face.

G95.1-   **Vascular myelopathies** — Functional disorders of the spinal cord caused by vascular hemorrhagic conditions.
Excludes ❷: intraspinal phlebitis and thrombophlebitis, except non-pyogenic (G08)

    MCC **G95.11**   **Acute infarction of spinal cord (embolic) (nonembolic)** —
Obstructive ischemic tissue necrosis of the spinal cord.
       Anoxia of spinal cord
       Arterial thrombosis of spinal cord

    MCC **G95.19**   **Other vascular myelopathies**
       Edema of spinal cord
       Hematomyelia
       Nonpyogenic intraspinal phlebitis and thrombophlebitis
       Subacute necrotic myelopathy

G95.2-   **Other and unspecified cord compression**

CC **G95.20**   **Unspecified cord compression**

CC **G95.29**   **Other cord compression**

G95.8-   **Other specified diseases of spinal cord**
Excludes 1:   neurogenic bladder NOS (N31.9)
           neurogenic bladder due to cauda equina syndrome (G83.4)
           neuromuscular dysfunction of bladder without spinal cord lesion (N31.-)

CC **G95.81**   **Conus medullaris syndrome**

CC **G95.89**   **Other specified diseases of spinal cord**
       Cord bladder NOS
       Drug-induced myelopathy
       Radiation-induced myelopathy
      Excludes 1:   myelopathy NOS (G95.9)

CC **G95.9**   **Disease of spinal cord, unspecified**
       Myelopathy NOS

G96-   **Other disorders of central nervous system**

CC **G96.0**   **Cerebrospinal fluid leak**
      Excludes 1:   cerebrospinal fluid leak from spinal puncture (G97.0)

G96.1-   **Disorders of meninges, not elsewhere classified**

CC **G96.11**   **Dural tear**
       AHA 14:4Q:p24 – Durotomy secondary to previous epidural injections
      Excludes 1:   accidental puncture or laceration of dura during a procedure (G97.41)

     G96.12   **Meningeal adhesions (cerebral) (spinal)**

     G96.19   **Other disorders of meninges, not elsewhere classified**

G96.8   **Other specified disorders of central nervous system**

G96.9   **Disorder of central nervous system, unspecified**

G97-   **Intraoperative and postprocedural complications** and disorders of nervous system, not elsewhere classified
Excludes ❷: intraoperative and postprocedural cerebrovascular infarction (I97.81-, I97.82-)

CC **G97.0**   **Cerebrospinal fluid leak from spinal puncture**

G97.1   **Other reaction to spinal and lumbar puncture**
       Headache due to lumbar puncture

CC **G97.2**   **Intracranial hypotension following ventricular shunting**

G97.3-   **Intraoperative hemorrhage and hematoma** of a nervous system organ or structure complicating a procedure
Excludes 1:   intraoperative hemorrhage and hematoma of a nervous system organ or structure due to accidental puncture and laceration during a procedure (G97.4-)

CC **G97.31**   **Intraoperative hemorrhage and hematoma of a nervous system organ or structure complicating a nervous system procedure**

CC **G97.32**   **Intraoperative hemorrhage and hematoma of a nervous system organ or structure complicating other procedure**

G97.4-   **Accidental puncture and laceration** of a nervous system organ or structure during a procedure

CC **G97.41**   **Accidental puncture or laceration of dura during a procedure**
       Incidental (inadvertent) durotomy

CC **G97.48**   **Accidental puncture and laceration of other nervous system organ or structure during a nervous system procedure**

CC **G97.49**   **Accidental puncture and laceration of other nervous system organ or structure during other procedure**

G97.5-   **Postprocedural hemorrhage** of a nervous system organ or structure following a procedure

CC **G97.51**   **Postprocedural hemorrhage of a nervous system organ or structure following a nervous system procedure**

CC **G97.52**   **Postprocedural hemorrhage of a nervous system organ or structure following other procedure**

G97.6-   **Postprocedural hematoma and seroma** of a nervous system organ or structure following a procedure

CC **G97.61**   **Postprocedural hematoma of a nervous system organ or structure following a nervous system procedure**

CC **G97.62**   **Postprocedural hematoma of a nervous system organ or structure following other procedure**

CC **G97.63**   **Postprocedural seroma of a nervous system organ or structure following a nervous system procedure**

CC **G97.64**   **Postprocedural seroma of a nervous system organ or structure following other procedure**

G97.8-   **Other intraoperative and postprocedural complications and disorders of nervous system**
       Use additional code to further specify disorder

CC **G97.81**   **Other intraoperative complications of nervous system**

CC **G97.82**   **Other postprocedural complications and disorders of nervous system**

G98-   **Other disorders of nervous system not elsewhere classified**
     Includes: Nervous system disorder NOS

G98.0   **Neurogenic arthritis, not elsewhere classified**
       Nonsyphilitic neurogenic arthropathy NEC
       Nonsyphilitic neurogenic spondylopathy NEC
      Excludes 1:   spondylopathy (in):
           syringomyelia and syringobulbia (G95.0)
           tabes dorsalis (A52.11)

G98.8   **Other disorders of nervous system**
       Nervous system disorder NOS

G93 - G98

Excludes 1: = NOT CODED HERE! (Do not code both)   **671**   *Excludes ❷:* = Not Included Here

G99- Other disorders of nervous system <u>in diseases classified elsewhere</u>

CC **G99.0** **Autonomic neuropathy in diseases classified elsewhere —**
[Not Allowed as PDX]
Code first underlying disease, such as:
Amyloidosis (E85.-)
Gout (M1A.-, M10.-)
Hyperthyroidism (E05.-)
Excludes 1: *diabetic autonomic neuropathy (E08-E14 with .43)*

CC **G99.2** **Myelopathy in diseases classified elsewhere —**
[Not Allowed as PDX]
Code first underlying disease, such as:
Neoplasm (C00-D49)
Excludes 1: *myelopathy in:*
intervertebral disease (M50.0-, M51.0-)
spondylosis (M47.0-, M47.1-)

G99.8 **Other specified disorders of nervous system in diseases classified elsewhere —** [Not Allowed as PDX]
Code first underlying disorder, such as:
Amyloidosis (E85.-)
Avitaminosis (E56.9)
Excludes 1: *nervous system involvement in:*
cysticercosis (B69.0)
rubella (B06.0-)
syphilis (A52.1-)

Chapter 7 – Diseases of the eye and adnexa (H00-H59)

Note: Use an external cause code following the code for the eye condition, if applicable, to identify the cause of the eye condition

Excludes ❷: *certain conditions originating in the perinatal period (P04-P96)*

certain infectious and parasitic diseases (A00-B99)

complications of pregnancy, childbirth and the puerperium (O00-O9A)

congenital malformations, deformations, and chromosomal abnormalities (Q00-Q99)

diabetes mellitus related eye conditions (E09.3-, E10.3-, E11.3-, E13.3-)

endocrine, nutritional and metabolic diseases (E00-E88)

injury (trauma) of eye and orbit (S05.-)

injury, poisoning and certain other consequences of external causes (S00-T88)

neoplasms (C00-D49)

symptoms, signs and abnormal clinical and laboratory findings, not elsewhere classified (R00-R94)

syphilis related eye disorders (A50.01, A50.3-, A51.43, A52.71)

This chapter contains the following blocks:
H00-H05	Disorders of eyelid, lacrimal system and orbit
H10-H11	Disorders of conjunctiva
H15-H22	Disorders of sclera, cornea, iris and ciliary body
H25-H28	Disorders of lens
H30-H36	Disorders of choroid and retina
H40-H42	Glaucoma
H43-H44	Disorders of vitreous body and globe
H46-H47	Disorders of optic nerve and visual pathways
H49-H52	Disorders of ocular muscles, binocular movement, accommodation and refraction
H53-H54	Visual disturbances and blindness
H55-H57	Other disorders of eye and adnexa
H59	Intraoperative and postprocedural complications and disorders of eye and adnexa, not elsewhere classified

Chapter-Specific Coding Guidelines

C.   Chapter-Specific Coding Guidelines

In addition to general coding guidelines, there are guidelines for specific diagnoses and/or conditions in the classification. Unless otherwise indicated, these guidelines apply to all health care settings. Please refer to Section II for guidelines on the selection of principal diagnosis.

7.   Chapter 7: Diseases of Eye and Adnexa (H00-H59)

a.   Glaucoma

1)   Assigning Glaucoma Codes
Assign as many codes from category H40, Glaucoma, as needed to identify the type of glaucoma, the affected eye, and the glaucoma stage.

2)   Bilateral glaucoma with same type and stage
When a patient has bilateral glaucoma and both eyes are documented as being the same type and stage, and there is a code for bilateral glaucoma, report only the code for the type of glaucoma, bilateral, with the seventh character for the stage.

When a patient has bilateral glaucoma and both eyes are documented as being the same type and stage, and the classification does not provide a code for bilateral glaucoma (i.e. subcategories H40.10, H40.11 and H40.20) report only one code for the type of glaucoma with the appropriate seventh character for the stage.

3)   Bilateral glaucoma stage with different types or stages
When a patient has bilateral glaucoma and each eye is documented as having a different type or stage, and the classification distinguishes laterality, assign the appropriate code for each eye rather than the code for bilateral glaucoma.

When a patient has bilateral glaucoma and each eye is documented as having a different type, and the classification does not distinguish laterality (i.e. subcategories H40.10, H40.11 and H40.20), assign one code for each type of glaucoma with the appropriate seventh character for the stage.
When a patient has bilateral glaucoma and each eye is documented as having the same type, but different stage, and the classification does not distinguish laterality (i.e. subcategories H40.10, H40.11 and H40.20), assign a code for the type of glaucoma for each eye with the seventh character for the specific glaucoma stage documented for each eye.

4)   Patient admitted with glaucoma and stage evolves during the admission
If a patient is admitted with glaucoma and the stage progresses during the admission, assign the code for highest stage documented.

5)   Indeterminate stage glaucoma
Assignment of the seventh character "4" for "indeterminate stage" should be based on the clinical documentation. The seventh character "4" is used for glaucomas whose stage cannot be clinically determined. This seventh character should not be confused with the seventh character "0", unspecified, which should be assigned when there is no documentation regarding the stage of the glaucoma.

Disorders of eyelid, lacrimal system and orbit (H00-H05)

Excludes ❷: *open wound of eyelid (S01.1-)*
superficial injury of eyelid (S00.1-, S00.2-)

H00-   Hordeolum and chalazion

H00.0-   <u>Hordeolum</u> (externum) (internum) of eyelid

H00.01- Hordeolum <u>externum</u> — Purulent inflammation of the sebaceous glands of the external eyelid surface, most often caused by Staphylococcus.
  Hordeolum NOS
  Stye

H00.011	Hordeolum externum <u>right</u> <u>upper</u> eyelid
H00.012	Hordeolum externum <u>right</u> <u>lower</u> eyelid
H00.013	Hordeolum externum <u>right</u> eye, <u>unspecified</u> eyelid
H00.014	Hordeolum externum <u>left</u> <u>upper</u> eyelid
H00.015	Hordeolum externum <u>left</u> <u>lower</u> eyelid
H00.016	Hordeolum externum <u>left</u> eye, <u>unspecified</u> eyelid
H00.019	Hordeolum externum <u>unspecified</u> eye, <u>unspecified</u> eyelid

H00.02- Hordeolum <u>internum</u> — Purulent inflammation of the sebaceous glands of the internal eyelid surface, most often caused by Staphylococcus.
  Infection of meibomian gland — A form affecting the meibomian glands of the conjunctiva of the eyelids.

H00.021	Hordeolum internum <u>right</u> <u>upper</u> eyelid
H00.022	Hordeolum internum <u>right</u> <u>lower</u> eyelid
H00.023	Hordeolum internum <u>right</u> eye, <u>unspecified</u> eyelid
H00.024	Hordeolum internum <u>left</u> <u>upper</u> eyelid
H00.025	Hordeolum internum <u>left</u> <u>lower</u> eyelid
H00.026	Hordeolum internum <u>left</u> eye, <u>unspecified</u> eyelid
H00.029	Hordeolum internum <u>unspecified</u> eye, <u>unspecified</u> eyelid

H00.03- <u>Abscess</u> of eyelid — A localized collection of pus caused by the disintegration of eyelid tissues.
  Furuncle of eyelid — An acute circumscribed inflammation of the subcutaneous tissue of the eyelid.

H00.031	Abscess of <u>right</u> <u>upper</u> eyelid
H00.032	Abscess of <u>right</u> <u>lower</u> eyelid
H00.033	Abscess of eyelid <u>right</u> eye, <u>unspecified</u> eyelid
H00.034	Abscess of <u>left</u> <u>upper</u> eyelid
H00.035	Abscess of <u>left</u> <u>lower</u> eyelid
H00.036	Abscess of eyelid <u>left</u> eye, <u>unspecified</u> eyelid
H00.039	Abscess of eyelid <u>unspecified</u> eye, <u>unspecified</u> eyelid

H00.1-   <u>Chalazion</u> — Chronic inflammation of a meibomian gland with formation of a granulomatous mass.
  Meibomian (gland) cyst
  Excludes ❷: *infected meibomian gland (H00.02-)*

H00.11	Chalazion <u>right</u> <u>upper</u> eyelid
H00.12	Chalazion <u>right</u> <u>lower</u> eyelid
H00.13	Chalazion <u>right</u> eye, <u>unspecified</u> eyelid
H00.14	Chalazion <u>left</u> <u>upper</u> eyelid
H00.15	Chalazion <u>left</u> <u>lower</u> eyelid
H00.16	Chalazion <u>left</u> eye, <u>unspecified</u> eyelid
H00.19	Chalazion <u>unspecified</u> eye, <u>unspecified</u> eyelid

H01-   Other inflammation of eyelid

H01.0-   <u>Blepharitis</u> — Inflammation of edges of the eyelids involving hair follicles and glands.
  Excludes 1:   *blepharoconjunctivitis (H10.5-)*

H01.00- <u>Unspecified</u> blepharitis

H01.001	Unspecified blepharitis <u>right</u> <u>upper</u> eyelid
H01.002	Unspecified blepharitis <u>right</u> <u>lower</u> eyelid
H01.003	Unspecified blepharitis <u>right</u> eye, <u>unspecified</u> eyelid

H00 - H01

H01.004   Unspecified blepharitis <u>left</u> <u>upper</u> eyelid

H01.005   Unspecified blepharitis <u>left</u> <u>lower</u> eyelid

H01.006   Unspecified blepharitis <u>left</u> eye, <u>unspecified</u> eyelid

H01.009   Unspecified blepharitis <u>unspecified</u> eye, <u>unspecified</u> eyelid

H01.01-   <u>Ulcerative</u> blepharitis — A form characterized by an eating away of a localized eyelid area.

H01.011   Ulcerative blepharitis <u>right</u> <u>upper</u> eyelid

H01.012   Ulcerative blepharitis <u>right</u> <u>lower</u> eyelid

H01.013   Ulcerative blepharitis <u>right</u> eye, <u>unspecified</u> eyelid

H01.014   Ulcerative blepharitis <u>left</u> <u>upper</u> eyelid

H01.015   Ulcerative blepharitis <u>left</u> <u>lower</u> eyelid

H01.016   Ulcerative blepharitis <u>left</u> eye, <u>unspecified</u> eyelid

H01.019   Ulcerative blepharitis <u>unspecified</u> eye, <u>unspecified</u> eyelid

H01.02-   <u>Squamous</u> blepharitis — A form characterized by the development of scales.

H01.021   Squamous blepharitis <u>right</u> <u>upper</u> eyelid

H01.022   Squamous blepharitis <u>right</u> <u>lower</u> eyelid

H01.023   Squamous blepharitis <u>right</u> eye, <u>unspecified</u> eyelid

H01.024   Squamous blepharitis <u>left</u> <u>upper</u> eyelid

H01.025   Squamous blepharitis <u>left</u> <u>lower</u> eyelid

H01.026   Squamous blepharitis <u>left</u> eye, <u>unspecified</u> eyelid

H01.029   Squamous blepharitis <u>unspecified</u> eye, <u>unspecified</u> eyelid

H01.1-   <u>Noninfectious dermatoses</u> of eyelid

H01.11-   <u>Allergic dermatitis</u> of eyelid — An inflammatory reaction caused by an allergen.

     Contact dermatitis of eyelid

H01.111   Allergic dermatitis of <u>right</u> <u>upper</u> eyelid

H01.112   Allergic dermatitis of <u>right</u> <u>lower</u> eyelid

H01.113   Allergic dermatitis of <u>right</u> eye, <u>unspecified</u> eyelid

H01.114   Allergic dermatitis of <u>left</u> <u>upper</u> eyelid

H01.115   Allergic dermatitis of <u>left</u> <u>lower</u> eyelid

H01.116   Allergic dermatitis of <u>left</u> eye, <u>unspecified</u> eyelid

H01.119   Allergic dermatitis of <u>unspecified</u> eye, <u>unspecified</u> eyelid

H01.12-   <u>Discoid lupus erythematosus</u> of eyelid — A superficial inflammation of the eyelids with red macules.

H01.121   Discoid lupus erythematosus of <u>right</u> <u>upper</u> eyelid

H01.122   Discoid lupus erythematosus of <u>right</u> <u>lower</u> eyelid

H01.123   Discoid lupus erythematosus of <u>right</u> eye, <u>unspecified</u> eyelid

H01.124   Discoid lupus erythematosus of <u>left</u> <u>upper</u> eyelid

H01.125   Discoid lupus erythematosus of <u>left</u> <u>lower</u> eyelid

H01.126   Discoid lupus erythematosus of <u>left</u> eye, <u>unspecified</u> eyelid

H01.129   Discoid lupus erythematosus of <u>unspecified</u> eye, <u>unspecified</u> eyelid

H01.13-   <u>Eczematous dermatitis</u> of eyelid — An inflammatory reaction involving the eyelids.

H01.131   Eczematous dermatitis of <u>right</u> <u>upper</u> eyelid

H01.132   Eczematous dermatitis of <u>right</u> <u>lower</u> eyelid

H01.133   Eczematous dermatitis of <u>right</u> eye, <u>unspecified</u> eyelid

H01.134   Eczematous dermatitis of <u>left</u> <u>upper</u> eyelid

H01.135   Eczematous dermatitis of <u>left</u> <u>lower</u> eyelid

H01.136   Eczematous dermatitis of <u>left</u> eye, <u>unspecified</u> eyelid

H01.139   Eczematous dermatitis of <u>unspecified</u> eye, <u>unspecified</u> eyelid

H01.14-   <u>Xeroderma</u> of eyelid — Dryness and roughness of the eyelid skin.

H01.141   Xeroderma of <u>right</u> <u>upper</u> eyelid

H01.142   Xeroderma of <u>right</u> <u>lower</u> eyelid

H01.143   Xeroderma of <u>right</u> eye, <u>unspecified</u> eyelid

H01.144   Xeroderma of <u>left</u> <u>upper</u> eyelid

H01.145   Xeroderma of <u>left</u> <u>lower</u> eyelid

H01.146   Xeroderma of <u>left</u> eye, <u>unspecified</u> eyelid

H01.149   Xeroderma of <u>unspecified</u> eye, <u>unspecified</u> eyelid

H01.8   Other specified inflammations of eyelid

H01.9   Unspecified inflammation of eyelid
     Inflammation of eyelid NOS

H02-   Other disorders of eyelid

   Excludes 1:   *congenital malformations of eyelid (Q10.0-Q10.3)*

H02.0-   <u>Entropion</u> and trichiasis of eyelid — The turning inward of the eyelid edge.

H02.00-   <u>Unspecified</u> entropion of eyelid

H02.001   Unspecified entropion of <u>right</u> <u>upper</u> eyelid

H02.002   Unspecified entropion of <u>right</u> <u>lower</u> eyelid

H02.003   Unspecified entropion of <u>right</u> eye, <u>unspecified</u> eyelid

H02.004   Unspecified entropion of <u>left</u> <u>upper</u> eyelid

H02.005   Unspecified entropion of <u>left</u> <u>lower</u> eyelid

H02.006   Unspecified entropion of <u>left</u> eye, <u>unspecified</u> eyelid

H02.009   Unspecified entropion of <u>unspecified</u> eye, <u>unspecified</u> eyelid

H02.01-   <u>Cicatricial</u> entropion of eyelid — A form caused by contraction of conjunctival scar tissue.

H02.011   Cicatricial entropion of <u>right</u> <u>upper</u> eyelid

H02.012   Cicatricial entropion of <u>right</u> <u>lower</u> eyelid

H02.013   Cicatricial entropion of <u>right</u> eye, <u>unspecified</u> eyelid

H02.014   Cicatricial entropion of <u>left</u> <u>upper</u> eyelid

H02.015   Cicatricial entropion of <u>left</u> <u>lower</u> eyelid

H02.016   Cicatricial entropion of <u>left</u> eye, <u>unspecified</u> eyelid

H02.019   Cicatricial entropion of <u>unspecified</u> eye, <u>unspecified</u> eyelid

H02.02-   <u>Mechanical</u> entropion of eyelid — A form caused by external forces.

H02.021   Mechanical entropion of <u>right</u> <u>upper</u> eyelid

H02.022   Mechanical entropion of <u>right</u> <u>lower</u> eyelid

H02.023   Mechanical entropion of <u>right</u> eye, <u>unspecified</u> eyelid

H02.024   Mechanical entropion of <u>left</u> <u>upper</u> eyelid

H02.025   Mechanical entropion of <u>left</u> <u>lower</u> eyelid

H02.026   Mechanical entropion of <u>left</u> eye, <u>unspecified</u> eyelid

H02.029   Mechanical entropion of <u>unspecified</u> eye, <u>unspecified</u> eyelid

H02.03-   <u>Senile</u> entropion of eyelid — A form caused by loss of tone of the obicularis oculi muscle.

H02.031   Senile entropion of <u>right</u> <u>upper</u> eyelid — [Age/15-124]

H02.032   Senile entropion of <u>right</u> <u>lower</u> eyelid — [Age/15-124]

H02.033   Senile entropion of <u>right</u> eye, <u>unspecified</u> eyelid — [Age/15-124]

H02.034   Senile entropion of <u>left</u> <u>upper</u> eyelid — [Age/15-124]

H02.035   Senile entropion of <u>left</u> <u>lower</u> eyelid — [Age/15-124]

H02.036   Senile entropion of <u>left</u> eye, <u>unspecified</u> eyelid — [Age/15-124]

H02.039   Senile entropion of <u>unspecified</u> eye, <u>unspecified</u> eyelid — [Age/15-124]

H02.04-   <u>Spastic</u> entropion of eyelid — A form caused by tonic spasm of the obicularis oculi muscle.

H02.041   Spastic entropion of <u>right</u> <u>upper</u> eyelid

H02.042   Spastic entropion of <u>right</u> <u>lower</u> eyelid

H02.043   Spastic entropion of <u>right</u> eye, <u>unspecified</u> eyelid

H02.044   Spastic entropion of <u>left</u> <u>upper</u> eyelid

H02.045   Spastic entropion of <u>left</u> <u>lower</u> eyelid

H02.046   Spastic entropion of <u>left</u> eye, <u>unspecified</u> eyelid

H02.049   Spastic entropion of <u>unspecified</u> eye, <u>unspecified</u> eyelid

---

Excludes 1: = NOT CODED HERE! (Do not code both)   **674**   *Excludes ❷:* = Not Included Here

H02.05- <u>Trichiasis without entropian</u> — The inward inversion of the eyelashes which rub against the cornea.

    H02.051 Trichiasis without entropian <u>right</u> <u>upper</u> eyelid

    H02.052 Trichiasis without entropian <u>right</u> <u>lower</u> eyelid

    H02.053 Trichiasis without entropian <u>right</u> eye, <u>unspecified</u> eyelid

    H02.054 Trichiasis without entropian <u>left</u> <u>upper</u> eyelid

    H02.055 Trichiasis without entropian <u>left</u> <u>lower</u> eyelid

    H02.056 Trichiasis without entropian <u>left</u> eye, <u>unspecified</u> eyelid

    H02.059 Trichiasis without entropian <u>unspecified</u> eye, <u>unspecified</u> eyelid

H02.1- <u>Ectropion</u> of eyelid — The turning outward of the eyelid edge.

  H02.10- <u>Unspecified</u> ectropion of eyelid

    H02.101 Unspecified ectropion of <u>right</u> <u>upper</u> eyelid

    H02.102 Unspecified ectropion of <u>right</u> <u>lower</u> eyelid

    H02.103 Unspecified ectropion of <u>right</u> eye, <u>unspecified</u> eyelid

    H02.104 Unspecified ectropion of <u>left</u> <u>upper</u> eyelid

    H02.105 Unspecified ectropion of <u>left</u> <u>lower</u> eyelid

    H02.106 Unspecified ectropion of <u>left</u> eye, <u>unspecified</u> eyelid

    H02.109 Unspecified ectropion of <u>unspecified</u> eye, <u>unspecified</u> eyelid

  H02.11- <u>Cicatricial</u> ectropion of eyelid — A form caused by contraction of conjunctival scar tissue.

    H02.111 Cicatricial ectropion of <u>right</u> <u>upper</u> eyelid

    H02.112 Cicatricial ectropion of <u>right</u> <u>lower</u> eyelid

    H02.113 Cicatricial ectropion of <u>right</u> eye, <u>unspecified</u> eyelid

    H02.114 Cicatricial ectropion of <u>left</u> <u>upper</u> eyelid

    H02.115 Cicatricial ectropion of <u>left</u> <u>lower</u> eyelid

    H02.116 Cicatricial ectropion of <u>left</u> eye, <u>unspecified</u> eyelid

    H02.119 Cicatricial ectropion of <u>unspecified</u> eye, <u>unspecified</u> eyelid

  H02.12- <u>Mechanical</u> ectropion of eyelid — A form caused by external forces.

    H02.121 Mechanical ectropion of <u>right</u> <u>upper</u> eyelid

    H02.122 Mechanical ectropion of <u>right</u> <u>lower</u> eyelid

    H02.123 Mechanical ectropion of <u>right</u> eye, <u>unspecified</u> eyelid

    H02.124 Mechanical ectropion of <u>left</u> <u>upper</u> eyelid

    H02.125 Mechanical ectropion of <u>left</u> <u>lower</u> eyelid

    H02.126 Mechanical ectropion of <u>left</u> eye, <u>unspecified</u> eyelid

    H02.129 Mechanical ectropion of <u>unspecified</u> eye, <u>unspecified</u> eyelid

  H02.13- <u>Senile</u> ectropion of eyelid — A form caused by loss of tone of the obicularis oculi muscle.

    H02.131 Senile ectropion of <u>right</u> <u>upper</u> eyelid — [Age/15-124]

    H02.132 Senile ectropion of <u>right</u> <u>lower</u> eyelid — [Age/15-124]

    H02.133 Senile ectropion of <u>right</u> eye, <u>unspecified</u> eyelid — [Age/15-124]

    H02.134 Senile ectropion of <u>left</u> <u>upper</u> eyelid — [Age/15-124]

    H02.135 Senile ectropion of <u>left</u> <u>lower</u> eyelid — [Age/15-124]

    H02.136 Senile ectropion of <u>left</u> eye, <u>unspecified</u> eyelid — [Age/15-124]

    H02.139 Senile ectropion of <u>unspecified</u> eye, <u>unspecified</u> eyelid — [Age/15-124]

  H02.14- <u>Spastic</u> ectropion of eyelid — A form caused by tonic spasm of the obicularis oculi muscle.

    H02.141 Spastic ectropion of <u>right</u> <u>upper</u> eyelid

    H02.142 Spastic ectropion of <u>right</u> <u>lower</u> eyelid

    H02.143 Spastic ectropion of <u>right</u> eye, <u>unspecified</u> eyelid

    H02.144 Spastic ectropion of <u>left</u> <u>upper</u> eyelid

    H02.145 Spastic ectropion of <u>left</u> <u>lower</u> eyelid

    H02.146 Spastic ectropion of <u>left</u> eye, <u>unspecified</u> eyelid

    H02.149 Spastic ectropion of <u>unspecified</u> eye, <u>unspecified</u> eyelid

H02.2- <u>Lagophthalmos</u> — Incomplete closure of the eyelids.

  H02.20- <u>Unspecified</u> lagophthalmos

    H02.201 Unspecified lagophthalmos <u>right</u> <u>upper</u> eyelid

    H02.202 Unspecified lagophthalmos <u>right</u> <u>lower</u> eyelid

    H02.203 Unspecified lagophthalmos <u>right</u> eye, <u>unspecified</u> eyelid

    H02.204 Unspecified lagophthalmos <u>left</u> <u>upper</u> eyelid

    H02.205 Unspecified lagophthalmos <u>left</u> <u>lower</u> eyelid

    H02.206 Unspecified lagophthalmos <u>left</u> eye, <u>unspecified</u> eyelid

    H02.209 Unspecified lagophthalmos <u>unspecified</u> eye, <u>unspecified</u> eyelid

  H02.21- <u>Cicatricial</u> lagophthalmos — A form caused by contraction of an eyelid scar.

    H02.211 Cicatricial lagophthalmos <u>right</u> <u>upper</u> eyelid

    H02.212 Cicatricial lagophthalmos <u>right</u> <u>lower</u> eyelid

    H02.213 Cicatricial lagophthalmos <u>right</u> eye, <u>unspecified</u> eyelid

    H02.214 Cicatricial lagophthalmos <u>left</u> <u>upper</u> eyelid

    H02.215 Cicatricial lagophthalmos <u>left</u> <u>lower</u> eyelid

    H02.216 Cicatricial lagophthalmos <u>left</u> eye, <u>unspecified</u> eyelid

    H02.219 Cicatricial lagophthalmos <u>unspecified</u> eye, <u>unspecified</u> eyelid

  H02.22- <u>Mechanical</u> lagophthalmos — A form caused by external forces.

    H02.221 Mechanical lagophthalmos <u>right</u> <u>upper</u> eyelid

    H02.222 Mechanical lagophthalmos <u>right</u> <u>lower</u> eyelid

    H02.223 Mechanical lagophthalmos <u>right</u> eye, <u>unspecified</u> eyelid

    H02.224 Mechanical lagophthalmos <u>left</u> <u>upper</u> eyelid

    H02.225 Mechanical lagophthalmos <u>left</u> <u>lower</u> eyelid

    H02.226 Mechanical lagophthalmos <u>left</u> eye, <u>unspecified</u> eyelid

    H02.229 Mechanical lagophthalmos <u>unspecified</u> eye, <u>unspecified</u> eyelid

  H02.23- <u>Paralytic</u> lagophthalmos — A form caused by impairment of the facial nerve.

    H02.231 Paralytic lagophthalmos <u>right</u> <u>upper</u> eyelid

    H02.232 Paralytic lagophthalmos <u>right</u> <u>lower</u> eyelid

    H02.233 Paralytic lagophthalmos <u>right</u> eye, <u>unspecified</u> eyelid

    H02.234 Paralytic lagophthalmos <u>left</u> <u>upper</u> eyelid

    H02.235 Paralytic lagophthalmos <u>left</u> <u>lower</u> eyelid

    H02.236 Paralytic lagophthalmos <u>left</u> eye, <u>unspecified</u> eyelid

    H02.239 Paralytic lagophthalmos <u>unspecified</u> eye, <u>unspecified</u> eyelid

H02.3- <u>Blepharochalasis</u> — Hypertrophy with loss of elasticity of the upper eyelids resulting in drooping.

    Pseudoptosis — Apparent ptosis of an eyelid resulting from a fold of skin or fat.

  H02.30 Blepharochalasis <u>unspecified</u> eye, <u>unspecified</u> eyelid

  H02.31 Blepharochalasis <u>right</u> <u>upper</u> eyelid

  H02.32 Blepharochalasis <u>right</u> <u>lower</u> eyelid

  H02.33 Blepharochalasis <u>right</u> eye, <u>unspecified</u> eyelid

  H02.34 Blepharochalasis <u>left</u> <u>upper</u> eyelid

  H02.35 Blepharochalasis <u>left</u> <u>lower</u> eyelid

  H02.36 Blepharochalasis <u>left</u> eye, <u>unspecified</u> eyelid

H02.4- <u>Ptosis</u> of eyelid — Prolapse or drooping of the upper eyelid.

  H02.40- <u>Unspecified</u> ptosis of eyelid

    H02.401 Unspecified ptosis of <u>right</u> eyelid

    H02.402 Unspecified ptosis of <u>left</u> eyelid

    H02.403 Unspecified ptosis of <u>bilateral</u> eyelids

    H02.409 Unspecified ptosis of <u>unspecified</u> eyelid

  H02.41- <u>Mechanical</u> ptosis of eyelid — A form caused by external forces.

    H02.411 Mechanical ptosis of <u>right</u> eyelid

    H02.412 Mechanical ptosis of <u>left</u> eyelid

H02 – H02

H02.413   Mechanical ptosis of <u>bilateral</u> eyelids

H02.419   Mechanical ptosis of <u>unspecified</u> eyelid

H02.42-   Myogenic ptosis of eyelid — A form caused by impairment of the ocular muscles.

H02.421   Myogenic ptosis of <u>right</u> eyelid

H02.422   Myogenic ptosis of <u>left</u> eyelid

H02.423   Myogenic ptosis of <u>bilateral</u> eyelids

H02.429   Myogenic ptosis of <u>unspecified</u> eyelid

H02.43-   Paralytic ptosis of eyelid — A form caused by severe impairment of the third nerve.

  Neurogenic ptosis of eyelid

H02.431   Paralytic ptosis of <u>right</u> eyelid

H02.432   Paralytic ptosis of <u>left</u> eyelid

H02.433   Paralytic ptosis of <u>bilateral</u> eyelids

H02.439   Paralytic ptosis <u>unspecified</u> eyelid

H02.5-   Other disorders affecting eyelid function

Excludes ❷: blepharospasm (G24.5)
                  organic tic (G25.69)
                  psychogenic tic (F95.-)

H02.51-   Abnormal innervation syndrome — Conditions due to crossed or fused ocular nerves.

H02.511   Abnormal innervation syndrome <u>right</u> <u>upper</u> eyelid

H02.512   Abnormal innervation syndrome <u>right</u> <u>lower</u> eyelid

H02.513   Abnormal innervation syndrome <u>right</u> eye, <u>unspecified</u> eyelid

H02.514   Abnormal innervation syndrome <u>left</u> <u>upper</u> eyelid

H02.515   Abnormal innervation syndrome <u>left</u> <u>lower</u> eyelid

H02.516   Abnormal innervation syndrome <u>left</u> eye, <u>unspecified</u> eyelid

H02.519   Abnormal innervation syndrome <u>unspecified</u> eye, <u>unspecified</u> eyelid

H02.52-   Blepharophimosis — Decreased width of the opening of the eyelids.

  Ankyloblepharon — The abnormal adhesion of the ciliary body edges to the eyelid.

H02.521   Blepharophimosis <u>right</u> <u>upper</u> eyelid

H02.522   Blepharophimosis <u>right</u> <u>lower</u> eyelid

H02.523   Blepharophimosis <u>right</u> eye, <u>unspecified</u> eyelid

H02.524   Blepharophimosis <u>left</u> <u>upper</u> eyelid

H02.525   Blepharophimosis <u>left</u> <u>lower</u> eyelid

H02.526   Blepharophimosis <u>left</u> eye, <u>unspecified</u> eyelid

H02.529   Blepharophimosis <u>unspecified</u> eye, <u>unspecified</u> lid

H02.53-   Eyelid retraction — The drawing-back of an eyelid.

  Eyelid lag

H02.531   Eyelid retraction <u>right</u> <u>upper</u> eyelid

H02.532   Eyelid retraction <u>right</u> <u>lower</u> eyelid

H02.533   Eyelid retraction <u>right</u> eye, <u>unspecified</u> eyelid

H02.534   Eyelid retraction <u>left</u> <u>upper</u> eyelid

H02.535   Eyelid retraction <u>left</u> <u>lower</u> eyelid

H02.536   Eyelid retraction <u>left</u> eye, <u>unspecified</u> eyelid

H02.539   Eyelid retraction <u>unspecified</u> eye, <u>unspecified</u> lid

H02.59-   Other disorders affecting eyelid function

  Deficient blink reflex — Impairment of the normal blink reflex.

  Sensory disorders — Abnormal conditions of eyelid function due to dysfunctional sensory stimulation.

H02.6-   Xanthelasma of eyelid — A fat deposit under the skin of the eyelid and usually toward the inner canthus.

H02.60   Xanthelasma of <u>unspecified</u> eye, <u>unspecified</u> eyelid

H02.61   Xanthelasma of <u>right</u> <u>upper</u> eyelid

H02.62   Xanthelasma of <u>right</u> <u>lower</u> eyelid

H02.63   Xanthelasma of <u>right</u> eye, <u>unspecified</u> eyelid

H02.64   Xanthelasma of <u>left</u> <u>upper</u> eyelid

H02.65   Xanthelasma of <u>left</u> <u>lower</u> eyelid

H02.66   Xanthelasma of <u>left</u> eye, <u>unspecified</u> eyelid

H02.7-   Other and unspecified degenerative disorders of eyelid and periocular area

H02.70   Unspecified degenerative disorders of eyelid and periocular area

H02.71-   Chloasma of eyelid and periocular area — Abnormal eyelid pigmentation with yellowish-brown spots or patches.

  Dyspigmentation of eyelid — Abnormal eyelid pigmentation.

  Hyperpigmentation of eyelid — The abnormal excessive pigmentation of an eyelid.

H02.711   Chloasma of <u>right</u> <u>upper</u> eyelid and periocular area

H02.712   Chloasma of <u>right</u> <u>lower</u> eyelid and periocular area

H02.713   Chloasma of <u>right</u> eye, <u>unspecified</u> eyelid and periocular area

H02.714   Chloasma of <u>left</u> <u>upper</u> eyelid and periocular area

H02.715   Chloasma of <u>left</u> <u>lower</u> eyelid and periocular area

H02.716   Chloasma of <u>left</u> eye, <u>unspecified</u> eyelid and periocular area

H02.719   Chloasma of <u>unspecified</u> eye, <u>unspecified</u> eyelid and periocular area

H02.72-   Madarosis of eyelid and periocular area — The abnormal loss of eyelashes.

  Hypotrichosis of eyelid — The abnormal reduction or lack of eyelid hair.

H02.721   Madarosis of <u>right</u> <u>upper</u> eyelid and periocular area

H02.722   Madarosis of <u>right</u> <u>lower</u> eyelid and periocular area

H02.723   Madarosis of <u>right</u> eye, <u>unspecified</u> eyelid and periocular area

H02.724   Madarosis of <u>left</u> <u>upper</u> eyelid and periocular area

H02.725   Madarosis of <u>left</u> <u>lower</u> eyelid and periocular area

H02.726   Madarosis of <u>left</u> eye, <u>unspecified</u> eyelid and periocular area

H02.729   Madarosis of <u>unspecified</u> eye, <u>unspecified</u> eyelid and periocular area

H02.73-   Vitiligo of eyelid and periocular area — A form marked by destruction of melanocytes.

  Hypopigmentation of eyelid — The abnormal lack of pigmentation of an eyelid.

H02.731   Vitiligo of <u>right</u> <u>upper</u> eyelid and periocular area

H02.732   Vitiligo of <u>right</u> <u>lower</u> eyelid and periocular area

H02.733   Vitiligo of <u>right</u> eye, <u>unspecified</u> eyelid and periocular area

H02.734   Vitiligo of <u>left</u> <u>upper</u> eyelid and periocular area

H02.735   Vitiligo of <u>left</u> <u>lower</u> eyelid and periocular area

H02.736   Vitiligo of <u>left</u> eye, <u>unspecified</u> eyelid and periocular area

H02.739   Vitiligo of <u>unspecified</u> eye, <u>unspecified</u> eyelid and periocular area

H02.79   Other degenerative disorders of eyelid and periocular area

H02.8-   Other specified disorders of <u>eyelid</u>

H02.81-   Retained foreign body in eyelid — The continued presence of foreign material in an eyelid.

  Use additional code to identify the type of retained foreign body (Z18.-)

  Excludes 1:   laceration of eyelid with foreign body (S01.12-)
                  retained intraocular foreign body (H44.6-, H44.7-)
                  superficial foreign body of eyelid and periocular area (S00.25-)

H02.811   Retained foreign body in <u>right</u> <u>upper</u> eyelid

H02.812   Retained foreign body in <u>right</u> <u>lower</u> eyelid

H02.813   Retained foreign body in <u>right</u> eye, <u>unspecified</u> eyelid

H02.814   Retained foreign body in <u>left</u> <u>upper</u> eyelid

H02.815   Retained foreign body in <u>left</u> <u>lower</u> eyelid

H02.816   Retained foreign body in <u>left</u> eye, <u>unspecified</u> eyelid

H02.819   Retained foreign body in <u>unspecified</u> eye, <u>unspecified</u> eyelid

H02.82-   Cysts of eyelid — An encapsulated, fluid-filled sac of an eyelid.

  Sebaceous cyst of eyelid — A cyst of a sebaceous gland.

H02.821   Cysts of <u>right</u> <u>upper</u> eyelid

H02.822   Cysts of <u>right</u> <u>lower</u> eyelid

H02-H02

H02.823　Cysts of <u>right</u> eye, <u>unspecified</u> eyelid
H02.824　Cysts of <u>left</u> <u>upper</u> eyelid
H02.825　Cysts of <u>left</u> <u>lower</u> eyelid
H02.826　Cysts of <u>left</u> eye, <u>unspecified</u> eyelid
H02.829　Cysts of <u>unspecified</u> eye, <u>unspecified</u> eyelid

H02.83- <u>Dermatochalasis</u> of eyelid — Excess and lax skin of the eyelids.
H02.831　Dermatochalasis of <u>right</u> <u>upper</u> eyelid
H02.832　Dermatochalasis of <u>right</u> <u>lower</u> eyelid
H02.833　Dermatochalasis of <u>right</u> eye, <u>unspecified</u> eyelid
H02.834　Dermatochalasis of <u>left</u> <u>upper</u> eyelid
H02.835　Dermatochalasis of <u>left</u> <u>lower</u> eyelid
H02.836　Dermatochalasis of <u>left</u> eye, <u>unspecified</u> eyelid
H02.839　Dermatochalasis of <u>unspecified</u> eye, <u>unspecified</u> eyelid

H02.84- <u>Edema</u> of eyelid — The abnormal accumulation of intercellular fluid of an eyelid.
　　　<u>Hyperemia</u> of eyelid — The abnormal congestion of blood of an eyelid.
H02.841　Edema of <u>right</u> <u>upper</u> eyelid
H02.842　Edema of <u>right</u> <u>lower</u> eyelid
H02.843　Edema of <u>right</u> eye, <u>unspecified</u> eyelid
H02.844　Edema of <u>left</u> <u>upper</u> eyelid
H02.845　Edema of <u>left</u> <u>lower</u> eyelid
H02.846　Edema of <u>left</u> eye, <u>unspecified</u> eyelid
H02.849　Edema of <u>unspecified</u> eye, <u>unspecified</u> eyelid

H02.85- <u>Elephantiasis</u> of eyelid — The massive hypertrophy of eyelid tissues.
H02.851　Elephantiasis of <u>right</u> <u>upper</u> eyelid
H02.852　Elephantiasis of <u>right</u> <u>lower</u> eyelid
H02.853　Elephantiasis of <u>right</u> eye, <u>unspecified</u> eyelid
H02.854　Elephantiasis of <u>left</u> <u>upper</u> eyelid
H02.855　Elephantiasis of <u>left</u> <u>lower</u> eyelid
H02.856　Elephantiasis of <u>left</u> eye, <u>unspecified</u> eyelid
H02.859　Elephantiasis of <u>unspecified</u> eye, <u>unspecified</u> eyelid

H02.86- <u>Hypertrichosis</u> of eyelid — The excessive growth of eyelid hair.
H02.861　Hypertrichosis of <u>right</u> <u>upper</u> eyelid
H02.862　Hypertrichosis of <u>right</u> <u>lower</u> eyelid
H02.863　Hypertrichosis of <u>right</u> eye, <u>unspecified</u> eyelid
H02.864　Hypertrichosis of <u>left</u> <u>upper</u> eyelid
H02.865　Hypertrichosis of <u>left</u> <u>lower</u> eyelid
H02.866　Hypertrichosis of <u>left</u> eye, <u>unspecified</u> eyelid
H02.869　Hypertrichosis of <u>unspecified</u> eye, <u>unspecified</u> eyelid

H02.87- <u>Vascular anomalies</u> of eyelid — Abnormal conditions of the eyelid blood vessels.
H02.871　Vascular anomalies of <u>right</u> <u>upper</u> eyelid
H02.872　Vascular anomalies of <u>right</u> <u>lower</u> eyelid
H02.873　Vascular anomalies of <u>right</u> eye, <u>unspecified</u> eyelid
H02.874　Vascular anomalies of <u>left</u> <u>upper</u> eyelid
H02.875　Vascular anomalies of <u>left</u> <u>lower</u> eyelid
H02.876　Vascular anomalies of <u>left</u> eye, <u>unspecified</u> eyelid
H02.879　Vascular anomalies of <u>unspecified</u> eye, <u>unspecified</u> eyelid

H02.89　Other specified disorders of eyelid
　　　Hemorrhage of eyelid — Bleeding from the eyelids.

H02.9　Unspecified disorder of eyelid
　　　Disorder of eyelid NOS

H04- Disorders of <u>lacrimal system</u>
　　Excludes 1:　*congenital malformations of lacrimal system (Q10.4-Q10.6)*
H04.0- <u>Dacryoadenitis</u> — Inflammation of a lacrimal gland.
H04.00- <u>Unspecified</u> dacryoadenitis
H04.001　Unspecified dacryoadenitis, <u>right</u> lacrimal gland
H04.002　Unspecified dacryoadenitis, <u>left</u> lacrimal gland
H04.003　Unspecified dacryoadenitis, <u>bilateral</u> lacrimal glands

H04.009　Unspecified dacryoadenitis, <u>unspecified</u> lacrimal gland
H04.01- <u>Acute</u> dacryoadenitis — A form characterized by sudden, severe onset.
H04.011　Acute dacryoadenitis, <u>right</u> lacrimal gland
H04.012　Acute dacryoadenitis, <u>left</u> lacrimal gland
H04.013　Acute dacryoadenitis, <u>bilateral</u> lacrimal glands
H04.019　Acute dacryoadenitis, <u>unspecified</u> lacrimal gland
H04.02- <u>Chronic</u> dacryoadenitis — A form characterized by slow development and persistence over a long period of time.
H04.021　Chronic dacryoadenitis, <u>right</u> lacrimal gland
H04.022　Chronic dacryoadenitis, <u>left</u> lacrimal gland
H04.023　Chronic dacryoadenitis, <u>bilateral</u> lacrimal gland
H04.029　Chronic dacryoadenitis, <u>unspecified</u> lacrimal gland
H04.03- <u>Chronic enlargement</u> of lacrimal gland — A form characterized by continued increased size.
H04.031　Chronic enlargement of <u>right</u> lacrimal gland
H04.032　Chronic enlargement of <u>left</u> lacrimal gland
H04.033　Chronic enlargement of <u>bilateral</u> lacrimal glands
H04.039　Chronic enlargement of <u>unspecified</u> lacrimal gland

H04.1-　Other disorders of <u>lacrimal gland</u>
H04.11- <u>Dacryops</u> — The constant flow of tears.
H04.111　Dacryops of <u>right</u> lacrimal gland
H04.112　Dacryops of <u>left</u> lacrimal gland
H04.113　Dacryops of <u>bilateral</u> lacrimal glands
H04.119　Dacryops of <u>unspecified</u> lacrimal gland
H04.12- <u>Dry eye</u> syndrome — The abnormal decrease of tear production.
　　　Tear film insufficiency, NOS
H04.121　Dry eye syndrome of <u>right</u> lacrimal gland
H04.122　Dry eye syndrome of <u>left</u> lacrimal gland
H04.123　Dry eye syndrome of <u>bilateral</u> lacrimal glands
H04.129　Dry eye syndrome of <u>unspecified</u> lacrimal gland
H04.13- Lacrimal <u>cyst</u> — Encapsulated, fluid-filled sacs of a lacrimal gland.
　　　Lacrimal cystic degeneration
H04.131　Lacrimal cyst, <u>right</u> lacrimal gland
H04.132　Lacrimal cyst, <u>left</u> lacrimal gland
H04.133　Lacrimal cyst, <u>bilateral</u> lacrimal glands
H04.139　Lacrimal cyst, <u>unspecified</u> lacrimal gland
H04.14- <u>Primary</u> lacrimal <u>gland atrophy</u> — The wasting-away of a lacrimal gland resulting from a lacrimal disorder.
H04.141　Primary lacrimal gland atrophy, <u>right</u> lacrimal gland
H04.142　Primary lacrimal gland atrophy, <u>left</u> lacrimal gland
H04.143　Primary lacrimal gland atrophy, <u>bilateral</u> lacrimal glands
H04.149　Primary lacrimal gland atrophy, <u>unspecified</u> lacrimal gland
H04.15- <u>Secondary</u> lacrimal <u>gland atrophy</u>
H04.151　Secondary lacrimal gland atrophy, <u>right</u> lacrimal gland
H04.152　Secondary lacrimal gland atrophy, <u>left</u> lacrimal gland
H04.153　Secondary lacrimal gland atrophy, <u>bilateral</u> lacrimal glands
H04.159　Secondary lacrimal gland atrophy, <u>unspecified</u> lacrimal gland
H04.16- Lacrimal gland <u>dislocation</u> — The wasting-away of a lacrimal gland resulting from another ocular disease.
H04.161　Lacrimal gland dislocation, <u>right</u> lacrimal gland
H04.162　Lacrimal gland dislocation, <u>left</u> lacrimal gland
H04.163　Lacrimal gland dislocation, <u>bilateral</u> lacrimal glands
H04.169　Lacrimal gland dislocation, <u>unspecified</u> lacrimal gland
H04.19　Other specified disorders of lacrimal gland
H04.2- <u>Epiphora</u> — The overflow of tears down the cheek.
H04.20- <u>Unspecified</u> epiphora

H02 - H04

H04.201 Unspecified epiphora, <u>right</u> lacrimal gland

H04.202 Unspecified epiphora, <u>left</u> lacrimal gland

H04.203 Unspecified epiphora, <u>bilateral</u> lacrimal glands

H04.209 Unspecified epiphora, <u>unspecified</u> lacrimal gland

H04.21- Epiphora due to <u>excess lacrimation</u> — A form caused by excessive tear production.

H04.211 Epiphora due to excess lacrimation, <u>right</u> lacrimal gland

H04.212 Epiphora due to excess lacrimation, <u>left</u> lacrimal gland

H04.213 Epiphora due to excess lacrimation, <u>bilateral</u> lacrimal glands

H04.219 Epiphora due to excess lacrimation, <u>unspecified</u> lacrimal gland

H04.22- Epiphora due to <u>insufficient drainage</u> — A form resulting from blocked drainage.

H04.221 Epiphora due to insufficient drainage, <u>right</u> lacrimal gland

H04.222 Epiphora due to insufficient drainage, <u>left</u> lacrimal gland

H04.223 Epiphora due to insufficient drainage, <u>bilateral</u> lacrimal glands

H04.229 Epiphora due to insufficient drainage, <u>unspecified</u> lacrimal gland

H04.3- <u>Acute and unspecified inflammation of lacrimal passages</u>
Excludes 1: *neonatal dacryocystitis (P39.1)*

H04.30- <u>Unspecified dacryocystitis</u>

H04.301 Unspecified dacryocystitis of <u>right</u> lacrimal passage

H04.302 Unspecified dacryocystitis of <u>left</u> lacrimal passage

H04.303 Unspecified dacryocystitis of <u>bilateral</u> lacrimal passages

H04.309 Unspecified dacryocystitis of <u>unspecified</u> lacrimal passage

H04.31- <u>Phlegmonous dacryocystitis</u> — Inflammation of the connective tissue of a lacrimal sac.

H04.311 Phlegmonous dacryocystitis of <u>right</u> lacrimal passage

H04.312 Phlegmonous dacryocystitis of <u>left</u> lacrimal passage

H04.313 Phlegmonous dacryocystitis of <u>bilateral</u> lacrimal passages

H04.319 Phlegmonous dacryocystitis of <u>unspecified</u> lacrimal passage

H04.32- <u>Acute dacryocystitis</u> — The sudden, severe onset of inflammation of a lacrimal sac.
Acute dacryopericystitis — A form affecting the tissues surrounding a lacrimal sac.

H04.321 Acute dacryocystitis of <u>right</u> lacrimal passage

H04.322 Acute dacryocystitis of <u>left</u> lacrimal passage

H04.323 Acute dacryocystitis of <u>bilateral</u> lacrimal passages

H04.329 Acute dacryocystitis of <u>unspecified</u> lacrimal passage

H04.33- <u>Acute lacrimal canaliculitis</u> — The sudden, severe onset of inflammation of the short passage between the lacrimal lake and the lacrimal sac.

H04.331 Acute lacrimal canaliculitis of <u>right</u> lacrimal passage

H04.332 Acute lacrimal canaliculitis of <u>left</u> lacrimal passage

H04.333 Acute lacrimal canaliculitis of <u>bilateral</u> lacrimal passages

H04.339 Acute lacrimal canaliculitis of <u>unspecified</u> lacrimal passage

H04.4- <u>Chronic</u> inflammation of lacrimal passages

H04.41- <u>Chronic dacryocystitis</u> — Inflammation of a lacrimal sac that develops slowly and persists over a long period of time.

H04.411 Chronic dacryocystitis of <u>right</u> lacrimal passage

H04.412 Chronic dacryocystitis of <u>left</u> lacrimal passage

H04.413 Chronic dacryocystitis of <u>bilateral</u> lacrimal passages

H04.419 Chronic dacryocystitis of <u>unspecified</u> lacrimal passage

H04.42- Chronic lacrimal <u>canaliculitis</u> — Inflammation of the short passage between the lacrimal lake and the lacrimal sac that develops slowly and persists over a long period of time.

H04.421 Chronic lacrimal canaliculitis of <u>right</u> lacrimal passage

H04.422 Chronic lacrimal canaliculitis of <u>left</u> lacrimal passage

H04.423 Chronic lacrimal canaliculitis of <u>bilateral</u> lacrimal passages

H04.429 Chronic lacrimal canaliculitis of <u>unspecified</u> lacrimal passage

H04.43- Chronic lacrimal <u>mucocele</u> — Dilatation with mucous secretion of the lacrimal passages.

H04.431 Chronic lacrimal mucocele of <u>right</u> lacrimal passage

H04.432 Chronic lacrimal mucocele of <u>left</u> lacrimal passage

H04.433 Chronic lacrimal mucocele of <u>bilateral</u> lacrimal passages

H04.439 Chronic lacrimal mucocele of <u>unspecified</u> lacrimal passage

H04.5- <u>Stenosis and insufficiency</u> of lacrimal passages

H04.51- <u>Dacryolith</u> — An abnormal concretion within the lacrimal passages.

H04.511 Dacryolith of <u>right</u> lacrimal passage

H04.512 Dacryolith of <u>left</u> lacrimal passage

H04.513 Dacryolith of <u>bilateral</u> lacrimal passages

H04.519 Dacryolith of <u>unspecified</u> lacrimal passage

H04.52- <u>Eversion</u> of lacrimal <u>punctum</u> — The turning outward of the eyelid lacrimal opening.

H04.521 Eversion of <u>right</u> lacrimal punctum

H04.522 Eversion of <u>left</u> lacrimal punctum

H04.523 Eversion of <u>bilateral</u> lacrimal punctum

H04.529 Eversion of <u>unspecified</u> lacrimal punctum

H04.53- <u>Neonatal obstruction</u> of <u>nasolacrimal duct</u> — The blockage of the nasal tear-draining duct that specifically develops after birth and is not due to a fetal distortion of the duct.
Excludes 1: *congenital stenosis and stricture of lacrimal duct (Q10.5)*

H04.531 Neonatal obstruction of <u>right</u> nasolacrimal duct — [Age/0]

H04.532 Neonatal obstruction of <u>left</u> nasolacrimal duct — [Age/0]

H04.533 Neonatal obstruction of <u>bilateral</u> nasolacrimal duct — [Age/0]

H04.539 Neonatal obstruction of <u>unspecified</u> nasolacrimal duct — [Age/0]

H04.54- <u>Stenosis</u> of lacrimal <u>canaliculi</u> — The narrowing of the passage between the punctum and the lacrimal sac.

H04.541 Stenosis of <u>right</u> lacrimal canaliculi

H04.542 Stenosis of <u>left</u> lacrimal canaliculi

H04.543 Stenosis of <u>bilateral</u> lacrimal canaliculi

H04.549 Stenosis of <u>unspecified</u> lacrimal canaliculi

H04.55- <u>Acquired stenosis</u> of <u>nasolacrimal duct</u> — The narrowing of the nasal tear-draining duct.

H04.551 Acquired stenosis of <u>right</u> nasolacrimal duct

H04.552 Acquired stenosis of <u>left</u> nasolacrimal duct

H04.553 Acquired stenosis of <u>bilateral</u> nasolacrimal duct

H04.559 Acquired stenosis of <u>unspecified</u> nasolacrimal duct

H04.56- <u>Stenosis</u> of lacrimal <u>punctum</u> — The narrowing of the eyelid lacrimal opening.

H04.561 Stenosis of <u>right</u> lacrimal punctum

H04.562 Stenosis of <u>left</u> lacrimal punctum

H04.563 Stenosis of <u>bilateral</u> lacrimal punctum

H04.569 Stenosis of <u>unspecified</u> lacrimal punctum

H04.57- <u>Stenosis</u> of lacrimal <u>sac</u> — The narrowing of the lacrimal sac.

H04.571 Stenosis of <u>right</u> lacrimal sac

H04.572 Stenosis of <u>left</u> lacrimal sac

H04 - H04

H04.573　Stenosis of _bilateral_ lacrimal sac

H04.579　Stenosis of _unspecified_ lacrimal sac

H04.6-　Other changes of lacrimal passages

H04.61- Lacrimal _fistula_ — An abnormal passage of the lacrimal passages.

H04.611　Lacrimal fistula _right_ lacrimal passage

H04.612　Lacrimal fistula _left_ lacrimal passage

H04.613　Lacrimal fistula _bilateral_ lacrimal passages

H04.619　Lacrimal fistula _unspecified_ lacrimal passage

H04.69　Other changes of lacrimal passages

H04.8-　Other disorders of lacrimal system

H04.81- _Granuloma_ of lacrimal passages — The formation of granular tissue within a lacrimal passage.

H04.811　Granuloma of _right_ lacrimal passage

H04.812　Granuloma of _left_ lacrimal passage

H04.813　Granuloma of _bilateral_ lacrimal passages

H04.819　Granuloma of _unspecified_ lacrimal passage

H04.89　Other disorders of lacrimal system

H04.9　Disorder of lacrimal system, unspecified

H05-　Disorders of _orbit_

　　Excludes 1:　_congenital malformation of orbit (Q10.7)_

H05.0- _Acute inflammation_ of orbit — The sudden, severe onset of inflammation of the cavity that contains the eyeball.

H05.00　_Unspecified_ acute inflammation of orbit

H05.01- _Cellulitis_ of orbit — A form marked by the inflammation of the cellular tissue.

　　Abscess of orbit — A form marked by the localized collection of pus caused by the disintegration of orbital tissues.

cc　H05.011　Cellulitis of _right_ orbit

cc　H05.012　Cellulitis of _left_ orbit

cc　H05.013　Cellulitis of _bilateral_ orbits

cc　H05.019　Cellulitis of _unspecified_ orbit

H05.02- _Osteomyelitis_ of orbit — A form characterized by inflammation of the orbital bone and bone marrow.

cc　H05.021　Osteomyelitis of _right_ orbit

cc　H05.022　Osteomyelitis of _left_ orbit

cc　H05.023　Osteomyelitis of _bilateral_ orbits

cc　H05.029　Osteomyelitis of _unspecified_ orbit

H05.03- _Periostitis_ of orbit — A form characterized by inflammation of the orbital periosteum.

cc　H05.031　Periostitis of _right_ orbit

cc　H05.032　Periostitis of _left_ orbit

cc　H05.033　Periostitis of _bilateral_ orbits

cc　H05.039　Periostitis of _unspecified_ orbit

H05.04- _Tenonitis_ of orbit — A form characterized by inflammation of the orbital tendons.

H05.041　Tenonitis of _right_ orbit

H05.042　Tenonitis of _left_ orbit

H05.043　Tenonitis of _bilateral_ orbits

H05.049　Tenonitis of _unspecified_ orbit

H05.1- _Chronic inflammatory disorders_ of orbit — Inflammatory disorders of the cavity that contains the eyeball which develop slowly and persist over a long period of time.

H05.10　_Unspecified_ chronic inflammatory disorders of orbit

H05.11- _Granuloma_ of orbit — A form characterized by the formation of granular tissue.

　　Pseudotumor (inflammatory) of orbit — A form marked by a mass of granular and fibrous inflammatory tissue.

H05.111　Granuloma of _right_ orbit

H05.112　Granuloma of _left_ orbit

H05.113　Granuloma of _bilateral_ orbits

H05.119　Granuloma of _unspecified_ orbit

H05.12- Orbital _myositis_ — A form characterized by inflammation of the orbital muscles.

H05.121　Orbital myositis, _right_ orbit

H05.122　Orbital myositis, _left_ orbit

H05.123　Orbital myositis, _bilateral_

H05.129　Orbital myositis, _unspecified_ orbit

H05.2- _Exophthalmic conditions_ — The abnormal protrusion of the eyeball.

H05.20　Unspecified exophthalmos

H05.21- _Displacement (lateral) of globe_ — A form characterized by the movement of the eyeball towards the side.

H05.211　Displacement (lateral) of globe, _right_ eye

H05.212　Displacement (lateral) of globe, _left_ eye

H05.213　Displacement (lateral) of globe, _bilateral_

H05.219　Displacement (lateral) of globe, _unspecified_ eye

H05.22- _Edema_ of orbit — A form characterized by the localized accumulation of intercellular orbital fluid.

　　Orbital congestion

H05.221　Edema of _right_ orbit

H05.222　Edema of _left_ orbit

H05.223　Edema of _bilateral_ orbit

H05.229　Edema of _unspecified_ orbit

H05.23- _Hemorrhage_ of orbit — A form characterized by bleeding from the orbit.

H05.231　Hemorrhage of _right_ orbit

H05.232　Hemorrhage of _left_ orbit

H05.233　Hemorrhage of _bilateral_ orbit

H05.239　Hemorrhage of _unspecified_ orbit

H05.24- _Constant_ exophthalmos — A form characterized by continued protrusion.

H05.241　Constant exophthalmos, _right_ eye

H05.242　Constant exophthalmos, _left_ eye

H05.243　Constant exophthalmos, _bilateral_

H05.249　Constant exophthalmos, _unspecified_ eye

H05.25- _Intermittent_ exophthalmos — A form characterized by the occurrence of protrusion at separated intervals.

H05.251　Intermittent exophthalmos, _right_ eye

H05.252　Intermittent exophthalmos, _left_ eye

H05.253　Intermittent exophthalmos, _bilateral_

H05.259　Intermittent exophthalmos, _unspecified_ eye

H05.26- _Pulsating_ exophthalmos — A form characterized by slight forward movement associated with vascular blood flow.

H05.261　Pulsating exophthalmos, _right_ eye

H05.262　Pulsating exophthalmos, _left_ eye

H05.263　Pulsating exophthalmos, _bilateral_

H05.269　Pulsating exophthalmos, _unspecified_ eye

H05.3- _Deformity_ of _orbit_ — The abnormal distortion of the normal orbital shape.

　　Excludes 1:　_congenital deformity of orbit (Q10.7)_

　　　　　　　　hypertelorism (Q75.2)

H05.30　_Unspecified_ deformity of orbit

H05.31- _Atrophy_ of orbit — A form resulting from the abnormal wasting-away of the orbital tissues.

H05.311　Atrophy of _right_ orbit

H05.312　Atrophy of _left_ orbit

H05.313　Atrophy of _bilateral_ orbit

H05.319　Atrophy of _unspecified_ orbit

H05.32- Deformity of orbit _due to bone disease_

　　Code also associated bone disease

H05.321　Deformity of _right_ orbit due to bone disease

H05.322　Deformity of _left_ orbit due to bone disease

H05.323　Deformity of _bilateral_ orbits due to bone disease

H05.329　Deformity of _unspecified_ orbit due to bone disease

H05.33- Deformity of orbit _due to trauma or surgery_

H05.331　Deformity of _right_ orbit due to trauma or surgery

H05.332　Deformity of _left_ orbit due to trauma or surgery

H05.333　Deformity of _bilateral_ orbits due to trauma or surgery

H05.339　Deformity of _unspecified_ orbit due to trauma or surgery

H05.34- _Enlargement_ of orbit — A form resulting from the abnormal increase in the size of the orbital tissues.

H05.341　Enlargement of _right_ orbit

H05.342　Enlargement of _left_ orbit

H04 | H05

H05.343   Enlargement of <u>bilateral</u> orbits

H05.349   Enlargement of <u>unspecified</u> orbit

H05.35- <u>Exostosis</u> of orbit — A form characterized by an abnormal bony growth the of the orbit.

H05.351   Exostosis of <u>right</u> orbit

H05.352   Exostosis of <u>left</u> orbit

H05.353   Exostosis of <u>bilateral</u> orbits

H05.359   Exostosis of <u>unspecified</u> orbit

H05.4- <u>Enophthalmos</u> — A backward displacement of the eyeball into the orbit.

H05.40- <u>Unspecified</u> enophthalmos

H05.401   Unspecified enophthalmos, <u>right</u> eye

H05.402   Unspecified enophthalmos, <u>left</u> eye

H05.403   Unspecified enophthalmos, <u>bilateral</u>

H05.409   Unspecified enophthalmos, <u>unspecified</u> eye

H05.41- Enophthalmos <u>due to atrophy</u> of orbital tissue — A form resulting from the wasting-away of orbital tissues.

H05.411   Enophthalmos due to atrophy of orbital tissue, <u>right</u> eye

H05.412   Enophthalmos due to atrophy of orbital tissue, <u>left</u> eye

H05.413   Enophthalmos due to atrophy of orbital tissue, <u>bilateral</u>

H05.419   Enophthalmos due to atrophy of orbital tissue, <u>unspecified</u> eye

H05.42- Enophthalmos <u>due to trauma or surgery</u>

H05.421   Enophthalmos due to trauma or surgery, <u>right</u> eye

H05.422   Enophthalmos due to trauma or surgery, <u>left</u> eye

H05.423   Enophthalmos due to trauma or surgery, <u>bilateral</u>

H05.429   Enophthalmos due to trauma or surgery, <u>unspecified</u> eye

H05.5- <u>Retained (old) foreign body</u> following penetrating wound of <u>orbit</u> — The continued presence of foreign material within the orbit.
Retrobulbar foreign body
Use additional code to identify the type of retained foreign body (Z18.-)
Excludes 1:   *current penetrating wound of orbit (S05.4-)*
Excludes ❷: *retained foreign body of eyelid (H02.81-)*
          retained intraocular foreign body (H44.6-, H44.7-)

H05.50   Retained (old) foreign body following penetrating wound of <u>unspecified</u> orbit

H05.51   Retained (old) foreign body following penetrating wound of <u>right</u> orbit

H05.52   Retained (old) foreign body following penetrating wound of <u>left</u> orbit

H05.53   Retained (old) foreign body following penetrating wound of <u>bilateral</u> orbits

H05.8- <u>Other</u> disorders of <u>orbit</u>

H05.81- <u>Cyst</u> of orbit — An encapsulated, fluid-filled sac of the orbit.
Encephalocele of orbit

H05.811   Cyst of <u>right</u> orbit

H05.812   Cyst of <u>left</u> orbit

H05.813   Cyst of <u>bilateral</u> orbits

H05.819   Cyst of <u>unspecified</u> orbit

H05.82- <u>Myopathy</u> of extraocular muscles — Abnormal disorders and conditions of the extraocular muscles.

H05.821   Myopathy of extraocular muscles, <u>right</u> orbit

H05.822   Myopathy of extraocular muscles, <u>left</u> orbit

H05.823   Myopathy of extraocular muscles, <u>bilateral</u>

H05.829   Myopathy of extraocular muscles, <u>unspecified</u> orbit

H05.89   Other disorders of orbit

H05.9   Unspecified disorder of orbit

Disorders of conjunctiva (H10-H11)

H10- <u>Conjunctivitis</u> — Inflammation of the conjunctiva.
Excludes 1:   *keratoconjunctivitis (H16.2-)*

H10.0- <u>Mucopurulent</u> conjunctivitis — A form characterized by mucous membrane pus formation.

H10.01- <u>Acute follicular</u> conjunctivitis — A form characterized by dense localized infiltrations of lymphoid tissue.

H10.011   Acute follicular conjunctivitis, <u>right</u> eye

H10.012   Acute follicular conjunctivitis, <u>left</u> eye

H10.013   Acute follicular conjunctivitis, <u>bilateral</u>

H10.019   Acute follicular conjunctivitis, <u>unspecified</u> eye

H10.02- <u>Other mucopurulent</u> conjunctivitis

H10.021   Other mucopurulent conjunctivitis, <u>right</u> eye

H10.022   Other mucopurulent conjunctivitis, <u>left</u> eye

H10.023   Other mucopurulent conjunctivitis, <u>bilateral</u>

H10.029   Other mucopurulent conjunctivitis, <u>unspecified</u> eye

H10.1- <u>Acute atopic</u> conjunctivitis — A form caused by an allergen.
Acute papillary conjunctivitis

H10.10   Acute atopic conjunctivitis, <u>unspecified</u> eye

H10.11   Acute atopic conjunctivitis, <u>right</u> eye

H10.12   Acute atopic conjunctivitis, <u>left</u> eye

H10.13   Acute atopic conjunctivitis, <u>bilateral</u>

H10.2- <u>Other acute</u> conjunctivitis

H10.21- <u>Acute toxic</u> conjunctivitis — A form caused by an external irritant (smoke, smog, cleaning chemical vapors, etc.), but not causing a burn, corrosion, or other injury to the conjunctival tissue.
Acute chemical conjunctivitis
Code first (T51-T65) to identify chemical and intent
Excludes 1:   *burn and corrosion of eye and adnexa (T26.-)*

H10.211   Acute toxic conjunctivitis, <u>right</u> eye

H10.212   Acute toxic conjunctivitis, <u>left</u> eye

H10.213   Acute toxic conjunctivitis, <u>bilateral</u>

H10.219   Acute toxic conjunctivitis, <u>unspecified</u> eye

H10.22- <u>Pseudomembranous</u> conjunctivitis — A form characterized by fibrous exudates which form a false membrane.

H10.221   Pseudomembranous conjunctivitis, <u>right</u> eye

H10.222   Pseudomembranous conjunctivitis, <u>left</u> eye

H10.223   Pseudomembranous conjunctivitis, <u>bilateral</u>

H10.229   Pseudomembranous conjunctivitis, <u>unspecified</u> eye

H10.23- <u>Serous</u> conjunctivitis, except viral — A form characterized by a watery discharge that is not viral in origin.
Excludes 1:   *viral conjunctivitis (B30.-)*

H10.231   Serous conjunctivitis, except viral, <u>right</u> eye

H10.232   Serous conjunctivitis, except viral, <u>left</u> eye

H10.233   Serous conjunctivitis, except viral, <u>bilateral</u>

H10.239   Serous conjunctivitis, except viral, <u>unspecified</u> eye

H10.3- <u>Unspecified acute</u> conjunctivitis
Excludes 1:   *ophthalmia neonatorum NOS (P39.1)*

H10.30   Unspecified acute conjunctivitis, <u>unspecified</u> eye

H10.31   Unspecified acute conjunctivitis, <u>right</u> eye

H10.32   Unspecified acute conjunctivitis, <u>left</u> eye

H10.33   Unspecified acute conjunctivitis, <u>bilateral</u>

H10.4- <u>Chronic</u> conjunctivitis — Inflammation of the conjunctiva that develops slowly and persists over a long period of time.

H10.40- <u>Unspecified chronic</u> conjunctivitis

H10.401   Unspecified chronic conjunctivitis, <u>right</u> eye

H10.402   Unspecified chronic conjunctivitis, <u>left</u> eye

H10.403   Unspecified chronic conjunctivitis, <u>bilateral</u>

H10.409   Unspecified chronic conjunctivitis, <u>unspecified</u> eye

H10.41- Chronic <u>giant papillary</u> conjunctivitis — A form that is characterized by groups of papillary inflammatory cells and caused by wearing of contact lenses.

H10.411   Chronic giant papillary conjunctivitis, <u>right</u> eye

H10.412   Chronic giant papillary conjunctivitis, <u>left</u> eye

H10.413   Chronic giant papillary conjunctivitis, <u>bilateral</u>

H10.419   Chronic giant papillary conjunctivitis, <u>unspecified</u> eye

H10.42- <u>Simple</u> chronic conjunctivitis — A form resulting from mild continuous acute symptoms.

H10.421   Simple chronic conjunctivitis, <u>right</u> eye

H10.422   Simple chronic conjunctivitis, <u>left</u> eye

H10.423   Simple chronic conjunctivitis, <u>bilateral</u>

H 0 5 - H 1 0

H10.429   Simple chronic conjunctivitis, <u>unspecified</u> eye

H10.43- Chronic <u>follicular</u> conjunctivitis — A form characterized by dense localized infiltrations of lymphoid tissue.

H10.431   Chronic follicular conjunctivitis, <u>right</u> eye

H10.432   Chronic follicular conjunctivitis, <u>left</u> eye

H10.433   Chronic follicular conjunctivitis, <u>bilateral</u>

H10.439   Chronic follicular conjunctivitis, <u>unspecified</u> eye

H10.44   <u>Vernal</u> conjunctivitis — A form characterized by onset during the spring and summer months.

    Excludes 1:   *vernal keratoconjunctivitis with limbar and corneal involvement (H16.26-)*

H10.45   <u>Other chronic allergic</u> conjunctivitis

H10.5-   <u>Blepharoconjunctivitis</u> — Inflammation of the eyelids and conjunctiva.

H10.50-   <u>Unspecified</u> blepharoconjunctivitis

H10.501   Unspecified blepharoconjunctivitis, <u>right</u> eye

H10.502   Unspecified blepharoconjunctivitis, <u>left</u> eye

H10.503   Unspecified blepharoconjunctivitis, <u>bilateral</u>

H10.509   Unspecified blepharoconjunctivitis, <u>unspecified</u> eye

H10.51-   <u>Ligneous</u> conjunctivitis — A form characterized by pseudomembranous lesions developing on the tarsal conjunctiva.

H10.511   Ligneous conjunctivitis, <u>right</u> eye

H10.512   Ligneous conjunctivitis, <u>left</u> eye

H10.513   Ligneous conjunctivitis, <u>bilateral</u>

H10.519   Ligneous conjunctivitis, <u>unspecified</u> eye

H10.52-   <u>Angular</u> blepharoconjunctivitis — A form affecting the canthal area.

H10.521   Angular blepharoconjunctivitis, <u>right</u> eye

H10.522   Angular blepharoconjunctivitis, <u>left</u> eye

H10.523   Angular blepharoconjunctivitis, <u>bilateral</u>

H10.529   Angular blepharoconjunctivitis, <u>unspecified</u> eye

H10.53-   <u>Contact</u> blepharoconjunctivitis — A form caused by various substances.

H10.531   Contact blepharoconjunctivitis, <u>right</u> eye

H10.532   Contact blepharoconjunctivitis, <u>left</u> eye

H10.533   Contact blepharoconjunctivitis, <u>bilateral</u>

H10.539   Contact blepharoconjunctivitis, <u>unspecified</u> eye

H10.8-   Other conjunctivitis

H10.81-   <u>Pingueculitis</u> — An inflammatory disorder of the pingueculae (yellowish, slightly raised, lipid-like deposits on the conjunctiva) characterized by acute inflammation, vascularized conjunctiva, redness, and irritation.

    Excludes 1:   *pinguecula (H11.15-)*

H10.811   Pingueculitis, <u>right</u> eye

H10.812   Pingueculitis, <u>left</u> eye

H10.813   Pingueculitis, <u>bilateral</u>

H10.819   Pingueculitis, <u>unspecified</u> eye

H10.89   Other conjunctivitis

H10.9   Unspecified conjunctivitis

H11-   <u>Other disorders of conjunctiva</u>

    Excludes 1:   *keratoconjunctivitis (H16.2-)*

H11.0-   <u>Pterygium</u> of eye — A triangular-shaped thickening of the conjunctiva extending from the inner canthus over the cornea towards the pupil.

    Excludes 1:   *pseudopterygium (H11.81-)*

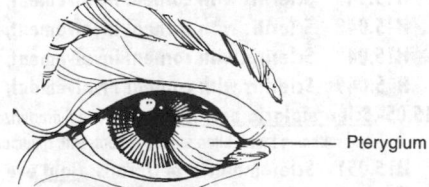

Pterygium

PTERYGIUM — RIGHT EYE

H11.00-   <u>Unspecified</u> pterygium of eye

H11.001   Unspecified pterygium of <u>right</u> eye

H11.002   Unspecified pterygium of <u>left</u> eye

H11.003   Unspecified pterygium of eye, <u>bilateral</u>

H11.009   Unspecified pterygium of <u>unspecified</u> eye

H11.01-   <u>Amyloid</u> pterygium — A form with amyloid deposition in blood vessel walls.

H11.011   Amyloid pterygium of <u>right</u> eye

H11.012   Amyloid pterygium of <u>left</u> eye

H11.013   Amyloid pterygium of eye, <u>bilateral</u>

H11.019   Amyloid pterygium of <u>unspecified</u> eye

H11.02-   <u>Central</u> pterygium of eye — A form which encroaches on the center of the cornea.

H11.021   Central pterygium of <u>right</u> eye

H11.022   Central pterygium of <u>left</u> eye

H11.023   Central pterygium of eye, <u>bilateral</u>

H11.029   Central pterygium of <u>unspecified</u> eye

H11.03-   <u>Double</u> pterygium of eye — Bilateral pterygiums occurring at the same time.

H11.031   Double pterygium of <u>right</u> eye

H11.032   Double pterygium of <u>left</u> eye

H11.033   Double pterygium of eye, <u>bilateral</u>

H11.039   Double pterygium of <u>unspecified</u> eye

H11.04-   <u>Peripheral</u> pterygium of eye, <u>stationary</u> — A stage in which the head of the pterygium remains permanently attached to the same point on the cornea.

H11.041   Peripheral pterygium, stationary, <u>right</u> eye

H11.042   Peripheral pterygium, stationary, <u>left</u> eye

H11.043   Peripheral pterygium, stationary, <u>bilateral</u>

H11.049   Peripheral pterygium, stationary, <u>unspecified</u> eye

H11.05-   <u>Peripheral</u> pterygium of eye, <u>progressive</u> — A stage in which the growth extends toward the center of the cornea.

H11.051   Peripheral pterygium, progressive, <u>right</u> eye

H11.052   Peripheral pterygium, progressive, <u>left</u> eye

H11.053   Peripheral pterygium, progressive, <u>bilateral</u>

H11.059   Peripheral pterygium, progressive, <u>unspecified</u> eye

H11.06-   <u>Recurrent</u> pterygium of eye — A form which returns after the initial condition has healed.

H11.061   Recurrent pterygium of <u>right</u> eye

H11.062   Recurrent pterygium of <u>left</u> eye

H11.063   Recurrent pterygium of eye, <u>bilateral</u>

H11.069   Recurrent pterygium of <u>unspecified</u> eye

H11.1-   Conjunctival degenerations and deposits

    Excludes ❷: *pseudopterygium (H11.81)*

H11.10   Unspecified conjunctival degenerations

H11.11-   <u>Conjunctival deposits</u> — Extraneous inorganic matter collected on the conjunctiva.

H11.111   Conjunctival deposits, <u>right</u> eye

H11.112   Conjunctival deposits, <u>left</u> eye

H11.113   Conjunctival deposits, <u>bilateral</u>

H11.119   Conjunctival deposits, <u>unspecified</u> eye

H11.12-   Conjunctival <u>concretions</u> — A condition marked by a hardening of the conjunctiva.

H11.121   Conjunctival concretions, <u>right</u> eye

H11.122   Conjunctival concretions, <u>left</u> eye

H11.123   Conjunctival concretions, <u>bilateral</u>

H11.129   Conjunctival concretions, <u>unspecified</u> eye

H11.13-   Conjunctival <u>pigmentations</u> — The pigmental discoloration of the conjunctiva.

    Conjunctival argyrosis [argyria] — A poisoning of the conjunctiva by silver, or a silver salt, causing a permanent ash gray discolorization.

H11.131   Conjunctival pigmentations, <u>right</u> eye

H11.132   Conjunctival pigmentations, <u>left</u> eye

H11.133   Conjunctival pigmentations, <u>bilateral</u>

H11.139   Conjunctival pigmentations, <u>unspecified</u> eye

H11.14-   Conjunctival <u>xerosis</u>, <u>unspecified</u> — An abnormal dryness of the conjunctiva.

    Excludes 1:   *xerosis of conjunctiva due to vitamin A deficiency (E50.0, E50.1)*

H11.141   Conjunctival xerosis, <u>unspecified</u>, <u>right</u> eye

H11.142   Conjunctival xerosis, <u>unspecified</u>, <u>left</u> eye

Excludes 1: = NOT CODED HERE! (Do not code both)

Excludes ❷: = Not Included Here

H10 - H11

H11.143   Conjunctival xerosis, <u>unspecified</u>, <u>bilateral</u>

H11.149   Conjunctival xerosis, <u>unspecified</u>, <u>unspecified</u> eye

H11.15-   <u>Pinguecula</u> — A yellowish thickening of the conjunctiva on the inner and outer margins of the cornea.

     Excludes 1:   *pingueculitis (H10.81-)*

     H11.151   Pinguecula, <u>right</u> eye

     H11.152   Pinguecula, <u>left</u> eye

     H11.153   Pinguecula, <u>bilateral</u>

     H11.159   Pinguecula, <u>unspecified</u> eye

H11.2-   <u>Conjunctival scars</u> — The dense healing tissue of the conjunctiva.

H11.21-   Conjunctival <u>adhesions and strands (localized)</u> — The formation of fibrous tissue of the conjunctiva.

     H11.211   Conjunctival adhesions and strands (localized), <u>right</u> eye

     H11.212   Conjunctival adhesions and strands (localized), <u>left</u> eye

     H11.213   Conjunctival adhesions and strands (localized), <u>bilateral</u>

     H11.219   Conjunctival adhesions and strands (localized), <u>unspecified</u> eye

H11.22-   Conjunctival <u>granuloma</u> — The formation of granulation tissue of the conjunctiva.

     H11.221   Conjunctival granuloma, <u>right</u> eye

     H11.222   Conjunctival granuloma, <u>left</u> eye

     H11.223   Conjunctival granuloma, <u>bilateral</u>

     H11.229   Conjunctival granuloma, <u>unspecified</u>

H11.23-   <u>Symblepharon</u> — The adhesion of the eyelid conjunctiva and the eyeball following an injury.

     H11.231   Symblepharon, <u>right</u> eye

     H11.232   Symblepharon, <u>left</u> eye

     H11.233   Symblepharon, <u>bilateral</u>

     H11.239   Symblepharon, <u>unspecified</u> eye

H11.24-   <u>Scarring</u> of conjunctiva — The dense post wound-healing tissue of the conjunctiva.

     H11.241   Scarring of conjunctiva, <u>right</u> eye

     H11.242   Scarring of conjunctiva, <u>left</u> eye

     H11.243   Scarring of conjunctiva, <u>bilateral</u>

     H11.249   Scarring of conjunctiva, <u>unspecified</u> eye

H11.3-   Conjunctival <u>hemorrhage</u> — Bleeding from the conjunctiva.

     Subconjunctival hemorrhage

H11.30   Conjunctival hemorrhage, <u>unspecified</u> eye

H11.31   Conjunctival hemorrhage, <u>right</u> eye

H11.32   Conjunctival hemorrhage, <u>left</u> eye

H11.33   Conjunctival hemorrhage, <u>bilateral</u>

H11.4-   <u>Other conjunctival vascular</u> disorders and cysts

H11.41-   <u>Vascular abnormalities</u> of conjunctiva

     Conjunctival aneurysm — The dilatation of a conjunctival artery.

     H11.411   Vascular abnormalities of conjunctiva, <u>right</u> eye

     H11.412   Vascular abnormalities of conjunctiva, <u>left</u> eye

     H11.413   Vascular abnormalities of conjunctiva, <u>bilateral</u> eye

     H11.419   Vascular abnormalities of conjunctiva, <u>unspecified</u> eye

H11.42-   Conjunctival <u>edema</u> — The excessive amount of fluid within the conjunctiva.

     H11.421   Conjunctival edema, <u>right</u> eye

     H11.422   Conjunctival edema, <u>left</u> eye

     H11.423   Conjunctival edema, <u>bilateral</u>

     H11.429   Conjunctival edema, <u>unspecified</u> eye

H11.43-   Conjunctival <u>hyperemia</u> — The abnormal excessive amount of blood in the conjunctiva.

     H11.431   Conjunctival hyperemia, <u>right</u> eye

     H11.432   Conjunctival hyperemia, <u>left</u> eye

     H11.433   Conjunctival hyperemia, <u>bilateral</u>

     H11.439   Conjunctival hyperemia, <u>unspecified</u> eye

---

H11.44-   Conjunctival <u>cysts</u> — An encapsulated, fluid-filled sac of the conjunctiva.

     H11.441   Conjunctival cysts, <u>right</u> eye

     H11.442   Conjunctival cysts, <u>left</u> eye

     H11.443   Conjunctival cysts, <u>bilateral</u>

     H11.449   Conjunctival cysts, <u>unspecified</u> eye

H11.8-   <u>Other specified disorders of conjunctiva</u>

H11.81-   <u>Pseudopterygium</u> of conjunctiva — A scar on the conjunctiva that is usually firmly attached to the underlying tissue.

     H11.811   Pseudopterygium of conjunctiva, <u>right</u> eye

     H11.812   Pseudopterygium of conjunctiva, <u>left</u> eye

     H11.813   Pseudopterygium of conjunctiva, <u>bilateral</u>

     H11.819   Pseudopterygium of conjunctiva, <u>unspecified</u> eye

H11.82-   <u>Conjunctivochalasis</u> — The formation of redundant conjunctival tissue which overlies the lower eyelid margin.

     H11.821   Conjunctivochalasis, <u>right</u> eye

     H11.822   Conjunctivochalasis, <u>left</u> eye

     H11.823   Conjunctivochalasis, <u>bilateral</u>

     H11.829   Conjunctivochalasis, <u>unspecified</u> eye

H11.89   Other specified disorders of conjunctiva

H11.9   Unspecified disorder of conjunctiva

Disorders of sclera, cornea, iris and ciliary body (H15-H22)

H15-   <u>Disorders of sclera</u>

H15.0-   <u>Scleritis</u> — Inflammation of the sclera.

H15.00-   <u>Unspecified</u> scleritis

     H15.001   Unspecified scleritis, <u>right</u> eye

     H15.002   Unspecified scleritis, <u>left</u> eye

     H15.003   Unspecified scleritis, <u>bilateral</u>

     H15.009   Unspecified scleritis, <u>unspecified</u> eye

H15.01-   <u>Anterior</u> scleritis — A form characterized by affecting that portion towards the front of the eye, including the corneal margins.

     H15.011   Anterior scleritis, <u>right</u> eye

     H15.012   Anterior scleritis, <u>left</u> eye

     H15.013   Anterior scleritis, <u>bilateral</u>

     H15.019   Anterior scleritis, <u>unspecified</u> eye

H15.02-   <u>Brawny</u> scleritis — A form characterized by thickening of the corneal margins.

     H15.021   Brawny scleritis, <u>right</u> eye

     H15.022   Brawny scleritis, <u>left</u> eye

     H15.023   Brawny scleritis, <u>bilateral</u>

     H15.029   Brawny scleritis, <u>unspecified</u> eye

H15.03-   <u>Posterior</u> scleritis — A form characterized by involvement of the underlying retina and choroid.

     Sclerotenonitis

     H15.031   Posterior scleritis, <u>right</u> eye

     H15.032   Posterior scleritis, <u>left</u> eye

     H15.033   Posterior scleritis, <u>bilateral</u>

     H15.039   Posterior scleritis, <u>unspecified</u> eye

H15.04-   <u>Scleritis with corneal involvement</u> — A form characterized by an inflammatory reaction in the cornea.

     H15.041   Scleritis with corneal involvement, <u>right</u> eye

     H15.042   Scleritis with corneal involvement, <u>left</u> eye

     H15.043   Scleritis with corneal involvement, <u>bilateral</u>

     H15.049   Scleritis with corneal involvement, <u>unspecified</u> eye

H15.05-   <u>Scleromalacia perforans</u> — A form characterized by degeneration and softening that is often seen in patients with rheumatoid arthritis.

     H15.051   Scleromalacia perforans, <u>right</u> eye

     H15.052   Scleromalacia perforans, <u>left</u> eye

     H15.053   Scleromalacia perforans, <u>bilateral</u>

     H15.059   Scleromalacia perforans, <u>unspecified</u> eye

H15.09-   <u>Other</u> scleritis

     Scleral abscess — A localized collection of pus, caused by the disintegration of scleral tissue.

     H15.091   Other scleritis, <u>right</u> eye

     H15.092   Other scleritis, <u>left</u> eye

H11-H15

H15.093   Other scleritis, **bilateral**
H15.099   Other scleritis, **unspecified** eye

H15.1-   Episcleritis — Inflammation of the loose connective tissue of the sclera.

H15.10- Unspecified episcleritis
H15.101   Unspecified episcleritis, **right** eye
H15.102   Unspecified episcleritis, **left** eye
H15.103   Unspecified episcleritis, **bilateral**
H15.109   Unspecified episcleritis, **unspecified** eye

H15.11- Episcleritis periodica fugax — A form characterized by the sudden accumulation of blood which lasts a short time.
H15.111   Episcleritis periodica fugax, **right** eye
H15.112   Episcleritis periodica fugax, **left** eye
H15.113   Episcleritis periodica fugax, **bilateral**
H15.119   Episcleritis periodica fugax, **unspecified** eye

H15.12- Nodular episcleritis — A form characterized by the formation of nodules.
H15.121   Nodular episcleritis, **right** eye
H15.122   Nodular episcleritis, **left** eye
H15.123   Nodular episcleritis, **bilateral**
H15.129   Nodular episcleritis, **unspecified** eye

H15.8-   Other disorders of sclera
Excludes ❷: *blue sclera (Q13.5)*
          degenerative myopia (H44.2-)

H15.81- Equatorial staphyloma — A form characterized by bulging at the equatorial region of the eye.
H15.811   Equatorial staphyloma, **right** eye
H15.812   Equatorial staphyloma, **left** eye
H15.813   Equatorial staphyloma, **bilateral**
H15.819   Equatorial staphyloma, **unspecified** eye

H15.82- Localized anterior staphyloma — A form characterized by protrusion in the anterior part of the eye.
H15.821   Localized anterior staphyloma, **right** eye
H15.822   Localized anterior staphyloma, **left** eye
H15.823   Localized anterior staphyloma, **bilateral**
H15.829   Localized anterior staphyloma, **unspecified** eye

H15.83- Staphyloma posticum — A form characterized by the backward bulging of the sclera.
H15.831   Staphyloma posticum, **right** eye
H15.832   Staphyloma posticum, **left** eye
H15.833   Staphyloma posticum, **bilateral**
H15.839   Staphyloma posticum, **unspecified** eye

H15.84- Scleral ectasia — The abnormal protrusion of the sclera and cornea.
H15.841   Scleral ectasia, **right** eye
H15.842   Scleral ectasia, **left** eye
H15.843   Scleral ectasia, **bilateral**
H15.849   Scleral ectasia, **unspecified** eye

H15.85- Ring staphyloma — A form characterized by bulging in a ring-like shape.
H15.851   Ring staphyloma, **right** eye
H15.852   Ring staphyloma, **left** eye
H15.853   Ring staphyloma, **bilateral**
H15.859   Ring staphyloma, **unspecified** eye

H15.89 Other disorders of sclera

H15.9 Unspecified disorder of sclera

H16-   Keratitis — Inflammation of the cornea.

H16.0-   Corneal ulcer — The abnormal erosion of the corneal tissue.

H16.00- Unspecified corneal ulcer
H16.001   Unspecified corneal ulcer, **right** eye
H16.002   Unspecified corneal ulcer, **left** eye
H16.003   Unspecified corneal ulcer, **bilateral**
H16.009   Unspecified corneal ulcer, **unspecified** eye

H16.01- Central corneal ulcer — A form situated in the central area of the cornea.
H16.011   Central corneal ulcer, **right** eye
H16.012   Central corneal ulcer, **left** eye
H16.013   Central corneal ulcer, **bilateral**
H16.019   Central corneal ulcer, **unspecified** eye

H16.02- Ring corneal ulcer — A form marked by the development of connected peripheral ulcers.
H16.021   Ring corneal ulcer, **right** eye
H16.022   Ring corneal ulcer, **left** eye
H16.023   Ring corneal ulcer, **bilateral**
H16.029   Ring corneal ulcer, **unspecified** eye

H16.03- Corneal ulcer with hypopyon — A form associated with pus in the anterior chamber.
H16.031   Corneal ulcer with hypopyon, **right** eye
H16.032   Corneal ulcer with hypopyon, **left** eye
H16.033   Corneal ulcer with hypopyon, **bilateral**
H16.039   Corneal ulcer with hypopyon, **unspecified** eye

H16.04- Marginal corneal ulcer — A form situated in the lateral margins of the cornea.
H16.041   Marginal corneal ulcer, **right** eye
H16.042   Marginal corneal ulcer, **left** eye
H16.043   Marginal corneal ulcer, **bilateral**
H16.049   Marginal corneal ulcer, **unspecified** eye

H16.05- Mooren's corneal ulcer — A form of a marginal, pus-forming ulcer usually seen in elderly patients.
H16.051   Mooren's corneal ulcer, **right** eye
H16.052   Mooren's corneal ulcer, **left** eye
H16.053   Mooren's corneal ulcer, **bilateral**
H16.059   Mooren's corneal ulcer, **unspecified** eye

H16.06- Mycotic corneal ulcer — A form caused by a fungus.
H16.061   Mycotic corneal ulcer, **right** eye
H16.062   Mycotic corneal ulcer, **left** eye
H16.063   Mycotic corneal ulcer, **bilateral**
H16.069   Mycotic corneal ulcer, **unspecified** eye

H16.07- Perforated corneal ulcer — A form involving the entire thickness of the cornea.
H16.071   Perforated corneal ulcer, **right** eye
H16.072   Perforated corneal ulcer, **left** eye
H16.073   Perforated corneal ulcer, **bilateral**
H16.079   Perforated corneal ulcer, **unspecified** eye

H16.1-   Other and unspecified superficial keratitis without conjunctivitis — Direct inflammation of the corneal epithelium, without associated conjunctivitis.

H16.10- Unspecified superficial keratitis
H16.101   Unspecified superficial keratitis, **right** eye
H16.102   Unspecified superficial keratitis, **left** eye
H16.103   Unspecified superficial keratitis, **bilateral**
H16.109   Unspecified superficial keratitis, **unspecified** eye

H16.11- Macular keratitis — A form characterized by circumscribed opacity of the cornea.
     Areolar keratitis — A form marked by small, circular spots.
     Nummular keratitis — A form marked by circular corneal deposits.
     Stellate keratitis — A form marked by star-shaped opacities.
     Striate keratitis — A form marked by lines of opacity on the cornea.
H16.111   Macular keratitis, **right** eye
H16.112   Macular keratitis, **left** eye
H16.113   Macular keratitis, **bilateral**
H16.119   Macular keratitis, **unspecified** eye

H16.12- Filamentary keratitis — A form characterized by twisted filaments of mucoid material on the surface of the cornea.
H16.121   Filamentary keratitis, **right** eye
H16.122   Filamentary keratitis, **left** eye
H16.123   Filamentary keratitis, **bilateral**
H16.129   Filamentary keratitis, **unspecified** eye

H16.13- Photokeratitis — A form characterized by fluorescein-positive infiltrates.
     Snow blindness — A form resulting from intensified, reflected sunlight off of snow.
     Welders keratitis — A form resulting from ultraviolet light from welding torches.
H16.131   Photokeratitis, **right** eye
H16.132   Photokeratitis, **left** eye

H15
–
H16

Excludes 1: = NOT CODED HERE! (Do not code both)   683   *Excludes ❷:* = Not Included Here

H16.133 Photokeratitis, <u>bilateral</u>

H16.139 Photokeratitis, <u>unspecified</u> eye

H16.14- <u>Punctate</u> keratitis — A form characterized by the formation of cellular and fibrous deposits on the cornea.

H16.141 Punctate keratitis, <u>right</u> eye

H16.142 Punctate keratitis, <u>left</u> eye

H16.143 Punctate keratitis, <u>bilateral</u>

H16.149 Punctate keratitis, <u>unspecified</u> eye

H16.2- <u>Keratoconjunctivitis</u> — Inflammation of the cornea and conjunctiva.

H16.20- <u>Unspecified</u> keratoconjunctivitis
    Superficial keratitis with conjunctivitis NOS

H16.201 Unspecified keratoconjunctivitis, <u>right</u> eye

H16.202 Unspecified keratoconjunctivitis, <u>left</u> eye

H16.203 Unspecified keratoconjunctivitis, <u>bilateral</u>

H16.209 Unspecified keratoconjunctivitis, <u>unspecified</u> eye

H16.21- <u>Exposure</u> keratoconjunctivitis — A form characterized by air exposure with drying of the conjunctiva and cornea.

H16.211 Exposure keratoconjunctivitis, <u>right</u> eye

H16.212 Exposure keratoconjunctivitis, <u>left</u> eye

H16.213 Exposure keratoconjunctivitis, <u>bilateral</u>

H16.219 Exposure keratoconjunctivitis, <u>unspecified</u> eye

H16.22- Keratoconjunctivitis <u>sicca, not specified as Sjögren's</u> — A form characterized by conjunctival blood congestion, lacrimal drying, and thickening of the cornea.

    Excludes 1:   *Sjögren's syndrome (M35.01)*

H16.221 Keratoconjunctivitis sicca, not specified as Sjögren's, <u>right</u> eye

H16.222 Keratoconjunctivitis sicca, not specified as Sjögren's, <u>left</u> eye

H16.223 Keratoconjunctivitis sicca, not specified as Sjögren's, <u>bilateral</u>

H16.229 Keratoconjunctivitis sicca, not specified as Sjögren's, <u>unspecified</u> eye

H16.23- <u>Neurotrophic</u> keratoconjunctivitis — A form of neurogenic origin.

H16.231 Neurotrophic keratoconjunctivitis, <u>right</u> eye

H16.232 Neurotrophic keratoconjunctivitis, <u>left</u> eye

H16.233 Neurotrophic keratoconjunctivitis, <u>bilateral</u>

H16.239 Neurotrophic keratoconjunctivitis, <u>unspecified</u> eye

H16.24- <u>Ophthalmia nodosa</u> — Inflammation of the conjunctiva produced by caterpillar hairs.

H16.241 Ophthalmia nodosa, <u>right</u> eye

H16.242 Ophthalmia nodosa, <u>left</u> eye

H16.243 Ophthalmia nodosa, <u>bilateral</u>

H16.249 Ophthalmia nodosa, <u>unspecified</u> eye

H16.25- <u>Phlyctenular</u> keratoconjunctivitis — A form characterized by small, gray, circumscribed lesions of the corneal limbus.

H16.251 Phlyctenular keratoconjunctivitis, <u>right</u> eye

H16.252 Phlyctenular keratoconjunctivitis, <u>left</u> eye

H16.253 Phlyctenular keratoconjunctivitis, <u>bilateral</u>

H16.259 Phlyctenular keratoconjunctivitis, <u>unspecified</u> eye

H16.26- <u>Vernal</u> keratoconjunctivitis, <u>with limbar and corneal involvement</u> — A form characterized by onset during the spring and summer months.

    Excludes 1:   *vernal conjunctivitis without limbar and corneal involvement (H10.44)*

H16.261 Vernal keratoconjunctivitis, with limbar and corneal involvement, <u>right</u> eye

H16.262 Vernal keratoconjunctivitis, with limbar and corneal involvement, <u>left</u> eye

H16.263 Vernal keratoconjunctivitis, with limbar and corneal involvement, <u>bilateral</u>

H16.269 Vernal keratoconjunctivitis, with limbar and corneal involvement, <u>unspecified</u> eye

H16.29- <u>Other</u> keratoconjunctivitis

H16.291 Other keratoconjunctivitis, <u>right</u> eye

H16.292 Other keratoconjunctivitis, <u>left</u> eye

H16.293 Other keratoconjunctivitis, <u>bilateral</u>

H16.299 Other keratoconjunctivitis, <u>unspecified</u> eye

H16.3- <u>Interstitial and deep</u> keratitis — Inflammation of the cornea with deposits deep in the layers of the cornea resulting in a ground-glass appearance.

H16.30- <u>Unspecified interstitial</u> keratitis

H16.301 Unspecified interstitial keratitis, <u>right</u> eye

H16.302 Unspecified interstitial keratitis, <u>left</u> eye

H16.303 Unspecified interstitial keratitis, <u>bilateral</u>

H16.309 Unspecified interstitial keratitis, <u>unspecified</u> eye

H16.31- <u>Corneal abscess</u> — A localized collection of pus, caused by the disintegration of corneal tissues.

H16.311 Corneal abscess, <u>right</u> eye

H16.312 Corneal abscess, <u>left</u> eye

H16.313 Corneal abscess, <u>bilateral</u>

H16.319 Corneal abscess, <u>unspecified</u> eye

H16.32- <u>Diffuse interstitial</u> keratitis — A form characterized by general involvement of the cornea.
    Cogan's syndrome

H16.321 Diffuse interstitial keratitis, <u>right</u> eye

H16.322 Diffuse interstitial keratitis, <u>left</u> eye

H16.323 Diffuse interstitial keratitis, <u>bilateral</u>

H16.329 Diffuse interstitial keratitis, <u>unspecified</u> eye

H16.33- <u>Sclerosing</u> keratitis — A form marked by deep opacity and associated with inflammation of the sclera.

H16.331 Sclerosing keratitis, <u>right</u> eye

H16.332 Sclerosing keratitis, <u>left</u> eye

H16.333 Sclerosing keratitis, <u>bilateral</u>

H16.339 Sclerosing keratitis, <u>unspecified</u> eye

H16.39- <u>Other interstitial</u> and deep keratitis

H16.391 Other interstitial and deep keratitis, <u>right</u> eye

H16.392 Other interstitial and deep keratitis, <u>left</u> eye

H16.393 Other interstitial and deep keratitis, <u>bilateral</u>

H16.399 Other interstitial and deep keratitis, <u>unspecified</u> eye

H16.4- <u>Corneal neovascularization</u> — The abnormal formation of new blood vessels.

H16.40- <u>Unspecified</u> corneal neovascularization

H16.401 Unspecified corneal neovascularization, <u>right</u> eye

H16.402 Unspecified corneal neovascularization, <u>left</u> eye

H16.403 Unspecified corneal neovascularization, <u>bilateral</u>

H16.409 Unspecified corneal neovascularization, <u>unspecified</u> eye

H16.41- <u>Ghost vessels (corneal)</u> — The presence of corneal blood vessels which have no blood flow.

H16.411 Ghost vessels (corneal), <u>right</u> eye

H16.412 Ghost vessels (corneal), <u>left</u> eye

H16.413 Ghost vessels (corneal), <u>bilateral</u>

H16.419 Ghost vessels (corneal), <u>unspecified</u> eye

H16.42- <u>Pannus (corneal)</u> — The superficial vascularization of the cornea with infiltration of granulation tissue.

H16.421 Pannus (corneal), <u>right</u> eye

H16.422 Pannus (corneal), <u>left</u> eye

H16.423 Pannus (corneal), <u>bilateral</u>

H16.429 Pannus (corneal), <u>unspecified</u> eye

H16.43- <u>Localized vascularization</u> of cornea — The formation of corneal blood vessels in a circumscribed area.

H16.431 Localized vascularization of cornea, <u>right</u> eye

H16.432 Localized vascularization of cornea, <u>left</u> eye

H16.433 Localized vascularization of cornea, <u>bilateral</u>

H16.439 Localized vascularization of cornea, <u>unspecified</u> eye

H16.44- <u>Deep vascularization</u> of cornea — The abnormal formation of blood vessels in the deep corneal layers.

H16.441 Deep vascularization of cornea, <u>right</u> eye

H16.442 Deep vascularization of cornea, <u>left</u> eye

H16.443 Deep vascularization of cornea, <u>bilateral</u>

H16.449 Deep vascularization of cornea, <u>unspecified</u> eye

H 1 6 - H 1 6

H16.8   Other keratitis — [Unacceptable PDX]

H16.9   Unspecified keratitis

H17-   Corneal scars and opacities — The dense post-healing tissue of the cornea, and the inability to pass light through the cornea.

H17.0-   Adherent leukoma — A form adhering to the iris.

H17.00 Adherent leukoma, unspecified eye

H17.01 Adherent leukoma, right eye

H17.02 Adherent leukoma, left eye

H17.03 Adherent leukoma, bilateral

H17.1-   Central corneal opacity — A form affecting the center of the cornea.

H17.10 Central corneal opacity, unspecified eye

H17.11 Central corneal opacity, right eye

H17.12 Central corneal opacity, left eye

H17.13 Central corneal opacity, bilateral

H17.8-   Other corneal scars and opacities

H17.81- Minor opacity of cornea — A form which is not severe enough to interfere with vision.
Corneal nebula — A form which can only be seen by oblique illumination.

H17.811 Minor opacity of cornea, right eye

H17.812 Minor opacity of cornea, left eye

H17.813 Minor opacity of cornea, bilateral

H17.819 Minor opacity of cornea, unspecified eye

H17.82- Peripheral opacity of cornea — A form affecting the noncentral margins of the cornea.

H17.821 Peripheral opacity of cornea, right eye

H17.822 Peripheral opacity of cornea, left eye

H17.823 Peripheral opacity of cornea, bilateral

H17.829 Peripheral opacity of cornea, unspecified eye

H17.89 Other corneal scars and opacities

H17.9   Unspecified corneal scar and opacity

H18-   Other disorders of cornea

H18.0-   Corneal pigmentations and deposits

H18.00- Unspecified corneal deposit

H18.001 Unspecified corneal deposit, right eye

H18.002 Unspecified corneal deposit, left eye

H18.003 Unspecified corneal deposit, bilateral

H18.009 Unspecified corneal deposit, unspecified eye

H18.01- Anterior corneal pigmentations — The deposition of colored matter in the outer layer of the cornea.
Staehli's line — A horizontal brown mark on the cornea that is seen in aged persons.

H18.011 Anterior corneal pigmentations, right eye

H18.012 Anterior corneal pigmentations, left eye

H18.013 Anterior corneal pigmentations, bilateral

H18.019 Anterior corneal pigmentations, unspecified eye

H18.02- Argentous corneal deposits — Silver corneal deposits.

H18.021 Argentous corneal deposits, right eye

H18.022 Argentous corneal deposits, left eye

H18.023 Argentous corneal deposits, bilateral

H18.029 Argentous corneal deposits, unspecified eye

H18.03- Corneal deposits in metabolic disorders
Code also associated metabolic disorder

H18.031 Corneal deposits in metabolic disorders, right eye

H18.032 Corneal deposits in metabolic disorders, left eye

H18.033 Corneal deposits in metabolic disorders, bilateral

H18.039 Corneal deposits in metabolic disorders, unspecified eye

H18.04- Kayser-Fleischer ring — A dark pigmented ring at the outer margin of the cornea.
Code also associated Wilson's disease (E83.01)

H18.041 Kayser-Fleischer ring, right eye

H18.042 Kayser-Fleischer ring, left eye

H18.043 Kayser-Fleischer ring, bilateral

H18.049 Kayser-Fleischer ring, unspecified eye

H18.05- Posterior corneal pigmentations — The deposition of colored matter in the innermost layer of the cornea.
Krukenberg's spindle — A vertical spindle-shaped, brownish-red opacity on the posterior surface of the cornea.

H18.051 Posterior corneal pigmentations, right eye

H18.052 Posterior corneal pigmentations, left eye

H18.053 Posterior corneal pigmentations, bilateral

H18.059 Posterior corneal pigmentations, unspecified eye

H18.06- Stromal corneal pigmentations — The deposition of colored matter in the main layers of the cornea.
Hematocornea — The presence of hematin deposits within the corneal layers.

H18.061 Stromal corneal pigmentations, right eye

H18.062 Stromal corneal pigmentations, left eye

H18.063 Stromal corneal pigmentations, bilateral

H18.069 Stromal corneal pigmentations, unspecified eye

H18.1-   Bullous keratopathy — A form contained in a small sac of tissue.

H18.10 Bullous keratopathy, unspecified eye

H18.11 Bullous keratopathy, right eye

H18.12 Bullous keratopathy, left eye

H18.13 Bullous keratopathy, bilateral

H18.2-   Other and unspecified corneal edema — Excessive fluid in the cornea.

H18.20 Unspecified corneal edema

H18.21- Corneal edema secondary to contact lens — A form caused by the irritating effects of contact lenses.
Excludes ❷: other corneal disorders due to contact lens (H18.82-)

H18.211 Corneal edema secondary to contact lens, right eye

H18.212 Corneal edema secondary to contact lens, left eye

H18.213 Corneal edema secondary to contact lens, bilateral

H18.219 Corneal edema secondary to contact lens, unspecified eye

H18.22- Idiopathic corneal edema — A form which is not associated with another disease.

H18.221 Idiopathic corneal edema, right eye

H18.222 Idiopathic corneal edema, left eye

H18.223 Idiopathic corneal edema, bilateral

H18.229 Idiopathic corneal edema, unspecified eye

H18.23- Secondary corneal edema — A form resulting from a disease or ocular injury.

H18.231 Secondary corneal edema, right eye

H18.232 Secondary corneal edema, left eye

H18.233 Secondary corneal edema, bilateral

H18.239 Secondary corneal edema, unspecified eye

H18.3-   Changes of corneal membranes — A change in the normal formation of the corneal membranes.

H18.30 Unspecified corneal membrane change

H18.31- Folds and rupture in Bowman's membrane — A form affecting the second-most outer corneal layer.

H18.311 Folds and rupture in Bowman's membrane, right eye

H18.312 Folds and rupture in Bowman's membrane, left eye

H18.313 Folds and rupture in Bowman's membrane, bilateral

H18.319 Folds and rupture in Bowman's membrane, unspecified eye

H18.32- Folds in Descemet's membrane — A doubling upon itself of the second-most inner corneal layer.

H18.321 Folds in Descemet's membrane, right eye

H18.322 Folds in Descemet's membrane, left eye

H18.323 Folds in Descemet's membrane, bilateral

H18.329 Folds in Descemet's membrane, unspecified eye

H18.33- Rupture In Descemet's membrane — A forcible tearing of the second-most inner corneal layer.

H18.331 Rupture in Descemet's membrane, right eye

H18.332 Rupture in Descemet's membrane, left eye

H18.333 Rupture in Descemet's membrane, bilateral

H16 - H18

H18.339 Rupture in Descemet's membrane, <u>unspecified</u> eye

H18.4- <u>Corneal degeneration</u> — Deterioration or loss of function of the corneal tissues.
> *Excludes 1:* *Mooren's ulcer (H16.0-)*
> *recurrent erosion of cornea (H18.83-)*

H18.40 <u>Unspecified</u> corneal degeneration

H18.41- <u>Arcus senilis</u> — Lipoid degeneration resulting in a gray-white ring on the cornea occurring with advancing age.
> Senile corneal changes — Corneal deteriorations occurring in advancing age.

H18.411 Arcus senilis, <u>right</u> eye

H18.412 Arcus senilis, <u>left</u> eye

H18.413 Arcus senilis, <u>bilateral</u>

H18.419 Arcus senilis, <u>unspecified</u> eye

H18.42- <u>Band keratopathy</u> — Band-like superficial gray-white flecks on the cornea.

H18.421 Band keratopathy, <u>right</u> eye

H18.422 Band keratopathy, <u>left</u> eye

H18.423 Band keratopathy, <u>bilateral</u>

H18.429 Band keratopathy, <u>unspecified</u> eye

H18.43 Other calcerous corneal degeneration

H18.44- <u>Keratomalacia</u> — Softening of the cornea.
> *Excludes 1:* *keratomalacia due to vitamin A deficiency (E50.4)*

H18.441 Keratomalacia, <u>right</u> eye

H18.442 Keratomalacia, <u>left</u> eye

H18.443 Keratomalacia, <u>bilateral</u>

H18.449 Keratomalacia, <u>unspecified</u> eye

H18.45- <u>Nodular</u> corneal degeneration — Nodular-like hypertrophy of the cornea.

H18.451 Nodular corneal degeneration, <u>right</u> eye

H18.452 Nodular corneal degeneration, <u>left</u> eye

H18.453 Nodular corneal degeneration, <u>bilateral</u>

H18.459 Nodular corneal degeneration, <u>unspecified</u> eye

H18.46- <u>Peripheral</u> corneal degeneration — Deterioration of the edges of the cornea.

H18.461 Peripheral corneal degeneration, <u>right</u> eye

H18.462 Peripheral corneal degeneration, <u>left</u> eye

H18.463 Peripheral corneal degeneration, <u>bilateral</u>

H18.469 Peripheral corneal degeneration, <u>unspecified</u> eye

H18.49 Other corneal degeneration

H18.5- <u>Hereditary corneal dystrophies</u> — An inherited corneal disorder of cellular abnormality.

H18.50 <u>Unspecified</u> hereditary corneal dystrophies

H18.51 Endothelial corneal dystrophy — A form affecting the innermost layer of the cornea.
> Fuchs' dystrophy

H18.52 Epithelial (juvenile) corneal dystrophy — A form affecting the epithelial layer occurring early in life.

H18.53 Granular corneal dystrophy — A form characterized by the presence of small opacities in the superficial layers of the cornea occurring during the first decade of life.

H18.54 Lattice corneal dystrophy — A form affecting the corneal lattice.

H18.55 Macular corneal dystrophy — A form affecting the corneal macula.

H18.59 Other hereditary corneal dystrophies

H18.6- <u>Keratoconus</u> — A conical protrusion of the center of the cornea without inflammation.

H18.60- Keratoconus, <u>unspecified</u>

H18.601 Keratoconus, unspecified, <u>right</u> eye

H18.602 Keratoconus, unspecified, <u>left</u> eye

H18.603 Keratoconus, unspecified, <u>bilateral</u>

H18.609 Keratoconus, unspecified, <u>unspecified</u> eye

H18.61- Keratoconus, <u>stable</u> — A form marked by slow, persistent progression.

H18.611 Keratoconus, stable, <u>right</u> eye

H18.612 Keratoconus, stable, <u>left</u> eye

H18.613 Keratoconus, stable, <u>bilateral</u>

H18.619 Keratoconus, stable, <u>unspecified</u> eye

H18.62- Keratoconus, <u>unstable</u> — A form marked by rapid progression.
> Acute hydrops — A form marked by sudden, severe onset.

H18.621 Keratoconus, unstable, <u>right</u> eye

H18.622 Keratoconus, unstable, <u>left</u> eye

H18.623 Keratoconus, unstable, <u>bilateral</u>

H18.629 Keratoconus, unstable, <u>unspecified</u> eye

H18.7- <u>Other and unspecified corneal deformities</u>
> *Excludes 1:* *congenital malformations of cornea (Q13.3-Q13.4)*

H18.70 Unspecified corneal deformity

H18.71- Corneal <u>ectasia</u> — The protrusion of a thinned, scarred cornea.

H18.711 Corneal ectasia, <u>right</u> eye

H18.712 Corneal ectasia, <u>left</u> eye

H18.713 Corneal ectasia, <u>bilateral</u>

H18.719 Corneal ectasia, <u>unspecified</u> eye

H18.72- Corneal <u>staphyloma</u> — The protrusion of the cornea.

H18.721 Corneal staphyloma, <u>right</u> eye

H18.722 Corneal staphyloma, <u>left</u> eye

H18.723 Corneal staphyloma, <u>bilateral</u>

H18.729 Corneal staphyloma, <u>unspecified</u> eye

H18.73- <u>Descemetocele</u> — Herniation of the Descemet membrane.

H18.731 Descemetocele, <u>right</u> eye

H18.732 Descemetocele, <u>left</u> eye

H18.733 Descemetocele, <u>bilateral</u>

H18.739 Descemetocele, <u>unspecified</u> eye

H18.79- <u>Other</u> corneal deformities

H18.791 Other corneal deformities, <u>right</u> eye

H18.792 Other corneal deformities, <u>left</u> eye

H18.793 Other corneal deformities, <u>bilateral</u>

H18.799 Other corneal deformities, <u>unspecified</u> eye

H18.8- Other specified disorders of cornea

H18.81- <u>Anesthesia and hypoesthesia</u> of cornea — Decreased sensitivity of the cornea.

H18.811 Anesthesia and hypoesthesia of cornea, <u>right</u> eye

H18.812 Anesthesia and hypoesthesia of cornea, <u>left</u> eye

H18.813 Anesthesia and hypoesthesia of cornea, <u>bilateral</u>

H18.819 Anesthesia and hypoesthesia of cornea, <u>unspecified</u> eye

H18.82- Corneal disorder due to contact lens — A form caused by the irritating effects of contact lenses.
> *Excludes ❷:* *corneal edema due to contact lens (H18.21-)*

H18.821 Corneal disorder due to contact lens, <u>right</u> eye

H18.822 Corneal disorder due to contact lens, <u>left</u> eye

H18.823 Corneal disorder due to contact lens, <u>bilateral</u>

H18.829 Corneal disorder due to contact lens, <u>unspecified</u> eye

H18.83- <u>Recurrent erosion</u> of cornea — The failure of the epithelial layer to fuse with the basement mambrane seen in recurring corneal ulcers.

H18.831 Recurrent erosion of cornea, <u>right</u> eye

H18.832 Recurrent erosion of cornea, <u>left</u> eye

H18.833 Recurrent erosion of cornea, <u>bilateral</u>

H18.839 Recurrent erosion of cornea, <u>unspecified</u> eye

H18.89- <u>Other specified</u> disorders of cornea

H18.891 Other specified disorders of cornea, <u>right</u> eye

H18.892 Other specified disorders of cornea, <u>left</u> eye

H18.893 Other specified disorders of cornea, <u>bilateral</u>

H18.899 Other specified disorders of cornea, <u>unspecified</u> eye

H18.9 Unspecified disorder of cornea

H18-H18

Excludes 1: = NOT CODED HERE! (Do not code both)   **686**   *Excludes ❷:* = Not Included Here

H20- **Iridocyclitis** — Inflammation of the iris and the ciliary body.

H20.0- **Acute and subacute** iridocyclitis — A sudden, severe onset of inflammation of the iris and the ciliary body.
> **Acute anterior uveitis** — A sudden, severe onset of inflammation of the iris and ciliary body.
> **Acute cyclitis** — A sudden, severe onset of inflammation of the ciliary body.
> **Acute iritis** — A sudden, severe onset of inflammation of the iris.
> **Subacute anterior uveitis** — A relatively sudden, severe onset of inflammation of the iris and ciliary body.
> **Subacute cyclitis** — A relatively sudden, severe onset of inflammation of the ciliary body.
> **Subacute iritis** — A relatively sudden, severe onset of inflammation of the iris.
> Excludes 1:   iridocyclitis, iritis, uveitis (due to) (in) diabetes mellitus (E08-E13 with .39)
> iridocyclitis, iritis, uveitis (due to) (in) diphtheria (A36.89)
> iridocyclitis, iritis, uveitis (due to) (in) gonococcal (A54.32)
> iridocyclitis, iritis, uveitis (due to) (in) herpes (simplex) (B00.51)
> iridocyclitis, iritis, uveitis (due to) (in) herpes zoster (B02.32)
> iridocyclitis, iritis, uveitis (due to) (in) late congenital syphilis (A50.39)
> iridocyclitis, iritis, uveitis (due to) (in) late syphilis (A52.71)
> iridocyclitis, iritis, uveitis (due to) (in) sarcoidosis (D86.83)
> iridocyclitis, iritis, uveitis (due to) (in) syphilis (A51.43)
> iridocyclitis, iritis, uveitis (due to) (in) toxoplasmosis (B58.09)
> iridocyclitis, iritis, uveitis (due to) (in) tuberculosis (A18.54)

cc **H20.00** **Unspecified** acute and subacute iridocyclitis

H20.01- **Primary** iridocyclitis — A form characterized by the infection originating within the iris and ciliary body.

cc **H20.011** Primary iridocyclitis, **right** eye
cc **H20.012** Primary iridocyclitis, **left** eye
cc **H20.013** Primary iridocyclitis, **bilateral**
cc **H20.019** Primary iridocyclitis, **unspecified** eye

H20.02- **Recurrent acute** iridocyclitis — A form characterized by the return of infection after it has healed.

cc **H20.021** Recurrent acute iridocyclitis, **right** eye
cc **H20.022** Recurrent acute iridocyclitis, **left** eye
cc **H20.023** Recurrent acute iridocyclitis, **bilateral**
cc **H20.029** Recurrent acute iridocyclitis, **unspecified** eye

H20.03- **Secondary infectious** iridocyclitis — A form characterized by the infection spreading from other ocular or periocular tissues.

cc **H20.031** Secondary infectious iridocyclitis, **right** eye
cc **H20.032** Secondary infectious iridocyclitis, **left** eye
cc **H20.033** Secondary infectious iridocyclitis, **bilateral**
cc **H20.039** Secondary infectious iridocyclitis, **unspecified** eye

H20.04- **Secondary noninfectious iridocyclitis** — A form characterized by an inflammatory reaction from other ocular or periocular infections.

H20.041 Secondary noninfectious iridocyclitis, **right** eye
H20.042 Secondary noninfectious iridocyclitis, **left** eye
H20.043 Secondary noninfectious iridocyclitis, **bilateral**
H20.049 Secondary noninfectious iridocyclitis, **unspecified** eye

H20.05- **Hypopyon** — An abnormal accumulation of pus in the anterior chamber of the eye.

H20.051 Hypopyon, **right** eye
H20.052 Hypopyon, **left** eye
H20.053 Hypopyon, **bilateral**
H20.059 Hypopyon, **unspecified** eye

H20.1- **Chronic** iridocyclitis — Inflammation of the iris and ciliary body which develops slowly and persists over a long period of time.
> Use additional code for any associated cataract (H26.21-)
> Excludes ❷: posterior cyclitis (H30.2-)

H20.10 Chronic iridocyclitis, **unspecified** eye
H20.11 Chronic iridocyclitis, **right** eye
H20.12 Chronic iridocyclitis, **left** eye

H20.13 Chronic iridocyclitis, **bilateral**

H20.2- **Lens-induced** iridocyclitis — A form characterized by secondary inflammatory reactions due to disorders of the lens.

H20.20 Lens-induced iridocyclitis, **unspecified** eye
H20.21 Lens-induced iridocyclitis, **right** eye
H20.22 Lens-induced iridocyclitis, **left** eye
H20.23 Lens-induced iridocyclitis, **bilateral**

H20.8- **Other iridocyclitis**
> Excludes ❷: glaucomatocyclitis crises (H40.4-)
> posterior cyclitis (H30.2-)
> sympathetic uveitis (H44.13-)

H20.81- **Fuchs' heterochromic** cyclitis — A form characterized by lightening of the iris color and a few keratic deposits on the cornea.

H20.811 Fuchs' heterochromic cyclitis, **right** eye
H20.812 Fuchs' heterochromic cyclitis, **left** eye
H20.813 Fuchs' heterochromic cyclitis, **bilateral**
H20.819 Fuchs' heterochromic cyclitis, **unspecified** eye

H20.82- **Vogt-Koyanagi syndrome** — A syndrome characterized by chronic iridocyclitis, exudative choroiditis, and patchy depigmentation of the skin and hair.

H20.821 Vogt-Koyanagi syndrome, **right** eye
H20.822 Vogt-Koyanagi syndrome, **left** eye
H20.823 Vogt-Koyanagi syndrome, **bilateral**
H20.829 Vogt-Koyanagi syndrome, **unspecified** eye

cc **H20.9** **Unspecified iridocyclitis**
> Uveitis NOS

H21- **Other disorders of iris and ciliary body**
> Excludes ❷: sympathetic uveitis (H44.1-)

H21.0- **Hyphema** — Hemorrhage within the anterior chamber of the eye.
> Excludes 1:   traumatic hyphema (S05.1-)

H21.00 Hyphema, **unspecified** eye
H21.01 Hyphema, **right** eye
H21.02 Hyphema, **left** eye
H21.03 Hyphema, **bilateral**

H21.1- **Other vascular disorders** of iris and ciliary body
> **Neovascularization of iris or ciliary body** — The formation of new abnormal blood vessels of the iris and ciliary body.
> **Rubeosis iridis** — An abnormal condition characterized by the new formation of vessels and connective tissue on the surface of the iris.
> **Rubeosis of iris**

H21.1x- **Other vascular disorders** of iris and ciliary body

H21.1x1 Other vascular disorders of iris and ciliary body, **right** eye
H21.1x2 Other vascular disorders of iris and ciliary body, **left** eye
H21.1x3 Other vascular disorders of iris and ciliary body, **bilateral**
H21.1x9 Other vascular disorders of iris and ciliary body, **unspecified** eye

H21.2- **Degeneration of iris and ciliary body** — Deteriorations of the iris and ciliary body.

H21.21- **Degeneration of chamber angle** — Loss of the normal ciliary body chamber angle.

H21.211 Degeneration of chamber angle, **right** eye
H21.212 Degeneration of chamber angle, **left** eye
H21.213 Degeneration of chamber angle, **bilateral**
H21.219 Degeneration of chamber angle, **unspecified** eye

H21.22- **Degeneration of ciliary body** — Deterioration of the ciliary body tissues.

H21.221 Degeneration of ciliary body, **right** eye
H21.222 Degeneration of ciliary body, **left** eye
H21.223 Degeneration of ciliary body, **bilateral**
H21.229 Degeneration of ciliary body, **unspecified** eye

H21.23- **Degeneration of iris (pigmentary)** — Abnormal deterioration of the iris pigment.
> **Translucency of iris** — A form marked by enough loss of pigment to allow light to pass through.

H21.231 Degeneration of iris (pigmentary), **right** eye
H21.232 Degeneration of iris (pigmentary), **left** eye

Excludes 1: = NOT CODED HERE! (Do not code both)   **687**   *Excludes ❷:* = Not Included Here

H21.233   Degeneration of iris (pigmentary), <u>bilateral</u>
H21.239   Degeneration of iris (pigmentary), <u>unspecified</u> eye

H21.24-   <u>Degeneration of pupillary margin</u> — Deterioration of the inner edge of the iris, surrounding the pupil.

H21.241   Degeneration of pupillary margin, <u>right</u> eye
H21.242   Degeneration of pupillary margin, <u>left</u> eye
H21.243   Degeneration of pupillary margin, <u>bilateral</u>
H21.249   Degeneration of pupillary margin, <u>unspecified</u> eye

H21.25-   <u>Iridoschisis</u> — Splitting of the iris into two layers.

H21.251   Iridoschisis, <u>right</u> eye
H21.252   Iridoschisis, <u>left</u> eye
H21.253   Iridoschisis, <u>bilateral</u>
H21.259   Iridoschisis, <u>unspecified</u> eye

H21.26-   <u>Iris atrophy</u> (essential) (progressive) — The wasting-away of the iris.

H21.261   Iris atrophy (essential) (progressive), <u>right</u> eye
H21.262   Iris atrophy (essential) (progressive), <u>left</u> eye
H21.263   Iris atrophy (essential) (progressive), <u>bilateral</u>
H21.269   Iris atrophy (essential) (progressive), <u>unspecified</u> eye

H21.27-   <u>Miotic pupillary cyst</u> — Serous filled sacs upon the pupillary margin of the iris.

H21.271   Miotic pupillary cyst, <u>right</u> eye
H21.272   Miotic pupillary cyst, <u>left</u> eye
H21.273   Miotic pupillary cyst, <u>bilateral</u>
H21.279   Miotic pupillary cyst, <u>unspecified</u> eye

H21.29   Other iris atrophy

H21.3-   <u>Cyst of iris, ciliary body and anterior chamber</u> — Encapsulated, fluid-filled sacs of the iris, ciliary body, and anterior chamber.

Excludes ❷: *miotic pupillary cyst (H21.27-)*

H21.30-   <u>Idiopathic</u> cysts of iris, ciliary body or anterior chamber — A form characterized by unknown etiology.
   Cyst of iris, ciliary body or anterior chamber NOS

H21.301   Idiopathic cysts of iris, ciliary body or anterior chamber, <u>right</u> eye
H21.302   Idiopathic cysts of iris, ciliary body or anterior chamber, <u>left</u> eye
H21.303   Idiopathic cysts of iris, ciliary body or anterior chamber, <u>bilateral</u>
H21.309   Idiopathic cysts of iris, ciliary body or anterior chamber, <u>unspecified</u> eye

H21.31-   <u>Exudative</u> cysts of iris or anterior chamber — A form characterized by cellular debris within the cysts.

H21.311   Exudative cysts of iris or anterior chamber, <u>right</u> eye
H21.312   Exudative cysts of iris or anterior chamber, <u>left</u> eye
H21.313   Exudative cysts of iris or anterior chamber, <u>bilateral</u>
H21.319   Exudative cysts of iris or anterior chamber, <u>unspecified</u> eye

H21.32-   <u>Implantation</u> cysts of iris, ciliary body or anterior chamber — A form characterized by down-growth of epithelium.

H21.321   Implantation cysts of iris, ciliary body or anterior chamber, <u>right</u> eye
H21.322   Implantation cysts of iris, ciliary body or anterior chamber, <u>left</u> eye
H21.323   Implantation cysts of iris, ciliary body or anterior chamber, <u>bilateral</u>
H21.329   Implantation cysts of iris, ciliary body or anterior chamber, <u>unspecified</u> eye

H21.33-   <u>Parasitic</u> cyst of iris, ciliary body or anterior chamber — A form characterized by infestation by a parasite.

cc H21.331   Parasitic cyst of iris, ciliary body or anterior chamber, <u>right</u> eye
cc H21.332   Parasitic cyst of iris, ciliary body or anterior chamber, <u>left</u> eye
cc H21.333   Parasitic cyst of iris, ciliary body or anterior chamber, <u>bilateral</u>

cc H21.339   Parasitic cyst of iris, ciliary body or anterior chamber, <u>unspecified</u> eye

H21.34-   <u>Primary cyst of pars plana</u> — A form characterized by development associated with ciliary body disorder of the ciliary ring.

H21.341   Primary cyst of pars plana, <u>right</u> eye
H21.342   Primary cyst of pars plana, <u>left</u> eye
H21.343   Primary cyst of pars plana, <u>bilateral</u>
H21.349   Primary cyst of pars plana, <u>unspecified</u> eye

H21.35-   <u>Exudative cyst of pars plana</u> — A form characterized by cellular debris within the cysts of the ciliary ring.

H21.351   Exudative cyst of pars plana, <u>right</u> eye
H21.352   Exudative cyst of pars plana, <u>left</u> eye
H21.353   Exudative cyst of pars plana, <u>bilateral</u>
H21.359   Exudative cyst of pars plana, <u>unspecified</u> eye

H21.4-   <u>Pupillary membranes</u> — Abnormal pupillary membrane formation.
   Iris bombé — The condition in which the iris is bowed forward with aqueous humor behind it.
   Pupillary occlusion — Complete closure of the pupillary opening.
   Pupillary seclusion — Complete covering of the iris and pupillary opening by the formation of a membrane.

Excludes 1:   *congenital pupillary membranes (Q13.8)*

H21.40   Pupillary membranes, <u>unspecified</u> eye
H21.41   Pupillary membranes, <u>right</u> eye
H21.42   Pupillary membranes, <u>left</u> eye
H21.43   Pupillary membranes, <u>bilateral</u>

H21.5-   Other and unspecified adhesions and disruptions of iris and ciliary body

Excludes 1:   *corectopia (Q13.2)*

H21.50-   <u>Unspecified adhesions of iris</u>
   Synechia (iris) NOS

H21.501   Unspecified adhesions of iris, <u>right</u> eye
H21.502   Unspecified adhesions of iris, <u>left</u> eye
H21.503   Unspecified adhesions of iris, <u>bilateral</u>
H21.509   Unspecified adhesions of iris and ciliary body, <u>unspecified</u> eye

H21.51-   <u>Anterior synechiae (iris)</u> — Adherence of the iris to the cornea.

H21.511   Anterior synechiae (iris), <u>right</u> eye
H21.512   Anterior synechiae (iris), <u>left</u> eye
H21.513   Anterior synechiae (iris), <u>bilateral</u>
H21.519   Anterior synechiae (iris), <u>unspecified</u> eye

H21.52-   <u>Goniosynechiae</u> — Adherence of the iris to the cornea at the angle of the anterior chamber.

H21.521   Goniosynechiae, <u>right</u> eye
H21.522   Goniosynechiae, <u>left</u> eye
H21.523   Goniosynechiae, <u>bilateral</u>
H21.529   Goniosynechiae, <u>unspecified</u> eye

H21.53-   <u>Iridodialysis</u> — The separation or loosening of the iris from its attachment.

H21.531   Iridodialysis, <u>right</u> eye
H21.532   Iridodialysis, <u>left</u> eye
H21.533   Iridodialysis, <u>bilateral</u>
H21.539   Iridodialysis, <u>unspecified</u> eye

H21.54-   <u>Posterior synechiae (iris)</u> — Adherence of the iris to the lens.

H21.541   Posterior synechiae (iris), <u>right</u> eye
H21.542   Posterior synechiae (iris), <u>left</u> eye
H21.543   Posterior synechiae (iris), <u>bilateral</u>
H21.549   Posterior synechiae (iris), <u>unspecified</u> eye

H21.55-   <u>Recession of chamber angle</u> — The drawing-back of the angle of the anterior chamber.

H21.551   Recession of chamber angle, <u>right</u> eye
H21.552   Recession of chamber angle, <u>left</u> eye
H21.553   Recession of chamber angle, <u>bilateral</u>
H21.559   Recession of chamber angle, <u>unspecified</u> eye

H21 - H21

Excludes 1: = NOT CODED HERE! (Do not code both)

Excludes ❷: = Not Included Here

© 2016 Channel Publishing, Ltd

H21.56- Pupillary abnormalities
Deformed pupil — A physically impaired pupil.
Ectopic pupil — Displacement of the pupil.
Rupture of sphincter, pupil — The forcible tearing of the pupil.
Excludes 1: congenital deformity of pupil (Q13.2-)
H21.561 Pupillary abnormality, right eye
H21.562 Pupillary abnormality, left eye
H21.563 Pupillary abnormality, bilateral
H21.569 Pupillary abnormality, unspecified eye
H21.8- Other specified disorders of iris and ciliary body
H21.81 Floppy iris syndrome — A potentially complicating condition, usually caused by a history of taking alpha-blockers, in which the iris does not stay properly dilated during cataract surgery.
Intraoperative floppy iris syndrome (IFIS)
Use additional code for adverse effect, if applicable, to identify drug (T36-T50 with fifth or sixth character 5)
H21.82 Plateau iris syndrome (post-iridectomy) (postprocedural) — The abnormal anatomical condition of angle crowding that may lead to acute angle-closure glaucoma.
H21.89 Other specified disorders of iris and ciliary body
H21.9 Unspecified disorder of iris and ciliary body
H22 Disorders of iris and ciliary body in diseases classified elsewhere — [Not Allowed as PDX]
Code first underlying disease, such as:
Gout (M1A.-, M10.-)
Leprosy (A30.-)
Parasitic disease (B89)

Disorders of lens (H25-H28)

H25- Age-related cataract — The opacity (inability to pass light through) of the crystalline lens of the eye with onset later in life.
AHA 16:1Q:p32 – Bilateral cataracts with separate surgical encounters
Senile cataract
Excludes ❷: capsular glaucoma with pseudoexfoliation of lens (H40.1-)
H25.0- Age-related incipient cataract — A form characterized by localized areas of opacity.
H25.01- Cortical age-related cataract — A form characterized by the opacity situated in the cortical layers of the lens.
H25.011 Cortical age-related cataract, right eye — [Age/15-124]
H25.012 Cortical age-related cataract, left eye — [Age/15-124]
H25.013 Cortical age-related cataract, bilateral — [Age/15-124]
H25.019 Cortical age-related cataract, unspecified eye — [Age/15-124]
H25.03- Anterior subcapsular polar age-related cataract — A form characterized by the opacity situated beneath the front, center portion of the capsule of the lens.
H25.031 Anterior subcapsular polar age-related cataract, right eye — [Age/15-124]
H25.032 Anterior subcapsular polar age-related cataract, left eye — [Age/15-124]
H25.033 Anterior subcapsular polar age-related cataract, bilateral — [Age/15-124]
H25.039 Anterior subcapsular polar age-related cataract, unspecified eye — [Age/15-124]
H25.04- Posterior subcapsular polar age-related cataract — A form characterized by the opacity situated beneath the back, center portion of the capsule of the lens.
H25.041 Posterior subcapsular polar age-related cataract, right eye — [Age/15-124]
H25.042 Posterior subcapsular polar age-related cataract, left eye — [Age/15-124]
H25.043 Posterior subcapsular polar age-related cataract, bilateral — [Age/15-124]
H25.049 Posterior subcapsular polar age-related cataract, unspecified eye — [Age/15-124]

H25.09- Other age-related incipient cataract
Coronary age-related cataract — A form marked by club-like opacities, with clear edges and center.
Punctate age-related cataract — A form marked by dot-like opacities.
Water clefts
H25.091 Other age-related incipient cataract, right eye — [Age/15-124]
H25.092 Other age-related incipient cataract, left eye — [Age/15-124]
H25.093 Other age-related incipient cataract, bilateral — [Age/15-124]
H25.099 Other age-related incipient cataract, unspecified eye — [Age/15-124]
H25.1- Age-related nuclear cataract — A form characterized by hardening opacity of the center of the lens.
Cataracta brunescens — A form marked by brown discoloration.
Nuclear sclerosis cataract — A form characterized by hardening opacity of the center of the lens.
H25.10 Age-related nuclear cataract, unspecified eye — [Age/15-124]
H25.11 Age-related nuclear cataract, right eye — [Age/15-124]
H25.12 Age-related nuclear cataract, left eye — [Age/15-124]
H25.13 Age-related nuclear cataract, bilateral — [Age/15-124]
H25.2- Age-related cataract, morgagnian type — A form characterized by a shrunken, soft, wrinkled, opaque lens.
Age-related hypermature cataract
H25.20 Age-related cataract, morgagnian type, unspecified eye — [Age/15-124]
H25.21 Age-related cataract, morgagnian type, right eye — [Age/15-124]
H25.22 Age-related cataract, morgagnian type, left eye — [Age/15-124]
H25.23 Age-related cataract, morgagnian type, bilateral — [Age/15-124]
H25.8- Other age-related cataract
H25.81- Combined forms of age-related cataract
H25.811 Combined forms of age-related cataract, right eye — [Age/15-124]
H25.812 Combined forms of age-related cataract, left eye — [Age/15-124]
H25.813 Combined forms of age-related cataract, bilateral — [Age/15-124]
H25.819 Combined forms of age-related cataract, unspecified eye — [Age/15-124]
H25.89 Other age-related cataract — [Age/15-124]
H25.9 Unspecified age-related cataract — [Age/15-124]
H26- Other cataract
Excludes 1: congenital cataract (Q12.0)
H26.0- Infantile and juvenile cataract — The opacity (inability to pass light through) of the crystalline lens of the eye characterized by onset early in life.
H26.00- Unspecified infantile and juvenile cataract
H26.001 Unspecified infantile and juvenile cataract, right eye — [Age/0-17]
H26.002 Unspecified infantile and juvenile cataract, left eye — [Age/0-17]
H26.003 Unspecified infantile and juvenile cataract, bilateral — [Age/0-17]
H26.009 Unspecified infantile and juvenile cataract, unspecified eye — [Age/0-17]
H26.01- Infantile and juvenile cortical, lamellar, or zonular cataract — A form characterized by the opacity affecting only the middle layers of the lens.
H26.011 Infantile and juvenile cortical, lamellar, or zonular cataract, right eye — [Age/0-17]
H26.012 Infantile and juvenile cortical, lamellar, or zonular cataract, left eye — [Age/0-17]
H26.013 Infantile and juvenile cortical, lamellar, or zonular cataract, bilateral — [Age/0-17]

H21-H26

Excludes 1: = NOT CODED HERE! (Do not code both)   689   *Excludes ❷:* = Not Included Here

© 2016 Channel Publishing, Ltd.

H26.019   **Infantile and juvenile cortical, lamellar, or zonular cataract, <u>unspecified</u> eye** — [Age/0-17]

H26.03-   **Infantile and juvenile <u>nuclear</u> cataract** — A form characterized by the opacity affecting the center of the lens.

    H26.031   **Infantile and juvenile nuclear cataract, <u>right</u> eye** — [Age/0-17]

    H26.032   **Infantile and juvenile nuclear cataract, <u>left</u> eye** — [Age/0-17]

    H26.033   **Infantile and juvenile nuclear cataract, <u>bilateral</u>** — [Age/0-17]

    H26.039   **Infantile and juvenile nuclear cataract, <u>unspecified</u> eye** — [Age/0-17]

H26.04-   **<u>Anterior</u> subcapsular polar infantile and juvenile cataract** — A form characterized by the opacity situated beneath the front, center portion of the capsule of the lens.

    H26.041   **Anterior subcapsular polar infantile and juvenile cataract, <u>right</u> eye** — [Age/0-17]

    H26.042   **Anterior subcapsular polar infantile and juvenile cataract, <u>left</u> eye** — [Age/0-17]

    H26.043   **Anterior subcapsular polar infantile and juvenile cataract, <u>bilateral</u>** — [Age/0-17]

    H26.049   **Anterior subcapsular polar infantile and juvenile cataract, <u>unspecified</u> eye** — [Age/0-17]

H26.05-   **<u>Posterior</u> subcapsular polar infantile and juvenile cataract** — A form characterized by the opacity situated beneath the back, center portion of the capsule of the lens.

    H26.051   **Posterior subcapsular polar infantile and juvenile cataract, <u>right</u> eye** — [Age/0-17]

    H26.052   **Posterior subcapsular polar infantile and juvenile cataract, <u>left</u> eye** — [Age/0-17]

    H26.053   **Posterior subcapsular polar infantile and juvenile cataract, <u>bilateral</u>** — [Age/0-17]

    H26.059   **Posterior subcapsular polar infantile and juvenile cataract, <u>unspecified</u> eye** — [Age/0-17]

H26.06-   **<u>Combined</u> forms of infantile and juvenile cataract**

    H26.061   **Combined forms of infantile and juvenile cataract, <u>right</u> eye** — [Age/0-17]

    H26.062   **Combined forms of infantile and juvenile cataract, <u>left</u> eye** — [Age/0-17]

    H26.063   **Combined forms of infantile and juvenile cataract, <u>bilateral</u>** — [Age/0-17]

    H26.069   **Combined forms of infantile and juvenile cataract, <u>unspecified</u> eye** — [Age/0-17]

H26.09   **Other infantile and juvenile cataract** — [Age/0-17]

H26.1-   **<u>Traumatic</u> cataract** — The opacity (inability to pass light through) of the crystalline lens of the eye due to an external injury.

    Use additional code (Chapter 20) to identify external cause

H26.10-   **<u>Unspecified</u> traumatic cataract**

    H26.101   **Unspecified traumatic cataract, <u>right</u> eye**

    H26.102   **Unspecified traumatic cataract, <u>left</u> eye**

    H26.103   **Unspecified traumatic cataract, <u>bilateral</u>**

    H26.109   **Unspecified traumatic cataract, <u>unspecified</u> eye**

H26.11-   **<u>Localized</u> traumatic opacities** — A form characterized by opacities appearing in small circumscribed areas.

    H26.111   **Localized traumatic opacities, <u>right</u> eye**

    H26.112   **Localized traumatic opacities, <u>left</u> eye**

    H26.113   **Localized traumatic opacities, <u>bilateral</u>**

    H26.119   **Localized traumatic opacities, <u>unspecified</u> eye**

H26.12-   **<u>Partially resolved</u> traumatic cataract** — A form characterized by partial clearing of the opacity.

    H26.121   **Partially resolved traumatic cataract, <u>right</u> eye**

    H26.122   **Partially resolved traumatic cataract, <u>left</u> eye**

    H26.123   **Partially resolved traumatic cataract, <u>bilateral</u>**

    H26.129   **Partially resolved traumatic cataract, <u>unspecified</u> eye**

H26.13-   **<u>Total</u> traumatic cataract** — A form characterized by complete opacity.

    H26.131   **Total traumatic cataract, <u>right</u> eye**

    H26.132   **Total traumatic cataract, <u>left</u> eye**

    H26.133   **Total traumatic cataract, <u>bilateral</u>**

    H26.139   **Total traumatic cataract, <u>unspecified</u> eye**

H26.2-   **<u>Complicated</u> cataract**

H26.20   **<u>Unspecified</u> complicated cataract**

    Cataracta complicata NOS

H26.21-   **Cataract <u>with neovascularization</u>** — A form characterized by the formation of new abnormal blood vessels.

    Code also associated condition, such as:

    Chronic iridocyclitis (H20.1-)

    H26.211   **Cataract with neovascularization, <u>right</u> eye**

    H26.212   **Cataract with neovascularization, <u>left</u> eye**

    H26.213   **Cataract with neovascularization, <u>bilateral</u>**

    H26.219   **Cataract with neovascularization, <u>unspecified</u> eye**

H26.22-   **Cataract <u>secondary to ocular disorders</u> (degenerative) (inflammatory)** — The opacity (inability to pass light through) of the crystalline lens of the eye due to ocular disorders and diseases.

    Code also associated ocular disorder

    H26.221   **Cataract secondary to ocular disorders (degenerative) (inflammatory), <u>right</u> eye**

    H26.222   **Cataract secondary to ocular disorders (degenerative) (inflammatory), <u>left</u> eye**

    H26.223   **Cataract secondary to ocular disorders (degenerative) (inflammatory), <u>bilateral</u>**

    H26.229   **Cataract secondary to ocular disorders (degenerative) (inflammatory), <u>unspecified</u> eye**

H26.23-   **<u>Glaucomatous flecks</u> (subcapsular)**

    Code first underlying glaucoma (H40-H42)

    H26.231   **Glaucomatous flecks (subcapsular), <u>right</u> eye**

    H26.232   **Glaucomatous flecks (subcapsular), <u>left</u> eye**

    H26.233   **Glaucomatous flecks (subcapsular), <u>bilateral</u>**

    H26.239   **Glaucomatous flecks (subcapsular), <u>unspecified</u> eye**

H26.3-   **<u>Drug-induced</u> cataract**

    Toxic cataract

    Use additional code for adverse effect, if applicable, to identify drug (T36-T50 with fifth or sixth character 5)

H26.30   **Drug-induced cataract, <u>unspecified</u> eye**

H26.31   **Drug-induced cataract, <u>right</u> eye**

H26.32   **Drug-induced cataract, <u>left</u> eye**

H26.33   **Drug-induced cataract, <u>bilateral</u>**

H26.4-   **<u>Secondary</u> cataract**

H26.40   **<u>Unspecified</u> secondary cataract**

H26.41-   **<u>Soemmering's ring</u>** — A recurrent doughnut-shaped opacity occurring after cataract surgery.

    H26.411   **Soemmering's ring, <u>right</u> eye**

    H26.412   **Soemmering's ring, <u>left</u> eye**

    H26.413   **Soemmering's ring, <u>bilateral</u>**

    H26.419   **Soemmering's ring, <u>unspecified</u> eye**

H26.49-   **<u>Other</u> secondary cataract**

    H26.491   **Other secondary cataract, <u>right</u> eye**

    H26.492   **Other secondary cataract, <u>left</u> eye**

    H26.493   **Other secondary cataract, <u>bilateral</u>**

    H26.499   **Other secondary cataract, <u>unspecified</u> eye**

H26.8   **Other specified cataract**

H26.9   **Unspecified cataract**

H27-   **Other disorders of lens**

    Excludes 1:   *congenital lens malformations (Q12.-)*
            mechanical complications of intraocular lens implant (T85.2)
            pseudophakia (Z96.1)

H27.0-   **<u>Aphakia</u>** — Absence of the crystalline lens of the eye.

    Acquired absence of lens

    Acquired aphakia

    Aphakia due to trauma

    Excludes 1:   *cataract extraction status (Z98.4-)*
            congenital absence of lens (Q12.3)
            congenital aphakia (Q12.3)

H27.00   **Aphakia, <u>unspecified</u> eye**

H27.01   **Aphakia, <u>right</u> eye**

H27.02   **Aphakia, <u>left</u> eye**

H27.03   **Aphakia, <u>bilateral</u>**

H26 - H27 (side tab)

H27.1- <u>Dislocation of lens</u> — Dislocation of the crystalline lens of the eye.

  H27.10 <u>Unspecified</u> dislocation of lens

  H27.11- <u>Subluxation</u> of lens — Partial dislocation of the crystalline lens of the eye.

    H27.111 Subluxation of lens, <u>right</u> eye

    H27.112 Subluxation of lens, <u>left</u> eye

    H27.113 Subluxation of lens, <u>bilateral</u>

    H27.119 Subluxation of lens, <u>unspecified</u> eye

  H27.12- <u>Anterior</u> dislocation of lens — The movement forward of the crystalline lens of the eye from its normal position.

    H27.121 Anterior dislocation of lens, <u>right</u> eye

    H27.122 Anterior dislocation of lens, <u>left</u> eye

    H27.123 Anterior dislocation of lens, <u>bilateral</u>

    H27.129 Anterior dislocation of lens, <u>unspecified</u> eye

  H27.13- <u>Posterior</u> dislocation of lens — The movement backward of the crystalline lens of the eye from its normal position.

    H27.131 Posterior dislocation of lens, <u>right</u> eye

    H27.132 Posterior dislocation of lens, <u>left</u> eye

    H27.133 Posterior dislocation of lens, <u>bilateral</u>

    H27.139 Posterior dislocation of lens, <u>unspecified</u> eye

H27.8 Other specified disorders of lens

H27.9 Unspecified disorder of lens

H28 Cataract <u>in diseases classified elsewhere</u> — [Not Allowed as PDX]
Code first underlying disease, such as:
Hypoparathyroidism (E20.-)
Myotonia (G71.1-)
Myxedema (E03.-)
Protein-calorie malnutrition (E40-E46)
  Excludes 1: cataract in diabetes mellitus (E08.36, E09.36, E10.36, E11.36, E13.36)

Disorders of choroid and retina (H30-H36)

H30- <u>Chorioretinal inflammation</u> — Inflammation of the retina and/or choroid.

  H30.0- <u>Focal</u> chorioretinal inflammation — Inflammation of the central retina and/or choroid.
Focal chorioretinitis
Focal choroiditis
Focal retinitis
Focal retinochoroiditis

  H30.00- <u>Unspecified</u> focal chorioretinal inflammation
Focal chorioretinitis NOS
Focal choroiditis NOS
Focal retinitis NOS
Focal retinochoroiditis NOS

    H30.001 Unspecified focal chorioretinal inflammation, <u>right</u> eye

    H30.002 Unspecified focal chorioretinal inflammation, <u>left</u> eye

    H30.003 Unspecified focal chorioretinal inflammation, <u>bilateral</u>

    H30.009 Unspecified focal chorioretinal inflammation, <u>unspecified</u> eye

  H30.01- Focal chorioretinal inflammation, <u>juxtapapillary</u>

    H30.011 Focal chorioretinal inflammation, juxtapapillary, <u>right</u> eye

    H30.012 Focal chorioretinal inflammation, juxtapapillary, <u>left</u> eye

    H30.013 Focal chorioretinal inflammation, juxtapapillary, <u>bilateral</u>

    H30.019 Focal chorioretinal inflammation, juxtapapillary, <u>unspecified</u> eye

  H30.02- Focal chorioretinal inflammation of <u>posterior pole</u>

    H30.021 Focal chorioretinal inflammation of posterior pole, <u>right</u> eye

    H30.022 Focal chorioretinal inflammation of posterior pole, <u>left</u> eye

    H30.023 Focal chorioretinal inflammation of posterior pole, <u>bilateral</u>

    H30.029 Focal chorioretinal inflammation of posterior pole, <u>unspecified</u> eye

H30.03- Focal chorioretinal inflammation, <u>peripheral</u>

  H30.031 Focal chorioretinal inflammation, peripheral, <u>right</u> eye

  H30.032 Focal chorioretinal inflammation, peripheral, <u>left</u> eye

  H30.033 Focal chorioretinal inflammation, peripheral, <u>bilateral</u>

  H30.039 Focal chorioretinal inflammation, peripheral, <u>unspecified</u> eye

H30.04- Focal chorioretinal inflammation, <u>macular or paramacular</u>

  H30.041 Focal chorioretinal inflammation, macular or paramacular, <u>right</u> eye

  H30.042 Focal chorioretinal inflammation, macular or paramacular, <u>left</u> eye

  H30.043 Focal chorioretinal inflammation, macular or paramacular, <u>bilateral</u>

  H30.049 Focal chorioretinal inflammation, macular or paramacular, <u>unspecified</u> eye

H30.1- <u>Disseminated</u> chorioretinal inflammation — Inflammation of multiple sites throughout the retina and choroid.
Disseminated chorioretinitis
Disseminated choroiditis
Disseminated retinitis
Disseminated retinochoroiditis
Excludes ❷: exudative retinopathy (H35.02-)

H30.10- <u>Unspecified</u> disseminated chorioretinal inflammation
Disseminated chorioretinitis NOS
Disseminated choroiditis NOS
Disseminated retinitis NOS
Disseminated retinochoroiditis NOS

  cc **H30.101** Unspecified disseminated chorioretinal inflammation, <u>right</u> eye

  cc **H30.102** Unspecified disseminated chorioretinal inflammation, <u>left</u> eye

  cc **H30.103** Unspecified disseminated chorioretinal inflammation, <u>bilateral</u>

  cc **H30.109** Unspecified disseminated chorioretinal inflammation, <u>unspecified</u> eye

H30.11- Disseminated chorioretinal inflammation of <u>posterior pole</u>

  cc **H30.111** Disseminated chorioretinal inflammation of posterior pole, <u>right</u> eye

  cc **H30.112** Disseminated chorioretinal inflammation of posterior pole, <u>left</u> eye

  cc **H30.113** Disseminated chorioretinal inflammation of posterior pole, <u>bilateral</u>

  cc **H30.119** Disseminated chorioretinal inflammation of posterior pole, <u>unspecified</u> eye

H30.12- Disseminated chorioretinal inflammation, <u>peripheral</u>

  cc **H30.121** Disseminated chorioretinal inflammation, peripheral <u>right</u> eye

  cc **H30.122** Disseminated chorioretinal inflammation, peripheral, <u>left</u> eye

  cc **H30.123** Disseminated chorioretinal inflammation, peripheral, <u>bilateral</u>

  cc **H30.129** Disseminated chorioretinal inflammation, peripheral, <u>unspecified</u> eye

H30.13- Disseminated chorioretinal inflammation, <u>generalized</u>

  cc **H30.131** Disseminated chorioretinal inflammation, generalized, <u>right</u> eye

  cc **H30.132** Disseminated chorioretinal inflammation, generalized, <u>left</u> eye

  cc **H30.133** Disseminated chorioretinal inflammation, generalized, <u>bilateral</u>

  cc **H30.139** Disseminated chorioretinal inflammation, generalized, <u>unspecified</u> eye

H30.14- <u>Acute posterior multifocal placoid pigment epitheliopathy</u>

  cc **H30.141** Acute posterior multifocal placoid pigment epitheliopathy, <u>right</u> eye

H27 - H30

cc H30.142   Acute posterior multifocal placoid pigment epitheliopathy, <u>left</u> eye

cc H30.143   Acute posterior multifocal placoid pigment epitheliopathy, <u>bilateral</u>

cc H30.149   Acute posterior multifocal placoid pigment epitheliopathy, <u>unspecified</u> eye

H30.2-   <u>Posterior cyclitis</u> — Specific inflammation of the peripheral retina characterized by "snowbanks" of inflammatory cells.
   Pars planitis

H30.20   Posterior cyclitis, <u>unspecified</u> eye

H30.21   Posterior cyclitis, <u>right</u> eye

H30.22   Posterior cyclitis, <u>left</u> eye

H30.23   Posterior cyclitis, <u>bilateral</u>

H30.8-   <u>Other</u> chorioretinal inflammations

H30.81-   <u>Harada's disease</u> — Inflammation of the choroid and retina associated with uveomeningitis.

H30.811   Harada's disease, <u>right</u> eye

H30.812   Harada's disease, <u>left</u> eye

H30.813   Harada's disease, <u>bilateral</u>

H30.819   Harada's disease, <u>unspecified</u> eye

H30.89-   <u>Other</u> chorioretinal inflammations

cc H30.891   Other chorioretinal inflammations, <u>right</u> eye

cc H30.892   Other chorioretinal inflammations, <u>left</u> eye

cc H30.893   Other chorioretinal inflammations, <u>bilateral</u>

cc H30.899   Other chorioretinal inflammations, <u>unspecified</u> eye

H30.9-   <u>Unspecified</u> chorioretinal inflammation
   Chorioretinitis NOS
   Choroiditis NOS
   Neuroretinitis NOS
   Retinitis NOS
   Retinochoroiditis NOS

cc H30.90   Unspecified chorioretinal inflammation, <u>unspecified</u> eye

cc H30.91   Unspecified chorioretinal inflammation, <u>right</u> eye

cc H30.92   Unspecified chorioretinal inflammation, <u>left</u> eye

cc H30.93   Unspecified chorioretinal inflammation, <u>bilateral</u>

H31-   <u>Other disorders of choroid</u>

H31.0-   <u>Chorioretinal scars</u> — Dense, wound-healing tissue of the choroid and retina.
   Excludes ❷: postsurgical chorioretinal scars (H59.81-)

H31.00-   <u>Unspecified</u> chorioretinal scars

H31.001   Unspecified chorioretinal scars, <u>right</u> eye

H31.002   Unspecified chorioretinal scars, <u>left</u> eye

H31.003   Unspecified chorioretinal scars, <u>bilateral</u>

H31.009   Unspecified chorioretinal scars, <u>unspecified</u> eye

H31.01-   <u>Macula scars</u> of posterior pole (postinflammatory) (post-traumatic) — A form affecting the macula.
   Excludes 1:   postprocedural chorioretinal scar (H59.81-)

H31.011   Macula scars of posterior pole (postinflammatory) (post-traumatic), <u>right</u> eye

H31.012   Macula scars of posterior pole (postinflammatory) (post-traumatic), <u>left</u> eye

H31.013   Macula scars of posterior pole (postinflammatory) (post-traumatic), <u>bilateral</u>

H31.019   Macula scars of posterior pole (postinflammatory) (post-traumatic), <u>unspecified</u> eye

H31.02-   <u>Solar retinopathy</u> — A form due to solar radiation affecting the macula.

H31.021   Solar retinopathy, <u>right</u> eye

H31.022   Solar retinopathy, <u>left</u> eye

H31.023   Solar retinopathy, <u>bilateral</u>

H31.029   Solar retinopathy, <u>unspecified</u> eye

H31.09-   <u>Other</u> chorioretinal scars

H31.091   Other chorioretinal scars, <u>right</u> eye

H31.092   Other chorioretinal scars, <u>left</u> eye

H31.093   Other chorioretinal scars, <u>bilateral</u>

H31.099   Other chorioretinal scars, <u>unspecified</u> eye

H31.1-   <u>Choroidal degeneration</u> — Deterioration of the choroid tissue.
   Excludes ❷: angioid streaks of macula (H35.33)

H31.10-   <u>Unspecified</u> choroidal degeneration
   Choroidal sclerosis NOS

H31.101   Choroidal degeneration, unspecified, <u>right</u> eye

H31.102   Choroidal degeneration, unspecified, <u>left</u> eye

H31.103   Choroidal degeneration, unspecified, <u>bilateral</u>

H31.109   Choroidal degeneration, unspecified, <u>unspecified</u> eye

H31.11-   <u>Age-related choroidal atrophy</u> — A form characterized by wasting-away of the choroid occurring in advancing age.

H31.111   Age-related choroidal atrophy, <u>right</u> eye — [Age/15-124]

H31.112   Age-related choroidal atrophy, <u>left</u> eye — [Age/15-124]

H31.113   Age-related choroidal atrophy, <u>bilateral</u> — [Age/15-124]

H31.119   Age-related choroidal atrophy, <u>unspecified</u> eye — [Age/15-124]

H31.12-   <u>Diffuse secondary atrophy</u> of choroid — A form due to systemic diseases and affecting the whole of the choroid.

H31.121   Diffuse secondary atrophy of choroid, <u>right</u> eye

H31.122   Diffuse secondary atrophy of choroid, <u>left</u> eye

H31.123   Diffuse secondary atrophy of choroid, <u>bilateral</u>

H31.129   Diffuse secondary atrophy of choroid, <u>unspecified</u> eye

H31.2-   <u>Hereditary choroidal dystrophy</u> — Inherited dystrophic and atrophic deteriorations of the choroid.
   *Excludes ❷: hyperornithinemia (E72.4)
            ornithinemia (E72.4)*

H31.20   Hereditary choroidal dystrophy, unspecified

H31.21   <u>Choroideremia</u> — A form characterized by primary choroidal degeneration with night blindness.

H31.22   <u>Choroidal dystrophy (central areolar) (generalized) (peripapillary)</u> — A form affecting the central portion of the choroid capillaries.

H31.23   <u>Gyrate atrophy, choroid</u> — A form affecting the whole of the choroid blood vessels.

H31.29   Other hereditary choroidal dystrophy

H31.3-   <u>Choroidal hemorrhage and rupture</u> — The escape of blood and forcible tearing of a blood vessel wall.

H31.30-   <u>Unspecified</u> choroidal hemorrhage

H31.301   Unspecified choroidal hemorrhage, <u>right</u> eye

H31.302   Unspecified choroidal hemorrhage, <u>left</u> eye

H31.303   Unspecified choroidal hemorrhage, <u>bilateral</u>

H31.309   Unspecified choroidal hemorrhage, <u>unspecified</u> eye

H31.31-   <u>Expulsive</u> choroidal hemorrhage — A form characterized by expulsion of blood into the choroid and retinal tissues.

H31.311   Expulsive choroidal hemorrhage, <u>right</u> eye

H31.312   Expulsive choroidal hemorrhage, <u>left</u> eye

H31.313   Expulsive choroidal hemorrhage, <u>bilateral</u>

H31.319   Expulsive choroidal hemorrhage, <u>unspecified</u> eye

H31.32-   Choroidal <u>rupture</u> — The forcible tearing of a choroid blood vessel.

cc H31.321   Choroidal rupture, <u>right</u> eye

cc H31.322   Choroidal rupture, <u>left</u> eye

cc H31.323   Choroidal rupture, <u>bilateral</u>

cc H31.329   Choroidal rupture, <u>unspecified</u> eye

H31.4-   Choroidal <u>detachment</u> — The separation of the choroid layers.

H31.40-   <u>Unspecified</u> choroidal detachment

cc H31.401   Unspecified choroidal detachment, <u>right</u> eye

cc H31.402   Unspecified choroidal detachment, <u>left</u> eye

cc H31.403   Unspecified choroidal detachment, <u>bilateral</u>

cc H31.409   Unspecified choroidal detachment, <u>unspecified</u> eye

H31.41-   <u>Hemorrhagic</u> choroidal detachment — A form characterized by blood within the separation.

cc H31.411   Hemorrhagic choroidal detachment, <u>right</u> eye

cc H31.412   Hemorrhagic choroidal detachment, <u>left</u> eye

© 2016 Channel Publishing, Ltd

Excludes 1: = NOT CODED HERE! (Do not code both)   **692**   *Excludes ❷: = Not Included Here*

cc **H31.413**   **Hemorrhagic choroidal detachment, <u>bilateral</u>**

cc **H31.419**   **Hemorrhagic choroidal detachment, <u>unspecified</u> eye**

H31.42- <u>Serous</u> choroidal detachment — *A form characterized by fluid within the separation.*

cc **H31.421**   **Serous choroidal detachment, <u>right</u> eye**

cc **H31.422**   **Serous choroidal detachment, <u>left</u> eye**

cc **H31.423**   **Serous choroidal detachment, <u>bilateral</u>**

cc **H31.429**   **Serous choroidal detachment, <u>unspecified</u> eye**

H31.8   **Other specified disorders of choroid**

H31.9   **Unspecified disorder of choroid**

H32   **Chorioretinal disorders <u>in diseases classified elsewhere</u>** —
[Not Allowed as PDX]
Code first underlying disease, such as:
Congenital toxoplasmosis (P37.1)
Histoplasmosis (B39.-)
Leprosy (A30.-)
Excludes 1:   *chorioretinitis (in):*
    toxoplasmosis (acquired) (B58.01)
    tuberculosis (A18.53)

H33-   **Retinal detachments and breaks** — *The separation of the retinal layer from the pigment epithelium, and the break in continuity of the retinal layer.*

Excludes 1:   *detachment of retinal pigment epithelium (H35.72-, H35.73-)*

H33.0-   <u>Retinal detachment with retinal break</u>
Rhegmatogenous retinal detachment
Excludes 1:   *serous retinal detachment (without retinal break) (H33.2-)*

H33.00- <u>Unspecified</u> retinal detachment with retinal break

  H33.001   **Unspecified retinal detachment with retinal break, <u>right</u> eye**

  H33.002   **Unspecified retinal detachment with retinal break, <u>left</u> eye**

  H33.003   **Unspecified retinal detachment with retinal break, <u>bilateral</u>**

  H33.009   **Unspecified retinal detachment with retinal break, <u>unspecified</u> eye**

H33.01- Retinal detachment with <u>single break</u> — *A form characterized by one current retinal break.*

  H33.011   **Retinal detachment with single break, <u>right</u> eye**

  H33.012   **Retinal detachment with single break, <u>left</u> eye**

  H33.013   **Retinal detachment with single break, <u>bilateral</u>**

  H33.019   **Retinal detachment with single break, <u>unspecified</u> eye**

H33.02- Retinal detachment with <u>multiple</u> breaks — *A form characterized by two or more current retinal breaks.*

  H33.021   **Retinal detachment with multiple breaks, <u>right</u> eye**

  H33.022   **Retinal detachment with multiple breaks, <u>left</u> eye**

  H33.023   **Retinal detachment with multiple breaks, <u>bilateral</u>**

  H33.029   **Retinal detachment with multiple breaks, <u>unspecified</u> eye**

H33.03- Retinal detachment with <u>giant retinal tear</u> — *A form characterized by a relatively large current break (tear).*

  H33.031   **Retinal detachment with giant retinal tear, <u>right</u> eye**

  H33.032   **Retinal detachment with giant retinal tear, <u>left</u> eye**

  H33.033   **Retinal detachment with giant retinal tear, <u>bilateral</u>**

  H33.039   **Retinal detachment with giant retinal tear, <u>unspecified</u> eye**

H33.04- Retinal detachment with <u>retinal dialysis</u> — *A form characterized by a demonstrable current break at the ora serrata.*

  H33.041   **Retinal detachment with retinal dialysis, <u>right</u> eye**

  H33.042   **Retinal detachment with retinal dialysis, <u>left</u> eye**

  H33.043   **Retinal detachment with retinal dialysis, <u>bilateral</u>**

  H33.049   **Retinal detachment with retinal dialysis, <u>unspecified</u> eye**

H33.05- <u>Total</u> retinal detachment — *A form characterized by a current complete, or almost complete, separation of the retinal layer.*

  H33.051   **Total retinal detachment, <u>right</u> eye**

H33.052   **Total retinal detachment, <u>left</u> eye**

H33.053   **Total retinal detachment, <u>bilateral</u>**

H33.059   **Total retinal detachment, <u>unspecified</u> eye**

H33.1-   <u>Retinoschisis</u> and retinal cysts — *Splitting of the retinal layers, and fluid-filled sacs of the retina.*
Excludes 1:   *congenital retinoschisis (Q14.1)*
    microcystoid degeneration of retina (H35.42-)

H33.10- <u>Unspecified</u> retinoschisis

H33.101   **Unspecified retinoschisis, <u>right</u> eye**

H33.102   **Unspecified retinoschisis, <u>left</u> eye**

H33.103   **Unspecified retinoschisis, <u>bilateral</u>**

H33.109   **Unspecified retinoschisis, <u>unspecified</u> eye**

H33.11- <u>Cyst of ora serrata</u> — *A form characterized by fluid-filled sacs in the serrated junction between the retina and the ciliary body.*

H33.111   **Cyst of ora serrata, <u>right</u> eye**

H33.112   **Cyst of ora serrata, <u>left</u> eye**

H33.113   **Cyst of ora serrata, <u>bilateral</u>**

H33.119   **Cyst of ora serrata, <u>unspecified</u> eye**

H33.12- Parasitic cyst of retina — *A form characterized by infestation of a parasite.*

cc **H33.121**   **Parasitic cyst of retina, <u>right</u> eye**

cc **H33.122**   **Parasitic cyst of retina, <u>left</u> eye**

cc **H33.123**   **Parasitic cyst of retina, <u>bilateral</u>**

cc **H33.129**   **Parasitic cyst of retina, <u>unspecified</u> eye**

H33.19- <u>Other</u> retinoschisis and retinal cysts
Pseudocyst of retina — *A dilated space of the retina.*

H33.191   **Other retinoschisis and retinal cysts, <u>right</u> eye**

H33.192   **Other retinoschisis and retinal cysts, <u>left</u> eye**

H33.193   **Other retinoschisis and retinal cysts, <u>bilateral</u>**

H33.199   **Other retinoschisis and retinal cysts, <u>unspecified</u> eye**

H33.2-   <u>Serous retinal detachment</u> — *The separation of the retinal layers from the pigment epithelium with serous fluid.*
Retinal detachment NOS
Retinal detachment without retinal break
Excludes 1:   *central serous chorioretinopathy (H35.71-)*

cc **H33.20**   **Serous retinal detachment, <u>unspecified</u> eye**

cc **H33.21**   **Serous retinal detachment, <u>right</u> eye**

cc **H33.22**   **Serous retinal detachment, <u>left</u> eye**

cc **H33.23**   **Serous retinal detachment, <u>bilateral</u>**

H33.3-   <u>Retinal breaks without detachment</u> — *A break, tear, or hole without separation of retinal layers.*
Excludes 1:   *chorioretinal scars after surgery for detachment (H59.81-)*
    peripheral retinal degeneration without break (H35.4-)

H33.30- <u>Unspecified</u> retinal break

H33.301   **Unspecified retinal break, <u>right</u> eye**

H33.302   **Unspecified retinal break, <u>left</u> eye**

H33.303   **Unspecified retinal break, <u>bilateral</u>**

H33.309   **Unspecified retinal break, <u>unspecified</u> eye**

H33.31- <u>Horseshoe tear</u> of retina without detachment — *A form characterized by a horseshoe-shaped tear of the retinal layer.*
Operculum of retina without detachment — *A form marked by the retinal tear completely free of the retinal surface.*

H33.311   **Horseshoe tear of retina without detachment, <u>right</u> eye**

H33.312   **Horseshoe tear of retina without detachment, <u>left</u> eye**

H33.313   **Horseshoe tear of retina without detachment, <u>bilateral</u>**

H33.319   **Horseshoe tear of retina without detachment, <u>unspecified</u> eye**

H33.32- <u>Round hole</u> of retina without detachment — *A form characterized by a round-shaped atrophic hole through the retinal layer.*

H33.321   **Round hole, <u>right</u> eye**

H33.322   **Round hole, <u>left</u> eye**

H33.323   **Round hole, <u>bilateral</u>**

H33.329   **Round hole, <u>unspecified</u> eye**

H31 - H33

H33.33- <u>Multiple defects</u> of retina without detachment — A form characterized by two or more breaks, tears, or holes.

    H33.331 Multiple defects of retina without detachment, <u>right</u> eye

    H33.332 Multiple defects of retina without detachment, <u>left</u> eye

    H33.333 Multiple defects of retina without detachment, <u>bilateral</u>

    H33.339 Multiple defects of retina without detachment, <u>unspecified</u> eye

H33.4- <u>Traction</u> detachment of retina — The separation of the retinal layer at its attachment due to the pulling force of the vitreous on the retina.

    Proliferative vitreo-retinopathy with retinal detachment

cc **H33.40** Traction detachment of retina, <u>unspecified</u> eye

cc **H33.41** Traction detachment of retina, <u>right</u> eye

cc **H33.42** Traction detachment of retina, <u>left</u> eye

cc **H33.43** Traction detachment of retina, <u>bilateral</u>

cc **H33.8** Other retinal detachments

H34- <u>Retinal vascular occlusions</u> — The obstruction of blood flow to and from the retina.

    Excludes 1:   *amaurosis fugax (G45.3)*

H34.0- <u>Transient retinal artery occlusion</u> — Temporary blockage of a retinal arterial branch.

cc **H34.00** Transient retinal artery occlusion, <u>unspecified</u> eye

cc **H34.01** Transient retinal artery occlusion, <u>right</u> eye

cc **H34.02** Transient retinal artery occlusion, <u>left</u> eye

cc **H34.03** Transient retinal artery occlusion, <u>bilateral</u>

H34.1- <u>Central retinal artery occlusion</u> — Blockage of the central retinal artery resulting in sudden and complete, or almost complete, loss of vision.

cc **H34.10** Central retinal artery occlusion, <u>unspecified</u> eye

cc **H34.11** Central retinal artery occlusion, <u>right</u> eye

cc **H34.12** Central retinal artery occlusion, <u>left</u> eye

cc **H34.13** Central retinal artery occlusion, <u>bilateral</u>

H34.2- Other retinal artery occlusions

    H34.21- <u>Partial retinal artery</u> occlusion — Incomplete blockage of the retinal artery and its branches.

        Hollenhorst's plaque — Erythromatous emboli deposits in the retinal arterioles.

        Retinal microembolism — A blood clot of a very minute size in a retinal artery.

cc **H34.211** Partial retinal artery occlusion, <u>right</u> eye

cc **H34.212** Partial retinal artery occlusion, <u>left</u> eye

cc **H34.213** Partial retinal artery occlusion, <u>bilateral</u>

cc **H34.219** Partial retinal artery occlusion, <u>unspecified</u> eye

    H34.23- <u>Retinal artery branch</u> occlusion — Blockage of a retinal arterial branch resulting in sudden partial loss of vision.

cc **H34.231** Retinal artery branch occlusion, <u>right</u> eye

cc **H34.232** Retinal artery branch occlusion, <u>left</u> eye

cc **H34.233** Retinal artery branch occlusion, <u>bilateral</u>

cc **H34.239** Retinal artery branch occlusion, <u>unspecified</u> eye

H34.8- Other retinal vascular occlusions

    H34.81- <u>Central retinal vein</u> occlusion — Blockage of the central retinal vein leading to increased intraocular pressure and retinal hemorrhages.

    One of the following 7th characters is to be assigned to codes in subcategory H34.81- to designate the severity of the occlusion:
    0   With macular edema
    1   With retinal neovascularization
    2   Stable
        Old retinal vein occlusion

CC-0-2 **H34.811-** Central retinal vein occlusion, <u>right</u> eye

CC-0-2 **H34.812-** Central retinal vein occlusion, <u>left</u> eye

CC-0-2 **H34.813-** Central retinal vein occlusion, <u>bilateral</u>

CC-0-2 **H34.819-** Central retinal vein occlusion, <u>unspecified</u> eye

    H34.82- <u>Venous engorgement</u> — The abnormal accumulation of venous blood in the retinal veins.

        Incipient retinal vein occlusion — A form marked by the beginning of blockage.

        Partial retinal vein occlusion — A form marked by incomplete blockage.

    H34.821 Venous engorgement, <u>right</u> eye

    H34.822 Venous engorgement, <u>left</u> eye

    H34.823 Venous engorgement, <u>bilateral</u>

    H34.829 Venous engorgement, <u>unspecified</u> eye

H34.83- <u>Tributary (branch) retinal vein occlusion</u> — Blockage of a tortuous retinal vein branch which may cause retinal hemorrhage.

    One of the following 7th characters is to be assigned to codes in subcategory H34.83- to designate the severity of the occlusion:
    0   With macular edema
    1   With retinal neovascularization
    2   Stable
        Old tributary (branch) retinal vein occlusion

H34.831- Tributary (branch) retinal vein occlusion, <u>right</u> eye

H34.832- Tributary (branch) retinal vein occlusion, <u>left</u> eye

H34.833- Tributary (branch) retinal vein occlusion, <u>bilateral</u>

H34.839- Tributary (branch) retinal vein occlusion, <u>unspecified</u> eye

cc **H34.9** Unspecified retinal vascular occlusion

H35- <u>Other retinal disorders</u>

    Excludes ❷: *diabetic retinal disorders (E08.311- E08.359, E09.311-E09.359, E10.311- E10.359, E11.311- E11.359, E13.311-E13.359)*

H35.0- <u>Background retinopathy</u> and retinal vascular changes — A disease of the retinal capillaries that is caused by some condition other than diabetes.

    Code also any associated hypertension (I10.)

H35.00 <u>Unspecified</u> background retinopathy

H35.01- <u>Changes in retinal vascular appearance</u> — New, abnormal vascular development.

    Retinal vascular sheathing — The white-line appearance of thickened retinal arterial walls.

    H35.011 Changes in retinal vascular appearance, <u>right</u> eye

    H35.012 Changes in retinal vascular appearance, <u>left</u> eye

    H35.013 Changes in retinal vascular appearance, <u>bilateral</u>

    H35.019 Changes in retinal vascular appearance, <u>unspecified</u> eye

H35.02- <u>Exudative</u> retinopathy — A disease of the retinal capillaries characterized by masses of white or yellowish exudate which deposit on the posterior part of the fundus oculi.

    Coats retinopathy

    H35.021 Exudative retinopathy, <u>right</u> eye

    H35.022 Exudative retinopathy, <u>left</u> eye

    H35.023 Exudative retinopathy, <u>bilateral</u>

    H35.029 Exudative retinopathy, <u>unspecified</u> eye

H35.03- <u>Hypertensive</u> retinopathy — A disease of the retinal capillaries due to the effects of hypertension.

    H35.031 Hypertensive retinopathy, <u>right</u> eye

    H35.032 Hypertensive retinopathy, <u>left</u> eye

    H35.033 Hypertensive retinopathy, <u>bilateral</u>

    H35.039 Hypertensive retinopathy, <u>unspecified</u> eye

H35.04- <u>Retinal micro-aneurysms</u>, unspecified — The presence of small dilated arterial sacs.

    H35.041 Retinal micro-aneurysms, unspecified, <u>right</u> eye

    H35.042 Retinal micro-aneurysms, unspecified, <u>left</u> eye

    H35.043 Retinal micro-aneurysms, unspecified, <u>bilateral</u>

    H35.049 Retinal micro-aneurysms, unspecified, <u>unspecified</u> eye

H35.05- <u>Retinal neovascularization</u>, unspecified — The abnormal development of new retinal blood vessels.

    H35.051 Retinal neovascularization, unspecified, <u>right</u> eye

    H35.052 Retinal neovascularization, unspecified, <u>left</u> eye

    H35.053 Retinal neovascularization, unspecified, <u>bilateral</u>

    H35.059 Retinal neovascularization, unspecified, <u>unspecified</u> eye

H35.06- <u>Retinal vasculitis</u> — Inflammation of the retinal blood vessels.

    Eales disease — A disease characterized by recurrent hemorrhages into the retina and vitreous.

    Retinal perivasculitis — Inflammation of the retinal perivascular sheaths.

    H35.061 Retinal vasculitis, <u>right</u> eye

H33 - H35

H35.062 Retinal vasculitis, <u>left</u> eye

H35.063 Retinal vasculitis, <u>bilateral</u>

H35.069 Retinal vasculitis, <u>unspecified</u> eye

H35.07- <u>Retinal telangiectasis</u> — The abnormal dilatation of a group of retinal capillaries.

H35.071 Retinal telangiectasis, <u>right</u> eye

H35.072 Retinal telangiectasis, <u>left</u> eye

H35.073 Retinal telangiectasis, <u>bilateral</u>

H35.079 Retinal telangiectasis, <u>unspecified</u> eye

H35.09 Other intraretinal microvascular abnormalities
Retinal varices — Enlarged, tortuous retinal capillary vessels.

H35.1- <u>Retinopathy of prematurity</u> — A developmental disorder of premature infants in which the normal development of the retinal vasculature is arrested and results in fibrovascular proliferation.

H35.10- Retinopathy of prematurity, <u>unspecified</u>
Retinopathy of prematurity NOS

H35.101 Retinopathy of prematurity, unspecified, <u>right</u> eye

H35.102 Retinopathy of prematurity, unspecified, <u>left</u> eye

H35.103 Retinopathy of prematurity, unspecified, <u>bilateral</u>

H35.109 Retinopathy of prematurity, unspecified, <u>unspecified</u> eye

H35.11- Retinopathy of prematurity, <u>stage 0</u> — The mildest form with no identifiable line of demarcation.

H35.111 Retinopathy of prematurity, stage 0, <u>right</u> eye

H35.112 Retinopathy of prematurity, stage 0, <u>left</u> eye

H35.113 Retinopathy of prematurity, stage 0, <u>bilateral</u>

H35.119 Retinopathy of prematurity, stage 0, <u>unspecified</u> eye

H35.12- Retinopathy of prematurity, <u>stage 1</u> — Blood vessel growth is mildly abnormal and a line of demarcation develops.

H35.121 Retinopathy of prematurity, stage 1, <u>right</u> eye

H35.122 Retinopathy of prematurity, stage 1, <u>left</u> eye

H35.123 Retinopathy of prematurity, stage 1, <u>bilateral</u>

H35.129 Retinopathy of prematurity, stage 1, <u>unspecified</u> eye

H35.13- Retinopathy of prematurity, <u>stage 2</u> — Blood vessel growth is moderately abnormal and the line becomes a ridge.

H35.131 Retinopathy of prematurity, stage 2, <u>right</u> eye

H35.132 Retinopathy of prematurity, stage 2, <u>left</u> eye

H35.133 Retinopathy of prematurity, stage 2, <u>bilateral</u>

H35.139 Retinopathy of prematurity, stage 2, <u>unspecified</u> eye

H35.14- Retinopathy of prematurity, <u>stage 3</u> — Blood vessel growth is severely abnormal and extra-retinal vascular proliferation occurs.

H35.141 Retinopathy of prematurity, stage 3, <u>right</u> eye

H35.142 Retinopathy of prematurity, stage 3, <u>left</u> eye

H35.143 Retinopathy of prematurity, stage 3, <u>bilateral</u>

H35.149 Retinopathy of prematurity, stage 3, <u>unspecified</u> eye

H35.15- Retinopathy of prematurity, <u>stage 4</u> — Blood vessel growth is severely abnormal and there is a partially detached retina.

H35.151 Retinopathy of prematurity, stage 4, <u>right</u> eye

H35.152 Retinopathy of prematurity, stage 4, <u>left</u> eye

H35.153 Retinopathy of prematurity, stage 4, <u>bilateral</u>

H35.159 Retinopathy of prematurity, stage 4, <u>unspecified</u> eye

H35.16- Retinopathy of prematurity, <u>stage 5</u> — There is a total retinal detachment.

H35.161 Retinopathy of prematurity, stage 5, <u>right</u> eye

H35.162 Retinopathy of prematurity, stage 5, <u>left</u> eye

H35.163 Retinopathy of prematurity, stage 5, <u>bilateral</u>

H35.169 Retinopathy of prematurity, stage 5, <u>unspecified</u> eye

H35.17- <u>Retrolental fibroplasia</u> — A condition in which the retina is already scarred.

H35.171 Retrolental fibroplasia, <u>right</u> eye

H35.172 Retrolental fibroplasia, <u>left</u> eye

H35.173 Retrolental fibroplasia, <u>bilateral</u>

H35.179 Retrolental fibroplasia, <u>unspecified</u> eye

H35.2- <u>Other non-diabetic proliferative retinopathy</u>
Proliferative vitreo-retinopathy
Excludes 1: *proliferative vitreo-retinopathy with retinal detachment (H33.4-)*

H35.20 Other non-diabetic proliferative retinopathy, <u>unspecified</u> eye

H35.21 Other non-diabetic proliferative retinopathy, <u>right</u> eye

H35.22 Other non-diabetic proliferative retinopathy, <u>left</u> eye

H35.23 Other non-diabetic proliferative retinopathy, <u>bilateral</u>

H35.3- Degeneration of macula and posterior pole — Deterioration of the yellow pigmented point of sharpest vision of the retina.

H35.30 Unspecified macular degeneration — [Age/15-124]
Age-related macular degeneration

H35.31- Nonexudative age-related macular degeneration — A form characterized by progressive cellular destruction and the lack of cellular debris.
Atrophic age-related macular degeneration
Dry age-related macular degeneration

One of the following 7th characters is to be assigned to codes in subcategory H35.31- to designate the stage of the disease:
0 Stage unspecified
1 Early dry stage
2 Intermediate dry stage
3 Advanced atrophic without subfoveal involvement
Advanced dry stage
4 Advanced atrophic with subfoveal involvement

H35.311- Nonexudative age-related macular degeneration, <u>right</u> eye — [Age/15-124]

H35.312- Nonexudative age-related macular degeneration, <u>left</u> eye — [Age/15-124]

H35.313- Nonexudative age-related macular degeneration, <u>bilateral</u> — [Age/15-124]

H35.319- Nonexudative age-related macular degeneration, <u>unspecified</u> eye — [Age/15-124]

H35.32- Exudative age-related macular degeneration — A form characterized by progressive cellular destruction and cellular debris.
Wet age-related macular degeneration

One of the following 7th characters is to be assigned to codes in subcategory H35.32- to designate the stage of the disease:
0 Stage unspecified
1 With active choroidal neovascularization
2 With inactive choroidal neovascularization
With involuted or regressed neovascularization
3 With inactive scar

H35.321- Exudative age-related macular degeneration, <u>right</u> eye — [Age/15-124]

H35.322- Exudative age-related macular degeneration, <u>left</u> eye — [Age/15-124]

H35.323- Exudative age-related macular degeneration, <u>bilateral</u> — [Age/15-124]

H35.329- Exudative age-related macular degeneration, <u>unspecified</u> eye — [Age/15-124]

H35.33 Angioid streaks of macula — A form characterized by dark brown pigmented streaks which anastomose and may be mistaken for blood vessels.

H35.34- <u>Macular cyst, hole, or pseudohole</u> — A form characterized by a membrane break of the macula.

H35.341 Macular cyst, hole, or pseudohole, <u>right</u> eye

H35.342 Macular cyst, hole, or pseudohole, <u>left</u> eye

H35.343 Macular cyst, hole, or pseudohole, <u>bilateral</u>

H35.349 Macular cyst, hole, or pseudohole, <u>unspecified</u> eye

H35.35- <u>Cystoid macular degeneration</u> — A form characterized by appearance of cyst-like macular and foveal cavities.
Excludes 1: *cystoid macular edema following cataract surgery (H59.03-)*

H35.351 Cystoid macular degeneration, <u>right</u> eye

H35.352 Cystoid macular degeneration, <u>left</u> eye

H35.353 Cystoid macular degeneration, <u>bilateral</u>

H3 5 - H3 5

Excludes 1: = NOT CODED HERE! (Do not code both)   *Excludes ❷:* = Not Included Here

H35.359 Cystoid macular degeneration, <u>unspecified</u> eye

H35.36- <u>Drusen (degenerative) of macula</u> — Hyaline excrescences of the Bruch's membrane of the choroid.

H35.361 Drusen (degenerative) of macula, <u>right</u> eye

H35.362 Drusen (degenerative) of macula, <u>left</u> eye

H35.363 Drusen (degenerative) of macula, <u>bilateral</u>

H35.369 Drusen (degenerative) of macula, <u>unspecified</u> eye

H35.37- <u>Puckering of macula</u> — A form characterized by wrinkling of the macular surface.

H35.371 Puckering of macula, <u>right</u> eye

H35.372 Puckering of macula, <u>left</u> eye

H35.373 Puckering of macula, <u>bilateral</u>

H35.379 Puckering of macula, <u>unspecified</u> eye

H35.38- <u>Toxic maculopathy</u> — A form caused by the effects of toxic substances.
Code first poisoning due to drug or toxin, if applicable (T36-T65 with fifth or sixth character 1-4 or 6)
Use additional code for adverse effect, if applicable, to identify drug (T36-T50 with fifth or sixth character 5)

H35.381 Toxic maculopathy, <u>right</u> eye

H35.382 Toxic maculopathy, <u>left</u> eye

H35.383 Toxic maculopathy, <u>bilateral</u>

H35.389 Toxic maculopathy, <u>unspecified</u> eye

H35.4- <u>Peripheral retinal degeneration</u> — Deterioration of the retina other than the macula.
Excludes 1: *hereditary retinal degeneration (dystrophy) (H35.5-)*
peripheral retinal degeneration with retinal break (H33.3-)

H35.40 <u>Unspecified</u> peripheral retinal degeneration

H35.41- <u>Lattice</u> degeneration of retina — A form characterized by atrophy of the retinal lattice.
Palisade degeneration of retina

H35.411 Lattice degeneration of retina, <u>right</u> eye

H35.412 Lattice degeneration of retina, <u>left</u> eye

H35.413 Lattice degeneration of retina, <u>bilateral</u>

H35.419 Lattice degeneration of retina, <u>unspecified</u> eye

H35.42- <u>Microcystoid</u> degeneration of retina — A form characterized by atrophic small cysts occurring in advancing age.

H35.421 Microcystoid degeneration of retina, <u>right</u> eye

H35.422 Microcystoid degeneration of retina, <u>left</u> eye

H35.423 Microcystoid degeneration of retina, <u>bilateral</u>

H35.429 Microcystoid degeneration of retina, <u>unspecified</u> eye

H35.43- <u>Paving stone</u> degeneration of retina — A form characterized by the paving stone appearance of the retina.

H35.431 Paving stone degeneration of retina, <u>right</u> eye

H35.432 Paving stone degeneration of retina, <u>left</u> eye

H35.433 Paving stone degeneration of retina, <u>bilateral</u>

H35.439 Paving stone degeneration of retina, <u>unspecified</u> eye

H35.44- Age-related reticular degeneration of retina — A form characterized by an atrophic net-like appearance.

H35.441 Age-related reticular degeneration of retina, <u>right</u> eye — [Age/15-124]

H35.442 Age-related reticular degeneration of retina, <u>left</u> eye — [Age/15-124]

H35.443 Age-related reticular degeneration of retina, <u>bilateral</u> — [Age/15-124]

H35.449 Age-related reticular degeneration of retina, <u>unspecified</u> eye — [Age/15-124]

H35.45- <u>Secondary pigmentary</u> degeneration — A form characterized by pigmentary changes due to nonocular diseases.

H35.451 Secondary pigmentary degeneration, <u>right</u> eye

H35.452 Secondary pigmentary degeneration, <u>left</u> eye

H35.453 Secondary pigmentary degeneration, <u>bilateral</u>

H35.459 Secondary pigmentary degeneration, <u>unspecified</u> eye

H35.46- <u>Secondary vitreoretinal</u> degeneration — A form characterized by destruction of vitreoretinal tissue due to nonocular diseases.

H35.461 Secondary vitreoretinal degeneration, <u>right</u> eye

H35.462 Secondary vitreoretinal degeneration, <u>left</u> eye

H35.463 Secondary vitreoretinal degeneration, <u>bilateral</u>

H35.469 Secondary vitreoretinal degeneration, <u>unspecified</u> eye

H35.5- <u>Hereditary retinal dystrophy</u> — Inherited dystrophic and atrophic retinal deteriorations.
Excludes 1: *dystrophies primarily involving Bruch's membrane (H31.1-)*

H35.50 Unspecified hereditary retinal dystrophy

H35.51 Vitreoretinal dystrophy — A form characterized by cystoid structure changes of the central retina.

H35.52 Pigmentary retinal dystrophy — A form characterized by retinal pigmentary atrophy.
Albipunctate retinal dystrophy
Retinitis pigmentosa
Tapetoretinal dystrophy

H35.53 Other dystrophies primarily involving the sensory retina
Stargardt's disease — A form marked by whitish foveal flecks and progressive foveal atrophy.

H35.54 Dystrophies primarily involving the retinal pigment epithelium
Vitelliform retinal dystrophy — A form marked by orange-yellow foveal disc.

H35.6- <u>Retinal hemorrhage</u> — The escape of blood into the retina.

H35.60 Retinal hemorrhage, <u>unspecified</u> eye

H35.61 Retinal hemorrhage, <u>right</u> eye

H35.62 Retinal hemorrhage, <u>left</u> eye

H35.63 Retinal hemorrhage, <u>bilateral</u>

H35.7- <u>Separation of retinal layers</u> — The abnormal separation of the pigment epithelium from the choroid.
Excludes 1: *retinal detachment (serous) (H33.2-)*
rhegmatogenous retinal detachment (H33.0-)

cc H35.70 Unspecified separation of retinal layers

H35.71- <u>Central</u> serous chorioretinopathy — A form characterized by serous fluid separation in the center of the retina.

H35.711 Central serous chorioretinopathy, <u>right</u> eye

H35.712 Central serous chorioretinopathy, <u>left</u> eye

H35.713 Central serous chorioretinopathy, <u>bilateral</u>

H35.719 Central serous chorioretinopathy, <u>unspecified</u> eye

H35.72- <u>Serous</u> detachment of retinal pigment epithelium — The separation of the retinal pigment epithelium from the choroid by serous fluid.

cc H35.721 Serous detachment of retinal pigment epithelium, <u>right</u> eye

cc H35.722 Serous detachment of retinal pigment epithelium, <u>left</u> eye

cc H35.723 Serous detachment of retinal pigment epithelium, <u>bilateral</u>

cc H35.729 Serous detachment of retinal pigment epithelium, <u>unspecified</u> eye

H35.73- <u>Hemorrhagic</u> detachment of retinal pigment epithelium — The separation of the retinal pigment epithelium from the choroid by the escape of blood into that separation.

cc H35.731 Hemorrhagic detachment of retinal pigment epithelium, <u>right</u> eye

cc H35.732 Hemorrhagic detachment of retinal pigment epithelium, <u>left</u> eye

cc H35.733 Hemorrhagic detachment of retinal pigment epithelium, <u>bilateral</u>

cc H35.739 Hemorrhagic detachment of retinal pigment epithelium, <u>unspecified</u> eye

H35.8- Other specified retinal disorders
Excludes ❷: *retinal hemorrhage (H35.6-)*

H35.81 Retinal edema — The accumulation of intercellular fluid.
Retinal cotton wool spots — The white or gray fluid opacities in the retina composed of cytoid bodies.

cc H35.82 Retinal ischemia — Deficiency of blood supply to the retina.

H35.89 Other specified retinal disorders

Excludes 1: = NOT CODED HERE! (Do not code both) 696 *Excludes ❷:* = Not Included Here

H35-H35

H35.9   **Unspecified retinal disorder**

H36   **Retinal disorders in diseases classified elsewhere** — [Not Allowed as PDX]
Code first underlying disease, such as:
    Lipid storage disorders (E75.-)
    Sickle-cell disorders (D57.-)
    Excludes 1:   *arteriosclerotic retinopathy (H35.0-)*
              diabetic retinopathy (E08.3-, E09.3-, E10.3-, E11.3-, E13.3-)

Glaucoma (H40-H42)

H40-   **Glaucoma** — An abnormal increase in intraocular pressure.
    Excludes 1:   *absolute glaucoma (H44.51-)*
              congenital glaucoma (Q15.0)
              traumatic glaucoma due to birth injury (P15.3)

H40.0-   **Glaucoma suspect** — A relatively low increase in intraocular pressure which does not meet all the criteria for the formal diagnosis of glaucoma.

    H40.00-   **Preglaucoma**, unspecified
       H40.001   **Preglaucoma, unspecified, right eye**
       H40.002   **Preglaucoma, unspecified, left eye**
       H40.003   **Preglaucoma, unspecified, bilateral**
       H40.009   **Preglaucoma, unspecified, unspecified eye**

    H40.01-   **Open angle with borderline findings, low risk** — A form with the angle of the anterior chamber open.
       Open angle, low risk
       H40.011   **Open angle with borderline findings, low risk, right eye**
       H40.012   **Open angle with borderline findings, low risk, left eye**
       H40.013   **Open angle with borderline findings, low risk, bilateral**
       H40.019   **Open angle with borderline findings, low risk, unspecified eye**

    H40.02-   **Open angle with borderline findings, high risk** — A form with the angle of the anterior chamber open.
       Open angle, high risk
       H40.021   **Open angle with borderline findings, high risk, right eye**
       H40.022   **Open angle with borderline findings, high risk, left eye**
       H40.023   **Open angle with borderline findings, high risk, bilateral**
       H40.029   **Open angle with borderline findings, high risk, unspecified eye**

    H40.03-   **Anatomical narrow angle** — A form characterized by the finding of a narrowed angle of the anterior chamber.
       Primary angle closure suspect
       H40.031   **Anatomical narrow angle, right eye**
       H40.032   **Anatomical narrow angle, left eye**
       H40.033   **Anatomical narrow angle, bilateral**
       H40.039   **Anatomical narrow angle, unspecified eye**

    H40.04-   **Steroid responder**
       H40.041   **Steroid responder, right eye**
       H40.042   **Steroid responder, left eye**
       H40.043   **Steroid responder, bilateral**
       H40.049   **Steroid responder, unspecified eye**

    H40.05-   **Ocular hypertension** — A form characterized by increased ocular blood pressure.
       H40.051   **Ocular hypertension, right eye**
       H40.052   **Ocular hypertension, left eye**
       H40.053   **Ocular hypertension, bilateral**
       H40.059   **Ocular hypertension, unspecified eye**

    H40.06-   **Primary angle closure without glaucoma damage** — An abnormal increase in intraocular pressure with the angle of the anterior chamber narrowed and without pre-existing ocular disease.
       H40.061   **Primary angle closure without glaucoma damage, right eye**
       H40.062   **Primary angle closure without glaucoma damage, left eye**
       H40.063   **Primary angle closure without glaucoma damage, bilateral**

       H40.069   **Primary angle closure without glaucoma damage, unspecified eye**

H40.1-   **Open-angle glaucoma** — An abnormal increase in intraocular pressure with the angle of the anterior chamber open.

    H40.10x-   **Unspecified open-angle glaucoma**
       One of the following 7th characters is to be assigned to code H40.10x- to designate the stage of glaucoma:
       0   **Stage unspecified**
       1   **Mild stage**
       2   **Moderate stage**
       3   **Severe stage**
       4   **Indeterminate stage**

    H40.11-   **Primary open-angle glaucoma** — A form without a pre-existing ocular disease.
       Chronic simple glaucoma
       One of the following 7th characters is to be assigned to each code in subcategory H40.11- to designate the stage of glaucoma:
       0   **Stage unspecified**
       1   **Mild stage**
       2   **Moderate stage**
       3   **Severe stage**
       4   **Indeterminate stage**
       H40.111-   **Primary open-angle glaucoma, right eye**
       H40.112-   **Primary open-angle glaucoma, left eye**
       H40.113-   **Primary open-angle glaucoma, bilateral**
       H40.119-   **Primary open-angle glaucoma, unspecified eye**

H40.12-   **Low-tension glaucoma** — A form marked by a relatively low increased intraocular pressure.
       One of the following 7th characters is to be assigned to code H40.12- to designate the stage of glaucoma:
       0   **Stage unspecified**
       1   **Mild stage**
       2   **Moderate stage**
       3   **Severe stage**
       4   **Indeterminate stage**
       H40.121-   **Low-tension glaucoma, right eye** — [Unacceptable PDX]
       H40.122-   **Low-tension glaucoma, left eye** — [Unacceptable PDX]
       H40.123-   **Low-tension glaucoma, bilateral** — [Unacceptable PDX]
       H40.129-   **Low-tension glaucoma, unspecified eye** — [Unacceptable PDX]

H40.13-   **Pigmentary glaucoma** — A form marked by an abnormal amount of pigment in the anterior chamber.
       One of the following 7th characters is to be assigned to code H40.13- to designate the stage of glaucoma:
       0   **Stage unspecified**
       1   **Mild stage**
       2   **Moderate stage**
       3   **Severe stage**
       4   **Indeterminate stage**
       H40.131-   **Pigmentary glaucoma, right eye** — [Unacceptable PDX]
       H40.132-   **Pigmentary glaucoma, left eye** — [Unacceptable PDX]
       H40.133-   **Pigmentary glaucoma, bilateral** — [Unacceptable PDX]
       H40.139-   **Pigmentary glaucoma, unspecified eye** — [Unacceptable PDX]

H40.14-   **Capsular glaucoma with pseudoexfoliation of lens** — A form marked by the presence of flakes or clumps of proteinaceous substance within the eye.
       One of the following 7th characters is to be assigned to code H40.14- to designate the stage of glaucoma:
       0   **Stage unspecified**
       1   **Mild stage**
       2   **Moderate stage**
       3   **Severe stage**
       4   **Indeterminate stage**
       H40.141-   **Capsular glaucoma with pseudoexfoliation of lens, right eye**
       H40.142-   **Capsular glaucoma with pseudoexfoliation of lens, left eye**
       H40.143-   **Capsular glaucoma with pseudoexfoliation of lens, bilateral**

H35 - H40

H40.149- Capsular glaucoma with pseudoexfoliation of lens, <u>unspecified</u> eye

H40.15- <u>Residual stage</u> of open-angle glaucoma

H40.151 Residual stage of open-angle glaucoma, <u>right</u> eye — [Unacceptable PDX]

H40.152 Residual stage of open-angle glaucoma, <u>left</u> eye — [Unacceptable PDX]

H40.153 Residual stage of open-angle glaucoma, <u>bilateral</u> — [Unacceptable PDX]

H40.159 Residual stage of open-angle glaucoma, <u>unspecified</u> eye — [Unacceptable PDX]

H40.2- <u>Primary angle-closure</u> glaucoma — An abnormal increase in intraocular pressure with the angle of the anterior chamber narrowed and without pre-existing ocular disease.

> *Excludes 1:*   *aqueous misdirection (H40.83-)*
>   *malignant glaucoma (H40.83-)*

H40.20x- <u>Unspecified</u> primary angle-closure glaucoma

One of the following 7th characters is to be assigned to code H40.20x- to designate the stage of glaucoma:
0   Stage unspecified
1   Mild stage
2   Moderate stage
3   Severe stage
4   Indeterminate stage

H40.21- <u>Acute</u> angle-closure glaucoma — A form marked by sudden, severe onset.
Acute angle-closure glaucoma attack
Acute angle-closure glaucoma crisis

CC **H40.211** Acute angle-closure glaucoma, <u>right</u> eye
CC **H40.212** Acute angle-closure glaucoma, <u>left</u> eye
CC **H40.213** Acute angle-closure glaucoma, <u>bilateral</u>
CC **H40.219** Acute angle-closure glaucoma, <u>unspecified</u> eye

H40.22- <u>Chronic</u> angle-closure glaucoma — A form marked by slow development, and persistence over a long period of time, often unnoticed.
Chronic primary angle-closure glaucoma

One of the following 7th characters is to be assigned to code H40.22- to designate the stage of glaucoma:
0   Stage unspecified
1   Mild stage
2   Moderate stage
3   Severe stage
4   Indeterminate stage

H40.221- Chronic angle-closure glaucoma, <u>right</u> eye
H40.222- Chronic angle-closure glaucoma, <u>left</u> eye
H40.223- Chronic angle-closure glaucoma, <u>bilateral</u>
H40.229- Chronic angle-closure glaucoma, <u>unspecified</u> eye

H40.23- <u>Intermittent</u> angle-closure glaucoma — A form occurring at separated intervals.

H40.231 Intermittent angle-closure glaucoma, <u>right</u> eye
H40.232 Intermittent angle-closure glaucoma, <u>left</u> eye
H40.233 Intermittent angle-closure glaucoma, <u>bilateral</u>
H40.239 Intermittent angle-closure glaucoma, <u>unspecified</u> eye

H40.24- <u>Residual stage</u> of angle-closure glaucoma

H40.241 Residual stage of angle-closure glaucoma, <u>right</u> eye
H40.242 Residual stage of angle-closure glaucoma, <u>left</u> eye
H40.243 Residual stage of angle-closure glaucoma, <u>bilateral</u>
H40.249 Residual stage of angle-closure glaucoma, <u>unspecified</u> eye

H40.3- Glaucoma <u>secondary to eye trauma</u>
Code also underlying condition

One of the following 7th characters is to be assigned to code H40.3- to designate the stage of glaucoma:
0   Stage unspecified
1   Mild stage
2   Moderate stage
3   Severe stage
4   Indeterminate stage

H40.30x- Glaucoma secondary to eye trauma, <u>unspecified</u> eye
H40.31x- Glaucoma secondary to eye trauma, <u>right</u> eye
H40.32x- Glaucoma secondary to eye trauma, <u>left</u> eye
H40.33x- Glaucoma secondary to eye trauma, <u>bilateral</u>

H40.4- Glaucoma <u>secondary to eye inflammation</u>
Code also underlying condition

One of the following 7th characters is to be assigned to code H40.4- to designate the stage of glaucoma:
0   Stage unspecified
1   Mild stage
2   Moderate stage
3   Severe stage
4   Indeterminate stage

H40.40x- Glaucoma secondary to eye inflammation, <u>unspecified</u> eye
H40.41x- Glaucoma secondary to eye inflammation, <u>right</u> eye
H40.42x- Glaucoma secondary to eye inflammation, <u>left</u> eye
H40.43x- Glaucoma secondary to eye inflammation, <u>bilateral</u>

H40.5- Glaucoma <u>secondary to other eye disorders</u>
Code also underlying eye disorder

One of the following 7th characters is to be assigned to code H40.5- to designate the stage of glaucoma:
0   Stage unspecified
1   Mild stage
2   Moderate stage
3   Severe stage
4   Indeterminate stage

H40.50x- Glaucoma secondary to other eye disorders, <u>unspecified</u> eye
H40.51x- Glaucoma secondary to other eye disorders, <u>right</u> eye
H40.52x- Glaucoma secondary to other eye disorders, <u>left</u> eye
H40.53x- Glaucoma secondary to other eye disorders, <u>bilateral</u>

H40.6- Glaucoma <u>secondary to drugs</u>
Use additional code for adverse effect, if applicable, to identify drug (T36-T50 with fifth or sixth character 5)

One of the following 7th characters is to be assigned to code H40.6- to designate the stage of glaucoma:
0   Stage unspecified
1   Mild stage
2   Moderate stage
3   Severe stage
4   Indeterminate stage

H40.60x- Glaucoma secondary to drugs, <u>unspecified</u> eye
H40.61x- Glaucoma secondary to drugs, <u>right</u> eye
H40.62x- Glaucoma secondary to drugs, <u>left</u> eye
H40.63x- Glaucoma secondary to drugs, <u>bilateral</u>

H40.8- <u>Other</u> glaucoma

H40.81- Glaucoma <u>with increased episcleral venous pressure</u> — A form due to increased venous pressure of the scleral vessels.

H40.811 Glaucoma with increased episcleral venous pressure, <u>right</u> eye
H40.812 Glaucoma with increased episcleral venous pressure, <u>left</u> eye
H40.813 Glaucoma with increased episcleral venous pressure, <u>bilateral</u>
H40.819 Glaucoma with increased episcleral venous pressure, <u>unspecified</u> eye

H40.82- <u>Hypersecretion</u> glaucoma — A form due to increased production of aqueous.

H40.821 Hypersecretion glaucoma, <u>right</u> eye
H40.822 Hypersecretion glaucoma, <u>left</u> eye

H40.823   Hypersecretion glaucoma, **bilateral**

H40.829   Hypersecretion glaucoma, **unspecified** eye

H40.83- **Aqueous misdirection** — An abnormal increase in intraocular pressure caused by the flow of aqueous back into the central cavity of eye, rather than forward.

   Malignant glaucoma

H40.831   Aqueous misdirection, **right** eye

H40.832   Aqueous misdirection, **left** eye

H40.833   Aqueous misdirection, **bilateral**

H40.839   Aqueous misdirection, **unspecified** eye

H40.89 Other specified glaucoma

H40.9   Unspecified glaucoma

H42   Glaucoma **in diseases classified elsewhere** — [Not Allowed as PDX]
Code first underlying condition, such as:
   Amyloidosis (E85.-)
   Aniridia (Q13.1)
   Lowe's syndrome (E72.03)
   Reiger's anomaly (Q13.81)
   Specified metabolic disorder (E70-E88)
Excludes 1:   *glaucoma (in) onchocerciasis (B73.02)*
         glaucoma (in) syphilis (A52.71)
         glaucoma (in) tuberculous (A18.59)
Excludes ❷: *glaucoma (in) diabetes mellitus (E08.39, E09.39, E10.39,*
         E11.39, E13.39)

Disorders of vitreous body and globe (H43-H44)

H43- **Disorders of vitreous body**

H43.0- Vitreous **prolapse** — The downward displacement of the vitreous body.
   Excludes 1:   *vitreous syndrome following cataract surgery (H59.0-)*
            traumatic vitreous prolapse (S05.2-)

H43.00 Vitreous prolapse, **unspecified** eye

H43.01 Vitreous prolapse, **right** eye

H43.02 Vitreous prolapse, **left** eye

H43.03 Vitreous prolapse, **bilateral**

H43.1- Vitreous **hemorrhage** — The abnormal escape of blood into the vitreous.

H43.10 Vitreous hemorrhage, **unspecified** eye

H43.11 Vitreous hemorrhage, **right** eye

H43.12 Vitreous hemorrhage, **left** eye

H43.13 Vitreous hemorrhage, **bilateral**

H43.2- **Crystalline deposits** in vitreous body — The deposition of angular solids within the vitreous.

H43.20 Crystalline deposits in vitreous body, **unspecified** eye

H43.21 Crystalline deposits in vitreous body, **right** eye

H43.22 Crystalline deposits In vitreous body, **left** eye

H43.23 Crystalline deposits in vitreous body, **bilateral**

H43.3- Other vitreous opacities

H43.31- **Vitreous membranes and strands** — The formation of abnormal vitreous membranes or strands of tissue.

H43.311   Vitreous membranes and strands, **right** eye

H43.312   Vitreous membranes and strands, **left** eye

H43.313   Vitreous membranes and strands, **bilateral**

H43.319   Vitreous membranes and strands, **unspecified** eye

H43.39- **Other** vitreous **opacities**
   Vitreous floaters — Small particles of proteins or cells which float in the vitreous body.

H43.391   Other vitreous opacities, **right** eye

H43.392   Other vitreous opacities, **left** eye

H43.393   Other vitreous opacities, **bilateral**

H43.399   Other vitreous opacities, **unspecified** eye

H43.8- Other disorders of vitreous body
   Excludes 1:   *proliferative vitreo-retinopathy with retinal detachment*
            (H33.4-)
   Excludes ❷: *vitreous abscess (H44.02-)*

H43.81- **Vitreous degeneration** — Deterioration of vitreous and its functional ability.
   Vitreous detachment — A form marked by separation of lining membrane from the retina.

H43.811   Vitreous degeneration, **right** eye

H43.812   Vitreous degeneration, **left** eye

H43.813   Vitreous degeneration, **bilateral**

H43.819   Vitreous degeneration, **unspecified** eye

H43.82- **Vitreomacular adhesion** — The abnormal persistent attachment of the membrane separating the vitreous gel and the macula (which normally separates during the aging process) that may result in retinal deformity or damage and cause visual impairment.
   Vitreomacular traction

H43.821   Vitreomacular adhesion, **right** eye — [Age/15-124]

H43.822   Vitreomacular adhesion, **left** eye — [Age/15-124]

H43.823   Vitreomacular adhesion, **bilateral** — [Age/15-124]

H43.829   Vitreomacular adhesion, **unspecified** eye —
         [Age/15-124]

H43.89 Other disorders of vitreous body

H43.9   Unspecified disorder of vitreous body

H44- **Disorders of globe**
   Includes: Disorders affecting multiple structures of eye

H44.0- **Purulent endophthalmitis** — A pus-producing inflammation of the ocular cavities.
   Use additional code to identify organism
   Excludes 1:   *bleb associated endophthalmitis (H59.4-)*

H44.00- **Unspecified** purulent endophthalmitis

cc H44.001   Unspecified purulent endophthalmitis, **right** eye

cc H44.002   Unspecified purulent endophthalmitis, **left** eye

cc H44.003   Unspecified purulent endophthalmitis, **bilateral**

cc H44.009   Unspecified purulent endophthalmitis, **unspecified** eye

H44.01- **Panophthalmitis (acute)** — Inflammation of all of the structures or tissues of the eye.

cc H44.011   Panophthalmitis (acute), **right** eye

cc H44.012   Panophthalmitis (acute), **left** eye

cc H44.013   Panophthalmitis (acute), **bilateral**

cc H44.019   Panophthalmitis (acute), **unspecified** eye

H44.02- **Vitreous abscess (chronic)** — A localized collection of pus caused by the disintegration of vitreous tissues.

cc H44.021   Vitreous abscess (chronic), **right** eye

cc H44.022   Vitreous abscess (chronic), **left** eye

cc H44.023   Vitreous abscess (chronic), **bilateral**

cc H44.029   Vitreous abscess (chronic), **unspecified** eye

H44.1- **Other** endophthalmitis
   Excludes 1:   *bleb associated endophthalmitis (H59.4-)*
   Excludes ❷: *ophthalmia nodosa (H16.2-)*

H44.11- **Panuveitis** — Inflammation of the entire uveal tract.

cc H44.111   Panuveitis, **right** eye

cc H44.112   Panuveitis, **left** eye

cc H44.113   Panuveitis, **bilateral**

cc H44.119   Panuveitis, **unspecified** eye

H44.12- **Parasitic endophthalmitis**, unspecified

cc H44.121   Parasitic endophthalmitis, unspecified, **right** eye

cc H44.122   Parasitic endophthalmitis, unspecified, **left** eye

cc H44.123   Parasitic endophthalmitis, unspecified, **bilateral**

cc H44.129   Parasitic endophthalmitis, unspecified, **unspecified** eye

H44.13- **Sympathetic uveitis** — Granulomatous inflammation of the uveal tract.

cc H44.131   Sympathetic uveitis, **right** eye

cc H44.132   Sympathetic uveitis, **left** eye

cc H44.133   Sympathetic uveitis, **bilateral**

cc H44.139   Sympathetic uveitis, **unspecified** eye

cc H44.19 Other endophthalmitis

H44.2- **Degenerative myopia** — Progressive nearsightedness leading to retinal detachment and blindness.
   Malignant myopia

H44.20 Degenerative myopia, **unspecified** eye

H44.21 Degenerative myopia, **right** eye

H44.22 Degenerative myopia, **left** eye

H44.23 Degenerative myopia, **bilateral**

H44.3- Other and unspecified degenerative disorders of globe

H44.30 Unspecified degenerative disorder of globe

H44.31- **Chalcosis** — The abnormal presence of copper in the globe.

H40 – H44

Excludes 1: = NOT CODED HERE! (Do not code both)   *Excludes ❷:* = Not Included Here

H44.311 Chalcosis, **right** eye

H44.312 Chalcosis, **left** eye

H44.313 Chalcosis, **bilateral**

H44.319 Chalcosis, **unspecified** eye

H44.32- **Siderosis** of eye — The abnormal deposit of iron in the conjunctiva marked by a rust-brown or yellowish discoloration.

H44.321 Siderosis of eye, **right** eye

H44.322 Siderosis of eye, **left** eye

H44.323 Siderosis of eye, **bilateral**

H44.329 Siderosis of eye, **unspecified** eye

H44.39- **Other** degenerative disorders of globe

H44.391 Other degenerative disorders of globe, **right** eye

H44.392 Other degenerative disorders of globe, **left** eye

H44.393 Other degenerative disorders of globe, **bilateral**

H44.399 Other degenerative disorders of globe, **unspecified** eye

H44.4- **Hypotony** of eye — Low intraocular pressure.

H44.40 **Unspecified** hypotony of eye

H44.41- **Flat anterior chamber** hypotony of eye — A condition characterized by loss of intraocular fluid within the anterior chamber resulting in compression of the chamber from surrounding tissues.

H44.411 Flat anterior chamber hypotony of **right** eye

H44.412 Flat anterior chamber hypotony of **left** eye

H44.413 Flat anterior chamber hypotony of eye, **bilateral**

H44.419 Flat anterior chamber hypotony of **unspecified** eye

H44.42- Hypotony of eye **due to ocular fistula** — An abnormal passage for the intraocular cavities resulting in decreased intraocular pressure.

H44.421 Hypotony of **right** eye due to ocular fistula

H44.422 Hypotony of **left** eye due to ocular fistula

H44.423 Hypotony of eye due to ocular fistula, **bilateral**

H44.429 Hypotony of **unspecified** eye due to ocular fistula

H44.43- Hypotony of eye **due to other ocular disorders**

H44.431 Hypotony of eye due to other ocular disorders, **right** eye

H44.432 Hypotony of eye due to other ocular disorders, **left** eye

H44.433 Hypotony of eye due to other ocular disorders, **bilateral**

H44.439 Hypotony of eye due to other ocular disorders, **unspecified** eye

H44.44- **Primary** hypotony of eye — Low intraocular pressure without a determinate cause.

H44.441 Primary hypotony of **right** eye

H44.442 Primary hypotony of **left** eye

H44.443 Primary hypotony of eye, **bilateral**

H44.449 Primary hypotony of **unspecified** eye

H44.5- **Degenerated conditions of globe**

H44.50 **Unspecified** degenerated conditions of globe

H44.51- **Absolute glaucoma** — The final stage of glaucoma characterized by pain in the eye and blindness.

H44.511 Absolute glaucoma, **right** eye

H44.512 Absolute glaucoma, **left** eye

H44.513 Absolute glaucoma, **bilateral**

H44.519 Absolute glaucoma, **unspecified** eye

H44.52- **Atrophy** of globe — A wasting-away of the globe tissues.
Phthisis bulbi

H44.521 Atrophy of globe, **right** eye

H44.522 Atrophy of globe, **left** eye

H44.523 Atrophy of globe, **bilateral**

H44.529 Atrophy of globe, **unspecified** eye

H44.53- **Leucocoria** — A reflection from the pupil due to the presence of a whitish mass in the pupillary area of the eye.

H44.531 Leucocoria, **right** eye

H44.532 Leucocoria, **left** eye

H44.533 Leucocoria, **bilateral**

H44.539 Leucocoria, **unspecified** eye

H44.6- **Retained (old) intraocular foreign body, magnetic** — The existing, noncurrent presence of a nonocular tissue particle that contains iron (or other magnetic elements), and is located within the intraocular tissues.

Use additional code to identify magnetic foreign body (Z18.11)

Excludes 1: *current intraocular foreign body (S05.-)*

Excludes ❷: *retained foreign body in eyelid (H02.81-)*
retained (old) foreign body following penetrating wound of orbit (H05.5-)
retained (old) intraocular foreign body, nonmagnetic (H44.7-)

H44.60- **Unspecified** retained (old) intraocular foreign body, **magnetic**

H44.601 Unspecified retained (old) intraocular foreign body, magnetic, **right** eye

H44.602 Unspecified retained (old) intraocular foreign body, magnetic, **left** eye

H44.603 Unspecified retained (old) intraocular foreign body, magnetic, **bilateral**

H44.609 Unspecified retained (old) intraocular foreign body, magnetic, **unspecified** eye

H44.61- Retained (old) **magnetic** foreign body **in anterior chamber**

H44.611 Retained (old) magnetic foreign body in anterior chamber, **right** eye

H44.612 Retained (old) magnetic foreign body in anterior chamber, **left** eye

H44.613 Retained (old) magnetic foreign body in anterior chamber, **bilateral**

H44.619 Retained (old) magnetic foreign body in anterior chamber, **unspecified** eye

H44.62- Retained (old) **magnetic** foreign body **in iris or ciliary body**

H44.621 Retained (old) magnetic foreign body in iris or ciliary body, **right** eye

H44.622 Retained (old) magnetic foreign body in iris or ciliary body, **left** eye

H44.623 Retained (old) magnetic foreign body in iris or ciliary body, **bilateral**

H44.629 Retained (old) magnetic foreign body in iris or ciliary body, **unspecified** eye

H44.63- Retained (old) **magnetic** foreign body **in lens**

H44.631 Retained (old) magnetic foreign body in lens, **right** eye

H44.632 Retained (old) magnetic foreign body in lens, **left** eye

H44.633 Retained (old) magnetic foreign body in lens, **bilateral**

H44.639 Retained (old) magnetic foreign body in lens, **unspecified** eye

H44.64- Retained (old) **magnetic** foreign body **in posterior wall of globe**

H44.641 Retained (old) magnetic foreign body in posterior wall of globe, **right** eye

H44.642 Retained (old) magnetic foreign body in posterior wall of globe, **left** eye

H44.643 Retained (old) magnetic foreign body in posterior wall of globe, **bilateral**

H44.649 Retained (old) magnetic foreign body in posterior wall of globe, **unspecified** eye

H44.65- Retained (old) **magnetic** foreign body **in vitreous body**

H44.651 Retained (old) magnetic foreign body in vitreous body, **right** eye

H44.652 Retained (old) magnetic foreign body in vitreous body, **left** eye

H44.653 Retained (old) magnetic foreign body in vitreous body, **bilateral**

H44.659 Retained (old) magnetic foreign body in vitreous body, **unspecified** eye

H44-H44

H44.69- Retained (old) intraocular foreign body, <u>magnetic, in other or multiple sites</u>

    H44.691 Retained (old) intraocular foreign body, magnetic, in other or multiple sites, <u>right</u> eye

    H44.692 Retained (old) intraocular foreign body, magnetic, in other or multiple sites, <u>left</u> eye

    H44.693 Retained (old) intraocular foreign body, magnetic, in other or multiple sites, <u>bilateral</u>

    H44.699 Retained (old) intraocular foreign body, magnetic, in other or multiple sites, <u>unspecified</u> eye

H44.7- <u>Retained (old) intraocular foreign body, nonmagnetic</u> — The existing, noncurrent presence of a nonocular tissue particle or mass that contains no iron (or other magnetic elements), and is located within the intraocular tissues.

  Use additional code to identify nonmagnetic foreign body (Z18.01-Z18.10, Z18.12, Z18.2-Z18.9)

  Excludes 1: *current intraocular foreign body (S05.-)*

  Excludes ❷: *retained foreign body in eyelid (H02.81-)*
    retained (old) foreign body following penetrating wound of orbit (H05.5-)
    retained (old) intraocular foreign body, magnetic (H44.6-)

H44.70- <u>Unspecified</u> retained (old) intraocular foreign body, <u>nonmagnetic</u>

    H44.701 Unspecified retained (old) intraocular foreign body, nonmagnetic, <u>right</u> eye

    H44.702 Unspecified retained (old) intraocular foreign body, nonmagnetic, <u>left</u> eye

    H44.703 Unspecified retained (old) intraocular foreign body, nonmagnetic, <u>bilateral</u>

    H44.709 Unspecified retained (old) intraocular foreign body, nonmagnetic, <u>unspecified</u> eye
        Retained (old) intraocular foreign body NOS

H44.71- Retained (<u>nonmagnetic</u>) (old) foreign body <u>in anterior chamber</u>

    H44.711 Retained (nonmagnetic) (old) foreign body in anterior chamber, <u>right</u> eye

    H44.712 Retained (nonmagnetic) (old) foreign body in anterior chamber, <u>left</u> eye

    H44.713 Retained (nonmagnetic) (old) foreign body in anterior chamber, <u>bilateral</u>

    H44.719 Retained (nonmagnetic) (old) foreign body in anterior chamber, <u>unspecified</u> eye

H44.72- Retained (<u>nonmagnetic</u>) (old) foreign body <u>in iris or ciliary body</u>

    H44.721 Retained (nonmagnetic) (old) foreign body in iris or ciliary body, <u>right</u> eye

    H44.722 Retained (nonmagnetic) (old) foreign body in iris or ciliary body, <u>left</u> eye

    H44.723 Retained (nonmagnetic) (old) foreign body in iris or ciliary body, <u>bilateral</u>

    H44.729 Retained (nonmagnetic) (old) foreign body in iris or ciliary body, <u>unspecified</u> eye

H44.73- Retained (<u>nonmagnetic</u>) (old) foreign body <u>in lens</u>

    H44.731 Retained (nonmagnetic) (old) foreign body in lens, <u>right</u> eye

    H44.732 Retained (nonmagnetic) (old) foreign body in lens, <u>left</u> eye

    H44.733 Retained (nonmagnetic) (old) foreign body in lens, <u>bilateral</u>

    H44.739 Retained (nonmagnetic) (old) foreign body in lens, <u>unspecified</u> eye

H44.74- Retained (<u>nonmagnetic</u>) (old) foreign body <u>in posterior wall of globe</u>

    H44.741 Retained (nonmagnetic) (old) foreign body in posterior wall of globe, <u>right</u> eye

    H44.742 Retained (nonmagnetic) (old) foreign body in posterior wall of globe, <u>left</u> eye

    H44.743 Retained (nonmagnetic) (old) foreign body in posterior wall of globe, <u>bilateral</u>

    H44.749 Retained (nonmagnetic) (old) foreign body in posterior wall of globe, <u>unspecified</u> eye

H44.75- Retained (<u>nonmagnetic</u>) (old) foreign body <u>in vitreous body</u>

    H44.751 Retained (nonmagnetic) (old) foreign body in vitreous body, <u>right</u> eye

    H44.752 Retained (nonmagnetic) (old) foreign body in vitreous body, <u>left</u> eye

    H44.753 Retained (nonmagnetic) (old) foreign body in vitreous body, <u>bilateral</u>

    H44.759 Retained (nonmagnetic) (old) foreign body in vitreous body, <u>unspecified</u> eye

H44.79- Retained (old) intraocular foreign body, <u>nonmagnetic, in other or multiple sites</u>

    H44.791 Retained (old) intraocular foreign body, nonmagnetic, in other or multiple sites, <u>right</u> eye

    H44.792 Retained (old) intraocular foreign body, nonmagnetic, in other or multiple sites, <u>left</u> eye

    H44.793 Retained (old) intraocular foreign body, nonmagnetic, in other or multiple sites, <u>bilateral</u>

    H44.799 Retained (old) intraocular foreign body, nonmagnetic, in other or multiple sites, <u>unspecified</u> eye

H44.8- Other disorders of globe

  H44.81- <u>Hemophthalmos</u> — Diffusion of blood into the eyeball.

    H44.811 Hemophthalmos, <u>right</u> eye

    H44.812 Hemophthalmos, <u>left</u> eye

    H44.813 Hemophthalmos, <u>bilateral</u>

    H44.819 Hemophthalmos, <u>unspecified</u> eye

  H44.82- <u>Luxation of globe</u> — The abnormal dislocation or displacement of the globe and its tissues.

    H44.821 Luxation of globe, <u>right</u> eye

    H44.822 Luxation of globe, <u>left</u> eye

    H44.823 Luxation of globe, <u>bilateral</u>

    H44.829 Luxation of globe, <u>unspecified</u> eye

  H44.89 Other disorders of globe

H44.9 Unspecified disorder of globe

Disorders of optic nerve and visual pathways (H46-H47)

H46- <u>Optic neuritis</u> — Inflammation of the optic nerve within the eyeball.
  Excludes ❷: *ischemic optic neuropathy (H47.01-)*
    neuromyelitis optica [Devic] (G36.0)

  H46.0- <u>Optic papillitis</u> — Inflammation of the optic disc.

  cc **H46.00** Optic papillitis, <u>unspecified</u> eye

  cc **H46.01** Optic papillitis, <u>right</u> eye

  cc **H46.02** Optic papillitis, <u>left</u> eye

  cc **H46.03** Optic papillitis, <u>bilateral</u>

  H46.1- <u>Retrobulbar neuritis</u> — The sudden, severe onset of inflammation of that portion of the optic nerve which is behind the eyeball.
    Retrobulbar neuritis NOS
    Excludes 1: *syphilitic retrobulbar neuritis (A52.15)*

  cc **H46.10** Retrobulbar neuritis, <u>unspecified</u> eye

  cc **H46.11** Retrobulbar neuritis, <u>right</u> eye

  cc **H46.12** Retrobulbar neuritis, <u>left</u> eye

  cc **H46.13** Retrobulbar neuritis, <u>bilateral</u>

  H46.2 Nutritional optic neuropathy — A disorder of the optic nerve due to a defect in nutrition.

  H46.3 Toxic optic neuropathy — A disorder of the optic nerve due to the toxic effect of substances.
    Code first (T51-T65) to identify cause

  cc **H46.8** Other optic neuritis

  cc **H46.9** Unspecified optic neuritis

H47- Other disorders of optic [2nd] nerve and visual pathways

  H47.0- Disorders of optic nerve, not elsewhere classified

    H47.01- <u>Ischemic optic neuropathy</u> — A disorder of the optic nerve due to a deficient blood supply.

      H47.011 Ischemic optic neuropathy, <u>right</u> eye

      H47.012 Ischemic optic neuropathy, <u>left</u> eye

      H47.013 Ischemic optic neuropathy, <u>bilateral</u>

H44 - H47

Excludes 1: = NOT CODED HERE! (Do not code both)   **701**   *Excludes ❷:* = Not Included Here

H47.019   Ischemic optic neuropathy, <u>unspecified</u> eye

H47.02- <u>Hemorrhage</u> in optic nerve sheath — The escape of blood within the covering of the optic nerve.

H47.021   Hemorrhage in optic nerve sheath, <u>right</u> eye

H47.022   Hemorrhage in optic nerve sheath, <u>left</u> eye

H47.023   Hemorrhage in optic nerve sheath, <u>bilateral</u>

H47.029   Hemorrhage in optic nerve sheath, <u>unspecified</u> eye

H47.03- Optic nerve <u>hypoplasia</u> — The congenital condition of underdevelopment of one or both optic nerves that results in varying degrees of vision loss.

H47.031   Optic nerve hypoplasia, <u>right</u> eye

H47.032   Optic nerve hypoplasia, <u>left</u> eye

H47.033   Optic nerve hypoplasia, <u>bilateral</u>

H47.039   Optic nerve hypoplasia, <u>unspecified</u> eye

H47.09- <u>Other disorders of optic nerve, not elsewhere classified</u>

Compression of optic nerve — The forced pressure upon the optic nerve.

H47.091   Other disorders of optic nerve, not elsewhere classified, <u>right</u> eye

H47.092   Other disorders of optic nerve, not elsewhere classified, <u>left</u> eye

H47.093   Other disorders of optic nerve, not elsewhere classified, <u>bilateral</u>

H47.099   Other disorders of optic nerve, not elsewhere classified, <u>unspecified</u> eye

H47.1- <u>Papilledema</u> — The abnormal accumulation of intercellular fluid of the optic nerve within the eyeball.

cc **H47.10**   Unspecified papilledema

cc **H47.11**   Papilledema associated with increased intracranial pressure

H47.12   Papilledema associated with decreased ocular pressure

H47.13   Papilledema associated with retinal disorder

H47.14- <u>Foster-Kennedy syndrome</u> — A form associated with optic neuritis and optic atrophy.

H47.141   Foster-Kennedy syndrome, <u>right</u> eye

H47.142   Foster-Kennedy syndrome, <u>left</u> eye

H47.143   Foster-Kennedy syndrome, <u>bilateral</u>

H47.149   Foster-Kennedy syndrome, <u>unspecified</u> eye

H47.2- <u>Optic atrophy</u> — The abnormal wasting-away of the optic nerve within the eyeball.

H47.20   <u>Unspecified</u> optic atrophy

H47.21- <u>Primary</u> optic atrophy — A form resulting from a condition of the optic nerve.

H47.211   Primary optic atrophy, <u>right</u> eye

H47.212   Primary optic atrophy, <u>left</u> eye

H47.213   Primary optic atrophy, <u>bilateral</u>

H47.219   Primary optic atrophy, <u>unspecified</u> eye

H47.22   <u>Hereditary</u> optic atrophy — A form inherited from one's parents.

Leber's optic atrophy — A form marked by progressive optic atrophy, with onset usually in males in their twenties.

H47.23- <u>Glaucomatous</u> optic atrophy — A form resulting from the continuous effects of glaucoma upon the optic disc.

H47.231   Glaucomatous optic atrophy, <u>right</u> eye

H47.232   Glaucomatous optic atrophy, <u>left</u> eye

H47.233   Glaucomatous optic atrophy, <u>bilateral</u>

H47.239   Glaucomatous optic atrophy, <u>unspecified</u> eye

H47.29- <u>Other</u> optic atrophy

Temporal pallor of optic disc — A form affecting only a portion of the optic disc.

H47.291   Other optic atrophy, <u>right</u> eye

H47.292   Other optic atrophy, <u>left</u> eye

H47.293   Other optic atrophy, <u>bilateral</u>

H47.299   Other optic atrophy, <u>unspecified</u> eye

H47.3- <u>Other disorders of optic disc</u>

H47.31- <u>Coloboma</u> of optic disc — A defect of the optic disc resulting from a failure of the fetal fissure to close.

H47.311   Coloboma of optic disc, <u>right</u> eye

H47.312   Coloboma of optic disc, <u>left</u> eye

H47.313   Coloboma of optic disc, <u>bilateral</u>

H47.319   Coloboma of optic disc, <u>unspecified</u> eye

H47.32- <u>Drusen</u> of optic disc — The whitish, hyaline lesions of the optic disc.

H47.321   Drusen of optic disc, <u>right</u> eye

H47.322   Drusen of optic disc, <u>left</u> eye

H47.323   Drusen of optic disc, <u>bilateral</u>

H47.329   Drusen of optic disc, <u>unspecified</u> eye

H47.33- <u>Pseudopapilledema</u> of optic disc — The abnormal elevation of the optic disc.

H47.331   Pseudopapilledema of optic disc, <u>right</u> eye

H47.332   Pseudopapilledema of optic disc, <u>left</u> eye

H47.333   Pseudopapilledema of optic disc, <u>bilateral</u>

H47.339   Pseudopapilledema of optic disc, <u>unspecified</u> eye

H47.39- <u>Other</u> disorders of optic disc

H47.391   Other disorders of optic disc, <u>right</u> eye

H47.392   Other disorders of optic disc, <u>left</u> eye

H47.393   Other disorders of optic disc, <u>bilateral</u>

H47.399   Other disorders of optic disc, <u>unspecified</u> eye

H47.4- Disorders of optic chiasm — Conditions resulting from effects upon the crossing of the optic nerves.

Code also underlying condition

cc **H47.41**   Disorders of optic chiasm in (due to) inflammatory disorders

cc **H47.42**   Disorders of optic chiasm in (due to) neoplasm

cc **H47.43**   Disorders of optic chiasm in (due to) vascular disorders

cc **H47.49**   Disorders of optic chiasm in (due to) other disorders

H47.5- <u>Disorders of other visual pathways</u> — Conditions resulting from disturbances of the optic nerve other than the optic chiasm.

Disorders of optic tracts, geniculate nuclei and optic radiations

Code also underlying condition

H47.51- Disorders of visual pathways <u>in (due to) inflammatory disorders</u>

cc **H47.511**   Disorders of visual pathways in (due to) inflammatory disorders, <u>right</u> side

cc **H47.512**   Disorders of visual pathways in (due to) inflammatory disorders, <u>left</u> side

cc **H47.519**   Disorders of visual pathways in (due to) inflammatory disorders, <u>unspecified</u> side

H47.52- Disorders of visual pathways <u>in (due to) neoplasm</u>

cc **H47.521**   Disorders of visual pathways in (due to) neoplasm, <u>right</u> side

cc **H47.522**   Disorders of visual pathways in (due to) neoplasm, <u>left</u> side

cc **H47.529**   Disorders of visual pathways in (due to) neoplasm, <u>unspecified</u> side

H47.53- Disorders of visual pathways <u>in (due to) vascular disorders</u>

cc **H47.531**   Disorders of visual pathways in (due to) vascular disorders, <u>right</u> side

cc **H47.532**   Disorders of visual pathways in (due to) vascular disorders, <u>left</u> side

cc **H47.539**   Disorders of visual pathways in (due to) vascular disorders, <u>unspecified</u> side

H47.6- <u>Disorders of visual cortex</u> — Conditions resulting from disturbances of the visual centers of the brain.

Code also underlying condition

Excludes 1:   injury to visual cortex S04.04

H47.61- <u>Cortical blindness</u> — Blindness resulting from a lesion of the visual area of the cerebral cortex.

H47.611   Cortical blindness, <u>right</u> side of brain

H47.612   Cortical blindness, <u>left</u> side of brain

H47.619   Cortical blindness, <u>unspecified</u> side of brain

H47.62- Disorders of visual cortex <u>in (due to) inflammatory disorders</u>

cc **H47.621**   Disorders of visual cortex in (due to) inflammatory disorders, <u>right</u> side of brain

cc **H47.622**   Disorders of visual cortex in (due to) inflammatory disorders, <u>left</u> side of brain

Side tab: **H47-H47**

cc **H47.629** Disorders of visual cortex in (due to) inflammatory disorders, <u>unspecified</u> side of brain

H47.63- Disorders of visual cortex <u>in (due to) neoplasm</u>

cc **H47.631** Disorders of visual cortex in (due to) neoplasm, <u>right</u> side of brain

cc **H47.632** Disorders of visual cortex in (due to) neoplasm, <u>left</u> side of brain

cc **H47.639** Disorders of visual cortex in (due to) neoplasm, <u>unspecified</u> side of brain

H47.64- Disorders of visual cortex <u>in (due to) vascular disorders</u>

cc **H47.641** Disorders of visual cortex in (due to) vascular disorders, <u>right</u> side of brain

cc **H47.642** Disorders of visual cortex in (due to) vascular disorders, <u>left</u> side of brain

cc **H47.649** Disorders of visual cortex in (due to) vascular disorders, <u>unspecified</u> side of brain

H47.9 Unspecified disorder of visual pathways

Disorders of ocular muscles, binocular movement, accommodation and refraction (H49-H52)

Excludes ❷: nystagmus and other irregular eye movements (H55)

H49- <u>Paralytic strabismus</u> — Deviation due to paralysis of an extraocular muscle.

Excludes ❷: internal ophthalmoplegia (H52.51-)
        internuclear ophthalmoplegia (H51.2-)
        progressive supranuclear ophthalmoplegia (G23.1)

H49.0- <u>Third</u> [oculomotor] nerve palsy

H49.00 Third [oculomotor] nerve palsy, <u>unspecified</u> eye

H49.01 Third [oculomotor] nerve palsy, <u>right</u> eye

H49.02 Third [oculomotor] nerve palsy, <u>left</u> eye

H49.03 Third [oculomotor] nerve palsy, <u>bilateral</u>

H49.1- <u>Fourth</u> [trochlear] nerve palsy

H49.10 Fourth [trochlear] nerve palsy, <u>unspecified</u> eye

H49.11 Fourth [trochlear] nerve palsy, <u>right</u> eye

H49.12 Fourth [trochlear] nerve palsy, <u>left</u> eye

H49.13 Fourth [trochlear] nerve palsy, <u>bilateral</u>

H49.2- <u>Sixth</u> [abducent] nerve palsy

H49.20 Sixth [abducent] nerve palsy, <u>unspecified</u> eye

H49.21 Sixth [abducent] nerve palsy, <u>right</u> eye

H49.22 Sixth [abducent] nerve palsy, <u>left</u> eye

H49.23 Sixth [abducent] nerve palsy, <u>bilateral</u>

H49.3- <u>Total</u> (external) ophthalmoplegia — Paralysis of the external and internal ocular muscles.

H49.30 Total (external) ophthalmoplegia, <u>unspecified</u> eye

H49.31 Total (external) ophthalmoplegia, <u>right</u> eye

H49.32 Total (external) ophthalmoplegia, <u>left</u> eye

H49.33 Total (external) ophthalmoplegia, <u>bilateral</u>

H49.4- <u>Progressive</u> external ophthalmoplegia — Paralysis which progresses from one extraocular muscle to another.

Excludes 1: Kearns-Sayre syndrome (H49.81-)

H49.40 Progressive external ophthalmoplegia, <u>unspecified</u> eye

H49.41 Progressive external ophthalmoplegia, <u>right</u> eye

H49.42 Progressive external ophthalmoplegia, <u>left</u> eye

H49.43 Progressive external ophthalmoplegia, <u>bilateral</u>

H49.8- Other paralytic strabismus

H49.81- <u>Kearns-Sayre syndrome</u> — A rare neuromuscular disorder that is characterized by paralysis which progresses from one extraocular muscle to another and is associated with pigmentary retinopathy.

Progressive external ophthalmoplegia with pigmentary retinopathy

Use additional code for other manifestation, such as:
Heart block (I45.9)

cc **H49.811** Kearns-Sayre syndrome, <u>right</u> eye

cc **H49.812** Kearns-Sayre syndrome, <u>left</u> eye

cc **H49.813** Kearns-Sayre syndrome, <u>bilateral</u>

cc **H49.819** Kearns-Sayre syndrome, <u>unspecified</u> eye

H49.88- <u>Other</u> paralytic strabismus — Paralysis of the external ocular muscles.

External ophthalmoplegia NOS

H49.881 Other paralytic strabismus, <u>right</u> eye

H49.882 Other paralytic strabismus, <u>left</u> eye

H49.883 Other paralytic strabismus, <u>bilateral</u>

H49.889 Other paralytic strabismus, <u>unspecified</u> eye

H49.9 Unspecified paralytic strabismus

H50- Other strabismus

H50.0- <u>Esotropia</u> — The turning inward of the eyes.

Convergent concomitant strabismus — Esotropia due to faulty insertion of eye muscles.

Excludes 1: intermittent esotropia (H50.31-, H50.32)

H50.00 <u>Unspecified</u> esotropia

H50.01- <u>Monocular</u> esotropia — A form characterized by affecting only one eye.

H50.011 Monocular esotropia, <u>right</u> eye

H50.012 Monocular esotropia, <u>left</u> eye

H50.02- Monocular esotropia <u>with A pattern</u>

H50.021 Monocular esotropia with A pattern, <u>right</u> eye

H50.022 Monocular esotropia with A pattern, <u>left</u> eye

H50.03- Monocular esotropia <u>with V pattern</u>

H50.031 Monocular esotropia with V pattern, <u>right</u> eye

H50.032 Monocular esotropia with V pattern, <u>left</u> eye

H50.04- Monocular esotropia <u>with other noncomitancies</u>

H50.041 Monocular esotropia with other noncomitancies, <u>right</u> eye

H50.042 Monocular esotropia with other noncomitancies, <u>left</u> eye

H50.05 Alternating esotropia — A form characterized by affecting each eye alternately.

H50.06 Alternating esotropia with A pattern

H50.07 Alternating esotropia with V pattern

H50.08 Alternating esotropia with other noncomitancies

H50.1- <u>Exotropia</u> — The turning outward of the eyes.

Divergent concomitant strabismus

Excludes 1: intermittent exotropia (H50.33-, H50.34)

H50.10 <u>Unspecified</u> exotropia

H50.11- <u>Monocular</u> exotropia — A form characterized by affecting only one eye.

H50.111 Monocular exotropia, <u>right</u> eye

H50.112 Monocular exotropia, <u>left</u> eye

H50.12- Monocular exotropia <u>with A pattern</u>

H50.121 Monocular exotropia with A pattern, <u>right</u> eye

H50.122 Monocular exotropia with A pattern, <u>left</u> eye

H50.13- Monocular exotropia <u>with V pattern</u>

H50.131 Monocular exotropia with V pattern, <u>right</u> eye

H50.132 Monocular exotropia with V pattern, <u>left</u> eye

H50.14- Monocular exotropia <u>with other noncomitancies</u>

H50.141 Monocular exotropia with other noncomitancies, <u>right</u> eye

H50.142 Monocular exotropia with other noncomitancies, <u>left</u> eye

H50.15 Alternating exotropia — A form characterized by affecting each eye alternately.

H50.16 Alternating exotropia with A pattern

H50.17 Alternating exotropia with V pattern

H50.18 Alternating exotropia with other noncomitancies

H50.2- <u>Vertical strabismus</u> — Upward deviation of an eye.

Hypertropia

H50.21 Vertical strabismus, <u>right</u> eye

H50.22 Vertical strabismus, <u>left</u> eye

H50.3- <u>Intermittent heterotropia</u> — Deviation of the eyes that occurs at intervals.

H50.30 <u>Unspecified</u> intermittent heterotropia

H50.31- Intermittent <u>monocular</u> esotropia — Inward deviation of one eye occurring at intervals.

H50.311 Intermittent monocular esotropia, <u>right</u> eye

H50.312 Intermittent monocular esotropia, <u>left</u> eye

H50.32 Intermittent alternating esotropia — Inward deviation of alternating eyes occurring at intervals.

H50.33- Intermittent <u>monocular</u> exotropia — Outward deviation of one eye occurring at intervals.

H50.331 Intermittent monocular exotropia, <u>right</u> eye

H50.332 Intermittent monocular exotropia, <u>left</u> eye

H50.34 Intermittent alternating <u>exotropia</u> — Outward deviation of alternating eyes occurring at intervals.

H50.4- Other and unspecified heterotropia

H50.40 Unspecified heterotropia

H50.41- <u>Cyclotropia</u> — Rotational deviation of an eye.

H50.411 Cyclotropia, right eye

H50.412 Cyclotropia, left eye

H50.42 Monofixation syndrome — The mild deviation of an eye, which does not cause diplopia.

H50.43 Accommodative component in esotropia

H50.5- Heterophoria — Deviation after visual alignment.

H50.50 Unspecified heterophoria

H50.51 Esophoria — A form characterized by turning inward.

H50.52 Exophoria — A form characterized by turning outward.

H50.53 Vertical heterophoria — A form characterized by turning upward.

H50.54 Cyclophoria — A form characterized by rotational turning.

H50.55 Alternating heterophoria — A form characterized by affecting each eye alternately.

H50.6- Mechanical strabismus — Deviation due to external forces.

H50.60 Mechanical strabismus, unspecified

H50.61- Brown's sheath syndrome — A form affecting the extraocular tendon sheaths.

H50.611 Brown's sheath syndrome, <u>right</u> eye

H50.612 Brown's sheath syndrome, <u>left</u> eye

H50.69 Other mechanical strabismus
Strabismus due to adhesions
Traumatic limitation of duction of eye muscle

H50.8- Other specified strabismus

H50.81- Duane's syndrome — An inherited syndrome characterized by limitation of abduction and deficient convergence.

H50.811 Duane's syndrome, <u>right</u> eye

H50.812 Duane's syndrome, <u>left</u> eye

H50.89 Other specified strabismus

H50.9 Unspecified strabismus

H51- Other disorders of binocular movement

H51.0 Palsy (spasm) of conjugate gaze

H51.1- Convergence insufficiency and excess

H51.11 Convergence insufficiency — Impairment of convergence.

H51.12 Convergence excess — Overcompensation of convergence.

H51.2- <u>Internuclear ophthalmoplegia</u> — Paralysis of extraocular muscles due to a lesion between the nuclei of the motor nerves of the eye.

H51.20 Internuclear ophthalmoplegia, <u>unspecified</u> eye

H51.21 Internuclear ophthalmoplegia, <u>right</u> eye

H51.22 Internuclear ophthalmoplegia, <u>left</u> eye

H51.23 Internuclear ophthalmoplegia, <u>bilateral</u>

H51.8 Other specified disorders of binocular movement

H51.9 Unspecified disorder of binocular movement

H52- Disorders of refraction and accommodation — REFRACTION — The deflection or change of direction of light as it passes through the lens. ACCOMMODATION — The adjustment in the shape and curvature of the lens when looking far away and near.

H52.0- <u>Hypermetropia</u> — An error of refraction in which the focal point is behind the retina causing near objects to be out of focus (farsightedness).

H52.00 Hypermetropia, <u>unspecified</u> eye

H52.01 Hypermetropia, <u>right</u> eye

H52.02 Hypermetropia, <u>left</u> eye

H52.03 Hypermetropia, <u>bilateral</u>

H52.1- <u>Myopia</u> — An error of refraction in which the focal point is in front of the retina causing objects far away not to be in focus (nearsightedness).
Excludes 1: degenerative myopia (H44.2-)

H52.10 Myopia, <u>unspecified</u> eye

H52.11 Myopia, <u>right</u> eye

H52.12 Myopia, <u>left</u> eye

H52.13 Myopia, <u>bilateral</u>

H52.2- <u>Astigmatism</u> — An error in refraction in which light is not sharply focused to a point on the retina, but to a diffuse area of the retina.

H52.20- <u>Unspecified</u> astigmatism

H52.201 Unspecified astigmatism, <u>right</u> eye

H52.202 Unspecified astigmatism, <u>left</u> eye

H52.203 Unspecified astigmatism, <u>bilateral</u>

H52.209 Unspecified astigmatism, <u>unspecified</u> eye

H52.21- <u>Irregular</u> astigmatism — A form in which the diffuse focus is different from one meridian to the other.

H52.211 Irregular astigmatism, <u>right</u> eye

H52.212 Irregular astigmatism, <u>left</u> eye

H52.213 Irregular astigmatism, <u>bilateral</u>

H52.219 Irregular astigmatism, <u>unspecified</u> eye

H52.22- <u>Regular</u> astigmatism — A form in which the diffuse focus is uniform from one meridian to the other.

H52.221 Regular astigmatism, <u>right</u> eye

H52.222 Regular astigmatism, <u>left</u> eye

H52.223 Regular astigmatism, <u>bilateral</u>

H52.229 Regular astigmatism, <u>unspecified</u> eye

H52.3- Anisometropia and aniseikonia

H52.31 Anisometropia — A condition in which refractive power of the eyes is unequal.

H52.32 Aniseikonia — A condition in which the size and shape of the ocular image of one differs from that of the other.

H52.4 Presbyopia — A defect of vision in advancing age involving loss of accommodation or recession of near points, due to a loss of elasticity of the crystalline lens.

H52.5- <u>Disorders of accommodation</u> — The adjustment in the shape and curvature of the lens when looking far away and near.

H52.51- <u>Internal ophthalmoplegia (complete) (total)</u> — Paralysis of the internal ocular muscles.

H52.511 Internal ophthalmoplegia (complete) (total), <u>right</u> eye

H52.512 Internal ophthalmoplegia (complete) (total), <u>left</u> eye

H52.513 Internal ophthalmoplegia (complete) (total), <u>bilateral</u>

H52.519 Internal ophthalmoplegia (complete) (total), <u>unspecified</u> eye

H52.52- <u>Paresis</u> of accommodation — A loss of accommodation due to a partial or complete paralysis of the ciliary muscle and lens.

H52.521 Paresis of accommodation, <u>right</u> eye

H52.522 Paresis of accommodation, <u>left</u> eye

H52.523 Paresis of accommodation, <u>bilateral</u>

H52.529 Paresis of accommodation, <u>unspecified</u> eye

H52.53- <u>Spasm</u> of accommodation — A sudden, involuntary contraction of the ciliary muscles producing excess of accommodation for near objects.

H52.531 Spasm of accommodation, <u>right</u> eye

H52.532 Spasm of accommodation, <u>left</u> eye

H52.533 Spasm of accommodation, <u>bilateral</u>

H52.539 Spasm of accommodation, <u>unspecified</u> eye

H52.6 Other disorders of refraction

H52.7 Unspecified disorder of refraction

Excludes 1: = NOT CODED HERE! (Do not code both)

Excludes ❷: = Not Included Here

Visual disturbances and blindness (H53-H54)

H53-   **Visual disturbances** — Impairment of the sense of sight.

   H53.0-   <u>Amblyopia ex anopsia</u> — Decreased visual acuity (reduction in clarity or sharpness of vision).

     Excludes 1:   *amblyopia due to vitamin A deficiency (E50.5)*

    H53.00- <u>Unspecified</u> amblyopia

      H53.001   Unspecified amblyopia, <u>right</u> eye

      H53.002   Unspecified amblyopia, <u>left</u> eye

      H53.003   Unspecified amblyopia, <u>bilateral</u>

      H53.009   Unspecified amblyopia, <u>unspecified</u> eye

    H53.01- <u>Deprivation</u> amblyopia — A form due to absence of light stimuli.

      H53.011   Deprivation amblyopia, <u>right</u> eye

      H53.012   Deprivation amblyopia, <u>left</u> eye

      H53.013   Deprivation amblyopia, <u>bilateral</u>

      H53.019   Deprivation amblyopia, <u>unspecified</u> eye

    H53.02- <u>Refractive</u> amblyopia — A form due to the deflection of light.

      H53.021   Refractive amblyopia, <u>right</u> eye

      H53.022   Refractive amblyopia, <u>left</u> eye

      H53.023   Refractive amblyopia, <u>bilateral</u>

      H53.029   Refractive amblyopia, <u>unspecified</u> eye

    H53.03- <u>Strabismic</u> amblyopia — A form due to suppression of vision in one eye to avoid diplopia.

      Excludes 1:   *strabismus (H50.-)*

      H53.031   Strabismic amblyopia, <u>right</u> eye

      H53.032   Strabismic amblyopia, <u>left</u> eye

      H53.033   Strabismic amblyopia, <u>bilateral</u>

      H53.039   Strabismic amblyopia, <u>unspecified</u> eye

    H53.04- Amblyopia suspect — Identified significant risk of amblyopia, but without certainty of diagnosis.

      H53.041   Amblyopia suspect, <u>right</u> eye

      H53.042   Amblyopia suspect, <u>left</u> eye

      H53.043   Amblyopia suspect, <u>bilateral</u>

      H53.049   Amblyopia suspect, <u>unspecified</u> eye

   H53.1-   **Subjective visual disturbances** — Impairment and distortion of sight as perceived by the patient.

     Excludes 1:   *subjective visual disturbances due to vitamin A deficiency (E50.5)*
            visual hallucinations (R44.1)

    H53.10 Unspecified subjective visual disturbances

    H53.11 Day blindness — Diminished vision in bright light.

      Hemeralopia

    H53.12- <u>Transient visual loss</u> — The temporary, complete loss of sight.

      Scintillating scotoma — Diminished vision with a luminous wall-like appearance.

     Excludes 1:   *amaurosis fugax (G45.3-)*
            transient retinal artery occlusion (H34.0-)

     CC **H53.121**   Transient visual loss, <u>right</u> eye

     CC **H53.122**   Transient visual loss, <u>left</u> eye

     CC **H53.123**   Transient visual loss, <u>bilateral</u>

     CC **H53.129**   Transient visual loss, <u>unspecified</u> eye

    H53.13- <u>Sudden</u> visual loss — The immediate, complete loss of sight.

     CC **H53.131**   Sudden visual loss, <u>right</u> eye

     CC **H53.132**   Sudden visual loss, <u>left</u> eye

     CC **H53.133**   Sudden visual loss, <u>bilateral</u>

     CC **H53.139**   Sudden visual loss, <u>unspecified</u> eye

    H53.14- Visual <u>discomfort</u> — Uneasiness and lack of comfort of the eyes.

      Asthenopia — Weakness or tiring of the eyes accompanied by pain, headache, and dimness of vision.

      Photophobia — An unusual intolerance of light.

      H53.141   Visual discomfort, <u>right</u> eye

      H53.142   Visual discomfort, <u>left</u> eye

      H53.143   Visual discomfort, <u>bilateral</u>

      H53.149   Visual discomfort, <u>unspecified</u>

    H53.15 Visual distortions of shape and size

      Metamorphopsia — Visual distortion of an object's size and shape.

    H53.16 Psychophysical visual disturbances — Impairment of sight due to emotional stimuli.

    H53.19   **Other subjective visual disturbances**

      Visual halos — The perception of a halo of light around an object.

   H53.2   **Diplopia** — The perception of two images of the same object.

      Double vision

   H53.3-   **Other and unspecified disorders of binocular vision**

    H53.30 Unspecified disorder of binocular vision

    H53.31 Abnormal retinal correspondence

    H53.32 Fusion with defective stereopsis

    H53.33 Simultaneous visual perception without fusion

    H53.34 Suppression of binocular vision

   H53.4-   **Visual field defects**

    H53.40 Unspecified visual field defects

    H53.41- <u>Scotoma involving central area</u> — Diminished vision at the center of the sighted object.

      Central scotoma

      H53.411   Scotoma involving central area, <u>right</u> eye

      H53.412   Scotoma involving central area, <u>left</u> eye

      H53.413   Scotoma involving central area, <u>bilateral</u>

      H53.419   Scotoma involving central area, <u>unspecified</u> eye

    H53.42- <u>Scotoma of blind spot area</u> — Diminished vision at some area other than the center of the sighted object.

      Enlarged blind spot

      H53.421   Scotoma of blind spot area, <u>right</u> eye

      H53.422   Scotoma of blind spot area, <u>left</u> eye

      H53.423   Scotoma of blind spot area, <u>bilateral</u>

      H53.429   Scotoma of blind spot area, <u>unspecified</u> eye

    H53.43- <u>Sector or arcuate defects</u> — An arc-shaped diminished vision area of the sighted object.

      Arcuate scotoma
      Bjerrum scotoma

      H53.431   Sector or arcuate defects, <u>right</u> eye

      H53.432   Sector or arcuate defects, <u>left</u> eye

      H53.433   Sector or arcuate defects, <u>bilateral</u>

      H53.439   Sector or arcuate defects, <u>unspecified</u> eye

    H53.45- <u>Other</u> localized visual field defect — Diminished vision within the visual field.

      Peripheral visual field defect
      Ring scotoma NOS
      Scotoma NOS

      H53.451   Other localized visual field defect, <u>right</u> eye

      H53.452   Other localized visual field defect, <u>left</u> eye

      H53.453   Other localized visual field defect, <u>bilateral</u>

      H53.459   Other localized visual field defect, <u>unspecified</u> eye

    H53.46- <u>Homonymous bilateral field defects</u> — Defective vision affecting the right and left halves of the eyes' visual field.

      Homonymous hemianopia
      Homonymous hemianopsia
      Quadrant anopia
      Quadrant anopsia

      H53.461   Homonymous bilateral field defects, <u>right</u> side

      H53.462   Homonymous bilateral field defects, <u>left</u> side

      H53.469   Homonymous bilateral field defects, <u>unspecified</u> side

        Homonymous bilateral field defects NOS

    H53.47 Heteronymous <u>bilateral</u> field defects — Defective vision affecting the nasal or temporal halves of the eyes' visual field.

      Heteronymous hemianop(s)ia

    H53.48- <u>Generalized contraction</u> of visual field

      H53.481   Generalized contraction of visual field, <u>right</u> eye

      H53.482   Generalized contraction of visual field, <u>left</u> eye

      H53.483   Generalized contraction of visual field, <u>bilateral</u>

      H53.489   Generalized contraction of visual field, <u>unspecified</u> eye

   H53.5-   **Color vision deficiencies** — Impairment of color perception.

      Color blindness

     Excludes ❷: *day blindness (H53.11)*

    H53.50 Unspecified color vision deficiencies

      Color blindness NOS

    H53.51 **Achromatopsia** — Inability to differentiate colors.

H53.52 Acquired color vision deficiency — A form developed after birth and not hereditary.

H53.53 Deuteranomaly — A form characterized by sensory loss of red-green colors without shortened spectrum.
  Deuteranopia

H53.54 Protanomaly — A form characterized by sensory loss of red-green colors with shortened spectrum.
  Protanopia

H53.55 Tritanomaly — A form characterized by sensory loss of blue and yellow colors.
  Tritanopia

H53.59 Other color vision deficiencies

H53.6- Night blindness — Impairment of vision at night or in dim light.
  Excludes 1: *night blindness due to vitamin A deficiency (E50.5)*

H53.60 Unspecified night blindness

H53.61 Abnormal dark adaptation curve — The abnormally slow adjustment from light to darkness.

H53.62 Acquired night blindness — A form developed after birth and not hereditary.

H53.63 Congenital night blindness — A form present at birth.

H53.69 Other night blindness

H53.7- Vision sensitivity deficiencies

H53.71 Glare sensitivity

H53.72 Impaired contrast sensitivity

H53.8 Other visual disturbances

H53.9 Unspecified visual disturbance

H54- Blindness and low vision
  Note: For definition of visual impairment categories see table below
  Code first any associated underlying cause of the blindness
  Excludes 1: *amaurosis fugax (G45.3)*

H54.0 Blindness, both eyes
  Visual impairment categories 3, 4, 5 in both eyes.

H54.1- Blindness, one eye, low vision other eye
  Visual impairment categories 3, 4, 5 in one eye, with categories 1 or 2 in the other eye

H54.10 Blindness, one eye, low vision other eye, <u>unspecified</u> eyes

H54.11 Blindness, <u>right</u> eye, low vision <u>left</u> eye

H54.12 Blindness, <u>left</u> eye, low vision <u>right</u> eye

H54.2 Low vision, both eyes
  Visual impairment categories 1 or 2 in both eyes.

H54.3 Unqualified visual loss, both eyes
  Visual impairment category 9 in both eyes.

H54.4- Blindness, one eye
  Visual impairment categories 3, 4, 5 in one eye [normal vision in other eye]

H54.40 Blindness, one eye, <u>unspecified</u> eye

H54.41 Blindness, <u>right</u> eye, normal vision <u>left</u> eye

H54.42 Blindness, <u>left</u> eye, normal vision <u>right</u> eye

H54.5- Low vision, one eye
  Visual impairment categories 1 or 2 in one eye [normal vision in other eye]

H54.50 Low vision, one eye, <u>unspecified</u> eye

H54.51 Low vision, <u>right</u> eye, normal vision <u>left</u> eye

H54.52 Low vision, <u>left</u> eye, normal vision <u>right</u> eye

H54.6- Unqualified visual loss, one eye
  Visual impairment category 9 in one eye [normal vision in other eye]

H54.60 Unqualified visual loss, one eye, <u>unspecified</u>

H54.61 Unqualified visual loss, <u>right</u> eye, normal vision <u>left</u> eye

H54.62 Unqualified visual loss, <u>left</u> eye, normal vision <u>right</u> eye

H54.7 Unspecified visual loss — [Unacceptable PDX]
  Visual impairment category 9 NOS

H54.8 Legal blindness, as defined in USA
  Blindness NOS according to USA definition
  Excludes 1: *legal blindness with specification of impairment level (H54.0-H54.7)*
  Note: The table below gives a classification of severity of visual impairment recommended by a WHO Study Group on the Prevention of Blindness, Geneva, 6-10 November 1972.
  The term "low vision" in category H54 comprises categories 1 and 2 of the table, the term "blindness" categories 3, 4 and 5, and the term "unqualified visual loss" category 9.
  If the extent of the visual field is taken into account, patients with a field no greater than 10 but greater than 5 around central fixation should be placed in category 3 and patients with a field no greater than 5 around central fixation should be placed in category 4, even if the central acuity is not impaired.

Category of Visual Impairment	Visual Acuity With Best Possible Correction	
	Maximum less than:	Minimum equal to or better than:
1	6/18 3/10 (0.3) 20/70	6/60 1/10 (0.1) 20/200
2	6/60 1/10 (0.1) 20/200	3/60 1/20 (0.5) 20/400
3	3/60 1/20 (0.05) 20/400	1/60 (finger counting at one meter) 1/50 (0.02) 5/300 (20/1200)
4	1/60 (finger counting at one meter) 1/50 (0.02) 5/300	Light perception
5	No light perception	—
9	Undetermined or unspecified	—

Other disorders of eye and adnexa (H55-H57)

H55- Nystagmus and other irregular eye movements

H55.0- Nystagmus — Constant, involuntary eyeball movements.

H55.00 Unspecified nystagmus

H55.01 Congenital nystagmus — A form characterized by presence at birth.

H55.02 Latent nystagmus — A form characterized by occurring only when one eye is covered.

H55.03 Visual deprivation nystagmus — A form characterized by occurring after being in a light-free environment.

H55.04 Dissociated nystagmus — A form characterized by dissimilar movements of both eyes.

H55.09 Other forms of nystagmus

H55.8- Other irregular eye movements

H55.81 Saccadic eye movements

H55.89 Other irregular eye movements

H57- Other disorders of eye and adnexa

H57.0- Anomalies of pupillary function

H57.00 Unspecified anomaly of pupillary function

H57.01 Argyll Robertson pupil, atypical — The absence of the pupillary light reflex, but no decrease in the power of accommodation.
  Excludes 1: *syphilitic Argyll Robertson pupil (A52.19)*

H57.02 Anisocoria — Inequality of the size of pupils (the open circular area formed by the iris).

H57.03 Miosis — The continued, abnormal contraction of the pupil.

H57.04 Mydriasis — The continued, abnormal dilation of the pupil.

H57.05- Tonic pupil — A condition which responds in a slow and delayed manner.

H57.051 Tonic pupil, <u>right</u> eye

H57.052 Tonic pupil, <u>left</u> eye

H57.053 Tonic pupil, <u>bilateral</u>

H57.059 Tonic pupil, <u>unspecified</u> eye

H57.09 Other anomalies of pupillary function

H57.1- Ocular pain

H57.10 Ocular pain, <u>unspecified</u> eye

H57.11 Ocular pain, <u>right</u> eye

H57.12 Ocular pain, <u>left</u> eye

H57.13   Ocular pain, <u>bilateral</u>
H57.8   Other specified disorders of eye and adnexa
H57.9   Unspecified disorder of eye and adnexa — [Unacceptable PDX]

Intraoperative and postprocedural complications and disorders of eye and adnexa, not elsewhere classified (H59)

H59-   Intraoperative and postprocedural complications and disorders of eye and adnexa, not elsewhere classified
   Excludes 1:   *mechanical complication of intraocular lens (T85.2)*
      mechanical complication of other ocular prosthetic devices, implants and grafts (T85.3)
      pseudophakia (Z96.1)
      secondary cataracts (H26.4-)

H59.0-   Disorders of the eye <u>following cataract surgery</u>
   H59.01- <u>Keratopathy (bullous aphakic)</u> following cataract surgery
      Vitreal corneal syndrome
      Vitreous (touch) syndrome
      cc **H59.011**   Keratopathy (bullous aphakic) following cataract surgery, <u>right</u> eye
      cc **H59.012**   Keratopathy (bullous aphakic) following cataract surgery, <u>left</u> eye
      cc **H59.013**   Keratopathy (bullous aphakic) following cataract surgery, <u>bilateral</u>
      cc **H59.019**   Keratopathy (bullous aphakic) following cataract surgery, <u>unspecified</u> eye
   H59.02- <u>Cataract (lens) fragments in eye</u> following cataract surgery
      H59.021   Cataract (lens) fragments in eye following cataract surgery, <u>right</u> eye
      H59.022   Cataract (lens) fragments in eye following cataract surgery, <u>left</u> eye
      H59.023   Cataract (lens) fragments in eye following cataract surgery, <u>bilateral</u>
      H59.029   Cataract (lens) fragments in eye following cataract surgery, <u>unspecified</u> eye
   H59.03- <u>Cystoid macular edema</u> following cataract surgery
      cc **H59.031**   Cystoid macular edema following cataract surgery, <u>right</u> eye
      cc **H59.032**   Cystoid macular edema following cataract surgery, <u>left</u> eye
      cc **H59.033**   Cystoid macular edema following cataract surgery, <u>bilateral</u>
      cc **H59.039**   Cystoid macular edema following cataract surgery, <u>unspecified</u> eye
   H59.09- <u>Other disorders of the eye</u> following cataract surgery
      cc **H59.091**   Other disorders of the <u>right</u> eye following cataract surgery
      cc **H59.092**   Other disorders of the <u>left</u> eye following cataract surgery
      cc **H59.093**   Other disorders of the eye following cataract surgery, <u>bilateral</u>
      cc **H59.099**   Other disorders of <u>unspecified</u> eye following cataract surgery

H59.1-   <u>Intraoperative hemorrhage and hematoma of eye and adnexa complicating a procedure</u>
   Excludes 1:   *intraoperative hemorrhage and hematoma of eye and adnexa due to accidental puncture or laceration during a procedure (H59.2-)*
   H59.11- <u>Intraoperative hemorrhage and hematoma</u> of eye and adnexa complicating <u>an ophthalmic procedure</u>
      cc **H59.111**   Intraoperative hemorrhage and hematoma of <u>right</u> eye and adnexa complicating an ophthalmic procedure
      cc **H59.112**   Intraoperative hemorrhage and hematoma of <u>left</u> eye and adnexa complicating an ophthalmic procedure
      cc **H59.113**   Intraoperative hemorrhage and hematoma of eye and adnexa complicating an ophthalmic procedure, <u>bilateral</u>

cc **H59.119**   Intraoperative hemorrhage and hematoma of <u>unspecified</u> eye and adnexa complicating an ophthalmic procedure
   H59.12- <u>Intraoperative hemorrhage and hematoma</u> of eye and adnexa complicating <u>other procedure</u>
      cc **H59.121**   Intraoperative hemorrhage and hematoma of <u>right</u> eye and adnexa complicating other procedure
      cc **H59.122**   Intraoperative hemorrhage and hematoma of <u>left</u> eye and adnexa complicating other procedure
      cc **H59.123**   Intraoperative hemorrhage and hematoma of eye and adnexa complicating other procedure, <u>bilateral</u>
      cc **H59.129**   Intraoperative hemorrhage and hematoma of <u>unspecified</u> eye and adnexa complicating other procedure

H59.2-   <u>Accidental puncture and laceration</u> of eye and adnexa during a procedure
   H59.21- Accidental puncture and laceration of eye and adnexa during an <u>ophthalmic procedure</u>
      cc **H59.211**   Accidental puncture and laceration of <u>right</u> eye and adnexa during an ophthalmic procedure
      cc **H59.212**   Accidental puncture and laceration of <u>left</u> eye and adnexa during an ophthalmic procedure
      cc **H59.213**   Accidental puncture and laceration of eye and adnexa during an ophthalmic procedure, <u>bilateral</u>
      cc **H59.219**   Accidental puncture and laceration of <u>unspecified</u> eye and adnexa during an ophthalmic procedure
   H59.22- Accidental puncture and laceration of eye and adnexa during <u>other procedure</u>
      cc **H59.221**   Accidental puncture and laceration of <u>right</u> eye and adnexa during other procedure
      cc **H59.222**   Accidental puncture and laceration of <u>left</u> eye and adnexa during other procedure
      cc **H59.223**   Accidental puncture and laceration of eye and adnexa during other procedure, <u>bilateral</u>
      cc **H59.229**   Accidental puncture and laceration of <u>unspecified</u> eye and adnexa during other procedure

H59.3-   <u>Postprocedural hemorrhage, hematoma and seroma</u> of eye and adnexa following a procedure
   H59.31- Postprocedural <u>hemorrhage</u> of eye and adnexa following an <u>ophthalmic procedure</u>
      cc **H59.311**   Postprocedural hemorrhage of <u>right</u> eye and adnexa following an ophthalmic procedure
      cc **H59.312**   Postprocedural hemorrhage of <u>left</u> eye and adnexa following an ophthalmic procedure
      cc **H59.313**   Postprocedural hemorrhage of eye and adnexa following an ophthalmic procedure, <u>bilateral</u>
      cc **H59.319**   Postprocedural hemorrhage of <u>unspecified</u> eye and adnexa following an ophthalmic procedure
   H59.32- Postprocedural <u>hemorrhage</u> of eye and adnexa following <u>other procedure</u>
      cc **H59.321**   Postprocedural hemorrhage of <u>right</u> eye and adnexa following other procedure
      cc **H59.322**   Postprocedural hemorrhage of <u>left</u> eye and adnexa following other procedure
      cc **H59.323**   Postprocedural hemorrhage of eye and adnexa following other procedure, <u>bilateral</u>
      cc **H59.329**   Postprocedural hemorrhage of <u>unspecified</u> eye and adnexa following other procedure
   H59.33- Postprocedural <u>hematoma</u> of eye and adnexa following an <u>ophthalmic procedure</u>
      cc **H59.331**   Postprocedural hematoma of <u>right</u> eye and adnexa following an ophthalmic procedure
      cc **H59.332**   Postprocedural hematoma of <u>left</u> eye and adnexa following an ophthalmic procedure
      cc **H59.333**   Postprocedural hematoma of eye and adnexa following an ophthalmic procedure, <u>bilateral</u>
      cc **H59.339**   Postprocedural hematoma of <u>unspecified</u> eye and adnexa following an ophthalmic procedure

H57 - H59

H59.34- Postprocedural <u>hematoma</u> of eye and adnexa following <u>other procedure</u>
 CC **H59.341**   Postprocedural hematoma of <u>right</u> eye and adnexa following other procedure
 CC **H59.342**   Postprocedural hematoma of <u>left</u> eye and adnexa following other procedure
 CC **H59.343**   Postprocedural hematoma of eye and adnexa following other procedure, <u>bilateral</u>
 CC **H59.349**   Postprocedural hematoma of <u>unspecified</u> eye and adnexa following other procedure

H59.35- Postprocedural <u>seroma</u> of eye and adnexa following an <u>ophthalmic procedure</u>
 CC **H59.351**   Postprocedural seroma of <u>right</u> eye and adnexa following an ophthalmic procedure
 CC **H59.352**   Postprocedural seroma of <u>left</u> eye and adnexa following an ophthalmic procedure
 CC **H59.353**   Postprocedural seroma of eye and adnexa following an ophthalmic procedure, <u>bilateral</u>
 CC **H59.359**   Postprocedural seroma of <u>unspecified</u> eye and adnexa following an ophthalmic procedure

H59.36- Postprocedural <u>seroma</u> of eye and adnexa following <u>other procedure</u>
 CC **H59.361**   Postprocedural seroma of <u>right</u> eye and adnexa following other procedure
 CC **H59.362**   Postprocedural seroma of <u>left</u> eye and adnexa following other procedure
 CC **H59.363**   Postprocedural seroma of eye and adnexa following other procedure, <u>bilateral</u>
 CC **H59.369**   Postprocedural seroma of <u>unspecified</u> eye and adnexa following other procedure

H59.4-   **Inflammation (infection) of postprocedural bleb**
   Postprocedural blebitis
   Excludes 1:   *filtering (vitreous) bleb after glaucoma surgery status (Z98.83)*

 H59.40   Inflammation (infection) of postprocedural bleb, unspecified
 H59.41   Inflammation (infection) of postprocedural bleb, stage 1
 H59.42   Inflammation (infection) of postprocedural bleb, stage 2
 H59.43   Inflammation (infection) of postprocedural bleb, stage 3
   Bleb endophthalmitis

H59.8-   **Other intraoperative and postprocedural complications and disorders of eye and adnexa, not elsewhere classified**
 H59.81- <u>Chorioretinal scars after surgery for detachment</u>
 CC **H59.811**   Chorioretinal scars after surgery for detachment, <u>right</u> eye
 CC **H59.812**   Chorioretinal scars after surgery for detachment, <u>left</u> eye
 CC **H59.813**   Chorioretinal scars after surgery for detachment, <u>bilateral</u>
 CC **H59.819**   Chorioretinal scars after surgery for detachment, <u>unspecified</u> eye
 CC **H59.88**   Other intraoperative complications of eye and adnexa, not elsewhere classified
 CC **H59.89**   Other postprocedural complications and disorders of eye and adnexa, not elsewhere classified

Chapter 8 – Diseases of the ear and mastoid process (H60-H95)

Note: Use an external cause code following the code for the ear condition, if applicable, to identify the cause of the ear condition

Excludes ❷: *certain conditions originating in the perinatal period (P04-P96)*
certain infectious and parasitic diseases (A00-B99)
complications of pregnancy, childbirth and the puerperium (O00-O9A)
congenital malformations, deformations and chromosomal abnormalities (Q00-Q99)
endocrine, nutritional and metabolic diseases (E00-E88)
injury, poisoning and certain other consequences of external causes (S00-T88)
neoplasms (C00-D49)
symptoms, signs and abnormal clinical and laboratory findings, not elsewhere classified (R00-R94)

This chapter contains the following blocks:

H60-H62	Diseases of external ear
H65-H75	Diseases of middle ear and mastoid
H80-H83	Diseases of inner ear
H90-H94	Other disorders of ear
H95	Intraoperative and postprocedural complications and disorders of ear and mastoid process, not elsewhere classified

Chapter-Specific Coding Guidelines

C.   Chapter-Specific Coding Guidelines
In addition to general coding guidelines, there are guidelines for specific diagnoses and/or conditions in the classification. Unless otherwise indicated, these guidelines apply to all health care settings. Please refer to Section II for guidelines on the selection of principal diagnosis.

8. Chapter 8: Diseases of Ear and Mastoid Process (H60-H95)

Reserved for future guideline expansion

Diseases of external ear (H60-H62)

H60-   Otitis externa — Inflammation of the external ear.

H60.0-   Abscess of external ear — A localized collection of pus caused by the disintegration of external ear tissue.
Boil of external ear
Carbuncle of auricle or external auditory canal — A necrotizing infection of the external ear and subcutaneous tissue composed of a cluster of boils (furuncles), with multiple formed or incipient draining sinuses.
Furuncle of external ear — A painful infectious nodule formed in the skin by circumscribed inflammation of the corium and subcutaneous tissue.

H60.00   Abscess of external ear, unspecified ear
H60.01   Abscess of right external ear
H60.02   Abscess of left external ear
H60.03   Abscess of external ear, bilateral

H60.1-   Cellulitis of external ear — Cellular tissue inflammation of the external ear.
Cellulitis of auricle
Cellulitis of external auditory canal

H60.10   Cellulitis of external ear, unspecified ear
H60.11   Cellulitis of right external ear
H60.12   Cellulitis of left external ear
H60.13   Cellulitis of external ear, bilateral

H60.2-   Malignant otitis externa — An extremely severe, necrotic bacterial inflammation of the external ear, often caused by Pseudomonas aeruginosa.

cc**H60.20   Malignant otitis externa, unspecified ear**
cc**H60.21   Malignant otitis externa, right ear**
cc**H60.22   Malignant otitis externa, left ear**
cc**H60.23   Malignant otitis externa, bilateral**

H60.3-   Other infective otitis externa — Inflammation of the external ear caused by invasion of microorganisms.

H60.31-   Diffuse otitis externa — A form which affects most of the external ear, including the external auditory canal.

H60.311   Diffuse otitis externa, right ear
H60.312   Diffuse otitis externa, left ear
H60.313   Diffuse otitis externa, bilateral

H60.319   Diffuse otitis externa, unspecified ear

H60.32-   Hemorrhagic otitis externa — A form marked by escape of blood at the infected areas.

H60.321   Hemorrhagic otitis externa, right ear
H60.322   Hemorrhagic otitis externa, left ear
H60.323   Hemorrhagic otitis externa, bilateral
H60.329   Hemorrhagic otitis externa, unspecified ear

H60.33-   Swimmer's ear — The sudden, severe onset of bacterial inflammation of the external ear, seen in warm humid weather and commonly precipitated by swimming.

H60.331   Swimmer's ear, right ear
H60.332   Swimmer's ear, left ear
H60.333   Swimmer's ear, bilateral
H60.339   Swimmer's ear, unspecified ear

H60.39-   Other infective otitis externa

H60.391   Other infective otitis externa, right ear
H60.392   Other infective otitis externa, left ear
H60.393   Other infective otitis externa, bilateral
H60.399   Other infective otitis externa, unspecified ear

H60.4-   Cholesteatoma of external ear — A cyst-like mass containing keratin debris and epithelial cells of the external ear.
Keratosis obturans of external ear (canal)
Excludes ❷: *cholesteatoma of middle ear (H71.-)*
recurrent cholesteatoma of postmastoidectomy cavity (H95.0-)

H60.40   Cholesteatoma of external ear, unspecified ear
H60.41   Cholesteatoma of right external ear
H60.42   Cholesteatoma of left external ear
H60.43   Cholesteatoma of external ear, bilateral

H60.5-   Acute noninfective otitis externa — The sudden, severe onset of inflammation of the external ear that is not caused by invasion of microorganisms.

H60.50-   Unspecified acute noninfective otitis externa
Acute otitis externa NOS

H60.501   Unspecified acute noninfective otitis externa, right ear
H60.502   Unspecified acute noninfective otitis externa, left ear
H60.503   Unspecified acute noninfective otitis externa, bilateral
H60.509   Unspecified acute noninfective otitis externa, unspecified ear

H60.51-   Acute actinic otitis externa — A form caused by the photochemical effects of sunlight and other high-intensity light.

H60.511   Acute actinic otitis externa, right ear
H60.512   Acute actinic otitis externa, left ear
H60.513   Acute actinic otitis externa, bilateral
H60.519   Acute actinic otitis externa, unspecified ear

H60.52-   Acute chemical otitis externa — A form caused by the effects of chemical substances.

H60.521   Acute chemical otitis externa, right ear
H60.522   Acute chemical otitis externa, left ear
H60.523   Acute chemical otitis externa, bilateral
H60.529   Acute chemical otitis externa, unspecified ear

H60.53-   Acute contact otitis externa — A form caused by the irritating effects of a substance in direct contact with the ear.

H60.531   Acute contact otitis externa, right ear
H60.532   Acute contact otitis externa, left ear
H60.533   Acute contact otitis externa, bilateral
H60.539   Acute contact otitis externa, unspecified ear

H60.54-   Acute eczematoid otitis externa — A form resembling eczema.

H60.541   Acute eczematoid otitis externa, right ear
H60.542   Acute eczematoid otitis externa, left ear
H60.543   Acute eczematoid otitis externa, bilateral
H60.549   Acute eczematoid otitis externa, unspecified ear

H60.55-   Acute reactive otitis externa

H60.551   Acute reactive otitis externa, right ear
H60.552   Acute reactive otitis externa, left ear

H60
-
H60

Excludes 1: = NOT CODED HERE! (Do not code both)   709   *Excludes ❷:* = Not Included Here

H60.553 Acute reactive otitis externa, <u>bilateral</u>

H60.559 Acute reactive otitis externa, <u>unspecified</u> ear

H60.59- <u>Other noninfective acute</u> otitis externa

H60.591 Other noninfective acute otitis externa, <u>right</u> ear

H60.592 Other noninfective acute otitis externa, <u>left</u> ear

H60.593 Other noninfective acute otitis externa, <u>bilateral</u>

H60.599 Other noninfective acute otitis externa, <u>unspecified</u> ear

H60.6- <u>Unspecified chronic</u> otitis externa — Inflammation of the external ear that is not caused by the invasion of microorganisms that develops slowly and persists over a long period of time.

H60.60 Unspecified chronic otitis externa, <u>unspecified</u> ear

H60.61 Unspecified chronic otitis externa, <u>right</u> ear

H60.62 Unspecified chronic otitis externa, <u>left</u> ear

H60.63 Unspecified chronic otitis externa, <u>bilateral</u>

H60.8- <u>Other</u> otitis externa

H60.8x- <u>Other</u> otitis externa

H60.8x1 Other otitis externa, <u>right</u> ear

H60.8x2 Other otitis externa, <u>left</u> ear

H60.8x3 Other otitis externa, <u>bilateral</u>

H60.8x9 Other otitis externa, <u>unspecified</u> ear

H60.9- <u>Unspecified</u> otitis externa

H60.90 Unspecified otitis externa, <u>unspecified</u> ear

H60.91 Unspecified otitis externa, <u>right</u> ear

H60.92 Unspecified otitis externa, <u>left</u> ear

H60.93 Unspecified otitis externa, <u>bilateral</u>

H61- <u>Other disorders of external ear</u> — Disorders of that portion to the outside of the tympanic membrane.

H61.0- <u>Chondritis and perichondritis</u> of external ear — The inflammation/infection of the fibrous connective tissue that covers the cartilage of the external ear.

AHA 15:1Q:p18 – Auricular chondritis due to Pseudomonas aeruginosa
Chondrodermatitis nodularis chronica helicis
Perichondritis of auricle
Perichondritis of pinna

H61.00- <u>Unspecified</u> perichondritis of external ear

H61.001 Unspecified perichondritis of <u>right</u> external ear

H61.002 Unspecified perichondritis of <u>left</u> external ear

H61.003 Unspecified perichondritis of external ear, <u>bilateral</u>

H61.009 Unspecified perichondritis of external ear, <u>unspecified</u> ear

H61.01- <u>Acute perichondritis</u> of external ear — The sudden, severe inflammation/infection of the fibrous connective tissue that covers the cartilage of the external ear.

H61.011 Acute perichondritis of <u>right</u> external ear

H61.012 Acute perichondritis of <u>left</u> external ear

H61.013 Acute perichondritis of external ear, <u>bilateral</u>

H61.019 Acute perichondritis of external ear, <u>unspecified</u> ear

H61.02- Chronic perichondritis of external ear — The inflammation/infection of the fibrous connective tissue that covers the cartilage of the external ear that is marked by slow development and persists over a long period of time.

H61.021 Chronic perichondritis of <u>right</u> external ear

H61.022 Chronic perichondritis of <u>left</u> external ear

H61.023 Chronic perichondritis of external ear, <u>bilateral</u>

H61.029 Chronic perichondritis of external ear, <u>unspecified</u> ear

H61.03- <u>Chondritis</u> of external ear — The inflammation/infection of the cartilage of the ear.

Chondritis of auricle
Chondritis of pinna

H61.031 Chondritis of <u>right</u> external ear

H61.032 Chondritis of <u>left</u> external ear

H61.033 Chondritis of external ear, <u>bilateral</u>

H61.039 Chondritis of external ear, <u>unspecified</u> ear

H61.1- Noninfective disorders of pinna

Excludes ❷: cauliflower ear (M95.1-)
gouty tophi of ear (M1A.-)

H61.10- <u>Unspecified noninfective disorders</u> of pinna

Disorder of pinna NOS

H61.101 Unspecified noninfective disorders of pinna, <u>right</u> ear

H61.102 Unspecified noninfective disorders of pinna, <u>left</u> ear

H61.103 Unspecified noninfective disorders of pinna, <u>bilateral</u>

H61.109 Unspecified noninfective disorders of pinna, <u>unspecified</u> ear

H61.11- <u>Acquired deformity</u> of pinna — A distortion of that portion of the external ear lying outside of the head which is not congenital.

Acquired deformity of auricle

Excludes ❷: cauliflower ear (M95.1-)

H61.111 Acquired deformity of pinna, <u>right</u> ear

H61.112 Acquired deformity of pinna, <u>left</u> ear

H61.113 Acquired deformity of pinna, <u>bilateral</u>

H61.119 Acquired deformity of pinna, <u>unspecified</u> ear

H61.12- <u>Hematoma</u> of pinna — The localized collection of blood within the tissues of that portion of the ear which lies outside of the head.

Hematoma of auricle

H61.121 Hematoma of pinna, <u>right</u> ear

H61.122 Hematoma of pinna, <u>left</u> ear

H61.123 Hematoma of pinna, <u>bilateral</u>

H61.129 Hematoma of pinna, <u>unspecified</u> ear

H61.19- <u>Other noninfective disorders</u> of pinna

H61.191 Noninfective disorders of pinna, <u>right</u> ear

H61.192 Noninfective disorders of pinna, <u>left</u> ear

H61.193 Noninfective disorders of pinna, <u>bilateral</u>

H61.199 Noninfective disorders of pinna, <u>unspecified</u> ear

H61.2- <u>Impacted cerumen</u> — The lodged or wedged accumulation of the wax-like secretion in the external auditory canal.

Wax in ear

H61.20 Impacted cerumen, <u>unspecified</u> ear — [Questionable Admission]

H61.21 Impacted cerumen, <u>right</u> ear — [Questionable Admission]

H61.22 Impacted cerumen, <u>left</u> ear — [Questionable Admission]

H61.23 Impacted cerumen, <u>bilateral</u> — [Questionable Admission]

H61.3- <u>Acquired stenosis</u> of external ear canal — The abnormal narrowing of the external auditory canal which is not inherited.

Collapse of external ear canal

Excludes 1: postprocedural stenosis of external ear canal (H95.81-)

H61.30- Acquired stenosis of external ear canal, <u>unspecified</u>

H61.301 Acquired stenosis of <u>right</u> external ear canal, unspecified

H61.302 Acquired stenosis of <u>left</u> external ear canal, unspecified

H61.303 Acquired stenosis of external ear canal, unspecified, <u>bilateral</u>

H61.309 Acquired stenosis of external ear canal, unspecified, <u>unspecified</u> ear

H61.31- <u>Acquired stenosis</u> of external ear canal <u>secondary to trauma</u> — A form due to external physical injury.

H61.311 Acquired stenosis of <u>right</u> external ear canal secondary to trauma

H61.312 Acquired stenosis of <u>left</u> external ear canal secondary to trauma

H61.313 Acquired stenosis of external ear canal secondary to trauma, <u>bilateral</u>

H61.319 Acquired stenosis of external ear canal secondary to trauma, <u>unspecified</u> ear

H61.32- <u>Acquired stenosis</u> of external ear canal <u>secondary to inflammation and infection</u> — A form resulting from the enlarging effects of inflammation/infection.

H61.321 Acquired stenosis of <u>right</u> external ear canal secondary to inflammation and infection

H61.322 Acquired stenosis of <u>left</u> external ear canal secondary to inflammation and infection

H61.323 Acquired stenosis of external ear canal secondary to inflammation and infection, <u>bilateral</u>

H61.329 Acquired stenosis of external ear canal secondary to inflammation and infection, <u>unspecified</u> ear

H61.39- Other acquired stenosis of external ear canal

H61.391 Other acquired stenosis of <u>right</u> external ear canal

H61.392 Other acquired stenosis of <u>left</u> external ear canal

H61.393 Other acquired stenosis of external ear canal, <u>bilateral</u>

H61.399 Other acquired stenosis of external ear canal, <u>unspecified</u> ear

H61.8- Other specified disorders of external ear

H61.81- <u>Exostosis</u> of external canal — A benign bony growth projecting from the external ear canal.

H61.811 Exostosis of <u>right</u> external canal

H61.812 Exostosis of <u>left</u> external canal

H61.813 Exostosis of external canal, <u>bilateral</u>

H61.819 Exostosis of external canal, <u>unspecified</u> ear

H61.89- <u>Other specified disorders</u> of external ear

H61.891 Other specified disorders of <u>right</u> external ear

H61.892 Other specified disorders of <u>left</u> external ear

H61.893 Other specified disorders of external ear, <u>bilateral</u>

H61.899 Other specified disorders of external ear, <u>unspecified</u> ear

H61.9- Disorder of external ear, unspecified

H61.90 Disorder of external ear, unspecified, <u>unspecified</u> ear

H61.91 Disorder of <u>right</u> external ear, unspecified

H61.92 Disorder of <u>left</u> external ear, unspecified

H61.93 Disorder of external ear, unspecified, <u>bilateral</u>

H62- Disorders of external ear <u>in diseases classified elsewhere</u>

H62.4- Otitis externa <u>in other diseases classified elsewhere</u>
Code first underlying disease, such as:
Erysipelas (A46)
Impetigo (L01.0)
Excludes 1: *otitis externa (in):*
candidiasis (B37.84)
herpes viral [herpes simplex] (B00.1)
herpes zoster (B02.8)

H62.40 Otitis externa in other diseases classified elsewhere, <u>unspecified</u> ear — [Not Allowed as PDX]

H62.41 Otitis externa in other diseases classified elsewhere, <u>right</u> ear — [Not Allowed as PDX]

H62.42 Otitis externa in other diseases classified elsewhere, <u>left</u> ear — [Not Allowed as PDX]

H62.43 Otitis externa in other diseases classified elsewhere, <u>bilateral</u> — [Not Allowed as PDX]

H62.8- Other disorders of external ear <u>in diseases classified elsewhere</u>
Code first underlying disease, such as:
Gout (M1A.-, M10.-)

H62.8x- Other disorders of external ear in diseases classified elsewhere

H62.8x1 Other disorders of <u>right</u> external ear in diseases classified elsewhere — [Not Allowed as PDX]

H62.8x2 Other disorders of <u>left</u> external ear in diseases classified elsewhere — [Not Allowed as PDX]

H62.8x3 Other disorders of external ear in diseases classified elsewhere, <u>bilateral</u> — [Not Allowed as PDX]

H62.8x9 Other disorders of external ear in diseases classified elsewhere, <u>unspecified</u> ear — [Not Allowed as PDX]

Diseases of middle ear and mastoid (H65-H75)

H65- <u>Nonsuppurative</u> <u>otitis media</u> — The inflammation of the middle ear, without pus formation.
Includes: Nonsuppurative otitis media with myringitis
Use additional code for any associated perforated tympanic membrane (H72.-)
Use additional code to identify:
Exposure to environmental tobacco smoke (Z77.22)
Exposure to tobacco smoke in the perinatal period (P96.81)
History of tobacco dependence (Z87.891)
Occupational exposure to environmental tobacco smoke (Z57.31)
Tobacco dependence (F17.-)
Tobacco use (Z72.0)

H65.0- <u>Acute serous</u> otitis media — The sudden, severe onset of inflammation of the middle ear that is characterized by serous exudation, without pus formation.
Acute and subacute secretory otitis

H65.00 Acute serous otitis media, <u>unspecified</u> ear

H65.01 Acute serous otitis media, <u>right</u> ear

H65.02 Acute serous otitis media, <u>left</u> ear

H65.03 Acute serous otitis media, <u>bilateral</u>

H65.04 Acute serous otitis media, <u>recurrent</u>, <u>right</u> ear

H65.05 Acute serous otitis media, <u>recurrent</u>, <u>left</u> ear

H65.06 Acute serous otitis media, <u>recurrent</u>, <u>bilateral</u>

H65.07 Acute serous otitis media, <u>recurrent</u>, <u>unspecified</u> ear

H65.1- <u>Other acute</u> nonsuppurative otitis media
Excludes 1: *otitic barotrauma (T70.0)*
otitis media (acute) NOS (H66.9)

H65.11- Acute and subacute <u>allergic</u> otitis media (mucoid) (sanguinous) (serous) — The sudden, severe onset of inflammation of the middle ear that is caused by an allergic reaction.

H65.111 Acute and subacute allergic otitis media (mucoid) (sanguinous) (serous), <u>right</u> ear

H65.112 Acute and subacute allergic otitis media (mucoid) (sanguinous) (serous), <u>left</u> ear

H65.113 Acute and subacute allergic otitis media (mucoid) (sanguinous) (serous), <u>bilateral</u>

H65.114 Acute and subacute allergic otitis media (mucoid) (sanguinous) (serous), <u>recurrent</u>, <u>right</u> ear

H65.115 Acute and subacute allergic otitis media (mucoid) (sanguinous) (serous), <u>recurrent</u>, <u>left</u> ear

H65.116 Acute and subacute allergic otitis media (mucoid) (sanguinous) (serous), <u>recurrent</u>, <u>bilateral</u>

H65.117 Acute and subacute allergic otitis media (mucoid) (sanguinous) (serous), <u>recurrent</u>, <u>unspecified</u> ear

H65.119 Acute and subacute allergic otitis media (mucoid) (sanguinous) (serous), <u>unspecified</u> ear

H65.19- <u>Other acute</u> nonsuppurative otitis media
Acute and subacute mucoid otitis media
Acute and subacute nonsuppurative otitis media NOS
Acute and subacute sanguinous otitis media
Acute and subacute seromucinous otitis media

H65.191 Other acute nonsuppurative otitis media, <u>right</u> ear

H65.192 Other acute nonsuppurative otitis media, <u>left</u> ear

H65.193 Other acute nonsuppurative otitis media, <u>bilateral</u>

H65.194 Other acute nonsuppurative otitis media, <u>recurrent</u>, <u>right</u> ear

H65.195 Other acute nonsuppurative otitis media, <u>recurrent</u>, <u>left</u> ear

H65.196 Other acute nonsuppurative otitis media, <u>recurrent</u>, <u>bilateral</u>

H65.197 Other acute nonsuppurative otitis media <u>recurrent</u>, <u>unspecified</u> ear

H65.199 Other acute nonsuppurative otitis media, <u>unspecified</u> ear

H65.2- <u>Chronic serous</u> otitis media — Inflammation of the middle ear that develops slowly and persists over a long period of time, without pus formation.
Chronic tubotympanal catarrh

H65.20 Chronic serous otitis media, <u>unspecified</u> ear

H65.21 Chronic serous otitis media, <u>right</u> ear

H65.22 Chronic serous otitis media, <u>left</u> ear

H65.23 Chronic serous otitis media, <u>bilateral</u>

5

H 6 1 - H 6 5

H65.3- <u>Chronic mucoid</u> otitis media — A form characterized by mucus-like substance in the middle ear, without pus formation.
    Chronic mucinous otitis media
    Chronic secretory otitis media
    Chronic transudative otitis media
    Glue ear
    Excludes 1:   *adhesive middle ear disease (H74.1)*

  H65.30 Chronic mucoid otitis media, <u>unspecified</u> ear

  H65.31 Chronic mucoid otitis media, <u>right</u> ear

  H65.32 Chronic mucoid otitis media, <u>left</u> ear

  H65.33 Chronic mucoid otitis media, <u>bilateral</u>

H65.4- <u>Other chronic nonsuppurative</u> otitis media

  H65.41- <u>Chronic allergic</u> otitis media — A form caused by an allergic reaction.

    H65.411   Chronic allergic otitis media, <u>right</u> ear

    H65.412   Chronic allergic otitis media, <u>left</u> ear

    H65.413   Chronic allergic otitis media, <u>bilateral</u>

    H65.419   Chronic allergic otitis media, <u>unspecified</u> ear

  H65.49- <u>Other chronic</u> nonsuppurative otitis media
    Chronic exudative otitis media
    Chronic nonsuppurative otitis media NOS
    Chronic otitis media with effusion (nonpurulent)
    Chronic seromucinous otitis media

    H65.491   Other chronic nonsuppurative otitis media, <u>right</u> ear

    H65.492   Other chronic nonsuppurative otitis media, <u>left</u> ear

    H65.493   Other chronic nonsuppurative otitis media, <u>bilateral</u>

    H65.499   Other chronic nonsuppurative otitis media, <u>unspecified</u> ear

H65.9- <u>Unspecified</u> nonsuppurative otitis media
    Allergic otitis media NOS
    Catarrhal otitis media NOS
    Exudative otitis media NOS
    Mucoid otitis media NOS
    Otitis media with effusion (nonpurulent) NOS
    Secretory otitis media NOS
    Seromucinous otitis media NOS
    Serous otitis media NOS
    Transudative otitis media NOS

  H65.90 Unspecified nonsuppurative otitis media, <u>unspecified</u> ear

  H65.91 Unspecified nonsuppurative otitis media, <u>right</u> ear

  H65.92 Unspecified nonsuppurative otitis media, <u>left</u> ear

  H65.93 Unspecified nonsuppurative otitis media, <u>bilateral</u>

H66- <u>Suppurative and unspecified</u> otitis media — The inflammation of the middle ear, with pus formation.
  Includes: Suppurative and unspecified otitis media with myringitis
  Use additional code to identify:
    Exposure to environmental tobacco smoke (Z77.22)
    Exposure to tobacco smoke in the perinatal period (P96.81)
    History of tobacco dependence (Z87.891)
    Occupational exposure to environmental tobacco smoke (Z57.31)
    Tobacco dependence (F17.-)
    Tobacco use (Z72.0)

H66.0- <u>Acute suppurative</u> otitis media — The sudden, severe onset of inflammation of the middle ear; with pus formation.

  H66.00- Acute suppurative otitis media <u>without</u> spontaneous rupture of ear drum

    H66.001   Acute suppurative otitis media without spontaneous rupture of ear drum, <u>right</u> ear

    H66.002   Acute suppurative otitis media without spontaneous rupture of ear drum, <u>left</u> ear

    H66.003   Acute suppurative otitis media without spontaneous rupture of ear drum, <u>bilateral</u>

    H66.004   Acute suppurative otitis media without spontaneous rupture of ear drum, <u>recurrent</u>, <u>right</u> ear

    H66.005   Acute suppurative otitis media without spontaneous rupture of ear drum, <u>recurrent</u>, <u>left</u> ear

    H66.006   Acute suppurative otitis media without spontaneous rupture of ear drum, <u>recurrent</u>, <u>bilateral</u>

    H66.007   Acute suppurative otitis media without spontaneous rupture of ear drum, <u>recurrent</u>, <u>unspecified</u> ear

    H66.009   Acute suppurative otitis media without spontaneous rupture of ear drum, <u>unspecified</u> ear

  H66.01- Acute suppurative otitis media <u>with spontaneous rupture of ear drum</u> — A form marked by the nontraumatic tearing open of the ear drum.

    H66.011   Acute suppurative otitis media with spontaneous rupture of ear drum, <u>right</u> ear

    H66.012   Acute suppurative otitis media with spontaneous rupture of ear drum, <u>left</u> ear

    H66.013   Acute suppurative otitis media with spontaneous rupture of ear drum, <u>bilateral</u>

    H66.014   Acute suppurative otitis media with spontaneous rupture of ear drum, <u>recurrent</u>, <u>right</u> ear

    H66.015   Acute suppurative otitis media with spontaneous rupture of ear drum, <u>recurrent</u>, <u>left</u> ear

    H66.016   Acute suppurative otitis media with spontaneous rupture of ear drum, <u>recurrent</u>, <u>bilateral</u>

    H66.017   Acute suppurative otitis media with spontaneous rupture of ear drum, <u>recurrent</u>, <u>unspecified</u> ear

    H66.019   Acute suppurative otitis media with spontaneous rupture of ear drum, <u>unspecified</u> ear

H66.1- <u>Chronic tubotympanic</u> suppurative otitis media — Inflammation of the tympanic cavity of the middle ear that develops slowly and persists over a long period of time, with pus formation.
    Benign chronic suppurative otitis media
    Chronic tubotympanic disease
  Use additional code for any associated perforated tympanic membrane (H72.-)

  H66.10 Chronic tubotympanic suppurative otitis media, <u>unspecified</u>

  H66.11 Chronic tubotympanic suppurative otitis media, <u>right</u> ear

  H66.12 Chronic tubotympanic suppurative otitis media, <u>left</u> ear

  H66.13 Chronic tubotympanic suppurative otitis media, <u>bilateral</u>

H66.2- <u>Chronic atticoantral</u> suppurative otitis media — Inflammation of the upper portion of the middle ear that develops slowly and persists over a long period of time, with pus formation that drains through a perforation of the tympanic membrane.
    Chronic atticoantral disease
  Use additional code for any associated perforated tympanic membrane (H72.-)

  H66.20 Chronic atticoantral suppurative otitis media, <u>unspecified</u> ear

  H66.21 Chronic atticoantral suppurative otitis media, <u>right</u> ear

  H66.22 Chronic atticoantral suppurative otitis media, <u>left</u> ear

  H66.23 Chronic atticoantral suppurative otitis media, <u>bilateral</u>

H66.3- <u>Other chronic</u> suppurative otitis media
    Chronic suppurative otitis media NOS
  Use additional code for any associated perforated tympanic membrane (H72.-)
    Excludes 1:   *tuberculous otitis media (A18.6)*

  H66.3x- <u>Other chronic</u> suppurative otitis media

    H66.3x1   Other chronic suppurative otitis media, <u>right</u> ear

    H66.3x2   Other chronic suppurative otitis media, <u>left</u> ear

    H66.3x3   Other chronic suppurative otitis media, <u>bilateral</u>

    H66.3x9   Other chronic suppurative otitis media, <u>unspecified</u> ear

H66.4- <u>Suppurative</u> otitis media, <u>unspecified</u>
    Purulent otitis media NOS
  Use additional code for any associated perforated tympanic membrane (H72.-)

  H66.40 Suppurative otitis media, unspecified, <u>unspecified</u> ear

  H66.41 Suppurative otitis media, unspecified, <u>right</u> ear

  H66.42 Suppurative otitis media, unspecified, <u>left</u> ear

  H66.43 Suppurative otitis media, unspecified, <u>bilateral</u>

H 65 I H 66

H66.9-   **Otitis media, <u>unspecified</u>**
> Otitis media NOS
> Acute otitis media NOS
> Chronic otitis media NOS
> Use additional code for any associated perforated tympanic membrane (H72.-)

   H66.90   Otitis media, unspecified, <u>unspecified</u> ear

   H66.91   Otitis media, unspecified, <u>right</u> ear

   H66.92   Otitis media, unspecified, <u>left</u> ear

   H66.93   Otitis media, unspecified, <u>bilateral</u>

H67-   **Otitis media <u>in diseases classified elsewhere</u>**
> Code first underlying disease, such as:
>   Viral disease NEC (B00-B34)
> Use additional code for any associated perforated tympanic membrane (H72.-)
> Excludes 1:   *otitis media in:*
>   *influenza (J09.X9, J10.83, J11.83)*
>   *measles (B05.3)*
>   *scarlet fever (A38.0)*
>   *tuberculosis (A18.6)*

   H67.1   Otitis media in diseases classified elsewhere, <u>right</u> ear — [Not Allowed as PDX]

   H67.2   Otitis media in diseases classified elsewhere, <u>left</u> ear — [Not Allowed as PDX]

   H67.3   Otitis media in diseases classified elsewhere, <u>bilateral</u> — [Not Allowed as PDX]

   H67.9   Otitis media in diseases classified elsewhere, <u>unspecified</u> ear — [Not Allowed as PDX]

H68-   **Eustachian salpingitis and obstruction**

   H68.0-   <u>Eustachian salpingitis</u> — Inflammation of the Eustachian (auditory) tube.

     H68.00- <u>Unspecified</u> Eustachian salpingitis

       H68.001   Unspecified Eustachian salpingitis, <u>right</u> ear

       H68.002   Unspecified Eustachian salpingitis, <u>left</u> ear

       H68.003   Unspecified Eustachian salpingitis, <u>bilateral</u>

       H68.009   Unspecified Eustachian salpingitis, <u>unspecified</u> ear

     H68.01- <u>Acute</u> Eustachian salpingitis — A form marked by sudden, severe onset.

       H68.011   Acute Eustachian salpingitis, <u>right</u> ear

       H68.012   Acute Eustachian salpingitis, <u>left</u> ear

       H68.013   Acute Eustachian salpingitis, <u>bilateral</u>

       H68.019   Acute Eustachian salpingitis, <u>unspecified</u> ear

     H68.02- <u>Chronic</u> Eustachian salpingitis — A form marked by slow development and persistence over a long period of time.

       H68.021   Chronic Eustachian salpingitis, <u>right</u> ear

       H68.022   Chronic Eustachian salpingitis, <u>left</u> ear

       H68.023   Chronic Eustachian salpingitis, <u>bilateral</u>

       H68.029   Chronic Eustachian salpingitis, <u>unspecified</u> ear

   H68.1-   <u>Obstruction</u> of Eustachian tube — Blockage of the Eustachian (auditory) tube.
> Stenosis of Eustachian tube — A reduction in the lumen of the Eustachian (auditory) tube.
> Stricture of Eustachian tube — A narrowing of the lumen of the Eustachian (auditory) tube.

     H68.10- <u>Unspecified</u> obstruction of Eustachian tube

       H68.101   Unspecified obstruction of Eustachian tube, <u>right</u> ear

       H68.102   Unspecified obstruction of Eustachian tube, <u>left</u> ear

       H68.103   Unspecified obstruction of Eustachian tube, <u>bilateral</u>

       H68.109   Unspecified obstruction of Eustachian tube, <u>unspecified</u> ear

     H68.11- <u>Osseous</u> obstruction of Eustachian tube — A form marked by bony overgrowth.

       H68.111   Osseous obstruction of Eustachian tube, <u>right</u> ear

       H68.112   Osseous obstruction of Eustachian tube, <u>left</u> ear

       H68.113   Osseous obstruction of Eustachian tube, <u>bilateral</u>

       H68.119   Osseous obstruction of Eustachian tube, <u>unspecified</u> ear

     H68.12- <u>Intrinsic cartilagenous</u> obstruction of Eustachian tube — A form marked by overgrowth of the Eustachian tube cartilage.

       H68.121   Intrinsic cartilagenous obstruction of Eustachian tube, <u>right</u> ear

       H68.122   Intrinsic cartilagenous obstruction of Eustachian tube, <u>left</u> ear

       H68.123   Intrinsic cartilagenous obstruction of Eustachian tube, <u>bilateral</u>

       H68.129   Intrinsic cartilagenous obstruction of Eustachian tube, <u>unspecified</u> ear

     H68.13- <u>Extrinsic cartilagenous</u> obstruction of Eustachian tube — A form marked by overgrowth of the cartilage surrounding the Eustachian tube.
> Compression of Eustachian tube

       H68.131   Extrinsic cartilagenous obstruction of Eustachian tube, <u>right</u> ear

       H68.132   Extrinsic cartilagenous obstruction of Eustachian tube, <u>left</u> ear

       H68.133   Extrinsic cartilagenous obstruction of Eustachian tube, <u>bilateral</u>

       H68.139   Extrinsic cartilagenous obstruction of Eustachian tube, <u>unspecified</u> ear

H69-   **Other and unspecified disorders of Eustachian tube**

   H69.0-   <u>Patulous</u> Eustachian tube — An abnormally wide, distended Eustachian (auditory) tube.

     H69.00   Patulous Eustachian tube, <u>unspecified</u> ear

     H69.01   Patulous Eustachian tube, <u>right</u> ear

     H69.02   Patulous Eustachian tube, <u>left</u> ear

     H69.03   Patulous Eustachian tube, <u>bilateral</u>

   H69.8-   <u>Other specified</u> disorders of Eustachian tube

     H69.80   Other specified disorders of Eustachian tube, <u>unspecified</u> ear

     H69.81   Other specified disorders of Eustachian tube, <u>right</u> ear

     H69.82   Other specified disorders of Eustachian tube, <u>left</u> ear

     H69.83   Other specified disorders of Eustachian tube, <u>bilateral</u>

   H69.9-   <u>Unspecified</u> Eustachian tube disorder

     H69.90   Unspecified Eustachian tube disorder, <u>unspecified</u> ear

     H69.91   Unspecified Eustachian tube disorder, <u>right</u> ear

     H69.92   Unspecified Eustachian tube disorder, <u>left</u> ear

     H69.93   Unspecified Eustachian tube disorder, <u>bilateral</u>

H70-   **Mastoiditis and related conditions**

   H70.0-   <u>Acute mastoiditis</u> — The sudden, severe onset of inflammation of the mastoid antrum (air cells) of the mastoid process of the temporal bone.
> Abscess of mastoid — A localized collection of pus caused by the disintegration of the mastoid antrum cells.
> Empyema of mastoid — The accumulation of pus within the mastoid antrum.

     H70.00- Acute mastoiditis <u>without</u> complications — A form without complications.

     CC **H70.001**   Acute mastoiditis without complications, <u>right</u> ear

     CC **H70.002**   Acute mastoiditis without complications, <u>left</u> ear

     CC **H70.003**   Acute mastoiditis without complications, <u>bilateral</u>

     CC **H70.009**   Acute mastoiditis without complications, <u>unspecified</u> ear

     H70.01- <u>Subperiosteal abscess</u> of mastoid — A localized collection of pus caused by the disintegration of mastoid antrum cells beneath the periosteum layer.

     CC **H70.011**   Subperiosteal abscess of mastoid, <u>right</u> ear

     CC **H70.012**   Subperiosteal abscess of mastoid, <u>left</u> ear

     CC **H70.013**   Subperiosteal abscess of mastoid, <u>bilateral</u>

     CC **H70.019**   Subperiosteal abscess of mastoid, <u>unspecified</u> ear

     H70.09- Acute mastoiditis <u>with other complications</u>

     CC **H70.091**   Acute mastoiditis with other complications, <u>right</u> ear

     CC **H70.092**   Acute mastoiditis with other complications, <u>left</u> ear

     CC **H70.093**   Acute mastoiditis with other complications, <u>bilateral</u>

     CC **H70.099**   Acute mastoiditis with other complications, <u>unspecified</u> ear

H66 - H70

Excludes 1: = NOT CODED HERE! (Do not code both)   **713**   *Excludes ❷:* = Not Included Here

H70.1-   <u>Chronic mastoiditis</u> — Inflammation of the mastoid antrum (air cells) of the mastoid process of the temporal bone which develops slowly and persists over a long period of time.
     Caries of mastoid — The decay of the mastoid bony substance.
     Fistula of mastoid — An abnormal passage of the mastoid.
     Excludes 1:   *tuberculous mastoiditis (A18.03)*

   H70.10   Chronic mastoiditis, <u>unspecified</u> ear
   H70.11   Chronic mastoiditis, <u>right</u> ear
   H70.12   Chronic mastoiditis, <u>left</u> ear
   H70.13   Chronic mastoiditis, <u>bilateral</u>

H70.2-   <u>Petrositis</u> — Inflammation of the petrous region of the temporal bone.
     Inflammation of petrous bone

   H70.20- <u>Unspecified</u> petrositis
     H70.201   Unspecified petrositis, <u>right</u> ear
     H70.202   Unspecified petrositis, <u>left</u> ear
     H70.203   Unspecified petrositis, <u>bilateral</u>
     H70.209   Unspecified petrositis, <u>unspecified</u> ear

   H70.21- <u>Acute</u> petrositis — A form characterized by sudden, severe onset.
     H70.211   Acute petrositis, <u>right</u> ear
     H70.212   Acute petrositis, <u>left</u> ear
     H70.213   Acute petrositis, <u>bilateral</u>
     H70.219   Acute petrositis, <u>unspecified</u> ear

   H70.22- <u>Chronic</u> petrositis — A form characterized by slow development and persistence over a long period of time.
     H70.221   Chronic petrositis, <u>right</u> ear
     H70.222   Chronic petrositis, <u>left</u> ear
     H70.223   Chronic petrositis, <u>bilateral</u>
     H70.229   Chronic petrositis, <u>unspecified</u> ear

H70.8-   Other mastoiditis and related conditions
     Excludes 1:   *preauricular sinus and cyst (Q18.1)*
                sinus, fistula, and cyst of branchial cleft (Q18.0)

   H70.81- <u>Postauricular fistula</u> — An abnormal passage just behind the mastoid cavity.
     H70.811   Postauricular fistula, <u>right</u> ear
     H70.812   Postauricular fistula, <u>left</u> ear
     H70.813   Postauricular fistula, <u>bilateral</u>
     H70.819   Postauricular fistula, <u>unspecified</u> ear

   H70.89- <u>Other mastoiditis and related conditions</u>
     H70.891   Other mastoiditis and related conditions, <u>right</u> ear
     H70.892   Other mastoiditis and related conditions, <u>left</u> ear
     H70.893   Other mastoiditis and related conditions, <u>bilateral</u>
     H70.899   Other mastoiditis and related conditions, <u>unspecified</u> ear

H70.9-   <u>Unspecified mastoiditis</u>
   H70.90   Unspecified mastoiditis, <u>unspecified</u> ear
   H70.91   Unspecified mastoiditis, <u>right</u> ear
   H70.92   Unspecified mastoiditis, <u>left</u> ear
   H70.93   Unspecified mastoiditis, <u>bilateral</u>

H71-   <u>Cholesteatoma</u> of <u>middle ear</u> — A cyst-like sac filled with keratin debris of the middle ear.
     Excludes ❷: *cholesteatoma of external ear (H60.4-)*
                 recurrent cholesteatoma of postmastoidectomy cavity (H95.0-)

H71.0-   <u>Cholesteatoma of attic</u> — A form located in the upper portion of the middle ear.
   H71.00   Cholesteatoma of attic, <u>unspecified</u> ear
   H71.01   Cholesteatoma of attic, <u>right</u> ear
   H71.02   Cholesteatoma of attic, <u>left</u> ear
   H71.03   Cholesteatoma of attic, <u>bilateral</u>

H71.1-   Cholesteatoma of <u>tympanum</u> — A form adjacent to the tympanic membrane.
   H71.10   Cholesteatoma of tympanum, <u>unspecified</u> ear
   H71.11   Cholesteatoma of tympanum, <u>right</u> ear
   H71.12   Cholesteatoma of tympanum, <u>left</u> ear
   H71.13   Cholesteatoma of tympanum, <u>bilateral</u>

H71.2-   Cholesteatoma of <u>mastoid</u> — A form located in the mastoid antrum.
   H71.20   Cholesteatoma of mastoid, <u>unspecified</u> ear
   H71.21   Cholesteatoma of mastoid, <u>right</u> ear

   H71.22   Cholesteatoma of mastoid, <u>left</u> ear
   H71.23   Cholesteatoma of mastoid, <u>bilateral</u>

H71.3-   <u>Diffuse</u> cholesteatosis — A form marked by the presence of cholesteatoma formation throughout the middle ear.
   H71.30   Diffuse cholesteatosis, <u>unspecified</u> ear
   H71.31   Diffuse cholesteatosis, <u>right</u> ear
   H71.32   Diffuse cholesteatosis, <u>left</u> ear
   H71.33   Diffuse cholesteatosis, <u>bilateral</u>

H71.9-   <u>Unspecified</u> cholesteatoma
   H71.90   Unspecified cholesteatoma, <u>unspecified</u> ear
   H71.91   Unspecified cholesteatoma, <u>right</u> ear
   H71.92   Unspecified cholesteatoma, <u>left</u> ear
   H71.93   Unspecified cholesteatoma, <u>bilateral</u>

H72-   <u>Perforation of tympanic membrane</u> — The tearing open of a hole in the tympanic membrane (ear drum).
     Includes: **Persistent post-traumatic perforation of ear drum** — A form which persists over a long period of time after healing by primary intent.
             Postinflammatory perforation of ear drum — A form which occurs as a sequelae to an inflammatory reaction of the ear drum.
     Code first any associated otitis media (H65.-, H66.1-, H66.2-, H66.3-, H66.4-, H66.9-, H67.-)
     Excludes 1:   *acute suppurative otitis media with rupture of the tympanic membrane (H66.01-)*
                traumatic rupture of ear drum (S09.2-)

H72.0-   <u>Central</u> perforation of tympanic membrane — A form in which the hole is in the approximate center of the tympanic membrane.
   H72.00   Central perforation of tympanic membrane, <u>unspecified</u> ear
   H72.01   Central perforation of tympanic membrane, <u>right</u> ear
   H72.02   Central perforation of tympanic membrane, <u>left</u> ear
   H72.03   Central perforation of tympanic membrane, <u>bilateral</u>

H72.1-   <u>Attic</u> perforation of tympanic membrane — A form in which the hole is to the uppermost margin of the tympanic membrane.
     Perforation of pars flaccida
   H72.10   Attic perforation of tympanic membrane, <u>unspecified</u> ear
   H72.11   Attic perforation of tympanic membrane, <u>right</u> ear
   H72.12   Attic perforation of tympanic membrane, <u>left</u> ear
   H72.13   Attic perforation of tympanic membrane, <u>bilateral</u>

H72.2-   Other marginal perforations of tympanic membrane
   H72.2x- <u>Other marginal perforations</u> of tympanic membrane
     H72.2x1   Other marginal perforations of tympanic membrane, <u>right</u> ear
     H72.2x2   Other marginal perforations of tympanic membrane, <u>left</u> ear
     H72.2x3   Other marginal perforations of tympanic membrane, <u>bilateral</u>
     H72.2x9   Other marginal perforations of tympanic membrane, <u>unspecified</u> ear

H72.8-   Other perforations of tympanic membrane
   H72.81- <u>Multiple</u> perforations of tympanic membrane
     H72.811   Multiple perforations of tympanic membrane, <u>right</u> ear
     H72.812   Multiple perforations of tympanic membrane, <u>left</u> ear
     H72.813   Multiple perforations of tympanic membrane, <u>bilateral</u>
     H72.819   Multiple perforations of tympanic membrane, <u>unspecified</u> ear

   H72.82- <u>Total</u> perforations of tympanic membrane — A form in which the entire tympanic membrane is obliterated.
     H72.821   Total perforations of tympanic membrane, <u>right</u> ear
     H72.822   Total perforations of tympanic membrane, <u>left</u> ear
     H72.823   Total perforations of tympanic membrane, <u>bilateral</u>
     H72.829   Total perforations of tympanic membrane, <u>unspecified</u> ear

H72.9-   <u>Unspecified</u> perforation of tympanic membrane
   H72.90   Unspecified perforation of tympanic membrane, <u>unspecified</u> ear

Excludes 1: = NOT CODED HERE! (Do not code both)   **714**   *Excludes ❷:* = Not Included Here

H70
–
H72

H72.91   Unspecified perforation of tympanic membrane, **right** ear
H72.92   Unspecified perforation of tympanic membrane, **left** ear
H72.93   Unspecified perforation of tympanic membrane, **bilateral**

H73-   Other disorders of tympanic membrane

H73.0-   <u>Acute myringitis</u> — The sudden, severe onset of inflammation of the ear drum.
     Excludes 1:   acute myringitis with otitis media (H65, H66)

   H73.00- <u>Unspecified</u> acute myringitis
     Acute tympanitis NOS
     H73.001   Acute myringitis, **right** ear
     H73.002   Acute myringitis, **left** ear
     H73.003   Acute myringitis, **bilateral**
     H73.009   Acute myringitis, **unspecified** ear

   H73.01- <u>Bullous</u> myringitis — A form marked by serous or hemorrhagic blebs.
     H73.011   Bullous myringitis, **right** ear
     H73.012   Bullous myringitis, **left** ear
     H73.013   Bullous myringitis, **bilateral**
     H73.019   Bullous myringitis, **unspecified** ear

   H73.09- <u>Other</u> acute myringitis
     H73.091   Other acute myringitis, **right** ear
     H73.092   Other acute myringitis, **left** ear
     H73.093   Other acute myringitis, **bilateral**
     H73.099   Other acute myringitis, **unspecified** ear

H73.1-   <u>Chronic myringitis</u> — Inflammation of the ear drum that develops slowly and persists over a long period of time.
     Chronic tympanitis
     Excludes 1:   chronic myringitis with otitis media (H65, H66)

   H73.10   Chronic myringitis, **unspecified** ear
   H73.11   Chronic myringitis, **right** ear
   H73.12   Chronic myringitis, **left** ear
   H73.13   Chronic myringitis, **bilateral**

H73.2-   <u>Unspecified</u> <u>myringitis</u>
   H73.20   Unspecified myringitis, **unspecified** ear
   H73.21   Unspecified myringitis, **right** ear
   H73.22   Unspecified myringitis, **left** ear
   H73.23   Unspecified myringitis, **bilateral**

H73.8-   Other specified disorders of tympanic membrane

   H73.81- <u>Atrophic flaccid tympanic membrane</u> — A wasting-away of the tympanic membrane with deterioration in the tone of the membrane.
     H73.811   Atrophic flaccid tympanic membrane, **right** ear
     H73.812   Atrophic flaccid tympanic membrane, **left** ear
     H73.813   Atrophic flaccid tympanic membrane, **bilateral**
     H73.819   Atrophic flaccid tympanic membrane, **unspecified** ear

   H73.82- <u>Atrophic nonflaccid tympanic membrane</u> — A wasting-away of the tympanic membrane without loss of tone of the membrane.
     H73.821   Atrophic nonflaccid tympanic membrane, **right** ear
     H73.822   Atrophic nonflaccid tympanic membrane, **left** ear
     H73.823   Atrophic nonflaccid tympanic membrane, **bilateral**
     H73.829   Atrophic nonflaccid tympanic membrane, **unspecified** ear

   H73.89- <u>Other specified</u> disorders of tympanic membrane
     H73.891   Other specified disorders of tympanic membrane, **right** ear
     H73.892   Other specified disorders of tympanic membrane, **left** ear
     H73.893   Other specified disorders of tympanic membrane, **bilateral**
     H73.899   Other specified disorders of tympanic membrane, **unspecified** ear

H73.9-   <u>Unspecified disorder of tympanic membrane</u>
   H73.90   Unspecified disorder of tympanic membrane, **unspecified** ear
   H73.91   Unspecified disorder of tympanic membrane, **right** ear
   H73.92   Unspecified disorder of tympanic membrane, **left** ear
   H73.93   Unspecified disorder of tympanic membrane, **bilateral**

H74-   Other disorders of middle ear mastoid
   Excludes ❷: mastoiditis (H70.-)

H74.0-   <u>Tympanosclerosis</u> — The formation and infiltration of hard fibrous tissue in the middle ear.
   H74.01   Tympanosclerosis, **right** ear
   H74.02   Tympanosclerosis, **left** ear
   H74.03   Tympanosclerosis, **bilateral**
   H74.09   Tympanosclerosis, **unspecified** ear

H74.1-   <u>Adhesive middle ear disease</u> — The abnormal adherence together of the middle ear structures by fibrous tissue which restricts their function.
     Adhesive otitis
     Excludes 1:   glue ear (H65.3-)
   H74.11   Adhesive **right** middle ear disease
   H74.12   Adhesive **left** middle ear disease
   H74.13   Adhesive middle ear disease, **bilateral**
   H74.19   Adhesive middle ear disease, **unspecified** ear

H74.2-   <u>Discontinuity and dislocation of ear ossicles</u> — The displacement of ear ossicles from their normal positions.
   H74.20   Discontinuity and dislocation of ear ossicles, **unspecified** ear
   H74.21   Discontinuity and dislocation of **right** ear ossicles
   H74.22   Discontinuity and dislocation of **left** ear ossicles
   H74.23   Discontinuity and dislocation of ear ossicles, **bilateral**

H74.3-   Other acquired abnormalities of ear ossicles

   H74.31- <u>Ankylosis</u> of ear ossicles — The abnormal fixation of the middle ear ossicles.
     H74.311   Ankylosis of ear ossicles, **right** ear
     H74.312   Ankylosis of ear ossicles, **left** ear
     H74.313   Ankylosis of ear ossicles, **bilateral**
     H74.319   Ankylosis of ear ossicles, **unspecified** ear

   H74.32- <u>Partial loss</u> of ear ossicles — The deterioration or partial destruction of ear ossicles.
     H74.321   Partial loss of ear ossicles, **right** ear
     H74.322   Partial loss of ear ossicles, **left** ear
     H74.323   Partial loss of ear ossicles, **bilateral**
     H74.329   Partial loss of ear ossicles, **unspecified** ear

   H74.39- <u>Other acquired abnormalities</u> of ear ossicles
     H74.391   Other acquired abnormalities of **right** ear ossicles
     H74.392   Other acquired abnormalities of **left** ear ossicles
     H74.393   Other acquired abnormalities of ear ossicles, **bilateral**
     H74.399   Other acquired abnormalities of ear ossicles, **unspecified** ear

H74.4-   <u>Polyp</u> of middle ear — A protruding growth of the middle ear.
   H74.40   Polyp of middle ear, **unspecified** ear
   H74.41   Polyp of **right** middle ear
   H74.42   Polyp of **left** middle ear
   H74.43   Polyp of middle ear, **bilateral**

H74.8-   <u>Other specified disorders of middle ear and mastoid</u>
   H74.8x- Other specified disorders of middle ear and mastoid
     H74.8x1   Other specified disorders of **right** middle ear and mastoid
     H74.8x2   Other specified disorders of **left** middle ear and mastoid
     H74.8x3   Other specified disorders of middle ear and mastoid, **bilateral**
     H74.8x9   Other specified disorders of middle ear and mastoid, **unspecified** ear

H74.9-   <u>Unspecified disorder of middle ear and mastoid</u>
   H74.90   Unspecified disorder of middle ear and mastoid, **unspecified** ear
   H74.91   Unspecified disorder of **right** middle ear and mastoid
   H74.92   Unspecified disorder of **left** middle ear and mastoid
   H74.93   Unspecified disorder of middle ear and mastoid, **bilateral**

H
7
2
-
H
7
4

Excludes 1: = NOT CODED HERE! (Do not code both)   **715**   *Excludes ❷:* = Not Included Here

H75- Other disorders of middle ear and mastoid <u>in diseases classified elsewhere</u>

Code first underlying disease

H75.0- Mastoiditis <u>in infectious and parasitic diseases classified elsewhere</u>

Excludes 1: mastoiditis (in):
 syphilis (A52.77)
 tuberculosis (A18.03)

H75.00 Mastoiditis in infectious and parasitic diseases classified elsewhere, <u>unspecified</u> ear — [Not Allowed as PDX]

H75.01 Mastoiditis in infectious and parasitic diseases classified elsewhere, <u>right</u> ear — [Not Allowed as PDX]

H75.02 Mastoiditis in infectious and parasitic diseases classified elsewhere, <u>left</u> ear — [Not Allowed as PDX]

H75.03 Mastoiditis in infectious and parasitic diseases classified elsewhere, <u>bilateral</u> — [Not Allowed as PDX]

H75.8- Other specified disorders of middle ear and mastoid <u>in diseases classified elsewhere</u>

H75.80 Other specified disorders of middle ear and mastoid in diseases classified elsewhere, <u>unspecified</u> ear — [Not Allowed as PDX]

H75.81 Other specified disorders of <u>right</u> middle ear and mastoid in diseases classified elsewhere — [Not Allowed as PDX]

H75.82 Other specified disorders of <u>left</u> middle ear and mastoid in diseases classified elsewhere — [Not Allowed as PDX]

H75.83 Other specified disorders of middle ear and mastoid in diseases classified elsewhere, <u>bilateral</u> — [Not Allowed as PDX]

Diseases of inner ear (H80-H83)

H80- <u>Otosclerosis</u> — The abnormal formation of spongy bone in the labyrinth of the ear.

Includes: Otospongiosis

H80.0- Otosclerosis involving <u>oval window</u>, <u>nonobliterative</u>

H80.00 Otosclerosis involving oval window, <u>nonobliterative</u>, <u>unspecified</u> ear

H80.01 Otosclerosis involving oval window, <u>nonobliterative</u>, <u>right</u> ear

H80.02 Otosclerosis involving oval window, <u>nonobliterative</u>, <u>left</u> ear

H80.03 Otosclerosis involving oval window, <u>nonobliterative</u>, <u>bilateral</u>

H80.1- Otosclerosis involving <u>oval window</u>, <u>obliterative</u> — A form resulting in complete replacement of the oval window by the spongy bone.

H80.10 Otosclerosis involving oval window, <u>obliterative</u>, <u>unspecified</u> ear

H80.11 Otosclerosis involving oval window, <u>obliterative</u>, <u>right</u> ear

H80.12 Otosclerosis involving oval window, <u>obliterative</u>, <u>left</u> ear

H80.13 Otosclerosis involving oval window, <u>obliterative</u>, <u>bilateral</u>

H80.2- <u>Cochlear</u> otosclerosis — A form affecting the cochlea of the inner ear.

Otosclerosis involving otic capsule — A form involving the enclosing skeletal portion of the inner ear.

Otosclerosis involving round window — A form affecting the round window of the inner ear.

H80.20 Cochlear otosclerosis, <u>unspecified</u> ear

H80.21 Cochlear otosclerosis, <u>right</u> ear

H80.22 Cochlear otosclerosis, <u>left</u> ear

H80.23 Cochlear otosclerosis, <u>bilateral</u>

H80.8- <u>Other</u> otosclerosis

H80.80 Other otosclerosis, <u>unspecified</u> ear

H80.81 Other otosclerosis, <u>right</u> ear

H80.82 Other otosclerosis, <u>left</u> ear

H80.83 Other otosclerosis, <u>bilateral</u>

H80.9- <u>Unspecified</u> otosclerosis

H80.90 Unspecified otosclerosis, <u>unspecified</u> ear

H80.91 Unspecified otosclerosis, <u>right</u> ear

H80.92 Unspecified otosclerosis, <u>left</u> ear

H80.93 Unspecified otosclerosis, <u>bilateral</u>

H81- Disorders of vestibular function

Excludes 1: epidemic vertigo (A88.1)
 vertigo NOS (R42)

H81.0- <u>Ménière's disease</u> — A disease of the inner ear characterized by deafness, ringing of the ears, dizziness, and a sensation of fullness or pressure in the ears.

Labyrinthine hydrops
Ménière's syndrome or vertigo

H81.01 Ménière's disease, <u>right</u> ear

H81.02 Ménière's disease, <u>left</u> ear

H81.03 Ménière's disease, <u>bilateral</u>

H81.09 Ménière's disease, <u>unspecified</u> ear

H81.1- <u>Benign paroxysmal vertigo</u> — An illusion of the external world moving due to disturbances of the vestibular centers or pathways in the central nervous system associated with a specific position of the head.

H81.10 Benign paroxysmal vertigo, <u>unspecified</u> ear

H81.11 Benign paroxysmal vertigo, <u>right</u> ear

H81.12 Benign paroxysmal vertigo, <u>left</u> ear

H81.13 Benign paroxysmal vertigo, <u>bilateral</u>

H81.2- <u>Vestibular neuronitis</u> — An illusion of the external world moving due to disturbances of the vestibular centers or pathways in the central nervous system due to inflammation of the vestibular nerves.

H81.20 Vestibular neuronitis, <u>unspecified</u> ear

H81.21 Vestibular neuronitis, <u>right</u> ear

H81.22 Vestibular neuronitis, <u>left</u> ear

H81.23 Vestibular neuronitis, <u>bilateral</u>

H81.3- <u>Other</u> peripheral vertigo — An illusion of the external world moving due to disturbances of the vestibular centers or pathways in the central nervous system.

H81.31- <u>Aural vertigo</u> — A form due to pressure of cerumen on the ear drum.

H81.311 Aural vertigo, <u>right</u> ear

H81.312 Aural vertigo, <u>left</u> ear

H81.313 Aural vertigo, <u>bilateral</u>

H81.319 Aural vertigo, <u>unspecified</u> ear

H81.39- <u>Other peripheral vertigo</u>

Lermoyez' syndrome
Otogenic vertigo
Peripheral vertigo NOS

H81.391 Other peripheral vertigo, <u>right</u> ear

H81.392 Other peripheral vertigo, <u>left</u> ear

H81.393 Other peripheral vertigo, <u>bilateral</u>

H81.399 Other peripheral vertigo, <u>unspecified</u> ear

H81.4- Vertigo of <u>central origin</u> — The illusion of true (rotational) vertigo due to a disease of the central nervous system.

Central positional nystagmus

H81.41 Vertigo of central origin, <u>right</u> ear

H81.42 Vertigo of central origin, <u>left</u> ear

H81.43 Vertigo of central origin, <u>bilateral</u>

H81.49 Vertigo of central origin, <u>unspecified</u> ear

H81.8- Other disorders of vestibular function

H81.8x- <u>Other disorders of vestibular function</u>

H81.8x1 Other disorders of vestibular function, <u>right</u> ear

H81.8x2 Other disorders of vestibular function, <u>left</u> ear

H81.8x3 Other disorders of vestibular function, <u>bilateral</u>

H81.8x9 Other disorders of vestibular function, <u>unspecified</u> ear

H81.9- <u>Unspecified</u> disorder of vestibular function

Vertiginous syndrome NOS

H81.90 Unspecified disorder of vestibular function, <u>unspecified</u> ear

H81.91 Unspecified disorder of vestibular function, <u>right</u> ear

H81.92 Unspecified disorder of vestibular function, <u>left</u> ear

H81.93 Unspecified disorder of vestibular function, <u>bilateral</u>

H82- Vertiginous syndromes <u>in diseases classified elsewhere</u>

Code first underlying disease

Excludes 1: epidemic vertigo (A88.1)

H82.1 Vertiginous syndromes in diseases classified elsewhere, <u>right</u> ear — [Not Allowed as PDX]

H82.2 Vertiginous syndromes in diseases classified elsewhere, <u>left</u> ear — [Not Allowed as PDX]

Excludes 1: = NOT CODED HERE! (Do not code both)

Excludes ❷: = Not Included Here

H82.3 Vertiginous syndromes in diseases classified elsewhere, <u>bilateral</u> — [Not Allowed as PDX]

H82.9 Vertiginous syndromes in diseases classified elsewhere, <u>unspecified</u> ear — [Not Allowed as PDX]

H83- Other diseases of inner ear

  H83.0- <u>Labyrinthitis</u> — Inflammation of the inner ear labyrinth.

   H83.01 Labyrinthitis, <u>right</u> ear

   H83.02 Labyrinthitis, <u>left</u> ear

   H83.03 Labyrinthitis, <u>bilateral</u>

   H83.09 Labyrinthitis, <u>unspecified</u> ear

  H83.1- <u>Labyrinthine fistula</u> — An abnormal passage communicating with the labyrinth.

   H83.11 Labyrinthine fistula, <u>right</u> ear

   H83.12 Labyrinthine fistula, <u>left</u> ear

   H83.13 Labyrinthine fistula, <u>bilateral</u>

   H83.19 Labyrinthine fistula, <u>unspecified</u> ear

  H83.2- <u>Labyrinthine dysfunction</u> — An abnormal impairment of function of the inner ear.
    Labyrinthine hypersensitivity
    Labyrinthine hypofunction
    Labyrinthine loss of function

  H83.2x- <u>Labyrinthine dysfunction</u>

   H83.2x1 Labyrinthine dysfunction, <u>right</u> ear

   H83.2x2 Labyrinthine dysfunction, <u>left</u> ear

   H83.2x3 Labyrinthine dysfunction, <u>bilateral</u>

   H83.2x9 Labyrinthine dysfunction, <u>unspecified</u> ear

  H83.3- Noise effects on inner ear
    Acoustic trauma of inner ear
    Noise-induced hearing loss of inner ear

  H83.3x- <u>Noise effects on inner ear</u>

   H83.3x1 Noise effects on <u>right</u> inner ear

   H83.3x2 Noise effects on <u>left</u> inner ear

   H83.3x3 Noise effects on inner ear, <u>bilateral</u>

   H83.3x9 Noise effects on inner ear, <u>unspecified</u> ear

  H83.8- Other specified diseases of inner ear

  H83.8x- <u>Other specified</u> diseases of inner ear

   H83.8x1 Other specified diseases of <u>right</u> inner ear

   H83.8x2 Other specified diseases of <u>left</u> inner ear

   H83.8x3 Other specified diseases of inner ear, <u>bilateral</u>

   H83.8x9 Other specified diseases of inner ear, <u>unspecified</u> ear

  H83.9- <u>Unspecified</u> disease of inner ear

   H83.90 Unspecified disease of inner ear, <u>unspecified</u> ear

   H83.91 Unspecified disease of <u>right</u> inner ear

   H83.92 Unspecified disease of <u>left</u> inner ear

   H83.93 Unspecified disease of inner ear, <u>bilateral</u>

Other disorders of ear (H90-H94)

H90- Conductive and sensorineural hearing loss — CONDUCTIVE HEARING LOSS — The decreased ability to perceive sounds due to a defect of the sound conducting apparatus of the ear. SENSORINEURAL HEARING LOSS — The decreased ability to perceive sounds due to a defect in the sensory mechanism of the ear or nerves.
  Excludes 1: *deaf nonspeaking NEC (H91.3)*
      deafness NOS (H91.9-)
      hearing loss NOS (H91.9-)
      noise-induced hearing loss (H83.3-)
      ototoxic hearing loss (H91.0-)
      sudden (idiopathic) hearing loss (H91.2-)
  AHA 15:2Q:p7x2 – Mixed hearing loss, bilateral

  H90.0 <u>Conductive</u> hearing loss, <u>bilateral</u>

  H90.1- <u>Conductive</u> hearing loss, <u>unilateral</u> with unrestricted hearing on the contralateral side

   H90.11 Conductive hearing loss, unilateral, <u>right</u> ear, with unrestricted hearing on the contralateral side

   H90.12 Conductive hearing loss, unilateral, <u>left</u> ear, with unrestricted hearing on the contralateral side

  H90.2 <u>Conductive</u> hearing loss, <u>unspecified</u>
    Conductive deafness NOS

  H90.3 <u>Sensorineural</u> hearing loss, <u>bilateral</u>

H90.4- <u>Sensorineural</u> hearing loss, <u>unilateral</u> with unrestricted hearing on the contralateral side

   H90.41 Sensorineural hearing loss, unilateral, <u>right</u> ear, with unrestricted hearing on the contralateral side

   H90.42 Sensorineural hearing loss, unilateral, <u>left</u> ear, with unrestricted hearing on the contralateral side

  H90.5 Unspecified <u>sensorineural</u> hearing loss
    Central hearing loss NOS
    Congenital deafness NOS
    Neural hearing loss NOS
    Perceptive hearing loss NOS
    Sensorineural deafness NOS
    Sensory hearing loss NOS
  Excludes 1: *abnormal auditory perception (H93.2-)*
      psychogenic deafness (F44.6)

  H90.6 <u>Mixed</u> conductive and sensorineural hearing loss, <u>bilateral</u>

  H90.7- <u>Mixed</u> conductive and sensorineural hearing loss, <u>unilateral</u> with unrestricted hearing on the contralateral side

   H90.71 Mixed conductive and sensorineural hearing loss, unilateral, <u>right</u> ear, with unrestricted hearing on the contralateral side

   H90.72 Mixed conductive and sensorineural hearing loss, unilateral, <u>left</u> ear, with unrestricted hearing on the contralateral side

  H90.8 Mixed conductive and sensorineural hearing loss, <u>unspecified</u>

  H90.A- Conductive and sensorineural hearing loss <u>with restricted hearing on the contralateral side</u>

   H90.A1- <u>Conductive</u> hearing loss, unilateral, with restricted hearing on the contralateral side

    H90.A11 Conductive hearing loss, unilateral, <u>right</u> ear, with restricted hearing on the contralateral side

    H90.A12 Conductive hearing loss, unilateral, <u>left</u> ear, with restricted hearing on the contralateral side

   H90.A2- <u>Sensorineural</u> hearing loss, unilateral, with restricted hearing on the contralateral side

    H90.A21 Sensorineural hearing loss, unilateral, <u>right</u> ear, with restricted hearing on the contralateral side

    H90.A22 Sensorineural hearing loss, unilateral, <u>left</u> ear, with restricted hearing on the contralateral side

   H90.A3- <u>Mixed</u> conductive and sensorineural hearing loss, unilateral, with restricted hearing on the contralateral side

    H90.A31 Mixed conductive and sensorineural hearing loss, unilateral, <u>right</u> ear, with restricted hearing on the contralateral side

    H90.A32 Mixed conductive and sensorineural hearing loss, unilateral, <u>left</u> ear, with restricted hearing on the contralateral side

H91- <u>Other and unspecified</u> <u>hearing loss</u>
  Excludes 1: *abnormal auditory perception (H93.2-)*
      hearing loss as classified in H90.-
      impacted cerumen (H61.2-)
      noise-induced hearing loss (H83.3-)
      psychogenic deafness (F44.6)
      transient ischemic deafness (H93.01-)

  H91.0- <u>Ototoxic hearing loss</u> — The decreased ability to perceive sounds due to a drug, toxin, or other external substance.
    Code first poisoning due to drug or toxin, if applicable (T36-T65 with fifth or sixth character 1-4 or 6)
    Use additional code for adverse effect, if applicable, to identify drug (T36-T50 with fift or sixth character 5)

   H91.01 Ototoxic hearing loss, <u>right</u> ear

   H91.02 Ototoxic hearing loss, <u>left</u> ear

   H91.03 Ototoxic hearing loss, <u>bilateral</u>

   H91.09 Ototoxic hearing loss, <u>unspecified</u> ear

  H91.1- <u>Presbycusis</u> — Progressive loss of hearing ability due to the normal aging process.
    Presbyacusia

   H91.10 Presbycusis, <u>unspecified</u> ear

   H91.11 Presbycusis, <u>right</u> ear

   H91.12 Presbycusis, <u>left</u> ear

   H91.13 Presbycusis, <u>bilateral</u>

H82 - H91

H91.2- **Sudden idiopathic** hearing loss — The sudden decreased ability to perceive sounds due to an unknown cause.
    Sudden hearing loss NOS
    H91.20 Sudden idiopathic hearing loss, **unspecified** ear
    H91.21 Sudden idiopathic hearing loss, **right** ear
    H91.22 Sudden idiopathic hearing loss, **left** ear
    H91.23 Sudden idiopathic hearing loss, **bilateral**

H91.3 **Deaf nonspeaking, not elsewhere classified**

H91.8- **Other specified hearing loss**
    H91.8x- **Other specified** hearing loss
      H91.8x1 Other specified hearing loss, **right** ear
      H91.8x2 Other specified hearing loss, **left** ear
      H91.8x3 Other specified hearing loss, **bilateral**
      H91.8x9 Other specified hearing loss, **unspecified** ear

H91.9- **Unspecified** hearing loss
    Deafness NOS
    High frequency deafness
    Low frequency deafness
    H91.90 Unspecified hearing loss, **unspecified** ear
    H91.91 Unspecified hearing loss, **right** ear
    H91.92 Unspecified hearing loss, **left** ear
    H91.93 Unspecified hearing loss, **bilateral**

H92- **Otalgia and effusion of ear**

H92.0- **Otalgia** — Pain in the ear.
    H92.01 Otalgia, **right** ear
    H92.02 Otalgia, **left** ear
    H92.03 Otalgia, **bilateral**
    H92.09 Otalgia, **unspecified** ear

H92.1- **Otorrhea** — Inflammation of the ear with purulent discharge.
    Excludes 1: **leakage of cerebrospinal fluid through ear (G96.0)**
    H92.10 Otorrhea, **unspecified** ear
    H92.11 Otorrhea, **right** ear
    H92.12 Otorrhea, **left** ear
    H92.13 Otorrhea, **bilateral**

H92.2- **Otorrhagia** — The abnormal discharge of blood from the ear.
    Excludes 1: **traumatic otorrhagia — code to injury**
    H92.20 Otorrhagia, **unspecified** ear
    H92.21 Otorrhagia, **right** ear
    H92.22 Otorrhagia, **left** ear
    H92.23 Otorrhagia, **bilateral**

H93- **Other disorders of ear, not elsewhere classified**

H93.0- **Degenerative and vascular disorders of ear**
    Excludes 1: **presbycusis (H91.1)**
    H93.01- **Transient ischemic deafness** — A temporary loss of hearing ability due to decreased blood flow to the ear.
      H93.011 Transient ischemic deafness, **right** ear
      H93.012 Transient ischemic deafness, **left** ear
      H93.013 Transient ischemic deafness, **bilateral**
      H93.019 Transient ischemic deafness, **unspecified** ear
    H93.09- **Unspecified degenerative and vascular disorders of ear**
      H93.091 Unspecified degenerative and vascular disorders of **right** ear
      H93.092 Unspecified degenerative and vascular disorders of **left** ear
      H93.093 Unspecified degenerative and vascular disorders of ear, **bilateral**
      H93.099 Unspecified degenerative and vascular disorders of **unspecified** ear

H93.1- **Tinnitus** — A ringing, buzzing, or clicking noise in the ear.
    H93.11 Tinnitus, **right** ear
    H93.12 Tinnitus, **left** ear
    H93.13 Tinnitus, **bilateral**
    H93.19 Tinnitus, **unspecified** ear

H93.A- **Pulsatile tinnitus** — A beating or pulsing sound in the ear that is synchronous with the heartbeat.
    H93.A1 Pulsatile tinnitus, **right** ear
    H93.A2 Pulsatile tinnitus, **left** ear
    H93.A3 Pulsatile tinnitus, **bilateral**
    H93.A9 Pulsatile tinnitus, **unspecified** ear

H93.2- **Other abnormal auditory perceptions**
    Excludes ❷: **auditory hallucinations (R44.0)**
    H93.21- **Auditory recruitment** — An abnormal increase in the perceived intensity of a sound out of proportion to the actual increase in the sound level.
      H93.211 Auditory recruitment, **right** ear
      H93.212 Auditory recruitment, **left** ear
      H93.213 Auditory recruitment, **bilateral**
      H93.219 Auditory recruitment, **unspecified** ear
    H93.22- **Diplacusis** — An abnormal perception of pitch characterized by hearing two tones for every sound produced.
      H93.221 Diplacusis, **right** ear
      H93.222 Diplacusis, **left** ear
      H93.223 Diplacusis, **bilateral**
      H93.229 Diplacusis, **unspecified** ear
    H93.23- **Hyperacusis** — The abnormal sensitivity to sound.
      H93.231 Hyperacusis, **right** ear
      H93.232 Hyperacusis, **left** ear
      H93.233 Hyperacusis, **bilateral**
      H93.239 Hyperacusis, **unspecified** ear
    H93.24- **Temporary auditory threshold shift** — A condition of temporary decreased auditory sensitivity to accommodate a higher decible environment.
      H93.241 Temporary auditory threshold shift, **right** ear
      H93.242 Temporary auditory threshold shift, **left** ear
      H93.243 Temporary auditory threshold shift, **bilateral**
      H93.249 Temporary auditory threshold shift, **unspecified** ear
    H93.25 **Central auditory processing disorder** — A disorder characterized by difficulty in the processing of auditory frequency, intensity, and temporal information in the central nervous system.
      Congenital auditory imperception
      Word deafness
      Excludes 1: **mixed receptive-expressive language disorder (F80.2)**
    H93.29- **Other** abnormal auditory perceptions
      H93.291 Other abnormal auditory perceptions, **right** ear
      H93.292 Other abnormal auditory perceptions, **left** ear
      H93.293 Other abnormal auditory perceptions, **bilateral**
      H93.299 Other abnormal auditory perceptions, **unspecified** ear

H93.3- **Disorders of acoustic nerve**
    Disorder of 8th cranial nerve
    Excludes 1: **acoustic neuroma (D33.3)**
             syphilitic acoustic neuritis (A52.15)
    H93.3x- **Disorders of acoustic nerve** — Dysfunction of the acoustic nerve.
      H93.3x1 Disorders of **right** acoustic nerve
      H93.3x2 Disorders of **left** acoustic nerve
      H93.3x3 Disorders of **bilateral** acoustic nerves
      H93.3x9 Disorders of **unspecified** acoustic nerve

H93.8- **Other specified disorders of ear**
    H93.8x- **Other specified disorders of ear**
      H93.8x1 Other specified disorders of **right** ear
      H93.8x2 Other specified disorders of **left** ear
      H93.8x3 Other specified disorders of ear, **bilateral**
      H93.8x9 Other specified disorders of ear, **unspecified** ear

H93.9- **Unspecified** disorder of ear
    H93.90 Unspecified disorder of ear, **unspecified** ear — [Unacceptable PDX]
    H93.91 Unspecified disorder of **right** ear — [Unacceptable PDX]
    H93.92 Unspecified disorder of **left** ear — [Unacceptable PDX]
    H93.93 Unspecified disorder of ear, **bilateral** — [Unacceptable PDX]

H
9
1
-
H
9
3

Excludes 1: = NOT CODED HERE! (Do not code both)

Excludes ❷: = Not Included Here

H94- Other disorders of ear in diseases classified elsewhere
H94.0- Acoustic neuritis in infectious and parasitic diseases classified elsewhere
Code first underlying disease, such as:
Parasitic disease (B65-B89)
Excludes 1:   acoustic neuritis (in):
herpes zoster (B02.29)
syphilis (A52.15)

H94.00 Acoustic neuritis in infectious and parasitic diseases classified elsewhere, <u>unspecified</u> ear — [Not Allowed as PDX]
H94.01 Acoustic neuritis in infectious and parasitic diseases classified elsewhere, <u>right</u> ear — [Not Allowed as PDX]
H94.02 Acoustic neuritis in infectious and parasitic diseases classified elsewhere, <u>left</u> ear — [Not Allowed as PDX]
H94.03 Acoustic neuritis in infectious and parasitic diseases classified elsewhere, <u>bilateral</u> — [Not Allowed as PDX]
H94.8- Other specified disorders of ear in diseases classified elsewhere
Code first underlying disease, such as:
Congenital syphilis (A50.0)
Excludes 1:   aural myiasis (B87.4)
syphilitic labyrinthitis (A52.79)

H94.80 Other specified disorders of ear in diseases classified elsewhere, <u>unspecified</u> ear — [Not Allowed as PDX]
H94.81 Other specified disorders of <u>right</u> ear in diseases classified elsewhere — [Not Allowed as PDX]
H94.82 Other specified disorders of <u>left</u> ear in diseases classified elsewhere — [Not Allowed as PDX]
H94.83 Other specified disorders of ear in diseases classified elsewhere, <u>bilateral</u> — [Not Allowed as PDX]

Intraoperative and postprocedural complications and disorders of ear and mastoid process, not elsewhere classified (H95)

H95- Intraoperative and postprocedural complications and disorders of ear and mastoid process, not elsewhere classified
H95.0- Recurrent cholesteatoma of postmastoidectomy cavity
H95.00 Recurrent cholesteatoma of postmastoidectomy cavity, <u>unspecified</u> ear
H95.01 Recurrent cholesteatoma of postmastoidectomy cavity, <u>right</u> ear
H95.02 Recurrent cholesteatoma of postmastoidectomy cavity, <u>left</u> ear
H95.03 Recurrent cholesteatoma of postmastoidectomy cavity, <u>bilateral</u> ears
H95.1- <u>Other</u> disorders of ear and mastoid process <u>following mastoidectomy</u>
H95.11- Chronic inflammation of postmastoidectomy cavity
H95.111 Chronic inflammation of postmastoidectomy cavity, <u>right</u> ear
H95.112 Chronic inflammation of postmastoidectomy cavity, <u>left</u> ear
H95.113 Chronic inflammation of postmastoidectomy cavity, <u>bilateral</u> ears
H95.119 Chronic inflammation of postmastoidectomy cavity, <u>unspecified</u> ear
H95.12- <u>Granulation</u> of <u>postmastoidectomy cavity</u>
H95.121 Granulation of postmastoidectomy cavity, <u>right</u> ear
H95.122 Granulation of postmastoidectomy cavity, <u>left</u> ear
H95.123 Granulation of postmastoidectomy cavity, <u>bilateral</u> ears
H95.129 Granulation of postmastoidectomy cavity, <u>unspecified</u> ear
H95.13- <u>Mucosal cyst</u> of <u>postmastoidectomy cavity</u>
H95.131 Mucosal cyst of postmastoidectomy cavity, <u>right</u> ear
H95.132 Mucosal cyst of postmastoidectomy cavity, <u>left</u> ear
H95.133 Mucosal cyst of postmastoidectomy cavity, <u>bilateral</u> ears

H95.139 Mucosal cyst of postmastoidectomy cavity, <u>unspecified</u> ear
H95.19- <u>Other</u> disorders <u>following mastoidectomy</u>
H95.191 Other disorders following mastoidectomy, <u>right</u> ear
H95.192 Other disorders following mastoidectomy, <u>left</u> ear
H95.193 Other disorders following mastoidectomy, <u>bilateral</u> ears
H95.199 Other disorders following mastoidectomy, <u>unspecified</u> ear
H95.2- <u>Intraoperative hemorrhage and hematoma</u> of ear and mastoid process complicating a procedure
Excludes 1:   intraoperative hemorrhage and hematoma of ear and mastoid process due to accidental puncture or laceration during a procedure (H95.3-)

cc **H95.21** Intraoperative hemorrhage and hematoma of ear and mastoid process complicating a <u>procedure on the ear and mastoid process</u>
cc **H95.22** Intraoperative hemorrhage and hematoma of ear and mastoid process complicating <u>other procedure</u>
H95.3- <u>Accidental puncture and laceration</u> of ear and mastoid process during a procedure
cc **H95.31** Accidental puncture and laceration of the ear and mastoid process during a <u>procedure on the ear and mastoid process</u>
cc **H95.32** Accidental puncture and laceration of the ear and mastoid process during <u>other procedure</u>
H95.4- <u>Postprocedural</u> <u>hemorrhage</u> of ear and mastoid process following a procedure
cc **H95.41** Postprocedural hemorrhage of ear and mastoid process following a <u>procedure on the ear and mastoid process</u>
cc **H95.42** Postprocedural hemorrhage of ear and mastoid process following <u>other procedure</u>
H95.5- <u>Postprocedural</u> <u>hematoma and seroma</u> of ear and mastoid process following a procedure
cc **H95.51** Postprocedural <u>hematoma</u> of ear and mastoid process following a <u>procedure on the ear and mastoid process</u>
cc **H95.52** Postprocedural <u>hematoma</u> of ear and mastoid process following <u>other procedure</u>
cc **H95.53** Postprocedural <u>seroma</u> of ear and mastoid process following a <u>procedure on the ear and mastoid process</u>
cc **H95.54** Postprocedural <u>seroma</u> of ear and mastoid process following <u>other procedure</u>
H95.8- Other intraoperative and postprocedural complications and disorders of the ear and mastoid process, not elsewhere classified
Excludes ❷: postprocedural complications and disorders following mastoidectomy (H95.0-, H95.1-)

H95.81- <u>Postprocedural stenosis</u> of external ear canal
cc **H95.811** Postprocedural stenosis of <u>right</u> external ear canal
cc **H95.812** Postprocedural stenosis of <u>left</u> external ear canal
cc **H95.813** Postprocedural stenosis of external ear canal, <u>bilateral</u>
cc **H95.819** Postprocedural stenosis of <u>unspecified</u> external ear canal
cc **H95.88** Other intraoperative complications and disorders of the ear and mastoid process, no telsewhere classified
Use additional code, if applicable, to further specify disorder
cc **H95.89** Other postprocedural complications and disorders of the ear and mastoid process, not elsewhere classified
Use additional code, if applicable, to further specify disorder

H
9
4
–
H
9
5

Chapter 9 – Diseases of the circulatory system (I00-I99)

Excludes ❷: *certain conditions originating in the perinatal period (P04-P96)*
certain infectious and parasitic diseases (A00-B99)
complications of pregnancy, childbirth and the puerperium (O00-O9A)
congenital malformations, deformations, and chromosomal abnormalities (Q00-Q99)
endocrine, nutritional and metabolic diseases (E00-E88)
injury, poisoning and certain other consequences of external causes (S00-T88)
neoplasms (C00-D49)
symptoms, signs and abnormal clinical and laboratory findings, not elsewhere classified (R00-R94)
systemic connective tissue disorders (M30-M36)
transient cerebral ischemic attacks and related syndromes (G45-)

This chapter contains the following blocks:

I00-I02   **Acute rheumatic fever**
I05-I09   **Chronic rheumatic heart diseases**
I10-I16   **Hypertensive diseases**
I20-I25   **Ischemic heart diseases**
I26-I28   **Pulmonary heart disease and diseases of pulmonary circulation**
I30-I52   **Other forms of heart disease**
I60-I69   **Cerebrovascular diseases**
I70-I79   **Diseases of arteries, arterioles and capillaries**
I80-I89   **Diseases of veins, lymphatic vessels and lymph nodes, not elsewhere classified**
I95-I99   **Other and unspecified disorders of the circulatory system**

Chapter-Specific Coding Guidelines

C.   Chapter-Specific Coding Guidelines
In addition to general coding guidelines, there are guidelines for specific diagnoses and/or conditions in the classification. Unless otherwise indicated, these guidelines apply to all health care settings. Please refer to Section II for guidelines on the selection of principal diagnosis.

9.   Chapter 9: Diseases of Circulatory System (I00-I99)

a.   Hypertension
The classification presumes a causal relationship between hypertension and heart involvement and between hypertension and kidney involvement, as the two conditions are linked by the term "with" in the Alphabetic Index. These conditions should be coded as related even in the absence of provider documentation explicitly linking them, unless the documentation clearly states the conditions are unrelated.

For hypertension and conditions not specifically linked by relational terms such as "with," "associated with" or "due to" in the classification, provider documentaton must link the conditions in order to code them as related.

1)   Hypertension with Heart Disease
Hypertension with heart conditions classified to I50.- or I51.4-I51.9, are assigned to, a code from category I11, Hypertensive heart disease, when a causal relationship is stated (due to hypertension) or implied (hypertensive). Use an additional code from category I50, Heart failure, to identify the type of heart failure in those patients with heart failure.

The same heart conditions (I50.-, I51.4-I51.9) with hypertension, ~~but without a stated causal relationship,~~ are coded separately if the provider has specifically documented a different cause. Sequence according to the circumstances of the admission/encounter.

2)   Hypertensive Chronic Kidney Disease
Assign codes from category I12, Hypertensive chronic kidney disease, when both hypertension and a condition classifiable to category N18, Chronic kidney disease (CKD), are present. ~~Unlike hypertension with heart disease, ICD-10-CM presumes a cause-and-effect relationship and classifies chronic kidney disease with hypertension as hypertensive chronic kidney disease.~~ CKD should not be coded as hypertensive if the physician has specifically documented a different cause.

The appropriate code from category N18 should be used as a secondary code with a code from category I12 to identify the stage of chronic kidney disease.

See Section I.C.14. Chronic kidney disease.

If a patient has hypertensive chronic kidney disease and acute renal failure, an additional code for the acute renal failure is required.

3)   Hypertensive Heart and Chronic Kidney Disease
Assign codes from combination category I13, Hypertensive heart and chronic kidney disease, when ~~both hypertensive kidney disease and hypertensive heart disease are stated in the diagnosis~~ there is hypertension with both heart and kidney involvement. ~~Assume a relationship between the hypertension and the chronic kidney disease, whether or not the condition is so designated.~~ If heart failure is present, assign an additional code from category I50 to identify the type of heart failure.

The appropriate code from category N18, Chronic kidney disease, should be used as a secondary code with a code from category I13 to identify the stage of chronic kidney disease.

See Section I.C.14. Chronic kidney disease.

The codes in category I13, Hypertensive heart and chronic kidney disease, are combination codes that include hypertension, heart disease and chronic kidney disease. The Includes note at I13 specifies that the conditions included at I11 and I12 are included together in I13. If a patient has hypertension, heart disease and chronic kidney disease then a code from I13 should be used, not individual codes for hypertension, heart disease and chronic kidney disease, or codes from I11 or I12.

For patients with both acute renal failure and chronic kidney disease, an additional code for acute renal failure is required.

4)   Hypertensive Cerebrovascular Disease
For hypertensive cerebrovascular disease, first assign the appropriate code from categories I60-I69, followed by the appropriate hypertension code.

5)   Hypertensive Retinopathy
Subcategory H35.0, Background retinopathy and retinal vascular changes, should be used with a code from category I10-I15, Hypertensive disease to include the systemic hypertension. The sequencing is based on the reason for the encounter.

6)   Hypertension, Secondary
Secondary hypertension is due to an underlying condition. Two codes are required: one to identify the underlying etiology and one from category I15 to identify the hypertension. Sequencing of codes is determined by the reason for admission/encounter.

7)   Hypertension, Transient
Assign code R03.0, Elevated blood pressure reading without diagnosis of hypertension, unless patient has an established diagnosis of hypertension. Assign code O13.-, Gestational [pregnancy-induced] hypertension without significant proteinuria, or O14.-, Pre-eclampsia, for transient hypertension of pregnancy.

8)   Hypertension, Controlled
This diagnostic statement usually refers to an existing state of hypertension under control by therapy. Assign the appropriate code from categories I10-I15, Hypertensive diseases.

9)   Hypertension, Uncontrolled
Uncontrolled hypertension may refer to untreated hypertension or hypertension not responding to current therapeutic regimen. In either case, assign the appropriate code from categories I10-I15, Hypertensive diseases.

10)   Hypertensive Crisis
Assign a code from category I16, Hypertensive crisis, for documented hypertensive urgency, hypertensive emergency or unspecified hypertensive crisis. Code also any identified hypertensive disease (I10-I15). The sequencing is based on the reason for the encounter.

b.   Atherosclerotic Coronary Artery Disease and Angina
ICD-10-CM has combination codes for atherosclerotic heart disease with angina pectoris. The subcategories for these codes are I25.11, Atherosclerotic heart disease of native coronary artery with angina pectoris and I25.7, Atherosclerosis of coronary artery bypass graft(s) and coronary artery of transplanted heart with angina pectoris.

When using one of these combination codes it is not necessary to use an additional code for angina pectoris. A causal relationship can be assumed in a patient with both atherosclerosis and angina pectoris, unless the documentation indicates the angina is due to something other than the atherosclerosis.

If a patient with coronary artery disease is admitted due to an acute myocardial infarction (AMI), the AMI should be sequenced before the coronary artery disease.

See Section I.C.9. Acute myocardial infarction (AMI).

c.   Intraoperative and Postprocedural Cerebrovascular Accident
Medical record documentation should clearly specify the cause-and-effect relationship between the medical intervention and the cerebrovascular accident in order to assign a code for intraoperative or postprocedural cerebrovascular accident.

I00-I00

Proper code assignment depends on whether it was an infarction or hemorrhage and whether it occurred intraoperatively or postoperatively. If it was a cerebral hemorrhage, code assignment depends on the type of procedure performed.

d.   Sequelae of Cerebrovascular Disease

1)   Category I69, Sequelae of Cerebrovascular disease
Category I69 is used to indicate conditions classifiable to categories I60-I67 as the causes of sequela (neurologic deficits), themselves classified elsewhere. These "late effects" include neurologic deficits that persist after initial onset of conditions classifiable to categories I60-I67. The neurologic deficits caused by cerebrovascular disease may be present from the onset or may arise at any time after the onset of the condition classifiable to categories I60-I67.

Codes from category I69, Sequelae of cerebrovascular disease, that specify hemiplegia, hemiparesis and monoplegia identify whether the dominant or nondominant side is affected. Should the affected side be documented, but not specified as dominant or nondominant, and the classification system does not indicate a default, code selection is as follows:
- For ambidextrous patients, the default should be dominant.
- If the left side is affected, the default is nondominant.
- If the right side is affected, the default is dominant.

2)   Codes from category I69 with codes from I60-I67
Codes from category I69 may be assigned on a health care record with codes from I60-I67, if the patient has a current cerebrovascular disease and deficits from an old cerebrovascular disease.

3)   Codes from category I69 and Personal history of transient ischemic attack (TIA) and cerebral infarction (Z86.73)
Codes from category I69 should not be assigned if the patient does not have neurologic deficits.

See Section I.C.21.c.4. History (of) for use of personal history codes.

e.   Acute myocardial infarction (AMI)

1)   ST elevation myocardial infarction (STEMI) and non ST elevation myocardial infarction (NSTEMI)
The ICD-10-CM codes for acute myocardial infarction (AMI) identify the site, such as anterolateral wall or true posterior wall. Subcategories I21.0-I21.2 and code I21.3 are used for ST elevation myocardial infarction (STEMI). Code I21.4, Non-ST elevation (NSTEMI) myocardial infarction, is used for non ST elevation myocardial infarction (NSTEMI) and nontransmural MIs.

If NSTEMI evolves to STEMI, assign the STEMI code. If STEMI converts to NSTEMI due to thrombolytic therapy, it is still coded as STEMI.

For encounters occurring while the myocardial infarction is equal to, or less than, four weeks old, including transfers to another acute setting or a postacute setting, and ~~the patient requires continued care for~~ the myocardial infarction meets the definition for "other diagnoses" (see Section III, Reporting Additional Diagnoses), codes from category I21 may continue to be reported. For encounters after the 4 week time frame and the   patient is still receiving care related to the myocardial infarction, the appropriate aftercare code should be assigned, rather than a code from category I21. For old or healed myocardial infarctions not requiring further care, code I25.2, Old myocardial infarction, may be assigned.

2)   Acute myocardial infarction, unspecified
Code I21.3, ST elevation (STEMI) myocardial infarction of unspecified site, is the default for the unspecified acute myocardial infarction. If only STEMI or transmural MI without the site is documented, assign code I21.3.

3)   AMI documented as nontransmural or subendocardial but site provided
If an AMI is documented as nontransmural or subendocardial, but the site is provided, it is still coded as a subendocardial AMI.

See Section I.C.21.3 for information on coding status post administration of tPA in a different facility within the last 24 hours.

4)   Subsequent acute myocardial infarction
A code from category I22, Subsequent ST elevation (STEMI) and non ST elevation (NSTEMI) myocardial infarction, is to be used when a patient who has suffered an AMI has a new AMI within the 4 week time frame of the initial AMI. A code from category I22 must be used in conjunction with a code from category I21. The sequencing of the I22 and I21 codes depends on the circumstances of the encounter.

Acute rheumatic fever (I00-I02)

I00   Rheumatic fever <u>without</u> heart involvement — A systemic inflammatory disease, with a severe onset, occurring as a delayed sequela of group A beta-hemolytic Streptococcus characterized by connective tissue inflammation, especially the blood vessels and joints.
Includes: Arthritis, rheumatic, acute or subacute
Excludes 1:   rheumatic fever with heart involvement (I01.0 - I01.9)

I01-   Rheumatic fever <u>with</u> heart involvement — A systemic inflammatory disease, with a severe onset, as a delayed sequela of group A beta-hemolytic Streptococcus characterized by connective tissue inflammation, specifically the heart, and of blood vessels and joints.
Excludes 1:   chronic diseases of rheumatic origin (I05-I09) unless rheumatic fever is also present or there is evidence of reactivation or activity of the rheumatic process

cc **I01.0   Acute rheumatic pericarditis** — A form characterized by inflammation of the outer fibrous and serous protective layers of the heart.
Any condition in I00 with pericarditis
Rheumatic pericarditis (acute)
Excludes 1:   acute pericarditis not specified as rheumatic (I30.-)

cc **I01.1   Acute rheumatic endocarditis** — A form characterized by inflammation of the inner serous lining membrane of the heart, including the valves of the heart.
Any condition in I00 with endocarditis or valvulitis
Acute rheumatic valvulitis

cc **I01.2   Acute rheumatic myocarditis** — A form characterized by inflammation of the cardiac muscle.
Any condition in I00 with myocarditis

cc **I01.8   Other acute rheumatic heart disease**
Any condition in I00 with other or multiple types of heart involvement
Acute rheumatic pancarditis — A form marked by inflammation of the pericardium and endocardium.

cc **I01.9   Acute rheumatic heart disease, unspecified**
Any condition in I00 with unspecified type of heart involvement
Rheumatic carditis, acute
Rheumatic heart disease, active or acute

I02-   Rheumatic <u>chorea</u> — Abrupt, involuntary, purposeless movements, muscular weakness, and emotional lability associated with rheumatic fever.
Includes: Sydenham's chorea
Excludes 1:   chorea NOS (G25.5)
Huntington's chorea (G10)

cc **I02.0   Rheumatic chorea with heart involvement** — A form marked by association with cardiac inflammation.
Chorea NOS with heart involvement
Rheumatic chorea with heart involvement of any type classifiable under I01.-

cc **I02.9   Rheumatic chorea without heart involvement**
Rheumatic chorea NOS

Chronic rheumatic heart diseases (I05-I09)

I05-   Rheumatic <u>mitral valve diseases</u> — Persistent, degenerative, rheumatic inflammatory lesions of the mitral valve.
Includes: Conditions classifiable to both I05.0 and I05.2-I05.9, whether specified as rheumatic or not
Excludes 1:   mitral valve disease specified as nonrheumatic (I34.-)
mitral valve disease with aortic and/or tricuspid valve involvement (I08.-)

I05.0   Rheumatic mitral stenosis — A form characterized by reduction in the mitral valve orifice size.
Mitral (valve) obstruction (rheumatic) — A form marked by blockage of the mitral valve orifice.

I05.1   Rheumatic mitral insufficiency — A form characterized by the inadequate function of the mitral valve.
Rheumatic mitral incompetence — A form marked by inadequate function of the mitral valve.
Rheumatic mitral regurgitation — A form marked by backflow of blood through the mitral valve.
Excludes 1:   mitral insufficiency not specified as rheumatic (I34.0)

I05.2   Rheumatic mitral stenosis <u>with insufficiency</u> — A form characterized by both reduction in the mitral valve orifice size and inadequate function and/or backflow of blood through the mitral valve.
Rheumatic mitral stenosis with incompetence or regurgitation

I05.8   Other rheumatic mitral valve diseases
Rheumatic mitral (valve) failure — A form characterized by the inability of the mitral valve to perform normally.

I
0
0
I
I
0
5

Excludes 1: = NOT CODED HERE! (Do not code both)   *Excludes ❷:* = Not Included Here

I05.9   **Rheumatic mitral valve disease, unspecified**
     Rheumatic mitral (valve) disorder (chronic) NOS

I06-   **Rheumatic aortic valve diseases** — Persistent, degenerative, rheumatic inflammatory lesions of the aortic valve.
    Excludes 1:   *aortic valve disease not specified as rheumatic (I35.-)*
              aortic valve disease with mitral and/or tricuspid valve involvement (I08.-)

I06.0   **Rheumatic aortic stenosis** — A form characterized by reduction in the aortic valve orifice size.
     Rheumatic aortic (valve) obstruction — A form marked by blockage of the aortic valve orifice size.

I06.1   **Rheumatic aortic insufficiency** — A form characterized by both reduction in the aortic valve orifice size and inadequate function.
     Rheumatic aortic incompetence — A form marked by inadequate function of the aortic valve.
     Rheumatic aortic regurgitation — A form marked by backflow of blood through the aortic valve.

I06.2   **Rheumatic aortic stenosis <u>with insufficiency</u>** — A form characterized by both reduction in the aortic valve orifice size and inadequate function and/or backflow of blood through the aortic valve.
     Rheumatic aortic stenosis with incompetence or regurgitation

I06.8   **Other rheumatic aortic valve diseases**

I06.9   **Rheumatic aortic valve disease, unspecified**
     Rheumatic aortic (valve) disease NOS

I07-   **Rheumatic tricuspid valve diseases** — Persistent, degenerative, rheumatic inflammatory lesions of the tricuspid valve.
    Includes: **Rheumatic tricuspid valve diseases specified as rheumatic or unspecified**
    Excludes 1:   *tricuspid valve disease specified as nonrheumatic (I36.-)*
              tricuspid valve disease with aortic and/or mitral valve involvement (I08.-)

I07.0   **Rheumatic tricuspid stenosis** — A form characterized by reduction in the tricuspid valve orifice size.
     Tricuspid (valve) stenosis (rheumatic)

I07.1   **Rheumatic tricuspid insufficiency** — A form characterized by the inadequate function of the tricuspid valve.
     Tricuspid (valve) insufficiency (rheumatic)

I07.2   **Rheumatic tricuspid stenosis and insufficiency** — A form characterized by both reduction in the tricuspid valve orifice size and inadequate function and/or backflow of blood through the tricuspid valve.

I07.8   **Other rheumatic tricuspid valve diseases**

I07.9   **Rheumatic tricuspid valve disease, unspecified**
     Rheumatic tricuspid valve disorder NOS

I08-   **Multiple valve diseases** — Persistent, degenerative, rheumatic inflammatory lesions of two or more heart valves.
    Includes: **Multiple valve diseases specified as rheumatic or unspecified**
    Excludes 1:   *endocarditis, valve unspecified (I38)*
              multiple valve disease specified a nonrheumatic (I34.-, I35.-, I36.-, I37.-, I38.-, Q22.-, Q23.-, Q24.8-)
              rheumatic valve disease NOS (I09.1)

I08.0   **Rheumatic disorders of both mitral and aortic valves**
     Involvement of both mitral and aortic valves specified as rheumatic or unspecified

I08.1   **Rheumatic disorders of both mitral and tricuspid valves**

I08.2   **Rheumatic disorders of both aortic and tricuspid valves**

I08.3   **Combined rheumatic disorders of mitral, aortic and tricuspid valves**

I08.8   **Other rheumatic multiple valve diseases**

I08.9   **Rheumatic multiple valve disease, unspecified**

I09-   **Other rheumatic heart diseases**

cc I09.0   **Rheumatic myocarditis** — Persistent, degenerative, rheumatic inflammatory lesions of the myocardium.
     Excludes 1:   *myocarditis not specified as rheumatic (I51.4)*

I09.1   **Rheumatic diseases of endocardium, valve unspecified**
     Rheumatic endocarditis (chronic)
     Rheumatic valvulitis (chronic)
     Excludes 1:   *endocarditis, valve unspecified (I38)*

cc I09.2   **Chronic rheumatic pericarditis** — Persistent, degenerative, rheumatic inflammatory lesions of the outer fibrous and serous protective layers of the heart.
     Adherent pericardium, rheumatic — A rheumatic degenerative condition characterized by increased friction and stickiness of the pericardium layers.
     Chronic rheumatic mediastinopericarditis — A rheumatic, degenerative, adhesive inflammation of the pericardium extending to the mediastinum.
     Chronic rheumatic myopericarditis — A rheumatic, degenerative inflammatory condition of the myocardium and pericardium.
     Excludes 1:   *chronic pericarditis not specified as rheumatic (I31.-)*

I09.8-   **Other specified rheumatic heart diseases**

cc I09.81   **Rheumatic heart failure** — A rheumatic condition resulting in markedly decreased cardiac output and marked by venocapillary congestion, hypertension, and edema.
     Use additional code to identify type of heart failure (I50.-)

I09.89   **Other specified rheumatic heart diseases**
     Rheumatic disease of pulmonary valve — Persistent, degenerative, rheumatic inflammatory lesions of the pulmonary valve.

I09.9   **Rheumatic heart disease, unspecified**
     Rheumatic carditis
     Excludes 1:   *rheumatoid carditis (M05.31)*

Hypertensive diseases (I10-I16)

Use additional code to identify:
    Exposure to environmental tobacco smoke (Z77.22)
    History of tobacco dependence (Z87.891)
    Occupational exposure to environmental tobacco smoke (Z57.31)
    Tobacco dependence (F17.-)
    Tobacco use (Z72.0)
    Excludes 1:   *neonatal hypertension (P29.2)*
              primary pulmonary hypertension (I27.0)
    Excludes ❷: *hypertensive disease complicating pregnancy, childbirth and the puerperium (O10-O11, O13-O16)*

I10   **Essential (primary) hypertension** — [Questionable Admission] — Persistently high arterial blood pressure, measuring above 140 mm Hg systolic and 90 mm Hg diastolic, and without a discoverable organic cause.
    Includes: **High blood pressure**
              Hypertension (arterial) (benign) (essential) (malignant) (primary) (systemic)
    Excludes 1:   *hypertensive disease complicating pregnancy, childbirth and the puerperium (O10-O11, O13-O16)*
    Excludes ❷: *essential (primary) hypertension involving vessels of brain (I60-I69)*
              essential (primary) hypertension involving vessels of eye (H35.0-)

I11-   **Hypertensive <u>heart</u> disease** — Heart function abnormality resulting from hypertension.
    Includes: **Any condition in I51.4-I51.9 due to hypertension**

I11.0   **Hypertensive heart disease <u>with heart failure</u>** — A form resulting in the decreased ability of the heart to pump enough blood to meet the needs of the body's tissues.
     Hypertensive heart failure
     Use additional code to identify type of heart failure (I50.-)

I11.9   **Hypertensive heart disease <u>without</u> heart failure**
     Hypertensive heart disease NOS

I12-   **Hypertensive <u>chronic kidney disease</u>** — Kidney damage and malfunction (usually parenchymal ischemia) that is associated with or resulting from hypertension.
    Includes: **Any condition in N18 and N26 due to hypertension**
              Arteriosclerosis of kidney — Thickening and loss of elasticity of the arterioles of the kidney.
              Arteriosclerotic nephritis (chronic) (interstitial) — Inflammation of the kidney due to arteriolar ischemia.
              Hypertensive nephropathy — Functional disease of the kidney due to hypertension.
              Nephrosclerosis — Inflammation of the kidney due to arteriolar ischemia.
    Excludes 1:   *hypertension due to kidney disease (I15.0, I15.1)*
              renovascular hypertension (I15.0)
              secondary hypertension (I15.-)
    Excludes ❷: *acute kidney failure (N17.-)*

cc I12.0   **Hypertensive chronic kidney disease with <u>stage 5</u> chronic kidney disease or end stage renal disease**
     Use additional code to identify the stage of chronic kidney disease (N18.5, N18.6)

I12.9   **Hypertensive chronic kidney disease with <u>stage 1 through stage 4</u> chronic kidney disease, or unspecified chronic kidney disease**
     Hypertensive chronic kidney disease NOS
     Hypertensive renal disease NOS
     Use additional code to identify the stage of chronic kidney disease (N18.1-N18.4, N18.9)

I05 - I12 (tab marker)

I13- **Hypertensive <u>heart and chronic kidney</u> disease** — Kidney damage with heart and kidney functional abnormalities resulting from hypertension.
Includes: Any condition in I11.- with any condition in I12.-
Cardiorenal disease
Cardiovascular renal disease — A form marked by hypertensive disease of the heart, blood vessels, and kidneys.

cc **I13.0** **Hypertensive heart and chronic kidney disease <u>with heart failure</u> and <u>stage 1 through stage 4</u> chronic kidney disease, or unspecified chronic kidney disease**
Use additional code to identify type of heart failure (I50.-)
Use additional code to identify stage of chronic kidney disease (N18.1-N18.4, N18.9)

I13.1- **Hypertensive heart and chronic kidney disease <u>without</u> heart failure**

I13.10 **Hypertensive heart and chronic kidney disease without heart failure, <u>with stage 1 through stage 4</u> chronic kidney disease, or unspecified chronic kidney disease**
Hypertensive heart disease and hypertensive chronic kidney disease NOS
Use additional code to identify the stage of chronic kidney disease (N18.1-N18.4, N18.9)

cc **I13.11** **Hypertensive heart and chronic kidney disease without heart failure, <u>with stage 5</u> chronic kidney disease, or end stage renal disease**
Use additional code to identify the stage of chronic kidney disease (N18.5, N18.6)

cc **I13.2** **Hypertensive heart and chronic kidney disease <u>with heart failure</u> and <u>with stage 5</u> chronic kidney disease, or end stage renal disease**
Use additional code to identify type of heart failure (I50.-)
Use additional code to identify the stage of chronic kidney disease (N18.5, N18.6)

I15- **<u>Secondary</u> hypertension** — Elevated arterial blood pressure due to various primary diseases.
Code also underlying condition
Excludes 1: *postprocedural hypertension (I97.3)*
Excludes ❷: *secondary hypertension involving vessels of brain (I60-I69)*
secondary hypertension involving vessels of eye (H35.0-)

I15.0 **Renovascular hypertension** — A form caused by primary renal disease.

I15.1 **Hypertension secondary to other renal disorders**

I15.2 **Hypertension secondary to endocrine disorders**

I15.8 **Other secondary hypertension**

I15.9 **Secondary hypertension, unspecified**

I16- **Hypertensive crisis** — The rapid elevation of blood pressure that is high enough to cause organ damage.
Code also any identified hypertensive disease (I10-I15)

I16.0 **Hypertensive urgency** — The rapid elevation of blood pressure without associated progressive organ dysfunction.

cc **I16.1** **Hypertensive emergency** — The rapid elevation of blood pressure that can lead to impending or progressive organ dysfunction.

cc **I16.9** **Hypertensive crisis, unspecified**

Ischemic heart diseases (I20-I25)

Use additional code to identify presence of hypertension (I10-I16)

I20- **Angina pectoris** — Severe, squeezing or pressure-like thoracic pain that is caused by reduced oxygenation of the cardiac muscle and often brought on by some form of exertion or stress.
Use additional code to identify:
Exposure to environmental tobacco smoke (Z77.22)
History of tobacco dependence (Z87.891)
Occupational exposure to environmental tobacco smoke (Z57.31)
Tobacco dependence (F17.-)
Tobacco use (Z72.0)
Excludes 1: *angina pectoris with atherosclerotic heart disease of native coronary arteries (I25.1-)*
atherosclerosis of coronary artery bypass graft(s) and coronary artery of transplanted heart with angina pectoris (I25.7-)
postinfarction angina (I23.7)

cc **I20.0** **<u>Unstable</u> angina** — Angina which is increased in frequency and duration, provoked with less than usual stimuli, occurs with abrupt onset (often while resting), and/or usual relief (rest and/or medication) does not help relieve it.
Accelerated angina
Crescendo angina
De novo effort angina
Intermediate coronary syndrome
Preinfarction syndrome
Worsening effort angina

cc **I20.1** **Angina pectoris <u>with documented spasm</u>** — A form with attacks associated with ST-segment elevations on EKG that often occur during rest.
Angiospastic angina
Prinzmetal angina
Spasm-induced angina
Variant angina

I20.8 **<u>Other forms</u> of angina pectoris**
Angina equivalent
Angina of effort
Coronary slow flow syndrome
Stable angina
Stenocardia
Use additional code(s) for symptoms associated with angina equivalent

I20.9 **Angina pectoris, <u>unspecified</u>**
Angina NOS
Anginal syndrome
Cardiac angina
Ischemic chest pain

I21- **ST elevation (STEMI) and non-ST elevation (NSTEMI) <u>myocardial infarction</u>** — A severe, sudden onset of myocardial necrosis due to obstruction of the coronary artery blood flow to an area of heart muscle.
AHA 12:4Q:p102 – Two STEMI myocardial infarctions a week apart in hospital
AHA 12:4Q:p103 – Two STEMI myocardial infarctions a week apart after discharge
AHA 13:1Q:p25 – Four-week time frame of the initial acute myocardial infarction
Includes: Cardiac infarction
Coronary (artery) embolism — An obstructing blood clot in the coronary arteries.
Coronary (artery) occlusion — An obstruction of a coronary artery by thrombosis or as a result of a spasm.
Coronary (artery) rupture — Forcible tearing of a coronary artery.
Coronary (artery) thrombosis — The formation or presence of an aggregation of blood factors, primarily platelets and fibrin forming a blood clot.
Infarction of heart, myocardium, or ventricle
Myocardial infarction specified as acute or with a stated duration of 4 weeks (28 days) or less from onset
Use additional code, if applicable, to identify:
Exposure to environmental tobacco smoke (Z77.22)
History of tobacco dependence (Z87.891)
Occupational exposure to environmental tobacco smoke (Z57.31)
Status post administration of tPA (rtPA) in a different facility within the last 24 hours prior to admission to current facility (Z92.82)
Tobacco dependence (F17.-)
Tobacco use (Z72.0)
Excludes ❷: *old myocardial infarction (I25.2)*
postmyocardial infarction syndrome (I24.1)
subsequent myocardial infarction (I22.-)

I21.0- **<u>ST elevation (STEMI)</u> myocardial infarction of <u>anterior wall</u>** — Infarction of the front portion of the heart that is defined by an ST segment elevation on EKG indicating a relatively large area of heart muscle is affected.

MCC **I21.01** **ST elevation (STEMI) myocardial infarction involving <u>left main</u> coronary artery** — A form identifying the obstruction in the left main coronary artery.

MCC **I21.02** **ST elevation (STEMI) myocardial infarction involving <u>left anterior descending</u> coronary artery** — A form identifying the obstruction in the left anterior descending coronary artery.
ST elevation (STEMI) myocardial infarction involving diagonal coronary artery

MCC **I21.09** **ST elevation (STEMI) myocardial infarction involving <u>other coronary artery</u> of anterior wall**
Acute transmural myocardial infarction of anterior wall — TRANSMURAL — A form involving the entire thickness of the heart muscle.
Anteroapical transmural (Q wave) infarction (acute)
Anterolateral transmural (Q wave) infarction (acute)
Anteroseptal transmural (Q wave) infarction (acute)
Transmural (Q wave) infarction (acute) (of) anterior (wall) NOS

I21.1- **<u>ST elevation (STEMI)</u> myocardial infarction of <u>inferior wall</u>** — Infarction of the lower portion of the heart that is defined by an ST segment elevation on EKG indicating a relatively large area of heart muscle is affected.

MCC **I21.11** **ST elevation (STEMI) myocardial infarction involving <u>right coronary</u> artery** — A form identifying the obstruction in the right coronary artery.
Inferoposterior transmural (Q wave) infarction (acute) — TRANSMURAL — A form involving the entire thickness of the heart muscle.

Excludes 1: = NOT CODED HERE! (Do not code both)   **724**   *Excludes ❷:* = Not Included Here

I 13 - I 21

© 2016 Channel Publishing, Ltd.

MCC **I21.19** **ST elevation (STEMI) myocardial infarction involving other coronary artery of inferior wall**
> Acute transmural myocardial infarction of inferior wall — TRANSMURAL – A form involving the entire thickness of the heart muscle.
> Inferolateral transmural (Q wave) infarction (acute)
> Transmural (Q wave) infarction (acute) (of) diaphragmatic wall
> Transmural (Q wave) infarction (acute) (of) inferior (wall) NOS
> *Excludes ❷: ST elevation (STEMI) myocardial infarction involving left circumflex coronary artery (I21.21)*

I21.2- **ST elevation (STEMI) myocardial infarction of other sites** — Infarction of the heart that is defined by an ST segment elevation on EKG indicating a relatively large area of heart muscle is affected.

MCC **I21.21** **ST elevation (STEMI) myocardial infarction involving left circumflex coronary artery** — A form identifying the obstruction in the left circumflex coronary artery.
> ST elevation (STEMI) myocardial infarction involving oblique marginal coronary artery

MCC **I21.29** **ST elevation (STEMI) myocardial infarction involving other sites**
> Acute transmural myocardial infarction of other sites — TRANSMURAL – A form involving the entire thickness of the heart muscle.
> Apical-lateral transmural (Q wave) infarction (acute)
> Basal-lateral transmural (Q wave) infarction (acute)
> High lateral transmural (Q wave) infarction (acute)
> Lateral (wall) NOS transmural (Q wave) infarction (acute)
> Posterior (true) transmural (Q wave) infarction (acute)
> Posterobasal transmural (Q wave) infarction (acute)
> Posterolateral transmural (Q wave) infarction (acute)
> Posteroseptal transmural (Q wave) infarction (acute)
> Septal transmural (Q wave) infarction (acute) NOS

MCC **I21.3** **ST elevation (STEMI) myocardial infarction of unspecified site** — Infarction of an unspecified area of the heart that is defined by an ST segment elevation on EKG indicating a relatively large area of heart muscle is affected.
> Acute transmural myocardial infarction of unspecified site
> Myocardial infarction (acute) NOS
> Transmural (Q wave) myocardial infarction NOS

MCC **I21.4** **Non-ST elevation (NSTEMI) myocardial infarction** — Infarction of the heart that is defined by NOT having an ST segment elevation on EKG and by a positive blood test for troponin (a protein released when the heart muscle is damaged) indicating a relatively small area of heart muscle is affected.
> Acute subendocardial myocardial infarction
> Non-Q wave myocardial infarction NOS
> Nontransmural myocardial infarction NOS

I22- **Subsequent ST elevation (STEMI) and non-ST elevation (NSTEMI) myocardial infarction** — See Includes Note below.
> AHA 12:4Q:p102 – Two STEMI myocardial infarctions a week apart in hospital
> AHA 12:4Q:p103 – Two STEMI myocardial infarctions a week apart after discharge
> AHA 13:1Q:p25 – Four-week time frame of the initial acute myocardial infarction
> Includes: Acute myocardial infarction occurring within four weeks (28 days) of a previous acute myocardial infarction, regardless of site
> Cardiac infarction
> Coronary (artery) embolism — An obstructing blood clot in the coronary arteries.
> Coronary (artery) occlusion — An obstruction of a coronary artery by thrombosis or as a result of a spasm.
> Coronary (artery) rupture — Forcible tearing of a coronary artery.
> Coronary (artery) thrombosis — The formation or presence of an aggregation of blood factors, primarily platelets and fibrin forming a blood clot.
> Infarction of heart, myocardium, or ventricle
> Recurrent myocardial infarction
> Reinfarction of myocardium
> Rupture of heart, myocardium, or ventricle
> Use additional code, if applicable, to identify:
> Exposure to environmental tobacco smoke (Z77.22)
> History of tobacco dependence (Z87.891)
> Occupational exposure to environmental tobacco smoke (Z57.31)
> Status post administration of tPA (rtPA) in a different facility within the last 24 hours prior to admission to current facility (Z92.82)
> Tobacco dependence (F17.-)
> Tobacco use (Z72.0)

MCC **I22.0** **Subsequent ST elevation (STEMI) myocardial infarction of anterior wall** — Infarction of the front portion of the heart that occurs within 4 weeks of a previous infarction that is defined by an ST segment elevation on EKG indicating a relatively large area of heart muscle is affected.
> Subsequent acute transmural myocardial infarction of anterior wall — TRANSMURAL – A form involving the entire thickness of the heart muscle.
> Subsequent transmural (Q wave) infarction (acute) (of) anterior (wall) NOS
> Subsequent anteroapical transmural (Q wave) infarction (acute)
> Subsequent anterolateral transmural (Q wave) infarction (acute)
> Subsequent anteroseptal transmural (Q wave) infarction (acute)

MCC **I22.1** **Subsequent ST elevation (STEMI) myocardial infarction of inferior wall** — Infarction of the lower portion of the heart that occurs within 4 weeks of a previous infarction that is defined by an ST segment elevation on EKG indicating a relatively large area of heart muscle is affected.
> Subsequent acute transmural myocardial infarction of inferior wall — TRANSMURAL – A form involving the entire thickness of the heart muscle.
> Subsequent transmural (Q wave) infarction (acute) (of) diaphragmatic wall
> Subsequent transmural (Q wave) infarction (acute) (of) inferior (wall) NOS
> Subsequent inferolateral transmural (Q wave) infarction (acute)
> Subsequent inferoposterior transmural (Q wave) infarction (acute)

MCC **I22.2** **Subsequent non-ST elevation (NSTEMI) myocardial infarction** — Infarction of the heart that occurs within 4 weeks of a previous infarction that is defined by NOT having an ST segment elevation on EKG and by a positive blood test for troponin (a protein released when the heart muscle is damaged) indicating a relatively small area of heart muscle is affected.
> Subsequent acute subendocardial myocardial infarction
> Subsequent non-Q wave myocardial infarction NOS
> Subsequent nontransmural myocardial infarction NOS

MCC **I22.8** **Subsequent ST elevation (STEMI) myocardial infarction of other sites** — Infarction of the heart that occurs within 4 weeks of a previous infarction that is defined by an ST segment elevation on EKG indicating a relatively large area of heart muscle is affected.
> Subsequent acute transmural myocardial infarction of other sites — TRANSMURAL – A form involving the entire thickness of the heart muscle.
> Subsequent apical-lateral transmural (Q wave) myocardial infarction (acute)
> Subsequent basal-lateral transmural (Q wave) myocardial infarction (acute)
> Subsequent high lateral transmural (Q wave) myocardial infarction (acute)
> Subsequent transmural (Q wave) myocardial infarction (acute) (of) lateral (wall) NOS
> Subsequent posterior (true)transmural (Q wave) myocardial infarction (acute)
> Subsequent posterobasal transmural (Q wave) myocardial infarction (acute)
> Subsequent posterolateral transmural (Q wave) myocardial infarction (acute)
> Subsequent posteroseptal transmural (Q wave) myocardial infarction (acute)
> Subsequent septal NOS transmural (Q wave) myocardial infarction (acute)

MCC **I22.9** **Subsequent ST elevation (STEMI) myocardial infarction of unspecified site** — Infarction of an unspecified area the heart that occurs within 4 weeks of a previous infarction that is defined by an ST segment elevation on EKG indicating a relatively large area of heart muscle is affected.
> Subsequent acute myocardial infarction of unspecified site
> Subsequent myocardial infarction (acute) NOS

I23- **Certain current complications following ST elevation (STEMI) and non-ST elevation (NSTEMI) myocardial infarction (within the 28 day period)**

CC **I23.0** **Hemopericardium as current complication following acute myocardial infarction** — [Age/15-124] — The abnormal presence of effused blood in the pericardial cavity.
> *Excludes 1:   hemopericardium not specified as current complication following acute myocardial infarction (I31.2)*

CC **I23.1** **Atrial septal defect as current complication following acute myocardial infarction** — [Age/15-124] — A break or opening in the atrial septum (wall).
> *Excludes 1:   acquired atrial septal defect not specified as current complication following acute myocardial infarction (I51.0)*

I 21 - I 23

Excludes 1: = NOT CODED HERE! (Do not code both)   **725**   *Excludes ❷:* = Not Included Here

cc **I23.2** <u>Ventricular septal defect</u> as current complication following acute myocardial infarction — [Age/15-124] – A break or opening in the ventricular septum (wall).
Excludes 1: *acquired ventricular septal defect not specified as current complication following acute myocardial infarction (I51.0)*

cc **I23.3** <u>Rupture of cardiac wall</u> without hemopericardium as current complication following acute myocardial infarction — [Age/15-124] – A tear of the heart muscle.

mcc **I23.4** <u>Rupture of chordae tendineae</u> as current complication following acute myocardial infarction – A forcible tearing of the strong, cord-like attachments of the heart valves to the papillary muscles.
Excludes 1: *rupture of chordae tendineae not specified as current complication following acute myocardial infarction (I51.1)*

mcc **I23.5** <u>Rupture of papillary muscle</u> as current complication following acute myocardial infarction – A forcible tearing of the conical intraventricular muscles attached to the chordae tendineae and heart wall.
Excludes 1: *rupture of papillary muscle not specified as current complication following acute myocardial infarction (I51.2)*

cc **I23.6** <u>Thrombosis of atrium, auricular appendage, and ventricle</u> as current complications following acute myocardial infarction — [Age/15-124] – The formation or presence of an aggregation of blood factors, primarily platelets and fibrin forming a blood clot.
Excludes 1: *thrombosis of atrium, auricular appendage, and ventricle not specified as current complication following acute myocardial infarction (I51.3)*

cc **I23.7** <u>Postinfarction angina</u> — [Age/15-124] – Angina occurring from a few hours and up to 30 days following an acute myocardial infarction.
AHA 15:2Q:p16 – Postinfarction angina

cc **I23.8** <u>Other current complications</u> following acute myocardial infarction — [Age/15-124]

I24- <u>Other acute</u> ischemic heart diseases
Excludes 1: *angina pectoris (I20.-)*
transient myocardial ischemia in newborn (P29.4)

cc **I24.0** <u>Acute coronary thrombosis</u> <u>not</u> resulting in myocardial infarction
Acute coronary (artery) (vein) embolism not resulting in myocardial infarction
Acute coronary (artery) (vein) occlusion not resulting in myocardial infarction
Acute coronary (artery) (vein) thromboembolism not resulting in myocardial infarction
Excludes 1: *atherosclerotic heart disease (I25.1-)*

cc **I24.1** <u>Dressler's syndrome</u> — Pericarditis with fever, leukocytosis, and pleurisy, occurring after an acute myocardial infarction.
Postmyocardial infarction syndrome
Excludes 1: *postinfarction angina (I23.7)*

cc **I24.8** Other forms of acute ischemic heart disease

cc **I24.9** Acute ischemic heart disease, unspecified
Excludes 1: *ischemic heart disease (chronic) NOS (I25.9)*

I25- <u>Chronic</u> ischemic heart disease
Use additional code to identify:
Chronic total occlusion of coronary artery (I25.82)
Exposure to environmental tobacco smoke (Z77.22)
History of tobacco dependence (Z87.891)
Occupational exposure to environmental tobacco smoke (Z57.31)
Tobacco dependence (F17.-)
Tobacco use (Z72.0)

I25.1- <u>Atherosclerotic heart disease</u> <u>of native</u> coronary artery — Coronary artery narrowing caused by deposition of plaque-forming cholesterol and other lipids within the lumen of those arteries.
Atherosclerotic cardiovascular disease
Coronary (artery) atheroma
Coronary (artery) atherosclerosis
Coronary (artery) disease
Coronary (artery) sclerosis
Use additional code, if applicable, to identify:
Coronary atherosclerosis due to calcified coronary lesion (I25.84)
Coronary atherosclerosis due to lipid rich plaque (I25.83)
Excludes ❷: *atheroembolism (I75.-)*
atherosclerosis of coronary artery bypass graft(s) and transplanted heart (I25.7-)

I25.10 Atherosclerotic heart disease of native coronary artery <u>without</u> angina pectoris — [Age/15-124]
Atherosclerotic heart disease NOS

I25.11- Atherosclerotic heart disease of native coronary artery <u>with angina pectoris</u> — A form with severe, squeezing or pressure-like thoracic pain that is caused by reduced oxygenation of the cardiac muscle and often brought on by some form of exertion or stress.
AHA 15:2Q:p16 – Postinfarction angina with atherosclerosis

cc **I25.110** Atherosclerotic heart disease of native coronary artery with <u>unstable</u> angina pectoris — [Age/15-124]
Excludes 1: *unstable angina without atherosclerotic heart disease (I20.0)*

I25.111 Atherosclerotic heart disease of native coronary artery with angina pectoris <u>with documented spasm</u> — [Age/15-124]
Excludes 1: *angina pectoris with documented spasm without atherosclerotic heart disease (I20.1)*

I25.118 Atherosclerotic heart disease of native coronary artery with <u>other forms</u> of angina pectoris — [Age/15-124]
Excludes 1: *other forms of angina pectoris without atherosclerotic heart disease (I20.8)*

I25.119 Atherosclerotic heart disease of native coronary artery with <u>unspecified</u> angina pectoris — [Age/15-124]
Atherosclerotic heart disease with angina NOS
Atherosclerotic heart disease with ischemic chest pain
Excludes 1: *unspecified angina pectoris without atherosclerotic heart disease (I20.9)*

I25.2 <u>Old</u> myocardial infarction — A known past myocardial infarction, not presenting any symptoms during the current episode of care.
Healed myocardial infarction
Past myocardial infarction diagnosed by ECG or other investigation, but currently presenting no symptoms

cc **I25.3** <u>Aneurysm</u> of heart — An abnormal enlargement and thinning of a portion of the heart wall.
Mural aneurysm
Ventricular aneurysm

I25.4- <u>Coronary artery aneurysm and dissection</u>

I25.41 <u>Coronary artery aneurysm</u> — An abnormal enlargement and thinning of a portion of a coronary artery wall.
Coronary arteriovenous fistula, acquired
Excludes 1: *congenital coronary (artery) aneurysm (Q24.5)*

mcc **I25.42** <u>Coronary artery dissection</u> — The splitting of the coronary artery wall that allows blood to flow within the wall layers.

I25.5 <u>Ischemic cardiomyopathy</u> — A weakened, dilated, and enlarged heart muscle that is caused by the decreased blood supply.
Excludes ❷: *coronary atherosclerosis (I25.1-, I25.7-)*

I25.6 <u>Silent myocardial ischemia</u> — Decreased blood supply to the heart muscle that isn't producing any symptoms.

I25.7- <u>Atherosclerosis</u> of coronary artery bypass graft(s) and coronary artery of transplanted heart <u>with angina pectoris</u>
Use additional code, if applicable, to identify:
Coronary atherosclerosis due to calcified coronary lesion (I25.84)
Coronary atherosclerosis due to lipid rich plaque (I25.83)
Excludes 1: *atherosclerosis of bypass graft(s) of transplanted heart without angina pectoris (I25.812)*
atherosclerosis of coronary artery bypass graft(s) without angina pectoris (I25.810)
atherosclerosis of native coronary artery of transplanted heart without angina pectoris (I25.811)
embolism or thrombus of coronary artery bypass graft(s) (T82.8-)

I25.70- Atherosclerosis of <u>coronary artery bypass graft(s), unspecified, with angina pectoris</u> — Narrowing of a coronary artery bypass graft caused by deposition of plaque-forming cholesterol and other lipids within the lumen of those arteries and severe, squeezing or pressure-like thoracic pain that is caused by reduced oxygenation of the cardiac muscle and often brought on by some form of exertion or stress.

cc **I25.700** Atherosclerosis of coronary artery bypass graft(s), unspecified, <u>with unstable</u> angina pectoris — [Age/15-124]
Excludes 1: *unstable angina pectoris without atherosclerosis of coronary artery bypass graft (I20.0)*

Excludes 1: = NOT CODED HERE! (Do not code both) **726** *Excludes ❷:* = Not Included Here

I25.701   Atherosclerosis of coronary artery bypass graft(s), unspecified, with angina pectoris <u>with documented spasm</u> — [Age/15-124]
> *Excludes 1:*   *angina pectoris with documented spasm without atherosclerosis of coronary artery bypass graft (I20.1)*

I25.708   Atherosclerosis of coronary artery bypass graft(s), unspecified, <u>with other forms</u> of angina pectoris — [Age/15-124]
> *Excludes 1:*   *other forms of angina pectoris without atherosclerosis of coronary artery bypass graft (I20.8)*

I25.709   Atherosclerosis of coronary artery bypass graft(s), unspecified, <u>with unspecified</u> angina pectoris — [Age/15-124]
> *Excludes 1:*   *unspecified angina pectoris without atherosclerosis of coronary artery bypass graft (I20.9)*

I25.71- Atherosclerosis of <u>autologous vein coronary artery bypass graft(s)</u> <u>with angina pectoris</u>

cc I25.710   Atherosclerosis of autologous <u>vein</u> coronary artery bypass graft(s) <u>with unstable</u> angina pectoris — [Age/15-124]
> *Excludes 1:*   *unstable angina without atherosclerosis of autologous vein coronary artery bypass graft(s) (I20.0)*

cc I25.711   Atherosclerosis of autologous <u>vein</u> coronary artery bypass graft(s) with angina pectoris <u>with documented spasm</u> — [Age/15-124]
> *Excludes 1:*   *angina pectoris with documented spasm without atherosclerosis of autologous vein coronary artery bypass graft(s) (I20.1)*

cc I25.718   Atherosclerosis of autologous <u>vein</u> coronary artery bypass graft(s) <u>with other forms</u> of angina pectoris — [Age/15-124]
> *Excludes 1:*   *other forms of angina pectoris without atherosclerosis of autologous vein coronary artery bypass graft(s) (I20.8)*

cc I25.719   Atherosclerosis of autologous <u>vein</u> coronary artery bypass graft(s) <u>with unspecified</u> angina pectoris — [Age/15-124]
> *Excludes 1:*   *unspecified angina pectoris without atherosclerosis of autologous vein coronary artery bypass graft(s) (I20.9)*

I25.72- Atherosclerosis of autologous <u>artery</u> coronary artery bypass graft(s) <u>with angina pectoris</u>
> Atherosclerosis of internal mammary artery graft with angina pectoris

cc I25.720   Atherosclerosis of autologous <u>artery</u> coronary artery bypass graft(s) <u>with unstable</u> angina pectoris — [Age/15-124]
> *Excludes 1:*   *unstable angina without atherosclerosis of autologous artery coronary artery bypass graft(s) (I20.0)*

cc I25.721   Atherosclerosis of autologous <u>artery</u> coronary artery bypass graft(s) with angina pectoris <u>with documented spasm</u> — [Age/15-124]
> *Excludes 1:*   *angina pectoris with documented spasm without atherosclerosis of autologous artery coronary artery bypass graft(s) (I20.1)*

cc I25.728   Atherosclerosis of autologous <u>artery</u> coronary artery bypass graft(s) <u>with other forms</u> of angina pectoris — [Age/15-124]
> *Excludes 1:*   *other forms of angina pectoris without atherosclerosis of autologous artery coronary artery bypass graft(s) (I20.8)*

cc I25.729   Atherosclerosis of autologous <u>artery</u> coronary artery bypass graft(s) <u>with unspecified</u> angina pectoris — [Age/15-124]
> *Excludes 1:*   *unspecified angina pectoris without atherosclerosis of autologous artery coronary artery bypass graft(s) (I20.9)*

I25.73- Atherosclerosis of <u>nonautologous biological</u> coronary artery bypass graft(s) <u>with angina pectoris</u>

cc I25.730   Atherosclerosis of <u>nonautologous biological</u> coronary artery bypass graft(s) <u>with unstable</u> angina pectoris — [Age/15-124]
> *Excludes 1:*   *unstable angina without atherosclerosis of nonautologous biological coronary artery bypass graft(s) (I20.0)*

cc I25.731   Atherosclerosis of <u>nonautologous biological</u> coronary artery bypass graft(s) with angina pectoris <u>with documented spasm</u> — [Age/15-124]
> *Excludes 1:*   *angina pectoris with documented spasm without atherosclerosis of nonautologous biological coronary artery bypass graft(s) (I20.1)*

cc I25.738   Atherosclerosis of <u>nonautologous biological</u> coronary artery bypass graft(s) <u>with other forms</u> of angina pectoris — [Age/15-124]
> *Excludes 1:*   *other forms of angina pectoris without atherosclerosis of nonautologous biological coronary artery bypass graft(s) (I20.8)*

cc I25.739   Atherosclerosis of <u>nonautologous biological</u> coronary artery bypass graft(s) <u>with unspecified</u> angina pectoris — [Age/15-124]
> *Excludes 1:*   *unspecified angina pectoris without atherosclerosis of nonautologous biological coronary artery bypass graft(s) (I20.9)*

I25.75- Atherosclerosis of <u>native coronary artery of transplanted heart</u> <u>with angina pectoris</u> — Narrowing of a native coronary artery of a transplanted heart caused by deposition of plaque-forming cholesterol and other lipids within the lumen of those arteries and severe, squeezing or pressure-like thoracic pain that is caused by reduced oxygenation of the cardiac muscle and often brought on by some form of exertion or stress.
> *Excludes 1:*   *atherosclerosis of native coronary artery of transplanted heart without angina pectoris (I25.811)*

cc I25.750   Atherosclerosis of native coronary artery of transplanted heart <u>with unstable</u> angina

cc I25.751   Atherosclerosis of native coronary artery of transplanted heart with angina pectoris <u>with documented spasm</u>

cc I25.758   Atherosclerosis of native coronary artery of transplanted heart <u>with other forms</u> of angina pectoris

cc I25.759   Atherosclerosis of native coronary artery of transplanted heart <u>with unspecified</u> angina pectoris

I25.76- Atherosclerosis of <u>bypass graft</u> of coronary artery of <u>transplanted heart</u> <u>with angina pectoris</u> — Narrowing of a coronary artery bypass graft of a transplanted heart caused by deposition of plaque-forming cholesterol and other lipids within the lumen of those arteries and severe, squeezing or pressure-like thoracic pain that is caused by reduced oxygenation of the cardiac muscle and often brought on by some form of exertion or stress.
> *Excludes 1:*   *atherosclerosis of bypass graft of coronary artery of transplanted heart without angina pectoris (I25.812)*

cc I25.760   Atherosclerosis of bypass graft of coronary artery of transplanted heart <u>with unstable angina</u> — [Age/15-124]

cc I25.761   Atherosclerosis of bypass graft of coronary artery of transplanted heart with angina pectoris <u>with documented spasm</u> — [Age/15-124]

cc I25.768   Atherosclerosis of bypass graft of coronary artery of transplanted heart <u>with other forms</u> of angina pectoris — [Age/15-124]

cc I25.769   Atherosclerosis of bypass graft of coronary artery of transplanted heart <u>with unspecified</u> angina pectoris — [Age/15-124]

I 2 5 - I 2 5

Excludes 1: = NOT CODED HERE! (Do not code both)   **727**   *Excludes ❷:* = Not Included Here

I25.79- Atherosclerosis of <u>other</u> coronary artery bypass graft(s) <u>with angina pectoris</u>

cc **I25.790** Atherosclerosis of other coronary artery bypass graft(s) <u>with unstable</u> angina pectoris — [Age/15-124]
  Excludes 1: unstable angina without atherosclerosis of other coronary artery bypassgraft(s) *(I20.0)*

cc **I25.791** Atherosclerosis of other coronary artery bypass graft(s) with angina pectoris <u>with documented spasm</u> — [Age/15-124]
  Excludes 1: angina pectoris with documented spasm without atherosclerosis of other coronary artery bypass graft(s) *(I20.1)*

cc **I25.798** Atherosclerosis of other coronary artery bypass graft(s) <u>with other forms</u> of angina pectoris — [Age/15-124]
  Excludes 1: other forms of angina pectoris without atherosclerosis of other coronary artery bypass graft(s) *(I20.8)*

cc **I25.799** Atherosclerosis of other coronary artery bypass graft(s) <u>with unspecified</u> angina pectoris — [Age/15-124]
  Excludes 1: unspecified angina pectoris without atherosclerosis of other coronary artery bypass graft(s) *(I20.9)*

I25.8- Other forms of chronic ischemic heart disease

I25.81- <u>Atherosclerosis of other coronary vessels</u> <u>without</u> angina pectoris — Coronary artery narrowing caused by deposition of plaque-forming cholesterol and other lipids within the lumen of those arteries without the symptoms of angina pectoris.
  Use additional code, if applicable, to identify:
    Coronary atherosclerosis due to calcified coronary lesion (I25.84)
    Coronary atherosclerosis due to lipid rich plaque (I25.83)
  Excludes 1: atherosclerotic heart disease of native coronary artery without angina pectoris *(I25.10)*

cc **I25.810** Atherosclerosis of <u>coronary artery bypass graft(s)</u> <u>without</u> angina pectoris — [Age/15-124] – A form occurring in a coronary artery bypass graft.
  Atherosclerosis of coronary artery bypass graft NOS
  Excludes 1: atherosclerosis of coronary bypass graft(s) with angina pectoris *(I25.70-I25.73-, I25.79-)*

cc **I25.811** Atherosclerosis of <u>native coronary artery of transplanted heart</u> <u>without</u> angina pectoris — A form occurring in a native coronary artery of a transplanted heart.
  Atherosclerosis of native coronary artery of transplanted heart NOS
  Excludes 1: atherosclerosis of native coronary artery of transplanted heart with angina pectoris *(I25.75-)*

cc **I25.812** Atherosclerosis of <u>bypass graft of coronary artery of transplanted heart</u> <u>without</u> angina pectoris — [Age/15-124] – A form occurring in a coronary artery bypass graft of a transplanted heart.
  Atherosclerosis of bypass graft of transplanted heart NOS
  Excludes 1: atherosclerosis of bypass graft of transplanted heart with angina pectoris *(I25.76)*

I25.82 <u>Chronic total occlusion of coronary artery</u> — [Unacceptable PDX] – A complete blockage of a coronary artery without an acute occlusion that has been present for an extended duration.
  Complete occlusion of coronary artery
  Total occlusion of coronary artery
  Code first coronary atherosclerosis (I25.1-, I25.7-, I25.81-)
  Excludes 1: acute coronary occulsion with myocardial infarction *(I21.-, I22.-)*
    acute coronary occulsion without myocardial infarction *(I24.0)*

I25.83 <u>Coronary atherosclerosis due to lipid rich plaque</u> — [Age/15-124] [Unacceptable PDX] – The identification of a coronary artery plaque that contains a greater than usual percentage of lipid material and results in a higher propensity to rupture than more fibrotic plaques.
  Code first coronary atherosclerosis (I25.1-, I25.7-, I25.81-)

I25.84 Coronary atherosclerosis <u>due to calcified coronary lesion</u> — [Unacceptable PDX] – The identification of a calcified coronary artery lesion that results in a higher propensity to rupture than more fibrotic plaques.
  Coronary atherosclerosis due to severely calcified coronary lesion
  Code first coronary atherosclerosis (I25.1-, I25.7-, I25.81-)

I25.89 Other forms of chronic ischemic heart disease

I25.9 Chronic ischemic heart disease, unspecified
  Ischemic heart disease (chronic) NOS

Pulmonary heart disease and diseases of pulmonary circulation (I26-I28)

I26- Pulmonary embolism — The closure of a pulmonary artery or one of its branches by a blood clot that traveled through the bloodstream to the lungs.
  Includes: Pulmonary (acute) (artery) (vein) infarction
    Pulmonary (acute) (artery) (vein) thromboembolism
    Pulmonary (acute) (artery) (vein) thrombosis
  Excludes ❷: chronic pulmonary embolism *(I27.82)*
    personal history of pulmonary embolism *(Z86.711)*
    pulmonary embolism complicating abortion, ectopic or molar pregnancy *(O00-O07, O08.2)*
    pulmonary embolism complicating pregnancy, childbirth and the puerperium *(O88.-)*
    pulmonary embolism due to complications of surgical and medical care *(T80.0, T81.7-, T82.8-)*
    pulmonary embolism due to trauma *(T79.0, T79.1)*
    septic (non-pulmonary) arterial embolism *(I76)*

I26.0- Pulmonary embolism <u>with acute cor pulmonale</u> — A relatively severe sudden onset of right heart decreased efficiency due to pulmonary hypertension caused by a pulmonary embolism.

MCC **I26.01** <u>Septic</u> pulmonary embolism with acute cor pulmonale — [Unacceptable PDX] – A form due to a localized collection of pus and bacteria that travels through the venous system to the heart and then continues into the pulmonary arterial system, where it lodges in a pulmonary vessel.
  Code first underlying infection

MCC **I26.02** <u>Saddle</u> embolus of pulmonary artery with acute cor pulmonale — A form characterized by a large embolism that straddles the bifurcation of the main pulmonary artery.

MCC **I26.09** <u>Other</u> pulmonary embolism with acute cor pulmonale
  AHA 14:4Q:p21 – Pulmonary hypertension with acute cor pulmonale
  Acute cor pulmonale NOS

I26.9- Pulmonary embolism <u>without</u> acute cor pulmonale

MCC **I26.90** <u>Septic</u> pulmonary embolism without acute cor pulmonale — [Unacceptable PDX]
  Code first underlying infection

MCC **I26.92** <u>Saddle</u> embolus of pulmonary artery without acute cor pulmonale

MCC **I26.99** <u>Other</u> pulmonary embolism without acute cor pulmonale
  Acute pulmonary embolism NOS
  Pulmonary embolism NOS

I27- Other pulmonary heart diseases

cc **I27.0** Primary pulmonary hypertension — Persistently high arterial blood pressure within the pulmonary circulation that is due to an organic cause.
  Excludes 1: pulmonary hypertension NOS *(I27.2)*
    secondary pulmonary hypertension *(I27.2)*

cc **I27.1** Kyphoscoliotic heart disease — Pulmonary hypertension due to severe hypoventilation that is caused by kyphoscoliosis (backward and lateral curvature of the spinal column).

I27.2 Other secondary pulmonary hypertension
  AHA 14:4Q:p21 – Pulmonary hypertension
  Pulmonary hypertension NOS
  Code also associated underlying condition

I27.8- Other specified pulmonary heart diseases

I27.81 Cor pulmonale (chronic) — Persistent pulmonary hypertension secondary to disease of the blood vessels of the lung.
  AHA 14:4Q:p21 – Cor pulmonale
  Cor pulmonale NOS
  Excludes 1: acute cor pulmonale *(I26.0-)*

I 2 5 - I 2 7

cc **I27.82** **Chronic pulmonary embolism** — A pulmonary vascular congestion condition characterized by the restriction or closure of the pulmonary artery or one of its branches by a blood clot(s) that persists over a long period of time.
Use additional code, if applicable, for associated long-term (current) use of anticoagulants (Z79.01)
Excludes 1:   *personal history of pulmonary embolism (Z86.711)*

I27.89 **Other specified pulmonary heart diseases**
Eisenmenger's complex
Eisenmenger's syndrome
Excludes 1:   *Eisenmenger's defect (Q21.8)*

I27.9 **Pulmonary heart disease, unspecified**
Chronic cardiopulmonary disease

I28- **Other diseases of pulmonary vessels**

cc **I28.0** **Arteriovenous fistula of pulmonary vessels** — An abnormal communication between a pulmonary artery and vein.
Excludes 1:   *congenital arteriovenous fistula (Q25.72)*

cc **I28.1** **Aneurysm of pulmonary artery** — A dilated sac in the wall of a pulmonary artery.
Excludes 1:   *congenital aneurysm (Q25.79)*
       congenital arteriovenous aneurysm (Q25.72)

I28.8 **Other diseases of pulmonary vessels**
Pulmonary arteritis — Inflammation of a pulmonary arterial wall.
Pulmonary endarteritis — Inflammation of the innermost lining of a pulmonary artery.
Rupture of pulmonary vessels — The forcible tearing of a pulmonary blood vessel wall.
Stenosis of pulmonary vessels — The narrowing of the lumen of a pulmonary blood vessel.
Stricture of pulmonary vessels — The decrease in caliber of a pulmonary blood vessel.

I28.9 **Disease of pulmonary vessels, unspecified**

Other forms of heart disease (I30-I52)

I30- **Acute pericarditis** — Inflammation of the outer fibrous and serous protective layers of the heart that is marked by a short and relatively severe course.
Includes: **Acute mediastinopericarditis** — A form marked by association with inflammation of the mediastinum.
       Acute myopericarditis — A form marked by association with inflammation of the myocardium.
       Acute pericardial effusion — The abnormal increase of pericardial fluids caused by the overproduction of fluid due to a disease affecting the pericardium.
       Acute pleuropericarditis — A form marked by association with inflammation of the pleura.
       Acute pneumopericarditis — A form marked by association with inflammation of the lung.
Excludes 1:   *Dressler's syndrome (I24.1)*
       rheumatic pericarditis (acute) (I01.0)

cc **I30.0** **Acute nonspecific idiopathic pericarditis** — Acute pericarditis of an unknown cause.

cc **I30.1** **Infective pericarditis** — A form caused by microorganisms.
Pneumococcal pericarditis — A form caused by pneumococcal microorganisms.
Pneumopyopericardium — A form marked by pus formation involving the pericardium and the lung.
Purulent pericarditis — A form marked by pus formation, indicating a bacterial infection.
Pyopericarditis — A form marked by pus formation within the pericardium.
Pyopericardium — A form marked by pus formation within the pericardium.
Pyopneumopericardium — A form marked by pus formation involving the pericardium and the lung.
Staphylococcal pericarditis — A form caused by staphylococcal microorganisms.
Streptococcal pericarditis — A form caused by streptococcal microorganisms.
Suppurative pericarditis — A form marked by the production of pus.
Viral pericarditis — A form caused by a virus.
Use additional code (B95-B97) to identify infectious agent

cc **I30.8** **Other forms of acute pericarditis**

cc **I30.9** **Acute pericarditis, unspecified**

I31- **Other diseases of pericardium**
Excludes 1:   *diseases of pericardium specified as rheumatic (I09.2)*
       postcardiotomy syndrome (I97.0)
       traumatic injury to pericardium (S26.-)

cc **I31.0** **Chronic adhesive pericarditis** — The condition of dense, fibrous tissue between the parietal and visceral layers of the pericardium.
Accretio cordis
Adherent pericardium
Adhesive mediastinopericarditis

cc **I31.1** **Chronic constrictive pericarditis** — Inflammation of the pericardium characterized by thickening and loss of elasticity.
Concretio cordis
Pericardial calcification

cc **I31.2** **Hemopericardium, not elsewhere classified** — The abnormal presence of effused blood in the pericardial cavity that is not due to trauma or a complication of a myocardial infarction.
Excludes 1:   *hemopericardium as current complication following acute myocardial infarction (I23.0)*

cc **I31.3** **Pericardial effusion (noninflammatory)** — The abnormal presence of excessive fluid in the pericardial cavity.
Chylopericardium — A form with chylous fluid.
Excludes 1:   *acute pericardial effusion (I30.9)*

cc **I31.4** **Cardiac tamponade** — [Unacceptable PDX] — The abnormal accumulation of fluid in the pericardium causing increased pressure on the heart so that ventricular filling is impaired and cardiac output is decreased.
Code first underlying cause

cc **I31.8** **Other specified diseases of pericardium**
Epicardial plaques
Focal pericardial adhesions

cc **I31.9** **Disease of pericardium, unspecified**
Pericarditis (chronic) NOS

I32 **Pericarditis in diseases classified elsewhere** — [Not Allowed as PDX]
cc **Code first underlying disease**
Excludes 1:   *pericarditis (in):*
       coxsackie (virus) (B33.23)
       gonococcal (A54.83)
       meningococcal (A39.53)
       rheumatoid (arthritis) (M05.31)
       syphilitic (A52.06)
       systemic lupus erythematosus (M32.12)
       tuberculosis (A18.84)

I33- **Acute and subacute endocarditis** — Inflammation of the endocardium, including the valves, with a sudden, severe onset or a more gradual and subtle development.
Excludes 1:   *acute rheumatic endocarditis (I01.1)*
       endocarditis NOS (I38)

MCC **I33.0** **Acute and subacute infective endocarditis** — Inflammation of the endocardium, including the valves, caused by a bacterial or fungal infection, and presenting with sudden, severe onset or a more gradual and subtle development.
Bacterial endocarditis (acute) (subacute)
Infective endocarditis (acute) (subacute) NOS
Endocarditis lenta (acute) (subacute)
Malignant endocarditis (acute) (subacute)
Purulent endocarditis (acute) (subacute)
Septic endocarditis (acute) (subacute)
Ulcerative endocarditis (acute) (subacute)
Vegetative endocarditis (acute) (subacute)
Use additional code (B95-B97) to identify infectious agent

MCC **I33.9** **Acute and subacute endocarditis, unspecified**
Acute endocarditis NOS
Acute myoendocarditis NOS
Acute periendocarditis NOS
Subacute endocarditis NOS
Subacute myoendocarditis NOS
Subacute periendocarditis NOS

I34- **Nonrheumatic mitral valve disorders** — Impaired function of the mitral valve that is not due to rheumatic fever.
Excludes 1:   *mitral valve disease (I05.9)*
       mitral valve failure (I05.8)
       mitral valve stenosis (I05.0)
       mitral valve disorder of unspecified cause with diseases of aortic and/or tricuspid valve(s) (I08.-)
       mitral valve disorder of unspecified cause with mitral stenosis or obstruction (I05.0)
       mitral valve disorder specified as congenital (Q23.2, Q23.3)
       mitral valve disorder specified as rheumatic (I05.-)

I34.0 **Nonrheumatic mitral (valve) insufficiency** — Inadequate function of the mitral valve.
Nonrheumatic mitral (valve) incompetence NOS — Synonym for Insufficiency.
Nonrheumatic mitral (valve) regurgitation NOS — The backflow of blood through the mitral valve.

I34.1 **Nonrheumatic mitral (valve) prolapse** — A form in which the valve leaflets do not close smoothly and evenly.
Floppy nonrheumatic mitral valve syndrome
Excludes 1:   *Marfan's syndrome (Q87.4-)*

I34.2 **Nonrheumatic mitral (valve) stenosis** — Reduction in the mitral valve orifice size.

I27 - I34

Excludes 1: = NOT CODED HERE! (Do not code both)   **729**   *Excludes ❷:* = Not Included Here

I34.8　Other nonrheumatic mitral valve disorders

I34.9　Nonrheumatic mitral valve disorder, unspecified

I35-　Nonrheumatic aortic valve disorders — Impaired function of the aortic valve that is not due to rheumatic fever.
> Excludes 1:　aortic valve disorder of unspecified cause but with diseases of mitral and/or tricuspid valve(s) (I08.-)
> aortic valve disorder specified as congenital (Q23.0, Q23.1)
> aortic valve disorder specified as rheumatic (I06.-)
> hypertrophic subaortic stenosis (I42.1)

I35.0　Nonrheumatic aortic (valve) stenosis — Reduction in the aortic valve orifice size.

I35.1　Nonrheumatic aortic (valve) insufficiency — Inadequate function of the aortic valve.
> Nonrheumatic aortic (valve) incompetence NOS — Synonym for Insufficiency.
> Nonrheumatic aortic (valve) regurgitation NOS — The backflow of blood through the aortic valve.

I35.2　Nonrheumatic aortic (valve) stenosis with insufficiency — Reduction in the aortic valve orifice size with dysfunction of the aortic valve.

I35.8　Other nonrheumatic aortic valve disorders

I35.9　Nonrheumatic aortic valve disorder, unspecified

I36-　Nonrheumatic tricuspid valve disorders — Impaired function of the tricuspid valve that is not due to rheumatic fever.
> Excludes 1:　tricuspid valve disorders of unspecified cause (I07.-)
> tricuspid valve disorders specified as congenital (Q22.4, Q22.8, Q22.9)
> tricuspid valve disorders specified as rheumatic (I07.-)
> tricuspid valve disorders with aortic and/or mitral valve involvement (I08.-)

I36.0　Nonrheumatic tricuspid (valve) stenosis — Reduction in the tricuspid valve orifice size.

I36.1　Nonrheumatic tricuspid (valve) insufficiency — Inadequate function of the tricuspid valve.
> Nonrheumatic tricuspid (valve) incompetence — Synonym for Insufficiency.
> Nonrheumatic tricuspid (valve) regurgitation — The backflow of blood through the tricuspid valve.

I36.2　Nonrheumatic tricuspid (valve) stenosis with insufficiency — Reduction in the tricuspid valve orifice size with inadequate function of the tricuspid valve.

I36.8　Other nonrheumatic tricuspid valve disorders

I36.9　Nonrheumatic tricuspid valve disorder, unspecified

I37-　Nonrheumatic pulmonary valve disorders — Impaired function of the pulmonary valve that is not due to rheumatic fever.
> Excludes 1:　pulmonary valve disorder specified as congenital (Q22.1, Q22.2, Q22.3)
> pulmonary valve disorder specified as rheumatic (I09.89)

I37.0　Nonrheumatic pulmonary valve stenosis — Reduction in the pulmonary valve orifice size.

I37.1　Nonrheumatic pulmonary valve insufficiency — Inadequate function of the pulmonary valve.
> Nonrheumatic pulmonary valve incompetence — Synonym for Insufficiency.
> Nonrheumatic pulmonary valve regurgitation

I37.2　Nonrheumatic pulmonary valve stenosis with insufficiency — Reduction in the pulmonary valve orifice size with inadequate function of the tricuspid valve.

I37.8　Other nonrheumatic pulmonary valve disorders

I37.9　Nonrheumatic pulmonary valve disorder, unspecified

I38　Endocarditis, valve unspecified
CC
> Includes:　Endocarditis (chronic) NOS
> Valvular incompetence NOS
> Valvular insufficiency NOS
> Valvular regurgitation NOS
> Valvular stenosis NOS
> Valvulitis (chronic) NOS
> Excludes 1:　congenital insufficiency of cardiac valve NOS (Q24.8)
> congenital stenosis of cardiac valve NOS (Q24.8)
> endocardial fibroelastosis (I42.4)
> endocarditis specified as rheumatic (I09.1)

I39　Endocarditis and heart valve disorders in diseases classified
CC　elsewhere — [Not Allowed as PDX]
> Code first underlying disease, such as:
> 　Q fever (A78)
> Excludes 1:　endocardial involvement in:
> 　candidiasis (B37.6)
> 　gonococcal infection (A54.83)
> 　Libman-Sacks disease (M32.11)
> 　listerosis (A32.82)
> 　meningococcal infection (A39.51)
> 　rheumatoid arthritis (M05.31)
> 　syphilis (A52.03)
> 　tuberculosis (A18.84)
> 　typhoid fever (A01.02)

I40-　Acute myocarditis — Inflammation of the myocardium with a sudden, severe onset.
> Includes:　Subacute myocarditis — A form with a more gradual and subtle development.
> Excludes 1:　acute rheumatic myocarditis (I01.2)

MCC **I40.0**　Infective myocarditis — Inflammation of the myocardium caused by bacterial microorganisms.
> Septic myocarditis
> Use additional code (B95-B97) to identify infectious agent

MCC **I40.1**　Isolated myocarditis — Inflammation of the myocardium chiefly affecting the interstitial fibrous tissue and of an unknown etiology.
> Fiedler's myocarditis
> Giant cell myocarditis
> Idiopathic myocarditis

MCC **I40.8**　Other acute myocarditis

MCC **I40.9**　Acute myocarditis, unspecified

I41　Myocarditis in diseases classified elsewhere — [Not Allowed as PDX]
MCC　Code first underlying disease, such as:
> 　Typhus (A75.0-A75.9)
> Excludes 1:　myocarditis (in):
> 　Chagas' disease (chronic) (B57.2)
> 　acute (B57.0)
> 　coxsackie (virus) infection (B33.22)
> 　diphtheritic (A36.81)
> 　gonococcal (A54.83)
> 　influenzal (J09.X9, J10.82, J11.82)
> 　meningococcal (A39.52)
> 　mumps (B26.82)
> 　rheumatoid arthritis (M05.31)
> 　sarcoid (D86.85)
> 　syphilis (A52.06)
> 　toxoplasmosis (B58.81)
> 　tuberculous (A18.84)

I42-　Cardiomyopathy — A disease of the heart muscle, usually of an unknown cause.
> Includes:　Myocardiopathy
> Code first pre-existing cardiomyopathy complicating pregnancy and puerperium (O99.4)
> Excludes ❷:　ischemic cardiomyopathy (I25.5)
> 　peripartum cardiomyopathy (O90.3)
> 　ventricular hypertrophy (I51.7)

CC **I42.0**　Dilated cardiomyopathy — The weakening and enlargement (dilation) of the left ventricular wall that leads to insufficient pumping function.
> Congestive cardiomyopathy

CC **I42.1**　Obstructive hypertrophic cardiomyopathy — A disease of unknown cause characterized by asymmetric hypertrophy of the left ventricle wall with variable obstruction of the left ventricle outflow tract.
> Hypertrophic subaortic stenosis (idiopathic)

CC **I42.2**　Other hypertrophic cardiomyopathy — Hypertrophy of the left ventricle wall.
> Nonobstructive hypertrophic cardiomyopathy

CC **I42.3**　Endomyocardial (eosinophilic) disease — A restrictive form left ventricular dysfunction associated with eosinophilia and fibrous tissue of the myocardium.
> Endomyocardial (tropical) fibrosis
> Löffler's endocarditis

CC **I42.4**　Endocardial fibroelastosis — A condition characterized by hypertrophy of the left ventricle wall caused by increased fibroelastic tissue production, often with increased ventricular capacity.
> Congenital cardiomyopathy
> Elastomyofibrosis

CC **I42.5**　Other restrictive cardiomyopathy — A form which progressively restricts the contractions of the ventricles.
> Constrictive cardiomyopathy NOS

Excludes 1: = NOT CODED HERE! (Do not code both)　　　**730**　　　Excludes ❷: = Not Included Here

I 3 4 - I 4 2

cc **I42.6   Alcoholic cardiomyopathy** — A disease of the heart muscle tissue due to the adverse chemical effects of excessive alcohol.
Code also presence of alcoholism (F10.-)

cc **I42.7   Cardiomyopathy <u>due to drug and external agent</u>**
Code first poisoning due to drug or toxin, if applicable (T36-T65 with fifth or sixth character 1-4 or 6)
Use additional code for adverse effect, if applicable, to identify drug (T36-T50 with fifth or sixth character 5)

cc **I42.8   Other cardiomyopathies**

cc **I42.9   Cardiomyopathy, unspecified**
Cardiomyopathy (primary) (secondary) NOS

I43   Cardiomyopathy <u>in diseases classified elsewhere</u> — [Not Allowed as PDX]
cc   Code first underlying disease, such as:
Amyloidosis (E85.-)
Glycogen storage disease (E74.0)
Gout (M10.0-)
Thyrotoxicosis (E05.0-E05.9-)
Excludes 1:   cardiomyopathy (in):
coxsackie (virus) (B33.24)
diphtheria (A36.81)
sarcoidosis (D86.85)
tuberculosis (A18.84)

I44-   <u>Atrioventricular</u> and left bundle-branch block

I44.0   Atrioventricular block, <u>first</u> degree — Impairment of conduction at the atrioventricular node which is prolonged, but the heart makes all of its beats.

I44.1   Atrioventricular block, <u>second</u> degree — Impairment of conduction at the atrioventricular node with partial progressive block and intermittent dropped beats.
Atrioventricular block, type I and II
Möbitz block block, type I and II
Second degree block, type I and II
Wenckebach's block

cc **I44.2   Atrioventricular block, <u>complete</u>** — Impairment of conduction at the atrioventricular node when no impulses are conducted.
Complete heart block NOS
Third degree block

I44.3-   Other and unspecified atrioventricular block
Atrioventricular block NOS

I44.30   <u>Unspecified</u> atrioventricular block

I44.39   <u>Other</u> atrioventricular block

I44.4   <u>Left anterior</u> fascicular block — [Questionable Admission] – Conduction impairment of the left anterior superior branch of the left bundle of His.

I44.5   <u>Left posterior</u> fascicular block — [Questionable Admission] – Conduction impairment of the left posterior inferior branch of the left bundle of His.

I44.6-   Other and unspecified fascicular block

I44.60   <u>Unspecified</u> fascicular block — [Questionable Admission]
Left bundle-branch hemiblock NOS

I44.69   <u>Other</u> fascicular block — [Questionable Admission]

I44.7   Left bundle-branch block, <u>unspecified</u> — [Questionable Admission]

I45-   Other conduction disorders

I45.0   <u>Right fascicular</u> block — [Questionable Admission] – Conduction impairment of the right branch of the bundle of His.

I45.1-   Other and unspecified right bundle-branch block

I45.10   Unspecified right bundle-branch block — [Questionable Admission]
Right bundle-branch block NOS

I45.19   Other right bundle-branch block — [Questionable Admission]

cc **I45.2   Bifascicular block** — Conduction impairment of the right branch and the left branch of the bundle of His.

cc **I45.3   Trifascicular block** — Conduction impairment of all three branches of the bundle of His.

I45.4   Nonspecific intraventricular block
Bundle-branch block NOS

I45.5   Other specified heart block
Sinoatrial block — Partial or complete conduction impairment of the sinoatrial node.
Sinoauricular block
Excludes 1:   heart block NOS (I45.9)

I45.6   Pre-excitation syndrome — A conductive cardiac disease that is characterized by the association of paroxysmal tachycardia and premature ventricular impulses.
Accelerated atrioventricular conduction
Accessory atrioventricular conduction
Anomalous atrioventricular excitation
Lown-Ganong-Levine syndrome
Pre-excitation atrioventricular conduction
Wolff-Parkinson-White syndrome

I45.8-   Other specified conduction disorders

I45.81   Long QT syndrome — A disorder (often hereditary) of the heart's electrical rhythm that is characterized by arrhythmia, syncope, dizziness, and sudden death.

cc **I45.89   Other specified conduction disorders**
AHA 13:2Q:p31 – Short QT syndrome
Atrioventricular [AV] dissociation
Interference dissociation
Isorhythmic dissociation
Nonparoxysmal AV nodal tachycardia

I45.9   Conduction disorder, unspecified
Heart block NOS
Stokes-Adams syndrome — A syndrome characterized by heart block and attacks of sudden loss of consciousness.

I46-   <u>Cardiac arrest</u> — The sudden cessation (stopping) of cardiac function, with disappearance of arterial blood pressure.
Excludes 1:   cardiogenic shock (R57.0)

MCC **I46.2   Cardiac arrest due to underlying <u>cardiac</u> condition**
Code first underlying cardiac condition

MCC **I46.8   Cardiac arrest due to <u>other</u> underlying condition**
Code first underlying condition

MCC **I46.9   Cardiac arrest, cause <u>unspecified</u>**

I47-   <u>Paroxysmal tachycardia</u> — A condition marked by attacks of rapid action of the heart having sudden onset and cessation.
Code first tachycardia complicating:
Abortion or ectopic or molar pregnancy (O00-O07, O08.8)
Obstetric surgery and procedures (O75.4)
Excludes 1:   sinoauricular tachycardia NOS (R00.0)
sinus [sinusal] tachycardia NOS (R00.0)
tachycardia NOS (R00.0)

cc **I47.0   Re-entry ventricular arrhythmia**

cc **I47.1   <u>Supraventricular</u> tachycardia** — An abnormally rapid atrial rhythm, usually in excess of 160 beats per minute resulting in decreased cardiac output.
Atrial (paroxysmal) tachycardia
Atrioventricular [AV] (paroxysmal) tachycardia
Atrioventricular re-entrant (nodal) tachycardia [AVNRT] [AVRT]
Junctional (paroxysmal) tachycardia
Nodal (paroxysmal) tachycardia

cc **I47.2   Ventricular tachycardia** — An abnormally rapid ventricular rhythm with aberrant ventricular excitation, usually in excess of 100 beats per minute, which is generated within the ventricle and is most commonly associated with atrioventricular dissociation.
AHA 13:3Q:p23 – Catecholaminergic polymorphic ventricular tachycardia (CPVT)

I47.9   Paroxysmal tachycardia, unspecified
Bouveret (-Hoffman) syndrome

I48-   <u>Atrial</u> fibrillation and flutter

I48.0   <u>Paroxysmal</u> atrial <u>fibrillation</u> — Atrial arrhythmia characterized by rapid, randomized contractions of the atria causing an irregular and often rapid ventricular rate that are classified as recurrent episodes that stops on its own in less than 7 days.

cc **I48.1   <u>Persistent</u> atrial <u>fibrillation</u>** — Atrial arrhythmia characterized by rapid, randomized contractions of the atria causing an irregular and often rapid ventricular rate that are classified as recurrent episodes that lasts more than 7 days.

I48.2   <u>Chronic</u> atrial <u>fibrillation</u> — Atrial arrhythmia characterized by rapid, randomized contractions of the atria causing an irregular and often rapid ventricular rate that is classified as an ongoing long-term episode.
Permanent atrial fibrillation

cc **I48.3   <u>Typical</u> atrial <u>flutter</u>** — A condition of cardiac arrhythmia in which the atrial contractions are rapid (200-300 per minute range). The ventricles are unable to respond to each atrial impulse, so that a partial block usually is present.
Type I atrial flutter

cc **I48.4   <u>Atypical</u> atrial <u>flutter</u>** — A condition of cardiac arrhythmia in which the atrial contractions are very rapid (300-400 per minute range). The ventricles are unable to respond to each atrial impulse, so that a partial block usually is present.
Type II atrial flutter

I 4 2 - I 4 8

Excludes 1: = NOT CODED HERE! (Do not code both)   **731**   *Excludes ❷:* = Not Included Here

I48.9- <u>Unspecified</u> atrial fibrillation and atrial flutter

I48.91 Unspecified atrial <u>fibrillation</u>

cc **I48.92** Unspecified atrial <u>flutter</u>

I49- **Other cardiac arrhythmias**
Code first cardiac arrhythmia complicating:
Abortion or ectopic or molar pregnancy (O00-O07, O08.8)
Obstetric surgery and procedures (O75.4)
Excludes 1: *bradycardia NOS (R00.1)*
neonatal dysrhythmia (P29.1-)
sinoatrial bradycardia (R00.1)
sinus bradycardia (R00.1)
vagal bradycardia (R00.1)

I49.0- <u>Ventricular</u> fibrillation and flutter

mcc **I49.01** **Ventricular fibrillation** — An arrhythmia characterized by quivering of the ventricle due to rapid repetitive excitation of myocardial fibers without coordinated contraction of the ventricle that results in the loss of the heart pumping and collapse of cardiac output and blood pressure.

mcc **I49.02** **Ventricular flutter** — A possible transition stage between ventricular tachycardia and ventricular fibrillation with the EKG showing rapid, uniform, and virtually regular oscillations, 180 or more per minute.

I49.1 **Atrial premature depolarization** — An early appearing cardiac beat originating in an atria.
Atrial premature beats

cc **I49.2** **Junctional premature depolarization** — An early appearing cardiac beat originating in the atrioventricular node.

I49.3 **Ventricular premature depolarization** — An early appearing cardiac beat originating in the Purkinje fibers of the ventricles.

I49.4- **Other and unspecified premature depolarization**

I49.40 **Unspecified premature depolarization**
Premature beats NOS

I49.49 **Other premature depolarization**
Ectopic beats — A heart beat originating at some point other than a sinus node.
Extrasystoles — A premature contraction of the heart that is independent of the normal rhythm and arises in response to an impulse in some part of the heart other than the sinoatrial node.
Extrasystolic arrhythmias
Premature contractions

I49.5 **Sick sinus syndrome** — Cardiac arrhythmia characterized by severe sinus bradycardia alone, sinus bradycardia alternating with tachycardia, or sinus bradycardia with atrioventricular block.
Tachycardia-bradycardia syndrome

I49.8 **Other specified cardiac arrhythmias**
Coronary sinus rhythm disorder
Ectopic rhythm disorder
Nodal rhythm disorder

I49.9 **Cardiac arrhythmia, unspecified**
Arrhythmia (cardiac) NOS

I50- <u>Heart failure</u> — The decreased ability of the heart to pump enough blood to meet the needs of the body's tissues.
AHA 14:1Q:p25 – Diastolic or systolic heart failure
AHA 14:4Q:p21 – Decompensated right heart failure
AHA 16:1Q:p10 – Diastolic or systolic heart failure (HFpEF, HFrEF)
Code first:
Heart failure complicating abortion or ectopic or molar pregnancy (O00-O07, O08.8)
Heart failure due to hypertension (I11.0)
Heart failure due to hypertension with chronic kidney disease (I13.-)
Heart failure following surgery (I97.13-)
Obstetric surgery and procedures (O75.4)
Rheumatic heart failure (I09.81)
Excludes 1: *neonatal cardiac failure (P29.0)*
Excludes ❷: *cardiac arrest (I46.-)*

cc **I50.1** **Left ventricular failure** — A condition of decreased cardiac output of the left ventricle.
Cardiac asthma
Edema of lung with heart disease NOS
Edema of lung with heart failure
Left heart failure
Pulmonary edema with heart disease NOS
Pulmonary edema with heart failure
Excludes 1: *edema of lung without heart disease or heart failure (J81.-)*
pulmonary edema without heart disease or failure (J81.-)

I50.2- <u>Systolic</u> (congestive) heart failure — A form caused by the left ventricle's inability to contract with enough force to pump adequate amounts of blood through the body that is characterized by excessive fluid retention, congestion in the lungs, and swelling of the legs and ankles.
Excludes 1: *combined systolic (congestive) and diastolic (congestive) heart failure (I50.4-)*

cc **I50.20** <u>Unspecified</u> systolic (congestive) heart failure

mcc **I50.21** <u>Acute</u> systolic (congestive) heart failure — A form marked by a sudden, severe onset.

cc **I50.22** <u>Chronic</u> systolic (congestive) heart failure — A form that persists over a long period of time.

mcc **I50.23** <u>Acute on chronic</u> systolic (congestive) heart failure — A form that persists over a long period of time and has a sudden, severe exacerbation of the condition.
AHA 13:2Q:p33 – Decompensated systolic heart failure

I50.3- <u>Diastolic</u> (congestive) heart failure — A form caused by the left ventricle's inability to relax properly and fill with blood as a result of stiffening of the heart muscle that is characterized by excessive fluid retention, congestion in the lungs, and swelling of the legs and ankles.
Excludes 1: *combined systolic (congestive) and diastolic (congestive) heart failure (I50.4-)*

cc **I50.30** <u>Unspecified</u> diastolic (congestive) heart failure

mcc **I50.31** <u>Acute</u> diastolic (congestive) heart failure — A form marked by a sudden, severe onset.

cc **I50.32** <u>Chronic</u> diastolic (congestive) heart failure — A form that persists over a long period of time.

mcc **I50.33** <u>Acute on chronic</u> diastolic (congestive) heart failure — A form that persists over a long period of time and has a sudden, severe exacerbation of the condition.

I50.4- <u>Combined</u> systolic (congestive) and diastolic (congestive) heart failure — A form in which the left ventricle's inability to contract and relax are both present.

cc **I50.40** <u>Unspecified</u> combined systolic (congestive) and diastolic (congestive) heart failure

mcc **I50.41** <u>Acute</u> combined systolic (congestive) and diastolic (congestive) heart failure — A form marked by a sudden, severe onset.

cc **I50.42** <u>Chronic</u> combined systolic (congestive) and diastolic (congestive) heart failure — A form that persists over a long period of time.

mcc **I50.43** <u>Acute on chronic</u> combined systolic (congestive) and diastolic (congestive) heart failure — A form that persists over a long period of time and has a sudden, severe exacerbation of the condition.

I50.9 **Heart failure, <u>unspecified</u>**
Biventricular (heart) failure NOS
Cardiac, heart or myocardial failure NOS
Congestive heart disease
Congestive heart failure NOS
Right ventricular failure (secondary to left heart failure)
Excludes ❷: *fluid overload (E87.70)*

I51- **Complications and ill-defined descriptions of heart disease**
Excludes 1: *any condition in I51.4-I51.9 due to hypertension (I11.-)*
any condition in I51.4-I51.9 due to hypertension and chronic kidney disease (I13.-)
heart disease specified as rheumatic (I00-I09)

cc **I51.0** **Cardiac septal defect, acquired** — [Age/15-124]
Acquired septal atrial defect (old)
Acquired septal auricular defect (old)
Acquired septal ventricular defect (old)
Excludes 1: *cardiac septal defect as current complication following acute myocardial infarction (I23.1, I23.2)*

mcc **I51.1** **Rupture of chordae tendineae, not elsewhere classified** — A forcible tearing of the strong, cord-like attachments of the heart valves to the papillary muscles.
Excludes 1: *rupture of chordae tendineae as current complication following acute myocardial infarction (I23.4)*

mcc **I51.2** **Rupture of papillary muscle, not elsewhere classified** — A forcible tearing of the conical intraventricular muscles attached to the chordae tendineae and heart wall.
Excludes 1: *rupture of papillary muscle as current complication following acute myocardial infarction (I23.5)*

Excludes 1: = NOT CODED HERE! (Do not code both)

Excludes ❷: = Not Included Here

I51.3   Intracardiac thrombosis, not elsewhere classified

AHA 13:1Q:p24 – Left atrial appendage thrombus
Apical thrombosis (old)
Atrial thrombosis (old)
Auricular thrombosis (old)
Mural thrombosis (old)
Ventricular thrombosis (old)

Excludes 1:   intracardiac thrombosis as current complication following acute myocardial infarction (I23.6)

I51.4   Myocarditis, unspecified — Inflammation of the heart muscle.
Chronic (interstitial) myocarditis
Myocardial fibrosis
Myocarditis NOS

Excludes 1:   acute or subacute myocarditis (I40.-)

I51.5   Myocardial degeneration — Deterioration of the heart muscle tissue.
Fatty degeneration of heart or myocardium
Myocardial disease
Senile degeneration of heart or myocardium

I51.7   Cardiomegaly — The abnormal enlargement of the heart.
Cardiac dilatation
Cardiac hypertrophy
Ventricular dilatation

I51.8-   Other ill-defined heart diseases

cc **I51.81   Takotsubo syndrome** — A reversible left ventricular dysfunction in patients without coronary disease that is precipitated by emotional or physiological stress.
Reversible left ventricular dysfunction following sudden emotional stress
Stress induced cardiomyopathy
Takotsubo cardiomyopathy
Transient left ventricular apical ballooning syndrome

I51.89   Other ill-defined heart diseases
Carditis (acute) (chronic)
Pancarditis (acute) (chronic)

I51.9   Heart disease, unspecified

I52   Other heart disorders in diseases classified elsewhere —
[Not Allowed as PDX]
Code first underlying disease, such as:
Congenital syphilis (A50.5)
Mucopolysaccharidosis (E76.3)
Schistosomiasis (B65.0-B65.9)

*Excludes 1:   heart disease (in):
gonococcal infection (A54.83)
meningococcal infection (A39.50)
rheumatoid arthritis (M05.31)
syphilis (A52.06)*

Cerebrovascular diseases (I60-I69)

Use additional code to identify presence of:
Alcohol abuse and dependence (F10.-)
Exposure to environmental tobacco smoke (Z77.22)
History of tobacco dependence (Z87.891)
Hypertension (I10-I15)
Occupational exposure to environmental tobacco smoke (Z57.31)
Tobacco dependence (F17.-)
Tobacco use (Z72.0)

*Excludes 1:   transient cerebral ischemic attacks and related syndromes (G45.-)
traumatic intracranial hemorrhage (S06.-)*

I60-   Nontraumatic subarachnoid hemorrhage — A hemorrhage into the subarachnoid (beneath the arachnoid layer of cerebral meninges) space.
Includes: Ruptured cerebral aneurysm
Excludes 1:   syphilitic ruptured cerebral aneurysm (A52.05)
Excludes ❷: sequelae of subarachnoid hemorrhage (I69.0-)

I60.0-   Nontraumatic subarachnoid hemorrhage from carotid siphon and bifurcation

MCC **I60.00   Nontraumatic subarachnoid hemorrhage from unspecified carotid siphon and bifurcation**

MCC **I60.01   Nontraumatic subarachnoid hemorrhage from right carotid siphon and bifurcation**

MCC **I60.02   Nontraumatic subarachnoid hemorrhage from left carotid siphon and bifurcation**

I60.1-   Nontraumatic subarachnoid hemorrhage from middle cerebral artery

MCC **I60.10   Nontraumatic subarachnoid hemorrhage from unspecified middle cerebral artery**

MCC **I60.11   Nontraumatic subarachnoid hemorrhage from right middle cerebral artery**

MCC **I60.12   Nontraumatic subarachnoid hemorrhage from left middle cerebral artery**

MCC **I60.2   Nontraumatic subarachnoid hemorrhage from anterior communicating artery**

I60.3-   Nontraumatic subarachnoid hemorrhage from posterior communicating artery

MCC **I60.30   Nontraumatic subarachnoid hemorrhage from unspecified posterior communicating artery**

MCC **I60.31   Nontraumatic subarachnoid hemorrhage from right posterior communicating artery**

MCC **I60.32   Nontraumatic subarachnoid hemorrhage from left posterior communicating artery**

MCC **I60.4   Nontraumatic subarachnoid hemorrhage from basilar artery**

I60.5-   Nontraumatic subarachnoid hemorrhage from vertebral artery

MCC **I60.50   Nontraumatic subarachnoid hemorrhage from unspecified vertebral artery**

MCC **I60.51   Nontraumatic subarachnoid hemorrhage from right vertebral artery**

MCC **I60.52   Nontraumatic subarachnoid hemorrhage from left vertebral artery**

MCC **I60.6   Nontraumatic subarachnoid hemorrhage from other intracranial arteries**

MCC **I60.7   Nontraumatic subarachnoid hemorrhage from unspecified intracranial artery**
Ruptured (congenital) berry aneurysm
Ruptured (congenital) cerebral aneurysm
Subarachnoid hemorrhage (nontraumatic) from cerebral artery NOS
Subarachnoid hemorrhage (nontraumatic) from communicating artery NOS

Excludes 1:   berry aneurysm, nonruptured (I67.1)

MCC **I60.8   Other nontraumatic subarachnoid hemorrhage**
Meningeal hemorrhage
Rupture of cerebral arteriovenous malformation

MCC **I60.9   Nontraumatic subarachnoid hemorrhage, unspecified**

I61-   Nontraumatic intracerebral hemorrhage — A hemorrhage within the brain.
Excludes ❷: sequelae of intracerebral hemorrhage (I69.1-)

MCC **I61.0   Nontraumatic intracerebral hemorrhage in hemisphere, subcortical** — A hemorrhage beneath the cerebral cortex.
Deep intracerebral hemorrhage (nontraumatic)

MCC **I61.1   Nontraumatic intracerebral hemorrhage in hemisphere, cortical** — A hemorrhage in the cerebral cortex.
Cerebral lobe hemorrhage (nontraumatic)
Superficial intracerebral hemorrhage (nontraumatic)

MCC **I61.2   Nontraumatic intracerebral hemorrhage in hemisphere, unspecified**

MCC **I61.3   Nontraumatic intracerebral hemorrhage in brain stem** — A hemorrhage in the brain stem.

MCC **I61.4   Nontraumatic intracerebral hemorrhage in cerebellum** — A hemorrhage in the cerebellum.

MCC **I61.5   Nontraumatic intracerebral hemorrhage, intraventricular** — A hemorrhage into the ventricles of the brain.

MCC **I61.6   Nontraumatic intracerebral hemorrhage, multiple localized** — A form marked by separate, distinct sites.

MCC **I61.8   Other nontraumatic intracerebral hemorrhage**

MCC **I61.9   Nontraumatic intracerebral hemorrhage, unspecified**

I62-   Other and unspecified nontraumatic intracranial hemorrhage
Excludes ❷: sequelae of intracranial hemorrhage (I69.2)

I62.0-   Nontraumatic subdural hemorrhage — A hemorrhage below the dura layer of meninges but does not involve the brain, but can compress on the brain.

MCC **I62.00   Nontraumatic subdural hemorrhage, unspecified**

MCC **I62.01   Nontraumatic acute subdural hemorrhage** — A form with a sudden, severe onset.

MCC **I62.02   Nontraumatic subacute subdural hemorrhage** — A form that develops over several days.

MCC **I62.03   Nontraumatic chronic subdural hemorrhage** — A form that develops over several weeks.

I51 - I62

Excludes 1: = NOT CODED HERE! (Do not code both)   **733**   *Excludes ❷: = Not Included Here*

MCC I62.1 Nontraumatic <u>extradural</u> hemorrhage — A hemorrhage between the skull and meninges which does not involve the brain.

Nontraumatic epidural hemorrhage — A hemorrhage situated upon or outside the dura (the outermost layer of cerebral meninges).

CC I62.9 Nontraumatic <u>intracranial</u> hemorrhage, <u>unspecified</u>

I63- <u>Cerebral infarction</u> — Local cerebral tissue ischemia that produces a neurological brain impairment.

Includes: Occlusion and stenosis of cerebral and precerebral arteries, resulting in cerebral infarction

Use additional code, if applicable, to identify status post administration of tPA (rtPA) in a different facility within the last 24 hours prior to admission to current facility (Z92.82)

Use additional code, if known, to indicate National Institutes of Health Stroke Scale (NIHSS) score (R29.7)

Excludes ❷: sequelae of cerebral infarction (I69.3-)

I63.0- Cerebral infarction <u>due to thrombosis of precerebral arteries</u> — A form marked by an abnormal aggregation of blood factors causing inadequate blood flow of the branched arteries before they anatomically branch into the brain.

MCC I63.00 Cerebral infarction due to <u>thrombosis</u> of <u>unspecified</u> precerebral artery

I63.01- Cerebral infarction due to <u>thrombosis</u> of <u>vertebral</u> artery

MCC I63.011 Cerebral infarction due to <u>thrombosis</u> of <u>right</u> vertebral artery

MCC I63.012 Cerebral infarction due to <u>thrombosis</u> of <u>left</u> vertebral artery

MCC I63.013 Cerebral infarction due to <u>thrombosis</u> of <u>bilateral</u> vertebral arteries

MCC I63.019 Cerebral infarction due to <u>thrombosis</u> of <u>unspecified</u> vertebral artery

MCC I63.02 Cerebral infarction due to <u>thrombosis</u> of <u>basilar</u> artery

I63.03- Cerebral infarction due to <u>thrombosis</u> of <u>carotid</u> artery

MCC I63.031 Cerebral infarction due to <u>thrombosis</u> of <u>right</u> carotid artery

MCC I63.032 Cerebral infarction due to <u>thrombosis</u> of <u>left</u> carotid artery

MCC I63.033 Cerebral infarction due to <u>thrombosis</u> of <u>bilateral</u> carotid arteries

MCC I63.039 Cerebral infarction due to <u>thrombosis</u> of <u>unspecified</u> carotid artery

MCC I63.09 Cerebral infarction due to <u>thrombosis</u> of <u>other</u> precerebral artery

I63.1- Cerebral infarction <u>due to embolism of precerebral arteries</u> — A form marked by obstruction caused by a blood clot or foreign substances of the branched arteries before they anatomically branch into the brain.

MCC I63.10 Cerebral infarction due to <u>embolism</u> of <u>unspecified</u> precerebral artery

I63.11- Cerebral infarction due to <u>embolism</u> of <u>vertebral</u> artery

MCC I63.111 Cerebral infarction due to <u>embolism</u> of <u>right</u> vertebral artery

MCC I63.112 Cerebral infarction due to <u>embolism</u> of <u>left</u> vertebral artery

MCC I63.113 Cerebral infarction due to <u>embolism</u> of <u>bilateral</u> vertebral arteries

MCC I63.119 Cerebral infarction due to <u>embolism</u> of <u>unspecified</u> vertebral artery

MCC I63.12 Cerebral infarction due to <u>embolism</u> of <u>basilar</u> artery

I63.13- Cerebral infarction due to <u>embolism</u> of <u>carotid</u> artery

MCC I63.131 Cerebral infarction due to <u>embolism</u> of <u>right</u> carotid artery

MCC I63.132 Cerebral infarction due to <u>embolism</u> of <u>left</u> carotid artery

MCC I63.133 Cerebral infarction due to <u>embolism</u> of <u>bilateral</u> carotid arteries

MCC I63.139 Cerebral infarction due to <u>embolism</u> of <u>unspecified</u> carotid artery

MCC I63.19 Cerebral infarction due to <u>embolism</u> of other <u>precerebral</u> artery

I63.2- Cerebral infarction due to <u>unspecified</u> <u>occlusion or stenosis</u> of precerebral arteries

MCC I63.20 Cerebral infarction due to <u>unspecified</u> occlusion or stenosis of <u>unspecified</u> precerebral arteries

I63.21- Cerebral infarction due to <u>unspecified</u> occlusion or stenosis of <u>vertebral</u> arteries

MCC I63.211 Cerebral infarction due to <u>unspecified</u> occlusion or stenosis of <u>right</u> vertebral arteries

MCC I63.212 Cerebral infarction due to <u>unspecified</u> occlusion or stenosis of <u>left</u> vertebral arteries

MCC I63.213 Cerebral infarction due to <u>unspecified</u> occlusion or stenosis of <u>bilateral</u> vertebral arteries

MCC I63.219 Cerebral infarction due to <u>unspecified</u> occlusion or stenosis of <u>unspecified</u> vertebral arteries

MCC I63.22 Cerebral infarction due to <u>unspecified</u> occlusion or stenosis of <u>basilar</u> arteries

I63.23- Cerebral infarction due to <u>unspecified</u> occlusion or stenosis of <u>carotid</u> arteries

MCC I63.231 Cerebral infarction due to <u>unspecified</u> occlusion or stenosis of <u>right</u> carotid arteries

MCC I63.232 Cerebral infarction due to <u>unspecified</u> occlusion or stenosis of <u>left</u> carotid arteries

MCC I63.233 Cerebral infarction due to <u>unspecified</u> occlusion or stenosis of <u>bilateral</u> carotid arteries

MCC I63.239 Cerebral infarction due to <u>unspecified</u> occlusion or stenosis of <u>unspecified</u> carotid arteries

MCC I63.29 Cerebral infarction due to <u>unspecified</u> occlusion or stenosis of other <u>precerebral</u> arteries

I63.3- Cerebral infarction <u>due to thrombosis of cerebral arteries</u> — A form marked by an abnormal aggregation of blood factors causing inadequate blood flow of the arteries within the brain.

MCC I63.30 Cerebral infarction due to <u>thrombosis</u> of <u>unspecified</u> <u>cerebral</u> artery

I63.31- Cerebral infarction due to <u>thrombosis</u> of <u>middle cerebral</u> artery

MCC I63.311 Cerebral infarction due to <u>thrombosis</u> of <u>right</u> middle cerebral artery

MCC I63.312 Cerebral infarction due to <u>thrombosis</u> of <u>left</u> middle cerebral artery

MCC I63.313 Cerebral infarction due to <u>thrombosis</u> of <u>bilateral</u> middle cerebral arteries

MCC I63.319 Cerebral infarction due to <u>thrombosis</u> of <u>unspecified</u> middle cerebral artery

I63.32- Cerebral infarction due to <u>thrombosis</u> of <u>anterior cerebral</u> artery

MCC I63.321 Cerebral infarction due to <u>thrombosis</u> of <u>right</u> anterior cerebral artery

MCC I63.322 Cerebral infarction due to <u>thrombosis</u> of <u>left</u> anterior cerebral artery

MCC I63.323 Cerebral infarction due to <u>thrombosis</u> of <u>bilateral</u> anterior arteries

MCC I63.329 Cerebral infarction due to <u>thrombosis</u> of <u>unspecified</u> anterior cerebral artery

I63.33- Cerebral infarction due to <u>thrombosis</u> of <u>posterior cerebral</u> artery

MCC I63.331 Cerebral infarction due to <u>thrombosis</u> of <u>right</u> posterior cerebral artery

MCC I63.332 Cerebral infarction due to <u>thrombosis</u> of <u>left</u> posterior cerebral artery

MCC I63.333 Cerebral infarction due to <u>thrombosis</u> of <u>bilateral</u> posterior arteries

MCC I63.339 Cerebral infarction due to <u>thrombosis</u> of <u>unspecified</u> posterior cerebral artery

I63.34- Cerebral infarction due to <u>thrombosis</u> of <u>cerebellar</u> artery

MCC I63.341 Cerebral infarction due to <u>thrombosis</u> of <u>right</u> cerebellar artery

MCC I63.342 Cerebral infarction due to <u>thrombosis</u> of <u>left</u> cerebellar artery

I
6
2
-
I
6
3

MCC **I63.343** Cerebral infarction due to <u>thrombosis</u> of <u>bilateral</u> cerebellar arteries

MCC **I63.349** Cerebral infarction due to <u>thrombosis</u> of <u>unspecified</u> cerebellar artery

MCC **I63.39** Cerebral infarction due to <u>thrombosis</u> of other <u>cerebral</u> artery

I63.4- Cerebral infarction due to <u>embolism</u> of <u>cerebral</u> arteries — A form marked by obstruction caused by a blood clot or foreign substances of the arteries within the brain.

MCC **I63.40** Cerebral infarction due to <u>embolism</u> of <u>unspecified</u> cerebral artery

I63.41- Cerebral infarction due to <u>embolism</u> of <u>middle</u> cerebral artery

MCC **I63.411** Cerebral infarction due to <u>embolism</u> of <u>right</u> middle cerebral artery

MCC **I63.412** Cerebral infarction due to <u>embolism</u> of <u>left</u> middle cerebral artery

MCC **I63.413** Cerebral infarction due to <u>embolism</u> of <u>bilateral</u> middle cerebral arteries

MCC **I63.419** Cerebral infarction due to <u>embolism</u> of <u>unspecified</u> middle cerebral artery

I63.42- Cerebral infarction due to <u>embolism</u> of <u>anterior</u> cerebral artery

MCC **I63.421** Cerebral infarction due to <u>embolism</u> of <u>right</u> anterior cerebral artery

MCC **I63.422** Cerebral infarction due to <u>embolism</u> of <u>left</u> anterior cerebral artery

MCC **I63.423** Cerebral infarction due to <u>embolism</u> of <u>bilateral</u> anterior cerebral arteries

MCC **I63.429** Cerebral infarction due to <u>embolism</u> of <u>unspecified</u> anterior cerebral artery

I63.43- Cerebral infarction due to <u>embolism</u> of <u>posterior</u> cerebral artery

MCC **I63.431** Cerebral infarction due to <u>embolism</u> of <u>right</u> posterior cerebral artery

MCC **I63.432** Cerebral infarction due to <u>embolism</u> of <u>left</u> posterior cerebral artery

MCC **I63.433** Cerebral infarction due to <u>embolism</u> of <u>bilateral</u> posterior cerebral arteries

MCC **I63.439** Cerebral infarction due to <u>embolism</u> of <u>unspecified</u> posterior cerebral artery

I63.44- Cerebral infarction due to <u>embolism</u> of <u>cerebellar</u> artery

MCC **I63.441** Cerebral infarction due to <u>embolism</u> of <u>right</u> cerebellar artery

MCC **I63.442** Cerebral infarction due to <u>embolism</u> of <u>left</u> cerebellar artery

MCC **I63.443** Cerebral infarction due to <u>embolism</u> of <u>bilateral</u> cerebellar arteries

MCC **I63.449** Cerebral infarction due to <u>embolism</u> of <u>unspecified</u> cerebellar artery

MCC **I63.49** Cerebral infarction due to <u>embolism</u> of <u>other cerebral</u> artery

I63.5- Cerebral infarction due to <u>unspecified occlusion or stenosis of cerebral arteries</u>

MCC **I63.50** Cerebral infarction due to <u>unspecified</u> occlusion or stenosis of unspecified cerebral artery

I63.51- Cerebral infarction due to <u>unspecified</u> occlusion or stenosis of <u>middle</u> cerebral artery

MCC **I63.511** Cerebral infarction due to <u>unspecified</u> occlusion or stenosis of <u>right</u> middle cerebral artery

MCC **I63.512** Cerebral infarction due to <u>unspecified</u> occlusion or stenosis of <u>left</u> middle cerebral artery

MCC **I63.513** Cerebral infarction due to <u>unspecified</u> occlusion or stenosis of <u>bilateral</u> middle arteries

MCC **I63.519** Cerebral infarction due to <u>unspecified</u> occlusion or stenosis of <u>unspecified</u> middle cerebral artery

I63.52- Cerebral infarction due to <u>unspecified</u> occlusion or stenosis of <u>anterior</u> cerebral artery

MCC **I63.521** Cerebral infarction due to <u>unspecified</u> occlusion or stenosis of <u>right</u> anterior cerebral artery

MCC **I63.522** Cerebral infarction due to <u>unspecified</u> occlusion or stenosis of <u>left</u> anterior cerebral artery

MCC **I63.523** Cerebral infarction due to <u>unspecified</u> occlusion or stenosis of <u>bilateral</u> anterior arteries

MCC **I63.529** Cerebral infarction due to <u>unspecified</u> occlusion or stenosis of <u>unspecified</u> anterior cerebral artery

I63.53- Cerebral infarction due to <u>unspecified</u> occlusion or stenosis of <u>posterior</u> cerebral artery

MCC **I63.531** Cerebral infarction due to <u>unspecified</u> occlusion or stenosis of <u>right</u> posterior cerebral artery

MCC **I63.532** Cerebral infarction due to <u>unspecified</u> occlusion or stenosis of <u>left</u> posterior cerebral artery

MCC **I63.533** Cerebral infarction due to <u>unspecified</u> occlusion or stenosis of <u>bilateral</u> posterior arteries

MCC **I63.539** Cerebral infarction due to <u>unspecified</u> occlusion or stenosis of <u>unspecified</u> posterior cerebral artery

I63.54- Cerebral infarction due to <u>unspecified</u> occlusion or stenosis of <u>cerebellar</u> artery

MCC **I63.541** Cerebral infarction due to <u>unspecified</u> occlusion or stenosis of <u>right</u> cerebellar artery

MCC **I63.542** Cerebral infarction due to <u>unspecified</u> occlusion or stenosis of <u>left</u> cerebellar artery

MCC **I63.543** Cerebral infarction due to <u>unspecified</u> occlusion or stenosis of <u>bilateral</u> cerebellar arteries

MCC **I63.549** Cerebral infarction due to <u>unspecified</u> occlusion or stenosis of <u>unspecified</u> cerebellar artery

MCC **I63.59** Cerebral infarction due to <u>unspecified</u> occlusion or stenosis of <u>other cerebral</u> artery

MCC **I63.6** Cerebral infarction due to <u>cerebral venous thrombosis</u>, nonpyogenic

MCC **I63.8** <u>Other</u> cerebral infarction

MCC **I63.9** Cerebral infarction, <u>unspecified</u>
   AHA 15:1Q:p25 – Cerebral infarction
   Stroke NOS

I65- <u>Occlusion and stenosis</u> of <u>precerebral</u> arteries, <u>not resulting in cerebral infarction</u> — Decreased blood flow conditions of the branched arteries before they anatomically branch into the brain.
   Includes: **Embolism of precerebral artery** — Obstruction caused by foreign substances or a blood clot.
      Narrowing of precerebral artery — Inadequate blood flow due to decreased lumenal patency.
      Obstruction (complete) (partial) of precerebral artery — Blockage by any means.
      Thrombosis of precerebral artery — An abnormal aggregation of blood factors causing inadequate blood flow.
   Excludes 1:   *insufficiency, NOS, of precerebral artery (G45.-)*
      insufficiency of precerebral arteries causing cerebral infarction (I63.0-I63.2)

I65.0- <u>Occlusion and stenosis</u> of <u>vertebral</u> artery

   I65.01 Occlusion and stenosis of <u>right</u> vertebral artery

   I65.02 Occlusion and stenosis of <u>left</u> vertebral artery

   I65.03 Occlusion and stenosis of <u>bilateral</u> vertebral arteries

   I65.09 Occlusion and stenosis of <u>unspecified</u> vertebral artery

I65.1 <u>Occlusion and stenosis</u> of <u>basilar</u> artery

I65.2- <u>Occlusion and stenosis</u> of <u>carotid</u> artery

   I65.21 Occlusion and stenosis of <u>right</u> carotid artery

   I65.22 Occlusion and stenosis of <u>left</u> carotid artery

   I65.23 Occlusion and stenosis of <u>bilateral</u> carotid arteries

   I65.29 Occlusion and stenosis of <u>unspecified</u> carotid artery

I65.8 <u>Occlusion and stenosis</u> of <u>other</u> precerebral arteries

I65.9 <u>Occlusion and stenosis</u> of <u>unspecified</u> precerebral artery
   Occlusion and stenosis of precerebral artery NOS

I63 - I65

Excludes 1: = NOT CODED HERE! (Do not code both)   735   *Excludes ❷:* = Not Included Here

I66- Occlusion and stenosis of cerebral arteries, not resulting in cerebral infarction — Blocked blood flow of the arteries within brain.

Includes: **Embolism of cerebral artery** — Obstruction caused by foreign substances or a blood clot.

        Narrowing of cerebral artery — Inadequate blood flow due to decreased lumenal patency.

        Obstruction (complete) (partial) of cerebral artery — Blockage by any means.

        Thrombosis of cerebral artery — An abnormal aggregation of blood factors causing inadequate blood flow.

Excludes 1:   *occlusion and stenosis of cerebral artery causing cerebral infarction (I63.3-I63.5)*

I66.0- Occlusion and stenosis of middle cerebral artery

    I66.01 Occlusion and stenosis of right middle cerebral artery

    I66.02 Occlusion and stenosis of left middle cerebral artery

    I66.03 Occlusion and stenosis of bilateral middle cerebral arteries

    I66.09 Occlusion and stenosis of unspecified middle cerebral artery

I66.1- Occlusion and stenosis of anterior cerebral artery

    I66.11 Occlusion and stenosis of right anterior cerebral artery

    I66.12 Occlusion and stenosis of left anterior cerebral artery

    I66.13 Occlusion and stenosis of bilateral anterior cerebral arteries

    I66.19 Occlusion and stenosis of unspecified anterior cerebral artery

I66.2- Occlusion and stenosis of posterior cerebral artery

    I66.21 Occlusion and stenosis of right posterior cerebral artery

    I66.22 Occlusion and stenosis of left posterior cerebral artery

    I66.23 Occlusion and stenosis of bilateral posterior cerebral arteries

    I66.29 Occlusion and stenosis of unspecified posterior cerebral artery

I66.3 Occlusion and stenosis of cerebellar arteries

I66.8 Occlusion and stenosis of other cerebral arteries

    Occlusion and stenosis of perforating arteries

I66.9 Occlusion and stenosis of unspecified cerebral artery

I67- Other cerebrovascular diseases

Excludes ❷: *sequelae of the listed conditions (I69.8)*

MCC **I67.0** Dissection of cerebral arteries, nonruptured — The tearing of the lining of a cerebral artery.

    Excludes 1: *ruptured cerebral arteries (I60.7)*

I67.1 Cerebral aneurysm, nonruptured — A sac formed by the dilatation of a cerebral arterial wall, in which the arterial wall has not torn open.

    Cerebral aneurysm NOS

    Cerebral arteriovenous fistula, acquired

    Internal carotid artery aneurysm, intracranial portion

    Internal carotid artery aneurysm, NOS

    Excludes 1: *congenital cerebral aneurysm, nonruptured (Q28.-)*

              ruptured cerebral aneurysm (I60.7)

I67.2 Cerebral atherosclerosis — [Age/15-124] — Narrowing of the cerebral an/or the precerebral arteries caused by deposition of plaque-forming cholesterol and other lipids within the lumen of those arteries.

    Atheroma of cerebral and precerebral arteries

CC **I67.3** Progressive vascular leukoencephalopathy

    Binswanger's disease

CC **I67.4** Hypertensive encephalopathy — A degenerative condition of the brain resulting from severe hypertension.

CC **I67.5** Moyamoya disease — The arterial graphic appearance of a filmy network of small vessels (resembling a puff of smoke) replacing the normal vascular pattern at the termination of the internal carotid artery; seen in patients with sudden cerebrovascular insufficiency.

CC **I67.6** Nonpyogenic thrombosis of intracranial venous system — An abnormal aggregation of blood factors causing obstruction of the intracranial venous sinus that is not formed by pus-producing organisms.

    Nonpyogenic thrombosis of cerebral vein

    Nonpyogenic thrombosis of intracranial venous sinus

    Excludes 1: *nonpyogenic thrombosis of intracranial venous system causing infarction (I63.6)*

CC **I67.7** Cerebral arteritis, not elsewhere classified

    Granulomatous angiitis of the nervous system

    Excludes 1: *allergic granulomatous angiitis (M30.1)*

I67.8- Other specified cerebrovascular diseases

CC **I67.81** Acute cerebrovascular insufficiency — Inadequate function of the cerebrovascular system, but not diagnostic of transient cerebral ischemia or stroke.

    Acute cerebrovascular insufficiency unspecified as to location or reversibility

CC **I67.82** Cerebral ischemia — Prolonged, persistent deficiency of blood supply to the brain.

    Chronic cerebral ischemia

MCC **I67.83** Posterior reversible encephalopathy syndrome — A syndrome characterized by headache, visual disturbance, and seizures that is often due to hypertension.

    PRES

I67.84- Cerebral vasospasm and vasoconstriction

CC **I67.841** Reversible cerebrovascular vasoconstriction syndrome — A cerebrovascular disorder associated with arterial dilation and constriction that is characterized by thunderclap headaches and sometime seizures.

    Call-Fleming syndrome

    Code first underlying condition, if applicable, such as eclampsia (O15.00-O15.9)

CC **I67.848** Other cerebral vasospasm and vasoconstriction

CC **I67.89** Other cerebrovascular disease

I67.9 Cerebrovascular disease, unspecified

I68- Cerebrovascular disorders in diseases classified elsewhere

I68.0 Cerebral amyloid angiopathy — [Not Allowed as PDX]

    Code first underlying amyloidosis (E85.-)

CC **I68.2** Cerebral arteritis in other diseases classified elsewhere — [Not Allowed as PDX]

    Code first underlying disease

    Excludes 1: *cerebral arteritis (in):*

              listerosis (A32.89)

              systemic lupus erythematosus (M32.19)

              syphilis (A52.04)

              tuberculosis (A18.89)

I68.8 Other cerebrovascular disorders in diseases classified elsewhere — [Not Allowed as PDX]

    Code first underlying disease

    Excludes 1: *syphilitic cerebral aneurysm (A52.05)*

I69- Sequelae of cerebrovascular disease

AHA 12:4Q:p106 – Affected side not specified (dominant and nondominant)

Note: Category I69 is to be used to indicate conditions in I60-I67 as the cause of sequelae. The "sequelae" include conditions specified as such or as residuals which may occur at any time after the onset of the causal condition.

Excludes 1: *personal history of cerebral infarction without residual deficit (Z86.73)*

              personal history of prolonged reversible ischemic neurologic deficit (PRIND) (Z86.73)

              personal history of reversible ischemic neurologcial deficit (RIND) (Z86.73)

              sequelae of traumatic intracranial injury (S06.-)

              transient ischemic attack (TIA) (G45.9)

I69.0- Sequelae of nontraumatic subarachnoid hemorrhage

    I69.00 Unspecified sequelae of nontraumatic subarachnoid hemorrhage

    I69.01- Cognitive deficits following nontraumatic subarachnoid hemorrhage

        I69.010 Attention and concentration deficit following nontraumatic subarachnoid hemorrhage

        I69.011 Memory deficit following nontraumatic subarachnoid hemorrhage

        I69.012 Visuospatial deficit and spatial neglect following nontraumatic subarachnoid hemorrhage

        I69.013 Psychomotor deficit following nontraumatic subarachnoid hemorrhage

        I69.014 Frontal lobe and executive function deficit following nontraumatic subarachnoid hemorrhage

        I69.015 Cognitive social or emotional deficit following nontraumatic subarachnoid hemorrhage

I66-I69

I69.018 **Other symptoms and signs** involving cognitive functions following nontraumatic subarachnoid hemorrhage

I69.019 **Unspecified symptoms and signs** involving cognitive functions following nontraumatic subarachnoid hemorrhage

I69.02- **Speech and language** deficits following nontraumatic subarachnoid hemorrhage

I69.020 **Aphasia** following nontraumatic subarachnoid hemorrhage

I69.021 **Dysphasia** following nontraumatic subarachnoid hemorrhage

I69.022 **Dysarthria** following nontraumatic subarachnoid hemorrhage

I69.023 **Fluency** disorder following nontraumatic subarachnoid hemorrhage
    Stuttering following nontraumatic subarachnoid hemorrhage

I69.028 **Other speech and language** deficits following nontraumatic subarachnoid hemorrhage

I69.03- **Monoplegia** of **upper limb** following nontraumatic subarachnoid hemorrhage

I69.031 Monoplegia of upper limb following nontraumatic subarachnoid hemorrhage affecting **right** dominant side

I69.032 Monoplegia of upper limb following nontraumatic subarachnoid hemorrhage affecting **left** dominant side

I69.033 Monoplegia of upper limb following nontraumatic subarachnoid hemorrhage affecting **right non**-dominant side

I69.034 Monoplegia of upper limb following nontraumatic subarachnoid hemorrhage affecting **left non**-dominant side

I69.039 Monoplegia of upper limb following nontraumatic subarachnoid hemorrhage affecting **unspecified side**

I69.04- **Monoplegia** of **lower limb** following nontraumatic subarachnoid hemorrhage

I69.041 Monoplegia of lower limb following nontraumatic subarachnoid hemorrhage affecting **right** dominant side

I69.042 Monoplegia of lower limb following nontraumatic subarachnoid hemorrhage affecting **left** dominant side

I69.043 Monoplegia of lower limb following nontraumatic subarachnoid hemorrhage affecting **right non**-dominant side

I69.044 Monoplegia of lower limb following nontraumatic subarachnoid hemorrhage affecting **left non**-dominant side

I69.049 Monoplegia of lower limb following nontraumatic subarachnoid hemorrhage affecting **unspecified side**

I69.05- **Hemiplegia and hemiparesis** following nontraumatic subarachnoid hemorrhage

cc **I69.051** **Hemiplegia and hemiparesis** following nontraumatic subarachnoid hemorrhage affecting **right** dominant side

cc **I69.052** **Hemiplegia and hemiparesis** following nontraumatic subarachnoid hemorrhage affecting **left** dominant side

cc **I69.053** **Hemiplegia and hemiparesis** following nontraumatic subarachnoid hemorrhage affecting **right non**-dominant side

cc **I69.054** **Hemiplegia and hemiparesis** following nontraumatic subarachnoid hemorrhage affecting **left non**-dominant side

cc **I69.059** **Hemiplegia and hemiparesis** following nontraumatic subarachnoid hemorrhage affecting **unspecified side**

I69.06- **Other paralytic** syndrome following nontraumatic subarachnoid hemorrhage
    Use additional code to identify type of paralytic syndrome, such as:
        Locked-in state (G83.5)
        Quadriplegia (G82.5-)
    Excludes 1:   hemiplegia/hemiparesis following nontraumatic subarachnoid hemorrhage (I69.05-)
            monoplegia of lower limb following nontraumatic subarachnoid hemorrhage (I69.04-)
            monoplegia of upper limb following nontraumatic subarachnoid hemorrhage (I69.03-)

I69.061 Other paralytic syndrome following nontraumatic subarachnoid hemorrhage affecting **right** dominant side

I69.062 Other paralytic syndrome following nontraumatic subarachnoid hemorrhage affecting **left** dominant side

I69.063 Other paralytic syndrome following nontraumatic subarachnoid hemorrhage affecting **right non**-dominant side

I69.064 Other paralytic syndrome following nontraumatic subarachnoid hemorrhage affecting **left non**-dominant side

I69.065 Other paralytic syndrome following nontraumatic subarachnoid hemorrhage, **bilateral**

I69.069 Other paralytic syndrome following nontraumatic subarachnoid hemorrhage affecting **unspecified side**

I69.09- **Other sequelae** of nontraumatic subarachnoid hemorrhage

I69.090 **Apraxia** following nontraumatic subarachnoid hemorrhage

I69.091 **Dysphagia** following nontraumatic subarachnoid hemorrhage
    Use additional code to identify the type of dysphagia, if known (R13.1-)

I69.092 **Facial weakness** following nontraumatic subarachnoid hemorrhage
    Facial droop following nontraumatic subarachnoid hemorrhage

I69.093 **Ataxia** following nontraumatic subarachnoid hemorrhage

I69.098 **Other sequelae** following nontraumatic subarachnoid hemorrhage
    Alterations of sensation following nontraumatic subarachnoid hemorrhage
    Disturbance of vision following nontraumatic subarachnoid hemorrhage
    Use additional code to identify the sequelae

I69.1- **Sequelae** of nontraumatic **intracerebral** hemorrhage

I69.10 **Unspecified** sequelae of nontraumatic **intracerebral** hemorrhage

I69.11- **Cognitive** deficits following nontraumatic **intracerebral** hemorrhage

I69.110 **Attention and concentration** deficit following nontraumatic **intracerebral** hemorrhage

I69.111 **Memory** deficit following nontraumatic **intracerebral** hemorrhage

I69.112 **Visuospatial deficit and spatial neglect** following nontraumatic **intracerebral** hemorrhage

I69.113 **Psychomotor** deficit following nontraumatic **intracerebral** hemorrhage

I69.114 **Frontal lobe and executive function** deficit following nontraumatic **intracerebral** hemorrhage

I69.115 Cognitive social or emotional deficit following nontraumatic **intracerebral** hemorrhage

I69.118 **Other symptoms and signs** involving cognitive functions following nontraumatic **intracerebral** hemorrhage

I 6 9 - I 6 9

Excludes 1: = NOT CODED HERE! (Do not code both)   737   *Excludes ❷:* = Not Included Here

I69.119 **Unspecified symptoms and signs** involving cognitive functions following nontraumatic **intracerebral** hemorrhage

I69.12- **Speech and language** deficits following nontraumatic **intracerebral** hemorrhage

I69.120 **Aphasia** following nontraumatic **intracerebral** hemorrhage

I69.121 **Dysphasia** following nontraumatic **intracerebral** hemorrhage

I69.122 **Dysarthria** following nontraumatic **intracerebral** hemorrhage

I69.123 **Fluency disorder** following nontraumatic **intracerebral** hemorrhage
  Stuttering following nontraumatic intracerebral hemorrhage

I69.128 **Other speech and language** deficits following nontraumatic **intracerebral** hemorrhage

I69.13- **Monoplegia** of **upper limb** following nontraumatic **intracerebral** hemorrhage

I69.131 Monoplegia of upper limb following nontraumatic **intracerebral** hemorrhage affecting **right** dominant side

I69.132 Monoplegia of upper limb following nontraumatic **intracerebral** hemorrhage affecting **left** dominant side

I69.133 Monoplegia of upper limb following nontraumatic **intracerebral** hemorrhage affecting **right non-**dominant side

I69.134 Monoplegia of upper limb following nontraumatic **intracerebral** hemorrhage affecting **left non-**dominant side

I69.139 Monoplegia of upper limb following nontraumatic **intracerebral** hemorrhage affecting **unspecified side**

I69.14- **Monoplegia** of **lower limb** following nontraumatic **intracerebral** hemorrhage

I69.141 Monoplegia of lower limb following nontraumatic **intracerebral** hemorrhage affecting **right** dominant side

I69.142 Monoplegia of lower limb following nontraumatic **intracerebral** hemorrhage affecting **left** dominant side

I69.143 Monoplegia of lower limb following nontraumatic **intracerebral** hemorrhage affecting **right non-**dominant side

I69.144 Monoplegia of lower limb following nontraumatic **intracerebral** hemorrhage affecting **left non-**dominant side

I69.149 Monoplegia of lower limb following nontraumatic **intracerebral** hemorrhage affecting **unspecified side**

I69.15- **Hemiplegia and hemiparesis** following nontraumatic **intracerebral** hemorrhage

CC **I69.151** **Hemiplegia and hemiparesis** following nontraumatic **intracerebral** hemorrhage affecting **right** dominant side

CC **I69.152** **Hemiplegia and hemiparesis** following nontraumatic **intracerebral** hemorrhage affecting **left** dominant side

CC **I69.153** **Hemiplegia and hemiparesis** following nontraumatic **intracerebral** hemorrhage affecting **right** non-dominant side

CC **I69.154** **Hemiplegia and hemiparesis** following nontraumatic **intracerebral** hemorrhage affecting **left non-**dominant side

CC **I69.159** **Hemiplegia and hemiparesis** following nontraumatic **intracerebral** hemorrhage affecting **unspecified side**

I69.16- **Other paralytic** syndrome following nontraumatic **intracerebral** hemorrhage
  Use additional code to identify type of paralytic syndrome, such as:
  Locked-in state (G83.5)
  Quadriplegia (G82.5-)
  Excludes 1: hemiplegia/hemiparesis following nontraumatic intracerebral hemorrhage (I69.15-)
  monoplegia of lower limb following nontraumatic intracerebral hemorrhage (I69.14-)
  monoplegia of upper limb following nontraumatic intracerebral hemorrhage (I69.13-)

I69.161 Other paralytic syndrome following nontraumatic **intracerebral** hemorrhage affecting **right** dominant side

I69.162 Other paralytic syndrome following nontraumatic **intracerebral** hemorrhage affecting **left** dominant side

I69.163 Other paralytic syndrome following nontraumatic **intracerebral** hemorrhage affecting **right non-**dominant side

I69.164 Other paralytic syndrome following nontraumatic **intracerebral** hemorrhage affecting **left non-**dominant side

I69.165 Other paralytic syndrome following nontraumatic **intracerebral** hemorrhage, **bilateral**

I69.169 Other paralytic syndrome following nontraumatic **intracerebral** hemorrhage affecting **unspecified side**

I69.19- **Other sequelae** of nontraumatic **intracerebral** hemorrhage

I69.190 **Apraxia** following nontraumatic **intracerebral** hemorrhage

I69.191 **Dysphagia** following nontraumatic **intracerebral** hemorrhage
  Use additional code to identify the type of dysphagia, if known (R13.1-)

I69.192 **Facial weakness** following nontraumatic **intracerebral** hemorrhage
  Facial droop following nontraumatic intracerebral hemorrhage

I69.193 **Ataxia** following nontraumatic **intracerebral** hemorrhage

I69.198 **Other sequelae** of nontraumatic **intracerebral** hemorrhage
  Alteration of sensations following nontraumatic intracerebral hemorrhage
  Disturbance of vision following nontraumatic intracerebral hemorrhage
  Use additional code to identify the sequelae

I69.2- **Sequelae** of other nontraumatic **intracranial** hemorrhage

I69.20 **Unspecified** sequelae of other nontraumatic **intracranial** hemorrhage

I69.21- **Cognitive** deficits following other nontraumatic **intracranial** hemorrhage

I69.210 **Attention and concentration** deficit following other nontraumatic **intracranial** hemorrhage

I69.211 **Memory** deficit following other nontraumatic **intracranial** hemorrhage

I69.212 **Visuospatial deficit and spatial neglect** following other nontraumatic **intracranial** hemorrhage

I69.213 **Psychomotor** deficit following other nontraumatic **intracranial** hemorrhage

I69.214 **Frontal lobe and executive function** deficit following other nontraumatic **intracranial** hemorrhage

I69.215 **Cognitive social or emotional** deficit following other nontraumatic **intracranial** hemorrhage

I69.218 **Other symptoms and signs** involving cognitive functions following other nontraumatic **intracranial** hemorrhage

I
6
9
-
I
6
9

I69.219   **Unspecified symptoms and signs** involving cognitive functions following other nontraumatic **intracranial** hemorrhage

I69.22-   **Speech and language** deficits following other nontraumatic **intracranial** hemorrhage

I69.220   **Aphasia** following other nontraumatic **intracranial** hemorrhage

I69.221   **Dysphasia** following other nontraumatic **intracranial** hemorrhage

I69.222   **Dysarthria** following other nontraumatic **intracranial** hemorrhage

I69.223   **Fluency disorder** following other nontraumatic **intracranial** hemorrhage
   Stuttering following other nontraumatic intracranial hemorrhage

I69.228   **Other speech and language** deficits following other nontraumatic **intracranial** hemorrhage

I69.23-   **Monoplegia** of **upper limb** following other nontraumatic **intracranial** hemorrhage

I69.231   Monoplegia of upper limb following other nontraumatic **intracranial** hemorrhage affecting **right** dominant side

I69.232   Monoplegia of upper limb following other nontraumatic **intracranial** hemorrhage affecting **left** dominant side

I69.233   Monoplegia of upper limb following other nontraumatic **intracranial** hemorrhage affecting **right non-**dominant side

I69.234   Monoplegia of upper limb following other nontraumatic **intracranial** hemorrhage affecting **left non-**dominant side

I69.239   Monoplegia of upper limb following other nontraumatic **intracranial** hemorrhage affecting **unspecified side**

I69.24-   **Monoplegia** of **lower limb** following other nontraumatic **intracranial** hemorrhage

I69.241   Monoplegia of lower limb following other nontraumatic **intracranial** hemorrhage affecting **right** dominant side

I69.242   Monoplegia of lower limb following other nontraumatic **intracranial** hemorrhage affecting **left** dominant side

I69.243   Monoplegia of lower limb following other nontraumatic **intracranial** hemorrhage affecting **right non-**dominant side

I69.244   Monoplegia of lower limb following other nontraumatic **intracranial** hemorrhage affecting **left non-**dominant side

I69.249   Monoplegia of lower limb following other nontraumatic **intracranial** hemorrhage affecting **unspecified side**

I69.25-   **Hemiplegia and hemiparesis** following other nontraumatic **intracranial** hemorrhage

cc I69.251   **Hemiplegia and hemiparesis** following other nontraumatic **intracranial** hemorrhage affecting **right** dominant side

cc I69.252   **Hemiplegia and hemiparesis** following other nontraumatic **intracranial** hemorrhage affecting **left** dominant side

cc I69.253   **Hemiplegia and hemiparesis** following other nontraumatic **intracranial** hemorrhage affecting **right non-**dominant side

cc I69.254   **Hemiplegia and hemiparesis** following other nontraumatic **intracranial** hemorrhage affecting **left non-**dominant side

cc I69.259   **Hemiplegia and hemiparesis** following other nontraumatic **intracranial** hemorrhage affecting **unspecified side**

I69.26-   **Other paralytic** syndrome following other nontraumatic **intracranial** hemorrhage
Use additional code to identify type of paralytic syndrome, such as:
   Locked-in state (G83.5)
   Quadriplegia (G82.5-)
Excludes 1:   *hemiplegia/hemiparesis following other nontraumatic intracranial hemorrhage (I69.25-)*
   monoplegia of lower limb following other nontraumatic intracranial hemorrhage (I69.24-)
   monoplegia of upper limb following other nontraumatic intracranial hemorrhage (I69.23-)

I69.261   Other paralytic syndrome following other nontraumatic **intracranial** hemorrhage affecting **right** dominant side

I69.262   Other paralytic syndrome following other nontraumatic **intracranial** hemorrhage affecting **left** dominant side

I69.263   Other paralytic syndrome following other nontraumatic **intracranial** hemorrhage affecting **right non-**dominant side

I69.264   Other paralytic syndrome following other nontraumatic **intracranial** hemorrhage affecting **left non-**dominant side

I69.265   Other paralytic syndrome following other nontraumatic **intracranial** hemorrhage, **bilateral**

I69.269   Other paralytic syndrome following other nontraumatic **intracranial** hemorrhage affecting **unspecified side**

I69.29-   **Other sequelae** of other nontraumatic **intracranial** hemorrhage

I69.290   **Apraxia** following other nontraumatic **intracranial** hemorrhage

I69.291   **Dysphagia** following other nontraumatic **intracranial** hemorrhage
Use additional code to identify the type of dysphagia, if known (R13.1-)

I69.292   **Facial weakness** following other nontraumatic **intracranial** hemorrhage
   Facial droop following other nontraumatic intracranial hemorrhage

I69.293   **Ataxia** following other nontraumatic **intracranial** hemorrhage

I69.298   **Other sequelae** of other nontraumatic **intracranial** hemorrhage
   Alteration of sensation following other nontraumatic intracranial hemorrhage
   Disturbance of vision following other nontraumatic intracranial hemorrhage
Use additional code to identify the sequelae

I69.3-   **Sequelae** of **cerebral infarction**
AHA 13:4Q:p127 – Admission to rehabilitation facility following an acute stroke
AHA 13:4Q:p128 – Residual aphasia and hemiplegia following acute cerebral infarction
AHA 15:1Q:p25 – Hemiplegia/hemiparesis of an old CVA
   Sequelae of stroke NOS

I69.30   **Unspecified** sequelae of cerebral **infarction**

I69.31-   **Cognitive** deficits following cerebral **infarction**

I69.310   **Attention and concentration** deficit following cerebral **infarction**

I69.311   **Memory** deficit following cerebral **infarction**

I69.312   **Visuospatial deficit and spatial neglect** following cerebral **infarction**

I69.313   **Psychomotor** deficit following cerebral **infarction**

I69.314   **Frontal lobe and executive function** deficit following cerebral **infarction**

I69.315   **Cognitive social or emotional** deficit following cerebral **infarction**

I69.318   <u>Other symptoms and signs</u> involving cognitive functions following cerebral <u>infarction</u>

I69.319   <u>Unspecified symptoms and signs</u> involving cognitive functions following cerebral <u>infarction</u>

I69.32-   <u>Speech and language</u> deficits following cerebral <u>infarction</u>

     I69.320   <u>Aphasia</u> following cerebral <u>infarction</u>

     I69.321   <u>Dysphasia</u> following cerebral <u>infarction</u>

     I69.322   <u>Dysarthria</u> following cerebral <u>infarction</u>

     I69.323   <u>Fluency disorder</u> following cerebral <u>infarction</u>
            Stuttering following cerebral infarction

     I69.328   <u>Other speech and language</u> deficits following cerebral <u>infarction</u>

I69.33-   <u>Monoplegia</u> of <u>upper limb</u> following cerebral infarction

     I69.331   Monoplegia of upper limb following cerebral <u>infarction</u> affecting <u>right</u> dominant side

     I69.332   Monoplegia of upper limb following cerebral <u>infarction</u> affecting <u>left</u> dominant side

     I69.333   Monoplegia of upper limb following cerebral <u>infarction</u> affecting <u>right</u> <u>non</u>-dominant side

     I69.334   Monoplegia of upper limb following cerebral <u>infarction</u> affecting <u>left</u> <u>non</u>-dominant side

     I69.339   Monoplegia of upper limb following cerebral <u>infarction</u> affecting <u>unspecified side</u>

I69.34-   <u>Monoplegia</u> of <u>lower limb</u> following cerebral <u>infarction</u>

     I69.341   Monoplegia of lower limb following cerebral <u>infarction</u> affecting <u>right</u> dominant side

     I69.342   Monoplegia of lower limb following cerebral <u>infarction</u> affecting <u>left</u> dominant side

     I69.343   Monoplegia of lower limb following cerebral <u>infarction</u> affecting <u>right</u> <u>non</u>-dominant side

     I69.344   Monoplegia of lower limb following cerebral <u>infarction</u> affecting <u>left</u> <u>non</u>-dominant side

     I69.349   Monoplegia of lower limb following cerebral <u>infarction</u> affecting <u>unspecified side</u>

I69.35-   <u>Hemiplegia and hemiparesis</u> following cerebral <u>infarction</u>

cc **I69.351**   <u>Hemiplegia and hemiparesis</u> following cerebral <u>infarction</u> affecting <u>right</u> dominant side

cc **I69.352**   <u>Hemiplegia and hemiparesis</u> following cerebral <u>infarction</u> affecting <u>left</u> dominant side

cc **I69.353**   <u>Hemiplegia and hemiparesis</u> following cerebral <u>infarction</u> affecting <u>right</u> <u>non</u>-dominant side

cc **I69.354**   <u>Hemiplegia and hemiparesis</u> following cerebral <u>infarction</u> affecting <u>left</u> <u>non</u>-dominant side

cc **I69.359**   <u>Hemiplegia and hemiparesis</u> following cerebral <u>infarction</u> affecting <u>unspecified side</u>

I69.36-   <u>Other paralytic</u> syndrome following cerebral <u>infarction</u>
     Use additional code to identify type of paralytic syndrome, such as:
         Locked-in state (G83.5)
         Quadriplegia (G82.5-)
     Excludes 1:   *hemiplegia/hemiparesis following cerebral infarction (I69.35-)*
                  monoplegia of lower limb following cerebral infarction (I69.34-)
                  monoplegia of upper limb following cerebral infarction (I69.33-)

     I69.361   Other paralytic syndrome following cerebral <u>infarction</u> affecting <u>right</u> dominant side

     I69.362   Other paralytic syndrome following cerebral <u>infarction</u> affecting <u>left</u> dominant side

     I69.363   Other paralytic syndrome following cerebral <u>infarction</u> affecting <u>right</u> <u>non</u>-dominant side

     I69.364   Other paralytic syndrome following cerebral <u>infarction</u> affecting <u>left</u> <u>non</u>-dominant side

     I69.365   Other paralytic syndrome following cerebral <u>infarction, bilateral</u>

     I69.369   Other paralytic syndrome following cerebral <u>infarction</u> affecting <u>unspecified side</u>

I69.39-   <u>Other sequelae</u> of cerebral <u>infarction</u>

     I69.390   <u>Apraxia</u> following cerebral <u>infarction</u>

     I69.391   <u>Dysphagia</u> following cerebral <u>infarction</u>
            Use additional code to identify the type of dysphagia, if known (R13.1-)

     I69.392   <u>Facial weakness</u> following cerebral <u>infarction</u>
            Facial droop following cerebral infarction

     I69.393   <u>Ataxia</u> following cerebral <u>infarction</u>

     I69.398   <u>Other sequelae</u> of cerebral <u>infarction</u>
            Alteration of sensation following cerebral infarction
            Disturbance of vision following cerebral infarction
            Use additional code to identify the sequelae

I69.8-   <u>Sequelae</u> of <u>other cerebrovascular diseases</u>
     Excludes 1:   *sequelae of traumatic intracranial injury (S06.-)*

I69.80   <u>Unspecified</u> sequelae of <u>other</u> cerebrovascular disease

I69.81-   <u>Cognitive</u> deficits following <u>other</u> cerebrovascular disease

     I69.810   <u>Attention and concentration</u> deficit following <u>other</u> cerebrovascular disease

     I69.811   <u>Memory</u> deficit following <u>other</u> cerebrovascular disease

     I69.812   <u>Visuospatial deficit and spatial neglect</u> following <u>other</u> cerebrovascular disease

     I69.813   <u>Psychomotor</u> deficit following <u>other</u> cerebrovascular disease

     I69.814   <u>Frontal lobe and executive function</u> deficit following <u>other</u> cerebrovascular disease

     I69.815   <u>Cognitive social or emotional</u> deficit following <u>other</u> cerebrovascular disease

     I69.818   <u>Other symptoms and signs</u> involving cognitive functions following <u>other</u> cerebrovascular disease

     I69.819   <u>Unspecified symptoms and signs</u> involving cognitive functions following <u>other</u> cerebrovascular disease

I69.82-   <u>Speech and language</u> deficits following <u>other</u> cerebrovascular disease

     I69.820   <u>Aphasia</u> following <u>other</u> cerebrovascular disease

     I69.821   <u>Dysphasia</u> following <u>other</u> cerebrovascular disease

     I69.822   <u>Dysarthria</u> following <u>other</u> cerebrovascular disease

     I69.823   <u>Fluency disorder</u> following <u>other</u> cerebrovascular disease
            Stuttering following other cerebrovascular disease

     I69.828   <u>Other speech and language</u> deficits following <u>other</u> cerebrovascular disease

I69.83-   <u>Monoplegia</u> of <u>upper limb</u> following <u>other</u> cerebrovascular disease

     I69.831   Monoplegia of upper limb following <u>other</u> cerebrovascular disease affecting <u>right</u> dominant side

     I69.832   Monoplegia of upper limb following <u>other</u> cerebrovascular disease affecting <u>left</u> dominant side

     I69.833   Monoplegia of upper limb following <u>other</u> cerebrovascular disease affecting <u>right</u> <u>non</u>-dominant side

     I69.834   Monoplegia of upper limb following <u>other</u> cerebrovascular disease affecting <u>left</u> <u>non</u>-dominant side

     I69.839   Monoplegia of upper limb following <u>other</u> cerebrovascular disease affecting <u>unspecified side</u>

I69.84-   <u>Monoplegia</u> of <u>lower limb</u> following <u>other</u> cerebrovascular disease

     I69.841   Monoplegia of lower limb following <u>other</u> cerebrovascular disease affecting <u>right</u> dominant side

     I69.842   Monoplegia of lower limb following <u>other</u> cerebrovascular disease affecting <u>left</u> dominant side

     I69.843   Monoplegia of lower limb following <u>other</u> cerebrovascular disease affecting <u>right</u> <u>non</u>-dominant side

I 69 - I 69

I69.844   Monoplegia of lower limb following <u>other</u> cerebrovascular disease affecting <u>left</u> <u>non-dominant side</u>

I69.849   Monoplegia of lower limb following <u>other</u> cerebrovascular disease affecting <u>unspecified side</u>

I69.85-   <u>Hemiplegia and hemiparesis</u> following <u>other</u> cerebrovascular disease

CC I69.851   <u>Hemiplegia and hemiparesis</u> following <u>other</u> cerebrovascular disease affecting <u>right</u> dominant side

CC I69.852   <u>Hemiplegia and hemiparesis</u> following <u>other</u> cerebrovascular disease affecting <u>left</u> dominant side

CC I69.853   <u>Hemiplegia and hemiparesis</u> following <u>other</u> cerebrovascular disease affecting <u>right</u> <u>non-dominant side</u>

CC I69.854   <u>Hemiplegia and hemiparesis</u> following <u>other</u> cerebrovascular disease affecting <u>left</u> <u>non-dominant side</u>

CC I69.859   <u>Hemiplegia and hemiparesis</u> following <u>other</u> cerebrovascular disease affecting <u>unspecified side</u>

I69.86-   <u>Other paralytic</u> syndrome following other cerebrovascular disease
Use additional code to identify type of paralytic syndrome, such as:
    Locked-in state (G83.5)
    Quadriplegia (G82.5-)
Excludes 1:   *hemiplegia/hemiparesis following other cerebrovascular disease (I69.85-)*
    monoplegia of lower limb following other cerebrovascular disease (I69.84-)
    monoplegia of upper limb following other cerebrovascular disease (I69.83-)

I69.861   Other paralytic syndrome following <u>other</u> cerebrovascular disease affecting <u>right</u> dominant side

I69.862   Other paralytic syndrome following <u>other</u> cerebrovascular disease affecting <u>left</u> dominant side

I69.863   Other paralytic syndrome following <u>other</u> cerebrovascular disease affecting <u>right</u> <u>non-dominant side</u>

I69.864   Other paralytic syndrome following <u>other</u> cerebrovascular disease affecting <u>left</u> <u>non-dominant side</u>

I69.865   Other paralytic syndrome following <u>other</u> cerebrovascular disease, <u>bilateral</u>

I69.869   Other paralytic syndrome following <u>other</u> cerebrovascular disease affecting <u>unspecified side</u>

I69.89-   <u>Other sequelae</u> of <u>other</u> cerebrovascular disease

I69.890   <u>Apraxia</u> following <u>other</u> cerebrovascular disease

I69.891   <u>Dysphagia</u> following <u>other</u> cerebrovascular disease
Use additional code to identify the type of dysphagia, if known (R13.1-)

I69.892   <u>Facial weakness</u> following <u>other</u> cerebrovascular disease
Facial droop following other cerebrovascular disease

I69.893   <u>Ataxia</u> following <u>other</u> cerebrovascular disease

I69.898   <u>Other sequelae</u> of <u>other</u> cerebrovascular disease
Alteration of sensation following other cerebrovascular disease
Disturbance of vision following other cerebrovascular disease
Use additional code to identify the sequelae

I69.9-   <u>Sequelae</u> of <u>unspecified</u> cerebrovascular diseases
Excludes 1:   *sequelae of stroke (I69.3)*
    sequelae of traumatic intracranial injury (S06.-)

I69.90   <u>Unspecified</u> sequelae of <u>unspecified</u> cerebrovascular disease

I69.91-   <u>Cognitive</u> deficits following <u>unspecified</u> cerebrovascular disease

I69.910   <u>Attention and concentration</u> deficit following <u>unspecified</u> cerebrovascular disease

I69.911   <u>Memory</u> deficit following <u>unspecified</u> cerebrovascular disease

I69.912   <u>Visuospatial deficit and spatial neglect</u> following <u>unspecified</u> cerebrovascular disease

I69.913   <u>Psychomotor</u> deficit following <u>unspecified</u> cerebrovascular disease

I69.914   <u>Frontal lobe and executive function</u> deficit following <u>unspecified</u> cerebrovascular disease

I69.915   <u>Cognitive social or emotional</u> deficit following <u>unspecified</u> cerebrovascular disease

I69.918   <u>Other symptoms and signs</u> involving cognitive functions following <u>unspecified</u> cerebrovascular disease

I69.919   <u>Unspecified symptoms and signs</u> involving cognitive functions following <u>unspecified</u> cerebrovascular disease

I69.92-   <u>Speech and language</u> deficits following <u>unspecified</u> cerebrovascular disease

I69.920   <u>Aphasia</u> following <u>unspecified</u> cerebrovascular disease

I69.921   <u>Dysphasia</u> following <u>unspecified</u> cerebrovascular disease

I69.922   <u>Dysarthria</u> following <u>unspecified</u> cerebrovascular disease

I69.923   <u>Fluency disorder</u> following <u>unspecified</u> cerebrovascular disease
Stuttering following unspecified cerebrovascular disease

I69.928   <u>Other speech and language</u> deficits following <u>unspecified</u> cerebrovascular disease

I69.93-   <u>Monoplegia</u> of <u>upper limb</u> following <u>unspecified</u> cerebrovascular disease

I69.931   Monoplegia of upper limb following <u>unspecified</u> cerebrovascular disease affecting <u>right</u> dominant side

I69.932   Monoplegia of upper limb following <u>unspecified</u> cerebrovascular disease affecting <u>left</u> dominant side

I69.933   Monoplegia of upper limb following <u>unspecified</u> cerebrovascular disease affecting <u>right</u> <u>non-dominant side</u>

I69.934   Monoplegia of upper limb following <u>unspecified</u> cerebrovascular disease affecting <u>left</u> <u>non-dominant side</u>

I69.939   Monoplegia of upper limb following <u>unspecified</u> cerebrovascular disease affecting <u>unspecified side</u>

I69.94-   <u>Monoplegia</u> of <u>lower limb</u> following <u>unspecified</u> cerebrovascular disease

I69.941   Monoplegia of lower limb following <u>unspecified</u> cerebrovascular disease affecting <u>right</u> dominant side

I69.942   Monoplegia of lower limb following <u>unspecified</u> cerebrovascular disease affecting <u>left</u> dominant side

I69.943   Monoplegia of lower limb following <u>unspecified</u> cerebrovascular disease affecting <u>right</u> <u>non-dominant side</u>

I69.944   Monoplegia of lower limb following <u>unspecified</u> cerebrovascular disease affecting <u>left</u> <u>non-dominant side</u>

I69.949   Monoplegia of lower limb following <u>unspecified</u> cerebrovascular disease affecting <u>unspecified side</u>

I69.95-   <u>Hemiplegia and hemiparesis</u> following <u>unspecified</u> cerebrovascular disease

CC I69.951   <u>Hemiplegia and hemiparesis</u> following <u>unspecified</u> cerebrovascular disease affecting <u>right</u> dominant side

CC I69.952   <u>Hemiplegia and hemiparesis</u> following <u>unspecified</u> cerebrovascular disease affecting <u>left</u> dominant side

I 69 - I 69

Excludes 1: = NOT CODED HERE! (Do not code both)   741   *Excludes ❷:* = Not Included Here

cc **I69.953** <u>Hemiplegia and hemiparesis</u> following <u>unspecified</u> cerebrovascular disease affecting <u>right</u> <u>non-dominant side</u>

cc **I69.954** <u>Hemiplegia and hemiparesis</u> following <u>unspecified</u> cerebrovascular disease affecting <u>left</u> <u>non-dominant side</u>

cc **I69.959** <u>Hemiplegia and hemiparesis</u> following <u>unspecified</u> cerebrovascular disease affecting <u>unspecified side</u>

I69.96- <u>Other paralytic</u> syndrome following <u>unspecified</u> cerebrovascular disease

Use additional code to identify type of paralytic syndrome, such as:
    Locked-in state (G83.5)
    Quadriplegia (G82.5-)

Excludes 1:   *hemiplegia/hemiparesis following unspecified cerebrovascular disease (I69.95-)*
       monoplegia of lower limb following unspecified cerebrovascular disease (I69.94-)
       monoplegia of upper limb following unspecified cerebrovascular disease (I69.93-)

I69.961 Other paralytic syndrome following <u>unspecified</u> cerebrovascular disease affecting <u>right</u> dominant side

I69.962 Other paralytic syndrome following <u>unspecified</u> cerebrovascular disease affecting <u>left</u> dominant side

I69.963 Other paralytic syndrome following <u>unspecified</u> cerebrovascular disease affecting <u>right</u> <u>non-dominant side</u>

I69.964 Other paralytic syndrome following <u>unspecified</u> cerebrovascular disease affecting <u>left</u> <u>non-dominant side</u>

I69.965 Other paralytic syndrome following <u>unspecified</u> cerebrovascular disease, <u>bilateral</u>

I69.969 Other paralytic syndrome following <u>unspecified</u> cerebrovascular disease affecting <u>unspecified side</u>

I69.99- <u>Other sequelae</u> of <u>unspecified</u> cerebrovascular disease

I69.990 <u>Apraxia</u> following <u>unspecified</u> cerebrovascular disease

I69.991 <u>Dysphagia</u> following <u>unspecified</u> cerebrovascular disease

Use additional code to identify the type of dysphagia, if known (R13.1-)

I69.992 <u>Facial weakness</u> following <u>unspecified</u> cerebrovascular disease

    Facial droop following unspecified cerebrovascular disease

I69.993 <u>Ataxia</u> following <u>unspecified</u> cerebrovascular disease

I69.998 <u>Other sequelae</u> following <u>unspecified</u> cerebrovascular disease

    Alteration in sensation following unspecified cerebrovascular disease
    Disturbance of vision following unspecified cerebrovascular disease

Use additional code to identify the sequelae

Diseases of arteries, arterioles and capillaries (I70-I79)

I70- <u>Atherosclerosis</u> — Narrowing of an arterial wall caused by deposition of plaque-forming cholesterol and other lipids within the lumen.

Includes: **Arteriolosclerosis** — Thickening, hardening, and loss of elasticity of the arteriole walls.
    Arterial degeneration — Deterioration and decrease in normal function of an artery.
    Arteriosclerosis — Thickening, hardening, and loss of elasticity of the arterial walls which in its severe form may cause complete obliteration of the lumen of the artery.
    Arteriosclerotic vascular disease — Thickening, hardening, and loss of elasticity of the arterial vascular system.
    Arteriovascular degeneration — Deterioration and decrease in normal function of an artery.
    Atheroma — The plaque of degenerated, thickened arterial intima with deposits of cholesterol and lipid material.
    Endarteritis deformans or obliterans — Inflammation of the inner lining of an artery resulting from fatty degeneration, lime salt deposits, and with narrowed or obliterated lumen.
    Senile arteritis — Prolonged inflammation of an artery.
    Senile endarteritis — Prolonged inflammation of the innermost lining of an artery.
    Vascular degeneration — Deterioration and decrease in normal function of an artery.

Use additional code to identify:
    Exposure to environmental tobacco smoke (Z77.22)
    History of tobacco dependence (Z87.891)
    Occupational exposure to environmental tobacco smoke (Z57.31)
    Tobacco dependence (F17.-)
    Tobacco use (Z72.0)

Excludes ❷: *arteriosclerotic cardiovascular disease (I25.1-)*
    arteriosclerotic heart disease (I25.1-)
    atheroembolism (I75.-)
    cerebral atherosclerosis (I67.2)
    coronary atherosclerosis (I25.1-)
    mesenteric atherosclerosis (K55.1)
    precerebral atherosclerosis (I67.2)
    primary pulmonary atherosclerosis (I27.0)

I70.0 **Atherosclerosis of aorta** — [Age/15-124]

I70.1 **Atherosclerosis of renal artery** — [Age/15-124]
    Goldblatt's kidney
    Excludes ❷: atherosclerosis of renal arterioles (I12.-)

I70.2- **Atherosclerosis of <u>native arteries of the extremities</u>**
    Mönckeberg's (medial) sclerosis
    Use additional code, if applicable, to identify chronic total occlusion of artery of extremity (I70.92)
    Excludes ❷: atherosclerosis of bypass graft of extremities (I70.30-I70.79)

I70.20- <u>Unspecified</u> atherosclerosis of <u>native</u> arteries of extremities

I70.201 <u>Unspecified</u> atherosclerosis of <u>native</u> arteries of extremities, <u>right</u> leg — [Age/15-124]

I70.202 <u>Unspecified</u> atherosclerosis of <u>native</u> arteries of extremities, <u>left</u> leg — [Age/15-124]

I70.203 <u>Unspecified</u> atherosclerosis of <u>native</u> arteries of extremities, <u>bilateral</u> legs — [Age/15-124]

I70.208 <u>Unspecified</u> atherosclerosis of <u>native</u> arteries of extremities, <u>other extremity</u> — [Age/15-124]

I70.209 <u>Unspecified</u> atherosclerosis of <u>native</u> arteries of extremities, <u>unspecified extremity</u> — [Age/15-124]

I70.21- Atherosclerosis of <u>native</u> arteries of extremities <u>with intermittent claudication</u>

I70.211 Atherosclerosis of <u>native</u> arteries of extremities <u>with intermittent claudication</u>, <u>right</u> leg — [Age/15-124]

I70.212 Atherosclerosis of <u>native</u> arteries of extremities <u>with intermittent claudication</u>, <u>left</u> leg — [Age/15-124]

I70.213 Atherosclerosis of <u>native</u> arteries of extremities <u>with intermittent claudication</u>, <u>bilateral</u> legs — [Age/15-124]

I70.218 Atherosclerosis of <u>native</u> arteries of extremities <u>with intermittent claudication</u>, <u>other extremity</u> — [Age/15-124]

I70.219 Atherosclerosis of <u>native</u> arteries of extremities <u>with intermittent claudication</u>, <u>unspecified extremity</u> — [Age/15-124]

I70.22- Atherosclerosis of <u>native</u> arteries of extremities <u>with rest pain</u>
Includes: Any condition classifiable to I70.21-

I70.221   Atherosclerosis of <u>native</u> arteries of extremities <u>with rest pain</u>, <u>right</u> leg — [Age/15-124]

I70.222   Atherosclerosis of <u>native</u> arteries of extremities <u>with rest pain</u>, <u>left</u> leg — [Age/15-124]

I70.223   Atherosclerosis of <u>native</u> arteries of extremities <u>with rest pain</u>, <u>bilateral</u> legs — [Age/15-124]

I70.228   Atherosclerosis of <u>native</u> arteries of extremities <u>with rest pain</u>, <u>other extremity</u> — [Age/15-124]

I70.229   Atherosclerosis of native arteries of extremities <u>with rest pain</u>, <u>unspecified extremity</u> — [Age/15-124]

I70.23- Atherosclerosis of <u>native</u> arteries of <u>right leg with ulceration</u>
Includes: Any condition classifiable to I70.211 and I70.221
Use additional code to identify severity of ulcer (L97.-)

I70.231   Atherosclerosis of <u>native</u> arteries of <u>right</u> leg <u>with ulceration</u> of <u>thigh</u> — [Age/15-124]

I70.232   Atherosclerosis of <u>native</u> arteries of <u>right</u> leg <u>with ulceration</u> of <u>calf</u> — [Age/15-124]

I70.233   Atherosclerosis of <u>native</u> arteries of <u>right</u> leg <u>with ulceration</u> of <u>ankle</u> — [Age/15-124]

I70.234   Atherosclerosis of <u>native</u> arteries of <u>right</u> leg <u>with ulceration</u> of <u>heel and midfoot</u> — [Age/15-124]
Atherosclerosis of native arteries of right leg with ulceration of plantar surface of midfoot

I70.235   Atherosclerosis of <u>native</u> arteries of <u>right</u> leg <u>with ulceration</u> of <u>other part of foot</u> — [Age/15-124]
Atherosclerosis of native arteries of right leg extremities with ulceration of toe

I70.238   Atherosclerosis of <u>native</u> arteries of <u>right</u> leg <u>with ulceration</u> of other part of <u>lower right leg</u> — [Age/15-124]

I70.239   Atherosclerosis of <u>native</u> arteries of <u>right</u> leg <u>with ulceration</u> of <u>unspecified site</u> — [Age/15-124]

I70.24- Atherosclerosis of <u>native</u> arteries of <u>left leg with ulceration</u>
Includes: Any condition classifiable to I70.212 and I70.222
Use additional code to identify severity of ulcer (L97.-)

I70.241   Atherosclerosis of <u>native</u> arteries of <u>left</u> leg <u>with ulceration</u> of <u>thigh</u> — [Age/15-124]

I70.242   Atherosclerosis of <u>native</u> arteries of <u>left</u> leg <u>with ulceration</u> of <u>calf</u> — [Age/15-124]

I70.243   Atherosclerosis of <u>native</u> arteries of <u>left</u> leg <u>with ulceration</u> of <u>ankle</u> — [Age/15-124]

I70.244   Atherosclerosis of <u>native</u> arteries of <u>left</u> leg <u>with ulceration</u> of <u>heel and midfoot</u> — [Age/15-124]
Atherosclerosis of native arteries of left leg with ulceration of plantar surface of midfoot

I70.245   Atherosclerosis of <u>native</u> arteries of <u>left</u> leg <u>with ulceration</u> of <u>other part of foot</u> — [Age/15-124]
Atherosclerosis of native arteries of left leg extremities with ulceration of toe

I70.248   Atherosclerosis of <u>native</u> arteries of <u>left</u> leg <u>with ulceration</u> of other part of <u>lower left leg</u> — [Age/15-124]

I70.249   Atherosclerosis of <u>native</u> arteries of <u>left</u> leg <u>with ulceration</u> of <u>unspecified site</u> — [Age/15-124]

I70.25   Atherosclerosis of <u>native</u> arteries of <u>other extremities with ulceration</u> — [Age/15-124]
Includes: Any condition classifiable to I70.218 and I70.228
Use additional code to identify the severity of the ulcer (L98.49-)

I70.26- Atherosclerosis of <u>native</u> arteries of extremities <u>with gangrene</u>
Includes: Any condition classifiable to I70.21-, I70.22-, I70.23-, I70.24-, and I70.25-
Use additional code to identify the severity of any ulcer (L97.-, L98.49-), if applicable

cc **I70.261**   Atherosclerosis of <u>native</u> arteries of extremities <u>with gangrene</u>, <u>right</u> leg — [Age/15-124]

cc **I70.262**   Atherosclerosis of <u>native</u> arteries of extremities <u>with gangrene</u>, <u>left</u> leg — [Age/15-124]

cc **I70.263**   Atherosclerosis of <u>native</u> arteries of extremities <u>with gangrene</u>, <u>bilateral</u> legs — [Age/15-124]

cc **I70.268**   Atherosclerosis of <u>native</u> arteries of extremities <u>with gangrene</u>, <u>other extremity</u> — [Age/15-124]

cc **I70.269**   Atherosclerosis of <u>native</u> arteries of extremities <u>with gangrene</u>, <u>unspecified extremity</u> — [Age/15-124]

I70.29- <u>Other</u> atherosclerosis of <u>native</u> arteries of extremities

I70.291   <u>Other</u> atherosclerosis of <u>native</u> arteries of extremities, <u>right</u> leg — [Age/15-124]

I70.292   <u>Other</u> atherosclerosis of <u>native</u> arteries of extremities, <u>left</u> leg — [Age/15-124]

I70.293   <u>Other</u> atherosclerosis of <u>native</u> arteries of extremities, <u>bilateral</u> legs — [Age/15-124]

I70.298   <u>Other</u> atherosclerosis of <u>native</u> arteries of extremities, <u>other extremity</u> — [Age/15-124]

I70.299   <u>Other</u> atherosclerosis of <u>native</u> arteries of extremities, <u>unspecified extremity</u> — [Age/15-124]

I70.3- Atherosclerosis of <u>unspecified type of bypass graft(s)</u> of the extremities
Use additional code, if applicable, to identify chronic total occlusion of artery of extremity (I70.92)
Excludes 1:   embolism or thrombus of bypass graft(s) of extremities (T82.8-)

I70.30- <u>Unspecified</u> atherosclerosis of <u>unspecified type of bypass graft(s) of the extremities</u>

I70.301   <u>Unspecified</u> atherosclerosis of unspecified type of bypass <u>graft(s)</u> of the extremities, <u>right</u> leg — [Age/15-124]

I70.302   <u>Unspecified</u> atherosclerosis of unspecified type of bypass <u>graft(s)</u> of the extremities, <u>left</u> leg — [Age/15-124]

I70.303   <u>Unspecified</u> atherosclerosis of unspecified type of bypass <u>graft(s)</u> of the extremities, <u>bilateral</u> legs — [Age/15-124]

I70.308   <u>Unspecified</u> atherosclerosis of unspecified type of bypass <u>graft(s)</u> of the extremities, <u>other extremity</u> — [Age/15-124]

I70.309   <u>Unspecified</u> atherosclerosis of unspecified type of bypass <u>graft(s)</u> of the extremities, <u>unspecified extremity</u> — [Age/15-124]

I70.31- Atherosclerosis of <u>unspecified type of bypass graft(s)</u> of the extremities <u>with intermittent claudication</u>

I70.311   Atherosclerosis of unspecified type of bypass <u>graft(s)</u> of the extremities <u>with intermittent claudication</u>, <u>right</u> leg — [Age/15-124]

I70.312   Atherosclerosis of unspecified type of bypass <u>graft(s)</u> of the extremities <u>with intermittent claudication</u>, <u>left</u> leg — [Age/15-124]

I70.313   Atherosclerosis of unspecified type of bypass <u>graft(s)</u> of the extremities <u>with intermittent claudication</u>, <u>bilateral</u> legs — [Age/15-124]

I70.318   Atherosclerosis of unspecified type of bypass <u>graft(s)</u> of the extremities <u>with intermittent claudication</u>, <u>other extremity</u> — [Age/15-124]

I70.319   Atherosclerosis of unspecified type of bypass <u>graft(s)</u> of the extremities <u>with intermittent claudication</u>, <u>unspecified extremity</u> — [Age/15-124]

I70.32- Atherosclerosis of <u>unspecified type of bypass graft(s)</u> of the extremities <u>with rest pain</u>
Includes: Any condition classifiable to I70.31-

I70.321   Atherosclerosis of unspecified type of bypass <u>graft(s)</u> of the extremities <u>with rest pain</u>, <u>right</u> leg — [Age/15-124]

I70.322   Atherosclerosis of unspecified type of bypass <u>graft(s)</u> of the extremities <u>with rest pain</u>, <u>left</u> leg — [Age/15-124]

I70 - I70

I70.323 Atherosclerosis of unspecified type of bypass graft(s) of the extremities with rest pain, bilateral legs — [Age/15-124]

I70.328 Atherosclerosis of unspecified type of bypass graft(s) of the extremities with rest pain, other extremity — [Age/15-124]

I70.329 Atherosclerosis of unspecified type of bypass graft(s) of the extremities with rest pain, unspecified extremity — [Age/15-124]

I70.33- Atherosclerosis of unspecified type of bypass graft(s) of the right leg with ulceration
Includes: Any condition classifiable to I70.311 and I70.321
Use additional code to identify severity of ulcer (L97.-)

cc **I70.331** Atherosclerosis of unspecified type of bypass graft(s) of the right leg with ulceration of thigh — [Age/15-124]

cc **I70.332** Atherosclerosis of unspecified type of bypass graft(s) of the right leg with ulceration of calf — [Age/15-124]

cc **I70.333** Atherosclerosis of unspecified type of bypass graft(s) of the right leg with ulceration of ankle — [Age/15-124]

cc **I70.334** Atherosclerosis of unspecified type of bypass graft(s) of the right leg with ulceration of heel and midfoot — [Age/15-124]
Atherosclerosis of unspecified type of bypass graft(s) of right leg with ulceration of plantar surface of midfoot

I70.335 Atherosclerosis of unspecified type of bypass graft(s) of the right leg with ulceration of other part of foot — [Age/15-124]
Atherosclerosis of unspecified type of bypass graft(s) of the right leg with ulceration of toe

cc **I70.338** Atherosclerosis of unspecified type of bypass graft(s) of the right leg with ulceration of other part of lower leg — [Age/15-124]

cc **I70.339** Atherosclerosis of unspecified type of bypass graft(s) of the right leg with ulceration of unspecified site — [Age/15-124]

I70.34- Atherosclerosis of unspecified type of bypass graft(s) of the left leg with ulceration
Includes: Any condition classifiable to I70.312 and I70.322
Use additional code to identify severity of ulcer (L97.-)

cc **I70.341** Atherosclerosis of unspecified type of bypass graft(s) of the left leg with ulceration of thigh — [Age/15-124]

cc **I70.342** Atherosclerosis of unspecified type of bypass graft(s) of the left leg with ulceration of calf — [Age/15-124]

cc **I70.343** Atherosclerosis of unspecified type of bypass graft(s) of the left leg with ulceration of ankle — [Age/15-124]

cc **I70.344** Atherosclerosis of unspecified type of bypass graft(s) of the left leg with ulceration of heel and midfoot — [Age/15-124]
Atherosclerosis of unspecified type of bypass graft(s) of left leg with ulceration of plantar surface of midfoot

I70.345 Atherosclerosis of unspecified type of bypass graft(s) of the left leg with ulceration of other part of foot — [Age/15-124]
Atherosclerosis of unspecified type of bypass graft(s) of the left leg with ulceration of toe

cc **I70.348** Atherosclerosis of unspecified type of bypass graft(s) of the left leg with ulceration of other part of lower leg — [Age/15-124]

cc **I70.349** Atherosclerosis of unspecified type of bypass graft(s) of the left leg with ulceration of unspecified site — [Age/15-124]

I70.35 Atherosclerosis of unspecified type of bypass graft(s) of other extremity with ulceration — [Age/15-124]
Includes: Any condition classifiable to I70.318 and I70.328
Use additional code to identify severity of ulcer (L98.49-)

I70.36- Atherosclerosis of unspecified type of bypass graft(s) of the extremities with gangrene
Includes: Any condition classifiable to I70.31-, I70.32-, I70.33-, I70.34-, I70.35
Use additional code to identify the severity of any ulcer (L97.-, L98.49-), if applicable

cc **I70.361** Atherosclerosis of unspecified type of bypass graft(s) of the extremities with gangrene, right leg — [Age/15-124]

cc **I70.362** Atherosclerosis of unspecified type of bypass graft(s) of the extremities with gangrene, left leg — [Age/15-124]

cc **I70.363** Atherosclerosis of unspecified type of bypass graft(s) of the extremities with gangrene, bilateral legs — [Age/15-124]

cc **I70.368** Atherosclerosis of unspecified type of bypass graft(s) of the extremities with gangrene, other extremity — [Age/15-124]

cc **I70.369** Atherosclerosis of unspecified type of bypass graft(s) of the extremities with gangrene, unspecified extremity — [Age/15-124]

I70.39- Other atherosclerosis of unspecified type of bypass graft(s) of the extremities

I70.391 Other atherosclerosis of unspecified type of bypass graft(s) of the extremities, right leg — [Age/15-124]

I70.392 Other atherosclerosis of unspecified type of bypass graft(s) of the extremities, left leg — [Age/15-124]

I70.393 Other atherosclerosis of unspecified type of bypass graft(s) of the extremities, bilateral legs — [Age/15-124]

I70.398 Other atherosclerosis of unspecified type of bypass graft(s) of the extremities, other extremity — [Age/15-124]

I70.399 Other atherosclerosis of unspecified type of bypass graft(s) of the extremities, unspecified extremity — [Age/15-124]

I70.4- Atherosclerosis of autologous vein bypass graft(s) of the extremities
Use additional code, if applicable, to identify chronic total occlusion of artery of extremity (I70.92)

I70.40- Unspecified atherosclerosis of autologous vein bypass graft(s) of the extremities

I70.401 Unspecified atherosclerosis of autologous vein bypass graft(s) of the extremities, right leg — [Age/15-124]

I70.402 Unspecified atherosclerosis of autologous vein bypass graft(s) of the extremities, left leg — [Age/15-124]

I70.403 Unspecified atherosclerosis of autologous vein bypass graft(s) of the extremities, bilateral legs — [Age/15-124]

I70.408 Unspecified atherosclerosis of autologous vein bypass graft(s) of the extremities, other extremity — [Age/15-124]

I70.409 Unspecified atherosclerosis of autologous vein bypass graft(s) of the extremities, unspecified extremity — [Age/15-124]

I70.41- Atherosclerosis of autologous vein bypass graft(s) of the extremities with intermittent claudication

I70.411 Atherosclerosis of autologous vein bypass graft(s) of the extremities with intermittent claudication, right leg — [Age/15-124]

I70.412 Atherosclerosis of autologous vein bypass graft(s) of the extremities with intermittent claudication, left leg — [Age/15-124]

I70.413 Atherosclerosis of autologous vein bypass graft(s) of the extremities with intermittent claudication, bilateral legs — [Age/15-124]

I70.418 Atherosclerosis of autologous vein bypass graft(s) of the extremities with intermittent claudication, other extremity — [Age/15-124]

I70-I70

I70.419 Atherosclerosis of autologous <u>vein</u> bypass graft(s) of the extremities <u>with intermittent claudication</u>, <u>unspecified extremity</u> — [Age/15-124]

I70.42- Atherosclerosis of autologous <u>vein</u> bypass graft(s) of the extremities <u>with rest pain</u>
Includes: Any condition classifiable to I70.41-

I70.421 Atherosclerosis of autologous vein bypass graft(s) of the extremities <u>with rest pain</u>, <u>right</u> leg — [Age/15-124]

I70.422 Atherosclerosis of autologous <u>vein</u> bypass graft(s) of the extremities <u>with rest pain</u>, <u>left</u> leg — [Age/15-124]

I70.423 Atherosclerosis of autologous vein bypass graft(s) of the extremities <u>with rest pain</u>, <u>bilateral</u> legs — [Age/15-124]

I70.428 Atherosclerosis of autologous <u>vein</u> bypass graft(s) of the extremities <u>with rest pain</u>, <u>other extremity</u> — [Age/15-124]

I70.429 Atherosclerosis of autologous <u>vein</u> bypass graft(s) of the extremities <u>with rest pain</u>, <u>unspecified extremity</u> — [Age/15-124]

I70.43- Atherosclerosis of autologous vein bypass graft(s) of the <u>right</u> leg <u>with ulceration</u>
Includes: Any condition classifiable to I70.411 and I70.421
Use additional code to identify severity of ulcer (L97.-)

cc **I70.431** Atherosclerosis of autologous <u>vein</u> bypass graft(s) of the <u>right</u> leg <u>with ulceration</u> of <u>thigh</u> — [Age/15-124]

cc **I70.432** Atherosclerosis of autologous <u>vein</u> bypass graft(s) of the <u>right</u> leg <u>with ulceration</u> of <u>calf</u> — [Age/15-124]

cc **I70.433** Atherosclerosis of autologous <u>vein</u> bypass graft(s) of the <u>right</u> leg <u>with ulceration</u> of <u>ankle</u> — [Age/15-124]

cc **I70.434** Atherosclerosis of autologous vein bypass graft(s) of the <u>right</u> leg <u>with ulceration</u> of <u>heel and midfoot</u> — [Age/15-124]
    Atherosclerosis of autologous vein bypass graft(s) of right leg with ulceration of plantar surface of midfoot

I70.435 Atherosclerosis of autologous <u>vein</u> bypass graft(s) of the <u>right</u> leg <u>with ulceration</u> of <u>other part of foot</u> — [Age/15-124]
    Atherosclerosis of autologous vein bypass graft(s) of right leg with ulceration of toe

cc **I70.438** Atherosclerosis of autologous <u>vein</u> bypass graft(s) of the <u>right</u> leg with ulceration of <u>other part of lower leg</u> — [Age/15-124]

cc **I70.439** Atherosclerosis of autologous <u>vein</u> bypass graft(s) of the <u>right</u> leg <u>with ulceration</u> of <u>unspecified site</u> — [Age/15-124]

I70.44- Atherosclerosis of autologous <u>vein</u> bypass graft(s) of the <u>left</u> leg <u>with ulceration</u>
Includes: Any condition classifiable to I70.412 and I70.422
Use additional code to identify severity of ulcer (L97.-)

cc **I70.441** Atherosclerosis of autologous <u>vein</u> bypass graft(s) of the <u>left</u> leg <u>with ulceration</u> of <u>thigh</u> — [Age/15-124]

cc **I70.442** Atherosclerosis of autologous <u>vein</u> bypass graft(s) of the <u>left</u> leg <u>with ulceration</u> of <u>calf</u> — [Age/15-124]

cc **I70.443** Atherosclerosis of autologous <u>vein</u> bypass graft(s) of the <u>left</u> leg <u>with ulceration</u> of <u>ankle</u> — [Age/15-124]

cc **I70.444** Atherosclerosis of autologous <u>vein</u> bypass graft(s) of the <u>left</u> leg <u>with ulceration</u> of <u>heel and midfoot</u> — [Age/15-124]
    Atherosclerosis of autologous vein bypass graft(s) of left leg with ulceration of plantar surface of midfoot

I70.445 Atherosclerosis of autologous <u>vein</u> bypass graft(s) of the <u>left</u> leg <u>with ulceration</u> of <u>other part of foot</u> — [Age/15-124]
    Atherosclerosis of autologous vein bypass graft(s) of left leg with ulceration of toe

cc **I70.448** Atherosclerosis of autologous <u>vein</u> bypass graft(s) of the <u>left</u> leg <u>with ulceration</u> of <u>other part of lower leg</u> — [Age/15-124]

cc **I70.449** Atherosclerosis of autologous <u>vein</u> bypass graft(s) of the <u>left</u> leg <u>with ulceration</u> of <u>unspecified site</u> — [Age/15-124]

I70.45 Atherosclerosis of autologous <u>vein</u> bypass graft(s) of <u>other extremity</u> <u>with ulceration</u> — [Age/15-124]
Includes: Any condition classifiable to I70.418, I70.428, and I70.438
Use additional code to identify severity of ulcer (L98.49)

I70.46- Atherosclerosis of autologous <u>vein</u> bypass graft(s) of the extremities <u>with gangrene</u>
Includes: Any condition classifiable to I70.41-, I70.42-, and I70.43-, I70.44-, I70.45
Use additional code to identify the severity of any ulcer (L97.-, L98.49-), if applicable

cc **I70.461** Atherosclerosis of autologous <u>vein</u> bypass graft(s) of the extremities <u>with gangrene</u>, <u>right</u> leg — [Age/15-124]

cc **I70.462** Atherosclerosis of autologous <u>vein</u> bypass graft(s) of the extremities <u>with gangrene</u>, <u>left</u> leg — [Age/15-124]

cc **I70.463** Atherosclerosis of autologous <u>vein</u> bypass graft(s) of the extremities <u>with gangrene</u>, <u>bilateral</u> legs — [Age/15-124]

cc **I70.468** Atherosclerosis of autologous <u>vein</u> bypass graft(s) of the extremities <u>with gangrene</u>, <u>other extremity</u> — [Age/15-124]

cc **I70.469** Atherosclerosis of autologous <u>vein</u> bypass graft(s) of the extremities <u>with gangrene</u>, <u>unspecified extremity</u> — [Age/15-124]

I70.49- <u>Other</u> atherosclerosis of autologous <u>vein</u> bypass graft(s) of the extremities

I70.491 <u>Other</u> atherosclerosis of autologous <u>vein</u> bypass graft(s) of the extremities, <u>right</u> leg — [Age/15-124]

I70.492 <u>Other</u> atherosclerosis of autologous <u>vein</u> bypass graft(s) of the extremities, <u>left</u> leg — [Age/15-124]

I70.493 <u>Other</u> atherosclerosis of autologous <u>vein</u> bypass graft(s) of the extremities, bilateral legs — [Age/15-124]

I70.498 <u>Other</u> atherosclerosis of autologous <u>vein</u> bypass graft(s) of the extremities, other extremity — [Age/15-124]

I70.499 <u>Other</u> atherosclerosis of autologous <u>vein</u> bypass graft(s) of the extremities, unspecified extremity — [Age/15-124]

I70.5- Atherosclerosis of nonautologous <u>biological</u> bypass graft(s) of the extremities
Use additional code, if applicable, to identify chronic total occlusion of artery of extremity (I70.92)

I70.50- <u>Unspecified</u> atherosclerosis of nonautologous <u>biological</u> bypass graft(s) of the extremities

I70.501 <u>Unspecified</u> atherosclerosis of nonautologous <u>biological</u> bypass graft(s) of the extremities, <u>right</u> leg — [Age/15-124]

I70.502 <u>Unspecified</u> atherosclerosis of nonautologous <u>biological</u> bypass graft(s) of the extremities, <u>left</u> leg — [Age/15-124]

I70.503 <u>Unspecified</u> atherosclerosis of nonautologous <u>biological</u> bypass graft(s) of the extremities, <u>bilateral</u> legs — [Age/15-124]

I70.508 <u>Unspecified</u> atherosclerosis of nonautologous <u>biological</u> bypass graft(s) of the extremities, <u>other extremity</u> — [Age/15-124]

I70.509 <u>Unspecified</u> atherosclerosis of nonautologous <u>biological</u> bypass graft(s) of the extremities, <u>unspecified extremity</u> — [Age/15-124]

I70 - I70

I70.51- Atherosclerosis of nonautologous <u>biological</u> bypass graft(s) of the extremities <u>with intermittent claudication</u>

    I70.511 Atherosclerosis of nonautologous <u>biological</u> bypass graft(s) of the extremities <u>with intermittent claudication</u>, <u>right</u> leg — [Age/15-124]

    I70.512 Atherosclerosis of nonautologous <u>biological</u> bypass graft(s) of the extremities <u>with intermittent claudication</u>, <u>left</u> leg — [Age/15-124]

    I70.513 Atherosclerosis of nonautologous <u>biological</u> bypass graft(s) of the extremities <u>with intermittent claudication</u>, <u>bilateral</u> legs — [Age/15-124]

    I70.518 Atherosclerosis of nonautologous <u>biological</u> bypass graft(s) of the extremities <u>with intermittent claudication</u>, <u>other extremity</u> — [Age/15-124]

    I70.519 Atherosclerosis of nonautologous <u>biological</u> bypass graft(s) of the extremities <u>with intermittent claudication</u>, <u>unspecified extremity</u> — [Age/15-124]

I70.52- Atherosclerosis of nonautologous <u>biological</u> bypass graft(s) of the extremities <u>with rest pain</u>
    Includes: Any condition classifiable to I70.51-

    I70.521 Atherosclerosis of nonautologous <u>biological</u> bypass graft(s) of the extremities <u>with rest pain</u>, <u>right</u> leg — [Age/15-124]

    I70.522 Atherosclerosis of nonautologous <u>biological</u> bypass graft(s) of the extremities <u>with rest pain</u>, <u>left</u> leg — [Age/15-124]

    I70.523 Atherosclerosis of nonautologous <u>biological</u> bypass graft(s) of the extremities <u>with rest pain</u>, <u>bilateral</u> legs — [Age/15-124]

    I70.528 Atherosclerosis of nonautologous <u>biological</u> bypass graft(s) of the extremities <u>with rest pain</u>, <u>other extremity</u> — [Age/15-124]

    I70.529 Atherosclerosis of nonautologous <u>biological</u> bypass graft(s) of the extremities <u>with rest pain</u>, <u>unspecified extremity</u> — [Age/15-124]

I70.53- Atherosclerosis of nonautologous <u>biological</u> bypass graft(s) of the <u>right</u> leg <u>with ulceration</u>
    Includes: Any condition classifiable to I70.511 and I70.521
    Use additional code to identify severity of ulcer (L97.-)

    cc **I70.531** Atherosclerosis of nonautologous <u>biological</u> bypass graft(s) of the <u>right</u> leg <u>with ulceration</u> of <u>thigh</u> — [Age/15-124]

    cc **I70.532** Atherosclerosis of nonautologous <u>biological</u> bypass graft(s) of the <u>right</u> leg <u>with ulceration</u> of <u>calf</u> — [Age/15-124]

    cc **I70.533** Atherosclerosis of nonautologous <u>biological</u> bypass graft(s) of the <u>right</u> leg <u>with ulceration</u> of <u>ankle</u> — [Age/15-124]

    cc **I70.534** Atherosclerosis of nonautologous <u>biological</u> bypass graft(s) of the <u>right</u> leg <u>with ulceration</u> of <u>heel and midfoot</u> — [Age/15-124]
        Atherosclerosis of nonautologous biological bypass graft(s) of right leg with ulceration of plantar surface of midfoot

    I70.535 Atherosclerosis of nonautologous <u>biological</u> bypass graft(s) of the <u>right</u> leg <u>with ulceration</u> of <u>other part of foot</u> — [Age/15-124]
        Atherosclerosis of nonautologous biological bypass graft(s) of the right leg with ulceration of toe

    cc **I70.538** Atherosclerosis of nonautologous <u>biological</u> bypass graft(s) of the <u>right</u> leg <u>with ulceration</u> of <u>other part of lower leg</u> — [Age/15-124]

    cc **I70.539** Atherosclerosis of nonautologous <u>biological</u> bypass graft(s) of the <u>right</u> leg <u>with ulceration</u> of <u>unspecified site</u> — [Age/15-124]

I70.54- Atherosclerosis of nonautologous <u>biological</u> bypass graft(s) of the <u>left</u> leg <u>with ulceration</u>
    Includes: Any condition classifiable to I70.512 and I70.522
    Use additional code to identify severity of ulcer (L97.-)

    cc **I70.541** Atherosclerosis of nonautologous <u>biological</u> bypass graft(s) of the <u>left</u> leg <u>with ulceration</u> of <u>thigh</u> — [Age/15-124]

    cc **I70.542** Atherosclerosis of nonautologous <u>biological</u> bypass graft(s) of the <u>left</u> leg <u>with ulceration</u> of <u>calf</u> — [Age/15-124]

    cc **I70.543** Atherosclerosis of nonautologous <u>biological</u> bypass graft(s) of the <u>left</u> leg <u>with ulceration</u> of <u>ankle</u> — [Age/15-124]

    cc **I70.544** Atherosclerosis of nonautologous <u>biological</u> bypass graft(s) of the <u>left</u> leg <u>with ulceration</u> of <u>heel and midfoot</u> — [Age/15-124]
        Atherosclerosis of nonautologous biological bypass graft(s) of left leg with ulceration of plantar surface of midfoot

    I70.545 Atherosclerosis of nonautologous <u>biological</u> bypass graft(s) of the <u>left</u> leg <u>with ulceration</u> of <u>other part of foot</u> — [Age/15-124]
        Atherosclerosis of nonautologous biological bypass graft(s) of the left leg with ulceration of toe

    cc **I70.548** Atherosclerosis of nonautologous <u>biological</u> bypass graft(s) of the <u>left</u> leg <u>with ulceration</u> of <u>other part of lower leg</u> — [Age/15-124]

    cc **I70.549** Atherosclerosis of nonautologous <u>biological</u> bypass graft(s) of the <u>left</u> leg <u>with ulceration</u> of <u>unspecified site</u> — [Age/15-124]

I70.55 Atherosclerosis of nonautologous <u>biological</u> bypass graft(s) of <u>other extremity</u> <u>with ulceration</u> — [Age/15-124]
    Includes: Any condition classifiable to I70.518, I70.528, and I70.538
    Use additional code to identify severity of ulcer (L98.49)

I70.56- Atherosclerosis of nonautologous <u>biological</u> bypass graft(s) of the extremities <u>with gangrene</u>
    Includes: Any condition classifiable to I70.51-, I70.52-, and I70.53-, I70.54-, I70.55
    Use additional code to identify the severity of any ulcer (L97.-, L98.49-), if applicable

    cc **I70.561** Atherosclerosis of nonautologous <u>biological</u> bypass graft(s) of the extremities <u>with gangrene</u>, <u>right</u> leg — [Age/15-124]

    cc **I70.562** Atherosclerosis of nonautologous <u>biological</u> bypass graft(s) of the extremities <u>with gangrene</u>, <u>left</u> leg — [Age/15-124]

    cc **I70.563** Atherosclerosis of nonautologous <u>biological</u> bypass graft(s) of the extremities <u>with gangrene</u>, <u>bilateral</u> legs — [Age/15-124]

    cc **I70.568** Atherosclerosis of nonautologous <u>biological</u> bypass graft(s) of the extremities <u>with gangrene</u>, <u>other extremity</u> — [Age/15-124]

    cc **I70.569** Atherosclerosis of nonautologous <u>biological</u> bypass graft(s) of the extremities <u>with gangrene</u>, <u>unspecified extremity</u> — [Age/15-124]

I70.59- <u>Other</u> atherosclerosis of nonautologous <u>biological</u> bypass graft(s) of the extremities

    I70.591 <u>Other</u> atherosclerosis of nonautologous <u>biological</u> bypass graft(s) of the extremities, <u>right</u> leg — [Age/15-124]

    I70.592 <u>Other</u> atherosclerosis of nonautologous <u>biological</u> bypass graft(s) of the extremities, <u>left</u> leg — [Age/15-124]

    I70.593 <u>Other</u> atherosclerosis of nonautologous <u>biological</u> bypass graft(s) of the extremities, <u>bilateral</u> legs — [Age/15-124]

    I70.598 <u>Other</u> atherosclerosis of nonautologous <u>biological</u> bypass graft(s) of the extremities, <u>other extremity</u> — [Age/15-124]

    I70.599 <u>Other</u> atherosclerosis of nonautologous <u>biological</u> bypass graft(s) of the extremities, <u>unspecified extremity</u> — [Age/15-124]

I 70 - I 70

I70.6-   Atherosclerosis of <u>nonbiological</u> bypass graft(s) of the extremities
    Use additional code, if applicable, to identify chronic total occlusion of artery of extremity (I70.92)

   I70.60-   <u>Unspecified</u> atherosclerosis of <u>nonbiological</u> bypass graft(s) of the extremities

     I70.601   <u>Unspecified</u> atherosclerosis of <u>nonbiological</u> bypass graft(s) of the extremities, <u>right</u> leg — [Age/15-124]

     I70.602   <u>Unspecified</u> atherosclerosis of <u>nonbiological</u> bypass graft(s) of the extremities, <u>left</u> leg — [Age/15-124]

     I70.603   <u>Unspecified</u> atherosclerosis of <u>nonbiological</u> bypass graft(s) of the extremities, <u>bilateral</u> legs — [Age/15-124]

     I70.608   <u>Unspecified</u> atherosclerosis of <u>nonbiological</u> bypass graft(s) of the extremities, <u>other</u> <u>extremity</u> — [Age/15-124]

     I70.609   <u>Unspecified</u> atherosclerosis of <u>nonbiological</u> bypass graft(s) of the extremities, <u>unspecified</u> <u>extremity</u> — [Age/15-124]

   I70.61-   Atherosclerosis of <u>nonbiological</u> bypass graft(s) of the extremities <u>with intermittent claudication</u>

     I70.611   Atherosclerosis of <u>nonbiological</u> bypass graft(s) of the extremities <u>with intermittent claudication</u>, <u>right</u> leg — [Age/15-124]

     I70.612   Atherosclerosis of <u>nonbiological</u> bypass graft(s) of the extremities <u>with intermittent claudication</u>, <u>left</u> leg — [Age/15-124]

     I70.613   Atherosclerosis of <u>nonbiological</u> bypass graft(s) of the extremities <u>with intermittent claudication</u>, <u>bilateral</u> legs — [Age/15-124]

     I70.618   Atherosclerosis of <u>nonbiological</u> bypass graft(s) of the extremities <u>with intermittent claudication</u>, <u>other extremity</u> — [Age/15-124]

     I70.619   Atherosclerosis of <u>nonbiological</u> bypass graft(s) of the extremities <u>with intermittent claudication</u>, <u>unspecified extremity</u> — [Age/15-124]

   I70.62-   Atherosclerosis of <u>nonbiological</u> bypass graft(s) of the extremities <u>with rest pain</u>
    Includes: Any condition classifiable to I70.61-

     I70.621   Atherosclerosis of <u>nonbiological</u> bypass graft(s) of the extremities <u>with rest pain</u>, <u>right</u> leg — [Age/15-124]

     I70.622   Atherosclerosis of <u>nonbiological</u> bypass graft(s) of the extremities <u>with rest pain</u>, <u>left</u> leg — [Age/15-124]

     I70.623   Atherosclerosis of <u>nonbiological</u> bypass graft(s) of the extremities <u>with rest pain</u>, <u>bilateral</u> legs — [Age/15-124]

     I70.628   Atherosclerosis of <u>nonbiological</u> bypass graft(s) of the extremities <u>with rest pain</u>, <u>other extremity</u> — [Age/15-124]

     I70.629   Atherosclerosis of <u>nonbiological</u> bypass graft(s) of the extremities <u>with rest pain</u>, <u>unspecified</u> <u>extremity</u> — [Age/15-124]

   I70.63-   Atherosclerosis of <u>nonbiological</u> bypass graft(s) of the <u>right</u> leg <u>with ulceration</u>
    Includes: Any condition classifiable to I70.611 and I70.621
    Use additional code to identify severity of ulcer (L97.-)

    CC **I70.631**   Atherosclerosis of <u>nonbiological</u> bypass graft(s) of the <u>right</u> leg <u>with ulceration</u> of <u>thigh</u> — [Age/15-124]

    CC **I70.632**   Atherosclerosis of <u>nonbiological</u> bypass graft(s) of the <u>right</u> leg <u>with ulceration</u> of <u>calf</u> — [Age/15-124]

    CC **I70.633**   Atherosclerosis of <u>nonbiological</u> bypass graft(s) of the <u>right</u> leg <u>with ulceration</u> of <u>ankle</u> — [Age/15-124]

    CC **I70.634**   Atherosclerosis of <u>nonbiological</u> bypass graft(s) of the <u>right</u> leg <u>with ulceration</u> of <u>heel and midfoot</u> — [Age/15-124]
     Atherosclerosis of nonbiological bypass graft(s) of right leg with ulceration of plantar surface of midfoot

    I70.635   Atherosclerosis of <u>nonbiological</u> bypass graft(s) of the <u>right</u> leg <u>with ulceration</u> of <u>other part of foot</u> — [Age/15-124]
     Atherosclerosis of nonbiological bypass graft(s) of the right leg with ulceration of toe

    CC **I70.638**   Atherosclerosis of <u>nonbiological</u> bypass graft(s) of the <u>right</u> leg <u>with ulceration</u> of <u>other part of lower leg</u> — [Age/15-124]

    CC **I70.639**   Atherosclerosis of <u>nonbiological</u> bypass graft(s) of the <u>right</u> leg <u>with ulceration</u> of <u>unspecified site</u> — [Age/15-124]

   I70.64-   Atherosclerosis of <u>nonbiological</u> bypass graft(s) of the <u>left</u> leg <u>with ulceration</u>
    Includes: Any condition classifiable to I70.612 and I70.622
    Use additional code to identify severity of ulcer (L97.-)

    CC **I70.641**   Atherosclerosis of <u>nonbiological</u> bypass graft(s) of the <u>left</u> leg <u>with ulceration</u> of <u>thigh</u> — [Age/15-124]

    CC **I70.642**   Atherosclerosis of <u>nonbiological</u> bypass graft(s) of the <u>left</u> leg <u>with ulceration</u> of <u>calf</u> — [Age/15-124]

    CC **I70.643**   Atherosclerosis of <u>nonbiological</u> bypass graft(s) of the <u>left</u> leg <u>with ulceration</u> of <u>ankle</u> — [Age/15-124]

    CC **I70.644**   Atherosclerosis of <u>nonbiological</u> bypass graft(s) of the <u>left</u> leg <u>with ulceration</u> of <u>heel and midfoot</u> — [Age/15-124]
     Atherosclerosis of nonbiological bypass graft(s) of left leg with ulceration of plantar surface of midfoot

    I70.645   Atherosclerosis of <u>nonbiological</u> bypass graft(s) of the <u>left</u> leg <u>with ulceration</u> of <u>other part of foot</u> — [Age/15-124]
     Atherosclerosis of nonbiological bypass graft(s) of the left leg with ulceration of toe

    CC **I70.648**   Atherosclerosis of <u>nonbiological</u> bypass graft(s) of the <u>left</u> leg <u>with ulceration</u> of <u>other part of lower leg</u> — [Age/15-124]

    CC **I70.649**   Atherosclerosis of <u>nonbiological</u> bypass graft(s) of the <u>left</u> leg <u>with ulceration</u> of <u>unspecified site</u> — [Age/15-124]

   I70.65   Atherosclerosis of <u>nonbiological</u> bypass graft(s) of <u>other extremity</u> with ulceration — [Age/15-124]
    Includes: Any condition classifiable to I70.618 and I70.628
    Use additional code to identify severity of ulcer (L98.49)

   I70.66-   Atherosclerosis of <u>nonbiological</u> bypass graft(s) of the extremities <u>with gangrene</u>
    Includes: Any condition classifiable to I70.61-, I70.62-, I70.63-, I70.64-, I70.65
    Use additional code to identify the severity of any ulcer (L97.-, L98.49-), if applicable

    CC **I70.661**   Atherosclerosis of <u>nonbiological</u> bypass graft(s) of the extremities <u>with gangrene</u>, <u>right</u> leg — [Age/15-124]

    CC **I70.662**   Atherosclerosis of <u>nonbiological</u> bypass graft(s) of the extremities <u>with gangrene</u>, <u>left</u> leg — [Age/15-124]

    CC **I70.663**   Atherosclerosis of <u>nonbiological</u> bypass graft(s) of the extremities <u>with gangrene</u>, <u>bilateral</u> legs — [Age/15-124]

    CC **I70.668**   Atherosclerosis of <u>nonbiological</u> bypass graft(s) of the extremities <u>with gangrene</u>, <u>other extremity</u> — [Age/15-124]

    CC **I70.669**   Atherosclerosis of <u>nonbiological</u> bypass graft(s) of the extremities <u>with gangrene</u>, <u>unspecified</u> <u>extremity</u> — [Age/15-124]

   I70.69-   <u>Other</u> atherosclerosis of <u>nonbiological</u> bypass graft(s) of the extremities

     I70.691   <u>Other</u> atherosclerosis of <u>nonbiological</u> bypass graft(s) of the extremities, <u>right</u> leg — [Age/15-124]

     I70.692   <u>Other</u> atherosclerosis of <u>nonbiological</u> bypass graft(s) of the extremities, <u>left</u> leg — [Age/15-124]

     I70.693   <u>Other</u> atherosclerosis of <u>nonbiological</u> bypass graft(s) of the extremities, <u>bilateral</u> legs — [Age/15-124]

I70 - I70

I70.698 Other atherosclerosis of nonbiological bypass graft(s) of the extremities, other extremity — [Age/15-124]

I70.699 Other atherosclerosis of nonbiological bypass graft(s) of the extremities, unspecified extremity — [Age/15-124]

I70.7- Atherosclerosis of other type of bypass graft(s) of the extremities
Use additional code, if applicable, to identify chronic total occlusion of artery of extremity (I70.92)

I70.70- Unspecified atherosclerosis of other type of bypass graft(s) of the extremities

I70.701 Unspecified atherosclerosis of other type of bypass graft(s) of the extremities, right leg — [Age/15-124]

I70.702 Unspecified atherosclerosis of other type of bypass graft(s) of the extremities, left leg — [Age/15-124]

I70.703 Unspecified atherosclerosis of other type of bypass graft(s) of the extremities, bilateral legs — [Age/15-124]

I70.708 Unspecified atherosclerosis of other type of bypass graft(s) of the extremities, other extremity — [Age/15-124]

I70.709 Unspecified atherosclerosis of other type of bypass graft(s) of the extremities, unspecified extremity — [Age/15-124]

I70.71- Atherosclerosis of other type of bypass graft(s) of the extremities with intermittent claudication

I70.711 Atherosclerosis of other type of bypass graft(s) of the extremities with intermittent claudication, right leg — [Age/15-124]

I70.712 Atherosclerosis of other type of bypass graft(s) of the extremities with intermittent claudication, left leg — [Age/15-124]

I70.713 Atherosclerosis of other type of bypass graft(s) of the extremities with intermittent claudication, bilateral legs — [Age/15-124]

I70.718 Atherosclerosis of other type of bypass graft(s) of the extremities with intermittent claudication, other extremity — [Age/15-124]

I70.719 Atherosclerosis of other type of bypass graft(s) of the extremities with intermittent claudication, unspecified extremity — [Age/15-124]

I70.72- Atherosclerosis of other type of bypass graft(s) of the extremities with rest pain
Includes: Any condition classifiable to I70.71-

I70.721 Atherosclerosis of other type of bypass graft(s) of the extremities with rest pain, right leg — [Age/15-124]

I70.722 Atherosclerosis of other type of bypass graft(s) of the extremities with rest pain, left leg — [Age/15-124]

I70.723 Atherosclerosis of other type of bypass graft(s) of the extremities with rest pain, bilateral legs — [Age/15-124]

I70.728 Atherosclerosis of other type of bypass graft(s) of the extremities with rest pain, other extremity — [Age/15-124]

I70.729 Atherosclerosis of other type of bypass graft(s) of the extremities with rest pain, unspecified extremity — [Age/15-124]

I70.73- Atherosclerosis of other type of bypass graft(s) of the right leg with ulceration
Includes: Any condition classifiable to I70.711 and I70.721
Use additional code to identify severity of ulcer (L97.-)

cc I70.731 Atherosclerosis of other type of bypass graft(s) of the right leg with ulceration of thigh — [Age/15-124]

cc I70.732 Atherosclerosis of other type of bypass graft(s) of the right leg with ulceration of calf — [Age/15-124]

cc I70.733 Atherosclerosis of other type of bypass graft(s) of the right leg with ulceration of ankle — [Age/15-124]

cc I70.734 Atherosclerosis of other type of bypass graft(s) of the right leg with ulceration of heel and midfoot — [Age/15-124]
Atherosclerosis of other type of bypass graft(s) of right leg with ulceration of plantar surface of midfoot

I70.735 Atherosclerosis of other type of bypass graft(s) of the right leg with ulceration of other part of foot — [Age/15-124]
Atherosclerosis of other type of bypass graft(s) of right leg with ulceration of toe

cc I70.738 Atherosclerosis of other type of bypass graft(s) of the right leg with ulceration of other part of lower leg — [Age/15-124]

cc I70.739 Atherosclerosis of other type of bypass graft(s) of the right leg with ulceration of unspecified site — [Age/15-124]

I70.74- Atherosclerosis of other type of bypass graft(s) of the left leg with ulceration
Includes: Any condition classifiable to I70.712 and I70.722
Use additional code to identify severity of ulcer (L97.-)

cc I70.741 Atherosclerosis of other type of bypass graft(s) of the left leg with ulceration of thigh — [Age/15-124]

cc I70.742 Atherosclerosis of other type of bypass graft(s) of the left leg with ulceration of calf — [Age/15-124]

cc I70.743 Atherosclerosis of other type of bypass graft(s) of the left leg with ulceration of ankle — [Age/15-124]

cc I70.744 Atherosclerosis of other type of bypass graft(s) of the left leg with ulceration of heel and midfoot — [Age/15-124]
Atherosclerosis of other type of bypass graft(s) of left leg with ulceration of plantar surface of midfoot

I70.745 Atherosclerosis of other type of bypass graft(s) of the left leg with ulceration of other part of foot — [Age/15-124]
Atherosclerosis of other type of bypass graft(s) of left leg with ulceration of toe

cc I70.748 Atherosclerosis of other type of bypass graft(s) of the left leg with ulceration of other part of lower leg — [Age/15-124]

cc I70.749 Atherosclerosis of other type of bypass graft(s) of the left leg with ulceration of unspecified site — [Age/15-124]

I70.75 Atherosclerosis of other type of bypass graft(s) of other extremity with ulceration — [Age/15-124]
Includes: Any condition classifiable to I70.718 and I70.728
Use additional code to identify severity of ulcer (L98.49)

I70.76- Atherosclerosis of other type of bypass graft(s) of the extremities with gangrene
Includes: Any condition classifiable to I70.71-, I70.72-, I70.73-, I70.74-, I70.75
Use additional code to identify the severity of any ulcer (L97.-, L98.49-), if applicable

cc I70.761 Atherosclerosis of other type of bypass graft(s) of the extremities with gangrene, right leg — [Age/15-124]

cc I70.762 Atherosclerosis of other type of bypass graft(s) of the extremities with gangrene, left leg — [Age/15-124]

cc I70.763 Atherosclerosis of other type of bypass graft(s) of the extremities with gangrene, bilateral legs — [Age/15-124]

cc I70.768 Atherosclerosis of other type of bypass graft(s) of the extremities with gangrene, other extremity — [Age/15-124]

cc I70.769 Atherosclerosis of other type of bypass graft(s) of the extremities with gangrene, unspecified extremity — [Age/15-124]

I70.79- Other atherosclerosis of other type of bypass graft(s) of the extremities

I70.791 Other atherosclerosis of other type of bypass graft(s) of the extremities, right leg — [Age/15-124]

I70.792 Other atherosclerosis of other type of bypass graft(s) of the extremities, left leg — [Age/15-124]

I70.793   Other atherosclerosis of other type of bypass graft(s) of the extremities, bilateral legs — [Age/15-124]

I70.798   Other atherosclerosis of other type of bypass graft(s) of the extremities, other extremity — [Age/15-124]

I70.799   Other atherosclerosis of other type of bypass graft(s) of the extremities, unspecified extremity — [Age/15-124]

I70.8   Atherosclerosis of other arteries — [Age/15-124]

I70.9-   Other and unspecified atherosclerosis

  I70.90   Unspecified atherosclerosis — [Age/15-124]

  I70.91   Generalized atherosclerosis — [Age/15-124]

cc **I70.92**   Chronic total occlusion of artery of the extremities — [Age/15-124] [Unacceptable PDX]
   Complete occlusion of artery of the extremities
   Total occlusion of artery of the extremities
   Code first atherosclerosis of arteries of the extremities (I70.2-, I70.3-, I70.4-, I70.5-, I70.6-, I70.7-)

I71-   Aortic aneurysm and dissection — AORTIC ANEURYSM – A sac formed by the dilatation of the aortic wall. AORTIC DISSECTION – A longitudinal splitting of the aortic arterial wall.

  Excludes 1:   aortic ectasia (I77.81-)
     syphilitic aortic aneurysm (A52.01)
     traumatic aortic aneurysm (S25.09, S35.09)

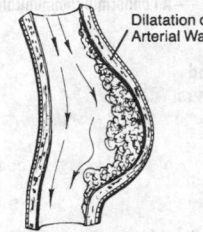
Dilatation of Arterial Wall

ARTERIAL ANEURYSM

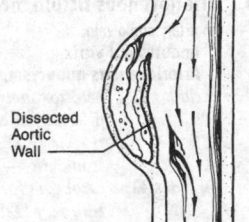
Dissected Aortic Wall

DISSECTING AORTIC ANEURYSM

I71.0-   Dissection of aorta — A longitudinal splitting of the aortic arterial wall.

MCC **I71.00**   Dissection of unspecified site of aorta

MCC **I71.01**   Dissection of thoracic aorta

MCC **I71.02**   Dissection of abdominal aorta

MCC **I71.03**   Dissection of thoracoabdominal aorta

MCC **I71.1**   Thoracic aortic aneurysm, ruptured — A form in the thoracic aorta in which the wall ruptures and results in a massive hemorrhage.

I71.2   Thoracic aortic aneurysm, without rupture

MCC **I71.3**   Abdominal aortic aneurysm, ruptured — A form in the abdominal aorta in which the wall ruptures, resulting in massive hemorrhage.

I71.4   Abdominal aortic aneurysm, without rupture

MCC **I71.5**   Thoracoabdominal aortic aneurysm, ruptured — A form in the thoracic and abdominal aorta in which the wall ruptures, resulting in massive hemorrhage.

I71.6   Thoracoabdominal aortic aneurysm, without rupture

MCC **I71.8**   Aortic aneurysm of unspecified site, ruptured
   Rupture of aorta NOS

I71.9   Aortic aneurysm of unspecified site, without rupture
   Aneurysm of aorta
   Dilatation of aorta
   Hyaline necrosis of aorta

I72-   Other aneurysm — A sac formed by the dilatation of an arterial wall.
  Includes: Aneurysm (cirsoid) (false) (ruptured) — CIRSOID – A form in which the blood vessels become dilated, lengthened, and tortuous. FALSE – A form in which the entire wall is injured and the blood is contained by the surrounding tissues, with eventual formation of a sac communicating with the artery. RUPTURED – A form in which the arterial wall ruptures resulting in massive hemorrhage.

  Excludes ❷: acquired aneurysm (I77.0)
     aneurysm (of) aorta (I71-)
     aneurysm (of) arteriovenous NOS (Q27.3-)
     carotid artery dissection (I77.71)
     cerebral (nonruptured) aneurysm (I67.1)
     coronary aneurysm (I25.4)
     coronary artery dissection (I25.42)
     dissection of artery NEC (I77.79)
     dissection of precerebral artery, congenital (nonruptured) (Q28.1)
     heart aneurysm (I25.3)
     iliac artery dissection (I77.72)
     pulmonary artery aneurysm (I28.1)
     renal artery dissection (I77.73)
     retinal aneurysm (H35.0)
     ruptured cerebral aneurysm (I60.7)
     varicose aneurysm (I77.0)
     vertebral artery dissection (I77.74)

I72.0   Aneurysm of carotid artery — A form affecting the carotid arteries which supply blood to the brain and head.
   Aneurysm of common carotid artery
   Aneurysm of external carotid artery
   Aneurysm of internal carotid artery, extracranial portion
  Excludes 1:   aneurysm of internal carotid artery, intracranial portion (I67.1)
     aneurysm of internal carotid artery NOS (I67.1)

I72.1   Aneurysm of artery of upper extremity

I72.2   Aneurysm of renal artery

I72.3   Aneurysm of iliac artery

I72.4   Aneurysm of artery of lower extremity

I72.5   Aneurysm of other precerebral arteries
   Aneurysm of basilar artery (trunk)
  Excludes ❷: aneurysm of carotid artery (I72.0)
     aneurysm of vertebral artery (I72.6)
     dissection of carotid artery (I77.71)
     dissection of other precerebral arteries (I77.75)
     dissection of vertebral artery (I77.74)

I72.6   Aneurysm of vertebral artery
  Excludes ❷: dissection of vertebral artery (I77.74)

I72.8   Aneurysm of other specified arteries

I72.9   Aneurysm of unspecified site

I73-   Other peripheral vascular diseases
  Excludes ❷: chilblains (T69.1)
     frostbite (T33-T34)
     immersion hand or foot (T69.0-)
     spasm of cerebral artery (G45.9)

I73.0-   Raynaud's syndrome — Paroxysmal digital cyanosis of an undetermined primary cause.
   Raynaud's disease
   Raynaud's phenomenon (secondary) — Paroxysmal digital cyanosis followed by redness of the skin of the digits which is precipitated by cold or emotional upset, and may be due to a number of regional or systemic disorders.

  I73.00   Raynaud's syndrome without gangrene

cc **I73.01**   Raynaud's syndrome with gangrene — A form with the death of tissue.

I73.1   Thromboangiitis obliterans [Buerger's disease] — Inflammatory occlusions of the more distal arteries, resulting in circulatory insufficiency of the toes and fingers, and thrombosis of superficial veins and is most commonly seen in young men who smoke.

I73.8-   Other specified peripheral vascular diseases
  Excludes 1:   diabetic (peripheral) angiopathy (E08-E13 with .51-.52)

  I73.81   Erythromelalgia — A rare condition of paroxysmal vasodilation with intense burning pain (most frequently in the extremities), severe redness, and increased temperature.

I 7 0 - I 7 3

© 2016 Channel Publishing, Ltd.

I73.89 Other specified peripheral vascular diseases
Acrocyanosis — Arteriolar vasoconstriction combined with dilatation of the subpapillary venous plexus of the skin resulting in symmetric coldness and cyanotic discoloration of the skin of the hands and feet.
Erythrocyanosis — Bluish-red discoloration on the legs and thighs associated with cyanosis.
Simple acroparesthesia [Schultze's type] — Tingling, numbness, and stiffness of the extremities of the simple form which tends to end in acrocyanosis.
Vasomotor acroparesthesia [Nothnagel's type] — Tingling, numbness, and stiffness in the extremities of the vasomotor or angiospastic form.

I73.9 Peripheral vascular disease, unspecified
Intermittent claudication — Pain, tension, and weakness while walking until it becomes impossible to continue.
Peripheral angiopathy NOS
Spasm of artery — A sudden, involuntary contraction of an arterial wall.
Excludes 1: *atherosclerosis of the extremities (I70.2- – I70.7-)*

I74- Arterial embolism and thrombosis — EMBOLISM — A blood clot or other substance blocking an artery. THROMBOSIS — An abnormal aggregation of blood factors causing an arterial obstruction.
Includes: **Embolic infarction** — A localized necrosis of tissue resulting from an arterial embolism.
Embolic occlusion — Blockage of an artery by an embolus.
Thrombotic infarction — A localized necrosis of tissue resulting from a thrombotic occlusion.
Thrombotic occlusion — Blockage of an artery by a thrombosis.
Code first embolism and thrombosis complicating abortion or ectopic or molar pregnancy (O00-O07, O08.2)
Code first embolism and thrombosis complicating pregnancy, childbirth and the puerperium (O88.-)
Excludes ❷: *atheroembolism (I75.-)*
basilar embolism and thrombosis (I63.0-I63.2, I65.1)
carotid embolism and thrombosis (I63.0-I63.2, I65.2)
cerebral embolism and thrombosis (I63.3-I63.5, I66.-)
coronary embolism and thrombosis (I21-I25)
mesenteric embolism and thrombosis (K55.0-)
ophthalmic embolism and thrombosis (H34-)
precerebral embolism and thrombosis NOS (I63.0-I63.2, I65.9)
pulmonary embolism and thrombosis (I26-)
renal embolism and thrombosis (N28.0)
retinal embolism and thrombosis (H34-)
septic embolism and thrombosis (I76)
vertebral embolism and thrombosis (I63.0-I63.2, I65.0)

I74.0- Embolism and thrombosis of abdominal aorta

MCC I74.01 Saddle embolism abdominal aorta — A form characterized by a large embolism that straddles the bifurcation of the abdominal aorta.

CC I74.09 Other arterial embolism and thrombosis of abdominal aorta
Aortic bifurcation syndrome
Aortoiliac obstruction — A form affecting the abdominal aorta and the iliac arteries.
Leriche's syndrome — A syndrome caused by obstruction of the terminal aorta characterized by muscle fatigue in the legs, absence of pulsation in the femoral arteries, and coldness of the lower extremities.

I74.1- Embolism and thrombosis of other and unspecified parts of aorta

CC I74.10 Embolism and thrombosis of unspecified parts of aorta

CC I74.11 Embolism and thrombosis of thoracic aorta

CC I74.19 Embolism and thrombosis of other parts of aorta

CC I74.2 Embolism and thrombosis of arteries of the upper extremities

CC I74.3 Embolism and thrombosis of arteries of the lower extremities

CC I74.4 Embolism and thrombosis of arteries of extremities, unspecified
Peripheral arterial embolism NOS

CC I74.5 Embolism and thrombosis of iliac artery

CC I74.8 Embolism and thrombosis of other arteries

CC I74.9 Embolism and thrombosis of unspecified artery

I75- Atheroembolism — The blockage of a terminal artery caused by the lodging of atheromatous (fatty) plaque debris in a terminal artery branch.
Includes: **Atherothrombotic microembolism**
Cholesterol embolism

I75.0- Atheroembolism of extremities

I75.01- Atheroembolism of upper extremity

CC I75.011 Atheroembolism of right upper extremity

CC I75.012 Atheroembolism of left upper extremity

CC I75.013 Atheroembolism of bilateral upper extremities

CC I75.019 Atheroembolism of unspecified upper extremity

I75.02- Atheroembolism of lower extremity

CC I75.021 Atheroembolism of right lower extremity

CC I75.022 Atheroembolism of left lower extremity

CC I75.023 Atheroembolism of bilateral lower extremities

CC I75.029 Atheroembolism of unspecified lower extremity

I75.8- Atheroembolism of other sites

CC I75.81 Atheroembolism of kidney
Use additional code for any associated acute kidney failure and chronic kidney disease (N17.-, N18.-)

CC I75.89 Atheroembolism of other site

I76 Septic arterial embolism — [Unacceptable PDX] — A localized collection of pus and bacteria that often originates in the heart or lungs and then travels through the systemic arterial system where it lodges in small vessels throughout the body, often in the brain, retina, and digits.
Code first underlying infection, such as:
Infective endocarditis (I33.0)
Lung abscess (J85.-)
Use additional code to identify the site of the embolism (I74.-)
Excludes ❷: *septic pulmonary embolism (I26.01, I26.90)*

I77- Other disorders of arteries and arterioles
Excludes ❷: *collagen (vascular) diseases (M30-M36)*
hypersensitivity angiitis (M31.0)
pulmonary artery (I28.-)

I77.0 Arteriovenous fistula, acquired — An abnormal communication between an artery and a vein.
Aneurysmal varix
Arteriovenous aneurysm, acquired
Excludes 1: *arteriovenous aneurysm NOS (Q27.3-)*
presence of arteriovenous shunt (fistula) for dialysis (Z99.2)
traumatic — see injury of blood vessel by body region
Excludes ❷: *cerebral (I67.1)*
coronary (I25.4)

I77.1 Stricture of artery — Decrease in caliber of an artery.
Narrowing of artery

CC I77.2 Rupture of artery — A forcible tearing of the arterial wall.
Erosion of artery — A wasting-away of the arterial wall.
Fistula of artery — An abnormal communication of an artery with another organ or tissue area.
Ulcer of artery — An eating-away of the arterial wall.
Excludes 1: *traumatic rupture of artery — see injury of blood vessel by body region*

I77.3 Arterial fibromuscular dysplasia — The abnormal multiplication or increase in the number of normal cells and the normal arrangement of the fibromuscular layers of an artery.
Fibromuscular hyperplasia (of) carotid artery
Fibromuscular hyperplasia (of) renal artery

CC I77.4 Celiac artery compression syndrome — Recurrent abdominal pain caused by the compression of the celiac artery by the median arcuate ligament of the diaphragm.

CC I77.5 Necrosis of artery — Death of the arterial wall tissue.

I77.6 Arteritis, unspecified
Aortitis NOS
Endarteritis NOS
Excludes 1: *arteritis or endarteritis:*
aortic arch (M31.4)
cerebral NEC (I67.7)
coronary (I25.89)
deformans (I70.-)
giant cell (M31.5., M31.6)
obliterans (I70.-)
senile (I70.-)

I77.7- Other arterial dissection — The splitting of an arterial wall that allows blood to flow within the wall layers.
Excludes ❷: *dissection of aorta (I71.0-)*
dissection of coronary artery (I25.42)

MCC I77.70 Dissection of unspecified artery

MCC I77.71 Dissection of carotid artery

MCC I77.72 Dissection of iliac artery

MCC I77.73 Dissection of renal artery

MCC I77.74 Dissection of vertebral artery
Excludes ❷: *aneurysm of vertebral artery (I72.6)*

I73 - I77

MCC I77.75   Dissection of other precerebral arteries
Dissection of basilar artery (trunk)
Excludes ❷: aneurysm of carotid artery (I72.0)
aneurysm of other precerebral arteries (I72.5)
aneurysm of vertebral artery (I72.6)
dissection of carotid artery (I77.71)
dissection of vertebral artery (I77.74)

MCC I77.76   Dissection of artery of upper extremity

MCC I77.77   Dissection of artery of lower extremitiy

MCC I77.79   Dissection of other specified artery

I77.8-   Other specified disorders of arteries and arterioles

I77.81-   Aortic ectasia — The abnormal widening of the aortic wall that is not diagnostic of an aneurysm.
Ectasis aorta
Excludes 1:   aortic aneurysm and dissection (I71.0-)

I77.810   Thoracic aortic ectasia

I77.811   Abdominal aortic ectasia

I77.812   Thoracoabdominal aortic ectasia

I77.819   Aortic ectasia, unspecified site

I77.89   Other specified disorders of arteries and arterioles

I77.9   Disorder of arteries and arterioles, unspecified

I78-   Diseases of capillaries

I78.0   Hereditary hemorrhagic telangiectasia — A hereditary disorder characterized by multiple telangiectatic lesions on the face, mouth, nose, and hand in association with epistaxis or gastrointestinal bleeding.
Rendu-Osler-Weber disease

I78.1   Nevus, non-neoplastic — Hypertrophy of the skin capillaries characterized by a reddish swelling or patch on the skin.
Araneus nevus
Senile nevus
Spider nevus
Stellar nevus
Excludes 1:   nevus NOS (D22.-)
vascular NOS (Q82.5)
Excludes ❷: blue nevus (D22.-)
flammeus nevus (Q82.5)
hairy nevus (D22.-)
melanocytic nevus (D22.-)
pigmented nevus (D22.-)
portwine nevus (Q82.5)
sanguineous nevus (Q82.5)
strawberry nevus (Q82.5)
verrucous nevus (Q82.5)

I78.8   Other diseases of capillaries

I78.9   Disease of capillaries, unspecified

I79-   Disorders of arteries, arterioles and capillaries in diseases classified elsewhere

I79.0   Aneurysm of aorta in diseases classified elsewhere — [Not Allowed as PDX]
Code first underlying disease
Excludes 1:   syphilitic aneurysm (A52.01)

I79.1   Aortitis in diseases classified elsewhere — [Not Allowed as PDX]
Code first underlying disease
Excludes 1:   syphilitic aortitis (A52.02)

I79.8   Other disorders of arteries, arterioles and capillaries in diseases classified elsewhere — [Not Allowed as PDX]
Code first underlying disease, such as:
Amyloidosis (E85.-)
Excludes 1:   diabetic (peripheral) angiopathy (E08-E13 with .51-.52)
syphilitic endarteritis (A52.09)
tuberculous endarteritis (A18.89)

Diseases of veins, lymphatic vessels and lymph nodes, not elsewhere classified (I80-I89)

I80-   Phlebitis and thrombophlebitis — PHLEBITIS – Inflammation of a vein attended by edema, stiffness, and pain at the site of inflammation. THROMBOPHLEBITIS – A partial or complete occlusion of a vein by a thrombus, with secondary inflammatory reaction in the wall of the vein.
Includes: **Endophlebitis** — Inflammation of the innermost lining of a vein.
Inflammation, vein — Tissue reaction to a venous condition or injury.
Periphlebitis — Inflammation of the external coat of the vein and the surrounding tissue.
Suppurative phlebitis — Pus-producing inflammation of a vein.
Code first phlebitis and thrombophlebitis complicating abortion, ectopic or molar pregnancy (O00-O07, O08.7)
Code first phlebitis and thrombophlebitis complicating pregnancy, childbirth and the puerperium (O22-, O87-)
Excludes 1:   venous embolism and thrombosis of lower extremities (I82.4-, I82.5-, I82.81-)

I80.0-   Phlebitis and thrombophlebitis of superficial vessels of lower extremities
Phlebitis and thrombophlebitis of femoropopliteal vein

I80.00   Phlebitis and thrombophlebitis of superficial vessels of unspecified lower extremity

I80.01   Phlebitis and thrombophlebitis of superficial vessels of right lower extremity

I80.02   Phlebitis and thrombophlebitis of superficial vessels of left lower extremity

I80.03   Phlebitis and thrombophlebitis of superficial vessels of lower extremities, bilateral

I80.1-   Phlebitis and thrombophlebitis of femoral vein

CC I80.10   Phlebitis and thrombophlebitis of unspecified femoral vein

CC I80.11   Phlebitis and thrombophlebitis of right femoral vein

CC I80.12   Phlebitis and thrombophlebitis of left femoral vein

CC I80.13   Phlebitis and thrombophlebitis of femoral vein, bilateral

I80.2-   Phlebitis and thrombophlebitis of other and unspecified deep vessels of lower extremities

I80.20-   Phlebitis and thrombophlebitis of unspecified deep vessels of lower extremities

CC I80.201   Phlebitis and thrombophlebitis of unspecified deep vessels of right lower extremity

CC I80.202   Phlebitis and thrombophlebitis of unspecified deep vessels of left lower extremlty

CC I80.203   Phlebitis and thrombophlebitis of unspecified deep vessels of lower extremities, bilateral

CC I80.209   Phlebitis and thrombophlebitis of unspecified deep vessels of unspecified lower extremity

I80.21-   Phlebitis and thrombophlebitis of iliac vein

CC I80.211   Phlebitis and thrombophlebitis of right iliac vein

CC I80.212   Phlebitis and thrombophlebitis of left iliac vein

CC I80.213   Phlebitis and thrombophlebitis of iliac vein, bilateral

CC I80.219   Phlebitis and thrombophlebitis of unspecified iliac vein

I80.22-   Phlebitis and thrombophlebitis of popliteal vein

CC I80.221   Phlebitis and thrombophlebitis of right popliteal vein

CC I80.222   Phlebitis and thrombophlebitis of left popliteal vein

CC I80.223   Phlebitis and thrombophlebitis of popliteal vein, bilateral

CC I80.229   Phlebitis and thrombophlebitis of unspecified popliteal vein

I80.23-   Phlebitis and thrombophlebitis of tibial vein

CC I80.231   Phlebitis and thrombophlebitis of right tibial vein

CC I80.232   Phlebitis and thrombophlebitis of left tibial vein

CC I80.233   Phlebitis and thrombophlebitis of tibial vein, bilateral

CC I80.239   Phlebitis and thrombophlebitis of unspecified tibial vein

I 7 7 - I 8 0

I80.29- Phlebitis and thrombophlebitis of <u>other deep</u> vessels of <u>lower</u> extremities

  CC **I80.291** Phlebitis and thrombophlebitis of <u>other deep</u> vessels of <u>right lower</u> extremity

  CC **I80.292** Phlebitis and thrombophlebitis of <u>other deep</u> vessels of <u>left lower</u> extremity

  CC **I80.293** Phlebitis and thrombophlebitis of <u>other deep</u> vessels of <u>lower</u> extremity, <u>bilateral</u>

  CC **I80.299** Phlebitis and thrombophlebitis of <u>other deep</u> vessels of <u>unspecified lower</u> extremity

I80.3 Phlebitis and thrombophlebitis of lower extremities, unspecified

I80.8 Phlebitis and thrombophlebitis of other sites

I80.9 Phlebitis and thrombophlebitis of unspecified site

I81 **Portal vein thrombosis** — An abnormal clotting aggregation of platelets and fibrin
MCC   in the portal vein causing obstruction.
    Portal (vein) obstruction — Blocking or clogging of the portal vein due to a thrombus.
    Excludes ❷: *hepatic vein thrombosis (I82.0)*
                   phlebitis of portal vein (K75.1)

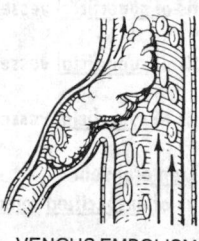 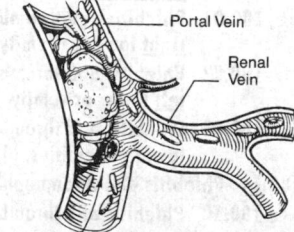

VENOUS EMBOLISM   PORTAL VEIN THROMBOSIS

I82- **Other venous embolism and thrombosis** — EMBOLISM — The blocking of a vein by a blood clot, or other substance, which has been brought to the site of obstruction by the blood flow. THROMBOSIS — An abnormal aggregation of blood factors causing an obstruction of a vein that remains in place at the site where it formed. ACUTE — A current episode with the sudden onset of symptoms. CHRONIC — A form that is not diagnosed as an acute episode (but often has had a previous acute episode) that is now being treated for the existing, non-acute condition.
  Code first venous embolism and thrombosis complicating:
    Abortion, ectopic or molar pregnancy (O00-O07, O08.7)
    Pregnancy, childbirth and the puerperium (O22-, O87-)
  Excludes ❷: *venous embolism and thrombosis (of):*
                  cerebral (I63.6, I67.6)
                  coronary (I21-I25)
                  intracranial and intraspinal, septic or NOS (G08)
                  intracranial, nonpyogenic (I67.6)
                  intraspinal, nonpyogenic (G95.1)
                  mesenteric (K55.0-)
                  portal (I81)
                  pulmonary (I26.-)

MCC **I82.0** **Budd-Chiari syndrome** — The symptomatic obstruction or occlusion of the hepatic veins (usually of unknown origin) causing enlargement and tenderness of the liver.
    Hepatic vein thrombosis — Formation of a thrombus in the hepatic vein causing obstruction.

CC **I82.1** **Thrombophlebitis migrans** — A recurring phlebitis affecting superficial peripheral veins and sometimes major and visceral veins.

I82.2- **Embolism and thrombosis of vena cava and other thoracic veins**

  I82.21- Embolism and thrombosis of <u>superior</u> vena cava

    CC **I82.210** <u>Acute</u> embolism and thrombosis of superior vena cava
          Embolism and thrombosis of superior vena cava NOS

    CC **I82.211** <u>Chronic</u> embolism and thrombosis of superior vena cava

  I82.22- Embolism and thrombosis of <u>inferior</u> vena cava

    MCC **I82.220** <u>Acute</u> embolism and thrombosis of inferior vena cava
          Embolism and thrombosis of inferior vena cava NOS

    MCC **I82.221** <u>Chronic</u> embolism and thrombosis of inferior vena cava

I82.29- Embolism and thrombosis of <u>other thoracic</u> veins
    Embolism and thrombosis of brachiocephalic (innominate) vein

  CC **I82.290** <u>Acute</u> embolism and thrombosis of other thoracic veins

  CC **I82.291** <u>Chronic</u> embolism and thrombosis of other thoracic veins

CC **I82.3** Embolism and thrombosis of renal vein

I82.4- <u>Acute</u> embolism and thrombosis of <u>deep veins</u> of <u>lower extremity</u>

  I82.40- Acute embolism and thrombosis of <u>unspecified deep</u> veins of lower extremity
    Deep vein thrombosis NOS
    DVT NOS
    Excludes 1:   *acute embolism and thrombosis of unspecified deep veins of distal lower extremity (I82.4Z-)*
                  acute embolism and thrombosis of unspecified deep veins of proximal lower extremity (I82.4Y-)

    CC **I82.401** Acute embolism and thrombosis of <u>unspecified deep</u> veins of <u>right</u> lower extremity

    CC **I82.402** Acute embolism and thrombosis of <u>unspecified deep</u> veins of <u>left</u> lower extremity

    CC **I82.403** Acute embolism and thrombosis of <u>unspecified deep</u> veins of lower extremity, <u>bilateral</u>

    CC **I82.409** Acute embolism and thrombosis of <u>unspecified deep</u> veins of <u>unspecified</u> lower extremity

  I82.41- Acute embolism and thrombosis of <u>femoral</u> vein

    CC **I82.411** Acute embolism and thrombosis of <u>right femoral</u> vein

    CC **I82.412** Acute embolism and thrombosis of <u>left femoral</u> vein

    CC **I82.413** Acute embolism and thrombosis of <u>femoral</u> vein, <u>bilateral</u>

    CC **I82.419** Acute embolism and thrombosis of <u>unspecified femoral</u> vein

  I82.42- Acute embolism and thrombosis of <u>iliac</u> vein

    CC **I82.421** Acute embolism and thrombosis of <u>right iliac</u> vein

    CC **I82.422** Acute embolism and thrombosis of <u>left iliac</u> vein

    CC **I82.423** Acute embolism and thrombosis of <u>iliac</u> vein, <u>bilateral</u>

    CC **I82.429** Acute embolism and thrombosis of <u>unspecified iliac</u> vein

  I82.43- Acute embolism and thrombosis of <u>popliteal</u> vein

    CC **I82.431** Acute embolism and thrombosis of <u>right popliteal</u> vein

    CC **I82.432** Acute embolism and thrombosis of <u>left popliteal</u> vein

    CC **I82.433** Acute embolism and thrombosis of <u>popliteal</u> vein, <u>bilateral</u>

    CC **I82.439** Acute embolism and thrombosis of <u>unspecified popliteal</u> vein

  I82.44- Acute embolism and thrombosis of <u>tibial</u> vein

    CC **I82.441** Acute embolism and thrombosis of <u>right tibial</u> vein

    CC **I82.442** Acute embolism and thrombosis of <u>left tibial</u> vein

    CC **I82.443** Acute embolism and thrombosis of <u>tibial</u> vein, <u>bilateral</u>

    CC **I82.449** Acute embolism and thrombosis of <u>unspecified tibial</u> vein

  I82.49- Acute embolism and thrombosis of <u>other specified</u> deep vein of lower extremity

    CC **I82.491** Acute embolism and thrombosis of <u>other specified</u> deep vein of <u>right</u> lower extremity

    CC **I82.492** Acute embolism and thrombosis of <u>other specified</u> deep vein of <u>left</u> lower extremity

    CC **I82.493** Acute embolism and thrombosis of <u>other specified</u> deep vein of lower extremity, <u>bilateral</u>

    CC **I82.499** Acute embolism and thrombosis of <u>other specified</u> deep vein of <u>unspecified</u> lower extremity

I80-I82

Excludes 1: = NOT CODED HERE! (Do not code both)   **752**   *Excludes ❷:* = Not Included Here

I82.4Y- Acute embolism and thrombosis of <u>unspecified</u> deep veins of <u>proximal</u> lower extremity
Acute embolism and thrombosis of deep vein of thigh NOS
Acute embolism and thrombosis of deep vein of upper leg NOS

cc **I82.4Y1** Acute embolism and thrombosis of <u>unspecified</u> deep veins of <u>right proximal</u> lower extremity

cc **I82.4Y2** Acute embolism and thrombosis of <u>unspecified</u> deep veins of <u>left proximal</u> lower extremity

cc **I82.4Y3** Acute embolism and thrombosis of <u>unspecified</u> deep veins of <u>proximal</u> lower extremity, <u>bilateral</u>

cc **I82.4Y9** Acute embolism and thrombosis of <u>unspecified</u> deep veins of <u>unspecified proximal</u> lower extremity

I82.4Z- Acute embolism and thrombosis of <u>unspecified</u> deep veins of <u>distal</u> lower extremity
Acute embolism and thrombosis of deep vein of calf NOS
Acute embolism and thrombosis of deep vein of lower leg NOS

cc **I82.4Z1** Acute embolism and thrombosis of <u>unspecified</u> deep veins of <u>right distal</u> lower extremity

cc **I82.4Z2** Acute embolism and thrombosis of <u>unspecified</u> deep veins of <u>left distal</u> lower extremity

cc **I82.4Z3** Acute embolism and thrombosis of <u>unspecified</u> deep veins of <u>distal</u> lower extremity, <u>bilateral</u>

cc **I82.4Z9** Acute embolism and thrombosis of <u>unspecified</u> deep veins of <u>unspecified distal</u> lower extremity

I82.5- <u>Chronic</u> embolism and thrombosis of deep veins of lower extremity
Use additional code, if applicable, for associated long-term (current) use of anticoagulants (Z79.01)
Excludes 1: *personal history of venous embolism and thrombosis (Z86.718)*

I82.50- <u>Chronic</u> embolism and thrombosis of <u>unspecified deep</u> veins of lower extremity
Excludes 1: *chronic embolism and thrombosis of unspecified deep veins of distal lower extremity (I82.5Z-)*
chronic embolism and thrombosis of unspecified deep veins of proximal lower extremity (I82.5Y-)

cc **I82.501** <u>Chronic</u> embolism and thrombosis of <u>unspecified</u> <u>deep</u> veins of <u>right</u> lower extremity

cc **I82.502** <u>Chronic</u> embolism and thrombosis of <u>unspecified</u> <u>deep</u> veins of <u>left</u> lower extremity

cc **I82.503** <u>Chronic</u> embolism and thrombosis of <u>unspecified</u> <u>deep</u> veins of lower extremity, <u>bilateral</u>

cc **I82.509** <u>Chronic</u> embolism and thrombosis of <u>unspecified</u> <u>deep</u> veins of <u>unspecified</u> lower extremity

I82.51- <u>Chronic</u> embolism and thrombosis of <u>femoral</u> vein

cc **I82.511** <u>Chronic</u> embolism and thrombosis of <u>right femoral</u> vein

cc **I82.512** <u>Chronic</u> embolism and thrombosis of <u>left femoral</u> vein

cc **I82.513** <u>Chronic</u> embolism and thrombosis of <u>femoral</u> vein, <u>bilateral</u>

cc **I82.519** <u>Chronic</u> embolism and thrombosis of <u>unspecified</u> <u>femoral</u> vein

I82.52- <u>Chronic</u> embolism and thrombosis of <u>iliac</u> vein

cc **I82.521** <u>Chronic</u> embolism and thrombosis of <u>right iliac</u> vein

cc **I82.522** <u>Chronic</u> embolism and thrombosis of <u>left iliac</u> vein

cc **I82.523** <u>Chronic</u> embolism and thrombosis of <u>iliac</u> vein, <u>bilateral</u>

cc **I82.529** <u>Chronic</u> embolism and thrombosis of <u>unspecified</u> <u>iliac</u> vein

I82.53- <u>Chronic</u> embolism and thrombosis of <u>popliteal</u> vein

cc **I82.531** <u>Chronic</u> embolism and thrombosis of <u>right popliteal</u> vein

cc **I82.532** <u>Chronic</u> embolism and thrombosis of <u>left popliteal</u> vein

cc **I82.533** <u>Chronic</u> embolism and thrombosis of <u>popliteal</u> vein, <u>bilateral</u>

cc **I82.539** <u>Chronic</u> embolism and thrombosis of <u>unspecified</u> <u>popliteal</u> vein

I82.54- <u>Chronic</u> embolism and thrombosis of <u>tibial</u> vein

cc **I82.541** <u>Chronic</u> embolism and thrombosis of <u>right tibial</u> vein

cc **I82.542** <u>Chronic</u> embolism and thrombosis of <u>left tibial</u> vein

cc **I82.543** <u>Chronic</u> embolism and thrombosis of <u>tibial</u> vein, <u>bilateral</u>

cc **I82.549** <u>Chronic</u> embolism and thrombosis of <u>unspecified</u> <u>tibial</u> vein

I82.59- <u>Chronic</u> embolism and thrombosis of <u>other specified</u> deep vein of lower extremity

cc **I82.591** <u>Chronic</u> embolism and thrombosis of <u>other</u> <u>specified</u> deep vein of <u>right</u> lower extremity

cc **I82.592** <u>Chronic</u> embolism and thrombosis of <u>other</u> <u>specified</u> deep vein of <u>left</u> lower extremity

cc **I82.593** <u>Chronic</u> embolism and thrombosis of <u>other</u> <u>specified</u> deep vein of lower extremity, <u>bilateral</u>

cc **I82.599** <u>Chronic</u> embolism and thrombosis of <u>other</u> <u>specified</u> deep vein of <u>unspecified</u> lower extremity

I82.5Y- <u>Chronic</u> embolism and thrombosis of <u>unspecified deep</u> veins of <u>proximal</u> lower extremity
Chronic embolism and thrombosis of deep veins of thigh NOS
Chronic embolism and thrombosis of deep veins of upper leg NOS

cc **I82.5Y1** <u>Chronic</u> embolism and thrombosis of <u>unspecified</u> <u>deep</u> veins of <u>right proximal</u> lower extremity

cc **I82.5Y2** <u>Chronic</u> embolism and thrombosis of <u>unspecified</u> <u>deep</u> veins of <u>left proximal</u> lower extremity

cc **I82.5Y3** <u>Chronic</u> embolism and thrombosis of <u>unspecified</u> <u>deep</u> veins of <u>proximal</u> lower extremity, <u>bilateral</u>

cc **I82.5Y9** <u>Chronic</u> embolism and thrombosis of <u>unspecified</u> <u>deep</u> veins of <u>unspecified proximal</u> lower extremity

I82.5Z- <u>Chronic</u> embolism and thrombosis of <u>unspecified deep</u> veins of <u>distal</u> lower extremity
Chronic embolism and thrombosis of deep veins of calf NOS
Chronic embolism and thrombosis of deep veins of lower leg NOS

cc **I82.5Z1** <u>Chronic</u> embolism and thrombosis of <u>unspecified</u> <u>deep</u> veins of <u>right distal</u> lower extremity

cc **I82.5Z2** <u>Chronic</u> embolism and thrombosis of <u>unspecified</u> <u>deep</u> veins of <u>left distal</u> lower extremity

cc **I82.5Z3** <u>Chronic</u> embolism and thrombosis of <u>unspecified</u> <u>deep</u> veins of <u>distal</u> lower extremity, bilateral

cc **I82.5Z9** <u>Chronic</u> embolism and thrombosis of <u>unspecified</u> deep veins of unspecified <u>distal</u> lower extremity

I82.6- Acute embolism and thrombosis of <u>veins</u> of <u>upper extremity</u>

I82.60- <u>Acute</u> embolism and thrombosis of <u>unspecified</u> veins of <u>upper</u> extremity

cc **I82.601** Acute embolism and thrombosis of <u>unspecified</u> veins of <u>right</u> upper extremity

cc **I82.602** Acute embolism and thrombosis of <u>unspecified</u> veins of <u>left</u> upper extremity

cc **I82.603** Acute embolism and thrombosis of <u>unspecified</u> veins of upper extremity, <u>bilateral</u>

cc **I82.609** Acute embolism and thrombosis of <u>unspecified</u> veins of <u>unspecified</u> upper extremity

I82.61- Acute embolism and thrombosis of <u>superficial</u> veins of <u>upper</u> extremity
Acute embolism and thrombosis of antecubital vein
Acute embolism and thrombosis of basilic vein
Acute embolism and thrombosis of cephalic vein

cc **I82.611** Acute embolism and thrombosis of <u>superficial</u> veins of <u>right</u> upper extremity

cc **I82.612** Acute embolism and thrombosis of <u>superficial</u> veins of <u>left</u> upper extremity

cc **I82.613** Acute embolism and thrombosis of <u>superficial</u> veins of upper extremity, <u>bilateral</u>

cc **I82.619** Acute embolism and thrombosis of <u>superficial</u> veins of <u>unspecified</u> upper extremity

I82 - I82

I82.62- Acute embolism and thrombosis of <u>deep</u> veins of <u>upper</u> extremity
   Acute embolism and thrombosis of brachial vein
   Acute embolism and thrombosis of radial vein
   Acute embolism and thrombosis of ulnar vein

cc **I82.621** Acute embolism and thrombosis of <u>deep</u> veins of <u>right</u> upper extremity

cc **I82.622** Acute embolism and thrombosis of <u>deep</u> veins of <u>left</u> upper extremity

cc **I82.623** Acute embolism and thrombosis of <u>deep</u> veins of upper extremity, <u>bilateral</u>

cc **I82.629** Acute embolism and thrombosis of <u>deep</u> veins of <u>unspecified</u> upper extremity

I82.7- <u>Chronic</u> embolism and thrombosis of veins of <u>upper</u> extremity
   Use additional code, if applicable, for associated long-term (current) use of anticoagulants (Z79.01)
   Excludes 1:   personal history of venous embolism and thrombosis (Z86.718)

I82.70- <u>Chronic</u> embolism and thrombosis of <u>unspecified</u> veins of <u>upper</u> extremity

cc **I82.701** <u>Chronic</u> embolism and thrombosis of <u>unspecified</u> veins of <u>right</u> upper extremity

cc **I82.702** <u>Chronic</u> embolism and thrombosis of <u>unspecified</u> veins of <u>left</u> upper extremity

cc **I82.703** <u>Chronic</u> embolism and thrombosis of <u>unspecified</u> veins of upper extremity, <u>bilateral</u>

cc **I82.709** <u>Chronic</u> embolism and thrombosis of <u>unspecified</u> veins of <u>unspecified</u> upper extremity

I82.71- <u>Chronic</u> embolism and thrombosis of <u>superficial</u> veins of <u>upper</u> extremity
   Chronic embolism and thrombosis of antecubital vein
   Chronic embolism and thrombosis of basilic vein
   Chronic embolism and thrombosis of cephalic vein

cc **I82.711** <u>Chronic</u> embolism and thrombosis of <u>superficial</u> veins of <u>right</u> upper extremity

cc **I82.712** <u>Chronic</u> embolism and thrombosis of <u>superficial</u> veins of <u>left</u> upper extremity

cc **I82.713** <u>Chronic</u> embolism and thrombosis of <u>superficial</u> veins of upper extremity, <u>bilateral</u>

cc **I82.719** <u>Chronic</u> embolism and thrombosis of <u>superficial</u> veins of <u>unspecified</u> upper extremity

I82.72- <u>Chronic</u> embolism and thrombosis of <u>deep</u> veins of <u>upper</u> extremity
   Chronic embolism and thrombosis of brachial vein
   Chronic embolism and thrombosis of radial vein
   Chronic embolism and thrombosis of ulnar vein

cc **I82.721** <u>Chronic</u> embolism and thrombosis of <u>deep</u> veins of <u>right</u> upper extremity

cc **I82.722** <u>Chronic</u> embolism and thrombosis of <u>deep</u> veins of <u>left</u> upper extremity

cc **I82.723** <u>Chronic</u> embolism and thrombosis of <u>deep</u> veins of upper extremity, <u>bilateral</u>

cc **I82.729** Chronic embolism and thrombosis of <u>deep</u> veins of <u>unspecified</u> upper extremity

I82.A- Embolism and thrombosis of axillary vein

I82.A1- <u>Acute</u> embolism and thrombosis of <u>axillary</u> vein

cc **I82.A11** Acute embolism and thrombosis of <u>right axillary</u> vein

cc **I82.A12** Acute embolism and thrombosis of <u>left axillary</u> vein

cc **I82.A13** Acute embolism and thrombosis of <u>axillary</u> vein, <u>bilateral</u>

cc **I82.A19** Acute embolism and thrombosis of <u>unspecified</u> <u>axillary</u> vein

I82.A2- <u>Chronic</u> embolism and thrombosis of <u>axillary</u> vein

cc **I82.A21** <u>Chronic</u> embolism and thrombosis of <u>right axillary</u> vein

cc **I82.A22** <u>Chronic</u> embolism and thrombosis of <u>left axillary</u> vein

cc **I82.A23** <u>Chronic</u> embolism and thrombosis of <u>axillary</u> vein, <u>bilateral</u>

cc **I82.A29** <u>Chronic</u> embolism and thrombosis of <u>unspecified</u> <u>axillary</u> vein

I82.B- Embolism and thrombosis of <u>subclavian</u> vein

I82.B1- <u>Acute</u> embolism and thrombosis of <u>subclavian</u> vein

cc **I82.B11** Acute embolism and thrombosis of <u>right subclavian</u> vein

cc **I82.B12** Acute embolism and thrombosis of <u>left subclavian</u> vein

cc **I82.B13** Acute embolism and thrombosis of <u>subclavian</u> vein, <u>bilateral</u>

cc **I82.B19** Acute embolism and thrombosis of <u>unspecified</u> <u>subclavian</u> vein

I82.B2- <u>Chronic</u> embolism and thrombosis of <u>subclavian</u> vein

cc **I82.B21** <u>Chronic</u> embolism and thrombosis of <u>right</u> <u>subclavian</u> vein

cc **I82.B22** <u>Chronic</u> embolism and thrombosis of <u>left</u> <u>subclavian</u> vein

cc **I82.B23** <u>Chronic</u> embolism and thrombosis of <u>subclavian</u> vein, <u>bilateral</u>

cc **I82.B29** <u>Chronic</u> embolism and thrombosis of <u>unspecified</u> <u>subclavian</u> vein

I82.C- Embolism and thrombosis of <u>internal jugular</u> vein

I82.C1- <u>Acute</u> embolism and thrombosis of <u>internal jugular</u> vein

cc **I82.C11** Acute embolism and thrombosis of <u>right internal jugular</u> vein

cc **I82.C12** Acute embolism and thrombosis of <u>left internal jugular</u> vein

cc **I82.C13** Acute embolism and thrombosis of <u>internal jugular</u> vein, <u>bilateral</u>

cc **I82.C19** Acute embolism and thrombosis of <u>unspecified</u> <u>internal jugular</u> vein

I82.C2- <u>Chronic</u> embolism and thrombosis of <u>internal jugular</u> vein

cc **I82.C21** <u>Chronic</u> embolism and thrombosis of <u>right internal jugular</u> vein

cc **I82.C22** <u>Chronic</u> embolism and thrombosis of <u>left internal jugular</u> vein

cc **I82.C23** <u>Chronic</u> embolism and thrombosis of <u>internal jugular</u> vein, <u>bilateral</u>

cc **I82.C29** <u>Chronic</u> embolism and thrombosis of <u>unspecified</u> <u>internal jugular</u> vein

I82.8- Embolism and thrombosis of <u>other specified veins</u>
   Use additional code, if applicable, for associated long-term (current) use of anticoagulants (Z79.01)

I82.81- Embolism and thrombosis of <u>superficial</u> veins of <u>lower</u> extremities
   Embolism and thrombosis of saphenous vein (greater) (lesser)

cc **I82.811** Embolism and thrombosis of <u>superficial</u> veins of <u>right</u> lower extremities

cc **I82.812** Embolism and thrombosis of <u>superficial</u> veins of <u>left</u> lower extremities

cc **I82.813** Embolism and thrombosis of <u>superficial</u> veins of lower extremities, <u>bilateral</u>

cc **I82.819** Embolism and thrombosis of <u>superficial</u> veins of <u>unspecified</u> lower extremities

I82.89- Embolism and thrombosis of <u>other specified veins</u>

cc **I82.890** <u>Acute</u> embolism and thrombosis of other specified veins

cc **I82.891** <u>Chronic</u> embolism and thrombosis of other specified veins

I82.9- Embolism and thrombosis of <u>unspecified</u> vein

cc **I82.90** <u>Acute</u> embolism and thrombosis of unspecified vein
   Embolism of vein NOS
   Thrombosis (vein) NOS

cc **I82.91** <u>Chronic</u> embolism and thrombosis of unspecified vein

I82
–
I82

Excludes 1: = NOT CODED HERE! (Do not code both)   **754**   *Excludes ❷:* = Not Included Here

I83- <u>Varicose veins</u> of <u>lower</u> extremities — Dilatated, tortuous superficial veins of the legs.

Excludes 1:   *varicose veins complicating pregnancy (O22.0-)*
varicose veins complicating the puerperium (O87.4)

I83.0- <u>Varicose veins</u> of <u>lower extremities</u> <u>with ulcer</u> — A form characterized by the sloughing of inflammatory necrotic tissue at the varicose vein site.
Use additional code to identify severity of ulcer (L97.-)

I83.00- Varicose veins of <u>unspecified</u> lower extremity with ulcer

I83.001   Varicose veins of <u>unspecified</u> lower extremity <u>with</u> <u>ulcer</u> of <u>thigh</u> — [Age/15-124]

I83.002   Varicose veins of <u>unspecified</u> lower extremity <u>with</u> <u>ulcer</u> of <u>calf</u> — [Age/15-124]

I83.003   Varicose veins of <u>unspecified</u> lower extremity <u>with</u> <u>ulcer</u> of <u>ankle</u> — [Age/15-124]

I83.004   Varicose veins of <u>unspecified</u> lower extremity <u>with</u> <u>ulcer</u> of <u>heel and midfoot</u> — [Age/15-124]
Varicose veins of unspecified lower extremity with ulcer of plantar surface of midfoot

I83.005   Varicose veins of <u>unspecified</u> lower extremity <u>with</u> <u>ulcer</u> <u>other part of foot</u> — [Age/15-124]
Varicose veins of unspecified lower extremity with ulcer of toe

I83.008   Varicose veins of <u>unspecified</u> lower extremity <u>with</u> <u>ulcer other part of lower leg</u> — [Age/15-124]

I83.009   Varicose veins of <u>unspecified</u> lower extremity <u>with</u> <u>ulcer</u> of <u>unspecified site</u> — [Age/15-124]

I83.01- Varicose veins of <u>right</u> lower extremity <u>with ulcer</u>

I83.011   Varicose veins of <u>right</u> lower extremity <u>with ulcer</u> of <u>thigh</u> — [Age/15-124]

I83.012   Varicose veins of <u>right</u> lower extremity <u>with ulcer</u> of <u>calf</u> — [Age/15-124]

I83.013   Varicose veins of <u>right</u> lower extremity <u>with ulcer</u> of <u>ankle</u> — [Age/15-124]

I83.014   Varicose veins of <u>right</u> lower extremity <u>with ulcer</u> of <u>heel and midfoot</u> — [Age/15-124]
Varicose veins of right lower extremity with ulcer of plantar surface of midfoot

I83.015   Varicose veins of <u>right</u> lower extremity <u>with ulcer</u> <u>other part of foot</u> — [Age/15-124]
Varicose veins of right lower extremity with ulcer of toe

I83.018   Varicose veins of <u>right</u> lower extremity <u>with ulcer</u> <u>other part of lower leg</u> — [Age/15-124]

I83.019   Varicose veins of <u>right</u> lower extremity <u>with ulcer</u> of <u>unspecified site</u> — [Age/15-124]

I83.02- Varicose veins of <u>left</u> lower extremity <u>with ulcer</u>

I83.021   Varicose veins of <u>left</u> lower extremity <u>with ulcer</u> of <u>thigh</u> — [Age/15-124]

I83.022   Varicose veins of <u>left</u> lower extremity <u>with ulcer</u> of <u>calf</u> — [Age/15-124]

I83.023   Varicose veins of <u>left</u> lower extremity <u>with ulcer</u> of <u>ankle</u> — [Age/15-124]

I83.024   Varicose veins of <u>left</u> lower extremity <u>with ulcer</u> of <u>heel and midfoot</u> — [Age/15-124]
Varicose veins of left lower extremity with ulcer of plantar surface of midfoot

I83.025   Varicose veins of <u>left</u> lower extremity <u>with ulcer</u> <u>other part of foot</u> — [Age/15-124]
Varicose veins of left lower extremity with ulcer of toe

I83.028   Varicose veins of <u>left</u> lower extremity <u>with ulcer</u> <u>other part of lower leg</u> — [Age/15-124]

I83.029   Varicose veins of <u>left</u> lower extremity <u>with ulcer</u> of <u>unspecified site</u> — [Age/15-124]

I83.1- <u>Varicose veins</u> of <u>lower extremities</u> <u>with inflammation</u> — A form characterized by massive tissue reaction and swelling.

I83.10   Varicose veins of <u>unspecified</u> lower extremity <u>with inflammation</u> — [Age/15-124]

I83.11   Varicose veins of <u>right</u> lower extremity <u>with inflammation</u> — [Age/15-124]

I83.12   Varicose veins of <u>left</u> lower extremity <u>with inflammation</u> — [Age/15-124]

I83.2- <u>Varicose veins</u> of <u>lower extremities</u> <u>with both ulcer and inflammation</u> — A form characterized by the sloughing of inflammatory necrotic tissue at the varicose vein site and inflammatory massive tissue reaction and swelling.
Use additional code to identify severity of ulcer (L97.-)

I83.20- Varicose veins of <u>unspecified</u> lower extremity <u>with both ulcer and inflammation</u>

cc **I83.201**   Varicose veins of <u>unspecified</u> lower extremity <u>with both ulcer</u> of <u>thigh</u> and <u>inflammation</u> — [Age/15-124]

cc **I83.202**   Varicose veins of <u>unspecified</u> lower extremity <u>with both ulcer</u> of <u>calf</u> and <u>inflammation</u> — [Age/15-124]

cc **I83.203**   Varicose veins of <u>unspecified</u> lower extremity <u>with both ulcer</u> of <u>ankle</u> and <u>inflammation</u> — [Age/15-124]

cc **I83.204**   Varicose veins of <u>unspecified</u> lower extremity <u>with both ulcer</u> of <u>heel and midfoot</u> and <u>inflammation</u> — [Age/15-124]
Varicose veins of unspecified lower extremity with both ulcer of plantar surface of midfoot and inflammation

cc **I83.205**   Varicose veins of <u>unspecified</u> lower extremity <u>with both ulcer</u> <u>other part of foot</u> and <u>inflammation</u> — [Age/15-124]
Varicose veins of unspecified lower extremity with both ulcer of toe and inflammation

cc **I83.208**   Varicose veins of <u>unspecified</u> lower extremity <u>with both ulcer</u> of <u>other part of lower extremity</u> and <u>inflammation</u> — [Age/15-124]

cc **I83.209**   Varicose veins of unspecified lower extremity <u>with both ulcer</u> of <u>unspecified site</u> and <u>inflammation</u> — [Age/15-124]

I83.21- Varicose veins of <u>right</u> lower extremity <u>with both ulcer and inflammation</u>

cc **I83.211**   Varicose veins of <u>right</u> lower extremity <u>with both ulcer</u> of <u>thigh</u> and <u>inflammation</u> — [Age/15-124]

cc **I83.212**   Varicose veins of <u>right</u> lower extremity <u>with both ulcer</u> of <u>calf</u> and <u>inflammation</u> — [Age/15-124]

cc **I83.213**   Varicose veins of <u>right</u> lower extremity <u>with both ulcer</u> of <u>ankle</u> and <u>inflammation</u> — [Age/15-124]

cc **I83.214**   Varicose veins of <u>right</u> lower extremity <u>with both ulcer</u> of <u>heel and midfoot</u> and <u>inflammation</u> — [Age/15-124]
Varicose veins of right lower extremity with both ulcer of plantar surface of midfoot and inflammation

cc **I83.215**   Varicose veins of <u>right</u> lower extremity <u>with both ulcer</u> <u>other part of foot</u> and <u>inflammation</u> — [Age/15-124]
Varicose veins of right lower extremity with both ulcer of toe and inflammation

cc **I83.218**   Varicose veins of <u>right</u> lower extremity <u>with both ulcer</u> of <u>other part of lower extremity</u> and <u>inflammation</u> — [Age/15-124]

cc **I83.219**   Varicose veins of <u>right</u> lower extremity <u>with both ulcer</u> of <u>unspecified site</u> and <u>inflammation</u> — [Age/15-124]

I83.22- Varicose veins of <u>left</u> lower extremity <u>with both ulcer and inflammation</u>

cc **I83.221**   Varicose veins of <u>left</u> lower extremity <u>with both ulcer</u> of <u>thigh</u> and <u>inflammation</u> — [Age/15-124]

cc **I83.222**   Varicose veins of <u>left</u> lower extremity <u>with both ulcer</u> of <u>calf</u> and <u>inflammation</u> — [Age/15-124]

cc **I83.223**   Varicose veins of <u>left</u> lower extremity <u>with both ulcer</u> of <u>ankle</u> and <u>inflammation</u> — [Age/15-124]

cc **I83.224**   Varicose veins of <u>left</u> lower extremity <u>with both ulcer</u> of <u>heel and midfoot</u> and <u>inflammation</u> — [Age/15-124]
Varicose veins of left lower extremity with both ulcer of plantar surface of midfoot and inflammation

cc **I83.225**   Varicose veins of <u>left</u> lower extremity <u>with both ulcer</u> <u>other part of foot</u> and <u>inflammation</u> — [Age/15-124]
Varicose veins of left lower extremity with both ulcer of toe and inflammation

I83 - I83

cc **I83.228** Varicose veins of <u>left</u> lower extremity <u>with both</u> <u>ulcer</u> of <u>other part of lower extremity</u> and <u>inflammation</u> — [Age/15-124]

cc **I83.229** Varicose veins of <u>left</u> lower extremity <u>with both</u> <u>ulcer</u> of <u>unspecified site</u> and <u>inflammation</u> — [Age/15-124]

I83.8- <u>Varicose veins</u> of <u>lower extremities with other complications</u>

I83.81- Varicose veins of lower extremities <u>with pain</u>

I83.811 Varicose veins of <u>right</u> lower extremities <u>with pain</u> — [Age/15-124]

I83.812 Varicose veins of <u>left</u> lower extremities <u>with pain</u> — [Age/15-124]

I83.813 Varicose veins of <u>bilateral</u> lower extremities <u>with pain</u> — [Age/15-124]

I83.819 Varicose veins of <u>unspecified</u> lower extremities <u>with pain</u> — [Age/15-124]

I83.89- Varicose veins of lower extremities <u>with other complications</u>
Varicose veins of lower extremities with edema — The accumulation of fluid in the intercellular spaces.
Varicose veins of lower extremities with swelling — The temporary enlargement of the tissues of a lower limb.

I83.891 Varicose veins of <u>right</u> lower extremities <u>with other complications</u> — [Age/15-124]

I83.892 Varicose veins of <u>left</u> lower extremities <u>with other complications</u> — [Age/15-124]

I83.893 Varicose veins of <u>bilateral</u> lower extremities <u>with other complications</u> — [Age/15-124]

I83.899 Varicose veins of <u>unspecified</u> lower extremities <u>with other complications</u> — [Age/15-124]

I83.9- <u>Asymptomatic</u> varicose veins of lower extremities
Phlebectasia of lower extremities
Varicose veins of lower extremities
Varix of lower extremities

I83.90 Asymptomatic varicose veins of <u>unspecified</u> lower extremity — [Age/15-124]
Varicose veins NOS

I83.91 Asymptomatic varicose veins of <u>right</u> lower extremity — [Age/15-124]

I83.92 Asymptomatic varicose veins of <u>left</u> lower extremity — [Age/15-124]

I83.93 Asymptomatic varicose veins of <u>bilateral</u> lower extremities — [Age/15-124]

I85- Esophageal varices
Use additional code to identify:
Alcohol abuse and dependence (F10.-)

I85.0- Esophageal varices — Dilatated, tortuous esophageal veins.
Idiopathic esophageal varices — A form without an identifiable cause.
Primary esophageal varices — A form arising within the esophageal vein tissue that is not due to another condition or disease.

cc **I85.00** Esophageal varices <u>without</u> bleeding
Esophageal varices NOS

mcc **I85.01** Esophageal varices <u>with bleeding</u> — Dilatated, tortuous esophageal veins with escape of blood.

I85.1- <u>Secondary</u> esophageal varices — A form due to another condition or disease.
Esophageal varices secondary to alcoholic liver disease
Esophageal varices secondary to cirrhosis of liver
Esophageal varices secondary to schistosomiasis
Esophageal varices secondary to toxic liver disease
Code first underlying disease

cc **I85.10** Secondary esophageal varices <u>without</u> bleeding

mcc **I85.11** Secondary esophageal varices <u>with bleeding</u>

I86- Varicose veins of other sites
Excludes 1: *varicose veins of unspecified site (I83.9-)*
Excludes ❷: *retinal varices (H35.0-)*

I86.0 Sublingual varices — Dilatated, tortuous veins under the tongue.

I86.1 Scrotal varices — [♂] – Dilatated, tortuous veins within the scrotum.
Varicocele — A condition of dilatated, tortuous veins of the testicles and epididymides.

I86.2 Pelvic varices — Dilatated, tortuous veins within the pelvic cavity.

I86.3 Vulval varices — [♀] – Dilatated, tortuous veins of the vulva.
Excludes 1: *vulval varices complicating childbirth and the puerperium (O87.8)*
vulval varices complicating pregnancy (O22.1-)

I86.4 Gastric varices — Dilatated, tortuous stomach veins.

I86.8 Varicose veins of other specified sites — [Age/15-124]
Varicose ulcer of nasal septum

I87- Other disorders of veins

I87.0- <u>Postthrombotic syndrome</u> — Conditions resulting from the destructive effects of thrombosis, including increased pressure in the deep and superficial veins, destruction of the valves of the deep veins, and obliteration in severe cases.
Chronic venous hypertension due to deep vein thrombosis
Postphlebitic syndrome
Excludes 1: *chronic venous hypertension without deep vein thrombosis (I87.3-)*

I87.00- Postthrombotic syndrome <u>without</u> complications
Asymptomatic Postthrombotic syndrome

I87.001 Postthrombotic syndrome without complications of <u>right</u> lower extremity

I87.002 Postthrombotic syndrome without complications of <u>left</u> lower extremity

I87.003 Postthrombotic syndrome without complications of <u>bilateral</u> lower extremity

I87.009 Postthrombotic syndrome without complications of <u>unspecified</u> extremity
Postthrombotic syndrome NOS

I87.01- Postthrombotic syndrome <u>with ulcer</u> — A form with necrotic tissue sites.
Use additional code to specify site and severity of ulcer (L97.-)

cc **I87.011** Postthrombotic syndrome <u>with ulcer</u> of <u>right</u> lower extremity

cc **I87.012** Postthrombotic syndrome <u>with ulcer</u> of <u>left</u> lower extremity

cc **I87.013** Postthrombotic syndrome <u>with ulcer</u> of <u>bilateral</u> lower extremity

cc **I87.019** Postthrombotic syndrome <u>with ulcer</u> of <u>unspecified</u> lower extremity

I87.02- Postthrombotic syndrome <u>with inflammation</u> — A form characterized by massive tissue infusion and swelling.

I87.021 Postthrombotic syndrome <u>with inflammation</u> of <u>right</u> lower extremity

I87.022 Postthrombotic syndrome <u>with inflammation</u> of <u>left</u> lower extremity

I87.023 Postthrombotic syndrome <u>with inflammation</u> of <u>bilateral</u> lower extremity

I87.029 Postthrombotic syndrome <u>with inflammation</u> of <u>unspecified</u> lower extremity

I87.03- Postthrombotic syndrome <u>with ulcer and inflammation</u> — A form with necrotic tissue sites and massive tissue infusion and swelling.
Use additional code to specify site and severity of ulcer (L97.-)

cc **I87.031** Postthrombotic syndrome <u>with ulcer and inflammation</u> of <u>right</u> lower extremity

cc **I87.032** Postthrombotic syndrome <u>with ulcer and inflammation</u> of <u>left</u> lower extremity

cc **I87.033** Postthrombotic syndrome <u>with ulcer and inflammation</u> of <u>bilateral</u> lower extremity

cc **I87.039** Postthrombotic syndrome <u>with ulcer and inflammation</u> of <u>unspecified</u> lower extremity

I87.09- Postthrombotic syndrome <u>with other complications</u>

I87.091 Postthrombotic syndrome <u>with other complications</u> of <u>right</u> lower extremity

I87.092 Postthrombotic syndrome <u>with other complications</u> of <u>left</u> lower extremity

I87.093 Postthrombotic syndrome <u>with other complications</u> of <u>bilateral</u> lower extremity

I87.099 Postthrombotic syndrome <u>with other complications</u> of <u>unspecified</u> lower extremity

I83 - I87

cc **I87.1** **Compression of vein** — The collapsing walls of a vein due to excessive external pressure around the vein.
>> **Stricture of vein** — Narrowing of the vein's lumen.
>> **Vena cava syndrome (inferior) (superior)** — Compression of the vena cava (usually superior) resulting in edema of the face, neck, and upper arm.
>> *Excludes ❷: compression of pulmonary vein (I28.8)*

I87.2 **Venous insufficiency (chronic) (peripheral)** — Impairment of the venous return, often due to defective venous valves.
>> **Stasis dermatitis** — Eczema and edema of the legs due to varicose veins.
>> *Excludes 1: stasis dermatitis with varicose veins of lower extremities (I83.1-, I83.2-)*

I87.3- **Chronic venous hypertension (idiopathic)** — Increased venous blood pressure in the deep and superficial veins that is not due to deep vein thrombosis.
>> **Stasis edema**
>> *Excludes 1: chronic venous hypertension due to deep vein thrombosis (I87.0-)*
>> *varicose veins of lower extremities (I83.-)*

I87.30- **Chronic venous hypertension (idiopathic) without complications**
>> **Asymptomatic chronic venous hypertension (idiopathic)**

I87.301 **Chronic venous hypertension (idiopathic) without complications of right lower extremity**

I87.302 **Chronic venous hypertension (idiopathic) without complications of left lower extremity**

I87.303 **Chronic venous hypertension (idiopathic) without complications of bilateral lower extremity**

I87.309 **Chronic venous hypertension (idiopathic) without complications of unspecified lower extremity**
>> **Chronic venous hypertension NOS**

I87.31- **Chronic venous hypertension (idiopathic) with ulcer** — A form with necrotic tissue sites.
>> **Use additional code to specify site and severity of ulcer (L97.-)**

cc **I87.311** **Chronic venous hypertension (idiopathic) with ulcer of right lower extremity**

cc **I87.312** **Chronic venous hypertension (idiopathic) with ulcer of left lower extremity**

cc **I87.313** **Chronic venous hypertension (idiopathic) with ulcer of bilateral lower extremity**

cc **I87.319** **Chronic venous hypertension (idiopathic) with ulcer of unspecified lower extremity**

I87.32- **Chronic venous hypertension (idiopathic) with inflammation** — A form characterized by massive tissue infusion and swelling.

I87.321 **Chronic venous hypertension (idiopathic) with inflammation of right lower extremity**

I87.322 **Chronic venous hypertension (idiopathic) with inflammation of left lower extremity**

I87.323 **Chronic venous hypertension (idiopathic) with inflammation of bilateral lower extremity**

I87.329 **Chronic venous hypertension (idiopathic) with inflammation of unspecified lower extremity**

I87.33- **Chronic venous hypertension (idiopathic) with ulcer and inflammation** — A form with necrotic tissue sites and massive tissue infusion and swelling.
>> **Use additional code to specify site and severity of ulcer (L97.-)**

cc **I87.331** **Chronic venous hypertension (idiopathic) with ulcer and inflammation of right lower extremity**

cc **I87.332** **Chronic venous hypertension (idiopathic) with ulcer and inflammation of left lower extremity**

cc **I87.333** **Chronic venous hypertension (idiopathic) with ulcer and inflammation of bilateral lower extremity**

cc **I87.339** **Chronic venous hypertension (idiopathic) with ulcer and inflammation of unspecified lower extremity**

I87.39- **Chronic venous hypertension (idiopathic) with other complications**

I87.391 **Chronic venous hypertension (idiopathic) with other complications of right lower extremity**

I87.392 **Chronic venous hypertension (idiopathic) with other complications of left lower extremity**

I87.393 **Chronic venous hypertension (idiopathic) with other complications of bilateral lower extremity**

I87.399 **Chronic venous hypertension (idiopathic) with other complications of unspecified lower extremity**

I87.8 **Other specified disorders of veins**
>> **Phlebosclerosis**
>> **Venofibrosis**

I87.9 **Disorder of vein, unspecified**

I88- **Nonspecific lymphadenitis** — Inflammation of lymph tissue causing mild swelling, pain, and tenderness.
>> *Excludes 1: acute lymphadenitis, except mesenteric (L04.-)*
>> *enlarged lymph nodes NOS (R59.-)*
>> *human immunodeficiency virus [HIV] disease resulting in generalized lymphadenopathy (B20)*

I88.0 **Nonspecific mesenteric lymphadenitis** — A form affecting the mesenteric (abdominal cavity) lymph nodes.
>> **Mesenteric lymphadenitis (acute) (chronic)**

I88.1 **Chronic lymphadenitis, except mesenteric** — A form that develops and persists over a relatively long period of time.
>> **Adenitis**
>> **Lymphadenitis**

I88.8 **Other nonspecific lymphadenitis**

I88.9 **Nonspecific lymphadenitis, unspecified**
>> **Lymphadenitis NOS**

I89- **Other noninfective disorders of lymphatic vessels and lymph nodes**
>> *Excludes 1: chylocele, tunica vaginalis (nonfilarial) NOS (N50.89)*
>> *enlarged lymph nodes NOS (R59.-)*
>> *filarial chylocele (B74.-)*
>> *hereditary lymphedema (Q82.0)*

I89.0 **Lymphedema, not elsewhere classified** — Accumulation of interstitial fluid of the lymphatic system.
>> **Elephantiasis (nonfilarial) NOS** — Edema and enlargement of an area due to lymphatic obstruction.
>> **Lymphangiectasis** — Dilatation of the lymphatic vessels.
>> **Obliteration, lymphatic vessel** — The complete destruction of a lymphatic vessel.
>> **Praecox lymphedema** — Puffiness and swelling of the lower limbs seen in girls at or near puberty.
>> **Secondary lymphedema** — Accumulation of interstitial fluid due to secondary obstruction of the lymphatic system.
>> *Excludes 1: postmastectomy lymphedema (I97.2)*

I89.1 **Lymphangitis** — Inflammation of the lymph vessels.
>> **Chronic lymphangitis**
>> **Lymphangitis NOS**
>> **Subacute lymphangitis**
>> *Excludes 1: acute lymphangitis (L03.-)*

I89.8 **Other specified noninfective disorders of lymphatic vessels and lymph nodes**
>> **Chylocele (nonfilarial)** — Severe, massive edema encapsulated by a sac.
>> **Chylous ascites** — The abnormal presence of chyle (triglycerides suspended in water) in the peritoneal cavity.
>> **Chylous cyst** — An abnormal mesenteric sac filled with chyle.
>> **Lipomelanotic reticulosis** — Lymph node hyperplasia of the reticular cells.
>> **Lymph node or vessel fistula** — An abnormal passage of chyle from a lymph duct.
>> **Lymph node or vessel infarction** — A localized area of necrosis due to the massive accumulation of chyle.
>> **Lymph node or vessel rupture** — A forcible tearing of the thoracic duct leaving chyle.

I89.9 **Noninfective disorder of lymphatic vessels and lymph nodes, unspecified**
>> **Disease of lymphatic vessels NOS**

I87 - I89

Other and unspecified disorders of the circulatory system (I95-I99)

I95- **Hypotension** — Abnormally low blood pressure.
Excludes 1:   cardiovascular collapse (R57.9)
maternal hypotension syndrome (O26.5-)
nonspecific low blood pressure reading NOS (R03.1)

I95.0 **Idiopathic hypotension** — A form of unknown etiology.

I95.1 **Orthostatic hypotension** — Syncope, or near syncope, due to abnormally low blood pressure when the person stands up.
Hypotension, postural
Excludes 1:   neurogenic orthostatic hypotension [Shy-Drager] (G90.3)
orthostatic hypotension due to drugs (I95.2)

I95.2 **Hypotension** <u>due to drugs</u>
Orthostatic hypotension due to drugs
Use additional code for adverse effect, if applicable, to identify drug (T36-T50 with fifth or sixth character 5)

I95.3 **Hypotension** <u>of hemodialysis</u> — A form occurring during, or as a result of, hemodialysis.
Intra-dialytic hypotension

I95.8- **Other hypotension**

I95.81 **Postprocedural hypotension** — A form occurring postoperatively.

I95.89 **Other hypotension**
Chronic hypotension

I95.9 **Hypotension, unspecified**

I96 **Gangrene,** <u>not elsewhere classified</u> — The death of tissue that is usually due to
cc   a loss of vascular supply.
AHA 13:2Q:p34 – Warfarin induced skin necrosis
Gangrenous cellulitis
Excludes 1:   gangrene in atherosclerosis of native arteries of the extremities (I70.26)
gangrene in diabetes mellitus (E08-E13 with .52)
gangrene in hernia (K40.1, K40.4, K41.1, K41.4, K42.1, K43.1-, K44.1, K45.1, K46.1)
gangrene in other peripheral vascular diseases (I73-)
gangrene of certain specified sites — see Alphabetical Index
gas gangrene (A48.0)
pyoderma gangrenosum (L88)

I97- <u>Intraoperative and postprocedural complications</u> and disorders of circulatory system, not elsewhere classified
Excludes 2:   postprocedural shock (T81.1-)

I97.0 **Postcardiotomy syndrome**

I97.1- **Other postprocedural cardiac functional disturbances**
Excludes 2:   acute pulmonary insufficiency following thoracic surgery (J95.1)
intraoperative cardiac functional disturbances (I97.7-)

I97.11- **Postprocedural cardiac insufficiency**

cc **I97.110** **Postprocedural cardiac insufficiency following cardiac surgery**

cc **I97.111** **Postprocedural cardiac insufficiency following other surgery**

I97.12- **Postprocedural cardiac arrest**

cc **I97.120** **Postprocedural cardiac arrest following cardiac surgery**

cc **I97.121** **Postprocedural cardiac arrest following other surgery**

I97.13- **Postprocedural heart failure**
Use additional code to identify the heart failure (I50.-)

cc **I97.130** **Postprocedural heart failure following cardiac surgery**

cc **I97.131** **Postprocedural heart failure following other surgery**

I97.19- **Other postprocedural cardiac functional disturbances**
Use additional code, if applicable, to further specify disorder

cc **I97.190** **Other postprocedural cardiac functional disturbances following cardiac surgery**

cc **I97.191** **Other postprocedural cardiac functional disturbances following other surgery**

I97.2 **Postmastectomy lymphedema syndrome** — [Age/15-124] – Edema of arm (same side as mastectomy) due to obliteration of lymph nodes and channels from the surgical procedure.
Elephantiasis due to mastectomy
Obliteration of lymphatic vessels

I97.3 **Postprocedural hypertension** — Elevated blood pressure occurring postoperatively.

I97.4- <u>Intraoperative hemorrhage and hematoma</u> of a circulatory system organ or structure complicating a procedure
Excludes 1:   intraoperative hemorrhage and hematoma of a circulatory system organ or structure due to accidental puncture and laceration during a procedure (I97.5-)
Excludes 2:   intraoperative cerebrovascular hemorrhage complicating a procedure (G97.3-)

I97.41- **Intraoperative hemorrhage and hematoma of a circulatory system organ or structure complicating a circulatory system procedure**

cc **I97.410** **Intraoperative hemorrhage and hematoma of a circulatory system organ or structure** <u>complicating a cardiac catheterization</u>

cc **I97.411** **Intraoperative hemorrhage and hematoma of a circulatory system organ or structure** <u>complicating a cardiac bypass</u>

cc **I97.418** **Intraoperative hemorrhage and hematoma of a circulatory system organ or structure** <u>complicating other circulatory system procedure</u>

cc **I97.42** **Intraoperative hemorrhage and hematoma of a circulatory system organ or structure** <u>complicating other procedure</u>

I97.5- <u>Accidental puncture and laceration</u> of a circulatory system organ or structure during a procedure
Excludes 2:   accidental puncture and laceration of brain during a procedure (G97.4-)

cc **I97.51** **Accidental puncture and laceration of a circulatory system organ or structure during a** <u>circulatory system procedure</u>

cc **I97.52** **Accidental puncture and laceration of a circulatory system organ or structure during** <u>other procedure</u>

I97.6- <u>Postprocedural hemorrhage, hematoma and seroma</u> of a circulatory system organ or structure following a procedure
Excludes 2:   postprocedural cerebrovascular hemorrhage complicating a procedure (G97.5-)

I97.61- **Postprocedural** <u>hemorrhage</u> of a circulatory system organ or structure following a circulatory system procedure

cc **I97.610** **Postprocedural** <u>hemorrhage</u> of a circulatory system organ or structure following a <u>cardiac catheterization</u>

cc **I97.611** **Postprocedural** <u>hemorrhage</u> of a circulatory system organ or structure following <u>cardiac bypass</u>

cc **I97.618** **Postprocedural** <u>hemorrhage</u> of a circulatory system organ or structure following <u>other circulatory system procedure</u>

I97.62- <u>Postprocedural hemorrhage, hematoma and seroma</u> of a circulatory system organ or structure <u>following other procedure</u>

cc **I97.620** **Postprocedural** <u>hemorrhage</u> of a circulatory system organ or structure following <u>other procedure</u>

cc **I97.621** **Postprocedural** <u>hematoma</u> of a circulatory system organ or structure following <u>other procedure</u>

cc **I97.622** **Postprocedural** <u>seroma</u> of a circulatory system organ or structure following <u>other procedure</u>

Excludes 1: = NOT CODED HERE! (Do not code both)   758   Excludes 2: = Not Included Here

I
9
5
-
I
9
7

© 2016 Channel Publishing Ltd

I97.63- <u>Postprocedural hematoma</u> of a circulatory system organ or structure <u>following a circulatory system procedure</u>

cc I97.630   Postprocedural <u>hematoma</u> of a circulatory system organ or structure following a <u>cardiac catheterization</u>

cc I97.631   Postprocedural <u>hematoma</u> of a circulatory system organ or structure following <u>cardiac bypass</u>

cc I97.638   Postprocedural <u>hematoma</u> of a circulatory system organ or structure following <u>other circulatory system procedure</u>

I97.64- <u>Postprocedural seroma</u> of a circulatory system organ or structure <u>following a circulatory system procedure</u>

cc I97.640   Postprocedural <u>seroma</u> of a circulatory system organ or structure following a <u>cardiac catheterization</u>

cc I97.641   Postprocedural <u>seroma</u> of a circulatory system organ or structure following <u>cardiac bypass</u>

cc I97.648   Postprocedural <u>seroma</u> of a circulatory system organ or structure following <u>other circulatory system procedure</u>

I97.7-   Intraoperative cardiac functional disturbances
Excludes ❷: acute pulmonary insufficiency following thoracic surgery (J95.1)
postprocedural cardiac functional disturbances (I97.1-)

I97.71- Intraoperative cardiac arrest

cc I97.710   Intraoperative cardiac arrest during <u>cardiac</u> surgery

cc I97.711   Intraoperative cardiac arrest during <u>other</u> surgery

I97.79- Other intraoperative cardiac functional disturbances
Use additional code, if applicable, to further specify disorder

cc I97.790   Other intraoperative cardiac functional disturbances during <u>cardiac</u> surgery

cc I97.791   Other intraoperative cardiac functional disturbances during <u>other</u> surgery

I97.8-   Other intraoperative and postprocedural complications and disorders of the circulatory system, not elsewhere classified
Use additional code, if applicable, to further specify disorder

I97.81- Intraoperative cerebrovascular infarction

cc I97.810   Intraoperative cerebrovascular infarction during <u>cardiac</u> surgery

cc I97.811   Intraoperative cerebrovascular infarction during <u>other</u> surgery

I97.82- Postprocedural cerebrovascular infarction

cc I97.820   Postprocedural cerebrovascular infarction following <u>cardiac</u> surgery

cc I97.821   Postprocedural cerebrovascular infarction following <u>other</u> surgery

cc I97.88   Other intraoperative complications of the circulatory system, <u>not elsewhere classified</u>

cc I97.89   Other postprocedural complications and disorders of the circulatory system, not elsewhere classified

I99-   Other and unspecified disorders of circulatory system

I99.8   Other disorder of circulatory system

I99.9   Unspecified disorder of circulatory system

I97 - I99

Excludes 1: = NOT CODED HERE! (Do not code both)   **759**   *Excludes ❷: =* Not Included Here

I99 - I99

Chapter 10 – Diseases of the respiratory system (J00-J99)

Note: When a respiratory condition is described as occurring in more than one site and is not specifically indexed, it should be classified to the lower anatomic site (e.g. tracheobronchitis to bronchitis in J40).

Use additional code, where applicable, to identify:

Exposure to environmental tobacco smoke (Z77.22)
Exposure to tobacco smoke in the perinatal period (P96.81)
History of tobacco dependence (Z87.891)
Occupational exposure to environmental tobacco smoke (Z57.31)
Tobacco dependence (F17.-)
Tobacco use (Z72.0)

Excludes ❷: *certain conditions originating in the perinatal period (P04-P96)*

certain infectious and parasitic diseases (A00-B99)

complications of pregnancy, childbirth and the puerperium (O00-O9A)

congenital malformations, deformations and chromosomal abnormalities (Q00-Q99)

endocrine, nutritional and metabolic diseases (E00-E88)

injury, poisoning and certain other consequences of external causes (S00-T88)

neoplasms (C00-D49)

smoke inhalation (T59.81-)

symptoms, signs and abnormal clinical and laboratory findings, not elsewhere classified (R00-R94)

This chapter contains the following blocks:

J00-J06	Acute upper respiratory infections
J09-J18	Influenza and pneumonia
J20-J22	Other acute lower respiratory infections
J30-J39	Other diseases of upper respiratory tract
J40-J47	Chronic lower respiratory diseases
J60-J70	Lung diseases due to external agents
J80-J84	Other respiratory diseases principally affecting the interstitium
J85-J86	Suppurative and necrotic conditions of the lower respiratory tract
J90-J94	Other diseases of the pleura
J95	Intraoperative and postprocedural complications and disorders of respiratory system, not elsewhere classified
J96-J99	Other diseases of the respiratory system

Chapter-Specific Coding Guidelines

C. Chapter-Specific Coding Guidelines

In addition to general coding guidelines, there are guidelines for specific diagnoses and/or conditions in the classification. Unless otherwise indicated, these guidelines apply to all health care settings. Please refer to Section II for guidelines on the selection of principal diagnosis.

10. Chapter 10: Diseases of the Respiratory System (J00-J99)

a. Chronic Obstructive Pulmonary Disease [COPD] and Asthma

1) Acute exacerbation of chronic obstructive bronchitis and asthma

The codes in categories J44 and J45 distinguish between uncomplicated cases and those in acute exacerbation. An acute exacerbation is a worsening or a decompensation of a chronic condition. An acute exacerbation is not equivalent to an infection superimposed on a chronic condition, though an exacerbation may be triggered by an infection.

b. Acute Respiratory Failure

1) Acute respiratory failure as principal diagnosis

A code from subcategory J96.0, Acute respiratory failure, or subcategory J96.2, Acute and chronic respiratory failure, may be assigned as a principal diagnosis when it is the condition established after study to be chiefly responsible for occasioning the admission to the hospital, and the selection is supported by the Alphabetic Index and Tabular List. However, chapter-specific coding guidelines (such as obstetrics, poisoning, HIV, newborn) that provide sequencing direction take precedence.

2) Acute respiratory failure as secondary diagnosis

Respiratory failure may be listed as a secondary diagnosis if it occurs after admission, or if it is present on admission, but does not meet the definition of principal diagnosis.

3) Sequencing of acute respiratory failure and another acute condition

When a patient is admitted with respiratory failure and another acute condition, (e.g., myocardial infarction, cerebrovascular accident, aspiration pneumonia), the principal diagnosis will not be the same in every situation. This applies whether the other acute condition is a respiratory or nonrespiratory condition. Selection of the principal diagnosis will be dependent on the circumstances of admission. If both the respiratory failure and the other acute condition are equally responsible for occasioning the admission to the hospital, and there are no chapter-specific sequencing rules, the guideline regarding two or more diagnoses that equally meet the definition for principal diagnosis *(Section II, C.)* may be applied in these situations.

If the documentation is not clear as to whether acute respiratory failure and another condition are equally responsible for occasioning the admission, query the provider for clarification.

c. Influenza due to certain identified influenza viruses

Code only confirmed cases of influenza due to certain identified influenza viruses (category J09), and due to other identified influenza virus (category J10). This is an exception to the hospital inpatient guideline Section II, H. (Uncertain Diagnosis).

In this context, "confirmation" does not require documentation of positive laboratory testing specific for avian or other novel influenza A or other identified influenza virus. However, coding should be based on the provider's diagnostic statement that the patient has avian influenza, or other novel influenza A, for category J09, or has another particular identified strain of influenza, such as H1N1 or H3N2, but not identified as novel or variant, for category J10.

If the provider records "suspected" or "possible" or "probable" avian influenza, or novel influenza, or other identified influenza, then the appropriate influenza code from category J11, Influenza due to unidentified influenza virus, should be assigned. A code from category J09, Influenza due to certain identified influenza viruses, should not be assigned nor should a code from category J10, Influenza due to other identified influenza virus.

d. Ventilator associated Pneumonia

1) Documentation of Ventilator associated Pneumonia

As with all procedural or postprocedural complications, code assignment is based on the provider's documentation of the relationship between the condition and the procedure.

Code J95.851, Ventilator associated pneumonia, should be assigned only when the provider has documented ventilator associated pneumonia (VAP). An additional code to identify the organism (e.g., Pseudomonas aeruginosa, code B96.5) should also be assigned. Do not assign an additional code from categories J12-J18 to identify the type of pneumonia.

Code J95.851 should not be assigned for cases where the patient has pneumonia and is on a mechanical ventilator and the provider has not specifically stated that the pneumonia is ventilator-associated pneumonia. If the documentation is unclear as to whether the patient has a pneumonia that is a complication attributable to the mechanical ventilator, query the provider.

2) Ventilator associated Pneumonia Develops after Admission

A patient may be admitted with one type of pneumonia (e.g., code J13, Pneumonia due to Streptococcus pneumonia) and subsequently develop VAP. In this instance, the principal diagnosis would be the appropriate code from categories J12-J18 for the pneumonia diagnosed at the time of admission. Code J95.851, Ventilator associated pneumonia, would be assigned as an additional diagnosis when the provider has also documented the presence of ventilator associated pneumonia.

Acute upper respiratory infections (J00-J06)

Excludes 1: *chronic obstructive pulmonary disease with acute lower respiratory infection (J44.0)*

influenza virus with other respiratory manifestations (J09.x2, J10.1, J11.1)

J00 Acute nasopharyngitis [common cold] — A sudden severe onset of mucous membrane inflammation of the nasopharynx that is marked by nasal congestion, continuous watery discharge, and malaise.

Acute rhinitis
Coryza (acute)
Infective nasopharyngitis NOS
Infective rhinitis
Nasal catarrh, acute
Nasopharyngitis NOS

Excludes 1: *acute pharyngitis (J02.-)*
acute sore throat NOS (J02.9)
pharyngitis NOS (J02.9)
rhinitis NOS (J31.0)
sore throat NOS (J02.9)

Excludes ❷: *allergic rhinitis (J30.1-J30.9)*
chronic pharyngitis (J31.2)
chronic rhinitis (J31.0)
chronic sore throat (J31.2)
nasopharyngitis, chronic (J31.1)
vasomotor rhinitis (J30.0)

J00 - J00 - J00

Excludes 1: = NOT CODED HERE! (Do not code both) **761** *Excludes ❷:* = Not Included Here

J01- **Acute sinusitis** — A sudden, severe onset of inflammation of the paranasal sinuses.
Includes: **Acute abscess of sinus** — A form marked by a localized collection of pus caused by the disintegration of sinus mucous membrane tissue.
Acute empyema of sinus — A form marked by an accumulation of pus within the sinus cavities.
Acute infection of sinus — A form caused by microorganisms.
Acute inflammation of sinus — A sudden, severe onset of inflammation of the paranasal sinuses.
Acute suppuration of sinus — A form marked by a pus-producing inflammation of the sinuses.
Use additional code (B95-B97) to identify infectious agent
Excludes 1: *sinusitis NOS (J32.9)*
Excludes ➋: *chronic sinusitis (J32.0-J32.8)*

J01.0- **Acute maxillary sinusitis** — A form affecting one of the paranasal sinuses, located in the body of the maxilla.
Acute antritis — A sudden, severe inflammation of the maxillary antrum.

J01.00 **Acute maxillary sinusitis, unspecified**

J01.01 **Acute recurrent maxillary sinusitis**

J01.1- **Acute frontal sinusitis** — A form affecting one of the paired paranasal sinuses, located in the frontal bone.

J01.10 **Acute frontal sinusitis, unspecified**

J01.11 **Acute recurrent frontal sinusitis**

J01.2- **Acute ethmoidal sinusitis** — A form affecting one of the grouped paranasal sinuses, located in the ethmoid bone.

J01.20 **Acute ethmoidal sinusitis, unspecified**

J01.21 **Acute recurrent ethmoidal sinusitis**

J01.3- **Acute sphenoidal sinusitis** — A form affecting one of the paired paranasal sinuses, located in the anterior part of the body of the sphenoid bone.

J01.30 **Acute sphenoidal sinusitis, unspecified**

J01.31 **Acute recurrent sphenoidal sinusitis**

J01.4- **Acute pansinusitis** — A sudden, severe inflammation involving all of the paranasal sinuses.

J01.40 **Acute pansinusitis, unspecified**

J01.41 **Acute recurrent pansinusitis**

J01.8- **Other acute sinusitis**

J01.80 **Other acute sinusitis**
Acute sinusitis involving more than one sinus but not pansinusitis

J01.81 **Other acute recurrent sinusitis**
Acute recurrent sinusitis involving more than one sinus but not pansinusitis

J01.9- **Acute sinusitis, unspecified**

J01.90 **Acute sinusitis, unspecified**

J01.91 **Acute recurrent sinusitis, unspecified**

J02- **Acute pharyngitis** — A sudden, severe inflammation of the pharynx.
Includes: **Acute sore throat** — A common term referring to acute pharyngitis.
Excludes 1: *acute laryngopharyngitis (J06.0)*
peritonsillar abscess (J36)
pharyngeal abscess (J39.1)
retropharyngeal abscess (J39.0)
Excludes ➋: *chronic pharyngitis (J31.2)*

J02.0 **Streptococcal pharyngitis** — An infectious disease caused by Streptococcus pyogenes, and characterized by severe sore throat, fever, vomiting, headache, and malaise.
Septic pharyngitis
Streptococcal sore throat
Excludes ➋: *scarlet fever (A38.-)*

J02.8 **Acute pharyngitis due to other specified organisms**
Use additional code (B95-B97) to identify infectious agent
Excludes 1: *acute pharyngitis due to coxsackie virus (B08.5)*
acute pharyngitis due to gonococcus (A54.5)
acute pharyngitis due to herpes [simplex] virus (B00.2)
acute pharyngitis due to infectious mononucleosis (B27.-)
enteroviral vesicular pharyngitis (B08.5)

J02.9 **Acute pharyngitis, unspecified**
Gangrenous pharyngitis (acute) — A form characterized by gangrenous patches.
Infective pharyngitis (acute) NOS
Pharyngitis (acute) NOS
Sore throat (acute) NOS
Suppurative pharyngitis (acute) — A form characterized by the production of pus.
Ulcerative pharyngitis (acute) — A form characterized by ulcers covered by a yellow, membrane-like deposit in the pharynx, with fever, pain, and prostration.

J03- **Acute tonsillitis** — A sudden, severe onset of inflammation of the tonsils, in which the tonsils are red and swollen.
Excludes 1: *acute sore throat (J02.-)*
hypertrophy of tonsils (J35.1)
peritonsillar abscess (J36)
sore throat NOS (J02.9)
streptococcal sore throat (J02.0)
Excludes ➋: *chronic tonsillitis (J35.0)*

J03.0- **Streptococcal tonsillitis** — A form caused by streptococcal microorganisms.

J03.00 **Acute streptococcal tonsillitis, unspecified**

J03.01 **Acute recurrent streptococcal tonsillitis**

J03.8- **Acute tonsillitis due to other specified organisms**
Use additional code (B95-B97) to identify infectious agent.
Excludes 1: *diphtheritic tonsillitis (A36.0)*
herpesviral pharyngotonsillitis (B00.2)
streptococcal tonsillitis (J03.0)
tuberculous tonsillitis (A15.8)
Vincent's tonsillitis (A69.1)

J03.80 **Acute tonsillitis due to other specified organisms**

J03.81 **Acute recurrent tonsillitis due to other specified organisms**

J03.9- **Acute tonsillitis, unspecified**
Follicular tonsillitis (acute) — A form characterized by affecting the crypts.
Gangrenous tonsillitis (acute) — A form characterized by gangrenous patches.
Infective tonsillitis (acute)
Tonsillitis (acute) NOS
Ulcerative tonsillitis (acute) — A form characterized by the eating-away and disintegration of the tonsil tissue.

J03.90 **Acute tonsillitis, unspecified**

J03.91 **Acute recurrent tonsillitis, unspecified**

J04- **Acute laryngitis and tracheitis** — A sudden, severe onset of inflammation of the larynx and/or trachea.
Use additional code (B95-B97) to identify infectious agent.
Excludes 1: *acute obstructive laryngitis [croup] and epiglottitis (J05.-)*
Excludes ➋: *laryngismus (stridulus) (J38.5)*

J04.0 **Acute laryngitis** — A sudden, severe onset of inflammation of the larynx.
Edematous laryngitis (acute) — A form characterized by abnormally large amounts of intercellular fluid of the laryngeal tissues.
Laryngitis (acute) NOS
Subglottic laryngitis (acute)
Suppurative laryngitis (acute) — A form caused by the production of pus.
Ulcerative laryngitis (acute) — A form characterized by the eating-away of laryngeal tissue.
Excludes 1: *acute obstructive laryngitis (J05.0)*
Excludes ➋: *chronic laryngitis (J37.0)*

J04.1- **Acute tracheitis** — A sudden, severe onset of inflammation of the trachea.
Acute viral tracheitis — A form caused by viral microorganisms.
Catarrhal tracheitis (acute) — A form caused by severe inflammation of the mucous membranes.
Tracheitis (acute) NOS
Excludes ➋: *chronic tracheitis (J42)*

J04.10 **Acute tracheitis without obstruction**

MCC **J04.11** **Acute tracheitis with obstruction** — A form marked by blockage of the airflow.

J04.2 **Acute laryngotracheitis** — A sudden, severe onset of inflammation of the larynx and trachea.
Laryngotracheitis NOS
Tracheitis (acute) with laryngitis (acute)
Excludes 1: *acute obstructive laryngotracheitis (J05.0)*
Excludes ➋: *chronic laryngotracheitis (J37.1)*

J04.3- **Supraglottitis, unspecified** — A form affecting the tissues just above the vocal cords.

J04.30 **Supraglottitis, unspecified, without obstruction**

MCC **J04.31** **Supraglottitis, unspecified, with obstruction** — A form marked by blockage of the airflow.

J05- **Acute obstructive laryngitis [croup] and epiglottitis**
Use additional code (B95-B97) to identify infectious agent.

J05.0 **Acute obstructive laryngitis [croup]** — A sudden, severe onset of obstruction of the larynx in infants and young children characterized by resonant barking cough, laryngeal spasm, difficult breathing, and hoarseness, usually due to an upper respiratory infection.
Obstructive laryngitis (acute) NOS
Obstructive laryngotracheitis NOS

J01 – J05

J05.1-   Acute _epiglottitis_ — A sudden, severe onset of inflammation of the flap of tissue at the opening to the larynx.
> **_Excludes ❷:_** _epiglottitis, chronic (J37.0)_

CC **J05.10   Acute epiglottitis _without_ obstruction**
> **Epiglottitis NOS**

MCC **J05.11   Acute epiglottitis _with obstruction_** — A form marked by blockage of the airflow.

J06-   Acute upper respiratory infections of multiple and unspecified sites
> **_Excludes 1:_** _acute respiratory infection NOS (J22)_
> _streptococcal pharyngitis (J02.0)_

J06.0   Acute laryngopharyngitis — A sudden, severe onset of inflammation of the larynx and pharynx.

J06.9   Acute upper respiratory infection, unspecified
> **Upper respiratory disease, acute**
> **Upper respiratory infection NOS**

Influenza and pneumonia (J09-J18)

> **_Excludes ❷:_** _allergic or eosinophilic pneumonia (J82)_
> _aspiration pneumonia NOS (J69.0)_
> _congenital pneumonia (P23.9)_
> _lipid pneumonia (J69.1)_
> _meconium pneumonia (P24.01)_
> _neonatal aspiration pneumonia (P24.-)_
> _pneumonia due to solids and liquids (J69.-)_
> _rheumatic pneumonia (I00)_
> _ventilator associated pneumonia (J95.851)_

J09-   Influenza due to certain identified influenza viruses — Infection of the respiratory tract by certain influenza viruses.
> **_Excludes 1:_** _influenza due to other identified influenza virus (J10-)_
> _influenza due to unidentified influenza virus (J11-)_
> _seasonal influenza due to other identified influenza virus (J10-)_
> _seasonal influenza due to unidentified influenza virus (J11-)_

J09.x-   Influenza due to _identified novel influenza A virus_ — Infection of the respiratory tract by novel influenza A viruses.
> **Avian influenza**
> **Bird influenza**
> **Influenza A/H5N1**
> **Influenza of other animal origin, not bird or swine**
> **Swine influenza virus (viruses that normally cause infections in pigs)**

MCC **J09.x1   Influenza due to identified novel influenza A virus _with pneumonia_** — A form marked by the concurring presence of inflammation of the lungs with exudate-filled air spaces.
> **Code also, if applicable, associated:**
> **Lung abscess (J85.1)**
> **Other specified type of pneumonia**

J09.x2   Influenza due to identified novel influenza A virus _with other respiratory_ manifestations — A form marked by fever, chills, malaise, cough, coryza, muscle aches, and prostration which may involve the upper respiratory organs.
> **Influenza due to identified novel influenza A virus NOS**
> **Influenza due to identified novel influenza A virus with laryngitis**
> **Influenza due to identified novel influenza A virus with pharyngitis**
> **Influenza due to identified novel influenza A virus with upper respiratory symptoms**
> **Use additional code, if applicable, for associated:**
> **Pleural effusion (J91.8)**
> **Sinusitis (J01.-)**

J09.x3   Influenza due to identified novel influenza A virus _with gastrointestinal manifestations_ — A form marked by infection of the gastrointestinal tract.
> **Influenza due to identified novel influenza A virus gastroenteritis**
> **_Excludes 1:_** _"intestinal flu" [viral gastroenteritis] (A08-)_

J09.x9   Influenza due to identified novel influenza A virus _with other_ manifestations
> **Influenza due to identified novel influenza A virus with encephalopathy**
> **Influenza due to identified novel influenza A virus with myocarditis**
> **Influenza due to identified novel influenza A virus with otitis media**
> **Use additional code to identify manifestation**

J10-   Influenza due to _other identified influenza_ virus — Infection of the respiratory tract by other (non novel influenza A viruses) influenza viruses.
> **_Excludes 1:_** _influenza due to avian influenza virus (J09.x-)_
> _influenza due to swine flu (J09.x-)_
> _influenza due to unidentifed influenza virus (J11-)_

J10.0-   Influenza due to _other_ identified influenza virus _with pneumonia_ — A form marked by the concurring presence of inflammation of the lungs with exudate-filled air spaces.
> **Code also associated lung abscess, if applicable (J85.1)**

MCC **J10.00   Influenza due to _other_ identified influenza virus _with unspecified type of pneumonia_**

MCC **J10.01   Influenza due to _other_ identified influenza virus _with the same other identified influenza virus pneumonia_**

MCC **J10.08   Influenza due to _other_ identified influenza virus _with other specified pneumonia_**
> **Code also other specified type of pneumonia**

J10.1   Influenza due to _other_ identified influenza virus _with other respiratory_ manifestations — A form marked by fever, chills, malaise, cough, coryza, muscle aches, and prostration which may involve the upper respiratory organs.
> **Influenza due to other identified influenza virus NOS**
> **Influenza due to other identified influenza virus with laryngitis**
> **Influenza due to other identified influenza virus with pharyngitis**
> **Influenza due to other identified influenza virus with upper respiratory symptoms**
> **Use additional code for associated pleural effusion, if applicable (J91.8)**
> **Use additional code for associated sinusitis, if applicable (J01.-)**

J10.2   Influenza due to _other_ identified influenza virus _with gastrointestinal manifestations_ — A form marked by infection of the gastrointestinal tract.
> **Influenza due to other identified influenza virus gastroenteritis**
> **_Excludes 1:_** _"intestinal flu" [viral gastroenteritis] (A08.-)_

J10.8-   Influenza due to _other_ identified influenza virus _with other manifestations_

J10.81   Influenza due to _other_ identified influenza virus _with encephalopathy_

J10.82   Influenza due to _other_ identified influenza virus _with myocarditis_

J10.83   Influenza due to _other_ identified influenza virus _with otitis media_
> **Use additional code for any associated perforated tympanic membrane (H72.-)**

J10.89   Influenza due to _other_ identified influenza virus _with other manifestations_
> **Use additional codes to identify the manifestations**

J11-   Influenza due to _unidentified influenza virus_

J11.0-   Influenza due to _unidentified_ influenza vIrus with pneumonia — A form marked by the concurring presence of inflammation of the lungs with exudate-filled air spaces.
> **Code also associated lung abscess, if applicable (J85.1)**

MCC **J11.00   Influenza due to _unidentified_ influenza virus _with unspecified type of pneumonia_**
> **Influenza with pneumonia NOS**

MCC **J11.08   Influenza due to _unidentified_ influenza virus _with specified pneumonia_**
> **Code also other specified type of pneumonia**

J11.1   Influenza due to _unidentified_ influenza virus _with other respiratory_ manifestations — A form marked by fever, chills, malaise, cough, coryza, muscle aches, and prostration which may involve the upper respiratory organs.
> **Influenza NOS**
> **Influenzal laryngitis NOS**
> **Influenzal pharyngitis NOS**
> **Influenza with upper respiratory symptoms NOS**
> **Use additional code for associated pleural effusion, if applicable (J91.8)**
> **Use additional code for associated sinusitis, if applicable (J01.-)**

J11.2   Influenza due to _unidentified_ influenza virus _with gastrointestinal manifestations_ — A form marked by infection of the gastrointestinal tract.
> **Influenza gastroenteritis NOS**
> **_Excludes 1:_** _"intestinal flu" [viral gastroenteritis] (A08.-)_

J05 - J11

J11.8-   Influenza due to <u>unidentified</u> influenza virus <u>with other manifestations</u>

> **J11.81   Influenza due to <u>unidentified</u> influenza virus <u>with encephalopathy</u>**
> Influenzal encephalopathy NOS

> **J11.82   Influenza due to <u>unidentified</u> influenza virus <u>with myocarditis</u>**
> Influenzal myocarditis NOS

> **J11.83   Influenza due to <u>unidentified</u> influenza virus <u>with otitis media</u>**
> Influenzal otitis media NOS
> Use additional code for any associated perforated tympanic membrane (H72.-)

> **J11.89   Influenza due to <u>unidentified</u> influenza virus <u>with other manifestations</u>**
> Use additional codes to identify the manifestations

J12-   Viral pneumonia, <u>not elsewhere classified</u> — Inflammation of the lung with exudate-filled air spaces caused by viral microorganisms.
Includes: Bronchopneumonia due to viruses other than influenza viruses
Code first associated influenza, if applicable (J09.x1, J10.0-, J11.0-)
Code also associated abscess, if applicable (J85.1)
Excludes 1:   *aspiration pneumonia due to anesthesia during labor and delivery (O74.0)*
aspiration pneumonia due to anesthesia during pregnancy (O29)
aspiration pneumonia due to anesthesia during puerperium (O89.0)
aspiration pneumonia due to solids and liquids (J69.-)
aspiration pneumonia NOS (J69.0)
congenital pneumonia (P23.0)
congenital rubella pneumonitis (P35.0)
interstitial pneumonia NOS (J84.9)
lipid pneumonia (J69.1)
neonatal aspiration pneumonia (P24.-)

MCC **J12.0   Adenoviral pneumonia** — A form caused by the group of adenovirus microorganisms.

MCC **J12.1   Respiratory syncytial virus pneumonia** — A form caused by the group of respiratory syncytial virus (RSV) microorganisms.

MCC **J12.2   Parainfluenza virus pneumonia** — A form caused by the group of parainfluenzal viral (HPIVs) microorganisms.

MCC **J12.3   Human metapneumovirus pneumonia** — A form caused by the group of human metapneumovirus (hMPV) microorganisms.

J12.8-   Other viral pneumonia

> MCC **J12.81   Pneumonia due to SARS-associated coronavirus** — A form caused by the group of SARS-associated coronavirus (SARS-CoV) microorganisms.
> Severe acute respiratory syndrome NOS

> MCC **J12.89   Other viral pneumonia**

MCC **J12.9   Viral pneumonia, unspecified**

J13   **Pneumonia due to Streptococcus pneumoniae** — Inflammation of the lungs
MCC   with exudate-filled air spaces caused by Streptococcal pneumoconiae microorganisms.
Bronchopneumonia due to S. pneumoniae
Code first associated influenza, if applicable (J09.x1, J10.0-, J11.0-)
Code also associated abscess, if applicable (J85.1)
Excludes 1:   *congenital pneumonia due to S. pneumoniae (P23.6)*
lobar pneumonia, unspecified organism (J18.1)
pneumonia due to other streptococci (J15.3-J15.4)

J14   **Pneumonia due to Hemophilus influenzae** — A form caused by the
MCC   microorganism Hemophilus influenzae, usually seen with chronic bronchopulmonary disease but may occur rarely as a primary infection.
Bronchopneumonia due to H. influenzae
Code first associated influenza, if applicable (J09.x1, J10.0-, J11.0-)
Code also associated abscess, if applicable (J85.1)
Excludes 1:   *congenital pneumonia due to H. influenzae (P23.6)*

J15-   Bacterial pneumonia, <u>not elsewhere classified</u>
Includes: Bronchopneumonia due to bacteria other than S. pneumoniae and H. influenzae
Code first associated influenza, if applicable (J09.x1, J10.0-, J11.0-)
Code also associated abscess, if applicable (J85.1)
Excludes 1:   *chlamydial pneumonia (J16.0)*
congenital pneumonia (P23.-)
Legionnaires' disease (A48.1)
spirochetal pneumonia (A69.8)

MCC **J15.0   Pneumonia due to Klebsiella pneumoniae** — A form caused by the microorganism Klebsiella pneumoniae and characterized by massive mucoid inflammatory exudates in the lung.

MCC **J15.1   Pneumonia due to Pseudomonas** — A form caused by the pseudomonas microorganisms, including Pseudomonas aeruginosa.

J15.2-   Pneumonia due to staphylococcus — A form caused by staphylococcal microorganisms, many strains of which are antibiotic resistant.

MCC **J15.20   Pneumonia due to staphylococcus, unspecified**

J15.21-   Pneumonia due to Staphylococcus aureus

> MCC **J15.211   Pneumonia due to methicillin susceptible Staphylococcus aureus** — A form caused by a form of the bacterium Staphylococcus aureus that is susceptible to antibiotic treatment.
> MSSA pneumonia
> Pneumonia due to Staphylococcus aureus NOS

> MCC **J15.212   Pneumonia due to methicillin resistant Staphylococcus aureus** — A form caused by a form of the bacterium Staphylococcus aureus that is resistant to treatment from beta-lactam class antibiotics.

MCC **J15.29   Pneumonia due to other staphylococcus**

MCC **J15.3   Pneumonia due to streptococcus, group B** — A form caused by Streptococcus agalactiae.

MCC **J15.4   Pneumonia due to other streptococci**
Excludes 1:   *pneumonia due to streptococcus, group B (J15.3)*
pneumonia due to Streptococcus pneumoniae (J13)

MCC **J15.5   Pneumonia due to Escherichia coli** — A form caused by Escherichia coli, normally present in intestinal flora, but pathogenic in the lungs.

MCC **J15.6   Pneumonia due to other aerobic Gram-negative bacteria**
Pneumonia due to Serratia marcescens — A form caused by the species Serratia marcescens.

MCC **J15.7   Pneumonia due to Mycoplasma pneumoniae** — The most common form of primary atypical pneumonia caused by the microorganism Mycoplasma pneumoniae.

MCC **J15.8   Pneumonia due to other specified bacteria**

MCC **J15.9   Unspecified bacterial pneumonia**
Pneumonia due to gram-positive bacteria

J16-   Pneumonia due to other infectious organisms, <u>not elsewhere classified</u>
Code first associated influenza, if applicable (J09.x1, J10.0-, J11.0-)
Code also associated abscess, if applicable (J85.1)
Excludes 1:   *congenital pneumonia (P23.-)*
ornithosis (A70)
pneumocystosis (B59)
pneumonia NOS (J18.9)

MCC **J16.0   Chlamydial pneumonia** — A form caused by the chlamydial gram-negative bacteria.

MCC **J16.8   Pneumonia due to other specified infectious organisms**

J17   Pneumonia <u>in diseases classified elsewhere</u> — [Not Allowed as PDX]
MCC   Code first underlying disease, such as:
     Q fever (A78)
     Rheumatic fever (I00)
     Schistosomiasis (B65.0-B65.9)
     Excludes 1:   *candidial pneumonia (B37.1)*
          chlamydial pneumonia (J16.0)
          gonorrheal pneumonia (A54.84)
          histoplasmosis pneumonia (B39.0-B39.2)
          measles pneumonia (B05.2)
          nocardiosis pneumonia (A43.0)
          pneumocystosis (B59)
          pneumonia due to Pneumocystis carinii (B59)
          pneumonia due to Pneumocystis jiroveci (B59)
          pneumonia in actinomycosis (A42.0)
          pneumonia in anthrax (A22.1)
          pneumonia in ascariasis (B77.81)
          pneumonia in aspergillosis (B44.0-B44.1)
          pneumonia in coccidioidomycosis (B38.0-B38.2)
          pneumonia in cytomegalovirus disease (B25.0)
          pneumonia in toxoplasmosis (B58.3)
          rubella pneumonia (B06.81)
          salmonella pneumonia (A02.22)
          spirochetal infection NEC with pneumonia (A69.8)
          tularemia pneumonia (A21.2)
          typhoid fever with pneumonia (A01.03)
          varicella pneumonia (B01.2)
          whooping cough with pneumonia (A37 with fifth-character 1)

J18-   Pneumonia, <u>unspecified organism</u>
     AHA 14:3Q:p4 – SIRS secondary to pneumonia
     Code first associated influenza, if applicable (J09.x1, J10.0-, J11.0-)
     Excludes 1:   *abscess of lung with pneumonia (J85.1)*
          aspiration pneumonia due to anesthesia during labor and delivery (O74.0)
          aspiration pneumonia due to anesthesia during pregnancy (O29)
          aspiration pneumonia due to anesthesia during puerperium (O89.0)
          aspiration pneumonia due to solids and liquids (J69.-)
          aspiration pneumonia NOS (J69.0)
          congenital pneumonia (P23.0)
          drug-induced interstitial lung disorder (J70.2-J70.4)
          interstitial pneumonia NOS (J84.9)
          lipid pneumonia (J69.1)
          neonatal aspiration pneumonia (P24.-)
          pneumonitis due to external agents (J67-J70)
          pneumonitis due to fumes and vapors (J68.0)
          usual interstitial pneumonia (J84.17)

MCC **J18.0**   **Bronchopneumonia, unspecified organism** — Inflammation of the lungs which usually begins in the terminal bronchioles and causes the air spaces to become filled with exudates.
        Excludes 1:   *hypostatic bronchopneumonia (J18.2)*
               lipid pneumonia (J69.1)
        Excludes ❷: *acute bronchiolitis (J21.-)*
               chronic bronchiolitis (J44.9)

MCC **J18.1**   **Lobar pneumonia, unspecified organism**

CC **J18.2**   **Hypostatic pneumonia, unspecified organism**
        Hypostatic bronchopneumonia
        Passive pneumonia

MCC **J18.8**   **Other pneumonia, unspecified organism**

MCC **J18.9**   **Pneumonia, unspecified organism**

Other acute lower respiratory infections (J20-J22)

Excludes ❷: *chronic obstructive pulmonary disease with acute lower respiratory infection (J44.0)*

J20-   **Acute bronchitis** — A sudden, severe onset of inflammation of the bronchi.
     Includes: **Acute and subacute bronchitis (with) bronchospasm** — A form marked by spasmodic contraction (tightening) of the muscles in the walls of the bronchioles.
          Acute and subacute bronchitis (with) tracheitis
          Acute and subacute bronchitis (with) tracheobronchitis, acute
          Acute and subacute fibrinous bronchitis
          Acute and subacute membranous bronchitis
          Acute and subacute purulent bronchitis
          Acute and subacute septic bronchitis
     Excludes 1:   *bronchitis NOS (J40)*
          tracheobronchitis NOS (J40)
     Excludes ❷: *acute bronchitis with bronchiectasis (J47.0)*
          acute bronchitis with chronic obstructive asthma (J44.0)
          acute bronchitis with chronic obstructive pulmonary disease (J44.0)
          allergic bronchitis NOS (J45.909-)
          bronchitis due to chemicals, fumes and vapors (J68.0)
          chronic bronchitis NOS (J42)
          chronic mucopurulent bronchitis (J41.1)
          chronic obstructive bronchitis (J44.-)
          chronic obstructive tracheobronchitis (J44.-)
          chronic simple bronchitis (J41.0)
          chronic tracheobronchitis (J42)

J20.0   **Acute bronchitis due to Mycoplasma pneumoniae**
J20.1   **Acute bronchitis due to Hemophilus influenzae**
J20.2   **Acute bronchitis due to streptococcus**
J20.3   **Acute bronchitis due to coxsackievirus**
J20.4   **Acute bronchitis due to parainfluenza virus**
J20.5   **Acute bronchitis due to respiratory syncytial virus**
J20.6   **Acute bronchitis due to rhinovirus**
J20.7   **Acute bronchitis due to echovirus**
J20.8   **Acute bronchitis due to other specified organisms**
J20.9   **Acute bronchitis, unspecified**

J21-   **Acute bronchiolitis** — A sudden, severe onset of inflammation of the bronchioles (the fine, small bronchial tubes).
     Includes: **Acute bronchiolitis with bronchospasm** — A form marked by spasmodic contraction (tightening) of the muscles in the walls of the bronchioles.
     Excludes ❷: *respiratory bronchiolitis interstitial lung disease (J84.115)*
CC **J21.0**   **Acute bronchiolitis due to respiratory syncytial virus**
CC **J21.1**   **Acute bronchiolitis due to human metapneumovirus**
CC **J21.8**   **Acute bronchiolitis due to other specified organisms**
CC **J21.9**   **Acute bronchiolitis, unspecified**
        Bronchiolitis (acute)
        Excludes 1:   *chronic bronchiolitis (J44.-)*

J22   **Unspecified acute lower respiratory infection**
     Acute (lower) respiratory (tract) infection NOS
     Excludes 1:   *upper respiratory infection (acute) (J06.9)*

Other diseases of upper respiratory tract (J30-J39)

J30-   **Vasomotor and allergic rhinitis** — ALLERGIC RHINITIS — Inflammation of the mucous membrane of the nose due to hypersensitivity of a particular allergen.
     Includes: **Spasmodic rhinorrhea**
     Excludes 1:   *allergic rhinitis with asthma (bronchial) (J45.909)*
          rhinitis NOS (J31.0)

J30.0   **Vasomotor rhinitis** — A non-allergic form without a known cause.
J30.1   **Allergic rhinitis due to pollens** — A form caused by the allergen pollen (the microspores of flowering plants).
        Allergy NOS due to pollen
        Hay fever
        Pollinosis
J30.2   **Other seasonal allergic rhinitis**
J30.5   **Allergic rhinitis due to food** — A form due to food allergens.
J30.8-   **Other allergic rhinitis**
     J30.81   **Allergic rhinitis due to animal (cat) (dog) hair and dander** — A form due to the old skin and hair cells of animals.
     J30.89   **Other allergic rhinitis**
          Perennial allergic rhinitis

J17 - J30

Excludes 1: = NOT CODED HERE! (Do not code both)   **765**   *Excludes ❷:* = Not Included Here

J30.9   Allergic rhinitis, unspecified

J31-   Chronic rhinitis, nasopharyngitis and pharyngitis
   Use additional code to identify:
   Exposure to environmental tobacco smoke (Z77.22)
   Exposure to tobacco smoke in the perinatal period (P96.81)
   History of tobacco dependence (Z87.891)
   Occupational exposure to environmental tobacco smoke (Z57.31)
   Tobacco dependence (F17.-)
   Tobacco use (Z72.0)

J31.0   Chronic rhinitis — Inflammation of the nasal mucous membrane which persists over a long period of time.
   Atrophic rhinitis (chronic) — A form marked by wasting of the mucous membrane and glands.
   Granulomatous rhinitis (chronic) — A form marked by the formation of granulomas.
   Hypertrophic rhinitis (chronic) — A form in which the mucous membrane swells and thickens.
   Obstructive rhinitis (chronic) — A form in which the mucous membrane swells sufficiently to obstruct the airflow.
   Ozena
   Purulent rhinitis (chronic) — A form marked by production of pus.
   Rhinitis (chronic) NOS
   Ulcerative rhinitis (chronic) — A form marked by the eating-away of the nasal mucous membrane.
   Excludes 1:   allergic rhinitis (J30.1-J30.9)
   *   vasomotor rhinitis (J30.0)*

J31.1   Chronic nasopharyngitis — Inflammation of the nasal and pharyngeal mucous membranes which develops slowly and persists over a long period of time.
   Excludes ❷: acute nasopharyngitis (J00)

J31.2   Chronic pharyngitis — Inflammation of the pharynx persisting over a long period of time.
   Chronic sore throat
   Atrophic pharyngitis (chronic)
   Granular pharyngitis (chronic)
   Hypertrophic pharyngitis (chronic)
   Excludes ❷: acute pharyngitis (J02.9)

J32-   Chronic sinusitis — Inflammation of one or more of the nasal sinuses which persists over a long period of time.
   Includes: **Sinus abscess** — The localized collection of pus within a sinus which persists over a long period of time.
   Sinus empyema — The accumulation of pus within a sinus cavity over a long period of time.
   Sinus infection
   Sinus suppuration — A form characterized by the production of pus.
   Use additional code to identify:
   Exposure to environmental tobacco smoke (Z77.22)
   Exposure to tobacco smoke in the perinatal period (P96.81)
   History of tobacco dependence (Z87.891)
   Infectious agent (B95-B97)
   Occupational exposure to environmental tobacco smoke (Z57.31)
   Tobacco dependence (F17-)
   Tobacco use (Z72.0)
   Excludes ❷: acute sinusitis (J01-)

J32.0   Chronic maxillary sinusitis — A form affecting one of the paired maxillary sinuses.
   Antritis (chronic) — A form affecting the maxillary antrum.
   Maxillary sinusitis NOS

J32.1   Chronic frontal sinusitis — A form affecting one of the paired frontal sinuses.
   Frontal sinusitis NOS

J32.2   Chronic ethmoidal sinusitis — A form affecting one of the paired groups of ethmoidal sinuses.
   Ethmoidal sinusitis NOS
   Excludes 1:   Woakes' ethmoiditis (J33.1)

J32.3   Chronic sphenoidal sinusitis — A form affecting one of the paired sphenoidal sinuses.
   Sphenoidal sinusitis NOS

J32.4   Chronic pansinusitis — A form affecting two or more of the sinuses at the same time.
   Pansinusitis NOS

J32.8   Other chronic sinusitis
   Sinusitis (chronic) involving more than one sinus but not pansinusitis

J32.9   Chronic sinusitis, unspecified
   Sinusitis (chronic) NOS

J33-   Nasal polyp — A protruding growth from the nasal mucous membrane.
   Use additional code to identify:
   Exposure to environmental tobacco smoke (Z77.22)
   Exposure to tobacco smoke in the perinatal period (P96.81)
   History of tobacco dependence (Z87.891)
   Occupational exposure to environmental tobacco smoke (Z57.31)
   Tobacco dependence (F17.-)
   Tobacco use (Z72.0)
   Excludes 1:   adenomatous polyps (D14.0)

J33.0   Polyp of nasal cavity — A protruding mucous membrane growth within the nose.
   Choanal polyp
   Nasopharyngeal polyp

J33.1   Polypoid sinus degeneration — Deterioration of the nasal sinus mucous membrane due to polypoid growth.
   Woakes' syndrome or ethmoiditis

J33.8   Other polyp of sinus
   Accessory polyp of sinus — A mucous membrane growth of one of the accessory sinuses.
   Ethmoidal polyp of sinus — A mucous membrane growth of the ethmoidal sinus.
   Maxillary polyp of sinus — A mucous membrane growth of the maxillary sinus.
   Sphenoidal polyp of sinus — A mucous membrane growth of the sphenoidal sinus.

J33.9   Nasal polyp, unspecified

J34-   Other and unspecified disorders of nose and nasal sinuses
   Excludes ❷: varicose ulcer of nasal septum (I86.8)

J34.0   Abscess, furuncle and carbuncle of nose — A localized collection of purulent fluid caused by the disintegration of nasal tissue.
   Cellulitis of nose — Cellular tissue Inflammation of the nose.
   Necrosis of nose — The localized death of nasal tissue cells.
   Ulceration of nose — An eating-away of the nasal tissue.

J34.1   Cyst and mucocele of nose and nasal sinus — The abnormal dilatation of a sinus cavity with accumulated mucous secretion.

J34.2   Deviated nasal septum — An abnormality of the nasoseptal cartilage characterized by a turning away from the midline to either side.
   Deflection or deviation of septum (nasal) (acquired)
   Excludes 1:   congenital deviated nasal septum (Q67.4)

J34.3   Hypertrophy of nasal turbinates — An enlargement of the turbinate bones of the nasal cavity and their lining membranes.

J34.8-   Other specified disorders of nose and nasal sinuses

J34.81   Nasal mucositis (ulcerative) — Inflammation and/or ulcerative sores of the nasal mucosal surfaces.
   Code also type of associated therapy, such as:
   Antineoplastic and immunosuppressive drugs (T45.1x-)
   Radiological procedure and radiotherapy (Y84.2)
   Excludes ❷: gastrointestinal mucositis (ulcerative) (K92.81)
   *   mucositis (ulcerative) of vagina and vulva (N76.81)*
   *   oral mucositis (ulcerative) (K12.3-)*

J34.89   Other specified disorders of nose and nasal sinuses
   Perforation of nasal septum NOS
   Rhinolith — A nasal stone or concretion.

J34.9   Unspecified disorder of nose and nasal sinuses

J35-   Chronic diseases of tonsils and adenoids
   Use additional code to identify:
   Exposure to environmental tobacco smoke (Z77.22)
   Exposure to tobacco smoke in the perinatal period (P96.81)
   History of tobacco dependence (Z87.891)
   Occupational exposure to environmental tobacco smoke (Z57.31)
   Tobacco dependence (F17.-)
   Tobacco use (Z72.0)

J35.0-   Chronic tonsillitis and adenoiditis — Inflammation of the palatine tonsils and/or the adenoids that persists over a long period of time.
   Excludes ❷: acute tonsillitis (J03.-)

J35.01   Chronic tonsillitis — A form affecting the palatine tonsils.

J35.02   Chronic adenoiditis — A form affecting the adenoids.

J35.03   Chronic tonsillitis and adenoiditis — A form affecting both the palatine tonsils and the adenoids.

J35.1   Hypertrophy of tonsils — The abnormal enlargement of the tonsils.
   Enlargement of tonsils
   Excludes 1:   hypertrophy of tonsils with tonsillitis (J35.0-)

J35.2   Hypertrophy of adenoids — The abnormal enlargement of the adenoids.
   Enlargement of adenoids
   Excludes 1:   hypertrophy of adenoids with adenoiditis (J35.0-)

J
3
0
-
J
3
5

J35.3 **Hypertrophy of tonsils with hypertrophy of adenoids**
> Excludes 1:   *hypertrophy of tonsils and adenoids with tonsillitis and adenoiditis (J35.03)*

J35.8 **Other chronic diseases of tonsils and adenoids**
Adenoid vegetations — A fungus-like growth of lymphoid tissue in the nasopharynx.
Amygdalolith — A chalky, hard mass within a tonsil.
Calculus, tonsil — A hard mass within a tonsil.
Cicatrix of tonsil (and adenoid) — The new healing tissue of tonsils and/or adenoids.
Tonsillar tag — A small appendage of tonsillar tissue.
Ulcer of tonsil — An eating-away of the tonsillar tissue.

J35.9 **Chronic disease of tonsils and adenoids, unspecified**
Disease (chronic) of tonsils and adenoids NOS

J36 **Peritonsillar abscess** — A localized collection of pus caused by the disintegration of
CC the connective tissue of the tonsil capsule.
Includes: **Abscess of tonsil** — A localized collection of pus caused by the disintegration of tonsillar lymphoid tissue.
Peritonsillar cellulitis
Quinsy
Use additional code (B95-B97) to identify infectious agent
> Excludes 1:   *acute tonsillitis (J03.-)*
> *chronic tonsillitis (J35.0)*
> *retropharyngeal abscess (J39.0)*
> *tonsillitis NOS (J03.9-)*

J37- **Chronic laryngitis and laryngotracheitis** — Inflammation of the larynx and/or
larynx and trachea which develops slowly and persists over a long period of time.
Use additional code to identify:
Exposure to environmental tobacco smoke (Z77.22)
Exposure to tobacco smoke in the perinatal period (P96.81)
History of tobacco dependence (Z87.891)
Infectious agent (B95-B97)
Occupational exposure to environmental tobacco smoke (Z57.31)
Tobacco dependence (F17.-)
Tobacco use (Z72.0)

J37.0 **Chronic laryngitis** — Inflammation of the larynx which develops slowly and
persists over a long period of time.
Catarrhal laryngitis — A form marked by atrophy of the mucous membrane.
Hypertrophic laryngitis — A form marked by the thickening and swelling of the mucous membrane.
Sicca laryngitis — A form marked by glue-like secretions.
> Excludes ❷: *acute laryngitis (J04.0)*
> *obstructive (acute) laryngitis (J05.0)*

J37.1 **Chronic laryngotracheitis** — Inflammation of the larynx and trachea which
develops slowly and persists over a long period of time.
Laryngitis, chronic, with tracheitis (chronic)
Tracheitis, chronic, with laryngitis
> Excludes 1: *chronic tracheitis (J42)*
> Excludes ❷: *acute laryngotracheitis (J04.2)*
> *acute tracheitis (J04.1)*

J38- **Diseases of vocal cords and larynx, not elsewhere classified**
Use additional code to identify:
Exposure to environmental tobacco smoke (Z77.22)
Exposure to tobacco smoke in the perinatal period (P96.81)
History of tobacco dependence (Z87.891)
Occupational exposure to environmental tobacco smoke (Z57.31)
Tobacco dependence (F17.-)
Tobacco use (Z72.0)
> Excludes 1: *congenital laryngeal stridor (P28.89)*
> *obstructive laryngitis (acute) (J05.0)*
> *postprocedural subglottic stenosis (J95.5)*
> *stridor (R06.1)*
> *ulcerative laryngitis (J04.0)*

J38.0- **Paralysis of vocal cords and larynx** — Loss of motor function of the
vocal cords or larynx.
Laryngoplegia — Paralysis of the larynx.
Paralysis of glottis — A loss of motor function of the vocal apparatus of the larynx.

J38.00 **Paralysis of vocal cords and larynx, unspecified**

J38.01 **Paralysis of vocal cords and larynx, unilateral**

J38.02 **Paralysis of vocal cords and larynx, bilateral**

J38.1 **Polyp of vocal cord and larynx** — A mucous membrane protruding
growth of the vocal cords or larynx.
> Excludes 1:   *adenomatous polyps (D14.1)*

J38.2 **Nodules of vocal cords** — Small, white nodules occurring on the vocal cords.
Chorditis (fibrinous) (nodosa) (tuberosa)
Singer's nodes
Teacher's nodes

J38.3 **Other diseases of vocal cords**
Abscess of vocal cords — A localized collection of pus caused by the disintegration of the vocal cord tissue.
Cellulitis of vocal cords — Inflammation of the cellular tissue of the vocal cords.
Granuloma of vocal cords — The formation of a granuloma on the vocal cords.
Leukokeratosis of vocal cords
Leukoplakia of vocal cords — White, thickened patches of the mucous membrane lining of the vocal cords.

J38.4 **Edema of larynx** — The accumulation of intercellular fluid of the laryngeal
tissues.
Edema (of) glottis — The accumulation of intercellular fluid of the vocal apparatus.
Subglottic edema — The accumulation of intercellular fluid of the tissues below the vocal cord apparatus.
Supraglottic edema — The accumulation of intercellular fluid in the tissues above the vocal apparatus.
> Excludes 1:   *acute obstructive laryngitis [croup] (J05.0)*
> *edematous laryngitis (J04.0)*

J38.5 **Laryngeal spasm** — A sudden, violent involuntary contraction of the laryngeal
muscles.
Laryngismus (stridulus)

J38.6 **Stenosis of larynx** — The abnormal reduction in the laryngeal orifice size.

J38.7 **Other diseases of larynx**
Abscess of larynx — A localized collection of pus caused by the disintegration of laryngeal tissue.
Cellulitis of larynx — Inflammation of the cellular tissue of the larynx.
Disease of larynx NOS
Necrosis of larynx — The death of a localized group of laryngeal cells.
Pachyderma of larynx — Localized, warty epithelial thickenings on the larynx.
Perichondritis of larynx — Inflammation of the dense connective tissue around the laryngeal cartilages.
Ulcer of larynx — An eating-away of the laryngeal tissue.

J39- **Other diseases of upper respiratory tract**
> Excludes 1:   *acute respiratory infection NOS (J22)*
> *acute upper respiratory infection (J06.9)*
> *upper respiratory inflammation due to chemicals, gases, fumes or vapors (J68.2)*

CC J39.0 **Retropharyngeal and parapharyngeal abscess** — A localized
collection of pus caused by the disintegration of the fascial tissue between the pharyngeal wall and the prevertebral fascia or the connective tissue within the pharynx.
Peripharyngeal abscess
> Excludes 1:   *peritonsillar abscess (J36)*

CC J39.1 **Other abscess of pharynx**
Cellulitis of pharynx — Inflammation of the cellular pharyngeal tissue.
Nasopharyngeal abscess — A localized collection of pus caused by the disintegration of the nasopharyngeal tissue.

J39.2 **Other diseases of pharynx**
Cyst of pharynx — A fluid-filled sac of the pharynx.
Edema of pharynx — The abnormal accumulation of intercellular fluid of the pharynx.
> Excludes ❷: *chronic pharyngitis (J31.2)*
> *ulcerative pharyngitis (J02.9)*

J39.3 **Upper respiratory tract hypersensitivity reaction, site
unspecified**
> Excludes 1:   *hypersensitivity reaction of upper respiratory tract, such as:*
> *extrinsic allergic alveolitis (J67.9)*
> *pneumoconiosis (J60-J67.9)*

J39.8 **Other specified diseases of upper respiratory tract**

J39.9 **Disease of upper respiratory tract, unspecified**

J
3
5
–
J
3
9

Chronic lower respiratory diseases (J40-J47)

Excludes 1:   *bronchitis due to chemicals, gases, fumes and vapors (J68.0)*
Excludes ❷: *cystic fibrosis (E84-)*

J40   **Bronchitis, <u>not specified as acute or chronic</u>**
     Bronchitis NOS
     Bronchitis with tracheitis NOS
     Catarrhal bronchitis
     Tracheobronchitis NOS
     Use additional code to identify:
     Exposure to environmental tobacco smoke (Z77.22)
     Exposure to tobacco smoke in the perinatal period (P96.81)
     History of tobacco dependence (Z87.891)
     Occupational exposure to environmental tobacco smoke (Z57.31)
     Tobacco dependence (F17-)
     Tobacco use (Z72.0)
     Excludes 1:   *acute bronchitis (J20.-)*
               allergic bronchitis NOS (J45.909-)
               asthmatic bronchitis NOS (J45.9-)
               bronchitis due to chemicals, gases, fumes and vapors (J68.0)

J41-   **Simple and mucopurulent chronic bronchitis**
     Use additional code to identify:
     Exposure to environmental tobacco smoke (Z77.22)
     Exposure to tobacco smoke in the perinatal period (P96.81)
     History of tobacco dependence (Z87.891)
     Occupational exposure to environmental tobacco smoke (Z57.31)
     Tobacco dependence (F17-)
     Tobacco use (Z72.0)
     Excludes 1:   *chronic bronchitis NOS (J42)*
               chronic obstructive bronchitis (J44-)

     J41.0   **Simple chronic bronchitis** — A form marked by mild, persistent symptoms of coughing and expectoration.

     J41.1   **Mucopurulent chronic bronchitis** — A form marked by persistent, significant mucopurulent discharge.

     J41.8   **Mixed simple and mucopurulent chronic bronchitis**

J42   **Unspecified chronic bronchitis**
     Chronic bronchitis NOS
     Chronic tracheitis
     Chronic tracheobronchitis
     Use additional code to identify:
     Exposure to environmental tobacco smoke (Z77.22)
     Exposure to tobacco smoke in the perinatal period (P96.81)
     History of tobacco dependence (Z87.891)
     Occupational exposure to environmental tobacco smoke (Z57.31)
     Tobacco dependence (F17-)
     Tobacco use (Z72.0)
     Excludes 1:   *chronic asthmatic bronchitis (J44-)*
               chronic bronchitis with airways obstruction (J44-)
               chronic emphysematous bronchitis (J44-)
               chronic obstructive pulmonary disease NOS (J44.9)
               simple and mucopurulent chronic bronchitis (J41-)

J43-   **Emphysema** — The abnormal increase in the size of the air spaces distal to the terminal bronchioles with destructive changes.
     Use additional code to identify:
     Exposure to environmental tobacco smoke (Z77.22)
     History of tobacco dependence (Z87.891)
     Occupational exposure to environmental tobacco smoke (Z57.31)
     Tobacco dependence (F17-)
     Tobacco use (Z72.0)
     Excludes 1:   *compensatory emphysema (J98.3)*
               emphysema due to inhalation of chemicals, gases, fumes or
                  vapors (J68.4)
               emphysema with chronic (obstructive) bronchitis (J44-)
               emphysematous (obstructive) bronchitis (J44-)
               interstitial emphysema (J98.2)
               mediastinal emphysema (J98.2)
               neonatal interstitial emphysema (P25.0)
               surgical (subcutaneous) emphysema (T81.82)
               traumatic subcutaneous emphysema (T79.7)

     J43.0   **Unilateral pulmonary emphysema [MacLeod's syndrome]** — A form with greater translucency over one lung.
         Swyer-James syndrome
         Unilateral emphysema
         Unilateral hyperlucent lung
         Unilateral pulmonary artery functional hypoplasia
         Unilateral transparency of lung

     J43.1   **Panlobular emphysema** — A form marked by generalized areas of destructive dilatations.
         Panacinar emphysema

     J43.2   **Centrilobular emphysema** — A form marked by localized areas of destructive dilatations.

     J43.8   **Other emphysema**

     J43.9   **Emphysema, unspecified**
         Bullous emphysema (lung) (pulmonary) — A form marked by large blebs.
         Emphysema (lung) (pulmonary) NOS
         Emphysematous bleb — A form characterized by single or multiple large cystic alveolar dilatations of the air spaces.
         Vesicular emphysema (lung) (pulmonary)

J44-   **<u>Other chronic obstructive pulmonary disease</u>** — A disease of decreased ability of the lungs to perform ventilation due to diffuse obstruction of the pulmonary system.
     AHA 13:4Q:p109 – Nicotine dependence and COPD
     AHA 13:4Q:p129 – Chronic hypoxic respiratory failure and COPD
     Includes: Asthma with chronic obstructive pulmonary disease
               Chronic asthmatic (obstructive) bronchitis
               Chronic bronchitis with airways obstruction
               Chronic bronchitis with emphysema
               Chronic emphysematous bronchitis
               Chronic obstructive asthma
               Chronic obstructive bronchitis
               Chronic obstructive tracheobronchitis
     Use additional code to identify:
     Exposure to environmental tobacco smoke (Z77.22)
     History of tobacco dependence (Z87.891)
     Occupational exposure to environmental tobacco smoke (Z57.31)
     Tobacco dependence (F17-)
     Tobacco use (Z72.0)
     Code also type of asthma, if applicable (J45.-)
     Excludes 1:   *bronchiectasis (J47-)*
               chronic bronchitis NOS (J42)
               chronic simple and mucopurulent bronchitis (J41-)
               chronic tracheitis (J42)
               chronic tracheobronchitis (J42)
               emphysema without chronic bronchitis (J43-)
     Excludes ❷: *lung diseases due to external agents (J60-J70)*

     cc **J44.0**   **Chronic obstructive pulmonary disease <u>with acute lower respiratory infection</u>**
         Use additional code to identify the infection

     cc **J44.1**   **Chronic obstructive pulmonary disease <u>with (acute) exacerbation</u>** — A form characterized by a sudden, severe increase in severity.
         Decompensated COPD
         Decompensated COPD with (acute) exacerbation
         Excludes ❷: *chronic obstructive pulmonary disease [COPD] with*
                     acute bronchitis (J44.0)

     J44.9   **Chronic obstructive pulmonary disease, unspecified**
         Chronic obstructive airway disease NOS
         Chronic obstructive lung disease NOS

J45-   **<u>Asthma</u>** — A chronic inflammatory disorder of the airways which results in narrowing of the airways and is characterized by difficult and labored breathing with coughing and wheezing.
     AHA 12:4Q:p99 – Acute exacerbation of asthma and status asthmaticus together
     Includes: Allergic (predominantly) asthma
               Allergic bronchitis NOS
               Allergic rhinitis with asthma
               Atopic asthma
               Extrinsic allergic asthma
               Hay fever with asthma
               Idiosyncratic asthma
               Intrinsic nonallergic asthma
               Nonallergic asthma
     Use additional code to identify:
     Exposure to environmental tobacco smoke (Z77.22)
     Exposure to tobacco smoke in the perinatal period (P96.81)
     History of tobacco dependence (Z87.891)
     Occupational exposure to environmental tobacco smoke (Z57.31)
     Tobacco dependence (F17.-)
     Tobacco use (Z72.0)
     Excludes 1:   *detergent asthma (J69.8)*
               eosinophilic asthma (J82)
               lung diseases due to external agents (J60-J70)
               miner's asthma (J60)
               wheezing NOS (R06.2)
               wood asthma (J67.8)
     Excludes ❷: *asthma with chronic obstructive pulmonary disease (J44.9)*
               chronic asthmatic (obstructive) bronchitis (J44.9)
               chronic obstructive asthma (J44.9)

     J45.2-   **Mild intermittent asthma** — A severity of symptoms frequency classification of two or fewer episodes per week.

         J45.20   **Mild intermittent asthma, uncomplicated**
                 Mild intermittent asthma NOS

J 40 - J 45

cc **J45.21   Mild intermittent asthma <u>with (acute) exacerbation</u>** — A form characterized by a sudden, severe increase in severity.

cc **J45.22   Mild intermittent asthma <u>with status asthmaticus</u>** — A continuous, obstructive asthmatic state unrelieved after initial therapy measures.

J45.3-   Mild persistent asthma — A severity of symptoms frequency classification of two or more episodes per week.

J45.30   Mild persistent asthma, uncomplicated
Mild persistent asthma NOS

cc **J45.31   Mild persistent asthma <u>with (acute) exacerbation</u>** — A form characterized by a sudden, severe increase in severity.

cc **J45.32   Mild persistent asthma <u>with status asthmaticus</u>** — A continuous, obstructive asthmatic state unrelieved after initial therapy measures.

J45.4-   Moderate persistent asthma — A severity of symptoms frequency classification of daily episodes.

J45.40   Moderate persistent asthma, uncomplicated
Moderate persistent asthma NOS

cc **J45.41   Moderate persistent asthma <u>with (acute) exacerbation</u>** — A form characterized by a sudden, severe increase in severity.

cc **J45.42   Moderate persistent asthma <u>with status asthmaticus</u>** — A continuous, obstructive asthmatic state unrelieved after initial therapy measures.

J45.5-   Severe persistent asthma — A severity of symptoms frequency classification of continuous episodes.

J45.50   Severe persistent asthma, uncomplicated
Severe persistent asthma NOS

cc **J45.51   Severe persistent asthma <u>with (acute) exacerbation</u>** — A form characterized by a sudden, severe increase in severity.

cc **J45.52   Severe persistent asthma <u>with status asthmaticus</u>** — A continuous, obstructive asthmatic state unrelieved after initial therapy measures.

J45.9-   Other and unspecified asthma

J45.90- Unspecified asthma
Asthmatic bronchitis NOS
Childhood asthma NOS
Late onset asthma

cc **J45.901   Unspecified asthma <u>with (acute) exacerbation</u>** — A form characterized by a sudden, severe increase in severity.

cc **J45.902   Unspecified asthma <u>with status asthmaticus</u>** — A continuous, obstructive asthmatic state unrelieved after initial therapy measures.

J45.909   Unspecified asthma, uncomplicated
Asthma NOS

J45.99- Other asthma

J45.990   Exercise induced bronchospasm — A form causing difficulty exhaling air that is triggered by exercise or strenuous activity.

J45.991   Cough variant asthma — A form in which coughing is the patient's only symptom.

J45.998   Other asthma

J47-   Bronchiectasis — Persistent dilatation of the bronchi with coughing, foul-smelling breath, and mucopurulent expectoration.
Includes: Bronchiolectasis
Use additional code to identify:
Exposure to environmental tobacco smoke (Z77.22)
Exposure to tobacco smoke in the perinatal period (P96.81)
History of tobacco dependence (Z87.891)
Occupational exposure to environmental tobacco smoke (Z57.31)
Tobacco dependence (F17-)
Tobacco use (Z72.0)
Excludes 1:   congenital bronchiectasis (Q33.4)
tuberculous bronchiectasis (current disease) (A15.0)

cc **J47.0   Bronchiectasis <u>with acute lower respiratory infection</u>**
Bronchiectasis with acute bronchitis
Use additional code to identify the infection

cc **J47.1   Bronchiectasis <u>with (acute) exacerbation</u>** — A form characterized by a sudden, severe increase in severity.

J47.9   Bronchiectasis, uncomplicated
Bronchiectasis NOS

Lung diseases due to external agents (J60-J70)

Excludes ❷: asthma (J45-)
malignant neoplasm of bronchus and lung (C34-)

J60   Coalworker's pneumoconiosis — [Age/15-124] — Destructive deposition of substantial amounts of coal dust particles in the lungs.
Anthracosilicosis
Anthracosis
Black lung disease
Coalworker's lung
Excludes 1:   coalworker pneumoconiosis with tuberculosis, any type in A15 (J65)

J61   Pneumoconiosis due to asbestos and other mineral fibers — [Age/15-124] — Destructive deposition of magnesium and calcium silicate in the lung tissues.
Asbestosis
Excludes 1:   pleural plaque with asbestosis (J92.0)
pneumoconiosis with tuberculosis, any type in A15 (J65)

J62-   Pneumoconiosis due to dust containing silica
Includes: Silicotic fibrosis (massive) of lung
Excludes 1:   pneumoconiosis with tuberculosis, any type in A15 (J65)

J62.0   Pneumoconiosis due to talc dust — Destructive deposition of magnesium silicate in the lung tissues.

J62.8   Pneumoconiosis due to other dust containing silica — Destructive deposition of silicon dioxide in the lung tissues.
Silicosis NOS

J63-   Pneumoconiosis due to other inorganic dusts
Excludes 1:   pneumoconiosis with tuberculosis, any type in A15 (J65)

J63.0   Aluminosis (of lung) — Destructive deposition of aluminum particles in the lung tissues.

J63.1   Bauxite fibrosis (of lung) — Destructive deposition of bauxite fumes containing fine particles of alumina and silica which lead to extreme pulmonary emphysema.

J63.2   Berylliosis — Destructive deposition of beryllium salts or dust in the lung tissues characterized by the formation of granulomas.

J63.3   Graphite fibrosis (of lung) — Fibrotic, destructive deposition of mineralized carbon in the lung tissues.

J63.4   Siderosis — Destructive deposition of iron particles in the lung tissue.

J63.5   Stannosis — Destructive deposition of tin oxide in the lung tissues.

J63.6   Pneumoconiosis due to other specified inorganic dusts

J64   Unspecified pneumoconiosis
Excludes 1:   pneumonoconiosis with tuberculosis, any type in A15 (J65)

J65   Pneumoconiosis associated with tuberculosis
Any condition in J60-J64 with tuberculosis, any type in A15
Silicotuberculosis

J66-   Airway disease due to specific organic dust
Excludes ❷: allergic alveolitis (J67.-)
asbestosis (J61)
bagassosis (J67.1)
farmer's lung (J67.0)
hypersensitivity pneumonitis due to organic dust (J67.-)
reactive airways dysfunction syndrome (J68.3)

J66.0   Byssinosis — A disease of the lung tissues caused by the inhalation of cotton dust.
Airway disease due to cotton dust

J66.1   Flax-dressers' disease — A disease of the lung tissue caused by the inhalation of flax plant particles.

J66.2   Cannabinosis — A disease of the lung caused by the inhalation of cannabis smoke.

J66.8   Airway disease due to other specific organic dusts

J67-   Hypersensitivity pneumonitis due to organic dust
Includes: Allergic alveolitis and pneumonitis due to inhaled organic dust and particles of fungal, actinomycetic or other origin
Excludes 1:   pneumonitis due to inhalation of chemicals, gases, fumes or vapors (J68.0)

J67.0   Farmer's lung — A form of hypersensitivity alveolitis caused by exposure to moldy hay that has fermented.
Harvester's lung
Haymaker's lung
Moldy hay disease

J 4 5 - J 6 7

J67.1 Bagassosis — A form of hypersensitivity pneumonitis due to inhalation of bagasse dust; the moldy, dusty fibrous waste of sugar cane after removal of the sugar-containing sap.
Bagasse disease
Bagasse pneumonitis

J67.2 Bird fancier's lung — A condition marked by cough, shortness of breath, fever, and chills caused by bird's excreta and seen in persons with extensive exposure to birds.
Budgerigar fancier's disease or lung — A form due to extensive exposure to an Australian parakeet (Budgerigar).
Pigeon fancier's disease or lung — A form due to extensive exposure to pigeons.

J67.3 Suberosis — Pneumoconiosis due to inhalation and tissue reaction to cork dust.
Corkhandler's disease or lung
Corkworker's disease or lung

J67.4 Maltworker's lung — A form of hypersensitivity alveolitis caused by working with germinated malt.
Alveolitis due to Aspergillus clavatus — A hypersensitivity from the organism Aspergillus clavatus.

J67.5 Mushroom-worker's lung — A form of hypersensitivity alveolitis caused by work involving the cultivating of mushrooms.

J67.6 Maple-bark-stripper's lung — A form of hypersensitivity alveolitis caused by work involving the stripping of bark from maple trees.
Alveolitis due to Cryptostroma corticale — A form of hypersensitivity alveolitis caused by Cryptostroma corticale, a fungi which grows under the bark of certain trees.
Cryptostromosis

CC **J67.7 Air conditioner and humidifier lung**
Allergic alveolitis due to fungal, thermophilic actinomycetes and other organisms growing in ventilation [air conditioning] systems

CC **J67.8 Hypersensitivity pneumonitis due to other organic dusts**
Cheese-washer's lung — A hypersensitivity lung disease caused by fungus released during cheese production.
Coffee-worker's lung — A hypersensitivity lung disease caused by work involving coffee bean processing dust.
Fish-meal worker's lung — A hypersensitivity lung disease caused by work involving the production of fish meal.
Furrier's lung — A hypersensitivity lung disease caused by work involving furs.
Sequoiosis — A hypersensitivity lung disease caused by sawdust.

CC **J67.9 Hypersensitivity pneumonitis due to unspecified organic dust**
Allergic alveolitis (extrinsic) NOS
Hypersensitivity pneumonitis NOS

J68- Respiratory conditions due to inhalation of chemicals, gases, fumes and vapors — Inflammation and other respiratory conditions due to the adverse effects of gaseous fumes and vapors.
Code first (T51-T65) to identify cause
Use additional code to identify associated respiratory conditions, such as:
Acute respiratory failure (J96.0-)

CC **J68.0 Bronchitis and pneumonitis due to chemicals, gases, fumes and vapors** — Inflammation of the bronchi and/or lungs due to the adverse effects of gaseous fumes and vapors.
Chemical bronchitis (acute)

MCC **J68.1 Pulmonary edema due to chemicals, gases, fumes and vapors** — A sudden, severe onset of an excessive amount of intercellular fluid due to the effects of gaseous fumes and vapors.
Chemical pulmonary edema (acute) (chronic)
Excludes 1:   pulmonary edema (acute) (chronic) NOS (J81-)

J68.2 Upper respiratory inflammation due to chemicals, gases, fumes and vapors, not elsewhere classified

J68.3 Other acute and subacute respiratory conditions due to chemicals, gases, fumes and vapors
Reactive airways dysfunction syndrome

J68.4 Chronic respiratory conditions due to chemicals, gases, fumes and vapors
Emphysema (diffuse) (chronic) due to inhalation of chemicals, gases, fumes and vapors — The prolonged, persistent increase in the size of the air spaces distal to the terminal bronchioles due to inhalation of chemical fumes and vapors.
Obliterative bronchiolitis (chronic) (subacute) due to inhalation of chemicals, gases, fumes and vapors — The destructive inflammation of the bronchi and bronchioles due to inhalation of chemical fumes and vapors.
Pulmonary fibrosis (chronic) due to inhalation of chemicals, gases, fumes and vapors — The prolonged, persistent development of fibrous tissue of the lung due to inhalation of chemical fumes and vapors.
Excludes 1:   chronic pulmonary edema due to chemicals, gases, fumes and vapors (J68.1)

J68.8 Other respiratory conditions due to chemicals, gases, fumes and vapors

J68.9 Unspecified respiratory condition due to chemicals, gases, fumes and vapors

J69- Pneumonitis due to solids and liquids — Inflammation of the lungs caused by the inhalation of solid and/or liquid matter.
Excludes 1:   neonatal aspiration syndromes (P24-)
postprocedural pneumonitis (J95.4)

MCC **J69.0 Pneumonitis due to inhalation of food and vomit**
Aspiration pneumonia NOS
Aspiration pneumonia (due to) food (regurgitated)
Aspiration pneumonia (due to) gastric secretions
Aspiration pneumonia (due to) milk
Aspiration pneumonia (due to) vomit
Code also any associated foreign body in respiratory tract (T17-)
Excludes 1:   chemical pneumonitis due to anesthesia (J95.4)
obstetric aspiration pneumonitis (O74.0)

MCC **J69.1 Pneumonitis due to inhalation of oils and essences**
Exogenous lipoid pneumonia
Lipid pneumonia NOS
Code first (T51-T65) to identify substance
Excludes 1:   endogenous lipoid pneumonia (J84.89)

MCC **J69.8 Pneumonitis due to inhalation of other solids and liquids**
Pneumonitis due to aspiration of blood
Pneumonitis due to aspiration of detergent
Code first (T51-T65) to identify substance

J70- Respiratory conditions due to other external agents

CC **J70.0 Acute pulmonary manifestations due to radiation** — Inflammation of the lungs due to the adverse effects of radiation.
Radiation pneumonitis
Use additional code (W88-W90, X39.0-) to identify the external cause

CC **J70.1 Chronic and other pulmonary manifestations due to radiation**
Fibrosis of lung following radiation — The fibrotic tissue reaction of the lung which develops slowly over a period of time and is caused by the adverse effects of radiation.
Use additional code (W88-W90, X39.0-) to identify the external cause

J70.2 Acute drug-induced interstitial lung disorders
Use additional code for adverse effect, if applicable, to identify drug (T36-T50 with fifth or sixth character 5)
Excludes 1:   interstitial pneumonia NOS (J84.9)
lymphoid interstitial pneumonia (J84.2)

J70.3 Chronic drug-induced interstitial lung disorders
Use additional code for adverse effect, if applicable, to identify drug (T36-T50 with fifth or sixth character 5)
Excludes 1:   interstitial pneumonia NOS (J84.9)
lymphoid interstitial pneumonia (J84.2)

J70.4 Drug-induced interstitial lung disorders, unspecified
Use additional code for adverse effect, if applicable, to identify drug (T36-T50 with fifth or sixth character 5)
Excludes 1:   interstitial pneumonia NOS (J84.9)
lymphoid interstitial pneumonia (J84.2)

J70.5 Respiratory conditions due to smoke inhalation
AHA 13:4Q:p121 – Acute respiratory failure due to smoke inhalation
Smoke inhalation NOS
Excludes 1:   smoke inhalation due to chemicals, gases, fumes and vapors (J68.9)

J70.8 Respiratory conditions due to other specified external agents
Code first (T51-T65) to identify the external agent

J70.9 Respiratory conditions due to unspecified external agent
Code first (T51-T65) to identify the external agent

J 67 - J 70

Other respiratory diseases principally affecting the interstitium (J80-J84)

J80 **Acute respiratory distress syndrome** — A syndrome characterized by damage to
CC the pulmonary capillary endothelium, alveolar hemorrhage, and interstitial edema following severe shock, trauma, or major thoracic surgery.
    Acute respiratory distress syndrome in adult or child
    Adult hyaline membrane disease
    Excludes 1:   *respiratory distress syndrome in newborn (perinatal) (P22.0)*

J81- **Pulmonary edema** — The severe, sudden accumulation of intercellular fluid of the lungs not due to heart disease.
    Use additional code to identify:
    Exposure to environmental tobacco smoke (Z77.22)
    History of tobacco dependence (Z87.891)
    Occupational exposure to environmental tobacco smoke (Z57.31)
    Tobacco dependence (F17-)
    Tobacco use (Z72.0)
    Excludes 1:   *chemical (acute) pulmonary edema (J68.1)*
         hypostatic pneumonia (J18.2)
         passive pneumonia (J18.2)
         pulmonary edema due to external agents (J60-J70)
         pulmonary edema with heart disease NOS (I50.1)
         pulmonary edema with heart failure (I50.1)

MCC **J81.0** **Acute** pulmonary edema — A sudden, severe onset.
    Acute edema of lung

CC **J81.1** **Chronic** pulmonary edema — A form that persists over a long period of time.
    Pulmonary congestion (chronic) (passive)
    Pulmonary edema NOS

J82 **Pulmonary eosinophilia, not elsewhere classified** — The abnormal
CC infiltration of the pulmonary tissues by eosinophils.
    Allergic pneumonia
    Eosinophilic asthma
    Eosinophilic pneumonia
    Löffler's pneumonia
    Tropical (pulmonary) eosinophilia NOS
    Excludes 1:   *pulmonary eosinophilia due to aspergillosis (B44-)*
         pulmonary eosinophilia due to drugs (J70.2-J70.4)
         pulmonary eosinophilia due to specified parasitic infection
          (B50-B83)
         pulmonary eosinophilia due to systemic connective tissue
          disorders (M30-M36)
         pulmonary infiltrate NOS (R91.8)

J84- **Other interstitial pulmonary diseases**
    Excludes 1:   *drug-induced interstitial lung disorders (J70.2-J70.4)*
         interstitial emphysema (J98.2)
         lung diseases due to external agents (J60-J70)

  J84.0- **Alveolar and parieto-alveolar conditions**
CC **J84.01** **Alveolar proteinosis** — The abnormal filling of the distal alveoli with proteinaceous material which prevents ventilation of the affected areas.

CC **J84.02** **Pulmonary alveolar microlithiasis** — The abnormal deposition of minute calculi in the alveoli of the lungs.

CC **J84.03** **Idiopathic pulmonary hemosiderosis** — [Not Allowed as PDX] – The abnormal deposition of iron pigment in the lung tissue.
    Essential brown induration of lung
    Code first underlying disease, such as:
    Disorders of iron metabolism (E83.1-)
    Excludes 1:   *acute idiopathic pulmonary hemorrhage in infants*
         [AIPHI] (R04.81)

CC **J84.09** **Other alveolar and parieto-alveolar conditions**

  J84.1- **Other interstitial pulmonary diseases with fibrosis**
    Excludes 1:   *pulmonary fibrosis (chronic) due to inhalation of*
         chemicals, gases, fumes or vapors (J68.4)
         pulmonary fibrosis (chronic) following radiation (J70.1)

  J84.10 **Pulmonary fibrosis, unspecified** — The progressive fibrous tissue replacement of the pulmonary alveolar walls leading to difficult or labored breathing.
    Capillary fibrosis of lung
    Cirrhosis of lung (chronic) NOS
    Fibrosis of lung (atrophic) (chronic) (confluent) (massive)
      (perialveolar) (peribronchial) NOS
    Induration of lung (chronic) NOS
    Postinflammatory pulmonary fibrosis — Progressive fibrosis of the pulmonary alveolar walls with difficult breathing following inflammatory reaction within the lung tissue.

  J84.11- **Idiopathic interstitial pneumonia** — The abnormal accumulation of damaged (e.g., fibrotic, inflammatory, plasma) cells in the space between the air sacs (alveoli) of the lungs that is not due to a known underlying cause and is primarily differentiated by histological appearance.
    Excludes 1:   *lymphoid interstitial pneumonia (J84.2)*
         pneumocystis pneumonia (B59)

  J84.111 **Idiopathic interstitial pneumonia, not otherwise specified**

  J84.112 **Idiopathic pulmonary fibrosis** — A progressive fibrotic lung disease that is limited to the lungs with the histological appearance of usual interstitial pneumonia (UIP).
    Cryptogenic fibrosing alveolitis
    Idiopathic fibrosing alveolitis

  J84.113 **Idiopathic non-specific interstitial pneumonitis** — A form marked by the histological appearance of diffuse inflammation with some degree of interstitial fibrosis.
    Excludes 1:   *non-specific interstitial pneumonia NOS,*
         or due to known underlying cause
         (J84.89)

CC **J84.114** **Acute interstitial pneumonitis** — A rapidly progressive, severe form with the histological appearance of organizing diffuse alveolar damage and without an identifiable underlying etiology.
    Hamman-Rich syndrome
    Excludes 1:   *pneumocystis pneumonia (B59)*

  J84.115 **Respiratory bronchiolitis interstitial lung disease** — A form marked by the patchy accumulation of macrophages in the peribronchiolar alveolar spaces and associated with the pathologic lesion of respiratory bronchiolitis with bronchiolocentric distribution.

CC **J84.116** **Cryptogenic organizing pneumonia** — A form marked by the proliferation of granulation tissue within small airways and alveolar ducts with the histological appearance of organizing pneumonia.
    Excludes 1:   *organizing pneumonia NOS, or due to*
         known underlying cause (J84.89)

CC **J84.117** **Desquamative interstitial pneumonia** — A form marked by the accumulation of macrophages in the alveoli that affects the lungs in a diffuse manner.

  J84.17 **Other interstitial pulmonary diseases with fibrosis in diseases classified elsewhere** — [Not Allowed as PDX]
    Interstitial pneumonia (nonspecific) (usual) due to collagen vascular disease
    Interstitial pneumonia (nonspecific) (usual) in diseases classified elsewhere
    Organizing pneumonia due to collagen vascular disease
    Organizing pneumonia in diseases classified elsewhere
    Code first underlying disease, such as:
    Progressive systemic sclerosis (M34.0)
    Rheumatoid arthritis (M05.00-M06.9)
    Systemic lupus erythematosis (M32.0-M32.9)

CC **J84.2** **Lymphoid interstitial pneumonia** — A form marked by lymphocytic and plasma cells in the interstitial spaces.
    Lymphoid interstitial pneumonitis

  J84.8- **Other specified interstitial pulmonary diseases**
    Excludes 1:   *exogenous lipoid pneumonia (J69.1)*
         unspecified lipoid pneumonia (J69.1)

MCC **J84.81** **Lymphangioleiomyomatosis** — [♀] – An obstructive lung disorder that affects women that is caused by the proliferation of smooth muscle cells surrounding the small airways and alveoli, and by cystic destruction of the lung tissue.
    Lymphangiomyomatosis

CC **J84.82** **Adult pulmonary Langerhans cell histiocytosis** — [Age/15-124] – An interstitial lung disorder that is characterized by focal Langerhans' cell granulomas that invade and destroy distal bronchioles.
    Adult PLCH

MCC **J84.83** **Surfactant mutations of the lung** — A severe form that decreases lung elasticity and results in alveolar collapse that is caused by a genetic abnormalty of the lung surfactant protein.

  J84.84- **Other interstitial lung diseases of childhood**
MCC **J84.841** **Neuroendocrine cell hyperplasia of infancy** — A form characterized by rapid breathing with the histological appearance of hyperplasia of neuroendocrine celss in the bronchioles.

MCC **J84.842** **Pulmonary interstitial glycogenosis** — A form marked by glycogen in the alveolar insterstitial spaces.

MCC **J84.843** **Alveolar capillary dysplasia with vein misalignment** — A developmental lung disorder characterized by abnormal development of the alveolar capillary vascular system.

MCC **J84.848** **Other interstitial lung diseases of childhood**

J 8 0 - J 8 4

J84.89 Other specified interstitial pulmonary diseases
Endogenous lipoid pneumonia — A pneumonia-like reaction of the lung tissue due to the aspiration of oils and fat tissues from the patient's own body.
Interstitial pneumonitis
Non-specific interstitial pneumonitis NOS
Organizing pneumonia NOS
Code first, if applicable:
Poisoning due to drug or toxin (T51-T65 with fifth or sixth character to indicate intent), for toxic pneumonopathy
Underlying cause of pneumonopathy, if known
Use additional code, for adverse effect, to identify drug (T36-T50 with fifth or sixth character 5), if drug-induced
Excludes 1:   *cryptogenic organizing pneumonia (J84.116)*
   idiopathic non-specific interstitial pneumonitis (J84.113)
   lipoid pneumonia, exogenous or unspecified (J69.1)
   lymphoid interstitial pneumonia (J84.2)

cc **J84.9 Interstitial pulmonary disease, unspecified**
Interstitial pneumonia NOS

Suppurative and necrotic conditions of the lower respiratory tract (J85-J86)

J85-   Abscess of lung and mediastinum
Use additional code (B95-B97) to identify infectious agent

mcc **J85.0   Gangrene and necrosis of lung** — The death of lung tissue cells.

mcc **J85.1   Abscess of lung with pneumonia** — A localized collection of pus caused by the disintegration of lung tissue with inflammation of the lung.
Code also the type of pneumonia

mcc **J85.2   Abscess of lung without pneumonia** — A localized collection of pus caused by the disintegration of lung tissue.
Abscess of lung NOS

mcc **J85.3   Abscess of mediastinum** — A localized collection of pus caused by the disintegration of mediastinal tissues.

J86-   Pyothorax — The accumulation of pus within the thoracic cavity.
Use additional code (B95-B97) to identify infectious agent
Excludes 1:   *abscess of lung (J85.-)*
   pyothorax due to tuberculosis (A15.6)

mcc **J86.0   Pyothorax with fistula** — A form associated with an abnormal passage of the thoracic cavity.
Any condition classifiable to J86.9 with fistula
Bronchocutaneous fistula — A form characterized by an abnormal passage between the bronchial region and the skin.
Bronchopleural fistula — A form characterized by an abnormal passage from the bronchial area to the pleura.
Hepatopleural fistula — A form characterized by an abnormal passage between the liver and the pleura.
Mediastinal fistula — A form characterized by an abnormal passage of the mediastinum.
Pleural fistula — A form characterized by an abnormal passage of the pleura.
Thoracic fistula — A form characterized by an abnormal passage of the thoracic cavity.

mcc **J86.9   Pyothorax without fistula**
Abscess of pleura — An abnormal localized accumulation of pus in the pleural cavity.
Abscess of thorax — An abnormal accumulation of pus within the thoracic cavity.
Empyema (chest) (lung) (pleura) — An abnormal localized accumulation of pus within the thoracic cavity.
Fibrinopurulent pleurisy — Inflammation of the pleura characterized by a localized collection of pus which contains fibrin.
Purulent pleurisy — Inflammation of the pleura with a localized collection of pus.
Pyopneumothorax — The abnormal massive collection of pus and air or gas in the pleural cavity.
Septic pleurisy — Inflammation of the pleura with a localized collection of pus caused by the decomposition of microorganisms.
Seropurulent pleurisy — Inflammation of the pleura with a localized collection of pus and serous fluid.
Suppurative pleurisy — Inflammation of the pleura with a localized collection of pus and serous fluid.

Other diseases of the pleura (J90-J94)

J90   Pleural effusion, _not elsewhere classified_ — Inflammation of the pleura with
cc   an abnormal accumulation of pleural fluid in the pleural space.
Encysted pleurisy — A form characterized by adhesions that localize the pleural effusion.
Pleural effusion NOS
Pleurisy with effusion (exudative) (serous)
Excludes 1:   *chylous (pleural) effusion (J94.0)*
   malignant pleural effusion (J91.0))
   pleurisy NOS (R09.1)
   tuberculous pleural effusion (A15.6)

J91-   Pleural effusion _in conditions classified elsewhere_
Excludes ❷: *pleural effusion in heart failure (I50.-)*
   pleural effusion in systemic lupus erythematosus (M32.13)

cc **J91.0   Malignant pleural effusion** — [Not Allowed as PDX] — The presence of malignant cells in the pleural fluid.
Code first underlying neoplasm

cc **J91.8   Pleural effusion in other conditions classified elsewhere** —
[Not Allowed as PDX]
AHA 15:2Q:p15 – Pleural effusion in congestive heart failure patients
Code first underlying disease, such as:
Filariasis (B74.0-B74.9)
Influenza (J09.x2, J10.1, J11.1)

J92-   Pleural plaque — The fibrous thickening of the pleura.
Includes: Pleural thickening

J92.0   Pleural plaque _with presence of asbestos_

J92.9   Pleural plaque _without_ asbestos
Pleural plaque NOS

J93-   Pneumothorax and air leak — The abnormal accumulation or presence of air or gas in the pleural space.
Excludes 1:   *congenital or perinatal pneumothorax (P25.1)*
   postprocedural air leak (J95.812)
   postprocedural pneumothorax (J95.811)
   traumatic pneumothorax (S27.0)
   tuberculous (current disease) pneumothorax (A15.-)
   pyopneumothorax (J86-)

mcc **J93.0   Spontaneous _tension_ pneumothorax** — A severe form of unknown cause in which a significant portion of the lung collapses and results in compression on the chest structures, including the major blood vessels, trachea, and heart.

J93.1-   Other _spontaneous_ pneumothorax

cc **J93.11   _Primary_ spontaneous pneumothorax** — A form of unknown cause that causes a partial collapse of the lung.

cc **J93.12   _Secondary_ spontaneous pneumothorax** —
[Unacceptable PDX] — A form due to another disease condition that causes a partial collapse of the lung.
Code first underlying condition, such as:
Catamenial pneumothorax due to endometriosis (N80.8)
Cystic fibrosis (E84-)
Eosinophilic pneumonia (J82)
Lymphangioleiomyomatosis (J84.81)
Malignant neoplasm of bronchus amd lung (C34-)
Marfan's syndrome (Q87.4)
Pneumonia due to Pneumocystis carinii (B59)
Secondary malignant neoplasm of lung (C78.0-)
Spontaneous rupture of the esophagus (K22.3)

J93.8-   Other pneumothorax and air leak

cc **J93.81   _Chronic_ pneumothorax** — A form marked by slow development, or persistence, over a period of time that causes a partial collapse of the lung.

cc **J93.82   Other _air leak_** — A form marked by the persistent escape of air from the lung into the pleural space without causing a partial collapse of the lung.
Persistent air leak

cc **J93.83   Other pneumothorax**
Acute pneumothorax — A form marked by sudden, severe onset that causes a partial collapse of the lung.
Spontaneous pneumothorax NOS

cc **J93.9   Pneumothorax, unspecified**
Pneumothorax NOS

J 8 4 - J 9 3

J94- Other pleural conditions
> *Excludes 1:* *pleurisy NOS (R09.1)*
> *traumatic hemopneumothorax (S27.2)*
> *traumatic hemothorax (S27.1)*
> *tuberculous pleural conditions (current disease) (A15.-)*

CC **J94.0 Chylous effusion** — An abnormal accumulation of chyle in the pleural space.
> **Chyliform effusion**

J94.1 Fibrothorax — An abnormal accumulation of fibrosis in the pleural space.

CC **J94.2 Hemothorax** — An abnormal accumulation of effused blood in the pleural space.
> **Hemopneumothorax** — An abnormal accumulation of effused blood and air in the pleural space.

CC **J94.8 Other specified pleural conditions**
> **Hydropneumothorax** — An abnormal accumulation of watery fluid and air in the pleural space.
> **Hydrothorax** — An abnormal accumulation of watery fluid in the pleural space.

J94.9 Pleural condition, unspecified

Intraoperative and postprocedural complications and disorders of respiratory system, not elsewhere classified (J95)

J95- Intraoperative and postprocedural complications and disorders of respiratory system, not elsewhere classified
> *Excludes ❷:* *aspiration pneumonia (J69.-)*
> *emphysema (subcutaneous) resulting from a procedure (T81.82)*
> *hypostatic pneumonia (J18.2)*
> *pulmonary manifestations due to radiation (J70.0-J70.1)*

J95.0- Tracheostomy complications

CC **J95.00 Unspecified tracheostomy complication**

CC **J95.01 Hemorrhage from tracheostomy stoma**

CC **J95.02 Infection of tracheostomy stoma**
> Use additional code to identify type of infection, such as:
> Cellulitis of neck (L03.8)
> Sepsis (A40, A41.-)

CC **J95.03 Malfunction of tracheostomy stoma**
> **Mechanical complication of tracheostomy stoma**
> **Obstruction of tracheostomy airway**
> **Tracheal stenosis due to tracheostomy**

CC **J95.04 Tracheo-esophageal fistula following tracheostomy**

CC **J95.09 Other tracheostomy complication**

MCC **J95.1 Acute pulmonary insufficiency following thoracic surgery**
> *Excludes ❷:* *functional disturbances following cardiac surgery (I97.0, I97.1-)*

MCC **J95.2 Acute pulmonary insufficiency following nonthoracic surgery**
> *Excludes ❷:* *functional disturbances following cardiac surgery (I97.0, I97.1-)*

MCC **J95.3 Chronic pulmonary insufficiency following surgery**
> *Excludes ❷:* *functional disturbances following cardiac surgery (I97.0, I97.1-)*

CC **J95.4 Chemical pneumonitis due to anesthesia**
> **Mendelson's syndrome**
> **Postprocedural aspiration pneumonia**
> Use additional code for adverse effect, if applicable, to identify drug (T41- with fifth or sixth character 5)
> *Excludes 1:* *aspiration pneumonitis due to anesthesia complicating labor and delivery (O74.0)*
> *aspiration pneumonitis due to anesthesia complicating pregnancy (O29)*
> *aspiration pneumonitis due to anesthesia complicating the puerperium (O89.01)*

CC **J95.5 Postprocedural subglottic stenosis**

J95.6- Intraoperative hemorrhage and hematoma of a respiratory system organ or structure complicating a procedure
> *Excludes 1:* *intraoperative hemorrhage and hematoma of a respiratory system organ or structure due to accidental puncture and laceration during procedure (J95.7-)*

CC **J95.61 Intraoperative hemorrhage and hematoma of a respiratory system organ or structure complicating a respiratory system procedure**

CC **J95.62 Intraoperative hemorrhage and hematoma of a respiratory system organ or structure complicating other procedure**

J95.7- Accidental puncture and laceration of a respiratory system organ or structure during a procedure
> *Excludes ❷:* *postprocedural pneumothorax (J95.811)*

CC **J95.71 Accidental puncture and laceration of a respiratory system organ or structure during a respiratory system procedure**

CC **J95.72 Accidental puncture and laceration of a respiratory system organ or structure during other procedure**

J95.8- Other intraoperative and postprocedural complications and disorders of respiratory system, not elsewhere classified

J95.81- Postprocedural pneumothorax and air leak

CC **J95.811 Postprocedural pneumothorax**

CC **J95.812 Postprocedural air leak**

J95.82- Postprocedural respiratory failure
> *Excludes 1:* *respiratory failure in other conditions (J96-)*

MCC **J95.821 Acute postprocedural respiratory failure**
> **Postprocedural respiratory failure NOS**

MCC **J95.822 Acute and chronic postprocedural respiratory failure**

J95.83- Postprocedural hemorrhage of a respiratory system organ or structure following a procedure

CC **J95.830 Postprocedural hemorrhage of a respiratory system organ or structure following a respiratory system procedure**

CC **J95.831 Postprocedural hemorrhage of a respiratory system organ or structure following other procedure**

CC **J95.84 Transfusion-related acute lung injury (TRALI)** — A pulmonary disorder occurring 1-6 hours post transfusion that is characterized by pulmonary distress, bilateral noncardiogenic pulmonary edema, hypotension, fever, and hypoxemia.

J95.85- Complication of respirator [ventilator]

CC **J95.850 Mechanical complication of respirator**
> *Excludes 1:* *encounter for respirator [ventilator] dependence during power failure (Z99.12)*

CC **J95.851 Ventilator associated pneumonia**
> **Ventilator associated pneumonitis**
> Use additional code to identify the organism, if known (B95-, B96-, B97-)
> *Excludes 1:* *ventilator lung in newborn (P27.8)*

CC **J95.859 Other complication of respirator [ventilator]**

J95.86- Postprocedural hematoma and seroma of a respiratory system organ or structure following a procedure

CC **J95.860 Postprocedural hematoma of a respiratory system organ or structure following a respiratory system procedure**

CC **J95.861 Postprocedural hematoma of a respiratory system organ or structure following other procedure**

CC **J95.862 Postprocedural seroma of a respiratory system organ or structure following a respiratory system procedure**

CC **J95.863 Postprocedural seroma of a respiratory system organ or structure following other procedure**

CC **J95.88 Other intraoperative complications of respiratory system, not elsewhere classified**

CC **J95.89 Other postprocedural complications and disorders of respiratory system, not elsewhere classified**
> Use additional code to identify disorder, such as:
> Aspiration pneumonia (J69.-)
> Bacterial or viral pneumonia (J12-J18)
> *Excludes ❷:* *acute pulmonary insufficiency following thoracic surgery (J95.1)*
> *postprocedural subglottic stenosis (J95.5)*

J 9 4 - J 9 5

Excludes 1: = NOT CODED HERE! (Do not code both)   773   *Excludes ❷:* = Not Included Here

Other diseases of the respiratory system (J96-J99)

J96- **Respiratory failure, not elsewhere classified**
   Excludes 1:   *acute respiratory distress syndrome (J80)*
              cardiorespiratory failure (R09.2)
              newborn respiratory distress syndrome (P22.0)
              postprocedural respiratory failure (J95.82-)
              respiratory arrest (R09.2)
              respiratory arrest of newborn (P28.81)
              respiratory failure of newborn (P28.5)

  J96.0-   <u>Acute respiratory failure</u> — A sudden, severe onset of decreased pulmonary function due to an abnormally low arterial oxygen level or an abnormally high arterial carbon dioxide level.
        AHA 13:4Q:p121 – Acute respiratory failure due to smoke inhalation

  MCC **J96.00**   **Acute respiratory failure, <u>unspecified</u> whether with hypoxia or hypercapnia**

  MCC **J96.01**   **Acute respiratory failure <u>with hypoxia</u>** — Insufficient level of oxygen reaching the tissues.

  MCC **J96.02**   **Acute respiratory failure <u>with hypercapnia</u>** — Abnormally high arterial carbon dioxide level.

  J96.1-   <u>**Chronic**</u> **respiratory failure**
        AHA 13:4Q:p129 – Chronic hypoxic respiratory failure and COPD

  cc **J96.10**   **Chronic respiratory failure, <u>unspecified</u> whether with hypoxia or hypercapnia**

  cc **J96.11**   **Chronic respiratory failure <u>with hypoxia</u>** — Insufficient level of oxygen reaching the tissues.

  cc **J96.12**   **Chronic respiratory failure <u>with hypercapnia</u>** — Abnormally high arterial carbon dioxide level.

  J96.2-   <u>**Acute and chronic**</u> **respiratory failure**
        Acute on chronic respiratory failure

  MCC **J96.20**   **Acute and chronic respiratory failure, <u>unspecified</u> whether with hypoxia or hypercapnia**

  MCC **J96.21**   **Acute and chronic respiratory failure <u>with hypoxia</u>** — Insufficient level of oxygen reaching the tissues.

  MCC **J96.22**   **Acute and chronic respiratory failure <u>with hypercapnia</u>** — Abnormally high arterial carbon dioxide level.

  J96.9-   **Respiratory failure, <u>unspecified</u>**

  MCC **J96.90**   **Respiratory failure, unspecified, <u>unspecified</u> whether with hypoxia or hypercapnia**

  MCC **J96.91**   **Respiratory failure, unspecified <u>with hypoxia</u>** — Insufficient level of oxygen reaching the tissues.

  MCC **J96.92**   **Respiratory failure, unspecified <u>with hypercapnia</u>** — Abnormally high arterial carbon dioxide level.

J98- **Other respiratory disorders**
   Use additional code to identify:
     Exposure to environmental tobacco smoke (Z77.22)
     Exposure to tobacco smoke in the perinatal period (P96.81)
     History of tobacco dependence (Z87.891)
     Occupational exposure to environmental tobacco smoke (Z57.31)
     Tobacco dependence (F17.-)
     Tobacco use (Z72.0)
   Excludes 1:   *newborn apnea (P28.4)*
             newborn sleep apnea (P28.3)
   Excludes ❷: *apnea NOS (R06.81)*
             sleep apnea (G47.3-)

  J98.0-   **Diseases of bronchus, <u>not elsewhere classified</u>**

    J98.01   **Acute bronchospasm** — The sudden, severe onset of narrowing of the bronchial airways.
       Excludes 1:   *acute bronchiolitis with bronchospasm (J21.-)*
                acute bronchitis with bronchospasm (J20.-)
                asthma (J45.-)
                exercise induced bronchospasm (J45.990)

    J98.09   **Other diseases of bronchus, not elsewhere classified**
       Broncholithiasis — The abnormal presence of calculi within the bronchial branches.
       Calcification of bronchus — The abnormal deposition of calcium salts in the bronchial tissues.
       Stenosis of bronchus — The abnormal reduction in the size of the bronchial airways.
       Tracheobronchial collapse — The abnormal reduction in the size of the bronchial or tracheal lumens.
       Tracheobronchial dyskinesia
       Ulcer of bronchus — A tissue-destroying sore of the bronchial tissues.

J98.1- **Pulmonary collapse** — An acute, airless state of all or part of a lung.
   Excludes 1:   *therapeutic collapse of lung status (Z98.3)*

  cc **J98.11**   **Atelectasis** — The airless collapse (alveolar deflation) of part or all of a lung.
       Excludes 1:   *newborn atelectasis*
                tuberculous atelectasis (current disease) (A15)

  cc **J98.19**   **Other pulmonary collapse**

  J98.2   **Interstitial emphysema** — The abnormal presence of air in the peribronchial and interstitial tissues of the lungs.
      Mediastinal emphysema — The abnormal presence of air in the mediastinal tissues.
    Excludes 1:   *emphysema NOS (J43.9)*
             emphysema in newborn (P25.0)
             surgical emphysema (subcutaneous) (T81.82)
             traumatic subcutaneous emphysema (T79.7)

  J98.3   **Compensatory emphysema** — Excessive inhalation of lung tissue following a morbid lung tissue condition.

  J98.4   **Other disorders of lung**
      Calcification of lung — The abnormal deposition of calcium salts within the pulmonary tissue.
      Cystic lung disease (acquired) — The abnormal presence of cystic air spaces.
      Lung disease NOS
      Pulmolithiasis — The abnormal presence of calculi within the pulmonary system.
    Excludes 1:   *acute interstitial pneumonitis (J84.114)*
             pulmonary insufficiency following surgery (J95.1-J95.2)

  J98.5-   **Diseases of mediastinum, <u>not elsewhere classified</u>**
    Excludes ❷: *abscess of mediastinum (J85.3)*

  MCC **J98.51**   **Mediastinitis** — Inflammation of the mediastinum.
       Code first underlying condition, if applicable, such as: postoperative mediastinitis (T81.-)

  MCC **J98.59**   **Other diseases of mediastinum, not elsewhere classified**
       Fibrosis of mediastinum — The abnormal presence of fibrous tissue within the mediastinum.
       Hernia of mediastinum — The abnormal protrusion of the mediastinum into other parts of the thoracic cavity.
       Retraction of mediastinum — The abnormal drawing-back of the normal mediastinal area.

  J98.6   **Disorders of diaphragm**
      Diaphragmatitis — Inflammation of the diaphragm.
      Paralysis of diaphragm — The abnormal loss or impairment of the motor function of the diaphragm.
      Relaxation of diaphragm — The abnormal decrease in the diaphragm tension.
    Excludes 1:   *congenital malformation of diaphragm NEC (Q79.1)*
             congenital diaphragmatic hernia (Q79.0)
    Excludes ❷: *diaphragmatic hernia (K44.-)*

  J98.8   **Other specified respiratory disorders**

  J98.9   **Respiratory disorder, unspecified**
      Respiratory disease (chronic) NOS

J99 **Respiratory disorders in diseases classified elsewhere** —
   [Not Allowed as PDX]
   Code first underlying disease, such as:
     Amyloidosis (E85.-)
     Ankylosing spondylitis (M45)
     Congenital syphilis (A50.5)
     Cryoglobulinemia (D89.1)
     Early congenital syphilis (A50.0)
     Schistosomiasis (B65.0-B65.9)
   Excludes 1:   *respiratory disorders in:*
          amebiasis (A06.5)
          blastomycosis (B40.0-B40.2)
          candidiasis (B37.1)
          coccidioidomycosis (B38.0-B38.2)
          cystic fibrosis with pulmonary manifestations (E84.0)
          dermatomyositis (M33.01, M33.11)
          histoplasmosis (B39.0-B39.2)
          late syphilis (A52.72, A52.73)
          polymyositis (M33.21)
          sicca syndrome (M35.02)
          systemic lupus erythematosus (M32.13)
          systemic sclerosis (M34.81)
          Wegener's granulomatosis (M31.30-M31.31)

J96-J99 (side tab)

Excludes 1: = NOT CODED HERE! (Do not code both)   **774**   *Excludes ❷:* = Not Included Here

Chapter 11 – Diseases of the digestive system (K00-K95)

Excludes ❷: certain conditions originating in the perinatal period (P04-P96)

certain infectious and parasitic diseases (A00-B99)

complications of pregnancy, childbirth and the puerperium (O00-O9A)

congenital malformations, deformations and chromosomal abnormalities (Q00-Q99)

endocrine, nutritional and metabolic diseases (E00-E88)

injury, poisoning and certain other consequences of external causes (S00-T88)

neoplasms (C00-D49)

symptoms, signs and abnormal clinical and laboratory findings, not elsewhere classified (R00-R94)

This chapter contains the following blocks:

K00-K14	Diseases of oral cavity and salivary glands
K20-K31	Diseases of esophagus, stomach and duodenum
K35-K38	Diseases of appendix
K40-K46	Hernia
K50-K52	Noninfective enteritis and colitis
K55-K64	Other diseases of intestines
K65-K68	Diseases of peritoneum and retroperitoneum
K70-K77	Diseases of liver
K80-K87	Disorders of gallbladder, biliary tract and pancreas
K90-K95	Other diseases of the digestive system

Chapter-Specific Coding Guidelines

C. Chapter-Specific Coding Guidelines

In addition to general coding guidelines, there are guidelines for specific diagnoses and/or conditions in the classification. Unless otherwise indicated, these guidelines apply to all health care settings. Please refer to Section II for guidelines on the selection of principal diagnosis.

11. Chapter 11: Diseases of the Digestive System (K00-K94)

Reserved for future guideline expansion

Diseases of oral cavity and salivary glands (K00-K14)

K00- Disorders of tooth development and eruption

Excludes ❷: embedded and impacted teeth (K01.-)

K00.0 Anodontia — Congenital absence of all or some of the teeth.

Hypodontia — Congenital absence of some of the teeth.

Oligodontia — The presence of less than the normal number of teeth, some of them being congenitally absent.

Excludes 1: acquired absence of teeth (K08.1-)

K00.1 Supernumerary teeth — An excess number of teeth.

Distomolar — Any tooth found distal to a third molar.

Fourth molar — A supernumerary molar distal to the third molar.

Mesiodens — A small supernumerary tooth situated palatally between the maxillary central incisor.

Paramolar — A supernumerary tooth appearing adjacent to a molar.

Supplementary teeth — Additional teeth.

Excludes ❷: supernumerary roots (K00.2)

K00.2 Abnormalities of size and form of teeth

Concrescence of teeth — The union of the roots of 2 approximating teeth by a deposit of cementum.

Dens evaginatus — The eruption of teeth before calcification is complete.

Dens in dente — A malformed tooth resulting from invagination of the crown before it is calcified.

Dens invaginatus — Synonym for Dens In Dente.

Enamel pearls — Tiny globules of enamel, firmly adherent to a tooth.

Fusion of teeth — The abnormal coherence of 2 or more teeth.

Gemination of teeth — The division of a tooth bud which results in the formation of 2 teeth, or of a double crown formed on a single root with a single pulp canal.

Macrodontia — An abnormal increase in the size of the teeth.

Microdontia — An abnormal smallness of the size of the teeth.

Peg-shaped [conical] teeth — Malformed teeth, with a characteristic peg-shaped appearance.

Supernumerary roots — An excess number of roots.

Taurodontism — An elongated variation in molar teeth form.

Tuberculum paramolare — A small nodule of tooth close to a molar.

Excludes 1: abnormalities of teeth due to congenital syphilis (A50.5)

tuberculum Carabelli, which is regarded as a normal variation and should not be coded

K00.3 Mottled teeth — A patchy discoloration of the teeth.

Dental fluorosis — A mottled discoloration of the enamel of the teeth resulting from ingestion of excessive amounts of fluorine during tooth development.

Mottling of enamel — A patchy or spotting of discoloration of the enamel.

Nonfluoride enamel opacities — An abnormal discoloration of the enamel by a nonfluoride cause.

Excludes ❷: deposits [accretions] on teeth (K03.6)

K00.4 Disturbances in tooth formation

Aplasia and hypoplasia of cementum — The lack or incomplete development of the bone-like connective tissue covering the root of a tooth.

Dilaceration of tooth — Developmental injury to a tooth characterized by a crease or band at the junction of the crown or root, or by tortuous roots with abnormal curvatures.

Enamel hypoplasia (neonatal) (postnatal) (prenatal) — Incomplete or defective development of the enamel of the teeth.

Regional odontodysplasia — The abnormal development of a group of teeth.

Turner's tooth — A permanent tooth enamel hypoplasia resulting from the spread of infection.

Excludes 1: Hutchinson's teeth and mulberry molars in congenital syphilis (A50.5)

Excludes ❷: mottled teeth (K00.3)

K00.5 Hereditary disturbances in tooth structure, not elsewhere classified

Amelogenesis imperfecta — An inherited condition resulting in defective development of the enamel of the teeth which is brown in color.

Dentinal dysplasia — An inherited condition affecting both the primary and secondary dentition, in which the teeth have short, distorted roots.

Dentinogenesis imperfecta — An inherited condition characterized by defective formation and calcification of the dentin, giving the teeth a brown or blue opalescent appearance.

Odontogenesis imperfecta — Synonym for Dentinogenesis, Imperfecta.

Shell teeth — An inherited condition in which the enamel appears essentially normal, the dentin is extremely thin, and the pulp chamber is enlarged.

K00.6 Disturbances in tooth eruption

Dentia praecox — A primary tooth that erupts during the neonatal period.

Natal tooth — A prematurely erupted deciduous tooth, visible in the jaw at birth.

Neonatal tooth — A primary tooth that erupts during the neonatal period.

Premature eruption of tooth — Appearance of a tooth before the proper time.

Premature shedding of primary [deciduous] tooth — The early loss of primary teeth before the proper time.

Prenatal teeth — Synonym for Natal Tooth.

Retained [persistent] primary tooth — The abnormal retention of primary teeth beyond the normal time.

Excludes ❷: embedded and impacted teeth (K01-)

K00.7 Teething syndrome — The uncomfortable symptoms associated with the process of erupting teeth.

K00.8 Other disorders of tooth development

Color changes during tooth formation

Intrinsic staining of teeth NOS

Excludes ❷: posteruptive color changes (K03.7)

K00.9 Disorder of tooth development, unspecified

Disorder of odontogenesis NOS

K01- Embedded and impacted teeth

Excludes 1: abnormal position of fully erupted teeth (M26.3-)

K01.0 Embedded teeth — An unerupted tooth, usually one completely covered by bone.

K01.1 Impacted teeth — A tooth so placed in the jaw that it is unable to erupt.

K02- Dental caries — The progressive decalcification of the hard, inorganic portion of a tooth caused by the action of microorganisms and followed by disintegration of the soft, organic portion.

Includes:	Caries of dentine
	Dental cavities
	Early childhood caries
	Pre-eruptive caries
	Recurrent caries (dentino enamel junction) (enamel) (to the pulp)
	Tooth decay

K02.3 Arrested dental caries — A form marked by the cessation of the decaying process.

Arrested coronal and root caries

K02.5- Dental caries on pit and fissure surface

Dental caries on chewing surface of tooth

K02.51 Dental caries on pit and fissure surface limited to enamel — A form involving the very hard, white substance that covers the dentin and forms the crown of a tooth.

White spot lesions [initial caries] on pit and fissure surface of tooth

---

K 0 0 - K 0 2

K02.52 Dental caries on pit and fissure surface penetrating into dentin — A form involving the primary, hard tooth substance which surrounds the root and is covered by enamel.
   Primary dental caries, cervical origin

K02.53 Dental caries on pit and fissure surface penetrating into pulp — A form involving the organic, viable center portion of a tooth.

K02.6- Dental caries on smooth surface

K02.61 Dental caries on smooth surface limited to enamel — A form involving the very hard, white substance that covers the dentin and forms the crown of a tooth.
   White spot lesions [initial caries] on smooth surface of tooth

K02.62 Dental caries on smooth surface penetrating into dentin — A form involving the primary, hard tooth substance which surrounds the root and is covered by enamel.

K02.63 Dental caries on smooth surface penetrating into pulp — A form involving the very hard, white substance that covers the dentin and forms the crown of a tooth.

K02.7 Dental root caries — A form involving the dental roots.

K02.9 Dental caries, unspecified

K03- Other diseases of hard tissues of teeth
   Excludes ❷: bruxism (F45.8)
   dental caries (K02.-)
   teeth-grinding NOS (F45.8)

K03.0 Excessive attrition of teeth — The abnormal wearing-away of the teeth in the course of normal use.
   Approximal wear of teeth
   Occlusal wear of teeth

K03.1 Abrasion of teeth — The mechanical or chemical friction process which wears away the substance of the teeth.
   Dentifrice abrasion of teeth
   Habitual abrasion of teeth
   Occupational abrasion of teeth
   Ritual abrasion of teeth
   Traditional abrasion of teeth
   Wedge defect NOS

K03.2 Erosion of teeth — The disintegration of tooth substance on surfaces free from attrition by mastication.
   Erosion of teeth due to diet
   Erosion of teeth due to drugs and medicaments
   Erosion of teeth due to persistent vomiting
   Erosion of teeth NOS
   Idiopathic erosion of teeth
   Occupational erosion of teeth

K03.3 Pathological resorption of teeth — The removal of enamel and other calcific portions of a tooth as a result of a pathological process.
   Internal granuloma of pulp
   Resorption of teeth (external)

K03.4 Hypercementosis — The abnormal, excessive growth of tooth cementum.
   Cementation hyperplasia — The excessive proliferation of normal cementum cells in normal arrangement leading to an overall increase in size.

K03.5 Ankylosis of teeth — The abnormal fusion of the root cementum with the adjacent alveolar bone.

K03.6 Deposits [accretions] on teeth — The abnormal addition of material growing on the teeth.
   Betel deposits [accretions] on teeth
   Black deposits [accretions] on teeth
   Extrinsic staining of teeth NOS
   Green deposits [accretions] on teeth
   Materia alba deposits [accretions] on teeth
   Orange deposits [accretions] on teeth
   Staining of teeth NOS
   Subgingival dental calculus
   Supragingival dental calculus
   Tobacco deposits [accretions] on teeth

K03.7 Posteruptive color changes of dental hard tissues — The abnormal discoloration of the teeth after they have broken out of the alveolar tissues.
   Excludes ❷: deposits [accretions] on teeth (K03.6)

K03.8- Other specified diseases of hard tissues of teeth

K03.81 Cracked tooth — The abnormal cracking or breaking of a tooth that is not due to trauma.
   Excludes 1: asymptomatic craze lines in enamel — omit code
   broken or fractured tooth due to trauma (S02.5)

K03.89 Other specified diseases of hard tissues of teeth

K03.9 Disease of hard tissues of teeth, unspecified

K04- Diseases of pulp and periapical tissues

K04.0- Pulpitis — Inflammation of the soft, neurovascular portion of the center of a tooth.
   Acute pulpitis — A form marked by sudden, severe onset.
   Chronic (hyperplastic) (ulcerative) pulpitis — A form marked by slow, progressive development.

cc **K04.01 Reversible pulpitis** — A form that can be restored.

cc **K04.02 Irreversible pulpitis** — A form with irreversible damage.

K04.1 Necrosis of pulp — The death of pulp tissue.
   Pulpal gangrene — The death of pulp tissue due to deficient or absent blood supply.

K04.2 Pulp degeneration — The deterioration of the pulp tissue and its function.
   Denticles — A relatively large, calcified growth within the pulp.
   Pulpal calcifications — Synonym for Denticles.
   Pulpal stones — Synonym for Denticles.

K04.3 Abnormal hard tissue formation in pulp — The abnormal replacement of the pulp tissue with hard tissue such as dentin.
   Secondary or irregular dentine

cc **K04.4 Acute apical periodontitis of pulpal origin** — A sudden, severe onset of inflammation of the dental periosteum, alveolar bone, and adjacent gingiva, originating from the pulp tissue.
   Acute apical periodontitis NOS
   Excludes 1: acute periodontitis (K05.2-)

K04.5 Chronic apical periodontitis — A progressive, slowly developing inflammation of the dental periosteum, alveolar bone, and adjacent gingiva.
   Apical or periapical granuloma — The abnormal formation of granulomas in the periapical tissues.
   Apical periodontitis NOS
   Excludes 1: chronic periodontitis (K05.3-)

K04.6 Periapical abscess with sinus — A localized collection of pus caused by the disintegration of the dental periosteum, alveolar bone, and adjacent gingiva, with a draining sinus outside of the area of inflammation.
   Dental abscess with sinus
   Dentoalveolar abscess with sinus

K04.7 Periapical abscess without sinus — A localized collection of pus caused by the disintegration of the dental periosteum, alveolar bone, and adjacent gingiva, without the formation of a draining sinus.
   Dental abscess without sinus
   Dentoalveolar abscess without sinus
   Periapical abscess without sinus

K04.8 Radicular cyst — An epithelium-lined sac at the apex of a tooth.
   Apical (periodontal) cyst
   Periapical cyst
   Residual radicular cyst
   Excludes ❷: lateral periodontal cyst (K09.0)

K04.9- Other and unspecified diseases of pulp and periapical tissues

K04.90 Unspecified diseases of pulp and periapical tissues

K04.99 Other diseases of pulp and periapical tissues

K05- Gingivitis and periodontal diseases
   Use additional code to identify:
   Alcohol abuse and dependence (F10.-)
   Exposure to environmental tobacco smoke (Z77.22)
   Exposure to tobacco smoke in the perinatal period (P96.81)
   History of tobacco dependence (Z87.891)
   Occupational exposure to environmental tobacco smoke (Z57.31)
   Tobacco dependence (F17.-)
   Tobacco use (Z72.0)

K05.0- Acute gingivitis — A sudden, severe onset of inflammation of the gums.
   Excludes 1: acute necrotizing ulcerative gingivitis (A69.1)
   herpesviral [herpes simplex] gingivostomatitis (B00.2)

K05.00 Acute gingivitis, plaque induced — A form that is due to the presence of plaque.
   Acute gingivitis NOS
   Plaque-induced gingival disease

K05.01 Acute gingivitis, non-plaque induced — A form that is due to conditions other than the presence of plaque.

K05.1-   Chronic gingivitis — Inflammation of the gums which develops slowly and persists over a long period of time.
> **Desquamative gingivitis (chronic)** — A form marked by the shedding of the gingival surface epithelium.
> **Gingivitis (chronic) NOS**
> **Hyperplastic gingivitis (chronic)** — A form marked by the abnormal increase in the size and arrangement of normal gingival cells.
> **Pregnancy associated gingivitis**
> **Simple marginal gingivitis (chronic)** — A form marked by engorgement of the gingiva with blood and edema.
> **Ulcerative gingivitis (chronic)** — A form marked by the eating-away of the gingival tissue.
>
> **Code first,** if applicable, diseases of the digestive system complicating pregnancy (O99.61-)

K05.10   Chronic gingivitis, plaque induced — A form that is due to the presence of plaque.
> **Chronic gingivitis NOS**
> **Gingivitis NOS**

K05.11   Chronic gingivitis, non-plaque induced — A form that is due to conditions other than the presence of plaque.

K05.2-   Aggressive periodontitis — A sudden, severe onset of inflammation of the supporting structure tissues of the teeth, including the gingival and alveolar bone.
> **Acute pericoronitis** — A form marked by the inflammation of the gingiva surrounding the crown of a partially erupted tooth, including the cementum, alveolar bone, and gingiva.
>
> *Excludes 1:   acute apical periodontitis (K04.4)*
> *periapical abscess (K04.7)*
> *periapical abscess with sinus (K04.6)*

K05.20   Aggressive periodontitis, unspecified

K05.21- Aggressive periodontitis, localized — A progressive inflammation with periodontal damage of the supporting structures of the teeth that is usually confined to the permanent first molars and incisors.
> **Periodontal abscess** — A localized collection of pus caused by the disintegration of the supporting structure tissues of the teeth.

> **K05.211   Aggressive periodontitis, localized, slight**

> **K05.212   Aggressive periodontitis, localized, moderate**

> **K05.213   Aggressive periodontitis, localized, severe**

> **K05.219   Aggressive periodontitis, localized, unspecified severity**

K05.22- Aggressive periodontitis, generalized — A progressive inflammation with periodontal damage of the supporting structures of the teeth that affects at least 3 permanent teeth other than the permanent first molars and incisors.

> **K05.221   Aggressive periodontitis, generalized, slight**

> **K05.222   Aggressive periodontitis, generalized, moderate**

> **K05.223   Aggressive periodontitis, generalized, severe**

> **K05.229   Aggressive periodontitis, generalized, unspecified severity**

K05.3-   Chronic periodontitis — Inflammation of the supporting tissues of the teeth including the cementum, alveolar bone, and gingiva, which develops slowly and persists over a long period of time.
> **Chronic pericoronitis** — A form marked by the inflammation of the gingiva surrounding the crown of a partially erupted tooth.
> **Complex periodontitis** — See Chronic Periodontitis above.
> **Periodontitis NOS**
> **Simplex periodontitis** — A form due to a variety of local irritants.
>
> *Excludes 1:   chronic apical periodontitis (K04.5)*

K05.30   Chronic periodontitis, unspecified

K05.31- Chronic periodontitis, localized — A form affecting the permanent first molars and incisors.

> **K05.311   Chronic periodontitis, localized, slight**

> **K05.312   Chronic periodontitis, localized, moderate**

> **K05.313   Chronic periodontitis, localized, severe**

> **K05.319   Chronic periodontitis, localized, unspecified severity**

K05.32- Chronic periodontitis, generalized — A form affecting at least 3 permanent teeth other than the permanent first molars and incisors.

> **K05.321   Chronic periodontitis, generalized, slight**

> **K05.322   Chronic periodontitis, generalized, moderate**

> **K05.323   Chronic periodontitis, generalized, severe**

> **K05.329   Chronic periodontitis, generalized, unspecified severity**

K05.4   Periodontosis — The noninflammatory degenerative destruction of the periodontal tissues.
> **Juvenile periodontosis**

K05.5   Other periodontal diseases
> **Combined periodontic-endodontic lesion**
> **Narrow gingival width (of periodontal soft tissue)**
>
> *Excludes ❷: leukoplakia of gingiva (K13.21)*

K05.6   Periodontal disease, unspecified

K06-   Other disorders of gingiva and edentulous alveolar ridge
> *Excludes ❷: acute gingivitis (K05.0)*
> *atrophy of edentulous alveolar ridge (K08.2)*
> *chronic gingivitis (K05.1)*
> *gingivitis NOS (K05.1)*

K06.0   Gingival recession — The abnormal receding of the gingival margin from the neck of a tooth.
> **Gingival recession (generalized) (localized) (postinfective) (postprocedural)**

K06.1   Gingival enlargement — The abnormal hypertrophy of the gums.
> **Gingival fibromatosis** — An inherited condition characterized by hypertrophy of the gums prior to the time of eruption of the teeth.

K06.2   Gingival and edentulous alveolar ridge lesions associated with trauma
> **Irritative hyperplasia of edentulous ridge [denture hyperplasia]**
> **Use additional code** (Chapter 20) to identify external cause or denture status (Z97.2)

K06.3   Horizontal alveolar bone loss

K06.8   Other specified disorders of gingiva and edentulous alveolar ridge
> **Fibrous epulis** — A fibrous tumor originating in the periosteum of the lower jaw and gingiva.
> **Flabby alveolar ridge**
> **Giant cell epulis** — A fibrous tumor originating in the periosteum of the lower jaw and gingiva.
> **Peripheral giant cell granuloma of gingiva** — A pedunculated lesion of the gingiva or alveolar ridge.
> **Pyogenic granuloma of gingiva**
> **Vertical ridge deficiency**
>
> *Excludes ❷: gingival cyst (K09.0)*

K06.9   Disorder of gingiva and edentulous alveolar ridge, unspecified

K08-   Other disorders of teeth and supporting structures
> *Excludes ❷: dentofacial anomalies [including malocclusion] (M26.-)*
> *disorders of jaw (M27.-)*

K08.0   Exfoliation of teeth due to systemic causes — The deterioration and loss of teeth due to systemic diseases which affect the development and support of the teeth.
> **Code also underlying systemic condition**

K08.1-   Complete loss of teeth — The acquired absence of some or all of the natural teeth.
> **Acquired loss of teeth, complete**
> *Excludes 1:   congenital absence of teeth (K00.0)*
> *exfoliation of teeth due to systemic causes (K08.0)*
> *partial loss of teeth (K08.4-)*

K08.10- Complete loss of teeth, unspecified cause

> **K08.101   Complete loss of teeth, unspecified cause, class I**

> **K08.102   Complete loss of teeth, unspecified cause, class II**

> **K08.103   Complete loss of teeth, unspecified cause, class III**

> **K08.104   Complete loss of teeth, unspecified cause, class IV**

> **K08.109   Complete loss of teeth, unspecified cause, unspecified class**
> > **Edentulism NOS**

K08.11- Complete loss of teeth due to trauma — Loss due to physical injury.

> **K08.111   Complete loss of teeth due to trauma, class I**

> **K08.112   Complete loss of teeth due to trauma, class II**

> **K08.113   Complete loss of teeth due to trauma, class III**

> **K08.114   Complete loss of teeth due to trauma, class IV**

> **K08.119   Complete loss of teeth due to trauma, unspecified class**

K08.12- Complete loss of teeth due to periodontal diseases — Loss due to a diseased condition of the teeth supporting structures.

> **K08.121   Complete loss of teeth due to periodontal diseases, class I**

> **K08.122   Complete loss of teeth due to periodontal diseases, class II**

K 0 5 I K 0 8

K08.123 Complete loss of teeth due to periodontal diseases, class III

K08.124 Complete loss of teeth due to periodontal diseases, class IV

K08.129 Complete loss of teeth due to periodontal diseases, unspecified class

K08.13- Complete loss of teeth <u>due to caries</u> — Loss due to cavities.

K08.131 Complete loss of teeth due to caries, class I

K08.132 Complete loss of teeth due to caries, class II

K08.133 Complete loss of teeth due to caries, class III

K08.134 Complete loss of teeth due to caries, class IV

K08.139 Complete loss of teeth due to caries, unspecified class

K08.19- Complete loss of teeth <u>due to other</u> specified cause

K08.191 Complete loss of teeth due to other specified cause, class I

K08.192 Complete loss of teeth due to other specified cause, class II

K08.193 Complete loss of teeth due to other specified cause, class III

K08.194 Complete loss of teeth due to other specified cause, class IV

K08.199 Complete loss of teeth due to other specified cause, unspecified class

K08.2- **Atrophy of edentulous alveolar ridge** — A wasting-away of a toothless alveolar ridge.

K08.20 **Unspecified atrophy of edentulous alveolar ridge**
Atrophy of the mandible NOS
Atrophy of the maxilla NOS

K08.21 **Minimal atrophy of the mandible**
Minimal atrophy of the edentulous mandible

K08.22 **Moderate atrophy of the mandible**
Moderate atrophy of the edentulous mandible

K08.23 **Severe atrophy of the mandible**
Severe atrophy of the edentulous mandible

K08.24 **Minimal atrophy of maxilla**
Minimal atrophy of the edentulous maxilla

K08.25 **Moderate atrophy of the maxilla**
Moderate atrophy of the edentulous maxilla

K08.26 **Severe atrophy of the maxilla**
Severe atrophy of the edentulous maxilla

K08.3 **Retained dental root** — A retained dental root fragment still present after loss of the rest of the tooth.

K08.4- **Partial loss** of teeth — The acquired absence of some of the natural teeth.
Acquired loss of teeth, partial
Excludes 1: *complete loss of teeth (K08.1-)*
congenital absence of teeth (K00.0)
Excludes ❷: *exfoliation of teeth due to systemic causes (K08.0)*

K08.40- Partial loss of teeth, <u>unspecified</u> cause

K08.401 Partial loss of teeth, unspecified cause, class I

K08.402 Partial loss of teeth, unspecified cause, class II

K08.403 Partial loss of teeth, unspecified cause, class III

K08.404 Partial loss of teeth, unspecified cause, class IV

K08.409 Partial loss of teeth, unspecified cause, unspecified class
Tooth extraction status NOS

K08.41- Partial loss of teeth <u>due to trauma</u> — Loss due to physical injury.

K08.411 Partial loss of teeth due to trauma, class I

K08.412 Partial loss of teeth due to trauma, class II

K08.413 Partial loss of teeth due to trauma, class III

K08.414 Partial loss of teeth due to trauma, class IV

K08.419 Partial loss of teeth due to trauma, unspecified class

K08.42- Partial loss of teeth <u>due to periodontal diseases</u> — Loss due to a diseased condition of the teeth supporting structures.

K08.421 Partial loss of teeth due to periodontal diseases, class I

K08.422 Partial loss of teeth due to periodontal diseases, class II

K08.423 Partial loss of teeth due to periodontal diseases, class III

K08.424 Partial loss of teeth due to periodontal diseases, class IV

K08.429 Partial loss of teeth due to periodontal diseases, unspecified class

K08.43- Partial loss of teeth <u>due to caries</u> — Loss due to cavities.

K08.431 Partial loss of teeth due to caries, class I

K08.432 Partial loss of teeth due to caries, class II

K08.433 Partial loss of teeth due to caries, class III

K08.434 Partial loss of teeth due to caries, class IV

K08.439 Partial loss of teeth due to caries, unspecified class

K08.49- Partial loss of teeth <u>due to other</u> specified cause

K08.491 Partial loss of teeth due to other specified cause, class I

K08.492 Partial loss of teeth due to other specified cause, class II

K08.493 Partial loss of teeth due to other specified cause, class III

K08.494 Partial loss of teeth due to other specified cause, class IV

K08.499 Partial loss of teeth due to other specified cause, unspecified class

K08.5- **Unsatisfactory restoration of tooth**
Defective bridge, crown, filling
Defective dental restoration
Excludes 1: *dental restoration status (Z98.811)*
Excludes ❷: *endosseous dental implant failure (M27.6-)*
unsatisfactory endodontic treatment (M27.5-)

K08.50 **Unsatisfactory restoration of tooth, unspecified**
Defective dental restoration NOS

K08.51 **Open restoration margins of tooth**
Dental restoration failure of marginal integrity
Open margin on tooth restoration
Poor gingival margin to tooth restoration

K08.52 **Unrepairable overhanging of dental restorative materials**
Overhanging of tooth restoration

K08.53- **Fractured dental restorative material**
Excludes 1: *cracked tooth (K03.81)*
traumatic fracture of tooth (S02.5)

K08.530 Fractured dental restorative material <u>without</u> loss of material

K08.531 Fractured dental restorative material <u>with loss of material</u>

K08.539 Fractured dental restorative material, <u>unspecified</u>

K08.54 **Contour of existing restoration of tooth biologically incompatible with oral health**
Dental restoration failure of periodontal anatomical integrity
Unacceptable contours of existing restoration of tooth
Unacceptable morphology of existing restoration of tooth

K08.55 **Allergy to existing dental restorative material**
Use additional code to identify the specific type of allergy

K08.56 **Poor aesthetic of existing restoration of tooth**
Dental restoration aesthetically inadequate or displeasing

K08.59 **Other unsatisfactory restoration of tooth**
Other defective dental restoration

K08.8- **Other specified disorders of teeth and supporting structures**

K08.81 **Primary occlusal trauma**

K08.82 **Secondary occlusal trauma**

K08.89 **Other specified disorders of teeth and supporting structures**
Enlargement of alveolar ridge NOS
Insufficient anatomic crown height
Insufficient clinical crown length
Irregular alveolar process
Toothache NOS

K08.9 **Disorder of teeth and supporting structures, unspecified**

K09-   Cysts of oral region, not elsewhere classified
Includes: Lesions showing histological features both of aneurysmal cyst
and of another fibro-osseous lesion
Excludes ❷: cysts of jaw (M27.0-, M27.4-)
radicular cyst (K04.8)

K09.0   Developmental odontogenic cysts — A cyst of the odontogenic
epithelium of the jaws.
Dentigerous cyst
Eruption cyst
Follicular cyst
Gingival cyst
Lateral periodontal cyst
Primordial cyst
Excludes ❷: keratocysts (D16.4, D16.5)
odontogenic keratocystic tumors (D16.4, D16.5)

K09.1   Developmental (nonodontogenic) cysts of oral region
Cyst (of) incisive canal
Cyst (of) palatine of papilla
Globulomaxillary cyst
Median palatal cyst
Nasoalveolar cyst
Nasolabial cyst
Nasopalatine duct cyst

K09.8   Other cysts of oral region, not elsewhere classified
Dermoid cyst
Epidermoid cyst
Lymphoepithelial cyst
Epstein's pearl

K09.9   Cyst of oral region, unspecified

K11-   Diseases of salivary glands
Use additional code to identify:
Alcohol abuse and dependence (F10.-)
Exposure to environmental tobacco smoke (Z77.22)
Exposure to tobacco smoke in the perinatal period (P96.81)
History of tobacco dependence (Z87.891)
Occupational exposure to environmental tobacco smoke (Z57.31)
Tobacco dependence (F17.-)
Tobacco use (Z72.0)

K11.0   Atrophy of salivary gland — A wasting-away of the salivary gland tissue.

K11.1   Hypertrophy of salivary gland — The abnormal enlargement of the
salivary glands and their tissues.

K11.2-   Sialoadenitis — Inflammation of a salivary gland.
Parotitis
Excludes 1:   epidemic parotitis (B26.-)
mumps (B26.-)
uveoparotid fever [Heerfordt] (D86.89)

K11.20   Sialoadenitis, unspecified

K11.21   Acute sialoadenitis — A form marked by sudden, severe onset.
Excludes 1:   acute recurrent sialoadenitis (K11.22)

K11.22   Acute recurrent sialoadenitis — A form marked by sudden, severe
onset following a previous episode.

K11.23   Chronic sialoadenitis — A form marked by slow, persistent progression.

cc **K11.3   Abscess of salivary gland** — A localized collection of pus caused by the
disintegration of salivary gland tissues.

cc **K11.4   Fistula of salivary gland** — An abnormal passage of a salivary gland.
Excludes 1:   congenital fistula of salivary gland (Q38.4)

K11.5   Sialolithiasis — The abnormal presence of a salivary calculi.
Calculus of salivary gland or duct
Stone of salivary gland or duct

K11.6   Mucocele of salivary gland — A mucous cyst of a salivary gland.
Mucous extravasation cyst of salivary gland — An encapsulated sac
containing blood of a salivary gland.
Mucous retention cyst of salivary gland — An encapsulated sac
containing glandular secretions of a salivary gland.
Ranula — A cystic tumor of a salivary gland.

K11.7   Disturbances of salivary secretion
Hypoptyalism — The abnormally decreased secretion of saliva.
Ptyalism — The abnormally excessive secretion of saliva.
Xerostomia — Dryness of the mouth caused by the decrease of normal salivary
secretion.
Excludes ❷: dry mouth NOS (R68.2)

K11.8   Other diseases of salivary glands
Benign lymphoepithelial lesion of salivary gland
Mikulicz' disease
Necrotizing sialometaplasia
Sialectasia
Stenosis of salivary duct
Stricture of salivary duct
Excludes 1:   sicca syndrome [Sjögren] (M35.0-)

K11.9   Disease of salivary gland, unspecified
Sialoadenopathy NOS

K12-   Stomatitis and related lesions — Inflammation and/or ulcerative sores of the oral
mucosal surfaces.
Use additional code to identify:
Alcohol abuse and dependence (F10.-)
Exposure to environmental tobacco smoke (Z77.22)
Exposure to tobacco smoke in the perinatal period (P96.81)
History of tobacco dependence (Z87.891)
Occupational exposure to environmental tobacco smoke (Z57.31)
Tobacco dependence (F17.-)
Tobacco use (Z72.0)
Excludes 1:   cancrum oris (A69.0)
cheilitis (K13.0)
gangrenous stomatitis (A69.0)
herpesviral [herpes simplex] gingivostomatitis (B00.2)
noma (A69.0)

K12.0   Recurrent oral aphthae — Small ulcers on the mucous membrane of the
mouth.
Aphthous stomatitis (major) (minor)
Bednar's aphthae
Periadenitis mucosa necrotica recurrens
Recurrent aphthous ulcer
Stomatitis herpetiformis

K12.1   Other forms of stomatitis
Stomatitis NOS
Denture stomatitis
Ulcerative stomatitis
Vesicular stomatitis
Excludes 1:   acute necrotizing ulcerative stomatitis (A69.1)
Vincent's stomatitis (A69.1)

cc **K12.2   Cellulitis and abscess of mouth** — CELLULITIS – Inflammation of the
oral cellular tissue. ABSCESS – A localized collection of pus, caused by the
disintegration of oral tissue.
Cellulitis of mouth (floor)
Submandibular abscess
Excludes ❷: abscess of salivary gland (K11.3)
abscess of tongue (K14.0)
periapical abscess (K04.6-K04.7)
periodontal abscess (K05.21)
peritonsillar abscess (J36)

K12.3-   Oral mucositis (ulcerative) — The eating-away of the oral mucosa.
Mucositis (oral) (oropharyneal)
Excludes ❷: gastrointestinal mucositis (ulcerative) (K92.81)
mucositis (ulcerative) of vagina and vulva (N76.81)
nasal mucositis (ulcerative) (J34.81)

K12.30   Oral mucositis (ulcerative), unspecified

K12.31   Oral mucositis (ulcerative) due to antineoplastic therapy
Use additional code for adverse effect, if applicable, to identify
antineoplastic and immunosuppressive drugs (T45.1x5)
Use additional code for other antineoplastic therapy, such as:
Radiological procedure and radiotherapy (Y84.2)

K12.32   Oral mucositis (ulcerative) due to other drugs
Use additional code for adverse effect, if applicable, to identify
drug (T36-T50 with fifth or sixth character 5)

K12.33   Oral mucositis (ulcerative) due to radiation
Use additional external cause code (W88-W90, X39.0-) to
identify cause

K12.39   Other oral mucositis (ulcerative)
Viral oral mucositis (ulcerative)

K
0
9
-
K
1
2

K13- **Other diseases of lip and oral mucosa**
Includes: Epithelial disturbances of tongue
Use additional code to identify:
Alcohol abuse and dependence (F10.-)
Exposure to environmental tobacco smoke (Z77.22)
Exposure to tobacco smoke in the perinatal period (P96.81)
History of tobacco dependence (Z87.891)
Occupational exposure to environmental tobacco smoke (Z57.31)
Tobacco dependence (F17.-)
Tobacco use (Z72.0)
Excludes ❷: certain disorders of gingiva and edentulous alveolar ridge
(K05-K06)
cysts of oral region (K09.-)
diseases of tongue (K14.-)
stomatitis and related lesions (K12.-)

K13.0 **Diseases of lips**
Abscess of lips — A localized collection of pus caused by the disintegration of the tissues of the lips.
Angular cheilitis — Superficial erosions and fissuring at the angles of the mouth.
Cellulitis of lips — Superficial erosions and fissuring of the lips.
Cheilitis NOS
Cheilodynia — Pain in the lips.
Cheilosis — The abnormal fissuring and dry scaling of the vermilion surface of the lips and the angles of the mouth.
Exfoliative cheilitis — Persistent peeling, dryness, and flaking of the lips.
Fistula of lips — An abnormal passage of the lip tissue.
Glandular cheilitis — Inflammation of the minor salivary glands of the lower lip.
Hypertrophy of lips — An abnormal enlargement of the lips.
Perlèche NEC — See Angular Cheilitis above.
Excludes 1: ariboflavinosis (E53.0)
cheilitis due to radiation-related disorders (L55-L59)
congenital fistula of lips (Q38.0)
congenital hypertrophy of lips (Q18.6)
Perlèche due to candidiasis (B37.83)
Perlèche due to riboflavin deficiency (E53.0)

K13.1 **Cheek and lip biting** — Habitual biting of the lip and oral mucosa that is usually seen in children with emotional issues.

K13.2- **Leukoplakia and other disturbances of oral epithelium, including tongue**
Excludes 1: carcinoma in situ of oral epithelium (D00.0-)
hairy leukoplakia (K13.3)
K13.21 **Leukoplakia of oral mucosa, including tongue** — Thick, whitish patches which develop upon the mucous membrane of the oral mucosa.
Leukokeratosis of oral mucosa
Leukoplakia of gingiva, lips, tongue
Excludes 1: hairy leukoplakia (K13.3)
leukokeratosis nicotina palati (K13.24)
K13.22 **Minimal keratinized residual ridge mucosa**
Minimal keratinization of alveolar ridge mucosa
K13.23 **Excessive keratinized residual ridge mucosa**
Excessive keratinization of alveolar ridge mucosa
K13.24 **Leukokeratosis nicotina palati** — The formation of whitish patches on the tongue due to the effects of cigarette smoking.
Smoker's palate
K13.29 **Other disturbances of oral epithelium, including tongue**
Erythroplakia of mouth or tongue
Focal epithelial hyperplasia of mouth or tongue
Leukoedema of mouth or tongue
Other oral epithelium disturbances

K13.3 **Hairy leukoplakia** — Whitish patches of the oral mucosa with a fuzzy appearance that are due to the Epstein-Barr virus and more often seen in immunocompromised pateints.

K13.4 **Granuloma and granuloma-like lesions of oral mucosa** — An oral mucosal granular growth.
Eosinophilic granuloma — Oral mucosal cystic lesions containing lipid and eosinophils.
Granuloma pyogenicum — An oral mucosal granular growth with the formation of pus.
Verrucous xanthoma — A wart-like growth of the oral mucosa.

K13.5 **Oral submucous fibrosis** — The formation of fibrous tissue in the oral tissue layers below the mucous membrane.
Submucous fibrosis of tongue

K13.6 **Irritative hyperplasia of oral mucosa** — The abnormal increase in the number of normal cells caused by irritative effects.
Excludes ❷: irritative hyperplasia of edentulous ridge [denture hyperplasia] (K06.2)

K13.7- **Other and unspecified lesions of oral mucosa**
K13.70 **Unspecified lesions of oral mucosa**
K13.79 **Other lesions of oral mucosa**
Focal oral mucinosis

K14- **Diseases of tongue**
Use additional code to identify:
Alcohol abuse and dependence (F10.-)
Exposure to environmental tobacco smoke (Z77.22)
History of tobacco dependence (Z87.891)
Occupational exposure to environmental tobacco smoke (Z57.31)
Tobacco dependence (F17.-)
Tobacco use (Z72.0)
Excludes ❷: erythroplakia (K13.29)
focal epithelial hyperplasia (K13.29)
leukedema of tongue (K13.29)
leukoplakia of tongue (K13.21)
hairy leukoplakia (K13.3)
macroglossia (congenital) (Q38.2)
submucous fibrosis of tongue (K13.5)

K14.0 **Glossitis** — Inflammation of the tongue.
Abscess of tongue — A localized collection of pus caused by the disintegration of glossal tissue.
Ulceration (traumatic) of tongue — A localized eating-away of glossal tissue.
Excludes 1: atrophic glossitis (K14.4)

K14.1 **Geographic tongue** — A condition characterized by white or yellowish plaque on the tongue gradually denuding to red patches with thickened white borders.
Benign migratory glossitis
Glossitis areata exfoliativa

K14.2 **Median rhomboid glossitis** — A congenital anomaly of the tongue characterized by reddish patches on the midline surface of the tongue.

K14.3 **Hypertrophy of tongue papillae** — Enlargement of the dorsal surface taste bud structures.
Black hairy tongue — A form marked by the presence of a brown, fur-like patch on the dorsal surface of the tongue.
Coated tongue — A form marked by a whitish or yellowish layer on the dorsal surface consisting of cellular debris.
Hypertrophy of foliate papillae — A form affecting the parallel mucosal folds on the margins of the tongue at the junction of its body and root.
Lingua villosa nigra — Synonym for Black Hairy Tongue.

K14.4 **Atrophy of tongue papillae** — A wasting-away of the dorsal surface taste bud structures.
Atrophic glossitis

K14.5 **Plicated tongue** — A disease characterized by cracks and divisions in the dorsal surface of the tongue.
Fissured tongue
Furrowed tongue
Scrotal tongue
Excludes 1: fissured tongue, congenital (Q38.3)

K14.6 **Glossodynia** — A painful tongue.
Glossopyrosis — A burning sensation in the tongue.
Painful tongue

K14.8 **Other diseases of tongue**
Atrophy of tongue — An abnormal wasting-away of the glossal tissue.
Crenated tongue — The abnormal notching of the surface of the tongue.
Enlargement of tongue — The abnormal increase in the size of the tongue.
Glossocele — The abnormal swelling and/or protrusion of the tongue.
Glossoptosis — The downward displacement of the tongue.
Hypertrophy of tongue — The abnormal overgrowth of the tongue.

K14.9 **Disease of tongue, unspecified**
Glossopathy NOS

K
1
3
-
K
1
4

Diseases of esophagus, stomach and duodenum (K20-K31)

Excludes ❷: *hiatus hernia (K44.-)*

K20- **Esophagitis** — Inflammation of the esophagus.
  Use additional code to identify:
   Alcohol abuse and dependence (F10.-)
  Excludes 1: *erosion of esophagus (K22.1-)*
    esophagitis with gastro-esophageal reflux disease (K21.0)
    reflux esophagitis (K21.0)
    ulcerative esophagitis (K22.1-)
  Excludes ❷: *eosinophilic gastritis or gastroenteritis (K52.81)*

 K20.0 **Eosinophilic esophagitis** — A condition involving eosinophil accumulation in the tissues lining the esophagus and characterized by severe inflammation that affects the ability to swallow.

 K20.8 **Other esophagitis**
   Abscess of esophagus — A localized collection of pus in the esophagus formed by the disintegration of tissues.

 K20.9 **Esophagitis, unspecified**
   Esophagitis NOS

K21- **Gastro-esophageal reflux disease** — A disease caused by a reflux of acid and pepsin from the stomach.
  AHA 16:1Q:p18 – Laryngopharyngeal reflux disease
  Excludes 1: *newborn esophageal reflux (P78.83)*

 K21.0 **Gastro-esophageal reflux disease with esophagitis** — A form with inflammation of the esophagus.
   Reflux esophagitis

 K21.9 **Gastro-esophageal reflux disease without esophagitis**
   Esophageal reflux NOS

K22- **Other diseases of esophagus**
  Excludes ❷: *esophageal varices (I85.-)*

 K22.0 **Achalasia of cardia** — Failure to relax the smooth muscle fibers of the esophagogastric sphincter due to degeneration of the ganglion cells in the wall of the esophagus.
   Achalasia NOS
   Cardiospasm
  Excludes 1: *congenital cardiospasm (Q39.5)*

 K22.1- **Ulcer of esophagus** — An open sore of the lining of the esophagus.
   Barrett's ulcer — See Ulcer of Esophagus above.
   Erosion of esophagus — The eating-away of the lining of the esophagus.
   Fungal ulcer of esophagus — A form caused by necrotic fungal infection.
   Peptic ulcer of esophagus — A form caused by the action of the acid gastric juice.
   Ulcer of esophagus due to ingestion of chemicals
   Ulcer of esophagus due to ingestion of drugs and medicaments
   Ulcerative esophagitis — See Ulcer of Esophagus above.
   Code first poisoning due to drug or toxin, if applicable (T36-T65 with fifth or sixth character 1-4 or 6)
   Use additional code for adverse effect, if applicable, to identify drug (T36-T50 with fifth or sixth character 5)
  Excludes 1: *Barrett's esophagus (K22.7-)*

  cc **K22.10** **Ulcer of esophagus without bleeding**
    Ulcer of esophagus NOS

  mcc **K22.11** **Ulcer of esophagus with bleeding** — A form with the escape of blood from the ulcer site.
    Excludes ❷: *bleeding esophageal varices (I85.01, I85.11)*

 K22.2 **Esophageal obstruction** — Blocking or clogging of the esophagus.
   Compression of esophagus — External pressure on the esophagus causing narrowing of the esophageal lumen.
   Constriction of esophagus — The narrowing of the esophagus.
   Stenosis of esophagus — The decrease in caliber of the esophagus.
   Stricture of esophagus — The narrowing of the esophagus.
  Excludes 1: *congenital stenosis or stricture of esophagus (Q39.3)*

 mcc **K22.3** **Perforation of esophagus** — A hole or opening through the esophageal wall.
   Rupture of esophagus — Forcible tearing or disruption through the esophageal wall.
  Excludes 1: *traumatic perforation of (thoracic) esophagus (S27.8-)*

 K22.4 **Dyskinesia of esophagus** — Impairment of the muscular control of the esophagus.
   Corkscrew esophagus — Esophageal spasm giving the appearance of a corkscrew.
   Diffuse esophageal spasm — The strong, painful, incoordinated, nonpropulsive contractions of the esophagus.
   Spasm of esophagus — The painful contractions of the esophagus.
  Excludes 1: *cardiospasm (K22.0)*

 K22.5 **Diverticulum of esophagus, acquired** — A defect in the esophagus creating a herniated sac or pouch of tissue.
   Esophageal pouch, acquired — A pocket-like space or sac in the esophagus.
  Excludes 1: *diverticulum of esophagus (congenital) (Q39.6)*

 mcc **K22.6** **Gastro-esophageal laceration-hemorrhage syndrome** — The slit-like bleeding lacerations of the esophagogastric junction following several days of severe vomiting.
   Mallory-Weiss syndrome

 K22.7- **Barrett's esophagus** — A metaplastic disorder of the lining of the lower esophagus caused by gastroesophageal reflux damage to the esophageal mucosa that is characterized by esophageal lining cells changing from squamous cells to goblet cells (usually found in the small intestine).
   Barrett's disease
   Barrett's syndrome
  Excludes 1: *Barrett's ulcer (K22.1)*
    malignant neoplasm of esophagus (C15.-)

  K22.70 **Barrett's esophagus without dysplasia**
    Barrett's esophagus NOS

  K22.71- **Barrett's esophagus with dysplasia** — A form with the development and presence of abnormal, potentially cancerous cells.

   K22.710 **Barrett's esophagus with low grade dysplasia**

   K22.711 **Barrett's esophagus with high grade dysplasia**

   K22.719 **Barrett's esophagus with dysplasia, unspecified**

 K22.8 **Other specified diseases of esophagus**
   Hemorrhage of esophagus NOS
  Excludes ❷: *esophageal varices (I85.-)*
    Paterson-Kelly syndrome (D50.1)

 K22.9 **Disease of esophagus, unspecified**

K23 **Disorders of esophagus in diseases classified elsewhere** —
  [Not Allowed as PDX]
  Code first underlying disease, such as:
   Congenital syphilis (A50.5)
  Excludes 1: *late syphilis (A52.79)*
    megaesophagus due to Chagas' disease (B57.31)
    tuberculosis (A18.83)

K25- **Gastric ulcer** — An inflammatory, necrotic, sloughing defect (open sore) in the gastric mucosa.
  Includes: **Erosion (acute) of stomach**
    Pylorus ulcer (peptic) — A form located in the pyloric antrum of the stomach.
    Stomach ulcer (peptic) — A form located in any portion of the stomach.
  Use additional code to identify:
   Alcohol abuse and dependence (F10.-)
  Excludes 1: *acute gastritis (K29.0-)*
    peptic ulcer NOS (K27.-)

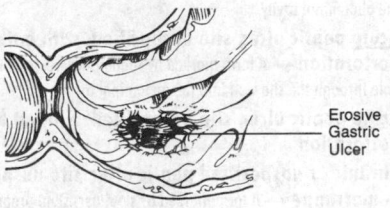

Erosive Gastric Ulcer

GASTRIC ULCER

 mcc **K25.0** **Acute gastric ulcer with hemorrhage** — A form marked by sudden, severe onset with hemorrhage at the site of the ulcer.

 mcc **K25.1** **Acute gastric ulcer with perforation** — A form marked by sudden, severe onset with the creation of a hole through the stomach wall into the abdominal cavity.

 mcc **K25.2** **Acute gastric ulcer with both hemorrhage and perforation** — A form marked by sudden, severe onset with hemorrhage and a hole through the stomach wall into the abdominal cavity.

 cc **K25.3** **Acute gastric ulcer without hemorrhage or perforation**

 mcc **K25.4** **Chronic or unspecified gastric ulcer with hemorrhage** — A form marked by slow, persistent progression with hemorrhage at the site of the ulcer.

 mcc **K25.5** **Chronic or unspecified gastric ulcer with perforation** — A form marked by slow, persistent progression with the creation of a hole through the stomach wall into the abdominal cavity.

 mcc **K25.6** **Chronic or unspecified gastric ulcer with both hemorrhage and perforation** — A form marked by slow, persistent progression with hemorrhage and a hole through the stomach wall into the abdominal cavity.

 K25.7 **Chronic gastric ulcer without hemorrhage or perforation**

K20 - K25

Excludes 1: = NOT CODED HERE! (Do not code both)   *Excludes ❷:* = Not Included Here

K25.9 Gastric ulcer, <u>unspecified as acute or chronic</u>, without hemorrhage or perforation

K26- <u>Duodenal ulcer</u> — An inflammatory, necrotic sloughing defect (open sore) in the duodenal mucosa.
  Includes: Duodenum ulcer (peptic)
      Erosion (acute) of duodenum
      Postpyloric ulcer (peptic)
  Use additional code to identify:
    Alcohol abuse and dependence (F10.-)
  Excludes 1:   peptic ulcer NOS (K27.-)

MCC **K26.0** <u>Acute</u> duodenal ulcer with hemorrhage — A form marked by sudden, severe onset with hemorrhage at the site of the ulcer.

MCC **K26.1** <u>Acute</u> duodenal ulcer with perforation — A form marked by sudden, severe onset with the creation of a hole through the duodenal wall into the abdominal cavity.

MCC **K26.2** <u>Acute</u> duodenal ulcer with both hemorrhage and perforation — A form marked by sudden, severe onset with hemorrhage and a hole through the duodenal wall into the abdominal cavity.

CC **K26.3** <u>Acute</u> duodenal ulcer without hemorrhage or perforation

MCC **K26.4** Chronic or unspecified duodenal ulcer with hemorrhage — A form marked by slow, persistent progression with hemorrhage at the site of the ulcer.
      AHA 16:1Q:p14 – Duodenal ulcer with hemorrhage due to Coumadin therapy

MCC **K26.5** Chronic or unspecified duodenal ulcer with perforation — A form marked by slow, persistent progression with the creation of a hole through the duodenal wall into the abdominal cavity.

MCC **K26.6** Chronic or unspecified duodenal ulcer with both hemorrhage and perforation — A form marked by slow, persistent progression with hemorrhage and a hole through the duodenal wall into the abdominal cavity.

K26.7 Chronic duodenal ulcer without hemorrhage or perforation

K26.9 Duodenal ulcer, <u>unspecified as acute or chronic</u>, without hemorrhage or perforation

K27- <u>Peptic ulcer</u>, site unspecified — An inflammatory, necrotic, sloughing defect (open sore) in an unspecified site of the gastroduodenal mucosa.
  Includes: Gastroduodenal ulcer NOS
      Peptic ulcer NOS
  Use additional code to identify:
    Alcohol abuse and dependence (F10.-)
  Excludes 1:   peptic ulcer of newborn (P78.82)

MCC **K27.0** <u>Acute</u> peptic ulcer, site unspecified, with hemorrhage — A form marked by sudden, severe onset with hemorrhage at the site of the ulcer.

MCC **K27.1** <u>Acute</u> peptic ulcer, site unspecified, with perforation — A form marked by sudden, severe onset with the creation of a hole through the site wall into the abdominal cavity.

MCC **K27.2** <u>Acute</u> peptic ulcer, site unspecified, with both hemorrhage and perforation — A form marked by sudden, severe onset with hemorrhage and a hole through the site wall into the abdominal cavity.

CC **K27.3** <u>Acute</u> peptic ulcer, site unspecified, without hemorrhage or perforation

MCC **K27.4** Chronic or unspecified peptic ulcer, site unspecified, with hemorrhage — A form marked by slow, persistent progression with hemorrhage at the site of the ulcer.

MCC **K27.5** Chronic or unspecified peptic ulcer, site unspecified, with perforation — A form marked by slow, persistent progression with hemorrhage and a hole through the site wall into the abdominal cavity.

MCC **K27.6** Chronic or unspecified peptic ulcer, site unspecified, with both hemorrhage and perforation — A form marked by slow, persistent progression with hemorrhage and a hole through the site wall into the abdominal cavity.

K27.7 Chronic peptic ulcer, site unspecified, without hemorrhage or perforation

K27.9 Peptic ulcer, site unspecified, <u>unspecified as acute or chronic</u>, without hemorrhage or perforation

K28- <u>Gastrojejunal ulcer</u> — An inflammatory, necrotic, sloughing defect (open sore) of the stomach and jejunum anastomotic site.
  Includes: Anastomotic ulcer (peptic) or erosion
      Gastrocolic ulcer (peptic) or erosion
      Gastrointestinal ulcer (peptic) or erosion
      Gastrojejunal ulcer (peptic) or erosion
      Jejunal ulcer (peptic) or erosion
      Marginal ulcer (peptic) or erosion
      Stomal ulcer (peptic) or erosion
  Use additional code to identify:
    Alcohol abuse and dependence (F10.-)
  Excludes 1:   primary ulcer of small intestine (K63.3)

MCC **K28.0** <u>Acute</u> gastrojejunal ulcer with hemorrhage — A form marked by sudden, severe onset with hemorrhage at the site of the ulcer.

MCC **K28.1** <u>Acute</u> gastrojejunal ulcer with perforation — A form marked by sudden, severe onset with the creation of a hole through the site wall into the abdominal cavity.

MCC **K28.2** <u>Acute</u> gastrojejunal ulcer with both hemorrhage and perforation — A form marked by sudden, severe onset with hemorrhage and a hole through the site wall into the abdominal cavity.

CC **K28.3** <u>Acute</u> gastrojejunal ulcer without hemorrhage or perforation

MCC **K28.4** Chronic or unspecified gastrojejunal ulcer with hemorrhage — A form marked by slow, persistent progression with hemorrhage at the site of the ulcer.

MCC **K28.5** Chronic or unspecified gastrojejunal ulcer with perforation — A form marked by slow, persistent progression with the creation of a hole through the site wall into the abdominal cavity.

MCC **K28.6** Chronic or unspecified gastrojejunal ulcer with both hemorrhage and perforation — A form marked by slow, persistent progression with hemorrhage and a hole through the site wall into the abdominal cavity.

K28.7 Chronic gastrojejunal ulcer without hemorrhage or perforation

K28.9 Gastrojejunal ulcer, <u>unspecified as acute or chronic</u>, without hemorrhage or perforation

K29- Gastritis and duodenitis
  Excludes 1:   eosinophilic gastritis or gastroenteritis (K52.81)
      Zollinger-Ellison syndrome (E16.4)

K29.0- <u>Acute gastritis</u> — The sudden, severe onset of inflammation of the stomach.
  Use additional code to identify:
    Alcohol abuse and dependence (F10.-)
  Excludes 1:   erosion (acute) of stomach (K25.-)

K29.00 Acute gastritis <u>without</u> bleeding

MCC **K29.01** Acute gastritis <u>with bleeding</u>

K29.2- <u>Alcoholic</u> gastritis — Inflammation of the stomach resulting from the overconsumption of alcoholic beverages.
  Use additional code to identify:
    Alcohol abuse and dependence (F10.-)

K29.20 Alcoholic gastritis <u>without</u> bleeding

MCC **K29.21** Alcoholic gastritis <u>with bleeding</u>

K29.3- <u>Chronic superficial</u> gastritis — Inflammation of the innermost layer of the stomach mucosa that persists over a period of time.

K29.30 Chronic superficial gastritis <u>without</u> bleeding

MCC **K29.31** Chronic superficial gastritis <u>with bleeding</u>

K29.4- <u>Chronic atrophic</u> gastritis — Gastritis which persists over a period of time resulting in a wasting-away of the stomach.
      Gastric atrophy

K29.40 Chronic atrophic gastritis <u>without</u> bleeding

MCC **K29.41** Chronic atrophic gastritis <u>with bleeding</u>

K29.5- <u>Unspecified chronic</u> gastritis
      Chronic antral gastritis
      Chronic fundal gastritis

K29.50 Unspecified chronic gastritis <u>without</u> bleeding

MCC **K29.51** Unspecified chronic gastritis <u>with bleeding</u>

K29.6- <u>Other</u> gastritis
      Giant hypertrophic gastritis — A form marked by gross hypertrophy of the stomach lining.
      Granulomatous gastritis — A form marked by granulomatous inflammation.
      Ménétrier's disease — See Giant Hypertrophic Gastritis above.

K29.60 Other gastritis <u>without</u> bleeding

MCC **K29.61** Other gastritis <u>with bleeding</u>

K25-K29

K29.7- Gastritis, <u>unspecified</u>

  K29.70 Gastritis, unspecified, <u>**without**</u> bleeding

MCC **K29.71** Gastritis, unspecified, <u>**with**</u> bleeding

K29.8- <u>Duodenitis</u> — Inflammation of the duodenum.

  K29.80 Duodenitis <u>**without**</u> bleeding

MCC **K29.81** Duodenitis <u>**with bleeding**</u>

K29.9- <u>Gastroduodenitis</u>, unspecified

  K29.90 Gastroduodenitis, unspecified, <u>**without**</u> bleeding

MCC **K29.91** Gastroduodenitis, unspecified, <u>**with**</u> bleeding

K30 **Functional dyspepsia** — The impairment of the power or function of digestion.

  Indigestion — The abnormal decrease of the stomach to break down food into absorbable substances.

  Excludes 1:   *dyspepsia NOS (R10.13)*
    heartburn (R12)
    nervous dyspepsia (F45.8)
    neurotic dyspepsia (F45.8)
    psychogenic dyspepsia (F45.8)

K31- **Other diseases of stomach and duodenum**

  Includes: **Functional disorders of stomach**

  Excludes ❷: *diabetic gastroparesis (E08.43, E09.43, E10.43, E11.43, E13.43)*
    diverticulum of duodenum (K57.00-K57.13)

CC **K31.0** **Acute dilatation of stomach** — The abnormal enlargement of the stomach.

  Acute distention of stomach

CC **K31.1** **Adult hypertrophic pyloric stenosis** — [Age/15-124] – Obstruction of the pyloric opening of the stomach into the duodenum associated with the abnormal increase in the size of the pyloric cells.

  Pyloric stenosis NOS

  Excludes 1:   *congenital or infantile pyloric stenosis (Q40.0)*

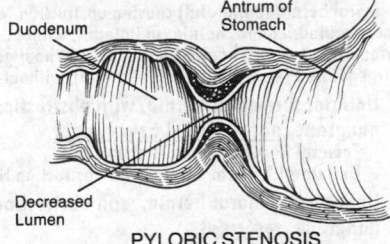

Duodenum

Antrum of Stomach

Decreased Lumen

PYLORIC STENOSIS

K31.2 **Hourglass stricture and stenosis of stomach** — A decrease in caliber at the middle of the stomach forming an hourglass appearance of the stomach.

  Excludes 1:   *congenital hourglass stomach (Q40.2)*
    hourglass contraction of stomach (K31.89)

K31.3 **Pylorospasm, <u>not elsewhere classified</u>** — The sudden, involuntary contraction of the pyloric muscles of the stomach.

  Excludes 1:   *congenital or infantile pylorospasm (Q40.0)*
    neurotic pylorospasm (F45.8)
    psychogenic pylorospasm (F45.8)

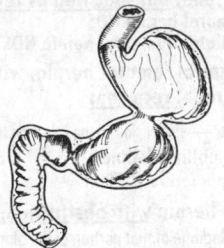

HOURGLASS STRICTURE OF STOMACH

K31.4 **Gastric diverticulum** — A protruding pouch of mucous membrane through a defect in the muscular wall of the stomach.

  Excludes 1:   *congenital diverticulum of stomach (Q40.2)*

CC **K31.5** **Obstruction of duodenum**

  Constriction of duodenum — A narrowing of the duodenum due to a loss in elasticity of the duodenal muscular walls.

  Duodenal ileus (chronic) — Obstruction and blockage of the duodenum which develops slowly and persists over a period of time.

  Stenosis of duodenum — A reduction in the size of the duodenal lumen.

  Stricture of duodenum — A decrease in caliber of the duodenal lumen.

  Volvulus of duodenum — Obstruction of the duodenum due to a knotting or twisting of the duodenum.

  Excludes 1:   *congenital stenosis of duodenum (Q41.0)*

CC **K31.6** **Fistula of stomach and duodenum** — An abnormal passage leading from the stomach or duodenum.

  Gastrocolic fistula — An abnormal passage between the stomach and the intestine.

  Gastrojejunocolic fistula — An abnormal passage between the stomach and the jejunum.

K31.7 **Polyp of stomach and duodenum** — A mucous membrane protruding growth.

  Excludes 1:   *adenomatous polyp of stomach (D13.1)*

K31.8- **Other specified diseases of stomach and duodenum**

  K31.81- **Angiodysplasia of stomach and duodenum** — The presence of small vascular abnormalities of the stomach or duodenum.

  MCC **K31.811** **Angiodysplasia of stomach and duodenum <u>with bleeding</u>**

  K31.819 **Angiodysplasia of stomach and duodenum <u>without bleeding</u>**

    Angiodysplasia of stomach and duodenum NOS

  MCC **K31.82** **Dieulafoy lesion (hemorrhagic) of stomach and duodenum** — A severe, often recurrent, hemorrhage from a pinpoint, non-ulcerated arterial lesion of the stomach or duodenum.

    Excludes ❷: *Dieulafoy lesion of intestine (K63.81)*

  K31.83 **Achlorhydria** — The decreased, or absent, production of hydrochloric stomach acid.

  K31.84 **Gastroparesis** — The condition of paralysis, or impaired contraction capacity of the stomach resulting in defective gastric emptying.

    AHA 13:4Q:p114 – Diabetic gastroparesis
    Gastroparalysis
    Code first undrlying disease, if known, such as:
      Anorexia nervosa (F50.0-)
      Diabetes mellitus (E08.43, E09.43, E10.43, E11.43, E13.43)
      Scleroderma (M34-)

  K31.89 **Other diseases of stomach and duodenum**

K31.9 **Disease of stomach and duodenum, unspecified**

Diseases of appendix (K35-K38)

K35- <u>Acute</u> **appendicitis** — The sudden, severe onset of inflammation of the appendix.

MCC **K35.2** **Acute appendicitis <u>with generalized peritonitis</u>** — A form resulting in the general inflammation of the lining membrane of the peritoneum.

  Appendicitis (acute) with generalized (diffuse) peritonitis following rupture or perforation of appendix
  Perforated appendix NOS
  Ruptured appendix NOS

MCC **K35.3** **Acute appendicitis <u>with localized peritonitis</u>** — A form resulting in the localized inflammation of the lining membrane of the peritoneum.

  Acute appendicitis with or without perforation or rupture with localized peritonitis
  Acute appendicitis with or without perforation or rupture with peritonitis NOS
  Acute appendicitis with peritoneal abscess — A form marked by the localized collection of pus caused by the disintegration of peritoneal tissue.

K35.8- **Other and unspecified acute appendicitis**

  CC **K35.80** **Unspecified acute appendicitis**
    Acute appendicitis NOS
    Acute appendicitis without (localized) (generalized) peritonitis

  CC **K35.89** **Other acute appendicitis**

K36 **Other appendicitis**

  Chronic appendicitis — Inflammation of the appendix which develops slowly and persists over a long period of time.

  Recurrent appendicitis — Inflammation of the appendix which returns periodically.

K37 **Unspecified appendicitis**

  Excludes 1:   *unspecified appendicitis with peritonitis (K35.2-K35.3)*

K38- **Other diseases of appendix**

  K38.0 **Hyperplasia of appendix**

  K38.1 **Appendicular concretions** — The presence of hardened tissue within the appendix.

    Fecalith of appendix — An appendiceal concretion formed around a center of fecal matter.
    Stercolith of appendix — Synonym for Fecalith of Appendix.

  K38.2 **Diverticulum of appendix** — A pouch of mucous membrane which protrudes through the appendiceal muscular wall.

  K38.3 **Fistula of appendix** — An abnormal passage leading outside of the appendix.

K
2
9
I
K
3
8

Excludes 1: = NOT CODED HERE! (Do not code both)   **783**   *Excludes ❷:* = Not Included Here

K38.8 Other specified diseases of appendix
Intussusception of appendix — The inward prolapse of the appendix into the intestine.

K38.9 Disease of appendix, unspecified

Hernia (K40-K46)

Note: Hernia with both gangrene and obstruction is classified to hernia with gangrene.
Includes: Acquired hernia
Congenital [except diaphragmatic or hiatus] hernia
Recurrent hernia

K40- Inguinal hernia — Protrusion of the intestine through the inguinal opening.
Includes: Bubonocele — See Indirect Inguinal Hernia below.
Direct inguinal hernia — Protrusion occurs directly through the abdominal wall.
Double inguinal hernia — Bilateral inguinal hernias.
Indirect inguinal hernia — Protrusion occurs through the internal inguinal ring into the inguinal canal.
Inguinal hernia NOS
Oblique inguinal hernia
Scrotal hernia — An inguinal hernia in which the herniated intestine descends into the scrotum.

K40.0- Bilateral inguinal hernia, with obstruction, without gangrene — A bilateral form marked by blockage of that portion of the alimentary tract, but without necrosis.
Inguinal hernia (bilateral) causing obstruction without gangrene
Incarcerated inguinal hernia (bilateral) without gangrene
Irreducible inguinal hernia (bilateral) without gangrene
Strangulated inguinal hernia (bilateral) without gangrene

cc **K40.00** Bilateral inguinal hernia, with obstruction, without gangrene, not specified as recurrent
Bilateral inguinal hernia, with obstruction, without gangrene NOS

cc **K40.01** Bilateral inguinal hernia, with obstruction, without gangrene, recurrent

K40.1- Bilateral inguinal hernia, with gangrene — A bilateral form marked by necrosis of the protruded segment due to deficient blood supply.

mcc **K40.10** Bilateral inguinal hernia, with gangrene, not specified as recurrent
Bilateral inguinal hernia, with gangrene NOS

mcc **K40.11** Bilateral inguinal hernia, with gangrene, recurrent

K40.2- Bilateral inguinal hernia, without obstruction or gangrene

K40.20 Bilateral inguinal hernia, without obstruction or gangrene, not specified as recurrent
Bilateral inguinal hernia NOS

K40.21 Bilateral inguinal hernia, without obstruction or gangrene, recurrent

K40.3- Unilateral inguinal hernia, with obstruction, without gangrene — A form marked by blockage of that portion of the alimentary tract, but without necrosis.
Inguinal hernia (unilateral) causing obstruction without gangrene
Incarcerated inguinal hernia (unilateral) without gangrene
Irreducible inguinal hernia (unilateral) without gangrene
Strangulated inguinal hernia (unilateral) without gangrene

cc **K40.30** Unilateral inguinal hernia, with obstruction, without gangrene, not specified as recurrent
Inguinal hernia, with obstruction NOS
Unilateral inguinal hernia, with obstruction, without gangrene NOS

cc **K40.31** Unilateral inguinal hernia, with obstruction, without gangrene, recurrent

K40.4- Unilateral inguinal hernia, with gangrene — A form marked by necrosis of the protruded segment due to deficient blood supply.

mcc **K40.40** Unilateral inguinal hernia, with gangrene, not specified as recurrent
Inguinal hernia with gangrene NOS
Unilateral inguinal hernia with gangrene NOS

mcc **K40.41** Unilateral inguinal hernia, with gangrene, recurrent

K40.9- Unilateral inguinal hernia, without obstruction or gangrene

K40.90 Unilateral inguinal hernia, without obstruction or gangrene, not specified as recurrent
Inguinal hernia NOS
Unilateral inguinal hernia NOS

K40.91 Unilateral inguinal hernia, without obstruction or gangrene, recurrent

K41- Femoral hernia — Protrusion of an abdominal organ through a defect in the femoral ring.

K41.0- Bilateral femoral hernia, with obstruction, without gangrene — A bilateral form marked by blockage of that portion of the alimentary tract, but without necrosis.
Femoral hernia (bilateral) causing obstruction, without gangrene
Incarcerated femoral hernia (bilateral), without gangrene
Irreducible femoral hernia (bilateral), without gangrene
Strangulated femoral hernia (bilateral), without gangrene

cc **K41.00** Bilateral femoral hernia, with obstruction, without gangrene, not specified as recurrent
Bilateral femoral hernia, with obstruction, without gangrene NOS

cc **K41.01** Bilateral femoral hernia, with obstruction, without gangrene, recurrent

K41.1- Bilateral femoral hernia, with gangrene — A bilateral form marked by necrosis of the protruded segment due to deficient blood supply.

mcc **K41.10** Bilateral femoral hernia, with gangrene, not specified as recurrent
Bilateral femoral hernia, with gangrene NOS

mcc **K41.11** Bilateral femoral hernia, with gangrene, recurrent

K41.2- Bilateral femoral hernia, without obstruction or gangrene

K41.20 Bilateral femoral hernia, without obstruction or gangrene, not specified as recurrent
Bilateral femoral hernia NOS

K41.21 Bilateral femoral hernia, without obstruction or gangrene, recurrent

K41.3- Unilateral femoral hernia, with obstruction, without gangrene — A form marked by blockage of that portion of the alimentary tract, but without necrosis.
Femoral hernia (unilateral) causing obstruction, without gangrene
Incarcerated femoral hernia (unilateral), without gangrene
Irreducible femoral hernia (unilateral), without gangrene
Strangulated femoral hernia (unilateral), without gangrene

cc **K41.30** Unilateral femoral hernia, with obstruction, without gangrene, not specified as recurrent
Femoral hernia, with obstruction NOS
Unilateral femoral hernia, with obstruction NOS

cc **K41.31** Unilateral femoral hernia, with obstruction, without gangrene, recurrent

K41.4- Unilateral femoral hernia, with gangrene — A form marked by necrosis of the protruded segment due to deficient blood supply.

mcc **K41.40** Unilateral femoral hernia, with gangrene, not specified as recurrent
Femoral hernia, with gangrene NOS
Unilateral femoral hernia, with gangrene NOS

mcc **K41.41** Unilateral femoral hernia, with gangrene, recurrent

K41.9- Unilateral femoral hernia, without obstruction or gangrene

K41.90 Unilateral femoral hernia, without obstruction or gangrene, not specified as recurrent
Femoral hernia NOS
Unilateral femoral hernia NOS

K41.91 Unilateral femoral hernia, without obstruction or gangrene, recurrent

K42- Umbilical hernia — Protrusion of the intestine through the umbilicus.
Includes: Paraumbilical hernia
Excludes 1: omphalocele (Q79.2)

cc **K42.0** Umbilical hernia with obstruction, without gangrene — A form marked by blockage of that portion of the alimentary tract, but without necrosis.
Umbilical hernia causing obstruction, without gangrene
Incarcerated umbilical hernia, without gangrene
Irreducible umbilical hernia, without gangrene
Strangulated umbilical hernia, without gangrene

mcc **K42.1** Umbilical hernia with gangrene — A form marked by necrosis of the protruded segment due to deficient blood supply.
Gangrenous umbilical hernia

K42.9 Umbilical hernia without obstruction or gangrene
Umbilical hernia NOS

K38 - K42

K43- __Ventral hernia__ — Protrusion of an abdominal organ through a defect in the abdominal wall.

CC **K43.0** **Incisional hernia __with obstruction, without gangrene__** — A form resulting from an incision in the abdominal wall with blockage of that organ's function, but without necrosis.
    Incarcerated incisional hernia, without gangrene
    Incisional hernia causing obstruction, without gangrene
    Irreducible incisional hernia, without gangrene
    Strangulated incisional hernia, without gangrene

MCC **K43.1** **Incisional hernia __with gangrene__** — A form resulting from an incision in the abdominal wall with necrosis.
    Gangrenous incisional hernia

K43.2 **Incisional hernia __without__ obstruction, __or gangrene__**
    Incisional hernia NOS

CC **K43.3** **Parastomal hernia __with obstruction, without gangrene__** — A form occurring at a stomal site in the abdominal wall with blockage of that organ's function, but without necrosis.
    Incarcerated parastomal hernia, without gangrene
    Irreducible parastomal hernia, without gangrene
    Parastomal hernia causing obstruction, without gangrene
    Strangulated parastomal hernia, without gangrene

MCC **K43.4** **Parastomal hernia __with gangrene__** — A form occurring at a stomal site in the abdominal wall with necrosis.
    Gangrenous parastomal hernia

K43.5 **Parastomal hernia __without__ obstruction, __or gangrene__**
    Parastomal hernia NOS

CC **K43.6** **Other and unspecified ventral hernia __with obstruction, without gangrene__**
    Epigastric hernia, without gangrene
    Hypogastric hernia causing obstruction, without gangrene
    Incarcerated epigastric hernia, without gangrene
    Incarcerated hypogastric hernia, without gangrene
    Incarcerated midline hernia, without gangrene
    Incarcerated spigelian hernia, without gangrene
    Incarcerated subxiphoid hernia, without gangrene
    Irreducible epigastric hernia, without gangrene
    Irreducible hypogastric hernia, without gangrene
    Irreducible midline hernia, without gangrene
    Irreducible spigelian hernia, without gangrene
    Irreducible subxiphoid hernia, without gangrene
    Midline hernia causing obstruction, without gangrene
    Spigelian hernia causing obstruction, without gangrene
    Strangulated epigastric hernia, without gangrene
    Strangulated hypogastric hernia, without gangrene
    Strangulated midline hernia, without gangrene
    Strangulated spigelian hernia, without gangrene
    Strangulated subxiphoid hernia, without gangrene
    Subxiphoid hernia causing obstruction, without gangrene

MCC **K43.7** **Other and unspecified ventral hernia __with gangrene__**
    Any condition listed under K43.6 specified as gangenous

K43.9 **Ventral hernia __without__ obstruction or gangrene**
    Epigastric hernia
    Ventral hernia NOS

K44- __Diaphragmatic hernia__ — Protrusion of an organ through the diaphragm.
    Includes: Hiatus hernia (esophageal) (sliding)
              Paraesophageal hernia
    Excludes 1: *congenital diaphragmatic hernia (Q79.0)*
                 congenital hiatus hernia (Q40.1)

CC **K44.0** **Diaphragmatic hernia __with obstruction, without gangrene__** — Protrusion of an organ through the diaphragm with blockage of that organ's function, but without necrosis.
    Diaphragmatic hernia causing obstruction
    Incarcerated diaphragmatic hernia
    Irreducible diaphragmatic hernia
    Strangulated diaphragmatic hernia

MCC **K44.1** **Diaphragmatic hernia __with gangrene__** — Protrusion of an organ through a defect in the diaphragm which has resulted in the necrosis of the herniated organ due to a deficient blood supply.
    Gangrenous diaphragmatic hernia

K44.9 **Diaphragmatic hernia __without__ obstruction or gangrene**
    Diaphragmatic hernia NOS

K45- __Other abdominal hernia__
    Includes: Abdominal hernia, specified site NEC
              Lumbar hernia
              Obturator hernia
              Pudendal hernia
              Retroperitoneal hernia
              Sciatic hernia

CC **K45.0** **Other specified abdominal hernia __with obstruction, without gangrene__**
    Other specified abdominal hernia causing obstruction
    Other specified incarcerated abdominal hernia
    Other specified irreducible abdominal hernia
    Other specified strangulated abdominal hernia

MCC **K45.1** **Other specified abdominal hernia __with gangrene__**
    Any condition listed under K45 specified as gangrenous

K45.8 **Other specified abdominal hernia __without__ obstruction or gangrene**

K46- __Unspecified abdominal__ hernia
    Includes: Enterocele
              Epiplocele
              Hernia NOS
              Interstitial hernia
              Intestinal hernia
              Intra-abdominal hernia
    Excludes 1: *vaginal enterocele (N81.5)*

CC **K46.0** **Unspecified abdominal hernia __with obstruction, without gangrene__**
    Unspecified abdominal hernia causing obstruction
    Unspecified incarcerated abdominal hernia
    Unspecified irreducible abdominal hernia
    Unspecified strangulated abdominal hernia

MCC **K46.1** **Unspecified abdominal hernia __with gangrene__**
    Any condition listed under K46 specified as gangrenous

K46.9 **Unspecified abdominal hernia __without__ obstruction or gangrene**
    Abdominal hernia NOS

Noninfective enteritis and colitis (K50-K52)

    Includes: Noninfective inflammatory bowel disease
    Excludes 1: *irritable bowel syndrome (K58.-)*
                 megacolon (K59.3-)

K50- __Crohn's disease [regional enteritis]__ — A chronic, granulomatous, inflammatory disease characterized by thickening of intestinal walls, low-grade fever, lymphoid hyperplasia, nonspecific granulomas, and mesenteric lymphadenitis.
    AHA 12:4Q:p104 – Crohn's disease of small intestine with abscess
    Includes: Granulomatous enteritis
    Use additional code to identify manifestations, such as:
       Pyoderma gangrenosum (L88)
    Excludes 1: *ulcerative colitis (K51.-)*

K50.0- **Crohn's disease of __small intestine__** — A chronic, granulomatous, inflammatory disease characterized by thickening of the small intestinal walls, low-grade fever, lymphoid hyperplasia, nonspecific granulomas, and mesenteric lymphadenitis.
    Crohn's disease [regional enteritis] of duodenum — A form affecting the duodenum.
    Crohn's disease [regional enteritis] of ileum — A form affecting the ileum.
    Crohn's disease [regional enteritis] of jejunum — A form affecting the jejunum.
    Regional ileitis
    Terminal ileitis
    Excludes 1: *Crohn's disease of both small and large intestine (K50.8-)*

CC **K50.00** **Crohn's disease of small intestine __without__ complications**

K50.01- **Crohn's disease of small intestine __with__ complications**

    CC **K50.011** **Crohn's disease of small intestine with __rectal bleeding__** — A form with the escape of blood from the rectum.

    CC **K50.012** **Crohn's disease of small intestine with __intestinal obstruction__** — A form with blockage of the intestine.

    CC **K50.013** **Crohn's disease of small intestine with __fistula__** — A form with a communicating passage from the small intestine.

    CC **K50.014** **Crohn's disease of small intestine with __abscess__** — A form with a localized collection of pus.

    CC **K50.018** **Crohn's disease of small intestine with __other__ complication**

K43 - K50

cc **K50.019**   **Crohn's disease of small intestine with <u>unspecified</u> complications**

K50.1-   **Crohn's disease of <u>large intestine</u>** — A chronic, granulomatous, inflammatory disease characterized by thickening of the large intestinal walls, low-grade fever, lymphoid hyperplasia, nonspecific granulomas, and mesenteric lymphadenitis.
> Crohn's disease [regional enteritis] of colon
> Crohn's disease [regional enteritis] of large bowel
> Crohn's disease [regional enteritis] of rectum
> Granulomatous colitis
> Regional colitis

> *Excludes 1:*   Crohn's disease of both small and large intestine (K50.8-)

cc **K50.10**   **Crohn's disease of large intestine <u>without</u> complications**

K50.11- **Crohn's disease of large intestine <u>with</u> complications**

cc **K50.111**   **Crohn's disease of large intestine with <u>rectal</u> <u>bleeding</u>** — A form with the escape of blood from the rectum.

cc **K50.112**   **Crohn's disease of large intestine with <u>intestinal</u> <u>obstruction</u>** — A form with blockage of the intestine.

cc **K50.113**   **Crohn's disease of large intestine with <u>fistula</u>** — A form with a communicating passage from the large intestine.

cc **K50.114**   **Crohn's disease of large intestine with <u>abscess</u>** — A form with a localized collection of pus.

cc **K50.118**   **Crohn's disease of large intestine with <u>other</u> complication**

cc **K50.119**   **Crohn's disease of large intestine with <u>unspecified</u> complications**

K50.8-   **Crohn's disease of <u>both small and large intestine</u>** — A chronic, granulomatous, inflammatory disease characterized by thickening of the small and large intestinal walls, low-grade fever, lymphoid hyperplasia, nonspecific granulomas, and mesenteric lymphadenitis.

cc **K50.80**   **Crohn's disease of both small and large intestine <u>without</u> complications**

K50.81- **Crohn's disease of both small and large intestine <u>with</u> complications**

cc **K50.811**   **Crohn's disease of both small and large intestine with <u>rectal bleeding</u>** — A form with the escape of blood from the rectum.

cc **K50.812**   **Crohn's disease of both small and large intestine with <u>intestinal obstruction</u>** — A form with blockage of the intestine.

cc **K50.813**   **Crohn's disease of both small and large intestine with <u>fistula</u>** — A form with a communicating passage from the small and/or large intestine.

cc **K50.814**   **Crohn's disease of both small and large intestine with <u>abscess</u>** — A form with a localized collection of pus.

cc **K50.818**   **Crohn's disease of both small and large intestine with <u>other</u> complication**

cc **K50.819**   **Crohn's disease of both small and large intestine with <u>unspecified</u> complications**

K50.9-   **Crohn's disease, <u>unspecified</u>**

cc **K50.90**   **Crohn's disease, unspecified, <u>without</u> complications**
> Crohn's disease NOS
> Regional enteritis NOS

K50.91- **Crohn's disease, unspecified, <u>with</u> complications**

cc **K50.911**   **Crohn's disease, unspecified, with <u>rectal</u> <u>bleeding</u>** — A form with the escape of blood from the rectum.

cc **K50.912**   **Crohn's disease, unspecified, with <u>intestinal</u> <u>obstruction</u>** — A form with blockage of the intestine.

cc **K50.913**   **Crohn's disease, unspecified, with <u>fistula</u>** — A form with a communicating passage from the small and/or large intestine.

cc **K50.914**   **Crohn's disease, unspecified, with <u>abscess</u>** — A form with a localized collection of pus.

cc **K50.918**   **Crohn's disease, unspecified, with other complication**

cc **K50.919**   **Crohn's disease, unspecified, with <u>unspecified</u> complications**

K51-   **<u>Ulcerative colitis</u>** — A chronic, recurrent, inflammatory, and ulcerative disease of the intestine that is characterized by bloody diarrhea, lower abdominal cramps, abdominal tenderness, and fever.
> **Use additional code to identify manifestations, such as:**
> Pyoderma gangrenosum (L88)

> *Excludes 1:*   Crohn's disease [regional enteritis] (K50.-)

K51.0-   **Ulcerative <u>(chronic) pancolitis</u>** — A chronic, recurrent, inflammatory, and ulcerative disease of the small and large intestine and rectum that is characterized by bloody diarrhea, lower abdominal cramps, abdominal tenderness, and fever.
> Backwash ileitis

cc **K51.00**   **Ulcerative (chronic) pancolitis <u>without</u> complications**
> Ulcerative (chronic) pancolitis NOS

K51.01- **Ulcerative (chronic) pancolitis <u>with</u> complications**

cc **K51.011**   **Ulcerative (chronic) pancolitis with <u>rectal</u> <u>bleeding</u>** — A form with the escape of blood from the rectum.

cc **K51.012**   **Ulcerative (chronic) pancolitis with <u>intestinal</u> <u>obstruction</u>** — A form with blockage of the intestine.

cc **K51.013**   **Ulcerative (chronic) pancolitis with <u>fistula</u>** — A form with a communicating passage from the intestine and/or rectum.

cc **K51.014**   **Ulcerative (chronic) pancolitis with <u>abscess</u>** — A form with a localized collection of pus.

cc **K51.018**   **Ulcerative (chronic) pancolitis with <u>other</u> complication**

cc **K51.019**   **Ulcerative (chronic) pancolitis with <u>unspecified</u> complications**

K51.2-   **Ulcerative <u>(chronic) proctitis</u>** — A chronic, recurrent, inflammatory, and ulcerative disease of the rectum that is characterized by bloody diarrhea, lower abdominal cramps, abdominal tenderness, and fever.

cc **K51.20**   **Ulcerative (chronic) proctitis <u>without</u> complications**
> Ulcerative (chronic) proctitis NOS

K51.21- **Ulcerative (chronic) proctitis <u>with</u> complications**

cc **K51.211**   **Ulcerative (chronic) proctitis with <u>rectal</u> <u>bleeding</u>** — A form with the escape of blood from the rectum.

cc **K51.212**   **Ulcerative (chronic) proctitis with <u>intestinal</u> <u>obstruction</u>** — A form with blockage of the intestine.

cc **K51.213**   **Ulcerative (chronic) proctitis with <u>fistula</u>** — A form with a communicating passage from the rectum.

cc **K51.214**   **Ulcerative (chronic) proctitis with <u>abscess</u>** — A form with a localized collection of pus.

cc **K51.218**   **Ulcerative (chronic) proctitis with <u>other</u> complication**

cc **K51.219**   **Ulcerative (chronic) proctitis with <u>unspecified</u> complications**

K51.3-   **Ulcerative <u>(chronic) rectosigmoiditis</u>** — A chronic, recurrent, inflammatory, and ulcerative disease of the sigmoid colon and rectum that is characterized by bloody diarrhea, lower abdominal cramps, abdominal tenderness, and fever.

cc **K51.30**   **Ulcerative (chronic) rectosigmoiditis <u>without</u> complications**
> Ulcerative (chronic) rectosigmoiditis NOS

K51.31- **Ulcerative (chronic) rectosigmoiditis <u>with</u> complications**

cc **K51.311**   **Ulcerative (chronic) rectosigmoiditis with <u>rectal</u> <u>bleeding</u>** — A form with the escape of blood from the rectum.

cc **K51.312**   **Ulcerative (chronic) rectosigmoiditis with <u>intestinal</u> <u>obstruction</u>** — A form with blockage of the intestine.

cc **K51.313**   **Ulcerative (chronic) rectosigmoiditis with <u>fistula</u>** — A form with a communicating passage from the sigmoid colon and/or rectum.

cc **K51.314**   **Ulcerative (chronic) rectosigmoiditis with <u>abscess</u>** — A form with a localized collection of pus.

cc **K51.318**   **Ulcerative (chronic) rectosigmoiditis with <u>other</u> complication**

cc **K51.319**   **Ulcerative (chronic) rectosigmoiditis with <u>unspecified</u> complications**

K51.4-   **<u>Inflammatory polyps of colon</u>** — A form with inflamed, protruding polyps.

> *Excludes 1:*   adenomatous polyp of colon (D12.6)
> polyposis of colon (D12.6)
> polyps of colon NOS (K63.5)

cc **K51.40**   **Inflammatory polyps of colon <u>without</u> complications**
> Inflammatory polyps of colon NOS

K50 - K51

K51.41- Inflammatory polyps of colon with complications

cc **K51.411** **Inflammatory polyps of colon with rectal bleeding** — A form with the escape of blood from the rectum.

cc **K51.412** **Inflammatory polyps of colon with intestinal obstruction** — A form with blockage of the intestine.

cc **K51.413** **Inflammatory polyps of colon with fistula** — A form with a communicating passage from the intestine.

cc **K51.414** **Inflammatory polyps of colon with abscess** — A form with a localized collection of pus.

cc **K51.418** **Inflammatory polyps of colon with other complication**

cc **K51.419** **Inflammatory polyps of colon with unspecified complications**

K51.5- **Left sided colitis** — A chronic, recurrent, inflammatory, and ulcerative disease of the transverse and sigmoid colon that is characterized by bloody diarrhea, lower abdominal cramps, abdominal tenderness, and fever.

Left hemicolitis

cc **K51.50** **Left sided colitis without complications**

Left sided colitis NOS

K51.51- Left sided colitis with complications

cc **K51.511** **Left sided colitis with rectal bleeding** — A form with the escape of blood from the rectum.

cc **K51.512** **Left sided colitis with intestinal obstruction** — A form with blockage of the intestine.

cc **K51.513** **Left sided colitis with fistula** — A form with a communicating passage from the transverse and/or sigmoid colon.

cc **K51.514** **Left sided colitis with abscess** — A form with a localized collection of pus.

cc **K51.518** **Left sided colitis with other complication**

cc **K51.519** **Left sided colitis with unspecified complications**

K51.8- **Other ulcerative colitis**

cc **K51.80** **Other ulcerative colitis without complications**

K51.81- Other ulcerative colitis with complications

cc **K51.811** **Other ulcerative colitis with rectal bleeding** — A form with the escape of blood from the rectum.

cc **K51.812** **Other ulcerative colitis with intestinal obstruction** — A form with blockage of the intestine.

cc **K51.813** **Other ulcerative colitis with fistula** — A form with a communicating passage from the intestine.

cc **K51.814** **Other ulcerative colitis with abscess** — A form with a localized collection of pus.

cc **K51.818** **Other ulcerative colitis with other complication**

cc **K51.819** **Other ulcerative colitis with unspecified complications**

K51.9- **Ulcerative colitis, unspecified**

cc **K51.90** **Ulcerative colitis, unspecified, without complications**

K51.91- Ulcerative colitis, unspecified, with complications

cc **K51.911** **Ulcerative colitis, unspecified with rectal bleeding** — A form with the escape of blood from the rectum.

cc **K51.912** **Ulcerative colitis, unspecified with intestinal obstruction** — A form with blockage of the intestine.

cc **K51.913** **Ulcerative colitis, unspecified with fistula** — A form with a communicating passage from the intestine.

cc **K51.914** **Ulcerative colitis, unspecified with abscess** — A form with a localized collection of pus.

cc **K51.918** **Ulcerative colitis, unspecified with other complication**

cc **K51.919** **Ulcerative colitis, unspecified with unspecified complications**

K52- **Other and unspecified noninfective gastroenteritis and colitis**

cc **K52.0** **Gastroenteritis and colitis due to radiation** — Inflammation of the stomach and small intestine and/or colon due to the adverse effects of radiation.

cc **K52.1** **Toxic gastroenteritis and colitis** — Inflammation of the stomach and small intestine and/or colon due to the chemically poisoning effects of toxic substances.

Drug-induced gastroenteritis and colitis — A form due to drugs.
Code first (T51-T65) to identify toxic agent
Use additional code for adverse effect, if applicable, to identify drug (T36-T50 with fifth or sixth character 5)

K52.2- **Allergic and dietetic gastroenteritis and colitis** — Inflammation of the stomach and small intestine and/or colon due to effects of an allergen.

Food hypersensitivity gastroenteritis or colitis
Use additional code to identify type of food allergy (Z91.01-, Z91.02-)

Excludes ❷: *allergic eosinophilic colitis (K52.82)*
allergic eosinophilic esophagitis (K20.0)
allergic eosinophilic gastritis (K52.81)
allergic eosinophilic gastroenteritis (K52.81)
food protein-induced proctocolitis (K52.82)

K52.21 **Food protein-induced enterocolitis syndrome**
Use additional code for hypovolemic shock, if present (R57.1)

K52.22 **Food protein-induced enteropathy**

K52.29 **Other allergic and dietetic gastroenteritis and colitis**
Food hypersensitivity gastroenteritis or colitis
Immediate gastrointestinal hypersensitivity

K52.3 **Indeterminate colitis**
Colonic inflammatory bowel disease unclassified (IBDU)
Excludes 1: *unspecified colitis (K52.9)*

K52.8- **Other specified noninfective gastroenteritis and colitis**

K52.81 **Eosinophilic gastritis or gastroenteritis** — A condition involving eosinophil accumulation in the tissues lining the stomach and intestines that is characterized by inflammation, vomiting, and severe abdominal pain.
Eosinophilic enteritis
Excludes ❷: *eosinophilic esophagitis (K20.0)*

K52.82 **Eosinophilic colitis** — A condition involving eosinophil accumulation in the tissues lining the large intestine that is characterized by inflammation, abdominal pain, diarrhea, and/or blood in the stool.
Allergic proctocolitis
Food-induced eosinophilic proctocolitis
Food protein-induced proctocolitis
Milk protein-induced proctocolitis

K52.83- **Microscopic colitis** — An inflammatory intestinal condition that is characterized by chronic nonbloody watery diarrhea with a normal appearing colon on colonoscopy, but some inflammatory changes on biopsy.

K52.831 **Collagenous colitis**

K52.832 **Lymphocytic colitis**

K52.838 **Other microscopic colitis**

K52.839 **Microscopic colitis, unspecified**

K52.89 **Other specified noninfective gastroenteritis and colitis**

K52.9 **Noninfective gastroenteritis and colitis, unspecified**
Colitis NOS
Enteritis NOS
Gastroenteritis NOS
Ileitis NOS
Jejunitis NOS
Sigmoiditis NOS
Excludes 1: *diarrhea NOS (R19.7)*
functional diarrhea (K59.1)
infectious gastroenteritis and colitis NOS (A09)
neonatal diarrhea (noninfective) (P78.3)
psychogenic diarrhea (F45.8)

K
5
1
-
K
5
2

Excludes 1: = NOT CODED HERE! (Do not code both)   *Excludes ❷:* = Not Included Here

Other diseases of intestines (K55-K64)

K55- <u>Vascular disorders</u> of intestine — The condition of an inadequate, functional decrease of blood flow to the intestine.
> Excludes 1:   *necrotizing enterocolitis of newborn (P77.-)*

K55.0- <u>Acute</u> vascular disorders of intestine — The sudden, severe onset of an inadequate, functional decrease of blood flow to the intestine.
> **Infarction of appendices epiploicae** — Ischemic necrosis of the intestinal, peritoneum-covered tabs of adipose tissue.
> **Mesenteric (artery) (vein) embolism** — The sudden blocking of the mesenteric artery by a blood clot or foreign material.
> **Mesenteric (artery) (vein) infarction** — Localized tissue necrosis of the mesentery resulting from obstruction of circulation in that area.
> **Mesenteric (artery) (vein) thrombosis** — The abnormal formation of a clot in a mesenteric artery or arteriole.

K55.01- Acute (reversible) <u>ischemia</u> of <u>small</u> intestine — The sudden, severe onset of inflammation of the small intestine due to and associated with a deficiency of blood supply.

MCC **K55.011** <u>Focal</u> (segmental) acute (reversible) ischemia of small intestine

MCC **K55.012** <u>Diffuse</u> acute (reversible) ischemia of small intestine

MCC **K55.019** Acute (reversible) ischemia of small intestine, extent <u>unspecified</u>

K55.02- Acute <u>infarction</u> of <u>small</u> intestine — Ischemic necrosis of the small intestine due to obstruction of the circulation to that area.
> Gangrene of small intestine
> Necrosis of small intestine

MCC **K55.021** <u>Focal</u> (segmental) acute infarction of small intestine

MCC **K55.022** <u>Diffuse</u> acute infarction of small intestine

MCC **K55.029** Acute infarction of small intestine, extent <u>unspecified</u>

K55.03- Acute (reversible) <u>ischemia</u> of <u>large</u> intestine — The sudden, severe onset of inflammation of the large intestine due to and associated with a deficiency of blood supply.
> Acute fulminant ischemic colitis
> Subacute ischemic colitis

MCC **K55.031** <u>Focal</u> (segmental) acute (reversible) ischemia of large intestine

MCC **K55.032** <u>Diffuse</u> acute (reversible) ischemia of large intestine

MCC **K55.039** Acute (reversible) ischemia of large intestine, extent <u>unspecified</u>

K55.04- Acute <u>infarction</u> of <u>large</u> intestine — Ischemic necrosis of the large intestine due to obstruction of the circulation to that area.
> Gangrene of large intestine
> Necrosis of large intestine

MCC **K55.041** <u>Focal</u> (segmental) acute infarction of large intestine

MCC **K55.042** <u>Diffuse</u> acute infarction of large intestine

MCC **K55.049** Acute infarction of large intestine, extent <u>unspecified</u>

K55.05- Acute (reversible) <u>ischemia</u> of intestine, <u>part unspecified</u>

MCC **K55.051** <u>Focal</u> (segmental) acute (reversible) ischemia of intestine, part unspecified

MCC **K55.052** <u>Diffuse</u> acute (reversible) ischemia of intestine, part unspecified

MCC **K55.059** Acute (reversible) ischemia of intestine, part and extent <u>unspecified</u>

K55.06- Acute <u>infarction</u> of intestine, part <u>unspecified</u>
> Acute intestinal infarction
> Gangrene of intestine
> Necrosis of intestine

MCC **K55.061** <u>Focal</u> (segmental) acute infarction of intestine, part unspecified

MCC **K55.062** <u>Diffuse</u> acute infarction of intestine, part unspecified

MCC **K55.069** Acute infarction of intestine, part and extent <u>unspecified</u>

CC **K55.1** <u>Chronic</u> vascular disorders of intestine — Inadequate, functional decrease of blood flow to the intestine which develops slowly and persists over a long period of time.
> **Chronic ischemic colitis** — Inflammation of the large intestine and associated with a deficiency of blood supply which develops slowly and persists over a long period of time.
> **Chronic ischemic enteritis** — Inflammation of the small intestine and associated with a deficiency of blood supply which develops slowly and persists over a long period of time.
> **Chronic ischemic enterocolitis** — Inflammation of the small and large intestine and associated with a deficiency of blood supply which develops slowly and persists over a long period of time.
> **Ischemic stricture of intestine** — The abnormal deficiency of blood supply to a localized area of the intestine resulting in contracture of the intestinal smooth muscles.
> **Mesenteric atherosclerosis** — The narrowing of the mesenteric arteries.
> **Mesenteric vascular insufficiency** — Abdominal pain after eating due to a deficiency of blood supply to the smooth muscle of the intestine.

K55.2- <u>Angiodysplasia</u> of colon — The presence of small, vascular abnormalities of the intestines.

K55.20 Angiodysplasia of colon <u>without</u> hemorrhage

MCC **K55.21** Angiodysplasia of colon <u>with hemorrhage</u>

K55.3- <u>Necrotizing enterocolitis</u> — A gastrointestinal disorder involving infection and inflammation that results in weakening and destruction of the intestinal tissues.
> Excludes 1:   *necrotizing enterocolitis of newborn (P77.-)*
> Excludes ❷: *necrotizing enterocolitis due to Clostridium difficile (A04.7)*

MCC **K55.30** Necrotizing enterocolitis, <u>unspecified</u>
> Necrotizing enterocolitis, NOS

MCC **K55.31** <u>Stage 1</u> necrotizing enterocolitis
> Necrotizing enterocolitis without pneumatosis, without perforation

MCC **K55.32** <u>Stage 2</u> necrotizing enterocolitis
> Necrotizing enterocolitis with pneumatosis, without perforation

MCC **K55.33** <u>Stage 3</u> necrotizing enterocolitis
> Necrotizing enterocolitis with perforation
> Necrotizing enterocolitis with pneumatosis and perforation

CC **K55.8** Other vascular disorders of intestine

CC **K55.9** Vascular disorder of intestine, unspecified
> Ischemic colitis
> Ischemic enteritis
> Ischemic enterocolitis

K56- Paralytic ileus and intestinal obstruction <u>without</u> hernia
> Excludes 1:   *congenital stricture or stenosis of intestine (Q41-Q42)*
> *cystic fibrosis with meconium ileus (E84.11)*
> *ischemic stricture of intestine (K55.1)*
> *meconium ileus NOS (P76.0)*
> *neonatal intestinal obstructions classifiable to P76.-*
> *obstruction of duodenum (K31.5)*
> *postprocedural intestinal obstruction (K91.3)*
> *stenosis of anus or rectum (K62.4)*
> *intestinal obstruction with hernia (K40-K46)*

CC **K56.0** <u>Paralytic ileus</u> — The neurogenic impairment of peristalsis.
> Paralysis of bowel
> Paralysis of colon
> Paralysis of intestine
> Excludes 1:   *gallstone ileus (K56.3)*
> *ileus NOS (K56.7)*
> *obstructive ileus NOS (K56.69)*

CC **K56.1** <u>Intussusception</u> — The prolapse (invagination, telescoping, sliding into) of one part of the intestine to an immediate adjacent part.
> Intussusception or invagination of bowel
> Intussusception or invagination of colon
> Intussusception or invagination of intestine
> Intussusception or invagination of rectum
> Excludes ❷: *intussusception of appendix (K38.8)*

MCC **K56.2** <u>Volvulus</u> — An intestinal obstruction due to a knotting or twisting of the intestine.
> Strangulation of colon or intestine
> Torsion of colon or intestine
> Twist of colon or intestine
> Excludes ❷: *volvulus of duodenum (K31.5)*

CC **K56.3** <u>Gallstone ileus</u> — An acute ileal obstruction due to the wedging or lodging of a gallstone in the small intestine.
> Obstruction of intestine by gallstone

K56.4-   **Other impaction of intestine**

    K56.41   **Fecal impaction** — An obstruction of the intestine due to the wedging or lodging of a fecal mass.
      Excludes 1:   *constipation (K59.0-)*
          incomplete defecation (R15.0)

   cc **K56.49**   **Other impaction of intestine**

cc **K56.5**   **Intestinal adhesions [bands] with obstruction (postprocedural) (postinfection)** — The blockage of the intestine resulting from the constricting effects of intestinal or peritoneal adhesions.
      Abdominal hernia due to adhesions with obstruction
      Peritoneal adhesions [bands] with intestinal obstruction (postprocedural) (postinfection)

K56.6-   **Other and unspecified intestinal obstruction**

cc **K56.60**   **Unspecified intestinal obstruction**
      Intestinal obstruction NOS
      Excludes 1:   *intestinal obstruction due to specified condition – code to condition*

cc **K56.69**   **Other intestinal obstruction**
      Enterostenosis NOS
      Obstructive ileus NOS
      Occlusion of colon or intestine NOS
      Stenosis of colon or intestine NOS
      Stricture of colon or intestine NOS
      Excludes 1:   *intestinal obstruction due to specified condition – code to condition*

cc **K56.7**   **Ileus, unspecified**
      Excludes 1:   *obstructive ileus (K56.69)*

K57-   **Diverticular disease of intestine** — A small mucosal pouch or sac (diverticula) which herniates through a defect in the muscular layer of the intestine. DIVERTICULOSIS – The presence of small mucosal pouches or sacs (diverticula) which herniate through defects in the muscular layer of the intestine. DIVERTICULITIS – Inflammation and/or infection of the diverticula, and if ruptured form abscesses.
   Excludes 1:   *congenital diverticulum of intestine (Q43.8)*
          Meckel's diverticulum (Q43.0)
   Excludes ❷: *diverticulum of appendix (K38.2)*

K57.0-   **Diverticulitis of small Intestine with perforation and abscess** — A form affecting the small intestine with ruptured diverticula and abscess formation.
      Diverticulitis of small intestine with peritonitis
      Excludes 1:   *diverticulitis of both small and large intestine with perforation and abscess (K57.4-)*

cc **K57.00**   **Diverticulitis of small intestine with perforation and abscess without bleeding**

mcc **K57.01**   **Diverticulitis of small intestine with perforation and abscess with bleeding** — A form with the escape of blood.

K57.1-   **Diverticular disease of small intestine without perforation or abscess**
      Excludes 1:   *diverticular disease of both small and large intestine without perforation or abscess (K57.5-)*

   K57.10   **Diverticulosis of small intestine without perforation or abscess without bleeding**
      Diverticular disease of small intestine NOS

mcc **K57.11**   **Diverticulosis of small intestine without perforation or abscess with bleeding** — A form with the escape of blood.

cc **K57.12**   **Diverticulitis of small intestine without perforation or abscess without bleeding**

mcc **K57.13**   **Diverticulitis of small intestine without perforation or abscess with bleeding** — A form with the escape of blood.

K57.2-   **Diverticulitis of large intestine with perforation and abscess** — A form affecting the large intestine with ruptured diverticula and abscess formation.
      Diverticulitis of colon with peritonitis
      Excludes 1:   *diverticulitis of both small and large intestine with perforation and abscess (K57.4-)*

cc **K57.20**   **Diverticulitis of large intestine with perforation and abscess without bleeding**

mcc **K57.21**   **Diverticulitis of large intestine with perforation and abscess with bleeding** — A form with the escape of blood.

K57.3-   **Diverticular disease of large intestine without perforation or abscess**
      Excludes 1:   *diverticular disease of both small and large intestine without perforation or abscess (K57.5-)*

   K57.30   **Diverticulosis of large intestine without perforation or abscess without bleeding**
      Diverticular disease of colon NOS

mcc **K57.31**   **Diverticulosis of large intestine without perforation or abscess with bleeding** — A form with the escape of blood.

cc **K57.32**   **Diverticulitis of large intestine without perforation or abscess without bleeding**

mcc **K57.33**   **Diverticulitis of large intestine without perforation or abscess with bleeding** — A form with the escape of blood.

K57.4-   **Diverticulitis of both small and large intestine with perforation and abscess** — A form affecting the small and large intestine with ruptured diverticula and abscess formation.
      Diverticulitis of both small and large intestine with peritonitis

cc **K57.40**   **Diverticulitis of both small and large intestine with perforation and abscess without bleeding**

mcc **K57.41**   **Diverticulitis of both small and large intestine with perforation and abscess with bleeding** — A form with the escape of blood.

K57.5-   **Diverticular disease of both small and large intestine without perforation or abscess**

   K57.50   **Diverticulosis of both small and large intestine without perforation or abscess without bleeding**
      Diverticular disease of both small and large intestine NOS

mcc **K57.51**   **Diverticulosis of both small and large intestine without perforation or abscess with bleeding** — A form with the escape of blood.

cc **K57.52**   **Diverticulitis of both small and large intestine without perforation or abscess without bleeding**

mcc **K57.53**   **Diverticulitis of both small and large intestine without perforation or abscess with bleeding** — A form with the escape of blood.

K57.8-   **Diverticulitis of intestine, part unspecified, with perforation and abscess** — A form affecting the intestine with ruptured diverticula and abscess formation.
      Diverticulitis of intestine NOS with peritonitis

cc **K57.80**   **Diverticulitis of intestine, part unspecified, with perforation and abscess without bleeding**

mcc **K57.81**   **Diverticulitis of intestine, part unspecified, with perforation and abscess with bleeding** — A form with the escape of blood.

K57.9-   **Diverticular disease of intestine, part unspecified, without perforation or abscess**

   K57.90   **Diverticulosis of intestine, part unspecified, without perforation or abscess without bleeding**
      Diverticular disease of intestine NOS

mcc **K57.91**   **Diverticulosis of intestine, part unspecified, without perforation or abscess with bleeding** — A form with the escape of blood.

cc **K57.92**   **Diverticulitis of intestine, part unspecified, without perforation or abscess without bleeding**

mcc **K57.93**   **Diverticulitis of intestine, part unspecified, without perforation or abscess with bleeding** — A form with the escape of blood.

K58-   **Irritable bowel syndrome** — A noninflammatory functional disorder of the intestine characterized by abdominal pain, diarrhea, constipation, passage of mucus, and/or bloating.
   Includes: Irritable colon
          Spastic colon

K58.0   **Irritable bowel syndrome with diarrhea**

K58.1   **Irritable bowel syndrome with constipation**

K58.2   **Mixed irritable bowel syndrome**

K58.8   **Other irritable bowel syndrome**

K58.9   **Irritable bowel syndrome without diarrhea**
      Irritable bowel syndrome NOS

K 5 6 I K 5 8

K59- **Other functional intestinal disorders**

Excludes 1:   change in bowel habit NOS (R19.4)
                intestinal malabsorption (K90.-)
                psychogenic intestinal disorders (F45.8)

Excludes ❷: functional disorders of stomach (K31.-)

K59.0- **Constipation** — Difficult and infrequent defecation.
Use additional code for adverse effect, if applicable, to identify drug (T36-T50 with fifth or sixth character 5)
Excludes 1:   fecal impaction (K56.41)
                incomplete defecation (R15.0)

K59.00 **Constipation, unspecified**

K59.01 <u>Slow transit</u> **constipation** — A form marked by a delay in the movement of fecal material throughout the colon secondary to smooth muscle dysfunction.

K59.02 <u>Outlet dysfunction</u> **constipation** — A form marked by dysfunction of the pelvic floor muscles during defecation.

K59.03 <u>Drug-induced</u> **constipation** — A form due to a drug that alters the nerve input to the gastrointestinal tract.
Use additional code for adverse effect, if applicable, to identify drug (T36-T50 with fifth or sixth character 5)

K59.04 <u>Chronic idiopathic</u> **constipation** — A form of unknown cause that is marked by its continued presence over a considerable period of time, usually more than 3 months.
Functional constipation

K59.09 **Other constipation**
Chronic constipation

K59.1 **Functional diarrhea** — The abnormal frequency and liquidity of feces due to a dysfunction of the gastrointestinal tract.
Excludes 1:   diarrhea NOS (R19.7)
                irritable bowel syndrome with diarrhea (K58.0)

cc **K59.2** **Neurogenic bowel, not elsewhere classified** — The neurologic disruption of normal defecation most commonly seen in patients with spinal cord dysfunction.

K59.3- **Megacolon, not elsewhere classified** — An abnormally large or dilated colon.
Dilatation of colon — The abnormal stretching of the colon beyond its normal dimensions.
Code first, if applicable, (T51-T65) to identify toxic agent
Excludes 1:   congenital megacolon (aganglionic) (Q43.1)
                megacolon (due to) (in) Chagas' disease (B57.32)
                megacolon (due to) (in) Clostridium difficile (A04.7)
                megacolon (due to) (in) Hirschsprung's disease (Q43.1)

cc **K59.31** **Toxic megacolon** — The significant dilatation of the colon with associated severe symptoms including fever, tachycardia, leukocytosis, and/or anemia.

cc **K59.39** **Other megacolon**
Megacolon NOS

K59.4 **Anal spasm** — A sudden, transitory constriction of the anal canal.
Proctalgia fugax — Spasmodic pain high in the rectum.

K59.8 **Other specified functional intestinal disorders**
Atony of colon — The lack of normal tone or strength of the colon.
Pseudo-obstruction (acute) (chronic) of intestine

K59.9 **Functional intestinal disorder, unspecified**

K60- **Fissure and fistula of anal and rectal regions**
Excludes 1:   fissure and fistula of anal and rectal regions with abscess or cellulitis (K61.-)
Excludes ❷: anal sphincter tear (healed) (nontraumatic) (old) (K62.81)

K60.0 **Acute anal fissure** — A sudden onset of a linear, ulcerative division of anal epithelium.

K60.1 **Chronic anal fissure** — A persistent linear, ulcerative division of anal epithelium.

K60.2 **Anal fissure, unspecified**

K60.3 **Anal fistula** — An abnormal passage from the anal canal.

K60.4 **Rectal fistula** — An abnormal passage from the rectum.
Fistula of rectum to skin — An abnormal passage from the rectum, usually rectal crypts, to the skin.
Excludes 1:   rectovaginal fistula (N82.3)
                vesicorectal fistual (N32.1)

K60.5 **Anorectal fistula** — An abnormal passage between the anus and the rectum.

K61- **Abscess of anal and rectal regions**
Includes: Abscess of anal and rectal regions
              Cellulitis of anal and rectal regions

cc **K61.0** **Anal abscess** — A localized collection of pus caused by the disintegration of the anal tissues.
Perianal abscess — A form located immediately beneath the skin adjacent to the anal canal.
Excludes 1:   intrasphincteric abscess (K61.4)

cc **K61.1** **Rectal abscess** — A localized collection of pus caused by the disintegration of the rectal tissues.
AHA 12:4Q:p104 – Rectal abscess with Crohn's disease of small intestine
Perirectal abscess — Purulent inflammation of the tissue immediately surrounding the rectum.
Excludes 1:   ischiorectal abscess (K61.3)

cc **K61.2** **Anorectal abscess** — A form localized to the anus and the rectum.

cc **K61.3** **Ischiorectal abscess** — A form localized to the ischium and the rectum.
Abscess of ischiorectal fossa

cc **K61.4** **Intrasphincteric abscess** — A form localized to the space between the interior and external anal sphincters.

K62- **Other diseases of anus and rectum**
Includes: Anal canal
Excludes ❷: colostomy and enterostomy malfunction (K94.0-, K94.1-)
                fecal incontinence (R15.-)
                hemorrhoids (K64-)

K62.0 **Anal polyp** — A protruding mucous membrane growth of the anus.

K62.1 **Rectal polyp** — A protruding mucous membrane growth of the rectum.
Excludes 1:   adenomatous polyp (D12.8)

K62.2 **Anal prolapse** — The abnormal protrusion of the anal mucosa through the anal opening.
Prolapse of anal canal

K62.3 **Rectal prolapse** — The abnormal protrusion of the rectal mucosa through the anus.
Prolapse of rectal mucosa

K62.4 **Stenosis of anus and rectum** — The abnormal decrease in caliber of the rectal and/or anal canal.
Stricture of anus (sphincter) — The abnormal decrease in the ability of the anal sphincter muscle to relax.

cc **K62.5** **Hemorrhage of anus and rectum** — The escape of blood from the anus and/or rectum.
Excludes 1:   gastrointestinal bleeding NOS (K92.2)
                melena (K92.1)
                neonatal rectal hemorrhage (P54.2)

cc **K62.6** **Ulcer of anus and rectum** — The abnormal eating-away of anal and/or rectal tissue.
Solitary ulcer of anus and rectum
Stercoral ulcer of anus and rectum
Excludes 1:   fissure and fistula of anus and rectum (K60-)
                ulcerative colitis (K51-)

K62.7 **Radiation proctitis** — Inflammation of the anus and/or rectum due to the effects of radiation.
Use additional code to identify the type of radiation (W90-)

K62.8- **Other specified diseases of anus and rectum**
Excludes ❷: ulcerative proctitis (K51.2)

K62.81 **Anal sphincter tear (healed) (nontraumatic) (old)** — The presence of a forceful disruption of the anal sphincter tissues that is not due to acute trauma.
Tear of anus, nontraumatic
Use additional code for any associated fecal incontinence (R15.-)
Excludes ❷: anal fissure (K60.-)
                anal sphincter tear (healed) (old) complicating delivery (O34.7-)
                traumatic tear of anal sphincter (S31.831)

K62.82 **Dysplasia of anus** — The abnormal shape and/or size of anal cells.
Anal intraepithelial neoplasia I and II (AIN I and II) (histologically confirmed)
Dysplasia of anus NOS
Mild and moderate dysplasia of anus (histologically confirmed)
Excludes 1:   abnormal results from anal cytologic examination without histologic confirmation (R85.61-)
                anal intraepithelial neoplasia III (D01.3)
                carcinoma in situ of anus (D01.3)
                HGSIL of anus (R85.613)
                severe dysplasia of anus (D01.3)

K
5
9
–
K
6
2

K62.89 Other specified diseases of anus and rectum
Proctitis NOS
Use additional code for any associated fecal incontinence (R15.-)

K62.9 Disease of anus and rectum, unspecified

K63- Other diseases of intestine

CC **K63.0 Abscess of intestine** — A localized collection of pus caused by the disintegration of intestinal tissue.
Excludes 1:   *abscess of intestine with Crohn's disease (K50.014, K50.114, K50.814, K50.914)*
abscess of intestine with diverticular disease (K57.0, K57.2, K57.4, K57.8)
abscess of intestine with ulcerative colitis (K51.014, K51.214, K51.314, K51.414, K51.514, K51.814, K51.914)
Excludes ❷: *abscess of anal and rectal regions (K61-)*
abscess of appendix (K35.3)

MCC **K63.1 Perforation of intestine (nontraumatic)** — The tearing open of an intestinal wall.
Perforation (nontraumatic) of rectum
Excludes 1:   *perforation (nontraumatic) of duodenum (K26.-)*
perforation (nontraumatic) of intestine with diverticular disease (K57.0, K57.2, K57.4, K57.8)
Excludes ❷: *perforation (nontraumatic) of appendix (K35.2, K35.3)*

CC **K63.2 Fistula of intestine** — The abnormal passage of the intestine.
Excludes 1:   *fistula of duodenum (K31.6)*
fistula of intestine with Crohn's disease (K50.013, K50.113, K50.813, K50.913)
fistula of intestine with ulcerative colitis (K51.013, K51.213, K51.313, K51.413, K51.513, K51.813, K51.913)
Excludes ❷: *fistula of anal and rectal regions (K60.-)*
fistula of appendix (K38.3)
intestinal-genital fistula, female (N82.2-N82.4)
vesicointestinal fistula (N32.1)

CC **K63.3 Ulcer of intestine** — The localized eating-away of intestinal tissue.
Primary ulcer of small intestine
Excludes 1:   *duodenal ulcer (K26-)*
gastrointestinal ulcer (K28-)
gastrojejunal ulcer (K28-)
jejunal ulcer (K28-)
peptic ulcer, site unspecified (K27-)
ulcer of intestine with perforation (K63.1)
ulcer of anus or rectum (K62.6)
ulcerative colitis (K51-)

K63.4 Enteroptosis — The downward displacement of the intestine in the abdominal cavity.

K63.5 Polyp of colon — A protruding mucous membrane growth of the large intestine.
AHA 15:2Q:p14 – Hyperplastic colon polyp
Excludes 1:   *adenomatous polyp of colon (D12.6)*
inflammatory polyp of colon (K51.4-)
polyposis of colon (D12.6)

K63.8- Other specified diseases of intestine

MCC **K63.81 Dieulafoy lesion of intestine** — A severe, often recurrent, hemorrhage from a pinpoint, non-ulcerated arterial lesion of the intestine.
Excludes ❷: *Dieulafoy lesion of stomach and duodenum (K31.82)*

K63.89 Other specified diseases of intestine

K63.9 Disease of intestine, unspecified

K64- Hemorrhoids and perianal venous thrombosis — HEMORRHOIDS – A varicose dilatation of one of the veins of the hemorrhoidal plexus.
Includes: Piles
Excludes 1:   *hemorrhoids complicating childbirth and the puerperium (O87.2)*
hemorrhoids complicating pregnancy (O22.4)

K64.0 First degree hemorrhoids
Grade/stage I hemorrhoids
Hemorrhoids (bleeding) without prolapse outside of anal canal

K64.1 Second degree hemorrhoids
Grade/stage II hemorrhoids
Hemorrhoids (bleeding) that prolapse with straining, but retract spontaneously

K64.2 Third degree hemorrhoids
Grade/stage III hemorrhoids
Hemorrhoids (bleeding) that prolapse with straining and require manual replacement back inside anal canal

K64.3 Fourth degree hemorrhoids
Grade/stage IV hemorrhoids
Hemorrhoids (bleeding) with prolapsed tissue that cannot be manually replaced

K64.4 Residual hemorrhoidal skin tags — Small, hemorrhoidal tissue walls remaining after primary treatment.
External hemorrhoids NOS
Skin tags of anus

K64.5 Perianal venous thrombosis
External hemorrhoids with thrombosis
Perianal hematoma
Thrombosed hemorrhoids NOS

K64.8 Other hemorrhoids
Internal hemorrhoids, without mention of degree
Prolapsed hemorrhoids, degree not specified

K64.9 Unspecified hemorrhoids
Hemorrhoids (bleeding) NOS
Hemorrhoids (bleeding) without mention of degree

Diseases of peritoneum and retroperitoneum (K65-K68)

K65- Peritonitis — Inflammation of the peritoneum.
AHA 13:2Q:p31 – Epiploic appendagitis
Use additional code (B95-B97), to identify infectious agent
Excludes 1:   *acute appendicitis with generalized peritonitis (K35.2)*
aseptic peritonitis (T81.6)
benign paroxysmal peritonitis (E85.0)
chemical peritonitis (T81.6)
diverticulitis of both small and large intestine with peritonitis (K57.4-)
diverticulitis of colon with peritonitis (K57.2-)
diverticulitis of intestine, NOS, with peritonitis (K57.8-)
diverticulitis of small intestine with peritonitis (K57.0-)
gonococcal peritonitis (A54.85)
neonatal peritonitis (P78.0-P78.1)
pelvic peritonitis, female (N73.3-N73.5)
periodic familial peritonitis (E85.0)
peritonitis due to talc or other foreign substance (T81.6)
peritonitis in chlamydia (A74.81)
peritonitis in diphtheria (A36.89)
peritonitis in syphilis (late) (A52.74)
peritonitis in tuberculosis (A18.31)
peritonitis with or following abortion or ectopic or molar pregnancy (O00-O07, O08.0)
peritonitis with or following appendicitis (K35-)
peritonitis with or following diverticular disease of intestine (K57-)
puerperal peritonitis (O85)
retroperitoneal infections (K68-)

MCC **K65.0 Generalized (acute) peritonitis** — A form that has spread to most of the peritoneal tissues.
Pelvic peritonitis (acute), male
Subphrenic peritonitis (acute)
Suppurative peritonitis (acute)

MCC **K65.1 Peritoneal abscess** — A form characterized by the localized collection of pus.
Abdominopelvic abscess
Abscess (of) omentum
Abscess (of) peritoneum
Mesenteric abscess
Retrocecal abscess
Subdiaphragmatic abscess
Subhepatic abscess
Subphrenic abscess

MCC **K65.2 Spontaneous bacterial peritonitis** — A form characterized by the lack of an identifiable source of infection that is often associated with ascites and cirrhosis.
Excludes 1:   *bacterial peritonitis NOS (K65.9)*

MCC **K65.3 Choleperitonitis** — A peritoneal inflammatory reaction resulting from the escape of bile into the peritoneum.
Peritonitis due to bile

CC **K65.4 Sclerosing mesenteritis** — A mesenteric inflammatory condition that is characterized by fat necrosis, inflammation, and fibrosis.
Fat necrosis of peritoneum
(Idiopathic) sclerosing mesenteric fibrosis
Mesenteric lipodystrophy
Mesenteric panniculitis
Retractile mesenteritis

MCC **K65.8 Other peritonitis**
Chronic proliferative peritonitis
Peritonitis due to urine

K62 - K65

MCC **K65.9 Peritonitis, unspecified**
Bacterial peritonitis NOS

K66- Other disorders of peritoneum
Excludes ❷: ascites (R18.-)
peritoneal effusion (chronic) (R18.8)

K66.0 Peritoneal adhesions (postprocedural) (postinfection) — The formation of fibrous bands within the peritoneum which abnormally restrict the function of the adhered organs.
AHA 14:1Q:p3 – Peritoneal adhesions
Adhesions (of) abdominal (wall)
Adhesions (of) diaphragm
Adhesions (of) intestine
Adhesions (of) male pelvis
Adhesions (of) omentum
Adhesions (of) stomach
Adhesive bands
Mesenteric adhesions
Excludes 1: female pelvic adhesions [bands] (N73.6)
peritoneal adhesions with intestinal obstruction (K56.5)

MCC **K66.1 Hemoperitoneum** — The abnormal escape of blood into the peritoneum.
Excludes 1: traumatic hemoperitoneum (S36.8-)

K66.8 Other specified disorders of peritoneum

K66.9 Disorder of peritoneum, unspecified

K67 Disorders of peritoneum in infectious diseases classified
MCC **elsewhere** — [Not Allowed as PDX]
Code first underlying disease, such as :
Congenital syphilis (A50.0)
Helminthiasis (B65.0-B83.9)
Excludes 1: peritonitis in chlamydia (A74.81)
peritonitis in diphtheria (A36.89)
peritonitis in gonococcal (A54.85)
peritonitis in syphilis (late) (A52.74)
peritonitis in tuberculosis (A18.31)

K68- Disorders of retroperitoneum
K68.1- Retroperitoneal abscess — The microorganism invasion of the tissues between the parietal peritoneum and the posterior abdominal wall that contains the kidneys, adrenal glands, ureters, and major abdominal vessels.

CC **K68.11 Postprocedural retroperitoneal abscess** — A form occurring following a procedure.

MCC **K68.12 Psoas muscle abscess** — The localized collection of pus of the psoas muscle.

MCC **K68.19 Other retroperitoneal abscess**

MCC **K68.9 Other disorders of retroperitoneum**

Diseases of liver (K70-K77)

Excludes 1: jaundice NOS (R17)
Excludes ❷: hemochromatosis (E83.11-)
Reye's syndrome (G93.7)
viral hepatitis (B15-B19)
Wilson's disease (E83.0)

K70- Alcoholic liver disease
Use additional code to identify:
Alcohol abuse and dependence (F10.-)

K70.0 Alcoholic fatty liver — [Age/15-124] — The abnormal accumulation of fat in the liver in persons with excessive chronic alcoholism.

K70.1- Alcoholic hepatitis — The sudden, severe onset of inflammation of the liver resulting from necrosis due to alcohol abuse.

K70.10 Alcoholic hepatitis without ascites — [Age/15-124]

K70.11 Alcoholic hepatitis with ascites — [Age/15-124] — The abnormal accumulation of fluid in the abdominal cavity.

K70.2 Alcoholic fibrosis and sclerosis of liver — [Age/15-124] — The degeneration of liver tissue with fibrosis due to chronic excessive exposure to alcohol as a hepatotoxin.

K70.3- Alcoholic cirrhosis of liver — The degeneration of liver tissue with scarring due to chronic excessive exposure to alcohol as a hepatotoxin.
Alcoholic cirrhosis NOS

K70.30 Alcoholic cirrhosis of liver without ascites — [Age/15-124]

K70.31 Alcoholic cirrhosis of liver with ascites — [Age/15-124] — The abnormal accumulation of fluid in the abdominal cavity.

K70.4- Alcoholic hepatic failure — Complete, or almost complete, loss of function of the liver due to chronic excessive exposure to alcohol as a hepatotoxin.
Acute alcoholic hepatic failure
Alcoholic hepatic failure NOS
Chronic alcoholic hepatic failure
Subacute alcoholic hepatic failure

K70.40 Alcoholic hepatic failure without coma — [Age/15-124]

MCC **K70.41 Alcoholic hepatic failure with coma** — [Age/15-124] — A form with loss of consciousness.

K70.9 Alcoholic liver disease, unspecified — [Age/15-124]

K71- Toxic liver disease — The degeneration of liver tissue due to a toxic substance other than alcohol.
Includes: Drug-induced idiosyncratic (unpredictable) liver disease
Drug-induced toxic (predictable) liver disease
Code first poisoning due to drug or toxin, if applicable (T36-T65 with fifth or sixth character 1-4 or 6)
Use additional code for adverse effect, if applicable, to identify drug (T36-T50 with fifth or sixth character 5)
Excludes ❷: alcoholic liver disease (K70.-)
Budd-Chiari syndrome (I82.0)

K71.0 Toxic liver disease with cholestasis — Damage to the liver that prevents the production and/or flow of bile from the liver.
Cholestasis with hepatocyte injury
"Pure" cholestasis

K71.1- Toxic liver disease with hepatic necrosis — The severe onset of liver dysfunction and localized tissue death of the hepatic tissues.
Hepatic failure (acute) (chronic) due to drugs

K71.10 Toxic liver disease with hepatic necrosis, without coma

MCC **K71.11 Toxic liver disease with hepatic necrosis, with coma** — A form with loss of consciousness.

K71.2 Toxic liver disease with acute hepatitis — The sudden, severe onset of an inflammatory reaction of the hepatic tissues.

K71.3 Toxic liver disease with chronic persistent hepatitis — An inflammatory reaction of the liver which is usually benign and characterized by little or no "piece-meal necrosis" of the liver cells.

K71.4 Toxic liver disease with chronic lobular hepatitis — A form affecting a lobe of the liver.

K71.5- Toxic liver disease with chronic active hepatitis — An inflammatory reaction of the liver which persists for more than six months' duration.
Toxic liver disease with lupoid hepatitis

K71.50 Toxic liver disease with chronic active hepatitis without ascites

K71.51 Toxic liver disease with chronic active hepatitis with ascites — The abnormal accumulation of fluid in the abdominal cavity.

K71.6 Toxic liver disease with hepatitis, not elsewhere classified

K71.7 Toxic liver disease with fibrosis and cirrhosis of liver — Degeneration of the liver tissue with fibrosis.

K71.8 Toxic liver disease with other disorders of liver
Toxic liver disease with focal nodular hyperplasia
Toxic liver disease with hepatic granulomas
Toxic liver disease with peliosis hepatis
Toxic liver disease with veno-occlusive disease of liver

K71.9 Toxic liver disease, unspecified

K72- Hepatic failure, not elsewhere classified
AHA 16:2Q:p35 – Hepatic failure with coma
Includes: Fulminant hepatitis NEC, with hepatic failure
Hepatic encephalopathy NOS
Liver (cell) necrosis with hepatic failure
Malignant hepatitis NEC, with hepatic failure
Yellow liver atrophy or dystrophy
Excludes 1: alcoholic hepatic failure (K70.4)
hepatic failure with toxic liver disease (K71.1-)
icterus of newborn (P55-P59)
postprocedural hepatic failure (K91.82)
Excludes ❷: hepatic failure complicating abortion or ectopic or molar pregnancy (O00-O07, O08.8)
hepatic failure complicating pregnancy, childbirth and the puerperium (O26.6-)
viral hepatitis with hepatic coma (B15-B19)

K72.0- Acute and subacute hepatic failure — Complete, or almost complete, loss of function of the liver.
AHA 14:2Q:p13 – Shock liver
AHA 15:2Q:p17 – Acute nonviral hepatitis
Acute non-viral hepatitis NOS

MCC **K72.00 Acute and subacute hepatic failure without coma**

K 6 5 - K 7 2

Excludes 1: = NOT CODED HERE! (Do not code both)   792   *Excludes ❷:* = Not Included Here

MCC **K72.01 Acute and subacute hepatic failure with coma** — A form with loss of consciousness.

K72.1- Chronic hepatic failure — The significantly ongoing loss of function of the liver.

   K72.10 Chronic hepatic failure without coma

MCC **K72.11 Chronic hepatic failure with coma** — A form with loss of consciousness.

K72.9- Hepatic failure, unspecified

   K72.90 Hepatic failure, unspecified without coma

MCC **K72.91 Hepatic failure, unspecified with coma** — A form with loss of consciousness.
      Hepatic coma NOS

K73- Chronic hepatitis, not elsewhere classified
   Excludes 1:   alcoholic hepatitis (chronic) (K70.1-)
   *   drug-induced hepatitis (chronic) (K71.-)*
   *   granulomatous hepatitis (chronic) NEC (K75.3)*
   *   reactive, nonspecific hepatitis (chronic) (K75.2)*
   *   viral hepatitis (chronic) (B15-B19)*

K73.0 Chronic persistent hepatitis, not elsewhere classified

K73.1 Chronic lobular hepatitis, not elsewhere classified

K73.2 Chronic active hepatitis, not elsewhere classified

K73.8 Other chronic hepatitis, not elsewhere classified

K73.9 Chronic hepatitis, unspecified

K74- Fibrosis and cirrhosis of liver
   Code also, if applicable, viral hepatitis (acute) (chronic) (B15-B19)
   Excludes 1:   alcoholic cirrhosis (of liver) (K70.3)
   *   alcoholic fibrosis of liver (K70.2)*
   *   cardiac sclerosis of liver (K76.1)*
   *   cirrhosis (of liver) with toxic liver disease (K71.7)*
   *   congenital cirrhosis (of liver) (P78.81)*
   *   pigmentary cirrhosis (of liver) (E83.110)*

K74.0 Hepatic fibrosis — Degeneration of the liver tissue with fibrosis.

K74.1 Hepatic sclerosis — Degeneration of the liver tissue with replacement by connective tissue.

K74.2 Hepatic fibrosis with hepatic sclerosis — Degeneration of the liver tissue with fibrosis and replacement by connective tissue.

K74.3 Primary biliary cirrhosis — Cirrhosis of the liver due to obstruction or infection of the major extrahepatic or intrahepatic bile ducts.
      Chronic nonsuppurative destructive cholangitis

K74.4 Secondary biliary cirrhosis — Cirrhosis of the liver due to obstruction or infection of the major extrahepatic or intrahepatic bile ducts that is caused by another disease or condition.

K74.6- Other and unspecified cirrhosis of liver

   K74.60 Unspecified cirrhosis of liver
         Cirrhosis (of liver) NOS

   K74.69 Other cirrhosis of liver — Degeneration of the liver tissue with fibrosis and inflammation.
         Cryptogenic cirrhosis (of liver)
         Macronodular cirrhosis (of liver)
         Micronodular cirrhosis (of liver)
         Mixed type cirrhosis (of liver)
         Portal cirrhosis (of liver)
         Postnecrotic cirrhosis (of liver)

K75- Other inflammatory liver diseases
   Excludes ❷: toxic liver disease (K71.-)

MCC **K75.0 Abscess of liver** — A localized collection of pus caused by the disintegration of hepatic tissue.
      Cholangitic hepatic abscess
      Hematogenic hepatic abscess
      Hepatic abscess NOS
      Lymphogenic hepatic abscess
      Pylephlebitic hepatic abscess
   Excludes 1:   amebic liver abscess (A06.4)
   *   cholangitis without liver abscess (K83.0)*
   *   pylephlebitis without liver abscess (K75.1)*
   Excludes ❷: acute or subacute hepatitis NOS (B17.9)
   *   acute or subacute non-viral hepatitis NOS (K72.0)*
   *   chronic hepatitis NEC (K73.8)*

MCC **K75.1 Phlebitis of portal vein** — Inflammation of the portal vein.
      Pylephlebitis
   Excludes 1:   pylephlebitic liver abscess (K75.0)

K75.2 Nonspecific reactive hepatitis
   Excludes 1:   acute or subacute hepatitis (K72.0-)
   *   chronic hepatitis NEC (K73.-)*
   *   viral hepatitis (B15-B19)*

K75.3 Granulomatous hepatitis, not elsewhere classified
   Excludes 1:   acute or subacute hepatitis (K72.0-)
   *   chronic hepatitis NEC (K73.-)*
   *   viral hepatitis (B15-B19)*

K75.4 Autoimmune hepatitis — An autoimmune disease (the body's immune system attacks itself) that is characterized by hepatocellular inflammation and necrosis which tends to progress to cirrhosis.
      Lupoid hepatitis NEC

K75.8- Other specified inflammatory liver diseases
   K75.81 Nonalcoholic steatohepatitis (NASH) — Inflammation of the liver caused by the buildup of fat in the liver, but is not associated with alcohol consumption.

   K75.89 Other specified inflammatory liver diseases

K75.9 Inflammatory liver disease, unspecified
      Hepatitis NOS
   Excludes 1:   acute or subacute hepatitis (K72.0-)
   *   chronic hepatitis NEC (K73.-)*
   *   viral hepatitis (B15-B19)*

K76- Other diseases of liver
   Excludes ❷: alcoholic liver disease (K70.-)
   *   amyloid degeneration of liver (E85.-)*
   *   cystic disease of liver (congenital) (Q44.6)*
   *   hepatic vein thrombosis (I82.0)*
   *   hepatomegaly NOS (R16.0)*
   *   pigmentary cirrhosis (of liver) (E83.110)*
   *   portal vein thrombosis (I81)*
   *   toxic liver disease (K71.-)*

K76.0 Fatty (change of) liver, not elsewhere classified — The abnormal accumulation of fat in the liver.
      Nonalcoholic fatty liver disease (NAFLD)
   Excludes 1:   nonalcoholic steatohepatitis (NASH) (K75.81)

K76.1 Chronic passive congestion of liver — The excessive accumulation of escaped blood in the liver tissues.
      Cardiac cirrhosis
      Cardiac sclerosis

MCC **K76.2 Central hemorrhagic necrosis of liver**
   Excludes 1:   liver necrosis with hepatic failure (K72-)

MCC **K76.3 Infarction of liver** — A localized area of necrosis due to obstruction of circulation to that area.

K76.4 Peliosis hepatis — A vascular condition of the liver that is characterized by multiple blood-filled cystic cavities.
      Hepatic angiomatosis

K76.5 Hepatic veno-occlusive disease — A syndrome characterized by hepatomegaly due to obstruction of the small veins of the liver (hepatic venules and hepatic sinusoids) that is most often seen in post stem cell and post chemotherapy patients (also called Sinusoidal Obstruction Syndrome (SOS)).
   Excludes 1:   Budd-Chiari syndrome (I82.0)

CC **K76.6 Portal hypertension** — An abnormally increased blood pressure in the portal venous system; a frequent complication of cirrhosis of the liver.
   Use additional code for any associated complications, such as:
      Portal hypertensive gastropathy (K31.89)

MCC **K76.7 Hepatorenal syndrome** — Renal failure associated with acute or chronic liver disease.
   Excludes 1:   hepatorenal syndrome following labor and delivery (O90.4)
   *   postprocedural hepatorenal syndrome (K91.83)*

K76.8- Other specified diseases of liver
   K76.81 Hepatopulmonary syndrome — [Unacceptable PDX] — A complication of liver disease that affects the lungs and is characterized by low blood oxygen levels and shortness of breath.
         Code first underlying disease, such as:
            Alcoholic cirrhosis of liver (K70.3-)
            Cirrhosis of liver without mention of alcohol (K74.6-)

   K76.89 Other specified diseases of liver
         Cyst (simple) of liver — The presence of a fluid-filled sac of the liver.
         Focal nodular hyperplasia of liver — The presence of benign vascular growth nodules of the liver.
         Hepatoptosis — The abnormal downward displacement of the liver.

K76.9 Liver disease, unspecified

K72 - K76

K77 **Liver disorders <u>in diseases classified elsewhere</u>** — [Not Allowed as PDX]
cc   Code first underlying disease, such as:
    Amyloidosis (E85.-)
    Congenital syphilis (A50.0, A50.5)
    Congenital toxoplasmosis (P37.1)
    Schistosomiasis (B65.0-B65.9)
  Excludes 1:   *alcoholic hepatitis (K70.1-)*
      alcoholic liver disease (K70.-)
      cytomegaloviral hepatitis (B25.1)
      herpesviral [herpes simplex] hepatitis (B00.81)
      infectious mononucleosis with liver disease (B27.0-B27.9
        with .9)
      mumps hepatitis (B26.81)
      sarcoidosis with liver disease (D86.89)
      secondary syphilis with liver disease (A51.45)
      syphilis (late) with liver disease (A52.74)
      toxoplasmosis (acquired) hepatitis (B58.1)
      tuberculosis with liver disease (A18.83)

Disorders of gallbladder, biliary tract and pancreas (K80-K87)

K80- <u>Cholelithiasis</u> — The formation and presence of gallbladder calculi.
  Excludes 1:   *retained cholelithiasis following cholecystectomy (K91.86)*
  K80.0- **Calculus of gallbladder <u>with acute</u> cholecystitis** — The presence of one or more gallstones associated with the severe, sudden onset of gallbladder inflammation.
    Any condition listed in K80.2 with acute cholecystitis
  cc **K80.00** **Calculus of gallbladder with acute cholecystitis <u>without</u> obstruction**
  cc **K80.01** **Calculus of gallbladder with acute cholecystitis <u>with obstruction</u>** — The blockage of a part of the biliary system.
  K80.1- **Calculus of gallbladder <u>with other</u> cholecystitis** — The presence of one or more gallstones with inflammation of the gallbladder of a chronic or unspecified intensity.
  cc **K80.10** **Calculus of gallbladder with <u>chronic</u> cholecystitis <u>without</u> obstruction**
    Cholelithiasis with cholecystitis NOS
  cc **K80.11** **Calculus of gallbladder with <u>chronic</u> cholecystitis <u>with obstruction</u>** — The blockage of a part of the biliary system.
  cc **K80.12** **Calculus of gallbladder with <u>acute and chronic</u> cholecystitis <u>without</u> obstruction**
  cc **K80.13** **Calculus of gallbladder with <u>acute and chronic</u> cholecystitis <u>with obstruction</u>** — The blockage of a part of the biliary system.
  cc **K80.18** **Calculus of gallbladder with <u>other</u> cholecystitis <u>without</u> obstruction**
  cc **K80.19** **Calculus of gallbladder with <u>other</u> cholecystitis <u>with obstruction</u>** — The blockage of a part of the biliary system.
  K80.2- **Calculus of gallbladder <u>without</u> cholecystitis** — The presence of one or more gallstones without associated inflammation of the gallbladder.
    Cholecystolithiasis without cholecystitis
    Cholelithiasis (without cholecystitis)
    Colic (recurrent) of gallbladder (without cholecystitis)
    Gallstone (impacted) of cystic duct (without cholecystitis)
    Gallstone (impacted) of gallbladder (without cholecystitis)
  K80.20 **Calculus of gallbladder without cholecystitis <u>without</u> obstruction**
  cc **K80.21** **Calculus of gallbladder without cholecystitis <u>with obstruction</u>** — The blockage of a part of the biliary system.
  K80.3- **Calculus of <u>bile duct with cholangitis</u>** — The presence of one or more gallstones in the bile duct with inflammation of the bile duct.
    Any condition listed in K80.5 with cholangitis
  cc **K80.30** **Calculus of bile duct with cholangitis, <u>unspecified</u>, <u>without</u> obstruction**
  cc **K80.31** **Calculus of bile duct with cholangitis, <u>unspecified</u>, <u>with obstruction</u>** — The blockage of a part of the biliary system.
  cc **K80.32** **Calculus of bile duct with <u>acute</u> cholangitis <u>without</u> obstruction**
  cc **K80.33** **Calculus of bile duct with <u>acute</u> cholangitis <u>with obstruction</u>** — The blockage of a part of the biliary system.
  cc **K80.34** **Calculus of bile duct with <u>chronic</u> cholangitis <u>without</u> obstruction**

cc **K80.35** **Calculus of bile duct with <u>chronic</u> cholangitis <u>with obstruction</u>** — The blockage of a part of the biliary system.
cc **K80.36** **Calculus of bile duct with <u>acute and chronic</u> cholangitis <u>without</u> obstruction**
cc **K80.37** **Calculus of bile duct with <u>acute and chronic</u> cholangitis <u>with obstruction</u>** — The blockage of a part of the biliary system.
K80.4- **Calculus of <u>bile duct with cholecystitis</u>** — The presence of one or more gallstones in the bile duct with gallbladder inflammation.
    Any condition listed in K80.5 with cholecystitis (with cholangitis)
cc **K80.40** **Calculus of bile duct with cholecystitis, <u>unspecified</u>, <u>without</u> obstruction**
cc **K80.41** **Calculus of bile duct with cholecystitis, <u>unspecified</u>, <u>with obstruction</u>** — The blockage of a part of the biliary system.
cc **K80.42** **Calculus of bile duct with <u>acute</u> cholecystitis <u>without</u> obstruction**
cc **K80.43** **Calculus of bile duct with <u>acute</u> cholecystitis <u>with obstruction</u>** — The blockage of a part of the biliary system.
cc **K80.44** **Calculus of bile duct with <u>chronic</u> cholecystitis <u>without</u> obstruction**
cc **K80.45** **Calculus of bile duct with <u>chronic</u> cholecystitis <u>with obstruction</u>** — The blockage of a part of the biliary system.
cc **K80.46** **Calculus of bile duct with <u>acute and chronic</u> cholecystitis <u>without</u> obstruction**
cc **K80.47** **Calculus of bile duct with <u>acute and chronic</u> cholecystitis <u>with obstruction</u>** — The blockage of a part of the biliary system.
K80.5- **Calculus of <u>bile duct without</u> cholangitis or cholecystitis** — The presence of one or more gallstones in the bile duct.
    Choledocholithiasis (without cholangitis or cholecystitis)
    Gallstone (impacted) of bile duct NOS (without cholangitis or cholecystitis)
    Gallstone (impacted) of common duct (without cholangitis or cholecystitis)
    Gallstone (impacted) of hepatic duct (without cholangitis or cholecystitis)
    Hepatic cholelithiasis (without cholangitis or cholecystitis)
    Hepatic colic (recurrent) (without cholangitis or cholecystitis)
  K80.50 **Calculus of bile duct without cholangitis or cholecystitis <u>without</u> obstruction**
cc **K80.51** **Calculus of bile duct without cholangitis or cholecystitis <u>with obstruction</u>** — The blockage of a part of the biliary system.
K80.6- **Calculus of <u>gallbladder and bile duct</u> with cholecystitis** — The presence of one or more gallstones in the gallbladder and bile duct with gallbladder inflammation.
cc **K80.60** **Calculus of gallbladder and bile duct with cholecystitis, <u>unspecified</u>, <u>without</u> obstruction**
cc **K80.61** **Calculus of gallbladder and bile duct with cholecystitis, <u>unspecified</u>, <u>with obstruction</u>** — The blockage of a part of the biliary system.
cc **K80.62** **Calculus of gallbladder and bile duct with <u>acute</u> cholecystitis <u>without</u> obstruction**
cc **K80.63** **Calculus of gallbladder and bile duct with <u>acute</u> cholecystitis <u>with obstruction</u>** — The blockage of a part of the biliary system.
cc **K80.64** **Calculus of gallbladder and bile duct with <u>chronic</u> cholecystitis <u>without</u> obstruction**
cc **K80.65** **Calculus of gallbladder and bile duct with <u>chronic</u> cholecystitis <u>with obstruction</u>** — The blockage of a part of the biliary system.
cc **K80.66** **Calculus of gallbladder and bile duct with <u>acute and chronic</u> cholecystitis <u>without</u> obstruction**
MCC **K80.67** **Calculus of gallbladder and bile duct with <u>acute and chronic</u> cholecystitis <u>with obstruction</u>** — The blockage of a part of the biliary system.
K80.7- **Calculus of gallbladder and bile duct <u>without</u> cholecystitis** — The presence of one or more gallstones in the gallbladder and bile duct.
  K80.70 **Calculus of gallbladder and bile duct without cholecystitis <u>without</u> obstruction**
cc **K80.71** **Calculus of gallbladder and bile duct without cholecystitis <u>with obstruction</u>** — The blockage of a part of the biliary system.
K80.8- **Other cholelithiasis**
  K80.80 **Other cholelithiasis <u>without</u> obstruction**

K77-K80

Excludes 1: = NOT CODED HERE! (Do not code both)

Excludes ❷: = Not Included Here

cc **K80.81**   **Other cholelithiasis <u>with obstruction</u>** — The blockage of a part of the biliary system.

K81-   <u>Cholecystitis</u>
Excludes 1:   *cholecystitis with cholelithiasis (K80.-)*

cc **K81.0**   **Acute cholecystitis** — The sudden, severe onset of inflammation of the gallbladder.
     Abscess of gallbladder — A localized collection of pus caused by the disintegration of gallbladder tissues.
     Angiocholecystitis — A form associated with an unusually vascular formation of the gallbladder.
     Emphysematous (acute) cholecystitis — A form caused by gas-producing organisms.
     Empyema of gallbladder — A form marked by the accumulation of pus within the gallbladder.
     Gangrene of gallbladder — A form marked by the death of gallbladder tissue due to decreased vascular supply.
     Gangrenous cholecystitis — A form marked by the death of gallbladder tissue due to decreased vascular supply.
     Suppurative cholecystitis — A form marked by the production of pus.

K81.1   **Chronic cholecystitis** — Inflammation of the gallbladder presenting with mild symptoms over a long period of time.

cc **K81.2**   **Acute cholecystitis with chronic cholecystitis** — Inflammation of the gallbladder with both persistent and severe, sudden onset.

K81.9   **Cholecystitis, unspecified**

K82-   Other diseases of gallbladder
Excludes 1:   *nonvisualization of gallbladder (R93.2)*
              postcholecystectomy syndrome (K91.5)

cc **K82.0**   **Obstruction of gallbladder** — The blockage of draining bile from the gallbladder.
     Occlusion of cystic duct or gallbladder without cholelithiasis
     Stenosis of cystic duct or gallbladder without cholelithiasis
     Stricture of cystic duct or gallbladder without cholelithiasis
     Excludes 1:   *obstruction of gallbladder with cholelithiasis (K80.-)*

cc **K82.1**   **Hydrops of gallbladder** — The abnormal accumulation of serous fluid within the gallbladder.
     Mucocele of gallbladder — The abnormal dilatation of the gallbladder with accumulated mucus secretion.

mcc **K82.2**   **Perforation of gallbladder** — The forcible tearing of the gallbladder wall.
     Rupture of cystic duct or gallbladder — The tearing-open of the cystic duct or gallbladder walls.

cc **K82.3**   **Fistula of gallbladder** — An abnormal passage of the gallbladder.
     Cholecystocolic fistula — An abnormal passage communicating the gallbladder with the intestine.
     Cholecystoduodenal fistula — An abnormal passage communicating the gallbladder with the duodenum.

K82.4   **Cholesterolosis of gallbladder** — The abnormal deposition of cholesterol in the gallbladder tissues.
     Strawberry gallbladder — The abnormal condition of cholesterol deposition in the gallbladder resulting in a strawberry-like appearance.
     Excludes 1:   *cholesterolosis of gallbladder with cholecystitis (K81-)*
              cholesterolosis of gallbladder with cholelithiasis (K80-)

K82.8   **Other specified diseases of gallbladder**
     Adhesions of cystic duct or gallbladder — The formation of fibrous bands of tissue of the gallbladder or cystic duct.
     Atrophy of cystic duct or gallbladder — The abnormal wasting-away of the gallbladder or cystic duct.
     Cyst of cystic duct or gallbladder — The abnormal accumulation of fluid contained in a sac of the gallbladder or cystic duct.
     Dyskinesia of cystic duct or gallbladder — The abnormal function of the filling and emptying mechanism of the gallbladder or cystic duct.
     Hypertrophy of cystic duct or gallbladder — The abnormal enlargement of constituent cells of the gallbladder or cystic duct.
     Nonfunctioning of cystic duct or gallbladder — The absence of normal gallbladder or cystic duct function.
     Ulcer of cystic duct or gallbladder — An eating-away of a localized area of the gallbladder or cystic duct.

K82.9   **Disease of gallbladder, unspecified**

K83-   Other diseases of biliary tract
Excludes 1:   *postcholecystectomy syndrome (K91.5)*
Excludes ❷: *conditions involving the gallbladder (K81-K82)*
              conditions involving the cystic duct (K81-K82)

cc **K83.0**   **Cholangitis** — Inflammation of a bile duct.
     Ascending cholangitis — A form affecting the upper bile ducts.
     Cholangitis NOS
     Primary cholangitis — A form resulting from direct invasion.
     Recurrent cholangitis — A form marked by the return of symptoms after a remission.
     Sclerosing cholangitis — A form marked by the hardening of the bile duct walls.
     Secondary cholangitis — A form caused by the effects of a systemic disease or toxin.
     Stenosing cholangitis — A form marked by a decrease in caliber of the bile duct's lumen.
     Suppurative cholangitis — A form marked by the production of pus.
     Excludes 1:   *cholangitic liver abscess (K75.0)*
              cholangitis with choledocholithiasis (K80.3-, K80.4-)
              chronic nonsuppurative destructive cholangitis (K74.3)

mcc **K83.1**   **Obstruction of bile duct** — The blockage of a bile duct.
     AHA 16:1Q:p18 – Biliary obstruction from neoplasm
     Occlusion of bile duct without cholelithiasis — The blockage of a bile duct.
     Stenosis of bile duct without cholelithiasis — The abnormal reduction in the size of a bile duct lumen.
     Stricture of bile duct without cholelithiasis — The decrease in caliber of a bile duct lumen.
     Excludes 1:   *congenital obstruction of bile duct (Q44.3)*
              obstruction of bile duct with cholelithiasis (K80.-)

mcc **K83.2**   **Perforation of bile duct** — The tearing-open of a bile duct wall.
     Rupture of bile duct

cc **K83.3**   **Fistula of bile duct** — An abnormal passage communicating from a bile duct.
     Choledochoduodenal fistula — An abnormal passage communicating a bile duct with the duodenum.

K83.4   **Spasm of sphincter of Oddi** — The abnormal function of the muscle fibers encircling the common bile duct as it enters the duodenum.

K83.5   **Biliary cyst** — An encapsulated, fluid-filled sac of a bile duct.

K83.8   **Other specified diseases of biliary tract**
     Adhesions of biliary tract — The formation of fibrous tissue bands affecting a bile duct.
     Atrophy of biliary tract — The abnormal wasting-away of bile duct tissues.
     Hypertrophy of biliary tract — The abnormal enlargement of the constituent cells of a bile duct.
     Ulcer of biliary tract — An abnormal eating-away of a localized area of a bile duct.

K83.9   **Disease of biliary tract, unspecified**

K85-   Acute pancreatitis — The sudden, severe onset of inflammation of the pancreas.
Includes: **Acute (recurrent) pancreatitis** — Multiple episodes of sudden, severe onset of inflammation of the pancreas.
              Subacute pancreatitis — A form marked by slightly milder onset and severity.

K85.0-   **<u>Idiopathic</u> acute pancreatitis** — The sudden, severe onset of inflammation of the pancreas without a known cause.

mcc **K85.00**   **Idiopathic acute pancreatitis <u>without</u> necrosis or infection**
mcc **K85.01**   **Idiopathic acute pancreatitis <u>with uninfected necrosis</u>**
mcc **K85.02**   **Idiopathic acute pancreatitis <u>with infected necrosis</u>**

K85.1-   **<u>Biliary</u> acute pancreatitis** — The sudden, severe onset of inflammation of the pancreas due to a disease or condition in the biliary system.
     Gallstone pancreatitis — The sudden, severe onset of inflammation of the pancreas due to effects of gallstones.

mcc **K85.10**   **Biliary acute pancreatitis <u>without</u> necrosis or infection**
mcc **K85.11**   **Biliary acute pancreatitis <u>with uninfected necrosis</u>**
mcc **K85.12**   **Biliary acute pancreatitis <u>with infected necrosis</u>**

K85.2-   **<u>Alcohol-induced</u> acute pancreatitis** — The sudden, severe onset of inflammation of the pancreas due to the effects of alcohol.
     Excludes ❷: *alcohol-induced chronic pancreatitis (K86.0)*

mcc **K85.20**   **Alcohol-induced acute pancreatitis <u>without</u> necrosis or infection**
mcc **K85.21**   **Alcohol-induced acute pancreatitis <u>with uninfected necrosis</u>**
mcc **K85.22**   **Alcohol-induced acute pancreatitis <u>with infected necrosis</u>**

K 8 0 - K 8 5

K85.3- <u>Drug-induced</u> acute pancreatitis — The sudden, severe onset of inflammation of the pancreas due to the effects of drugs.
Use additional code for adverse effect, if applicable, to identify drug (T36-T50 with fifth or sixth character 5)
Use additional code to identify drug abuse and dependence (F11.- – F17.-)

мсс **K85.30** Drug-induced acute pancreatitis <u>without</u> necrosis or infection

мсс **K85.31** Drug-induced acute pancreatitis <u>with uninfected necrosis</u>

мсс **K85.32** Drug-induced acute pancreatitis <u>with infected necrosis</u>

K85.8- <u>Other</u> acute pancreatitis

мсс **K85.80** Other acute pancreatitis <u>without</u> necrosis or infection

мсс **K85.81** Other acute pancreatitis <u>with uninfected necrosis</u>

мсс **K85.82** Other acute pancreatitis <u>with infected necrosis</u>

K85.9- Acute pancreatitis, <u>unspecified</u>
Pancreatitis NOS

мсс **K85.90** Acute pancreatitis <u>without</u> necrosis or infection, unspecified

мсс **K85.91** Acute pancreatitis <u>with uninfected necrosis</u>, unspecified

мсс **K85.92** Acute pancreatitis <u>with infected necrosis</u>, unspecified

K86- **Other diseases of pancreas**
Excludes ❷: *fibrocystic disease of pancreas (E84-)*
islet cell tumor (of pancreas) (D13.7)
pancreatic steatorrhea (K90.3)

cc **K86.0** **Alcohol-induced chronic pancreatitis** — Inflammation of the pancreas which persists over a long period of time that results in the loss of exocrine and endocrine function due to the effects of alcohol.
Code also exocrine pancreatic insufficiency (K86.81)
Use additional code to identify:
Alcohol abuse and dependence (F10-)
Excludes ❷: *alcohol induced acute pancreatitis (K85.2-)*

cc **K86.1** **Other chronic pancreatitis**
Chronic pancreatitis NOS
Infectious chronic pancreatitis — Inflammation of the pancreas which persists over a long period of time that results in the loss of exocrine and endocrine function due to invading microorganisms.
Recurrent chronic pancreatitis — Inflammation of the pancreas which persists over a long period of time that results in the loss of exocrine and endocrine function that recurs but is not diagnostic of acute pancreatitis.
Relapsing chronic pancreatitis — Inflammation of the pancreas which persists over a long period of time that results in the loss of exocrine and endocrine function that recurs but is not diagnostic of acute pancreatitis.
Code also exocrine pancreatic insufficiency (K86.81)

cc **K86.2** **Cyst of pancreas** — The abnormal presence of a fluid-filled sac in the pancreas.

cc **K86.3** **Pseudocyst of pancreas** — The abnormal presence of a pancreatic juice-filled sac in the abdomen.

K86.8- **Other specified diseases of pancreas**
K86.81 **Exocrine pancreatic insufficiency** — The inadequate production of pancreatic enzymes resulting in maldigestion, malabsorption, and nutrient deficiencies.

K86.89 **Other specified diseases of pancreas**
Aseptic pancreatic necrosis, unrelated to acute pancreatitis — The localized death of pancreatic tissue cells which is not associated with invading microorganisms.
Atrophy of pancreas — An abnormal wasting-away of the pancreas.
Calculus of pancreas — An abnormal concretion within the pancreas.
Cirrhosis of pancreas — The loss of normal microscopic tissue formation.
Fibrosis of pancreas — The abnormal formation of fibrous tissue which replaces the pancreatic tissue.
Pancreatic fat necrosis, unrelated to acute pancreatitis — The localized death of pancreatic tissue due to the splitting of neutral fats into fatty acids and glycerol.
Pancreatic infantilism — A condition affecting normal growth caused by defective pancreatic function.
Pancreatic necrosis NOS, unrelated to acute pancreatitis

K86.9 **Disease of pancreas, unspecified**

K87 **Disorders of gallbladder, biliary tract and pancreas <u>in diseases classified elsewhere</u>** — [Not Allowed as PDX]
Code first underlying disease
Excludes 1: *cytomegaloviral pancreatitis(B25.2)*
mumps pancreatitis (B26.3)
syphilitic gallbladder (A52.74)
syphilitic pancreas (A52.74)
tuberculosis of gallbladder (A18.83)
tuberculosis of pancreas (A18.83)

Other diseases of the digestive system (K90-K95)

K90- **Intestinal malabsorption** — Inadequate absorption of nutrients from the intestinal tract.
Excludes 1: *intestinal malabsorption following gastrointestinal surgery (K91.2)*

K90.0 **Celiac disease** — Inadequate absorption of nutrients from the intestinal tract precipitated by ingestion of gluten-containing (a protein of wheat) foods, and characterized by the degeneration of intestinal cells and fatty stools.
Celiac disease with steatorrhea
Gluten-sensitive enteropathy
Nontropical sprue
Code also exocrine pancreatic insufficiency (K86.81)
Use additional code for associated disorders including:
Dermatitis herpetiformis (L13.0)
Gluten ataxia (G32.81)

cc **K90.1** **Tropical sprue** — Inadequate absorption of nutrients from the intestinal tract occurring in the tropics and associated with anemia due to folic acid deficiency.
Sprue NOS
Tropical steatorrhea

cc **K90.2** **Blind loop syndrome, not elsewhere classified** — Inadequate intestinal absorption due to changes in the anatomy of the small intestine.
Blind loop syndrome NOS
Excludes 1: *congenital blind loop syndrome (Q43.8)*
postsurgical blind loop syndrome (K91.2)

cc **K90.3** **Pancreatic steatorrhea** — The excessive amount of fat in the feces, of pancreatic origin.

K90.4- **Other malabsorption due to intolerance**
Excludes ❷: *gluten-sensitive enteropathy (K90.0)*
lactose intolerance (E73.-)

cc **K90.41** **Non-celiac gluten sensitivity** — The condition of difficulty tolerating the ingestion of gluten-containing (a protein of wheat) foods that produce gastrointestinal symptoms, headaches, "foggy mind," joint pain, and chronic fatigue, but is not diagnostic of celiac disease.
Gluten-sensitivity NOS
Non-celiac gluten-sensitive enteropathy

cc **K90.49** **Malabsorption due to intolerance, not elsewhere classified**
Malabsorption due to intolerance to carbohydrate
Malabsorption due to intolerance to fat
Malabsorption due to intolerance to protein
Malabsorption due to intolerance to starch

K90.8- **Other intestinal malabsorption**
cc **K90.81** **Whipple's disease** — A disease caused by infection with Tropheryma whipplei that is characterized by "foamy" appearing enlarged mesenteric lymph nodes, malabsorption, progressive debility, and articular abnormalities.

cc **K90.89** **Other intestinal malabsorption**

cc **K90.9** **Intestinal malabsorption, unspecified**

K91- **<u>Intraoperative and postprocedural complications</u> and disorders of digestive system, not elsewhere classified**
Excludes ❷: *complications of artificial opening of digestive system (K94-)*
complications of bariatric procedures (K95-)
gastrojejunal ulcer (K28-)
postprocedural (radiation) retroperitoneal abscess (K68.11)
radiation colitis (K52.0)
radiation gastroenteritis (K52.0)
radiation proctitis (K62.7)

K91.0 **Vomiting following gastrointestinal surgery** — The forcible expulsion of the stomach contents through the mouth following gastrointestinal surgery.

K91.1 **Postgastric surgery syndromes**
Dumping syndrome — A symptom complex marked by nausea, weakness, sweating, tachycardia, vomiting, diarrhea, and syncope that occurs after ingestion of food by postgastrectomy or gastrojejunostomy patients.
Postgastrectomy syndrome — Synonym for Dumping Syndrome.
Postvagotomy syndrome — A form of dumping syndrome following a vagotomy.

cc **K91.2** **Postsurgical malabsorption, not elsewhere classified**
Postsurgical blind loop syndrome — Inadequate intestinal absorption following a surgical procedure.
Excludes 1: *malabsorption osteomalacia in adults (M83.2)*
malabsorption osteoporosis, postsurgical (M80.8-, M81.8)

cc **K91.3** **Postprocedural intestinal obstruction** — The blockage of the intestine following a surgical procedure.

K91.5 **Postcholecystectomy syndrome** — A syndrome characterized by abdominal pain or jaundice following a cholecystectomy.

Excludes 1: = NOT CODED HERE! (Do not code both) 796 *Excludes* ❷: = Not Included Here

K 8 5 – K 9 1

K91.6- <u>Intraoperative hemorrhage and hematoma</u> of a digestive system organ or structure complicating a procedure
Excludes 1: *intraoperative hemorrhage and hematoma of a digestive system organ or structure due to accidental puncture and laceration during a procedure (K91.7-)*

CC **K91.61** Intraoperative hemorrhage and hematoma of a digestive system organ or structure complicating a <u>digestive system procedure</u>

CC **K91.62** Intraoperative hemorrhage and hematoma of a digestive system organ or structure complicating <u>other procedure</u>

K91.7- <u>Accidental puncture and laceration</u> of a digestive system organ or structure during a procedure

CC **K91.71** Accidental puncture and laceration of a digestive system organ or structure during a <u>digestive system procedure</u>

CC **K91.72** Accidental puncture and laceration of a digestive system organ or structure during <u>other procedure</u>

K91.8- Other intraoperative and postprocedural complications and disorders of digestive system

CC **K91.81** Other intraoperative complications of digestive system

CC **K91.82** Postprocedural hepatic failure

CC **K91.83** Postprocedural hepatorenal syndrome

K91.84- <u>Postprocedural hemorrhage</u> of a digestive system organ or structure following a procedure

CC **K91.840** Postprocedural hemorrhage of a digestive system organ or structure following a <u>digestive system procedure</u>

CC **K91.841** Postprocedural hemorrhage of a digestive system organ or structure following <u>other procedure</u>

K91.85- Complications of intestinal pouch — The abnormal function or condition of a surgically created intestinal pouch.

CC **K91.850** Pouchitis — Inflammation of the surgically created pouch with symptoms that may include diarrhea, bloody stool, urgency, incontinence, abdominal pain, and fever.
Inflammation of internal ileoanal pouch

CC **K91.858** Other complications of intestinal pouch

CC **K91.86** Retained cholelithiasis following cholecystectomy

K91.87- <u>Postprocedural hematoma and seroma</u> of a digestive system organ or structure following a procedure

CC **K91.870** Postprocedural <u>hematoma</u> of a digestive system organ or structure following a <u>digestive system procedure</u>

CC **K91.871** Postprocedural <u>hematoma</u> of a digestive system organ or structure following <u>other procedure</u>

CC **K91.872** Postprocedural <u>seroma</u> of a digestive system organ or structure following a <u>digestive system procedure</u>

CC **K91.873** Postprocedural <u>seroma</u> of a digestive system organ or structure following <u>other procedure</u>

CC **K91.89** Other postprocedural complications and disorders of digestive system
Use additional code, if applicable, to further specify disorder
Excludes ❷: *postprocedural retroperitoneal abscess (K68.11)*

K92- Other diseases of digestive system
Excludes 1: *neonatal gastrointestinal hemorrhage (P54.0-P54.3)*

CC **K92.0** Hematemesis — The abnormal presence of blood in the vomitus.

CC **K92.1** Melena — Black, tarry-colored feces due to the abnormal escape of blood into the fecal material.
Excludes 1: *occult blood in feces (R19.5)*

CC **K92.2** Gastrointestinal hemorrhage, unspecified — The abnormal escape of blood from the gastrointestinal tract.
Gastric hemorrhage NOS
Intestinal hemorrhage NOS
Excludes 1: *acute hemorrhagic gastritis (K29.01)*
hemorrhage of anus and rectum (K62.5)
angiodysplasia of stomach with hemorrhage (K31.811)
diverticular disease with hemorrhage (K57.-)
gastritis and duodenitis with hemorrhage (K29.-)
peptic ulcer with hemorrhage (K25-K28)

K92.8- Other specified diseases of the digestive system

CC **K92.81** Gastrointestinal mucositis (ulcerative) — Inflammation and/or ulcerative sores of the gastrointestinal mucosal surfaces.
Code also type of associated therapy, such as:
Antineoplastic and immunosuppressive drugs (T45.1x-)
Radiological procedure and radiotherapy (Y84.2)
Excludes ❷: *mucositis (ulcerative) of vagina and vulva (N76.81)*
nasal mucositis (ulcerative) (J34.81)
oral mucositis (ulcerative) (K12.3-)

K92.89 Other specified diseases of the digestive system

K92.9 Disease of digestive system, unspecified

K94- Complications of artificial openings of the digestive system

K94.0- <u>Colostomy</u> complications — The abnormal function or condition of a colostomy.

K94.00 Colostomy complication, unspecified

CC **K94.01** Colostomy hemorrhage — A form with the abnormal escape of blood.

CC **K94.02** Colostomy infection — A form characterized by cellular inflammation that is caused by microorganisms.
Use additional code to specify type of infection, such as:
Cellulitis of abdominal wall (L03.311)
Sepsis (A40.-, A41.-)

CC **K94.03** Colostomy malfunction — The abnormal, or cessation of, function of a colostomy.
Mechanical complication of colostomy

CC **K94.09** Other complications of colostomy

K94.1- <u>Enterostomy</u> complications — The abnormal function or condition of an enterostomy.

K94.10 Enterostomy complication, unspecified

CC **K94.11** Enterostomy hemorrhage — A form with the abnormal escape of blood.

CC **K94.12** Enterostomy infection — A form characterized by cellular inflammation that is caused by microorganisms.
Use additional code to specify type of infection, such as:
Cellulitis of abdominal wall (L03.311)
Sepsis (A40.-, A41.-)

CC **K94.13** Enterostomy malfunction — The abnormal, or cessation of, function of an enterostomy.
Mechanical complication of enterostomy

CC **K94.19** Other complications of enterostomy

K94.2- <u>Gastrostomy</u> complications — The abnormal function or condition of a gastrostomy.

K94.20 Gastrostomy complication, unspecified

K94.21 Gastrostomy hemorrhage — A form with the abnormal escape of blood.

CC **K94.22** Gastrostomy infection — A form characterized by cellular inflammation that is caused by microorganisms.
Use additional code to specify type of infection, such as:
Cellulitis of abdominal wall (L03.311)
Sepsis (A40.-, A41.-)

CC **K94.23** Gastrostomy malfunction — The abnormal, or cessation of, function of a gastrostomy.
Mechanical complication of gastrostomy

K94.29 Other complications of gastrostomy

K94.3- <u>Esophagostomy</u> complications — The abnormal function or condition of an esophagostomy.

CC **K94.30** Esophagostomy complications, unspecified

CC **K94.31** Esophagostomy hemorrhage — A form with the abnormal escape of blood.

CC **K94.32** Esophagostomy infection — A form characterized by cellular inflammation that is caused by microorganisms.
Use additional code to identify the infection

CC **K94.33** Esophagostomy malfunction — The abnormal, or cessation of, function of an esophagostomy.
Mechanical complication of esophagostomy

CC **K94.39** Other complications of esophagostomy

K91-K94

K95   Complications of bariatric procedures

  K95.0-   Complications of gastric band procedure

  cc **K95.01   Infection due to gastric band procedure** — A form characterized by cellular inflammation that is caused by microorganisms.
Use additional code to specify type of infection or organism, such as:
  Bacterial and viral infectious agents (B95.-, B96.-)
  Cellulitis of abdominal wall (L03.311)
  Sepsis (A40-, A41-)

  cc **K95.09   Other complications of gastric band procedure**
Use additional code, if applicable, to further specify complication

  K95.8-   Complications of other bariatric procedure

  Excludes 1:   complications of gastric band surgery (K95.0-)

  cc **K95.81   Infection due to other bariatric procedure** — A form characterized by cellular inflammation that is caused by microorganisms.
Use additional code to specify type of infection or organism, such as:
  Bacterial and viral infectious agents (B95.-, B96.-)
  Cellulitis of abdominal wall (L03.311)
  Sepsis (A04-, A41-)

  cc **K95.89   Other complications of other bariatric procedure**
Use additional code, if applicable, to further specify complication

Chapter 12 – Diseases of the skin and subcutaneous tissue (L00-L99)

Excludes ❷: *certain conditions originating in the perinatal period (P04-P96)*
    certain infectious and parasitic diseases (A00-B99)
    complications of pregnancy, childbirth and the puerperium (O00-O9A)
    congenital malformations, deformations, and chromosomal abnormalities (Q00-Q99)
    endocrine, nutritional and metabolic diseases (E00-E88)
    lipomelanotic reticulosis (I89.8)
    neoplasms (C00-D49)
    symptoms, signs and abnormal clinical and laboratory findings, not elsewhere classified (R00-R94)
    systemic connective tissue disorders (M30-M36)
    viral warts (B07-)

This chapter contains the following blocks:

L00-L08	Infections of the skin and subcutaneous tissue
L10-L14	Bullous disorders
L20-L30	Dermatitis and eczema
L40-L45	Papulosquamous disorders
L49-L54	Urticaria and erythema
L55-L59	Radiation-related disorders of the skin and subcutaneous tissue
L60-L75	Disorders of skin appendages
L76	Intraoperative and postprocedural complications of skin and subcutaneous tissue
L80-L99	Other disorders of the skin and subcutaneous tissue

Chapter-Specific Coding Guidelines

C.   Chapter-Specific Coding Guidelines
In addition to general coding guidelines, there are guidelines for specific diagnoses and/or conditions in the classification. Unless otherwise indicated, these guidelines apply to all health care settings. Please refer to Section II for guidelines on the selection of principal diagnosis.

12.   Chapter 12: Diseases of the Skin and Subcutaneous Tissue (L00-L99)

a.   Pressure ulcer stage codes

1)   Pressure ulcer stages
Codes from category L89, Pressure ulcer, ~~are combination codes that~~ identify the site of the pressure ulcer as well as the stage of the ulcer.

The ICD-10-CM classifies pressure ulcer stages based on severity, which is designated by stages 1-4, unspecified stage and unstageable.

Assign as many codes from category L89 as needed to identify all the pressure ulcers the patient has, if applicable.

2)   Unstageable pressure ulcers
Assignment of the code for unstageable pressure ulcer (L89.--0) should be based on the clinical documentation. These codes are used for pressure ulcers whose stage cannot be clinically determined (e.g., the ulcer is covered by eschar or has been treated with a skin or muscle graft) and pressure ulcers that are documented as deep tissue injury but not documented as due to trauma. This code should not be confused with the codes for unspecified stage (L89.--9). When there is no documentation regarding the stage of the pressure ulcer, assign the appropriate code for unspecified stage (L89.--9).

3)   Documented pressure ulcer stage
Assignment of the pressure ulcer stage code should be guided by clinical documentation of the stage or documentation of the terms found in the Alphabetic Index. For clinical terms describing the stage that are not found in the Alphabetic Index, and there is no documentation of the stage, the provider should be queried.

4)   Patients admitted with pressure ulcers documented as healed
No code is assigned if the documentation states that the pressure ulcer is completely healed.

5)   Patients admitted with pressure ulcers documented as healing
Pressure ulcers described as healing should be assigned the appropriate pressure ulcer stage code based on the documentation in the medical record. If the documentation does not provide information about the stage of the healing pressure ulcer, assign the appropriate code for unspecified stage.

If the documentation is unclear as to whether the patient has a current (new) pressure ulcer or if the patient is being treated for a healing pressure ulcer, query the provider.

For ulcers that were present on admission but healed at the time of discharge, assign the code for the site and stage of the pressure ulcer at the time of admission.

6)   Patient admitted with pressure ulcer evolving into another stage during the admission
If a patient is admitted with a pressure ulcer at one stage and it progresses to a higher stage, ~~assign the code for the highest stage reported for that site~~ two separate codes should be assigned: one code for the site and stage of the ulcer on admission and a second code for the same ulcer site and the highest stage reported during the stay.

Infections of the skin and subcutaneous tissue (L00-L08)

Use additional code (B95-B97) to identify infectious agent
Excludes ❷: *hordeolum (H00.0)*
    infective dermatitis (L30.3)
    local infections of skin classified in Chapter 1
    lupus panniculitis (L93.2)
    panniculitis NOS (M79.3)
    panniculitis of neck and back (M54.0-)
    Perlèche NOS (K13.0)
    Perlèche due to candidiasis (B37.0)
    Perlèche due to riboflavin deficiency (E53.0)
    pyogenic granuloma (L98.0)
    relapsing panniculitis [Weber-Christian] (M35.6)
    viral warts (B07.-)
    zoster (B02.-)

L00   Staphylococcal scalded skin syndrome — A blistering skin disease caused by a toxin produced from a Staphylococcus bacterial infection.
    Ritter's disease
    Use additional code to identify percentage of skin exfoliation (L49.-)
    Excludes 1:   *bullous impetigo (L01.03)*
        pemphigus neonatorum (L01.03)
        toxic epidermal necrolysis [Lyell] (L51.2)

L01-   Impetigo
    Excludes 1:   *impetigo herpetiformis (L40.1)*

   L01.0-   Impetigo — A contagious skin infection characterized by vesicles and pustules that rupture and form a yellow crust, usually caused by Streptococcus.
        Impetigo contagiosa
        Impetigo vulgaris

      L01.00   Impetigo, unspecified
          Impetigo NOS

      L01.01   Non-bullous impetigo — A form caused by Staphylococcus or Streptococcus that is usually caused by a break in the skin and smaller blisters.

      L01.02   Bockhart's impetigo — A form marked by Inflammation of the hair follicles with pus formation.
          Impetigo follicularis
          Perifolliculitis NOS
          Superficial pustular perifolliculitis

      L01.03   Bullous impetigo — A form caused by Staphylococcus that occurs in infants and children and forms larger blisters.
          Impetigo neonatorum
          Pemphigus neonatorum

      L01.09   Other impetigo
          Ulcerative impetigo — A form with an open sore.

   L01.1   Impetiginization of other dermatoses

L02-   Cutaneous abscess, furuncle and carbuncle — ABSCESS – A localized collection of pus caused by the disintegration of skin tissue. CARBUNCLE – A necrotizing infection of the skin and subcutaneous tissue composed of a cluster of boils (furuncles), with multiple formed or incipient draining sinuses. FURUNCLE (BOIL) – A painful nodule formed in the skin characterized by circumscribed inflammation of the corium and subcutaneous tissue.
    Use additional code to identify organism (B95-B96)
    Excludes ❷: *abscess of anus and rectal regions (K61.-)*
        abscess of female genital organs (external) (N76.4)
        abscess of male genital organs (external) (N48.2, N49.-)

   L02.0-   Cutaneous abscess, furuncle and carbuncle of face
        Excludes ❷: *abscess of ear, external (H60.0)*
            abscess of eyelid (H00.0)
            abscess of head [any part, except face] (L02.8)
            abscess of lacrimal gland (H04.0)
            abscess of lacrimal passages (H04.3)
            abscess of mouth (K12.2)
            abscess of nose (J34.0)
            abscess of orbit (H05.0)
            submandibular abscess (K12.2)

   CC **L02.01   Cutaneous abscess of face**

L00 - L02

© 2016 Channel Publishing, Ltd.

L02.02   Furuncle of face
    Boil of face
    Folliculitis of face

L02.03   Carbuncle of face

L02.1-   Cutaneous abscess, furuncle and carbuncle of neck

cc **L02.11**   Cutaneous abscess of neck

L02.12   Furuncle of neck
    Boil of neck
    Folliculitis of neck

L02.13   Carbuncle of neck

L02.2-   Cutaneous abscess, furuncle and carbuncle of trunk
    Excludes 1:   non-newborn omphalitis (L08.82)
                omphalitis of newborn (P38.-)
    Excludes ❷: abscess of breast (N61.1)
                abscess of buttocks (L02.3)
                abscess of female external genital organs (N76.4)
                abscess of male external genital organs (N48.2, N49.-)
                abscess of hip (L02.4)

L02.21-   Cutaneous abscess of trunk

cc **L02.211**   Cutaneous abscess of abdominal wall

cc **L02.212**   Cutaneous abscess of back [any part, except buttock]

cc **L02.213**   Cutaneous abscess of chest wall

cc **L02.214**   Cutaneous abscess of groin

cc **L02.215**   Cutaneous abscess of perineum

cc **L02.216**   Cutaneous abscess of umbilicus

cc **L02.219**   Cutaneous abscess of trunk, unspecified

L02.22-   Furuncle of trunk
    Boil of trunk
    Folliculitis of trunk

L02.221   Furuncle of abdominal wall

L02.222   Furuncle of back [any part, except buttock]

L02.223   Furuncle of chest wall

L02.224   Furuncle of groin

L02.225   Furuncle of perineum

L02.226   Furuncle of umbilicus

L02.229   Furuncle of trunk, unspecified

L02.23-   Carbuncle of trunk

L02.231   Carbuncle of abdominal wall

L02.232   Carbuncle of back [any part, except buttock]

L02.233   Carbuncle of chest wall

L02.234   Carbuncle of groin

L02.235   Carbuncle of perineum

L02.236   Carbuncle of umbilicus

L02.239   Carbuncle of trunk, unspecified

L02.3-   Cutaneous abscess, furuncle and carbuncle of buttock
    Excludes 1:   pilonidal cyst with abscess (L05.01)

cc **L02.31**   Cutaneous abscess of buttock
    Cutaneous abscess of gluteal region

L02.32   Furuncle of buttock
    Boil of buttock
    Folliculitis of buttock
    Furuncle of gluteal region

L02.33   Carbuncle of buttock
    Carbuncle of gluteal region

L02.4-   Cutaneous abscess, furuncle and carbuncle of limb
    Excludes ❷: cutaneous abscess, furuncle and carbuncle of groin
                (L02.214, L02.224, L02.234)
                cutaneous abscess, furuncle and carbuncle of hand
                (L02.5-)
                cutaneous abscess, furuncle and carbuncle of foot
                (L02.6-)

L02.41-   Cutaneous abscess of limb

cc **L02.411**   Cutaneous abscess of right axilla

cc **L02.412**   Cutaneous abscess of left axilla

cc **L02.413**   Cutaneous abscess of right upper limb

cc **L02.414**   Cutaneous abscess of left upper limb

cc **L02.415**   Cutaneous abscess of right lower limb

cc **L02.416**   Cutaneous abscess of left lower limb

cc **L02.419**   Cutaneous abscess of limb, unspecified

L02.42-   Furuncle of limb
    Boil of limb
    Folliculitis of limb

L02.421   Furuncle of right axilla

L02.422   Furuncle of left axilla

L02.423   Furuncle of right upper limb

L02.424   Furuncle of left upper limb

L02.425   Furuncle of right lower limb

L02.426   Furuncle of left lower limb

L02.429   Furuncle of limb, unspecified

L02.43-   Carbuncle of limb

L02.431   Carbuncle of right axilla

L02.432   Carbuncle of left axilla

L02.433   Carbuncle of right upper limb

L02.434   Carbuncle of left upper limb

L02.435   Carbuncle of right lower limb

L02.436   Carbuncle of left lower limb

L02.439   Carbuncle of limb, unspecified

L02.5-   Cutaneous abscess, furuncle and carbuncle of hand

L02.51-   Cutaneous abscess of hand

cc **L02.511**   Cutaneous abscess of right hand

cc **L02.512**   Cutaneous abscess of left hand

cc **L02.519**   Cutaneous abscess of unspecified hand

L02.52-   Furuncle hand
    Boil of hand
    Folliculitis of hand

L02.521   Furuncle right hand

L02.522   Furuncle left hand

L02.529   Furuncle unspecified hand

L02.53-   Carbuncle of hand

L02.531   Carbuncle of right hand

L02.532   Carbuncle of left hand

L02.539   Carbuncle of unspecified hand

L02.6-   Cutaneous abscess, furuncle and carbuncle of foot

L02.61-   Cutaneous abscess of foot

cc **L02.611**   Cutaneous abscess of right foot

cc **L02.612**   Cutaneous abscess of left foot

cc **L02.619**   Cutaneous abscess of unspecified foot

L02.62-   Furuncle of foot
    Boil of foot
    Folliculitis of foot

L02.621   Furuncle of right foot

L02.622   Furuncle of left foot

L02.629   Furuncle of unspecified foot

L02.63-   Carbuncle of foot

L02.631   Carbuncle of right foot

L02.632   Carbuncle of left foot

L02.639   Carbuncle of unspecified foot

L02.8-   Cutaneous abscess, furuncle and carbuncle of other sites

L02.81-   Cutaneous abscess of other sites

cc **L02.811**   Cutaneous abscess of head [any part, except face]

cc **L02.818**   Cutaneous abscess of other sites

L02.82-   Furuncle of other sites
    Boil of other sites
    Folliculitis of other sites

L02.821   Furuncle of head [any part, except face]

L02.828   Furuncle of other sites

L02.83-   Carbuncle of other sites

L02.831   Carbuncle of head [any part, except face]

L02.838   Carbuncle of other sites

L02.9-   Cutaneous abscess, furuncle and carbuncle, unspecified

cc **L02.91**   Cutaneous abscess, unspecified

L02.92   Furuncle, unspecified
    Boil NOS
    Furunculosis NOS

L02.93   Carbuncle, unspecified

L02 - L02

Excludes 1: = NOT CODED HERE! (Do not code both)   **800**   *Excludes ❷:* = Not Included Here

L03- **Cellulitis and acute lymphangitis** — CELLULITIS – Cellular tissue inflammation.
ACUTE LYMPHANGITIS – The sudden, severe onset of inflammation of a lymphatic vessel.

Excludes ❷: cellulitis of anal and rectal region (K61.-)
cellulitis of external auditory canal (H60.1)
cellulitis of eyelid (H00.0)
cellulitis of female external genital organs (N76.4)
cellulitis of lacrimal apparatus (H04.3)
cellulitis of male external genital organs (N48.2, N49.-)
cellulitis of mouth (K12.2)
cellulitis of nose (J34.0)
eosinophilic cellulitis [Wells] (L98.3)
febrile neutrophilic dermatosis [Sweet] (L98.2)
lymphangitis (chronic) (subacute) (I89.1)

L03.0- **Cellulitis and acute lymphangitis of finger and toe**
Infection of nail
Onychia — Inflammation of the nail matrix, resulting in the shedding of the nail.
Paronychia — Inflammation of the folds of tissue surrounding the fingernail.
Perionychia — Inflammation of the folds of tissue surrounding the fingernail.

L03.01- **Cellulitis of finger**
Felon
Whitlow

Excludes 1: herpetic whitlow (B00.89)

L03.011 **Cellulitis of right finger**
L03.012 **Cellulitis of left finger**
L03.019 **Cellulitis of unspecified finger**

L03.02- **Acute lymphangitis of finger**
Hangnail with lymphangitis of finger

L03.021 **Acute lymphangitis of right finger**
L03.022 **Acute lymphangitis of left finger**
L03.029 **Acute lymphangitis of unspecified finger**

L03.03- **Cellulitis of toe**
L03.031 **Cellulitis of right toe**
L03.032 **Cellulitis of left toe**
L03.039 **Cellulitis of unspecified toe**

L03.04- **Acute lymphangitis of toe**
Hangnail with lymphangitis of toe

L03.041 **Acute lymphangitis of right toe**
L03.042 **Acute lymphangitis of left toe**
L03.049 **Acute lymphangitis of unspecified toe**

L03.1- **Cellulitis and acute lymphangitis of other parts of limb**

L03.11- **Cellulitis of other parts of limb**
Excludes ❷: cellulitis of fingers (L03.01-)
cellulitis of toes (L03.03-)
groin (L03.314)

cc **L03.111** **Cellulitis of right axilla**
cc **L03.112** **Cellulitis of left axilla**
cc **L03.113** **Cellulitis of right upper limb**
cc **L03.114** **Cellulitis of left upper limb**
cc **L03.115** **Cellulitis of right lower limb**
cc **L03.116** **Cellulitis of left lower limb**
cc **L03.119** **Cellulitis of unspecified part of limb**

L03.12- **Acute lymphangitis of other parts of limb**
Excludes ❷: acute lymphangitis of fingers (L03.2-)
acute lymphangitis of toes (L03.04-)
acute lymphangitis of groin (L03.324)

cc **L03.121** **Acute lymphangitis of right axilla**
cc **L03.122** **Acute lymphangitis of left axilla**
cc **L03.123** **Acute lymphangitis of right upper limb**
cc **L03.124** **Acute lymphangitis of left upper limb**
cc **L03.125** **Acute lymphangitis of right lower limb**
cc **L03.126** **Acute lymphangitis of left lower limb**
cc **L03.129** **Acute lymphangitis of unspecified part of limb**

L03.2- **Cellulitis and acute lymphangitis of face and neck**

L03.21- **Cellulitis and acute lymphangitis of face**

cc **L03.211** **Cellulitis of face**
Excludes ❷: abscess of orbit (H05.01-)
cellulitis of ear (H60.1-)
cellulitis of eyelid (H00.0-)
cellulitis of head (L03.81)
cellulitis of lacrimal apparatus (H04.3)
cellulitis of lip (K13.0)
cellulitis of mouth (K12.2)
cellulitis of nose (internal) (J34.0)
cellulitis of orbit (H05.0T-)
cellulitis of scalp (L03.81)

cc **L03.212** **Acute lymphangitis of face**
cc **L03.213** **Periorbital cellulitis**
Preseptal cellulitis

L03.22- **Cellulitis and acute lymphangitis of neck**
cc **L03.221** **Cellulitis of neck**
cc **L03.222** **Acute lymphangitis of neck**

L03.3- **Cellulitis and acute lymphangitis of trunk**

L03.31- **Cellulitis of trunk**
Excludes ❷: cellulitis of anal and rectal regions (K61.-)
cellulitis of breast NOS (N61.0)
cellulitis of female external genital organs (N76.4)
cellulitis of male external genital organs (N48.2, N49.-)
omphalitis of newborn (P38.-)
puerperal cellulitis of breast (O91.2)

cc **L03.311** **Cellulitis of abdominal wall**
Excludes ❷: cellulitis of umbilicus (L03.316)
cellulitis of groin (L03.314)

cc **L03.312** **Cellulitis of back [any part except buttock]**
cc **L03.313** **Cellulitis of chest wall**
cc **L03.314** **Cellulitis of groin**
cc **L03.315** **Cellulitis of perineum**
cc **L03.316** **Cellulitis of umbilicus**
cc **L03.317** **Cellulitis of buttock**
cc **L03.319** **Cellulitis of trunk, unspecified**

L03.32- **Acute lymphangitis of trunk**
cc **L03.321** **Acute lymphangitis of abdominal wall**
cc **L03.322** **Acute lymphangitis of back [any part except buttock]**
cc **L03.323** **Acute lymphangitis of chest wall**
cc **L03.324** **Acute lymphangitis of groin**
cc **L03.325** **Acute lymphangitis of perineum**
cc **L03.326** **Acute lymphangitis of umbilicus**
cc **L03.327** **Acute lymphangitis of buttock**
cc **L03.329** **Acute lymphangitis of trunk, unspecified**

L03.8- **Cellulitis and acute lymphangitis of other sites**

L03.81- **Cellulitis of other sites**
cc **L03.811** **Cellulitis of head [any part, except face]**
Cellulitis of scalp
Excludes ❷: cellulitis of face (L03.211)

cc **L03.818** **Cellulitis of other sites**

L03.89- **Acute lymphangitis of other sites**
cc **L03.891** **Acute lymphangitis of head [any part, except face]**
cc **L03.898** **Acute lymphangitis of other sites**

L03.9- **Cellulitis and acute lymphangitis, unspecified**
cc **L03.90** **Cellulitis, unspecified**
cc **L03.91** **Acute lymphangitis, unspecified**
Excludes 1: lymphangitis NOS (I89.1)

L
0
3
-
L
0
3

L04-   **Acute lymphadenitis** — The sudden, severe onset of infectious inflammation of the lymph glands or nodes.
   Includes: Abscess (acute) of lymph nodes, except mesenteric
               Acute lymphadenitis, except mesenteric
   Excludes 1:   *chronic or subacute lymphadenitis, except mesenteric (I88.1)*
               enlarged lymph nodes (R59.-)
               human immunodeficiency virus [HIV] disease resulting in
                  generalized lymphadenopathy (B20)
               lymphadenitis NOS (I88.9)
               nonspecific mesenteric lymphadenitis (I88.0)

   L04.0   **Acute lymphadenitis of face, head and neck**
   L04.1   **Acute lymphadenitis of trunk**
   L04.2   **Acute lymphadenitis of upper limb**
            Acute lymphadenitis of axilla
            Acute lymphadenitis of shoulder
   L04.3   **Acute lymphadenitis of lower limb**
            Acute lymphadenitis of hip
            Excludes ❷: *acute lymphadenitis of groin (L04.1)*
   L04.8   **Acute lymphadenitis of other sites**
   L04.9   **Acute lymphadenitis, unspecified**

L05-   **Pilonidal cyst and sinus** — A hair-containing sacrococcygeal dermoid cyst or sinus that often opens at a postanal dimple.

   L05.0-   **Pilonidal cyst and sinus with abscess** — A form with a localized collection of pus.
      CC **L05.01**   **Pilonidal cyst <u>with</u> abscess**
               Pilonidal abscess
               Pilonidal dimple with abscess
               Postanal dimple with abscess
               Excludes ❷: *congenital sacral dimple (Q82.6)*
                        parasacral dimple (Q82.6)

      CC **L05.02**   **Pilonidal sinus <u>with</u> abscess**
               Coccygeal fistula with abscess
               Coccygeal sinus with abscess
               Pilonidal fistula with abscess

   L05.9-   **Pilonidal cyst and sinus without abscess**
      L05.91   **Pilonidal cyst <u>without</u> abscess**
               Pilonidal dimple
               Postanal dimple
               Pilonidal cyst NOS
               Excludes ❷: *congenital sacral dimple (Q82.6)*
                        parasacral dimple (Q82.6)

      L05.92   **Pilonidal sinus <u>without</u> abscess**
               Coccygeal fistula
               Coccygeal sinus without abscess
               Pilonidal fistula

L08-   **Other local infections of skin and subcutaneous tissue**
   L08.0   **Pyoderma** — A nonspecific purulent skin infection.
            Dermatitis gangrenosa — A form characterized by unique skin lesions, and often associated with an underlying systemic disease.
            Purulent dermatitis — Inflammation of the skin with pus.
            Septic dermatitis — Inflammation of the skin with decomposition of microorganisms.
            Suppurative dermatitis — Inflammation of the skin with production of pus.
            Excludes 1:   *pyoderma gangrenosum (L88)*
                     pyoderma vegetans (L08.81)

   CC **L08.1**   **Erythrasma** — A chronic bacterial skin infection caused by Corynebacterium minutissimum that occurs primarily in the folds of the skin.

   L08.8-   **Other specified local infections of the skin and subcutaneous tissue**
      L08.81   **Pyoderma vegetans** — A purulent skin infection that is characterized by large verrucous plaques and elevated borders with an unknown cause.
               Excludes 1:   *pyoderma gangrenosum (L88)*
                        pyoderma NOS (L08.0)
      L08.82   **Omphalitis not of newborn** — Infection of the umbilical stump.
               Excludes 1:   *omphalitis of newborn (P38.-)*
      L08.89   **Other specified local infections of the skin and subcutaneous tissue**

   L08.9   **Local infection of the skin and subcutaneous tissue, unspecified**

Bullous disorders (L10-L14)

   Excludes 1:   *benign familial pemphigus [Hailey-Hailey] (Q82.8)*
               staphylococcal scalded skin syndrome (L00)
               toxic epidermal necrolysis [Lyell] (L51.2)

L10-   **Pemphigus** — A group of distinctive autoimmune diseases marked by successive crops of bullae.
   Excludes 1:   *pemphigus neonatorum (L01.03)*

   CC **L10.0**   **Pemphigus vulgaris** — A form manifested by suprabasal, intraepidermal bullae of the skin and mucous membranes with sores often in the mouth.
   CC **L10.1**   **Pemphigus vegetans** — A mild, pustular variant of pemphigus.
   CC **L10.2**   **Pemphigus foliaceous** — A form characterized by generalized vesicular and scaling skin eruption.
   CC **L10.3**   **Brazilian pemphigus [fogo selvagem]** — A form endemic to some South American countries that is transmitted by an insect.
   CC **L10.4**   **Pemphigus erythematosus** — Chronic pemphigus characterized by lesions limited to the face and chest, and resembling those of disseminated lupus erythematosus.
               Senear-Usher syndrome
   CC **L10.5**   **Drug-induced pemphigus**
               Use additional code for adverse effect, if applicable, to identify drug (T36-T50 with fifth or sixth character 5)
   L10.8-   **Other pemphigus**
      CC **L10.81**   **Paraneoplastic pemphigus** — A form characterized by painful sores in the mouth, lips, and esophagus that is a complication of cancer, usually a lymphoma.
      CC **L10.89**   **Other pemphigus**
   CC **L10.9**   **Pemphigus, unspecified**

L11-   **Other acantholytic disorders**
   L11.0   **Acquired keratosis follicularis**
            Excludes 1:   *keratosis follicularis (congenital) [Darier-White] (Q82.8)*
   L11.1   **Transient acantholytic dermatosis [Grover]**
   L11.8   **Other specified acantholytic disorders**
   L11.9   **Acantholytic disorder, unspecified**

L12-   **Pemphigoid** — A group of bullous connective tissue autoimmune skin diseases that are similar but clearly distinguishable from those of the pemphigus group.
   Excludes 1:   *herpes gestationis (O26.4-)*
               impetigo herpetiformis (L40.1)

   CC **L12.0**   **Bullous pemphigoid** — A chronic, generalized bullous eruption that usually occurs in elderly adults, but rarely the mouth.
   L12.1   **Cicatricial pemphigoid** — A form affecting mucous membranes, but not the skin.
            Benign mucous membrane pemphigoid
   L12.2   **Chronic bullous disease of childhood** — [Age/0-17]
            Juvenile dermatitis herpetiformis
   L12.3-   **Acquired epidermolysis bullosa**
            Excludes 1:   *epidermolysis bullosa (congenital) (Q81.-)*
      CC **L12.30**   **Acquired epidermolysis bullosa, unspecified**
      CC **L12.31**   **Epidermolysis bullosa due to drug**
               Use additional code for adverse effect, if applicable, to identify drug (T36-T50 with fifth or sixth character 5)
      CC **L12.35**   **Other acquired epidermolysis bullosa**
   CC **L12.8**   **Other pemphigoid**
   CC **L12.9**   **Pemphigoid, unspecified**

L13-   **Other bullous disorders**
   L13.0   **Dermatitis herpetiformis** — A chronic dermatitis characterized by grouped, symmetrical erythematous, papular, vesicular eczematous, or bullous lesions that occur in successive crops in varied combinations and accompanied by burning and itching.
            Duhring's disease
            Hydroa herpetiformis
            Excludes 1:   *juvenile dermatitis herpetiformis (L12.2)*
                     senile dermatitis herpetiformis (L12.0)
   L13.1   **Subcorneal pustular dermatitis** — A chronic, pustular disease that is characterized by a relapsing course with sterile, pustular blebs and chiefly affecting women in middle life.
            Sneddon-Wilkinson disease
   L13.8   **Other specified bullous disorders**
   L13.9   **Bullous disorder, unspecified**

L
0
4
–
L
13

L14   Bullous disorders in diseases classified elsewhere —
[Not Allowed as PDX]
Code first underlying disease

Dermatitis and eczema (L20-L30)

Note: In this block the terms dermatitis and eczema are used synonymously and interchangeably.
Excludes ❷: chronic (childhood) granulomatous disease (D71)
dermatitis gangrenosa (L08.0)
dermatitis herpetiformis (L13.0)
dry skin dermatitis (L85.3)
factitial dermatitis (L98.1)
perioral dermatitis (L71.0)
radiation-related disorders of the skin and subcutaneous tissue (L55-L59)
stasis dermatitis (I87.2)

L20-   Atopic dermatitis — A chronic skin disease of unknown etiology that is characterized by dry and itchy skin, and rash on the face, inside of the elbows, and behind the knees.

L20.0   Besnier's prurigo

L20.8-   Other atopic dermatitis
Excludes ❷: circumscribed neurodermatitis (L28.0)

   L20.81   Atopic neurodermatitis
Diffuse neurodermatitis

   L20.82   Flexural eczema

   L20.83   Infantile (acute) (chronic) eczema — [Age/0-17]

   L20.84   Intrinsic (allergic) eczema

   L20.89   Other atopic dermatitis

L20.9   Atopic dermatitis, unspecified

L21-   Seborrheic dermatitis — A chronic inflammatory skin disease of unknown etiology that is characterized by scaly, stubborn dandruff, and itchy and red skin.
Excludes ❷: infective dermatitis (L30.3)
seborrheic keratosis (L82.-)

L21.0   Seborrhea capitis — [Age/0-17]
Cradle cap

L21.1   Seborrheic infantile dermatitis — [Age/0-17]

L21.8   Other seborrheic dermatitis

L21.9   Seborrheic dermatitis, unspecified
Seborrhea NOS

L22   Diaper dermatitis — A cutaneous reaction in an infant (or one who wears a diaper) that is localized to the areas ordinarily covered by, and in contact with, the diaper.
Diaper erythema
Diaper rash
Psoriasiform diaper rash

L23-   Allergic contact dermatitis — An acute, allergic response inflammation of the skin caused by contact with various substances to which a delayed hypersensitivity has been acquired.
Excludes 1:   allergy NOS (T78.40)
contact dermatitis NOS (L25.9)
dermatitis NOS (L30.9)
Excludes ❷: dermatitis due to substances taken internally (L27.-)
dermatitis of eyelid (H01.1-)
diaper dermatitis (L22)
eczema of external ear (H60.5-)
irritant contact dermatitis (L24.-)
perioral dermatitis (L71.0)
radiation-related disorders of the skin and subcutaneous tissue (L55-L59)

L23.0   Allergic contact dermatitis due to metals
Allergic contact dermatitis due to chromium
Allergic contact dermatitis due to nickel

L23.1   Allergic contact dermatitis due to adhesives

L23.2   Allergic contact dermatitis due to cosmetics

L23.3   Allergic contact dermatitis due to drugs in contact with skin
Use additional code for adverse effect, if applicable, to identify drug (T36-T50 with fifth or sixth character 5)
Excludes ❷: dermatitis due to ingested drugs and medicaments (L27.0-L27.1)

L23.4   Allergic contact dermatitis due to dyes

L23.5   Allergic contact dermatitis due to other chemical products
Allergic contact dermatitis due to cement
Allergic contact dermatitis due to insecticide
Allergic contact dermatitis due to plastic
Allergic contact dermatitis due to rubber

L23.6   Allergic contact dermatitis due to food in contact with the skin
Excludes ❷: dermatitis due to ingested food (L27.2)

L23.7   Allergic contact dermatitis due to plants, except food
Excludes ❷: allergy NOS due to pollen (J30.1)

L23.8-   Allergic contact dermatitis due to other agents

   L23.81   Allergic contact dermatitis due to animal (cat) (dog) dander
Allergic contact dermatitis due to animal (cat) (dog) hair

   L23.89   Allergic contact dermatitis due to other agents

L23.9   Allergic contact dermatitis, unspecified cause
Allergic contact eczema NOS

L24-   Irritant contact dermatitis — An acute inflammation of the skin caused by contact with various substances.
Excludes 1:   allergy NOS (T78.40)
contact dermatitis NOS (L25.9)
dermatitis NOS (L30.9)
Excludes ❷: allergic contact dermatitis (L23.-)
dermatitis due to substances taken internally (L27.-)
dermatitis of eyelid (H01.1-)
diaper dermatitis (L22)
eczema of external ear (H60.5-)
perioral dermatitis (L71.0)
radiation-related disorders of the skin and subcutaneous tissue (L55-L59)

L24.0   Irritant contact dermatitis due to detergents

L24.1   Irritant contact dermatitis due to oils and greases

L24.2   Irritant contact dermatitis due to solvents
Irritant contact dermatitis due to chlorocompound
Irritant contact dermatitis due to cyclohexane
Irritant contact dermatitis due to ester
Irritant contact dermatitis due to glycol
Irritant contact dermatitis due to hydrocarbon
Irritant contact dermatitis due to ketone

L24.3   Irritant contact dermatitis due to cosmetics

L24.4   Irritant contact dermatitis due to drugs in contact with skin
Use additional code for adverse effect, if applicable, to identify drug (T36-T50 with fifth or sixth character 5)

L24.5   Irritant contact dermatitis due to other chemical products
Irritant contact dermatitis due to cement
Irritant contact dermatitis due to insecticide
Irritant contact dermatitis due to plastic
Irritant contact dermatitis due to rubber

L24.6   Irritant contact dermatitis due to food in contact with skin
Excludes ❷: dermatitis due to ingested food (L27.2)

L24.7   Irritant contact dermatitis due to plants, except food
Excludes ❷: allergy NOS to pollen (J30.1)

L24.8-   Irritant contact dermatitis due to other agents

   L24.81   Irritant contact dermatitis due to metals
Irritant contact dermatitis due to chromium
Irritant contact dermatitis due to nickel

   L24.89   Irritant contact dermatitis due to other agents
Irritant contact dermatitis due to dyes

L24.9   Irritant contact dermatitis, unspecified cause
Irritant contact eczema NOS

L25-   Unspecified contact dermatitis
Excludes 1:   allergic contact dermatitis (L23.-)
allergy NOS (T78.40)
dermatitis NOS (L30.9)
irritant contact dermatitis (L24.-)
Excludes ❷: dermatitis due to ingested substances (L27.-)
dermatitis of eyelid (H01.1-)
eczema of external ear (H60.5-)
perioral dermatitis (L71.0)
radiation-related disorders of the skin and subcutaneous tissue (L55-L59)

L25.0   Unspecified contact dermatitis due to cosmetics

L25.1   Unspecified contact dermatitis due to drugs in contact with skin
Use additional code for adverse effect, if applicable, to identify drug (T36-T50 with fifth or sixth character 5)
Excludes ❷: dermatitis due to ingested drugs and medicaments (L27.0-L27.1)

L25.2   Unspecified contact dermatitis due to dyes

L
1
4
-
L
2
5

L25.3 Unspecified contact dermatitis due to <u>other chemical products</u>
Unspecified contact dermatitis due to cement
Unspecified contact dermatitis due to insecticide

L25.4 Unspecified contact dermatitis due to <u>food in contact with skin</u>

Excludes ❷: dermatitis due to ingested food (L27.2)

L25.5 Unspecified contact dermatitis due to <u>plants, except food</u>

Excludes 1: nettle rash (L50.9)
Excludes ❷: allergy NOS due to pollen (J30.1)

L25.8 Unspecified contact dermatitis due to <u>other</u> agents

L25.9 Unspecified contact dermatitis, <u>unspecified</u> cause
Contact dermatitis (occupational) NOS
Contact eczema (occupational) NOS

L26 Exfoliative dermatitis — An inflammatory skin disease that is characterized by excessive shedding or peeling of the nonviable outer layer of the skin caused by excessive growth of the basal layer of the skin.
Hebra's pityriasis

Excludes 1: Ritter's disease (L00)

L27- Dermatitis <u>due to substances taken internally</u> — Inflammation of the skin due to substances taken internally.

Excludes 1: allergy NOS (T78.40)
Excludes ❷: adverse food reaction, except dermatitis (T78.0-T78.1)
contact dermatitis (L23-L25)
drug photoallergic response (L56.1)
drug phototoxic response (L56.0)
urticaria (L50.-)

L27.0 <u>Generalized</u> skin eruption due to drugs and medicaments taken internally
Use additional code for adverse effect, if applicable, to identify drug (T36-T50 with fifth or sixth character 5)

L27.1 <u>Localized</u> skin eruption due to drugs and medicaments taken internally
Use additional code for adverse effect, if applicable, to identify drug (T36-T50 with fifth or sixth character 5)

L27.2 Dermatitis due to ingested <u>food</u>

Excludes ❷: dermatitis due to food in contact with skin (L23.6, L24.6, L25.4)

L27.8 Dermatitis due to <u>other</u> substances taken internally

L27.9 Dermatitis due to <u>unspecified</u> substance taken internally

L28- Lichen simplex chronicus and prurigo

L28.0 Lichen simplex chronicus — A skin disorder that is characterized by chronic itching and scratching, by the self-perpetuating scratch-itch cycle.
Circumscribed neurodermatitis
Lichen NOS

L28.1 Prurigo nodularis — A form of neurodermatitis with discrete, firm, rough-surfaced, intensely itchy nodules occurring on extensor surfaces of the extremities.

L28.2 Other prurigo
Prurigo NOS
Prurigo Hebra
Prurigo mitis
Urticaria papulosa

L29- Pruritus

Excludes 1: neurotic excoriation (L98.1)
psychogenic pruritus (F45.8)

L29.0 Pruritus ani — The intense, chronic itching of the anal region.

L29.1 Pruritus scroti — [♂] — The intense, chronic itching of the scrotal region.

L29.2 Pruritus vulvae — [♀] — The intense, chronic itching of the vulvar region.

L29.3 Anogenital pruritus, unspecified

L29.8 Other pruritus

L29.9 Pruritus, unspecified
Itch NOS

L30- <u>Other and unspecified</u> dermatitis

Excludes ❷: contact dermatitis (L23-L25)
dry skin dermatitis (L85.3)
small plaque parapsoriasis (L41.3)
stasis dermatitis (I87.2)

L30.0 Nummular dermatitis — A skin eruption condition characterized by distinct, coin-shaped (nummular) sores.

L30.1 Dyshidrosis [pompholyx] — A skin eruption condition characterized by vesicular eruption on the palms and soles, and is accompanied by intense itching.

L30.2 Cutaneous autosensitization — A skin eruption condition characterized by widespread eruption from a distant local focus.
Candidid [levurid]
Dermatophytid
Eczematid

L30.3 Infective dermatitis
Infectious eczematoid dermatitis

L30.4 Erythema intertrigo — A superficial inflammatory skin disease characterized by macerated, erythematous patches on opposing skin surfaces, such as under pendulous breasts.

L30.5 Pityriasis alba — A common skin disorder characterized by hypopigmented, round to oval scaling patches on the face, neck, and shoulders.

L30.8 Other specified dermatitis

L30.9 Dermatitis, unspecified
Eczema NOS

Papulosquamous disorders (L40-L45)

L40- Psoriasis

L40.0 Psoriasis vulgaris — A chronic, recurrent inflammatory skin disease characterized by rounded, circumscribed, erythematous, dry scaling patches that are covered with silvery-white lamellated scales.
Nummular psoriasis
Plaque psoriasis

L40.1 Generalized pustular psoriasis — A form marked by pus-filled blisters.
Impetigo herpetiformis
Von Zumbusch's disease

L40.2 Acrodermatitis continua

L40.3 Pustulosis palmaris et plantaris — A form marked by pus-filled blisters of the fingers and toes.

L40.4 Guttate psoriasis — A form marked by teardrop shaped lesions.

L40.5- Arthropathic psoriasis — Psoriasis associated with arthritis, especially of the distal interphalangeal joints.

L40.50 Arthropathic psoriasis, unspecified

L40.51 Distal interphalangeal psoriatic arthropathy

L40.52 Psoriatic arthritis mutilans

L40.53 Psoriatic spondylitis

L40.54 Psoriatic juvenile arthropathy

L40.59 Other psoriatic arthropathy

L40.8 Other psoriasis
Flexural psoriasis

L40.9 Psoriasis, unspecified

L41- Parapsoriasis — A group of maculopapular, scaly erythrodermas of slow development.

Excludes 1: poikiloderma vasculare atrophicans (L94.5)

L41.0 Pityriasis lichenoides et varioliformis acuta — A form marked by a polymorphous eruption composed of macules, papules, and occasional vesicles.
Mucha-Habermann disease

L41.1 Pityriasis lichenoides chronica — A form marked by erythematous, yellowish, scaly macules.

L41.3 Small plaque parapsoriasis

L41.4 Large plaque parapsoriasis

L41.5 Retiform parapsoriasis

L41.8 Other parapsoriasis

L41.9 Parapsoriasis, unspecified

L42 Pityriasis rosea — A mild inflammatory exanthem characterized by salmon-colored papular and macular lesions that are usually seen parallel to the lines of cleavage of the skin.

L43- Lichen planus — An inflammatory skin disease characterized by wide, flat, itchy papules that have a distinctive sheen and occur in circumscribed patches.

Excludes 1: lichen planopilaris (L66.1)

L43.0 Hypertrophic lichen planus

L43.1 Bullous lichen planus

L43.2 Lichenoid drug reaction
Use additional code for adverse effect, if applicable, to identify drug (T36-T50 with fifth or sixth character 5)

L43.3 Subacute (active) lichen planus
Lichen planus tropicus

L43.8 Other lichen planus

L43.9 Lichen planus, unspecified

L25 - L43

L44- Other papulosquamous disorders

L44.0 Pityriasis rubra pilaris — A rare, chronic inflammatory skin disease characterized by small follicular papules, and disseminated yellowish-pink scaling patches.

L44.1 Lichen nitidus — A rare skin disease characterized by numerous, pinhead-size, flat, glistening discrete papules.

L44.2 Lichen striatus — A skin disorder characterized by linear lichenoid papules, usually occurring in young children.

L44.3 Lichen ruber moniliformis

L44.4 Infantile papular acrodermatitis [Gianotti-Crosti] — [Age/0-17]

L44.8 Other specified papulosquamous disorders

L44.9 Papulosquamous disorder, unspecified

L45 Papulosquamous disorders in diseases classified elsewhere — [Not Allowed as PDX]
Code first underlying disease

Urticaria and erythema (L49-L54)

Excludes 1: *Lyme disease (A69.2-)*
rosacea (L71.-)

L49- Exfoliation due to erythematous conditions according to extent of body surface involved
Code first erythematous condition causing exfoliation, such as:
Ritter's disease (L00)
(Staphylococcal) scalded skin syndrom (L00)
Stevens-Johnson syndrome (L51.1)
Stevens-Johnson syndrome-toxic epidermal necrolysis overlap syndrome (L51.3)
Toxic epidermal necrolysis (L51.2)

L49.0 Exfoliation due to erythematous condition involving less than 10 percent of body surface — [Unacceptable PDX]
Exfoliation due to erythematous condition NOS

L49.1 Exfoliation due to erythematous condition involving 10-19 percent of body surface — [Unacceptable PDX]

L49.2 Exfoliation due to erythematous condition involving 20-29 percent of body surface — [Unacceptable PDX]

cc **L49.3 Exfoliation due to erythematous condition involving 30-39 percent of body surface** — [Unacceptable PDX]

cc **L49.4 Exfoliation due to erythematous condition involving 40-49 percent of body surface** — [Unacceptable PDX]

cc **L49.5 Exfoliation due to erythematous condition involving 50-59 percent of body surface** — [Unacceptable PDX]

cc **L49.6 Exfoliation due to erythematous condition involving 60-69 percent of body surface** — [Unacceptable PDX]

cc **L49.7 Exfoliation due to erythematous condition involving 70-79 percent of body surface** — [Unacceptable PDX]

cc **L49.8 Exfoliation due to erythematous condition involving 80-89 percent of body surface** — [Unacceptable PDX]

cc **L49.9 Exfoliation due to erythematous condition involving 90 or more percent of body surface** — [Unacceptable PDX]

L50- Urticaria — A vascular reaction of the skin characterized by elevated wheals, welts, or reddened patches and associated with severe itching or stinging.

Excludes 1: *allergic contact dermatitis (L23-)*
angioneurotic edema (T78.3)
giant urticaria (T78.3)
hereditary angio-edema (D84.1)
Quincke's edema (T78.3)
serum urticaria (T80.6-)
solar urticaria (L56.3)
urticaria neonatorum (P83.8)
urticaria papulosa (L28.2)
urticaria pigmentosa (Q82.2)

L50.0 Allergic urticaria — A form due to a hypersensitive reaction to an allergen.

L50.1 Idiopathic urticaria — A form of unknown origin.

L50.2 Urticaria due to cold and heat — A form due to the exposure effects of cold or heat.
Excludes ❷: *familial cold urticaria (M04.2)*

L50.3 Dermatographic urticaria — A form due to the skin's hypersensitivity to the minor trauma of daily life that is characterized by raised and inflamed skin where the object disrupted the skin.

L50.4 Vibratory urticaria — A form occurring after contact with vibratory equipment.

L50.5 Cholinergic urticaria — A form produced by the action of internal acetylcholine or mast cells that are released in increased amounts during emotional stress or increased environmental heat.

L50.6 Contact urticaria — A form due to contact with an item or substance.

L50.8 Other urticaria
Chronic urticaria — A form that persists and recurs over a long period of time.
Recurrent periodic urticaria

L50.9 Urticaria, unspecified

L51- Erythema multiforme — An inflammatory skin disease characterized by a variety of skin eruptions including rashes, red welts, and/or purple or blistered areas that is often due to a herpes virus or response to medications or illness.
Use additional code for adverse effect, if applicable, to identify drug (T36-T50 with fifth or sixth character 5)
Use additional code to identify associated manifestations, such as:
Arthropathy associated with dermatological disorders (M14.8-)
Conjunctival edema (H11.42)
Conjunctivitis (H10.22-)
Corneal scars and opacities (H17-)
Corneal ulcer (H16.0-)
Edema of eyelid (H02.84)
Inflammation of eyelid (H01.8)
Keratoconjunctivitis sicca (H16.22-)
Mechanical lagophthalmos (H02.22-)
Stomatitis (K12-)
Symblepharon (H11.23-)
Use additional code to identify percentage of skin exfoliation (L49.-)
Excludes 1: *staphylococcal scalded skin syndrome (L00)*
Ritter's disease (L00)

L51.0 Nonbullous erythema multiforme

cc **L51.1 Stevens-Johnson syndrome** — A form within the same spectrum as toxic epidermal necrolysis that is characterized by severe, extensive skin lesions, involvement of the mucous membranes, and generally involves less than 10% of the body surface.

cc **L51.2 Toxic epidermal necrolysis [Lyell]** — A form within the same spectrum as Stevens-Johnson syndrome that is characterized by severe, extensive skin lesions, involvement of the mucous membranes with multiple large blisters, and generally involves more than 30% of the body surface.

cc **L51.3 Stevens-Johnson syndrome-toxic epidermal necrolysis overlap syndrome** — A form within the same spectrum as toxic epidermal necrolysis that is characterized by severe, extensive skin lesions, involvement of the mucous membranes, and generally involves 10% to 30% of the body surface.
SJS-TEN overlap syndrome

L51.8 Other erythema multiforme

L51.9 Erythema multiforme, unspecified
Erythema iris — A form marked by the formation of concentric rings, producing a target-like appearance.
Erythema multiforme major NOS — A form marked by typical target-like rashes or raised, edematous papules with involvement of one or more mucous membranes but not diagnostic of Stevens-Johnson syndrome or toxic epidermal necrolysis.
Erythema multiforme minor NOS — A form marked by typical target-like rashes or raised, edematous papules.
Herpes iris — A form marked by vesicular lesions.

L52 Erythema nodosum — An acute skin disease characterized by tender, red nodules that are due to exudation of blood and serum.
Excludes 1: *tuberculous erythema nodosum (A18.4)*

L53- Other erythematous conditions
Excludes 1: *erythema ab igne (L59.0)*
erythema due to external agents in contact with skin (L23-L25)
erythema intertrigo (L30.4)

cc **L53.0 Toxic erythema** — A generalized, diffuse erythematous eruption that is due to a drug or toxin.
Code first poisoning due to drug or toxin, if applicable (T36-T65 with fifth or sixth character 1-4 or 6)
Use additional code for adverse effect, if applicable, to identify drug (T36-T50 with fifth or sixth character 5)
Excludes 1: *neonatal erythema toxicum (P83.1)*

cc **L53.1 Erythema annulare centrifugum**

cc **L53.2 Erythema marginatum**

cc **L53.3 Other chronic figurate erythema**

L53.8 Other specified erythematous conditions

L53.9 Erythematous condition, unspecified
Erythema NOS
Erythroderma NOS

L44 – L53

L54 **Erythema in diseases classified elsewhere** — [Not Allowed as PDX]
Code first underlying disease

Radiation-related disorders of the skin and subcutaneous tissue (L55-L59)

L55- **Sunburn** — An injury to the skin following excessive exposure to the ultraviolet rays of sunlight.

L55.0 **Sunburn of first degree** — A form affecting the outer layer (epidermis) of the skin causing redness, tenderness, and mild pain.

L55.1 **Sunburn of second degree** — A form affecting the outer layer (epidermis) and a portion of the inner layer (dermis) of the skin causing blisters.

L55.2 **Sunburn of third degree** — A form affecting the full-thickness of the skin (epidermis and dermis) and often the underlying subcutaneous tissues.

L55.9 **Sunburn, unspecified**

L56- **Other acute skin changes due to ultraviolet radiation** — An injury to the skin following excessive exposure to ultraviolet rays (sunlight).
Use additional code to identify the source of the ultraviolet radiation (W89, X32)

L56.0 **Drug phototoxic response** — A form caused by a nonimmunologic type of photosensitivity.
Use additional code for adverse effect, if applicable, to identify drug (T36-T50 with fifth or sixth character 5)

L56.1 **Drug photoallergic response** — A form caused by an immunologic type of photosensitivity.
Use additional code for adverse effect, if applicable, to identify drug (T36-T50 with fifth or sixth character 5)

L56.2 **Photocontact dermatitis [berloque dermatitis]** — A form aggravated by oil found in perfumes and colognes.

L56.3 **Solar urticaria** — A form causing acute inflammation of the skin.

L56.4 **Polymorphous light eruption** — A form characterized by skin lesions.

L56.5 **Disseminated superficial actinic porokeratosis (DSAP)** — An autosomal dominantly inherited skin disorder induced by ultraviolet light causing dry patches on the arms and legs.

L56.8 **Other specified acute skin changes due to ultraviolet radiation**

L56.9 **Acute skin change due to ultraviolet radiation, unspecified**

L57- **Skin changes due to chronic exposure to nonionizing radiation**
Use additional code to identify the source of the ultraviolet radiation (W89, X32)

L57.0 **Actinic keratosis** — A premalignant skin lesion characterized by sharply outlined, reddened growth that is caused by excessive exposure to the sun.
Keratosis NOS
Senile keratosis
Solar keratosis

L57.1 **Actinic reticuloid** — A photosensitivity dermatitis that is characterized by itchy, red, inflamed skin that resembles reticulosis on biopsy.

L57.2 **Cutis rhomboidalis nuchae**

L57.3 **Poikiloderma of Civatte**

L57.4 **Cutis laxa senilis**
Elastosis senilis

L57.5 **Actinic granuloma**

L57.8 **Other skin changes due to chronic exposure to nonionizing radiation**
Farmer's skin
Sailor's skin
Solar dermatitis

L57.9 **Skin changes due to chronic exposure to nonionizing radiation, unspecified**

L58- **Radiodermatitis** — Damage to the skin from ionizing radiation.
Use additional code to identify the source of the radiation (W88, W90)

L58.0 **Acute radiodermatitis**

L58.1 **Chronic radiodermatitis**

L58.9 **Radiodermatitis, unspecified**

L59- **Other disorders of skin and subcutaneous tissue related to radiation**

L59.0 **Erythema ab igne [dermatitis ab igne]** — Localized areas of erythema and/or hyperpigmentation caused by repeated exposure to infrared (heat) radiation.

L59.8 **Other specified disorders of the skin and subcutaneous tissue related to radiation**

L59.9 **Disorder of the skin and subcutaneous tissue related to radiation, unspecified**

Disorders of skin appendages (L60-L75)

Excludes 1: congenital malformations of integument (Q84.-)

L60- **Nail disorders**
Excludes ❷: clubbing of nails (R68.3)
onychia and paronychia (L03.0-)

L60.0 **Ingrowing nail** — The inward growing of the nail into the soft tissues.

L60.1 **Onycholysis** — The loosening of the nails from their nailbeds.

L60.2 **Onychogryphosis** — An abnormal overgrowth of the nails with an inward curvature.

L60.3 **Nail dystrophy** — Abnormal changes in nail texture, structure, or color.

L60.4 **Beau's lines** — Ridges or indentations in the nail plate.

L60.5 **Yellow nail syndrome** — Yellow coloring of the nails due to an underlying disease, usually lyphedema.

L60.8 **Other nail disorders**

L60.9 **Nail disorder, unspecified**

L62 **Nail disorders in diseases classified elsewhere** — [Not Allowed as PDX]
Code first underlying disease, such as:
Pachydermoperiostosis (M89.4-)

L63- **Alopecia areata** — An abnormal autoimmune loss of hair in sharply defined patches usually on the beard or scalp.

L63.0 **Alopecia (capitis) totalis** — A form losing all the hair on the scalp.

L63.1 **Alopecia universalis** — A form losing all the hair on the body, including pubic hair.

L63.2 **Ophiasis** — A form marked by involvement of the temporal and occipital margins of the scalp in a continuous band.

L63.8 **Other alopecia areata**

L63.9 **Alopecia areata, unspecified**

L64- **Androgenic alopecia** — The loss of hair on the scalp caused by diminished hair follicles.
Includes: Male-pattern baldness

L64.0 **Drug-induced androgenic alopecia**
Use additional code for adverse effect, if applicable, to identify drug (T36-T50 with fifth or sixth character 5)

L64.8 **Other androgenic alopecia**

L64.9 **Androgenic alopecia, unspecified**

L65- **Other nonscarring hair loss**
Use additional code for adverse effect, if applicable, to identify drug (T36-T50 with fifth or sixth character 5)
Excludes 1: trichotillomania (F63.3)

L65.0 **Telogen effluvium**

L65.1 **Anagen effluvium**

L65.2 **Alopecia mucinosa**

L65.8 **Other specified nonscarring hair loss**

L65.9 **Nonscarring hair loss, unspecified**
Alopecia NOS

L66- **Cicatricial alopecia [scarring hair loss]**

L66.0 **Pseudopelade**

L66.1 **Lichen planopilaris**
Follicular lichen planus

L66.2 **Folliculitis decalvans**

L66.3 **Perifolliculitis capitis abscedens**

L66.4 **Folliculitis ulerythematosa reticulata**

L66.8 **Other cicatricial alopecia**
AHA 15:1Q:p19 – Cicatricial alopecia due to second degree burns

L66.9 **Cicatricial alopecia, unspecified**

L67- **Hair color and hair shaft abnormalities**
Excludes 1: monilethrix (Q84.1)
pili annulati (Q84.1)
telogen effluvium (L65.0)

L67.0 **Trichorrhexis nodosa**

L67.1 **Variations in hair color**
Canities
Greyness, hair (premature)
Heterochromia of hair
Poliosis circumscripta, acquired
Poliosis NOS

L 5 4 – L 6 7

L67.8   **Other hair color and hair shaft abnormalities**
Fragilitas crinium

L67.9   **Hair color and hair shaft abnormality, unspecified**

L68-   Hypertrichosis — The excessive growth or coverage of hair.
Includes: Excess hair
Excludes 1:   congenital hypertrichosis (Q84.2)
persistent lanugo (Q84.2)

L68.0   **Hirsutism**

L68.1   **Acquired hypertrichosis lanuginosa**

L68.2   **Localized hypertrichosis**

L68.3   **Polytrichia**

L68.8   **Other hypertrichosis**

L68.9   **Hypertrichosis, unspecified**

L70-   Acne — An inflammatory pilosebaceous disease.
Excludes ❷: acne keloid (L73.0)

L70.0   **Acne vulgaris** — A form characterized by comedones, papules, pustules, cysts, and nodules occurring chiefly on the face, neck, upper trunk, and upper arms.

L70.1   **Acne conglobata** — A form characterized by numerous comedones, pus, and cyst and sinus formation with severe scarring.

L70.2   **Acne varioliformis** — A form characterized by superficial, brownish-red papulopustules occurring on the forehead and scalp.
Acne necrotica miliaris

L70.3   **Acne tropica** — A severe form occurring in the tropics.

L70.4   **Infantile acne** — [Age/0-17] – A form presenting in the first year of life.

L70.5   **Acné excoriée** — Hyperpigmentation of healed acne sites that have been exacerbated by the individual applying pressure.
Acné excoriée des jeunes filles
Picker's acne

L70.8   **Other acne**

L70.9   **Acne, unspecified**

L71-   Rosacea — A chronic inflammatory disease of the capillary-rich areas of the face that is characterized by erythema, pustules, and telangiectasia.
Use additional code for adverse effect, if applicable, to identify drug (T36-T50 with fifth or sixth character 5)

L71.0   **Perioral dermatitis** — A papular, sometimes pustular eruption of the area surrounding the mouth, and occurring almost exclusively in women between the ages of 20 and 35.

L71.1   **Rhinophyma** — A form of rosacea marked by nodular swelling, redness, sebaceous hyperplasia, and congestion of the distal portion of the nose.

L71.8   **Other rosacea**

L71.9   **Rosacea, unspecified**

L72-   Follicular cysts of skin and subcutaneous tissue

L72.0   **Epidermal cyst** — An encapsulated keratin-filled sac of the epidermis that has implanted into the dermis.

L72.1-   Pilar and trichodermal cyst

L72.11   Pilar cyst — An encapsulated keratin-filled sac of the epidermis that is derived from the outer root sheath of a hair follicle.

L72.12   Trichodermal cyst — Pilar cyst(s) that grow extensively and rapidly, multiplying into a tumor-like mass.
Trichilemmal (proliferating) cyst

L72.2   **Steatocystoma multiplex** — A skin disorder characterized by the development of multiple cysts.

L72.3   **Sebaceous cyst** — An encapsulated, keratin and sebum-filled sac of a pilosebaceous unit.
Excludes ❷: pilar cyst (L72.11)
trichilemmal (proliferating) cyst (L72.12)

L72.8   **Other follicular cysts of the skin and subcutaneous tissue**

L72.9   **Follicular cyst of the skin and subcutaneous tissue, unspecified**

L73-   Other follicular disorders

L73.0   **Acne keloid** — A keloid-like scar from a follicular-based pustule.

L73.1   **Pseudofolliculitis barbae** — An inflammatory skin condition of shaved hair (usually facial) in which the hair curls back into the skin causing a foreign body like reaction.

L73.2   **Hidradenitis suppurativa** — Inflammation of the apocrine sweat glands with secondary infection marked by abscessed cutaneous nodules and sinus formation.

L73.8   **Other specified follicular disorders**
Sycosis barbae

L73.9   **Follicular disorder, unspecified**

L74-   Eccrine sweat disorders
Excludes ❷: generalized hyperhidrosis (R61)

L74.0   **Miliaria rubra** — A condition caused by the obstruction of the sweat ducts that is characterized by discrete, pruritic, erythematous papulovesicles.

L74.1   **Miliaria crystallina**

L74.2   **Miliaria profunda**
Miliaria tropicalis

L74.3   **Miliaria, unspecified**

L74.4   **Anhidrosis** — The diminished or complete absence of sweat secretion.
Hypohidrosis

L74.5-   Focal hyperhidrosis — Excessive sweating involving one or more specific locations on the body.

L74.51-   Primary focal hyperhidrosis — A form not related to an underlying condition.

L74.510   Primary focal hyperhidrosis, axilla

L74.511   Primary focal hyperhidrosis, face

L74.512   Primary focal hyperhidrosis, palms

L74.513   Primary focal hyperhidrosis, soles

L74.519   Primary focal hyperhidrosis, unspecified

L74.52   Secondary focal hyperhidrosis — A form due to an underlying condition or medical treatment.
Frey's syndrome — A form characterized by warmth and sweating in the face due to eating certain foods and often associated as a consequence of parotid gland damage.

L74.8   **Other eccrine sweat disorders**

L74.9   **Eccrine sweat disorder, unspecified**
Sweat gland disorder NOS

L75-   Apocrine sweat disorders
Excludes 1:   dyshidrosis (L30.1)
hidradenitis suppurativa (L73.2)

L75.0   **Bromhidrosis** — Foul-smelling sweat due to the decomposition of microorganisms of the apocrine sweat glands.

L75.1   **Chromhidrosis** — The abnormal coloration of sweat.

L75.2   **Apocrine miliaria** — A skin disease characterized by conical, flesh-colored, or grayish, intensely pruritic, discrete follicular papules.
Fox-Fordyce disease

L75.8   **Other apocrine sweat disorders**

L75.9   **Apocrine sweat disorder, unspecified**

Intraoperative and postprocedural complications of skin and subcutaneous tissue (L76)

L76-   Intraoperative and postprocedural complications of skin and subcutaneous tissue

L76.0-   Intraoperative hemorrhage and hematoma of skin and subcutaneous tissue complicating a procedure
Excludes 1:   intraoperative hemorrhage and hematoma of skin and subcutaneous tissue due to accidental puncture and laceration during a procedure (L76.1-)

cc **L76.01   Intraoperative hemorrhage and hematoma of skin and subcutaneous tissue complicating a dermatologic procedure**

cc **L76.02   Intraoperative hemorrhage and hematoma of skin and subcutaneous tissue complicating other procedure**

L76.1-   Accidental puncture and laceration of skin and subcutaneous tissue during a procedure

cc **L76.11   Accidental puncture and laceration of skin and subcutaneous tissue during a dermatologic procedure**

cc **L76.12   Accidental puncture and laceration of skin and subcutaneous tissue during other procedure**

L76.2-   Postprocedural hemorrhage of skin and subcutaneous tissue following a procedure

cc **L76.21   Postprocedural hemorrhage of skin and subcutaneous tissue following a dermatologic procedure**

cc **L76.22   Postprocedural hemorrhage of skin and subcutaneous tissue following other procedure**

L 6 7 - L 7 6

L76.3- Postprocedural hematoma and seroma of skin and subcutaneous tissue following a procedure

cc **L76.31** Postprocedural hematoma of skin and subcutaneous tissue following a dermatologic procedure

cc **L76.32** Postprocedural hematoma of skin and subcutaneous tissue following other procedure

cc **L76.33** Postprocedural seroma of skin and subcutaneous tissue following a dermatologic procedure

cc **L76.34** Postprocedural seroma of skin and subcutaneous tissue following other procedure

L76.8- Other intraoperative and postprocedural complications of skin and subcutaneous tissue

Use additional code, if applicable, to further specify disorder

L76.81 Other intraoperative complications of skin and subcutaneous tissue

L76.82 Other postprocedural complications of skin and subcutaneous tissue

Other disorders of the skin and subcutaneous tissue (L80-L99)

L80 Vitiligo — An epidermal pigment cell destructive disorder of an unknown etiology marked by paper-white macules and patches and usually affecting the skin over bony prominences.

Excludes ❷: vitiligo of eyelids (H02.73-)
vitiligo of vulva (N90.89)

L81- Other disorders of pigmentation

Excludes 1: birthmark NOS (Q82.5)
Peutz-Jeghers syndrome (Q85.8)

Excludes ❷: nevus — see Alphabetical Index

L81.0 Postinflammatory hyperpigmentation

L81.1 Chloasma

L81.2 Freckles

L81.3 Café au lait spots

L81.4 Other melanin hyperpigmentation
Lentigo

L81.5 Leukoderma, not elsewhere classified

L81.6 Other disorders of diminished melanin formation

L81.7 Pigmented purpuric dermatosis
Angioma serpiginosum

L81.8 Other specified disorders of pigmentation
Iron pigmentation
Tattoo pigmentation

L81.9 Disorder of pigmentation, unspecified

L82- Seborrheic keratosis — A benign skin tumor of epidermal origin that forms numerous yellow or brown raised lesions.
Includes: Basal cell papilloma
Dermatosis papulosa nigra
Leser-Trélat disease

Excludes ❷: seborrheic dermatitis (L21.-)

L82.0 Inflamed seborrheic keratosis — A form marked by symptomatic inflammation of the lesion.

L82.1 Other seborrheic keratosis
Seborrheic keratosis NOS

L83 Acanthosis nigricans — A hypertrophic skin disease characterized by hyperpigmentation and papillary hypertrophy of the body fold regions.
Confluent and reticulated papillomatosis

L84 Corns and callosities — CORN – The inward thickening of the outer layer of the skin caused by friction and pressure. CALLOSITIES – The localized thickening of the skin caused by abnormal friction or pressure.
Callus
Clavus

L85- Other epidermal thickening

Excludes ❷: hypertrophic disorders of the skin (L91.-)

L85.0 Acquired ichthyosis — A generalized skin disorder marked by dryness, roughness, and scaliness that is due to hypertrophy of the outer layer of the skin.

Excludes 1: congenital ichthyosis (Q80.-)

L85.1 Acquired keratosis [keratoderma] palmaris et plantaris — A hypertrophic skin disorder marked by thickening of the outer layer of the skin of the palms and soles.

Excludes 1: inherited keratosis palmaris et plantaris (Q82.8)

L85.2 Keratosis punctata (palmaris et plantaris)

L85.3 Xerosis cutis
Dry skin dermatitis

L85.8 Other specified epidermal thickening
Cutaneous horn

L85.9 Epidermal thickening, unspecified

L86 Keratoderma in diseases classified elsewhere — [Not Allowed as PDX]
Code first underlying disease, such as:
Reiter's disease (M02.3-)

Excludes 1: gonococcal keratoderma (A54.89)
gonococcal keratosis (A54.89)
keratoderma due to vitamin A deficiency (E50.8)
keratosis due to vitamin A deficiency (E50.8)
xeroderma due to vitamin A deficiency (E50.8)

L87- Transepidermal elimination disorders

Excludes 1: granuloma annulare (perforating) (L92.0)

L87.0 Keratosis follicularis et parafollicularis in cutem penetrans — A hypertrophic, follicular skin disease characterized by keratotic pegs of the hair follicles and eccrine ducts that extend down into the corium.
Kyrle disease
Hyperkeratosis follicularis penetrans

L87.1 Reactive perforating collagenosis

L87.2 Elastosis perforans serpiginosa — A hypertrophic skin disorder marked by loss of the normal elasticity of the skin.

L87.8 Other transepidermal elimination disorders

L87.9 Transepidermal elimination disorder, unspecified

L88 Pyoderma gangrenosum — A fungating, pedunculated growth of the skin in which
cc the granulations consist of masses of pyogenic organisms.
Phagedenic pyoderma

Excludes 1: dermatitis gangrenosa (L08.0)

L89- Pressure ulcer — A localized, inflammatory, necrotic skin defect that develops slowly and persists over a period of time that is caused by prolonged pressure at the site.
Includes: Bed sore
Decubitus ulcer
Plaster ulcer
Pressure area
Pressure sore
Code first any associated gangrene (I96)

Excludes ❷: decubitus (trophic) ulcer of cervix (uteri) (N86)
diabetic ulcers (E08.621, E08.622, E09.621, E09.622, E10.621,
E10.622, E11.621, E11.622, E13.621, E13.622)
non-pressure chronic ulcer of skin (L97.-)
skin infections (L00-L08)
varicose ulcer (I83.0, I83.2)

L89.0- Pressure ulcer of elbow

L89.00- Pressure ulcer of unspecified elbow

L89.000 Pressure ulcer of unspecified elbow, unstageable

L89.001 Pressure ulcer of unspecified elbow, stage 1
Healing pressure ulcer of unspecified elbow, stage 1
Pressure pre-ulcer skin changes limited to persistent focal edema, unspecified elbow

L89.002 Pressure ulcer of unspecified elbow, stage 2
Healing pressure ulcer of unspecified elbow, stage 2
Pressure ulcer with abrasion, blister, partial thickness skin loss involving epidermis and/or dermis, unspecified elbow

mcc **L89.003 Pressure ulcer of unspecified elbow, stage 3**
Healing pressure ulcer of unspecified elbow, stage 3
Pressure ulcer with full thickness skin loss involving damage or necrosis of subcutaneous tissue, unspecified elbow

mcc **L89.004 Pressure ulcer of unspecified elbow, stage 4**
Healing pressure ulcer of unspecified elbow, stage 4
Pressure ulcer with necrosis of soft tissues through to underlying muscle, tendon, or bone, unspecified elbow

L89.009 Pressure ulcer of unspecified elbow, unspecified stage
Healing pressure ulcer of elbow NOS
Healing pressure ulcer of unspecified elbow, unspecified stage

Excludes 1: = NOT CODED HERE! (Do not code both)

Excludes ❷: = Not Included Here

L 7 6 - L 8 9

© 2016 Channel Publishing Ltd

L89.01- Pressure ulcer of <u>right</u> <u>elbow</u>

L89.010 Pressure ulcer of <u>right</u> <u>elbow</u>, unstageable

L89.011 Pressure ulcer of <u>right</u> <u>elbow</u>, stage 1
  Healing pressure ulcer of right elbow, stage 1
  Pressure pre-ulcer skin changes limited to persistent focal edema, right elbow

L89.012 Pressure ulcer of <u>right</u> <u>elbow</u>, stage 2
  Healing pressure ulcer of right elbow, stage 2
  Pressure ulcer with abrasion, blister, partial thickness skin loss involving epidermis and/or dermis, right elbow

ᴹᶜᶜ**L89.013** Pressure ulcer of <u>right</u> <u>elbow</u>, stage 3
  Healing pressure ulcer of right elbow, stage 3
  Pressure ulcer with full thickness skin loss involving damage or necrosis of subcutaneous tissue, right elbow

ᴹᶜᶜ**L89.014** Pressure ulcer of <u>right</u> <u>elbow</u>, stage 4
  Healing pressure ulcer of right elbow, stage 4
  Pressure ulcer with necrosis of soft tissues through to underlying muscle, tendon, or bone, right elbow

L89.019 Pressure ulcer of <u>right</u> <u>elbow</u>, unspecified stage
  Healing pressure right of elbow NOS
  Healing pressure ulcer of unspecified elbow, unspecified stage

L89.02- Pressure ulcer of <u>left</u> <u>elbow</u>

L89.020 Pressure ulcer of <u>left</u> <u>elbow</u>, unstageable

L89.021 Pressure ulcer of <u>left</u> <u>elbow</u>, stage 1
  Healing pressure ulcer of left elbow, stage 1
  Pressure pre-ulcer skin changes limited to persistent focal edema, left elbow

L89.022 Pressure ulcer of <u>left</u> <u>elbow</u>, stage 2
  Healing pressure ulcer of left elbow, stage 2
  Pressure ulcer with abrasion, blister, partial thickness skin loss involving epidermis and/or dermis, left elbow

ᴹᶜᶜ**L89.023** Pressure ulcer of <u>left</u> <u>elbow</u>, stage 3
  Healing pressure ulcer of left elbow, stage 3
  Pressure ulcer with full thickness skin loss involving damage or necrosis of subcutaneous tissue, left elbow

ᴹᶜᶜ**L89.024** Pressure ulcer of <u>left</u> <u>elbow</u>, stage 4
  Healing pressure ulcer of left elbow, stage 4
  Pressure ulcer with necrosis of soft tissues through to underlying muscle, tendon, or bone, left elbow

L89.029 Pressure ulcer of <u>left</u> <u>elbow</u>, unspecified stage
  Healing pressure ulcer of left of elbow NOS
  Healing pressure ulcer of unspecified elbow, unspecified stage

L89.1- <u>Pressure ulcer</u> of <u>back</u>

L89.10- Pressure ulcer of <u>unspecified</u> part of <u>back</u>

L89.100 Pressure ulcer of <u>unspecified</u> part of <u>back</u>, unstageable

L89.101 Pressure ulcer of <u>unspecified</u> part of <u>back</u>, stage 1
  Healing pressure ulcer of unspecified part of back, stage 1
  Pressure pre-ulcer skin changes limited to persistent focal edema, unspecified part of back

L89.102 Pressure ulcer of <u>unspecified</u> part of <u>back</u>, stage 2
  Healing pressure ulcer of unspecified part of back, stage 2
  Pressure ulcer with abrasion, blister, partial thickness skin loss involving epidermis and/or dermis, unspecified part of back

ᴹᶜᶜ**L89.103** Pressure ulcer of <u>unspecified</u> part of <u>back</u>, stage 3
  Healing pressure ulcer of unspecified part of back, stage 3
  Pressure ulcer with full thickness skin loss involving damage or necrosis of subcutaneous tissue, unspecified part of back

ᴹᶜᶜ**L89.104** Pressure ulcer of <u>unspecified</u> part of <u>back</u>, stage 4
  Healing pressure ulcer of unspecified part of back, stage 4
  Pressure ulcer with necrosis of soft tissues through to underlying muscle, tendon, or bone, unspecified part of back

L89.109 Pressure ulcer of <u>unspecified</u> part of <u>back</u>, unspecified stage
  Healing pressure ulcer of unspecified part of back NOS
  Healing pressure ulcer of unspecified part of back, unspecified stage

L89.11- Pressure ulcer of <u>right</u> <u>upper back</u>
  Pressure ulcer of right shoulder blade

L89.110 Pressure ulcer of <u>right</u> <u>upper back</u>, unstageable

L89.111 Pressure ulcer of <u>right</u> <u>upper back</u>, stage 1
  Healing pressure ulcer of right upper back, stage 1
  Pressure pre-ulcer skin changes limited to persistent focal edema, right upper back

L89.112 Pressure ulcer of <u>right</u> <u>upper back</u>, stage 2
  Healing pressure ulcer of right upper back, stage 2
  Pressure ulcer with abrasion, blister, partial thickness skin loss involving epidermis and/or dermis, right upper back

ᴹᶜᶜ**L89.113** Pressure ulcer of <u>right</u> <u>upper back</u>, stage 3
  Healing pressure ulcer of right upper back, stage 3
  Pressure ulcer with full thickness skin loss involving damage or necrosis of subcutaneous tissue, right upper back

ᴹᶜᶜ**L89.114** Pressure ulcer of <u>right</u> <u>upper back</u>, stage 4
  Healing pressure ulcer of right upper back, stage 4
  Pressure ulcer with necrosis of soft tissues through to underlying muscle, tendon, or bone, right upper back

L89.119 Pressure ulcer of <u>right</u> <u>upper back</u>, unspecified stage
  Healing pressure ulcer of right upper back NOS
  Healing pressure ulcer of right upper back, unspecified stage

L89.12- Pressure ulcer of <u>left upper back</u>
  Pressure ulcer of left shoulder blade

L89.120 Pressure ulcer of <u>left upper back</u>, unstageable

L89.121 Pressure ulcer of <u>left upper back</u>, stage 1
  Healing pressure ulcer of left upper back, stage 1
  Pressure pre-ulcer skin changes limited to persistent focal edema, left upper back

L89.122 Pressure ulcer of <u>left upper back</u>, stage 2
  Healing pressure ulcer of left upper back, stage 2
  Pressure ulcer with abrasion, blister, partial thickness skin loss involving epidermis and/or dermis, left upper back

ᴹᶜᶜ**L89.123** Pressure ulcer of <u>left upper back</u>, stage 3
  Healing pressure ulcer of left upper back, stage 3
  Pressure ulcer with full thickness skin loss involving damage or necrosis of subcutaneous tissue, left upper back

ᴹᶜᶜ**L89.124** Pressure ulcer of <u>left upper back</u>, stage 4
  Healing pressure ulcer of left upper back, stage 4
  Pressure ulcer with necrosis of soft tissues through to underlying muscle, tendon, or bone, left upper back

L89.129 Pressure ulcer of <u>left upper back</u>, unspecified stage
  Healing pressure ulcer of left upper back NOS
  Healing pressure ulcer of left upper back, unspecified stage

L89.13- Pressure ulcer of <u>right lower back</u>

L89.130 Pressure ulcer of <u>right lower back</u>, unstageable

L89.131 Pressure ulcer of <u>right lower back</u>, stage 1
  Healing pressure ulcer of right lower back, stage 1
  Pressure pre-ulcer skin changes limited to persistent focal edema, right lower back

L89.132 Pressure ulcer of <u>right lower back</u>, stage 2
  Healing pressure ulcer of right lower back, stage 2
  Pressure ulcer with abrasion, blister, partial thickness skin loss involving epidermis and/or dermis, right lower back

ᴹᶜᶜ**L89.133** Pressure ulcer of <u>right lower back</u>, stage 3
  Healing pressure ulcer of right lower back, stage 3
  Pressure ulcer with full thickness skin loss involving damage or necrosis of subcutaneous tissue, right lower back

ᴹᶜᶜ**L89.134** Pressure ulcer of <u>right lower back</u>, stage 4
  Healing pressure ulcer of right lower back, stage 4
  Pressure ulcer with necrosis of soft tissues through to underlying muscle, tendon, or bone, right lower back

L89.139 Pressure ulcer of <u>right lower back</u>, unspecified stage
  Healing pressure ulcer of right lower back NOS
  Healing pressure ulcer of right lower back, unspecified stage

L89.14- Pressure ulcer of <u>left lower back</u>

L89.140 Pressure ulcer of <u>left lower back</u>, unstageable

L89.141 Pressure ulcer of <u>left lower back</u>, stage 1
Healing pressure ulcer of left lower back, stage 1
Pressure pre-ulcer skin changes limited to persistent focal edema, left lower back

L89.142 Pressure ulcer of <u>left lower back</u>, stage 2
Healing pressure ulcer of left lower back, stage 2
Pressure ulcer with abrasion, blister, partial thickness skin loss involving epidermis and/or dermis, left lower back

MCC L89.143 Pressure ulcer of <u>left lower back</u>, stage 3
Healing pressure ulcer of left lower back, stage 3
Pressure ulcer with full thickness skin loss involving damage or necrosis of subcutaneous tissue, left lower back

MCC L89.144 Pressure ulcer of <u>left lower back</u>, stage 4
Healing pressure ulcer of left lower back, stage 4
Pressure ulcer with necrosis of soft tissues through to underlying muscle, tendon, or bone, left lower back

L89.149 Pressure ulcer of <u>left lower back</u>, unspecified stage
Healing pressure ulcer of left lower back NOS
Healing pressure ulcer of left lower back, unspecified stage

L89.15- Pressure ulcer of <u>sacral</u> region
Pressure ulcer of coccyx
Pressure ulcer of tailbone

L89.150 Pressure ulcer of <u>sacral</u> region, unstageable

L89.151 Pressure ulcer of <u>sacral</u> region, stage 1
Healing pressure ulcer of sacral region, stage 1
Pressure pre-ulcer skin changes limited to persistent focal edema, sacral region

L89.152 Pressure ulcer of <u>sacral</u> region, stage 2
Healing pressure ulcer of sacral region, stage 2
Pressure ulcer with abrasion, blister, partial thickness skin loss involving epidermis and/or dermis, sacral region

MCC L89.153 Pressure ulcer of <u>sacral</u> region, stage 3
Healing pressure ulcer of sacral region, stage 3
Pressure ulcer with full thickness skin loss involving damage or necrosis of subcutaneous tissue, sacral region

MCC L89.154 Pressure ulcer of <u>sacral</u> region, stage 4
Healing pressure ulcer of sacral region, stage 4
Pressure ulcer with necrosis of soft tissues through to underlying muscle, tendon, or bone, sacral region

L89.159 Pressure ulcer of <u>sacral</u> region, unspecified stage
Healing pressure ulcer of sacral region NOS
Healing pressure ulcer of sacral region, unspecified stage

L89.2- <u>Pressure ulcer</u> of hip

L89.20- Pressure ulcer of <u>unspecified</u> hip

L89.200 Pressure ulcer of <u>unspecified</u> hip, unstageable

L89.201 Pressure ulcer of <u>unspecified</u> hip, stage 1
Healing pressure ulcer of unspecified hip back, stage 1
Pressure pre-ulcer skin changes limited to persistent focal edema, unspecified hip

L89.202 Pressure ulcer of <u>unspecified</u> hip, stage 2
Healing pressure ulcer of unspecified hip, stage 2
Pressure ulcer with abrasion, blister, partial thickness skin loss involving epidermis and/or dermis, unspecified hip

MCC L89.203 Pressure ulcer of <u>unspecified</u> hip, stage 3
Healing pressure ulcer of unspecified hip, stage 3
Pressure ulcer with full thickness skin loss involving damage or necrosis of subcutaneous tissue, unspecified hip

MCC L89.204 Pressure ulcer of <u>unspecified</u> hip, stage 4
Healing pressure ulcer of unspecified hip, stage 4
Pressure ulcer with necrosis of soft tissues through to underlying muscle, tendon, or bone, unspecified hip

L89.209 Pressure ulcer of <u>unspecified</u> hip, unspecified stage
Healing pressure ulcer of unspecified hip NOS
Healing pressure ulcer of unspecified hip, unspecified stage

L89.21- Pressure ulcer of <u>right hip</u>

L89.210 Pressure ulcer of <u>right hip</u>, unstageable

L89.211 Pressure ulcer of <u>right hip</u>, stage 1
Healing pressure ulcer of right hip back, stage 1
Pressure pre-ulcer skin changes limited to persistent focal edema, right hip

L89.212 Pressure ulcer of <u>right hip</u>, stage 2
Healing pressure ulcer of right hip, stage 2
Pressure ulcer with abrasion, blister, partial thickness skin loss involving epidermis and/or dermis, right hip

MCC L89.213 Pressure ulcer of <u>right hip</u>, stage 3
Healing pressure ulcer of right hip, stage 3
Pressure ulcer with full thickness skin loss involving damage or necrosis of subcutaneous tissue, right hip

MCC L89.214 Pressure ulcer of <u>right hip</u>, stage 4
Healing pressure ulcer of right hip, stage 4
Pressure ulcer with necrosis of soft tissues through to underlying muscle, tendon, or bone, right hip

L89.219 Pressure ulcer of <u>right hip</u>, unspecified stage
Healing pressure ulcer of right hip NOS
Healing pressure ulcer of right hip, unspecified stage

L89.22- Pressure ulcer of <u>left hip</u>

L89.220 Pressure ulcer of <u>left hip</u>, unstageable

L89.221 Pressure ulcer of <u>left hip</u>, stage 1
Healing pressure ulcer of left hip back, stage 1
Pressure pre-ulcer skin changes limited to persistent focal edema, left hip

L89.222 Pressure ulcer of <u>left hip</u>, stage 2
Healing pressure ulcer of left hip, stage 2
Pressure ulcer with abrasion, blister, partial thickness skin loss involving epidermis and/or dermis, left hip

MCC L89.223 Pressure ulcer of <u>left hip</u>, stage 3
Healing pressure ulcer of left hip, stage 3
Pressure ulcer with full thickness skin loss involving damage or necrosis of subcutaneous tissue, left hip

MCC L89.224 Pressure ulcer of <u>left hip</u>, stage 4
Healing pressure ulcer of left hip, stage 4
Pressure ulcer with necrosis of soft tissues through to underlying muscle, tendon, or bone, left hip

L89.229 Pressure ulcer of <u>left hip</u>, unspecified stage
Healing pressure ulcer of left hip NOS
Healing pressure ulcer of left hip, unspecified stage

L89.3- <u>Pressure ulcer</u> of buttock

L89.30- Pressure ulcer of <u>unspecified</u> buttock

L89.300 Pressure ulcer of <u>unspecified</u> buttock, unstageable

L89.301 Pressure ulcer of <u>unspecified</u> buttock, stage 1
Healing pressure ulcer of unspecified buttock, stage 1
Pressure pre-ulcer skin changes limited to persistent focal edema, unspecified buttock

L89.302 Pressure ulcer of <u>unspecified</u> buttock, stage 2
Healing pressure ulcer of unspecified buttock, stage 2
Pressure ulcer with abrasion, blister, partial thickness skin loss involving epidermis and/or dermis, unspecified buttock

MCC L89.303 Pressure ulcer of <u>unspecified</u> buttock, stage 3
Healing pressure ulcer of unspecified buttock, stage 3
Pressure ulcer with full thickness skin loss involving damage or necrosis of subcutaneous tissue, unspecified buttock

MCC L89.304 Pressure ulcer of <u>unspecified</u> buttock, stage 4
Healing pressure ulcer of unspecified buttock, stage 4
Pressure ulcer with necrosis of soft tissues through to underlying muscle, tendon, or bone, unspecified buttock

L89.309 Pressure ulcer of <u>unspecified</u> buttock, unspecified stage
Healing pressure ulcer of unspecified buttock NOS
Healing pressure ulcer of unspecified buttock, unspecified stage

L89.31- Pressure ulcer of <u>right buttock</u>

L89.310 Pressure ulcer of <u>right buttock</u>, unstageable

L89.311 Pressure ulcer of <u>right buttock</u>, stage 1
Healing pressure ulcer of right buttock, stage 1
Pressure pre-ulcer skin changes limited to persistent focal edema, right buttock

---

Excludes 1: = NOT CODED HERE! (Do not code both)   810   *Excludes ❷:* = Not Included Here

L89.312   Pressure ulcer of <u>right buttock</u>, stage 2
   Healing pressure ulcer of right buttock, stage 2
   Pressure ulcer with abrasion, blister, partial thickness skin loss involving epidermis and/or dermis, right buttock

мcc L89.313   Pressure ulcer of <u>right buttock</u>, stage 3
   Healing pressure ulcer of right buttock, stage 3
   Pressure ulcer with full thickness skin loss involving damage or necrosis of subcutaneous tissue, right buttock

мcc L89.314   Pressure ulcer of <u>right buttock</u>, stage 4
   Healing pressure ulcer of right buttock, stage 4
   Pressure ulcer with necrosis of soft tissues through to underlying muscle, tendon, or bone, right buttock

L89.319   Pressure ulcer of <u>right buttock</u>, unspecified stage
   Healing pressure ulcer of right buttock NOS
   Healing pressure ulcer of right buttock, unspecified stage

L89.32-   Pressure ulcer of <u>left buttock</u>

L89.320   Pressure ulcer of <u>left buttock</u>, unstageable

L89.321   Pressure ulcer of <u>left buttock</u>, stage 1
   Healing pressure ulcer of left buttock, stage 1
   Pressure pre-ulcer skin changes limited to persistent focal edema, left buttock

L89.322   Pressure ulcer of <u>left buttock</u>, stage 2
   Healing pressure ulcer of left buttock, stage 2
   Pressure ulcer with abrasion, blister, partial thickness skin loss involving epidermis and/or dermis, left buttock

мcc L89.323   Pressure ulcer of <u>left buttock</u>, stage 3
   Healing pressure ulcer of left buttock, stage 3
   Pressure ulcer with full thickness skin loss involving damage or necrosis of subcutaneous tissue, left buttock

мcc L89.324   Pressure ulcer of <u>left buttock</u>, stage 4
   Healing pressure ulcer of left buttock, stage 4
   Pressure ulcer with necrosis of soft tissues through to underlying muscle, tendon, or bone, left buttock

L89.329   Pressure ulcer of <u>left buttock</u>, unspecified stage
   Healing pressure ulcer of left buttock NOS
   Healing pressure ulcer of left buttock, unspecified stage

L89.4-   <u>Pressure ulcer</u> of contiguous site of back, buttock and hip

L89.40   Pressure ulcer of <u>contiguous site of back, buttock and hip</u>, unspecified stage
   Healing pressure ulcer of contiguous site of back, buttock and hip NOS
   Healing pressure ulcer of contiguous site of back, buttock and hip, unspecified stage

L89.41   Pressure ulcer of <u>contiguous site of back, buttock and hip</u>, stage 1
   Healing pressure ulcer of contiguous site of back, buttock and hip, stage 1
   Pressure pre-ulcer skin changes limited to persistent focal edema, contiguous site of back, buttock and hip

L89.42   Pressure ulcer of <u>contiguous site of back, buttock and hip</u>, stage 2
   Healing pressure ulcer of contiguous site of back, buttock and hip, stage 2
   Pressure ulcer with abrasion, blister, partial thickness skin loss involving epidermis and/or dermis, contiguous site of back, buttock and hip

мcc L89.43   Pressure ulcer of <u>contiguous site of back, buttock and hip</u>, stage 3
   Healing pressure ulcer of contiguous site of back, buttock and hip, stage 3
   Pressure ulcer with full thickness skin loss involving damage or necrosis of subcutaneous tissue, contiguous site of back, buttock and hip

мcc L89.44   Pressure ulcer of <u>contiguous site of back, buttock and hip</u>, stage 4
   Healing pressure ulcer of contiguous site of back, buttock and hip, stage 4
   Pressure ulcer with necrosis of soft tissues through to underlying muscle, tendon, or bone, contiguous site of back, buttock and hip

L89.45   Pressure ulcer of <u>contiguous site of back, buttock and hip</u>, unstageable

L89.5-   <u>Pressure ulcer</u> of ankle

L89.50-   Pressure ulcer of <u>unspecified ankle</u>

L89.500   Pressure ulcer of <u>unspecified ankle</u>, unstageable

L89.501   Pressure ulcer of <u>unspecified ankle</u>, stage 1
   Healing pressure ulcer of unspecified ankle, stage 1
   Pressure pre-ulcer skin changes limited to persistent focal edema, unspecified ankle

L89.502   Pressure ulcer of <u>unspecified ankle</u>, stage 2
   Healing pressure ulcer of unspecified ankle, stage 2
   Pressure ulcer with abrasion, blister, partial thickness skin loss involving epidermis and/or dermis, unspecified ankle

мcc L89.503   Pressure ulcer of <u>unspecified ankle</u>, stage 3
   Healing pressure ulcer of unspecified ankle, stage 3
   Pressure ulcer with full thickness skin loss involving damage or necrosis of subcutaneous tissue, unspecified ankle

мcc L89.504   Pressure ulcer of <u>unspecified ankle</u>, stage 4
   Healing pressure ulcer of unspecified ankle, stage 4
   Pressure ulcer with necrosis of soft tissues through to underlying muscle, tendon, or bone, unspecified ankle

L89.509   Pressure ulcer of <u>unspecified ankle</u>, unspecified stage
   Healing pressure ulcer of unspecified ankle NOS
   Healing pressure ulcer of unspecified ankle, unspecified stage

L89.51-   Pressure ulcer of <u>right ankle</u>

L89.510   Pressure ulcer of <u>right ankle</u>, unstageable

L89.511   Pressure ulcer of <u>right ankle</u>, stage 1
   Healing pressure ulcer of right ankle, stage 1
   Pressure pre-ulcer skin changes limited to persistent focal edema, right ankle

L89.512   Pressure ulcer of <u>right ankle</u>, stage 2
   Healing pressure ulcer of right ankle, stage 2
   Pressure ulcer with abrasion, blister, partial thickness skin loss involving epidermis and/or dermis, right ankle

мcc L89.513   Pressure ulcer of <u>right ankle</u>, stage 3
   Healing pressure ulcer of right ankle, stage 3
   Pressure ulcer with full thickness skin loss involving damage or necrosis of subcutaneous tissue, right ankle

мcc L89.514   Pressure ulcer of <u>right ankle</u>, stage 4
   Healing pressure ulcer of right ankle, stage 4
   Pressure ulcer with necrosis of soft tissues through to underlying muscle, tendon, or bone, right ankle

L89.519   Pressure ulcer of <u>right ankle</u>, unspecified stage
   Healing pressure ulcer of right ankle NOS
   Healing pressure ulcer of right ankle, unspecified stage

L89.52-   Pressure ulcer of <u>left ankle</u>

L89.520   Pressure ulcer of <u>left ankle</u>, unstageable

L89.521   Pressure ulcer of <u>left ankle</u>, stage 1
   Healing pressure ulcer of left ankle, stage 1
   Pressure pre-ulcer skin changes limited to persistent focal edema, left ankle

L89.522   Pressure ulcer of <u>left ankle</u>, stage 2
   Healing pressure ulcer of left ankle, stage 2
   Pressure ulcer with abrasion, blister, partial thickness skin loss involving epidermis and/or dermis, left ankle

мcc L89.523   Pressure ulcer of <u>left ankle</u>, stage 3
   Healing pressure ulcer of left ankle, stage 3
   Pressure ulcer with full thickness skin loss involving damage or necrosis of subcutaneous tissue, left ankle

мcc L89.524   Pressure ulcer of <u>left ankle</u>, stage 4
   Healing pressure ulcer of left ankle, stage 4
   Pressure ulcer with necrosis of soft tissues through to underlying muscle, tendon, or bone, left ankle

L89.529   Pressure ulcer of <u>left ankle</u>, unspecified stage
   Healing pressure ulcer of left ankle NOS
   Healing pressure ulcer of left ankle, unspecified stage

L89 - L89

L89.6- ~~Pressure ulcer~~ of heel
  L89.60- Pressure ulcer of ~~unspecified heel~~
    L89.600 Pressure ulcer of ~~unspecified heel~~, unstageable
    L89.601 Pressure ulcer of ~~unspecified heel~~, stage 1
      Healing pressure ulcer of unspecified heel, stage 1
      Pressure pre-ulcer skin changes limited to persistent focal edema, unspecified heel
    L89.602 Pressure ulcer of ~~unspecified heel~~, stage 2
      Healing pressure ulcer of unspecified heel, stage 2
      Pressure ulcer with abrasion, blister, partial thickness skin loss involving epidermis and/or dermis, unspecified heel
    ᴹᶜᶜ**L89.603** Pressure ulcer of ~~unspecified heel~~, stage 3
      Healing pressure ulcer of unspecified heel, stage 3
      Pressure ulcer with full thickness skin loss involving damage or necrosis of subcutaneous tissue, unspecified heel
    ᴹᶜᶜ**L89.604** Pressure ulcer of ~~unspecified heel~~, stage 4
      Healing pressure ulcer of unspecified heel, stage 4
      Pressure ulcer with necrosis of soft tissues through to underlying muscle, tendon, or bone, unspecified heel
    L89.609 Pressure ulcer of ~~unspecified heel~~, unspecified stage
      Healing pressure ulcer of unspecified heel NOS
      Healing pressure ulcer of unspecified heel, unspecified stage
  L89.61- Pressure ulcer of ~~right heel~~
    L89.610 Pressure ulcer of ~~right heel~~, unstageable
    L89.611 Pressure ulcer of ~~right heel~~, stage 1
      Healing pressure ulcer of right heel, stage 1
      Pressure pre-ulcer skin changes limited to persistent focal edema, right heel
    L89.612 Pressure ulcer of ~~right heel~~, stage 2
      Healing pressure ulcer of right heel, stage 2
      Pressure ulcer with abrasion, blister, partial thickness skin loss involving epidermis and/or dermis, right heel
    ᴹᶜᶜ**L89.613** Pressure ulcer of ~~right heel~~, stage 3
      Healing pressure ulcer of right heel, stage 3
      Pressure ulcer with full thickness skin loss involving damage or necrosis of subcutaneous tissue, right heel
    ᴹᶜᶜ**L89.614** Pressure ulcer of ~~right heel~~, stage 4
      Healing pressure ulcer of right heel, stage 4
      Pressure ulcer with necrosis of soft tissues through to underlying muscle, tendon, or bone, right heel
    L89.619 Pressure ulcer of ~~right heel~~, unspecified stage
      Healing pressure ulcer of right heel NOS
      Healing pressure ulcer of unspecified heel, right stage
  L89.62- Pressure ulcer of ~~left heel~~
    L89.620 Pressure ulcer of ~~left heel~~, unstageable
    L89.621 Pressure ulcer of ~~left heel~~, stage 1
      Healing pressure ulcer of left heel, stage 1
      Pressure pre-ulcer skin changes limited to persistent focal edema, left heel
    L89.622 Pressure ulcer of ~~left heel~~, stage 2
      Healing pressure ulcer of left heel, stage 2
      Pressure ulcer with abrasion, blister, partial thickness skin loss involving epidermis and/or dermis, left heel
    ᴹᶜᶜ**L89.623** Pressure ulcer of ~~left heel~~, stage 3
      Healing pressure ulcer of left heel, stage 3
      Pressure ulcer with full thickness skin loss involving damage or necrosis of subcutaneous tissue, left heel
    ᴹᶜᶜ**L89.624** Pressure ulcer of ~~left heel~~, stage 4
      Healing pressure ulcer of left heel, stage 4
      Pressure ulcer with necrosis of soft tissues through to underlying muscle, tendon, or bone, left heel
    L89.629 Pressure ulcer of ~~left heel~~, unspecified stage
      Healing pressure ulcer of left heel NOS
      Healing pressure ulcer of left heel, unspecified stage

L89.8- ~~Pressure ulcer~~ of other site
  L89.81- Pressure ulcer of ~~head~~
    Pressure ulcer of face
    L89.810 Pressure ulcer of ~~head~~, unstageable
    L89.811 Pressure ulcer of ~~head~~, stage 1
      Healing pressure ulcer of head, stage 1
      Pressure pre-ulcer skin changes limited to persistent focal edema, head
    L89.812 Pressure ulcer of ~~head~~, stage 2
      Healing pressure ulcer of head, stage 2
      Pressure ulcer with abrasion, blister, partial thickness skin loss involving epidermis and/or dermis, head
    ᴹᶜᶜ**L89.813** Pressure ulcer of ~~head~~, stage 3
      Healing pressure ulcer of head, stage 3
      Pressure ulcer with full thickness skin loss involving damage or necrosis of subcutaneous tissue, head
    ᴹᶜᶜ**L89.814** Pressure ulcer of ~~head~~, stage 4
      Healing pressure ulcer of head, stage 4
      Pressure ulcer with necrosis of soft tissues through to underlying muscle, tendon, or bone, head
    L89.819 Pressure ulcer of ~~head~~, unspecified stage
      Healing pressure ulcer of head NOS
      Healing pressure ulcer of head, unspecified stage
  L89.89- Pressure ulcer of other site
    L89.890 Pressure ulcer of ~~other~~ site, unstageable
    L89.891 Pressure ulcer of ~~other~~ site, stage 1
      Healing pressure ulcer of other site, stage 1
      Pressure pre-ulcer skin changes limited to persistent focal edema, other site
    L89.892 Pressure ulcer of ~~other~~ site, stage 2
      Healing pressure ulcer of other site, stage 2
      Pressure ulcer with abrasion, blister, partial thickness skin loss involving epidermis and/or dermis, other site
    ᴹᶜᶜ**L89.893** Pressure ulcer of ~~other~~ site, stage 3
      Healing pressure ulcer of other site, stage 3
      Pressure ulcer with full thickness skin loss involving damage or necrosis of subcutaneous tissue, other site
    ᴹᶜᶜ**L89.894** Pressure ulcer of ~~other~~ site, stage 4
      Healing pressure ulcer of other site, stage 4
      Pressure ulcer with necrosis of soft tissues through to underlying muscle, tendon, or bone, other site
    L89.899 Pressure ulcer of ~~other~~ site, unspecified stage
      Healing pressure ulcer of other site NOS
      Healing pressure ulcer of other site, unspecified stage

L89.9- ~~Pressure ulcer~~ of unspecified site
  L89.90 Pressure ulcer of ~~unspecified site~~, unspecified stage
    Healing pressure ulcer of unspecified site NOS
    Healing pressure ulcer of unspecified site, unspecified stage
  L89.91 Pressure ulcer of ~~unspecified site~~, stage 1
    Healing pressure ulcer of unspecified site, stage 1
    Pressure pre-ulcer skin changes limited to persistent focal edema, unspecified site
  L89.92 Pressure ulcer of ~~unspecified site~~, stage 2
    Healing pressure ulcer of unspecified site, stage 2
    Pressure ulcer with abrasion, blister, partial thickness skin loss involving epidermis and/or dermis, unspecified site
  ᴹᶜᶜ**L89.93** Pressure ulcer of ~~unspecified site~~, stage 3
    Healing pressure ulcer of unspecified site, stage 3
    Pressure ulcer with full thickness skin loss involving damage or necrosis of subcutaneous tissue, unspecified site
  ᴹᶜᶜ**L89.94** Pressure ulcer of ~~unspecified site~~, stage 4
    Healing pressure ulcer of unspecified site, stage 4
    Pressure ulcer with necrosis of soft tissues through to underlying muscle, tendon, or bone, unspecified site
  L89.95 Pressure ulcer of ~~unspecified site~~, unstageable

L90- **Atrophic disorders of skin** — Skin diseases characterized by wasting-away of the skin tissue.

L90.0 **Lichen sclerosus et atrophicus**
Excludes ❷: lichen sclerosus of external female genital organs (N90.4)
lichen sclerosus of external male genital organs (N48.0)

L90.1 **Anetoderma of Schweninger-Buzzi**

L90.2 **Anetoderma of Jadassohn-Pellizzari**

L90.3 **Atrophoderma of Pasini and Pierini**

L90.4 **Acrodermatitis chronica atrophicans**

L90.5 **Scar conditions and fibrosis of skin**
AHA 15:1Q:p19 – Skin contracture due to third degree burns
Adherent scar (skin)
Cicatrix
Disfigurement of skin due to scar
Fibrosis of skin NOS
Scar NOS
Excludes ❷: hypertrophic scar (L91.0)
keloid scar (L91.0)

L90.6 **Striae atrophicae**

L90.8 **Other atrophic disorders of skin**

L90.9 **Atrophic disorder of skin, unspecified**

L91- **Hypertrophic disorders of skin**

L91.0 **Hypertrophic scar** — A firm, elevated, irregularly-shaped growth of the skin due to excessive amounts of collagen in the skin during healing of a wound. It may also appear without a history of trauma.
Keloid
Keloid scar
Excludes ❷: acne keloid (L73.0)
scar NOS (L90.5)

L91.8 **Other hypertrophic disorders of the skin**

L91.9 **Hypertrophic disorder of the skin, unspecified**

L92- **Granulomatous disorders of skin and subcutaneous tissue** — Skin diseases characterized by the development of granulomatous tissue.
Excludes ❷: actinic granuloma (L57.5)

L92.0 **Granuloma annulare**
Perforating granuloma annulare

L92.1 **Necrobiosis lipoidica, not elsewhere classified**
Excludes 1: necrobiosis lipoidica associated with diabetes mellitus (E08-E13 with .620)

L92.2 **Granuloma faciale [eosinophilic granuloma of skin]**

L92.3 **Foreign body granuloma of the skin and subcutaneous tissue**
Use additional code to identify the type of retained foreign body (Z18.-)

L92.8 **Other granulomatous disorders of the skin and subcutaneous tissue**

L92.9 **Granulomatous disorder of the skin and subcutaneous tissue, unspecified**

L93- **Lupus erythematosus** — A superficial autimmune skin disorder characterized by inflammation, red macules, adherent scales, and patulous follicles that fall off, leaving scars.
Use additional code for adverse effect, if applicable, to identify drug (T36-T50 with fifth or sixth character 5)
Excludes 1: lupus exedens (A18.4)
lupus vulgaris (A18.4)
scleroderma (M34.-)
systemic lupus erythematosus (M32.-)

L93.0 **Discoid lupus erythematosus** — A form primarily affecting the face, ears, and scalp.
Lupus erythematosus NOS

L93.1 **Subacute cutaneous lupus erythematosus** — A form primarily affecting women that is characterized by scaly annular lesions and plaques.

L93.2 **Other local lupus erythematosus**
Lupus erythematosus profundus
Lupus panniculitis — A form marked by subcutaneous nodules.

L94- **Other localized connective tissue disorders**
Excludes 1: systemic connective tissue disorders (M30-M36)

L94.0 **Localized scleroderma [morphea]** — A chronic, atrophic skin disease characterized by replacement of localized areas of the skin and subcutaneous tissues with constricting connective tissue.
Circumscribed scleroderma

L94.1 **Linear scleroderma** — A form marked by a line of thickened skin that affects the muscle and bone below it, often causing the arm or leg to not grow at the same pace as the other.
En coup de sabre lesion

L94.2 **Calcinosis cutis** — The abnormal deposition of calcium salts forming nodules in the skin.

L94.3 **Sclerodactyly** — A chronic, atrophic skin disease characterized by replacement of localized areas of the skin and subcutaneous tissues with constricting connective tissue.

L94.4 **Gottron's papules** — A connective tissue disease that is characterized by inflammation of the skin and often the underlying muscles.

L94.5 **Poikiloderma vasculare atrophicans** — A skin disorder characterized by mottled dispigmentation, telangiectasia, and atrophy.

L94.6 **Ainhum** — The growth of constricting fibrous tissue around the base of a toe that eventually leads to loss of the digit.

L94.8 **Other specified localized connective tissue disorders**

L94.9 **Localized connective tissue disorder, unspecified**

L95- **Vasculitis limited to skin, not elsewhere classified**
Excludes 1: angioma serpiginosum (L81.7)
Henoch(-Schönlein) purpura (D69.0)
hypersensitivity angiitis (M31.0)
lupus panniculitis (L93.2)
panniculitis NOS (M79.3)
panniculitis of neck and back (M54.0-)
polyarteritis nodosa (M30.0)
relapsing panniculitis (M35.6)
rheumatoid vasculitis (M05.2)
serum sickness (T80.6-)
urticaria (L50-)
Wegener's granulomatosis (M31.3-)

L95.0 **Livedoid vasculitis** — A chronic skin and vascular disorder characterized by painful purple marks and ulcers of the lower extremities.
Atrophie blanche (en plaque)

L95.1 **Erythema elevatum diutinum** — A chronic skin and vascular disorder characterized by red, purple, brown, or yellow nodules of the extremities.

L95.8 **Other vasculitis limited to the skin**

L95.9 **Vasculitis limited to the skin, unspecified**

L97- **Non-pressure chronic ulcer** of lower limb, not elsewhere classified — A localized, inflammatory, necrotic skin defect of the lower extermity that develops slowly and persists over a period of time and is NOT caused by prolonged pressure at the site.
Includes: Chronic ulcer of skin of lower limb NOS
Non-healing ulcer of skin
Non-infected sinus of skin
Trophic ulcer NOS
Tropical ulcer NOS
Ulcer of skin of lower limb NOS
Code first any associated underlying condition, such as:
Any associated gangrene (I96)
Atherosclerosis of the lower extremities (I70.23-, I70.24-, I70.33-, I70.34-, I70.43-, I70.44-, I70.53-, I70.54-, I70.63-, I70.64-, I70.73-, I70.74-)
Chronic venous hypertension (I87.31-, I87.33-)
Diabetic ulcers (E08.621, E08.622, E09.621, E09.622, E10.621, E10.622, E11.621, E11.622, E13.621, E13.622)
Postphlebitic syndrome (I87.01-, I87.03-)
Postthrombotic syndrome (I87.01-, I87.03-)
Varicose ulcer (I83.0-, I83.2-)
Excludes ❷: pressure ulcer (pressure area) (L89.-)
skin infections (L00-L08)
specific infections classified to A00-B99

L97.1- **Non-pressure chronic ulcer** of thigh

L97.10- **Non-pressure chronic ulcer of unspecified thigh**

cc **L97.101** **Non-pressure chronic ulcer of unspecified thigh limited to breakdown of skin**

cc **L97.102** **Non-pressure chronic ulcer of unspecified thigh with fat layer exposed**

cc **L97.103** **Non-pressure chronic ulcer of unspecified thigh with necrosis of muscle**

cc **L97.104** **Non-pressure chronic ulcer of unspecified thigh with necrosis of bone**

cc **L97.109** **Non-pressure chronic ulcer of unspecified thigh with unspecified severity**

L97.11- **Non-pressure chronic ulcer of right thigh**

cc **L97.111** **Non-pressure chronic ulcer of right thigh limited to breakdown of skin**

cc **L97.112** **Non-pressure chronic ulcer of right thigh with fat layer exposed**

L90 - L97

cc **L97.113** Non-pressure chronic ulcer of <u>right</u> thigh <u>with</u> <u>necrosis of muscle</u>

cc **L97.114** Non-pressure chronic ulcer of <u>right</u> thigh <u>with</u> <u>necrosis of bone</u>

cc **L97.119** Non-pressure chronic ulcer of <u>right</u> thigh with <u>unspecified</u> severity

L97.12- Non-pressure chronic ulcer of <u>left</u> thigh

cc **L97.121** Non-pressure chronic ulcer of <u>left</u> thigh limited to <u>breakdown of skin</u>

cc **L97.122** Non-pressure chronic ulcer of <u>left</u> thigh <u>with fat layer exposed</u>

cc **L97.123** Non-pressure chronic ulcer of <u>left</u> thigh <u>with</u> <u>necrosis of muscle</u>

cc **L97.124** Non-pressure chronic ulcer of <u>left</u> thigh <u>with</u> <u>necrosis of bone</u>

cc **L97.129** Non-pressure chronic ulcer of <u>left</u> thigh with <u>unspecified</u> severity

L97.2- <u>Non-pressure chronic ulcer</u> of calf

L97.20- Non-pressure chronic ulcer of <u>unspecified</u> <u>calf</u>

cc **L97.201** Non-pressure chronic ulcer of <u>unspecified</u> calf limited to <u>breakdown of skin</u>

cc **L97.202** Non-pressure chronic ulcer of <u>unspecified</u> calf <u>with</u> <u>fat layer exposed</u>

cc **L97.203** Non-pressure chronic ulcer of <u>unspecified</u> calf <u>with</u> <u>necrosis of muscle</u>

cc **L97.204** Non-pressure chronic ulcer of <u>unspecified</u> calf <u>with</u> <u>necrosis of bone</u>

cc **L97.209** Non-pressure chronic ulcer of <u>unspecified</u> calf with <u>unspecified</u> severity

L97.21- Non-pressure chronic ulcer of <u>right</u> calf

cc **L97.211** Non-pressure chronic ulcer of <u>right</u> calf limited to <u>breakdown of skin</u>

cc **L97.212** Non-pressure chronic ulcer of <u>right</u> calf <u>with fat</u> <u>layer exposed</u>

cc **L97.213** Non-pressure chronic ulcer of <u>right</u> calf <u>with</u> <u>necrosis of muscle</u>

cc **L97.214** Non-pressure chronic ulcer of <u>right</u> calf <u>with</u> <u>necrosis of bone</u>

cc **L97.219** Non-pressure chronic ulcer of <u>right</u> calf with <u>unspecified</u> severity

L97.22- Non-pressure chronic ulcer of <u>left</u> calf

cc **L97.221** Non-pressure chronic ulcer of <u>left</u> calf limited to <u>breakdown of skin</u>

cc **L97.222** Non-pressure chronic ulcer of <u>left</u> calf <u>with fat</u> <u>layer exposed</u>

cc **L97.223** Non-pressure chronic ulcer of <u>left</u> calf <u>with necrosis</u> <u>of muscle</u>

cc **L97.224** Non-pressure chronic ulcer of <u>left</u> calf <u>with necrosis</u> <u>of bone</u>

cc **L97.229** Non-pressure chronic ulcer of <u>left</u> calf with <u>unspecified</u> severity

L97.3- <u>Non-pressure chronic ulcer</u> of ankle

L97.30- Non-pressure chronic ulcer of <u>unspecified</u> <u>ankle</u>

cc **L97.301** Non-pressure chronic ulcer of <u>unspecified</u> ankle limited to <u>breakdown of skin</u>

cc **L97.302** Non-pressure chronic ulcer of <u>unspecified</u> ankle <u>with fat layer exposed</u>

cc **L97.303** Non-pressure chronic ulcer of <u>unspecified</u> ankle <u>with necrosis of muscle</u>

cc **L97.304** Non-pressure chronic ulcer of <u>unspecified</u> ankle <u>with necrosis of bone</u>

cc **L97.309** Non-pressure chronic ulcer of <u>unspecified</u> ankle with <u>unspecified</u> severity

L97.31- Non-pressure chronic ulcer of <u>right</u> ankle

cc **L97.311** Non-pressure chronic ulcer of <u>right</u> ankle limited to <u>breakdown of skin</u>

cc **L97.312** Non-pressure chronic ulcer of <u>right</u> ankle <u>with fat</u> <u>layer exposed</u>

cc **L97.313** Non-pressure chronic ulcer of <u>right</u> ankle <u>with</u> <u>necrosis of muscle</u>

cc **L97.314** Non-pressure chronic ulcer of <u>right</u> ankle <u>with</u> <u>necrosis of bone</u>

cc **L97.319** Non-pressure chronic ulcer of <u>right</u> ankle with <u>unspecified</u> severity

L97.32- Non-pressure chronic ulcer of <u>left</u> ankle

cc **L97.321** Non-pressure chronic ulcer of <u>left</u> ankle limited to <u>breakdown of skin</u>

cc **L97.322** Non-pressure chronic ulcer of <u>left</u> ankle <u>with fat</u> <u>layer exposed</u>

cc **L97.323** Non-pressure chronic ulcer of <u>left</u> ankle <u>with</u> <u>necrosis of muscle</u>

cc **L97.324** Non-pressure chronic ulcer of <u>left</u> ankle <u>with</u> <u>necrosis of bone</u>

cc **L97.329** Non-pressure chronic ulcer of <u>left</u> ankle with <u>unspecified</u> severity

L97.4- <u>Non-pressure chronic ulcer</u> of heel and midfoot
  Non-pressure chronic ulcer of plantar surface of midfoot

L97.40- Non-pressure chronic ulcer of <u>unspecified</u> heel and <u>midfoot</u>

cc **L97.401** Non-pressure chronic ulcer of <u>unspecified</u> heel and midfoot limited to <u>breakdown of skin</u>

cc **L97.402** Non-pressure chronic ulcer of <u>unspecified</u> heel and midfoot <u>with fat layer exposed</u>

cc **L97.403** Non-pressure chronic ulcer of <u>unspecified</u> heel and midfoot <u>with necrosis of muscle</u>

cc **L97.404** Non-pressure chronic ulcer of <u>unspecified</u> heel and midfoot <u>with necrosis of bone</u>

cc **L97.409** Non-pressure chronic ulcer of unspecified heel and midfoot with <u>unspecified</u> severity

L97.41- Non-pressure chronic ulcer of <u>right</u> <u>heel and midfoot</u>

cc **L97.411** Non-pressure chronic ulcer of <u>right</u> heel and midfoot limited to <u>breakdown of skin</u>

cc **L97.412** Non-pressure chronic ulcer of <u>right</u> heel and midfoot <u>with fat layer exposed</u>

cc **L97.413** Non-pressure chronic ulcer of <u>right</u> heel and midfoot <u>with necrosis of muscle</u>

cc **L97.414** Non-pressure chronic ulcer of <u>right</u> heel and midfoot <u>with necrosis of bone</u>

cc **L97.419** Non-pressure chronic ulcer of <u>right</u> heel and midfoot with <u>unspecified</u> severity

L97.42- Non-pressure chronic ulcer of <u>left</u> <u>heel and midfoot</u>

cc **L97.421** Non-pressure chronic ulcer of <u>left</u> heel and midfoot limited to <u>breakdown of skin</u>

cc **L97.422** Non-pressure chronic ulcer of <u>left</u> heel and midfoot <u>with fat layer exposed</u>

cc **L97.423** Non-pressure chronic ulcer of <u>left</u> heel and midfoot <u>with necrosis of muscle</u>

cc **L97.424** Non-pressure chronic ulcer of <u>left</u> heel and midfoot <u>with necrosis of bone</u>

cc **L97.429** Non-pressure chronic ulcer of <u>left</u> heel and midfoot with <u>unspecified</u> severity

L97.5- <u>Non-pressure chronic ulcer</u> of <u>other part of foot</u>
  Non-pressure chronic ulcer of toe

L97.50- Non-pressure chronic ulcer of <u>other part of unspecified</u> <u>foot</u>

L97.501 Non-pressure chronic ulcer of <u>other part of</u> <u>unspecified foot</u> limited to <u>breakdown of skin</u>

L97.502 Non-pressure chronic ulcer of <u>other part of</u> <u>unspecified foot</u> <u>with fat layer exposed</u>

L97.503 Non-pressure chronic ulcer of <u>other part of</u> <u>unspecified foot</u> <u>with necrosis of muscle</u>

L97.504 Non-pressure chronic ulcer of <u>other part of</u> <u>unspecified foot</u> <u>with necrosis of bone</u>

L97.509 Non-pressure chronic ulcer of <u>other part of</u> <u>unspecified foot</u> with <u>unspecified</u> severity

L97.51- Non-pressure chronic ulcer of <u>other part</u> of <u>right</u> <u>foot</u>

L97.511   Non-pressure chronic ulcer of <u>other part</u> of <u>right</u> foot limited to <u>breakdown of skin</u>

L97.512   Non-pressure chronic ulcer of <u>other part</u> of <u>right</u> foot <u>with fat layer exposed</u>

L97.513   Non-pressure chronic ulcer of <u>other part</u> of <u>right</u> foot <u>with necrosis of muscle</u>

L97.514   Non-pressure chronic ulcer of <u>other part</u> of <u>right</u> foot <u>with necrosis of bone</u>

L97.519   Non-pressure chronic ulcer of <u>other part</u> of <u>right</u> foot with <u>unspecified</u> severity

L97.52- Non-pressure chronic ulcer of other part of <u>left</u> <u>foot</u>

L97.521   Non-pressure chronic ulcer of <u>other part</u> of <u>left</u> foot limited to <u>breakdown of skin</u>

L97.522   Non-pressure chronic ulcer of <u>other part</u> of <u>left</u> foot <u>with fat layer exposed</u>

L97.523   Non-pressure chronic ulcer of <u>other part</u> of <u>left</u> foot <u>with necrosis of muscle</u>

L97.524   Non-pressure chronic ulcer of <u>other part</u> of <u>left</u> foot <u>with necrosis of bone</u>

L97.529   Non-pressure chronic ulcer of <u>other part</u> of <u>left</u> foot with <u>unspecified</u> severity

L97.8-   <u>Non-pressure chronic ulcer</u> of other part of lower leg

L97.80   Non-pressure chronic ulcer of <u>other part of unspecified lower leg</u>

cc L97.801   Non-pressure chronic ulcer of other part of unspecified <u>lower leg</u> limited to <u>breakdown of skin</u>

cc L97.802   Non-pressure chronic ulcer of other part of unspecified <u>lower leg</u> <u>with fat layer exposed</u>

cc L97.803   Non-pressure chronic ulcer of other part of unspecified <u>lower leg</u> <u>with necrosis of muscle</u>

cc L97.804   Non-pressure chronic ulcer of other part of unspecified <u>lower leg</u> <u>with necrosis of bone</u>

cc L97.809   Non-pressure chronic ulcer of other part of unspecified <u>lower leg</u> with <u>unspecified</u> severity

L97.81- Non-pressure chronic ulcer of <u>other part of right</u> <u>lower leg</u>

cc L97.811   Non-pressure chronic ulcer of other part of <u>right</u> lower leg limited to <u>breakdown of skin</u>

cc L97.812   Non-pressure chronic ulcer of other part of <u>right</u> lower leg <u>with fat layer exposed</u>

cc L97.813   Non-pressure chronic ulcer of other part of <u>right</u> lower leg <u>with necrosis of muscle</u>

cc L97.814   Non-pressure chronic ulcer of other part of <u>right</u> lower leg <u>with necrosis of bone</u>

cc L97.819   Non-pressure chronic ulcer of other part of <u>right</u> lower leg with <u>unspecified</u> severity

L97.82- Non-pressure chronic ulcer of <u>other part of</u> <u>left</u> lower leg

cc L97.821   Non-pressure chronic ulcer of other part of <u>left</u> lower leg limited to <u>breakdown of skin</u>

cc L97.822   Non-pressure chronic ulcer of other part of <u>left</u> lower leg <u>with fat layer exposed</u>

cc L97.823   Non-pressure chronic ulcer of other part of <u>left</u> lower leg <u>with necrosis of muscle</u>

cc L97.824   Non-pressure chronic ulcer of other part of <u>left</u> lower leg <u>with necrosis of bone</u>

cc L97.829   Non-pressure chronic ulcer of other part of <u>left</u> lower leg with <u>unspecified</u> severity

L97.9-   <u>Non-pressure chronic ulcer</u> of <u>unspecified part of lower leg</u>

L97.90- Non-pressure chronic ulcer of <u>unspecified part of</u> <u>unspecified lower leg</u>

cc L97.901   Non-pressure chronic ulcer of unspecified part of <u>unspecified</u> lower leg limited to <u>breakdown of skin</u>

cc L97.902   Non-pressure chronic ulcer of unspecified part of <u>unspecified</u> lower leg <u>with fat layer exposed</u>

cc L97.903   Non-pressure chronic ulcer of unspecified part of <u>unspecified</u> lower leg <u>with necrosis of muscle</u>

cc L97.904   Non-pressure chronic ulcer of unspecified part of <u>unspecified</u> lower leg <u>with necrosis of bone</u>

cc L97.909   Non-pressure chronic ulcer of unspecified part of <u>unspecified</u> lower leg with <u>unspecified</u> severity

L97.91- Non-pressure chronic ulcer of <u>unspecified part of</u> <u>right</u> lower leg

cc L97.911   Non-pressure chronic ulcer of unspecified part of <u>right</u> lower leg limited to <u>breakdown of skin</u>

cc L97.912   Non-pressure chronic ulcer of unspecified part of <u>right</u> lower leg <u>with fat layer exposed</u>

cc L97.913   Non-pressure chronic ulcer of unspecified part of <u>right</u> lower leg <u>with necrosis of muscle</u>

cc L97.914   Non-pressure chronic ulcer of unspecified part of <u>right</u> lower leg <u>with necrosis of bone</u>

cc L97.919   Non-pressure chronic ulcer of unspecified part of <u>right</u> lower leg with <u>unspecified</u> severity

L97.92- Non-pressure chronic ulcer of <u>unspecified part of</u> <u>left</u> lower leg

cc L97.921   Non-pressure chronic ulcer of unspecified part of <u>left</u> lower leg limited to <u>breakdown of skin</u>

cc L97.922   Non-pressure chronic ulcer of unspecified part of <u>left</u> lower leg <u>with fat layer exposed</u>

cc L97.923   Non-pressure chronic ulcer of unspecified part of <u>left</u> lower leg <u>with necrosis of muscle</u>

cc L97.924   Non-pressure chronic ulcer of unspecified part of <u>left</u> lower leg <u>with necrosis of bone</u>

cc L97.929   Non-pressure chronic ulcer of unspecified part of <u>left</u> lower leg with <u>unspecified</u> severity

L98-   Other disorders of skin and subcutaneous tissue, <u>not elsewhere classified</u>

L98.0   **Pyogenic granuloma** — A fungating, pedunculated growth of the skin in which the granulations consist of masses of pyogenic organisms.

Excludes ❷: *pyogenic granuloma of gingiva (K06.8)*
     pyogenic granuloma of maxillary alveolar ridge (K04.5)
     pyogenic granuloma of oral mucosa (K13.4)

L98.1   **Factitial dermatitis** — Self-inflicted skin lesions.

Neurotic excoriation

Excludes 1:   *excoriation (skin-picking) disorder (F42.4)*

L98.2   **Febrile neutrophilic dermatosis [Sweet]** — A reactive skin disorder characterized by tender papules that develop into plaques and fever.

cc **L98.3**   **Eosinophilic cellulitis [Wells]** — A granulomatous skin disorder characterized by tender cellulitis-like plaques and eosinophils in the dermis.

L98.4-   <u>Non-pressure chronic ulcer of skin</u>, <u>not elsewhere classified</u> — A localized, inflammatory, necrotic skin defect that develops slowly and persists over a period of time that is NOT of the lower extermity and that is NOT caused by prolonged pressure at the site.

Chronic ulcer of skin NOS
Tropical ulcer NOS
Ulcer of skin NOS

Excludes ❷: *pressure ulcer (pressure area) (L89.-)*
     gangrene (I96)
     skin infections (L00-L08)
     specific infections classified to A00-B99
     ulcer of lower limb NEC (L97.-)
     varicose ulcer (I83.0-I82.2)

L98.41- Non-pressure chronic ulcer of <u>buttock</u>

L98.411   Non-pressure chronic ulcer of buttock limited to <u>breakdown of skin</u>

L98.412   Non-pressure chronic ulcer of buttock <u>with fat layer exposed</u>

L98.413   Non-pressure chronic ulcer of buttock <u>with necrosis of muscle</u>

L98.414   Non-pressure chronic ulcer of buttock <u>with necrosis of bone</u>

L98.419   Non-pressure chronic ulcer of buttock with <u>unspecified</u> severity

L 9 7 - L 9 8

Excludes 1: = NOT CODED HERE! (Do not code both)   *Excludes ❷:* = Not Included Here

L98.42- Non-pressure chronic ulcer of <u>back</u>

L98.421 Non-pressure chronic ulcer of back limited to <u>breakdown of skin</u>

L98.422 Non-pressure chronic ulcer of back <u>with fat layer exposed</u>

L98.423 Non-pressure chronic ulcer of back <u>with necrosis of muscle</u>

L98.424 Non-pressure chronic ulcer of back <u>with necrosis of bone</u>

L98.429 Non-pressure chronic ulcer of back with <u>unspecified</u> severity

L98.49- Non-pressure chronic ulcer of skin of <u>other sites</u>
Non-pressure chronic ulcer of skin NOS

L98.491 Non-pressure chronic ulcer of skin of <u>other sites</u> limited to <u>breakdown of skin</u>

L98.492 Non-pressure chronic ulcer of skin of <u>other sites</u> <u>with fat layer exposed</u>

L98.493 Non-pressure chronic ulcer of skin of <u>other sites</u> <u>with necrosis of muscle</u>

L98.494 Non-pressure chronic ulcer of skin of <u>other sites</u> <u>with necrosis of bone</u>

L98.499 Non-pressure chronic ulcer of skin of <u>other sites</u> with <u>unspecified</u> severity

L98.5 **Mucinosis of the skin** — A skin disorder characterized by the abnormal accumulation of mucin in the skin.
Focal mucinosis
Lichen myxedematosus
Reticular erythematous mucinosis
Excludes 1: *focal oral mucinosis (K13.79)*
myxedema (E03.9)

L98.6 **Other infiltrative disorders of the skin and subcutaneous tissue**
Excludes 1: *hyalinosis cutis et mucosae (E78.89)*

L98.7 **Excessive and redundant skin and subcutaneous tissue**
Loose or sagging skin following bariatric surgery weight loss
Loose or sagging skin following dietary weight loss
Loose or sagging skin, NOS
Excludes ❷: *acquired excess or redundant skin of eyelid (H02.3-)*
congenital excess or redundant skin of eyelid (Q10.3)
skin changes due to chronic exposure to nonionizing radiation (L57.-)

L98.8 **Other specified disorders of the skin and subcutaneous tissue**
AHA 13:2Q:p32 – Acrokeratosis paraneoplastica

L98.9 **Disorder of the skin and subcutaneous tissue, unspecified**

L99 **Other disorders of skin and subcutaneous tissue in diseases classified elsewhere** — [Not Allowed as PDX]
Code first underlying disease, such as:
Amyloidosis (E85.-)
Excludes 1: *skin disorders in diabetes (E08-E13 with .62)*
skin disorders in gonorrhea (A54.89)
skin disorders in syphilis (A51.31, A52.79)

L98 - L99

Chapter 13 – Diseases of the musculoskeletal system and connective tissue (M00-M99)

Note: Use an external cause code following the code for the musculoskeletal condition, if applicable, to identify the cause of the musculoskeletal condition

Excludes ❷: *arthropathic psoriasis (L40.5-)*
certain conditions originating in the perinatal period (P04-P96)
certain infectious and parasitic diseases (A00-B99)
compartment syndrome (traumatic) (T79.A-)
complications of pregnancy, childbirth and the puerperium (O00-O9A)
congenital malformations, deformations, and chromosomal abnormalities (Q00-Q99)
endocrine, nutritional and metabolic diseases (E00-E88)
injury, poisoning and certain other consequences of external causes (S00-T88)
neoplasms (C00-D49)
symptoms, signs and abnormal clinical and laboratory findings, not elsewhere classified (R00-R94)

This chapter contains the following blocks:

M00-M02	Infectious arthropathies
M04	Autoinflammatory syndromes
M05-M14	Inflammatory polyarthropathies
M15-M19	Osteoarthritis
M20-M25	Other joint disorders
M26-M27	Dentofacial anomalies [including malocclusion] and other disorders of jaw
M30-M36	Systemic connective tissue disorders
M40-M43	Deforming dorsopathies
M45-M49	Spondylopathies
M50-M54	Other dorsopathies
M60-M63	Disorders of muscles
M65-M67	Disorders of synovium and tendon
M70-M79	Other soft tissue disorders
M80-M85	Disorders of bone density and structure
M86-M90	Other osteopathies
M91-M94	Chondropathies
M95	Other disorders of the musculoskeletal system and connective tissue
M96	Intraoperative and postprocedural complications and disorders of musculoskeletal system, not elsewhere classified
M97	Periprosthetic fracture around internal prosthetic joint
M99	Biomechanical lesions, not elsewhere classified

Chapter-Specific Coding Guidelines

C. Chapter-Specific Coding Guidelines
In addition to general coding guidelines, there are guidelines for specific diagnoses and/or conditions in the classification. Unless otherwise indicated, these guidelines apply to all health care settings. Please refer to Section II for guidelines on the selection of principal diagnosis.

13. Chapter 13: Diseases of the Musculoskeletal System and Connective Tissue (M00-M99)

a. Site and laterality
Most of the codes within Chapter 13 have site and laterality designations. The site represents the bone, joint or the muscle involved. For some conditions where more than one bone, joint or muscle is usually involved, such as osteoarthritis, there is a "multiple sites" code available. For categories where no multiple site code is provided and more than one bone, joint or muscle is involved, multiple codes should be used to indicate the different sites involved.

1) Bone versus joint
For certain conditions, the bone may be affected at the upper or lower end, (e.g., avascular necrosis of bone, M87, Osteoporosis, M80, M81). Though the portion of the bone affected may be at the joint, the site designation will be the bone, not the joint.

b. Acute traumatic versus chronic or recurrent musculoskeletal conditions
Many musculoskeletal conditions are a result of previous injury or trauma to a site, or are recurrent conditions. Bone, joint or muscle conditions that are the result of a healed injury are usually found in chapter 13. Recurrent bone, joint or muscle conditions are also usually found in chapter 13. Any current, acute injury should be coded to the appropriate injury code from chapter 19. Chronic or recurrent conditions should generally be coded with a code from chapter 13. If it is difficult to determine from the documentation in the record which code is best to describe a condition, query the provider.

c. Coding of Pathologic Fractures
7th character A is for use as long as the patient is receiving active treatment for the fracture. ~~Examples of active treatment are: surgical treatment, emergency department encounter, evaluation and continuing treatment by the same or a different physician.~~ While the patient may be seen by a new or different provider over the course of treatment for a pathological fracture, assignment of the 7th character is based on whether the patient is undergoing active treatment and not whether the provider is seeing the patient for the first time.

7th character D is to be used for encounters after the patient has completed active treatment. The other 7th characters, listed under each subcategory in the Tabular List, are to be used for subsequent encounters for routine care of fractures during the healing and recovery phase as well as treatment of problems associated with the healing, such as malunions, nonunions, and sequelae.

Care for complications of surgical treatment for fracture repairs during the healing or recovery phase should be coded with the appropriate complication codes.

See Section I.C.19. Coding of traumatic fractures.

d. Osteoporosis
Osteoporosis is a systemic condition, meaning that all bones of the musculoskeletal system are affected. Therefore, site is not a component of the codes under category M81, Osteoporosis without current pathological fracture. The site codes under category M80, Osteoporosis with current pathological fracture, identify the site of the fracture, not the osteoporosis.

1) Osteoporosis without pathological fracture
Category M81, Osteoporosis without current pathological fracture, is for use for patients with osteoporosis who do not currently have a pathologic fracture due to the osteoporosis, even if they have had a fracture in the past. For patients with a history of osteoporosis fractures, status code Z87.310, Personal history of (healed) osteoporosis fracture, should follow the code from M81.

2) Osteoporosis with current pathological fracture
Category M80, Osteoporosis with current pathological fracture, is for patients who have a current pathologic fracture at the time of an encounter. The codes under M80 identify the site of the fracture. A code from category M80, not a traumatic fracture code, should be used for any patient with known osteoporosis who suffers a fracture, even if the patient had a minor fall or trauma, if that fall or trauma would not usually break a normal, healthy bone.

Arthropathies (M00-M25)

Includes: Disorders affecting predominantly peripheral (limb) joints

Infectious arthropathies (M00-M02)

Note: This block comprises arthropathies due to microbiological agents. Distinction is made between the following types of etiological relationship:
  a) **direct infection of joint**, where organisms invade synovial tissue and microbial antigen is present in the joint;
  b) **indirect infection**, which may be of two types: a reactive arthropathy, where microbial infection of the body is established but neither organisms nor antigens can be identified in the joint, and a postinfective arthropathy, where microbial antigen is present but recovery of an organism is inconstant and evidence of local multiplication is lacking.

M00- Pyogenic arthritis — An acute inflammation within the joint with pus formation that is due to infection by microorganisms.

M00.0- Staphylococcal arthritis and polyarthritis — A form caused by staphylococcal microorganisms.
Use additional code (B95.61-B95.8) to identify bacterial agent
Excludes ❷: *infection and inflammatory reaction due to internal joint prosthesis (T84.5-)*

cc **M00.00 Staphylococcal arthritis, unspecified joint**
M00.01-Staphylococcal arthritis, shoulder
  cc **M00.011   Staphylococcal arthritis, right shoulder**
  cc **M00.012   Staphylococcal arthritis, left shoulder**
  cc **M00.019   Staphylococcal arthritis, unspecified shoulder**
M00.02-Staphylococcal arthritis, elbow
  cc **M00.021   Staphylococcal arthritis, right elbow**
  cc **M00.022   Staphylococcal arthritis, left elbow**
  cc **M00.029   Staphylococcal arthritis, unspecified elbow**
M00.03-Staphylococcal arthritis, wrist
      Staphylococcal arthritis of carpal bones
  cc **M00.031   Staphylococcal arthritis, right wrist**

M00 – M00

cc M00.032 Staphylococcal arthritis, <u>left</u> wrist
cc M00.039 Staphylococcal arthritis, <u>unspecified</u> wrist
M00.04-Staphylococcal arthritis, <u>hand</u>
    Staphylococcal arthritis of metacarpus and phalanges
cc M00.041 Staphylococcal arthritis, <u>right</u> hand
cc M00.042 Staphylococcal arthritis, <u>left</u> hand
cc M00.049 Staphylococcal arthritis, <u>unspecified</u> hand
M00.05-Staphylococcal arthritis, <u>hip</u>
cc M00.051 Staphylococcal arthritis, <u>right</u> hip
cc M00.052 Staphylococcal arthritis, <u>left</u> hip
cc M00.059 Staphylococcal arthritis, <u>unspecified</u> hip
M00.06-Staphylococcal arthritis, <u>knee</u>
cc M00.061 Staphylococcal arthritis, <u>right</u> knee
cc M00.062 Staphylococcal arthritis, <u>left</u> knee
cc M00.069 Staphylococcal arthritis, <u>unspecified</u> knee
M00.07-Staphylococcal arthritis, <u>ankle and foot</u>
    Staphylococcal arthritis, tarsus, metatarsus and phalanges
cc M00.071 Staphylococcal arthritis, <u>right</u> ankle and foot
cc M00.072 Staphylococcal arthritis, <u>left</u> ankle and foot
cc M00.079 Staphylococcal arthritis, <u>unspecified</u> ankle and foot
cc M00.08 Staphylococcal arthritis, <u>vertebrae</u>
cc M00.09 Staphylococcal <u>polyarthritis</u>
M00.1- <u>Pneumococcal</u> arthritis and polyarthritis — A form caused by pneumococcal microorganisms.
cc M00.10 Pneumococcal arthritis, <u>unspecified</u> joint
M00.11-Pneumococcal arthritis, <u>shoulder</u>
cc M00.111 Pneumococcal arthritis, <u>right</u> shoulder
cc M00.112 Pneumococcal arthritis, <u>left</u> shoulder
cc M00.119 Pneumococcal arthritis, <u>unspecified</u> shoulder
M00.12-Pneumococcal arthritis, <u>elbow</u>
cc M00.121 Pneumococcal arthritis, <u>right</u> elbow
cc M00.122 Pneumococcal arthritis, <u>left</u> elbow
cc M00.129 Pneumococcal arthritis, <u>unspecified</u> elbow
M00.13-Pneumococcal arthritis, <u>wrist</u>
    Pneumococcal arthritis of carpal bones
cc M00.131 Pneumococcal arthritis, <u>right</u> wrist
cc M00.132 Pneumococcal arthritis, <u>left</u> wrist
cc M00.139 Pneumococcal arthritis, <u>unspecified</u> wrist
M00.14-Pneumococcal arthritis, <u>hand</u>
    Pneumococcal arthritis of metacarpus and phalanges
cc M00.141 Pneumococcal arthritis, <u>right</u> hand
cc M00.142 Pneumococcal arthritis, <u>left</u> hand
cc M00.149 Pneumococcal arthritis, <u>unspecified</u> hand
M00.15-Pneumococcal arthritis, <u>hip</u>
cc M00.151 Pneumococcal arthritis, <u>right</u> hip
cc M00.152 Pneumococcal arthritis, <u>left</u> hip
cc M00.159 Pneumococcal arthritis, <u>unspecified</u> hip
M00.16-Pneumococcal arthritis, <u>knee</u>
cc M00.161 Pneumococcal arthritis, <u>right</u> knee
cc M00.162 Pneumococcal arthritis, <u>left</u> knee
cc M00.169 Pneumococcal arthritis, <u>unspecified</u> knee
M00.17-Pneumococcal arthritis, <u>ankle and foot</u>
    Pneumococcal arthritis, tarsus, metatarsus and phalanges
cc M00.171 Pneumococcal arthritis, <u>right</u> ankle and foot
cc M00.172 Pneumococcal arthritis, <u>left</u> ankle and foot
cc M00.179 Pneumococcal arthritis, <u>unspecified</u> ankle and foot
cc M00.18 Pneumococcal arthritis, <u>vertebrae</u>
cc M00.19 Pneumococcal <u>polyarthritis</u>
M00.2- <u>Other streptococcal</u> arthritis and polyarthritis — A form caused by streptococcal microorganisms.
    Use additional code (B95.0-B95.2, B95.4-B95.5) to identify bacterial agent
cc M00.20 Other streptococcal arthritis, <u>unspecified</u> joint
M00.21-Other streptococcal arthritis, <u>shoulder</u>
cc M00.211 Other streptococcal arthritis, <u>right</u> shoulder
cc M00.212 Other streptococcal arthritis, <u>left</u> shoulder

cc M00.219 Other streptococcal arthritis, <u>unspecified</u> shoulder
M00.22-Other streptococcal arthritis, <u>elbow</u>
cc M00.221 Other streptococcal arthritis, <u>right</u> elbow
cc M00.222 Other streptococcal arthritis, <u>left</u> elbow
cc M00.229 Other streptococcal arthritis, <u>unspecified</u> elbow
M00.23-Other streptococcal arthritis, <u>wrist</u>
    Other streptococcal arthritis of carpal bones
cc M00.231 Other streptococcal arthritis, <u>right</u> wrist
cc M00.232 Other streptococcal arthritis, <u>left</u> wrist
cc M00.239 Other streptococcal arthritis, <u>unspecified</u> wrist
M00.24-Other streptococcal arthritis, <u>hand</u>
    Other streptococcal arthritis metacarpus and phalanges
cc M00.241 Other streptococcal arthritis, <u>right</u> hand
cc M00.242 Other streptococcal arthritis, <u>left</u> hand
cc M00.249 Other streptococcal arthritis, <u>unspecified</u> hand
M00.25-Other streptococcal arthritis, <u>hip</u>
cc M00.251 Other streptococcal arthritis, <u>right</u> hip
cc M00.252 Other streptococcal arthritis, <u>left</u> hip
cc M00.259 Other streptococcal arthritis, <u>unspecified</u> hip
M00.26-Other streptococcal arthritis, <u>knee</u>
cc M00.261 Other streptococcal arthritis, <u>right</u> knee
cc M00.262 Other streptococcal arthritis, <u>left</u> knee
cc M00.269 Other streptococcal arthritis, <u>unspecified</u> knee
M00.27-Other streptococcal arthritis, <u>ankle and foot</u>
    Other streptococcal arthritis, tarsus, metatarsus and phalanges
cc M00.271 Other streptococcal arthritis, <u>right</u> ankle and foot
cc M00.272 Other streptococcal arthritis, <u>left</u> ankle and foot
cc M00.279 Other streptococcal arthritis, <u>unspecified</u> ankle and foot
cc M00.28 Other streptococcal arthritis, <u>vertebrae</u>
cc M00.29 Other streptococcal <u>polyarthritis</u>
M00.8- Arthritis and polyarthritis <u>due to other bacteria</u>
    Use additional code (B96) to identify bacteria
cc M00.80 Arthritis due to other bacteria, <u>unspecified</u> joint
M00.81-Arthritis due to other bacteria, <u>shoulder</u>
cc M00.811 Arthritis due to other bacteria, <u>right</u> shoulder
cc M00.812 Arthritis due to other bacteria, <u>left</u> shoulder
cc M00.819 Arthritis due to other bacteria, <u>unspecified</u> shoulder
M00.82-Arthritis due to other bacteria, <u>elbow</u>
cc M00.821 Arthritis due to other bacteria, <u>right</u> elbow
cc M00.822 Arthritis due to other bacteria, <u>left</u> elbow
cc M00.829 Arthritis due to other bacteria, <u>unspecified</u> elbow
M00.83-Arthritis due to other bacteria, <u>wrist</u>
    Arthritis due to other bacteria, carpal bones
cc M00.831 Arthritis due to other bacteria, <u>right</u> wrist
cc M00.832 Arthritis due to other bacteria, <u>left</u> wrist
cc M00.839 Arthritis due to other bacteria, <u>unspecified</u> wrist
M00.84-Arthritis due to other bacteria, <u>hand</u>
    Arthritis due to other bacteria, metacarpus and phalanges
cc M00.841 Arthritis due to other bacteria, <u>right</u> hand
cc M00.842 Arthritis due to other bacteria, <u>left</u> hand
cc M00.849 Arthritis due to other bacteria, <u>unspecified</u> hand
M00.85-Arthritis due to other bacteria, <u>hip</u>
cc M00.851 Arthritis due to other bacteria, <u>right</u> hip
cc M00.852 Arthritis due to other bacteria, <u>left</u> hip
cc M00.859 Arthritis due to other bacteria, <u>unspecified</u> hip
M00.86-Arthritis due to other bacteria, <u>knee</u>
cc M00.861 Arthritis due to other bacteria, <u>right</u> knee
cc M00.862 Arthritis due to other bacteria, <u>left</u> knee
cc M00.869 Arthritis due to other bacteria, <u>unspecified</u> knee
M00.87-Arthritis due to other bacteria, <u>ankle and foot</u>
    Arthritis due to other bacteria, tarsus, metatarsus, and phalanges
cc M00.871 Arthritis due to other bacteria, <u>right</u> ankle and foot
cc M00.872 Arthritis due to other bacteria, <u>left</u> ankle and foot

M O 0 - M O 0

cc **M00.879** Arthritis due to other bacteria, <u>unspecified</u> ankle and foot

cc **M00.88** Arthritis due to other bacteria, <u>vertebrae</u>

cc **M00.89** <u>Polyarthritis</u> due to other bacteria

cc **M00.9** Pyogenic arthritis, <u>unspecified</u>
Infective arthritis NOS

M01- Direct infections of joint <u>in infectious and parasitic diseases classified elsewhere</u> — An acute inflammation within the joint caused by the infectious or parasitic organism in an underlying disease.
Code first underlying disease, such as:
Leprosy [Hansen's disease] (A30.-)
Mycoses (B35-B49)
O'nyong-nyong fever (A92.1)
Paratyphoid fever (A01.1-A01.4)
Excludes 1:   *arthropathy in Lyme disease (A69.23)*
gonococcal arthritis (A54.42)
meningococcal arthritis (A39.83)
mumps arthritis (B26.85)
postinfective arthropathy (M02.-)
postmeningococcal arthritis (A39.84)
reactive arthritis (M02.3-)
rubella arthritis (B06.82)
sarcoidosis arthritis (D86.86)
typhoid fever arthritis (A01.04)
tuberculosis arthritis (A18.01-A18.02)

M01.x- Direct infection of joint in infectious and parasitic diseases classified elsewhere

cc **M01.x0** Direct infection of <u>unspecified</u> joint in infectious and parasitic diseases classified elsewhere — [Not Allowed as PDX]

M01.x1- Direct infection of <u>shoulder</u> joint in infectious and parasitic diseases classified elsewhere

cc **M01.x11** Direct infection of <u>right</u> shoulder in infectious and parasitic diseases classified elsewhere — [Not Allowed as PDX]

cc **M01.x12** Direct infection of <u>left</u> shoulder in infectious and parasitic diseases classified elsewhere — [Not Allowed as PDX]

cc **M01.x19** Direct infection of <u>unspecified</u> shoulder in infectious and parasitic diseases classified elsewhere — [Not Allowed as PDX]

M01.x2- Direct infection of <u>elbow</u> in infectious and parasitic diseases classified elsewhere

cc **M01.x21** Direct infection of <u>right</u> elbow in infectious and parasitic diseases classified elsewhere — [Not Allowed as PDX]

cc **M01.x22** Direct infection of <u>left</u> elbow in infectious and parasitic diseases classified elsewhere — [Not Allowed as PDX]

cc **M01.x29** Direct infection of <u>unspecified</u> elbow in infectious and parasitic diseases classified elsewhere — [Not Allowed as PDX]

M01.x3- Direct infection of <u>wrist</u> in infectious and parasitic diseases classified elsewhere
Direct infection of carpal bones in infectious and parasitic diseases classified elsewhere

cc **M01.x31** Direct infection of <u>right</u> wrist in infectious and parasitic diseases classified elsewhere — [Not Allowed as PDX]

cc **M01.x32** Direct infection of <u>left</u> wrist in infectious and parasitic diseases classified elsewhere — [Not Allowed as PDX]

cc **M01.x39** Direct infection of <u>unspecified</u> wrist in infectious and parasitic diseases classified elsewhere — [Not Allowed as PDX]

M01.x4- Direct infection of <u>hand</u> in infectious and parasitic diseases classified elsewhere
Direct infection of metacarpus and phalanges in infectious and parasitic diseases classified elsewhere

cc **M01.x41** Direct infection of <u>right</u> hand in infectious and parasitic diseases classified elsewhere — [Not Allowed as PDX]

cc **M01.x42** Direct infection of <u>left</u> hand in infectious and parasitic diseases classified elsewhere — [Not Allowed as PDX]

cc **M01.x49** Direct infection of <u>unspecified</u> hand in infectious and parasitic diseases classified elsewhere — [Not Allowed as PDX]

M01.x5- Direct infection of <u>hip</u> in infectious and parasitic diseases classified elsewhere

cc **M01.x51** Direct infection of <u>right</u> hip in infectious and parasitic diseases classified elsewhere — [Not Allowed as PDX]

cc **M01.x52** Direct infection of <u>left</u> hip in infectious and parasitic diseases classified elsewhere — [Not Allowed as PDX]

cc **M01.x59** Direct infection of <u>unspecified</u> hip in infectious and parasitic diseases classified elsewhere — [Not Allowed as PDX]

M01.x6- Direct infection of <u>knee</u> in infectious and parasitic diseases classified elsewhere

cc **M01.x61** Direct infection of <u>right</u> knee in infectious and parasitic diseases classified elsewhere — [Not Allowed as PDX]

cc **M01.x62** Direct infection of <u>left</u> knee in infectious and parasitic diseases classified elsewhere — [Not Allowed as PDX]

cc **M01.x69** Direct infection of <u>unspecified</u> knee in infectious and parasitic diseases classified elsewhere — [Not Allowed as PDX]

M01.x7- Direct infection of <u>ankle and foot</u> in infectious and parasitic diseases classified elsewhere
Direct infection of tarsus, metatarsus and phalanges in infectious and parasitic diseases classified elsewhere

cc **M01.x71** Direct infection of <u>right</u> ankle and foot in infectious and parasitic diseases classified elsewhere — [Not Allowed as PDX]

cc **M01.x72** Direct infection of <u>left</u> ankle and foot in infectious and parasitic diseases classified elsewhere — [Not Allowed as PDX]

cc **M01.x79** Direct infection of <u>unspecified</u> ankle and foot in infectious and parasitic diseases classified elsewhere — [Not Allowed as PDX]

cc **M01.x8** Direct infection of <u>vertebrae</u> in infectious and parasitic diseases classified elsewhere — [Not Allowed as PDX]

cc **M01.x9** Direct infection of <u>multiple joints</u> in infectious and parasitic diseases classified elsewhere — [Not Allowed as PDX]

M02- <u>Postinfective and reactive arthropathies</u> — Inflammation of the joint following an infection or as a reactive response to an infection elsewhere in the body.
Code first underlying disease, such as:
Congenital syphilis [Clutton's joints] (A50.5)
Enteritis due to Yersinia enterocolitica (A04.6)
Infective endocarditis (I33.0)
Viral hepatitis (B15-B19)
Excludes 1:   *Behçet's disease (M35.2)*
direct infections of joint in infectious and parasitic diseases classified elsewhere (M01.-)
postmeningococcal arthritis (A39.84)
mumps arthritis (B26.85)
rubella arthritis (B06.82)
syphilis arthritis (late) (A52.77)
rheumatic fever (I00)
tabetic arthropathy [Charcot's] (A52.16)

M02.0- Arthropathy <u>following intestinal bypass</u> — A form following an intestinal bypass surgery.

M02.00 Arthropathy following intestinal bypass, <u>unspecified</u> site

M02.01- Arthropathy following intestinal bypass, <u>shoulder</u>

M02.011 Arthropathy following intestinal bypass, <u>right</u> shoulder

M02.012 Arthropathy following intestinal bypass, <u>left</u> shoulder

M02.019 Arthropathy following intestinal bypass, <u>unspecified</u> shoulder

M00 – M02

M02.02- Arthropathy following intestinal bypass, <u>elbow</u>
  M02.021 Arthropathy following intestinal bypass, <u>right</u> elbow
  M02.022 Arthropathy following intestinal bypass, <u>left</u> elbow
  M02.029 Arthropathy following intestinal bypass, <u>unspecified</u> elbow
M02.03- Arthropathy following intestinal bypass, <u>wrist</u>
  Arthropathy following intestinal bypass, carpal bones
  M02.031 Arthropathy following intestinal bypass, <u>right</u> wrist
  M02.032 Arthropathy following intestinal bypass, <u>left</u> wrist
  M02.039 Arthropathy following intestinal bypass, <u>unspecified</u> wrist
M02.04- Arthropathy following intestinal bypass, <u>hand</u>
  Arthropathy following intestinal bypass, metacarpals and phalanges
  M02.041 Arthropathy following intestinal bypass, <u>right</u> hand
  M02.042 Arthropathy following intestinal bypass, <u>left</u> hand
  M02.049 Arthropathy following intestinal bypass, <u>unspecified</u> hand
M02.05- Arthropathy following intestinal bypass, <u>hip</u>
  M02.051 Arthropathy following intestinal bypass, <u>right</u> hip
  M02.052 Arthropathy following intestinal bypass, <u>left</u> hip
  M02.059 Arthropathy following intestinal bypass, <u>unspecified</u> hip
M02.06- Arthropathy following intestinal bypass, <u>knee</u>
  M02.061 Arthropathy following intestinal bypass, <u>right</u> knee
  M02.062 Arthropathy following intestinal bypass, <u>left</u> knee
  M02.069 Arthropathy following intestinal bypass, <u>unspecified</u> knee
M02.07- Arthropathy following intestinal bypass, <u>ankle and foot</u>
  Arthropathy following intestinal bypass, tarsus, metatarsus and phalanges
  M02.071 Arthropathy following intestinal bypass, <u>right</u> ankle and foot
  M02.072 Arthropathy following intestinal bypass, <u>left</u> ankle and foot
  M02.079 Arthropathy following intestinal bypass, <u>unspecified</u> ankle and foot
  M02.08 Arthropathy following intestinal bypass, <u>vertebrae</u>
  M02.09 Arthropathy following intestinal bypass, <u>multiple sites</u>
M02.1- <u>Postdysenteric</u> arthropathy — A form following a dysentery infection.
cc M02.10 Postdysenteric arthropathy, <u>unspecified</u> site
M02.11- Postdysenteric arthropathy, <u>shoulder</u>
  cc M02.111 Postdysenteric arthropathy, <u>right</u> shoulder
  cc M02.112 Postdysenteric arthropathy, <u>left</u> shoulder
  cc M02.119 Postdysenteric arthropathy, <u>unspecified</u> shoulder
M02.12- Postdysenteric arthropathy, <u>elbow</u>
  cc M02.121 Postdysenteric arthropathy, <u>right</u> elbow
  cc M02.122 Postdysenteric arthropathy, <u>left</u> elbow
  cc M02.129 Postdysenteric arthropathy, <u>unspecified</u> elbow
M02.13- Postdysenteric arthropathy, <u>wrist</u>
  Postdysenteric arthropathy, carpal bones
  cc M02.131 Postdysenteric arthropathy, <u>right</u> wrist
  cc M02.132 Postdysenteric arthropathy, <u>left</u> wrist
  cc M02.139 Postdysenteric arthropathy, <u>unspecified</u> wrist
M02.14- Postdysenteric arthropathy, <u>hand</u>
  Postdysenteric arthropathy, metacarpus and phalanges
  cc M02.141 Postdysenteric arthropathy, <u>right</u> hand
  cc M02.142 Postdysenteric arthropathy, <u>left</u> hand
  cc M02.149 Postdysenteric arthropathy, <u>unspecified</u> hand
M02.15- Postdysenteric arthropathy, <u>hip</u>
  cc M02.151 Postdysenteric arthropathy, <u>right</u> hip
  cc M02.152 Postdysenteric arthropathy, <u>left</u> hip
  cc M02.159 Postdysenteric arthropathy, <u>unspecified</u> hip
M02.16- Postdysenteric arthropathy, <u>knee</u>
  cc M02.161 Postdysenteric arthropathy, <u>right</u> knee
  cc M02.162 Postdysenteric arthropathy, <u>left</u> knee

cc M02.169 Postdysenteric arthropathy, <u>unspecified</u> knee
M02.17- Postdysenteric arthropathy, <u>ankle and foot</u>
  Postdysenteric arthropathy, tarsus, metatarsus and phalanges
  cc M02.171 Postdysenteric arthropathy, <u>right</u> ankle and foot
  cc M02.172 Postdysenteric arthropathy, <u>left</u> ankle and foot
  cc M02.179 Postdysenteric arthropathy, <u>unspecified</u> ankle and foot
cc M02.18 Postdysenteric arthropathy, <u>vertebrae</u>
cc M02.19 Postdysenteric arthropathy, <u>multiple sites</u>
M02.2- <u>Postimmunization</u> arthropathy — A form following an immunization.
  M02.20 Postimmunization arthropathy, <u>unspecified</u> site
M02.21- Postimmunization arthropathy, <u>shoulder</u>
  M02.211 Postimmunization arthropathy, <u>right</u> shoulder
  M02.212 Postimmunization arthropathy, <u>left</u> shoulder
  M02.219 Postimmunization arthropathy, <u>unspecified</u> shoulder
M02.22- Postimmunization arthropathy, <u>elbow</u>
  M02.221 Postimmunization arthropathy, <u>right</u> elbow
  M02.222 Postimmunization arthropathy, <u>left</u> elbow
  M02.229 Postimmunization arthropathy, <u>unspecified</u> elbow
M02.23- Postimmunization arthropathy, <u>wrist</u>
  Postimmunization arthropathy, carpal bones
  M02.231 Postimmunization arthropathy, <u>right</u> wrist
  M02.232 Postimmunization arthropathy, <u>left</u> wrist
  M02.239 Postimmunization arthropathy, <u>unspecified</u> wrist
M02.24- Postimmunization arthropathy, <u>hand</u>
  Postimmunization arthropathy, metacarpus and phalanges
  M02.241 Postimmunization arthropathy, <u>right</u> hand
  M02.242 Postimmunization arthropathy, <u>left</u> hand
  M02.249 Postimmunization arthropathy, <u>unspecified</u> hand
M02.25- Postimmunization arthropathy, <u>hip</u>
  M02.251 Postimmunization arthropathy, <u>right</u> hip
  M02.252 Postimmunization arthropathy, <u>left</u> hip
  M02.259 Postimmunization arthropathy, <u>unspecified</u> hip
M02.26- Postimmunization arthropathy, <u>knee</u>
  M02.261 Postimmunization arthropathy, <u>right</u> knee
  M02.262 Postimmunization arthropathy, <u>left</u> knee
  M02.269 Postimmunization arthropathy, <u>unspecified</u> knee
M02.27- Postimmunization arthropathy, <u>ankle and foot</u>
  Postimmunization arthropathy, tarsus, metatarsus and phalanges
  M02.271 Postimmunization arthropathy, <u>right</u> ankle and foot
  M02.272 Postimmunization arthropathy, <u>left</u> ankle and foot
  M02.279 Postimmunization arthropathy, <u>unspecified</u> ankle and foot
  M02.28 Postimmunization arthropathy, <u>vertebrae</u>
  M02.29 Postimmunization arthropathy, <u>multiple sites</u>
M02.3- <u>Reiter's disease</u> — An autoimmune form that is characterized by inflammation of the large joints, eyes, and genitals or urinary tract.
  Reactive arthritis
cc M02.30 Reiter's disease, <u>unspecified</u> site
M02.31- Reiter's disease, <u>shoulder</u>
  cc M02.311 Reiter's disease, <u>right</u> shoulder
  cc M02.312 Reiter's disease, <u>left</u> shoulder
  cc M02.319 Reiter's disease, <u>unspecified</u> shoulder
M02.32- Reiter's disease, <u>elbow</u>
  cc M02.321 Reiter's disease, <u>right</u> elbow
  cc M02.322 Reiter's disease, <u>left</u> elbow
  cc M02.329 Reiter's disease, <u>unspecified</u> elbow
M02.33- Reiter's disease, <u>wrist</u>
  Reiter's disease, carpal bones
  cc M02.331 Reiter's disease, <u>right</u> wrist
  cc M02.332 Reiter's disease, <u>left</u> wrist
  cc M02.339 Reiter's disease, <u>unspecified</u> wrist

M02-M02

M02.34-Reiter's disease, <u>hand</u>
Reiter's disease, metacarpus and phalanges
cc **M02.341** Reiter's disease, <u>right</u> hand
cc **M02.342** Reiter's disease, <u>left</u> hand
cc **M02.349** Reiter's disease, <u>unspecified</u> hand

M02.35-Reiter's disease, <u>hip</u>
cc **M02.351** Reiter's disease, <u>right</u> hip
cc **M02.352** Reiter's disease, <u>left</u> hip
cc **M02.359** Reiter's disease, <u>unspecified</u> hip

M02.36-Reiter's disease, <u>knee</u>
cc **M02.361** Reiter's disease, <u>right</u> knee
cc **M02.362** Reiter's disease, <u>left</u> knee
cc **M02.369** Reiter's disease, <u>unspecified</u> knee

M02.37-Reiter's disease, <u>ankle and foot</u>
Reiter's disease, tarsus, metatarsus and phalanges
cc **M02.371** Reiter's disease, <u>right</u> ankle and foot
cc **M02.372** Reiter's disease, <u>left</u> ankle and foot
cc **M02.379** Reiter's disease, <u>unspecified</u> ankle and foot
cc **M02.38** Reiter's disease, <u>vertebrae</u>
cc **M02.39** Reiter's disease, <u>multiple sites</u>

M02.8- <u>Other reactive</u> arthropathies
cc **M02.80** Other reactive arthropathies, <u>unspecified</u> site — [Not Allowed as PDX]

M02.81-Other reactive arthropathies, <u>shoulder</u>
cc **M02.811** Other reactive arthropathies, <u>right</u> shoulder — [Not Allowed as PDX]
cc **M02.812** Other reactive arthropathies, <u>left</u> shoulder — [Not Allowed as PDX]
cc **M02.819** Other reactive arthropathies, <u>unspecified</u> shoulder — [Not Allowed as PDX]

M02.82-Other reactive arthropathies, <u>elbow</u>
cc **M02.821** Other reactive arthropathies, <u>right</u> elbow — [Not Allowed as PDX]
cc **M02.822** Other reactive arthropathies, <u>left</u> elbow — [Not Allowed as PDX]
cc **M02.829** Other reactive arthropathies, <u>unspecified</u> elbow — [Not Allowed as PDX]

M02.83-Other reactive arthropathies, <u>wrist</u>
Other reactive arthropathies, carpal bones
cc **M02.831** Other reactive arthropathies, <u>right</u> wrist — [Not Allowed as PDX]
cc **M02.832** Other reactive arthropathies, <u>left</u> wrist — [Not Allowed as PDX]
cc **M02.839** Other reactive arthropathies, <u>unspecified</u> wrist — [Not Allowed as PDX]

M02.84-Other reactive arthropathies, <u>hand</u>
Other reactive arthropathies, metacarpus and phalanges
cc **M02.841** Other reactive arthropathies, <u>right</u> hand — [Not Allowed as PDX]
cc **M02.842** Other reactive arthropathies, <u>left</u> hand — [Not Allowed as PDX]
cc **M02.849** Other reactive arthropathies, <u>unspecified</u> hand — [Not Allowed as PDX]

M02.85-Other reactive arthropathies, <u>hip</u>
cc **M02.851** Other reactive arthropathies, <u>right</u> hip — [Not Allowed as PDX]
cc **M02.852** Other reactive arthropathies, <u>left</u> hip — [Not Allowed as PDX]
cc **M02.859** Other reactive arthropathies, <u>unspecified</u> hip — [Not Allowed as PDX]

M02.86-Other reactive arthropathies, <u>knee</u>
cc **M02.861** Other reactive arthropathies, <u>right</u> knee — [Not Allowed as PDX]
cc **M02.862** Other reactive arthropathies, <u>left</u> knee — [Not Allowed as PDX]
cc **M02.869** Other reactive arthropathies, <u>unspecified</u> knee — [Not Allowed as PDX]

M02.87-Other reactive arthropathies, <u>ankle and foot</u>
Other reactive arthropathies, tarsus, metatarsus and phalanges
cc **M02.871** Other reactive arthropathies, <u>right</u> ankle and foot — [Not Allowed as PDX]
cc **M02.872** Other reactive arthropathies, <u>left</u> ankle and foot — [Not Allowed as PDX]
cc **M02.879** Other reactive arthropathies, <u>unspecified</u> ankle and foot — [Not Allowed as PDX]
cc **M02.88** Other reactive arthropathies, <u>vertebrae</u> — [Not Allowed as PDX]
cc **M02.89** Other reactive arthropathies, <u>multiple sites</u> — [Not Allowed as PDX]
M02.9 Reactive arthropathy, <u>unspecified</u> — [Not Allowed as PDX]

Autoinflammatory syndromes (M04)

M04- <u>Autoinflammatory syndromes</u> — Disorders involving regulation of the immune system that are caused by genetic mutations and are generally characterized by recurrent systemic inflammation, fever, rashes, arthritis, ophthalmic inflammation, headaches, and lymphadenopathy, and some may lead to secondary amyloidosis.
Excludes ❷: Crohn's disease (K50.-)

M04.1 **Periodic fever syndromes** — A form involving recurrent fever episodes.
Familial Mediterranean fever — A form caused by the mutation of the MEFV gene that is characterized by brief episodes of fever, arthritis, rash on the lower legs, and in some cases pleuritis and peritonitis.
Hyperimmunoglobin D syndrome — A form caused by the mutation of the MVK gene that is characterized by episodes of fever, cervical lymphadenopathy, diffuse rash, headache, arthritis, and abdominal pain.
Mevalonate kinase deficiency — A form caused by the mutation of the MVK gene that is characterized by episodes of fever, enlarged spleen, diffuse rash, central nervous system conditions, arthritis, and abdominal pain.
Tumor necrosis factor receptor associated periodic syndrome [TRAPS] — A form caused by the mutation of the TNFRSF1A gene that is characterized by episodes of fever, migrating rash with deep pain under the rash, periorbital edema, myalgia, arthritis, and abdominal and chest pain.

M04.2 **Cryopyrin-associated periodic syndromes** — A form caused by the mutation of the NLRP3 gene that is characterized by recurrent episodes of fever, urticarial rash, arthralgias, non-infectious conjunctivitis, and headaches.
Chronic infantile neurological, cutaneous and articular syndrome [CINCA] — A severe form characterized by an ever-present rash, aseptic meningitis, and papilledema.
Familial cold autoinflammatory syndrome — A milder form triggered by cold exposure.
Familial cold urticaria — A milder form triggered by cold exposure.
Muckle-Wells syndrome — A more severe form with more frequent and prolonged episodes and may include headaches from aseptic meningitis.
Neonatal onset multisystemic inflammatory disorder [NOMID] — A severe form characterized by an ever-present rash, aseptic meningitis, and papilledema.

M04.8 **Other autoinflammatory syndromes**
Blau syndrome — A form caused by the mutation of the NOD2 gene that is characterized by daily intermittent fevers, rash, granulomatosis, arthritis, and uveitis.
Deficiency of interleukin 1 receptor antagonist [DIRA] — A form caused by the mutation of the IR1RN gene that is characterized by a severe pustular rash, osteitis, and joint swelling.
Majeed syndrome — A form caused by the mutation of the LPIN2 gene that is characterized by high fevers, chronic recurrent multifocal osteomyelitis, inflammatory dermatosis, and dyserythropoietic anemia.
Periodic fever, aphthous stomatitis, pharyngitis, and adenopathy syndrome [PFAPA] — A form caused by the mutation of an unknown gene that is characterized by periodic fever, aphthous stomatitis, pharyngitis, and adenopathy.
Pyogenic arthritis, pyoderma gangrenosum, and acne syndrome [PAPA] — A form caused by the mutation of the PSTPIP1 gene that is characterized by periodic non-infectious pyogenic arthritis, pyoderma gangrenosum, and cystic acne.

M04.9 **Autoinflammatory syndrome, unspecified**

M02 I M04

Inflammatory polyarthropathies (M05-M14)

M05- <u>Rheumatoid arthritis with rheumatoid factor</u> — A chronic, systemic autoimmune inflammatory disease characterized by inflammation of the joint structures with resultant crippling deformities that may affect organs throughout the body with the presence of the rheumatoid factor autoantibody in the blood.

Excludes 1:   *juvenile rheumatoid arthritis (M08-)*
rheumatic fever (I00)
rheumatoid arthritis of spine (M45-)

M05.0- <u>Felty's syndrome</u> — A form with an enlarged spleen, abnormally low white blood cell count, and repeated infections.

Rheumatoid arthritis with splenoadenomegaly and leukopenia

M05.00 Felty's syndrome, <u>unspecified</u> site

M05.01- Felty's syndrome, <u>shoulder</u>

  M05.011 Felty's syndrome, <u>right</u> shoulder

  M05.012 Felty's syndrome, <u>left</u> shoulder

  M05.019 Felty's syndrome, <u>unspecified</u> shoulder

M05.02- Felty's syndrome, <u>elbow</u>

  M05.021 Felty's syndrome, <u>right</u> elbow

  M05.022 Felty's syndrome, <u>left</u> elbow

  M05.029 Felty's syndrome, <u>unspecified</u> elbow

M05.03- Felty's syndrome, <u>wrist</u>

  Felty's syndrome, carpal bones

  M05.031 Felty's syndrome, <u>right</u> wrist

  M05.032 Felty's syndrome, <u>left</u> wrist

  M05.039 Felty's syndrome, <u>unspecified</u> wrist

M05.04- Felty's syndrome, <u>hand</u>

  Felty's syndrome, metacarpus and phalanges

  M05.041 Felty's syndrome, <u>right</u> hand

  M05.042 Felty's syndrome, <u>left</u> hand

  M05.049 Felty's syndrome, <u>unspecified</u> hand

M05.05- Felty's syndrome, <u>hip</u>

  M05.051 Felty's syndrome, <u>right</u> hip

  M05.052 Felty's syndrome, <u>left</u> hip

  M05.059 Felty's syndrome, <u>unspecified</u> hip

M05.06- Felty's syndrome, <u>knee</u>

  M05.061 Felty's syndrome, <u>right</u> knee

  M05.062 Felty's syndrome, <u>left</u> knee

  M05.069 Felty's syndrome, <u>unspecified</u> knee

M05.07- Felty's syndrome, <u>ankle and foot</u>

  Felty's syndrome, tarsus, metatarsus and phalanges

  M05.071 Felty's syndrome, <u>right</u> ankle and foot

  M05.072 Felty's syndrome, <u>left</u> ankle and foot

  M05.079 Felty's syndrome, <u>unspecified</u> ankle and foot

M05.09 Felty's syndrome, <u>multiple sites</u>

M05.1- Rheumatoid <u>lung disease</u> with rheumatoid <u>arthritis</u> — A form with pulmonary disorders that may include bronchiolitis, pleural effusion, nodules, and interstitial lung disease.

M05.10 Rheumatoid lung disease with rheumatoid arthritis of <u>unspecified</u> site

M05.11- Rheumatoid lung disease with rheumatoid arthritis of <u>shoulder</u>

  M05.111 Rheumatoid lung disease with rheumatoid arthritis of <u>right</u> shoulder

  M05.112 Rheumatoid lung disease with rheumatoid arthritis of <u>left</u> shoulder

  M05.119 Rheumatoid lung disease with rheumatoid arthritis of <u>unspecified</u> shoulder

M05.12- Rheumatoid lung disease with rheumatoid arthritis of <u>elbow</u>

  M05.121 Rheumatoid lung disease with rheumatoid arthritis of <u>right</u> elbow

  M05.122 Rheumatoid lung disease with rheumatoid arthritis of <u>left</u> elbow

  M05.129 Rheumatoid lung disease with rheumatoid arthritis of <u>unspecified</u> elbow

M05.13- Rheumatoid lung disease with rheumatoid arthritis of <u>wrist</u>

  Rheumatoid lung disease with rheumatoid arthritis, carpal bones

  M05.131 Rheumatoid lung disease with rheumatoid arthritis of <u>right</u> wrist

  M05.132 Rheumatoid lung disease with rheumatoid arthritis of <u>left</u> wrist

  M05.139 Rheumatoid lung disease with rheumatoid arthritis of <u>unspecified</u> wrist

M05.14- Rheumatoid lung disease with rheumatoid arthritis of <u>hand</u>

  Rheumatoid lung disease with rheumatoid arthritis, metacarpus and phalanges

  M05.141 Rheumatoid lung disease with rheumatoid arthritis of <u>right</u> hand

  M05.142 Rheumatoid lung disease with rheumatoid arthritis of <u>left</u> hand

  M05.149 Rheumatoid lung disease with rheumatoid arthritis of <u>unspecified</u> hand

M05.15- Rheumatoid lung disease with rheumatoid arthritis of <u>hip</u>

  M05.151 Rheumatoid lung disease with rheumatoid arthritis of <u>right</u> hip

  M05.152 Rheumatoid lung disease with rheumatoid arthritis of <u>left</u> hip

  M05.159 Rheumatoid lung disease with rheumatoid arthritis of <u>unspecified</u> hip

M05.16- Rheumatoid lung disease with rheumatoid arthritis of <u>knee</u>

  M05.161 Rheumatoid lung disease with rheumatoid arthritis of <u>right</u> knee

  M05.162 Rheumatoid lung disease with rheumatoid arthritis of <u>left</u> knee

  M05.169 Rheumatoid lung disease with rheumatoid arthritis of <u>unspecified</u> knee

M05.17- Rheumatoid lung disease with rheumatoid arthritis of <u>ankle and foot</u>

  Rheumatoid lung disease with rheumatoid arthritis, tarsus, metatarsus and phalanges

  M05.171 Rheumatoid lung disease with rheumatoid arthritis of <u>right</u> ankle and foot

  M05.172 Rheumatoid lung disease with rheumatoid arthritis of <u>left</u> ankle and foot

  M05.179 Rheumatoid lung disease with rheumatoid arthritis of <u>unspecified</u> ankle and foot

M05.19 Rheumatoid lung disease with rheumatoid arthritis of <u>multiple sites</u>

M05.2- Rheumatoid <u>vasculitis</u> with rheumatoid <u>arthritis</u> — A form with vascular disorders involving inflammation of the medium and small arteries throughout the body causing rashes, numbness, tingling, and/or loss of sensation.

M05.20 Rheumatoid vasculitis with rheumatoid arthritis of <u>unspecified</u> site

M05.21- Rheumatoid vasculitis with rheumatoid arthritis of <u>shoulder</u>

  M05.211 Rheumatoid vasculitis with rheumatoid arthritis of <u>right</u> shoulder

  M05.212 Rheumatoid vasculitis with rheumatoid arthritis of <u>left</u> shoulder

  M05.219 Rheumatoid vasculitis with rheumatoid arthritis of <u>unspecified</u> shoulder

M05.22- Rheumatoid vasculitis with rheumatoid arthritis of <u>elbow</u>

  M05.221 Rheumatoid vasculitis with rheumatoid arthritis of <u>right</u> elbow

  M05.222 Rheumatoid vasculitis with rheumatoid arthritis of <u>left</u> elbow

  M05.229 Rheumatoid vasculitis with rheumatoid arthritis of <u>unspecified</u> elbow

M05-M05

M05.23- Rheumatoid vasculitis with rheumatoid arthritis of <u>wrist</u>
Rheumatoid vasculitis with rheumatoid arthritis, carpal bones

M05.231 Rheumatoid vasculitis with rheumatoid arthritis of <u>right</u> wrist

M05.232 Rheumatoid vasculitis with rheumatoid arthritis of <u>left</u> wrist

M05.239 Rheumatoid vasculitis with rheumatoid arthritis of <u>unspecified</u> wrist

M05.24- Rheumatoid vasculitis with rheumatoid arthritis of <u>hand</u>
Rheumatoid vasculitis with rheumatoid arthritis, metacarpus and phalanges

M05.241 Rheumatoid vasculitis with rheumatoid arthritis of <u>right</u> hand

M05.242 Rheumatoid vasculitis with rheumatoid arthritis of <u>left</u> hand

M05.249 Rheumatoid vasculitis with rheumatoid arthritis of <u>unspecified</u> hand

M05.25- Rheumatoid vasculitis with rheumatoid arthritis of <u>hip</u>

M05.251 Rheumatoid vasculitis with rheumatoid arthritis of <u>right</u> hip

M05.252 Rheumatoid vasculitis with rheumatoid arthritis of <u>left</u> hip

M05.259 Rheumatoid vasculitis with rheumatoid arthritis of <u>unspecified</u> hip

M05.26- Rheumatoid vasculitis with rheumatoid arthritis of <u>knee</u>

M05.261 Rheumatoid vasculitis with rheumatoid arthritis of <u>right</u> knee

M05.262 Rheumatoid vasculitis with rheumatoid arthritis of <u>left</u> knee

M05.269 Rheumatoid vasculitis with rheumatoid arthritis of <u>unspecified</u> knee

M05.27- Rheumatoid vasculitis with rheumatoid arthritis of <u>ankle and foot</u>
Rheumatoid vasculitis with rheumatoid arthritis, tarsus, metatarsus and phalanges

M05.271 Rheumatoid vasculitis with rheumatoid arthritis of <u>right</u> ankle and foot

M05.272 Rheumatoid vasculitis with rheumatoid arthritis of <u>left</u> ankle and foot

M05.279 Rheumatoid vasculitis with rheumatoid arthritis of <u>unspecified</u> ankle and foot

M05.29 Rheumatoid vasculitis with rheumatoid arthritis of <u>multiple sites</u>

M05.3- Rheumatoid <u>heart</u> disease <u>with</u> rheumatoid <u>arthritis</u> — A form with heart disorders.
Rheumatoid carditis
Rheumatoid endocarditis
Rheumatoid myocarditis
Rheumatoid pericarditis

M05.30 Rheumatoid heart disease with rheumatoid arthritis of <u>unspecified</u> site

M05.31- Rheumatoid heart disease with rheumatoid arthritis of <u>shoulder</u>

M05.311 Rheumatoid heart disease with rheumatoid arthritis of <u>right</u> shoulder

M05.312 Rheumatoid heart disease with rheumatoid arthritis of <u>left</u> shoulder

M05.319 Rheumatoid heart disease with rheumatoid arthritis of <u>unspecified</u> shoulder

M05.32- Rheumatoid heart disease with rheumatoid arthritis of <u>elbow</u>

M05.321 Rheumatoid heart disease with rheumatoid arthritis of <u>right</u> elbow

M05.322 Rheumatoid heart disease with rheumatoid arthritis of <u>left</u> elbow

M05.329 Rheumatoid heart disease with rheumatoid arthritis of <u>unspecified</u> elbow

M05.33- Rheumatoid heart disease with rheumatoid arthritis of <u>wrist</u>
Rheumatoid heart disease with rheumatoid arthritis, carpal bones

M05.331 Rheumatoid heart disease with rheumatoid arthritis of <u>right</u> wrist

M05.332 Rheumatoid heart disease with rheumatoid arthritis of <u>left</u> wrist

M05.339 Rheumatoid heart disease with rheumatoid arthritis of <u>unspecified</u> wrist

M05.34- Rheumatoid heart disease with rheumatoid arthritis of <u>hand</u>
Rheumatoid heart disease with rheumatoid arthritis, metacarpus and phalanges

M05.341 Rheumatoid heart disease with rheumatoid arthritis of <u>right</u> hand

M05.342 Rheumatoid heart disease with rheumatoid arthritis of <u>left</u> hand

M05.349 Rheumatoid heart disease with rheumatoid arthritis of <u>unspecified</u> hand

M05.35- Rheumatoid heart disease with rheumatoid arthritis of <u>hip</u>

M05.351 Rheumatoid heart disease with rheumatoid arthritis of <u>right</u> hip

M05.352 Rheumatoid heart disease with rheumatoid arthritis of <u>left</u> hip

M05.359 Rheumatoid heart disease with rheumatoid arthritis of <u>unspecified</u> hip

M05.36- Rheumatoid heart disease with rheumatoid arthritis of <u>knee</u>

M05.361 Rheumatoid heart disease with rheumatoid arthritis of <u>right</u> knee

M05.362 Rheumatoid heart disease with rheumatoid arthritis of <u>left</u> knee

M05.369 Rheumatoid heart disease with rheumatoid arthritis of <u>unspecified</u> knee

M05.37- Rheumatoid heart disease with rheumatoid arthritis of <u>ankle and foot</u>
Rheumatoid heart disease with rheumatoid arthritis, tarsus, metatarsus and phalanges

M05.371 Rheumatoid heart disease with rheumatoid arthritis of <u>right</u> ankle and foot

M05.372 Rheumatoid heart disease with rheumatoid arthritis of <u>left</u> ankle and foot

M05.379 Rheumatoid heart disease with rheumatoid arthritis of <u>unspecified</u> ankle and foot

M05.39 Rheumatoid heart disease with rheumatoid arthritis of <u>multiple sites</u>

M05.4- Rheumatoid <u>myopathy</u> <u>with</u> rheumatoid <u>arthritis</u> — A form involving the muscles causing inflammation and weakness.

cc **M05.40** Rheumatoid myopathy with rheumatoid arthritis of <u>unspecified</u> site

M05.41- Rheumatoid myopathy with rheumatoid arthritis of <u>shoulder</u>

cc **M05.411** Rheumatoid myopathy with rheumatoid arthritis of <u>right</u> shoulder

cc **M05.412** Rheumatoid myopathy with rheumatoid arthritis of <u>left</u> shoulder

cc **M05.419** Rheumatoid myopathy with rheumatoid arthritis of <u>unspecified</u> shoulder

M05.42- Rheumatoid myopathy with rheumatoid arthritis of <u>elbow</u>

cc **M05.421** Rheumatoid myopathy with rheumatoid arthritis of <u>right</u> elbow

cc **M05.422** Rheumatoid myopathy with rheumatoid arthritis of <u>left</u> elbow

cc **M05.429** Rheumatoid myopathy with rheumatoid arthritis of <u>unspecified</u> elbow

M 0 5 I M 0 5

M05.43- Rheumatoid myopathy with rheumatoid arthritis of <u>wrist</u>
Rheumatoid myopathy with rheumatoid arthritis, carpal bones

cc **M05.431** Rheumatoid myopathy with rheumatoid arthritis of <u>right</u> wrist

cc **M05.432** Rheumatoid myopathy with rheumatoid arthritis of <u>left</u> wrist

cc **M05.439** Rheumatoid myopathy with rheumatoid arthritis of <u>unspecified</u> wrist

M05.44- Rheumatoid myopathy with rheumatoid arthritis of <u>hand</u>
Rheumatoid myopathy with rheumatoid arthritis, metacarpus and phalanges

cc **M05.441** Rheumatoid myopathy with rheumatoid arthritis of <u>right</u> hand

cc **M05.442** Rheumatoid myopathy with rheumatoid arthritis of <u>left</u> hand

cc **M05.449** Rheumatoid myopathy with rheumatoid arthritis of <u>unspecified</u> hand

M05.45- Rheumatoid myopathy with rheumatoid arthritis of <u>hip</u>

cc **M05.451** Rheumatoid myopathy with rheumatoid arthritis of <u>right</u> hip

cc **M05.452** Rheumatoid myopathy with rheumatoid arthritis of <u>left</u> hip

cc **M05.459** Rheumatoid myopathy with rheumatoid arthritis of <u>unspecified</u> hip

M05.46- Rheumatoid myopathy with rheumatoid arthritis of <u>knee</u>

cc **M05.461** Rheumatoid myopathy with rheumatoid arthritis of <u>right</u> knee

cc **M05.462** Rheumatoid myopathy with rheumatoid arthritis of <u>left</u> knee

cc **M05.469** Rheumatoid myopathy with rheumatoid arthritis of <u>unspecified</u> knee

M05.47- Rheumatoid myopathy with rheumatoid arthritis of <u>ankle and foot</u>
Rheumatoid myopathy with rheumatoid arthritis, tarsus, metatarsus and phalanges

cc **M05.471** Rheumatoid myopathy with rheumatoid arthritis of <u>right</u> ankle and foot

cc **M05.472** Rheumatoid myopathy with rheumatoid arthritis of <u>left</u> ankle and foot

cc **M05.479** Rheumatoid myopathy with rheumatoid arthritis of <u>unspecified</u> ankle and foot

cc **M05.49** Rheumatoid myopathy with rheumatoid arthritis of <u>multiple sites</u>

M05.5- Rheumatoid <u>polyneuropathy</u> <u>with</u> rheumatoid <u>arthritis</u> — A form affecting the peripheral nervous system causing inflammation, damage to the nerves, and pain.

M05.50 Rheumatoid polyneuropathy with rheumatoid arthritis of <u>unspecified</u> site

M05.51- Rheumatoid polyneuropathy with rheumatoid arthritis of <u>shoulder</u>

M05.511 Rheumatoid polyneuropathy with rheumatoid arthritis of <u>right</u> shoulder

M05.512 Rheumatoid polyneuropathy with rheumatoid arthritis of <u>left</u> shoulder

M05.519 Rheumatoid polyneuropathy with rheumatoid arthritis of <u>unspecified</u> shoulder

M05.52- Rheumatoid polyneuropathy with rheumatoid arthritis of <u>elbow</u>

M05.521 Rheumatoid polyneuropathy with rheumatoid arthritis of <u>right</u> elbow

M05.522 Rheumatoid polyneuropathy with rheumatoid arthritis of <u>left</u> elbow

M05.529 Rheumatoid polyneuropathy with rheumatoid arthritis of <u>unspecified</u> elbow

M05.53- Rheumatoid polyneuropathy with rheumatoid arthritis of <u>wrist</u>
Rheumatoid polyneuropathy with rheumatoid arthritis, carpal bones

M05.531 Rheumatoid polyneuropathy with rheumatoid arthritis of <u>right</u> wrist

M05.532 Rheumatoid polyneuropathy with rheumatoid arthritis of <u>left</u> wrist

M05.539 Rheumatoid polyneuropathy with rheumatoid arthritis of <u>unspecified</u> wrist

M05.54- Rheumatoid polyneuropathy with rheumatoid arthritis of <u>hand</u>
Rheumatoid polyneuropathy with rheumatoid arthritis, metacarpus and phalanges

M05.541 Rheumatoid polyneuropathy with rheumatoid arthritis of <u>right</u> hand

M05.542 Rheumatoid polyneuropathy with rheumatoid arthritis of <u>left</u> hand

M05.549 Rheumatoid polyneuropathy with rheumatoid arthritis of <u>unspecified</u> hand

M05.55- Rheumatoid polyneuropathy with rheumatoid arthritis of <u>hip</u>

M05.551 Rheumatoid polyneuropathy with rheumatoid arthritis of <u>right</u> hip

M05.552 Rheumatoid polyneuropathy with rheumatoid arthritis of <u>left</u> hip

M05.559 Rheumatoid polyneuropathy with rheumatoid arthritis of <u>unspecified</u> hip

M05.56- Rheumatoid polyneuropathy with rheumatoid arthritis of <u>knee</u>

M05.561 Rheumatoid polyneuropathy with rheumatoid arthritis of <u>right</u> knee

M05.562 Rheumatoid polyneuropathy with rheumatoid arthritis of <u>left</u> knee

M05.569 Rheumatoid polyneuropathy with rheumatoid arthritis of <u>unspecified</u> knee

M05.57- Rheumatoid polyneuropathy with rheumatoid arthritis of <u>ankle and foot</u>
Rheumatoid polyneuropathy with rheumatoid arthritis, tarsus, metatarsus and phalanges

M05.571 Rheumatoid polyneuropathy with rheumatoid arthritis of <u>right</u> ankle and foot

M05.572 Rheumatoid polyneuropathy with rheumatoid arthritis of <u>left</u> ankle and foot

M05.579 Rheumatoid polyneuropathy with rheumatoid arthritis of <u>unspecified</u> ankle and foot

M05.59 Rheumatoid polyneuropathy with rheumatoid arthritis of <u>multiple sites</u>

M05.6- Rheumatoid <u>arthritis</u> <u>with</u> involvement of <u>other organs and systems</u>

M05.60 Rheumatoid arthritis of <u>unspecified</u> site with involvement of other organs and systems

M05.61- Rheumatoid arthritis of <u>shoulder</u> with involvement of other organs and systems

M05.611 Rheumatoid arthritis of <u>right</u> shoulder with involvement of other organs and systems

M05.612 Rheumatoid arthritis of <u>left</u> shoulder with involvement of other organs and systems

M05.619 Rheumatoid arthritis of <u>unspecified</u> shoulder with involvement of other organs and systems

M05.62- Rheumatoid arthritis of <u>elbow</u> with involvement of other organs and systems

M05.621 Rheumatoid arthritis of <u>right</u> elbow with involvement of other organs and systems

M05.622 Rheumatoid arthritis of <u>left</u> elbow with involvement of other organs and systems

M05.629 Rheumatoid arthritis of <u>unspecified</u> elbow with involvement of other organs and systems

M05-M05

M05.63- Rheumatoid arthritis of <u>wrist</u> with involvement of other organs and systems
    Rheumatoid arthritis of carpal bones with involvement of other organs and systems

M05.631 Rheumatoid arthritis of <u>right</u> wrist with involvement of other organs and systems

M05.632 Rheumatoid arthritis of <u>left</u> wrist with involvement of other organs and systems

M05.639 Rheumatoid arthritis of <u>unspecified</u> wrist with involvement of other organs and systems

M05.64- Rheumatoid arthritis of <u>hand</u> with involvement of other organs and systems
    Rheumatoid arthritis of metacarpus and phalanges with involvement of other organs and systems

M05.641 Rheumatoid arthritis of <u>right</u> hand with involvement of other organs and systems

M05.642 Rheumatoid arthritis of <u>left</u> hand with involvement of other organs and systems

M05.649 Rheumatoid arthritis of <u>unspecified</u> hand with involvement of other organs and systems

M05.65- Rheumatoid arthritis of <u>hip</u> with involvement of other organs and systems

M05.651 Rheumatoid arthritis of <u>right</u> hip with involvement of other organs and systems

M05.652 Rheumatoid arthritis of <u>left</u> hip with involvement of other organs and systems

M05.659 Rheumatoid arthritis of <u>unspecified</u> hip with involvement of other organs and systems

M05.66- Rheumatoid arthritis of <u>knee</u> with involvement of other organs and systems

M05.661 Rheumatoid arthritis of <u>right</u> knee with involvement of other organs and systems

M05.662 Rheumatoid arthritis of <u>left</u> knee with involvement of other organs and systems

M05.669 Rheumatoid arthritis of <u>unspecified</u> knee with involvement of other organs and systems

M05.67- Rheumatoid arthritis of <u>ankle and foot</u> with involvement of other organs and systems
    Rheumatoid arthritis of tarsus, metatarsus and phalanges with involvement of other organs and systems

M05.671 Rheumatoid arthritis of <u>right</u> ankle and foot with involvement of other organs and systems

M05.672 Rheumatoid arthritis of <u>left</u> ankle and foot with involvement of other organs and systems

M05.679 Rheumatoid arthritis of <u>unspecified</u> ankle and foot with involvement of other organs and systems

M05.69 Rheumatoid arthritis of <u>multiple sites</u> with involvement of other organs and systems

M05.7- Rheumatoid <u>arthritis</u> <u>with</u> rheumatoid <u>factor without</u> organ or systems involvement — A form without the known involvement of other organs or tissues.

M05.70 Rheumatoid arthritis with rheumatoid factor of <u>unspecified</u> site without organ or systems involvement

M05.71- Rheumatoid arthritis with rheumatoid factor of <u>shoulder</u> without organ or systems involvement

M05.711 Rheumatoid arthritis with rheumatoid factor of <u>right</u> shoulder without organ or systems involvement

M05.712 Rheumatoid arthritis with rheumatoid factor of <u>left</u> shoulder without organ or systems involvement

M05.719 Rheumatoid arthritis with rheumatoid factor of <u>unspecified</u> shoulder without organ or systems involvement

M05.72- Rheumatoid arthritis with rheumatoid factor of <u>elbow</u> without organ or systems involvement

M05.721 Rheumatoid arthritis with rheumatoid factor of <u>right</u> elbow without organ or systems involvement

M05.722 Rheumatoid arthritis with rheumatoid factor of <u>left</u> elbow without organ or systems involvement

M05.729 Rheumatoid arthritis with rheumatoid factor of <u>unspecified</u> elbow without organ or systems involvement

M05.73- Rheumatoid arthritis with rheumatoid factor of <u>wrist</u> without organ or systems involvement

M05.731 Rheumatoid arthritis with rheumatoid factor of <u>right</u> wrist without organ or systems involvement

M05.732 Rheumatoid arthritis with rheumatoid factor of <u>left</u> wrist without organ or systems involvement

M05.739 Rheumatoid arthritis with rheumatoid factor of <u>unspecified</u> wrist without organ or systems involvement

M05.74- Rheumatoid arthritis with rheumatoid factor of <u>hand</u> without organ or systems involvement

M05.741 Rheumatoid arthritis with rheumatoid factor of <u>right</u> hand without organ or systems involvement

M05.742 Rheumatoid arthritis with rheumatoid factor of <u>left</u> hand without organ or systems involvement

M05.749 Rheumatoid arthritis with rheumatoid factor of <u>unspecified</u> hand without organ or systems involvement

M05.75- Rheumatoid arthritis with rheumatoid factor of <u>hip</u> without organ or systems involvement

M05.751 Rheumatoid arthritis with rheumatoid factor of <u>right</u> hip without organ or systems involvement

M05.752 Rheumatoid arthritis with rheumatoid factor of <u>left</u> hip without organ or systems involvement

M05.759 Rheumatoid arthritis with rheumatoid factor of <u>unspecified</u> hip without organ or systems involvement

M05.76- Rheumatoid arthritis with rheumatoid factor of <u>knee</u> without organ or systems involvement

M05.761 Rheumatoid arthritis with rheumatoid factor of <u>right</u> knee without organ or systems involvement

M05.762 Rheumatoid arthritis with rheumatoid factor of <u>left</u> knee without organ or systems involvement

M05.769 Rheumatoid arthritis with rheumatoid factor of <u>unspecified</u> knee without organ or systems involvement

M05.77- Rheumatoid arthritis with rheumatoid factor of <u>ankle and foot</u> without organ or systems involvement

M05.771 Rheumatoid arthritis with rheumatoid factor of <u>right</u> ankle and foot without organ or systems involvement

M05.772 Rheumatoid arthritis with rheumatoid factor of <u>left</u> ankle and foot without organ or systems involvement

M05.779 Rheumatoid arthritis with rheumatoid factor of <u>unspecified</u> ankle and foot without organ or systems involvement

M05.79 Rheumatoid arthritis with rheumatoid factor of <u>multiple sites</u> without organ or systems involvement

M05.8- <u>Other</u> rheumatoid arthritis <u>with</u> rheumatoid <u>factor</u>

M05.80 Other rheumatoid arthritis with rheumatoid factor of <u>unspecified</u> site

M05.81- Other rheumatoid arthritis with rheumatoid factor of <u>shoulder</u>

M05.811 Other rheumatoid arthritis with rheumatoid factor of <u>right</u> shoulder

M05.812 Other rheumatoid arthritis with rheumatoid factor of <u>left</u> shoulder

M05.819 Other rheumatoid arthritis with rheumatoid factor of <u>unspecified</u> shoulder

M0 5 I M0 5

Excludes 1: = NOT CODED HERE! (Do not code both)

Excludes ❷: = Not Included Here

M05.82-Other rheumatoid arthritis with rheumatoid factor of elbow

M05.821   Other rheumatoid arthritis with rheumatoid factor of <u>right</u> elbow

M05.822   Other rheumatoid arthritis with rheumatoid factor of <u>left</u> elbow

M05.829   Other rheumatoid arthritis with rheumatoid factor of <u>unspecified</u> elbow

M05.83-Other rheumatoid arthritis with rheumatoid factor of <u>wrist</u>

M05.831   Other rheumatoid arthritis with rheumatoid factor of <u>right</u> wrist

M05.832   Other rheumatoid arthritis with rheumatoid factor of <u>left</u> wrist

M05.839   Other rheumatoid arthritis with rheumatoid factor of <u>unspecified</u> wrist

M05.84-Other rheumatoid arthritis with rheumatoid factor of hand

M05.841   Other rheumatoid arthritis with rheumatoid factor of <u>right</u> hand

M05.842   Other rheumatoid arthritis with rheumatoid factor of <u>left</u> hand

M05.849   Other rheumatoid arthritis with rheumatoid factor of <u>unspecified</u> hand

M05.85-Other rheumatoid arthritis with rheumatoid factor of <u>hip</u>

M05.851   Other rheumatoid arthritis with rheumatoid factor of <u>right</u> hip

M05.852   Other rheumatoid arthritis with rheumatoid factor of <u>left</u> hip

M05.859   Other rheumatoid arthritis with rheumatoid factor of <u>unspecified</u> hip

M05.86-Other rheumatoid arthritis with rheumatoid factor of knee

M05.861   Other rheumatoid arthritis with rheumatoid factor of <u>right</u> knee

M05.862   Other rheumatoid arthritis with rheumatoid factor of <u>left</u> knee

M05.869   Other rheumatoid arthritis with rheumatoid factor of <u>unspecified</u> knee

M05.87-Other rheumatoid arthritis with rheumatoid factor of ankle and foot

M05.871   Other rheumatoid arthritis with rheumatoid factor of <u>right</u> ankle and foot

M05.872   Other rheumatoid arthritis with rheumatoid factor of <u>left</u> ankle and foot

M05.879   Other rheumatoid arthritis with rheumatoid factor of <u>unspecified</u> ankle and foot

M05.89 Other rheumatoid arthritis with rheumatoid factor of <u>multiple sites</u>

M05.9 Rheumatoid arthritis with rheumatoid factor, <u>unspecified</u>

M06- Other rheumatoid arthritis

M06.0- Rheumatoid <u>arthritis</u> <u>without</u> rheumatoid <u>factor</u> — A chronic, systemic autoimmune inflammatory disease characterized by inflammation of the joint structures with resultant crippling deformities that may affect organs throughout the body WITHOUT the presence of the rheumatoid factor autoantibody in the blood.

M06.00 Rheumatoid arthritis without rheumatoid factor, <u>unspecified</u> site

M06.01-Rheumatoid arthritis without rheumatoid factor, <u>shoulder</u>

M06.011   Rheumatoid arthritis without rheumatoid factor, <u>right</u> shoulder

M06.012   Rheumatoid arthritis without rheumatoid factor, <u>left</u> shoulder

M06.019   Rheumatoid arthritis without rheumatoid factor, <u>unspecified</u> shoulder

M06.02-Rheumatoid arthritis without rheumatoid factor, <u>elbow</u>

M06.021   Rheumatoid arthritis without rheumatoid factor, <u>right</u> elbow

M06.022   Rheumatoid arthritis without rheumatoid factor, <u>left</u> elbow

M06.029   Rheumatoid arthritis without rheumatoid factor, <u>unspecified</u> elbow

M06.03-Rheumatoid arthritis without rheumatoid factor, <u>wrist</u>

M06.031   Rheumatoid arthritis without rheumatoid factor, <u>right</u> wrist

M06.032   Rheumatoid arthritis without rheumatoid factor, <u>left</u> wrist

M06.039   Rheumatoid arthritis without rheumatoid factor, <u>unspecified</u> wrist

M06.04-Rheumatoid arthritis without rheumatoid factor, <u>hand</u>

M06.041   Rheumatoid arthritis without rheumatoid factor, <u>right</u> hand

M06.042   Rheumatoid arthritis without rheumatoid factor, <u>left</u> hand

M06.049   Rheumatoid arthritis without rheumatoid factor, <u>unspecified</u> hand

M06.05-Rheumatoid arthritis without rheumatoid factor, <u>hip</u>

M06.051   Rheumatoid arthritis without rheumatoid factor, <u>right</u> hip

M06.052   Rheumatoid arthritis without rheumatoid factor, <u>left</u> hip

M06.059   Rheumatoid arthritis without rheumatoid factor, <u>unspecified</u> hip

M06.06-Rheumatoid arthritis without rheumatoid factor, <u>knee</u>

M06.061   Rheumatoid arthritis without rheumatoid factor, <u>right</u> knee

M06.062   Rheumatoid arthritis without rheumatoid factor, <u>left</u> knee

M06.069   Rheumatoid arthritis without rheumatoid factor, <u>unspecified</u> knee

M06.07-Rheumatoid arthritis without rheumatoid factor, <u>ankle and foot</u>

M06.071   Rheumatoid arthritis without rheumatoid factor, <u>right</u> ankle and foot

M06.072   Rheumatoid arthritis without rheumatoid factor, <u>left</u> ankle and foot

M06.079   Rheumatoid arthritis without rheumatoid factor, <u>unspecified</u> ankle and foot

M06.08 Rheumatoid arthritis without rheumatoid factor, <u>vertebrae</u>

M06.09 Rheumatoid arthritis without rheumatoid factor, <u>multiple sites</u>

M06.1 **Adult-onset Still's disease** — [Age/15-124] – A form characterized by high fevers, salmon-colored rash, and joint pain.
  Excludes 1:   *Still's disease NOS (M08.2-)*

M06.2- <u>Rheumatoid bursitis</u> — A form characterized by inflammation of the bursae and tendons.

M06.20 Rheumatoid bursitis, <u>unspecified</u> site

M06.21-Rheumatoid bursitis, <u>shoulder</u>

M06.211   Rheumatoid bursitis, <u>right</u> shoulder

M06.212   Rheumatoid bursitis, <u>left</u> shoulder

M06.219   Rheumatoid bursitis, <u>unspecified</u> shoulder

M06.22-Rheumatoid bursitis, <u>elbow</u>

M06.221   Rheumatoid bursitis, <u>right</u> elbow

M06.222   Rheumatoid bursitis, <u>left</u> elbow

M06.229   Rheumatoid bursitis, <u>unspecified</u> elbow

M06.23-Rheumatoid bursitis, <u>wrist</u>

M06.231   Rheumatoid bursitis, <u>right</u> wrist

M06.232   Rheumatoid bursitis, <u>left</u> wrist

M06.239   Rheumatoid bursitis, <u>unspecified</u> wrist

Excludes 1: = NOT CODED HERE! (Do not code both)   826   *Excludes ❷:* = Not Included Here

M06.24-Rheumatoid bursitis, **hand**
   M06.241 Rheumatoid bursitis, **right** hand
   M06.242 Rheumatoid bursitis, **left** hand
   M06.249 Rheumatoid bursitis, **unspecified** hand
M06.25-Rheumatoid bursitis, **hip**
   M06.251 Rheumatoid bursitis, **right** hip
   M06.252 Rheumatoid bursitis, **left** hip
   M06.259 Rheumatoid bursitis, **unspecified** hip
M06.26-Rheumatoid bursitis, **knee**
   M06.261 Rheumatoid bursitis, **right** knee
   M06.262 Rheumatoid bursitis, **left** knee
   M06.269 Rheumatoid bursitis, **unspecified** knee
M06.27-Rheumatoid bursitis, **ankle and foot**
   M06.271 Rheumatoid bursitis, **right** ankle and foot
   M06.272 Rheumatoid bursitis, **left** ankle and foot
   M06.279 Rheumatoid bursitis, **unspecified** ankle and foot
M06.28 Rheumatoid bursitis, **vertebrae**
M06.29 Rheumatoid bursitis, **multiple sites**
M06.3- **Rheumatoid nodule** — A form characterized by soft tissue masses that are usually found in the subcutaneous tissue of the hands and arms.
M06.30 Rheumatoid nodule, **unspecified** site
M06.31-Rheumatoid nodule, **shoulder**
   M06.311 Rheumatoid nodule, **right** shoulder
   M06.312 Rheumatoid nodule, **left** shoulder
   M06.319 Rheumatoid nodule, **unspecified** shoulder
M06.32-Rheumatoid nodule, **elbow**
   M06.321 Rheumatoid nodule, **right** elbow
   M06.322 Rheumatoid nodule, **left** elbow
   M06.329 Rheumatoid nodule, **unspecified** elbow
M06.33-Rheumatoid nodule, **wrist**
   M06.331 Rheumatoid nodule, **right** wrist
   M06.332 Rheumatoid nodule, **left** wrist
   M06.339 Rheumatoid nodule, **unspecified** wrist
M06.34 Rheumatoid nodule, **hand**
   M06.341 Rheumatoid nodule, **right** hand
   M06.342 Rheumatoid nodule, **left** hand
   M06.349 Rheumatoid nodule, **unspecified** hand
M06.35-Rheumatoid nodule, **hip**
   M06.351 Rheumatoid nodule, **right** hip
   M06.352 Rheumatoid nodule, **left** hip
   M06.359 Rheumatoid nodule, **unspecified** hip
M06.36-Rheumatoid nodule, **knee**
   M06.361 Rheumatoid nodule, **right** knee
   M06.362 Rheumatoid nodule, **left** knee
   M06.369 Rheumatoid nodule, **unspecified** knee
M06.37-Rheumatoid nodule, **ankle and foot**
   M06.371 Rheumatoid nodule, **right** ankle and foot
   M06.372 Rheumatoid nodule, **left** ankle and foot
   M06.379 Rheumatoid nodule, **unspecified** ankle and foot
M06.38 Rheumatoid nodule, **vertebrae**
M06.39 Rheumatoid nodule, **multiple sites**
M06.4 **Inflammatory polyarthropathy** — A form affecting many joints and often symmetrically.
   Excludes 1: *polyarthritis NOS (M13.0)*
M06.8- **Other specified** rheumatoid arthritis
M06.80 Other specified rheumatoid arthritis, **unspecified** site
M06.81-Other specified rheumatoid arthritis, **shoulder**
   M06.811 Other specified rheumatoid arthritis, **right** shoulder
   M06.812 Other specified rheumatoid arthritis, **left** shoulder
   M06.819 Other specified rheumatoid arthritis, **unspecified** shoulder

M06.82-Other specified rheumatoid arthritis, **elbow**
   M06.821 Other specified rheumatoid arthritis, **right** elbow
   M06.822 Other specified rheumatoid arthritis, **left** elbow
   M06.829 Other specified rheumatoid arthritis, **unspecified** elbow
M06.83-Other specified rheumatoid arthritis, **wrist**
   M06.831 Other specified rheumatoid arthritis, **right** wrist
   M06.832 Other specified rheumatoid arthritis, **left** wrist
   M06.839 Other specified rheumatoid arthritis, **unspecified** wrist
M06.84-Other specified rheumatoid arthritis, **hand**
   M06.841 Other specified rheumatoid arthritis, **right** hand
   M06.842 Other specified rheumatoid arthritis, **left** hand
   M06.849 Other specified rheumatoid arthritis, **unspecified** hand
M06.85-Other specified rheumatoid arthritis, **hip**
   M06.851 Other specified rheumatoid arthritis, **right** hip
   M06.852 Other specified rheumatoid arthritis, **left** hip
   M06.859 Other specified rheumatoid arthritis, **unspecified** hip
M06.86-Other specified rheumatoid arthritis, **knee**
   M06.861 Other specified rheumatoid arthritis, **right** knee
   M06.862 Other specified rheumatoid arthritis, **left** knee
   M06.869 Other specified rheumatoid arthritis, **unspecified** knee
M06.87-Other specified rheumatoid arthritis, **ankle and foot**
   M06.871 Other specified rheumatoid arthritis, **right** ankle and foot
   M06.872 Other specified rheumatoid arthritis, **left** ankle and foot
   M06.879 Other specified rheumatoid arthritis, **unspecified** ankle and foot
M06.88 Other specified rheumatoid arthritis, **vertebrae**
M06.89 Other specified rheumatoid arthritis, **multiple sites**
M06.9 Rheumatoid arthritis, **unspecified**
M07- **Enteropathic arthropathies** — An inflammatory joint disease that is linked with gastrointestinal pathology.
   Code also associated enteropathy, such as:
    Regional enteritis [Crohn's disease] (K50.-)
    Ulcerative colitis (K51.-)
   Excludes 1: *psoriatic arthropathies (L40.5-)*
M07.6- **Enteropathic arthropathies**
M07.60 Enteropathic arthropathies, **unspecified** site
M07.61-Enteropathic arthropathies, **shoulder**
   M07.611 Enteropathic arthropathies, **right** shoulder
   M07.612 Enteropathic arthropathies, **left** shoulder
   M07.619 Enteropathic arthropathies, **unspecified** shoulder
M07.62-Enteropathic arthropathies, **elbow**
   M07.621 Enteropathic arthropathies, **right** elbow
   M07.622 Enteropathic arthropathies, **left** elbow
   M07.629 Enteropathic arthropathies, **unspecified** elbow
M07.63-Enteropathic arthropathies, **wrist**
   M07.631 Enteropathic arthropathies, **right** wrist
   M07.632 Enteropathic arthropathies, **left** wrist
   M07.639 Enteropathic arthropathies, **unspecified** wrist
M07.64-Enteropathic arthropathies, **hand**
   M07.641 Enteropathic arthropathies, **right** hand
   M07.642 Enteropathic arthropathies, **left** hand
   M07.649 Enteropathic arthropathies, **unspecified** hand
M07.65-Enteropathic arthropathies, **hip**
   M07.651 Enteropathic arthropathies, **right** hip
   M07.652 Enteropathic arthropathies, **left** hip
   M07.659 Enteropathic arthropathies, **unspecified** hip

M06 | M07

M07.66- Enteropathic arthropathies, <u>knee</u>
    M07.661 Enteropathic arthropathies, <u>right</u> knee
    M07.662 Enteropathic arthropathies, <u>left</u> knee
    M07.669 Enteropathic arthropathies, <u>unspecified</u> knee
M07.67- Enteropathic arthropathies, <u>ankle and foot</u>
    M07.671 Enteropathic arthropathies, <u>right</u> ankle and foot
    M07.672 Enteropathic arthropathies, <u>left</u> ankle and foot
    M07.679 Enteropathic arthropathies, <u>unspecified</u> ankle and foot
  M07.68 Enteropathic arthropathies, <u>vertebrae</u>
  M07.69 Enteropathic arthropathies, <u>multiple sites</u>

M08- <u>Juvenile arthritis</u> — An autoimmune or inflammatory disease of the synovium of the joints that presents prior to 16-17 years of age that is usually characterized by joint swelling, joint pain, and redness and warmth over the affected joints.
  Code also any associated underlying condition, such as:
    Regional enteritis [Crohn's disease] (K50.-)
    Ulcerative colitis (K51.-)
  Excludes 1:   arthropathy in Whipple's disease (M14.8)
           Felty's syndrome (M05.0)
           juvenile dermatomyositis (M33.0-)
           psoriatic juvenile arthropathy (L40.54)

M08.0- <u>Unspecified</u> juvenile rheumatoid arthritis — A form specified as juvenile rheumatoid arthritis with or without the identification of the rheumatoid factor in the blood.
    Juvenile rheumatoid arthritis with or without rheumatoid factor
  M08.00 Unspecified juvenile rheumatoid arthritis of <u>unspecified</u> site
  M08.01- Unspecified juvenile rheumatoid arthritis, <u>shoulder</u>
    M08.011 Unspecified juvenile rheumatoid arthritis, <u>right</u> shoulder
    M08.012 Unspecified juvenile rheumatoid arthritis, <u>left</u> shoulder
    M08.019 Unspecified juvenile rheumatoid arthritis, <u>unspecified</u> shoulder
  M08.02- Unspecified juvenile rheumatoid arthritis of <u>elbow</u>
    M08.021 Unspecified juvenile rheumatoid arthritis, <u>right</u> elbow
    M08.022 Unspecified juvenile rheumatoid arthritis, <u>left</u> elbow
    M08.029 Unspecified juvenile rheumatoid arthritis, <u>unspecified</u> elbow
  M08.03- Unspecified juvenile rheumatoid arthritis, <u>wrist</u>
    M08.031 Unspecified juvenile rheumatoid arthritis, <u>right</u> wrist
    M08.032 Unspecified juvenile rheumatoid arthritis, <u>left</u> wrist
    M08.039 Unspecified juvenile rheumatoid arthritis, <u>unspecified</u> wrist
  M08.04- Unspecified juvenile rheumatoid arthritis, <u>hand</u>
    M08.041 Unspecified juvenile rheumatoid arthritis, <u>right</u> hand
    M08.042 Unspecified juvenile rheumatoid arthritis, <u>left</u> hand
    M08.049 Unspecified juvenile rheumatoid arthritis, <u>unspecified</u> hand
  M08.05- Unspecified juvenile rheumatoid arthritis, <u>hip</u>
    M08.051 Unspecified juvenile rheumatoid arthritis, <u>right</u> hip
    M08.052 Unspecified juvenile rheumatoid arthritis, <u>left</u> hip
    M08.059 Unspecified juvenile rheumatoid arthritis, <u>unspecified</u> hip
  M08.06- Unspecified juvenile rheumatoid arthritis, <u>knee</u>
    M08.061 Unspecified juvenile rheumatoid arthritis, <u>right</u> knee
    M08.062 Unspecified juvenile rheumatoid arthritis, <u>left</u> knee
    M08.069 Unspecified juvenile rheumatoid arthritis, <u>unspecified</u> knee
  M08.07- Unspecified juvenile rheumatoid arthritis, <u>ankle and foot</u>
    M08.071 Unspecified juvenile rheumatoid arthritis, <u>right</u> ankle and foot
    M08.072 Unspecified juvenile rheumatoid arthritis, <u>left</u> ankle and foot

    M08.079 Unspecified juvenile rheumatoid arthritis, <u>unspecified</u> ankle and foot
  M08.08 Unspecified juvenile rheumatoid arthritis, <u>vertebrae</u>
  M08.09 Unspecified juvenile rheumatoid arthritis, <u>multiple sites</u>
M08.1 Juvenile ankylosing spondylitis — A form affecting the vertebral joints and the muscles, tendons, and ligaments of the spine that cause the stiffening of the spine.
  Excludes 1:   ankylosing spondylitis in adults (M45.0-)
M08.2- Juvenile rheumatoid arthritis <u>with systemic onset</u> — A juvenile idiopathic arthritis that is characterized by fever and rash in addition to the inflammation of the joints.
    Still's disease NOS
  Excludes 1:   adult-onset Still's disease (M06.1-)
  M08.20 Juvenile rheumatoid arthritis with systemic onset, <u>unspecified</u> site
  M08.21- Juvenile rheumatoid arthritis with systemic onset, <u>shoulder</u>
    M08.211 Juvenile rheumatoid arthritis with systemic onset, <u>right</u> shoulder
    M08.212 Juvenile rheumatoid arthritis with systemic onset, <u>left</u> shoulder
    M08.219 Juvenile rheumatoid arthritis with systemic onset, <u>unspecified</u> shoulder
  M08.22- Juvenile rheumatoid arthritis with systemic onset, <u>elbow</u>
    M08.221 Juvenile rheumatoid arthritis with systemic onset, <u>right</u> elbow
    M08.222 Juvenile rheumatoid arthritis with systemic onset, <u>left</u> elbow
    M08.229 Juvenile rheumatoid arthritis with systemic onset, <u>unspecified</u> elbow
  M08.23- Juvenile rheumatoid arthritis with systemic onset, <u>wrist</u>
    M08.231 Juvenile rheumatoid arthritis with systemic onset, <u>right</u> wrist
    M08.232 Juvenile rheumatoid arthritis with systemic onset, <u>left</u> wrist
    M08.239 Juvenile rheumatoid arthritis with systemic onset, <u>unspecified</u> wrist
  M08.24- Juvenile rheumatoid arthritis with systemic onset, <u>hand</u>
    M08.241 Juvenile rheumatoid arthritis with systemic onset, <u>right</u> hand
    M08.242 Juvenile rheumatoid arthritis with systemic onset, <u>left</u> hand
    M08.249 Juvenile rheumatoid arthritis with systemic onset, <u>unspecified</u> hand
  M08.25- Juvenile rheumatoid arthritis with systemic onset, <u>hip</u>
    M08.251 Juvenile rheumatoid arthritis with systemic onset, <u>right</u> hip
    M08.252 Juvenile rheumatoid arthritis with systemic onset, <u>left</u> hip
    M08.259 Juvenile rheumatoid arthritis with systemic onset, <u>unspecified</u> hip
  M08.26- Juvenile rheumatoid arthritis with systemic onset, <u>knee</u>
    M08.261 Juvenile rheumatoid arthritis with systemic onset, <u>right</u> knee
    M08.262 Juvenile rheumatoid arthritis with systemic onset, <u>left</u> knee
    M08.269 Juvenile rheumatoid arthritis with systemic onset, <u>unspecified</u> knee
  M08.27- Juvenile rheumatoid arthritis with systemic onset, <u>ankle and foot</u>
    M08.271 Juvenile rheumatoid arthritis with systemic onset, <u>right</u> ankle and foot
    M08.272 Juvenile rheumatoid arthritis with systemic onset, <u>left</u> ankle and foot
    M08.279 Juvenile rheumatoid arthritis with systemic onset, <u>unspecified</u> ankle and foot
  M08.28 Juvenile rheumatoid arthritis with systemic onset, <u>vertebrae</u>

M07-M08

M08.29 Juvenile rheumatoid arthritis with systemic onset, <u>multiple sites</u>

M08.3 **Juvenile rheumatoid polyarthritis (seronegative)** — An autoimmune disorder form that is characterized by inflammation of 5 or more joints with soreness, swelling, and stiffness and without the identification of the rheumatoid factor in the blood.

M08.4- <u>**Pauciarticular**</u> **juvenile rheumatoid arthritis** — An autoimmune disorder form that is characterized by inflammation of 4 or less joints with soreness, swelling, and stiffness and usually with the identification of the rheumatoid factor in the blood.

M08.40 Pauciarticular juvenile rheumatoid arthritis, <u>unspecified</u> site

M08.41- Pauciarticular juvenile rheumatoid arthritis, <u>shoulder</u>

   M08.411 Pauciarticular juvenile rheumatoid arthritis, <u>right</u> shoulder

   M08.412 Pauciarticular juvenile rheumatoid arthritis, <u>left</u> shoulder

   M08.419 Pauciarticular juvenile rheumatoid arthritis, <u>unspecified</u> shoulder

M08.42- Pauciarticular juvenile rheumatoid arthritis, <u>elbow</u>

   M08.421 Pauciarticular juvenile rheumatoid arthritis, <u>right</u> elbow

   M08.422 Pauciarticular juvenile rheumatoid arthritis, <u>left</u> elbow

   M08.429 Pauciarticular juvenile rheumatoid arthritis, <u>unspecified</u> elbow

M08.43- Pauciarticular juvenile rheumatoid arthritis, <u>wrist</u>

   M08.431 Pauciarticular juvenile rheumatoid arthritis, <u>right</u> wrist

   M08.432 Pauciarticular juvenile rheumatoid arthritis, <u>left</u> wrist

   M08.439 Pauciarticular juvenile rheumatoid arthritis, <u>unspecified</u> wrist

M08.44- Pauciarticular juvenile rheumatoid arthritis, <u>hand</u>

   M08.441 Pauciarticular juvenile rheumatoid arthritis, <u>right</u> hand

   M08.442 Pauciarticular juvenile rheumatoid arthritis, <u>left</u> hand

   M08.449 Pauciarticular juvenile rheumatoid arthritis, <u>unspecified</u> hand

M08.45- Pauciarticular juvenile rheumatoid arthritis, <u>hip</u>

   M08.451 Pauciarticular juvenile rheumatoid arthritis, <u>right</u> hip

   M08.452 Pauciarticular juvenile rheumatoid arthritis, <u>left</u> hip

   M08.459 Pauciarticular juvenile rheumatoid arthritis, <u>unspecified</u> hip

M08.46- Pauciarticular juvenile rheumatoid arthritis, <u>knee</u>

   M08.461 Pauciarticular juvenile rheumatoid arthritis, <u>right</u> knee

   M08.462 Pauciarticular juvenile rheumatoid arthritis, <u>left</u> knee

   M08.469 Pauciarticular juvenile rheumatoid arthritis, <u>unspecified</u> knee

M08.47- Pauciarticular juvenile rheumatoid arthritis, <u>ankle and foot</u>

   M08.471 Pauciarticular juvenile rheumatoid arthritis, <u>right</u> ankle and foot

   M08.472 Pauciarticular juvenile rheumatoid arthritis, <u>left</u> ankle and foot

   M08.479 Pauciarticular juvenile rheumatoid arthritis, <u>unspecified</u> ankle and foot

M08.48 Pauciarticular juvenile rheumatoid arthritis, vertebrae

M08.8- <u>Other</u> juvenile arthritis

M08.80 Other juvenile arthritis, <u>unspecified</u> site

M08.81- Other juvenile arthritis, <u>shoulder</u>

   M08.811 Other juvenile arthritis, <u>right</u> shoulder

   M08.812 Other juvenile arthritis, <u>left</u> shoulder

   M08.819 Other juvenile arthritis, <u>unspecified</u> shoulder

M08.82- Other juvenile arthritis, <u>elbow</u>

   M08.821 Other juvenile arthritis, <u>right</u> elbow

   M08.822 Other juvenile arthritis, <u>left</u> elbow

   M08.829 Other juvenile arthritis, <u>unspecified</u> elbow

M08.83- Other juvenile arthritis, <u>wrist</u>

   M08.831 Other juvenile arthritis, <u>right</u> wrist

   M08.832 Other juvenile arthritis, <u>left</u> wrist

   M08.839 Other juvenile arthritis, <u>unspecified</u> wrist

M08.84- Other juvenile arthritis, <u>hand</u>

   M08.841 Other juvenile arthritis, <u>right</u> hand

   M08.842 Other juvenile arthritis, <u>left</u> hand

   M08.849 Other juvenile arthritis, <u>unspecified</u> hand

M08.85- Other juvenile arthritis, <u>hip</u>

   M08.851 Other juvenile arthritis, <u>right</u> hip

   M08.852 Other juvenile arthritis, <u>left</u> hip

   M08.859 Other juvenile arthritis, <u>unspecified</u> hip

M08.86- Other juvenile arthritis, <u>knee</u>

   M08.861 Other juvenile arthritis, <u>right</u> knee

   M08.862 Other juvenile arthritis, <u>left</u> knee

   M08.869 Other juvenile arthritis, <u>unspecified</u> knee

M08.87- Other juvenile arthritis, <u>ankle and foot</u>

   M08.871 Other juvenile arthritis, <u>right</u> ankle and foot

   M08.872 Other juvenile arthritis, <u>left</u> ankle and foot

   M08.879 Other juvenile arthritis, <u>unspecified</u> ankle and foot

M08.88 Other juvenile arthritis, <u>other specified site</u>
     Other juvenile arthritis, vertebrae

M08.89 Other juvenile arthritis, <u>multiple sites</u>

M08.9- Juvenile arthritis, <u>unspecified</u>
   Excludes 1:   *juvenile rheumatoid arthritis, unspecified (M08.0-)*

M08.90 Juvenile arthritis, unspecified, <u>unspecified</u> site

M08.91- Juvenile arthritis, unspecified, <u>shoulder</u>

   M08.911 Juvenile arthritis, unspecified, <u>right</u> shoulder

   M08.912 Juvenile arthritis, unspecified, <u>left</u> shoulder

   M08.919 Juvenile arthritis, unspecified, <u>unspecified</u> shoulder

M08.92- Juvenile arthritis, unspecified, <u>elbow</u>

   M08.921 Juvenile arthritis, unspecified, <u>right</u> elbow

   M08.922 Juvenile arthritis, unspecified, <u>left</u> elbow

   M08.929 Juvenile arthritis, unspecified, <u>unspecified</u> elbow

M08.93- Juvenile arthritis, unspecified, <u>wrist</u>

   M08.931 Juvenile arthritis, unspecified, <u>right</u> wrist

   M08.932 Juvenile arthritis, unspecified, <u>left</u> wrist

   M08.939 Juvenile arthritis, unspecified, <u>unspecified</u> wrist

M08.94- Juvenile arthritis, unspecified, <u>hand</u>

   M08.941 Juvenile arthritis, unspecified, <u>right</u> hand

   M08.942 Juvenile arthritis, unspecified, <u>left</u> hand

   M08.949 Juvenile arthritis, unspecified, <u>unspecified</u> hand

M08.95- Juvenile arthritis, unspecified, <u>hip</u>

   M08.951 Juvenile arthritis, unspecified, <u>right</u> hip

   M08.952 Juvenile arthritis, unspecified, <u>left</u> hip

   M08.959 Juvenile arthritis, unspecified, <u>unspecified</u> hip

M08.96- Juvenile arthritis, unspecified, <u>knee</u>

   M08.961 Juvenile arthritis, unspecified, <u>right</u> knee

   M08.962 Juvenile arthritis, unspecified, <u>left</u> knee

   M08.969 Juvenile arthritis, unspecified, <u>unspecified</u> knee

M08.97- Juvenile arthritis, unspecified, <u>ankle and foot</u>

   M08.971 Juvenile arthritis, unspecified, <u>right</u> ankle and foot

   M08.972 Juvenile arthritis, unspecified, <u>left</u> ankle and foot

   M08.979 Juvenile arthritis, unspecified, <u>unspecified</u> ankle and foot

M08.98 Juvenile arthritis, unspecified, <u>vertebrae</u>

M08.99 Juvenile arthritis, unspecified, <u>multiple sites</u>

M08 I M08

Excludes 1: = NOT CODED HERE! (Do not code both)   **829**   *Excludes ❷:* = Not Included Here

M1A- Chronic gout — A form of arthritis that is characterized by the deposition of urate crystals in and around the joints that causes inflammation and degenerative changes that persists over a long period of time with repeated episodes of soreness and aching.

  Use additional code to identify:
    Autonomic neuropathy in diseases classified elsewhere (G99.0)
    Calculus of urinary tract in diseases classified elsewhere (N22)
    Cardiomyopathy in diseases classified elsewhere (I43)
    Disorders of external ear in diseases classified elsewhere (H61.1-, H62.8-)
    Disorders of iris and ciliary body in diseases classified elsewhere (H22)
    Glomerular disorders in diseases classified elsewhere (N08)
  Excludes 1:   gout NOS (M10.-)
  Excludes ❷: acute gout (M10.-)

  The appropriate 7th character is to be added to each code from category M1A:
  0   Without tophus (tophi)
  1   With tophus (tophi) — The appearance of enlarged joints due to nodular monosodium urate crystal deposits.

M1A.0- Idiopathic chronic gout — A form that is of a primary cause (versus due to another condition or disease) or unknown cause.
      Chronic gouty bursitis
      Primary chronic gout
  M1A.00x- Idiopathic chronic gout, unspecified site
  M1A.01- Idiopathic chronic gout, shoulder
    M1A.011- Idiopathic chronic gout, right shoulder
    M1A.012- Idiopathic chronic gout, left shoulder
    M1A.019- Idiopathic chronic gout, unspecified shoulder
  M1A.02- Idiopathic chronic gout, elbow
    M1A.021- Idiopathic chronic gout, right elbow
    M1A.022- Idiopathic chronic gout, left elbow
    M1A.029- Idiopathic chronic gout, unspecified elbow
  M1A.03- Idiopathic chronic gout, wrist
    M1A.031- Idiopathic chronic gout, right wrist
    M1A.032- Idiopathic chronic gout, left wrist
    M1A.039- Idiopathic chronic gout, unspecified wrist
  M1A.04- Idiopathic chronic gout, hand
    M1A.041- Idiopathic chronic gout, right hand
    M1A.042- Idiopathic chronic gout, left hand
    M1A.049- Idiopathic chronic gout, unspecified hand
  M1A.05- Idiopathic chronic gout, hip
    M1A.051- Idiopathic chronic gout, right hip
    M1A.052- Idiopathic chronic gout, left hip
    M1A.059- Idiopathic chronic gout, unspecified hip
  M1A.06- Idiopathic chronic gout, knee
    M1A.061- Idiopathic chronic gout, right knee
    M1A.062- Idiopathic chronic gout, left knee
    M1A.069- Idiopathic chronic gout, unspecified knee
  M1A.07- Idiopathic chronic gout, ankle and foot
    M1A.071- Idiopathic chronic gout, right ankle and foot
    M1A.072- Idiopathic chronic gout, left ankle and foot
    M1A.079- Idiopathic chronic gout, unspecified ankle and foot
  M1A.08x- Idiopathic chronic gout, vertebrae
  M1A.09x- Idiopathic chronic gout, multiple sites

M1A.1- Lead-induced chronic gout — A form that is due to the toxic effects of lead and its compounds.
    Code first toxic effects of lead and its compounds (T56.0-)
  M1A.10x- Lead-induced chronic gout, unspecified site
  M1A.11- Lead-induced chronic gout, shoulder
    M1A.111- Lead-induced chronic gout, right shoulder
    M1A.112- Lead-induced chronic gout, left shoulder
    M1A.119- Lead-induced chronic gout, unspecified shoulder
  M1A.12- Lead-induced chronic gout, elbow
    M1A.121- Lead-induced chronic gout, right elbow
    M1A.122- Lead-induced chronic gout, left elbow
    M1A.129- Lead-induced chronic gout, unspecified elbow
  M1A.13- Lead-induced chronic gout, wrist
    M1A.131- Lead-induced chronic gout, right wrist
    M1A.132- Lead-induced chronic gout, left wrist
    M1A.139- Lead-induced chronic gout, unspecified wrist

M1A.14- Lead-induced chronic gout, hand
    M1A.141- Lead-induced chronic gout, right hand
    M1A.142- Lead-induced chronic gout, left hand
    M1A.149- Lead-induced chronic gout, unspecified hand
  M1A.15- Lead-induced chronic gout, hip
    M1A.151- Lead-induced chronic gout, right hip
    M1A.152- Lead-induced chronic gout, left hip
    M1A.159- Lead-induced chronic gout, unspecified hip
  M1A.16- Lead-induced chronic gout, knee
    M1A.161- Lead-induced chronic gout, right knee
    M1A.162- Lead-induced chronic gout, left knee
    M1A.169- Lead-induced chronic gout, unspecified knee
  M1A.17- Lead-induced chronic gout, ankle and foot
    M1A.171- Lead-induced chronic gout, right ankle and foot
    M1A.172- Lead-induced chronic gout, left ankle and foot
    M1A.179- Lead-induced chronic gout, unspecified ankle and foot
  M1A.18x- Lead-induced chronic gout, vertebrae
  M1A.19x- Lead-induced chronic gout, multiple sites

M1A.2- Drug-induced chronic gout — A form that is due to medications and their effects.
    Use additional code for adverse effect, if applicable, to identify drug (T36-T50 with fifth or sixth character 5)
  M1A.20x- Drug-induced chronic gout, unspecified site
  M1A.21- Drug-induced chronic gout, shoulder
    M1A.211- Drug-induced chronic gout, right shoulder
    M1A.212- Drug-induced chronic gout, left shoulder
    M1A.219- Drug-induced chronic gout, unspecified shoulder
  M1A.22- Drug-induced chronic gout, elbow
    M1A.221- Drug-induced chronic gout, right elbow
    M1A.222- Drug-induced chronic gout, left elbow
    M1A.229- Drug-induced chronic gout, unspecified elbow
  M1A.23- Drug-induced chronic gout, wrist
    M1A.231- Drug-induced chronic gout, right wrist
    M1A.232- Drug-induced chronic gout, left wrist
    M1A.239- Drug-induced chronic gout, unspecified wrist
  M1A.24- Drug-induced chronic gout, hand
    M1A.241- Drug-induced chronic gout, right hand
    M1A.242- Drug-induced chronic gout, left hand
    M1A.249- Drug-induced chronic gout, unspecified hand
  M1A.25- Drug-induced chronic gout, hip
    M1A.251- Drug-induced chronic gout, right hip
    M1A.252- Drug-induced chronic gout, left hip
    M1A.259- Drug-induced chronic gout, unspecified hip
  M1A.26- Drug-induced chronic gout, knee
    M1A.261- Drug-induced chronic gout, right knee
    M1A.262- Drug-induced chronic gout, left knee
    M1A.269- Drug-induced chronic gout, unspecified knee
  M1A.27- Drug-induced chronic gout, ankle and foot
    M1A.271- Drug-induced chronic gout, right ankle and foot
    M1A.272- Drug-induced chronic gout, left ankle and foot
    M1A.279- Drug-induced chronic gout, unspecified ankle and foot
  M1A.28x- Drug-induced chronic gout, vertebrae
  M1A.29x- Drug-induced chronic gout, multiple sites

M1A.3- Chronic gout due to renal impairment — A form that is due to the decreased function of the kidney resulting in inadequate removal of uric acid from the blood.
    Code first associated renal disease
  M1A.30x- Chronic gout due to renal impairment, unspecified site
  M1A.31- Chronic gout due to renal impairment, shoulder
    M1A.311- Chronic gout due to renal impairment, right shoulder
    M1A.312- Chronic gout due to renal impairment, left shoulder

M1A.319- Chronic gout due to renal impairment, <u>unspecified</u> shoulder

M1A.32-   Chronic gout due to renal impairment, <u>elbow</u>

M1A.321- Chronic gout due to renal impairment, <u>right</u> elbow

M1A.322- Chronic gout due to renal impairment, <u>left</u> elbow

M1A.329- Chronic gout due to renal impairment, <u>unspecified</u> elbow

M1A.33-   Chronic gout due to renal impairment, <u>wrist</u>

M1A.331- Chronic gout due to renal impairment, <u>right</u> wrist

M1A.332- Chronic gout due to renal impairment, <u>left</u> wrist

M1A.339- Chronic gout due to renal impairment, <u>unspecified</u> wrist

M1A.34-   Chronic gout due to renal impairment, <u>hand</u>

M1A.341- Chronic gout due to renal impairment, <u>right</u> hand

M1A.342- Chronic gout due to renal impairment, <u>left</u> hand

M1A.349- Chronic gout due to renal impairment, <u>unspecified</u> hand

M1A.35-   Chronic gout due to renal impairment, <u>hip</u>

M1A.351- Chronic gout due to renal impairment, <u>right</u> hip

M1A.352- Chronic gout due to renal impairment, <u>left</u> hip

M1A.359- Chronic gout due to renal impairment, <u>unspecified</u> hip

M1A.36-   Chronic gout due to renal impairment, <u>knee</u>

M1A.361- Chronic gout due to renal impairment, <u>right</u> knee

M1A.362- Chronic gout due to renal impairment, <u>left</u> knee

M1A.369- Chronic gout due to renal impairment, <u>unspecified</u> knee

M1A.37-   Chronic gout due to renal impairment, <u>ankle and foot</u>

M1A.371- Chronic gout due to renal impairment, <u>right</u> ankle and foot

M1A.372- Chronic gout due to renal impairment, <u>left</u> ankle and foot

M1A.379- Chronic gout due to renal impairment, <u>unspecified</u> ankle and foot

M1A.38x- Chronic gout due to renal impairment, <u>vertebrae</u>

M1A.39x- Chronic gout due to renal impairment, <u>multiple sites</u>

M1A.4- <u>Other secondary</u> chronic gout
Code first associated condition

M1A.40x- Other secondary chronic gout, <u>unspecified</u> site

M1A.41-   Other secondary chronic gout, <u>shoulder</u>

M1A.411- Other secondary chronic gout, <u>right</u> shoulder

M1A.412- Other secondary chronic gout, <u>left</u> shoulder

M1A.419- Other secondary chronic gout, <u>unspecified</u> shoulder

M1A.42-   Other secondary chronic gout, <u>elbow</u>

M1A.421- Other secondary chronic gout, <u>right</u> elbow

M1A.422- Other secondary chronic gout, <u>left</u> elbow

M1A.429- Other secondary chronic gout, <u>unspecified</u> elbow

M1A.43-   Other secondary chronic gout, <u>wrist</u>

M1A.431- Other secondary chronic gout, <u>right</u> wrist

M1A.432- Other secondary chronic gout, <u>left</u> wrist

M1A.439- Other secondary chronic gout, <u>unspecified</u> wrist

M1A.44-   Other secondary chronic gout, <u>hand</u>

M1A.441- Other secondary chronic gout, <u>right</u> hand

M1A.442- Other secondary chronic gout, <u>left</u> hand

M1A.449- Other secondary chronic gout, <u>unspecified</u> hand

M1A.45-   Other secondary chronic gout, <u>hip</u>

M1A.451- Other secondary chronic gout, <u>right</u> hip

M1A.452- Other secondary chronic gout, <u>left</u> hip

M1A.459- Other secondary chronic gout, <u>unspecified</u> hip

M1A.46-   Other secondary chronic gout, <u>knee</u>

M1A.461- Other secondary chronic gout, <u>right</u> knee

M1A.462- Other secondary chronic gout, <u>left</u> knee

M1A.469- Other secondary chronic gout, <u>unspecified</u> knee

M1A.47-   Other secondary chronic gout, <u>ankle and foot</u>

M1A.471- Other secondary chronic gout, <u>right</u> ankle and foot

M1A.472- Other secondary chronic gout, <u>left</u> ankle and foot

M1A.479- Other secondary chronic gout, <u>unspecified</u> ankle and foot

M1A.48x- Other secondary chronic gout, <u>vertebrae</u>

M1A.49x- Other secondary chronic gout, <u>multiple sites</u>

M1A.9xx- Chronic gout, <u>unspecified</u>

M10- <u>Gout</u> — A form of arthritis that is characterized by the deposition of urate crystals in and around the joints that causes inflammation and degenerative changes that presents as a sudden, severe onset of sharp pain, swelling, redness, and tenderness of the affected joint.
<u>Acute</u> gout
Gout <u>attack</u>
Gout <u>flare</u>
Gout <u>NOS</u>
Podagra — A form affecting the big toe.
Use additional code to identify:
Autonomic neuropathy in diseases classified elsewhere (G99.0)
Calculus of urinary tract in diseases classified elsewhere (N22)
Cardiomyopathy in diseases classified elsewhere (I43)
Disorders of external ear in diseases classified elsewhere (H61.1-, H62.8-)
Disorders of iris and ciliary body in diseases classified elsewhere (H22)
Glomerular disorders in diseases classified elsewhere (N08)
Excludes ❷: chronic gout (M1A.-)

M10.0- Idiopathic gout — A form that is of a primary cause (versus due to another condition or disease) or unknown cause.
Gouty bursitis
Primary gout

M10.00 Idiopathic gout, <u>unspecified</u> site

M10.01- Idiopathic gout, <u>shoulder</u>

M10.011 Idiopathic gout, <u>right</u> shoulder

M10.012 Idiopathic gout, <u>left</u> shoulder

M10.019 Idiopathic gout, <u>unspecified</u> shoulder

M10.02- Idiopathic gout, <u>elbow</u>

M10.021 Idiopathic gout, <u>right</u> elbow

M10.022 Idiopathic gout, <u>left</u> elbow

M10.029 Idiopathic gout, <u>unspecified</u> elbow

M10.03- Idiopathic gout, <u>wrist</u>

M10.031 Idiopathic gout, <u>right</u> wrist

M10.032 Idiopathic gout, <u>left</u> wrist

M10.039 Idiopathic gout, <u>unspecified</u> wrist

M10.04- Idiopathic gout, <u>hand</u>

M10.041 Idiopathic gout, <u>right</u> hand

M10.042 Idiopathic gout, <u>left</u> hand

M10.049 Idiopathic gout, <u>unspecified</u> hand

M10.05- Idiopathic gout, <u>hip</u>

M10.051 Idiopathic gout, <u>right</u> hip

M10.052 Idiopathic gout, <u>left</u> hip

M10.059 Idiopathic gout, <u>unspecified</u> hip

M10.06- Idiopathic gout, <u>knee</u>

M10.061 Idiopathic gout, <u>right</u> knee

M10.062 Idiopathic gout, <u>left</u> knee

M10.069 Idiopathic gout, <u>unspecified</u> knee

M10.07- Idiopathic gout, <u>ankle and foot</u>

M10.071 Idiopathic gout, <u>right</u> ankle and foot

M10.072 Idiopathic gout, <u>left</u> ankle and foot

M10.079 Idiopathic gout, <u>unspecified</u> ankle and foot

M10.08 Idiopathic gout, <u>vertebrae</u>

M10.09 Idiopathic gout, <u>multiple sites</u>

M10.1- <u>Lead-induced</u> gout — A form that is due to the toxic effects of lead and its compounds.
Code first toxic effects of lead and its compounds (T56.0-).

M10.10 Lead-induced gout, <u>unspecified</u> site

M10.11- Lead-induced gout, <u>shoulder</u>

M10.111 Lead-induced gout, <u>right</u> shoulder

M10.112 Lead-induced gout, <u>left</u> shoulder

M10.119 Lead-induced gout, <u>unspecified</u> shoulder

M 1 A - M 1 0

M10.12- Lead-induced gout, <u>elbow</u>
    M10.121　Lead-induced gout, <u>right</u> elbow
    M10.122　Lead-induced gout, <u>left</u> elbow
    M10.129　Lead-induced gout, <u>unspecified</u> elbow
M10.13- Lead-induced gout, <u>wrist</u>
    M10.131　Lead-induced gout, <u>right</u> wrist
    M10.132　Lead-induced gout, <u>left</u> wrist
    M10.139　Lead-induced gout, <u>unspecified</u> wrist
M10.14- Lead-induced gout, <u>hand</u>
    M10.141　Lead-induced gout, <u>right</u> hand
    M10.142　Lead-induced gout, <u>left</u> hand
    M10.149　Lead-induced gout, <u>unspecified</u> hand
M10.15- Lead-induced gout, <u>hip</u>
    M10.151　Lead-induced gout, <u>right</u> hip
    M10.152　Lead-induced gout, <u>left</u> hip
    M10.159　Lead-induced gout, <u>unspecified</u> hip
M10.16- Lead-induced gout, <u>knee</u>
    M10.161　Lead-induced gout, <u>right</u> knee
    M10.162　Lead-induced gout, <u>left</u> knee
    M10.169　Lead-induced gout, <u>unspecified</u> knee
M10.17- Lead-induced gout, <u>ankle and foot</u>
    M10.171　Lead-induced gout, <u>right</u> ankle and foot
    M10.172　Lead-induced gout, <u>left</u> ankle and foot
    M10.179　Lead-induced gout, <u>unspecified</u> ankle and foot
M10.18　Lead-induced gout, <u>vertebrae</u>
M10.19　Lead-induced gout, <u>multiple sites</u>
M10.2-　<u>Drug-induced</u> gout — A form that is due to medications and their effects.
    Use additional code for adverse effect, if applicable, to identify drug
    (T36-T50 with fifth or sixth character 5)
M10.20　Drug-induced gout, <u>unspecified</u> site
M10.21- Drug-induced gout, <u>shoulder</u>
    M10.211　Drug-induced gout, <u>right</u> shoulder
    M10.212　Drug-induced gout, <u>left</u> shoulder
    M10.219　Drug-induced gout, <u>unspecified</u> shoulder
M10.22- Drug-induced gout, <u>elbow</u>
    M10.221　Drug-induced gout, <u>right</u> elbow
    M10.222　Drug-induced gout, <u>left</u> elbow
    M10.229　Drug-induced gout, <u>unspecified</u> elbow
M10.23- Drug-induced gout, <u>wrist</u>
    M10.231　Drug-induced gout, <u>right</u> wrist
    M10.232　Drug-induced gout, <u>left</u> wrist
    M10.239　Drug-induced gout, <u>unspecified</u> wrist
M10.24- Drug-induced gout, <u>hand</u>
    M10.241　Drug-induced gout, <u>right</u> hand
    M10.242　Drug-induced gout, <u>left</u> hand
    M10.249　Drug-induced gout, <u>unspecified</u> hand
M10.25- Drug-induced gout, <u>hip</u>
    M10.251　Drug-induced gout, <u>right</u> hip
    M10.252　Drug-induced gout, <u>left</u> hip
    M10.259　Drug-induced gout, <u>unspecified</u> hip
M10.26- Drug-induced gout, <u>knee</u>
    M10.261　Drug-induced gout, <u>right</u> knee
    M10.262　Drug-induced gout, <u>left</u> knee
    M10.269　Drug-induced gout, <u>unspecified</u> knee
M10.27- Drug-induced gout, <u>ankle and foot</u>
    M10.271　Drug-induced gout, <u>right</u> ankle and foot
    M10.272　Drug-induced gout, <u>left</u> ankle and foot
    M10.279　Drug-induced gout, <u>unspecified</u> ankle and foot
M10.28　Drug-induced gout, <u>vertebrae</u>
M10.29　Drug-Induced gout, <u>multiple sites</u>

M10.3-　Gout <u>due to renal impairment</u> — A form that is due to the decreased
    function of the kidney resulting in inadequate removal of uric acid from the blood.
    Code first associated renal disease
M10.30　Gout due to renal impairment, <u>unspecified</u> site
M10.31- Gout due to renal impairment, <u>shoulder</u>
    M10.311　Gout due to renal impairment, <u>right</u> shoulder
    M10.312　Gout due to renal impairment, <u>left</u> shoulder
    M10.319　Gout due to renal impairment, <u>unspecified</u> shoulder
M10.32- Gout due to renal impairment, <u>elbow</u>
    M10.321　Gout due to renal impairment, <u>right</u> elbow
    M10.322　Gout due to renal impairment, <u>left</u> elbow
    M10.329　Gout due to renal impairment, <u>unspecified</u> elbow
M10.33- Gout due to renal impairment, <u>wrist</u>
    M10.331　Gout due to renal impairment, <u>right</u> wrist
    M10.332　Gout due to renal impairment, <u>left</u> wrist
    M10.339　Gout due to renal impairment, <u>unspecified</u> wrist
M10.34- Gout due to renal impairment, <u>hand</u>
    M10.341　Gout due to renal impairment, <u>right</u> hand
    M10.342　Gout due to renal impairment, <u>left</u> hand
    M10.349　Gout due to renal impairment, <u>unspecified</u> hand
M10.35- Gout due to renal impairment, <u>hip</u>
    M10.351　Gout due to renal impairment, <u>right</u> hip
    M10.352　Gout due to renal impairment, <u>left</u> hip
    M10.359　Gout due to renal impairment, <u>unspecified</u> hip
M10.36- Gout due to renal impairment, <u>knee</u>
    M10.361　Gout due to renal impairment, <u>right</u> knee
    M10.362　Gout due to renal impairment, <u>left</u> knee
    M10.369　Gout due to renal impairment, <u>unspecified</u> knee
M10.37- Gout due to renal impairment, <u>ankle and foot</u>
    M10.371　Gout due to renal impairment, <u>right</u> ankle and foot
    M10.372　Gout due to renal impairment, <u>left</u> ankle and foot
    M10.379　Gout due to renal impairment, <u>unspecified</u> ankle and foot
M10.38　Gout due to renal impairment, <u>vertebrae</u>
M10.39　Gout due to renal impairment, <u>multiple sites</u>
M10.4-　<u>Other secondary</u> gout
    Code first associated condition
M10.40　Other secondary gout, <u>unspecified</u> site
M10.41- Other secondary gout, <u>shoulder</u>
    M10.411　Other secondary gout, <u>right</u> shoulder
    M10.412　Other secondary gout, <u>left</u> shoulder
    M10.419　Other secondary gout, <u>unspecified</u> shoulder
M10.42- Other secondary gout, <u>elbow</u>
    M10.421　Other secondary gout, <u>right</u> elbow
    M10.422　Other secondary gout, <u>left</u> elbow
    M10.429　Other secondary gout, <u>unspecified</u> elbow
M10.43- Other secondary gout, <u>wrist</u>
    M10.431　Other secondary gout, <u>right</u> wrist
    M10.432　Other secondary gout, <u>left</u> wrist
    M10.439　Other secondary gout, <u>unspecified</u> wrist
M10.44- Other secondary gout, <u>hand</u>
    M10.441　Other secondary gout, <u>right</u> hand
    M10.442　Other secondary gout, <u>left</u> hand
    M10.449　Other secondary gout, <u>unspecified</u> hand
M10.45- Other secondary gout, <u>hip</u>
    M10.451　Other secondary gout, <u>right</u> hip
    M10.452　Other secondary gout, <u>left</u> hip
    M10.459　Other secondary gout, <u>unspecified</u> hip
M10.46- Other secondary gout, <u>knee</u>
    M10.461　Other secondary gout, <u>right</u> knee
    M10.462　Other secondary gout, <u>left</u> knee
    M10.469　Other secondary gout, <u>unspecified</u> knee

M10-M10

M10.47- Other secondary gout, <u>ankle and foot</u>
 M10.471 Other secondary gout, <u>right</u> ankle and foot
 M10.472 Other secondary gout, <u>left</u> ankle and foot
 M10.479 Other secondary gout, <u>unspecified</u> ankle and foot
M10.48 Other secondary gout, <u>vertebrae</u>
M10.49 Other secondary gout, <u>multiple sites</u>

M10.9 Gout, <u>unspecified</u>
 Gout NOS

M11- <u>Other crystal arthropathies</u> — A group of joint diseases characterized by the deposition of crystals in the joints.

M11.0- <u>Hydroxyapatite deposition</u> disease — A form caused the deposition of hydroxyapatite crystals in the joints.

M11.00 Hydroxyapatite deposition disease, <u>unspecified</u> site
M11.01- Hydroxyapatite deposition disease, <u>shoulder</u>
 M11.011 Hydroxyapatite deposition disease, <u>right</u> shoulder
 M11.012 Hydroxyapatite deposition disease, <u>left</u> shoulder
 M11.019 Hydroxyapatite deposition disease, <u>unspecified</u> shoulder
M11.02- Hydroxyapatite deposition disease, <u>elbow</u>
 M11.021 Hydroxyapatite deposition disease, <u>right</u> elbow
 M11.022 Hydroxyapatite deposition disease, <u>left</u> elbow
 M11.029 Hydroxyapatite deposition disease, <u>unspecified</u> elbow
M11.03- Hydroxyapatite deposition disease, <u>wrist</u>
 M11.031 Hydroxyapatite deposition disease, <u>right</u> wrist
 M11.032 Hydroxyapatite deposition disease, <u>left</u> wrist
 M11.039 Hydroxyapatite deposition disease, <u>unspecified</u> wrist
M11.04- Hydroxyapatite deposition disease, <u>hand</u>
 M11.041 Hydroxyapatite deposition disease, <u>right</u> hand
 M11.042 Hydroxyapatite deposition disease, <u>left</u> hand
 M11.049 Hydroxyapatite deposition disease, <u>unspecified</u> hand
M11.05- Hydroxyapatite deposition disease, <u>hip</u>
 M11.051 Hydroxyapatite deposition disease, <u>right</u> hip
 M11.052 Hydroxyapatite deposition disease, <u>left</u> hip
 M11.059 Hydroxyapatite deposition disease, <u>unspecified</u> hip
M11.06- Hydroxyapatite deposition disease, <u>knee</u>
 M11.061 Hydroxyapatite deposition disease, <u>right</u> knee
 M11.062 Hydroxyapatite deposition disease, <u>left</u> knee
 M11.069 Hydroxyapatite deposition disease, <u>unspecified</u> knee
M11.07- Hydroxyapatite deposition disease, <u>ankle and foot</u>
 M11.071 Hydroxyapatite deposition disease, <u>right</u> ankle and foot
 M11.072 Hydroxyapatite deposition disease, <u>left</u> ankle and foot
 M11.079 Hydroxyapatite deposition disease, <u>unspecified</u> ankle and foot
M11.08 Hydroxyapatite deposition disease, <u>vertebrae</u>
M11.09 Hydroxyapatite deposition disease, <u>multiple sites</u>

M11.1- <u>Familial chondrocalcinosis</u> — A form caused the deposition of calcium pyrophosphate dihydrate crystals in the joints.

M11.10 Familial chondrocalcinosis, <u>unspecified</u> site
M11.11- Familial chondrocalcinosis, <u>shoulder</u>
 M11.111 Familial chondrocalcinosis, <u>right</u> shoulder
 M11.112 Familial chondrocalcinosis, <u>left</u> shoulder
 M11.119 Familial chondrocalcinosis, <u>unspecified</u> shoulder
M11.12- Familial chondrocalcinosis, <u>elbow</u>
 M11.121 Familial chondrocalcinosis, <u>right</u> elbow
 M11.122 Familial chondrocalcinosis, <u>left</u> elbow
 M11.129 Familial chondrocalcinosis, <u>unspecified</u> elbow
M11.13- Familial chondrocalcinosis, <u>wrist</u>
 M11.131 Familial chondrocalcinosis, <u>right</u> wrist
 M11.132 Familial chondrocalcinosis, <u>left</u> wrist
 M11.139 Familial chondrocalcinosis, <u>unspecified</u> wrist

M11.14- Familial chondrocalcinosis, <u>hand</u>
 M11.141 Familial chondrocalcinosis, <u>right</u> hand
 M11.142 Familial chondrocalcinosis, <u>left</u> hand
 M11.149 Familial chondrocalcinosis, <u>unspecified</u> hand
M11.15- Familial chondrocalcinosis, <u>hip</u>
 M11.151 Familial chondrocalcinosis, <u>right</u> hip
 M11.152 Familial chondrocalcinosis, <u>left</u> hip
 M11.159 Familial chondrocalcinosis, <u>unspecified</u> hip
M11.16- Familial chondrocalcinosis, <u>knee</u>
 M11.161 Familial chondrocalcinosis, <u>right</u> knee
 M11.162 Familial chondrocalcinosis, <u>left</u> knee
 M11.169 Familial chondrocalcinosis, <u>unspecified</u> knee
M11.17- Familial chondrocalcinosis, <u>ankle and foot</u>
 M11.171 Familial chondrocalcinosis, <u>right</u> ankle and foot
 M11.172 Familial chondrocalcinosis, <u>left</u> ankle and foot
 M11.179 Familial chondrocalcinosis, <u>unspecified</u> ankle and foot
M11.18 Familial chondrocalcinosis, <u>vertebrae</u>
M11.19 Familial chondrocalcinosis, <u>multiple sites</u>

M11.2- <u>Other chondrocalcinosis</u> — A chronic inherited form caused by the deposition of calcium pyrophosphate dihydrate crystals in the joints.
 Chondrocalcinosis NOS

M11.20 Other chondrocalcinosis, <u>unspecified</u> site
M11.21- Other chondrocalcinosis, <u>shoulder</u>
 M11.211 Other chondrocalcinosis, <u>right</u> shoulder
 M11.212 Other chondrocalcinosis, <u>left</u> shoulder
 M11.219 Other chondrocalcinosis, <u>unspecified</u> shoulder
M11.22- Other chondrocalcinosis, <u>elbow</u>
 M11.221 Other chondrocalcinosis, <u>right</u> elbow
 M11.222 Other chondrocalcinosis, <u>left</u> elbow
 M11.229 Other chondrocalcinosis, <u>unspecified</u> elbow
M11.23- Other chondrocalcinosis, <u>wrist</u>
 M11.231 Other chondrocalcinosis, <u>right</u> wrist
 M11.232 Other chondrocalcinosis, <u>left</u> wrist
 M11.239 Other chondrocalcinosis, <u>unspecified</u> wrist
M11.24- Other chondrocalcinosis, <u>hand</u>
 M11.241 Other chondrocalcinosis, <u>right</u> hand
 M11.242 Other chondrocalcinosis, <u>left</u> hand
 M11.249 Other chondrocalcinosis, <u>unspecified</u> hand
M11.25- Other chondrocalcinosis, <u>hip</u>
 M11.251 Other chondrocalcinosis, <u>right</u> hip
 M11.252 Other chondrocalcinosis, <u>left</u> hip
 M11.259 Other chondrocalcinosis, <u>unspecified</u> hip
M11.26- Other chondrocalcinosis, <u>knee</u>
 M11.261 Other chondrocalcinosis, <u>right</u> knee
 M11.262 Other chondrocalcinosis, <u>left</u> knee
 M11.269 Other chondrocalcinosis, <u>unspecified</u> knee
M11.27- Other chondrocalcinosis, <u>ankle and foot</u>
 M11.271 Other chondrocalcinosis, <u>right</u> ankle and foot
 M11.272 Other chondrocalcinosis, <u>left</u> ankle and foot
 M11.279 Other chondrocalcinosis, <u>unspecified</u> ankle and foot
M11.28 Other chondrocalcinosis, <u>vertebrae</u>
M11.29 Other chondrocalcinosis, <u>multiple sites</u>

M11.8- <u>Other specified crystal</u> arthropathies
M11.80 Other specified crystal arthropathies, <u>unspecified</u> site
M11.81- Other specified crystal arthropathies, <u>shoulder</u>
 M11.811 Other specified crystal arthropathies, <u>right</u> shoulder
 M11.812 Other specified crystal arthropathies, <u>left</u> shoulder
 M11.819 Other specified crystal arthropathies, <u>unspecified</u> shoulder

M10 - M11

M11.82- Other specified crystal arthropathies, <u>elbow</u>
    M11.821 Other specified crystal arthropathies, <u>right</u> elbow
    M11.822 Other specified crystal arthropathies, <u>left</u> elbow
    M11.829 Other specified crystal arthropathies, <u>unspecified</u> elbow
M11.83- Other specified crystal arthropathies, <u>wrist</u>
    M11.831 Other specified crystal arthropathies, <u>right</u> wrist
    M11.832 Other specified crystal arthropathies, <u>left</u> wrist
    M11.839 Other specified crystal arthropathies, <u>unspecified</u> wrist
M11.84- Other specified crystal arthropathies, <u>hand</u>
    M11.841 Other specified crystal arthropathies, <u>right</u> hand
    M11.842 Other specified crystal arthropathies, <u>left</u> hand
    M11.849 Other specified crystal arthropathies, <u>unspecified</u> hand
M11.85- Other specified crystal arthropathies, <u>hip</u>
    M11.851 Other specified crystal arthropathies, <u>right</u> hip
    M11.852 Other specified crystal arthropathies, <u>left</u> hip
    M11.859 Other specified crystal arthropathies, <u>unspecified</u> hip
M11.86- Other specified crystal arthropathies, <u>knee</u>
    M11.861 Other specified crystal arthropathies, <u>right</u> knee
    M11.862 Other specified crystal arthropathies, <u>left</u> knee
    M11.869 Other specified crystal arthropathies, <u>unspecified</u> knee
M11.87- Other specified crystal arthropathies, <u>ankle and foot</u>
    M11.871 Other specified crystal arthropathies, <u>right</u> ankle and foot
    M11.872 Other specified crystal arthropathies, <u>left</u> ankle and foot
    M11.879 Other specified crystal arthropathies, <u>unspecified</u> ankle and foot
M11.88 Other specified crystal arthropathies, <u>vertebrae</u>
M11.89 Other specified crystal arthropathies, <u>multiple sites</u>
M11.9 Crystal arthropathy, <u>unspecified</u>

M12- <u>Other and unspecified</u> arthropathy
  Excludes 1:   *arthrosis (M15-M19)*
                 cricoarytenoid arthropathy (J38.7)
M12.0- <u>Chronic postrheumatic arthropathy [Jaccoud]</u> — Chronic inflammation of the joints that follows patients with previous rheumatoid arthritis attacks and the rheumatoid factor is not present in the blood.
  M12.00 Chronic postrheumatic arthropathy [Jaccoud], <u>unspecified</u> site
  M12.01- Chronic postrheumatic arthropathy [Jaccoud], <u>shoulder</u>
    M12.011 Chronic postrheumatic arthropathy [Jaccoud], <u>right</u> shoulder
    M12.012 Chronic postrheumatic arthropathy [Jaccoud], <u>left</u> shoulder
    M12.019 Chronic postrheumatic arthropathy [Jaccoud], <u>unspecified</u> shoulder
  M12.02- Chronic postrheumatic arthropathy [Jaccoud], <u>elbow</u>
    M12.021 Chronic postrheumatic arthropathy [Jaccoud], <u>right</u> elbow
    M12.022 Chronic postrheumatic arthropathy [Jaccoud], <u>left</u> elbow
    M12.029 Chronic postrheumatic arthropathy [Jaccoud], <u>unspecified</u> elbow
  M12.03- Chronic postrheumatic arthropathy [Jaccoud], <u>wrist</u>
    M12.031 Chronic postrheumatic arthropathy [Jaccoud], <u>right</u> wrist
    M12.032 Chronic postrheumatic arthropathy [Jaccoud], <u>left</u> wrist
    M12.039 Chronic postrheumatic arthropathy [Jaccoud], <u>unspecified</u> wrist

M12.04- Chronic postrheumatic arthropathy [Jaccoud], <u>hand</u>
    M12.041 Chronic postrheumatic arthropathy [Jaccoud], <u>right</u> hand
    M12.042 Chronic postrheumatic arthropathy [Jaccoud], <u>left</u> hand
    M12.049 Chronic postrheumatic arthropathy [Jaccoud], <u>unspecified</u> hand
M12.05- Chronic postrheumatic arthropathy [Jaccoud], <u>hip</u>
    M12.051 Chronic postrheumatic arthropathy [Jaccoud], <u>right</u> hip
    M12.052 Chronic postrheumatic arthropathy [Jaccoud], <u>left</u> hip
    M12.059 Chronic postrheumatic arthropathy [Jaccoud], <u>unspecified</u> hip
M12.06- Chronic postrheumatic arthropathy [Jaccoud], <u>knee</u>
    M12.061 Chronic postrheumatic arthropathy [Jaccoud], <u>right</u> knee
    M12.062 Chronic postrheumatic arthropathy [Jaccoud], <u>left</u> knee
    M12.069 Chronic postrheumatic arthropathy [Jaccoud], <u>unspecified</u> knee
M12.07- Chronic postrheumatic arthropathy [Jaccoud], <u>ankle and foot</u>
    M12.071 Chronic postrheumatic arthropathy [Jaccoud], <u>right</u> ankle and foot
    M12.072 Chronic postrheumatic arthropathy [Jaccoud], <u>left</u> ankle and foot
    M12.079 Chronic postrheumatic arthropathy [Jaccoud], <u>unspecified</u> ankle and foot
M12.08 Chronic postrheumatic arthropathy [Jaccoud], <u>other specified site</u>
    Chronic postrheumatic arthropathy [Jaccoud], vertebrae
M12.09 Chronic postrheumatic arthropathy [Jaccoud], <u>multiple sites</u>
M12.1- <u>Kaschin-Beck</u> disease — A chronic osteochondropathy that is characterized by joint pain, stiffness, shortened limb length, and enlarged joints of the fingers that is found primarily in southern China and surrounding areas.
    Osteochondroarthrosis deformans endemica
M12.10 Kaschin-Beck disease, <u>unspecified</u> site
M12.11- Kaschin-Beck disease, <u>shoulder</u>
    M12.111 Kaschin-Beck disease, <u>right</u> shoulder
    M12.112 Kaschin-Beck disease, <u>left</u> shoulder
    M12.119 Kaschin-Beck disease, <u>unspecified</u> shoulder
M12.12- Kaschin-Beck disease, <u>elbow</u>
    M12.121 Kaschin-Beck disease, <u>right</u> elbow
    M12.122 Kaschin-Beck disease, <u>left</u> elbow
    M12.129 Kaschin-Beck disease, <u>unspecified</u> elbow
M12.13- Kaschin-Beck disease, <u>wrist</u>
    M12.131 Kaschin-Beck disease, <u>right</u> wrist
    M12.132 Kaschin-Beck disease, <u>left</u> wrist
    M12.139 Kaschin-Beck disease, <u>unspecified</u> wrist
M12.14- Kaschin-Beck disease, <u>hand</u>
    M12.141 Kaschin-Beck disease, <u>right</u> hand
    M12.142 Kaschin-Beck disease, <u>left</u> hand
    M12.149 Kaschin-Beck disease, <u>unspecified</u> hand
M12.15- Kaschin-Beck disease, <u>hip</u>
    M12.151 Kaschin-Beck disease, <u>right</u> hip
    M12.152 Kaschin-Beck disease, <u>left</u> hip
    M12.159 Kaschin-Beck disease, <u>unspecified</u> hip
M12.16- Kaschin-Beck disease, <u>knee</u>
    M12.161 Kaschin-Beck disease, <u>right</u> knee
    M12.162 Kaschin-Beck disease, <u>left</u> knee
    M12.169 Kaschin-Beck disease, <u>unspecified</u> knee

M12.17- **Kaschin-Beck disease, <u>ankle and foot</u>**
   M12.171 Kaschin-Beck disease, <u>right</u> ankle and foot
   M12.172 Kaschin-Beck disease, <u>left</u> ankle and foot
   M12.179 Kaschin-Beck disease, <u>unspecified</u> ankle and foot
M12.18 **Kaschin-Beck disease, <u>vertebrae</u>**
M12.19 **Kaschin-Beck disease, <u>multiple sites</u>**
M12.2- <u>**Villonodular synovitis (pigmented)**</u> — A chronic synovial joint disorder that is characterized by nodular lesions.
M12.20 **Villonodular synovitis (pigmented), <u>unspecified</u> site**
M12.21- **Villonodular synovitis (pigmented), <u>shoulder</u>**
   M12.211 Villonodular synovitis (pigmented), <u>right</u> shoulder
   M12.212 Villonodular synovitis (pigmented), <u>left</u> shoulder
   M12.219 Villonodular synovitis (pigmented), <u>unspecified</u> shoulder
M12.22- **Villonodular synovitis (pigmented), <u>elbow</u>**
   M12.221 Villonodular synovitis (pigmented), <u>right</u> elbow
   M12.222 Villonodular synovitis (pigmented), <u>left</u> elbow
   M12.229 Villonodular synovitis (pigmented), <u>unspecified</u> elbow
M12.23- **Villonodular synovitis (pigmented), <u>wrist</u>**
   M12.231 Villonodular synovitis (pigmented), <u>right</u> wrist
   M12.232 Villonodular synovitis (pigmented), <u>left</u> wrist
   M12.239 Villonodular synovitis (pigmented), <u>unspecified</u> wrist
M12.24- **Villonodular synovitis (pigmented), <u>hand</u>**
   M12.241 Villonodular synovitis (pigmented), <u>right</u> hand
   M12.242 Villonodular synovitis (pigmented), <u>left</u> hand
   M12.249 Villonodular synovitis (pigmented), <u>unspecified</u> hand
M12.25- **Villonodular synovitis (pigmented), <u>hip</u>**
   M12.251 Villonodular synovitis (pigmented), <u>right</u> hip
   M12.252 Villonodular synovitis (pigmented), <u>left</u> hip
   M12.259 Villonodular synovitis (pigmented), <u>unspecified</u> hip
M12.26- **Villonodular synovitis (pigmented), <u>knee</u>**
   M12.261 Villonodular synovitis (pigmented), <u>right</u> knee
   M12.262 Villonodular synovitis (pigmented), <u>left</u> knee
   M12.269 Villonodular synovitis (pigmented), <u>unspecified</u> knee
M12.27- **Villonodular synovitis (pigmented), <u>ankle and foot</u>**
   M12.271 Villonodular synovitis (pigmented), <u>right</u> ankle and foot
   M12.272 Villonodular synovitis (pigmented), <u>left</u> ankle and foot
   M12.279 Villonodular synovitis (pigmented), <u>unspecified</u> ankle and foot
M12.28 **Villonodular synovitis (pigmented), <u>other specified site</u>**
   Villonodular synovitis (pigmented), vertebrae
M12.29 **Villonodular synovitis (pigmented), <u>multiple sites</u>**
M12.3- <u>**Palindromic rheumatism**</u> — A chronic arthropathy that is characterized by sudden attacks of acute pain, swelling, and stiffness that come and go but do not show signs of permanent damage to the joints.
M12.30 **Palindromic rheumatism, <u>unspecified</u> site**
M12.31- **Palindromic rheumatism, <u>shoulder</u>**
   M12.311 Palindromic rheumatism, <u>right</u> shoulder
   M12.312 Palindromic rheumatism, <u>left</u> shoulder
   M12.319 Palindromic rheumatism, <u>unspecified</u> shoulder
M12.32- **Palindromic rheumatism, <u>elbow</u>**
   M12.321 Palindromic rheumatism, <u>right</u> elbow
   M12.322 Palindromic rheumatism, <u>left</u> elbow
   M12.329 Palindromic rheumatism, <u>unspecified</u> elbow
M12.33- **Palindromic rheumatism, <u>wrist</u>**
   M12.331 Palindromic rheumatism, <u>right</u> wrist
   M12.332 Palindromic rheumatism, <u>left</u> wrist
   M12.339 Palindromic rheumatism, <u>unspecified</u> wrist
M12.34- **Palindromic rheumatism, <u>hand</u>**
   M12.341 Palindromic rheumatism, <u>right</u> hand

M12.342 Palindromic rheumatism, <u>left</u> hand
M12.349 Palindromic rheumatism, <u>unspecified</u> hand
M12.35- **Palindromic rheumatism, <u>hip</u>**
   M12.351 Palindromic rheumatism, <u>right</u> hip
   M12.352 Palindromic rheumatism, <u>left</u> hip
   M12.359 Palindromic rheumatism, <u>unspecified</u> hip
M12.36- **Palindromic rheumatism, <u>knee</u>**
   M12.361 Palindromic rheumatism, <u>right</u> knee
   M12.362 Palindromic rheumatism, <u>left</u> knee
   M12.369 Palindromic rheumatism, <u>unspecified</u> knee
M12.37- **Palindromic rheumatism, <u>ankle and foot</u>**
   M12.371 Palindromic rheumatism, <u>right</u> ankle and foot
   M12.372 Palindromic rheumatism, <u>left</u> ankle and foot
   M12.379 Palindromic rheumatism, <u>unspecified</u> ankle and foot
M12.38 **Palindromic rheumatism, <u>other specified site</u>**
   Palindromic rheumatism, vertebrae
M12.39 **Palindromic rheumatism, <u>multiple sites</u>**
M12.4- <u>**Intermittent hydrarthrosis**</u> — A rare arthropathy that usually affects women that is characterized by symmetric joint effusions of the knees and often occurring around the menses period.
M12.40 **Intermittent hydrarthrosis, <u>unspecified</u> site**
M12.41- **Intermittent hydrarthrosis, <u>shoulder</u>**
   M12.411 Intermittent hydrarthrosis, <u>right</u> shoulder
   M12.412 Intermittent hydrarthrosis, <u>left</u> shoulder
   M12.419 Intermittent hydrarthrosis, <u>unspecified</u> shoulder
M12.42- **Intermittent hydrarthrosis, <u>elbow</u>**
   M12.421 Intermittent hydrarthrosis, <u>right</u> elbow
   M12.422 Intermittent hydrarthrosis, <u>left</u> elbow
   M12.429 Intermittent hydrarthrosis, <u>unspecified</u> elbow
M12.43- **Intermittent hydrarthrosis, <u>wrist</u>**
   M12.431 Intermittent hydrarthrosis, <u>right</u> wrist
   M12.432 Intermittent hydrarthrosis, <u>left</u> wrist
   M12.439 Intermittent hydrarthrosis, <u>unspecified</u> wrist
M12.44- **Intermittent hydrarthrosis, <u>hand</u>**
   M12.441 Intermittent hydrarthrosis, <u>right</u> hand
   M12.442 Intermittent hydrarthrosis, <u>left</u> hand
   M12.449 Intermittent hydrarthrosis, <u>unspecified</u> hand
M12.45- **Intermittent hydrarthrosis, <u>hip</u>**
   M12.451 Intermittent hydrarthrosis, <u>right</u> hip
   M12.452 Intermittent hydrarthrosis, <u>left</u> hip
   M12.459 Intermittent hydrarthrosis, <u>unspecified</u> hip
M12.46- **Intermittent hydrarthrosis, <u>knee</u>**
   M12.461 Intermittent hydrarthrosis, <u>right</u> knee
   M12.462 Intermittent hydrarthrosis, <u>left</u> knee
   M12.469 Intermittent hydrarthrosis, <u>unspecified</u> knee
M12.47- **Intermittent hydrarthrosis, <u>ankle and foot</u>**
   M12.471 Intermittent hydrarthrosis, <u>right</u> ankle and foot
   M12.472 Intermittent hydrarthrosis, <u>left</u> ankle and foot
   M12.479 Intermittent hydrarthrosis, <u>unspecified</u> ankle and foot
M12.48 **Intermittent hydrarthrosis, <u>other site</u>**
M12.49 **Intermittent hydrarthrosis, <u>multiple sites</u>**
M12.5- <u>**Traumatic arthropathy**</u> — An arthropathy that is due to a traumatic injury to a joint.
   AHA 15:1Q:p17 – Traumatic arthritis of hip secondary to femur fracture
   Excludes 1: *current injury — see Alphabetic Index*
       post-traumatic osteoarthritis of first carpometacarpal joint (M18.2-M18.3)
       post-traumatic osteoarthritis of hip (M16.4-M16.5)
       post-traumatic osteoarthritis of knee (M17.2-M17.3)
       post-traumatic osteoarthritis NOS (M19.1-)
       post-traumatic osteoarthritis of other single joints (M19.1-)
M12.50 **Traumatic arthropathy, <u>unspecified</u> site**

M 1 2 - M 1 2

M12.51- Traumatic arthropathy, <u>shoulder</u>
  M12.511 Traumatic arthropathy, <u>right</u> shoulder
  M12.512 Traumatic arthropathy, <u>left</u> shoulder
  M12.519 Traumatic arthropathy, <u>unspecified</u> shoulder
M12.52- Traumatic arthropathy, <u>elbow</u>
  M12.521 Traumatic arthropathy, <u>right</u> elbow
  M12.522 Traumatic arthropathy, <u>left</u> elbow
  M12.529 Traumatic arthropathy, <u>unspecified</u> elbow
M12.53- Traumatic arthropathy, <u>wrist</u>
  M12.531 Traumatic arthropathy, <u>right</u> wrist
  M12.532 Traumatic arthropathy, <u>left</u> wrist
  M12.539 Traumatic arthropathy, <u>unspecified</u> wrist
M12.54- Traumatic arthropathy, <u>hand</u>
  M12.541 Traumatic arthropathy, <u>right</u> hand
  M12.542 Traumatic arthropathy, <u>left</u> hand
  M12.549 Traumatic arthropathy, <u>unspecified</u> hand
M12.55- Traumatic arthropathy, <u>hip</u>
  M12.551 Traumatic arthropathy, <u>right</u> hip
  M12.552 Traumatic arthropathy, <u>left</u> hip
  M12.559 Traumatic arthropathy, <u>unspecified</u> hip
M12.56- Traumatic arthropathy, <u>knee</u>
  M12.561 Traumatic arthropathy, <u>right</u> knee
  M12.562 Traumatic arthropathy, <u>left</u> knee
  M12.569 Traumatic arthropathy, <u>unspecified</u> knee
M12.57- Traumatic arthropathy, <u>ankle and foot</u>
  M12.571 Traumatic arthropathy, <u>right</u> ankle and foot
  M12.572 Traumatic arthropathy, <u>left</u> ankle and foot
  M12.579 Traumatic arthropathy, <u>unspecified</u> ankle and foot
M12.58 Traumatic arthropathy, <u>other specified site</u>
    Traumatic arthropathy, vertebrae
M12.59 Traumatic arthropathy, <u>multiple sites</u>
M12.8- <u>Other specific arthropathies</u>, <u>not elsewhere classified</u>
    Transient arthropathy
M12.80 Other specific arthropathies, not elsewhere classified, <u>unspecified</u> site
M12.81- Other specific arthropathies, not elsewhere classified, <u>shoulder</u>
  M12.811 Other specific arthropathies, not elsewhere classified, <u>right</u> shoulder
  M12.812 Other specific arthropathies, not elsewhere classified, <u>left</u> shoulder
  M12.819 Other specific arthropathies, not elsewhere classified, <u>unspecified</u> shoulder
M12.82- Other specific arthropathies, not elsewhere classified, <u>elbow</u>
  M12.821 Other specific arthropathies, not elsewhere classified, <u>right</u> elbow
  M12.822 Other specific arthropathies, not elsewhere classified, <u>left</u> elbow
  M12.829 Other specific arthropathies, not elsewhere classified, <u>unspecified</u> elbow
M12.83- Other specific arthropathies, not elsewhere classified, <u>wrist</u>
  M12.831 Other specific arthropathies, not elsewhere classified, <u>right</u> wrist
  M12.832 Other specific arthropathies, not elsewhere classified, <u>left</u> wrist
  M12.839 Other specific arthropathies, not elsewhere classified, <u>unspecified</u> wrist
M12.84- Other specific arthropathies, not elsewhere classified, <u>hand</u>
  M12.841 Other specific arthropathies, not elsewhere classified, <u>right</u> hand
  M12.842 Other specific arthropathies, not elsewhere classified, <u>left</u> hand
  M12.849 Other specific arthropathies, not elsewhere classified, <u>unspecified</u> hand

M12.85- Other specific arthropathies, not elsewhere classified, <u>hip</u>
  M12.851 Other specific arthropathies, not elsewhere classified, <u>right</u> hip
  M12.852 Other specific arthropathies, not elsewhere classified, <u>left</u> hip
  M12.859 Other specific arthropathies, not elsewhere classified, <u>unspecified</u> hip
M12.86- Other specific arthropathies, not elsewhere classified, <u>knee</u>
  M12.861 Other specific arthropathies, not elsewhere classified, <u>right</u> knee
  M12.862 Other specific arthropathies, not elsewhere classified, <u>left</u> knee
  M12.869 Other specific arthropathies, not elsewhere classified, <u>unspecified</u> knee
M12.87- Other specific arthropathies, not elsewhere classified, <u>ankle and foot</u>
  M12.871 Other specific arthropathies, not elsewhere classified, <u>right</u> ankle and foot
  M12.872 Other specific arthropathies, not elsewhere classified, <u>left</u> ankle and foot
  M12.879 Other specific arthropathies, not elsewhere classified, <u>unspecified</u> ankle and foot
M12.88 Other specific arthropathies, not elsewhere classified, <u>other specified site</u>
    Other specific arthropathies, not elsewhere classified, vertebrae
M12.89 Other specific arthropathies, not elsewhere classified, <u>multiple sites</u>
M12.9 Arthropathy, <u>unspecified</u>

M13- <u>Other arthritis</u>
  Excludes 1: *arthrosis (M15-M19)*
              osteoarthritis (M15-M19)
M13.0 <u>Polyarthritis</u>, <u>unspecified</u> — A form affecting multiple joints and of an unknown cause.
M13.1- <u>Monoarthritis</u>, <u>not elsewhere classified</u> — A form affecting a single joint and of an unknown cause.
  M13.10 Monoarthritis, not elsewhere classified, <u>unspecified</u> site
  M13.11- Monoarthritis, not elsewhere classified, <u>shoulder</u>
    M13.111 Monoarthritis, not elsewhere classified, <u>right</u> shoulder
    M13.112 Monoarthritis, not elsewhere classified, <u>left</u> shoulder
    M13.119 Monoarthritis, not elsewhere classified, <u>unspecified</u> shoulder
  M13.12- Monoarthritis, not elsewhere classified, <u>elbow</u>
    M13.121 Monoarthritis, not elsewhere classified, <u>right</u> elbow
    M13.122 Monoarthritis, not elsewhere classified, <u>left</u> elbow
    M13.129 Monoarthritis, not elsewhere classified, <u>unspecified</u> elbow
  M13.13- Monoarthritis, not elsewhere classified, <u>wrist</u>
    M13.131 Monoarthritis, not elsewhere classified, <u>right</u> wrist
    M13.132 Monoarthritis, not elsewhere classified, <u>left</u> wrist
    M13.139 Monoarthritis, not elsewhere classified, <u>unspecified</u> wrist
  M13.14- Monoarthritis, not elsewhere classified, <u>hand</u>
    M13.141 Monoarthritis, not elsewhere classified, <u>right</u> hand
    M13.142 Monoarthritis, not elsewhere classified, <u>left</u> hand
    M13.149 Monoarthritis, not elsewhere classified, <u>unspecified</u> hand
  M13.15- Monoarthritis, not elsewhere classified, <u>hip</u>
    M13.151 Monoarthritis, not elsewhere classified, <u>right</u> hip
    M13.152 Monoarthritis, not elsewhere classified, <u>left</u> hip
    M13.159 Monoarthritis, not elsewhere classified, <u>unspecified</u> hip
  M13.16- Monoarthritis, not elsewhere classified, <u>knee</u>
    M13.161 Monoarthritis, not elsewhere classified, <u>right</u> knee

M12 – M13

M13.162   Monoarthritis, not elsewhere classified, <u>left</u> knee

M13.169   Monoarthritis, not elsewhere classified, <u>unspecified</u> knee

M13.17- Monoarthritis, not elsewhere classified, <u>ankle and foot</u>

M13.171   Monoarthritis, not elsewhere classified, <u>right</u> ankle and foot

M13.172   Monoarthritis, not elsewhere classified, <u>left</u> ankle and foot

M13.179   Monoarthritis, not elsewhere classified, <u>unspecified</u> ankle and foot

M13.8-   <u>Other specified arthritis</u>

    Allergic arthritis — Inflammation of a joint(s) that is due to an allergen.

    Excludes 1:   osteoarthritis (M15-M19)

M13.80   Other specified arthritis, <u>unspecified</u> site

M13.81- Other specified arthritis, <u>shoulder</u>

M13.811   Other specified arthritis, <u>right</u> shoulder

M13.812   Other specified arthritis, <u>left</u> shoulder

M13.819   Other specified arthritis, <u>unspecified</u> shoulder

M13.82- Other specified arthritis, <u>elbow</u>

M13.821   Other specified arthritis, <u>right</u> elbow

M13.822   Other specified arthritis, <u>left</u> elbow

M13.829   Other specified arthritis, <u>unspecified</u> elbow

M13.83- Other specified arthritis, <u>wrist</u>

M13.831   Other specified arthritis, <u>right</u> wrist

M13.832   Other specified arthritis, <u>left</u> wrist

M13.839   Other specified arthritis, <u>unspecified</u> wrist

M13.84- Other specified arthritis, <u>hand</u>

M13.841   Other specified arthritis, <u>right</u> hand

M13.842   Other specified arthritis, <u>left</u> hand

M13.849   Other specified arthritis, <u>unspecified</u> hand

M13.85- Other specified arthritis, <u>hip</u>

M13.851   Other specified arthritis, <u>right</u> hip

M13.852   Other specified arthritis, <u>left</u> hip

M13.859   Other specified arthritis, <u>unspecified</u> hip

M13.86- Other specified arthritis, <u>knee</u>

M13.861   Other specified arthritis, <u>right</u> knee

M13.862   Other specified arthritis, <u>left</u> knee

M13.869   Other specified arthritis, <u>unspecified</u> knee

M13.87- Other specified arthritis, <u>ankle and foot</u>

M13.871   Other specified arthritis, <u>right</u> ankle and foot

M13.872   Other specified arthritis, <u>left</u> ankle and foot

M13.879   Other specified arthritis, <u>unspecified</u> ankle and foot

M13.88   Other specified arthritis, <u>other site</u>

M13.89   Other specified arthritis, <u>multiple sites</u>

M14-   Arthropathies <u>in other diseases classified elsewhere</u>

    Excludes 1:   *arthropathy in:*

       diabetes mellitus (E08-E13 with .61-)

       hematological disorders (M36.2-M36.3)

       hypersensitivity reactions (M36.4)

       neoplastic disease (M36.1)

       neurosyphillis (A52.16)

       sarcoidosis (D86.86)

       enteropathic arthropathies (M07.-)

       juvenile psoriatic arthropathy (L40.54)

       lipoid dermatoarthritis (E78.81)

M14.6-   <u>Charcot's joint</u> — An arthropathy that is characterized by decreased sensation at the site (usually a weight bearing joint) that leads to bony abnormalities, deformity, and ulceration.

    Neuropathic arthropathy

    Excludes 1:   *Charcot's joint in diabetes mellitus (E08-E13 with .610)*

       Charcot's joint in tabes dorsalis (A52.16)

M14.60   Charcot's joint, <u>unspecified</u> site

M14.61- Charcot's joint, <u>shoulder</u>

M14.611   Charcot's joint, <u>right</u> shoulder

M14.612   Charcot's joint, <u>left</u> shoulder

M14.619   Charcot's joint, <u>unspecified</u> shoulder

M14.62- Charcot's joint, <u>elbow</u>

M14.621   Charcot's joint, <u>right</u> elbow

M14.622   Charcot's joint, <u>left</u> elbow

M14.629   Charcot's joint, <u>unspecified</u> elbow

M14.63- Charcot's joint, <u>wrist</u>

M14.631   Charcot's joint, <u>right</u> wrist

M14.632   Charcot's joint, <u>left</u> wrist

M14.639   Charcot's joint, <u>unspecified</u> wrist

M14.64- Charcot's joint, <u>hand</u>

M14.641   Charcot's joint, <u>right</u> hand

M14.642   Charcot's joint, <u>left</u> hand

M14.649   Charcot's joint, <u>unspecified</u> hand

M14.65- Charcot's joint, <u>hip</u>

M14.651   Charcot's joint, <u>right</u> hip

M14.652   Charcot's joint, <u>left</u> hip

M14.659   Charcot's joint, <u>unspecified</u> hip

M14.66- Charcot's joint, <u>knee</u>

M14.661   Charcot's joint, <u>right</u> knee

M14.662   Charcot's joint, <u>left</u> knee

M14.669   Charcot's joint, <u>unspecified</u> knee

M14.67- Charcot's joint, <u>ankle and foot</u>

M14.671   Charcot's joint, <u>right</u> ankle and foot

M14.672   Charcot's joint, <u>left</u> ankle and foot

M14.679   Charcot's joint, <u>unspecified</u> ankle and foot

M14.68   Charcot's joint, <u>vertebrae</u>

M14.69   Charcot's joint, <u>multiple sites</u>

M14.8-   Arthropathies <u>in other specified diseases classified elsewhere</u>

    Code first underlying disease, such as:

       Amyloidosis (E85.-)

       Erythema multiforme (L51-)

       Erythema nodosum (L52)

       Hemochromatosis (E83.11-)

       Hyperparathyroidism (E21-)

       Hypothyroidism (E00-E03)

       Sickle-cell disorders (D57-)

       Thyrotoxicosis [hyperthyroidism] (E05-)

       Whipple's disease (K90.81)

M14.80   Arthropathies in other specified diseases classified elsewhere, <u>unspecified</u> site — [Not Allowed as PDX]

M14.81- Arthropathies in other specified diseases classified elsewhere, <u>shoulder</u>

M14.811   Arthropathies in other specified diseases classified elsewhere, <u>right</u> shoulder — [Not Allowed as PDX]

M14.812   Arthropathies in other specified diseases classified elsewhere, <u>left</u> shoulder — [Not Allowed as PDX]

M14.819   Arthropathies in other specified diseases classified elsewhere, <u>unspecified</u> shoulder — [Not Allowed as PDX]

M14.82- Arthropathies in other specified diseases classified elsewhere, <u>elbow</u>

M14.821   Arthropathies in other specified diseases classified elsewhere, <u>right</u> elbow — [Not Allowed as PDX]

M14.822   Arthropathies in other specified diseases classified elsewhere, <u>left</u> elbow — [Not Allowed as PDX]

M14.829   Arthropathies in other specified diseases classified elsewhere, <u>unspecified</u> elbow — [Not Allowed as PDX]

M14.83- Arthropathies in other specified diseases classified elsewhere, <u>wrist</u>

M14.831   Arthropathies in other specified diseases classified elsewhere, <u>right</u> wrist — [Not Allowed as PDX]

M14.832   Arthropathies in other specified diseases classified elsewhere, <u>left</u> wrist — [Not Allowed as PDX]

M14.839   Arthropathies in other specified diseases classified elsewhere, <u>unspecified</u> wrist — [Not Allowed as PDX]

M14.84- Arthropathies in other specified diseases classified elsewhere, <u>hand</u>

M14.841   Arthropathies in other specified diseases classified elsewhere, <u>right</u> hand — [Not Allowed as PDX]

M14.842   Arthropathies in other specified diseases classified elsewhere, <u>left</u> hand — [Not Allowed as PDX]

M14.849 Arthropathies in other specified diseases classified elsewhere, **unspecified** hand — [Not Allowed as PDX]

M14.85- Arthropathies in other specified diseases classified elsewhere, **hip**

M14.851 Arthropathies in other specified diseases classified elsewhere, **right** hip — [Not Allowed as PDX]

M14.852 Arthropathies in other specified diseases classified elsewhere, **left** hip — [Not Allowed as PDX]

M14.859 Arthropathies in other specified diseases classified elsewhere, **unspecified** hip — [Not Allowed as PDX]

M14.86- Arthropathies in other specified diseases classified elsewhere, **knee**

M14.861 Arthropathies in other specified diseases classified elsewhere, **right** knee — [Not Allowed as PDX]

M14.862 Arthropathies in other specified diseases classified elsewhere, **left** knee — [Not Allowed as PDX]

M14.869 Arthropathies in other specified diseases classified elsewhere, **unspecified** knee — [Not Allowed as PDX]

M14.87- Arthropathies in other specified diseases classified elsewhere, **ankle and foot**

M14.871 Arthropathies in other specified diseases classified elsewhere, **right** ankle and foot — [Not Allowed as PDX]

M14.872 Arthropathies in other specified diseases classified elsewhere, **left** ankle and foot — [Not Allowed as PDX]

M14.879 Arthropathies in other specified diseases classified elsewhere, **unspecified** ankle and foot — [Not Allowed as PDX]

M14.88 Arthropathies in other specified diseases classified elsewhere, **vertebrae** — [Not Allowed as PDX]

M14.89 Arthropathies in other specified diseases classified elsewhere, **multiple sites** — [Not Allowed as PDX]

Osteoarthritis (M15-M19)

Excludes ❷: *osteoarthritis of spine (M47.-)*

M15- **Polyosteoarthritis** — A degenerative inflammation of the joints that is caused by the breakdown, weardown, or erosion of the joint cartilage and results in damage to the underlying bone.

Includes: Arthritis of multiple sites

Excludes 1: *bilateral involvement of single joint (M16-M19)*

M15.0 **Primary generalized (osteo)arthritis** — A form occurring without any known secondary cause.

M15.1 **Heberden's nodes (with arthropathy)** — A form marked by the formation of hard nodules in the distal interphalangeal joints of the fingers and toes.

Interphalangeal distal osteoarthritis

M15.2 **Bouchard's nodes (with arthropathy)** — A form marked by the formation of hard or gelatinous nodules in the proximal interphalangeal joints of the fingers and toes.

Juxtaphalangeal distal osteoarthritis

M15.3 **Secondary multiple arthritis** — A form caused by another underlying disease or condition.

Post-traumatic polyosteoarthritis

M15.4 **Erosive (osteo)arthritis** — A form marked by "saw-tooth" deformities of the interphalangeal joints of the hand.

M15.8 **Other polyosteoarthritis**

M15.9 **Polyosteoarthritis, unspecified**

Generalized osteoarthritis NOS

M16- **Osteoarthritis of hip**

M16.0 **Bilateral primary osteoarthritis of hip**

M16.1- **Unilateral primary osteoarthritis of hip**

Primary osteoarthritis of hip NOS

M16.10 Unilateral primary osteoarthritis, **unspecified** hip

M16.11 Unilateral primary osteoarthritis, **right** hip

M16.12 Unilateral primary osteoarthritis, **left** hip

M16.2 **Bilateral osteoarthritis resulting from hip dysplasia**

M16.3- **Unilateral osteoarthritis resulting from hip dysplasia**

Dysplastic osteoarthritis of hip NOS

M16.30 Unilateral osteoarthritis resulting from hip dysplasia, **unspecified** hip

M16.31 Unilateral osteoarthritis resulting from hip dysplasia, **right** hip

M16.32 Unilateral osteoarthritis resulting from hip dysplasia, **left** hip

M16.4 **Bilateral post-traumatic osteoarthritis of hip**

M16.5- **Unilateral post-traumatic osteoarthritis of hip**

Post-traumatic osteoarthritis of hip NOS

M16.50 Unilateral post-traumatic osteoarthritis, **unspecified** hip

M16.51 Unilateral post-traumatic osteoarthritis, **right** hip

M16.52 Unilateral post-traumatic osteoarthritis, **left** hip

M16.6 **Other bilateral secondary osteoarthritis of hip**

M16.7 **Other unilateral secondary osteoarthritis of hip**

Secondary osteoarthritis of hip NOS

M16.9 **Osteoarthritis of hip, unspecified**

M17- **Osteoarthritis of knee**

M17.0 **Bilateral primary osteoarthritis of knee**

M17.1- **Unilateral primary osteoarthritis of knee**

Primary osteoarthritis of knee NOS

M17.10 Unilateral primary osteoarthritis, **unspecified** knee

M17.11 Unilateral primary osteoarthritis, **right** knee

M17.12 Unilateral primary osteoarthritis, **left** knee

M17.2 **Bilateral post-traumatic osteoarthritis of knee**

M17.3- **Unilateral post-traumatic osteoarthritis of knee**

Post-traumatic osteoarthritis of knee NOS

M17.30 Unilateral post-traumatic osteoarthritis, **unspecified** knee

M17.31 Unilateral post-traumatic osteoarthritis, **right** knee

M17.32 Unilateral post-traumatic osteoarthritis, **left** knee

M17.4 **Other bilateral secondary osteoarthritis of knee**

M17.5 **Other unilateral secondary osteoarthritis of knee**

Secondary osteoarthritis of knee NOS

M17.9 **Osteoarthritis of knee, unspecified**

M18- **Osteoarthritis of first carpometacarpal joint**

M18.0 **Bilateral primary osteoarthritis of first carpometacarpal joints**

M18.1- **Unilateral primary osteoarthritis of first carpometacarpal joint**

Primary osteoarthritis of first carpometacarpal joint NOS

M18.10 Unilateral primary osteoarthritis of first carpometacarpal joint, **unspecified** hand

M18.11 Unilateral primary osteoarthritis of first carpometacarpal joint, **right** hand

M18.12 Unilateral primary osteoarthritis of first carpometacarpal joint, **left** hand

M18.2 **Bilateral post-traumatic osteoarthritis of first carpometacarpal joints**

M18.3- **Unilateral post-traumatic osteoarthritis of first carpometacarpal joint**

Post-traumatic osteoarthritis of first carpometacarpal joint NOS

M18.30 Unilateral post-traumatic osteoarthritis of first carpometacarpal joint, **unspecified** hand

M18.31 Unilateral post-traumatic osteoarthritis of first carpometacarpal joint, **right** hand

M18.32 Unilateral post-traumatic osteoarthritis of first carpometacarpal joint, **left** hand

M18.4 **Other bilateral secondary osteoarthritis of first carpometacarpal joints**

M18.5- **Other unilateral secondary osteoarthritis of first carpometacarpal joint**

Secondary osteoarthritis of first carpometacarpal joint NOS

M18.50 Other unilateral secondary osteoarthritis of first carpometacarpal joint, **unspecified** hand

M18.51 Other unilateral secondary osteoarthritis of first carpometacarpal joint, **right** hand

M18.52 Other unilateral secondary osteoarthritis of first carpometacarpal joint, **left** hand

M18.9 **Osteoarthritis of first carpometacarpal joint, unspecified**

M14
-
M18

M19   Other and unspecified osteoarthritis
> *Excludes 1:*   polyarthritis (M15.-)
> *Excludes ❷:*   arthrosis of spine (M47.-)
>   hallux rigidus (M20.2)
>   osteoarthritis of spine (M47.-)

M19.0- Primary osteoarthritis of other joints
  M19.01- Primary osteoarthritis, shoulder
    M19.011   Primary osteoarthritis, right shoulder
    M19.012   Primary osteoarthritis, left shoulder
    M19.019   Primary osteoarthritis, unspecified shoulder
  M19.02- Primary osteoarthritis, elbow
    M19.021   Primary osteoarthritis, right elbow
    M19.022   Primary osteoarthritis, left elbow
    M19.029   Primary osteoarthritis, unspecified elbow
  M19.03- Primary osteoarthritis, wrist
    M19.031   Primary osteoarthritis, right wrist
    M19.032   Primary osteoarthritis, left wrist
    M19.039   Primary osteoarthritis, unspecified wrist
  M19.04- Primary osteoarthritis, hand
> *Excludes ❷:*   primary osteoarthritis of first carpometacarpal joint (M18.0-, M18.1-)

    M19.041   Primary osteoarthritis, right hand
    M19.042   Primary osteoarthritis, left hand
    M19.049   Primary osteoarthritis, unspecified hand
  M19.07- Primary osteoarthritis ankle and foot
    M19.071   Primary osteoarthritis, right ankle and foot
    M19.072   Primary osteoarthritis, left ankle and foot
    M19.079   Primary osteoarthritis, unspecified ankle and foot

M19.1- Post-traumatic osteoarthritis of other joints
  M19.11- Post-traumatic osteoarthritis, shoulder
    M19.111   Post-traumatic osteoarthritis, right shoulder
    M19.112   Post-traumatic osteoarthritis, left shoulder
    M19.119   Post-traumatic osteoarthritis, unspecified shoulder
  M19.12- Post-traumatic osteoarthritis, elbow
    M19.121   Post-traumatic osteoarthritis, right elbow
    M19.122   Post-traumatic osteoarthritis, left elbow
    M19.129   Post-traumatic osteoarthritis, unspecified elbow
  M19.13- Post-traumatic osteoarthritis, wrist
    M19.131   Post-traumatic osteoarthritis, right wrist
    M19.132   Post-traumatic osteoarthritis, left wrist
    M19.139   Post-traumatic osteoarthritis, unspecified wrist
  M19.14- Post-traumatic osteoarthritis, hand
> *Excludes ❷:*   post-traumatic osteoarthritis of first carpometacarpal joint (M18.2-, M18.3-)

    M19.141   Post-traumatic osteoarthritis, right hand
    M19.142   Post-traumatic osteoarthritis, left hand
    M19.149   Post-traumatic osteoarthritis, unspecified hand
  M19.17- Post-traumatic osteoarthritis, ankle and foot
    M19.171   Post-traumatic osteoarthritis, right ankle and foot
    M19.172   Post-traumatic osteoarthritis, left ankle and foot
    M19.179   Post-traumatic osteoarthritis, unspecified ankle and foot

M19.2- Secondary osteoarthritis of other joints
  M19.21- Secondary osteoarthritis, shoulder
    M19.211   Secondary osteoarthritis, right shoulder
    M19.212   Secondary osteoarthritis, left shoulder
    M19.219   Secondary osteoarthritis, unspecified shoulder
  M19.22- Secondary osteoarthritis, elbow
    M19.221   Secondary osteoarthritis, right elbow
    M19.222   Secondary osteoarthritis, left elbow
    M19.229   Secondary osteoarthritis, unspecified elbow
  M19.23- Secondary osteoarthritis, wrist
    M19.231   Secondary osteoarthritis, right wrist
    M19.232   Secondary osteoarthritis, left wrist
    M19.239   Secondary osteoarthritis, unspecified wrist

  M19.24- Secondary osteoarthritis, hand
    M19.241   Secondary osteoarthritis, right hand
    M19.242   Secondary osteoarthritis, left hand
    M19.249   Secondary osteoarthritis, unspecified hand
  M19.27- Secondary osteoarthritis, ankle and foot
    M19.271   Secondary osteoarthritis, right ankle and foot
    M19.272   Secondary osteoarthritis, left ankle and foot
    M19.279   Secondary osteoarthritis, unspecified ankle and foot

M19.9- Osteoarthritis, unspecified site
  M19.90   Unspecified osteoarthritis, unspecified site
    Arthrosis NOS
    Arthritis NOS
    Osteoarthritis NOS
  M19.91   Primary osteoarthritis, unspecified site
    Primary osteoarthritis NOS
  M19.92   Post-traumatic osteoarthritis, unspecified site
    Post-traumatic osteoarthritis NOS
  M19.93   Secondary osteoarthritis, unspecified site
    Secondary osteoarthritis NOS

Other joint disorders (M20-M25)

> *Excludes ❷:*   joints of the spine (M40-M54)

M20- Acquired deformities of fingers and toes — The deviation of the normal anatomical structure and alignment of the fingers and toes.
> *Excludes 1:*   acquired absence of fingers and toes (Z89.-)
>   congenital absence of fingers and toes (Q71.3-, Q72.3-)
>   congenital deformities and malformations of fingers and toes (Q66.-, Q68-Q70, Q74.-)

M20.0- Deformity of finger(s)
> *Excludes 1:*   clubbing of fingers (R68.3)
>   palmar fascial fibromatosis [Dupuytren] (M72.0)
>   trigger finger (M65.3)

  M20.00- Unspecified deformity of finger(s)
    M20.001   Unspecified deformity of right finger(s)
    M20.002   Unspecified deformity of left finger(s)
    M20.009   Unspecified deformity of unspecified finger(s)
  M20.01- Mallet finger — The permanent flexion of a distal phalanx.
    M20.011   Mallet finger of right finger(s)
    M20.012   Mallet finger of left finger(s)
    M20.019   Mallet finger of unspecified finger(s)
  M20.02- Boutonnière deformity — Flexion of the proximal phalanx and hyperextension of the distal joint.
    M20.021   Boutonnière deformity of right finger(s)
    M20.022   Boutonnière deformity of left finger(s)
    M20.029   Boutonnière deformity of unspecified finger(s)
  M20.03- Swan-neck deformity — Hyperextended proximal interphalangeal joint and flexion of the distal interphalangeal joint.
    M20.031   Swan-neck deformity of right finger(s)
    M20.032   Swan-neck deformity of left finger(s)
    M20.039   Swan-neck deformity of unspecified finger(s)
  M20.09- Other deformity of finger(s)
    M20.091   Other deformity of right finger(s)
    M20.092   Other deformity of left finger(s)
    M20.099   Other deformity of finger(s), unspecified finger(s)
M20.1- Hallux valgus (acquired) — Angulation of the great toe towards other toes of that foot.
> *Excludes ❷:*   bunion (M21.6-)

  M20.10 Hallux valgus (acquired), unspecified foot
  M20.11 Hallux valgus (acquired), right foot
  M20.12 Hallux valgus (acquired), left foot
M20.2- Hallux rigidus — Painful restriction of joint motion of the great toe.
  M20.20 Hallux rigidus, unspecified foot
  M20.21 Hallux rigidus, right foot
  M20.22 Hallux rigidus, left foot

M19
-
M20

M20.3- <u>Hallux varus (acquired)</u> — Angulation of the great toe away from the other toes of that foot.

M20.30 Hallux varus (acquired), <u>unspecified</u> foot

M20.31 Hallux varus (acquired), <u>right</u> foot

M20.32 Hallux varus (acquired), <u>left</u> foot

M20.4- <u>Other hammer toe(s) (acquired)</u> — The claw-like deformity of a toe, other than a great toe.

M20.40 Other hammer toe(s) (acquired), <u>unspecified</u> foot

M20.41 Other hammer toe(s) (acquired), <u>right</u> foot

M20.42 Other hammer toe(s) (acquired), <u>left</u> foot

M20.5- <u>Other deformities of toe(s) (acquired)</u>

M20.5x- Other deformities of toe(s) (acquired)

M20.5x1 Other deformities of toe(s) (acquired), <u>right</u> foot

M20.5x2 Other deformities of toe(s) (acquired), <u>left</u> foot

M20.5x9 Other deformities of toe(s) (acquired), <u>unspecified</u> foot

M20.6- <u>Acquired</u> deformities of toe(s), <u>unspecified</u>

M20.60 Acquired deformities of toe(s), <u>unspecified</u>, <u>unspecified</u> foot

M20.61 Acquired deformities of toe(s), <u>unspecified</u>, <u>right</u> foot

M20.62 Acquired deformities of toe(s), <u>unspecified</u>, <u>left</u> foot

M21- <u>Other acquired deformities of limbs</u> — The deviation of the normal anatomical structure and alignment of the limbs, except of the fingers and toes.

Excludes 1:   acquired absence of limb (Z89.-)
             congenital absence of limbs (Q71-Q73)
             congenital deformities and malformations of limbs (Q65-Q66, Q68-Q74)

Excludes ❷: acquired deformities of fingers or toes (M20.-)
             coxa plana (M91.2)

M21.0- <u>Valgus</u> deformity, <u>not elsewhere classified</u> — Angulation away from the body.

Excludes 1:   metatarsus valgus (Q66.6)
             talipes calcaneovalgus (Q66.4)

M21.00 Valgus deformity, not elsewhere classified, <u>unspecified</u> site

M21.02- Valgus deformity, not elsewhere classified, <u>elbow</u>

Cubitus valgus — Angulation of the forearm away from the body.

M21.021 Valgus deformity, not elsewhere classified, <u>right</u> elbow

M21.022 Valgus deformity, not elsewhere classified, <u>left</u> elbow

M21.029 Valgus deformity, not elsewhere classified, <u>unspecified</u> elbow

M21.05- Valgus deformity, not elsewhere classified, <u>hip</u>

M21.051 Valgus deformity, not elsewhere classified, <u>right</u> hip

M21.052 Valgus deformity, not elsewhere classified, <u>left</u> hip

M21.059 Valgus deformity, not elsewhere classified, <u>unspecified</u> hip

M21.06- Valgus deformity, not elsewhere classified, <u>knee</u>

Genu valgum — The deformity in which the knees are close together.
Knock knee

M21.061 Valgus deformity, not elsewhere classified, <u>right</u> knee

M21.062 Valgus deformity, not elsewhere classified, <u>left</u> knee

M21.069 Valgus deformity, not elsewhere classified, <u>unspecified</u> knee

M21.07- Valgus deformity, not elsewhere classified, <u>ankle</u>

M21.071 Valgus deformity, not elsewhere classified, <u>right</u> ankle

M21.072 Valgus deformity, not elsewhere classified, <u>left</u> ankle

M21.079 Valgus deformity, not elsewhere classified, <u>unspecified</u> ankle

M21.1- <u>Varus</u> deformity, <u>not elsewhere classified</u> — Angulation towards the body.

Excludes 1:   metatarsus varus (Q66.22)
             tibia vara (M92.5)

M21.10 Varus deformity, not elsewhere classified, <u>unspecified</u> site

M21.12- Varus deformity, not elsewhere classified, <u>elbow</u>

Cubitus varus, elbow — Angulation of the forearm towards the body.

M21.121 Varus deformity, not elsewhere classified, <u>right</u> elbow

M21.122 Varus deformity, not elsewhere classified, <u>left</u> elbow

M21.129 Varus deformity, not elsewhere classified, <u>unspecified</u> elbow

M21.15- Varus deformity, not elsewhere classified, <u>hip</u>

M21.151 Varus deformity, not elsewhere classified, <u>right</u> hip

M21.152 Varus deformity, not elsewhere classified, <u>left</u> hip

M21.159 Varus deformity, not elsewhere classified, <u>unspecified</u> hip

M21.16- Varus deformity, not elsewhere classified, <u>knee</u>

Bow leg
Genu varum — The deformity in which the knees are more separated.

M21.161 Varus deformity, not elsewhere classified, <u>right</u> knee

M21.162 Varus deformity, not elsewhere classified, <u>left</u> knee

M21.169 Varus deformity, not elsewhere classified, <u>unspecified</u> knee

M21.17- Varus deformity, not elsewhere classified, <u>ankle</u>

M21.171 Varus deformity, not elsewhere classified, <u>right</u> ankle

M21.172 Varus deformity, not elsewhere classified, <u>left</u> ankle

M21.179 Varus deformity, not elsewhere classified, <u>unspecified</u> ankle

M21.2- <u>Flexion deformity</u> — The inability to straighten the joint to its normal range of motion postion.

M21.20 Flexion deformity, <u>unspecified</u> site

M21.21- Flexion deformity, <u>shoulder</u>

M21.211 Flexion deformity, <u>right</u> shoulder

M21.212 Flexion deformity, <u>left</u> shoulder

M21.219 Flexion deformity, <u>unspecified</u> shoulder

M21.22- Flexion deformity, <u>elbow</u>

M21.221 Flexion deformity, <u>right</u> elbow

M21.222 Flexion deformity, <u>left</u> elbow

M21.229 Flexion deformity, <u>unspecified</u> elbow

M21.23- Flexion deformity, <u>wrist</u>

M21.231 Flexion deformity, <u>right</u> wrist

M21.232 Flexion deformity, <u>left</u> wrist

M21.239 Flexion deformity, <u>unspecified</u> wrist

M21.24- Flexion deformity, <u>finger joints</u>

M21.241 Flexion deformity, <u>right</u> finger joints

M21.242 Flexion deformity, <u>left</u> finger joints

M21.249 Flexion deformity, <u>unspecified</u> finger joints

M21.25- Flexion deformity, <u>hip</u>

M21.251 Flexion deformity, <u>right</u> hip

M21.252 Flexion deformity, <u>left</u> hip

M21.259 Flexion deformity, <u>unspecified</u> hip

M21.26- Flexion deformity, <u>knee</u>

M21.261 Flexion deformity, <u>right</u> knee

M21.262 Flexion deformity, <u>left</u> knee

M21.269 Flexion deformity, <u>unspecified</u> knee

M21.27- Flexion deformity, <u>ankle and toes</u>

M21.271 Flexion deformity, <u>right</u> ankle and toes

M21.272 Flexion deformity, <u>left</u> ankle and toes

M21.279 Flexion deformity, <u>unspecified</u> ankle and toes

M20 - M21

M21.3- Wrist or foot drop (acquired)

M21.33- <u>Wrist drop (acquired)</u> — Paralysis of the extensor muscles with a dropping deformity of the hand.

M21.331 Wrist drop, <u>right</u> wrist

M21.332 Wrist drop, <u>left</u> wrist

M21.339 Wrist drop, <u>unspecified</u> wrist

M21.37- <u>Foot drop (acquired)</u> — Paralysis of the extensor muscles with a dropping deformity of the foot.

M21.371 Foot drop, <u>right</u> foot

M21.372 Foot drop, <u>left</u> foot

M21.379 Foot drop, <u>unspecified</u> foot

M21.4- <u>Flat foot</u> [pes planus] (acquired) — The flattened-out arch of a foot.

  Excludes 1:   *congenital pes planus (Q66.5-)*

M21.40 Flat foot [pes planus] (acquired), <u>unspecified</u> foot

M21.41 Flat foot [pes planus] (acquired), <u>right</u> foot

M21.42 Flat foot [pes planus] (acquired), <u>left</u> foot

M21.5- <u>Acquired</u> clawhand, clubhand, clawfoot and clubfoot

  Excludes 1:   *clubfoot, not specified as acquired (Q66.89)*

M21.51- Acquired <u>clawhand</u> — A deformity with extension of the 4th and 5th metacarpophalangeal joints with flexion of the 4th and 5th fingers that is caused by damage to the ulnar nerve.

M21.511 Acquired clawhand, <u>right</u> hand

M21.512 Acquired clawhand, <u>left</u> hand

M21.519 Acquired clawhand, <u>unspecified</u> hand

M21.52- Acquired <u>clubhand</u> — A twisting deformity of the hand.

M21.521 Acquired clubhand, <u>right</u> hand

M21.522 Acquired clubhand, <u>left</u> hand

M21.529 Acquired clubhand, <u>unspecified</u> hand

M21.53- Acquired <u>clawfoot</u> — The increased arch of the foot with deformity of the toes.

M21.531 Acquired clawfoot, <u>right</u> foot

M21.532 Acquired clawfoot, <u>left</u> foot

M21.539 Acquired clawfoot, <u>unspecified</u> foot

M21.54- Acquired <u>clubfoot</u> — The turning inward of the heel with turning upward of the inner edge of the foot.

M21.541 Acquired clubfoot, <u>right</u> foot

M21.542 Acquired clubfoot, <u>left</u> foot

M21.549 Acquired clubfoot, <u>unspecified</u> foot

M21.6- Other acquired deformities of foot

  Excludes ❷: *deformities of toe (acquired) (M20.1-M20.6-)*

M21.61- <u>Bunion</u> — Hypertrophy/edema/bursitis of the medial eminence of the first metatarsal head.

M21.611 Bunion of <u>right</u> foot

M21.612 Bunion of <u>left</u> foot

M21.619 Bunion of <u>unspecified</u> foot

M21.62- <u>Bunionette</u> — Hypertrophy/edema/bursitis of the lateral condyle of the fifth metatarsal head.

M21.621 Bunionette of <u>right</u> foot

M21.622 Bunionette of <u>left</u> foot

M21.629 Bunionette of <u>unspecified</u> foot

M21.6x- <u>Other acquired</u> deformities of <u>foot</u>

M21.6x1 Other acquired deformities of <u>right</u> foot

M21.6x2 Other acquired deformities of <u>left</u> foot

M21.6x9 Other acquired deformities of <u>unspecified</u> foot

M21.7- <u>Unequal limb length (acquired)</u>

  Note: The site used should correspond to the shorter limb

M21.70 Unequal limb length (acquired), <u>unspecified</u> site

M21.72- Unequal limb length (acquired), <u>humerus</u>

M21.721 Unequal limb length (acquired), <u>right</u> humerus

M21.722 Unequal limb length (acquired), <u>left</u> humerus

M21.729 Unequal limb length (acquired), <u>unspecified</u> humerus

M21.73- Unequal limb length (acquired), <u>ulna and radius</u>

M21.731 Unequal limb length (acquired), <u>right</u> ulna

M21.732 Unequal limb length (acquired), <u>left</u> ulna

M21.733 Unequal limb length (acquired), <u>right</u> radius

M21.734 Unequal limb length (acquired), <u>left</u> radius

M21.739 Unequal limb length (acquired), <u>unspecified</u> ulna and radius

M21.75- Unequal limb length (acquired), <u>femur</u>

M21.751 Unequal limb length (acquired), <u>right</u> femur

M21.752 Unequal limb length (acquired), <u>left</u> femur

M21.759 Unequal limb length (acquired), <u>unspecified</u> femur

M21.76- Unequal limb length (acquired), <u>tibia and fibula</u>

M21.761 Unequal limb length (acquired), <u>right</u> tibia

M21.762 Unequal limb length (acquired), <u>left</u> tibia

M21.763 Unequal limb length (acquired), <u>right</u> fibula

M21.764 Unequal limb length (acquired), <u>left</u> fibula

M21.769 Unequal limb length (acquired), <u>unspecified</u> tibia and fibula

M21.8- <u>Other specified acquired</u> deformities of limbs

  Excludes ❷: *coxa plana (M91.2)*

M21.80 Other specified acquired deformities of <u>unspecified</u> limb

M21.82- Other specified acquired deformities of <u>upper arm</u>

M21.821 Other specified acquired deformities of <u>right</u> upper arm

M21.822 Other specified acquired deformities of <u>left</u> upper arm

M21.829 Other specified acquired deformities of <u>unspecified</u> upper arm

M21.83- Other specified acquired deformities of <u>forearm</u>

M21.831 Other specified acquired deformities of <u>right</u> forearm

M21.832 Other specified acquired deformities of <u>left</u> forearm

M21.839 Other specified acquired deformities of <u>unspecified</u> forearm

M21.85- Other specified acquired deformities of <u>thigh</u>

M21.851 Other specified acquired deformities of <u>right</u> thigh

M21.852 Other specified acquired deformities of <u>left</u> thigh

M21.859 Other specified acquired deformities of <u>unspecified</u> thigh

M21.86- Other specified acquired deformities of <u>lower leg</u>

M21.861 Other specified acquired deformities of <u>right</u> lower leg

M21.862 Other specified acquired deformities of <u>left</u> lower leg

M21.869 Other specified acquired deformities of <u>unspecified</u> lower leg

M21.9- <u>Unspecified acquired deformity</u> of limb and hand

M21.90 Unspecified acquired deformity of <u>unspecified</u> limb

M21.92- Unspecified acquired deformity of <u>upper arm</u>

M21.921 Unspecified acquired deformity of <u>right</u> upper arm

M21.922 Unspecified acquired deformity of <u>left</u> upper arm

M21.929 Unspecified acquired deformity of <u>unspecified</u> upper arm

M21.93- Unspecified acquired deformity of <u>forearm</u>

M21.931 Unspecified acquired deformity of <u>right</u> forearm

M21.932 Unspecified acquired deformity of <u>left</u> forearm

M21.939 Unspecified acquired deformity of <u>unspecified</u> forearm

M21.94- Unspecified acquired deformity of <u>hand</u>

M21.941 Unspecified acquired deformity of hand, <u>right</u> hand

M21.942 Unspecified acquired deformity of hand, <u>left</u> hand

M21.949 Unspecified acquired deformity of hand, <u>unspecified</u> hand

M21.95- Unspecified acquired deformity of <u>thigh</u>

M21.951 Unspecified acquired deformity of <u>right</u> thigh

M21.952 Unspecified acquired deformity of <u>left</u> thigh

M21.959 Unspecified acquired deformity of <u>unspecified</u> thigh

M21-M21

M21.96- Unspecified acquired deformity of <u>lower leg</u>
    M21.961   Unspecified acquired deformity of <u>right</u> lower leg
    M21.962   Unspecified acquired deformity of <u>left</u> lower leg
    M21.969   Unspecified acquired deformity of <u>unspecified</u> lower leg

M22-   Disorder of <u>patella</u>
   Excludes 1:   *traumatic dislocation of patella (S83.0-)*
   M22.0-   <u>Recurrent dislocation</u> of patella — The current dislocation of the patella that is due to previous tissue damage or defect, but is not due to a current traumatic event.
     M22.00   Recurrent dislocation of patella, <u>unspecified</u> knee
     M22.01   Recurrent dislocation of patella, <u>right</u> knee
     M22.02   Recurrent dislocation of patella, <u>left</u> knee
   M22.1-   <u>Recurrent subluxation</u> of patella — Partial dislocation of the patella.
       Incomplete dislocation of patella
     M22.10   Recurrent subluxation of patella, <u>unspecified</u> knee
     M22.11   Recurrent subluxation of patella, <u>right</u> knee
     M22.12   Recurrent subluxation of patella, <u>left</u> knee
   M22.2-   Patellofemoral disorders
     M22.2x-   <u>Patellofemoral disorders</u>
       M22.2x1   Patellofemoral disorders, <u>right</u> knee
       M22.2x2   Patellofemoral disorders, <u>left</u> knee
       M22.2x9   Patellofemoral disorders, <u>unspecified</u> knee
   M22.3-   Other derangements of patella
     M22.3x-   <u>Other derangements</u> of patella
       M22.3x1   Other derangements of patella, <u>right</u> knee
       M22.3x2   Other derangements of patella, <u>left</u> knee
       M22.3x9   Other derangements of patella, <u>unspecified</u> knee
   M22.4-   <u>Chondromalacia</u> patellae — The softening of the patellar cartilage tissue.
     M22.40   Chondromalacia patellae, <u>unspecified</u> knee
     M22.41   Chondromalacia patellae, <u>right</u> knee
     M22.42   Chondromalacia patellae, <u>left</u> knee
   M22.8-   Other disorders of patella
     M22.8x-   <u>Other disorders</u> of patella
       M22.8x1   Other disorders of patella, <u>right</u> knee
       M22.8x2   Other disorders of patella, <u>left</u> knee
       M22.8x9   Other disorders of patella, <u>unspecified</u> knee
   M22.9-   <u>Unspecified disorder</u> of patella
     M22.90   Unspecified disorder of patella, <u>unspecified</u> knee
     M22.91   Unspecified disorder of patella, <u>right</u> knee
     M22.92   Unspecified disorder of patella, <u>left</u> knee

M23-   <u>Internal derangement</u> of <u>knee</u> — The instability disorders of the knee joint ligaments and menisci due to the malfunctioning disarrangement of the knee joint structures that is due to a previous direct trauma or an injury (wearing) of repetitive use, but not the result of an acute trauma.
   Excludes 1:   *ankylosis (M24.66)*
       current injury — see injury of knee and lower leg (S80-S89)
       deformity of knee (M21.-)
       osteochondritis dissecans (M93.2)
       recurrent dislocation or subluxation of joints (M24.4)
       recurrent dislocation or subluxation of patella (M22.0-M22.1)
   M23.0-   <u>Cystic meniscus</u>
     M23.00-   Cystic meniscus, <u>unspecified meniscus</u>
       Cystic meniscus, unspecified lateral meniscus
       Cystic meniscus, unspecified medial meniscus
       M23.000   Cystic meniscus, <u>unspecified lateral</u> meniscus, <u>right</u> knee
       M23.001   Cystic meniscus, <u>unspecified lateral</u> meniscus, <u>left</u> knee
       M23.002   Cystic meniscus, <u>unspecified lateral</u> meniscus, <u>unspecified</u> knee
       M23.003   Cystic meniscus, <u>unspecified medial</u> meniscus, <u>right</u> knee
       M23.004   Cystic meniscus, <u>unspecified medial</u> meniscus, <u>left</u> knee
       M23.005   Cystic meniscus, <u>unspecified medial</u> meniscus, <u>unspecified</u> knee

M23.006   Cystic meniscus, <u>unspecified</u> meniscus, <u>right</u> knee
M23.007   Cystic meniscus, <u>unspecified</u> meniscus, <u>left</u> knee
M23.009   Cystic meniscus, <u>unspecified</u> meniscus, <u>unspecified</u> knee
M23.01- Cystic meniscus, <u>anterior horn</u> of <u>medial</u> meniscus
   M23.011   Cystic meniscus, anterior horn of medial meniscus, <u>right</u> knee
   M23.012   Cystic meniscus, anterior horn of medial meniscus, <u>left</u> knee
   M23.019   Cystic meniscus, anterior horn of medial meniscus, <u>unspecified</u> knee
M23.02- Cystic meniscus, <u>posterior horn</u> of <u>medial</u> meniscus
   M23.021   Cystic meniscus, posterior horn of medial meniscus, <u>right</u> knee
   M23.022   Cystic meniscus, posterior horn of medial meniscus, <u>left</u> knee
   M23.029   Cystic meniscus, posterior horn of medial meniscus, <u>unspecified</u> knee
M23.03- Cystic meniscus, <u>other medial meniscus</u>
   M23.031   Cystic meniscus, other medial meniscus, <u>right</u> knee
   M23.032   Cystic meniscus, other medial meniscus, <u>left</u> knee
   M23.039   Cystic meniscus, other medial meniscus, <u>unspecified</u> knee
M23.04- Cystic meniscus, <u>anterior horn</u> of <u>lateral</u> meniscus
   M23.041   Cystic meniscus, anterior horn of lateral meniscus, <u>right</u> knee
   M23.042   Cystic meniscus, anterior horn of lateral meniscus, <u>left</u> knee
   M23.049   Cystic meniscus, anterior horn of lateral meniscus, <u>unspecified</u> knee
M23.05- Cystic meniscus, <u>posterior horn</u> of <u>lateral</u> meniscus
   M23.051   Cystic meniscus, posterior horn of lateral meniscus, <u>right</u> knee
   M23.052   Cystic meniscus, posterior horn of lateral meniscus, <u>left</u> knee
   M23.059   Cystic meniscus, posterior horn of lateral meniscus, <u>unspecified</u> knee
M23.06- Cystic meniscus, <u>other lateral</u> meniscus
   M23.061   Cystic meniscus, other lateral meniscus, <u>right</u> knee
   M23.062   Cystic meniscus, other lateral meniscus, <u>left</u> knee
   M23.069   Cystic meniscus, other lateral meniscus, <u>unspecified</u> knee
M23.2-   Derangement of meniscus <u>due to old tear or injury</u>
     Old bucket-handle tear
M23.20- Derangement of <u>unspecified</u> meniscus due to old tear or injury
     Derangement of unspecified lateral meniscus due to old tear or injury
     Derangement of unspecified medial meniscus due to old tear or injury
   M23.200   Derangement of <u>unspecified lateral</u> meniscus due to old tear or injury, <u>right</u> knee
   M23.201   Derangement of <u>unspecified lateral</u> meniscus due to old tear or injury, <u>left</u> knee
   M23.202   Derangement of <u>unspecified lateral</u> meniscus due to old tear or injury, <u>unspecified</u> knee
   M23.203   Derangement of <u>unspecified medial</u> meniscus due to old tear or injury, <u>right</u> knee
   M23.204   Derangement of <u>unspecified medial</u> meniscus due to old tear or injury, <u>left</u> knee
   M23.205   Derangement of <u>unspecified medial</u> meniscus due to old tear or injury, <u>unspecified</u> knee
   M23.206   Derangement of <u>unspecified</u> meniscus due to old tear or injury, <u>right</u> knee
   M23.207   Derangement of <u>unspecified</u> meniscus due to old tear or injury, <u>left</u> knee
   M23.209   Derangement of <u>unspecified</u> meniscus due to old tear or injury, <u>unspecified</u> knee

M23.21- Derangement of <u>anterior horn</u> of medial meniscus due to old tear or injury

   M23.211 Derangement of anterior horn of medial meniscus due to old tear or injury, <u>right</u> knee

   M23.212 Derangement of anterior horn of medial meniscus due to old tear or injury, <u>left</u> knee

   M23.219 Derangement of anterior horn of medial meniscus due to old tear or injury, <u>unspecified</u> knee

M23.22- Derangement of <u>posterior horn</u> of <u>medial</u> meniscus due to old tear or injury

   M23.221 Derangement of posterior horn of medial meniscus due to old tear or injury, <u>right</u> knee

   M23.222 Derangement of posterior horn of medial meniscus due to old tear or injury, <u>left</u> knee

   M23.229 Derangement of posterior horn of medial meniscus due to old tear or injury, <u>unspecified</u> knee

M23.23- Derangement of other medial meniscus due to old tear or injury

   M23.231 Derangement of other medial meniscus due to old tear or injury, <u>right</u> knee

   M23.232 Derangement of other medial meniscus due to old tear or injury, <u>left</u> knee

   M23.239 Derangement of other medial meniscus due to old tear or injury, <u>unspecified</u> knee

M23.24- Derangement of <u>anterior horn</u> of <u>lateral</u> meniscus due to old tear or injury

   M23.241 Derangement of anterior horn of lateral meniscus due to old tear or injury, <u>right</u> knee

   M23.242 Derangement of anterior horn of lateral meniscus due to old tear or injury, <u>left</u> knee

   M23.249 Derangement of anterior horn of lateral meniscus due to old tear or injury, <u>unspecified</u> knee

M23.25- Derangement of <u>posterior horn</u> of <u>lateral</u> meniscus due to old tear or injury

   M23.251 Derangement of posterior horn of lateral meniscus due to old tear or injury, <u>right</u> knee

   M23.252 Derangement of posterior horn of lateral meniscus due to old tear or injury, <u>left</u> knee

   M23.259 Derangement of posterior horn of lateral meniscus due to old tear or injury, <u>unspecified</u> knee

M23.26- Derangement of <u>other lateral</u> meniscus due to old tear or injury

   M23.261 Derangement of other lateral meniscus due to old tear or injury, <u>right</u> knee

   M23.262 Derangement of other lateral meniscus due to old tear or injury, <u>left</u> knee

   M23.269 Derangement of other lateral meniscus due to old tear or injury, <u>unspecified</u> knee

M23.3- <u>Other meniscus derangements</u>
    Degenerate meniscus
    Detached meniscus
    Retained meniscus

M23.30- Other meniscus derangements, <u>unspecified</u> meniscus
    Other meniscus derangements, unspecified lateral meniscus
    Other meniscus derangements, unspecified medial meniscus

   M23.300 Other meniscus derangements, <u>unspecified</u> <u>lateral</u> meniscus, <u>right</u> knee

   M23.301 Other meniscus derangements, <u>unspecified</u> <u>lateral</u> meniscus, <u>left</u> knee

   M23.302 Other meniscus derangements, <u>unspecified</u> <u>lateral</u> meniscus, <u>unspecified</u> knee

   M23.303 Other meniscus derangements, <u>unspecified</u> <u>medial</u> meniscus, <u>right</u> knee

   M23.304 Other meniscus derangements, <u>unspecified</u> <u>medial</u> meniscus, <u>left</u> knee

   M23.305 Other meniscus derangements, <u>unspecified</u> <u>medial</u> meniscus, <u>unspecified</u> knee

   M23.306 Other meniscus derangements, <u>unspecified</u> meniscus, <u>right</u> knee

   M23.307 Other meniscus derangements, <u>unspecified</u> meniscus, <u>left</u> knee

   M23.309 Other meniscus derangements, <u>unspecified</u> meniscus, <u>unspecified</u> knee

M23.31- Other meniscus derangements, <u>anterior horn</u> of <u>medial</u> meniscus

   M23.311 Other meniscus derangements, anterior horn of medial meniscus, <u>right</u> knee

   M23.312 Other meniscus derangements, anterior horn of medial meniscus, <u>left</u> knee

   M23.319 Other meniscus derangements, anterior horn of medial meniscus, <u>unspecified</u> knee

M23.32- Other meniscus derangements, <u>posterior horn</u> of <u>medial</u> meniscus

   M23.321 Other meniscus derangements, posterior horn of medial meniscus, <u>right</u> knee

   M23.322 Other meniscus derangements, posterior horn of medial meniscus, <u>left</u> knee

   M23.329 Other meniscus derangements, posterior horn of medial meniscus, <u>unspecified</u> knee

M23.33- Other meniscus derangements, <u>other medial</u> meniscus

   M23.331 Other meniscus derangements, other medial meniscus, <u>right</u> knee

   M23.332 Other meniscus derangements, other medial meniscus, <u>left</u> knee

   M23.339 Other meniscus derangements, other medial meniscus, <u>unspecified</u> knee

M23.34- Other meniscus derangements, <u>anterior horn</u> of <u>lateral</u> meniscus

   M23.341 Other meniscus derangements, anterior horn of lateral meniscus, <u>right</u> knee

   M23.342 Other meniscus derangements, anterior horn of lateral meniscus, <u>left</u> knee

   M23.349 Other meniscus derangements, anterior horn of lateral meniscus, <u>unspecified</u> knee

M23.35- Other meniscus derangements, posterior horn of <u>lateral</u> meniscus

   M23.351 Other meniscus derangements, posterior horn of lateral meniscus, <u>right</u> knee

   M23.352 Other meniscus derangements, posterior horn of lateral meniscus, <u>left</u> knee

   M23.359 Other meniscus derangements, posterior horn of lateral meniscus, <u>unspecified</u> knee

M23.36- Other meniscus derangements, <u>other lateral</u> meniscus

   M23.361 Other meniscus derangements, other lateral meniscus, <u>right</u> knee

   M23.362 Other meniscus derangements, other lateral meniscus, <u>left</u> knee

   M23.369 Other meniscus derangements, other lateral meniscus, <u>unspecified</u> knee

M23.4- <u>Loose body</u> in <u>knee</u> — The presence of nonattached pieces of joint tissue in the knee joint.

   M23.40 Loose body in knee, <u>unspecified</u> knee

   M23.41 Loose body in knee, <u>right</u> knee

   M23.42 Loose body in knee, <u>left</u> knee

M23.5- <u>Chronic instability</u> of <u>knee</u>

   M23.50 Chronic instability of knee, <u>unspecified</u> knee

   M23.51 Chronic instability of knee, <u>right</u> knee

   M23.52 Chronic instability of knee, <u>left</u> knee

M23.6- <u>Other spontaneous disruption of ligament(s)</u> of <u>knee</u>

M23.60- Other spontaneous disruption of <u>unspecified</u> <u>ligament</u> of knee

   M23.601 Other spontaneous disruption of <u>unspecified</u> ligament of <u>right</u> knee

   M23.602 Other spontaneous disruption of <u>unspecified</u> ligament of <u>left</u> knee

   M23.609 Other spontaneous disruption of <u>unspecified</u> ligament of <u>unspecified</u> knee

M23 - M23

M23.61- Other spontaneous disruption of <u>anterior cruciate ligament</u> of knee

    M23.611   Other spontaneous disruption of anterior cruciate ligament of <u>right</u> knee

    M23.612   Other spontaneous disruption of anterior cruciate ligament of <u>left</u> knee

    M23.619   Other spontaneous disruption of anterior cruciate ligament of <u>unspecified</u> knee

M23.62- Other spontaneous disruption of <u>posterior cruciate ligament</u> of knee

    M23.621   Other spontaneous disruption of posterior cruciate ligament of <u>right</u> knee

    M23.622   Other spontaneous disruption of posterior cruciate ligament of <u>left</u> knee

    M23.629   Other spontaneous disruption of posterior cruciate ligament of <u>unspecified</u> knee

M23.63- Other spontaneous disruption of <u>medial collateral ligament</u> of knee

    M23.631   Other spontaneous disruption of medial collateral ligament of <u>right</u> knee

    M23.632   Other spontaneous disruption of medial collateral ligament of <u>left</u> knee

    M23.639   Other spontaneous disruption of medial collateral ligament of <u>unspecified</u> knee

M23.64- Other spontaneous disruption of <u>lateral collateral ligament</u> of knee

    M23.641   Other spontaneous disruption of lateral collateral ligament of <u>right</u> knee

    M23.642   Other spontaneous disruption of lateral collateral ligament of <u>left</u> knee

    M23.649   Other spontaneous disruption of lateral collateral ligament of <u>unspecified</u> knee

M23.67- Other spontaneous disruption of <u>capsular ligament</u> of knee

    M23.671   Other spontaneous disruption of capsular ligament of <u>right</u> knee

    M23.672   Other spontaneous disruption of capsular ligament of <u>left</u> knee

    M23.679   Other spontaneous disruption of capsular ligament of <u>unspecified</u> knee

M23.8-   Other internal derangements of knee
    Laxity of ligament of knee
    Snapping knee

M23.8x- <u>Other internal derangements</u> of knee

    M23.8x1   Other internal derangements of <u>right</u> knee

    M23.8x2   Other internal derangements of <u>left</u> knee

    M23.8x9   Other internal derangements of <u>unspecified</u> knee

M23.9-   <u>Unspecified</u> internal derangement of knee

    M23.90   Unspecified internal derangement of <u>unspecified</u> knee

    M23.91   Unspecified internal derangement of <u>right</u> knee

    M23.92   Unspecified internal derangement of <u>left</u> knee

M24-   Other specific joint derangements
    Excludes 1:   *current injury — see injury of joint by body region*
    Excludes ❷: *ganglion (M67.4)*
        snapping knee (M23.8-)
        temporomandibular joint disorders (M26.6-)

M24.0-   <u>Loose body in joint</u> — The presence of nonattached pieces of joint tissue in the joint.
    Excludes ❷: *loose body in knee (M23.4)*

    M24.00   Loose body in <u>unspecified</u> joint

M24.01- Loose body in <u>shoulder</u>

    M24.011   Loose body in <u>right</u> shoulder

    M24.012   Loose body in <u>left</u> shoulder

    M24.019   Loose body in <u>unspecified</u> shoulder

M24.02- Loose body in <u>elbow</u>

    M24.021   Loose body in <u>right</u> elbow

    M24.022   Loose body in <u>left</u> elbow

    M24.029   Loose body in <u>unspecified</u> elbow

M24.03- Loose body in <u>wrist</u>

    M24.031   Loose body in <u>right</u> wrist

    M24.032   Loose body in <u>left</u> wrist

    M24.039   Loose body in <u>unspecified</u> wrist

M24.04- Loose body in <u>finger</u> joints

    M24.041   Loose body in <u>right</u> finger joint(s)

    M24.042   Loose body in <u>left</u> finger joint(s)

    M24.049   Loose body in <u>unspecified</u> finger joint(s)

M24.05- Loose body in <u>hip</u>

    M24.051   Loose body in <u>right</u> hip

    M24.052   Loose body in <u>left</u> hip

    M24.059   Loose body in <u>unspecified</u> hip

M24.07- Loose body in <u>ankle and toe</u> joints

    M24.071   Loose body in <u>right</u> ankle

    M24.072   Loose body in <u>left</u> ankle

    M24.073   Loose body in <u>unspecified</u> ankle

    M24.074   Loose body in <u>right</u> toe joint(s)

    M24.075   Loose body in <u>left</u> toe joint(s)

    M24.076   Loose body in <u>unspecified</u> toe joints

M24.08   Loose body, <u>other site</u>

M24.1-   <u>Other articular cartilage disorders</u>
    Excludes ❷: *chondrocalcinosis (M11.1, M11.2-)*
        internal derangement of knee (M23.-)
        metastatic calcification (E83.5)
        ochronosis (E70.2)

M24.10   Other articular cartilage disorders, <u>unspecified</u> site

M24.11- Other articular cartilage disorders, <u>shoulder</u>

    M24.111   Other articular cartilage disorders, <u>right</u> shoulder

    M24.112   Other articular cartilage disorders, <u>left</u> shoulder

    M24.119   Other articular cartilage disorders, <u>unspecified</u> shoulder

M24.12- Other articular cartilage disorders, <u>elbow</u>

    M24.121   Other articular cartilage disorders, <u>right</u> elbow

    M24.122   Other articular cartilage disorders, <u>left</u> elbow

    M24.129   Other articular cartilage disorders, <u>unspecified</u> elbow

M24.13- Other articular cartilage disorders, <u>wrist</u>

    M24.131   Other articular cartilage disorders, <u>right</u> wrist

    M24.132   Other articular cartilage disorders, <u>left</u> wrist

    M24.139   Other articular cartilage disorders, <u>unspecified</u> wrist

M24.14- Other articular cartilage disorders, <u>hand</u>

    M24.141   Other articular cartilage disorders, <u>right</u> hand

    M24.142   Other articular cartilage disorders, <u>left</u> hand

    M24.149   Other articular cartilage disorders, <u>unspecified</u> hand

M24.15- Other articular cartilage disorders, <u>hip</u>

    M24.151   Other articular cartilage disorders, <u>right</u> hip

    M24.152   Other articular cartilage disorders, <u>left</u> hip

    M24.159   Other articular cartilage disorders, <u>unspecified</u> hip

M24.17- Other articular cartilage disorders, <u>ankle and foot</u>

    M24.171   Other articular cartilage disorders, <u>right</u> ankle

    M24.172   Other articular cartilage disorders, <u>left</u> ankle

    M24.173   Other articular cartilage disorders, <u>unspecified</u> ankle

    M24.174   Other articular cartilage disorders, <u>right</u> foot

    M24.175   Other articular cartilage disorders, <u>left</u> foot

    M24.176   Other articular cartilage disorders, <u>unspecified</u> foot

M24.2-   <u>Disorder of ligament</u>
    Instability secondary to old ligament injury
    Ligamentous laxity NOS
    Excludes 1:   *familial ligamentous laxity (M35.7)*
    Excludes ❷: *internal derangement of knee (M23.5-M23.89)*

M24.20   Disorder of ligament, <u>unspecified</u> site

M24.21- Disorder of ligament, <u>shoulder</u>

    M24.211   Disorder of ligament, <u>right</u> shoulder

    M24.212   Disorder of ligament, <u>left</u> shoulder

M23
-
M24

M24.219   Disorder of ligament, <u>unspecified</u> shoulder

M24.22- Disorder of ligament, <u>elbow</u>

M24.221   Disorder of ligament, <u>right</u> elbow

M24.222   Disorder of ligament, <u>left</u> elbow

M24.229   Disorder of ligament, <u>unspecified</u> elbow

M24.23- Disorder of ligament, <u>wrist</u>

M24.231   Disorder of ligament, <u>right</u> wrist

M24.232   Disorder of ligament, <u>left</u> wrist

M24.239   Disorder of ligament, <u>unspecified</u> wrist

M24.24- Disorder of ligament, <u>hand</u>

M24.241   Disorder of ligament, <u>right</u> hand

M24.242   Disorder of ligament, <u>left</u> hand

M24.249   Disorder of ligament, <u>unspecified</u> hand

M24.25- Disorder of ligament, <u>hip</u>

M24.251   Disorder of ligament, <u>right</u> hip

M24.252   Disorder of ligament, <u>left</u> hip

M24.259   Disorder of ligament, <u>unspecified</u> hip

M24.27- Disorder of ligament, <u>ankle and foot</u>

M24.271   Disorder of ligament, <u>right</u> ankle

M24.272   Disorder of ligament, <u>left</u> ankle

M24.273   Disorder of ligament, <u>unspecified</u> ankle

M24.274   Disorder of ligament, <u>right</u> foot

M24.275   Disorder of ligament, <u>left</u> foot

M24.276   Disorder of ligament, <u>unspecified</u> foot

M24.28   Disorder of ligament, <u>vertebrae</u>

M24.3-   <u>Pathological dislocation of joint</u>, <u>not elsewhere classified</u> —
The dislocation of a joint that is due to the effects of a disease process.

> *Excludes 1:*   *congenital dislocation or displacement of joint — see congenital malformations and deformations of the musculoskeletal system (Q65-Q79)*
> *current injury — see injury of joints and ligaments by body region*
> *recurrent dislocation of joint (M24.4-)*

M24.30   Pathological dislocation of <u>unspecified</u> joint, not elsewhere classified

M24.31- Pathological dislocation of <u>shoulder</u>, not elsewhere classified

M24.311   Pathological dislocation of <u>right</u> shoulder, not elsewhere classified

M24.312   Pathological dislocation of <u>left</u> shoulder, not elsewhere classified

M24.319   Pathological dislocation of <u>unspecified</u> shoulder, not elsewhere classified

M24.32- Pathological dislocation of <u>elbow</u>, not elsewhere classified

M24.321   Pathological dislocation of <u>right</u> elbow, not elsewhere classified

M24.322   Pathological dislocation of <u>left</u> elbow, not elsewhere classified

M24.329   Pathological dislocation of <u>unspecified</u> elbow, not elsewhere classified

M24.33- Pathological dislocation of <u>wrist</u>, not elsewhere classified

M24.331   Pathological dislocation of <u>right</u> wrist, not elsewhere classified

M24.332   Pathological dislocation of <u>left</u> wrist, not elsewhere classified

M24.339   Pathological dislocation of <u>unspecified</u> wrist, not elsewhere classified

M24.34- Pathological dislocation of <u>hand</u>, not elsewhere classified

M24.341   Pathological dislocation of <u>right</u> hand, not elsewhere classified

M24.342   Pathological dislocation of <u>left</u> hand, not elsewhere classified

M24.349   Pathological dislocation of <u>unspecified</u> hand, not elsewhere classified

M24.35- Pathological dislocation of <u>hip</u>, not elsewhere classified

M24.351   Pathological dislocation of <u>right</u> hip, not elsewhere classified

M24.352   Pathological dislocation of <u>left</u> hip, not elsewhere classified

M24.359   Pathological dislocation of <u>unspecified</u> hip, not elsewhere classified

M24.36- Pathological dislocation of <u>knee</u>, not elsewhere classified

M24.361   Pathological dislocation of <u>right</u> knee, not elsewhere classified

M24.362   Pathological dislocation of <u>left</u> knee, not elsewhere classified

M24.369   Pathological dislocation of <u>unspecified</u> knee, not elsewhere classified

M24.37- Pathological dislocation of <u>ankle and foot</u>, not elsewhere classified

M24.371   Pathological dislocation of <u>right</u> ankle, not elsewhere classified

M24.372   Pathological dislocation of <u>left</u> ankle, not elsewhere classified

M24.373   Pathological dislocation of <u>unspecified</u> ankle, not elsewhere classified

M24.374   Pathological dislocation of <u>right</u> foot, not elsewhere classified

M24.375   Pathological dislocation of <u>left</u> foot, not elsewhere classified

M24.376   Pathological dislocation of <u>unspecified</u> foot, not elsewhere classified

M24.4-   <u>Recurrent</u> <u>dislocation</u> of joint — *The redislocation of a joint following a period of proper location.*

> *Recurrent subluxation of joint*
> *Excludes ❷:*   *recurrent dislocation of patella (M22.0-M22.1)*
> *recurrent vertebral dislocation (M43.3-, M43.4, M43.5-)*

M24.40   Recurrent dislocation, <u>unspecified</u> joint

M24.41- Recurrent dislocation, <u>shoulder</u>

M24.411   Recurrent dislocation, <u>right</u> shoulder

M24.412   Recurrent dislocation, <u>left</u> shoulder

M24.419   Recurrent dislocation, <u>unspecified</u> shoulder

M24.42- Recurrent dislocation, <u>elbow</u>

M24.421   Recurrent dislocation, <u>right</u> elbow

M24.422   Recurrent dislocation, <u>left</u> elbow

M24.429   Recurrent dislocation, <u>unspecified</u> elbow

M24.43- Recurrent dislocation, <u>wrist</u>

M24.431   Recurrent dislocation, <u>right</u> wrist

M24.432   Recurrent dislocation, <u>left</u> wrist

M24.439   Recurrent dislocation, <u>unspecified</u> wrist

M24.44- Recurrent dislocation, <u>hand and finger(s)</u>

M24.441   Recurrent dislocation, <u>right</u> hand

M24.442   Recurrent dislocation, <u>left</u> hand

M24.443   Recurrent dislocation, <u>unspecified</u> hand

M24.444   Recurrent dislocation, <u>right</u> finger

M24.445   Recurrent dislocation, <u>left</u> finger

M24.446   Recurrent dislocation, <u>unspecified</u> finger

M24.45- Recurrent dislocation, <u>hip</u>

M24.451   Recurrent dislocation, <u>right</u> hip

M24.452   Recurrent dislocation, <u>left</u> hip

M24.459   Recurrent dislocation, <u>unspecified</u> hip

M24.46- Recurrent dislocation, <u>knee</u>

M24.461   Recurrent dislocation, <u>right</u> knee

M24.462   Recurrent dislocation, <u>left</u> knee

M24.469   Recurrent dislocation, <u>unspecified</u> knee

M24.47- Recurrent dislocation, <u>ankle, foot and toes</u>

M24.471   Recurrent dislocation, <u>right</u> ankle

M24.472   Recurrent dislocation, <u>left</u> ankle

M24.473   Recurrent dislocation, <u>unspecified</u> ankle

M24.474   Recurrent dislocation, <u>right</u> foot

M24.475   Recurrent dislocation, <u>left</u> foot

M24.476   Recurrent dislocation, <u>unspecified</u> foot

M24.477   Recurrent dislocation, <u>right</u> toe(s)

M24 - M24

M24.478 Recurrent dislocation, <u>left</u> toe(s)

M24.479 Recurrent dislocation, <u>unspecified</u> toe(s)

M24.5- <u>Contracture</u> of joint — The condition of decreased flexibility of a joint.
Excludes 1: contracture of muscle without contracture of joint (M62.4-)
contracture of tendon (sheath) without contracture of joint (M62.4-)
Dupuytren's contracture (M72.0)
Excludes ❷: acquired deformities of limbs (M20-M21)

M24.50 Contracture, <u>unspecified</u> joint

M24.51- Contracture, <u>shoulder</u>

M24.511 Contracture, <u>right</u> shoulder

M24.512 Contracture, <u>left</u> shoulder

M24.519 Contracture, <u>unspecified</u> shoulder

M24.52- Contracture, <u>elbow</u>

M24.521 Contracture, <u>right</u> elbow

M24.522 Contracture, <u>left</u> elbow

M24.529 Contracture, <u>unspecified</u> elbow

M24.53- Contracture, <u>wrist</u>

M24.531 Contracture, <u>right</u> wrist

M24.532 Contracture, <u>left</u> wrist

M24.539 Contracture, <u>unspecified</u> wrist

M24.54- Contracture, <u>hand</u>

M24.541 Contracture, <u>right</u> hand

M24.542 Contracture, <u>left</u> hand

M24.549 Contracture, <u>unspecified</u> hand

M24.55- Contracture, <u>hip</u>

M24.551 Contracture, <u>right</u> hip

M24.552 Contracture, <u>left</u> hip

M24.559 Contracture, <u>unspecified</u> hip

M24.56- Contracture, <u>knee</u>

M24.561 Contracture, <u>right</u> knee

M24.562 Contracture, <u>left</u> knee

M24.569 Contracture, <u>unspecified</u> knee

M24.57- Contracture, <u>ankle and foot</u>

M24.571 Contracture, <u>right</u> ankle

M24.572 Contracture, <u>left</u> ankle

M24.573 Contracture, <u>unspecified</u> ankle

M24.574 Contracture, <u>right</u> foot

M24.575 Contracture, <u>left</u> foot

M24.576 Contracture, <u>unspecified</u> foot

M24.6- <u>Ankylosis</u> of joint — The condition of significant stiffness or immobility of a joint.
Excludes 1: stiffness of joint without ankylosis (M25.6-)
Excludes ❷: spine (M43.2-)

M24.60 Ankylosis, <u>unspecified</u> joint

M24.61- Ankylosis, <u>shoulder</u>

M24.611 Ankylosis, <u>right</u> shoulder

M24.612 Ankylosis, <u>left</u> shoulder

M24.619 Ankylosis, <u>unspecified</u> shoulder

M24.62- Ankylosis, <u>elbow</u>

M24.621 Ankylosis, <u>right</u> elbow

M24.622 Ankylosis, <u>left</u> elbow

M24.629 Ankylosis, <u>unspecified</u> elbow

M24.63- Ankylosis, <u>wrist</u>

M24.631 Ankylosis, <u>right</u> wrist

M24.632 Ankylosis, <u>left</u> wrist

M24.639 Ankylosis, <u>unspecified</u> wrist

M24.64- Ankylosis, <u>hand</u>

M24.641 Ankylosis, <u>right</u> hand

M24.642 Ankylosis, <u>left</u> hand

M24.649 Ankylosis, <u>unspecified</u> hand

M24.65- Ankylosis, <u>hip</u>

M24.651 Ankylosis, <u>right</u> hip

M24.652 Ankylosis, <u>left</u> hip

M24.659 Ankylosis, <u>unspecified</u> hip

M24.66- Ankylosis, <u>knee</u>

M24.661 Ankylosis, <u>right</u> knee

M24.662 Ankylosis, <u>left</u> knee

M24.669 Ankylosis, <u>unspecified</u> knee

M24.67- Ankylosis, <u>ankle and foot</u>

M24.671 Ankylosis, <u>right</u> ankle

M24.672 Ankylosis, <u>left</u> ankle

M24.673 Ankylosis, <u>unspecified</u> ankle

M24.674 Ankylosis, <u>right</u> foot

M24.675 Ankylosis, <u>left</u> foot

M24.676 Ankylosis, <u>unspecified</u> foot

M24.7 Protrusio acetabuli

M24.8- <u>Other specific</u> joint derangements, <u>not elsewhere classified</u>
Excludes ❷: iliotibial band syndrome (M76.3)

M24.80 Other specific joint derangements of <u>unspecified</u> joint, not elsewhere classified

M24.81- Other specific joint derangements of <u>shoulder</u>, not elsewhere classified

M24.811 Other specific joint derangements of <u>right</u> shoulder, not elsewhere classified

M24.812 Other specific joint derangements of <u>left</u> shoulder, not elsewhere classified

M24.819 Other specific joint derangements of <u>unspecified</u> shoulder, not elsewhere classified

M24.82- Other specific joint derangements of <u>elbow</u>, not elsewhere classified

M24.821 Other specific joint derangements of <u>right</u> elbow, not elsewhere classified

M24.822 Other specific joint derangements of <u>left</u> elbow, not elsewhere classified

M24.829 Other specific joint derangements of <u>unspecified</u> elbow, not elsewhere classified

M24.83- Other specific joint derangements of wrist, not elsewhere classified

M24.831 Other specific joint derangements of <u>right</u> wrist, not elsewhere classified

M24.832 Other specific joint derangements of <u>left</u> wrist, not elsewhere classified

M24.839 Other specific joint derangements of <u>unspecified</u> wrist, not elsewhere classified

M24.84- Other specific joint derangements of <u>hand</u>, not elsewhere classified

M24.841 Other specific joint derangements of <u>right</u> hand, not elsewhere classified

M24.842 Other specific joint derangements of <u>left</u> hand, not elsewhere classified

M24.849 Other specific joint derangements of <u>unspecified</u> hand, not elsewhere classified

M24.85- Other specific joint derangements of <u>hip</u>, not elsewhere classified
Irritable hip

M24.851 Other specific joint derangements of <u>right</u> hip, not elsewhere classified

M24.852 Other specific joint derangements of <u>left</u> hip, not elsewhere classified

M24.859 Other specific joint derangements of <u>unspecified</u> hip, not elsewhere classified

M24.87- Other specific joint derangements of <u>ankle and foot</u>, not elsewhere classified

M24.871 Other specific joint derangements of <u>right</u> ankle, not elsewhere classified

M24.872 Other specific joint derangements of <u>left</u> ankle, not elsewhere classified

M24.873 Other specific joint derangements of <u>unspecified</u> ankle, not elsewhere classified

M24.874 Other specific joint derangements of <u>right</u> foot, not elsewhere classified

M24 - M24

M24.875   Other specific joint derangements <u>left</u> foot, not elsewhere classified

M24.876   Other specific joint derangements of <u>unspecified</u> foot, not elsewhere classified

M24.9   Joint derangement, <u>unspecified</u>

M25-   <u>Other joint disorder</u>, <u>not elsewhere classified</u>
Excludes ❷: *abnormality of gait and mobility (R26.-)*
acquired deformities of limb (M20-M21)
calcification of bursa (M71.4-)
calcification of shoulder (joint) (M75.3)
calcification of tendon (M65.2-)
difficulty in walking (R26.2)
temporomandibular joint disorder (M26.6-)

M25.0-   <u>Hemarthrosis</u> — The abnormal presence of free blood in a joint.
Excludes 1:   *current injury — see injury of joint by body region*
hemophilic arthropathy (M36.2)

cc **M25.00**   Hemarthrosis, <u>unspecified</u> joint

M25.01- Hemarthrosis, <u>shoulder</u>
cc **M25.011**   Hemarthrosis, <u>right</u> shoulder
cc **M25.012**   Hemarthrosis, <u>left</u> shoulder
cc **M25.019**   Hemarthrosis, <u>unspecified</u> shoulder

M25.02- Hemarthrosis, <u>elbow</u>
cc **M25.021**   Hemarthrosis, <u>right</u> elbow
cc **M25.022**   Hemarthrosis, <u>left</u> elbow
cc **M25.029**   Hemarthrosis, <u>unspecified</u> elbow

M25.03- Hemarthrosis, <u>wrist</u>
cc **M25.031**   Hemarthrosis, <u>right</u> wrist
cc **M25.032**   Hemarthrosis, <u>left</u> wrist
cc **M25.039**   Hemarthrosis, <u>unspecified</u> wrist

M25.04- Hemarthrosis, <u>hand</u>
cc **M25.041**   Hemarthrosis, <u>right</u> hand
cc **M25.042**   Hemarthrosis, <u>left</u> hand
cc **M25.049**   Hemarthrosis, <u>unspecified</u> hand

M25.05- Hemarthrosis, <u>hip</u>
cc **M25.051**   Hemarthrosis, <u>right</u> hip
cc **M25.052**   Hemarthrosis, <u>left</u> hip
cc **M25.059**   Hemarthrosis, <u>unspecified</u> hip

M25.06- Hemarthrosis, <u>knee</u>
cc **M25.061**   Hemarthrosis, <u>right</u> knee
cc **M25.062**   Hemarthrosis, <u>left</u> knee
cc **M25.069**   Hemarthrosis, <u>unspecified</u> knee

M25.07- Hemarthrosis, <u>ankle and foot</u>
cc **M25.071**   Hemarthrosis, <u>right</u> ankle
cc **M25.072**   Hemarthrosis, <u>left</u> ankle
cc **M25.073**   Hemarthrosis, <u>unspecified</u> ankle
cc **M25.074**   Hemarthrosis, <u>right</u> foot
cc **M25.075**   Hemarthrosis, <u>left</u> foot
cc **M25.076**   Hemarthrosis, <u>unspecified</u> foot

cc **M25.08**   Hemarthrosis, <u>other specified site</u>
Hemarthrosis, vertebrae

M25.1-   <u>Fistula of joint</u> — The presence of an abnormal communicating passage of a joint.
M25.10   Fistula, <u>unspecified</u> joint

M25.11- Fistula, <u>shoulder</u>
M25.111   Fistula, <u>right</u> shoulder
M25.112   Fistula, <u>left</u> shoulder
M25.119   Fistula, <u>unspecified</u> shoulder

M25.12- Fistula, <u>elbow</u>
M25.121   Fistula, <u>right</u> elbow
M25.122   Fistula, <u>left</u> elbow
M25.129   Fistula, <u>unspecified</u> elbow

M25.13- Fistula, wrist
M25.131   Fistula, <u>right</u> wrist
M25.132   Fistula, <u>left</u> wrist
M25.139   Fistula, <u>unspecified</u> wrist

M25.14- Fistula, <u>hand</u>
M25.141   Fistula, <u>right</u> hand

M25.142   Fistula, <u>left</u> hand
M25.149   Fistula, <u>unspecified</u> hand

M25.15- Fistula, <u>hip</u>
M25.151   Fistula, <u>right</u> hip
M25.152   Fistula, <u>left</u> hip
M25.159   Fistula, <u>unspecified</u> hip

M25.16- Fistula, <u>knee</u>
M25.161   Fistula, <u>right</u> knee
M25.162   Fistula, <u>left</u> knee
M25.169   Fistula, <u>unspecified</u> knee

M25.17- Fistula, <u>ankle and foot</u>
M25.171   Fistula, <u>right</u> ankle
M25.172   Fistula, <u>left</u> ankle
M25.173   Fistula, <u>unspecified</u> ankle
M25.174   Fistula, <u>right</u> foot
M25.175   Fistula, <u>left</u> foot
M25.176   Fistula, <u>unspecified</u> foot

M25.18   Fistula, <u>other specified site</u>
Fistula, vertebrae

M25.2-   <u>Flail joint</u> — The condition of abnormal mobility of a joint.
M25.20   Flail joint, <u>unspecified</u> joint

M25.21- Flail joint, <u>shoulder</u>
M25.211   Flail joint, <u>right</u> shoulder
M25.212   Flail joint, <u>left</u> shoulder
M25.219   Flail joint, <u>unspecified</u> shoulder

M25.22- Flail joint, <u>elbow</u>
M25.221   Flail joint, <u>right</u> elbow
M25.222   Flail joint, <u>left</u> elbow
M25.229   Flail joint, <u>unspecified</u> elbow

M25.23- Flail joint, <u>wrist</u>
M25.231   Flail joint, <u>right</u> wrist
M25.232   Flail joint, <u>left</u> wrist
M25.239   Flail joint, <u>unspecified</u> wrist

M25.24- Flail joint, <u>hand</u>
M25.241   Flail joint, <u>right</u> hand
M25.242   Flail joint, <u>left</u> hand
M25.249   Flail joint, <u>unspecified</u> hand

M25.25- Flail joint, <u>hip</u>
M25.251   Flail joint, <u>right</u> hip
M25.252   Flail joint, <u>left</u> hip
M25.259   Flail joint, <u>unspecified</u> hip

M25.26- Flail joint, <u>knee</u>
M25.261   Flail joint, <u>right</u> knee
M25.262   Flail joint, <u>left</u> knee
M25.269   Flail joint, <u>unspecified</u> knee

M25.27- Flail joint, <u>ankle and foot</u>
M25.271   Flail joint, <u>right</u> ankle and foot
M25.272   Flail joint, <u>left</u> ankle and foot
M25.279   Flail joint, <u>unspecified</u> ankle and foot

M25.28   Flail joint, <u>other site</u>

M25.3-   <u>Other instability</u> of joint
Excludes 1:   *instability of joint secondary to old ligament injury (M24.2-)*
instability of joint secondary to removal of joint prosthesis (M96.8-)
Excludes ❷: *spinal instabilities (M53.2-)*

M25.30   Other instability, <u>unspecified</u> joint

M25.31- Other instability, <u>shoulder</u>
M25.311   Other instability, <u>right</u> shoulder
M25.312   Other instability, <u>left</u> shoulder
M25.319   Other instability, <u>unspecified</u> shoulder

M25.32- Other instability, <u>elbow</u>
M25.321   Other instability, <u>right</u> elbow
M25.322   Other instability, <u>left</u> elbow
M25.329   Other instability, <u>unspecified</u> elbow

M24 - M25

Excludes 1: = NOT CODED HERE! (Do not code both)   847   *Excludes ❷:* = Not Included Here

M25.33- Other instability, <u>wrist</u>
  M25.331 Other instability, <u>right</u> wrist
  M25.332 Other instability, <u>left</u> wrist
  M25.339 Other instability, <u>unspecified</u> wrist
M25.34- Other instability, <u>hand</u>
  M25.341 Other instability, <u>right</u> hand
  M25.342 Other instability, <u>left</u> hand
  M25.349 Other instability, <u>unspecified</u> hand
M25.35- Other instability, <u>hip</u>
  M25.351 Other instability, <u>right</u> hip
  M25.352 Other instability, <u>left</u> hip
  M25.359 Other instability, <u>unspecified</u> hip
M25.36- Other instability, <u>knee</u>
  M25.361 Other instability, <u>right</u> knee
  M25.362 Other instability, <u>left</u> knee
  M25.369 Other instability, <u>unspecified</u> knee
M25.37- Other instability, <u>ankle and foot</u>
  M25.371 Other instability, <u>right</u> ankle
  M25.372 Other instability, <u>left</u> ankle
  M25.373 Other instability, <u>unspecified</u> ankle
  M25.374 Other instability, <u>right</u> foot
  M25.375 Other instability, <u>left</u> foot
  M25.376 Other instability, <u>unspecified</u> foot
M25.4- <u>Effusion</u> of joint — The abnormal increased amount of fluid in a joint.
  Excludes 1: *hydrarthrosis in yaws (A66.6)*
         intermittent hydrarthrosis (M12.4-)
         other infective (teno)synovitis (M65.1-)
  M25.40 Effusion, <u>unspecified</u> joint
  M25.41- Effusion, <u>shoulder</u>
    M25.411 Effusion, <u>right</u> shoulder
    M25.412 Effusion, <u>left</u> shoulder
    M25.419 Effusion, <u>unspecified</u> shoulder
  M25.42- Effusion, <u>elbow</u>
    M25.421 Effusion, <u>right</u> elbow
    M25.422 Effusion, <u>left</u> elbow
    M25.429 Effusion, <u>unspecified</u> elbow
  M25.43- Effusion, <u>wrist</u>
    M25.431 Effusion, <u>right</u> wrist
    M25.432 Effusion, <u>left</u> wrist
    M25.439 Effusion, <u>unspecified</u> wrist
  M25.44- Effusion, <u>hand</u>
    M25.441 Effusion, <u>right</u> hand
    M25.442 Effusion, <u>left</u> hand
    M25.449 Effusion, <u>unspecified</u> hand
  M25.45- Effusion, <u>hip</u>
    M25.451 Effusion, <u>right</u> hip
    M25.452 Effusion, <u>left</u> hip
    M25.459 Effusion, <u>unspecified</u> hip
  M25.46- Effusion, <u>knee</u>
    M25.461 Effusion, <u>right</u> knee
    M25.462 Effusion, <u>left</u> knee
    M25.469 Effusion, <u>unspecified</u> knee
  M25.47- Effusion, <u>ankle and foot</u>
    M25.471 Effusion, <u>right</u> ankle
    M25.472 Effusion, <u>left</u> ankle
    M25.473 Effusion, <u>unspecified</u> ankle
    M25.474 Effusion, <u>right</u> foot
    M25.475 Effusion, <u>left</u> foot
    M25.476 Effusion, <u>unspecified</u> foot
  M25.48 Effusion, <u>other site</u>

M25.5- <u>Pain in joint</u> — The condition of discomfort of a joint.
  Excludes ❷: *pain in hand (M79.64-)*
         pain in fingers (M79.64-)
         pain in foot (M79.67-)
         pain in limb (M79.6-)
         pain in toes (M79.67-)
  M25.50 Pain in <u>unspecified</u> joint
  M25.51- Pain in <u>shoulder</u>
    M25.511 Pain in <u>right</u> shoulder
    M25.512 Pain in <u>left</u> shoulder
    M25.519 Pain in <u>unspecified</u> shoulder
  M25.52- Pain in <u>elbow</u>
    M25.521 Pain in <u>right</u> elbow
    M25.522 Pain in <u>left</u> elbow
    M25.529 Pain in <u>unspecified</u> elbow
  M25.53- Pain in <u>wrist</u>
    M25.531 Pain in <u>right</u> wrist
    M25.532 Pain in <u>left</u> wrist
    M25.539 Pain in <u>unspecified</u> wrist
  M25.54- Pain in <u>joints of hand</u>
    M25.541 Pain in joints of hand of <u>right</u> hand
    M25.542 Pain in joints of hand of <u>left</u> hand
    M25.559 Pain in joints of hand of <u>unspecified</u> hand
           Pain in joints of hand NOS
  M25.55- Pain in <u>hip</u>
    M25.551 Pain in <u>right</u> hip
    M25.552 Pain in <u>left</u> hip
    M25.559 Pain in <u>unspecified</u> hip
  M25.56- Pain in <u>knee</u>
    M25.561 Pain in <u>right</u> knee
    M25.562 Pain in <u>left</u> knee
    M25.569 Pain in <u>unspecified</u> knee
  M25.57- Pain in <u>ankle and joints of foot</u>
    M25.571 Pain in <u>right</u> ankle and joints of right foot
    M25.572 Pain in <u>left</u> ankle and joints of left foot
    M25.579 Pain in <u>unspecified</u> ankle and joints of unspecified foot

M25.6- <u>Stiffness</u> of joint, <u>not elsewhere classified</u>
  Excludes 1: *ankylosis of joint (M24.6-)*
         contracture of joint (M24.5-)
  M25.60 Stiffness of <u>unspecified</u> joint, not elsewhere classified
  M25.61- Stiffness of <u>shoulder</u>, not elsewhere classified
    M25.611 Stiffness of <u>right</u> shoulder, not elsewhere classified
    M25.612 Stiffness of <u>left</u> shoulder, not elsewhere classified
    M25.619 Stiffness of <u>unspecified</u> shoulder, not elsewhere classified
  M25.62- Stiffness of <u>elbow</u>, not elsewhere classified
    M25.621 Stiffness of <u>right</u> elbow, not elsewhere classified
    M25.622 Stiffness of <u>left</u> elbow, not elsewhere classified
    M25.629 Stiffness of <u>unspecified</u> elbow, not elsewhere classified
  M25.63- Stiffness of <u>wrist</u>, not elsewhere classified
    M25.631 Stiffness of <u>right</u> wrist, not elsewhere classified
    M25.632 Stiffness of <u>left</u> wrist, not elsewhere classified
    M25.639 Stiffness of <u>unspecified</u> wrist, not elsewhere classified
  M25.64- Stiffness of <u>hand</u>, not elsewhere classified
    M25.641 Stiffness of <u>right</u> hand, not elsewhere classified
    M25.642 Stiffness of <u>left</u> hand, not elsewhere classified
    M25.649 Stiffness of <u>unspecified</u> hand, not elsewhere classified
  M25.65- Stiffness of <u>hip</u>, not elsewhere classified
    M25.651 Stiffness of <u>right</u> hip, not elsewhere classified
    M25.652 Stiffness of <u>left</u> hip, not elsewhere classified
    M25.659 Stiffness of <u>unspecified</u> hip, not elsewhere classified

M25 - M25

M25.66- Stiffness of <u>knee</u>, not elsewhere classified
    M25.661 Stiffness of <u>right</u> knee, not elsewhere classified
    M25.662 Stiffness of <u>left</u> knee, not elsewhere classified
    M25.669 Stiffness of <u>unspecified</u> knee, not elsewhere classified
M25.67- Stiffness of <u>ankle and foot</u>, not elsewhere classified
    M25.671 Stiffness of <u>right</u> ankle, not elsewhere classified
    M25.672 Stiffness of <u>left</u> ankle, not elsewhere classified
    M25.673 Stiffness of <u>unspecified</u> ankle, not elsewhere classified
    M25.674 Stiffness of <u>right</u> foot, not elsewhere classified
    M25.675 Stiffness of <u>left</u> foot, not elsewhere classified
    M25.676 Stiffness of <u>unspecified</u> foot, not elsewhere classified

M25.7- <u>Osteophyte</u> — The bony tissue growth along the margins of a joint.
  M25.70 Osteophyte, <u>unspecified</u> joint
  M25.71- Osteophyte, <u>shoulder</u>
    M25.711 Osteophyte, <u>right</u> shoulder
    M25.712 Osteophyte, <u>left</u> shoulder
    M25.719 Osteophyte, <u>unspecified</u> shoulder
  M25.72- Osteophyte, <u>elbow</u>
    M25.721 Osteophyte, <u>right</u> elbow
    M25.722 Osteophyte, <u>left</u> elbow
    M25.729 Osteophyte, <u>unspecified</u> elbow
  M25.73- Osteophyte, <u>wrist</u>
    M25.731 Osteophyte, <u>right</u> wrist
    M25.732 Osteophyte, <u>left</u> wrist
    M25.739 Osteophyte, <u>unspecified</u> wrist
  M25.74- Osteophyte, <u>hand</u>
    M25.741 Osteophyte, <u>right</u> hand
    M25.742 Osteophyte, <u>left</u> hand
    M25.749 Osteophyte, <u>unspecified</u> hand
  M25.75- Osteophyte, <u>hip</u>
    M25.751 Osteophyte, <u>right</u> hip
    M25.752 Osteophyte, <u>left</u> hip
    M25.759 Osteophyte, <u>unspecified</u> hip
  M25.76- Osteophyte, <u>knee</u>
    M25.761 Osteophyte, <u>right</u> knee
    M25.762 Osteophyte, <u>left</u> knee
    M25.769 Osteophyte, <u>unspecified</u> knee
  M25.77- Osteophyte, <u>ankle and foot</u>
    M25.771 Osteophyte, <u>right</u> ankle
    M25.772 Osteophyte, <u>left</u> ankle
    M25.773 Osteophyte, <u>unspecified</u> ankle
    M25.774 Osteophyte, <u>right</u> foot
    M25.775 Osteophyte, <u>left</u> foot
    M25.776 Osteophyte, <u>unspecified</u> foot
  M25.78 Osteophyte, <u>vertebrae</u>

M25.8- <u>Other specified</u> joint disorders
    AHA 14:4Q:p25 – Femoroacetabular impingement
  M25.80 Other specified joint disorders, <u>unspecified</u> joint
  M25.81- Other specified joint disorders, <u>shoulder</u>
    M25.811 Other specified joint disorders, <u>right</u> shoulder
    M25.812 Other specified joint disorders, <u>left</u> shoulder
    M25.819 Other specified joint disorders, <u>unspecified</u> shoulder
  M25.82- Other specified joint disorders, <u>elbow</u>
    M25.821 Other specified joint disorders, <u>right</u> elbow
    M25.822 Other specified joint disorders, <u>left</u> elbow
    M25.829 Other specified joint disorders, <u>unspecified</u> elbow
  M25.83- Other specified joint disorders, <u>wrist</u>
    M25.831 Other specified joint disorders, <u>right</u> wrist
    M25.832 Other specified joint disorders, <u>left</u> wrist
    M25.839 Other specified joint disorders, <u>unspecified</u> wrist

M25.84- Other specified joint disorders, <u>hand</u>
    M25.841 Other specified joint disorders, <u>right</u> hand
    M25.842 Other specified joint disorders, <u>left</u> hand
    M25.849 Other specified joint disorders, <u>unspecified</u> hand
M25.85- Other specified joint disorders, <u>hip</u>
    M25.851 Other specified joint disorders, <u>right</u> hip
    M25.852 Other specified joint disorders, <u>left</u> hip
    M25.859 Other specified joint disorders, <u>unspecified</u> hip
M25.86- Other specified joint disorders, <u>knee</u>
    M25.861 Other specified joint disorders, <u>right</u> knee
    M25.862 Other specified joint disorders, <u>left</u> knee
    M25.869 Other specified joint disorders, <u>unspecified</u> knee
M25.87- Other specified joint disorders, <u>ankle and foot</u>
    M25.871 Other specified joint disorders, <u>right</u> ankle and foot
    M25.872 Other specified joint disorders, <u>left</u> ankle and foot
    M25.879 Other specified joint disorders, <u>unspecified</u> ankle and foot
M25.9   Joint disorder, <u>unspecified</u>

Dentofacial anomalies [including malocclusion] and other disorders of jaw (M26-M27)

    Excludes 1:   *hemifacial atrophy or hypertrophy (Q67.4)*
                   unilateral condylar hyperplasia or hypoplasia (M27.8)

M26- <u>Dentofacial anomalies</u> [including malocclusion]
  M26.0- <u>Major</u> anomalies of jaw size — The functionally significant deviation of normal jaw size.
    Excludes 1:   *acromegaly (E22.0)*
                   Robin's syndrome (Q87.0)
  M26.00 Unspecified anomaly of jaw size
  M26.01 Maxillary hyperplasia — The abnormal, developmental enlargement of the upper jaw bone (maxilla).
  M26.02 Maxillary hypoplasia — The abnormal, developmental smallness of the upper jaw bone (maxilla).
    AHA 14:3Q:p23 – Maxillary hypoplasia
  M26.03 Mandibular hyperplasia — The abnormal, developmental enlargement of the lower jaw bone (mandible).
  M26.04 Mandibular hypoplasia — The abnormal, developmental smallness of the lower jaw bone (mandible).
  M26.05 Macrogenia — The abnormal, developmental enlargement of the chin (mandible).
  M26.06 Microgenia — The abnormal, developmental smallness of the chin (mandible).
  M26.07 Excessive tuberosity of jaw — The abnormal presence of excessive bone and/or soft tissue of the jaw.
    Entire maxillary tuberosity
  M26.09 Other specified anomalies of jaw size
  M26.1- Anomalies of <u>jaw-cranial base</u> relationship — The functionally significant deviation of the anatomical location of the jaw in relation to the skull.
  M26.10 Unspecified anomaly of jaw-cranial base relationship
  M26.11 Maxillary asymmetry — The dissimilar position of the upper jaw to the skull.
  M26.12 Other jaw asymmetry
  M26.19 Other specified anomalies of jaw-cranial base relationship
  M26.2- Anomalies of <u>dental arch</u> relationship — The malposition of the teeth and alveolar process creating a functionally significant abnormality of the dental arch.
  M26.20 Unspecified anomaly of dental arch relationship
  M26.21- Malocclusion, Angle's class
    M26.211 Malocclusion, Angle's class I
        Neutro-occlusion
    M26.212 Malocclusion, Angle's class II
        Disto-occlusion Division I
        Disto-occlusion Division II
    M26.213 Malocclusion, Angle's class III
        Mesio-occlusion
    M26.219 Malocclusion, Angle's class, unspecified

M25 - M26

M26.22- <u>Open occlusal</u> relationship
    M26.220 **Open anterior occlusal relationship**
        Anterior openbite
    M26.221 **Open posterior occlusal relationship**
        Posterior openbite

M26.23 <u>Excessive horizontal overlap</u>
    Excessive horizontal overjet

M26.24 <u>Reverse articulation</u>
    Crossbite (anterior) (posterior)

M26.25 Anomalies of interarch distance

M26.29 Other anomalies of dental arch relationship
    Midline deviation of dental arch
    Overbite (excessive) deep
    Overbite (excessive) horizontal
    Overbite (excessive) vertical
    Posterior lingual occlusion of mandibular teeth

M26.3- Anomalies of <u>tooth position</u> of fully erupted tooth or teeth
    Excludes ❷: embedded and impacted teeth (K01.-)

    M26.30 Unspecified anomaly of tooth position of fully erupted tooth or teeth
        Abnormal spacing of fully erupted tooth or teeth NOS
        Displacement of fully erupted tooth or teeth NOS
        Transposition of fully erupted tooth or teeth NOS

    M26.31 Crowding of fully erupted teeth

    M26.32 Excessive spacing of fully erupted teeth
        Diastema of fully erupted tooth or teeth NOS

    M26.33 Horizontal displacement of fully erupted tooth or teeth
        Tipped tooth or teeth
        Tipping of fully erupted tooth

    M26.34 Vertical displacement of fully erupted tooth or teeth
        Extruded tooth
        Infraeruption of tooth or teeth
        Supraeruption of tooth or teeth

    M26.35 Rotation of fully erupted tooth or teeth

    M26.36 Insufficient interocclusal distance of fully erupted teeth (ridge)
        Lack of adequate intermaxillary vertical dimension of fully erupted teeth

    M26.37 Excessive interocclusal distance of fully erupted teeth
        Excessive intermaxillary vertical dimension of fully erupted teeth
        Loss of occlusal vertical dimension of fully erupted teeth

    M26.39 Other anomalies of tooth position of fully erupted tooth or teeth

M26.4   Malocclusion, unspecified

M26.5- Dentofacial <u>functional abnormalities</u>
    Excludes 1:   bruxism (F45.8)
             teeth-grinding NOS (F45.8)

    M26.50 Dentofacial functional abnormalities, unspecified

    M26.51 Abnormal jaw closure

    M26.52 Limited mandibular range of motion

    M26.53 Deviation in opening and closing of the mandible

    M26.54 Insufficient anterior guidance
        Insufficient anterior occlusal guidance

    M26.55 Centric occlusion maximum intercuspation discrepancy
        Excludes 1: centric occlusion NOS (M26.59)

    M26.56 Non-working side interference
        Balancing side interference

    M26.57 Lack of posterior occlusal support

    M26.59 Other dentofacial functional abnormalities
        Centric occlusion (of teeth) NOS
        Malocclusion due to abnormal swallowing
        Malocclusion due to mouth breathing
        Malocclusion due to tongue, lip or finger habits

M26.6- <u>Temporomandibular joint disorders</u> — The abnormal function of the temporomandibular joint.
    Excludes ❷: current temporomandibular joint dislocation (S03.0)
            current temporomandibular joint sprain (S03.4)

    M26.60- Temporomandibular joint disorder, <u>unspecified</u>
        M26.601 <u>Right</u> temporomandibular joint disorder, unspecified
        M26.602 <u>Left</u> temporomandibular joint disorder, unspecified

        M26.603 <u>Bilateral</u> temporomandibular joint disorder, unspecified
        M26.609 Unspecified temporomandibular joint disorder, <u>unspecified side</u>
            Temporomandibular joint disorder NOS

    M26.61- <u>Adhesions and ankylosis</u> of temporomandibular joint — The immobility and/or fixation of the temporomandibular joint.
        M26.611 Adhesions and ankylosis of <u>right</u> temporomandibular joint
        M26.612 Adhesions and ankylosis of <u>left</u> temporomandibular joint
        M26.613 Adhesions and ankylosis of <u>bilateral</u> temporomandibular joint
        M26.619 Adhesions and ankylosis of temporomandibular joint, <u>unspecified side</u>

    M26.62- <u>Arthralgia</u> of temporomandibular joint — A condition characterized by discomfort and pain of the temporomandibular joint.
        M26.621 Arthralgia of <u>right</u> temporomandibular joint
        M26.622 Arthralgia of <u>left</u> temporomandibular joint
        M26.623 Arthralgia of <u>bilateral</u> temporomandibular joint
        M26.629 Arthralgia of temporomandibular joint, <u>unspecified side</u>

    M26.63- <u>Articular disc disorder</u> of temporomandibular joint — Dysfunction of the temporomandibular joint caused by the deterioration of the temporomandibular articular disc.
        M26.631 Articular disc disorder of <u>right</u> temporomandibular joint
        M26.632 Articular disc disorder of <u>left</u> temporomandibular joint
        M26.633 Articular disc disorder of <u>bilateral</u> temporomandibular joint
        M26.639 Articular disc disorder of temporomandibular joint, <u>unspecified side</u>

    M26.69 Other specified disorders of temporomandibular joint

M26.7- <u>Dental alveolar</u> anomalies

    M26.70 Unspecified alveolar anomaly

    M26.71 Alveolar maxillary hyperplasia — The abnormal developmental enlargement of the upper jaw alveolar process cavities.

    M26.72 Alveolar mandibular hyperplasia — The abnormal developmental enlargement of the lower jaw alveolar process cavities.

    M26.73 Alveolar maxillary hypoplasia — The abnormal developmental smallness of the upper jaw alveolar process cavities.

    M26.74 Alveolar mandibular hypoplasia — The abnormal developmental smallness of the lower jaw alveolar process cavities.

    M26.79 Other specified alveolar anomalies

M26.8- <u>Other</u> dentofacial anomalies

    M26.81 Anterior soft tissue impingement
        Anterior soft tissue impingement on teeth

    M26.82 Posterior soft tissue impingement
        Posterior soft tissue impingement on teeth

    M26.89 Other dentofacial anomalies

M26.9   Dentofacial anomaly, <u>unspecified</u>

M27- Other diseases of jaws

    M27.0 Developmental disorders of jaws
        Latent bone cyst of jaw
        Stafne's cyst
        Torus mandibularis
        Torus palatinus

    M27.1 Giant cell granuloma, central — An abnormal, benign reparative reaction to an injury of the jaw characterized by the proliferation of numerous fibroplastic giant cells.
        Giant cell granuloma NOS
        Excludes 1: peripheral giant cell granuloma (K06.8)

Excludes 1: = NOT CODED HERE! (Do not code both)   **850**   *Excludes ❷: = Not Included Here*

M 2 6 - M 2 7

M27.2 Inflammatory conditions of jaws
Osteitis of jaw(s)
Osteomyelitis (neonatal) jaw(s)
Osteoradionecrosis jaw(s)
Periostitis jaw(s)
Sequestrum of jaw bone
Use additional code (W88-W90, X39.0) to identify radiation, if radiation-induced
Excludes ❷: osteonecrosis of jaw due to drug (M87.180)

M27.3 Alveolitis of jaws — Inflammation of the bony cavities or sockets of the mandible and maxilla.
Alveolar osteitis
Dry socket — A form resulting from exposure of the bone after tooth extraction.

M27.4- Other and unspecified cysts of jaw
Excludes 1: cysts of oral region (K09.-)
latent bone cyst of jaw (M27.0)
Stafne's cyst (M27.0)

M27.40 Unspecified cyst of jaw
Cyst of jaw NOS

M27.49 Other cysts of jaw
Aneurysmal cyst of jaw — The bulging of the jaw cortex resembling an arterial aneurysm in shape.
Hemorrhagic cyst of jaw — A cyst of the jaw caused by the escape of blood within a jaw bone.
Traumatic cyst of jaw — A cyst of the jaw resulting from trauma to the jaw bone.

M27.5- Periradicular pathology associated with previous endodontic treatment

M27.51 Perforation of root canal space due to endodontic treatment

M27.52 Endodontic overfill

M27.53 Endodontic underfill

M27.59 Other periradicular pathology associated with previous endodontic treatment

M27.6- Endosseous dental implant failure

M27.61 Osseointegration failure of dental implant
Hemorrhagic complications of dental implant placement
Iatrogenic osseointegration failure of dental implant
Osseointegration failure of dental implant due to complications of systemic disease
Osseointegration failure of dental implant due to poor bone quality
Pre-Integration failure of dental implant NOS
Pre-osseointegration failure of dental implant

M27.62 Post-osseointegration biological failure of dental implant
Failure of dental implant due to lack of attached gingiva
Failure of dental implant due to occlusal trauma (caused by poor prosthetic design)
Failure of dental implant due to parafunctional habits
Failure of dental implant due to periodontal infection (peri-implantitis)
Failure of dental implant due to poor oral hygiene
Iatrogenic post-osseointegration failure of dental implant
Post-osseointegration failure of dental implant due to complications of systemic disease

M27.63 Post-osseointegration mechanical failure of dental implant
Failure of dental prosthesis causing loss of dental implant
Fracture of dental implant
Excludes ❷: cracked tooth (K03.81)
fractured dental restorative material with loss of material (K08.531)
fractured dental restorative material without loss of material (K08.530)
fractured tooth (S02.5)

M27.69 Other endosseous dental implant failure
Dental implant failure NOS

M27.8 Other specified diseases of jaws
Cherubism
Exostosis
Fibrous dysplasia
Unilateral condylar hyperplasia
Unilateral condylar hypoplasia
Excludes 1: jaw pain (R68.84)

M27.9 Disease of jaws, unspecified

Systemic connective tissue disorders (M30-M36)

Includes: Autoimmune disease NOS
Collagen (vascular) disease NOS
Systemic autoimmune disease
Systemic collagen (vascular) disease
Excludes 1: autoimmune disease, single organ or single cell-type — code to relevant condition category

M30- Polyarteritis nodosa and related conditions
Excludes 1: microscopic polyarteritis (M31.7)

cc M30.0 Polyarteritis nodosa — A systemic vasculitis that is characterized by acute necrotizing inflammation of the small- to medium-sized arteries and microaneurysm formation.

cc M30.1 Polyarteritis with lung involvement [Churg-Strauss] — A form involving the pulmonary circulation.
Allergic granulomatous angiitis

cc M30.2 Juvenile polyarteritis — A form affecting infants and young children that often has a neurologic component.

cc M30.3 Mucocutaneous lymph node syndrome [Kawasaki] — A form marked by tender lymph nodes and skin and mucous membrane inflammation that usually affects young children.

cc M30.8 Other conditions related to polyarteritis nodosa
Polyangiitis overlap syndrome

M31- Other necrotizing vasculopathies
cc M31.0 Hypersensitivity angiitis — A group of necrotizing inflammatory diseases affecting primarily the small blood vessels and characterized by palpable purpura.
Goodpasture's syndrome — Severe, acute glomerulonephritis accompanied by diffuse hemorrhagic inflammation of the lungs.

mcc M31.1 Thrombotic microangiopathy — The formation of thrombi in the arterioles and capillaries.
Thrombotic thrombocytopenic purpura — Thrombotic microangiopathy associated with thrombocytopenia, hemolytic anemia, azotemia, and fever.

cc M31.2 Lethal midline granuloma — A necrotizing tumor-like granuloma which results in destruction of the mid-face and invariably in death.

M31.3- Wegener's granulomatosis — Focal necrotizing arteriolitis, and granulomatous lesions of the respiratory tract with widespread inflammation of all of the organs of the body.
Necrotizing respiratory granulomatosis

cc M31.30 Wegener's granulomatosis without renal involvement
Wegener's granulomatosis NOS

cc M31.31 Wegener's granulomatosis with renal involvement

cc M31.4 Aortic arch syndrome [Takayasu] — An occlusive polyarteritis of unknown cause usually affecting the branches of the aortic arch.

M31.5 Giant cell arteritis with polymyalgia rheumatica

M31.6 Other giant cell arteritis — Chronic inflammation of the large arteries, usually the temporal, occipital, or ophthalmic arteries, accompanied by the presence of giant cells which cause thickening of the intima with narrowing and eventual occlusion of the lumen.

cc M31.7 Microscopic polyangiitis — A form of polyarteritis nodosa affecting the smallest vessels.
Microscopic polyarteritis
Excludes 1: polyarteritis nodosa (M30.0)

cc M31.8 Other specified necrotizing vasculopathies
Hypocomplementemic vasculitis
Septic vasculitis

cc M31.9 Necrotizing vasculopathy, unspecified

M32- Systemic lupus erythematosus (SLE) — An inflammatory autoimmune disorder of the connective tissue that is characterized by rash, joint pain, leukopenia, fever, malaise, and in severe cases organ involvement.
Excludes 1: lupus erythematosus (discoid) (NOS) (L93.0)

M32.0 Drug-induced systemic lupus erythematosus
Use additional code for adverse effect, if applicable, to identify drug (T36-T50 with fifth or sixth character 5)

M32.1- Systemic lupus erythematosus with organ or system involvement

M32.10 Systemic lupus erythematosus, organ or system involvement unspecified

cc M32.11 Endocarditis in systemic lupus erythematosus
Libman-Sacks disease

cc M32.12 Pericarditis in systemic lupus erythematosus
Lupus pericarditis

M32.13 Lung involvement in systemic lupus erythematosus
Pleural effusion due to systemic lupus erythematosus

M27-M32

M32.14 <u>Glomerular</u> disease in systemic lupus erythematosus
AHA 13:4Q:p125 – Lupus complicated by lupus nephritis
Lupus renal disease NOS

M32.15 <u>Tubulo-interstitial nephropathy</u> in systemic lupus erythematosus

M32.19 <u>Other</u> organ or system involvement in systemic lupus erythematosus

M32.8 Other forms of systemic lupus erythematosus

M32.9 Systemic lupus erythematosus, unspecified
SLE NOS
Systemic lupus erythematosus NOS
Systemic lupus erythematosus without organ involvement

M33- <u>Dermatopolymyositis</u> — A connective tissue disease characterized by inflammation of the skin, edema, and inflammation of the muscles.

M33.0- <u>Juvenile</u> dermatopolymyositis

CC M33.00 Juvenile dermatopolymyositis, organ involvement <u>unspecified</u>

CC M33.01 Juvenile dermatopolymyositis <u>with respiratory involvement</u>

CC M33.02 Juvenile dermatopolymyositis <u>with myopathy</u>

CC M33.09 Juvenile dermatopolymyositis <u>with other organ involvement</u>

M33.1- <u>Other</u> dermatopolymyositis

CC M33.10 Other dermatopolymyositis, organ involvement <u>unspecified</u>

CC M33.11 Other dermatopolymyositis <u>with respiratory involvement</u>

CC M33.12 Other dermatopolymyositis <u>with myopathy</u>

CC M33.19 Other dermatopolymyositis <u>with other organ involvement</u>

M33.2- <u>Polymyositis</u> — A connective tissue disease characterized by inflammation and degeneration of the muscles, edema, and without skin changes.

CC M33.20 Polymyositis, organ involvement <u>unspecified</u>

CC M33.21 Polymyositis <u>with respiratory involvement</u>

CC M33.22 Polymyositis <u>with myopathy</u>

CC M33.29 Polymyositis <u>with other organ involvement</u>

M33.9- Dermatopolymyositis, <u>unspecified</u>

CC M33.90 Dermatopolymyositis, unspecified, organ involvement unspecified

CC M33.91 Dermatopolymyositis, unspecified <u>with respiratory involvement</u>

CC M33.92 Dermatopolymyositis, unspecified <u>with myopathy</u>

CC M33.99 Dermatopolymyositis, unspecified <u>with other organ involvement</u>

M34- Systemic sclerosis [scleroderma] — A chronic disease characterized by diffuse fibrous hardening of the skin and internal organs, loss of elasticity, and deposition of melanin in the basal cells.
Excludes 1: circumscribed scleroderma (L94.0)
neonatal scleroderma (P83.8)

M34.0 Progressive systemic sclerosis

M34.1 CR(E)ST syndrome
Combination of calcinosis, Raynaud's phenomenon, esophageal dysfunction, sclerodactyly, telangiectasia

M34.2 Systemic sclerosis induced by drug and chemical
Code first poisoning due to drug or toxin, if applicable (T36-T65 with fifth or sixth character 1-4 or 6)
Use additional code for adverse effect, if applicable, to identify drug (T36-T50 with fifth or sixth character 5)

M34.8- Other forms of systemic sclerosis

CC M34.81 Systemic sclerosis <u>with lung involvement</u>

CC M34.82 Systemic sclerosis <u>with myopathy</u>

M34.83 Systemic sclerosis <u>with polyneuropathy</u>

M34.89 Other systemic sclerosis

M34.9 Systemic sclerosis, unspecified

M35- Other systemic involvement of connective tissue
Excludes 1: reactive perforating collagenosis (L87.1)

M35.0- <u>Sicca syndrome</u> [Sjögren] — An autoimmune disorder characterized by drying of the mucous membranes and eyes, enlargement of the parotid glands, and chronic polyarthritis.

M35.00 Sicca syndrome, <u>unspecified</u>

M35.01 Sicca syndrome <u>with keratoconjunctivitis</u>

M35.02 Sicca syndrome <u>with lung involvement</u>

CC M35.03 Sicca syndrome <u>with myopathy</u>

M35.04 Sicca syndrome <u>with tubulo-interstitial nephropathy</u>
Renal tubular acidosis in sicca syndrome

M35.09 Sicca syndrome <u>with other organ involvement</u>

CC M35.1 Other overlap syndromes
Mixed connective tissue disease
Excludes 1: polyangiitis overlap syndrome (M30.8)

CC M35.2 Behçet's disease — An autoinflammatory disorder that is characterized by oral ulcers, genital ulcers, and uveitis.

M35.3 Polymyalgia rheumatica — An inflammatory disease characterized by pain and stiffness of the shoulder, upper arms, hips, and neck and elevated erythrocyte sedimentation rate.
Excludes 1: polymyalgia rheumatica with giant cell arteritis (M31.5)

M35.4 Diffuse (eosinophilic) fasciitis — An inflammatory disease affecting the fascia that is usually limited to the arms and legs.

CC M35.5 Multifocal fibrosclerosis

M35.6 Relapsing panniculitis [Weber-Christian] — Inflammation of the subcutaneous fat with associated relapsing fever.
Excludes 1: lupus panniculitis (L93.2)
panniculitis NOS (M79.3-)

M35.7 Hypermobility syndrome — Joints that can move beyond the normal range of motion.
Familial ligamentous laxity
Excludes 1: Ehlers-Danlos syndrome (Q79.6)
ligamentous laxity, NOS (M24.2-)

CC M35.8 Other specified systemic involvement of connective tissue

M35.9 Systemic involvement of connective tissue, unspecified
Autoimmune disease (systemic) NOS
Collagen (vascular) disease NOS

M36- Systemic disorders of connective tissue in diseases classified elsewhere
Excludes ❷: arthropathies in diseases classified elsewhere (M14.-)

CC M36.0 Dermato(poly)myositis in neoplastic disease —
[Not Allowed as PDX]
Code first underlying neoplasm (C00-D49)

M36.1 Arthropathy in neoplastic disease — [Not Allowed as PDX]
Code first underlying neoplasm, such as:
Leukemia (C91-C95)
Malignant histiocytosis (C96.A)
Multiple myeloma (C90.0)

M36.2 Hemophilic arthropathy — [Not Allowed as PDX]
Hemarthrosis in hemophilic arthropathy
Code first underlying disease, such as:
Factor VIII deficiency (D66)
With vascular defect (D68.0)
Factor IX deficiency (D67)
Hemophilia (classical) (D66)
Hemophilia B (D67)
Hemophilia C (D68.1)

M36.3 Arthropathy in other blood disorders — [Not Allowed as PDX]

M36.4 Arthropathy in hypersensitivity reactions classified elsewhere — [Not Allowed as PDX]
Code first underlying disease, such as:
Henoch (-Schönlein) purpura (D69.0)
Serum sickness (T80.6-)

M36.8 Systemic disorders of connective tissue <u>in other diseases classified elsewhere</u> — [Not Allowed as PDX]
Code first underlying disease, such as:
Alkaptonuria (E70.2)
Hypogammaglobulinemia (D80.-)
Ochronosis (E70.2)

Dorsopathies (M40-M54)

Deforming dorsopathies (M40-M43)

M40- <u>Kyphosis and lordosis</u>
Excludes 1: congenital kyphosis and lordosis (Q76.4)
kyphoscoliosis (M41.-)
postprocedural kyphosis and lordosis (M96.-)

M40.0- <u>Postural kyphosis</u> — The increased convexity of the spinal position that is due to improper posture.
Excludes 1: osteochondrosis of spine (M42.-)

M40.00 Postural kyphosis, site <u>unspecified</u>

M40.03 Postural kyphosis, <u>cervicothoracic</u> region

Excludes 1: = NOT CODED HERE! (Do not code both)

Excludes ❷: = Not Included Here

M 3 2 - M 4 0

M40.04 Postural kyphosis, <u>thoracic</u> region

M40.05 Postural kyphosis, <u>thoracolumbar</u> region

M40.1- <u>Other secondary</u> kyphosis

M40.10 Other secondary kyphosis, site <u>unspecified</u>

M40.12 Other secondary kyphosis, <u>cervical</u> region

M40.13 Other secondary kyphosis, <u>cervicothoracic</u> region

M40.14 Other secondary kyphosis, <u>thoracic</u> region

M40.15 Other secondary kyphosis, <u>thoracolumbar</u> region

M40.2- Other and unspecified kyphosis

M40.20-<u>Unspecified</u> kyphosis

M40.202 Unspecified kyphosis, cervical region

M40.203 Unspecified kyphosis, <u>cervicothoracic</u> region

M40.204 Unspecified kyphosis, <u>thoracic</u> region

M40.205 Unspecified kyphosis, <u>thoracolumbar</u> region

M40.209 Unspecified kyphosis, <u>site unspecified</u>

M40.29-<u>Other</u> kyphosis

M40.292 Other kyphosis, <u>cervical</u> region

M40.293 Other kyphosis, <u>cervicothoracic</u> region

M40.294 Other kyphosis, <u>thoracic</u> region

M40.295 Other kyphosis, <u>thoracolumbar</u> region

M40.299 Other kyphosis, site <u>unspecified</u>

M40.3- <u>Flatback syndrome</u> — The abnormal alignment of the spine in which the spine appears flat versus naturally curved.

M40.30 Flatback syndrome, <u>site unspecified</u>

M40.35 Flatback syndrome, <u>thoracolumbar</u> region

M40.36 Flatback syndrome, <u>lumbar</u> region

M40.37 Flatback syndrome, <u>lumbosacral</u> region

M40.4- <u>Postural</u> lordosis — The increased concavity of the spinal position that is due to improper posture.

Acquired lordosis

M40.40 Postural lordosis, <u>site unspecified</u>

M40.45 Postural lordosis, <u>thoracolumbar</u> region

M40.46 Postural lordosis, <u>lumbar</u> region

M40.47 Postural lordosis, <u>lumbosacral</u> region

M40.5- <u>Lordosis, unspecified</u>

M40.50 Lordosis, unspecified, site <u>unspecified</u>

M40.55 Lordosis, unspecified, <u>thoracolumbar</u> region

M40.56 Lordosis, unspecified, <u>lumbar</u> region

M40.57 Lordosis, unspecified, <u>lumbosacral</u> region

M41- <u>Scoliosis</u> — The lateral curvature of the spine.

Includes: **Kyphoscoliosis** — The backward and lateral curvature of the spine.

Excludes 1: *congenital scoliosis NOS (Q67.5)*
congenital scoliosis due to bony malformation (Q76.3)
postural congenital scoliosis (Q67.5)
kyphoscoliotic heart disease (I27.1)
postprocedural scoliosis (M96.-)

M41.0- <u>Infantile idiopathic</u> scoliosis — A form usually diagnosed before the age of 3 and with an unknown cause.

M41.00 Infantile idiopathic scoliosis, <u>site unspecified</u>

M41.02 Infantile idiopathic scoliosis, <u>cervical</u> region

M41.03 Infantile idiopathic scoliosis, <u>cervicothoracic</u> region

M41.04 Infantile idiopathic scoliosis, <u>thoracic</u> region

M41.05 Infantile idiopathic scoliosis, <u>thoracolumbar</u> region

M41.06 Infantile idiopathic scoliosis, <u>lumbar</u> region

M41.07 Infantile idiopathic scoliosis, <u>lumbosacral</u> region

M41.08 Infantile idiopathic scoliosis, <u>sacral and sacrococcygeal</u> region

M41.1- Juvenile and adolescent idiopathic scoliosis

M41.11-<u>Juvenile idiopathic</u> scoliosis — A form usually diagnosed between the ages of 4 and 10 and with an unknown cause.

M41.112 Juvenile idiopathic scoliosis, <u>cervical</u> region

M41.113 Juvenile idiopathic scoliosis, <u>cervicothoracic</u> region

M41.114 Juvenile idiopathic scoliosis, <u>thoracic</u> region

M41.115 Juvenile idiopathic scoliosis, <u>thoracolumbar</u> region

M41.116 Juvenile idiopathic scoliosis, <u>lumbar</u> region

M41.117 Juvenile idiopathic scoliosis, <u>lumbosacral</u> region

M41.119 Juvenile idiopathic scoliosis, <u>site unspecified</u>

M41.12-<u>Adolescent</u> scoliosis — A form usually diagnosed between the ages of 10 and 18 and with an unknown cause.

M41.122 Adolescent idiopathic scoliosis, <u>cervical</u> region

M41.123 Adolescent idiopathic scoliosis, <u>cervicothoracic</u> region

M41.124 Adolescent idiopathic scoliosis, <u>thoracic</u> region

M41.125 Adolescent idiopathic scoliosis, <u>thoracolumbar</u> region

M41.126 Adolescent idiopathic scoliosis, <u>lumbar</u> region

M41.127 Adolescent idiopathic scoliosis, <u>lumbosacral</u> region

M41.129 Adolescent idiopathic scoliosis, <u>site unspecified</u>

M41.2- <u>Other idiopathic</u> scoliosis

M41.20 Other idiopathic scoliosis, <u>site unspecified</u>

M41.22 Other idiopathic scoliosis, <u>cervical</u> region

M41.23 Other idiopathic scoliosis, <u>cervicothoracic</u> region

M41.24 Other idiopathic scoliosis, <u>thoracic</u> region

M41.25 Other idiopathic scoliosis, <u>thoracolumbar</u> region

M41.26 Other idiopathic scoliosis, <u>lumbar</u> region

M41.27 Other idiopathic scoliosis, <u>lumbosacral</u> region

M41.3- <u>Thoracogenic</u> scoliosis — A form due to disease or operative trauma to the thoracic cage.

M41.30 Thoracogenic scoliosis, <u>site unspecified</u>

M41.34 Thoracogenic scoliosis, <u>thoracic</u> region

M41.35 Thoracogenic scoliosis, <u>thoracolumbar</u> region

M41.4- <u>Neuromuscular</u> scoliosis — A form due to a neurologic or muscular disease.

Scoliosis secondary to cerebral palsy, Friedreich's ataxia, poliomyelitis and other neuromuscular disorders

Code also underlying condition

M41.40 Neuromuscular scoliosis, <u>site unspecified</u>

M41.41 Neuromuscular scoliosis, <u>occipito-atlanto-axial</u> region

M41.42 Neuromuscular scoliosis, <u>cervical</u> region

M41.43 Neuromuscular scoliosis, <u>cervicothoracic</u> region

M41.44 Neuromuscular scoliosis, <u>thoracic</u> region

M41.45 Neuromuscular scoliosis, <u>thoracolumbar</u> region

M41.46 Neuromuscular scoliosis, <u>lumbar</u> region

M41.47 Neuromuscular scoliosis, <u>lumbosacral</u> region

M41.5- <u>Other secondary</u> scoliosis

M41.50 Other secondary scoliosis, <u>site unspecified</u>

M41.52 Other secondary scoliosis, <u>cervical</u> region

M41.53 Other secondary scoliosis, <u>cervicothoracic</u> region

M41.54 Other secondary scoliosis, <u>thoracic</u> region

M41.55 Other secondary scoliosis, <u>thoracolumbar</u> region

M41.56 Other secondary scoliosis, <u>lumbar</u> region

M41.57 Other secondary scoliosis, <u>lumbosacral</u> region

M41.8- <u>Other forms</u> of scoliosis

M41.80 Other forms of scoliosis, <u>site unspecified</u>

M41.82 Other forms of scoliosis, <u>cervical</u> region

M41.83 Other forms of scoliosis, <u>cervicothoracic</u> region

M41.84 Other forms of scoliosis, <u>thoracic</u> region

M41.85 Other forms of scoliosis, <u>thoracolumbar</u> region

M41.86 Other forms of scoliosis, <u>lumbar</u> region

M41.87 Other forms of scoliosis, <u>lumbosacral</u> region

M41.9 Scoliosis, unspecified

M42- <u>Spinal osteochondrosis</u> — Diseases affecting both the bone and cartilage of the spine.

M42.0- <u>Juvenile osteochondrosis of spine</u> — A developmental disease of the vertebral bone-growth centers characterized by degeneration and recalcification of the vertebrae with resultant deformity of the spine.

Calvé's disease

Scheuermann's disease

Excludes 1: *postural kyphosis (M40.0)*

M42.00 Juvenile osteochondrosis of spine, <u>site unspecified</u>

M42.01 Juvenile osteochondrosis of spine, <u>occipito-atlanto-axial</u> region

M42.02 Juvenile osteochondrosis of spine, <u>cervical region</u>

M40 - M42

M42.03 Juvenile osteochondrosis of spine, <u>cervicothoracic</u> region

M42.04 Juvenile osteochondrosis of spine, <u>thoracic</u> region

M42.05 Juvenile osteochondrosis of spine, <u>thoracolumbar</u> region

M42.06 Juvenile osteochondrosis of spine, <u>lumbar</u> region

M42.07 Juvenile osteochondrosis of spine, <u>lumbosacral</u> region

M42.08 Juvenile osteochondrosis of spine, <u>sacral and sacrococcygeal</u> region

M42.09 Juvenile osteochondrosis of spine, <u>multiple sites</u> in spine

M42.1- <u>Adult</u> osteochondrosis of spine — Degeneration and recalcification of the vertebrae in adults.

M42.10 Adult osteochondrosis of spine, <u>site unspecified</u> — [Age/15-124]

M42.11 Adult osteochondrosis of spine, <u>occipito-atlanto-axial</u> region — [Age/15-124]

M42.12 Adult osteochondrosis of spine, <u>cervical</u> region — [Age/15-124]

M42.13 Adult osteochondrosis of spine, <u>cervicothoracic</u> region — [Age/15-124]

M42.14 Adult osteochondrosis of spine, <u>thoracic</u> region — [Age/15-124]

M42.15 Adult osteochondrosis of spine, <u>thoracolumbar</u> region — [Age/15-124]

M42.16 Adult osteochondrosis of spine, <u>lumbar</u> region — [Age/15-124]

M42.17 Adult osteochondrosis of spine, <u>lumbosacral</u> region — [Age/15-124]

M42.18 Adult osteochondrosis of spine, <u>sacral and sacrococcygeal</u> region — [Age/15-124]

M42.19 Adult osteochondrosis of spine, <u>multiple sites</u> in spine — [Age/15-124]

M42.9   Spinal osteochondrosis, unspecified

M43- <u>Other deforming dorsopathies</u>

Excludes 1:   congenital spondylolysis and spondylolisthesis (Q76.2)
hemivertebra (Q76.3-Q76.4)
Klippel-Feil syndrome (Q76.1)
lumbarization and sacralization (Q76.4)
platyspondylisis (Q76.4)
spina bifida occulta (Q76.0)
spinal curvature in osteoporosis (M80.-)
spinal curvature in Paget's disease of bone [osteitis deformans] (M88.-)

M43.0- <u>Spondylolysis</u> — A defect in the connection between vertebrae.

Excludes 1:   congenital spondylolysis (Q76.2)
spondylolisthesis (M43.1)

M43.00 Spondylolysis, <u>site unspecified</u>

M43.01 Spondylolysis, <u>occipito-atlanto-axial</u> region

M43.02 Spondylolysis, <u>cervical</u> region

M43.03 Spondylolysis, <u>cervicothoracic</u> region

M43.04 Spondylolysis, <u>thoracic</u> region

M43.05 Spondylolysis, <u>thoracolumbar</u> region

M43.06 Spondylolysis, <u>lumbar</u> region

M43.07 Spondylolysis, <u>lumbosacral</u> region

M43.08 Spondylolysis, <u>sacral and sacrococcygeal</u> region

M43.09 Spondylolysis, <u>multiple sites</u> in spine

M43.1- <u>Spondylolisthesis</u> — The forward displacement of a vertebra.

Excludes 1:   acute traumatic of lumbosacral region (S33.1)
acute traumatic of sites other than lumbosacral — code to Fracture, vertebra, by region
congenital spondylolisthesis (Q76.2)

M43.10 Spondylolisthesis, <u>site unspecified</u>

M43.11 Spondylolisthesis, <u>occipito-atlanto-axial</u> region

M43.12 Spondylolisthesis, <u>cervical</u> region

M43.13 Spondylolisthesis, <u>cervicothoracic</u> region

M43.14 Spondylolisthesis, <u>thoracic</u> region

M43.15 Spondylolisthesis, <u>thoracolumbar</u> region

M43.16 Spondylolisthesis, <u>lumbar</u> region

M43.17 Spondylolisthesis, <u>lumbosacral</u> region

M43.18 Spondylolisthesis, <u>sacral and sacrococcygeal</u> region

M43.19 Spondylolisthesis, <u>multiple sites</u> in spine

M43.2- <u>Fusion of spine</u> — Inflammation of the spinal joints that causes the vertebrae to fuse together.

Ankylosis of spinal joint

Excludes 1:   ankylosing spondylitis (M45.0-)
congenital fusion of spine (Q76.4)

Excludes ❷: arthrodesis status (Z98.1)
pseudoarthrosis after fusion or arthrodesis (M96.0)

M43.20 Fusion of spine, <u>site unspecified</u>

M43.21 Fusion of spine, <u>occipito-atlanto-axial</u> region

M43.22 Fusion of spine, <u>cervical</u> region

M43.23 Fusion of spine, <u>cervicothoracic</u> region

M43.24 Fusion of spine, <u>thoracic</u> region

M43.25 Fusion of spine, <u>thoracolumbar</u> region

M43.26 Fusion of spine, <u>lumbar</u> region

M43.27 Fusion of spine, <u>lumbosacral</u> region

M43.28 Fusion of spine, <u>sacral and sacrococcygeal</u> region

M43.3   Recurrent atlantoaxial dislocation with myelopathy

M43.4   Other recurrent atlantoaxial dislocation

M43.5- Other recurrent vertebral dislocation

Excludes 1:   biomechanical lesions NEC (M99.-)

M43.5x- <u>Other recurrent vertebral dislocation</u>

M43.5x2 Other recurrent vertebral dislocation, <u>cervical</u> region

M43.5x3 Other recurrent vertebral dislocation, <u>cervicothoracic</u> region

M43.5x4 Other recurrent vertebral dislocation, <u>thoracic</u> region

M43.5x5 Other recurrent vertebral dislocation, <u>thoracolumbar</u> region

M43.5x6 Other recurrent vertebral dislocation, <u>lumbar</u> region

M43.5x7 Other recurrent vertebral dislocation, <u>lumbosacral</u> region

M43.5x8 Other recurrent vertebral dislocation, <u>sacral and sacrococcygeal</u> region

M43.5x9 Other recurrent vertebral dislocation, <u>site unspecified</u>

M43.6   Torticollis — The contracted state of the neck muscles causing the characteristic head tilt.

Excludes 1:   congenital (sternomastoid) torticollis (Q68.0)
current injury — see Injury, of spine, by body region
ocular torticollis (R29.891)
psychogenic torticollis (F45.8)
spasmodic torticollis (G24.3)
torticollis due to birth injury (P15.2)

M43.8- Other specified deforming dorsopathies

Excludes ❷: kyphosis and lordosis (M40.-)
scoliosis (M41.-)

M43.8x- <u>Other specified deforming dorsopathies</u>

M43.8x1 Other specified deforming dorsopathies, <u>occipito-atlanto-axial</u> region

M43.8x2 Other specified deforming dorsopathies, <u>cervical</u> region

M43.8x3 Other specified deforming dorsopathies, <u>cervicothoracic</u> region

M43.8x4 Other specified deforming dorsopathies, <u>thoracic</u> region

M43.8x5 Other specified deforming dorsopathies, <u>thoracolumbar</u> region

M43.8x6 Other specified deforming dorsopathies, <u>lumbar</u> region

M43.8x7 Other specified deforming dorsopathies, <u>lumbosacral</u> region

M43.8x8 Other specified deforming dorsopathies, <u>sacral and sacrococcygeal</u> region

M43.8x9 Other specified deforming dorsopathies, <u>site unspecified</u>

M43.9   Deforming dorsopathy, unspecified

Curvature of spine NOS

Spondylopathies (M45-M49)

M45- <u>Ankylosing spondylitis</u> — Inflammation of the spinal joints that causes the spine to become stiff and inflexible.
    Rheumatoid arthritis of spine — A form of rheumatoid arthritis that affects the vertebrae and marked by immobility, pain, and calcification.
    Excludes 1:   *arthropathy in Reiter's disease (M02.3-)*
                      juvenile (ankylosing) spondylitis (M08.1)
    Excludes ❷: *Behçet's disease (M35.2)*

  M45.0   Ankylosing spondylitis of <u>multiple sites</u> in spine
  M45.1   Ankylosing spondylitis of <u>occipito-atlanto-axial</u> region
  M45.2   Ankylosing spondylitis of <u>cervical</u> region
  M45.3   Ankylosing spondylitis of <u>cervicothoracic</u> region
  M45.4   Ankylosing spondylitis of <u>thoracic</u> region
  M45.5   Ankylosing spondylitis of <u>thoracolumbar</u> region
  M45.6   Ankylosing spondylitis of <u>lumbar</u> region
  M45.7   Ankylosing spondylitis of <u>lumbosacral</u> region
  M45.8   Ankylosing spondylitis <u>sacral and sacrococcygeal</u> region
  M45.9   Ankylosing spondylitis of <u>unspecified</u> sites in spine

M46- Other inflammatory spondylopathies
  M46.0- <u>Spinal enthesopathy</u> — A disorder of the spinal ligamentous or muscular attachments.
      Disorder of ligamentous or muscular attachments of spine
    M46.00 Spinal enthesopathy, <u>site unspecified</u>
    M46.01 Spinal enthesopathy, <u>occipito-atlanto-axial</u> region
    M46.02 Spinal enthesopathy, <u>cervical</u> region
    M46.03 Spinal enthesopathy, <u>cervicothoracic</u> region
    M46.04 Spinal enthesopathy, <u>thoracic</u> region
    M46.05 Spinal enthesopathy, <u>thoracolumbar</u> region
    M46.06 Spinal enthesopathy, <u>lumbar</u> region
    M46.07 Spinal enthesopathy, <u>lumbosacral</u> region
    M46.08 Spinal enthesopathy, <u>sacral and sacrococcygeal</u> region
    M46.09 Spinal enthesopathy, <u>multiple sites</u> in spine
  M46.1   Sacroiliitis, not elsewhere classified
  M46.2- <u>Osteomyelitis</u> of vertebra — Inflammation of the vertebrae caused by microorganisms.
    cc **M46.20** Osteomyelitis of vertebra, <u>site unspecified</u>
    cc **M46.21** Osteomyelitis of vertebra, <u>occipito-atlanto-axial</u> region
    cc **M46.22** Osteomyelitis of vertebra, <u>cervical</u> region
    cc **M46.23** Osteomyelitis of vertebra, <u>cervicothoracic</u> region
    cc **M46.24** Osteomyelitis of vertebra, <u>thoracic</u> region
    cc **M46.25** Osteomyelitis of vertebra, <u>thoracolumbar</u> region
    cc **M46.26** Osteomyelitis of vertebra, <u>lumbar</u> region
    cc **M46.27** Osteomyelitis of vertebra, <u>lumbosacral</u> region
    cc **M46.28** Osteomyelitis of vertebra, <u>sacral and sacrococcygeal</u> region
  M46.3- <u>Infection of intervertebral disc (pyogenic)</u> — Inflammation of an intervertebral disc with pus formation that is due to infection by microorganisms.
    Use additional code (B95-B97) to identify infectious agent
    cc **M46.30** Infection of intervertebral disc (pyogenic), <u>site unspecified</u>
    cc **M46.31** Infection of intervertebral disc (pyogenic), <u>occipito-atlanto-axial</u> region
    cc **M46.32** Infection of intervertebral disc (pyogenic), <u>cervical</u> region
    cc **M46.33** Infection of intervertebral disc (pyogenic), <u>cervicothoracic</u> region
    cc **M46.34** Infection of intervertebral disc (pyogenic), <u>thoracic</u> region
    cc **M46.35** Infection of intervertebral disc (pyogenic), <u>thoracolumbar</u> region
    cc **M46.36** Infection of intervertebral disc (pyogenic), <u>lumbar</u> region
    cc **M46.37** Infection of intervertebral disc (pyogenic), <u>lumbosacral</u> region
    cc **M46.38** Infection of intervertebral disc (pyogenic), <u>sacral and sacrococcygeal</u> region
    cc **M46.39** Infection of intervertebral disc (pyogenic), <u>multiple sites</u> in spine

M46.4- <u>Discitis, unspecified</u>
  M46.40 Discitis, unspecified, <u>site unspecified</u>
  M46.41 Discitis, unspecified, <u>occipito-atlanto-axial</u> region
  M46.42 Discitis, unspecified, <u>cervical</u> region
  M46.43 Discitis, unspecified, <u>cervicothoracic</u> region
  M46.44 Discitis, unspecified, <u>thoracic</u> region
  M46.45 Discitis, unspecified, <u>thoracolumbar</u> region
  M46.46 Discitis, unspecified, <u>lumbar</u> region
  M46.47 Discitis, unspecified, <u>lumbosacral</u> region
  M46.48 Discitis, unspecified, <u>sacral and sacrococcygeal</u> region
  M46.49 Discitis, unspecified, <u>multiple sites</u> in spine

M46.5- <u>Other infective</u> spondylopathies
  M46.50 Other infective spondylopathies, <u>site unspecified</u>
  M46.51 Other infective spondylopathies, <u>occipito-atlanto-axial</u> region
  M46.52 Other infective spondylopathies, <u>cervical</u> region
  M46.53 Other infective spondylopathies, <u>cervicothoracic</u> region
  M46.54 Other infective spondylopathies, <u>thoracic</u> region
  M46.55 Other infective spondylopathies, <u>thoracolumbar</u> region
  M46.56 Other infective spondylopathies, <u>lumbar</u> region
  M46.57 Other infective spondylopathies, <u>lumbosacral</u> region
  M46.58 Other infective spondylopathies, <u>sacral and sacrococcygeal</u> region
  M46.59 Other infective spondylopathies, <u>multiple sites</u> in spine

M46.8- <u>Other specified inflammatory</u> spondylopathies
  M46.80 Other specified inflammatory spondylopathies, <u>site unspecified</u>
  M46.81 Other specified inflammatory spondylopathies, <u>occipito-atlanto-axial</u> region
  M46.82 Other specified inflammatory spondylopathies, <u>cervical</u> region
  M46.83 Other specified inflammatory spondylopathies, <u>cervicothoracic</u> region
  M46.84 Other specified inflammatory spondylopathies, <u>thoracic</u> region
  M46.85 Other specified inflammatory spondylopathies, <u>thoracolumbar</u> region
  M46.86 Other specified inflammatory spondylopathies, <u>lumbar</u> region
  M46.87 Other specified inflammatory spondylopathies, <u>lumbosacral</u> region
  M46.88 Other specified inflammatory spondylopathies, <u>sacral and sacrococcygeal</u> region
  M46.89 Other specified inflammatory spondylopathies, <u>multiple sites</u> in spine

M46.9- <u>Unspecified</u> inflammatory spondylopathy
  M46.90 Unspecified inflammatory spondylopathy, <u>site unspecified</u>
  M46.91 Unspecified inflammatory spondylopathy, <u>occipito-atlanto-axial</u> region
  M46.92 Unspecified inflammatory spondylopathy, <u>cervical</u> region
  M46.93 Unspecified inflammatory spondylopathy, <u>cervicothoracic</u> region
  M46.94 Unspecified inflammatory spondylopathy, <u>thoracic</u> region
  M46.95 Unspecified inflammatory spondylopathy, <u>thoracolumbar</u> region
  M46.96 Unspecified inflammatory spondylopathy, <u>lumbar</u> region
  M46.97 Unspecified inflammatory spondylopathy, <u>lumbosacral</u> region
  M46.98 Unspecified inflammatory spondylopathy, <u>sacral and sacrococcygeal</u> region
  M46.99 Unspecified inflammatory spondylopathy, <u>multiple sites</u> in spine

M 4 5 I M 4 6

M47- Spondylosis — Degenerative joint disease of the spine.
Includes: Arthrosis or osteoarthritis of spine
Degeneration of facet joints

M47.0- Anterior spinal and vertebral artery compression syndromes

M47.01- Anterior spinal artery compression syndromes — A form resulting in the restriction of blood flow through the anterior spinal artery.

cc **M47.011 Anterior spinal artery compression syndromes, occipito-atlanto-axial region**

cc **M47.012 Anterior spinal artery compression syndromes, cervical region**

cc **M47.013 Anterior spinal artery compression syndromes, cervicothoracic region**

cc **M47.014 Anterior spinal artery compression syndromes, thoracic region**

cc **M47.015 Anterior spinal artery compression syndromes, thoracolumbar region**

cc **M47.016 Anterior spinal artery compression syndromes, lumbar region**

cc **M47.019 Anterior spinal artery compression syndromes, site unspecified**

M47.02- Vertebral artery compression syndromes — A form resulting in the restriction of blood flow through the vertebral artery.

cc **M47.021 Vertebral artery compression syndromes, occipito-atlanto-axial region**

cc **M47.022 Vertebral artery compression syndromes, cervical region**

cc **M47.029 Vertebral artery compression syndromes, site unspecified**

M47.1- Other spondylosis with myelopathy — Degenerative joint disease of the spine that results in a disorder of the spinal cord.
Spondylogenic compression of spinal cord

Excludes 1:   vertebral subluxation (M43.3-M43.59)

cc **M47.10 Other spondylosis with myelopathy, site unspecified**

cc **M47.11 Other spondylosis with myelopathy, occipito-atlanto-axial region**

cc **M47.12 Other spondylosis with myelopathy, cervical region**

cc **M47.13 Other spondylosis with myelopathy, cervicothoracic region**

cc **M47.14 Other spondylosis with myelopathy, thoracic region**

cc **M47.15 Other spondylosis with myelopathy, thoracolumbar region**

cc **M47.16 Other spondylosis with myelopathy, lumbar region**

M47.2- Other spondylosis with radiculopathy

M47.20 Other spondylosis with radiculopathy, site unspecified

M47.21 Other spondylosis with radiculopathy, occipito-atlanto-axial region

M47.22 Other spondylosis with radiculopathy, cervical region

M47.23 Other spondylosis with radiculopathy, cervicothoracic region

M47.24 Other spondylosis with radiculopathy, thoracic region

M47.25 Other spondylosis with radiculopathy, thoracolumbar region

M47.26 Other spondylosis with radiculopathy, lumbar region

M47.27 Other spondylosis with radiculopathy, lumbosacral region

M47.28 Other spondylosis with radiculopathy, sacral and sacrococcygeal region

M47.8- Other spondylosis

M47.81- Spondylosis without myelopathy or radiculopathy

M47.811 Spondylosis without myelopathy or radiculopathy, occipito-atlanto-axial region

M47.812 Spondylosis without myelopathy or radiculopathy, cervical region

M47.813 Spondylosis without myelopathy or radiculopathy, cervicothoracic region

M47.814 Spondylosis without myelopathy or radiculopathy, thoracic region

M47.815 Spondylosis without myelopathy or radiculopathy, thoracolumbar region

M47.816 Spondylosis without myelopathy or radiculopathy, lumbar region

M47.817 Spondylosis without myelopathy or radiculopathy, lumbosacral region

M47.818 Spondylosis without myelopathy or radiculopathy, sacral and sacrococcygeal region

M47.819 Spondylosis without myelopathy or radiculopathy, site unspecified

M47.89- Other spondylosis

M47.891 Other spondylosis, occipito-atlanto-axial region

M47.892 Other spondylosis, cervical region

M47.893 Other spondylosis, cervicothoracic region

M47.894 Other spondylosis, thoracic region

M47.895 Other spondylosis, thoracolumbar region

M47.896 Other spondylosis, lumbar region

M47.897 Other spondylosis, lumbosacral region

M47.898 Other spondylosis, sacral and sacrococcygeal region

M47.899 Other spondylosis, site unspecified

M47.9 Spondylosis, unspecified

M48- Other spondylopathies

M48.0- Spinal stenosis — The narrowing of the spinal column with compression of the spinal nerve roots.
Caudal stenosis

M48.00 Spinal stenosis, site unspecified

M48.01 Spinal stenosis, occipito-atlanto-axial region

M48.02 Spinal stenosis, cervical region

M48.03 Spinal stenosis, cervicothoracic region

M48.04 Spinal stenosis, thoracic region

M48.05 Spinal stenosis, thoracolumbar region

M48.06 Spinal stenosis, lumbar region

M48.07 Spinal stenosis, lumbosacral region

M48.08 Spinal stenosis, sacral and sacrococcygeal region

M48.1- Ankylosing hyperostosis [Forestier] — The spinal arthropathy that is characterized by ossification of the ligaments and connective tissue of the spine.
Diffuse idiopathic skeletal hyperostosis [DISH]

M48.10 Ankylosing hyperostosis [Forestier], site unspecified

M48.11 Ankylosing hyperostosis [Forestier], occipito-atlanto-axial region

M48.12 Ankylosing hyperostosis [Forestier], cervical region

M48.13 Ankylosing hyperostosis [Forestier], cervicothoracic region

M48.14 Ankylosing hyperostosis [Forestier], thoracic region

M48.15 Ankylosing hyperostosis [Forestier], thoracolumbar region

M48.16 Ankylosing hyperostosis [Forestier], lumbar region

M48.17 Ankylosing hyperostosis [Forestier], lumbosacral region

M48.18 Ankylosing hyperostosis [Forestier], sacral and sacrococcygeal region

M48.19 Ankylosing hyperostosis [Forestier], multiple sites in spine

M48.2- Kissing spine — A disorder in which the spinal processes of adjacent vertebrae are in contact.

M48.20 Kissing spine, site unspecified

M48.21 Kissing spine, occipito-atlanto-axial region

M48.22 Kissing spine, cervical region

M48.23 Kissing spine, cervicothoracic region

M48.24 Kissing spine, thoracic region

M48.25 Kissing spine, thoracolumbar region

M48.26 Kissing spine, lumbar region

M48.27 Kissing spine, lumbosacral region

M48.3- Traumatic spondylopathy — A disorder of the spine as a result of trauma.

cc **M48.30 Traumatic spondylopathy, site unspecified**

cc **M48.31 Traumatic spondylopathy, occipito-atlanto-axial region**

cc **M48.32 Traumatic spondylopathy, cervical region**

cc **M48.33 Traumatic spondylopathy, cervicothoracic region**

cc **M48.34 Traumatic spondylopathy, thoracic region**

cc **M48.35 Traumatic spondylopathy, thoracolumbar region**

cc **M48.36 Traumatic spondylopathy, lumbar region**

cc **M48.37 Traumatic spondylopathy, lumbosacral region**

M47 - M48 (side tab)

Excludes 1: = NOT CODED HERE! (Do not code both)   **Excludes ❷:** = Not Included Here

CC M48.38   Traumatic spondylopathy, <u>sacral and sacrococcygeal</u> region

M48.4-   <u>Fatigue fracture</u> of <u>vertebra</u> — A break of a diseased or weakened bone by a minor injury that would otherwise not break a healthy bone.

Stress fracture of vertebra

Excludes 1:   *pathological fracture NOS (M84.4-)*
pathological fracture of vertebra due to neoplasm (M84.58)
pathological fracture of vertebra due to other diagnosis (M84.68)
pathological fracture of vertebra due to osteoporosis (M80-)
traumatic fracture of vertebrae (S12.0-S12.3-, S22.0-, S32.0-)

The appropriate 7th character is to be added to each code from subcategory M48.4:
A   Initial encounter for fracture
D   Subsequent encounter for fracture with routine healing
G   Subsequent encounter for fracture with delayed healing
S   Sequela of fracture

M48.40x-   Fatigue fracture of vertebra, <u>site unspecified</u>
M48.41x-   Fatigue fracture of vertebra, <u>occipito-atlanto-axial</u> region
M48.42x-   Fatigue fracture of vertebra, <u>cervical</u> region
M48.43x-   Fatigue fracture of vertebra, <u>cervicothoracic</u> region
M48.44x-   Fatigue fracture of vertebra, <u>thoracic</u> region
M48.45x-   Fatigue fracture of vertebra, <u>thoracolumbar</u> region
M48.46x-   Fatigue fracture of vertebra, <u>lumbar</u> region
M48.47x-   Fatigue fracture of vertebra, <u>lumbosacral</u> region
M48.48x-   Fatigue fracture of vertebra, <u>sacral and sacrococcygeal</u> region

M48.5-   <u>Collapsed vertebra</u>, <u>not elsewhere classified</u>
Collapsed vertebra NOS
Compression fracture of vertebra NOS
Wedging of vertebra NOS

Excludes 1:   *current injury — see Injury of spine, by body region*
fatigue fracture of vertebra (M48.4)
pathological fracture of vertebra due to neoplasm (M84.58)
pathological fracture of vertebra due to other diagnosis (M84.68)
pathological fracture of vertebra due to osteoporosis (M80.-)
pathological fracture NOS (M84.4-)
stress fracture of vertebra (M48.4-)
traumatic fracture of vertebra (S12.-, S22.-, S32.-)

The appropriate 7th character is to be added to each code from subcategory M48.5:
A   Initial encounter for fracture
D   Subsequent encounter for fracture with routine healing
G   Subsequent encounter for fracture with delayed healing
S   Sequela of fracture

CC-A M48.50x-   Collapsed vertebra, not elsewhere classified, <u>site unspecified</u>
CC-A M48.51x-   Collapsed vertebra, not elsewhere classified, <u>occipito-atlanto-axial</u> region
CC-A M48.52x-   Collapsed vertebra, not elsewhere classified, <u>cervical</u> region
CC-A M48.53x-   Collapsed vertebra, not elsewhere classified, <u>cervicothoracic</u> region
CC-A M48.54x-   Collapsed vertebra, not elsewhere classified, <u>thoracic</u> region
CC-A M48.55x-   Collapsed vertebra, not elsewhere classified, <u>thoracolumbar</u> region
CC-A M48.56x-   Collapsed vertebra, not elsewhere classified, <u>lumbar</u> region
CC-A M48.57x-   Collapsed vertebra, not elsewhere classified, <u>lumbosacral</u> region
CC-A M48.58x-   Collapsed vertebra, not elsewhere classified, <u>sacral and sacrococcygeal</u> region

M48.8-   Other specified spondylopathies
Ossification of posterior longitudinal ligament

M48.8x-   <u>Other specified spondylopathies</u>
M48.8x1   Other specified spondylopathies, <u>occipito-atlanto-axial</u> region
M48.8x2   Other specified spondylopathies, <u>cervical</u> region
M48.8x3   Other specified spondylopathies, <u>cervicothoracic</u> region
M48.8x4   Other specified spondylopathies, <u>thoracic</u> region
M48.8x5   Other specified spondylopathies, <u>thoracolumbar</u> region
M48.8x6   Other specified spondylopathies, <u>lumbar</u> region
M48.8x7   Other specified spondylopathies, <u>lumbosacral</u> region
M48.8x8   Other specified spondylopathies, <u>sacral and sacrococcygeal</u> region
M48.8x9   Other specified spondylopathies, <u>site unspecified</u>

M48.9   Spondylopathy, <u>unspecified</u>

M49-   Spondylopathies <u>in diseases classified elsewhere</u>
Includes: Curvature of spine in diseases classified elsewhere
Deformity of spine in diseases classified elsewhere
Kyphosis in diseases classified elsewhere
Scoliosis in diseases classified elsewhere
Spondylopathy in diseases classified elsewhere

Code first underlying disease, such as:
Brucellosis (A23.-)
Charcot-Marie-Tooth disease (G60.0)
Enterobacterial infections (A01-A04)
Osteitis fibrosa cystica (E21.0)

Excludes 1:   *curvature of spine in tuberculosis [Pott's] (A18.01)*
enteropathic arthropathies (M07.-)
gonococcal spondylitis (A54.41)
neuropathic spondylopathy in syringomyelia (G95.0)
neuropathic spondylopathy in tabes dorsalis (A52.11)
neuropathic [tabes dorsalis] spondylitis (A52.11)
nonsyphilitic neuropathic spondylopathy NEC (G98.0)
spondylitis in syphilis (acquired) (A52.77)
tuberculosis spondylitis (A18.01)
typhoid fever spondylitis (A01.05)

M49.8-   <u>Spondylopathy</u> <u>in diseases classified elsewhere</u>
M49.80   Spondylopathy in diseases classified elsewhere, <u>site unspecified</u> — [Not Allowed as PDX]
M49.81   Spondylopathy in diseases classified elsewhere, <u>occipito-atlanto-axial</u> region — [Not Allowed as PDX]
M49.82   Spondylopathy in diseases classified elsewhere, <u>cervical</u> region — [Not Allowed as PDX]
M49.83   Spondylopathy in diseases classified elsewhere, <u>cervicothoracic</u> region — [Not Allowed as PDX]
M49.84   Spondylopathy in diseases classified elsewhere, <u>thoracic</u> region — [Not Allowed as PDX]
M49.85   Spondylopathy in diseases classified elsewhere, <u>thoracolumbar</u> region — [Not Allowed as PDX]
M49.86   Spondylopathy in diseases classified elsewhere, <u>lumbar</u> region — [Not Allowed as PDX]
M49.87   Spondylopathy in diseases classified elsewhere, <u>lumbosacral</u> region — [Not Allowed as PDX]
M49.88   Spondylopathy in diseases classified elsewhere, <u>sacral and sacrococcygeal</u> region — [Not Allowed as PDX]
M49.89   Spondylopathy in diseases classified elsewhere, <u>multiple sites</u> in spine — [Not Allowed as PDX]

Other dorsopathies (M50-M54)

Excludes 1:   *current injury — see injury of spine by body region*
discitis NOS (M46.4-)

M50-   <u>Cervical disc disorders</u> — The abnormal condition of a cervical disc.
AHA 16:1Q:p17 – Code to the most superior level of disorder
Note: Code to the most superior level of disorder
Includes: Cervicothoracic disc disorders with cervicalgia
Cervicothoracic disc disorders

M50.0-   Cervical disc disorder <u>with myelopathy</u> — A form that results in a disorder of the spinal cord.

CC M50.00   Cervical disc disorder with myelopathy, <u>unspecified cervical region</u>

Excludes 1: = NOT CODED HERE! (Do not code both)   **857**   *Excludes ❷:* = Not Included Here

cc **M50.01** Cervical disc disorder with myelopathy, <u>high cervical</u> region
C2-C3 disc disorder with myelopathy
C3-C4 disc disorder with myelopathy

M50.02-Cervical disc disorder with myelopathy, <u>mid-cervical</u> region

cc **M50.020** Cervical disc disorder with myelopathy, mid-cervical region, <u>unspecified level</u>

cc **M50.021** Cervical disc disorder at <u>C4-C5 level</u> with myelopathy
C4-C5 disc disorder with myelopathy

cc **M50.022** Cervical disc disorder at <u>C5-C6 level</u> with myelopathy
C5-C6 disc disorder with myelopathy

cc **M50.023** Cervical disc disorder at <u>C6-C7 level</u> with myelopathy
C6-C7 disc disorder with myelopathy

cc **M50.03** Cervical disc disorder with myelopathy, <u>cervicothoracic</u> region
C7-T1 disc disorder with myelopathy

M50.1- Cervical disc disorder <u>with radiculopathy</u> — A form with injury (compression and/or inflammation) to the spinal nerve root.
Excludes 2: *brachial radiculitis NOS (M54.13)*

M50.10 Cervical disc disorder with radiculopathy, <u>unspecified cervical</u> region

M50.11 Cervical disc disorder with radiculopathy, <u>high cervical</u> region
C2-C3 disc disorder with radiculopathy
C3 radiculopathy due to disc disorder
C3-C4 disc disorder with radiculopathy
C4 radiculopathy due to disc disorder

M50.12-Cervical disc disorder with radiculopathy, <u>mid-cervical</u> region

M50.120 Mid-cervical disc disorder, <u>unspecified</u>

M50.121 Cervical disc disorder at <u>C4-C5 level</u> with radiculopathy
C4-C5 disc disorder with radiculopathy
C5 radiculopathy due to disc disorder

M50.122 Cervical disc disorder at <u>C5-C6 level</u> with radiculopathy
C5-C6 disc disorder with radiculopathy
C6 radiculopathy due to disc disorder

M50.123 Cervical disc disorder at <u>C6-C7 level</u> with radiculopathy
C6-C7 disc disorder with radiculopathy
C7 radiculopathy due to disc disorder

M50.13 Cervical disc disorder with radiculopathy, <u>cervicothoracic</u> region
C7-T1 disc disorder with radiculopathy
C8 radiculopathy due to disc disorder

M50.2- <u>Other cervical disc displacement</u> — The dislocation of a cervical intervertebral disc.

M50.20 Other cervical disc displacement, <u>unspecified cervical</u> region

M50.21 Other cervical disc displacement, <u>high cervical</u> region
Other C2-C3 cervical disc displacement
Other C3-C4 cervical disc displacement

M50.22-Other cervical disc displacement, <u>mid-cervical</u> region

M50.220 Other cervical disc displacement, mid-cervical region, <u>unspecified level</u>

M50.221 Other cervical disc displacement at <u>C4-C5 level</u>
Other C4-C5 cervical disc displacement

M50.222 Other cervical disc displacement at <u>C5-C6 level</u>
Other C5-C6 cervical disc displacement

M50.223 Other cervical disc displacement at <u>C6-C7 level</u>
Other C6-C7 cervical disc displacement

M50.23 Other cervical disc displacement, <u>cervicothoracic</u> region
Other C7-T1 cervical disc displacement

M50.3- <u>Other cervical disc degeneration</u> — The deterioration of a cervical intervertebral disc.

M50.30 Other cervical disc degeneration, <u>unspecified cervical</u> region

M50.31 Other cervical disc degeneration, <u>high cervical</u> region
Other C2-C3 cervical disc degeneration
Other C3-C4 cervical disc degeneration

M50.32-Other cervical disc degeneration, <u>mid-cervical</u> region

M50.320 Other cervical disc degeneration, mid-cervical region, <u>unspecified level</u>

M50.321 Other cervical disc degeneration at <u>C4-C5 level</u>
Other C4-C5 cervical disc degeneration

M50.322 Other cervical disc degeneration at <u>C5-C6 level</u>
Other C5-C6 cervical disc degeneration

M50.323 Other cervical disc degeneration at <u>C6-C7 level</u>
Other C6-C7 cervical disc degeneration

M50.33 Other cervical disc degeneration, <u>cervicothoracic</u> region
Other C7-T1 cervical disc degeneration

M50.8- <u>Other cervical disc disorders</u>

M50.80 Other cervical disc disorders, <u>unspecified cervical</u> region

M50.81 Other cervical disc disorders, <u>high cervical</u> region
Other C2-C3 cervical disc disorders
Other C3-C4 cervical disc disorders

M50.82-Other cervical disc disorders, <u>mid-cervical</u> region

M50.820 Other cervical disc disorders, mid-cervical region, <u>unspecified level</u>

M50.821 Other cervical disc disorders at <u>C4-C5 level</u>
Other C4-C5 cervical disc disorders

M50.822 Other cervical disc disorders at <u>C5-C6 level</u>
Other C5-C6 cervical disc disorders

M50.823 Other cervical disc disorders at <u>C6-C7 level</u>
Other C6-C7 cervical disc disorders

M50.83 Other cervical disc disorders, <u>cervicothoracic</u> region
Other C7-T1 cervical disc disorders

M50.9- <u>Cervical disc disorder, unspecified</u>

M50.90 Cervical disc disorder, unspecified, <u>unspecified cervical</u> region

M50.91 Cervical disc disorder, unspecified, <u>high cervical</u> region
C2-C3 cervical disc disorder, unspecified
C3-C4 cervical disc disorder, unspecified

M50.92-Cervical disc disorder, unspecified, <u>mid-cervical</u> region

M50.920 Unspecified cervical disc disorder, mid-cervical region, <u>unspecified level</u>

M50.921 Unspecified cervical disc disorder at <u>C4-C5 level</u>
Unspecified C4-C5 cervical disc disorder

M50.922 Unspecified cervical disc disorder at <u>C5-C6 level</u>
Unspecified C5-C6 cervical disc disorder

M50.923 Unspecified cervical disc disorder at <u>C6-C7 level</u>
Unspecified C6-C7 cervical disc disorder

M50.93 Cervical disc disorder, unspecified, <u>cervicothoracic</u> region
C7-T1 cervical disc disorder, unspecified

M51- <u>Thoracic, thoracolumbar, and lumbosacral intervertebral disc disorders</u> — The abnormal condition of a thoracic, thoracolumbar, or lumbosacral disc.
Excludes 2: *cervical and cervicothoracic disc disorders (M50.-)*
sacral and sacrococcygeal disorders (M53.3)

M51.0- Thoracic, thoracolumbar and lumbosacral intervertebral disc disorders <u>with myelopathy</u> — A form that results in a disorder of the spinal cord.

cc **M51.04** Intervertebral disc disorders with myelopathy, <u>thoracic</u> region

cc **M51.05** Intervertebral disc disorders with myelopathy, <u>thoracolumbar</u> region

cc **M51.06** Intervertebral disc disorders with myelopathy, <u>lumbar</u> region

M51.1- Thoracic, thoracolumbar and lumbosacral intervertebral disc disorders <u>with radiculopathy</u> — A form with injury (compression and/or inflammation) to the spinal nerve root.
Sciatica due to intervertebral disc disorder
Excludes 1: *lumbar radiculitis NOS (M54.16)*
sciatica NOS (M54.3)

M51.14 Intervertebral disc disorders with radiculopathy, <u>thoracic</u> region

M51.15 Intervertebral disc disorders with radiculopathy, <u>thoracolumbar</u> region

M50-M51

M51.16 Intervertebral disc disorders with radiculopathy, <u>lumbar</u> region

M51.17 Intervertebral disc disorders with radiculopathy, <u>lumbosacral</u> region

M51.2- <u>Other</u> thoracic, thoracolumbar and lumbosacral intervertebral disc <u>displacement</u> — The dislocation of a thoracic, thoracolumbar, or lumbosacral intervertebral disc.

    Lumbago due to displacement of intervertebral disc

M51.24 Other intervertebral disc displacement, <u>thoracic</u> region

M51.25 Other intervertebral disc displacement, <u>thoracolumbar</u> region

M51.26 Other intervertebral disc displacement, <u>lumbar</u> region

M51.27 Other intervertebral disc displacement, <u>lumbosacral</u> region

M51.3- <u>Other</u> thoracic, thoracolumbar and lumbosacral intervertebral disc <u>degeneration</u> — The deterioration of a thoracic, thoracolumbar, or lumbosacral intervertebral disc.

M51.34 Other intervertebral disc degeneration, <u>thoracic</u> region

M51.35 Other intervertebral disc degeneration, <u>thoracolumbar</u> region

M51.36 Other intervertebral disc degeneration, <u>lumbar</u> region

M51.37 Other intervertebral disc degeneration, <u>lumbosacral</u> region

M51.4- <u>Schmorl's nodes</u> — A bony defect of a spinal vertebra.

M51.44 Schmorl's nodes, <u>thoracic</u> region

M51.45 Schmorl's nodes, <u>thoracolumbar</u> region

M51.46 Schmorl's nodes, <u>lumbar</u> region

M51.47 Schmorl's nodes, <u>lumbosacral</u> region

M51.8- <u>Other</u> thoracic, thoracolumbar and lumbosacral intervertebral disc <u>disorders</u>

M51.84 Other intervertebral disc disorders, <u>thoracic</u> region

M51.85 Other intervertebral disc disorders, <u>thoracolumbar</u> region

M51.86 Other intervertebral disc disorders, <u>lumbar</u> region

M51.87 Other intervertebral disc disorders, <u>lumbosacral</u> region

M51.9 <u>Unspecified</u> thoracic, thoracolumbar and lumbosacral intervertebral disc disorder

M53- <u>Other</u> and <u>unspecified</u> dorsopathies, <u>not elsewhere classified</u>

M53.0 **Cervicocranial syndrome** — The neurological dysfunction of the upper portion of the cervical spinal cord and associated nerve roots that is caused by misalignment of the cervical vertebrae and characterized by dizziness, headache, tinnitis, and sinus or ear pain.

    Posterior cervical sympathetic syndrome

M53.1 **Cervicobrachial syndrome** — The neurological dysfunction of the lower portion of the cervical spinal cord and associated nerve roots that is characterized by neck pain with numbness and tingling, and pain down the arm.
    Excludes ❷: cervical disc disorder (M50.-)
              thoracic outlet syndrome (G54.0)

M53.2- **Spinal instabilities** — The abnormal excessive movement of the spinal vertebrae.

M53.2x- <u>Spinal instabilities</u>

M53.2x1 Spinal instabilities, <u>occipito-atlanto-axial</u> region

M53.2x2 Spinal instabilities, <u>cervical</u> region

M53.2x3 Spinal instabilities, <u>cervicothoracic</u> region

M53.2x4 Spinal instabilities, <u>thoracic</u> region

M53.2x5 Spinal instabilities, <u>thoracolumbar</u> region

M53.2x6 Spinal instabilities, <u>lumbar</u> region

M53.2x7 Spinal instabilities, <u>lumbosacral</u> region

M53.2x8 Spinal instabilities, <u>sacral and sacrococcygeal</u> region

M53.2x9 Spinal instabilities, <u>site unspecified</u>

M53.3 Sacrococcygeal disorders, not elsewhere classified
    Coccygodynia

M53.8- <u>Other specified dorsopathies</u>

M53.80 Other specified dorsopathies, <u>site unspecified</u>

M53.81 Other specified dorsopathies, <u>occipito-atlanto-axial</u> region

M53.82 Other specified dorsopathies, <u>cervical</u> region

M53.83 Other specified dorsopathies, <u>cervicothoracic</u> region

M53.84 Other specified dorsopathies, <u>thoracic</u> region

M53.85 Other specified dorsopathies, <u>thoracolumbar</u> region

M53.86 Other specified dorsopathies, <u>lumbar</u> region

M53.87 Other specified dorsopathies, <u>lumbosacral</u> region

M53.88 Other specified dorsopathies, <u>sacral and sacrococcygeal</u> region

M53.9 Dorsopathy, <u>unspecified</u>

M54- <u>Dorsalgia</u> — Back pain.
    Excludes 1:   psychogenic dorsalgia (F45.41)

M54.0- <u>Panniculitis affecting regions of neck and back</u> — Inflammation of the subcutaneous fat of the sacral or back region.
    Excludes 1:   lupus panniculitis (L93.2)
              panniculitis NOS (M79.3)
              relapsing [Weber-Christian] panniculitis (M35.6)

M54.00 Panniculitis affecting regions of neck and back, <u>site unspecified</u>

M54.01 Panniculitis affecting regions of neck and back, <u>occipito-atlanto-axial</u> region

M54.02 Panniculitis affecting regions of neck and back, <u>cervical</u> region

M54.03 Panniculitis affecting regions of neck and back, cervicothoracic region

M54.04 Panniculitis affecting regions of neck and back, <u>thoracic</u> region

M54.05 Panniculitis affecting regions of neck and back, <u>thoracolumbar</u> region

M54.06 Panniculitis affecting regions of neck and back, <u>lumbar</u> region

M54.07 Panniculitis affecting regions of neck and back, <u>lumbosacral</u> region

M54.08 Panniculitis affecting regions of neck and back, <u>sacral and sacrococcygeal</u> region

M54.09 Panniculitis affecting regions, neck and back, <u>multiple sites</u> in spine

M54.1- <u>Radiculopathy</u> — Irritation, compression, or inflammation of a spinal nerve root.
    Brachial neuritis or radiculitis NOS
    Lumbar neuritis or radiculitis NOS
    Lumbosacral neuritis or radiculitis NOS
    Thoracic neuritis or radiculitis NOS
    Radiculitis NOS
    Excludes 1:   neuralgia and neuritis NOS (M79.2)
              radiculopathy with cervical disc disorder (M50.1)
              radiculopathy with lumbar and other intervertebral disc disorder (M51.1-)
              radiculopathy with spondylosis (M47.2-)

M54.10 Radiculopathy, <u>site unspecified</u>

M54.11 Radiculopathy, <u>occipito-atlanto-axial</u> region

M54.12 Radiculopathy, <u>cervical</u> region

M54.13 Radiculopathy, <u>cervicothoracic</u> region

M54.14 Radiculopathy, <u>thoracic</u> region

M54.15 Radiculopathy, <u>thoracolumbar</u> region

M54.16 Radiculopathy, <u>lumbar</u> region

M54.17 Radiculopathy, <u>lumbosacral</u> region

M54.18 Radiculopathy, <u>sacral and sacrococcygeal</u> region

M54.2 **Cervicalgia** — Neck pain.
    Excludes 1:   cervicalgia due to intervertebral cervical disc disorder (M50.-)

M54.3- <u>Sciatica</u> — Sciatic nerve pain radiating to the buttock and leg.
    Excludes 1:   lesion of sciatic nerve (G57.0)
              sciatica due to intervertebral disc disorder (M51.1-)
              sciatica with lumbago (M54.4-)

M54.30 Sciatica, <u>unspecified</u> side

M54.31 Sciatica, <u>right</u> side

M54.32 Sciatica, <u>left</u> side

M54.4- <u>Lumbago with sciatica</u> — Pain in the lumbar region with sciatic nerve pain radiating to the buttock and leg.
    Excludes 1:   lumbago with sciatica due to intervertebral disc disorder (M51.1-)

M54.40 Lumbago with sciatica, <u>unspecified</u> side

M54.41 Lumbago with sciatica, <u>right</u> side

M51 - M54

Excludes 1: = NOT CODED HERE! (Do not code both)

Excludes ❷: = Not Included Here

M54.42 **Lumbago with sciatica,** <u>left</u> side

M54.5 **Low back pain** — Pain in the lumbar region.
　　Loin pain
　　Lumbago NOS
　　Excludes 1:　low back strain (S39.012)
　　　　lumbago due to intervertebral disc displacement
　　　　(M51.2-)
　　　　lumbago with sciatica (M54.4-)

M54.6 **Pain in thoracic spine**
　　Excludes 1:　pain in thoracic spine due to intervertebral disc
　　　　disorder (M51.-)

M54.8- **Other dorsalgia**
　　Excludes 1:　dorsalgia in thoracic region (M54.6)
　　　　low back pain (M54.5)

　M54.81 **Occipital neuralgia** — A neck and back of the head pain disorder with
　　the pain sometimes radiating to the face or side of the face.

　M54.89 **Other dorsalgia**

M54.9 **Dorsalgia, unspecified**
　　Backache NOS
　　Back pain NOS

Soft tissue disorders (M60-M79)

Disorders of muscles (M60-M63)

Excludes 1:　dermatopolymyositis (M33-)
　　muscular dystrophies and myopathies (G71-G72)
　　myopathy in amyloidosis (E85.-)
　　myopathy in polyarteritis nodosa (M30.0)
　　myopathy in rheumatoid arthritis (M05.32)
　　myopathy in scleroderma (M34.-)
　　myopathy in Sjögren's syndrome (M35.03)
　　myopathy in systemic lupus erythematosus (M32.-)

M60- <u>Myositis</u> — Inflammation of the muscles.
　　Excludes ❷:　inclusion body myositis [IBM] (G72.41)

　M60.0- <u>Infective</u> myositis — A form caused by microorganisms.
　　Tropical pyomyositis
　　Use additional code (B95-B97) to identify infectious agent

　　M60.00-**Infective myositis,** <u>unspecified</u> site
　　cc M60.000 Infective myositis, unspecified <u>right arm</u>
　　　　Infective myositis, right upper limb NOS
　　cc M60.001 Infective myositis, unspecified <u>left arm</u>
　　　　Infective myositis, left upper limb NOS
　　cc M60.002 Infective myositis, unspecified <u>arm</u>
　　　　Infective myositis, upper limb NOS
　　cc M60.003 Infective myositis, unspecified <u>right leg</u>
　　　　Infective myositis, right lower limb NOS
　　cc M60.004 Infective myositis, unspecified <u>left leg</u>
　　　　Infective myositis, left lower limb NOS
　　cc M60.005 Infective myositis, unspecified <u>leg</u>
　　　　Infective myositis, lower limb NOS
　　cc M60.009 Infective myositis, unspecified <u>site</u>

　　M60.01-**Infective myositis,** <u>shoulder</u>
　　cc M60.011 Infective myositis, <u>right</u> shoulder
　　cc M60.012 Infective myositis, <u>left</u> shoulder
　　cc M60.019 Infective myositis, <u>unspecified</u> shoulder

　　M60.02-**Infective myositis,** <u>upper arm</u>
　　cc M60.021 Infective myositis, <u>right</u> upper arm
　　cc M60.022 Infective myositis, <u>left</u> upper arm
　　cc M60.029 Infective myositis, <u>unspecified</u> upper arm

　　M60.03-**Infective myositis,** <u>forearm</u>
　　cc M60.031 Infective myositis, <u>right</u> forearm
　　cc M60.032 Infective myositis, <u>left</u> forearm
　　cc M60.039 Infective myositis, <u>unspecified</u> forearm

　　M60.04-**Infective myositis,** <u>hand and fingers</u>
　　cc M60.041 Infective myositis, <u>right</u> hand
　　cc M60.042 Infective myositis, <u>left</u> hand
　　cc M60.043 Infective myositis, <u>unspecified</u> hand
　　cc M60.044 Infective myositis, <u>right</u> finger(s)
　　cc M60.045 Infective myositis, <u>left</u> finger(s)
　　cc M60.046 Infective myositis, <u>unspecified</u> finger(s)

M60.05-**Infective myositis,** <u>thigh</u>
　cc M60.051 Infective myositis, <u>right</u> thigh
　cc M60.052 Infective myositis, <u>left</u> thigh
　cc M60.059 Infective myositis, <u>unspecified</u> thigh

M60.06-**Infective myositis,** <u>lower leg</u>
　cc M60.061 Infective myositis, <u>right</u> lower leg
　cc M60.062 Infective myositis, <u>left</u> lower leg
　cc M60.069 Infective myositis, <u>unspecified</u> lower leg

M60.07-**Infective myositis,** <u>ankle, foot and toes</u>
　cc M60.070 Infective myositis, <u>right</u> ankle
　cc M60.071 Infective myositis, <u>left</u> ankle
　cc M60.072 Infective myositis, <u>unspecified</u> ankle
　cc M60.073 Infective myositis, <u>right</u> foot
　cc M60.074 Infective myositis, <u>left</u> foot
　cc M60.075 Infective myositis, <u>unspecified</u> foot
　cc M60.076 Infective myositis, <u>right</u> toe(s)
　cc M60.077 Infective myositis, <u>left</u> toe(s)
　cc M60.078 Infective myositis, <u>unspecified</u> toe(s)

cc M60.08 Infective myositis, <u>other</u> site
cc M60.09 Infective myositis, <u>multiple sites</u>

M60.1- <u>Interstitial myositis</u> — A form with fibrous degeneration of muscle tissue.
　M60.10 Interstitial myositis of <u>unspecified</u> site
　M60.11-**Interstitial myositis,** <u>shoulder</u>
　　M60.111 Interstitial myositis, <u>right</u> shoulder
　　M60.112 Interstitial myositis, <u>left</u> shoulder
　　M60.119 Interstitial myositis, <u>unspecified</u> shoulder
　M60.12-**Interstitial myositis,** <u>upper arm</u>
　　M60.121 Interstitial myositis, <u>right</u> upper arm
　　M60.122 Interstitial myositis, <u>left</u> upper arm
　　M60.129 Interstitial myositis, <u>unspecified</u> upper arm
　M60.13-**Interstitial myositis,** <u>forearm</u>
　　M60.131 Interstitial myositis, <u>right</u> forearm
　　M60.132 Interstitial myositis, <u>left</u> forearm
　　M60.139 Interstitial myositis, <u>unspecified</u> forearm
　M60.14-**Interstitial myositis,** <u>hand</u>
　　M60.141 Interstitial myositis, <u>right</u> hand
　　M60.142 Interstitial myositis, <u>left</u> hand
　　M60.149 Interstitial myositis, <u>unspecified</u> hand
　M60.15-**Interstitial myositis,** <u>thigh</u>
　　M60.151 Interstitial myositis, <u>right</u> thigh
　　M60.152 Interstitial myositis, <u>left</u> thigh
　　M60.159 Interstitial myositis, <u>unspecified</u> thigh
　M60.16-**Interstitial myositis,** <u>lower leg</u>
　　M60.161 Interstitial myositis, <u>right</u> lower leg
　　M60.162 Interstitial myositis, <u>left</u> lower leg
　　M60.169 Interstitial myositis, <u>unspecified</u> lower leg
　M60.17-**Interstitial myositis,** <u>ankle and foot</u>
　　M60.171 Interstitial myositis, <u>right</u> ankle and foot
　　M60.172 Interstitial myositis, <u>left</u> ankle and foot
　　M60.179 Interstitial myositis, <u>unspecified</u> ankle and foot
　M60.18 Interstitial myositis, <u>other</u> site
　M60.19 Interstitial myositis, <u>multiple sites</u>

M60.2- <u>Foreign body granuloma of soft tissue</u>, <u>not elsewhere</u>
　<u>classified</u> — The formation of a tumor-like mass of fibroblast tissue with a
　foreign body reaction.
　　Use additional code to identify the type of retained foreign body
　　(Z18.-)
　　Excludes 1:　foreign body granuloma of skin and subcutaneous
　　　　tissue (L92.3)
　M60.20 Foreign body granuloma of soft tissue, not elsewhere
　　classified, <u>unspecified site</u>
　M60.21-**Foreign body granuloma of soft tissue, not elsewhere**
　　classified, <u>shoulder</u>
　　M60.211 Foreign body granuloma of soft tissue, not
　　　elsewhere classified, <u>right</u> shoulder

M 5 4 - M 6 0

M60.212 Foreign body granuloma of soft tissue, not elsewhere classified, <u>left</u> shoulder

M60.219 Foreign body granuloma of soft tissue, not elsewhere classified, <u>unspecified</u> shoulder

M60.22- Foreign body granuloma of soft tissue, not elsewhere classified, <u>upper arm</u>

M60.221 Foreign body granuloma of soft tissue, not elsewhere classified, <u>right</u> upper arm

M60.222 Foreign body granuloma of soft tissue, not elsewhere classified, <u>left</u> upper arm

M60.229 Foreign body granuloma of soft tissue, not elsewhere classified, <u>unspecified</u> upper arm

M60.23- Foreign body granuloma of soft tissue, not elsewhere classified, <u>forearm</u>

M60.231 Foreign body granuloma of soft tissue, not elsewhere classified, <u>right</u> forearm

M60.232 Foreign body granuloma of soft tissue, not elsewhere classified, <u>left</u> forearm

M60.239 Foreign body granuloma of soft tissue, not elsewhere classified, <u>unspecified</u> forearm

M60.24- Foreign body granuloma of soft tissue, not elsewhere classified, <u>hand</u>

M60.241 Foreign body granuloma of soft tissue, not elsewhere classified, <u>right</u> hand

M60.242 Foreign body granuloma of soft tissue, not elsewhere classified, <u>left</u> hand

M60.249 Foreign body granuloma of soft tissue, not elsewhere classified, <u>unspecified</u> hand

M60.25- Foreign body granuloma of soft tissue, not elsewhere classified, <u>thigh</u>

M60.251 Foreign body granuloma of soft tissue, not elsewhere classified, <u>right</u> thigh

M60.252 Foreign body granuloma of soft tissue, not elsewhere classified, <u>left</u> thigh

M60.259 Foreign body granuloma of soft tissue, not elsewhere classified, <u>unspecified</u> thigh

M60.26- Foreign body granuloma of soft tissue, not elsewhere classified, <u>lower leg</u>

M60.261 Foreign body granuloma of soft tissue, not elsewhere classified, <u>right</u> lower leg

M60.262 Foreign body granuloma of soft tissue, not elsewhere classified, <u>left</u> lower leg

M60.269 Foreign body granuloma of soft tissue, not elsewhere classified, <u>unspecified</u> lower leg

M60.27- Foreign body granuloma of soft tissue, not elsewhere classified, <u>ankle and foot</u>

M60.271 Foreign body granuloma of soft tissue, not elsewhere classified, <u>right</u> ankle and foot

M60.272 Foreign body granuloma of soft tissue, not elsewhere classified, <u>left</u> ankle and foot

M60.279 Foreign body granuloma of soft tissue, not elsewhere classified, <u>unspecified</u> ankle and foot

M60.28 Foreign body granuloma of soft tissue, not elsewhere classified, <u>other</u> <u>site</u>

M60.8- <u>Other myositis</u>

M60.80 Other myositis, <u>unspecified site</u>

M60.81- Other myositis <u>shoulder</u>

M60.811 Other myositis, <u>right</u> shoulder

M60.812 Other myositis, <u>left</u> shoulder

M60.819 Other myositis, <u>unspecified</u> shoulder

M60.82- Other myositis, <u>upper arm</u>

M60.821 Other myositis, <u>right</u> upper arm

M60.822 Other myositis, <u>left</u> upper arm

M60.829 Other myositis, <u>unspecified</u> upper arm

M60.83- Other myositis, <u>forearm</u>

M60.831 Other myositis, <u>right</u> forearm

M60.832 Other myositis, <u>left</u> forearm

M60.839 Other myositis, <u>unspecified</u> forearm

M60.84- Other myositis, <u>hand</u>

M60.841 Other myositis, <u>right</u> hand

M60.842 Other myositis, <u>left</u> hand

M60.849 Other myositis, <u>unspecified</u> hand

M60.85- Other myositis, <u>thigh</u>

M60.851 Other myositis, <u>right</u> thigh

M60.852 Other myositis, <u>left</u> thigh

M60.859 Other myositis, <u>unspecified</u> thigh

M60.86- Other myositis, <u>lower leg</u>

M60.861 Other myositis, <u>right</u> lower leg

M60.862 Other myositis, <u>left</u> lower leg

M60.869 Other myositis, <u>unspecified</u> lower leg

M60.87- Other myositis, <u>ankle and foot</u>

M60.871 Other myositis, <u>right</u> ankle and foot

M60.872 Other myositis, <u>left</u> ankle and foot

M60.879 Other myositis, <u>unspecified</u> ankle and foot

M60.88 Other myositis, <u>other site</u>

M60.89 Other myositis, <u>multiple sites</u>

M60.9 Myositis, <u>unspecified</u>

M61- <u>Calcification and ossification of muscle</u> — The deposition of calcium, or the conversion into bony tissue, of the muscle.

M61.0- Myositis ossificans <u>traumatica</u> — The conversion of traumatized muscular tissue into bony tissue.

M61.00 Myositis ossificans traumatica, <u>unspecified</u> <u>site</u>

M61.01- Myositis ossificans traumatica, <u>shoulder</u>

M61.011 Myositis ossificans traumatica, <u>right</u> shoulder

M61.012 Myositis ossificans traumatica, <u>left</u> shoulder

M61.019 Myositis ossificans traumatica, <u>unspecified</u> shoulder

M61.02- Myositis ossificans traumatica, <u>upper arm</u>

M61.021 Myositis ossificans traumatica, <u>right</u> upper arm

M61.022 Myositis ossificans traumatica, <u>left</u> upper arm

M61.029 Myositis ossificans traumatica, <u>unspecified</u> upper arm

M61.03- Myositis ossificans traumatica, <u>forearm</u>

M61.031 Myositis ossificans traumatica, <u>right</u> forearm

M61.032 Myositis ossificans traumatica, <u>left</u> forearm

M61.039 Myositis ossificans traumatica, <u>unspecified</u> forearm

M61.04- Myositis ossificans traumatica, <u>hand</u>

M61.041 Myositis ossificans traumatica, <u>right</u> hand

M61.042 Myositis ossificans traumatica, <u>left</u> hand

M61.049 Myositis ossificans traumatica, <u>unspecified</u> hand

M61.05- Myositis ossificans traumatica, <u>thigh</u>

M61.051 Myositis ossificans traumatica, <u>right</u> thigh

M61.052 Myositis ossificans traumatica, <u>left</u> thigh

M61.059 Myositis ossificans traumatica, <u>unspecified</u> thigh

M61.06- Myositis ossificans traumatica, <u>lower leg</u>

M61.061 Myositis ossificans traumatica, <u>right</u> lower leg

M61.062 Myositis ossificans traumatica, <u>left</u> lower leg

M61.069 Myositis ossificans traumatica, <u>unspecified</u> lower leg

M61.07- Myositis ossificans traumatica, <u>ankle and foot</u>

M61.071 Myositis ossificans traumatica, <u>right</u> ankle and foot

M61.072 Myositis ossificans traumatica, <u>left</u> ankle and foot

M61.079 Myositis ossificans traumatica, <u>unspecified</u> ankle and foot

M61.08 Myositis ossificans traumatica, <u>other site</u>

M61.09 Myositis ossificans traumatica, <u>multiple sites</u>

M61.1- Myositis ossificans <u>progressiva</u> — A chronic, progressive conversion of muscle tissue to bony tissue that begins early in life.
Fibrodysplasia ossificans progressiva

M61.10 Myositis ossificans progressiva, <u>unspecified</u> site

M61.11- Myositis ossificans progressiva, <u>shoulder</u>

M61.111 Myositis ossificans progressiva, <u>right</u> shoulder

M61.112 Myositis ossificans progressiva, <u>left</u> shoulder

M 60 – M 61

M61.119   Myositis ossificans progressiva, <u>unspecified</u> shoulder

M61.12- Myositis ossificans progressiva, <u>upper arm</u>

M61.121   Myositis ossificans progressiva, <u>right</u> upper arm

M61.122   Myositis ossificans progressiva, <u>left</u> upper arm

M61.129   Myositis ossificans progressiva, <u>unspecified</u> arm

M61.13- Myositis ossificans progressiva, <u>forearm</u>

M61.131   Myositis ossificans progressiva, <u>right</u> forearm

M61.132   Myositis ossificans progressiva, <u>left</u> forearm

M61.139   Myositis ossificans progressiva, <u>unspecified</u> forearm

M61.14- Myositis ossificans progressiva, <u>hand and finger(s)</u>

M61.141   Myositis ossificans progressiva, <u>right</u> hand

M61.142   Myositis ossificans progressiva, <u>left</u> hand

M61.143   Myositis ossificans progressiva, <u>unspecified</u> hand

M61.144   Myositis ossificans progressiva, <u>right</u> finger(s)

M61.145   Myositis ossificans progressiva, <u>left</u> finger(s)

M61.146   Myositis ossificans progressiva, <u>unspecified</u> finger(s)

M61.15- Myositis ossificans progressiva, <u>thigh</u>

M61.151   Myositis ossificans progressiva, <u>right</u> thigh

M61.152   Myositis ossificans progressiva, <u>left</u> thigh

M61.159   Myositis ossificans progressiva, <u>unspecified</u> thigh

M61.16- Myositis ossificans progressiva, <u>lower leg</u>

M61.161   Myositis ossificans progressiva, <u>right</u> lower leg

M61.162   Myositis ossificans progressiva, <u>left</u> lower leg

M61.169   Myositis ossificans progressiva, <u>unspecified</u> lower leg

M61.17- Myositis ossificans progressiva, <u>ankle, foot and toe(s)</u>

M61.171   Myositis ossificans progressiva, <u>right</u> ankle

M61.172   Myositis ossificans progressiva, <u>left</u> ankle

M61.173   Myositis ossificans progressiva, <u>unspecified</u> ankle

M61.174   Myositis ossificans progressiva, <u>right</u> foot

M61.175   Myositis ossificans progressiva, <u>left</u> foot

M61.176   Myositis ossificans progressiva, <u>unspecified</u> foot

M61.177   Myositis ossificans progressiva, <u>right</u> toe(s)

M61.178   Myositis ossificans progressiva, <u>left</u> toe(s)

M61.179   Myositis ossificans progressiva, <u>unspecified</u> toe(s)

M61.18   Myositis ossificans progressiva, <u>other site</u>

M61.19   Myositis ossificans progressiva, <u>multiple sites</u>

M61.2- <u>Paralytic calcification and ossification of muscle</u>
Myositis ossificans associated with quadriplegia or paraplegia

M61.20   Paralytic calcification and ossification of muscle, <u>unspecified site</u>

M61.21- Paralytic calcification and ossification of muscle, <u>shoulder</u>

M61.211   Paralytic calcification and ossification of muscle, <u>right</u> shoulder

M61.212   Paralytic calcification and ossification of muscle, <u>left</u> shoulder

M61.219   Paralytic calcification and ossification of muscle, <u>unspecified</u> shoulder

M61.22- Paralytic calcification and ossification of muscle, <u>upper arm</u>

M61.221   Paralytic calcification and ossification of muscle, <u>right</u> upper arm

M61.222   Paralytic calcification and ossification of muscle, <u>left</u> upper arm

M61.229   Paralytic calcification and ossification of muscle, <u>unspecified</u> upper arm

M61.23- Paralytic calcification and ossification of muscle, <u>forearm</u>

M61.231   Paralytic calcification and ossification of muscle, <u>right</u> forearm

M61.232   Paralytic calcification and ossification of muscle, <u>left</u> forearm

M61.239   Paralytic calcification and ossification of muscle, <u>unspecified</u> forearm

M61.24- Paralytic calcification and ossification of muscle, <u>hand</u>

M61.241   Paralytic calcification and ossification of muscle, <u>right</u> hand

M61.242   Paralytic calcification and ossification of muscle, <u>left</u> hand

M61.249   Paralytic calcification and ossification of muscle, <u>unspecified</u> hand

M61.25- Paralytic calcification and ossification of muscle, <u>thigh</u>

M61.251   Paralytic calcification and ossification of muscle, <u>right</u> thigh

M61.252   Paralytic calcification and ossification of muscle, <u>left</u> thigh

M61.259   Paralytic calcification and ossification of muscle, <u>unspecified</u> thigh

M61.26- Paralytic calcification and ossification of muscle, <u>lower leg</u>

M61.261   Paralytic calcification and ossification of muscle, <u>right</u> lower leg

M61.262   Paralytic calcification and ossification of muscle, <u>left</u> lower leg

M61.269   Paralytic calcification and ossification of muscle, <u>unspecified</u> lower leg

M61.27- Paralytic calcification and ossification of muscle, <u>ankle and foot</u>

M61.271   Paralytic calcification and ossification of muscle, <u>right</u> ankle and foot

M61.272   Paralytic calcification and ossification of muscle, <u>left</u> ankle and foot

M61.279   Paralytic calcification and ossification of muscle, <u>unspecified</u> ankle and foot

M61.28   Paralytic calcification and ossification of muscle, <u>other site</u>

M61.29   Paralytic calcification and ossification of muscle, <u>multiple sites</u>

M61.3- Calcification and ossification of muscles associated <u>with burns</u>
Myositis ossificans associated with burns

M61.30   Calcification and ossification of muscles associated with burns, <u>unspecified site</u>

M61.31- Calcification and ossification of muscles associated with burns, <u>shoulder</u>

M61.311   Calcification and ossification of muscles associated with burns, <u>right</u> shoulder

M61.312   Calcification and ossification of muscles associated with burns, <u>left</u> shoulder

M61.319   Calcification and ossification of muscles associated with burns, <u>unspecified</u> shoulder

M61.32- Calcification and ossification of muscles associated with burns, <u>upper arm</u>

M61.321   Calcification and ossification of muscles associated with burns, <u>right</u> upper arm

M61.322   Calcification and ossification of muscles associated with burns, <u>left</u> upper arm

M61.329   Calcification and ossification of muscles associated with burns, <u>unspecified</u> upper arm

M61.33- Calcification and ossification of muscles associated with burns, <u>forearm</u>

M61.331   Calcification and ossification of muscles associated with burns, <u>right</u> forearm

M61.332   Calcification and ossification of muscles associated with burns, <u>left</u> forearm

M61.339   Calcification and ossification of muscles associated with burns, <u>unspecified</u> forearm

M61.34- Calcification and ossification of muscles associated with burns, <u>hand</u>

M61.341   Calcification and ossification of muscles associated with burns, <u>right</u> hand

M61.342   Calcification and ossification of muscles associated with burns, <u>left</u> hand

M
6
1
I
M
6
1

M61.349 Calcification and ossification of muscles associated with burns, <u>unspecified</u> hand

M61.35- Calcification and ossification of muscles associated with burns, <u>thigh</u>

M61.351 Calcification and ossification of muscles associated with burns, <u>right</u> thigh

M61.352 Calcification and ossification of muscles associated with burns, <u>left</u> thigh

M61.359 Calcification and ossification of muscles associated with burns, <u>unspecified</u> thigh

M61.36- Calcification and ossification of muscles associated with burns, <u>lower leg</u>

M61.361 Calcification and ossification of muscles associated with burns, <u>right</u> lower leg

M61.362 Calcification and ossification of muscles associated with burns, <u>left</u> lower leg

M61.369 Calcification and ossification of muscles associated with burns, <u>unspecified</u> lower leg

M61.37- Calcification and ossification of muscles associated with burns, <u>ankle and foot</u>

M61.371 Calcification and ossification of muscles associated with burns, <u>right</u> ankle and foot

M61.372 Calcification and ossification of muscles associated with burns, <u>left</u> ankle and foot

M61.379 Calcification and ossification of muscles associated with burns, <u>unspecified</u> ankle and foot

M61.38 Calcification and ossification of muscles associated with burns, <u>other site</u>

M61.39 Calcification and ossification of muscles associated with burns, <u>multiple sites</u>

M61.4- <u>Other calcification</u> of muscle
> *Excludes 1:   calcific tendinitis NOS (M65.2-)*
> *calcific tendinitis of shoulder (M75.3)*

M61.40 Other calcification of muscle, <u>unspecified site</u>

M61.41- Other calcification of muscle, <u>shoulder</u>

M61.411 Other calcification of muscle, <u>right</u> shoulder

M61.412 Other calcification of muscle, <u>left</u> shoulder

M61.419 Other calcification of muscle, <u>unspecified</u> shoulder

M61.42- Other calcification of muscle, <u>upper arm</u>

M61.421 Other calcification of muscle, <u>right</u> upper arm

M61.422 Other calcification of muscle, <u>left</u> upper arm

M61.429 Other calcification of muscle, <u>unspecified</u> upper arm

M61.43- Other calcification of muscle, <u>forearm</u>

M61.431 Other calcification of muscle, <u>right</u> forearm

M61.432 Other calcification of muscle, <u>left</u> forearm

M61.439 Other calcification of muscle, <u>unspecified</u> forearm

M61.44- Other calcification of muscle, <u>hand</u>

M61.441 Other calcification of muscle, <u>right</u> hand

M61.442 Other calcification of muscle, <u>left</u> hand

M61.449 Other calcification of muscle, <u>unspecified</u> hand

M61.45- Other calcification of muscle, <u>thigh</u>

M61.451 Other calcification of muscle, <u>right</u> thigh

M61.452 Other calcification of muscle, <u>left</u> thigh

M61.459 Other calcification of muscle, <u>unspecified</u> thigh

M61.46- Other calcification of muscle, <u>lower leg</u>

M61.461 Other calcification of muscle, <u>right</u> lower leg

M61.462 Other calcification of muscle, <u>left</u> lower leg

M61.469 Other calcification of muscle, <u>unspecified</u> lower leg

M61.47- Other calcification of muscle, <u>ankle and foot</u>

M61.471 Other calcification of muscle, <u>right</u> ankle and foot

M61.472 Other calcification of muscle, <u>left</u> ankle and foot

M61.479 Other calcification of muscle, <u>unspecified</u> ankle and foot

M61.48 Other calcification of muscle, other site

M61.49 Other calcification of muscle, <u>multiple sites</u>

M61.5- <u>Other ossification</u> of muscle

M61.50 Other ossification of muscle, <u>unspecified site</u>

M61.51- Other ossification of muscle, <u>shoulder</u>

M61.511 Other ossification of muscle, <u>right</u> shoulder

M61.512 Other ossification of muscle, <u>left</u> shoulder

M61.519 Other ossification of muscle, <u>unspecified</u> shoulder

M61.52- Other ossification of muscle, <u>upper arm</u>

M61.521 Other ossification of muscle, <u>right</u> upper arm

M61.522 Other ossification of muscle, <u>left</u> upper arm

M61.529 Other ossification of muscle, <u>unspecified</u> upper arm

M61.53- Other ossification of muscle, <u>forearm</u>

M61.531 Other ossification of muscle, <u>right</u> forearm

M61.532 Other ossification of muscle, <u>left</u> forearm

M61.539 Other ossification of muscle, <u>unspecified</u> forearm

M61.54- Other ossification of muscle, <u>hand</u>

M61.541 Other ossification of muscle, <u>right</u> hand

M61.542 Other ossification of muscle, <u>left</u> hand

M61.549 Other ossification of muscle, <u>unspecified</u> hand

M61.55- Other ossification of muscle, <u>thigh</u>

M61.551 Other ossification of muscle, <u>right</u> thigh

M61.552 Other ossification of muscle, <u>left</u> thigh

M61.559 Other ossification of muscle, <u>unspecified</u> thigh

M61.56- Other ossification of muscle, <u>lower leg</u>

M61.561 Other ossification of muscle, <u>right</u> lower leg

M61.562 Other ossification of muscle, <u>left</u> lower leg

M61.569 Other ossification of muscle, <u>unspecified</u> lower leg

M61.57- Other ossification of muscle, <u>ankle and foot</u>

M61.571 Other ossification of muscle, <u>right</u> ankle and foot

M61.572 Other ossification of muscle, <u>left</u> ankle and foot

M61.579 Other ossification of muscle, <u>unspecified</u> ankle and foot

M61.58 Other ossification of muscle, <u>other site</u>

M61.59 Other ossification of muscle, <u>multiple sites</u>

M61.9 Calcification and ossification of muscle, <u>unspecified</u>

M62- Other disorders of muscle
> *Excludes 1:   alcoholic myopathy (G72.1)*
> *cramp and spasm (R25.2)*
> *drug-induced myopathy (G72.0)*
> *myalgia (M79.1)*
> *stiff-man syndrome (G25.82)*
> *Excludes ❷: nontraumatic hematoma of muscle (M79.81)*

M62.0- <u>Separation of muscle (nontraumatic)</u> — The nontraumatic disruption of a muscle attachment or groups of muscles from each other.
> Diastasis of muscle
> *Excludes 1:   diastasis recti complicating pregnancy, labor and delivery (O71.8)*
> *traumatic separation of muscle — see strain of muscle by body region*

M62.00 Separation of muscle (nontraumatic), <u>unspecified site</u>

M62.01- Separation of muscle (nontraumatic), <u>shoulder</u>

M62.011 Separation of muscle (nontraumatic), <u>right</u> shoulder

M62.012 Separation of muscle (nontraumatic), <u>left</u> shoulder

M62.019 Separation of muscle (nontraumatic), <u>unspecified</u> shoulder

M62.02- Separation of muscle (nontraumatic), <u>upper arm</u>

M62.021 Separation of muscle (nontraumatic), <u>right</u> upper arm

M62.022 Separation of muscle (nontraumatic), <u>left</u> upper arm

M62.029 Separation of muscle (nontraumatic), <u>unspecified</u> upper arm

M62.03- Separation of muscle (nontraumatic), <u>forearm</u>

M62.031 Separation of muscle (nontraumatic), <u>right</u> forearm

M62.032 Separation of muscle (nontraumatic), <u>left</u> forearm

M62.039 Separation of muscle (nontraumatic), <u>unspecified</u> forearm

M61 - M62

M62.04- Separation of muscle (nontraumatic), <u>hand</u>
- M62.041 Separation of muscle (nontraumatic), <u>right</u> hand
- M62.042 Separation of muscle (nontraumatic), <u>left</u> hand
- M62.049 Separation of muscle (nontraumatic), <u>unspecified</u> hand

M62.05- Separation of muscle (nontraumatic), <u>thigh</u>
- M62.051 Separation of muscle (nontraumatic), <u>right</u> thigh
- M62.052 Separation of muscle (nontraumatic), <u>left</u> thigh
- M62.059 Separation of muscle (nontraumatic), <u>unspecified</u> thigh

M62.06- Separation of muscle (nontraumatic), <u>lower leg</u>
- M62.061 Separation of muscle (nontraumatic), <u>right</u> lower leg
- M62.062 Separation of muscle (nontraumatic), <u>left</u> lower leg
- M62.069 Separation of muscle (nontraumatic), <u>unspecified</u> lower leg

M62.07- Separation of muscle (nontraumatic), <u>ankle and foot</u>
- M62.071 Separation of muscle (nontraumatic), <u>right</u> ankle and foot
- M62.072 Separation of muscle (nontraumatic), <u>left</u> ankle and foot
- M62.079 Separation of muscle (nontraumatic), <u>unspecified</u> ankle and foot

M62.08 Separation of muscle (nontraumatic), <u>other site</u>

M62.1- <u>Other rupture</u> of muscle (nontraumatic) — The nontraumatic disruption of a muscle tissue.
- Excludes 1:   traumatic rupture of muscle — see strain of muscle by body region
- Excludes ❷: rupture of tendon (M66.-)

M62.10 Other rupture of muscle (nontraumatic), <u>unspecified site</u>

M62.11- Other rupture of muscle (nontraumatic), <u>shoulder</u>
- M62.111 Other rupture of muscle (nontraumatic), <u>right</u> shoulder
- M62.112 Other rupture of muscle (nontraumatic), <u>left</u> shoulder
- M62.119 Other rupture of muscle (nontraumatic), <u>unspecified</u> shoulder

M62.12- Other rupture of muscle (nontraumatic), <u>upper arm</u>
- M62.121 Other rupture of muscle (nontraumatic), <u>right</u> upper arm
- M62.122 Other rupture of muscle (nontraumatic), <u>left</u> upper arm
- M62.129 Other rupture of muscle (nontraumatic), <u>unspecified</u> upper arm

M62.13- Other rupture of muscle (nontraumatic), <u>forearm</u>
- M62.131 Other rupture of muscle (nontraumatic), <u>right</u> forearm
- M62.132 Other rupture of muscle (nontraumatic), <u>left</u> forearm
- M62.139 Other rupture of muscle (nontraumatic), <u>unspecified</u> forearm

M62.14- Other rupture of muscle (nontraumatic), <u>hand</u>
- M62.141 Other rupture of muscle (nontraumatic), <u>right</u> hand
- M62.142 Other rupture of muscle (nontraumatic), <u>left</u> hand
- M62.149 Other rupture of muscle (nontraumatic), <u>unspecified</u> hand

M62.15- Other rupture of muscle (nontraumatic), <u>thigh</u>
- M62.151 Other rupture of muscle (nontraumatic), <u>right</u> thigh
- M62.152 Other rupture of muscle (nontraumatic), <u>left</u> thigh
- M62.159 Other rupture of muscle (nontraumatic), <u>unspecified</u> thigh

M62.16- Other rupture of muscle (nontraumatic), <u>lower leg</u>
- M62.161 Other rupture of muscle (nontraumatic), <u>right</u> lower leg
- M62.162 Other rupture of muscle (nontraumatic), <u>left</u> lower leg
- M62.169 Other rupture of muscle (nontraumatic), <u>unspecified</u> lower leg

M62.17- Other rupture of muscle (nontraumatic), <u>ankle and foot</u>
- M62.171 Other rupture of muscle (nontraumatic), <u>right</u> ankle and foot
- M62.172 Other rupture of muscle (nontraumatic), <u>left</u> ankle and foot
- M62.179 Other rupture of muscle (nontraumatic), <u>unspecified</u> ankle and foot

M62.18 Other rupture of muscle (nontraumatic), <u>other site</u>

M62.2- <u>Nontraumatic ischemic infarction</u> of muscle — The nontraumatic localized area of muscle necrosis due to obstruction of circulation to that muscle.
- Excludes 1:   compartment syndrome (traumatic) (T79.A-)
  - nontraumatic compartment syndrome (M79.A-)
  - traumatic ischemia of muscle (T79.6)
  - rhabdomyolysis (M62.82)
  - Volkmann's ischemic contracture (T79.6)

M62.20 Nontraumatic ischemic infarction of muscle, <u>unspecified site</u>

M62.21- Nontraumatic ischemic infarction of muscle, <u>shoulder</u>
- M62.211 Nontraumatic ischemic infarction of muscle, <u>right</u> shoulder
- M62.212 Nontraumatic ischemic infarction of muscle, <u>left</u> shoulder
- M62.219 Nontraumatic ischemic infarction of muscle, <u>unspecified</u> shoulder

M62.22- Nontraumatic ischemic infarction of muscle, <u>upper arm</u>
- M62.221 Nontraumatic ischemic infarction of muscle, <u>right</u> upper arm
- M62.222 Nontraumatic ischemic infarction of muscle, <u>left</u> upper arm
- M62.229 Nontraumatic ischemic infarction of muscle, <u>unspecified</u> upper arm

M62.23- Nontraumatic ischemic infarction of muscle, <u>forearm</u>
- M62.231 Nontraumatic ischemic infarction of muscle, <u>right</u> forearm
- M62.232 Nontraumatic ischemic infarction of muscle, <u>left</u> forearm
- M62.239 Nontraumatic ischemic infarction of muscle, <u>unspecified</u> forearm

M62.24- Nontraumatic ischemic infarction of muscle, <u>hand</u>
- M62.241 Nontraumatic ischemic infarction of muscle, <u>right</u> hand
- M62.242 Nontraumatic ischemic infarction of muscle, <u>left</u> hand
- M62.249 Nontraumatic ischemic infarction of muscle, <u>unspecified</u> hand

M62.25- Nontraumatic ischemic infarction of muscle, <u>thigh</u>
- M62.251 Nontraumatic ischemic infarction of muscle, <u>right</u> thigh
- M62.252 Nontraumatic ischemic infarction of muscle, <u>left</u> thigh
- M62.259 Nontraumatic ischemic infarction of muscle, <u>unspecified</u> thigh

M62.26- Nontraumatic ischemic infarction of muscle, <u>lower leg</u>
- M62.261 Nontraumatic ischemic infarction of muscle, <u>right</u> lower leg
- M62.262 Nontraumatic ischemic infarction of muscle, <u>left</u> lower leg
- M62.269 Nontraumatic ischemic infarction of muscle, <u>unspecified</u> lower leg

M62.27- Nontraumatic ischemic infarction of muscle, <u>ankle and foot</u>
- M62.271 Nontraumatic ischemic infarction of muscle, <u>right</u> ankle and foot
- M62.272 Nontraumatic ischemic infarction of muscle, <u>left</u> ankle and foot
- M62.279 Nontraumatic ischemic infarction of muscle, <u>unspecified</u> ankle and foot

M62.28 Nontraumatic ischemic infarction of muscle, <u>other site</u>

M62 - M62

M62.3   Immobility syndrome (paraplegic) — The condition of muscular dysfunction caused by prolonged immobility and disuse of the muscles.

M62.4-   Contracture of muscle — The abnormal tightening of a muscle.
      Contracture of tendon (sheath)
      Excludes 1:   contracture of joint (M24.5-)

M62.40   Contracture of muscle, unspecified site

M62.41- Contracture of muscle, shoulder
      M62.411   Contracture of muscle, right shoulder
      M62.412   Contracture of muscle, left shoulder
      M62.419   Contracture of muscle, unspecified shoulder

M62.42- Contracture of muscle, upper arm
      M62.421   Contracture of muscle, right upper arm
      M62.422   Contracture of muscle, left upper arm
      M62.429   Contracture of muscle, unspecified upper arm

M62.43- Contracture of muscle, forearm
      M62.431   Contracture of muscle, right forearm
      M62.432   Contracture of muscle, left forearm
      M62.439   Contracture of muscle, unspecified forearm

M62.44- Contracture of muscle, hand
      M62.441   Contracture of muscle, right hand
      M62.442   Contracture of muscle, left hand
      M62.449   Contracture of muscle, unspecified hand

M62.45- Contracture of muscle, thigh
      M62.451   Contracture of muscle, right thigh
      M62.452   Contracture of muscle, left thigh
      M62.459   Contracture of muscle, unspecified thigh

M62.46- Contracture of muscle, lower leg
      M62.461   Contracture of muscle, right lower leg
      M62.462   Contracture of muscle, left lower leg
      M62.469   Contracture of muscle, unspecified lower leg

M62.47- Contracture of muscle, ankle and foot
      M62.471   Contracture of muscle, right ankle and foot
      M62.472   Contracture of muscle, left ankle and foot
      M62.479   Contracture of muscle, unspecified ankle and foot

M62.48   Contracture of muscle, other site

M62.49   Contracture of muscle, multiple sites

M62.5-   Muscle wasting and atrophy, not elsewhere classified —
      MUSCLE WASTING — The disintegration of the muscle cells. MUSCLE ATROPHY — The abnormal decrease in muscle mass.
      Disuse atrophy NEC
      Excludes 1:   neuralgic amyotrophy (G54.5)
                        progressive muscular atrophy (G12.29)
                        sarcopenia (M62.84)
      Excludes ❷: pelvic muscle wasting (N81.84)

M62.50   Muscle wasting and atrophy, not elsewhere classified, unspecified site

M62.51- Muscle wasting and atrophy, not elsewhere classified, shoulder
      M62.511   Muscle wasting and atrophy, not elsewhere classified, right shoulder
      M62.512   Muscle wasting and atrophy, not elsewhere classified, left shoulder
      M62.519   Muscle wasting and atrophy, not elsewhere classified, unspecified shoulder

M62.52- Muscle wasting and atrophy, not elsewhere classified, upper arm
      M62.521   Muscle wasting and atrophy, not elsewhere classified, right upper arm
      M62.522   Muscle wasting and atrophy, not elsewhere classified, left upper arm
      M62.529   Muscle wasting and atrophy, not elsewhere classified, unspecified upper arm

M62.53- Muscle wasting and atrophy, not elsewhere classified, forearm
      M62.531   Muscle wasting and atrophy, not elsewhere classified, right forearm

M62.532   Muscle wasting and atrophy, not elsewhere classified, left forearm

M62.539   Muscle wasting and atrophy, not elsewhere classified, unspecified forearm

M62.54- Muscle wasting and atrophy, not elsewhere classified, hand
      M62.541   Muscle wasting and atrophy, not elsewhere classified, right hand
      M62.542   Muscle wasting and atrophy, not elsewhere classified, left hand
      M62.549   Muscle wasting and atrophy, not elsewhere classified, unspecified hand

M62.55- Muscle wasting and atrophy, not elsewhere classified, thigh
      M62.551   Muscle wasting and atrophy, not elsewhere classified, right thigh
      M62.552   Muscle wasting and atrophy, not elsewhere classified, left thigh
      M62.559   Muscle wasting and atrophy, not elsewhere classified, unspecified thigh

M62.56- Muscle wasting and atrophy, not elsewhere classified, lower leg
      M62.561   Muscle wasting and atrophy, not elsewhere classified, right lower leg
      M62.562   Muscle wasting and atrophy, not elsewhere classified, left lower leg
      M62.569   Muscle wasting and atrophy, not elsewhere classified, unspecified lower leg

M62.57- Muscle wasting and atrophy, not elsewhere classified, ankle and foot
      M62.571   Muscle wasting and atrophy, not elsewhere classified, right ankle and foot
      M62.572   Muscle wasting and atrophy, not elsewhere classified, left ankle and foot
      M62.579   Muscle wasting and atrophy, not elsewhere classified, unspecified ankle and foot

M62.58   Muscle wasting and atrophy, not elsewhere classified, other site

M62.59   Muscle wasting and atrophy, not elsewhere classified, multiple sites

M62.8-   Other specified disorders of muscle
      Excludes ❷: nontraumatic hematoma of muscle (M79.81)

M62.81   Muscle weakness (generalized) — A decrease in a patient's normal muscle strength.
      Excludes 1:   muscle weakness in sarcopenia (M62.84)

CC **M62.82   Rhabdomyolysis** — A condition characterized by the destruction of skeletal muscle that releases potentially toxic muscle cell components into the circulation.
      Excludes 1:   traumatic rhabdomyolysis (T79.6)

M62.83- Muscle spasm — The sudden involuntary contraction of a muscle.
      M62.830   Muscle spasm of back
      M62.831   Muscle spasm of calf
            Charley-horse
      M62.838   Other muscle spasm

M62.84   Sarcopenia
      Age-related sarcopenia
      Code first underlying disease, if applicable, such as:
            Disorders of myoneural junction and muscle disease in diseases classified elsewhere (G73.-)
            Other and unspecified myopathies (G72.-)
            Primary disorders of muscles (G71.-)

M62.89   Other specified disorders of muscle
      Muscle (sheath) hernia

M62.9   Disorder of muscle, unspecified

M63- Disorders of muscle <u>in diseases classified elsewhere</u>
Code first underlying disease, such as:
Leprosy (A30.-)
Neoplasm (C49.-, C79.89, D21.-, D48.1)
Schistosomiasis (B65.-)
Trichinellosis (B75)

Excludes 1:   myopathy in cysticercosis (B69.81)
myopathy in endocrine diseases (G73.7)
myopathy in metabolic diseases (G73.7)
myopathy in sarcoidosis (D86.87)
myopathy in secondary syphilis (A51.49)
myopathy in syphilis (late) (A52.78)
myopathy in toxoplasmosis (B58.82)
myopathy in tuberculosis (A18.09)

M63.8- Disorders of muscle in diseases classified elsewhere

M63.80 Disorders of muscle in diseases classified elsewhere, <u>unspecified</u> <u>site</u> — [Not Allowed as PDX]

M63.81- Disorders of muscle in diseases classified elsewhere, <u>shoulder</u>

M63.811   Disorders of muscle in diseases classified elsewhere, <u>right</u> shoulder — [Not Allowed as PDX]

M63.812   Disorders of muscle in diseases classified elsewhere, <u>left</u> shoulder — [Not Allowed as PDX]

M63.819   Disorders of muscle in diseases classified elsewhere, <u>unspecified</u> shoulder — [Not Allowed as PDX]

M63.82- Disorders of muscle in diseases classified elsewhere, <u>upper arm</u>

M63.821   Disorders of muscle in diseases classified elsewhere, <u>right</u> upper arm — [Not Allowed as PDX]

M63.822   Disorders of muscle in diseases classified elsewhere, <u>left</u> upper arm — [Not Allowed as PDX]

M63.829   Disorders of muscle in diseases classified elsewhere, <u>unspecified</u> upper arm — [Not Allowed as PDX]

M63.83- Disorders of muscle in diseases classified elsewhere, <u>forearm</u>

M63.831   Disorders of muscle in diseases classified elsewhere, <u>right</u> forearm — [Not Allowed as PDX]

M63.832   Disorders of muscle in diseases classified elsewhere, <u>left</u> forearm — [Not Allowed as PDX]

M63.839   Disorders of muscle in diseases classified elsewhere, <u>unspecified</u> forearm — [Not Allowed as PDX]

M63.84- Disorders of muscle in diseases classified elsewhere, <u>hand</u>

M63.841   Disorders of muscle in diseases classified elsewhere, <u>right</u> hand — [Not Allowed as PDX]

M63.842   Disorders of muscle in diseases classified elsewhere, <u>left</u> hand — [Not Allowed as PDX]

M63.849   Disorders of muscle in diseases classified elsewhere, <u>unspecified</u> hand — [Not Allowed as PDX]

M63.85- Disorders of muscle in diseases classified elsewhere, <u>thigh</u>

M63.851   Disorders of muscle in diseases classified elsewhere, <u>right</u> thigh — [Not Allowed as PDX]

M63.852   Disorders of muscle in diseases classified elsewhere, <u>left</u> thigh — [Not Allowed as PDX]

M63.859   Disorders of muscle in diseases classified elsewhere, <u>unspecified</u> thigh — [Not Allowed as PDX]

M63.86- Disorders of muscle in diseases classified elsewhere, <u>lower leg</u>

M63.861   Disorders of muscle in diseases classified elsewhere, <u>right</u> lower leg — [Not Allowed as PDX]

M63.862   Disorders of muscle in diseases classified elsewhere, <u>left</u> lower leg — [Not Allowed as PDX]

M63.869   Disorders of muscle in diseases classified elsewhere, <u>unspecified</u> lower leg — [Not Allowed as PDX]

M63.87- Disorders of muscle in diseases classified elsewhere, <u>ankle and foot</u>

M63.871   Disorders of muscle in diseases classified elsewhere, <u>right</u> ankle and foot — [Not Allowed as PDX]

M63.872   Disorders of muscle in diseases classified elsewhere, <u>left</u> ankle and foot — [Not Allowed as PDX]

M63.879   Disorders of muscle in diseases classified elsewhere, <u>unspecified</u> ankle and foot — [Not Allowed as PDX]

M63.88   Disorders of muscle in diseases classified elsewhere, <u>other site</u> — [Not Allowed as PDX]

M63.89   Disorders of muscle in diseases classified elsewhere, <u>multiple sites</u> — [Not Allowed as PDX]

Disorders of synovium and tendon (M65-M67)

M65- <u>Synovitis and tenosynovitis</u> — Inflammation of the synovial membrane or tendon sheath.
Excludes 1:   *chronic crepitant synovitis of hand and wrist (M70.0-)*
current injury — see injury of ligament or tendon by body region
soft tissue disorders related to use, overuse and pressure (M70.-)

M65.0- <u>Abscess of tendon sheath</u> — A localized collection of pus caused by the disintegration of a tendon sheath.
Use additional code (B95-B96) to identify bacterial agent.

M65.00 Abscess of tendon sheath, <u>unspecified</u> <u>site</u>

M65.01- Abscess of tendon sheath, <u>shoulder</u>

M65.011   Abscess of tendon sheath, <u>right</u> shoulder

M65.012   Abscess of tendon sheath, <u>left</u> shoulder

M65.019   Abscess of tendon sheath, <u>unspecified</u> shoulder

M65.02- Abscess of tendon sheath, <u>upper arm</u>

M65.021   Abscess of tendon sheath, <u>right</u> upper arm

M65.022   Abscess of tendon sheath, <u>left</u> upper arm

M65.029   Abscess of tendon sheath, <u>unspecified</u> upper arm

M65.03- Abscess of tendon sheath, <u>forearm</u>

M65.031   Abscess of tendon sheath, <u>right</u> forearm

M65.032   Abscess of tendon sheath, <u>left</u> forearm

M65.039   Abscess of tendon sheath, <u>unspecified</u> forearm

M65.04- Abscess of tendon sheath, <u>hand</u>

M65.041   Abscess of tendon sheath, <u>right</u> hand

M65.042   Abscess of tendon sheath, <u>left</u> hand

M65.049   Abscess of tendon sheath, <u>unspecified</u> hand

M65.05- Abscess of tendon sheath, thigh

M65.051   Abscess of tendon sheath, <u>right</u> thigh

M65.052   Abscess of tendon sheath, <u>left</u> thigh

M65.059   Abscess of tendon sheath, <u>unspecified</u> thigh

M65.06- Abscess of tendon sheath, <u>lower leg</u>

M65.061   Abscess of tendon sheath, <u>right</u> lower leg

M65.062   Abscess of tendon sheath, <u>left</u> lower leg

M65.069   Abscess of tendon sheath, <u>unspecified</u> lower leg

M65.07- Abscess of tendon sheath, <u>ankle and foot</u>

M65.071   Abscess of tendon sheath, <u>right</u> ankle and foot

M65.072   Abscess of tendon sheath, <u>left</u> ankle and foot

M65.079   Abscess of tendon sheath, <u>unspecified</u> ankle and foot

M65.08 Abscess of tendon sheath, <u>other site</u>

M65.1- <u>Other infective (teno)synovitis</u>

M65.10 Other infective (teno)synovitis, <u>unspecified</u> <u>site</u>

M65.11- Other infective (teno)synovitis, <u>shoulder</u>

M65.111   Other infective (teno)synovitis, <u>right</u> shoulder

M65.112   Other infective (teno)synovitis, <u>left</u> shoulder

M65.119   Other infective (teno)synovitis, <u>unspecified</u> shoulder

M65.12- Other infective (teno)synovitis, <u>elbow</u>

M65.121   Other infective (teno)synovitis, <u>right</u> elbow

M65.122   Other infective (teno)synovitis, <u>left</u> elbow

M65.129   Other infective (teno)synovitis, <u>unspecified</u> elbow

M65.13- Other infective (teno)synovitis, <u>wrist</u>

M65.131   Other infective (teno)synovitis, <u>right</u> wrist

M65.132   Other infective (teno)synovitis, <u>left</u> wrist

Excludes 1: = NOT CODED HERE! (Do not code both)

Excludes ❷: = Not Included Here

M65.139 Other infective (teno)synovitis, <u>unspecified</u> wrist
M65.14- Other infective (teno)synovitis, <u>hand</u>
    M65.141 Other infective (teno)synovitis, <u>right</u> hand
    M65.142 Other infective (teno)synovitis, <u>left</u> hand
    M65.149 Other infective (teno)synovitis, <u>unspecified</u> hand
M65.15- Other infective (teno)synovitis, <u>hip</u>
    M65.151 Other infective (teno)synovitis, <u>right</u> hip
    M65.152 Other infective (teno)synovitis, <u>left</u> hip
    M65.159 Other infective (teno)synovitis, <u>unspecified</u> hip
M65.16- Other infective (teno)synovitis, <u>knee</u>
    M65.161 Other infective (teno)synovitis, <u>right</u> knee
    M65.162 Other infective (teno)synovitis, <u>left</u> knee
    M65.169 Other infective (teno)synovitis, <u>unspecified</u> knee
M65.17- Other infective (teno)synovitis, <u>ankle and foot</u>
    M65.171 Other infective (teno)synovitis, <u>right</u> ankle and foot
    M65.172 Other infective (teno)synovitis, <u>left</u> ankle and foot
    M65.179 Other infective (teno)synovitis, <u>unspecified</u> ankle and foot
M65.18 Other infective (teno)synovitis, <u>other site</u>
M65.19 Other infective (teno)synovitis, <u>multiple sites</u>
M65.2- <u>Calcific tendinitis</u> — The deposition of calcium and its salts in a tendon.
    Excludes 1:   *tendinitis as classified in M75-M77*
                calcified tendinitis of shoulder (M75.3)
M65.20 Calcific tendinitis, <u>unspecified site</u>
M65.22- Calcific tendinitis, <u>upper arm</u>
    M65.221 Calcific tendinitis, <u>right</u> upper arm
    M65.222 Calcific tendinitis, <u>left</u> upper arm
    M65.229 Calcific tendinitis, <u>unspecified</u> upper arm
M65.23- Calcific tendinitis, <u>forearm</u>
    M65.231 Calcific tendinitis, <u>right</u> forearm
    M65.232 Calcific tendinitis, <u>left</u> forearm
    M65.239 Calcific tendinitis, <u>unspecified</u> forearm
M65.24- Calcific tendinitis, <u>hand</u>
    M65.241 Calcific tendinitis, <u>right</u> hand
    M65.242 Calcific tendinitis, <u>left</u> hand
    M65.249 Calcific tendinitis, <u>unspecified</u> hand
M65.25- Calcific tendinitis, <u>thigh</u>
    M65.251 Calcific tendinitis, <u>right</u> thigh
    M65.252 Calcific tendinitis, <u>left</u> thigh
    M65.259 Calcific tendinitis, <u>unspecified</u> thigh
M65.26- Calcific tendinitis, <u>lower leg</u>
    M65.261 Calcific tendinitis, <u>right</u> lower leg
    M65.262 Calcific tendinitis, <u>left</u> lower leg
    M65.269 Calcific tendinitis, <u>unspecified</u> lower leg
M65.27- Calcific tendinitis, <u>ankle and foot</u>
    M65.271 Calcific tendinitis, <u>right</u> ankle and foot
    M65.272 Calcific tendinitis, <u>left</u> ankle and foot
    M65.279 Calcific tendinitis, <u>unspecified</u> ankle and foot
M65.28 Calcific tendinitis, <u>other site</u>
M65.29 Calcific tendinitis, <u>multiple sites</u>
M65.3- <u>Trigger finger</u> — The temporary arrest of flexion or extension of a finger with subsequent snapping into place.
      Nodular tendinous disease
M65.30 Trigger finger, <u>unspecified</u> finger
M65.31- Trigger <u>thumb</u>
    M65.311 Trigger thumb, <u>right</u> thumb
    M65.312 Trigger thumb, <u>left</u> thumb
    M65.319 Trigger thumb, <u>unspecified</u> thumb
M65.32- Trigger finger, <u>index</u> finger
    M65.321 Trigger finger, <u>right</u> index finger
    M65.322 Trigger finger, <u>left</u> index finger
    M65.329 Trigger finger, <u>unspecified</u> index finger
M65.33- Trigger finger, <u>middle</u> finger
    M65.331 Trigger finger, <u>right</u> middle finger
    M65.332 Trigger finger, <u>left</u> middle finger

M65.339 Trigger finger, <u>unspecified</u> middle finger
M65.34- Trigger finger, <u>ring</u> finger
    M65.341 Trigger finger, <u>right</u> ring finger
    M65.342 Trigger finger, <u>left</u> ring finger
    M65.349 Trigger finger, <u>unspecified</u> ring finger
M65.35- Trigger finger, <u>little</u> finger
    M65.351 Trigger finger, <u>right</u> little finger
    M65.352 Trigger finger, <u>left</u> little finger
    M65.359 Trigger finger, <u>unspecified</u> little finger
M65.4 Radial styloid tenosynovitis [de Quervain] — Inflammation of the radial styloid tendon sheath.
M65.8- <u>Other synovitis and tenosynovitis</u>
M65.80 Other synovitis and tenosynovitis, <u>unspecified</u> site
M65.81- Other synovitis and tenosynovitis, <u>shoulder</u>
    M65.811 Other synovitis and tenosynovitis, <u>right</u> shoulder
    M65.812 Other synovitis and tenosynovitis, <u>left</u> shoulder
    M65.819 Other synovitis and tenosynovitis, <u>unspecified</u> shoulder
M65.82- Other synovitis and tenosynovitis, <u>upper arm</u>
    M65.821 Other synovitis and tenosynovitis, <u>right</u> upper arm
    M65.822 Other synovitis and tenosynovitis, <u>left</u> upper arm
    M65.829 Other synovitis and tenosynovitis, <u>unspecified</u> upper arm
M65.83- Other synovitis and tenosynovitis, <u>forearm</u>
    M65.831 Other synovitis and tenosynovitis, <u>right</u> forearm
    M65.832 Other synovitis and tenosynovitis, <u>left</u> forearm
    M65.839 Other synovitis and tenosynovitis, <u>unspecified</u> forearm
M65.84- Other synovitis and tenosynovitis, <u>hand</u>
    M65.841 Other synovitis and tenosynovitis, <u>right</u> hand
    M65.842 Other synovitis and tenosynovitis, <u>left</u> hand
    M65.849 Other synovitis and tenosynovitis, <u>unspecified</u> hand
M65.85- Other synovitis and tenosynovitis, <u>thigh</u>
    M65.851 Other synovitis and tenosynovitis, <u>right</u> thigh
    M65.852 Other synovitis and tenosynovitis, <u>left</u> thigh
    M65.859 Other synovitis and tenosynovitis, <u>unspecified</u> thigh
M65.86- Other synovitis and tenosynovitis, <u>lower leg</u>
    M65.861 Other synovitis and tenosynovitis, <u>right</u> lower leg
    M65.862 Other synovitis and tenosynovitis, <u>left</u> lower leg
    M65.869 Other synovitis and tenosynovitis, <u>unspecified</u> lower leg
M65.87- Other synovitis and tenosynovitis, <u>ankle and foot</u>
    M65.871 Other synovitis and tenosynovitis, <u>right</u> ankle and foot
    M65.872 Other synovitis and tenosynovitis, <u>left</u> ankle and foot
    M65.879 Other synovitis and tenosynovitis, <u>unspecified</u> ankle and foot
M65.88 Other synovitis and tenosynovitis, <u>other site</u>
M65.89 Other synovitis and tenosynovitis, multiple sites
M65.9 Synovitis and tenosynovitis, <u>unspecified</u>
M66- <u>Spontaneous rupture of synovium and tendon</u>
    Includes: Rupture that occurs when a normal force is applied to tissues that are inferred to have less than normal strength
    Excludes ❷: *rotator cuff syndrome (M75.1-)*
                rupture where an abnormal force is applied to normal tissue — see injury of tendon by body region
M66.0 Rupture of popliteal cyst — An accumulation of effused synovial fluid behind the knee that has ruptured.
M66.1- Rupture of <u>synovium</u> — An accumulation of effused synovial fluid that has ruptured.
      Rupture of synovial cyst
    Excludes ❷: *rupture of popliteal cyst (M66.0)*
M66.10 Rupture of synovium, <u>unspecified</u> joint
M66.11- Rupture of synovium, <u>shoulder</u>
    M66.111 Rupture of synovium, <u>right</u> shoulder
    M66.112 Rupture of synovium, <u>left</u> shoulder

M65 - M66

M66.119 Rupture of synovium, <u>unspecified</u> shoulder
M66.12-Rupture of synovium, <u>elbow</u>
    M66.121 Rupture of synovium, <u>right</u> elbow
    M66.122 Rupture of synovium, <u>left</u> elbow
    M66.129 Rupture of synovium, <u>unspecified</u> elbow
M66.13-Rupture of synovium, <u>wrist</u>
    M66.131 Rupture of synovium, <u>right</u> wrist
    M66.132 Rupture of synovium, <u>left</u> wrist
    M66.139 Rupture of synovium, <u>unspecified</u> wrist
M66.14-Rupture of synovium, <u>hand and fingers</u>
    M66.141 Rupture of synovium, <u>right</u> hand
    M66.142 Rupture of synovium, <u>left</u> hand
    M66.143 Rupture of synovium, <u>unspecified</u> hand
    M66.144 Rupture of synovium, <u>right</u> finger(s)
    M66.145 Rupture of synovium, <u>left</u> finger(s)
    M66.146 Rupture of synovium, <u>unspecified</u> finger(s)
M66.15-Rupture of synovium, <u>hip</u>
    M66.151 Rupture of synovium, <u>right</u> hip
    M66.152 Rupture of synovium, <u>left</u> hip
    M66.159 Rupture of synovium, <u>unspecified</u> hip
M66.17-Rupture of synovium, <u>ankle, foot and toes</u>
    M66.171 Rupture of synovium, <u>right</u> ankle
    M66.172 Rupture of synovium, <u>left</u> ankle
    M66.173 Rupture of synovium, <u>unspecified</u> ankle
    M66.174 Rupture of synovium, <u>right</u> foot
    M66.175 Rupture of synovium, <u>left</u> foot
    M66.176 Rupture of synovium, <u>unspecified</u> foot
    M66.177 Rupture of synovium, <u>right</u> toe(s)
    M66.178 Rupture of synovium, <u>left</u> toe(s)
    M66.179 Rupture of synovium, <u>unspecified</u> toe(s)
M66.18 Rupture of synovium, <u>other site</u>
M66.2- Spontaneous rupture of <u>extensor</u> tendons
M66.20 Spontaneous rupture of extensor tendons, <u>unspecified site</u>
M66.21-Spontaneous rupture of extensor tendons, <u>shoulder</u>
    M66.211 Spontaneous rupture of extensor tendons, <u>right</u> shoulder
    M66.212 Spontaneous rupture of extensor tendons, <u>left</u> shoulder
    M66.219 Spontaneous rupture of extensor tendons, <u>unspecified</u> shoulder
M66.22-Spontaneous rupture of extensor tendons, <u>upper arm</u>
    M66.221 Spontaneous rupture of extensor tendons, <u>right</u> upper arm
    M66.222 Spontaneous rupture of extensor tendons, <u>left</u> upper arm
    M66.229 Spontaneous rupture of extensor tendons, <u>unspecified</u> upper arm
M66.23-Spontaneous rupture of extensor tendons, <u>forearm</u>
    M66.231 Spontaneous rupture of extensor tendons, <u>right</u> forearm
    M66.232 Spontaneous rupture of extensor tendons, <u>left</u> forearm
    M66.239 Spontaneous rupture of extensor tendons, <u>unspecified</u> forearm
M66.24-Spontaneous rupture of extensor tendons, <u>hand</u>
    M66.241 Spontaneous rupture of extensor tendons, <u>right</u> hand
    M66.242 Spontaneous rupture of extensor tendons, <u>left</u> hand
    M66.249 Spontaneous rupture of extensor tendons, <u>unspecified</u> hand
M66.25-Spontaneous rupture of extensor tendons, <u>thigh</u>
    M66.251 Spontaneous rupture of extensor tendons, <u>right</u> thigh
    M66.252 Spontaneous rupture of extensor tendons, <u>left</u> thigh
    M66.259 Spontaneous rupture of extensor tendons, <u>unspecified</u> thigh

M66.26-Spontaneous rupture of extensor tendons, <u>lower leg</u>
    M66.261 Spontaneous rupture of extensor tendons, <u>right</u> lower leg
    M66.262 Spontaneous rupture of extensor tendons, <u>left</u> lower leg
    M66.269 Spontaneous rupture of extensor tendons, <u>unspecified</u> lower leg
M66.27-Spontaneous rupture of extensor tendons, <u>ankle and foot</u>
    M66.271 Spontaneous rupture of extensor tendons, <u>right</u> ankle and foot
    M66.272 Spontaneous rupture of extensor tendons, <u>left</u> ankle and foot
    M66.279 Spontaneous rupture of extensor tendons, <u>unspecified</u> ankle and foot
M66.28 Spontaneous rupture of extensor tendons, <u>other site</u>
M66.29 Spontaneous rupture of extensor tendons, <u>multiple sites</u>
M66.3- Spontaneous rupture of <u>flexor</u> tendons
M66.30 Spontaneous rupture of flexor tendons, <u>unspecified site</u>
M66.31-Spontaneous rupture of flexor tendons, <u>shoulder</u>
    M66.311 Spontaneous rupture of flexor tendons, <u>right</u> shoulder
    M66.312 Spontaneous rupture of flexor tendons, <u>left</u> shoulder
    M66.319 Spontaneous rupture of flexor tendons, <u>unspecified</u> shoulder
M66.32-Spontaneous rupture of flexor tendons, <u>upper arm</u>
    M66.321 Spontaneous rupture of flexor tendons, <u>right</u> upper arm
    M66.322 Spontaneous rupture of flexor tendons, <u>left</u> upper arm
    M66.329 Spontaneous rupture of flexor tendons, <u>unspecified</u> upper arm
M66.33-Spontaneous rupture of flexor tendons, <u>forearm</u>
    M66.331 Spontaneous rupture of flexor tendons, <u>right</u> forearm
    M66.332 Spontaneous rupture of flexor tendons, <u>left</u> forearm
    M66.339 Spontaneous rupture of flexor tendons, <u>unspecified</u> forearm
M66.34-Spontaneous rupture of flexor tendons, <u>hand</u>
    M66.341 Spontaneous rupture of flexor tendons, <u>right</u> hand
    M66.342 Spontaneous rupture of flexor tendons, <u>left</u> hand
    M66.349 Spontaneous rupture of flexor tendons, <u>unspecified</u> hand
M66.35-Spontaneous rupture of flexor tendons, <u>thigh</u>
    M66.351 Spontaneous rupture of flexor tendons, <u>right</u> thigh
    M66.352 Spontaneous rupture of flexor tendons, <u>left</u> thigh
    M66.359 Spontaneous rupture of flexor tendons, <u>unspecified</u> thigh
M66.36-Spontaneous rupture of flexor tendons, <u>lower leg</u>
    M66.361 Spontaneous rupture of flexor tendons, <u>right</u> lower leg
    M66.362 Spontaneous rupture of flexor tendons, <u>left</u> lower leg
    M66.369 Spontaneous rupture of flexor tendons, <u>unspecified</u> lower leg
M66.37-Spontaneous rupture of flexor tendons, <u>ankle and foot</u>
    M66.371 Spontaneous rupture of flexor tendons, <u>right</u> ankle and foot
    M66.372 Spontaneous rupture of flexor tendons, <u>left</u> ankle and foot
    M66.379 Spontaneous rupture of flexor tendons, <u>unspecified</u> ankle and foot
M66.38 Spontaneous rupture of flexor tendons, <u>other site</u>
M66.39 Spontaneous rupture of flexor tendons, <u>multiple sites</u>
M66.8- Spontaneous rupture of <u>other</u> tendons
M66.80 Spontaneous rupture of other tendons, <u>unspecified site</u>
M66.81-Spontaneous rupture of other tendons, <u>shoulder</u>

M66.811   Spontaneous rupture of other tendons, <u>right</u> shoulder

M66.812   Spontaneous rupture of other tendons, <u>left</u> shoulder

M66.819   Spontaneous rupture of other tendons, <u>unspecified</u> shoulder

M66.82- Spontaneous rupture of other tendons, <u>upper arm</u>

M66.821   Spontaneous rupture of other tendons, <u>right</u> upper arm

M66.822   Spontaneous rupture of other tendons, <u>left</u> upper arm

M66.829   Spontaneous rupture of other tendons, <u>unspecified</u> upper arm

M66.83- Spontaneous rupture of other tendons, <u>forearm</u>

M66.831   Spontaneous rupture of other tendons, <u>right</u> forearm

M66.832   Spontaneous rupture of other tendons, <u>left</u> forearm

M66.839   Spontaneous rupture of other tendons, <u>unspecified</u> forearm

M66.84- Spontaneous rupture of other tendons, <u>hand</u>

M66.841   Spontaneous rupture of other tendons, <u>right</u> hand

M66.842   Spontaneous rupture of other tendons, <u>left</u> hand

M66.849   Spontaneous rupture of other tendons, <u>unspecified</u> hand

M66.85- Spontaneous rupture of other tendons, <u>thigh</u>

M66.851   Spontaneous rupture of other tendons, <u>right</u> thigh

M66.852   Spontaneous rupture of other tendons, <u>left</u> thigh

M66.859   Spontaneous rupture of other tendons, <u>unspecified</u> thigh

M66.86- Spontaneous rupture of other tendons, <u>lower leg</u>

M66.861   Spontaneous rupture of other tendons, <u>right</u> lower leg

M66.862   Spontaneous rupture of other tendons, <u>left</u> lower leg

M66.869   Spontaneous rupture of other tendons, <u>unspecified</u> lower leg

M66.87- Spontaneous rupture of other tendons, <u>ankle and foot</u>

M66.871   Spontaneous rupture of other tendons, <u>right</u> ankle and foot

M66.872   Spontaneous rupture of other tendons, <u>left</u> ankle and foot

M66.879   Spontaneous rupture of other tendons, <u>unspecified</u> ankle and foot

M66.88   Spontaneous rupture of other tendons, <u>other</u>

M66.89   Spontaneous rupture of other tendons, <u>multiple sites</u>

M66.9   Spontaneous rupture of <u>unspecified</u> tendon

Rupture at musculotendinous junction, nontraumatic

M67-   <u>Other disorders</u> of synovium and tendon

Excludes 1:   *palmar fascial fibromatosis [Dupuytren] (M72.0)*
tendinitis NOS (M77.9-)
xanthomatosis localized to tendons (E78.2)

M67.0-   <u>Short Achilles tendon (acquired)</u> — The abnormally reduced length of the Achilles tendon.

M67.00   Short Achilles tendon (acquired), <u>unspecified</u> ankle

M67.01   Short Achilles tendon (acquired), <u>right</u> ankle

M67.02   Short Achilles tendon (acquired), <u>left</u> ankle

M67.2-   <u>Synovial hypertrophy, not elsewhere classified</u>

Excludes 1:   *villonodular synovitis (pigmented) (M12.2-)*

M67.20   Synovial hypertrophy, not elsewhere classified, <u>unspecified</u> site

M67.21- Synovial hypertrophy, not elsewhere classified, <u>shoulder</u>

M67.211   Synovial hypertrophy, not elsewhere classified, <u>right</u> shoulder

M67.212   Synovial hypertrophy, not elsewhere classified, <u>left</u> shoulder

M67.219   Synovial hypertrophy, not elsewhere classified, <u>unspecified</u> shoulder

M67.22- Synovial hypertrophy, not elsewhere classified, <u>upper arm</u>

M67.221   Synovial hypertrophy, not elsewhere classified, <u>right</u> upper arm

M67.222   Synovial hypertrophy, not elsewhere classified, <u>left</u> upper arm

M67.229   Synovial hypertrophy, not elsewhere classified, <u>unspecified</u> upper arm

M67.23- Synovial hypertrophy, not elsewhere classified, <u>forearm</u>

M67.231   Synovial hypertrophy, not elsewhere classified, <u>right</u> forearm

M67.232   Synovial hypertrophy, not elsewhere classified, <u>left</u> forearm

M67.239   Synovial hypertrophy, not elsewhere classified, <u>unspecified</u> forearm

M67.24- Synovial hypertrophy, not elsewhere classified, <u>hand</u>

M67.241   Synovial hypertrophy, not elsewhere classified, <u>right</u> hand

M67.242   Synovial hypertrophy, not elsewhere classified, <u>left</u> hand

M67.249   Synovial hypertrophy, not elsewhere classified, <u>unspecified</u> hand

M67.25- Synovial hypertrophy, not elsewhere classified, <u>thigh</u>

M67.251   Synovial hypertrophy, not elsewhere classified, <u>right</u> thigh

M67.252   Synovial hypertrophy, not elsewhere classified, <u>left</u> thigh

M67.259   Synovial hypertrophy, not elsewhere classified, <u>unspecified</u> thigh

M67.26- Synovial hypertrophy, not elsewhere classified, <u>lower leg</u>

M67.261   Synovial hypertrophy, not elsewhere classified, <u>right</u> lower leg

M67.262   Synovial hypertrophy, not elsewhere classified, <u>left</u> lower leg

M67.269   Synovial hypertrophy, not elsewhere classified, <u>unspecified</u> lower leg

M67.27- Synovial hypertrophy, not elsewhere classified, <u>ankle and foot</u>

M67.271   Synovial hypertrophy, not elsewhere classified, <u>right</u> ankle and foot

M67.272   Synovial hypertrophy, not elsewhere classified, <u>left</u> ankle and foot

M67.279   Synovial hypertrophy, not elsewhere classified, <u>unspecified</u> ankle and foot

M67.28   Synovial hypertrophy, not elsewhere classified, <u>other site</u>

M67.29   Synovial hypertrophy, not elsewhere classified, <u>multiple sites</u>

M67.3-   <u>Transient</u> synovitis — Inflammation of the synovial membrane that only lasts a few days or weeks, has no known cause (traumatic or medical), and most often affects children.

Toxic synovitis

Excludes 1:   *palindromic rheumatism (M12.3-)*

M67.30   Transient synovitis, <u>unspecified</u> <u>site</u>

M67.31- Transient synovitis, <u>shoulder</u>

M67.311   Transient synovitis, <u>right</u> shoulder

M67.312   Transient synovitis, <u>left</u> shoulder

M67.319   Transient synovitis, <u>unspecified</u> shoulder

M67.32- Transient synovitis, <u>elbow</u>

M67.321   Transient synovitis, <u>right</u> elbow

M67.322   Transient synovitis, <u>left</u> elbow

M67.329   Transient synovitis, <u>unspecified</u> elbow

M67.33- Transient synovitis, <u>wrist</u>

M67.331   Transient synovitis, <u>right</u> wrist

M67.332   Transient synovitis, <u>left</u> wrist

M67.339   Transient synovitis, <u>unspecified</u> wrist

M67.34- Transient synovitis, <u>hand</u>

M67.341   Transient synovitis, <u>right</u> hand

M67.342   Transient synovitis, <u>left</u> hand

M67.349   Transient synovitis, <u>unspecified</u> hand

M66
–
M67

M67.35- Transient synovitis, <u>hip</u>
    M67.351 Transient synovitis, <u>right</u> hip
    M67.352 Transient synovitis, <u>left</u> hip
    M67.359 Transient synovitis, <u>unspecified</u> hip
M67.36- Transient synovitis, <u>knee</u>
    M67.361 Transient synovitis, <u>right</u> knee
    M67.362 Transient synovitis, <u>left</u> knee
    M67.369 Transient synovitis, <u>unspecified</u> knee
M67.37- Transient synovitis, <u>ankle and foot</u>
    M67.371 Transient synovitis, <u>right</u> ankle and foot
    M67.372 Transient synovitis, <u>left</u> ankle and foot
    M67.379 Transient synovitis, <u>unspecified</u> ankle and foot
M67.38 Transient synovitis, <u>other site</u>
M67.39 Transient synovitis, <u>multiple sites</u>
M67.4- <u>Ganglion</u> — A cystic tumor of joint tissue or a tendon sheath.
    Ganglion of joint or tendon (sheath)
    Excludes 1:   *ganglion in yaws (A66.6)*
    Excludes ❷: *cyst of bursa (M71.2-M71.3)*
                  cyst of synovium (M71.2-M71.3)
M67.40 Ganglion, <u>unspecified site</u>
M67.41- Ganglion, <u>shoulder</u>
    M67.411 Ganglion, <u>right</u> shoulder
    M67.412 Ganglion, <u>left</u> shoulder
    M67.419 Ganglion, <u>unspecified</u> shoulder
M67.42- Ganglion, <u>elbow</u>
    M67.421 Ganglion, <u>right</u> elbow
    M67.422 Ganglion, <u>left</u> elbow
    M67.429 Ganglion, <u>unspecified</u> elbow
M67.43- Ganglion, <u>wrist</u>
    M67.431 Ganglion, <u>right</u> wrist
    M67.432 Ganglion, <u>left</u> wrist
    M67.439 Ganglion, <u>unspecified</u> wrist
M67.44- Ganglion, <u>hand</u>
    M67.441 Ganglion, <u>right</u> hand
    M67.442 Ganglion, <u>left</u> hand
    M67.449 Ganglion, <u>unspecified</u> hand
M67.45- Ganglion, <u>hip</u>
    M67.451 Ganglion, <u>right</u> hip
    M67.452 Ganglion, <u>left</u> hip
    M67.459 Ganglion, <u>unspecified</u> hip
M67.46- Ganglion, <u>knee</u>
    M67.461 Ganglion, <u>right</u> knee
    M67.462 Ganglion, <u>left</u> knee
    M67.469 Ganglion, <u>unspecified</u> knee
M67.47- Ganglion, <u>ankle and foot</u>
    M67.471 Ganglion, <u>right</u> ankle and foot
    M67.472 Ganglion, <u>left</u> ankle and foot
    M67.479 Ganglion, <u>unspecified</u> ankle and foot
M67.48 Ganglion, <u>other site</u>
M67.49 Ganglion, <u>multiple sites</u>
M67.5- <u>Plica syndrome</u> — An inflammatory disorder of the remnants of synovial tissue characterized by swelling, a clicking sensation, and weakness.
    Plica knee
M67.50 Plica syndrome, <u>unspecified</u> knee
M67.51 Plica syndrome, <u>right</u> knee
M67.52 Plica syndrome, <u>left</u> knee
M67.8- <u>Other specified</u> disorders of synovium and tendon
M67.80 Other specified disorders of synovium and tendon, <u>unspecified</u> site
M67.81- Other specified disorders of synovium and tendon, <u>shoulder</u>
    M67.811 Other specified disorders of synovium, <u>right</u> shoulder
    M67.812 Other specified disorders of synovium, <u>left</u> shoulder

    M67.813 Other specified disorders of tendon, <u>right</u> shoulder
    M67.814 Other specified disorders of tendon, <u>left</u> shoulder
    M67.819 Other specified disorders of synovium and tendon, <u>unspecified</u> shoulder
M67.82- Other specified disorders of synovium and tendon, <u>elbow</u>
    M67.821 Other specified disorders of synovium, <u>right</u> elbow
    M67.822 Other specified disorders of synovium, <u>left</u> elbow
    M67.823 Other specified disorders of tendon, <u>right</u> elbow
    M67.824 Other specified disorders of tendon, <u>left</u> elbow
    M67.829 Other specified disorders of synovium and tendon, <u>unspecified</u> elbow
M67.83- Other specified disorders of synovium and tendon, <u>wrist</u>
    M67.831 Other specified disorders of synovium, <u>right</u> wrist
    M67.832 Other specified disorders of synovium, <u>left</u> wrist
    M67.833 Other specified disorders of tendon, <u>right</u> wrist
    M67.834 Other specified disorders of tendon, <u>left</u> wrist
    M67.839 Other specified disorders of synovium and tendon, <u>unspecified</u> forearm
M67.84- Other specified disorders of synovium and tendon, <u>hand</u>
    M67.841 Other specified disorders of synovium, <u>right</u> hand
    M67.842 Other specified disorders of synovium, <u>left</u> hand
    M67.843 Other specified disorders of tendon, <u>right</u> hand
    M67.844 Other specified disorders of tendon, <u>left</u> hand
    M67.849 Other specified disorders of synovium and tendon, <u>unspecified</u> hand
M67.85- Other specified disorders of synovium and tendon, <u>hip</u>
    M67.851 Other specified disorders of synovium, <u>right</u> hip
    M67.852 Other specified disorders of synovium, <u>left</u> hip
    M67.853 Other specified disorders of tendon, <u>right</u> hip
    M67.854 Other specified disorders of tendon, <u>left</u> hip
    M67.859 Other specified disorders of synovium and tendon, <u>unspecified</u> hip
M67.86- Other specified disorders of synovium and tendon, <u>knee</u>
    M67.861 Other specified disorders of synovium, <u>right</u> knee
    M67.862 Other specified disorders of synovium, <u>left</u> knee
    M67.863 Other specified disorders of tendon, <u>right</u> knee
    M67.864 Other specified disorders of tendon, <u>left</u> knee
    M67.869 Other specified disorders of synovium and tendon, <u>unspecified</u> knee
M67.87- Other specified disorders of synovium and tendon, <u>ankle and foot</u>
    M67.871 Other specified disorders of synovium, <u>right</u> ankle and foot
    M67.872 Other specified disorders of synovium, <u>left</u> ankle and foot
    M67.873 Other specified disorders of tendon, <u>right</u> ankle and foot
    M67.874 Other specified disorders of tendon, <u>left</u> ankle and foot
    M67.879 Other specified disorders of synovium and tendon, <u>unspecified</u> ankle and foot
M67.88 Other specified disorders of synovium and tendon, <u>other site</u>
M67.89 Other specified disorders of synovium and tendon, <u>multiple sites</u>
M67.9- <u>Unspecified disorder</u> of synovium and tendon
M67.90 Unspecified disorder of synovium and tendon, <u>unspecified site</u>
M67.91- Unspecified disorder of synovium and tendon, <u>shoulder</u>
    M67.911 Unspecified disorder of synovium and tendon, <u>right</u> shoulder
    M67.912 Unspecified disorder of synovium and tendon, <u>left</u> shoulder
    M67.919 Unspecified disorder of synovium and tendon, <u>unspecified</u> shoulder

M 6 7 - M 6 7

M67.92- Unspecified disorder of synovium and tendon, <u>upper arm</u>

   M67.921   Unspecified disorder of synovium and tendon, <u>right</u> upper arm

   M67.922   Unspecified disorder of synovium and tendon, <u>left</u> upper arm

   M67.929   Unspecified disorder of synovium and tendon, <u>unspecified</u> upper arm

M67.93- Unspecified disorder of synovium and tendon, <u>forearm</u>

   M67.931   Unspecified disorder of synovium and tendon, <u>right</u> forearm

   M67.932   Unspecified disorder of synovium and tendon, <u>left</u> forearm

   M67.939   Unspecified disorder of synovium and tendon, <u>unspecified</u> forearm

M67.94- Unspecified disorder of synovium and tendon, <u>hand</u>

   M67.941   Unspecified disorder of synovium and tendon, <u>right</u> hand

   M67.942   Unspecified disorder of synovium and tendon, <u>left</u> hand

   M67.949   Unspecified disorder of synovium and tendon, <u>unspecified</u> hand

M67.95- Unspecified disorder of synovium and tendon, <u>thigh</u>

   M67.951   Unspecified disorder of synovium and tendon, <u>right</u> thigh

   M67.952   Unspecified disorder of synovium and tendon, <u>left</u> thigh

   M67.959   Unspecified disorder of synovium and tendon, <u>unspecified</u> thigh

M67.96- Unspecified disorder of synovium and tendon, <u>lower leg</u>

   M67.961   Unspecified disorder of synovium and tendon, <u>right</u> lower leg

   M67.962   Unspecified disorder of synovium and tendon, <u>left</u> lower leg

   M67.969   Unspecified disorder of synovium and tendon, <u>unspecified</u> lower leg

M67.97- Unspecified disorder of synovium and tendon, <u>ankle and foot</u>

   M67.971   Unspecified disorder of synovium and tendon, <u>right</u> ankle and foot

   M67.972   Unspecified disorder of synovium and tendon, <u>left</u> ankle and foot

   M67.979   Unspecified disorder of synovium and tendon, <u>unspecified</u> ankle and foot

M67.98 Unspecified disorder of synovium and tendon, <u>other site</u>

M67.99 Unspecified disorder of synovium and tendon, <u>multiple sites</u>

Other soft tissue disorders (M70-M79)

M70- <u>Soft tissue disorders related to use, overuse and pressure</u> —
Inflammation and/or irritation of the soft tissues (synovial membranes, bursae, muscles, tendons) due to use (usual or unusual), overuse, and/or pressure.
Includes: Soft tissue disorders of occupational origin
Use additional external cause code to identify activity causing disorder (Y93.-)
Excludes 1:   *bursitis NOS (M71.9-)*
Excludes ❷: *bursitis of shoulder (M75.5)*
         enthesopathies (M76-M77)
         pressure ulcer (pressure area) (L89.-)

M70.0- <u>Crepitant synovitis</u> (acute) (chronic) of hand and wrist

  M70.03- Crepitant synovitis (acute) (chronic), <u>wrist</u>

    M70.031   Crepitant synovitis (acute) (chronic), <u>right</u> wrist

    M70.032   Crepitant synovitis (acute) (chronic), <u>left</u> wrist

    M70.039   Crepitant synovitis (acute) (chronic), <u>unspecified</u> wrist

  M70.04- Crepitant synovitis (acute) (chronic), <u>hand</u>

    M70.041   Crepitant synovitis (acute) (chronic), <u>right</u> hand

    M70.042   Crepitant synovitis (acute) (chronic), <u>left</u> hand

    M70.049   Crepitant synovitis (acute) (chronic), <u>unspecified</u> hand

M70.1- <u>Bursitis</u> of hand

  M70.10 Bursitis, <u>unspecified</u> hand

  M70.11 Bursitis, <u>right</u> hand

  M70.12 Bursitis, <u>left</u> hand

M70.2- <u>Olecranon</u> bursitis

  M70.20 Olecranon bursitis, <u>unspecified</u> elbow

  M70.21 Olecranon bursitis, <u>right</u> elbow

  M70.22 Olecranon bursitis, <u>left</u> elbow

M70.3- <u>Other</u> bursitis of <u>elbow</u>

  M70.30 Other bursitis of elbow, <u>unspecified</u> elbow

  M70.31 Other bursitis of elbow, <u>right</u> elbow

  M70.32 Other bursitis of elbow, <u>left</u> elbow

M70.4- <u>Prepatellar</u> bursitis

  M70.40 Prepatellar bursitis, <u>unspecified</u> knee

  M70.41 Prepatellar bursitis, <u>right</u> knee

  M70.42 Prepatellar bursitis, <u>left</u> knee

M70.5- <u>Other</u> bursitis of <u>knee</u>

  M70.50 Other bursitis of knee, <u>unspecified</u> knee

  M70.51 Other bursitis of knee, <u>right</u> knee

  M70.52 Other bursitis of knee, <u>left</u> knee

M70.6- <u>Trochanteric</u> bursitis
       Trochanteric tendinitis

  M70.60 Trochanteric bursitis, <u>unspecified</u> hip

  M70.61 Trochanteric bursitis, <u>right</u> hip

  M70.62 Trochanteric bursitis, <u>left</u> hip

M70.7- Other bursitis of <u>hip</u>
       Ischial bursitis

  M70.70 Other bursitis of hip, <u>unspecified</u> hip

  M70.71 Other bursitis of hip, <u>right</u> hip

  M70.72 Other bursitis of hip, <u>left</u> hip

M70.8- <u>Other soft tissue disorders</u> related to use, overuse and pressure

  M70.80 Other soft tissue disorders related to use, overuse and pressure of <u>unspecified</u> site

  M70.81- Other soft tissue disorders related to use, overuse and pressure of <u>shoulder</u>

    M70.811   Other soft tissue disorders related to use, overuse and pressure, <u>right</u> shoulder

    M70.812   Other soft tissue disorders related to use, overuse and pressure, <u>left</u> shoulder

    M70.819   Other soft tissue disorders related to use, overuse and pressure, <u>unspecified</u> shoulder

  M70.82- Other soft tissue disorders related to use, overuse and pressure of <u>upper arm</u>

    M70.821   Other soft tissue disorders related to use, overuse and pressure, <u>right</u> upper arm

    M70.822   Other soft tissue disorders related to use, overuse and pressure, <u>left</u> upper arm

    M70.829   Other soft tissue disorders related to use, overuse and pressure, <u>unspecified</u> upper arms

  M70.83- Other soft tissue disorders related to use, overuse and pressure of <u>forearm</u>

    M70.831   Other soft tissue disorders related to use, overuse and pressure, <u>right</u> forearm

    M70.832   Other soft tissue disorders related to use, overuse and pressure, <u>left</u> forearm

    M70.839   Other soft tissue disorders related to use, overuse and pressure, <u>unspecified</u> forearm

  M70.84- Other soft tissue disorders related to use, overuse and pressure of <u>hand</u>

    M70.841   Other soft tissue disorders related to use, overuse and pressure, <u>right</u> hand

    M70.842   Other soft tissue disorders related to use, overuse and pressure, <u>left</u> hand

    M70.849   Other soft tissue disorders related to use, overuse and pressure, <u>unspecified</u> hand

M 6 7 I M 7 0

M70.85- Other soft tissue disorders related to use, overuse and pressure of <u>thigh</u>

  M70.851 Other soft tissue disorders related to use, overuse and pressure, <u>right</u> thigh

  M70.852 Other soft tissue disorders related to use, overuse and pressure, <u>left</u> thigh

  M70.859 Other soft tissue disorders related to use, overuse and pressure, <u>unspecified</u> thigh

M70.86 Other soft tissue disorders related to use, overuse and pressure <u>lower leg</u>

  M70.861 Other soft tissue disorders related to use, overuse and pressure, <u>right</u> lower leg

  M70.862 Other soft tissue disorders related to use, overuse and pressure, <u>left</u> lower leg

  M70.869 Other soft tissue disorders related to use, overuse and pressure, <u>unspecified</u> leg

M70.87- Other soft tissue disorders related to use, overuse and pressure of <u>ankle and foot</u>

  M70.871 Other soft tissue disorders related to use, overuse and pressure, <u>right</u> ankle and foot

  M70.872 Other soft tissue disorders related to use, overuse and pressure, <u>left</u> ankle and foot

  M70.879 Other soft tissue disorders related to use, overuse and pressure, <u>unspecified</u> ankle and foot

M70.88 Other soft tissue disorders related to use, overuse and pressure <u>other site</u>

M70.89 Other soft tissue disorders related to use, overuse and pressure <u>multiple sites</u>

M70.9- <u>Unspecified</u> soft tissue disorder related to use, overuse and pressure

M70.90 Unspecified soft tissue disorder related to use, overuse and pressure of <u>unspecified site</u>

M70.91- Unspecified soft tissue disorder related to use, overuse and pressure of <u>shoulder</u>

  M70.911 Unspecified soft tissue disorder related to use, overuse and pressure, <u>right</u> shoulder

  M70.912 Unspecified soft tissue disorder related to use, overuse and pressure, <u>left</u> shoulder

  M70.919 Unspecified soft tissue disorder related to use, overuse and pressure, <u>unspecified</u> shoulder

M70.92- Unspecified soft tissue disorder related to use, overuse and pressure of <u>upper arm</u>

  M70.921 Unspecified soft tissue disorder related to use, overuse and pressure, <u>right</u> upperarm

  M70.922 Unspecified soft tissue disorder related to use, overuse and pressure, <u>left</u> upperarm

  M70.929 Unspecified soft tissue disorder related to use, overuse and pressure, <u>unspecified</u> upper arm

M70.93- Unspecified soft tissue disorder related to use, overuse and pressure of <u>forearm</u>

  M70.931 Unspecified soft tissue disorder related to use, overuse and pressure, <u>right</u> forearm

  M70.932 Unspecified soft tissue disorder related to use, overuse and pressure, <u>left</u> forearm

  M70.939 Unspecified soft tissue disorder related to use, overuse and pressure, <u>unspecified</u> forearm

M70.94- Unspecified soft tissue disorder related to use, overuse and pressure of <u>hand</u>

  M70.941 Unspecified soft tissue disorder related to use, overuse and pressure, <u>right</u> hand

  M70.942 Unspecified soft tissue disorder related to use, overuse and pressure, <u>left</u> hand

  M70.949 Unspecified soft tissue disorder related to use, overuse and pressure, <u>unspecified</u> hand

M70.95- Unspecified soft tissue disorder related to use, overuse and pressure of <u>thigh</u>

  M70.951 Unspecified soft tissue disorder related to use, overuse and pressure, <u>right</u> thigh

  M70.952 Unspecified soft tissue disorder related to use, overuse and pressure, <u>left</u> thigh

  M70.959 Unspecified soft tissue disorder related to use, overuse and pressure, <u>unspecified</u> thigh

M70.96- Unspecified soft tissue disorder related to use, overuse and pressure <u>lower leg</u>

  M70.961 Unspecified soft tissue disorder related to use, overuse and pressure, <u>right</u> lower leg

  M70.962 Unspecified soft tissue disorder related to use, overuse and pressure, <u>left</u> lower leg

  M70.969 Unspecified soft tissue disorder related to use, overuse and pressure, <u>unspecified</u> lower leg

M70.97- Unspecified soft tissue disorder related to use, overuse and pressure of <u>ankle and foot</u>

  M70.971 Unspecified soft tissue disorder related to use, overuse and pressure, <u>right</u> ankle and foot

  M70.972 Unspecified soft tissue disorder related to use, overuse and pressure, <u>left</u> ankle and foot

  M70.979 Unspecified soft tissue disorder related to use, overuse and pressure, <u>unspecified</u> ankle and foot

M70.98 Unspecified soft tissue disorder related to use, overuse and pressure <u>other</u>

M70.99 Unspecified soft tissue disorder related to use, overuse and pressure <u>multiple sites</u>

M71- Other bursopathies

  Excludes 1: *bunion (M20.1)*

      bursitis related to use, overuse or pressure (M70.-)

      enthesopathies (M76-M77)

M71.0- <u>Abscess of bursa</u> — A localized collection of pus caused by the disintegration of bursal tissue.

  Use additional code (B95.-, B96.-) to identify causative organism

M71.00 Abscess of bursa, <u>unspecified site</u>

M71.01- Abscess of bursa, <u>shoulder</u>

  M71.011 Abscess of bursa, <u>right</u> shoulder

  M71.012 Abscess of bursa, <u>left</u> shoulder

  M71.019 Abscess of bursa, <u>unspecified</u> shoulder

M71.02- Abscess of bursa, <u>elbow</u>

  M71.021 Abscess of bursa, <u>right</u> elbow

  M71.022 Abscess of bursa, <u>left</u> elbow

  M71.029 Abscess of bursa, <u>unspecified</u> elbow

M71.03- Abscess of bursa, <u>wrist</u>

  M71.031 Abscess of bursa, <u>right</u> wrist

  M71.032 Abscess of bursa, <u>left</u> wrist

  M71.039 Abscess of bursa, <u>unspecified</u> wrist

M71.04- Abscess of bursa, <u>hand</u>

  M71.041 Abscess of bursa, <u>right</u> hand

  M71.042 Abscess of bursa, <u>left</u> hand

  M71.049 Abscess of bursa, <u>unspecified</u> hand

M71.05- Abscess of bursa, <u>hip</u>

  M71.051 Abscess of bursa, <u>right</u> hip

  M71.052 Abscess of bursa, <u>left</u> hip

  M71.059 Abscess of bursa, <u>unspecified</u> hip

M71.06- Abscess of bursa, <u>knee</u>

  M71.061 Abscess of bursa, <u>right</u> knee

  M71.062 Abscess of bursa, <u>left</u> knee

  M71.069 Abscess of bursa, <u>unspecified</u> knee

M71.07- Abscess of bursa, <u>ankle and foot</u>

  M71.071 Abscess of bursa, <u>right</u> ankle and foot

  M71.072 Abscess of bursa, <u>left</u> ankle and foot

  M71.079 Abscess of bursa, <u>unspecified</u> ankle and foot

M71.08 Abscess of bursa, other site

M71.09 Abscess of bursa, <u>multiple sites</u>

M71.1- <u>Other infective</u> bursitis

  Use additional code (B95.-, B96.-) to identify causative organism

M71.10 Other infective bursitis, <u>unspecified site</u>

M71.11- Other infective bursitis, <u>shoulder</u>

M71.111   Other infective bursitis, **right** shoulder
M71.112   Other infective bursitis, **left** shoulder
M71.119   Other infective bursitis, **unspecified** shoulder
M71.12- Other infective bursitis, **elbow**
M71.121   Other infective bursitis, **right** elbow
M71.122   Other infective bursitis, **left** elbow
M71.129   Other infective bursitis, **unspecified** elbow
M71.13- Other infective bursitis, **wrist**
M71.131   Other infective bursitis, **right** wrist
M71.132   Other infective bursitis, **left** wrist
M71.139   Other infective bursitis, **unspecified** wrist
M71.14- Other infective bursitis, **hand**
M71.141   Other infective bursitis, **right** hand
M71.142   Other infective bursitis, **left** hand
M71.149   Other infective bursitis, **unspecified** hand
M71.15- Other infective bursitis, **hip**
M71.151   Other infective bursitis, **right** hip
M71.152   Other infective bursitis, **left** hip
M71.159   Other infective bursitis, **unspecified** hip
M71.16- Other infective bursitis, **knee**
M71.161   Other infective bursitis, **right** knee
M71.162   Other infective bursitis, **left** knee
M71.169   Other infective bursitis, **unspecified** knee
M71.17- Other infective bursitis, **ankle and foot**
M71.171   Other infective bursitis, **right** ankle and foot
M71.172   Other infective bursitis, **left** ankle and foot
M71.179   Other infective bursitis, **unspecified** ankle and foot
M71.18   Other infective bursitis, other site
M71.19   Other infective bursitis, **multiple sites**
M71.2- **Synovial cyst of popliteal space [Baker]** — An accumulation of effused synovial fluid behind the knee that is contained by a membrane.
  Excludes 1:   synovial cyst of popliteal space with rupture (M66.0)
M71.20   Synovial cyst of popliteal space [Baker], **unspecified** knee
M71.21   Synovial cyst of popliteal space [Baker], **right** knee
M71.22   Synovial cyst of popliteal space [Baker], **left** knee
M71.3- **Other bursal cyst** — An accumulation of effused synovial fluid that is contained by a membrane.
    Synovial cyst NOS
  Excludes 1:   synovial cyst with rupture (M66.1-)
M71.30   Other bursal cyst, **unspecified** site
M71.31- Other bursal cyst, **shoulder**
M71.311   Other bursal cyst, **right** shoulder
M71.312   Other bursal cyst, **left** shoulder
M71.319   Other bursal cyst, **unspecified** shoulder
M71.32- Other bursal cyst, **elbow**
M71.321   Other bursal cyst, **right** elbow
M71.322   Other bursal cyst, **left** elbow
M71.329   Other bursal cyst, **unspecified** elbow
M71.33- Other bursal cyst, **wrist**
M71.331   Other bursal cyst, **right** wrist
M71.332   Other bursal cyst, **left** wrist
M71.339   Other bursal cyst, **unspecified** wrist
M71.34- Other bursal cyst, **hand**
M71.341   Other bursal cyst, **right** hand
M71.342   Other bursal cyst, **left** hand
M71.349   Other bursal cyst, **unspecified** hand
M71.35- Other bursal cyst, **hip**
M71.351   Other bursal cyst, **right** hip
M71.352   Other bursal cyst, **left** hip
M71.359   Other bursal cyst, **unspecified** hip
M71.37- Other bursal cyst, **ankle and foot**
M71.371   Other bursal cyst, **right** ankle and foot
M71.372   Other bursal cyst, **left** ankle and foot
M71.379   Other bursal cyst, **unspecified** ankle and foot
M71.38   Other bursal cyst, **other site**

M71.39   Other bursal cyst, **multiple sites**
M71.4- **Calcium deposit in bursa** — The deposition of calcium and its salts in the bursae.
  Excludes ❷: calcium deposit in bursa of shoulder (M75.3)
M71.40   Calcium deposit in bursa, **unspecified** site
M71.42- Calcium deposit in bursa, **elbow**
M71.421   Calcium deposit in bursa, **right** elbow
M71.422   Calcium deposit in bursa, **left** elbow
M71.429   Calcium deposit in bursa, **unspecified** elbow
M71.43- Calcium deposit in bursa, wrist
M71.431   Calcium deposit in bursa, **right** wrist
M71.432   Calcium deposit in bursa, **left** wrist
M71.439   Calcium deposit in bursa, **unspecified** wrist
M71.44- Calcium deposit in bursa, hand
M71.441   Calcium deposit in bursa, **right** hand
M71.442   Calcium deposit in bursa, **left** hand
M71.449   Calcium deposit in bursa, **unspecified** hand
M71.45- Calcium deposit in bursa, **hip**
M71.451   Calcium deposit in bursa, **right** hip
M71.452   Calcium deposit in bursa, **left** hip
M71.459   Calcium deposit in bursa, **unspecified** hip
M71.46- Calcium deposit in bursa, **knee**
M71.461   Calcium deposit in bursa, **right** knee
M71.462   Calcium deposit in bursa, **left** knee
M71.469   Calcium deposit in bursa, **unspecified** knee
M71.47- Calcium deposit in bursa, **ankle and foot**
M71.471   Calcium deposit in bursa, **right** ankle and foot
M71.472   Calcium deposit in bursa, **left** ankle and foot
M71.479   Calcium deposit in bursa, **unspecified** ankle and foot
M71.48   Calcium deposit in bursa, **other site**
M71.49   Calcium deposit in bursa, **multiple sites**
M71.5- **Other** bursitis, **not elsewhere classified**
  Excludes 1:   bursitis NOS (M71.9-)
  Excludes ❷: bursitis of shoulder (M75.5)
              bursitis of tibial collateral [Pellegrini-Stieda] (M76.4-)
M71.50   Other bursitis, not elsewhere classified, **unspecified** site
M71.52- Other bursitis, not elsewhere classified, **elbow**
M71.521   Other bursitis, not elsewhere classified, **right** elbow
M71.522   Other bursitis, not elsewhere classified, **left** elbow
M71.529   Other bursitis, not elsewhere classified, **unspecified** elbow
M71.53- Other bursitis, not elsewhere classified, **wrist**
M71.531   Other bursitis, not elsewhere classified, **right** wrist
M71.532   Other bursitis, not elsewhere classified, **left** wrist
M71.539   Other bursitis, not elsewhere classified, **unspecified** wrist
M71.54- Other bursitis, not elsewhere classified, **hand**
M71.541   Other bursitis, not elsewhere classified, **right** hand
M71.542   Other bursitis, not elsewhere classified, **left** hand
M71.549   Other bursitis, not elsewhere classified, **unspecified** hand
M71.55- Other bursitis, not elsewhere classified, **hip**
M71.551   Other bursitis, not elsewhere classified, **right** hip
M71.552   Other bursitis, not elsewhere classified, **left** hip
M71.559   Other bursitis, not elsewhere classified, **unspecified** hip
M71.56- Other bursitis, not elsewhere classified, **knee**
M71.561   Other bursitis, not elsewhere classified, **right** knee
M71.562   Other bursitis, not elsewhere classified, **left** knee
M71.569   Other bursitis, not elsewhere classified, **unspecified** knee
M71.57- Other bursitis, not elsewhere classified, **ankle and foot**
M71.571   Other bursitis, not elsewhere classified, **right** ankle and foot

M71-M71

Excludes 1: = NOT CODED HERE! (Do not code both)   873   *Excludes ❷:* = Not Included Here

M71.572 Other bursitis, not elsewhere classified, <u>left</u> ankle and foot

M71.579 Other bursitis, not elsewhere classified, <u>unspecified</u> ankle and foot

M71.58 Other bursitis, not elsewhere classified, <u>other site</u>

M71.8- <u>Other specified bursopathies</u>

M71.80 Other specified bursopathies, <u>unspecified site</u>

M71.81- Other specified bursopathies, <u>shoulder</u>

M71.811 Other specified bursopathies, <u>right</u> shoulder

M71.812 Other specified bursopathies, <u>left</u> shoulder

M71.819 Other specified bursopathies, <u>unspecified</u> shoulder

M71.82- Other specified bursopathies, <u>elbow</u>

M71.821 Other specified bursopathies, <u>right</u> elbow

M71.822 Other specified bursopathies, <u>left</u> elbow

M71.829 Other specified bursopathies, <u>unspecified</u> elbow

M71.83- Other specified bursopathies, <u>wrist</u>

M71.831 Other specified bursopathies, <u>right</u> wrist

M71.832 Other specified bursopathies, <u>left</u> wrist

M71.839 Other specified bursopathies, <u>unspecified</u> wrist

M71.84- Other specified bursopathies, <u>hand</u>

M71.841 Other specified bursopathies, <u>right</u> hand

M71.842 Other specified bursopathies, <u>left</u> hand

M71.849 Other specified bursopathies, <u>unspecified</u> hand

M71.85- Other specified bursopathies, <u>hip</u>

M71.851 Other specified bursopathies, <u>right</u> hip

M71.852 Other specified bursopathies, <u>left</u> hip

M71.859 Other specified bursopathies, <u>unspecified</u> hip

M71.86- Other specified bursopathies, <u>knee</u>

M71.861 Other specified bursopathies, <u>right</u> knee

M71.862 Other specified bursopathies, <u>left</u> knee

M71.869 Other specified bursopathies, <u>unspecified</u> knee

M71.87- Other specified bursopathies, <u>ankle and foot</u>

M71.871 Other specified bursopathies, <u>right</u> ankle and foot

M71.872 Other specified bursopathies, <u>left</u> ankle and foot

M71.879 Other specified bursopathies, <u>unspecified</u> ankle and foot

M71.88 Other specified bursopathies, <u>other site</u>

M71.89 Other specified bursopathies, <u>multiple sites</u>

M71.9 Bursopathy, <u>unspecified</u>
Bursitis NOS

M72- Fibroblastic disorders
Excludes ❷: *retroperitoneal fibromatosis (D48.3)*

M72.0 Palmar fascial fibromatosis [Dupuytren] — [Age/15-124] — The formation of a fibrous nodule in the palmar fascia.

M72.1 Knuckle pads — The formation of nodular fibrous masses on the knuckles of the hands.

M72.2 Plantar fascial fibromatosis — The formation of a fibrous nodule in the plantar fascia.
Plantar fasciitis — Inflammation of the plantar fascia.

M72.4 Pseudosarcomatous fibromatosis — A sarcoma-like appearing proliferation of fibroblasts in the subcutaneous tissue.
Nodular fasciitis — The formation of nodular fibrous masses of the fascia.

MCC **M72.6 Necrotizing fasciitis** — A fulminating infection of the fascia characterized by cellulitis and thrombosis of the subcutaneous vessels and gangrene of the underlying tissue.
Use additional code (B95.-, B96.-) to identify causative organism

M72.8 Other fibroblastic disorders
Abscess of fascia — A localized collection of pus caused by the disintegration of fascial tissue.
Fasciitis NEC
Other infective fasciitis
Use additional code to (B95.-, B96.-) identify causative organism
Excludes 1: *diffuse (eosinophilic) fasciitis (M35.4)*
necrotizing fasciitis (M72.6)
nodular fasciitis (M72.4)
perirenal fasciitis NOS (N13.5)
perirenal fasciitis with infection (N13.6)
plantar fasciitis (M72.2)

M72.9 Fibroblastic disorder, unspecified
Fasciitis NOS
Fibromatosis NOS

M75- Shoulder lesions
Excludes ❷: *shoulder-hand syndrome (M89.0-)*

M75.0- <u>Adhesive capsulitis</u> of shoulder — The adhesive inflammation of the shoulder joint capsule with progressive stiffness.
AHA 15:2Q:p23 Frozen shoulder
Frozen shoulder
Periarthritis of shoulder

M75.00 Adhesive capsulitis of <u>unspecified</u> shoulder

M75.01 Adhesive capsulitis of <u>right</u> shoulder

M75.02 Adhesive capsulitis of <u>left</u> shoulder

M75.1- <u>Rotator cuff tear or rupture, not specified as traumatic</u> — The non-traumatic injury of the tendons and/or muscles of the shoulder that hold the humeral head in the shallow glenohumeral joint socket.
Rotator cuff syndrome
Supraspinatus syndrome
Supraspinatus tear or rupture, not specified as traumatic
Excludes 1: *tear of rotator cuff, traumatic (S46.01-)*

M75.10- <u>Unspecified</u> rotator cuff tear or rupture, not specified as traumatic

M75.100 Unspecified rotator cuff tear or rupture of <u>unspecified</u> shoulder, not specified as traumatic

M75.101 Unspecified rotator cuff tear or rupture of <u>right</u> shoulder, not specified as traumatic

M75.102 Unspecified rotator cuff tear or rupture of <u>left</u> shoulder, not specified as traumatic

M75.11- <u>Incomplete</u> rotator cuff tear or rupture, not specified as traumatic — A form where the tendon(s) have a partial tear but remain intact.

M75.110 Incomplete rotator cuff tear or rupture of <u>unspecified</u> shoulder, not specified as traumatic

M75.111 Incomplete rotator cuff tear or rupture of <u>right</u> shoulder, not specified as traumatic

M75.112 Incomplete rotator cuff tear or rupture of <u>left</u> shoulder, not specified as traumatic

M75.12- <u>Complete</u> rotator cuff tear or rupture, not specified as traumatic — A form where the tendon(s) have a full-thickness tear and often become detached.

M75.120 Complete rotator cuff tear or rupture of <u>unspecified</u> shoulder, not specified as traumatic

M75.121 Complete rotator cuff tear or rupture of <u>right</u> shoulder, not specified as traumatic

M75.122 Complete rotator cuff tear or rupture of <u>left</u> shoulder, not specified as traumatic

M75.2- <u>Bicipital</u> tendinitis — Inflammation of the long head of the biceps tendon.

M75.20 Bicipital tendinitis, <u>unspecified</u> shoulder

M75.21 Bicipital tendinitis, <u>right</u> shoulder

M75.22 Bicipital tendinitis, <u>left</u> shoulder

M75.3- <u>Calcific</u> tendinitis of shoulder — The deposition of calcium in the inflamed tendons of the shoulder.
Calcified bursa of shoulder

M75.30 Calcific tendinitis of <u>unspecified</u> shoulder

M75.31 Calcific tendinitis of <u>right</u> shoulder

M75.32 Calcific tendinitis of <u>left</u> shoulder

M75.4- <u>Impingement syndrome</u> of shoulder — The downward compression of the bursa and/or tendons of the shoulder from the acromion process.

M75.40 Impingement syndrome of <u>unspecified</u> shoulder

M75.41 Impingement syndrome of <u>right</u> shoulder

M75.42 Impingement syndrome of <u>left</u> shoulder

M75.5- <u>Bursitis</u> of shoulder — Inflammation of the shoulder bursa.

M75.50 Bursitis of <u>unspecified</u> shoulder

M75.51 Bursitis of <u>right</u> shoulder

M75.52 Bursitis of <u>left</u> shoulder

M75.8- <u>Other</u> shoulder lesions

M75.80 Other shoulder lesions, <u>unspecified</u> shoulder

M75.81 Other shoulder lesions, <u>right</u> shoulder

M75.82 Other shoulder lesions, <u>left</u> shoulder

M75.9- Shoulder lesion, <u>unspecified</u>

    M75.90 Shoulder lesion, unspecified, <u>unspecified</u> shoulder

    M75.91 Shoulder lesion, unspecified, <u>right</u> shoulder

    M75.92 Shoulder lesion, unspecified, <u>left</u> shoulder

M76- Enthesopathies, lower limb, excluding foot
Excludes ❷: *bursitis due to use, overuse and pressure (M70-)*
      enthesopathies of ankle and foot (M77.5-)

M76.0- <u>Gluteal</u> tendinitis — Inflammation of the tendons that attach the gluteal muscles to the femur.

    M76.00 Gluteal tendinitis, <u>unspecified</u> hip

    M76.01 Gluteal tendinitis, <u>right</u> hip

    M76.02 Gluteal tendinitis, <u>left</u> hip

M76.1- <u>Psoas</u> tendinitis — Inflammation of the iliopsoas tendons.

    M76.10 Psoas tendinitis, <u>unspecified</u> hip

    M76.11 Psoas tendinitis, <u>right</u> hip

    M76.12 Psoas tendinitis, <u>left</u> hip

M76.2- <u>Iliac crest spur</u> — A mass of bony tissue projecting from the iliac crest.

    M76.20 Iliac crest spur, <u>unspecified</u> hip

    M76.21 Iliac crest spur, <u>right</u> hip

    M76.22 Iliac crest spur, <u>left</u> hip

M76.3- <u>Iliotibial band syndrome</u> — Inflammation of the iliotibial fascia band of the upper leg and knee.

    M76.30 Iliotibial band syndrome, <u>unspecified</u> leg

    M76.31 Iliotibial band syndrome, <u>right</u> leg

    M76.32 Iliotibial band syndrome, <u>left</u> leg

M76.4- <u>Tibial collateral bursitis [Pellegrini-Stieda]</u> — Inflammation of the bursa over the tibial collateral ligament.

    M76.40 Tibial collateral bursitis [Pellegrini-Stieda], <u>unspecified</u> leg

    M76.41 Tibial collateral bursitis [Pellegrini-Stieda], <u>right</u> leg

    M76.42 Tibial collateral bursitis [Pellegrini-Stieda], <u>left</u> leg

M76.5- <u>Patellar</u> tendinitis — Inflammation of the patellar tendon.

    M76.50 Patellar tendinitis, <u>unspecified</u> knee

    M76.51 Patellar tendinitis, <u>right</u> knee

    M76.52 Patellar tendinitis, <u>left</u> knee

M76.6- <u>Achilles</u> tendinitis — Inflammation of the Achilles tendon.
    Achilles bursitis — Inflammation of the Achilles bursa.

    M76.60 Achilles tendinitis, <u>unspecified</u> leg

    M76.61 Achilles tendinitis, <u>right</u> leg

    M76.62 Achilles tendinitis, <u>left</u> leg

M76.7- <u>Peroneal</u> tendinitis — Inflammation of the peroneal tendon.

    M76.70 Peroneal tendinitis, <u>unspecified</u> leg

    M76.71 Peroneal tendinitis, <u>right</u> leg

    M76.72 Peroneal tendinitis, <u>left</u> leg

M76.8- <u>Other specified</u> enthesopathies of lower limb, excluding foot

    M76.81-<u>Anterior tibial syndrome</u>

        M76.811 Anterior tibial syndrome, <u>right</u> leg

        M76.812 Anterior tibial syndrome, <u>left</u> leg

        M76.819 Anterior tibial syndrome, <u>unspecified</u> leg

    M76.82-<u>Posterior tibial tendinitis</u>

        M76.821 Posterior tibial tendinitis, <u>right</u> leg

        M76.822 Posterior tibial tendinitis, <u>left</u> leg

        M76.829 Posterior tibial tendinitis, <u>unspecified</u> leg

    M76.89-Other specified enthesopathies of <u>lower limb</u>, excluding foot

        M76.891 Other specified enthesopathies of <u>right</u> lower limb, excluding foot

        M76.892 Other specified enthesopathies of <u>left</u> lower limb, excluding foot

        M76.899 Other specified enthesopathies of <u>unspecified</u> lower limb, excluding foot

M76.9 Unspecified enthesopathy, lower limb, excluding foot

M77- Other enthesopathies
Excludes 1: *bursitis NOS (M71.9-)*
Excludes ❷: *bursitis due to use, overuse and pressure (M70.-)*
      osteophyte (M25.7)
      spinal enthesopathy (M46.0-)

M77.0- <u>Medial</u> epicondylitis — Inflammation of the medial epicondyle of the humerus and its surrounding tissue.

    M77.00 Medial epicondylitis, <u>unspecified</u> elbow

    M77.01 Medial epicondylitis, <u>right</u> elbow

    M77.02 Medial epicondylitis, <u>left</u> elbow

M77.1- <u>Lateral</u> epicondylitis — Inflammation of the lateral epicondyle of the humerus and its surrounding tissue.
    Tennis elbow

    M77.10 Lateral epicondylitis, <u>unspecified</u> elbow

    M77.11 Lateral epicondylitis, <u>right</u> elbow

    M77.12 Lateral epicondylitis, <u>left</u> elbow

M77.2- <u>Periarthritis</u> of <u>wrist</u> — Inflammation of the tissue surrounding the wrist joint.

    M77.20 Periarthritis, <u>unspecified</u> wrist

    M77.21 Periarthritis, <u>right</u> wrist

    M77.22 Periarthritis, <u>left</u> wrist

M77.3- <u>Calcaneal spur</u> — A bony tissue projection on the calcaneous.

    M77.30 Calcaneal spur, <u>unspecified</u> foot

    M77.31 Calcaneal spur, <u>right</u> foot

    M77.32 Calcaneal spur, <u>left</u> foot

M77.4- <u>Metatarsalgia</u>
Excludes 1: *Morton's metatarsalgia (G57.6)*

    M77.40 Metatarsalgia, <u>unspecified</u> foot

    M77.41 Metatarsalgia, <u>right</u> foot

    M77.42 Metatarsalgia, <u>left</u> foot

M77.5- <u>Other</u> enthesopathy of foot

    M77.50 Other enthesopathy of <u>unspecified</u> foot

    M77.51 Other enthesopathy of <u>right</u> foot

    M77.52 Other enthesopathy of <u>left</u> foot

M77.8 Other enthesopathies, not elsewhere classified

M77.9 Enthesopathy, unspecified
    Bone spur NOS
    Capsulitis NOS
    Periarthritis NOS
    Tendinitis NOS

M79- Other and unspecified soft tissue disorders, <u>not elsewhere classified</u>
Excludes 1: *psychogenic rheumatism (F45.8)*
      soft tissue pain, psychogenic (F45.41)

M79.0 Rheumatism, unspecified — A connective tissue disease marked by inflammation, degeneration, and metabolic changes.
Excludes 1: *fibromyalgia (M79.7)*
      palindromic rheumatism (M12.3-)

M79.1 Myalgia — Pain or inflammation of the muscles.
    Myofascial pain syndrome
Excludes 1: *fibromyalgia (M79.7)*
      myositis (M60.-)

M79.2 Neuralgia and neuritis, unspecified — Pain or inflammation of the nerves or nerve roots.
Excludes 1: *brachial radiculitis NOS (M54.1)*
      lumbosacral radiculitis NOS (M54.1)
      mononeuropathies (G56-G58)
      radiculitis NOS (M54.1)
      sciatica (M54.3-M54.4)

M79.3 Panniculitis, unspecified — Inflammation of the subcutaneous fat.
Excludes 1: *lupus panniculitis (L93.2)*
      neck and back panniculitis (M54.0-)
      relapsing [Weber-Christian] panniculitis (M35.6)

M79.4 Hypertrophy of (infrapatellar) fat pad — The enlargement of the fat pad of the knee.

M79.5 Residual foreign body in soft tissue — The retention of a foreign body in the soft tissue following healing of the primary injury.
Excludes 1: *foreign body granuloma of skin and subcutaneous tissue (L92.3)*
      foreign body granuloma of soft tissue (M60.2-)

M75-M79

M79.6- **Pain in limb, hand, foot, fingers and toes**
  Excludes ❷: *pain in joint (M25.5-)*
  M79.60- **Pain in limb, unspecified**
    M79.601 **Pain in right arm**
      Pain in right upper limb NOS
    M79.602 **Pain in left arm**
      Pain in left upper limb NOS
    M79.603 **Pain in arm, unspecified**
      Pain in upper limb NOS
    M79.604 **Pain in right leg**
      Pain in right lower limb NOS
    M79.605 **Pain in left leg**
      Pain in left lower limb NOS
    M79.606 **Pain in leg, unspecified**
      Pain in lower limb NOS
    M79.609 **Pain in unspecified limb**
      Pain in limb NOS
  M79.62- **Pain in upper arm**
      Pain in axillary region
    M79.621 **Pain in right upper arm**
    M79.622 **Pain in left upper arm**
    M79.629 **Pain in unspecified upper arm**
  M79.63- **Pain in forearm**
    M79.631 **Pain in right forearm**
    M79.632 **Pain in left forearm**
    M79.639 **Pain in unspecified forearm**
  M79.64- **Pain in hand and fingers**
    M79.641 **Pain in right hand**
    M79.642 **Pain in left hand**
    M79.643 **Pain in unspecified hand**
    M79.644 **Pain in right finger(s)**
    M79.645 **Pain in left finger(s)**
    M79.646 **Pain in unspecified finger(s)**
  M79.65- **Pain in thigh**
    M79.651 **Pain in right thigh**
    M79.652 **Pain in left thigh**
    M79.659 **Pain in unspecified thigh**
  M79.66- **Pain in lower leg**
    M79.661 **Pain in right lower leg**
    M79.662 **Pain in left lower leg**
    M79.669 **Pain in unspecified lower leg**
  M79.67- **Pain in foot and toes**
    M79.671 **Pain in right foot**
    M79.672 **Pain in left foot**
    M79.673 **Pain in unspecified foot**
    M79.674 **Pain in right toe(s)**
    M79.675 **Pain in left toe(s)**
    M79.676 **Pain in unspecified toe(s)**
M79.7 **Fibromyalgia** — A condition of widespread pain of the soft tissues and muscles that is characterized by muscle pain, fatigue, sleep, and hypersensitivity to localized pressure.
      Fibromyositis
      Fibrositis
      Myofibrositis
M79.A- **Nontraumatic compartment syndrome** — An abnormal condition characterized by increased pressure within a closed tissue space containing muscles and nerves that compromises circulation and may lead to tissue necrosis.
    Code first, if applicable, associated postprocedural complication
    Excludes 1: *compartment syndrome NOS (T79.A-)*
                fibromyalgia (M79.7)
                nontraumatic ischemic infarction of muscle (M62.2-)
                traumatic compartment syndrome (T79.A-)
  M79.A1- **Nontraumatic compartment syndrome of upper extremity**
      Nontraumatic compartment syndrome of shoulder, arm, forearm, wrist, hand, and fingers
  cc M79.A11 **Nontraumatic compartment syndrome of right upper extremity**

  cc M79.A12 **Nontraumatic compartment syndrome of left upper extremity**
  cc M79.A19 **Nontraumatic compartment syndrome of unspecified upper extremity**
  M79.A2- **Nontraumatic compartment syndrome of lower extremity**
      Nontraumatic compartment syndrome of hip, buttock, thigh, leg, foot, and toes
  cc M79.A21 **Nontraumatic compartment syndrome of right lower extremity**
  cc M79.A22 **Nontraumatic compartment syndrome of left lower extremity**
  cc M79.A29 **Nontraumatic compartment syndrome of unspecified lower extremity**
  cc M79.A3 **Nontraumatic compartment syndrome of abdomen**
  cc M79.A9 **Nontraumatic compartment syndrome of other sites**
M79.8- **Other specified soft tissue disorders**
  M79.81 **Nontraumatic hematoma of soft tissue** — A localized swelling mass of clotted blood within a soft tissue site that is not due to an identified injury.
      Nontraumatic hematoma of muscle
      Nontraumatic seroma of muscle and soft tissue
  M79.89 **Other specified soft tissue disorders**
      Polyalgia — Pain in several of the soft tissues at the same time.
M79.9 **Soft tissue disorder, unspecified**

Osteopathies and chondropathies (M80-M94)

Disorders of bone density and structure (M80-M85)

M80- **Osteoporosis with current pathological fracture** — A break of a diseased or weakened bone by a minor injury that would not otherwise break a healthy bone due to a degenerative bone disease of increased porosity of the bone with resultant softening.
    Includes: Osteoporosis with current fragility fracture
    Use additional code to identify major osseous defect, if applicable (M89.7-)
    Excludes 1:   *collapsed vertebra NOS (M48.5)*
                pathological fracture NOS (M84.4)
                wedging of vertebra NOS (M48.5)
    Excludes ❷: *personal history of (healed) osteoporosis fracture (Z87.310)*

    The appropriate 7th character is to be added to each code from category M80:
    A   Initial encounter for fracture
    D   Subsequent encounter for fracture with routine healing
    G   Subsequent encounter for fracture with delayed healing
    K   Subsequent encounter for fracture with nonunion
    P   Subsequent encounter for fracture with malunion
    S   Sequela

  M80.0- **Age-related osteoporosis with current pathological fracture**
      Involutional osteoporosis with current pathological fracture
      Osteoporosis NOS with current pathological fracture
      Postmenopausal osteoporosis with current pathological fracture
      Senile osteoporosis with current pathological fracture
  CC-A,K,P M80.00x- **Age-related osteoporosis with current pathological fracture, unspecified site [Age/15-124]**
  M80.01- **Age-related osteoporosis with current pathological fracture, shoulder**
  CC-A,K,P M80.011- **Age-related osteoporosis with current pathological fracture, right shoulder** — [Age/15-124]
  CC-A,K,P M80.012- **Age-related osteoporosis with current pathological fracture, left shoulder** — [Age/15-124]
  CC-A,K,P M80.019- **Age-related osteoporosis with current pathological fracture, unspecified shoulder** — [Age/15-124]
  M80.02- **Age-related osteoporosis with current pathological fracture, humerus**
  CC-A,K,P M80.021- **Age-related osteoporosis with current pathological fracture, right humerus** — [Age/15-124]
  CC-A,K,P M80.022- **Age-related osteoporosis with current pathological fracture, left humerus** — [Age/15-124]
  CC-A,K,P M80.029- **Age-related osteoporosis with current pathological fracture, unspecified humerus** — [Age/15-124]

M79-M80

M80.03- Age-related osteoporosis with current pathological fracture, <u>forearm</u>
Age-related osteoporosis with current pathological fracture of wrist

CC-A,K,P **M80.031-** Age-related osteoporosis with current pathological fracture, <u>right</u> forearm — [Age/15-124]

CC-A,K,P **M80.032-** Age-related osteoporosis with current pathological fracture, <u>left</u> forearm — [Age/15-124]

CC-A,K,P **M80.039-** Age-related osteoporosis with current pathological fracture, <u>unspecified</u> forearm — [Age/15-124]

M80.04- Age-related osteoporosis with current pathological fracture, <u>hand</u>

CC-A,K,P **M80.041-** Age-related osteoporosis with current pathological fracture, <u>right</u> hand — [Age/15-124]

CC-A,K,P **M80.042-** Age-related osteoporosis with current pathological fracture, <u>left</u> hand — [Age/15-124]

CC-A,K,P **M80.049-** Age-related osteoporosis with current pathological fracture, <u>unspecified</u> hand — [Age/15-124]

M80.05- Age-related osteoporosis with current pathological fracture, <u>femur</u>
Age-related osteoporosis with current pathological fracture of hip

CC-A,K,P **M80.051-** Age-related osteoporosis with current pathological fracture, <u>right</u> femur — [Age/15-124]

CC-A,K,P **M80.052-** Age-related osteoporosis with current pathological fracture, <u>left</u> femur — [Age/15-124]

CC-A,K,P **M80.059-** Age-related osteoporosis with current pathological fracture, <u>unspecified</u> femur — [Age/15-124]

M80.06- Age-related osteoporosis with current pathological fracture, <u>lower leg</u>

CC-A,K,P **M80.061-** Age-related osteoporosis with current pathological fracture, <u>right</u> lower leg — [Age/15-124]

CC-A,K,P **M80.062-** Age-related osteoporosis with current pathological fracture, <u>left</u> lower leg — [Age/15-124]

CC-A,K,P **M80.069-** Age-related osteoporosis with current pathological fracture, <u>unspecified</u> lower leg — [Age/15-124]

M80.07- Age-related osteoporosis with current pathological fracture, <u>ankle and foot</u>

CC-A,K,P **M80.071-** Age-related osteoporosis with current pathological fracture, <u>right</u> ankle and foot — [Age/15-124]

CC-A,K,P **M80.072-** Age-related osteoporosis with current pathological fracture, <u>left</u> ankle and foot — [Age/15-124]

CC-A,K,P **M80.079-** Age-related osteoporosis with current pathological fracture, <u>unspecified</u> ankle and foot — [Age/15-124]

CC-A,K,P **M80.08x-** Age-related osteoporosis with current pathological fracture, <u>vertebra(e)</u> — [Age/15-124]

M80.8- <u>Other</u> osteoporosis <u>with current pathological fracture</u>
Drug-induced osteoporosis with current pathological fracture
Idiopathic osteoporosis with current pathological fracture
Osteoporosis of disuse with current pathological fracture
Postoophorectomy osteoporosis with current pathological fracture
Postsurgical malabsorption osteoporosis with current pathological fracture
Post-traumatic osteoporosis with current pathological fracture
Use additional code for adverse effect, if applicable, to identify drug (T36-T50 with fifth or sixth character 5)

CC-A,K,P **M80.80x-** Other osteoporosis with current pathological fracture, <u>unspecified site</u>

M80.81- Other osteoporosis with pathological fracture, <u>shoulder</u>

CC-A,K,P **M80.811-** Other osteoporosis with current pathological fracture, <u>right</u> shoulder

CC-A,K,P **M80.812-** Other osteoporosis with current pathological fracture, <u>left</u> shoulder

CC-A,K,P **M80.819-** Other osteoporosis with current pathological fracture, <u>unspecified</u> shoulder

M80.82- Other osteoporosis with current pathological fracture, <u>humerus</u>

CC-A,K,P **M80.821-** Other osteoporosis with current pathological fracture, <u>right</u> humerus

CC-A,K,P **M80.822-** Other osteoporosis with current pathological fracture, <u>left</u> humerus

CC-A,K,P **M80.829-** Other osteoporosis with current pathological fracture, <u>unspecified</u> humerus

M80.83- Other osteoporosis with current pathological fracture, <u>forearm</u>
Other osteoporosis with current pathological fracture of wrist

CC-A,K,P **M80.831-** Other osteoporosis with current pathological fracture, <u>right</u> forearm

CC-A,K,P **M80.832-** Other osteoporosis with current pathological fracture, <u>left</u> forearm

CC-A,K,P **M80.839-** Other osteoporosis with current pathological fracture, <u>unspecified</u> forearm

M80.84- Other osteoporosis with current pathological fracture, <u>hand</u>

CC-A,K,P **M80.841-** Other osteoporosis with current pathological fracture, <u>right</u> hand

CC-A,K,P **M80.842-** Other osteoporosis with current pathological fracture, <u>left</u> hand

CC-A,K,P **M80.849-** Other osteoporosis with current pathological fracture, <u>unspecified</u> hand

M80.85- Other osteoporosis with current pathological fracture, <u>femur</u>
Other osteoporosis with current pathological fracture of hip

CC-A,K,P **M80.851-** Other osteoporosis with current pathological fracture, <u>right</u> femur

CC-A,K,P **M80.852-** Other osteoporosis with current pathological fracture, <u>left</u> femur

CC-A,K,P **M80.859-** Other osteoporosis with current pathological fracture, <u>unspecified</u> femur

M80.86- Other osteoporosis with current pathological fracture, <u>lower leg</u>

CC-A,K,P **M80.861-** Other osteoporosis with current pathological fracture, <u>right</u> lower leg

CC-A,K,P **M80.862-** Other osteoporosis with current pathological fracture, <u>left</u> lower leg

CC-A,K,P **M80.869-** Other osteoporosis with current pathological fracture, <u>unspecified</u> lower leg

M80.87- Other osteoporosis with current pathological fracture, <u>ankle and foot</u>

CC-A,K,P **M80.871-** Other osteoporosis with current pathological fracture, <u>right</u> ankle and foot

CC-A,K,P **M80.872-** Other osteoporosis with current pathological fracture, <u>left</u> ankle and foot

CC-A,K,P **M80.879-** Other osteoporosis with current pathological fracture, <u>unspecified</u> ankle and foot

CC-A,K,P **M80.88x-** Other osteoporosis with current pathological fracture, vertebra(e)

M81- Osteoporosis <u>without</u> current pathological fracture — A degenerative bone disorder due to bone loss and characterized by porosity, softening, decreased bone strength, and susceptibility to relatively minor force fractures.
Use additional code to identify:
Major osseous defect, if applicable (M89.7-)
Personal history of (healed) osteoporosis fracture, if applicable (Z87.310)
Excludes 1: osteoporosis with current pathological fracture (M80.-)
Sudeck's atrophy (M89.0)

M81.0 <u>Age-related</u> osteoporosis without current pathological fracture — [Age/15-124]
Involutional osteoporosis without current pathological fracture
Osteoporosis NOS
Postmenopausal osteoporosis without current pathological fracture
Senile osteoporosis without current pathological fracture

M81.6 <u>Localized</u> osteoporosis [Lequesne]
Excludes 1: Sudeck's atrophy (M89.0)

M80
|
M81

M81.8 **Other** osteoporosis without current pathological fracture
Drug-induced osteoporosis without current pathological fracture
Idiopathic osteoporosis without current pathological fracture
Osteoporosis of disuse without current pathological fracture
Postoophorectomy osteoporosis without current pathological fracture
Postsurgical malabsorption osteoporosis without current pathological fracture
Post-traumatic osteoporosis without current pathological fracture
Use additional code for adverse effect, if applicable, to identify drug (T36-T50 with fifth or sixth character 5)

M83- **Adult osteomalacia** — Softening of the bone.
Excludes 1: infantile and juvenile osteomalacia (E55.0)
renal osteodystrophy (N25.0)
rickets (active) (E55.0)
rickets (active) sequelae (E64.3)
vitamin D-resistant osteomalacia (E83.3)
vitamin D-resistant rickets (active) (E83.3)

M83.0 **Puerperal osteomalacia** — [♀, Age/12-55] — A form following pregnancy.

M83.1 **Senile osteomalacia** — [Age/15-124] — A form that is age-related.

M83.2 **Adult osteomalacia due to malabsorption** — [Age/15-124] — A form due to the body's decreased ability to absorb nutrients.
Postsurgical malabsorption osteomalacia in adults

M83.3 **Adult osteomalacia due to malnutrition** — [Age/15-124] — A form due to the decreased intake of nutrients.

M83.4 **Aluminum bone disease** — A form due to aluminum toxicity.

M83.5 **Other drug-induced osteomalacia in adults** — [Age/15-124]
Use additional code for adverse effect, if applicable, to identify drug (T36-T50 with fifth or sixth character 5)

M83.8 **Other adult osteomalacia** — [Age/15-124]

M83.9 **Adult osteomalacia, unspecified** — [Age/15-124]

M84- **Disorder of continuity of bone**
Excludes ❷: traumatic fracture of bone-see fracture, by site

M84.3- **Stress fracture** — A fracture that is due to multiple/repetitive stress forces as opposed to an isolated acute traumatic injury event.
Fatigue fracture
March fracture
Stress fracture NOS
Stress reaction
Use additional external cause code(s) to identify the cause of the stress fracture
Excludes 1: pathological fracture NOS (M84.4.-)
pathological fracture due to osteoporosis (M80.-)
traumatic fracture (S12.-, S22.-, S32.-, S42.-, S52.-, S62.-, S72.-, S82.-, S92.-)
Excludes ❷: personal history of (healed) stress (fatigue) fracture (Z87.312)
stress fracture of vertebra (M48.4-)

The appropriate 7th character is to be added to each code from subcategory M84.3:
A   Initial encounter for fracture
D   Subsequent encounter for fracture with routine healing
G   Subsequent encounter for fracture with delayed healing
K   Subsequent encounter for fracture with nonunion
P   Subsequent encounter for fracture with malunion
S   Sequela

CC-K,P **M84.30x-** Stress fracture, **unspecified** **site**

M84.31- Stress fracture, **shoulder**

CC-K,P **M84.311-** Stress fracture, **right** shoulder

CC-K,P **M84.312-** Stress fracture, **left** shoulder

CC-K,P **M84.319-** Stress fracture, **unspecified** shoulder

M84.32- Stress fracture, **humerus**

CC-K,P **M84.321-** Stress fracture, **right** humerus

CC-K,P **M84.322-** Stress fracture, **left** humerus

CC-K,P **M84.329-** Stress fracture, **unspecified** humerus

M84.33- Stress fracture, **ulna and radius**

CC-K,P **M84.331-** Stress fracture, **right** ulna

CC-K,P **M84.332-** Stress fracture, **left** ulna

CC-K,P **M84.333-** Stress fracture, **right** radius

CC-K,P **M84.334-** Stress fracture, **left** radius

CC-K,P **M84.339-** Stress fracture, **unspecified** ulna and radius

M84.34- Stress fracture, **hand and fingers**

CC-K,P **M84.341-** Stress fracture, **right** hand

CC-K,P **M84.342-** Stress fracture, **left** hand

CC-K,P **M84.343-** Stress fracture, **unspecified** hand

CC-K,P **M84.344-** Stress fracture, **right** finger(s)

CC-K,P **M84.345-** Stress fracture, **left** finger(s)

CC-K,P **M84.346-** Stress fracture, **unspecified** finger(s)

M84.35- Stress fracture, **pelvis and femur**
Stress fracture, hip

CC-K,P **M84.350-** Stress fracture, pelvis

CC-K,P **M84.351-** Stress fracture, **right** femur

CC-K,P **M84.352-** Stress fracture, **left** femur

CC-K,P **M84.353-** Stress fracture, **unspecified** femur

CC-K,P **M84.359-** Stress fracture, hip, **unspecified**

M84.36- Stress fracture, **tibia and fibula**

CC-K,P **M84.361-** Stress fracture, **right** tibia

CC-K,P **M84.362-** Stress fracture, **left** tibia

CC-K,P **M84.363-** Stress fracture, **right** fibula

CC-K,P **M84.364-** Stress fracture, **left** fibula

CC-K,P **M84.369-** Stress fracture, **unspecified** tibia and fibula

M84.37- Stress fracture, **ankle, foot and toes**

CC-K,P **M84.371-** Stress fracture, **right** ankle

CC-K,P **M84.372-** Stress fracture, **left** ankle

CC-K,P **M84.373-** Stress fracture, **unspecified** ankle

CC-K,P **M84.374-** Stress fracture, **right** foot

CC-K,P **M84.375-** Stress fracture, **left** foot

CC-K,P **M84.376-** Stress fracture, **unspecified** foot

CC-K,P **M84.377-** Stress fracture, **right** toe(s)

CC-K,P **M84.378-** Stress fracture, **left** toe(s)

CC-K,P **M84.379-** Stress fracture, **unspecified** toe(s)

CC-K,P **M84.38x-** Stress fracture, **other site**
Excludes ❷: stress fracture of vertebra (M48.4-)

M84.4- **Pathological fracture, not elsewhere classified** — A break of a diseased or weakened bone by a minor injury that would not otherwise break a healthy bone and that is NOT due to osteoporosis.
Chronic fracture
Pathological fracture NOS
Excludes 1: collapsed vertebra NEC (M48.5)
pathological fracture in neoplastic disease (M84.5-)
pathological fracture in osteoporosis (M80.-)
pathological fracture in other disease (M84.6-)
stress fracture (M84.3-)
traumatic fracture (S12.-, S22.-, S32.-, S42.-, S52.-, S62.-, S72.-, S82.-, S92.-)
Excludes ❷: personal history of (healed) pathological fracture (Z87.311)

The appropriate 7th character is to be added to each code from subcategory M84.4:
A   Initial encounter for fracture
D   Subsequent encounter for fracture with routine healing
G   Subsequent encounter for fracture with delayed healing
K   Subsequent encounter for fracture with nonunion
P   Subsequent encounter for fracture with malunion
S   Sequela

CC-A,K,P **M84.40x-** Pathological fracture, **unspecified** site

M84.41- Pathological fracture, **shoulder**

CC-A,K,P **M84.411-** Pathological fracture, **right** shoulder

CC-A,K,P **M84.412-** Pathological fracture, **left** shoulder

CC-A,K,P **M84.419-** Pathological fracture, **unspecified** shoulder

M84.42- Pathological fracture, **humerus**

CC-A,K,P **M84.421-** Pathological fracture, **right** humerus

CC-A,K,P **M84.422-** Pathological fracture, **left** humerus

CC-A,K,P **M84.429-** Pathological fracture, **unspecified** humerus

M84.43- Pathological fracture, **ulna and radius**

CC-A,K,P **M84.431-** Pathological fracture, **right** ulna

CC-A,K,P **M84.432-** Pathological fracture, **left** ulna

CC-A,K,P **M84.433-** Pathological fracture, **right** radius

CC-A,K,P **M84.434-** Pathological fracture, **left** radius

CC-A,K,P **M84.439-** Pathological fracture, **unspecified** ulna and radius

M84.44- Pathological fracture, **hand and fingers**

CC-A,K,P **M84.441-** Pathological fracture, **right** hand

Excludes 1: = NOT CODED HERE! (Do not code both)   **Excludes ❷:** = Not Included Here

CC-A,K,P **M84.442-** Pathological fracture, <u>left</u> hand

CC-A,K,P **M84.443-** Pathological fracture, <u>unspecified</u> hand

CC-A,K,P **M84.444-** Pathological fracture, <u>right</u> finger(s)

CC-A,K,P **M84.445-** Pathological fracture, <u>left</u> finger(s)

CC-A,K,P **M84.446-** Pathological fracture, <u>unspecified</u> finger(s)

M84.45- Pathological fracture, <u>femur and pelvis</u>

CC-A,K,P **M84.451-** Pathological fracture, <u>right</u> femur

CC-A,K,P **M84.452-** Pathological fracture, <u>left</u> femur

CC-A,K,P **M84.453-** Pathological fracture, <u>unspecified</u> femur

CC-A,K,P **M84.454-** Pathological fracture, pelvis

CC-A,K,P **M84.459-** Pathological fracture, hip, <u>unspecified</u>

M84.46- Pathological fracture, <u>tibia and fibula</u>

CC-A,K,P **M84.461-** Pathological fracture, <u>right</u> tibia

CC-A,K,P **M84.462-** Pathological fracture, <u>left</u> tibia

CC-A,K,P **M84.463-** Pathological fracture, <u>right</u> fibula

CC-A,K,P **M84.464-** Pathological fracture, <u>left</u> fibula

CC-A,K,P **M84.469-** Pathological fracture, <u>unspecified</u> tibia and fibula

M84.47- Pathological fracture, <u>ankle, foot and toes</u>

CC-A,K,P **M84.471-** Pathological fracture, <u>right</u> ankle

CC-A,K,P **M84.472-** Pathological fracture, <u>left</u> ankle

CC-A,K,P **M84.473-** Pathological fracture, <u>unspecified</u> ankle

CC-A,K,P **M84.474-** Pathological fracture, <u>right</u> foot

CC-A,K,P **M84.475-** Pathological fracture, <u>left</u> foot

CC-A,K,P **M84.476-** Pathological fracture, <u>unspecified</u> foot

CC-A,K,P **M84.477-** Pathological fracture, <u>right</u> toe(s)

CC-A,K,P **M84.478-** Pathological fracture, <u>left</u> toe(s)

CC-A,K,P **M84.479-** Pathological fracture, <u>unspecified</u> toe(s)

CC-A,K,P **M84.48x-** Pathological fracture, <u>other site</u>

M84.5- Pathological fracture <u>in neoplastic disease</u>
Code also underlying neoplasm

The appropriate 7th character is to be added to each code from subcategory M84.5:
- **A**   Initial encounter for fracture
- **D**   Subsequent encounter for fracture with routine healing
- **G**   Subsequent encounter for fracture with delayed healing
- **K**   Subsequent encounter for fracture with nonunion
- **P**   Subsequent encounter for fracture with malunion
- **S**   Sequela

CC-A,K,P **M84.50x-** Pathological fracture in neoplastic disease, <u>unspecified</u> <u>site</u>

M84.51- Pathological fracture in neoplastic disease, <u>shoulder</u>

CC-A,K,P **M84.511-** Pathological fracture in neoplastic disease, <u>right</u> shoulder

CC-A,K,P **M84.512-** Pathological fracture in neoplastic disease, <u>left</u> shoulder

CC-A,K,P **M84.519-** Pathological fracture in neoplastic disease, <u>unspecified</u> shoulder

M84.52- Pathological fracture in neoplastic disease, <u>humerus</u>

CC-A,K,P **M84.521-** Pathological fracture in neoplastic disease, <u>right</u> humerus

CC-A,K,P **M84.522-** Pathological fracture in neoplastic disease, <u>left</u> humerus

CC-A,K,P **M84.529-** Pathological fracture in neoplastic disease, <u>unspecified</u> humerus

M84.53- Pathological fracture in neoplastic disease, <u>ulna and radius</u>

CC-A,K,P **M84.531-** Pathological fracture in neoplastic disease, <u>right</u> ulna

CC-A,K,P **M84.532-** Pathological fracture in neoplastic disease, <u>left</u> ulna

CC-A,K,P **M84.533-** Pathological fracture in neoplastic disease, <u>right</u> radius

CC-A,K,P **M84.534-** Pathological fracture in neoplastic disease, <u>left</u> radius

CC-A,K,P **M84.539-** Pathological fracture in neoplastic disease, <u>unspecified</u> ulna and radius

M84.54- Pathological fracture in neoplastic disease, <u>hand</u>

CC-A,K,P **M84.541-** Pathological fracture in neoplastic disease, <u>right</u> hand

CC-A,K,P **M84.542-** Pathological fracture in neoplastic disease, <u>left</u> hand

CC-A,K,P **M84.549-** Pathological fracture in neoplastic disease, <u>unspecified</u> hand

M84.55- Pathological fracture in neoplastic disease, <u>pelvis and femur</u>

CC-A,K,P **M84.550-** Pathological fracture in neoplastic disease, pelvis

CC-A,K,P **M84.551-** Pathological fracture in neoplastic disease, <u>right</u> femur

CC-A,K,P **M84.552-** Pathological fracture in neoplastic disease, <u>left</u> femur

CC-A,K,P **M84.553-** Pathological fracture in neoplastic disease, <u>unspecified</u> femur

CC-A,K,P **M84.559-** Pathological fracture in neoplastic disease, hip, <u>unspecified</u>

M84.56- Pathological fracture in neoplastic disease, <u>tibia and fibula</u>

CC-A,K,P **M84.561-** Pathological fracture in neoplastic disease, <u>right</u> tibia

CC-A,K,P **M84.562-** Pathological fracture in neoplastic disease, <u>left</u> tibia

CC-A,K,P **M84.563-** Pathological fracture in neoplastic disease, <u>right</u> fibula

CC-A,K,P **M84.564-** Pathological fracture in neoplastic disease, <u>left</u> fibula

CC-A,K,P **M84.569-** Pathological fracture in neoplastic disease, <u>unspecified</u> tibia and fibula

M84.57- Pathological fracture in neoplastic disease, <u>ankle and foot</u>

CC-A,K,P **M84.571-** Pathological fracture in neoplastic disease, <u>right</u> ankle

CC-A,K,P **M84.572-** Pathological fracture in neoplastic disease, <u>left</u> ankle

CC-A,K,P **M84.573-** Pathological fracture in neoplastic disease, <u>unspecified</u> ankle

CC-A,K,P **M84.574-** Pathological fracture in neoplastic disease, <u>right</u> foot

CC-A,K,P **M84.575-** Pathological fracture in neoplastic disease, <u>left</u> foot

CC-A,K,P **M84.576-** Pathological fracture in neoplastic disease, <u>unspecified</u> foot

CC-A,K,P **M84.58x-** Pathological fracture in neoplastic disease, <u>other specified site</u>
Pathological fracture in neoplastic disease, vertebrae

M84.6- Pathological fracture <u>in other disease</u>
Code also underlying condition
Excludes 1:   *pathological fracture in osteoporosis (M80.-)*

The appropriate 7th character is to be added to each code from subcategory M84.6:
- **A**   Initial encounter for fracture
- **D**   Subsequent encounter for fracture with routine healing
- **G**   Subsequent encounter for fracture with delayed healing
- **K**   Subsequent encounter for fracture with nonunion
- **P**   Subsequent encounter for fracture with malunion
- **S**   Sequela

CC-A,K,P **M84.60x-** Pathological fracture in other disease, <u>unspecified</u> site

M84.61- Pathological fracture in other disease, <u>shoulder</u>

CC-A,K,P **M84.611-** Pathological fracture in other disease, <u>right</u> shoulder

CC-A,K,P **M84.612-** Pathological fracture in other disease, <u>left</u> shoulder

CC-A,K,P **M84.619-** Pathological fracture in other disease, <u>unspecified</u> shoulder

M84.62- Pathological fracture in other disease, <u>humerus</u>

CC-A,K,P **M84.621** Pathological fracture in other disease, <u>right</u> humerus

CC-A,K,P **M84.622-** Pathological fracture in other disease, <u>left</u> humerus

M84 - M84

CC-A,K,P **M84.629-** Pathological fracture in other disease, <u>unspecified</u> humerus

M84.63- Pathological fracture in other disease, <u>ulna and radius</u>

CC-A,K,P **M84.631-** Pathological fracture in other disease, <u>right</u> ulna

CC-A,K,P **M84.632-** Pathological fracture in other disease, <u>left</u> ulna

CC-A,K,P **M84.633-** Pathological fracture in other disease, <u>right</u> radius

CC-A,K,P **M84.634-** Pathological fracture in other disease, <u>left</u> radius

CC-A,K,P **M84.639-** Pathological fracture in other disease, <u>unspecified</u> ulna and radius

M84.64- Pathological fracture in other disease, <u>hand</u>

CC-A,K,P **M84.641-** Pathological fracture in other disease, <u>right</u> hand

CC-A,K,P **M84.642-** Pathological fracture in other disease, <u>left</u> hand

CC-A,K,P **M84.649-** Pathological fracture in other disease, <u>unspecified</u> hand

M84.65- Pathological fracture in other disease, <u>pelvis and femur</u>

CC-A,K,P **M84.650-** Pathological fracture in other disease, pelvis

CC-A,K,P **M84.651-** Pathological fracture in other disease, <u>right</u> femur

CC-A,K,P **M84.652-** Pathological fracture in other disease, <u>left</u> femur

CC-A,K,P **M84.653-** Pathological fracture in other disease, <u>unspecified</u> femur

CC-A,K,P **M84.659-** Pathological fracture in other disease, hip, <u>unspecified</u>

M84.66- Pathological fracture in other disease, <u>tibia and fibula</u>

CC-A,K,P **M84.661-** Pathological fracture in other disease, <u>right</u> tibia

CC-A,K,P **M84.662-** Pathological fracture in other disease, <u>left</u> tibia

CC-A,K,P **M84.663-** Pathological fracture in other disease, <u>right</u> fibula

CC-A,K,P **M84.664-** Pathological fracture in other disease, <u>left</u> fibula

CC-A,K,P **M84.669-** Pathological fracture in other disease, <u>unspecified</u> tibia and fibula

M84.67 Pathological fracture in other disease, ankle and foot

CC-A,K,P **M84.671-** Pathological fracture in other disease, <u>right</u> ankle

CC-A,K,P **M84.672-** Pathological fracture in other disease, <u>left</u> ankle

CC-A,K,P **M84.673-** Pathological fracture in other disease, <u>unspecified</u> ankle

CC-A,K,P **M84.674-** Pathological fracture in other disease, <u>right</u> foot

CC-A,K,P **M84.675-** Pathological fracture in other disease, <u>left</u> foot

CC-A,K,P **M84.676-** Pathological fracture in other disease, <u>unspecified</u> foot

CC-A,K,P **M84.68x-** Pathological fracture in other disease, <u>other site</u>

M84.7- Nontraumatic fracture, not elsewhere classified

M84.75- Atypical femoral fracture

> **The appropriate 7th character is to be added to each code from M84.75:**
> **A** Initial encounter for fracture
> **D** Subsequent encounter for fracture with routine healing
> **G** Subsequent encounter for fracture with delayed healing
> **K** Subsequent encounter for fracture with nonunion
> **P** Subsequent encounter for fracture with malunion
> **S** Sequela

CC-A,K,P **M84.750-** Atypical femoral fracture, <u>unspecified</u>

CC-A,K,P **M84.751-** <u>Incomplete</u> atypical femoral fracture, <u>right</u> leg

CC-A,K,P **M84.752-** <u>Incomplete</u> atypical femoral fracture, <u>left</u> leg

CC-A,K,P **M84.753-** <u>Incomplete</u> atypical femoral fracture, <u>unspecified</u> leg

CC-A,K,P **M84.754-** <u>Complete</u> transverse atypical femoral fracture, <u>right</u> leg

CC-A,K,P **M84.755-** <u>Complete</u> transverse atypical femoral fracture, <u>left</u> leg

CC-A,K,P **M84.756-** <u>Complete</u> transverse atypical femoral fracture, <u>unspecified</u> leg

CC-A,K,P **M84.757-** <u>Complete</u> oblique atypical femoral fracture, <u>right</u> leg

CC-A,K,P **M84.758-** <u>Complete</u> oblique atypical femoral fracture, <u>left</u> leg

CC-A,K,P **M84.759-** <u>Complete</u> oblique atypical femoral fracture, <u>unspecified</u> leg

M84.8- <u>Other disorders of continuity of bone</u>

M84.80 Other disorders of continuity of bone, <u>unspecified</u> <u>site</u>

M84.81- Other disorders of continuity of bone, <u>shoulder</u>

M84.811 Other disorders of continuity of bone, <u>right</u> shoulder

M84.812 Other disorders of continuity of bone, <u>left</u> shoulder

M84.819 Other disorders of continuity of bone, <u>unspecified</u> shoulder

M84.82- Other disorders of continuity of bone, <u>humerus</u>

M84.821 Other disorders of continuity of bone, <u>right</u> humerus

M84.822 Other disorders of continuity of bone, <u>left</u> humerus

M84.829 Other disorders of continuity of bone, <u>unspecified</u> humerus

M84.83- Other disorders of continuity of bone, <u>ulna and radius</u>

M84.831 Other disorders of continuity of bone, <u>right</u> ulna

M84.832 Other disorders of continuity of bone, <u>left</u> ulna

M84.833 Other disorders of continuity of bone, <u>right</u> radius

M84.834 Other disorders of continuity of bone, <u>left</u> radius

M84.839 Other disorders of continuity of bone, <u>unspecified</u> ulna and radius

M84.84- Other disorders of continuity of bone, <u>hand</u>

M84.841 Other disorders of continuity of bone, <u>right</u> hand

M84.842 Other disorders of continuity of bone, <u>left</u> hand

M84.849 Other disorders of continuity of bone, <u>unspecified</u> hand

M84.85- Other disorders of continuity of bone, <u>pelvic region and thigh</u>

M84.851 Other disorders of continuity of bone, <u>right</u> pelvic region and thigh

M84.852 Other disorders of continuity of bone, <u>left</u> pelvic region and thigh

M84.859 Other disorders of continuity of bone, <u>unspecified</u> pelvic region and thigh

M84.86- Other disorders of continuity of bone, <u>tibia and fibula</u>

M84.861 Other disorders of continuity of bone, <u>right</u> tibia

M84.862 Other disorders of continuity of bone, <u>left</u> tibia

M84.863 Other disorders of continuity of bone, <u>right</u> fibula

M84.864 Other disorders of continuity of bone, <u>left</u> fibula

M84.869 Other disorders of continuity of bone, <u>unspecified</u> tibia and fibula

M84.87- Other disorders of continuity of bone, <u>ankle and foot</u>

M84.871 Other disorders of continuity of bone, <u>right</u> ankle and foot

M84.872 Other disorders of continuity of bone, <u>left</u> ankle and foot

M84.879 Other disorders of continuity of bone, <u>unspecified</u> ankle and foot

M84.88 Other disorders of continuity of bone, <u>other site</u>

M84.9 Disorder of continuity of bone, <u>unspecified</u>

M85- <u>Other disorders of bone density and structure</u>
> *Excludes 1:* osteogenesis imperfecta (Q78.0)
> osteopetrosis (Q78.2)
> osteopoikilosis (Q78.8)
> polyostotic fibrous dysplasia (Q78.1)

M85.0- <u>Fibrous dysplasia (monostotic)</u> — The replacement the bone marrow with fibrous tissue that is limited to a single bone.
> *Excludes ❷:* fibrous dysplasia of jaw (M27.8)

M85.00 Fibrous dysplasia (monostotic), <u>unspecified</u> site

M85.01- Fibrous dysplasia (monostotic), <u>shoulder</u>

M85.011 Fibrous dysplasia (monostotic), <u>right</u> shoulder

M85.012 Fibrous dysplasia (monostotic), <u>left</u> shoulder

M85.019 Fibrous dysplasia (monostotic), <u>unspecified</u> shoulder

M85.02- Fibrous dysplasia (monostotic), <u>upper arm</u>

M85.021 Fibrous dysplasia (monostotic), <u>right</u> upper arm

M85.022 Fibrous dysplasia (monostotic), <u>left</u> upper arm

M84 - M85

M85.029   Fibrous dysplasia (monostotic), <u>unspecified</u> upper arm

M85.03- Fibrous dysplasia (monostotic), <u>forearm</u>
- M85.031   Fibrous dysplasia (monostotic), <u>right</u> forearm
- M85.032   Fibrous dysplasia (monostotic), <u>left</u> forearm
- M85.039   Fibrous dysplasia (monostotic), <u>unspecified</u> forearm

M85.04- Fibrous dysplasia (monostotic), <u>hand</u>
- M85.041   Fibrous dysplasia (monostotic), <u>right</u> hand
- M85.042   Fibrous dysplasia (monostotic), <u>left</u> hand
- M85.049   Fibrous dysplasia (monostotic), <u>unspecified</u> hand

M85.05- Fibrous dysplasia (monostotic), <u>thigh</u>
- M85.051   Fibrous dysplasia (monostotic), <u>right</u> thigh
- M85.052   Fibrous dysplasia (monostotic), <u>left</u> thigh
- M85.059   Fibrous dysplasia (monostotic), <u>unspecified</u> thigh

M85.06- Fibrous dysplasia (monostotic), <u>lower leg</u>
- M85.061   Fibrous dysplasia (monostotic), <u>right</u> lower leg
- M85.062   Fibrous dysplasia (monostotic), <u>left</u> lower leg
- M85.069   Fibrous dysplasia (monostotic), <u>unspecified</u> lower leg

M85.07   Fibrous dysplasia (monostotic), <u>ankle and foot</u>
- M85.071   Fibrous dysplasia (monostotic), <u>right</u> ankle and foot
- M85.072   Fibrous dysplasia (monostotic), <u>left</u> ankle and foot
- M85.079   Fibrous dysplasia (monostotic), <u>unspecified</u> ankle and foot

M85.08   Fibrous dysplasia (monostotic), <u>other site</u>

M85.09   Fibrous dysplasia (monostotic), <u>multiple sites</u>

M85.1-   Skeletal fluorosis — A bone disease marked by excessive fluoride accumulation in the bones.

M85.10   Skeletal fluorosis, <u>unspecified</u> <u>site</u>

M85.11- Skeletal fluorosis, <u>shoulder</u>
- M85.111   Skeletal fluorosis, <u>right</u> shoulder
- M85.112   Skeletal fluorosis, <u>left</u> shoulder
- M85.119   Skeletal fluorosis, <u>unspecified</u> shoulder

M85.12- Skeletal fluorosis, <u>upper arm</u>
- M85.121   Skeletal fluorosis, <u>right</u> upper arm
- M85.122   Skeletal fluorosis, <u>left</u> upper arm
- M85.129   Skeletal fluorosis, <u>unspecified</u> upper arm

M85.13- Skeletal fluorosis, <u>forearm</u>
- M85.131   Skeletal fluorosis, <u>right</u> forearm
- M85.132   Skeletal fluorosis, <u>left</u> forearm
- M85.139   Skeletal fluorosis, <u>unspecified</u> forearm

M85.14- Skeletal fluorosis, <u>hand</u>
- M85.141   Skeletal fluorosis, <u>right</u> hand
- M85.142   Skeletal fluorosis, <u>left</u> hand
- M85.149   Skeletal fluorosis, <u>unspecified</u> hand

M85.15- Skeletal fluorosis, <u>thigh</u>
- M85.151   Skeletal fluorosis, <u>right</u> thigh
- M85.152   Skeletal fluorosis, <u>left</u> thigh
- M85.159   Skeletal fluorosis, <u>unspecified</u> thigh

M85.16- Skeletal fluorosis, <u>lower leg</u>
- M85.161   Skeletal fluorosis, <u>right</u> lower leg
- M85.162   Skeletal fluorosis, <u>left</u> lower leg
- M85.169   Skeletal fluorosis, <u>unspecified</u> lower leg

M85.17- Skeletal fluorosis, <u>ankle and foot</u>
- M85.171   Skeletal fluorosis, <u>right</u> ankle and foot
- M85.172   Skeletal fluorosis, <u>left</u> ankle and foot
- M85.179   Skeletal fluorosis, <u>unspecified</u> ankle and foot

M85.18   Skeletal fluorosis, <u>other site</u>

M85.19   Skeletal fluorosis, <u>multiple sites</u>

M85.2   **Hyperostosis of skull** — The abnormal formation of new bone on the inner side of the cranial bones.

M85.3-   <u>Osteitis condensans</u> — Inflammation of the bone with the marrow cavity filled with osseous tissue.

M85.30   Osteitis condensans, <u>unspecified</u> <u>site</u>

M85.31- Osteitis condensans, shoulder
- M85.311   Osteitis condensans, <u>right</u> shoulder
- M85.312   Osteitis condensans, <u>left</u> shoulder
- M85.319   Osteitis condensans, <u>unspecified</u> shoulder

M85.32- Osteitis condensans, <u>upper arm</u>
- M85.321   Osteitis condensans, <u>right</u> upper arm
- M85.322   Osteitis condensans, <u>left</u> upper arm
- M85.329   Osteitis condensans, <u>unspecified</u> upper arm

M85.33- Osteitis condensans, <u>forearm</u>
- M85.331   Osteitis condensans, <u>right</u> forearm
- M85.332   Osteitis condensans, <u>left</u> forearm
- M85.339   Osteitis condensans, <u>unspecified</u> forearm

M85.34- Osteitis condensans, <u>hand</u>
- M85.341   Osteitis condensans, <u>right</u> hand
- M85.342   Osteitis condensans, <u>left</u> hand
- M85.349   Osteitis condensans, <u>unspecified</u> hand

M85.35- Osteitis condensans, <u>thigh</u>
- M85.351   Osteitis condensans, <u>right</u> thigh
- M85.352   Osteitis condensans, <u>left</u> thigh
- M85.359   Osteitis condensans, <u>unspecified</u> thigh

M85.36- Osteitis condensans, <u>lower leg</u>
- M85.361   Osteitis condensans, <u>right</u> lower leg
- M85.362   Osteitis condensans, <u>left</u> lower leg
- M85.369   Osteitis condensans, <u>unspecified</u> lower leg

M85.37- Osteitis condensans, <u>ankle and foot</u>
- M85.371   Osteitis condensans, <u>right</u> ankle and foot
- M85.372   Osteitis condensans, <u>left</u> ankle and foot
- M85.379   Osteitis condensans, <u>unspecified</u> ankle and foot

M85.38   Osteitis condensans, <u>other site</u>

M85.39   Osteitis condensans, <u>multiple sites</u>

M85.4-   <u>Solitary bone cyst</u> — An encapsulated space within bone tissue usually occurring in the metaphyses of long bones of children and adolescents.
    Excludes ❷: solitary cyst of jaw (M27.4)

M85.40   Solitary bone cyst, <u>unspecified</u> <u>site</u>

M85.41- Solitary bone cyst, <u>shoulder</u>
- M85.411   Solitary bone cyst, <u>right</u> shoulder
- M85.412   Solitary bone cyst, <u>left</u> shoulder
- M85.419   Solitary bone cyst, <u>unspecified</u> shoulder

M85.42- Solitary bone cyst, <u>humerus</u>
- M85.421   Solitary bone cyst, <u>right</u> humerus
- M85.422   Solitary bone cyst, <u>left</u> humerus
- M85.429   Solitary bone cyst, <u>unspecified</u> humerus

M85.43- Solitary bone cyst, <u>ulna and radius</u>
- M85.431   Solitary bone cyst, <u>right</u> ulna and radius
- M85.432   Solitary bone cyst, <u>left</u> ulna and radius
- M85.439   Solitary bone cyst, <u>unspecified</u> ulna and radius

M85.44- Solitary bone cyst, <u>hand</u>
- M85.441   Solitary bone cyst, <u>right</u> hand
- M85.442   Solitary bone cyst, <u>left</u> hand
- M85.449   Solitary bone cyst, <u>unspecified</u> hand

M85.45- Solitary bone cyst, <u>pelvis</u>
- M85.451   Solitary bone cyst, <u>right</u> pelvis
- M85.452   Solitary bone cyst, <u>left</u> pelvis
- M85.459   Solitary bone cyst, <u>unspecified</u> pelvis

M85.46- Solitary bone cyst, <u>tibia and fibula</u>
- M85.461   Solitary bone cyst, <u>right</u> tibia and fibula
- M85.462   Solitary bone cyst, <u>left</u> tibia and fibula
- M85.469   Solitary bone cyst, <u>unspecified</u> tibia and fibula

M85.47- Solitary bone cyst, <u>ankle and foot</u>
- M85.471   Solitary bone cyst, <u>right</u> ankle and foot
- M85.472   Solitary bone cyst, <u>left</u> ankle and foot
- M85.479   Solitary bone cyst, <u>unspecified</u> ankle and foot

M85 - M85

© 2016 Channel Publishing, Ltd.

M85.48 Solitary bone cyst, <u>other site</u>

M85.5- Aneurysmal bone cyst — A form producing a bulge in the bone cortex and appearing similar to an aneurysm.

 Excludes ❷: aneurysmal cyst of jaw (M27.4)

M85.50 Aneurysmal bone cyst, <u>unspecified</u> <u>site</u>

M85.51- Aneurysmal bone cyst, <u>shoulder</u>

 M85.511 Aneurysmal bone cyst, <u>right</u> shoulder

 M85.512 Aneurysmal bone cyst, <u>left</u> shoulder

 M85.519 Aneurysmal bone cyst, <u>unspecified</u> shoulder

M85.52- Aneurysmal bone cyst, <u>upper arm</u>

 M85.521 Aneurysmal bone cyst, <u>right</u> upper arm

 M85.522 Aneurysmal bone cyst, <u>left</u> upper arm

 M85.529 Aneurysmal bone cyst, <u>unspecified</u> upper arm

M85.53- Aneurysmal bone cyst, <u>forearm</u>

 M85.531 Aneurysmal bone cyst, <u>right</u> forearm

 M85.532 Aneurysmal bone cyst, <u>left</u> forearm

 M85.539 Aneurysmal bone cyst, <u>unspecified</u> forearm

M85.54- Aneurysmal bone cyst, <u>hand</u>

 M85.541 Aneurysmal bone cyst, <u>right</u> hand

 M85.542 Aneurysmal bone cyst, <u>left</u> hand

 M85.549 Aneurysmal bone cyst, <u>unspecified</u> hand

M85.55- Aneurysmal bone cyst, <u>thigh</u>

 M85.551 Aneurysmal bone cyst, <u>right</u> thigh

 M85.552 Aneurysmal bone cyst, <u>left</u> thigh

 M85.559 Aneurysmal bone cyst, <u>unspecified</u> thigh

M85.56- Aneurysmal bone cyst, <u>lower leg</u>

 M85.561 Aneurysmal bone cyst, <u>right</u> lower leg

 M85.562 Aneurysmal bone cyst, <u>left</u> lower leg

 M85.569 Aneurysmal bone cyst, <u>unspecified</u> lower leg

M85.57- Aneurysmal bone cyst, <u>ankle and foot</u>

 M85.571 Aneurysmal bone cyst, <u>right</u> ankle and foot

 M85.572 Aneurysmal bone cyst, <u>left</u> ankle and foot

 M85.579 Aneurysmal bone cyst, <u>unspecified</u> ankle and foot

M85.58 Aneurysmal bone cyst, <u>other site</u>

M85.59 Aneurysmal bone cyst, <u>multiple sites</u>

M85.6- <u>Other cyst</u> of bone

 Excludes 1: cyst of jaw NEC (M27.4)

  osteitis fibrosa cystica generalisata [von Recklinghausen's disease of bone] (E21.0)

M85.60 Other cyst of bone, <u>unspecified site</u>

M85.61- Other cyst of bone, <u>shoulder</u>

 M85.611 Other cyst of bone, <u>right</u> shoulder

 M85.612 Other cyst of bone, <u>left</u> shoulder

 M85.619 Other cyst of bone, <u>unspecified</u> shoulder

M85.62- Other cyst of bone, <u>upper arm</u>

 M85.621 Other cyst of bone, <u>right</u> upper arm

 M85.622 Other cyst of bone, <u>left</u> upper arm

 M85.629 Other cyst of bone, <u>unspecified</u> upper arm

M85.63- Other cyst of bone, <u>forearm</u>

 M85.631 Other cyst of bone, <u>right</u> forearm

 M85.632 Other cyst of bone, <u>left</u> forearm

 M85.639 Other cyst of bone, <u>unspecified</u> forearm

M85.64- Other cyst of bone, <u>hand</u>

 M85.641 Other cyst of bone, <u>right</u> hand

 M85.642 Other cyst of bone, <u>left</u> hand

 M85.649 Other cyst of bone, <u>unspecified</u> hand

M85.65- Other cyst of bone, <u>thigh</u>

 M85.651 Other cyst of bone, <u>right</u> thigh

 M85.652 Other cyst of bone, <u>left</u> thigh

 M85.659 Other cyst of bone, <u>unspecified</u> thigh

M85.66- Other cyst of bone, <u>lower leg</u>

 M85.661 Other cyst of bone, <u>right</u> lower leg

 M85.662 Other cyst of bone, <u>left</u> lower leg

 M85.669 Other cyst of bone, <u>unspecified</u> lower leg

M85.67- Other cyst of bone, <u>ankle and foot</u>

 M85.671 Other cyst of bone, <u>right</u> ankle and foot

 M85.672 Other cyst of bone, <u>left</u> ankle and foot

 M85.679 Other cyst of bone, <u>unspecified</u> ankle and foot

M85.68 Other cyst of bone, <u>other site</u>

M85.69 Other cyst of bone, <u>multiple sites</u>

M85.8- <u>Other specified</u> disorders of bone density and structure

 Hyperostosis of bones, except skull

 Osteosclerosis, acquired

 Excludes 1: diffuse idiopathic skeletal hyperostosis [DISH] (M48.1)

  osteosclerosis congenita (Q77.4)

  osteosclerosis fragilitas (generalista) (Q78.2)

  osteosclerosis myelofibrosis (D75.81)

M85.80 Other specified disorders of bone density and structure, <u>unspecified site</u>

M85.81- Other specified disorders of bone density and structure, <u>shoulder</u>

 M85.811 Other specified disorders of bone density and structure, <u>right</u> shoulder

 M85.812 Other specified disorders of bone density and structure, <u>left</u> shoulder

 M85.819 Other specified disorders of bone density and structure, <u>unspecified</u> shoulder

M85.82- Other specified disorders of bone density and structure, <u>upper arm</u>

 M85.821 Other specified disorders of bone density and structure, <u>right</u> upper arm

 M85.822 Other specified disorders of bone density and structure, <u>left</u> upper arm

 M85.829 Other specified disorders of bone density and structure, <u>unspecified</u> upper arm

M85.83- Other specified disorders of bone density and structure, <u>forearm</u>

 M85.831 Other specified disorders of bone density and structure, <u>right</u> forearm

 M85.832 Other specified disorders of bone density and structure, <u>left</u> forearm

 M85.839 Other specified disorders of bone density and structure, <u>unspecified</u> forearm

M85.84- Other specified disorders of bone density and structure, <u>hand</u>

 M85.841 Other specified disorders of bone density and structure, <u>right</u> hand

 M85.842 Other specified disorders of bone density and structure, <u>left</u> hand

 M85.849 Other specified disorders of bone density and structure, <u>unspecified</u> hand

M85.85- Other specified disorders of bone density and structure, <u>thigh</u>

 M85.851 Other specified disorders of bone density and structure, <u>right</u> thigh

 M85.852 Other specified disorders of bone density and structure, <u>left</u> thigh

 M85.859 Other specified disorders of bone density and structure, <u>unspecified</u> thigh

M85.86- Other specified disorders of bone density and structure, <u>lower leg</u>

 M85.861 Other specified disorders of bone density and structure, <u>right</u> lower leg

 M85.862 Other specified disorders of bone density and structure, <u>left</u> lower leg

 M85.869 Other specified disorders of bone density and structure, <u>unspecified</u> lower leg

M85.87- Other specified disorders of bone density and structure, <u>ankle and foot</u>

 M85.871 Other specified disorders of bone density and structure, <u>right</u> ankle and foot

 M85.872 Other specified disorders of bone density and structure, <u>left</u> ankle and foot

M 8 5 – M 8 5

Excludes 1: = NOT CODED HERE! (Do not code both)

Excludes ❷: = Not Included Here

M85.879　Other specified disorders of bone density and structure, <u>unspecified</u> ankle and foot

M85.88　Other specified disorders of bone density and structure, <u>other site</u>

M85.89　Other specified disorders of bone density and structure, <u>multiple sites</u>

M85.9　Disorder of bone density and structure, <u>unspecified</u>

Other osteopathies (M86-M90)

Excludes 1:　postprocedural osteopathies (M96.-)

M86-　<u>Osteomyelitis</u> — Inflammation of the bone or bone marrow.
Use additional code (B95-B97) to identify infectious agent
Use additional code to identify major osseous defect, if applicable (M89.7-)
Excludes 1:　osteomyelitis due to:
　　　　echinococcus (B67.2)
　　　　gonococcus (A54.43)
　　　　salmonella (A02.24)
Excludes ❷:　ostemyelitis of:
　　　　orbit (H05.0-)
　　　　petrous bone (H70.2-)
　　　　vertebra (M46.2-)

M86.0-　<u>Acute hematogenous</u> osteomyelitis — The sudden, severe onset of inflammation of the bone caused by microorganisms that invade through the bloodstream.

cc **M86.00**　Acute hematogenous osteomyelitis, <u>unspecified</u> <u>site</u>

M86.01-Acute hematogenous osteomyelitis, <u>shoulder</u>

cc **M86.011**　Acute hematogenous osteomyelitis, <u>right</u> shoulder

cc **M86.012**　Acute hematogenous osteomyelitis, <u>left</u> shoulder

cc **M86.019**　Acute hematogenous osteomyelitis, <u>unspecified</u> shoulder

M86.02-Acute hematogenous osteomyelitis, <u>humerus</u>

cc **M86.021**　Acute hematogenous osteomyelitis, <u>right</u> humerus

cc **M86.022**　Acute hematogenous osteomyelitis, <u>left</u> humerus

cc **M86.029**　Acute hematogenous osteomyelitis, <u>unspecified</u> humerus

M86.03-Acute hematogenous osteomyelitis, <u>radius and ulna</u>

cc **M86.031**　Acute hematogenous osteomyelitis, <u>right</u> radius and ulna

cc **M86.032**　Acute hematogenous osteomyelitis, <u>left</u> radius and ulna

cc **M86.039**　Acute hematogenous osteomyelitis, <u>unspecified</u> radius and ulna

M86.04-Acute hematogenous osteomyelitis, <u>hand</u>

cc **M86.041**　Acute hematogenous osteomyelitis, <u>right</u> hand

cc **M86.042**　Acute hematogenous osteomyelitis, <u>left</u> hand

cc **M86.049**　Acute hematogenous osteomyelitis, <u>unspecified</u> hand

M86.05-Acute hematogenous osteomyelitis, <u>femur</u>

cc **M86.051**　Acute hematogenous osteomyelitis, <u>right</u> femur

cc **M86.052**　Acute hematogenous osteomyelitis, <u>left</u> femur

cc **M86.059**　Acute hematogenous osteomyelitis, <u>unspecified</u> femur

M86.06-Acute hematogenous osteomyelitis, <u>tibia and fibula</u>

cc **M86.061**　Acute hematogenous osteomyelitis, <u>right</u> tibia and fibula

cc **M86.062**　Acute hematogenous osteomyelitis, <u>left</u> tibia and fibula

cc **M86.069**　Acute hematogenous osteomyelitis, <u>unspecified</u> tibia and fibula

M86.07-Acute hematogenous osteomyelitis, <u>ankle and foot</u>

cc **M86.071**　Acute hematogenous osteomyelitis, <u>right</u> ankle and foot

cc **M86.072**　Acute hematogenous osteomyelitis, <u>left</u> ankle and foot

cc **M86.079**　Acute hematogenous osteomyelitis, <u>unspecified</u> ankle and foot

cc **M86.08**　Acute hematogenous osteomyelitis, <u>other sites</u>

cc **M86.09**　Acute hematogenous osteomyelitis, <u>multiple sites</u>

M86.1-　<u>Other acute</u> osteomyelitis

cc **M86.10**　Other acute osteomyelitis, <u>unspecified</u> <u>site</u>

M86.11-Other acute osteomyelitis, <u>shoulder</u>

cc **M86.111**　Other acute osteomyelitis, <u>right</u> shoulder

cc **M86.112**　Other acute osteomyelitis, <u>left</u> shoulder

cc **M86.119**　Other acute osteomyelitis, <u>unspecified</u> shoulder

M86.12-Other acute osteomyelitis, <u>humerus</u>

cc **M86.121**　Other acute osteomyelitis, <u>right</u> humerus

cc **M86.122**　Other acute osteomyelitis, <u>left</u> humerus

cc **M86.129**　Other acute osteomyelitis, <u>unspecified</u> humerus

M86.13-Other acute osteomyelitis, <u>radius and ulna</u>

cc **M86.131**　Other acute osteomyelitis, <u>right</u> radius and ulna

cc **M86.132**　Other acute osteomyelitis, <u>left</u> radius and ulna

cc **M86.139**　Other acute osteomyelitis, <u>unspecified</u> radius and ulna

M86.14-Other acute osteomyelitis, <u>hand</u>

cc **M86.141**　Other acute osteomyelitis, <u>right</u> hand

cc **M86.142**　Other acute osteomyelitis, <u>left</u> hand

cc **M86.149**　Other acute osteomyelitis, <u>unspecified</u> hand

M86.15-Other acute osteomyelitis, <u>femur</u>

cc **M86.151**　Other acute osteomyelitis, <u>right</u> femur

cc **M86.152**　Other acute osteomyelitis, <u>left</u> femur

cc **M86.159**　Other acute osteomyelitis, <u>unspecified</u> femur

M86.16-Other acute osteomyelitis, <u>tibia and fibula</u>

cc **M86.161**　Other acute osteomyelitis, <u>right</u> tibia and fibula

cc **M86.162**　Other acute osteomyelitis, <u>left</u> tibia and fibula

cc **M86.169**　Other acute osteomyelitis, <u>unspecified</u> tibia and fibula

M86.17-Other acute osteomyelitis, <u>ankle and foot</u>

cc **M86.171**　Other acute osteomyelitis, <u>right</u> ankle and foot

cc **M86.172**　Other acute osteomyelitis, <u>left</u> ankle and foot

cc **M86.179**　Other acute osteomyelitis, <u>unspecified</u> ankle and foot

cc **M86.18**　Other acute osteomyelitis, <u>other site</u>

cc **M86.19**　Other acute osteomyelitis, <u>multiple sites</u>

M86.2-　<u>Subacute</u> osteomyelitis

cc **M86.20**　Subacute osteomyelitis, <u>unspecified</u> <u>site</u>

M86.21-Subacute osteomyelitis, <u>shoulder</u>

cc **M86.211**　Subacute osteomyelitis, <u>right</u> shoulder

cc **M86.212**　Subacute osteomyelitis, <u>left</u> shoulder

cc **M86.219**　Subacute osteomyelitis, <u>unspecified</u> shoulder

M86.22-Subacute osteomyelitis, <u>humerus</u>

cc **M86.221**　Subacute osteomyelitis, <u>right</u> humerus

cc **M86.222**　Subacute osteomyelitis, <u>left</u> humerus

cc **M86.229**　Subacute osteomyelitis, <u>unspecified</u> humerus

M86.23-Subacute osteomyelitis, <u>radius and ulna</u>

cc **M86.231**　Subacute osteomyelitis, <u>right</u> radius and ulna

cc **M86.232**　Subacute osteomyelitis, <u>left</u> radius and ulna

cc **M86.239**　Subacute osteomyelitis, <u>unspecified</u> radius and ulna

M86.24-Subacute osteomyelitis, <u>hand</u>

cc **M86.241**　Subacute osteomyelitis, <u>right</u> hand

cc **M86.242**　Subacute osteomyelitis, <u>left</u> hand

cc **M86.249**　Subacute osteomyelitis, <u>unspecified</u> hand

M86.25-Subacute osteomyelitis, <u>femur</u>

cc **M86.251**　Subacute osteomyelitis, <u>right</u> femur

cc **M86.252**　Subacute osteomyelitis, <u>left</u> femur

cc **M86.259**　Subacute osteomyelitis, <u>unspecified</u> femur

M86.26-Subacute osteomyelitis, <u>tibia and fibula</u>

cc **M86.261**　Subacute osteomyelitis, <u>right</u> tibia and fibula

cc **M86.262**　Subacute osteomyelitis, <u>left</u> tibia and fibula

cc **M86.269**　Subacute osteomyelitis, <u>unspecified</u> tibia and fibula

M86.27-Subacute osteomyelitis, <u>ankle and foot</u>

cc **M86.271**　Subacute osteomyelitis, <u>right</u> ankle and foot

M85 | M86

cc M86.272   Subacute osteomyelitis, <u>left</u> ankle and foot

cc M86.279   Subacute osteomyelitis, <u>unspecified</u> ankle and foot

cc M86.28   Subacute osteomyelitis, <u>other site</u>

cc M86.29   Subacute osteomyelitis, <u>multiple sites</u>

M86.3-   <u>Chronic multifocal</u> osteomyelitis — An autoinflammatory recurrent disease of the bone that is characterized by inflammation, bone lesions, periodic fevers, and bone pain.

cc M86.30   Chronic multifocal osteomyelitis, <u>unspecified site</u>

M86.31-   Chronic multifocal osteomyelitis, <u>shoulder</u>

   cc M86.311   Chronic multifocal osteomyelitis, <u>right</u> shoulder

   cc M86.312   Chronic multifocal osteomyelitis, <u>left</u> shoulder

   cc M86.319   Chronic multifocal osteomyelitis, <u>unspecified</u> shoulder

M86.32-   Chronic multifocal osteomyelitis, <u>humerus</u>

   cc M86.321   Chronic multifocal osteomyelitis, <u>right</u> humerus

   cc M86.322   Chronic multifocal osteomyelitis, <u>left</u> humerus

   cc M86.329   Chronic multifocal osteomyelitis, <u>unspecified</u> humerus

M86.33-   Chronic multifocal osteomyelitis, <u>radius and ulna</u>

   cc M86.331   Chronic multifocal osteomyelitis, <u>right</u> radius and ulna

   cc M86.332   Chronic multifocal osteomyelitis, <u>left</u> radius and ulna

   cc M86.339   Chronic multifocal osteomyelitis, <u>unspecified</u> radius and ulna

M86.34-   Chronic multifocal osteomyelitis, <u>hand</u>

   cc M86.341   Chronic multifocal osteomyelitis, <u>right</u> hand

   cc M86.342   Chronic multifocal osteomyelitis, <u>left</u> hand

   cc M86.349   Chronic multifocal osteomyelitis, <u>unspecified</u> hand

M86.35-   Chronic multifocal osteomyelitis, <u>femur</u>

   cc M86.351   Chronic multifocal osteomyelitis, <u>right</u> femur

   cc M86.352   Chronic multifocal osteomyelitis, <u>left</u> femur

   cc M86.359   Chronic multifocal osteomyelitis, <u>unspecified</u> femur

M86.36-   Chronic multifocal osteomyelitis, <u>tibia and fibula</u>

   cc M86.361   Chronic multifocal osteomyelitis, <u>right</u> tibia and fibula

   cc M86.362   Chronic multifocal osteomyelitis, <u>left</u> tibia and fibula

   cc M86.369   Chronic multifocal osteomyelitis, <u>unspecified</u> tibia and fibula

M86.37-   Chronic multifocal osteomyelitis, <u>ankle and foot</u>

   cc M86.371   Chronic multifocal osteomyelitis, <u>right</u> ankle and foot

   cc M86.372   Chronic multifocal osteomyelitis, <u>left</u> ankle and foot

   cc M86.379   Chronic multifocal osteomyelitis, <u>unspecified</u> ankle and foot

cc M86.38   Chronic multifocal osteomyelitis, <u>other site</u>

cc M86.39   Chronic multifocal osteomyelitis, <u>multiple sites</u>

M86.4-   <u>Chronic</u> osteomyelitis <u>with draining sinus</u> — Inflammation of the bone caused by microorganisms that develops slowly and persists over a long period of time and creates a suppuration passage to the skin or other tissues.

cc M86.40   Chronic osteomyelitis with draining sinus, <u>unspecified site</u>

M86.41-   Chronic osteomyelitis with draining sinus, <u>shoulder</u>

   cc M86.411   Chronic osteomyelitis with draining sinus, <u>right</u> shoulder

   cc M86.412   Chronic osteomyelitis with draining sinus, <u>left</u> shoulder

   cc M86.419   Chronic osteomyelitis with draining sinus, <u>unspecified</u> shoulder

M86.42-   Chronic osteomyelitis with draining sinus, <u>humerus</u>

   cc M86.421   Chronic osteomyelitis with draining sinus, <u>right</u> humerus

   cc M86.422   Chronic osteomyelitis with draining sinus, <u>left</u> humerus

   cc M86.429   Chronic osteomyelitis with draining sinus, <u>unspecified</u> humerus

M86.43-   Chronic osteomyelitis with draining sinus, <u>radius and ulna</u>

   cc M86.431   Chronic osteomyelitis with draining sinus, <u>right</u> radius and ulna

   cc M86.432   Chronic osteomyelitis with draining sinus, <u>left</u> radius and ulna

   cc M86.439   Chronic osteomyelitis with draining sinus, <u>unspecified</u> radius and ulna

M86.44-   Chronic osteomyelitis with draining sinus, <u>hand</u>

   cc M86.441   Chronic osteomyelitis with draining sinus, <u>right</u> hand

   cc M86.442   Chronic osteomyelitis with draining sinus, <u>left</u> hand

   cc M86.449   Chronic osteomyelitis with draining sinus, <u>unspecified</u> hand

M86.45-   Chronic osteomyelitis with draining sinus, <u>femur</u>

   cc M86.451   Chronic osteomyelitis with draining sinus, <u>right</u> femur

   cc M86.452   Chronic osteomyelitis with draining sinus, <u>left</u> femur

   cc M86.459   Chronic osteomyelitis with draining sinus, <u>unspecified</u> femur

M86.46-   Chronic osteomyelitis with draining sinus, <u>tibia and fibula</u>

   cc M86.461   Chronic osteomyelitis with draining sinus, <u>right</u> tibia and fibula

   cc M86.462   Chronic osteomyelitis with draining sinus, <u>left</u> tibia and fibula

   cc M86.469   Chronic osteomyelitis with draining sinus, <u>unspecified</u> tibia and fibula

M86.47-   Chronic osteomyelitis with draining sinus, <u>ankle and foot</u>

   cc M86.471   Chronic osteomyelitis with draining sinus, <u>right</u> ankle and foot

   cc M86.472   Chronic osteomyelitis with draining sinus, <u>left</u> ankle and foot

   cc M86.479   Chronic osteomyelitis with draining sinus, <u>unspecified</u> ankle and foot

cc M86.48   Chronic osteomyelitis with draining sinus, <u>other site</u>

cc M86.49   Chronic osteomyelitis with draining sinus, <u>multiple sites</u>

M86.5-   <u>Other chronic hematogenous</u> osteomyelitis — Inflammation of the bone caused by microorganisms that invade through the bloodstream and that develops slowly and persists over a long period of time.

cc M86.50   Other chronic hematogenous osteomyelitis, <u>unspecified site</u>

M86.51-   Other chronic hematogenous osteomyelitis, <u>shoulder</u>

   cc M86.511   Other chronic hematogenous osteomyelitis, <u>right</u> shoulder

   cc M86.512   Other chronic hematogenous osteomyelitis, <u>left</u> shoulder

   cc M86.519   Other chronic hematogenous osteomyelitis, <u>unspecified</u> shoulder

M86.52-   Other chronic hematogenous osteomyelitis, <u>humerus</u>

   cc M86.521   Other chronic hematogenous osteomyelitis, <u>right</u> humerus

   cc M86.522   Other chronic hematogenous osteomyelitis, <u>left</u> humerus

   cc M86.529   Other chronic hematogenous osteomyelitis, <u>unspecified</u> humerus

M86.53-   Other chronic hematogenous osteomyelitis, <u>radius and ulna</u>

   cc M86.531   Other chronic hematogenous osteomyelitis, <u>right</u> radius and ulna

   cc M86.532   Other chronic hematogenous osteomyelitis, <u>left</u> radius and ulna

   cc M86.539   Other chronic hematogenous osteomyelitis, <u>unspecified</u> radius and ulna

M86.54-   Other chronic hematogenous osteomyelitis, <u>hand</u>

   cc M86.541   Other chronic hematogenous osteomyelitis, <u>right</u> hand

M86 - M86

cc M86.542   Other chronic hematogenous osteomyelitis, <u>left</u> hand

cc M86.549   Other chronic hematogenous osteomyelitis, <u>unspecified</u> hand

M86.55- Other chronic hematogenous osteomyelitis, <u>femur</u>

    cc M86.551   Other chronic hematogenous osteomyelitis, <u>right</u> femur

    cc M86.552   Other chronic hematogenous osteomyelitis, <u>left</u> femur

    cc M86.559   Other chronic hematogenous osteomyelitis, <u>unspecified</u> femur

M86.56- Other chronic hematogenous osteomyelitis, <u>tibia and fibula</u>

    cc M86.561   Other chronic hematogenous osteomyelitis, <u>right</u> tibia and fibula

    cc M86.562   Other chronic hematogenous osteomyelitis, <u>left</u> tibia and fibula

    cc M86.569   Other chronic hematogenous osteomyelitis, <u>unspecified</u> tibia and fibula

M86.57- Other chronic hematogenous osteomyelitis, <u>ankle and foot</u>

    cc M86.571   Other chronic hematogenous osteomyelitis, <u>right</u> ankle and foot

    cc M86.572   Other chronic hematogenous osteomyelitis, <u>left</u> ankle and foot

    cc M86.579   Other chronic hematogenous osteomyelitis, <u>unspecified</u> ankle and foot

cc M86.58   Other chronic hematogenous osteomyelitis, <u>other site</u>

cc M86.59   Other chronic hematogenous osteomyelitis, <u>multiple sites</u>

M86.6-   <u>Other chronic</u> osteomyelitis

cc M86.60   Other chronic osteomyelitis, <u>unspecified site</u>

M86.61- Other chronic osteomyelitis, <u>shoulder</u>

    cc M86.611   Other chronic osteomyelitis, <u>right</u> shoulder

    cc M86.612   Other chronic osteomyelitis, <u>left</u> shoulder

    cc M86.619   Other chronic osteomyelitis, <u>unspecified</u> shoulder

M86.62- Other chronic osteomyelitis, <u>humerus</u>

    cc M86.621   Other chronic osteomyelitis, <u>right</u> humerus

    cc M86.622   Other chronic osteomyelitis, <u>left</u> humerus

    cc M86.629   Other chronic osteomyelitis, <u>unspecified</u> humerus

M86.63- Other chronic osteomyelitis, <u>radius and ulna</u>

    cc M86.631   Other chronic osteomyelitis, <u>right</u> radius and ulna

    cc M86.632   Other chronic osteomyelitis, <u>left</u> radius and ulna

    cc M86.639   Other chronic osteomyelitis, <u>unspecified</u> radius and ulna

M86.64- Other chronic osteomyelitis, <u>hand</u>

    cc M86.641   Other chronic osteomyelitis, <u>right</u> hand

    cc M86.642   Other chronic osteomyelitis, <u>left</u> hand

    cc M86.649   Other chronic osteomyelitis, <u>unspecified</u> hand

M86.65- Other chronic osteomyelitis, <u>thigh</u>

    cc M86.651   Other chronic osteomyelitis, <u>right</u> thigh

    cc M86.652   Other chronic osteomyelitis, <u>left</u> thigh

    cc M86.659   Other chronic osteomyelitis, <u>unspecified</u> thigh

M86.66- Other chronic osteomyelitis, <u>tibia and fibula</u>

    cc M86.661   Other chronic osteomyelitis, <u>right</u> tibia and fibula

    cc M86.662   Other chronic osteomyelitis, <u>left</u> tibia and fibula

    cc M86.669   Other chronic osteomyelitis, <u>unspecified</u> tibia and fibula

M86.67- Other chronic osteomyelitis, <u>ankle and foot</u>

    cc M86.671   Other chronic osteomyelitis, <u>right</u> ankle and foot

    cc M86.672   Other chronic osteomyelitis, <u>left</u> ankle and foot

    cc M86.679   Other chronic osteomyelitis, <u>unspecified</u> ankle and foot

cc M86.68   Other chronic osteomyelitis, <u>other site</u>

cc M86.69   Other chronic osteomyelitis, <u>multiple sites</u>

M86.8-   Other osteomyelitis
    Brodie's abscess — A localized necrosis of bone.

M86.8x- <u>Other</u> osteomyelitis

    cc M86.8x0   Other osteomyelitis, multiple sites

    cc M86.8x1   Other osteomyelitis, shoulder

    cc M86.8x2   Other osteomyelitis, upper arm

    cc M86.8x3   Other osteomyelitis, forearm

    cc M86.8x4   Other osteomyelitis, hand

    cc M86.8x5   Other osteomyelitis, thigh

    cc M86.8x6   Other osteomyelitis, lower leg

    cc M86.8x7   Other osteomyelitis, ankle and foot

    cc M86.8x8   Other osteomyelitis, other site

    cc M86.8x9   Other osteomyelitis, unspecified sites

cc M86.9   Osteomyelitis, <u>unspecified</u>
    Infection of bone NOS
    Periostitis without osteomyelitis

M87-   <u>Osteonecrosis</u> — The condition of progressive sclerosis and death of bone tissue that is due to decreased blood flow to the bone.
    Includes: Avascular necrosis of bone
    Use additional code to identify major osseous defect, if applicable (M89.7-)
    Excludes 1:   *juvenile osteonecrosis (M91-M92)*
                 osteochondropathies (M90-M93)

M87.0-   <u>Idiopathic aseptic necrosis of bone</u> — A form of unknown etiology.

cc M87.00   Idiopathic aseptic necrosis of <u>unspecified</u> <u>bone</u>

M87.01- Idiopathic aseptic necrosis of <u>shoulder</u>
    Idiopathic aseptic necrosis of clavicle and scapula

    cc M87.011   Idiopathic aseptic necrosis of <u>right</u> shoulder

    cc M87.012   Idiopathic aseptic necrosis of <u>left</u> shoulder

    cc M87.019   Idiopathic aseptic necrosis of <u>unspecified</u> shoulder

M87.02- Idiopathic aseptic necrosis of <u>humerus</u>

    cc M87.021   Idiopathic aseptic necrosis of <u>right</u> humerus

    cc M87.022   Idiopathic aseptic necrosis of <u>left</u> humerus

    cc M87.029   Idiopathic aseptic necrosis of <u>unspecified</u> humerus

M87.03- Idiopathic aseptic necrosis of <u>radius, ulna and carpus</u>

    cc M87.031   Idiopathic aseptic necrosis of <u>right</u> radius

    cc M87.032   Idiopathic aseptic necrosis of <u>left</u> radius

    cc M87.033   Idiopathic aseptic necrosis of <u>unspecified</u> radius

    cc M87.034   Idiopathic aseptic necrosis of <u>right</u> ulna

    cc M87.035   Idiopathic aseptic necrosis of <u>left</u> ulna

    cc M87.036   Idiopathic aseptic necrosis of <u>unspecified</u> ulna

    cc M87.037   Idiopathic aseptic necrosis of <u>right</u> carpus

    cc M87.038   Idiopathic aseptic necrosis of <u>left</u> carpus

    cc M87.039   Idiopathic aseptic necrosis of <u>unspecified</u> carpus

M87.04- Idiopathic aseptic necrosis of <u>hand and fingers</u>
    Idiopathic aseptic necrosis of metacarpals and phalanges of hands

    cc M87.041   Idiopathic aseptic necrosis of <u>right</u> hand

    cc M87.042   Idiopathic aseptic necrosis of <u>left</u> hand

    cc M87.043   Idiopathic aseptic necrosis of <u>unspecified</u> hand

    cc M87.044   Idiopathic aseptic necrosis of <u>right</u> finger(s)

    cc M87.045   Idiopathic aseptic necrosis of <u>left</u> finger(s)

    cc M87.046   Idiopathic aseptic necrosis of <u>unspecified</u> finger(s)

M87.05- Idiopathic aseptic necrosis of <u>pelvis and femur</u>

    cc M87.050   Idiopathic aseptic necrosis of pelvis

    cc M87.051   Idiopathic aseptic necrosis of <u>right</u> femur

    cc M87.052   Idiopathic aseptic necrosis of <u>left</u> femur

    cc M87.059   Idiopathic aseptic necrosis of <u>unspecified</u> femur
          Idiopathic aseptic necrosis of hip NOS

M87.06- Idiopathic aseptic necrosis of <u>tibia and fibula</u>

    cc M87.061   Idiopathic aseptic necrosis of <u>right</u> tibia

    cc M87.062   Idiopathic aseptic necrosis of <u>left</u> tibia

    cc M87.063   Idiopathic aseptic necrosis of <u>unspecified</u> tibia

    cc M87.064   Idiopathic aseptic necrosis of <u>right</u> fibula

    cc M87.065   Idiopathic aseptic necrosis of <u>left</u> fibula

    cc M87.066   Idiopathic aseptic necrosis of <u>unspecified</u> fibula

M86 - M87

Excludes 1: = NOT CODED HERE! (Do not code both)   885   *Excludes ❷:* = Not Included Here

M87.07- Idiopathic aseptic necrosis of <u>ankle, foot and toes</u>
Idiopathic aseptic necrosis of metatarsus, tarsus, and phalanges of toes

cc **M87.071** Idiopathic aseptic necrosis of <u>right</u> ankle

cc **M87.072** Idiopathic aseptic necrosis of <u>left</u> ankle

cc **M87.073** Idiopathic aseptic necrosis of <u>unspecified</u> ankle

cc **M87.074** Idiopathic aseptic necrosis of <u>right</u> foot

cc **M87.075** Idiopathic aseptic necrosis of <u>left</u> foot

cc **M87.076** Idiopathic aseptic necrosis of <u>unspecified</u> foot

cc **M87.077** Idiopathic aseptic necrosis of <u>right</u> toe(s)

cc **M87.078** Idiopathic aseptic necrosis of <u>left</u> toe(s)

cc **M87.079** Idiopathic aseptic necrosis of <u>unspecified</u> toe(s)

cc **M87.08** Idiopathic aseptic necrosis of bone, <u>other site</u>

cc **M87.09** Idiopathic aseptic necrosis of bone, <u>multiple sites</u>

M87.1- Osteonecrosis <u>due to drugs</u>
Use additional code for adverse effect, if applicable, to identify drug (T36-T50 with fifth or sixth character 5)

cc **M87.10** Osteonecrosis due to drugs, <u>unspecified</u> <u>bone</u>

M87.11- Osteonecrosis due to drugs, <u>shoulder</u>

cc **M87.111** Osteonecrosis due to drugs, <u>right</u> shoulder

cc **M87.112** Osteonecrosis due to drugs, <u>left</u> shoulder

cc **M87.119** Osteonecrosis due to drugs, <u>unspecified</u> shoulder

M87.12- Osteonecrosis due to drugs, <u>humerus</u>

cc **M87.121** Osteonecrosis due to drugs, <u>right</u> humerus

cc **M87.122** Osteonecrosis due to drugs, <u>left</u> humerus

cc **M87.129** Osteonecrosis due to drugs, <u>unspecified</u> humerus

M87.13- Osteonecrosis due to drugs of <u>radius, ulna and carpus</u>

cc **M87.131** Osteonecrosis due to drugs of <u>right</u> radius

cc **M87.132** Osteonecrosis due to drugs of <u>left</u> radius

cc **M87.133** Osteonecrosis due to drugs of <u>unspecified</u> radius

cc **M87.134** Osteonecrosis due to drugs of <u>right</u> ulna

cc **M87.135** Osteonecrosis due to drugs of <u>left</u> ulna

cc **M87.136** Osteonecrosis due to drugs of <u>unspecified</u> ulna

cc **M87.137** Osteonecrosis due to drugs of <u>right</u> carpus

cc **M87.138** Osteonecrosis due to drugs of <u>left</u> carpus

cc **M87.139** Osteonecrosis due to drugs of <u>unspecified</u> carpus

M87.14- Osteonecrosis due to drugs, <u>hand and fingers</u>

cc **M87.141** Osteonecrosis due to drugs, <u>right</u> hand

cc **M87.142** Osteonecrosis due to drugs, <u>left</u> hand

cc **M87.143** Osteonecrosis due to drugs, <u>unspecified</u> hand

cc **M87.144** Osteonecrosis due to drugs, <u>right</u> finger(s)

cc **M87.145** Osteonecrosis due to drugs, <u>left</u> finger(s)

cc **M87.146** Osteonecrosis due to drugs, <u>unspecified</u> finger(s)

M87.15- Osteonecrosis due to drugs, <u>pelvis and femur</u>

cc **M87.150** Osteonecrosis due to drugs, pelvis

cc **M87.151** Osteonecrosis due to drugs, <u>right</u> femur

cc **M87.152** Osteonecrosis due to drugs, <u>left</u> femur

cc **M87.159** Osteonecrosis due to drugs, <u>unspecified</u> femur

M87.16- Osteonecrosis due to drugs, <u>tibia and fibula</u>

cc **M87.161** Osteonecrosis due to drugs, <u>right</u> tibia

cc **M87.162** Osteonecrosis due to drugs, <u>left</u> tibia

cc **M87.163** Osteonecrosis due to drugs, <u>unspecified</u> tibia

cc **M87.164** Osteonecrosis due to drugs, <u>right</u> fibula

cc **M87.165** Osteonecrosis due to drugs, <u>left</u> fibula

cc **M87.166** Osteonecrosis due to drugs, <u>unspecified</u> fibula

M87.17- Osteonecrosis due to drugs, <u>ankle, foot and toes</u>

cc **M87.171** Osteonecrosis due to drugs, <u>right</u> ankle

cc **M87.172** Osteonecrosis due to drugs, <u>left</u> ankle

cc **M87.173** Osteonecrosis due to drugs, <u>unspecified</u> ankle

cc **M87.174** Osteonecrosis due to drugs, <u>right</u> foot

cc **M87.175** Osteonecrosis due to drugs, <u>left</u> foot

cc **M87.176** Osteonecrosis due to drugs, <u>unspecified</u> foot

cc **M87.177** Osteonecrosis due to drugs, <u>right</u> toe(s)

cc **M87.178** Osteonecrosis due to drugs, <u>left</u> toe(s)

cc **M87.179** Osteonecrosis due to drugs, <u>unspecified</u> toe(s)

M87.18- Osteonecrosis due to drugs, <u>other site</u>

cc **M87.180** Osteonecrosis due to drugs, <u>jaw</u>

cc **M87.188** Osteonecrosis due to drugs, <u>other site</u>

cc **M87.19** Osteonecrosis due to drugs, <u>multiple sites</u>

M87.2- Osteonecrosis <u>due to previous trauma</u>

cc **M87.20** Osteonecrosis due to previous trauma, <u>unspecified</u> <u>bone</u>

M87.21- Osteonecrosis due to previous trauma, <u>shoulder</u>

cc **M87.211** Osteonecrosis due to previous trauma, <u>right</u> shoulder

cc **M87.212** Osteonecrosis due to previous trauma, <u>left</u> shoulder

cc **M87.219** Osteonecrosis due to previous trauma, <u>unspecified</u> shoulder

M87.22- Osteonecrosis due to previous trauma, <u>humerus</u>

cc **M87.221** Osteonecrosis due to previous trauma, <u>right</u> humerus

cc **M87.222** Osteonecrosis due to previous trauma, <u>left</u> humerus

cc **M87.229** Osteonecrosis due to previous trauma, <u>unspecified</u> humerus

M87.23- Osteonecrosis due to previous trauma of <u>radius, ulna and carpus</u>

cc **M87.231** Osteonecrosis due to previous trauma of <u>right</u> radius

cc **M87.232** Osteonecrosis due to previous trauma of <u>left</u> radius

cc **M87.233** Osteonecrosis due to previous trauma of <u>unspecified</u> radius

cc **M87.234** Osteonecrosis due to previous trauma of <u>right</u> ulna

cc **M87.235** Osteonecrosis due to previous trauma of <u>left</u> ulna

cc **M87.236** Osteonecrosis due to previous trauma of <u>unspecified</u> ulna

cc **M87.237** Osteonecrosis due to previous trauma of <u>right</u> carpus

cc **M87.238** Osteonecrosis due to previous trauma of <u>left</u> carpus

cc **M87.239** Osteonecrosis due to previous trauma of <u>unspecified</u> carpus

M87.24- Osteonecrosis due to previous trauma, <u>hand and fingers</u>

cc **M87.241** Osteonecrosis due to previous trauma, <u>right</u> hand

cc **M87.242** Osteonecrosis due to previous trauma, <u>left</u> hand

cc **M87.243** Osteonecrosis due to previous trauma, <u>unspecified</u> hand

cc **M87.244** Osteonecrosis due to previous trauma, <u>right</u> finger(s)

cc **M87.245** Osteonecrosis due to previous trauma, <u>left</u> finger(s)

cc **M87.246** Osteonecrosis due to previous trauma, <u>unspecified</u> finger(s)

M87.25- Osteonecrosis due to previous trauma, <u>pelvis and femur</u>

cc **M87.250** Osteonecrosis due to previous trauma, pelvis

cc **M87.251** Osteonecrosis due to previous trauma, <u>right</u> femur

cc **M87.252** Osteonecrosis due to previous trauma, <u>left</u> femur

cc **M87.256** Osteonecrosis due to previous trauma, <u>unspecified</u> femur

M87.26- Osteonecrosis due to previous trauma, <u>tibia and fibula</u>

cc **M87.261** Osteonecrosis due to previous trauma, <u>right</u> tibia

cc **M87.262** Osteonecrosis due to previous trauma, <u>left</u> tibia

cc **M87.263** Osteonecrosis due to previous trauma, <u>unspecified</u> tibia

cc **M87.264** Osteonecrosis due to previous trauma, <u>right</u> fibula

cc **M87.265** Osteonecrosis due to previous trauma, <u>left</u> fibula

cc **M87.266** Osteonecrosis due to previous trauma, <u>unspecified</u> fibula

M87.27- Osteonecrosis due to previous trauma, <u>ankle, foot and toes</u>

cc **M87.271** Osteonecrosis due to previous trauma, <u>right</u> ankle

cc **M87.272** Osteonecrosis due to previous trauma, <u>left</u> ankle

cc **M87.273** Osteonecrosis due to previous trauma, <u>unspecified</u> ankle

cc **M87.274** Osteonecrosis due to previous trauma, <u>right</u> foot

---

Excludes 1: = NOT CODED HERE! (Do not code both)

Excludes ❷: = Not Included Here

cc M87.275   Osteonecrosis due to previous trauma, <u>left</u> foot

cc M87.276   Osteonecrosis due to previous trauma, <u>unspecified</u> foot

cc M87.277   Osteonecrosis due to previous trauma, <u>right</u> toe(s)

cc M87.278   Osteonecrosis due to previous trauma, <u>left</u> toe(s)

cc M87.279   Osteonecrosis due to previous trauma, <u>unspecified</u> toe(s)

cc M87.28   Osteonecrosis due to previous trauma, <u>other site</u>

cc M87.29   Osteonecrosis due to previous trauma, <u>multiple sites</u>

M87.3-   <u>Other secondary</u> osteonecrosis

cc M87.30   Other secondary osteonecrosis, <u>unspecified bone</u>

M87.31- Other secondary osteonecrosis, <u>shoulder</u>

cc M87.311   Other secondary osteonecrosis, <u>right</u> shoulder

cc M87.312   Other secondary osteonecrosis, <u>left</u> shoulder

cc M87.319   Other secondary osteonecrosis, <u>unspecified</u> shoulder

M87.32- Other secondary osteonecrosis, <u>humerus</u>

cc M87.321   Other secondary osteonecrosis, <u>right</u> humerus

cc M87.322   Other secondary osteonecrosis, <u>left</u> humerus

cc M87.329   Other secondary osteonecrosis, <u>unspecified</u> humerus

M87.33- Other secondary osteonecrosis of <u>radius, ulna and carpus</u>

cc M87.331   Other secondary osteonecrosis of <u>right</u> radius

cc M87.332   Other secondary osteonecrosis of <u>left</u> radius

cc M87.333   Other secondary osteonecrosis of <u>unspecified</u> radius

cc M87.334   Other secondary osteonecrosis of <u>right</u> ulna

cc M87.335   Other secondary osteonecrosis of <u>left</u> ulna

cc M87.336   Other secondary osteonecrosis of <u>unspecified</u> ulna

cc M87.337   Other secondary osteonecrosis of <u>right</u> carpus

cc M87.338   Other secondary osteonecrosis of <u>left</u> carpus

cc M87.339   Other secondary osteonecrosis of <u>unspecified</u> carpus

M87.34- Other secondary osteonecrosis, <u>hand and fingers</u>

cc M87.341   Other secondary osteonecrosis, <u>right</u> hand

cc M87.342   Other secondary osteonecrosis, <u>left</u> hand

cc M87.343   Other secondary osteonecrosis, <u>unspecified</u> hand

cc M87.344   Other secondary osteonecrosis, <u>right</u> finger(s)

cc M87.345   Other secondary osteonecrosis, <u>left</u> finger(s)

cc M87.346   Other secondary osteonecrosis, <u>unspecified</u> finger(s)

M87.35- Other secondary osteonecrosis, <u>pelvis and femur</u>

cc M87.350   Other secondary osteonecrosis, pelvis

cc M87.351   Other secondary osteonecrosis, <u>right</u> femur

cc M87.352   Other secondary osteonecrosis, <u>left</u> femur

cc M87.353   Other secondary osteonecrosis, <u>unspecified</u> femur

M87.36- Other secondary osteonecrosis, <u>tibia and fibula</u>

cc M87.361   Other secondary osteonecrosis, <u>right</u> tibia

cc M87.362   Other secondary osteonecrosis, <u>left</u> tibia

cc M87.363   Other secondary osteonecrosis, <u>unspecified</u> tibia

cc M87.364   Other secondary osteonecrosis, <u>right</u> fibula

cc M87.365   Other secondary osteonecrosis, <u>left</u> fibula

cc M87.366   Other secondary osteonecrosis, <u>unspecified</u> fibula

M87.37- Other secondary osteonecrosis, <u>ankle and foot</u>

cc M87.371   Other secondary osteonecrosis, <u>right</u> ankle

cc M87.372   Other secondary osteonecrosis, <u>left</u> ankle

cc M87.373   Other secondary osteonecrosis, <u>unspecified</u> ankle

cc M87.374   Other secondary osteonecrosis, <u>right</u> foot

cc M87.375   Other secondary osteonecrosis, <u>left</u> foot

cc M87.376   Other secondary osteonecrosis, <u>unspecified</u> foot

cc M87.377   Other secondary osteonecrosis, <u>right</u> toe(s)

cc M87.378   Other secondary osteonecrosis, <u>left</u> toe(s)

cc M87.379   Other secondary osteonecrosis, <u>unspecified</u> toe(s)

cc M87.38   Other secondary osteonecrosis, <u>other site</u>

cc M87.39   Other secondary osteonecrosis, <u>multiple sites</u>

M87.8-   <u>Other</u> osteonecrosis

cc M87.80   Other osteonecrosis, <u>unspecified bone</u>

M87.81- Other osteonecrosis, <u>shoulder</u>

cc M87.811   Other osteonecrosis, <u>right</u> shoulder

cc M87.812   Other osteonecrosis, <u>left</u> shoulder

cc M87.819   Other osteonecrosis, <u>unspecified</u> shoulder

M87.82- Other osteonecrosis, <u>humerus</u>

cc M87.821   Other osteonecrosis, <u>right</u> humerus

cc M87.822   Other osteonecrosis, <u>left</u> humerus

cc M87.829   Other osteonecrosis, <u>unspecified</u> humerus

M87.83- Other osteonecrosis of <u>radius, ulna and carpus</u>

cc M87.831   Other osteonecrosis of <u>right</u> radius

cc M87.832   Other osteonecrosis of <u>left</u> radius

cc M87.833   Other osteonecrosis of <u>unspecified</u> radius

cc M87.834   Other osteonecrosis of <u>right</u> ulna

cc M87.835   Other osteonecrosis of <u>left</u> ulna

cc M87.836   Other osteonecrosis of <u>unspecified</u> ulna

cc M87.837   Other osteonecrosis of <u>right</u> carpus

cc M87.838   Other osteonecrosis of <u>left</u> carpus

cc M87.839   Other osteonecrosis of <u>unspecified</u> carpus

M87.84- Other osteonecrosis, <u>hand and fingers</u>

cc M87.841   Other osteonecrosis, <u>right</u> hand

cc M87.842   Other osteonecrosis, <u>left</u> hand

cc M87.843   Other osteonecrosis, <u>unspecified</u> hand

cc M87.844   Other osteonecrosis, <u>right</u> finger(s)

cc M87.845   Other osteonecrosis, <u>left</u> finger(s)

cc M87.849   Other osteonecrosis, <u>unspecified</u> finger(s)

M87.85- Other osteonecrosis, <u>pelvis and femur</u>

cc M87.850   Other osteonecrosis, pelvis

cc M87.851   Other osteonecrosis, <u>right</u> femur

cc M87.852   Other osteonecrosis, <u>left</u> femur

cc M87.859   Other osteonecrosis, <u>unspecified</u> femur

M87.86- Other osteonecrosis, <u>tibia and fibula</u>

cc M87.861   Other osteonecrosis, <u>right</u> tibia

cc M87.862   Other osteonecrosis, <u>left</u> tibia

cc M87.863   Other osteonecrosis, <u>unspecified</u> tibia

cc M87.864   Other osteonecrosis, <u>right</u> fibula

cc M87.865   Other osteonecrosis, <u>left</u> fibula

cc M87.869   Other osteonecrosis, <u>unspecified</u> fibula

M87.87- Other osteonecrosis, <u>ankle, foot and toes</u>

cc M87.871   Other osteonecrosis, <u>right</u> ankle

cc M87.872   Other osteonecrosis, <u>left</u> ankle

cc M87.873   Other osteonecrosis, <u>unspecified</u> ankle

cc M87.874   Other osteonecrosis, <u>right</u> foot

cc M87.875   Other osteonecrosis, <u>left</u> foot

cc M87.876   Other osteonecrosis, <u>unspecified</u> foot

cc M87.877   Other osteonecrosis, <u>right</u> toe(s)

cc M87.878   Other osteonecrosis, <u>left</u> toe(s)

cc M87.879   Other osteonecrosis, <u>unspecified</u> toe(s)

cc M87.88   Other osteonecrosis, <u>other site</u>

cc M87.89   Other osteonecrosis, <u>multiple sites</u>

cc M87.9   Osteonecrosis, <u>unspecified</u>

     Necrosis of bone NOS

M88-   <u>Osteitis deformans [Paget's disease of bone]</u> — Inflammation of the bone with softening and deformity, especially bowing of the long bones.

     Excludes 1:   *osteitis deformans in neoplastic disease (M90.6)*

M88.0   Osteitis deformans of <u>skull</u>

M88.1   Osteitis deformans of <u>vertebrae</u>

M88.8-   Osteitis deformans of <u>other bones</u>

     M88.81- Osteitis deformans of <u>shoulder</u>

         M88.811   Osteitis deformans of <u>right</u> shoulder

         M88.812   Osteitis deformans of <u>left</u> shoulder

         M88.819   Osteitis deformans of <u>unspecified</u> shoulder

M87 - M88

M88.82- Osteitis deformans of <u>upper arm</u>

    M88.821 Osteitis deformans of <u>right</u> upper arm

    M88.822 Osteitis deformans of <u>left</u> upper arm

    M88.829 Osteitis deformans of <u>unspecified</u> upper arm

M88.83- Osteitis deformans of <u>forearm</u>

    M88.831 Osteitis deformans of <u>right</u> forearm

    M88.832 Osteitis deformans of <u>left</u> forearm

    M88.839 Osteitis deformans of <u>unspecified</u> forearm

M88.84- Osteitis deformans of <u>hand</u>

    M88.841 Osteitis deformans of <u>right</u> hand

    M88.842 Osteitis deformans of <u>left</u> hand

    M88.849 Osteitis deformans of <u>unspecified</u> hand

M88.85- Osteitis deformans of <u>thigh</u>

    M88.851 Osteitis deformans of <u>right</u> thigh

    M88.852 Osteitis deformans of <u>left</u> thigh

    M88.859 Osteitis deformans of <u>unspecified</u> thigh

M88.86- Osteitis deformans of <u>lower leg</u>

    M88.861 Osteitis deformans of <u>right</u> lower leg

    M88.862 Osteitis deformans of <u>left</u> lower leg

    M88.869 Osteitis deformans of <u>unspecified</u> lower leg

M88.87- Osteitis deformans of <u>ankle and foot</u>

    M88.871 Osteitis deformans of <u>right</u> ankle and foot

    M88.872 Osteitis deformans of <u>left</u> ankle and foot

    M88.879 Osteitis deformans of <u>unspecified</u> ankle and foot

M88.88 Osteitis deformans of <u>other bones</u>

    Excludes ❷: *osteitis deformans of skull (M88.0)*

                    osteitis deformans of vertebrae (M88.1)

M88.89 Osteitis deformans of <u>multiple sites</u>

M88.9 Osteitis deformans of <u>unspecified</u> bone

M89- Other disorders of bone

M89.0- <u>Algoneurodystrophy</u> — Bone deterioration that is due to damage of the supplying nerve.

    Shoulder-hand syndrome

    Sudeck's atrophy

    Excludes 1:   *causalgia, lower limb (G57.7-)*

                    causalgia, upper limb (G56.4-)

                    complex regional pain syndrome II, lower limb (G57.7-)

                    complex regional pain syndrome II, upper limb (G56.4-)

                    reflex sympathetic dystrophy (G90.5-)

M89.00 Algoneurodystrophy, <u>unspecified</u> <u>site</u>

M89.01- Algoneurodystrophy, <u>shoulder</u>

    M89.011 Algoneurodystrophy, <u>right</u> shoulder

    M89.012 Algoneurodystrophy, <u>left</u> shoulder

    M89.019 Algoneurodystrophy, <u>unspecified</u> shoulder

M89.02- Algoneurodystrophy, <u>upper arm</u>

    M89.021 Algoneurodystrophy, <u>right</u> upper arm

    M89.022 Algoneurodystrophy, <u>left</u> upper arm

    M89.029 Algoneurodystrophy, <u>unspecified</u> upper arm

M89.03- Algoneurodystrophy, <u>forearm</u>

    M89.031 Algoneurodystrophy, <u>right</u> forearm

    M89.032 Algoneurodystrophy, <u>left</u> forearm

    M89.039 Algoneurodystrophy, <u>unspecified</u> forearm

M89.04- Algoneurodystrophy, <u>hand</u>

    M89.041 Algoneurodystrophy, <u>right</u> hand

    M89.042 Algoneurodystrophy, <u>left</u> hand

    M89.049 Algoneurodystrophy, <u>unspecified</u> hand

M89.05- Algoneurodystrophy, <u>thigh</u>

    M89.051 Algoneurodystrophy, <u>right</u> thigh

    M89.052 Algoneurodystrophy, <u>left</u> thigh

    M89.059 Algoneurodystrophy, <u>unspecified</u> thigh

M89.06- Algoneurodystrophy, <u>lower leg</u>

    M89.061 Algoneurodystrophy, <u>right</u> lower leg

    M89.062 Algoneurodystrophy, <u>left</u> lower leg

    M89.069 Algoneurodystrophy, <u>unspecified</u> lower leg

M89.07- Algoneurodystrophy, <u>ankle and foot</u>

    M89.071 Algoneurodystrophy, <u>right</u> ankle and foot

M89.072 Algoneurodystrophy, <u>left</u> ankle and foot

M89.079 Algoneurodystrophy, <u>unspecified</u> ankle and foot

M89.08 Algoneurodystrophy, <u>other site</u>

M89.09 Algoneurodystrophy, <u>multiple sites</u>

M89.1- <u>Physeal arrest</u> — The cessation of the normal epiphyseal bone growth.

    Arrest of growth plate

    Epiphyseal arrest

    Growth plate arrest

M89.12- Physeal arrest, <u>humerus</u>

    M89.121 <u>Complete</u> physeal arrest, <u>right</u> proximal humerus

    M89.122 <u>Complete</u> physeal arrest, <u>left</u> proximal humerus

    M89.123 Partial physeal arrest, <u>right</u> proximal humerus

    M89.124 Partial physeal arrest, <u>left</u> proximal humerus

    M89.125 <u>Complete</u> physeal arrest, <u>right</u> distal humerus

    M89.126 <u>Complete</u> physeal arrest, <u>left</u> distal humerus

    M89.127 Partial physeal arrest, <u>right</u> distal humerus

    M89.128 Partial physeal arrest, <u>left</u> distal humerus

    M89.129 Physeal arrest, humerus, <u>unspecified</u>

M89.13- Physeal arrest, <u>forearm</u>

    M89.131 <u>Complete</u> physeal arrest, <u>right</u> distal radius

    M89.132 <u>Complete</u> physeal arrest, <u>left</u> distal radius

    M89.133 Partial physeal arrest, <u>right</u> distal radius

    M89.134 Partial physeal arrest, <u>left</u> distal radius

    M89.138 Other physeal arrest of forearm

    M89.139 Physeal arrest, forearm, <u>unspecified</u>

M89.15- Physeal arrest, <u>femur</u>

    M89.151 <u>Complete</u> physeal arrest, <u>right</u> proximal femur

    M89.152 <u>Complete</u> physeal arrest, <u>left</u> proximal femur

    M89.153 Partial physeal arrest, <u>right</u> proximal femur

    M89.154 Partial physeal arrest, <u>left</u> proximal femur

    M89.155 <u>Complete</u> physeal arrest, <u>right</u> distal femur

    M89.156 <u>Complete</u> physeal arrest, <u>left</u> distal femur

    M89.157 Partial physeal arrest, <u>right</u> distal femur

    M89.158 Partial physeal arrest, <u>left</u> distal femur

    M89.159 Physeal arrest, femur, <u>unspecified</u>

M89.16- Physeal arrest, <u>lower leg</u>

    M89.160 <u>Complete</u> physeal arrest, <u>right</u> proximal tibia

    M89.161 <u>Complete</u> physeal arrest, <u>left</u> proximal tibia

    M89.162 Partial physeal arrest, <u>right</u> proximal tibia

    M89.163 Partial physeal arrest, <u>left</u> proximal tibia

    M89.164 <u>Complete</u> physeal arrest, <u>right</u> distal tibia

    M89.165 <u>Complete</u> physeal arrest, <u>left</u> distal tibia

    M89.166 Partial physeal arrest, <u>right</u> distal tibia

    M89.167 Partial physeal arrest, <u>left</u> distal tibia

    M89.168 Other physeal arrest of lower leg

    M89.169 Physeal arrest, lower leg, <u>unspecified</u>

M89.18 Physeal arrest, other site

M89.2- <u>Other disorders of bone development and growth</u>

M89.20 Other disorders of bone development and growth, <u>unspecified site</u>

M89.21- Other disorders of bone development and growth, <u>shoulder</u>

    M89.211 Other disorders of bone development and growth, <u>right</u> shoulder

    M89.212 Other disorders of bone development and growth, <u>left</u> shoulder

    M89.219 Other disorders of bone development and growth, <u>unspecified</u> shoulder

M89.22- Other disorders of bone development and growth, <u>humerus</u>

    M89.221 Other disorders of bone development and growth, <u>right</u> humerus

    M89.222 Other disorders of bone development and growth, <u>left</u> humerus

    M89.229 Other disorders of bone development and growth, <u>unspecified</u> humerus

M88 - M89 *(side tab)*

M89.23- Other disorders of bone development and growth, <u>ulna and radius</u>
  M89.231 Other disorders of bone development and growth, <u>right</u> ulna
  M89.232 Other disorders of bone development and growth, <u>left</u> ulna
  M89.233 Other disorders of bone development and growth, <u>right</u> radius
  M89.234 Other disorders of bone development and growth, <u>left</u> radius
  M89.239 Other disorders of bone development and growth, <u>unspecified</u> ulna and radius
M89.24- Other disorders of bone development and growth, <u>hand</u>
  M89.241 Other disorders of bone development and growth, <u>right</u> hand
  M89.242 Other disorders of bone development and growth, <u>left</u> hand
  M89.249 Other disorders of bone development and growth, <u>unspecified</u> hand
M89.25- Other disorders of bone development and growth, <u>femur</u>
  M89.251 Other disorders of bone development and growth, <u>right</u> femur
  M89.252 Other disorders of bone development and growth, <u>left</u> femur
  M89.259 Other disorders of bone development and growth, <u>unspecified</u> femur
M89.26- Other disorders of bone development and growth, <u>tibia and fibula</u>
  M89.261 Other disorders of bone development and growth, <u>right</u> tibia
  M89.262 Other disorders of bone development and growth, <u>left</u> tibia
  M89.263 Other disorders of bone development and growth, <u>right</u> fibula
  M89.264 Other disorders of bone development and growth, <u>left</u> fibula
  M89.269 Other disorders of bone development and growth, <u>unspecified</u> lower leg
M89.27- Other disorders of bone development and growth, <u>ankle and foot</u>
  M89.271 Other disorders of bone development and growth, <u>right</u> ankle and foot
  M89.272 Other disorders of bone development and growth, <u>left</u> ankle and foot
  M89.279 Other disorders of bone development and growth, <u>unspecified</u> ankle and foot
M89.28 Other disorders of bone development and growth, <u>other site</u>
M89.29 Other disorders of bone development and growth, <u>multiple sites</u>
M89.3- <u>Hypertrophy</u> of bone — Enlargement of a bone.
M89.30 Hypertrophy of bone, <u>unspecified site</u>
M89.31- Hypertrophy of bone, <u>shoulder</u>
  M89.311 Hypertrophy of bone, <u>right</u> shoulder
  M89.312 Hypertrophy of bone, <u>left</u> shoulder
  M89.319 Hypertrophy of bone, <u>unspecified</u> shoulder
M89.32- Hypertrophy of bone, <u>humerus</u>
  M89.321 Hypertrophy of bone, <u>right</u> humerus
  M89.322 Hypertrophy of bone, <u>left</u> humerus
  M89.329 Hypertrophy of bone, <u>unspecified</u> humerus
M89.33- Hypertrophy of bone, <u>ulna and radius</u>
  M89.331 Hypertrophy of bone, <u>right</u> ulna
  M89.332 Hypertrophy of bone, <u>left</u> ulna
  M89.333 Hypertrophy of bone, <u>right</u> radius
  M89.334 Hypertrophy of bone, <u>left</u> radius
  M89.339 Hypertrophy of bone, <u>unspecified</u> ulna and radius

M89.34- Hypertrophy of bone, <u>hand</u>
  M89.341 Hypertrophy of bone, <u>right</u> hand
  M89.342 Hypertrophy of bone, <u>left</u> hand
  M89.349 Hypertrophy of bone, <u>unspecified</u> hand
M89.35- Hypertrophy of bone, <u>femur</u>
  M89.351 Hypertrophy of bone, <u>right</u> femur
  M89.352 Hypertrophy of bone, <u>left</u> femur
  M89.359 Hypertrophy of bone, <u>unspecified</u> femur
M89.36- Hypertrophy of bone, <u>tibia and fibula</u>
  M89.361 Hypertrophy of bone, <u>right</u> tibia
  M89.362 Hypertrophy of bone, <u>left</u> tibia
  M89.363 Hypertrophy of bone, <u>right</u> fibula
  M89.364 Hypertrophy of bone, <u>left</u> fibula
  M89.369 Hypertrophy of bone, <u>unspecified</u> tibia and fibula
M89.37- Hypertrophy of bone, <u>ankle and foot</u>
  M89.371 Hypertrophy of bone, <u>right</u> ankle and foot
  M89.372 Hypertrophy of bone, <u>left</u> ankle and foot
  M89.379 Hypertrophy of bone, <u>unspecified</u> ankle and foot
M89.38 Hypertrophy of bone, <u>other site</u>
M89.39 Hypertrophy of bone, <u>multiple sites</u>
M89.4- <u>Other hypertrophic</u> osteoarthropathy
    Marie-Bamberger disease — Inflammation and enlargement of the distal fingers and toes that is due to pulmonary disorders.
    Pachydermoperiostosis
M89.40 Other hypertrophic osteoarthropathy, <u>unspecified site</u>
M89.41- Other hypertrophic osteoarthropathy, <u>shoulder</u>
  M89.411 Other hypertrophic osteoarthropathy, <u>right</u> shoulder
  M89.412 Other hypertrophic osteoarthropathy, <u>left</u> shoulder
  M89.419 Other hypertrophic osteoarthropathy, <u>unspecified</u> shoulder
M89.42- Other hypertrophic osteoarthropathy, <u>upper arm</u>
  M89.421 Other hypertrophic osteoarthropathy, <u>right</u> upper arm
  M89.422 Other hypertrophic osteoarthropathy, <u>left</u> upper arm
  M89.429 Other hypertrophic osteoarthropathy, <u>unspecified</u> upper arm
M89.43- Other hypertrophic osteoarthropathy, <u>forearm</u>
  M89.431 Other hypertrophic osteoarthropathy, <u>right</u> forearm
  M89.432 Other hypertrophic osteoarthropathy, <u>left</u> forearm
  M89.439 Other hypertrophic osteoarthropathy, <u>unspecified</u> forearm
M89.44- Other hypertrophic osteoarthropathy, <u>hand</u>
  M89.441 Other hypertrophic osteoarthropathy, <u>right</u> hand
  M89.442 Other hypertrophic osteoarthropathy, <u>left</u> hand
  M89.449 Other hypertrophic osteoarthropathy, <u>unspecified</u> hand
M89.45- Other hypertrophic osteoarthropathy, <u>thigh</u>
  M89.451 Other hypertrophic osteoarthropathy, <u>right</u> thigh
  M89.452 Other hypertrophic osteoarthropathy, <u>left</u> thigh
  M89.459 Other hypertrophic osteoarthropathy, <u>unspecified</u> thigh
M89.46- Other hypertrophic osteoarthropathy, <u>lower leg</u>
  M89.461 Other hypertrophic osteoarthropathy, <u>right</u> lower leg
  M89.462 Other hypertrophic osteoarthropathy, <u>left</u> lower leg
  M89.469 Other hypertrophic osteoarthropathy, <u>unspecified</u> lower leg
M89.47- Other hypertrophic osteoarthropathy, <u>ankle and foot</u>
  M89.471 Other hypertrophic osteoarthropathy, <u>right</u> ankle and foot
  M89.472 Other hypertrophic osteoarthropathy, <u>left</u> ankle and foot
  M89.479 Other hypertrophic osteoarthropathy, <u>unspecified</u> ankle and foot
M89.48 Other hypertrophic osteoarthropathy, <u>other site</u>

M89
M89
M89

M89.49 Other hypertrophic osteoarthropathy, <u>multiple sites</u>

M89.5- <u>Osteolysis</u> — Resorption of bone.
Use additional code to identify major osseous defect, if applicable (M89.7-)
Excludes ❷: periprosthetic osteolysis of internal prosthetic joint (T84.05-)

    M89.50 Osteolysis, <u>unspecified site</u>

    M89.51- Osteolysis, <u>shoulder</u>
        M89.511 Osteolysis, <u>right</u> shoulder
        M89.512 Osteolysis, <u>left</u> shoulder
        M89.519 Osteolysis, <u>unspecified</u> shoulder

    M89.52- Osteolysis, <u>upper arm</u>
        M89.521 Osteolysis, <u>right</u> upper arm
        M89.522 Osteolysis, <u>left</u> upper arm
        M89.529 Osteolysis, <u>unspecified</u> upper arm

    M89.53- Osteolysis, <u>forearm</u>
        M89.531 Osteolysis, <u>right</u> forearm
        M89.532 Osteolysis, <u>left</u> forearm
        M89.539 Osteolysis, <u>unspecified</u> forearm

    M89.54- Osteolysis, <u>hand</u>
        M89.541 Osteolysis, <u>right</u> hand
        M89.542 Osteolysis, <u>left</u> hand
        M89.549 Osteolysis, <u>unspecified</u> hand

    M89.55- Osteolysis, <u>thigh</u>
        M89.551 Osteolysis, <u>right</u> thigh
        M89.552 Osteolysis, <u>left</u> thigh
        M89.559 Osteolysis, <u>unspecified</u> thigh

    M89.56- Osteolysis, <u>lower leg</u>
        M89.561 Osteolysis, <u>right</u> lower leg
        M89.562 Osteolysis, <u>left</u> lower leg
        M89.569 Osteolysis, <u>unspecified</u> lower leg

    M89.57- Osteolysis, <u>ankle and foot</u>
        M89.571 Osteolysis, <u>right</u> ankle and foot
        M89.572 Osteolysis, <u>left</u> ankle and foot
        M89.579 Osteolysis, <u>unspecified</u> ankle and foot

    M89.58 Osteolysis, <u>other site</u>

    M89.59 Osteolysis, <u>multiple sites</u>

M89.6- <u>Osteopathy after poliomyelitis</u>
Use additional code (B91) to identify previous poliomyelitis
Excludes 1: postpolio syndrome (G14)

    M89.60 Osteopathy after poliomyelitis, <u>unspecified site</u>

    M89.61- Osteopathy after poliomyelitis, <u>shoulder</u>
        M89.611 Osteopathy after poliomyelitis, <u>right</u> shoulder
        M89.612 Osteopathy after poliomyelitis, <u>left</u> shoulder
        M89.619 Osteopathy after poliomyelitis, <u>unspecified</u> shoulder

    M89.62- Osteopathy after poliomyelitis, <u>upper arm</u>
        M89.621 Osteopathy after poliomyelitis, <u>right</u> upper arm
        M89.622 Osteopathy after poliomyelitis, <u>left</u> upper arm
        M89.629 Osteopathy after poliomyelitis, <u>unspecified</u> upper arm

    M89.63- Osteopathy after poliomyelitis, <u>forearm</u>
        M89.631 Osteopathy after poliomyelitis, <u>right</u> forearm
        M89.632 Osteopathy after poliomyelitis, <u>left</u> forearm
        M89.639 Osteopathy after poliomyelitis, <u>unspecified</u> forearm

    M89.64- Osteopathy after poliomyelitis, <u>hand</u>
        M89.641 Osteopathy after poliomyelitis, <u>right</u> hand
        M89.642 Osteopathy after poliomyelitis, <u>left</u> hand
        M89.649 Osteopathy after poliomyelitis, <u>unspecified</u> hand

    M89.65- Osteopathy after poliomyelitis, <u>thigh</u>
        M89.651 Osteopathy after poliomyelitis, <u>right</u> thigh
        M89.652 Osteopathy after poliomyelitis, <u>left</u> thigh
        M89.659 Osteopathy after poliomyelitis, <u>unspecified</u> thigh

    M89.66- Osteopathy after poliomyelitis, <u>lower leg</u>
        M89.661 Osteopathy after poliomyelitis, <u>right</u> lower leg

        M89.662 Osteopathy after poliomyelitis, <u>left</u> lower leg
        M89.669 Osteopathy after poliomyelitis, <u>unspecified</u> lower leg

    M89.67- Osteopathy after poliomyelitis, <u>ankle and foot</u>
        M89.671 Osteopathy after poliomyelitis, <u>right</u> ankle and foot
        M89.672 Osteopathy after poliomyelitis, <u>left</u> ankle and foot
        M89.679 Osteopathy after poliomyelitis, <u>unspecified</u> ankle and foot

    M89.68 Osteopathy after poliomyelitis, <u>other site</u>

    M89.69 Osteopathy after poliomyelitis, <u>multiple sites</u>

M89.7- <u>Major osseous defect</u> — A condition of extensive, localized bone loss that has important implications regarding future diagnosis and restoration options.
Code first underlying disease, if known, such as:
    Aseptic necrosis of bone (M87.-)
    Malignant neoplasm of bone (C40.-)
    Osteolysis (M89.5)
    Osteomyelitis (M86.-)
    Osteonecrosis (M87.-)
    Osteoporosis (M80.-, M81.-)
    Periprosthetic osteolysis (T84.05-)

    M89.70 Major osseous defect, <u>unspecified site</u>

    M89.71- Major osseous defect, <u>shoulder region</u>
        Major osseous defect clavicle or scapula
        M89.711 Major osseous defect, <u>right</u> shoulder region
        M89.712 Major osseous defect, <u>left</u> shoulder region
        M89.719 Major osseous defect, <u>unspecified</u> shoulder region

    M89.72- Major osseous defect, <u>humerus</u>
        M89.721 Major osseous defect, <u>right</u> humerus
        M89.722 Major osseous defect, <u>left</u> humerus
        M89.729 Major osseous defect, <u>unspecified</u> humerus

    M89.73- Major osseous defect, <u>forearm</u>
        Major osseous defect of radius and ulna
        M89.731 Major osseous defect, <u>right</u> forearm
        M89.732 Major osseous defect, <u>left</u> forearm
        M89.739 Major osseous defect, <u>unspecified</u> forearm

    M89.74- Major osseous defect, <u>hand</u>
        Major osseous defect of carpus, fingers, metacarpus
        M89.741 Major osseous defect, <u>right</u> hand
        M89.742 Major osseous defect, <u>left</u> hand
        M89.749 Major osseous defect, <u>unspecified</u> hand

    M89.75- Major osseous defect, <u>pelvic region and thigh</u>
        Major osseous defect of femur and pelvis
        M89.751 Major osseous defect, <u>right</u> pelvic region and thigh
        M89.752 Major osseous defect, <u>left</u> pelvic region and thigh
        M89.759 Major osseous defect, <u>unspecified</u> pelvic region and thigh

    M89.76- Major osseous defect, <u>lower leg</u>
        Major osseous defect of fibula and tibia
        M89.761 Major osseous defect, <u>right</u> lower leg
        M89.762 Major osseous defect, <u>left</u> lower leg
        M89.769 Major osseous defect, <u>unspecified</u> lower leg

    M89.77- Major osseous defect, <u>ankle and foot</u>
        Major osseous defect of metatarsus, tarsus, toes
        M89.771 Major osseous defect, <u>right</u> ankle and foot
        M89.772 Major osseous defect, <u>left</u> ankle and foot
        M89.779 Major osseous defect, <u>unspecified</u> ankle and foot

    M89.78 Major osseous defect, <u>other site</u>

    M89.79 Major osseous defect, <u>multiple sites</u>

M89.8- <u>Other specified</u> disorders of bone
    Infantile cortical hyperostoses
    Post-traumatic subperiosteal ossification

    M89.8x- Other specified disorders of bone
        M89.8x0 Other specified disorders of bone, multiple sites
        M89.8x1 Other specified disorders of bone, shoulder
        M89.8x2 Other specified disorders of bone, upper arm
        M89.8x3 Other specified disorders of bone, forearm
        M89.8x4 Other specified disorders of bone, hand

M89.8x5   **Other specified disorders of bone, thigh**

M89.8x6   **Other specified disorders of bone, lower leg**

M89.8x7   **Other specified disorders of bone, ankle and foot**

M89.8x8   **Other specified disorders of bone, other site**

M89.8x9   **Other specified disorders of bone, unspecified site**

M89.9   Disorder of bone, <u>unspecified</u>

M90-   Osteopathies <u>in diseases classified elsewhere</u>

Excludes 1:   osteochondritis, osteomyelitis, and osteopathy (in):
cryptococcosis (B45.3)
diabetes mellitus (E08-E13 with .69-)
gonococcal (A54.43)
neurogenic syphilis (A52.11)
renal osteodystrophy (N25.0)
salmonellosis (A02.24)
secondary syphilis (A51.46)
syphilis (late) (A52.77)

M90.5-   Osteonecrosis <u>in diseases classified elsewhere</u>
Code first underlying disease, such as:
Caisson disease (T70.3)
Hemoglobinopathy (D50-D64)

cc **M90.50   Osteonecrosis in diseases classified elsewhere, <u>unspecified site</u>** — [Not Allowed as PDX]

M90.51-Osteonecrosis in diseases classified elsewhere, <u>shoulder</u>

cc **M90.511   Osteonecrosis in diseases classified elsewhere, <u>right</u> shoulder** — [Not Allowed as PDX]

cc **M90.512   Osteonecrosis in diseases classified elsewhere, <u>left</u> shoulder** — [Not Allowed as PDX]

cc **M90.519   Osteonecrosis in diseases classified elsewhere, <u>unspecified</u> shoulder** — [Not Allowed as PDX]

M90.52-Osteonecrosis in diseases classified elsewhere, <u>upper arm</u>

cc **M90.521   Osteonecrosis in diseases classified elsewhere, <u>right</u> upper arm** — [Not Allowed as PDX]

cc **M90.522   Osteonecrosis in diseases classified elsewhere, <u>left</u> upper arm** — [Not Allowed as PDX]

cc **M90.529   Osteonecrosis in diseases classified elsewhere, <u>unspecified</u> upper arm** — [Not Allowed as PDX]

M90.53-Osteonecrosis in diseases classified elsewhere, <u>forearm</u>

cc **M90.531   Osteonecrosis in diseases classified elsewhere, <u>right</u> forearm** — [Not Allowed as PDX]

cc **M90.532   Osteonecrosis in diseases classified elsewhere, <u>left</u> forearm** — [Not Allowed as PDX]

cc **M90.539   Osteonecrosis in diseases classified elsewhere, <u>unspecified</u> forearm** — [Not Allowed as PDX]

M90.54-Osteonecrosis in diseases classified elsewhere, <u>hand</u>

cc **M90.541   Osteonecrosis in diseases classified elsewhere, <u>right</u> hand** — [Not Allowed as PDX]

cc **M90.542   Osteonecrosis in diseases classified elsewhere, <u>left</u> hand** — [Not Allowed as PDX]

cc **M90.549   Osteonecrosis in diseases classified elsewhere, <u>unspecified</u> hand** — [Not Allowed as PDX]

M90.55-Osteonecrosis in diseases classified elsewhere, <u>thigh</u>

cc **M90.551   Osteonecrosis in diseases classified elsewhere, <u>right</u> thigh** — [Not Allowed as PDX]

cc **M90.552   Osteonecrosis in diseases classified elsewhere, <u>left</u> thigh** — [Not Allowed as PDX]

cc **M90.559   Osteonecrosis in diseases classified elsewhere, <u>unspecified</u> thigh** — [Not Allowed as PDX]

M90.56-Osteonecrosis in diseases classified elsewhere, <u>lower leg</u>

cc **M90.561   Osteonecrosis in diseases classified elsewhere, <u>right</u> lower leg** — [Not Allowed as PDX]

cc **M90.562   Osteonecrosis in diseases classified elsewhere, <u>left</u> lower leg** — [Not Allowed as PDX]

cc **M90.569   Osteonecrosis in diseases classified elsewhere, <u>unspecified</u> lower leg** — [Not Allowed as PDX]

M90.57-Osteonecrosis in diseases classified elsewhere, <u>ankle and foot</u>

cc **M90.571   Osteonecrosis in diseases classified elsewhere, <u>right</u> ankle and foot** — [Not Allowed as PDX]

cc **M90.572   Osteonecrosis in diseases classified elsewhere, <u>left</u> ankle and foot** — [Not Allowed as PDX]

---

cc **M90.579   Osteonecrosis in diseases classified elsewhere, <u>unspecified</u> ankle and foot** — [Not Allowed as PDX]

cc **M90.58   Osteonecrosis in diseases classified elsewhere, <u>other</u> site** — [Not Allowed as PDX]

cc **M90.59   Osteonecrosis in diseases classified elsewhere, <u>multiple</u> sites** — [Not Allowed as PDX]

M90.6-   Osteitis deformans <u>in neoplastic diseases</u>
Osteitis deformans in malignant neoplasm of bone
Code first the neoplasm (C40.-, C41.-)

Excludes 1:   osteitis deformans [Paget's disease of bone] (M88.-)

M90.60   Osteitis deformans in neoplastic diseases, <u>unspecified</u> site — [Not Allowed as PDX]

M90.61-Osteitis deformans in neoplastic diseases, <u>shoulder</u>

M90.611   Osteitis deformans in neoplastic diseases, <u>right</u> shoulder — [Not Allowed as PDX]

M90.612   Osteitis deformans in neoplastic diseases, <u>left</u> shoulder — [Not Allowed as PDX]

M90.619   Osteitis deformans in neoplastic diseases, <u>unspecified</u> shoulder — [Not Allowed as PDX]

M90.62-Osteitis deformans in neoplastic diseases, <u>upper arm</u>

M90.621   Osteitis deformans in neoplastic diseases, <u>right</u> upper arm — [Not Allowed as PDX]

M90.622   Osteitis deformans in neoplastic diseases, <u>left</u> upper arm — [Not Allowed as PDX]

M90.629   Osteitis deformans in neoplastic diseases, <u>unspecified</u> upper arm — [Not Allowed as PDX]

M90.63-Osteitis deformans in neoplastic diseases, <u>forearm</u>

M90.631   Osteitis deformans in neoplastic diseases, <u>right</u> forearm — [Not Allowed as PDX]

M90.632   Osteitis deformans in neoplastic diseases, <u>left</u> forearm — [Not Allowed as PDX]

M90.639   Osteitis deformans in neoplastic diseases, <u>unspecified</u> forearm — [Not Allowed as PDX]

M90.64-Osteitis deformans in neoplastic diseases, <u>hand</u>

M90.641   Osteitis deformans in neoplastic diseases, <u>right</u> hand — [Not Allowed as PDX]

M90.642   Osteitis deformans in neoplastic diseases, <u>left</u> hand — [Not Allowed as PDX]

M90.649   Osteitis deformans in neoplastic diseases, <u>unspecified</u> hand — [Not Allowed as PDX]

M90.65-Osteitis deformans in neoplastic diseases, <u>thigh</u>

M90.651   Osteitis deformans in neoplastic diseases, <u>right</u> thigh — [Not Allowed as PDX]

M90.652   Osteitis deformans in neoplastic diseases, <u>left</u> thigh — [Not Allowed as PDX]

M90.659   Osteitis deformans in neoplastic diseases, <u>unspecified</u> thigh — [Not Allowed as PDX]

M90.66-Osteitis deformans in neoplastic diseases, <u>lower leg</u>

M90.661   Osteitis deformans in neoplastic diseases, <u>right</u> lower leg — [Not Allowed as PDX]

M90.662   Osteitis deformans in neoplastic diseases, <u>left</u> lower leg — [Not Allowed as PDX]

M90.669   Osteitis deformans in neoplastic diseases, <u>unspecified</u> lower leg — [Not Allowed as PDX]

M90.67-Osteitis deformans in neoplastic diseases, <u>ankle and foot</u>

M90.671   Osteitis deformans in neoplastic diseases, <u>right</u> ankle and foot — [Not Allowed as PDX]

M90.672   Osteitis deformans in neoplastic diseases, <u>left</u> ankle and foot — [Not Allowed as PDX]

M90.679   Osteitis deformans in neoplastic diseases, <u>unspecified</u> ankle and foot — [Not Allowed as PDX]

M90.68   Osteitis deformans in neoplastic diseases, <u>other site</u> — [Not Allowed as PDX]

M90.69   Osteitis deformans in neoplastic diseases, <u>multiple</u> sites — [Not Allowed as PDX]

M 8 9 - M 9 0

Excludes 1: = NOT CODED HERE! (Do not code both)   **891**   *Excludes ❷:* = Not Included Here

M90.8-   Osteopathy in diseases classified elsewhere
Code first underlying disease, such as:
Rickets (E55.0)
Vitamin-D-resistant rickets (E83.3)

M90.80   Osteopathy in diseases classified elsewhere, unspecified site — [Not Allowed as PDX]

M90.81- Osteopathy in diseases classified elsewhere, shoulder

M90.811   Osteopathy in diseases classified elsewhere, right shoulder — [Not Allowed as PDX]

M90.812   Osteopathy in diseases classified elsewhere, left shoulder — [Not Allowed as PDX]

M90.819   Osteopathy in diseases classified elsewhere, unspecified shoulder — [Not Allowed as PDX]

M90.82- Osteopathy in diseases classified elsewhere, upper arm

M90.821   Osteopathy in diseases classified elsewhere, right upper arm — [Not Allowed as PDX]

M90.822   Osteopathy in diseases classified elsewhere, left upper arm — [Not Allowed as PDX]

M90.829   Osteopathy in diseases classified elsewhere, unspecified upper arm — [Not Allowed as PDX]

M90.83- Osteopathy in diseases classified elsewhere, forearm

M90.831   Osteopathy in diseases classified elsewhere, right forearm — [Not Allowed as PDX]

M90.832   Osteopathy in diseases classified elsewhere, left forearm — [Not Allowed as PDX]

M90.839   Osteopathy in diseases classified elsewhere, unspecified forearm — [Not Allowed as PDX]

M90.84- Osteopathy in diseases classified elsewhere, hand

M90.841   Osteopathy in diseases classified elsewhere, right hand — [Not Allowed as PDX]

M90.842   Osteopathy in diseases classified elsewhere, left hand — [Not Allowed as PDX]

M90.849   Osteopathy in diseases classified elsewhere, unspecified hand — [Not Allowed as PDX]

M90.85- Osteopathy in diseases classified elsewhere, thigh

M90.851   Osteopathy in diseases classified elsewhere, right thigh — [Not Allowed as PDX]

M90.852   Osteopathy in diseases classified elsewhere, left thigh — [Not Allowed as PDX]

M90.859   Osteopathy in diseases classified elsewhere, unspecified thigh — [Not Allowed as PDX]

M90.86- Osteopathy in diseases classified elsewhere, lower leg

M90.861   Osteopathy in diseases classified elsewhere, right lower leg — [Not Allowed as PDX]

M90.862   Osteopathy in diseases classified elsewhere, left lower leg — [Not Allowed as PDX]

M90.869   Osteopathy in diseases classified elsewhere, unspecified lower leg — [Not Allowed as PDX]

M90.87- Osteopathy in diseases classified elsewhere, ankle and foot

M90.871   Osteopathy in diseases classified elsewhere, right ankle and foot — [Not Allowed as PDX]

M90.872   Osteopathy in diseases classified elsewhere, left ankle and foot — [Not Allowed as PDX]

M90.879   Osteopathy in diseases classified elsewhere, unspecified ankle and foot — [Not Allowed as PDX]

M90.88   Osteopathy in diseases classified elsewhere, other site — [Not Allowed as PDX]

M90.89   Osteopathy in diseases classified elsewhere, multiple sites — [Not Allowed as PDX]

Chondropathies (M91-M94)

Excludes 1:   postprocedural chondropathies (M96.-)

M91-   Juvenile osteochondrosis of hip and pelvis — A developmental disease of the hip and pelvis bone-growth centers characterized by degeneration and recalcification of the hip or pelvis with resultant deformity.

Excludes 1:   slipped upper femoral epiphysis (nontraumatic) (M93.0)

M91.0   Juvenile osteochondrosis of pelvis
Osteochondrosis (juvenile) of acetabulum
Osteochondrosis (juvenile) of iliac crest [Buchanan]
Osteochondrosis (juvenile) of ischiopubic synchondrosis [van Neck]
Osteochondrosis (juvenile) of symphysis pubis [Pierson]

M91.1-   Juvenile osteochondrosis of head of femur [Legg-Calvé-Perthes]

M91.10   Juvenile osteochondrosis of head of femur [Legg-Calvé-Perthes], unspecified leg

M91.11   Juvenile osteochondrosis of head of femur [Legg-Calvé-Perthes], right leg

M91.12   Juvenile osteochondrosis of head of femur [Legg-Calvé-Perthes], left leg

M91.2-   Coxa plana
Hip deformity due to previous juvenile osteochondrosis

M91.20   Coxa plana, unspecified hip

M91.21   Coxa plana, right hip

M91.22   Coxa plana, left hip

M91.3-   Pseudocoxalgia

M91.30   Pseudocoxalgia, unspecified hip

M91.31   Pseudocoxalgia, right hip

M91.32   Pseudocoxalgia, left hip

M91.4-   Coxa magna

M91.40   Coxa magna, unspecified hip

M91.41   Coxa magna, right hip

M91.42   Coxa magna, left hip

M91.8-   Other juvenile osteochondrosis of hip and pelvis
Juvenile osteochondrosis after reduction of congenital dislocation of hip

M91.80   Other juvenile osteochondrosis of hip and pelvis, unspecified leg

M91.81   Other juvenile osteochondrosis of hip and pelvis, right leg

M91.82   Other juvenile osteochondrosis of hip and pelvis, left leg

M91.9-   Juvenile osteochondrosis of hip and pelvis, unspecified

M91.90   Juvenile osteochondrosis of hip and pelvis, unspecified, unspecified leg

M91.91   Juvenile osteochondrosis of hip and pelvis, unspecified, right leg

M91.92   Juvenile osteochondrosis of hip and pelvis, unspecified, left leg

M92-   Other juvenile osteochondrosis

M92.0-   Juvenile osteochondrosis of humerus
Osteochondrosis (juvenile) of capitulum of humerus [Panner]
Osteochondrosis (juvenile) of head of humerus [Haas]

M92.00   Juvenile osteochondrosis of humerus, unspecified arm

M92.01   Juvenile osteochondrosis of humerus, right arm

M92.02   Juvenile osteochondrosis of humerus, left arm

M92.1-   Juvenile osteochondrosis of radius and ulna
Osteochondrosis (juvenile) of lower ulna [Burns]
Osteochondrosis (juvenile) of radial head [Brailsford]

M92.10   Juvenile osteochondrosis of radius and ulna, unspecified arm

M92.11   Juvenile osteochondrosis of radius and ulna, right arm

M92.12   Juvenile osteochondrosis of radius and ulna, left arm

M92.2-   Juvenile osteochondrosis, hand

M92.20- Unspecified juvenile osteochondrosis, hand

M92.201   Unspecified juvenile osteochondrosis, right hand

M92.202   Unspecified juvenile osteochondrosis, left hand

M92.209   Unspecified juvenile osteochondrosis, unspecified hand

M92.21-Osteochondrosis (juvenile) of <u>carpal lunate [Kienböck]</u>

  M92.211 Osteochondrosis (juvenile) of carpal lunate [Kienböck], <u>right</u> hand

  M92.212 Osteochondrosis (juvenile) of carpal lunate [Kienböck], <u>left</u> hand

  M92.219 Osteochondrosis (juvenile) of carpal lunate [Kienböck], <u>unspecified</u> hand

M92.22-Osteochondrosis (juvenile) of <u>metacarpal heads [Mauclaire]</u>

  M92.221 Osteochondrosis (juvenile) of metacarpal heads [Mauclaire], <u>right</u> hand

  M92.222 Osteochondrosis (juvenile) of metacarpal heads [Mauclaire], <u>left</u> hand

  M92.229 Osteochondrosis (juvenile) of metacarpal heads [Mauclaire], <u>unspecified</u> hand

M92.29-<u>Other</u> juvenile osteochondrosis, <u>hand</u>

  M92.291 Other juvenile osteochondrosis, <u>right</u> hand

  M92.292 Other juvenile osteochondrosis, <u>left</u> hand

  M92.299 Other juvenile osteochondrosis, <u>unspecified</u> hand

M92.3- <u>Other</u> juvenile osteochondrosis, <u>upper limb</u>

  M92.30 Other juvenile osteochondrosis, <u>unspecified</u> upper limb

  M92.31 Other juvenile osteochondrosis, <u>right</u> upper limb

  M92.32 Other juvenile osteochondrosis, <u>left</u> upper limb

M92.4- Juvenile osteochondrosis of <u>patella</u>

  Osteochondrosis (juvenile) of primary patellar center [Köhler]
  Osteochondrosis (juvenile) of secondary patellar centre [Sinding Larsen]

  M92.40 Juvenile osteochondrosis of patella, <u>unspecified</u> knee

  M92.41 Juvenile osteochondrosis of patella, <u>right</u> knee

  M92.42 Juvenile osteochondrosis of patella, <u>left</u> knee

M92.5- Juvenile osteochondrosis of <u>tibia and fibula</u>

  Osteochondrosis (juvenile) of proximal tibia [Blount]
  Osteochondrosis (juvenile) of tibial tubercle [Osgood-Schlatter]
  Tibia vara

  M92.50 Juvenile osteochondrosis of tibia and fibula, <u>unspecified</u> leg

  M92.51 Juvenile osteochondrosis of tibia and fibula, <u>right</u> leg

  M92.52 Juvenile osteochondrosis of tibia and fibula, <u>left</u> leg

M92.6- Juvenile osteochondrosis of <u>tarsus</u>

  Osteochondrosis (juvenile) of calcaneum [Sever]
  Osteochondrosis (juvenile) of os tibiale externum [Haglund]
  Osteochondrosis (juvenile) of talus [Diaz]
  Osteochondrosis (juvenile) of tarsal navicular [Köhler]

  M92.60 Juvenile osteochondrosis of tarsus, <u>unspecified</u> ankle

  M92.61 Juvenile osteochondrosis of tarsus, <u>right</u> ankle

  M92.62 Juvenile osteochondrosis of tarsus, <u>left</u> ankle

M92.7- Juvenile osteochondrosis of <u>metatarsus</u>

  Osteochondrosis (juvenile) of fifth metatarsus [Iselin]
  Osteochondrosis (juvenile) of second metatarsus [Freiberg]

  M92.70 Juvenile osteochondrosis of metatarsus, <u>unspecified</u> foot

  M92.71 Juvenile osteochondrosis of metatarsus, <u>right</u> foot

  M92.72 Juvenile osteochondrosis of metatarsus, <u>left</u> foot

M92.8 <u>Other specified</u> juvenile osteochondrosis

  Calcaneal apophysitis

M92.9 Juvenile osteochondrosis, <u>unspecified</u>

  Juvenile apophysitis NOS
  Juvenile epiphysitis NOS
  Juvenile osteochondritis NOS
  Juvenile osteochondrosis NOS

M93- Other osteochondropathies

  Excludes ❷: *osteochondrosis of spine (M42.-)*

M93.0- <u>Slipped upper femoral epiphysis (nontraumatic)</u> — The partial dislocation of the hip that is not due to trauma.

  Use additional code for associated chondrolysis (M94.3)

  M93.00-<u>Unspecified</u> slipped upper femoral epiphysis (nontraumatic)

    M93.001 Unspecified slipped upper femoral epiphysis (nontraumatic), <u>right</u> hip

    M93.002 Unspecified slipped upper femoral epiphysis (nontraumatic), <u>left</u> hip

    M93.003 Unspecified slipped upper femoral epiphysis (nontraumatic), <u>unspecified</u> hip

  M93.01-<u>Acute</u> slipped upper femoral epiphysis (nontraumatic)

    M93.011 Acute slipped upper femoral epiphysis (nontraumatic), <u>right</u> hip

    M93.012 Acute slipped upper femoral epiphysis (nontraumatic), <u>left</u> hip

    M93.013 Acute slipped upper femoral epiphysis (nontraumatic), <u>unspecified</u> hip

  M93.02-<u>Chronic</u> slipped upper femoral epiphysis (nontraumatic)

    M93.021 Chronic slipped upper femoral epiphysis (nontraumatic), <u>right</u> hip

    M93.022 Chronic slipped upper femoral epiphysis (nontraumatic), <u>left</u> hip

    M93.023 Chronic slipped upper femoral epiphysis (nontraumatic), <u>unspecified</u> hip

  M93.03-<u>Acute on chronic</u> slipped upper femoral epiphysis (nontraumatic)

    M93.031 Acute on chronic slipped upper femoral epiphysis (nontraumatic), <u>right</u> hip

    M93.032 Acute on chronic slipped upper femoral epiphysis (nontraumatic), <u>left</u> hip

    M93.033 Acute on chronic slipped upper femoral epiphysis (nontraumatic), <u>unspecified</u> hip

M93.1 Kienböck's disease of adults — [Age/15-124] — Degeneration and recalcification of the bones in adults.

  Adult osteochondrosis of carpal lunates

M93.2- <u>Osteochondritis dissecans</u> — Inflammation of both the bone and cartilage with fragmenting pieces of cartilage into the joint.

  M93.20 Osteochondritis dissecans of <u>unspecified site</u>

  M93.21-Osteochondritis dissecans of <u>shoulder</u>

    M93.211 Osteochondritis dissecans, <u>right</u> shoulder

    M93.212 Osteochondritis dissecans, <u>left</u> shoulder

    M93.219 Osteochondritis dissecans, <u>unspecified</u> shoulder

  M93.22-Osteochondritis dissecans of <u>elbow</u>

    M93.221 Osteochondritis dissecans, <u>right</u> elbow

    M93.222 Osteochondritis dissecans, <u>left</u> elbow

    M93.229 Osteochondritis dissecans, <u>unspecified</u> elbow

  M93.23-Osteochondritis dissecans of <u>wrist</u>

    M93.231 Osteochondritis dissecans, <u>right</u> wrist

    M93.232 Osteochondritis dissecans, <u>left</u> wrist

    M93.239 Osteochondritis dissecans, <u>unspecified</u> wrist

  M93.24-Osteochondritis dissecans of <u>joints of hand</u>

    M93.241 Osteochondritis dissecans, joints of <u>right</u> hand

    M93.242 Osteochondritis dissecans, joints of <u>left</u> hand

    M93.249 Osteochondritis dissecans, joints of <u>unspecified</u> hand

  M93.25-Osteochondritis dissecans of <u>hip</u>

    M93.251 Osteochondritis dissecans, <u>right</u> hip

    M93.252 Osteochondritis dissecans, <u>left</u> hip

    M93.259 Osteochondritis dissecans, <u>unspecified</u> hip

  M93.26-Osteochondritis dissecans <u>knee</u>

    M93.261 Osteochondritis dissecans, <u>right</u> knee

    M93.262 Osteochondritis dissecans, <u>left</u> knee

    M93.269 Osteochondritis dissecans, <u>unspecified</u> knee

  M93.27-Osteochondritis dissecans of <u>ankle and joints of foot</u>

    M93.271 Osteochondritis dissecans, <u>right</u> ankle and joints of <u>right</u> foot

    M93.272 Osteochondritis dissecans, <u>left</u> ankle and joints of <u>left</u> foot

    M93.279 Osteochondritis dissecans, <u>unspecified</u> ankle and joints of foot

  M93.28 Osteochondritis dissecans <u>other site</u>

  M93.29 Osteochondritis dissecans <u>multiple sites</u>

M93.8- <u>Other specified</u> osteochondropathies

  M93.80 Other specified osteochondropathies of <u>unspecified site</u>

M92
|
M93

M93.81- Other specified osteochondropathies of <u>shoulder</u>
- M93.811   Other specified osteochondropathies, <u>right</u> shoulder
- M93.812   Other specified osteochondropathies, <u>left</u> shoulder
- M93.819   Other specified osteochondropathies, <u>unspecified</u> shoulder

M93.82- Other specified osteochondropathies of <u>upper arm</u>
- M93.821   Other specified osteochondropathies, <u>right</u> upper arm
- M93.822   Other specified osteochondropathies, <u>left</u> upper arm
- M93.829   Other specified osteochondropathies, <u>unspecified</u> upper arm

M93.83- Other specified osteochondropathies of <u>forearm</u>
- M93.831   Other specified osteochondropathies, <u>right</u> forearm
- M93.832   Other specified osteochondropathies, <u>left</u> forearm
- M93.839   Other specified osteochondropathies, <u>unspecified</u> forearm

M93.84- Other specified osteochondropathies of <u>hand</u>
- M93.841   Other specified osteochondropathies, <u>right</u> hand
- M93.842   Other specified osteochondropathies, <u>left</u> hand
- M93.849   Other specified osteochondropathies, <u>unspecified</u> hand

M93.85- Other specified osteochondropathies of <u>thigh</u>
- M93.851   Other specified osteochondropathies, <u>right</u> thigh
- M93.852   Other specified osteochondropathies, <u>left</u> thigh
- M93.859   Other specified osteochondropathies, <u>unspecified</u> thigh

M93.86- Other specified osteochondropathies <u>lower leg</u>
- M93.861   Other specified osteochondropathies, <u>right</u> lower leg
- M93.862   Other specified osteochondropathies, <u>left</u> lower leg
- M93.869   Other specified osteochondropathies, <u>unspecified</u> lower leg

M93.87- Other specified osteochondropathies of <u>ankle and foot</u>
- M93.871   Other specified osteochondropathies, <u>right</u> ankle and foot
- M93.872   Other specified osteochondropathies, <u>left</u> ankle and foot
- M93.879   Other specified osteochondropathies, <u>unspecified</u> ankle and foot

M93.88   Other specified osteochondropathies <u>other</u>

M93.89   Other specified osteochondropathies <u>multiple sites</u>

M93.9-   Osteochondropathy, <u>unspecified</u>
     Apophysitis NOS
     Epiphysitis NOS
     Osteochondritis NOS
     Osteochondrosis NOS

M93.90   Osteochondropathy, unspecified of <u>unspecified</u> <u>site</u>

M93.91- Osteochondropathy, unspecified of <u>shoulder</u>
- M93.911   Osteochondropathy, unspecified, <u>right</u> shoulder
- M93.912   Osteochondropathy, unspecified, <u>left</u> shoulder
- M93.919   Osteochondropathy, unspecified, <u>unspecified</u> shoulder

M93.92- Osteochondropathy, unspecified of <u>upper arm</u>
- M93.921   Osteochondropathy, unspecified, <u>right</u> upper arm
- M93.922   Osteochondropathy, unspecified, <u>left</u> upper arm
- M93.929   Osteochondropathy, unspecified, <u>unspecified</u> upper arm

M93.93- Osteochondropathy, unspecified of <u>forearm</u>
- M93.931   Osteochondropathy, unspecified, <u>right</u> forearm
- M93.932   Osteochondropathy, unspecified, <u>left</u> forearm
- M93.939   Osteochondropathy, unspecified, <u>unspecified</u> forearm

M93.94- Osteochondropathy, unspecified of <u>hand</u>
- M93.941   Osteochondropathy, unspecified, <u>right</u> hand
- M93.942   Osteochondropathy, unspecified, <u>left</u> hand

M93.949   Osteochondropathy, unspecified, <u>unspecified</u> hand

M93.95- Osteochondropathy, unspecified of <u>thigh</u>
- M93.951   Osteochondropathy, unspecified, <u>right</u> thigh
- M93.952   Osteochondropathy, unspecified, <u>left</u> thigh
- M93.959   Osteochondropathy, unspecified, <u>unspecified</u> thigh

M93.96- Osteochondropathy, unspecified <u>lower leg</u>
- M93.961   Osteochondropathy, unspecified, <u>right</u> lower leg
- M93.962   Osteochondropathy, unspecified, <u>left</u> lower leg
- M93.969   Osteochondropathy, unspecified, <u>unspecified</u> lower leg

M93.97- Osteochondropathy, unspecified of <u>ankle and foot</u>
- M93.971   Osteochondropathy, unspecified, <u>right</u> ankle and foot
- M93.972   Osteochondropathy, unspecified, <u>left</u> ankle and foot
- M93.979   Osteochondropathy, unspecified, <u>unspecified</u> ankle and foot

M93.98   Osteochondropathy, unspecified <u>other</u>

M93.99   Osteochondropathy, unspecified <u>multiple sites</u>

M94-   <u>Other disorders of cartilage</u>

M94.0   **Chondrocostal junction syndrome [Tietze]** — Inflammation of the costal cartilages of the ribs with chest pain similar to coronary artery disease.
     Costochondritis

M94.1   **Relapsing polychondritis** — Inflammation and degeneration of various cartilaginous structures.

M94.2-   <u>Chondromalacia</u> — The softening of the articular cartilage.
     Excludes 1:   chondromalacia patellae (M22.4)

M94.20   Chondromalacia, <u>unspecified</u> site

M94.21- Chondromalacia, <u>shoulder</u>
- M94.211   Chondromalacia, <u>right</u> shoulder
- M94.212   Chondromalacia, <u>left</u> shoulder
- M94.219   Chondromalacia, <u>unspecified</u> shoulder

M94.22- Chondromalacia, <u>elbow</u>
- M94.221   Chondromalacia, <u>right</u> elbow
- M94.222   Chondromalacia, <u>left</u> elbow
- M94.229   Chondromalacia, <u>unspecified</u> elbow

M94.23- Chondromalacia, <u>wrist</u>
- M94.231   Chondromalacia, <u>right</u> wrist
- M94.232   Chondromalacia, <u>left</u> wrist
- M94.239   Chondromalacia, <u>unspecified</u> wrist

M94.24- Chondromalacia, joints of <u>hand</u>
- M94.241   Chondromalacia, joints of <u>right</u> hand
- M94.242   Chondromalacia, joints of <u>left</u> hand
- M94.249   Chondromalacia, joints of <u>unspecified</u> hand

M94.25- Chondromalacia, <u>hip</u>
- M94.251   Chondromalacia, <u>right</u> hip
- M94.252   Chondromalacia, <u>left</u> hip
- M94.259   Chondromalacia, <u>unspecified</u> hip

M94.26- Chondromalacia, <u>knee</u>
- M94.261   Chondromalacia, <u>right</u> knee
- M94.262   Chondromalacia, <u>left</u> knee
- M94.269   Chondromalacia, <u>unspecified</u> knee

M94.27- Chondromalacia, <u>ankle and joints of foot</u>
- M94.271   Chondromalacia, <u>right</u> ankle and joints of <u>right</u> foot
- M94.272   Chondromalacia, <u>left</u> ankle and joints of <u>left</u> foot
- M94.279   Chondromalacia, <u>unspecified</u> ankle and joints of foot

M94.28   Chondromalacia, <u>other site</u>

M94.29   Chondromalacia, <u>multiple sites</u>

M93 - M94

M94.3- <u>Chondrolysis</u> — Resorption of cartilage.
Code first any associated slipped upper femoral epiphysis (nontraumatic) (M93.0-)

    M94.35- Chondrolysis, <u>hip</u>

        M94.351 Chondrolysis, <u>right</u> hip

        M94.352 Chondrolysis, <u>left</u> hip

        M94.359 Chondrolysis, <u>unspecified</u> hip

M94.8- Other specified disorders of cartilage

    M94.8x- <u>Other specified disorders of cartilage</u>

        M94.8x0 Other specified disorders of cartilage, multiple sites

        M94.8x1 Other specified disorders of cartilage, shoulder

        M94.8x2 Other specified disorders of cartilage, upper arm

        M94.8x3 Other specified disorders of cartilage, forearm

        M94.8x4 Other specified disorders of cartilage, hand

        M94.8x5 Other specified disorders of cartilage, thigh

        M94.8x6 Other specified disorders of cartilage, lower leg

        M94.8x7 Other specified disorders of cartilage, ankle and foot

        M94.8x8 Other specified disorders of cartilage, other site

        M94.8x9 Other specified disorders of cartilage, unspecified sites

    M94.9 Disorder of cartilage, <u>unspecified</u>

Other disorders of the musculoskeletal system and connective tissue (M95)

M95- Other acquired deformities of musculoskeletal system and connective tissue

    Excludes ❷: *acquired absence of limbs and organs (Z89-Z90)*
          acquired deformities of limbs (M20-M21)
          congenital malformations and deformations of the
            musculoskeletal system (Q65-Q79)
          deforming dorsopathies (M40-M43)
          dentofacial anomalies [including malocclusion] (M26.-)
          postprocedural musculoskeletal disorders (M96.-)

    M95.0 Acquired deformity of nose

        Excludes ❷: *deviated nasal septum (J34.2)*

    M95.1- <u>Cauliflower</u> ear — Formation of fibrous tissue at the site of damaged cartilage of the ear.

        Excludes ❷: *other acquired deformities of ear (H61.1)*

        M95.10 Cauliflower ear, <u>unspecified</u> ear

        M95.11 Cauliflower ear, <u>right</u> ear

        M95.12 Cauliflower ear, <u>left</u> ear

    M95.2 Other acquired deformity of <u>head</u>

    M95.3 Acquired deformity of <u>neck</u>

    M95.4 Acquired deformity of <u>chest and rib</u>

        AHA 14:4Q:p26 – Rib deformity associated with congenital scoliosis

    M95.5 Acquired deformity of <u>pelvis</u>

        Excludes 1:   *maternal care for known or suspected disproportion (O33.-)*

    M95.8 Other specified acquired deformities of musculoskeletal system

    M95.9 Acquired deformity of musculoskeletal system, <u>unspecified</u>

Intraoperative and postprocedural complications and disorders of musculoskeletal system, not elsewhere classified (M96)

M96- <u>Intraoperative and postprocedural complications</u> and disorders of musculoskeletal system, not elsewhere classified

    Excludes ❷: *arthropathy following intestinal bypass (M02.0-)*
          complications of internal orthopedic prosthetic devices,
            implants and grafts (T84.-)
          disorders associated with osteoporosis (M80)
          periprosthetic fracture around internal prosthetic joint (M97.-)
          presence of functional implants and other devices (Z96-Z97)

  cc **M96.0** Pseudarthrosis after fusion or arthrodesis

    M96.1 Postlaminectomy syndrome, not elsewhere classified

    M96.2 Postradiation kyphosis

    M96.3 Postlaminectomy kyphosis

    M96.4 Postsurgical lordosis

    M96.5 Postradiation scoliosis

    M96.6- <u>Fracture of bone following insertion of orthopedic implant, joint prosthesis, or bone plate</u>

        Intraoperative fracture of bone during insertion of orthopedic implant, joint prosthesis, or bone plate

        Excludes ❷: *complication of internal orthopedic devices, implants or grafts (T84.-)*

    M96.62- Fracture of <u>humerus</u> following insertion of orthopedic implant, joint prosthesis, or bone plate

    cc **M96.621** Fracture of humerus following insertion of orthopedic implant, joint prosthesis, or bone plate, <u>right</u> arm

    cc **M96.622** Fracture of humerus following insertion of orthopedic implant, joint prosthesis, or bone plate, <u>left</u> arm

    cc **M96.629** Fracture of humerus following insertion of orthopedic implant, joint prosthesis, or bone plate, <u>unspecified</u> arm

    M96.63- Fracture of <u>radius or ulna</u> following insertion of orthopedic implant, joint prosthesis, or bone plate

    cc **M96.631** Fracture of radius or ulna following insertion of orthopedic implant, joint prosthesis, or bone plate, <u>right</u> arm

    cc **M96.632** Fracture of radius or ulna following insertion of orthopedic implant, joint prosthesis, or bone plate, <u>left</u> arm

    cc **M96.639** Fracture of radius or ulna following insertion of orthopedic implant, joint prosthesis, or bone plate, <u>unspecified</u> arm

  cc **M96.65** Fracture of <u>pelvis</u> following insertion of orthopedic implant, joint prosthesis, or bone plate

    M96.66- Fracture of <u>femur</u> following insertion of orthopedic implant, joint prosthesis, or bone plate

    cc **M96.661** Fracture of femur following insertion of orthopedic implant, joint prosthesis, or bone plate, <u>right</u> leg

    cc **M96.662** Fracture of femur following insertion of orthopedic implant, joint prosthesis, or bone plate, <u>left</u> leg

    cc **M96.669** Fracture of femur following insertion of orthopedic implant, joint prosthesis, or bone plate, <u>unspecified</u> leg

    M96.67- Fracture of <u>tibia or fibula</u> following insertion of orthopedic implant, joint prosthesis, or bone plate

    cc **M96.671** Fracture of tibia or fibula following insertion of orthopedic implant, joint prosthesis, or bone plate, <u>right</u> leg

    cc **M96.672** Fracture of tibia or fibula following insertion of orthopedic implant, joint prosthesis, or bone plate, <u>left</u> leg

    cc **M96.679** Fracture of tibia or fibula following insertion of orthopedic implant, joint prosthesis, or bone plate, <u>unspecified</u> leg

  cc **M96.69** Fracture of <u>other bone</u> following insertion of orthopedic implant, joint prosthesis, or bone plate

M94 - M96

Excludes 1: = NOT CODED HERE! (Do not code both)   *Excludes ❷: = Not Included Here*

M96.8- <u>Other</u> intraoperative and postprocedural complications and disorders of musculoskeletal system, not elsewhere classified

M96.81- <u>Intraoperative hemorrhage and hematoma</u> of a musculoskeletal structure complicating a procedure

> Excludes 1:   intraoperative hemorrhage and hematoma of a musculoskeletal structure due to accidental puncture and laceration during a procedure (M96.82-)

cc **M96.810** Intraoperative hemorrhage and hematoma of a musculoskeletal structure complicating a <u>musculoskeletal system procedure</u>

cc **M96.811** Intraoperative hemorrhage and hematoma of a musculoskeletal structure complicating <u>other procedure</u>

M96.82- <u>Accidental puncture and laceration</u> of a musculoskeletal structure during a procedure

cc **M96.820** Accidental puncture and laceration of a musculoskeletal structure during a <u>musculoskeletal system procedure</u>

cc **M96.821** Accidental puncture and laceration of a musculoskeletal structure during <u>other procedure</u>

M96.83- <u>Postprocedural hemorrhage</u> of a musculoskeletal structure following a procedure

cc **M96.830** Postprocedural <u>hemorrhage</u> of a musculoskeletal structure following a <u>musculoskeletal system procedure</u>

cc **M96.831** Postprocedural <u>hemorrhage</u> of a musculoskeletal structure following <u>other procedure</u>

M96.84- <u>Postprocedural hematoma and seroma</u> of a musculoskeletal structure following a procedure

cc **M96.840** Postprocedural <u>hematoma</u> of a musculoskeletal structure following a <u>musculoskeletal system procedure</u>

cc **M96.841** Postprocedural <u>hematoma</u> of a musculoskeletal structure following <u>other procedure</u>

cc **M96.842** Postprocedural <u>seroma</u> of a musculoskeletal structure following a <u>musculoskeletal system procedure</u>

cc **M96.843** Postprocedural <u>seroma</u> of a musculoskeletal structure following <u>other procedure</u>

cc **M96.89** Other intraoperative and postprocedural complications and disorders of the musculoskeletal system

> Instability of joint secondary to removal of joint prosthesis
> Use additional code, if applicable, to further specify disorder

Periprosthetic fracture around internal prosthetic joint (M97)

M97- <u>Periprosthetic</u> fracture around internal prosthetic joint

> *Excludes ❷:*   breakage (fracture) of prosthetic joint (T84.01-)
> fracture of bone following insertion of orthopedic implant, joint prosthesis or bone plate (M96.6-)

The appropriate 7th character is to be added to each code from category M97:
A   Initial encounter
D   Subsequent encounter
S   Sequela

M97.0- Periprosthetic fracture around internal prosthetic <u>hip</u> joint

cc-a **M97.01x-** Periprosthetic fracture around internal prosthetic <u>right</u> hip joint

cc-a **M97.02x-** Periprosthetic fracture around internal prosthetic <u>left</u> hip joint

M97.1- Periprosthetic fracture around internal prosthetic <u>knee</u> joint

cc-a **M97.11x-** Periprosthetic fracture around internal prosthetic <u>right</u> knee joint

cc-a **M97.12x-** Periprosthetic fracture around internal prosthetic <u>left</u> knee joint

M97.2- Periprosthetic fracture around internal prosthetic <u>ankle</u> joint

cc-a **M97.21x-** Periprosthetic fracture around internal prosthetic <u>right</u> ankle joint

cc-a **M97.22x-** Periprosthetic fracture around internal prosthetic <u>left</u> ankle joint

M97.3- Periprosthetic fracture around internal prosthetic <u>shoulder</u> joint

cc-a **M97.31x-** Periprosthetic fracture around internal prosthetic <u>right</u> shoulder joint

cc-a **M97.32x-** Periprosthetic fracture around internal prosthetic <u>left</u> shoulder joint

M97.4- Periprosthetic fracture around internal prosthetic <u>elbow</u> joint

cc-a **M97.41x-** Periprosthetic fracture around internal prosthetic <u>right</u> elbow joint

cc-a **M97.42x-** Periprosthetic fracture around internal prosthetic <u>left</u> elbow joint

cc-a **M97.8xx-** Periprosthetic fracture around <u>other</u> internal prosthetic joint

> Periprosthetic fracture around internal prosthetic finger joint
> Periprosthetic fracture around internal prosthetic spinal joint
> Periprosthetic fracture around internal prosthetic toe joint
> Periprosthetic fracture around internal prosthetic wrist joint
> Use additional code to identify the joint (Z96.6-)

cc-a **M97.9xx-** Periprosthetic fracture around <u>unspecified</u> internal prosthetic joint

M 9 5 - M 9 7

Biomechanical lesions, not elsewhere classified (M99)

M99- Biomechanical lesions, <u>not elsewhere classified</u>
   Note: This category should not be used if the condition can be classified elsewhere.

M99.0- <u>Segmental and somatic dysfunction</u>
   M99.00 Segmental and somatic dysfunction of head region
   M99.01 Segmental and somatic dysfunction of cervical region
   M99.02 Segmental and somatic dysfunction of thoracic region
   M99.03 Segmental and somatic dysfunction of lumbar region
   M99.04 Segmental and somatic dysfunction of sacral region
   M99.05 Segmental and somatic dysfunction of pelvic region
   M99.06 Segmental and somatic dysfunction of lower extremity
   M99.07 Segmental and somatic dysfunction of upper extremity
   M99.08 Segmental and somatic dysfunction of rib cage
   M99.09 Segmental and somatic dysfunction of abdomen and other regions

M99.1- <u>Subluxation complex (vertebral)</u>
   cc **M99.10** Subluxation complex (vertebral) of head region
   cc **M99.11** Subluxation complex (vertebral) of cervical region
   M99.12 Subluxation complex (vertebral) of thoracic region
   M99.13 Subluxation complex (vertebral) of lumbar region
   M99.14 Subluxation complex (vertebral) of sacral region
   M99.15 Subluxation complex (vertebral) of pelvic region
   M99.16 Subluxation complex (vertebral) of lower extremity
   M99.17 Subluxation complex (vertebral) of upper extremity
   cc **M99.18** Subluxation complex (vertebral) of rib cage
   M99.19 Subluxation complex (vertebral) of abdomen and other regions

M99.2- <u>Subluxation stenosis</u> of neural canal
   M99.20 Subluxation stenosis of neural canal of head region
   M99.21 Subluxation stenosis of neural canal of cervical region
   M99.22 Subluxation stenosis of neural canal of thoracic region
   M99.23 Subluxation stenosis of neural canal of lumbar region
   M99.24 Subluxation stenosis of neural canal of sacral region
   M99.25 Subluxation stenosis of neural canal of pelvic region
   M99.26 Subluxation stenosis of neural canal of lower extremity
   M99.27 Subluxation stenosis of neural canal of upper extremity
   M99.28 Subluxation stenosis of neural canal of rib cage
   M99.29 Subluxation stenosis of neural canal of abdomen and other regions

M99.3- <u>Osseous stenosis</u> of neural canal
   M99.30 Osseous stenosis of neural canal of head region
   M99.31 Osseous stenosis of neural canal of cervical region
   M99.32 Osseous stenosis of neural canal of thoracic region
   M99.33 Osseous stenosis of neural canal of lumbar region
   M99.34 Osseous stenosis of neural canal of sacral region
   M99.35 Osseous stenosis of neural canal of pelvic region
   M99.36 Osseous stenosis of neural canal of lower extremity
   M99.37 Osseous stenosis of neural canal of upper extremity
   M99.38 Osseous stenosis of neural canal of rib cage
   M99.39 Osseous stenosis of neural canal of abdomen and other regions

M99.4- <u>Connective tissue stenosis</u> of neural canal
   M99.40 Connective tissue stenosis of neural canal of head region
   M99.41 Connective tissue stenosis of neural canal of cervical region
   M99.42 Connective tissue stenosis of neural canal of thoracic region
   M99.43 Connective tissue stenosis of neural canal of lumbar region
   M99.44 Connective tissue stenosis of neural canal of sacral region
   M99.45 Connective tissue stenosis of neural canal of pelvic region
   M99.46 Connective tissue stenosis of neural canal of lower extremity
   M99.47 Connective tissue stenosis of neural canal of upper extremity
   M99.48 Connective tissue stenosis of neural canal of rib cage
   M99.49 Connective tissue stenosis of neural canal of abdomen and other regions

M99.5- <u>Intervertebral disc stenosis</u> of neural canal
   M99.50 Intervertebral disc stenosis of neural canal of head region
   M99.51 Intervertebral disc stenosis of neural canal of cervical region
   M99.52 Intervertebral disc stenosis of neural canal of thoracic region
   M99.53 Intervertebral disc stenosis of neural canal of lumbar region
   M99.54 Intervertebral disc stenosis of neural canal of sacral region
   M99.55 Intervertebral disc stenosis of neural canal of pelvic region
   M99.56 Intervertebral disc stenosis of neural canal of lower extremity
   M99.57 Intervertebral disc stenosis of neural canal of upper extremity
   M99.58 Intervertebral disc stenosis of neural canal of rib cage
   M99.59 Intervertebral disc stenosis of neural canal of abdomen and other regions

M99.6- <u>Osseous and subluxation stenosis</u> of intervertebral foramina
   M99.60 Osseous and subluxation stenosis of intervertebral foramina of head region
   M99.61 Osseous and subluxation stenosis of intervertebral foramina of cervical region
   M99.62 Osseous and subluxation stenosis of intervertebral foramina of thoracic region
   M99.63 Osseous and subluxation stenosis of intervertebral foramina of lumbar region
   M99.64 Osseous and subluxation stenosis of intervertebral foramina of sacral region
   M99.65 Osseous and subluxation stenosis of intervertebral foramina of pelvic region
   M99.66 Osseous and subluxation stenosis of intervertebral foramina of lower extremity
   M99.67 Osseous and subluxation stenosis of intervertebral foramina of upper extremity
   M99.68 Osseous and subluxation stenosis of intervertebral foramina of rib cage
   M99.69 Osseous and subluxation stenosis of intervertebral foramina of abdomen and other regions

M99 - M99

M99.7- <u>Connective tissue and disc stenosis</u> of intervertebral foramina

    M99.70 Connective tissue and disc stenosis of intervertebral foramina of head region

    M99.71 Connective tissue and disc stenosis of intervertebral foramina of cervical region

    M99.72 Connective tissue and disc stenosis of intervertebral foramina of thoracic region

    M99.73 Connective tissue and disc stenosis of intervertebral foramina of lumbar region

    M99.74 Connective tissue and disc stenosis of intervertebral foramina of sacral region

    M99.75 Connective tissue and disc stenosis of intervertebral foramina of pelvic region

    M99.76 Connective tissue and disc stenosis of intervertebral foramina of lower extremity

    M99.77 Connective tissue and disc stenosis of intervertebral foramina of upper extremity

    M99.78 Connective tissue and disc stenosis of intervertebral foramina of rib cage

    M99.79 Connective tissue and disc stenosis of intervertebral foramina of abdomen and other regions

M99.8- <u>Other</u> biomechanical lesions

    M99.80 Other biomechanical lesions of head region

    M99.81 Other biomechanical lesions of cervical region

    M99.82 Other biomechanical lesions of thoracic region

    M99.83 Other biomechanical lesions of lumbar region

    M99.84 Other biomechanical lesions of sacral region

    M99.85 Other biomechanical lesions of pelvic region

    M99.86 Other biomechanical lesions of lower extremity

    M99.87 Other biomechanical lesions of upper extremity

    M99.88 Other biomechanical lesions of rib cage

    M99.89 Other biomechanical lesions of abdomen and other regions

M99.9 Biomechanical lesion, <u>unspecified</u>

M 9 9 - M 9 9

Chapter 14 – Diseases of the genitourinary system (N00-N99)

Excludes ❷: certain conditions originating in the perinatal period (P04-P96)
certain infectious and parasitic diseases (A00-B99)
complications of pregnancy, childbirth and the puerperium (O00-O9A)
congenital malformations, deformations and chromosomal abnormalities (Q00-Q99)
endocrine, nutritional and metabolic diseases (E00-E88)
injury, poisoning and certain other consequences of external causes (S00-T88)
neoplasms (C00-D49)
symptoms, signs and abnormal clinical and laboratory findings, not elsewhere classified (R00-R94)

This chapter contains the following blocks:
N00-N08   Glomerular diseases
N10-N16   Renal tubulo-interstitial diseases
N17-N19   Acute kidney failure and chronic kidney disease
N20-N23   Urolithiasis
N25-N29   Other disorders of kidney and ureter
N30-N39   Other diseases of the urinary system
N40-N53   Diseases of male genital organs
N60-N65   Disorders of breast
N70-N77   Inflammatory diseases of female pelvic organs
N80-N98   Noninflammatory disorders of female genital tract
N99   Intraoperative and postprocedural complications and disorders of genitourinary system, not elsewhere classified

Chapter-Specific Coding Guidelines

C. Chapter-Specific Coding Guidelines
In addition to general coding guidelines, there are guidelines for specific diagnoses and/or conditions in the classification. Unless otherwise indicated, these guidelines apply to all health care settings. Please refer to Section II for guidelines on the selection of principal diagnosis.

14. Chapter 14: Diseases of Genitourinary System (N00-N99)

a. Chronic kidney disease

1) Stages of chronic kidney disease (CKD)
The ICD-10-CM classifies CKD based on severity. The severity of CKD is designated by stages 1-5. Stage 2, code N18.2, equates to mild CKD; stage 3, code N18.3, equates to moderate CKD; and stage 4, code N18.4, equates to severe CKD. Code N18.6, End stage renal disease (ESRD), is assigned when the provider has documented end-stage-renal disease (ESRD).

If both a stage of CKD and ESRD are documented, assign code N18.6 only.

2) Chronic kidney disease and kidney transplant status
Patients who have undergone kidney transplant may still have some form of chronic kidney disease (CKD) because the kidney transplant may not fully restore kidney function. Therefore, the presence of CKD alone does not constitute a transplant complication. Assign the appropriate N18 code for the patient's stage of CKD and code Z94.0, Kidney transplant status. If a transplant complication such as failure or rejection or other transplant complication is documented, see section I.C.19.g for information on coding complications of a kidney transplant. If the documentation is unclear as to whether the patient has a complication of the transplant, query the provider.

3) Chronic kidney disease with other conditions
Patients with CKD may also suffer from other serious conditions, most commonly diabetes mellitus and hypertension. The sequencing of the CKD code in relationship to codes for other contributing conditions is based on the conventions in the Tabular List.

See I.C.9. Hypertensive chronic kidney disease.
See I.C.19. Chronic kidney disease and kidney transplant complications.

Glomerular diseases (N00-N08)

Excludes 1:   hypertensive chronic kidney disease (I12.-)
Code also any associated kidney failure (N17-N19).

N00-   Acute nephritic syndrome — The sudden, sever onset of inflammation of the glomeruli of the kidney of various causes including following a streptococcal infection of the throat or skin.
Includes: Acute glomerular disease
Acute glomerulonephritis — The sudden, severe onset of inflammation and proliferation of the glomeruli of the kidney that is characterized by hematuria, proteinuria, and red blood cell casts.
Acute nephritis — The sudden, severe onset of inflammation of the kidney.
Excludes 1:   acute tubulo-interstitial nephritis (N10)
nephritic syndrome NOS (N05.-)

MCC **N00.0   Acute nephritic syndrome with minor glomerular abnormality**
Acute nephritic syndrome with minimal change lesion

MCC **N00.1   Acute nephritic syndrome with focal and segmental glomerular lesions**
Acute nephritic syndrome with focal and segmental hyalinosis
Acute nephritic syndrome with focal and segmental sclerosis
Acute nephritic syndrome with focal glomerulonephritis

MCC **N00.2   Acute nephritic syndrome with diffuse membranous glomerulonephritis**

MCC **N00.3   Acute nephritic syndrome with diffuse mesangial proliferative glomerulonephritis**

MCC **N00.4   Acute nephritic syndrome with diffuse endocapillary proliferative glomerulonephritis**

MCC **N00.5   Acute nephritic syndrome with diffuse mesangiocapillary glomerulonephritis**
Acute nephritic syndrome with membranoproliferative glomerulonephritis, types 1 and 3, or NOS

MCC **N00.6   Acute nephritic syndrome with dense deposit disease**
Acute nephritic syndrome with membranoproliferative glomerulonephritis, type 2

MCC **N00.7   Acute nephritic syndrome with diffuse crescentic glomerulonephritis**
Acute nephritic syndrome with extracapillary glomerulonephritis

MCC **N00.8   Acute nephritic syndrome with other morphologic changes**
Acute nephritic syndrome with proliferative glomerulonephritis NOS

MCC **N00.9   Acute nephritic syndrome with unspecified morphologic changes**

N01-   Rapidly progressive nephritic syndrome — A form characterized by a rapid downhill course, rapid decrease in the glomerular filtration rate, and glomerular crescent formation.
Includes: Rapidly progressive glomerular disease
Rapidly progressive glomerulonephritis
Rapidly progressive nephritis
Excludes 1:   nephritic syndrome NOS (N05.-)

MCC **N01.0   Rapidly progressive nephritic syndrome with minor glomerular abnormality**
Rapidly progressive nephritic syndrome with minimal change lesion

MCC **N01.1   Rapidly progressive nephritic syndrome with focal and segmental glomerular lesions**
Rapidly progressive nephritic syndrome with focal and segmental hyalinosis
Rapidly progressive nephritic syndrome with focal and segmental sclerosis
Rapidly progressive nephritic syndrome with focal glomerulonephritis

MCC **N01.2   Rapidly progressive nephritic syndrome with diffuse membranous glomerulonephritis**

MCC **N01.3   Rapidly progressive nephritic syndrome with diffuse mesangial proliferative glomerulonephritis**

MCC **N01.4   Rapidly progressive nephritic syndrome with diffuse endocapillary proliferative glomerulonephritis**

MCC **N01.5   Rapidly progressive nephritic syndrome with diffuse mesangiocapillary glomerulonephritis**
Rapidly progressive nephritic syndrome with membranoproliferative glomerulonephritis, types 1 and 3, or NOS

MCC **N01.6   Rapidly progressive nephritic syndrome with dense deposit disease**
Rapidly progressive nephritic syndrome with membranoproliferative glomerulonephritis, type 2

N00-N01

MCC **N01.7 Rapidly progressive nephritic syndrome with diffuse crescentic glomerulonephritis**
Rapidly progressive nephritic syndrome with extracapillary glomerulonephritis

MCC **N01.8 Rapidly progressive nephritic syndrome with other morphologic changes**
Rapidly progressive nephritic syndrome with proliferative glomerulonephritis NOS

MCC **N01.9 Rapidly progressive nephritic syndrome with unspecified morphologic changes**

N02- Recurrent and persistent hematuria
Excludes 1: *acute cystitis with hematuria (N30.01)*
hematuria NOS (R31.9)
hematuria not associated with specified morphologic lesions (R31.-)

CC **N02.0 Recurrent and persistent hematuria with minor glomerular abnormality**
Recurrent and persistent hematuria with minimal change lesion

CC **N02.1 Recurrent and persistent hematuria with focal and segmental glomerular lesions**
Recurrent and persistent hematuria with focal and segmental hyalinosis
Recurrent and persistent hematuria with focal and segmental sclerosis
Recurrent and persistent hematuria with focal glomerulonephritis

CC **N02.2 Recurrent and persistent hematuria with diffuse membranous glomerulonephritis**

CC **N02.3 Recurrent and persistent hematuria with diffuse mesangial proliferative glomerulonephritis**

CC **N02.4 Recurrent and persistent hematuria with diffuse endocapillary proliferative glomerulonephritis**

CC **N02.5 Recurrent and persistent hematuria with diffuse mesangiocapillary glomerulonephritis**
Recurrent and persistent hematuria with membranoproliferative glomerulonephritis, types 1 and 3, or NOS

CC **N02.6 Recurrent and persistent hematuria with dense deposit disease**
Recurrent and persistent hematuria with membranoproliferative glomerulonephritis, type 2

CC **N02.7 Recurrent and persistent hematuria with diffuse crescentic glomerulonephritis**
Recurrent and persistent hematuria with extracapillary glomerulonephritis

CC **N02.8 Recurrent and persistent hematuria with other morphologic changes**
Recurrent and persistent hematuria with proliferative glomerulonephritis NOS

CC **N02.9 Recurrent and persistent hematuria with unspecified morphologic changes**

N03- Chronic nephritic syndrome — A form that persists over a long period of time.
Includes: Chronic glomerular disease
Chronic glomerulonephritis
Chronic nephritis
Excludes 1: *chronic tubulo-interstitial nephritis (N11.-)*
diffuse sclerosing glomerulonephritis (N05.8-)
nephritic syndrome NOS (N05.-)

CC **N03.0 Chronic nephritic syndrome with minor glomerular abnormality**
Chronic nephritic syndrome with minimal change lesion

CC **N03.1 Chronic nephritic syndrome with focal and segmental glomerular lesions**
Chronic nephritic syndrome with focal and segmental hyalinosis
Chronic nephritic syndrome with focal and segmental sclerosis
Chronic nephritic syndrome with focal glomerulonephritis

CC **N03.2 Chronic nephritic syndrome with diffuse membranous glomerulonephritis**

CC **N03.3 Chronic nephritic syndrome with diffuse mesangial proliferative glomerulonephritis**

CC **N03.4 Chronic nephritic syndrome with diffuse endocapillary proliferative glomerulonephritis**

CC **N03.5 Chronic nephritic syndrome with diffuse mesangiocapillary glomerulonephritis**
Chronic nephritic syndrome with membranoproliferative glomerulonephritis, types 1 and 3, or NOS

CC **N03.6 Chronic nephritic syndrome with dense deposit disease**
Chronic nephritic syndrome with membranoproliferative glomerulonephritis, type 2

CC **N03.7 Chronic nephritic syndrome with diffuse crescentic glomerulonephritis**
Chronic nephritic syndrome with extracapillary glomerulonephritis

CC **N03.8 Chronic nephritic syndrome with other morphologic changes**
Chronic nephritic syndrome with proliferative glomerulonephritis NOS

CC **N03.9 Chronic nephritic syndrome with unspecified morphologic changes**

N04- Nephrotic syndrome — A kidney disease syndrome characterized by massive edema, marked proteinuria, hypoalbuminemia, and hyperlipidemia.
Includes: Congenital nephrotic syndrome
Lipoid nephrosis

CC **N04.0 Nephrotic syndrome with minor glomerular abnormality**
Nephrotic syndrome with minimal change lesion

CC **N04.1 Nephrotic syndrome with focal and segmental glomerular lesions**
Nephrotic syndrome with focal and segmental hyalinosis
Nephrotic syndrome with focal and segmental sclerosis
Nephrotic syndrome with focal glomerulonephritis

CC **N04.2 Nephrotic syndrome with diffuse membranous glomerulonephritis**

CC **N04.3 Nephrotic syndrome with diffuse mesangial proliferative glomerulonephritis**

CC **N04.4 Nephrotic syndrome with diffuse endocapillary proliferative glomerulonephritis**

CC **N04.5 Nephrotic syndrome with diffuse mesangiocapillary glomerulonephritis**
Nephrotic syndrome with membranoproliferative glomerulonephritis, types 1 and 3, or NOS

CC **N04.6 Nephrotic syndrome with dense deposit disease**
Nephrotic syndrome with membranoproliferative glomerulonephritis, type 2

CC **N04.7 Nephrotic syndrome with diffuse crescentic glomerulonephritis**
Nephrotic syndrome with extracapillary glomerulonephritis

CC **N04.8 Nephrotic syndrome with other morphologic changes**
Nephrotic syndrome with proliferative glomerulonephritis NOS

CC **N04.9 Nephrotic syndrome with unspecified morphologic changes**

N05- Unspecified nephritic syndrome
Includes: Glomerular disease NOS
Glomerulonephritis NOS
Nephritis NOS
Nephropathy NOS and renal disease NOS with morphological lesion specified in .0-.8
Excludes 1: *nephropathy NOS with no stated morphological lesion (N28.9)*
renal disease NOS with no stated morphological lesion (N28.9)
tubulo-interstitial nephritis NOS (N12)

N05.0 Unspecified nephritic syndrome with minor glomerular abnormality
Unspecified nephritic syndrome with minimal change lesion

N05.1 Unspecified nephritic syndrome with focal and segmental glomerular lesions
Unspecified nephritic syndrome with focal and segmental hyalinosis
Unspecified nephritic syndrome with focal and segmental sclerosis
Unspecified nephritic syndrome with focal glomerulonephritis

CC **N05.2 Unspecified nephritic syndrome with diffuse membranous glomerulonephritis**

CC **N05.3 Unspecified nephritic syndrome with diffuse mesangial proliferative glomerulonephritis**

CC **N05.4 Unspecified nephritic syndrome with diffuse endocapillary proliferative glomerulonephritis**

CC **N05.5 Unspecified nephritic syndrome with diffuse mesangiocapillary glomerulonephritis**
Unspecified nephritic syndrome with membranoproliferative glomerulonephritis, types 1 and 3, or NOS

N05.6 Unspecified nephritic syndrome with dense deposit disease
Unspecified nephritic syndrome with membranoproliferative glomerulonephritis, type 2

N05.7 Unspecified nephritic syndrome with diffuse crescentic glomerulonephritis
Unspecified nephritic syndrome with extracapillary glomerulonephritis

Excludes 1: = NOT CODED HERE! (Do not code both)   Excludes ❷: = Not Included Here

N05.8   Unspecified nephritic syndrome <u>with</u> other morphologic changes
> Unspecified nephritic syndrome with proliferative glomerulonephritis NOS

N05.9   Unspecified nephritic syndrome <u>with</u> unspecified morphologic changes

N06-   <u>Isolated proteinuria with specified morphological lesion</u>
> *Excludes 1:   proteinuria not associated with specific morphologic lesions (R80.0)*

N06.0   Isolated proteinuria <u>with</u> minor glomerular abnormality
> Isolated proteinuria with minimal change lesion

N06.1   Isolated proteinuria <u>with</u> focal and segmental glomerular lesions
> Isolated proteinuria with focal and segmental hyalinosis
> Isolated proteinuria with focal and segmental sclerosis
> Isolated proteinuria with focal glomerulonephritis

CC N06.2   Isolated proteinuria <u>with</u> <u>diffuse</u> membranous glomerulonephritis

CC N06.3   Isolated proteinuria <u>with</u> <u>diffuse</u> mesangial proliferative glomerulonephritis

CC N06.4   Isolated proteinuria <u>with</u> <u>diffuse</u> endocapillary proliferative glomerulonephritis

CC N06.5   Isolated proteinuria <u>with</u> <u>diffuse</u> mesangiocapillary glomerulonephritis
> Isolated proteinuria with membranoproliferative glomerulonephritis, types 1 and 3, or NOS

N06.6   Isolated proteinuria <u>with</u> dense deposit disease
> Isolated proteinuria with membranoproliferative glomerulonephritis, type 2

N06.7   Isolated proteinuria <u>with</u> <u>diffuse</u> crescentic glomerulonephritis
> Isolated proteinuria with extracapillary glomerulonephritis

N06.8   Isolated proteinuria <u>with</u> other morphologic lesion
> Isolated proteinuria with proliferative glomerulonephritis NOS

N06.9   Isolated proteinuria <u>with</u> unspecified morphologic lesion

N07-   <u>Hereditary nephropathy, not elsewhere classified</u>
> *Excludes ❷: Alport's syndrome (Q87.81-)*
> *hereditary amyloid nephropathy (E85.-)*
> *nail patella syndrome (Q87.2)*
> *non-neuropathic heredofamilial amyloidosis (E85.-)*

N07.0   Hereditary nephropathy, not elsewhere classified <u>with</u> minor glomerular abnormality
> Hereditary nephropathy, not elsewhere classified with minimal change lesion

N07.1   Hereditary nephropathy, not elsewhere classified <u>with</u> focal and segmental glomerular lesions
> Hereditary nephropathy, not elsewhere classified with focal and segmental hyalinosis
> Hereditary nephropathy, not elsewhere classified with focal and segmental sclerosis
> Hereditary nephropathy, not elsewhere classified with focal glomerulonephritis

CC N07.2   Hereditary nephropathy, not elsewhere classified <u>with</u> <u>diffuse</u> membranous glomerulonephritis

CC N07.3   Hereditary nephropathy, not elsewhere classified <u>with</u> <u>diffuse</u> mesangial proliferative glomerulonephritis

CC N07.4   Hereditary nephropathy, not elsewhere classified <u>with</u> <u>diffuse</u> endocapillary proliferative glomerulonephritis

CC N07.5   Hereditary nephropathy, not elsewhere classified <u>with</u> <u>diffuse</u> mesangiocapillary glomerulonephritis
> Hereditary nephropathy, not elsewhere classified with membranoproliferative glomerulonephritis, types 1 and 3, or NOS

N07.6   Hereditary nephropathy, not elsewhere classified <u>with</u> dense deposit disease
> Hereditary nephropathy, not elsewhere classified with membranoproliferative glomerulonephritis, type 2

N07.7   Hereditary nephropathy, not elsewhere classified <u>with</u> <u>diffuse</u> crescentic glomerulonephritis
> Hereditary nephropathy, not elsewhere classified with extracapillary glomerulonephritis

N07.8   Hereditary nephropathy, not elsewhere classified <u>with</u> other morphologic lesions
> Hereditary nephropathy, not elsewhere classified with proliferative glomerulonephritis NOS

N07.9   Hereditary nephropathy, not elsewhere classified <u>with</u> unspecified morphologic lesions

N08   Glomerular disorders <u>in diseases classified elsewhere</u> —
> [Not Allowed as PDX]
> Glomerulonephritis
> Nephritis
> Nephropathy
> Code first underlying disease, such as:
> Amyloidosis (E85.-)
> Congenital syphilis (A50.5)
> Cryoglobulinemia (D89.1)
> Disseminated intravascular coagulation (D65)
> Gout (M1A.-, M10.-)
> Microscopic polyangiitis (M31.7)
> Multiple myeloma (C90.0-)
> Sepsis (A40.0-A41.9)
> Sickle-cell disease (D57.0-D57.8)
> *Excludes 1:   glomerulonephritis, nephritis and nephropathy (in):*
> *antiglomerular basement membrane disease (M31.0)*
> *diabetes (E08-E13 with .21)*
> *gonococcal (A54.21)*
> *Goodpasture's syndrome (M31.0)*
> *hemolytic-uremic syndrome (D59.3)*
> *lupus (M32.14)*
> *mumps (B26.83)*
> *syphilis (A52.75)*
> *systemic lupus erythematosus (M32.14)*
> *Wegener's granulomatosis (M31.31)*
> *pyelonephritis in diseases classified elsewhere (N16)*
> *renal tubulo-interstitial disorders classified elsewhere (N16)*

Renal tubulo-interstitial diseases (N10-N16)

> Includes: Pyelonephritis
> *Excludes 1:   pyeloureteritis cystica (N28.85)*

N10   <u>Acute</u> tubulo-interstitial nephritis — Inflammation of the kidney tissue between
CC   the tubules (interstitial) that has a sudden, severe onset.
> Acute infectious interstitial nephritis
> Acute pyelitis
> Acute tubulo-interstitial nephritis
> Hemoglobin nephrosis
> Myoglobin nephrosis
> Use additional code (B95-B97), to identify infectious agent.

N11-   <u>Chronic</u> tubulo-interstitial nephritis — Inflammation and fibrosis of the kidney
> tissue between the tubules (interstitial) that persists over a long period of time.
> Includes: Chronic infectious interstitial nephritis
> Chronic pyelitis
> Chronic pyelonephritis
> Use additional code (B95-B97), to identify infectious agent.

N11.0   Nonobstructive reflux-associated chronic pyelonephritis
> Pyelonephritis (chronic) associated with (vesicoureteral) reflux
> *Excludes 1:   vesicoureteral reflux NOS (N13.70)*

CC N11.1   Chronic obstructive pyelonephritis
> Pyelonephritis (chronic) associated with anomaly of pelviureteric junction
> Pyelonephritis (chronic) associated with anomaly of pyeloureteric junction
> Pyelonephritis (chronic) associated with crossing of vessel
> Pyelonephritis (chronic) associated with kinking of ureter
> Pyelonephritis (chronic) associated with obstruction of ureter
> Pyelonephritis (chronic) associated with stricture of pelviureteric junction
> Pyelonephritis (chronic) associated with stricture of ureter
> *Excludes 1:   calculous pyelonephritis (N20.9)*
> *obstructive uropathy (N13.-)*

CC N11.8   Other chronic tubulo-interstitial nephritis
> Nonobstructive chronic pyelonephritis NOS

CC N11.9   Chronic tubulo-interstitial nephritis, unspecified
> Chronic interstitial nephritis NOS
> Chronic pyelitis NOS
> Chronic pyelonephritis NOS

N12   Tubulo-interstitial nephritis, <u>not specified as acute or chronic</u>
CC   Interstitial nephritis NOS
> Pyelitis NOS
> Pyelonephritis NOS
> *Excludes 1:   calculous pyelonephritis (N20.9)*

Excludes 1: = NOT CODED HERE! (Do not code both)   **901**   *Excludes ❷: = Not Included Here*

N13- **Obstructive and reflux uropathy** — HYDRONEPHROSIS —The abnormal accumulation of urine in the renal pelvis due to obstruction of the renal outflow.

> *Excludes ❷:* *calculus of kidney and ureter without hydronephrosis (N20.-)*
> *congenital obstructive defects of renal pelvis and ureter (Q62.0-Q62.3)*
> *hydronephrosis with ureteropelvic junction obstruction (Q62.1)*
> *obstructive pyelonephritis (N11.1)*

CC **N13.0** **Hydronephrosis** <u>with ureteropelvic obstruction</u>

Hydronephrosis due to acquired occlusion of ureteropelvic junction

> *Excludes ❷:* *hydronephrosis with ureteropelvic junction obstruction due to calculus (N13.2)*

CC **N13.1** **Hydronephrosis** <u>with ureteral stricture</u>, not elsewhere classified

> *Excludes 1:* *hydronephrosis with ureteral stricture with infection (N13.6)*

CC **N13.2** **Hydronephrosis** <u>with renal and ureteral calculous obstruction</u>

> *Excludes 1:* *hydronephrosis with renal and ureteral calculous obstruction with infection (N13.6)*

N13.3- **Other and unspecified hydronephrosis**

> *Excludes 1:* *hydronephrosis with infection (N13.6)*

CC **N13.30** **Unspecified hydronephrosis**

CC **N13.39** **Other hydronephrosis**

CC **N13.4** **Hydroureter** — Distention of a ureter with fluid due to obstruction.

> *Excludes 1:* *congenital hydroureter (Q62.3-)*
> *hydroureter with infection (N13.6)*
> *vesicoureteral-reflux with hydroureter (N13.73-)*

N13.5 **Crossing vessel and stricture of ureter without hydronephrosis** — The decrease in the usual ureteral lumen diameter that is often due to external forces (compression by blood vessels, abnormal growths).

Kinking and stricture of ureter without hydronephrosis

> *Excludes 1:* *crossing vessel and stricture of ureter without hydronephrosis with infection (N13.6)*

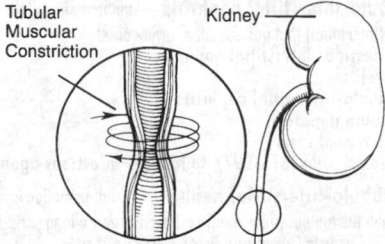

Tubular Muscular Constriction
Kidney

URETERAL CONSTRICTION

CC **N13.6** **Pyonephrosis** — The abnormal accumulation of pus in the renal pelvis due to obstruction of the renal outflow.

Conditions in N13.0-N13.5 with infection
Obstructive uropathy with infection
Use additional code (B95-B97), to identify infectious agent

N13.7- <u>Vesicoureteral-reflux</u> — The abnormal backward flow of urine from the bladder into the ureters and kidneys.

> *Excludes 1:* *reflux-associated pyelonephritis (N11.0)*

N13.70 **Vesicoureteral-reflux,** <u>unspecified</u>

Vesicoureteral-reflux NOS

N13.71 **Vesicoureteral-reflux** <u>without</u> **reflux nephropathy**

N13.72- **Vesicoureteral-reflux** <u>with reflux nephropathy</u> <u>without</u> **hydroureter**

N13.721 **Vesicoureteral-reflux with reflux nephropathy without hydroureter, unilateral**

N13.722 **Vesicoureteral-reflux with reflux nephropathy without hydroureter, bilateral**

N13.729 **Vesicoureteral-reflux with reflux nephropathy without hydroureter, unspecified**

N13.73- **Vesicoureteral-reflux** <u>with reflux nephropathy</u> <u>with</u> **hydroureter**

N13.731 **Vesicoureteral-reflux with reflux nephropathy with hydroureter, unilateral**

N13.732 **Vesicoureteral-reflux with reflux nephropathy with hydroureter, bilateral**

N13.739 **Vesicoureteral-reflux with reflux nephropathy with hydroureter, unspecified**

CC **N13.8** **Other obstructive and reflux uropathy**

Urinary tract obstruction due to specified cause
Code first, if applicable, any causal condition, such as:
Enlarged prostate (N40.1)

N13.9 **Obstructive and reflux uropathy, unspecified**

Urinary tract obstruction NOS

N14- **Drug- and heavy-metal-induced tubulo-interstitial and tubular conditions**

Code first poisoning due to drug or toxin, if applicable (T36-T65 with fifth or sixth character 1-4 or 6)
Use additional code for adverse effect, if applicable, to identify drug (T36-T50 with fifth or sixth character 5)

N14.0 **Analgesic nephropathy** — A form caused by the effects of long term analgesic medication use.

N14.1 **Nephropathy induced by other drugs, medicaments and biological substances**

N14.2 **Nephropathy induced by unspecified drug, medicament or biological substance**

N14.3 **Nephropathy induced by heavy metals**

N14.4 **Toxic nephropathy, not elsewhere classified**

N15- **Other renal tubulo-interstitial diseases**

N15.0 **Balkan nephropathy** — A form of chronic tubulointerstitial disease that is commonly seen in southeastern Europe and marked by urothelial atypia.

Balkan endemic nephropathy

MCC **N15.1** **Renal and perinephric abscess**

N15.8 **Other specified renal tubulo-interstitial diseases**

N15.9 **Renal tubulo-interstitial disease, unspecified**

Infection of kidney NOS

> *Excludes 1:* *urinary tract infection NOS (N39.0)*

N16 **Renal tubulo-interstitial disorders** <u>in diseases classified elsewhere</u> — [Not Allowed as PDX]

Pyelonephritis
Tubulo-interstitial nephritis
Code first underlying disease, such as:
Brucellosis (A23.0-A23.9)
Cryoglobulinemia (D89.1)
Glycogen storage disease (E74.0)
Leukemia (C91-C95)
Lymphoma (C81.0-C85.9, C96.0-C96.9)
Multiple myeloma (C90.0-)
Sepsis (A40.0-A41.9)
Wilson's disease (E83.0)

> *Excludes 1:* *diphtheritic pyelonephritis and tubulo-interstitial nephritis (A36.84)*
> *pyelonephritis and tubulo-interstitial nephritis in candidiasis (B37.49)*
> *pyelonephritis and tubulo-interstitial nephritis in cystinosis (E72.0)*
> *pyelonephritis and tubulo-interstitial nephritis in salmonella infection (A02.25)*
> *pyelonephritis and tubulo-interstitial nephritis in sarcoidosis (D86.84)*
> *pyelonephritis and tubulo-interstitial nephritis in sicca syndrome [Sjogren's] (M35.04)*
> *pyelonephritis and tubulo-interstitial nephritis in systemic lupus erythematosus (M32.15)*
> *pyelonephritis and tubulo-interstitial nephritis in toxoplasmosis (B58.83)*
> *renal tubular degeneration in diabetes (E08-E13 with .29)*
> *syphilitic pyelonephritis and tubulo-interstitial nephritis (A52.75)*

**N
1
3
-
N
1
6**

Acute kidney failure and chronic kidney disease (N17-N19)

Excludes ❷: congenital renal failure (P96.0)
drug- and heavy-metal-induced tubulo-interstitial and tubular conditions (N14.-)
extrarenal uremia (R39.2)
hemolytic-uremic syndrome (D59.3)
hepatorenal syndrome (K76.7)
postpartum hepatorenal syndrome (O90.4)
posttraumatic renal failure (T79.5)
prerenal uremia (R39.2)
renal failure complicating abortion or ectopic or molar pregnancy (O00-O07, O08.4)
renal failure following labor and delivery (O90.4)
renal failure postprocedural (N99.0)

N17- Acute kidney failure — The sudden, severe onset of inadequate kidney function.
Code also associated underlying condition
Excludes 1: posttraumatic renal failure (T79.5)

MCC N17.0 Acute kidney failure with tubular necrosis — A form characterized by the destruction of renal tubules.
Acute tubular necrosis
Renal tubular necrosis
Tubular necrosis NOS

MCC N17.1 Acute kidney failure with acute cortical necrosis — A form characterized by the destruction of the renal cortex.
Acute cortical necrosis
Cortical necrosis NOS
Renal cortical necrosis

MCC N17.2 Acute kidney failure with medullary necrosis — A form characterized by the destruction of the renal medulla.
Medullary [papillary] necrosis NOS
Acute medullary [papillary] necrosis
Renal medullary [papillary] necrosis

CC N17.8 Other acute kidney failure

CC N17.9 Acute kidney failure, unspecified
Acute kidney injury (nontraumatic)
Excludes ❷: traumatic kidney injury (S37.0-)

N18- Chronic kidney disease (CKD) — Kidney damage marked by the persistent and usually progressive reduction in the glomerular filtration rate and albuminuria. The stages of chronic kidney disease listed below are based on the level of kidney function (glomerular filtration rate).
Code first any associated:
Diabetic chronic kidney disease (E08.22, E09.22, E10.22, E11.22, E13.22)
Hypertensive chronic kidney disease (I12.-, I13.-)
Use additional code to identify kidney transplant status, if applicable, (Z94.0)

N18.1 Chronic kidney disease, stage 1

N18.2 Chronic kidney disease, stage 2 (mild)

N18.3 Chronic kidney disease, stage 3 (moderate)

CC N18.4 Chronic kidney disease, stage 4 (severe)
AHA 13:1Q:p24 – Kidney transplant failure with stage IV chronic kidney disease

CC N18.5 Chronic kidney disease, stage 5
Excludes 1: chronic kidney disease, stage 5 requiring chronic dialysis (N18.6)

MCC N18.6 End stage renal disease — A severe form requiring dialysis or kidney transplantation.
AHA 13:4Q:p124 – Encounter for hemodialysis
AHA 13:4Q:p125 – End stage renal disease
Chronic kidney disease requiring chronic dialysis
Use additional code to identify dialysis status (Z99.2)

N18.9 Chronic kidney disease, unspecified
Chronic renal disease
Chronic renal failure NOS
Chronic renal insufficiency
Chronic uremia

N19 Unspecified kidney failure
Uremia NOS
Excludes 1: acute kidney failure (N17.-)
chronic kidney disease (N18.-)
chronic uremia (N18.9)
extrarenal uremia (R39.2)
prerenal uremia (R39.2)
renal insufficiency (acute) (N28.9)
uremia of newborn (P96.0)

Urolithiasis (N20-N23)

N20- Calculus of kidney and ureter
Calculous pyelonephritis
Excludes 1: nephrocalcinosis (E83.5)
that with hydronephrosis (N13.2)

N20.0 Calculus of kidney — An abnormal concretion occurring within the kidney.
Nephrolithiasis NOS
Renal calculus
Renal stone
Staghorn calculus
Stone in kidney

CC N20.1 Calculus of ureter — An abnormal concretion occurring within the ureter.
Ureteric stone

CC N20.2 Calculus of kidney with calculus of ureter

N20.9 Urinary calculus, unspecified

N21- Calculus of lower urinary tract
Includes: Calculus of lower urinary tract with cystitis and urethritis

N21.0 Calculus in bladder — An abnormal concretion occurring within the bladder.
Calculus in diverticulum of bladder
Urinary bladder stone
Excludes ❷: staghorn calculus (N20.0)

N21.1 Calculus in urethra — An abnormal concretion occurring within the urethra.
Excludes ❷: calculus of prostate (N42.0)

N21.8 Other lower urinary tract calculus

N21.9 Calculus of lower urinary tract, unspecified
Excludes 1: calculus of urinary tract NOS (N20.9)

N22 Calculus of urinary tract in diseases classified elsewhere —
[Not Allowed as PDX]
Code first underlying disease, such as:
Gout (M1A.-, M10.-)
Schistosomiasis (B65.0-B65.9)

N23 Unspecified renal colic

Other disorders of kidney and ureter (N25-N29)

Excludes ❷: disorders of kidney and ureter with urolithiasis (N20-N23)

N25- Disorders resulting from impaired renal tubular function
Excludes 1: metabolic disorders classifiable to E70-E88

N25.0 Renal osteodystrophy — Various developmental bone formation disorders caused by the hypocalcemic, hyperphosphatemic effects of renal disease.
Azotemic osteodystrophy
Phosphate-losing tubular disorders
Renal rickets
Renal short stature

CC N25.1 Nephrogenic diabetes insipidus — Failure of the renal tubules to reabsorb water and with failure to respond to excessive production of antidiuretic hormone.
Excludes 1: diabetes insipidus NOS (E23.2)

N25.8- Other disorders resulting from impaired renal tubular function

CC N25.81 Secondary hyperparathyroidism of renal origin — A form of hyperparathyroidism due to a renal disease that lowers the serum calcium levels and results in the overstimulation of the parathyroid glands.
Excludes 1: secondary hyperparathyroidism, non-renal (E21.1)

N25.89 Other disorders resulting from impaired renal tubular function
Hypokalemic nephropathy — Dysfunction of the kidney associated with low potassium blood levels.
Lightwood-Albright syndrome
Renal tubular acidosis NOS

N25.9 Disorder resulting from impaired renal tubular function, unspecified

N26- Unspecified contracted kidney — The abnormal reduction in size of the kidney.
Excludes 1: contracted kidney due to hypertension (I12.-)
diffuse sclerosing glomerulonephritis (N05.8.-)
hypertensive nephrosclerosis (arteriolar) (arteriosclerotic) (I12.-)
small kidney of unknown cause (N27.-)

N26.1 Atrophy of kidney (terminal) — The abnormal wasting-away of the kidney.

N26.2 Page kidney — External compression of the kidney (often by a hematoma) causing decreased blood flow to the kidney that results in hypertension.

N26.9 Renal sclerosis, unspecified

N17-N26

N27- **Small kidney of unknown cause** — The abnormally diminished size of the kidney, of an unknown origin.

    Includes: Oligonephronia

N27.0   **Small kidney, <u>unilateral</u>**

N27.1   **Small kidney, <u>bilateral</u>**

N27.9   **Small kidney, <u>unspecified</u>**

N28- **Other disorders of kidney and ureter, not elsewhere classified**

cc N28.0   **Ischemia and infarction of kidney**

    Renal artery embolism — Blockage of the renal artery due to a clot of blood.

    Renal artery obstruction — Blockage of the renal artery.

    Renal artery occlusion — Narrowing, or complete closure, of the renal artery.

    Renal artery thrombosis — An abnormal aggregation of blood factors causing a renal artery obstruction.

    Renal infarct — Obstructive ischemic tissue necrosis of the kidney.

    Excludes 1:   *atherosclerosis of renal artery (extrarenal part) (I70.1)*
            congenital stenosis of renal artery (Q27.1)
            Goldblatt's kidney (I70.1)

N28.1   **Cyst of kidney, acquired** — A closed sac or pouch in a kidney, with a definite wall that contains fluid or semisolid material.

    Cyst (multiple) (solitary) of kidney, acquired

    Excludes 1:   *cystic kidney disease (congenital) (Q61.-)*

N28.8- **Other specified disorders of kidney and ureter**

    Excludes 1:   *hydroureter (N13.4)*
            ureteric stricture with hydronephrosis (N13.1)
            ureteric stricture without hydronephrosis (N13.5)

N28.81   **Hypertrophy of kidney** — Abnormal enlargement of a kidney.

N28.82   **Megaloureter** — The abnormal enlargment of the lumen of a ureter.

N28.83   **Nephroptosis** — Downward displacement of a kidney.

cc N28.84   **Pyelitis cystica** — Inflammation of the kidney pelvis with the formation of multiple submucosal cysts.

cc N28.85   **Pyeloureteritis cystica** — Inflammation of the kidney pelvis and ureter with the formation of multiple submucosal cysts.

cc N28.86   **Ureteritis cystica** — Inflammation of the ureters with formation of multiple submucosal cysts.

N28.89   **Other specified disorders of kidney and ureter**

N28.9   **Disorder of kidney and ureter, unspecified**

    Nephropathy NOS

    Renal disease (acute) NOS

    Renal insufficiency (acute)

    Excludes 1:   *chronic renal insufficiency (N18.9)*
            unspecified nephritic syndrome (N05.-)

N29 **Other disorders of kidney and ureter <u>in diseases classified elsewhere</u>** — [Not Allowed as PDX]

    Code first underlying disease, such as:

    Amyloidosis (E85.-)

    Nephrocalcinosis (E83.5)

    Schistosomiasis (B65.0-B65.9)

    Excludes 1:   *disorders of kidney and ureter in:*
            cystinosis (E72.0)
            gonorrhea (A54.21)
            syphilis (A52.75)
            tuberculosis (A18.11)

Other diseases of the urinary system (N30-N39)

    Excludes 1:   *urinary infection (complicating):*
            abortion or ectopic or molar pregnancy (O00-O07, O08.8)
            pregnancy, childbirth and the puerperium (O23.-, O75.3, O86.2-)

N30- **<u>Cystitis</u>** — Inflammation of the bladder.

    Use additional code to identify infectious agent (B95-B97)

    Excludes 1:   *prostatocystitis (N41.3)*

N30.0- **<u>Acute</u> cystitis** — A severe, sudden onset of inflammation of the bladder.

    Excludes 1:   *irradiation cystitis (N30.4-)*
            trigonitis (N30.3-)

cc N30.00   **Acute cystitis <u>without</u> hematuria**

cc N30.01   **Acute cystitis <u>with hematuria</u>** — Blood in the urine.

N30.1- **<u>Interstitial</u> cystitis (chronic)** — A persistent inflammatory lesion involving the entire thickness of the bladder, seen most often in women.

N30.10   **Interstitial cystitis (chronic) <u>without</u> hematuria**

N30.11   **Interstitial cystitis (chronic) <u>with hematuria</u>** — Blood in the urine.

N30.2- **Other chronic cystitis**

N30.20   **Other chronic cystitis <u>without</u> hematuria**

N30.21   **Other chronic cystitis <u>with hematuria</u>** — Blood in the urine.

N30.3- **<u>Trigonitis</u>** — Inflammation or localized hyperemia of the trigone area of the bladder.

    Urethrotrigonitis — Inflammation of the urethra and bladder trigone area.

N30.30   **Trigonitis <u>without</u> hematuria**

N30.31   **Trigonitis <u>with hematuria</u>** — Blood in the urine.

N30.4- **<u>Irradiation</u> cystitis** — Inflammation of the bladder due to the effects of radiation.

cc N30.40   **Irradiation cystitis <u>without</u> hematuria**

cc N30.41   **Irradiation cystitis <u>with hematuria</u>** — Blood in the urine.

N30.8- **<u>Other</u> cystitis**

    Abscess of bladder — A localized collection of pus caused by the disintegration of bladder tissues.

N30.80   **Other cystitis <u>without</u> hematuria**

N30.81   **Other cystitis <u>with hematuria</u>** — Blood in the urine.

N30.9- **Cystitis, <u>unspecified</u>**

N30.90   **Cystitis, unspecified <u>without</u> hematuria**

N30.91   **Cystitis, unspecified <u>with hematuria</u>** — Blood in the urine.

N31- **Neuromuscular dysfunction of bladder, <u>not elsewhere classified</u>**

    Use additional code to identify any associated urinary incontinence (N39.3-N39.4-)

    Excludes 1:   *cord bladder NOS (G95.89)*
            neurogenic bladder due to cauda equina syndrome (G83.4)
            neuromuscular dysfunction due to spinal cord lesion (G95.89)

N31.0   **Uninhibited neuropathic bladder, not elsewhere classified**

N31.1   **Reflex neuropathic bladder, not elsewhere classified**

N31.2   **Flaccid neuropathic bladder, not elsewhere classified**

    Atonic (motor) (sensory) neuropathic bladder

    Autonomous neuropathic bladder

    Nonreflex neuropathic bladder

N31.8   **Other neuromuscular dysfunction of bladder**

N31.9   **Neuromuscular dysfunction of bladder, unspecified**

    Neurogenic bladder dysfunction NOS

N32- **Other disorders of bladder**

    Excludes ❷: *calculus of bladder (N21.0)*
            cystocele (N81.1-)
            hernia or prolapse of bladder, female (N81.1-)

N32.0   **Bladder-neck obstruction** — Blockage of the urethral opening of the bladder.

    Bladder-neck stenosis (acquired)

    Excludes 1:   *congenital bladder-neck obstruction (Q64.3-)*

cc N32.1   **Vesicointestinal fistula** — An abnormal passage between the bladder and the intestine.

    Vesicorectal fistula — An abnormal passage between the bladder and the rectum.

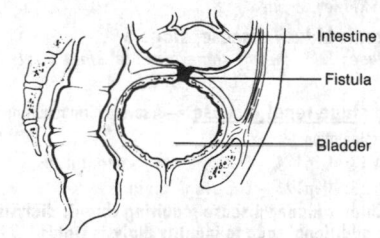

VESICOENTERIC FISTULA

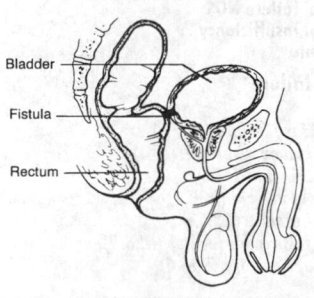

VESICORECTAL FISTULA

N 27 - N 32

cc **N32.2** **Vesical fistula, not elsewhere classified**
  Excludes 1: *fistula between bladder and female genital tract (N82.0-N82.1)*

N32.3 **Diverticulum of bladder** — A pouch created by the herniation of bladder-lining mucous membrane through a defect in the bladder muscular wall.
  Excludes 1: *congenital diverticulum of bladder (Q64.6)*
  diverticulitis of bladder (N30.8-)

N32.8- **Other specified disorders of bladder**
  N32.81 **Overactive bladder** — A condition of abnormal bladder muscle contraction causing symptoms of urinary frequency, urgency, and/or urge incontinence.
      Detrusor muscle hyperactivity
      Excludes 1: *frequent urination due to specified bladder condition — code to condition*

  N32.89 **Other specified disorders of bladder**
      Bladder hemorrhage — The abnormal escape of blood from the bladder tissues.
      Bladder hypertrophy — The abnormal enlargement of constituent bladder tissue.
      Calcified bladder — The abnormal deposition of calcium in the bladder tissues.
      Contracted bladder — The abnormal tightening and drawing inward of the bladder tissues.

N32.9 **Bladder disorder, unspecified**

N33 **Bladder disorders in diseases classified elsewhere** —
  [Not Allowed as PDX]
  Code first underlying disease, such as:
    Schistosomiasis (B65.0-B65.9)
  Excludes 1: *bladder disorder in syphilis (A52.76)*
    bladder disorder in tuberculosis (A18.12)
    candidal cystitis (B37.41)
    chlamydial cystitis (A56.01)
    cystitis in gonorrhea (A54.01)
    cystitis in neurogenic bladder (N31.-)
    diphtheritic cystitis (A36.85)
    syphilitic cystitis (A52.76)
    trichomonal cystitis (A59.03)

N34- **Urethritis and urethral syndrome**
  Use additional code (B95-B97), to identify infectious agent
  Excludes ❷: *Reiter's disease (M02.3-)*
    urethritis in diseases with a predominantly sexual mode of transmission (A50-A64)
    urethrotrigonitis (N30.3-)

cc **N34.0** **Urethral abscess** — A localized collection of pus caused by the disintegration of the urethral tissue.
      Abscess (of) Cowper's gland
      Abscess (of) Littré's gland
      Abscess (of) urethral (gland)
      Periurethral abscess
      Excludes 1: *urethral caruncle (N36.2)*

N34.1 **Nonspecific urethritis** — Inflammation of the urethra.
      Nongonococcal urethritis
      Nonvenereal urethritis

N34.2 **Other urethritis**
      Meatitis, urethral — Inflammation of the external urethral opening.
      Postmenopausal urethritis
      Ulcer of urethra (meatus)
      Urethritis NOS

N34.3 **Urethral syndrome, unspecified**

N35- **Urethral stricture** — A decrease in the diameter of the urethral lumen.
  Excludes 1: *congenital urethral stricture (Q64.3-)*
    postprocedural urethral stricture (N99.1-)

N35.0- **Post-traumatic urethral stricture**
      Urethral stricture due to injury
      Excludes 1: *postprocedural urethral stricture (N99.1-)*

  N35.01- **Post-traumatic urethral stricture, male**
      N35.010 **Post-traumatic urethral stricture, male, meatal —** [♂]
      N35.011 **Post-traumatic bulbous urethral stricture**
      N35.012 **Post-traumatic membranous urethral stricture**
      N35.013 **Post-traumatic anterior urethral stricture**
      N35.014 **Post-traumatic urethral stricture, male, unspecified —** [♂]

N35.02- **Post-traumatic urethral stricture, female**
      N35.021 **Urethral stricture due to childbirth —** [♀]
      N35.028 **Other post-traumatic urethral stricture, female —** [♀]

N35.1- **Postinfective urethral stricture, not elsewhere classified**
      Excludes 1: *urethral stricture associated with schistosomiasis (B65.-, N29)*
        gonococcal urethral stricture (A54.01)
        syphilitic urethral stricture (A52.76)

  N35.11- **Postinfective urethral stricture, not elsewhere classified, male**
      N35.111 **Postinfective urethral stricture, not elsewhere classified, male, meatal —** [♂]
      N35.112 **Postinfective bulbous urethral stricture, not elsewhere classified**
      N35.113 **Postinfective membranous urethral stricture, not elsewhere classified**
      N35.114 **Postinfective anterior urethral stricture, not elsewhere classified**
      N35.119 **Postinfective urethral stricture, not elsewhere classified, male, unspecified —** [♂]

  N35.12 **Postinfective urethral stricture, not elsewhere classified, female —** [♀]

N35.8 **Other urethral stricture**
      Excludes 1: *postprocedural urethral stricture (N99.1-)*

N35.9 **Urethral stricture, unspecified**

N36- **Other disorders of urethra**
  cc **N36.0** **Urethral fistula** — An abnormal passage involving the urethra.
      Urethroperineal fistula
      Urethrorectal fistula
      Urinary fistula NOS
      Excludes 1: *urethroscrotal fistula (N50.89)*
        urethrovaginal fistula (N82.1)
        urethrovesicovaginal fistula (N82.1)

N36.1 **Urethral diverticulum** — A circumscribed pouch or sac of mucous membrane lining through a defect in the muscular layer.

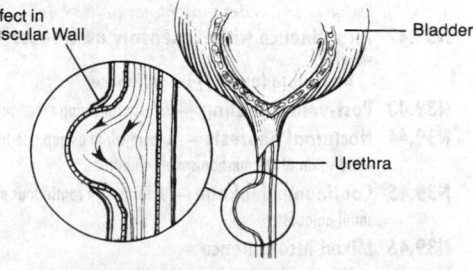

Defect in Muscular Wall
Bladder
Urethra

URETHRAL DIVERTICULUM

N36.2 **Urethral caruncle** — A small fleshy projection of the urethra.

N36.4- **Urethral functional and muscular disorders**
  Use additional code to identify associated urinary stress incontinence (N39.3)
  N36.41 **Hypermobility of urethra** — The abnormal displacement of the urethra due to anatomical changes that may lead to urine leakage.
  N36.42 **Intrinsic sphincter deficiency (ISD)** — Weakening of the urethral spincter musculature.
  N36.43 **Combined hypermobility of urethra and intrinsic sphincter deficiency**
  N36.44 **Muscular disorders of urethra**
      Bladder sphincter dyssynergy

N36.5 **Urethral false passage** — The presence of non-urethral passage that transports urine.

N36.8 **Other specified disorders of urethra**
      Excludes 1: *congenital urethrocele (Q64.7)*
        female urethrocele (N81.0)

N36.9 **Urethral disorder, unspecified**

N 3 2 – N 3 6

Excludes 1: = NOT CODED HERE! (Do not code both)
Excludes ❷: = Not Included Here

N37   Urethral disorders <u>in diseases classified elsewhere</u> —
[Not Allowed as PDX]
Code first underlying disease
Excludes 1:   urethritis (in):
          candidal infection (B37.41)
          chlamydial (A56.01)
          gonorrhea (A54.01)
          syphilis (A52.76)
          trichomonal infection (A59.03)
          tuberculosis (A18.13)

N39-   Other disorders of urinary system
Excludes ❷: hematuria NOS (R31.-)
       recurrent or persistent hematuria (N02.-)
       recurrent or persistent hematuria with specified morphological
         lesion (N02.-)
       proteinuria NOS (R80.-)

CC **N39.0**   Urinary tract infection, site not specified — The abnormal presence
of microorganisms in the urine indicating an infection of the urinary tract.
Use additional code (B95-B97), to identify infectious agent.
Excludes 1:   candidiasis of urinary tract (B37.4-)
       neonatal urinary tract infection (P39.3)
       urinary tract infection of specified site, such as:
         cystitis (N30.-)
         urethritis (N34.-)

N39.3   Stress incontinence (female) (male) — The involuntary passage of
urine during physical exertion or activity, laughing, coughing, or sneezing.
Code also any associated overactive bladder (N32.81)
Excludes 1:   mixed incontinence (N39.46)

N39.4-   Other specified urinary incontinence — The involuntary passage of
urine.
Code also any associated overactive bladder (N32.81)
Excludes 1:   enuresis NOS (R32)
       functional urinary incontinence (R39.81)
       urinary incontinence associated with cognitive
         impairment (R39.81)
       urinary incontinence NOS (R32)
       urinary incontinence of nonorganic origin (F98.0)

    N39.41   Urge incontinence — A form associated with a strong, sudden desire to
void.
       Excludes 1:   mixed incontinence (N39.46)

    N39.42   Incontinence without sensory awareness — A form without
warning.
       Insensible (urinary) incontinence

    N39.43   Post-void dribbling — A form following emptying of the bladder.

    N39.44   Nocturnal enuresis — A form while asleep due to a delay in
maturation of the mechanism of inhibition.

    N39.45   Continuous leakage — A form with continuous passage of urine in
small amounts.

    N39.46   Mixed incontinence
       Urge and stress incontinence

    N39.49- Other specified urinary incontinence
      N39.490   Overflow incontinence — A form in which the bladder is
overfilled and leaks a small amount of urine continuously, and does
not completely empty even after voiding.

      N39.491   Coital incontinence — A form occurring during sexual
intercourse or orgasm.

      N39.492   Postural (urinary) incontinence — A form occurring as a
result of change of body position.

      N39.498   Other specified urinary incontinence
         Reflex incontinence — A form in which the micturation reflex
          is interrupted.
         Total incontinence — A form in which control is lost.

N39.8   Other specified disorders of urinary system

N39.9   Disorder of urinary system, unspecified

Diseases of male genital organs (N40-N53)

N40-   <u>Benign prostatic hyperplasia</u> — The abnormal proliferation and/or growth of
prostate cellular tissues.
   Includes: Adenofibromatous hypertrophy of prostate
            Benign hypertrophy of the prostate
            Benign prostatic hypertrophy
            BPH
            Enlarged prostate
            Nodular prostate
            Polyp of prostate
   Excludes 1:   benign neoplasms of prostate (adenoma, benign)
            (fibroadenoma) (fibroma) (myoma) (D29.1)
   Excludes ❷: malignant neoplasm of prostate (C61)

N40.0   Benign prostatic hyperplasia <u>without lower urinary tract</u>
<u>symptoms</u> — [♂, Age/15-124]
       Enlarged prostate NOS
       Enlarged prostate without LUTS

N40.1   Benign prostatic hyperplasia <u>with lower urinary tract</u>
<u>symptoms</u> — [♂, Age/15-124]
       Enlarged prostate with LUTS
   Use additional code for associated symptoms, when specified:
       Incomplete bladder emptying (R39.14)
       Nocturia (R35.1)
       Straining on urination (R39.16)
       Urinary frequency (R35.0)
       Urinary hesitancy (R39.11)
       Urinary incontinence (N39.4-)
       Urinary obstruction (N13.8)
       Urinary retention (R33.8)
       Urinary urgency (R39.15)
       Weak urinary stream (R39.12)

N40.2   Nodular prostate <u>without</u> lower urinary tract symptoms —
[♂, Age/15-124] — A form with the presence of nodule(s).
       Nodular prostate without LUTS

N40.3   Nodular prostate <u>with lower urinary tract symptoms</u> —
[♂, Age/15-124]
   Use additional code for associated symptoms, when specified:
       Incomplete bladder emptying (R39.14)
       Nocturia (R35.1)
       Straining on urination (R39.16)
       Urinary frequency (R35.0)
       Urinary hesitancy (R39.11)
       Urinary incontinence (N39.4-)
       Urinary obstruction (N13.8)
       Urinary retention (R33.8)
       Urinary urgency (R39.15)
       Weak urinary stream (R39.12)

N41-   <u>Inflammatory</u> diseases of prostate
   Use additional code (B95-B97), to identify infectious agent

CC **N41.0**   <u>Acute</u> prostatitis — [♂, Age/15-124] — The sudden, severe onset of
inflammation of the prostate.

N41.1   <u>Chronic</u> prostatitis — [♂, Age/15-124] — Inflammation of the prostate which
develops slowly and persists over a long period of time.

CC **N41.2**   Abscess of prostate — [♂, Age/15-124] — A localized collection of pus
caused by the disintegration of prostatic tissue.

N41.3   Prostatocystitis — [♂, Age/15-124] — Inflammation of the prostate gland
and bladder.

N41.4   Granulomatous prostatitis — [♂, Age/15-124] — Inflammation of the
prostate with the formation of granular tissue.

N41.8   Other inflammatory diseases of prostate — [♂, Age/15-124]

N41.9   Inflammatory disease of prostate, unspecified — [♂, Age/15-124]
       Prostatitis NOS

N42-   Other and unspecified disorders of prostate

N42.0   Calculus of prostate — [♂, Age/15-124] — A concretion within the prostate
gland.
       Prostatic stone

N42.1   Congestion and hemorrhage of prostate — [♂, Age/15-124] — An
abnormal accumulation or escape of blood within the prostate.
   Excludes 1:   enlarged prostate (N40.-)
       hematuria (R31.-)
       hyperplasia of prostate (N40.-)
       inflammatory diseases of prostate (N41.-)

Left margin tab: N37-N42

N42.3- Dysplasia of prostate — The abnormal shape and/or size of prostatic cells.

N42.30 Unspecified dysplasia of prostate — [♂]

N42.31 Prostatic intraepithelial neoplasia — [♂]
PIN
Prostatic intraepithelial neoplasia I (PIN I)
Prostatic intraepithelial neoplasia II (PIN II)
*Excludes 1:   prostatic intraepithelial neoplasia III (PIN III)
(D07.5)*

N42.32 Atypical small acinar proliferation of prostate — [♂]

N42.39 Other dysplasia of prostate — [♂]

N42.8- Other specified disorders of prostate

N42.81 Prostatodynia syndrome — [♂, Age/15-124]
Painful prostate syndrome

N42.82 Prostatosis syndrome — [♂, Age/15-124]

N42.83 Cyst of prostate — [♂, Age/15-124] — An encapsulated, fluid-filled sac of the prostate.

N42.89 Other specified disorders of prostate — [♂, Age/15-124]

N42.9 Disorder of prostate, unspecified — [♂, Age/15-124]

N43- Hydrocele and spermatocele
Includes: Hydrocele of spermatic cord, testis or tunica vaginalis
Excludes 1:   congenital hydrocele (P83.5)

N43.0 Encysted hydrocele — [♂] — The abnormal accumulation of serous fluid which occurs outside the cavity of the tunica vaginalis testes.

CC **N43.1 Infected hydrocele** — [♂] — The abnormal accumulation of serous fluid within the scrotum marked by the invasion of microorganisms.
Use additional code (B95-B97), to identify infectious agent

N43.2 Other hydrocele — [♂]

N43.3 Hydrocele, unspecified — [♂]

N43.4- Spermatocele of epididymis — A cystic mass of the epididymis containing spermatozoa.
Spermatic cyst

N43.40 Spermatocele of epididymis, unspecified — [♂]

N43.41 Spermatocele of epididymis, single — [♂]

N43.42 Spermatocele of epididymis, multiple — [♂]

N44- Noninflammatory disorders of testis

N44.0- Torsion of testis — The abnormal twisting of a testis within the scrotum.

CC **N44.00 Torsion of testis, unspecified** — [♂]

CC **N44.01 Extravaginal torsion of spermatic cord** — [♂] — A form in which the spermatic cord is twisted, proximal to the attachments of the tunica vaginalis.

CC **N44.02 Intravaginal torsion of spermatic cord** — [♂] — A form in which the spermatic cord is twisted, within the tunica vaginalis.
Torsion of spermatic cord NOS

CC **N44.03 Torsion of appendix testis** — [♂] — The abnormal twisting of the remnant of the embryologic müllerian duct.

CC **N44.04 Torsion of appendix epididymis** — [♂] — The abnormal twisting of the remnant of the mesonephros.

N44.1 Cyst of tunica albuginea testis — [♂] — An encapsulated, fluid-filled sac of the tunica albuginea.

N44.2 Benign cyst of testis — [♂] — An encapsulated, fluid-filled sac of the testis.

N44.8 Other noninflammatory disorders of the testis — [♂]

N45- Orchitis and epididymitis
Use additional code (B95-B97), to identify infectious agent.

N45.1 Epididymitis — [♂] — Inflammation of the epididymis.

N45.2 Orchitis — [♂] — Inflammation of the testis.

N45.3 Epididymo-orchitis — [♂] — Inflammation of the epididymis and testis.

CC **N45.4 Abscess of epididymis or testis** — [♂] — A localized collection of pus caused by the disintegration of tissue.

N46- Male infertility — The inability or diminished ability of the male to produce offspring.
Excludes 1:   vasectomy status (Z98.52)

N46.0- Azoospermia — The absence of spermatozoa in the semen.
Absolute male infertility
Male infertility due to germinal (cell) aplasia
Male infertility due to spermatogenic arrest (complete)

N46.01 Organic azoospermia — [♂, Age/15-124] — A form caused by the diseases or conditions of the sperm-producing testes.
Azoospermia NOS

N46.02- Azoospermia due to extratesticular causes
Code also associated cause

N46.021 Azoospermia due to drug therapy — [♂, Age/15-124]

N46.022 Azoospermia due to infection — [♂, Age/15-124]

N46.023 Azoospermia due to obstruction of efferent ducts — [♂, Age/15-124]

N46.024 Azoospermia due to radiation — [♂, Age/15-124]

N46.025 Azoospermia due to systemic disease — [♂, Age/15-124]

N46.029 Azoospermia due to other extratesticular causes — [♂, Age/15-124]

N46.1- Oligospermia — The diminished amount of spermatozoa in the seminal fluid.
Male infertility due to germinal cell desquamation
Male infertility due to hypospermatogenesis
Male infertility due to incomplete spermatogenic arrest

N46.11 Organic oligospermia — [♂, Age/15-124] — A form caused by the diseases or conditions of the sperm-producing testes.
Oligospermia NOS

N46.12- Oligospermia due to extratesticular causes
Code also associated cause

N46.121 Oligospermia due to drug therapy — [♂, Age/15-124]

N46.122 Oligospermia due to infection — [♂, Age/15-124]

N46.123 Oligospermia due to obstruction of efferent ducts — [♂, Age/15-124]

N46.124 Oligospermia due to radiation — [♂, Age/15-124]

N46.125 Oligospermia due to systemic disease — [♂, Age/15-124]

N46.129 Oligospermia due to other extratesticular causes — [♂, Age/15-124]

N46.8 Other male infertility — [♂, Age/15-124]

N46.9 Male infertility, unspecified — [♂, Age/15-124]

N47- Disorders of prepuce

N47.0 Adherent prepuce, newborn — [♂, Age/0]

N47.1 Phimosis — [♂] — The inability to draw the foreskin back from over the glans.

N47.2 Paraphimosis — [♂] — The condition in which the retracted foreskin cannot be pulled back into its normal position causing constriction.

N47.3 Deficient foreskin — [♂]

N47.4 Benign cyst of prepuce — [♂] — An encapsulated, fluid-filled sac of the prepuce.

N47.5 Adhesions of prepuce and glans penis — [♂] — The formation of fibrous bands of the prepuce and/or glans penis.

N47.6 Balanoposthitis — [♂] — Inflammation of the glans penis and prepuce.
Use additional code (B95-B97), to identify infectious agent
Excludes 1:   balanitis (N48.1)

N47.7 Other inflammatory diseases of prepuce — [♂]
Use additional code (B95-B97), to identify infectious agent

N47.8 Other disorders of prepuce — [♂]

N48- Other disorders of penis

N48.0 Leukoplakia of penis — [♂] — A disease characterized by the shriveled, white, and glossy appearance of the glans penis with the meatus stenosed.
Balanitis xerotica obliterans
Kraurosis of penis
Lichen sclerosus of external male genital organs
Excludes 1:   carcinoma in situ of penis (D07.4)

N48.1 Balanitis — [♂] — Inflammation of the glans penis.
Use additional code (B95-B97), to identify infectious agent
*Excludes 1:   amebic balanitis (A06.8)
balanitis xerotica obliterans (N48.0)
candidal balanitis (B37.42)
gonococcal balanitis (A54.23)
herpesviral [herpes simplex] balanitis (A60.01)*

N48.2- Other inflammatory disorders of penis
Use additional code (B95-B97), to identify infectious agent.
*Excludes 1:   balanitis (N48.1)
balanitis xerotica obliterans (N48.0)
balanoposthitis (N47.6)*

N48.21 Abscess of corpus cavernosum and penis — [♂] — A localized collection of pus caused by the disintegration of corpus cavernosum and/or penile tissue.

N48.22 Cellulitis of corpus cavernosum and penis — [♂]

N
4
2
–
N
4
8

N48.29 **Other inflammatory disorders of penis** — [♂]

N48.3- **Priapism** — An abnormal, persistent erection of the penis which is accompanied by pain and tenderness.
Painful erection
Code first underlying cause

cc N48.30 **Priapism, unspecified** — [♂]

cc N48.31 **Priapism due to trauma** — [♂]

cc N48.32 **Priapism due to disease classified elsewhere** — [♂]
[Not Allowed as PDX]

cc N48.33 **Priapism, drug-induced** — [♂]

cc N48.39 **Other priapism** — [♂]

N48.5 **Ulcer of penis** — [♂] — The eating-away of penile tissue.

N48.6 **Induration penis plastica** — [♂] — The abnormal curvature of the penis caused by fibrous tissue that results in painful erection.
Peyronie's disease
Plastic induration of penis

N48.8- **Other specified disorders of penis**

N48.81 **Thrombosis of superficial vein of penis** — [♂] — An abnormal aggregation of blood factors causing an obstruction of the superficial vein of the penis.

N48.82 **Acquired torsion of penis** — [♂]
Acquired torsion of penis NOS
Excludes 1: congenital torsion of penis (Q55.63)

N48.83 **Acquired buried penis** — [♂] — The condition of the penis being hidden underneath the skin.
Excludes 1: congenital hidden penis (Q55.64)

N48.89 **Other specified disorders of penis** — [♂]

N48.9 **Disorder of penis, unspecified** — [♂]

N49- **Inflammatory disorders of male genital organs, not elsewhere classified**
Use additional code (B95-B97), to identify infectious agent
Excludes 1: inflammation of penis (N48.1, N48.2-)
orchitis and epididymitis (N45.-)

N49.0 **Inflammatory disorders of seminal vesicle** — [♂]
Vesiculitis NOS

N49.1 **Inflammatory disorders of spermatic cord, tunica vaginalis and vas deferens** — [♂]
Vasitis

N49.2 **Inflammatory disorders of scrotum** — [♂]

N49.3 **Fournier gangrene** — [♂]

N49.8 **Inflammatory disorders of other specified male genital organs** — [♂]
Inflammation of multiple sites in male genital organs

N49.9 **Inflammatory disorder of unspecified male genital organ** — [♂]
Abscess of unspecified male genital organ
Boil of unspecified male genital organ
Carbuncle of unspecified male genital organ
Cellulitis of unspecified male genital organ

N50- **Other and unspecified disorders of male genital organs**
Excludes ❷: torsion of testis (N44.0-)

N50.0 **Atrophy of testis** — [♂] — The abnormal wasting away of the testis.

N50.1 **Vascular disorders of male genital organs** — [♂]
Hematocele, NOS, of male genital organs
Hemorrhage of male genital organs
Thrombosis of male genital organs

N50.3 **Cyst of epididymis** — [♂] — An encapsulated, fluid-filled sac of the epididymis.

N50.8- **Other specified disorders of male genital organs**

N50.81- **Testicular pain**

N50.811- **Right testicular pain** — [♂]

N50.812- **Left testicular pain** — [♂]

N50.819- **Testicular pain, unspecified** — [♂]

N50.82 **Scrotal pain** — [♂]

N50.89 **Other specified disorders of male genital organs** — [♂]
Atrophy of scrotum, seminal vesicle, spermatic cord, tunica vaginalis and vas deferens
Chylocele, tunica vaginalis (nonfilarial) NOS
Edema of scrotum, seminal vesicle, spermatic cord, tunica vaginalis and vas deferens
Hypertrophy of scrotum, seminal vesicle, spermatic cord, tunica vaginalis and vas deferens
Stricture of spermatic cord, tunica vaginalis, and vas deferens
Ulcer of scrotum, seminal vesicle, spermatic cord, testis, tunica vaginalis and vas deferens
Urethroscrotal fistula

N50.9 **Disorder of male genital organs, unspecified** — [♂]

N51 **Disorders of male genital organs in diseases classified elsewhere** — [♂] [Not Allowed as PDX]
Code first underlying disease, such as:
Filariasis (B74.0-B74.9)
Excludes 1: amebic balanitis (A06.8)
candidal balanitis (B37.42)
gonococcal balanitis (A54.23)
gonococcal prostatitis (A54.22)
herpesviral [herpes simplex] balanitis (A60.01)
trichomonal prostatitis (A59.02)
tuberculous prostatitis (A18.14)

N52- **Male erectile dysfunction** — Inability to achieve or maintain erection of the penis, caused by an anatomical condition.
Excludes 1: psychogenic impotence (F52.21)

N52.0- **Vasculogenic erectile dysfunction** — A form of vascular origin.

N52.01 **Erectile dysfunction due to arterial insufficiency** — [♂, Age/15-124]

N52.02 **Corporo-venous occlusive erectile dysfunction** — [♂, Age/15-124]

N52.03 **Combined arterial insufficiency and corporo-venous occlusive erectile dysfunction** — [♂, Age/15-124]

N52.1 **Erectile dysfunction due to diseases classified elsewhere** — [♂, Age/15-124] [Not Allowed as PDX]
Code first underlying disease

N52.2 **Drug-induced erectile dysfunction** — [♂, Age/15-124]

N52.3- **Postprocedural erectile dysfunction**

N52.31 **Erectile dysfunction following radical prostatectomy** — [♂, Age/15-124]

N52.32 **Erectile dysfunction following radical cystectomy** — [♂, Age/15-124]

N52.33 **Erectile dysfunction following urethral surgery** — [♂, Age/15-124]

N52.34 **Erectile dysfunction following simple prostatectomy** — [♂, Age/15-124]

N52.35 **Erectile dysfunction following radiation therapy** — [♂, Age/15-124]

N52.36 **Erectile dysfunction following interstitial seed therapy** — [♂, Age/15-124]

N52.37 **Erectile dysfunction following prostate ablative therapy** — [♂, Age/15-124]
Erectile dysfunction following cryotherapy
Erectile dysfunction following other prostate ablative therapies
Erectile dysfunction following ultrasound ablative therapies

N52.39 **Other and unspecified postprocedural erectile dysfunction** — [♂, Age/15-124]

N52.8 **Other male erectile dysfunction** — [♂, Age/15-124]

N52.9 **Male erectile dysfunction, unspecified** — [♂, Age/15-124]
Impotence NOS

N48 – N52

N53-   **Other male sexual dysfunction**
> *Excludes 1:*   *psychogenic sexual dysfunction (F52.-)*

N53.1-   **Ejaculatory dysfunction** — The abnormal release of the ejaculate.
> *Excludes 1:*   *premature ejaculation (F52.4)*

N53.11   **Retarded ejaculation** — [♂] – A form that is slow to occur.

N53.12   **Painful ejaculation** — [♂] – A form that causes pain.

N53.13   **Anejaculatory orgasm** — [♂] – A male orgasm that occurs with ejaculation.

N53.14   **Retrograde ejaculation** — [♂] – A condition in which the ejaculate is released into the bladder instead of through the urethra.

N53.19   **Other ejaculatory dysfunction** — [♂]
> Ejaculatory dysfunction NOS

N53.8   **Other male sexual dysfunction** — [♂]

N53.9   **Unspecified male sexual dysfunction** — [♂]

Disorders of breast (N60-N65)

> *Excludes 1:*   *disorders of breast associated with childbirth (O91-O92)*

N60-   **Benign mammary dysplasia** — Abnormal development of breast tissue.
> Includes: Fibrocystic mastopathy

N60.0-   **Solitary cyst of breast** — A single, encapsulated, fluid-filled sac of the breast.
> Cyst of breast

N60.01   **Solitary cyst of <u>right</u> breast**

N60.02   **Solitary cyst of <u>left</u> breast**

N60.09   **Solitary cyst of <u>unspecified</u> breast**

N60.1-   **Diffuse cystic mastopathy** — A disease of the breast characterized by nodular cyst formation, tenderness, fluctuation of size, and ductal epithelial hyperplasia.
> Cystic breast
> Fibrocystic disease of breast
> *Excludes 1:*   *diffuse cystic mastopathy with epithelial proliferation (N60.3-)*

N60.11   **Diffuse cystic mastopathy of <u>right</u> breast** — [Age/15-124]

N60.12   **Diffuse cystic mastopathy of <u>left</u> breast** — [Age/15-124]

N60.19   **Diffuse cystic mastopathy of <u>unspecified</u> breast** — [Age/15-124]

N60.2-   **Fibroadenosis of breast** — A non-neoplastic nodular breast condition with fibrous tissue formation.
> Adenofibrosis of breast
> *Excludes ❷:*   *fibroadenoma of breast (D24.-)*

N60.21   **Fibroadenosis of <u>right</u> breast**

N60.22   **Fibroadenosis of <u>left</u> breast**

N60.29   **Fibroadenosis of <u>unspecified</u> breast**

N60.3-   **Fibrosclerosis of breast** — Fibrosis and sclerosis of the breast.
> Cystic mastopathy with epithelial proliferation

N60.31   **Fibrosclerosis of <u>right</u> breast**

N60.32   **Fibrosclerosis of <u>left</u> breast**

N60.39   **Fibrosclerosis of unspecified breast**

N60.4-   **Mammary duct ectasia** — A disease characterized by dilatation of the mammary gland ducts, intraductal inflammation, and interstitial inflammatory reaction.

N60.41   **Mammary duct ectasia of <u>right</u> breast**

N60.42   **Mammary duct ectasia of <u>left</u> breast**

N60.49   **Mammary duct ectasia of <u>unspecified</u> breast**

N60.8-   **Other benign mammary dysplasias**

N60.81   **Other benign mammary dysplasias of <u>right</u> breast**

N60.82   **Other benign mammary dysplasias of <u>left</u> breast**

N60.89   **Other benign mammary dysplasias of <u>unspecified</u> breast**

N60.9-   **Unspecified benign mammary dysplasia**

N60.91   **Unspecified benign mammary dysplasia of <u>right</u> breast**

N60.92   **Unspecified benign mammary dysplasia of <u>left</u> breast**

N60.99   **Unspecified benign mammary dysplasia of unspecified breast**

N61-   **Inflammatory disorders of breast**
> *Excludes 1:*   *inflammatory carcinoma of breast (C50.9)*
> *inflammatory disorder of breast associated with childbirth (O91.-)*
> *neonatal infective mastitis (P39.0)*
> *thrombophlebitis of breast [Mondor's disease] (I80.8)*

N61.0   **Mastitis <u>without</u> abscess** — Inflammation of the breast.
> **Cellulitis (acute) (nonpuerperal) (subacute) of breast NOS**
> **Cellulitis (acute) (nonpuerperal) (subacute) of nipple NOS**
> **Infective mastitis (acute) (nonpuerperal) (subacute)** — Inflammation of the breast due to the invasion and multiplication of microorganisms.
> **Mastitis (acute) (nonpuerperal) (subacute) NOS**

N61.1   **Abscess of the breast and nipple** — A localized collection of pus caused by the disintegration of mammary or areola tissue.
> **Abscess (acute) (chronic) (nonpuerperal) of areola**
> **Abscess (acute) (chronic) (nonpuerperal) of breast**
> **Carbuncle of breast** — A necrotizing infection of the breast composed of a cluster of boils.
> **Mastitis with abscess**

N62   **Hypertrophy of breast** — The abnormal enlargement of the breast.
> **Gynecomastia** — An abnormally large mammary gland in the male which may sometimes secrete milk.
> **Hypertrophy of breast NOS**
> **Massive pubertal hypertrophy of breast**
> *Excludes 1:*   *breast engorgement of newborn (P83.4)*
> *disproportion of reconstructed breast (N65.1)*

N63   **Unspecified lump in breast**
> **Nodule(s) NOS in breast**

N64-   **Other disorders of breast**
> *Excludes ❷:*   *mechanical complication of breast prosthesis and implant (T85.4-)*

N64.0   **Fissure and fistula of nipple** — A crack-like sore of the nipple.

N64.1   **Fat necrosis of breast** — [Unacceptable PDX] – Necrosis of the fatty tissue of the breast.
> **Fat necrosis (segmental) of breast**
> Code first breast necrosis due to breast graft (T85.898)

N64.2   **Atrophy of breast** — The abnormal wasting-away of the breast.

N64.3   **Galactorrhea not associated with childbirth** — The abnormal flow of milk from the breasts.

N64.4   **Mastodynia** — Pain and discomfort of the breast.

N64.5-   **Other signs and symptoms in breast**
> *Excludes ❷:*   *abnormal findings on diagnostic imaging of breast (R92.-)*

N64.51   **Induration of breast** — The abnormal hardening of the breast tissue.

N64.52   **Nipple discharge** — The abnormal drainage of fluid from the nipple.
> *Excludes 1:*   *abnormal findings in nipple discharge (R89.-)*

N64.53   **Retraction of nipple** — The drawing-back of the nipple.

N64.59   **Other signs and symptoms in breast**

N64.8-   **Other specified disorders of breast**

N64.81   **Ptosis of breast** — [Age/15-124] – The condition of sagging or drooping of the breast.
> *Excludes 1:*   *ptosis of native breast in relation to reconstructed breast (N65.1)*

N64.82   **Hypoplasia of breast** — [Age/15-124] – The condition of postpubertal underdevelopment of the breast.
> **Micromastia**
> *Excludes 1:*   *congenital absence of breast (Q83.0)*
> *hypoplasia of native breast in relation to reconstructed breast (N65.1)*

N64.89   **Other specified disorders of breast**
> **Galactocele** — A breast mass caused by the occlusion of a milk duct and containing a milk-like liquid.
> **Subinvolution of breast (postlactational)** — The failure of the breast to return to normal size after enlargement.

N64.9   **Disorder of breast, unspecified**

N65-   **Deformity and disproportion of reconstructed breast**

N65.0   **Deformity of reconstructed breast** — [Age/15-124] – The condition of a displeasing shape of the reconstructed breast.
> **Contour irregularity in reconstructed breast**
> **Excess tissue in reconstructed breast**
> **Misshapen reconstructed breast**

N65.1   **Disproportion of reconstructed breast** — [Age/15-124] – The condition of a displeasing balance of proportion of the reconstructed breast to the other breast.
> **Breast asymmetry between native breast and reconstructed breast**
> **Disproportion between native breast and reconstructed breast**

Excludes 1: = NOT CODED HERE! (Do not code both)   **909**   *Excludes ❷:* = Not Included Here

Inflammatory diseases of female pelvic organs (N70-N77)

Excludes 1: *inflammatory diseases of female pelvic organs complicating: abortion or ectopic or molar pregnancy (O00-O07, O08.0) pregnancy, childbirth and the puerperium (O23.-, O75.3, O85, O86.-)*

N70- <u>Salpingitis and oophoritis</u> — Inflammation of the fallopian tube and the ovary.
Includes: **Abscess (of) fallopian tube** — A localized collection of pus caused by the disintegration of fallopian tube tissue.
Abscess (of) ovary — A localized collection of pus caused by the disintegration of ovarian tissue.
Pyosalpinx — The presence of pus within the fallopian tube.
Salpingo-oophoritis — Inflammation of the fallopian tube and ovary.
Tubo-ovarian abscess — A localized collection of pus caused by the disintegration of tubal and ovarian tissues.
Tubo-ovarian inflammatory disease — Inflammation of the fallopian tube and ovary.
Use additional code (B95-B97), to identify infectious agent
Excludes 1: *gonococcal infection (A54.24)*
tuberculous infection (A18.17)

N70.0- <u>Acute</u> salpingitis and oophoritis — The sudden, severe onset of inflammation of the fallopian tube and the ovary.

CC **N70.01** Acute salpingitis — [♀]

CC **N70.02** Acute oophoritis — [♀]

CC **N70.03** Acute salpingitis and oophoritis — [♀]

N70.1- <u>Chronic</u> salpingitis and oophoritis — Inflammation of the fallopian tube and ovary that develops slowly and persists over a long period of time.
Hydrosalpinx

N70.11 Chronic salpingitis — [♀]

N70.12 Chronic oophoritis — [♀]

N70.13 Chronic salpingitis and oophoritis — [♀]

N70.9- Salpingitis and oophoritis, <u>unspecified</u>

N70.91 Salpingitis, unspecified — [♀]

N70.92 Oophoritis, unspecified — [♀]

N70.93 Salpingitis and oophoritis, unspecified — [♀]

N71- <u>Inflammatory disease of uterus</u>, except cervix — Inflammation of the uterus.
Includes: **Endo (myo) metritis** — Inflammation of the mucous membrane lining of the uterus.
Metritis — Inflammation of the uterus.
Myometritis — Inflammation of the muscular wall of the uterus.
Pyometra — The abnormal accumulation of pus within the uterine cavity.
Uterine abscess — A localized collection of pus caused by the disintegration of uterine tissues.
Use additional code (B95-B97), to identify infectious agent
Excludes 1: *hyperplastic endometritis (N85.0-)*
infection of uterus following delivery (O85, O86.-)

CC **N71.0** <u>Acute</u> inflammatory disease of uterus — [♀] — The sudden, severe onset.

N71.1 <u>Chronic</u> inflammatory disease of uterus — [♀] — Develops slowly and persists over a long period of time.

N71.9 Inflammatory disease of uterus, <u>unspecified</u> — [♀]

N72 Inflammatory disease of cervix uteri — [♀] — Inflammation of the neck of the uterus.
Includes: **Cervicitis (with or without erosion or ectropion)**
Endocervicitis (with or without erosion or ectropion)
Exocervicitis (with or without erosion or ectropion)
Use additional code (B95-B97), to identify infectious agent
Excludes 1: *erosion and ectropion of cervix without cervicitis (N86)*

N73- Other female pelvic inflammatory diseases
Use additional code (B95-B97), to identify infectious agent

CC **N73.0** Acute parametritis and pelvic cellulitis — [♀] — The sudden, severe onset of inflammation of the cellular tissue adjacent to the uterus, and inflammation of the cellular tissue in the pelvic cavity.
Abscess of broad ligament
Abscess of parametrium
Pelvic cellulitis, female

N73.1 Chronic parametritis and pelvic cellulitis — [♀] — Inflammation of the cellular tissue adjacent to the uterus, and pelvic cellular tissue that develops slowly and persists over a long period of time.
Any condition in N73.0 specified as chronic
Excludes 1: *tuberculous parametritis and pelvic cellultis (A18.17)*

N73.2 Unspecified parametritis and pelvic cellulitis — [♀]
Any condition in N73.0 unspecified whether acute or chronic

MCC **N73.3** Female acute pelvic peritonitis — [♀] — The sudden, severe onset of inflammation of the pelvic cavity cellular tissue.

CC **N73.4** Female chronic pelvic peritonitis — [♀] – Inflammation of the pelvic cavity cellular tissue in the female that develops slowly and persists over a long period of time.
Excludes 1: *tuberculous pelvic (female) peritonitis (A18.17)*

N73.5 Female pelvic peritonitis, unspecified — [♀]

N73.6 Female pelvic peritoneal adhesions (postinfective) — [♀] – The formation of fibrotic adhesive bands within the female pelvic peritoneum.
AHA 14:1Q:p3 – Peritoneal adhesions
Excludes ❷: *postprocedural pelvic peritoneal adhesions (N99.4)*

N73.8 Other specified female pelvic inflammatory diseases — [♀]

N73.9 Female pelvic inflammatory disease, unspecified — [♀]
Female pelvic infection or inflammation NOS

N74 Female pelvic inflammatory disorders <u>in diseases classified elsewhere</u> — [♀] [Not Allowed as PDX]
Code first underlying disease
Excludes 1: *chlamydial cervicitis (A56.02)*
chlamydial pelvic inflammatory disease (A56.11)
gonococcal cervicitis (A54.03)
gonococcal pelvic inflammatory disease (A54.24)
herpesviral [herpes simplex] cervicitis (A60.03)
herpesviral [herpes simplex] pelvic inflammatory disease (A60.09)
syphilitic cervicitis (A52.76)
syphilitic pelvic inflammatory disease (A52.76)
trichomonal cervicitis (A59.09)
tuberculous cervicitis (A18.16)
tuberculous pelvic inflammatory disease (A18.17)

N75- Diseases of Bartholin's gland

N75.0 Cyst of Bartholin's gland — [♀] – An encapsulated, fluid-filled sac of the small glands on either side of the vaginal orifice.

CC **N75.1** Abscess of Bartholin's gland — [♀] – A localized collection of pus caused by the disintegration of Bartholin's gland tissue.

N75.8 Other diseases of Bartholin's gland — [♀]
Bartholinitis

N75.9 Disease of Bartholin's gland, unspecified — [♀]

N76- Other inflammation of vagina and vulva
Use additional code (B95-B97), to identify infectious agent
Excludes ❷: *senile (atrophic) vaginitis (N95.2)*
vulvar vestibulitis (N94.810)

N76.0 Acute vaginitis — [♀] – The sudden, severe onset of inflammation of the vagina.
Acute vulvovaginitis
Vaginitis NOS
Vulvovaginitis NOS

N76.1 Subacute and chronic vaginitis — [♀] – Inflammation of the vagina that develops slower than an acute infection and persists over a long period of time.
Chronic vulvovaginitis
Subacute vulvovaginitis

N76.2 Acute vulvitis — [♀] – The sudden, severe onset of inflammation of the vulva.
Vulvitis NOS

N76.3 Subacute and chronic vulvitis — [♀] – Inflammation of the vulva that develops slower than an acute infection and persists over a long period of time.

CC **N76.4** Abscess of vulva — [♀] – A localized collection of pus caused by the disintegration of vulva tissue.
Furuncle of vulva — An inflammatory subcutaneous nodule of the vulva.

N76.5 Ulceration of vagina — [♀] – The localized eating-away of vaginal tissue.

N76.6 Ulceration of vulva — [♀] – The localized eating-away of vulvar tissue.

N76.8- Other specified inflammation of vagina and vulva

CC **N76.81** Mucositis (ulcerative) of vagina and vulva — [♀] – Inflammation and/or ulcerative sores of the mucous membranes of the vagina and/or vulva.
Code also type of associated therapy, such as:
Antineoplastic and immunosuppressive drugs (T45.1x-)
Radiological procedure and radiotherapy (Y84.2)
Excludes ❷: *gastrointestinal mucositis (ulcerative) (K92.81)*
nasal mucositis (ulcerative) (J34.81)
oral mucositis (ulcerative) (K12.3-)

N76.89 Other specified inflammation of vagina and vulva — [♀]

Excludes 1: = NOT CODED HERE! (Do not code both)   **910**   **Excludes ❷:** = Not Included Here

N77- Vulvovaginal ulceration and inflammation <u>in diseases classified</u> <u>elsewhere</u>

N77.0 Ulceration of vulva in diseases classified elsewhere — [♀]
[Not Allowed as PDX]
Code first underlying disease, such as:
Behçet's disease (M35.2)
Excludes 1:   ulceration of vulva in gonococcal infection (A54.02)
ulceration of vulva in herpesviral [herpes simplex]
infection (A60.04)
ulceration of vulva in syphilis (A51.0)
ulceration of vulva in tuberculosis (A18.18)

N77.1 Vaginitis, vulvitis and vulvovaginitis in diseases classified elsewhere — [♀] [Not Allowed as PDX]
Code first underlying disease, such as:
Pinworm (B80)
Excludes 1:   candidal vulvovaginitis (B37.3)
chlamydial vulvovaginitis (A56.02)
gonococcal vulvovaginitis (A54.02)
herpesviral [herpes simplex] vulvovaginitis (A60.04)
trichomonal vulvovaginitis (A59.01)
tuberculous vulvovaginitis (A18.18)
vulvovaginitis in early syphilis (A51.0)
vulvovaginitis in late syphilis (A52.76)

Noninflammatory disorders of female genital tract (N80-N98)

N80- <u>Endometriosis</u> — A condition of endometrial tissue growth outside of the uterus.

N80.0 Endometriosis of uterus — [♀] – A form affecting the endometrium of the uterus.
Adenomyosis — A form characterized by in-growth of the endometrium into the uterine muscle layer.
Excludes 1:   stromal endometriosis (D39.0)

N80.1 Endometriosis of ovary — [♀] – A form affecting the ovary.

N80.2 Endometriosis of fallopian tube — [♀] – A form affecting the fallopian tube.

N80.3 Endometriosis of pelvic peritoneum — [♀] – A form affecting the pelvic peritoneum.

N80.4 Endometriosis of rectovaginal septum and vagina — [♀] – A form affecting the tissue between the rectum and the vagina.

N80.5 Endometriosis of intestine — [♀] – A form affecting the intestine.

N80.6 Endometriosis in cutaneous scar — [♀] – A form appearing in the scar healing tissue of the skin.

N80.8 Other endometriosis — [♀]

N80.9 Endometriosis, unspecified — [♀]

N81- <u>Female genital prolapse</u>
Excludes 1:   genital prolapse complicating pregnancy, labor or delivery
(O34.5-)
prolapse and hernia of ovary and fallopian tube (N83.4-)
prolapse of vaginal vault after hysterectomy (N99.3)

N81.0 Urethrocele — [♀] – A hernia of the urethral wall that protrudes into the vagina.
Excludes 1:   urethrocele with cystocele (N81.1-)
urethrocele with prolapse of uterus (N81.2-N81.4)

N81.1- Cystocele — A hernia of the bladder that protrudes into the vagina.
Cystocele with urethrocele
Cystourethrocele — A hernia of the bladder and bladder neck/upper urethra that protrudes into the vagina.
Excludes 1:   cystocele with prolapse of uterus (N81.2-N81.4)

N81.10 Cystocele, unspecified — [♀]
Prolapse of (anterior) vaginal wall NOS

N81.11 Cystocele, midline — [♀] – A hernia of the bladder that protrudes into the vagina due to damage to the central portion of the pubocervical fascia.

N81.12 Cystocele, lateral — [♀] – A hernia of the bladder that protrudes into the vagina due to disruption of the lateral vaginal attachments to the arcus tendineus.
Paravaginal cystocele

N81.2 Incomplete uterovaginal prolapse — [♀] – The downward displacement of the uterus and vaginal walls in which the uterus descends into the introitus.
First degree uterine prolapse — A form with protrusion past the cervical os.
Prolapse of cervix NOS
Second degree uterine prolapse — A form with protrusion into the vaginal orifice.
Excludes 1:   cervical stump prolaspe (N81.85)

N81.3 Complete uterovaginal prolapse — [♀] – The downward displacement of the uterus and vaginal walls in which the uterus descends and protrudes beyond the introitus.
Procidentia (uteri) NOS
Third degree uterine prolapse — A form with protrusion beyond the vaginal orifice.

N81.4 Uterovaginal prolapse, unspecified — [♀]
Prolapse of uterus NOS

N81.5 Vaginal enterocele — [♀] – A herniation of the intestine into the rectal vaginal pouch
Excludes 1:   enterocele with prolapse of uterus (N81.2-N81.4)

N81.6 Rectocele — [♀] – A hernia of the anterior wall of the rectum that protrudes into the vagina.
Prolapse of posterior vaginal wall
Use additional code for any associated fecal incontinence, if applicable (R15.-)
Excludes ❷: perineocele (N81.81)
rectal prolapse (K62.3)
rectocele with prolapse of uterus (N81.2-N81.4)

N81.8- Other female genital prolapse

N81.81 Perineocele — [♀] – A hernia between the rectum and vagina that protrudes into the vagina

N81.82 Incompetence or weakening of pubocervical tissue — [♀]

N81.83 Incompetence or weakening of rectovaginal tissue — [♀]

N81.84 Pelvic muscle wasting — [♀]
Disuse atrophy of pelvic muscles and anal sphincter

N81.85 Cervical stump prolapse — [♀] – The downward displacement of the posthysterectomy cervical stump.

N81.89 Other female genital prolapse — [♀]
Deficient perineum
Old laceration of muscles of pelvic floor — Lacerations of pelvic floor muscles which have healed per primam.

N81.9 Female genital prolapse, unspecified — [♀]

N82- Fistulae involving female genital tract
Excludes 1:   vesicointestinal fistulae (N32.1)

cc N82.0 Vesicovaginal fistula — [♀] – An abnormal passage communicating the bladder with the vagina.

cc N82.1 Other female urinary-genital tract fistulae — [♀]
Cervicovesical fistula — An abnormal passage communicating the cervix with the bladder.
Ureterovaginal fistula — An abnormal passage communicating the ureter with the vagina.
Urethrovaginal fistula — An abnormal passage communicating the urethra with the vagina.
Uteroureteric fistula — An abnormal passage communicating a ureter with the uterus.
Uterovesical fistula — An abnormal passage communicating the uterus with the bladder.

cc N82.2 Fistula of vagina to small intestine — [♀] – An abnormal passage communicating the samll intestine with the vagina.

cc N82.3 Fistula of vagina to large intestine — [♀] – An abnormal passage communicating the large intestine with the vagina.
Rectovaginal fistula

cc N82.4 Other female intestinal-genital tract fistulae — [♀]
Intestinouterine fistula — An abnormal passage communicating the intestine with the vagina.

cc N82.5 Female genital tract-skin fistulae — [♀] – An abnormal passage communicating the female genital tract with the skin.
Uterus to abdominal wall fistula — An abnormal passage communicating the uterus with the abdominal wall.
Vaginoperineal fistula — An abnormal passage communicating the vagina with the perineum.

cc N82.8 Other female genital tract fistulae — [♀]

cc N82.9 Female genital tract fistula, unspecified — [♀]

N83- Noninflammatory disorders of ovary, fallopian tube and broad ligament
Excludes ❷: hydrosalpinx (N70.1-)

N83.0- <u>Follicular cyst of ovary</u> — An encapsulated, enlarged graafian follicle filled with accumulated transudate.
Cyst of graafian follicle
Hemorrhagic follicular cyst (of ovary)

N83.00 Follicular cyst of ovary, <u>unspecified</u> side — [♀]

N83.01 Follicular cyst of <u>right</u> ovary — [♀]

N83.02 Follicular cyst of <u>left</u> ovary — [♀]

Excludes 1: = NOT CODED HERE! (Do not code both)

Excludes ❷: = Not Included Here

N83.1- <u>Corpus luteum</u> cyst — An encapsulated, enlarged serous-filled corpus luteum, or a localized swelling of clotted blood within a corpus luteum.
> **Hemorrhagic corpus luteum cyst** — The escape of blood from, or forcible tearing of the wall of a corpus luteum cyst.

N83.10 Corpus luteum cyst of ovary, <u>unspecified</u> side — [♀]

N83.11 Corpus luteum cyst of <u>right</u> ovary — [♀]

N83.12 Corpus luteum cyst of <u>left</u> ovary — [♀]

N83.2- Other and unspecified ovarian cysts
> Excludes 1:   developmental ovarian cyst (Q50.1)
>   neoplastic ovarian cyst (D27.-)
>   polycystic ovarian syndrome (E28.2)
>   Stein-Leventhal syndrome (E28.2)

N83.20- <u>Unspecified</u> ovarian cysts

N83.201 Unspecified ovarian cyst, <u>right</u> side — [♀]

N83.202 Unspecified ovarian cyst, <u>left</u> side — [♀]

N83.209 Unspecified ovarian cyst, <u>unspecified</u> side — [♀]
> Ovarian cyst, NOS

N83.29- <u>Other</u> ovarian cysts
> Retention cyst of ovary
> Simple cyst of ovary

N83.291 Other ovarian cyst, <u>right</u> side — [♀]

N83.292 Other ovarian cyst, <u>left</u> side — [♀]

N83.299 Other ovarian cyst, <u>unspecified</u> side — [♀]

N83.3- <u>Acquired atrophy</u> of ovary and fallopian tube

N83.31- Acquired atrophy of <u>ovary</u> — An abnormal wasting-away of an ovary.

N83.311 Acquired atrophy of <u>right</u> ovary — [♀]

N83.312 Acquired atrophy of <u>left</u> ovary — [♀]

N83.319 Acquired atrophy of ovary, <u>unspecified</u> side — [♀]
> Acquired atrophy of ovary, NOS

N83.32- Acquired atrophy of <u>fallopian tube</u> — An abnormal wasting-away of a fallopian tube.

N83.321 Acquired atrophy of <u>right</u> fallopian tube — [♀]

N83.322 Acquired atrophy of <u>left</u> fallopian tube — [♀]

N83.329 Acquired atrophy of fallopian tube, <u>unspecified</u> side — [♀]
> Acquired atrophy of fallopian tube, NOS

N83.33- Acquired atrophy of <u>ovary and fallopian tube</u> — An abnormal wasting-away of an ovary and a fallopian tube.

N83.331 Acquired atrophy of <u>right</u> ovary and fallopian tube — [♀]

N83.332 Acquired atrophy of <u>left</u> ovary and fallopian tube — [♀]

N83.339 Acquired atrophy of ovary and fallopian tube, <u>unspecified</u> side — [♀]
> Acquired atrophy of ovary and fallopian tube, NOS

N83.4- <u>Prolapse and hernia</u> of ovary and fallopian tube — An abnormal protrusion or displacement from the normal position of an ovary or fallopian tube.

N83.40 Prolapse and hernia of ovary and fallopian tube, <u>unspecified</u> side — [♀]
> Prolapse and hernia of ovary and fallopian tube, NOS

N83.41 Prolapse and hernia of <u>right</u> ovary and fallopian tube — [♀]

N83.42 Prolapse and hernia of <u>left</u> ovary and fallopian tube — [♀]

N83.5- <u>Torsion</u> of ovary, ovarian pedicle and fallopian tube
> Torsion of accessory tube

N83.51- Torsion of <u>ovary and ovarian pedicle</u> — The abnormal twisting of an ovary and/or an ovarian pedicle.

cc **N83.511** Torsion of <u>right</u> ovary and ovarian pedicle — [♀]

cc **N83.512** Torsion of <u>left</u> ovary and ovarian pedicle — [♀]

cc **N83.519** Torsion of ovary and ovarian pedicle, <u>unspecified</u> side — [♀]
> Torsion of ovary and ovarian pedicle, NOS

N83.52- Torsion of <u>fallopian tube</u> — The abnormal twisting of a fallopian tube.
> **Torsion of hydatid of Morgagni** — The abnormal twisting of a cyst-like remnant of the oviduct.

cc **N83.521** Torsion of <u>right</u> fallopian tube — [♀]

cc **N83.522** Torsion of <u>left</u> fallopian tube — [♀]

cc **N83.529** Torsion of fallopian tube, <u>unspecified</u> side — [♀]
> Torsion of fallopian tube, NOS

cc **N83.53** Torsion of ovary, ovarian pedicle and fallopian tube — [♀] — The abnormal twisting of an ovary, ovarian pedicle and fallopian tube.

N83.6 Hematosalpinx — [♀] — The abnormally retained menstrual fluid in a fallopian tube.
> Excludes 1:   hematosalpinx (with) (in):
>   hematocolpos (N89.7)
>   hematometra (N85.7)
>   tubal pregnancy (O00.1-)

N83.7 Hematoma of broad ligament — [♀] — A localized swelling mass of clotted blood in the broad ligament, caused by a break in a blood vessel.

N83.8 Other noninflammatory disorders of ovary, fallopian tube and broad ligament — [♀]
> **Broad ligament laceration syndrome [Allen-Masters]** — A forceful disruption of the broad ligament.

N83.9 Noninflammatory disorder of ovary, fallopian tube and broad ligament, unspecified — [♀]

N84- Polyp of female genital tract
> Excludes 1:   adenomatous polyp (D28.-)
>   placental polyp (O90.89)

N84.0 Polyp of corpus uteri — [♀] — A protruding mucous membrane growth of that portion of the uterus above the isthmus and below the fallopian tube orifices.
> **Polyp of endometrium** — A sessile benign projecting mass on the endometrium.
> **Polyp of uterus NOS**
> Excludes 1:   polypoid endometrial hyperplasia (N85.0-)

N84.1 Polyp of cervix uteri — [♀] — A protruding mucous membrane growth of the cervix.
> **Mucous polyp of cervix**

N84.2 Polyp of vagina — [♀] — A protruding mucous membrane growth of the vagina.

N84.3 Polyp of vulva — [♀] — A protruding mucous membrane growth of the labia and vulva.
> **Polyp of labia**

N84.8 Polyp of other parts of female genital tract — [♀]

N84.9 Polyp of female genital tract, unspecified — [♀]

N85- Other noninflammatory disorders of uterus, except cervix
> Excludes 1:   endometriosis (N80.-)
>   inflammatory diseases of uterus (N71.-)
>   noninflammatory disorders of cervix, except malposition (N86-N88)
>   polyp of corpus uteri (N84.0)
>   uterine prolapse (N81.-)

N85.0- Endometrial hyperplasia — The abnormal overgrowth of the endometrium.

N85.00 Endometrial hyperplasia, unspecified — [♀]
> **Hyperplasia (adenomatous) (cystic) (glandular) of endometrium**
> **Hyperplastic endometritis** — The abnormal overgrowth of an inflamed endometrium.

N85.01 Benign endometrial hyperplasia — [♀] — A form caused by the hormonal effects of unopposed estrogens.
> **Endometrial hyperplasia (complex) (simple) without atypia**

N85.02 Endometrial intraepithelial neoplasia [EIN] — [♀] — A form indicating an emergent neoplastic precancerous lesion.
> **Endometrial hyperplasia with atypia**
> Excludes 1:   malignant neoplasm of endometrium (with endometrial intraepithelial neoplasia [EIN]) (C54.1)

N85.2 Hypertrophy of uterus — [♀] — The abnormal enlargement of the uterus.
> **Bulky or enlarged uterus**
> Excludes 1:   puerperal hypertrophy of uterus (O90.89)

N85.3 Subinvolution of uterus — [♀] — A diffuse, symmetrical uterine enlargement with failure to return to its normal size and position.
> Excludes 1:   puerperal subinvolution of uterus (O90.89)

N85.4 Malposition of uterus — [♀] — The abnormal position of the uterus.
> **Anteversion of uterus** — The abnormal forward displacement of the uterus.
> **Retroflexion of uterus** — The abnormal bending backward of the uterus at the cervix.
> **Retroversion of uterus** — The abnormal displacement of the uterus backward, including the cervix.
> Excludes 1:   malposition of uterus complicating pregnancy, labor or delivery (O34.5-, O65.5)

N 8 3 - N 8 5

Excludes 1: = NOT CODED HERE! (Do not code both)

Excludes ❷: = Not Included Here

N85.5 **Inversion of uterus** — [♀] – The abnormal, persistent turning inside out of the uterus.
    Excludes 1:   *current obstetric trauma (O71.2)*
                    postpartum inversion of uterus (O71.2)

N85.6 **Intrauterine synechiae** — [♀] – The abnormal adherence and adhesions of the uterus.

N85.7 **Hematometra** — [♀] – The abnormal accumulation of blood within the uterus.
    Hematosalpinx with hematometra
    Excludes 1:   *hematometra with hematocolpos (N89.7)*

N85.8 **Other specified noninflammatory disorders of uterus** — [♀]
    Atrophy of uterus, acquired —— An abnormal wasting-away of the uterus.
    Fibrosis of uterus NOS

N85.9 **Noninflammatory disorder of uterus, unspecified** — [♀]
    Disorder of uterus NOS

N86 **Erosion and ectropion of cervix uteri** — [♀]
    Decubitus (trophic) ulcer of cervix —— The abnormal, localized eating-away of cervical tissue.
    Eversion of cervix —— The abnormal turning inside out of the cervix.
    Excludes 1:   *erosion and ectropion of cervix with cervicitis (N72)*

N87- <u>Dysplasia of cervix uteri</u> —— The cellular deviation of the cervical epithelium.
    Excludes 1:   *abnormal results from cervical cytologic examination without histologic confirmation (R87.61-)*
                 carcinoma in situ of cervix uteri (D06.-)
                 cervical intraepithelial neoplasia III [CIN III] (D06.-)
                 HGSIL of cervix (R87.613)
                 severe dysplasia of cervix uteri (D06.-)

N87.0 <u>Mild</u> **cervical dysplasia** — [♀]
    Cervical intraepithelial neoplasia I [CIN I]

N87.1 <u>Moderate</u> **cervical dysplasia** — [♀]
    Cervical intraepithelial neoplasia II [CIN II]

N87.9 **Dysplasia of cervix uteri, <u>unspecified</u>** — [♀]
    Anaplasia of cervix
    Cervical atypism
    Cervical dysplasia NOS

N88- **Other noninflammatory disorders of cervix uteri**
    Excludes ❷: *inflammatory disease of cervix (N72)*
                 polyp of cervix (N84.1)

N88.0 **Leukoplakia of cervix uteri** — [♀] – The abnormal development of white, thickened patches of the mucous membrane of the cervix.

N88.1 **Old laceration of cervix uteri** — [♀] – The presence of a healed lacerated wound of the cervix.
    Adhesions of cervix
    Excludes 1:   *current obstetric trauma (O71.3)*

N88.2 **Stricture and stenosis of cervix uteri** — [♀] – An abnormal narrowing of the cervical opening.
    Excludes 1:   *stricture and stenosis of cervix uteri complicating labor (O65.5)*

N88.3 **Incompetence of cervix uteri** — [♀] – The abnormal widening of the cervical opening due to inadequate function.
    Investigation and management of (suspected) cervical incompetence in a nonpregnant woman
    Excludes 1:   *cervical incompetence complicating pregnancy (O34.3-)*

N88.4 **Hypertrophic elongation of cervix uteri** — [♀] – The abnormal increased length of the cervix into the vagina due to enlargement of the cervical tissues.

N88.8 **Other specified noninflammatory disorders of cervix uteri** — [♀]
    Excludes 1:   *current obstetric trauma (O71.3)*

N88.9 **Noninflammatory disorder of cervix uteri, unspecified** — [♀]

N89- **Other noninflammatory disorders of vagina**
    Excludes 1:   *abnormal results from vaginal cytologic examination without histologic confirmation (R87.62-)*
                 carcinoma in situ of vagina (D07.2)
                 HGSIL of vagina (R87.623)
                 inflammation of vagina (N76.-)
                 senile (atrophic) vaginitis (N95.2)
                 severe dysplasia of vagina (D07.2)
                 trichomonal leukorrhea (A59.00)
                 vaginal intraepithelial neoplasia [VAIN], grade III (D07.2)

N89.0 <u>Mild</u> **vaginal dysplasia** — [♀] – The abnormal development of vaginal cellular tissue.
    Vaginal intraepithelial neoplasia [VAIN], grade I

N89.1 <u>Moderate</u> **<u>vaginal</u> dysplasia** — [♀] – The abnormal development of vaginal cellular tissue.
    Vaginal intraepithelial neoplasia [VAIN], grade II

N89.3 **Dysplasia of <u>vagina</u>, <u>unspecified</u>** — [♀]

N89.4 **Leukoplakia of vagina** — [♀] – The abnormal development of white, thickened patches on the mucous membrane of the vagina.

N89.5 **Stricture and atresia of vagina** — [♀] – The abnormal narrowing, or complete blockage of the vagina.
    Vaginal adhesions —— The abnormal development of fibrotic tissue in the vagina.
    Vaginal stenosis —— An abnormal decrease in caliber of the vaginal canal.
    Excludes 1:   *congenital atresia or stricture (Q52.4)*
                 postprocedural adhesions of vagina (N99.2)

N89.6 **Tight hymenal ring** — [♀] – An abnormally thick, or impenetrable membranous fold of the vaginal orifice.
    Rigid hymen
    Tight introitus
    Excludes 1:   *imperforate hymen (Q52.3)*

N89.7 **Hematocolpos** — [♀] – The abnormal filling of the vagina with menstrual blood.
    Hematocolpos with hematometra or hematosalpinx

N89.8 **Other specified noninflammatory disorders of vagina** — [♀]
    Leukorrhea NOS
    Old vaginal laceration —— The presence of a healed vaginal laceration.
    Pessary ulcer of vagina
    Excludes 1:   *current obstetric trauma (O70.-, O71.4, O71.7-O71.8)*
                 old laceration involving muscles of pelvic floor (N81.8)

N89.9 **Noninflammatory disorder of vagina, unspecified** — [♀]

N90- **Other noninflammatory disorders of vulva and perineum**
    Excludes 1:   *anogenital (venereal) warts (A63.0)*
                 carcinoma in situ of vulva (D07.1)
                 condyloma acuminatum (A63.0)
                 current obstetric trauma (O70.-, O71.7-O71.8)
                 inflammation of vulva (N76.-)
                 severe dysplasia of vulva (D07.1)
                 vulvar intraepithelial neoplasm III [VIN III] (D07.1)

N90.0 <u>Mild</u> **<u>vulvar</u> dysplasia** — [♀] – The abnormal development of vulvar cellular tissue.
    Vulvar intrepithelial neoplasia [VIN], grade I

N90.1 <u>Moderate</u> **<u>vulvar</u> dysplasia** — [♀] – The abnormal development of vulvar cellular tissue.
    Vulvar intraepithelial neoplasia [VIN], grade II

N90.3 **Dysplasia of <u>vulva</u>, <u>unspecified</u>** — [♀]

N90.4 **Leukoplakia of vulva** — [♀] – A vulvar dystrophic condition characterized by the development of white, thickened patches.
    Dystrophy of vulva —— Abnormal hypertrophic cellular changes of the vulva.
    Kraurosis of vulva —— A vulvar dystrophic condition characterized by a dry, shriveled vulva with leukoplakic patches and intense itching.
    Lichen sclerosus of external female genital organs

N90.5 **Atrophy of vulva** — [♀] – An abnormal wasting-away of the vulva.
    Stenosis of vulva

N90.6- **Hypertrophy of vulva** —— An abnormal enlargement of the vulva.

   N90.60 **Unspecified hypertrophy of vulva** — [♀]
      Unspecified hypertrophy of labia

   N90.61 **Childhood asymmetric labium majus enlargement** — [♀, Age/0-17] – An abnormal enlargement of one side of the vulva due to excessive tissue growth and occurring during pre- and early puberty.
      CALME

   N90.69 **Other specified hypertrophy of vulva** — [♀]
      Other specified hypertrophy of labia

N90.7 **Vulvar cyst** — [♀] – An encapsulated, fluid-filled sac of the vulva.

N 8 5 - N 9 0

Excludes 1: = NOT CODED HERE! (Do not code both)   **913**   *Excludes ❷:* = Not Included Here

N90.8- **Other specified noninflammatory disorders of vulva and perineum**

N90.81- **Female genital mutilation status** — The condition of having the female genitalia removed, in all or part, as a cultural practice performed in Africa, the Middle East, and part of Asia.
Female genital cutting status

N90.810 **Female genital mutilation status, unspecified** — [♀]
Female genital cutting status, unspecified
Female genital mutilation status NOS

N90.811 **Female genital mutilation Type I status** — [♀]
Clitorectomy status
Female genital cutting Type I status

N90.812 **Female genital mutilation Type II status** — [♀]
Clitorectomy with excision of labia minora status
Female genital cutting Type II status

N90.813 **Female genital mutilation Type III status** — [♀]
Female genital cutting Type III status
Infibulation status

N90.818 **Other female genital mutilation status** — [♀]
Female genital cutting Type IV status
Female genital mutilation Type IV status
Other female genital cutting status

N90.89 **Other specified noninflammatory disorders of vulva and perineum** — [♀]
Adhesions of vulva
Hypertrophy of clitoris

N90.9 **Noninflammatory disorder of vulva and perineum, unspecified** — [♀]

N91- **Absent, scanty and rare menstruation**
Excludes 1: *ovarian dysfunction (E28.-)*

N91.0 **Primary amenorrhea** — [♀] — The absence of menstruation prior to age 16 years.

N91.1 **Secondary amenorrhea** — [♀] — The absence of menstruation for a period of 6 months or greater.

N91.2 **Amenorrhea, unspecified** — [♀]

N91.3 **Primary oligomenorrhea** — [♀] — The decreased frequency of menstruation.

N91.4 **Secondary oligomenorrhea** — [♀] — The decreased frequency of menstruation that is due to another disease or condition.

N91.5 **Oligomenorrhea, unspecified** — [♀]
Hypomenorrhea NOS

N92- **Excessive, frequent and irregular menstruation**
Excludes 1: *postmenopausal bleeding (N95.0)*
precocious puberty (menstruation) (E30.1)

N92.0 **Excessive and frequent menstruation with regular cycle** — [♀] — The abnormal increase or increased number of cycles of menstruation.
Heavy periods NOS — The increased volume of menstrual flow.
Menorrhagia NOS — The excessive uterine bleeding occurring at the regular intervals of menstruation.
Polymenorrhea — Abnormally frequent menstruation.

N92.1 **Excessive and frequent menstruation with irregular cycle** — [♀] — A menstrual cycle which is different than the average four-week interval.
Irregular intermenstrual bleeding — Nonmenstrual uterine bleeding unrelated to menstrual cycle.
Irregular, shortened intervals between menstrual bleeding
Menometrorrhagia
Metrorrhagia

N92.2 **Excessive menstruation at puberty** — [♀, Age/0-17]
Excessive bleeding associated with onset of menstrual periods
Pubertal menorrhagia
Puberty bleeding

N92.3 **Ovulation bleeding** — [♀] — Uterine bleeding associated with ovulation.
Regular intermenstrual bleeding

N92.4 **Excessive bleeding in the premenopausal period** — [♀]
Climacteric menorrhagia or metrorrhagia
Menopausal menorrhagia or metrorrhagia
Preclimacteric menorrhagia or metrorrhagia
Premenopausal menorrhagia or metrorrhagia

N92.5 **Other specified irregular menstruation** — [♀]

N92.6 **Irregular menstruation, unspecified** — [♀]
Irregular bleeding NOS
Irregular periods NOS
Excludes 1: *irregular menstruation with:*
lengthened intervals or scanty bleeding (N91.3-N91.5)
shortened intervals or excessive bleeding (N92.1)

N93- **Other abnormal uterine and vaginal bleeding**
Excludes 1: *neonatal vaginal hemorrhage (P54.6)*
precocious puberty (menstruation) (E30.1)
pseudomenses (P54.6)

N93.0 **Postcoital and contact bleeding** — [♀] — Abnormal bleeding following sexual intercourse.

N93.1 **Pre-pubertal vaginal bleeding** — [♀, Age/0-17] — Abnormal pre-pubertal vaginal bleeding of an unknown cause, including not due to menstruation.

N93.8 **Other specified abnormal uterine and vaginal bleeding** — [♀]
Dysfunctional or functional uterine or vaginal bleeding NOS

N93.9 **Abnormal uterine and vaginal bleeding, unspecified** — [♀]

N94- **Pain and other conditions associated with female genital organs and menstrual cycle**

N94.0 **Mittelschmerz** — [♀] — Abdominal pain occurring at the time of ovulation.

N94.1- **Dyspareunia** — The occurrence of pain during sexual intercourse.
Excludes 1: *psychogenic dyspareunia (F52.6)*

N94.10 **Unspecified dyspareunia** — [♀]

N94.11 **Superficial (introital) dyspareunia** — [♀] — A form occurring on vaginal entry.

N94.12 **Deep dyspareunia** — [♀] — A form occurring with mid or upper vaginal penetration.

N94.19 **Other specified dyspareunia** — [♀]

N94.2 **Vaginismus** — [♀] — The painful spasm of the muscles surrounding the vagina.
Excludes 1: *psychogenic vaginismus (F52.5)*

N94.3 **Premenstrual tension syndrome** — [♀] — A syndrome of various symptoms occurring in the days preceding menstruation marked by emotional instability, irritability, insomnia, and headache.
Premenstrual dysphoric disorder — A severe form of premenstrual tension syndrome that significantly disrupts a woman's day-to-day activities.
Code also associated menstrual migraine (G43.82-, G43.83-)
Excludes 1: *premenstrual dysphoric disorder (F32.81)*

N94.4 **Primary dysmenorrhea** — [♀] — The excessively painful uterine cramps that accompany menstruation.

N94.5 **Secondary dysmenorrhea** — [♀] — A form that is associated with another medical condition.

N94.6 **Dysmenorrhea, unspecified** — [♀]
Excludes 1: *psychogenic dysmenorrhea (F45.8)*

N94.8- **Other specified conditions associated with female genital organs and menstrual cycle**

N94.81- **Vulvodynia** — The condition of persistent pain in the vulva that is characterized by burning, soreness, itching, rawness, and painful intercourse.

N94.810 **Vulvar vestibulitis** — [♀] — A form marked by pain with symptoms generally limited to the vaginal opening that results in painful vaginal entry (tampons or intercourse) and/or pain associated with sitting or wearing tight clothing.

N94.818 **Other vulvodynia** — [♀]

N94.819 **Vulvodynia, unspecified** — [♀]
Vulvodynia NOS

N94.89 **Other specified conditions associated with female genital organs and menstrual cycle** — [♀]

N94.9 **Unspecified condition associated with female genital organs and menstrual cycle** — [♀]

N90-N94

N95- Menopausal and other perimenopausal disorders
     Menopausal and other perimenopausal disorders due to naturally occurring (age-related) menopause and perimenopause
     Excludes 1:   *excessive bleeding in the premenopausal period (N92.4)*
           menopausal and perimenopausal disorders due to artificial or premature menopause (E89.4-, E28.31-)
           premature menopause (E28.31-)
     Excludes ❷: *postmenopausal osteoporosis (M81.0-)*
           postmenopausal osteoporosis with current pathological fracture (M80.0-)
           postmenopausal urethritis (N34.2)

N95.0   Postmenopausal bleeding — [♀] – Abnormal bleeding following menopause.

N95.1   Menopausal and female climacteric states — [♀]
     Symptoms such as flushing, sleeplessness, headache, lack of concentration, associated with natural (age-related) menopause
     Use additional code for associated symptoms
     Excludes 1:   *asymptomatic menopausal state (Z78.0)*
           symptoms associated with artificial menopause (E89.41)
           symptoms associated with premature menopause (E28.310)

N95.2   Postmenopausal atrophic vaginitis — [♀] – The wasting-away of the vaginal tissues associated with the cessation of menstruation.
     Senile (atrophic) vaginitis

N95.8   Other specified menopausal and perimenopausal disorders — [♀]

N95.9   Unspecified menopausal and perimenopausal disorder — [♀]

N96   Recurrent pregnancy loss — [♀]
     Investigation or care in a nonpregnant woman with history of recurrent pregnancy loss
     Excludes 1:   *recurrent pregancy loss with current pregnancy (O26.2-)*

N97-   Female infertility — Inability, or diminished ability, of a female to produce offspring.
     Includes: Inability to achieve a pregnancy
           Sterility, female NOS
     Excludes 1:   *female infertility associated with:*
           hypopituitarism (E23.0)
           Stein-Leventhal syndrome (E28.2)
     Excludes ❷: *incompetence of cervix uteri (N88.3)*

N97.0   Female infertility associated with anovulation — [♀] – A form characterized by absence of ovulation.

N97.1   Female infertility of tubal origin — [♀] – A form resulting from dysfunctional fallopian tube conditions.
     Female infertility associated with congenital anomaly of tube
     Female infertility due to tubal block
     Female infertility due to tubal occlusion
     Female infertility due to tubal stenosis

N97.2   Female infertility of uterine origin — [♀] – A form resulting from dysfunctional uterine conditions.
     Female infertility associated with congenital anomaly of uterus
     Female infertility due to nonimplantation of ovum

N97.8   Female infertility of other origin — [♀]

N97.9   Female infertility, unspecified — [♀]

N98-   Complications associated with artificial fertilization

cc **N98.0   Infection associated with artificial insemination** — [♀]

cc **N98.1   Hyperstimulation of ovaries** — [♀]
     Hyperstimulation of ovaries NOS
     Hyperstimulation of ovaries associated with induced ovulation

cc **N98.2   Complications of attempted introduction of fertilized ovum following in vitro fertilization** — [♀]

cc **N98.3   Complications of attempted introduction of embryo in embryo transfer** — [♀]

cc **N98.8   Other complications associated with artificial fertilization** — [♀]

cc **N98.9   Complication associated with artificial fertilization, unspecified** — [♀]

Intraoperative and postprocedural complications and disorders of genitourinary system, not elsewhere classified (N99)

N99-   Intraoperative and postprocedural complications and disorders of genitourinary system, not elsewhere classified
     Excludes ❷: *irradiation cystitis (N30.4-)*
           postoophorectomy osteoporosis with current pathological fracture (M80.8-)
           postoophorectomy osteoporosis without current pathological fracture (M81.8)

N99.0   Postprocedural (acute) (chronic) kidney failure
     Use additional code to type of kidney disease

N99.1-   Postprocedural urethral stricture
     Postcatheterization urethral stricture

N99.11- Postprocedural urethral stricture, male

N99.110   Postprocedural urethral stricture, male, meatal — [♂]

N99.111   Postprocedural bulbous urethral stricture — [♂]

N99.112   Postprocedural membranous urethral stricture — [♂]

N99.113   Postprocedural anterior bulbous urethral stricture — [♂]

N99.114   Postprocedural urethral stricture, male, unspecified — [♂]

N99.115   Postprocedural fossa navicularis urethral stricture

N99.12   Postprocedural urethral stricture, female — [♀]

N99.2   Postprocedural adhesions of vagina — [♀]

N99.3   Prolapse of vaginal vault after hysterectomy — [♀]

N99.4   Postprocedural pelvic peritoneal adhesions
     Excludes ❷: *pelvic peritoneal adhesions NOS (N73.6)*
           postinfective pelvic peritoneal adhesions (N73.6)

N99.5-   Complications of stoma of urinary tract
     Excludes ❷: *mechanical complication of urinary catheter (T83.0-)*

N99.51- Complication of cystostomy

cc **N99.510   Cystostomy hemorrhage**

cc **N99.511   Cystostomy infection**

cc **N99.512   Cystostomy malfunction**

cc **N99.518   Other cystostomy complication**

N99.52- Complication of incontinent external stoma of urinary tract

N99.520   Hemorrhage of incontinent external stoma of urinary tract

N99.521   Infection of incontinent external stoma of urinary tract

N99.522   Malfunction of incontinent external stoma of urinary tract

N99.523   Herniation of incontinent stoma of urinary tract

N99.524   Stenosis of incontinent stoma of urinary tract

N99.528   Other complication of incontinent external stoma of urinary tract

N99.53- Complication of continent stoma of urinary tract

N99.530   Hemorrhage of continent stoma of urinary tract

N99.531   Infection of continent stoma of urinary tract

N99.532   Malfunction of continent stoma of urinary tract

N99.533   Herniation of continent stoma of urinary tract

N99.534   Stenosis of continent stoma of urinary tract

N99.538   Other complication of continent stoma of urinary tract

N95 - N99

N99.6- <u>Intraoperative hemorrhage and hematoma</u> of a genitourinary system organ or structure complicating a procedure
Excludes 1: intraoperative hemorrhage and hematoma of a genitourinary system organ or structure due to accidental puncture or laceration during a procedure (N99.7-)

cc **N99.61** Intraoperative hemorrhage and hematoma of a genitourinary system organ or structure complicating a <u>genitourinary system procedure</u>

cc **N99.62** Intraoperative hemorrhage and hematoma of a genitourinary system organ or structure complicating <u>other procedure</u>

N99.7- Accidental puncture and laceration of a genitourinary system organ or structure during a procedure

cc **N99.71** Accidental puncture and laceration of a genitourinary system organ or structure during a <u>genitourinary system procedure</u>

cc **N99.72** Accidental puncture and laceration of a genitourinary system organ or structure during <u>other procedure</u>

N99.8- Other intraoperative and postprocedural complications and disorders of genitourinary system

N99.81 Other intraoperative complications of genitourinary system

N99.82- <u>Postprocedural hemorrhage</u> of a genitourinary system organ or structure following a procedure

cc **N99.820** Postprocedural hemorrhage of a genitourinary system organ or structure following a <u>genitourinary system procedure</u>

cc **N99.821** Postprocedural hemorrhage of a genitourinary system organ or structure following <u>other procedure</u>

N99.83 Residual ovary syndrome —[♀]

N99.84- <u>Postprocedural hematoma and seroma</u> of a genitourinary system organ or structure following a procedure

cc **N99.840** Postprocedural <u>hematoma</u> of a genitourinary system organ or structure following a <u>genitourinary system procedure</u>

cc **N99.841** Postprocedural <u>hematoma</u> of a genitourinary system organ or structure following <u>other procedure</u>

cc **N99.842** Postprocedural <u>seroma</u> of a genitourinary system organ or structure following a <u>genitourinary system procedure</u>

cc **N99.843** Postprocedural <u>seroma</u> of a genitourinary system organ or structure following <u>other procedure</u>

N99.89 Other postprocedural complications and disorders of genitourinary system

N99–N99

Chapter 15 – Pregnancy, childbirth and the puerperium (O00-O9A)

Note: **CODES FROM THIS CHAPTER ARE FOR USE ONLY ON MATERNAL RECORDS, NEVER ON NEWBORN RECORDS.** Codes from this chapter are for use for conditions related to or aggravated by the pregnancy, childbirth, or by the puerperium (maternal causes or obstetric causes)

Use additional code from category Z3A, Weeks of gestation, to identify the specific week of the pregnancy, if known.

Trimesters are counted from the first day of the last menstrual period. They are defined as follows:

1st trimester- less than 14 weeks 0 days
2nd trimester- 14 weeks 0 days to less than 28 weeks 0 days
3rd trimester- 28 weeks 0 days until delivery

Excludes 1:　*supervision of normal pregnancy (Z34.-)*
Excludes ❷:　*mental and behavioral disorders associated with the puerperium (F53)*
　　　　　　　obstetrical tetanus (A34)
　　　　　　　postpartum necrosis of pituitary gland (E23.0)
　　　　　　　puerperal osteomalacia (M83.0)

This chapter contains the following blocks:

O00-O08	Pregnancy with abortive outcome
O09	Supervision of high risk pregnancy
O10-O16	Edema, proteinuria and hypertensive disorders in pregnancy, childbirth and the puerperium
O20-O29	Other maternal disorders predominantly related to pregnancy
O30-O48	Maternal care related to the fetus and amniotic cavity and possible delivery problems
O60-O77	Complications of labor and delivery
O80-O82	Encounter for delivery
O85-O92	Complications predominantly related to the puerperium
O94-O9A	Other obstetric conditions, not elsewhere classified

Chapter-Specific Coding Guidelines

C.　Chapter-Specific Coding Guidelines

In addition to general coding guidelines, there are guidelines for specific diagnoses and/or conditions in the classification. Unless otherwise indicated, these guidelines apply to all health care settings. Please refer to Section II for guidelines on the selection of principal diagnosis.

15.　Chapter 15: Pregnancy, Childbirth, and the Puerperium (O00-O9A)

a.　General Rules for Obstetric Cases

1)　Codes from chapter 15 and sequencing priority
Obstetric cases require codes from chapter 15, codes in the range O00-O9A, Pregnancy, Childbirth, and the Puerperium. Chapter 15 codes have sequencing priority over codes from other chapters. Additional codes from other chapters may be used in conjunction with chapter 15 codes to further specify conditions. Should the provider document that the pregnancy is incidental to the encounter, then code Z33.1, Pregnant state, incidental, should be used in place of any chapter 15 codes. It is the provider's responsibility to state that the condition being treated is not affecting the pregnancy.

2)　Chapter 15 codes used only on the maternal record
Chapter 15 codes are to be used only on the maternal record, never on the record of the newborn.

3)　Final character for trimester
The majority of codes in Chapter 15 have a final character indicating the trimester of pregnancy. The timeframes for the trimesters are indicated at the beginning of the chapter. If trimester is not a component of a code it is because the condition always occurs in a specific trimester, or the concept of trimester of pregnancy is not applicable. Certain codes have characters for only certain trimesters because the condition does not occur in all trimesters, but it may occur in more than just one.

Assignment of the final character for trimester should be based on the provider's documentation of the trimester (or number of weeks) for the current admission/encounter. This applies to the assignment of trimester for pre-existing conditions as well as those that develop during or are due to the pregnancy. The provider's documentation of the number of weeks may be used to assign the appropriate code identifying the trimester.

Whenever delivery occurs during the current admission, and there is an "in childbirth" option for the obstetric complication being coded, the "in childbirth" code should be assigned.

4)　Selection of trimester for inpatient admissions that encompass more than one trimesters
In instances when a patient is admitted to a hospital for complications of pregnancy during one trimester and remains in the hospital into a subsequent trimester, the trimester character for the antepartum complication code should be assigned on the basis of the trimester when the complication developed, not the trimester of the discharge. If the condition developed prior to the current admission/encounter or represents a pre-existing condition, the trimester character for the trimester at the time of the admission/encounter should be assigned.

5)　Unspecified trimester
Each category that includes codes for trimester has a code for "unspecified trimester." The "unspecified trimester" code should rarely be used, such as when the documentation in the record is insufficient to determine the trimester and it is not possible to obtain clarification.

6)　7th character for Fetus Identification
Where applicable, a 7th character is to be assigned for certain categories (O31, O32, O33.3 - O33.6, O35, O36, O40, O41, O60.1, O60.2, O64, and O69) to identify the fetus for which the complication code applies.

Assign 7th character "0":
• For single gestations
• When the documentation in the record is insufficient to determine the fetus affected and it is not possible to obtain clarification.
• When it is not possible to clinically determine which fetus is affected.

b.　Selection of OB Principal or First-listed Diagnosis

1)　Routine outpatient prenatal visits
For routine outpatient prenatal visits when no complications are present, a code from category Z34, Encounter for supervision of normal pregnancy, should be used as the first-listed diagnosis. These codes should not be used in conjunction with chapter 15 codes.

2)　*Supervision of High-Risk Pregnancy*
Codes from category O09, Supervision of high-risk pregnancy, are intended for use only during the prenatal period. For complications during the labor or delivery episode as a result of a high-risk pregnancy, assign the applicable complication codes from Chapter 15. If there are no complications during the labor and delivery episode, assign code O80, Encounter for full-term uncomplicated delivery.

For routine prenatal outpatient visits for patients with high-risk pregnancies, a code from category O09, Supervision of high-risk pregnancy, should be used as the first-listed diagnosis. Secondary chapter 15 codes may be used in conjunction with these codes if appropriate.

3)　Episodes when no delivery occurs
In episodes when no delivery occurs, the principal diagnosis should correspond to the principal complication of the pregnancy which necessitated the encounter. Should more than one complication exist, all of which are treated or monitored, any of the complications codes may be sequenced first.

4)　When a delivery occurs
~~When a delivery occurs, the principal diagnosis should correspond to the main circumstances or complication of the delivery.~~ When an obstetric patient is admitted and delivers during that admission, the condition that prompted the admission should be sequenced as the principal diagnosis. If multiple conditions prompted the admission, sequence the one most related to the delivery as the principal diagnosis. A code for any complication of the delivery should be assigned as an additional diagnosis. In cases of cesarean delivery, ~~the selection of the principal diagnosis should be the condition established after study that was responsible for the patient's admission.~~ If if the patient was admitted with a condition that resulted in the performance of a cesarean procedure, that condition should be selected as the principal diagnosis. If the reason for the admission/~~encounter~~ was unrelated to the condition resulting in the cesarean delivery, the condition related to the reason for the admission/~~encounter~~ should be selected as the principal diagnosis.

5)　Outcome of delivery
A code from category Z37, Outcome of delivery, should be included on every maternal record when a delivery has occurred. These codes are not to be used on subsequent records or on the newborn record.

c.　Pre-existing conditions versus conditions due to the pregnancy
Certain categories in Chapter 15 distinguish between conditions of the mother that existed prior to pregnancy (pre-existing) and those that are a direct result of pregnancy. When assigning codes from Chapter 15, it is important to assess if a condition was pre-existing prior to pregnancy or developed during or due to the pregnancy in order to assign the correct code.

O00 | O00

Categories that do not distinguish between pre-existing and pregnancy-related conditions may be used for either. It is acceptable to use codes specifically for the puerperium with codes complicating pregnancy and childbirth if a condition arises postpartum during the delivery encounter.

d. Pre-existing hypertension in pregnancy

Category O10, Pre-existing hypertension complicating pregnancy, childbirth and the puerperium, includes codes for hypertensive heart and hypertensive chronic kidney disease. When assigning one of the O10 codes that includes hypertensive heart disease or hypertensive chronic kidney disease, it is necessary to add a secondary code from the appropriate hypertension category to specify the type of heart failure or chronic kidney disease.

See Section I.C.9. Hypertension.

e. Fetal Conditions Affecting the Management of the Mother

1) Codes from categories O35 and O36

Codes from categories O35, Maternal care for known or suspected fetal abnormality and damage, and O36, Maternal care for other fetal problems, are assigned only when the fetal condition is actually responsible for modifying the management of the mother, i.e., by requiring diagnostic studies, additional observation, special care, or termination of pregnancy. The fact that the fetal condition exists does not justify assigning a code from this series to the mother's record.

2) In utero surgery

In cases when surgery is performed on the fetus, a diagnosis code from category O35, Maternal care for known or suspected fetal abnormality and damage, should be assigned identifying the fetal condition. Assign the appropriate procedure code for the procedure performed.

No code from Chapter 16, the perinatal codes, should be used on the mother's record to identify fetal conditions. Surgery performed in utero on a fetus is still to be coded as an obstetric encounter.

f. HIV Infection in Pregnancy, Childbirth and the Puerperium

During pregnancy, childbirth or the puerperium, a patient admitted because of an HIV-related illness should receive a principal diagnosis from subcategory O98.7-, Human immunodeficiency [HIV] disease complicating pregnancy, childbirth and the puerperium, followed by the code(s) for the HIV-related illness(es).

Patients with asymptomatic HIV infection status admitted during pregnancy, childbirth, or the puerperium should receive codes of O98.7- and Z21, Asymptomatic human immunodeficiency virus [HIV] infection status.

g. Diabetes mellitus in pregnancy

Diabetes mellitus is a significant complicating factor in pregnancy. Pregnant women who are diabetic should be assigned a code from category O24, Diabetes mellitus in pregnancy, childbirth, and the puerperium, first, followed by the appropriate diabetes code(s) (E08-E13) from Chapter 4.

h. Long-term use of insulin *and oral hypoglycemics*

Code Z79.4, Long-term (current) use of insulin, or code Z79.84, Long-term (current) use of oral hypoglycemic drugs, should also be assigned if the diabetes mellitus is being treated with insulin or oral medications. If the patient is treated with both oral medications and insulin, only the code for insulin-controlled should be assigned.

i. Gestational (pregnancy induced) diabetes

Gestational (pregnancy induced) diabetes can occur during the second and third trimester of pregnancy in women who were not diabetic prior to pregnancy. Gestational diabetes can cause complications in the pregnancy similar to those of pre-existing diabetes mellitus. It also puts the woman at greater risk of developing diabetes after the pregnancy. Codes for gestational diabetes are in subcategory O24.4, Gestational diabetes mellitus. No other code from category O24, Diabetes mellitus in pregnancy, childbirth, and the puerperium, should be used with a code from O24.4.

The codes under subcategory O24.4 include diet controlled, ~~and~~ insulin controlled, and controlled by oral hypoglycemic drugs. If a patient with gestational diabetes is treated with both diet and insulin, only the code for insulin-controlled is required. If a patient with gestational diabetes is treated with both diet and oral hypoglycemic medications, only the code for "controlled by oral hypoglycemic drugs" is required. Code Z79.4, Long-term (current) use of insulin or code Z79.84, Long-term (current) use of oral hypoglycemic drugs, should not be assigned with codes from subcategory O24.4.

An abnormal glucose tolerance in pregnancy is assigned a code from subcategory O99.81, Abnormal glucose complicating pregnancy, childbirth, and the puerperium.

j. Sepsis and septic shock complicating abortion, pregnancy, childbirth and the puerperium

When assigning a chapter 15 code for sepsis complicating abortion, pregnancy, childbirth, and the puerperium, a code for the specific type of infection should be assigned as an additional diagnosis. If severe sepsis is present, a code from subcategory R65.2, Severe sepsis, and code(s) for associated organ dysfunction(s) should also be assigned as additional diagnoses.

k. Puerperal sepsis

Code O85, Puerperal sepsis, should be assigned with a secondary code to identify the causal organism (e.g., for a bacterial infection, assign a code from category B95-B96, Bacterial infections in conditions classified elsewhere). A code from category A40, Strepto-coccal sepsis, or A41, Other sepsis, should not be used for puerperal sepsis. If applicable, use additional codes to identify severe sepsis (R65.2-) and any associated acute organ dysfunction.

l. Alcohol and tobacco use during pregnancy, childbirth and the puerperium

1) Alcohol use during pregnancy, childbirth and the puerperium

Codes under subcategory O99.31, Alcohol use complicating pregnancy, childbirth, and the puerperium, should be assigned for any pregnancy case when a mother uses alcohol during the pregnancy or postpartum. A secondary code from category F10, Alcohol related disorders, should also be assigned to identify manifestations of the alcohol use.

2) Tobacco use during pregnancy, childbirth and the puerperium

Codes under subcategory O99.33, Smoking (tobacco) complicating pregnancy, childbirth, and the puerperium, should be assigned for any pregnancy case when a mother uses any type of tobacco product during the pregnancy or postpartum. A secondary code from category F17, Nicotine dependence, Tobacco use, should also be assigned to identify the type of nicotine dependence.

m. Poisoning, toxic effects, adverse effects and underdosing in a pregnant patient

A code from subcategory O9A.2, Injury, poisoning and certain other consequences of external causes complicating pregnancy, childbirth, and the puerperium, should be sequenced first, followed by the appropriate injury, poisoning, toxic effect, adverse effect or underdosing code, and then the additional code(s) that specifies the condition caused by the poisoning, toxic effect, adverse effect or underdosing.

See Section I.C.19. Adverse effects, poisoning, underdosing and toxic effects.

n. Normal Delivery, Code O80

1) Encounter for full term uncomplicated delivery

Code O80 should be assigned when a woman is admitted for a full-term normal delivery and delivers a single, healthy infant without any complications antepartum, during the delivery, or postpartum during the delivery episode. Code O80 is always a principal diagnosis. It is not to be used if any other code from chapter 15 is needed to describe a current complication of the antenatal, delivery, or perinatal period. Additional codes from other chapters may be used with code O80 if they are not related to or are in any way complicating the pregnancy.

2) Uncomplicated delivery with resolved antepartum complication

Code O80 may be used if the patient had a complication at some point during the pregnancy, but the complication is not present at the time of the admission for delivery.

3) Outcome of delivery for O80

Z37.0, Single live birth, is the only outcome of delivery code appropriate for use with O80.

o. The Peripartum and Postpartum Periods

1) Peripartum and Postpartum periods

The postpartum period begins immediately after delivery and continues for six weeks following delivery. The peripartum period is defined as the last month of pregnancy to five months postpartum.

2) Peripartum and postpartum complication

A postpartum complication is any complication occurring within the six-week period.

3) Pregnancy-related complications after 6 week period

Chapter 15 codes may also be used to describe pregnancy-related complications after the peripartum or postpartum period if the provider documents that a condition is pregnancy related.

4) Admission for routine postpartum care following delivery outside hospital

When the mother delivers outside the hospital prior to admission and is admitted for routine postpartum care and no complications are noted, code Z39.0, Encounter for care and examination of mother immediately after delivery, should be assigned as the principal diagnosis.

5) Pregnancy associated cardiomyopathy
Pregnancy associated cardiomyopathy, code O90.3, is unique in that it may be diagnosed in the third trimester of pregnancy but may continue to progress months after delivery. For this reason, it is referred to as peripartum cardiomyopathy. Code O90.3 is only for use when the cardiomyopathy develops as a result of pregnancy in a woman who did not have pre-existing heart disease.

p. Code O94, Sequelae of complication of pregnancy, childbirth, and the puerperium

1) Code O94
Code O94, Sequelae of complication of pregnancy, childbirth, and the puerperium, is for use in those cases when an initial complication of a pregnancy develops a sequelae requiring care or treatment at a future date.

2) After the initial postpartum period
This code may be used at any time after the initial postpartum period.

3) Sequencing of Code O94
This code, like all sequela codes, is to be sequenced following the code describing the sequelae of the complication.

q. Termination of Pregnancy and Spontaneous abortions

1) Abortion with Liveborn Fetus
When an attempted termination of pregnancy results in a liveborn fetus, assign code Z33.2, Encounter for elective termination of pregnancy and a code from category Z37, Outcome of Delivery.

2) Retained Products of Conception following an abortion
Subsequent encounters for retained products of conception following a spontaneous abortion or elective termination of pregnancy are assigned the appropriate code from category O03, Spontaneous abortion, or codes O07.4, Failed attempted termination of pregnancy without complication and Z33.2, Encounter for elective termination of pregnancy. This advice is appropriate even when the patient was discharged previously with a discharge diagnosis of complete abortion.

3) Complications leading to abortion
Codes from Chapter 15 may be used as additional codes to identify any documented complications of the pregnancy in conjunction with codes in categories in O07 and O08.

r. Abuse in a pregnant patient
For suspected or confirmed cases of abuse of a pregnant patient, a code(s) from subcategories O9A.3, Physical abuse complicating pregnancy, childbirth, and the puerperium, O9A.4, Sexual abuse complicating pregnancy, childbirth, and the puerperium, and O9A.5, Psychological abuse complicating pregnancy, childbirth, and the puerperium, should be sequenced first, followed by the appropriate codes (if applicable) to identify any associated current injury due to physical abuse, sexual abuse, and the perpetrator of abuse.

See Section I.C.19.f. Adult and child abuse, neglect and other maltreatment.

Pregnancy with abortive outcome (O00-O08)

Excludes 1:   *continuing pregnancy in multiple gestation after abortion of one fetus or more (O31.1-, O31.3-)*

O00- Ectopic pregnancy — The development of a fertilized ovum outside of the uterus.
Includes: Ruptured ectopic pregnancy — A breaking open of a fertilized ovum that lies outside of the uterus.
Use additional code from category O08 to identify any associated complication

O00.0- Abdominal pregnancy — The development of a fertilized ovum within the abdominal cavity.
Excludes 1:   *maternal care for viable fetus in abdominal pregnancy (O36.7-)*

cc **O00.00 Abdominal pregnancy *without* intrauterine pregnancy** — [♀, Age/12-55]
Abdominal pregnancy NOS

cc **O00.01 Abdominal pregnancy *with* intrauterine pregnancy** — [♀, Age/12-55]

O00.1- Tubal pregnancy — The development of a fertilized ovum within the fallopian tube.
Fallopian pregnancy
Rupture of (fallopian) tube due to pregnancy — The forcible tearing of a fallopian tube wall due to a tubal pregnancy.
Tubal abortion — The expulsion of a tubal pregnancy through the open end (abdominal) of a fallopian tube.

cc **O00.10 Tubal pregnancy *without* intrauterine pregnancy** — [♀, Age/12-55]
Tubal pregnancy NOS

cc **O00.11 Tubal pregnancy *with* intrauterine pregnancy** — [♀, Age/12-55]

O00.2- Ovarian pregnancy — The development of a fertilized ovum within an ovary.

cc **O00.20 Ovarian pregnancy *without* intrauterine pregnancy** — [♀, Age/12-55]
Ovarian pregnancy NOS

cc **O00.21 Ovarian pregnancy *with* intrauterine pregnancy** — [♀, Age/12-55]

O00.8- Other ectopic pregnancy
Cervical pregnancy — The development of a fertilized ovum within the cervical canal.
Cornual pregnancy — The development of a fertilized ovum within one of the horns of a bicornate uterus.
Intraligamentous pregnancy — The development of a fertilized ovum within the broad ligament.
Mural pregnancy — The development of a fertilized ovum within a fallopian tube uterine orifice.

cc **O00.80 Other ectopic pregnancy *without* intrauterine pregnancy** — [♀, Age/12-55]
Other ectopic pregnancy NOS

cc **O00.81 Other ectopic pregnancy *with* intrauterine pregnancy** — [♀, Age/12-55]

O00.9- Ectopic pregnancy, *unspecified*

cc **O00.90 Unspecified ectopic pregnancy *without* intrauterine pregnancy** — [♀, Age/12-55]
Ectopic pregnancy NOS

cc **O00.91 Unspecified ectopic pregnancy *with* intrauterine pregnancy** — [♀, Age/12-55]

O01- Hydatidiform mole — An abnormal pregnancy characterized by the cystic degeneration of the chorionic villi, with the appearance of a grape-like mass.
Use additional code from category O08 to identify any associated complication
**Excludes 1:   *chorioadenoma (destruens) (D39.2)*
   *malignant hydatidiform mole (D39.2)***

O01.0 Classical hydatidiform mole — [♀, Age/12-55]
Complete hydatidiform mole

O01.1 Incomplete and partial hydatidiform mole — [♀, Age/12-55]

O01.9 Hydatidiform mole, unspecified — [♀, Age/12-55]
Trophoblastic disease NOS
Vesicular mole NOS

O00-O01

O02- Other abnormal products of conception
   Use additional code from category O08 to identify any associated
      complication
   Excludes 1:   papyraceous fetus (O31.0-)
   O02.0   Blighted ovum and nonhydatidiform mole — [♀, Age/12-55] – A
      fertilized ovum that fails to develop.
         Carneous mole
         Fleshy mole
         Intrauterine mole NOS
         Molar pregnancy NEC
         Pathological ovum
   O02.1   Missed abortion — [♀, Age/12-55]
      Early fetal death, before completion of 20 weeks of gestation, with
         retention of dead fetus
      Excludes 1:   failed induced abortion (O07-)
                        fetal death (intrauterine) (late) (O36.4)
                        missed abortion with blighted ovum (O02.0)
                        missed abortion with hydatidiform mole (O01-)
                        missed abortion with nonhydatidiform (O02.0)
                        missed abortion with other abnormal products of
                           conception (O02.8-)
                        missed delivery (O36.4)
                        stillbirth (P95)
   O02.8-   Other specified abnormal products of conception
      Excludes 1:   abnormal products of conception with blighted ovum
                           (O02.0)
                        abnormal products of conception with hydatidiform
                           mole (O01.-)
                        abnormal products of conception with nonhydatidiform
                           mole (O02.0)
      **O02.81   Inappropriate change in quantitative human chorionic
         gonadotropin (hCG) in early pregnancy** — [♀, Age/12-55]
            Biochemical pregnancy
            Chemical pregnancy
            Inappropriate level of quantitative human chorionic
               gonadotropin (hCG) for gestational age in early
               pregnancy
      O02.89   Other specified abnormal products of conception —
            [♀, Age/12-55]
   O02.9   Abnormal product of conception, unspecified — [♀, Age/12-55]

O03- Spontaneous abortion — The premature expulsion of the fetus that occurs naturally
   and without an apparent cause.
   **Note: Incomplete abortion includes retained products of conception
      following spontaneous abortion**
   Includes: Miscarriage
   cc **O03.0   Genital tract and pelvic infection following incomplete
      spontaneous abortion** — [♀, Age/12-55]
         Endometritis following incomplete spontaneous abortion
         Oophoritis following incomplete spontaneous abortion
         Parametritis following incomplete spontaneous abortion
         Pelvic peritonitis following incomplete spontaneous abortion
         Salpingitis following incomplete spontaneous abortion
         Salpingo-oophoritis following incomplete spontaneous abortion
      Excludes 1:   sepsis following incomplete spontaneous abortion
                           (O03.37)
                        urinary tract infection following incomplete
                           spontaneous abortion (O03.38)
   **O03.1   Delayed or excessive hemorrhage following incomplete
      spontaneous abortion** — [♀, Age/12-55]
         Afibrinogenemia following incomplete spontaneous abortion
         Defibrination syndrome following incomplete spontaneous
            abortion
         Hemolysis following incomplete spontaneous abortion
         Intravascular coagulation following incomplete spontaneous
            abortion
   mcc **O03.2   Embolism following incomplete spontaneous abortion** —
      [♀, Age/12-55]
         Air embolism following incomplete spontaneous abortion
         Amniotic fluid embolism following incomplete spontaneous
            abortion
         Blood-clot embolism following incomplete spontaneous abortion
         Embolism NOS following incomplete spontaneous abortion
         Fat embolism following incomplete spontaneous abortion
         Pulmonary embolism following incomplete spontaneous abortion
         Pyemic embolism following incomplete spontaneous abortion
         Septic or septicopyemic embolism following incomplete
            spontaneous abortion
         Soap embolism following incomplete spontaneous abortion

**O03.3- Other and unspecified complications following incomplete
   spontaneous abortion**
   cc **O03.30   Unspecified complication following incomplete
      spontaneous abortion** — [♀, Age/12-55]
   mcc **O03.31   Shock following incomplete spontaneous abortion** —
         [♀, Age/12-55]
            Circulatory collapse following incomplete spontaneous
               abortion
            Shock (postprocedural) following incomplete spontaneous
               abortion
         Excludes 1:   shock due to infection following incomplete
                              spontaneous abortion (O03.37)
   mcc **O03.32   Renal failure following incomplete spontaneous
      abortion** — [♀, Age/12-55]
            Kidney failure (acute) following incomplete spontaneous
               abortion
            Oliguria following incomplete spontaneous abortion
            Renal shutdown following incomplete spontaneous abortion
            Renal tubular necrosis following incomplete spontaneous
               abortion
            Uremia following incomplete spontaneous abortion
   cc **O03.33   Metabolic disorder following incomplete spontaneous
      abortion** — [♀, Age/12-55]
   cc **O03.34   Damage to pelvic organs following incomplete
      spontaneous abortion** — [♀, Age/12-55]
            Laceration, perforation, tear or chemical damage of bladder
               following incomplete spontaneous abortion
            Laceration, perforation, tear or chemical damage of bowel
               following incomplete spontaneous abortion
            Laceration, perforation, tear or chemical damage of broad
               ligament following incomplete spontaneous abortion
            Laceration, perforation, tear or chemical damage of cervix
               following incomplete spontaneous abortion
            Laceration, perforation, tear or chemical damage of
               periurethral tissue following incomplete spontaneous
               abortion
            Laceration, perforation, tear or chemical damage of uterus
               following incomplete spontaneous abortion
            Laceration, perforation, tear or chemical damage of vagina
               following incomplete spontaneous abortion
   cc **O03.35   Other venous complications following incomplete
      spontaneous abortion** — [♀, Age/12-55]
   cc **O03.36   Cardiac arrest following incomplete spontaneous
      abortion** — [♀, Age/12-55]
   cc **O03.37   Sepsis following incomplete spontaneous abortion** —
      [♀, Age/12-55]
         Use additional code to identify infectious agent (B95-B97)
         Use additional code to identify severe sepsis, if applicable
            (R65.2-)
         Excludes 1:   septic or septicopyemic embolism following
                              incomplete spontaneous abortion (O03.2)
   cc **O03.38   Urinary tract infection following incomplete spontaneous
      abortion** — [♀, Age/12-55]
            Cystitis following incomplete spontaneous abortion
   cc **O03.39   Incomplete spontaneous abortion with other
      complications** — [♀, Age/12-55]
   O03.4   Incomplete spontaneous abortion without complication —
      [♀, Age/12-55]
   cc **O03.5   Genital tract and pelvic infection following complete or
      unspecified spontaneous abortion** — [♀, Age/12-55]
         Endometritis following complete or unspecified spontaneous
            abortion
         Oophoritis following complete or unspecified spontaneous abortion
         Parametritis following complete or unspecified spontaneous
            abortion
         Pelvic peritonitis following complete or unspecified spontaneous
            abortion
         Salpingitis following complete or unspecified spontaneous abortion
         Salpingo-oophoritis following complete or unspecified
            spontaneous abortion
      Excludes 1:   sepsis following complete or unspecified spontaneous
                           abortion (O03.87)
                        urinary tract infection following complete or
                           unspecified spontaneous abortion (O03.88)

O 0 2 - O 0 3

O03.6 <u>Delayed or excessive hemorrhage following complete or unspecified</u> spontaneous abortion — [♀, Age/12-55]
- Afibrinogenemia following complete or unspecified spontaneous abortion
- Defibrination syndrome following complete or unspecified spontaneous abortion
- Hemolysis following complete or unspecified spontaneous abortion
- Intravascular coagulation following complete or unspecified spontaneous abortion

CC **O03.7** <u>Embolism following complete or unspecified</u> spontaneous abortion — [♀, Age/12-55]
- Air embolism following complete or unspecified spontaneous abortion
- Amniotic fluid embolism following complete or unspecified spontaneous abortion
- Blood-clot embolism following complete or unspecified spontaneous abortion
- Embolism NOS following complete or unspecified spontaneous abortion
- Fat embolism following complete or unspecified spontaneous abortion
- Pulmonary embolism following complete or unspecified spontaneous complications
- Pyemic embolism following complete or unspecified spontaneous abortion
- Septic or septicopyemic embolism following complete or unspecified spontaneous abortion
- Soap embolism following complete or unspecified spontaneous abortion

O03.8- <u>Other</u> and unspecified complications following <u>complete or unspecified</u> spontaneous abortion

CC **O03.80** <u>Unspecified complication following complete or unspecified</u> spontaneous abortion — [♀, Age/12-55]

MCC **O03.81** <u>Shock following complete or unspecified</u> spontaneous abortion — [♀, Age/12-55]
- Circulatory collapse following complete or unspecified spontaneous abortion
- Shock (postprocedural) following complete or unspecified spontaneous abortion
- *Excludes 1:*   *shock due to infection following complete or unspecified spontaneous abortion (O03.87)*

MCC **O03.82** <u>Renal failure following complete or unspecified</u> spontaneous abortion — [♀, Age/12-55]
- Kidney failure (acute) following complete or unspecified spontaneous abortion
- Oliguria following complete or unspecified spontaneous abortion
- Renal shutdown following complete or unspecified spontaneous abortion
- Renal tubular necrosis following complete or unspecified spontaneous abortion
- Uremia following complete or unspecified spontaneous abortion

CC **O03.83** <u>Metabolic disorder following complete or unspecified</u> spontaneous abortion — [♀, Age/12-55]

CC **O03.84** <u>Damage to pelvic organs following complete or unspecified</u> spontaneous abortion — [♀, Age/12-55]
- Laceration, perforation, tear or chemical damage of bladder following complete or unspecified spontaneous abortion
- Laceration, perforation, tear or chemical damage of bowel following complete or unspecified spontaneous abortion
- Laceration, perforation, tear or chemical damage of broad ligament following complete or unspecified spontaneous abortion
- Laceration, perforation, tear or chemical damage of cervix following complete or unspecified spontaneous abortion
- Laceration, perforation, tear or chemical damage of periurethral tissue following complete or unspecified spontaneous abortion
- Laceration, perforation, tear or chemical damage of uterus following complete or unspecified spontaneous abortion
- Laceration, perforation, tear or chemical damage of vagina following complete or unspecified spontaneous abortion

CC **O03.85** <u>Other venous complications following complete or unspecified</u> spontaneous abortion — [♀, Age/12-55]

CC **O03.86** <u>Cardiac arrest following complete or unspecified</u> spontaneous abortion — [♀, Age/12-55]

CC **O03.87** <u>Sepsis following complete or unspecified</u> spontaneous abortion — [♀, Age/12-55]
- Use additional code to identify infectious agent (B95-B97)
- Use additional code to identify severe sepsis, if applicable (R65.2-)
- *Excludes 1:*   *septic or septicopyemic embolism following complete or unspecified spontaneousabortion (O03.7)*

CC **O03.88** <u>Urinary tract infection following complete or unspecified</u> spontaneous abortion — [♀, Age/12-55]
- Cystitis following complete or unspecified spontaneous abortion

CC **O03.89** <u>Complete or unspecified</u> spontaneous abortion <u>with other complications</u> — [♀, Age/12-55]

O03.9 <u>Complete or unspecified</u> spontaneous abortion <u>without complication</u> — [♀, Age/12-55]
- Miscarriage NOS
- Spontaneous abortion NOS

O04- <u>Complications following (induced) termination of pregnancy</u> — The expulsion of the fetus that is brought on intentionally by authorized medical professionals.
- Includes: Complications following (induced) termination of pregnancy
- *Excludes 1:*   *encounter for elective termination of pregnancy, uncomplicated (Z33.2)*
  - *failed attempted termination of pregnancy (O07.-)*

CC **O04.5** <u>Genital tract and pelvic infection following (induced) termination</u> of pregnancy — [♀, Age/12-55]
- Endometritis following (induced) termination of pregnancy
- Oophoritis following (induced) termination of pregnancy
- Parametritis following (induced) termination of pregnancy
- Pelvic peritonitis following (induced) termination of pregnancy
- Salpingitis following (induced) termination of pregnancy
- Salpingo-oophoritis following (induced) termination of pregnancy
- *Excludes 1:*   *sepsis following (induced) termination of pregnancy (O04.87)*
  - *urinary tract infection following (induced) termination of pregnancy (O04.88)*

O04.6 <u>Delayed or excessive hemorrhage following (induced) termination</u> of pregnancy — [♀, Age/12-55]
- Afibrinogenemia following (induced) termination of pregnancy
- Defibrination syndrome following (induced) termination of pregnancy
- Hemolysis following (induced) termination of pregnancy
- Intravascular coagulation following (induced) termination of pregnancy

MCC **O04.7** <u>Embolism following (induced) termination</u> of pregnancy — [♀, Age/12-55]
- Air embolism following (induced) termination of pregnancy
- Amniotic fluid embolism following (induced) termination of pregnancy
- Blood-clot embolism following (induced) termination of pregnancy
- Embolism NOS following (induced) termination of pregnancy
- Fat embolism following (induced) termination of pregnancy
- Pulmonary embolism following (induced) termination of pregnancy
- Pyemic embolism following (induced) termination of pregnancy
- Septic or septicopyemic embolism following (induced) termination of pregnancy
- Soap embolism following (induced) termination of pregnancy

O04.8- <u>(Induced) termination</u> of pregnancy <u>with other</u> and unspecified complications

CC **O04.80** <u>(Induced) termination</u> of pregnancy <u>with unspecified complications</u> — [♀, Age/12-55]

MCC **O04.81** <u>Shock following (induced) termination</u> of pregnancy — [♀, Age/12-55]
- Circulatory collapse following (induced) termination of pregnancy
- Shock (postprocedural) following (induced) termination of pregnancy
- *Excludes 1:*   *shock due to infection following (induced) termination of pregnancy (O04.87)*

MCC **O04.82** <u>Renal failure following (induced) termination</u> of pregnancy — [♀, Age/12-55]
- Kidney failure (acute) following (induced) termination of pregnancy
- Oliguria following (induced) termination of pregnancy
- Renal shutdown following (induced) termination of pregnancy
- Renal tubular necrosis following (induced) termination of pregnancy
- Uremia following (induced) termination of pregnancy

O03 - O04

CC **O04.83** Metabolic disorder following (induced) termination of pregnancy — [♀, Age/12-55]

CC **O04.84** Damage to pelvic organs following (induced) termination of pregnancy — [♀, Age/12-55]
Laceration, perforation, tear or chemical damage of bladder following (induced) termination of pregnancy
Laceration, perforation, tear or chemical damage of bowel following (induced) termination of pregnancy
Laceration, perforation, tear or chemical damage of broad ligament following (induced) termination of pregnancy
Laceration, perforation, tear or chemical damage of cervix following (induced) termination of pregnancy
Laceration, perforation, tear or chemical damage of periurethral tissue following (induced) termination of pregnancy
Laceration, perforation, tear or chemical damage of uterus following (induced) termination of pregnancy
Laceration, perforation, tear or chemical damage of vagina following (induced) termination of pregnancy

CC **O04.85** Other venous complications following (induced) termination of pregnancy — [♀, Age/12-55]

CC **O04.86** Cardiac arrest following (induced) termination of pregnancy — [♀, Age/12-55]

CC **O04.87** Sepsis following (induced) termination of pregnancy — [♀, Age/12-55]
Use additional code to identify infectious agent (B95-B97)
Use additional code to identify severe sepsis, if applicable (R65.2-)
Excludes 1: *septic or septicopyemic embolism following (induced) termination of pregnancy (O04.7)*

CC **O04.88** Urinary tract infection following (induced) termination of pregnancy — [♀, Age/12-55]
Cystitis following (induced) termination of pregnancy

CC **O04.89** (Induced) termination of pregnancy with other complications — [♀, Age/12-55]

O07- Failed attempted termination of pregnancy — The inability of authorized medical professionals to induce the expulsion of the fetus.
Includes: Failure of attempted induction of termination of pregnancy
Incomplete elective abortion
Excludes 1: *incomplete spontaneous abortion (O03.0-)*

CC **O07.0** Genital tract and pelvic infection following failed attempted termination of pregnancy — [♀, Age/12-55]
Endometritis following failed attempted termination of pregnancy
Oophoritis following failed attempted termination of pregnancy
Parametritis following failed attempted termination of pregnancy
Pelvic peritonitis following failed attempted termination of pregnancy
Salpingitis following failed attempted termination of pregnancy
Salpingo-oophoritis following failed attempted termination of pregnancy
Excludes 1: *sepsis following failed attempted termination of pregnancy (O07.37)*
urinary tract infection following failed attempted termination of pregnancy (O07.38)

CC **O07.1** Delayed or excessive hemorrhage following failed attempted termination of pregnancy — [♀, Age/12-55]
Afibrinogenemia following failed attempted termination of pregnancy
Defibrination syndrome following failed attempted termination of pregnancy
Hemolysis following failed attempted termination of pregnancy
Intravascular coagulation following failed attempted termination of pregnancy

MCC **O07.2** Embolism following failed attempted termination of pregnancy — [♀, Age/12-55]
Air embolism following failed attempted termination of pregnancy
Amniotic fluid embolism following failed attempted termination of pregnancy
Blood-clot embolism following failed attempted termination of pregnancy
Embolism NOS following failed attempted termination of pregnancy
Fat embolism following failed attempted termination of pregnancy
Pulmonary embolism following failed attempted termination of pregnancy
Pyemic embolism following failed attempted termination of pregnancy
Septic or septicopyemic embolism following failed attempted termination of pregnancy
Soap embolism following failed attempted termination of pregnancy

O07.3- Failed attempted termination of pregnancy with other and unspecified complications

CC **O07.30** Failed attempted termination of pregnancy with unspecified complications — [♀, Age/12-55]

MCC **O07.31** Shock following failed attempted termination of pregnancy — [♀, Age/12-55]
Circulatory collapse following failed attempted termination of pregnancy
Shock (postprocedural) following failed attempted termination of pregnancy
Excludes 1: *shock due to infection following failed attempted termination of pregnancy (O07.37)*

MCC **O07.32** Renal failure following failed attempted termination of pregnancy — [♀, Age/12-55]
Kidney failure (acute) following failed attempted termination of pregnancy
Oliguria following failed attempted termination of pregnancy
Renal shutdown following failed attempted termination of pregnancy
Renal tubular necrosis following failed attempted termination of pregnancy
Uremia following failed attempted termination of pregnancy

CC **O07.33** Metabolic disorder following failed attempted termination of pregnancy — [♀, Age/12-55]

CC **O07.34** Damage to pelvic organs following failed attempted termination of pregnancy — [♀, Age/12-55]
Laceration, perforation, tear or chemical damage of bladder following failed attempted termination of pregnancy
Laceration, perforation, tear or chemical damage of bowel following failed attempted termination of pregnancy
Laceration, perforation, tear or chemical damage of broad ligament following failed attempted termination of pregnancy
Laceration, perforation, tear or chemical damage of cervix following failed attempted termination of pregnancy
Laceration, perforation, tear or chemical damage of periurethral tissue following failed attempted termination of pregnancy
Laceration, perforation, tear or chemical damage of uterus following failed attempted termination of pregnancy
Laceration, perforation, tear or chemical damage of vagina following failed attempted termination of pregnancy

CC **O07.35** Other venous complications following failed attempted termination of pregnancy — [♀, Age/12-55]

CC **O07.36** Cardiac arrest following failed attempted termination of pregnancy — [♀, Age/12-55]

CC **O07.37** Sepsis following failed attempted termination of pregnancy — [♀, Age/12-55]
Use additional code (B95-B97), to identify infectious agent
Use additional code (R65.2-) to identify severe sepsis, if applicable
Excludes 1: *septic or septicopyemic embolism following failed attempted termination of pregnancy (O07.2)*

CC **O07.38** Urinary tract infection following failed attempted termination of pregnancy — [♀, Age/12-55]
Cystitis following failed attempted termination of pregnancy

CC **O07.39** Failed attempted termination of pregnancy with other complications — [♀, Age/12-55]

O07.4 Failed attempted termination of pregnancy without complication — [♀, Age/12-55]

O08- Complications following ectopic and molar pregnancy
This category is for use with categories O00-O02 to identify any associated complications

CC **O08.0** Genital tract and pelvic infection following ectopic and molar pregnancy — [♀, Age/12-55]
Endometritis following ectopic and molar pregnancy
Oophoritis following ectopic and molar pregnancy
Parametritis following ectopic and molar pregnancy
Pelvic peritonitis following ectopic and molar pregnancy
Salpingitis following ectopic and molar pregnancy
Salpingo-oophoritis following ectopic and molar pregnancy
Excludes 1: *sepsis following ectopic and molar pregnancy (O08.82)*
urinary tract infection (O08.83)

CC **O08.1** <u>Delayed or excessive hemorrhage following ectopic</u> and molar pregnancy — [♀, Age/12-55]

    Afibrinogenemia following ectopic and molar pregnancy
    Defibrination syndrome following ectopic and molar pregnancy
    Hemolysis following ectopic and molar pregnancy
    Intravascular coagulation following ectopic and molar pregnancy

    Excludes 1:   *delayed or excessive hemorrhage due to incomplete abortion (O03.1)*

MCC **O08.2** <u>Embolism following ectopic</u> and molar pregnancy — [♀, Age/12-55]

    Air embolism following ectopic and molar pregnancy
    Amniotic fluid embolism following ectopic and molar pregnancy
    Blood-clot embolism following ectopic and molar pregnancy
    Embolism NOS following ectopic and molar pregnancy
    Fat embolism following ectopic and molar pregnancy
    Pulmonary embolism following ectopic and molar pregnancy
    Pyemic embolism following ectopic and molar pregnancy
    Septic or septicopyemic embolism following ectopic and molar pregnancy
    Soap embolism following ectopic and molar pregnancy

MCC **O08.3** <u>Shock following ectopic</u> and molar pregnancy — [♀, Age/12-55]

    Circulatory collapse following ectopic and molar pregnancy
    Shock (postprocedural) following ectopic and molar pregnancy

    Excludes 1:   *shock due to infection following ectopic and molar pregnancy (O08.82)*

MCC **O08.4** <u>Renal failure following ectopic</u> and molar pregnancy — [♀, Age/12-55]

    Kidney failure (acute) following ectopic and molar pregnancy
    Oliguria following ectopic and molar pregnancy
    Renal shutdown following ectopic and molar pregnancy
    Renal tubular necrosis following ectopic and molar pregnancy
    Uremia following ectopic and molar pregnancy

CC **O08.5** <u>Metabolic disorders following</u> an <u>ectopic</u> and molar pregnancy — [♀, Age/12-55]

CC **O08.6** <u>Damage to pelvic organs and tissues following</u> an <u>ectopic</u> and molar pregnancy — [♀, Age/12-55]

    Laceration, perforation, tear or chemical damage of bladder following an ectopic and molar pregnancy
    Laceration, perforation, tear or chemical damage of bowel following an ectopic and molar pregnancy
    Laceration, perforation, tear or chemical damage of broad ligament following an ectopic and molar pregnancy
    Laceration, perforation, tear or chemical damage of cervix following an ectopic and molar pregnancy
    Laceration, perforation, tear or chemical damage of periurethral tissue following an ectopic and molar pregnancy
    Laceration, perforation, tear or chemical damage of uterus following an ectopic and molar pregnancy
    Laceration, perforation, tear or chemical damage of vagina following an ectopic and molar pregnancy

CC **O08.7** Other venous complications following an <u>ectopic</u> and molar pregnancy — [♀, Age/12-55]

O08.8- <u>Other</u> complications following an <u>ectopic</u> and molar pregnancy

CC **O08.81** <u>Cardiac arrest following</u> an <u>ectopic</u> and molar pregnancy — [♀, Age/12-55]

CC **O08.82** <u>Sepsis following ectopic</u> and molar pregnancy — [♀, Age/12-55]

    Use additional code (B95-B97), to identify infectious agent
    Use additional code (R65.2-) to identify severe sepsis, if applicable

    Excludes 1:   *septic or septicopyemic embolism following ectopic and molar pregnancy (O08.2)*

CC **O08.83** <u>Urinary tract infection following</u> an <u>ectopic</u> and molar pregnancy — [♀, Age/12-55]

    Cystitis following an ectopic and molar pregnancy

CC **O08.89** <u>Other</u> complications following an <u>ectopic</u> and molar pregnancy — [♀, Age/12-55]

CC **O08.9** <u>Unspecified</u> complication following an <u>ectopic</u> and molar pregnancy — [♀, Age/12-55]

Supervision of high risk pregnancy (O09)

O09- <u>Supervision of high risk pregnancy</u> — Conditions (medical and lifestyle) that are present before pregnancy, or present during pregnancy, that prompt providers to provide special monitoring and/or care during the pregnancy.

O09.0- Supervision of pregnancy <u>with history of infertility</u>

  O09.00 Supervision of pregnancy with history of infertility, <u>unspecified</u> trimester — [♀, Age/12-55] [Unacceptable PDX]

  O09.01 Supervision of pregnancy with history of infertility, <u>first</u> trimester — [♀, Age/12-55] [Unacceptable PDX]

  O09.02 Supervision of pregnancy with history of infertility, <u>second</u> trimester — [♀, Age/12-55] [Unacceptable PDX]

  O09.03 Supervision of pregnancy with history of infertility, <u>third</u> trimester — [♀, Age/12-55] [Unacceptable PDX]

O09.1- Supervision of pregnancy <u>with history of ectopic pregnancy</u>

  O09.10 Supervision of pregnancy with history of ectopic pregnancy, <u>unspecified</u> trimester — [♀, Age/12-55] [Unacceptable PDX]

  O09.11 Supervision of pregnancy with history of ectopic pregnancy, <u>first</u> trimester — [♀, Age/12-55] [Unacceptable PDX]

  O09.12 Supervision of pregnancy with history of ectopic pregnancy, <u>second</u> trimester — [♀, Age/12-55] [Unacceptable PDX]

  O09.13 Supervision of pregnancy with history of ectopic pregnancy, <u>third</u> trimester — [♀, Age/12-55] [Unacceptable PDX]

O09.A- Supervision of pregnancy <u>with history of molar pregnancy</u>

  O09.A0 Supervision of pregnancy with history of molar pregnancy, <u>unspecified</u> trimester — [♀, Age/12-55] [Unacceptable PDX]

  O09.A1 Supervision of pregnancy with history of molar pregnancy, <u>first</u> trimester — [♀, Age/12-55] [Unacceptable PDX]

  O09.A2 Supervision of pregnancy with history of molar pregnancy, <u>second</u> trimester — [♀, Age/12-55] [Unacceptable PDX]

  O09.A3 Supervision of pregnancy with history of molar pregnancy, <u>third</u> trimester — [♀, Age/12-55] [Unacceptable PDX]

O09.2- Supervision of pregnancy <u>with other poor reproductive or obstetric history</u>

    Excludes ❷: *pregnancy care for patient with history of recurrent pregnancy loss (O26.2-)*

  O09.21-   Supervision of pregnancy <u>with history of pre-term labor</u>

    O09.211 Supervision of pregnancy with history of pre-term labor, <u>first</u> trimester — [♀, Age/12-55] [Unacceptable PDX]

    O09.212 Supervision of pregnancy with history of pre-term labor, <u>second</u> trimester — [♀, Age/12-55] [Unacceptable PDX]

    O09.213 Supervision of pregnancy with history of pre-term labor, <u>third</u> trimester — [♀, Age/12-55] [Unacceptable PDX]

    O09.219 Supervision of pregnancy with history of pre-term labor, unspecified trimester — [♀, Age/12-55] [Unacceptable PDX]

  O09.29-   Supervision of pregnancy <u>with other poor reproductive or obstetric history</u>

    Supervision of pregnancy with history of neonatal death
    Supervision of pregnancy with history of stillbirth

    O09.291 Supervision of pregnancy with other poor reproductive or obstetric history, <u>first</u> trimester — [♀, Age/12-55] [Unacceptable PDX]

    O09.292 Supervision of pregnancy with other poor reproductive or obstetric history, <u>second</u> trimester — [♀, Age/12-55] [Unacceptable PDX]

    O09.293 Supervision of pregnancy with other poor reproductive or obstetric history, <u>third</u> trimester — [♀, Age/12-55] [Unacceptable PDX]

    O09.299 Supervision of pregnancy with other poor reproductive or obstetric history, <u>unspecified</u> trimester — [♀, Age/12-55] [Unacceptable PDX]

O08 - O09

O09.3- Supervision of pregnancy <u>with insufficient antenatal care</u>
Supervision of concealed pregnancy
Supervision of hidden pregnancy

O09.30 Supervision of pregnancy with insufficient antenatal care, <u>unspecified</u> trimester — [♀, Age/12-55] [Unacceptable PDX]

O09.31 Supervision of pregnancy with insufficient antenatal care, <u>first</u> trimester — [♀, Age/12-55] [Unacceptable PDX]

O09.32 Supervision of pregnancy with insufficient antenatal care, <u>second</u> trimester — [♀, Age/12-55] [Unacceptable PDX]

O09.33 Supervision of pregnancy with insufficient antenatal care, <u>third</u> trimester — [♀, Age/12-55] [Unacceptable PDX]

O09.4- Supervision of pregnancy <u>with grand multiparity</u>

O09.40 Supervision of pregnancy with grand multiparity, <u>unspecified</u> trimester — [♀, Age/12-55] [Unacceptable PDX]

O09.41 Supervision of pregnancy with grand multiparity, <u>first</u> trimester — [♀, Age/12-55] [Unacceptable PDX]

O09.42 Supervision of pregnancy with grand multiparity, <u>second</u> trimester — [♀, Age/12-55] [Unacceptable PDX]

O09.43 Supervision of pregnancy with grand multiparity, <u>third</u> trimester — [♀, Age/12-55] [Unacceptable PDX]

O09.5- Supervision of elderly primigravida and multigravida
Pregnancy for a female 35 years and older at expected date of delivery

O09.51- <u>Supervision of elderly primigravida</u>

O09.511 Supervision of elderly primigravida, <u>first</u> trimester — [♀, Age/12-55] [Unacceptable PDX]

O09.512 Supervision of elderly primigravida, <u>second</u> trimester — [♀, Age/12-55] [Unacceptable PDX]

O09.513 Supervision of elderly primigravida, <u>third</u> trimester — [♀, Age/12-55] [Unacceptable PDX]

O09.519 Supervision of elderly primigravida, <u>unspecified</u> trimester — [♀, Age/12-55] [Unacceptable PDX]

O09.52- <u>Supervision of elderly multigravida</u>

O09.521 Supervision of elderly multigravida, <u>first</u> trimester — [♀, Age/12-55] [Unacceptable PDX]

O09.522 Supervision of elderly multigravida, <u>second</u> trimester — [♀, Age/12-55] [Unacceptable PDX]

O09.523 Supervision of elderly multigravida, <u>third</u> trimester — [♀, Age/12-55] [Unacceptable PDX]

O09.529 Supervision of elderly multigravida, <u>unspecified</u> trimester — [♀, Age/12-55] [Unacceptable PDX]

O09.6- Supervision of young primigravida and multigravida
Supervision of pregnancy for a female less than 16 years old at expected date of delivery

O09.61- <u>Supervision of young primigravida</u>

O09.611 Supervision of young primigravida, <u>first</u> trimester — [♀, Age/12-55] [Unacceptable PDX]

O09.612 Supervision of young primigravida, <u>second</u> trimester — [♀, Age/12-55] [Unacceptable PDX]

O09.613 Supervision of young primigravida, <u>third</u> trimester — [♀, Age/12-55] [Unacceptable PDX]

O09.619 Supervision of young primigravida, <u>unspecified</u> trimester — [♀, Age/12-55] [Unacceptable PDX]

O09.62- <u>Supervision of young multigravida</u>

O09.621 Supervision of young multigravida, <u>first</u> trimester — [♀, Age/12-55] [Unacceptable PDX]

O09.622 Supervision of young multigravida, <u>second</u> trimester — [♀, Age/12-55] [Unacceptable PDX]

O09.623 Supervision of young multigravida, <u>third</u> trimester — [♀, Age/12-55] [Unacceptable PDX]

O09.629 Supervision of young multigravida, <u>unspecified</u> trimester — [♀, Age/12-55] [Unacceptable PDX]

O09.7- <u>Supervision of high risk pregnancy due to social problems</u>

O09.70 Supervision of high risk pregnancy due to social problems, <u>unspecified</u> trimester — [♀, Age/12-55] [Unacceptable PDX]

O09.71 Supervision of high risk pregnancy due to social problems, <u>first</u> trimester — [♀, Age/12-55] [Unacceptable PDX]

O09.72 Supervision of high risk pregnancy due to social problems, <u>second</u> trimester — [♀, Age/12-55] [Unacceptable PDX]

O09.73 Supervision of high risk pregnancy due to social problems, <u>third</u> trimester — [♀, Age/12-55] [Unacceptable PDX]

O09.8- Supervision of other high risk pregnancies

O09.81- Supervision of pregnancy <u>resulting from assisted reproductive technology</u>
Supervision of pregnancy resulting from in-vitro fertilization
Excludes ❷: gestational carrier status (Z33.3)

O09.811 Supervision of pregnancy resulting from assisted reproductive technology, <u>first</u> trimester — [♀, Age/12-55] [Unacceptable PDX]

O09.812 Supervision of pregnancy resulting from assisted reproductive technology, <u>second</u> trimester — [♀, Age/12-55] [Unacceptable PDX]

O09.813 Supervision of pregnancy resulting from assisted reproductive technology, <u>third</u> trimester — [♀, Age/12-55] [Unacceptable PDX]

O09.819 Supervision of pregnancy resulting from assisted reproductive technology, <u>unspecified</u> trimester — [♀, Age/12-55] [Unacceptable PDX]

O09.82- Supervision of pregnancy <u>with history of in utero procedure during previous pregnancy</u>

O09.821 Supervision of pregnancy with history of in utero procedure during previous pregnancy, <u>first</u> trimester — [♀, Age/12-55] [Unacceptable PDX]

O09.822 Supervision of pregnancy with history of in utero procedure during previous pregnancy, <u>second</u> trimester — [♀, Age/12-55] [Unacceptable PDX]

O09.823 Supervision of pregnancy with history of in utero procedure during previous pregnancy, <u>third</u> trimester — [♀, Age/12-55] [Unacceptable PDX]

O09.829 Supervision of pregnancy with history of in utero procedure during previous pregnancy, <u>unspecified</u> trimester — [♀, Age/12-55] [Unacceptable PDX]
Excludes 1: supervision of pregnancy affected by in utero procedure during current pregnancy (O35.7)

O09.89- Supervision of other high risk pregnancies

O09.891 Supervision of other high risk pregnancies, <u>first</u> trimester — [♀, Age/12-55] [Unacceptable PDX]

O09.892 Supervision of other high risk pregnancies, <u>second</u> trimester — [♀, Age/12-55] [Unacceptable PDX]

O09.893 Supervision of other high risk pregnancies, <u>third</u> trimester — [♀, Age/12-55] [Unacceptable PDX]

O09.899 Supervision of other high risk pregnancies, <u>unspecified</u> trimester — [♀, Age/12-55] [Unacceptable PDX]

O09.9- Supervision of high risk pregnancy, <u>unspecified</u>

O09.90 Supervision of high risk pregnancy, unspecified, <u>unspecified</u> trimester — [♀, Age/12-55] [Unacceptable PDX]

O09.91 Supervision of high risk pregnancy, unspecified, <u>first</u> trimester — [♀, Age/12-55] [Unacceptable PDX]

O09.92 Supervision of high risk pregnancy, unspecified, <u>second</u> trimester — [♀, Age/12-55] [Unacceptable PDX]

O09.93 Supervision of high risk pregnancy, unspecified, <u>third</u> trimester — [♀, Age/12-55] [Unacceptable PDX]

Edema, proteinuria and hypertensive disorders in pregnancy, childbirth and the puerperium (O10-O16)

O10- <u>Pre-existing hypertension</u> complicating pregnancy, childbirth and the puerperium — Persistently high arterial blood pressure.
    Includes: Pre-existing hypertension with pre-existing proteinuria complicating pregnancy, childbirth and the puerperium
    Excludes ❷: pre-existing hypertension with superimposed pre-eclampsia complicating pregnancy, childbirth and the puerperium (O11.-)

O10.0- **Pre-existing <u>essential</u> hypertension complicating pregnancy, childbirth and the puerperium** — Persistently high arterial blood pressure of a relatively mild degree.
    Any condition in I10 specified as a reason for obstetric care during pregnancy, childbirth or the puerperium

   O10.01- **Pre-existing essential hypertension <u>complicating pregnancy</u>,**

    cc **O10.011** **Pre-existing essential hypertension complicating pregnancy, <u>first</u> trimester** — [♀, Age/12-55]

    cc **O10.012** **Pre-existing essential hypertension complicating pregnancy, <u>second</u> trimester** — [♀, Age/12-55]

    cc **O10.013** **Pre-existing essential hypertension complicating pregnancy, <u>third</u> trimester** — [♀, Age/12-55]

    O10.019 **Pre-existing essential hypertension complicating pregnancy, <u>unspecified</u> trimester** — [♀, Age/12-55]

   cc **O10.02** **Pre-existing essential hypertension <u>complicating childbirth</u>** — [♀, Age/12-55]

   O10.03 **Pre-existing essential hypertension <u>complicating the puerperium</u>** — [♀, Age/12-55]

O10.1- **Pre-existing <u>hypertensive heart disease</u> complicating pregnancy, childbirth and the puerperium** — Persistently high arterial blood pressure resulting in functional cardiac abnormalities.
    Any condition in I11 specified as a reason for obstetric care during pregnancy, childbirth or the puerperium
    Use additional code from I11 to identify the type of hypertensive heart disease

   O10.11- **Pre-existing hypertensive heart disease <u>complicating pregnancy</u>**

    O10.111 **Pre-existing hypertensive heart disease complicating pregnancy, <u>first</u> trimester** — [♀, Age/12-55]

    O10.112 **Pre-existing hypertensive heart disease complicating pregnancy, <u>second</u> trimester** — [♀, Age/12-55]

    O10.113 **Pre-existing hypertensive heart disease complicating pregnancy, <u>third</u> trimester** — [♀, Age/12-55]

    O10.119 **Pre-existing hypertensive heart disease complicating pregnancy, <u>unspecified</u> trimester** — [♀, Age/12-55]

   O10.12 **Pre-existing hypertensive heart disease <u>complicating childbirth</u>** — [♀, Age/12-55]

   O10.13 **Pre-existing hypertensive heart disease <u>complicating the puerperium</u>** — [♀, Age/12-55]

O10.2- **Pre-existing <u>hypertensive chronic kidney disease</u> complicating pregnancy, childbirth and the puerperium** — Persistently high arterial blood pressure resulting in functional kidney abnormalities.
    Any condition in I12 specified as a reason for obstetric care during pregnancy, childbirth or the puerperium
    Use additional code from I12 to identify the type of hypertensive chronic kidney disease

   O10.21- **Pre-existing hypertensive chronic kidney disease complicating pregnancy**

    O10.211 **Pre-existing hypertensive chronic kidney disease complicating pregnancy, <u>first</u> trimester** — [♀, Age/12-55]

    O10.212 **Pre-existing hypertensive chronic kidney disease complicating pregnancy, <u>second</u> trimester** — [♀, Age/12-55]

    O10.213 **Pre-existing hypertensive chronic kidney disease complicating pregnancy, <u>third</u> trimester** — [♀, Age/12-55]

    O10.219 **Pre-existing hypertensive chronic kidney disease complicating pregnancy, <u>unspecified</u> trimester** — [♀, Age/12-55]

   O10.22 **Pre-existing hypertensive chronic kidney disease <u>complicating childbirth</u>** — [♀, Age/12-55]

   O10.23 **Pre-existing hypertensive chronic kidney disease <u>complicating the puerperium</u>** — [♀, Age/12-55]

O10.3- **Pre-existing <u>hypertensive heart and chronic kidney disease</u> complicating pregnancy, childbirth and the puerperium** — Persistently high arterial blood pressure resulting in heart and kidney functional abnormalities.
    Any condition in I13 specified as a reason for obstetric care during pregnancy, childbirth or the puerperium
    Use additional code from I13 to identify the type of hypertensive heart and chronic kidney disease

   O10.31- **Pre-existing hypertensive heart and chronic kidney disease <u>complicating pregnancy</u>**

    O10.311 **Pre-existing hypertensive heart and chronic kidney disease complicating pregnancy, <u>first</u> trimester** — [♀, Age/12-55]

    O10.312 **Pre-existing hypertensive heart and chronic kidney disease complicating pregnancy, <u>second</u> trimester** — [♀, Age/12-55]

    O10.313 **Pre-existing hypertensive heart and chronic kidney disease complicating pregnancy, <u>third</u> trimester** — [♀, Age/12-55]

    O10.319 **Pre-existing hypertensive heart and chronic kidney disease complicating pregnancy, <u>unspecified</u> trimester** — [♀, Age/12-55]

   O10.32 **Pre-existing hypertensive heart and chronic kidney disease <u>complicating childbirth</u>** — [♀, Age/12-55]

   O10.33 **Pre-existing hypertensive heart and chronic kidney disease <u>complicating the puerperium</u>** — [♀, Age/12-55]

O10.4- **Pre-existing <u>secondary</u> hypertension complicating pregnancy, childbirth and the puerperium** — Persistently high arterial blood pressure resulting in functional cardiac abnormalities.
    Any condition in I15 specified as a reason for obstetric care during pregnancy, childbirth or the puerperium
    Use additional code from I15 to identify the type of secondary hypertension

   O10.41- **Pre-existing secondary hypertension <u>complicating pregnancy</u>**

    cc **O10.411** **Pre-existing secondary hypertension complicating pregnancy, <u>first</u> trimester** — [♀, Age/12-55]

    cc **O10.412** **Pre-existing secondary hypertension complicating pregnancy, <u>second</u> trimester** — [♀, Age/12-55]

    cc **O10.413** **Pre-existing secondary hypertension complicating pregnancy, <u>third</u> trimester** — [♀, Age/12-55]

    O10.419 **Pre-existing secondary hypertension complicating pregnancy, <u>unspecified</u> trimester** — [♀, Age/12-55]

   MCC **O10.42** **Pre-existing secondary hypertension <u>complicating childbirth</u>** — [♀, Age/12-55]

   cc **O10.43** **Pre-existing secondary hypertension <u>complicating the puerperium</u>** — [♀, Age/12-55]

O10.9- **<u>Unspecified</u> pre-existing <u>hypertension</u> complicating pregnancy, childbirth and the puerperium**

   O10.91- **Unspecified pre-existing hypertension <u>complicating pregnancy</u>**

    cc **O10.911** **Unspecified pre-existing hypertension complicating pregnancy, <u>first</u> trimester** — [♀, Age/12-55]

    cc **O10.912** **Unspecified pre-existing hypertension complicating pregnancy, <u>second</u> trimester** — [♀, Age/12-55]

    cc **O10.913** **Unspecified pre-existing hypertension complicating pregnancy, <u>third</u> trimester** — [♀, Age/12-55]

    O10.919 **Unspecified pre-existing hypertension complicating pregnancy, <u>unspecified</u> trimester** — [♀, Age/12-55]

   cc **O10.92** **Unspecified pre-existing hypertension <u>complicating childbirth</u>** — [♀, Age/12-55]

   O10.93 **Unspecified pre-existing hypertension <u>complicating the puerperium</u>** — [♀, Age/12-55]

O10 - O10

Excludes 1: = NOT CODED HERE! (Do not code both)   **925**   *Excludes ❷: = Not Included Here*

O11- Pre-existing hypertension with pre-eclampsia
Includes: Conditions in O10 complicated by pre-eclampsia
Pre-eclampsia superimposed pre-existing hypertension
Use additional code from O10 to identify the type of hypertension

MCC **O11.1   Pre-existing hypertension with pre-eclampsia, first trimester** — [♀, Age/12-55]

MCC **O11.2   Pre-existing hypertension with pre-eclampsia, second trimester** — [♀, Age/12-55]

MCC **O11.3   Pre-existing hypertension with pre-eclampsia, third trimester** — [♀, Age/12-55]

O11.4   Pre-existing hypertension with pre-eclampsia, complicating childbirth — [♀, Age/12-55]

O11.5   Pre-existing hypertension with pre-eclampsia, complicating the puerperium — [♀, Age/12-55]

O11.9   Pre-existing hypertension with pre-eclampsia, unspecified trimester — [♀, Age/12-55]

O12- Gestational [pregnancy-induced] edema and proteinuria without hypertension

O12.0- Gestational edema — The excessive accumulation of interstitial fluid and venous congestion of the legs that occurs during pregnancy without hypertension.

O12.00 Gestational edema, unspecified trimester — [♀, Age/12-55]

O12.01 Gestational edema, first trimester — [♀, Age/12-55]

O12.02 Gestational edema, second trimester — [♀, Age/12-55]

O12.03 Gestational edema, third trimester — [♀, Age/12-55]

O12.04 Gestational edema, complicating childbirth — [♀, Age/12-55]

O12.05 Gestational edema, complicating the puerperium — [♀, Age/12-55]

O12.1- Gestational proteinuria — The abnormal volume of proteins in the urine that occurs during pregnancy without hypertension.

O12.10 Gestational proteinuria, unspecified trimester — [♀, Age/12-55]

CC **O12.11 Gestational proteinuria, first trimester** — [♀, Age/12-55]

CC **O12.12 Gestational proteinuria, second trimester** — [♀, Age/12-55]

CC **O12.13 Gestational proteinuria, third trimester** — [♀, Age/12-55]

O12.14 Gestational proteinuria, complicating childbirth — [♀, Age/12-55]

O12.15 Gestational proteinuria, complicating the puerperium — [♀, Age/12-55]

O12.2- Gestational edema with proteinuria — The excessive accumulation of interstitial fluid and venous congestion of the legs and the abnormal volume of proteins in the urine that occurs during pregnancy without hypertension.

O12.20 Gestational edema with proteinuria, unspecified trimester — [♀, Age/12-55]

CC **O12.21 Gestational edema with proteinuria, first trimester** — [♀, Age/12-55]

CC **O12.22 Gestational edema with proteinuria, second trimester** — [♀, Age/12-55]

CC **O12.23 Gestational edema with proteinuria, third trimester** — [♀, Age/12-55]

O12.24 Gestational edema with proteinuria, complicating childbirth — [♀, Age/12-55]

O12.25 Gestational edema with proteinuria, complicating the puerperium — [♀, Age/12-55]

O13- Gestational [pregnancy-induced] hypertension without significant proteinuria — Temporary elevated arterial blood pressure noted during pregnancy.
AHA 16:1Q:p5 – Gestational hypertension
Includes: Gestational hypertension NOS
Transient hypertension of pregnancy

O13.1   Gestational [pregnancy-induced] hypertension without significant proteinuria, first trimester — [♀, Age/12-55]

O13.2   Gestational [pregnancy-induced] hypertension without significant proteinuria, second trimester — [♀, Age/12-55]

O13.3   Gestational [pregnancy-induced] hypertension without significant proteinuria, third trimester — [♀, Age/12-55]

O13.4   Gestational [pregnancy-induced] hypertension without significant proteinuria, complicating childbirth — [♀, Age/12-55]

O13.5   Gestational [pregnancy-induced] hypertension without significant proteinuria, complicating the puerperium — [♀, Age/12-55]

O13.9   Gestational [pregnancy-induced] hypertension without significant proteinuria, unspecified trimester — [♀, Age/12-55]

O14- Pre-eclampsia — A pregnancy-induced hypertensive condition characterized by a large volume of proteins in the urine and edema.
Excludes 1:   pre-existing hypertension with pre-eclampsia (O11)

O14.0- Mild to moderate pre-eclampsia

O14.00 Mild to moderate pre-eclampsia, unspecified trimester — [♀, Age/12-55]

CC **O14.02 Mild to moderate pre-eclampsia, second trimester** — [♀, Age/12-55]

CC **O14.03 Mild to moderate pre-eclampsia, third trimester** — [♀, Age/12-55]

O14.04 Mild to moderate pre-eclampsia, complicating childbirth — [♀, Age/12-55]

O14.05 Mild to moderate pre-eclampsia, complicating the puerperium — [♀, Age/12-55]

O14.1- Severe pre-eclampsia
Excludes 1:   HELLP syndrome (O14.2-)

O14.10 Severe pre-eclampsia, unspecified trimester — [♀, Age/12-55]

MCC **O14.12 Severe pre-eclampsia, second trimester** — [♀, Age/12-55]

MCC **O14.13 Severe pre-eclampsia, third trimester** — [♀, Age/12-55]

O14.14 Severe pre-eclampsia, complicating childbirth — [♀, Age/12-55]

O14.15 Severe pre-eclampsia, complicating the puerperium — [♀, Age/12-55]

O14.2- HELLP syndrome
Severe pre-eclampsia with hemolysis, elevated liver enzymes and low platelet count (HELLP)

O14.20 HELLP syndrome (HELLP), unspecified trimester — [♀, Age/12-55]

MCC **O14.22 HELLP syndrome (HELLP), second trimester** — [♀, Age/12-55]

MCC **O14.23 HELLP syndrome (HELLP), third trimester** — [♀, Age/12-55]

O14.24 HELLP syndrome, complicating childbirth — [♀, Age/12-55]

O14.25 HELLP syndrome, complicating the puerperium — [♀, Age/12-55]

O14.9- Unspecified pre-eclampsia

O14.90 Unspecified pre-eclampsia, unspecified trimester — [♀, Age/12-55]

CC **O14.92 Unspecified pre-eclampsia, second trimester** — [♀, Age/12-55]

CC **O14.93 Unspecified pre-eclampsia, third trimester** — [♀, Age/12-55]

O14.94 Unspecified pre-eclampsia, complicating childbirth — [♀, Age/12-55]

O14.95 Unspecified pre-eclampsia, complicating the puerperium — [♀, Age/12-55]

O15- Eclampsia — The onset of seizures in a women with pre-eclapmsia or pre-existing hypertension conditions.
Includes: Convulsions following conditions in O10-O14 and O16

O15.0- Eclampsia complicating pregnancy

O15.00 Eclampsia complicating pregnancy, unspecified trimester — [♀, Age/12-55]

MCC **O15.02 Eclampsia complicating pregnancy, second trimester** — [♀, Age/12-55]

MCC **O15.03 Eclampsia complicating pregnancy, third trimester** — [♀, Age/12-55]

MCC **O15.1   Eclampsia complicating labor** — [♀, Age/12-55]

MCC **O15.2   Eclampsia complicating the puerperium** — [♀, Age/12-55]

O15.9   Eclampsia, unspecified as to time period — [♀, Age/12-55]
Eclampsia NOS

O16- Unspecified maternal hypertension

CC **O16.1   Unspecified maternal hypertension, first trimester** — [♀, Age/12-55]

CC **O16.2   Unspecified maternal hypertension, second trimester** — [♀, Age/12-55]

CC **O16.3   Unspecified maternal hypertension, third trimester** — [♀, Age/12-55]

Excludes 1: = NOT CODED HERE! (Do not code both)   *Excludes ❷:* = Not Included Here

O11-O16

© 2016 Channel Publishing, Ltd.

O16.4 Unspecified maternal hypertension, <u>complicating childbirth</u> — [♀, Age/12-55]

O16.5 Unspecified maternal hypertension, <u>complicating the puerperium</u> — [♀, Age/12-55]

O16.9 Unspecified maternal hypertension, <u>unspecified</u> trimester — [♀, Age/12-55]

Other maternal disorders predominantly related to pregnancy (O20-O29)

Excludes ❷: *maternal care related to the fetus and amniotic cavity and possible delivery problems (O30-O48)*
   maternal diseases classifiable elsewhere but complicating pregnancy, labor and delivery, and the puerperium (O98-O99)

O20- Hemorrhage in early pregnancy
   Includes: Hemorrhage before completion of 20 weeks gestation
   Excludes 1:   *pregnancy with abortive outcome (O00-O08)*

cc **O20.0** Threatened abortion — [♀, Age/12-55]
      Hemorrhage specified as due to threatened abortion

O20.8 Other hemorrhage in early pregnancy — [♀, Age/12-55]

cc **O20.9** Hemorrhage in early pregnancy, unspecified — [♀, Age/12-55]

O21- Excessive vomiting in pregnancy

O21.0 Mild hyperemesis gravidarum — [♀, Age/12-55]
      Hyperemesis gravidarum, mild or unspecified, starting before the end of the 20th week of gestation

O21.1 Hyperemesis gravidarum <u>with metabolic disturbance</u> — [♀, Age/12-55]
      Hyperemesis gravidarum, starting before the end of the 20th week of gestation, with metabolic disturbance such as carbohydrate depletion
      Hyperemesis gravidarum, starting before the end of the 20th week of gestation, with metabolic disturbance such as dehydration
      Hyperemesis gravidarum, starting before the end of the 20th week of gestation, with metabolic disturbance such as electrolyte imbalance

O21.2 Late vomiting of pregnancy — [♀, Age/12-55]
      Excessive vomiting starting after 20 completed weeks of gestation

O21.8 Other vomiting complicating pregnancy — [♀, Age/12-55]
      Vomiting due to diseases classified elsewhere, complicating pregnancy
      Use additional code, to identify cause.

O21.9 Vomiting of pregnancy, unspecified — [♀, Age/12-55]

O22- Venous complications and hemorrhoids <u>in pregnancy</u>
   Excludes 1:   *venous complications of:*
         abortion NOS (O03.9)
         ectopic or molar pregnancy (O08.7)
         failed attempted abortion (O07.35)
         induced abortion (O04.85)
         spontaneous abortion (O03.89)
   Excludes ❷: *obstetric pulmonary embolism (O88-)*
         venous complications and hemorrhoids of childbirth and the puerperium (O87-)

O22.0- <u>Varicose veins of lower extremity</u> in pregnancy — Dilated, tortuous leg veins presenting symptoms during pregnancy.
      Varicose veins NOS in pregnancy

O22.00 Varicose veins of lower extremity in pregnancy, <u>unspecified</u> trimester — [♀, Age/12-55]

O22.01 Varicose veins of lower extremity in pregnancy, <u>first</u> trimester — [♀, Age/12-55]

O22.02 Varicose veins of lower extremity in pregnancy, <u>second</u> trimester — [♀, Age/12-55]

O22.03 Varicose veins of lower extremity in pregnancy, <u>third</u> trimester — [♀, Age/12-55]

O22.1- <u>Genital varices</u> in pregnancy — Dilated, tortuous genital veins presenting symptoms during pregnancy.
      Perineal varices in pregnancy
      Vaginal varices in pregnancy
      Vulval varices in pregnancy

O22.10 Genital varices in pregnancy, <u>unspecified</u> trimester — [♀, Age/12-55]

O22.11 Genital varices in pregnancy, <u>first</u> trimester — [♀, Age/12-55]

O22.12 Genital varices in pregnancy, <u>second</u> trimester — [♀, Age/12-55]

O22.13 Genital varices in pregnancy, <u>third</u> trimester — [♀, Age/12-55]

O22.2- <u>Superficial thrombophlebitis</u> in pregnancy — Inflammation of a superficial vein with thrombus formation during pregnancy.
      Phlebitis in pregnancy NOS
      Thrombophlebitis of legs in pregnancy
      Thrombosis in pregnancy NOS
   Use additional code to identify the superficial thrombophlebitis (I80.0-)

cc **O22.20** Superficial thrombophlebitis in pregnancy, <u>unspecified</u> trimester — [♀, Age/12-55]

cc **O22.21** Superficial thrombophlebitis in pregnancy, <u>first</u> trimester — [♀, Age/12-55]

cc **O22.22** Superficial thrombophlebitis in pregnancy, <u>second</u> trimester — [♀, Age/12-55]

cc **O22.23** Superficial thrombophlebitis in pregnancy, <u>third</u> trimester — [♀, Age/12-55]

O22.3- <u>Deep phlebothrombosis</u> in pregnancy — Inflammation of a deep vein with thrombus formation during pregnancy.
      Deep vein thrombosis, antepartum
   Use additional code to identify the deep vein thrombosis (I82.4-, I82.5-, I82.62-. I82.72-)
   Use additional code, if applicable, for associated long-term (current) use of anticoagulants (Z79.01)

cc **O22.30** Deep phlebothrombosis in pregnancy, <u>unspecified</u> trimester — [♀, Age/12-55]

mcc **O22.31** Deep phlebothrombosis in pregnancy, <u>first</u> trimester — [♀, Age/12-55]

mcc **O22.32** Deep phlebothrombosis in pregnancy, <u>second</u> trimester — [♀, Age/12-55]

mcc **O22.33** Deep phlebothrombosis in pregnancy, <u>third</u> trimester — [♀, Age/12-55]

O22.4- <u>Hemorrhoids</u> in pregnancy — The varicose dilatation of a vein of the hemorrhoidal plexus during pregnancy.

cc **O22.40** Hemorrhoids in pregnancy, <u>unspecified</u> trimester — [♀, Age/12-55]

cc **O22.41** Hemorrhoids in pregnancy, <u>first</u> trimester — [♀, Age/12-55]

cc **O22.42** Hemorrhoids in pregnancy, <u>second</u> trimester — [♀, Age/12-55]

cc **O22.43** Hemorrhoids in pregnancy, <u>third</u> trimester — [♀, Age/12-55]

O22.5- <u>Cerebral venous thrombosis</u> in pregnancy — The formation of a thrombus in a cerebral vessel during pregnancy.
      Cerebrovenous sinus thrombosis in pregnancy

cc **O22.50** Cerebral venous thrombosis in pregnancy, <u>unspecified</u> trimester — [♀, Age/12-55]

cc **O22.51** Cerebral venous thrombosis in pregnancy, <u>first</u> trimester — [♀, Age/12-55]

cc **O22.52** Cerebral venous thrombosis in pregnancy, <u>second</u> trimester — [♀, Age/12-55]

cc **O22.53** Cerebral venous thrombosis in pregnancy, <u>third</u> trimester — [♀, Age/12-55]

O22.8- <u>Other venous complications</u> in pregnancy

O22.8x- Other venous complications in pregnancy

cc **O22.8x1** Other venous complications in pregnancy, <u>first</u> trimester — [♀, Age/12-55]

cc **O22.8x2** Other venous complications in pregnancy, <u>second</u> trimester — [♀, Age/12-55]

cc **O22.8x3** Other venous complications in pregnancy, <u>third</u> trimester — [♀, Age/12-55]

cc **O22.8x9** Other venous complications in pregnancy, <u>unspecified</u> trimester — [♀, Age/12-55]

O22.9- Venous complication in pregnancy, <u>unspecified</u>
      Gestational phlebitis NOS
      Gestational phlebopathy NOS
      Gestational thrombosis NOS

cc **O22.90** Venous complication in pregnancy, unspecified, <u>unspecified</u> trimester — [♀, Age/12-55]

O22.91 Venous complication in pregnancy, unspecified, <u>first</u> trimester — [♀, Age/12-55]

O 1 6 - O 2 2

O22.92 Venous complication in pregnancy, unspecified, <u>second</u> trimester — [♀, Age/12-55]

O22.93 Venous complication in pregnancy, unspecified, <u>third</u> trimester — [♀, Age/12-55]

O23- <u>Infections of genitourinary tract</u> in pregnancy
Use additional code to identify organism (B95-, B96-)
*Excludes ❷: gonococcal infections complicating pregnancy, childbirth and the puerperium (O98.2)
infections with a predominantly sexual mode of transmission NOS complicating pregnancy, childbirth and the puerperium (O98.3)
syphilis complicating pregnancy, childbirth and the puerperium (O98.1)
tuberculosis of genitourinary system complicating pregnancy, childbirth and the puerperium (O98.0)
venereal disease NOS complicating pregnancy, childbirth and the puerperium (O98.3)*

O23.0- <u>Infections of kidney</u> in pregnancy
Pyelonephritis in pregnancy

O23.00 Infections of kidney in pregnancy, <u>unspecified</u> trimester — [♀, Age/12-55]

cc **O23.01** Infections of kidney in pregnancy, <u>first</u> trimester — [♀, Age/12-55]

cc **O23.02** Infections of kidney in pregnancy, <u>second</u> trimester — [♀, Age/12-55]

cc **O23.03** Infections of kidney in pregnancy, <u>third</u> trimester — [♀, Age/12-55]

O23.1- <u>Infections of bladder</u> in pregnancy

O23.10 Infections of bladder in pregnancy, <u>unspecified</u> trimester — [♀, Age/12-55]

cc **O23.11** Infections of bladder in pregnancy, <u>first</u> trimester — [♀, Age/12-55]

cc **O23.12** Infections of bladder in pregnancy, <u>second</u> trimester — [♀, Age/12-55]

cc **O23.13** Infections of bladder in pregnancy, <u>third</u> trimester — [♀, Age/12-55]

O23.2- <u>Infections of urethra</u> in pregnancy

O23.20 Infections of urethra in pregnancy, <u>unspecified</u> trimester — [♀, Age/12-55]

cc **O23.21** Infections of urethra in pregnancy, <u>first</u> trimester — [♀, Age/12-55]

cc **O23.22** Infections of urethra in pregnancy, <u>second</u> trimester — [♀, Age/12-55]

cc **O23.23** Infections of urethra in pregnancy, <u>third</u> trimester — [♀, Age/12-55]

O23.3- <u>Infections of other parts of urinary tract</u> in pregnancy

O23.30 Infections of other parts of urinary tract in pregnancy, <u>unspecified</u> trimester — [♀, Age/12-55]

cc **O23.31** Infections of other parts of urinary tract in pregnancy, <u>first</u> trimester — [♀, Age/12-55]

cc **O23.32** Infections of other parts of urinary tract in pregnancy, <u>second</u> trimester — [♀, Age/12-55]

cc **O23.33** Infections of other parts of urinary tract in pregnancy, <u>third</u> trimester — [♀, Age/12-55]

O23.4- <u>Unspecified</u> infection of urinary tract in pregnancy

O23.40 Unspecified infection of urinary tract in pregnancy, <u>unspecified</u> trimester — [♀, Age/12-55]

cc **O23.41** Unspecified infection of urinary tract in pregnancy, <u>first</u> trimester — [♀, Age/12-55]

cc **O23.42** Unspecified infection of urinary tract in pregnancy, <u>second</u> trimester — [♀, Age/12-55]

cc **O23.43** Unspecified infection of urinary tract in pregnancy, <u>third</u> trimester — [♀, Age/12-55]

O23.5- <u>Infections of the genital tract</u> in pregnancy

O23.51- Infection of <u>cervix</u> in pregnancy

cc **O23.511** Infections of cervix in pregnancy, <u>first</u> trimester — [♀, Age/12-55]

cc **O23.512** Infections of cervix in pregnancy, <u>second</u> trimester — [♀, Age/12-55]

cc **O23.513** Infections of cervix in pregnancy, <u>third</u> trimester — [♀, Age/12-55]

O23.519 Infections of cervix in pregnancy, <u>unspecified</u> trimester — [♀, Age/12-55]

O23.52- <u>Salpingo-oophoritis</u> in pregnancy
Oophoritis in pregnancy
Salpingitis in pregnancy

cc **O23.521** Salpingo-oophoritis in pregnancy, <u>first</u> trimester — [♀, Age/12-55]

cc **O23.522** Salpingo-oophoritis in pregnancy, <u>second</u> trimester — [♀, Age/12-55]

cc **O23.523** Salpingo-oophoritis in pregnancy, <u>third</u> trimester — [♀, Age/12-55]

O23.529 Salpingo-oophoritis in pregnancy, <u>unspecified</u> trimester — [♀, Age/12-55]

O23.59- Infection of <u>other part of genital tract</u> in pregnancy

cc **O23.591** Infection of other part of genital tract in pregnancy, <u>first</u> trimester — [♀, Age/12-55]

cc **O23.592** Infection of other part of genital tract in pregnancy, <u>second</u> trimester — [♀, Age/12-55]

cc **O23.593** Infection of other part of genital tract in pregnancy, <u>third</u> trimester — [♀, Age/12-55]

O23.599 Infection of other part of genital tract in pregnancy, <u>unspecified</u> trimester — [♀, Age/12-55]

O23.9- <u>Unspecified</u> genitourinary tract infection in pregnancy
Genitourinary tract infection in pregnancy NOS

O23.90 Unspecified genitourinary tract infection in pregnancy, <u>unspecified</u> trimester — [♀, Age/12-55]

cc **O23.91** Unspecified genitourinary tract infection in pregnancy, <u>first</u> trimester — [♀, Age/12-55]

cc **O23.92** Unspecified genitourinary tract infection in pregnancy, <u>second</u> trimester — [♀, Age/12-55]

cc **O23.93** Unspecified genitourinary tract infection in pregnancy, <u>third</u> trimester — [♀, Age/12-55]

O24- <u>Diabetes mellitus</u> in pregnancy, childbirth, and the puerperium

O24.0- <u>Pre-existing type 1 diabetes mellitus</u>, in pregnancy, childbirth and the puerperium
Juvenile onset diabetes mellitus, in pregnancy, childbirth and the puerperium
Ketosis-prone diabetes mellitus in pregnancy, childbirth and the puerperium
Use additional code from category E10 to further identify any manifestations

O24.01- Pre-existing <u>type 1</u> diabetes mellitus, <u>in pregnancy</u>

cc **O24.011** Pre-existing type 1 diabetes mellitus, in pregnancy, <u>first</u> trimester — [♀, Age/12-55]

cc **O24.012** Pre-existing type 1 diabetes mellitus, in pregnancy, <u>second</u> trimester — [♀, Age/12-55]

cc **O24.013** Pre-existing type 1 diabetes mellitus, in pregnancy, <u>third</u> trimester — [♀, Age/12-55]

cc **O24.019** Pre-existing type 1 diabetes mellitus, in pregnancy, <u>unspecified</u> trimester — [♀, Age/12-55]

MCC **O24.02** Pre-existing <u>type 1</u> diabetes mellitus, <u>in childbirth</u> — [♀, Age/12-55]

cc **O24.03** Pre-existing <u>type 1</u> diabetes mellitus, <u>in the puerperium</u> — [♀, Age/12-55]

O24.1- Pre-existing <u>type 2</u> diabetes mellitus in pregnancy, childbirth and the puerperium
Insulin-resistant diabetes mellitus in pregnancy, childbirth and the puerperium
Use additional code (for):
From category E11 to further identify any manifestations
Long-term (current) use of insulin (Z79.4)

O24.11- Pre-existing <u>type 2</u> diabetes mellitus, <u>in pregnancy</u>

cc **O24.111** Pre-existing type 2 diabetes mellitus, in pregnancy, <u>first</u> trimester — [♀, Age/12-55]

cc **O24.112** Pre-existing type 2 diabetes mellitus, in pregnancy, <u>second</u> trimester — [♀, Age/12-55]

cc **O24.113** Pre-existing type 2 diabetes mellitus, in pregnancy, <u>third</u> trimester — [♀, Age/12-55]

O 22 - O 24

CC **O24.119** Pre-existing type 2 diabetes mellitus, in pregnancy, <u>unspecified</u> trimester — [♀, Age/12-55]

MCC **O24.12** Pre-existing <u>type 2</u> diabetes mellitus, <u>in childbirth</u> — [♀, Age/12-55]

CC **O24.13** Pre-existing <u>type 2</u> diabetes mellitus, <u>in the</u> <u>puerperium</u> — [♀, Age/12-55]

O24.3- <u>Unspecified</u> pre-existing diabetes mellitus in pregnancy, childbirth and the puerperium
Use additional code (for):
   From category E11 to further identify any manifestation
   Long-term (current) use of insulin (Z79.4)

O24.31- <u>Unspecified</u> pre-existing diabetes mellitus in pregnancy

CC **O24.311** Unspecified pre-existing diabetes mellitus in pregnancy, <u>first</u> trimester — [♀, Age/12-55]

CC **O24.312** Unspecified pre-existing diabetes mellitus in pregnancy, <u>second</u> trimester — [♀, Age/12-55]

CC **O24.313** Unspecified pre-existing diabetes mellitus in pregnancy, <u>third</u> trimester — [♀, Age/12-55]

CC **O24.319** Unspecified pre-existing diabetes mellitus in pregnancy, <u>unspecified</u> trimester — [♀, Age/12-55]

MCC **O24.32** <u>Unspecified</u> pre-existing diabetes mellitus <u>in childbirth</u> — [♀, Age/12-55]

CC **O24.33** <u>Unspecified</u> pre-existing diabetes mellitus <u>in the</u> <u>puerperium</u> — [♀, Age/12-55]

O24.4- <u>Gestational diabetes mellitus</u>
AHA 16:1Q:p5 – Delivery complicated by gestational diabetes
   Diabetes mellitus arising in pregnancy
   Gestational diabetes mellitus NOS

O24.41- Gestational diabetes mellitus <u>in pregnancy</u>

O24.410 Gestational diabetes mellitus in pregnancy, <u>diet</u> <u>controlled</u> — [♀, Age/12-55]

O24.414 Gestational diabetes mellitus in pregnancy, <u>insulin</u> <u>controlled</u> — [♀, Age/12-55]

O24.415 Gestational diabetes mellitus in pregnancy, <u>controlled by oral hypoglycemic drugs</u> — [♀, Age/12-55]
   Gestational diabetes mellitus in pregnancy, controlled by oral antidiabetic drugs

O24.419 Gestational diabetes mellitus in pregnancy, <u>unspecified control</u> — [♀, Age/12-55]
AHA 15:4Q:p34 – Oral medication control of gestational diabetes

O24.42- Gestational diabetes mellitus <u>in childbirth</u>

O24.420 Gestational diabetes mellitus in childbirth, <u>diet</u> <u>controlled</u> — [♀, Age/12-55]

O24.424 Gestational diabetes mellitus in childbirth, <u>insulin</u> <u>controlled</u> — [♀, Age/12-55]

O24.425 Gestational diabetes mellitus in childbirth, <u>controlled by oral hypoglycemic drugs</u> — [♀, Age/12-55]
   Gestational diabetes mellitus in childbirth, controlled by oral antidiabetic drugs

O24.429 Gestational diabetes mellitus in childbirth, <u>unspecified control</u> — [♀, Age/12-55]

O24.43- Gestational diabetes mellitus <u>in the puerperium</u>

O24.430 Gestational diabetes mellitus in the puerperium, <u>diet controlled</u> — [♀, Age/12-55]

O24.434 Gestational diabetes mellitus in the puerperium, <u>insulin controlled</u> — [♀, Age/12-55]

O24.435 Gestational diabetes mellitus in puerperium, <u>controlled by oral hypoglycemic drugs</u> — [♀, Age/12-55]
   Gestational diabetes mellitus in puerperium, controlled by oral antidiabetic drugs

O24.439 Gestational diabetes mellitus in the puerperium, <u>unspecified control</u> — [♀, Age/12-55]

O24.8- <u>Other pre-existing diabetes mellitus</u> in pregnancy, childbirth, and the puerperium
Use additional code (for):
   From categories E08, E09 and E13 to further identify any manifestation
   Long-term (current) use of insulin (Z79.4)

O24.81- Other pre-existing diabetes mellitus <u>in pregnancy</u>

CC **O24.811** Other pre-existing diabetes mellitus in pregnancy, <u>first</u> trimester — [♀, Age/12-55]

CC **O24.812** Other pre-existing diabetes mellitus in pregnancy, <u>second</u> trimester — [♀, Age/12-55]

CC **O24.813** Other pre-existing diabetes mellitus in pregnancy, <u>third</u> trimester — [♀, Age/12-55]

CC **O24.819** Other pre-existing diabetes mellitus in pregnancy, <u>unspecified</u> trimester — [♀, Age/12-55]

MCC **O24.82** Other pre-existing diabetes mellitus <u>in childbirth</u> — [♀, Age/12-55]

CC **O24.83** Other pre-existing diabetes mellitus <u>in the puerperium</u> — [♀, Age/12-55]

O24.9- <u>Unspecified</u> diabetes mellitus in pregnancy, childbirth and the puerperium
Use additional code for long-term (current) use of insulin (Z79.4)

O24.91- Unspecified diabetes mellitus <u>in pregnancy</u>

CC **O24.911** Unspecified diabetes mellitus in pregnancy, <u>first</u> trimester — [♀, Age/12-55]

CC **O24.912** Unspecified diabetes mellitus in pregnancy, <u>second</u> trimester — [♀, Age/12-55]

CC **O24.913** Unspecified diabetes mellitus in pregnancy, <u>third</u> trimester — [♀, Age/12-55]

CC **O24.919** Unspecified diabetes mellitus in pregnancy, <u>unspecified</u> trimester — [♀, Age/12-55]

O24.92 Unspecified diabetes mellitus <u>in childbirth</u> — [♀, Age/12-55]

CC **O24.93** Unspecified diabetes mellitus <u>in the puerperium</u> — [♀, Age/12-55]

O25- <u>Malnutrition</u> in pregnancy, childbirth and the puerperium

O25.1- Malnutrition in pregnancy — The inadequate intake of nutrients during pregnancy.

O25.10 Malnutrition in pregnancy, <u>unspecified</u> trimester — [♀, Age/12-55]

O25.11 Malnutrition in pregnancy, <u>first</u> trimester — [♀, Age/12-55]

O25.12 Malnutrition in pregnancy, <u>second</u> trimester — [♀, Age/12-55]

O25.13 Malnutrition in pregnancy, <u>third</u> trimester — [♀, Age/12-55]

O25.2 Malnutrition <u>in childbirth</u> — [♀, Age/12-55]

O25.3 Malnutrition <u>in the puerperium</u> — [♀, Age/12-55]

O26- Maternal care for other conditions predominantly related to pregnancy

O26.0- <u>Excessive weight gain</u> in pregnancy
Excludes ❷: gestational edema (O12.0, O12.2)

O26.00 Excessive weight gain in pregnancy, <u>unspecified</u> trimester — [♀, Age/12-55]

O26.01 Excessive weight gain in pregnancy, <u>first</u> trimester — [♀, Age/12-55]

O26.02 Excessive weight gain in pregnancy, <u>second</u> trimester — [♀, Age/12-55]

O26.03 Excessive weight gain in pregnancy, <u>third</u> trimester — [♀, Age/12-55]

O26.1- <u>Low weight gain</u> in pregnancy

O26.10 Low weight gain in pregnancy, <u>unspecified</u> trimester — [♀, Age/12-55]

O26.11 Low weight gain in pregnancy, <u>first</u> trimester — [♀, Age/12-55]

O26.12 Low weight gain in pregnancy, <u>second</u> trimester — [♀, Age/12-55]

O26.13 Low weight gain in pregnancy, <u>third</u> trimester — [♀, Age/12-55]

O26.2- Pregnancy care for patient <u>with recurrent pregnancy loss</u>

O26.20 Pregnancy care for patient with recurrent pregnancy loss, <u>unspecified</u> trimester — [♀, Age/12-55]

O24 - O26

O26.21 Pregnancy care for patient with recurrent pregnancy loss, first trimester — [♀, Age/12-55]

O26.22 Pregnancy care for patient with recurrent pregnancy loss, second trimester — [♀, Age/12-55]

O26.23 Pregnancy care for patient with recurrent pregnancy loss, third trimester — [♀, Age/12-55]

O26.3- Retained intrauterine contraceptive device in pregnancy

O26.30 Retained intrauterine contraceptive device in pregnancy, unspecified trimester — [♀, Age/12-55]

O26.31 Retained intrauterine contraceptive device in pregnancy, first trimester — [♀, Age/12-55]

O26.32 Retained intrauterine contraceptive device in pregnancy, second trimester — [♀, Age/12-55]

O26.33 Retained intrauterine contraceptive device in pregnancy, third trimester — [♀, Age/12-55]

O26.4- Herpes gestationis — A form of dermatitis herpetiformis that occurs during pregnancy that clears upon delivery.

O26.40 Herpes gestationis, unspecified trimester — [♀, Age/12-55]

O26.41 Herpes gestationis, first trimester — [♀, Age/12-55]

O26.42 Herpes gestationis, second trimester — [♀, Age/12-55]

O26.43 Herpes gestationis, third trimester — [♀, Age/12-55]

O26.5- Maternal hypotension syndrome — Abnormally low blood pressure during pregnancy.
    Supine hypotensive syndrome

O26.50 Maternal hypotension syndrome, unspecified trimester — [♀, Age/12-55]

O26.51 Maternal hypotension syndrome, first trimester — [♀, Age/12-55]

O26.52 Maternal hypotension syndrome, second trimester — [♀, Age/12-55]

O26.53 Maternal hypotension syndrome, third trimester — [♀, Age/12-55]

O26.6- Liver and biliary tract disorders in pregnancy, childbirth and the puerperium
Use additional code to identify the specific disorder
Excludes ❷: *hepatorenal syndrome following labor and delivery (O90.4)*

O26.61- Liver and biliary tract disorders in pregnancy

CC **O26.611 Liver and biliary tract disorders in pregnancy, first trimester** — [♀, Age/12-55]

CC **O26.612 Liver and biliary tract disorders in pregnancy, second trimester** — [♀, Age/12-55]

CC **O26.613 Liver and biliary tract disorders in pregnancy, third trimester** — [♀, Age/12-55]

O26.619 Liver and biliary tract disorders in pregnancy, unspecified trimester — [♀, Age/12-55]

CC **O26.62 Liver and biliary tract disorders in childbirth** — [♀, Age/12-55]

O26.63 Liver and biliary tract disorders in the puerperium — [♀, Age/12-55]

O26.7- Subluxation of symphysis (pubis) in pregnancy, childbirth and the puerperium — The abnormal displacement or movement of the symphysis pubis during pregnancy.
Excludes 1:   *traumatic separation of symphysis (pubis) during childbirth (O71.6)*

O26.71- Subluxation of symphysis (pubis) in pregnancy

O26.711 Subluxation of symphysis (pubis) in pregnancy, first trimester — [♀, Age/12-55]

O26.712 Subluxation of symphysis (pubis) in pregnancy, second trimester — [♀, Age/12-55]

O26.713 Subluxation of symphysis (pubis) in pregnancy, third trimester — [♀, Age/12-55]

O26.719 Subluxation of symphysis (pubis) in pregnancy, unspecified trimester — [♀, Age/12-55]

O26.72 Subluxation of symphysis (pubis) in childbirth — [♀, Age/12-55]

O26.73 Subluxation of symphysis (pubis) in the puerperium — [♀, Age/12-55]

O26.8- Other specified pregnancy related conditions

O26.81- Pregnancy related exhaustion and fatigue

O26.811 Pregnancy related exhaustion and fatigue, first trimester — [♀, Age/12-55]

O26.812 Pregnancy related exhaustion and fatigue, second trimester — [♀, Age/12-55]

O26.813 Pregnancy related exhaustion and fatigue, third trimester — [♀, Age/12-55]

O26.819 Pregnancy related exhaustion and fatigue, unspecified trimester — [♀, Age/12-55]

O26.82- Pregnancy related peripheral neuritis

O26.821 Pregnancy related peripheral neuritis, first trimester — [♀, Age/12-55]

O26.822 Pregnancy related peripheral neuritis, second trimester — [♀, Age/12-55]

O26.823 Pregnancy related peripheral neuritis, third trimester — [♀, Age/12-55]

O26.829 Pregnancy related peripheral neuritis, unspecified trimester — [♀, Age/12-55]

O26.83- Pregnancy related renal disease
Use additional code to identify the specific disorder

CC **O26.831 Pregnancy related renal disease, first trimester** — [♀, Age/12-55]

CC **O26.832 Pregnancy related renal disease, second trimester** — [♀, Age/12-55]

CC **O26.833 Pregnancy related renal disease, third trimester** — [♀, Age/12-55]

O26.839 Pregnancy related renal disease, unspecified trimester — [♀, Age/12-55]

O26.84- Uterine size-date discrepancy complicating pregnancy
Excludes 1:   *encounter for suspected problem with fetal growth ruled out (Z03.74)*

O26.841 Uterine size-date discrepancy, first trimester — [♀, Age/12-55]

O26.842 Uterine size-date discrepancy, second trimester — [♀, Age/12-55]

O26.843 Uterine size-date discrepancy, third trimester — [♀, Age/12-55]

O26.849 Uterine size-date discrepancy, unspecified trimester — [♀, Age/12-55]

O26.85- Spotting complicating pregnancy — The presence of light vaginal bleeding during pregnancy.

O26.851 Spotting complicating pregnancy, first trimester — [♀, Age/12-55]

O26.852 Spotting complicating pregnancy, second trimester — [♀, Age/12-55]

O26.853 Spotting complicating pregnancy, third trimester — [♀, Age/12-55]

O26.859 Spotting complicating pregnancy, unspecified trimester — [♀, Age/12-55]

O26.86 Pruritic urticarial papules and plaques of pregnancy (PUPPP) — [♀, Age/12-55]
Polymorphic eruption of pregnancy

O26.87- Cervical shortening — The premature effacing and dilation of the cervix during pregnancy.
Excludes 1:   *encounter for suspected cervical shortening ruled out (Z03.75)*

CC **O26.872 Cervical shortening, second trimester** — [♀, Age/12-55]

CC **O26.873 Cervical shortening, third trimester** — [♀, Age/12-55]

CC **O26.879 Cervical shortening, unspecified trimester** — [♀, Age/12-55]

O26.89- Other specified pregnancy related conditions

O26.891 Other specified pregnancy related conditions, first trimester — [♀, Age/12-55]

O26.892 Other specified pregnancy related conditions, second trimester — [♀, Age/12-55]

O26.893 Other specified pregnancy related conditions, <u>third</u> trimester — [♀, Age/12-55]
AHA 15:3Q:p40 – Prophylactic Rhogam

O26.899 Other specified pregnancy related conditions, <u>unspecified</u> trimester — [♀, Age/12-55]

O26.9- Pregnancy related conditions, <u>unspecified</u>

O26.90 Pregnancy related conditions, unspecified, <u>unspecified</u> trimester — [♀, Age/12-55]

O26.91 Pregnancy related conditions, unspecified, <u>first</u> trimester — [♀, Age/12-55]

O26.92 Pregnancy related conditions, unspecified, <u>second</u> trimester — [♀, Age/12-55]

O26.93 Pregnancy related conditions, unspecified, <u>third</u> trimester — [♀, Age/12-55]

O28- <u>Abnormal findings</u> on antenatal screening of mother
Excludes 1: diagnostic findings classified elsewhere — see Alphabetical Index

O28.0 Abnormal hematological finding on antenatal screening of mother — [♀, Age/12-55]

O28.1 Abnormal biochemical finding on antenatal screening of mother — [♀, Age/12-55]

O28.2 Abnormal cytological finding on antenatal screening of mother — [♀, Age/12-55]

O28.3 Abnormal ultrasonic finding on antenatal screening of mother — [♀, Age/12-55]

O28.4 Abnormal radiological finding on antenatal screening of mother — [♀, Age/12-55]

O28.5 Abnormal chromosomal and genetic finding on antenatal screening of mother — [♀, Age/12-55]

O28.8 Other abnormal findings on antenatal screening of mother — [♀, Age/12-55]

O28.9 Unspecified abnormal findings on antenatal screening of mother — [♀, Age/12-55]

O29- <u>Complications of anesthesia during pregnancy</u>
Includes: Maternal complications arising from the administration of a general, regional or local anesthetic, analgesic or other sedation during pregnancy
Use additional code, if necessary, to identify the complication
Excludes ❷: complications of anesthesia during labor and delivery (O74.-)
complicatios of anesthesia during the puerperium (O89.-)

O29.0- <u>Pulmonary complications</u> of anesthesia during pregnancy

O29.01- <u>Aspiration pneumonitis</u> due to anesthesia during pregnancy
Inhalation of stomach contents or secretions NOS due to anesthesia during pregnancy
Mendelson's syndrome due to anesthesia during pregnancy

O29.011 Aspiration pneumonitis due to anesthesia during pregnancy, <u>first</u> trimester — [♀, Age/12-55]

O29.012 Aspiration pneumonitis due to anesthesia during pregnancy, <u>second</u> trimester — [♀, Age/12-55]

O29.013 Aspiration pneumonitis due to anesthesia during pregnancy, <u>third</u> trimester — [♀, Age/12-55]

O29.019 Aspiration pneumonitis due to anesthesia during pregnancy, <u>unspecified</u> trimester — [♀, Age/12-55]

O29.02- <u>Pressure collapse of lung</u> due to anesthesia during pregnancy

O29.021 Pressure collapse of lung due to anesthesia during pregnancy, <u>first</u> trimester — [♀, Age/12-55]

O29.022 Pressure collapse of lung due to anesthesia during pregnancy, <u>second</u> trimester — [♀, Age/12-55]

O29.023 Pressure collapse of lung due to anesthesia during pregnancy, <u>third</u> trimester — [♀, Age/12-55]

O29.029 Pressure collapse of lung due to anesthesia during pregnancy, <u>unspecified</u> trimester — [♀, Age/12-55]

O29.09- <u>Other pulmonary</u> complications of anesthesia during pregnancy

O29.091 Other pulmonary complications of anesthesia during pregnancy, <u>first</u> trimester — [♀, Age/12-55]

O29.092 Other pulmonary complications of anesthesia during pregnancy, <u>second</u> trimester — [♀, Age/12-55]

O29.093 Other pulmonary complications of anesthesia during pregnancy, <u>third</u> trimester — [♀, Age/12-55]

O29.099 Other pulmonary complications of anesthesia during pregnancy, <u>unspecified</u> trimester — [♀, Age/12-55]

O29.1- <u>Cardiac complications</u> of anesthesia during pregnancy

O29.11- <u>Cardiac arrest</u> due to anesthesia during pregnancy

O29.111 Cardiac arrest due to anesthesia during pregnancy, <u>first</u> trimester — [♀, Age/12-55]

O29.112 Cardiac arrest due to anesthesia during pregnancy, <u>second</u> trimester — [♀, Age/12-55]

O29.113 Cardiac arrest due to anesthesia during pregnancy, <u>third</u> trimester — [♀, Age/12-55]

O29.119 Cardiac arrest due to anesthesia during pregnancy, <u>unspecified</u> trimester — [♀, Age/12-55]

O29.12- <u>Cardiac failure</u> due to anesthesia during pregnancy

O29.121 Cardiac failure due to anesthesia during pregnancy, <u>first</u> trimester — [♀, Age/12-55]

O29.122 Cardiac failure due to anesthesia during pregnancy, <u>second</u> trimester — [♀, Age/12-55]

O29.123 Cardiac failure due to anesthesia during pregnancy, <u>third</u> trimester — [♀, Age/12-55]

O29.129 Cardiac failure due to anesthesia during pregnancy, <u>unspecified</u> trimester — [♀, Age/12-55]

O29.19- <u>Other cardiac complications</u> of anesthesia during pregnancy

O29.191 Other cardiac complications of anesthesia during pregnancy, <u>first</u> trimester — [♀, Age/12-55]

O29.192 Other cardiac complications of anesthesia during pregnancy, <u>second</u> trimester — [♀, Age/12-55]

O29.193 Other cardiac complications of anesthesia during pregnancy, <u>third</u> trimester — [♀, Age/12-55]

O29.199 Other cardiac complications of anesthesia during pregnancy, <u>unspecified</u> trimester — [♀, Age/12-55]

O29.2- <u>Central nervous system complications</u> of anesthesia during pregnancy

O29.21- <u>Cerebral anoxia</u> due to anesthesia during pregnancy

O29.211 Cerebral anoxia due to anesthesia during pregnancy, <u>first</u> trimester — [♀, Age/12-55]

O29.212 Cerebral anoxia due to anesthesia during pregnancy, <u>second</u> trimester — [♀, Age/12-55]

O29.213 Cerebral anoxia due to anesthesia during pregnancy, <u>third</u> trimester — [♀, Age/12-55]

O29.219 Cerebral anoxia due to anesthesia during pregnancy, <u>unspecified</u> trimester — [♀, Age/12-55]

O29.29- <u>Other central nervous system complications</u> of anesthesia during pregnancy

O29.291 Other central nervous system complications of anesthesia during pregnancy, <u>first</u> trimester — [♀, Age/12-55]

O29.292 Other central nervous system complications of anesthesia during pregnancy, <u>second</u> trimester — [♀, Age/12-55]

O29.293 Other central nervous system complications of anesthesia during pregnancy, <u>third</u> trimester — [♀, Age/12-55]

O29.299 Other central nervous system complications of anesthesia during pregnancy, <u>unspecified</u> trimester — [♀, Age/12-55]

O29.3- <u>Toxic reaction to local anesthesia</u> during pregnancy

O29.3x- Toxic reaction to local anesthesia during pregnancy

O29.3x1 Toxic reaction to local anesthesia during pregnancy, <u>first</u> trimester — [♀, Age/12-55]

O29.3x2 Toxic reaction to local anesthesia during pregnancy, <u>second</u> trimester — [♀, Age/12-55]

O29.3x3 Toxic reaction to local anesthesia during pregnancy, <u>third</u> trimester — [♀, Age/12-55]

O29.3x9 Toxic reaction to local anesthesia during pregnancy, <u>unspecified</u> trimester — [♀, Age/12-55]

O26 - O29

O29.4- <u>Spinal and epidural anesthesia induced headache</u> during pregnancy

O29.40 Spinal and epidural anesthesia induced headache during pregnancy, <u>unspecified</u> trimester — [♀, Age/12-55]

O29.41 Spinal and epidural anesthesia induced headache during pregnancy, <u>first</u> trimester — [♀, Age/12-55]

O29.42 Spinal and epidural anesthesia induced headache during pregnancy, <u>second</u> trimester — [♀, Age/12-55]

O29.43 Spinal and epidural anesthesia induced headache during pregnancy, <u>third</u> trimester — [♀, Age/12-55]

O29.5- <u>Other complications of spinal and epidural anesthesia</u> during pregnancy

O29.5x Other complications of spinal and epidural anesthesia during pregnancy

O29.5x1 Other complications of spinal and epidural anesthesia during pregnancy, <u>first</u> trimester — [♀, Age/12-55]

O29.5x2 Other complications of spinal and epidural anesthesia during pregnancy, <u>second</u> trimester — [♀, Age/12-55]

O29.5x3 Other complications of spinal and epidural anesthesia during pregnancy, <u>third</u> trimester — [♀, Age/12-55]

O29.5x9 Other complications of spinal and epidural anesthesia during pregnancy, <u>unspecified</u> trimester — [♀, Age/12-55]

O29.6- <u>Failed or difficult intubation for anesthesia</u> during pregnancy

O29.60 Failed or difficult intubation for anesthesia during pregnancy, <u>unspecified</u> trimester — [♀, Age/12-55]

O29.61 Failed or difficult intubation for anesthesia during pregnancy, <u>first</u> trimester — [♀, Age/12-55]

O29.62 Failed or difficult intubation for anesthesia during pregnancy, <u>second</u> trimester — [♀, Age/12-55]

O29.63 Failed or difficult intubation for anesthesia during pregnancy, <u>third</u> trimester — [♀, Age/12-55]

O29.8- <u>Other complications of anesthesia</u> during pregnancy

O29.8x Other complications of anesthesia during pregnancy

O29.8x1 Other complications of anesthesia during pregnancy, <u>first</u> trimester — [♀, Age/12-55]

O29.8x2 Other complications of anesthesia during pregnancy, <u>second</u> trimester — [♀, Age/12-55]

O29.8x3 Other complications of anesthesia during pregnancy, <u>third</u> trimester — [♀, Age/12-55]

O29.8x9 Other complications of anesthesia during pregnancy, <u>unspecified</u> trimester — [♀, Age/12-55]

O29.9- <u>Unspecified</u> complication of anesthesia during pregnancy

O29.90 Unspecified complication of anesthesia during pregnancy, <u>unspecified</u> trimester — [♀, Age/12-55]

O29.91 Unspecified complication of anesthesia during pregnancy, <u>first</u> trimester — [♀, Age/12-55]

O29.92 Unspecified complication of anesthesia during pregnancy, <u>second</u> trimester — [♀, Age/12-55]

O29.93 Unspecified complication of anesthesia during pregnancy, <u>third</u> trimester — [♀, Age/12-55]

Maternal care related to the fetus and amniotic cavity and possible delivery problems (O30-O48)

O30- <u>Multiple gestation</u> — The presence of more than one developing fetus within the uterus.

Code also any complications specific to multiple gestation

O30.0- <u>Twin</u> pregnancy — The presence of two fetuses.

O30.00- Twin pregnancy, <u>unspecified number</u> of placenta and <u>unspecified number</u> of amniotic sacs

O30.001 Twin pregnancy, unspecified number of placenta and unspecified number of amniotic sacs, <u>first</u> trimester — [♀, Age/12-55]

O30.002 Twin pregnancy, unspecified number of placenta and unspecified number of amniotic sacs, <u>second</u> trimester — [♀, Age/12-55]

O30.003 Twin pregnancy, unspecified number of placenta and unspecified number of amniotic sacs, <u>third</u> trimester — [♀, Age/12-55]

O30.009 Twin pregnancy, unspecified number of placenta and unspecified number of amniotic sacs, <u>unspecified</u> trimester — [♀, Age/12-55]

O30.01- Twin pregnancy, <u>monochorionic/monoamniotic</u>

Twin pregnancy, one placenta, one amniotic sac

Excludes 1:   conjoined twins (O30.02-)

O30.011 Twin pregnancy, monochorionic/monoamniotic, <u>first</u> trimester — [♀, Age/12-55]

O30.012 Twin pregnancy, monochorionic/monoamniotic, <u>second</u> trimester — [♀, Age/12-55]

O30.013 Twin pregnancy, monochorionic/monoamniotic, <u>third</u> trimester — [♀, Age/12-55]

O30.019 Twin pregnancy, monochorionic/monoamniotic, <u>unspecified</u> trimester — [♀, Age/12-55]

O30.02- <u>Conjoined</u> twin pregnancy

O30.021 Conjoined twin pregnancy, <u>first</u> trimester — [♀, Age/12-55]

O30.022 Conjoined twin pregnancy, <u>second</u> trimester — [♀, Age/12-55]

O30.023 Conjoined twin pregnancy, <u>third</u> trimester — [♀, Age/12-55]

O30.029 Conjoined twin pregnancy, <u>unspecified</u> trimester — [♀, Age/12-55]

O30.03- Twin pregnancy, <u>monochorionic/diamniotic</u>

Twin pregnancy, one placenta, two amniotic sacs

O30.031 Twin pregnancy, monochorionic/diamniotic, <u>first</u> trimester — [♀, Age/12-55]

O30.032 Twin pregnancy, monochorionic/diamniotic, <u>second</u> trimester — [♀, Age/12-55]

O30.033 Twin pregnancy, monochorionic/diamniotic, <u>third</u> trimester — [♀, Age/12-55]

O30.039 Twin pregnancy, monochorionic/diamniotic, <u>unspecified</u> trimester — [♀, Age/12-55]

O30.04- Twin pregnancy, <u>dichorionic/diamniotic</u>

Twin pregnancy, two placentae, two amniotic sacs

O30.041 Twin pregnancy, dichorionic/diamniotic, <u>first</u> trimester — [♀, Age/12-55]

O30.042 Twin pregnancy, dichorionic/diamniotic, <u>second</u> trimester — [♀, Age/12-55]

O30.043 Twin pregnancy, dichorionic/diamniotic, <u>third</u> trimester — [♀, Age/12-55]

O30.049 Twin pregnancy, dichorionic/diamniotic, <u>unspecified</u> trimester — [♀, Age/12-55]

O30.09- Twin pregnancy, <u>unable to determine number</u> of placenta and number of amniotic sacs

O30.091 Twin pregnancy, unable to determine number of placenta and number of amniotic sacs, <u>first</u> trimester — [♀, Age/12-55]

O30.092 Twin pregnancy, unable to determine number of placenta and number of amniotic sacs, <u>second</u> trimester — [♀, Age/12-55]

O30.093 Twin pregnancy, unable to determine number of placenta and number of amniotic sacs, <u>third</u> trimester — [♀, Age/12-55]

O30.099 Twin pregnancy, unable to determine number of placenta and number of amniotic sacs, <u>unspecified</u> trimester — [♀, Age/12-55]

O30.1- **Triplet** pregnancy — The presence of three fetuses.
AHA 16:2Q:p8 – Triamniotic trichorionic triplet pregnancy

O30.10- Triplet pregnancy, <u>unspecified number</u> of placenta and <u>unspecified number</u> of amniotic sacs

cc **O30.101** Triplet pregnancy, unspecified number of placenta and unspecified number of amniotic sacs, <u>first</u> trimester — [♀, Age/12-55]

cc **O30.102** Triplet pregnancy, unspecified number of placenta and unspecified number of amniotic sacs, <u>second</u> trimester — [♀, Age/12-55]

cc **O30.103** Triplet pregnancy, unspecified number of placenta and unspecified number of amniotic sacs, <u>third</u> trimester — [♀, Age/12-55]

O30.109 Triplet pregnancy, unspecified number of placenta and unspecified number of amniotic sacs, <u>unspecified</u> trimester — [♀, Age/12-55]

O30.11- Triplet pregnancy <u>with two or more</u> <u>monochorionic</u> fetuses

cc **O30.111** Triplet pregnancy with two or more monochorionic fetuses, <u>first</u> trimester — [♀, Age/12-55]

cc **O30.112** Triplet pregnancy with two or more monochorionic fetuses, <u>second</u> trimester — [♀, Age/12-55]

cc **O30.113** Triplet pregnancy with two or more monochorionic fetuses, <u>third</u> trimester — [♀, Age/12-55]

O30.119 Triplet pregnancy with two or more monochorionic fetuses, <u>unspecified</u> trimester — [♀, Age/12-55]

O30.12- Triplet pregnancy <u>with two or more monoamniotic</u> fetuses

cc **O30.121** Triplet pregnancy with two or more monoamniotic fetuses, <u>first</u> trimester — [♀, Age/12-55]

cc **O30.122** Triplet pregnancy with two or more monoamniotic fetuses, <u>second</u> trimester — [♀, Age/12-55]

cc **O30.123** Triplet pregnancy with two or more monoamniotic fetuses, <u>third</u> trimester — [♀, Age/12-55]

O30.129 Triplet pregnancy with two or more monoamniotic fetuses, <u>unspecified</u> trimester — [♀, Age/12-55]

O30.19- Triplet pregnancy, <u>unable to determine number</u> of placenta and number of amniotic sacs

cc **O30.191** Triplet pregnancy, unable to determine number of placenta and number of amniotic sacs, <u>first</u> trimester — [♀, Age/12-55]

cc **O30.192** Triplet pregnancy, unable to determine number of placenta and number of amniotic sacs, <u>second</u> trimester — [♀, Age/12-55]

cc **O30.193** Triplet pregnancy, unable to determine number of placenta and number of amniotic sacs, <u>third</u> trimester — [♀, Age/12-55]

O30.199 Triplet pregnancy, unable to determine number of placenta and number of amniotic sacs, <u>unspecified</u> trimester — [♀, Age/12-55]

O30.2- <u>Quadruplet</u> pregnancy — The presence of four fetuses.

O30.20- Quadruplet pregnancy, <u>unspecified number</u> of placenta and <u>unspecified number</u> of amnioticsacs

cc **O30.201** Quadruplet pregnancy, unspecified number of placenta and unspecified number of amniotic sacs, <u>first</u> trimester — [♀, Age/12-55]

cc **O30.202** Quadruplet pregnancy, unspecified number of placenta and unspecified number of amniotic sacs, <u>second</u> trimester — [♀, Age/12-55]

cc **O30.203** Quadruplet pregnancy, unspecified number of placenta and unspecified number of amniotic sacs, <u>third</u> trimester — [♀, Age/12-55]

O30.209 Quadruplet pregnancy, unspecified number of placenta and unspecified number of amniotic sacs, <u>unspecified</u> trimester — [♀, Age/12-55]

O30.21- Quadruplet pregnancy <u>with two or more</u> <u>monochorionic</u> fetuses

cc **O30.211** Quadruplet pregnancy with two or more monochorionic fetuses, <u>first</u> trimester — [♀, Age/12-55]

cc **O30.212** Quadruplet pregnancy with two or more monochorionic fetuses, <u>second</u> trimester — [♀, Age/12-55]

cc **O30.213** Quadruplet pregnancy with two or more monochorionic fetuses, <u>third</u> trimester — [♀, Age/12-55]

O30.219 Quadruplet pregnancy with two or more monochorionic fetuses, <u>unspecified</u> trimester — [♀, Age/12-55]

O30.22- Quadruplet pregnancy <u>with two or more</u> <u>monoamniotic</u> fetuses

cc **O30.221** Quadruplet pregnancy with two or more monoamniotic fetuses, <u>first</u> trimester — [♀, Age/12-55]

cc **O30.222** Quadruplet pregnancy with two or more monoamniotic fetuses, <u>second</u> trimester — [♀, Age/12-55]

cc **O30.223** Quadruplet pregnancy with two or more monoamniotic fetuses, <u>third</u> trimester — [♀, Age/12-55]

O30.229 Quadruplet pregnancy with two or more monoamniotic fetuses, <u>unspecified</u> trimester — [♀, Age/12-55]

O30.29- Quadruplet pregnancy, <u>unable to determine number</u> of placenta and number of amniotic sacs

cc **O30.291** Quadruplet pregnancy, unable to determine number of placenta and number of amniotic sacs, <u>first</u> trimester — [♀, Age/12-55]

cc **O30.292** Quadruplet pregnancy, unable to determine number of placenta and number of amniotic sacs, <u>second</u> trimester — [♀, Age/12-55]

O30.293 Quadruplet pregnancy, unable to determine number of placenta and number of amniotic sacs, <u>third</u> trimester — [♀, Age/12-55]

O30.299 Quadruplet pregnancy, unable to determine number of placenta and number of amniotic sacs, <u>unspecified</u> trimester — [♀, Age/12-55]

O30.8- <u>Other specified</u> multiple gestation
Multiple gestation pregnancy greater then quadruplets

O30.80- Other specified multiple gestation, <u>unspecified</u> <u>number</u> of placenta and <u>unspecified number</u> of amniotic sacs

cc **O30.801** Other specified multiple gestation, unspecified number of placenta and unspecified number of amniotic sacs, <u>first</u> trimester — [♀, Age/12-55]

cc **O30.802** Other specified multiple gestation, unspecified number of placenta and unspecified number of amniotic sacs, <u>second</u> trimester — [♀, Age/12-55]

cc **O30.803** Other specified multiple gestation, unspecified number of placenta and unspecified number of amniotic sacs, <u>third</u> trimester — [♀, Age/12-55]

O30.809 Other specified multiple gestation, unspecified number of placenta and unspecified number of amniotic sacs, <u>unspecified</u> trimester — [♀, Age/12-55]

O30 I O30

Excludes 1: = NOT CODED HERE! (Do not code both)   933   *Excludes ❷:* = Not Included Here

O30.81- Other specified multiple gestation <u>with two or more monochorionic</u> fetuses

CC **O30.811** Other specified multiple gestation with two or more monochorionic fetuses, <u>first</u> trimester — [♀, Age/12-55]

CC **O30.812** Other specified multiple gestation with two or more monochorionic fetuses, <u>second</u> trimester — [♀, Age/12-55]

CC **O30.813** Other specified multiple gestation with two or more monochorionic fetuses, <u>third</u> trimester — [♀, Age/12-55]

O30.819 Other specified multiple gestation with two or more monochorionic fetuses, <u>unspecified</u> trimester — [♀, Age/12-55]

O30.82- Other specified multiple gestation <u>with two or more monoamniotic</u> fetuses

CC **O30.821** Other specified multiple gestation with two or more monoamniotic fetuses, <u>first</u> trimester — [♀, Age/12-55]

CC **O30.822** Other specified multiple gestation with two or more monoamniotic fetuses, <u>second</u> trimester — [♀, Age/12-55]

CC **O30.823** Other specified multiple gestation with two or more monoamniotic fetuses, <u>third</u> trimester — [♀, Age/12-55]

O30.829 Other specified multiple gestation with two or more monoamniotic fetuses, <u>unspecified</u> trimester — [♀, Age/12-55]

O30.89- Other specified multiple gestation, <u>unable to determine number</u> of placenta and number of amniotic sacs

CC **O30.891** Other specified multiple gestation, unable to determine number of placenta and number of amniotic sacs, <u>first</u> trimester — [♀, Age/12-55]

CC **O30.892** Other specified multiple gestation, unable to determine number of placenta and number of amniotic sacs, <u>second</u> trimester — [♀, Age/12-55]

CC **O30.893** Other specified multiple gestation, unable to determine number of placenta and number of amniotic sacs, <u>third</u> trimester — [♀, Age/12-55]

O30.899 Other specified multiple gestation, unable to determine number of placenta and number of amniotic sacs, <u>unspecified</u> trimester — [♀, Age/12-55]

O30.9- Multiple gestation, <u>unspecified</u>
  Multiple pregnancy NOS

O30.90 Multiple gestation, unspecified, <u>unspecified</u> trimester — [♀, Age/12-55]

O30.91 Multiple gestation, unspecified, <u>first</u> trimester — [♀, Age/12-55]

O30.92 Multiple gestation, unspecified, <u>second</u> trimester — [♀, Age/12-55]

O30.93 Multiple gestation, unspecified, <u>third</u> trimester — [♀, Age/12-55]

O31- <u>Complications specific to multiple gestation</u>
  AHA 12:4Q:p107 – Fetus A and B same as fetus 1 and 2
  Excludes ②: delayed delivery of second twin, triplet, etc. (O63.2)
     malpresentation of one fetus or more (O32.9)
     placental transfusion syndromes (O43.0-)

One of the following 7th characters is to be assigned to each code under category O31. 7th character 0 is for single gestations and multiple gestations where the fetus is unspecified. 7th characters 1 through 9 are for cases of multiple gestations to identify the fetus for which the code applies. The appropriate code from category O30, Multiple gestation, must also be assigned when assigning a code from category O31 that has a 7th character of 1 through 9.
0   Not applicable or unspecified
1   Fetus 1
2   Fetus 2
3   Fetus 3
4   Fetus 4
5   Fetus 5
9   Other fetus

O31.0- <u>Papyraceous fetus</u> — The dead fetus that is pressed flat by the development of the living twin.
  Fetus compressus

O31.00x- Papyraceous fetus, <u>unspecified</u> trimester — [♀, Age/12-55]

O31.01x- Papyraceous fetus, <u>first</u> trimester — [♀, Age/12-55]

O31.02x- Papyraceous fetus, <u>second</u> trimester — [♀, Age/12-55]

O31.03x- Papyraceous fetus, <u>third</u> trimester — [♀, Age/12-55]

O31.1- <u>Continuing pregnancy after spontaneous abortion</u> of one fetus or more

O31.10x- Continuing pregnancy after spontaneous abortion of one fetus or more, <u>unspecified</u> trimester — [♀, Age/12-55]

O31.11x- Continuing pregnancy after spontaneous abortion of one fetus or more, <u>first</u> trimester — [♀, Age/12-55]

O31.12x- Continuing pregnancy after spontaneous abortion of one fetus or more, <u>second</u> trimester — [♀, Age/12-55]

O31.13x- Continuing pregnancy after spontaneous abortion of one fetus or more, <u>third</u> trimester — [♀, Age/12-55]

O31.2- <u>Continuing pregnancy after intrauterine death</u> of one fetus or more

O31.20x- Continuing pregnancy after intrauterine death of one fetus or more, <u>unspecified</u> trimester — [♀, Age/12-55]

O31.21x- Continuing pregnancy after intrauterine death of one fetus or more, <u>first</u> trimester — [♀, Age/12-55]

O31.22x- Continuing pregnancy after intrauterine death of one fetus or more, <u>second</u> trimester — [♀, Age/12-55]

O31.23x- Continuing pregnancy after intrauterine death of one fetus or more, <u>third</u> trimester — [♀, Age/12-55]

O31.3- Continuing pregnancy <u>after elective fetal reduction</u> of one fetus or more
  Continuing pregnancy after selective termination of one fetus or more

O31.30x- Continuing pregnancy after elective fetal reduction of one fetus or more, <u>unspecified</u> trimester — [♀, Age/12-55]

O31.31x- Continuing pregnancy after elective fetal reduction of one fetus or more, <u>first</u> trimester — [♀, Age/12-55]

O31.32x- Continuing pregnancy after elective fetal reduction of one fetus or more, <u>second</u> trimester — [♀, Age/12-55]

O31.33x- Continuing pregnancy after elective fetal reduction of one fetus or more, <u>third</u> trimester — [♀, Age/12-55]

O31.8- Other complications specific to multiple gestation

O31.8x- <u>Other complications specific to multiple gestation</u>

CC-0-9 **O31.8x1-** Other complications specific to multiple gestation, <u>first</u> trimester — [♀, Age/12-55]

CC-0-9 **O31.8x2-** Other complications specific to multiple gestation, <u>second</u> trimester — [♀, Age/12-55]

CC-0-9 **O31.8x3-** Other complications specific to multiple gestation, <u>third</u> trimester — [♀, Age/12-55]

O31.8x9- Other complications specific to multiple gestation, <u>unspecified</u> trimester — [♀, Age/12-55]

O 30 - O 31

Excludes 1: = NOT CODED HERE! (Do not code both)

Excludes ②: = Not Included Here

O32- Maternal care for malpresentation of fetus
AHA 12:4Q:p107 – Fetus A and B same as fetus 1 and 2
Includes: The listed conditions as a reason for observation, hospitalization or other obstetric care of the mother, or for cesarean delivery before onset of labor
Excludes 1:   malpresentation of fetus with obstructed labor (O64.-)

One of the following 7th characters is to be assigned to each code under category O32. 7th character 0 is for single gestations and multiple gestations where the fetus is unspecified. 7th characters 1 through 9 are for cases of multiple gestations to identify the fetus for which the code applies. The appropriate code from category O30, Multiple gestation, must also be assigned when assigning a code from category O32 that has a 7th character of 1 through 9.
0   Not applicable or unspecified
1   Fetus 1
2   Fetus 2
3   Fetus 3
4   Fetus 4
5   Fetus 5
9   Other fetus

O32.0xx- Maternal care for unstable lie — [♀, Age/12-55] – A fetal position which is changes repeatedly.

O32.1xx- Maternal care for breech presentation — [♀, Age/12-55] – Presentation of the buttocks in the birth canal during labor.
Maternal care for buttocks presentation
Maternal care for complete breech
Maternal care for frank breech
Excludes 1:   footling presentation (O32.8)
incomplete breech (O32.8)

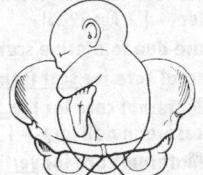

BREECH PRESENTATION

O32.2xx- Maternal care for transverse and oblique lie — [♀, Age/12-55] – Presentation of the body (trunk) in the birth canal during labor.
Maternal care for oblique presentation
Maternal care for transverse presentation

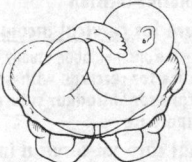

TRANSVERSE LIE

O32.3xx- Maternal care for face, brow and chin presentation — [♀, Age/12-55] – Presentation of the fetal face, brow (forehead), or chin (mentum) in the birth canal during labor.

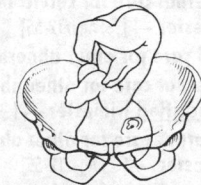

FACE/BROW PRESENTATION

O32.4xx- Maternal care for high head at term — [♀, Age/12-55] – The situation of the fetus at term with its head in a cephalic position, but not presenting into the pelvic brim.
Maternal care for failure of head to enter pelvic brim

O32.6xx- Maternal care for compound presentation — [♀, Age/12-55] – Presentation of the fetus with a prolapsed arm or leg alongside the head or alongside a breech.

O32.8xx- Maternal care for other malpresentation of fetus — [♀, Age/12-55]
Maternal care for footling presentation — Presentation of one or both feet in the birth canal during labor.
Maternal care for incomplete breech — Breech presentation with only one of the legs bent at the knees in the birth canal during labor.

O32.9xx- Maternal care for malpresentation of fetus, unspecified — [♀, Age/12-55]

O33- Maternal care for disproportion — The relative difference in size between the fetal head and the pelvis.
AHA 12:4Q:p107 – Fetus A and B same as fetus 1 and 2
Includes: The listed conditions as a reason for observation, hospitalization or other obstetric care of the mother, or for cesarean delivery before onset of labor
Excludes 1:   disproportion with obstructed labor (O65-O66)

cc **O33.0 Maternal care for disproportion due to deformity of maternal pelvic bones** — [♀, Age/12-55]
Maternal care for disproportion due to pelvic deformity causing disproportion NOS

O33.1 Maternal care for disproportion due to generally contracted pelvis — [♀, Age/12-55] – A pelvic opening that is reduced more than 2 cm in diameter.
Maternal care for disproportion due to contracted pelvis NOS causing disproportion

O33.2 Maternal care for disproportion due to inlet contraction of pelvis — [♀, Age/12-55] – The reduced upper opening of the pelvis.
Maternal care for disproportion due to inlet contraction (pelvis) causing disproportion

O33.3xx- Maternal care for disproportion due to outlet contraction of pelvis — [♀, Age/12-55] – The reduced lower opening of the pelvis.
Maternal care for disproportion due to mid-cavity contraction (pelvis)
Maternal care for disproportion due to outlet contraction (pelvis)

One of the following 7th characters is to be assigned to code O33.3. 7th character 0 is for single gestations and multiple gestations where the fetus is unspecified. 7th characters 1 through 9 are for cases of multiple gestations to identify the fetus for which the code applies. The appropriate code from category O30, Multiple gestation, must also be assigned when assigning code O33.3 with a 7th character of 1 through 9.
0   Not applicable or unspecified
1   Fetus 1
2   Fetus 2
3   Fetus 3
4   Fetus 4
5   Fetus 5
9   Other fetus

O33.4xx- Maternal care for disproportion of mixed maternal and fetal origin — [♀, Age/12-55]

One of the following 7th characters is to be assigned to code O33.4. 7th character 0 is for single gestations and multiple gestations where the fetus is unspecified. 7th characters 1 through 9 are for cases of multiple gestations to identify the fetus for which the code applies. The appropriate code from category O30, Multiple gestation, must also be assigned when assigning code O33.4 with a 7th character of 1 through 9.
0   Not applicable or unspecified
1   Fetus 1
2   Fetus 2
3   Fetus 3
4   Fetus 4
5   Fetus 5
9   Other fetus

O 3 2 - O 3 3

Excludes 1: = NOT CODED HERE! (Do not code both)

Excludes ❷: = Not Included Here

O33.5xx-   Maternal care for disproportion due to <u>unusually large fetus</u> — [♀, Age/12-55] – A larger than average fetus that is too large for the normal maternal pelvis.
> Maternal care for disproportion due to disproportion of fetal origin with normally formed fetus
> Maternal care for disproportion due to fetal disproportion NOS

> One of the following 7th characters is to be assigned to code O33.5. 7th character 0 is for single gestations and multiple gestations where the fetus is unspecified. 7th characters 1 through 9 are for cases of multiple gestations to identify the fetus for which the code applies. The appropriate code from category O30, Multiple gestation, must also be assigned when assigning code O33.5 with a 7th character of 1 through 9.
>
> 0   Not applicable or unspecified
> 1   Fetus 1
> 2   Fetus 2
> 3   Fetus 3
> 4   Fetus 4
> 5   Fetus 5
> 9   Other fetus

O33.6xx-   Maternal care for disproportion due to <u>hydrocephalic fetus</u> — [♀, Age/12-55] – The abnormal massive accumulation of fluid within the fetal cranial vault.

> One of the following 7th characters is to be assigned to code O33.6. 7th character 0 is for single gestations and multiple gestations where the fetus is unspecified. 7th characters 1 through 9 are for cases of multiple gestations to identify the fetus for which the code applies. The appropriate code from category O30, Multiple gestation, must also be assigned when assigning code O33.6 with a 7th character of 1 through 9.
>
> 0   Not applicable or unspecified
> 1   Fetus 1
> 2   Fetus 2
> 3   Fetus 3
> 4   Fetus 4
> 5   Fetus 5
> 9   Other fetus

O33.7xx-   Maternal care for disproportion due to other <u>fetal deformities</u> — [♀, Age/12-55]
> Maternal care for disproportion due to fetal ascites
> Maternal care for disproportion due to fetal hydrops
> Maternal care for disproportion due to fetal meningomyelocele
> Maternal care for disproportion due to fetal sacral teratoma
> Maternal care for disproportion due to fetal tumor
>
> *Excludes 1:*   obstructed labor due to other fetal deformities (O66.3)

> One of the following 7th characters is to be assigned to code O33.7. 7th character 0 is for single gestations and multiple gestations where the fetus is unspecified. 7th characters 1 through 9 are for cases of multiple gestations to identify the fetus for which the code applies. The appropriate code from category O30, Multiple gestation, must also be assigned when assigning code O33.7 with a 7th character of 1 through 9.
>
> 0   Not applicable or unspecified
> 1   Fetus 1
> 2   Fetus 2
> 3   Fetus 3
> 4   Fetus 4
> 5   Fetus 5
> 9   Other fetus

O33.8   Maternal care for disproportion of <u>other</u> origin — [♀, Age/12-55]

O33.9   Maternal care for disproportion, <u>unspecified</u> — [♀, Age/12-55]
> Maternal care for disproportion due to cephalopelvic disproportion NOS
> Maternal care for disproportion due to fetopelvic disproportion NOS

O34-   Maternal care for <u>abnormality of pelvic organs</u>
Includes: The listed conditions as a reason for hospitalization or other obstetric care of the mother, or for cesarean delivery before onset of labor
Code first any associated obstructed labor (O65.5)
Use additional code for specific condition

O34.0-   Maternal care for <u>congenital malformation of uterus</u> — Maternal uterine conditions that have been present since birth.
> Maternal care for double uterus
> Maternal care for uterus bicornis

> **O34.00** Maternal care for unspecified congenital malformation of uterus, <u>unspecified</u> trimester — [♀, Age/12-55]
>
> **O34.01** Maternal care for unspecified congenital malformation of uterus, <u>first</u> trimester — [♀, Age/12-55]
>
> **O34.02** Maternal care for unspecified congenital malformation of uterus, <u>second</u> trimester — [♀, Age/12-55]
>
> **O34.03** Maternal care for unspecified congenital malformation of uterus, <u>third</u> trimester — [♀, Age/12-55]

O34.1-   Maternal care for <u>benign tumor of corpus uteri</u> — Abnormal growths of the uterus.
> *Excludes ❷:*   maternal care for benign tumor of cervix (O34.4-)
> maternal care for malignant neoplasm of uterus (O9A.1-)

> **O34.10** Maternal care for benign tumor of corpus uteri, <u>unspecified</u> trimester — [♀, Age/12-55]
>
> **O34.11** Maternal care for benign tumor of corpus uteri, <u>first</u> trimester — [♀, Age/12-55]
>
> **O34.12** Maternal care for benign tumor of corpus uteri, <u>second</u> trimester — [♀, Age/12-55]
>
> **O34.13** Maternal care for benign tumor of corpus uteri, <u>third</u> trimester — [♀, Age/12-55]

O34.2-   Maternal care due to uterine scar from previous surgery
> **O34.21-**   Maternal care for <u>scar from previous cesarean delivery</u>
>
> > **O34.211** Maternal care for <u>low transverse</u> scar from previous cesarean delivery — [♀, Age/12-55]
> >
> > **O34.212** Maternal care for <u>vertical</u> scar from previous cesarean delivery — [♀, Age/12-55]
> > Maternal care for classical scar from previous cesarean delivery
> >
> > **O34.219** Maternal care for <u>unspecified</u> type scar from previous cesarean delivery — [♀, Age/12-55]
>
> **O34.29** Maternal care due to <u>uterine scar from other previous surgery</u> — [♀, Age/12-55]
> Maternal care due to uterine scar from other transmural uterine incision

O34.3-   Maternal care for <u>cervical incompetence</u> — The abnormal dilation of the cervix before the onset of labor, usually during the second trimester.
> Maternal care for cerclage with or without cervical incompetence
> Maternal care for Shirodkar suture with or without cervical incompetence

> **O34.30** Maternal care for cervical incompetence, <u>unspecified</u> trimester — [♀, Age/12-55]
>
> ᴍᴄᴄ **O34.31** Maternal care for cervical incompetence, <u>first</u> trimester — [♀, Age/12-55]
>
> ᴍᴄᴄ **O34.32** Maternal care for cervical incompetence, <u>second</u> trimester — [♀, Age/12-55]
>
> ᴍᴄᴄ **O34.33** Maternal care for cervical incompetence, <u>third</u> trimester — [♀, Age/12-55]

O34.4-   Maternal care for other abnormalities of cervix
> **O34.40** Maternal care for other abnormalities of cervix, <u>unspecified</u> trimester — [♀, Age/12-55]
>
> **O34.41** Maternal care for other abnormalities of cervix, <u>first</u> trimester — [♀, Age/12-55]
>
> **O34.42** Maternal care for other abnormalities of cervix, <u>second</u> trimester — [♀, Age/12-55]
>
> **O34.43** Maternal care for other abnormalities of cervix, <u>third</u> trimester — [♀, Age/12-55]

O33 - O34

O34.5- Maternal care for other abnormalities of gravid uterus

O34.51- Maternal care for <u>incarceration of gravid uterus</u> — The abnormal confinement of the uterus.

O34.511 Maternal care for incarceration of gravid uterus, <u>first</u> trimester — [♀, Age/12-55]

O34.512 Maternal care for incarceration of gravid uterus, <u>second</u> trimester — [♀, Age/12-55]

O34.513 Maternal care for incarceration of gravid uterus, <u>third</u> trimester — [♀, Age/12-55]

O34.519 Maternal care for incarceration of gravid uterus, <u>unspecified</u> trimester — [♀, Age/12-55]

O34.52- Maternal care for <u>prolapse of gravid uterus</u> — The downward displacement of the gravid uterus.

O34.521 Maternal care for prolapse of gravid uterus, <u>first</u> trimester — [♀, Age/12-55]

O34.522 Maternal care for prolapse of gravid uterus, <u>second</u> trimester — [♀, Age/12-55]

O34.523 Maternal care for prolapse of gravid uterus, <u>third</u> trimester — [♀, Age/12-55]

O34.529 Maternal care for prolapse of gravid uterus, <u>unspecified</u> trimester — [♀, Age/12-55]

O34.53- Maternal care for <u>retroversion of gravid uterus</u> — The abnormal turning backwards of the uterus.

O34.531 Maternal care for retroversion of gravid uterus, <u>first</u> trimester — [♀, Age/12-55]

O34.532 Maternal care for retroversion of gravid uterus, <u>second</u> trimester — [♀, Age/12-55]

O34.533 Maternal care for retroversion of gravid uterus, <u>third</u> trimester — [♀, Age/12-55]

O34.539 Maternal care for retroversion of gravid uterus, <u>unspecified</u> trimester — [♀, Age/12-55]

O34.59- Maternal care for <u>other</u> abnormalities of gravid uterus

O34.591 Maternal care for other abnormalities of gravid uterus, <u>first</u> trimester — [♀, Age/12-55]

O34.592 Maternal care for other abnormalities of gravid uterus, <u>second</u> trimester — [♀, Age/12-55]

O34.593 Maternal care for other abnormalities of gravid uterus, <u>third</u> trimester — [♀, Age/12-55]

O34.599 Maternal care for other abnormalities of gravid uterus, <u>unspecified</u> trimester — [♀, Age/12-55]

O34.6- Maternal care for <u>abnormality of vagina</u>
Excludes ❷: maternal care for vaginal varices in pregnancy (O22.1-)

O34.60 Maternal care for abnormality of vagina, <u>unspecified</u> trimester — [♀, Age/12-55]

O34.61 Maternal care for abnormality of vagina, <u>first</u> trimester — [♀, Age/12-55]

O34.62 Maternal care for abnormality of vagina, <u>second</u> trimester — [♀, Age/12-55]

O34.63 Maternal care for abnormality of vagina, <u>third</u> trimester — [♀, Age/12-55]

O34.7- Maternal care for <u>abnormality of vulva and perineum</u>
Excludes ❷: maternal care for perineal and vulval varices in pregnancy (O22.1-)

O34.70 Maternal care for abnormality of vulva and perineum, <u>unspecified</u> trimester — [♀, Age/12-55]

O34.71 Maternal care for abnormality of vulva and perineum, <u>first</u> trimester — [♀, Age/12-55]

O34.72 Maternal care for abnormality of vulva and perineum, <u>second</u> trimester — [♀, Age/12-55]

O34.73 Maternal care for abnormality of vulva and perineum, <u>third</u> trimester — [♀, Age/12-55]

O34.8- Maternal care for <u>other</u> abnormalities of <u>pelvic organs</u>

O34.80 Maternal care for other abnormalities of pelvic organs, <u>unspecified</u> trimester — [♀, Age/12-55]

O34.81 Maternal care for other abnormalities of pelvic organs, <u>first</u> trimester — [♀, Age/12-55]

O34.82 Maternal care for other abnormalities of pelvic organs, <u>second</u> trimester — [♀, Age/12-55]

O34.83 Maternal care for other abnormalities of pelvic organs, <u>third</u> trimester — [♀, Age/12-55]

O34.9- Maternal care for abnormality of pelvic organ, <u>unspecified</u>

O34.90 Maternal care for abnormality of pelvic organ, unspecified, <u>unspecified</u> trimester — [♀, Age/12-55]

O34.91 Maternal care for abnormality of pelvic organ, unspecified, <u>first</u> trimester — [♀, Age/12-55]

O34.92 Maternal care for abnormality of pelvic organ, unspecified, <u>second</u> trimester — [♀, Age/12-55]

O34.93 Maternal care for abnormality of pelvic organ, unspecified, <u>third</u> trimester — [♀, Age/12-55]

O35- Maternal care for <u>known or suspected fetal abnormality and damage</u>
AHA 12:4Q:p107 – Fetus A and B same as fetus 1 and 2
Includes: The listed conditions in the fetus as a reason for hospitalization or other obstetric care to the mother, or for termination of pregnancy
Code also any associated maternal condition
Excludes 1:   encounter for suspected maternal and fetal conditions ruled out (Z03.7-)

One of the following 7th characters is to be assigned to each code under category O35. 7th character 0 is for single gestations and multiple gestations where the fetus is unspecified. 7th characters 1 through 9 are for cases of multiple gestations to identify the fetus for which the code applies. The appropriate code from category O30, Multiple gestation, must also be assigned when assigning a code from category O35 that has a 7th character of 1 through 9.
0   Not applicable or unspecified
1   Fetus 1
2   Fetus 2
3   Fetus 3
4   Fetus 4
5   Fetus 5
9   Other fetus

O35.0xx- Maternal care for (suspected) <u>central nervous system malformation in fetus</u> — [♀, Age/12-55]
Maternal care for fetal anencephaly
Maternal care for fetal hydrocephalus
Maternal care for fetal spina bifida
Excludes ❷: chromosomal abnormality in fetus (O35.1)

O35.1xx- Maternal care for (suspected) <u>chromosomal abnormality in fetus</u> — [♀, Age/12-55]

O35.2xx- Maternal care for (suspected) <u>hereditary disease in fetus</u> — [♀, Age/12-55]
Excludes ❷: chromosomal abnormality in fetus (O35.1)

O35.3xx- Maternal care for (suspected) <u>damage to fetus from viral disease in mother</u> — [♀, Age/12-55]
Maternal care for damage to fetus from maternal cytomegalovirus infection
Maternal care for damage to fetus from maternal rubella

O35.4xx- Maternal care for (suspected) damage to fetus <u>from alcohol</u> — [♀, Age/12-55]

O35.5xx- Maternal care for (suspected) damage to fetus <u>by drugs</u> — [♀, Age/12-55]
Maternal care for damage to fetus from drug addiction

O35.6xx- Maternal care for (suspected) damage to fetus <u>by radiation</u> — [♀, Age/12-55]

O35.7xx- Maternal care for (suspected) damage to fetus <u>by other medical procedures</u> — [♀, Age/12-55]
Maternal care for damage to fetus by amniocentesis
Maternal care for damage to fetus by biopsy procedures
Maternal care for damage to fetus by hematological investigation
Maternal care for damage to fetus by intrauterine contraceptive device
Maternal care for damage to fetus by intrauterine surgery

O35.8xx- Maternal care for <u>other</u> (suspected) fetal abnormality and damage — [♀, Age/12-55]
Maternal care for damage to fetus from maternal listeriosis
Maternal care for damage to fetus from maternal toxoplasmosis

O 3 4 - O 3 5

Excludes 1: = NOT CODED HERE! (Do not code both)   937   *Excludes ❷: = Not Included Here*

O35.9xx- Maternal care for (suspected) fetal abnormality and damage, <u>unspecified</u> — [♀, Age/12-55]

O36- Maternal care <u>for other fetal problems</u>
AHA 12:4Q:p107 – Fetus A and B same as fetus 1 and 2
Includes: The listed conditions in the fetus as a reason for hospitalization or other obstetric care of the mother, or for termination of pregnancy
Excludes 1: encounter for suspected maternal and fetal conditions ruled out (Z03.7-)
placental transfusion syndromes (O43.0-)
Excludes ❷: labor and delivery complicated by fetal stress (O77.-)

One of the following 7th characters is to be assigned to each code under category O36. 7th character 0 is for single gestations and multiple gestations where the fetus is unspecified. 7th characters 1 through 9 are for cases of multiple gestations to identify the fetus for which the code applies. The appropriate code from category O30, Multiple gestation, must also be assigned when assigning a code from category O36 that has a 7th character of 1 through 9.
0   Not applicable or unspecified
1   Fetus 1
2   Fetus 2
3   Fetus 3
4   Fetus 4
5   Fetus 5
9   Other fetus

O36.0- Maternal care for rhesus isoimmunization — The development of Rh-negative agglutinins in an Rh-negative mother in response to the development of Rh-positive fetal agglutinins.
Maternal care for Rh incompatibility (with hydrops fetalis)

O36.01- Maternal care for <u>anti-D [Rh] antibodies</u>
AHA 14:4Q:p17x2 – Maternal care for anti-D [RH] antibodies

CC-0-9 **O36.011-** Maternal care for anti-D [Rh] antibodies, <u>first</u> trimester — [♀, Age/12-55]

CC-0-9 **O36.012-** Maternal care for anti-D [Rh] antibodies, <u>second</u> trimester — [♀, Age/12-55]

CC-0-9 **O36.013-** Maternal care for anti-D [Rh] antibodies, <u>third</u> trimester — [♀, Age/12-55]

O36.019- Maternal care for anti-D [Rh] antibodies, <u>unspecified</u> trimester — [♀, Age/12-55]

O36.09- Maternal care for other <u>rhesus isoimmunization</u>

CC-0-9 **O36.091-** Maternal care for other rhesus isoimmunization, <u>first</u> trimester — [♀, Age/12-55]

CC-0-9 **O36.092-** Maternal care for other rhesus isoimmunization, <u>second</u> trimester — [♀, Age/12-55]

CC-0-9 **O36.093-** Maternal care for other rhesus isoimmunization, <u>third</u> trimester — [♀, Age/12-55]

O36.099- Maternal care for other rhesus <u>isoimmunization, unspecified</u> trimester — [♀, Age/12-55]

O36.1- Maternal care for other isoimmunization — The development of agglutinins due to a blood-group incompatibility.
Maternal care for ABO isoimmunization

O36.11- Maternal care for <u>Anti-A sensitization</u>
Maternal care for isoimmunization NOS (with hydrops fetalis)

O36.111- Maternal care for Anti-A sensitization, <u>first</u> trimester — [♀, Age/12-55]

O36.112- Maternal care for Anti-A sensitization, <u>second</u> trimester — [♀, Age/12-55]

O36.113- Maternal care for Anti-A sensitization, <u>third</u> trimester — [♀, Age/12-55]

O36.119- Maternal care for Anti-A sensitization, <u>unspecified</u> trimester — [♀, Age/12-55]

O36.19- Maternal care for <u>other isoimmunization</u>
Maternal care for Anti-B sensitization

O36.191- Maternal care for other isoimmunization, <u>first</u> trimester — [♀, Age/12-55]

O36.192- Maternal care for other isoimmunization, <u>second</u> trimester — [♀, Age/12-55]

O36.193- Maternal care for other isoimmunization, <u>third</u> trimester — [♀, Age/12-55]

O36.199- Maternal care for other isoimmunization, <u>unspecified</u> trimester — [♀, Age/12-55]

O36.2- Maternal care for <u>hydrops fetalis</u> — The presence of whole body edema of the fetus.
Maternal care for hydrops fetalis NOS
Maternal care for hydrops fetalis not associated with isoimmunization
Excludes 1: hydrops fetalis associated with ABO isoimmunization (O36.1-)
hydrops fetalis associated with rhesus isoimmunization (O36.0-)

O36.20x- Maternal care for hydrops fetalis, <u>unspecified</u> trimester — [♀, Age/12-55]

O36.21x- Maternal care for hydrops fetalis, <u>first</u> trimester — [♀, Age/12-55]

O36.22x- Maternal care for hydrops fetalis, <u>second</u> trimester — [♀, Age/12-55]

O36.23x- Maternal care for hydrops fetalis, <u>third</u> trimester — [♀, Age/12-55]

O36.4xx- Maternal care for intrauterine death — [♀, Age/12-55]
CC-0-9 Maternal care for intrauterine fetal death NOS
Maternal care for intrauterine fetal death after completion of 20 weeks of gestation
Maternal care for late fetal death
Maternal care for missed delivery
Excludes 1: missed abortion (O02.1)
stillbirth (P95)

O36.5- Maternal care for <u>known or suspected poor fetal growth</u> — The abnormally low fetal weight/size in comparison to gestational age.

O36.51- Maternal care for known or suspected <u>placental insufficiency</u>

O36.511- Maternal care for known or suspected placental insufficiency, <u>first</u> trimester — [♀, Age/12-55]

O36.512- Maternal care for known or suspected placental insufficiency, <u>second</u> trimester — [♀, Age/12-55]

O36.513- Maternal care for known or suspected placental insufficiency, <u>third</u> trimester — [♀, Age/12-55]

O36.519- Maternal care for known or suspected placental insufficiency, <u>unspecified</u> trimester — [♀, Age/12-55]

O36.59- Maternal care for <u>other</u> known or suspected poor fetal growth
Maternal care for known or suspected light-for-dates NOS
Maternal care for known or suspected small-for-dates NOS

O36.591- Maternal care for other known or suspected poor fetal growth, <u>first</u> trimester — [♀, Age/12-55]

O36.592- Maternal care for other known or suspected poor fetal growth, <u>second</u> trimester — [♀, Age/12-55]

O36.593- Maternal care for other known or suspected poor fetal growth, <u>third</u> trimester — [♀, Age/12-55]

O36.599- Maternal care for other known or suspected poor fetal growth, <u>unspecified</u> trimester — [♀, Age/12-55]

O36.6- Maternal care for <u>excessive fetal growth</u> — The abnormally high fetal weight/size in comparison to gestational age.
Maternal care for known or suspected large-for-dates

O36.60x- Maternal care for excessive fetal growth, <u>unspecified</u> trimester — [♀, Age/12-55]

O36.61x- Maternal care for excessive fetal growth, <u>first</u> trimester — [♀, Age/12-55]

O36.62x- Maternal care for excessive fetal growth, <u>second</u> trimester — [♀, Age/12-55]

O36.63x- Maternal care for excessive fetal growth, <u>third</u> trimester — [♀, Age/12-55]

O36.7- Maternal care for <u>viable fetus in abdominal</u> pregnancy

O36.70x- Maternal care for viable fetus in abdominal pregnancy, <u>unspecified</u> trimester — [♀, Age/12-55]

O36.71x- Maternal care for viable fetus in abdominal pregnancy, <u>first</u> trimester — [♀, Age/12-55]

O36.72x- Maternal care for viable fetus in abdominal pregnancy, <u>second</u> trimester — [♀, Age/12-55]

O36.73x- Maternal care for viable fetus in abdominal pregnancy, <u>third</u> trimester — [♀, Age/12-55]

O
3
5
-
O
3
6

O36.8- Maternal care for other specified fetal problems

O36.80x- Pregnancy with <u>inconclusive fetal viability</u> — [♀, Age/12-55] [Unacceptable PDX]
Encounter to determine fetal viability of pregnancy

O36.81- <u>Decreased fetal movements</u>

O36.812- Decreased fetal movements, <u>second</u> trimester — [♀, Age/12-55]

O36.813- Decreased fetal movements, <u>third</u> trimester — [♀, Age/12-55]

O36.819- Decreased fetal movements, <u>unspecified</u> trimester — [♀, Age/12-55]

O36.82- <u>Fetal anemia and thrombocytopenia</u>

O36.821- Fetal anemia and thrombocytopenia, <u>first</u> trimester — [♀, Age/12-55]

O36.822- Fetal anemia and thrombocytopenia, <u>second</u> trimester — [♀, Age/12-55]

O36.823- Fetal anemia and thrombocytopenia, <u>third</u> trimester — [♀, Age/12-55]

O36.829- Fetal anemia and thrombocytopenia, <u>unspecified</u> trimester — [♀, Age/12-55]

O36.89- Maternal care for <u>other specified</u> fetal problems

O36.891- Maternal care for other specified fetal problems, <u>first</u> trimester — [♀, Age/12-55]

O36.892- Maternal care for other specified fetal problems, <u>second</u> trimester — [♀, Age/12-55]

O36.893- Maternal care for other specified fetal problems, <u>third</u> trimester — [♀, Age/12-55]

O36.899- Maternal care for other specified fetal problems, <u>unspecified</u> trimester — [♀, Age/12-55]

O36.9- Maternal care for fetal problem, <u>unspecified</u>

O36.90x- Maternal care for fetal problem, unspecified, <u>unspecified</u> trimester — [♀, Age/12-55]

O36.91x- Maternal care for fetal problem, unspecified, <u>first</u> trimester — [♀, Age/12-55]

O36.92x- Maternal care for fetal problem, unspecified, <u>second</u> trimester — [♀, Age/12-55]

O36.93x- Maternal care for fetal problem, unspecified, <u>third</u> trimester — [♀, Age/12-55]

O40- <u>Polyhydramnios</u> — The excessive amount of amniotic fluid.
AHA 12:4Q:p107 – Fetus A and B same as fetus 1 and 2
AHA 16:1Q:p4 – Polyhydramnios and laceration
Includes: Hydramnios
Excludes 1: encounter for suspected maternal and fetal conditions ruled out (Z03.7-)

One of the following 7th characters is to be assigned to each code under category O40. 7th character 0 is for single gestations and multiple gestations where the fetus is unspecified. 7th characters 1 through 9 are for cases of multiple gestations to identify the fetus for which the code applies. The appropriate code from category O30, Multiple gestation, must also be assigned when assigning a code from category O40 that has a 7th character of 1 through 9.
0   Not applicable or unspecified
1   Fetus 1
2   Fetus 2
3   Fetus 3
4   Fetus 4
5   Fetus 5
9   Other fetus

O40.1xx- Polyhydramnios, <u>first</u> trimester — [♀, Age/12-55]
O40.2xx- Polyhydramnios, <u>second</u> trimester — [♀, Age/12-55]
O40.3xx- Polyhydramnios, <u>third</u> trimester — [♀, Age/12-55]
O40.9xx- Polyhydramnios, <u>unspecified</u> trimester — [♀, Age/12-55]

O41- Other disorders of amniotic fluid and membranes
AHA 12:4Q:p107 – Fetus A and B same as fetus 1 and 2
Excludes 1: encounter for suspected maternal and fetal conditions ruled out (Z03.7-)

One of the following 7th characters is to be assigned to each code under category O41. 7th character 0 is for single gestations and multiple gestations where the fetus is unspecified. 7th characters 1 through 9 are for cases of multiple gestations to identify the fetus for which the code applies. The appropriate code from category O30, Multiple gestation, must also be assigned when assigning a code from category O41 that has a 7th character of 1 through 9.
0   Not applicable or unspecified
1   Fetus 1
2   Fetus 2
3   Fetus 3
4   Fetus 4
5   Fetus 5
9   Other fetus

O41.0- <u>Oligohydramnios</u> — The abnormally low amount of amniotic fluid. Oligohydramnios without rupture of membranes

O41.00x- Oligohydramnios, <u>unspecified</u> trimester — [♀, Age/12-55]
CC-0-9 **O41.01x-** Oligohydramnios, <u>first</u> trimester — [♀, Age/12-55]
CC-0-9 **O41.02x-** Oligohydramnios, <u>second</u> trimester — [♀, Age/12-55]
CC-0-9 **O41.03x-** Oligohydramnios, <u>third</u> trimester — [♀, Age/12-55]

O41.1- Infection of amniotic sac and membranes — Invasion of microorganisms of the amniotic cavity.

O41.10- <u>Infection of amniotic sac and membranes, unspecified</u>

MCC-0-9 **O41.101-** Infection of amniotic sac and membranes, unspecified, <u>first</u> trimester — [♀, Age/12-55]

MCC-0-9 **O41.102-** Infection of amniotic sac and membranes, unspecified, <u>second</u> trimester — [♀, Age/12-55]

MCC-0-9 **O41.103-** Infection of amniotic sac and membranes, unspecified, <u>third</u> trimester — [♀, Age/12-55]

O41.109- Infection of amniotic sac and membranes, unspecified, <u>unspecified</u> trimester — [♀, Age/12-55]

O41.12- <u>Chorioamnionitis</u> — Inflammation of the fetal amniotic membranes caused by microorganisms.

MCC-0-9 **O41.121-** Chorioamnionitis, <u>first</u> trimester — [♀, Age/12-55]
MCC-0-9 **O41.122-** Chorioamnionitis, <u>second</u> trimester — [♀, Age/12-55]
MCC-0-9 **O41.123-** Chorioamnionitis, <u>third</u> trimester — [♀, Age/12-55]
O41.129- Chorioamnionitis, <u>unspecified</u> trimester — [♀, Age/12-55]

O41.14- <u>Placentitis</u> — Inflammation of the placenta caused by microorganisms.

MCC-0-9 **O41.141-** Placentitis, <u>first</u> trimester — [♀, Age/12-55]
MCC-0-9 **O41.142-** Placentitis, <u>second</u> trimester — [♀, Age/12-55]
MCC-0-9 **O41.143-** Placentitis, <u>third</u> trimester — [♀, Age/12-55]
O41.149- Placentitis, <u>unspecified</u> trimester — [♀, Age/12-55]

O41.8- Other specified disorders of amniotic fluid and membranes

O41.8x- <u>Other specified</u> disorders of amniotic fluid and membranes

O41.8x1- Other specified disorders of amniotic fluid and membranes, <u>first</u> trimester — [♀, Age/12-55]

O41.8x2- Other specified disorders of amniotic fluid and membranes, <u>second</u> trimester — [♀, Age/12-55]

O41.8x3- Other specified disorders of amniotic fluid and membranes, <u>third</u> trimester — [♀, Age/12-55]

O41.8x9- Other specified disorders of amniotic fluid and membranes, <u>unspecified</u> trimester — [♀, Age/12-55]

O41.9- Disorder of amniotic fluid and membranes, <u>unspecified</u>

O41.90x- Disorder of amniotic fluid and membranes, unspecified, <u>unspecified</u> trimester — [♀, Age/12-55]

O41.91x- Disorder of amniotic fluid and membranes, unspecified, <u>first</u> trimester — [♀, Age/12-55]

O41.92x- Disorder of amniotic fluid and membranes, unspecified, <u>second</u> trimester — [♀, Age/12-55]

O36 - O41

O41.93x- Disorder of amniotic fluid and membranes, unspecified, <u>third</u> trimester — [♀, Age/12-55]

O42- <u>Premature rupture of membranes</u> — The rupture or tear of the amniotic sac prior to the onset of labor.
AHA 16:1Q:p3,5 – Premature rupture of membranes and laceration

O42.0- Premature rupture of membranes, <u>onset of labor within 24 hours of rupture</u>

O42.00 Premature rupture of membranes, onset of labor within 24 hours of rupture, <u>unspecified</u> weeks of gestation — [♀, Age/12-55]

O42.01- <u>Preterm</u> premature rupture of membranes, onset of labor within 24 hours of rupture
Premature rupture of membranes before 37 completed weeks of gestation

O42.011 Preterm premature rupture of membranes, onset of labor within 24 hours of rupture, <u>first</u> trimester — [♀, Age/12-55]

O42.012 Preterm premature rupture of membranes, onset of labor within 24 hours of rupture, <u>second</u> trimester — [♀, Age/12-55]

O42.013 Preterm premature rupture of membranes, onset of labor within 24 hours of rupture, <u>third</u> trimester — [♀, Age/12-55]

O42.019 Preterm premature rupture of membranes, onset of labor within 24 hours of rupture, <u>unspecified</u> trimester — [♀, Age/12-55]

O42.02 <u>Full-term</u> premature rupture of membranes, onset of labor within 24 hours of rupture — [♀, Age/12-55]
Premature rupture of membranes at or after 37 completed weeks of gestation, onset of labor within 24 hours of rupture

O42.1- Premature rupture of membranes, onset of labor <u>more than 24</u> hours following rupture

O42.10 Premature rupture of membranes, onset of labor more than 24 hours following rupture, unspecified weeks of gestation — [♀, Age/12-55]

O42.11- Preterm premature rupture of membranes, onset of labor more than 24 hours following rupture
Premature rupture of membranes before 37 completed weeks of gestation

O42.111 Preterm premature rupture of membranes, onset of labor more than 24 hours following rupture, <u>first</u> trimester — [♀, Age/12-55]

O42.112 Preterm premature rupture of membranes, onset of labor more than 24 hours following rupture, <u>second</u> trimester — [♀, Age/12-55]

O42.113 Preterm premature rupture of membranes, onset of labor more than 24 hours following rupture, <u>third</u> trimester — [♀, Age/12-55]

O42.119 Preterm premature rupture of membranes, onset of labor more than 24 hours following rupture, <u>unspecified</u> trimester — [♀, Age/12-55]

O42.12 <u>Full-term</u> premature rupture of membranes, onset of labor more than 24 hours following rupture — [♀, Age/12-55]
Premature rupture of membranes at or after 37 completed weeks of gestation, onset of labor more than 24 hours following rupture

O42.9- Premature rupture of membranes, <u>unspecified as to length of time</u> between rupture and onset of labor

O42.90 Premature rupture of membranes, unspecified as to length of time between rupture and onset of labor, unspecified weeks of gestation — [♀, Age/12-55]

O42.91- <u>Preterm</u> premature rupture of membranes, unspecified as to length of time between rupture and onset of labor
Premature rupture of membranes before 37 completed weeks of gestation

O42.911 Preterm premature rupture of membranes, unspecified as to length of time between rupture and onset of labor, <u>first</u> trimester — [♀, Age/12-55]

O42.912 Preterm premature rupture of membranes, unspecified as to length of time between rupture and onset of labor, <u>second</u> trimester — [♀, Age/12-55]

O42.913 Preterm premature rupture of membranes, unspecified as to length of time between rupture and onset of labor, <u>third</u> trimester — [♀, Age/12-55]

O42.919 Preterm premature rupture of membranes, unspecified as to length of time between rupture and onset of labor, <u>unspecified</u> trimester — [♀, Age/12-55]

O42.92 <u>Full-term</u> premature rupture of membranes, unspecified as to length of time between rupture and onset of labor — [♀, Age/12-55]
Premature rupture of membranes at or after 37 completed weeks of gestation, unspecified as to length of time between rupture and onset of labor

O43- Placental disorders
Excludes ❷: maternal care for poor fetal growth due to placental insufficiency (O36.5-)
placenta previa (O44.-)
placental polyp (O90.89)
placentitis (O41.14-)
premature separation of placenta [abruptio placentae] (O45.-)

O43.0- <u>Placental transfusion syndromes</u> — The abnormal flow of blood to the fetus.

O43.01- <u>Fetomaternal</u> placental transfusion syndrome— The abnormal flow of fetal blood cells to the mother through a defect in the placental membranes.
Maternofetal placental transfusion syndrome

O43.011 Fetomaternal placental transfusion syndrome, <u>first</u> trimester — [♀, Age/12-55]

O43.012 Fetomaternal placental transfusion syndrome, <u>second</u> trimester — [♀, Age/12-55]

O43.013 Fetomaternal placental transfusion syndrome, <u>third</u> trimester — [♀, Age/12-55]

O43.019 Fetomaternal placental transfusion syndrome, <u>unspecified</u> trimester — [♀, Age/12-55]

O43.02- <u>Fetus-to-fetus</u> placental transfusion syndrome — The disproportionate flow of blood to one fetus versus the other.

O43.021 Fetus-to-fetus placental transfusion syndrome, <u>first</u> trimester — [♀, Age/12-55]

O43.022 Fetus-to-fetus placental transfusion syndrome, <u>second</u> trimester — [♀, Age/12-55]

O43.023 Fetus-to-fetus placental transfusion syndrome, <u>third</u> trimester — [♀, Age/12-55]

O43.029 Fetus-to-fetus placental transfusion syndrome, <u>unspecified</u> trimester — [♀, Age/12-55]

O43.1- Malformation of placenta — The abnormal development of the placenta.

O43.10- <u>Malformation</u> of placenta, <u>unspecified</u>
Abnormal placenta NOS

O43.101 Malformation of placenta, unspecified, <u>first</u> trimester — [♀, Age/12-55]

O43.102 Malformation of placenta, unspecified, <u>second</u> trimester — [♀, Age/12-55]

O43.103 Malformation of placenta, unspecified, <u>third</u> trimester — [♀, Age/12-55]

O43.109 Malformation of placenta, unspecified, <u>unspecified</u> trimester — [♀, Age/12-55]

O43.11- <u>Circumvallate</u> placenta — A condition in which the layers of the placenta fold into an abnormal position.

O43.111 Circumvallate placenta, <u>first</u> trimester — [♀, Age/12-55]

O43.112 Circumvallate placenta, <u>second</u> trimester — [♀, Age/12-55]

O43.113 Circumvallate placenta, <u>third</u> trimester — [♀, Age/12-55]

O43.119 Circumvallate placenta, <u>unspecified</u> trimester — [♀, Age/12-55]

O43.12-   <u>Velamentous</u> insertion of umbilical cord — The abnormal insertion of the umbilical cord in the placenta.

     O43.121   Velamentous insertion of umbilical cord, <u>first</u> trimester — [♀, Age/12-55]

     O43.122   Velamentous insertion of umbilical cord, <u>second</u> trimester — [♀, Age/12-55]

     O43.123   Velamentous insertion of umbilical cord, <u>third</u> trimester — [♀, Age/12-55]

     O43.129   Velamentous insertion of umbilical cord, <u>unspecified</u> trimester — [♀, Age/12-55]

O43.19-   <u>Other</u> malformation of placenta

     O43.191   Other malformation of placenta, <u>first</u> trimester — [♀, Age/12-55]

     O43.192   Other malformation of placenta, <u>second</u> trimester — [♀, Age/12-55]

     O43.193   Other malformation of placenta, <u>third</u> trimester — [♀, Age/12-55]

     O43.199   Other malformation of placenta, <u>unspecified</u> trimester — [♀, Age/12-55]

O43.2-   Morbidly adherent placenta

   Code also associated third stage postpartum hemorrhage, if applicable (O72.0)

     Excludes 1:   retained placenta (O73.-)

O43.21-   Placenta <u>accreta</u> — The abnormally deep attachment of the placenta onto the myometrium instead of the endometrium of pregnancy (decidua).

     O43.211   Placenta accreta, <u>first</u> trimester — [♀, Age/12-55]

     O43.212   Placenta accreta, <u>second</u> trimester — [♀, Age/12-55]

     O43.213   Placenta accreta, <u>third</u> trimester — [♀, Age/12-55]

     O43.219   Placenta accreta, <u>unspecified</u> trimester — [♀, Age/12-55]

O43.22-   Placenta <u>increta</u> — The abnormally deep attachment of the placenta into the myometrium.

     O43.221   Placenta increta, <u>first</u> trimester — [♀, Age/12-55]

     O43.222   Placenta increta, <u>second</u> trimester — [♀, Age/12-55]

     O43.223   Placenta increta, <u>third</u> trimester — [♀, Age/12-55]

     O43.229   Placenta increta, <u>unspecified</u> trimester — [♀, Age/12-55]

O43.23-   Placenta <u>percreta</u> — The abnormally deep attachment of the placenta and through the myometrium.

     O43.231   Placenta percreta, <u>first</u> trimester — [♀, Age/12-55]

     O43.232   Placenta percreta, <u>second</u> trimester — [♀, Age/12-55]

     O43.233   Placenta percreta, <u>third</u> trimester — [♀, Age/12-55]

     O43.239   Placenta percreta, <u>unspecified</u> trimester — [♀, Age/12-55]

O43.8-   Other placental disorders

O43.81-   Placental <u>infarction</u> — Ischemic placental tissue necrosis due to obstruction of a placental vessel.

     O43.811   Placental infarction, <u>first</u> trimester — [♀, Age/12-55]

     O43.812   Placental infarction, <u>second</u> trimester — [♀, Age/12-55]

     O43.813   Placental infarction, <u>third</u> trimester — [♀, Age/12-55]

     O43.819   Placental infarction, <u>unspecified</u> trimester — [♀, Age/12-55]

O43.89-   <u>Other</u> placental disorders

   Placental dysfunction

     O43.891   Other placental disorders, <u>first</u> trimester — [♀, Age/12-55]

     O43.892   Other placental disorders, <u>second</u> trimester — [♀, Age/12-55]

     O43.893   Other placental disorders, <u>third</u> trimester — [♀, Age/12-55]

     O43.899   Other placental disorders, <u>unspecified</u> trimester — [♀, Age/12-55]

O43.9-   <u>Unspecified</u> placental disorder

     O43.90   Unspecified placental disorder, <u>unspecified</u> trimester — [♀, Age/12-55]

     O43.91   Unspecified placental disorder, <u>first</u> trimester — [♀, Age/12-55]

     O43.92   Unspecified placental disorder, <u>second</u> trimester — [♀, Age/12-55]

     O43.93   Unspecified placental disorder, <u>third</u> trimester — [♀, Age/12-55]

O44-   <u>Placenta previa</u> — The implantation of the placenta in the lower uterine segment.

O44.0-   <u>Complete</u> placenta previa <u>NOS or without hemorrhage</u>

   Placenta previa NOS

     O44.00   Complete placenta previa NOS or without hemorrhage, <u>unspecified</u> trimester — [♀, Age/12-55]

   cc **O44.01**   Complete placenta previa NOS or without hemorrhage, <u>first</u> trimester — [♀, Age/12-55]

   cc **O44.02**   Complete placenta previa NOS or without hemorrhage, <u>second</u> trimester — [♀, Age/12-55]

   cc **O44.03**   Complete placenta previa NOS or without hemorrhage, <u>third</u> trimester — [♀, Age/12-55]

O44.1-   <u>Complete</u> placenta previa <u>with hemorrhage</u>

     Excludes 1:   labor and delivery complicated by hemorrhage from vasa previa (O69.4)

     O44.10   Complete placenta previa with hemorrhage, <u>unspecified</u> trimester — [♀, Age/12-55]

   MCC **O44.11**   Complete placenta previa with hemorrhage, <u>first</u> trimester — [♀, Age/12-55]

   MCC **O44.12**   Complete placenta previa with hemorrhage, <u>second</u> trimester — [♀, Age/12-55]

   MCC **O44.13**   Complete placenta previa with hemorrhage, <u>third</u> trimester — [♀, Age/12-55]

O44.2-   <u>Partial</u> placenta previa <u>without hemorrhage</u>

   Marginal placenta previa, NOS or without hemorrhage

     O44.20   Partial placenta previa NOS or without hemorrhage, <u>unspecified</u> trimester — [♀, Age/12-55]

   cc **O44.21**   Partial placenta previa NOS or without hemorrhage, <u>first</u> trimester — [♀, Age/12-55]

   cc **O44.22**   Partial placenta previa NOS or without hemorrhage, <u>second</u> trimester — [♀, Age/12-55]

   cc **O44.23**   Partial placenta previa NOS or without hemorrhage, <u>third</u> trimester — [♀, Age/12-55]

O44.3-   <u>Partial</u> placenta previa <u>with hemorrhage</u>

   Marginal placenta previa with hemorrhage

     O44.30   Partial placenta previa with hemorrhage, <u>unspecified</u> trimester — [♀, Age/12-55]

   MCC **O44.31**   Partial placenta previa with hemorrhage, <u>first</u> trimester — [♀, Age/12-55]

   MCC **O44.32**   Partial placenta previa with hemorrhage, <u>second</u> trimester — [♀, Age/12-55]

   MCC **O44.33**   Partial placenta previa with hemorrhage, <u>third</u> trimester — [♀, Age/12-55]

O44.4-   <u>Low lying</u> placenta <u>NOS or without hemorrhage</u>

   Low implantation of placenta NOS or without hemorrhage

     O44.40   Low lying placenta NOS or without hemorrhage, <u>unspecified</u> trimester — [♀, Age/12-55]

   cc **O44.41**   Low lying placenta NOS or without hemorrhage, <u>first</u> trimester — [♀, Age/12-55]

   cc **O44.42**   Low lying placenta NOS or without hemorrhage, <u>second</u> trimester — [♀, Age/12-55]

   cc **O44.43**   Low lying placenta NOS or without hemorrhage, <u>third</u> trimester — [♀, Age/12-55]

O44.5-   <u>Low lying</u> placenta <u>with hemorrhage</u>

   Low implantation of placenta with hemorrhage

     O44.50   Low lying placenta with hemorrhage, <u>unspecified</u> trimester — [♀, Age/12-55]

   MCC **O44.51**   Low lying placenta with hemorrhage, <u>first</u> trimester — [♀, Age/12-55]

   MCC **O44.52**   Low lying placenta with hemorrhage, <u>second</u> trimester — [♀, Age/12-55]

   MCC **O44.53**   Low lying placenta with hemorrhage, <u>third</u> trimester — [♀, Age/12-55]

O 43 - O 44

O45- <u>Premature separation of placenta [abruptio placentae]</u> — The premature detachment of the placenta from the uterus.

O45.0- Premature separation of placenta <u>with coagulation defect</u>

O45.00- Premature separation of placenta with coagulation defect, <u>unspecified</u>

MCC **O45.001** Premature separation of placenta with coagulation defect, unspecified, <u>first</u> trimester — [♀, Age/12-55]

MCC **O45.002** Premature separation of placenta with coagulation defect, unspecified, <u>second</u> trimester — [♀, Age/12-55]

MCC **O45.003** Premature separation of placenta with coagulation defect, unspecified, <u>third</u> trimester — [♀, Age/12-55]

O45.009 Premature separation of placenta with coagulation defect, unspecified, <u>unspecified</u> trimester — [♀, Age/12-55]

O45.01- Premature separation of placenta <u>with afibrinogenemia</u> — A form caused by the decreased ability of the blood to coagulate due to the decrease or absence of fibrinogen in the blood plasma.

Premature separation of placenta with hypofibrinogenemia

MCC **O45.011** Premature separation of placenta with afibrinogenemia, <u>first</u> trimester — [♀, Age/12-55]

MCC **O45.012** Premature separation of placenta with afibrinogenemia, <u>second</u> trimester — [♀, Age/12-55]

MCC **O45.013** Premature separation of placenta with afibrinogenemia, <u>third</u> trimester — [♀, Age/12-55]

O45.019 Premature separation of placenta with afibrinogenemia, <u>unspecified</u> trimester — [♀, Age/12-55]

O45.02- Premature separation of placenta <u>with disseminated intravascular coagulation</u> — The condition of abnormal blood clotting and compromised blood flow.

MCC **O45.021** Premature separation of placenta with disseminated intravascular coagulation, <u>first</u> trimester — [♀, Age/12-55]

MCC **O45.022** Premature separation of placenta with disseminated intravascular coagulation, <u>second</u> trimester — [♀, Age/12-55]

MCC **O45.023** Premature separation of placenta with disseminated intravascular coagulation, <u>third</u> trimester — [♀, Age/12-55]

O45.029 Premature separation of placenta with disseminated intravascular coagulation, <u>unspecified</u> trimester — [♀, Age/12-55]

O45.09- Premature separation of placenta <u>with other coagulation defect</u>

MCC **O45.091** Premature separation of placenta with other coagulation defect, <u>first</u> trimester — [♀, Age/12-55]

MCC **O45.092** Premature separation of placenta with other coagulation defect, <u>second</u> trimester — [♀, Age/12-55]

MCC **O45.093** Premature separation of placenta with other coagulation defect, <u>third</u> trimester — [♀, Age/12-55]

O45.099 Premature separation of placenta with other coagulation defect, <u>unspecified</u> trimester — [♀, Age/12-55]

O45.8- Other premature separation of placenta

O45.8x-<u>Other</u> premature separation of placenta

MCC **O45.8x1** Other premature separation of placenta, <u>first</u> trimester — [♀, Age/12-55]

MCC **O45.8x2** Other premature separation of placenta, <u>second</u> trimester — [♀, Age/12-55]

MCC **O45.8x3** Other premature separation of placenta, <u>third</u> trimester — [♀, Age/12-55]

O45.8x9 Other premature separation of placenta, <u>unspecified</u> trimester — [♀, Age/12-55]

O45.9- Premature separation of placenta, <u>unspecified</u>
Abruptio placentae NOS

O45.90 Premature separation of placenta, unspecified, <u>unspecified</u> trimester — [♀, Age/12-55]

MCC **O45.91** Premature separation of placenta, unspecified, <u>first</u> trimester — [♀, Age/12-55]

MCC **O45.92** Premature separation of placenta, unspecified, <u>second</u> trimester — [♀, Age/12-55]

MCC **O45.93** Premature separation of placenta, unspecified, <u>third</u> trimester — [♀, Age/12-55]

O46- <u>Antepartum hemorrhage, not elsewhere classified</u>

Excludes 1: hemorrhage in early pregnancy (O20.-)
intrapartum hemorrhage NEC (O67.-)
placenta previa (O44.-)
premature separation of placenta [abruptio placentae] (O45.-)

O46.0- Antepartum hemorrhage with coagulation defect — Bloody uterine discharge due to impairment of the blood to normally coagulate.

O46.00- Antepartum hemorrhage <u>with coagulation defect</u>, <u>unspecified</u>

MCC **O46.001** Antepartum hemorrhage with coagulation defect, unspecified, <u>first</u> trimester — [♀, Age/12-55]

MCC **O46.002** Antepartum hemorrhage with coagulation defect, unspecified, <u>second</u> trimester — [♀, Age/12-55]

MCC **O46.003** Antepartum hemorrhage with coagulation defect, unspecified, <u>third</u> trimester — [♀, Age/12-55]

O46.009 Antepartum hemorrhage with coagulation defect, unspecified, <u>unspecified</u> trimester — [♀, Age/12-55]

O46.01- Antepartum hemorrhage <u>with afibrinogenemia</u> — A form caused by the decreased ability of the blood to coagulate due to the decrease or absence of fibrinogen in the blood plasma.

Antepartum hemorrhage with hypofibrinogenemia

MCC **O46.011** Antepartum hemorrhage with afibrinogenemia, <u>first</u> trimester — [♀, Age/12-55]

MCC **O46.012** Antepartum hemorrhage with afibrinogenemia, <u>second</u> trimester — [♀, Age/12-55]

MCC **O46.013** Antepartum hemorrhage with afibrinogenemia, <u>third</u> trimester — [♀, Age/12-55]

O46.019 Antepartum hemorrhage with afibrinogenemia, <u>unspecified</u> trimester — [♀, Age/12-55]

O46.02- Antepartum hemorrhage <u>with disseminated intravascular coagulation</u> — The condition of abnormal blood clotting and compromised blood flow.

MCC **O46.021** Antepartum hemorrhage with disseminated intravascular coagulation, <u>first</u> trimester — [♀, Age/12-55]

MCC **O46.022** Antepartum hemorrhage with disseminated intravascular coagulation, <u>second</u> trimester — [♀, Age/12-55]

MCC **O46.023** Antepartum hemorrhage with disseminated intravascular coagulation, <u>third</u> trimester — [♀, Age/12-55]

O46.029 Antepartum hemorrhage with disseminated intravascular coagulation, <u>unspecified</u> trimester — [♀, Age/12-55]

O46.09- Antepartum hemorrhage <u>with other coagulation defect</u>

MCC **O46.091** Antepartum hemorrhage with other coagulation defect, <u>first</u> trimester — [♀, Age/12-55]

MCC **O46.092** Antepartum hemorrhage with other coagulation defect, <u>second</u> trimester — [♀, Age/12-55]

MCC **O46.093** Antepartum hemorrhage with other coagulation defect, <u>third</u> trimester — [♀, Age/12-55]

O46.099 Antepartum hemorrhage with other coagulation defect, <u>unspecified</u> trimester — [♀, Age/12-55]

O46.8- Other antepartum hemorrhage

O46.8x-<u>Other antepartum hemorrhage</u>

O46.8x1 Other antepartum hemorrhage, <u>first</u> trimester — [♀, Age/12-55]

O46.8x2 Other antepartum hemorrhage, <u>second</u> trimester — [♀, Age/12-55]

O46.8x3 Other antepartum hemorrhage, <u>third</u> trimester — [♀, Age/12-55]

O46.8x9 Other antepartum hemorrhage, unspecified trimester — [♀, Age/12-55]

O
4
5
-
O
4
6

O46.9-   Antepartum hemorrhage, <u>unspecified</u>

    O46.90   Antepartum hemorrhage, unspecified, <u>unspecified</u> trimester — [♀, Age/12-55]

    O46.91   Antepartum hemorrhage, unspecified, <u>first</u> trimester — [♀, Age/12-55]

    O46.92   Antepartum hemorrhage, unspecified, <u>second</u> trimester — [♀, Age/12-55]

    O46.93   Antepartum hemorrhage, unspecified, <u>third</u> trimester — [♀, Age/12-55]

O47-   <u>False labor</u> — Labor symptoms occurring before the actual onset of labor.
    Includes: Braxton Hicks contractions
             Threatened labor
    Excludes 1:   preterm labor (O60.-)

    O47.0-   False labor before 37 completed weeks of gestation

        O47.00   False labor before 37 completed weeks of gestation, unspecified trimester — [♀, Age/12-55]

   cc   O47.02   False labor before 37 completed weeks of gestation, <u>second</u> trimester — [♀, Age/12-55]

   cc   O47.03   False labor before 37 completed weeks of gestation, <u>third</u> trimester — [♀, Age/12-55]

  cc   O47.1   False labor at or after 37 completed weeks of gestation — [♀, Age/12-55]

    O47.9   False labor, unspecified — [♀, Age/12-55]

O48-   <u>Late pregnancy</u>

    O48.0   Post-term pregnancy — [♀, Age/12-55]
        AHA 16:1Q:p5 – Delivery complicated by post-term pregnancy
        Pregnancy over 40 completed weeks to 42 completed weeks gestation

    O48.1   Prolonged pregnancy — [♀, Age/12-55]
        Pregnancy which has advanced beyond 42 completed weeks gestation

Complications of labor and delivery (O60-O77)

O60-   <u>Preterm labor</u>
    AHA 12:4Q:p107 – Fetus A and B same as fetus 1 and 2
    Includes: Onset (spontaneous) of labor before 37 completed weeks of gestation
    Excludes 1:   false labor (O47.0-)
                 threatened labor NOS (O47.0-)

    O60.0-   Preterm labor <u>without</u> delivery — The onset of labor before the pregnancy has reached term, and without delivery.

        O60.00   Preterm labor without delivery, <u>unspecified</u> trimester — [♀, Age/12-55]

   MCC   O60.02   Preterm labor without delivery, <u>second</u> trimester — [♀, Age/12-55]

   MCC   O60.03   Preterm labor without delivery, <u>third</u> trimester — [♀, Age/12-55]

    O60.1-   Preterm labor <u>with preterm delivery</u> — The onset of labor before the pregnancy has reached term, and with delivery before term.
        AHA 16:2Q:p10 – Twin pregnancy, preterm delivery

> One of the following 7th characters is to be assigned to each code under subcategory O60.1. 7th character 0 is for single gestations and multiple gestations where the fetus is unspecified. 7th characters 1 through 9 are for cases of multiple gestations to identify the fetus for which the code applies. The appropriate code from category O30, Multiple gestation, must also be assigned when assigning a code from subcategory O60.1 that has a 7th character of 1 through 9.
> 0   Not applicable or unspecified
> 1   Fetus 1
> 2   Fetus 2
> 3   Fetus 3
> 4   Fetus 4
> 5   Fetus 5
> 9   Other fetus

  CC-0-9   O60.10x-   Preterm labor with preterm delivery, <u>unspecified</u> trimester — [♀, Age/12-55]
           Preterm labor with delivery NOS

  MCC-0-9   O60.12x-   Preterm labor <u>second</u> trimester with preterm delivery <u>second</u> trimester — [♀, Age/12-55]

  MCC-0-9   O60.13x-   Preterm labor <u>second</u> trimester with preterm delivery <u>third</u> trimester — [♀, Age/12-55]

  MCC-0-9   O60.14x-   Preterm labor <u>third</u> trimester with preterm delivery <u>third</u> trimester — [♀, Age/12-55]

    O60.2-   <u>Term delivery with preterm labor</u> — The onset of labor before the pregnancy has reached term, and with delivery at term.

> One of the following 7th characters is to be assigned to each code under subcategory O60.2. 7th character 0 is for single gestations and multiple gestations where the fetus is unspecified. 7th characters 1 through 9 are for cases of multiple gestations to identify the fetus for which the code applies. The appropriate code from category O30, Multiple gestation, must also be assigned when assigning a code from subcategory O60.2 that has a 7th character of 1 through 9.
> 0   Not applicable or unspecified
> 1   Fetus 1
> 2   Fetus 2
> 3   Fetus 3
> 4   Fetus 4
> 5   Fetus 5
> 9   Other fetus

  CC-0-9   O60.20x-   Term delivery with preterm labor, <u>unspecified</u> trimester — [♀, Age/12-55]

  MCC-0-9   O60.22x-   Term delivery with preterm labor, <u>second</u> trimester — [♀, Age/12-55]

  MCC-0-9   O60.23x-   Term delivery with preterm labor, <u>third</u> trimester — [♀, Age/12-55]

O61-   <u>Failed induction of labor</u>

    O61.0   Failed medical induction of labor — [♀, Age/12-55] – Failure of induction of labor by medical methods, such as oxytocic drugs.
        Failed induction (of labor) by oxytocin
        Failed induction (of labor) by prostaglandins

    O61.1-   Failed instrumental induction of labor — [♀, Age/12-55] – Failure of induction of labor by surgical or other instrumental methods.
        Failed mechanical induction (of labor)
        Failed surgical induction (of labor)

    O61.8   Other failed induction of labor — [♀, Age/12-55]

    O61.9   Failed induction of labor, unspecified — [♀, Age/12-55]

O62-   <u>Abnormalities of forces of labor</u>

    O62.0   Primary inadequate contractions — [♀, Age/12-55] – Dysfunction and weakness of uterine contractions during the first stage of labor.
        Failure of cervical dilatation
        Primary hypotonic uterine dysfunction
        Uterine inertia during latent phase of labor

    O62.1   Secondary uterine inertia — [♀, Age/12-55] – Dysfunction and weakness of uterine contractions during the second stage of labor.
        Arrested active phase of labor
        Secondary hypotonic uterine dysfunction

    O62.2   Other uterine inertia — [♀, Age/12-55]
        Atony of uterus without hemorrhage — The loss of normal uterine muscle tone, without any associated hemorrhage.
        Atony of uterus NOS
        Desultory labor — Random uterine contractions.
        Hypotonic uterine dysfunction NOS
        Irregular labor — Varying intensity of uterine contractions.
        Poor contractions — Weak uterine contractions.
        Slow slope active phase of labor — Less than the normal intensity of contractions and progression of labor.
        Uterine inertia NOS
    Excludes 1:   atony of uterus with hemorrhage (postpartum) (O72.1)
                 postpartum atony of uterus without hemorrhage (O75.89)

    O62.3   Precipitate labor — [♀, Age/12-55] – Frequent, intense contractions with rapid delivery.

O 4 6 – O 6 2

O62.4 Hypertonic, incoordinate, and prolonged uterine contractions — [♀, Age/12-55] – The increased resting tone and uncoordinated, or abnormally long uterine contractions.
  Cervical spasm — The abnormally intense contraction of the cervix.
  Contraction ring dystocia — The ring-like circular muscle contraction of the uterus.
  Dyscoordinate labor — Uncoordinated uterine contractions.
  Hour-glass contraction of uterus — The ring-like circular muscle contraction of the uterus.
  Hypertonic uterine dysfunction — The increased resting tone of the uterus.
  Incoordinate uterine action — Uncoordinated uterine contractions.
  Tetanic contractions — The abnormal sustained contraction of the uterus.
  Uterine dystocia NOS
  Uterine spasm — The abnormally intense contraction of the uterus.
  Excludes 1: dystocia (fetal) (maternal) NOS (O66.9)

O62.8 Other abnormalities of forces of labor — [♀, Age/12-55]

O62.9 Abnormality of forces of labor, unspecified — [♀, Age/12-55]

O63- Long labor — Labor prolonged beyond the normal length of time, generally considered more than 18 hours.

O63.0 Prolonged first stage (of labor) — [♀, Age/12-55]

O63.1 Prolonged second stage (of labor) — [♀, Age/12-55]

O63.2 Delayed delivery of second twin, triplet, etc. — [♀, Age/12-55]

cc **O63.9 Long labor, unspecified** — [♀, Age/12-55]
  Prolonged labor NOS

O64- Obstructed labor due to malposition and malpresentation of fetus
  AHA 12:4Q:p107 – Fetus A and B same as fetus 1 and 2

  One of the following 7th characters is to be assigned to each code under category O64. 7th character 0 is for single gestations and multiple gestations where the fetus is unspecified. 7th characters 1 through 9 are for cases of multiple gestations to identify the fetus for which the code applies. The appropriate code from category O30, Multiple gestation, must also be assigned when assigning a code from category O64 that has a 7th character of 1 through 9.
  0   Not applicable or unspecified
  1   Fetus 1
  2   Fetus 2
  3   Fetus 3
  4   Fetus 4
  5   Fetus 5
  9   Other fetus

O64.0xx- Obstructed labor due to incomplete rotation of fetal head — [♀, Age/12-55]
  Deep transverse arrest
  Obstructed labor due to persistent occipitoiliac (position)
  Obstructed labor due to persistent occipitoposterior (position)
  Obstructed labor due to persistent occipitosacral (position)
  Obstructed labor due to persistent occipitotransverse (position)

O64.1xx- Obstructed labor due to breech presentation — [♀, Age/12-55]
  Obstructed labor due to buttocks presentation
  Obstructed labor due to complete breech presentation
  Obstructed labor due to frank breech presentation

O64.2xx- Obstructed labor due to face presentation — [♀, Age/12-55]
  Obstructed labor due to chin presentation

O64.3xx- Obstructed labor due to brow presentation — [♀, Age/12-55]

O64.4xx- Obstructed labor due to shoulder presentation — [♀, Age/12-55]
  Prolapsed arm
  Excludes 1: impacted shoulders (O66.0)
    shoulder dystocia (O66.0)

O64.5xx- Obstructed labor due to compound presentation — [♀, Age/12-55]

O64.8xx- Obstructed labor due to other malposition and malpresentation — [♀, Age/12-55]
  Obstructed labor due to footling presentation
  Obstructed labor due to incomplete breech presentation

O64.9xx- Obstructed labor due to malposition and malpresentation, unspecified — [♀, Age/12-55]

O65- Obstructed labor due to maternal pelvic abnormality

O65.0 Obstructed labor due to deformed pelvis — [♀, Age/12-55]

O65.1 Obstructed labor due to generally contracted pelvis — [♀, Age/12-55] – A pelvic opening that is reduced more than 2 cm in diameter.

O65.2 Obstructed labor due to pelvic inlet contraction — [♀, Age/12-55] – The reduced upper opening of the pelvis.

O65.3 Obstructed labor due to pelvic outlet and mid-cavity contraction — [♀, Age/12-55] – The reduced lower opening of the pelvis.

O65.4 Obstructed labor due to fetopelvic disproportion, unspecified — [♀, Age/12-55]
  Excludes 1: dystocia due to abnormality of fetus (O66.2-O66.3)

O65.5 Obstructed labor due to abnormality of maternal pelvic organs — [♀, Age/12-55]
  Obstructed labor due to conditions listed in O34.-
  Use additional code to identify abnormality of pelvic organs O34.-

O65.8 Obstructed labor due to other maternal pelvic abnormalities — [♀, Age/12-55]

O65.9 Obstructed labor due to maternal pelvic abnormality, unspecified — [♀, Age/12-55]

O66- Other obstructed labor

O66.0 Obstructed labor due to shoulder dystocia — [♀, Age/12-55] – Obstructed labor due to impaction of the shoulders at the pelvic brim.
  Impacted shoulders

O66.1 Obstructed labor due to locked twins — [♀, Age/12-55] – Obstructed labor due to entwined necks of twins.

O66.2 Obstructed labor due to unusually large fetus — [♀, Age/12-55]

O66.3 Obstructed labor due to other abnormalities of fetus — [♀, Age/12-55]
  Dystocia due to fetal ascites
  Dystocia due to fetal hydrops
  Dystocia due to fetal meningomyelocele
  Dystocia due to fetal sacral teratoma
  Dystocia due to fetal tumor
  Dystocia due to hydrocephalic fetus
  Use additional code to identify cause of obstruction

O66.4- Failed trial of labor

  O66.40 Failed trial of labor, unspecified — [♀, Age/12-55]

  O66.41 Failed attempted vaginal birth after previous cesarean delivery — [♀, Age/12-55]
    Code first rupture of uterus, if applicable (O71.0-, O71.1)

O66.5 Attempted application of vacuum extractor and forceps — [♀, Age/12-55]
  Attempted application of vacuum or forceps, with subsequent delivery by forceps or cesarean delivery

O66.6 Obstructed labor due to other multiple fetuses — [♀, Age/12-55]

O66.8 Other specified obstructed labor — [♀, Age/12-55]
  Use additional code to identify cause of obstruction

O66.9 Obstructed labor, unspecified — [♀, Age/12-55]
  Dystocia NOS
  Fetal dystocia NOS
  Maternal dystocia NOS

O67- Labor and delivery complicated by intrapartum hemorrhage, not elsewhere classified
  Excludes 1: antepartum hemorrhage NEC (O46.-)
    placenta previa (O44.-)
    premature separation of placenta [abruptio placentae] (O45.-)
  Excludes ❷: postpartum hemorrhage (O72.-)

MCC **O67.0 Intrapartum hemorrhage with coagulation defect** — [♀, Age/12-55]
  Intrapartum hemorrhage (excessive) associated with afibrinogenemia
  Intrapartum hemorrhage (excessive) associated with disseminated intravascular coagulation
  Intrapartum hemorrhage (excessive) associated with hyperfibrinolysis
  Intrapartum hemorrhage (excessive) associated with hypofibrinogenemia

O67.8 Other intrapartum hemorrhage — [♀, Age/12-55]
  Excessive intrapartum hemorrhage

O67.9 Intrapartum hemorrhage, unspecified — [♀, Age/12-55]

O62-O67

O68 Labor and delivery complicated by abnormality of fetal acid-base

CC balance — [♀, Age/12-55]
Fetal acidemia complicating labor and delivery
Fetal acidosis complicating labor and delivery
Fetal alkalosis complicating labor and delivery
Fetal metabolic acidemia complicating labor and delivery
Excludes 1: *fetal stress NOS (O77.9)*
labor and delivery complicated by electrocardiographic evidence of fetal stress (O77.8)
labor and delivery complicated by ultrasonic evidence of fetal stress (O77.8)
Excludes ❷: *abnormality in fetal heart rate or rhythm (O76)*
labor and delivery complicated by meconium in amniotic fluid (O77.0)

O69- Labor and delivery complicated by umbilical cord complications

AHA 12:4Q:p107 – Fetus A and B same as fetus 1 and 2

One of the following 7th characters is to be assigned to each code under category O69. 7th character 0 is for single gestations and multiple gestations where the fetus is unspecified. 7th characters 1 through 9 are for cases of multiple gestations to identify the fetus for which the code applies. The appropriate code from category O30, Multiple gestation, must also be assigned when assigning a code from category O69 that has a 7th character of 1 through 9.

0 Not applicable or unspecified
1 Fetus 1
2 Fetus 2
3 Fetus 3
4 Fetus 4
5 Fetus 5
9 Other fetus

O69.0xx- Labor and delivery complicated by prolapse of cord —
[♀, Age/12-55] – The abnormal presentation of the umbilical cord in the vagina.

O69.1xx- Labor and delivery complicated by cord around neck, with compression — [♀, Age/12-55] – The abnormal presence of the umbilical cord wrapped around the fetal neck, with constricting tension on the neck.
Excludes 1: *labor and delivery complicated by cord around neck, without compression (O69.81)*

O69.2xx- Labor and delivery complicated by other cord entanglement, with compression — [♀, Age/12-55] – Umbilical cord entanglement with the fetus, other than wrapped around the neck, and with constricting tension to the affected part.
Labor and delivery complicated by compression of cord NOS
Labor and delivery complicated by entanglement of cords of twins in monoamniotic sac
Labor and delivery complicated by knot in cord
Excludes 1: *labor and delivery complicated by other cord entanglement, without compression (O69.82)*

O69.3xx- Labor and delivery complicated by short cord —
[♀, Age/12-55] – The abnormally small length of the umbilical cord.

O69.4xx- Labor and delivery complicated by vasa previa —
[♀, Age/12-55] – The abnormal presentation of the umbilical vessels in front of the fetal head.
Labor and delivery complicated by hemorrhage from vasa previa

O69.5xx- Labor and delivery complicated by vascular lesion of cord — [♀, Age/12-55] – Damage to or medical condition of the umbilical cord vessels.
Labor and delivery complicated by cord bruising
Labor and delivery complicated by cord hematoma
Labor and delivery complicated by thrombosis of umbilical vessels

O69.8- Labor and delivery complicated by other cord complications

O69.81x- Labor and delivery complicated by cord around neck, without compression — [♀, Age/12-55]

O69.82x- Labor and delivery complicated by other cord entanglement, without compression — [♀, Age/12-55]

O69.89x- Labor and delivery complicated by other cord complications — [♀, Age/12-55]

O69.9xx- Labor and delivery complicated by cord complication, unspecified — [♀, Age/12-55]

O70- Perineal laceration during delivery
AHA 16:1Q:p6-8 – Perineal lacerations
AHA 16:1Q:p4 – Polyhydramnios and laceration
AHA 16:1Q:p3,5 – Premature rupture of membranes and laceration
Includes: Episiotomy extended by laceration — The tearing continuance of the surgical incision of the vulvar orifice.
Excludes 1: *obstetric high vaginal laceration alone (O71.4)*

O70.0 First degree perineal laceration during delivery —
[♀, Age/12-55] – A tear of the superficial layers of the perineal organs.
Perineal laceration, rupture or tear involving fourchette during delivery
Perineal laceration, rupture or tear involving labia during delivery
Perineal laceration, rupture or tear involving skin during delivery
Perineal laceration, rupture or tear involving vagina during delivery
Perineal laceration, rupture or tear involving vulva during delivery
Slight perineal laceration, rupture or tear during delivery

O70.1 Second degree perineal laceration during delivery —
[♀, Age/12-55] – A tear of the inner and muscular layers of the perineal organs.
AHA 16:2Q:p34 – Second degree perineal laceration
Perineal laceration, rupture or tear during delivery as in O70.0, also involving pelvic floor
Perineal laceration, rupture or tear during delivery as in O70.0, also involving perineal muscles
Perineal laceration, rupture or tear during delivery as in O70.0, also involving vaginal muscles
Excludes 1: *perineal laceration involving anal sphincter (O70.2)*

O70.2- Third degree perineal laceration during delivery — A tear of the tissues between the vaginal and perineal muscular layers and the rectal mucosa/sphincter.
Perineal laceration, rupture or tear during delivery as in O70.1, also involving anal sphincter
Perineal laceration, rupture or tear during delivery as in O70.1, also involving rectovaginal septum
Perineal laceration, rupture or tear during delivery as in O70.1, also involving sphincter NOS
Excludes 1: *anal sphincter tear during delivery without third degree perineal laceration (O70.4)*
perineal laceration involving anal or rectal mucosa (O70.3)

CC **O70.20** Third degree perineal laceration during delivery, unspecified — [♀, Age/12-55]

CC **O70.21** Third degree perineal laceration during delivery, IIIa — [♀, Age/12-55]
Third degree perineal laceration during delivery with less than 50% of external anal sphincter (EAS) thickness torn

CC **O70.22** Third degree perineal laceration during delivery, IIIb — [♀, Age/12-55]
Third degree perineal laceration during delivery with more than 50% of external anal sphincter (EAS) thickness torn

CC **O70.23** Third degree perineal laceration during delivery, IIIc — [♀, Age/12-55]
Third degree perineal laceration during delivery with both external anal sphincter (EAS) and internal anal sphincter (IAS) torn

CC **O70.3** Fourth degree perineal laceration during delivery —
[♀, Age/12-55] – A tear that extends into the anal and rectal mucosa.
Perineal laceration, rupture or tear during delivery as in O70.2, also involving anal mucosa
Perineal laceration, rupture or tear during delivery as in O70.2, also involving rectal mucosa

CC **O70.4** Anal sphincter tear complicating delivery, not associated with third degree laceration — [♀, Age/12-55]
Excludes 1: *anal sphincter tear with third degree perineal laceration (O70.2)*

O70.9 Perineal laceration during delivery, unspecified —
[♀, Age/12-55]

O71- Other obstetric trauma
Includes: Obstetric damage from instruments

O71.0- Rupture of uterus (spontaneous) before onset of labor — The tearing-open of the uterus wall, before the onset of labor.
Excludes 1: *disruption of (current) cesarean delivery wound (O90.0)*
laceration of uterus, NEC (O71.81)

O71.00 Rupture of uterus before onset of labor, unspecified trimester — [♀, Age/12-55]

MCC **O71.02** Rupture of uterus before onset of labor, second trimester — [♀, Age/12-55]

O 6 8 - O 7 1

© 2016 Channel Publishing, Ltd.

MCC O71.03 Rupture of uterus before onset of labor, <u>third</u> trimester — [♀, Age/12-55]

MCC O71.1 Rupture of uterus <u>during labor</u> — [♀, Age/12-55] – The tearing-open of the uterus wall, during and after labor.

Rupture of uterus not stated as occurring before onset of labor

Excludes 1: *disruption of cesarean delivery wound (O90.0)*
laceration of uterus, NEC (O71.81)

CC O71.2 Postpartum inversion of uterus — [♀, Age/12-55] – The turning inside out of the uterus.

CC O71.3 Obstetric laceration of cervix — [♀, Age/12-55] – A tear of the cervix.
Annular detachment of cervix

CC O71.4 Obstetric high vaginal laceration alone — [♀, Age/12-55] – Laceration of vaginal wall or sulcus without mention of perineal laceration.

Laceration of vaginal wall without perineal laceration

Excludes 1: *obstetric high vaginal laceration with perineal laceration (O70.-)*

CC O71.5 Other obstetric injury to pelvic organs — [♀, Age/12-55]

AHA 14:4Q:p18 – Periurethral laceration during delivery

AHA 16:1Q:p4 – Periurethral laceration during delivery
Obstetric injury to bladder — Traumatic damage to the bladder.
Obstetric injury to urethra — Traumatic damage to the urethra.

Excludes ❷: *obstetric periurethral trauma (O71.82)*

CC O71.6 Obstetric damage to pelvic joints and ligaments — [♀, Age/12-55]

Obstetric avulsion of inner symphyseal cartilage — The tearing detachment of the cartilage of the symphysis pubis.
Obstetric damage to coccyx — Injury to the small bone at the end of the sacrum.
Obstetric traumatic separation of symphysis (pubis) — The separating detachment of the symphysis pubis.

CC O71.7 Obstetric hematoma of pelvis — [♀, Age/12-55] – A localized swelling mass of clotted blood caused by a break in a blood vessel.
Obstetric hematoma of perineum
Obstetric hematoma of vagina
Obstetric hematoma of vulva

O71.8- Other specified obstetric trauma

O71.81 Laceration of uterus, not elsewhere classified — [♀, Age/12-55]

O71.82 Other specified trauma to perineum and vulva — [♀, Age/12-55]

AHA 14:4Q:p18 – Periurethral laceration during delivery
Obstetric periurethral trauma

O71.89 Other specified obstetric trauma — [♀, Age/12-55]

O71.9 Obstetric trauma, unspecified — [♀, Age/12-55]

O72- <u>Postpartum hemorrhage</u>

Includes: Hemorrhage after delivery of fetus or infant

CC O72.0 Third-stage hemorrhage — [♀, Age/12-55]
Hemorrhage associated with retained, trapped or adherent placenta
Retained placenta NOS
Code also type of adherent placenta (O43.2-)

CC O72.1 Other immediate postpartum hemorrhage — [♀, Age/12-55]
AHA 16:1Q:p4 – Uterine atony with hemorrhage
Hemorrhage following delivery of placenta
Postpartum hemorrhage (atonic) NOS
Uterine atony with hemorrhage

Excludes 1: *uterine atony NOS (O62.2)*
uterine atony without hemorrhage (O62.2)
postpartum atony of uterus without hemorrhage (O75.89)

CC O72.2 Delayed and secondary postpartum hemorrhage — [♀, Age/12-55]
Hemorrhage associated with retained portions of placenta or membranes after the first 24 hours following delivery of placenta
Retained products of conception NOS, following delivery

O72.3 Postpartum coagulation defects — [♀, Age/12-55]
Postpartum afibrinogenemia
Postpartum fibrinolysis

O73- <u>Retained placenta and membranes</u>, <u>without</u> hemorrhage

Excludes 1: *placenta accreta (O43.21-)*
placenta increta (O43.22-)
placenta percreta (O43.23-)

O73.0 Retained placenta without hemorrhage — [♀, Age/12-55]
Adherent placenta, without hemorrhage
Trapped placenta without hemorrhage

O73.1 Retained portions of placenta and membranes, without hemorrhage — [♀, Age/12-55]
Retained products of conception following delivery, without hemorrhage

O74- <u>Complications of anesthesia during labor and delivery</u>

Includes: Maternal complications arising from the administration of a general, regional or local anesthetic, analgesic or other sedation during labor and delivery

Use additional code, if applicable, to identify specific complication

O74.0 <u>Aspiration pneumonitis</u> due to anesthesia during labor and delivery — [♀, Age/12-55]
Inhalation of stomach contents or secretions NOS due to anesthesia during labor and delivery
Mendelson's syndrome due to anesthesia during labor and delivery

O74.1 Other pulmonary complications of anesthesia during labor and delivery — [♀, Age/12-55]

O74.2 <u>Cardiac complications</u> of anesthesia during labor and delivery — [♀, Age/12-55]

O74.3 <u>Central nervous system</u> complications of anesthesia during labor and delivery — [♀, Age/12-55]

O74.4 Toxic reaction to local anesthesia during labor and delivery — [♀, Age/12-55]

O74.5 <u>Spinal and epidural anesthesia-induced headache</u> during labor and delivery — [♀, Age/12-55]

O74.6 <u>Other complications of spinal and epidural anesthesia</u> during labor and delivery — [♀, Age/12-55]

O74.7 <u>Failed or difficult intubation for anesthesia</u> during labor and delivery — [♀, Age/12-55]

O74.8 <u>Other</u> complications of anesthesia during labor and delivery — [♀, Age/12-55]

O74.9 Complication of anesthesia during labor and delivery, <u>unspecified</u> — [♀, Age/12-55]

O75- Other complications of labor and delivery, <u>not elsewhere classified</u>

Excludes ❷: *puerperal (postpartum) infection (O86.-)*
puerperal (postpartum) sepsis (O85)

O75.0 Maternal distress during labor and delivery — [♀, Age/12-55]

MCC O75.1 Shock during or following labor and delivery — [♀, Age/12-55]
Obstetric shock following labor and delivery

CC O75.2 Pyrexia during labor, not elsewhere classified — [♀, Age/12-55]

MCC O75.3 Other infection during labor — [♀, Age/12-55]
Sepsis during labor
Use additional code (B95-B97), to identify infectious agent

O75.4 Other complications of obstetric surgery and procedures — [♀, Age/12-55]
Cardiac arrest following obstetric surgery or procedures
Cardiac failure following obstetric surgery or procedures
Cerebral anoxia following obstetric surgery or procedures
Pulmonary edema following obstetric surgery or procedures
Use additional code to identify specific complication

Excludes ❷: *complications of anesthesia during labor and delivery (O74.-)*
disruption of obstetrical (surgical) wound (O90.0-O90.1)
hematoma of obstetrical (surgical) wound (O90.2)
infection of obstetrical (surgical) wound (O86.0)

O75.5 Delayed delivery after artificial rupture of membranes — [♀, Age/12-55]

O75.8- Other specified complications of labor and delivery

O75.81 Maternal exhaustion complicating labor and delivery — [♀, Age/12-55]

O75.82 Onset (spontaneous) of labor after 37 completed weeks of gestation but before 39 completed weeks of gestation, with delivery by (planned) cesarean section — [♀, Age/12-55]
Delivery by (planned) cesarean section occurring after 37 completed weeks of gestation but before 39 completed weeks gestation due to (spontaneous) onset of labor
Code first to specify reason for planned cesarean section, such as:
Cephalopelvic disproportion (normally formed fetus) (O33.9)
Previous cesarean delivery (O34.21)

O75.89 Other specified complications of labor and delivery — [♀, Age/12-55]

O75.9 Complication of labor and delivery, unspecified — [♀, Age/12-55]

Excludes 1: = NOT CODED HERE! (Do not code both)

Excludes ❷: = Not Included Here

O76 <u>Abnormality in fetal heart rate</u> and rhythm complicating labor and delivery — [♀, Age/12-55]
    AHA 13:4Q:p118 – Meconium amniotic fluid and fetal decelerations
    Depressed fetal heart rate tones complicating labor and delivery
    Fetal bradycardia complicating labor and delivery
    Fetal heart rate decelerations complicating labor and delivery
    Fetal heart rate irregularity complicating labor and delivery
    Fetal heart rate abnormal variability complicating labor and delivery
    Fetal tachycardia complicating labor and delivery
    Non-reassuring fetal heart rate or rhythm complicating labor and delivery
    Excludes 1:   *fetal stress NOS (O77.9)*
                 labor and delivery complicated by electrocardiographic evidence of fetal stress (O77.8)
                  labor and delivery complicated by ultrasonic evidence of fetal stress (O77.8)
    Excludes ❷: *fetal metabolic acidemia (O68)*
                 other fetal stress (O77.0-O77.1)

O77- <u>Other fetal stress</u> complicating labor and delivery
  O77.0 **Labor and delivery complicated by meconium in amniotic fluid** — [♀, Age/12-55] – The unusual presence of fetal bowel meconium in the amniotic fluid.
      AHA 13:4Q:p117 – Delivery complicated by meconium in amniotic fluid
      AHA 13:4Q:p118 – Meconium amniotic fluid and fetal decelerations
  O77.1 **Fetal stress in labor or delivery due to drug administration** — [♀, Age/12-55]
  O77.8 **Labor and delivery complicated by other evidence of fetal stress** — [♀, Age/12-55]
      Labor and delivery complicated by electrocardiographic evidence of fetal stress
      Labor and delivery complicated by ultrasonic evidence of fetal stress
      Excludes 1:   *abnormality of fetal acid-base balance (O68)*
                  abnormality in fetal heart rate or rhythm (O76)
                  fetal metabolic acidemia (O68)
  O77.9 **Labor and delivery complicated by fetal stress, unspecified** — [♀, Age/12-55]
      Excludes 1:   *abnormality of fetal acid-base balance (O68)*
                  abnormality in fetal heart rate or rhythm (O76)
                  fetal metabolic acidemia (O68)

Encounter for delivery (O80-O82)

O80 **Encounter for full-term uncomplicated delivery** — [♀, Age/12-55]
    AHA 14:2Q:p9 – Uncomplicated delivery with Pitocin to augment active labor
    Delivery requiring minimal or no assistance, with or without episiotomy, without fetal manipulation [e.g., rotation version] or instrumentation [forceps] of a spontaneous, cephalic, vaginal, full-term, single, live-born infant. This code is for use as a single diagnosis code and is not to be used with any other code from chapter 15.
    Use additional code to indicate outcome of delivery (Z37.0)
O82 **Encounter for cesarean delivery without indication** — [♀, Age/12-55]
    Use additional code to indicate outcome of delivery (Z37.0)

Complications predominantly related to the puerperium (O85-O92)

    Excludes ❷: *mental and behavioral disorders associated with the puerperium (F53)*
                 obstetrical tetanus (A34)
                 puerperal osteomalacia (M83.0)

O85 **Puerperal sepsis** — [♀, Age/12-55] – Postpartum infection of the bloodstream, including the toxins produced.
MCC
    Postpartum sepsis
    Puerperal peritonitis
    Puerperal pyemia
    Use additional code (B95-B97), to identify infectious agent
    Use additional code (R65.2-) to identify severe sepsis, if applicable
    Excludes 1:   *fever of unknown origin following delivery (O86.4)*
                 genital tract infection following delivery (O86.1-)
                 obstetric pyemic and septic embolism (O88.3-)
                 puerperal septic thrombophlebitis (O86.81)
                 urinary tract infection following delivery (O86.2-)
    Excludes ❷: *sepsis during labor (O75.3)*

O86- <u>Other puerperal infections</u>
    Use additional code (B95-B97), to identify infectious agent
    Excludes ❷: *infection during labor (O75.3)*
                 obstetrical tetanus (A34)
  O86.0 **Infection of <u>obstetric surgical wound</u>** — [♀, Age/12-55]
      Infected cesarean delivery wound following delivery
      Infected perineal repair following delivery
  O86.1- **Other infection of <u>genital tract</u> following delivery**
    cc **O86.11 Cervicitis following delivery** — [♀, Age/12-55]
    cc **O86.12 Endometritis following delivery** — [♀, Age/12-55]
    cc **O86.13 Vaginitis following delivery** — [♀, Age/12-55]
    cc **O86.19 Other infection of genital tract following delivery** — [♀, Age/12-55]
  O86.2- **<u>Urinary tract</u> infection following delivery**
    cc **O86.20 Urinary tract infection following delivery, unspecified** — [♀, Age/12-55]
      Puerperal urinary tract infection NOS
    cc **O86.21 Infection of kidney following delivery** — [♀, Age/12-55]
    cc **O86.22 Infection of bladder following delivery** — [♀, Age/12-55]
      Infection of urethra following delivery
    cc **O86.29 Other urinary tract infection following delivery** — [♀, Age/12-55]
  cc **O86.4** **<u>Pyrexia</u> of unknown origin following delivery** — [♀, Age/12-55]
      Puerperal infection NOS following delivery
      Puerperal pyrexia NOS following delivery
      Excludes ❷: *pyrexia during labor (O75.2)*
  O86.8- **<u>Other</u> specified puerperal infections**
    MCC **O86.81 Puerperal septic thrombophlebitis** — [♀, Age/12-55]
    MCC **O86.89 Other specified puerperal infections** — [♀, Age/12-55]

O87- <u>Venous complications and hemorrhoids</u> in the puerperium
    Includes: Venous complications in labor, delivery and the puerperium
    Excludes ❷: *obstetric embolism (O88-)*
                 puerperal septic thrombophlebitis (O86.81)
                 venous complications in pregnancy (O22-)
  cc **O87.0** **<u>Superficial</u> thrombophlebitis in the puerperium** — [♀, Age/12-55] – Inflammation of a superficial vein with thrombus formation following delivery.
      Puerperal phlebitis NOS
      Puerperal thrombosis NOS
  MCC **O87.1** **<u>Deep</u> phlebothrombosis In the puerperium** — [♀, Age/12-55] – Inflammation of a deep vein with thrombus following delivery.
      Deep vein thrombosis, postpartum
      Pelvic thrombophlebitis, postpartum
      Use additional code to identify the deep vein thrombosis (I82.4-, I82.5-, I82.62-. I82.72-)
      Use additional code, if applicable, for associated long-term (current) use of anticoagulants (Z79.01)
  cc **O87.2** **<u>Hemorrhoids</u> in the puerperium** — [♀, Age/12-55] – A varicose dilatation of a vein of the hemorrhoidal plexus following delivery.
  cc **O87.3** **<u>Cerebral venous thrombosis</u> in the puerperium** — [♀, Age/12-55] – Formation of a thrombus in a cerebral vessel following delivery.
      Cerebrovenous sinus thrombosis in the puerperium
  O87.4 **<u>Varicose veins</u> of lower extremity in the puerperium** — [♀, Age/12-55] – Dilated, tortuous leg veins presenting symptoms following delivery.
  cc **O87.8** **Other venous complications in the puerperium** — [♀, Age/12-55]
      Genital varices in the puerperium — Dilated, tortuous vulvar and perineal veins following delivery.
  O87.9 **Venous complication in the puerperium, unspecified** — [♀, Age/12-55]
      Puerperal phlebopathy NOS

O88- <u>Obstetric embolism</u>
    Excludes 1:   *embolism complicating abortion NOS (O03.2)*
                 embolism complicating ectopic or molar pregnancy (O08.2)
                 embolism complicating failed attempted abortion (O07.2)
                 embolism complicating induced abortion (O04.7)
                 embolism complicating spontaneous abortion (O03.2, O03.7)
  O88.0- **Obstetric <u>air</u> embolism** — The blockage of an artery with an embolism of air or bubbles of nitrogen.
    O88.01-   **Obstetric air embolism <u>in pregnancy</u>**
      MCC **O88.011 Air embolism in pregnancy, <u>first</u> trimester** — [♀, Age/12-55]

O76 - O88

мсс **O88.012 Air embolism in pregnancy, second trimester** — [♀, Age/12-55]

мсс **O88.013 Air embolism in pregnancy, third trimester** — [♀, Age/12-55]

O88.019 Air embolism in pregnancy, unspecified trimester — [♀, Age/12-55]

мсс **O88.02 Air embolism in childbirth** — [♀, Age/12-55]

мсс **O88.03 Air embolism in the puerperium** — [♀, Age/12-55]

O88.1- Amniotic fluid embolism — The blockage of an artery with an embolism composed of amniotic fluid.

> Anaphylactoid syndrome in pregnancy

O88.11- Amniotic fluid embolism in pregnancy

мсс **O88.111 Amniotic fluid embolism in pregnancy, first trimester** — [♀, Age/12-55]

мсс **O88.112 Amniotic fluid embolism in pregnancy, second trimester** — [♀, Age/12-55]

мсс **O88.113 Amniotic fluid embolism in pregnancy, third trimester** — [♀, Age/12-55]

O88.119 Amniotic fluid embolism in pregnancy, unspecified trimester — [♀, Age/12-55]

мсс **O88.12 Amniotic fluid embolism in childbirth** — [♀, Age/12-55]

мсс **O88.13 Amniotic fluid embolism in the puerperium** — [♀, Age/12-55]

O88.2- Obstetric thromboembolism — The blockage of an artery with an embolism composed of clotted blood.

O88.21- Thromboembolism in pregnancy
> Obstetric (pulmonary) embolism NOS

мсс **O88.211 Thromboembolism in pregnancy, first trimester** — [♀, Age/12-55]

мсс **O88.212 Thromboembolism in pregnancy, second trimester** — [♀, Age/12-55]

мсс **O88.213 Thromboembolism in pregnancy, third trimester** — [♀, Age/12-55]

O88.219 Thromboembolism in pregnancy, unspecified trimester — [♀, Age/12-55]

мсс **O88.22 Thromboembolism in childbirth** — [♀, Age/12-55]

мсс **O88.23 Thromboembolism in the puerperium** — [♀, Age/12-55]
> Puerperal (pulmonary) embolism NOS — The blockage of a pulmonary artery with an embolism composed of clotted blood.

O88.3- Obstetric pyemic and septic embolism

O88.31- Pyemic and septic embolism in pregnancy — The blockage of an artery with an embolism composed of pus or septic debris.

мсс **O88.311 Pyemic and septic embolism in pregnancy, first trimester** — [♀, Age/12-55]

мсс **O88.312 Pyemic and septic embolism in pregnancy, second trimester** — [♀, Age/12-55]

мсс **O88.313 Pyemic and septic embolism in pregnancy, third trimester** — [♀, Age/12-55]

сс **O88.319 Pyemic and septic embolism in pregnancy, unspecified trimester** — [♀, Age/12-55]

мсс **O88.32 Pyemic and septic embolism in childbirth** — [♀, Age/12-55]

мсс **O88.33 Pyemic and septic embolism in the puerperium** — [♀, Age/12-55]

O88.8- Other obstetric embolism
> Obstetric fat embolism

O88.81- Other embolism in pregnancy

мсс **O88.811 Other embolism in pregnancy, first trimester** — [♀, Age/12-55]

мсс **O88.812 Other embolism in pregnancy, second trimester** — [♀, Age/12-55]

мсс **O88.813 Other embolism in pregnancy, third trimester** — [♀, Age/12-55]

O88.819 Other embolism in pregnancy, unspecified trimester — [♀, Age/12-55]

мсс **O88.82 Other embolism in childbirth** — [♀, Age/12-55]

мсс **O88.83 Other embolism in the puerperium** — [♀, Age/12-55]

O89- Complications of anesthesia during the puerperium
Includes: Maternal complications arising from the administration of a general, regional or local anesthetic, analgesic or other sedation during the puerperium
Use additional code, if applicable, to identify specific complication

O89.0- Pulmonary complications of anesthesia during the puerperium

O89.01 Aspiration pneumonitis due to anesthesia during the puerperium — [♀, Age/12-55]
> Inhalation of stomach contents or secretions NOS due to anesthesia during the puerperium
> Mendelson's syndrome due to anesthesia during the puerperium

O89.09 Other pulmonary complications of anesthesia during the puerperium — [♀, Age/12-55]

O89.1 Cardiac complications of anesthesia during the puerperium — [♀, Age/12-55]

O89.2 Central nervous system complications of anesthesia during the puerperium — [♀, Age/12-55]

O89.3 Toxic reaction to local anesthesia during the puerperium — [♀, Age/12-55]

O89.4 Spinal and epidural anesthesia-induced headache during the puerperium — [♀, Age/12-55]

O89.5 Other complications of spinal and epidural anesthesia during the puerperium — [♀, Age/12-55]

O89.6 Failed or difficult intubation for anesthesia during the puerperium — [♀, Age/12-55]

O89.8 Other complications of anesthesia during the puerperium — [♀, Age/12-55]

O89.9 Complication of anesthesia during the puerperium, unspecified — [♀, Age/12-55]

O90- Complications of the puerperium, not elsewhere classified

O90.0 Disruption of cesarean delivery wound — [♀, Age/12-55] – The separation of the surgical incision layers.
> Dehiscence of cesarean delivery wound
> *Excludes 1:* *rupture of uterus (spontaneous) before onset of labor (O71.0-)*
> *rupture of uterus during labor (O71.1)*

O90.1 Disruption of perineal obstetric wound — [♀, Age/12-55] – The separation of the surgical layers of a perineal wound.
> Disruption of wound of episiotomy
> Disruption of wound of perineal laceration
> Secondary perineal tear

O90.2 Hematoma of obstetric wound — [♀, Age/12-55] – A localized swelling mass of blood of a cesarean section or perineal wound.

мсс **O90.3 Peripartum cardiomyopathy** — [♀, Age/12-55] – A condition of cardiac enlargement and congestive heart failure that develops late in pregnancy or in the months following delivery in women without pre-existing heart disease.
> Conditions in I42.- arising during pregnancy and the puerperium
> *Excludes 1:* *pre-existing heart disease complicating pregnancy and the puerperium (O99.4-)*

мсс **O90.4 Postpartum acute kidney failure** — [♀, Age/12-55]
> Hepatorenal syndrome following labor and delivery

O90.5 Postpartum thyroiditis — [♀, Age/12-55]

O90.6 Postpartum mood disturbance — [♀, Age/12-55]
> Postpartum blues
> Postpartum dysphoria
> Postpartum sadness
> *Excludes 1:* *postpartum depression (F53)*
> *puerperal psychosis (F53)*

O90.8- Other complications of the puerperium, not elsewhere classified

O90.81 Anemia of the puerperium — [♀, Age/12-55]
> Postpartum anemia NOS
> *Excludes 1:* *pre-existing anemia complicating the puerperium (O99.03)*

O90.89 Other complications of the puerperium, not elsewhere classified — [♀, Age/12-55]
> Placental polyp

O90.9 Complication of the puerperium, unspecified — [♀, Age/12-55]

O88-O90

Excludes 1: = NOT CODED HERE! (Do not code both)   **948**   *Excludes ❷:* = Not Included Here

O91- Infections of breast associated with pregnancy, the puerperium and lactation
Use additional code to identify infection

O91.0- Infection of nipple associated with pregnancy, the puerperium and lactation — Cellular injury of the nipple due to invasion of microorganisms.

     O91.01-   Infection of nipple associated with pregnancy
       Gestational abscess of nipple

       O91.011 Infection of nipple associated with pregnancy, first trimester — [♀, Age/12-55]

       O91.012 Infection of nipple associated with pregnancy, second trimester — [♀, Age/12-55]

       O91.013 Infection of nipple associated with pregnancy, third trimester — [♀, Age/12-55]

       O91.019 Infection of nipple associated with pregnancy, unspecified trimester — [♀, Age/12-55]

     O91.02 Infection of nipple associated with the puerperium — [♀, Age/12-55]
       Puerperal abscess of nipple

     O91.03 Infection of nipple associated with lactation — [♀, Age/12-55]
       Abscess of nipple associated with lactation

O91.1- Abscess of breast associated with pregnancy, the puerperium and lactation — A localized collection of pus caused by the disintegration of breast tissue.

     O91.11-   Abscess of breast associated with pregnancy
       Gestational mammary abscess
       Gestational purulent mastitis
       Gestational subareolar abscess

       O91.111 Abscess of breast associated with pregnancy, first trimester — [♀, Age/12-55]

       O91.112 Abscess of breast associated with pregnancy, second trimester — [♀, Age/12-55]

       O91.113 Abscess of breast associated with pregnancy, third trimester — [♀, Age/12-55]

       O91.119 Abscess of breast associated with pregnancy, unspecified trimester — [♀, Age/12-55]

     O91.12 Abscess of breast associated with the puerperium — [♀, Age/12-55]
       Puerperal mammary abscess
       Puerperal purulent mastitis
       Puerperal subareolar abscess

     O91.13 Abscess of breast associated with lactation — [♀, Age/12-55]
       Mammary abscess associated with lactation
       Purulent mastitis associated with lactation
       Subareolar abscess associated with lactation

O91.2- Nonpurulent mastitis associated with pregnancy, the puerperium and lactation — Inflammation of the breast without the presence or formation of pus.

     O91.21-   Nonpurulent mastitis associated with pregnancy
       Gestational interstitial mastitis
       Gestational lymphangitis of breast
       Gestational mastitis NOS
       Gestational parenchymatous mastitis

       O91.211 Nonpurulent mastitis associated with pregnancy, first trimester — [♀, Age/12-55]

       O91.212 Nonpurulent mastitis associated with pregnancy, second trimester — [♀, Age/12-55]

       O91.213 Nonpurulent mastitis associated with pregnancy, third trimester — [♀, Age/12-55]

       O91.219 Nonpurulent mastitis associated with pregnancy, unspecified trimester — [♀, Age/12-55]

     O91.22 Nonpurulent mastitis associated with the puerperium — [♀, Age/12-55]
       Puerperal interstitial mastitis
       Puerperal lymphangitis of breast
       Puerperal mastitis NOS
       Puerperal parenchymatous mastitis

     O91.23 Nonpurulent mastitis associated with lactation — [♀, Age/12-55]
       Interstitial mastitis associated with lactation
       Lymphangitis of breast associated with lactation
       Mastitis NOS associated with lactation
       Parenchymatous mastitis associated with lactation

O92- Other disorders of breast and disorders of lactation associated with pregnancy and the puerperium

    O92.0- Retracted nipple associated with pregnancy, the puerperium, and lactation — A condition in which the nipple is drawn back from its normal position.

     O92.01-   Retracted nipple associated with pregnancy

       O92.011 Retracted nipple associated with pregnancy, first trimester — [♀, Age/12-55]

       O92.012 Retracted nipple associated with pregnancy, second trimester — [♀, Age/12-55]

       O92.013 Retracted nipple associated with pregnancy, third trimester — [♀, Age/12-55]

       O92.019 Retracted nipple associated with pregnancy, unspecified trimester — [♀, Age/12-55]

     O92.02 Retracted nipple associated with the puerperium — [♀, Age/12-55]

     O92.03 Retracted nipple associated with lactation — [♀, Age/12-55]

    O92.1- Cracked nipple associated with pregnancy, the puerperium, and lactation — A condition in which the nipple is split or partially fissured.
     Fissure of nipple, gestational or puerperal

     O92.11-   Cracked nipple associated with pregnancy

       O92.111 Cracked nipple associated with pregnancy, first trimester — [♀, Age/12-55]

       O92.112 Cracked nipple associated with pregnancy, second trimester — [♀, Age/12-55]

       O92.113 Cracked nipple associated with pregnancy, third trimester — [♀, Age/12-55]

       O92.119 Cracked nipple associated with pregnancy, unspecified trimester — [♀, Age/12-55]

     O92.12 Cracked nipple associated with the puerperium — [♀, Age/12-55]

     O92.13 Cracked nipple associated with lactation — [♀, Age/12-55]

    O92.2- Other and unspecified disorders of breast associated with pregnancy and the puerperium

     O92.20 Unspecified disorder of breast associated with pregnancy and the puerperium — [♀, Age/12-55]

     O92.29 Other disorders of breast associated with pregnancy and the puerperium — [♀, Age/12-55]

    O92.3 Agalactia — [♀, Age/12-55] – Absence or failure of the secretion of milk.
     Primary agalactia
     Excludes 1:   *elective agalactia (O92.5)*
             secondary agalactia (O92.5)
             therapeutic agalactia (O92.5)

    O92.4 Hypogalactia — [♀, Age/12-55] – The abnormally low volume of the secretion of milk.

    O92.5 Suppressed lactation — [♀, Age/12-55] – The sudden stoppage of milk secretion.
     Elective agalactia
     Secondary agalactia
     Therapeutic agalactia
     Excludes 1:   *primary agalactia (O92.3)*

    O92.6 Galactorrhea — [♀, Age/12-55] – Persistent secretion of milk, irrespective of nursing.

    O92.7- Other and unspecified disorders of lactation

     O92.70 Unspecified disorders of lactation — [♀, Age/12-55]

     O92.79 Other disorders of lactation — [♀, Age/12-55]
       Puerperal galactocele — The cystic enlargement of a mammary gland containing milk.

Other obstetric conditions, not elsewhere classified (O94-O9A)

O94 Sequelae of complication of pregnancy, childbirth, and the puerperium — [♀, Age/12-55]
Note: This category is to be used to indicate conditions in O00-O77-, O85-O94 and O98-O9A- as the cause of late effects. The sequelae include conditions specified as such, or as late effects, which may occur at any time after the puerperium.
Code first condition resulting from (sequela) of complication of pregnancy, childbirth, and the puerperium

Side tab: O91-O94

© 2016 Channel Publishing, Ltd.

O98- **Maternal infectious and parasitic diseases classifiable elsewhere but complicating pregnancy, childbirth and the puerperium**
Includes: The listed conditions when complicating the pregnant state, when aggravated by the pregnancy, or as a reason for obstetric care
Use additional code (Chapter 1), to identify specific infectious or parasitic disease
Excludes ❷: herpes gestationis (O26.4-)
infectious carrier state (O99.82-, O99.83-)
obstetrical tetanus (A34)
puerperal infection (O86.-)
puerperal sepsis (O85)
when the reason for maternal care is that the disease is known or suspected to have affected the fetus (O35-O36)

O98.0- **Tuberculosis complicating pregnancy, childbirth and the puerperium**
Conditions in A15-A19

O98.01-   **Tuberculosis complicating pregnancy**

cc **O98.011** **Tuberculosis complicating pregnancy, first** trimester — [♀, Age/12-55]

cc **O98.012** **Tuberculosis complicating pregnancy, second** trimester — [♀, Age/12-55]

cc **O98.013** **Tuberculosis complicating pregnancy, third** trimester — [♀, Age/12-55]

O98.019 **Tuberculosis complicating pregnancy, unspecified** trimester — [♀, Age/12-55]

cc **O98.02 Tuberculosis complicating childbirth** — [♀, Age/12-55]

cc **O98.03 Tuberculosis complicating the puerperium** — [♀, Age/12-55]

O98.1- **Syphilis complicating pregnancy, childbirth and the puerperium**
Conditions in A50-A53

O98.11-   **Syphilis complicating pregnancy**

cc **O98.111 Syphilis complicating pregnancy, first trimester** — [♀, Age/12-55]

cc **O98.112 Syphilis complicating pregnancy, second** trimester — [♀, Age/12-55]

cc **O98.113 Syphilis complicating pregnancy, third trimester** — [♀, Age/12-55]

O98.119 Syphilis complicating pregnancy, unspecified trimester — [♀, Age/12-55]

cc **O98.12 Syphilis complicating childbirth** — [♀, Age/12-55]

cc **O98.13 Syphilis complicating the puerperium** — [♀, Age/12-55]

O98.2- **Gonorrhea complicating pregnancy, childbirth and the puerperium**
Conditions in A54.-

O98.21-   **Gonorrhea complicating pregnancy**

cc **O98.211 Gonorrhea complicating pregnancy, first** trimester — [♀, Age/12-55]

cc **O98.212 Gonorrhea complicating pregnancy, second** trimester — [♀, Age/12-55]

cc **O98.213 Gonorrhea complicating pregnancy, third** trimester — [♀, Age/12-55]

O98.219 Gonorrhea complicating pregnancy, unspecified trimester — [♀, Age/12-55]

cc **O98.22 Gonorrhea complicating childbirth** — [♀, Age/12-55]

cc **O98.23 Gonorrhea complicating the puerperium** — [♀, Age/12-55]

O98.3- **Other infections with a predominantly sexual mode of transmission complicating pregnancy, childbirth and the puerperium**
Conditions in A55-A64

O98.31-   **Other infections with a predominantly sexual mode of transmission complicating pregnancy**

cc **O98.311 Other infections with a predominantly sexual mode of transmission complicating pregnancy, first** trimester — [♀, Age/12-55]

cc **O98.312 Other infections with a predominantly sexual mode of transmission complicating pregnancy, second** trimester — [♀, Age/12-55]

cc **O98.313 Other infections with a predominantly sexual mode of transmission complicating pregnancy, third** trimester — [♀, Age/12-55]

cc **O98.319** **Other infections with a predominantly sexual mode of transmission complicating pregnancy, unspecified** trimester — [♀, Age/12-55]

cc **O98.32 Other infections with a predominantly sexual mode of transmission complicating childbirth** — [♀, Age/12-55]

cc **O98.33 Other infections with a predominantly sexual mode of transmission complicating the puerperium** — [♀, Age/12-55]

O98.4- **Viral hepatitis complicating pregnancy, childbirth and the puerperium**
Conditions in B15-B19

O98.41-   **Viral hepatitis complicating pregnancy**

cc **O98.411 Viral hepatitis complicating pregnancy, first** trimester — [♀, Age/12-55]

cc **O98.412 Viral hepatitis complicating pregnancy, second** trimester — [♀, Age/12-55]

cc **O98.413 Viral hepatitis complicating pregnancy, third** trimester — [♀, Age/12-55]

O98.419 **Viral hepatitis complicating pregnancy, unspecified** trimester — [♀, Age/12-55]

cc **O98.42 Viral hepatitis complicating childbirth** — [♀, Age/12-55]

cc **O98.43 Viral hepatitis complicating the puerperium** — [♀, Age/12-55]

O98.5- **Other viral diseases complicating pregnancy, childbirth and the puerperium**
Conditions in A80-B09, B25-B34, R87.81-, R87.82-
Excludes 1:   human immunodeficiency virus [HIV] disease complicating pregnancy, childbirth and the puerperium (O98.7-)

O98.51-   **Other viral diseases complicating pregnancy**

cc **O98.511 Other viral diseases complicating pregnancy, first** trimester — [♀, Age/12-55]

cc **O98.512 Other viral diseases complicating pregnancy, second trimester** — [♀, Age/12-55]

cc **O98.513 Other viral diseases complicating pregnancy, third** trimester — [♀, Age/12-55]

O98.519 Other viral diseases complicating pregnancy, unspecified trimester — [♀, Age/12-55]

cc **O98.52 Other viral diseases complicating childbirth** — [♀, Age/12-55]

cc **O98.53 Other viral diseases complicating the puerperium** — [♀, Age/12-55]

O98.6- **Protozoal diseases complicating pregnancy, childbirth and the puerperium**
Conditions in B50-B64

O98.61-   **Protozoal diseases complicating pregnancy**

cc **O98.611 Protozoal diseases complicating pregnancy, first** trimester — [♀, Age/12-55]

cc **O98.612 Protozoal diseases complicating pregnancy, second** trimester — [♀, Age/12-55]

cc **O98.613 Protozoal diseases complicating pregnancy, third** trimester — [♀, Age/12-55]

O98.619 **Protozoal diseases complicating pregnancy, unspecified** trimester — [♀, Age/12-55]

cc **O98.62 Protozoal diseases complicating childbirth** — [♀, Age/12-55]

cc **O98.63 Protozoal diseases complicating the puerperium** — [♀, Age/12-55]

O98.7- **Human immunodeficiency virus [HIV] disease complicating pregnancy, childbirth and the puerperium**
Use additional code to identify the type of HIV disease:
Acquired immune deficiency syndrome (AIDS) (B20)
Asymptomatic HIV status (Z21)
HIV positive NOS (Z21)
Symptomatic HIV disease (B20)

O98.71-   **Human immunodeficiency virus [HIV] disease complicating pregnancy**

cc **O98.711 Human immunodeficiency virus [HIV] disease complicating pregnancy, first** trimester — [♀, Age/12-55] cc **O98.712** Human immunodeficiency virus [HIV] disease complicating pregnancy, <u>second</u> trimester — [♀, Age/12-55]

cc **O98.713** Human immunodeficiency virus [HIV] disease complicating pregnancy, <u>third</u> trimester — [♀, Age/12-55]

O98.719 Human immunodeficiency virus [HIV] disease complicating pregnancy, <u>unspecified</u> trimester — [♀, Age/12-55]

cc **O98.72** Human immunodeficiency virus [HIV] disease complicating <u>childbirth</u> — [♀, Age/12-55]

cc **O98.73** Human immunodeficiency virus [HIV] disease complicating <u>the puerperium</u> — [♀, Age/12-55]

O98.8- <u>Other</u> maternal infectious and parasitic diseases complicating pregnancy, childbirth and the puerperium

O98.81- Other maternal infectious and parasitic diseases complicating <u>pregnancy</u>

cc **O98.811** Other maternal infectious and parasitic diseases complicating pregnancy, <u>first</u> trimester — [♀, Age/12-55]

cc **O98.812** Other maternal infectious and parasitic diseases complicating pregnancy, <u>second</u> trimester — [♀, Age/12-55]

cc **O98.813** Other maternal infectious and parasitic diseases complicating pregnancy, <u>third</u> trimester — [♀, Age/12-55]

O98.819 Other maternal infectious and parasitic diseases complicating pregnancy, <u>unspecified</u> trimester — [♀, Age/12-55]

cc **O98.82** Other maternal infectious and parasitic diseases complicating <u>childbirth</u> — [♀, Age/12-55]

cc **O98.83** Other maternal infectious and parasitic diseases complicating <u>the puerperium</u> — [♀, Age/12-55]

O98.9- <u>Unspecified</u> maternal infectious and parasitic disease complicating pregnancy, childbirth and the puerperium

O98.91- Unspecified maternal infectious and parasitic disease complicating <u>pregnancy</u>

cc **O98.911** Unspecified maternal Infectious and parasitic disease complicating pregnancy, <u>first</u> trimester — [♀, Age/12-55]

cc **O98.912** Unspecified maternal infectious and parasitic disease complicating pregnancy, <u>second</u> trimester — [♀, Age/12-55]

cc **O98.913** Unspecified maternal infectious and parasitic disease complicating pregnancy, <u>third</u> trimester — [♀, Age/12-55]

O98.919 Unspecified maternal infectious and parasitic disease complicating pregnancy, <u>unspecified</u> trimester — [♀, Age/12-55]

cc **O98.92** Unspecified maternal infectious and parasitic disease complicating <u>childbirth</u> — [♀, Age/12-55]

cc **O98.93** Unspecified maternal infectious and parasitic disease complicating <u>the puerperium</u> — [♀, Age/12-55]

O99- <u>Other maternal diseases classifiable elsewhere</u> but complicating pregnancy, childbirth and the puerperium
Includes: Conditions which complicate the pregnant state, are aggravated by the pregnancy or are a main reason for obstetric care
Use additional code to identify specific condition
Excludes ❷: when the reason for maternal care is that the condition is known or suspected to have affected the fetus (O35-O36)

O99.0- <u>Anemia</u> complicating pregnancy, childbirth and the puerperium
AHA 16:1Q:p4 – Pregnancy complicated by anemia
Conditions in D50-D64
Excludes 1: anemia arising in the puerperium (O90.81)
postpartum anemia NOS (O90.81)

O99.01- Anemia complicating <u>pregnancy</u>

O99.011 Anemia complicating pregnancy, <u>first</u> trimester — [♀, Age/12-55]

O99.012 Anemia complicating pregnancy, <u>second</u> trimester — [♀, Age/12-55]

O99.013 Anemia complicating pregnancy, <u>third</u> trimester — [♀, Age/12-55]

O99.019 Anemia complicating pregnancy, <u>unspecified</u> trimester — [♀, Age/12-55]

O99.02 Anemia complicating <u>childbirth</u> — [♀, Age/12-55]

O99.03 Anemia complicating <u>the puerperium</u> — [♀, Age/12-55]
Excludes 1: postpartum anemia not pre-existing prior to delivery (O90.81)

O99.1- <u>Other diseases of the blood and blood-forming organs and certain disorders involving the immune mechanism</u> complicating pregnancy, childbirth and the puerperium
Conditions in D65-D89
Excludes ❷: hemorrhage with coagulation defects (O45.-, O46.0-, O67.0, O72.3)

O99.11- Other diseases of the blood and blood-forming organs and certain disorders involving the immune mechanism complicating <u>pregnancy</u>

cc **O99.111** Other diseases of the blood and blood-forming organs and certain disorders involving the immune mechanism complicating pregnancy, <u>first</u> trimester — [♀, Age/12-55]

cc **O99.112** Other diseases of the blood and blood-forming organs and certain disorders involving the immune mechanism complicating pregnancy, <u>second</u> trimester — [♀, Age/12-55]

cc **O99.113** Other diseases of the blood and blood-forming organs and certain disorders involving the immune mechanism complicating pregnancy, <u>third</u> trimester — [♀, Age/12-55]

cc **O99.119** Other diseases of the blood and blood-forming organs and certain disorders involving the immune mechanism complicating pregnancy, <u>unspecified</u> trimester — [♀, Age/12-55]

cc **O99.12** Other diseases of the blood and blood-forming organs and certain disorders involving the immune mechanism complicating <u>childbirth</u> — [♀, Age/12-55]

cc **O99.13** Other diseases of the blood and blood-forming organs and certain disorders involving the immune mechanism complicating <u>the puerperium</u> — [♀, Age/12-55]

O99.2- <u>Endocrine, nutritional and metabolic diseases</u> complicating pregnancy, childbirth and the puerperium
Conditions in E00-E88
Excludes ❷: diabetes mellitus (O24.-)
malnutrition (O25.-)
postpartum thyroiditis (O90.5)

O99.21- <u>Obesity</u> complicating pregnancy, childbirth, and the puerperium
Use additional code to identify the type of obesity (E66.-)

O99.210 Obesity complicating <u>pregnancy</u>, <u>unspecified</u> trimester — [♀, Age/12-55]

O99.211 Obesity complicating <u>pregnancy</u>, <u>first</u> trimester — [♀, Age/12-55]

O99.212 Obesity complicating <u>pregnancy</u>, <u>second</u> trimester — [♀, Age/12-55]

O99.213 Obesity complicating <u>pregnancy</u>, <u>third</u> trimester — [♀, Age/12-55]

O99.214 Obesity complicating <u>childbirth</u> — [♀, Age/12-55]

O99.215 Obesity complicating <u>the puerperium</u> — [♀, Age/12-55]

O99.28- <u>Other</u> endocrine, nutritional and metabolic diseases complicating pregnancy, childbirth and the puerperium

O99.280 Endocrine, nutritional and metabolic diseases complicating <u>pregnancy</u>, <u>unspecified</u> trimester — [♀, Age/12-55]

O99.281 Endocrine, nutritional and metabolic diseases complicating <u>pregnancy</u>, <u>first</u> trimester — [♀, Age/12-55]

© 2016 Channel Publishing, Ltd.

098 - 099

O99.282 Endocrine, nutritional and metabolic diseases complicating pregnancy, second trimester — [♀, Age/12-55]

O99.283 Endocrine, nutritional and metabolic diseases complicating pregnancy, third trimester — [♀, Age/12-55]

O99.284 Endocrine, nutritional and metabolic diseases complicating childbirth — [♀, Age/12-55]

O99.285 Endocrine, nutritional and metabolic diseases complicating the puerperium — [♀, Age/12-55]

O99.3- Mental disorders and diseases of the nervous system complicating pregnancy, childbirth and the puerperium

O99.31- Alcohol use complicating pregnancy, childbirth, and the puerperium
Use additional code(s) from F10 to identify manifestations of the alcohol use

O99.310 Alcohol use complicating pregnancy, unspecified trimester — [♀, Age/12-55]

O99.311 Alcohol use complicating pregnancy, first trimester — [♀, Age/12-55]

O99.312 Alcohol use complicating pregnancy, second trimester — [♀, Age/12-55]

O99.313 Alcohol use complicating pregnancy, third trimester — [♀, Age/12-55]

O99.314 Alcohol use complicating childbirth — [♀, Age/12-55]

O99.315 Alcohol use complicating the puerperium — [♀, Age/12-55]

O99.32- Drug use complicating pregnancy, childbirth, and the puerperium
Use additional code(s) from F11-F16 and F18-F19 to identify manifestations of the drug use

O99.320 Drug use complicating pregnancy, unspecified trimester — [♀, Age/12-55]

cc **O99.321 Drug use complicating pregnancy, first trimester —** [♀, Age/12-55]

cc **O99.322 Drug use complicating pregnancy, second trimester —** [♀, Age/12-55]

cc **O99.323 Drug use complicating pregnancy, third trimester —** [♀, Age/12-55]

cc **O99.324 Drug use complicating childbirth —** [♀, Age/12-55]

cc **O99.325 Drug use complicating the puerperium —** [♀, Age/12-55]

O99.33- Tobacco use disorder complicating pregnancy, childbirth, and the puerperium
Smoking complicating pregnancy, childbirth, and the puerperium
Use additional code from category F17 to identify type of tobacco nicotine dependence

O99.330 Smoking (tobacco) complicating pregnancy, unspecified trimester — [♀, Age/12-55]

O99.331 Smoking (tobacco) complicating pregnancy, first trimester — [♀, Age/12-55]

O99.332 Smoking (tobacco) complicating pregnancy, second trimester — [♀, Age/12-55]

O99.333 Smoking (tobacco) complicating pregnancy, third trimester — [♀, Age/12-55]

O99.334 Smoking (tobacco) complicating childbirth — [♀, Age/12-55]

O99.335 Smoking (tobacco) complicating the puerperium — [♀, Age/12-55]

O99.34- Other mental disorders complicating pregnancy, childbirth, and the puerperium
Conditions in F01-F09 and F20-F99
Excludes ❷: postpartum mood disturbance (O90.6)
postnatal psychosis (F53)
puerperal psychosis (F53)

O99.340 Other mental disorders complicating pregnancy, unspecified trimester — [♀, Age/12-55]

O99.341 Other mental disorders complicating pregnancy, first trimester — [♀, Age/12-55]

O99.342 Other mental disorders complicating pregnancy, second trimester — [♀, Age/12-55]

O99.343 Other mental disorders complicating pregnancy, third trimester — [♀, Age/12-55]

O99.344 Other mental disorders complicating childbirth — [♀, Age/12-55]

O99.345 Other mental disorders complicating the puerperium — [♀, Age/12-55]

O99.35- Diseases of the nervous system complicating pregnancy, childbirth, and the puerperium
Conditions in G00-G99
Excludes ❷: pregnancy related peripheral neuritis (O26.8-)

O99.350 Diseases of the nervous system complicating pregnancy, unspecified trimester — [♀, Age/12-55]

O99.351 Diseases of the nervous system complicating pregnancy, first trimester — [♀, Age/12-55]

O99.352 Diseases of the nervous system complicating pregnancy, second trimester — [♀, Age/12-55]

O99.353 Diseases of the nervous system complicating pregnancy, third trimester — [♀, Age/12-55]

cc **O99.354 Diseases of the nervous system complicating childbirth —** [♀, Age/12-55]

cc **O99.355 Diseases of the nervous system complicating the puerperium —** [♀, Age/12-55]

O99.4- Diseases of the circulatory system complicating pregnancy, childbirth and the puerperium
AHA 16:2Q:p8 – Preexisting pulmonary hypertension complicating pregnancy
Conditions in I00-I99
Excludes 1: peripartum cardiomyopathy (O90.3)
Excludes ❷: hypertensive disorders (O10-O16)
obstetric embolism (O88.-)
venous complications and cerebrovenous sinus thrombosis in labor, childbirth and the puerperium (O87-)
venous complications and cerebrovenous sinus thrombosis in pregnancy (O22-)

O99.41- Diseases of the circulatory system complicating pregnancy

cc **O99.411 Diseases of the circulatory system complicating pregnancy, first trimester —** [♀, Age/12-55]

cc **O99.412 Diseases of the circulatory system complicating pregnancy, second trimester —** [♀, Age/12-55]

cc **O99.413 Diseases of the circulatory system complicating pregnancy, third trimester —** [♀, Age/12-55]

O99.419 Diseases of the circulatory system complicating pregnancy, unspecified trimester — [♀, Age/12-55]

MCC **O99.42 Diseases of the circulatory system complicating childbirth —** [♀, Age/12-55]

cc **O99.43 Diseases of the circulatory system complicating the puerperium —** [♀, Age/12-55]

O99.5- Diseases of the respiratory system complicating pregnancy, childbirth and the puerperium
Conditions in J00-J99

O99.51- Diseases of the respiratory system complicating pregnancy

O99.511 Diseases of the respiratory system complicating pregnancy, first trimester — [♀, Age/12-55]

O99.512 Diseases of the respiratory system complicating pregnancy, second trimester — [♀, Age/12-55]

O99.513 Diseases of the respiratory system complicating pregnancy, third trimester — [♀, Age/12-55]

O99.519 Diseases of the respiratory system complicating pregnancy, unspecified trimester — [♀, Age/12-55]

O99.52 Diseases of the respiratory system complicating childbirth — [♀, Age/12-55]

O99.53 Diseases of the respiratory system complicating the puerperium — [♀, Age/12-55]

O99-O99

Excludes 1: = NOT CODED HERE! (Do not code both)   **952**   *Excludes ❷:* = Not Included Here

O99.6- <u>Diseases of the digestive system</u> complicating pregnancy, childbirth and the puerperium
 AHA 16:1Q:p4 – Pregnancy complicated by gallstones
 Conditions in K00-K93
 Excludes ❷: *hemorrhoids in pregnancy (O22.4-)*
  liver and biliary tract disorders in pregnancy, childbirth and the puerperium (O26.6-)

 O99.61- Diseases of the digestive system complicating <u>pregnancy</u>

  O99.611 Diseases of the digestive system complicating pregnancy, <u>first</u> trimester — [♀, Age/12-55]

  O99.612 Diseases of the digestive system complicating pregnancy, <u>second</u> trimester — [♀, Age/12-55]

  O99.613 Diseases of the digestive system complicating pregnancy, <u>third</u> trimester — [♀, Age/12-55]

  O99.619 Diseases of the digestive system complicating pregnancy, <u>unspecified</u> trimester — [♀, Age/12-55]

 O99.62 Diseases of the digestive system complicating <u>childbirth</u> — [♀, Age/12-55]

 O99.63 Diseases of the digestive system complicating <u>the puerperium</u> — [♀, Age/12-55]

O99.7- <u>Diseases of the skin and subcutaneous tissue</u> complicating pregnancy, childbirth and the puerperium
 Conditions in L00-L99
 Excludes ❷: *herpes gestationis (O26.4)*
  pruritic urticarial papules and plaques of pregnancy (PUPPP) (O26.86)

 O99.71- Diseases of the skin and subcutaneous tissue complicating <u>pregnancy</u>

  O99.711 Diseases of the skin and subcutaneous tissue complicating pregnancy, <u>first</u> trimester — [♀, Age/12-55]

  O99.712 Diseases of the skin and subcutaneous tissue complicating pregnancy, <u>second</u> trimester — [♀, Age/12-55]

  O99.713 Diseases of the skin and subcutaneous tissue complicating pregnancy, <u>third</u> trimester — [♀, Age/12-55]

  O99.719 Diseases of the skin and subcutaneous tissue complicating pregnancy, <u>unspecified</u> trimester — [♀, Age/12-55]

 O99.72 Diseases of the skin and subcutaneous tissue complicating <u>childbirth</u> — [♀, Age/12-55]

 O99.73 Diseases of the skin and subcutaneous tissue complicating <u>the puerperium</u> — [♀, Age/12-55]

O99.8- <u>Other specified diseases and conditions</u> complicating pregnancy, childbirth and the puerperium
 Conditions in D00-D48, H00-H95, M00-N99, and Q00-Q99
 Use additional code to identify condition
 Excludes ❷: *genitourinary infections in pregnancy (O23-)*
  infection of genitourinary tract following delivery (O86.1-O86.3)
  malignant neoplasm complicating pregnancy, childbirth and the puerperium (O9A.1-)
  maternal care for known or suspected abnormality of maternal pelvic organs (O34-)
  postpartum acute kidney failure (O90.4)
  traumatic injuries in pregnancy (O9A.2-)

 O99.81- <u>Abnormal glucose</u> complicating pregnancy, childbirth and the puerperium
  Excludes 1: *gestational diabetes (O24.4-)*

  O99.810 Abnormal glucose complicating <u>pregnancy</u> — [♀, Age/12-55]

  O99.814 Abnormal glucose complicating <u>childbirth</u> — [♀, Age/12-55]

  O99.815 Abnormal glucose complicating <u>the puerperium</u> — [♀, Age/12-55]

O99.82- <u>Streptococcus B carrier state</u> complicating pregnancy, childbirth and the puerperium
 Excludes 1: *carrier of streptococcus group B (GBS) in a nonpregnant woman (Z22.330)*

 O99.820 Streptococcus B carrier state complicating <u>pregnancy</u> — [♀, Age/12-55] [Unacceptable PDX]

 O99.824 Streptococcus B carrier state complicating <u>childbirth</u> — [♀, Age/12-55]

 O99.825 Streptococcus B carrier state complicating <u>the puerperium</u> — [♀, Age/12-55] [Unacceptable PDX]

O99.83- <u>Other infection carrier state</u> complicating pregnancy, childbirth and the puerperium
 Use additional code to identify the carrier state (Z22.-)

 cc **O99.830** Other infection carrier state complicating <u>pregnancy</u> — [♀, Age/12-55]

 cc **O99.834** Other infection carrier state complicating <u>childbirth</u> — [♀, Age/12-55]

 cc **O99.835** Other infection carrier state complicating <u>the puerperium</u> — [♀, Age/12-55]

O99.84- <u>Bariatric surgery status</u> complicating pregnancy, childbirth and the puerperium
 Gastric banding status complicating pregnancy, childbirth and the puerperium
 Gastric bypass status for obesity complicating pregnancy, childbirth and the puerperium
 Obesity surgery status complicating pregnancy, childbirth and the puerperium

 O99.840 Bariatric surgery status complicating <u>pregnancy, unspecified</u> trimester — [♀, Age/12-55]

 O99.841 Bariatric surgery status complicating <u>pregnancy, first</u> trimester — [♀, Age/12-55]

 O99.842 Bariatric surgery status complicating <u>pregnancy, second</u> trimester — [♀, Age/12-55]

 O99.843 Bariatric surgery status complicating <u>pregnancy, third</u> trimester — [♀, Age/12-55]

 O99.844 Bariatric surgery status complicating <u>childbirth</u> — [♀, Age/12-55]

 O99.845 Bariatric surgery status complicating <u>the puerperium</u> — [♀, Age/12-55]

O99.89 <u>Other specified</u> diseases and conditions complicating pregnancy, childbirth and the puerperium — [♀, Age/12-55]

O9A- Maternal malignant neoplasms, traumatic injuries and abuse classifiable elsewhere but complicating pregnancy, childbirth and the puerperium

 O9A.1- <u>Malignant neoplasm</u> complicating pregnancy, childbirth and the puerperium
  Conditions in C00-C96
  Use additional code to identify neoplasm
  Excludes ❷: *maternal care for benign tumor of corpus uteri (O34.1-)*
   maternal care for benign tumor of cervix (O34.4-)

  O9A.11- Malignant neoplasm complicating <u>pregnancy</u>

   O9A.111 Malignant neoplasm complicating pregnancy, <u>first</u> trimester — [♀, Age/12-55]

   O9A.112 Malignant neoplasm complicating pregnancy, <u>second</u> trimester — [♀, Age/12-55]

   O9A.113 Malignant neoplasm complicating pregnancy, <u>third</u> trimester — [♀, Age/12-55]

   O9A.119 Malignant neoplasm complicating pregnancy, <u>unspecified</u> trimester — [♀, Age/12-55]

  O9A.12 Malignant neoplasm complicating <u>childbirth</u> — [♀, Age/12-55]

  O9A.13 Malignant neoplasm complicating <u>the puerperium</u> — [♀, Age/12-55]
   AHA 15:3Q:p19 – Malignant neoplasm complicating puerperium

O99 - O9A

O9A.2- <u>Injury, poisoning and certain other consequences of external causes</u> complicating pregnancy, childbirth and the puerperium
> Conditions in S00-T88, except T74 and T76
> Use additional code(s) to identify the injury or poisoning
> *Excludes ❷: physical, sexual and psychological abuse complicating pregnancy, childbirth and the puerperium (O9A.3-, O9A.4-, O9A.5-)*

O9A.21- Injury, poisoning and certain other consequences of external causes complicating <u>pregnancy</u>

O9A.211 Injury, poisoning and certain other consequences of external causes complicating pregnancy, <u>first</u> trimester — [♀, Age/12-55]

O9A.212 Injury, poisoning and certain other consequences of external causes complicating pregnancy, <u>second</u> trimester — [♀, Age/12-55]

O9A.213 Injury, poisoning and certain other consequences of external causes complicating pregnancy, <u>third</u> trimester — [♀, Age/12-55]

O9A.219 Injury, poisoning and certain other consequences of external causes complicating pregnancy, <u>unspecified</u> trimester — [♀, Age/12-55]

O9A.22 Injury, poisoning and certain other consequences of external causes complicating <u>childbirth</u> — [♀, Age/12-55]

O9A.23 Injury, poisoning and certain other consequences of external causes complicating <u>the puerperium</u> — [♀, Age/12-55]

O9A.3- <u>Physical abuse</u> complicating pregnancy, childbirth and the puerperium
> Conditions in T74.11 or T76.11
> Use additional code (if applicable):
> To identify any associated current injury due to physical abuse
> To identify the perpetrator of abuse (Y07.-)
> *Excludes ❷: sexual abuse complicating pregnancy, childbirth and the puerperium (O9A.4-)*

O9A.31- Physical abuse complicating <u>pregnancy</u>

O9A.311 Physical abuse complicating pregnancy, <u>first</u> trimester — [♀, Age/12-55]

O9A.312 Physical abuse complicating pregnancy, <u>second</u> trimester — [♀, Age/12-55]

O9A.313 Physical abuse complicating pregnancy, <u>third</u> trimester — [♀, Age/12-55]

O9A.319 Physical abuse complicating pregnancy, <u>unspecified</u> trimester — [♀, Age/12-55]

O9A.32 Physical abuse complicating <u>childbirth</u> — [♀, Age/12-55]

O9A.33 Physical abuse complicating <u>the puerperium</u> — [♀, Age/12-55]

O9A.4- <u>Sexual abuse</u> complicating pregnancy, childbirth and the puerperium
> Conditions in T74.21 or T76.21
> Use additional code (if applicable):
> To identify any associated current injury due to sexual abuse
> To identify the perpetrator of abuse (Y07.-)

O9A.41- Sexual abuse complicating <u>pregnancy</u>

O9A.411 Sexual abuse complicating pregnancy, <u>first</u> trimester — [♀, Age/12-55]

O9A.412 Sexual abuse complicating pregnancy, <u>second</u> trimester — [♀, Age/12-55]

O9A.413 Sexual abuse complicating pregnancy, <u>third</u> trimester — [♀, Age/12-55]

O9A.419 Sexual abuse complicating pregnancy, <u>unspecified</u> trimester — [♀, Age/12-55]

O9A.42 Sexual abuse complicating <u>childbirth</u> — [♀, Age/12-55]

O9A.43 Sexual abuse complicating <u>the puerperium</u> — [♀, Age/12-55]

O9A.5- <u>Psychological abuse</u> complicating pregnancy, childbirth and the puerperium
> Conditions in T74.31 or T76.31
> Use additional code to identify the perpetrator of abuse (Y07.-)

O9A.51- Psychological abuse complicating <u>pregnancy</u>

O9A.511 Psychological abuse complicating pregnancy, <u>first</u> trimester — [♀, Age/12-55]

O9A.512 Psychological abuse complicating pregnancy, <u>second</u> trimester — [♀, Age/12-55]

O9A.513 Psychological abuse complicating pregnancy, <u>third</u> trimester — [♀, Age/12-55]

O9A.519 Psychological abuse complicating pregnancy, <u>unspecified</u> trimester — [♀, Age/12-55]

O9A.52 Psychological abuse complicating <u>childbirth</u> — [♀, Age/12-55]

O9A.53 Psychological abuse complicating <u>the puerperium</u> — [♀, Age/12-55]

O9A – O9A

Chapter 16 – Certain conditions originating in the perinatal period (P00-P96)

Note: Codes from this chapter are for use on newborn records only, never on maternal records

Includes: Conditions that have their origin in the fetal or perinatal period (before birth through the first 28 days after birth) even if morbidity occurs later

Excludes ❷: congenital malformations, deformations and chromosomal abnormalities (Q00-Q99)

endocrine, nutritional and metabolic diseases (E00-E88)

injury, poisoning and certain other consequences of external causes (S00-T88)

neoplasms (C00-D49)

tetanus neonatorum (A33)

This chapter contains the following blocks:

P00-P04	Newborn affected by maternal factors and by complications of pregnancy, labor, and delivery
P05-P08	Disorders of newborn related to length of gestation and fetal growth
P09	Abnormal findings on neonatal screening
P10-P15	Birth trauma
P19-P29	Respiratory and cardiovascular disorders specific to the perinatal period
P35-P39	Infections specific to the perinatal period
P50-P61	Hemorrhagic and hematological disorders of newborn
P70-P74	Transitory endocrine and metabolic disorders specific to newborn
P76-P78	Digestive system disorders of newborn
P80-P83	Conditions involving the integument and temperature regulation of newborn
P84	Other problems with newborn
P90-P96	Other disorders originating in the perinatal period

Chapter-Specific Coding Guidelines

C. Chapter-Specific Coding Guidelines

In addition to general coding guidelines, there are guidelines for specific diagnoses and/or conditions in the classification. Unless otherwise indicated, these guidelines apply to all health care settings. Please refer to Section II for guidelines on the selection of principal diagnosis.

16. Chapter 16: Certain Conditions Originating in the Perinatal Period (P00-P96)

For coding and reporting purposes the perinatal period is defined as before birth through the 28th day following birth. The following guidelines are provided for reporting purposes

a. General Perinatal Rules

1) Use of Chapter 16 Codes
Codes in this chapter are <u>never</u> for use on the maternal record.

Codes from Chapter 15, the obstetric chapter, are never permitted on the newborn record. Chapter 16 codes may be used throughout the life of the patient if the condition is still present.

2) Principal Diagnosis for Birth Record
When coding the birth episode in a newborn record, assign a code from category Z38, Liveborn infants according to place of birth and type of delivery, as the principal diagnosis. A code from category Z38 is assigned only once, to a newborn at the time of birth. If a newborn is transferred to another institution, a code from category Z38 should not be used at the receiving hospital.

A code from category Z38 is used only on the newborn record, not on the mother's record.

3) Use of Codes from other Chapters with Codes from Chapter 16
Codes from other chapters may be used with codes from chapter 16 if the codes from the other chapters provide more specific detail. Codes for signs and symptoms may be assigned when a definitive diagnosis has not been established. If the reason for the encounter is a perinatal condition, the code from chapter 16 should be sequenced first.

4) Use of Chapter 16 Codes after the Perinatal Period
Should a condition originate in the perinatal period, and continue throughout the life of the patient, the perinatal code should continue to be used regardless of the patient's age.

5) Birth process or community acquired conditions
If a newborn has a condition that may be either due to the birth process or community acquired and the documentation does not indicate which it is, the default is due to the birth process and the code from Chapter 16 should be used. If the condition is community-acquired, a code from Chapter 16 should not be assigned.

6) Code all clinically significant conditions
All clinically significant conditions noted on routine newborn examination should be coded. A condition is clinically significant if it requires:
- clinical evaluation; or
- therapeutic treatment; or
- diagnostic procedures; or
- extended length of hospital stay; or
- increased nursing care and/or monitoring; or
- has implications for future health care needs

Note: The perinatal guidelines listed above are the same as the general coding guidelines for "additional diagnoses", except for the final point regarding implications for future health care needs. Codes should be assigned for conditions that have been specified by the provider as having implications for future health care needs.

b. Observation and Evaluation of Newborns for Suspected Conditions not Found
~~Reserved for future expansion~~

1) Assign a code from category Z05, Observation and evaluation of newborns and infants for suspected conditions ruled out, to identify those instances when a healthy newborn is evaluated for a suspected condition that is determined after study not to be present. Do not use a code from category Z05 when the patient has identified signs or symptoms of a suspected problem; in such cases code the sign or symptom.

2) A code from category Z05 may also be assigned as a principal or first-listed code for readmissions or encounters when the code from category Z38 code no longer applies. Codes from category Z05 are for use only for healthy newborns and infants for which no condition after study is found to be present.

3) Z05 on a birth record
A code from category Z05 is to be used as a secondary code after the code from category Z38, Liveborn infants according to place of birth and type of delivery.

c. Coding Additional Perinatal Diagnoses

1) Assigning codes for conditions that require treatment
Assign codes for conditions that require treatment or further investigation, prolong the length of stay, or require resource utilization.

2) Codes for conditions specified as having implications for future health care needs
Assign codes for conditions that have been specified by the provider as having implications for future health care needs.

Note: This guideline should not be used for adult patients.

d. Prematurity and Fetal Growth Retardation
Providers utilize different criteria in determining prematurity. A code for prematurity should not be assigned unless it is documented. Assignment of codes in categories P05, Disorders of newborn related to slow fetal growth and fetal malnutrition, and P07, Disorders of newborn related to short gestation and low birth weight, not elsewhere classified, should be based on the recorded birth weight and estimated gestational age. Codes from category P05 should not be assigned with codes from category P07.

When both birth weight and gestational age are available, two codes from category P07 should be assigned, with the code for birth weight sequenced before the code for gestational age.

e. Low birth weight and immaturity status
Codes from category P07, Disorders of newborn related to short gestation and low birth weight, not elsewhere classified, are for use for a child or adult who was premature or had a low birth weight as a newborn and this is affecting the patient's current health status.

See Section I.C.21. Factors influencing health status and contact with health services, Status.

f. Bacterial Sepsis of Newborn
Category P36, Bacterial sepsis of newborn, includes congenital sepsis. If a perinate is documented as having sepsis without documentation of congenital or community acquired, the default is congenital and a code from category P36 should be assigned. If the P36 code includes the causal organism, an additional code from category B95, Streptococcus, Staphylococcus, and Enterococcus as the cause of diseases classified elsewhere, or B96, Other bacterial agents as the cause of diseases classified elsewhere, should not be assigned. If the P36 code does not include the causal organism, assign an additional code from category B96. If applicable, use additional codes to identify severe sepsis (R65.2-) and any associated acute organ dysfunction.

g. Stillbirth
Code P95, Stillbirth, is only for use in institutions that maintain separate records for stillbirths. No other code should be used with P95. Code P95 should not be used on the mother's record.

Excludes 1: = NOT CODED HERE! (Do not code both)   *Excludes ❷:* = Not Included Here

Newborn affected by maternal factors and by complications of pregnancy, labor, and delivery (P00-P04)

Note: These codes are for use when the listed maternal conditions are specified as the cause of confirmed morbidity or potential morbidity which have their origin in the perinatal period (before birth through the first 28 days after birth).

P00- Newborn affected by <u>maternal conditions</u> that may be <u>unrelated</u> to present pregnancy

Code first any current condition in newborn

Excludes ❷: encounter for observation of newborn for suspected diseases and conditions ruled out (Z05.-)
newborn affected by maternal complications of pregnancy (P01.-)
newborn affected by maternal endocrine and metabolic disorders (P70-P74)
newborn affected by noxious substances transmitted via placenta or breast milk (P04.-)

P00.0 Newborn affected by maternal hypertensive disorders
Newborn affected by maternal conditions classifiable to O10-O11, O13-O16

P00.1 Newborn affected by maternal renal and urinary tract diseases
Newborn affected by maternal conditions classifiable to N00-N39

P00.2 Newborn affected by maternal infectious and parasitic diseases
AHA 15:3Q:p20 – Suspected sepsis in newborn, ruled out
Newborn affected by maternal infectious disease classifiable to A00-B99, J09 and J10
Excludes 1:   infections specific to the perinatal period (P35-P39)
maternal genital tract or other localized infections (P00.8)

P00.3 Newborn affected by other maternal circulatory and respiratory diseases
Newborn affected by maternal conditions classifiable to I00-I99, J00-J99, Q20-Q34 and not included in P00.0, P00.2

P00.4 Newborn affected by maternal nutritional disorders
Newborn affected by maternal disorders classifiable to E40-E64
Maternal malnutrition NOS

P00.5 Newborn affected by maternal injury
Newborn affected by maternal conditions classifiable to O9A.2-

P00.6 Newborn affected by surgical procedure on mother
Newborn affected by amniocentesis
Excludes 1:   cesarean delivery for present delivery (P03.4)
damage to placenta from amniocentesis, cesarean delivery or surgical induction (P02.1)
previous surgery to uterus or pelvic organs (P03.89)
Excludes ❷: newborn affected by complication of (fetal) intrauterine procedure (P96.5)

P00.7 Newborn affected by other medical procedures on mother, not elsewhere classified
Newborn affected by radiation to mother
Excludes 1:   damage to placenta from amniocentesis, cesarean delivery or surgical induction (P02.1)
newborn affected by other complications of labor and delivery (P03.-)

P00.8- Newborn affected by other maternal conditions

P00.81 Newborn affected by periodontal disease in mother

P00.89 Newborn affected by other maternal conditions
Newborn affected by conditions classifiable to T80-T88
Newborn affected by maternal genital tract or other localized infections
Newborn affected by maternal systemic lupus erythematosus

P00.9 Newborn affected by unspecified maternal condition

P01- <u>Newborn affected by maternal complications</u> of pregnancy
Code first any current condition in newborn
Excludes ❷: encounter for observation of newborn for suspected diseases and conditions ruled out (Z05.-)

P01.0 Newborn affected by incompetent cervix

P01.1 Newborn affected by premature rupture of membranes

P01.2 Newborn affected by oligohydramnios
Excludes 1:   oligohydramnios due to premature rupture of membranes (P01.1)

P01.3 Newborn affected by polyhydramnios
Newborn affected by hydramnios

P01.4 Newborn affected by ectopic pregnancy
Newborn affected by abdominal pregnancy

P01.5 Newborn affected by multiple pregnancy
Newborn affected by triplet (pregnancy)
Newborn affected by twin (pregnancy)

P01.6 Newborn affected by maternal death

P01.7 Newborn affected by malpresentation before labor
Newborn affected by breech presentation before labor
Newborn affected by external version before labor
Newborn affected by face presentation before labor
Newborn affected by transverse lie before labor
Newborn affected by unstable lie before labor

P01.8 Newborn affected by other maternal complications of pregnancy

P01.9 Newborn affected by maternal complication of pregnancy, unspecified

P02- <u>Newborn affected by complications</u> of placenta, cord and membranes
Code first any current condition in newborn
Excludes ❷: encounter for observation of newborn for suspected diseases and conditions ruled out (Z05.-)

P02.0 Newborn affected by placenta previa

P02.1 Newborn affected by other forms of placental separation and hemorrhage
Newborn affected by abruptio placenta
Newborn affected by accidental hemorrhage
Newborn affected by antepartum hemorrhage
Newborn affected by damage to placenta from amniocentesis, cesarean delivery or surgical induction
Newborn affected by maternal blood loss
Newborn affected by premature separation of placenta

P02.2- Newborn affected by other and unspecified morphological and functional abnormalities of placenta

P02.20 Newborn affected by unspecified morphological and functional abnormalities of placenta

P02.29 Newborn affected by other morphological and functional abnormalities of placenta
Newborn affected by placental dysfunction
Newborn affected by placental infarction
Newborn affected by placental insufficiency

P02.3 Newborn affected by placental transfusion syndromes
Newborn affected by placental and cord abnormalities resulting in twin-to-twin or other transplacental transfusion

P02.4 Newborn affected by prolapsed cord

P02.5 Newborn affected by other compression of umbilical cord
Newborn affected by umbilical cord (tightly) around neck
Newborn affected by entanglement of umbilical cord
Newborn affected by knot in umbilical cord

P02.6- Newborn affected by other and unspecified conditions of umbilical cord

P02.60 Newborn affected by unspecified conditions of umbilical cord

P02.69 Newborn affected by other conditions of umbilical cord
Newborn affected by short umbilical cord
Newborn affected by vasa previa
Excludes 1:   newborn affected by single umbilical artery (Q27.0)

P02.7 Newborn affected by chorioamnionitis
Newborn affected by amnionitis
Newborn affected by membranitis
Newborn affected by placentitis

P02.8 Newborn affected by other abnormalities of membranes

P02.9 Newborn affected by abnormality of membranes, unspecified

P00 - P02

Excludes 1: = NOT CODED HERE! (Do not code both)   **956**   *Excludes ❷:* = Not Included Here

P03-   Newborn affected by other complications of labor and delivery
Code first any current condition in newborn
Excludes ❷: encounter for observation of newborn for suspected diseases and conditions ruled out (Z05.-)

P03.0   Newborn affected by breech delivery and extraction

P03.1   Newborn affected by other malpresentation, malposition and disproportion during labor and delivery
Newborn affected by contracted pelvis
Newborn affected by conditions classifiable to O64-O66
Newborn affected by persistent occipitoposterior
Newborn affected by transverse lie

P03.2   Newborn affected by forceps delivery

P03.3   Newborn affected by delivery by vacuum extractor [ventouse]

P03.4   Newborn affected by cesarean delivery

P03.5   Newborn affected by precipitate delivery
Newborn affected by rapid second stage

P03.6   Newborn affected by abnormal uterine contractions
Newborn affected by conditions classifiable to O62.-, except O62.3
Newborn affected by hypertonic labor
Newborn affected by uterine inertia

P03.8-   Newborn affected by other specified complications of labor and delivery

P03.81-   Newborn affected by abnormality in fetal (intrauterine) heart rate or rhythm
Excludes 1:   neonatal cardiac dysrhythmia (P29.1-)

P03.810   Newborn affected by abnormality in fetal (intrauterine) heart rate or rhythm before the onset of labor

P03.811   Newborn affected by abnormality in fetal (intrauterine) heart rate or rhythm during labor

P03.819   Newborn affected by abnormality in fetal (intrauterine) heart rate or rhythm, unspecified as to time of onset

P03.82   Meconium passage during delivery — The presence of meconium at delivery without the presence of the distinctive mixing of meconium staining that is indicative of a stress on the fetus.
Excludes 1:   meconium aspiration (P24.00, P24.01)
meconium staining (P96.83)

P03.89   Newborn affected by other specified complications of labor and delivery
Newborn affected by abnormality of maternal soft tissues
Newborn affected by conditions classifiable to O60-O75 and by procedures used in labor and delivery not included in P02.- and P03.0-P03.6
Newborn affected by induction of labor

P03.9   Newborn affected by complication of labor and delivery, unspecified

P04-   Newborn affected by noxious substances transmitted via placenta or breast milk
Includes: Nonteratogenic effects of substances transmitted via placenta
Excludes ❷: congenital malformations (Q00-Q99)
encounter for observation of newborn for suspected diseases and conditions ruled out (Z05.-)
neonatal jaundice from excessive hemolysis due to drugs or toxins transmitted from mother (P58.4)
newborn in contact with and (suspected) exposures hazardous to health not transmitted via placenta or breast milk (Z77.-)

P04.0   Newborn affected by maternal anesthesia and analgesia in pregnancy, labor and delivery
Newborn affected by reactions and intoxications from maternal opiates and tranquilizers administered during labor and delivery

P04.1   Newborn affected by other maternal medication
Newborn affected by cancer chemotherapy
Newborn affected by cytotoxic drugs
Excludes 1:   dysmorphism due to warfarin (Q86.2)
fetal hydantoin syndrome (Q86.1)
maternal use of drugs of addiction (P04.4-)

P04.2   Newborn affected by maternal use of tobacco
Newborn affected by exposure in utero to tobacco smoke
Excludes ❷: newborn exposure to environmental tobacco smoke (P96.81)

P04.3   Newborn affected by maternal use of alcohol
Excludes 1:   fetal alcohol syndrome (Q86.0)

P04.4-   Newborn affected by maternal use of drugs of addiction

P04.41   Newborn affected by maternal use of cocaine
"Crack baby"

P04.49   Newborn affected by maternal use of other drugs of addiction
Excludes ❷: newborn affected by maternal anesthesia and analgesia (P04.0)
withdrawal symptoms from maternal use of drugs of addiction (P96.1)

P04.5   Newborn affected by maternal use of nutritional chemical substances

P04.6   Newborn affected by maternal exposure to environmental chemical substances

P04.8   Newborn affected by other maternal noxious substances

P04.9   Newborn affected by maternal noxious substance, unspecified

Disorders of newborn related to length of gestation and fetal growth (P05-P08)

P05-   Disorders of newborn related to slow fetal growth and fetal malnutrition

P05.0-   Newborn light for gestational age
Newborn light-for-dates
Weight below but length above 10th percentile for gestational age

P05.00   Newborn light for gestational age, unspecified weight

P05.01   Newborn light for gestational age, less than 500 grams

P05.02   Newborn light for gestational age, 500-749 grams

P05.03   Newborn light for gestational age, 750-999 grams

P05.04   Newborn light for gestational age, 1000-1249 grams

P05.05   Newborn light for gestational age, 1250-1499 grams

P05.06   Newborn light for gestational age, 1500-1749 grams

P05.07   Newborn light for gestational age, 1750-1999 grams

P05.08   Newborn light for gestational age, 2000-2499 grams

P05.09   Newborn light for gestational age, 2500 grams and over
Newborn light for gestational age, other

P05.1-   Newborn small for gestational age
Newborn small-and-light-for-dates
Newborn small-for-dates
Weight and length below 10th percentile for gestational age

P05.10   Newborn small for gestational age, unspecified weight

P05.11   Newborn small for gestational age, less than 500 grams

P05.12   Newborn small for gestational age, 500-749 grams

P05.13   Newborn small for gestational age, 750-999 grams

P05.14   Newborn small for gestational age, 1000-1249 grams

P05.15   Newborn small for gestational age, 1250-1499 grams

P05.16   Newborn small for gestational age, 1500-1749 grams

P05.17   Newborn small for gestational age, 1750-1999 grams

P05.18   Newborn small for gestational age, 2000-2499 grams

P05.19   Newborn small for gestational age, other
Newborn small for gestational age, 2500 grams and over

P05.2   Newborn affected by fetal (intrauterine) malnutrition not light or small for gestational age
Infant, not light or small for gestational age, showing signs of fetal malnutrition, such as dry, peeling skin and loss of subcutaneous tissue
Excludes 1:   newborn affected by fetal malnutrition with light for gestational age (P05.0-)
newborn affected by fetal malnutrition with small for gestational age (P05.1-)

P05.9   Newborn affected by slow intrauterine growth, unspecified
Newborn affected by fetal growth retardation NOS

P03 - P05

P07- **Disorders of newborn related to short gestation and low birth weight, not elsewhere classified**
    Note: When both birth weight and gestational age of the newborn are available, both should be coded with birth weight sequenced before gestational age
    Includes: The listed conditions, without further specification, as the cause of morbidity or additional care, in newborn

P07.0- <u>Extremely low birth weight</u> newborn
    Newborn birth weight 999 g. or less
    Excludes 1: low birth weight due to slow fetal growth and fetal malnutrition (P05.-)

P07.00 Extremely low birth weight newborn, unspecified weight

P07.01 Extremely low birth weight newborn, less than 500 grams

P07.02 Extremely low birth weight newborn, 500-749 grams

P07.03 Extremely low birth weight newborn, 750-999 grams

P07.1- <u>Other low birth weight</u> newborn
    Newborn birth weight 1000-2499 g.
    Excludes 1: low birth weight due to slow fetal growth and fetal malnutrition (P05.-)

P07.10 Other low birth weight newborn, unspecified weight

P07.14 Other low birth weight newborn, 1000-1249 grams

P07.15 Other low birth weight newborn, 1250-1499 grams

P07.16 Other low birth weight newborn, 1500-1749 grams

P07.17 Other low birth weight newborn, 1750-1999 grams

P07.18 Other low birth weight newborn, 2000-2499 grams

P07.2- <u>Extreme immaturity</u> of newborn
    Less than 28 completed weeks (less than 196 completed days) of gestation

P07.20 Extreme immaturity of newborn, unspecified weeks of gestation
    Gestational age less than 28 completed weeks NOS

P07.21 Extreme immaturity of newborn, gestational age less than 23 completed weeks
    Extreme immaturity of newborn, gestational age less than 23 weeks, 0 days

P07.22 Extreme immaturity of newborn, gestational age 23 completed weeks
    Extreme immaturity of newborn, gestational age 23 weeks, 0 days through 23 weeks, 6 days

P07.23 Extreme immaturity of newborn, gestational age 24 completed weeks
    Extreme immaturity of newborn, gestational age 24 weeks, 0 days through 24 weeks, 6 days

P07.24 Extreme immaturity of newborn, gestational age 25 completed weeks
    Extreme immaturity of newborn, gestational age 25 weeks, 0 days through 25 weeks, 6 days

P07.25 Extreme immaturity of newborn, gestational age 26 completed weeks
    Extreme immaturity of newborn, gestational age 26 weeks, 0 days through 26 weeks, 6 days

P07.26 Extreme immaturity of newborn, gestational age 27 completed weeks
    Extreme immaturity of newborn, gestational age 27 weeks, 0 days through 27 weeks, 6 days

P07.3- <u>Preterm [premature] newborn [other]</u>
    28 completed weeks or more but less than 37 completed weeks (196 completed days but less than 259 completed days) of gestation.
    Prematurity NOS

P07.30 Preterm newborn, unspecified weeks of gestation

P07.31 Preterm newborn, gestational age 28 completed weeks
    Preterm newborn, gestational age 28 weeks, 0 days through 28 weeks, 6 days

P07.32 Preterm newborn, gestational age 29 completed weeks
    Preterm newborn, gestational age 29 weeks, 0 days through 29 weeks, 6 days

P07.33 Preterm newborn, gestational age 30 completed weeks
    Preterm newborn, gestational age 30 weeks, 0 days through 30 weeks, 6 days

P07.34 Preterm newborn, gestational age 31 completed weeks
    Preterm newborn, gestational age 31 weeks, 0 days through 31 weeks, 6 days

P07.35 Preterm newborn, gestational age 32 completed weeks
    Preterm newborn, gestational age 32 weeks, 0 days through 32 weeks, 6 days

P07.36 Preterm newborn, gestational age 33 completed weeks
    Preterm newborn, gestational age 33 weeks, 0 days through 33 weeks, 6 days

P07.37 Preterm newborn, gestational age 34 completed weeks
    Preterm newborn, gestational age 34 weeks, 0 days through 34 weeks, 6 days

P07.38 Preterm newborn, gestational age 35 completed weeks
    Preterm newborn, gestational age 35 weeks, 0 days through 35 weeks, 6 days

P07.39 Preterm newborn, gestational age 36 completed weeks
    Preterm newborn, gestational age 36 weeks, 0 days through 36 weeks, 6 days

P08- **Disorders of newborn related to <u>long gestation and high birth weight</u>**
    Note: When both birth weight and gestational age of the newborn are available, priority of assignment should be given to birth weight
    Includes: The listed conditions, without further specification, as causes of morbidity or additional care, in newborn

P08.0 **Exceptionally large newborn baby**
    Usually implies a birth weight of 4500 g. or more
    Excludes 1: syndrome of infant of diabetic mother (P70.1)
    syndrome of infant of mother with gestational diabetes (P70.0)

P08.1 **Other heavy for gestational age newborn**
    Other newborn heavy- or large-for-dates regardless of period of gestation
    Usually implies a birth weight of 4000 g. to 4499 g.
    Excludes 1: newborn with a birth weight of 4500 or more (P08.0)
    syndrome of infant of diabetic mother (P70.1)
    syndrome of infant of mother with gestational diabetes (P70.0)

P08.2- **Late newborn, not heavy for gestational age**
    AHA 14:1Q:p14 – Post-term newborn

P08.21 **Post-term newborn**
    Newborn with gestation period over 40 completed weeks to 42 completed weeks

P08.22 **Prolonged gestation of newborn**
    Newborn with gestation period over 42 completed weeks (294 days or more), not heavy- or large-for-dates
    Postmaturity NOS

Abnormal findings on neonatal screening (P09)

P09 **Abnormal findings on neonatal screening**
    Use additional code to identify signs, symptoms and conditions associated with the screening
    Excludes ❷: nonspecific serologic evidence of human immunodeficiency virus [HIV] (R75)

P07-P09

Birth trauma (P10-P15)

P10- <u>Intracranial laceration and hemorrhage due to birth injury</u>
Excludes 1:   *intracranial hemorrhage of newborn NOS (P52.9)*
                  intracranial hemorrhage of newborn due to anoxia or hypoxia (P52.-)
                  nontraumatic intracranial hemorrhage of newborn (P52.-)

MCC **P10.0**   **Subdural hemorrhage due to birth injury** — The escape of blood below the dura of the infant.
            Subdural hematoma (localized) due to birth injury
            Excludes 1:   subdural hemorrhage accompanying tentorial tear (P10.4)

MCC **P10.1**   **Cerebral hemorrhage due to birth injury** — The escape of blood within the cerebrum of the infant.

CC **P10.2**   **Intraventricular hemorrhage due to birth injury** — The escape of blood within the cerebral ventricles of the infant.

MCC **P10.3**   **Subarachnoid hemorrhage due to birth injury** — The escape of blood below the subarachnoid layer of the meninges of the infant.

MCC **P10.4**   **Tentorial tear due to birth injury** — The disruption of the dura that covers the cerebellum and supports the occipital lobes.

MCC **P10.8**   **Other intracranial lacerations and hemorrhages due to birth injury**

MCC **P10.9**   **Unspecified intracranial laceration and hemorrhage due to birth injury**

P11- <u>Other</u> birth injuries to <u>central nervous system</u>

MCC **P11.0**   **Cerebral edema due to birth injury** — The accumulation of fluid on the brain.

P11.1   **Other specified brain damage due to birth injury**

MCC **P11.2**   **Unspecified brain damage due to birth injury**

P11.3   **Birth injury to facial nerve** — Traumatic damage to a facial nerve during, or due to, birth.
            Facial palsy due to birth injury

P11.4   **Birth injury to other cranial nerves**

P11.5   **Birth injury to spine and spinal cord** — Traumatic damage to the spine and spinal cord during, or due to, birth.
            Fracture of spine due to birth injury

MCC **P11.9**   **Birth injury to central nervous system, unspecified**

P12- **Birth injury to** <u>scalp</u> — The traumatic damage to the infant's scalp during, or due to, birth.

P12.0   **Cephalhematoma due to birth injury** — The subcutaneous swelling of the head with blood, often from the application of forceps during delivery.

P12.1   **Chignon (from vacuum extraction) due to birth injury** — The temporary swelling of the scalp due to the suction from the vacuum cap.

CC **P12.2**   **Epicranial subaponeurotic hemorrhage due to birth injury** — The accumulation of blood due to the rupture of blood vessels in the dense connective tissue of the scalp.
            Subgaleal hemorrhage

P12.3   **Bruising of scalp due to birth injury**

P12.4   **Injury of scalp of newborn due to monitoring equipment**
            Sampling incision of scalp of newborn
            Scalp clip (electrode) injury of newborn

P12.8-   **Other birth injuries to scalp**

     P12.81   **Caput succedaneum** — The swelling edema of the scalp produced during labor.

     P12.89   **Other birth injuries to scalp**

P12.9   **Birth injury to scalp, unspecified**

P13- **Birth injury to** <u>skeleton</u>
Excludes ❷: birth injury to spine (P11.5)

P13.0   **Fracture of skull due to birth injury**

P13.1   **Other birth injuries to skull**
            Excludes 1:   cephalhematoma (P12.0)

P13.2   **Birth injury to femur**

P13.3   **Birth injury to other long bones**

P13.4   **Fracture of clavicle due to birth injury**

P13.8   **Birth injuries to other parts of skeleton**

P13.9   **Birth injury to skeleton, unspecified**

P14- **Birth injury to** <u>peripheral nervous system</u>

P14.0   **Erb's paralysis due to birth injury** — The loss of the function of small muscles in the hand, due to injury to the fifth and sixth cervical roots.

P14.1   **Klumpke's paralysis due to birth injury** — The loss of muscular control of the arm due to injury of the eighth cervical and first dorsal nerve roots.

P14.2   **Phrenic nerve paralysis due to birth injury** — The loss or impairment of function of the nerve that innervates the pleura, pericardium, diaphragm, peritoneum, and sympathetic plexuses.

P14.3   **Other brachial plexus birth injuries**

P14.8   **Birth injuries to other parts of peripheral nervous system**

P14.9   **Birth injury to peripheral nervous system, unspecified**

P15- <u>Other birth injuries</u>

P15.0   **Birth injury to liver**
            Rupture of liver due to birth injury

P15.1   **Birth injury to spleen**
            Rupture of spleen due to birth injury

P15.2   **Sternomastoid injury due to birth injury**

P15.3   **Birth injury to eye**
            Subconjunctival hemorrhage due to birth injury
            Traumatic glaucoma due to birth injury

P15.4   **Birth injury to face**
            Facial congestion due to birth injury

P15.5   **Birth injury to external genitalia**

P15.6   **Subcutaneous fat necrosis due to birth injury**

P15.8   **Other specified birth injuries**

P15.9   **Birth injury, unspecified**

Respiratory and cardiovascular disorders specific to the perinatal period (P19-P29)

P19- **Metabolic acidemia in newborn** — The metabolic disturbance of the normal acid-base balance of the fetus or infant.
            Includes: Metabolic acidemia in newborn

P19.0   **Metabolic acidemia in newborn first noted before onset of labor**

P19.1   **Metabolic acidemia in newborn first noted during labor**

P19.2   **Metabolic acidemia noted at birth**

P19.9   **Metabolic acidemia, unspecified**

P22- <u>Respiratory distress of newborn</u>
Excludes 1:   respiratory arrest of newborn (P28.81)
                respiratory failure of newborn NOS (P28.5)

MCC **P22.0**   **Respiratory distress syndrome of newborn** — The acute lung underdevelopment condition of the newborn that is characterized by airless alveoli, inelastic lungs, cyanosis, and rapid respirations.
            Cardiorespiratory distress syndrome of newborn
            Hyaline membrane disease
            Idiopathic respiratory distress syndrome [IRDS or RDS] of newborn
            Pulmonary hypoperfusion syndrome
            Respiratory distress syndrome, type I

P22.1   **Transient tachypnea of newborn** — The nonsustained excessive rapidity of respiration.
            Idiopathic tachypnea of newborn
            Respiratory distress syndrome, type II
            Wet lung syndrome — The condition of pulmonary impairment due to excessive and delayed absorption of fluid in the lungs.

P22.8   **Other respiratory distress of newborn**

P22.9   **Respiratory distress of newborn, unspecified**

P10 - P22

P23- <u>Congenital pneumonia</u> — The inflammation of the lungs with exudate-filled air spaces that is present at birth.

Includes: Infective pneumonia acquired in utero or during birth

Excludes 1: *neonatal pneumonia resulting from aspiration (P24.-)*

MCC **P23.0** **Congenital pneumonia due to viral agent**
Use additional code (B97) to identify organism

Excludes 1: *congenital rubella pneumonitis (P35.0)*

MCC **P23.1** **Congenital pneumonia due to Chlamydia**

MCC **P23.2** **Congenital pneumonia due to staphylococcus**

MCC **P23.3** **Congenital pneumonia due to streptococcus, group B**

MCC **P23.4** **Congenital pneumonia due to Escherichia coli**

MCC **P23.5** **Congenital pneumonia due to Pseudomonas**

MCC **P23.6** **Congenital pneumonia due to other bacterial agents**
Congenital pneumonia due to Hemophilus influenzae
Congenital pneumonia due to Klebsiella pneumoniae
Congenital pneumonia due to Mycoplasma
Congenital pneumonia due to Streptococcus, except group B
Use additional code (B95-B96) to identify organism

MCC **P23.8** **Congenital pneumonia due to other organisms**

MCC **P23.9** **Congenital pneumonia, unspecified**

P24- <u>Neonatal aspiration</u> — The inhalation of fluid into the lungs that may result in a significant respiratory compromise.

Includes: Aspiration in utero and during delivery

P24.0- <u>Meconium aspiration</u> — The inhalation of fetal intestinal meconium.

Excludes 1: *meconium passage (without aspiration) during delivery (P03.82)*
meconium staining (P96.83)

P24.00 **Meconium aspiration <u>without</u> respiratory symptoms**
Meconium aspiration NOS

MCC **P24.01** **Meconium aspiration <u>with respiratory symptoms</u>**
Meconium aspiration pneumonia
Meconium aspiration pneumonitis
Meconium aspiration syndrome NOS
Use additional code to identify any secondary pulmonary hypertension, if applicable (I27.2)

P24.1- **Neonatal aspiration of (clear) <u>amniotic fluid</u> and mucus** — The inhalation of the non-meconium stained amniotic fluid.
Neonatal aspiration of liquor (amnii)

P24.10 **Neonatal aspiration of (clear) amniotic fluid and mucus <u>without</u> respiratory symptoms**
Neonatal aspiration of amniotic fluid and mucus NOS

MCC **P24.11** **Neonatal aspiration of (clear) amniotic fluid and mucus <u>with respiratory symptoms</u>**
Neonatal aspiration of amniotic fluid and mucus with pneumonia
Neonatal aspiration of amniotic fluid and mucus with pneumonitis
Use additional code to identify any secondary pulmonary hypertension, if applicable (I27.2)

P24.2- **Neonatal aspiration of <u>blood</u>** — The inhalation of blood.

P24.20 **Neonatal aspiration of blood <u>without</u> respiratory symptoms**
Neonatal aspiration of blood NOS

MCC **P24.21** **Neonatal aspiration of blood <u>with respiratory symptoms</u>**
Neonatal aspiration of blood with pneumonia
Neonatal aspiration of blood with pneumonitis
Use additional code to identify any secondary pulmonary hypertension, if applicable (I27.2)

P24.3- **Neonatal aspiration of <u>milk and regurgitated food</u>**
Neonatal aspiration of stomach contents

P24.30 **Neonatal aspiration of milk and regurgitated food <u>without</u> respiratory symptoms**
Neonatal aspiration of milk and regurgitated food NOS

MCC **P24.31** **Neonatal aspiration of milk and regurgitated food <u>with respiratory symptoms</u>**
Neonatal aspiration of milk and regurgitated food with pneumonia
Neonatal aspiration of milk and regurgitated food with pneumonitis
Use additional code to identify any secondary pulmonary hypertension, if applicable (I27.2)

P24.8- <u>Other</u> neonatal aspiration

P24.80 **Other neonatal aspiration <u>without</u> respiratory symptoms**
Neonatal aspiration NEC

MCC **P24.81** **Other neonatal aspiration <u>with respiratory symptoms</u>**
Neonatal aspiration pneumonia NEC
Neonatal aspiration with pneumonitis NEC
Neonatal aspiration with pneumonia NOS
Neonatal aspiration with pneumonitis NOS
Use additional code to identify any secondary pulmonary hypertension, if applicable (I27.2)

P24.9 **Neonatal aspiration, <u>unspecified</u>**

P25- <u>Interstitial emphysema</u> and related conditions originating in the perinatal period

MCC **P25.0** **Interstitial emphysema originating in the perinatal period** — The presence of air in the peribronchial and interstitial tissues of the lungs.

MCC **P25.1** **Pneumothorax originating in the perinatal period** — The accumulation of air or gas in the pleural space.

MCC **P25.2** **Pneumomediastinum originating in the perinatal period** — The presence of air or gas in the mediastinum.

MCC **P25.3** **Pneumopericardium originating in the perinatal period** — The presence of air or gas in the pericardium.

MCC **P25.8** **Other conditions related to interstitial emphysema originating in the perinatal period**

P26- <u>Pulmonary hemorrhage</u> originating in the perinatal period — The escape of blood from the lungs.

Excludes 1: *acute idiopathic hemorrhage in infants over 28 days old (R04.81)*

MCC **P26.0** **Tracheobronchial hemorrhage originating in the perinatal period**

MCC **P26.1** **Massive pulmonary hemorrhage originating in the perinatal period**

MCC **P26.8** **Other pulmonary hemorrhages originating in the perinatal period**

MCC **P26.9** **Unspecified pulmonary hemorrhage originating in the perinatal period**

P27- <u>Chronic respiratory disease</u> originating in the perinatal period

Excludes 1: *respiratory distress of newborn (P22.0-P22.9)*

MCC **P27.0** **Wilson-Mikity syndrome** — Pulmonary insufficiency caused by the presence of multiple cyst-like areas of hyperaeration with thickening of the interstitial tissues.
Pulmonary dysmaturity

MCC **P27.1** **Bronchopulmonary dysplasia originating in the perinatal period**

MCC **P27.8** **Other chronic respiratory diseases originating in the perinatal period**
Congenital pulmonary fibrosis — The formation of fibrous tissue around the pulmonary alveolar walls.
Ventilator lung in newborn

MCC **P27.9** **Unspecified chronic respiratory disease originating in the perinatal period**

P23-P27

P28- <u>Other respiratory conditions</u> originating in the perinatal period
Excludes 1:   congenital malformations of the respiratory system (Q30-Q34)

cc **P28.0**   **Primary atelectasis of newborn** — The imperfect expansion of the lungs immediately after birth.
Primary failure to expand terminal respiratory units
Pulmonary hypoplasia associated with short gestation
Pulmonary immaturity NOS

P28.1-   **Other and unspecified atelectasis of newborn**

cc **P28.10**   **Unspecified atelectasis of newborn**
Atelectasis of newborn NOS

cc **P28.11**   **Resorption atelectasis without respiratory distress syndrome**
Excludes 1:   resorption atelectasis with respiratory distress syndrome (P22.0)

cc **P28.19**   **Other atelectasis of newborn**
Partial atelectasis of newborn
Secondary atelectasis of newborn

cc **P28.2**   **Cyanotic attacks of newborn** — The sudden, severe condition of reduced hemoglobin concentration in the blood characterized by bluish or purple skin discoloration.
Excludes 1:   apnea of newborn (P28.3-P28.4)

cc **P28.3**   **Primary sleep apnea of newborn** — The abnormal, periodic cessation of breathing due to a lack of sufficient neural impulses to the respiratory system.
Central sleep apnea of newborn
Obstructive sleep apnea of newborn
Sleep apnea of newborn NOS

cc **P28.4**   **Other apnea of newborn**
Apnea of prematurity
Obstructive apnea of newborn
Excludes 1:   obstructive sleep apnea of newborn (P28.3)

mcc **P28.5**   **Respiratory failure of newborn** — The sudden onset of severely decreased pulmonary function.
Excludes 1:   respiratory arrest of newborn (P28.81)
respiratory distress of newborn (P22.0-)

P28.8-   **Other specified respiratory conditions of newborn**

mcc **P28.81**   **Respiratory arrest of newborn** — The cessation of breathing.

P28.89   **Other specified respiratory conditions of newborn**
Congenital laryngeal stridor
Sniffles in newborn
Snuffles in newborn
Excludes 1:   early congenital syphilitic rhinitis (A50.05)

P28.9   **Respiratory condition of newborn, unspecified**
Respiratory depression in newborn

P29- <u>Cardiovascular disorders</u> originating in the perinatal period
Excludes 1:   congenital malformations of the circulatory system (Q20-Q28)

P29.0   **Neonatal cardiac failure** — The decreased ability of the heart to pump enough blood to meet the needs of the body's tissues.

P29.1-   **Neonatal cardiac dysrhythmia**

P29.11   **Neonatal tachycardia** — An abnormal, persistent rapid fetal heart rate.

P29.12   **Neonatal bradycardia** — An abnormal, persistent slow fetal heart rate.

P29.2   **Neonatal hypertension** — Abnormally elevated blood pressure.

mcc **P29.3**   **Persistent fetal circulation** — The progressive, severe decrease in the oxygenation of the blood due to the failure of the newborn's circulation to change from the fetal circulation to the normal air-breathing circulation.
Delayed closure of ductus arteriosus
(Persistent) pulmonary hypertension of newborn

P29.4   **Transient myocardial ischemia in newborn**

P29.8-   **Other cardiovascular disorders originating in the perinatal period**

mcc **P29.81**   **Cardiac arrest of newborn** — The cessation of cardiac function.

P29.89   **Other cardiovascular disorders originating in the perinatal period**
AHA 14:4Q:p23 – Possible systolic ejection murmur

P29.9   **Cardiovascular disorder originating in the perinatal period, unspecified**

Infections specific to the perinatal period (P35-P39)

Infections acquired in utero, during birth via the umbilicus, or during the first 28 days after birth
Excludes ❷: asymptomatic human immunodeficiency virus [HIV] infection status (Z21)
congenital gonococcal infection (A54.-)
congenital pneumonia (P23.-)
congenital syphilis (A50.-)
human immunodeficiency virus [HIV] disease (B20)
infant botulism (A48.51)
infectious diseases not specific to the perinatal period (A00-B99, J09, J10.-)
intestinal infectious disease (A00-A09)
laboratory evidence of human immunodeficiency virus [HIV] (R75)
tetanus neonatorum (A33)

P35- <u>Congenital viral diseases</u>
Includes: Infections acquired in utero or during birth

cc **P35.0**   **Congenital rubella syndrome**
Congenital rubella pneumonitis

mcc **P35.1**   **Congenital cytomegalovirus infection**

mcc **P35.2**   **Congenital herpesviral [herpes simplex] infection**

mcc **P35.3**   **Congenital viral hepatitis**

mcc **P35.8**   **Other congenital viral diseases**
Congenital varicella [chickenpox]

mcc **P35.9**   **Congenital viral disease, unspecified**

P36- <u>Bacterial sepsis</u> of newborn — The infectious disease of the newborn that is due to the accumulation and persistence of bacteria and/or their toxins in the blood.
Includes: Congenital sepsis
Use additional code(s), if applicable, to identify severe sepsis (R65.2-) and associated acute organ dysfunction(s)

mcc **P36.0**   **Sepsis of newborn due to streptococcus, group B**

P36.1-   **Sepsis of newborn due to other and unspecified streptococci**

mcc **P36.10**   **Sepsis of newborn due to unspecified streptococci**

mcc **P36.19**   **Sepsis of newborn due to other streptococci**

mcc **P36.2**   **Sepsis of newborn due to Staphylococcus aureus**

P36.3-   **Sepsis of newborn due to other and unspecified staphylococci**

mcc **P36.30**   **Sepsis of newborn due to unspecified staphylococci**

mcc **P36.39**   **Sepsis of newborn due to other staphylococci**

mcc **P36.4**   **Sepsis of newborn due to Escherichia coli**

mcc **P36.5**   **Sepsis of newborn due to anaerobes**

mcc **P36.8**   **Other bacterial sepsis of newborn**
Use additional code from category B96 to identify organism

mcc **P36.9**   **Bacterial sepsis of newborn, unspecified**

P37- <u>Other congenital</u> infectious and parasitic diseases
Excludes ❷: congenital syphilis (A50.-)
infectious neonatal diarrhea (A00-A09)
necrotizing enterocolitis in newborn (P77.-)
noninfectious neonatal diarrhea (P78.3)
ophthalmia neonatorum due to gonococcus (A54.31)
tetanus neonatorum (A33)

mcc **P37.0**   **Congenital tuberculosis**

mcc **P37.1**   **Congenital toxoplasmosis**
Hydrocephalus due to congenital toxoplasmosis

mcc **P37.2**   **Neonatal (disseminated) listeriosis**

mcc **P37.3**   **Congenital falciparum malaria**

mcc **P37.4**   **Other congenital malaria**

P37.5   **Neonatal candidiasis**

mcc **P37.8**   **Other specified congenital infectious and parasitic diseases**

mcc **P37.9**   **Congenital infectious or parasitic disease, unspecified**

P28 – P37

Excludes 1: = NOT CODED HERE! (Do not code both)   **961**   Excludes ❷: = Not Included Here

P38- <u>Omphalitis</u> of newborn — Inflamation of the umbilicus.
Excludes 1:   omphalitis not of newborn (L08.82)
          tetanus omphalitis (A33)
          umbilical hemorrhage of newborn (P51.-)

CC **P38.1**   **Omphalitis with mild hemorrhage**

CC **P38.9**   **Omphalitis without hemorrhage**
          Omphalitis of newborn NOS

P39- <u>Other infections</u> specific to the perinatal period
Use additional code to identify organism or specific infection

CC **P39.0**   **Neonatal infective mastitis** — Inflammation of the newborn breast.
          Excludes 1:   breast engorgement of newborn (P83.4)
                    noninfective mastitis of newborn (P83.4)

P39.1   **Neonatal conjunctivitis and dacryocystitis** — Inflammation of the
          conjunctiva and/or lacrimal sac.
          Neonatal chlamydial conjunctivitis
          Ophthalmia neonatorum NOS
          Excludes 1:   gonococcal conjunctivitis (A54.31)

CC **P39.2**   **Intra-amniotic infection affecting newborn, not elsewhere
          classified**

CC **P39.3**   **Neonatal urinary tract infection**

CC **P39.4**   **Neonatal skin infection**
          Neonatal pyoderma
          Excludes 1:   pemphigus neonatorum (L00)
                    staphylococcal scalded skin syndrome (L00)

CC **P39.8**   **Other specified infections specific to the perinatal period**

CC **P39.9**   **Infection specific to the perinatal period, unspecified**

Hemorrhagic and hematological disorders of newborn (P50-P61)

Excludes 1:   congenital stenosis and stricture of bile ducts (Q44.3)
          Crigler-Najjar syndrome (E80.5)
          Dubin-Johnson syndrome (E80.6)
          Gilbert syndrome (E80.4)
          hereditary hemolytic anemias (D55-D58)

P50- **Newborn affected by** <u>intrauterine (fetal) blood loss</u> — The diminished
blood volume of the fetus that affects the fetus and newborn.
Excludes 1:   congenital anemia from intrauterine (fetal) blood loss (P61.3)

P50.0   **Newborn affected by intrauterine (fetal) blood loss from vasa
          previa**

P50.1   **Newborn affected by intrauterine (fetal) blood loss from
          ruptured cord**

P50.2   **Newborn affected by intrauterine (fetal) blood loss from
          placenta**

P50.3   **Newborn affected by hemorrhage into co-twin**

P50.4   **Newborn affected by hemorrhage into maternal circulation**

P50.5   **Newborn affected by intrauterine (fetal) blood loss from cut
          end of co-twin's cord**

P50.8   **Newborn affected by other intrauterine (fetal) blood loss**

P50.9   **Newborn affected by intrauterine (fetal) blood loss,
          unspecified**
          Newborn affected by fetal hemorrhage NOS

P51- <u>Umbilical hemorrhage</u> of newborn — The escape of blood from the umbilicus.
Excludes 1:   omphalitis with mild hemorrhage (P38.1)
          umbilical hemorrhage from cut end of co-twins cord (P50.5)

P51.0   **Massive umbilical hemorrhage of newborn**

P51.8   **Other umbilical hemorrhages of newborn**
          Slipped umbilical ligature NOS

P51.9   **Umbilical hemorrhage of newborn, unspecified**

P52- <u>Intracranial nontraumatic hemorrhage</u> of newborn — The escape of blood
within the skull.
Includes: Intracranial hemorrhage due to anoxia or hypoxia
Excludes 1:   intracranial hemorrhage due to birth injury (P10.-)
          intracranial hemorrhage due to other injury (S06.-)

CC **P52.0**   **Intraventricular (nontraumatic) hemorrhage, grade 1, of
          newborn**
          Subependymal hemorrhage (without intraventricular extension)
          Bleeding into germinal matrix

CC **P52.1**   **Intraventricular (nontraumatic) hemorrhage, grade 2, of
          newborn** — The escape of blood into the ventricles of the brain.
          Subependymal hemorrhage with intraventricular extension
          Bleeding into ventricle

P52.2-   **Intraventricular (nontraumatic) hemorrhage, grade 3 and
          grade 4, of newborn**

MCC **P52.21**   **Intraventricular (nontraumatic) hemorrhage, grade 3, of
          newborn**
          **Subependymal hemorrhage with intraventricular extension
          with enlargement of ventricle**

MCC **P52.22**   **Intraventricular (nontraumatic) hemorrhage, grade 4, of
          newborn**
          Bleeding into cerebral cortex
          Subependymal hemorrhage with intracerebral extension

CC **P52.3**   **Unspecified intraventricular (nontraumatic) hemorrhage of
          newborn**

MCC **P52.4**   **Intracerebral (nontraumatic) hemorrhage of newborn** — The
          escape of blood within the brain.

MCC **P52.5**   **Subarachnoid (nontraumatic) hemorrhage of newborn** — The
          escape of blood into the subarachnoid space.

MCC **P52.6**   **Cerebellar (nontraumatic) and posterior fossa hemorrhage of
          newborn**

MCC **P52.8**   **Other intracranial (nontraumatic) hemorrhages of newborn**

MCC **P52.9**   **Intracranial (nontraumatic) hemorrhage of newborn,
          unspecified**

P53 **Hemorrhagic disease of newborn** — A bleeding disorder of the
CC newborn that is caused by a transient vitamin K deficiency.
     Vitamin K deficiency of newborn

P54- <u>Other neonatal hemorrhages</u>
Excludes 1:   newborn affected by (intrauterine) blood loss (P50.-)
          pulmonary hemorrhage originating in the perinatal period
          (P26.-)

P54.0   **Neonatal hematemesis** — The presence of blood in the vomitus.
          Excludes 1:   neonatal hematemesis due to swallowed maternal
                    blood (P78.2)

MCC **P54.1**   **Neonatal melena** — The presence of black, tarry stools due to blood in the
          feces.
          Excludes 1:   neonatal melena due to swallowed maternal blood
                    (P78.2)

MCC **P54.2**   **Neonatal rectal hemorrhage** — The escape of blood from the rectum.

MCC **P54.3**   **Other neonatal gastrointestinal hemorrhage** — The escape of blood
          from the gastrointestinal tract.

CC **P54.4**   **Neonatal adrenal hemorrhage** — The escape of blood from the
          adrenals.

P54.5   **Neonatal cutaneous hemorrhage** — The escape of blood from the skin.
          Neonatal bruising
          Neonatal ecchymoses
          Neonatal petechiae
          Neonatal superficial hematoma
          Excludes ❷: bruising of scalp due to birth injury (P12.3)
                    cephalhematoma due to birth injury (P12.0)

P54.6   **Neonatal vaginal hemorrhage** — [♀] — The escape of blood from the
          vagina.
          Neonatal pseudomenses

P54.8   **Other specified neonatal hemorrhages**

P54.9   **Neonatal hemorrhage, unspecified**

P
3
8
|
P
5
4

P55- Hemolytic disease of newborn — The premature destruction of red blood cells of the fetus or newborn.

P55.0 Rh isoimmunization of newborn — The premature destruction of red blood cells of the fetus or newborn that is caused by an antigen-antibody reaction of fetal/maternal blood group incompatibility.

P55.1 ABO isoimmunization of newborn — The premature destruction of mature red blood cells due to an ABO fetal/maternal blood group incompatibility.
AHA 15:3Q:p20 – ABO incompatibility and Coombs test

P55.8 Other hemolytic diseases of newborn

P55.9 Hemolytic disease of newborn, unspecified

P56- Hydrops fetalis due to hemolytic disease
Excludes 1: hydrops fetalis NOS (P83.2)

MCC **P56.0 Hydrops fetalis due to isoimmunization** — The accumulation of massive edema of the newborn that is usually associated with erythroblastosis.

P56.9- Hydrops fetalis due to other and unspecified hemolytic disease

MCC **P56.90 Hydrops fetalis due to unspecified hemolytic disease**

MCC **P56.99 Hydrops fetalis due to other hemolytic disease**

P57- Kernicterus

MCC **P57.0 Kernicterus due to isoimmunization** — The toxic accumulation of bilirubin in the brain that is due to isoimmunization.

MCC **P57.8 Other specified kernicterus**
Excludes 1: Crigler-Najjar syndrome (E80.5)

MCC **P57.9 Kernicterus, unspecified**

P58- Neonatal jaundice due to other excessive hemolysis — The deposition of yellow bile pigment in the skin due to the premature destruction of blood cells.
Excludes 1: jaundice due to isoimmunization (P55-P57)

P58.0 Neonatal jaundice due to bruising

P58.1 Neonatal jaundice due to bleeding

P58.2 Neonatal jaundice due to infection

P58.3 Neonatal jaundice due to polycythemia

P58.4- Neonatal jaundice due to drugs or toxins transmitted from mother or given to newborn
Code first poisoning due to drug or toxin, if applicable (T36-T65 with fifth or sixth character 1-4 or 6)
Use additional code for adverse effect, if applicable, to identify drug (T36-T50 with fifth or sixth character 5)

P58.41 Neonatal jaundice due to drugs or toxins transmitted from mother

P58.42 Neonatal jaundice due to drugs or toxins given to newborn

P58.5 Neonatal jaundice due to swallowed maternal blood

P58.8 Neonatal jaundice due to other specified excessive hemolysis

P58.9 Neonatal jaundice due to excessive hemolysis, unspecified

P59- Neonatal jaundice from other and unspecified causes
AHA 15:3Q:p20 – Hyperbilirubinemia documentation
Excludes 1: jaundice due to inborn errors of metabolism (E70-E88)
kernicterus (P57.-)

P59.0 Neonatal jaundice associated with preterm delivery — The deposition of yellow bile pigment in the skin that occurs in preterm infants.
Hyperbilirubinemia of prematurity
Jaundice due to delayed conjugation associated with preterm delivery

MCC **P59.1 Inspissated bile syndrome** — The deposition of yellow bile pigment in the skin due to an obstruction of the biliary system.

P59.2- Neonatal jaundice from other and unspecified hepatocellular damage — The deposition of yellow bile pigment in the skin due to an injury to the liver tissue.
Excludes 1: congenital viral hepatitis (P35.3)

MCC **P59.20 Neonatal jaundice from unspecified hepatocellular damage**

MCC **P59.29 Neonatal jaundice from other hepatocellular damage**
Neonatal giant cell hepatitis
Neonatal (idiopathic) hepatitis

P59.3 Neonatal jaundice from breast milk inhibitor

P59.8 Neonatal jaundice from other specified causes

P59.9 Neonatal jaundice, unspecified
Neonatal physiological jaundice (intense) (prolonged) NOS

P60 Disseminated intravascular coagulation of newborn — A blood
MCC coagulation disorder in the newborn that is associated with fibrinolysis.
Defibrination syndrome of newborn

P61- Other perinatal hematological disorders
Excludes 1: transient hypogammaglobulinemia of infancy (D80.7)

MCC **P61.0 Transient neonatal thrombocytopenia** — The temporary decrease in the number of blood platelets in the newborn.
Neonatal thrombocytopenia due to exchange transfusion
Neonatal thrombocytopenia due to idiopathic maternal thrombocytopenia
Neonatal thrombocytopenia due to isoimmunization

P61.1 Polycythemia neonatorum — An abnormally increased red blood cell mass in the newborn.

CC **P61.2 Anemia of prematurity** — An abnormal reduction of red blood cells in a premature infant.

CC **P61.3 Congenital anemia from fetal blood loss** — An abnormal reduction of red blood cells in the newborn due to hemorrhage or other loss of fetal blood.

CC **P61.4 Other congenital anemias, not elsewhere classified**
Congenital anemia NOS

MCC **P61.5 Transient neonatal neutropenia** — A temporary reduction in the number of neutrophilic leukocytes in the newborn.
Excludes 1: congenital neutropenia (nontransient) (D70.0)

CC **P61.6 Other transient neonatal disorders of coagulation**

P61.8 Other specified perinatal hematological disorders

P61.9 Perinatal hematological disorder, unspecified

Transitory endocrine and metabolic disorders specific to newborn (P70-P74)

Includes: Transitory endocrine and metabolic disturbances caused by the infant's response to maternal endocrine and metabolic factors, or its adjustment to extrauterine environment

P70- Transitory disorders of carbohydrate metabolism specific to newborn

P70.0 Syndrome of infant of mother with gestational diabetes
Newborn (with hypoglycemia) affected by maternal gestational diabetes
Excludes 1: newborn (with hypoglycemia) affected by maternal (pre-existing) diabetes mellitus (P70.1)
syndrome of infant of a diabetic mother (P70.1)

P70.1 Syndrome of infant of a diabetic mother
Newborn (with hypoglycemia) affected by maternal (pre-existing) diabetes mellitus
Excludes 1: newborn (with hypoglycemia) affected by maternal gestational diabetes (P70.0)
syndrome of infant of mother with gestational diabetes (P70.0)

CC **P70.2 Neonatal diabetes mellitus** — The metabolic syndrome of faulty pancreatic activity of the newborn.

P70.3 Iatrogenic neonatal hypoglycemia

P70.4 Other neonatal hypoglycemia
Transitory neonatal hypoglycemia — The abnormally low glucose level of the newborn.

CC **P70.8 Other transitory disorders of carbohydrate metabolism of newborn**

P70.9 Transitory disorder of carbohydrate metabolism of newborn, unspecified

P71- Transitory neonatal disorders of calcium and magnesium metabolism

CC **P71.0 Cow's milk hypocalcemia in newborn** — The abnormally low levels of calcium in the newborn due the excessive amount of phosphates in cow's milk.

CC **P71.1 Other neonatal hypocalcemia**
Excludes 1: neonatal hypoparathyroidism (P71.4)

CC **P71.2 Neonatal hypomagnesemia** — The abnormally low levels of magnesium in the newborn.

CC **P71.3 Neonatal tetany without calcium or magnesium deficiency**
Neonatal tetany NOS

CC **P71.4 Transitory neonatal hypoparathyroidism**

CC **P71.8 Other transitory neonatal disorders of calcium and magnesium metabolism**

CC **P71.9 Transitory neonatal disorder of calcium and magnesium metabolism, unspecified**

P55 - P71

P72-   Other transitory neonatal endocrine disorders
  Excludes 1:   congenital hypothyroidism with or without goiter (E03.0-E03.1)
              dyshormogenetic goiter (E07.1)
              Pendred's syndrome (E07.1)

cc **P72.0   Neonatal goiter, not elsewhere classified**
        Transitory congenital goiter with normal functioning

cc **P72.1   Transitory neonatal hyperthyroidism** — The disorder of excessive circulating thyroid hormones of the newborn.
        Neonatal thyrotoxicosis

cc **P72.2   Other transitory neonatal disorders of thyroid function, not elsewhere classified**
        Transitory neonatal hypothyroidism

cc **P72.8   Other specified transitory neonatal endocrine disorders**

P72.9   Transitory neonatal endocrine disorder, unspecified

P74-   Other transitory neonatal electrolyte and metabolic disturbances

mcc **P74.0   Late metabolic acidosis of newborn** — The disturbance of the acid-base status of the newborn.
        Excludes 1:   (fetal) metabolic acidosis of newborn (P19)

P74.1   Dehydration of newborn

P74.2   Disturbances of sodium balance of newborn

P74.3   Disturbances of potassium balance of newborn

P74.4   Other transitory electrolyte disturbances of newborn

cc **P74.5   Transitory tyrosinemia of newborn**

cc **P74.6   Transitory hyperammonemia of newborn**

cc **P74.8   Other transitory metabolic disturbances of newborn**
        Amino-acid metabolic disorders described as transitory

P74.9   Transitory metabolic disturbance of newborn, unspecified

Digestive system disorders of newborn (P76-P78)

P76-   Other intestinal obstruction of newborn

P76.0   Meconium plug syndrome — The blocking of the intestine that is due to unusually thick or hard meconium.
        Meconium ileus NOS
        Excludes 1:   meconium ileus in cystic fibrosis (E84.11)

cc **P76.1   Transitory ileus of newborn** — The temporary obstruction of the newborn's intestine.
        Excludes 1:   Hirschsprung's disease (Q43.1)

P76.2   Intestinal obstruction due to inspissated milk — The blocking of the intestine that is due to unusual thickening of the milk in the intestine.

P76.8   Other specified intestinal obstruction of newborn
        Excludes 1:   intestinal obstruction classifiable to K56.-

P76.9   Intestinal obstruction of newborn, unspecified

P77-   Necrotizing enterocolitis of newborn — A gastrointestinal disorder involving infection and inflammation that mostly affects premature infants and results in weakening and destruction of the intestinal tissues.

mcc **P77.1   Stage 1 necrotizing enterocolitis in newborn**
        Necrotizing enterocolitis without pneumatosis, without perforation

mcc **P77.2   Stage 2 necrotizing enterocolitis in newborn**
        Necrotizing enterocolitis with pneumatosis, without perforation

mcc **P77.3   Stage 3 necrotizing enterocolitis in newborn**
        Necrotizing enterocolitis with perforation
        Necrotizing enterocolitis with pneumatosis and perforation

mcc **P77.9   Necrotizing enterocolitis in newborn, unspecified**
        Necrotizing enterocolitis in newborn, NOS

P78-   Other perinatal digestive system disorders
  Excludes 1:   cystic fibrosis (E84.0-E84.9)
              neonatal gastrointestinal hemorrhages (P54.0-P54.3)

mcc **P78.0   Perinatal intestinal perforation** — The tearing through the wall of the intestine.
        Meconium peritonitis — Inflammation of the peritoneum in the newborn due to escaped meconium.

P78.1   Other neonatal peritonitis
        Neonatal peritonitis NOS

P78.2   Neonatal hematemesis and melena due to swallowed maternal blood

P78.3   Noninfective neonatal diarrhea
        Neonatal diarrhea NOS

P78.8-   Other specified perinatal digestive system disorders

P78.81   Congenital cirrhosis (of liver)

P78.82   Peptic ulcer of newborn

P78.83   Newborn esophageal reflux
        Neonatal esophageal reflux

P78.89   Other specified perinatal digestive system disorders

P78.9   Perinatal digestive system disorder, unspecified

Conditions involving the integument and temperature regulation of newborn (P80-P83)

P80-   Hypothermia of newborn

P80.0   Cold injury syndrome
        Severe and usually chronic hypothermia associated with a pink flushed appearance, edema and neurological and biochemical abnormalities
        Excludes 1:   mild hypothermia of newborn (P80.8)

P80.8   Other hypothermia of newborn
        Mild hypothermia of newborn

P80.9   Hypothermia of newborn, unspecified

P81-   Other disturbances of temperature regulation of newborn

P81.0   Environmental hyperthermia of newborn

P81.8   Other specified disturbances of temperature regulation of newborn

P81.9   Disturbance of temperature regulation of newborn, unspecified
        Fever of newborn NOS

P83-   Other conditions of integument specific to newborn
  Excludes 1:   congenital malformations of skin and integument (Q80-Q84)
              hydrops fetalis due to hemolytic disease (P56.-)
              neonatal skin infection (P39.4)
              staphylococcal scalded skin syndrome (L00)
  Excludes ❷: cradle cap (L21.0)
              diaper [napkin] dermatitis (L22)

cc **P83.0   Sclerema neonatorum** — The abnormal hardening of the subcutaneous fat that occurs in infants with other neonatal diseases.

P83.1   Neonatal erythema toxicum — The skin condition of small erythematous patches that develop in different locations.

mcc **P83.2   Hydrops fetalis not due to hemolytic disease** — The presence of whole body edema of the newborn that is not due to isoimmunization.
        Hydrops fetalis NOS

P83.3-   Other and unspecified edema specific to newborn — The presence of increased amounts of intercellular fluid in the newborn.

cc **P83.30   Unspecified edema specific to newborn**

cc **P83.39   Other edema specific to newborn**

P83.4   Breast engorgement of newborn — The excessive fullness of the breast tissues with a fluid.
        Noninfective mastitis of newborn

P83.5   Congenital hydrocele — [♂] — The accumulation of fluid within the unclosed vaginal process.

P83.6   Umbilical polyp of newborn — The presence of a polypoid nodule of the umbilicus.

P83.8   Other specified conditions of integument specific to newborn
        Bronze baby syndrome
        Neonatal scleroderma
        Urticaria neonatorum

P83.9   Condition of the integument specific to newborn, unspecified

---

Excludes 1: = NOT CODED HERE! (Do not code both)   **964**   *Excludes ❷:* = Not Included Here

P72 - P83

Other problems with newborn (P84)

P84   Other problems with newborn
   Acidemia of newborn
   Acidosis of newborn
   Anoxia of newborn NOS
   Asphyxia of newborn NOS
   Hypercapnia of newborn
   Hypoxemia of newborn
   Hypoxia of newborn NOS
   Mixed metabolic and respiratory acidosis of newborn
   Excludes 1:   *intracranial hemorrhage due to anoxia or hypoxia (P52.-)*
         hypoxic ischemic encephalopathy [HIE] (P91.6-)
         late metabolic acidosis of newborn (P74.0)

Other disorders originating in the perinatal period (P90-P96)

P90   Convulsions of newborn — The involuntary contraction, or series of
MCC   contractions, of the voluntary muscles.
   Excludes 1:   *benign myoclonic epilepsy in infancy (G40.3-)*
         benign neonatal convulsions (familial) (G40.3-)

P91-   Other disturbances of cerebral status of newborn
MCC **P91.0   Neonatal cerebral ischemia**
MCC **P91.1   Acquired periventricular cysts of newborn**
MCC **P91.2   Neonatal cerebral leukomalacia**
      Periventricular leukomalacia
MCC **P91.3   Neonatal cerebral irritability**
MCC **P91.4   Neonatal cerebral depression**
MCC **P91.5   Neonatal coma**
P91.6-   Hypoxic ischemic encephalopathy [HIE] — The condition of cellular brain damage due to the insufficient supply of oxygenated blood to the cerebral tissues.

   CC **P91.60   Hypoxic ischemic encephalopathy [HIE], unspecified**
   CC **P91.61   Mild hypoxic ischemic encephalopathy [HIE]**
   CC **P91.62   Moderate hypoxic ischemic encephalopathy [HIE]**
   MCC **P91.63   Severe hypoxic ischemic encephalopathy [HIE]**
P91.8   Other specified disturbances of cerebral status of newborn
P91.9   Disturbance of cerebral status of newborn, unspecified

P92-   Feeding problems of newborn
   Excludes 1:   *feeding problems in child over 28 days old (R63.3)*
P92.0-   Vomiting of newborn
      Excludes 1:   *vomiting of child over 28 days old (R11.-)*
   MCC **P92.01   Bilious vomiting of newborn**
         Excludes 1:   *bilious vomiting in child over 28 days old (R11.14)*
   P92.09   Other vomiting of newborn
         Excludes 1:   *regurgitation of food in newborn (P92.1)*
P92.1   Regurgitation and rumination of newborn
P92.2   Slow feeding of newborn
P92.3   Underfeeding of newborn
P92.4   Overfeeding of newborn
P92.5   Neonatal difficulty in feeding at breast
P92.6   Failure to thrive in newborn
      Excludes 1:   *failure to thrive in child over 28 days old (R62.51)*
P92.8   Other feeding problems of newborn
P92.9   Feeding problem of newborn, unspecified

P93-   Reactions and intoxications due to drugs administered to newborn
   Includes: Reactions and intoxications due to drugs administered to fetus affecting newborn
   Excludes 1:   *jaundice due to drugs or toxins transmitted from mother or given to newborn (P58.4-)*
         reactions and intoxications from maternal opiates, tranquilizers and other medication (P04.0-P04.1,P04.4)
         withdrawal symptoms from maternal use of drugs of addiction (P96.1)
         withdrawal symptoms from therapeutic use of drugs in newborn (P96.2)
   CC **P93.0   Grey baby syndrome**
         Grey syndrome from chloramphenicol administration in newborn
   CC **P93.8   Other reactions and intoxications due to drugs administered to newborn**
         Use additional code for adverse effect, if applicable, to identify drug (T36-T50 with fifth or sixth character 5)

P94-   Disorders of muscle tone of newborn
   CC **P94.0   Transient neonatal myasthenia gravis** — The autoimmune disorder of progressive muscular weakness of the newborn.
      Excludes 1:   *myasthenia gravis (G70.0)*
   P94.1   Congenital hypertonia
   P94.2   Congenital hypotonia
      Floppy baby syndrome, unspecified
   P94.8   Other disorders of muscle tone of newborn
   P94.9   Disorder of muscle tone of newborn, unspecified

P95   Stillbirth
   Deadborn fetus NOS
   Fetal death of unspecified cause
   Stillbirth NOS
   Excludes 1:   *maternal care for intrauterine death (O36.4)*
         missed abortion (O02.1)
         outcome of delivery, stillbirth (Z37.1, Z37.3, Z37.4, Z37.7)

P96-   Other conditions originating in the perinatal period
   P96.0   Congenital renal failure — The complete, or significantly decreased, kidney function.
      Uremia of newborn
   CC **P96.1   Neonatal withdrawal symptoms from maternal use of drugs of addiction**
      Drug withdrawal syndrome in infant of dependent mother
      Neonatal abstinence syndrome
      Excludes 1:   *reactions and intoxications from maternal opiates and tranquilizers administered during labor and delivery (P04.0)*
   CC **P96.2   Withdrawal symptoms from therapeutic use of drugs in newborn**
   P96.3   Wide cranial sutures of newborn — The larger than expected soft spots between the bony plates of the skull.
      Neonatal craniotabes
   P96.5   Complication to newborn due to (fetal) intrauterine procedure
      Excludes ❷: *newborn affected by amniocentesis (P00.6)*
   P96.8-   Other specified conditions originating in the perinatal period
      P96.81   Exposure to (parental) (environmental) tobacco smoke in the perinatal period
         Excludes ❷: *newborn affected by in utero exposure to tobacco (P04.2)*
               exposure to environmental tobacco smoke after the perinatal period (Z77.22)
      P96.82   Delayed separation of umbilical cord
      P96.83   Meconium staining — The presence of the distinctive mixing of the amniotic fluid and the passed fetal meconium that has occurred prior to delivery.
         Excludes 1:   *meconium aspiration (P24.00, P24.01)*
               meconium passage during delivery (P03.82)
      P96.89   Other specified conditions originating in the perinatal period
         Use additional code to specify condition
   P96.9   Condition originating in the perinatal period, unspecified
      Congenital debility NOS

P84 - P96

Excludes 1: = NOT CODED HERE! (Do not code both)   965   *Excludes ❷:* = Not Included Here

Chapter 17 – Congenital malformations, deformations and chromosomal abnormalities (Q00-Q99)

Note: Codes from this chapter are not for use on maternal or fetal records
Excludes ❷: inborn errors of metabolism (E70-E88)

This chapter contains the following blocks:

Q00-Q07	Congenital malformations of the nervous system
Q10-Q18	Congenital malformations of eye, ear, face and neck
Q20-Q28	Congenital malformations of the circulatory system
Q30-Q34	Congenital malformations of the respiratory system
Q35-Q37	Cleft lip and cleft palate
Q38-Q45	Other congenital malformations of the digestive system
Q50-Q56	Congenital malformations of genital organs
Q60-Q64	Congenital malformations of the urinary system
Q65-Q79	Congenital malformations and deformations of the musculoskeletal system
Q80-Q89	Other congenital malformations
Q90-Q99	Chromosomal abnormalities, not elsewhere classified

Chapter-Specific Coding Guidelines

C. Chapter-Specific Coding Guidelines

In addition to general coding guidelines, there are guidelines for specific diagnoses and/or conditions in the classification. Unless otherwise indicated, these guidelines apply to all health care settings. Please refer to Section II for guidelines on the selection of principal diagnosis.

17. Chapter 17: Congenital Malformations, Deformations, and Chromosomal Abnormalities (Q00-Q99)

Assign an appropriate code(s) from categories Q00-Q99, Congenital malformations, deformations, and chromosomal abnormalities when a malformation/deformation or chromosomal abnormality is documented. A malformation/deformation/or chromosomal abnormality may be the principal/first-listed diagnosis on a record or a secondary diagnosis.

When a malformation/deformation/or chromosomal abnormality does not have a unique code assignment, assign additional code(s) for any manifestations that may be present.

When the code assignment specifically identifies the malformation/deformation/or chromosomal abnormality, manifestations that are an inherent component of the anomaly should not be coded separately. Additional codes should be assigned for manifestations that are not an inherent component.

Codes from Chapter 17 may be used throughout the life of the patient. If a congenital malformation or deformity has been corrected, a personal history code should be used to identify the history of the malformation or deformity. Although present at birth, malformation/deformation/or chromosomal abnormality may not be identified until later in life. Whenever the condition is diagnosed by the physician, it is appropriate to assign a code from codes Q00-Q99.

For the birth admission, the appropriate code from category Z38, Liveborn infants, according to place of birth and type of delivery, should be sequenced as the principal diagnosis, followed by any congenital anomaly codes, Q00-Q99.

Congenital malformations of the nervous system (Q00-Q07)

Q00- Anencephaly and similar malformations

MCC Q00.0 Anencephaly — The congenital absence of part of the skull, brain, and spinal cord.
    Acephaly — The congenital absence of the head.
    Acrania — The congenital absence of part of the skull.
    Amyelencephaly — The congenital absence of part of the brain and spinal cord.
    Hemianencephaly — The congenital absence of one half of the brain.
    Hemicephaly — The congenital absence of a portion of the cerebrum.

MCC Q00.1 Craniorachischisis — The congenital fissure of the skull and spinal column.

MCC Q00.2 Iniencephaly — The congenital enlargement of the foramen magnum of the base of the skull with the anomalous formation of the vertebrae.

Q01- **Encephalocele** — The protrusion of the brain substance through a defect in the skull.
    Includes: **Arnold-Chiari syndrome, type III** — The protrusion of the brain substance and spinal cord through a foramen magnum defect.
    Encephalocystocele — The protrusion of the brain substance through a skull defect with an accumulation of fluid.
    Encephalomyelocele — The protrusion of the brain substance and spinal cord through a foramen magnum defect.
    Hydroencephalocele — The protrusion of the brain substance through a skull defect with an accumulation of fluid.
    Hydromeningocele, cranial — The protrusion of a cerebrospinal fluid-filled meningeal sac through a skull defect.
    Meningocele, cerebral — The protrusion of the cerebral meninges through a skull defect.
    Meningoencephalocele — The protrusion of the brain substance and cerebral meninges through a skull defect.
    Excludes 1: Meckel-Gruber syndrome (Q61.9)

CC Q01.0 Frontal encephalocele — A form with a frontal bone defect.

CC Q01.1 Nasofrontal encephalocele — A form with a frontal/nasal bone defect.

CC Q01.2 Occipital encephalocele — A form with an occipital bone defect.

CC Q01.8 Encephalocele of other sites

CC Q01.9 Encephalocele, unspecified

Q02 Microcephaly — The congenital smallness of the head.
    Includes: **Hydromicrocephaly** — A form of microcephalus with an abnormally large amount of cerebrospinal fluid.
    Micrencephalon
    Excludes 1: Meckel-Gruber syndrome (Q61.9)

Q03- **Congenital hydrocephalus** — The congenital abnormal accumulation of fluid within the head.
    Includes: **Hydrocephalus in newborn**
    Excludes 1: Arnold-Chiari syndrome, type II (Q07.0-)
    acquired hydrocephalus (G91.-)
    hydrocephalus due to congenital toxoplasmosis (P37.1)
    hydrocephalus with spina bifida (Q05.0-Q05.4)

Q03.0 Malformations of aqueduct of Sylvius — The developmental deviation of the aqueduct of Sylvius.
    Anomaly of aqueduct of Sylvius
    Obstruction of aqueduct of Sylvius, congenital
    Stenosis of aqueduct of Sylvius

Q03.1 Atresia of foramina of Magendie and Luschka — The absence or closure of the foramina of Magendie and Luschka.
    Dandy-Walker syndrome

Q03.8 Other congenital hydrocephalus

Q03.9 Congenital hydrocephalus, unspecified

Q04- Other congenital malformations of brain
    Excludes 1: cyclopia (Q87.0)
    macrocephaly (Q75.3)

MCC Q04.0 Congenital malformations of corpus callosum
    Agenesis of corpus callosum — The failure of embryonic development of a portion of the corpus callosum.

MCC Q04.1 Arhinencephaly — The absence of the rhinencephalon.

MCC Q04.2 Holoprosencephaly — The malformation of the prosencephalon.

MCC Q04.3 Other reduction deformities of brain
  Absence of part of brain — The nonexistence of a portion of the brain.
  Agenesis of part of brain — The failure of embryonic development of a portion of the brain.
  Agyria — A brain malformation that is marked by abnormally developed convolutions of the cerebral cortex that leads to a small brain.
  Aplasia of part of brain — The lack of development of a portion of the brain.
  Hydranencephaly — The lack of development of a portion of the cerebrum and the intracranial cavity is filled with fluid.
  Hypoplasia of part of brain — The incomplete development of a portion of the brain.
  Lissencephaly — The lack of development of folds of the cerebrum.
  Microgyria — The malformation of the brain that is characterized by the development of small convolutions in the cerebrum.
  Pachygyria — The malformation of the brain that is characterized by the development of thick convolutions of the brain.
  Excludes 1: congenital malformations of corpus callosum (Q04.0)

CC Q04.4 Septo-optic dysplasia of brain — The underdevelopment of the optic nerve, pituitary gland, and a midline portion of the brain.

CC Q04.5 Megalencephaly — The excessive size of the head.

CC Q04.6 Congenital cerebral cysts — An encapsulated, fluid-filled sac of the cerebrum.
  Porencephaly — The presence of cysts or cavities in the brain substance.
  Schizencephaly — The presence of cysts or cavities in the clefts of the brain.
  Excludes 1: acquired porencephalic cyst (G93.0)

CC Q04.8 Other specified congenital malformations of brain
  Arnold-Chiari syndrome, type IV — The lack of development of the cerebellum.
  Macrogyria — The excessive size of the convolutions of the brain.

Q04.9 Congenital malformation of brain, unspecified
  Congenital anomaly NOS of brain
  Congenital deformity NOS of brain
  Congenital disease or lesion NOS of brain
  Multiple anomalies NOS of brain, congenital

Q05- Spina bifida — The congenital defective closure of the bony portion of the spinal column with protrusion of the spinal cord and meninges.
  Includes: **Hydromeningocele (spinal)** — The protrusion of the cerebrospinal fluid-filled meninges through a vertebral column defect.
    Meningocele (spinal) — The protrusion of the meninges through a vertebral column defect.
    Meningomyelocele — The protrusion of the meninges and part of the spinal cord substance through a vertebral column defect.
    Myelocele — The protrusion of the spinal cord substance through a vertebral column defect.
    Myelomeningocele — The protrusion of the meninges and part of the spinal cord substance through a vertebral column defect.
    Rachischisis — The congenital fissure of the vertebral column.
    Spina bifida (aperta) (cystica) — The protrusion of spinal tissue through a vertebral column defect.
    Syringomyelocele — The protrusion of the spinal cord through a vertebral column defect while remaining connected to the central cord.
  Use additional code for any associated paraplegia (paraparesis) (G82.2-)
  Excludes 1: Arnold-Chiari syndrome, type II (Q07.0-)
    spina bifida occulta (Q76.0)

CC Q05.0 Cervical spina bifida with hydrocephalus — A form affecting the cervical spinal cord with accumulation of fluid within the cranial meninges.

CC Q05.1 Thoracic spina bifida with hydrocephalus — A form affecting the thoracic spinal cord with accumulation of fluid within the cranial meninges.
  Dorsal spina bifida with hydrocephalus
  Thoracolumbar spina bifida with hydrocephalus

CC Q05.2 Lumbar spina bifida with hydrocephalus — A form affecting the lumbar spinal cord with accumulation of fluid within the cranial meninges.
  Lumbosacral spina bifida with hydrocephalus

CC Q05.3 Sacral spina bifida with hydrocephalus — A form affecting the sacral spinal cord with accumulation of fluid within the cranial meninges.

CC Q05.4 Unspecified spina bifida with hydrocephalus

Q05.5 Cervical spina bifida without hydrocephalus

Q05.6 Thoracic spina bifida without hydrocephalus
  Dorsal spina bifida NOS
  Thoracolumbar spina bifida NOS

Q05.7 Lumbar spina bifida without hydrocephalus
  Lumbosacral spina bifida NOS

Q05.8 Sacral spina bifida without hydrocephalus

Q05.9 Spina bifida, unspecified

Q06- Other congenital malformations of spinal cord

Q06.0 Amyelia — The absence of the spinal cord.

Q06.1 Hypoplasia and dysplasia of spinal cord
  Atelomyelia — The incomplete development of the spinal cord.
  Myelatelia — The imperfect development of the spinal cord.
  Myelodysplasia of spinal cord — The deviation of normal development of the spinal cord.

Q06.2 Diastematomyelia — The congenital splitting of the spinal cord by a bony projection.

Q06.3 Other congenital cauda equina malformations

Q06.4 Hydromyelia — The congenital accumulation of fluid in the central portion of the spinal cord.
  Hydrorachis — The accumulation of water in the spinal column.

Q06.8 Other specified congenital malformations of spinal cord

Q06.9 Congenital malformation of spinal cord, unspecified
  Congenital anomaly NOS of spinal cord
  Congenital deformity NOS of spinal cord
  Congenital disease or lesion NOS of spinal cord

Q07- Other congenital malformations of nervous system
  Excludes ❷: congenital central alveolar hypoventilation syndrome (G47.35)
    familial dysautonomia [Riley-Day] (G90.1)
    neurofibromatosis (nonmalignant) (Q85.0-)

Q07.0- Arnold-Chiari syndrome — The protrusion of the cerebellum down into the spinal canal.
  Arnold-Chiari syndrome, type II — The protrusion of the cerebellum and medulla oblongata down into the spinal canal.
  Excludes 1: Arnold-Chiari syndrome, type III (Q01.-)
    Arnold-Chiari syndrome, type IV (Q04.8)

Q07.00 Arnold-Chiari syndrome without spina bifida or hydrocephalus

Q07.01 Arnold-Chiari syndrome with spina bifida

CC Q07.02 Arnold-Chiari syndrome with hydrocephalus — A form with accumulation of fluid within the cranial meninges.

CC Q07.03 Arnold-Chiari syndrome with spina bifida and hydrocephalus

Q07.8 Other specified congenital malformations of nervous system
  Agenesis of nerve — The failure of embryonic development of a nerve.
  Displacement of brachial plexus — The developmental dislocation of the brachial plexus.
  Jaw-winking syndrome — A congenital unilateral ptosis of the eyelid that is of nervous system origin and is momentarily improved by movement of the jaw.
  Marcus Gunn's syndrome

Q07.9 Congenital malformation of nervous system, unspecified
  Congenital anomaly NOS of nervous system
  Congenital deformity NOS of nervous system
  Congenital disease or lesion NOS of nervous system

Q04 - Q07

Congenital malformations of eye, ear, face and neck (Q10-Q18)

Excludes ❷: *cleft lip and cleft palate (Q35-Q37)*
congenital malformation of cervical spine (Q05.0, Q05.5, Q67.5, Q76.0-Q76.4)
congenital malformation of larynx (Q31.-)
congenital malformation of lip NEC (Q38.0)
congenital malformation of nose (Q30.-)
congenital malformation of parathyroid gland (Q89.2)
congenital malformation of thyroid gland (Q89.2)

Q10- Congenital malformations of eyelid, lacrimal apparatus and orbit

Excludes 1:   *cryptophthalmos NOS (Q11.2)*
cryptophthalmos syndrome (Q87.0)

Q10.0   Congenital ptosis — The congenital drooping of the upper eyelid.

Q10.1   Congenital ectropion — The congenital turning outward of the eyelid margin.

Q10.2   Congenital entropion — The congenital turning inward of the eyelid margin.

Q10.3   Other congenital malformations of eyelid
Ablepharon — The partial or complete absence of the eyelids.
Blepharophimosis, congenital — The reduced size of the eyelids.
Coloboma of eyelid — A full-thickness defect in the eyelid.
Congenital absence or agenesis of cilia — The failure of embryonic development of the cilia.
Congenital absence or agenesis of eyelid — The failure of embryonic development of the eyelid.
Congenital accessory eyelid — The presence of a supplementary eyelid.
Congenital accessory eye muscle — The development of supplementary eye muscles.
Congenital malformation of eyelid NOS

Q10.4   Absence and agenesis of lacrimal apparatus — The failure of embryonic development of the lacrimal apparatus.
Congenital absence of punctum lacrimale

Q10.5   Congenital stenosis and stricture of lacrimal duct — The congenital narrowing of the lacrimal ducts.

Q10.6   Other congenital malformations of lacrimal apparatus
Congenital malformation of lacrimal apparatus NOS

Q10.7   Congenital malformation of orbit

Q11- Anophthalmos, microphthalmos and macrophthalmos

Q11.0   Cystic eyeball — The congenital cystic malformation of the eyeball.

Q11.1   Other anophthalmos — The failure of embryonic development of the eye.
Anophthalmos NOS
Agenesis of eye
Aplasia of eye

Q11.2   Microphthalmos — The congenital smallness of the eye without associated developmental defects.
Cryptophthalmos NOS
Dysplasia of eye
Hypoplasia of eye
Rudimentary eye

Excludes 1:   cryptophthalmos syndrome (Q87.0)

Q11.3   Macrophthalmos — The larger than normal eyeball.

Excludes 1:   macrophthalmos in congenital glaucoma (Q15.0)

Q12- Congenital lens malformations

Q12.0   Congenital cataract — The congenital opacity of the crystalline lens.

Q12.1   Congenital displaced lens — The congenital improper position of the lens.

Q12.2   Coloboma of lens — A defect in the lens.

Q12.3   Congenital aphakia — The congenital absence of the lens.

Q12.4   Spherophakia — The abnormal roundness of the lens.

Q12.8   Other congenital lens malformations
Microphakia — The abnormal smallness of the lens.

Q12.9   Congenital lens malformation, unspecified

Q13- Congenital malformations of anterior segment of eye

Q13.0   Coloboma of iris — The fissure of the iris.
Coloboma NOS

Q13.1   Absence of iris — The congenital absence of the iris.
Aniridia
Use additional code for associated glaucoma (H42)

Q13.2   Other congenital malformations of iris
Anisocoria, congenital — The inequality of the pupillary diameters.
Atresia of pupil — The absence or closure of the pupil.
Congenital malformation of iris NOS
Corectopia — The abnormal placement of the pupil.

Q13.3   Congenital corneal opacity — The congenital nontransparency of the cornea.

Q13.4   Other congenital corneal malformations
Congenital malformation of cornea NOS
Microcornea — The abnormal smallness of the cornea.
Peter's anomaly

Q13.5   Blue sclera

Q13.8- Other congenital malformations of anterior segment of eye

Q13.81   Rieger's anomaly
Use additional code for associated glaucoma (H42)

Q13.89   Other congenital malformations of anterior segment of eye

Q13.9   Congenital malformation of anterior segment of eye, unspecified

Q14- Congenital malformations of posterior segment of eye

Excludes ❷: optic nerve hypoplasia (H47.03-)

Q14.0   Congenital malformation of vitreous humor
Congenital vitreous opacity — The nontransparency of the vitreous.

Q14.1   Congenital malformation of retina
Congenital retinal aneurysm — The sac-like dilatation of a retinal artery.

Q14.2   Congenital malformation of optic disc
Coloboma of optic disc — The optic disc defect that is due to the incomplete closure of the fetal optic stalk.

Q14.3   Congenital malformation of choroid

Q14.8   Other congenital malformations of posterior segment of eye
Coloboma of the fundus — The congenital defect of the fundus.

Q14.9   Congenital malformation of posterior segment of eye, unspecified

Q15- Other congenital malformations of eye

Excludes 1:   *congenital nystagmus (H55.01)*
ocular albinism (E70.31-)
optic nerve hypoplasia (H47.03-)
retinitis pigmentosa (H35.52)

Q15.0   Congenital glaucoma — The increased intraocular pressure resulting in thickening of the cornea.
Axenfeld's anomaly — The inherited developmental deviation of the iris and angular structures in the anterior chamber.
Buphthalmos — The congenital thickening and enlargement of the fibrous coats of the eye.
Glaucoma of childhood
Glaucoma of newborn
Hydrophthalmos
Keratoglobus, congenital, with glaucoma — The bilateral enlargement of the corneas with a globular shape.
Macrocornea with glaucoma
Macrophthalmos in congenital glaucoma
Megalocornea with glaucoma — The increase in thickness of the cornea.

Q15.8   Other specified congenital malformations of eye

Q15.9   Congenital malformation of eye, unspecified
Congenital anomaly of eye
Congenital deformity of eye

Q16- Congenital malformations of ear causing impairment of hearing

Excludes 1:   congenital deafness (H90.-)

Q16.0   Congenital absence of (ear) auricle

Q16.1   Congenital absence, atresia and stricture of auditory canal (external)
Congenital atresia or stricture of osseous meatus — The absence or closure of the osseous meatus.

Q16.2   Absence of eustachian tube

Q16.3   Congenital malformation of ear ossicles
Congenital fusion of ear ossicles — The immobilizing malformation of the ear ossicles.

Q16.4   Other congenital malformations of middle ear
Congenital malformation of middle ear NOS

Q16.5   Congenital malformation of inner ear
Congenital anomaly of membranous labyrinth — The developmental deviation of the membranous labyrinth.
Congenital anomaly of organ of Corti — The developmental deviation of the organ of Corti.

Q16.9   Congenital malformation of ear causing impairment of hearing, unspecified
Congenital absence of ear NOS

Q10 - Q16

Excludes 1: = NOT CODED HERE! (Do not code both)   *Excludes ❷: = Not Included Here*

Q17- Other congenital malformations of ear
> Excludes 1:   congenital malformations of ear with impairment of hearing
> (Q16.0-Q16.9)
> preauricular sinus (Q18.1)

Q17.0   Accessory auricle — The congenital supplementary auricle.
Accessory tragus — The supplementary cartilaginous projection of the external opening of the ear.
Polyotia — The development of more than two ears.
Preauricular appendage or tag — The development of a supplementary preauricular appendage.
Supernumerary ear — The congenital supplementary auricle.
Supernumerary lobule — The development of a supplementary ear lobe.

Q17.1   Macrotia — The congenital enlargement of the external ear.

Q17.2   Microtia — The congenital incomplete development of the external ear.

Q17.3   Other misshapen ear
Pointed ear — A developmental deviation of the external ear in which the ear is pointed.

Q17.4   Misplaced ear — The abnormal location of the ear.
Low-set ears — The lower than usual location of the ear.
> Excludes 1:   cervical auricle (Q18.2)

Q17.5   Prominent ear — A developmental deviation of the external ear in which it protrudes away from the head abnormally.
Bat ear — A developmental deviation of the external ear in which it grows at a right angle to the head.

Q17.8   Other specified congenital malformations of ear
Congenital absence of lobe of ear

Q17.9   Congenital malformation of ear, unspecified
Congenital anomaly of ear NOS

Q18- Other congenital malformations of face and neck
> Excludes 1:   cleft lip and cleft palate (Q35-Q37)
> conditions classified to Q67.0-Q67.4
> congenital malformations of skull and face bones (Q75.-)
> cyclopia (Q87.0)
> dentofacial anomalies [including malocclusion] (M26.-)
> malformation syndromes affecting facial appearance (Q87.0)
> persistent thyroglossal duct (Q89.2)

Q18.0   Sinus, fistula and cyst of branchial cleft — The congenital failure of the fetal branchial cleft passage to close.
Branchial vestige

Q18.1   Preauricular sinus and cyst — PREAURICULAR SINUS OR FISTULA – The congenital passage of the pit-like depression of the external ear. PREAURICULAR CYST – The congenital fluid-filled sac resulting from the imperfect fusion of the first and second branchial arches.
Fistula of auricle, congenital
Cervicoaural fistula

Q18.2   Other branchial cleft malformations
Branchial cleft malformation NOS
Cervical auricle — The congenital flap of skin and yellow cartilage sometimes seen on the side of the neck at the external opening of a persistent branchial cleft.
Otocephaly — The lack of development of the lower jaw.

Q18.3   Webbing of neck — The congenital web-like tissue that spans the neck to the shoulder.
Pterygium colli — The thick fold of skin on the side of the neck.

Q18.4   Macrostomia — The congenital exaggeration of the width of the mouth.

Q18.5   Microstomia — The congenital smallness of the width of the mouth.

Q18.6   Macrocheilia — The congenital excessive size of the lips.
Hypertrophy of lip, congenital

Q18.7   Microcheilia — The congenital smallness of the lips.

Q18.8   Other specified congenital malformations of face and neck
Medial cyst of face and neck
Medial fistula of face and neck
Medial sinus of face and neck

Q18.9   Congenital malformation of face and neck, unspecified
Congenital anomaly NOS of face and neck

Congenital malformations of the circulatory system (Q20-Q28)

Q20- Congenital malformations of cardiac chambers and connections
> Excludes 1:   dextrocardia with situs inversus (Q89.3)
> mirror-image atrial arrangement with situs inversus (Q89.3)

MCC **Q20.0   Common arterial trunk** — The congenital absence of a separating septum between the aorta and pulmonary artery.
Persistent truncus arteriosus
> Excludes 1:   aortic septal defect (Q21.4)

MCC **Q20.1   Double outlet right ventricle** — The congenital malformation of the great vessels in which both the aorta and the pulmonary artery arise from the right ventricle; almost always associated with a ventricular septal defect.
Taussig-Bing syndrome

MCC **Q20.2   Double outlet left ventricle** — The congenital malformation of the great vessels in which both the aorta and the pulmonary artery arise from the left ventricle.

MCC **Q20.3   Discordant ventriculoarterial connection** — The congenital malformation in which the aorta arises from the right ventricle and the pulmonary artery arises from the left ventricle; opposite of normal.
Dextrotransposition of aorta — The abnormal formation of the aorta in which it arises from the right ventricle.
Transposition of great vessels (complete)

MCC **Q20.4   Double inlet ventricle** — The congenital malformation of a three-chambered heart consisting of two atria and one ventricle.
Common ventricle
Cor triloculare biatriatum
Single ventricle

CC **Q20.5   Discordant atrioventricular connection** — The transposition of the great vessels with inversion of the ventricles.
Corrected transposition
Levotransposition
Ventricular inversion

Q20.6   Isomerism of atrial appendages
Isomerism of atrial appendages with asplenia or polysplenia

Q20.8   Other congenital malformations of cardiac chambers and connections
Cor binoculare — The congenital malformation of the heart in which there is a single atrium and a single ventricle.

Q20.9   Congenital malformation of cardiac chambers and connections, unspecified

Q21- Congenital malformations of cardiac septa
> Excludes 1:   acquired cardiac septal defect (I51.0)

CC **Q21.0   Ventricular septal defect** — The congenital malformation of the ventricular septum in which there is persistent patency between the ventricles.
Roger's disease

CC **Q21.1   Atrial septal defect** — The congenital malformation of the atrial septum in which there is a patency between the two atria with a rim of septum completely around the defect.
Coronary sinus defect
Patent or persistent foramen ovale
Patent or persistent ostium secundum defect (type II)
Patent or persistent sinus venosus defect

CC **Q21.2   Atrioventricular septal defect** — The persistent fetal opening between the atrium and ventricle.
Common atrioventricular canal
Endocardial cushion defect
Ostium primum atrial septal defect (type I)

MCC **Q21.3   Tetralogy of Fallot**
AHA 14:3Q:p16 – Tetralogy of Fallot
Ventricular septal defect with pulmonary stenosis or atresia, dextroposition of aorta and hypertrophy of right ventricle

Q21.4   Aortopulmonary septal defect — The developmental deviation of the atrial septum that allows communication between the aorta and the pulmonary artery.
Aortic septal defect
Aortopulmonary window

Q21.8   Other congenital malformations of cardiac septa
Eisenmenger's defect — A form with severe pulmonary hypertension and hypertrophy of the right ventricle.
Pentalogy of Fallot
> Excludes 1:   Eisenmenger's complex (I27.8)
> Eisenmenger's syndrome (I27.8)

Q21.9   Congenital malformation of cardiac septum, unspecified
Septal (heart) defect NOS

Excludes 1: = NOT CODED HERE! (Do not code both)   *Excludes ❷: = Not Included Here*

Q22- Congenital malformations of pulmonary and tricuspid valves

MCC **Q22.0 Pulmonary valve atresia** — The absence or closure of the pulmonary valve.

CC **Q22.1 Congenital pulmonary valve stenosis** — The reduction in the size of the pulmonary valve orifice.

CC **Q22.2 Congenital pulmonary valve insufficiency** — The developmental deviation in which the pulmonary valve does not completely close.
     Congenital pulmonary valve regurgitation

CC **Q22.3 Other congenital malformations of pulmonary valve**
     Congenital malformation of pulmonary valve NOS
     Supernumerary cusps of pulmonary valve

MCC **Q22.4 Congenital tricuspid stenosis** — The congenital incomplete development of the tricuspid valve.
     Congenital tricuspid atresia

MCC **Q22.5 Ebstein's anomaly** — The congenital malformation of the tricuspid valve attachments.

MCC **Q22.6 Hypoplastic right heart syndrome** — The incomplete development of the right ventricle.

MCC **Q22.8 Other congenital malformations of tricuspid valve**

MCC **Q22.9 Congenital malformation of tricuspid valve, unspecified**

Q23- Congenital malformations of aortic and mitral valves

CC **Q23.0 Congenital stenosis of aortic valve** — The congenital reduction in the size of the aortic valve orifice.
     Congenital aortic atresia
     Congenital aortic stenosis NOS
     Excludes 1:   *congenital stenosis of aortic valve in hypoplastic left heart syndrome (Q23.4)*
                 congenital subaortic stenosis (Q24.4)
                 supravalvular aortic stenosis (congenital) (Q25.3)

CC **Q23.1 Congenital insufficiency of aortic valve** — The congenital failure of the aortic valve to close completely.
     Bicuspid aortic valve — The presence of two leaflets instead of three.
     Congenital aortic insufficiency

CC **Q23.2 Congenital mitral stenosis** — The congenital reduction in the size of the mitral valve orifice.
     Congenital mitral atresia

CC **Q23.3 Congenital mitral insufficiency** — The congenital failure of the mitral valve to close completely.

MCC **Q23.4 Hypoplastic left heart syndrome** — The incomplete development of the left ventricle.

Q23.8 Other congenital malformations of aortic and mitral valves

Q23.9 Congenital malformation of aortic and mitral valves, unspecified

Q24- Other congenital malformations of heart
     Excludes 1:   *endocardial fibroelastosis (I42.4)*

CC **Q24.0 Dextrocardia** — The malforming displacement of the heart with the heart displaced into the abdomen.
     Excludes 1:   *dextrocardia with situs inversus (Q89.3)*
                 isomerism of atrial appendages (with asplenia or polysplenia) (Q20.6)
                 mirror-image atrial arrangement with situs inversus (Q89.3)

CC **Q24.1 Levocardia** — The malforming displacement of the heart with the heart in its normal position while the other viscera are transposed.

MCC **Q24.2 Cor triatriatum** — The congenital formation of an accessory atrium into which the pulmonary veins empty.

CC **Q24.3 Pulmonary infundibular stenosis** — The congenital formation of a defective infundibulum of the right ventricle which causes a reduction in the pulmonic valve capacity.
     Subvalvular pulmonic stenosis

MCC **Q24.4 Congenital subaortic stenosis** — The congenital formation of a left ventricle obstructive lesion which causes a pressure gradient in the ventricle.

CC **Q24.5 Malformation of coronary vessels** — The developmental deviation of a coronary artery.
     Congenital coronary (artery) aneurysm

MCC **Q24.6 Congenital heart block** — The congenital impairment of heart conduction.

Q24.8 Other specified congenital malformations of heart
     Congenital diverticulum of left ventricle — The sac-like dilatation of the left ventricle.
     Congenital malformation of myocardium — The developmental deviation of the myocardium.
     Congenital malformation of pericardium — The developmental deviation of the pericardium.
     Malposition of heart — The malforming displacement of the heart.
     Uhl's disease — The development of a paper-thin right ventricular wall that dilates easily.

Q24.9 Congenital malformation of heart, unspecified
     Congenital anomaly of heart
     Congenital disease of heart

Q25- Congenital malformations of great arteries

CC **Q25.0 Patent ductus arteriosus** — The congenital persistence of the vessel in the fetus that connects the pulmonary artery and the aorta.
     Patent ductus Botallo
     Persistent ductus arteriosus

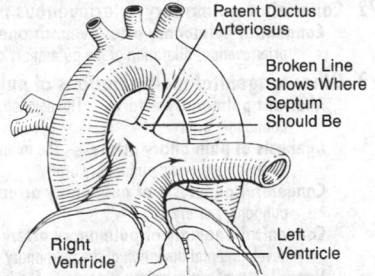

PATENT DUCTUS ARTERIOSUS

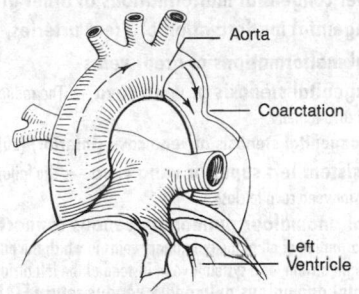

COARCTATION OF AORTA

CC **Q25.1 Coarctation of aorta** — The congenital discrete narrowing of the aortic arch.
     Coarctation of aorta (preductal) (postductal)
     Stenosis of aorta

Q25.2- Atresia of aorta — The congenital abnormality in size of the aorta.

CC **Q25.21 Interruption of aortic arch** — The congenital discontinuation of a portion of the aortic arch.
     Atresia of aortic arch

CC **Q25.29 Other atresia of aorta**
     Atresia of aorta — The congenital reduction in size of the aorta.

CC **Q25.3 Supravalvular aortic stenosis** — The reduction in size of that portion of the aorta just above the mitral valve.
     Excludes 1:   *congenital aortic stenosis NOS (Q23.0)*
                 congenital stenosis of aortic valve (Q23.0)

Q25.4- Other congenital malformations of aorta
     Excludes 1:   *hypoplasia of aorta in hypoplastic left heart syndrome (Q23.4)*

CC **Q25.40 Congenital malformation of aorta, unspecified**

CC **Q25.41 Absence and aplasia of aorta** — The nonexistence or lack of development of the aorta.

CC **Q25.42 Hypoplasia of aorta** — The incomplete development of the aorta.

CC **Q25.43 Congenital aneurysm of aorta** — The arterial wall dilatation of the aorta.
     Congenital aneurysm of aortic root
     Congenital aneurysm of aortic sinus

CC **Q25.44 Congenital dilation of aorta** — The widening of the aorta.

CC **Q25.45 Double aortic arch** — The malformation of the aorta consisting of two aortic arches.
     Vascular ring of aorta

Q22-Q25

cc **Q25.46** **Tortuous aortic arch**— An anomalous aortic arch.
> **Persistent convolutions of aortic arch** — An anomalous aortic arch which infolds upon itself.

cc **Q25.47** **Right aortic arch** — An anomalous aortic arch which passes over the right, rather than the left, bronchus.
> **Persistent right aortic arch**

cc **Q25.48** **Anomalous origin of subclavian artery**

cc **Q25.49** **Other congenital malformations of aorta**

MCC **Q25.5** **Atresia of pulmonary artery** — The absence or closure of the pulmonary artery.

MCC **Q25.6** **Stenosis of pulmonary artery** — The reduction in the size of the pulmonary artery lumen.
> **Supravalvular pulmonary stenosis**

Q25.7- **Other congenital malformations of pulmonary artery**

MCC **Q25.71** **Coarctation of pulmonary artery** — The discrete narrowing of the pulmonary artery.

MCC **Q25.72** **Congenital pulmonary arteriovenous malformation**
> **Congenital pulmonary arteriovenous aneurysm** — The arteriovenous dilatation of the pulmonary artery.

MCC **Q25.79** **Other congenital malformations of pulmonary artery**
> **Aberrant pulmonary artery** — The developmental deviation of the pulmonary artery.
> **Agenesis of pulmonary artery** — The failure of embryonic development of the pulmonary artery.
> **Congenital aneurysm of pulmonary artery** — The dilatation of the pulmonary artery.
> **Congenital anomaly of pulmonary artery** — The congenital developmental deviation of the pulmonary artery.
> **Hypoplasia of pulmonary artery** — The incomplete development of the pulmonary artery.

cc **Q25.8** **Other congenital malformations of other great arteries**

cc **Q25.9** **Congenital malformation of great arteries, unspecified**

Q26- **Congenital malformations of great veins**

cc **Q26.0** **Congenital stenosis of vena cava** — The reduction in the size of the vena cava lumen.
> **Congenital stenosis of vena cava (inferior) (superior)**

cc **Q26.1** **Persistent left superior vena cava** — The failure of the fetal left superior vena cava to close.

cc **Q26.2** **Total anomalous pulmonary venous connection** — The congenital malformation of all of the pulmonary veins in which the pulmonary veins empty into the right atrium, or a systemic vein, instead of the left atrium.
> **Total anomalous pulmonary venous return [TAPVR], subdiaphragmatic** — A form contained within the thoracic cavity.
> **Total anomalous pulmonary venous return [TAPVR], supradiaphragmatic** — A form connecting to systemic veins in the abdominal cavity.

cc **Q26.3** **Partial anomalous pulmonary venous connection** — The congenital malformation in which some, but not all, of the pulmonary veins empty into the right atrium instead of the left atrium.
> **Partial anomalous pulmonary venous return**

cc **Q26.4** **Anomalous pulmonary venous connection, unspecified**

Q26.5 **Anomalous portal venous connection**

Q26.6 **Portal vein-hepatic artery fistula**

cc **Q26.8** **Other congenital malformations of great veins**
> **Absence of vena cava (inferior) (superior)** — The nonexistence of the vena cava.
> **Azygos continuation of inferior vena cava**
> **Persistent left posterior cardinal vein** — The failure of the fetal left posterior cardinal vein to close.
> **Scimitar syndrome** — The complete or partial venous drainage of the right lung into the inferior vena cava.

cc **Q26.9** **Congenital malformation of great vein, unspecified**
> **Congenital anomaly of vena cava (inferior) (superior) NOS**

Q27- **Other congenital malformations of peripheral vascular system**
> *Excludes ❷:* *anomalies of cerebral and precerebral vessels (Q28.0-Q28.3)*
> *anomalies of coronary vessels (Q24.5)*
> *anomalies of pulmonary artery (Q25.5-Q25.7)*
> *congenital retinal aneurysm (Q14.1)*
> *hemangioma and lymphangioma (D18.-)*

Q27.0 **Congenital absence and hypoplasia of umbilical artery** — The congenital nonexistence or incomplete development of the umbilical artery.
> **Single umbilical artery** — The presence of one umbilical artery instead of the normal two.

Q27.1 **Congenital renal artery stenosis** — The reduction in the size of the renal artery lumen.

Q27.2 **Other congenital malformations of renal artery**
> **Congenital malformation of renal artery NOS**
> **Multiple renal arteries**

Q27.3- **Arteriovenous malformation (peripheral)** — The abnormally developed arteries and veins of the peripheral vascular system.
> **Arteriovenous aneurysm** — The presence of an abnormal arteriovenous connection of peripheral blood vessels.
> *Excludes 1:* *acquired arteriovenous aneurysm (I77.0)*
> *Excludes ❷:* *arteriovenous malformation of cerebral vessels (Q28.2)*
> *arteriovenous malformation of precerebral vessels (Q28.0)*

cc **Q27.30** **Arteriovenous malformation, site unspecified**

Q27.31 **Arteriovenous malformation of vessel of upper limb**

Q27.32 **Arteriovenous malformation of vessel of lower limb**

Q27.33 **Arteriovenous malformation of digestive system vessel**

Q27.34 **Arteriovenous malformation of renal vessel**

Q27.39 **Arteriovenous malformation, other site**

cc **Q27.4** **Congenital phlebectasia** — The presence of a dilatated vein.

Q27.8 **Other specified congenital malformations of peripheral vascular system**
> **Absence of peripheral vascular system**
> **Atresia of peripheral vascular system**
> **Congenital aneurysm (peripheral)**
> **Congenital stricture, artery**
> **Congenital varix**
> *Excludes 1:* *arteriovenous malformation (Q27.3-)*

Q27.9 **Congenital malformation of peripheral vascular system, unspecified**
> **Anomaly of artery or vein NOS**

Q28- **Other congenital malformations of circulatory system**
> *Excludes 1:* *congenital aneurysm NOS (Q27.8)*
> *congenital coronary aneurysm (Q24.5)*
> *ruptured cerebral arteriovenous malformation (I60.8)*
> *ruptured malformation of precerebral vessels (I72.0)*
> *Excludes ❷:* *congenital peripheral aneurysm (Q27.8)*
> *congenital pulmonary aneurysm (Q25.79)*
> *congenital retinal aneurysm (Q14.1)*

cc **Q28.0** **Arteriovenous malformation of precerebral vessels** — The presence of an abnormal precerebral arteriovenous connection.
> **Congenital arteriovenous precerebral aneurysm (nonruptured)**

cc **Q28.1** **Other malformations of precerebral vessels** — The abnormally developed precerebral arteries and veins.
> **Congenital malformation of precerebral vessels NOS**
> **Congenital precerebral aneurysm (nonruptured)**

MCC **Q28.2** **Arteriovenous malformation of cerebral vessels** — The presence of an abnormal cerebral arteriovenous connection.
> **Arteriovenous malformation of brain NOS**
> **Congenital arteriovenous cerebral aneurysm (nonruptured)**

MCC **Q28.3** **Other malformations of cerebral vessels** — The abnormally developed arteries and veins of the brain.
> **Congenital cerebral aneurysm (nonruptured)**
> **Congenital malformation of cerebral vessels NOS**
> **Developmental venous anomaly**

cc **Q28.8** **Other specified congenital malformations of circulatory system**
> **Congenital aneurysm, specified site NEC**
> **Spinal vessel anomaly** — The abnormally developed arteries and veins of the spinal vessels.

cc **Q28.9** **Congenital malformation of circulatory system, unspecified**

Congenital malformations of the respiratory system (Q30-Q34)

Q30- **Congenital malformations of nose**
> *Excludes 1:* *congenital deviation of nasal septum (Q67.4)*

Q30.0 **Choanal atresia** — The congenital occlusion of the nasal choanae that is due to the failure of the embryonic bucconasal membrane to rupture.
> **Atresia of nares (anterior) (posterior)**
> **Congenital stenosis of nares (anterior) (posterior)**

Q30.1 **Agenesis and underdevelopment of nose** — The failure of embryonic development of the nose.
> **Congenital absent of nose** — The nonexistence of the nose.

Q30.2 **Fissured, notched and cleft nose** — The developmental deviation of the nose resulting from the incomplete union of the paired nasal primordia.

Q25-Q30

Q30.3 **Congenital perforated nasal septum** — The developmental deviation of the nose marked by turning away from the midline.

Q30.8 **Other congenital malformations of nose**
    Accessory nose — The condition of a supplementary nose.
    Congenital anomaly of nasal sinus wall — The malformation of the wall of a nasal sinus.

Q30.9 **Congenital malformation of nose, unspecified**

Q31- **Congenital malformations of larynx**
    Excludes 1:   *congenital laryngeal stridor NOS (P28.89)*

Q31.0 **Web of larynx** — The congenital formation of a membrane between the vocal cords.
    Glottic web of larynx
    Subglottic web of larynx
    Web of larynx NOS

cc **Q31.1** **Congenital subglottic stenosis** — The narrowing of the larynx just below the vocal cords.

cc **Q31.2** **Laryngeal hypoplasia** — The incomplete development of the larynx.

cc **Q31.3** **Laryngocele** — The air-sac herniation of the larynx.

cc **Q31.5** **Congenital laryngomalacia** — The congenital softening of the larynx.

cc **Q31.8** **Other congenital malformations of larynx**
    Absence of larynx — The failure of embryonic development of the larynx.
    Agenesis of larynx — The failure of embryonic development of the larynx.
    Atresia of larynx — The absence or closure of the larynx.
    Congenital cleft thyroid cartilage — The fissure of the thyroid cartilage resulting from the failure of the parts to fuse during embryonic development.
    Congenital fissure of epiglottis — An abnormal groove in the epiglottis.
    Congenital stenosis of larynx NEC
    Posterior cleft of cricoid cartilage — The fissure of the posterior portion of the cricoid cartilage.

cc **Q31.9** **Congenital malformation of larynx, unspecified**

Q32- **Congenital malformations of trachea and bronchus**
    Excludes 1:   *congenital bronchiectasis (Q33.4)*

cc **Q32.0** **Congenital tracheomalacia** — The congenital softening of the trachea.

cc **Q32.1** **Other congenital malformations of trachea**
    Atresia of trachea — The absence or closure of the trachea.
    Congenital anomaly of tracheal cartilage — The developmental deviation of the tracheal cartilage.
    Congenital dilatation of trachea — The increased width of the trachea
    Congenital malformation of trachea — The developmental deviation of the trachea.
    Congenital stenosis of trachea — The narrowing of the trachea.
    Congenital tracheocele — The protrusion of the tracheal mucous membrane through the tracheal wall.

cc **Q32.2** **Congenital bronchomalacia** — The congenital softening of the bronchus.

cc **Q32.3** **Congenital stenosis of bronchus** — The narrowing of the bronchus.

cc **Q32.4** **Other congenital malformations of bronchus**
    Absence of bronchus — The failure of embryonic development of the bronchus.
    Agenesis of bronchus — The failure of embryonic development of the bronchus.
    Atresia of bronchus — The absence or closure of the bronchus.
    Congenital diverticulum of bronchus — The mucous membrane herniation of the bronchus.
    Congenital malformation of bronchus NOS

Q33- **Congenital malformations of lung**

cc **Q33.0** **Congenital cystic lung** — The congenital development of multiple, small cysts in the lungs.
    Congenital cystic lung disease
    Congenital honeycomb lung — A form marked by the appearance of honeycomb-like, radiolucent shadows on x-ray.
    Congenital polycystic lung disease
    Excludes 1:   *cystic fibrosis (E84.0)*
                   cystic lung disease, acquired or unspecified (J98.4)

Q33.1 **Accessory lobe of lung** — The condition of a supplementary lobe.
    Azygos lobe (fissured), lung

mcc **Q33.2** **Sequestration of lung** — The separation of a lung segment from the bronchial airways.

mcc **Q33.3** **Agenesis of lung** — The failure of embryonic development of the lung.
    Congenital absence of lung (lobe) — The nonexistence of a portion of a lung.

cc **Q33.4** **Congenital bronchiectasis** — The congenital dilatation of the bronchi.

Q33.5 **Ectopic tissue in lung**

mcc **Q33.6** **Congenital hypoplasia and dysplasia of lung**
    Excludes 1:   *pulmonary hypoplasia associated with short gestation (P28.0)*

Q33.8 **Other congenital malformations of lung**

Q33.9 **Congenital malformation of lung, unspecified**

Q34- **Other congenital malformations of respiratory system**
    Excludes ❷: *congenital central alveolar hypoventilation syndrome (G47.35)*

Q34.0 **Anomaly of pleura** — The developmental deviation of the pleura.

Q34.1 **Congenital cyst of mediastinum** — The fluid-filled sac of the mediastinum.

Q34.8 **Other specified congenital malformations of respiratory system**
    Atresia of nasopharynx — The absence or closure of the nasopharynx.

Q34.9 **Congenital malformation of respiratory system, unspecified**
    Congenital absence of respiratory system
    Congenital anomaly of respiratory system NOS

Cleft lip and cleft palate (Q35-Q37)

Use additional code to identify associated malformation of the nose (Q30.2)
Excludes 1:   *Robin's syndrome (Q87.0)*

Q35- **Cleft palate** — The congenital failure of the palate to fuse properly, forming a grooved or fissured depression in the roof of the mouth.
    Includes: **Fissure of palate**
               Palatoschisis
    Excludes 1:   *cleft palate with cleft lip (Q37-)*

Q35.1 **Cleft hard palate**

Q35.3 **Cleft soft palate**

Q35.5 **Cleft hard palate with cleft soft palate**

Q35.7 **Cleft uvula**

Q35.9 **Cleft palate, unspecified**
    Cleft palate NOS

Q36- **Cleft lip** — The congenital failure of the maxillary and median nasal processes to fuse, forming a groove or fissure in the lip.
    Includes: **Cheiloschisis**
               Congenital fissure of lip
               Harelip
               Labium leporinum
    Excludes 1:   *cleft lip with cleft palate (Q37.-)*

Q36.0 **Cleft lip, bilateral**

Q36.1 **Cleft lip, median**

Q36.9 **Cleft lip, unilateral**
    Cleft lip NOS

Q37- **Cleft palate with cleft lip** — The congenital failure of the palate and lip to fuse properly, forming a grooved or fissured palate and lip.
    Includes: **Cheilopalatoschisis**

Q37.0 **Cleft hard palate with bilateral cleft lip**

Q37.1 **Cleft hard palate with unilateral cleft lip**
    Cleft hard palate with cleft lip NOS

Q37.2 **Cleft soft palate with bilateral cleft lip**

Q37.3 **Cleft soft palate with unilateral cleft lip**
    Cleft soft palate with cleft lip NOS

Q37.4 **Cleft hard and soft palate with bilateral cleft lip**

Q37.5 **Cleft hard and soft palate with unilateral cleft lip**
    Cleft hard and soft palate with cleft lip NOS

Q37.8 **Unspecified cleft palate with bilateral cleft lip**

Q37.9 **Unspecified cleft palate with unilateral cleft lip**
    Cleft palate with cleft lip NOS

Other congenital malformations of the digestive system (Q38-Q45)

Q38- **Other congenital malformations of tongue, mouth and pharynx**
    Excludes 1:   *dentofacial anomalies (M26.-)*
                   macrostomia (Q18.4)
                   microstomia (Q18.5)

Q38.0 **Congenital malformations of lips, not elsewhere classified**
    Congenital fistula of lip
    Congenital malformation of lip NOS
    Van der Woude's syndrome
    Excludes 1:   *cleft lip (Q36.-)*
                   cleft lip with cleft palate (Q37.-)
                   macrocheilia (Q18.6)
                   microcheilia (Q18.7)

Excludes 1: = NOT CODED HERE! (Do not code both)   **973**   *Excludes ❷:* = Not Included Here

Q38.1 **Ankyloglossia** — The congenital shortness of the tongue frenulum.
Tongue tie

Q38.2 **Macroglossia** — The congenital largeness of the tongue.
Congenital hypertrophy of tongue

Q38.3 **Other congenital malformations of tongue**
Aglossia — The congenital absence of the tongue.
Bifid tongue — The anterior division of the tongue.
Congenital adhesion of tongue — The congenital restricting fibrous tissue bands of the tongue.
Congenital fissure of tongue — The congenital groove of the tongue.
Congenital malformation of tongue NOS
Double tongue — The anterior division of the tongue.
Hypoglossia — The incomplete development of the tongue.
Hypoplasia of tongue — The incomplete development of the tongue.
Microglossia — The congenital smallness of the tongue.

Q38.4 **Congenital malformations of salivary glands and ducts**
Atresia of salivary glands and ducts — The absence or closure of a salivary duct.
Congenital absence of salivary glands and ducts — The congenital nonexistence of a salivary gland.
Congenital accessory salivary glands and ducts — The congenital presence of a supplementary salivary gland.
Congenital fistula of salivary gland — The congenital abnormal passage of a salivary duct.

Q38.5 **Congenital malformations of palate, not elsewhere classified**
Congenital absence of uvula — The congenital nonexistence of the uvula.
Congenital malformation of palate NOS
Congenital high arched palate
Excludes 1:   *cleft palate (Q35.-)*
cleft palate with cleft lip (Q37.-)

Q38.6 **Other congenital malformations of mouth**
Congenital malformation of mouth NOS

Q38.7 **Congenital pharyngeal pouch** — The congenital sac-like pouch of pharyngeal mucous membrane tissue.
Congenital diverticulum of pharynx
Excludes 1:   *pharyngeal pouch syndrome (D82.1)*

Q38.8 **Other congenital malformations of pharynx**
Congenital malformation of pharynx NOS
Imperforate pharynx — The abnormally closed pharygeal opening.

Q39- **Congenital malformations of esophagus**

MCC **Q39.0** **Atresia of esophagus without fistula** — The absence or closure of the esophagus.
Atresia of esophagus NOS

MCC **Q39.1** **Atresia of esophagus with tracheo-esophageal fistula** — The absence or closure of the esophagus with the abnormal passage between the esophagus and the trachea.
Atresia of esophagus with broncho-esophageal fistula

MCC **Q39.2** **Congenital tracheo-esophageal fistula without atresia** — The abnormal passage between the esophagus and the trachea.
Congenital tracheo-esophageal fistula NOS

MCC **Q39.3** **Congenital stenosis and stricture of esophagus** — The reduction in the size of the esophageal orifice or the decrease in caliber of the esophageal lumen.

MCC **Q39.4** **Esophageal web** — The presence of a web-like structure in the lower esophagus.

CC **Q39.5** **Congenital dilatation of esophagus** — The increased size of the esophageal lumen.
Congenital cardiospasm

CC **Q39.6** **Congenital diverticulum of esophagus** — The sac-like pouch of esophageal mucous membrane tissue.
Congenital esophageal pouch

CC **Q39.8** **Other congenital malformations of esophagus**
Congenital absence of esophagus — The absence or closure of the esophagus.
Congenital displacement of esophagus — The abnormal anatomical location of the esophagus.
Congenital duplication of esophagus — The presence of a supplementary esophagus.

CC **Q39.9** **Congenital malformation of esophagus, unspecified**

Q40- **Other congenital malformations of upper alimentary tract**

Q40.0 **Congenital hypertrophic pyloric stenosis** — The congenital obstruction of the pyloric orifice.
Congenital or infantile constriction — The narrowing of the pyloric orifice.
Congenital or infantile hypertrophy — The enlargement of the pylorus, resulting in the narrowing of the pyloric orifice.
Congenital or infantile spasm — The involuntary contraction of the muscle surrounding the pyloric orifice.
Congenital or infantile stenosis — The failure of the pylorus to open completely.
Congenital or infantile stricture — The decrease in caliber of the pyloric orifice.

Q40.1 **Congenital hiatus hernia** — The congenital displacement of an organ through the esophageal hiatus in the diaphragm.
Congenital displacement of cardia through esophageal hiatus
Excludes 1:   *congenital diaphragmatic hernia (Q79.0)*

Q40.2 **Other specified congenital malformations of stomach**
Congenital displacement of stomach — The abnormal anatomical location of the stomach.
Congenital diverticulum of stomach — The sac-like pouch of stomach mucous membrane tissue.
Congenital hourglass stomach — The constriction of the smooth muscle of the stomach, forming an hourglass-shaped appearance.
Congenital duplication of stomach — The presence of a supplementary stomach.
Megalogastria — The excessive largeness of the stomach.
Microgastria — The smallness of the stomach.

Q40.3 **Congenital malformation of stomach, unspecified**

Q40.8 **Other specified congenital malformations of upper alimentary tract**

Q40.9 **Congenital malformation of upper alimentary tract, unspecified**
Congenital anomaly of upper alimentary tract
Congenital deformity of upper alimentary tract

Q41- **Congenital absence, atresia and stenosis of small intestine**
Includes: Congenital obstruction, occlusion or stricture of small intestine or intestine NOS
Excludes 1:   *cystic fibrosis with intestinal manifestation (E84.11)*
meconium ileus NOS (without cystic fibrosis) (P76.0)

CC **Q41.0** **Congenital absence, atresia and stenosis of duodenum**

CC **Q41.1** **Congenital absence, atresia and stenosis of jejunum**
Apple peel syndrome — The abnormal development of the small bowel marked by the jejunum ending in a blind pouch and the small intestine wrapping itself around.
Imperforate jejunum — The abnormally closed jejunal lumen.

CC **Q41.2** **Congenital absence, atresia and stenosis of ileum**

CC **Q41.8** **Congenital absence, atresia and stenosis of other specified parts of small intestine**

CC **Q41.9** **Congenital absence, atresia and stenosis of small intestine, part unspecified**
Congenital absence, atresia and stenosis of intestine NOS

Q42- **Congenital absence, atresia and stenosis of large intestine**
Includes: Congenital obstruction, occlusion and stricture of large intestine

CC **Q42.0** **Congenital absence, atresia and stenosis of rectum with fistula** — A form with an abnormal passage.

CC **Q42.1** **Congenital absence, atresia and stenosis of rectum without fistula**
Imperforate rectum — The abnormally closed rectum.

CC **Q42.2** **Congenital absence, atresia and stenosis of anus with fistula** — A form with an abnormal passage.

CC **Q42.3** **Congenital absence, atresia and stenosis of anus without fistula**
Imperforate anus — The abnormally closed anus.

CC **Q42.8** **Congenital absence, atresia and stenosis of other parts of large intestine**

CC **Q42.9** **Congenital absence, atresia and stenosis of large intestine, part unspecified**

Q43- **Other congenital malformations of intestine**

Q43.0 **Meckel's diverticulum (displaced) (hypertrophic)** — The congenital sacculation of the ileum.
Persistent omphalomesenteric duct
Persistent vitelline duct

Q
3
8
-
Q
4
3

Excludes 1: = NOT CODED HERE! (Do not code both)   *Excludes ❷:* = Not Included Here

cc **Q43.1**   **Hirschsprung's disease** — The congenital largeness or dilatation of the colon that is due to absence of ganglion nerve cells of the large intestine.
    Aganglionosis
    Congenital (aganglionic) megacolon

cc **Q43.2**   **Other congenital functional disorders of colon**
    Congenital dilatation of colon — The increase in the lumenal width of the colon.

cc **Q43.3**   **Congenital malformations of intestinal fixation**
    Congenital omental, anomalous adhesions [bands] — The fibrous tissue abnormally adhering to the omentum.
    Congenital peritoneal adhesions [bands] — The fibrous tissue abnormally adhering to the peritoneum.
    Incomplete rotation of cecum and colon
    Insufficient rotation of cecum and colon
    Jackson's membrane — The fibrous web-like tissue layer that may obstruct the bowel.
    Malrotation of colon — The abnormal rotational displacement of the colon.
    Rotation failure of cecum and colon
    Universal mesentery

cc **Q43.4**   **Duplication of intestine** — The presence of an additional intestine.

cc **Q43.5**   **Ectopic anus** — The malposition of the anus.

cc **Q43.6**   **Congenital fistula of rectum and anus** — The presence of an abnormal passage.
    Excludes 1:   *congenital fistula of anus with absence, atresia and stenosis (Q42.2)*
          congenital fistula of rectum with absence, atresia and stenosis (Q42.0)
          congenital rectovaginal fistula (Q52.2)
          congenital urethrorectal fistula (Q64.73)
          pilonidal fistula or sinus (L05.-)

cc **Q43.7**   **Persistent cloaca** — The persistence of the fetal cavity into which the intestinal, urinary, and reproductive ducts open.
    Cloaca NOS

cc **Q43.8**   **Other specified congenital malformations of intestine**
    AHA 13:2Q:p31 – Epiploic appendagitis
    Congenital blind loop syndrome
    Congenital diverticulitis, colon
    Congenital diverticulum, intestine — The sac-like pouch of mucous membrane tissue of the colon.
    Dolichocolon — An abnormally long colon.
    Megaloappendix — The abnormal largeness of the appendix.
    Megaloduodenum — The abnormal largeness of the duodenum.
    Microcolon — The abnormal smallness of the colon.
    Transposition of appendix — The malposition of the appendix.
    Transposition of colon — The malposition of the colon.
    Transposition of intestine — The malposition of the intestine.

cc **Q43.9**   **Congenital malformation of intestine, unspecified**

Q44-   **Congenital malformations of gallbladder, bile ducts and liver**

cc **Q44.0**   **Agenesis, aplasia and hypoplasia of gallbladder** — The failure of embryonic development of the gallbladder.
    Congenital absence of gallbladder — The nonexistence of the gallbladder.

cc **Q44.1**   **Other congenital malformations of gallbladder**
    Congenital malformation of gallbladder NOS
    Intrahepatic gallbladder — The malposition of the gallbladder within the liver.

MCC **Q44.2**   **Atresia of bile ducts** — The congenital absence or closure of a biliary duct.

MCC **Q44.3**   **Congenital stenosis and stricture of bile ducts** — The decrease in caliber of a bile duct or passage.

cc **Q44.4**   **Choledochal cyst** — The congenital cystic dilatation of the common bile duct.

cc **Q44.5**   **Other congenital malformations of bile ducts**
    Accessory hepatic duct — The formation of additional hepatic ducts.
    Biliary duct duplication — The formation of an additional biliary duct.
    Congenital malformation of bile duct NOS
    Cystic duct duplication — The formation of an additional cystic duct.

cc **Q44.6**   **Cystic disease of liver** — The congenital formation of multiple cysts in the liver.
    Fibrocystic disease of liver

cc **Q44.7**   **Other congenital malformations of liver**
    Accessory liver — The formation of additional liver tissue.
    Alagille's syndrome
    Congenital absence of liver — The nonexistence of part, or all, of the liver.
    Congenital hepatomegaly — The enlargement of the liver.
    Congenital malformation of liver NOS

Q45-   **Other congenital malformations of digestive system**
    Excludes ❷: *congenital diaphragmatic hernia (Q79.0)*
          congenital hiatus hernia (Q40.1)

cc **Q45.0**   **Agenesis, aplasia and hypoplasia of pancreas** — The failure of embryonic development of the pancreas.
    Congenital absence of pancreas — The nonexistence of the pancreas.

cc **Q45.1**   **Annular pancreas** — The developmental deviation in which the pancreas forms a complete ring around the duodenum.

cc **Q45.2**   **Congenital pancreatic cyst**

cc **Q45.3**   **Other congenital malformations of pancreas and pancreatic duct**
    Accessory pancreas — The inconstant separate part of the head of the pancreas.
    Congenital malformation of pancreas or pancreatic duct NOS
    Excludes 1:   *congenital diabetes mellitus (E10.-)*
          cystic fibrosis (E84.0-E84.9)
          fibrocystic disease of pancreas (E84.-)
          neonatal diabetes mellitus (P70.2)

Q45.8   **Other specified congenital malformations of digestive system**
    Absence (complete) (partial) of alimentary tract NOS
    Duplication of digestive system
    Malposition, congenital of digestive system

Q45.9   **Congenital malformation of digestive system, unspecified**
    Congenital anomaly of digestive system
    Congenital deformity of digestive system

Congenital malformations of genital organs (Q50-Q56)

    Excludes 1:   *androgen insensitivity syndrome (E34.5-)*
          syndromes associated with anomalies in the number and form of chromosomes (Q90-Q99)

Q50-   **Congenital malformations of ovaries, fallopian tubes and broad ligaments**

Q50.0-   **Congenital absence of ovary** — The nonexistence of an ovary.
    Excludes 1:   *Turner's syndrome (Q96.-)*

    Q50.01   **Congenital absence of ovary, unilateral** — [♀]

    Q50.02   **Congenital absence of ovary, bilateral** — [♀]

Q50.1   **Developmental ovarian cyst** — [♀] – The fluid-filled sac formed by the vestigal structure associated with an ovary.

Q50.2   **Congenital torsion of ovary** — [♀] – The abnormal twisting of an ovary.

Q50.3-   **Other congenital malformations of ovary**

    Q50.31   **Accessory ovary** — [♀] – The formation of an additional ovary.

    Q50.32   **Ovarian streak** — [♀]
         46, XX with streak gonads

    Q50.39   **Other congenital malformation of ovary** — [♀]
         Congenital malformation of ovary NOS

Q50.4   **Embryonic cyst of fallopian tube** — [♀] – The congenital development of a fluid-filled sac of embryonic tissue of the fallopian tubes or broad ligaments.
    Fimbrial cyst

Q50.5   **Embryonic cyst of broad ligament** — [♀]
    Epoophoron cyst — The fluid-filled sac formed by the vestigal structure associated with an ovary.
    Parovarian cyst

Q50.6   **Other congenital malformations of fallopian tube and broad ligament** — [♀]
    Absence of fallopian tube and broad ligament — The nonexistence of a fallopian tube or broad ligament.
    Accessory fallopian tube and broad ligament — The formation of an additional fallopian tube or broad ligament.
    Atresia of fallopian tube and broad ligament — The absence or closure of a fallopian tube or broad ligament.
    Congenital malformation of fallopian tube or broad ligament NOS

Q51-   **Congenital malformations of uterus and cervix**

Q51.0   **Agenesis and aplasia of uterus** — [♀] – The failure of embryonic development of the uterus.
    Congenital absence of uterus — The nonexistence of the uterus.

Q51.1-   **Doubling of uterus with doubling of cervix and vagina** — The congenital malformation of the uterus forming two uterine cavities, cervices, and vaginas.

    Q51.10   **Doubling of uterus with doubling of cervix and vagina without obstruction** — [♀]
         Doubling of uterus with doubling of cervix and vagina NOS

    Q51.11   **Doubling of uterus with doubling of cervix and vagina with obstruction** — [♀]

Q43 – Q51

Q51.2 **Other doubling of uterus** — [♀] – The congenital malformation of the uterus forming two uterine cavities.
Doubling of uterus NOS
Septate uterus, complete or partial — The presence of a muscular or fibrous uterine fundus tissue septum that is caused by the failure of the embryonic tissue to be resorbed between the two uterine horns during development.

Q51.3 **Bicornate uterus** — [♀] – The malformation of the two uterine horns.
Bicornate uterus, complete or partial

Q51.4 **Unicornate uterus** — [♀] – The malformation in which the uterus has one horn.
Unicornate uterus with or without a separate uterine horn
Uterus with only one functioning horn

Q51.5 **Agenesis and aplasia of cervix** — [♀] – The failure of embryonic development of the cervix.
Congenital absence of cervix

Q51.6 **Embryonic cyst of cervix** — [♀] – The congenital fluid-filled sac of embryonic tissue of the cervix.

Q51.7 **Congenital fistulae between uterus and digestive and urinary tracts** — [♀] – The abnormal passage between the uterus and/or the digestive and urinary tracts.

Q51.8- **Other congenital malformations of uterus and cervix**

Q51.81- **Other congenital malformations of uterus**

Q51.810 **Arcuate uterus** — [♀] – The presence of a malformed uterine fundus marked by a slightly convex uterine fundus.
Arcuatus uterus

Q51.811 **Hypoplasia of uterus** — [♀] – The incomplete embryonic development of the uterus.

Q51.818 **Other congenital malformations of uterus** — [♀]
Müllerian anomaly of uterus NEC

Q51.82- **Other congenital malformations of cervix**

Q51.820 **Cervical duplication** — [♀] – The congenital presence of two cervices often associated with a didelphys uterus.

Q51.821 **Hypoplasia of cervix** — [♀] – The incomplete embryonic development of the cervix.

Q51.828 **Other congenital malformations of cervix** — [♀]

Q51.9 **Congenital malformation of uterus and cervix, unspecified** — [♀]

Q52- **Other congenital malformations of female genitalia**

Q52.0 **Congenital absence of vagina** — [♀] – The nonexistence of the vagina.
Vaginal agenesis, total or partial

Q52.1- **Doubling of vagina** – The congenital malformation of the vagina forming two vaginal canals.
Excludes 1: *doubling of vagina with doubling of uterus and cervix (Q51.1-)*

Q52.10 **Doubling of vagina, unspecified** — [♀]
Septate vagina NOS

Q52.11 **Transverse vaginal septum** — [♀] – The congenital presence of a fibrous horizontal tissue wall in the vaginal cavity that results in a partial or complete blockage of the vagina.

Q52.12- **Longitudinal vaginal septum** — The congenital presence of a fibrous vertical tissue wall in the vaginal cavity that essentially creates two vaginal cavities.

Q52.120 **Longitudinal vaginal septum, nonobstructing** — [♀]

Q52.121 **Longitudinal vaginal septum, obstructing, right side** — [♀]

Q52.122 **Longitudinal vaginal septum, obstructing, left side** — [♀]

Q52.123 **Longitudinal vaginal septum, microperforate, right side** — [♀]

Q52.124 **Longitudinal vaginal septum, microperforate, left side** — [♀]

Q52.129 **Other and unspecified longitudinal vaginal septum** — [♀]

Q52.2 **Congenital rectovaginal fistula** — [♀] – The presence of an abnormal passage between the vagina and rectum.
Excludes 1: *cloaca (Q43.7)*

Q52.3 **Imperforate hymen** — [♀] – The abnormally closed vaginal opening.

Q52.4 **Other congenital malformations of vagina** — [♀]
Canal of Nuck cyst, congenital — The fluid-filled sac formed from the fetal peritoneal membrane that extends down into the inguinal canal.
Congenital malformation of vagina NOS
Embryonic vaginal cyst — The fluid-filled sac of embryonal vaginal tissue.
Gartner's duct cyst — The fluid-filled sac formed in the embryonic remnant of the mesonephric ducts in female development.

Q52.5 **Fusion of labia** — [♀] – The abnormal anatomical connection of the vulvar folds.

Q52.6 **Congenital malformation of clitoris** — [♀] – The incomplete embryonic development of the clitoris.

Q52.7- **Other and unspecified congenital malformations of vulva**

Q52.70 **Unspecified congenital malformations of vulva** — [♀]
Congenital malformation of vulva NOS

Q52.71 **Congenital absence of vulva** — [♀]

Q52.79 **Other congenital malformations of vulva** — [♀]
Congenital cyst of vulva — The fluid-filled sac of the vulva.

Q52.8 **Other specified congenital malformations of female genitalia** — [♀]

Q52.9 **Congenital malformation of female genitalia, unspecified** — [♀]

Q53- **Undescended and ectopic testicle**

Q53.0- **Ectopic testis** — The malposition of a testis.

Q53.00 **Ectopic testis, unspecified** — [♂]

Q53.01 **Ectopic testis, unilateral** — [♂]

Q53.02 **Ectopic testes, bilateral** — [♂]

Q53.1- **Undescended testicle, unilateral** — The congenital failure of the testis to descend into the scrotum.

Q53.10 **Unspecified undescended testicle, unilateral** — [♂]

Q53.11 **Abdominal testis, unilateral** — [♂]

Q53.12 **Ectopic perineal testis, unilateral** — [♂]

Q53.2- **Undescended testicle, bilateral**

Q53.20 **Undescended testicle, unspecified, bilateral** — [♂]

Q53.21 **Abdominal testis, bilateral** — [♂]

Q53.22 **Ectopic perineal testis, bilateral** — [♂]

Q53.9 **Undescended testicle, unspecified** — [♂]
Cryptorchism NOS

Q54- **Hypospadias** — The congenital opening of the urethra on the under side of the penis.
Excludes 1: *epispadias (Q64.0)*

Q54.0 **Hypospadias, balanic** — [♂] – A form opening from the glans of the penis.
Hypospadias, coronal
Hypospadias, glandular

Q54.1 **Hypospadias, penile** — [♂] – A form opening from the under side of the shaft of the penis.

Q54.2 **Hypospadias, penoscrotal** — [♂] – A form opening from where the penis and scrotum meet.

Q54.3 **Hypospadias, perineal** — [♂] – A form opening from the perineum.

Q54.4 **Congenital chordee** — [♂] – The downward bowing of the penis that is usually due to hypospadias.
Chordee without hypospadias

Q54.8 **Other hypospadias** — [♂]
Hypospadias with intersex state

Q54.9 **Hypospadias, unspecified** — [♂]

Q55- **Other congenital malformations of male genital organs**
Excludes 1: *congenital hydrocele (P83.5)*
hypospadias (Q54.-)

Q55.0 **Absence and aplasia of testis** — [♂] – The nonexistence, or failure of embryonic development of the testis.
Monorchism — The development of only one testicle.

Q55.1 **Hypoplasia of testis and scrotum** — [♂] – The incomplete embryonic development of the testis and/or scrotum.
Fusion of testes — The abnormal anatomical connection of the testes.

Q55.2- **Other and unspecified congenital malformations of testis and scrotum**

Q55.20 **Unspecified congenital malformations of testis and scrotum** — [♂]
Congenital malformation of testis or scrotum NOS

Q55.21 **Polyorchism** — [♂] – The presence of more than two testicles.

Q
5
1
-
Q
5
5

Excludes 1: = NOT CODED HERE! (Do not code both)   **976**   **Excludes ❷:** = Not Included Here

Q55.22 Retractile testis — [♂] – The condition characterized by the testis periodically disappearing from the scrotum.

Q55.23 Scrotal transposition — [♂] – The condition characterized by the scrotum (and testes) being located above the penis.

Q55.29 Other congenital malformations of testis and scrotum — [♂]

Q55.3 Atresia of vas deferens — [♂] – The absence or closure of the vas deferens.
> **Code first any associated cystic fibrosis (E84.-)**

Q55.4 Other congenital malformations of vas deferens, epididymis, seminal vesicles and prostate — [♂]
> **Absence or aplasia of prostate** — The nonexistence, or failure of embryonic development of the prostate.
> **Absence or aplasia of spermatic cord** — The incomplete embryonic development of the spermatic cord.
> **Congenital malformation of vas deferens, epididymis, seminal vesicles or prostate NOS**

Q55.5 Congenital absence and aplasia of penis — [♂] – The nonexistence, or failure of embryonic development of the penis.

Q55.6- Other congenital malformations of penis

Q55.61 Curvature of penis (lateral) — [♂] – The developmental deviation of the penis.

Q55.62 Hypoplasia of penis — [♂] – The incomplete embryonic development of the penis.
> **Micropenis** — An abnormally small penis.

Q55.63 Congenital torsion of penis — [♂]
> *Excludes 1:   acquired torsion of penis (N48.82)*

Q55.64 Hidden penis — [♂] – The developmental deviation of the penis marked by being beneath the skin.
> **Buried penis**
> **Concealed penis**
> *Excludes 1:   acquired buried penis (N48.83)*

Q55.69 Other congenital malformation of penis — [♂]
> **Congenital malformation of penis NOS**

Q55.7 Congenital vasocutaneous fistula — [♂] – An abnormal passage between the vas deferens and the skin.

Q55.8 Other specified congenital malformations of male genital organs — [♂]

Q55.9 Congenital malformation of male genital organ, unspecified — [♂]
> **Congenital anomaly of male genital organ**
> **Congenital deformity of male genital organ**

Q56- Indeterminate sex and pseudohermaphroditism
> *Excludes 1:   46,XX true hermaphrodite (Q99.1)*
> *androgen insensitivity syndrome (E34.5-)*
> *chimera 46,XX/46,XY true hermaphrodite (Q99.0)*
> *female pseudohermaphroditism with adrenocortical disorder (E25.-)*
> *pseudohermaphroditism with specified chromosomal anomaly (Q96-Q99)*
> *pure gonadal dysgenesis (Q99.1)*

Q56.0 Hermaphroditism, not elsewhere classified — The anomaly in which there is both ovarian and testicular tissue.
> **Ovotestis** — A gonad containing both ovarian and testicular tissue.

Q56.1 Male pseudohermaphroditism, not elsewhere classified — [♂] – A form when testicular tissue is present.
> **46, XY with streak gonads**
> **Male pseudohermaphroditism NOS**

Q56.2 Female pseudohermaphroditism, not elsewhere classified — [♀] – A form when ovarian tissue is present.
> **Female pseudohermaphroditism NOS**

Q56.3 Pseudohermaphroditism, unspecified

Q56.4 Indeterminate sex, unspecified
> **Ambiguous genitalia**

Congenital malformations of the urinary system (Q60-Q64)

Q60- Renal agenesis and other reduction defects of kidney — The failure, or deviation, of embryonic development of the kidney.
> **Includes: Congenital absence of kidney** — The nonexistence of the kidney.
> **Congenital atrophy of kidney** — The wasting of the kidney.
> **Infantile atrophy of kidney** — A protein-calorie malnutrition of the kidney.

cc **Q60.0 Renal agenesis, unilateral**

cc **Q60.1 Renal agenesis, bilateral**

cc **Q60.2 Renal agenesis, unspecified**

cc **Q60.3 Renal hypoplasia, unilateral**

cc **Q60.4 Renal hypoplasia, bilateral**

cc **Q60.5 Renal hypoplasia, unspecified**

cc **Q60.6 Potter's syndrome** — The failure of embryonic development of the kidney that leads to oligohydramnios.

Q61- Cystic kidney disease — The presence of congenital cysts of the kidneys.
> *Excludes 1:   acquired cyst of kidney (N28.1)*
> *Potter's syndrome (Q60.6)*

Q61.0- Congenital renal cyst — The presence of a renal cyst, that is not diagnostic of a specified cystic kidney disease.

cc **Q61.00 Congenital renal cyst, unspecified**
> **Cyst of kidney NOS (congenital)**

cc **Q61.01 Congenital single renal cyst**

cc **Q61.02 Congenital multiple renal cysts**

Q61.1- Polycystic kidney, infantile type — A disease characterized by the formation of multiple cysts throughout both kidneys, and carried by both members of a pair of homologous chromosomes.
> **Polycystic kidney, autosomal recessive**

cc **Q61.11 Cystic dilatation of collecting ducts**

cc **Q61.19 Other polycystic kidney, infantile type**

cc **Q61.2 Polycystic kidney, adult type** — A disease characterized by the formation of multiple cysts throughout both kidneys, and carried by only one of a pair of homologous chromosomes.
> **Polycystic kidney, autosomal dominant**

cc **Q61.3 Polycystic kidney, unspecified**

cc **Q61.4 Renal dysplasia** — A form characterized by the abnormal development of kidney tissue.
> **Multicystic dysplastic kidney**
> **Multicystic kidney (development)**
> **Multicystic kidney disease** — The presence of multiple renal cysts, that is not diagnostic of a specified cystic kidney disease.
> **Multicystic renal dysplasia**
> *Excludes 1:   polycystic kidney disease (Q61.11-Q61.3)*

cc **Q61.5 Medullary cystic kidney** — A form characterized by the deteriorization of the medullary tissues of the kidney in which the kidney has a spongy, or porous appearance and feeling.
> **Nephronophthisis**
> **Sponge kidney NOS**

cc **Q61.8 Other cystic kidney diseases**
> **Fibrocystic kidney**
> **Fibrocystic renal degeneration or disease**

cc **Q61.9 Cystic kidney disease, unspecified**
> **Meckel-Gruber syndrome**

Q62- Congenital obstructive defects of renal pelvis and congenital malformations of ureter

cc **Q62.0 Congenital hydronephrosis** — The congenital accumulation of urine in the kidney pelvis.

Q62.1- Congenital occlusion of ureter — The congenital blocking of the renal pelvis or ureter.
> **Atresia and stenosis of ureter** — The decrease in caliber of a ureter.

cc **Q62.10 Congenital occlusion of ureter, unspecified**

cc **Q62.11 Congenital occlusion of ureteropelvic junction** — The congenital blocking of the ureteropelvic junction.

cc **Q62.12 Congenital occlusion of ureterovesical orifice** — The congenital blocking of the ureterovesical junction.

cc **Q62.2 Congenital megaureter** — The developmental dilatation of the ureteral lumen diameter.
> **Congenital dilatation of ureter**

Q55-Q62

Q62.3- Other obstructive defects of renal pelvis and ureter

cc **Q62.31 Congenital ureterocele, orthotopic**

cc **Q62.32 Cecoureterocele**
    Ectopic ureterocele

cc **Q62.39 Other obstructive defects of renal pelvis and ureter**
    Ureteropelvic junction obstruction NOS

Q62.4 Agenesis of ureter — The failure of embryonic development of the ureter.
    Congenital absence ureter

Q62.5 Duplication of ureter — The developmental deviation in which there are two ureters on the same side.
    Accessory ureter — The supplemental formation of an ureter.
    Double ureter

Q62.6- Malposition of ureter — The developmental malposition of the ureter.

Q62.60 Malposition of ureter, unspecified

Q62.61 Deviation of ureter

Q62.62 Displacement of ureter

Q62.63 Anomalous implantation of ureter
    Ectopia of ureter
    Ectopic ureter

Q62.69 Other malposition of ureter

Q62.7 Congenital vesico-uretero-renal reflux

Q62.8 Other congenital malformations of ureter
    Anomaly of ureter NOS

Q63- Other congenital malformations of kidney
    Excludes 1:   congenital nephrotic syndrome (N04.-)

Q63.0 Accessory kidney — The supplemental formation of kidney tissue.

Q63.1 Lobulated, fused and horseshoe kidney — LOBULATED – The developmental deviation in which the kidney forms several lobules. FUSED – The developmental deviation in which both kidneys are connected anatomically. HORSESHOE KIDNEY – The developmental deviation in which the kidneys fuse together and have a horseshoe appearance.

Q63.2 Ectopic kidney — The developmental malposition of the kidney.
    Congenital displaced kidney
    Malrotation of kidney

Q63.3 Hyperplastic and giant kidney — The excessive development of normal cells of the kidney.
    Compensatory hypertrophy of kidney

Q63.8 Other specified congenital malformations of kidney
    Congenital renal calculi — The formation of a concretion in the kidney.

Q63.9 Congenital malformation of kidney, unspecified

Q64- Other congenital malformations of urinary system

Q64.0 Epispadias — [♂] – The congenital opening of the urethra on the upper side of the penis.
    Excludes 1:   hypospadias (Q54.-)

Q64.1- Exstrophy of urinary bladder — The congenital malformation of the bladder and abdominal wall in which the bladder appears to be turned inside out.

cc **Q64.10 Exstrophy of urinary bladder, unspecified**
    Ectopia vesicae

cc **Q64.11 Supravesical fissure of urinary bladder**

cc **Q64.12 Cloacal extrophy of urinary bladder**

cc **Q64.19 Other exstrophy of urinary bladder**
    Extroversion of bladder

cc **Q64.2 Congenital posterior urethral valves** — The developmental formation of an obstructing urethral tissue valve.

Q64.3- Other atresia and stenosis of urethra and bladder neck

cc **Q64.31 Congenital bladder neck obstruction** — The blocking of the bladder neck.
    Congenital obstruction of vesicourethral orifice

cc **Q64.32 Congenital stricture of urethra** — The narrowing of the urethral lumen.

cc **Q64.33 Congenital stricture of urinary meatus** — The narrowing of the urethral opening.

cc **Q64.39 Other atresia and stenosis of urethra and bladder neck**
    Atresia and stenosis of urethra and bladder neck NOS

Q64.4 Malformation of urachus — The developmental deviation of the urachus.
    Cyst of urachus
    Patent urachus
    Prolapse of urachus

Q64.5 Congenital absence of bladder and urethra — The nonexistence of the bladder or urethra.

Q64.6 Congenital diverticulum of bladder — The sac-like pouch of bladder tissue.

Q64.7- Other and unspecified congenital malformations of bladder and urethra
    Excludes 1:   congenital prolapse of bladder (mucosa) (Q79.4)

Q64.70 Unspecified congenital malformation of bladder and urethra
    Malformation of bladder or urethra NOS

Q64.71 Congenital prolapse of urethra — The downward displacement of the urethra.

Q64.72 Congenital prolapse of urinary meatus — The downward displacement of the urethral orifice.

Q64.73 Congenital urethrorectal fistula — The abnormal passage between the urethra and the rectum.

Q64.74 Double urethra — The malformation of the urethra in which two normal passages exist.

Q64.75 Double urinary meatus — The malformation of the urinary meatus in which two normal openings exist.

Q64.79 Other congenital malformations of bladder and urethra

Q64.8 Other specified congenital malformations of urinary system

Q64.9 Congenital malformation of urinary system, unspecified
    Congenital anomaly NOS of urinary system
    Congenital deformity NOS of urinary system

Congenital malformations and deformations of the musculoskeletal system (Q65-Q79)

Q65- Congenital deformities of hip
    Excludes 1:   clicking hip (R29.4)

Q65.0- Congenital dislocation of hip, unilateral — The congenital displacement of the hip joint (slipping out of the normal socket position).

Q65.00 Congenital dislocation of unspecified hip, unilateral

Q65.01 Congenital dislocation of right hip, unilateral

Q65.02 Congenital dislocation of left hip, unilateral

Q65.1 Congenital dislocation of hip, bilateral

Q65.2 Congenital dislocation of hip, unspecified

Q65.3- Congenital partial dislocation of hip, unilateral — The congenital partial displacement of the hip joint from its normal position.

Q65.30 Congenital partial dislocation of unspecified hip, unilateral

Q65.31 Congenital partial dislocation of right hip, unilateral

Q65.32 Congenital partial dislocation of left hip, unilateral

Q65.4 Congenital partial dislocation of hip, bilateral

Q65.5 Congenital partial dislocation of hip, unspecified

Q65.6 Congenital unstable hip
    Congenital dislocatable hip

Q65.8- Other congenital deformities of hip

Q65.81 Congenital coxa valga — The congenital increase in the angle formed by the head of the femur and the shaft of the femur.

Q65.82 Congenital coxa vara — The congenital decrease in the angle formed by the head of the femur and the shaft of the femur.

Q65.89 Other specified congenital deformities of hip
    Anteversion of femoral neck — The forward displacement of the head of the femur.
    Congenital acetabular dysplasia — The impairment of embryonic development of the acetabulum.

Q65.9 Congenital deformity of hip, unspecified

Q66- Congenital deformities of feet
    Excludes 1:   reduction defects of feet (Q72.-)
    valgus deformities (acquired) (M21.0-)
    varus deformities (acquired) (M21.1-)

Q66.0 Congenital talipes equinovarus — The congenital turning inward of the heel with turning upward of the inner edge of the foot.

Q66.1 Congenital talipes calcaneovarus — The turning inward of the heel with the turning upward of the toes and forefoot.

Q66.2- Congenital metatarsus (primus) varus — The congenital turning inward of the metatarsals.

Q66.21 Congenital metatarsus primus varus — The congenital turning inward of the first metatarsal.

Q 6 2 - Q 6 6

Q66.22 Congenital metatarsus adductus — The congenital turning inward of all the metatarsals.
　　Congenital metatarsus varus

Q66.3 Other congenital varus deformities of feet
　　Hallux varus, congenital

Q66.4 Congenital talipes calcaneovalgus — The congenital turning outward of the foot with the turning upward of the toes and forefoot.

Q66.5- Congenital pes planus — The congenital malformation of the bones of the foot causing the arch to flatten (also known as flatfoot).
　　Congenital flat foot
　　Congenital rigid flat foot
　　Congenital spastic (everted) flat foot
　　Excludes 1:　pes planus, acquired (M21.4)

Q66.50 Congenital pes planus, unspecified foot

Q66.51 Congenital pes planus, _right_ foot

Q66.52 Congenital pes planus, _left_ foot

Q66.6 Other congenital valgus deformities of feet
　　Congenital metatarsus valgus

Q66.7 Congenital pes cavus

Q66.8- Other congenital deformities of feet

Q66.80 Congenital vertical talus deformity, unspecified foot

Q66.81 Congenital vertical talus deformity, _right_ foot

Q66.82 Congenital vertical talus deformity, _left_ foot

Q66.89 Other congenital deformities of feet
　　Congenital asymmetric talipes
　　Congenital clubfoot NOS
　　Congenital talipes NOS
　　Congenital tarsal coalition
　　Hammer toe, congenital

Q66.9 Congenital deformity of feet, unspecified

Q67- Congenital musculoskeletal deformities of head, face, spine and chest
　　Excludes 1:　congenital malformation syndromes classified to Q87.-
　　　　Potter's syndrome (Q60.6)

Q67.0 Congenital facial asymmetry — The dissimilarity of the facial bones.

Q67.1 Congenital compression facies

Q67.2 Dolichocephaly — The elongation of the head.

Q67.3 Plagiocephaly — The unsymmetrical formation of the head.

Q67.4 Other congenital deformities of skull, face and jaw
　　Congenital depressions in skull — The inward displacement of an area of the skull.
　　Congenital hemifacial atrophy or hypertrophy
　　Deviation of nasal septum, congenital — The displacement of the nasal septum towards one side.
　　Squashed or bent nose, congenital
　　Excludes 1:　dentofacial anomalies [including malocclusion] (M26.-)
　　　　syphilitic saddle nose (A50.5)

cc **Q67.5 Congenital deformity of spine**
　　AHA 14:4Q:p26 – Congenital scoliosis
　　Congenital postural scoliosis
　　Congenital scoliosis NOS
　　Excludes 1:　infantile idiopathic scoliosis (M41.0)
　　　　scoliosis due to congenital bony malformation (Q76.3)

Q67.6 Pectus excavatum — The congenital depression of the sternum.
　　Congenital funnel chest

Q67.7 Pectus carinatum — The congenital prominence of the sternum.
　　Congenital pigeon chest

cc **Q67.8 Other congenital deformities of chest**
　　Congenital deformity of chest wall NOS

Q68- Other congenital musculoskeletal deformities
　　Excludes 1:　reduction defects of limb(s) (Q71-Q73)
　　Excludes ❷:　congenital myotonic chondrodystrophy (G71.13)

Q68.0 Congenital deformity of sternocleidomastoid muscle — The congenital malformation of the sternocleidomastoid muscle.
　　Congenital contracture of sternocleidomastoid (muscle)
　　Congenital (sternomastoid) torticollis — The twisting condition of the neck that is due to malformation of the sternocleidomastoid muscle.
　　Sternomastoid tumor (congenital) — The abnormal growth of the sternomastoid region.

cc **Q68.1 Congenital deformity of finger(s) and hand**
　　Congenital clubfinger — The turning inward of a finger.
　　Spade-like hand (congenital) — The thickened, square-shaped appearance of the hand.

Q68.2 Congenital deformity of knee — The congenital malformation of the knee joint.
　　Congenital dislocation of knee — The congenital displacement of the knee joint from its normal position.
　　Congenital genu recurvatum — The congenital hyperextension of the knee.

Q68.3 Congenital bowing of femur — The congenital bending of the femur.
　　Excludes 1:　anteversion of femur (neck) (Q65.89)

Q68.4 Congenital bowing of tibia and fibula — The congenital bending of the tibia or fibula.

Q68.5 Congenital bowing of long bones of leg, unspecified

Q68.6 Discoid meniscus — A thickened, oval (instead of crescent shaped) mass of the meniscus.

Q68.8 Other specified congenital musculoskeletal deformities
　　Congenital deformity of clavicle
　　Congenital deformity of elbow
　　Congenital deformity of forearm
　　Congenital deformity of scapula
　　Congenital deformity of wrist
　　Congenital dislocation of elbow
　　Congenital dislocation of shoulder
　　Congenital dislocation of wrist

Q69- Polydactyly — The congenital developmental deviation in which there are supernumerary digits.

Q69.0 Accessory finger(s) — The congenital formation of supernumerary fingers of the hand.

Q69.1 Accessory thumb(s) — The congenital formation of the supernumerary thumb of the hand.

Q69.2 Accessory toe(s) — The congenital formation of supernumerary digits of the foot.
　　Accessory hallux

Q69.9 Polydactyly, unspecified
　　Supernumerary digit(s) NOS

Q70- Syndactyly — The congenital formation of a tissue web between digits.

Q70.0- _Fused fingers_ — The complete fusion of the bones of one digit to another.
　　Complex syndactyly of fingers with synostosis

Q70.00 Fused fingers, _unspecified_ hand

Q70.01 Fused fingers, _right_ hand

Q70.02 Fused fingers, _left_ hand

Q70.03 Fused fingers, _bilateral_

Q70.1- _Webbed fingers_ — The congenital formation of a tissue web between digits.
　　Simple syndactyly of fingers without synostosis

Q70.10 Webbed fingers, _unspecified_ hand

Q70.11 Webbed fingers, _right_ hand

Q70.12 Webbed fingers, _left_ hand

Q70.13 Webbed fingers, _bilateral_

Q70.2- _Fused toes_ — The complete fusion of the bones of one digit to another.
　　Complex syndactyly of toes with synostosis

Q70.20 Fused toes, _unspecified_ foot

Q70.21 Fused toes, _right_ foot

Q70.22 Fused toes, _left_ foot

Q70.23 Fused toes, _bilateral_

Q70.3- _Webbed toes_ — The congenital formation of a tissue web between digits.
　　Simple syndactyly of toes without synostosis

Q70.30 Webbed toes, _unspecified_ foot

Q70.31 Webbed toes, _right_ foot

Q70.32 Webbed toes, _left_ foot

Q70.33 Webbed toes, _bilateral_

Q70.4 Polysyndactyly, unspecified
　　Excludes 1:　specified syndactyly of hand and feet — code to
　　　　specified conditions (Q70.0-Q70.3-)

Q70.9 Syndactyly, unspecified
　　Symphalangy NOS

Q71- Reduction defects of upper limb — The congenital absence of a portion of the upper limb.

Q71.0- Congenital _complete absence_ of _upper_ limb

Q71.00 Congenital complete absence of _unspecified_ upper limb

Q71.01 Congenital complete absence of _right_ upper limb

Q71.02 Congenital complete absence of _left_ upper limb

Q71.03 Congenital complete absence of upper limb, _bilateral_

Q66 - Q71

Excludes 1: = NOT CODED HERE! (Do not code both)　　　　**979**　　　　*Excludes ❷:* = Not Included Here

Q71.1- Congenital <u>absence of upper arm and forearm with hand</u> <u>present</u>

Q71.10 Congenital absence of <u>unspecified</u> upper arm and forearm with hand present

Q71.11 Congenital absence of <u>right</u> upper arm and forearm with hand present

Q71.12 Congenital absence of <u>left</u> upper arm and forearm with hand present

Q71.13 Congenital absence of upper arm and forearm with hand present, <u>bilateral</u>

Q71.2- Congenital <u>absence of both forearm and hand</u>

Q71.20 Congenital absence of both forearm and hand, <u>unspecified</u> upper limb

Q71.21 Congenital absence of both forearm and hand, <u>right</u> upper limb

Q71.22 Congenital absence of both forearm and hand, <u>left</u> upper limb

Q71.23 Congenital absence of both forearm and hand, <u>bilateral</u>

Q71.3- Congenital <u>absence of hand and finger</u>

Q71.30 Congenital absence of <u>unspecified</u> hand and finger

Q71.31 Congenital absence of <u>right</u> hand and finger

Q71.32 Congenital absence of <u>left</u> hand and finger

Q71.33 Congenital absence of hand and finger, <u>bilateral</u>

Q71.4- <u>Longitudinal reduction</u> defect of <u>radius</u> — The congenital decreased length, or absence, of the radius.

    Clubhand (congenital)
    Radial clubhand

Q71.40 Longitudinal reduction defect of <u>unspecified</u> radius

Q71.41 Longitudinal reduction defect of <u>right</u> radius

Q71.42 Longitudinal reduction defect of <u>left</u> radius

Q71.43 Longitudinal reduction defect of radius, <u>bilateral</u>

Q71.5- <u>Longitudinal reduction</u> defect of <u>ulna</u> — The congenital decreased length, or absence, of the ulna.

Q71.50 Longitudinal reduction defect of <u>unspecified</u> ulna

Q71.51 Longitudinal reduction defect of <u>right</u> ulna

Q71.52 Longitudinal reduction defect of <u>left</u> ulna

Q71.53 Longitudinal reduction defect of ulna, <u>bilateral</u>

Q71.6- <u>Lobster-claw hand</u> — The absence of one or more of the middle digits of the hand.

Q71.60 Lobster-claw hand, <u>unspecified</u> hand

Q71.61 Lobster-claw <u>right</u> hand

Q71.62 Lobster-claw <u>left</u> hand

Q71.63 Lobster-claw hand, <u>bilateral</u>

Q71.8- Other reduction defects of upper limb

Q71.81- Congenital <u>shortening</u> of <u>upper</u> limb — The decreased length of the arm.

Q71.811 Congenital shortening of <u>right</u> upper limb

Q71.812 Congenital shortening of <u>left</u> upper limb

Q71.813 Congenital shortening of upper limb, <u>bilateral</u>

Q71.819 Congenital shortening of <u>unspecified</u> upper limb

Q71.89- <u>Other reduction</u> defects of <u>upper</u> limb

Q71.891 Other reduction defects of <u>right</u> upper limb

Q71.892 Other reduction defects of <u>left</u> upper limb

Q71.893 Other reduction defects of upper limb, <u>bilateral</u>

Q71.899 Other reduction defects of <u>unspecified</u> upper limb

Q71.9- <u>Unspecified reduction</u> defect of upper limb

Q71.90 Unspecified reduction defect of <u>unspecified</u> upper limb

Q71.91 Unspecified reduction defect of <u>right</u> upper limb

Q71.92 Unspecified reduction defect of <u>left</u> upper limb

Q71.93 Unspecified reduction defect of upper limb, <u>bilateral</u>

Q72- Reduction defects of lower limb — The congenital absence of a portion of the lower limb.

Q72.0- Congenital <u>complete absence</u> of <u>lower</u> limb

Q72.00 Congenital complete absence of <u>unspecified</u> lower limb

Q72.01 Congenital complete absence of <u>right</u> lower limb

Q72.02 Congenital complete absence of <u>left</u> lower limb

Q72.03 Congenital complete absence of lower limb, <u>bilateral</u>

Q72.1- Congenital <u>absence of thigh and lower leg with foot present</u>

Q72.10 Congenital absence of <u>unspecified</u> thigh and lower leg with foot present

Q72.11 Congenital absence of <u>right</u> thigh and lower leg with foot present

Q72.12 Congenital absence of <u>left</u> thigh and lower leg with foot present

Q72.13 Congenital absence of thigh and lower leg with foot present, <u>bilateral</u>

Q72.2- Congenital <u>absence of both lower leg and foot</u>

Q72.20 Congenital absence of both lower leg and foot, <u>unspecified</u> lower limb

Q72.21 Congenital absence of both lower leg and foot, <u>right</u> lower limb

Q72.22 Congenital absence of both lower leg and foot, <u>left</u> lower limb

Q72.23 Congenital absence of both lower leg and foot, <u>bilateral</u>

Q72.3- Congenital <u>absence of foot and toe(s)</u>

Q72.30 Congenital absence of unspecified foot and toe(s)

Q72.31 Congenital absence of <u>right</u> foot and toe(s)

Q72.32 Congenital absence of <u>left</u> foot and toe(s)

Q72.33 Congenital absence of foot and toe(s), <u>bilateral</u>

Q72.4- <u>Longitudinal reduction</u> defect of <u>femur</u> — The congenital decreased length, or absence, of the femur.

    Proximal femoral focal deficiency

Q72.40 Longitudinal reduction defect of <u>unspecified</u> femur

Q72.41 Longitudinal reduction defect of <u>right</u> femur

Q72.42 Longitudinal reduction defect of <u>left</u> femur

Q72.43 Longitudinal reduction defect of femur, <u>bilateral</u>

Q72.5- <u>Longitudinal reduction</u> defect of <u>tibia</u> — The congenital decreased length, or absence, of the tibia.

Q72.50 Longitudinal reduction defect of <u>unspecified</u> tibia

Q72.51 Longitudinal reduction defect of <u>right</u> tibia

Q72.52 Longitudinal reduction defect of <u>left</u> tibia

Q72.53 Longitudinal reduction defect of tibia, <u>bilateral</u>

Q72.6- <u>Longitudinal reduction</u> defect of <u>fibula</u> — The congenital decreased length, or absence, of the fibula.

Q72.60 Longitudinal reduction defect of <u>unspecified</u> fibula

Q72.61 Longitudinal reduction defect of <u>right</u> fibula

Q72.62 Longitudinal reduction defect of <u>left</u> fibula

Q72.63 Longitudinal reduction defect of fibula, <u>bilateral</u>

Q72.7- <u>Split foot</u> — The absence of one or more of the middle digits of the hand.

Q72.70 Split foot, <u>unspecified</u> lower limb

Q72.71 Split foot, <u>right</u> lower limb

Q72.72 Split foot, <u>left</u> lower limb

Q72.73 Split foot, <u>bilateral</u>

Q72.8- <u>Other reduction</u> defects of <u>lower</u> limb

Q72.81- Congenital <u>shortening</u> of <u>lower</u> limb

Q72.811 Congenital shortening of <u>right</u> lower limb

Q72.812 Congenital shortening of <u>left</u> lower limb

Q72.813 Congenital shortening of lower limb, <u>bilateral</u>

Q72.819 Congenital shortening of <u>unspecified</u> lower limb

Q72.89- <u>Other reduction</u> defects of <u>lower</u> limb

Q72.891 Other reduction defects of <u>right</u> lower limb

Q72.892 Other reduction defects of <u>left</u> lower limb

Q72.893 Other reduction defects of lower limb, <u>bilateral</u>

Q72.899 Other reduction defects of <u>unspecified</u> lower limb

Q72.9- <u>Unspecified reduction</u> defect of lower limb

Q72.90 Unspecified reduction defect of <u>unspecified</u> lower limb

Q72.91 Unspecified reduction defect of <u>right</u> lower limb

Q72.92 Unspecified reduction defect of <u>left</u> lower limb

Q72.93 Unspecified reduction defect of lower limb, <u>bilateral</u>

Q71 - Q72

Excludes 1: = NOT CODED HERE! (Do not code both)

Excludes ❷: = Not Included Here

Q73- Reduction defects of unspecified limb

Q73.0 **Congenital absence of unspecified limb(s)**
Amelia NOS

Q73.1 **Phocomelia, unspecified limb(s)**
Phocomelia NOS

Q73.8 **Other reduction defects of unspecified limb(s)**
Longitudinal reduction deformity of unspecified limb(s)
Ectromelia of limb NOS
Hemimelia of limb NOS
Reduction defect of limb NOS

Q74- **Other congenital malformations of limb(s)**
Excludes 1: *polydactyly (Q69.-)*
reduction defect of limb (Q71-Q73)
syndactyly (Q70.-)

Q74.0 **Other congenital malformations of upper limb(s), including shoulder girdle**
Accessory carpal bones — The congenital formation of supplementary carpal bones of the hand.
Cleidocranial dysostosis — The failure of bony development of the cranial bones with absence of part, or all, of the clavicles.
Congenital pseudarthrosis of clavicle — The congenital malformation of the clavicle.
Macrodactylia (fingers) — The congenital largeness of the fingers.
Madelung's deformity — The congenital overgrowth of the distal ulna resulting in deviation of the hand.
Radioulnar synostosis — The congenital fusion of the proximal ends of the radius and ulna.
Sprengel's deformity — The congenital malposition of the scapula above its normal position.
Triphalangeal thumb — The formation of three phalanges of the thumb versus the usual two.

Q74.1 **Congenital malformation of knee**
Congenital absence of patella — The nonexistence of the patella.
Congenital dislocation of patella — The displacement of the patella.
Congenital genu valgum — The deformity in which the knees are close together.
Congenital genu varum — The deformity in which the knees are more separated.
Rudimentary patella — An imperfectly developed patella.
Excludes 1: *congenital dislocation of knee (Q68.2)*
congenital genu recurvatum (Q68.2)
nail patella syndrome (Q87.2)

Q74.2 **Other congenital malformations of lower limb(s), including pelvic girdle**
Congenital fusion of sacroiliac joint
Congenital malformation of ankle joint
Congenital malformation of sacroiliac joint
Excludes 1: *anteversion of femur (neck) (Q65.89)*

cc **Q74.3** **Arthrogryposis multiplex congenita**

Q74.8 **Other specified congenital malformations of limb(s)**

Q74.9 **Unspecified congenital malformation of limb(s)**
Congenital anomaly of limb(s) NOS

Q75- **Other congenital malformations of skull and face bones**
Excludes 1: *congenital malformation of face NOS (Q18-)*
congenital malformation syndromes classified to Q87-
dentofacial anomalies [including malocclusion] (M26-)
musculoskeletal deformities of head and face (Q67.0-Q67.4)
skull defects associated with congenital anomalies of brain such as:
anencephaly (Q00.0)
encephalocele (Q01-)
hydrocephalus (Q03-)
microcephaly (Q02)

Q75.0 **Craniosynostosis** — The premature closure of the skull sutures.
Acrocephaly — The malformation of the skull in which the top of the head is pointed.
Imperfect fusion of skull — The abnormal coherence of the skull bones.
Oxycephaly — The malformation of the skull in which the top of the head is pointed.
Trigonocephaly — The malformation of the skull at the suture of the frontal bones.

Q75.1 **Craniofacial dysostosis** — The craniofacial malformation consisting of widely-spaced eyes, exophthalmos, optic atrophy, strabismus, acrocephaly, and a beak-shaped nose.
Crouzon's disease

Q75.2 **Hypertelorism** — The malformation in which the eyes are widely spaced.

Q75.3 **Macrocephaly** — An overly large head.

Q75.4 **Mandibulofacial dysostosis** — The craniofacial malformation marked by absent cheek bones, an undersized jaw, and/or an undersized zygoma bone.
Franceschetti syndrome
Treacher Collins syndrome

Q75.5 **Oculomandibular dysostosis**

Q75.8 **Other specified congenital malformations of skull and face bones**
Absence of skull bone, congenital — The nonexistence of skull bone(s).
Congenital deformity of forehead — The malformation of the forehead.
Platybasia — The malformation of the occipital and upper vertebral bones in which the base of the skull appears pushed up into the head.

Q75.9 **Congenital malformation of skull and face bones, unspecified**
Congenital anomaly of face bones NOS
Congenital anomaly of skull NOS

Q76- **Congenital malformations of spine and bony thorax**
Excludes 1: *congenital musculoskeletal deformities of spine and chest (Q67.5-Q67.8)*

Q76.0 **Spina bifida occulta** — The congenital malformation of the bony spinal canal without impingement upon the spinal cord.
Excludes 1: *meningocele (spinal) (Q05.-)*
spina bifida (aperta) (cystica) (Q05.-)

Q76.1 **Klippel-Feil syndrome** — The congenital reduction in the neck height resulting from absence or incomplete development of cervical vertebrae.
Cervical fusion syndrome

Q76.2 **Congenital spondylolisthesis** — The congenital forward displacement of a vertebra.
Congenital spondylolysis
Excludes 1: *spondylolisthesis (acquired) (M43.1-)*
spondylolysis (acquired) (M43.0-)

cc **Q76.3** **Congenital scoliosis due to congenital bony malformation**
Hemivertebra fusion or failure of segmentation with scoliosis

Q76.4- **Other congenital malformations of spine, not associated with scoliosis**

Q76.41- **Congenital kyphosis** — The congenital increased convexity of the spinal position.
Q76.411 **Congenital kyphosis, occipito-atlanto-axial region**
Q76.412 **Congenital kyphosis, cervical region**
Q76.413 **Congenital kyphosis, cervicothoracic region**
Q76.414 **Congenital kyphosis, thoracic region**
Q76.415 **Congenital kyphosis, thoracolumbar region**
Q76.419 **Congenital kyphosis, unspecified region**

Q76.42- **Congenital lordosis** — The congenital increased concavity of the spinal position.
cc **Q76.425** **Congenital lordosis, thoracolumbar region**
cc **Q76.426** **Congenital lordosis, lumbar region**
cc **Q76.427** **Congenital lordosis, lumbosacral region**
cc **Q76.428** **Congenital lordosis, sacral and sacrococcygeal region**
cc **Q76.429** **Congenital lordosis, unspecified region**

Q76.49 **Other congenital malformations of spine, not associated with scoliosis**
Congenital absence of vertebra NOS
Congenital fusion of spine NOS
Congenital malformation of lumbosacral (joint) (region) NOS
Congenital malformation of spine NOS
Hemivertebra NOS
Malformation of spine NOS
Platyspondylisis NOS
Supernumerary vertebra NOS

Q76.5 **Cervical rib** — The congenital formation of an additional rib bone arising from a cervical vertebra.
Supernumerary rib in cervical region

cc **Q76.6** **Other congenital malformations of ribs**
Accessory rib — The formation of a supplementary rib.
Congenital absence of rib — The nonexistence of a rib.
Congenital fusion of ribs — The abnormal anatomical connection of the ribs.
Congenital malformation of ribs NOS
Excludes 1: *short rib syndrome (Q77.2)*

cc **Q76.7** **Congenital malformation of sternum**
Congenital absence of sternum — The nonexistence of the sternum.
Sternum bifidum — The malforming separation of the sternum into 2 parts.

cc **Q76.8** **Other congenital malformations of bony thorax**

cc **Q76.9** **Congenital malformation of bony thorax, unspecified**

Q73-Q76

Q77- **Osteochondrodysplasia with defects of growth of tubular bones and spine**
  Excludes 1: *mucopolysaccharidosis (E76.0-E76.3)*
  Excludes ❷: *congenital myotonic chondrodystrophy (G71.13)*
 Q77.0 **Achondrogenesis** — The lack of embryonic development of the bony cartilage.
  Hypochondrogenesis
 Q77.1 **Thanatophoric short stature** — The skeletal deformity marked by extremely short limbs, narrow chest, and underdeveloped lungs.
 cc **Q77.2** **Short rib syndrome** — The impairment of embryonic development of the rib cage.
  Asphyxiating thoracic dysplasia [Jeune]
 Q77.3 **Chondrodysplasia punctata**
  Excludes 1: *Rhizomelic chondrodysplasia punctata (E71.43)*
 Q77.4 **Achondroplasia** — The impairment of embryonic development of the bony cartilage.
  Hypochondroplasia
  Osteosclerosis congenita
 Q77.5 **Diastrophic dysplasia**
 Q77.6 **Chondroectodermal dysplasia** — The congenital malformation of the bony cartilage that is associated with defective development of the skin, hair, and teeth.
  Ellis-van Creveld syndrome
 Q77.7 **Spondyloepiphyseal dysplasia**
 Q77.8 **Other osteochondrodysplasia with defects of growth of tubular bones and spine**
 Q77.9 **Osteochondrodysplasia with defects of growth of tubular bones and spine, unspecified**

Q78- **Other osteochondrodysplasias**
  Excludes ❷: *congenital myotonic chondrodystrophy (G71.13)*
 cc **Q78.0** **Osteogenesis imperfecta** — The congenital brittleness of the bones.
  Fragilitas ossium
  Osteopsathyrosis
 Q78.1 **Polyostotic fibrous dysplasia** — The congenital fibrous displacement of bony tissue.
  Albright(-McCune)(-Sternberg) syndrome — The fibrous dysplasia of the bone in association with melanotic pigmentation of the skin.
 cc **Q78.2** **Osteopetrosis** — The congenital excessive calcification of the bones.
  Albers-Schönberg syndrome
  Osteosclerosis NOS
 Q78.3 **Progressive diaphyseal dysplasia** — The congenital excessive thickness of the bones, especially the long bones.
  Camurati-Engelmann syndrome
 Q78.4 **Enchondromatosis** — The overgrowth of cartilage resulting in a thinned cortex of the affected bone.
  Maffucci's syndrome
  Ollier's disease
 Q78.5 **Metaphyseal dysplasia** — The congenital thinning of the long bones.
  Pyle's syndrome
 Q78.6 **Multiple congenital exostoses** — The congenital development of multiple bony spurs.
  Diaphyseal aclasis
 Q78.8 **Other specified osteochondrodysplasias**
  Osteopoikilosis — The congenital excessive calcification of spots of bones.
 Q78.9 **Osteochondrodysplasia, unspecified**
  Chondrodystrophy NOS
  Osteodystrophy NOS

Q79- **Congenital malformations of musculoskeletal system, not elsewhere classified**
  Excludes ❷: *congenital (sternomastoid) torticollis (Q68.0)*
 MCC **Q79.0** **Congenital diaphragmatic hernia** — The protrusion of an organ through a defect in the diaphragm.
  Excludes 1: *congenital hiatus hernia (Q40.1)*
 MCC **Q79.1** **Other congenital malformations of diaphragm**
  Absence of diaphragm — The nonexistence of the diaphragm.
  Congenital malformation of diaphragm NOS
  Eventration of diaphragm — The elevation of the diaphragm from abdominal organ pressure.
 MCC **Q79.2** **Exomphalos** — The protrusion of an abdominal organ into the umbilicus.
  Omphalocele — The congenital protrusion of the intestine at the umbilicus.
  Excludes 1: *umbilical hernia (K42.-)*
 MCC **Q79.3** **Gastroschisis** — A congenital fissure of the abdominal wall with protrusion of the intestine.

MCC **Q79.4** **Prune belly syndrome** — The absence of the lower abdominal rectus and oblique muscles.
  Congenital prolapse of bladder mucosa
  Eagle-Barrett syndrome
Q79.5- **Other congenital malformations of abdominal wall**
  Excludes 1: *umbilical hernia (K42.-)*
 MCC **Q79.51** **Congenital hernia of bladder** — The protrusion of the bladder through a defect in the abdominal wall.
 MCC **Q79.59** **Other congenital malformations of abdominal wall**
 cc **Q79.6** **Ehlers-Danlos syndrome** — The congenital syndrome characterized by fragile and hyperelastic tissue, hyperextensibility of joints, visceral malformations, and calcified subcutaneous cysts.
 Q79.8 **Other congenital malformations of musculoskeletal system**
  Absence of muscle — The congenital nonexistence of a muscle.
  Absence of tendon — The congenital nonexistence of a tendon.
  Accessory muscle — The congenital formation of an additional muscle.
  Amyotrophia congenita — The incomplete development of a muscle.
  Congenital constricting bands
  Congenital shortening of tendon
  Poland syndrome
 Q79.9 **Congenital malformation of musculoskeletal system, unspecified**
  Congenital anomaly of musculoskeletal system NOS
  Congenital deformity of musculoskeletal system NOS

Other congenital malformations (Q80-Q89)

Q80- **Congenital ichthyosis** — The congenital development of rough, dry, and scaly skin.
  Excludes 1: *Refsum's disease (G60.1)*
 Q80.0 **Ichthyosis vulgaris**
 Q80.1 **X-linked ichthyosis**
 Q80.2 **Lamellar ichthyosis**
  Collodion baby
 Q80.3 **Congenital bullous ichthyosiform erythroderma**
 Q80.4 **Harlequin fetus** — The severe form that is marked by thick, horny scales covering the fetus.
 Q80.8 **Other congenital ichthyosis**
 Q80.9 **Congenital ichthyosis, unspecified**

Q81- **Epidermolysis bullosa** — The hereditary disease marked by the development of bullae and vesicles on the skin.
 Q81.0 **Epidermolysis bullosa simplex**
  Excludes 1: *Cockayne's syndrome (Q87.1)*
 Q81.1 **Epidermolysis bullosa letalis**
  Herlitz' syndrome
 Q81.2 **Epidermolysis bullosa dystrophica**
 Q81.8 **Other epidermolysis bullosa**
 Q81.9 **Epidermolysis bullosa, unspecified**

Q82- **Other congenital malformations of skin**
  Excludes 1: *acrodermatitis enteropathica (E83.2)*
     congenital erythropoietic porphyria (E80.0)
     pilonidal cyst or sinus (L05.-)
     Sturge-Weber (-Dimitri) syndrome (Q85.8)
 Q82.0 **Hereditary lymphedema** — Edema of the legs resulting from obstruction of the lymphatic system.
 Q82.1 **Xeroderma pigmentosum** — The extreme sensitivity of the skin and eyes to light.
 Q82.2 **Mastocytosis** — The presence of pink to brown areas on the skin that are caused by abnormal masses of mast cells.
  Urticaria pigmentosa
  Excludes 1: *malignant mastocytosis (C96.2)*
 Q82.3 **Incontinentia pigmenti** — The congenital developmental deviation of the skin pigment.
 Q82.4 **Ectodermal dysplasia (anhidrotic)** — The congenital malformation in which the skin is smooth and glossy, absence of sweat glands, and defective development of the hair.
  Excludes 1: *Ellis-van Creveld syndrome (Q77.6)*

Excludes 1: = NOT CODED HERE! (Do not code both)

Excludes ❷: = Not Included Here

Q82.5 Congenital non-neoplastic nevus
Birthmark NOS
Flammeus nevus — A congenital malformation of capillary blood vessels within the skin.
Portwine nevus — A diffuse area of overgrowth of new blood vessels within the skin.
Sanguineous nevus
Strawberry nevus — An excessive overgrowth of blood vessels and connective tissue within the skin.
Vascular nevus NOS
Verrucous nevus
Excludes ❷: café au lait spots (L81.3)
lentigo (L81.4)
nevus NOS (D22.-)
araneus nevus (I78.1)
melanocytic nevus (D22.-)
pigmented nevus (D22.-)
spider nevus (I78.1)
stellar nevus (I78.1)

Q82.6 Congenital sacral dimple — A congenital indentation of the skin in the lower back just above the crease between the buttocks.
Parasacaral dimple
Excludes ❷: pilonidal cyst with abscess (L05.01)
pilonidal cyst without abscess (L05.91)

Q82.8 Other specified congenital malformations of skin
AHA 16:1Q:p17 – Sacral dimple
Abnormal palmar creases
Accessory skin tags
Benign familial pemphigus [Hailey-Hailey]
Congenital poikiloderma
Cutis laxa (hyperelastica)
Dermatoglyphic anomalies
Inherited keratosis palmaris et plantaris
Keratosis follicularis [Darier-White]
Excludes 1: Ehlers-Danlos syndrome (Q79.6)

Q82.9 Congenital malformation of skin, unspecified

Q83- Congenital malformations of breast
Excludes ❷: absence of pectoral muscle (Q79.8)
hypoplasia of breast (N64.82)
micromastia (N64.82)

Q83.0 Congenital absence of breast with absent nipple — The congenital nonexistence of a breast and nipple.

Q83.1 Accessory breast — The formation of an additional breast.
Supernumerary breast

Q83.2 Absent nipple — The congenital nonexistence of a nipple.

Q83.3 Accessory nipple — The formation of an additional nipple.
Supernumerary nipple

Q83.8 Other congenital malformations of breast

Q83.9 Congenital malformation of breast, unspecified

Q84- Other congenital malformations of integument
Q84.0 Congenital alopecia — The absence of hair, most commonly of the scalp.
Congenital atrichosis

Q84.1 Congenital morphological disturbances of hair, not elsewhere classified
Beaded hair — The swelling and constrictions in the hair shafts.
Monilethrix — An inherited disease marked by brittle, beaded hair.
Pili annulati — The banded appearance discoloration of the hair.
Excludes 1: Menkes' kinky hair syndrome (E83.0)

Q84.2 Other congenital malformations of hair
Congenital hypertrichosis — The excessive growth of hair.
Congenital malformation of hair NOS
Persistent lanugo — The continued presence of the fine hair of the fetus.

Q84.3 Anonychia — The absence of a nail or nails.
Excludes 1: nail patella syndrome (Q87.2)

Q84.4 Congenital leukonychia — The whitish discoloration of the nails.

Q84.5 Enlarged and hypertrophic nails
Congenital onychauxis — The overgrowth of the nails.
Pachyonychia — The thickening of the nails.

Q84.6 Other congenital malformations of nails
Congenital clubnail — The clubbed appearance of the nails.
Congenital koilonychia — The formation of thin, concave nails.
Congenital malformation of nail NOS

Q84.8 Other specified congenital malformations of integument
Aplasia cutis congenita — The congenital absence of a portion of the epidermis.

Q84.9 Congenital malformation of integument, unspecified
Congenital anomaly of integument NOS
Congenital deformity of integument NOS

Q85- Phakomatoses, not elsewhere classified
Excludes 1: ataxia telangiectasia [Louis-Bar] (G11.3)
familial dysautonomia [Riley-Day] (G90.1)

Q85.0- Neurofibromatosis (nonmalignant)
Q85.00 Neurofibromatosis, unspecified
Q85.01 Neurofibromatosis, type 1
Von Recklinghausen disease
Q85.02 Neurofibromatosis, type 2
Acoustic neurofibromatosis
Q85.03 Schwannomatosis
Q85.09 Other neurofibromatosis

cc **Q85.1 Tuberous sclerosis** — A syndrome characterized by sclerotic patches on the brain and tumors on the lateral ventricles with resultant mental deterioration and epileptic convulsions.
Bourneville's disease
Epiloia

cc **Q85.8 Other phakomatoses, not elsewhere classified**
Peutz-Jeghers Syndrome
Sturge-Weber(-Dimitri) syndrome
von Hippel-Lindau syndrome
Excludes 1: Meckel-Gruber syndrome (Q61.9)

cc **Q85.9 Phakomatosis, unspecified**
Hamartosis NOS

Q86- Congenital malformation syndromes due to known exogenous causes, not elsewhere classified
Excludes ❷: iodine-deficiency-related hypothyroidism (E00-E02)
nonteratogenic effects of substances transmitted via placenta or breast milk (P04.-)

Q86.0 Fetal alcohol syndrome (dysmorphic)

Q86.1 Fetal hydantoin syndrome
Meadow's syndrome

Q86.2 Dysmorphism due to warfarin

Q86.8 Other congenital malformation syndromes due to known exogenous causes

Q87- Other specified congenital malformation syndromes affecting multiple systems
Use additional code(s) to identify all associated manifestations
Q87.0 Congenital malformation syndromes predominantly affecting facial appearance
Acrocephalopolysyndactyly
Acrocephalosyndactyly [Apert]
Cryptophthalmos syndrome
Cyclopia
Goldenhar syndrome
Moebius syndrome
Oro-facial-digital syndrome
Robin syndrome
Whistling face

cc **Q87.1 Congenital malformation syndromes predominantly associated with short stature**
Aarskog syndrome
Cockayne syndrome
De Lange syndrome
Dubowitz syndrome
Noonan syndrome
Prader-Willi syndrome
Robinow-Silverman-Smith syndrome
Russell-Silver syndrome
Seckel syndrome
Excludes 1: Ellis-van Creveld syndrome (Q77.6)
Smith-Lemli-Opitz syndrome (E78.72)

cc **Q87.2 Congenital malformation syndromes predominantly involving limbs**
Holt-Oram syndrome
Klippel-Trenaunay-Weber syndrome
Nail patella syndrome
Rubinstein-Taybi syndrome
Sirenomelia syndrome
Thrombocytopenia with absent radius [TAR] syndrome
VATER syndrome

Q82 - Q87

cc **Q87.3** **Congenital malformation syndromes involving early overgrowth**
Beckwith-Wiedemann syndrome
Sotos syndrome
Weaver syndrome

Q87.4- **Marfan's syndrome** — A hereditary syndrome characterized by long extremities, dislocation of the optic lens, and dilatation of the ascending aorta.

cc **Q87.40** **Marfan's syndrome, unspecified**

Q87.41- **Marfan's syndrome with cardiovascular manifestations**

cc **Q87.410** **Marfan's syndrome with aortic dilation**

cc **Q87.418** **Marfan's syndrome with other cardiovascular manifestations**

cc **Q87.42** **Marfan's syndrome with ocular manifestations**

cc **Q87.43** **Marfan's syndrome with skeletal manifestation**

cc **Q87.5** **Other congenital malformation syndromes with other skeletal changes**

Q87.8- **Other specified congenital malformation syndromes, not elsewhere classified**
Excludes 1: *Zellweger syndrome (E71.510)*

cc **Q87.81** **Alport syndrome** — A hereditary syndrome characterized by damaged small blood vessels in the kidneys that can lead to kidney disease and failure.
Use additional code to identify stage of chronic kidney disease (N18.1-N18.6)

cc **Q87.82** **Arterial tortuosity syndrome** — A congenital malformation syndrome characterized by elongation and deformation of the pulmonary and systemic arteries.

cc **Q87.89** **Other specified congenital malformation syndromes, not elsewhere classified**
Laurence-Moon (-Bardet)-Biedl syndrome

Q89- **Other congenital malformations, not elsewhere classified**

Q89.0- **Congenital absence and malformations of spleen**
Excludes 1: *isomerism of atrial appendages (with asplenia or polysplenia) (Q20.6)*

cc **Q89.01** **Asplenia (congenital)** — The nonexistence of the spleen.

cc **Q89.09** **Congenital malformations of spleen** — The congenital developmental deviation of the spleen.
Congenital splenomegaly — The abnormal largeness of the spleen.

Q89.1 **Congenital malformations of adrenal gland** — The congenital developmental deviation of the adrenal glands.
Excludes 1: *adrenogenital disorders (E25.-)*
congenital adrenal hyperplasia (E25.0)

Q89.2 **Congenital malformations of other endocrine glands**
Congenital malformation of parathyroid or thyroid gland — The congenital developmental deviation of the parathyroid or thyroid gland.
Persistent thyroglossal duct — The abnormal continued patency of the thyroglossal or thyrolingual ducts.
Thyroglossal cyst — The formation of a fluid-filled sac in the thyroglossal duct.
Excludes 1: *congenital goiter (E03.0)*
congenital hypothyroidism (E03.1)

cc **Q89.3** **Situs inversus** — The lateral transposition of the thoracic or abdominal viscera.
Dextrocardia with situs inversus
Mirror-image atrial arrangement with situs inversus
Situs inversus or transversus abdominalis
Situs inversus or transversus thoracis
Transposition of abdominal viscera
Transposition of thoracic viscera
Excludes 1: *dextrocardia NOS (Q24.0)*

mcc **Q89.4** **Conjoined twins** — Congenital physically joined twins.
Craniopagus — A form united at the heads.
Dicephaly — A form with two heads and the body of one.
Pygopagus — A form united at the sacrum.
Thoracopagus — A form united at the sternum.

cc **Q89.7** **Multiple congenital malformations, not elsewhere classified**
Multiple congenital anomalies NOS
Multiple congenital deformities NOS
Excludes 1: *congenital malformation syndromes affecting multiple systems (Q87.-)*

cc **Q89.8** **Other specified congenital malformations**
Use additional code(s) to identify all associated manifestations

Q89.9 **Congenital malformation, unspecified**
Congenital anomaly NOS
Congenital deformity NOS

Chromosomal abnormalities, not elsewhere classified (Q90-Q99)

Excludes ❷: *mitochondrial metabolic disorders (E88.4-)*

Q90- **Down syndrome** — The chromosomal abnormality that is characterized by moderate-to-severe mental retardation, sloping forehead, small ear canals, flat-bridged nose, and short phalanges.
Use additional code(s) to identify any associated physical conditions and degree of intellectual disabilities (F70-F79)

Q90.0 **Trisomy 21, nonmosaicism (meiotic nondisjunction)**

Q90.1 **Trisomy 21, mosaicism (mitotic nondisjunction)**

Q90.2 **Trisomy 21, translocation**

Q90.9 **Down syndrome, unspecified**
Trisomy 21 NOS

Q91- **Trisomy 18 and Trisomy 13**

cc **Q91.0** **Trisomy 18, nonmosaicism (meiotic nondisjunction)**

cc **Q91.1** **Trisomy 18, mosaicism (mitotic nondisjunction)**

cc **Q91.2** **Trisomy 18, translocation**

cc **Q91.3** **Trisomy 18, unspecified** — The chromosomal abnormality that is characterized by mental retardation, neonatal hepatitis, low-set ears, skull malformation, and short digits.

cc **Q91.4** **Trisomy 13, nonmosaicism (meiotic nondisjunction)**

cc **Q91.5** **Trisomy 13, mosaicism (mitotic nondisjunction)**

cc **Q91.6** **Trisomy 13, translocation**

cc **Q91.7** **Trisomy 13, unspecified** — The chromosomal abnormality that is characterized by impaired midline facial development, cleft lip and palate, polydactyly, and mental retardation.

Q92- **Other trisomies and partial trisomies of the autosomes, not elsewhere classified**
Includes: Unbalanced translocations and insertions
Excludes 1: *trisomies of chromosomes 13, 18, 21 (Q90-Q91)*

Q92.0 **Whole chromosome trisomy, nonmosaicism (meiotic nondisjunction)**

Q92.1 **Whole chromosome trisomy, mosaicism (mitotic nondisjunction)**

Q92.2 **Partial trisomy**
Less than whole arm duplicated
Whole arm or more duplicated
Excludes 1: *partial trisomy due to unbalanced translocation (Q92.5)*

Q92.5 **Duplications with other complex rearrangements**
Partial trisomy due to unbalanced translocations
Code also any associated deletions due to unbalanced translocations, inversions and insertions (Q93.7)

Q92.6- **Marker chromosomes**
Trisomies due to dicentrics
Trisomies due to extra rings
Trisomies due to isochromosomes
Individual with marker heterochromatin

Q92.61 **Marker chromosomes in normal individual**

Q92.62 **Marker chromosomes in abnormal individual**

Q92.7 **Triploidy and polyploidy**

Q92.8 **Other specified trisomies and partial trisomies of autosomes**
Duplications identified by fluorescence in situ hybridization (FISH)
Duplications identified by in situ hybridization (ISH)
Duplications seen only at prometaphase

Q92.9 **Trisomy and partial trisomy of autosomes, unspecified**

Q93- **Monosomies and deletions from the autosomes, not elsewhere classified**

Q93.0 **Whole chromosome monosomy, nonmosaicism (meiotic nondisjunction)**

Q93.1 **Whole chromosome monosomy, mosaicism (mitotic nondisjunction)**

Q93.2 **Chromosome replaced with ring, dicentric or isochromosome**

cc **Q93.3** **Deletion of short arm of chromosome 4**
Wolff-Hirschorn syndrome

cc **Q93.4** **Deletion of short arm of chromosome 5** — The chromosomal abnormality that is characterized by a cat-like cry, widely-spaced eyes, microcephaly, mental retardation, and laryngeal defects.
Cri-du-chat syndrome

cc **Q93.5** **Other deletions of part of a chromosome**
Angelman syndrome

Q87-Q93

cc **Q93.7   Deletions with other complex rearrangements**
Deletions due to unbalanced translocations, inversions and insertions
Code also any associated duplications due to unbalanced translocations, inversions and insertions (Q92.5)

Q93.8-   Other deletions from the autosomes

MCC **Q93.81   Velo-cardio-facial syndrome** — A condition caused by the deletion of a small segment of the long arm of chromosome 22 that is associated with over thirty different features; most common are cleft palate, heart defects, and characteristic facial appearance.
Deletion 22q11.2

cc **Q93.88   Other microdeletions**
Miller-Dieker syndrome — A neurodevelopmental disorder caused by the mutation in the LIS1 gene that is characterized by seizures, mental retardation, and early death.
Smith-Magenis syndrome — A condition caused by the deletion of a small segment of chromosome 17 that is characterized by a variety of features including some degree of self injury, sleep disturbances, short stature, and flat facial features.

cc **Q93.89   Other deletions from the autosomes**
Deletions identified by fluorescence in situ hybridization (FISH)
Deletions identified by in situ hybridization (ISH)
Deletions seen only at prometaphase

cc **Q93.9   Deletion from autosomes, unspecified**

Q95-   Balanced rearrangements and structural markers, not elsewhere classified
Includes: Robertsonian and balanced reciprocal translocations and insertions

Q95.0   Balanced translocation and insertion in normal individual

Q95.1   Chromosome inversion in normal individual

Q95.2   Balanced autosomal rearrangement in abnormal individual

Q95.3   Balanced sex/autosomal rearrangement in abnormal individual

Q95.5   Individual with autosomal fragile site

Q95.8   Other balanced rearrangements and structural markers

Q95.9   Balanced rearrangement and structural marker, unspecified

Q96-   Turner's syndrome — The condition of a defective or absent second X chromosome resulting in short stature and undifferentiated gonads with a female phenotype.
Excludes 1:   Noonan syndrome (Q87.1)

Q96.0   Karyotype 45, X — [♀]

Q96.1   Karyotype 46, X iso (Xq) — [♀]
Karyotype 46, isochromosome Xq

Q96.2   Karyotype 46, X with abnormal sex chromosome, except iso (Xq) — [♀]
Karyotype 46, X with abnormal sex chromosome, except isochromosome Xq

Q96.3   Mosaicism, 45, X/46, XX or XY — [♀]

Q96.4   Mosaicism, 45, X/other cell line(s) with abnormal sex chromosome — [♀]

Q96.8   Other variants of Turner's syndrome — [♀]

Q96.9   Turner's syndrome, unspecified — [♀]

Q97-   Other sex chromosome abnormalities, female phenotype, not elsewhere classified
Excludes 1:   Turner's syndrome (Q96.-)

Q97.0   Karyotype 47, XXX — [♀]

Q97.1   Female with more than three X chromosomes — [♀]

Q97.2   Mosaicism, lines with various numbers of X chromosomes — [♀]

Q97.3   Female with 46, XY karyotype — [♀]

Q97.8   Other specified sex chromosome abnormalities, female phenotype — [♀]

Q97.9   Sex chromosome abnormality, female phenotype, unspecified — [♀]

Q98-   Other sex chromosome abnormalities, male phenotype, not elsewhere classified

Q98.0   Klinefelter syndrome karyotype 47, XXY — [♂] – The condition of an extra X chromosome resulting in the presence of small testes, abnormal Leydig cells, long legs, and a slightly subnormal intelligence.

Q98.1   Klinefelter syndrome, male with more than two X chromosomes — [♂]

Q98.3   Other male with 46, XX karyotype — [♂]

Q98.4   Klinefelter syndrome, unspecified — [♂]

Q98.5   Karyotype 47, XYY

Q98.6   Male with structurally abnormal sex chromosome — [♂]

Q98.7   Male with sex chromosome mosaicism — [♂]

Q98.8   Other specified sex chromosome abnormalities, male phenotype — [♂]

Q98.9   Sex chromosome abnormality, male phenotype, unspecified — [♂]

Q99-   Other chromosome abnormalities, not elsewhere classified

Q99.0   Chimera 46, XX/46, XY
Chimera 46, XX/46, XY true hermaphrodite

Q99.1   46, XX true hermaphrodite
46, XX with streak gonads
46, XY with streak gonads
Pure gonadal dysgenesis

Q99.2   Fragile X chromosome
Fragile X syndrome

Q99.8   Other specified chromosome abnormalities

Q99.9   Chromosomal abnormality, unspecified

Q93 - Q99

Q93.7 Deletions with other complex rearrangements
Deletions due to unbalanced translocations, inversions and insertions
Code also any associated duplications due to unbalanced translocations, inversions and insertions (Q92.-)

Q93.8- Other deletions from the autosomes
Q93.81 Velo-cardio-facial syndrome — A condition caused by the deletion of a small segment of the long arm of chromosome 22 that is associated with characteristic facial appearance.
Deletion 22q11.2

Q93.88 Other microdeletions
Miller-Dieker syndrome — A neurodevelopmental disorder marked by the mutation in the LIS1 gene that is characterized by seizures, mental retardation and early death.
Smith-Magenis syndrome — A condition caused by the deletion of a small segment of chromosome 17 that is characterized by a variety of features including coarse facies, short stature, sleep disturbance, short stature and behavioral features.

Q93.89 Other deletions from the autosomes
Deletions identified by fluorescence in situ hybridization (FISH)
Deletions identified by micro hybridization (ish)
Deletions seen only at prometaphase

Q93.9 Deletion from autosomes, unspecified

Q95- Balanced rearrangements and structural markers, not elsewhere classified
Includes: Robertsonian and balanced reciprocal translocations and insertions

Q95.0 Balanced translocation and insertion in normal individual
Q95.1 Chromosome inversion in normal individual
Q95.2 Balanced autosomal rearrangement in abnormal individual
Q95.3 Balanced sex/autosomal rearrangement in abnormal individual
Q95.5 Individual with autosomal fragile site
Q95.8 Other balanced rearrangements and structural markers
Q95.9 Balanced rearrangement and structural marker, unspecified

Q96- Turner's syndrome — The condition of a genetically monosomic X chromosome resulting in short stature and multimutilated gonads with sterile phenotype.

Q96.0 Karyotype 45, X — [1]
Q96.1 Karyotype 46, X iso (Xq) — [1]
Karyotype 46, isochromosome Xq
Q96.2 Karyotype 46, X with abnormal sex chromosome, except iso (Xq) — [1]
Karyotype 46, X with abnormal sex chromosome, except isochromosome Xq
Q96.3 Mosaicism, 45, X/46, XX or XY — [1]
Q96.4 Mosaicism, 45, X/other cell line(s) with abnormal sex chromosome — [1]
Q96.8 Other variants of Turner's syndrome — [1]
Q96.9 Turner's syndrome, unspecified — [1]

Q97- Other sex chromosome abnormalities, female phenotype, not elsewhere classified

Q97.0 Karyotype 47, XXX — [1]
Q97.1 Female with more than three X chromosomes — [1]
Q97.2 Mosaicism, lines with various numbers of X chromosomes — [1]
Q97.3 Female with 46, XY karyotype — [1]
Q97.8 Other specified sex chromosome abnormalities, female phenotype — [1]
Q97.9 Sex chromosome abnormality, female phenotype, unspecified — [1]

Q98- Other sex chromosome abnormalities, male phenotype, not elsewhere classified
Q98.0 Klinefelter syndrome karyotype 47, XXY — [1] — The condition of an extra Z chromosome resulting in the presence of small testes, abnormal Leydig cells, long legs, and a slightly decreased fetal sperm.
Q98.1 Klinefelter syndrome, male with more than two X chromosomes — [1]
Q98.3 Other male with 46, XX karyotype — [1]
Q98.4 Klinefelter syndrome, unspecified — [1]
Q98.5 Karyotype 47, XYY
Q98.6 Male with structurally abnormal sex chromosome — [1]
Q98.7 Male with sex chromosome mosaicism — [1]
Q98.8- Other specified sex chromosome abnormalities, male phenotype — [1]
Q98.9 Sex chromosome abnormality, male phenotype, unspecified — [1]

Q99- Other chromosome abnormalities, not elsewhere classified
Q99.0 Chimera 46, XX/46, XY
Chimera 46, XX/46, XY true hermaphrodite
Q99.1 46, XX true hermaphrodite
46, XX with streak gonads
46, XY with streak gonads
Pure gonadal dysgenesis
Q99.2 Fragile X chromosome
Fragile X syndrome
Q99.8 Other specified chromosome abnormalities
Q99.9 Chromosomal abnormality, unspecified

Chapter 18 – Symptoms, signs and abnormal clinical and laboratory findings, not elsewhere classified (R00-R99)

Note: This chapter includes symptoms, signs, abnormal results of clinical or other investigative procedures, and ill-defined conditions regarding which no diagnosis classifiable elsewhere is recorded. Signs and symptoms that point rather definitely to a given diagnosis have been assigned to a category in other chapters of the classification. In general, categories in this chapter include the less well-defined conditions and symptoms that, without the necessary study of the case to establish a final diagnosis, point perhaps equally to two or more diseases or to two or more systems of the body. Practically all categories in the chapter could be designated "not otherwise specified", "unknown etiology" or "transient". The Alphabetical Index should be consulted to determine which symptoms and signs are to be allocated here and which to other chapters. The residual subcategories, numbered .8, are generally provided for other relevant symptoms that cannot be allocated elsewhere in the classification.

The conditions and signs or symptoms included in categories R00-R94 consist of:

(a) cases for which no more specific diagnosis can be made even after all the facts bearing on the case have been investigated;

(b) signs or symptoms existing at the time of initial encounter that proved to be transient and whose causes could not be determined;

(c) provisional diagnosis in a patient who failed to return for further investigation or care;

(d) cases referred elsewhere for investigation or treatment before the diagnosis was made;

(e) cases in which a more precise diagnosis was not available for any other reason;

(f) certain symptoms, for which supplementary information is provided, that represent important problems in medical care in their own right.

Excludes ②: *abnormal findings on antenatal screening of mother (O28-)*
certain conditions originating in the perinatal period (P04-P96)
signs and symptoms classified in the body system chapters
signs and symptoms of breast (N63, N64.5)

This chapter contains the following blocks:

R00-R09	Symptoms and signs involving the circulatory and respiratory systems
R10-R19	Symptoms and signs involving the digestive system and abdomen
R20-R23	Symptoms and signs involving the skin and subcutaneous tissue
R25-R29	Symptoms and signs involving the nervous and musculoskeletal systems
R30-R39	Symptoms and signs involving the genitourinary system
R40-R46	Symptoms and signs involving cognition, perception, emotional state and behavior
R47-R49	Symptoms and signs involving speech and voice
R50-R69	General symptoms and signs
R70-R79	Abnormal findings on examination of blood, without diagnosis
R80-R82	Abnormal findings on examination of urine, without diagnosis
R83-R89	Abnormal findings on examination of other body fluids, substances and tissues, without diagnosis
R90-R94	Abnormal findings on diagnostic imaging and in function studies, without diagnosis
R97	Abnormal tumor markers
R99	Ill-defined and unknown cause of mortality

Chapter-Specific Coding Guidelines

C. Chapter-Specific Coding Guidelines
In addition to general coding guidelines, there are guidelines for specific diagnoses and/or conditions in the classification. Unless otherwise indicated, these guidelines apply to all health care settings. Please refer to Section II for guidelines on the selection of principal diagnosis.

18. Chapter 18: Symptoms, Signs, and Abnormal Clinical and Laboratory Findings, Not Elsewhere Classified (R00-R99)

Chapter 18 includes symptoms, signs, abnormal results of clinical or other investigative procedures, and ill-defined conditions regarding which no diagnosis classifiable elsewhere is recorded. Signs and symptoms that point to a specific diagnosis have been assigned to a category in other chapters of the classification.

a. Use of symptom codes
Codes that describe symptoms and signs are acceptable for reporting purposes when a related definitive diagnosis has not been established (confirmed) by the provider.

b. Use of a symptom code with a definitive diagnosis code
Codes for signs and symptoms may be reported in addition to a related definitive diagnosis when the sign or symptom is not routinely associated with that diagnosis, such as the various signs and symptoms associated with complex syndromes. The definitive diagnosis code should be sequenced before the symptom code.

Signs or symptoms that are associated routinely with a disease process should not be assigned as additional codes, unless otherwise instructed by the classification.

c. Combination codes that include symptoms
ICD-10-CM contains a number of combination codes that identify both the definitive diagnosis and common symptoms of that diagnosis. When using one of these combination codes, an additional code should not be assigned for the symptom.

d. Repeated falls
Code R29.6, Repeated falls, is for use for encounters when a patient has recently fallen and the reason for the fall is being investigated.

Code Z91.81, History of falling, is for use when a patient has fallen in the past and is at risk for future falls. When appropriate, both codes R29.6 and Z91.81 may be assigned together.

e. Coma scale
The coma scale codes (R40.2-) can be used in conjunction with traumatic brain injury codes, acute cerebrovascular disease or sequelae of cerebrovascular disease codes. These codes are primarily for use by trauma registries, but they may be used in any setting where this information is collected. The coma scale may also be used to assess the status of the central nervous system for other non-trauma conditions, such as monitoring patients in the intensive care unit regardless of medical condition. The coma scale codes should be sequenced after the diagnosis code(s).

These codes, one from each subcategory, are needed to complete the scale. The 7th character indicates when the scale was recorded. The 7th character should match for all three codes.

At a minimum, report the initial score documented on presentation at your facility. This may be a score from the emergency medicine technician (EMT) or in the emergency department. If desired, a facility may choose to capture multiple coma scale scores.

Assign code R40.24, Glasgow coma scale, total score, when only the total score is documented in the medical record and not the individual score(s).

f. Functional quadriplegia
Functional quadriplegia (code R53.2) is the lack of ability to use one's limbs or to ambulate due to extreme debility. It is not associated with neurologic deficit or injury, and code R53.2 should not be used for cases of neurologic quadriplegia. It should only be assigned if functional quadriplegia is specifically documented in the medical record.

g. SIRS due to Non-Infectious Process
The systemic inflammatory response syndrome (SIRS) can develop as a result of certain non-infectious disease processes, such as trauma, malignant neoplasm, or pancreatitis. When SIRS is documented with a noninfectious condition, and no subsequent infection is documented, the code for the underlying condition, such as an injury, should be assigned, followed by code R65.10, Systemic inflammatory response syndrome (SIRS) of non-infectious origin without acute organ dysfunction, or code R65.11, Systemic inflammatory response syndrome (SIRS) of non-infectious origin with acute organ dysfunction. If an associated acute organ dysfunction is documented, the appropriate code(s) for the specific type of organ dysfunction(s) should be assigned in addition to code R65.11. If acute organ dysfunction is documented, but it cannot be determined if the acute organ dysfunction is associated with SIRS or due to another condition (e.g., directly due to the trauma), the provider should be queried.

h. Death NOS
Code R99, Ill-defined and unknown cause of mortality, is only for use in the very limited circumstance when a patient who has already died is brought into an emergency department or other healthcare facility and is pronounced dead upon arrival. It does not represent the discharge disposition of death.

i. NIHSS Stroke Scale
The NIH stroke scale (NIHSS) codes (R29.7- -) can be used in conjunction with acute stroke codes (I63) to identify the patient's neurological status and the severity of the stroke. The stroke scale codes should be sequenced after the acute stroke diagnosis code(s).

At a minimum, report the initial score documented. If desired, a facility may choose to capture multiple stroke scale scores.

See Section I.B.14. for information concerning the medical record documentation that may be used for assignment of the NIHSS codes.

R00
I
R00

Symptoms and signs involving the circulatory and respiratory systems (R00-R09)

R00- Abnormalities of heart beat

> Excludes 1:   *abnormalities originating in the perinatal period (P29.1-)*
> Excludes ❷: *specified arrhythmias (I47-I49)*

R00.0   Tachycardia, unspecified
 Rapid heart beat
 Sinoauricular tachycardia NOS
 Sinus [sinusal] tachycardia NOS

> Excludes 1:   *neonatal tachycardia (P29.11)*
>   *paroxysmal tachycardia (I47.-)*

R00.1   Bradycardia, unspecified
 Sinoatrial bradycardia
 Sinus bradycardia
 Slow heart beat
 Vagal bradycardia
Use additional code for adverse effect, if applicable, to identify drug (T36-T50 with fifth or sixth character 5)

> Excludes 1:   *neonatal bradycardia (P29.12)*

R00.2   Palpitations — The rapid, throbbing pulsation of the heart.
 Awareness of heart beat

R00.8   Other abnormalities of heart beat

R00.9   Unspecified abnormalities of heart beat

R01- Cardiac murmurs and other cardiac sounds

> Excludes 1:   *cardiac murmurs and sounds originating in the perinatal period (P29.8)*

R01.0   Benign and innocent cardiac murmurs — The extra or unusal sound of blood moving through the heart and heart valves.
 Functional cardiac murmur

R01.1   Cardiac murmur, unspecified
 Cardiac bruit NOS
 Heart murmur NOS
 Systolic murmur NOS

R01.2   Other cardiac sounds
 Cardiac dullness, increased or decreased — The diminished resonance of the heart sounds.
 Precordial friction — The rubbing sound of the lower part of the heart.

R03- Abnormal blood-pressure reading, without diagnosis

R03.0   Elevated blood-pressure reading, without diagnosis of hypertension — [Questionable Admission]
 Note: This category is to be used to record an episode of elevated blood pressure in a patient in whom no formal diagnosis of hypertension has been made, or as an isolated incidental finding.

R03.1   Nonspecific low blood-pressure reading

> Excludes 1:   *hypotension (I95-)*
>   *maternal hypotension syndrome (O26.5-)*
>   *neurogenic orthostatic hypotension (G90.3)*

R04- Hemorrhage from respiratory passages

R04.0   Epistaxis — Bleeding from the nostrils.
 Hemorrhage from nose
 Nosebleed

R04.1   Hemorrhage from throat — Bleeding from the throat.

> Excludes ❷: *hemoptysis (R04.2)*

cc **R04.2   Hemoptysis** — The coughing-up of blood or bloodstained sputum.

 AHA 13:4Q:p118 – Hemoptysis with pneumonia
 Blood-stained sputum
 Cough with hemorrhage

R04.8- Hemorrhage from other sites in respiratory passages

cc **R04.81 Acute idiopathic pulmonary hemorrhage in infants** — [Age/0-17] – The presence of blood in the airway of infants without an identifiable cause, and in severe cases with sudden onset of overt bleeding and acute respiratory distress or failure.
  AIPHI
  Acute idiopathic hemorrhage in infants over 28 days old

> Excludes 1:   *perinatal pulmonary hemorrhage (P26.-)*
>   *von Willebrand's disease (D68.0)*

cc **R04.89 Hemorrhage from other sites in respiratory passages**
 Pulmonary hemorrhage NOS

cc **R04.9   Hemorrhage from respiratory passages, unspecified**

R05   Cough

> Excludes 1:   *cough with hemorrhage (R04.2)*
>   *smoker's cough (J41.0)*

R06- Abnormalities of breathing

> Excludes 1:   *acute respiratory distress syndrome (J80)*
>   *respiratory arrest (R09.2)*
>   *respiratory arrest of newborn (P28.81)*
>   *respiratory distress syndrome of newborn (P22.-)*
>   *respiratory failure (J96.-)*
>   *respiratory failure of newborn (P28.5)*

R06.0- Dyspnea — Difficult or labored breathing, breathlessness.

> Excludes 1:   *tachypnea NOS (R06.82)*
>   *transient tachypnea of newborn (P22.1)*

R06.00 Dyspnea, unspecified

R06.01 Orthopnea — The condition of difficult breathing except when in an upright position.

R06.02 Shortness of breath — The inability to adequately inspirate the lungs.

R06.09 Other forms of dyspnea

R06.1   Stridor — The high-pitched inspiratory sound from the larynx.

> Excludes 1:   *congenital laryngeal stridor (P28.89)*
>   *laryngismus (stridulus) (J38.5)*

R06.2   Wheezing — The whistling sound made during breathing.
AHA 16:2Q:p33 – Wheezing due to exposure to electronic cigarette vapors

> Excludes 1:   *asthma (J45-)*

cc **R06.3   Periodic breathing** — The condition marked by increasing and decreasing rates of respiration with periods of apnea.
 Cheyne-Stokes breathing

R06.4   Hyperventilation — The abnormally increased breathing resulting in too much oxygen and not enough carbon dioxide in the blood.

> Excludes 1:   *psychogenic hyperventilation (F45.8)*

R06.5   Mouth breathing — Breathing predominantly through the mouth instead of the through the nose, often during sleep.

> Excludes ❷: *dry mouth NOS (R68.2)*

R06.6   Hiccough — The involuntary, rapid spasm of the diaphragm and lungs with closure of the glottis.

> Excludes 1:   *psychogenic hiccough (F45.8)*

R06.7   Sneezing — The extremely rapid expulsion of air from the lungs caused by the irritation of the mucous membrane of the tract.

R06.8- Other abnormalities of breathing

R06.81 Apnea, not elsewhere classified — The abnormal, periodic cessation of breathing.
 Apnea NOS

> Excludes 1:   *apnea (of) newborn (P28.4)*
>   *sleep apnea (G47.3-)*
>   *sleep apnea of newborn (primary) (P28.3)*

R06.82 Tachypnea, not elsewhere classified — The condition of quick, shallow breathing.
 Tachypnea NOS

> Excludes 1:   *transitory tachypnea of newborn (P22.1)*

R06.83 Snoring

R06.89 Other abnormalities of breathing
 Breath-holding (spells)
 Sighing

R06.9   Unspecified abnormalities of breathing

R07- Pain in throat and chest

> Excludes 1:   *epidemic myalgia (B33.0)*
> Excludes ❷: *jaw pain R68.84*
>   *pain in breast (N64.4)*

R07.0   Pain in throat

> Excludes 1:   *chronic sore throat (J31.2)*
>   *sore throat (acute) NOS (J02.9)*
> Excludes ❷: *dysphagia (R13.1-)*
>   *pain in neck (M54.2)*

R07.1   Chest pain on breathing
 Painful respiration

R07.2   Precordial pain — Chest pain in the area that overlies the heart and lower thorax.

R00 - R07

Excludes 1: = NOT CODED HERE! (Do not code both)   **988**   Excludes ❷: = Not Included Here

R07.8-   Other chest pain

R07.81   Pleurodynia — Paroxysmal pain in the intercostal muscles.
   Pleurodynia NOS
   Excludes 1:   epidemic pleurodynia (B33.0)

R07.82   Intercostal pain

R07.89   Other chest pain
   Anterior chest-wall pain NOS

R07.9   Chest pain, unspecified

R09-   Other symptoms and signs involving the circulatory and respiratory system
   Excludes 1:   acute respiratory distress syndrome (J80)
      respiratory arrest of newborn (P28.81)
      respiratory distress syndrome of newborn (P22.0)
      respiratory failure (J96.-)
      respiratory failure of newborn (P28.5)

R09.0-   Asphyxia and hypoxemia
   Excludes 1:   asphyxia due to carbon monoxide (T58.-)
      asphyxia due to foreign body in respiratory tract (T17.-)
      birth (intrauterine) asphyxia (P84)
      hypercapnia (R06.4)
      hyperventilation (R06.4)
      traumatic asphyxia (T71.-)

cc **R09.01   Asphyxia** — The life threatening, severely deficient supply of oxygenated blood to the body's tissues (also refers to stopping of the pulse).

R09.02   Hypoxemia — The abnormal condition of deficient oxygenation of the blood.

R09.1   Pleurisy — Inflammation of the pleura.
   Excludes 1:   pleurisy with effusion (J90)

MCC **R09.2   Respiratory arrest** — The cessation of breathing.
   Cardiorespiratory failure — The inability of the heart and lungs to perform adequately.
   Excludes 1:   cardiac arrest (I46.-)
      respiratory arrest of newborn (P28.81)
      respiratory distress of newborn (P22.0)
      respiratory failure (J96.-)
      respiratory failure of newborn (P28.5)
      respiratory insufficiency (R06.89)
      respiratory insufficiency of newborn (P28.5)

R09.3   Abnormal sputum
   Abnormal amount of sputum
   Abnormal color of sputum
   Abnormal odor of sputum
   Excessive sputum
   Excludes 1:   blood-stained sputum (R04.2)

R09.8-   Other specified symptoms and signs involving the circulatory and respiratory systems

R09.81   Nasal congestion

R09.82   Postnasal drip

R09.89   Other specified symptoms and signs involving the circulatory and respiratory systems
   Bruit (arterial)
   Abnormal chest percussion
   Feeling of foreign body in throat
   Friction sounds in chest
   Chest tympany
   Choking sensation
   Rales
   Weak pulse
   Excludes ❷: foreign body in throat (T17.2-)
      wheezing (R06.2)

Symptoms and signs involving the digestive system and abdomen (R10-R19)

Excludes ❷: congenital or infantile pylorospasm (Q40.0)
   gastrointestinal hemorrhage (K92.0-K92.2)
   intestinal obstruction (K56.-)
   newborn gastrointestinal hemorrhage (P54.0-P54.3)
   newborn intestinal obstruction (P76.-)
   pylorospasm (K31.3)
   signs and symptoms involving the urinary system (R30-R39)
   symptoms referable to female genital organs (N94.-)
   symptoms referable to male genital organs male (N48-N50)

R10-   Abdominal and pelvic pain
   Excludes 1:   renal colic (N23)
   Excludes ❷: dorsalgia (M54.-)
      flatulence and related conditions (R14.-)

R10.0   Acute abdomen
   Severe abdominal pain (generalized) (with abdominal rigidity)
   Excludes 1:   abdominal rigidity NOS (R19.3)
      generalized abdominal pain NOS (R10.84)
      localized abdominal pain (R10.1-R10.3-)

R10.1-   Pain localized to upper abdomen

R10.10   Upper abdominal pain, unspecified

R10.11   Right upper quadrant pain

R10.12   Left upper quadrant pain

R10.13   Epigastric pain
   Dyspepsia
   Excludes 1:   functional dyspepsia (K30)

R10.2   Pelvic and perineal pain
   Excludes 1:   vulvodynia (N94.81)

R10.3-   Pain localized to other parts of lower abdomen

R10.30   Lower abdominal pain, unspecified

R10.31   Right lower quadrant pain

R10.32   Left lower quadrant pain

R10.33   Periumbilical pain

R10.8-   Other abdominal pain

R10.81-   Abdominal tenderness
   Abdominal tenderness NOS

R10.811   Right upper quadrant abdominal tenderness

R10.812   Left upper quadrant abdominal tenderness

R10.813   Right lower quadrant abdominal tenderness

R10.814   Left lower quadrant abdominal tenderness

R10.815   Periumbilic abdominal tenderness

R10.816   Epigastric abdominal tenderness

R10.817   Generalized abdominal tenderness

R10.819   Abdominal tenderness, unspecified site

R10.82-   Rebound abdominal tenderness — A form felt upon the release of applied pressure.

R10.821   Right upper quadrant rebound abdominal tenderness

R10.822   Left upper quadrant rebound abdominal tenderness

R10.823   Right lower quadrant rebound abdominal tenderness

R10.824   Left lower quadrant rebound abdominal tenderness

R10.825   Periumbilic rebound abdominal tenderness

R10.826   Epigastric rebound abdominal tenderness

R10.827   Generalized rebound abdominal tenderness

R10.829   Rebound abdominal tenderness, unspecified site

R10.83   Colic — [Age/0-17] – The greater frequency and duration of crying and apparent discomfort.
   Colic NOS
   Infantile colic
   Excludes 1:   colic in adult and child over 12 months old (R10.84)

R10.84   Generalized abdominal pain
   Excludes 1:   generalized abdominal pain associated with acute abdomen (R10.0)

R10.9   Unspecified abdominal pain

R07-R10

R11- Nausea and vomiting
> Excludes 1:   cyclical vomiting associated with migraine (G43.A-)
> excessive vomiting in pregnancy (O21-)
> hematemesis (K92.0)
> neonatal hematemesis (P54.0)
> newborn vomiting (P92.0-)
> psychogenic vomiting (F50.89)
> vomiting associated with bulimia nervosa (F50.2)
> vomiting following gastrointestinal surgery (K91.0)

R11.0   Nausea
Nausea NOS
Nausea without vomiting

R11.1- Vomiting

R11.10   Vomiting, unspecified
Vomiting NOS

R11.11   Vomiting without nausea

R11.12   Projectile vomiting — Vomiting with great force.

R11.13   Vomiting of fecal matter

R11.14   Bilious vomiting — Vomitus with bile.
Bilious emesis

R11.2   Nausea with vomiting, unspecified
Persistent nausea with vomiting NOS

R12   Heartburn — The burning sensation in the esophagus.
> Excludes 1:   dyspepsia NOS (R10.13)
> functional dyspepsia (K30)

R13- Aphagia and dysphagia

R13.0   Aphagia
Inability to swallow
> Excludes 1:   psychogenic aphagia (F50.9)

R13.1- Dysphagia — Difficulty in swallowing.
Code first, if applicable, dysphagia following cerebrovascular disease (I69. with final characters -91)
> Excludes 1:   psychogenic dysphagia (F45.8)

R13.10   Dysphagia, unspecified
Difficulty in swallowing NOS

R13.11   Dysphagia, oral phase — A form involving the cheeks, lips, palate, and tongue in which the food/liquid is chewed in preparation for swallowing.

R13.12   Dysphagia, oropharyngeal phase — A form involving the tongue base and pharyngeal walls in which the tongue pushes the food or liquid to the back of the mouth, beginning the swallowing process.

R13.13   Dysphagia, pharyngeal phase — A form involving the pharynx and larynx in which the food or liquid quickly passes through the pharynx.

R13.14   Dysphagia, pharyngoesophageal phase — A form involving the upper esophageal sphincter in which the food or liquid moves through the esophagus and into the stomach.

R13.19   Other dysphagia
Cervical dysphagia
Neurogenic dysphagia — A form caused by disease or impairment of the nervous system.

R14- Flatulence and related conditions
> Excludes 1:   psychogenic aerophagy (F45.8)

R14.0   Abdominal distension (gaseous)
Bloating
Tympanites (abdominal) (intestinal)

R14.1   Gas pain

R14.2   Eructation

R14.3   Flatulence

R15- Fecal incontinence — The inability to control the excretion of feces.
Includes: Encopresis NOS
> Excludes 1:   fecal incontinence of nonorganic origin (F98.1)

R15.0   Incomplete defecation
> Excludes 1:   constipation (K59.0-)
> fecal impaction (K56.41)

R15.1   Fecal smearing
Fecal soiling

R15.2   Fecal urgency

R15.9   Full incontinence of feces
Fecal incontinence NOS

R16-   Hepatomegaly and splenomegaly, not elsewhere classified

R16.0   Hepatomegaly, not elsewhere classified — The abnormal enlargement of the liver.
Hepatomegaly NOS

R16.1   Splenomegaly, not elsewhere classified — The abnormal enlargement of the spleen.
Splenomegaly NOS

R16.2   Hepatomegaly with splenomegaly, not elsewhere classified — The abnormal enlargement of the liver and spleen.
Hepatosplenomegaly NOS

R17   Unspecified jaundice — The abnormal deposition of bilirubin in the skin resulting in the yellowish skin discoloration.
CC
> Excludes 1:   neonatal jaundice (P55, P57-P59)

R18-   Ascites — The abnormal accumulation of serous fluid in the abdominal cavity.
Includes: Fluid in peritoneal cavity
> Excludes 1:   ascites in alcoholic cirrhosis (K70.31)
> ascites in alcoholic hepatitis (K70.11)
> ascites in toxic liver disease with chronic active hepatitis (K71.51)

CC **R18.0   Malignant ascites** — [Unacceptable PDX] – A form due to a malignant neoplasm.
Code first malignancy, such as:
Malignant neoplasm of ovary (C56.-)
Secondary malignant neoplasm of retroperitoneum and peritoneum (C78.6)

CC **R18.8   Other ascites**
Ascites NOS
Peritoneal effusion (chronic)

R19-   Other symptoms and signs involving the digestive system and abdomen
> Excludes 1:   acute abdomen (R10.0)

R19.0-   Intra-abdominal and pelvic swelling, mass and lump
> Excludes 1:   abdominal distension (gaseous) (R14.-)
> ascites (R18.-)

R19.00   Intra-abdominal and pelvic swelling, mass and lump, unspecified site

R19.01   Right upper quadrant abdominal swelling, mass and lump

R19.02   Left upper quadrant abdominal swelling, mass and lump

R19.03   Right lower quadrant abdominal swelling, mass and lump

R19.04   Left lower quadrant abdominal swelling, mass and lump

R19.05   Periumbilic swelling, mass or lump
Diffuse or generalized umbilical swelling or mass

R19.06   Epigastric swelling, mass or lump

R19.07   Generalized intra-abdominal and pelvic swelling, mass and lump
Diffuse or generalized intra-abdominal swelling or mass NOS
Diffuse or generalized pelvic swelling or mass NOS

R19.09   Other intra-abdominal and pelvic swelling, mass and lump

R19.1-   Abnormal bowel sounds

R19.11   Absent bowel sounds

R19.12   Hyperactive bowel sounds

R19.15   Other abnormal bowel sounds
Abnormal bowel sounds NOS

R19.2   Visible peristalsis
Hyperperistalsis — An abnormal increase in the wave-like motion of the intestines.

R19.3-   Abdominal rigidity — The abnormal stiffness of the abdomen.
> Excludes 1:   abdominal rigidity with severe abdominal pain (R10.0)

R19.30   Abdominal rigidity, unspecified site

R19.31   Right upper quadrant abdominal rigidity

R19.32   Left upper quadrant abdominal rigidity

R19.33   Right lower quadrant abdominal rigidity

R19.34   Left lower quadrant abdominal rigidity

R19.35   Periumbilic abdominal rigidity

R19.36   Epigastric abdominal rigidity

R19.37   Generalized abdominal rigidity

Excludes 1: = NOT CODED HERE! (Do not code both)

Excludes ❷: = Not Included Here

R19.4   Change in bowel habit
     Excludes 1:   *constipation (K59.0-)*
                functional diarrhea (K59.1)

R19.5   Other fecal abnormalities
     Abnormal stool color
     Bulky stools
     Mucus in stools
     Occult blood in feces
     Occult blood in stools
     Excludes 1:   *melena (K92.1)*
                neonatal melena (P54.1)

R19.6   Halitosis — The condition of offensive or bad breath.

R19.7   Diarrhea, unspecified
     Diarrhea NOS
     Excludes 1:   *functional diarrhea (K59.1)*
                neonatal diarrhea (P78.3)
                psychogenic diarrhea (F45.8)

R19.8   Other specified symptoms and signs involving the digestive system and abdomen

Symptoms and signs involving the skin and subcutaneous tissue (R20-R23)

     Excludes ❷: *symptoms relating to breast (N64.4-N64.5)*

R20-   Disturbances of skin sensation
     Excludes 1:   *dissociative anesthesia and sensory loss (F44.6)*
                psychogenic disturbances (F45.8)

R20.0   Anesthesia of skin — The loss of sensation of the skin.

R20.1   Hypoesthesia of skin — The abnormally decreased sensitivity of the skin.

R20.2   Paresthesia of skin — The abnormal or perverted sensation of the skin.
     Formication
     Pins and needles
     Tingling skin
     Excludes 1:   *acroparesthesia (I73.8)*

R20.3   Hyperesthesia — The abnormally increased sensitivity of the skin.

R20.8   Other disturbances of skin sensation

R20.9   Unspecified disturbances of skin sensation

R21   Rash and other nonspecific skin eruption
     Includes: Rash NOS
     Excludes 1:   *specified type of rash — code to condition*
                vesicular eruption (R23.8)

R22-   <u>Localized swelling, mass and lump</u> of skin and subcutaneous tissue
     Includes: Subcutaneous nodules (localized) (superficial)
     Excludes 1:   *abnormal findings on diagnostic imaging (R90-R93)*
                edema (R60-)
                enlarged lymph nodes (R59-)
                localized adiposity (E65)
                swelling of joint (M25.4-)

R22.0   Localized swelling, mass and lump, <u>head</u>

R22.1   Localized swelling, mass and lump, <u>neck</u>

R22.2   Localized swelling, mass and lump, <u>trunk</u>
     Excludes 1:   *intra-abdominal or pelvic mass and lump (R19.0-)*
                intra-abdominal or pelvic swelling (R19.0-)
     Excludes ❷: *breast mass and lump (N63)*

R22.3-   Localized swelling, mass and lump, <u>upper limb</u>

    R22.30   Localized swelling, mass and lump, <u>unspecified</u> upper limb

    R22.31   Localized swelling, mass and lump, <u>right</u> upper limb

    R22.32   Localized swelling, mass and lump, <u>left</u> upper limb

    R22.33   Localized swelling, mass and lump, upper limb, <u>bilateral</u>

R22.4-   Localized swelling, mass and lump, <u>lower limb</u>

    R22.40   Localized swelling, mass and lump, <u>unspecified</u> lower limb

    R22.41   Localized swelling, mass and lump, <u>right</u> lower limb

    R22.42   Localized swelling, mass and lump, <u>left</u> lower limb

    R22.43   Localized swelling, mass and lump, lower limb, <u>bilateral</u>

R22.9   Localized swelling, mass and lump, <u>unspecified</u>

R23-   Other skin changes

R23.0   Cyanosis — The condition of reduced hemoglobin concentration in the blood resulting in the bluish or purple skin discoloration.
     Excludes 1:   *acrocyanosis (I73.8)*
                cyanotic attacks of newborn (P28.2)

R23.1   Pallor — Paleness of the skin.
     Clammy skin

R23.2   Flushing — The sudden redness of the skin.
     Excessive blushing
     Code first, if applicable, menopausal and female climacteric states (N95.1)

R23.3   Spontaneous ecchymoses — Small, hemorrhagic spots on the skin.
     Petechiae
     Excludes 1:   *ecchymoses of newborn (P54.5)*
                purpura (D69.-)

R23.4   Changes in skin texture
     Desquamation of skin
     Induration of skin
     Scaling of skin
     Excludes 1:   *epidermal thickening NOS (L85.9)*

R23.8   Other skin changes

R23.9   Unspecified skin changes

Symptoms and signs involving the nervous and musculoskeletal systems (R25-R29)

R25-   Abnormal involuntary movements — The condition of bodily movements that are not voluntarily controlled.
     Excludes 1:   *specific movement disorders (G20-G26)*
                stereotyped movement disorders (F98.4)
                tic disorders (F95.-)

R25.0   Abnormal head movements

R25.1   Tremor, unspecified — The condition of muscles contracting involuntarily in a rhythmic, oscillating-like pattern in one or more body parts.
     Excludes 1:   *chorea NOS (G25.5)*
                essential tremor (G25.0)
                hysterical tremor (F44.4)
                intention tremor (G25.2)

R25.2   Cramp and spasm
     Excludes ❷: *carpopedal spasm (R29.0)*
                charley-horse (M62.831)
                infantile spasms (G40.4-)
                muscle spasm of back (M62.830)
                muscle spasm of calf (M62.831)

R25.3   Fasciculation — The condition of small, local muscles contracting involuntarily.
     Twitching NOS

R25.8   Other abnormal involuntary movements

R25.9   Unspecified abnormal involuntary movements

R26-   Abnormalities of gait and mobility — The abnormal deviation of the manner or style of walking.
     Excludes 1:   *ataxia NOS (R27.0)*
                hereditary ataxia (G11.-)
                locomotor (syphilitic) ataxia (A52.11)
                immobility syndrome (paraplegic) (M62.3)

R26.0   Ataxic gait — A form marked by unsteadiness and uncoordinated walk.
     Staggering gait — A form marked by swaying and apparent loss (with recovery) of balance.

R26.1   Paralytic gait — A form marked by loss of motor ability while walking.
     Spastic gait — A form marked by the legs being held together and moving in a stiff manner.

R26.2   Difficulty in walking, <u>not elsewhere classified</u>
     Excludes 1:   *falling (R29.6)*
                unsteadiness on feet (R26.81)

R26.8-   Other abnormalities of gait and mobility

    R26.81   Unsteadiness on feet

    R26.89   Other abnormalities of gait and mobility

R26.9   Unspecified abnormalities of gait and mobility

R
19
-
R
26

Excludes 1: = NOT CODED HERE! (Do not code both)   *Excludes ❷: =* Not Included Here

R27- **Other lack of coordination** — The lack of harmonious functioning of the body parts.
  Excludes 1:   *ataxic gait (R26.0)*
     hereditary ataxia (G11.-)
     vertigo NOS (R42)
  R27.0 **Ataxia, unspecified**
    Excludes 1:   *ataxia following cerebrovascular disease (I69. with final characters -93)*
  R27.8 **Other lack of coordination**
  R27.9 **Unspecified lack of coordination**

R29- **Other symptoms and signs involving the nervous and musculoskeletal systems**
  cc **R29.0** **Tetany** — The condition of intermittent tonic spasms involving the extremities.
    Carpopedal spasm — The spasm of the hand or foot, or of the thumbs and great toes.
    Excludes 1:   *hysterical tetany (F44.5)*
       neonatal tetany (P71.3)
       parathyroid tetany (E20.9)
       post-thyroidectomy tetany (E89.2)
  cc **R29.1** **Meningismus** — The irritation of the brain and spinal cord with symptoms simulating meningitis, but without actual inflammation.
  R29.2 **Abnormal reflex**
    Excludes ❷: *abnormal pupillary reflex (H57.0)*
       hyperactive gag reflex (J39.2)
       vasovagal reaction or syncope (R55)
  R29.3 **Abnormal posture**
  R29.4 **Clicking hip**
    Excludes 1:   *congenital deformities of hip (Q65.-)*
  cc **R29.5** **Transient paralysis** — The temporary loss of motor function.
    Code first any associated spinal cord injury (S14.0, S14.1-, S24.0, S24.1-, S34.0-, S34.1-)
    Excludes 1:   *transient ischemic attack (G45.9)*
  R29.6 **Repeated falls**
    Falling
    Tendency to fall
    Excludes ❷: *at risk for falling (Z91.81)*
       history of falling (Z91.81)
  R29.7- **National Institutes of Health Stroke Scale (NIHSS) score**
    Code first the type of cerebral infarction (I63.-)
    R29.70- NIHSS score 0-9
      R29.700 **NIHSS score 0** — [Unacceptable PDX]
      R29.701 **NIHSS score 1** — [Unacceptable PDX]
      R29.702 **NIHSS score 2** — [Unacceptable PDX]
      R29.703 **NIHSS score 3** — [Unacceptable PDX]
      R29.704 **NIHSS score 4** — [Unacceptable PDX]
      R29.705 **NIHSS score 5** — [Unacceptable PDX]
      R29.706 **NIHSS score 6** — [Unacceptable PDX]
      R29.707 **NIHSS score 7** — [Unacceptable PDX]
      R29.708 **NIHSS score 8** — [Unacceptable PDX]
      R29.709 **NIHSS score 9** — [Unacceptable PDX]
    R29.71- NIHSS score 10-19
      R29.710 **NIHSS score 10** — [Unacceptable PDX]
      R29.711 **NIHSS score 11** — [Unacceptable PDX]
      R29.712 **NIHSS score 12** — [Unacceptable PDX]
      R29.713 **NIHSS score 13** — [Unacceptable PDX]
      R29.714 **NIHSS score 14** — [Unacceptable PDX]
      R29.715 **NIHSS score 15** — [Unacceptable PDX]
      R29.716 **NIHSS score 16** — [Unacceptable PDX]
      R29.717 **NIHSS score 17** — [Unacceptable PDX]
      R29.718 **NIHSS score 18** — [Unacceptable PDX]
      R29.719 **NIHSS score 19** — [Unacceptable PDX]

R29.72- NIHSS score 20-29
  R29.720 **NIHSS score 20** — [Unacceptable PDX]
  R29.721 **NIHSS score 21** — [Unacceptable PDX]
  R29.722 **NIHSS score 22** — [Unacceptable PDX]
  R29.723 **NIHSS score 23** — [Unacceptable PDX]
  R29.724 **NIHSS score 24** — [Unacceptable PDX]
  R29.725 **NIHSS score 25** — [Unacceptable PDX]
  R29.726 **NIHSS score 26** — [Unacceptable PDX]
  R29.727 **NIHSS score 27** — [Unacceptable PDX]
  R29.728 **NIHSS score 28** — [Unacceptable PDX]
  R29.729 **NIHSS score 29** — [Unacceptable PDX]
R29.73- NIHSS score 30-39
  R29.730 **NIHSS score 30** — [Unacceptable PDX]
  R29.731 **NIHSS score 31** — [Unacceptable PDX]
  R29.732 **NIHSS score 32** — [Unacceptable PDX]
  R29.733 **NIHSS score 33** — [Unacceptable PDX]
  R29.734 **NIHSS score 34** — [Unacceptable PDX]
  R29.735 **NIHSS score 35** — [Unacceptable PDX]
  R29.736 **NIHSS score 36** — [Unacceptable PDX]
  R29.737 **NIHSS score 37** — [Unacceptable PDX]
  R29.738 **NIHSS score 38** — [Unacceptable PDX]
  R29.739 **NIHSS score 39** — [Unacceptable PDX]
R29.74- NIHSS score 40-42
  R29.740 **NIHSS score 40** — [Unacceptable PDX]
  R29.741 **NIHSS score 41** — [Unacceptable PDX]
  R29.742 **NIHSS score 42** — [Unacceptable PDX]
R29.8- **Other symptoms and signs involving the nervous and musculoskeletal systems**
  R29.81- **Other symptoms and signs involving the nervous system**
    R29.810 **Facial weakness** — The loss or impairment of normal facial muscle control.
      Facial droop
      Excludes 1:   *Bell's palsy (G51.0)*
         facial weakness following cerebrovascular disease (I69. with final characters-92)
    R29.818 **Other symptoms and signs involving the nervous system**
  R29.89- **Other symptoms and signs involving the musculoskeletal system**
    Excludes ❷: *pain in limb (M79.6-)*
    R29.890 **Loss of height** — The relatively recent loss of a patient's normal height.
      Excludes 1:   *osteoporosis (M80-M81)*
    R29.891 **Ocular torticollis** — The abnormal tilting of the head caused by vision problems.
      Excludes 1:   *congenital (sternomastoid) torticollis Q68.0*
         psychogenic torticollis (F45.8)
         spasmodic torticollis (G24.3)
         torticollis due to birth injury (P15.8)
         torticollis NOS M43.6
    R29.898 **Other symptoms and signs involving the musculoskeletal system**
  R29.9- **Unspecified symptoms and signs involving the nervous and musculoskeletal systems**
    R29.90 **Unspecified symptoms and signs involving the nervous system**
    R29.91 **Unspecified symptoms and signs involving the musculoskeletal system**

Symptoms and signs involving the genitourinary system (R30-R39)

R30- Pain associated with micturition
> Excludes 1: *psychogenic pain associated with micturition (F45.8)*

R30.0 Dysuria — The condition of painful urination.
> **Strangury**

R30.1 Vesical tenesmus — The sensation of bladder fullness after voiding.

R30.9 Painful micturition, unspecified
> **Painful urination NOS**

R31- Hematuria — The abnormal presence of blood in the urine.
> Excludes 1: *hematuria included with underlying conditions, such as:*
> *acute cystitis with hematuria (N30.01)*
> *recurrent and persistent hematuria in glomerular diseases (N02.-)*

R31.0 Gross hematuria — A form that is visible in the urine.

R31.1 Benign essential microscopic hematuria

R31.2- Other microscopic hematuria

R31.21 Asymptomatic microscopic hematuria
> **AMH**

R31.29 Other microscopic hematuria

R31.9 Hematuria, unspecified

R32 Unspecified urinary incontinence
> **Enuresis NOS**
> Excludes 1: *functional urinary incontinence (R39.81)*
> *nonorganic enuresis (F98.0)*
> *stress incontinence and other specified urinary incontinence (N39.3-N39.4-)*
> *urinary incontinence associated with cognitive impairment (R39.81)*

R33- Retention of urine — The abnormal accumulation of urine in the bladder due to the inability to urinate.
> Excludes 1: *psychogenic retention of urine (F45.8)*

R33.0 Drug-induced retention of urine
> Use additional code for adverse effect, if applicable, to identify drug (T36-T50 with fifth or sixth character 5)

R33.8 Other retention of urine
> Code first, if applicable, any causal condition, such as:
> **Enlarged prostate (N40.1)**

R33.9 Retention of urine, unspecified

R34 Anuria and oliguria — The lack, or significantly decreased normal amount, of urine.
> Excludes 1: *anuria and oliguria complicating abortion or ectopic or molar pregnancy (O00-O07, O08.4)*
> *anuria and oliguria complicating pregnancy (O26.83-)*
> *anuria and oliguria complicating the puerperium (O90.4)*

R35- Polyuria — The condition of passing a large volume of urine in a given period.
> Code first, if applicable, any causal condition, such as:
> **Enlarged prostate (N40.1)**
> Excludes 1: *psychogenic polyuria (F45.8)*

R35.0 Frequency of micturition — The condition of urination at short intervals without increase in daily volume of urinary output.

R35.1 Nocturia — The condition of excessive urination at night.

R35.8 Other polyuria
> **Polyuria NOS**

R36- Urethral discharge

R36.0 Urethral discharge without blood

R36.1 Hematospermia — [♂] — The abnormal presence of blood in the ejaculate.

R36.9 Urethral discharge, unspecified
> **Penile discharge NOS**
> **Urethrorrhea**

R37 Sexual dysfunction, unspecified

R39- Other and unspecified symptoms and signs involving the genitourinary system

CC **R39.0 Extravasation of urine** — The escape of urine into the tissues.

R39.1- Other difficulties with micturition
> Code first, if applicable, any causal condition, such as:
> **Enlarged prostate (N40.1)**

R39.11 Hesitancy of micturition

R39.12 Poor urinary stream
> **Weak urinary steam**

R39.13 Splitting of urinary stream

R39.14 Feeling of incomplete bladder emptying

R39.15 Urgency of urination
> Excludes 1: *urge incontinence (N39.41, N39.46)*

R39.16 Straining to void

R39.19- Other difficulties with micturition

R39.191 Need to immediately re-void

R39.192 Position dependent micturition

R39.198 Other difficulties with micturition

R39.2 Extrarenal uremia — The retention of by-products normally excreted in the urine that is due to non-kidney disorders.
> **Prerenal uremia**
> Excludes 1: *uremia NOS (N19)*

R39.8- Other symptoms and signs involving the genitourinary system

R39.81 Functional urinary incontinence
> Urinary incontinence due to cognitive impairment, or severe physical disability or immobility
> Excludes 1: *stress incontinence and other specified urinary incontinence (N39.3-N39.4-)*
> *urinary incontinence NOS (R32)*

R39.82 Chronic bladder pain

R39.89 Other symptoms and signs involving the genitourinary system

R39.9 Unspecified symptoms and signs involving the genitourinary system

Symptoms and signs involving cognition, perception, emotional state and behavior (R40-R46)

> Excludes ❷: *symptoms and signs constituting part of a pattern of mental disorder (F01-F99)*

R40- Somnolence, stupor and coma
> Excludes 1: *neonatal coma (P91.5)*
> *somnolence, stupor and coma in diabetes (E08-E13)*
> *somnolence, stupor and coma in hepatic failure (K72-)*
> *somnolence, stupor and coma in hypoglycemia (nondiabetic) (E15)*

R40.0 Somnolence
> **Drowsiness**
> Excludes 1: *coma (R40.2-)*

R40.1 Stupor — The partial or nearly complete state of unconsciousness.
> **Catatonic stupor**
> **Semicoma**
> Excludes 1: *catatonic schizophrenia (F20.2)*
> *coma (R40.2-)*
> *depressive stupor (F31-F33)*
> *dissociative stupor (F44.2)*
> *manic stupor (F30.2)*

R40.2- Coma — A state of profound unconsciousness that is characterized by the inability to be aroused, absence of spontaneous eye movements, response to painful stimuli, and vocalization.
> AHA 14:1Q:p19 – Glasgow coma scale (GCS) score
> Code first any associated:
> **Fracture of skull (S02.-)**
> **Intracranial injury (S06.-)**
> Note: One code from each subcategory, R40.21-R40.23, is required to complete the coma scale

MCC **R40.20 Unspecified coma**
> **Coma NOS**
> **Unconsciousness NOS**

R40.21- Coma scale, eyes open
> The following appropriate 7th character is to be added to subcategory R40.21-:
> **0 - Unspecified time**
> **1 - In the field [EMT or ambulance]**
> **2 - At arrival to emergency department**
> **3 - At hospital admission**
> **4 - 24 hours or more after hospital admission**

MCC-0-4 **R40.211- Coma scale, eyes open, never**

MCC-0-4 **R40.212- Coma scale, eyes open, to pain**

R40.213- Coma scale, eyes open, to sound

R40.214- Coma scale, eyes open, spontaneous

R 3 0 | R 4 0

R40.22- Coma scale, <u>best verbal response</u>

The following appropriate 7th character is to be added to subcategory R40.22-:
- 0 - Unspecified time
- 1 - In the field [EMT or ambulance]
- 2 - At arrival to emergency department
- 3 - At hospital admission
- 4 - 24 hours or more after hospital admission

MCC-0-4 **R40.221-** Coma scale, best verbal response, <u>none</u>

MCC-0-4 **R40.222-** Coma scale, best verbal response, <u>incomprehensible words</u>

R40.223- Coma scale, best verbal response, <u>inappropriate words</u>

R40.224- Coma scale, best verbal response, <u>confused conversation</u>

R40.225- Coma scale, best verbal response, <u>oriented</u>

R40.23- Coma scale, <u>best motor response</u>

The following appropriate 7th character is to be added to subcategory R40.23-:
- 0 - Unspecified time
- 1 - In the field [EMT or ambulance]
- 2 - At arrival to emergency department
- 3 - At hospital admission
- 4 - 24 hours or more after hospital admission

MCC-0-4 **R40.231-** Coma scale, best motor response, <u>none</u>

MCC-0-4 **R40.232-** Coma scale, best motor response, <u>extension</u>

R40.233- Coma scale, best motor response, <u>abnormal</u>

MCC-0-4 **R40.234-** Coma scale, best motor response, <u>flexion withdrawal</u>

R40.235- Coma scale, best motor response, <u>localizes pain</u>

R40.236- Coma scale, best motor response, <u>obeys commands</u>

R40.24- Glasgow coma scale, total score

AHA 15:2Q:p17 – Glasgow coma numeric scores

Note: Assign a code from subcategory R40.24, when only the total coma score is documented

The following appropriate 7th character is to be added to subcategory R40.24-:
- 0 - Unspecified time
- 1 - In the field [EMT or ambulance]
- 2 - At arrival to emergency department
- 3 - At hospital admission
- 4 - 24 hours or more after hospital admission

R40.241 Glasgow coma scale score 13-15

R40.242 Glasgow coma scale score 9-12

R40.243 Glasgow coma scale score 3-8

R40.244 Other coma, without documented Glasgow coma scale score, or with partial score reported

CC **R40.3** Persistent vegetative state — A condition characterized by a permanent state of wakefulness without awareness (an eyes-open unconsciousness).

R40.4 Transient alteration of awareness — A condition characterized by staring spells or temporary loss of awareness.

R41- Other symptoms and signs involving cognitive functions and awareness

Excludes 1: *dissociative [conversion] disorders (F44-)*
mild cognitive impairment, so stated (G31.84)

R41.0 Disorientation, unspecified
Confusion NOS
Delirium NOS

R41.1 Anterograde amnesia — The lack of memory for recent events after an amnesia episode.

R41.2 Retrograde amnesia — The lack of memory for events preceding the trauma or condition.

R41.3 Other amnesia
Amnesia NOS
Memory loss NOS

Excludes 1: *amnestic disorder due to known physiologic condition (F04)*
amnestic syndrome due to psychoactive substance use (F10-F19 with 5th character .6)
mild memory disturbance due to known physiological condition (F06.8)
transient global amnesia (G45.4)

CC **R41.4** Neurologic neglect syndrome — The condition of neurologically originating behavioral abnormalities that are usually the result of dysfunctional sensory stimuli recognition.
Asomatognosia
Hemi-akinesia
Hemi-inattention
Hemispatial neglect
Left-sided neglect
Sensory neglect
Visuospatial neglect

Excludes 1: *visuospatial deficit (R41.842)*

R41.8- Other symptoms and signs involving cognitive functions and awareness

R41.81 Age-related cognitive decline — [Age/15-124] — The condition of mental deterioration associated with old age, without mention of psychosis.
Senility NOS

R41.82 Altered mental status, unspecified
Change in mental status NOS

Excludes 1: *altered level of consciousness (R40.-)*
altered mental status due to known condition — code to condition
delirium NOS (R41.0)

R41.83 Borderline intellectual functioning — [Unacceptable PDX]
IQ level 71 to 84

Excludes 1: *intellectual disabilities (F70-F79)*

R41.84- Other specified cognitive deficit

Excludes 1: *cognitive deficits as sequelae of cerebrovascular disease (I69.01-, I69.11-, I69.21-, I69.31-, I69.81-, I69.91-)*

R41.840 Attention and concentration deficit
Excludes 1: *attention-deficit hyperactivity disorders (F90.-)*

R41.841 Cognitive communication deficit

R41.842 Visuospatial deficit

R41.843 Psychomotor deficit

R41.844 Frontal lobe and executive function deficit

R41.89 Other symptoms and signs involving cognitive functions and awareness
Anosognosia

R41.9 Unspecified symptoms and signs involving cognitive functions and awareness

R42 Dizziness and giddiness — The disturbed sense of balance and steadiness.
Light-headedness
Vertigo NOS

Excludes 1: *vertiginous syndromes (H81.-)*
vertigo from infrasound (T75.23)

R43- Disturbances of smell and taste

R43.0 Anosmia — The loss of the sense of smell.

R43.1 Parosmia — The abnormal deviation of the sense of smell.

R43.2 Parageusia — The abnormal deviation of the sense of taste, or a bad taste in the mouth.

R43.8 Other disturbances of smell and taste
Mixed disturbance of smell and taste

R43.9 Unspecified disturbances of smell and taste

R44- Other symptoms and signs involving general sensations and perceptions

Excludes 1: *alcoholic hallucinations (F1.5)*
hallucinations in drug psychosis (F11-F19 with .5)
hallucinations in mood disorders with psychotic symptoms (F30.2, F31.5, F32.3, F33.3)
hallucinations in schizophrenia, schizotypal and delusional disorders (F20-F29)

Excludes ❷: *disturbances of skin sensation (R20.-)*

CC **R44.0** Auditory hallucinations — A sensory perception disorder of sensing external sounds that does not result from an external stimulus.

R44.1 Visual hallucinations — A sensory perception disorder of sensing visual images that does not result from an external stimulus.

CC **R44.2** Other hallucinations

CC **R44.3** Hallucinations, unspecified

R44.8 Other symptoms and signs involving general sensations and perceptions

R44.9 Unspecified symptoms and signs involving general sensations and perceptions

---

Excludes 1: = NOT CODED HERE! (Do not code both)

Excludes ❷: = Not Included Here

R45- **Symptoms and signs involving emotional state**

R45.0 **Nervousness**
 Nervous tension

R45.1 **Restlessness and agitation**

R45.2 **Unhappiness**

R45.3 **Demoralization and apathy**
 Excludes 1: *anhedonia (R45.84)*

R45.4 **Irritability and anger**

R45.5 **Hostility**

R45.6 **Violent behavior**

R45.7 **State of emotional shock and stress, unspecified**

R45.8- **Other symptoms and signs involving emotional state**

 R45.81 **Low self-esteem**

 R45.82 **Worries**

 R45.83 **Excessive crying of child, adolescent or adult**
 Excludes 1: *excessive crying of infant (baby) R68.11*

 R45.84 **Anhedonia**

 R45.85- **Homicidal and suicidal ideations**
 Excludes 1: *suicide attempt (T14.91)*

  R45.850 **Homicidal ideations** — [Unacceptable PDX]

 cc **R45.851** **Suicidal ideations**

 R45.86 **Emotional lability**

 R45.87 **Impulsiveness**

 R45.89 **Other symptoms and signs involving emotional state**

R46- **Symptoms and signs involving appearance and behavior**
 Excludes 1: *appearance and behavior in schizophrenia, schizotypal and delusional disorders (F20-F29)*
 mental and behavioral disorders (F01-F99)

R46.0 **Very low level of personal hygiene**

R46.1 **Bizarre personal appearance**

R46.2 **Strange and inexplicable behavior**

R46.3 **Overactivity**

R46.4 **Slowness and poor responsiveness**
 Excludes 1: *stupor (R40.1)*

R46.5 **Suspiciousness and marked evasiveness**

R46.6 **Undue concern and preoccupation with stressful events**

R46.7 **Verbosity and circumstantial detail obscuring reason for contact**

R46.8- **Other symptoms and signs involving appearance and behavior**

 R46.81 **Obsessive-compulsive behavior** — [Unacceptable PDX]
 Excludes 1: *obsessive-compulsive disorder (F42.-)*

 R46.89 **Other symptoms and signs involving appearance and behavior** — [Unacceptable PDX]

Symptoms and signs involving speech and voice (R47-R49)

R47- **Speech disturbances, not elsewhere classified**
 Excludes 1: *autism (F84.0)*
 cluttering (F80.81)
 specific developmental disorders of speech and language (F80.-)
 stuttering (F80.81)

R47.0- **Dysphasia and aphasia**

 cc **R47.01** **Aphasia** — The absence or impairment of the ability to communicate through speech, writing, or signs.
 Excludes 1: *aphasia following cerebrovascular disease (I69. with final characters -20)*
 progressive isolated aphasia (G31.01)

 R47.02 **Dysphasia** — The lack of coordination to arrange words in their proper order.
 Excludes 1: *dysphasia following cerebrovascular disease (I69. with final characters -21)*

R47.1 **Dysarthria and anarthria** — Difficulty articulating words of speech.
 Excludes 1: *dysarthria following cerebrovascular disease (I69. with final characters -22)*

R47.8- **Other speech disturbances**
 Excludes 1: *dysarthria following cerebrovascular disease (I69. with final characters -28)*

 R47.81 **Slurred speech** — Slow and distorted speech.

R47.82 **Fluency disorder in conditions classified elsewhere** —
 [Not Allowed as PDX]
 Stuttering in conditions classified elsewhere
 Code first underlying disease or condition, such as:
 Parkinson's disease (G20)
 Excludes 1: *adult onset fluency disorder (F98.5)*
 childhood onset fluency disorder (F80.81)
 fluency disorder (stuttering) following cerebrovascular disease (I69. with final characters-23)

R47.89 **Other speech disturbances**

R47.9 **Unspecified speech disturbances**

R48- **Dyslexia and other symbolic dysfunctions, not elsewhere classified**
 Excludes 1: *specific developmental disorders of scholastic skills (F81-)*

R48.0 **Dyslexia and alexia** — The inability to read that is due to an organic disorder.

R48.1 **Agnosia** — The loss of comprehension of sensory stimuli.
 Astereognosia (astereognosis)
 Autotopagnosia
 Excludes 1: *visual object agnosia (R48.3)*

R48.2 **Apraxia** — The inability to perform voluntary movements without any organic cause.
 Excludes 1: *apraxia following cerebrovascular disease (I69. with final characters -90)*

R48.3 **Visual agnosia** — The inability to interpret images that are seen.
 Prosopagnosia — The impairment of the ability to recognize familiar faces.
 Simultanagnosia (asimultagnosia) — The inability to recognize two or more objects at the same time.

R48.8 **Other symbolic dysfunctions**
 Acalculia — The inability to perform simple arithmetical calculations.
 Agraphia — The difficulty with writing.

R48.9 **Unspecified symbolic dysfunctions**

R49- **Voice and resonance disorders**
 Excludes 1: *psychogenic voice and resonance disorders (F44.4)*

R49.0 **Dysphonia** — The impairment of speaking.
 Hoarseness — The rougher than usual quality of the voice.

R49.1 **Aphonia** — The loss of the ability to produce sounds.
 Loss of voice

R49.2- **Hypernasality and hyponasality**

 R49.21 **Hypernasality** — The Increased nasal resonance of the voice.

 R49.22 **Hyponasality** — The decreased nasal resonance of the voice.

R49.8 **Other voice and resonance disorders**

R49.9 **Unspecified voice and resonance disorder**
 Change in voice NOS
 Resonance disorder NOS

General symptoms and signs (R50-R69)

R50- **Fever of other and unknown origin** — The abnormal elevation of the body's temperature.
 Excludes 1: *chills without fever (R68.83)*
 febrile convulsions (R56.0-)
 fever of unknown origin during labor (O75.2)
 fever of unknown origin in newborn (P81.9)
 hypothermia due to illness (R68.0)
 malignant hyperthermia due to anesthesia (T88.3)
 puerperal pyrexia NOS (O86.4)

R50.2 **Drug-induced fever**
 Use additional code for adverse effect, if applicable, to identify drug (T36-T50 with fifth or sixth character 5)
 Excludes 1: *postvaccination (postimmunization) fever (R50.83)*

R50.8- **Other specified fever**

 R50.81 **Fever presenting with conditions classified elsewhere** —
 [Not Allowed as PDX]
 Code first underlying condition when associated fever is present, such as with:
 Leukemia (C91-C95)
 Neutropenia (D70-)
 Sickle-cell disease (D57-)

 R50.82 **Postprocedural fever** — A form that is associated/due to a procedure.
 Excludes 1: *postprocedural infection (T81.4-)*
 posttransfusion fever (R50.84)
 postvaccination (postimmunization) fever (R50.83)

R 4 5 - R 5 0

R50.83 Postvaccination fever — A form that is associated/due to a vaccination.
Postimmunization fever

R50.84 Febrile nonhemolytic transfusion reaction — A form that is associated/due to a transfusion, but not due to hemolysis.
FNHTR
Posttransfusion fever

R50.9 Fever, unspecified
Fever NOS
Fever of unknown origin [FUO]
Fever with chills
Fever with rigors
Hyperpyrexia NOS
Persistent fever
Pyrexia NOS

R51 Headache
Facial pain NOS
Excludes 1: *atypical face pain (G50.1)*
migraine and other headache syndromes (G43-G44)
trigeminal neuralgia (G50.0)

R52 Pain, unspecified
Acute pain NOS
Generalized pain NOS
Pain NOS
Excludes 1: *acute and chronic pain, not elsewhere classified (G89-)*
localized pain, unspecified type — code to pain by site, such as:
abdomen pain (R10-)
back pain (M54.9)
breast pain (N64.4)
chest pain (R07.1-R07.9)
ear pain (H92.0-)
eye pain (H57.1)
headache (R51)
joint pain (M25.5-)
limb pain (M79.6-)
lumbar region pain (M54.5)
pelvic and perineal pain (R10.2)
shoulder pain (M25.51-)
spine pain (M54-)
throat pain (R07.0)
tongue pain (K14.6)
tooth pain (K08.8)
pain disorders exclusively related to psychological factors (F45.41)
renal colic (N23)

R53- Malaise and fatigue — MALAISE – The vague feeling of bodily discomfort. FATIGUE – The state of decreased bodily efficiency usually resulting from prolonged or excessive exertion.

R53.0 Neoplastic (malignant) related fatigue
Code first associated neoplasm

R53.1 Weakness
Asthenia NOS
Excludes 1: *age-related weakness (R54)*
muscle weakness (M62.8-)
sarcopenia (M62.84)
senile asthenia (R54)

MCC **R53.2 Functional quadriplegia** — The condition of loss or impairment of function of the limbs that is not due to a neurological or psychological condition.
Complete immobility due to severe physical disability or frailty
Excludes 1: *frailty NOS (R54)*
hysterical paralysis (F44.4)
immobility syndrome (M62.3)
neurologic quadriplegia (G82.5-)
quadriplegia (G82.50)

R53.8- Other malaise and fatigue
Excludes 1: *combat exhaustion and fatigue (F43.0)*
congenital debility (P96.9)
exhaustion and fatigue due to depressive episode (F32.-)
exhaustion and fatigue due to excessive exertion (T73.3)
exhaustion and fatigue due to exposure (T73.2)
exhaustion and fatigue due to heat (T67.-)
exhaustion and fatigue due to pregnancy (O26.8-)
exhaustion and fatigue due to recurrent depressive episode (F33)
exhaustion and fatigue due to senile debility (R54)

R53.81 Other malaise
Chronic debility
Debility NOS
General physical deterioration
Malaise NOS
Nervous debility
Excludes 1: *age-related physical debility (R54)*

R53.82 Chronic fatigue, unspecified
Chronic fatigue syndrome NOS — The abnormal condition of persistent, debilitating fatigue characterized by decreased physical activity, muscle weakness, headaches and depression.
Excludes 1: *postviral fatigue syndrome (G93.3)*

R53.83 Other fatigue
Fatigue NOS
Lack of energy
Lethargy
Tiredness

R54 Age-related physical debility — [Age/15-124]
Frailty
Old age
Senescence
Senile asthenia
Senile debility
Excludes 1: *age-related cognitive decline (R41.81)*
sarcopenia (M62.84)
senile psychosis (F03)
senility NOS (R41.81)

R55 Syncope and collapse — SYNCOPE – A brief lapse of consciousness caused by a temporary lack of arterial oxygen to the brain. COLLAPSE – The state of prostration and weakness due to decreased circulation.
Blackout — A form of syncope that is accompanied by failure of vision.
Fainting
Vasovagal attack — A form of syncope associated with abrupt emotional stress.
Excludes 1: *cardiogenic shock (R57.0)*
carotid sinus syncope (G90.01)
heat syncope (T67.1)
neurocirculatory asthenia (F45.8)
neurogenic orthostatic hypotension (G90.3)
orthostatic hypotension (I95.1)
postprocedural shock (T81.1-)
psychogenic syncope (F48.8)
shock NOS (R57.9)
shock complicating or following abortion or ectopic or molar pregnancy (O00-O07, O08.3)
shock complicating or following labor and delivery (O75.1)
Stokes-Adams attack (I45.9)
unconsciousness NOS (R40.2-)

R56- Convulsions, <u>not elsewhere classified</u> — A sudden, violent contraction of the voluntary muscle groups.
Excludes 1: *dissociative convulsions and seizures (F44.5)*
epileptic convulsions and seizures (G40.-)
newborn convulsions and seizures (P90)

R56.0- Febrile convulsions

CC **R56.00 Simple febrile convulsions** — A form brought on by a high body temperature.
Febrile convulsion NOS
Febrile seizure NOS

CC **R56.01 Complex febrile convulsions** — Fever-associated seizures that are prolonged (usually more than 15 minutes) or reoccur with 24 hours, and usually focus on one part of the body.
Atypical febrile seizure
Complex febrile seizure
Complicated febrile seizure
Excludes 1: *status epilepticus (G40.901)*

CC **R56.1 Post traumatic seizures**
Excludes 1: *post traumatic epilepsy (G40.-)*

R50 - R56

Excludes 1: = NOT CODED HERE! (Do not code both)

Excludes ❷: = Not Included Here

R56.9 Unspecified convulsions
Convulsion disorder
Fit NOS
Recurrent convulsions
Seizure(s) (convulsive) NOS

R57- Shock, not elsewhere classified
Excludes 1: *anaphylactic reaction or shock due to adverse food reaction (T78.0-)*
anaphylactic shock due to adverse effect of correct drug or medicament properly administered (T88.6)
anaphylactic shock due to serum (T80.5-)
anaphylactic shock NOS (T78.2)
anesthetic shock (T88.3)
electric shock (T75.4)
obstetric shock (O75.1)
postprocedural shock (T81.1-)
psychic shock (F43.0)
septic shock (R65.21)
shock complicating or following ectopic or molar pregnancy (O00-O07, O08.3)
shock due to lightning (T75.01)
traumatic shock (T79.4)
toxic shock syndrome (A48.3)

MCC **R57.0 Cardiogenic shock** — The failure of peripheral circulation that is due to a decreased cardiac output.

MCC **R57.1 Hypovolemic shock** — The failure of peripheral circulation that is due to a decreased blood volume.

MCC **R57.8 Other shock**

CC **R57.9 Shock, unspecified**
Failure of peripheral circulation NOS

R58 Hemorrhage, not elsewhere classified
Hemorrhage NOS
Excludes 1: *hemorrhage included with underlying conditions, such as:*
acute duodenal ulcer with hemorrhage (K26.0)
acute gastritis with bleeding (K29.01)
ulcerative enterocolitis with rectal bleeding (K51.01)

R59- Enlarged lymph nodes
Includes: swollen glands
Excludes 1: *lymphadenitis NOS (I88.9)*
acute lymphadenitis (L04.-)
chronic lymphadenitis (I88.1)
mesenteric (acute) (chronic) lymphadenitis (I88.0)

R59.0 Localized enlarged lymph nodes

R59.1 Generalized enlarged lymph nodes
Lymphadenopathy NOS

R59.9 Enlarged lymph nodes, unspecified

R60- Edema, not elsewhere classified — The accumulation of fluid in the intercellular spaces.
Excludes 1: *angioneurotic edema (T78.3)*
ascites (R18-)
cerebral edema (G93.6)
cerebral edema due to birth injury (P11.0)
edema of larynx (J38.4)
edema of nasopharynx (J39.2)
edema of pharynx (J39.2)
gestational edema (O12.0-)
hereditary edema (Q82.0)
hydrops fetalis NOS (P83.2)
hydrothorax (J94.8)
newborn edema (P83.3)
nutritional edema (E40-E46)
pulmonary edema (J81-)

R60.0 Localized edema

R60.1 Generalized edema

R60.9 Edema, unspecified
Fluid retention NOS

R61 Generalized hyperhidrosis — Excessive sweating occurring over the entire body.
Excessive sweating
Night sweats
Secondary hyperhidrosis
Code first, if applicable, menopausal and female climacteric states (N95.1)
Excludes 1: *focal (primary) (secondary) hyperhidrosis (L74.5-)*
Frey's syndrome (L74.52)
localized (primary) (secondary) hyperhidrosis (L74.5-)

R62- Lack of expected normal physiological development in childhood and adults
Excludes 1: *delayed puberty (E30.0)*
gonadal dysgenesis (Q99.1)
hypopituitarism (E23.0)

R62.0 Delayed milestone in childhood — [Age/0-17]
Delayed attainment of expected physiological developmental stage
Late talker
Late walker

R62.5- Other and unspecified lack of expected normal physiological development in childhood — The abnormal condition in children that fail to meet the standardized growth and developmental chart progress.
Excludes 1: *HIV disease resulting in failure to thrive (B20)*
physical retardation due to malnutrition (E45)

R62.50 Unspecified lack of expected normal physiological development in childhood
Infantilism NOS

R62.51 Failure to thrive (child) — [Age/0-17] – A form in which a child loses weight or fails to gain weight.
Failure to gain weight
Excludes 1: *failure to thrive in child under 28 days old (P92.6)*

R62.52 Short stature (child) — A form in which a child has a slower than normal rate maturation of bone/height for his/her age.
Lack of growth
Physical retardation
Short stature NOS
Excludes 1: *short stature due to endocrine disorder (E34.3)*

R62.59 Other lack of expected normal physiological development in childhood

R62.7 Adult failure to thrive — [Age/15-124] – The abnormal condition of an adult patient whose health status is deteriorating or not improving.

R63- Symptoms and signs concerning food and fluid intake
Excludes 1: *bulimia NOS (F50.2)*
eating disorders of nonorganic origin (F50.-)
malnutrition (E40-E46)

R63.0 Anorexia — The lack or loss of appetite for food.
Loss of appetite
Excludes 1: *anorexia nervosa (F50.0-)*
loss of appetite of nonorganic origin (F50.89)

R63.1 Polydipsia
Excessive thirst

R63.2 Polyphagia
Excessive eating
Hyperalimentation NOS

R63.3 Feeding difficulties
Feeding problem (elderly) (infant) NOS
Excludes 1: *feeding problems of newborn (P92.-)*
infant feeding disorder of nonorganic origin (F98.2-)

R63.4 Abnormal weight loss — The relatively recent loss of a patient's usual weight.

R63.5 Abnormal weight gain — The relatively recent increase in a patient's usual weight.
Excludes 1: *excessive weight gain in pregnancy (O26.0-)*
obesity (E66.-)

R63.6 Underweight — The condition of weighing less than a person's standard weight for his/her height.
Use additional code to identify body mass index (BMI), if known (Z68.-)
Excludes 1: *abnormal weight loss (R63.4)*
anorexia nervosa (F50.0-)
malnutrition (E40-E46)

R63.8 Other symptoms and signs concerning food and fluid intake

R64 Cachexia — The state of general ill health and malnutrition.
CC Wasting syndrome
Code first underlying condition, if known
Excludes 1: *abnormal weight loss (R63.4)*
nutritional marasmus (E41)

R
5
6
I
R
6
4

R65- **Symptoms and signs specifically associated with systemic inflammation and infection**
AHA 14:3Q:p4 – SIRS secondary to pneumonia

R65.1- **Systemic inflammatory response syndrome (SIRS) of non-infectious origin**
Code first underlying condition, such as:
Heatstroke (T67.0)
Injury and trauma (S00-T88)
Excludes 1: *sepsis — code to infection*
severe sepsis (R65.2)

CC **R65.10** **Systemic inflammatory response syndrome (SIRS) of non-infectious origin without acute organ dysfunction**
Systemic inflammatory response syndrome (SIRS) NOS

MCC **R65.11** **Systemic inflammatory response syndrome (SIRS) of non-infectious origin with acute organ dysfunction**
Use additional code to identify specific acute organ dysfunction, such as:
Acute kidney failure (N17.-)
Acute respiratory failure (J96.0-)
Critical illness myopathy (G72.81)
Critical illness polyneuropathy (G62.81)
Disseminated intravascular coagulopathy [DIC] (D65)
Encephalopathy (metabolic) (septic) (G93.41)
Hepatic failure (K72.0-)

R65.2- **Severe sepsis**
Infection with associated acute organ dysfunction
Sepsis with acute organ dysfunction
Sepsis with multiple organ dysfunction
Systemic inflammatory response syndrome due to infectious process with acute organ dysfunction
Code first underlying infection, such as:
Infection following a procedure (T81.4-)
Infections following infusion, transfusion and therapeutic injection (T80.2-)
Puerperal sepsis (O85)
Sepsis following complete or unspecified spontaneous abortion (O03.87)
Sepsis following ectopic and molar pregnancy (O08.82)
Sepsis following incomplete spontaneous abortion (O03.37)
Sepsis following (induced) termination of pregnancy (O04.87)
Sepsis NOS (A41.9)
Use additional code to identify specific acute organ dysfunction, such as:
Acute kidney failure (N17.-)
Acute respiratory failure (J96.0-)
Critical illness myopathy (G72.81)
Critical illness polyneuropathy (G62.81)
Disseminated intravascular coagulopathy [DIC] (D65)
Encephalopathy (metabolic) (septic) (G93.41)
Hepatic failure (K72.0-)

MCC **R65.20** **Severe sepsis without septic shock**
Severe sepsis NOS

MCC **R65.21** **Severe sepsis with septic shock** — Sepsis with sepsis-induced hypotension despite fluid resuscitation and inadequate tissue perfusion (failure of peripheral circulation). Septic shock is the final stage in the SIRS-sepsis-severe sepsis-septic shock continuum.

R68- **Other general symptoms and signs**

R68.0 **Hypothermia, not associated with low environmental temperature**
Excludes 1: *hypothermia NOS (accidental) (T68)*
hypothermia due to anesthesia (T88.51)
hypothermia due to low environmental temperature (T68)
newborn hypothermia (P80.-)

R68.1- **Nonspecific symptoms peculiar to infancy**
Excludes 1: *colic, infantile (R10.83)*
neonatal cerebral irritability (P91.3)
teething syndrome (K00.7)

R68.11 **Excessive crying of infant (baby)** — [Age/0-17]
Excludes 1: *excessive crying of child, adolescent, or adult (R45.83)*

R68.12 **Fussy infant (baby)** — [Age/0-17]
Irritable infant

R68.13 **Apparent life threatening event in infant (ALTE)** — [Age/0-17] — A condition that is frightening to the observer that is characterized by various symptoms including cyanosis, apnea, color change, muscle tone change, limb jerking, and choking that is not due to an identifiable diagnosis.
Apparent life threatening event in newborn
Code first confirmed diagnosis, if known
Use additional code(s) for associated signs and symptoms if no confirmed diagnosis established, or if signs and symptoms are not associated routinely with confirmed diagnosis, or provide additional information for cause of ALTE

R68.19 **Other nonspecific symptoms peculiar to infancy** — [Age/0-17]

R68.2 **Dry mouth, unspecified**
Excludes 1: *dry mouth due to dehydration (E86.0)*
dry mouth due to sicca syndrome [Sjögren] (M35.0-)
salivary gland hyposecretion (K11.7)

R68.3 **Clubbing of fingers** — The distortional enlargement of the fingers.
Clubbing of nails
Excludes 1: *congenital clubfinger (Q68.1)*

R68.8- **Other general symptoms and signs**

R68.81 **Early satiety**

R68.82 **Decreased libido** — [Age/15-124]
Decreased sexual desire

R68.83 **Chills (without fever)**
Chills NOS
Excludes 1: *chills with fever (R50.9)*

R68.84 **Jaw pain**
Mandibular pain
Maxilla pain
Excludes 1: *temporomandibular joint arthralgia (M26.62-)*

R68.89 **Other general symptoms and signs**

R69 **Illness, unspecified**
Unknown and unspecified cases of morbidity

Abnormal findings on examination of blood, without diagnosis (R70-R79)

Excludes ❷: *abnormal findings on antenatal screening of mother (O28.-)*
abnormalities of lipids (E78.-)
abnormalities of platelets and thrombocytes (D69.-)
abnormalities of white blood cells classified elsewhere (D70-D72)
coagulation hemorrhagic disorders (D65-D68)
diagnostic abnormal findings classified elsewhere — see Alphabetical Index
hemorrhagic and hematological disorders of newborn (P50-P61)

R70- **Elevated erythrocyte sedimentation rate and abnormality of plasma viscosity**

R70.0 **Elevated erythrocyte sedimentation rate**

R70.1 **Abnormal plasma viscosity**

R71- **Abnormality of red blood cells**
Excludes 1: *anemias (D50-D64)*
anemia of premature infant (P61.2)
benign (familial) polycythemia (D75.0)
congenital anemias (P61.2-P61.4)
newborn anemia due to isoimmunization (P55.-)
polycythemia neonatorum (P61.1)
polycythemia NOS (D75.1)
polycythemia vera (D45)
secondary polycythemia (D75.1)

CC **R71.0** **Precipitous drop in hematocrit** — A relatively recent, significant, comparative lowering of a patient's hematocrit.
Drop (precipitous) in hemoglobin
Drop in hematocrit

R71.8 **Other abnormality of red blood cells**
Abnormal red-cell morphology NOS
Abnormal red-cell volume NOS
Anisocytosis — The condition of an excessive variation in the size of erythrocytes in the blood.
Poikilocytosis — The condition of a variation in size of red corpuscles in the blood.

R73- Elevated blood glucose level
> *Excludes 1:*   *diabetes mellitus (E08-E13)*
> *diabetes mellitus in pregnancy, childbirth and the puerperium (O24.-)*
> *neonatal disorders (P70.0-P70.2)*
> *postsurgical hypoinsulinemia (E89.1)*

R73.0- Abnormal glucose
> *Excludes 1:*   *abnormal glucose in pregnancy (O99.81-)*
> *diabetes mellitus (E08-E13)*
> *dysmetabolic syndrome X (E88.81)*
> *gestational diabetes (O24.4-)*
> *glycosuria (R81)*
> *hypoglycemia (E16.2)*

R73.01 Impaired fasting glucose
Elevated fasting glucose

R73.02 Impaired glucose tolerance (oral)
Elevated glucose tolerance

R73.03 Prediabetes
Latent diabetes

R73.09 Other abnormal glucose
Abnormal glucose NOS
Abnormal non-fasting glucose tolerance

R73.9 Hyperglycemia, unspecified

R74- Abnormal serum enzyme levels

R74.0 Nonspecific elevation of levels of transaminase and lactic acid dehydrogenase [LDH]

R74.8 Abnormal levels of other serum enzymes
Abnormal level of acid phosphatase
Abnormal level of alkaline phosphatase
Abnormal level of amylase
Abnormal level of lipase [triacylglycerol lipase]

R74.9 Abnormal serum enzyme level, unspecified

R75 Inconclusive laboratory evidence of human immunodeficiency virus [HIV]
Nonconclusive HIV-test finding in infants
> *Excludes 1:*   *asymptomatic human immunodeficiency virus [HIV] infection status (Z21)*
> *human immunodeficiency virus [HIV] disease (B20)*

R76- Other abnormal immunological findings in serum

R76.0 Raised antibody titer
> *Excludes 1:*   *isoimmunization in pregnancy (O36.0-O36.1)*
> *isoimmunization affecting newborn (P55-)*

R76.1- Nonspecific reaction to test for tuberculosis

R76.11 Nonspecific reaction to tuberculin skin test without active tuberculosis
Abnormal result of Mantoux test
PPD positive
Tuberculin (skin test) positive
Tuberculin (skin test) reactor
> *Excludes 1:*   *nonspecific reaction to cell mediated immunity measurement of gamma interferon antigen response without active tuberculosis (R76.12)*

R76.12 Nonspecific reaction to cell mediated immunity measurement of gamma interferon antigen response without active tuberculosis
Nonspecific reaction to QuantiFERON-TB test (QFT) without active tuberculosis
> *Excludes 1:*   *nonspecific reaction to tuberculin skin test without active tuberculosis (R76.11)*
> *positive tuberculin skin test (R76.11)*

R76.8 Other specified abnormal immunological findings in serum
Raised level of immunoglobulins NOS

R76.9 Abnormal immunological finding in serum, unspecified

R77- Other abnormalities of plasma proteins
> *Excludes 1:*   *disorders of plasma-protein metabolism (E88.0)*

R77.0 Abnormality of albumin

R77.1 Abnormality of globulin
Hyperglobulinemia NOS

R77.2 Abnormality of alphafetoprotein

R77.8 Other specified abnormalities of plasma proteins

R77.9 Abnormality of plasma protein, unspecified

R78- Findings of drugs and other substances, not normally found in blood
Use additional code to identify the any retained foreign body, if applicable (Z18.-)
> *Excludes 1:*   *mental or behavioral disorders due to psychoactive substance use (F10-F19)*

R78.0 Finding of alcohol in blood
Use additional external cause code (Y90.-), for detail regarding alcohol level

R78.1 Finding of opiate drug in blood

R78.2 Finding of cocaine in blood

R78.3 Finding of hallucinogen in blood

R78.4 Finding of other drugs of addictive potential in blood

R78.5 Finding of other psychotropic drug in blood

R78.6 Finding of steroid agent in blood

R78.7- Finding of abnormal level of heavy metals in blood

R78.71 Abnormal lead level in blood
> *Excludes 1:*   *lead poisoning (T56.0-)*

R78.79 Finding of abnormal level of heavy metals in blood

R78.8- Finding of other specified substances, not normally found in blood

CC **R78.81 Bacteremia**
> *Excludes 1:*   *sepsis-code to specified infection*

R78.89 Finding of other specified substances, not normally found in blood
Finding of abnormal level of lithium in blood

R78.9 Finding of unspecified substance, not normally found in blood

R79- Other abnormal findings of blood chemistry
Use additional code to identify any retained foreign body, if applicable (Z18-)
> *Excludes 1:*   *abnormality of fluid, electrolyte or acid-base balance (E86-E87)*
> *asymptomatic hyperuricemia (E79.0)*
> *hyperglycemia NOS (R73.9)*
> *hypoglycemia NOS (E16.2)*
> *neonatal hypoglycemia (P70.3-P70.4)*
> *specific findings indicating disorder of amino-acid metabolism (E70-E72)*
> *specific findings indicating disorder of carbohydrate metabolism (E73-E74)*
> *specific findings indicating disorder of lipid metabolism (E75.-)*

R79.0 Abnormal level of blood mineral
Abnormal blood level of cobalt
Abnormal blood level of copper
Abnormal blood level of iron
Abnormal blood level of magnesium
Abnormal blood level of mineral NEC
Abnormal blood level of zinc
> *Excludes 1:*   *abnormal level of lithium (R78.89)*
> *disorders of mineral metabolism (E83.-)*
> *neonatal hypomagnesemia (P71.2)*
> *nutritional mineral deficiency (E58-E61)*

R79.1 Abnormal coagulation profile
Abnormal or prolonged bleeding time
Abnormal or prolonged coagulation time
Abnormal or prolonged partial thromboplastin time [PTT]
Abnormal or prolonged prothrombin time [PT]
> *Excludes 1:*   *coagulation defects (D68.-)*

R79.8- Other specified abnormal findings of blood chemistry

R79.81 Abnormal blood-gas level

R79.82 Elevated C-reactive protein (CRP)

R79.89 Other specified abnormal findings of blood chemistry

R79.9 Abnormal finding of blood chemistry, unspecified

R 7 3 - R 7 9

Excludes 1: = NOT CODED HERE! (Do not code both)   *Excludes ❷:* = Not Included Here

Abnormal findings on examination of urine, without diagnosis (R80-R82)

Excludes 1: abnormal findings on antenatal screening of mother (O28.-)
diagnostic abnormal findings classified elsewhere — see Alphabetical Index
specific findings indicating disorder of amino-acid metabolism (E70-E72)
specific findings indicating disorder of carbohydrate metabolism (E73-E74)

R80- **Proteinuria** — The presence of excess serum proteins in the urine.
Excludes 1: gestational proteinuria (O12.1-)

R80.0 **Isolated proteinuria**
Idiopathic proteinuria
Excludes 1: isolated proteinuria with specific morphological lesion (N06.-)

R80.1 **Persistent proteinuria, unspecified**

R80.2 **Orthostatic proteinuria, unspecified**
Postural proteinuria

R80.3 **Bence Jones proteinuria** — The presence of Bence-Jones protein in the urine.

R80.8 **Other proteinuria**

R80.9 **Proteinuria, unspecified**
Albuminuria NOS

R81 **Glycosuria** — The presence of glucose in the urine.
Excludes 1: renal glycosuria (E74.8)

R82- **Other and unspecified abnormal findings in urine**
Includes: Chromoabnormalities in urine
Use additional code to identify any retained foreign body, if applicable (Z18.-)
Excludes ❷: hematuria (R31.-)

cc R82.0 **Chyluria** — The presence of chyle in the urine.
Excludes 1: filarial chyluria (B74.-)

cc R82.1 **Myoglobinuria** — The presence of myoglobin in the urine.

R82.2 **Biliuria** — The presence of bile in the urine.

R82.3 **Hemoglobinuria** — The presence of hemoglobin in the urine.
Excludes 1: hemoglobinuria due to hemolysis from external causes NEC (D59.6)
hemoglobinuria due to paroxysmal nocturnal [Marchiafava-Micheli] (D59.5)

R82.4 **Acetonuria** — The presence of acetone in the urine.
Ketonuria — The presence of ketone bodies in the urine.

R82.5 **Elevated urine levels of drugs, medicaments and biological substances**
Elevated urine levels of catecholamines
Elevated urine levels of indoleacetic acid
Elevated urine levels of 17-ketosteroids
Elevated urine levels of steroids

R82.6 **Abnormal urine levels of substances chiefly nonmedicinal as to source**
Abnormal urine level of heavy metals

R82.7- **Abnormal findings on microbiological examination of urine**
Excludes 1: colonization status (Z22.-)

R82.71 **Bacteriuria**

R82.79 **Other abnormal findings on microbiological examination of urine**
Positive culture findings of urine

R82.8 **Abnormal findings on cytological and histological examination of urine**

R82.9- **Other and unspecified abnormal findings in urine**

R82.90 **Unspecified abnormal findings in urine**

R82.91 **Other chromoabnormalities of urine**
Chromoconversion (dipstick)
Idiopathic dipstick converts positive for blood with no cellular forms in sediment
Excludes 1: hemoglobinuria (R82.3)
myoglobinuria (R82.1)

R82.99 **Other abnormal findings in urine**
Cells and casts in urine
Crystalluria
Melanuria

Abnormal findings on examination of other body fluids, substances and tissues, without diagnosis (R83-R89)

Excludes 1: abnormal findings on antenatal screening of mother (O28.-)
diagnostic abnormal findings classified elsewhere — see Alphabetical Index
Excludes ❷: abnormal findings on examination of blood, without diagnosis (R70-R79)
abnormal findings on examination of urine, without diagnosis (R80-R82)
abnormal tumor markers (R97.-)

R83- **Abnormal findings in cerebrospinal fluid**

R83.0 **Abnormal level of enzymes in cerebrospinal fluid**

R83.1 **Abnormal level of hormones in cerebrospinal fluid**

R83.2 **Abnormal level of other drugs, medicaments and biological substances in cerebrospinal fluid**

R83.3 **Abnormal level of substances chiefly nonmedicinal as to source in cerebrospinal fluid**

R83.4 **Abnormal immunological findings in cerebrospinal fluid**

R83.5 **Abnormal microbiological findings in cerebrospinal fluid**
Positive culture findings in cerebrospinal fluid
Excludes 1: colonization status (Z22.-)

R83.6 **Abnormal cytological findings in cerebrospinal fluid**

R83.8 **Other abnormal findings in cerebrospinal fluid**
Abnormal chromosomal findings in cerebrospinal fluid

R83.9 **Unspecified abnormal finding in cerebrospinal fluid**

R84- **Abnormal findings in specimens from respiratory organs and thorax**
Includes: Abnormal findings in bronchial washings
Abnormal findings in nasal secretions
Abnormal findings in pleural fluid
Abnormal findings in sputum
Abnormal findings in throat scrapings
Excludes 1: blood-stained sputum (R04.2)

R84.0 **Abnormal level of enzymes in specimens from respiratory organs and thorax**

R84.1 **Abnormal level of hormones in specimens from respiratory organs and thorax**

R84.2 **Abnormal level of other drugs, medicaments and biological substances in specimens from respiratory organs and thorax**

R84.3 **Abnormal level of substances chiefly nonmedicinal as to source in specimens from respiratory organs and thorax**

R84.4 **Abnormal immunological findings in specimens from respiratory organs and thorax**

R84.5 **Abnormal microbiological findings in specimens from respiratory organs and thorax**
Positive culture findings in specimens from respiratory organs and thorax
Excludes 1: colonization status (Z22.-)

R84.6 **Abnormal cytological findings in specimens from respiratory organs and thorax**

R84.7 **Abnormal histological findings in specimens from respiratory organs and thorax**

R84.8 **Other abnormal findings in specimens from respiratory organs and thorax**
Abnormal chromosomal findings in specimens from respiratory organs and thorax

R84.9 **Unspecified abnormal finding in specimens from respiratory organs and thorax**

R85- **Abnormal findings in specimens from digestive organs and abdominal cavity**
Includes: Abnormal findings in peritoneal fluid
Abnormal findings in saliva
Excludes 1: cloudy peritoneal dialysis effluent (R88.0)
fecal abnormalities (R19.5)

R85.0 **Abnormal level of enzymes in specimens from digestive organs and abdominal cavity**

R85.1 **Abnormal level of hormones in specimens from digestive organs and abdominal cavity**

R85.2 **Abnormal level of other drugs, medicaments and biological substances in specimens from digestive organs and abdominal cavity**

R85.3 Abnormal level of substances chiefly nonmedicinal as to source in specimens from digestive organs and abdominal cavity

R85.4 Abnormal immunological findings in specimens from digestive organs and abdominal cavity

R85.5 Abnormal microbiological findings in specimens from digestive organs and abdominal cavity
   Positive culture findings in specimens from digestive organs and abdominal cavity
   Excludes 1:   colonization status (Z22.-)

R85.6- Abnormal cytological findings in specimens from digestive organs and abdominal cavity

   R85.61- Abnormal cytologic smear of anus
      Excludes 1:   abnormal cytological findings in specimens from other digestive organs and abdominal cavity (R85.69)
      anal intraepithelial neoplasia I [AIN I] (K62.82)
      anal intraepithelial neoplasia II [AIN II] (K62.82)
      anal intraepithelial neoplasia III [AIN III] (D01.3)
      carcinoma in situ of anus (histologically confirmed) (D01.3)
      dysplasia (mild) (moderate) of anus (histologically confirmed) (K62.82)
      severe dysplasia of anus (histologically confirmed) (D01.3)
      Excludes ❷: anal high risk human papillomavirus (HPV) DNA test positive (R85.81)
      anal low risk human papillomavirus (HPV) DNA test positive (R85.82)

      R85.610 Atypical squamous cells of undetermined significance on cytologic smear of anus (ASC-US)

      R85.611 Atypical squamous cells cannot exclude high grade squamous intraepithelial lesion on cytologic smear of anus (ASC-H)

      R85.612 Low grade squamous intraepithelial lesion on cytologic smear of anus (LGSIL)

      R85.613 High grade squamous intraepithelial lesion on cytologic smear of anus (HGSIL)

      R85.614 Cytologic evidence of malignancy on smear of anus

      R85.615 Unsatisfactory cytologic smear of anus
         Inadequate sample of cytologic smear of anus

      R85.616 Satisfactory anal smear but lacking transformation zone

      R85.618 Other abnormal cytological findings on specimens from anus

      R85.619 Unspecified abnormal cytological findings in specimens from anus
         Abnormal anal cytology NOS
         Atypical glandular cells of anus NOS

   R85.69 Abnormal cytological findings in specimens from other digestive organs and abdominal cavity

R85.7 Abnormal histological findings in specimens from digestive organs and abdominal cavity

R85.8- Other abnormal findings in specimens from digestive organs and abdominal cavity

   R85.81 Anal high risk human papillomavirus (HPV) DNA test positive
      Excludes 1:   anogenital warts due to human papillomavirus (HPV) (A63.0)
      condyloma acuminatum (A63.0)

   R85.82 Anal low risk human papillomavirus (HPV) DNA test positive
      Use additional code for associated human papillomavirus (B97.7)

   R85.89 Other abnormal findings in specimens from digestive organs and abdominal cavity
      Abnormal chromosomal findings in specimens from digestive organs and abdominal cavity

R85.9 Unspecified abnormal finding in specimens from digestive organs and abdominal cavity

R86- Abnormal findings in specimens from male genital organs
   Includes: Abnormal findings in prostatic secretions
   Abnormal findings in semen, seminal fluid
   Abnormal spermatozoa
   Excludes 1:   azoospermia (N46.0-)
   oligospermia (N46.1-)

R86.0 Abnormal level of enzymes in specimens from male genital organs — [♂]

R86.1 Abnormal level of hormones in specimens from male genital organs — [♂]

R86.2 Abnormal level of other drugs, medicaments and biological substances in specimens from male genital organs — [♂]

R86.3 Abnormal level of substances chiefly nonmedicinal as to source in specimens from male genital organs — [♂]

R86.4 Abnormal immunological findings in specimens from male genital organs — [♂]

R86.5 Abnormal microbiological findings in specimens from male genital organs — [♂]
   Positive culture findings in specimens from male genital organs
   Excludes 1:   colonization status (Z22.-)

R86.6 Abnormal cytological findings in specimens from male genital organs — [♂]

R86.7 Abnormal histological findings in specimens from male genital organs — [♂]

R86.8 Other abnormal findings in specimens from male genital organs — [♂]
   Abnormal chromosomal findings in specimens from male genital organs

R86.9 Unspecified abnormal finding in specimens from male genital organs — [♂]

R87- Abnormal findings in specimens from female genital organs
   Includes: Abnormal findings in secretion and smears from cervix uteri
   Abnormal findings in secretion and smears from vagina
   Abnormal findings in secretion and smears from vulva

R87.0 Abnormal level of enzymes in specimens from female genital organs — [♀]

R87.1 Abnormal level of hormones in specimens from female genital organs — [♀]

R87.2 Abnormal level of other drugs, medicaments and biological substances in specimens from female genital organs — [♀]

R87.3 Abnormal level of substances chiefly nonmedicinal as to source in specimens from female genital organs — [♀]

R87.4 Abnormal immunological findings in specimens from female genital organs — [♀]

R87.5 Abnormal microbiological findings in specimens from female genital organs — [♀]
   Positive culture findings in specimens from female genital organs
   Excludes 1:   colonization status (Z22.-)

R87.6- Abnormal cytological findings in specimens from female genital organs

   R87.61- Abnormal cytological findings in specimens from cervix uteri
      Excludes 1:   abnormal cytological findings in specimens from other female genital organs (R87.69)
      abnormal cytological findings in specimens from vagina (R87.62-)
      carcinoma in situ of cervix uteri (histologically confirmed) (D06.-)
      cervical intraepithelial neoplasia I [CIN I] (N87.0)
      cervical intraepithelial neoplasia II [CIN II] (N87.1)
      cervical intraepithelial neoplasia III [CIN III] (D06.-)
      dysplasia (mild) (moderate) of cervix uteri (histologically confirmed) (N87.-)
      severe dysplasia of cervix uteri (histologically confirmed) (D06.-)
      Excludes ❷: cervical high risk human papillomavirus (HPV) DNA test positive (R87.810)
      cervical low risk human papillomavirus (HPV) DNA test positive (R87.820)

      R87.610 Atypical squamous cells of undetermined significance on cytologic smear of cervix (ASC-US) — [♀]

R87.611 Atypical squamous cells cannot exclude high grade squamous intraepithelial lesion on cytologic smear of cervix (ASC-H) — [♀]

R87.612 Low grade squamous intraepithelial lesion on cytologic smear of cervix (LGSIL) — [♀]

R87.613 High grade squamous intraepithelial lesion on cytologic smear of cervix (HGSIL) — [♀]

R87.614 Cytologic evidence of malignancy on smear of cervix — [♀]

R87.615 Unsatisfactory cytologic smear of cervix — [♀]
　　Inadequate sample of cytologic smear of cervix

R87.616 Satisfactory cervical smear but lacking transformation zone — [♀]

R87.618 Other abnormal cytological findings on specimens from cervix uteri — [♀]

R87.619 Unspecified abnormal cytological findings in specimens from cervix uteri — [♀]
　　Abnormal cervical cytology NOS
　　Abnormal Papanicolaou smear of cervix NOS
　　Abnormal thin preparation smear of cervix NOS
　　Atypical endocervical cells of cervix NOS
　　Atypical endometrial cells of cervix NOS
　　Atypical glandular cells of cervix NOS

R87.62- Abnormal cytological findings in specimens from vagina
　Use additional code to identify acquired absence of uterus and cervix, if applicable (Z90.71-)
　Excludes 1: 　*abnormal cytological findings in specimens from cervix uteri (R87.61-)*
　　　abnormal cytological findings in specimens from other female genital organs (R87.69)
　　　carcinoma in situ of vagina (histologically confirmed) (D07.2)
　　　dysplasia (mild) (moderate) of vagina (histologically confirmed) (N89.-)
　　　severe dysplasia of vagina (histologically confirmed) (D07.2)
　　　vaginal intraepithelial neoplasia I [VAIN I] (N89.0)
　　　vaginal intraepithelial neoplasia II [VAIN II] (N89.1)
　　　vaginal intraepithelial neoplasia III [VAIN III] (D07.2)
　Excludes ❷: 　*vaginal high risk human papillomavirus (HPV) DNA test positive (R87.811)*
　　　vaginal low risk human papillomavirus (HPV) DNA test positive (R87.821)

R87.620 Atypical squamous cells of undetermined significance on cytologic smear of vagina (ASC-US) — [♀]

R87.621 Atypical squamous cells cannot exclude high grade squamous intraepithelial lesion on cytologic smear of vagina (ASC-H) — [♀]

R87.622 Low grade squamous intraepithelial lesion on cytologic smear of vagina (LGSIL) — [♀]

R87.623 High grade squamous intraepithelial lesion on cytologic smear of vagina (HGSIL) — [♀]

R87.624 Cytologic evidence of malignancy on smear of vagina — [♀]

R87.625 Unsatisfactory cytologic smear of vagina — [♀]
　　Inadequate sample of cytologic smear of vagina

R87.628 Other abnormal cytological findings on specimens from vagina — [♀]

R87.629 Unspecified abnormal cytological findings in specimens from vagina — [♀]
　　Abnormal Papanicolaou smear of vagina NOS
　　Abnormal thin preparation smear of vagina NOS
　　Abnormal vaginal cytology NOS
　　Atypical endocervical cells of vagina NOS
　　Atypical endometrial cells of vagina NOS
　　Atypical glandular cells of vagina NOS

R87.69 Abnormal cytological findings in specimens from other female genital organs — [♀]
　　Abnormal cytological findings in specimens from female genital organs NOS
　Excludes 1: 　*dysplasia of vulva (histologically confirmed) (N90.0-N90.3)*

R87.7 Abnormal histological findings in specimens from female genital organs — [♀]
　Excludes 1: 　*carcinoma in situ (histologically confirmed) of female genital organs (D06-D07.3)*
　　　cervical intraepithelial neoplasia I [CIN I] (N87.0)
　　　cervical intraepithelial neoplasia II [CIN II] (N87.1)
　　　cervical intraepithelial neoplasia III [CIN III] (D06.-)
　　　dysplasia (mild) (moderate) of cervix uteri (histologically confirmed) (N87.-)
　　　dysplasia (mild) (moderate) of vagina (histologically confirmed) (N89.-)
　　　severe dysplasia of cervix uteri (histologically confirmed) (D06.-)
　　　severe dysplasia of vagina (histologically confirmed) (D07.2)
　　　vaginal intraepithelial neoplasia I [VAIN I] (N89.0)
　　　vaginal intraepithelial neoplasia II [VAIN II] (N89.1)
　　　vaginal intraepithelial neoplasia III [VAIN III] (D07.2)

R87.8- Other abnormal findings in specimens from female genital organs

　R87.81- High risk human papillomavirus (HPV) DNA test positive from female genital organs
　　Excludes 1: 　*anogenital warts due to human papillomavirus (HPV) (A63.0)*
　　　condyloma acuminatum (A63.0)

　　R87.810 Cervical high risk human papillomavirus (HPV) DNA test positive — [♀]

　　R87.811 Vaginal high risk human papillomavirus (HPV) DNA test positive — [♀]

　R87.82- Low risk human papillomavirus (HPV) DNA test positive from female genital organs
　　Use additional code for associated human papillomavirus (B97.7)

　　R87.820 Cervical low risk human papillomavirus (HPV) DNA test positive — [♀]

　　R87.821 Vaginal low risk human papillomavirus (HPV) DNA test positive — [♀]

　R87.89 Other abnormal findings in specimens from female genital organs — [♀]
　　Abnormal chromosomal findings in specimens from female genital organs

R87.9 Unspecified abnormal finding in specimens from female genital organs — [♀]

R88- Abnormal findings in other body fluids and substances

R88.0 Cloudy (hemodialysis) (peritoneal) dialysis effluent

R88.8 Abnormal findings in other body fluids and substances

R89- Abnormal findings in specimens from other organs, systems and tissues
　Includes: 　Abnormal findings in nipple discharge
　　Abnormal findings in synovial fluid
　　Abnormal findings in wound secretions

R89.0 Abnormal level of enzymes in specimens from other organs, systems and tissues

R89.1 Abnormal level of hormones in specimens from other organs, systems and tissues

R89.2 Abnormal level of other drugs, medicaments and biological substances in specimens from other organs, systems and tissues

R89.3 Abnormal level of substances chiefly nonmedicinal as to source in specimens from other organs, systems and tissues

R89.4 Abnormal immunological findings in specimens from other organs, systems and tissues

R89.5 Abnormal microbiological findings in specimens from other organs, systems and tissues
　　Positive culture findings in specimens from other organs, systems and tissues
　Excludes 1: 　colonization status (Z22.-)

R89.6 Abnormal cytological findings in specimens from other organs, systems and tissues

R89.7 Abnormal histological findings in specimens from other organs, systems and tissues

R87 - R89

R89.8   Other abnormal findings in specimens from other organs, systems and tissues
> Abnormal chromosomal findings in specimens from other organs, systems and tissues

R89.9   Unspecified abnormal finding in specimens from other organs, systems and tissues

Abnormal findings on diagnostic imaging and in function studies, without diagnosis (R90-R94)

Includes: Nonspecific abnormal findings on diagnostic imaging by computerized axial tomography [CAT scan]
Nonspecific abnormal findings on diagnostic imaging by magnetic resonance imaging [MRI] [NMR]
Nonspecific abnormal findings on diagnostic imaging by positron emission tomography [PET scan]
Nonspecific abnormal findings on diagnostic imaging by thermography
Nonspecific abnormal findings on diagnostic imaging by ultrasound [echogram]
Nonspecific abnormal findings on diagnostic imaging by X-ray examination

Excludes 1:   *abnormal findings on antenatal screening of mother (O28.-)*
diagnostic abnormal findings classified elsewhere — see Alphabetical Index

R90-   Abnormal findings on diagnostic imaging of central nervous system

R90.0   Intracranial space-occupying lesion found on diagnostic imaging of central nervous system

R90.8-   Other abnormal findings on diagnostic imaging of central nervous system

     R90.81   Abnormal echoencephalogram

     R90.82   White matter disease, unspecified

     R90.89   Other abnormal findings on diagnostic imaging of central nervous system
> Other cerebrovascular abnormality found on diagnostic imaging of central nervous system

R91-   Abnormal findings on diagnostic imaging of lung

R91.1   Solitary pulmonary nodule
> Coin lesion lung
> Solitary pulmonary nodule, subsegmental branch of the bronchial tree

R91.8   Other nonspecific abnormal finding of lung field
> Lung mass NOS found on diagnostic imaging of lung
> Pulmonary infiltrate NOS
> Shadow, lung

R92-   Abnormal and inconclusive findings on diagnostic imaging of breast

R92.0   Mammographic microcalcification found on diagnostic imaging of breast — The presence of tiny granule-like deposits of calcium within the breast tissue that is identified by mammography.
> *Excludes 2:*   *mammographic calcification (calculus) found on diagnostic imaging of breast (R92.1)*

R92.1   Mammographic calcification found on diagnostic imaging of breast — The presence of multiple calcium deposits within the breast tissue that is identified by mammography.
> Mammographic calculus found on diagnostic imaging of breast

R92.2   Inconclusive mammogram — A mammogram that has not found an abnormal condition, but requires further testing to rule out abnormal conditions.
> AHA 15:1Q:p24 – Dense breasts on mammogram
> Dense breasts NOS
> Inconclusive mammogram NEC
> Inconclusive mammography due to dense breasts
> Inconclusive mammography NEC

R92.8   Other abnormal and inconclusive findings on diagnostic imaging of breast

R93-   Abnormal findings on diagnostic imaging of other body structures

R93.0   Abnormal findings on diagnostic imaging of skull and head, not elsewhere classified
> *Excludes 1:*   *intracranial space-occupying lesion found on diagnostic imaging (R90.0)*

R93.1   Abnormal findings on diagnostic imaging of heart and coronary circulation
> Abnormal echocardiogram NOS
> Abnormal heart shadow

R93.2   Abnormal findings on diagnostic imaging of liver and biliary tract
> Nonvisualization of gallbladder

R93.3   Abnormal findings on diagnostic imaging of other parts of digestive tract

R93.4-   Abnormal findings on diagnostic imaging of urinary organs
> *Excludes 2:*   *hypertrophy of kidney (N28.81)*

     R93.41   Abnormal radiologic findings on diagnostic imaging of renal pelvis, ureter, or bladder
> Filling defect of bladder found on diagnostic imaging
> Filling defect of renal pelvis found on diagnostic imaging
> Filling defect of ureter found on diagnostic imaging

     R93.42-   Abnormal radiologic findings on diagnostic imaging of kidney

         R93.421   Abnormal radiologic findings on diagnostic imaging of right kidney

         R93.422   Abnormal radiologic findings on diagnostic imaging of left kidney

         R93.429   Abnormal radiologic findings on diagnostic imaging of unspecified kidney

     R93.49   Abnormal radiologic findings on diagnostic imaging of other urinary organs

R93.5   Abnormal findings on diagnostic imaging of other abdominal regions, including retroperitoneum

R93.6   Abnormal findings on diagnostic imaging of limbs
> *Excludes 2:*   *abnormal finding in skin and subcutaneous tissue (R93.8)*

R93.7   Abnormal findings on diagnostic imaging of other parts of musculoskeletal system
> *Excludes 2:*   *abnormal findings on diagnostic imaging of skull (R93.0)*

R93.8   Abnormal findings on diagnostic imaging of other specified body structures
> Abnormal finding by radioisotope localization of placenta
> Abnormal radiological finding in skin and subcutaneous tissue
> Mediastinal shift

R93.9   Diagnostic imaging inconclusive due to excess body fat of patient

R94-   Abnormal results of function studies
Includes: Abnormal results of radionuclide [radioisotope] uptake studies
Abnormal results of scintigraphy

R94.0-   Abnormal results of function studies of central nervous system

     R94.01   Abnormal electroencephalogram [EEG]

     R94.02   Abnormal brain scan

     R94.09   Abnormal results of other function studies of central nervous system

R94.1-   Abnormal results of function studies of peripheral nervous system and special senses

     R94.11-   Abnormal results of function studies of eye

         R94.110   Abnormal electro-oculogram [EOG]

         R94.111   Abnormal electroretinogram [ERG]
> Abnormal retinal function study

         R94.112   Abnormal visually evoked potential [VEP]

         R94.113   Abnormal oculomotor study

         R94.118   Abnormal results of other function studies of eye

     R94.12-   Abnormal results of function studies of ear and other special senses

         R94.120   Abnormal auditory function study

         R94.121   Abnormal vestibular function study

         R94.128   Abnormal results of other function studies of ear and other special senses

     R94.13-   Abnormal results of function studies of peripheral nervous system

         R94.130   Abnormal response to nerve stimulation, unspecified

         R94.131   Abnormal electromyogram [EMG]
> *Excludes 1:*   *electromyogram of eye (R94.113)*

         R94.138   Abnormal results of other function studies of peripheral nervous system

R94.2 **Abnormal results of pulmonary function studies**
Reduced ventilatory capacity
Reduced vital capacity

R94.3- **Abnormal results of cardiovascular function studies**

R94.30 **Abnormal result of cardiovascular function study, unspecified**

R94.31 **Abnormal electrocardiogram [ECG] [EKG]**
Excludes 1:   long QT syndrome (I45.81)

R94.39 **Abnormal result of other cardiovascular function study**
Abnormal electrophysiological intracardiac studies
Abnormal phonocardiogram
Abnormal vectorcardiogram

R94.4 **Abnormal results of kidney function studies**
Abnormal renal function test

R94.5 **Abnormal results of liver function studies**

R94.6 **Abnormal results of thyroid function studies**

R94.7 **Abnormal results of other endocrine function studies**
Excludes ❷: abnormal glucose (R73.0-)

R94.8 **Abnormal results of function studies of other organs and systems**
Abnormal basal metabolic rate [BMR]
Abnormal bladder function test
Abnormal splenic function test

Abnormal tumor markers (R97)

R97- **Abnormal tumor markers** — The presence of substances that are produced by tumor cells, or by other cells, in response to neoplastic conditions.
Elevated tumor associated antigens [TAA] — The increased presence of antigens that are relatively restricted to tumor cells.
Elevated tumor specific antigens [TSA] — The increased presence of antigens that are unique to tumor cells.

R97.0 **Elevated carcinoembryonic antigen [CEA]**

R97.1 **Elevated cancer antigen 125 [CA 125]** — [♀]

R97.2- **Elevated prostate specific antigen [PSA]**

R97.20 **Elevated prostate specific antigen [PSA]** — [♂, Age/15-124]
[Questionable Admission]

R97.21 **Rising PSA following treatment for malignant neoplasm of prostate** — [♂, Age/15-124] [Questionable Admission]

R97.8 **Other abnormal tumor markers**

Ill-defined and unknown cause of mortality (R99)

R99 **Ill-defined and unknown cause of mortality**
Death (unexplained) NOS
Unspecified cause of mortality

Chapter 19 – Injury, poisoning and certain other consequences of external causes (S00-T88)

<u>**EDUCATIONAL ANNOTATIONS — ILLUSTRATIONS AND DEFINITIONS**</u>

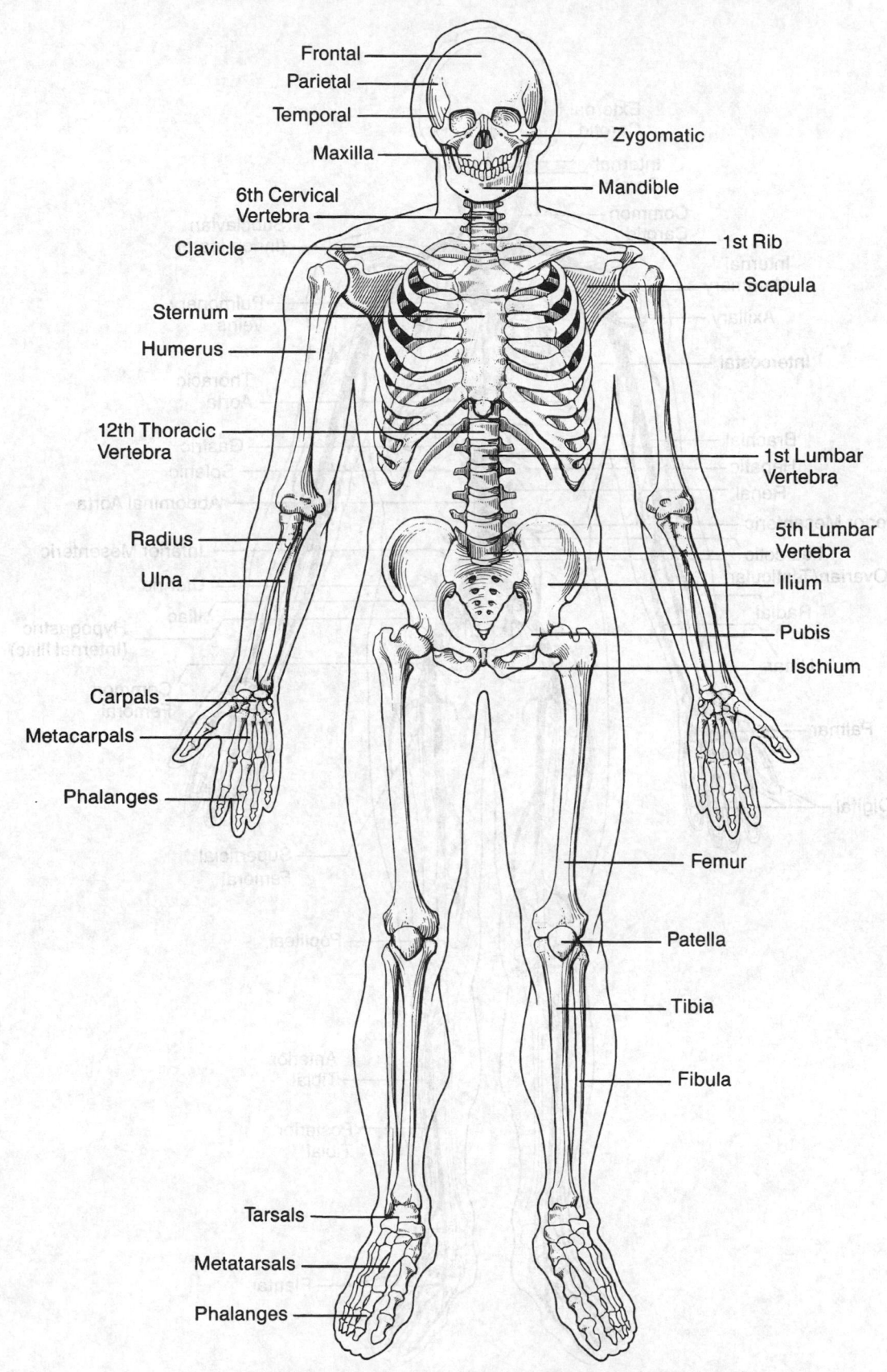

Frontal

Parietal

Temporal

Maxilla

Zygomatic

Mandible

6th Cervical Vertebra

Clavicle

1st Rib

Scapula

Sternum

Humerus

12th Thoracic Vertebra

1st Lumbar Vertebra

5th Lumbar Vertebra

Radius

Ulna

Ilium

Pubis

Ischium

Carpals

Metacarpals

Phalanges

Femur

Patella

Tibia

Fibula

Tarsals

Metatarsals

Phalanges

ANTERIOR VIEW OF HUMAN SKELETON

S00 - S00

Excludes 1: = NOT CODED HERE! (Do not code both)   **1005**   *Excludes ❷:* = Not Included Here

Chapter 19 – Injury, poisoning and certain other consequences of external causes (S00-T88)
EDUCATIONAL ANNOTATIONS — ILLUSTRATIONS AND DEFINITIONS

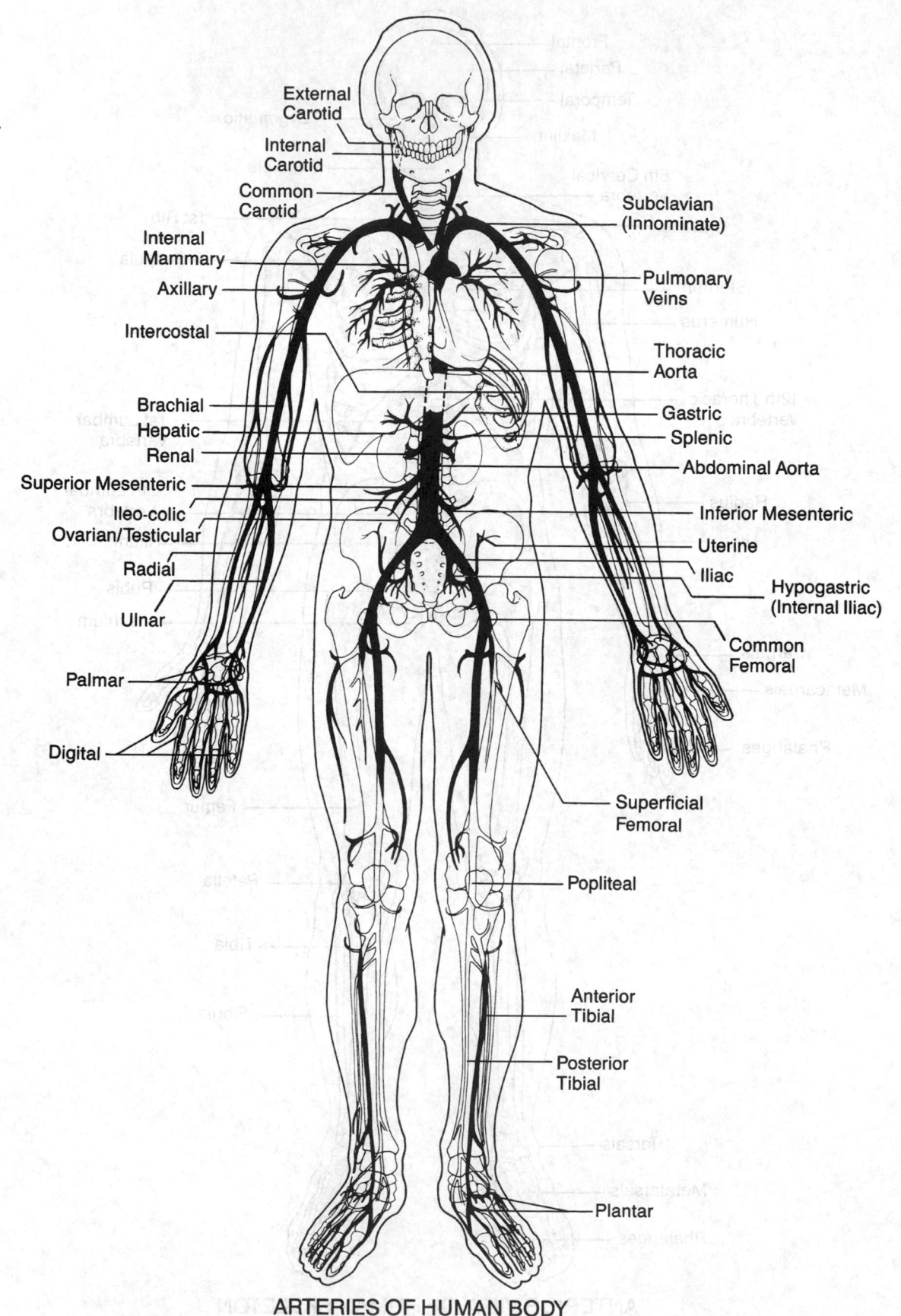

ARTERIES OF HUMAN BODY

S00-S00

Chapter 19 – Injury, poisoning and certain other consequences of external causes (S00-T88)
EDUCATIONAL ANNOTATIONS — ILLUSTRATIONS AND DEFINITIONS

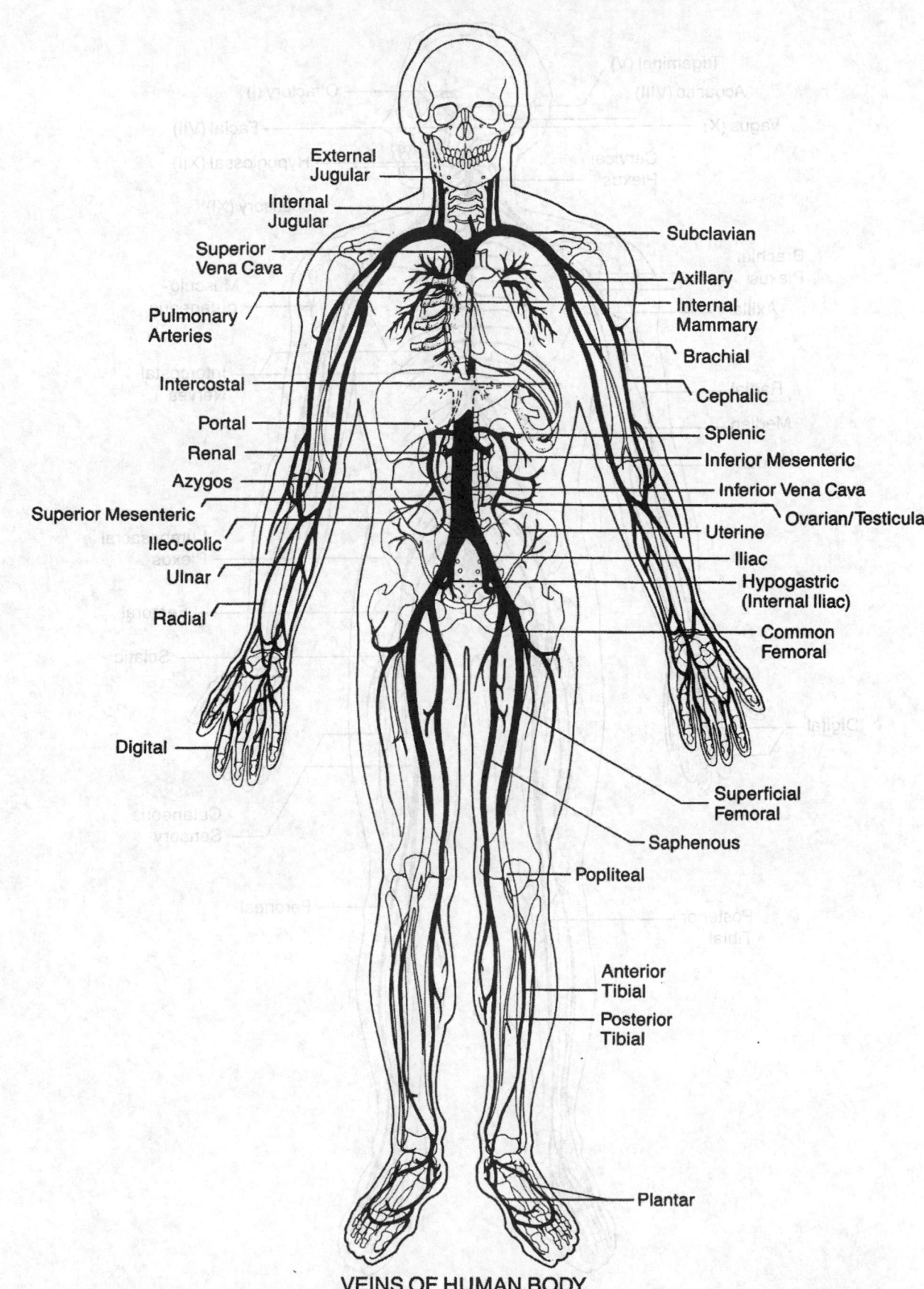

External Jugular
Internal Jugular
Superior Vena Cava
Pulmonary Arteries
Intercostal
Portal
Renal
Azygos
Superior Mesenteric
Ileo-colic
Ulnar
Radial
Digital

Subclavian
Axillary
Internal Mammary
Brachial
Cephalic
Splenic
Inferior Mesenteric
Inferior Vena Cava
Ovarian/Testicular
Uterine
Iliac
Hypogastric (Internal Iliac)
Common Femoral
Superficial Femoral
Saphenous
Popliteal
Anterior Tibial
Posterior Tibial
Plantar

VEINS OF HUMAN BODY

S00 - S00

Excludes 1: = NOT CODED HERE! (Do not code both)   **1007**   *Excludes ❷:* = Not Included Here

Chapter 19 – Injury, poisoning and certain other consequences of external causes (S00-T88)
EDUCATIONAL ANNOTATIONS — ILLUSTRATIONS AND DEFINITIONS

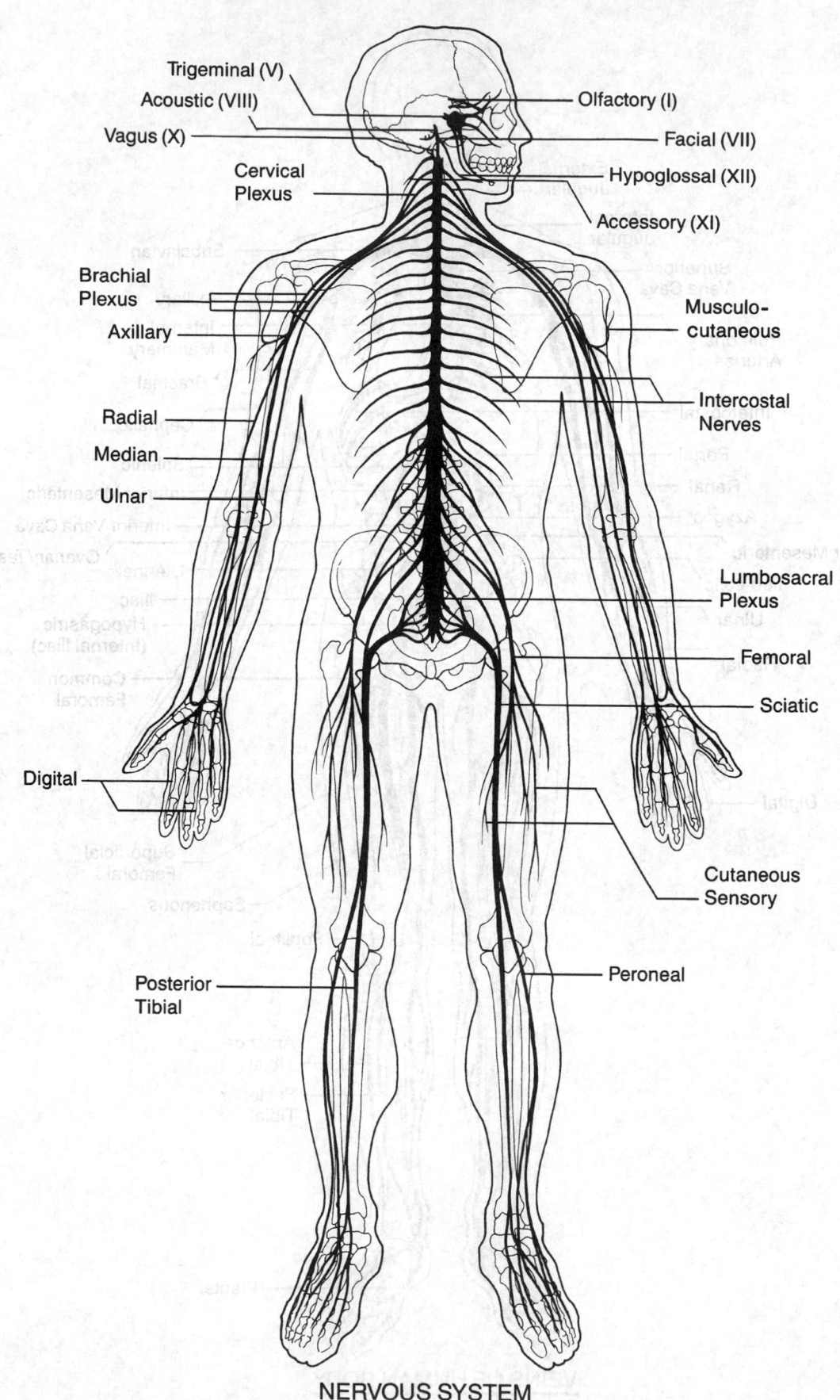

NERVOUS SYSTEM

Chapter 19 – Injury, poisoning and certain other consequences of external causes (S00-T88)
EDUCATIONAL ANNOTATIONS — ILLUSTRATIONS AND DEFINITIONS

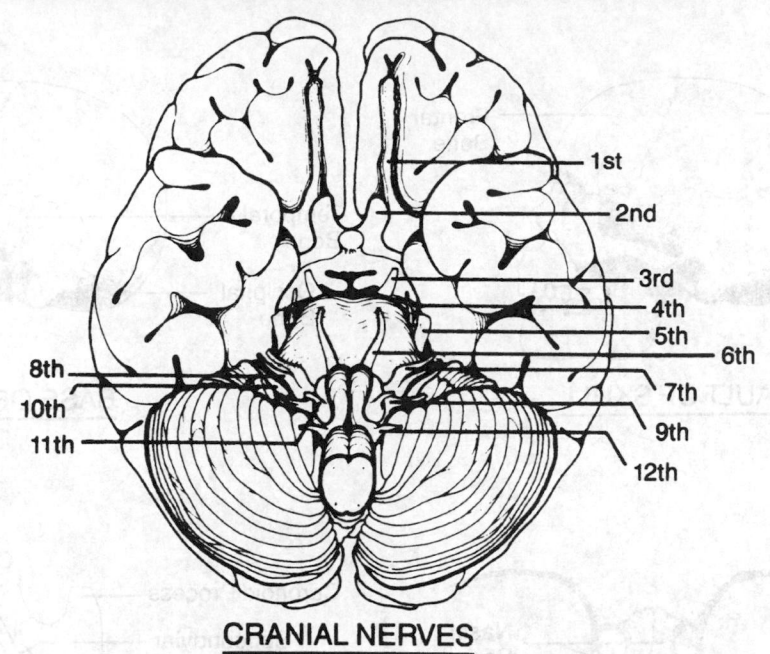

CRANIAL NERVES

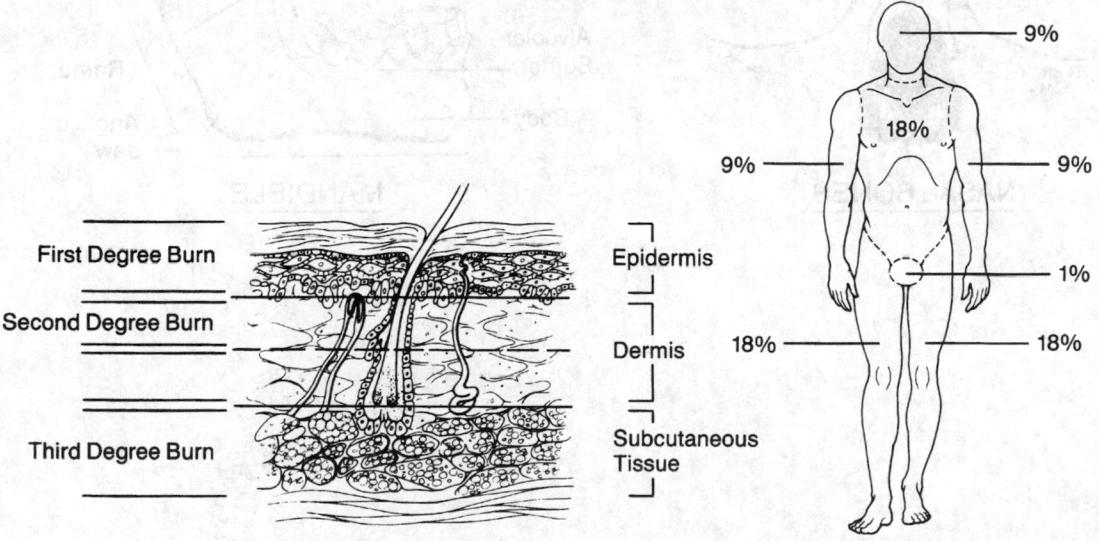

First Degree Burn

Second Degree Burn

Third Degree Burn

Epidermis

Dermis

Subcutaneous Tissue

EXTENT OF SKIN BURN

9%

18%

9%   9%

1%

18%   18%

BODY SURFACE RULE OF NINES

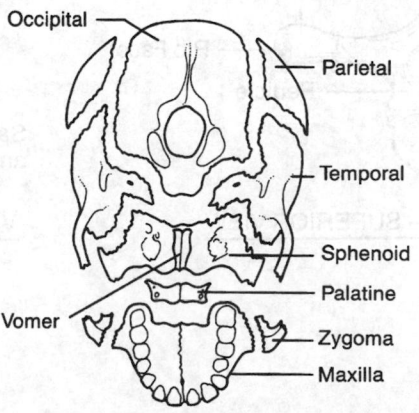

Occipital

Parietal

Temporal

Sphenoid

Palatine

Vomer

Zygoma

Maxilla

ORBITAL FLOOR AND MALAR BONES

S00-S00

Excludes 1: **= NOT CODED HERE! (Do not code both)**   **1009**   ***Excludes ❷:*** **= Not Included Here**

Chapter 19 – Injury, poisoning and certain other consequences of external causes (S00-T88)
<u>EDUCATIONAL ANNOTATIONS — ILLUSTRATIONS AND DEFINITIONS</u>

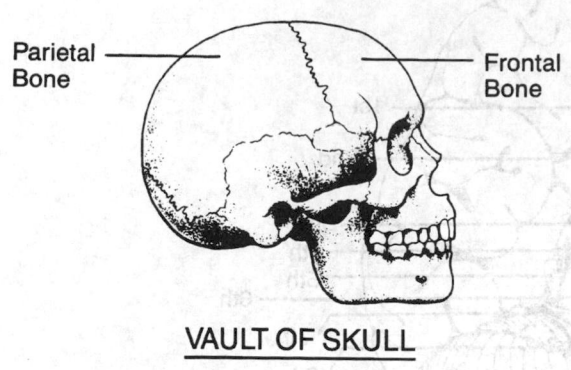

Parietal Bone

Frontal Bone

<u>VAULT OF SKULL</u>

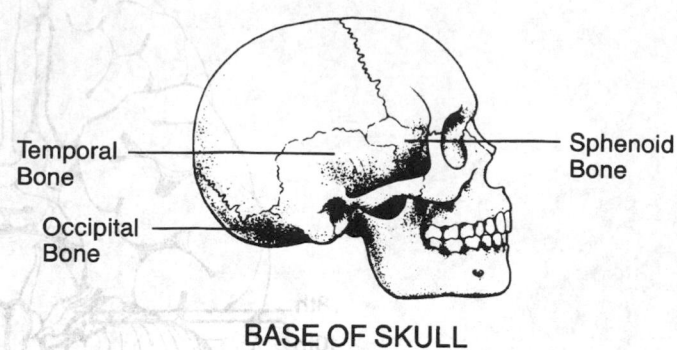

Temporal Bone

Occipital Bone

Sphenoid Bone

<u>BASE OF SKULL</u>

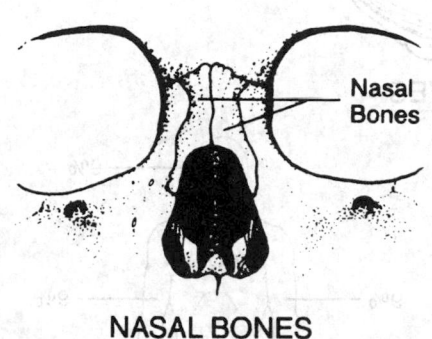

Nasal Bones

<u>NASAL BONES</u>

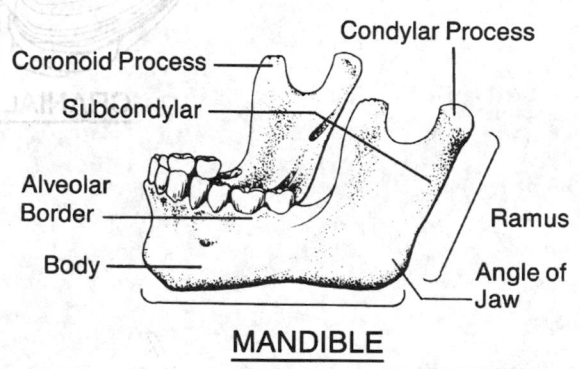

Coronoid Process

Condylar Process

Subcondylar

Alveolar Border

Body

Ramus

Angle of Jaw

<u>MANDIBLE</u>

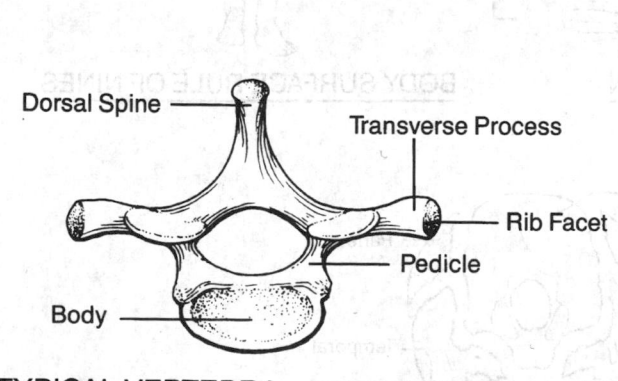

Dorsal Spine

Transverse Process

Rib Facet

Pedicle

Body

<u>TYPICAL VERTEBRA</u> — <u>SUPERIOR VIEW</u>

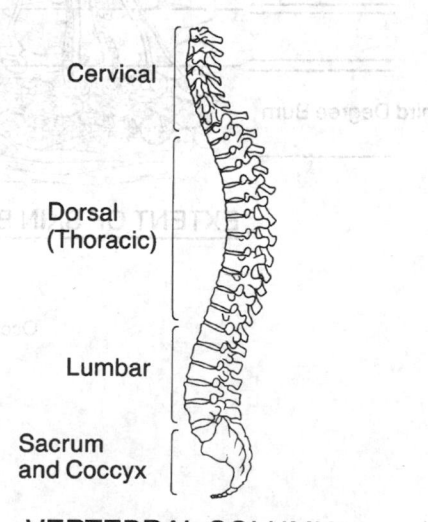

Cervical

Dorsal (Thoracic)

Lumbar

Sacrum and Coccyx

<u>VERTEBRAL COLUMN</u>

S00-S00

Chapter 19 – Injury, poisoning and certain other consequences of external causes (S00-T88)
EDUCATIONAL ANNOTATIONS — ILLUSTRATIONS AND DEFINITIONS

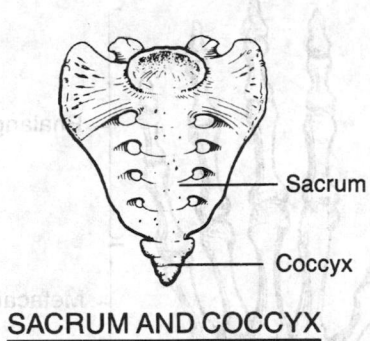

SACRUM AND COCCYX

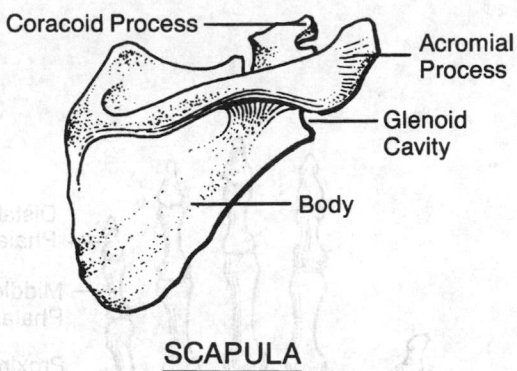

SCAPULA

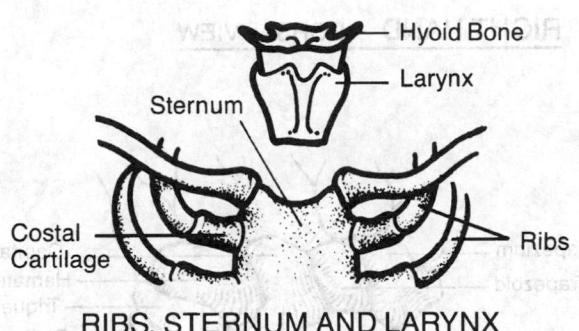

RIBS, STERNUM AND LARYNX

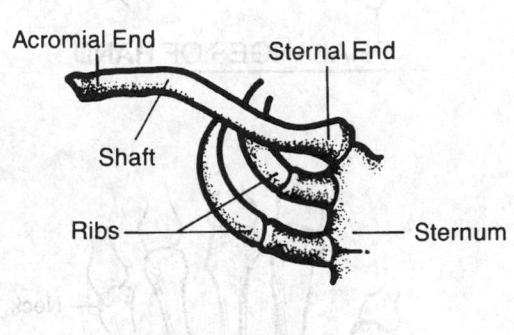

CLAVICLE

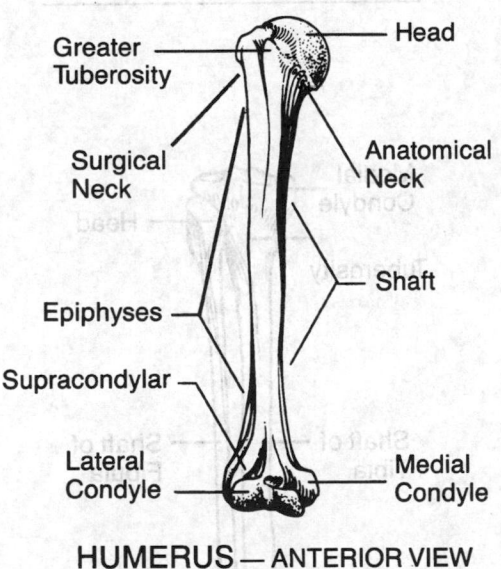

HUMERUS — ANTERIOR VIEW

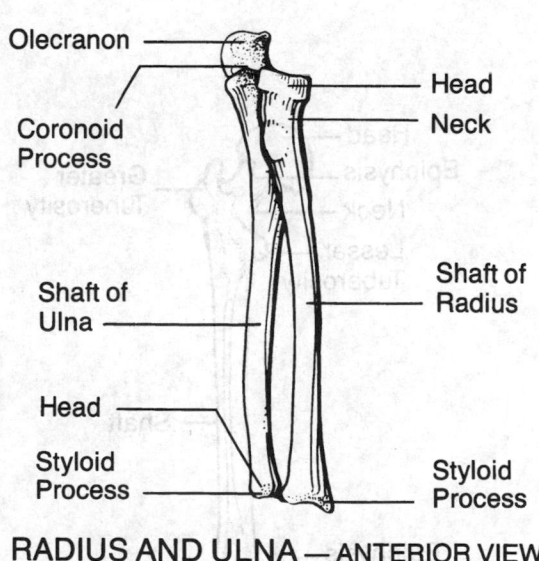

RADIUS AND ULNA — ANTERIOR VIEW

S00-S00

Excludes 1: = NOT CODED HERE! (Do not code both)   **1011**   *Excludes ❷:* = Not Included Here

Chapter 19 – Injury, poisoning and certain other consequences of external causes (S00-T88)
EDUCATIONAL ANNOTATIONS — ILLUSTRATIONS AND DEFINITIONS

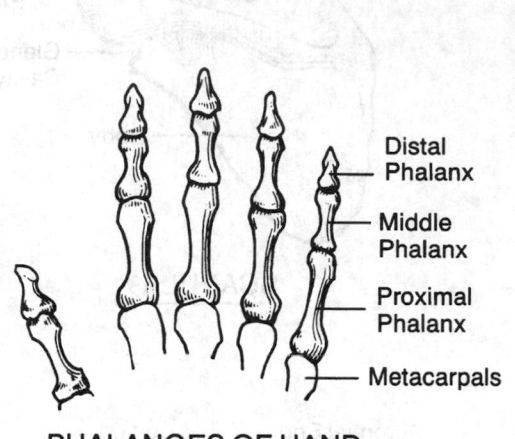

PHALANGES OF HAND

Distal Phalanx
Middle Phalanx
Proximal Phalanx
Metacarpals

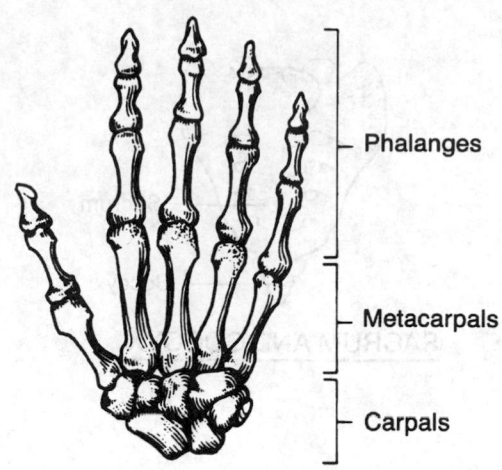

RIGHT HAND — DORSAL VIEW

Phalanges
Metacarpals
Carpals

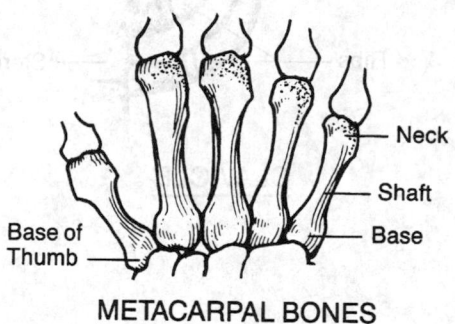

METACARPAL BONES

Base of Thumb
Neck
Shaft
Base

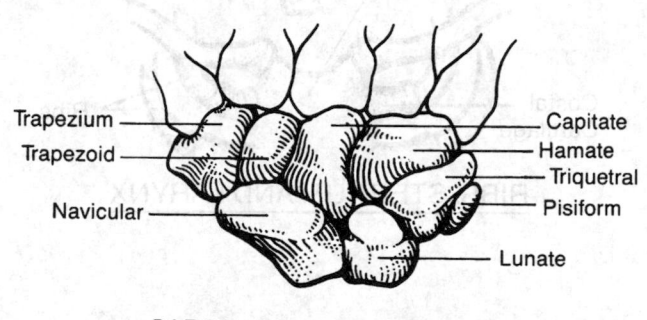

CARPAL BONES — DORSAL VIEW

Trapezium
Trapezoid
Navicular
Capitate
Hamate
Triquetral
Pisiform
Lunate

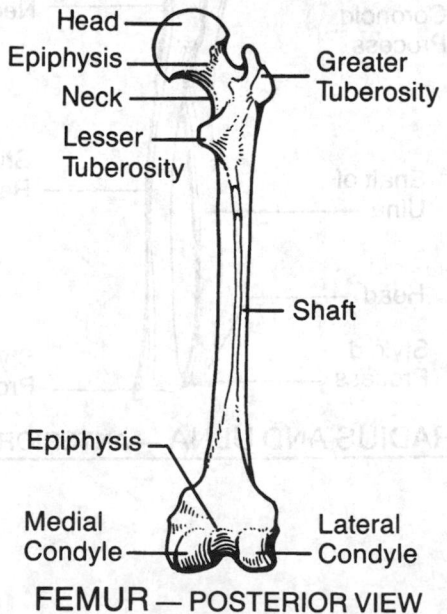

FEMUR — POSTERIOR VIEW

Head
Epiphysis
Neck
Lesser Tuberosity
Greater Tuberosity
Shaft
Epiphysis
Medial Condyle
Lateral Condyle

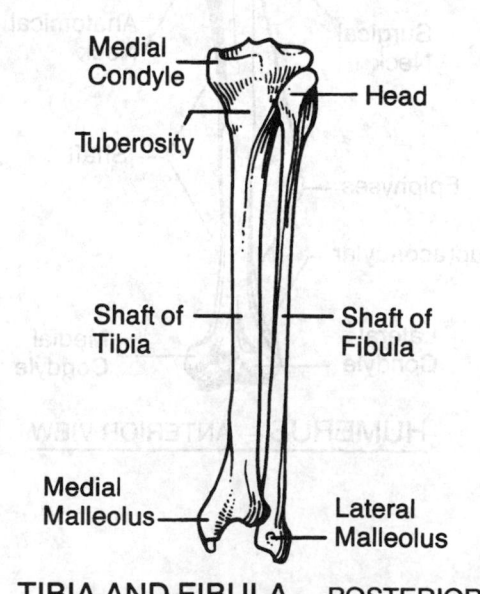

TIBIA AND FIBULA — POSTERIOR VIEW

Medial Condyle
Tuberosity
Head
Shaft of Tibia
Shaft of Fibula
Medial Malleolus
Lateral Malleolus

S00-S00

© 2016 Channel Publishing, Ltd.

Chapter 19 – Injury, poisoning and certain other consequences of external causes (S00-T88)
<u>**EDUCATIONAL ANNOTATIONS — ILLUSTRATIONS AND DEFINITIONS**</u>

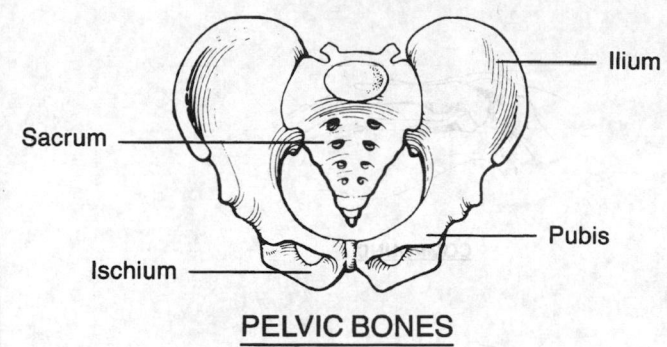

<u>PELVIC BONES</u>

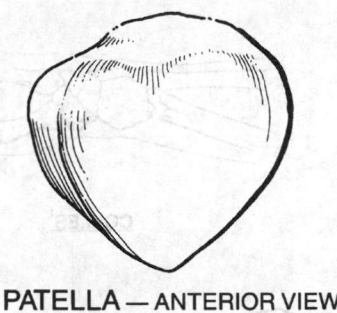

<u>PATELLA</u> — ANTERIOR VIEW

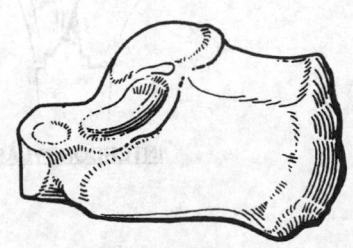

<u>CALCANEUS</u> — MEDIAL VIEW

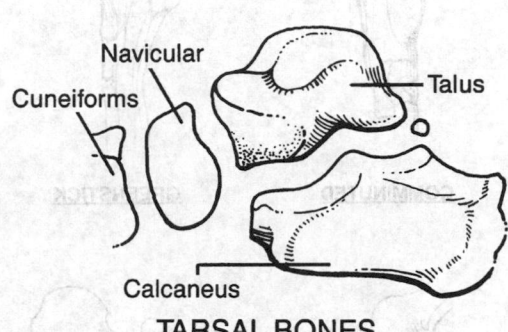

<u>TARSAL BONES</u>

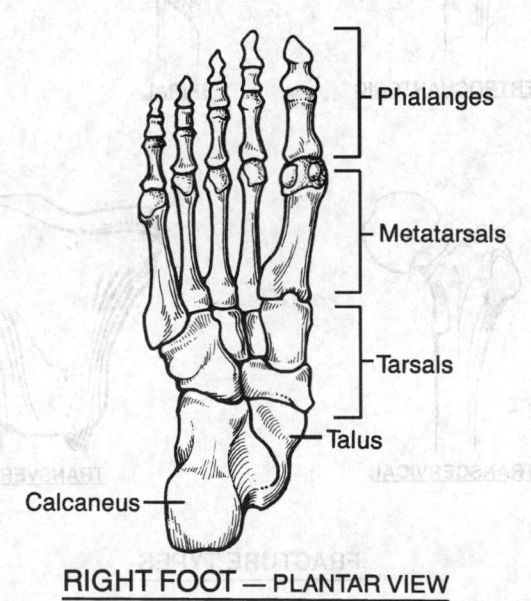

<u>RIGHT FOOT</u> — PLANTAR VIEW

S00 – S00

Chapter 19 – Injury, poisoning and certain other consequences of external causes (S00-T88)
EDUCATIONAL ANNOTATIONS — ILLUSTRATIONS AND DEFINITIONS

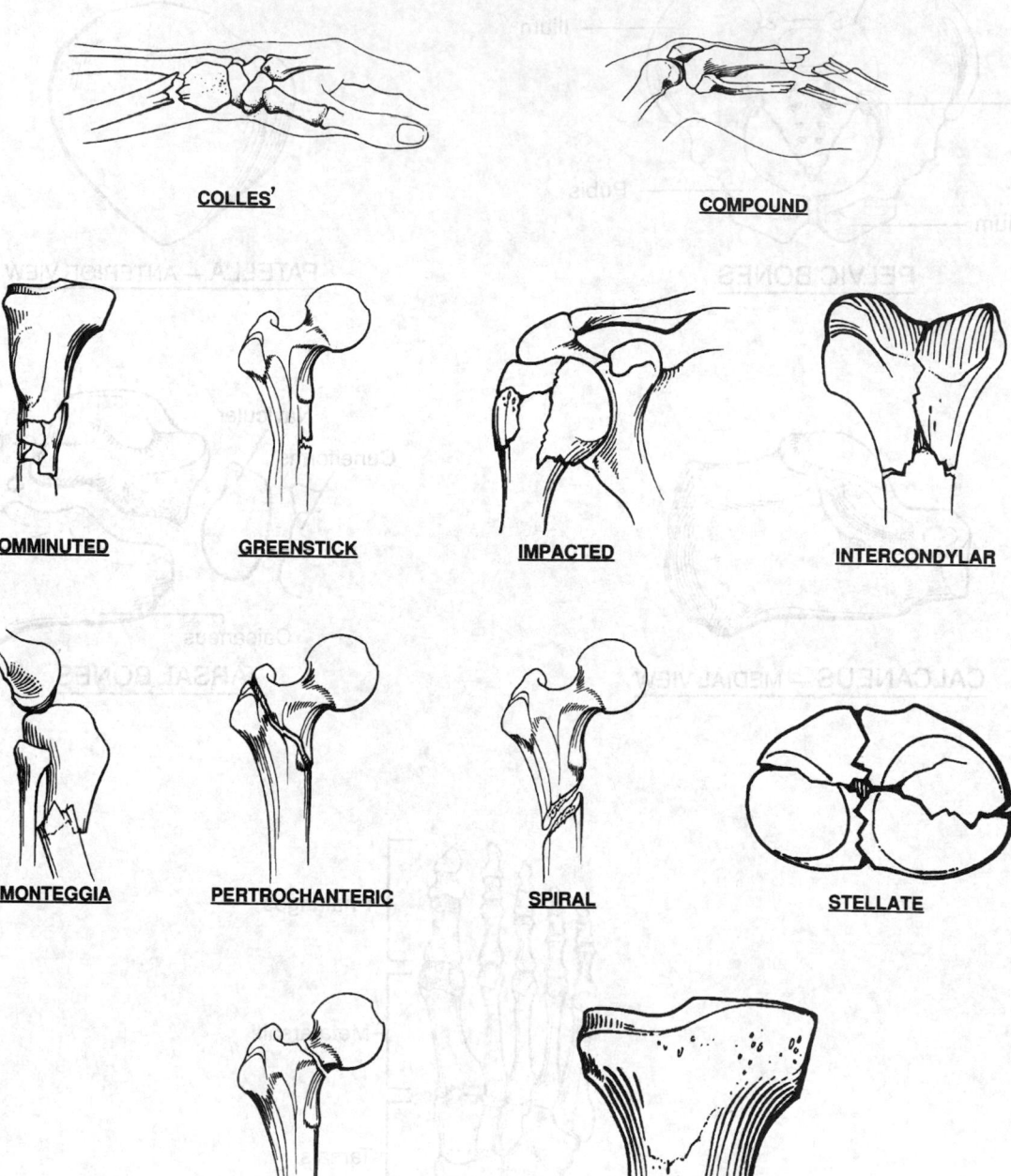

COLLES'   COMPOUND

COMMINUTED   GREENSTICK   IMPACTED   INTERCONDYLAR

MONTEGGIA   PERTROCHANTERIC   SPIRAL   STELLATE

TRANSCERVICAL   TRANSVERSE

FRACTURE TYPES

S00-S00

Chapter 19 – Injury, poisoning and certain other consequences of external causes (S00-T88)
EDUCATIONAL ANNOTATIONS — ILLUSTRATIONS AND DEFINITIONS

Acetabulum – The round, concave depression in the pelvic bone that articulates with the femoral head forming the hip joint.

Aorta, Abdominal – The abdominal aorta is continuous from the thoracic aorta artery and ends by branching into the right and left common iliac arteries. Many abdominal arteries branch off from the abdominal aorta.

Aorta, Thoracic – The upper most portion of the aorta that lies within the thoracic cavity.

Azygos Vein – The azygos vein drains to the superior vena cava and drains blood from the right side of the posterior thorax.

Carpal – The 8 compact bones of the wrist, forming 2 rows of 4 bones each. The proximal row contains the scaphoid, lunate, pisiform, and triquetrum. The distal row contains the trapezium, trapezoid, capitate, and hamate.

Celiac Artery – The celiac artery (also known as the celiac trunk) branches from the abdominal aorta and then almost immediately (1-2cm) branches into the common hepatic artery, the splenic artery, and left gastric artery.

Clavicle – The paired, straightened S-shaped bones (also known as the collarbones) that connect the sternum with the scapula.

Coccyx – The small wedge-shaped bone (also known as the tailbone) at the end of the spinal column.

Conchae Bone – The 2 small paired bones of the nasal cavity that are attached to the maxilla.

Ethmoid Bone – The single bone located between the orbits that forms the roof of the nasal cavity, part of the floor of the cranial cavity, and part of the orbit.

Facial Bone – Any one of the 14 bones of the facial area below the cranium (2 nasal bones, vomer, 2 conchae, 2 maxilla, mandible, 2 palatine bones, 2 zygomatic bones, 2 lacrimal bones).

Femoral Artery – The femoral artery branches from the external iliac artery and serves the legs.

Femoral Shaft – The middle long portion of the femur.

Femur – The paired long bones (also known as the thigh bone) that articulate at the hip and the knee. It is the longest bone in the body.

Fibula – The paired long slender bones of the lower leg located toward the outside of the lower leg that articulate at the knee and the ankle.

Frontal Bone – The single bone in the front of the skull that also forms part of the roof of the nasal cavity and part of the orbit.

Glenoid Cavity – The shallow, round depression of the scapula that articulates with the humeral head.

Humeral Head – The upper end of the humerus that is part of the shoulder joint.

Humeral Shaft – The middle, long portion of the humerus.

Humerus – The paired, long bones of the upper arm that articulate at the shoulder and the elbow. The capitulum of the humerus articulates with the head of the radius, and the trochlea of the humerus articulates with the trochlear notch of the ulna.

Hyoid Bone – The single horseshoe-shaped bone that lies in the front of the neck and just under the chin and aids in tongue movement and swallowing. It is not directly articulated with any other bone and not considered part of the skull.

Iliac Artery, Common – The common iliac artery branches from the aortic bifurcation of the abdominal aorta and branches almost immediately (4 cm in length) into the internal and external iliac arteries.

Iliac Artery, External – The external iliac artery branches from the common iliac artery and serves the legs.

Inferior Mesenteric Artery – The inferior mesenteric artery branches from the abdominal aorta and serves the descending colon, part of the transverse colon, sigmoid colon, and the upper part of the rectum.

Inferior Vena Cava – The inferior vena cava drains to the right atrium of the heart and drains blood from the common iliac veins.

Innominate Artery – The innominate artery (also known as the brachiocephalic artery) branches from the aortic arch and branches to the right common carotid artery, the internal mammary artery, and the subclavian artery.

Lacrimal Bone – The 2 small paired bones that form the medial side of the orbit and the nasolacrimal canal.

Lower Femur – The distal end of the femur that articulates with the knee joint.

Mandible – The single horseshoe-shaped bone forming the lower jaw.

Maxilla – The 2 fused irregularly-shaped bones that form the upper jaw, the roof of the mouth, and a part of the orbit.

Metacarpal – One of the 5 cylindrical bones of the palm of the hand connecting the carpals to the phalanges of the hand.

Metatarsal – One of the 5 cylindrical bones connecting the tarsals and the phalanges of the foot.

Nasal Bone – The 2 small paired bones that form the bridge of the nose.

S00 – S00

© 2016 Channel Publishing, Ltd.

Excludes 1: = NOT CODED HERE! (Do not code both)   **1015**   *Excludes ❷:* = Not Included Here

Chapter 19 – Injury, poisoning and certain other consequences of external causes (S00-T88)
<u>EDUCATIONAL ANNOTATIONS — ILLUSTRATIONS AND DEFINITIONS</u>

Occipital Bone – The single bone of the base and back of the skull.

Orbit – The bones (7) which form the orbit (eye socket): Zygomatic, sphenoid, ethmoid, maxilla, lacrimal, palatine, and frontal.

Palatine Bone – The 2 small paired bones at the back of the nasal cavity that form the floor and lateral wall of the nasal cavity, part of the roof of the mouth, and part of the floor of the orbit.

Parietal Bone – The 2 paired bones that form the top and sides of the skull.

Patella – The paired triangular-shaped bones situated at the front of the knee.

Pelvic Bone – Any of the three bones (ilium, ischium, pubis) that connect with the sacrum to form the pelvic girdle.

Phalanx, Finger – The digital bones of the fingers. Each finger contains three bones: Proximal phalanx, intermediate (middle) phalanx, and distal phalanx.

Phalanx, Thumb – The digital bones of the thumb. The thumb contains two bones: Proximal phalanx and distal phalanx.

Phalanx, Toe – The digital bones of the toes. Each toe contains three bones: Proximal phalanx, intermediate (middle) phalanx, and distal phalanx, except the great toe which only has proximal and distal phalanx bones.

Pneumothorax, Traumatic – The traumatic entry of air, blood, or fluid into the pleural space.

Portal Vein – The portal vein drains to the hepatic vein and drains blood from the gastrointestinal tract and liver.

Renal Vein – The renal vein drains to the inferior vena cava and drains blood from the kidney.

Rib – The 12 paired arched bones of the rib cage that partially enclose and protect the chest cavity.

Sacrum – The large wedge-shaped vertebra at the lower end of the spine that connects with S5.

Scapula – The paired flat, triangular bones located in the upper back behind the shoulder (also called the shoulder blade).

Skull – The skull consists of all (22) of the cranial and facial bones. Eight of these bones form the cranium (occipital bone, frontal bone, 2 temporal bones, 2 parietal bones, sphenoid bone, ethmoid bone), and 14 of these bones form the skull below the cranium (2 nasal bones, vomer, 2 conchae, 2 maxilla, mandible, 2 palatine bones, 2 zygomatic bones, 2 lacrimal bones).

Sphenoid Bone – The single winged-shaped bone of the skull floor that forms part of the base of the cranial cavity, sides of the skull, and part of the orbital floor and side.

Splenic Vein – The splenic vein drains to the portal vein and drains blood from the spleen and pancreas.

Sternum – The long flat bone (also known as the breast bone) of the chest that connects to the clavicles and most of the ribs.

Subclavian Artery – The left subclavian artery branches from the aortic arch and serves the thorax, head, and left upper limb. The right subclavian artery branches from the innominate artery (also known as the brachiocephalic artery) and serves the thorax, head, and right upper limb.

Subclavian Vein – The subclavian vein drains to the innominate vein and drains blood from the axillary vein and external jugular vein.

Superior Mesenteric Artery – The superior mesenteric artery branches from the abdominal aorta and serves the duodenum, ascending colon, part of the transverse colon, and pancreas.

Superior Mesenteric Vein – The superior mesenteric vein drains to the portal vein and drains blood from the small intestine.

Superior Vena Cava – The major vein transporting de-oxygenated blood from the upper body and head that empties into the right atrium.

Tarsal – The seven bones of the foot (calcaneus, talus, cuboid, navicular, and the medial, intermediate, and lateral cuneiform bones) distal to the tibia and fibula and proximal to the metatarsal bones.

Temporal Bone – The 2 paired bones that form the lower sides and base of the skull and contain the internal organs and structures of hearing.

Tibia – The paired long bones of the lower leg (also known as the shin bone) that is the innermost bone of the lower leg supporting and articulating with the knee and with the ankle.

Ulna – The paired long bones of the forearms that are closer to the side of the body than the radii.

Vertebra, Cervical – The cervical section of the spinal vertebral column comprised of 7 vertebra, C1-C7.

Vertebra, Lumbar – The lumbar section of the spinal vertebral column comprised of 5 vertebra, S1-S5.

Vertebra, Thoracic – The thoracic section of the spinal vertebral column comprised of 12 vertebra, T1-T12.

Vomer Bone – The single bone of the inferior nasal septum.

Zygomatic Bone – The 2 paired quadrangular bones of the cheeks (also known as the malar bones) that form the cheek prominence and lower-outer part of the orbit.

S00 - S00

Chapter 19 – Injury, poisoning and certain other consequences of external causes (S00-T88)

Use additional code to identify any retained foreign body, if applicable (Z18-)

Excludes 1:   *birth trauma (P10-P15)*
                 obstetric trauma (O70-O71)

This chapter contains the following blocks:

S00-S09	Injuries to the head
S10-S19	Injuries to the neck
S20-S29	Injuries to the thorax
S30-S39	Injuries to the abdomen, lower back, lumbar spine, pelvis and external genitals
S40-S49	Injuries to the shoulder and upper arm
S50-S59	Injuries to the elbow and forearm
S60-S69	Injuries to the wrist, hand and fingers
S70-S79	Injuries to the hip and thigh
S80-S89	Injuries to the knee and lower leg
S90-S99	Injuries to the ankle and foot
T07	Injuries involving multiple body regions
T14	Injury of unspecified body region
T15-T19	Effects of foreign body entering through natural orifice
T20-T25	Burns and corrosions of external body surface, specified by site
T26-T28	Burns and corrosions confined to eye and internal organs
T30-T32	Burns and corrosions of multiple and unspecified body regions
T33-T34	Frostbite
T36-T50	Poisoning by, adverse effects of and underdosing of drugs, medicaments and biological substances
T51-T65	Toxic effects of substances chiefly nonmedicinal as to source
T66-T78	Other and unspecified effects of external causes
T79	Certain early complications of trauma
T80-T88	Complications of surgical and medical care, not elsewhere classified

Note: Use secondary code(s) from Chapter 20, External causes of morbidity, to indicate cause of injury. Codes within the T section that include the external cause do not require an additional external cause code

The chapter uses the S-section for coding different types of injuries related to single body regions and the T-section to cover injuries to unspecified body regions as well as poisoning and certain other consequences of external causes.

Chapter-Specific Coding Guidelines

C.   Chapter-Specific Coding Guidelines
In addition to general coding guidelines, there are guidelines for specific diagnoses and/or conditions in the classification. Unless otherwise indicated, these guidelines apply to all health care settings. Please refer to Section II for guidelines on the selection of principal diagnosis.

19.   Chapter 19: Injury, Poisoning, and Certain Other Consequences of External Causes (S00-T88)

a.   Application of 7th Characters in Chapter 19
Most categories in chapter 19 have a 7th character requirement for each applicable code. Most categories in this chapter have three 7th character values (with the exception of fractures): A, initial encounter and D, subsequent encounter and S, sequela. Categories for traumatic fractures have additional 7th character values. While the patient may be seen by a new or different provider over the course of treatment for an injury, assignment of the 7th character is based on whether the patient is undergoing active treatment and not whether the provider is seeing the patient for the first time.

For complication codes, active treatment refers to treatment for the condition described by the code, even though it may be related to an earlier precipitating problem. For example, code T84.50xA, Infection and inflammatory reaction due to unspecified internal joint prosthesis, initial encounter, is used when active treatment is provided for the infection, even though the condition relates to the prosthetic device, implant or graft that was placed at a previous encounter.

7th character "A" initial encounter is used ~~while~~ for each encounter where the patient is receiving active treatment for the condition. ~~Examples of active treatment are: surgical treatment, emergency department encounter, and evaluation and continuing treatment by the same or a different physician.~~

7th character "D" subsequent encounter is used for encounters after the patient has ~~received~~ completed active treatment of the condition and is receiving routine care for the condition during the healing or recovery phase. ~~Examples of subsequent care are: cast change or removal, an x ray to check healing status of fracture, removal of external or internal fixation device, medication adjustment, other aftercare and follow up visits following treatment of the injury or condition.~~

The aftercare Z codes should not be used for aftercare for conditions such as injuries or poisonings, where 7th characters are provided to identify subsequent care. For example, for aftercare of an injury, assign the acute injury code with the 7th character "D" (subsequent encounter).

7th character "S", sequela, is for use for complications or conditions that arise as a direct result of an condition, such as scar formation after a burn. The scars are sequelae of the burn. When using 7th character "S", it is necessary to use both the injury code that precipitated the sequela and the code for the sequela itself. The "S" is added only to the injury code, not the sequela code. The 7th character "S" identifies the injury responsible for the sequela. The specific type of sequela (e.g., scar) is sequenced first, followed by the injury code.

See Section I.B.10 Sequela (Late Effects).

b.   Coding of Injuries
When coding injuries, assign separate codes for each injury unless a combination code is provided, in which case the combination code is assigned. Code T07, Unspecified multiple injuries should not be assigned in the inpatient setting unless information for a more specific code is not available. Traumatic injury codes (S00-T14.9) are not to be used for normal, healing surgical wounds or to identify complications of surgical wounds.

The code for the most serious injury, as determined by the provider and the focus of treatment, is sequenced first.

1)   Superficial injuries
Superficial injuries such as abrasions or contusions are not coded when associated with more severe injuries of the same site.

2)   Primary injury with damage to nerves/blood vessels
When a primary injury results in minor damage to peripheral nerves or blood vessels, the primary injury is sequenced first with additional code(s) for injuries to nerves and spinal cord (such as category S04), and/or injury to blood vessels (such as category S15). When the primary injury is to the blood vessels or nerves, that injury should be sequenced first.

c.   Coding of Traumatic Fractures
The principles of multiple coding of injuries should be followed in coding fractures. Fractures of specified sites are coded individually by site in accordance with both the provisions within categories S02, S12, S22, S32, S42, S49, S52, S59, S62, S72, S79, S82, S89, S92 and the level of detail furnished by medical record content.

A fracture not indicated as open or closed should be coded to closed. A fracture not indicated whether displaced or not displaced should be coded to displaced.

More specific guidelines are as follows:

1)   Initial vs. Subsequent Encounter for Fractures
Traumatic fractures are coded using the appropriate 7th character for initial encounter (A, B, C) ~~while~~ for each encounter where the patient is receiving active treatment for the fracture. ~~Examples of active treatment are: surgical treatment, emergency department encounter, and evaluation and continuing (ongoing) treatment by the same or different physician.~~ The appropriate 7th character for initial encounter should also be assigned for a patient who delayed seeking treatment for the fracture or nonunion.

Fractures are coded using the appropriate 7th character for subsequent care for encounters after the patient has completed active treatment of the fracture and is receiving routine care for the fracture during the healing or recovery phase. ~~Examples of fracture aftercare are: cast change or removal, an x ray to check healing status of fracture, removal of external or internal fixation device, medication adjustment, and follow up visits following fracture treatment.~~

Care for complications of surgical treatment for fracture repairs during the healing or recovery phase should be coded with the appropriate complication codes.

Care of complications of fractures, such as malunion and nonunion, should be reported with the appropriate 7th character for subsequent care with nonunion (K, M, N,) or subsequent care with malunion (P, Q, R).

Malunion/nonunion: The appropriate 7th character for initial encounter should also be assigned for a patient who delayed seeking treatment for the fracture or nonunion.

The open fracture designations in the assignment of the 7th character for fractures of the forearm, femur and lower leg, including ankle are based on the Gustilo open fracture classification. When the Gustilo classification type is not specified for an open fracture, the 7th character for open fracture type I or II should be assigned (B, E, H, M, Q).

A code from category M80, not a traumatic fracture code, should be used for any patient with known osteoporosis who suffers a fracture, even if the patient had a minor fall or trauma, if that fall or trauma would not usually break a normal, healthy bone.

See Section I.C.13. Osteoporosis.
The aftercare Z codes should not be used for aftercare for traumatic fractures. For aftercare of a traumatic fracture, assign the acute fracture code with the appropriate 7th character.

Excludes 1: = NOT CODED HERE! (Do not code both)   **1017**   *Excludes* ❷: = Not Included Here

S00-S00

2) Multiple fractures sequencing

Multiple fractures are sequenced in accordance with the severity of the fracture.

d. Coding of Burns and Corrosions

The ICD-10-CM makes a distinction between burns and corrosions. The burn codes are for thermal burns, except sunburns, that come from a heat source, such as a fire or hot appliance. The burn codes are also for burns resulting from electricity and radiation. Corrosions are burns due to chemicals. The guidelines are the same for burns and corrosions.

Current burns (T20-T25) are classified by depth, extent and by agent (X code). Burns are classified by depth as first degree (erythema), second degree (blistering), and third degree (full-thickness involvement). Burns of the eye and internal organs (T26-T28) are classified by site, but not by degree.

1) Sequencing of burn and related condition codes

Sequence first the code that reflects the highest degree of burn when more than one burn is present.

a. When the reason for the admission or encounter is for treatment of external multiple burns, sequence first the code that reflects the burn of the highest degree.

b. When a patient has both internal and external burns, the circumstances of admission govern the selection of the principal diagnosis or first-listed diagnosis.

c. When a patient is admitted for burn injuries and other related conditions such as smoke inhalation and/or respiratory failure, the circumstances of admission govern the selection of the principal or first-listed diagnosis.

2) Burns of the same local site

Classify burns of the same local site (three-character category level, T20-T28) but of different degrees to the subcategory identifying the highest degree recorded in the diagnosis.

3) Non-healing burns

Non-healing burns are coded as acute burns.

Necrosis of burned skin should be coded as a non-healed burn.

4) Infected Burn

For any documented infected burn site, use an additional code for the infection.

5) Assign separate codes for each burn site

When coding burns, assign separate codes for each burn site. Category T30, Burn and corrosion, body region unspecified is extremely vague and should rarely be used.

6) Burns and Corrosions Classified According to Extent of Body Surface Involved

Assign codes from category T31, Burns classified according to extent of body surface involved, or T32, Corrosions classified according to extent of body surface involved, when the site of the burn is not specified or when there is a need for additional data. It is advisable to use category T31 as additional coding when needed to provide data for evaluating burn mortality, such as that needed by burn units. It is also advisable to use category T31 as an additional code for reporting purposes when there is mention of a third-degree burn involving 20 percent or more of the body surface.

Categories T31 and T32 are based on the classic "rule of nines" in estimating body surface involved: head and neck are assigned nine percent, each arm nine percent, each leg 18 percent, the anterior trunk 18 percent, posterior trunk 18 percent, and genitalia one percent. Providers may change these percentage assignments where necessary to accommodate infants and children who have proportionately larger heads than adults, and patients who have large buttocks, thighs, or abdomen that involve burns.

7) Encounters for treatment of sequela of burns

Encounters for the treatment of the late effects of burns or corrosions (i.e., scars or joint contractures) should be coded with a burn or corrosion code with the 7th character "S" for sequela.

8) Sequelae with a late effect code and current burn

When appropriate, both a code for a current burn or corrosion with 7th character "A" or "D" and a burn or corrosion code with 7th character "S" may be assigned on the same record (when both a current burn and sequelae of an old burn exist). Burns and corrosions do not heal at the same rate and a current healing wound may still exist with sequela of a healed burn or corrosion.

See Section I.B.10 Sequela (Late Effects).

9) Use of an external cause code with burns and corrosions

An external cause code should be used with burns and corrosions to identify the source and intent of the burn, as well as the place where it occurred.

e. Adverse Effects, Poisoning, Underdosing and Toxic Effects

Codes in categories T36-T65 are combination codes that include the substance that was taken as well as the intent. No additional external cause code is required for poisonings, toxic effects, adverse effects and underdosing codes.

1) Do not code directly from the Table of Drugs

Do not code directly from the Table of Drugs and Chemicals. Always refer back to the Tabular List.

2) Use as many codes as necessary to describe

Use as many codes as necessary to describe completely all drugs, medicinal or biological substances.

3) If the same code would describe the causative agent

If the same code would describe the causative agent for more than one adverse reaction, poisoning, toxic effect or underdosing, assign the code only once.

4) If two or more drugs, medicinal or biological substances

If two or more drugs, medicinal or biological substances are reported, code each individually unless a combination code is listed in the Table of Drugs and Chemicals.

5) The occurrence of drug toxicity is classified in ICD-10-CM as follows:

(a) Adverse Effect

When coding an adverse effect of a drug that has been correctly prescribed and properly administered, assign the appropriate code for the nature of the adverse effect followed by the appropriate code for the adverse effect of the drug (T36-T50). The code for the drug should have a 5th or 6th character "5" (for example T36.0X5-). Examples of the nature of an adverse effect are tachycardia, delirium, gastrointestinal hemorrhaging, vomiting, hypokalemia, hepatitis, renal failure, or respiratory failure.

(b) Poisoning

When coding a poisoning or reaction to the improper use of a medication (e.g., overdose, wrong substance given or taken in error, wrong route of administration), first assign the appropriate code from categories T36-T50. The poisoning codes have an associated intent as their 5th or 6th character accidental, intentional self-harm, assault and undetermined. If the intent of the poisoning is unknown or unspecified, code the intent as accidental intent. The undetermined intent is only for use if the documentation in the record specifies that the intent cannot be determined. Use additional code(s) for all manifestations of poisonings.

If there is also a diagnosis of abuse or dependence of the substance, the abuse or dependence is assigned as an additional code.

Examples of poisoning include:

(i) Error was made in drug prescription
Errors made in drug prescription or in the administration of the drug by provider, nurse, patient, or other person.

(ii) Overdose of a drug intentionally taken
If an overdose of a drug was intentionally taken or administered and resulted in drug toxicity, it would be coded as a poisoning.

(iii) Nonprescribed drug taken with correctly prescribed and properly administered drug
If a nonprescribed drug or medicinal agent was taken in combination with a correctly prescribed and properly administered drug, any drug toxicity or other reaction resulting from the interaction of the two drugs would be classified as a poisoning.

(iv) Interaction of drug(s) and alcohol
When a reaction results from the interaction of a drug(s) and alcohol, this would be classified as poisoning.

See Section I.C.4. if poisoning is the result of insulin pump malfunctions.

(c) Underdosing

Underdosing refers to taking less of a medication than is prescribed by a provider or a manufacturer's instruction. For underdosing, assign the code from categories T36-T50 (fifth or sixth character "6").

Codes for underdosing should never be assigned as principal or first-listed codes. If a patient has a relapse or exacerbation of the medical condition for which the drug is prescribed because of the reduction in dose, then the medical condition itself should be coded.

Noncompliance (Z91.12-, Z91.13-) or complication of care (Y63.61, Y63.6-Y63.9) codes are to be used with an underdosing code to indicate intent, if known.

(d) Toxic Effects

When a harmful substance is ingested or comes in contact with a person, this is classified as a toxic effect. The toxic effect codes are in categories T51-T65.

Toxic effect codes have an associated intent: accidental, intentional self-harm, assault and undetermined.

f.　Adult and child abuse, neglect and other maltreatment

Sequence first the appropriate code from categories T74.- (Adult and child abuse, neglect and other maltreatment, confirmed) or T76.- (Adult and child abuse, neglect and other maltreatment, suspected) for abuse, neglect and other maltreatment, followed by any accompanying mental health or injury code(s).

If the documentation in the medical record states abuse or neglect it is coded as confirmed (T74.-). It is coded as suspected if it is documented as suspected (T76.-).

For cases of confirmed abuse or neglect an external cause code from the assault section (X92-Y09) should be added to identify the cause of any physical injuries. A perpetrator code (Y07) should be added when the perpetrator of the abuse is known. For suspected cases of abuse or neglect, do not report external cause or perpetrator code.

If a suspected case of abuse, neglect or mistreatment is ruled out during an encounter code Z04.71, Encounter for examination and observation following alleged physical adult abuse, ruled out, or code Z04.72, Encounter for examination and observation following alleged physical child abuse, ruled out, should be used, not a code from T76.

If a suspected case of alleged rape or sexual abuse is ruled out during an encounter code Z04.41, Encounter for examination and observation following alleged ~~physical~~ adult rape ~~abuse, ruled out,~~ or code Z04.42, Encounter for examination and observation following alleged child rape ~~or sexual abuse, ruled out,~~ should be used, not a code from T76.

See Section I.C.15. Abuse in a pregnant patient.

g.　Complications of care

1)　General guidelines for complications of care

(a)　Documentation of complications of care

See section I.B.16. for information on documentation of complications of care.

2)　Pain due to medical devices

Pain associated with devices, implants or grafts left in a surgical site (for example painful hip prosthesis) is assigned to the appropriate code(s) found in Chapter 19, Injury, poisoning, and certain other consequences of external causes. Specific codes for pain due to medical devices are found in the T code section of the ICD-10-CM. Use additional code(s) from category G89 to identify acute or chronic pain due to presence of the device, implant or graft (G89.18 or G89.28).

3)　Transplant complications

(a)　Transplant complications other than kidney

Codes under category T86, Complications of transplanted organs and tissues, are for use for both complications and rejection of transplanted organs. A transplant complication code is only assigned if the complication affects the function of the transplanted organ. Two codes are required to fully describe a transplant complication: the appropriate code from category T86 and a secondary code that identifies the complication.

Pre-existing conditions or conditions that develop after the transplant are not coded as complications unless they affect the function of the transplanted organs.

See I.C.21. for transplant organ removal status.
See I.C.2. for malignant neoplasm associated with transplanted organ.

(b)　Kidney transplant complications

Patients who have undergone kidney transplant may still have some form of chronic kidney disease (CKD) because the kidney transplant may not fully restore kidney function. Code T86.1- should be assigned for documented complications of a kidney transplant, such as transplant failure or rejection or other transplant complication. Code T86.1- should not be assigned for post kidney transplant patients who have chronic kidney (CKD) unless a transplant complication such as transplant failure or rejection is documented. If the documentation is unclear as to whether the patient has a complication of the transplant, query the provider.

Conditions that affect the function of the transplanted kidney, other than CKD, should be assigned a code from subcategory T86.1, Complications of transplanted organ, kidney, and a secondary code that identifies the complication.

For patients with CKD following a kidney transplant, but who do not have a complication such as failure or rejection, *see section I.C.14. Chronic kidney disease and kidney transplant status.*

4)　Complication codes that include the external cause

As with certain other T codes, some of the complications of care codes have the external cause included in the code. The code includes the nature of the complication as well as the type of procedure that caused the complication. No external cause code indicating the type of procedure is necessary for these codes.

5)　Complications of care codes within the body system chapters

Intraoperative and postprocedural complication codes are found within the body system chapters with codes specific to the organs and structures of that body system. These codes should be sequenced first, followed by a code(s) for the specific complication, if applicable.

Injuries to the head (S00-S09)

Includes:　Injuries of ear
　　　　　Injuries of eye
　　　　　Injuries of face [any part]
　　　　　Injuries of gum
　　　　　Injuries of jaw
　　　　　Injuries of oral cavity
　　　　　Injuries of palate
　　　　　Injuries of periocular area
　　　　　Injuries of scalp
　　　　　Injuries of temporomandibular joint area
　　　　　Injuries of tongue
　　　　　Injuries of tooth

Code also for any associated infection

Excludes ❷:　burns and corrosions (T20-T32)
　　　　　effects of foreign body in ear (T16)
　　　　　effects of foreign body in larynx (T17.3)
　　　　　effects of foreign body in mouth NOS (T18.0)
　　　　　effects of foreign body in nose (T17.0-T17.1)
　　　　　effects of foreign body in pharynx (T17.2)
　　　　　effects of foreign body on external eye (T15.-)
　　　　　frostbite (T33-T34)
　　　　　insect bite or sting, venomous (T63.4)

S00-　Superficial injury of head

Excludes 1:　diffuse cerebral contusion (S06.2-)
　　　　　focal cerebral contusion (S06.3-)
　　　　　injury of eye and orbit (S05.-)
　　　　　open wound of head (S01.-)

The appropriate 7th character is to be added to each code from category S00:
　A　**Initial** encounter
　D　**Subsequent** encounter
　S　**Sequela**

S00.0-　Superficial injury of scalp

S00.00x-　Unspecified superficial injury of scalp

S00.01x-　Abrasion of scalp

S00.02x-　Blister (nonthermal) of scalp

S00.03x-　Contusion of scalp
　　　　Bruise of scalp
　　　　Hematoma of scalp

S00.04x-　External constriction of part of scalp

S00.05x-　Superficial foreign body of scalp
　　　　Splinter in the scalp

S00.06x-　Insect bite (nonvenomous) of scalp

S00.07x-　Other superficial bite of scalp
　　　　Excludes 1:　open bite of scalp (S01.05)

S00.1-　Contusion of eyelid and periocular area
　　　Black eye
　　　Excludes ❷:　contusion of eyeball and orbital tissues (S05.1)

S00.10x-　Contusion of unspecified eyelid and periocular area

S00.11x-　Contusion of right eyelid and periocular area

S00.12x-　Contusion of left eyelid and periocular area

S00.2-　Other and unspecified superficial injuries of eyelid and periocular area
　　　Excludes ❷:　superficial injury of conjunctiva and cornea (S05.0-)

S00.20-　Unspecified superficial injury of eyelid and periocular area

　S00.201-　Unspecified superficial injury of right eyelid and periocular area

　S00.202-　Unspecified superficial injury of left eyelid and periocular area

S 0 0 l S 0 0

S00.209- Unspecified superficial injury of <u>unspecified</u> eyelid and periocular area

S00.21- <u>Abrasion</u> of eyelid and periocular area

S00.211- Abrasion of <u>right</u> eyelid and periocular area

S00.212- Abrasion of <u>left</u> eyelid and periocular area

S00.219- Abrasion of <u>unspecified</u> eyelid and periocular area

S00.22- <u>Blister</u> (nonthermal) of eyelid and periocular area

S00.221- Blister (nonthermal) of <u>right</u> eyelid and periocular area

S00.222- Blister (nonthermal) of <u>left</u> eyelid and periocular area

S00.229- Blister (nonthermal) of <u>unspecified</u> eyelid and periocular area

S00.24- <u>External constriction</u> of eyelid and periocular area

S00.241- External constriction of <u>right</u> eyelid and periocular area

S00.242- External constriction of <u>left</u> eyelid and periocular area

S00.249- External constriction of <u>unspecified</u> eyelid and periocular area

S00.25- <u>Superficial foreign body</u> of eyelid and periocular area
  Splinter of eyelid and periocular area
  Excludes ❷: retained foreign body in eyelid (H02.81-)

S00.251- Superficial foreign body of <u>right</u> eyelid and periocular area

S00.252- Superficial foreign body of <u>left</u> eyelid and periocular area

S00.259- Superficial foreign body of <u>unspecified</u> eyelid and periocular area

S00.26- <u>Insect bite (nonvenomous)</u> of eyelid and periocular area

S00.261- Insect bite (nonvenomous) of <u>right</u> eyelid and periocular area

S00.262- Insect bite (nonvenomous) of <u>left</u> eyelid and periocular area

S00.269- Insect bite (nonvenomous) of <u>unspecified</u> eyelid and periocular area

S00.27- <u>Other superficial bite</u> of eyelid and periocular area
  Excludes 1:   open bite of eyelid and periocular area (S01.15)

S00.271- Other superficial bite of <u>right</u> eyelid and periocular area

S00.272- Other superficial bite of <u>left</u> eyelid and periocular area

S00.279- Other superficial bite of <u>unspecified</u> eyelid and periocular area

S00.3- Superficial injury of <u>nose</u>

S00.30x- Unspecified superficial injury of nose

S00.31x- Abrasion of nose

S00.32x- Blister (nonthermal) of nose

S00.33x- Contusion of nose
  Bruise of nose
  Hematoma of nose

S00.34x- External constriction of nose

S00.35x- Superficial foreign body of nose
  Splinter in the nose

S00.36x- Insect bite (nonvenomous) of nose

S00.37x- Other superficial bite of nose
  Excludes 1:   open bite of nose (S01.25)

S00.4- Superficial injury of <u>ear</u>

S00.40- <u>Unspecified</u> superficial injury of ear

S00.401- Unspecified superficial injury of <u>right</u> ear

S00.402- Unspecified superficial injury of <u>left</u> ear

S00.409- Unspecified superficial injury of <u>unspecified</u> ear

S00.41- <u>Abrasion</u> of ear

S00.411- Abrasion of <u>right</u> ear

S00.412- Abrasion of <u>left</u> ear

S00.419- Abrasion of <u>unspecified</u> ear

S00.42- <u>Blister</u> (nonthermal) of ear

S00.421- Blister (nonthermal) of <u>right</u> ear

S00.422- Blister (nonthermal) of <u>left</u> ear

S00.429- Blister (nonthermal) of <u>unspecified</u> ear

S00.43- <u>Contusion</u> of ear
  Bruise of ear
  Hematoma of ear

S00.431- Contusion of <u>right</u> ear

S00.432- Contusion of <u>left</u> ear

S00.439- Contusion of <u>unspecified</u> ear

S00.44- <u>External constriction</u> of ear

S00.441- External constriction of <u>right</u> ear

S00.442- External constriction of <u>left</u> ear

S00.449- External constriction of <u>unspecified</u> ear

S00.45- <u>Superficial foreign body</u> of ear
  Splinter in the ear

S00.451- Superficial foreign body of <u>right</u> ear

S00.452- Superficial foreign body of <u>left</u> ear

S00.459- Superficial foreign body of <u>unspecified</u> ear

S00.46- <u>Insect bite (nonvenomous)</u> of ear

S00.461- Insect bite (nonvenomous) of <u>right</u> ear

S00.462- Insect bite (nonvenomous) of <u>left</u> ear

S00.469- Insect bite (nonvenomous) of <u>unspecified</u> ear

S00.47- <u>Other superficial bite</u> of ear
  Excludes 1:   open bite of ear (S01.35)

S00.471- Other superficial bite of <u>right</u> ear

S00.472- Other superficial bite of <u>left</u> ear

S00.479- Other superficial bite of <u>unspecified</u> ear

S00.5- Superficial injury of <u>lip and oral cavity</u>

S00.50- <u>Unspecified</u> superficial injury of lip and oral cavity

S00.501- Unspecified superficial injury of <u>lip</u>

S00.502- Unspecified superficial injury of <u>oral cavity</u>

S00.51- <u>Abrasion</u> of lip and oral cavity

S00.511- Abrasion of lip

S00.512- Abrasion of oral <u>cavity</u>

S00.52- <u>Blister</u> (nonthermal) of lip and oral cavity

S00.521- Blister (nonthermal) of <u>lip</u>

S00.522- Blister (nonthermal) of <u>oral cavity</u>

S00.53- <u>Contusion</u> of lip and oral cavity

S00.531- Contusion of <u>lip</u>
  Bruise of lip
  Hematoma of oral cavity

S00.532- Contusion of <u>oral cavity</u>
  Bruise of lip
  Hematoma of oral cavity

S00.54- <u>External constriction</u> of lip and oral cavity

S00.541- External constriction of <u>lip</u>

S00.542- External constriction of <u>oral cavity</u>

S00.55- <u>Superficial foreign body</u> of lip and oral cavity

S00.551- Superficial foreign body of <u>lip</u>
  Splinter of lip and oral cavity

S00.552- Superficial foreign body of <u>oral cavity</u>
  Splinter of lip and oral cavity

S00.56- <u>Insect bite (nonvenomous)</u> of lip and oral cavity

S00.561- Insect bite (nonvenomous) of <u>lip</u>

S00.562- Insect bite (nonvenomous) of <u>oral cavity</u>

S00.57- <u>Other superficial bite</u> of lip and oral cavity

S00.571- Other superficial bite of <u>lip</u>
  Excludes 1:   open bite of lip (S01.551)

S00.572- Other superficial bite of <u>oral cavity</u>
  Excludes 1:   open bite of oral cavity (S01.552)

S00.8- <u>Superficial injury of other parts of head</u>
  Superficial injuries of face [any part]

S00.80x- Unspecified superficial injury of other part of head

S00.81x- Abrasion of other part of head

S00.82x- Blister (nonthermal) of other part of head

S00.83x- Contusion of other part of head
    Bruise of other part of head
    Hematoma of other part of head

S00.84x- External constriction of other part of head

S00.85x- Superficial foreign body of other part of head
    Splinter in other part of head

S00.86x- Insect bite (nonvenomous) of other part of head

S00.87x- Other superficial bite of other part of head
    Excludes 1:   *open bite of other part of head (S01.85)*

S00.9- Superficial injury of unspecified part of head

S00.90x- Unspecified superficial injury of unspecified part of head

S00.91x- Abrasion of unspecified part of head

S00.92x- Blister (nonthermal) of unspecified part of head

S00.93x- Contusion of unspecified part of head
    Bruise of head
    Hematoma of head

S00.94x- External constriction of unspecified part of head

S00.95x- Superficial foreign body of unspecified part of head
    Splinter of head

S00.96x- Insect bite (nonvenomous) of unspecified part of head

S00.97x- Other superficial bite of unspecified part of head
    Excludes 1:   *open bite of head (S01.95)*

S01- Open wound of head
Code also any associated:
    Injury of cranial nerve (S04.-)
    Injury of muscle and tendon of head (S09.1-)
    Intracranial injury (S06.-)
    Wound infection
    Excludes 1:   *open skull fracture (S02.- with 7th character B)*
    Excludes ❷: *injury of eye and orbit (S05.-)*
               traumatic amputation of part of head (S08.-)

> The appropriate 7th character is to be added to each code from category S01:
> **A**   Initial encounter
> **D**   Subsequent encounter
> **S**   Sequela

S01.0- Open wound of scalp
    Excludes 1:   *avulsion of scalp (S08.0)*

S01.00x- Unspecified open wound of scalp

S01.01x- Laceration without foreign body of scalp

S01.02x- Laceration with foreign body of scalp
    AHA 15:1Q:p5 – Laceration with foreign body of scalp

S01.03x- Puncture wound without foreign body of scalp

S01.04x- Puncture wound with foreign body of scalp

S01.05x- Open bite of scalp
    Bite of scalp NOS
    Excludes 1:   *superficial bite of scalp (S00.06, S00.07-)*

S01.1- Open wound of eyelid and periocular area
    Open wound of eyelid and periocular area with or without involvement of lacrimal passages

S01.10- Unspecified open wound of eyelid and periocular area

CC-A S01.101- Unspecified open wound of right eyelid and periocular area

CC-A S01.102- Unspecified open wound of left eyelid and periocular area

CC-A S01.109- Unspecified open wound of unspecified eyelid and periocular area

S01.11- Laceration without foreign body of eyelid and periocular area

    S01.111- Laceration without foreign body of right eyelid and periocular area

    S01.112- Laceration without foreign body of left eyelid and periocular area

    S01.119- Laceration without foreign body of unspecified eyelid and periocular area

S01.12- Laceration with foreign body of eyelid and periocular area

    S01.121- Laceration with foreign body of right eyelid and periocular area

    S01.122- Laceration with foreign body of left eyelid and periocular area

    S01.129- Laceration with foreign body of unspecified eyelid and periocular area

S01.13- Puncture wound without foreign body of eyelid and periocular area

    S01.131- Puncture wound without foreign body of right eyelid and periocular area

    S01.132- Puncture wound without foreign body of left eyelid and periocular area

    S01.139- Puncture wound without foreign body of unspecified eyelid and periocular area

S01.14- Puncture wound with foreign body of eyelid and periocular area

    S01.141- Puncture wound with foreign body of right eyelid and periocular area

    S01.142- Puncture wound with foreign body of left eyelid and periocular area

    S01.149- Puncture wound with foreign body of unspecified eyelid and periocular area

S01.15- Open bite of eyelid and periocular area
    Bite of eyelid and periocular area NOS
    Excludes 1:   *superficial bite of eyelid and periocular area (S00.26, S00.27)*

    S01.151- Open bite of right eyelid and periocular area

    S01.152- Open bite of left eyelid and periocular area

    S01.159- Open bite of unspecified eyelid and periocular area

S01.2- Open wound of nose

S01.20x- Unspecified open wound of nose

S01.21x- Laceration without foreign body of nose
    AHA 15:1Q:p5 – Laceration body of nose

S01.22x- Laceration with foreign body of nose

S01.23x- Puncture wound without foreign body of nose

S01.24x- Puncture wound with foreign body of nose

S01.25x- Open bite of nose
    Bite of nose NOS
    Excludes 1:   *superficial bite of nose (S00.36, S00.37)*

S01.3- Open wound of ear

S01.30- Unspecified open wound of ear

    S01.301- Unspecified open wound of right ear

    S01.302- Unspecified open wound of left ear

    S01.309- Unspecified open wound of unspecified ear

S01.31- Laceration without foreign body of ear

    S01.311- Laceration without foreign body of right ear

    S01.312- Laceration without foreign body of left ear

    S01.319- Laceration without foreign body of unspecified ear

S01.32- Laceration with foreign body of ear

    S01.321- Laceration with foreign body of right ear

    S01.322- Laceration with foreign body of left ear

    S01.329- Laceration with foreign body of unspecified ear

S01.33- Puncture wound without foreign body of ear

    S01.331- Puncture wound without foreign body of right ear

    S01.332- Puncture wound without foreign body of left ear

    S01.339- Puncture wound without foreign body of unspecified ear

S01.34- Puncture wound with foreign body of ear

    S01.341- Puncture wound with foreign body of right ear

    S01.342- Puncture wound with foreign body of left ear

    S01.349- Puncture wound with foreign body of unspecified ear

S01.35- Open bite of ear
    Bite of ear NOS
    Excludes 1:   *superficial bite of ear (S00.46, S00.47)*

    S01.351- Open bite of right ear

    S01.352- Open bite of left ear

    S01.359- Open bite of unspecified ear

S00 - S01

S01.4- Open wound of <u>cheek and temporomandibular area</u>

S01.40- <u>Unspecified</u> open wound of cheek and temporomandibular area

S01.401- Unspecified open wound of <u>right</u> cheek and temporomandibular area

S01.402- Unspecified open wound of <u>left</u> cheek and temporomandibular area

S01.409- Unspecified open wound of <u>unspecified</u> cheek and temporomandibular area

S01.41- <u>Laceration</u> <u>without</u> foreign body of cheek and temporomandibular area

S01.411- Laceration <u>without</u> foreign body of <u>right</u> cheek and temporomandibular area
AHA 15:1Q:p5 – Laceration of cheek

S01.412- Laceration <u>without</u> foreign body of <u>left</u> cheek and temporomandibular area

S01.419- Laceration <u>without</u> foreign body of <u>unspecified</u> cheek and temporomandibular area

S01.42- <u>Laceration</u> <u>with foreign body</u> of cheek and temporomandibular area

S01.421- Laceration <u>with foreign body</u> of <u>right</u> cheek and temporomandibular area

S01.422- Laceration <u>with foreign body</u> of <u>left</u> cheek and temporomandibular area

S01.429- Laceration <u>with foreign body</u> of <u>unspecified</u> cheek and temporomandibular area

S01.43- <u>Puncture</u> wound <u>without</u> foreign body of cheek and temporomandibular area

S01.431- Puncture wound <u>without</u> foreign body of <u>right</u> cheek and temporomandibular area

S01.432- Puncture wound <u>without</u> foreign body of <u>left</u> cheek and temporomandibular area

S01.439- Puncture wound <u>without</u> foreign body of <u>unspecified</u> cheek andtemporomandibular area

S01.44- <u>Puncture</u> wound <u>with foreign body</u> of cheek and temporomandibular area

S01.441- Puncture wound <u>with foreign body</u> of <u>right</u> cheek and temporomandibular area

S01.442- Puncture wound <u>with foreign body</u> of <u>left</u> cheek and temporomandibular area

S01.449- Puncture wound <u>with foreign body</u> of <u>unspecified</u> cheek and temporomandibular area

S01.45- <u>Open bite</u> of cheek and temporomandibular area
Bite of cheek and temporomandibular area NOS
Excludes ❷: superficial bite of cheek and temporomandibular area (S00.86, S00.87)

S01.451- Open bite of <u>right</u> cheek and temporomandibular area

S01.452- Open bite of <u>left</u> cheek and temporomandibular area

S01.459- Open bite of <u>unspecified</u> cheek and temporomandibular area

S01.5- Open wound of <u>lip and oral cavity</u>
Excludes ❷: tooth dislocation (S03.2)
tooth fracture (S02.5)

S01.50- <u>Unspecified</u> open wound of lip and oral cavity

S01.501- Unspecified open wound of <u>lip</u>

S01.502- Unspecified open wound of <u>oral cavity</u>

S01.51- <u>Laceration</u> of lip and oral cavity <u>without</u> foreign body

S01.511- Laceration <u>without</u> foreign body of <u>lip</u>

S01.512- Laceration <u>without</u> foreign body of <u>oral cavity</u>

S01.52- <u>Laceration</u> of lip and oral cavity <u>with foreign body</u>

S01.521- Laceration <u>with foreign body</u> of <u>lip</u>

S01.522- Laceration <u>with foreign body</u> of <u>oral cavity</u>

S01.53- <u>Puncture</u> wound of lip and oral cavity <u>without</u> foreign body

S01.531- Puncture wound <u>without</u> foreign body of <u>lip</u>

S01.532- Puncture wound <u>without</u> foreign body of <u>oral cavity</u>

S01.54- <u>Puncture</u> wound of lip and oral cavity <u>with foreign body</u>

S01.541- Puncture wound <u>with foreign body</u> of <u>lip</u>

S01.542- Puncture wound <u>with foreign body</u> of <u>oral cavity</u>

S01.55- <u>Open bite</u> of lip and oral cavity

S01.551- Open bite of <u>lip</u>
Bite of lip NOS
Excludes 1: superficial bite of lip (S00.571)

S01.552- Open bite of <u>oral cavity</u>
Bite of oral cavity NOS
Excludes 1: superficial bite of oral cavity (S00.572)

S01.8- Open wound of <u>other parts of head</u>

S01.80x- Unspecified open wound of other part of head

S01.81x- Laceration <u>without</u> foreign body of other part of head

S01.82x- Laceration <u>with foreign body</u> of other part of head

S01.83x- Puncture wound <u>without</u> foreign body of other part of head

S01.84x- Puncture wound <u>with foreign body</u> of other part of head

S01.85x- Open bite of other part of head
Bite of other part of head NOS
Excludes 1: superficial bite of other part of head (S00.85)

S01.9- Open wound of <u>unspecified part of head</u>

S01.90x- Unspecified open wound of unspecified part of head

S01.91x- Laceration <u>without</u> foreign body of unspecified part of head

S01.92x- Laceration <u>with foreign body</u> of unspecified part of head

S01.93x- Puncture wound <u>without</u> foreign body of unspecified part of head

S01.94x- Puncture wound <u>with foreign body</u> of unspecified part of head

S01.95x- Open bite of unspecified part of head
Bite of head NOS
Excludes 1: superficial bite of head NOS (S00.97)

S02- <u>Fracture of skull and facial bones</u>
Note: A fracture not indicated as open or closed should be coded to closed
Code also any associated intracranial injury (S06.-)

The appropriate 7th character is to be added to each code from category S02:
A <u>Initial</u> encounter for <u>closed</u> fracture
B <u>Initial</u> encounter for <u>open</u> fracture
D <u>Subsequent</u> encounter for fracture <u>with routine healing</u>
G <u>Subsequent</u> encounter for fracture <u>with delayed healing</u>
K <u>Subsequent</u> encounter for fracture <u>with nonunion</u>
S <u>Sequela</u>

S02.0xx- Fracture of <u>vault</u> of skull
CC-A,K MCC-B Fracture of frontal bone
Fracture of parietal bone

S02.1- Fracture of <u>base</u> of skull
Excludes 1: orbit NOS (S02.8)
Excludes ❷: orbital floor (S02.3-)

S02.10- <u>Unspecified</u> fracture of base of skull
CC-A,K MCC-B **S02.101-** Fracture of base of skull, <u>right</u> side
CC-A,K MCC-B **S02.102-** Fracture of base of skull, <u>left</u> side
CC-A,K MCC-B **S02.109-** Fracture of base of skull, <u>unspecified</u> side

S02.11- Fracture of <u>occiput</u>
CC-A,K MCC-B **S02.110-** Type I occipital condyle fracture, <u>unspecified</u> side
CC-A,K MCC-B **S02.111-** Type II occipital condyle fracture, <u>unspecified</u> side
CC-A,K MCC-B **S02.112-** Type III occipital condyle fracture, <u>unspecified</u> side
CC-A,K MCC-B **S02.113-** Unspecified occipital condyle fracture
CC-A,K MCC-B **S02.118-** Other fracture of occiput, <u>unspecified</u> side
CC-A,K MCC-B **S02.119-** Unspecified fracture of occiput
CC-A,K MCC-B **S02.11A-** Type I occipital condyle fracture, <u>right</u> side
CC-A,K MCC-B **S02.11B-** Type I occipital condyle fracture, <u>left</u> side
CC-A,K MCC-B **S02.11C-** Type II occipital condyle fracture, <u>right</u> side
CC-A,K MCC-B **S02.11D-** Type II occipital condyle fracture, <u>left</u> side
CC-A,K MCC-B **S02.11E-** Type III occipital condyle fracture, <u>right</u> side
CC-A,K MCC-B **S02.11F-** Type III occipital condyle fracture, <u>left</u> side
CC-A,K MCC-B **S02.11G-** Other fracture of occiput, <u>right</u> side

S01 -S02

CC-A,K MCC-B **S02.11H-** Other fracture of occiput, **left** side

S02.19x- **Other** fracture of **base** of skull

CC-A,K MCC-B Fracture of anterior fossa of base of skull
Fracture of ethmoid sinus
Fracture of frontal sinus
Fracture of middle fossa of base of skull
Fracture of orbital roof
Fracture of posterior fossa of base of skull
Fracture of sphenoid
Fracture of temporal bone

S02.2xx- Fracture of **nasal bones**
CC-B,K

S02.3- Fracture of **orbital floor**
Excludes 1: *orbit NOS (S02.8)*
Excludes ❷: *orbital roof (S02.1-)*

CC-A,B,K **S02.30x-** Fracture of orbital floor, **unspecified** side

CC-A,B,K **S02.31x-** Fracture of orbital floor, **right** side

CC-A,B,K **S02.32x-** Fracture of orbital floor, **left** side

S02.4- Fracture of **malar, maxillary and zygoma bones**
Fracture of superior maxilla
Fracture of upper jaw (bone)
Fracture of zygomatic process of temporal bone

S02.40- Fracture of malar, maxillary and zygoma bones, **unspecified**

CC-A,B,K **S02.400-** Malar fracture, **unspecified** side

CC-A,B,K **S02.401-** Maxillary fracture, **unspecified** side

CC-A,B,K **S02.402-** Zygomatic fracture, **unspecified** side

CC-A,B,K **S02.40A-** Malar fracture, **right** side

CC-A,B,K **S02.40B-** Malar fracture, **left** side

CC-A,B,K **S02.40C-** Maxillary fracture, **right** side

CC-A,B,K **S02.40D-** Maxillary fracture, **left** side

CC-A,B,K **S02.40E-** Zygomatic fracture, **right** side

CC-A,B,K **S02.40F-** Zygomatic fracture, **left** side

S02.41- **LeFort** fracture

CC-A,B,K **S02.411-** LeFort I fracture

CC-A,B,K **S02.412-** LeFort II fracture

CC-A,B,K **S02.413-** LeFort III fracture

CC-A,B,K **S02.42x-** Fracture of **alveolus of maxilla**

S02.5xx- Fracture of **tooth (traumatic)**
CC-K Broken tooth
Excludes 1: *cracked tooth (nontraumatic) (K03.81)*

S02.6- Fracture of **mandible**
Fracture of lower jaw (bone)

S02.60- Fracture of mandible, unspecified

CC-A,B,K **S02.600-** Fracture of **unspecified part of body** of mandible, **unspecified** side

CC-A,B,K **S02.601-** Fracture of **unspecified part of body** of **right** mandible

CC-A,B,K **S02.602-** Fracture of **unspecified part of body** of **left** mandible

CC-A,B,K **S02.609-** Fracture of mandible, **unspecified**

S02.61- Fracture of **condylar process** of mandible

CC-A,B,K **S02.610-** Fracture of condylar process of mandible, **unspecified** side

CC-A,B,K **S02.611-** Fracture of condylar process of **right** mandible

CC-A,B,K **S02.612-** Fracture of condylar process of **left** mandible

S02.62- Fracture of **subcondylar process** of mandible

CC-A,B,K **S02.620-** Fracture of subcondylar process of mandible, **unspecified** side

CC-A,B,K **S02.621-** Fracture of subcondylar process of **right** mandible

CC-A,B,K **S02.622-** Fracture of subcondylar process of **left** mandible

S02.63- Fracture of **coronoid process** of mandible

CC-A,B,K **S02.630-** Fracture of coronoid process of mandible, **unspecified** side

CC-A,B,K **S02.631-** Fracture of coronoid process of **right** mandible

CC-A,B,K **S02.632-** Fracture of coronoid process of **left** mandible

S02.64- Fracture of **ramus** of mandible

CC-A,B,K **S02.640-** Fracture of ramus of mandible, **unspecified** side

CC-A,B,K **S02.641-** Fracture of ramus of **right** mandible

CC-A,B,K **S02.642-** Fracture of ramus of **left** mandible

S02.65- Fracture of **angle** of mandible

CC-A,B,K **S02.650-** Fracture of angle of mandible, **unspecified** side

CC-A,B,K **S02.651-** Fracture of angle of **right** mandible

CC-A,B,K **S02.652-** Fracture of angle of **left** mandible

CC-A,B,K **S02.66x-** Fracture of symphysis of mandible

S02.67- Fracture of **alveolus** of mandible

CC-A,B,K **S02.670-** Fracture of alveolus of mandible, **unspecified** side

CC-A,B,K **S02.671-** Fracture of alveolus of **right** mandible

CC-A,B,K **S02.672-** Fracture of alveolus of **left** mandible

CC-A,B,K **S02.69x-** Fracture of mandible of other specified site

S02.8- Fractures of **other specified skull and facial bones**
Fracture of orbit NOS
Fracture of palate
Excludes 1: *fracture of orbital floor (S02.3-)*
fracture of orbital roof (S02.1-)

CC-A,B,K **S02.80x-** Fracture of other specified skull and facial bones, **unspecified** side

CC-A,B,K **S02.81x-** Fracture of other specified skull and facial bones, **right** side

CC-A,B,K **S02.82x-** Fracture of other specified skull and facial bones, **left** side

S02.9- Fracture of **unspecified** skull and facial bones

S02.91x- Unspecified fracture of **skull**
CC-A,K MCC-B

S02.92x- Unspecified fracture of **facial bones**
CC-A,B,K

S03- **Dislocation and sprain** of joints and ligaments of **head**
Includes: Avulsion of joint (capsule) or ligament of head
Laceration of cartilage, joint (capsule) or ligament of head
Sprain of cartilage, joint (capsule) or ligament of head
Traumatic hemarthrosis of joint or ligament of head
Traumatic rupture of joint or ligament of head
Traumatic subluxation of joint or ligament of head
Traumatic tear of joint or ligament of head
Code also any associated open wound
Excludes ❷: *Strain of muscle or tendon of head (S09.1)*

The appropriate 7th character is to be added to each code from category S03:
A **Initial** encounter
D **Subsequent** encounter
S **Sequela**

S03.0- **Dislocation** of **jaw**
Dislocation of jaw (cartilage) (meniscus)
Dislocation of mandible
Dislocation of temporomandibular (joint)

S03.00x- Dislocation of jaw, **unspecified** side

S03.01x- Dislocation of jaw, **right** side

S03.02x- Dislocation of jaw, **left** side

S03.03x- Dislocation of jaw, **bilateral**

S03.1xx- Dislocation of septal cartilage of nose

S03.2xx- Dislocation of tooth

S03.4- **Sprain** of **jaw**
Sprain of temporomandibular (joint) (ligament)

S03.40x- Sprain of jaw, **unspecified** side

S03.41x- Sprain of jaw, **right** side

S03.42x- Sprain of jaw, **left** side

S03.43x- Sprain of jaw, **bilateral**

S03.8xx- Sprain of joints and ligaments of **other** parts of head

S03.9xx- Sprain of joints and ligaments of **unspecified** parts of head

S 0 2 - S 0 3

S04- **Injury** of <u>cranial nerve</u>
The selection of side should be based on the side of the body being affected
Code first any associated intracranial injury (S06.-)
Code also any associated:
Open wound of head (S01.-)
Skull fracture (S02.-)

The appropriate 7th character is to be added to each code from category S04:
- **A** <u>Initial</u> encounter
- **D** <u>Subsequent</u> encounter
- **S** <u>Sequela</u>

S04.0- **Injury** of <u>optic nerve and pathways</u>
Use additional code to identify any visual field defect or blindness (H53.4-, H54)

S04.01- Injury of <u>optic nerve</u>
Injury of <u>2nd</u> cranial nerve

CC-A **S04.011-** Injury of optic nerve, <u>right</u> eye

CC-A **S04.012-** Injury of optic nerve, <u>left</u> eye

CC-A **S04.019-** Injury of optic nerve, <u>unspecified</u> eye
Injury of optic nerve NOS

CC-A **S04.02x-** Injury of <u>optic chiasm</u>

S04.03- Injury of <u>optic tract and pathways</u>
Injury of optic radiation

CC-A **S04.031-** Injury of optic tract and pathways, <u>right</u> eye

CC-A **S04.032-** Injury of optic tract and pathways, <u>left</u> eye

CC-A **S04.039-** Injury of optic tract and pathways, <u>unspecified</u> eye
Injury of optic tract and pathways NOS

S04.04- Injury of <u>visual cortex</u>

CC-A **S04.041-** Injury of visual cortex, <u>right</u> eye

CC-A **S04.042-** Injury of visual cortex, <u>left</u> eye

CC-A **S04.049-** Injury of visual cortex, <u>unspecified</u> eye
Injury of visual cortex NOS

S04.1- Injury of <u>oculomotor nerve</u>
Injury of <u>3rd</u> cranial nerve

CC-A **S04.10x-** Injury of oculomotor nerve, <u>unspecified</u> side

CC-A **S04.11x-** Injury of oculomotor nerve, <u>right</u> side

CC-A **S04.12x-** Injury of oculomotor nerve, <u>left</u> side

S04.2- Injury of <u>trochlear nerve</u>
Injury of <u>4th</u> cranial nerve

CC-A **S04.20x-** Injury of trochlear nerve, <u>unspecified</u> side

CC-A **S04.21x-** Injury of trochlear nerve, <u>right</u> side

CC-A **S04.22x-** Injury of trochlear nerve, <u>left</u> side

S04.3- Injury of <u>trigeminal nerve</u>
Injury of <u>5th</u> cranial nerve

CC-A **S04.30x-** Injury of trigeminal nerve, <u>unspecified</u> side

CC-A **S04.31x-** Injury of trigeminal nerve, <u>right</u> side

CC-A **S04.32x-** Injury of trigeminal nerve, <u>left</u> side

S04.4- Injury of <u>abducent nerve</u>
Injury of <u>6th</u> cranial nerve

CC-A **S04.40x-** Injury of abducent nerve, <u>unspecified</u> side

CC-A **S04.41x-** Injury of abducent nerve, <u>right</u> side

CC-A **S04.42x-** Injury of abducent nerve, <u>left</u> side

S04.5- Injury of <u>facial nerve</u>
Injury of <u>7th</u> cranial nerve

CC-A **S04.50x-** Injury of facial nerve, <u>unspecified</u> side

CC-A **S04.51x-** Injury of facial nerve, <u>right</u> side

CC-A **S04.52x-** Injury of facial nerve, <u>left</u> side

S04.6- Injury of <u>acoustic nerve</u>
Injury of auditory nerve
Injury of <u>8th</u> cranial nerve

CC-A **S04.60x-** Injury of acoustic nerve, <u>unspecified</u> side

CC-A **S04.61x-** Injury of acoustic nerve, <u>right</u> side

CC-A **S04.62x-** Injury of acoustic nerve, <u>left</u> side

S04.7- Injury of <u>accessory nerve</u>
Injury of <u>11th</u> cranial nerve

CC-A **S04.70x-** Injury of accessory nerve, <u>unspecified</u> side

CC-A **S04.71x-** Injury of accessory nerve, <u>right</u> side

CC-A **S04.72x-** Injury of accessory nerve, <u>left</u> side

S04.8- Injury of other cranial nerves

S04.81- Injury of <u>olfactory [1st] nerve</u>

CC-A **S04.811-** Injury of olfactory [1st] nerve, <u>right</u> side

CC-A **S04.812-** Injury of olfactory [1st] nerve, <u>left</u> side

CC-A **S04.819-** Injury of olfactory [1st] nerve, <u>unspecified</u> side

S04.89- Injury of <u>other cranial nerves</u>
Injury of vagus [10th] nerve

CC-A **S04.891-** Injury of other cranial nerves, <u>right</u> side

CC-A **S04.892-** Injury of other cranial nerves, <u>left</u> side

CC-A **S04.899-** Injury of other cranial nerves, <u>unspecified</u> side

S04.9xx- Injury of <u>unspecified</u> cranial nerve
CC-A

S05- Injury of <u>eye and orbit</u>
Includes: Open wound of eye and orbit
Excludes ❷: 2nd cranial [optic] nerve injury (S04.0-)
3rd cranial [oculomotor] nerve injury (S04.1-)
open wound of eyelid and periocular area (S01.1-)
orbital bone fracture (S02.1-, S02.3-, S02.8-)
superficial injury of eyelid (S00.1-S00.2)

The appropriate 7th character is to be added to each code from category S05:
- **A** <u>Initial</u> encounter
- **D** <u>Subsequent</u> encounter
- **S** <u>Sequela</u>

S05.0- Injury of <u>conjunctiva and corneal abrasion</u> <u>without</u> foreign body
Excludes 1: foreign body in conjunctival sac (T15.1)
foreign body in cornea (T15.0)

S05.00x- Injury of conjunctiva and corneal abrasion <u>without</u> foreign body, <u>unspecified</u> eye

S05.01x- Injury of conjunctiva and corneal abrasion <u>without</u> foreign body, <u>right</u> eye

S05.02x- Injury of conjunctiva and corneal abrasion <u>without</u> foreign body, <u>left</u> eye

S05.1- <u>Contusion</u> of <u>eyeball and orbital tissues</u>
Traumatic hyphema
Excludes ❷: black eye NOS (S00.1)
contusion of eyelid and periocular area (S00.1)

S05.10x- Contusion of eyeball and orbital tissues, <u>unspecified</u> eye

S05.11x- Contusion of eyeball and orbital tissues, <u>right</u> eye

S05.12x- Contusion of eyeball and orbital tissues, <u>left</u> eye

S05.2- <u>Ocular laceration and rupture</u> <u>with prolapse or loss of intraocular tissue</u>

CC-A **S05.20x-** Ocular laceration and rupture with prolapse or loss of intraocular tissue, <u>unspecified</u> eye

CC-A **S05.21x-** Ocular laceration and rupture with prolapse or loss of intraocular tissue, <u>right</u> eye

CC-A **S05.22x-** Ocular laceration and rupture with prolapse or loss of intraocular tissue, <u>left</u> eye

S05.3- <u>Ocular laceration</u> <u>without</u> prolapse or loss of intraocular tissue
Laceration of eye NOS

CC-A **S05.30x-** Ocular laceration <u>without</u> prolapse or loss of intraocular tissue, <u>unspecified</u> eye

CC-A **S05.31x-** Ocular laceration <u>without</u> prolapse or loss of intraocular tissue, <u>right</u> eye

CC-A **S05.32x-** Ocular laceration <u>without</u> prolapse or loss of intraocular tissue, <u>left</u> eye

S05.4- <u>Penetrating wound</u> of orbit <u>with or without</u> foreign body
Excludes ❷: retained (old) foreign body following penetrating wound in orbit (H05.5-)

CC-A **S05.40x-** Penetrating wound of orbit with or <u>without</u> foreign body, <u>unspecified</u> eye

CC-A **S05.41x-** Penetrating wound of orbit with or <u>without</u> foreign body, <u>right</u> eye

CC-A **S05.42x-** Penetrating wound of orbit with or <u>without</u> foreign body, <u>left</u> eye

S04
-
S05

© 2016 Channel Publishing Ltd

S05.5-   <u>Penetrating wound</u> <u>with foreign body of eyeball</u>
     Excludes ❷: retained (old) intraocular foreign body (H44.6-, H44.7)

CC-A **S05.50x-**   Penetrating wound <u>with foreign body</u> of <u>unspecified</u> eyeball

CC-A **S05.51x-**   Penetrating wound <u>with foreign body</u> of <u>right</u> eyeball

CC-A **S05.52x-**   Penetrating wound <u>with foreign body</u> of <u>left</u> eyeball

S05.6-   <u>Penetrating wound</u> <u>without</u> foreign body of eyeball
     Ocular penetration NOS

     S05.60x-   Penetrating wound <u>without</u> foreign body of <u>unspecified</u> eyeball

     S05.61x-   Penetrating wound <u>without</u> foreign body of <u>right</u> eyeball

     S05.62x-   Penetrating wound <u>without</u> foreign body of <u>left</u> eyeball

S05.7-   <u>Avulsion</u> of eye
     Traumatic enucleation

CC-A **S05.70x-**   Avulsion of <u>unspecified</u> eye

CC-A **S05.71x-**   Avulsion of <u>right</u> eye

CC-A **S05.72x-**   Avulsion of <u>left</u> eye

S05.8-   <u>Other injuries</u> of eye and orbit
     Lacrimal duct injury

     S05.8x-   <u>Other</u> injuries of eye and orbit

CC-A **S05.8x1-**   Other injuries of <u>right</u> eye and orbit

CC-A **S05.8x2-**   Other injuries of <u>left</u> eye and orbit

CC-A **S05.8x9-**   Other injuries of <u>unspecified</u> eye and orbit

S05.9-   <u>Unspecified</u> injury of eye and orbit
     Injury of eye NOS

     S05.90x-   Unspecified injury of <u>unspecified</u> eye and orbit

CC-A **S05.91x-**   Unspecified injury of <u>right</u> eye and orbit

CC-A **S05.92x-**   Unspecified injury of <u>left</u> eye and orbit

S06-   <u>Intracranial injury</u>
     Includes: Traumatic brain injury
     Code also any associated:
       Open wound of head (S01.-)
       Skull fracture (S02.-)
     Excludes 1:   head injury NOS (S09.90)

The appropriate 7th character is to be added to each code from category S06:
     A   <u>Initial</u> **encounter**
     D   <u>Subsequent</u> **encounter**
     S   <u>Sequela</u>

S06.0-   <u>Concussion</u>
     Commotio cerebri
     Excludes 1:   concussion with other intracranial injuries classified in subcategories S06.1- to S06.6-, S06.81- and S06.82- code to specified intracranial injury

     S06.0x-   Concussion

       S06.0x0-   Concussion <u>without</u> loss of consciousness

CC-A   **S06.0x1-**   Concussion <u>with</u> loss of consciousness of <u>30 minutes or less</u>

CC-A   **S06.0x9-**   Concussion <u>with</u> loss of consciousness of <u>unspecified</u> duration
         Concussion NOS

S06.1-   Traumatic cerebral edema
     Diffuse traumatic cerebral edema
     Focal traumatic cerebral edema

     S06.1x-   <u>Traumatic cerebral edema</u>
       AHA 15:1Q:p12 – Traumatic cerebral edema

MCC-A **S06.1x0-**   Traumatic cerebral edema <u>without</u> loss of consciousness

MCC-A **S06.1x1-**   Traumatic cerebral edema <u>with</u> loss of consciousness of <u>30 minutes or less</u>

MCC-A **S06.1x2-**   Traumatic cerebral edema <u>with</u> loss of consciousness of <u>31 minutes to 59 minutes</u>

MCC-A **S06.1x3-**   Traumatic cerebral edema <u>with</u> loss of consciousness of <u>1 hour to 5 hours 59 minutes</u>

MCC-A **S06.1x4-**   Traumatic cerebral edema <u>with</u> loss of consciousness of <u>6 hours to 24 hours</u>

MCC-A **S06.1x5-**   Traumatic cerebral edema <u>with</u> loss of consciousness <u>greater than 24</u> hours <u>with return</u> to pre-existing conscious level

MCC-A **S06.1x6-**   Traumatic cerebral edema <u>with</u> loss of consciousness <u>greater than 24</u> hours <u>without</u> return to pre-existing conscious level <u>with patient surviving</u>

MCC-A **S06.1x7-**   Traumatic cerebral edema <u>with</u> loss of consciousness of <u>any duration with death</u> due to <u>brain injury</u> prior to regaining consciousness

MCC-A **S06.1x8-**   Traumatic cerebral edema <u>with</u> loss of consciousness of <u>any duration with death</u> due to <u>other cause</u> prior to regaining consciousness

MCC-A **S06.1x9-**   Traumatic cerebral edema with loss of consciousness of <u>unspecified</u> duration
         Traumatic cerebral edema NOS

S06.2-   Diffuse traumatic brain injury
     Diffuse axonal brain injury
     Excludes 1:   traumatic diffuse cerebral edema (S06.1x-)

     S06.2x-   <u>Diffuse traumatic brain injury</u>

       S06.2x0-   Diffuse traumatic brain injury <u>without</u> loss of consciousness

CC-A **S06.2x1-**   Diffuse traumatic brain injury <u>with</u> loss of consciousness of <u>30 minutes or less</u>

CC-A **S06.2x2-**   Diffuse traumatic brain injury <u>with</u> loss of consciousness of <u>31 minutes to 59 minutes</u>

CC-A **S06.2x3-**   Diffuse traumatic brain injury <u>with</u> loss of consciousness of <u>1 hour to 5 hours 59 minutes</u>

CC-A **S06.2x4-**   Diffuse traumatic brain injury <u>with</u> loss of consciousness of <u>6 hours to 24 hours</u>

CC-A **S06.2x5-**   Diffuse traumatic brain injury <u>with</u> loss of consciousness <u>greater than 24</u> hours <u>with return</u> to pre-existing conscious levels

MCC-A **S06.2x6-**   Diffuse traumatic brain injury <u>with</u> loss of consciousness <u>greater than 24</u> hours <u>without return</u> to pre-existing conscious level <u>with patient surviving</u>

MCC-A **S06.2x7-**   Diffuse traumatic brain injury <u>with</u> loss of consciousness of <u>any duration with death</u> due to <u>brain injury</u> prior to regaining consciousness

MCC-A **S06.2x8-**   Diffuse traumatic brain injury <u>with</u> loss of consciousness of <u>any duration with death</u> due to <u>other cause</u> prior to regaining consciousness

CC-A **S06.2x9-**   Diffuse traumatic brain injury <u>with</u> loss of consciousness of <u>unspecified</u> duration
         Diffuse traumatic brain injury NOS

S06.3-   <u>Focal traumatic brain injury</u>
     Excludes 1:   any condition classifiable to S06.4-S06.6
           focal cerebral edema (S06.1)

     S06.30-   <u>Unspecified</u> focal traumatic brain injury

       S06.300-   Unspecified focal traumatic brain injury <u>without</u> loss of consciousness

CC-A **S06.301-**   Unspecified focal traumatic brain injury <u>with</u> loss of consciousness of <u>30 minutes or less</u>

CC-A **S06.302-**   Unspecified focal traumatic brain injury <u>with</u> loss of consciousness of <u>31 minutes to 59 minutes</u>

CC-A **S06.303-**   Unspecified focal traumatic brain injury <u>with</u> loss of consciousness of <u>1 hour to 5 hours 59 minutes</u>

CC-A **S06.304-**   Unspecified focal traumatic brain injury <u>with</u> loss of consciousness of <u>6 hours to 24 hours</u>

CC-A **S06.305-**   Unspecified focal traumatic brain injury <u>with</u> loss of consciousness <u>greater than 24</u> hours <u>with return</u> to pre-existing conscious level

MCC-A **S06.306-**   Unspecified focal traumatic brain injury <u>with</u> loss of consciousness <u>greater than 24</u> hours <u>without return</u> to pre-existing conscious level <u>with patient surviving</u>

MCC-A **S06.307-**   Unspecified focal traumatic brain injury <u>with</u> loss of consciousness of <u>any duration with death</u> due to <u>brain injury</u> prior to regaining consciousness

MCC-A **S06.308-**   Unspecified focal traumatic brain injury <u>with</u> loss of consciousness of <u>any duration with death</u> due to <u>other cause</u> prior to regaining consciousness

---

Excludes 1: = NOT CODED HERE! (Do not code both)   **1025**   *Excludes ❷:* = Not Included Here

CC-A **S06.309-** Unspecified focal traumatic brain injury <u>with</u> loss of consciousness of <u>unspecified</u> duration
Unspecified focal traumatic brain injury NOS

S06.31- <u>Contusion and laceration</u> of <u>right</u> cerebrum

MCC-A **S06.310-** Contusion and laceration of <u>right</u> cerebrum <u>without</u> loss of consciousness

MCC-A **S06.311-** Contusion and laceration of <u>right</u> cerebrum <u>with</u> loss of consciousness of <u>30 minutes or less</u>

MCC-A **S06.312-** Contusion and laceration of <u>right</u> cerebrum <u>with</u> loss of consciousness of <u>31minutes to 59 minutes</u>

MCC-A **S06.313-** Contusion and laceration of <u>right</u> cerebrum <u>with</u> loss of consciousness of <u>1 hour to 5 hours 59 minutes</u>

MCC-A **S06.314-** Contusion and laceration of <u>right</u> cerebrum <u>with</u> loss of consciousness of <u>6 hours to 24 hours</u>

MCC-A **S06.315-** Contusion and laceration of <u>right</u> cerebrum <u>with</u> loss of consciousness <u>greater than 24</u> hours <u>with return</u> to pre-existing conscious level

MCC-A **S06.316-** Contusion and laceration of <u>right</u> cerebrum <u>with</u> loss of consciousness <u>greater than 24</u> hours <u>without return</u> to pre-existing conscious level <u>with patient surviving</u>

MCC-A **S06.317-** Contusion and laceration of <u>right</u> cerebrum <u>with</u> loss of consciousness of <u>any duration with death</u> due to <u>brain injury</u> prior to regaining consciousness

MCC-A **S06.318-** Contusion and laceration of <u>right</u> cerebrum <u>with</u> loss of consciousness of <u>any duration with death</u> due to <u>other cause</u> prior to regaining consciousness

MCC-A **S06.319-** Contusion and laceration of <u>right</u> cerebrum <u>with</u> loss of consciousness of <u>unspecified</u> duration
Contusion and laceration of right cerebrum NOS

S06.32- <u>Contusion and laceration</u> of <u>left</u> cerebrum

MCC-A **S06.320-** Contusion and laceration of <u>left</u> cerebrum <u>without</u> loss of consciousness

MCC-A **S06.321-** Contusion and laceration of <u>left</u> cerebrum <u>with</u> loss of consciousness of <u>30 minutes or less</u>

MCC-A **S06.322-** Contusion and laceration of <u>left</u> cerebrum <u>with</u> loss of consciousness of <u>31 minutes to 59 minutes</u>

MCC-A **S06.323-** Contusion and laceration of <u>left</u> cerebrum <u>with</u> loss of consciousness of <u>1 hour to 5 hours 59 minutes</u>

MCC-A **S06.324-** Contusion and laceration of <u>left</u> cerebrum <u>with</u> loss of consciousness of <u>6 hours to 24 hours</u>

MCC-A **S06.325-** Contusion and laceration of <u>left</u> cerebrum <u>with</u> loss of consciousness <u>greater than 24</u> hours <u>with return</u> to pre-existing conscious level

MCC-A **S06.326-** Contusion and laceration of <u>left</u> cerebrum <u>with</u> loss of consciousness <u>greater than 24</u> hours <u>without return</u> to pre-existing conscious level <u>with patient surviving</u>

MCC-A **S06.327-** Contusion and laceration of <u>left</u> cerebrum <u>with</u> loss of consciousness of <u>any duration with death</u> due to <u>brain injury</u> prior to regaining consciousness

MCC-A **S06.328-** Contusion and laceration of <u>left</u> cerebrum <u>with</u> loss of consciousness of <u>any duration with death</u> due to <u>other cause</u> prior to regaining consciousness

MCC-A **S06.329-** Contusion and laceration of <u>left</u> cerebrum <u>with</u> loss of consciousness of <u>unspecified</u> duration
Contusion and laceration of left cerebrum NOS

S06.33- <u>Contusion and laceration</u> of cerebrum, <u>unspecified</u>

MCC-A **S06.330-** Contusion and laceration of cerebrum, <u>unspecified</u>, <u>without</u> loss of consciousness

MCC-A **S06.331-** Contusion and laceration of cerebrum, <u>unspecified</u>, <u>with</u> loss of consciousness of <u>30 minutes or less</u>

MCC-A **S06.332-** Contusion and laceration of cerebrum, <u>unspecified</u>, <u>with</u> loss of consciousness of <u>31 minutes to 59 minutes</u>

MCC-A **S06.333-** Contusion and laceration of cerebrum, <u>unspecified</u>, <u>with</u> loss of consciousness of <u>1 hour to 5 hours 59 minutes</u>

MCC-A **S06.334-** Contusion and laceration of cerebrum, <u>unspecified</u>, <u>with</u> loss of consciousness of <u>6 hours to 24 hours</u>

MCC-A **S06.335-** Contusion and laceration of cerebrum, <u>unspecified</u>, <u>with</u> loss of consciousness <u>greater than 24</u> hours <u>with return</u> to pre-existing conscious level

MCC-A **S06.336-** Contusion and laceration of cerebrum, <u>unspecified</u>, <u>with</u> loss of consciousness <u>greater than 24</u> hours <u>without return</u> to pre-existing conscious level <u>with patient surviving</u>

MCC-A **S06.337-** Contusion and laceration of cerebrum, <u>unspecified</u>, <u>with</u> loss of consciousness of <u>any duration with death</u> due to <u>brain injury</u> prior to regaining consciousness

MCC-A **S06.338-** Contusion and laceration of cerebrum, <u>unspecified</u>, <u>with</u> loss of consciousness of <u>any duration with death</u> due to <u>other cause</u> prior to regaining consciousness

MCC-A **S06.339-** Contusion and laceration of cerebrum, <u>unspecified</u>, <u>with</u> loss of consciousness of <u>unspecified</u> duration
Contusion and laceration of cerebrum NOS

S06.34- <u>Traumatic hemorrhage</u> of <u>right</u> cerebrum
AHA 15:1Q:p12 – Right frontal intracranial hemorrhage
Traumatic intracerebral hemorrhage and hematoma of right cerebrum

MCC-A **S06.340-** Traumatic hemorrhage of <u>right</u> cerebrum <u>without</u> loss of consciousness

MCC-A **S06.341-** Traumatic hemorrhage of <u>right</u> cerebrum <u>with</u> loss of consciousness of <u>30 minutes or less</u>

MCC-A **S06.342-** Traumatic hemorrhage of <u>right</u> cerebrum <u>with</u> loss of consciousness of <u>31 minutes to 59 minutes</u>

MCC-A **S06.343-** Traumatic hemorrhage of <u>right</u> cerebrum <u>with</u> loss of consciousness of <u>1 hours to 5 hours 59 minutes</u>

MCC-A **S06.344-** Traumatic hemorrhage of <u>right</u> cerebrum <u>with</u> loss of consciousness of <u>6 hours to 24 hours</u>

MCC-A **S06.345-** Traumatic hemorrhage of <u>right</u> cerebrum <u>with</u> loss of consciousness greater than 24 hours <u>with return</u> to pre-existing conscious level

MCC-A **S06.346-** Traumatic hemorrhage of <u>right</u> cerebrum <u>with</u> loss of consciousness <u>greater than 24</u> hours <u>without return</u> to pre-existing conscious level <u>with patient surviving</u>

MCC-A **S06.347-** Traumatic hemorrhage of <u>right</u> cerebrum <u>with</u> loss of consciousness of <u>any duration with death</u> due to <u>brain injury</u> prior to regaining consciousness

MCC-A **S06.348-** Traumatic hemorrhage of <u>right</u> cerebrum <u>with</u> loss of consciousness of <u>any duration with death</u> due to <u>other cause</u> prior to regaining consciousness

MCC-A **S06.349-** Traumatic hemorrhage of <u>right</u> cerebrum <u>with</u> loss of consciousness of <u>unspecified</u> duration
Traumatic hemorrhage of right cerebrum NOS

S06.35- <u>Traumatic hemorrhage</u> of <u>left</u> cerebrum
Traumatic intracerebral hemorrhage and hematoma of left cerebrum

MCC-A **S06.350-** Traumatic hemorrhage of <u>left</u> cerebrum <u>without</u> loss of consciousness

MCC-A **S06.351-** Traumatic hemorrhage of <u>left</u> cerebrum <u>with</u> loss of consciousness of <u>30 minutes or less</u>

MCC-A **S06.352-** Traumatic hemorrhage of <u>left</u> cerebrum <u>with</u> loss of consciousness of <u>31 minutes to 59 minutes</u>

MCC-A **S06.353-** Traumatic hemorrhage of <u>left</u> cerebrum <u>with</u> loss of consciousness of <u>1 hours to 5 hours 59 minutes</u>

MCC-A **S06.354-** Traumatic hemorrhage of <u>left</u> cerebrum <u>with</u> loss of consciousness of <u>6 hours to 24 hours</u>

MCC-A **S06.355-** Traumatic hemorrhage of <u>left</u> cerebrum <u>with</u> loss of consciousness <u>greater than 24</u> hours <u>with return</u> to pre-existing conscious level

MCC-A **S06.356-** Traumatic hemorrhage of <u>left</u> cerebrum <u>with</u> loss of consciousness greater than 24 hours <u>without</u> return to pre-existing conscious level <u>with patient surviving</u>

MCC-A **S06.357-** Traumatic hemorrhage of <u>left</u> cerebrum <u>with</u> loss of consciousness of <u>any duration with death</u> due to <u>brain injury</u> prior to regaining consciousness

MCC-A **S06.358-** Traumatic hemorrhage of <u>left</u> cerebrum <u>with</u> loss of consciousness of <u>any duration with death</u> due to <u>other cause</u> prior to regaining consciousness

MCC-A **S06.359-** Traumatic hemorrhage of <u>left</u> cerebrum <u>with</u> loss of consciousness of <u>unspecified</u> duration
     Traumatic hemorrhage of left cerebrum NOS

S06.36- <u>Traumatic hemorrhage</u> of cerebrum, <u>unspecified</u>
     Traumatic intracerebral hemorrhage and hematoma, unspecified

MCC-A **S06.360-** Traumatic hemorrhage of cerebrum, <u>unspecified</u>, <u>without</u> loss of consciousness

MCC-A **S06.361-** Traumatic hemorrhage of cerebrum, <u>unspecified</u>, <u>with</u> loss of consciousness of <u>30 minutes or less</u>

MCC-A **S06.362-** Traumatic hemorrhage of cerebrum, <u>unspecified</u>, <u>with</u> loss of consciousness of <u>31 minutes to 59 minutes</u>

MCC-A **S06.363-** Traumatic hemorrhage of cerebrum, <u>unspecified</u>, <u>with</u> loss of consciousness of <u>1 hours to 5 hours 59 minutes</u>

MCC-A **S06.364-** Traumatic hemorrhage of cerebrum, <u>unspecified</u>, <u>with</u> loss of consciousness of <u>6 hours to 24 hours</u>

MCC-A **S06.365-** Traumatic hemorrhage of cerebrum, <u>unspecified</u>, <u>with</u> loss of consciousness <u>greater than 24</u> hours <u>with return</u> to pre-existing conscious level

MCC-A **S06.366-** Traumatic hemorrhage of cerebrum, <u>unspecified</u>, <u>with</u> loss of consciousness <u>greater than 24</u> hours <u>without return</u> to pre-existing conscious level <u>with patient surviving</u>

MCC-A **S06.367-** Traumatic hemorrhage of cerebrum, <u>unspecified</u>, <u>with</u> loss of consciousness of <u>any duration with death</u> due to <u>brain injury</u> prior to regaining consciousness

MCC-A **S06.368-** Traumatic hemorrhage of cerebrum, <u>unspecified</u>, with loss of consciousness of <u>any duration with death</u> due to <u>other cause</u> prior to regaining consciousness

MCC-A **S06.369-** Traumatic hemorrhage of cerebrum, <u>unspecified</u>, <u>with</u> loss of consciousness of <u>unspecified</u> duration
     Traumatic hemorrhage of cerebrum NOS

S06.37- <u>Contusion, laceration, and hemorrhage</u> of <u>cerebellum</u>

MCC-A **S06.370-** Contusion, laceration, and hemorrhage of cerebellum <u>without</u> loss of consciousness

CC-A **S06.371-** Contusion, laceration, and hemorrhage of cerebellum <u>with</u> loss of consciousness of <u>30 minutes or less</u>

CC-A **S06.372-** Contusion, laceration, and hemorrhage of cerebellum <u>with</u> loss of consciousness of <u>31 minutes to 59 minutes</u>

CC-A **S06.373-** Contusion, laceration, and hemorrhage of cerebellum <u>with</u> loss of consciousness of <u>1 hour to 5 hours 59</u> minutes

CC-A **S06.374-** Contusion, laceration, and hemorrhage of cerebellum <u>with</u> loss of consciousness of <u>6 hours to 24 hours</u>

CC-A **S06.375-** Contusion, laceration, and hemorrhage of cerebellum <u>with</u> loss of consciousness <u>greater than 24</u> hours <u>with return</u> to pre-existing conscious level

MCC-A **S06.376-** Contusion, laceration, and hemorrhage of cerebellum <u>with</u> loss of consciousness <u>greater than 24</u> hours <u>without return</u> to pre-existing conscious level <u>with patient surviving</u>

MCC-A **S06.377-** Contusion, laceration, and hemorrhage of cerebellum <u>with</u> loss of consciousness of <u>any duration with death</u> due to <u>brain injury</u> prior to regaining consciousness

MCC-A **S06.378-** Contusion, laceration, and hemorrhage of cerebellum <u>with</u> loss of consciousness of <u>any duration with death</u> due to <u>other cause</u> prior to regaining consciousness

CC-A **S06.379-** Contusion, laceration, and hemorrhage of cerebellum <u>with</u> loss of consciousness of <u>unspecified</u> duration
     Contusion, laceration, and hemorrhage of cerebellum NOS

S06.38- <u>Contusion, laceration, and hemorrhage</u> of <u>brainstem</u>

MCC-A **S06.380-** Contusion, laceration, and hemorrhage of brainstem <u>without</u> loss of consciousness

CC-A **S06.381-** Contusion, laceration, and hemorrhage of brainstem <u>with</u> loss of consciousness of <u>30 minutes or less</u>

CC-A **S06.382-** Contusion, laceration, and hemorrhage of brainstem <u>with</u> loss of consciousness of <u>31 minutes to 59 minutes</u>

CC-A **S06.383-** Contusion, laceration, and hemorrhage of brainstem <u>with</u> loss of consciousness of <u>1 hour to 5 hours 59</u> minutes

CC-A **S06.384-** Contusion, laceration, and hemorrhage of brainstem <u>with</u> loss of consciousness of <u>6 hours to 24 hours</u>

CC-A **S06.385-** Contusion, laceration, and hemorrhage of brainstem <u>with</u> loss of consciousness <u>greater than 24</u> hours <u>with return</u> to pre-existing conscious level

MCC-A **S06.386-** Contusion, laceration, and hemorrhage of brainstem <u>with</u> loss of consciousness <u>greater than 24</u> hours <u>without return</u> to pre-existing conscious level <u>with patient surviving</u>

MCC-A **S06.387-** Contusion, laceration, and hemorrhage of brainstem <u>with</u> loss of consciousness of <u>any duration with death</u> due to <u>brain injury</u> prior to regaining consciousness

MCC-A **S06.388-** Contusion, laceration, and hemorrhage of brainstem <u>with</u> loss of consciousness of <u>any duration with death</u> due to <u>other cause</u> prior to regaining consciousness

CC-A **S06.389-** Contusion, laceration, and hemorrhage of brainstem <u>with</u> loss of consciousness of <u>unspecified</u> duration
     Contusion, laceration, and hemorrhage of brainstem NOS

S06.4-   **Epidural hemorrhage**
     Extradural hemorrhage NOS
     Extradural hemorrhage (traumatic)

S06.4x-   <u>Epidural hemorrhage</u>

MCC-A **S06.4x0-** Epidural hemorrhage <u>without</u> loss of consciousness

MCC-A **S06.4x1-** Epidural hemorrhage <u>with</u> loss of consciousness of <u>30 minutes or less</u>

MCC-A **S06.4x2-** Epidural hemorrhage <u>with</u> loss of consciousness of <u>31 minutes to 59 minutes</u>

MCC-A **S06.4x3-** Epidural hemorrhage <u>with</u> loss of consciousness of <u>1 hour to 5 hours 59 minutes</u>

MCC-A **S06.4x4-** Epidural hemorrhage <u>with</u> loss of consciousness of <u>6 hours to 24 hours</u>

MCC-A **S06.4x5-** Epidural hemorrhage <u>with</u> loss of consciousness <u>greater than 24</u> hours <u>with return</u> to pre-existing conscious level

MCC-A **S06.4x6-** Epidural hemorrhage <u>with</u> loss of consciousness <u>greater than 24</u> hours <u>without return</u> to pre-existing conscious level <u>with patient surviving</u>

MCC-A **S06.4x7-** Epidural hemorrhage <u>with</u> loss of consciousness of <u>any duration with death</u> due to <u>brain injury</u> prior to regaining consciousness

MCC-A **S06.4x8-** Epidural hemorrhage <u>with</u> loss of consciousness of <u>any duration with death</u> due to <u>other causes</u> prior to regaining consciousness

MCC-A **S06.4x9-** Epidural hemorrhage <u>with</u> loss of consciousness of <u>unspecified</u> duration
     Epidural hemorrhage NOS

S06 | S06 | S06

Excludes 1: = NOT CODED HERE! (Do not code both)   **1027**   *Excludes ❷:* = Not Included Here

S06.5-   **Traumatic subdural hemorrhage**

  S06.5x-   <u>Traumatic subdural hemorrhage</u>

MCC-A **S06.5x0-**   Traumatic subdural hemorrhage <u>without</u> loss of consciousness

MCC-A **S06.5x1-**   Traumatic subdural hemorrhage <u>with</u> loss of consciousness of <u>30 minutes or less</u>

MCC-A **S06.5x2-**   Traumatic subdural hemorrhage <u>with</u> loss of consciousness of <u>31 minutes to 59 minutes</u>

MCC-A **S06.5x3-**   Traumatic subdural hemorrhage <u>with</u> loss of consciousness of <u>1 hour to 5 hours 59 minutes</u>

MCC-A **S06.5x4-**   Traumatic subdural hemorrhage <u>with</u> loss of consciousness of <u>6 hours to 24 hours</u>

MCC-A **S06.5x5-**   Traumatic subdural hemorrhage <u>with</u> loss of consciousness <u>greater than 24</u> hours <u>with return</u> to pre-existing conscious level

MCC-A **S06.5x6-**   Traumatic subdural hemorrhage <u>with</u> loss of consciousness <u>greater than 24</u> hours <u>without return</u> to pre-existing conscious level <u>with patient surviving</u>

MCC-A **S06.5x7-**   Traumatic subdural hemorrhage <u>with</u> loss of consciousness of <u>any duration with death</u> due to <u>brain injury</u> before regaining consciousness

MCC-A **S06.5x8-**   Traumatic subdural hemorrhage <u>with</u> loss of consciousness of <u>any duration with death</u> due to <u>other cause</u> before regaining consciousness

MCC-A **S06.5x9-**   Traumatic subdural hemorrhage <u>with</u> loss of consciousness of <u>unspecified</u> duration
    Traumatic subdural hemorrhage NOS

S06.6-   **Traumatic subarachnoid hemorrhage**

  S06.6x-   <u>Traumatic subarachnoid hemorrhage</u>

MCC-A **S06.6x0-**   Traumatic subarachnoid hemorrhage <u>without</u> loss of consciousness

MCC-A **S06.6x1-**   Traumatic subarachnoid hemorrhage <u>with</u> loss of consciousness of <u>30 minutes or less</u>

MCC-A **S06.6x2-**   Traumatic subarachnoid hemorrhage <u>with</u> loss of consciousness of <u>31 minutes to 59 minutes</u>

MCC-A **S06.6x3-**   Traumatic subarachnoid hemorrhage <u>with</u> loss of consciousness of <u>1 hour to 5 hours 59 minutes</u>

MCC-A **S06.6x4-**   Traumatic subarachnoid hemorrhage <u>with</u> loss of consciousness of <u>6 hours to 24 hours</u>

MCC-A **S06.6x5-**   Traumatic subarachnoid hemorrhage <u>with</u> loss of consciousness <u>greater than 24</u> hours <u>with return</u> to pre-existing conscious level

MCC-A **S06.6x6-**   Traumatic subarachnoid hemorrhage <u>with</u> loss of consciousness <u>greater than 24</u> hours <u>without return</u> to pre-existing conscious level <u>with patient surviving</u>

MCC-A **S06.6x7-**   Traumatic subarachnoid hemorrhage <u>with</u> loss of consciousness of <u>any duration with death</u> due to <u>brain injury</u> prior to regaining consciousness

MCC-A **S06.6x8-**   Traumatic subarachnoid hemorrhage <u>with</u> loss of consciousness of <u>any duration with death</u> due to <u>other cause</u> prior to regaining consciousness

MCC-A **S06.6x9-**   Traumatic subarachnoid hemorrhage <u>with</u> loss of consciousness of <u>unspecified</u> duration
    Traumatic subarachnoid hemorrhage NOS

S06.8-   **Other specified intracranial injuries**

  S06.81-   Injury of <u>right internal carotid artery, intracranial portion, not elsewhere classified</u>

    S06.810-   Injury of <u>right</u> internal carotid artery, intracranial portion, not elsewhere classified <u>without</u> loss of consciousness

CC-A **S06.811-**   Injury of <u>right</u> internal carotid artery, intracranial portion, not elsewhere classified <u>with</u> loss of consciousness of <u>30 minutes or less</u>

CC-A **S06.812-**   Injury of <u>right</u> internal carotid artery, intracranial portion, not elsewhere classified <u>with</u> loss of consciousness of <u>31 minutes to 59 minutes</u>

CC-A **S06.813-**   Injury of <u>right</u> internal carotid artery, intracranial portion, not elsewhere classified <u>with</u> loss of consciousness of <u>1 hour to 5 hours 59 minutes</u>

CC-A **S06.814-**   Injury of <u>right</u> internal carotid artery, intracranial portion, not elsewhere classified <u>with</u> loss of consciousness of <u>6 hours to 24 hours</u>

CC-A **S06.815-**   Injury of <u>right</u> internal carotid artery, intracranial portion, not elsewhere classified <u>with</u> loss of consciousness <u>greater than 24</u> hours <u>with return</u> to pre-existing conscious level

MCC-A **S06.816-**   Injury of <u>right</u> internal carotid artery, intracranial portion, not elsewhere classified <u>with</u> loss of consciousness <u>greater than 24</u> hours <u>without return</u> to pre-existing conscious level <u>with patient surviving</u>

MCC-A **S06.817-**   Injury of <u>right</u> internal carotid artery, intracranial portion, not elsewhere classified <u>with</u> loss of consciousness of <u>any duration with death</u> due to <u>brain injury</u> prior to regaining consciousness

MCC-A **S06.818-**   Injury of <u>right</u> internal carotid artery, intracranial portion, not elsewhere classified <u>with</u> loss of consciousness of <u>any duration with death</u> due to <u>other cause</u> prior to regaining consciousness

CC-A **S06.819-**   Injury of <u>right</u> internal carotid artery, intracranial portion, not elsewhere classified <u>with</u> loss of consciousness of <u>unspecified</u> duration
    Injury of right internal carotid artery, intracranial portion, not elsewhere classified NOS

  S06.82-   Injury of <u>left internal carotid artery, intracranial portion, not elsewhere classified</u>

    S06.820-   Injury of <u>left</u> internal carotid artery, intracranial portion, not elsewhere classified <u>without</u> loss of consciousness

CC-A **S06.821-**   Injury of <u>left</u> internal carotid artery, intracranial portion, not elsewhere classified <u>with</u> loss of consciousness of <u>30 minutes or less</u>

CC-A **S06.822-**   Injury of <u>left</u> internal carotid artery, intracranial portion, not elsewhere classified <u>with</u> loss of consciousness of <u>31 minutes to 59 minutes</u>

CC-A **S06.823-**   Injury of <u>left</u> internal carotid artery, intracranial portion, not elsewhere classified <u>with</u> loss of consciousness of <u>1 hour to 5 hours 59 minutes</u>

CC-A **S06.824-**   Injury of <u>left</u> internal carotid artery, intracranial portion, not elsewhere classified <u>with</u> loss of consciousness of <u>6 hours to 24 hours</u>

CC-A **S06.825-**   Injury of <u>left</u> internal carotid artery, intracranial portion, not elsewhere classified <u>with</u> loss of consciousness <u>greater than 24</u> hours <u>with return</u> to pre-existing conscious level

MCC-A **S06.826-**   Injury of <u>left</u> internal carotid artery, intracranial portion, not elsewhere classified <u>with</u> loss of consciousness <u>greater than 24</u> hours <u>without return</u> to pre-existing conscious level <u>with patient surviving</u>

MCC-A **S06.827-**   Injury of <u>left</u> internal carotid artery, intracranial portion, not elsewhere classified <u>with</u> loss of consciousness of <u>any duration with death</u> due to <u>brain injury</u> prior to regaining consciousness

MCC-A **S06.828-**   Injury of <u>left</u> internal carotid artery, intracranial portion, not elsewhere classified <u>with</u> loss of consciousness of <u>any duration with death</u> due to <u>other cause</u> prior to regaining consciousness

CC-A **S06.829-**   Injury of <u>left</u> internal carotid artery, intracranial portion, not elsewhere classified <u>with</u> loss of consciousness of <u>unspecified</u> duration
    Injury of left internal carotid artery, intracranial portion, not elsewhere classified NOS

  S06.89-   <u>Other specified intracranial injury</u>
    Excludes 1:   concussion (S06.0x-)

    S06.890-   Other specified intracranial injury <u>without</u> loss of consciousness

S06 - S06

S06

CC-A **S06.891-** Other specified intracranial injury <u>with</u> loss of consciousness of <u>30 minutes or less</u>

CC-A **S06.892-** Other specified intracranial injury <u>with</u> loss of consciousness of <u>31 minutes to 59 minutes</u>

CC-A **S06.893-** Other specified intracranial injury <u>with</u> loss of consciousness of <u>1 hour to 5 hours 59 minutes</u>

CC-A **S06.894-** Other specified intracranial injury <u>with</u> loss of consciousness of <u>6 hours to 24 hours</u>

CC-A **S06.895-** Other specified intracranial injury <u>with</u> loss of consciousness <u>greater than 24</u> hours <u>with return</u> to pre-existing conscious level

MCC-A **S06.896-** Other specified intracranial injury <u>with</u> loss of consciousness <u>greater than 24</u> hours <u>without return</u> to pre-existing conscious level <u>with patient surviving</u>

MCC-A **S06.897-** Other specified intracranial injury <u>with</u> loss of consciousness of <u>any duration with death</u> due to <u>brain injury</u> prior to regaining consciousness

MCC-A **S06.898-** Other specified intracranial injury <u>with</u> loss of consciousness of <u>any duration with death</u> due to <u>other cause</u> prior to regaining consciousness

CC-A **S06.899-** Other specified intracranial injury <u>with</u> loss of consciousness of <u>unspecified</u> duration

S06.9- Unspecified intracranial injury
    Brain injury NOS
    Head injury NOS with loss of consciousness
    Traumatic brain injury NOS
    Excludes 1:   *conditions classifiable to S06.0- to S06.8- code to specified intracranial injury*
        head injury NOS (S09.90)

S06.9x- <u>Unspecified intracranial injury</u>

S06.9x0- Unspecified intracranial injury <u>without</u> loss of consciousness

CC-A **S06.9x1-** Unspecified intracranial injury <u>with</u> loss of consciousness of <u>30 minutes or less</u>

CC-A **S06.9x2-** Unspecified intracranial injury <u>with</u> loss of consciousness of <u>31 minutes to 59 minutes</u>

CC-A **S06.9x3-** Unspecified intracranial injury <u>with</u> loss of consciousness of <u>1 hour to 5 hours 59 minutes</u>

CC-A **S06.9x4-** Unspecified intracranial injury <u>with</u> loss of consciousness of <u>6 hours to 24 hours</u>

CC-A **S06.9x5-** Unspecified intracranial injury <u>with</u> loss of consciousness <u>greater than 24</u> hours <u>with return</u> to pre-existing conscious level

MCC-A **S06.9x6-** Unspecified intracranial injury <u>with</u> loss of consciousness <u>greater than 24</u> hours <u>without return</u> to pre-existing conscious level <u>with patient surviving</u>

MCC-A **S06.9x7-** Unspecified intracranial injury <u>with</u> loss of consciousness of <u>any duration with death</u> due to <u>brain injury</u> prior to regaining consciousness

MCC-A **S06.9x8-** Unspecified intracranial injury <u>with</u> loss of consciousness of <u>any duration with death</u> due to <u>other cause</u> prior to regaining consciousness

CC-A **S06.9x9-** Unspecified intracranial injury <u>with</u> loss of consciousness of <u>unspecified</u> duration

S07- <u>Crushing injury</u> of <u>head</u>
Use additional code for all associated injuries, such as:
    Intracranial injuries (S06.-)
    Skull fractures (S02.-)

The appropriate 7th character is to be added to each code from category S07:
A   <u>Initial</u> encounter
D   <u>Subsequent</u> encounter
S   <u>Sequela</u>

S07.0xx- Crushing injury of face
CC-A

S07.1xx- Crushing injury of skull
CC-A

S07.8xx- Crushing injury of other parts of head
CC-A

S07.9xx- Crushing injury of head, part <u>unspecified</u>
CC-A

S08- <u>Avulsion and traumatic amputation</u> of <u>part of head</u>
Note: An amputation not identified as partial or complete should be coded to complete

The appropriate 7th character is to be added to each code from category S08:
A   <u>Initial</u> encounter
D   <u>Subsequent</u> encounter
S   <u>Sequela</u>

S08.0xx- Avulsion of scalp

S08.1- <u>Traumatic amputation</u> of <u>ear</u>
  S08.11- <u>Complete</u> traumatic amputation of ear
    S08.111- Complete traumatic amputation of <u>right</u> ear
    S08.112- Complete traumatic amputation of <u>left</u> ear
    S08.119- Complete traumatic amputation of <u>unspecified</u> ear
  S08.12- <u>Partial</u> traumatic amputation of ear
    S08.121- Partial traumatic amputation of <u>right</u> ear
    S08.122- Partial traumatic amputation of <u>left</u> ear
    S08.129- Partial traumatic amputation of <u>unspecified</u> ear

S08.8- Traumatic amputation of other parts of head
  S08.81- Traumatic amputation of <u>nose</u>
    S08.811- Complete traumatic amputation of nose
    S08.812- Partial traumatic amputation of nose
  S08.89x- Traumatic amputation of other parts of head

S09- <u>Other and unspecified</u> injuries of head

The appropriate 7th character is to be added to each code from category S09:
A   <u>Initial</u> encounter
D   <u>Subsequent</u> encounter
S   <u>Sequela</u>

S09.0xx- Injury of blood vessels of head, <u>not elsewhere classified</u>
CC-A   *Excludes 1:*   *injury of cerebral blood vessels (S06.-)*
        injury of precerebral blood vessels (S15.-)

S09.1- <u>Injury of muscle and tendon</u> of <u>head</u>
Code also any associated open wound (S01.-)
Excludes ❷: *sprain to joints and ligament of head (S03.9)*
  S09.10x- Unspecified injury of muscle and tendon of head
    Injury of muscle and tendon of head NOS
  S09.11x- Strain of muscle and tendon of head
  S09.12x- Laceration of muscle and tendon of head
  S09.19x- Other specified injury of muscle and tendon of head

S09.2- <u>Traumatic rupture</u> of <u>ear drum</u>
Excludes 1:   *traumatic rupture of ear drum due to blast injury (S09.31-)*
CC-A **S09.20x-** Traumatic rupture of <u>unspecified</u> ear drum
CC-A **S09.21x-** Traumatic rupture of <u>right</u> ear drum
CC-A **S09.22x-** Traumatic rupture of <u>left</u> ear drum

S09.3- Other specified and unspecified injury of <u>middle and inner ear</u>
Excludes 1:   *injury to ear NOS (S09.91-)*
Excludes ❷: *injury to external ear (S00.4-, S01.3-, S08.1-)*
  S09.30- <u>Unspecified</u> injury of middle and inner ear
CC-A **S09.301-** Unspecified injury of <u>right</u> middle and inner ear
CC-A **S09.302-** Unspecified injury of <u>left</u> middle and inner ear
CC-A **S09.309-** Unspecified injury of <u>unspecified</u> middle and inner ear
  S09.31- <u>Primary blast</u> injury of ear
    Blast injury of ear NOS
CC-A **S09.311-** Primary blast injury of <u>right</u> ear
CC-A **S09.312-** Primary blast injury of <u>left</u> ear
CC-A **S09.313-** Primary blast injury of ear, <u>bilateral</u>
CC-A **S09.319-** Primary blast injury of <u>unspecified</u> ear
  S09.39- <u>Other specified injury</u> of middle and inner ear
    Secondary blast injury to ear
CC-A **S09.391-** Other specified injury of <u>right</u> middle and inner ear
CC-A **S09.392-** Other specified injury of <u>left</u> middle and inner ear

S06 – S09

CC-A **S09.399-**   Other specified injury of <u>unspecified</u> middle and inner ear

S09.8xx-   <u>Other</u> specified injuries of head

S09.9-   <u>Unspecified</u> injury of face and head

   S09.90x-   Unspecified injury of <u>head</u>
      Head injury NOS
      Excludes 1:   *brain injury NOS (S06.9-)*
                head injury NOS with loss of consciousness (S06.9-)
                intracranial injury NOS (S06.9-)

   S09.91x-   Unspecified injury of <u>ear</u>
      Injury of ear NOS

   S09.92x-   Unspecified injury of <u>nose</u>
      Injury of nose NOS

   S09.93x-   Unspecified injury of <u>face</u>
      Injury of face NOS

Injuries to the neck (S10-S19)

Includes: Injuries of nape
              Injuries of supraclavicular region
              Injuries of throat
Excludes ❷: *burns and corrosions (T20-T32)*
             effects of foreign body in esophagus (T18.1)
             effects of foreign body in larynx (T17.3)
             effects of foreign body in pharynx (T17.2)
             effects of foreign body in trachea (T17.4)
             frostbite (T33-T34)
             insect bite or sting, venomous (T63.4)

S10-   <u>Superficial Injury</u> of <u>neck</u>
   The appropriate 7th character is to be added to each code from category S10:
    A   <u>Initial</u> encounter
    D   <u>Subsequent</u> encounter
    S   <u>Sequela</u>

  S10.0xx-   <u>Contusion</u> of throat
      Contusion of cervical esophagus
      Contusion of larynx
      Contusion of pharynx
      Contusion of trachea

  S10.1-   <u>Other and unspecified</u> superficial injuries of throat

   S10.10x-   Unspecified superficial injuries of throat

   S10.11x-   Abrasion of throat

   S10.12x-   Blister (nonthermal) of throat

   S10.14x-   External constriction of part of throat

   S10.15x-   Superficial foreign body of throat
      Splinter in the throat

   S10.16x-   Insect bite (nonvenomous) of throat

   S10.17x-   Other superficial bite of throat
      Excludes 1:   *open bite of throat (S11.85)*

  S10.8-   Superficial injury of <u>other specified parts</u> of neck

   S10.80x-   Unspecified superficial injury of other specified part of neck

   S10.81x-   Abrasion of other specified part of neck

   S10.82x-   Blister (nonthermal) of other specified part of neck

   S10.83x-   Contusion of other specified part of neck

   S10.84x-   External constriction of other specified part of neck

   S10.85x-   Superficial foreign body of other specified part of neck
      Splinter in other specified part of neck

   S10.86x-   Insect bite of other specified part of neck

   S10.87x-   Other superficial bite of other specified part of neck
      Excludes 1:   *open bite of other specified parts of neck (S11.85)*

  S10.9-   Superficial injury of <u>unspecified</u> part of neck

   S10.90x-   Unspecified superficial injury of unspecified part of neck

   S10.91x-   Abrasion of unspecified part of neck

   S10.92x-   Blister (nonthermal) of unspecified part of neck

   S10.93x-   Contusion of unspecified part of neck

   S10.94x-   External constriction of unspecified part of neck

   S10.95x-   Superficial foreign body of unspecified part of neck

   S10.96x-   Insect bite of unspecified part of neck

S10.97x-   Other superficial bite of unspecified part of neck

S11-   <u>Open wound</u> of <u>neck</u>
   Code also any associated:
      Spinal cord injury (S14.0, S14.1-)
      Wound infection
   Excludes ❷: *open fracture of vertebra (S12.- with 7th character B)*
   The appropriate 7th character is to be added to each code from category S11:
    A   <u>Initial</u> encounter
    D   <u>Subsequent</u> encounter
    S   <u>Sequela</u>

  S11.0-   Open wound of <u>larynx and trachea</u>

   S11.01-   Open wound of <u>larynx</u>
      Excludes ❷: *open wound of vocal cord (S11.03)*

MCC-A **S11.011-**   Laceration <u>without</u> foreign body of larynx

MCC-A **S11.012-**   Laceration <u>with foreign body</u> of larynx

MCC-A **S11.013-**   <u>Puncture</u> wound <u>without</u> foreign body of larynx

MCC-A **S11.014-**   <u>Puncture</u> wound <u>with foreign body</u> of larynx

MCC-A **S11.015-**   Open bite of larynx
      Bite of larynx NOS

MCC-A **S11.019-**   Unspecified open wound of larynx

   S11.02-   Open wound of <u>trachea</u>
      Open wound of cervical trachea
      Open wound of trachea NOS
      Excludes ❷: *open wound of thoracic trachea (S27.5-)*

MCC-A **S11.021-**   <u>Laceration</u> <u>without</u> foreign body of trachea

MCC-A **S11.022-**   <u>Laceration</u> <u>with foreign body</u> of trachea

MCC-A **S11.023-**   <u>Puncture</u> wound <u>without</u> foreign body of trachea

MCC-A **S11.024-**   <u>Puncture</u> wound <u>with foreign body</u> of trachea

MCC-A **S11.025-**   Open bite of trachea
      Bite of trachea NOS

MCC-A **S11.029-**   Unspecified open wound of trachea

   S11.03-   Open wound of <u>vocal cord</u>

MCC-A **S11.031-**   <u>Laceration</u> <u>without</u> foreign body of vocal cord

MCC-A **S11.032-**   <u>Laceration</u> <u>with foreign body</u> of vocal cord

MCC-A **S11.033-**   <u>Puncture</u> wound <u>without</u> foreign body of vocal cord

MCC-A **S11.034-**   <u>Puncture</u> wound <u>with foreign body</u> of vocal cord

MCC-A **S11.035-**   Open bite of vocal cord
      Bite of vocal cord NOS

MCC-A **S11.039-**   Unspecified open wound of vocal cord

  S11.1-   Open wound of <u>thyroid gland</u>

CC-A **S11.10x-**   Unspecified open wound of thyroid gland

CC-A **S11.11x-**   Laceration <u>without</u> foreign body of thyroid gland

CC-A **S11.12x-**   <u>Laceration</u> <u>with foreign body</u> of thyroid gland

CC-A **S11.13x-**   <u>Puncture</u> wound <u>without</u> foreign body of thyroid gland

CC-A **S11.14x-**   <u>Puncture</u> wound <u>with foreign body</u> of thyroid gland

CC-A **S11.15x-**   Open bite of thyroid gland
      Bite of thyroid gland NOS

  S11.2-   Open wound of <u>pharynx and cervical esophagus</u>
      Excludes 1: *open wound of esophagus NOS (S27.8-)*

CC-A **S11.20x-**   Unspecified open wound of pharynx and cervical esophagus

CC-A **S11.21x-**   <u>Laceration</u> <u>without</u> foreign body of pharynx and cervical esophagus

CC-A **S11.22x-**   <u>Laceration</u> <u>with foreign body</u> of pharynx and cervical esophagus

CC-A **S11.23x-**   <u>Puncture</u> wound <u>without</u> foreign body of pharynx and cervical esophagus

CC-A **S11.24x-**   <u>Puncture</u> wound <u>with foreign body</u> of pharynx and cervical esophagus

CC-A **S11.25x-**   Open bite of pharynx and cervical esophagus
      Bite of pharynx and cervical esophagus NOS

  S11.8-   Open wound of <u>other specified parts</u> of neck

   S11.80x-   Unspecified open wound of other specified part of neck

   S11.81x-   <u>Laceration</u> <u>without</u> foreign body of other specified part of neck

   S11.82x-   <u>Laceration</u> <u>with foreign body</u> of other specified part of neck

S09 - S11

S11.83x- Puncture wound without foreign body of other specified part of neck

S11.84x- Puncture wound with foreign body of other specified part of neck

S11.85x- Open bite of other specified part of neck
Bite of other specified part of neck NOS
Excludes 1: *superficial bite of other specified part of neck (S10.87)*

S11.89x- Other open wound of other specified part of neck

S11.9- Open wound of unspecified part of neck

S11.90x- Unspecified open wound of unspecified part of neck

S11.91x- Laceration without foreign body of unspecified part of neck

S11.92x- Laceration with foreign body of unspecified part of neck

S11.93x- Puncture wound without foreign body of unspecified part of neck

S11.94x- Puncture wound with foreign body of unspecified part of neck

S11.95x- Open bite of unspecified part of neck
Bite of neck NOS
Excludes 1: *superficial bite of neck (S10.97)*

S12- Fracture of cervical vertebra and other parts of neck
Note: A fracture not indicated as nondisplaced or displaced should be classified to displaced
Note: A fracture not indicated as open or closed should be coded to closed
Includes: Fracture of cervical neural arch
Fracture of cervical spine
Fracture of cervical spinous process
Fracture of cervical transverse process
Fracture of cervical vertebral arch
Fracture of neck
Code first any associated cervical spinal cord injury (S14.0, S14.1-)

The appropriate 7th character is to be added to all codes from subcategories S12.0-S12.6:
A   Initial encounter for closed fracture
B   Initial encounter for open fracture
D   Subsequent encounter for fracture with routine healing
G   Subsequent encounter for fracture with delayed healing
K   Subsequent encounter for fracture with nonunion
S   Sequela

S12.0- Fracture of first cervical vertebra
Atlas

S12.00- Unspecified fracture of first cervical vertebra

CC-A,K MCC-B **S12.000-** Unspecified displaced fracture of first cervical vertebra

CC-A,K MCC-B **S12.001-** Unspecified nondisplaced fracture of first cervical vertebra

S12.01x- Stable burst fracture of first cervical vertebra
CC-A,K MCC-B

S12.02x- Unstable burst fracture of first cervical vertebra
CC-A,K MCC-B

S12.03- Posterior arch fracture of first cervical vertebra

CC-A,K MCC-B **S12.030-** Displaced posterior arch fracture of first cervical vertebra

CC-A,K MCC-B **S12.031-** Nondisplaced posterior arch fracture of first cervical vertebra

S12.04- Lateral mass fracture of first cervical vertebra

CC-A,K MCC-B **S12.040-** Displaced lateral mass fracture of first cervical vertebra

CC-A,K MCC-B **S12.041-** Nondisplaced lateral mass fracture of first cervical vertebra

S12.09- Other fracture of first cervical vertebra

CC-A,K MCC-B **S12.090-** Other displaced fracture of first cervical vertebra

CC-A,K MCC-B **S12.091-** Other nondisplaced fracture of first cervical vertebra

S12.1- Fracture of second cervical vertebra
Axis

S12.10- Unspecified fracture of second cervical vertebra

CC-A,K MCC-B **S12.100-** Unspecified displaced fracture of second cervical vertebra

CC-A,K MCC-B **S12.101-** Unspecified nondisplaced fracture of second cervical vertebra

S12.11- Type II dens fracture

CC-A,K MCC-B **S12.110-** Anterior displaced Type II dens fracture

CC-A,K MCC-B **S12.111-** Posterior displaced Type II dens fracture

CC-A,K MCC-B **S12.112-** Nondisplaced Type II dens fracture

S12.12- Other dens fracture

CC-A,K MCC-B **S12.120-** Other displaced dens fracture

CC-A,K MCC-B **S12.121-** Other nondisplaced dens fracture

S12.13- Unspecified traumatic spondylolisthesis of second cervical vertebra

CC-A,K MCC-B **S12.130-** Unspecified traumatic displaced spondylolisthesis of second cervical vertebra

CC-A,K MCC-B **S12.131-** Unspecified traumatic nondisplaced spondylolisthesis of second cervical vertebra

S12.14x- Type III traumatic spondylolisthesis of second cervical vertebra
CC-A,K MCC-B

S12.15- Other traumatic spondylolisthesis of second cervical vertebra

CC-A,K MCC-B **S12.150-** Other traumatic displaced spondylolisthesis of second cervical vertebra

CC-A,K MCC-B **S12.151-** Other traumatic nondisplaced spondylolisthesis of second cervical vertebra

S12.19- Other fracture of second cervical vertebra

CC-A,K MCC-B **S12.190-** Other displaced fracture of second cervical vertebra

CC-A,K MCC-B **S12.191-** Other nondisplaced fracture of second cervical vertebra

S12.2- Fracture of third cervical vertebra

S12.20- Unspecified fracture of third cervical vertebra

CC-A,K MCC-B **S12.200-** Unspecified displaced fracture of third cervical vertebra

CC-A,K MCC-B **S12.201-** Unspecified nondisplaced fracture of third cervical vertebra

S12.23- Unspecified traumatic spondylolisthesis of third cervical vertebra

CC-A,K MCC-B **S12.230-** Unspecified traumatic displaced spondylolisthesis of third cervical vertebra

CC-A,K MCC-B **S12.231-** Unspecified traumatic nondisplaced spondylolisthesis of third cervical vertebra

S12.24x- Type III traumatic spondylolisthesis of third cervical vertebra
CC-A,K MCC-B

S12.25- Other traumatic spondylolisthesis of third cervical vertebra

CC-A,K MCC-B **S12.250-** Other traumatic displaced spondylolisthesis of third cervical vertebra

CC-A,K MCC-B **S12.251-** Other traumatic nondisplaced spondylolisthesis of third cervical vertebra

S12.29- Other fracture of third cervical vertebra

CC-A,K MCC-B **S12.290-** Other displaced fracture of third cervical vertebra

CC-A,K MCC-B **S12.291-** Other nondisplaced fracture of third cervical vertebra

S12.3- Fracture of fourth cervical vertebra

S12.30- Unspecified fracture of fourth cervical vertebra

CC-A,K MCC-B **S12.300-** Unspecified displaced fracture of fourth cervical vertebra

CC-A,K MCC-B **S12.301-** Unspecified nondisplaced fracture of fourth cervical vertebra

S12.33- Unspecified traumatic spondylolisthesis of fourth cervical vertebra

CC-A,K MCC-B **S12.330-** Unspecified traumatic displaced spondylolisthesis of fourth cervical vertebra

CC-A,K MCC-B **S12.331-** Unspecified traumatic nondisplaced spondylolisthesis of fourth cervical vertebra

S12.34x- Type III traumatic spondylolisthesis of fourth cervical vertebra
CC-A,K MCC-B

S12.35- Other traumatic spondylolisthesis of fourth cervical vertebra

S11 - S12

CC-A,K MCC-B **S12.350-** Other traumatic <u>displaced</u> spondylolisthesis of fourth cervical vertebra

CC-A,K MCC-B **S12.351-** Other traumatic <u>nondisplaced</u> spondylolisthesis of fourth cervical vertebra

S12.39- <u>Other fracture</u> of fourth cervical vertebra

CC-A,K MCC-B **S12.390-** Other <u>displaced</u> fracture of fourth cervical vertebra

CC-A,K MCC-B **S12.391-** Other <u>nondisplaced</u> fracture of fourth cervical vertebra

S12.4- <u>Fracture</u> of <u>fifth</u> cervical vertebra

S12.40- <u>Unspecified fracture</u> of fifth cervical vertebra

CC-A,K MCC-B **S12.400-** Unspecified <u>displaced</u> fracture of fifth cervical vertebra

CC-A,K MCC-B **S12.401-** Unspecified <u>nondisplaced</u> fracture of fifth cervical vertebra

S12.43- <u>Unspecified traumatic spondylolisthesis</u> of fifth cervical vertebra

CC-A,K MCC-B **S12.430-** Unspecified traumatic <u>displaced</u> spondylolisthesis of fifth cervical vertebra

CC-A,K MCC-B **S12.431-** Unspecified traumatic <u>nondisplaced</u> spondylolisthesis of fifth cervical vertebra

S12.44x- <u>Type III traumatic spondylolisthesis</u> of fifth cervical
CC-A,K MCC-B vertebra

S12.45- <u>Other traumatic spondylolisthesis</u> of fifth cervical vertebra

CC-A,K MCC-B **S12.450-** Other traumatic <u>displaced</u> spondylolisthesis of fifth cervical vertebra

CC-A,K MCC-B **S12.451-** Other traumatic <u>nondisplaced</u> spondylolisthesis of fifth cervical vertebra

S12.49- <u>Other fracture</u> of fifth cervical vertebra

CC-A,K MCC-B **S12.490-** Other <u>displaced</u> fracture of fifth cervical vertebra

CC-A,K MCC-B **S12.491-** Other <u>nondisplaced</u> fracture of fifth cervical vertebra

S12.5- <u>Fracture</u> of <u>sixth</u> cervical vertebra

S12.50- <u>Unspecified fracture</u> of sixth cervical vertebra

CC-A,K MCC-B **S12.500-** Unspecified <u>displaced</u> fracture of sixth cervical vertebra

CC-A,K MCC-B **S12.501-** Unspecified <u>nondisplaced</u> fracture of sixth cervical vertebra

S12.53- <u>Unspecified traumatic spondylolisthesis</u> of sixth cervical vertebra

CC-A,K MCC-B **S12.530-** Unspecified traumatic <u>displaced</u> spondylolisthesis of sixth cervical vertebra

CC-A,K MCC-B **S12.531-** Unspecified traumatic <u>nondisplaced</u> spondylolisthesis of sixth cervical vertebra

S12.54x- <u>Type III traumatic spondylolisthesis</u> of sixth cervical
CC-A,K MCC-B vertebra

S12.55- <u>Other traumatic spondylolisthesis</u> of sixth cervical vertebra

CC-A,K MCC-B **S12.550-** Other traumatic <u>displaced</u> spondylolisthesis of sixth cervical vertebra

CC-A,K MCC-B **S12.551-** Other traumatic <u>nondisplaced</u> spondylolisthesis of sixth cervical vertebra

S12.59- <u>Other fracture</u> of sixth cervical vertebra

CC-A,K MCC-B **S12.590-** Other <u>displaced</u> fracture of sixth cervical vertebra

CC-A,K MCC-B **S12.591-** Other <u>nondisplaced</u> fracture of sixth cervical vertebra

S12.6- <u>Fracture</u> of <u>seventh</u> cervical vertebra

S12.60- <u>Unspecified fracture</u> of seventh cervical vertebra

CC-A,K MCC-B **S12.600-** Unspecified <u>displaced</u> fracture of seventh cervical vertebra

CC-A,K MCC-B **S12.601-** Unspecified <u>nondisplaced</u> fracture of seventh cervical vertebra

S12.63- <u>Unspecified traumatic spondylolisthesis</u> of seventh cervical vertebra

CC-A,K MCC-B **S12.630-** Unspecified traumatic <u>displaced</u> spondylolisthesis of seventh cervical vertebra

CC-A,K MCC-B **S12.631-** Unspecified traumatic <u>nondisplaced</u> spondylolisthesis of seventh cervical vertebra

S12.64x- <u>Type III traumatic spondylolisthesis</u> of seventh cervical
CC-A,K MCC-B vertebra

S12.65- <u>Other traumatic spondylolisthesis</u> of seventh cervical vertebra

CC-A,K MCC-B **S12.650-** Other traumatic <u>displaced</u> spondylolisthesis of seventh cervical vertebra

CC-A,K MCC-B **S12.651-** Other traumatic <u>nondisplaced</u> spondylolisthesis of seventh cervical vertebra

S12.69- <u>Other fracture</u> of seventh cervical vertebra

CC-A,K MCC-B **S12.690-** Other <u>displaced</u> fracture of seventh cervical vertebra

CC-A,K MCC-B **S12.691-** Other <u>nondisplaced</u> fracture of seventh cervical vertebra

S12.8xx- <u>Fracture</u> of <u>other parts of neck</u>
MCC-A Hyoid bone
  Larynx
  Thyroid cartilage
  Trachea

The appropriate 7th character is to be added to code S12.8:
A <u>Initial</u> encounter
D <u>Subsequent</u> encounter
S <u>Sequela</u>

S12.9xx- <u>Fracture</u> of <u>neck, unspecified</u>
CC-A Fracture of neck NOS
  Fracture of cervical spine NOS
  Fracture of cervical vertebra NOS

The appropriate 7th character is to be added to code S12.9:
A <u>Initial</u> encounter
D <u>Subsequent</u> encounter
S <u>Sequela</u>

S13- <u>Dislocation and sprain</u> of joints and ligaments at <u>neck</u> level
Includes: Avulsion of joint or ligament at neck level
  Laceration of cartilage, joint or ligament at neck level
  Sprain of cartilage, joint or ligament at neck level
  Traumatic hemarthrosis of joint or ligament at neck level
  Traumatic rupture of joint or ligament at neck level
  Traumatic subluxation of joint or ligament at neck level
  Traumatic tear of joint or ligament at neck level
Code also any associated open wound
Excludes ❷: *strain of muscle or tendon at neck level (S16.1)*

The appropriate 7th character is to be added to each code from category S13:
A <u>Initial</u> encounter
D <u>Subsequent</u> encounter
S <u>Sequela</u>

S13.0xx- <u>Traumatic rupture</u> of <u>cervical intervertebral disc</u>
CC-A *Excludes 1:* *rupture or displacement (nontraumatic) of cervical intervertebral disc NOS (M50.-)*

S13.1- <u>Subluxation and dislocation</u> of <u>cervical vertebrae</u>
Code also any associated:
  Open wound of neck (S11.-)
  Spinal cord injury (S14.1-)
Excludes ❷: *fracture of cervical vertebrae (S12.0-S12.3-)*

S13.10- Subluxation and dislocation of <u>unspecified</u> cervical vertebrae

CC-A **S13.100-** <u>Subluxation</u> of unspecified cervical vertebrae

CC-A **S13.101-** <u>Dislocation</u> of unspecified cervical vertebrae

S13.11- Subluxation and dislocation of <u>C0/C1</u> cervical vertebrae
  Subluxation and dislocation of atlantooccipital joint
  Subluxation and dislocation of atloidooccipital joint
  Subluxation and dislocation of occipitoatloid joint

CC-A **S13.110-** <u>Subluxation</u> of C0/C1 cervical vertebrae

CC-A **S13.111-** <u>Dislocation</u> of C0/C1 cervical vertebrae

S13.12- Subluxation and dislocation of <u>C1/C2</u> cervical vertebrae
  Subluxation and dislocation of atlantoaxial joint

CC-A **S13.120-** <u>Subluxation</u> of C1/C2 cervical vertebrae

CC-A **S13.121-** <u>Dislocation</u> of C1/C2 cervical vertebrae

S13.13- Subluxation and dislocation of <u>C2/C3</u> cervical vertebrae

CC-A **S13.130-** <u>Subluxation</u> of C2/C3 cervical vertebrae

CC-A **S13.131-** <u>Dislocation</u> of C2/C3 cervical vertebrae

S13.14- Subluxation and dislocation of <u>C3/C4</u> cervical vertebrae

CC-A **S13.140-** <u>Subluxation</u> of C3/C4 cervical vertebrae

CC-A **S13.141-** <u>Dislocation</u> of C3/C4 cervical vertebrae

S12 - S13

S13.15- Subluxation and dislocation of <u>C4/C5</u> cervical vertebrae
CC-A **S13.150-** <u>Subluxation</u> of C4/C5 cervical vertebrae
CC-A **S13.151-** <u>Dislocation</u> of C4/C5 cervical vertebrae
S13.16- Subluxation and dislocation of <u>C5/C6</u> cervical vertebrae
CC-A **S13.160-** <u>Subluxation</u> of C5/C6 cervical vertebrae
CC-A **S13.161-** <u>Dislocation</u> of C5/C6 cervical vertebrae
S13.17- Subluxation and dislocation of <u>C6/C7</u> cervical vertebrae
CC-A **S13.170-** <u>Subluxation</u> of C6/C7 cervical vertebrae
CC-A **S13.171-** <u>Dislocation</u> of C6/C7 cervical vertebrae
S13.18- Subluxation and dislocation of <u>C7/T1</u> cervical vertebrae
CC-A **S13.180-** <u>Subluxation</u> of C7/T1 cervical vertebrae
CC-A **S13.181-** <u>Dislocation</u> of C7/T1 cervical vertebrae
S13.2- Dislocation of other and <u>unspecified</u> parts of neck
CC-A **S13.20x-** Dislocation of <u>unspecified</u> parts of neck
CC-A **S13.29x-** Dislocation of <u>other</u> parts of neck
S13.4xx- <u>Sprain of ligaments</u> of cervical spine
    Sprain of anterior longitudinal (ligament), cervical
    Sprain of atlanto-axial (joints)
    Sprain of atlanto-occipital (joints)
    Whiplash injury of cervical spine
S13.5xx- Sprain of thyroid region
    Sprain of cricoarytenoid (joint) (ligament)
    Sprain of cricothyroid (joint) (ligament)
    Sprain of thyroid cartilage
S13.8xx- Sprain of joints and ligaments of <u>other</u> parts of neck
S13.9xx- Sprain of joints and ligaments of <u>unspecified</u> parts of neck

S14- <u>Injury of nerves and spinal cord</u> at <u>neck</u> level
Note: Code to highest level of cervical cord injury
Code also any associated:
    Fracture of cervical vertebra (S12.0- -S12.6.-)
    Open wound of neck (S11.-)
    Transient paralysis (R29.5)
The appropriate 7th character is to be added to each code from
    category S14:
A   <u>Initial</u> encounter
D   <u>Subsequent</u> encounter
S   <u>Sequela</u>
S14.0xx- <u>Concussion and edema</u> of cervical spinal cord
MCC-A
S14.1- Other and unspecified injuries of cervical spinal cord
S14.10- <u>Unspecified injury</u> of cervical spinal cord
MCC-A **S14.101-** Unspecified injury at <u>C1</u> level of cervical spinal cord
MCC-A **S14.102-** Unspecified injury at <u>C2</u> level of cervical spinal cord
MCC-A **S14.103-** Unspecified injury at <u>C3</u> level of cervical spinal cord
MCC-A **S14.104-** Unspecified injury at <u>C4</u> level of cervical spinal cord
MCC-A **S14.105-** Unspecified injury at <u>C5</u> level of cervical spinal cord
MCC-A **S14.106-** Unspecified injury at <u>C6</u> level of cervical spinal cord
MCC-A **S14.107-** Unspecified injury at <u>C7</u> level of cervical spinal cord
MCC-A **S14.108-** Unspecified injury at <u>C8</u> level of cervical spinal cord
S14.109- Unspecified injury at <u>unspecified</u> level of cervical spinal cord
    Injury of cervical spinal cord NOS
S14.11- <u>Complete lesion</u> of cervical spinal cord
MCC-A **S14.111-** Complete lesion at <u>C1</u> level of cervical spinal cord
MCC-A **S14.112-** Complete lesion at <u>C2</u> level of cervical spinal cord
MCC-A **S14.113-** Complete lesion at <u>C3</u> level of cervical spinal cord
MCC-A **S14.114-** Complete lesion at <u>C4</u> level of cervical spinal cord
MCC-A **S14.115-** Complete lesion at <u>C5</u> level of cervical spinal cord
MCC-A **S14.116-** Complete lesion at <u>C6</u> level of cervical spinal cord
MCC-A **S14.117-** Complete lesion at <u>C7</u> level of cervical spinal cord
MCC-A **S14.118-** Complete lesion at <u>C8</u> level of cervical spinal cord

S14.119- Complete lesion at <u>unspecified</u> level of cervical spinal cord
S14.12- <u>Central cord syndrome</u> of cervical spinal cord
MCC-A **S14.121-** Central cord syndrome at <u>C1</u> level of cervical spinal cord
MCC-A **S14.122-** Central cord syndrome at <u>C2</u> level of cervical spinal cord
MCC-A **S14.123-** Central cord syndrome at <u>C3</u> level of cervical spinal cord
MCC-A **S14.124-** Central cord syndrome at <u>C4</u> level of cervical spinal cord
MCC-A **S14.125-** Central cord syndrome at <u>C5</u> level of cervical spinal cord
MCC-A **S14.126-** Central cord syndrome at <u>C6</u> level of cervical spinal cord
MCC-A **S14.127-** Central cord syndrome at <u>C7</u> level of cervical spinal cord
MCC-A **S14.128-** Central cord syndrome at <u>C8</u> level of cervical spinal cord
S14.129- Central cord syndrome at <u>unspecified</u> level of cervical spinal cord
S14.13- <u>Anterior cord syndrome</u> of cervical spinal cord
MCC-A **S14.131-** Anterior cord syndrome at <u>C1</u> level of cervical spinal cord
MCC-A **S14.132-** Anterior cord syndrome at <u>C2</u> level of cervical spinal cord
MCC-A **S14.133-** Anterior cord syndrome at <u>C3</u> level of cervical spinal cord
MCC-A **S14.134-** Anterior cord syndrome at <u>C4</u> level of cervical spinal cord
MCC-A **S14.135-** Anterior cord syndrome at <u>C5</u> level of cervical spinal cord
MCC-A **S14.136-** Anterior cord syndrome at <u>C6</u> level of cervical spinal cord
MCC-A **S14.137-** Anterior cord syndrome at <u>C7</u> level of cervical spinal cord
MCC-A **S14.138-** Anterior cord syndrome at <u>C8</u> level of cervical spinal cord
S14.139- Anterior cord syndrome at <u>unspecified</u> level of cervical spinal cord
S14.14- <u>Brown-Séquard syndrome</u> of cervical spinal cord
MCC-A **S14.141-** Brown-Séquard syndrome at <u>C1</u> level of cervical spinal cord
MCC-A **S14.142-** Brown-Séquard syndrome at <u>C2</u> level of cervical spinal cord
MCC-A **S14.143-** Brown-Séquard syndrome at <u>C3</u> level of cervical spinal cord
MCC-A **S14.144-** Brown-Séquard syndrome at <u>C4</u> level of cervical spinal cord
MCC-A **S14.145-** Brown-Séquard syndrome at <u>C5</u> level of cervical spinal cord
MCC-A **S14.146-** Brown-Séquard syndrome at <u>C6</u> level of cervical spinal cord
MCC-A **S14.147-** Brown-Séquard syndrome at <u>C7</u> level of cervical spinal cord
MCC-A **S14.148-** Brown-Séquard syndrome at <u>C8</u> level of cervical spinal cord
S14.149- Brown-Séquard syndrome at <u>unspecified</u> level of cervical spinal cord
S14.15- <u>Other incomplete lesions</u> of cervical spinal cord
    Incomplete lesion of cervical spinal cord NOS
    Posterior cord syndrome of cervical spinal cord
MCC-A **S14.151-** Other incomplete lesion at <u>C1</u> level of cervical spinal cord
MCC-A **S14.152-** Other incomplete lesion at <u>C2</u> level of cervical spinal cord
MCC-A **S14.153-** Other incomplete lesion at <u>C3</u> level of cervical spinal cord

S13 - S14

MCC-A **S14.154-** Other incomplete lesion at <u>C4</u> level of cervical spinal cord

MCC-A **S14.155-** Other incomplete lesion at <u>C5</u> level of cervical spinal cord

MCC-A **S14.156-** Other incomplete lesion at <u>C6</u> level of cervical spinal cord

MCC-A **S14.157-** Other incomplete lesion at <u>C7</u> level of cervical spinal cord

MCC-A **S14.158-** Other incomplete lesion at <u>C8</u> level of cervical spinal cord

S14.159- Other incomplete lesion at <u>unspecified</u> level of cervical spinal cord

S14.2xx- Injury of nerve root of cervical spine

S14.3xx- Injury of brachial plexus

S14.4xx- Injury of peripheral nerves of neck

S14.5xx- Injury of cervical sympathetic nerves

S14.8xx- Injury of <u>other</u> specified nerves of neck

S14.9xx- Injury of <u>unspecified</u> nerves of neck

S15- <u>Injury of blood vessels</u> at <u>neck</u> level

Code also any associated open wound (S11.-)

The appropriate 7th character is to be added to each code from category S15:
- **A**   <u>Initial</u> encounter
- **D**   <u>Subsequent</u> encounter
- **S**   <u>Sequela</u>

S15.0- Injury of <u>carotid artery</u> of neck

Injury of carotid artery (common) (external) (internal, extracranial portion)

Injury of carotid artery NOS

Excludes 1:   injury of internal carotid artery, intracranial portion (S06.8)

S15.00- <u>Unspecified</u> injury of carotid artery

CC-A **S15.001-** Unspecified injury of <u>right</u> carotid artery

CC-A **S15.002-** Unspecified injury of <u>left</u> carotid artery

CC-A **S15.009-** Unspecified injury of <u>unspecified</u> carotid artery

S15.01- <u>Minor laceration</u> of carotid artery

Incomplete transection of carotid artery

Laceration of carotid artery NOS

Superficial laceration of carotid artery

CC-A **S15.011-** Minor laceration of <u>right</u> carotid artery

CC-A **S15.012-** Minor laceration of <u>left</u> carotid artery

CC-A **S15.019-** Minor laceration of <u>unspecified</u> carotid artery

S15.02- <u>Major laceration</u> of carotid artery

Complete transection of carotid artery

Traumatic rupture of carotid artery

CC-A **S15.021-** Major laceration of <u>right</u> carotid artery

CC-A **S15.022-** Major laceration of <u>left</u> carotid artery

CC-A **S15.029-** Major laceration of <u>unspecified</u> carotid artery

S15.09- <u>Other specified</u> injury of carotid artery

CC-A **S15.091-** Other specified injury of <u>right</u> carotid artery

CC-A **S15.092-** Other specified injury of <u>left</u> carotid artery

CC-A **S15.099-** Other specified injury of <u>unspecified</u> carotid artery

S15.1- Injury of <u>vertebral artery</u>

S15.10- <u>Unspecified</u> injury of vertebral artery

CC-A **S15.101-** Unspecified injury of <u>right</u> vertebral artery

CC-A **S15.102-** Unspecified injury of <u>left</u> vertebral artery

CC-A **S15.109-** Unspecified injury of <u>unspecified</u> vertebral artery

S15.11- <u>Minor laceration</u> of vertebral artery

Incomplete transection of vertebral artery

Laceration of vertebral artery NOS

Superficial laceration of vertebral artery

CC-A **S15.111-** Minor laceration of <u>right</u> vertebral artery

CC-A **S15.112-** Minor laceration of <u>left</u> vertebral artery

CC-A **S15.119-** Minor laceration of <u>unspecified</u> vertebral artery

S15.12- <u>Major laceration</u> of vertebral artery

Complete transection of vertebral artery

Traumatic rupture of vertebral artery

CC-A **S15.121-** Major laceration of <u>right</u> vertebral artery

CC-A **S15.122-** Major laceration of <u>left</u> vertebral artery

CC-A **S15.129-** Major laceration of <u>unspecified</u> vertebral artery

S15.19- <u>Other specified</u> injury of vertebral artery

CC-A **S15.191-** Other specified injury of <u>right</u> vertebral artery

CC-A **S15.192-** Other specified injury of <u>left</u> vertebral artery

CC-A **S15.199-** Other specified injury of <u>unspecified</u> vertebral artery

S15.2- Injury of <u>external jugular vein</u>

S15.20- <u>Unspecified</u> injury of external jugular vein

CC-A **S15.201-** Unspecified injury of <u>right</u> external jugular vein

CC-A **S15.202-** Unspecified injury of <u>left</u> external jugular vein

CC-A **S15.209-** Unspecified injury of <u>unspecified</u> external jugular vein

S15.21- <u>Minor laceration</u> of external jugular vein

Incomplete transection of external jugular vein

Laceration of external jugular vein NOS

Superficial laceration of external jugular vein

CC-A **S15.211-** Minor laceration of <u>right</u> external jugular vein

CC-A **S15.212-** Minor laceration of <u>left</u> external jugular vein

CC-A **S15.219-** Minor laceration of <u>unspecified</u> external jugular vein

S15.22- <u>Major laceration</u> of external jugular vein

Complete transection of external jugular vein

Traumatic rupture of external jugular vein

CC-A **S15.221-** Major laceration of <u>right</u> external jugular vein

CC-A **S15.222-** Major laceration of <u>left</u> external jugular vein

CC-A **S15.229-** Major laceration of <u>unspecified</u> external jugular vein

S15.29- <u>Other specified</u> injury of external jugular vein

CC-A **S15.291-** Other specified injury of <u>right</u> external jugular vein

CC-A **S15.292-** Other specified injury of <u>left</u> external jugular vein

CC-A **S15.299-** Other specified injury of <u>unspecified</u> external jugular vein

S15.3- Injury of <u>internal jugular vein</u>

S15.30- <u>Unspecified</u> injury of internal jugular vein

CC-A **S15.301-** Unspecified injury of <u>right</u> internal jugular vein

CC-A **S15.302-** Unspecified injury of <u>left</u> internal jugular vein

CC-A **S15.309-** Unspecified injury of <u>unspecified</u> internal jugular vein

S15.31- <u>Minor laceration</u> of internal jugular vein

Incomplete transection of internal jugular vein

Laceration of internal jugular vein NOS

Superficial laceration of internal jugular vein

CC-A **S15.311-** Minor laceration of <u>right</u> internal jugular vein

CC-A **S15.312-** Minor laceration of <u>left</u> internal jugular vein

CC-A **S15.319-** Minor laceration of <u>unspecified</u> internal jugular vein

S15.32- <u>Major laceration</u> of internal jugular vein

Complete transection of internal jugular vein

Traumatic rupture of internal jugular vein

CC-A **S15.321-** Major laceration of <u>right</u> internal jugular vein

CC-A **S15.322-** Major laceration of <u>left</u> internal jugular vein

CC-A **S15.329-** Major laceration of <u>unspecified</u> internal jugular vein

S15.39- <u>Other specified</u> injury of internal jugular vein

CC-A **S15.391-** Other specified injury of <u>right</u> internal jugular vein

CC-A **S15.392-** Other specified injury of <u>left</u> internal jugular vein

CC-A **S15.399-** Other specified injury of <u>unspecified</u> internal jugular vein

S15.8xx- Injury of <u>other</u> specified blood vessels at neck level
CC-A

S15.9xx- Injury of <u>unspecified</u> blood vessel at neck level
CC-A

S16- <u>Injury of muscle, fascia and tendon</u> at <u>neck</u> level

Code also any associated open wound (S11.-)

Excludes ❷: sprain of joint or ligament at neck level (S13.9)

The appropriate 7th character is to be added to each code from category S16:
- **A**   <u>Initial</u> encounter
- **D**   <u>Subsequent</u> encounter
- **S**   <u>Sequela</u>

S16.1xx- <u>Strain</u> of muscle, fascia and tendon at neck level

S16.2xx- <u>Laceration</u> of muscle, fascia and tendon at neck level

S16.8xx- <u>Other</u> specified injury of muscle, fascia and tendon at neck level

S16.9xx- <u>Unspecified</u> injury of muscle, fascia and tendon at neck level

S17- <u>Crushing</u> injury of neck
Use additional code for all associated injuries, such as:
Injury of blood vessels (S15.-)
Open wound of neck (S11.-)
Spinal cord injury (S14.0, S14.1-)
Vertebral fracture (S12.0--S12.3-)

The appropriate 7th character is to be added to each code from category S17:
A   <u>Initial</u> encounter
D   <u>Subsequent</u> encounter
S   <u>Sequela</u>

S17.0xx- Crushing injury of <u>larynx and trachea</u>
CC-A

S17.8xx- Crushing injury of <u>other</u> specified parts of neck
CC-A

S17.9xx- Crushing injury of neck, part <u>unspecified</u>
CC-A

S19- Other specified and unspecified injuries of neck
The appropriate 7th character is to be added to each code from category S19:
A   <u>Initial</u> encounter
D   <u>Subsequent</u> encounter
S   <u>Sequela</u>

S19.8- <u>Other specified</u> injuries of neck
S19.80x- Other specified injuries of <u>unspecified</u> part of neck
S19.81x- Other specified injuries of <u>larynx</u>
S19.82x- Other specified injuries of <u>cervical trachea</u>
Excludes ❷: other specified injury of thoracic trachea (S27.5-)
S19.83x- Other specified injuries of <u>vocal cord</u>
S19.84x- Other specified injuries of <u>thyroid gland</u>
S19.85x- Other specified injuries of <u>pharynx and cervical esophagus</u>
S19.89x- Other specified injuries of <u>other specified</u> part of neck
S19.9xx- <u>Unspecified</u> injury of neck

Injuries to the thorax (S20-S29)

Includes: Injuries of breast
Injuries of chest (wall)
Injuries of interscapular area
Excludes ❷: burns and corrosions (T20-T32)
effects of foreign body in bronchus (T17.5)
effects of foreign body in esophagus (T18.1)
effects of foreign body in lung (T17.8)
effects of foreign body in trachea (T17.4)
frostbite (T33-T34)
injuries of axilla
injuries of clavicle
injuries of scapular region
injuries of shoulder
insect bite or sting, venomous (T63.4)

S20- <u>Superficial injury</u> of <u>thorax</u>
The appropriate 7th character is to be added to each code from category S20:
A   <u>Initial</u> encounter
D   <u>Subsequent</u> encounter
S   <u>Sequela</u>

S20.0- <u>Contusion</u> of <u>breast</u>
S20.00x- Contusion of breast, <u>unspecified</u> breast
S20.01x- Contusion of <u>right</u> breast
S20.02x- Contusion of <u>left</u> breast
S20.1- Other and unspecified superficial injuries of <u>breast</u>
S20.10- <u>Unspecified</u> superficial injuries of breast
S20.101- Unspecified superficial injuries of breast, <u>right</u> breast
S20.102- Unspecified superficial injuries of breast, <u>left</u> breast

S20.109- Unspecified superficial injuries of breast, <u>unspecified</u> breast
S20.11- <u>Abrasion</u> of breast
S20.111- Abrasion of breast, <u>right</u> breast
S20.112- Abrasion of breast, <u>left</u> breast
S20.119- Abrasion of breast, <u>unspecified</u> breast
S20.12- <u>Blister</u> (nonthermal) of breast
S20.121- Blister (nonthermal) of breast, <u>right</u> breast
S20.122- Blister (nonthermal) of breast, <u>left</u> breast
S20.129- Blister (nonthermal) of breast, <u>unspecified</u> breast
S20.14- <u>External constriction</u> of part of breast
S20.141- External constriction of part of breast, <u>right</u> breast
S20.142- External constriction of part of breast, <u>left</u> breast
S20.149- External constriction of part of breast, <u>unspecified</u> breast
S20.15- <u>Superficial foreign body</u> of breast
Splinter in the breast
S20.151- Superficial foreign body of breast, <u>right</u> breast
S20.152- Superficial foreign body of breast, <u>left</u> breast
S20.159- Superficial foreign body of breast, <u>unspecified</u> breast
S20.16- <u>Insect bite (nonvenomous)</u> of breast
S20.161- Insect bite (nonvenomous) of breast, <u>right</u> breast
S20.162- Insect bite (nonvenomous) of breast, <u>left</u> breast
S20.169- Insect bite (nonvenomous) of breast, <u>unspecified</u> breast
S20.17- <u>Other superficial bite</u> of breast
Excludes 1: open bite of breast (S21.05-)
S20.171- Other superficial bite of breast, <u>right</u> breast
S20.172- Other superficial bite of breast, <u>left</u> breast
S20.179- Other superficial bite of breast, <u>unspecified</u> breast
S20.2- <u>Contusion</u> of <u>thorax</u>
S20.20x- Contusion of thorax, <u>unspecified</u>
S20.21- Contusion of <u>front wall</u> of thorax
S20.211- Contusion of <u>right</u> front wall of thorax
S20.212- Contusion of <u>left</u> front wall of thorax
S20.219- Contusion of <u>unspecified</u> front wall of thorax
S20.22- Contusion of <u>back wall</u> of thorax
S20.221- Contusion of <u>right</u> back wall of thorax
S20.222- Contusion of <u>left</u> back wall of thorax
S20.229- Contusion of <u>unspecified</u> back wall of thorax
S20.3- Other and unspecified superficial injuries of <u>front wall</u> of thorax
S20.30- <u>Unspecified</u> superficial injuries of <u>front wall</u> of thorax
S20.301- Unspecified superficial injuries of <u>right</u> front wall of thorax
S20.302- Unspecified superficial injuries of <u>left</u> front wall of thorax
S20.309- Unspecified superficial injuries of <u>unspecified</u> front wall of thorax
S20.31- <u>Abrasion</u> of <u>front wall</u> of thorax
S20.311- Abrasion of <u>right</u> front wall of thorax
S20.312- Abrasion of <u>left</u> front wall of thorax
S20.319- Abrasion of <u>unspecified</u> front wall of thorax
S20.32- <u>Blister</u> (nonthermal) of <u>front wall</u> of thorax
S20.321- Blister (nonthermal) of <u>right</u> front wall of thorax
S20.322- Blister (nonthermal) of <u>left</u> front wall of thorax
S20.329- Blister (nonthermal) of <u>unspecified</u> front wall of thorax
S20.34- <u>External constriction</u> of <u>front wall</u> of thorax
S20.341- External constriction of <u>right</u> front wall of thorax
S20.342- External constriction of <u>left</u> front wall of thorax
S20.349- External constriction of <u>unspecified</u> front wall of thorax

S16-S20

S20.35- Superficial foreign body of front wall of thorax
Splinter in front wall of thorax

S20.351- Superficial foreign body of right front wall of thorax

S20.352- Superficial foreign body of left front wall of thorax

S20.359- Superficial foreign body of unspecified front wall of thorax

S20.36- Insect bite (nonvenomous) of front wall of thorax

S20.361- Insect bite (nonvenomous) of right front wall of thorax

S20.362- Insect bite (nonvenomous) of left front wall of thorax

S20.369- Insect bite (nonvenomous) of unspecified front wall of thorax

S20.37- Other superficial bite of front wall of thorax
Excludes 1:   open bite of front wall of thorax (S21.14)

S20.371- Other superficial bite of right front wall of thorax

S20.372- Other superficial bite of left front wall of thorax

S20.379- Other superficial bite of unspecified front wall of thorax

S20.4- Other and unspecified superficial injuries of back wall of thorax

S20.40- Unspecified superficial injuries of back wall of thorax

S20.401- Unspecified superficial injuries of right back wall of thorax

S20.402- Unspecified superficial injuries of left back wall of thorax

S20.409- Unspecified superficial injuries of unspecified back wall of thorax

S20.41- Abrasion of back wall of thorax

S20.411- Abrasion of right back wall of thorax

S20.412- Abrasion of left back wall of thorax

S20.419- Abrasion of unspecified back wall of thorax

S20.42- Blister (nonthermal) of back wall of thorax

S20.421- Blister (nonthermal) of right back wall of thorax

S20.422- Blister (nonthermal) of left back wall of thorax

S20.429- Blister (nonthermal) of unspecified back wall of thorax

S20.44- External constriction of back wall of thorax

S20.441- External constriction of right back wall of thorax

S20.442- External constriction of left back wall of thorax

S20.449- External constriction of unspecified back wall of thorax

S20.45- Superficial foreign body of back wall of thorax
Splinter of back wall of thorax

S20.451- Superficial foreign body of right back wall of thorax

S20.452- Superficial foreign body of left back wall of thorax

S20.459- Superficial foreign body of unspecified back wall of thorax

S20.46- Insect bite (nonvenomous) of back wall of thorax

S20.461- Insect bite (nonvenomous) of right back wall of thorax

S20.462- Insect bite (nonvenomous) of left back wall of thorax

S20.469- Insect bite (nonvenomous) of unspecified back wall of thorax

S20.47- Other superficial bite of back wall of thorax
Excludes 1:   open bite of back wall of thorax (S21.24)

S20.471- Other superficial bite of right back wall of thorax

S20.472- Other superficial bite of left back wall of thorax

S20.479- Other superficial bite of unspecified back wall of thorax

S20.9- Superficial injury of unspecified parts of thorax
Excludes 1:   contusion of thorax NOS (S20.20)

S20.90x- Unspecified superficial injury of unspecified parts of thorax
Superficial injury of thoracic wall NOS

S20.91x- Abrasion of unspecified parts of thorax

S20.92x- Blister (nonthermal) of unspecified parts of thorax

S20.94x- External constriction of unspecified parts of thorax

S20.95x- Superficial foreign body of unspecified parts of thorax
Splinter in thorax NOS

S20.96x- Insect bite (nonvenomous) of unspecified parts of thorax

S20.97x- Other superficial bite of unspecified parts of thorax
Excludes 1:   open bite of thorax NOS (S21.95)

S21- Open wound of thorax
Code also any associated injury, such as :
Injury of heart (S26.-)
Injury of intrathoracic organs (S27.-)
Rib fracture (S22.3-, S22.4-)
Spinal cord injury (S24.0-, S24.1-)
Traumatic hemothorax (S27.1)
Traumatic hemopneumothorax (S27.3)
Traumatic pneumothorax (S27.0)
Wound infection
Excludes 1:   traumatic amputation (partial) of thorax (S28.1)

The appropriate 7th character is to be added to each code from category S21:
A   Initial encounter
D   Subsequent encounter
S   Sequela

S21.0- Open wound of breast

S21.00- Unspecified open wound of breast

S21.001- Unspecified open wound of right breast

S21.002- Unspecified open wound of left breast

S21.009- Unspecified open wound of unspecified breast

S21.01- Laceration without foreign body of breast

S21.011- Laceration without foreign body of right breast

S21.012- Laceration without foreign body of left breast

S21.019- Laceration without foreign body of unspecified breast

S21.02- Laceration with foreign body of breast

S21.021- Laceration with foreign body of right breast

S21.022- Laceration with foreign body of left breast

S21.029- Laceration with foreign body of unspecified breast

S21.03- Puncture wound without foreign body of breast

S21.031- Puncture wound without foreign body of right breast

S21.032- Puncture wound without foreign body of left breast

S21.039- Puncture wound without foreign body of unspecified breast

S21.04- Puncture wound with foreign body of breast

S21.041- Puncture wound with foreign body of right breast

S21.042- Puncture wound with foreign body of left breast

S21.049- Puncture wound with foreign body of unspecified breast

S21.05- Open bite of breast
Bite of breast NOS
Excludes 1:   superficial bite of breast (S20.17)

S21.051- Open bite of right breast

S21.052- Open bite of left breast

S21.059- Open bite of unspecified breast

S21.1- Open wound of front wall of thorax without penetration into thoracic cavity
Open wound of chest without penetration into thoracic cavity

S21.10- Unspecified open wound of front wall of thorax without penetration into thoracic cavity

CC-A **S21.101-** Unspecified open wound of right front wall of thorax without penetration into thoracic cavity

CC-A **S21.102-** Unspecified open wound of <u>left</u> front wall of thorax <u>without</u> penetration into thoracic cavity

CC-A **S21.109-** Unspecified open wound of <u>unspecified</u> front wall of thorax <u>without</u> penetration into thoracic cavity

S21.11- <u>Laceration</u> <u>without</u> foreign body of front wall of thorax <u>without</u> penetration into thoracic cavity

CC-A **S21.111-** Laceration <u>without</u> foreign body of <u>right</u> front wall of thorax <u>without</u> penetration into thoracic cavity

CC-A **S21.112-** Laceration <u>without</u> foreign body of <u>left</u> front wall of thorax <u>without</u> penetration into thoracic cavity

CC-A **S21.119-** Laceration <u>without</u> foreign body of <u>unspecified</u> front wall of thorax <u>without</u> penetration into thoracic cavity

S21.12- Laceration <u>with foreign body</u> of front wall of thorax <u>without</u> penetration into thoracic cavity

CC-A **S21.121-** Laceration <u>with foreign body</u> of <u>right</u> front wall of thorax <u>without</u> penetration into thoracic cavity

CC-A **S21.122-** Laceration <u>with foreign body</u> of <u>left</u> front wall of thorax <u>without</u> penetration into thoracic cavity

CC-A **S21.129-** Laceration <u>with foreign body</u> of <u>unspecified</u> front wall of thorax <u>without</u> penetration into thoracic cavity

S21.13- <u>Puncture</u> wound <u>without</u> foreign body of front wall of thorax <u>without</u> penetration into thoracic cavity

CC-A **S21.131-** Puncture wound <u>without</u> foreign body of <u>right</u> front wall of thorax <u>without</u> penetration into thoracic cavity

CC-A **S21.132-** Puncture wound <u>without</u> foreign body of <u>left</u> front wall of thorax <u>without</u> penetration into thoracic cavity

CC-A **S21.139-** Puncture wound <u>without</u> foreign body of <u>unspecified</u> front wall of thorax <u>without</u> penetration into thoracic cavity

S21.14- <u>Puncture</u> wound <u>with foreign body</u> of front wall of thorax <u>without</u> penetration into thoracic cavity

CC-A **S21.141-** Puncture wound <u>with foreign body</u> of <u>right</u> front wall of thorax <u>without</u> penetration into thoracic cavity

CC-A **S21.142-** Puncture wound <u>with foreign body</u> of <u>left</u> front wall of thorax <u>without</u> penetration into thoracic cavity

CC-A **S21.149-** Puncture wound <u>with foreign body</u> of <u>unspecified</u> front wall of thorax <u>without</u> penetration into thoracic cavity

S21.15- <u>Open bite</u> of front wall of thorax <u>without</u> penetration into thoracic cavity

    Bite of front wall of thorax NOS

    Excludes 1:   *superficial bite of front wall of thorax (S20.37)*

CC-A **S21.151-** Open bite of <u>right</u> front wall of thorax <u>without</u> penetration into thoracic cavity

CC-A **S21.152-** Open bite of <u>left</u> front wall of thorax <u>without</u> penetration into thoracic cavity

CC-A **S21.159-** Open bite of <u>unspecified</u> front wall of thorax <u>without</u> penetration into thoracic cavity

S21.2- <u>Open wound</u> of <u>back wall</u> of <u>thorax</u> <u>without</u> penetration into thoracic cavity

S21.20- <u>Unspecified</u> open wound of <u>back wall</u> of thorax <u>without</u> penetration into thoracic cavity

S21.201- Unspecified open wound of <u>right</u> back wall of thorax <u>without</u> penetration into thoracic cavity

S21.202- Unspecified open wound of <u>left</u> back wall of thorax <u>without</u> penetration into thoracic cavity

S21.209- Unspecified open wound of <u>unspecified</u> back wall of thorax <u>without</u> penetration into thoracic cavity

S21.21- <u>Laceration</u> <u>without</u> foreign body of <u>back wall</u> of thorax <u>without</u> penetration into thoracic cavity

S21.211- Laceration <u>without</u> foreign body of <u>right</u> back wall of thorax <u>without</u> penetration into thoracic cavity

S21.212- Laceration <u>without</u> foreign body of <u>left</u> back wall of thorax <u>without</u> penetration into thoracic cavity

S21.219- Laceration <u>without</u> foreign body of <u>unspecified</u> back wall of thorax <u>without</u> penetration into thoracic cavity

S21.22- <u>Laceration</u> <u>with foreign body</u> of <u>back wall</u> of thorax <u>without</u> penetration into thoracic cavity

S21.221- Laceration <u>with foreign body</u> of <u>right</u> back wall of thorax <u>without</u> penetration into thoracic cavity

S21.222- Laceration <u>with foreign body</u> of <u>left</u> back wall of thorax <u>without</u> penetration into thoracic cavity

S21.229- Laceration <u>with foreign body</u> of <u>unspecified</u> back wall of thorax <u>without</u> penetration into thoracic cavity

S21.23- <u>Puncture</u> wound <u>without</u> foreign body of <u>back wall</u> of thorax <u>without</u> penetration into thoracic cavity

S21.231- Puncture wound <u>without</u> foreign body of <u>right</u> back wall of thorax <u>without</u> penetration into thoracic cavity

S21.232- Puncture wound <u>without</u> foreign body of <u>left</u> back wall of thorax <u>without</u> penetration into thoracic cavity

S21.239- Puncture wound <u>without</u> foreign body of <u>unspecified</u> back wall of thorax <u>without</u> penetration into thoracic cavity

S21.24- <u>Puncture</u> wound <u>with foreign body</u> of <u>back wall</u> of thorax <u>without</u> penetration into thoracic cavity

S21.241- Puncture wound <u>with foreign body</u> of <u>right</u> back wall of thorax <u>without</u> penetration into thoracic cavity

S21.242- Puncture wound <u>with foreign body</u> of <u>left</u> back wall of thorax <u>without</u> penetration into thoracic cavity

S21.249- Puncture wound <u>with foreign body</u> of <u>unspecified</u> back wall of thorax <u>without</u> penetration into thoracic cavity

S21.25- <u>Open bite</u> of <u>back wall</u> of thorax <u>without</u> penetration into thoracic cavity

    Bite of back wall of thorax NOS

    Excludes 1:   *superficial bite of back wall of thorax (S20.47)*

S21.251- Open bite of <u>right</u> back wall of thorax <u>without</u> penetration into thoracic cavity

S21.252- Open bite of <u>left</u> back wall of thorax <u>without</u> penetration into thoracic cavity

S21.259- Open bite of <u>unspecified</u> back wall of thorax <u>without</u> penetration into thoracic cavity

S21.3- <u>Open wound</u> of <u>front wall</u> of <u>thorax</u> <u>with penetration into thoracic cavity</u>

    Open wound of chest with penetration into thoracic cavity

S21.30- <u>Unspecified</u> open wound of <u>front wall</u> of thorax <u>with penetration into thoracic cavity</u>

MCC-A **S21.301-** Unspecified open wound of <u>right</u> front wall of thorax <u>with penetration</u> into thoracic cavity

MCC-A **S21.302-** Unspecified open wound of <u>left</u> front wall of thorax <u>with penetration</u> into thoracic cavity

MCC-A **S21.309-** Unspecified open wound of <u>unspecified</u> front wall of thorax <u>with penetration</u> into thoracic cavity

S21.31- <u>Laceration</u> <u>without</u> foreign body of <u>front wall</u> of thorax <u>with penetration into thoracic cavity</u>

MCC-A **S21.311-** Laceration <u>without</u> foreign body of <u>right</u> front wall of thorax <u>with penetration</u> into thoracic cavity

MCC-A **S21.312-** Laceration <u>without</u> foreign body of <u>left</u> front wall of thorax <u>with penetration</u> into thoracic cavity

MCC-A **S21.319-** Laceration <u>without</u> foreign body of <u>unspecified</u> front wall of thorax <u>with penetration</u> into thoracic cavity

S21.32- <u>Laceration</u> <u>with foreign body</u> of <u>front wall</u> of thorax <u>with penetration into thoracic cavity</u>

MCC-A **S21.321-** Laceration <u>with foreign body</u> of <u>right</u> front wall of thorax <u>with penetration</u> into thoracic cavity

MCC-A **S21.322-** Laceration <u>with foreign body</u> of <u>left</u> front wall of thorax <u>with penetration</u> into thoracic cavity

MCC-A **S21.329-** Laceration <u>with foreign body</u> of <u>unspecified</u> front wall of thorax <u>with penetration</u> into thoracic cavity

S21.33- <u>Puncture</u> wound <u>without</u> foreign body of front wall of thorax <u>with penetration into thoracic cavity</u>

MCC-A **S21.331-** Puncture wound <u>without</u> foreign body of <u>right</u> front wall of thorax <u>with penetration</u> into thoracic cavity

MCC-A **S21.332-** Puncture wound <u>without</u> foreign body of <u>left</u> front wall of thorax <u>with penetration</u> into thoracic cavity

MCC-A **S21.339-** Puncture wound <u>without</u> foreign body of <u>unspecified</u> front wall of thorax <u>with penetration</u> into thoracic cavity

S21.34- <u>Puncture</u> wound <u>with foreign body</u> of <u>front wall</u> of thorax <u>with penetration into thoracic cavity</u>

MCC-A **S21.341-** Puncture wound <u>with foreign body</u> of <u>right</u> front wall of thorax <u>with penetration</u> into thoracic cavity

MCC-A **S21.342-** Puncture wound <u>with foreign body</u> of <u>left</u> front wall of thorax <u>with penetration</u> into thoracic cavity

MCC-A **S21.349-** Puncture wound <u>with foreign body</u> of <u>unspecified</u> front wall of thorax <u>with penetration</u> into thoracic cavity

S21.35- <u>Open bite</u> of <u>front wall</u> of thorax <u>with penetration into thoracic cavity</u>
    Excludes 1:   *superficial bite of front wall of thorax (S20.37)*

MCC-A **S21.351-** Open bite of <u>right</u> front wall of thorax <u>with penetration</u> into thoracic cavity

MCC-A **S21.352-** Open bite of <u>left</u> front wall of thorax <u>with penetration</u> into thoracic cavity

MCC-A **S21.359-** Open bite of <u>unspecified</u> front wall of thorax <u>with penetration</u> into thoracic cavity

S21.4- <u>Open wound</u> of <u>back wall</u> of thorax <u>with penetration into thoracic cavity</u>

S21.40- <u>Unspecified</u> open wound of <u>back wall</u> of thorax <u>with penetration into thoracic cavity</u>

MCC-A **S21.401-** Unspecified open wound of <u>right</u> back wall of thorax <u>with penetration</u> into thoracic cavity

MCC-A **S21.402-** Unspecified open wound of <u>left</u> back wall of thorax <u>with penetration</u> into thoracic cavity

MCC-A **S21.409-** Unspecified open wound of <u>unspecified</u> back wall of thorax <u>with penetration</u> into thoracic cavity

S21.41- <u>Laceration</u> <u>without</u> foreign body of <u>back wall</u> of thorax <u>with penetration into thoracic cavity</u>

MCC-A **S21.411-** Laceration <u>without</u> foreign body of <u>right</u> back wall of thorax <u>with penetration</u> into thoracic cavity

MCC-A **S21.412-** Laceration <u>without</u> foreign body of <u>left</u> back wall of thorax <u>with penetration</u> into thoracic cavity

MCC-A **S21.419-** Laceration <u>without</u> foreign body of <u>unspecified</u> back wall of thorax <u>with penetration</u> into thoracic cavity

S21.42- <u>Laceration</u> <u>with foreign body</u> of <u>back wall</u> of thorax <u>with penetration into thoracic cavity</u>

MCC-A **S21.421-** Laceration <u>with foreign body</u> of <u>right</u> back wall of thorax <u>with penetration</u> into thoracic cavity

MCC-A **S21.422-** Laceration <u>with foreign body</u> of <u>left</u> back wall of thorax <u>with penetration</u> into thoracic cavity

MCC-A **S21.429-** Laceration <u>with foreign body</u> of <u>unspecified</u> back wall of thorax <u>with penetration</u> into thoracic cavity

S21.43- <u>Puncture</u> wound <u>without</u> foreign body of <u>back wall</u> of thorax <u>with penetration into thoracic cavity</u>

MCC-A **S21.431-** Puncture wound <u>without</u> foreign body of <u>right</u> back wall of thorax <u>with penetration</u> into thoracic cavity

MCC-A **S21.432-** Puncture wound <u>without</u> foreign body of <u>left</u> back wall of thorax <u>with penetration</u> into thoracic cavity

MCC-A **S21.439-** Puncture wound <u>without</u> foreign body of <u>unspecified</u> back wall of thorax <u>with penetration</u> into thoracic cavity

S21.44- <u>Puncture</u> wound <u>with foreign body</u> of <u>back wall</u> of thorax <u>with penetration into thoracic cavity</u>

MCC-A **S21.441-** Puncture wound <u>with foreign body</u> of <u>right</u> back wall of thorax <u>with penetration</u> into thoracic cavity

MCC-A **S21.442-** Puncture wound <u>with foreign body</u> of <u>left</u> back wall of thorax <u>with penetration</u> into thoracic cavity

MCC-A **S21.449-** Puncture wound <u>with foreign body</u> of <u>unspecified</u> back wall of thorax <u>with penetration</u> into thoracic cavity

S21.45- <u>Open bite</u> of <u>back wall</u> of thorax <u>with penetration into thoracic cavity</u>
    Bite of back wall of thorax NOS
    Excludes 1:   *superficial bite of back wall of thorax (S20.47)*

MCC-A **S21.451-** Open bite of <u>right</u> back wall of thorax <u>with penetration</u> into thoracic cavity

MCC-A **S21.452-** Open bite of <u>left</u> back wall of thorax <u>with penetration</u> into thoracic cavity

MCC-A **S21.459-** Open bite of <u>unspecified</u> back wall of thorax <u>with penetration</u> into thoracic cavity

S21.9- <u>Open wound</u> of <u>unspecified</u> part of thorax
    Open wound of thoracic wall NOS

CC-A **S21.90x-** <u>Unspecified</u> open wound of <u>unspecified</u> part of thorax

CC-A **S21.91x-** <u>Laceration</u> <u>without</u> foreign body of <u>unspecified</u> part of thorax

CC-A **S21.92x-** <u>Laceration</u> <u>with foreign body</u> of <u>unspecified</u> part of thorax

CC-A **S21.93x-** <u>Puncture</u> wound <u>without</u> foreign body of <u>unspecified</u> part of thorax

CC-A **S21.94x-** <u>Puncture</u> wound <u>with foreign body</u> of <u>unspecified</u> part of thorax

CC-A **S21.95x-** <u>Open bite</u> of <u>unspecified</u> part of thorax
    Excludes 1:   *superficial bite of thorax (S20.97)*

S22- <u>Fracture</u> of <u>rib(s), sternum and thoracic spine</u>
  Note: A fracture not indicated as nondisplaced or displaced should be classified to displaced
  Note: A fracture not indicated as open or closed should be coded to closed
  Includes: Fracture of thoracic neural arch
            Fracture of thoracic spinous process
            Fracture of thoracic transverse process
            Fracture of thoracic vertebra
            Fracture of thoracic vertebral arch
  Code first any associated:
    Injury of intrathoracic organ (S27.-)
    Spinal cord injury (S24.0-, S24.1-)
  Excludes 1:   *transection of thorax (S28.1)*
  Excludes ❷: *fracture of clavicle (S42.0-)*
                fracture of scapula (S42.1-)

> The appropriate 7th character is to be added to each code from category S22:
> **A**   <u>Initial</u> encounter for <u>closed</u> fracture
> **B**   <u>Initial</u> encounter for <u>open</u> fracture
> **D**   <u>Subsequent</u> encounter for fracture <u>with routine healing</u>
> **G**   <u>Subsequent</u> encounter for fracture <u>with delayed healing</u>
> **K**   <u>Subsequent</u> encounter for fracture <u>with nonunion</u>
> **S**   <u>Sequela</u>

S22.0- <u>Fracture</u> of <u>thoracic vertebra</u>

S22.00- Fracture of <u>unspecified</u> thoracic vertebra

CC-A,K MCC-B **S22.000-** <u>Wedge</u> compression fracture of unspecified thoracic vertebra

CC-A,K MCC-B **S22.001-** <u>Stable burst</u> fracture of unspecified thoracic vertebra

CC-A,K MCC-B **S22.002-** <u>Unstable burst</u> fracture of unspecified thoracic vertebra

CC-A,K MCC-B **S22.008-** <u>Other</u> fracture of unspecified thoracic vertebra

CC-A,K MCC-B **S22.009-** <u>Unspecified</u> fracture of unspecified thoracic vertebra

S22.01- Fracture of <u>first</u> thoracic vertebra

CC-A,K MCC-B **S22.010-** <u>Wedge</u> compression fracture of first thoracic vertebra

CC-A,K MCC-B **S22.011-** <u>Stable burst</u> fracture of first thoracic vertebra

CC-A,K MCC-B **S22.012-** <u>Unstable burst</u> fracture of first thoracic vertebra

CC-A,K MCC-B **S22.018-** <u>Other</u> fracture of first thoracic vertebra

CC-A,K MCC-B **S22.019-** <u>Unspecified</u> fracture of first thoracic vertebra

S21-S22 *(side tab)*

S22.02-   Fracture of <u>second</u> thoracic vertebra

CC-A,K MCC-B S22.020-   <u>Wedge</u> compression fracture of second thoracic vertebra

CC-A,K MCC-B S22.021-   <u>Stable burst</u> fracture of second thoracic vertebra

CC-A,K MCC-B S22.022-   <u>Unstable burst</u> fracture of second thoracic vertebra

CC-A,K MCC-B S22.028-   <u>Other</u> fracture of second thoracic vertebra

CC-A,K MCC-B S22.029-   <u>Unspecified</u> fracture of second thoracic vertebra

S22.03-   Fracture of <u>third</u> thoracic vertebra

CC-A,K MCC-B S22.030-   <u>Wedge</u> compression fracture of third thoracic vertebra

CC-A,K MCC-B S22.031-   <u>Stable burst</u> fracture of third thoracic vertebra

CC-A,K MCC-B S22.032-   <u>Unstable burst</u> fracture of third thoracic vertebra

CC-A,K MCC-B S22.038-   <u>Other</u> fracture of third thoracic vertebra

CC-A,K MCC-B S22.039-   <u>Unspecified</u> fracture of third thoracic vertebra

S22.04-   Fracture of <u>fourth</u> thoracic vertebra

CC-A,K MCC-B S22.040-   <u>Wedge</u> compression fracture of fourth thoracic vertebra

CC-A,K MCC-B S22.041-   <u>Stable burst</u> fracture of fourth thoracic vertebra

CC-A,K MCC-B S22.042-   <u>Unstable burst</u> fracture of fourth thoracic vertebra

CC-A,K MCC-B S22.048-   <u>Other</u> fracture of fourth thoracic vertebra

CC-A,K MCC-B S22.049-   <u>Unspecified</u> fracture of fourth thoracic vertebra

S22.05-   Fracture of <u>T5-T6</u> vertebra

CC-A,K MCC-B S22.050-   <u>Wedge</u> compression fracture of T5-T6 vertebra

CC-A,K MCC-B S22.051-   <u>Stable burst</u> fracture of T5-T6 vertebra

CC-A,K MCC-B S22.052-   <u>Unstable burst</u> fracture of T5-T6 vertebra

CC-A,K MCC-B S22.058-   <u>Other</u> fracture of T5-T6 vertebra

CC-A,K MCC-B S22.059-   <u>Unspecified</u> fracture of T5-T6 vertebra

S22.06-   Fracture of <u>T7-T8</u> vertebra

CC-A,K MCC-B S22.060-   <u>Wedge</u> compression fracture of T7-T8 vertebra

CC-A,K MCC-B S22.061-   <u>Stable burst</u> fracture of T7-T8 vertebra

CC-A,K MCC-B S22.062-   <u>Unstable burst</u> fracture of T7-T8 vertebra

CC-A,K MCC-B S22.068-   <u>Other</u> fracture of T7-T8 thoracic vertebra

CC-A,K MCC-B S22.069-   <u>Unspecified</u> fracture of T7-T8 vertebra

S22.07-   Fracture of <u>T9-T10</u> vertebra

CC-A,K MCC-B S22.070-   <u>Wedge</u> compression fracture of T9-T10 vertebra

CC-A,K MCC-B S22.071-   Stable burst fracture of T9-T10 vertebra

CC-A,K MCC-B S22.072-   <u>Unstable burst</u> fracture of T9-T10 vertebra

CC-A,K MCC-B S22.078-   Other fracture of T9-T10 vertebra

CC-A,K MCC-B S22.079-   <u>Unspecified</u> fracture of T9-T10 vertebra

S22.08-   Fracture of <u>T11-T12</u> vertebra

CC-A,K MCC-B S22.080-   <u>Wedge</u> compression fracture of T11-T12 vertebra

CC-A,K MCC-B S22.081-   <u>Stable burst</u> fracture of T11-T12 vertebra

CC-A,K MCC-B S22.082-   <u>Unstable burst</u> fracture of T11-T12 vertebra

CC-A,K MCC-B S22.088-   <u>Other</u> fracture of T11-T12 vertebra

CC-A,K MCC-B S22.089-   <u>Unspecified</u> fracture of T11-T12 vertebra

S22.2-   Fracture of <u>sternum</u>

S22.20x-   <u>Unspecified</u> fracture of sternum
CC-A,K MCC-B

S22.21x-   Fracture of <u>manubrium</u>
CC-A,K MCC-B

S22.22x-   Fracture of <u>body</u> of sternum
CC-A,K MCC-B

S22.23x-   Sternal <u>manubrial dissociation</u>
CC-A,K MCC-B

S22.24x-   Fracture of <u>xiphoid process</u>
CC-A,K MCC-B

S22.3-   Fracture of <u>one rib</u>

S22.31x-   Fracture of one rib, <u>right</u> side
CC-A,K MCC-B

S22.32x-   Fracture of one rib, <u>left</u> side
CC-A,K MCC-B

S22.39x-   Fracture of one rib, <u>unspecified</u> side
CC-A,K MCC-B

S22.4-   <u>Multiple</u> fractures of <u>ribs</u>
    Fractures of two or more ribs
    Excludes 1:   flail chest (S22.5-)

S22.41x-   Multiple fractures of ribs, <u>right</u> side
CC-A,K MCC-B

S22.42x-   Multiple fractures of ribs, <u>left</u> side
CC-A,K MCC-B

S22.43x-   Multiple fractures of ribs, <u>bilateral</u>
CC-A,K MCC-B

S22.49x-   Multiple fractures of ribs, <u>unspecified</u> side
CC-A,K MCC-B

S22.5xx-   <u>Flail chest</u>
CC-K MCC-A,B

S22.9xx-   Fracture of <u>bony</u> <u>thorax</u>, part <u>unspecified</u>
CC-A,K MCC-B

S23-   <u>Dislocation and sprain</u> of joints and ligaments of <u>thorax</u>
   Includes: Avulsion of joint or ligament of thorax
         Laceration of cartilage, joint or ligament of thorax
         Sprain of cartilage, joint or ligament of thorax
         Traumatic hemarthrosis of joint or ligament of thorax
         Traumatic rupture of joint or ligament of thorax
         Traumatic subluxation of joint or ligament of thorax
         Traumatic tear of joint or ligament of thorax
   Code also any associated open wound
   Excludes ❷: dislocation, sprain of sternoclavicular joint (S43.2, S43.6)
         strain of muscle or tendon of thorax (S29.01-)

The appropriate 7th character is to be added to each code from category S23:
A   <u>Initial</u> encounter
D   <u>Subsequent</u> encounter
S   <u>Sequela</u>

S23.0xx-   <u>Traumatic rupture</u> of <u>thoracic intervertebral disc</u>
   Excludes 1:   rupture or displacement (nontraumatic) of thoracic intervertebral disc NOS (M51.- with fifth character 4)

S23.1-   <u>Subluxation and dislocation</u> of <u>thoracic vertebra</u>
   Code also any associated:
     Open wound of thorax (S21.-)
     Spinal cord injury (S24.0-, S24.1-)
   Excludes ❷: fracture of thoracic vertebrae (S22.0-)

S23.10-   Subluxation and dislocation of <u>unspecified</u> thoracic vertebra

S23.100-   <u>Subluxation</u> of unspecified thoracic vertebra

S23.101-   <u>Dislocation</u> of unspecified thoracic vertebra

S23.11-   Subluxation and dislocation of <u>T1/T2</u> thoracic vertebra

S23.110-   <u>Subluxation</u> of T1/T2 thoracic vertebra

S23.111-   <u>Dislocation</u> of T1/T2 thoracic vertebra

S23.12-   Subluxation and dislocation of T2/T3-T3/T4 thoracic vertebra

S23.120-   <u>Subluxation</u> of <u>T2/T3</u> thoracic vertebra

S23.121-   <u>Dislocation</u> of <u>T2/T3</u> thoracic vertebra

S23.122-   <u>Subluxation</u> of <u>T3/T4</u> thoracic vertebra

S23.123-   <u>Dislocation</u> of <u>T3/T4</u> thoracic vertebra

S23.13-   Subluxation and dislocation of T4/T5-T5/T6 thoracic vertebra

S23.130-   <u>Subluxation</u> of <u>T4/T5</u> thoracic vertebra

S23.131-   <u>Dislocation</u> of <u>T4/T5</u> thoracic vertebra

S23.132-   <u>Subluxation</u> of <u>T5/T6</u> thoracic vertebra

S23.133-   <u>Dislocation</u> of <u>T5/T6</u> thoracic vertebra

S23.14-   Subluxation and dislocation of T6/T7-T7/T8 thoracic vertebra

S23.140-   <u>Subluxation</u> of <u>T6/T7</u> thoracic vertebra

S23.141-   <u>Dislocation</u> of <u>T6/T7</u> thoracic vertebra

S23.142-   <u>Subluxation</u> of <u>T7/T8</u> thoracic vertebra

S23.143-   <u>Dislocation</u> of <u>T7/T8</u> thoracic vertebra

S23.15-   Subluxation and dislocation of T8/T9-T9/T10 thoracic vertebra

S23.150-   <u>Subluxation</u> of <u>T8/T9</u> thoracic vertebra

S23.151-   <u>Dislocation</u> of <u>T8/T9</u> thoracic vertebra

S23.152-   <u>Subluxation</u> of <u>T9/T10</u> thoracic vertebra

S23.153-   <u>Dislocation</u> of <u>T9/T10</u> thoracic vertebra

S23.16-   Subluxation and dislocation of T10/T11-T11/T12 thoracic vertebra

S23.160-   <u>Subluxation</u> of <u>T10/T11</u> thoracic vertebra

S23.161-   <u>Dislocation</u> of <u>T10/T11</u> thoracic vertebra

S23.162-   <u>Subluxation</u> of <u>T11/T12</u> thoracic vertebra

S22 - S23

S23.163- Dislocation of T11/T12 thoracic vertebra

S23.17- Subluxation and dislocation of T12/L1 thoracic vertebra

S23.170- Subluxation of T12/L1 thoracic vertebra

S23.171- Dislocation of T12/L1 thoracic vertebra

S23.2- Dislocation of other and unspecified parts of thorax

S23.20x- Dislocation of unspecified part of thorax

S23.29x- Dislocation of other parts of thorax

S23.3xx- Sprain of ligaments of thoracic spine

S23.4- Sprain of ribs and sternum

S23.41x- Sprain of ribs

S23.42- Sprain of sternum

S23.420- Sprain of sternoclavicular (joint) (ligament)

S23.421- Sprain of chondrosternal joint

S23.428- Other sprain of sternum

S23.429- Unspecified sprain of sternum

S23.8xx- Sprain of other specified parts of thorax

S23.9xx- Sprain of unspecified parts of thorax

S24- Injury of nerves and spinal cord at thorax level
    Note: Code to highest level of thoracic spinal cord injury
        Injuries to the spinal cord (S24.0 and S24.1) refer to the cord level and not bone level injury, and can affect nerve roots at and below the level given.
    Code also any associated:
        Fracture of thoracic vertebra (S22.0-)
        Open wound of thorax (S21.-)
        Transient paralysis (R29.5)
    Excludes ❷: injury of brachial plexus (S14.3)

The appropriate 7th character is to be added to each code from category S24:
  A Initial encounter
  D Subsequent encounter
  S Sequela

S24.0xx- Concussion and edema of thoracic spinal cord
MCC-A

S24.1- Other and unspecified injuries of thoracic spinal cord

S24.10- Unspecified injury of thoracic spinal cord

MCC-A S24.101- Unspecified injury at T1 level of thoracic spinal cord

MCC-A S24.102- Unspecified injury at T2-T6 level of thoracic spinal cord

MCC-A S24.103- Unspecified injury at T7-T10 level of thoracic spinal cord

MCC-A S24.104- Unspecified injury at T11-T12 level of thoracic spinal cord

S24.109- Unspecified injury at unspecified level of thoracic spinal cord
    Injury of thoracic spinal cord NOS

S24.11- Complete lesion of thoracic spinal cord

MCC-A S24.111- Complete lesion at T1 level of thoracic spinal cord

MCC-A S24.112- Complete lesion at T2-T6 level of thoracic spinal cord

MCC-A S24.113- Complete lesion at T7-T10 level of thoracic spinal cord

MCC-A S24.114- Complete lesion at T11-T12 level of thoracic spinal cord

S24.119- Complete lesion at unspecified level of thoracic spinal cord

S24.13- Anterior cord syndrome of thoracic spinal cord

MCC-A S24.131- Anterior cord syndrome at T1 level of thoracic spinal cord

MCC-A S24.132- Anterior cord syndrome at T2-T6 level of thoracic spinal cord

MCC-A S24.133- Anterior cord syndrome at T7-T10 level of thoracic spinal cord

MCC-A S24.134- Anterior cord syndrome at T11-T12 level of thoracic spinal cord

S24.139- Anterior cord syndrome at unspecified level of thoracic spinal cord

S24.14- Brown-Séquard syndrome of thoracic spinal cord

MCC-A S24.141- Brown-Séquard syndrome at T1 level of thoracic spinal cord

MCC-A S24.142- Brown-Séquard syndrome at T2-T6 level of thoracic spinal cord

MCC-A S24.143- Brown-Séquard syndrome at T7-T10 level of thoracic spinal cord

MCC-A S24.144- Brown-Séquard syndrome at T11-T12 level of thoracic spinal cord

S24.149- Brown-Séquard syndrome at unspecified level of thoracic spinal cord

S24.15- Other incomplete lesions of thoracic spinal cord
    Incomplete lesion of thoracic spinal cord NOS
    Posterior cord syndrome of thoracic spinal cord

MCC-A S24.151- Other incomplete lesion at T1 level of thoracic spinal cord

MCC-A S24.152- Other incomplete lesion at T2-T6 level of thoracic spinal cord

MCC-A S24.153- Other incomplete lesion at T7-T10 level of thoracic spinal cord

MCC-A S24.154- Other incomplete lesion at T11-T12 level of thoracic spinal cord

S24.159- Other incomplete lesion at unspecified level of thoracic spinal cord

S24.2xx- Injury of nerve root of thoracic spine

S24.3xx- Injury of peripheral nerves of thorax

S24.4xx- Injury of thoracic sympathetic nervous system
    Injury of cardiac plexus
    Injury of esophageal plexus
    Injury of pulmonary plexus
    Injury of stellate ganglion
    Injury of thoracic sympathetic ganglion

S24.8xx- Injury of other specified nerves of thorax

S24.9xx- Injury of unspecified nerve of thorax

S25- Injury of blood vessels of thorax
    Code also any associated open wound (S21.-)

The appropriate 7th character is to be added to each code from category S25:
  A Initial encounter
  D Subsequent encounter
  S Sequela

S25.0- Injury of thoracic aorta
    Injury of aorta NOS

MCC-A S25.00x- Unspecified injury of thoracic aorta

MCC-A S25.01x- Minor laceration of thoracic aorta
    Incomplete transection of thoracic aorta
    Laceration of thoracic aorta NOS
    Superficial laceration of thoracic aorta

MCC-A S25.02x- Major laceration of thoracic aorta
    Complete transection of thoracic aorta
    Traumatic rupture of thoracic aorta

MCC-A S25.09x- Other specified injury of thoracic aorta

S25.1- Injury of innominate or subclavian artery

S25.10- Unspecified injury of innominate or subclavian artery

MCC-A S25.101- Unspecified injury of right innominate or subclavian artery

MCC-A S25.102- Unspecified injury of left innominate or subclavian artery

MCC-A S25.109- Unspecified injury of unspecified innominate or subclavian artery

S25.11- Minor laceration of innominate or subclavian artery
    Incomplete transection of innominate or subclavian artery
    Laceration of innominate or subclavian artery NOS
    Superficial laceration of innominate or subclavian artery

MCC-A S25.111- Minor laceration of right innominate or subclavian artery

MCC-A S25.112- Minor laceration of left innominate or subclavian artery

MCC-A S25.119- Minor laceration of unspecified innominate or subclavian artery

S23 - S25

S25.12-   Major laceration of innominate or subclavian artery
Complete transection of innominate or subclavian artery
Traumatic rupture of innominate or subclavian artery

MCC-A **S25.121-**   Major laceration of right innominate or subclavian artery

MCC-A **S25.122-**   Major laceration of left innominate or subclavian artery

MCC-A **S25.129-**   Major laceration of unspecified innominate or subclavian artery

S25.19-   Other specified injury of innominate or subclavian artery

MCC-A **S25.191-**   Other specified injury of right innominate or subclavian artery

MCC-A **S25.192-**   Other specified injury of left innominate or subclavian artery

MCC-A **S25.199-**   Other specified injury of unspecified innominate or subclavian artery

S25.2-   Injury of superior vena cava
Injury of vena cava NOS

MCC-A **S25.20x-**   Unspecified injury of superior vena cava

MCC-A **S25.21x-**   Minor laceration of superior vena cava
Incomplete transection of superior vena cava
Laceration of superior vena cava NOS
Superficial laceration of superior vena cava

MCC-A **S25.22x-**   Major laceration of superior vena cava
Complete transection of superior vena cava
Traumatic rupture of superior vena cava

MCC-A **S25.29x-**   Other specified injury of superior vena cava

S25.3-   Injury of innominate or subclavian vein

S25.30-   Unspecified injury of innominate or subclavian vein

MCC-A **S25.301-**   Unspecified injury of right innominate or subclavian vein

MCC-A **S25.302-**   Unspecified injury of left innominate or subclavian vein

MCC-A **S25.309-**   Unspecified injury of unspecified innominate or subclavian vein

S25.31-   Minor laceration of innominate or subclavian vein
Incomplete transection of innominate or subclavian vein
Laceration of innominate or subclavian vein NOS
Superficial laceration of innominate or subclavian vein

MCC-A **S25.311-**   Minor laceration of right innominate or subclavian vein

MCC-A **S25.312-**   Minor laceration of left innominate or subclavian vein

MCC-A **S25.319-**   Minor laceration of unspecified innominate or subclavian vein

S25.32-   Major laceration of innominate or subclavian vein
Complete transection of innominate or subclavian vein
Traumatic rupture of innominate or subclavian vein

MCC-A **S25.321-**   Major laceration of right innominate or subclavian vein

MCC-A **S25.322-**   Major laceration of left innominate or subclavian vein

MCC-A **S25.329-**   Major laceration of unspecified innominate or subclavian vein

S25.39-   Other specified injury of innominate or subclavian vein

MCC-A **S25.391-**   Other specified injury of right innominate or subclavian vein

MCC-A **S25.392-**   Other specified injury of left innominate or subclavian vein

MCC-A **S25.399-**   Other specified injury of unspecified innominate or subclavian vein

S25.4-   Injury of pulmonary blood vessels

S25.40-   Unspecified injury of pulmonary blood vessels

MCC-A **S25.401-**   Unspecified injury of right pulmonary blood vessels

MCC-A **S25.402-**   Unspecified injury of left pulmonary blood vessels

MCC-A **S25.409-**   Unspecified injury of unspecified pulmonary blood vessels

S25.41-   Minor laceration of pulmonary blood vessels
Incomplete transection of pulmonary blood vessels
Laceration of pulmonary blood vessels NOS
Superficial laceration of pulmonary blood vessels

MCC-A **S25.411-**   Minor laceration of right pulmonary blood vessels

MCC-A **S25.412-**   Minor laceration of left pulmonary blood vessels

MCC-A **S25.419-**   Minor laceration of unspecified pulmonary blood vessels

S25.42-   Major laceration of pulmonary blood vessels
Complete transection of pulmonary blood vessels
Traumatic rupture of pulmonary blood vessels

MCC-A **S25.421-**   Major laceration of right pulmonary blood vessels

MCC-A **S25.422-**   Major laceration of left pulmonary blood vessels

MCC-A **S25.429-**   Major laceration of unspecified pulmonary blood vessels

S25.49-   Other specified injury of pulmonary blood vessels

MCC-A **S25.491-**   Other specified injury of right pulmonary blood vessels

MCC-A **S25.492-**   Other specified injury of left pulmonary blood vessels

MCC-A **S25.499-**   Other specified injury of unspecified pulmonary blood vessels

S25.5-   Injury of intercostal blood vessels

S25.50-   Unspecified injury of intercostal blood vessels

CC-A **S25.501-**   Unspecified injury of intercostal blood vessels, right side

CC-A **S25.502-**   Unspecified injury of intercostal blood vessels, left side

CC-A **S25.509-**   Unspecified injury of intercostal blood vessels, unspecified side

S25.51-   Laceration of intercostal blood vessels

CC-A **S25.511-**   Laceration of intercostal blood vessels, right side

CC-A **S25.512-**   Laceration of intercostal blood vessels, left side

CC-A **S25.519-**   Laceration of intercostal blood vessels, unspecified side

S25.59-   Other specified injury of intercostal blood vessels

CC-A **S25.591-**   Other specified injury of intercostal blood vessels, right side

CC-A **S25.592-**   Other specified injury of intercostal blood vessels, left side

CC-A **S25.599-**   Other specified injury of intercostal blood vessels, unspecified side

S25.8-   Injury of other blood vessels of thorax
Injury of azygos vein
Injury of mammary artery or vein

S25.80-   Unspecified injury of other blood vessels of thorax

CC-A **S25.801-**   Unspecified injury of other blood vessels of thorax, right side

CC-A **S25.802-**   Unspecified injury of other blood vessels of thorax, left side

CC-A **S25.809-**   Unspecified injury of other blood vessels of thorax, unspecified side

S25.81-   Laceration of other blood vessels of thorax

CC-A **S25.811-**   Laceration of other blood vessels of thorax, right side

CC-A **S25.812-**   Laceration of other blood vessels of thorax, left side

CC-A **S25.819-**   Laceration of other blood vessels of thorax, unspecified side

S25.89-   Other specified injury of other blood vessels of thorax

CC-A **S25.891-**   Other specified injury of other blood vessels of thorax, right side

CC-A **S25.892-**   Other specified injury of other blood vessels of thorax, left side

CC-A **S25.899-**   Other specified injury of other blood vessels of thorax, unspecified side

S25.9-   Injury of unspecified blood vessel of thorax

CC-A **S25.90x-**   Unspecified injury of unspecified blood vessel of thorax

CC-A **S25.91x-**   Laceration of unspecified blood vessel of thorax

S25-S25

CC-A S25.99x- <u>Other</u> specified injury of <u>unspecified</u> <u>blood vessel of thorax</u>

S26- Injury of <u>heart</u>
Code also any associated:
    Open wound of thorax (S21.-)
    Traumatic hemopneumothorax (S27.2)
    Traumatic hemothorax (S27.1)
    Traumatic pneumothorax (S27.0)

The appropriate 7th character is to be added to each code from category S26:
  A <u>Initial</u> encounter
  D <u>Subsequent</u> encounter
  S <u>Sequela</u>

S26.0- Injury of <u>heart with hemopericardium</u>
CC-A S26.00x- <u>Unspecified</u> injury of heart with hemopericardium
CC-A S26.01x- <u>Contusion</u> of heart with hemopericardium
S26.02- <u>Laceration</u> of heart <u>with hemopericardium</u>
MCC-A S26.020- <u>Mild</u> laceration of heart <u>with hemopericardium</u>
    Laceration of heart without penetration of heart chamber
MCC-A S26.021- <u>Moderate</u> laceration of heart <u>with hemopericardium</u>
    Laceration of heart with penetration of heart chamber
MCC-A S26.022- <u>Major</u> laceration of heart <u>with hemopericardium</u>
    Laceration of heart with penetration of multiple heart chambers
CC-A S26.09x- <u>Other</u> injury of heart <u>with hemopericardium</u>
S26.1- Injury of <u>heart</u> <u>without</u> hemopericardium
CC-A S26.10x- <u>Unspecified</u> injury of heart <u>without</u> hemopericardium
CC-A S26.11x- <u>Contusion</u> of heart <u>without</u> hemopericardium
MCC-A S26.12x- <u>Laceration</u> of heart <u>without</u> hemopericardium
CC-A S26.19x- <u>Other</u> injury of heart <u>without</u> hemopericardium
S26.9- Injury of heart, <u>unspecified with or without</u> hemopericardium
CC-A S26.90x- <u>Unspecified</u> injury of heart, <u>unspecified with or without</u> hemopericardium
CC-A S26.91x- <u>Contusion</u> of heart, <u>unspecified with or without</u> hemopericardium
MCC-A S26.92x- <u>Laceration</u> of heart, <u>unspecified with or without</u> hemopericardium
    Laceration of heart NOS
CC-A S26.99x- <u>Other</u> injury of heart, <u>unspecified with or without</u> hemopericardium

S27- Injury of <u>other and unspecified</u> <u>intrathoracic organs</u>
Code also any associated open wound of thorax (S21.-)
Excludes ❷: *injury of cervical esophagus (S10-S19)*
         injury of trachea (cervical) (S10-S19)

The appropriate 7th character is to be added to each code from category S27:
  A <u>Initial</u> encounter
  D <u>Subsequent</u> encounter
  S <u>Sequela</u>

S27.0xx- Traumatic <u>pneumothorax</u>
CC-A   *Excludes 1:* *spontaneous pneumothorax (J93.-)*
S27.1xx- Traumatic <u>hemothorax</u>
MCC-A
S27.2xx- Traumatic <u>hemopneumothorax</u>
MCC-A
S27.3- Other and unspecified injuries of <u>lung</u>
S27.30- <u>Unspecified</u> injury of lung
CC-A S27.301- Unspecified injury of lung, <u>unilateral</u>
CC-A S27.302- Unspecified injury of lung, <u>bilateral</u>
CC-A S27.309- Unspecified injury of lung, <u>unspecified</u>
S27.31- <u>Primary blast</u> injury of lung
    Blast injury of lung NOS
CC-A S27.311- Primary blast injury of lung, <u>unilateral</u>
CC-A S27.312- Primary blast injury of lung, <u>bilateral</u>
CC-A S27.319- Primary blast injury of lung, <u>unspecified</u>
S27.32- <u>Contusion</u> of lung
CC-A S27.321- Contusion of lung, <u>unilateral</u>
CC-A S27.322- Contusion of lung, <u>bilateral</u>

CC-A S27.329- Contusion of lung, <u>unspecified</u>
S27.33- <u>Laceration</u> of lung
MCC-A S27.331- Laceration of lung, <u>unilateral</u>
MCC-A S27.332- Laceration of lung, <u>bilateral</u>
MCC-A S27.339- Laceration of lung, <u>unspecified</u>
S27.39- <u>Other</u> injuries of lung
    Secondary blast injury of lung
CC-A S27.391- Other injuries of lung, <u>unilateral</u>
CC-A S27.392- Other injuries of lung, <u>bilateral</u>
CC-A S27.399- Other injuries of lung, <u>unspecified</u>
S27.4- Injury of <u>bronchus</u>
S27.40- <u>Unspecified</u> injury of bronchus
MCC-A S27.401- Unspecified injury of bronchus, <u>unilateral</u>
MCC-A S27.402- Unspecified injury of bronchus, <u>bilateral</u>
MCC-A S27.409- Unspecified injury of bronchus, <u>unspecified</u>
S27.41- <u>Primary blast</u> injury of bronchus
    Blast injury of bronchus NOS
MCC-A S27.411- Primary blast injury of bronchus, <u>unilateral</u>
MCC-A S27.412- Primary blast injury of bronchus, <u>bilateral</u>
MCC-A S27.419- Primary blast injury of bronchus, <u>unspecified</u>
S27.42- <u>Contusion</u> of bronchus
MCC-A S27.421- Contusion of bronchus, <u>unilateral</u>
MCC-A S27.422- Contusion of bronchus, <u>bilateral</u>
MCC-A S27.429- Contusion of bronchus, <u>unspecified</u>
S27.43- <u>Laceration</u> of bronchus
MCC-A S27.431- Laceration of bronchus, <u>unilateral</u>
MCC-A S27.432- Laceration of bronchus, <u>bilateral</u>
MCC-A S27.439- Laceration of bronchus, <u>unspecified</u>
S27.49- <u>Other</u> injury of bronchus
    Secondary blast injury of bronchus
MCC-A S27.491- Other injury of bronchus, <u>unilateral</u>
MCC-A S27.492- Other injury of bronchus, <u>bilateral</u>
MCC-A S27.499- Other injury of bronchus, <u>unspecified</u>
S27.5- Injury of <u>thoracic trachea</u>
CC-A S27.50x- <u>Unspecified</u> injury of thoracic trachea
CC-A S27.51x- <u>Primary blast</u> injury of thoracic trachea
    Blast injury of thoracic trachea NOS
CC-A S27.52x- <u>Contusion</u> of thoracic trachea
CC-A S27.53x- <u>Laceration</u> of thoracic trachea
CC-A S27.59x- <u>Other</u> injury of thoracic trachea
    Secondary blast injury of thoracic trachea
S27.6- Injury of <u>pleura</u>
CC-A S27.60x- <u>Unspecified</u> injury of pleura
CC-A S27.63x- <u>Laceration</u> of pleura
CC-A S27.69x- <u>Other</u> injury of pleura
S27.8- Injury of <u>other specified</u> intrathoracic organs
S27.80- Injury of <u>diaphragm</u>
CC-A S27.802- <u>Contusion</u> of diaphragm
CC-A S27.803- <u>Laceration</u> of diaphragm
CC-A S27.808- <u>Other</u> injury of diaphragm
CC-A S27.809- <u>Unspecified</u> injury of diaphragm
S27.81- Injury of <u>esophagus (thoracic part)</u>
MCC-A S27.812- <u>Contusion</u> of esophagus (thoracic part)
MCC-A S27.813- <u>Laceration</u> of esophagus (thoracic part)
MCC-A S27.818- <u>Other</u> injury of esophagus (thoracic part)
MCC-A S27.819- <u>Unspecified</u> injury of esophagus (thoracic part)
S27.89- Injury of <u>other specified</u> intrathoracic organs
    Injury of lymphatic thoracic duct
    Injury of thymus gland
CC-A S27.892- <u>Contusion</u> of other specified intrathoracic organs
CC-A S27.893- <u>Laceration</u> of other specified intrathoracic organs
CC-A S27.898- <u>Other</u> injury of other specified intrathoracic organs
CC-A S27.899- <u>Unspecified</u> injury of other specified intrathoracic organs
S27.9xx- Injury of <u>unspecified</u> intrathoracic organ
CC-A

Excludes 1: = NOT CODED HERE! (Do not code both)   **1042**   *Excludes ❷:* = Not Included Here

S28- Crushing injury of <u>thorax</u>, and traumatic amputation of part of thorax

The appropriate 7th character is to be added to each code from category S28:
A <u>Initial</u> encounter
D <u>Subsequent</u> encounter
S <u>Sequela</u>

S28.0xx- <u>Crushed</u> chest
Use additional code for all associated injuries
Excludes 1: flail chest (S22.5)

S28.1xx- <u>Traumatic amputation</u> (partial) of <u>part of thorax</u>, except
CC-A breast

S28.2- <u>Traumatic amputation</u> of <u>breast</u>
S28.21- <u>Complete</u> traumatic amputation of breast
Traumatic amputation of breast NOS
S28.211- Complete traumatic amputation of <u>right</u> breast
S28.212- Complete traumatic amputation of <u>left</u> breast
S28.219- Complete traumatic amputation of <u>unspecified</u> breast
S28.22- <u>Partial</u> traumatic amputation of <u>breast</u>
S28.221- Partial traumatic amputation of <u>right</u> breast
S28.222- Partial traumatic amputation of <u>left</u> breast
S28.229- Partial traumatic amputation of <u>unspecified</u> breast

S29- Other and <u>unspecified</u> injuries of thorax
Code also any associated open wound (S21.-)
The appropriate 7th character is to be added to each code from category S29:
A <u>Initial</u> encounter
D <u>Subsequent</u> encounter
S <u>Sequela</u>

S29.0- Injury of <u>muscle and tendon</u> at <u>thorax</u> level
S29.00- <u>Unspecified</u> injury of muscle and tendon of thorax
S29.001- Unspecified injury of muscle and tendon of <u>front wall</u> of thorax
S29.002- Unspecified injury of muscle and tendon of <u>back wall</u> of thorax
S29.009- Unspecified injury of muscle and tendon of <u>unspecified</u> wall of thorax
S29.01- <u>Strain</u> of muscle and tendon of thorax
S29.011- Strain of muscle and tendon of <u>front wall</u> of thorax
S29.012- Strain of muscle and tendon of <u>back wall</u> of thorax
S29.019- Strain of muscle and tendon of <u>unspecified</u> wall of thorax
S29.02- <u>Laceration</u> of muscle and tendon of thorax
CC-A **S29.021-** Laceration of muscle and tendon of <u>front wall</u> of thorax
S29.022- Laceration of muscle and tendon of <u>back wall</u> of thorax
CC-A **S29.029-** Laceration of muscle and tendon of <u>unspecified</u> wall of thorax
S29.09- <u>Other</u> injury of muscle and tendon of thorax
S29.091- Other injury of muscle and tendon of <u>front wall</u> of thorax
S29.092- Other injury of muscle and tendon of <u>back wall</u> of thorax
S29.099- Other injury of muscle and tendon of <u>unspecified</u> wall of thorax
S29.8xx- <u>Other</u> specified injuries of thorax
S29.9xx- <u>Unspecified</u> injury of thorax

Injuries to the abdomen, lower back, lumbar spine, pelvis and external genitals (S30-S39)

Includes: Injuries to the abdominal wall
Injuries to the anus
Injuries to the buttock
Injuries to the external genitalia
Injuries to the flank
Injuries to the groin
Excludes ❷: burns and corrosions (T20-T32)
effects of foreign body in anus and rectum (T18.5)
effects of foreign body in genitourinary tract (T19.-)
effects of foreign body in stomach, small intestine and colon (T18.2-T18.4)
frostbite (T33-T34)
insect bite or sting, venomous (T63.4)

S30- <u>Superficial</u> injury of <u>abdomen, lower back, pelvis and external genitals</u>
Excludes ❷: superficial injury of hip (S70.-)
The appropriate 7th character is to be added to each code from category S30:
A <u>Initial</u> encounter
D <u>Subsequent</u> encounter
S <u>Sequela</u>

S30.0xx- <u>Contusion</u> of <u>lower back and pelvis</u>
Contusion of buttock
S30.1xx- <u>Contusion</u> of <u>abdominal wall</u>
Contusion of flank
Contusion of groin
S30.2- <u>Contusion</u> of <u>external genital organs</u>
S30.20- Contusion of <u>unspecified</u> external genital organ
S30.201- Contusion of unspecified external genital organ, <u>male</u> — [♂]
S30.202- Contusion of unspecified external genital organ, <u>female</u> — [♀]
S30.21x- Contusion of penis — [♂]
S30.22x- Contusion of scrotum and testes — [♂]
S30.23x- Contusion of vagina and vulva — [♀]
S30.3xx- Contusion of anus
S30.8- <u>Other</u> superficial injuries of abdomen, lower back, pelvis and external genitals
S30.81- <u>Abrasion</u> of abdomen, lower back, pelvis and external genitals
S30.810- Abrasion of lower back and pelvis
S30.811- Abrasion of abdominal wall
S30.812- Abrasion of penis — [♂]
S30.813- Abrasion of scrotum and testes — [♂]
S30.814- Abrasion of vagina and vulva — [♀]
S30.815- Abrasion of <u>unspecified</u> external genital organs, <u>male</u> — [♂]
S30.816- Abrasion of <u>unspecified</u> external genital organs, <u>female</u> — [♀]
S30.817- Abrasion of anus
S30.82- <u>Blister</u> (nonthermal) of abdomen, lower back, pelvis and external genitals
S30.820- Blister (nonthermal) of lower back and pelvis
S30.821- Blister (nonthermal) of abdominal wall
S30.822- Blister (nonthermal) of penis — [♂]
S30.823- Blister (nonthermal) of scrotum and testes — [♂]
S30.824- Blister (nonthermal) of vagina and vulva — [♀]
S30.825- Blister (nonthermal) of <u>unspecified</u> external genital organs, <u>male</u> — [♂]
S30.826- Blister (nonthermal) of <u>unspecified</u> external genital organs, <u>female</u> — [♀]
S30.827- Blister (nonthermal) of anus
S30.84- <u>External constriction</u> of abdomen, lower back, pelvis and external genitals
S30.840- External constriction of lower back and pelvis
S30.841- External constriction of abdominal wall

S28 - S30

S30.842- External constriction of penis —[♂]
　　　　 Hair tourniquet syndrome of penis
　　　　 Use additional cause code to identify the constricting
　　　　 item (W49.0-)

S30.843- External constriction of scrotum and testes —[♂]

S30.844- External constriction of vagina and vulva —[♀]

S30.845- External constriction of <u>unspecified</u> external genital
　　　　 organs, <u>male</u> —[♂]

S30.846- External constriction of <u>unspecified</u> external genital
　　　　 organs, <u>female</u> —[♀]

S30.85- <u>Superficial foreign body</u> of abdomen, lower back, pelvis
　　　　 and external genitals
　　　　　 Splinter in the abdomen, lower back, pelvis and external
　　　　　 genitals

S30.850- Superficial foreign body of lower back and pelvis

S30.851- Superficial foreign body of abdominal wall

S30.852- Superficial foreign body of penis —[♂]

S30.853- Superficial foreign body of scrotum and testes —
　　　　 [♂]

S30.854- Superficial foreign body of vagina and vulva —[♀]

S30.855- Superficial foreign body of <u>unspecified</u> external
　　　　 genital organs, <u>male</u> —[♂]

S30.856- Superficial foreign body of <u>unspecified</u> external
　　　　 genital organs, <u>female</u> —[♀]

S30.857- Superficial foreign body of anus

S30.86- <u>Insect bite (nonvenomous)</u> of abdomen, lower back,
　　　　 pelvis and external genitals

S30.860- Insect bite (nonvenomous) of lower back and pelvis

S30.861- Insect bite (nonvenomous) of abdominal wall

S30.862- Insect bite (nonvenomous) of penis —[♂]

S30.863- Insect bite (nonvenomous) of scrotum and testes —
　　　　 [♂]

S30.864- Insect bite (nonvenomous) of vagina and vulva —
　　　　 [♀]

S30.865- Insect bite (nonvenomous) of <u>unspecified</u> external
　　　　 genital organs, <u>male</u> —[♂]

S30.866- Insect bite (nonvenomous) of <u>unspecified</u> external
　　　　 genital organs, <u>female</u> —[♀]

S30.867- Insect bite (nonvenomous) of anus

S30.87- <u>Other superficial bite</u> of abdomen, lower back, pelvis and
　　　　 external genitals
　　　　　 Excludes 1:　open bite of abdomen, lower back, pelvis and
　　　　　　　　　　　 external genitals (S31.05, S31.15, S31.25,
　　　　　　　　　　　 S31.35, S31.45, S31.55)

S30.870- Other superficial bite of lower back and pelvis

S30.871- Other superficial bite of abdominal wall

S30.872- Other superficial bite of penis —[♂]

S30.873- Other superficial bite of scrotum and testes —[♂]

S30.874- Other superficial bite of vagina and vulva —[♀]

S30.875- Other superficial bite of <u>unspecified</u> external
　　　　 genital organs, <u>male</u> —[♂]

S30.876- Other superficial bite of <u>unspecified</u> external
　　　　 genital organs, <u>female</u> —[♀]

S30.877- Other superficial bite of anus

S30.9- <u>Unspecified superficial injury</u> of abdomen, lower back, pelvis
　　　　 and external genitals

S30.91x- Unspecified superficial injury of lower back and pelvis

S30.92x- Unspecified superficial injury of abdominal wall

S30.93x- Unspecified superficial injury of penis —[♂]

S30.94x- Unspecified superficial injury of scrotum and testes —
　　　　 [♂]

S30.95x- Unspecified superficial injury of vagina and vulva —
　　　　 [♀]

S30.96x- Unspecified superficial injury of <u>unspecified</u> external
　　　　 genital organs, <u>male</u> —[♂]

S30.97x- Unspecified superficial injury of <u>unspecified</u> external
　　　　 genital organs, <u>female</u> —[♀]

S30.98x- Unspecified superficial injury of anus

S31- <u>Open wound</u> of <u>abdomen, lower back, pelvis and external genitals</u>
Code also any associated:
　Spinal cord injury (S24.0, S24.1-, S34.0-, S34.1-)
　Wound infection
Excludes 1:　traumatic amputation of part of abdomen, lower back and
　　　　　　 pelvis (S38.2-, S38.3)
Excludes ❷:　open wound of hip (S71.00-S71.02)
　　　　　　 open fracture of pelvis (S32.1- -S32.9 with 7th character B)

The appropriate 7th character is to be added to each code from
category S31:
A　<u>Initial</u> encounter
D　<u>Subsequent</u> encounter
S　<u>Sequela</u>

S31.0- Open wound of <u>lower back and pelvis</u>

S31.00- <u>Unspecified</u> open wound of lower back and pelvis

S31.000- Unspecified open wound of lower back and pelvis
　　　　 <u>without</u> penetration into retroperitoneum
　　　　　 Unspecified open wound of lower back and pelvis NOS

MCC-A **S31.001-** Unspecified open wound of lower back and pelvis
　　　　 <u>with penetration</u> into retroperitoneum

S31.01- <u>Laceration</u> <u>without</u> foreign body of lower back and pelvis

S31.010- Laceration <u>without</u> foreign body of lower back and
　　　　 pelvis <u>without</u> penetration into retroperitoneum
　　　　　 Laceration without foreign body of lower back and
　　　　　 pelvis NOS

MCC-A **S31.011-** Laceration <u>without</u> foreign body of lower back and
　　　　 pelvis <u>with penetration</u> into retroperitoneum

S31.02- <u>Laceration</u> <u>with foreign body</u> of lower back and pelvis

S31.020- Laceration <u>with foreign body</u> of lower back and
　　　　 pelvis <u>without</u> penetration into retroperitoneum
　　　　　 Laceration with foreign body of lower back and pelvis
　　　　　 NOS

MCC-A **S31.021-** Laceration <u>with foreign body</u> of lower back and
　　　　 pelvis <u>with penetration</u> into retroperitoneum

S31.03- <u>Puncture</u> wound <u>without</u> foreign body of lower back and
　　　　 pelvis

S31.030- Puncture wound <u>without</u> foreign body of lower back
　　　　 and pelvis <u>without</u> penetration into
　　　　 retroperitoneum
　　　　　 Puncture wound without foreign body of lower back
　　　　　 and pelvis NOS

MCC-A **S31.031-** Puncture wound <u>without</u> foreign body of lower back
　　　　 and pelvis <u>with penetration</u> into retroperitoneum

S31.04- <u>Puncture</u> wound <u>with foreign body</u> of lower back and
　　　　 pelvis

S31.040- Puncture wound <u>with foreign body</u> of lower back
　　　　 and pelvis <u>without</u> penetration into
　　　　 retroperitoneum
　　　　　 Puncture wound with foreign body of lower back and
　　　　　 pelvis NOS

MCC-A **S31.041-** Puncture wound <u>with foreign body</u> of lower back
　　　　 and pelvis <u>with penetration</u> into retroperitoneum

S31.05- <u>Open bite</u> of lower back and pelvis
　　　　　 Bite of lower back and pelvis NOS
　　　　　 Excludes 1:　superficial bite of lower back and pelvis (S30.860,
　　　　　　　　　　　 S30.870)

S31.050- Open bite of lower back and pelvis <u>without</u>
　　　　 penetration into retroperitoneum
　　　　　 Open bite of lower back and pelvis NOS

MCC-A **S31.051-** Open bite of lower back and pelvis <u>with</u>
　　　　 <u>penetration</u> into retroperitoneum

S31.1- <u>Open wound</u> of <u>abdominal wall</u> <u>without</u> penetration into
　　　　 peritoneal cavity
　　　　　 Open wound of abdominal wall NOS
　　　　 Excludes ❷:　open wound of abdominal wall with penetration into
　　　　　　　　　　　 peritoneal cavity (S31.6-)

S31.10- <u>Unspecified</u> open wound of abdominal wall <u>without</u>
　　　　 penetration into peritoneal cavity

S31.100- Unspecified open wound of abdominal wall, <u>right</u>
　　　　 <u>upper</u> quadrant <u>without</u> penetration into
　　　　 peritoneal cavity

S30 - S31

S31.101- Unspecified open wound of abdominal wall, <u>left</u> <u>upper</u> quadrant <u>without</u> penetration into peritoneal cavity

S31.102- Unspecified open wound of abdominal wall, <u>epigastric region</u> <u>without</u> penetration into peritoneal cavity

S31.103- Unspecified open wound of abdominal wall, <u>right</u> <u>lower</u> quadrant <u>without</u> penetration into peritoneal cavity

S31.104- Unspecified open wound of abdominal wall, <u>left</u> <u>lower</u> quadrant <u>without</u> penetration into peritoneal cavity

S31.105- Unspecified open wound of abdominal wall, <u>periumbilic region</u> <u>without</u> penetration into peritoneal cavity

S31.109- Unspecified open wound of abdominal wall, <u>unspecified</u> <u>quadrant</u> <u>without</u> penetration into peritoneal cavity
    Unspecified open wound of abdominal wall NOS

S31.11- <u>Laceration</u> <u>without</u> foreign body of abdominal wall <u>without</u> penetration into peritoneal cavity

S31.110- Laceration <u>without</u> foreign body of abdominal wall, <u>right</u> <u>upper</u> quadrant <u>without</u> penetration into peritoneal cavity

S31.111- Laceration <u>without</u> foreign body of abdominal wall, <u>left</u> <u>upper</u> quadrant <u>without</u> penetration into peritoneal cavity

S31.112- Laceration <u>without</u> foreign body of abdominal wall, <u>epigastric region</u> <u>without</u> penetration into peritoneal cavity

S31.113- Laceration <u>without</u> foreign body of abdominal wall, <u>right</u> <u>lower</u> quadrant <u>without</u> penetration into peritoneal cavity

S31.114- Laceration <u>without</u> foreign body of abdominal wall, <u>left</u> <u>lower</u> quadrant <u>without</u> penetration into peritoneal cavity

S31.115- Laceration <u>without</u> foreign body of abdominal wall, <u>periumbilic region</u> <u>without</u> penetration into peritoneal cavity

S31.119- Laceration <u>without</u> foreign body of abdominal wall, <u>unspecified</u> <u>quadrant</u> <u>without</u> penetration into peritoneal cavity

S31.12- <u>Laceration with foreign body</u> of abdominal wall <u>without</u> penetration into peritoneal cavity

S31.120- Laceration of abdominal wall <u>with foreign body</u>, <u>right</u> <u>upper</u> quadrant <u>without</u> penetration into peritoneal cavity

S31.121- Laceration of abdominal wall <u>with foreign body</u>, <u>left</u> <u>upper</u> quadrant <u>without</u> penetration into peritoneal cavity

S31.122- Laceration of abdominal wall <u>with foreign body</u>, <u>epigastric region</u> <u>without</u> penetration into peritoneal cavity

S31.123- Laceration of abdominal wall <u>with foreign body</u>, <u>right</u> <u>lower</u> quadrant <u>without</u> penetration into peritoneal cavity

S31.124- Laceration of abdominal wall <u>with foreign body</u>, <u>left</u> <u>lower</u> quadrant <u>without</u> penetration into peritoneal cavity

S31.125- Laceration of abdominal wall <u>with foreign body</u>, <u>periumbilic</u> region <u>without</u> penetration into peritoneal cavity

S31.129- Laceration of abdominal wall <u>with foreign body</u>, <u>unspecified</u> <u>quadrant</u> <u>without</u> penetration into peritoneal cavity

S31.13- <u>Puncture</u> wound of abdominal wall <u>without</u> foreign body <u>without</u> penetration into peritoneal cavity

S31.130- Puncture wound of abdominal wall <u>without</u> foreign body, <u>right</u> <u>upper</u> quadrant <u>without</u> penetration into peritoneal cavity

S31.131- Puncture wound of abdominal wall <u>without</u> foreign body, <u>left</u> <u>upper</u> quadrant <u>without</u> penetration into peritoneal cavity

S31.132- Puncture wound of abdominal wall <u>without</u> foreign body, <u>epigastric region</u> <u>without</u> penetration into peritoneal cavity

S31.133- Puncture wound of abdominal wall <u>without</u> foreign body, <u>right</u> <u>lower</u> quadrant <u>without</u> penetration into peritoneal cavity

S31.134- Puncture wound of abdominal wall <u>without</u> foreign body, <u>left</u> <u>lower</u> quadrant <u>without</u> penetration into peritoneal cavity

S31.135- Puncture wound of abdominal wall <u>without</u> foreign body, periumbilic region <u>without</u> penetration into peritoneal cavity

S31.139- Puncture wound of abdominal wall <u>without</u> foreign body, <u>unspecified</u> <u>quadrant</u> <u>without</u> penetration into peritoneal cavity

S31.14- <u>Puncture</u> wound of abdominal wall <u>with foreign body</u> <u>without</u> penetration into peritoneal cavity

S31.140- Puncture wound of abdominal wall <u>with foreign body</u>, <u>right</u> <u>upper</u> quadrant <u>without</u> penetration into peritoneal cavity

S31.141- Puncture wound of abdominal wall <u>with foreign body</u>, <u>left</u> <u>upper</u> quadrant <u>without</u> penetration into peritoneal cavity

S31.142- Puncture wound of abdominal wall <u>with foreign body</u>, <u>epigastric region</u> <u>without</u> penetration into peritoneal cavity

S31.143- Puncture wound of abdominal wall <u>with foreign body</u>, <u>right</u> <u>lower</u> quadrant <u>without</u> penetration into peritoneal cavity

S31.144- Puncture wound of abdominal wall <u>with foreign body</u>, <u>left</u> <u>lower</u> quadrant <u>without</u> penetration into peritoneal cavity

S31.145- Puncture wound of abdominal wall <u>with foreign body</u>, <u>periumbilic region</u> <u>without</u> penetration into peritoneal cavity

S31.149- Puncture wound of abdominal wall <u>with foreign body</u>, <u>unspecified</u> <u>quadrant</u> <u>without</u> penetration into peritoneal cavity

S31.15- <u>Open bite</u> of abdominal wall <u>without</u> penetration into peritoneal cavity
    Bite of abdominal wall NOS
    Excludes 1:   *superficial bite of abdominal wall (S30.871)*

S31.150- Open bite of abdominal wall, <u>right</u> <u>upper</u> quadrant <u>without</u> penetration into peritoneal cavity

S31.151- Open bite of abdominal wall, <u>left</u> <u>upper</u> quadrant <u>without</u> penetration into peritoneal cavity

S31.152- Open bite of abdominal wall, <u>epigastric region</u> <u>without</u> penetration into peritoneal cavity

S31.153- Open bite of abdominal wall, <u>right</u> <u>lower</u> quadrant <u>without</u> penetration into peritoneal cavity

S31.154- Open bite of abdominal wall, <u>left</u> <u>lower</u> quadrant <u>without</u> penetration into peritoneal cavity

S31.155- Open bite of abdominal wall, <u>periumbilic region</u> <u>without</u> penetration into peritoneal cavity

S31.159- Open bite of abdominal wall, <u>unspecified</u> <u>quadrant</u> <u>without</u> penetration into peritoneal cavity

S31.2- Open wound of <u>penis</u>

S31.20x- Unspecified open wound of penis — [♂]

S31.21x- Laceration <u>without</u> foreign body of penis — [♂]

S31.22x- Laceration <u>with foreign body</u> of penis — [♂]

S31.23x- Puncture wound <u>without</u> foreign body of penis — [♂]

S31.24x- Puncture wound <u>with foreign body</u> of penis — [♂]

S31.25x- Open bite of penis — [♂]
    Bite of penis NOS
    Excludes 1:   *superficial bite of penis (S30.862, S30.872)*

S 3 1 - S 3 1

S31.3-   Open wound of <u>scrotum and testes</u>

    S31.30x-   Unspecified open wound of scrotum and testes — [♂]

    S31.31x-   Laceration <u>without</u> foreign body of scrotum and testes — [♂]

    S31.32x-   Laceration <u>with foreign body</u> of scrotum and testes — [♂]

    S31.33x-   Puncture wound <u>without</u> foreign body of scrotum and testes — [♂]

    S31.34x-   Puncture wound <u>with foreign body</u> of scrotum and testes — [♂]

    S31.35x-   Open bite of scrotum and testes — [♂]
        Bite of scrotum and testes NOS
        Excludes 1:   *superficial bite of scrotum and testes (S30.863, S30.873)*

S31.4-   Open wound of <u>vagina and vulva</u>
    Excludes 1:   *injury to vagina and vulva during delivery (O70.-, O71.4)*

    S31.40x-   Unspecified open wound of vagina and vulva — [♀]

    S31.41x-   Laceration <u>without</u> foreign body of vagina and vulva — [♀]

    S31.42x-   Laceration <u>with foreign body</u> of vagina and vulva — [♀]

    S31.43x-   Puncture wound <u>without</u> foreign body of vagina and vulva — [♀]

    S31.44x-   Puncture wound <u>with foreign body</u> of vagina and vulva — [♀]

    S31.45x-   Open bite of vagina and vulva — [♀]
        Bite of vagina and vulva NOS
        Excludes 1:   *superficial bite of vagina and vulva (S30.864, S30.874)*

S31.5-   Open wound of <u>unspecified external genital organs</u>
    Excludes 1:   *traumatic amputation of external genital organs (S38.21, S38.22)*

    S31.50-   <u>Unspecified</u> open wound of <u>unspecified</u> external genital organs

        S31.501-   Unspecified open wound of <u>unspecified</u> external genital organs, <u>male</u> — [♂]

        S31.502-   Unspecified open wound of <u>unspecified</u> external genital organs, <u>female</u> — [♀]

    S31.51-   <u>Laceration without</u> foreign body of <u>unspecified</u> external genital organs

        S31.511-   Laceration <u>without</u> foreign body of <u>unspecified</u> external genital organs, <u>male</u> — [♂]

        S31.512-   Laceration <u>without</u> foreign body of <u>unspecified</u> external genital organs, <u>female</u> — [♀]

    S31.52-   <u>Laceration with foreign body</u> of <u>unspecified</u> external genital organs

        S31.521-   Laceration <u>with foreign body</u> of <u>unspecified</u> external genital organs, <u>male</u> — [♂]

        S31.522-   Laceration <u>with foreign body</u> of <u>unspecified</u> external genital organs, <u>female</u> — [♀]

    S31.53-   <u>Puncture</u> wound <u>without</u> foreign body of <u>unspecified</u> external genital organs

        S31.531-   Puncture wound <u>without</u> foreign body of <u>unspecified</u> external genital organs, <u>male</u> — [♂]

        S31.532-   Puncture wound <u>without</u> foreign body of <u>unspecified</u> external genital organs, <u>female</u> — [♀]

    S31.54-   <u>Puncture</u> wound <u>with foreign body</u> of <u>unspecified</u> external genital organs

        S31.541-   Puncture wound <u>with foreign body</u> of <u>unspecified</u> external genital organs, <u>male</u> — [♂]

        S31.542-   Puncture wound <u>with foreign body</u> of <u>unspecified</u> external genital organs, <u>female</u> — [♀]

    S31.55-   <u>Open bite</u> of <u>unspecified external genital organs</u>
        Bite of unspecified external genital organs NOS
        Excludes 1:   *superficial bite of unspecified external genital organs (S30.865, S30.866, S30.875, S30.876)*

        S31.551-   Open bite of <u>unspecified</u> external genital organs, <u>male</u> — [♂]

        S31.552-   Open bite of <u>unspecified</u> external genital organs, <u>female</u> — [♀]

S31.6-   Open wound of <u>abdominal wall</u> <u>with penetration</u> into peritoneal cavity

    S31.60-   <u>Unspecified</u> open wound of <u>abdominal wall</u> <u>with penetration</u> into peritoneal cavity

    MCC-A **S31.600-**   Unspecified open wound of abdominal wall, <u>right upper</u> quadrant <u>with penetration</u> into peritoneal cavity

    MCC-A **S31.601-**   Unspecified open wound of abdominal wall, <u>left upper</u> quadrant <u>with penetration</u> into peritoneal cavity

    MCC-A **S31.602-**   Unspecified open wound of abdominal wall, <u>epigastric region</u> <u>with penetration</u> into peritoneal cavity

    MCC-A **S31.603-**   Unspecified open wound of abdominal wall, <u>right lower</u> quadrant <u>with penetration</u> into peritoneal cavity

    MCC-A **S31.604-**   Unspecified open wound of abdominal wall, <u>left lower</u> quadrant <u>with penetration</u> into peritoneal cavity

    MCC-A **S31.605-**   Unspecified open wound of abdominal wall, <u>periumbilic region</u> <u>with penetration</u> into peritoneal cavity

    MCC-A **S31.609-**   Unspecified open wound of abdominal wall, <u>unspecified quadrant</u> <u>with penetration</u> into peritoneal cavity

    S31.61-   <u>Laceration without</u> foreign body of abdominal wall <u>with penetration</u> into peritoneal cavity

    MCC-A **S31.610-**   Laceration <u>without</u> foreign body of abdominal wall, <u>right upper</u> quadrant <u>with penetration</u> into peritoneal cavity

    MCC-A **S31.611-**   Laceration <u>without</u> foreign body of abdominal wall, <u>left upper</u> quadrant <u>with penetration</u> into peritoneal cavity

    MCC-A **S31.612-**   Laceration <u>without</u> foreign body of abdominal wall, <u>epigastric region</u> <u>with penetration</u> into peritoneal cavity

    MCC-A **S31.613-**   Laceration <u>without</u> foreign body of abdominal wall, <u>right lower</u> quadrant <u>with penetration</u> into peritoneal cavity

    MCC-A **S31.614-**   Laceration <u>without</u> foreign body of abdominal wall, <u>left lower</u> quadrant <u>with penetration</u> into peritoneal cavity

    MCC-A **S31.615-**   Laceration <u>without</u> foreign body of abdominal wall, <u>periumbilic region</u> <u>with penetration</u> into peritoneal cavity

    MCC-A **S31.619-**   Laceration <u>without</u> foreign body of abdominal wall, <u>unspecified quadrant</u> <u>with penetration</u> into peritoneal cavity

    S31.62-   <u>Laceration with foreign body</u> of abdominal wall <u>with penetration</u> into peritoneal cavity

    MCC-A **S31.620-**   Laceration <u>with foreign body</u> of abdominal wall, <u>right upper</u> quadrant <u>with penetration</u> into peritoneal cavity

    MCC-A **S31.621-**   Laceration <u>with foreign body</u> of abdominal wall, <u>left upper</u> quadrant <u>with penetration</u> into peritoneal cavity

    MCC-A **S31.622-**   Laceration <u>with foreign body</u> of abdominal wall, <u>epigastric region</u> <u>with penetration</u> into peritoneal cavity

    MCC-A **S31.623-**   Laceration <u>with foreign body</u> of abdominal wall, <u>right lower</u> quadrant <u>with penetration</u> into peritoneal cavity

    MCC-A **S31.624-**   Laceration <u>with foreign body</u> of abdominal wall, <u>left lower</u> quadrant <u>with penetration</u> into peritoneal cavity

    MCC-A **S31.625-**   Laceration <u>with foreign body</u> of abdominal wall, <u>periumbilic region</u> <u>with penetration</u> into peritoneal cavity

Excludes 1: = NOT CODED HERE! (Do not code both)

Excludes 2: = Not Included Here

S31 - S31

MCC-A **S31.629-** Laceration with foreign body of abdominal wall, unspecified quadrant with penetration into peritoneal cavity

S31.63- Puncture wound without foreign body of abdominal wall with penetration into peritoneal cavity

MCC-A **S31.630-** Puncture wound without foreign body of abdominal wall, right upper quadrant with penetration into peritoneal cavity

MCC-A **S31.631-** Puncture wound without foreign body of abdominal wall, left upper quadrant with penetration into peritoneal cavity

MCC-A **S31.632-** Puncture wound without foreign body of abdominal wall, epigastric region with penetration into peritoneal cavity

MCC-A **S31.633-** Puncture wound without foreign body of abdominal wall, right lower quadrant with penetration into peritoneal cavity

MCC-A **S31.634-** Puncture wound without foreign body of abdominal wall, left lower quadrant with penetration into peritoneal cavity

MCC-A **S31.635-** Puncture wound without foreign body of abdominal wall, periumbilic region with penetration into peritoneal cavity

MCC-A **S31.639-** Puncture wound without foreign body of abdominal wall, unspecified quadrant with penetration into peritoneal cavity

S31.64- Puncture wound with foreign body of abdominal wall with penetration into peritoneal cavity

MCC-A **S31.640-** Puncture wound with foreign body of abdominal wall, right upper quadrant with penetration into peritoneal cavity

MCC-A **S31.641-** Puncture wound with foreign body of abdominal wall, left upper quadrant with penetration into peritoneal cavity

MCC-A **S31.642-** Puncture wound with foreign body of abdominal wall, epigastric region with penetration into peritoneal cavity

MCC-A **S31.643-** Puncture wound with foreign body of abdominal wall, right lower quadrant with penetration into peritoneal cavity

MCC-A **S31.644-** Puncture wound with foreign body of abdominal wall, left lower quadrant with penetration into peritoneal cavity

MCC-A **S31.645-** Puncture wound with foreign body of abdominal wall, periumbilic region with penetration into peritoneal cavity

MCC-A **S31.649-** Puncture wound with foreign body of abdominal wall, unspecified quadrant with penetration into peritoneal cavity

S31.65- Open bite of abdominal wall with penetration into peritoneal cavity
 Excludes 1:   *superficial bite of abdominal wall (S30.861, S30.871)*

MCC-A **S31.650-** Open bite of abdominal wall, right upper quadrant with penetration into peritoneal cavity

MCC-A **S31.651-** Open bite of abdominal wall, left upper quadrant with penetration into peritoneal cavity

MCC-A **S31.652-** Open bite of abdominal wall, epigastric region with penetration into peritoneal cavity

MCC-A **S31.653-** Open bite of abdominal wall, right lower quadrant with penetration into peritoneal cavity

MCC-A **S31.654-** Open bite of abdominal wall, left lower quadrant with penetration into peritoneal cavity

MCC-A **S31.655-** Open bite of abdominal wall, periumbilic region with penetration into peritoneal cavity

MCC-A **S31.659-** Open bite of abdominal wall, unspecified quadrant with penetration into peritoneal cavity

S31.8- Open wound of other parts of abdomen, lower back and pelvis

S31.80- Open wound of unspecified buttock

S31.801- Laceration without foreign body of unspecified buttock

S31.802- Laceration with foreign body of unspecified buttock

S31.803- Puncture wound without foreign body of unspecified buttock

S31.804- Puncture wound with foreign body of unspecified buttock

S31.805- Open bite of unspecified buttock
 Bite of buttock NOS
 Excludes 1:   *superficial bite of buttock (S30.870)*

S31.809- Unspecified open wound of unspecified buttock

S31.81- Open wound of right buttock

S31.811- Laceration without foreign body of right buttock

S31.812- Laceration with foreign body of right buttock

S31.813- Puncture wound without foreign body of right buttock

S31.814- Puncture wound with foreign body of right buttock

S31.815- Open bite of right buttock
 Bite of right buttock NOS
 Excludes 1:   *superficial bite of buttock (S30.870)*

S31.819- Unspecified open wound of right buttock

S31.82- Open wound of left buttock

S31.821- Laceration without foreign body of left buttock

S31.822- Laceration with foreign body of left buttock

S31.823- Puncture wound without foreign body of left buttock

S31.824- Puncture wound with foreign body of left buttock

S31.825- Open bite of left buttock
 Bite of left buttock NOS
 Excludes 1:   *superficial bite of buttock (S30.870)*

S31.829- Unspecified open wound of left buttock

S31.83- Open wound of anus

S31.831- Laceration without foreign body of anus

S31.832- Laceration with foreign body of anus

S31.833- Puncture wound without foreign body of anus

S31.834- Puncture wound with foreign body of anus

S31.835- Open bite of anus
 Bite of anus NOS
 Excludes 1:   *superficial bite of anus (S30.877)*

S31.839- Unspecified open wound of anus

S32- Fracture of lumbar spine and pelvis
 Note: A fracture not indicated as displaced or nondisplaced should be coded to displaced
 Note: A fracture not indicated as opened or closed should be coded to closed
 Includes: Fracture of lumbosacral neural arch
     Fracture of lumbosacral spinous process
     Fracture of lumbosacral transverse process
     Fracture of lumbosacral vertebra
     Fracture of lumbosacral vertebral arch
 Code first any associated spinal cord and spinal nerve injury (S34.-)
 Excludes 1:   *transection of abdomen (S38.3)*
 Excludes ❷: *fracture of hip NOS (S72.0-)*

The appropriate 7th character is to be added to each code from category S32:
  A   Initial encounter for closed fracture
  B   Initial encounter for open fracture
  D   Subsequent encounter for fracture with routine healing
  G   Subsequent encounter for fracture with delayed healing
  K   Subsequent encounter for fracture with nonunion
  S   Sequela

S32.0- Fracture of lumbar vertebra
 Fracture of lumbar spine NOS

S32.00- Fracture of unspecified lumbar vertebra

CC-A,K MCC-B **S32.000-** Wedge compression fracture of unspecified lumbar vertebra

S31 | **S32**

CC-A,K MCC-B **S32.001-** <u>Stable burst</u> fracture of <u>unspecified</u> lumbar vertebra

CC-A,K MCC-B **S32.002-** <u>Unstable burst</u> fracture of <u>unspecified</u> lumbar vertebra

CC-A,K MCC-B **S32.008-** <u>Other</u> fracture of <u>unspecified</u> lumbar vertebra

CC-A,K MCC-B **S32.009-** <u>Unspecified</u> fracture of <u>unspecified</u> lumbar vertebra

S32.01- Fracture of <u>first</u> lumbar vertebra

CC-A,K MCC-B **S32.010-** <u>Wedge</u> compression fracture of first lumbar vertebra

CC-A,K MCC-B **S32.011-** <u>Stable burst</u> fracture of first lumbar vertebra

CC-A,K MCC-B **S32.012-** <u>Unstable burst</u> fracture of first lumbar vertebra

CC-A,K MCC-B **S32.018-** <u>Other</u> fracture of first lumbar vertebra

CC-A,K MCC-B **S32.019-** <u>Unspecified</u> fracture of first lumbar vertebra

S32.02- Fracture of <u>second</u> lumbar vertebra

CC-A,K MCC-B **S32.020-** <u>Wedge</u> compression fracture of second lumbar vertebra

CC-A,K MCC-B **S32.021-** <u>Stable burst</u> fracture of second lumbar vertebra

CC-A,K MCC-B **S32.022-** <u>Unstable burst</u> fracture of second lumbar vertebra

CC-A,K MCC-B **S32.028-** <u>Other</u> fracture of second lumbar vertebra

CC-A,K MCC-B **S32.029-** <u>Unspecified</u> fracture of second lumbar vertebra

S32.03- Fracture of <u>third</u> lumbar vertebra

CC-A,K MCC-B **S32.030-** <u>Wedge</u> compression fracture of third lumbar vertebra

CC-A,K MCC-B **S32.031-** <u>Stable burst</u> fracture of third lumbar vertebra

CC-A,K MCC-B **S32.032-** <u>Unstable burst</u> fracture of third lumbar vertebra

CC-A,K MCC-B **S32.038-** <u>Other</u> fracture of third lumbar vertebra

CC-A,K MCC-B **S32.039-** <u>Unspecified</u> fracture of third lumbar vertebra

S32.04- Fracture of <u>fourth</u> lumbar vertebra

CC-A,K MCC-B **S32.040-** <u>Wedge</u> compression fracture of fourth lumbar vertebra

CC-A,K MCC-B **S32.041-** <u>Stable burst</u> fracture of fourth lumbar vertebra

CC-A,K MCC-B **S32.042-** <u>Unstable burst</u> fracture of fourth lumbar vertebra

CC-A,K MCC-B **S32.048-** <u>Other</u> fracture of fourth lumbar vertebra

CC-A,K MCC-B **S32.049-** <u>Unspecified</u> fracture of fourth lumbar vertebra

S32.05- Fracture of <u>fifth</u> lumbar vertebra

CC-A,K MCC-B **S32.050-** <u>Wedge</u> compression fracture of fifth lumbar vertebra

CC-A,K MCC-B **S32.051-** <u>Stable burst</u> fracture of fifth lumbar vertebra

CC-A,K MCC-B **S32.052-** <u>Unstable burst</u> fracture of fifth lumbar vertebra

CC-A,K MCC-B **S32.058-** <u>Other</u> fracture of fifth lumbar vertebra

CC-A,K MCC-B **S32.059-** <u>Unspecified</u> fracture of fifth lumbar vertebra

S32.1- Fracture of <u>sacrum</u>

Note: For vertical fractures, code to most medial fracture extension

Note: Use two codes if both a vertical and transverse fracture are present

Code also any associated fracture of pelvic ring (S32.8-)

S32.10x- <u>Unspecified</u> fracture of sacrum
CC-A,K MCC-B

S32.11- Zone I fracture of sacrum

Vertical sacral ala fracture of sacrum

CC-A,K MCC-B **S32.110-** <u>Nondisplaced</u> Zone I fracture of sacrum

CC-A,K MCC-B **S32.111-** <u>Minimally</u> <u>displaced</u> Zone I fracture of sacrum

CC-A,K MCC-B **S32.112-** <u>Severely</u> <u>displaced</u> Zone I fracture of sacrum

CC-A,K MCC-B **S32.119-** <u>Unspecified</u> Zone I fracture of sacrum

S32.12- Zone II fracture of sacrum

Vertical foraminal region fracture of sacrum

CC-A,K MCC-B **S32.120-** <u>Nondisplaced</u> Zone II fracture of sacrum

CC-A,K MCC-B **S32.121-** <u>Minimally</u> <u>displaced</u> Zone II fracture of sacrum

CC-A,K MCC-B **S32.122-** <u>Severely</u> <u>displaced</u> Zone II fracture of sacrum

CC-A,K MCC-B **S32.129-** <u>Unspecified</u> Zone II fracture of sacrum

S32.13- Zone III fracture of sacrum

Vertical fracture into spinal canal region of sacrum

CC-A,K MCC-B **S32.130-** <u>Nondisplaced</u> Zone III fracture of sacrum

CC-A,K MCC-B **S32.131-** <u>Minimally</u> <u>displaced</u> Zone III fracture of sacrum

CC-A,K MCC-B **S32.132-** <u>Severely</u> <u>displaced</u> Zone III fracture of sacrum

CC-A,K MCC-B **S32.139-** <u>Unspecified</u> Zone III fracture of sacrum

S32.14x- Type 1 fracture of sacrum

CC-A,K MCC-B Transverse flexion fracture of sacrum without displacement

S32.15x- Type 2 fracture of sacrum

CC-A,K MCC-B Transverse flexion fracture of sacrum with posterior displacement

S32.16x- Type 3 fracture of sacrum

CC-A,K MCC-B Transverse extension fracture of sacrum with anterior displacement

S32.17x- Type 4 fracture of sacrum

CC-A,K MCC-B Transverse segmental comminution of upper sacrum

S32.19x- <u>Other</u> fracture of sacrum
CC-A,K MCC-B

S32.2xx- Fracture of coccyx
CC-A,K MCC-B

S32.3- Fracture of <u>ilium</u>

Excludes 1: *fracture of ilium with associated disruption of pelvic ring (S32.8-)*

S32.30- <u>Unspecified</u> fracture of ilium

CC-A,K MCC-B **S32.301-** Unspecified fracture of <u>right</u> ilium

CC-A,K MCC-B **S32.302-** Unspecified fracture of <u>left</u> ilium

CC-A,K MCC-B **S32.309-** Unspecified fracture of <u>unspecified</u> ilium

S32.31- <u>Avulsion</u> fracture of ilium

CC-A,K MCC-B **S32.311-** <u>Displaced</u> avulsion fracture of <u>right</u> ilium

CC-A,K MCC-B **S32.312-** <u>Displaced</u> avulsion fracture of <u>left</u> ilium

CC-A,K MCC-B **S32.313-** <u>Displaced</u> avulsion fracture of <u>unspecified</u> ilium

CC-A,K MCC-B **S32.314-** <u>Nondisplaced</u> avulsion fracture of <u>right</u> ilium

CC-A,K MCC-B **S32.315-** <u>Nondisplaced</u> avulsion fracture of <u>left</u> ilium

CC-A,K MCC-B **S32.316-** <u>Nondisplaced</u> avulsion fracture of <u>unspecified</u> ilium

S32.39- <u>Other</u> fracture of ilium

CC-A,K MCC-B **S32.391-** Other fracture of <u>right</u> ilium

CC-A,K MCC-B **S32.392-** Other fracture of <u>left</u> ilium

CC-A,K MCC-B **S32.399-** Other fracture of <u>unspecified</u> ilium

S32.4- Fracture of <u>acetabulum</u>

Code also any associated fracture of pelvic ring (S32.8-)

S32.40- <u>Unspecified</u> fracture of acetabulum

CC-K MCC-A,B **S32.401-** Unspecified fracture of <u>right</u> acetabulum

CC-K MCC-A,B **S32.402-** Unspecified fracture of <u>left</u> acetabulum

CC-K MCC-A,B **S32.409-** Unspecified fracture of <u>unspecified</u> acetabulum

S32.41- Fracture of <u>anterior wall</u> of acetabulum

CC-K MCC-A,B **S32.411-** <u>Displaced</u> fracture of anterior wall of <u>right</u> acetabulum

CC-K MCC-A,B **S32.412-** <u>Displaced</u> fracture of anterior wall of <u>left</u> acetabulum

CC-K MCC-A,B **S32.413-** <u>Displaced</u> fracture of anterior wall of <u>unspecified</u> acetabulum

CC-K MCC-A,B **S32.414-** <u>Nondisplaced</u> fracture of anterior wall of <u>right</u> acetabulum

CC-K MCC-A,B **S32.415-** <u>Nondisplaced</u> fracture of anterior wall of <u>left</u> acetabulum

CC-K MCC-A,B **S32.416-** <u>Nondisplaced</u> fracture of anterior wall of <u>unspecified</u> acetabulum

S32.42- Fracture of <u>posterior wall</u> of acetabulum

CC-K MCC-A,B **S32.421-** <u>Displaced</u> fracture of posterior wall of <u>right</u> acetabulum

CC-K MCC-A,B **S32.422-** <u>Displaced</u> fracture of posterior wall of <u>left</u> acetabulum

CC-K MCC-A,B **S32.423-** <u>Displaced</u> fracture of posterior wall of <u>unspecified</u> acetabulum

CC-K MCC-A,B **S32.424-** <u>Nondisplaced</u> fracture of posterior wall of <u>right</u> acetabulum

CC-K MCC-A,B **S32.425-** <u>Nondisplaced</u> fracture of posterior wall of <u>left</u> acetabulum

CC-K MCC-A,B **S32.426-** <u>Nondisplaced</u> fracture of posterior wall of <u>unspecified</u> acetabulum

S32.43- Fracture of <u>anterior column [iliopubic]</u> of acetabulum

CC-K MCC-A,B **S32.431-** <u>Displaced</u> fracture of anterior column [iliopubic] of <u>right</u> acetabulum

CC-K MCC-A,B **S32.432-** <u>Displaced</u> fracture of anterior column [iliopubic] of <u>left</u> acetabulum

S32 - S32

CC-K MCC-A,B **S32.433-** <u>Displaced</u> fracture of anterior column [iliopubic] of <u>unspecified</u> acetabulum

CC-K MCC-A,B **S32.434-** <u>Nondisplaced</u> fracture of anterior column [iliopubic] of <u>right</u> acetabulum

CC-K MCC-A,B **S32.435-** <u>Nondisplaced</u> fracture of anterior column [iliopubic] of <u>left</u> acetabulum

CC-K MCC-A,B **S32.436-** <u>Nondisplaced</u> fracture of anterior column [iliopubic] of <u>unspecified</u> acetabulum

S32.44- Fracture of <u>posterior column [ilioischial]</u> of acetabulum

CC-K MCC-A,B **S32.441-** <u>Displaced</u> fracture of posterior column [ilioischial] of <u>right</u> acetabulum

CC-K MCC-A,B **S32.442-** <u>Displaced</u> fracture of posterior column [ilioischial] of <u>left</u> acetabulum

CC-K MCC-A,B **S32.443-** <u>Displaced</u> fracture of posterior column [ilioischial] of <u>unspecified</u> acetabulum

CC-K MCC-A,B **S32.444-** <u>Nondisplaced</u> fracture of posterior column [ilioischial] of <u>right</u> acetabulum

CC-K MCC-A,B **S32.445-** <u>Nondisplaced</u> fracture of posterior column [ilioischial] of <u>left</u> acetabulum

CC-K MCC-A,B **S32.446-** <u>Nondisplaced</u> fracture of posterior column [ilioischial] of <u>unspecified</u> acetabulum

S32.45- <u>Transverse</u> fracture of acetabulum

CC-K MCC-A,B **S32.451-** <u>Displaced</u> transverse fracture of <u>right</u> acetabulum

CC-K MCC-A,B **S32.452-** <u>Displaced</u> transverse fracture of <u>left</u> acetabulum

CC-K MCC-A,B **S32.453-** <u>Displaced</u> transverse fracture of <u>unspecified</u> acetabulum

CC-K MCC-A,B **S32.454-** <u>Nondisplaced</u> transverse fracture of <u>right</u> acetabulum

CC-K MCC-A,B **S32.455-** <u>Nondisplaced</u> transverse fracture of <u>left</u> acetabulum

CC-K MCC-A,B **S32.456-** <u>Nondisplaced</u> transverse fracture of <u>unspecified</u> acetabulum

S32.46- <u>Associated transverse-posterior</u> fracture of acetabulum

CC-K MCC-A,B **S32.461-** <u>Displaced</u> associated transverse-posterior fracture of <u>right</u> acetabulum

CC-K MCC-A,B **S32.462-** <u>Displaced</u> associated transverse-posterior fracture of <u>left</u> acetabulum

CC-K MCC-A,B **S32.463-** <u>Displaced</u> associated transverse-posterior fracture of <u>unspecified</u> acetabulum

CC-K MCC-A,B **S32.464-** <u>Nondisplaced</u> associated transverse-posterior fracture of <u>right</u> acetabulum

CC-K MCC-A,B **S32.465-** <u>Nondisplaced</u> associated transverse-posterior fracture of <u>left</u> acetabulum

CC-K MCC-A,B **S32.466-** <u>Nondisplaced</u> associated transverse-posterior fracture of <u>unspecified</u> acetabulum

S32.47- Fracture of <u>medial wall</u> of acetabulum

CC-K MCC-A,B **S32.471-** <u>Displaced</u> fracture of medial wall of <u>right</u> acetabulum

CC-K MCC-A,B **S32.472-** <u>Displaced</u> fracture of medial wall of <u>left</u> acetabulum

CC-K MCC-A,B **S32.473-** <u>Displaced</u> fracture of medial wall of <u>unspecified</u> acetabulum

CC-K MCC-A,B **S32.474-** <u>Nondisplaced</u> fracture of medial wall of <u>right</u> acetabulum

CC-K MCC-A,B **S32.475-** <u>Nondisplaced</u> fracture of medial wall of <u>left</u> acetabulum

CC-K MCC-A,B **S32.476-** <u>Nondisplaced</u> fracture of medial wall of <u>unspecified</u> acetabulum

S32.48- <u>Dome</u> fracture of acetabulum

CC-K MCC-A,B **S32.481-** <u>Displaced</u> dome fracture of <u>right</u> acetabulum

CC-K MCC-A,B **S32.482-** <u>Displaced</u> dome fracture of <u>left</u> acetabulum

CC-K MCC-A,B **S32.483-** <u>Displaced</u> dome fracture of <u>unspecified</u> acetabulum

CC-K MCC-A,B **S32.484-** <u>Nondisplaced</u> dome fracture of <u>right</u> acetabulum

CC-K MCC-A,B **S32.485-** <u>Nondisplaced</u> dome fracture of <u>left</u> acetabulum

CC-K MCC-A,B **S32.486-** <u>Nondisplaced</u> dome fracture of <u>unspecified</u> acetabulum

S32.49- <u>Other specified</u> fracture of acetabulum

CC-K MCC-A,B **S32.491-** Other specified fracture of <u>right</u> acetabulum

CC-K MCC-A,B **S32.492-** Other specified fracture of <u>left</u> acetabulum

CC-K MCC-A,B **S32.499-** Other specified fracture of <u>unspecified</u> acetabulum

S32.5- Fracture of <u>pubis</u>

　Excludes 1:　fracture of pubis with associated disruption of pelvic ring (S32.8-)

S32.50- <u>Unspecified</u> fracture of pubis

CC-A,K MCC-B **S32.501-** Unspecified fracture of <u>right</u> pubis

CC-A,K MCC-B **S32.502-** Unspecified fracture of <u>left</u> pubis

CC-A,K MCC-B **S32.509-** Unspecified fracture of <u>unspecified</u> pubis

S32.51- Fracture of <u>superior rim</u> of pubis

CC-A,K MCC-B **S32.511-** Fracture of superior rim of <u>right</u> pubis

CC-A,K MCC-B **S32.512-** Fracture of superior rim of <u>left</u> pubis

CC-A,K MCC-B **S32.519-** Fracture of superior rim of <u>unspecified</u> pubis

S32.59- <u>Other specified</u> fracture of pubis

CC-A,K MCC-B **S32.591-** Other specified fracture of <u>right</u> pubis

CC-A,K MCC-B **S32.592-** Other specified fracture of <u>left</u> pubis

CC-A,K MCC-B **S32.599-** Other specified fracture of <u>unspecified</u> pubis

S32.6- Fracture of <u>ischium</u>

　Excludes 1:　fracture of ischium with associated disruption of pelvic ring (S32.8-)

S32.60- <u>Unspecified</u> fracture of ischium

CC-A,K MCC-B **S32.601-** Unspecified fracture of <u>right</u> ischium

CC-A,K MCC-B **S32.602-** Unspecified fracture of <u>left</u> ischium

CC-A,K MCC-B **S32.609-** Unspecified fracture of <u>unspecified</u> ischium

S32.61- <u>Avulsion</u> fracture of ischium

CC-A,K MCC-B **S32.611-** <u>Displaced</u> avulsion fracture of <u>right</u> ischium

CC-A,K MCC-B **S32.612-** <u>Displaced</u> avulsion fracture of <u>left</u> ischium

CC-A,K MCC-B **S32.613-** <u>Displaced</u> avulsion fracture of <u>unspecified</u> ischium

CC-A,K MCC-B **S32.614-** <u>Nondisplaced</u> avulsion fracture of <u>right</u> ischium

CC-A,K MCC-B **S32.615-** <u>Nondisplaced</u> avulsion fracture of <u>left</u> ischium

CC-A,K MCC-B **S32.616-** <u>Nondisplaced</u> avulsion fracture of <u>unspecified</u> ischium

S32.69- <u>Other specified</u> fracture of ischium

CC-A,K MCC-B **S32.691-** Other specified fracture of <u>right</u> ischium

CC-A,K MCC-B **S32.692-** Other specified fracture of <u>left</u> ischium

CC-A,K MCC-B **S32.699-** Other specified fracture of <u>unspecified</u> ischium

S32.8- Fracture of <u>other parts of pelvis</u>

　Code also any associated:
　　Fracture of acetabulum (S32.4-)
　　Sacral fracture (S32.1-)

S32.81- <u>Multiple</u> fractures of pelvis <u>with disruption of pelvic ring</u>

　Multiple pelvic fractures with disruption of pelvic circle

CC-A,K MCC-B **S32.810-** Multiple fractures of pelvis with <u>stable</u> disruption of pelvic ring

CC-A,K MCC-B **S32.811-** Multiple fractures of pelvis with <u>unstable</u> disruption of pelvic ring

S32.82x- <u>Multiple</u> fractures of pelvis <u>without</u> disruption of pelvic ring
CC-A,K MCC-B

　Multiple pelvic fractures without disruption of pelvic circle

S32.89x- Fracture of <u>other</u> parts of pelvis
CC-A,K MCC-B

S32.9xx- Fracture of <u>unspecified</u> parts of lumbosacral spine and pelvis
CC-A,K MCC-B

　Fracture of lumbosacral spine NOS
　Fracture of pelvis NOS

S32 - S32

S33   Dislocation and sprain of joints and ligaments of lumbar spine and pelvis
   Includes: Avulsion of joint or ligament of lumbar spine and pelvis
      Laceration of cartilage, joint or ligament of lumbar spine and pelvis
      Sprain of cartilage, joint or ligament of lumbar spine and pelvis
      Traumatic hemarthrosis of joint or ligament of lumbar spine and pelvis
      Traumatic rupture of joint or ligament of lumbar spine and pelvis
      Traumatic subluxation of joint or ligament of lumbar spine and pelvis
      Traumatic tear of joint or ligament of lumbar spine and pelvis
   Code also any associated open wound
   Excludes 1:   nontraumatic rupture or displacement of lumbar intervertebral disc NOS (M51.-)
      obstetric damage to pelvic joints and ligaments (O71.6)
   Excludes ❷: dislocation and sprain of joints and ligaments of hip (S73.-)
      strain of muscle of lower back and pelvis (S39.01-)

   The appropriate 7th character is to be added to each code from category S33:
   A   Initial encounter
   D   Subsequent encounter
   S   Sequela

S33.0xx-   Traumatic rupture of lumbar intervertebral disc
      Excludes 1:   rupture or displacement (nontraumatic) of lumbar intervertebral disc NOS (M51.- with fifth character 6)

S33.1-   Subluxation and dislocation of lumbar vertebra
      Code also any associated:
         Open wound of abdomen, lower back and pelvis (S31)
         Spinal cord injury (S24.0, S24.1-, S34.0-, S34.1-)
      Excludes ❷: fracture of lumbar vertebrae (S32.0-)

   S33.10- Subluxation and dislocation of unspecified lumbar vertebra
      S33.100-   Subluxation of unspecified lumbar vertebra
      S33.101-   Dislocation of unspecified lumbar vertebra
   S33.11- Subluxation and dislocation of L1/L2 lumbar vertebra
      S33.110-   Subluxation of L1/L2 lumbar vertebra
      S33.111-   Dislocation of L1/L2 lumbar vertebra
   S33.12- Subluxation and dislocation of L2/L3 lumbar vertebra
      S33.120-   Subluxation of L2/L3 lumbar vertebra
      S33.121-   Dislocation of L2/L3 lumbar vertebra
   S33.13- Subluxation and dislocation of L3/L4 lumbar vertebra
      S33.130-   Subluxation of L3/L4 lumbar vertebra
      S33.131-   Dislocation of L3/L4 lumbar vertebra
   S33.14- Subluxation and dislocation of L4/L5 lumbar vertebra
      S33.140-   Subluxation of L4/L5 lumbar vertebra
      S33.141-   Dislocation of L4/L5 lumbar vertebra

S33.2xx-   Dislocation of sacroiliac and sacrococcygeal joint
S33.3-   Dislocation of other and unspecified parts of lumbar spine and pelvis
   S33.30x-   Dislocation of unspecified parts of lumbar spine and pelvis
   S33.39x-   Dislocation of other parts of lumbar spine and pelvis
S33.4xx-   Traumatic rupture of symphysis pubis
S33.5xx-   Sprain of ligaments of lumbar spine
S33.6xx-   Sprain of sacroiliac joint
S33.8xx-   Sprain of other parts of lumbar spine and pelvis
S33.9xx-   Sprain of unspecified parts of lumbar spine and pelvis

S34-   Injury of lumbar and sacral spinal cord and nerves at abdomen, lower back and pelvis level
   Note: Code to highest level of lumbar cord injury
      Injuries to the spinal cord (S34.0 and S34.1) refer to the cord level and not bone level injury, and can affect nerve roots at and below the level given.
   Code also any associated:
      Fracture of vertebra (S22.0-, S32.0-)
      Open wound of abdomen, lower back and pelvis (S31.-)
      Transient paralysis (R29.5)

   The appropriate 7th character is to be added to each code from category S34:
   A   Initial encounter
   D   Subsequent encounter
   S   Sequela

S34.0-   Concussion and edema of lumbar and sacral spinal cord
MCC-A   **S34.01x-**   Concussion and edema of lumbar spinal cord
MCC-A   **S34.02x-**   Concussion and edema of sacral spinal cord
      Concussion and edema of conus medullaris
S34.1-   Other and unspecified injury of lumbar and sacral spinal cord
   S34.10-   Unspecified injury to lumbar spinal cord
   MCC-A   **S34.101-**   Unspecified injury to L1 level of lumbar spinal cord
      Unspecified injury to lumbar spinal cord level 1
   MCC-A   **S34.102-**   Unspecified injury to L2 level of lumbar spinal cord
      Unspecified injury to lumbar spinal cord level 2
   MCC-A   **S34.103-**   Unspecified injury to L3 level of lumbar spinal cord
      Unspecified injury to lumbar spinal cord level 3
   MCC-A   **S34.104-**   Unspecified injury to L4 level of lumbar spinal cord
      Unspecified injury to lumbar spinal cord level 4
   MCC-A   **S34.105-**   Unspecified injury to L5 level of lumbar spinal cord
      Unspecified injury to lumbar spinal cord level 5
   MCC-A   **S34.109-**   Unspecified injury to unspecified level of lumbar spinal cord
   S34.11-   Complete lesion of lumbar spinal cord
   MCC-A   **S34.111-**   Complete lesion of L1 level of lumbar spinal cord
      Complete lesion of lumbar spinal cord level 1
   MCC-A   **S34.112-**   Complete lesion of L2 level of lumbar spinal cord
      Complete lesion of lumbar spinal cord level 2
   MCC-A   **S34.113-**   Complete lesion of L3 level of lumbar spinal cord
      Complete lesion of lumbar spinal cord level 3
   MCC-A   **S34.114-**   Complete lesion of L4 level of lumbar spinal cord
      Complete lesion of lumbar spinal cord level 4
   MCC-A   **S34.115-**   Complete lesion of L5 level of lumbar spinal cord
      Complete lesion of lumbar spinal cord level 5
   MCC-A   **S34.119-**   Complete lesion of unspecified level of lumbar spinal cord
   S34.12-   Incomplete lesion of lumbar spinal cord
   MCC-A   **S34.121-**   Incomplete lesion of L1 level of lumbar spinal cord
      Incomplete lesion of lumbar spinal cord level 1
   MCC-A   **S34.122-**   Incomplete lesion of L2 level of lumbar spinal cord
      Incomplete lesion of lumbar spinal cord level 2
   MCC-A   **S34.123-**   Incomplete lesion of L3 level of lumbar spinal cord
      Incomplete lesion of lumbar spinal cord level 3
   MCC-A   **S34.124-**   Incomplete lesion of L4 level of lumbar spinal cord
      Incomplete lesion of lumbar spinal cord level 4
   MCC-A   **S34.125-**   Incomplete lesion of L5 level of lumbar spinal cord
      Incomplete lesion of lumbar spinal cord level 5
   MCC-A   **S34.129-**   Incomplete lesion of unspecified level of lumbar spinal cord
   S34.13-   Other and unspecified injury to sacral spinal cord
      Other injury to conus medullaris
   MCC-A   **S34.131-**   Complete lesion of sacral spinal cord
      Complete lesion of conus medullaris
   MCC-A   **S34.132-**   Incomplete lesion of sacral spinal cord
      Incomplete lesion of conus medullaris
   MCC-A   **S34.139-**   Unspecified injury to sacral spinal cord
      Unspecified injury of conus medullaris
S34.2-   Injury of nerve root of lumbar and sacral spine
   S34.21x-   Injury of nerve root of lumbar spine
   S34.22x-   Injury of nerve root of sacral spine

S33 - S34

S34.3xx-   Injry of cauda equina
MCC-A

S34.4xx-   Injury of lumbosacral plexus

S34.5xx-   Injury of lumbar, sacral and pelvic sympathetic nerves
Injury of celiac ganglion or plexus
Injury of hypogastric plexus
Injury of mesenteric plexus (inferior) (superior)
Injury of splanchnic nerve

S34.6xx-   Injury of peripheral nerve(s) at abdomen, lower back and pelvis level

S34.8xx-   Injury of other nerves at abdomen, lower back and pelvis level

S34.9xx-   Injury of unspecified nerves at abdomen, lower back and pelvis level

S35-   Injury of blood vessels at abdomen, lower back and pelvis level
Code also any associated open wound (S31.-)
The appropriate 7th character is to be added to each code from category S35:
A   Initial encounter
D   Subsequent encounter
S   Sequela

S35.0-   Injury of abdominal aorta
Excludes 1:   injury of aorta NOS (S25.0)

MCC-A **S35.00x-**   Unspecified injury of abdominal aorta

MCC-A **S35.01x-**   Minor laceration of abdominal aorta
Incomplete transection of abdominal aorta
Laceration of abdominal aorta NOS
Superficial laceration of abdominal aorta

MCC-A **S35.02x-**   Major laceration of abdominal aorta
Complete transection of abdominal aorta
Traumatic rupture of abdominal aorta

MCC-A **S35.09x-**   Other injury of abdominal aorta

S35.1-   Injury of inferior vena cava
Injury of hepatic vein
Excludes 1:   injury of vena cava NOS (S25.2)

MCC-A **S35.10x-**   Unspecified injury of inferior vena cava

MCC-A **S35.11x-**   Minor laceration of inferior vena cava
Incomplete transection of inferior vena cava
Laceration of inferior vena cava NOS
Superficial laceration of inferior vena cava

MCC-A **S35.12x-**   Major laceration of inferior vena cava
Complete transection of inferior vena cava
Traumatic rupture of inferior vena cava

MCC-A **S35.19x-**   Other injury of inferior vena cava

S35.2-   Injury of celiac or mesenteric artery and branches

S35.21-   Injury of celiac artery

MCC-A **S35.211-**   Minor laceration of celiac artery
Incomplete transection of celiac artery
Laceration of celiac artery NOS
Superficial laceration of celiac artery

MCC-A **S35.212-**   Major laceration of celiac artery
Complete transection of celiac artery
Traumatic rupture of celiac artery

MCC-A **S35.218-**   Other injury of celiac artery

MCC-A **S35.219-**   Unspecified injury of celiac artery

S35.22-   Injury of superior mesenteric artery

MCC-A **S35.221-**   Minor laceration of superior mesenteric artery
Incomplete transection of superior mesenteric artery
Laceration of superior mesenteric artery NOS
Superficial laceration of superior mesenteric artery

MCC-A **S35.222-**   Major laceration of superior mesenteric artery
Complete transection of superior mesenteric artery
Traumatic rupture of superior mesenteric artery

MCC-A **S35.228-**   Other injury of superior mesenteric artery

MCC-A **S35.229-**   Unspecified injury of superior mesenteric artery

S35.23-   Injury of inferior mesenteric artery

MCC-A **S35.231-**   Minor laceration of inferior mesenteric artery
Incomplete transection of inferior mesenteric artery
Laceration of inferior mesenteric artery NOS
Superficial laceration of inferior mesenteric artery

MCC-A **S35.232-**   Major laceration of inferior mesenteric artery
Complete transection of inferior mesenteric artery
Traumatic rupture of inferior mesenteric artery

MCC-A **S35.238-**   Other injury of inferior mesenteric artery

MCC-A **S35.239-**   Unspecified injury of inferior mesenteric artery

S35.29-   Injury of branches of celiac and mesenteric artery
Injury of gastric artery
Injury of gastroduodenal artery
Injury of hepatic artery
Injury of splenic artery

MCC-A **S35.291-**   Minor laceration of branches of celiac and mesenteric artery
Incomplete transection of branches of celiac and mesenteric artery
Laceration of branches of celiac and mesenteric artery NOS
Superficial laceration of branches of celiac and mesenteric artery

MCC-A **S35.292-**   Major laceration of branches of celiac and mesenteric artery
Complete transection of branches of celiac and mesenteric artery
Traumatic rupture of branches of celiac and mesenteric artery

MCC-A **S35.298-**   Other injury of branches of celiac and mesenteric artery

MCC-A **S35.299-**   Unspecified injury of branches of celiac and mesenteric artery

S35.3-   Injury of portal or splenic vein and branches

S35.31-   Injury of portal vein

MCC-A **S35.311-**   Laceration of portal vein

MCC-A **S35.318-**   Other specified injury of portal vein

MCC-A **S35.319-**   Unspecified injury of portal vein

S35.32-   Injury of splenic vein

MCC-A **S35.321-**   Laceration of splenic vein

MCC-A **S35.328-**   Other specified injury of splenic vein

MCC-A **S35.329-**   Unspecified injury of splenic vein

S35.33-   Injury of superior mesenteric vein

MCC-A **S35.331-**   Laceration of superior mesenteric vein

MCC-A **S35.338-**   Other specified injury of superior mesenteric vein

MCC-A **S35.339-**   Unspecified injury of superior mesenteric vein

S35.34-   Injury of inferior mesenteric vein

MCC-A **S35.341-**   Laceration of inferior mesenteric vein

MCC-A **S35.348-**   Other specified injury of inferior mesenteric vein

MCC-A **S35.349-**   Unspecified injury of inferior mesenteric vein

S35.4-   Injury of renal blood vessels

S35.40-   Unspecified injury of renal blood vessel

MCC-A **S35.401-**   Unspecified injury of right renal artery

MCC-A **S35.402-**   Unspecified injury of left renal artery

MCC-A **S35.403-**   Unspecified injury of unspecified renal artery

MCC-A **S35.404-**   Unspecified injury of right renal vein

MCC-A **S35.405-**   Unspecified injury of left renal vein

MCC-A **S35.406-**   Unspecified injury of unspecified renal vein

S35.41-   Laceration of renal blood vessel

MCC-A **S35.411-**   Laceration of right renal artery

MCC-A **S35.412-**   Laceration of left renal artery

MCC-A **S35.413-**   Laceration of unspecified renal artery

MCC-A **S35.414-**   Laceration of right renal vein

MCC-A **S35.415-**   Laceration of left renal vein

MCC-A **S35.416-**   Laceration of unspecified renal vein

S35.49-   Other specified injury of renal blood vessel

MCC-A **S35.491-**   Other specified injury of right renal artery

MCC-A **S35.492-**   Other specified injury of left renal artery

MCC-A **S35.493-**   Other specified injury of unspecified renal artery

MCC-A **S35.494-**   Other specified injury of right renal vein

MCC-A **S35.495-**   Other specified injury of left renal vein

MCC-A **S35.496-**   Other specified injury of unspecified renal vein

S35.5-   Injury of iliac blood vessels

MCC-A **S35.50x-**   Injury of unspecified iliac blood vessel(s)

S35.51-   Injury of iliac artery or vein
Injury of hypogastric artery or vein

MCC-A **S35.511-**   Injury of right iliac artery

S 3 4 - S 3 5

MCC-A **S35.512-** Injury of <u>left iliac</u> <u>artery</u>

MCC-A **S35.513-** Injury of <u>unspecified</u> iliac <u>artery</u>

MCC-A **S35.514-** Injury of <u>right</u> iliac <u>vein</u>

MCC-A **S35.515-** Injury of <u>left</u> iliac <u>vein</u>

MCC-A **S35.516-** Injury of <u>unspecified</u> iliac <u>vein</u>

S35.53- Injury of <u>uterine</u> artery or vein

CC-A **S35.531-** Injury of <u>right</u> uterine <u>artery</u> — [♀]

CC-A **S35.532-** Injury of <u>left</u> uterine <u>artery</u> — [♀]

CC-A **S35.533-** Injury of <u>unspecified</u> uterine <u>artery</u> — [♀]

CC-A **S35.534-** Injury of <u>right</u> uterine <u>vein</u> — [♀]

CC-A **S35.535-** Injury of <u>left</u> uterine <u>vein</u> — [♀]

CC-A **S35.536-** Injury of <u>unspecified</u> uterine <u>vein</u> — [♀]

MCC-A **S35.59x-** Injury of <u>other iliac blood vessels</u>

S35.8- Injury of <u>other blood vessels</u> at <u>abdomen, lower back and pelvis level</u>

    Injury of ovarian artery or vein

S35.8x- Injury of <u>other blood vessels</u> at abdomen, lower back and pelvis level

CC-A **S35.8x1-** <u>Laceration</u> of <u>other</u> blood vessels at abdomen, lower back and pelvis level

CC-A **S35.8x8-** <u>Other</u> specified injury of <u>other</u> blood vessels at abdomen, lower back and pelvis level

CC-A **S35.8x9-** <u>Unspecified</u> injury of <u>other</u> blood vessels at abdomen, lower back and pelvis level

S35.9- Injury of <u>unspecified blood vessel</u> at <u>abdomen, lower back and pelvis level</u>

CC-A **S35.90x-** <u>Unspecified</u> injury of <u>unspecified</u> blood vessel at abdomen, lower back and pelvis level

CC-A **S35.91x-** <u>Laceration</u> of <u>unspecified</u> blood vessel at abdomen, lower back and pelvis level

CC-A **S35.99x-** <u>Other</u> specified injury of <u>unspecified</u> blood vessel at abdomen, lower back and pelvis level

S36- Injury of <u>intra-abdominal organs</u>

    Code also any associated open wound (S31.-)

> The appropriate 7th character is to be added to each code from category S36:
> **A** <u>Initial</u> encounter
> **D** <u>Subsequent</u> encounter
> **S** <u>Sequela</u>

S36.0- Injury of <u>spleen</u>

CC-A **S36.00x-** <u>Unspecified</u> injury of spleen

S36.02- <u>Contusion</u> of spleen

    AHA 15:1Q:p10 – Perisplenic hematoma

    AHA 15:2Q:p36 – Official Correction of 15:1Q:p10

CC-A **S36.020-** <u>Minor</u> contusion of spleen

    Contusion of spleen less than 2 cm

CC-A **S36.021-** <u>Major</u> contusion of spleen

    Contusion of spleen greater than 2 cm

CC-A **S36.029-** <u>Unspecified</u> contusion of spleen

S36.03- <u>Laceration</u> of spleen

    AHA 15:1Q:p10 – Delayed splenic rupture, grade 3 splenic laceration

    AHA 15:2Q:p36 – Official Correction of 15:1Q:p10

CC-A **S36.030-** <u>Superficial</u> (capsular) laceration of spleen

    Laceration of spleen less than 1 cm

    Minor laceration of spleen

MCC-A **S36.031-** <u>Moderate</u> laceration of spleen

    Laceration of spleen 1 to 3 cm

MCC-A **S36.032-** <u>Major</u> laceration of spleen

    Avulsion of spleen

    Laceration of spleen greater than 3 cm

    Massive laceration of spleen

    Multiple moderate lacerations of spleen

    Stellate laceration of spleen

CC-A **S36.039-** <u>Unspecified</u> laceration of spleen

CC-A **S36.09x-** <u>Other</u> injury of spleen

S36.1- Injury of <u>liver and gallbladder and bile duct</u>

S36.11- Injury of <u>liver</u>

CC-A **S36.112-** <u>Contusion</u> of liver

CC-A **S36.113-** <u>Laceration</u> of liver, <u>unspecified</u> degree

CC-A **S36.114-** <u>Minor</u> laceration of liver

    Laceration involving capsule only, or, without significant involvement of hepatic parenchyma [i.e., less than 1 cm deep]

MCC-A **S36.115-** <u>Moderate</u> laceration of liver

    Laceration involving parenchyma but without major disruption of parenchyma [i.e., less than 10 cm long and less than 3 cm deep]

MCC-A **S36.116-** <u>Major</u> laceration of liver

    Laceration with significant disruption of hepatic parenchyma [i.e., greater than 10 cm long and 3 cm deep]

    Multiple moderate lacerations, with or without hematoma

    Stellate laceration of liver

CC-A **S36.118-** <u>Other</u> injury of liver

CC-A **S36.119-** <u>Unspecified</u> injury of liver

S36.12- Injury of <u>gallbladder</u>

CC-A **S36.122-** <u>Contusion</u> of gallbladder

CC-A **S36.123-** <u>Laceration</u> of gallbladder

CC-A **S36.128-** <u>Other</u> injury of gallbladder

CC-A **S36.129-** <u>Unspecified</u> injury of gallbladder

CC-A **S36.13x-** Injury of <u>bile duct</u>

S36.2- Injury of <u>pancreas</u>

S36.20- <u>Unspecified</u> injury of pancreas

CC-A **S36.200-** Unspecified injury of <u>head</u> of pancreas

CC-A **S36.201-** Unspecified injury of <u>body</u> of pancreas

CC-A **S36.202-** Unspecified injury of <u>tail</u> of pancreas

CC-A **S36.209-** Unspecified injury of <u>unspecified</u> part of pancreas

S36.22- <u>Contusion</u> of pancreas

CC-A **S36.220-** Contusion of <u>head</u> of pancreas

CC-A **S36.221-** Contusion of <u>body</u> of pancreas

CC-A **S36.222-** Contusion of <u>tail</u> of pancreas

CC-A **S36.229-** Contusion of <u>unspecified</u> part of pancreas

S36.23- <u>Laceration</u> of pancreas, <u>unspecified</u> degree

CC-A **S36.230-** Laceration of <u>head</u> of pancreas, <u>unspecified</u> degree

CC-A **S36.231-** Laceration of <u>body</u> of pancreas, <u>unspecified</u> degree

CC-A **S36.232-** Laceration of <u>tail</u> of pancreas, <u>unspecified</u> degree

CC-A **S36.239-** Laceration of <u>unspecified</u> part of pancreas, <u>unspecified</u> degree

S36.24- <u>Minor</u> laceration of pancreas

CC-A **S36.240-** Minor laceration of <u>head</u> of pancreas

CC-A **S36.241-** Minor laceration of <u>body</u> of pancreas

CC-A **S36.242-** Minor laceration of <u>tail</u> of pancreas

CC-A **S36.249-** Minor laceration of <u>unspecified</u> part of pancreas

S36.25- <u>Moderate</u> laceration of pancreas

CC-A **S36.250-** Moderate laceration of <u>head</u> of pancreas

CC-A **S36.251-** Moderate laceration of <u>body</u> of pancreas

CC-A **S36.252-** Moderate laceration of <u>tail</u> of pancreas

CC-A **S36.259-** Moderate laceration of <u>unspecified</u> part of pancreas

S36.26- <u>Major</u> laceration of pancreas

CC-A **S36.260-** Major laceration of <u>head</u> of pancreas

CC-A **S36.261-** Major laceration of <u>body</u> of pancreas

CC-A **S36.262-** Major laceration of <u>tail</u> of pancreas

CC-A **S36.269-** Major laceration of <u>unspecified</u> part of pancreas

S36.29- <u>Other</u> injury of pancreas

CC-A **S36.290-** Other injury of <u>head</u> of pancreas

CC-A **S36.291-** Other injury of <u>body</u> of pancreas

CC-A **S36.292-** Other injury of <u>tail</u> of pancreas

CC-A **S36.299-** Other injury of <u>unspecified</u> part of pancreas

S36.3- Injury of <u>stomach</u>

CC-A **S36.30x-** <u>Unspecified</u> injury of stomach

CC-A **S36.32x-** <u>Contusion</u> of stomach

CC-A **S36.33x-** <u>Laceration</u> of stomach

CC-A **S36.39x-** <u>Other</u> injury of stomach

S35–S36

S36.4- Injury of small intestine
S36.40- Unspecified injury of small intestine
CC-A **S36.400- Unspecified injury of duodenum**
CC-A **S36.408- Unspecified injury of other part of small intestine**
CC-A **S36.409- Unspecified injury of unspecified part of small intestine**
S36.41- Primary blast injury of small intestine
      Blast injury of small intestine NOS
CC-A **S36.410- Primary blast injury of duodenum**
CC-A **S36.418- Primary blast injury of other part of small intestine**
CC-A **S36.419- Primary blast injury of unspecified part of small intestine**
S36.42- Contusion of small intestine
CC-A **S36.420- Contusion of duodenum**
CC-A **S36.428- Contusion of other part of small intestine**
CC-A **S36.429- Contusion of unspecified part of small intestine**
S36.43- Laceration of small intestine
CC-A **S36.430- Laceration of duodenum**
CC-A **S36.438- Laceration of other part of small intestine**
CC-A **S36.439- Laceration of unspecified part of small intestine**
S36.49- Other injury of small intestine
CC-A **S36.490- Other injury of duodenum**
CC-A **S36.498- Other injury of other part of small intestine**
CC-A **S36.499- Other injury of unspecified part of small intestine**
S36.5- Injury of colon
      Excludes ❷: injury of rectum (S36.6-)
S36.50- Unspecified injury of colon
CC-A **S36.500- Unspecified injury of ascending [right] colon**
CC-A **S36.501- Unspecified injury of transverse colon**
CC-A **S36.502- Unspecified injury of descending [left] colon**
CC-A **S36.503- Unspecified injury of sigmoid colon**
CC-A **S36.508- Unspecified injury of other part of colon**
CC-A **S36.509- Unspecified injury of unspecified part of colon**
S36.51- Primary blast injury of colon
         Blast injury of colon NOS
CC-A **S36.510- Primary blast injury of ascending [right] colon**
CC-A **S36.511- Primary blast injury of transverse colon**
CC-A **S36.512- Primary blast injury of descending [left] colon**
CC-A **S36.513- Primary blast injury of sigmoid colon**
CC-A **S36.518- Primary blast injury of other part of colon**
CC-A **S36.519- Primary blast injury of unspecified part of colon**
S36.52- Contusion of colon
CC-A **S36.520- Contusion of ascending [right] colon**
CC-A **S36.521- Contusion of transverse colon**
CC-A **S36.522- Contusion of descending [left] colon**
CC-A **S36.523- Contusion of sigmoid colon**
CC-A **S36.528- Contusion of other part of colon**
CC-A **S36.529- Contusion of unspecified part of colon**
S36.53- Laceration of colon
CC-A **S36.530- Laceration of ascending [right] colon**
CC-A **S36.531- Laceration of transverse colon**
CC-A **S36.532- Laceration of descending [left] colon**
CC-A **S36.533- Laceration of sigmoid colon**
CC-A **S36.538- Laceration of other part of colon**
CC-A **S36.539- Laceration of unspecified part of colon**
S36.59- Other injury of colon
         Secondary blast injury of colon
CC-A **S36.590- Other injury of ascending [right] colon**
CC-A **S36.591- Other injury of transverse colon**
CC-A **S36.592- Other injury of descending [left] colon**
CC-A **S36.593- Other injury of sigmoid colon**
CC-A **S36.598- Other injury of other part of colon**
CC-A **S36.599- Other injury of unspecified part of colon**
S36.6- Injury of rectum
CC-A **S36.60x- Unspecified injury of rectum**

CC-A **S36.61x- Primary blast injury of rectum**
         Blast injury of rectum NOS
CC-A **S36.62x- Contusion of rectum**
CC-A **S36.63x- Laceration of rectum**
CC-A **S36.69x- Other injury of rectum**
         Secondary blast injury of rectum
S36.8- Injury of other intra-abdominal organs
CC-A **S36.81x- Injury of peritoneum**
S36.89- Injury of other intra-abdominal organs
         Injury of retroperitoneum
CC-A **S36.892- Contusion of other intra-abdominal organs**
CC-A **S36.893- Laceration of other intra-abdominal organs**
CC-A **S36.898- Other injury of other intra-abdominal organs**
CC-A **S36.899- Unspecified injury of other intra-abdominal organs**
S36.9- Injury of unspecified intra-abdominal organ
CC-A **S36.90x- Unspecified injury of unspecified intra-abdominal organ**
CC-A **S36.92x- Contusion of unspecified intra-abdominal organ**
CC-A **S36.93x- Laceration of unspecified intra-abdominal organ**
CC-A **S36.99x- Other injury of unspecified intra-abdominal organ**

S37- Injury of urinary and pelvic organs
      Code also any associated open wound (S31.-)
      Excludes 1:   obstetric trauma to pelvic organs (O71.-)
      Excludes ❷: injury of peritoneum (S36.81)
                  injury of retroperitoneum (S36.89-)
The appropriate 7th character is to be added to each code from category S37:
   A   Initial encounter
   D   Subsequent encounter
   S   Sequela
S37.0- Injury of kidney
      Excludes ❷: acute kidney injury (nontraumatic) (N17.9)
S37.00- Unspecified injury of kidney
CC-A **S37.001- Unspecified injury of right kidney**
CC-A **S37.002- Unspecified injury of left kidney**
CC-A **S37.009- Unspecified injury of unspecified kidney**
S37.01- Minor contusion of kidney
         Contusion of kidney less than 2 cm
         Contusion of kidney NOS
CC-A **S37.011- Minor contusion of right kidney**
CC-A **S37.012- Minor contusion of left kidney**
CC-A **S37.019- Minor contusion of unspecified kidney**
S37.02- Major contusion of kidney
         Contusion of kidney greater than 2 cm
CC-A **S37.021- Major contusion of right kidney**
CC-A **S37.022- Major contusion of left kidney**
CC-A **S37.029- Major contusion of unspecified kidney**
S37.03- Laceration of kidney, unspecified degree
CC-A **S37.031- Laceration of right kidney, unspecified degree**
CC-A **S37.032- Laceration of left kidney, unspecified degree**
CC-A **S37.039- Laceration of unspecified kidney, unspecified degree**
S37.04- Minor laceration of kidney
         Laceration of kidney less than 1 cm
CC-A **S37.041- Minor laceration of right kidney**
CC-A **S37.042- Minor laceration of left kidney**
CC-A **S37.049- Minor laceration of unspecified kidney**
S37.05- Moderate laceration of kidney
         Laceration of kidney 1 to 3 cm
CC-A **S37.051- Moderate laceration of right kidney**
CC-A **S37.052- Moderate laceration of left kidney**
CC-A **S37.059- Moderate laceration of unspecified kidney**
S37.06- Major laceration of kidney
         Avulsion of kidney
         Laceration of kidney greater than 3 cm
         Massive laceration of kidney
         Multiple moderate lacerations of kidney
         Stellate laceration of kidney
MCC-A **S37.061- Major laceration of right kidney**

S36 – S37

MCC-A **S37.062-** Major laceration of <u>left</u> kidney
MCC-A **S37.069-** Major laceration of <u>unspecified</u> kidney
S37.09- <u>Other</u> injury of kidney
MCC-A **S37.091-** Other injury of <u>right</u> kidney
MCC-A **S37.092-** Other injury of <u>left</u> kidney
MCC-A **S37.099-** Other injury of <u>unspecified</u> kidney
S37.1- Injury of <u>ureter</u>
CC-A **S37.10x-** <u>Unspecified</u> injury of ureter
CC-A **S37.12x-** <u>Contusion</u> of ureter
CC-A **S37.13x-** <u>Laceration</u> of ureter
CC-A **S37.19x-** Other injury of ureter
S37.2- Injury of <u>bladder</u>
CC-A **S37.20x-** <u>Unspecified</u> injury of bladder
CC-A **S37.22x-** <u>Contusion</u> of bladder
CC-A **S37.23x-** <u>Laceration</u> of bladder
CC-A **S37.29x-** <u>Other</u> injury of bladder
S37.3- Injury of <u>urethra</u>
CC-A **S37.30x-** <u>Unspecified</u> injury of urethra
CC-A **S37.32x-** <u>Contusion</u> of urethra
CC-A **S37.33x-** <u>Laceration</u> of urethra
CC-A **S37.39x-** <u>Other</u> injury of urethra
S37.4- Injury of <u>ovary</u>
  S37.40- <u>Unspecified</u> injury of ovary
    S37.401- Unspecified injury of ovary, <u>unilateral</u> — [♀]
    S37.402- Unspecified injury of ovary, <u>bilateral</u> — [♀]
    S37.409- Unspecified injury of ovary, <u>unspecified</u> — [♀]
  S37.42- <u>Contusion</u> of ovary
    S37.421- Contusion of ovary, <u>unilateral</u> — [♀]
    S37.422- Contusion of ovary, <u>bilateral</u> — [♀]
    S37.429- Contusion of ovary, <u>unspecified</u> — [♀]
  S37.43- <u>Laceration</u> of ovary
    S37.431- Laceration of ovary, <u>unilateral</u> — [♀]
    S37.432- Laceration of ovary, <u>bilateral</u> — [♀]
    S37.439- Laceration of ovary, <u>unspecified</u> — [♀]
  S37.49- <u>Other</u> injury of ovary
    S37.491- Other injury of ovary, <u>unilateral</u> — [♀]
    S37.492- Other injury of ovary, <u>bilateral</u> — [♀]
    S37.499- Other injury of ovary, <u>unspecified</u> — [♀]
S37.5- Injury of <u>fallopian tube</u>
  S37.50- <u>Unspecified</u> injury of fallopian tube
    S37.501- Unspecified injury of fallopian tube, <u>unilateral</u> — [♀]
    S37.502- Unspecified injury of fallopian tube, <u>bilateral</u> — [♀]
    S37.509- Unspecified injury of fallopian tube, <u>unspecified</u> — [♀]
  S37.51- <u>Primary blast</u> injury of fallopian tube
    Blast injury of fallopian tube NOS
    S37.511- Primary blast injury of fallopian tube, <u>unilateral</u> — [♀]
    S37.512- Primary blast injury of fallopian tube, <u>bilateral</u> — [♀]
    S37.519- Primary blast injury of fallopian tube, <u>unspecified</u> — [♀]
  S37.52- <u>Contusion</u> of fallopian tube
    S37.521- Contusion of fallopian tube, <u>unilateral</u> — [♀]
    S37.522- Contusion of fallopian tube, <u>bilateral</u> — [♀]
    S37.529- Contusion of fallopian tube, <u>unspecified</u> — [♀]
  S37.53- <u>Laceration</u> of fallopian tube
    S37.531- Laceration of fallopian tube, <u>unilateral</u> — [♀]
    S37.532- Laceration of fallopian tube, <u>bilateral</u> — [♀]
    S37.539- Laceration of fallopian tube, <u>unspecified</u> — [♀]
  S37.59- <u>Other</u> injury of fallopian tube
    Secondary blast injury of fallopian tube
    S37.591- Other injury of fallopian tube, <u>unilateral</u> — [♀]

S37.592- Other injury of fallopian tube, <u>bilateral</u> — [♀]
S37.599- Other injury of fallopian tube, <u>unspecified</u> — [♀]
S37.6- Injury of <u>uterus</u>
  Excludes 1:   *injury to gravid uterus (O9A.2-)*
          injury to uterus during delivery (O71.-)
CC-A **S37.60x-** <u>Unspecified</u> injury of uterus — [♀]
CC-A **S37.62x-** <u>Contusion</u> of uterus — [♀]
CC-A **S37.63x-** <u>Laceration</u> of uterus — [♀]
CC-A **S37.69x-** <u>Other</u> injury of uterus — [♀]
S37.8- Injury of <u>other urinary and pelvic organs</u>
  S37.81- Injury of <u>adrenal gland</u>
CC-A   **S37.812-** <u>Contusion</u> of adrenal gland
CC-A   **S37.813-** <u>Laceration</u> of adrenal gland
CC-A   **S37.818-** <u>Other</u> injury of adrenal gland
CC-A   **S37.819-** <u>Unspecified</u> injury of adrenal gland
  S37.82- Injury of <u>prostate</u>
    S37.822- <u>Contusion</u> of prostate — [♂]
    S37.823- <u>Laceration</u> of prostate — [♂]
    S37.828- <u>Other</u> injury of prostate — [♂]
    S37.829- <u>Unspecified</u> injury of prostate — [♂]
  S37.89- Injury of other urinary and pelvic organ
CC-A   **S37.892-** <u>Contusion</u> of other urinary and pelvic organ
CC-A   **S37.893-** <u>Laceration</u> of other urinary and pelvic organ
CC-A   **S37.898-** <u>Other</u> injury of other urinary and pelvic organ
CC-A   **S37.899-** <u>Unspecified</u> injury of other urinary and pelvic organ
S37.9- Injury of <u>unspecified urinary and pelvic organ</u>
CC-A **S37.90x-** <u>Unspecified</u> injury of unspecified urinary and pelvic organ
CC-A **S37.92x-** <u>Contusion</u> of unspecified urinary and pelvic organ
CC-A **S37.93x-** <u>Laceration</u> of unspecified urinary and pelvic organ
CC-A **S37.99x-** <u>Other</u> injury of unspecified urinary and pelvic organ
S38- <u>Crushing injury</u> and <u>traumatic amputation</u> of <u>abdomen, lower back, pelvis and external genitals</u>
  Note: An amputation not identified as partial or complete should be coded to complete

> **The appropriate 7th character is to be added to each code from category S38:**
> **A**   <u>Initial</u> encounter
> **D**   <u>Subsequent</u> encounter
> **S**   <u>Sequela</u>

S38.0- <u>Crushing injury</u> of <u>external genital organs</u>
  Use additional code for any associated injuries
  S38.00- Crushing injury of <u>unspecified external genital organs</u>
    S38.001- Crushing injury of <u>unspecified</u> external genital organs, <u>male</u> — [♂]
    S38.002- Crushing injury of <u>unspecified</u> external genital organs, <u>female</u> — [♀]
  S38.01x- Crushing injury of <u>penis</u> — [♂]
  S38.02x- Crushing injury of <u>scrotum and testis</u> — [♂]
  S38.03x- Crushing injury of <u>vulva</u> — [♀]
S38.1xx- Crushing injury of <u>abdomen, lower back, and pelvis</u>
  Use additional code for all associated injuries, such as:
    Fracture of thoracic or lumbar spine and pelvis (S22.0-, S32.-)
    Injury to intra-abdominal organs (S36.-)
    Injury to urinary and pelvic organs (S37.-)
    Open wound of abdominal wall (S31.-)
    Spinal cord injury (S34.0, S34.1-)
  Excludes ❷: crushing injury of external genital organs (S38.0-)
S38.2- <u>Traumatic amputation</u> of <u>external genital organs</u>
  S38.21- Traumatic amputation of <u>female external genital organs</u>
    Traumatic amputation of clitoris
    Traumatic amputation of labium (majus) (minus)
    Traumatic amputation of vulva
    S38.211- <u>Complete</u> traumatic amputation of female external genital organs — [♀]
    S38.212- <u>Partial</u> traumatic amputation of female external genital organs — [♀]

S37 – S38

S38.22- Traumatic amputation of <u>penis</u>
 S38.221- <u>Complete</u> traumatic amputation of penis — [♂]
 S38.222- <u>Partial</u> traumatic amputation of penis — [♂]
S38.23- Traumatic amputation of <u>scrotum and testis</u>
 S38.231- <u>Complete</u> traumatic amputation of scrotum and testis — [♂]
 S38.232- <u>Partial</u> traumatic amputation of scrotum and testis — [♂]
S38.3xx- Transection (partial) of <u>abdomen</u>

S39- <u>Other and unspecified</u> injuries of <u>abdomen, lower back, pelvis and external genitals</u>
Code also any associated open wound (S31.-)
Excludes ❷: sprain of joints and ligaments of lumbar spine and pelvis (S33.-)

The appropriate 7th character is to be added to each code from category S39:
 A <u>Initial</u> encounter
 D <u>Subsequent</u> encounter
 S <u>Sequela</u>

S39.0- Injury of <u>muscle, fascia and tendon</u> of <u>abdomen, lower back and pelvis</u>
 S39.00- <u>Unspecified</u> injury of muscle, fascia and tendon of abdomen, lower back and pelvis
  S39.001- Unspecified injury of muscle, fascia and tendon of <u>abdomen</u>
  S39.002- Unspecified injury of muscle, fascia and tendon of <u>lower back</u>
  S39.003- Unspecified injury of muscle, fascia and tendon of <u>pelvis</u>
 S39.01- <u>Strain</u> of muscle, fascia and tendon of abdomen, lower back and pelvis
  S39.011- Strain of muscle, fascia and tendon of <u>abdomen</u>
  S39.012- Strain of muscle, fascia and tendon of <u>lower back</u>
  S39.013- Strain of muscle, fascia and tendon of <u>pelvis</u>
 S39.02- <u>Laceration</u> of muscle, fascia and tendon of abdomen, lower back and pelvis
  S39.021- Laceration of muscle, fascia and tendon of <u>abdomen</u>
  S39.022- Laceration of muscle, fascia and tendon of <u>lower back</u>
  S39.023- Laceration of muscle, fascia and tendon of <u>pelvis</u>
 S39.09- <u>Other injury</u> of muscle, fascia and tendon of abdomen, lower back and pelvis
  S39.091- Other injury of muscle, fascia and tendon of <u>abdomen</u>
  S39.092- Other injury of muscle, fascia and tendon of <u>lower back</u>
  S39.093- Other injury of muscle, fascia and tendon of <u>pelvis</u>
S39.8- <u>Other specified</u> injuries of abdomen, lower back, pelvis and external genitals
 S39.81x- Other specified injuries of <u>abdomen</u>
 S39.82x- Other specified injuries of <u>lower back</u>
 S39.83x- Other specified injuries of <u>pelvis</u>
 S39.84- Other specified injuries of <u>external genitals</u>
  S39.840- <u>Fracture</u> of <u>corpus cavernosum penis</u> — [♂]
  S39.848- <u>Other</u> specified injuries of external genitals
S39.9- <u>Unspecified</u> injury of abdomen, lower back, pelvis and external genitals
 S39.91x- Unspecified injury of <u>abdomen</u>
 S39.92x- Unspecified injury of <u>lower back</u>
 S39.93x- Unspecified injury of <u>pelvis</u>
 S39.94x- Unspecified injury of <u>external genitals</u>

Injuries to the shoulder and upper arm (S40-S49)

Includes: Injuries of axilla
    Injuries of scapular region
Excludes ❷: burns and corrosions (T20-T32)
     frostbite (T33-T34)
     injuries of elbow (S50-S59)
     insect bite or sting, venomous (T63.4)

S40- <u>Superficial injury</u> of <u>shoulder and upper arm</u>
The appropriate 7th character is to be added to each code from category S40:
 A <u>Initial</u> encounter
 D <u>Subsequent</u> encounter
 S <u>Sequela</u>
S40.0- <u>Contusion</u> of shoulder and upper arm
 S40.01- <u>Contusion</u> of <u>shoulder</u>
  S40.011- Contusion of <u>right</u> shoulder
  S40.012- Contusion of <u>left</u> shoulder
  S40.019- Contusion of <u>unspecified</u> shoulder
 S40.02- Contusion of <u>upper arm</u>
  S40.021- Contusion of <u>right</u> upper arm
  S40.022- Contusion of <u>left</u> upper arm
  S40.029- Contusion of <u>unspecified</u> upper arm
S40.2- Other superficial injuries of shoulder
 S40.21- <u>Abrasion</u> of <u>shoulder</u>
  S40.211- Abrasion of <u>right</u> shoulder
  S40.212- Abrasion of <u>left</u> shoulder
  S40.219- Abrasion of <u>unspecified</u> shoulder
 S40.22- <u>Blister</u> (nonthermal) of <u>shoulder</u>
  S40.221- Blister (nonthermal) of <u>right</u> shoulder
  S40.222- Blister (nonthermal) of <u>left</u> shoulder
  S40.229- Blister (nonthermal) of <u>unspecified</u> shoulder
 S40.24- <u>External constriction</u> of <u>shoulder</u>
  S40.241- External constriction of <u>right</u> shoulder
  S40.242- External constriction of <u>left</u> shoulder
  S40.249- External constriction of <u>unspecified</u> shoulder
 S40.25- <u>Superficial foreign body</u> of <u>shoulder</u>
   Splinter in the shoulder
  S40.251- Superficial foreign body of <u>right</u> shoulder
  S40.252- Superficial foreign body of <u>left</u> shoulder
  S40.259- Superficial foreign body of <u>unspecified</u> shoulder
 S40.26- <u>Insect bite (nonvenomous)</u> of <u>shoulder</u>
  S40.261- Insect bite (nonvenomous) of <u>right</u> shoulder
  S40.262- Insect bite (nonvenomous) of <u>left</u> shoulder
  S40.269- Insect bite (nonvenomous) of <u>unspecified</u> shoulder
 S40.27- <u>Other superficial bite</u> of <u>shoulder</u>
   Excludes 1: open bite of shoulder (S41.05)
  S40.271- Other superficial bite of <u>right</u> shoulder
  S40.272- Other superficial bite of <u>left</u> shoulder
  S40.279- Other superficial bite of <u>unspecified</u> shoulder
S40.8- Other superficial injuries of <u>upper arm</u>
 S40.81- <u>Abrasion</u> of <u>upper arm</u>
  S40.811- Abrasion of <u>right</u> upper arm
  S40.812- Abrasion of <u>left</u> upper arm
  S40.819- Abrasion of <u>unspecified</u> upper arm
 S40.82- <u>Blister</u> (nonthermal) of <u>upper arm</u>
  S40.821- Blister (nonthermal) of <u>right</u> upper arm
  S40.822- Blister (nonthermal) of <u>left</u> upper arm
  S40.829- Blister (nonthermal) of <u>unspecified</u> upper arm
 S40.84- <u>External constriction</u> of <u>upper arm</u>
  S40.841- External constriction of <u>right</u> upper arm
  S40.842- External constriction of <u>left</u> upper arm
  S40.849- External constriction of <u>unspecified</u> upper arm
 S40.85- <u>Superficial foreign body</u> of <u>upper arm</u>
   Splinter in the upper arm
  S40.851- Superficial foreign body of <u>right</u> upper arm
  S40.852- Superficial foreign body of <u>left</u> upper arm

S38 – S40

S40.859- Superficial foreign body of <u>unspecified</u> upper arm

S40.86- <u>Insect bite (nonvenomous)</u> of <u>upper arm</u>

   S40.861- Insect bite (nonvenomous) of <u>right</u> upper arm

   S40.862- Insect bite (nonvenomous) of <u>left</u> upper arm

   S40.869- Insect bite (nonvenomous) of <u>unspecified</u> upper arm

S40.87- <u>Other superficial bite</u> of <u>upper arm</u>
   Excludes 1: *open bite of upper arm (S41.14)*
   Excludes ❷: *other superficial bite of shoulder (S40.27-)*

   S40.871- Other superficial bite of <u>right</u> upper arm

   S40.872- Other superficial bite of <u>left</u> upper arm

   S40.879- Other superficial bite of <u>unspecified</u> upper arm

S40.9- Unspecified superficial injury of shoulder and upper arm

S40.91- <u>Unspecified superficial injury</u> of <u>shoulder</u>

   S40.911- Unspecified superficial injury of <u>right</u> shoulder

   S40.912- Unspecified superficial injury of <u>left</u> shoulder

   S40.919- Unspecified superficial injury of <u>unspecified</u> shoulder

S40.92- <u>Unspecified superficial injury</u> of <u>upper arm</u>

   S40.921- Unspecified superficial injury of <u>right</u> upper arm

   S40.922- Unspecified superficial injury of <u>left</u> upper arm

   S40.929- Unspecified superficial injury of <u>unspecified</u> upper arm

S41- Open wound of <u>shoulder and upper arm</u>
  Code also any associated wound infection
  Excludes 1: *traumatic amputation of shoulder and upper arm (S48.-)*
  Excludes ❷: *open fracture of shoulder and upper arm (S42.- with 7th character B or C)*

The appropriate 7th character is to be added to each code from category S41:
  A <u>Initial</u> encounter
  D <u>Subsequent</u> encounter
  S <u>Sequela</u>

S41.0- <u>Open wound</u> of <u>shoulder</u>

S41.00- <u>Unspecified</u> open wound of <u>shoulder</u>

   S41.001- Unspecified open wound of <u>right</u> shoulder

   S41.002- Unspecified open wound of <u>left</u> shoulder

   S41.009- Unspecified open wound of <u>unspecified</u> shoulder

S41.01- <u>Laceration</u> <u>without</u> foreign body of <u>shoulder</u>

   S41.011- Laceration <u>without</u> foreign body of <u>right</u> shoulder

   S41.012- Laceration <u>without</u> foreign body of <u>left</u> shoulder

   S41.019- Laceration <u>without</u> foreign body of <u>unspecified</u> shoulder

S41.02- <u>Laceration</u> <u>with foreign body</u> of <u>shoulder</u>

   S41.021- Laceration <u>with foreign body</u> of <u>right</u> shoulder

   S41.022- Laceration <u>with foreign body</u> of <u>left</u> shoulder

   S41.029- Laceration <u>with foreign body</u> of <u>unspecified</u> shoulder

S41.03- <u>Puncture</u> wound <u>without</u> foreign body of <u>shoulder</u>

   S41.031- Puncture wound <u>without</u> foreign body of <u>right</u> shoulder

   S41.032- Puncture wound <u>without</u> foreign body of <u>left</u> shoulder

   S41.039- Puncture wound <u>without</u> foreign body of <u>unspecified</u> shoulder

S41.04- <u>Puncture</u> wound <u>with foreign body</u> of shoulder

   S41.041- Puncture wound <u>with foreign body</u> of <u>right</u> shoulder

   S41.042- Puncture wound <u>with foreign body</u> of <u>left</u> shoulder

   S41.049- Puncture wound <u>with foreign body</u> of <u>unspecified</u> shoulder

S41.05- Open bite of <u>shoulder</u>
   Bite of shoulder NOS
   Excludes 1: *superficial bite of shoulder (S40.27)*

   S41.051- Open bite of <u>right</u> shoulder

   S41.052- Open bite of <u>left</u> shoulder

   S41.059- Open bite of <u>unspecified</u> shoulder

S41.1- <u>Open wound</u> of <u>upper arm</u>

S41.10- <u>Unspecified</u> open wound of <u>upper arm</u>

   S41.101- Unspecified open wound of <u>right</u> upper arm

   S41.102- Unspecified open wound of <u>left</u> upper arm

   S41.109- Unspecified open wound of <u>unspecified</u> upper arm

S41.11- <u>Laceration</u> <u>without</u> foreign body of <u>upper arm</u>

   S41.111- Laceration <u>without</u> foreign body of <u>right</u> upper arm

   S41.112- Laceration <u>without</u> foreign body of <u>left</u> upper arm

   S41.119- Laceration <u>without</u> foreign body of <u>unspecified</u> upper arm

S41.12- <u>Laceration</u> <u>with foreign body</u> of <u>upper arm</u>

   S41.121- Laceration <u>with foreign body</u> of <u>right</u> upper arm

   S41.122- Laceration <u>with foreign body</u> of <u>left</u> upper arm

   S41.129- Laceration <u>with foreign body</u> of <u>unspecified</u> upper arm

S41.13- <u>Puncture</u> wound <u>without</u> foreign body of <u>upper arm</u>

   S41.131- Puncture wound <u>without</u> foreign body of <u>right</u> upper arm

   S41.132- Puncture wound <u>without</u> foreign body of <u>left</u> upper arm

   S41.139- Puncture wound <u>without</u> foreign body of <u>unspecified</u> upper arm

S41.14- <u>Puncture</u> wound <u>with foreign body</u> of <u>upper arm</u>

   S41.141- Puncture wound <u>with foreign body</u> of <u>right</u> upper arm

   S41.142- Puncture wound <u>with foreign body</u> of <u>left</u> upper arm

   S41.149- Puncture wound <u>with foreign body</u> of <u>unspecified</u> upper arm

S41.15- <u>Open bite</u> of <u>upper arm</u>
   Bite of upper arm NOS
   Excludes 1: *superficial bite of upper arm (S40.87)*

   S41.151- Open bite of <u>right</u> upper arm

   S41.152- Open bite of <u>left</u> upper arm

   S41.159- Open bite of <u>unspecified</u> upper arm

S42- <u>Fracture of shoulder and upper arm</u>
  Note: A fracture not indicated as displaced or nondisplaced should be coded to displaced
  Note: A fracture not indicated as open or closed should be coded to closed
  Excludes 1: *traumatic amputation of shoulder and upper arm (S48.-)*

The appropriate 7th character is to be added to all codes from category S42:
  A <u>Initial</u> encounter for <u>closed</u> fracture
  B <u>Initial</u> encounter for <u>open</u> fracture
  D <u>Subsequent</u> encounter for fracture <u>with routine healing</u>
  G <u>Subsequent</u> encounter for fracture <u>with delayed healing</u>
  K <u>Subsequent</u> encounter for fracture <u>with nonunion</u>
  P <u>Subsequent</u> encounter for fracture <u>with malunion</u>
  S <u>Sequela</u>

S42.0- <u>Fracture</u> of <u>clavicle</u>

S42.00- <u>Fracture</u> of <u>unspecified</u> part of <u>clavicle</u>

  CC-B,K,P **S42.001-** Fracture of <u>unspecified</u> part of <u>right</u> clavicle

  CC-B,K,P **S42.002-** Fracture of <u>unspecified</u> part of <u>left</u> clavicle

  CC-B,K,P **S42.009-** Fracture of <u>unspecified</u> part of <u>unspecified</u> clavicle

S42.01- Fracture of <u>sternal end</u> of <u>clavicle</u>

  CC-B,K,P **S42.011-** <u>Anterior</u> displaced fracture of sternal end of <u>right</u> clavicle

  CC-B,K,P **S42.012-** <u>Anterior</u> displaced fracture of sternal end of <u>left</u> clavicle

  CC-B,K,P **S42.013-** <u>Anterior</u> displaced fracture of sternal end of <u>unspecified</u> clavicle
       Displaced fracture of sternal end of clavicle NOS

  CC-B,K,P **S42.014-** <u>Posterior</u> displaced fracture of sternal end of <u>right</u> clavicle

  CC-B,K,P **S42.015-** <u>Posterior</u> displaced fracture of sternal end of <u>left</u> clavicle

  CC-B,K,P **S42.016-** <u>Posterior</u> displaced fracture of sternal end of <u>unspecified</u> clavicle

CC-B,K,P **S42.017-** <u>Nondisplaced</u> fracture of sternal end of <u>right</u> clavicle

CC-B,K,P **S42.018-** <u>Nondisplaced</u> fracture of sternal end of <u>left</u> clavicle

CC-B,K,P **S42.019-** <u>Nondisplaced</u> fracture of sternal end of <u>unspecified</u> clavicle

S42.02- Fracture of <u>shaft</u> of <u>clavicle</u>

CC-B,K,P **S42.021-** <u>Displaced</u> fracture of shaft of <u>right</u> clavicle

CC-B,K,P **S42.022-** <u>Displaced</u> fracture of shaft of <u>left</u> clavicle

CC-B,K,P **S42.023-** <u>Displaced</u> fracture of shaft of <u>unspecified</u> clavicle

CC-B,K,P **S42.024-** <u>Nondisplaced</u> fracture of shaft of <u>right</u> clavicle

CC-B,K,P **S42.025-** <u>Nondisplaced</u> fracture of shaft of <u>left</u> clavicle

CC-B,K,P **S42.026-** <u>Nondisplaced</u> fracture of shaft of <u>unspecified</u> clavicle

S42.03- Fracture of <u>lateral end</u> of <u>clavicle</u>
Fracture of acromial end of clavicle

CC-B,K,P **S42.031-** <u>Displaced</u> fracture of lateral end of <u>right</u> clavicle

CC-B,K,P **S42.032-** <u>Displaced</u> fracture of lateral end of <u>left</u> clavicle

CC-B,K,P **S42.033-** <u>Displaced</u> fracture of lateral end of <u>unspecified</u> clavicle

CC-B,K,P **S42.034-** <u>Nondisplaced</u> fracture of lateral end of <u>right</u> clavicle

CC-B,K,P **S42.035-** <u>Nondisplaced</u> fracture of lateral end of <u>left</u> clavicle

CC-B,K,P **S42.036-** <u>Nondisplaced</u> fracture of lateral end of <u>unspecified</u> clavicle

S42.1- Fracture of <u>scapula</u>

S42.10- Fracture of <u>unspecified</u> part of <u>scapula</u>

CC-B,K,P **S42.101-** Fracture of <u>unspecified</u> part of scapula, <u>right</u> shoulder

CC-B,K,P **S42.102-** Fracture of <u>unspecified</u> part of scapula, <u>left</u> shoulder

CC-B,K,P **S42.109-** Fracture of <u>unspecified</u> part of scapula, <u>unspecified</u> shoulder

S42.11- Fracture of <u>body</u> of <u>scapula</u>

CC-B,K,P **S42.111-** <u>Displaced</u> fracture of body of scapula, <u>right</u> shoulder

CC-B,K,P **S42.112-** <u>Displaced</u> fracture of body of scapula, <u>left</u> shoulder

CC-B,K,P **S42.113-** <u>Displaced</u> fracture of body of scapula, <u>unspecified</u> shoulder

CC-B,K,P **S42.114-** <u>Nondisplaced</u> fracture of body of scapula, <u>right</u> shoulder

CC-B,K,P **S42.115-** <u>Nondisplaced</u> fracture of body of scapula, <u>left</u> shoulder

CC-B,K,P **S42.116-** <u>Nondisplaced</u> fracture of body of scapula, <u>unspecified</u> shoulder

S42.12- Fracture of <u>acromial process</u>

CC-B,K,P **S42.121-** <u>Displaced</u> fracture of acromial process, <u>right</u> shoulder

CC-B,K,P **S42.122-** <u>Displaced</u> fracture of acromial process, <u>left</u> shoulder

CC-B,K,P **S42.123-** <u>Displaced</u> fracture of acromial process, <u>unspecified</u> shoulder

CC-B,K,P **S42.124-** <u>Nondisplaced</u> fracture of acromial process, <u>right</u> shoulder

CC-B,K,P **S42.125-** <u>Nondisplaced</u> fracture of acromial process, <u>left</u> shoulder

CC-B,K,P **S42.126-** <u>Nondisplaced</u> fracture of acromial process, <u>unspecified</u> shoulder

S42.13- Fracture of <u>coracoid process</u>

CC-B,K,P **S42.131-** <u>Displaced</u> fracture of coracoid process, <u>right</u> shoulder

CC-B,K,P **S42.132-** <u>Displaced</u> fracture of coracoid process, <u>left</u> shoulder

CC-B,K,P **S42.133-** <u>Displaced</u> fracture of coracoid process, <u>unspecified</u> shoulder

CC-B,K,P **S42.134-** <u>Nondisplaced</u> fracture of coracoid process, <u>right</u> shoulder

CC-B,K,P **S42.135-** <u>Nondisplaced</u> fracture of coracoid process, <u>left</u> shoulder

CC-B,K,P **S42.136-** <u>Nondisplaced</u> fracture of coracoid process, <u>unspecified</u> shoulder

S42.14- Fracture of <u>glenoid cavity</u> of <u>scapula</u>

CC-B,K,P **S42.141-** <u>Displaced</u> fracture of glenoid cavity of scapula, <u>right</u> shoulder

CC-B,K,P **S42.142-** <u>Displaced</u> fracture of glenoid cavity of scapula, <u>left</u> shoulder

CC-B,K,P **S42.143-** <u>Displaced</u> fracture of glenoid cavity of scapula, <u>unspecified</u> shoulder

CC-B,K,P **S42.144-** <u>Nondisplaced</u> fracture of glenoid cavity of scapula, <u>right</u> shoulder

CC-B,K,P **S42.145-** <u>Nondisplaced</u> fracture of glenoid cavity of scapula, <u>left</u> shoulder

CC-B,K,P **S42.146-** <u>Nondisplaced</u> fracture of glenoid cavity of scapula, <u>unspecified</u> shoulder

S42.15- Fracture of <u>neck</u> of <u>scapula</u>

CC-B,K,P **S42.151-** <u>Displaced</u> fracture of neck of scapula, <u>right</u> shoulder

CC-B,K,P **S42.152-** <u>Displaced</u> fracture of neck of scapula, <u>left</u> shoulder

CC-B,K,P **S42.153-** <u>Displaced</u> fracture of neck of scapula, <u>unspecified</u> shoulder

CC-B,K,P **S42.154-** <u>Nondisplaced</u> fracture of neck of scapula, <u>right</u> shoulder

CC-B,K,P **S42.155-** <u>Nondisplaced</u> fracture of neck of scapula, <u>left</u> shoulder

CC-B,K,P **S42.156-** <u>Nondisplaced</u> fracture of neck of scapula, <u>unspecified</u> shoulder

S42.19- Fracture of other part of <u>scapula</u>

CC-B,K,P **S42.191-** Fracture of other part of scapula, <u>right</u> shoulder

CC-B,K,P **S42.192-** Fracture of other part of scapula, <u>left</u> shoulder

CC-B,K,P **S42.199-** Fracture of other part of scapula, <u>unspecified</u> shoulder

S42.2- <u>Fracture</u> of <u>upper end</u> of <u>humerus</u>
Fracture of proximal end of humerus
Excludes ❷:　*fracture of shaft of humerus (S42.3-)*
physeal fracture of upper end of humerus (S49.0-)

S42.20- <u>Unspecified</u> fracture of <u>upper end</u> of <u>humerus</u>

S42.201- Unspecified fracture of upper end of <u>right</u> humerus
CC-A,K,P MCC-B

S42.202- Unspecified fracture of upper end of <u>left</u> humerus
CC-A,K,P MCC-B

S42.209- Unspecified fracture of upper end of <u>unspecified</u>
CC-A,K,P MCC-B humerus

S42.21- <u>Unspecified</u> fracture of <u>surgical neck</u> of <u>humerus</u>
Fracture of neck of humerus NOS

S42.211- Unspecified <u>displaced</u> fracture of surgical neck of
CC-A,K,P MCC-B <u>right</u> humerus

S42.212- Unspecified <u>displaced</u> fracture of surgical neck of
CC-A,K,P MCC-B <u>left</u> humerus

S42.213- Unspecified <u>displaced</u> fracture of surgical neck of
CC-A,K,P MCC-B <u>unspecified</u> humerus

S42.214- Unspecified <u>nondisplaced</u> fracture of surgical neck
CC-A,K,P MCC-B of <u>right</u> humerus

S42.215- Unspecified <u>nondisplaced</u> fracture of surgical neck
CC-A,K,P MCC-B of <u>left</u> humerus

S42.216- Unspecified <u>nondisplaced</u> fracture of surgical neck
CC-A,K,P MCC-B of <u>unspecified</u> humerus

S42.22- <u>2-part</u> fracture of <u>surgical neck</u> of <u>humerus</u>

S42.221- 2-part <u>displaced</u> fracture of surgical neck of <u>right</u>
CC-A,K,P MCC-B humerus

S42.222- 2-part <u>displaced</u> fracture of surgical neck of <u>left</u>
CC-A,K,P MCC-B humerus

S42.223- 2-part <u>displaced</u> fracture of surgical neck of
CC-A,K,P MCC-B <u>unspecified</u> humerus

S42.224- 2-part <u>nondisplaced</u> fracture of surgical neck of
CC-A,K,P MCC-B <u>right</u> humerus

S42.225- 2-part <u>nondisplaced</u> fracture of surgical neck of <u>left</u>
CC-A,K,P MCC-B humerus

S
4
2
-
S
4
2

S42.226- 2-part nondisplaced fracture of surgical neck of unspecified humerus
CC-A,K,P MCC-B

S42.23- 3-part fracture of surgical neck of humerus

S42.231- 3-part fracture of surgical neck of right humerus
CC-A,K,P MCC-B

S42.232- 3-part fracture of surgical neck of left humerus
CC-A,K,P MCC-B

S42.239- 3-part fracture of surgical neck of unspecified humerus
CC-A,K,P MCC-B

S42.24- 4-part fracture of surgical neck of humerus

S42.241- 4-part fracture of surgical neck of right humerus
CC-A,K,P MCC-B

S42.242- 4-part fracture of surgical neck of left humerus
CC-A,K,P MCC-B

S42.249- 4-part fracture of surgical neck of unspecified humerus
CC-A,K,P MCC-B

S42.25- Fracture of greater tuberosity of humerus

S42.251- Displaced fracture of greater tuberosity of right humerus
CC-A,K,P MCC-B

S42.252- Displaced fracture of greater tuberosity of left humerus
CC-A,K,P MCC-B

S42.253- Displaced fracture of greater tuberosity of unspecified humerus
CC-A,K,P MCC-B

S42.254- Nondisplaced fracture of greater tuberosity of right humerus
CC-A,K,P MCC-B

S42.255- Nondisplaced fracture of greater tuberosity of left humerus
CC-A,K,P MCC-B

S42.256- Nondisplaced fracture of greater tuberosity of unspecified humerus
CC-A,K,P MCC-B

S42.26- Fracture of lesser tuberosity of humerus

S42.261- Displaced fracture of lesser tuberosity of right humerus
CC-A,K,P MCC-B

S42.262- Displaced fracture of lesser tuberosity of left humerus
CC-A,K,P MCC-B

S42.263- Displaced fracture of lesser tuberosity of unspecified humerus
CC-A,K,P MCC-B

S42.264- Nondisplaced fracture of lesser tuberosity of right humerus
CC-A,K,P MCC-B

S42.265- Nondisplaced fracture of lesser tuberosity of left humerus
CC-A,K,P MCC-B

S42.266- Nondisplaced fracture of lesser tuberosity of unspecified humerus
CC-A,K,P MCC-B

S42.27- Torus fracture of upper end of humerus

The appropriate 7th character is to be added to all codes in subcategory S42.27:
A   Initial encounter for closed fracture
D   Subsequent encounter for fracture with routine healing
G   Subsequent encounter for fracture with delayed healing
K   Subsequent encounter for fracture with nonunion
P   Subsequent encounter for fracture with malunion
S   Sequela

S42.271- Torus fracture of upper end of right humerus
CC-A,K,P

S42.272- Torus fracture of upper end of left humerus
CC-A,K,P

S42.279- Torus fracture of upper end of unspecified humerus
CC-A,K,P

S42.29- Other fracture of upper end of humerus
Fracture of anatomical neck of humerus
Fracture of articular head of humerus

S42.291- Other displaced fracture of upper end of right humerus
CC-A,K,P MCC-B

S42.292- Other displaced fracture of upper end of left humerus
CC-A,K,P MCC-B

S42.293- Other displaced fracture of upper end of unspecified humerus
CC-A,K,P MCC-B

S42.294- Other nondisplaced fracture of upper end of right humerus
CC-A,K,P MCC-B

S42.295- Other nondisplaced fracture of upper end of left humerus
CC-A,K,P MCC-B

S42.296- Other nondisplaced fracture of upper end of unspecified humerus
CC-A,K,P MCC-B

S42.3- Fracture of shaft of humerus
Fracture of humerus NOS
Fracture of upper arm NOS
Excludes ❷: physeal fractures of upper end of humerus (S49.0-)
physeal fractures of lower end of humerus (S49.1-)

S42.30- Unspecified fracture of shaft of humerus

S42.301- Unspecified fracture of shaft of humerus, right arm
CC-A,K,P MCC-B

S42.302- Unspecified fracture of shaft of humerus, left arm
CC-A,K,P MCC-B

S42.309- Unspecified fracture of shaft of humerus, unspecified arm
CC-A,K,P MCC-B

S42.31- Greenstick fracture of shaft of humerus

The appropriate 7th character is to be added to all codes in subcategory S42.31:
A   Initial encounter for closed fracture
D   Subsequent encounter for fracture with routine healing
G   Subsequent encounter for fracture with delayed healing
K   Subsequent encounter for fracture with nonunion
P   Subsequent encounter for fracture with malunion
S   Sequela

S42.311- Greenstick fracture of shaft of humerus, right arm
CC-A,K,P

S42.312- Greenstick fracture of shaft of humerus, left arm
CC-A,K,P

S42.319- Greenstick fracture of shaft of humerus, unspecified arm
CC-A,K,P

S42.32- Transverse fracture of shaft of humerus

S42.321- Displaced transverse fracture of shaft of humerus, right arm
CC-A,K,P MCC-B

S42.322- Displaced transverse fracture of shaft of humerus, left arm
CC-A,K,P MCC-B

S42.323- Displaced transverse fracture of shaft of humerus, unspecified arm
CC-A,K,P MCC-B

S42.324- Nondisplaced transverse fracture of shaft of humerus, right arm
CC-A,K,P MCC-B

S42.325- Nondisplaced transverse fracture of shaft of humerus, left arm
CC-A,K,P MCC-B

S42.326- Nondisplaced transverse fracture of shaft of humerus, unspecified arm
CC-A,K,P MCC-B

S42.33- Oblique fracture of shaft of humerus

S42.331- Displaced oblique fracture of shaft of humerus, right arm
CC-A,K,P MCC-B

S42.332- Displaced oblique fracture of shaft of humerus, left arm
CC-A,K,P MCC-B

S42.333- Displaced oblique fracture of shaft of humerus, unspecified arm
CC-A,K,P MCC-B

S42.334- Nondisplaced oblique fracture of shaft of humerus, right arm
CC-A,K,P MCC-B

S42.335- Nondisplaced oblique fracture of shaft of humerus, left arm
CC-A,K,P MCC-B

S42.336- Nondisplaced oblique fracture of shaft of humerus, unspecified arm
CC-A,K,P MCC-B

S42.34- Spiral fracture of shaft of humerus

S42.341- Displaced spiral fracture of shaft of humerus, right arm
CC-A,K,P MCC-B

S42.342- Displaced spiral fracture of shaft of humerus, left arm
CC-A,K,P MCC-B

S42.343- Displaced spiral fracture of shaft of humerus, unspecified arm
CC-A,K,P MCC-B

S42.344- Nondisplaced spiral fracture of shaft of humerus, right arm
CC-A,K,P MCC-B

S42.345- Nondisplaced spiral fracture of shaft of humerus, left arm
CC-A,K,P MCC-B

S42 - S42

S42.346- Nondisplaced spiral fracture of shaft of humerus,
CC-A,K,P MCC-B unspecified arm

S42.35- Comminuted fracture of shaft of humerus

S42.351- Displaced comminuted fracture of shaft of
CC-A,K,P MCC-B humerus, right arm

S42.352- Displaced comminuted fracture of shaft of
CC-A,K,P MCC-B humerus, left arm

S42.353- Displaced comminuted fracture of shaft of
CC-A,K,P MCC-B humerus, unspecified arm

S42.354- Nondisplaced comminuted fracture of shaft of
CC-A,K,P MCC-B humerus, right arm

S42.355- Nondisplaced comminuted fracture of shaft of
CC-A,K,P MCC-B humerus, left arm

S42.356- Nondisplaced comminuted fracture of shaft of
CC-A,K,P MCC-B humerus, unspecified arm

S42.36- Segmental fracture of shaft of humerus

S42.361- Displaced segmental fracture of shaft of humerus,
CC-A,K,P MCC-B right arm

S42.362- Displaced segmental fracture of shaft of humerus,
CC-A,K,P MCC-B left arm

S42.363- Displaced segmental fracture of shaft of humerus,
CC-A,K,P MCC-B unspecified arm

S42.364- Nondisplaced segmental fracture of shaft of
CC-A,K,P MCC-B humerus, right arm

S42.365- Nondisplaced segmental fracture of shaft of
CC-A,K,P MCC-B humerus, left arm

S42.366- Nondisplaced segmental fracture of shaft of
CC-A,K,P MCC-B humerus, unspecified arm

S42.39- Other fracture of shaft of humerus

S42.391- Other fracture of shaft of right humerus
CC-A,K,P MCC-B

S42.392- Other fracture of shaft of left humerus
CC-A,K,P MCC-B

S42.399- Other fracture of shaft of unspecified humerus
CC-A,K,P MCC-B

S42.4- Fracture of lower end of humerus
Fracture of distal end of humerus
Excludes ❷: fracture of shaft of humerus (S42.3-)
physeal fracture of lower end of humerus (S49.1-)

S42.40- Unspecified fracture of lower end of humerus
Fracture of elbow NOS

S42.401- Unspecified fracture of lower end of right humerus
CC-A,K,P MCC-B

S42.402- Unspecified fracture of lower end of left humerus
CC-A,K,P MCC-B

S42.409- Unspecified fracture of lower end of unspecified
CC-A,K,P MCC-B humerus

S42.41- Simple supracondylar fracture without intercondylar
fracture of humerus

S42.411- Displaced simple supracondylar fracture without
CC-A,K,P MCC-B intercondylar fracture of right humerus

S42.412- Displaced simple supracondylar fracture without
CC-A,K,P MCC-B intercondylar fracture of left humerus

S42.413- Displaced simple supracondylar fracture without
CC-A,K,P MCC-B intercondylar fracture of unspecified humerus

S42.414- Nondisplaced simple supracondylar fracture
CC-A,K,P MCC-B without intercondylar fracture of right humerus

S42.415- Nondisplaced simple supracondylar fracture
CC-A,K,P MCC-B without intercondylar fracture of left humerus

S42.416- Nondisplaced simple supracondylar fracture
CC-A,K,P MCC-B without intercondylar fracture of unspecified
humerus

S42.42- Comminuted supracondylar fracture without intercondylar
fracture of humerus

S42.421- Displaced comminuted supracondylar fracture
CC-A,K,P MCC-B without intercondylar fracture of right humerus

S42.422- Displaced comminuted supracondylar fracture
CC-A,K,P MCC-B without intercondylar fracture of left humerus

S42.423- Displaced comminuted supracondylar fracture
CC-A,K,P MCC-B without intercondylar fracture of unspecified
humerus

S42.424- Nondisplaced comminuted supracondylar fracture
CC-A,K,P MCC-B without intercondylar fracture of right humerus

S42.425- Nondisplaced comminuted supracondylar fracture
CC-A,K,P MCC-B without intercondylar fracture of left humerus

S42.426- Nondisplaced comminuted supracondylar fracture
CC-A,K,P MCC-B without intercondylar fracture of unspecified
humerus

S42.43- Fracture (avulsion) of lateral epicondyle of humerus

S42.431- Displaced fracture (avulsion) of lateral epicondyle
CC-A,K,P MCC-B of right humerus

S42.432- Displaced fracture (avulsion) of lateral epicondyle
CC-A,K,P MCC-B of left humerus

S42.433- Displaced fracture (avulsion) of lateral epicondyle
CC-A,K,P MCC-B of unspecified humerus

S42.434- Nondisplaced fracture (avulsion) of lateral
CC-A,K,P MCC-B epicondyle of right humerus

S42.435- Nondisplaced fracture (avulsion) of lateral
CC-A,K,P MCC-B epicondyle of left humerus

S42.436- Nondisplaced fracture (avulsion) of lateral
CC-A,K,P MCC-B epicondyle of unspecified humerus

S42.44- Fracture (avulsion) of medial epicondyle of humerus

S42.441- Displaced fracture (avulsion) of medial epicondyle
CC-A,K,P MCC-B of right humerus

S42.442- Displaced fracture (avulsion) of medial epicondyle
CC-A,K,P MCC-B of left humerus

S42.443- Displaced fracture (avulsion) of medial epicondyle
CC-A,K,P MCC-B of unspecified humerus

S42.444- Nondisplaced fracture (avulsion) of medial
CC-A,K,P MCC-B epicondyle of right humerus

S42.445- Nondisplaced fracture (avulsion) of medial
CC-A,K,P MCC-B epicondyle of left humerus

S42.446- Nondisplaced fracture (avulsion) of medial
CC-A,K,P MCC-B epicondyle of unspecified humerus

S42.447- Incarcerated fracture (avulsion) of medial
CC-A,K,P MCC-B epicondyle of right humerus

S42.448- Incarcerated fracture (avulsion) of medial
CC-A,K,P MCC-B epicondyle of left humerus

S42.449- Incarcerated fracture (avulsion) of medial
CC-A,K,P MCC-B epicondyle of unspecified humerus

S42.45- Fracture of lateral condyle of humerus
Fracture of capitellum of humerus

S42.451- Displaced fracture of lateral condyle of right
CC-A,K,P MCC-B humerus

S42.452- Displaced fracture of lateral condyle of left
CC-A,K,P MCC-B humerus

S42.453- Displaced fracture of lateral condyle of unspecified
CC-A,K,P MCC-B humerus

S42.454- Nondisplaced fracture of lateral condyle of right
CC-A,K,P MCC-B humerus

S42.455- Nondisplaced fracture of lateral condyle of left
CC-A,K,P MCC-B humerus

S42.456- Nondisplaced fracture of lateral condyle of
CC-A,K,P MCC-B unspecified humerus

S42.46- Fracture of medial condyle of humerus
Trochlea fracture of humerus

S42.461- Displaced fracture of medial condyle of right
CC-A,K,P MCC-B humerus

S42.462- Displaced fracture of medial condyle of left
CC-A,K,P MCC-B humerus

S42.463- Displaced fracture of medial condyle of unspecified
CC-A,K,P MCC-B humerus

S42.464- Nondisplaced fracture of medial condyle of right
CC-A,K,P MCC-B humerus

S42.465- Nondisplaced fracture of medial condyle of left
CC-A,K,P MCC-B humerus

S
4
2
-
S
4
2

S42.466- Nondisplaced fracture of medial condyle of
CC-A,K,P MCC-B   unspecified humerus

S42.47- Transcondylar fracture of humerus

S42.471- Displaced transcondylar fracture of right humerus
CC-A,K,P MCC-B

S42.472- Displaced transcondylar fracture of left humerus
CC-A,K,P MCC-B

S42.473- Displaced transcondylar fracture of unspecified
CC-A,K,P MCC-B   humerus

S42.474- Nondisplaced transcondylar fracture of right
CC-A,K,P MCC-B   humerus

S42.475- Nondisplaced transcondylar fracture of left
CC-A,K,P MCC-B   humerus

S42.476- Nondisplaced transcondylar fracture of unspecified
CC-A,K,P MCC-B   humerus

S42.48- Torus fracture of lower end of humerus

> The appropriate 7th character is to be added to all codes
> in subcategory S42.48:
> - **A** Initial encounter for closed fracture
> - **D** Subsequent encounter for fracture with routine healing
> - **G** Subsequent encounter for fracture with delayed healing
> - **K** Subsequent encounter for fracture with nonunion
> - **P** Subsequent encounter for fracture with malunion
> - **S** Sequela

CC-A,K,P **S42.481-** Torus fracture of lower end of right humerus

CC-A,K,P **S42.482-** Torus fracture of lower end of left humerus

CC-A,K,P **S42.489-** Torus fracture of lower end of unspecified humerus

S42.49- Other fracture of lower end of humerus

S42.491- Other displaced fracture of lower end of right
CC-A,K,P MCC-B   humerus

S42.492- Other displaced fracture of lower end of left
CC-A,K,P MCC-B   humerus

S42.493- Other displaced fracture of lower end of
CC-A,K,P MCC-B   unspecified humerus

S42.494- Other nondisplaced fracture of lower end of right
CC-A,K,P MCC-B   humerus

S42.495- Other nondisplaced fracture of lower end of left
CC-A,K,P MCC-B   humerus

S42.496- Other nondisplaced fracture of lower end of
CC-A,K,P MCC-B   unspecified humerus

S42.9- Fracture of shoulder girdle, part unspecified
Fracture of shoulder NOS

S42.90x- Fracture of unspecified shoulder girdle, part
CC-A,K,P MCC-B   unspecified

S42.91x- Fracture of right shoulder girdle, part unspecified
CC-A,K,P MCC-B

S42.92x- Fracture of left shoulder girdle, part unspecified
CC-A,K,P MCC-B

S43- Dislocation and sprain of joints and ligaments of shoulder girdle
Includes: Avulsion of joint or ligament of shoulder girdle
Laceration of cartilage, joint or ligament of shoulder girdle
Sprain of cartilage, joint or ligament of shoulder girdle
Traumatic hemarthrosis of joint or ligament of shoulder girdle
Traumatic rupture of joint or ligament of shoulder girdle
Traumatic subluxation of joint or ligament of shoulder girdle
Traumatic tear of joint or ligament of shoulder girdle
Code also any associated open wound
Excludes ❷: strain of muscle, fascia and tendon of shoulder and upper arm (S46.-)

> The appropriate 7th character is to be added to each code from
> category S43:
> - **A** Initial encounter
> - **D** Subsequent encounter
> - **S** Sequela

S43.0- Subluxation and dislocation of shoulder joint
Dislocation of glenohumeral joint
Subluxation of glenohumeral joint

S43.00- Unspecified subluxation and dislocation of shoulder joint
Dislocation of humerus NOS
Subluxation of humerus NOS

S43.001- Unspecified subluxation of right shoulder joint

S43.002- Unspecified subluxation of left shoulder joint

S43.003- Unspecified subluxation of unspecified shoulder joint

S43.004- Unspecified dislocation of right shoulder joint

S43.005- Unspecified dislocation of left shoulder joint

S43.006- Unspecified dislocation of unspecified shoulder joint

S43.01- Anterior subluxation and dislocation of humerus

S43.011- Anterior subluxation of right humerus

S43.012- Anterior subluxation of left humerus

S43.013- Anterior subluxation of unspecified humerus

S43.014- Anterior dislocation of right humerus

S43.015- Anterior dislocation of left humerus

S43.016- Anterior dislocation of unspecified humerus

S43.02- Posterior subluxation and dislocation of humerus

S43.021- Posterior subluxation of right humerus

S43.022- Posterior subluxation of left humerus

S43.023- Posterior subluxation of unspecified humerus

S43.024- Posterior dislocation of right humerus

S43.025- Posterior dislocation of left humerus

S43.026- Posterior dislocation of unspecified humerus

S43.03- Inferior subluxation and dislocation of humerus

S43.031- Inferior subluxation of right humerus

S43.032- Inferior subluxation of left humerus

S43.033- Inferior subluxation of unspecified humerus

S43.034- Inferior dislocation of right humerus

S43.035- Inferior dislocation of left humerus

S43.036- Inferior dislocation of unspecified humerus

S43.08- Other subluxation and dislocation of shoulder joint

S43.081- Other subluxation of right shoulder joint

S43.082- Other subluxation of left shoulder joint

S43.083- Other subluxation of unspecified shoulder joint

S43.084- Other dislocation of right shoulder joint

S43.085- Other dislocation of left shoulder joint

S43.086- Other dislocation of unspecified shoulder joint

S43.1- Subluxation and dislocation of acromioclavicular joint

S43.10- Unspecified dislocation of acromioclavicular joint

S43.101- Unspecified dislocation of right acromioclavicular joint

S43.102- Unspecified dislocation of left acromioclavicular joint

S43.109- Unspecified dislocation of unspecified acromioclavicular joint

S43.11- Subluxation of acromioclavicular joint

S43.111- Subluxation of right acromioclavicular joint

S43.112- Subluxation of left acromioclavicular joint

S43.119- Subluxation of unspecified acromioclavicular joint

S43.12- Dislocation of acromioclavicular joint, 100%-200% displacement

S43.121- Dislocation of right acromioclavicular joint, 100%-200% displacement

S43.122- Dislocation of left acromioclavicular joint, 100%-200% displacement

S43.129- Dislocation of unspecified acromioclavicular joint, 100%-200% displacement

S43.13- Dislocation of acromioclavicular joint, greater than 200% displacement

S43.131- Dislocation of right acromioclavicular joint, greater than 200% displacement

S43.132- Dislocation of left acromioclavicular joint, greater than 200% displacement

S43.139- Dislocation of unspecified acromioclavicular joint, greater than 200% displacement

S43.14- Inferior dislocation of acromioclavicular joint

S43.141- Inferior dislocation of right acromioclavicular joint

S43.142- Inferior dislocation of left acromioclavicular joint

S42 - S43 (side tab)

S43.149- Inferior dislocation of <u>unspecified</u> acromioclavicular joint

S43.15- <u>Posterior</u> dislocation of <u>acromioclavicular joint</u>

S43.151- Posterior dislocation of <u>right</u> acromioclavicular joint

S43.152- Posterior dislocation of <u>left</u> acromioclavicular joint

S43.159- Posterior dislocation of <u>unspecified</u> acromioclavicular joint

S43.2- <u>Subluxation and dislocation</u> of <u>sternoclavicular joint</u>

S43.20- <u>Unspecified subluxation and dislocation</u> of <u>sternoclavicular joint</u>

CC-A S43.201- Unspecified <u>subluxation</u> of <u>right</u> sternoclavicular joint

CC-A S43.202- Unspecified <u>subluxation</u> of <u>left</u> sternoclavicular joint

CC-A S43.203- Unspecified <u>subluxation</u> of <u>unspecified</u> sternoclavicular joint

CC-A S43.204- Unspecified <u>dislocation</u> of <u>right</u> sternoclavicular joint

CC-A S43.205- Unspecified <u>dislocation</u> of <u>left</u> sternoclavicular joint

CC-A S43.206- Unspecified <u>dislocation</u> of <u>unspecified</u> sternoclavicular joint

S43.21- <u>Anterior</u> subluxation and dislocation of <u>sternoclavicular joint</u>

CC-A S43.211- Anterior <u>subluxation</u> of <u>right</u> sternoclavicular joint

CC-A S43.212- Anterior <u>subluxation</u> of <u>left</u> sternoclavicular joint

CC-A S43.213- Anterior <u>subluxation</u> of <u>unspecified</u> sternoclavicular joint

CC-A S43.214- Anterior <u>dislocation</u> of <u>right</u> sternoclavicular joint

CC-A S43.215- Anterior <u>dislocation</u> of <u>left</u> sternoclavicular joint

CC-A S43.216- Anterior <u>dislocation</u> of <u>unspecified</u> sternoclavicular joint

S43.22- <u>Posterior</u> subluxation and dislocation of sternoclavicular joint

CC-A S43.221- Posterior <u>subluxation</u> of <u>right</u> sternoclavicular joint

CC-A S43.222- Posterior <u>subluxation</u> of <u>left</u> sternoclavicular joint

CC-A S43.223- Posterior <u>subluxation</u> of <u>unspecified</u> sternoclavicular joint

CC-A S43.224- Posterior <u>dislocation</u> of <u>right</u> sternoclavicular joint

CC-A S43.225- Posterior <u>dislocation</u> of <u>left</u> sternoclavicular joint

CC-A S43.226- Posterior <u>dislocation</u> of <u>unspecified</u> sternoclavicular joint

S43.3- <u>Subluxation and dislocation</u> of <u>other and unspecified</u> parts of <u>shoulder girdle</u>

S43.30- <u>Subluxation and dislocation</u> of <u>unspecified</u> parts of <u>shoulder girdle</u>

Dislocation of shoulder girdle NOS
Subluxation of shoulder girdle NOS

S43.301- <u>Subluxation</u> of <u>unspecified</u> parts of <u>right</u> shoulder girdle

S43.302- <u>Subluxation</u> of <u>unspecified</u> parts of <u>left</u> shoulder girdle

S43.303- <u>Subluxation</u> of <u>unspecified</u> parts of <u>unspecified</u> shoulder girdle

S43.304- <u>Dislocation</u> of <u>unspecified</u> parts of <u>right</u> shoulder girdle

S43.305- <u>Dislocation</u> of <u>unspecified</u> parts of <u>left</u> shoulder girdle

S43.306- <u>Dislocation</u> of <u>unspecified</u> parts of <u>unspecified</u> shoulder girdle

S43.31- Subluxation and dislocation of <u>scapula</u>

S43.311- <u>Subluxation</u> of <u>right</u> scapula

S43.312- <u>Subluxation</u> of <u>left</u> scapula

S43.313- <u>Subluxation</u> of <u>unspecified</u> scapula

S43.314- <u>Dislocation</u> of <u>right</u> scapula

S43.315- <u>Dislocation</u> of <u>left</u> scapula

S43.316- <u>Dislocation</u> of <u>unspecified</u> scapula

S43.39- Subluxation and dislocation of <u>other parts</u> of <u>shoulder girdle</u>

S43.391- <u>Subluxation</u> of other parts of <u>right</u> shoulder girdle

S43.392- <u>Subluxation</u> of other parts of <u>left</u> shoulder girdle

S43.393- <u>Subluxation</u> of other parts of <u>unspecified</u> shoulder girdle

S43.394- <u>Dislocation</u> of other parts of <u>right</u> shoulder girdle

S43.395- <u>Dislocation</u> of other parts of <u>left</u> shoulder girdle

S43.396- <u>Dislocation</u> of other parts of <u>unspecified</u> shoulder girdle

S43.4- <u>Sprain</u> of <u>shoulder joint</u>

S43.40- <u>Unspecified</u> sprain of <u>shoulder joint</u>

S43.401- Unspecified sprain of <u>right</u> shoulder joint

S43.402- Unspecified sprain of <u>left</u> shoulder joint

S43.409- Unspecified sprain of <u>unspecified</u> shoulder joint

S43.41- <u>Sprain</u> of <u>coracohumeral (ligament)</u>

S43.411- Sprain of <u>right</u> coracohumeral (ligament)

S43.412- Sprain of <u>left</u> coracohumeral (ligament)

S43.419- Sprain of <u>unspecified</u> coracohumeral (ligament)

S43.42- <u>Sprain</u> of <u>rotator cuff capsule</u>

Excludes 1: rotator cuff syndrome (complete) (incomplete), not specified as traumatic (M75.1-)
Excludes ❷: injury of tendon of rotator cuff (S46.0-)

S43.421- Sprain of <u>right</u> rotator cuff capsule

S43.422- Sprain of <u>left</u> rotator cuff capsule

S43.429- Sprain of <u>unspecified</u> rotator cuff capsule

S43.43- <u>Superior glenoid labrum lesion</u>

SLAP lesion

S43.431- Superior glenoid labrum lesion of <u>right</u> shoulder

S43.432- Superior glenoid labrum lesion of <u>left</u> shoulder

S43.439- Superior glenoid labrum lesion of <u>unspecified</u> shoulder

S43.49- <u>Other sprain</u> of <u>shoulder joint</u>

S43.491- Other sprain of <u>right</u> shoulder joint

S43.492- Other sprain of <u>left</u> shoulder joint

S43.499- Other sprain of <u>unspecified</u> shoulder joint

S43.5- <u>Sprain</u> of <u>acromioclavicular joint</u>

Sprain of acromioclavicular ligament

S43.50x- Sprain of <u>unspecified</u> acromioclavicular joint

S43.51x- Sprain of <u>right</u> acromioclavicular joint

S43.52x- Sprain of <u>left</u> acromioclavicular joint

S43.6- <u>Sprain</u> of <u>sternoclavicular joint</u>

S43.60x- Sprain of <u>unspecified</u> sternoclavicular joint

S43.61x- Sprain of <u>right</u> sternoclavicular joint

S43.62x- Sprain of <u>left</u> sternoclavicular joint

S43.8- <u>Sprain</u> of <u>other specified parts</u> of <u>shoulder girdle</u>

S43.80x- Sprain of other specified parts of <u>unspecified</u> shoulder girdle

S43.81x- Sprain of other specified parts of <u>right</u> shoulder girdle

S43.82x- Sprain of other specified parts of <u>left</u> shoulder girdle

S43.9- <u>Sprain</u> of <u>unspecified parts</u> of <u>shoulder girdle</u>

S43.90x- Sprain of <u>unspecified</u> parts of <u>unspecified</u> shoulder girdle

Sprain of shoulder girdle NOS

S43.91x- Sprain of <u>unspecified</u> parts of <u>right</u> shoulder girdle

S43.92x- Sprain of <u>unspecified</u> parts of <u>left</u> shoulder girdle

S43 | S43

S44-   Injury of nerves at shoulder and upper arm level
Code also any associated open wound (S41.-)
Excludes ❷: *injury of brachial plexus (S14.3-)*

The appropriate 7th character is to be added to each code from category S44:
A   Initial encounter
D   Subsequent encounter
S   Sequela

S44.0-   Injury of ulnar nerve at upper arm level
Excludes 1:   *ulnar nerve NOS (S54.0)*

S44.00x-   Injury of ulnar nerve at upper arm level, unspecified arm

S44.01x-   Injury of ulnar nerve at upper arm level, right arm

S44.02x-   Injury of ulnar nerve at upper arm level, left arm

S44.1-   Injury of median nerve at upper arm level
Excludes 1:   *median nerve NOS (S54.1)*

S44.10x-   Injury of median nerve at upper arm level, unspecified arm

S44.11x-   Injury of median nerve at upper arm level, right arm

S44.12x-   Injury of median nerve at upper arm level, left arm

S44.2-   Injury of radial nerve at upper arm level
Excludes 1:   *radial nerve NOS (S54.2)*

S44.20x-   Injury of radial nerve at upper arm level, unspecified arm

S44.21x-   Injury of radial nerve at upper arm level, right arm

S44.22x-   Injury of radial nerve at upper arm level, left arm

S44.3-   Injury of axillary nerve

S44.30x-   Injury of axillary nerve, unspecified arm

S44.31x-   Injury of axillary nerve, right arm

S44.32x-   Injury of axillary nerve, left arm

S44.4-   Injury of musculocutaneous nerve

S44.40x-   Injury of musculocutaneous nerve, unspecified arm

S44.41x-   Injury of musculocutaneous nerve, right arm

S44.42x-   Injury of musculocutaneous nerve, left arm

S44.5-   Injury of cutaneous sensory nerve at shoulder and upper arm level

S44.50x-   Injury of cutaneous sensory nerve at shoulder and upper arm level, unspecified arm

S44.51x-   Injury of cutaneous sensory nerve at shoulder and upper arm level, right arm

S44.52x-   Injury of cutaneous sensory nerve at shoulder and upper arm level, left arm

S44.8-   Injury of other nerves at shoulder and upper arm level

S44.8x-   Injury of other nerves at shoulder and upper arm level

S44.8x1-   Injury of other nerves at shoulder and upper arm level, right arm

S44.8x2-   Injury of other nerves at shoulder and upper arm level, left arm

S44.8x9-   Injury of other nerves at shoulder and upper arm level, unspecified arm

S44.9-   Injury of unspecified nerve at shoulder and upper arm level

S44.90x-   Injury of unspecified nerve at shoulder and upper arm level, unspecified arm

S44.91x-   Injury of unspecified nerve at shoulder and upper arm level, right arm

S44.92x-   Injury of unspecified nerve at shoulder and upper arm level, left arm

S45-   Injury of blood vessels at shoulder and upper arm level
Code also any associated open wound (S41.-)
Excludes ❷: *injury of subclavian artery (S25.1)*
      injury of subclavian vein (S25.3)

The appropriate 7th character is to be added to each code from category S45:
A   Initial encounter
D   Subsequent encounter
S   Sequela

S45.0-   Injury of axillary artery

S45.00-   Unspecified injury of axillary artery

MCC-A **S45.001-**   Unspecified injury of axillary artery, right side

MCC-A **S45.002-**   Unspecified injury of axillary artery, left side

MCC-A **S45.009-**   Unspecified injury of axillary artery, unspecified side

S45.01-   Laceration of axillary artery

MCC-A **S45.011-**   Laceration of axillary artery, right side

MCC-A **S45.012-**   Laceration of axillary artery, left side

MCC-A **S45.019-**   Laceration of axillary artery, unspecified side

S45.09-   Other specified injury of axillary artery

MCC-A **S45.091-**   Other specified injury of axillary artery, right side

MCC-A **S45.092-**   Other specified injury of axillary artery, left side

MCC-A **S45.099-**   Other specified injury of axillary artery, unspecified side

S45.1-   Injury of brachial artery

S45.10-   Unspecified injury of brachial artery

CC-A **S45.101-**   Unspecified injury of brachial artery, right side

CC-A **S45.102-**   Unspecified injury of brachial artery, left side

CC-A **S45.109-**   Unspecified injury of brachial artery, unspecified side

S45.11-   Laceration of brachial artery

CC-A **S45.111-**   Laceration of brachial artery, right side

CC-A **S45.112-**   Laceration of brachial artery, left side

CC-A **S45.119-**   Laceration of brachial artery, unspecified side

S45.19-   Other specified injury of brachial artery

CC-A **S45.191-**   Other specified injury of brachial artery, right side

CC-A **S45.192-**   Other specified injury of brachial artery, left side

CC-A **S45.199-**   Other specified injury of brachial artery, unspecified side

S45.2-   Injury of axillary or brachial vein

S45.20-   Unspecified injury of axillary or brachial vein

CC-A **S45.201-**   Unspecified injury of axillary or brachial vein, right side

CC-A **S45.202-**   Unspecified injury of axillary or brachial vein, left side

CC-A **S45.209-**   Unspecified injury of axillary or brachial vein, unspecified side

S45.21-   Laceration of axillary or brachial vein

CC-A **S45.211-**   Laceration of axillary or brachial vein, right side

CC-A **S45.212-**   Laceration of axillary or brachial vein, left side

CC-A **S45.219-**   Laceration of axillary or brachial vein, unspecified side

S45.29-   Other specified injury of axillary or brachial vein

CC-A **S45.291-**   Other specified injury of axillary or brachial vein, right side

CC-A **S45.292-**   Other specified injury of axillary or brachial vein, left side

CC-A **S45.299-**   Other specified injury of axillary or brachial vein, unspecified side

S45.3-   Injury of superficial vein at shoulder and upper arm level

S45.30-   Unspecified injury of superficial vein at shoulder and upper arm level

CC-A **S45.301-**   Unspecified injury of superficial vein at shoulder and upper arm level, right arm

CC-A **S45.302-**   Unspecified injury of superficial vein at shoulder and upper arm level, left arm

S44 - S45

CC-A **S45.309-** Unspecified injury of superficial vein at shoulder and upper arm level, <u>unspecified</u> arm

S45.31- <u>Laceration</u> of <u>superficial vein</u> at shoulder and upper arm level

CC-A **S45.311-** Laceration of superficial vein at shoulder and upper arm level, <u>right</u> arm

CC-A **S45.312-** Laceration of superficial vein at shoulder and upper arm level, <u>left</u> arm

CC-A **S45.319-** Laceration of superficial vein at shoulder and upper arm level, <u>unspecified</u> arm

S45.39- <u>Other specified</u> injury of <u>superficial vein</u> at shoulder and upper arm level

CC-A **S45.391-** Other specified injury of superficial vein at shoulder and upper arm level, <u>right</u> arm

CC-A **S45.392-** Other specified injury of superficial vein at shoulder and upper arm level, <u>left</u> arm

CC-A **S45.399-** Other specified injury of superficial vein at shoulder and upper arm level, <u>unspecified</u> arm

S45.8- Injury of <u>other specified blood vessels</u> at shoulder and upper arm level

S45.80- <u>Unspecified</u> injury of <u>other specified blood vessels</u> at shoulder and upper arm level

CC-A **S45.801-** Unspecified injury of other specified blood vessels at shoulder and upper arm level, <u>right</u> arm

CC-A **S45.802-** Unspecified injury of other specified blood vessels at shoulder and upper arm level, <u>left</u> arm

CC-A **S45.809-** Unspecified injury of other specified blood vessels at shoulder and upper arm level, <u>unspecified</u> arm

S45.81- <u>Laceration</u> of <u>other specified blood vessels</u> at shoulder and upper arm level

CC-A **S45.811-** Laceration of other specified blood vessels at shoulder and upper arm level, <u>right</u> arm

CC-A **S45.812-** Laceration of other specified blood vessels at shoulder and upper arm level, <u>left</u> arm

CC-A **S45.819-** Laceration of other specified blood vessels at shoulder and upper arm level, <u>unspecified</u> arm

S45.89- <u>Other specified injury</u> of <u>other specified blood vessels</u> <u>at shoulder and upper arm level</u>

CC-A **S45.891-** Other specified injury of other specified blood vessels at shoulder and upper arm level, <u>right</u> arm

CC-A **S45.892-** Other specified injury of other specified blood vessels at shoulder and upper arm level, <u>left</u> arm

CC-A **S45.899-** Other specified injury of other specified blood vessels at shoulder and upper arm level, <u>unspecified</u> arm

S45.9- Injury of <u>unspecified blood vessel</u> at shoulder and upper arm level

S45.90- <u>Unspecified</u> injury of <u>unspecified blood vessel</u> at shoulder and upper arm level

CC-A **S45.901-** Unspecified injury of unspecified blood vessel at shoulder and upper arm level, <u>right</u> arm

CC-A **S45.902-** Unspecified injury of unspecified blood vessel at shoulder and upper arm level, <u>left</u> arm

CC-A **S45.909-** Unspecified injury of unspecified blood vessel at shoulder and upper arm level, <u>unspecified</u> arm

S45.91- <u>Laceration</u> of <u>unspecified blood vessel</u> at shoulder and upper arm level

CC-A **S45.911-** Laceration of unspecified blood vessel at shoulder and upper arm level, <u>right</u> arm

CC-A **S45.912-** Laceration of unspecified blood vessel at shoulder and upper arm level, <u>left</u> arm

CC-A **S45.919-** Laceration of unspecified blood vessel at shoulder and upper arm level, <u>unspecified</u> arm

S45.99- <u>Other specified injury</u> of <u>unspecified blood vessel</u> at shoulder and upper arm level

CC-A **S45.991-** Other specified injury of unspecified blood vessel at shoulder and upper arm level, <u>right</u> arm

CC-A **S45.992-** Other specified injury of unspecified blood vessel at shoulder and upper arm level, <u>left</u> arm

---

CC-A **S45.999-** Other specified injury of unspecified blood vessel at shoulder and upper arm level, <u>unspecified</u> arm

S46- Injury of <u>muscle, fascia and tendon</u> <u>at shoulder and upper arm level</u>
Code also any associated open wound (S41.-)
Excludes ❷: injury of muscle, fascia and tendon at elbow (S56.-)
sprain of joints and ligaments of shoulder girdle (S43.9)

The appropriate 7th character is to be added to each code from category S46:
A <u>Initial</u> encounter
D <u>Subsequent</u> encounter
S <u>Sequela</u>

S46.0- Injury of <u>muscle(s) and tendon(s)</u> of the <u>rotator cuff of shoulder</u>

S46.00- <u>Unspecified</u> injury of <u>muscle(s) and tendon(s)</u> of the <u>rotator cuff of shoulder</u>

S46.001- Unspecified injury of muscle(s) and tendon(s) of the rotator cuff of <u>right</u> shoulder

S46.002- Unspecified injury of muscle(s) and tendon(s) of the rotator cuff of <u>left</u> shoulder

S46.009- Unspecified injury of muscle(s) and tendon(s) of the rotator cuff of <u>unspecified</u> shoulder

S46.01- <u>Strain</u> of <u>muscle(s) and tendon(s)</u> of the <u>rotator cuff of shoulder</u>

S46.011- Strain of muscle(s) and tendon(s) of the rotator cuff of <u>right</u> shoulder

S46.012- Strain of muscle(s) and tendon(s) of the rotator cuff of <u>left</u> shoulder

S46.019- Strain of muscle(s) and tendon(s) of the rotator cuff of <u>unspecified</u> shoulder

S46.02- <u>Laceration</u> of <u>muscle(s) and tendon(s)</u> of the <u>rotator cuff of shoulder</u>

CC-A **S46.021-** Laceration of muscle(s) and tendon(s) of the rotator cuff of <u>right</u> shoulder

CC-A **S46.022-** Laceration of muscle(s) and tendon(s) of the rotator cuff of <u>left</u> shoulder

CC-A **S46.029-** Laceration of muscle(s) and tendon(s) of the rotator cuff of <u>unspecified</u> shoulder

S46.09- <u>Other injury</u> of <u>muscle(s) and tendon(s)</u> of the <u>rotator cuff of shoulder</u>

S46.091- Other injury of muscle(s) and tendon(s) of the rotator cuff of <u>right</u> shoulder

S46.092- Other injury of muscle(s) and tendon(s) of the rotator cuff of <u>left</u> shoulder

S46.099- Other injury of muscle(s) and tendon(s) of the rotator cuff of <u>unspecified</u> shoulder

S46.1- Injury of <u>muscle, fascia and tendon</u> of <u>long head of biceps</u>

S46.10- <u>Unspecified</u> injury of <u>muscle, fascia and tendon</u> of <u>long head of biceps</u>

S46.101- Unspecified injury of muscle, fascia and tendon of long head of biceps, <u>right</u> arm

S46.102- Unspecified injury of muscle, fascia and tendon of long head of biceps, <u>left</u> arm

S46.109- Unspecified injury of muscle, fascia and tendon of long head of biceps, <u>unspecified</u> arm

S46.11- <u>Strain</u> of <u>muscle, fascia and tendon</u> of <u>long head of biceps</u>

S46.111- Strain of muscle, fascia and tendon of long head of biceps, <u>right</u> arm

S46.112- Strain of muscle, fascia and tendon of long head of biceps, <u>left</u> arm

S46.119- Strain of muscle, fascia and tendon of long head of biceps, <u>unspecified</u> arm

S46.12- <u>Laceration</u> of <u>muscle, fascia and tendon</u> of <u>long head of biceps</u>

CC-A **S46.121-** Laceration of muscle, fascia and tendon of long head of biceps, <u>right</u> arm

CC-A **S46.122-** Laceration of muscle, fascia and tendon of long head of biceps, <u>left</u> arm

S45 - S46

CC-A S46.129- Laceration of muscle, fascia and tendon of long head of biceps, <u>unspecified</u> arm

S46.19- <u>Other</u> injury of <u>muscle, fascia and tendon</u> of <u>long head of biceps</u>

 S46.191- Other injury of muscle, fascia and tendon of long head of biceps, <u>right</u> arm

 S46.192- Other injury of muscle, fascia and tendon of long head of biceps, <u>left</u> arm

 S46.199- Other injury of muscle, fascia and tendon of long head of biceps, <u>unspecified</u> arm

S46.2- Injury of <u>muscle, fascia and tendon</u> of <u>other parts of biceps</u>

 S46.20- <u>Unspecified</u> injury of <u>muscle, fascia and tendon</u> of <u>other parts of biceps</u>

  S46.201- Unspecified injury of muscle, fascia and tendon of other parts of biceps, <u>right</u> arm

  S46.202- Unspecified injury of muscle, fascia and tendon of other parts of biceps, <u>left</u> arm

  S46.209- Unspecified injury of muscle, fascia and tendon of other parts of biceps, <u>unspecified</u> arm

 S46.21- <u>Strain</u> of <u>muscle, fascia and tendon</u> of <u>other parts of biceps</u>

  S46.211- Strain of muscle, fascia and tendon of other parts of biceps, <u>right</u> arm

  S46.212- Strain of muscle, fascia and tendon of other parts of biceps, <u>left</u> arm

  S46.219- Strain of muscle, fascia and tendon of other parts of biceps, <u>unspecified</u> arm

 S46.22- <u>Laceration</u> of <u>muscle, fascia and tendon</u> of <u>other parts of biceps</u>

CC-A S46.221- Laceration of muscle, fascia and tendon of other parts of biceps, <u>right</u> arm

CC-A S46.222- Laceration of muscle, fascia and tendon of other parts of biceps, <u>left</u> arm

CC-A S46.229- Laceration of muscle, fascia and tendon of other parts of biceps, <u>unspecified</u> arm

 S46.29- <u>Other</u> injury of <u>muscle, fascia and tendon</u> of <u>other parts of biceps</u>

  S46.291- Other injury of muscle, fascia and tendon of other parts of biceps, <u>right</u> arm

  S46.292- Other injury of muscle, fascia and tendon of other parts of biceps, <u>left</u> arm

  S46.299- Other injury of muscle, fascia and tendon of other parts of biceps, <u>unspecified</u> arm

S46.3- Injury of <u>muscle, fascia and tendon</u> of <u>triceps</u>

 S46.30- <u>Unspecified</u> injury of <u>muscle, fascia and tendon</u> of <u>triceps</u>

  S46.301- Unspecified injury of muscle, fascia and tendon of triceps, <u>right</u> arm

  S46.302- Unspecified injury of muscle, fascia and tendon of triceps, <u>left</u> arm

  S46.309- Unspecified injury of muscle, fascia and tendon of triceps, <u>unspecified</u> arm

 S46.31- <u>Strain</u> of <u>muscle, fascia and tendon</u> of <u>triceps</u>

  S46.311- Strain of muscle, fascia and tendon of triceps, <u>right</u> arm

  S46.312- Strain of muscle, fascia and tendon of triceps, <u>left</u> arm

  S46.319- Strain of muscle, fascia and tendon of triceps, <u>unspecified</u> arm

 S46.32- <u>Laceration</u> of <u>muscle, fascia and tendon</u> of <u>triceps</u>

CC-A S46.321- Laceration of muscle, fascia and tendon of triceps, <u>right</u> arm

CC-A S46.322- Laceration of muscle, fascia and tendon of triceps, <u>left</u> arm

CC-A S46.329- Laceration of muscle, fascia and tendon of triceps, <u>unspecified</u> arm

 S46.39- <u>Other injury</u> of muscle, fascia and tendon of <u>triceps</u>

  S46.391- Other injury of muscle, fascia and tendon of triceps, <u>right</u> arm

S46.392- Other injury of muscle, fascia and tendon of triceps, <u>left</u> arm

S46.399- Other injury of muscle, fascia and tendon of triceps, <u>unspecified</u> arm

S46.8- <u>Injury</u> of <u>other muscles, fascia and tendons</u> <u>at shoulder and upper arm level</u>

 S46.80- <u>Unspecified</u> injury of <u>other muscles, fascia and tendons</u> <u>at shoulder and upper arm level</u>

  S46.801- Unspecified injury of other muscles, fascia and tendons at shoulder and upper arm level, <u>right</u> arm

  S46.802- Unspecified injury of other muscles, fascia and tendons at shoulder and upper arm level, <u>left</u> arm

  S46.809- Unspecified injury of other muscles, fascia and tendons at shoulder and upper arm level, <u>unspecified</u> arm

 S46.81- <u>Strain</u> of <u>other muscles, fascia and tendons</u> <u>at shoulder and upper arm level</u>

  S46.811- Strain of other muscles, fascia and tendons at shoulder and upper arm level, <u>right</u> arm

  S46.812- Strain of other muscles, fascia and tendons at shoulder and upper arm level, <u>left</u> arm

  S46.819- Strain of other muscles, fascia and tendons at shoulder and upper arm level, <u>unspecified</u> arm

 S46.82- <u>Laceration</u> of <u>other muscles, fascia and tendons</u> <u>at shoulder and upper arm level</u>

CC-A S46.821- Laceration of other muscles, fascia and tendons at shoulder and upper arm level, <u>right</u> arm

CC-A S46.822- Laceration of other muscles, fascia and tendons at shoulder and upper arm level, <u>left</u> arm

CC-A S46.829- Laceration of other muscles, fascia and tendons at shoulder and upper arm level, <u>unspecified</u> arm

 S46.89- <u>Other injury</u> of <u>other muscles, fascia and tendons</u> <u>at shoulder and upper arm level</u>

  S46.891- Other injury of other muscles, fascia and tendons at shoulder and upper arm level, <u>right</u> arm

  S46.892- Other injury of other muscles, fascia and tendons at shoulder and upper arm level, <u>left</u> arm

  S46.899- Other injury of other muscles, fascia and tendons at shoulder and upper arm level, <u>unspecified</u> arm

S46.9- Injury of <u>unspecified</u> <u>muscle, fascia and tendon</u> <u>at shoulder and upper arm level</u>

 S46.90- <u>Unspecified</u> injury of <u>unspecified</u> <u>muscle, fascia and tendon</u> <u>at shoulder and upper arm level</u>

  S46.901- Unspecified injury of unspecified muscle, fascia and tendon at shoulder and upper arm level, <u>right</u> arm

  S46.902- Unspecified injury of unspecified muscle, fascia and tendon at shoulder and upper arm level, <u>left</u> arm

  S46.909- Unspecified injury of <u>unspecified</u> muscle, fascia and tendon at shoulder and upper arm level, <u>unspecified</u> arm

 S46.91- <u>Strain</u> of <u>unspecified</u> <u>muscle, fascia and tendon</u> <u>at shoulder and upper arm level</u>

  S46.911- Strain of unspecified muscle, fascia and tendon at shoulder and upper arm level, <u>right</u> arm

  S46.912- Strain of unspecified muscle, fascia and tendon at shoulder and upper arm level, <u>left</u> arm

  S46.919- Strain of unspecified muscle, fascia and tendon at shoulder and upper arm level, <u>unspecified</u> arm

 S46.92- <u>Laceration</u> of <u>unspecified</u> <u>muscle, fascia and tendon</u> <u>at shoulder and upper arm level</u>

CC-A S46.921- Laceration of unspecified muscle, fascia and tendon at shoulder and upper arm level, <u>right</u> arm

CC-A S46.922- Laceration of unspecified muscle, fascia and tendon at shoulder and upper arm level, <u>left</u> arm

CC-A S46.929- Laceration of unspecified muscle, fascia and tendon at shoulder and upper arm level, <u>unspecified</u> arm

S44-S46

S46.99- Other injury of unspecified muscle, fascia and tendon at shoulder and upper arm level

S46.991- Other injury of unspecified muscle, fascia and tendon at shoulder and upper arm level, right arm

S46.992- Other injury of unspecified muscle, fascia and tendon at shoulder and upper arm level, left arm

S46.999- Other injury of unspecified muscle, fascia and tendon at shoulder and upper arm level, unspecified arm

S47- Crushing injury of shoulder and upper arm
Use additional code for all associated injuries
Excludes ❷: crushing injury of elbow (S57.0-)
The appropriate 7th character is to be added to each code from category S47:
A   Initial encounter
D   Subsequent encounter
S   Sequela

S47.1xx- Crushing injury of right shoulder and upper arm

S47.2xx- Crushing injury of left shoulder and upper arm

S47.9xx- Crushing injury of shoulder and upper arm, unspecified arm

S48- Traumatic amputation of shoulder and upper arm
Note: An amputation not identified as partial or complete should be coded to complete
Excludes 1: traumatic amputation at elbow level (S58.0)
The appropriate 7th character is to be added to each code from category S48:
A   Initial encounter
D   Subsequent encounter
S   Sequela

S48.0- Traumatic amputation at shoulder joint

S48.01- Complete traumatic amputation at shoulder joint

CC-A S48.011- Complete traumatic amputation at right shoulder joint

CC-A S48.012- Complete traumatic amputation at left shoulder joint

CC-A S48.019- Complete traumatic amputation at unspecified shoulder joint

S48.02- Partial traumatic amputation at shoulder joint

CC-A S48.021- Partial traumatic amputation at right shoulder joint

CC-A S48.022- Partial traumatic amputation at left shoulder joint

CC-A S48.029- Partial traumatic amputation at unspecified shoulder joint

S48.1- Traumatic amputation at level between shoulder and elbow

S48.11- Complete traumatic amputation at level between shoulder and elbow

CC-A S48.111- Complete traumatic amputation at level between right shoulder and elbow

CC-A S48.112- Complete traumatic amputation at level between left shoulder and elbow

CC-A S48.119- Complete traumatic amputation at level between unspecified shoulder and elbow

S48.12- Partial traumatic amputation at level between shoulder and elbow

CC-A S48.121- Partial traumatic amputation at level between right shoulder and elbow

CC-A S48.122- Partial traumatic amputation at level between left shoulder and elbow

CC-A S48.129- Partial traumatic amputation at level between unspecified shoulder and elbow

S48.9- Traumatic amputation of shoulder and upper arm, level unspecified

S48.91- Complete traumatic amputation of shoulder and upper arm, level unspecified

CC-A S48.911- Complete traumatic amputation of right shoulder and upper arm, level unspecified

CC-A S48.912- Complete traumatic amputation of left shoulder and upper arm, level unspecified

CC-A S48.919- Complete traumatic amputation of unspecified shoulder and upper arm, level unspecified

S48.92- Partial traumatic amputation of shoulder and upper arm, level unspecified

CC-A S48.921- Partial traumatic amputation of right shoulder and upper arm, level unspecified

CC-A S48.922- Partial traumatic amputation of left shoulder and upper arm, level unspecified

CC-A S48.929- Partial traumatic amputation of unspecified shoulder and upper arm, level unspecified

S49- Other and unspecified injuries of shoulder and upper arm
The appropriate 7th character is to be added to each code from subcategories S49.0 and S49.1:
A   Initial encounter for closed fracture
D   Subsequent encounter for fracture with routine healing
G   Subsequent encounter for fracture with delayed healing
K   Subsequent encounter for fracture with nonunion
P   Subsequent encounter for fracture with malunion
S   Sequela

S49.0- Physeal fracture of upper end of humerus

S49.00- Unspecified physeal fracture of upper end of humerus

CC-A,K,P S49.001- Unspecified physeal fracture of upper end of humerus, right arm

CC-A,K,P S49.002- Unspecified physeal fracture of upper end of humerus, left arm

CC-A,K,P S49.009- Unspecified physeal fracture of upper end of humerus, unspecified arm

S49.01- Salter-Harris Type I physeal fracture of upper end of humerus

CC-A,K,P S49.011- Salter-Harris Type I physeal fracture of upper end of humerus, right arm

CC-A,K,P S49.012- Salter-Harris Type I physeal fracture of upper end of humerus, left arm

CC-A,K,P S49.019- Salter-Harris Type I physeal fracture of upper end of humerus, unspecified arm

S49.02- Salter-Harris Type II physeal fracture of upper end of humerus

CC-A,K,P S49.021- Salter-Harris Type II physeal fracture of upper end of humerus, right arm

CC-A,K,P S49.022- Salter-Harris Type II physeal fracture of upper end of humerus, left arm

CC-A,K,P S49.029- Salter-Harris Type II physeal fracture of upper end of humerus, unspecified arm

S49.03- Salter-Harris Type III physeal fracture of upper end of humerus

CC-A,K,P S49.031- Salter-Harris Type III physeal fracture of upper end of humerus, right arm

CC-A,K,P S49.032- Salter-Harris Type III physeal fracture of upper end of humerus, left arm

CC-A,K,P S49.039- Salter-Harris Type III physeal fracture of upper end of humerus, unspecified arm

S49.04- Salter-Harris Type IV physeal fracture of upper end of humerus

CC-A,K,P S49.041- Salter-Harris Type IV physeal fracture of upper end of humerus, right arm

CC-A,K,P S49.042- Salter-Harris Type IV physeal fracture of upper end of humerus, left arm

CC-A,K,P S49.049- Salter-Harris Type IV physeal fracture of upper end of humerus, unspecified arm

S49.09- Other physeal fracture of upper end of humerus

CC-A,K,P S49.091- Other physeal fracture of upper end of humerus, right arm

CC-A,K,P S49.092- Other physeal fracture of upper end of humerus, left arm

CC-A,K,P S49.099- Other physeal fracture of upper end of humerus, unspecified arm

S46-S49

S49.1- Physeal fracture of lower end of humerus
- S49.10- Unspecified physeal fracture of lower end of humerus
- CC-A,K,P S49.101- Unspecified physeal fracture of lower end of humerus, right arm
- CC-A,K,P S49.102- Unspecified physeal fracture of lower end of humerus, left arm
- CC-A,K,P S49.109- Unspecified physeal fracture of lower end of humerus, unspecified arm
- S49.11- Salter-Harris Type I physeal fracture of lower end of humerus
- CC-A,K,P S49.111- Salter-Harris Type I physeal fracture of lower end of humerus, right arm
- CC-A,K,P S49.112- Salter-Harris Type I physeal fracture of lower end of humerus, left arm
- CC-A,K,P S49.119- Salter-Harris Type I physeal fracture of lower end of humerus, unspecified arm
- S49.12- Salter-Harris Type II physeal fracture of lower end of humerus
- CC-A,K,P S49.121- Salter-Harris Type II physeal fracture of lower end of humerus, right arm
- CC-A,K,P S49.122- Salter-Harris Type II physeal fracture of lower end of humerus, left arm
- CC-A,K,P S49.129- Salter-Harris Type II physeal fracture of lower end of humerus, unspecified arm
- S49.13- Salter-Harris Type III physeal fracture of lower end of humerus
- CC-A,K,P S49.131- Salter-Harris Type III physeal fracture of lower end of humerus, right arm
- CC-A,K,P S49.132- Salter-Harris Type III physeal fracture of lower end of humerus, left arm
- CC-A,K,P S49.139- Salter-Harris Type III physeal fracture of lower end of humerus, unspecified arm
- S49.14- Salter-Harris Type IV physeal fracture of lower end of humerus
- CC-A,K,P S49.141- Salter-Harris Type IV physeal fracture of lower end of humerus, right arm
- CC-A,K,P S49.142- Salter-Harris Type IV physeal fracture of lower end of humerus, left arm
- CC-A,K,P S49.149- Salter-Harris Type IV physeal fracture of lower end of humerus, unspecified arm
- S49.19- Other physeal fracture of lower end of humerus
- CC-A,K,P S49.191- Other physeal fracture of lower end of humerus, right arm
- CC-A,K,P S49.192- Other physeal fracture of lower end of humerus, left arm
- CC-A,K,P S49.199- Other physeal fracture of lower end of humerus, unspecified arm

S49.8- Other specified injuries of shoulder and upper arm
The appropriate 7th character is to be added to each code in subcategory S49.8:
- A Initial encounter
- D Subsequent encounter
- S Sequela
- S49.80x- Other specified injuries of shoulder and upper arm, unspecified arm
- S49.81x- Other specified injuries of right shoulder and upper arm
- S49.82x- Other specified injuries of left shoulder and upper arm

S49.9- Unspecified injury of shoulder and upper arm
The appropriate 7th character is to be added to each code in subcategory S49.9:
- A Initial encounter
- D Subsequent encounter
- S Sequela
- S49.90x- Unspecified injury of shoulder and upper arm, unspecified arm
- S49.91x- Unspecified injury of right shoulder and upper arm
- S49.92x- Unspecified injury of left shoulder and upper arm

Injuries to the elbow and forearm (S50-S59)

Excludes ❷: burns and corrosions (T20-T32)
frostbite (T33-T34)
injuries of wrist and hand (S60-S69)
insect bite or sting, venomous (T63.4)

S50- Superficial injury of elbow and forearm
Excludes ❷: superficial injury of wrist and hand (S60.-)
The appropriate 7th character is to be added to each code from category S50:
- A Initial encounter
- D Subsequent encounter
- S Sequela
- S50.0- Contusion of elbow
  - S50.00x- Contusion of unspecified elbow
  - S50.01x- Contusion of right elbow
  - S50.02x- Contusion of left elbow
- S50.1- Contusion of forearm
  - S50.10x- Contusion of unspecified forearm
  - S50.11x- Contusion of right forearm
  - S50.12x- Contusion of left forearm
- S50.3- Other superficial injuries of elbow
  - S50.31- Abrasion of elbow
    - S50.311- Abrasion of right elbow
    - S50.312- Abrasion of left elbow
    - S50.319- Abrasion of unspecified elbow
  - S50.32- Blister (nonthermal) of elbow
    - S50.321- Blister (nonthermal) of right elbow
    - S50.322- Blister (nonthermal) of left elbow
    - S50.329- Blister (nonthermal) of unspecified elbow
  - S50.34- External constriction of elbow
    - S50.341- External constriction of right elbow
    - S50.342- External constriction of left elbow
    - S50.349- External constriction of unspecified elbow
  - S50.35- Superficial foreign body of elbow
    Splinter in the elbow
    - S50.351- Superficial foreign body of right elbow
    - S50.352- Superficial foreign body of left elbow
    - S50.359- Superficial foreign body of unspecified elbow
  - S50.36- Insect bite (nonvenomous) of elbow
    - S50.361- Insect bite (nonvenomous) of right elbow
    - S50.362- Insect bite (nonvenomous) of left elbow
    - S50.369- Insect bite (nonvenomous) of unspecified elbow
  - S50.37- Other superficial bite of elbow
    Excludes 1: open bite of elbow (S51.04)
    - S50.371- Other superficial bite of right elbow
    - S50.372- Other superficial bite of left elbow
    - S50.379- Other superficial bite of unspecified elbow
- S50.8- Other superficial injuries of forearm
  - S50.81- Abrasion of forearm
    - S50.811- Abrasion of right forearm
    - S50.812- Abrasion of left forearm
    - S50.819- Abrasion of unspecified forearm
  - S50.82- Blister (nonthermal) of forearm
    - S50.821- Blister (nonthermal) of right forearm
    - S50.822- Blister (nonthermal) of left forearm
    - S50.829- Blister (nonthermal) of unspecified forearm
  - S50.84- External constriction of forearm
    - S50.841- External constriction of right forearm
    - S50.842- External constriction of left forearm
    - S50.849- External constriction of unspecified forearm
  - S50.85- Superficial foreign body of forearm
    Splinter in the forearm
    - S50.851- Superficial foreign body of right forearm
    - S50.852- Superficial foreign body of left forearm
    - S50.859- Superficial foreign body of unspecified forearm

S49 - S50

S50.86- Insect bite (nonvenomous) of forearm
  S50.861- Insect bite (nonvenomous) of right forearm
  S50.862- Insect bite (nonvenomous) of left forearm
  S50.869- Insect bite (nonvenomous) of unspecified forearm
S50.87- Other superficial bite of forearm
    Excludes 1:   open bite of forearm (S51.84)
  S50.871- Other superficial bite of right forearm
  S50.872- Other superficial bite of left forearm
  S50.879- Other superficial bite of unspecified forearm
S50.9- Unspecified superficial injury of elbow and forearm
  S50.90- Unspecified superficial injury of elbow
    S50.901- Unspecified superficial injury of right elbow
    S50.902- Unspecified superficial injury of left elbow
    S50.909- Unspecified superficial injury of unspecified elbow
  S50.91- Unspecified superficial injury of forearm
    S50.911- Unspecified superficial injury of right forearm
    S50.912- Unspecified superficial injury of left forearm
    S50.919- Unspecified superficial injury of unspecified forearm

S51- Open wound of elbow and forearm
  AHA 12:4Q:p108 – Open anterior dislocation of the right elbow
  Code also any associated wound infection
  Excludes 1:   open fracture of elbow and forearm (S52.- with open fracture 7th character)
  *   traumatic amputation of elbow and forearm (S58.-)*
  Excludes ❷: open wound of wrist and hand (S61.-)
  The appropriate 7th character is to be added to each code from category S51:
    A   Initial encounter
    D   Subsequent encounter
    S   Sequela
  S51.0- Open wound of elbow
    S51.00- Unspecified open wound of elbow
      S51.001- Unspecified open wound of right elbow
      S51.002- Unspecified open wound of left elbow
      S51.009- Unspecified open wound of unspecified elbow
              Open wound of elbow NOS
    S51.01- Laceration without foreign body of elbow
      S51.011- Laceration without foreign body of right elbow
      S51.012- Laceration without foreign body of left elbow
      S51.019- Laceration without foreign body of unspecified elbow
    S51.02- Laceration with foreign body of elbow
      S51.021- Laceration with foreign body of right elbow
      S51.022- Laceration with foreign body of left elbow
      S51.029- Laceration with foreign body of unspecified elbow
    S51.03- Puncture wound without foreign body of elbow
      S51.031- Puncture wound without foreign body of right elbow
      S51.032- Puncture wound without foreign body of left elbow
      S51.039- Puncture wound without foreign body of unspecified elbow
    S51.04- Puncture wound with foreign body of elbow
      S51.041- Puncture wound with foreign body of right elbow
      S51.042- Puncture wound with foreign body of left elbow
      S51.049- Puncture wound with foreign body of unspecified elbow
    S51.05- Open bite of elbow
            Bite of elbow NOS
        Excludes 1:   superficial bite of elbow (S50.36, S50.37)
      S51.051- Open bite, right elbow
      S51.052- Open bite, left elbow
      S51.059- Open bite, unspecified elbow

S51.8- Open wound of forearm
    Excludes ❷: open wound of elbow (S51.0-)
  S51.80- Unspecified open wound of forearm
    S51.801- Unspecified open wound of right forearm
    S51.802- Unspecified open wound of left forearm
    S51.809- Unspecified open wound of unspecified forearm
            Open wound of forearm NOS
  S51.81- Laceration without foreign body of forearm
    S51.811- Laceration without foreign body of right forearm
    S51.812- Laceration without foreign body of left forearm
    S51.819- Laceration without foreign body of unspecified forearm
  S51.82- Laceration with foreign body of forearm
    S51.821- Laceration with foreign body of right forearm
    S51.822- Laceration with foreign body of left forearm
    S51.829- Laceration with foreign body of unspecified forearm
  S51.83- Puncture wound without foreign body of forearm
    S51.831- Puncture wound without foreign body of right forearm
    S51.832- Puncture wound without foreign body of left forearm
    S51.839- Puncture wound without foreign body of unspecified forearm
  S51.84- Puncture wound with foreign body of forearm
    S51.841- Puncture wound with foreign body of right forearm
    S51.842- Puncture wound with foreign body of left forearm
    S51.849- Puncture wound with foreign body of unspecified forearm
  S51.85- Open bite of forearm
            Bite of forearm NOS
        Excludes 1:   superficial bite of forearm (S50.86, S50.87)
    S51.851- Open bite of right forearm
    S51.852- Open bite of left forearm
    S51.859- Open bite of unspecified forearm

Excludes 1: = NOT CODED HERE! (Do not code both)   **1067**   *Excludes ❷:* = Not Included Here

S52-   Fracture of forearm

Note: A fracture not indicated as displaced or nondisplaced should be coded to displaced

Note: A fracture not indicated as open or closed should be coded to closed

Note: The open fracture designations are based on the Gustilo open fracture classification

Excludes 1:   traumatic amputation of forearm (S58.-)

Excludes ❷: fracture at wrist and hand level (S62.-)

The appropriate 7th character is to be added to all codes from category S52:

- A   Initial encounter for closed fracture
- B   Initial encounter for open fracture type I or II
  Initial encounter for open fracture NOS
- C   Initial encounter for open fracture type IIIA, IIIB, or IIIC
- D   Subsequent encounter for closed fracture with routine healing
- E   Subsequent encounter for open fracture type I or II with routine healing
- F   Subsequent encounter for open fracture type IIIA, IIIB, or IIIC with routine healing
- G   Subsequent encounter for closed fracture with delayed healing
- H   Subsequent encounter for open fracture type I or II with delayed healing
- J   Subsequent encounter for open fracture type IIIA, IIIB, or IIIC with delayed healing
- K   Subsequent encounter for closed fracture with nonunion
- M   Subsequent encounter for open fracture type I or II with nonunion
- N   Subsequent encounter for open fracture type IIIA, IIIB, or IIIC with nonunion
- P   Subsequent encounter for closed fracture with malunion
- Q   Subsequent encounter for open fracture type I or II with malunion
- R   Subsequent encounter for open fracture type IIIA, IIIB, or IIIC with malunion
- S   Sequela

S52.0-   Fracture of upper end of ulna

Fracture of proximal end of ulna

Excludes ❷: fracture of elbow NOS (S42.40-)
fractures of shaft of ulna (S52.2-)

S52.00-   Unspecified fracture of upper end of ulna

S52.001-   Unspecified fracture of upper end of right ulna
CC-K,M,N,P,Q,R MCC-B,C

S52.002-   Unspecified fracture of upper end of left ulna
CC-K,M,N,P,Q,R MCC-B,C

S52.009-   Unspecified fracture of upper end of unspecified ulna
CC-K,M,N,P,Q,R MCC-B,C

S52.01-   Torus fracture of upper end of ulna

The appropriate 7th character is to be added to all codes in subcategory S52.01:

- A   Initial encounter for closed fracture
- D   Subsequent encounter for fracture with routine healing
- G   Subsequent encounter for fracture with delayed healing
- K   Subsequent encounter for fracture with nonunion
- P   Subsequent encounter for fracture with malunion
- S   Sequela

CC-A,K,P **S52.011-**   Torus fracture of upper end of right ulna

CC-A,K,P **S52.012-**   Torus fracture of upper end of left ulna

CC-A,K,P **S52.019-**   Torus fracture of upper end of unspecified ulna

S52.02-   Fracture of olecranon process without intraarticular extension of ulna

S52.021-   Displaced fracture of olecranon process without intraarticular extension of right ulna
CC-K,M,N,P,Q,R MCC-B,C

S52.022-   Displaced fracture of olecranon process without intraarticular extension of left ulna
CC-K,M,N,P,Q,R MCC-B,C

S52.023-   Displaced fracture of olecranon process without intraarticular extension of unspecified ulna
CC-K,M,N,P,Q,R MCC-B,C

S52.024-   Nondisplaced fracture of olecranon process without intraarticular extension of right ulna
CC-K,M,N,P,Q,R MCC-B,C

S52.025-   Nondisplaced fracture of olecranon process without intraarticular extension of left ulna
CC-K,M,N,P,Q,R MCC-B,C

S52.026-   Nondisplaced fracture of olecranon process without intraarticular extension of unspecified ulna
CC-K,M,N,P,Q,R MCC-B,C

S52.03-   Fracture of olecranon process with intraarticular extension of ulna

S52.031-   Displaced fracture of olecranon process with intraarticular extension of right ulna
CC-K,M,N,P,Q,R MCC-B,C

S52.032-   Displaced fracture of olecranon process with intraarticular extension of left ulna
CC-K,M,N,P,Q,R MCC-B,C

S52.033-   Displaced fracture of olecranon process with intraarticular extension of unspecified ulna
CC-K,M,N,P,Q,R MCC-B,C

S52.034-   Nondisplaced fracture of olecranon process with intraarticular extension of right ulna
CC-K,M,N,P,Q,R MCC-B,C

S52.035-   Nondisplaced fracture of olecranon process with intraarticular extension of left ulna
CC-K,M,N,P,Q,R MCC-B,C

S52.036-   Nondisplaced fracture of olecranon process with intraarticular extension of unspecified ulna
CC-K,M,N,P,Q,R MCC-B,C

S52.04-   Fracture of coronoid process of ulna

S52.041-   Displaced fracture of coronoid process of right ulna
CC-K,M,N,P,Q,R MCC-B,C

S52.042-   Displaced fracture of coronoid process of left ulna
CC-K,M,N,P,Q,R MCC-B,C

S52.043-   Displaced fracture of coronoid process of unspecified ulna
CC-K,M,N,P,Q,R MCC-B,C

S52.044-   Nondisplaced fracture of coronoid process of right ulna
CC-K,M,N,P,Q,R MCC-B,C

S52.045-   Nondisplaced fracture of coronoid process of left ulna
CC-K,M,N,P,Q,R MCC-B,C

S52.046-   Nondisplaced fracture of coronoid process of unspecified ulna
CC-K,M,N,P,Q,R MCC-B,C

S52.09-   Other fracture of upper end of ulna

S52.091-   Other fracture of upper end of right ulna
CC-K,M,N,P,Q,R MCC-B,C

S52.092-   Other fracture of upper end of left ulna
CC-K,M,N,P,Q,R MCC-B,C

S52.099-   Other fracture of upper end of unspecified ulna
CC-K,M,N,P,Q,R MCC-B,C

S52.1-   Fracture of upper end of radius

Fracture of proximal end of radius

Excludes ❷: physeal fractures of upper end of radius (S59.2-)
fracture of shaft of radius (S52.3-)

S52.10-   Unspecified fracture of upper end of radius

S52.101-   Unspecified fracture of upper end of right radius
CC-K,M,N,P,Q,R MCC-B,C

S52.102-   Unspecified fracture of upper end of left radius
CC-K,M,N,P,Q,R MCC-B,C

S52.109-   Unspecified fracture of upper end of unspecified radius
CC-K,M,N,P,Q,R MCC-B,C

S52 - S52

© 2016 Channel Publishing, Ltd.

S52.11- Torus fracture of upper end of radius

The appropriate 7th character is to be added to all codes in subcategory S52.11:
A   Initial encounter for closed fracture
D   Subsequent encounter for fracture with routine healing
G   Subsequent encounter for fracture with delayed healing
K   Subsequent encounter for fracture with nonunion
P   Subsequent encounter for fracture with malunion
S   Sequela

CC-A,K,P S52.111- Torus fracture of upper end of right radius
CC-A,K,P S52.112- Torus fracture of upper end of left radius
CC-A,K,P S52.119- Torus fracture of upper end of unspecified radius

S52.12- Fracture of head of radius
S52.121- Displaced fracture of head of right radius
CC-K,M,N,P,Q,R MCC-B,C
S52.122- Displaced fracture of head of left radius
CC-K,M,N,P,Q,R MCC-B,C
S52.123- Displaced fracture of head of unspecified radius
CC-K,M,N,P,Q,R MCC-B,C
S52.124- Nondisplaced fracture of head of right radius
CC-K,M,N,P,Q,R MCC-B,C
S52.125- Nondisplaced fracture of head of left radius
CC-K,M,N,P,Q,R MCC-B,C
S52.126- Nondisplaced fracture of head of unspecified radius
CC-K,M,N,P,Q,R MCC-B,C

S52.13- Fracture of neck of radius
S52.131- Displaced fracture of neck of right radius
CC-K,M,N,P,Q,R MCC-B,C
S52.132- Displaced fracture of neck of left radius
CC-K,M,N,P,Q,R MCC-B,C
S52.133- Displaced fracture of neck of unspecified radius
CC-K,M,N,P,Q,R MCC-B,C
S52.134- Nondisplaced fracture of neck of right radius
CC-K,M,N,P,Q,R MCC-B,C
S52.135- Nondisplaced fracture of neck of left radius
CC-K,M,N,P,Q,R MCC-B,C
S52.136- Nondisplaced fracture of neck of unspecified radius
CC-K,M,N,P,Q,R MCC-B,C

S52.18- Other fracture of upper end of radius
S52.181- Other fracture of upper end of right radius
CC-K,M,N,P,Q,R MCC-B,C
S52.182- Other fracture of upper end of left radius
CC-K,M,N,P,Q,R MCC-B,C
S52.189- Other fracture of upper end of unspecified radius
CC-K,M,N,P,Q,R MCC-B,C

S52.2- Fracture of shaft of ulna
S52.20- Unspecified fracture of shaft of ulna
Fracture of ulna NOS
S52.201- Unspecified fracture of shaft of right ulna
CC-A,K,M,N,P,Q,R MCC-B,C
S52.202- Unspecified fracture of shaft of left ulna
CC-A,K,M,N,P,Q,R MCC-B,C
S52.209- Unspecified fracture of shaft of unspecified ulna
CC-A,K,M,N,P,Q,R MCC-B,C

S52.21- Greenstick fracture of shaft of ulna

The appropriate 7th character is to be added to all codes in subcategory S52.21:
A   Initial encounter for closed fracture
D   Subsequent encounter for fracture with routine healing
G   Subsequent encounter for fracture with delayed healing
K   Subsequent encounter for fracture with nonunion
P   Subsequent encounter for fracture with malunion
S   Sequela

CC-A,K,P S52.211- Greenstick fracture of shaft of right ulna
CC-A,K,P S52.212- Greenstick fracture of shaft of left ulna
CC-A,K,P S52.219- Greenstick fracture of shaft of unspecified ulna

S52.22- Transverse fracture of shaft of ulna
S52.221- Displaced transverse fracture of shaft of right ulna
CC-A,K,M,N,P,Q,R MCC-B,C
S52.222- Displaced transverse fracture of shaft of left ulna
CC-A,K,M,N,P,Q,R MCC-B,C
S52.223- Displaced transverse fracture of shaft of unspecified ulna
CC-A,K,M,N,P,Q,R MCC-B,C
S52.224- Nondisplaced transverse fracture of shaft of right ulna
CC-A,K,M,N,P,Q,R MCC-B,C
S52.225- Nondisplaced transverse fracture of shaft of left ulna
CC-A,K,M,N,P,Q,R MCC-B,C
S52.226- Nondisplaced transverse fracture of shaft of unspecified ulna
CC-A,K,M,N,P,Q,R MCC-B,C

S52.23- Oblique fracture of shaft of ulna
S52.231- Displaced oblique fracture of shaft of right ulna
CC-A,K,M,N,P,Q,R MCC-B,C
S52.232- Displaced oblique fracture of shaft of left ulna
CC-A,K,M,N,P,Q,R MCC-B,C
S52.233- Displaced oblique fracture of shaft of unspecified ulna
CC-A,K,M,N,P,Q,R MCC-B,C
S52.234- Nondisplaced oblique fracture of shaft of right ulna
CC-A,K,M,N,P,Q,R MCC-B,C
S52.235- Nondisplaced oblique fracture of shaft of left ulna
CC-A,K,M,N,P,Q,R MCC-B,C
S52.236- Nondisplaced oblique fracture of shaft of unspecified ulna
CC-A,K,M,N,P,Q,R MCC-B,C

S52.24- Spiral fracture of shaft of ulna
S52.241- Displaced spiral fracture of shaft of ulna, right arm
CC-A,K,M,N,P,Q,R MCC-B,C
S52.242- Displaced spiral fracture of shaft of ulna, left arm
CC-A,K,M,N,P,Q,R MCC-B,C
S52.243- Displaced spiral fracture of shaft of ulna, unspecified arm
CC-A,K,M,N,P,Q,R MCC-B,C
S52.244- Nondisplaced spiral fracture of shaft of ulna, right arm
CC-A,K,M,N,P,Q,R MCC-B,C
S52.245- Nondisplaced spiral fracture of shaft of ulna, left arm
CC-A,K,M,N,P,Q,R MCC-B,C
S52.246- Nondisplaced spiral fracture of shaft of ulna, unspecified arm
CC-A,K,M,N,P,Q,R MCC-B,C

S52.25- Comminuted fracture of shaft of ulna
S52.251- Displaced comminuted fracture of shaft of ulna, right arm
CC-A,K,M,N,P,Q,R MCC-B,C
S52.252- Displaced comminuted fracture of shaft of ulna, left arm
CC-A,K,M,N,P,Q,R MCC-B,C
S52.253- Displaced comminuted fracture of shaft of ulna, unspecified arm
CC-A,K,M,N,P,Q,R MCC-B,C
S52.254- Nondisplaced comminuted fracture of shaft of ulna, right arm
CC-A,K,M,N,P,Q,R MCC-B,C
S52.255- Nondisplaced comminuted fracture of shaft of ulna, left arm
CC-A,K,M,N,P,Q,R MCC-B,C
S52.256- Nondisplaced comminuted fracture of shaft of ulna, unspecified arm
CC-A,K,M,N,P,Q,R MCC-B,C

S52
I
S52

S52.26- Segmental fracture of shaft of ulna

S52.261- Displaced segmental fracture of shaft of ulna, right arm
CC-A,K,M,N,P,Q,R MCC-B,C

S52.262- Displaced segmental fracture of shaft of ulna, left arm
CC-A,K,M,N,P,Q,R MCC-B,C

S52.263- Displaced segmental fracture of shaft of ulna, unspecified arm
CC-A,K,M,N,P,Q,R MCC-B,C

S52.264- Nondisplaced segmental fracture of shaft of ulna, right arm
CC-A,K,M,N,P,Q,R MCC-B,C

S52.265- Nondisplaced segmental fracture of shaft of ulna, left arm
CC-A,K,M,N,P,Q,R MCC-B,C

S52.266- Nondisplaced segmental fracture of shaft of ulna, unspecified arm
CC-A,K,M,N,P,Q,R MCC-B,C

S52.27- Monteggia's fracture of ulna
Fracture of upper shaft of ulna with dislocation of radial head

S52.271- Monteggia's fracture of right ulna
CC-K,M,N,P,Q,R MCC-B,C

S52.272- Monteggia's fracture of left ulna
CC-K,M,N,P,Q,R MCC-B,C

S52.279- Monteggia's fracture of unspecified ulna
CC-K,M,N,P,Q,R MCC-B,C

S52.28- Bent bone of ulna

S52.281- Bent bone of right ulna
CC-A,K,M,N,P,Q,R MCC-B,C

S52.282- Bent bone of left ulna
CC-A,K,M,N,P,Q,R MCC-B,C

S52.283- Bent bone of unspecified ulna
CC-A,K,M,N,P,Q,R MCC-B,C

S52.29- Other fracture of shaft of ulna

S52.291- Other fracture of shaft of right ulna
CC-A,K,M,N,P,Q,R MCC-B,C

S52.292- Other fracture of shaft of left ulna
CC-A,K,M,N,P,Q,R MCC-B,C

S52.299- Other fracture of shaft of unspecified ulna
CC-A,K,M,N,P,Q,R MCC-B,C

S52.3- Fracture of shaft of radius

S52.30- Unspecified fracture of shaft of radius

S52.301- Unspecified fracture of shaft of right radius
CC-A,K,M,N,P,Q,R MCC-B,C

S52.302- Unspecified fracture of shaft of left radius
CC-A,K,M,N,P,Q,R MCC-B,C

S52.309- Unspecified fracture of shaft of unspecified radius
CC-A,K,M,N,P,Q,R MCC-B,C

S52.31- Greenstick fracture of shaft of radius

> The appropriate 7th character is to be added to all codes in subcategory S52.31:
> A   Initial encounter for closed fracture
> D   Subsequent encounter for fracture with routine healing
> G   Subsequent encounter for fracture with delayed healing
> K   Subsequent encounter for fracture with nonunion
> P   Subsequent encounter for fracture with malunion
> S   Sequela

CC-A,K,P **S52.311-** Greenstick fracture of shaft of radius, right arm

CC-A,K,P **S52.312-** Greenstick fracture of shaft of radius, left arm

CC-A,K,P **S52.319-** Greenstick fracture of shaft of radius, unspecified arm

S52.32- Transverse fracture of shaft of radius

S52.321- Displaced transverse fracture of shaft of right radius
CC-A,K,M,N,P,Q,R MCC-B,C

S52.322- Displaced transverse fracture of shaft of left radius
CC-A,K,M,N,P,Q,R MCC-B,C

S52.323- Displaced transverse fracture of shaft of unspecified radius
CC-A,K,M,N,P,Q,R MCC-B,C

S52.324- Nondisplaced transverse fracture of shaft of right radius
CC-A,K,M,N,P,Q,R MCC-B,C

S52.325- Nondisplaced transverse fracture of shaft of left radius
CC-A,K,M,N,P,Q,R MCC-B,C

S52.326- Nondisplaced transverse fracture of shaft of unspecified radius
CC-A,K,M,N,P,Q,R MCC-B,C

S52.33- Oblique fracture of shaft of radius

S52.331- Displaced oblique fracture of shaft of right radius
CC-A,K,M,N,P,Q,R MCC-B,C

S52.332- Displaced oblique fracture of shaft of left radius
CC-A,K,M,N,P,Q,R MCC-B,C

S52.333- Displaced oblique fracture of shaft of unspecified radius
CC-A,K,M,N,P,Q,R MCC-B,C

S52.334- Nondisplaced oblique fracture of shaft of right radius
CC-A,K,M,N,P,Q,R MCC-B,C

S52.335- Nondisplaced oblique fracture of shaft of left radius
CC-A,K,M,N,P,Q,R MCC-B,C

S52.336- Nondisplaced oblique fracture of shaft of unspecified radius
CC-A,K,M,N,P,Q,R MCC-B,C

S52.34- Spiral fracture of shaft of radius

S52.341- Displaced spiral fracture of shaft of radius, right arm
CC-A,K,M,N,P,Q,R MCC-B,C

S52.342- Displaced spiral fracture of shaft of radius, left arm
CC-A,K,M,N,P,Q,R MCC-B,C

S52.343- Displaced spiral fracture of shaft of radius, unspecified arm
CC-A,K,M,N,P,Q,R MCC-B,C

S52.344- Nondisplaced spiral fracture of shaft of radius, right arm
CC-A,K,M,N,P,Q,R MCC-B,C

S52.345- Nondisplaced spiral fracture of shaft of radius, left arm
CC-A,K,M,N,P,Q,R MCC-B,C

S52.346- Nondisplaced spiral fracture of shaft of radius, unspecified arm
CC-A,K,M,N,P,Q,R MCC-B,C

S52.35- Comminuted fracture of shaft of radius

S52.351- Displaced comminuted fracture of shaft of radius, right arm
CC-A,K,M,N,P,Q,R MCC-B,C

S52.352- Displaced comminuted fracture of shaft of radius, left arm
CC-A,K,M,N,P,Q,R MCC-B,C

S52.353- Displaced comminuted fracture of shaft of radius, unspecified arm
CC-A,K,M,N,P,Q,R MCC-B,C

S52.354- Nondisplaced comminuted fracture of shaft of radius, right arm
CC-A,K,M,N,P,Q,R MCC-B,C

S52.355- Nondisplaced comminuted fracture of shaft of radius, left arm
CC-A,K,M,N,P,Q,R MCC-B,C

S52.356- Nondisplaced comminuted fracture of shaft of radius, unspecified arm
CC-A,K,M,N,P,Q,R MCC-B,C

S52.36- Segmental fracture of shaft of radius

S52.361- Displaced segmental fracture of shaft of radius, right arm
CC-A,K,M,N,P,Q,R MCC-B,C

S52.362- Displaced segmental fracture of shaft of radius, left arm
CC-A,K,M,N,P,Q,R MCC-B,C

S52.363- Displaced segmental fracture of shaft of radius, unspecified arm
CC-A,K,M,N,P,Q,R MCC-B,C

S52.364- Nondisplaced segmental fracture of shaft of radius, right arm
CC-A,K,M,N,P,Q,R MCC-B,C

S52 - S52

S52.365- <u>Nondisplaced</u> segmental fracture of shaft of radius, <u>left</u> arm
CC-A,K,M,N,P,Q,R MCC-B,C

S52.366- <u>Nondisplaced</u> segmental fracture of shaft of radius, <u>unspecified</u> arm
CC-A,K,M,N,P,Q,R MCC-B,C

S52.37- <u>Galeazzi's</u> fracture
Fracture of lower shaft of radius with radioulnar joint dislocation

S52.371- Galeazzi's fracture of <u>right</u> radius
CC-A,K,M,N,P,Q,R MCC-B,C

S52.372- Galeazzi's fracture of <u>left</u> radius
CC-A,K,M,N,P,Q,R MCC-B,C

S52.379- Galeazzi's fracture of <u>unspecified</u> radius
CC-A,K,M,N,P,Q,R MCC-B,C

S52.38- <u>Bent bone</u> of <u>radius</u>

S52.381- Bent bone of <u>right</u> radius
CC-A,K,M,N,P,Q,R MCC-B,C

S52.382- Bent bone of <u>left</u> radius
CC-A,K,M,N,P,Q,R MCC-B,C

S52.389- Bent bone of <u>unspecified</u> radius
CC-A,K,M,N,P,Q,R MCC-B,C

S52.39- <u>Other</u> fracture of <u>shaft</u> of <u>radius</u>

S52.391- Other fracture of shaft of radius, <u>right</u> arm
CC-A,K,M,N,P,Q,R MCC-B,C

S52.392- Other fracture of shaft of radius, <u>left</u> arm
CC-A,K,M,N,P,Q,R MCC-B,C

S52.399- Other fracture of shaft of radius, <u>unspecified</u> arm
CC-A,K,M,N,P,Q,R MCC-B,C

S52.5- Fracture of <u>lower end</u> of <u>radius</u>
Fracture of distal end of radius
Excludes ❷: physeal fractures of lower end of radius (S59.2-)

S52.50- <u>Unspecified</u> fracture of the <u>lower end</u> of <u>radius</u>

S52.501- Unspecified fracture of the lower end of <u>right</u> radius
CC-A,K,M,N,P,Q,R MCC-B,C

S52.502- Unspecified fracture of the lower end of <u>left</u> radius
CC-A,K,M,N,P,Q,R MCC-B,C

S52.509- Unspecified fracture of the lower end of <u>unspecified</u> radius
CC-A,K,M,N,P,Q,R MCC-B,C

S52.51- <u>Fracture</u> of <u>radial styloid process</u>

S52.511- <u>Displaced</u> fracture of <u>right</u> radial styloid process
CC-A,K,M,N,P,Q,R MCC-B,C

S52.512- <u>Displaced</u> fracture of <u>left</u> radial styloid process
CC-A,K,M,N,P,Q,R MCC-B,C

S52.513- <u>Displaced</u> fracture of <u>unspecified</u> radial styloid process
CC-A,K,M,N,P,Q,R MCC-B,C

S52.514- <u>Nondisplaced</u> fracture of <u>right</u> radial styloid process
CC-A,K,M,N,P,Q,R MCC-B,C

S52.515- <u>Nondisplaced</u> fracture of <u>left</u> radial styloid process
CC-A,K,M,N,P,Q,R MCC-B,C

S52.516- <u>Nondisplaced</u> fracture of <u>unspecified</u> radial styloid process
CC-A,K,M,N,P,Q,R MCC-B,C

S52.52- <u>Torus</u> fracture of <u>lower end</u> of <u>radius</u>
The appropriate 7th character is to be added to all codes in subcategory S52.52:
A <u>Initial</u> encounter for <u>closed</u> fracture
D <u>Subsequent</u> encounter for fracture <u>with routine healing</u>
G <u>Subsequent</u> encounter for fracture <u>with delayed healing</u>
K <u>Subsequent</u> encounter for fracture <u>with nonunion</u>
P <u>Subsequent</u> encounter for fracture <u>with malunion</u>
S <u>Sequela</u>

CC-A,K,P **S52.521-** Torus fracture of lower end of <u>right</u> radius
CC-A,K,P **S52.522-** Torus fracture of lower end of <u>left</u> radius
CC-A,K,P **S52.529-** Torus fracture of lower end of <u>unspecified</u> radius

S52.53- <u>Colles'</u> fracture

S52.531- Colles' fracture of <u>right</u> radius
CC-A,K,M,N,P,Q,R MCC-B,C

S52.532- Colles' fracture of <u>left</u> radius
CC-A,K,M,N,P,Q,R MCC-B,C

S52.539- Colles' fracture of <u>unspecified</u> radius
CC-A,K,M,N,P,Q,R MCC-B,C

S52.54- <u>Smith's</u> fracture

S52.541- Smith's fracture of <u>right</u> radius
CC-A,K,M,N,P,Q,R MCC-B,C

S52.542- Smith's fracture of <u>left</u> radius
CC-A,K,M,N,P,Q,R MCC-B,C

S52.549- Smith's fracture of <u>unspecified</u> radius
CC-A,K,M,N,P,Q,R MCC-B,C

S52.55- <u>Other extraarticular</u> fracture of <u>lower end</u> of <u>radius</u>

S52.551- Other extraarticular fracture of lower end of <u>right</u> radius
CC-A,K,M,N,P,Q,R MCC-B,C

S52.552- Other extraarticular fracture of lower end of <u>left</u> radius
CC-A,K,M,N,P,Q,R MCC-B,C

S52.559- Other extraarticular fracture of lower end of <u>unspecified</u> radius
CC-A,K,M,N,P,Q,R MCC-B,C

S52.56- <u>Barton's</u> fracture

S52.561- Barton's fracture of <u>right</u> radius
CC-A,K,M,N,P,Q,R MCC-B,C

S52.562- Barton's fracture of <u>left</u> radius
CC-A,K,M,N,P,Q,R MCC-B,C

S52.569- Barton's fracture of <u>unspecified</u> radius
CC-A,K,M,N,P,Q,R MCC-B,C

S52.57- <u>Other intraarticular</u> fracture of <u>lower end</u> of <u>radius</u>

S52.571- Other intraarticular fracture of lower end of <u>right</u> radius
CC-A,K,M,N,P,Q,R MCC-B,C

S52.572- Other intraarticular fracture of lower end of <u>left</u> radius
CC-A,K,M,N,P,Q,R MCC-B,C

S52.579- Other intraarticular fracture of lower end of <u>unspecified</u> radius
CC-A,K,M,N,P,Q,R MCC-B,C

S52.59- <u>Other</u> fractures of <u>lower end</u> of <u>radius</u>

S52.591- Other fractures of lower end of <u>right</u> radius
CC-A,K,M,N,P,Q,R MCC-B,C

S52.592- Other fractures of lower end of <u>left</u> radius
CC-A,K,M,N,P,Q,R MCC-B,C

S52.599- Other fractures of lower end of <u>unspecified</u> radius
CC-A,K,M,N,P,Q,R MCC-B,C

S52.6- Fracture of <u>lower end</u> of <u>ulna</u>

S52.60- <u>Unspecified</u> fracture of <u>lower end</u> of <u>ulna</u>

S52.601- Unspecified fracture of lower end of <u>right</u> ulna
CC-A,K,M,N,P,Q,R MCC-B,C

S52.602- Unspecified fracture of lower end of <u>left</u> ulna
CC-A,K,M,N,P,Q,R MCC-B,C

S52.609- Unspecified fracture of lower end of <u>unspecified</u> ulna
CC-A,K,M,N,P,Q,R MCC-B,C

S52.61- Fracture of <u>ulna styloid process</u>

S52.611- <u>Displaced</u> fracture of <u>right</u> ulna styloid process
CC-A,K,M,N,P,Q,R MCC-B,C

S52.612- <u>Displaced</u> fracture of <u>left</u> ulna styloid process
CC-A,K,M,N,P,Q,R MCC-B,C

S52.613- <u>Displaced</u> fracture of <u>unspecified</u> ulna styloid process
CC-A,K,M,N,P,Q,R MCC-B,C

S52.614- <u>Nondisplaced</u> fracture of <u>right</u> ulna styloid process
CC-A,K,M,N,P,Q,R MCC-B,C

S52.615- <u>Nondisplaced</u> fracture of <u>left</u> ulna styloid process
CC-A,K,M,N,P,Q,R MCC-B,C

S52.616- <u>Nondisplaced</u> fracture of <u>unspecified</u> ulna styloid process
CC-A,K,M,N,P,Q,R MCC-B,C

S52 - S52 - S52

S52.62- Torus fracture of <u>lower end</u> of <u>ulna</u>
The appropriate 7th character is to be added to all codes in subcategory S52.62:
A   <u>Initial</u> encounter for <u>closed</u> fracture
D   <u>Subsequent</u> encounter for fracture <u>with routine healing</u>
G   <u>Subsequent</u> encounter for fracture <u>with delayed healing</u>
K   <u>Subsequent</u> encounter for fracture <u>with nonunion</u>
P   <u>Subsequent</u> encounter for fracture <u>with malunion</u>
S   <u>Sequela</u>

CC-A,K,P S52.621- Torus fracture of lower end of <u>right</u> ulna
CC-A,K,P S52.622- Torus fracture of lower end of <u>left</u> ulna
CC-A,K,P S52.629- Torus fracture of lower end of <u>unspecified</u> ulna

S52.69- <u>Other</u> fracture of <u>lower end</u> of <u>ulna</u>
S52.691- Other fracture of lower end of <u>right</u> ulna
CC-A,K,M,N,P,Q,R MCC-B,C
S52.692- Other fracture of lower end of <u>left</u> ulna
CC-A,K,M,N,P,Q,R MCC-B,C
S52.699- Other fracture of lower end of <u>unspecified</u> ulna
CC-A,K,M,N,P,Q,R MCC-B,C

S52.9- <u>Unspecified</u> fracture of <u>forearm</u>
S52.90x- Unspecified fracture of <u>unspecified</u> forearm
CC-A,K,M,N,P,Q,R MCC-B,C
S52.91x- Unspecified fracture of <u>right</u> forearm
CC-A,K,M,N,P,Q,R MCC-B,C
S52.92x- Unspecified fracture of <u>left</u> forearm
CC-A,K,M,N,P,Q,R MCC-B,C

S53- <u>Dislocation and sprain</u> of joints and ligaments of <u>elbow</u>
AHA 12:4Q:p108 – Open anterior dislocation of the right elbow
Includes: Avulsion of joint or ligament of elbow
Laceration of cartilage, joint or ligament of elbow
Sprain of cartilage, joint or ligament of elbow
Traumatic hemarthrosis of joint or ligament of elbow
Traumatic rupture of joint or ligament of elbow
Traumatic subluxation of joint or ligament of elbow
Traumatic tear of joint or ligament of elbow
Code also any associated open wound
Excludes ❷: strain of muscle, fascia and tendon at forearm level (S56.-)

The appropriate 7th character is to be added to each code from category S53:
A   <u>Initial</u> encounter
D   <u>Subsequent</u> encounter
S   <u>Sequela</u>

S53.0- <u>Subluxation and dislocation</u> of <u>radial head</u>
Dislocation of radiohumeral joint
Subluxation of radiohumeral joint
Excludes 1:   Monteggia's fracture-dislocation (S52.27-)

S53.00- <u>Unspecified</u> subluxation and dislocation of <u>radial head</u>
S53.001- Unspecified <u>subluxation</u> of <u>right</u> radial head
S53.002- Unspecified <u>subluxation</u> of <u>left</u> radial head
S53.003- Unspecified <u>subluxation</u> of <u>unspecified</u> radial head
S53.004- Unspecified <u>dislocation</u> of <u>right</u> radial head
S53.005- Unspecified <u>dislocation</u> of <u>left</u> radial head
S53.006- Unspecified <u>dislocation</u> of <u>unspecified</u> radial head

S53.01- <u>Anterior</u> subluxation and dislocation of <u>radial head</u>
Anteriomedial subluxation and dislocation of radial head
S53.011- Anterior <u>subluxation</u> of <u>right</u> radial head
S53.012- Anterior <u>subluxation</u> of <u>left</u> radial head
S53.013- Anterior <u>subluxation</u> of <u>unspecified</u> radial head
S53.014- Anterior <u>dislocation</u> of <u>right</u> radial head
S53.015- Anterior <u>dislocation</u> of <u>left</u> radial head
S53.016- Anterior <u>dislocation</u> of <u>unspecified</u> radial head

S53.02- <u>Posterior</u> subluxation and dislocation of <u>radial head</u>
Posteriolateral subluxation and dislocation of radial head
S53.021- Posterior <u>subluxation</u> of <u>right</u> radial head
S53.022- Posterior <u>subluxation</u> of <u>left</u> radial head
S53.023- Posterior <u>subluxation</u> of <u>unspecified</u> radial head
S53.024- Posterior <u>dislocation</u> of <u>right</u> radial head
S53.025- Posterior <u>dislocation</u> of <u>left</u> radial head
S53.026- Posterior <u>dislocation</u> of <u>unspecified</u> radial head

S53.03- <u>Nursemaid's</u> elbow
AHA 15:1Q:p7 – Right radial head subluxation
S53.031- Nursemaid's elbow, <u>right</u> elbow
S53.032- Nursemaid's elbow, <u>left</u> elbow
S53.033- Nursemaid's elbow, <u>unspecified</u> elbow

S53.09- <u>Other</u> subluxation and dislocation of <u>radial head</u>
S53.091- Other <u>subluxation</u> of <u>right</u> radial head
S53.092- Other <u>subluxation</u> of <u>left</u> radial head
S53.093- Other <u>subluxation</u> of <u>unspecified</u> radial head
S53.094- Other <u>dislocation</u> of <u>right</u> radial head
S53.095- Other <u>dislocation</u> of <u>left</u> radial head
S53.096- Other <u>dislocation</u> of <u>unspecified</u> radial head

S53.1- Subluxation and dislocation of <u>ulnohumeral joint</u>
Subluxation and dislocation of elbow NOS
Excludes 1:   dislocation of radial head alone (S53.0-)

S53.10- <u>Unspecified</u> subluxation and dislocation of <u>ulnohumeral joint</u>
S53.101- Unspecified <u>subluxation</u> of <u>right</u> ulnohumeral joint
S53.102- Unspecified <u>subluxation</u> of <u>left</u> ulnohumeral joint
S53.103- Unspecified <u>subluxation</u> of <u>unspecified</u> ulnohumeral joint
S53.104- Unspecified <u>dislocation</u> of <u>right</u> ulnohumeral joint
S53.105- Unspecified <u>dislocation</u> of <u>left</u> ulnohumeral joint
S53.106- Unspecified <u>dislocation</u> of <u>unspecified</u> ulnohumeral joint

S53.11- <u>Anterior</u> subluxation and dislocation of <u>ulnohumeral joint</u>
S53.111- Anterior <u>subluxation</u> of <u>right</u> ulnohumeral joint
S53.112- Anterior <u>subluxation</u> of <u>left</u> ulnohumeral joint
S53.113- Anterior <u>subluxation</u> of <u>unspecified</u> ulnohumeral joint
S53.114- Anterior <u>dislocation</u> of <u>right</u> ulnohumeral joint
S53.115- Anterior <u>dislocation</u> of <u>left</u> ulnohumeral joint
S53.116- Anterior <u>dislocation</u> of <u>unspecified</u> ulnohumeral joint

S53.12- <u>Posterior</u> subluxation and dislocation of <u>ulnohumeral joint</u>
S53.121- Posterior <u>subluxation</u> of <u>right</u> ulnohumeral joint
S53.122- Posterior <u>subluxation</u> of <u>left</u> ulnohumeral joint
S53.123- Posterior <u>subluxation</u> of <u>unspecified</u> ulnohumeral joint
S53.124- Posterior <u>dislocation</u> of <u>right</u> ulnohumeral joint
S53.125- Posterior <u>dislocation</u> of <u>left</u> ulnohumeral joint
S53.126- Posterior <u>dislocation</u> of <u>unspecified</u> ulnohumeral joint

S53.13- <u>Medial</u> subluxation and dislocation of <u>ulnohumeral joint</u>
S53.131- Medial <u>subluxation</u> of <u>right</u> ulnohumeral joint
S53.132- Medial <u>subluxation</u> of <u>left</u> ulnohumeral joint
S53.133- Medial <u>subluxation</u> of <u>unspecified</u> ulnohumeral joint
S53.134- Medial <u>dislocation</u> of <u>right</u> ulnohumeral joint
S53.135- Medial <u>dislocation</u> of <u>left</u> ulnohumeral joint
S53.136- Medial <u>dislocation</u> of <u>unspecified</u> ulnohumeral joint

S53.14- <u>Lateral</u> subluxation and dislocation of <u>ulnohumeral joint</u>
S53.141- Lateral <u>subluxation</u> of <u>right</u> ulnohumeral joint
S53.142- Lateral <u>subluxation</u> of <u>left</u> ulnohumeral joint
S53.143- Lateral <u>subluxation</u> of <u>unspecified</u> ulnohumeral joint
S53.144- Lateral <u>dislocation</u> of <u>right</u> ulnohumeral joint
S53.145- Lateral <u>dislocation</u> of <u>left</u> ulnohumeral joint
S53.146- Lateral <u>dislocation</u> of <u>unspecified</u> ulnohumeral joint

S53.19- <u>Other</u> subluxation and dislocation of <u>ulnohumeral joint</u>
S53.191- Other <u>subluxation</u> of <u>right</u> ulnohumeral joint
S53.192- Other <u>subluxation</u> of <u>left</u> ulnohumeral joint
S53.193- Other <u>subluxation</u> of <u>unspecified</u> ulnohumeral joint

S53.194- Other <u>dislocation</u> of <u>right</u> ulnohumeral joint
S53.195- Other <u>dislocation</u> of <u>left</u> ulnohumeral joint
S53.196- Other <u>dislocation</u> of <u>unspecified</u> ulnohumeral joint

S53.2- <u>Traumatic rupture</u> of <u>radial collateral ligament</u>
  Excludes 1: sprain of radial collateral ligament NOS (S53.43-)
  S53.20x- **Traumatic rupture** of <u>unspecified</u> radial collateral ligament
  S53.21x- **Traumatic rupture** of <u>right</u> radial collateral ligament
  S53.22x- **Traumatic rupture** of <u>left</u> radial collateral ligament

S53.3- <u>Traumatic rupture</u> of <u>ulnar collateral ligament</u>
  Excludes 1: sprain of ulnar collateral ligament (S53.44-)
  S53.30x- **Traumatic rupture** of <u>unspecified</u> ulnar collateral ligament
  S53.31x- **Traumatic rupture** of <u>right</u> ulnar collateral ligament
  S53.32x- **Traumatic rupture** of <u>left</u> ulnar collateral ligament

S53.4- <u>Sprain</u> of <u>elbow</u>
  Excludes ❷: traumatic rupture of radial collateral ligament (S53.2-)
  traumatic rupture of ulnar collateral ligament (S53.3-)
  S53.40- <u>Unspecified</u> sprain of <u>elbow</u>
    S53.401- **Unspecified** sprain of <u>right</u> elbow
    S53.402- **Unspecified** sprain of <u>left</u> elbow
    S53.409- **Unspecified** sprain of <u>unspecified</u> elbow
      Sprain of elbow NOS
  S53.41- <u>Radiohumeral</u> (joint) <u>sprain</u>
    S53.411- **Radiohumeral** (joint) sprain of <u>right</u> elbow
    S53.412- **Radiohumeral** (joint) sprain of <u>left</u> elbow
    S53.419- **Radiohumeral** (joint) sprain of <u>unspecified</u> elbow
  S53.42- <u>Ulnohumeral</u> (joint) <u>sprain</u>
    S53.421- **Ulnohumeral** (joint) sprain of <u>right</u> elbow
    S53.422- **Ulnohumeral** (joint) sprain of <u>left</u> elbow
    S53.429- **Ulnohumeral** (joint) sprain of <u>unspecified</u> elbow
  S53.43- <u>Radial collateral ligament</u> <u>sprain</u>
    S53.431- **Radial collateral ligament** sprain of <u>right</u> elbow
    S53.432- **Radial collateral ligament** sprain of <u>left</u> elbow
    S53.439- **Radial collateral ligament** sprain of <u>unspecified</u> elbow
  S53.44- <u>Ulnar collateral ligament</u> <u>sprain</u>
    S53.441- **Ulnar collateral ligament** sprain of <u>right</u> elbow
    S53.442- **Ulnar collateral ligament** sprain of <u>left</u> elbow
    S53.449- **Ulnar collateral ligament** sprain of <u>unspecified</u> elbow
  S53.49- <u>Other</u> sprain of <u>elbow</u>
    S53.491- **Other** sprain of <u>right</u> elbow
    S53.492- **Other** sprain of <u>left</u> elbow
    S53.499- **Other** sprain of <u>unspecified</u> elbow

S54- Injury of <u>nerves</u> at <u>forearm level</u>
  Code also any associated open wound (S51.-)
  Excludes ❷: injury of nerves at wrist and hand level (S64.-)
  The appropriate 7th character is to be added to each code from category S54:
  A <u>Initial</u> encounter
  D <u>Subsequent</u> encounter
  S <u>Sequela</u>

S54.0- Injury of <u>ulnar</u> nerve at <u>forearm level</u>
    Injury of ulnar nerve NOS
  S54.00x- Injury of ulnar nerve at forearm level, <u>unspecified</u> arm
  S54.01x- Injury of ulnar nerve at forearm level, <u>right</u> arm
  S54.02x- Injury of ulnar nerve at forearm level, <u>left</u> arm

S54.1- Injury of <u>median</u> nerve at <u>forearm level</u>
    Injury of median nerve NOS
  S54.10x- Injury of median nerve at forearm level, <u>unspecified</u> arm
  S54.11x- Injury of median nerve at forearm level, <u>right</u> arm
  S54.12x- Injury of median nerve at forearm level, <u>left</u> arm

S54.2- Injury of <u>radial</u> nerve at <u>forearm level</u>
    Injury of radial nerve NOS
  S54.20x- Injury of radial nerve at forearm level, <u>unspecified</u> arm

S54.21x- Injury of radial nerve at forearm level, <u>right</u> arm
S54.22x- Injury of radial nerve at forearm level, <u>left</u> arm

S54.3- Injury of <u>cutaneous sensory</u> nerve at <u>forearm level</u>
  S54.30x- Injury of cutaneous sensory nerve at forearm level, <u>unspecified</u> arm
  S54.31x- Injury of cutaneous sensory nerve at forearm level, <u>right</u> arm
  S54.32x- Injury of cutaneous sensory nerve at forearm level, <u>left</u> arm

S54.8- Injury of <u>other nerves</u> at <u>forearm level</u>
  S54.8x- Injury of other nerves at forearm level
    S54.8x1- Injury of other nerves at forearm level, <u>right</u> arm
    S54.8x2- Injury of other nerves at forearm level, <u>left</u> arm
    S54.8x9- Injury of other nerves at forearm level, <u>unspecified</u> arm

S54.9- Injury of <u>unspecified nerve</u> at <u>forearm level</u>
  S54.90x- Injury of unspecified nerve at forearm level, <u>unspecified</u> arm
  S54.91x- Injury of unspecified nerve at forearm level, <u>right</u> arm
  S54.92x- Injury of unspecified nerve at forearm level, <u>left</u> arm

S55- <u>Injury of blood vessels</u> at <u>forearm level</u>
  Code also any associated open wound (S51.-)
  Excludes ❷: injury of blood vessels at wrist and hand level (S65.-)
  injury of brachial vessels (S45.1-S45.2)
  The appropriate 7th character is to be added to each code from category S55:
  A <u>Initial</u> encounter
  D <u>Subsequent</u> encounter
  S <u>Sequela</u>

S55.0- Injury of <u>ulnar artery</u> at <u>forearm level</u>
  S55.00- <u>Unspecified</u> injury of <u>ulnar artery</u> at <u>forearm level</u>
    CC-A S55.001- Unspecified injury of ulnar artery at forearm level, <u>right</u> arm
    CC-A S55.002- Unspecified injury of ulnar artery at forearm level, <u>left</u> arm
    CC-A S55.009- Unspecified injury of ulnar artery at forearm level, <u>unspecified</u> arm
  S55.01- <u>Laceration</u> of <u>ulnar artery</u> at <u>forearm level</u>
    CC-A S55.011- Laceration of ulnar artery at forearm level, <u>right</u> arm
    CC-A S55.012- Laceration of ulnar artery at forearm level, <u>left</u> arm
    CC-A S55.019- Laceration of ulnar artery at forearm level, <u>unspecified</u> arm
  S55.09- <u>Other</u> specified injury of <u>ulnar artery</u> at <u>forearm level</u>
    CC-A S55.091- Other specified injury of ulnar artery at forearm level, <u>right</u> arm
    CC-A S55.092- Other specified injury of ulnar artery at forearm level, <u>left</u> arm
    CC-A S55.099- Other specified injury of ulnar artery at forearm level, <u>unspecified</u> arm

S55.1- Injury of <u>radial artery</u> at <u>forearm level</u>
  S55.10- Unspecified injury of radial artery at forearm level
    CC-A S55.101- Unspecified injury of radial artery at forearm level, <u>right</u> arm
    CC-A S55.102- Unspecified injury of radial artery at forearm level, <u>left</u> arm
    CC-A S55.109- Unspecified injury of radial artery at forearm level, <u>unspecified</u> arm
  S55.11- <u>Laceration</u> of <u>radial artery</u> at <u>forearm level</u>
    CC-A S55.111- Laceration of radial artery at forearm level, <u>right</u> arm
    CC-A S55.112- Laceration of radial artery at forearm level, <u>left</u> arm
    CC-A S55.119- Laceration of radial artery at forearm level, <u>unspecified</u> arm
  S55.19- <u>Other</u> specified injury of <u>radial artery</u> at <u>forearm level</u>
    CC-A S55.191- Other specified injury of radial artery at forearm level, <u>right</u> arm

S
5
3
–
S
5
5

Excludes 1: = NOT CODED HERE! (Do not code both)   **1073**   *Excludes ❷:* = Not Included Here

CC-A **S55.192-** Other specified injury of radial artery at forearm level, <u>left</u> arm

CC-A **S55.199-** Other specified injury of radial artery at forearm level, <u>unspecified</u> arm

S55.2- Injury of <u>vein</u> at <u>forearm level</u>

S55.20- <u>Unspecified</u> injury of <u>vein</u> at <u>forearm level</u>

CC-A **S55.201-** Unspecified injury of vein at forearm level, <u>right</u> arm

CC-A **S55.202-** Unspecified injury of vein at forearm level, <u>left</u> arm

CC-A **S55.209-** Unspecified injury of vein at forearm level, <u>unspecified</u> arm

S55.21- <u>Laceration</u> of <u>vein</u> at <u>forearm level</u>

CC-A **S55.211-** Laceration of vein at forearm level, <u>right</u> arm

CC-A **S55.212-** Laceration of vein at forearm level, <u>left</u> arm

CC-A **S55.219-** Laceration of vein at forearm level, <u>unspecified</u> arm

S55.29- <u>Other specified injury</u> of <u>vein</u> at <u>forearm level</u>

CC-A **S55.291-** Other specified injury of vein at forearm level, <u>right</u> arm

CC-A **S55.292-** Other specified injury of vein at forearm level, <u>left</u> arm

CC-A **S55.299-** Other specified injury of vein at forearm level, <u>unspecified</u> arm

S55.8- Injury of <u>other blood vessels</u> at <u>forearm level</u>

S55.80- <u>Unspecified</u> injury of <u>other blood vessels</u> at <u>forearm level</u>

CC-A **S55.801-** Unspecified injury of other blood vessels at forearm level, <u>right</u> arm

CC-A **S55.802-** Unspecified injury of other blood vessels at forearm level, <u>left</u> arm

CC-A **S55.809-** Unspecified injury of other blood vessels at forearm level, <u>unspecified</u> arm

S55.81- <u>Laceration</u> of <u>other blood vessels</u> at <u>forearm level</u>

CC-A **S55.811-** Laceration of other blood vessels at forearm level, <u>right</u> arm

CC-A **S55.812-** Laceration of other blood vessels at forearm level, <u>left</u> arm

CC-A **S55.819-** Laceration of other blood vessels at forearm level, <u>unspecified</u> arm

S55.89- <u>Other specified injury</u> of <u>other blood vessels</u> at <u>forearm level</u>

CC-A **S55.891-** Other specified injury of other blood vessels at forearm level, <u>right</u> arm

CC-A **S55.892-** Other specified injury of other blood vessels at forearm level, <u>left</u> arm

CC-A **S55.899-** Other specified injury of other blood vessels at forearm level, <u>unspecified</u> arm

S55.9- Injury of <u>unspecified blood vessel</u> at <u>forearm level</u>

S55.90- <u>Unspecified</u> injury of <u>unspecified blood vessel</u> at <u>forearm level</u>

CC-A **S55.901-** Unspecified injury of unspecified blood vessel at forearm level, <u>right</u> arm

CC-A **S55.902-** Unspecified injury of unspecified blood vessel at forearm level, <u>left</u> arm

CC-A **S55.909-** Unspecified injury of unspecified blood vessel at forearm level, <u>unspecified</u> arm

S55.91- <u>Laceration</u> of <u>unspecified blood vessel</u> at <u>forearm level</u>

CC-A **S55.911-** Laceration of unspecified blood vessel at forearm level, <u>right</u> arm

CC-A **S55.912-** Laceration of unspecified blood vessel at forearm level, <u>left</u> arm

CC-A **S55.919-** Laceration of unspecified blood vessel at forearm level, <u>unspecified</u> arm

S55.99- <u>Other specified injury</u> of <u>unspecified blood vessel</u> at <u>forearm level</u>

CC-A **S55.991-** Other specified injury of <u>unspecified</u> blood vessel at forearm level, <u>right</u> arm

CC-A **S55.992-** Other specified injury of <u>unspecified</u> blood vessel at forearm level, <u>left</u> arm

CC-A **S55.999-** Other specified injury of <u>unspecified</u> blood vessel at forearm level, <u>unspecified</u> arm

S56- <u>Injury of muscle, fascia and tendon</u> at <u>forearm level</u>
Code also any associated open wound (S51.-)
Excludes ❷: *injury of muscle, fascia and tendon at or below wrist (S66.-)*
sprain of joints and ligaments of elbow (S53.4-)

The appropriate 7th character is to be added to each code from category S56:
A   <u>Initial</u> encounter
D   <u>Subsequent</u> encounter
S   <u>Sequela</u>

S56.0- Injury of <u>flexor</u> muscle, fascia and tendon of <u>thumb</u> at <u>forearm level</u>

S56.00- <u>Unspecified</u> injury of <u>flexor</u> muscle, fascia and tendon of <u>thumb</u> at <u>forearm level</u>

S56.001- Unspecified injury of flexor muscle, fascia and tendon of <u>right</u> thumb at forearm level

S56.002- Unspecified injury of flexor muscle, fascia and tendon of <u>left</u> thumb at forearm level

S56.009- Unspecified injury of flexor muscle, fascia and tendon of <u>unspecified</u> thumb at forearm level

S56.01- <u>Strain</u> of <u>flexor</u> muscle, fascia and tendon of <u>thumb</u> at <u>forearm level</u>

S56.011- Strain of flexor muscle, fascia and tendon of <u>right</u> thumb at forearm level

S56.012- Strain of flexor muscle, fascia and tendon of <u>left</u> thumb at forearm level

S56.019- Strain of flexor muscle, fascia and tendon of <u>unspecified</u> thumb at forearm level

S56.02- <u>Laceration</u> of <u>flexor</u> muscle, fascia and tendon of <u>thumb</u> at <u>forearm level</u>

CC-A **S56.021-** Laceration of flexor muscle, fascia and tendon of <u>right</u> thumb at forearm level

CC-A **S56.022-** Laceration of flexor muscle, fascia and tendon of <u>left</u> thumb at forearm level

CC-A **S56.029-** Laceration of flexor muscle, fascia and tendon of <u>unspecified</u> thumb at forearm level

S56.09- <u>Other injury</u> of <u>flexor</u> muscle, fascia and tendon of <u>thumb</u> at <u>forearm level</u>

S56.091- Other injury of flexor muscle, fascia and tendon of <u>right</u> thumb at forearm level

S56.092- Other injury of flexor muscle, fascia and tendon of <u>left</u> thumb at forearm level

S56.099- Other injury of flexor muscle, fascia and tendon of <u>unspecified</u> thumb at forearm level

S56.1- Injury of <u>flexor</u> muscle, fascia and tendon <u>of other and unspecified</u> <u>finger</u> at <u>forearm level</u>

S56.10- <u>Unspecified</u> injury of <u>flexor</u> muscle, fascia and tendon of other and unspecified <u>finger</u> at <u>forearm level</u>

S56.101- Unspecified injury of flexor muscle, fascia and tendon of <u>right index</u> finger at forearm level

S56.102- Unspecified injury of flexor muscle, fascia and tendon of <u>left index</u> finger at forearm level

S56.103- Unspecified injury of flexor muscle, fascia and tendon of <u>right middle</u> finger at forearm level

S56.104- Unspecified injury of flexor muscle, fascia and tendon of <u>left middle</u> finger at forearm level

S56.105- Unspecified injury of flexor muscle, fascia and tendon of <u>right ring</u> finger at forearm level

S56.106- Unspecified injury of flexor muscle, fascia and tendon of <u>left ring</u> finger at forearm level

S56.107- Unspecified injury of flexor muscle, fascia and tendon of <u>right little</u> finger at forearm level

S56.108- Unspecified injury of flexor muscle, fascia and tendon of <u>left little</u> finger at forearm level

S56.109- Unspecified injury of flexor muscle, fascia and tendon of <u>unspecified finger</u> at forearm level

S55 – S56

S56.11- Strain of flexor muscle, fascia and tendon of other and unspecified finger at forearm level

S56.111- Strain of flexor muscle, fascia and tendon of right index finger at forearm level

S56.112- Strain of flexor muscle, fascia and tendon of left index finger at forearm level

S56.113- Strain of flexor muscle, fascia and tendon of right middle finger at forearm level

S56.114- Strain of flexor muscle, fascia and tendon of left middle finger at forearm level

S56.115- Strain of flexor muscle, fascia and tendon of right ring finger at forearm level

S56.116- Strain of flexor muscle, fascia and tendon of left ring finger at forearm level

S56.117- Strain of flexor muscle, fascia and tendon of right little finger at forearm level

S56.118- Strain of flexor muscle, fascia and tendon of left little finger at forearm level

S56.119- Strain of flexor muscle, fascia and tendon of finger of unspecified finger at forearm level

S56.12- Laceration of flexor muscle, fascia and tendon of other and unspecified finger at forearm level

CC-A **S56.121-** Laceration of flexor muscle, fascia and tendon of right index finger at forearm level

CC-A **S56.122-** Laceration of flexor muscle, fascia and tendon of left index finger at forearm level

CC-A **S56.123-** Laceration of flexor muscle, fascia and tendon of right middle finger at forearm level

CC-A **S56.124-** Laceration of flexor muscle, fascia and tendon of left middle finger at forearm level

CC-A **S56.125-** Laceration of flexor muscle, fascia and tendon of right ring finger at forearm level

CC-A **S56.126-** Laceration of flexor muscle, fascia and tendon of left ring finger at forearm level

CC-A **S56.127-** Laceration of flexor muscle, fascia and tendon of right little finger at forearm level

CC-A **S56.128-** Laceration of flexor muscle, fascia and tendon of left little finger at forearm level

CC-A **S56.129-** Laceration of flexor muscle, fascia and tendon of unspecified finger at forearm level

S56.19- Other injury of flexor muscle, fascia and tendon of other and unspecified finger at forearm level

S56.191- Other injury of flexor muscle, fascia and tendon of right index finger at forearm level

S56.192- Other injury of flexor muscle, fascia and tendon of left index finger at forearm level

S56.193- Other injury of flexor muscle, fascia and tendon of right middle finger at forearm level

S56.194- Other injury of flexor muscle, fascia and tendon of left middle finger at forearm level

S56.195- Other injury of flexor muscle, fascia and tendon of right ring finger at forearm level

S56.196- Other injury of flexor muscle, fascia and tendon of left ring finger at forearm level

S56.197- Other injury of flexor muscle, fascia and tendon of right little finger at forearm level

S56.198- Other injury of flexor muscle, fascia and tendon of left little finger at forearm level

S56.199- Other injury of flexor muscle, fascia and tendon of unspecified finger at forearm level

S56.2- Injury of other flexor muscle, fascia and tendon at forearm level

S56.20- Unspecified injury of other flexor muscle, fascia and tendon at forearm level

S56.201- Unspecified injury of other flexor muscle, fascia and tendon at forearm level, right arm

S56.202- Unspecified injury of other flexor muscle, fascia and tendon at forearm level, left arm

S56.209- Unspecified injury of other flexor muscle, fascia and tendon at forearm level, unspecified arm

S56.21- Strain of other flexor muscle, fascia and tendon at forearm level

S56.211- Strain of other flexor muscle, fascia and tendon at forearm level, right arm

S56.212- Strain of other flexor muscle, fascia and tendon at forearm level, left arm

S56.219- Strain of other flexor muscle, fascia and tendon at forearm level, unspecified arm

S56.22- Laceration of other flexor muscle, fascia and tendon at forearm level

CC-A **S56.221-** Laceration of other flexor muscle, fascia and tendon at forearm level, right arm

CC-A **S56.222-** Laceration of other flexor muscle, fascia and tendon at forearm level, left arm

CC-A **S56.229-** Laceration of other flexor muscle, fascia and tendon at forearm level, unspecified arm

S56.29- Other injury of other flexor muscle, fascia and tendon at forearm level

S56.291- Other injury of other flexor muscle, fascia and tendon at forearm level, right arm

S56.292- Other injury of other flexor muscle, fascia and tendon at forearm level, left arm

S56.299- Other injury of other flexor muscle, fascia and tendon at forearm level, unspecified arm

S56.3- Injury of extensor or abductor muscles, fascia and tendons of thumb at forearm level

S56.30- Unspecified injury of extensor or abductor muscles, fascia and tendons of thumb at forearm level

S56.301- Unspecified injury of extensor or abductor muscles, fascia and tendons of right thumb at forearm level

S56.302- Unspecified injury of extensor or abductor muscles, fascia and tendons of left thumb at forearm level

S56.309- Unspecified injury of extensor or abductor muscles, fascia and tendons of unspecified thumb at forearm level

S56.31- Strain of extensor or abductor muscles, fascia and tendons of thumb at forearm level

S56.311- Strain of extensor or abductor muscles, fascia and tendons of right thumb at forearm level

S56.312- Strain of extensor or abductor muscles, fascia and tendons of left thumb at forearm level

S56.319- Strain of extensor or abductor muscles, fascia and tendons of unspecified thumb at forearm level

S56.32- Laceration of extensor or abductor muscles, fascia and tendons of thumb at forearm level

CC-A **S56.321-** Laceration of extensor or abductor muscles, fascia and tendons of right thumb at forearm level

CC-A **S56.322-** Laceration of extensor or abductor muscles, fascia and tendons of left thumb at forearm level

CC-A **S56.329-** Laceration of extensor or abductor muscles, fascia and tendons of unspecified thumb at forearm level

S56.39- Other injury of extensor or abductor muscles, fascia and tendons of thumb at forearm level

S56.391- Other injury of extensor or abductor muscles, fascia and tendons of right thumb at forearm level

S56.392- Other injury of extensor or abductor muscles, fascia and tendons of left thumb at forearm level

S56.399- Other injury of extensor or abductor muscles, fascia and tendons of unspecified thumb at forearm level

S56.4- Injury of extensor muscle, fascia and tendon of other and unspecified finger at forearm level

S56.40- Unspecified injury of extensor muscle, fascia and tendon of other and unspecified finger at forearm level

S56.401- Unspecified injury of extensor muscle, fascia and tendon of right index finger at forearm level

S56.402- Unspecified injury of extensor muscle, fascia and tendon of left index finger at forearm level

S56 | S56 | S56

S56.403- Unspecified injury of extensor muscle, fascia and tendon of <u>right middle</u> finger at forearm level

S56.404- Unspecified injury of extensor muscle, fascia and tendon of <u>left middle</u> finger at forearm level

S56.405- Unspecified injury of extensor muscle, fascia and tendon of <u>right ring</u> finger at forearm level

S56.406- Unspecified injury of extensor muscle, fascia and tendon of <u>left ring</u> finger at forearm level

S56.407- Unspecified injury of extensor muscle, fascia and tendon of <u>right little</u> finger at forearm level

S56.408- Unspecified injury of extensor muscle, fascia and tendon of <u>left little</u> finger at forearm level

S56.409- Unspecified injury of extensor muscle, fascia and tendon of <u>unspecified finger</u> at forearm level

S56.41- <u>Strain</u> of <u>extensor</u> muscle, fascia and tendon of other and unspecified <u>finger</u> at <u>forearm level</u>

S56.411- Strain of extensor muscle, fascia and tendon of <u>right index</u> finger at forearm level

S56.412- Strain of extensor muscle, fascia and tendon of <u>left index</u> finger at forearm level

S56.413- Strain of extensor muscle, fascia and tendon of <u>right middle</u> finger at forearm level

S56.414- Strain of extensor muscle, fascia and tendon of <u>left middle</u> finger at forearm level

S56.415- Strain of extensor muscle, fascia and tendon of <u>right ring</u> finger at forearm level

S56.416- Strain of extensor muscle, fascia and tendon of <u>left ring</u> finger at forearm level

S56.417- Strain of extensor muscle, fascia and tendon of <u>right little</u> finger at forearm level

S56.418- Strain of extensor muscle, fascia and tendon of <u>left little</u> finger at forearm level

S56.419- Strain of extensor muscle, fascia and tendon of finger, <u>unspecified finger</u> at forearm level

S56.42- <u>Laceration</u> of <u>extensor</u> muscle, fascia and tendon of other and unspecified <u>finger</u> at forearm level

CC-A S56.421- Laceration of extensor muscle, fascia and tendon of <u>right index</u> finger at forearm level

CC-A S56.422- Laceration of extensor muscle, fascia and tendon of <u>left index</u> finger at forearm level

CC-A S56.423- Laceration of extensor muscle, fascia and tendon of <u>right middle</u> finger at forearm level

CC-A S56.424- Laceration of extensor muscle, fascia and tendon of <u>left middle</u> finger at forearm level

CC-A S56.425- Laceration of extensor muscle, fascia and tendon of <u>right ring</u> finger at forearm level

CC-A S56.426- Laceration of extensor muscle, fascia and tendon of <u>left ring</u> finger at forearm level

CC-A S56.427- Laceration of extensor muscle, fascia and tendon of <u>right little</u> finger at forearm level

CC-A S56.428- Laceration of extensor muscle, fascia and tendon of <u>left little</u> finger at forearm level

CC-A S56.429- Laceration of extensor muscle, fascia and tendon of <u>unspecified finger</u> at forearm level

S56.49- <u>Other injury</u> of <u>extensor</u> muscle, fascia and tendon of other and unspecified <u>finger</u> at <u>forearm level</u>

S56.491- Other injury of extensor muscle, fascia and tendon of <u>right index</u> finger at forearm level

S56.492- Other injury of extensor muscle, fascia and tendon of <u>left index</u> finger at forearm level

S56.493- Other injury of extensor muscle, fascia and tendon of <u>right middle</u> finger at forearm level

S56.494- Other injury of extensor muscle, fascia and tendon of <u>left middle</u> finger at forearm level

S56.495- Other injury of extensor muscle, fascia and tendon of <u>right ring</u> finger at forearm level

S56.496- Other injury of extensor muscle, fascia and tendon of <u>left ring</u> finger at forearm level

S56.497- Other injury of extensor muscle, fascia and tendon of <u>right little</u> finger at forearm level

S56.498- Other injury of extensor muscle, fascia and tendon of <u>left little</u> finger at forearm level

S56.499- Other injury of extensor muscle, fascia and tendon of <u>unspecified finger</u> at forearm level

S56.5- <u>Injury</u> of <u>other extensor</u> muscle, fascia and tendon at forearm level

S56.50- <u>Unspecified</u> injury of <u>other extensor</u> muscle, fascia and tendon at <u>forearm level</u>

S56.501- Unspecified injury of other extensor muscle, fascia and tendon at forearm level, <u>right arm</u>

S56.502- Unspecified injury of other extensor muscle, fascia and tendon at forearm level, <u>left arm</u>

S56.509- Unspecified injury of other extensor muscle, fascia and tendon at forearm level, <u>unspecified</u> arm

S56.51- <u>Strain</u> of <u>other extensor</u> muscle, fascia and tendon at <u>forearm level</u>

S56.511- Strain of other extensor muscle, fascia and tendon at forearm level, <u>right arm</u>

S56.512- Strain of other extensor muscle, fascia and tendon at forearm level, <u>left arm</u>

S56.519- Strain of other extensor muscle, fascia and tendon at forearm level, <u>unspecified</u> arm

S56.52- <u>Laceration</u> of <u>other extensor</u> muscle, fascia and tendon at <u>forearm level</u>

CC-A S56.521- Laceration of other extensor muscle, fascia and tendon at forearm level, <u>right arm</u>

CC-A S56.522- Laceration of other extensor muscle, fascia and tendon at forearm level, <u>left arm</u>

CC-A S56.529- Laceration of other extensor muscle, fascia and tendon at forearm level, <u>unspecified</u> arm

S56.59- <u>Other injury</u> of <u>other extensor</u> muscle, fascia and tendon at <u>forearm level</u>

S56.591- Other injury of other extensor muscle, fascia and tendon at forearm level, <u>right arm</u>

S56.592- Other injury of other extensor muscle, fascia and tendon at forearm level, <u>left arm</u>

S56.599- Other injury of other extensor muscle, fascia and tendon at forearm level, <u>unspecified</u> arm

S56.8- <u>Injury</u> of <u>other</u> muscles, fascia and tendons at <u>forearm level</u>

S56.80- <u>Unspecified</u> injury of <u>other</u> muscles, fascia and tendons at <u>forearm level</u>

S56.801- Unspecified injury of other muscles, fascia and tendons at forearm level, <u>right arm</u>

S56.802- Unspecified injury of other muscles, fascia and tendons at forearm level, <u>left arm</u>

S56.809- Unspecified injury of other muscles, fascia and tendons at forearm level, <u>unspecified</u> arm

S56.81- <u>Strain</u> of <u>other</u> muscles, fascia and tendons at <u>forearm level</u>

S56.811- Strain of other muscles, fascia and tendons at forearm level, <u>right arm</u>

S56.812- Strain of other muscles, fascia and tendons at forearm level, <u>left arm</u>

S56.819- Strain of other muscles, fascia and tendons at forearm level, <u>unspecified</u> arm

S56.82- <u>Laceration</u> of <u>other</u> muscles, fascia and tendons at <u>forearm level</u>

CC-A S56.821- Laceration of other muscles, fascia and tendons at forearm level, <u>right arm</u>

CC-A S56.822- Laceration of other muscles, fascia and tendons at forearm level, <u>left arm</u>

CC-A S56.829- Laceration of other muscles, fascia and tendons at forearm level, <u>unspecified</u> arm

S56.89- <u>Other injury</u> of <u>other</u> muscles, fascia and tendons at <u>forearm level</u>

S56.891- Other injury of other muscles, fascia and tendons at forearm level, <u>right arm</u>

Excludes 1: = NOT CODED HERE! (Do not code both)   1076   *Excludes ❷:* = Not Included Here

S55–S56

S56.892- Other injury of other muscles, fascia and tendons at forearm level, <u>left</u> arm

S56.899- Other injury of other muscles, fascia and tendons at forearm level, <u>unspecified</u> arm

S56.9- <u>Injury</u> of <u>unspecified</u> muscles, fascia and tendons at <u>forearm level</u>

    S56.90- <u>Unspecified</u> injury of <u>unspecified</u> muscles, fascia and tendons at <u>forearm level</u>

      S56.901- Unspecified injury of unspecified muscles, fascia and tendons at forearm level, <u>right</u> arm

      S56.902- Unspecified injury of unspecified muscles, fascia and tendons at forearm level, <u>left</u> arm

      S56.909- Unspecified injury of unspecified muscles, fascia and tendons at forearm level, <u>unspecified</u> arm

    S56.91- <u>Strain</u> of <u>unspecified</u> muscles, fascia and tendons at <u>forearm level</u>

      S56.911- Strain of unspecified muscles, fascia and tendons at forearm level, <u>right</u> arm

      S56.912- Strain of unspecified muscles, fascia and tendons at forearm level, <u>left</u> arm

      S56.919- Strain of unspecified muscles, fascia and tendons at forearm level, <u>unspecified</u> arm

    S56.92- <u>Laceration</u> of <u>unspecified</u> muscles, fascia and tendons at <u>forearm level</u>

  CC-A **S56.921-** Laceration of unspecified muscles, fascia and tendons at forearm level, <u>right</u> arm

  CC-A **S56.922-** Laceration of unspecified muscles, fascia and tendons at forearm level, <u>left</u> arm

  CC-A **S56.929-** Laceration of unspecified muscles, fascia and tendons at forearm level, <u>unspecified</u> arm

    S56.99- <u>Other injury</u> of <u>unspecified</u> muscles, fascia and tendons at <u>forearm level</u>

      S56.991- Other injury of unspecified muscles, fascia and tendons at forearm level, <u>right</u> arm

      S56.992- Other injury of unspecified muscles, fascia and tendons at forearm level, <u>left</u> arm

      S56.999- Other injury of unspecified muscles, fascia and tendons at forearm level, <u>unspecified</u> arm

S57- <u>Crushing</u> injury of <u>elbow and forearm</u>
Use additional code(s) for all associated injuries
Excludes ❷: crushing injury of wrist and hand (S67.-)

The appropriate 7th character is to be added to each code from category S57:
A <u>Initial</u> encounter
D <u>Subsequent</u> encounter
S <u>Sequela</u>

  S57.0- <u>Crushing</u> injury of <u>elbow</u>

    S57.00x- Crushing injury of <u>unspecified</u> elbow

    S57.01x- Crushing injury of <u>right</u> elbow

    S57.02x- Crushing injury of <u>left</u> elbow

  S57.8- <u>Crushing</u> injury of <u>forearm</u>

    S57.80x- Crushing injury of <u>unspecified</u> forearm

    S57.81x- Crushing injury of <u>right</u> forearm

    S57.82x- Crushing injury of <u>left</u> forearm

S58- <u>Traumatic amputation</u> of <u>elbow and forearm</u>
Note: An amputation not identified as partial or complete should be coded to complete
Excludes 1: traumatic amputation of wrist and hand (S68.-)

The appropriate 7th character is to be added to each code from category S58:
A <u>Initial</u> encounter
D <u>Subsequent</u> encounter
S <u>Sequela</u>

  S58.0- <u>Traumatic amputation</u> at <u>elbow level</u>

    S58.01- <u>Complete</u> traumatic amputation at <u>elbow level</u>

  CC-A **S58.011-** Complete traumatic amputation at elbow level, <u>right</u> arm

  CC-A **S58.012-** Complete traumatic amputation at elbow level, <u>left</u> arm

  CC-A **S58.019-** Complete traumatic amputation at elbow level, <u>unspecified</u> arm

    S58.02- <u>Partial</u> traumatic amputation at <u>elbow level</u>

  CC-A **S58.021-** Partial traumatic amputation at elbow level, <u>right</u> arm

  CC-A **S58.022-** Partial traumatic amputation at elbow level, <u>left</u> arm

  CC-A **S58.029-** Partial traumatic amputation at elbow level, <u>unspecified</u> arm

  S58.1- <u>Traumatic amputation</u> at <u>level between elbow and wrist</u>

    S58.11- <u>Complete</u> traumatic amputation at <u>level between elbow and wrist</u>

  CC-A **S58.111-** Complete traumatic amputation at level between elbow and wrist, <u>right</u> arm

  CC-A **S58.112-** Complete traumatic amputation at level between elbow and wrist, <u>left</u> arm

  CC-A **S58.119-** Complete traumatic amputation at level between elbow and wrist, <u>unspecified</u> arm

    S58.12- <u>Partial</u> traumatic amputation at <u>level between elbow and wrist</u>

  CC-A **S58.121-** Partial traumatic amputation at level between elbow and wrist, <u>right</u> arm

  CC-A **S58.122-** Partial traumatic amputation at level between elbow and wrist, <u>left</u> arm

  CC-A **S58.129-** Partial traumatic amputation at level between elbow and wrist, <u>unspecified</u> arm

  S58.9- <u>Traumatic amputation</u> of forearm, <u>level unspecified</u>
Excludes 1: traumatic amputation of wrist (S68.-)

    S58.91- <u>Complete</u> traumatic amputation of forearm, <u>level unspecified</u>

  CC-A **S58.911-** Complete traumatic amputation of <u>right</u> forearm, level unspecified

  CC-A **S58.912-** Complete traumatic amputation of <u>left</u> forearm, level unspecified

  CC-A **S58.919-** Complete traumatic amputation of <u>unspecified</u> forearm, level unspecified

    S58.92- <u>Partial</u> traumatic amputation of forearm, <u>level unspecified</u>

  CC-A **S58.921-** Partial traumatic amputation of <u>right</u> forearm, level unspecified

  CC-A **S58.922-** Partial traumatic amputation of <u>left</u> forearm, level unspecified

  CC-A **S58.929-** Partial traumatic amputation of <u>unspecified</u> forearm, level unspecified

S59- <u>Other and unspecified injuries</u> of <u>elbow and forearm</u>
Excludes ❷: other and unspecified injuries of wrist and hand (S69.-)

The appropriate 7th character is to be added to each code from subcategories S59.0, S59.1, and S59.2:
A <u>Initial</u> encounter for <u>closed</u> fracture
D <u>Subsequent</u> encounter for fracture <u>with routine healing</u>
G <u>Subsequent</u> encounter for fracture <u>with delayed healing</u>
K <u>Subsequent</u> encounter for fracture <u>with nonunion</u>
P <u>Subsequent</u> encounter for fracture <u>with malunion</u>
S <u>Sequela</u>

  S59.0- <u>Physeal</u> fracture of <u>lower end</u> of <u>ulna</u>

    S59.00- <u>Unspecified physeal</u> fracture of <u>lower end</u> of <u>ulna</u>

  CC-A,K,P **S59.001-** Unspecified physeal fracture of lower end of ulna, <u>right</u> arm

  CC-A,K,P **S59.002-** Unspecified physeal fracture of lower end of ulna, <u>left</u> arm

  CC-A,K,P **S59.009-** Unspecified physeal fracture of lower end of ulna, <u>unspecified</u> arm

    S59.01- <u>Salter-Harris Type I</u> physeal fracture of <u>lower end</u> of <u>ulna</u>

  CC-A,K,P **S59.011-** Salter-Harris Type I physeal fracture of lower end of ulna, <u>right</u> arm

  CC-A,K,P **S59.012-** Salter-Harris Type I physeal fracture of lower end of ulna, <u>left</u> arm

  CC-A,K,P **S59.019-** Salter-Harris Type I physeal fracture of lower end of ulna, <u>unspecified</u> arm

S59.02- Salter-Harris Type II physeal fracture of lower end of ulna
CC-A,K,P **S59.021-** Salter-Harris Type II physeal fracture of lower end of ulna, right arm
CC-A,K,P **S59.022-** Salter-Harris Type II physeal fracture of lower end of ulna, left arm
CC-A,K,P **S59.029-** Salter-Harris Type II physeal fracture of lower end of ulna, unspecified arm
S59.03- Salter-Harris Type III physeal fracture of lower end of ulna
CC-A,K,P **S59.031-** Salter-Harris Type III physeal fracture of lower end of ulna, right arm
CC-A,K,P **S59.032-** Salter-Harris Type III physeal fracture of lower end of ulna, left arm
CC-A,K,P **S59.039-** Salter-Harris Type III physeal fracture of lower end of ulna, unspecified arm
S59.04- Salter-Harris Type IV physeal fracture of lower end of ulna
CC-A,K,P **S59.041-** Salter-Harris Type IV physeal fracture of lower end of ulna, right arm
CC-A,K,P **S59.042-** Salter-Harris Type IV physeal fracture of lower end of ulna, left arm
CC-A,K,P **S59.049-** Salter-Harris Type IV physeal fracture of lower end of ulna, unspecified arm
S59.09- Other physeal fracture of lower end of ulna
CC-A,K,P **S59.091-** Other physeal fracture of lower end of ulna, right arm
CC-A,K,P **S59.092-** Other physeal fracture of lower end of ulna, left arm
CC-A,K,P **S59.099-** Other physeal fracture of lower end of ulna, unspecified arm
S59.1- Physeal fracture of upper end of radius
S59.10- Unspecified physeal fracture of upper end of radius
CC-K,P **S59.101-** Unspecified physeal fracture of upper end of radius, right arm
CC-K,P **S59.102-** Unspecified physeal fracture of upper end of radius, left arm
CC-K,P **S59.109-** Unspecified physeal fracture of upper end of radius, unspecified arm
S59.11- Salter-Harris Type I physeal fracture of upper end of radius
CC-K,P **S59.111-** Salter-Harris Type I physeal fracture of upper end of radius, right arm
CC-K,P **S59.112-** Salter-Harris Type I physeal fracture of upper end of radius, left arm
CC-K,P **S59.119-** Salter-Harris Type I physeal fracture of upper end of radius, unspecified arm
S59.12- Salter-Harris Type II physeal fracture of upper end of radius
CC-K,P **S59.121-** Salter-Harris Type II physeal fracture of upper end of radius, right arm
CC-K,P **S59.122-** Salter-Harris Type II physeal fracture of upper end of radius, left arm
CC-K,P **S59.129-** Salter-Harris Type II physeal fracture of upper end of radius, unspecified arm
S59.13- Salter-Harris Type III physeal fracture of upper end of radius
CC-K,P **S59.131-** Salter-Harris Type III physeal fracture of upper end of radius, right arm
CC-K,P **S59.132-** Salter-Harris Type III physeal fracture of upper end of radius, left arm
CC-K,P **S59.139-** Salter-Harris Type III physeal fracture of upper end of radius, unspecified arm
S59.14- Salter-Harris Type IV physeal fracture of upper end of radius
CC-K,P **S59.141-** Salter-Harris Type IV physeal fracture of upper end of radius, right arm
CC-K,P **S59.142-** Salter-Harris Type IV physeal fracture of upper end of radius, left arm

CC-K,P **S59.149-** Salter-Harris Type IV physeal fracture of upper end of radius, unspecified arm
S59.19- Other physeal fracture of upper end of radius
CC-K,P **S59.191-** Other physeal fracture of upper end of radius, right arm
CC-K,P **S59.192-** Other physeal fracture of upper end of radius, left arm
CC-K,P **S59.199-** Other physeal fracture of upper end of radius, unspecified arm
S59.2- Physeal fracture of lower end of radius
S59.20- Unspecified physeal fracture of lower end of radius
CC-A,K,P **S59.201-** Unspecified physeal fracture of lower end of radius, right arm
CC-A,K,P **S59.202-** Unspecified physeal fracture of lower end of radius, left arm
CC-A,K,P **S59.209-** Unspecified physeal fracture of lower end of radius, unspecified arm
S59.21- Salter-Harris Type I physeal fracture of lower end of radius
CC-A,K,P **S59.211-** Salter-Harris Type I physeal fracture of lower end of radius, right arm
CC-A,K,P **S59.212-** Salter-Harris Type I physeal fracture of lower end of radius, left arm
CC-A,K,P **S59.219-** Salter-Harris Type I physeal fracture of lower end of radius, unspecified arm
S59.22- Salter-Harris Type II physeal fracture of lower end of radius
CC-A,K,P **S59.221-** Salter-Harris Type II physeal fracture of lower end of radius, right arm
CC-A,K,P **S59.222-** Salter-Harris Type II physeal fracture of lower end of radius, left arm
CC-A,K,P **S59.229-** Salter-Harris Type II physeal fracture of lower end of radius, unspecified arm
S59.23- Salter-Harris Type III physeal fracture of lower end of radius
CC-A,K,P **S59.231-** Salter-Harris Type III physeal fracture of lower end of radius, right arm
CC-A,K,P **S59.232-** Salter-Harris Type III physeal fracture of lower end of radius, left arm
CC-A,K,P **S59.239-** Salter-Harris Type III physeal fracture of lower end of radius, unspecified arm
S59.24- Salter-Harris Type IV physeal fracture of lower end of radius
CC-A,K,P **S59.241-** Salter-Harris Type IV physeal fracture of lower end of radius, right arm
CC-A,K,P **S59.242-** Salter-Harris Type IV physeal fracture of lower end of radius, left arm
CC-A,K,P **S59.249-** Salter-Harris Type IV physeal fracture of lower end of radius, unspecified arm
S59.29- Other physeal fracture of lower end of radius
CC-A,K,P **S59.291-** Other physeal fracture of lower end of radius, right arm
CC-A,K,P **S59.292-** Other physeal fracture of lower end of radius, left arm
CC-A,K,P **S59.299-** Other physeal fracture of lower end of radius, unspecified arm
S59.8- Other specified injuries of elbow and forearm

> The appropriate 7th character is to be added to each code in subcategory S59.8:
> A   Initial encounter
> D   Subsequent encounter
> S   Sequela

S59.80- Other specified injuries of elbow
S59.801- Other specified injuries of right elbow
S59.802- Other specified injuries of left elbow
S59.809- Other specified injuries of unspecified elbow
S59.81- Other specified injuries of forearm
S59.811- Other specified injuries right forearm

S59 - S59

S59.812-　Other specified injuries <u>left</u> forearm
S59.819-　Other specified injuries <u>unspecified</u> forearm

S59.9-　<u>Unspecified injury</u> of <u>elbow and forearm</u>
　　The appropriate 7th character is to be added to each code in
　　　subcategory S59.9:
　　A　<u>Initial</u> encounter
　　D　<u>Subsequent</u> encounter
　　S　<u>Sequela</u>

　S59.90-　<u>Unspecified injury</u> of <u>elbow</u>
　　S59.901-　Unspecified injury of <u>right</u> elbow
　　S59.902-　Unspecified injury of <u>left</u> elbow
　　S59.909-　Unspecified injury of <u>unspecified</u> elbow

　S59.91-　<u>Unspecified injury</u> of <u>forearm</u>
　　S59.911-　Unspecified injury of <u>right</u> forearm
　　S59.912-　Unspecified injury of <u>left</u> forearm
　　S59.919-　Unspecified injury of <u>unspecified</u> forearm

Injuries to the wrist, hand and fingers (S60-S69)

Excludes ❷:　burns and corrosions (T20-T32)
　　　　　　frostbite (T33-T34)
　　　　　　insect bite or sting, venomous (T63.4)

S60-　<u>Superficial injury</u> of <u>wrist, hand and fingers</u>
　　The appropriate 7th character is to be added to each code from
　　　category S60:
　　A　<u>Initial</u> encounter
　　D　<u>Subsequent</u> encounter
　　S　<u>Sequela</u>

　S60.0-　<u>Contusion</u> of <u>finger</u> <u>without</u> damage to nail
　　　Excludes 1:　contusion involving nail (matrix) (S60.1)
　　S60.00x-　<u>Contusion</u> of <u>unspecified</u> finger <u>without</u> damage to nail
　　　　Contusion of finger(s) NOS
　　S60.01-　<u>Contusion</u> of <u>thumb</u> <u>without</u> damage to nail
　　　S60.011-　Contusion of <u>right</u> thumb without damage to nail
　　　S60.012-　Contusion of <u>left</u> thumb without damage to nail
　　　S60.019-　Contusion of <u>unspecified</u> thumb without damage to nail
　　S60.02-　<u>Contusion</u> of <u>index</u> finger <u>without</u> damage to nail
　　　S60.021-　Contusion of <u>right</u> index finger without damage to nail
　　　S60.022-　Contusion of <u>left</u> index finger without damage to nail
　　　S60.029-　Contusion of <u>unspecified</u> index finger without damage to nail
　　S60.03-　<u>Contusion</u> of <u>middle</u> finger <u>without</u> damage to nail
　　　S60.031-　Contusion of <u>right</u> middle finger without damage to nail
　　　S60.032-　Contusion of <u>left</u> middle finger without damage to nail
　　　S60.039-　Contusion of <u>unspecified</u> middle finger without damage to nail
　　S60.04-　<u>Contusion</u> of <u>ring</u> finger <u>without</u> damage to nail
　　　S60.041-　Contusion of <u>right</u> ring finger without damage to nail
　　　S60.042-　Contusion of <u>left</u> ring finger without damage to nail
　　　S60.049-　Contusion of <u>unspecified</u> ring finger without damage to nail
　　S60.05-　<u>Contusion</u> of <u>little</u> finger <u>without</u> damage to nail
　　　S60.051-　Contusion of <u>right</u> little finger without damage to nail
　　　S60.052-　Contusion of <u>left</u> little finger without damage to nail
　　　S60.059-　Contusion of <u>unspecified</u> little finger without damage to nail
　S60.1-　<u>Contusion</u> of <u>finger</u> <u>with damage to nail</u>
　　S60.10x-　<u>Contusion</u> of <u>unspecified</u> finger <u>with damage to nail</u>
　　S60.11-　<u>Contusion</u> of <u>thumb</u> <u>with damage to nail</u>
　　　S60.111-　Contusion of <u>right</u> thumb with damage to nail

　　　S60.112-　Contusion of <u>left</u> thumb with damage to nail
　　　S60.119-　Contusion of <u>unspecified</u> thumb with damage to nail
　　S60.12-　<u>Contusion</u> of <u>index</u> finger <u>with damage to nail</u>
　　　S60.121-　Contusion of <u>right</u> index finger with damage to nail
　　　S60.122-　Contusion of <u>left</u> index finger with damage to nail
　　　S60.129-　Contusion of <u>unspecified</u> index finger with damage to nail
　　S60.13-　<u>Contusion</u> of <u>middle</u> finger <u>with damage to nail</u>
　　　S60.131-　Contusion of <u>right</u> middle finger with damage to nail
　　　S60.132-　Contusion of <u>left</u> middle finger with damage to nail
　　　S60.139-　Contusion of <u>unspecified</u> middle finger with damage to nail
　　S60.14-　<u>Contusion</u> of <u>ring</u> finger <u>with damage to nail</u>
　　　S60.141-　Contusion of <u>right</u> ring finger with damage to nail
　　　S60.142-　Contusion of <u>left</u> ring finger with damage to nail
　　　S60.149-　Contusion of <u>unspecified</u> ring finger with damage to nail
　　S60.15-　<u>Contusion</u> of <u>little</u> finger <u>with damage to nail</u>
　　　S60.151-　Contusion of <u>right</u> little finger with damage to nail
　　　S60.152-　Contusion of <u>left</u> little finger with damage to nail
　　　S60.159-　Contusion of <u>unspecified</u> little finger with damage to nail

　S60.2-　<u>Contusion</u> of <u>wrist and hand</u>
　　　Excludes ❷:　contusion of fingers (S60.0-, S60.1-)
　　S60.21-　<u>Contusion</u> of <u>wrist</u>
　　　S60.211-　Contusion of <u>right</u> wrist
　　　S60.212-　Contusion of <u>left</u> wrist
　　　S60.219-　Contusion of <u>unspecified</u> wrist
　　S60.22-　<u>Contusion</u> of <u>hand</u>
　　　S60.221-　Contusion of <u>right</u> hand
　　　S60.222-　Contusion of <u>left</u> hand
　　　S60.229-　Contusion of <u>unspecified</u> hand

　S60.3-　<u>Other superficial injuries</u> of <u>thumb</u>
　　S60.31-　<u>Abrasion</u> of <u>thumb</u>
　　　S60.311-　Abrasion of <u>right</u> thumb
　　　S60.312-　Abrasion of <u>left</u> thumb
　　　S60.319-　Abrasion of <u>unspecified</u> thumb
　　S60.32-　<u>Blister</u> (nonthermal) of <u>thumb</u>
　　　S60.321-　Blister (nonthermal) of <u>right</u> thumb
　　　S60.322-　Blister (nonthermal) of <u>left</u> thumb
　　　S60.329-　Blister (nonthermal) of <u>unspecified</u> thumb
　　S60.34-　<u>External constriction</u> of <u>thumb</u>
　　　　Hair tourniquet syndrome of thumb
　　　　Use additional cause code to identify the constricting item
　　　　　(W49.0-)
　　　S60.341-　External constriction of <u>right</u> thumb
　　　S60.342-　External constriction of <u>left</u> thumb
　　　S60.349-　External constriction of <u>unspecified</u> thumb
　　S60.35-　<u>Superficial foreign body</u> of <u>thumb</u>
　　　　Splinter in the thumb
　　　S60.351-　Superficial foreign body of <u>right</u> thumb
　　　S60.352-　Superficial foreign body of <u>left</u> thumb
　　　S60.359-　Superficial foreign body of <u>unspecified</u> thumb
　　S60.36-　<u>Insect bite (nonvenomous)</u> of <u>thumb</u>
　　　S60.361-　Insect bite (nonvenomous) of <u>right</u> thumb
　　　S60.362-　Insect bite (nonvenomous) of <u>left</u> thumb
　　　S60.369-　Insect bite (nonvenomous) of <u>unspecified</u> thumb
　　S60.37-　<u>Other superficial bite</u> of <u>thumb</u>
　　　　Excludes 1:　open bite of thumb (S61.05-, S61.15-)
　　　S60.371-　Other superficial bite of <u>right</u> thumb
　　　S60.372-　Other superficial bite of <u>left</u> thumb
　　　S60.379-　Other superficial bite of <u>unspecified</u> thumb

---

Excludes 1: = NOT CODED HERE! (Do not code both)　　　**1079**　　　*Excludes ❷:* = Not Included Here

S60.39- Other superficial injuries of thumb
    S60.391- Other superficial injuries of right thumb
    S60.392- Other superficial injuries of left thumb
    S60.399- Other superficial injuries of unspecified thumb
S60.4- Other superficial injuries of other fingers
  S60.41- Abrasion of fingers
    S60.410- Abrasion of right index finger
    S60.411- Abrasion of left index finger
    S60.412- Abrasion of right middle finger
    S60.413- Abrasion of left middle finger
    S60.414- Abrasion of right ring finger
    S60.415- Abrasion of left ring finger
    S60.416- Abrasion of right little finger
    S60.417- Abrasion of left little finger
    S60.418- Abrasion of other finger
        Abrasion of specified finger with unspecified laterality
    S60.419- Abrasion of unspecified finger
  S60.42- Blister (nonthermal) of fingers
    S60.420- Blister (nonthermal) of right index finger
    S60.421- Blister (nonthermal) of left index finger
    S60.422- Blister (nonthermal) of right middle finger
    S60.423- Blister (nonthermal) of left middle finger
    S60.424- Blister (nonthermal) of right ring finger
    S60.425- Blister (nonthermal) of left ring finger
    S60.426- Blister (nonthermal) of right little finger
    S60.427- Blister (nonthermal) of left little finger
    S60.428- Blister (nonthermal) of other finger
        Blister (nonthermal) of specified finger with unspecified laterality
    S60.429- Blister (nonthermal) of unspecified finger
  S60.44- External constriction of fingers
        Hair tourniquet syndrome of finger
        Use additional cause code to identify the constricting item (W49.0-)
    S60.440- External constriction of right index finger
    S60.441- External constriction of left index finger
    S60.442- External constriction of right middle finger
    S60.443- External constriction of left middle finger
    S60.444- External constriction of right ring finger
    S60.445- External constriction of left ring finger
    S60.446- External constriction of right little finger
    S60.447- External constriction of left little finger
    S60.448- External constriction of other finger
        External constriction of specified finger with unspecified laterality
    S60.449- External constriction of unspecified finger
  S60.45- Superficial foreign body of fingers
        Splinter in the finger(s)
    S60.450- Superficial foreign body of right index finger
    S60.451- Superficial foreign body of left index finger
    S60.452- Superficial foreign body of right middle finger
    S60.453- Superficial foreign body of left middle finger
    S60.454- Superficial foreign body of right ring finger
    S60.455- Superficial foreign body of left ring finger
    S60.456- Superficial foreign body of right little finger
    S60.457- Superficial foreign body of left little finger
    S60.458- Superficial foreign body of other finger
        Superficial foreign body of specified finger with unspecified laterality
    S60.459- Superficial foreign body of unspecified finger
  S60.46- Insect bite (nonvenomous) of fingers
    S60.460- Insect bite (nonvenomous) of right index finger
    S60.461- Insect bite (nonvenomous) of left index finger
    S60.462- Insect bite (nonvenomous) of right middle finger
    S60.463- Insect bite (nonvenomous) of left middle finger
    S60.464- Insect bite (nonvenomous) of right ring finger
    S60.465- Insect bite (nonvenomous) of left ring finger

S60.466- Insect bite (nonvenomous) of right little finger
S60.467- Insect bite (nonvenomous) of left little finger
S60.468- Insect bite (nonvenomous) of other finger
    Insect bite (nonvenomous) of specified finger with unspecified laterality
S60.469- Insect bite (nonvenomous) of unspecified finger
  S60.47- Other superficial bite of fingers
    Excludes 1: open bite of fingers (S61.25-, S61.35-)
    S60.470- Other superficial bite of right index finger
    S60.471- Other superficial bite of left index finger
    S60.472- Other superficial bite of right middle finger
    S60.473- Other superficial bite of left middle finger
    S60.474- Other superficial bite of right ring finger
    S60.475- Other superficial bite of left ring finger
    S60.476- Other superficial bite of right little finger
    S60.477- Other superficial bite of left little finger
    S60.478- Other superficial bite of other finger
        Other superficial bite of specified finger with unspecified laterality
    S60.479- Other superficial bite of unspecified finger
S60.5- Other superficial injuries of hand
    Excludes ❷: superficial injuries of fingers (S60.3-, S60.4-)
  S60.51- Abrasion of hand
    S60.511- Abrasion of right hand
    S60.512- Abrasion of left hand
    S60.519- Abrasion of unspecified hand
  S60.52- Blister (nonthermal) of hand
    S60.521- Blister (nonthermal) of right hand
    S60.522- Blister (nonthermal) of left hand
    S60.529- Blister (nonthermal) of unspecified hand
  S60.54- External constriction of hand
    S60.541- External constriction of right hand
    S60.542- External constriction of left hand
    S60.549- External constriction of unspecified hand
  S60.55- Superficial foreign body of hand
        Splinter in the hand
    S60.551- Superficial foreign body of right hand
    S60.552- Superficial foreign body of left hand
    S60.559- Superficial foreign body of unspecified hand
  S60.56- Insect bite (nonvenomous) of hand
    S60.561- Insect bite (nonvenomous) of right hand
    S60.562- Insect bite (nonvenomous) of left hand
    S60.569- Insect bite (nonvenomous) of unspecified hand
  S60.57- Other superficial bite of hand
    Excludes 1: open bite of hand (S61.45-)
    S60.571- Other superficial bite of hand of right hand
    S60.572- Other superficial bite of hand of left hand
    S60.579- Other superficial bite of hand of unspecified hand
S60.8- Other superficial injuries of wrist
  S60.81- Abrasion of wrist
    S60.811- Abrasion of right wrist
    S60.812- Abrasion of left wrist
    S60.819- Abrasion of unspecified wrist
  S60.82- Blister (nonthermal) of wrist
    S60.821- Blister (nonthermal) of right wrist
    S60.822- Blister (nonthermal) of left wrist
    S60.829- Blister (nonthermal) of unspecified wrist
  S60.84- External constriction of wrist
    S60.841- External constriction of right wrist
    S60.842- External constriction of left wrist
    S60.849- External constriction of unspecified wrist
  S60.85- Superficial foreign body of wrist
        Splinter in the wrist
    S60.851- Superficial foreign body of right wrist
    S60.852- Superficial foreign body of left wrist
    S60.859- Superficial foreign body of unspecified wrist

S60 – S60

Excludes 1: = NOT CODED HERE! (Do not code both)   **1080**   *Excludes ❷:* = Not Included Here

S60.86- Insect bite (nonvenomous) of wrist
    S60.861- Insect bite (nonvenomous) of right wrist
    S60.862- Insect bite (nonvenomous) of left wrist
    S60.869- Insect bite (nonvenomous) of unspecified wrist
  S60.87- Other superficial bite of wrist
     Excludes 1:   open bite of wrist (S61.55)
    S60.871- Other superficial bite of right wrist
    S60.872- Other superficial bite of left wrist
    S60.879- Other superficial bite of unspecified wrist
S60.9- Unspecified superficial injury of wrist, hand and fingers
  S60.91- Unspecified superficial injury of wrist
    S60.911- Unspecified superficial injury of right wrist
    S60.912- Unspecified superficial injury of left wrist
    S60.919- Unspecified superficial injury of unspecified wrist
  S60.92- Unspecified superficial injury of hand
    S60.921- Unspecified superficial injury of right hand
    S60.922- Unspecified superficial injury of left hand
    S60.929- Unspecified superficial injury of unspecified hand
  S60.93- Unspecified superficial injury of thumb
    S60.931- Unspecified superficial injury of right thumb
    S60.932- Unspecified superficial injury of left thumb
    S60.939- Unspecified superficial injury of unspecified thumb
  S60.94- Unspecified superficial injury of other fingers
    S60.940- Unspecified superficial injury of right index finger
    S60.941- Unspecified superficial injury of left index finger
    S60.942- Unspecified superficial injury of right middle finger
    S60.943- Unspecified superficial injury of left middle finger
    S60.944- Unspecified superficial injury of right ring finger
    S60.945- Unspecified superficial injury of left ring finger
    S60.946- Unspecified superficial injury of right little finger
    S60.947- Unspecified superficial injury of left little finger
    S60.948- Unspecified superficial injury of other finger
      Unspecified superficial injury of specified finger with unspecified laterality
    S60.949- Unspecified superficial injury of unspecified finger

S61- Open wound of wrist, hand and fingers
  Code also any associated wound infection
  Excludes 1:   open fracture of wrist, hand and finger (S62.- with 7th character B)
         traumatic amputation of wrist and hand (S68.-)

The appropriate 7th character is to be added to each code from category S61:
  A Initial encounter
  D Subsequent encounter
  S Sequela

S61.0- Open wound of thumb without damage to nail
    Excludes 1:   open wound of thumb with damage to nail (S61.1-)
  S61.00- Unspecified open wound of thumb without damage to nail
    S61.001- Unspecified open wound of right thumb without damage to nail
    S61.002- Unspecified open wound of left thumb without damage to nail
    S61.009- Unspecified open wound of unspecified thumb without damage to nail
  S61.01- Laceration without foreign body of thumb without damage to nail
    S61.011- Laceration without foreign body of right thumb without damage to nail
    S61.012- Laceration without foreign body of left thumb without damage to nail
    S61.019- Laceration without foreign body of unspecified thumb without damage to nail
  S61.02- Laceration with foreign body of thumb without damage to nail
    S61.021- Laceration with foreign body of right thumb without damage to nail

S61.022- Laceration with foreign body of left thumb without damage to nail
S61.029- Laceration with foreign body of unspecified thumb without damage to nail
  S61.03- Puncture wound without foreign body of thumb without damage to nail
    S61.031- Puncture wound without foreign body of right thumb without damage to nail
    S61.032- Puncture wound without foreign body of left thumb without damage to nail
    S61.039- Puncture wound without foreign body of unspecified thumb without damage to nail
  S61.04- Puncture wound with foreign body of thumb without damage to nail
    S61.041- Puncture wound with foreign body of right thumb without damage to nail
    S61.042- Puncture wound with foreign body of left thumb without damage to nail
    S61.049- Puncture wound with foreign body of unspecified thumb without damage to nail
  S61.05- Open bite of thumb without damage to nail
     Bite of thumb NOS
     Excludes 1:   superficial bite of thumb (S60.36-, S60.37-)
    S61.051- Open bite of right thumb without damage to nail
    S61.052- Open bite of left thumb without damage to nail
    S61.059- Open bite of unspecified thumb without damage to nail
S61.1- Open wound of thumb with damage to nail
  S61.10- Unspecified open wound of thumb with damage to nail
    S61.101- Unspecified open wound of right thumb with damage to nail
    S61.102- Unspecified open wound of left thumb with damage to nail
    S61.109- Unspecified open wound of unspecified thumb with damage to nail
  S61.11- Laceration without foreign body of thumb with damage to nail
    S61.111- Laceration without foreign body of right thumb with damage to nail
    S61.112- Laceration without foreign body of left thumb with damage to nail
    S61.119- Laceration without foreign body of unspecified thumb with damage to nail
  S61.12- Laceration with foreign body of thumb with damage to nail
    S61.121- Laceration with foreign body of right thumb with damage to nail
    S61.122- Laceration with foreign body of left thumb with damage to nail
    S61.129- Laceration with foreign body of unspecified thumb with damage to nail
  S61.13- Puncture wound without foreign body of thumb with damage to nail
    S61.131- Puncture wound without foreign body of right thumb with damage to nail
    S61.132- Puncture wound without foreign body of left thumb with damage to nail
    S61.139- Puncture wound without foreign body of unspecified thumb with damage to nail
  S61.14- Puncture wound with foreign body of thumb with damage to nail
    S61.141- Puncture wound with foreign body of right thumb with damage to nail
    S61.142- Puncture wound with foreign body of left thumb with damage to nail
    S61.149- Puncture wound with foreign body of unspecified thumb with damage to nail

S 6 0 I S 6 1

S61.15- Open bite of thumb with damage to nail
    Bite of thumb with damage to nail NOS
    Excludes 1:   superficial bite of thumb (S60.36-, S60.37-)

S61.151- Open bite of right thumb with damage to nail

S61.152- Open bite of left thumb with damage to nail

S61.159- Open bite of unspecified thumb with damage to nail

S61.2- Open wound of other finger without damage to nail
    Excludes 1:   open wound of finger involving nail (matrix) (S61.3-)
    Excludes ❷: open wound of thumb without damage to nail (S61.0-)

S61.20- Unspecified open wound of other finger without damage to nail

S61.200- Unspecified open wound of right index finger without damage to nail

S61.201- Unspecified open wound of left index finger without damage to nail

S61.202- Unspecified open wound of right middle finger without damage to nail

S61.203- Unspecified open wound of left middle finger without damage to nail

S61.204- Unspecified open wound of right ring finger without damage to nail

S61.205- Unspecified open wound of left ring finger without damage to nail

S61.206- Unspecified open wound of right little finger without damage to nail

S61.207- Unspecified open wound of left little finger without damage to nail

S61.208- Unspecified open wound of other finger without damage to nail
    Unspecified open wound of specified finger with unspecified laterality without damage to nail

S61.209- Unspecified open wound of unspecified finger without damage to nail

S61.21- Laceration without foreign body of finger without damage to nail

S61.210- Laceration without foreign body of right index finger without damage to nail

S61.211- Laceration without foreign body of left index finger without damage to nail

S61.212- Laceration without foreign body of right middle finger without damage to nail

S61.213- Laceration without foreign body of left middle finger without damage to nail

S61.214- Laceration without foreign body of right ring finger without damage to nail

S61.215- Laceration without foreign body of left ring finger without damage to nail

S61.216- Laceration without foreign body of right little finger without damage to nail

S61.217- Laceration without foreign body of left little finger without damage to nail

S61.218- Laceration without foreign body of other finger without damage to nail
    Laceration without foreign body of specified finger with unspecified laterality without damage to nail

S61.219- Laceration without foreign body of unspecified finger without damage to nail

S61.22- Laceration with foreign body of finger without damage to nail

S61.220- Laceration with foreign body of right index finger without damage to nail

S61.221- Laceration with foreign body of left index finger without damage to nail

S61.222- Laceration with foreign body of right middle finger without damage to nail

S61.223- Laceration with foreign body of left middle finger without damage to nail

S61.224- Laceration with foreign body of right ring finger without damage to nail

S61.225- Laceration with foreign body of left ring finger without damage to nail

S61.226- Laceration with foreign body of right little finger without damage to nail

S61.227- Laceration with foreign body of left little finger without damage to nail

S61.228- Laceration with foreign body of other finger without damage to nail
    Laceration with foreign body of specified finger with unspecified laterality without damage to nail

S61.229- Laceration with foreign body of unspecified finger without damage to nail

S61.23- Puncture wound without foreign body of finger without damage to nail

S61.230- Puncture wound without foreign body of right index finger without damage to nail

S61.231- Puncture wound without foreign body of left index finger without damage to nail

S61.232- Puncture wound without foreign body of right middle finger without damage to nail

S61.233- Puncture wound without foreign body of left middle finger without damage to nail

S61.234- Puncture wound without foreign body of right ring finger without damage to nail

S61.235- Puncture wound without foreign body of left ring finger without damage to nail

S61.236- Puncture wound without foreign body of right little finger without damage to nail

S61.237- Puncture wound without foreign body of left little finger without damage to nail

S61.238- Puncture wound without foreign body of other finger without damage to nail
    Puncture wound without foreign body of specified finger with unspecified laterality without damage to nail

S61.239- Puncture wound without foreign body of unspecified finger without damage to nail

S61.24- Puncture wound with foreign body of finger without damage to nail

S61.240- Puncture wound with foreign body of right index finger without damage to nail

S61.241- Puncture wound with foreign body of left index finger without damage to nail

S61.242- Puncture wound with foreign body of right middle finger without damage to nail

S61.243- Puncture wound with foreign body of left middle finger without damage to nail

S61.244- Puncture wound with foreign body of right ring finger without damage to nail

S61.245- Puncture wound with foreign body of left ring finger without damage to nail

S61.246- Puncture wound with foreign body of right little finger without damage to nail

S61.247- Puncture wound with foreign body of left little finger without damage to nail

S61.248- Puncture wound with foreign body of other finger without damage to nail
    Puncture wound with foreign body of specified finger with unspecified laterality without damage to nail

S61.249- Puncture wound with foreign body of unspecified finger without damage to nail

S61.25- Open bite of finger without damage to nail
    Bite of finger without damage to nail NOS
    Excludes 1:   superficial bite of finger (S60.46-, S60.47-)

S61.250- Open bite of right index finger without damage to nail

S61.251- Open bite of left index finger without damage to nail

S61.252- Open bite of right middle finger without damage to nail

S61.253- Open bite of <u>left</u> <u>middle</u> finger <u>without</u> damage to nail

S61.254- Open bite of <u>right</u> <u>ring</u> finger <u>without</u> damage to nail

S61.255- Open bite of <u>left</u> <u>ring</u> finger <u>without</u> damage to nail

S61.256- Open bite of <u>right</u> <u>little</u> finger <u>without</u> damage to nail

S61.257- Open bite of <u>left</u> <u>little</u> finger <u>without</u> damage to nail

S61.258- Open bite of other <u>finger</u> <u>without</u> damage to nail
　　Open bite of specified finger with unspecified laterality without damage to nail

S61.259- Open bite of <u>unspecified</u> finger <u>without</u> damage to nail

S61.3- <u>Open wound</u> of other finger <u>with damage to nail</u>

　S61.30- <u>Unspecified open wound</u> of <u>finger</u> <u>with damage to nail</u>

　　S61.300- Unspecified open wound of <u>right</u> <u>index</u> finger <u>with damage to nail</u>

　　S61.301- Unspecified open wound of <u>left</u> <u>index</u> finger <u>with damage to nail</u>

　　S61.302- Unspecified open wound of <u>right</u> <u>middle</u> finger <u>with damage to nail</u>

　　S61.303- Unspecified open wound of <u>left</u> <u>middle</u> finger <u>with damage to nail</u>

　　S61.304- Unspecified open wound of <u>right</u> <u>ring</u> finger <u>with damage to nail</u>

　　S61.305- Unspecified open wound of <u>left</u> <u>ring</u> finger <u>with damage to nail</u>

　　S61.306- Unspecified open wound of <u>right</u> <u>little</u> finger <u>with damage to nail</u>

　　S61.307- Unspecified open wound of <u>left</u> <u>little</u> finger <u>with damage to nail</u>

　　S61.308- Unspecified open wound of <u>other</u> finger <u>with damage to nail</u>
　　　Unspecified open wound of specified finger with unspecified laterality with damage to nail

　　S61.309- Unspecified open wound of <u>unspecified</u> finger <u>with damage to nail</u>

　S61.31- <u>Laceration</u> <u>without</u> foreign body of <u>finger</u> <u>with damage to nail</u>

　　S61.310- Laceration <u>without</u> foreign body of <u>right</u> <u>index</u> finger <u>with damage to nail</u>

　　S61.311- Laceration <u>without</u> foreign body of <u>left</u> <u>index</u> finger <u>with damage to nail</u>

　　S61.312- Laceration <u>without</u> foreign body of <u>right</u> <u>middle</u> finger <u>with damage to nail</u>

　　S61.313- Laceration <u>without</u> foreign body of <u>left</u> <u>middle</u> finger <u>with damage to nail</u>

　　S61.314- Laceration <u>without</u> foreign body of <u>right</u> <u>ring</u> finger <u>with damage to nail</u>

　　S61.315- Laceration <u>without</u> foreign body of <u>left</u> <u>ring</u> finger <u>with damage to nail</u>

　　S61.316- Laceration <u>without</u> foreign body of <u>right</u> <u>little</u> finger <u>with damage to nail</u>

　　S61.317- Laceration <u>without</u> foreign body of <u>left</u> <u>little</u> finger <u>with damage to nail</u>

　　S61.318- Laceration <u>without</u> foreign body of <u>other</u> finger <u>with damage to nail</u>
　　　Laceration without foreign body of specified finger with unspecified laterality with damage to nail

　　S61.319- Laceration <u>without</u> foreign body of <u>unspecified</u> finger <u>with damage to nail</u>

　S61.32- <u>Laceration</u> <u>with foreign body</u> of <u>finger</u> <u>with damage to nail</u>

　　S61.320- Laceration <u>with foreign body</u> of <u>right</u> <u>index</u> finger <u>with damage to nail</u>

　　S61.321- Laceration <u>with foreign body</u> of <u>left</u> <u>index</u> finger <u>with damage to nail</u>

S61.322- Laceration <u>with foreign body</u> of <u>right</u> <u>middle</u> finger <u>with damage to nail</u>

S61.323- Laceration <u>with foreign body</u> of <u>left</u> <u>middle</u> finger <u>with damage to nail</u>

S61.324- Laceration <u>with foreign body</u> of <u>right</u> <u>ring</u> finger <u>with damage to nail</u>

S61.325- Laceration <u>with foreign body</u> of <u>left</u> <u>ring</u> finger <u>with damage to nail</u>

S61.326- Laceration <u>with foreign body</u> of <u>right</u> <u>little</u> finger <u>with damage to nail</u>

S61.327- Laceration <u>with foreign body</u> of <u>left</u> <u>little</u> finger <u>with damage to nail</u>

S61.328- Laceration <u>with foreign body</u> of <u>other</u> finger <u>with damage to nail</u>
　Laceration with foreign body of specified finger with unspecified laterality with damage to nail

S61.329- Laceration <u>with foreign body</u> of <u>unspecified</u> finger <u>with damage to nail</u>

S61.33- <u>Puncture</u> wound <u>without</u> foreign body of <u>finger</u> <u>with damage to nail</u>

　S61.330- Puncture wound <u>without</u> foreign body of <u>right</u> <u>index</u> finger <u>with damage to nail</u>

　S61.331- Puncture wound <u>without</u> foreign body of <u>left</u> <u>index</u> finger <u>with damage to nail</u>

　S61.332- Puncture wound <u>without</u> foreign body of <u>right</u> <u>middle</u> finger <u>with damage to nail</u>

　S61.333- Puncture wound <u>without</u> foreign body of <u>left</u> <u>middle</u> finger <u>with damage to nail</u>

　S61.334- Puncture wound <u>without</u> foreign body of <u>right</u> <u>ring</u> finger <u>with damage to nail</u>

　S61.335- Puncture wound <u>without</u> foreign body of <u>left</u> <u>ring</u> finger <u>with damage to nail</u>

　S61.336- Puncture wound <u>without</u> foreign body of <u>right</u> <u>little</u> finger <u>with damage to nail</u>

　S61.337- Puncture wound <u>without</u> foreign body of <u>left</u> <u>little</u> finger <u>with damage to nail</u>

　S61.338- Puncture wound <u>without</u> foreign body of <u>other</u> finger <u>with damage to nail</u>
　　Puncture wound without foreign body of specified finger with unspecified laterality with damage to nail

　S61.339- Puncture wound <u>without</u> foreign body of <u>unspecified</u> finger <u>with damage to nail</u>

S61.34- <u>Puncture</u> wound <u>with foreign body</u> of <u>finger</u> <u>with damage to nail</u>

　S61.340- Puncture wound <u>with foreign body</u> of <u>right</u> <u>index</u> finger <u>with damage to nail</u>

　S61.341- Puncture wound <u>with foreign body</u> of <u>left</u> <u>index</u> finger <u>with damage to nail</u>

　S61.342- Puncture wound <u>with foreign body</u> of <u>right</u> <u>middle</u> finger <u>with damage to nail</u>

　S61.343- Puncture wound <u>with foreign body</u> of <u>left</u> <u>middle</u> finger <u>with damage to nail</u>

　S61.344- Puncture wound <u>with foreign body</u> of <u>right</u> <u>ring</u> finger <u>with damage to nail</u>

　S61.345- Puncture wound <u>with foreign body</u> of <u>left</u> <u>ring</u> finger <u>with damage to nail</u>

　S61.346- Puncture wound <u>with foreign body</u> of <u>right</u> <u>little</u> finger <u>with damage to nail</u>

　S61.347- Puncture wound <u>with foreign body</u> of <u>left</u> <u>little</u> finger <u>with damage to nail</u>

　S61.348- Puncture wound <u>with foreign body</u> of <u>other</u> finger <u>with damage to nail</u>
　　Puncture wound with foreign body of specified finger with unspecified laterality with damage to nail

　S61.349- Puncture wound <u>with foreign body</u> of <u>unspecified</u> finger <u>with damage to nail</u>

S61 - S61

S61.35- Open bite of finger with damage to nail
Bite of finger with damage to nail NOS
Excludes 1: superficial bite of finger (S60.46-, S60.47-)
S61.350- Open bite of right index finger with damage to nail
S61.351- Open bite of left index finger with damage to nail
S61.352- Open bite of right middle finger with damage to nail
S61.353- Open bite of left middle finger with damage to nail
S61.354- Open bite of right ring finger with damage to nail
S61.355- Open bite of left ring finger with damage to nail
S61.356- Open bite of right little finger with damage to nail
S61.357- Open bite of left little finger with damage to nail
S61.358- Open bite of other finger with damage to nail
Open bite of specified finger with unspecified laterality with damage to nail
S61.359- Open bite of unspecified finger with damage to nail
S61.4- Open wound of hand
S61.40- Unspecified open wound of hand
S61.401- Unspecified open wound of right hand
S61.402- Unspecified open wound of left hand
S61.409- Unspecified open wound of unspecified hand
S61.41- Laceration without foreign body of hand
S61.411- Laceration without foreign body of right hand
S61.412- Laceration without foreign body of left hand
S61.419- Laceration without foreign body of unspecified hand
S61.42- Laceration with foreign body of hand
S61.421- Laceration with foreign body of right hand
S61.422- Laceration with foreign body of left hand
S61.429- Laceration with foreign body of unspecified hand
S61.43- Puncture wound without foreign body of hand
S61.431- Puncture wound without foreign body of right hand
S61.432- Puncture wound without foreign body of left hand
S61.439- Puncture wound without foreign body of unspecified hand
S61.44- Puncture wound with foreign body of hand
S61.441- Puncture wound with foreign body of right hand
S61.442- Puncture wound with foreign body of left hand
S61.449- Puncture wound with foreign body of unspecified hand
S61.45- Open bite of hand
Bite of hand NOS
Excludes 1: superficial bite of hand (S60.56-, S60.57-)
S61.451- Open bite of right hand
S61.452- Open bite of left hand
S61.459- Open bite of unspecified hand
S61.5- Open wound of wrist
S61.50- Unspecified open wound of wrist
S61.501- Unspecified open wound of right wrist
S61.502- Unspecified open wound of left wrist
S61.509- Unspecified open wound of unspecified wrist
S61.51- Laceration without foreign body of wrist
S61.511- Laceration without foreign body of right wrist
S61.512- Laceration without foreign body of left wrist
S61.519- Laceration without foreign body of unspecified wrist
S61.52- Laceration with foreign body of wrist
S61.521- Laceration with foreign body of right wrist
S61.522- Laceration with foreign body of left wrist
S61.529- Laceration with foreign body of unspecified wrist
S61.53- Puncture wound without foreign body of wrist
S61.531- Puncture wound without foreign body of right wrist
S61.532- Puncture wound without foreign body of left wrist
S61.539- Puncture wound without foreign body of unspecified wrist

S61.54- Puncture wound with foreign body of wrist
S61.541- Puncture wound with foreign body of right wrist
S61.542- Puncture wound with foreign body of left wrist
S61.549- Puncture wound with foreign body of unspecified wrist
S61.55- Open bite of wrist
Bite of wrist NOS
Excludes 1: superficial bite of wrist (S60.86-, S60.87-)
S61.551- Open bite of right wrist
S61.552- Open bite of left wrist
S61.559- Open bite of unspecified wrist

S62- Fracture at wrist and hand level
Note: A fracture not indicated as displaced or nondisplaced should be coded to displaced
Note: A fracture not indicated as open or closed should be coded to closed
Excludes 1: traumatic amputation of wrist and hand (S68.-)
Excludes 2: fracture of distal parts of ulna and radius (S52.-)

The appropriate 7th character is to be added to each code from category S62:
A   Initial encounter for closed fracture
B   Initial encounter for open fracture
D   Subsequent encounter for fracture with routine healing
G   Subsequent encounter for fracture with delayed healing
K   Subsequent encounter for fracture with nonunion
P   Subsequent encounter for fracture with malunion
S   Sequela

S62.0- Fracture of navicular [scaphoid] bone of wrist
S62.00- Unspecified fracture of navicular [scaphoid] bone of wrist
CC-B,K,P **S62.001-** Unspecified fracture of navicular [scaphoid] bone of right wrist
CC-B,K,P **S62.002-** Unspecified fracture of navicular [scaphoid] bone of left wrist
CC-B,K,P **S62.009-** Unspecified fracture of navicular [scaphoid] bone of unspecified wrist
S62.01- Fracture of distal pole of navicular [scaphoid] bone of wrist
Fracture of volar tuberosity of navicular [scaphoid] bone of wrist
CC-B,K,P **S62.011-** Displaced fracture of distal pole of navicular [scaphoid] bone of right wrist
CC-B,K,P **S62.012-** Displaced fracture of distal pole of navicular [scaphoid] bone of left wrist
CC-B,K,P **S62.013-** Displaced fracture of distal pole of navicular [scaphoid] bone of unspecified wrist
CC-B,K,P **S62.014-** Nondisplaced fracture of distal pole of navicular [scaphoid] bone of right wrist
CC-B,K,P **S62.015-** Nondisplaced fracture of distal pole of navicular [scaphoid] bone of left wrist
CC-B,K,P **S62.016-** Nondisplaced fracture of distal pole of navicular [scaphoid] bone of unspecified wrist
S62.02- Fracture of middle third of navicular [scaphoid] bone of wrist
CC-B,K,P **S62.021-** Displaced fracture of middle third of navicular [scaphoid] bone of right wrist
CC-B,K,P **S62.022-** Displaced fracture of middle third of navicular [scaphoid] bone of left wrist
CC-B,K,P **S62.023-** Displaced fracture of middle third of navicular [scaphoid] bone of unspecified wrist
CC-B,K,P **S62.024-** Nondisplaced fracture of middle third of navicular [scaphoid] bone of right wrist
CC-B,K,P **S62.025-** Nondisplaced fracture of middle third of navicular [scaphoid] bone of left wrist
CC-B,K,P **S62.026-** Nondisplaced fracture of middle third of navicular [scaphoid] bone of unspecified wrist
S62.03- Fracture of proximal third of navicular [scaphoid] bone of wrist
CC-B,K,P **S62.031-** Displaced fracture of proximal third of navicular [scaphoid] bone of right wrist
CC-B,K,P **S62.032-** Displaced fracture of proximal third of navicular [scaphoid] bone of left wrist

S61 - S62

CC-B,K,P **S62.033-** <u>Displaced</u> fracture of proximal third of navicular [scaphoid] bone of <u>unspecified</u> wrist

CC-B,K,P **S62.034-** <u>Nondisplaced</u> fracture of proximal third of navicular [scaphoid] bone of <u>right</u> wrist

CC-B,K,P **S62.035-** <u>Nondisplaced</u> fracture of proximal third of navicular [scaphoid] bone of <u>left</u> wrist

CC-B,K,P **S62.036-** <u>Nondisplaced</u> fracture of proximal third of navicular [scaphoid] bone of <u>unspecified</u> wrist

S62.1- Fracture of <u>other and unspecified</u> carpal bone(s)
    Excludes ❷: fracture of scaphoid of wrist (S62.0-)

S62.10- Fracture of <u>unspecified</u> carpal bone
    Fracture of wrist NOS

CC-B,K,P **S62.101-** Fracture of <u>unspecified</u> carpal bone, <u>right</u> wrist

CC-B,K,P **S62.102-** Fracture of <u>unspecified</u> carpal bone, <u>left</u> wrist

CC-B,K,P **S62.109-** Fracture of <u>unspecified</u> carpal bone, <u>unspecified</u> wrist

S62.11- Fracture of <u>triquetrum [cuneiform]</u> bone of <u>wrist</u>

CC-B,K,P **S62.111-** <u>Displaced</u> fracture of triquetrum [cuneiform] bone, <u>right</u> wrist

CC-B,K,P **S62.112-** <u>Displaced</u> fracture of triquetrum [cuneiform] bone, <u>left</u> wrist

CC-B,K,P **S62.113-** <u>Displaced</u> fracture of triquetrum [cuneiform] bone, <u>unspecified</u> wrist

CC-B,K,P **S62.114-** <u>Nondisplaced</u> fracture of triquetrum [cuneiform] bone, <u>right</u> wrist

CC-B,K,P **S62.115-** <u>Nondisplaced</u> fracture of triquetrum [cuneiform] bone, <u>left</u> wrist

CC-B,K,P **S62.116-** <u>Nondisplaced</u> fracture of triquetrum [cuneiform] bone, <u>unspecified</u> wrist

S62.12- Fracture of <u>lunate [semilunar]</u>

CC-B,K,P **S62.121-** <u>Displaced</u> fracture of lunate [semilunar], <u>right</u> wrist

CC-B,K,P **S62.122-** <u>Displaced</u> fracture of lunate [semilunar], <u>left</u> wrist

CC-B,K,P **S62.123-** <u>Displaced</u> fracture of lunate [semilunar], <u>unspecified</u> wrist

CC-B,K,P **S62.124-** <u>Nondisplaced</u> fracture of lunate [semilunar], <u>right</u> wrist

CC-B,K,P **S62.125-** <u>Nondisplaced</u> fracture of lunate [semilunar], <u>left</u> wrist

CC-B,K,P **S62.126-** <u>Nondisplaced</u> fracture of lunate [semilunar], <u>unspecified</u> wrist

S62.13- Fracture of <u>capitate [os magnum]</u> bone

CC-B,K,P **S62.131-** <u>Displaced</u> fracture of capitate [os magnum] bone, <u>right</u> wrist

CC-B,K,P **S62.132-** <u>Displaced</u> fracture of capitate [os magnum] bone, <u>left</u> wrist

CC-B,K,P **S62.133-** <u>Displaced</u> fracture of capitate [os magnum] bone, <u>unspecified</u> wrist

CC-B,K,P **S62.134-** <u>Nondisplaced</u> fracture of capitate [os magnum] bone, <u>right</u> wrist

CC-B,K,P **S62.135-** <u>Nondisplaced</u> fracture of capitate [os magnum] bone, <u>left</u> wrist

CC-B,K,P **S62.136-** <u>Nondisplaced</u> fracture of capitate [os magnum] bone, <u>unspecified</u> wrist

S62.14- Fracture of body of <u>hamate [unciform]</u> bone
    Fracture of hamate [unciform] bone NOS

CC-B,K,P **S62.141-** <u>Displaced</u> fracture of body of hamate [unciform] bone, <u>right</u> wrist

CC-B,K,P **S62.142-** <u>Displaced</u> fracture of body of hamate [unciform] bone, <u>left</u> wrist

CC-B,K,P **S62.143-** <u>Displaced</u> fracture of body of hamate [unciform] bone, <u>unspecified</u> wrist

CC-B,K,P **S62.144-** <u>Nondisplaced</u> fracture of body of hamate [unciform] bone, <u>right</u> wrist

CC-B,K,P **S62.145-** <u>Nondisplaced</u> fracture of body of hamate [unciform] bone, <u>left</u> wrist

CC-B,K,P **S62.146-** <u>Nondisplaced</u> fracture of body of hamate [unciform] bone, <u>unspecified</u> wrist

S62.15- Fracture of <u>hook process</u> of hamate [unciform] bone
    Fracture of unciform process of hamate [unciform] bone

CC-B,K,P **S62.151-** <u>Displaced</u> fracture of hook process of hamate [unciform] bone, <u>right</u> wrist

CC-B,K,P **S62.152-** <u>Displaced</u> fracture of hook process of hamate [unciform] bone, <u>left</u> wrist

CC-B,K,P **S62.153-** <u>Displaced</u> fracture of hook process of hamate [unciform] bone, <u>unspecified</u> wrist

CC-B,K,P **S62.154-** <u>Nondisplaced</u> fracture of hook process of hamate [unciform] bone, <u>right</u> wrist

CC-B,K,P **S62.155-** <u>Nondisplaced</u> fracture of hook process of hamate [unciform] bone, <u>left</u> wrist

CC-B,K,P **S62.156-** <u>Nondisplaced</u> fracture of hook process of hamate [unciform] bone, <u>unspecified</u> wrist

S62.16- Fracture of <u>pisiform</u>

CC-B,K,P **S62.161-** <u>Displaced</u> fracture of pisiform, <u>right</u> wrist

CC-B,K,P **S62.162-** <u>Displaced</u> fracture of pisiform, <u>left</u> wrist

CC-B,K,P **S62.163-** <u>Displaced</u> fracture of pisiform, <u>unspecified</u> wrist

CC-B,K,P **S62.164-** <u>Nondisplaced</u> fracture of pisiform, <u>right</u> wrist

CC-B,K,P **S62.165-** <u>Nondisplaced</u> fracture of pisiform, <u>left</u> wrist

CC-B,K,P **S62.166-** <u>Nondisplaced</u> fracture of pisiform, <u>unspecified</u> wrist

S62.17- Fracture of <u>trapezium [larger multangular]</u>

CC-B,K,P **S62.171-** <u>Displaced</u> fracture of trapezium [larger multangular], <u>right</u> wrist

CC-B,K,P **S62.172-** <u>Displaced</u> fracture of trapezium [larger multangular], <u>left</u> wrist

CC-B,K,P **S62.173-** <u>Displaced</u> fracture of trapezium [larger multangular], <u>unspecified</u> wrist

CC-B,K,P **S62.174-** <u>Nondisplaced</u> fracture of trapezium [larger multangular], <u>right</u> wrist

CC-B,K,P **S62.175-** <u>Nondisplaced</u> fracture of trapezium [larger multangular], <u>left</u> wrist

CC-B,K,P **S62.176-** <u>Nondisplaced</u> fracture of trapezium [larger multangular], <u>unspecified</u> wrist

S62.18- Fracture of <u>trapezoid [smaller multangular]</u>

CC-B,K,P **S62.181-** <u>Displaced</u> fracture of trapezoid [smaller multangular], <u>right</u> wrist

CC-B,K,P **S62.182-** <u>Displaced</u> fracture of trapezoid [smaller multangular], <u>left</u> wrist

CC-B,K,P **S62.183-** <u>Displaced</u> fracture of trapezoid [smaller multangular], <u>unspecified</u> wrist

CC-B,K,P **S62.184-** <u>Nondisplaced</u> fracture of trapezoid [smaller multangular], <u>right</u> wrist

CC-B,K,P **S62.185-** <u>Nondisplaced</u> fracture of trapezoid [smaller multangular], <u>left</u> wrist

CC-B,K,P **S62.186-** <u>Nondisplaced</u> fracture of trapezoid [smaller multangular], <u>unspecified</u> wrist

S62.2- Fracture of <u>first</u> metacarpal bone

S62.20- <u>Unspecified</u> fracture of <u>first</u> metacarpal bone

CC-B,K,P **S62.201-** Unspecified fracture of first metacarpal bone, <u>right</u> hand

CC-B,K,P **S62.202-** Unspecified fracture of first metacarpal bone, <u>left</u> hand

CC-B,K,P **S62.209-** Unspecified fracture of first metacarpal bone, <u>unspecified</u> hand

S62.21- <u>Bennett's</u> fracture

CC-B,K,P **S62.211-** Bennett's fracture, <u>right</u> hand

CC-B,K,P **S62.212-** Bennett's fracture, <u>left</u> hand

CC-B,K,P **S62.213-** Bennett's fracture, <u>unspecified</u> hand

S62.22- <u>Rolando's</u> fracture

CC-B,K,P **S62.221-** <u>Displaced</u> Rolando's fracture, <u>right</u> hand

CC-B,K,P **S62.222-** <u>Displaced</u> Rolando's fracture, <u>left</u> hand

CC-B,K,P **S62.223-** <u>Displaced</u> Rolando's fracture, <u>unspecified</u> hand

CC-B,K,P **S62.224-** <u>Nondisplaced</u> Rolando's fracture, <u>right</u> hand

CC-B,K,P **S62.225-** <u>Nondisplaced</u> Rolando's fracture, <u>left</u> hand

CC-B,K,P **S62.226-** <u>Nondisplaced</u> Rolando's fracture, <u>unspecified</u> hand

S 6 2 I S 6 2

Excludes 1: = NOT CODED HERE! (Do not code both)   *Excludes ❷:* = Not Included Here

S62.23- Other fracture of base of first metacarpal bone

CC-B,K,P **S62.231-** Other displaced fracture of base of first metacarpal bone, right hand

CC-B,K,P **S62.232-** Other displaced fracture of base of first metacarpal bone, left hand

CC-B,K,P **S62.233-** Other displaced fracture of base of first metacarpal bone, unspecified hand

CC-B,K,P **S62.234-** Other nondisplaced fracture of base of first metacarpal bone, right hand

CC-B,K,P **S62.235-** Other nondisplaced fracture of base of first metacarpal bone, left hand

CC-B,K,P **S62.236-** Other nondisplaced fracture of base of first metacarpal bone, unspecified hand

S62.24- Fracture of shaft of first metacarpal bone

CC-B,K,P **S62.241-** Displaced fracture of shaft of first metacarpal bone, right hand

CC-B,K,P **S62.242-** Displaced fracture of shaft of first metacarpal bone, left hand

CC-B,K,P **S62.243-** Displaced fracture of shaft of first metacarpal bone, unspecified hand

CC-B,K,P **S62.244-** Nondisplaced fracture of shaft of first metacarpal bone, right hand

CC-B,K,P **S62.245-** Nondisplaced fracture of shaft of first metacarpal bone, left hand

CC-B,K,P **S62.246-** Nondisplaced fracture of shaft of first metacarpal bone, unspecified hand

S62.25- Fracture of neck of first metacarpal bone

CC-B,K,P **S62.251-** Displaced fracture of neck of first metacarpal bone, right hand

CC-B,K,P **S62.252-** Displaced fracture of neck of first metacarpal bone, left hand

CC-B,K,P **S62.253-** Displaced fracture of neck of first metacarpal bone, unspecified hand

CC-B,K,P **S62.254-** Nondisplaced fracture of neck of first metacarpal bone, right hand

CC-B,K,P **S62.255-** Nondisplaced fracture of neck of first metacarpal bone, left hand

CC-B,K,P **S62.256-** Nondisplaced fracture of neck of first metacarpal bone, unspecified hand

S62.29- Other fracture of first metacarpal bone

CC-B,K,P **S62.291-** Other fracture of first metacarpal bone, right hand

CC-B,K,P **S62.292-** Other fracture of first metacarpal bone, left hand

CC-B,K,P **S62.299-** Other fracture of first metacarpal bone, unspecified hand

S62.3- Fracture of other and unspecified metacarpal bone
Excludes ❷: fracture of first metacarpal bone (S62.2-)

S62.30- Unspecified fracture of other metacarpal bone

CC-B,K,P **S62.300-** Unspecified fracture of second metacarpal bone, right hand

CC-B,K,P **S62.301-** Unspecified fracture of second metacarpal bone, left hand

CC-B,K,P **S62.302-** Unspecified fracture of third metacarpal bone, right hand

CC-B,K,P **S62.303-** Unspecified fracture of third metacarpal bone, left hand

CC-B,K,P **S62.304-** Unspecified fracture of fourth metacarpal bone, right hand

CC-B,K,P **S62.305-** Unspecified fracture of fourth metacarpal bone, left hand

CC-B,K,P **S62.306-** Unspecified fracture of fifth metacarpal bone, right hand

CC-B,K,P **S62.307-** Unspecified fracture of fifth metacarpal bone, left hand

CC-B,K,P **S62.308-** Unspecified fracture of other metacarpal bone
Unspecified fracture of specified metacarpal bone with unspecified laterality

CC-B,K,P **S62.309-** Unspecified fracture of unspecified metacarpal bone

S62.31- Displaced fracture of base of other metacarpal bone

CC-B,K,P **S62.310-** Displaced fracture of base of second metacarpal bone, right hand

CC-B,K,P **S62.311-** Displaced fracture of base of second metacarpal bone. left hand

CC-B,K,P **S62.312-** Displaced fracture of base of third metacarpal bone, right hand

CC-B,K,P **S62.313-** Displaced fracture of base of third metacarpal bone, left hand

CC-B,K,P **S62.314-** Displaced fracture of base of fourth metacarpal bone, right hand

CC-B,K,P **S62.315-** Displaced fracture of base of fourth metacarpal bone, left hand

CC-B,K,P **S62.316-** Displaced fracture of base of fifth metacarpal bone, right hand

CC-B,K,P **S62.317-** Displaced fracture of base of fifth metacarpal bone. left hand

CC-B,K,P **S62.318-** Displaced fracture of base of other metacarpal bone
Displaced fracture of base of specified metacarpal bone with unspecified laterality

CC-B,K,P **S62.319-** Displaced fracture of base of unspecified metacarpal bone

S62.32- Displaced fracture of shaft of other metacarpal bone

CC-B,K,P **S62.320-** Displaced fracture of shaft of second metacarpal bone, right hand

CC-B,K,P **S62.321-** Displaced fracture of shaft of second metacarpal bone, left hand

CC-B,K,P **S62.322-** Displaced fracture of shaft of third metacarpal bone, right hand

CC-B,K,P **S62.323-** Displaced fracture of shaft of third metacarpal bone, left hand

CC-B,K,P **S62.324-** Displaced fracture of shaft of fourth metacarpal bone, right hand

CC-B,K,P **S62.325-** Displaced fracture of shaft of fourth metacarpal bone, left hand

CC-B,K,P **S62.326-** Displaced fracture of shaft of fifth metacarpal bone, right hand

CC-B,K,P **S62.327-** Displaced fracture of shaft of fifth metacarpal bone, left hand

CC-B,K,P **S62.328-** Displaced fracture of shaft of other metacarpal bone
Displaced fracture of shaft of specified metacarpal bone with unspecified laterality

CC-B,K,P **S62.329-** Displaced fracture of shaft of unspecified metacarpal bone

S62.33- Displaced fracture of neck of other metacarpal bone

CC-B,K,P **S62.330-** Displaced fracture of neck of second metacarpal bone, right hand

CC-B,K,P **S62.331-** Displaced fracture of neck of second metacarpal bone, left hand

CC-B,K,P **S62.332-** Displaced fracture of neck of third metacarpal bone, right hand

CC-B,K,P **S62.333-** Displaced fracture of neck of third metacarpal bone, left hand

CC-B,K,P **S62.334-** Displaced fracture of neck of fourth metacarpal bone, right hand

CC-B,K,P **S62.335-** Displaced fracture of neck of fourth metacarpal bone, left hand

CC-B,K,P **S62.336-** Displaced fracture of neck of fifth metacarpal bone, right hand

CC-B,K,P **S62.337-** Displaced fracture of neck of fifth metacarpal bone, left hand

CC-B,K,P **S62.338-** Displaced fracture of neck of other metacarpal bone
Displaced fracture of neck of specified metacarpal bone with unspecified laterality

CC-B,K,P **S62.339-** Displaced fracture of neck of unspecified metacarpal bone

S62-S62

S62.34- <u>Nondisplaced</u> fracture of <u>base</u> of <u>other</u> <u>metacarpal</u> bone

CC-B,K,P **S62.340-** <u>Nondisplaced</u> fracture of <u>base</u> of <u>second</u> metacarpal bone, <u>right</u> hand

CC-B,K,P **S62.341-** <u>Nondisplaced</u> fracture of <u>base</u> of <u>second</u> metacarpal bone, <u>left</u> hand

CC-B,K,P **S62.342-** <u>Nondisplaced</u> fracture of <u>base</u> of <u>third</u> metacarpal bone, <u>right</u> hand

CC-B,K,P **S62.343-** <u>Nondisplaced</u> fracture of <u>base</u> of <u>third</u> metacarpal bone, <u>left</u> hand

CC-B,K,P **S62.344-** <u>Nondisplaced</u> fracture of <u>base</u> of <u>fourth</u> metacarpal bone, <u>right</u> hand

CC-B,K,P **S62.345-** <u>Nondisplaced</u> fracture of <u>base</u> of <u>fourth</u> metacarpal bone, <u>left</u> hand

CC-B,K,P **S62.346-** <u>Nondisplaced</u> fracture of <u>base</u> of <u>fifth</u> metacarpal bone, <u>right</u> hand

CC-B,K,P **S62.347-** <u>Nondisplaced</u> fracture of <u>base</u> of <u>fifth</u> metacarpal bone. <u>left</u> hand

CC-B,K,P **S62.348-** <u>Nondisplaced</u> fracture of <u>base</u> of <u>other</u> metacarpal bone
Nondisplaced fracture of base of specified metacarpal bone with unspecified laterality

CC-B,K,P **S62.349-** <u>Nondisplaced</u> fracture of <u>base</u> of <u>unspecified</u> metacarpal bone

S62.35- <u>Nondisplaced</u> fracture of <u>shaft</u> of <u>other</u> <u>metacarpal</u> bone

CC-B,K,P **S62.350-** <u>Nondisplaced</u> fracture of <u>shaft</u> of <u>second</u> metacarpal bone, <u>right</u> hand

CC-B,K,P **S62.351-** <u>Nondisplaced</u> fracture of <u>shaft</u> of <u>second</u> metacarpal bone, <u>left</u> hand

CC-B,K,P **S62.352-** <u>Nondisplaced</u> fracture of <u>shaft</u> of <u>third</u> metacarpal bone, <u>right</u> hand

CC-B,K,P **S62.353-** <u>Nondisplaced</u> fracture of <u>shaft</u> of <u>third</u> metacarpal bone, <u>left</u> hand

CC-B,K,P **S62.354-** <u>Nondisplaced</u> fracture of <u>shaft</u> of <u>fourth</u> metacarpal bone, <u>right</u> hand

CC-B,K,P **S62.355-** <u>Nondisplaced</u> fracture of <u>shaft</u> of <u>fourth</u> metacarpal bone, <u>left</u> hand

CC-B,K,P **S62.356-** <u>Nondisplaced</u> fracture of <u>shaft</u> of <u>fifth</u> metacarpal bone, <u>right</u> hand

CC-B,K,P **S62.357-** <u>Nondisplaced</u> fracture of <u>shaft</u> of <u>fifth</u> metacarpal bone, <u>left</u> hand

CC-B,K,P **S62.358-** <u>Nondisplaced</u> fracture of <u>shaft</u> of <u>other</u> metacarpal bone
Nondisplaced fracture of shaft of specified metacarpal bone with unspecified laterality

CC-B,K,P **S62.359-** <u>Nondisplaced</u> fracture of <u>shaft</u> of <u>unspecified</u> metacarpal bone

S62.36- <u>Nondisplaced</u> fracture of <u>neck</u> of <u>other</u> <u>metacarpal</u> bone

CC-B,K,P **S62.360-** <u>Nondisplaced</u> fracture of <u>neck</u> of <u>second</u> metacarpal bone, <u>right</u> hand

CC-B,K,P **S62.361-** <u>Nondisplaced</u> fracture of <u>neck</u> of <u>second</u> metacarpal bone, <u>left</u> hand

CC-B,K,P **S62.362-** <u>Nondisplaced</u> fracture of <u>neck</u> of <u>third</u> metacarpal bone, <u>right</u> hand

CC-B,K,P **S62.363-** <u>Nondisplaced</u> fracture of <u>neck</u> of <u>third</u> metacarpal bone, <u>left</u> hand

CC-B,K,P **S62.364-** <u>Nondisplaced</u> fracture of <u>neck</u> of <u>fourth</u> metacarpal bone, <u>right</u> hand

CC-B,K,P **S62.365-** <u>Nondisplaced</u> fracture of <u>neck</u> of <u>fourth</u> metacarpal bone, <u>left</u> hand

CC-B,K,P **S62.366-** <u>Nondisplaced</u> fracture of <u>neck</u> of <u>fifth</u> metacarpal bone, <u>right</u> hand

CC-B,K,P **S62.367-** <u>Nondisplaced</u> fracture of <u>neck</u> of <u>fifth</u> metacarpal bone, <u>left</u> hand

CC-B,K,P **S62.368-** <u>Nondisplaced</u> fracture of <u>neck</u> of <u>other</u> metacarpal bone
Nondisplaced fracture of neck of specified metacarpal bone with unspecified laterality

CC-B,K,P **S62.369-** <u>Nondisplaced</u> fracture of <u>neck</u> of <u>unspecified</u> metacarpal bone

S62.39- <u>Other fracture</u> of <u>other</u> <u>metacarpal</u> bone

CC-B,K,P **S62.390-** Other fracture of <u>second</u> metacarpal bone, <u>right</u> hand

CC-B,K,P **S62.391-** Other fracture of <u>second</u> metacarpal bone, <u>left</u> hand

CC-B,K,P **S62.392-** Other fracture of <u>third</u> metacarpal bone, <u>right</u> hand

CC-B,K,P **S62.393-** Other fracture of <u>third</u> metacarpal bone, <u>left</u> hand

CC-B,K,P **S62.394-** Other fracture of <u>fourth</u> metacarpal bone, <u>right</u> hand

CC-B,K,P **S62.395-** Other fracture of <u>fourth</u> metacarpal bone, <u>left</u> hand

CC-B,K,P **S62.396-** Other fracture of <u>fifth</u> metacarpal bone, <u>right</u> hand

CC-B,K,P **S62.397-** Other fracture of <u>fifth</u> metacarpal bone, <u>left</u> hand

CC-B,K,P **S62.398-** Other fracture of <u>other</u> metacarpal bone
Other fracture of specified metacarpal bone with unspecified laterality

CC-B,K,P **S62.399-** Other fracture of <u>unspecified</u> metacarpal bone

S62.5- <u>Fracture</u> of <u>thumb</u>

S62.50- Fracture of <u>unspecified phalanx</u> of <u>thumb</u>

CC-B,K,P **S62.501-** Fracture of unspecified phalanx of <u>right</u> thumb

CC-B,K,P **S62.502-** Fracture of unspecified phalanx of <u>left</u> thumb

CC-B,K,P **S62.509-** Fracture of unspecified phalanx of <u>unspecified</u> thumb

S62.51- Fracture of <u>proximal phalanx</u> of <u>thumb</u>

CC-B,K,P **S62.511-** <u>Displaced</u> fracture of <u>proximal</u> phalanx of <u>right</u> thumb

CC-B,K,P **S62.512-** <u>Displaced</u> fracture of <u>proximal</u> phalanx of <u>left</u> thumb

CC-B,K,P **S62.513-** <u>Displaced</u> fracture of <u>proximal</u> phalanx of <u>unspecified</u> thumb

CC-B,K,P **S62.514-** <u>Nondisplaced</u> fracture of <u>proximal</u> phalanx of <u>right</u> thumb

CC-B,K,P **S62.515-** <u>Nondisplaced</u> fracture of <u>proximal</u> phalanx of <u>left</u> thumb

CC-B,K,P **S62.516-** <u>Nondisplaced</u> fracture of <u>proximal</u> phalanx of <u>unspecified</u> thumb

S62.52- Fracture of <u>distal phalanx</u> of <u>thumb</u>

CC-B,K,P **S62.521-** <u>Displaced</u> fracture of <u>distal</u> phalanx of <u>right</u> thumb

CC-B,K,P **S62.522-** <u>Displaced</u> fracture of <u>distal</u> phalanx of <u>left</u> thumb

CC-B,K,P **S62.523-** <u>Displaced</u> fracture of <u>distal</u> phalanx of <u>unspecified</u> thumb

CC-B,K,P **S62.524-** <u>Nondisplaced</u> fracture of <u>distal</u> phalanx of <u>right</u> thumb

CC-B,K,P **S62.525-** <u>Nondisplaced</u> fracture of <u>distal</u> phalanx of <u>left</u> thumb

CC-B,K,P **S62.526-** <u>Nondisplaced</u> fracture of <u>distal</u> phalanx of <u>unspecified</u> thumb

S62.6- Fracture of <u>other and unspecified finger(s)</u>
Excludes ❷: fracture of thumb (S62.5-)

S62.60- Fracture of <u>unspecified phalanx</u> of <u>finger</u>

CC-B,K,P **S62.600-** Fracture of <u>unspecified</u> phalanx of <u>right</u> <u>index</u> finger

CC-B,K,P **S62.601-** Fracture of <u>unspecified</u> phalanx of <u>left</u> <u>index</u> finger

CC-B,K,P **S62.602-** Fracture of <u>unspecified</u> phalanx of <u>right</u> <u>middle</u> finger

CC-B,K,P **S62.603-** Fracture of <u>unspecified</u> phalanx of <u>left</u> <u>middle</u> finger

CC-B,K,P **S62.604-** Fracture of <u>unspecified</u> phalanx of <u>right</u> <u>ring</u> finger

CC-B,K,P **S62.605-** Fracture of <u>unspecified</u> phalanx of <u>left</u> <u>ring</u> finger

CC-B,K,P **S62.606-** Fracture of <u>unspecified</u> phalanx of <u>right</u> <u>little</u> finger

CC-B,K,P **S62.607-** Fracture of <u>unspecified</u> phalanx of <u>left</u> <u>little</u> finger

CC-B,K,P **S62.608-** Fracture of <u>unspecified</u> phalanx of <u>other</u> finger
Fracture of unspecified phalanx of specified finger with unspecified laterality

CC-B,K,P **S62.609-** Fracture of <u>unspecified</u> phalanx of <u>unspecified</u> finger

S62.61- <u>Displaced</u> fracture of <u>proximal phalanx</u> of <u>finger</u>

CC-B,K,P **S62.610-** <u>Displaced</u> fracture of <u>proximal</u> phalanx of <u>right</u> index finger

S62 - S62

CC-B,K,P **S62.611-** <u>Displaced</u> fracture of <u>proximal</u> phalanx of <u>left</u> <u>index</u> finger

CC-B,K,P **S62.612-** <u>Displaced</u> fracture of <u>proximal</u> phalanx of <u>right</u> <u>middle</u> finger

CC-B,K,P **S62.613-** <u>Displaced</u> fracture of <u>proximal</u> phalanx of <u>left</u> <u>middle</u> finger

CC-B,K,P **S62.614-** <u>Displaced</u> fracture of <u>proximal</u> phalanx of <u>right</u> <u>ring</u> finger

CC-B,K,P **S62.615-** <u>Displaced</u> fracture of <u>proximal</u> phalanx of <u>left</u> <u>ring</u> finger

CC-B,K,P **S62.616-** <u>Displaced</u> fracture of <u>proximal</u> phalanx of <u>right</u> <u>little</u> finger

CC-B,K,P **S62.617-** <u>Displaced</u> fracture of <u>proximal</u> phalanx of <u>left</u> <u>little</u> finger

CC-B,K,P **S62.618-** <u>Displaced</u> fracture of <u>proximal</u> phalanx of <u>other</u> finger
Displaced fracture of proximal phalanx of specified finger with unspecified laterality

CC-B,K,P **S62.619-** <u>Displaced</u> fracture of proximal phalanx of <u>unspecified</u> finger

S62.62- <u>Displaced</u> fracture of <u>medial</u> <u>phalanx</u> of <u>finger</u>

CC-B,K,P **S62.620-** <u>Displaced</u> fracture of <u>medial</u> phalanx of <u>right</u> <u>index</u> finger

CC-B,K,P **S62.621-** <u>Displaced</u> fracture of <u>medial</u> phalanx of <u>left</u> <u>index</u> finger

CC-B,K,P **S62.622-** <u>Displaced</u> fracture of <u>medial</u> phalanx of <u>right</u> <u>middle</u> finger

CC-B,K,P **S62.623-** <u>Displaced</u> fracture of <u>medial</u> phalanx of <u>left</u> <u>middle</u> finger

CC-B,K,P **S62.624-** <u>Displaced</u> fracture of <u>medial</u> phalanx of <u>right</u> <u>ring</u> finger

CC-B,K,P **S62.625-** <u>Displaced</u> fracture of <u>medial</u> phalanx of <u>left</u> <u>ring</u> finger

CC-B,K,P **S62.626-** <u>Displaced</u> fracture of <u>medial</u> phalanx of <u>right</u> <u>little</u> finger

CC-B,K,P **S62.627-** <u>Displaced</u> fracture of <u>medial</u> phalanx of <u>left</u> <u>little</u> finger

CC-B,K,P **S62.628-** <u>Displaced</u> fracture of <u>medial</u> phalanx of <u>other</u> finger
Displaced fracture of medial phalanx of specified finger with unspecified laterality

CC-B,K,P **S62.629-** <u>Displaced</u> fracture of <u>medial</u> phalanx of <u>unspecified</u> finger

S62.63- <u>Displaced</u> fracture of <u>distal</u> <u>phalanx</u> of <u>finger</u>

CC-B,K,P **S62.630-** <u>Displaced</u> fracture of <u>distal</u> phalanx of <u>right</u> <u>index</u> finger

CC-B,K,P **S62.631-** <u>Displaced</u> fracture of <u>distal</u> phalanx of <u>left</u> <u>index</u> finger

CC-B,K,P **S62.632-** <u>Displaced</u> fracture of <u>distal</u> phalanx of <u>right</u> <u>middle</u> finger

CC-B,K,P **S62.633-** <u>Displaced</u> fracture of <u>distal</u> phalanx of <u>left</u> <u>middle</u> finger

CC-B,K,P **S62.634-** <u>Displaced</u> fracture of <u>distal</u> phalanx of <u>right</u> <u>ring</u> finger

CC-B,K,P **S62.635-** <u>Displaced</u> fracture of <u>distal</u> phalanx of <u>left</u> <u>ring</u> finger

CC-B,K,P **S62.636-** <u>Displaced</u> fracture of <u>distal</u> phalanx of <u>right</u> <u>little</u> finger

CC-B,K,P **S62.637-** <u>Displaced</u> fracture of <u>distal</u> phalanx of <u>left</u> <u>little</u> finger

CC-B,K,P **S62.638-** <u>Displaced</u> fracture of <u>distal</u> phalanx of <u>other</u> finger
Displaced fracture of distal phalanx of specified finger with unspecified laterality

CC-B,K,P **S62.639-** <u>Displaced</u> fracture of <u>distal</u> phalanx of <u>unspecified</u> finger

S62.64- <u>Nondisplaced</u> fracture of <u>proximal</u> <u>phalanx</u> of <u>finger</u>

CC-B,K,P **S62.640-** <u>Nondisplaced</u> fracture of <u>proximal</u> phalanx of <u>right</u> <u>index</u> finger

CC-B,K,P **S62.641-** <u>Nondisplaced</u> fracture of <u>proximal</u> phalanx of <u>left</u> <u>index</u> finger

CC-B,K,P **S62.642-** <u>Nondisplaced</u> fracture of <u>proximal</u> phalanx of <u>right</u> <u>middle</u> finger

CC-B,K,P **S62.643-** <u>Nondisplaced</u> fracture of <u>proximal</u> phalanx of <u>left</u> <u>middle</u> finger

CC-B,K,P **S62.644-** <u>Nondisplaced</u> fracture of <u>proximal</u> phalanx of <u>right</u> <u>ring</u> finger

CC-B,K,P **S62.645-** <u>Nondisplaced</u> fracture of <u>proximal</u> phalanx of <u>left</u> <u>ring</u> finger

CC-B,K,P **S62.646-** <u>Nondisplaced</u> fracture of <u>proximal</u> phalanx of <u>right</u> <u>little</u> finger

CC-B,K,P **S62.647-** <u>Nondisplaced</u> fracture of <u>proximal</u> phalanx of <u>left</u> <u>little</u> finger

CC-B,K,P **S62.648-** <u>Nondisplaced</u> fracture of <u>proximal</u> phalanx of <u>other</u> finger
Nondisplaced fracture of proximal phalanx of specified finger with unspecified laterality

CC-B,K,P **S62.649-** <u>Nondisplaced</u> fracture of <u>proximal</u> phalanx of <u>unspecified</u> finger

S62.65- <u>Nondisplaced</u> fracture of <u>medial</u> <u>phalanx</u> of <u>finger</u>

CC-B,K,P **S62.650-** <u>Nondisplaced</u> fracture of <u>medial</u> phalanx of <u>right</u> <u>index</u> finger

CC-B,K,P **S62.651-** <u>Nondisplaced</u> fracture of <u>medial</u> phalanx of <u>left</u> <u>index</u> finger

CC-B,K,P **S62.652-** <u>Nondisplaced</u> fracture of <u>medial</u> phalanx of <u>right</u> <u>middle</u> finger

CC-B,K,P **S62.653-** <u>Nondisplaced</u> fracture of <u>medial</u> phalanx of <u>left</u> <u>middle</u> finger

CC-B,K,P **S62.654-** <u>Nondisplaced</u> fracture of <u>medial</u> phalanx of <u>right</u> <u>ring</u> finger

CC-B,K,P **S62.655-** <u>Nondisplaced</u> fracture of <u>medial</u> phalanx of <u>left</u> <u>ring</u> finger

CC-B,K,P **S62.656-** <u>Nondisplaced</u> fracture of <u>medial</u> phalanx of <u>right</u> <u>little</u> finger

CC-B,K,P **S62.657-** <u>Nondisplaced</u> fracture of <u>medial</u> phalanx of <u>left</u> <u>little</u> finger

CC-B,K,P **S62.658-** <u>Nondisplaced</u> fracture of <u>medial</u> phalanx of <u>other</u> finger
Nondisplaced fracture of medial phalanx of specified finger with unspecified laterality

CC-B,K,P **S62.659-** <u>Nondisplaced</u> fracture of <u>medial</u> phalanx of <u>unspecified</u> finger

S62.66- <u>Nondisplaced</u> fracture of <u>distal</u> <u>phalanx</u> of <u>finger</u>

CC-B,K,P **S62.660-** <u>Nondisplaced</u> fracture of <u>distal</u> phalanx of <u>right</u> <u>index</u> finger

CC-B,K,P **S62.661-** <u>Nondisplaced</u> fracture of <u>distal</u> phalanx of <u>left</u> <u>index</u> finger

CC-B,K,P **S62.662-** <u>Nondisplaced</u> fracture of <u>distal</u> phalanx of <u>right</u> <u>middle</u> finger

CC-B,K,P **S62.663-** <u>Nondisplaced</u> fracture of <u>distal</u> phalanx of <u>left</u> <u>middle</u> finger

CC-B,K,P **S62.664-** <u>Nondisplaced</u> fracture of <u>distal</u> phalanx of <u>right</u> <u>ring</u> finger

CC-B,K,P **S62.665-** <u>Nondisplaced</u> fracture of <u>distal</u> phalanx of <u>left</u> <u>ring</u> finger

CC-B,K,P **S62.666-** <u>Nondisplaced</u> fracture of <u>distal</u> phalanx of <u>right</u> <u>little</u> finger

CC-B,K,P **S62.667-** <u>Nondisplaced</u> fracture of <u>distal</u> phalanx of <u>left</u> <u>little</u> finger

CC-B,K,P **S62.668-** <u>Nondisplaced</u> fracture of <u>distal</u> phalanx of <u>other</u> finger
Nondisplaced fracture of distal phalanx of specified finger with unspecified laterality

CC-B,K,P **S62.669-** <u>Nondisplaced</u> fracture of <u>distal</u> phalanx of <u>unspecified</u> finger

S62.9- <u>Unspecified</u> <u>fracture</u> of <u>wrist and hand</u>

CC-B,K,P **S62.90x-** Unspecified fracture of <u>unspecified</u> wrist and hand

CC-B,K,P **S62.91x-** Unspecified fracture of <u>right</u> wrist and hand

CC-B,K,P **S62.92x-** Unspecified fracture of <u>left</u> wrist and hand

S62 - S62

Excludes 1: = NOT CODED HERE! (Do not code both)   **1088**   *Excludes ❷:* = Not Included Here

S63-   Dislocation and sprain of joints and ligaments at wrist and hand level

Includes: Avulsion of joint or ligament at wrist and hand level
             Laceration of cartilage, joint or ligament at wrist and hand level
             Sprain of cartilage, joint or ligament at wrist and hand level
             Traumatic hemarthrosis of joint or ligament at wrist and hand level
             Traumatic rupture of joint or ligament at wrist and hand level
             Traumatic subluxation of joint or ligament at wrist and hand level
             Traumatic tear of joint or ligament at wrist and hand level

Code also any associated open wound

Excludes ❷: strain of muscle, fascia and tendon of wrist and hand (S66.-)

The appropriate 7th character is to be added to each code from category S63:
A   Initial encounter
D   Subsequent encounter
S   Sequela

S63.0-   Subluxation and dislocation of wrist and hand joints

S63.00- Unspecified subluxation and dislocation of wrist and hand
             Dislocation of carpal bone NOS
             Dislocation of distal end of radius NOS
             Subluxation of carpal bone NOS
             Subluxation of distal end of radius NOS

S63.001- Unspecified subluxation of right wrist and hand

S63.002- Unspecified subluxation of left wrist and hand

S63.003- Unspecified subluxation of unspecified wrist and hand

S63.004- Unspecified dislocation of right wrist and hand

S63.005- Unspecified dislocation of left wrist and hand

S63.006- Unspecified dislocation of unspecified wrist and hand

S63.01- Subluxation and dislocation of distal radioulnar joint

S63.011- Subluxation of distal radioulnar joint of right wrist

S63.012- Subluxation of distal radioulnar joint of left wrist

S63.013- Subluxation of distal radioulnar joint of unspecified wrist

S63.014- Dislocation of distal radioulnar joint of right wrist

S63.015- Dislocation of distal radioulnar joint of left wrist

S63.016- Dislocation of distal radioulnar joint of unspecified wrist

S63.02- Subluxation and dislocation of radiocarpal joint

S63.021- Subluxation of radiocarpal joint of right wrist

S63.022- Subluxation of radiocarpal joint of left wrist

S63.023- Subluxation of radiocarpal joint of unspecified wrist

S63.024- Dislocation of radiocarpal joint of right wrist

S63.025- Dislocation of radiocarpal joint of left wrist

S63.026- Dislocation of radiocarpal joint of unspecified wrist

S63.03- Subluxation and dislocation of midcarpal joint

S63.031- Subluxation of midcarpal joint of right wrist

S63.032- Subluxation of midcarpal joint of left wrist

S63.033- Subluxation of midcarpal joint of unspecified wrist

S63.034- Dislocation of midcarpal joint of right wrist

S63.035- Dislocation of midcarpal joint of left wrist

S63.036- Dislocation of midcarpal joint of unspecified wrist

S63.04- Subluxation and dislocation of carpometacarpal joint of thumb

Excludes ❷: interphalangeal subluxation and dislocation of thumb (S63.1-)

S63.041- Subluxation of carpometacarpal joint of right thumb

S63.042- Subluxation of carpometacarpal joint of left thumb

S63.043- Subluxation of carpometacarpal joint of unspecified thumb

S63.044- Dislocation of carpometacarpal joint of right thumb

S63.045- Dislocation of carpometacarpal joint of left thumb

S63.046- Dislocation of carpometacarpal joint of unspecified thumb

S63.05- Subluxation and dislocation of other carpometacarpal joint

Excludes ❷: subluxation and dislocation of carpometacarpal joint of thumb (S63.04-)

S63.051- Subluxation of other carpometacarpal joint of right hand

S63.052- Subluxation of other carpometacarpal joint of left hand

S63.053- Subluxation of other carpometacarpal joint of unspecified hand

S63.054- Dislocation of other carpometacarpal joint of right hand

S63.055- Dislocation of other carpometacarpal joint of left hand

S63.056- Dislocation of other carpometacarpal joint of unspecified hand

S63.06- Subluxation and dislocation of metacarpal (bone), proximal end

S63.061- Subluxation of metacarpal (bone), proximal end of right hand

S63.062- Subluxation of metacarpal (bone), proximal end of left hand

S63.063- Subluxation of metacarpal (bone), proximal end of unspecified hand

S63.064- Dislocation of metacarpal (bone), proximal end of right hand

S63.065- Dislocation of metacarpal (bone), proximal end of left hand

S63.066- Dislocation of metacarpal (bone), proximal end of unspecified hand

S63.07- Subluxation and dislocation of distal end of ulna

S63.071- Subluxation of distal end of right ulna

S63.072- Subluxation of distal end of left ulna

S63.073- Subluxation of distal end of unspecified ulna

S63.074- Dislocation of distal end of right ulna

S63.075- Dislocation of distal end of left ulna

S63.076- Dislocation of distal end of unspecified ulna

S63.09- Other subluxation and dislocation of wrist and hand

S63.091- Other subluxation of right wrist and hand

S63.092- Other subluxation of left wrist and hand

S63.093- Other subluxation of unspecified wrist and hand

S63.094- Other dislocation of right wrist and hand

S63.095- Other dislocation of left wrist and hand

S63.096- Other dislocation of unspecified wrist and hand

S63.1-   Subluxation and dislocation of thumb

S63.10- Unspecified subluxation and dislocation of thumb

S63.101- Unspecified subluxation of right thumb

S63.102- Unspecified subluxation of left thumb

S63.103- Unspecified subluxation of unspecified thumb

S63.104- Unspecified dislocation of right thumb

S63.105- Unspecified dislocation of left thumb

S63.106- Unspecified dislocation of unspecified thumb

S63.11- Subluxation and dislocation of metacarpophalangeal joint of thumb

S63.111- Subluxation of metacarpophalangeal joint of right thumb

S63.112- Subluxation of metacarpophalangeal joint of left thumb

S63.113- Subluxation of metacarpophalangeal joint of unspecified thumb

S63.114- Dislocation of metacarpophalangeal joint of right thumb

S63.115- Dislocation of metacarpophalangeal joint of left thumb

S63.116- Dislocation of metacarpophalangeal joint of unspecified thumb

S 6 3 - S 6 3

S63.12- Subluxation and dislocation of <u>unspecified</u> <u>interphalangeal joint</u> of <u>thumb</u>

S63.121- <u>Subluxation</u> of unspecified interphalangeal joint of <u>right</u> thumb

S63.122- <u>Subluxation</u> of unspecified interphalangeal joint of <u>left</u> thumb

S63.123- <u>Subluxation</u> of unspecified interphalangeal joint of <u>unspecified</u> thumb

S63.124- <u>Dislocation</u> of unspecified interphalangeal joint of <u>right</u> thumb

S63.125- <u>Dislocation</u> of unspecified interphalangeal joint of <u>left</u> thumb

S63.126- <u>Dislocation</u> of unspecified interphalangeal joint of <u>unspecified</u> thumb

S63.13- Subluxation and dislocation of <u>proximal interphalangeal joint</u> of <u>thumb</u>

S63.131- <u>Subluxation</u> of proximal interphalangeal joint of <u>right</u> thumb

S63.132- <u>Subluxation</u> of proximal interphalangeal joint of <u>left</u> thumb

S63.133- <u>Subluxation</u> of proximal interphalangeal joint of <u>unspecified</u> thumb

S63.134- <u>Dislocation</u> of proximal interphalangeal joint of <u>right</u> thumb

S63.135- <u>Dislocation</u> of proximal interphalangeal joint of <u>left</u> thumb

S63.136- <u>Dislocation</u> of proximal interphalangeal joint of <u>unspecified</u> thumb

S63.14- Subluxation and dislocation of <u>distal interphalangeal joint</u> of <u>thumb</u>

S63.141- <u>Subluxation</u> of distal interphalangeal joint of <u>right</u> thumb

S63.142- <u>Subluxation</u> of distal interphalangeal joint of <u>left</u> thumb

S63.143- <u>Subluxation</u> of distal interphalangeal joint of <u>unspecified</u> thumb

S63.144- <u>Dislocation</u> of distal interphalangeal joint of <u>right</u> thumb

S63.145- <u>Dislocation</u> of distal interphalangeal joint of <u>left</u> thumb

S63.146- <u>Dislocation</u> of distal interphalangeal joint of <u>unspecified</u> thumb

S63.2- Subluxation and dislocation of <u>other finger(s)</u>
Excludes ❷: *subluxation and dislocation of thumb (S63.1-)*

S63.20- <u>Unspecified subluxation</u> of other <u>finger</u>

S63.200- Unspecified subluxation of <u>right</u> <u>index</u> finger

S63.201- Unspecified subluxation of <u>left</u> <u>index</u> finger

S63.202- Unspecified subluxation of <u>right</u> <u>middle</u> finger

S63.203- Unspecified subluxation of <u>left</u> <u>middle</u> finger

S63.204- Unspecified subluxation of <u>right</u> <u>ring</u> finger

S63.205- Unspecified subluxation of <u>left</u> <u>ring</u> finger

S63.206- Unspecified subluxation of <u>right</u> <u>little</u> finger

S63.207- Unspecified subluxation of <u>left</u> <u>little</u> finger

S63.208- Unspecified subluxation of <u>other</u> finger
Unspecified subluxation of specified finger with unspecified laterality

S63.209- Unspecified subluxation of <u>unspecified</u> finger

S63.21- <u>Subluxation</u> of <u>metacarpophalangeal joint</u> of <u>finger</u>

S63.210- Subluxation of metacarpophalangeal joint of <u>right</u> <u>index</u> finger

S63.211- Subluxation of metacarpophalangeal joint of <u>left</u> <u>index</u> finger

S63.212- Subluxation of metacarpophalangeal joint of <u>right</u> <u>middle</u> finger

S63.213- Subluxation of metacarpophalangeal joint of <u>left</u> <u>middle</u> finger

S63.214- Subluxation of metacarpophalangeal joint of <u>right</u> <u>ring</u> finger

S63.215- Subluxation of metacarpophalangeal joint of <u>left</u> <u>ring</u> finger

S63.216- Subluxation of metacarpophalangeal joint of <u>right</u> <u>little</u> finger

S63.217- Subluxation of metacarpophalangeal joint of <u>left</u> <u>little</u> finger

S63.218- Subluxation of metacarpophalangeal joint of <u>other</u> finger
Subluxation of metacarpophalangeal joint of specified finger with unspecified laterality

S63.219- Subluxation of metacarpophalangeal joint of <u>unspecified</u> finger

S63.22- <u>Subluxation</u> of <u>unspecified interphalangeal joint</u> of <u>finger</u>

S63.220- Subluxation of unspecified interphalangeal joint of <u>right</u> <u>index</u> finger

S63.221- Subluxation of unspecified interphalangeal joint of <u>left</u> <u>index</u> finger

S63.222- Subluxation of unspecified interphalangeal joint of <u>right</u> <u>middle</u> finger

S63.223- Subluxation of unspecified interphalangeal joint of <u>left</u> <u>middle</u> finger

S63.224- Subluxation of unspecified interphalangeal joint of <u>right</u> <u>ring</u> finger

S63.225- Subluxation of unspecified interphalangeal joint of <u>left</u> <u>ring</u> finger

S63.226- Subluxation of unspecified interphalangeal joint of <u>right</u> <u>little</u> finger

S63.227- Subluxation of unspecified interphalangeal joint of <u>left</u> <u>little</u> finger

S63.228- Subluxation of unspecified interphalangeal joint of <u>other</u> finger
Subluxation of unspecified interphalangeal joint of specified finger with unspecified laterality

S63.229- Subluxation of unspecified interphalangeal joint of <u>unspecified</u> finger

S63.23- <u>Subluxation</u> of <u>proximal interphalangeal joint</u> of <u>finger</u>

S63.230- Subluxation of proximal interphalangeal joint of <u>right</u> <u>index</u> finger

S63.231- Subluxation of proximal interphalangeal joint of <u>left</u> <u>index</u> finger

S63.232- Subluxation of proximal interphalangeal joint of <u>right</u> <u>middle</u> finger

S63.233- Subluxation of proximal interphalangeal joint of <u>left</u> <u>middle</u> finger

S63.234- Subluxation of proximal interphalangeal joint of <u>right</u> <u>ring</u> finger

S63.235- Subluxation of proximal interphalangeal joint of <u>left</u> <u>ring</u> finger

S63.236- Subluxation of proximal interphalangeal joint of <u>right</u> <u>little</u> finger

S63.237- Subluxation of proximal interphalangeal joint of <u>left</u> <u>little</u> finger

S63.238- Subluxation of proximal interphalangeal joint of <u>other</u> finger
Subluxation of proximal interphalangeal joint of specified finger with unspecified laterality

S63.239- Subluxation of proximal interphalangeal joint of <u>unspecified</u> finger

S63.24- <u>Subluxation</u> of <u>distal interphalangeal joint</u> of <u>finger</u>

S63.240- Subluxation of distal interphalangeal joint of <u>right</u> <u>index</u> finger

S63.241- Subluxation of distal interphalangeal joint of <u>left</u> <u>index</u> finger

S63.242- Subluxation of distal interphalangeal joint of <u>right</u> <u>middle</u> finger

S63.243- Subluxation of distal interphalangeal joint of <u>left</u> <u>middle</u> finger

S63.244- Subluxation of distal interphalangeal joint of <u>right</u> <u>ring</u> finger

S63.245- Subluxation of distal interphalangeal joint of <u>left</u> <u>ring</u> finger

S63.246- Subluxation of distal interphalangeal joint of <u>right</u> <u>little</u> finger

S63.247- Subluxation of distal interphalangeal joint of <u>left</u> <u>little</u> finger

S63.248- Subluxation of distal interphalangeal joint of <u>other</u> finger
    Subluxation of distal interphalangeal joint of specified finger with unspecified laterality

S63.249- Subluxation of distal interphalangeal joint of <u>unspecified</u> finger

S63.25- <u>Unspecified</u> <u>dislocation</u> of <u>other</u> <u>finger</u>

S63.250- Unspecified dislocation of <u>right</u> <u>index</u> finger

S63.251- Unspecified dislocation of <u>left</u> <u>index</u> finger

S63.252- Unspecified dislocation of <u>right</u> <u>middle</u> finger

S63.253- Unspecified dislocation of <u>left</u> <u>middle</u> finger

S63.254- Unspecified dislocation of <u>right</u> <u>ring</u> finger

S63.255- Unspecified dislocation of <u>left</u> <u>ring</u> finger

S63.256- Unspecified dislocation of <u>right</u> <u>little</u> finger

S63.257- Unspecified dislocation of <u>left</u> <u>little</u> finger

S63.258- Unspecified dislocation of <u>other</u> finger
    Unspecified dislocation of specified finger with unspecified laterality

S63.259- Unspecified dislocation of <u>unspecified</u> finger
    Unspecified dislocation of specified finger with unspecified laterality

S63.26- <u>Dislocation</u> of <u>metacarpophalangeal joint</u> of <u>finger</u>

S63.260- Dislocation of metacarpophalangeal joint of <u>right</u> <u>index</u> finger

S63.261- Dislocation of metacarpophalangeal joint of <u>left</u> <u>index</u> finger

S63.262- Dislocation of metacarpophalangeal joint of <u>right</u> <u>middle</u> finger

S63.263- Dislocation of metacarpophalangeal joint of <u>left</u> <u>middle</u> finger

S63.264- Dislocation of metacarpophalangeal joint of <u>right</u> <u>ring</u> finger

S63.265- Dislocation of metacarpophalangeal joint of <u>left</u> <u>ring</u> finger

S63.266- Dislocation of metacarpophalangeal joint of <u>right</u> <u>little</u> finger

S63.267- Dislocation of metacarpophalangeal joint of <u>left</u> <u>little</u> finger

S63.268- Dislocation of metacarpophalangeal joint of <u>other</u> finger
    Dislocation of metacarpophalangeal joint of specified finger with unspecified laterality

S63.269- Dislocation of metacarpophalangeal joint of <u>unspecified</u> finger

S63.27- <u>Dislocation</u> of <u>unspecified interphalangeal joint</u> of <u>finger</u>

S63.270- Dislocation of unspecified interphalangeal joint of <u>right</u> <u>index</u> finger

S63.271- Dislocation of unspecified interphalangeal joint of <u>left</u> <u>index</u> finger

S63.272- Dislocation of unspecified interphalangeal joint of <u>right</u> <u>middle</u> finger

S63.273- Dislocation of unspecified interphalangeal joint of <u>left</u> <u>middle</u> finger

S63.274- Dislocation of unspecified interphalangeal joint of <u>right</u> <u>ring</u> finger

S63.275- Dislocation of unspecified interphalangeal joint of <u>left</u> <u>ring</u> finger

S63.276- Dislocation of unspecified interphalangeal joint of <u>right</u> <u>little</u> finger

S63.277- Dislocation of unspecified interphalangeal joint of <u>left</u> <u>little</u> finger

S63.278- Dislocation of unspecified interphalangeal joint of <u>other</u> finger
    Dislocation of unspecified interphalangeal joint of specified finger with unspecified laterality

S63.279- Dislocation of unspecified interphalangeal joint of <u>unspecified</u> finger
    Dislocation of unspecified interphalangeal joint of specified finger without specified laterality

S63.28- Dislocation of <u>proximal interphalangeal joint</u> of <u>finger</u>

S63.280- Dislocation of proximal interphalangeal joint of <u>right</u> <u>index</u> finger

S63.281- Dislocation of proximal interphalangeal joint of <u>left</u> <u>index</u> finger

S63.282- Dislocation of proximal interphalangeal joint of <u>right</u> <u>middle</u> finger

S63.283- Dislocation of proximal interphalangeal joint of <u>left</u> <u>middle</u> finger

S63.284- Dislocation of proximal interphalangeal joint of <u>right</u> <u>ring</u> finger

S63.285- Dislocation of proximal interphalangeal joint of <u>left</u> <u>ring</u> finger

S63.286- Dislocation of proximal interphalangeal joint of <u>right</u> <u>little</u> finger

S63.287- Dislocation of proximal interphalangeal joint of <u>left</u> <u>little</u> finger

S63.288- Dislocation of proximal interphalangeal joint of <u>other</u> finger
    Dislocation of proximal interphalangeal joint of specified finger with unspecified laterality

S63.289- Dislocation of proximal interphalangeal joint of <u>unspecified</u> finger

S63.29- <u>Dislocation</u> of <u>distal interphalangeal joint</u> of <u>finger</u>

S63.290- Dislocation of distal interphalangeal joint of <u>right</u> <u>index</u> finger

S63.291- Dislocation of distal interphalangeal joint of <u>left</u> <u>index</u> finger

S63.292- Dislocation of distal interphalangeal joint of <u>right</u> <u>middle</u> finger

S63.293- Dislocation of distal interphalangeal joint of <u>left</u> <u>middle</u> finger

S63.294- Dislocation of distal interphalangeal joint of <u>right</u> <u>ring</u> finger

S63.295- Dislocation of distal interphalangeal joint of <u>left</u> <u>ring</u> finger

S63.296- Dislocation of distal interphalangeal joint of <u>right</u> <u>little</u> finger

S63.297- Dislocation of distal interphalangeal joint of <u>left</u> <u>little</u> finger

S63.298- Dislocation of distal interphalangeal joint of <u>other</u> finger
    Dislocation of distal interphalangeal joint of specified finger with unspecified laterality

S63.299- Dislocation of distal interphalangeal joint of <u>unspecified</u> finger

S63.3- <u>Traumatic rupture</u> of <u>ligament</u> of <u>wrist</u>

S63.30- <u>Traumatic rupture</u> of <u>unspecified ligament</u> of <u>wrist</u>

S63.301- Traumatic rupture of unspecified ligament of <u>right</u> wrist

S63.302- Traumatic rupture of unspecified ligament of <u>left</u> wrist

S63.309- Traumatic rupture of unspecified ligament of <u>unspecified</u> wrist

S63.31- <u>Traumatic rupture</u> of <u>collateral</u> ligament of <u>wrist</u>

S63.311- Traumatic rupture of collateral ligament of <u>right</u> wrist

S63.312- Traumatic rupture of collateral ligament of <u>left</u> wrist

S63.319- Traumatic rupture of collateral ligament of <u>unspecified</u> wrist

S63 | S63

S63.32- Traumatic rupture of radiocarpal ligament

  S63.321- Traumatic rupture of right radiocarpal ligament

  S63.322- Traumatic rupture of left radiocarpal ligament

  S63.329- Traumatic rupture of unspecified radiocarpal ligament

S63.33- Traumatic rupture of ulnocarpal (palmar) ligament

  S63.331- Traumatic rupture of right ulnocarpal (palmar) ligament

  S63.332- Traumatic rupture of left ulnocarpal (palmar) ligament

  S63.339- Traumatic rupture of unspecified ulnocarpal (palmar) ligament

S63.39- Traumatic rupture of other ligament of wrist

  S63.391- Traumatic rupture of other ligament of right wrist

  S63.392- Traumatic rupture of other ligament of left wrist

  S63.399- Traumatic rupture of other ligament of unspecified wrist

S63.4- Traumatic rupture of ligament of finger at metacarpophalangeal and interphalangeal joint(s)

  S63.40- Traumatic rupture of unspecified ligament of finger at metacarpophalangeal and interphalangeal joint

   S63.400- Traumatic rupture of unspecified ligament of right index finger at metacarpophalangeal and interphalangeal joint

   S63.401- Traumatic rupture of unspecified ligament of left index finger at metacarpophalangeal and interphalangeal joint

   S63.402- Traumatic rupture of unspecified ligament of right middle finger at metacarpophalangeal and interphalangeal joint

   S63.403- Traumatic rupture of unspecified ligament of left middle finger at metacarpophalangeal and interphalangeal joint

   S63.404- Traumatic rupture of unspecified ligament of right ring finger at metacarpophalangeal and interphalangeal joint

   S63.405- Traumatic rupture of unspecified ligament of left ring finger at metacarpophalangeal and interphalangeal joint

   S63.406- Traumatic rupture of unspecified ligament of right little finger at metacarpophalangeal and interphalangeal joint

   S63.407- Traumatic rupture of unspecified ligament of left little finger at metacarpophalangeal and interphalangeal joint

   S63.408- Traumatic rupture of unspecified ligament of other finger at metacarpophalangeal and interphalangeal joint
   Traumatic rupture of unspecified ligament of specified finger with unspecified laterality at metacarpophalangeal and interphalangeal joint

   S63.409- Traumatic rupture of unspecified ligament of unspecified finger at metacarpophalangeal and interphalangeal joint

  S63.41- Traumatic rupture of collateral ligament of finger at metacarpophalangeal and interphalangeal joint

   S63.410- Traumatic rupture of collateral ligament of right index finger at metacarpophalangeal and interphalangeal joint

   S63.411- Traumatic rupture of collateral ligament of left index finger at metacarpophalangeal and interphalangeal joint

   S63.412- Traumatic rupture of collateral ligament of right middle finger at metacarpophalangeal and interphalangeal joint

   S63.413- Traumatic rupture of collateral ligament of left middle finger at metacarpophalangeal and interphalangeal joint

   S63.414- Traumatic rupture of collateral ligament of right ring finger at metacarpophalangeal and interphalangeal joint

   S63.415- Traumatic rupture of collateral ligament of left ring finger at metacarpophalangeal and interphalangeal joint

   S63.416- Traumatic rupture of collateral ligament of right little finger at metacarpophalangeal and interphalangeal joint

   S63.417- Traumatic rupture of collateral ligament of left little finger at metacarpophalangeal and interphalangeal joint

   S63.418- Traumatic rupture of collateral ligament of other finger at metacarpophalangeal and interphalangeal joint
   Traumatic rupture of collateral ligament of specified finger with unspecified laterality at metacarpophalangeal and interphalangeal joint

   S63.419- Traumatic rupture of collateral ligament of unspecified finger at metacarpophalangeal and interphalangeal joint

  S63.42- Traumatic rupture of palmar ligament of finger at metacarpophalangeal and interphalangeal joint

   S63.420- Traumatic rupture of palmar ligament of right index finger at metacarpophalangeal and interphalangeal joint

   S63.421- Traumatic rupture of palmar ligament of left index finger at metacarpophalangeal and interphalangeal joint

   S63.422- Traumatic rupture of palmar ligament of right middle finger at metacarpophalangeal and interphalangeal joint

   S63.423- Traumatic rupture of palmar ligament of left middle finger at metacarpophalangeal and interphalangeal joint

   S63.424- Traumatic rupture of palmar ligament of right ring finger at metacarpophalangeal and interphalangeal joint

   S63.425- Traumatic rupture of palmar ligament of left ring finger at metacarpophalangeal and interphalangeal joint

   S63.426- Traumatic rupture of palmar ligament of right little finger at metacarpophalangeal and interphalangeal joint

   S63.427- Traumatic rupture of palmar ligament of left little finger at metacarpophalangeal and interphalangeal joint

   S63.428- Traumatic rupture of palmar ligament of other finger at metacarpophalangeal and interphalangeal joint
   Traumatic rupture of palmar ligament of specified finger with unspecified laterality at metacarpophalangeal and interphalangeal joint

   S63.429- Traumatic rupture of palmar ligament of unspecified finger at metacarpophalangeal and interphalangeal joint

  S63.43- Traumatic rupture of volar plate of finger at metacarpophalangeal and interphalangeal joint

   S63.430- Traumatic rupture of volar plate of right index finger at metacarpophalangeal and interphalangeal joint

   S63.431- Traumatic rupture of volar plate of left index finger at metacarpophalangeal and interphalangeal joint

   S63.432- Traumatic rupture of volar plate of right middle finger at metacarpophalangeal and interphalangeal joint

   S63.433- Traumatic rupture of volar plate of left middle finger at metacarpophalangeal and interphalangeal joint

S63 - S63

S63.434- Traumatic rupture of volar plate of <u>right</u> <u>ring</u> finger at metacarpophalangeal and interphalangeal joint

S63.435- Traumatic rupture of volar plate of <u>left</u> <u>ring</u> finger at metacarpophalangeal and interphalangeal joint

S63.436- Traumatic rupture of volar plate of <u>right</u> <u>little</u> finger at metacarpophalangeal and interphalangeal joint

S63.437- Traumatic rupture of volar plate of <u>left</u> <u>little</u> finger at metacarpophalangeal and interphalangeal joint

S63.438- Traumatic rupture of volar plate of <u>other</u> finger at metacarpophalangeal and interphalangeal joint
Traumatic rupture of volar plate of specified finger with unspecified laterality at metacarpophalangeal and interphalangeal joint

S63.439- Traumatic rupture of volar plate of <u>unspecified</u> finger at metacarpophalangeal and interphalangeal joint

S63.49- <u>Traumatic rupture</u> of <u>other ligament</u> of <u>finger</u> at <u>metacarpophalangeal and interphalangeal joint</u>

S63.490- Traumatic rupture of other ligament of <u>right</u> <u>index</u> finger at metacarpophalangeal and interphalangeal joint

S63.491- Traumatic rupture of other ligament of <u>left</u> <u>index</u> finger at metacarpophalangeal and interphalangeal joint

S63.492- Traumatic rupture of other ligament of <u>right</u> <u>middle</u> finger at metacarpophalangeal and interphalangeal joint

S63.493- Traumatic rupture of other ligament of <u>left</u> <u>middle</u> finger at metacarpophalangeal and interphalangeal joint

S63.494- Traumatic rupture of other ligament of <u>right</u> <u>ring</u> finger at metacarpophalangeal and interphalangeal joint

S63.495- Traumatic rupture of other ligament of <u>left</u> <u>ring</u> finger at metacarpophalangeal and interphalangeal joint

S63.496- Traumatic rupture of other ligament of <u>right</u> <u>little</u> finger at metacarpophalangeal and Interphalangeal joint

S63.497- Traumatic rupture of other ligament of <u>left</u> <u>little</u> finger at metacarpophalangeal and interphalangeal joint

S63.498- Traumatic rupture of other ligament of <u>other</u> finger at metacarpophalangeal and interphalangeal joint
Traumatic rupture of ligament of specified finger with unspecified laterality at metacarpophalangeal and interphalangeal joint

S63.499- Traumatic rupture of other ligament of <u>unspecified</u> finger at metacarpophalangeal and interphalangeal joint

S63.5- <u>Other and unspecified</u> <u>sprain</u> of <u>wrist</u>

S63.50- <u>Unspecified</u> sprain of <u>wrist</u>

S63.501- Unspecified sprain of <u>right</u> wrist

S63.502- Unspecified sprain of <u>left</u> wrist

S63.509- Unspecified sprain of <u>unspecified</u> wrist

S63.51- <u>Sprain</u> of <u>carpal (joint)</u>

S63.511- Sprain of carpal joint of <u>right</u> wrist

S63.512- Sprain of carpal joint of <u>left</u> wrist

S63.519- Sprain of carpal joint of <u>unspecified</u> wrist

S63.52- <u>Sprain</u> of <u>radiocarpal joint</u>
Excludes 1: *traumatic rupture of radiocarpal ligament (S63.32-)*

S63.521- Sprain of radiocarpal joint of <u>right</u> wrist

S63.522- Sprain of radiocarpal joint of <u>left</u> wrist

S63.529- Sprain of radiocarpal joint of <u>unspecified</u> wrist

S63.59- <u>Other specified sprain</u> of <u>wrist</u>

S63.591- Other specified sprain of <u>right</u> wrist

S63.592- Other specified sprain of <u>left</u> wrist

S63.599- Other specified sprain of <u>unspecified</u> wrist

S63.6- <u>Other and unspecified</u> <u>sprain</u> of <u>finger(s)</u>
Excludes 1: *traumatic rupture of ligament of finger at metacarpophalangeal and interphalangeal joint(s) (S63.4-)*

S63.60- <u>Unspecified</u> <u>sprain</u> of <u>thumb</u>

S63.601- Unspecified sprain of <u>right</u> thumb

S63.602- Unspecified sprain of <u>left</u> thumb

S63.609- Unspecified sprain of <u>unspecified</u> thumb

S63.61- <u>Unspecified</u> <u>sprain</u> of other and <u>unspecified</u> <u>finger(s)</u>

S63.610- Unspecified sprain of <u>right</u> <u>index</u> finger

S63.611- Unspecified sprain of <u>left</u> <u>index</u> finger

S63.612- Unspecified sprain of <u>right</u> <u>middle</u> finger

S63.613- Unspecified sprain of <u>left</u> <u>middle</u> finger

S63.614- Unspecified sprain of <u>right</u> <u>ring</u> finger

S63.615- Unspecified sprain of <u>left</u> <u>ring</u> finger

S63.616- Unspecified sprain of <u>right</u> <u>little</u> finger

S63.617- Unspecified sprain of <u>left</u> <u>little</u> finger

S63.618- Unspecified sprain of other <u>finger</u>
Unspecified sprain of specified finger with unspecified laterality

S63.619- Unspecified sprain of <u>unspecified</u> finger

S63.62- <u>Sprain</u> of <u>interphalangeal joint</u> of <u>thumb</u>

S63.621- Sprain of interphalangeal joint of <u>right</u> thumb

S63.622- Sprain of interphalangeal joint of <u>left</u> thumb

S63.629- Sprain of interphalangeal joint of <u>unspecified</u> thumb

S63.63- <u>Sprain</u> of <u>interphalangeal joint</u> of <u>other and unspecified</u> <u>finger(s)</u>

S63.630- Sprain of interphalangeal joint of <u>right</u> <u>index</u> finger

S63.631- Sprain of interphalangeal joint of <u>left</u> <u>index</u> finger

S63.632- Sprain of interphalangeal joint of <u>right</u> <u>middle</u> finger

S63.633- Sprain of interphalangeal joint of <u>left</u> <u>middle</u> finger

S63.634- Sprain of interphalangeal joint of <u>right</u> <u>ring</u> finger

S63.635- Sprain of interphalangeal joint of <u>left</u> <u>ring</u> finger

S63.636- Sprain of interphalangeal joint of <u>right</u> <u>little</u> finger

S63.637- Sprain of interphalangeal joint of <u>left</u> <u>little</u> finger

S63.638- Sprain of interphalangeal joint of <u>other</u> finger

S63.639- Sprain of interphalangeal joint of <u>unspecified</u> finger

S63.64- <u>Sprain</u> of <u>metacarpophalangeal joint</u> of <u>thumb</u>

S63.641- Sprain of metacarpophalangeal joint of <u>right</u> thumb

S63.642- Sprain of metacarpophalangeal joint of <u>left</u> thumb

S63.649- Sprain of metacarpophalangeal joint of <u>unspecified</u> thumb

S63.65- <u>Sprain</u> of <u>metacarpophalangeal joint</u> of <u>other and unspecified</u> <u>finger(s)</u>

S63.650- Sprain of metacarpophalangeal joint of <u>right</u> <u>index</u> finger

S63.651- Sprain of metacarpophalangeal joint of <u>left</u> <u>index</u> finger

S63.652- Sprain of metacarpophalangeal joint of <u>right</u> <u>middle</u> finger

S63.653- Sprain of metacarpophalangeal joint of <u>left</u> <u>middle</u> finger

S63.654- Sprain of metacarpophalangeal joint of <u>right</u> <u>ring</u> finger

S63.655- Sprain of metacarpophalangeal joint of <u>left</u> <u>ring</u> finger

S63.656- Sprain of metacarpophalangeal joint of <u>right</u> <u>little</u> finger

S63.657- Sprain of metacarpophalangeal joint of <u>left</u> <u>little</u> finger

S63 - S63

S63.658- Sprain of metacarpophalangeal joint of other finger
Sprain of metacarpophalangeal joint of specified finger with unspecified laterality

S63.659- Sprain of metacarpophalangeal joint of unspecified finger

S63.68- Other sprain of thumb

S63.681- Other sprain of right thumb

S63.682- Other sprain of left thumb

S63.689- Other sprain of unspecified thumb

S63.69- Other sprain of other and unspecified finger(s)

S63.690- Other sprain of right index finger

S63.691- Other sprain of left index finger

S63.692- Other sprain of right middle finger

S63.693- Other sprain of left middle finger

S63.694- Other sprain of right ring finger

S63.695- Other sprain of left ring finger

S63.696- Other sprain of right little finger

S63.697- Other sprain of left little finger

S63.698- Other sprain of other finger
Other sprain of specified finger with unspecified laterality

S63.699- Other sprain of unspecified finger

S63.8- Sprain of other part of wrist and hand

S63.8x- Sprain of other part of wrist and hand

S63.8x1- Sprain of other part of right wrist and hand

S63.8x2- Sprain of other part of left wrist and hand

S63.8x9- Sprain of other part of unspecified wrist and hand

S63.9- Sprain of unspecified part of wrist and hand

S63.90x- Sprain of unspecified part of unspecified wrist and hand

S63.91x- Sprain of unspecified part of right wrist and hand

S63.92x- Sprain of unspecified part of left wrist and hand

S64- Injury of nerves at wrist and hand level
Code also any associated open wound (S61.-)

The appropriate 7th character is to be added to each code from category S64:
A   Initial encounter
D   Subsequent encounter
S   Sequela

S64.0- Injury of ulnar nerve at wrist and hand level

S64.00x- Injury of ulnar nerve at wrist and hand level of unspecified arm

S64.01x- Injury of ulnar nerve at wrist and hand level of right arm

S64.02x- Injury of ulnar nerve at wrist and hand level of left arm

S64.1- Injury of median nerve at wrist and hand level

S64.10x- Injury of median nerve at wrist and hand level of unspecified arm

S64.11x- Injury of median nerve at wrist and hand level of right arm

S64.12x- Injury of median nerve at wrist and hand level of left arm

S64.2- Injury of radial nerve at wrist and hand level

S64.20x- Injury of radial nerve at wrist and hand level of unspecified arm

S64.21x- Injury of radial nerve at wrist and hand level of right arm

S64.22x- Injury of radial nerve at wrist and hand level of left arm

S64.3- Injury of digital nerve of thumb

S64.30x- Injury of digital nerve of unspecified thumb

S64.31x- Injury of digital nerve of right thumb

S64.32x- Injury of digital nerve of left thumb

S64.4- Injury of digital nerve of other and unspecified finger

S64.40x- Injury of digital nerve of unspecified finger

S64.49- Injury of digital nerve of other finger

S64.490- Injury of digital nerve of right index finger

S64.491- Injury of digital nerve of left index finger

S64.492- Injury of digital nerve of right middle finger

S64.493- Injury of digital nerve of left middle finger

S64.494- Injury of digital nerve of right ring finger

S64.495- Injury of digital nerve of left ring finger

S64.496- Injury of digital nerve of right little finger

S64.497- Injury of digital nerve of left little finger

S64.498- Injury of digital nerve of other finger
Injury of digital nerve of specified finger with unspecified laterality

S64.8- Injury of other nerves at wrist and hand level

S64.8x- Injury of other nerves at wrist and hand level

S64.8x1- Injury of other nerves at wrist and hand level of right arm

S64.8x2- Injury of other nerves at wrist and hand level of left arm

S64.8x9- Injury of other nerves at wrist and hand level of unspecified arm

S64.9- Injury of unspecified nerve at wrist and hand level

S64.90x- Injury of unspecified nerve at wrist and hand level of unspecified arm

S64.91x- Injury of unspecified nerve at wrist and hand level of right arm

S64.92x- Injury of unspecified nerve at wrist and hand level of left arm

S65- Injury of blood vessels at wrist and hand level
Code also any associated open wound (S61.-)

The appropriate 7th character is to be added to each code from category S65:
A   Initial encounter
D   Subsequent encounter
S   Sequela

S65.0- Injury of ulnar artery at wrist and hand level

S65.00- Unspecified injury of ulnar artery at wrist and hand level

CC-A S65.001- Unspecified injury of ulnar artery at wrist and hand level of right arm

CC-A S65.002- Unspecified injury of ulnar artery at wrist and hand level of left arm

CC-A S65.009- Unspecified injury of ulnar artery at wrist and hand level of unspecified arm

S65.01- Laceration of ulnar artery at wrist and hand level

CC-A S65.011- Laceration of ulnar artery at wrist and hand level of right arm

CC-A S65.012- Laceration of ulnar artery at wrist and hand level of left arm

CC-A S65.019- Laceration of ulnar artery at wrist and hand level of unspecified arm

S65.09- Other specified injury of ulnar artery at wrist and hand level

CC-A S65.091- Other specified injury of ulnar artery at wrist and hand level of right arm

CC-A S65.092- Other specified injury of ulnar artery at wrist and hand level of left arm

CC-A S65.099- Other specified injury of ulnar artery at wrist and hand level of unspecified arm

S65.1- Injury of radial artery at wrist and hand level

S65.10- Unspecified injury of radial artery at wrist and hand level

CC-A S65.101- Unspecified injury of radial artery at wrist and hand level of right arm

CC-A S65.102- Unspecified injury of radial artery at wrist and hand level of left arm

CC-A S65.109- Unspecified injury of radial artery at wrist and hand level of unspecified arm

S65.11- Laceration of radial artery at wrist and hand level

CC-A S65.111- Laceration of radial artery at wrist and hand level of right arm

CC-A **S65.112-** Laceration of radial artery at wrist and hand level of <u>left</u> arm

CC-A **S65.119-** Laceration of radial artery at wrist and hand level of <u>unspecified</u> arm

S65.19- <u>Other specified injury</u> of <u>radial artery</u> at <u>wrist and hand level</u>

CC-A **S65.191-** Other specified injury of radial artery at wrist and hand level of <u>right</u> arm

CC-A **S65.192-** Other specified injury of radial artery at wrist and hand level of <u>left</u> arm

CC-A **S65.199-** Other specified injury of radial artery at wrist and hand level of <u>unspecified</u> arm

S65.2- <u>Injury of superficial palmar arch</u>

S65.20- <u>Unspecified</u> injury of <u>superficial palmar arch</u>

CC-A **S65.201-** Unspecified injury of superficial palmar arch of <u>right</u> hand

CC-A **S65.202-** Unspecified injury of superficial palmar arch of <u>left</u> hand

CC-A **S65.209-** Unspecified injury of superficial palmar arch of <u>unspecified</u> hand

S65.21- <u>Laceration</u> of <u>superficial palmar arch</u>

CC-A **S65.211-** Laceration of superficial palmar arch of <u>right</u> hand

CC-A **S65.212-** Laceration of superficial palmar arch of <u>left</u> hand

CC-A **S65.219-** Laceration of superficial palmar arch of <u>unspecified</u> hand

S65.29- <u>Other specified injury</u> of <u>superficial palmar arch</u>

CC-A **S65.291-** Other specified injury of superficial palmar arch of <u>right</u> hand

CC-A **S65.292-** Other specified injury of superficial palmar arch of <u>left</u> hand

CC-A **S65.299-** Other specified injury of superficial palmar arch of <u>unspecified</u> hand

S65.3- <u>Injury of deep palmar arch</u>

S65.30- <u>Unspecified</u> injury of <u>deep palmar arch</u>

CC-A **S65.301-** Unspecified injury of deep palmar arch of <u>right</u> hand

CC-A **S65.302-** Unspecified injury of deep palmar arch of <u>left</u> hand

CC-A **S65.309-** Unspecified injury of deep palmar arch of <u>unspecified</u> hand

S65.31- <u>Laceration</u> of <u>deep palmar arch</u>

CC-A **S65.311-** Laceration of deep palmar arch of <u>right</u> hand

CC-A **S65.312-** Laceration of deep palmar arch of <u>left</u> hand

CC-A **S65.319-** Laceration of deep palmar arch of <u>unspecified</u> hand

S65.39- <u>Other specified injury</u> of <u>deep palmar arch</u>

CC-A **S65.391-** Other specified injury of deep palmar arch of <u>right</u> hand

CC-A **S65.392-** Other specified injury of deep palmar arch of <u>left</u> hand

CC-A **S65.399-** Other specified injury of deep palmar arch of <u>unspecified</u> hand

S65.4- <u>Injury of blood vessel</u> of <u>thumb</u>

S65.40- <u>Unspecified</u> injury of <u>blood vessel</u> of <u>thumb</u>

CC-A **S65.401-** Unspecified injury of blood vessel of <u>right</u> thumb

CC-A **S65.402-** Unspecified injury of blood vessel of <u>left</u> thumb

CC-A **S65.409-** Unspecified injury of blood vessel of <u>unspecified</u> thumb

S65.41- <u>Laceration</u> of <u>blood vessel</u> of <u>thumb</u>

CC-A **S65.411-** Laceration of blood vessel of <u>right</u> thumb

CC-A **S65.412-** Laceration of blood vessel of <u>left</u> thumb

CC-A **S65.419-** Laceration of blood vessel of <u>unspecified</u> thumb

S65.49- <u>Other specified injury</u> of <u>blood vessel</u> of <u>thumb</u>

CC-A **S65.491-** Other specified injury of blood vessel of <u>right</u> thumb

CC-A **S65.492-** Other specified injury of blood vessel of <u>left</u> thumb

CC-A **S65.499-** Other specified injury of blood vessel of <u>unspecified</u> thumb

S65.5- <u>Injury of blood vessel</u> of <u>other and unspecified</u> <u>finger</u>

S65.50- <u>Unspecified</u> injury of <u>blood vessel</u> of <u>other and unspecified</u> <u>finger</u>

CC-A **S65.500-** Unspecified injury of blood vessel of <u>right</u> <u>index</u> finger

CC-A **S65.501-** Unspecified injury of blood vessel of <u>left</u> <u>index</u> finger

CC-A **S65.502-** Unspecified injury of blood vessel of <u>right</u> <u>middle</u> finger

CC-A **S65.503-** Unspecified injury of blood vessel of <u>left</u> <u>middle</u> finger

CC-A **S65.504-** Unspecified injury of blood vessel of <u>right</u> <u>ring</u> finger

CC-A **S65.505-** Unspecified injury of blood vessel of <u>left</u> <u>ring</u> finger

CC-A **S65.506-** Unspecified injury of blood vessel of <u>right</u> <u>little</u> finger

CC-A **S65.507-** Unspecified injury of blood vessel of <u>left</u> <u>little</u> finger

CC-A **S65.508-** Unspecified injury of blood vessel of <u>other</u> finger
Unspecified injury of blood vessel of specified finger with unspecified laterality

CC-A **S65.509-** Unspecified injury of blood vessel of <u>unspecified</u> finger

S65.51- <u>Laceration</u> of <u>blood vessel</u> of <u>other and unspecified</u> <u>finger</u>

CC-A **S65.510-** Laceration of blood vessel of <u>right</u> <u>index</u> finger

CC-A **S65.511-** Laceration of blood vessel of <u>left</u> <u>index</u> finger

CC-A **S65.512-** Laceration of blood vessel of <u>right</u> <u>middle</u> finger

CC-A **S65.513-** Laceration of blood vessel of <u>left</u> <u>middle</u> finger

CC-A **S65.514-** Laceration of blood vessel of <u>right</u> <u>ring</u> finger

CC-A **S65.515-** Laceration of blood vessel of <u>left</u> <u>ring</u> finger

CC-A **S65.516-** Laceration of blood vessel of <u>right</u> <u>little</u> finger

CC-A **S65.517-** Laceration of blood vessel of <u>left</u> <u>little</u> finger

CC-A **S65.518-** Laceration of blood vessel of <u>other</u> finger
Laceration of blood vessel of specified finger with unspecified laterality

CC-A **S65.519-** Laceration of blood vessel of <u>unspecified</u> finger

S65.59- <u>Other specified injury</u> of <u>blood vessel</u> of <u>other and unspecified</u> <u>finger</u>

CC-A **S65.590-** Other specified injury of blood vessel of <u>right</u> <u>index</u> finger

CC-A **S65.591-** Other specified injury of blood vessel of <u>left</u> <u>index</u> finger

CC-A **S65.592-** Other specified injury of blood vessel of <u>right</u> <u>middle</u> finger

CC-A **S65.593-** Other specified injury of blood vessel of <u>left</u> <u>middle</u> finger

CC-A **S65.594-** Other specified injury of blood vessel of <u>right</u> <u>ring</u> finger

CC-A **S65.595-** Other specified injury of blood vessel of <u>left</u> <u>ring</u> finger

CC-A **S65.596-** Other specified injury of blood vessel of <u>right</u> <u>little</u> finger

CC-A **S65.597-** Other specified injury of blood vessel of <u>left</u> <u>little</u> finger

CC-A **S65.598-** Other specified injury of blood vessel of <u>other</u> finger
Other specified injury of blood vessel of specified finger with unspecified laterality

CC-A **S65.599-** Other specified injury of blood vessel of <u>unspecified</u> finger

S65.8- Injury of <u>other blood vessels</u> at <u>wrist and hand level</u>

S65.80- <u>Unspecified</u> injury of <u>other blood vessels</u> at <u>wrist and hand level</u>

CC-A **S65.801-** Unspecified injury of other blood vessels at wrist and hand level of <u>right</u> arm

CC-A **S65.802-** Unspecified injury of other blood vessels at wrist and hand level of <u>left</u> arm

---

Excludes 1: = NOT CODED HERE! (Do not code both)   **1095**   *Excludes* ❷: = Not Included Here

S65 - S65

CC-A **S65.809-** Unspecified injury of other blood vessels at wrist and hand level of unspecified arm

S65.81- Laceration of other blood vessels at wrist and hand level

CC-A **S65.811-** Laceration of other blood vessels at wrist and hand level of right arm

CC-A **S65.812-** Laceration of other blood vessels at wrist and hand level of left arm

CC-A **S65.819-** Laceration of other blood vessels at wrist and hand level of unspecified arm

S65.89- Other specified injury of other blood vessels at wrist and hand level

CC-A **S65.891-** Other specified injury of other blood vessels at wrist and hand level of right arm

CC-A **S65.892-** Other specified injury of other blood vessels at wrist and hand level of left arm

CC-A **S65.899-** Other specified injury of other blood vessels at wrist and hand level of unspecified arm

S65.9- Injury of unspecified blood vessel at wrist and hand level

S65.90- Unspecified injury of unspecified blood vessel at wrist and hand level

CC-A **S65.901-** Unspecified injury of unspecified blood vessel at wrist and hand level of right arm

CC-A **S65.902-** Unspecified injury of unspecified blood vessel at wrist and hand level of left arm

CC-A **S65.909-** Unspecified injury of unspecified blood vessel at wrist and hand level of unspecified arm

S65.91- Laceration of unspecified blood vessel at wrist and hand level

CC-A **S65.911-** Laceration of unspecified blood vessel at wrist and hand level of right arm

CC-A **S65.912-** Laceration of unspecified blood vessel at wrist and hand level of left arm

CC-A **S65.919-** Laceration of unspecified blood vessel at wrist and hand level of unspecified arm

S65.99- Other specified injury of unspecified blood vessel at wrist and hand level

CC-A **S65.991-** Other specified injury of unspecified blood vessel at wrist and hand of right arm

CC-A **S65.992-** Other specified injury of unspecified blood vessel at wrist and hand of left arm

CC-A **S65.999-** Other specified injury of unspecified blood vessel at wrist and hand of unspecified arm

S66- Injury of muscle, fascia and tendon at wrist and hand level
Code also any associated open wound (S61.-)
Excludes ❷: sprain of joints and ligaments of wrist and hand (S63.-)
The appropriate 7th character is to be added to each code from category S66:
A   Initial encounter
D   Subsequent encounter
S   Sequela

S66.0- Injury of long flexor muscle, fascia and tendon of thumb at wrist and hand level

S66.00- Unspecified injury of long flexor muscle, fascia and tendon of thumb at wrist and hand level

S66.001- Unspecified injury of long flexor muscle, fascia and tendon of right thumb at wrist and hand level

S66.002- Unspecified injury of long flexor muscle, fascia and tendon of left thumb at wrist and hand level

S66.009- Unspecified injury of long flexor muscle, fascia and tendon of unspecified thumb at wrist and hand level

S66.01- Strain of long flexor muscle, fascia and tendon of thumb at wrist and hand level

S66.011- Strain of long flexor muscle, fascia and tendon of right thumb at wrist and hand level

S66.012- Strain of long flexor muscle, fascia and tendon of left thumb at wrist and hand level

S66.019- Strain of long flexor muscle, fascia and tendon of unspecified thumb at wrist and hand level

S66.02- Laceration of long flexor muscle, fascia and tendon of thumb at wrist and hand level

CC-A **S66.021-** Laceration of long flexor muscle, fascia and tendon of right thumb at wrist and hand level

CC-A **S66.022-** Laceration of long flexor muscle, fascia and tendon of left thumb at wrist and hand level

CC-A **S66.029-** Laceration of long flexor muscle, fascia and tendon of unspecified thumb at wrist and hand level

S66.09- Other specified injury of long flexor muscle, fascia and tendon of thumb at wrist and hand level

S66.091- Other specified injury of long flexor muscle, fascia and tendon of right thumb at wrist and hand level

S66.092- Other specified injury of long flexor muscle, fascia and tendon of left thumb at wrist and hand level

S66.099- Other specified injury of long flexor muscle, fascia and tendon of unspecified thumb at wrist and hand level

S66.1- Injury of flexor muscle, fascia and tendon of other and unspecified finger at wrist and hand level
Excludes ❷: Injury of long flexor muscle, fascia and tendon of thumb at wrist and hand level (S66.0-)

S66.10- Unspecified injury of flexor muscle, fascia and tendon of other and unspecified finger at wrist and hand level

S66.100- Unspecified injury of flexor muscle, fascia and tendon of right index finger at wrist and hand level

S66.101- Unspecified injury of flexor muscle, fascia and tendon of left index finger at wrist and hand level

S66.102- Unspecified injury of flexor muscle, fascia and tendon of right middle finger at wrist and hand level

S66.103- Unspecified injury of flexor muscle, fascia and tendon of left middle finger at wrist and hand level

S66.104- Unspecified injury of flexor muscle, fascia and tendon of right ring finger at wrist and hand level

S66.105- Unspecified injury of flexor muscle, fascia and tendon of left ring finger at wrist and hand level

S66.106- Unspecified injury of flexor muscle, fascia and tendon of right little finger at wristand hand level

S66.107- Unspecified injury of flexor muscle, fascia and tendon of left little finger at wristand hand level

S66.108- Unspecified injury of flexor muscle, fascia and tendon of other finger at wrist and hand level
Unspecified injury of flexor muscle, fascia and tendon of specified finger with unspecified laterality at wrist and hand level

S66.109- Unspecified injury of flexor muscle, fascia and tendon of unspecified finger at wrist and hand level

S66.11- Strain of flexor muscle, fascia and tendon of other and unspecified finger at wrist and hand level

S66.110- Strain of flexor muscle, fascia and tendon of right index finger at wrist and hand level

S66.111- Strain of flexor muscle, fascia and tendon of left index finger at wrist and hand level

S66.112- Strain of flexor muscle, fascia and tendon of right middle finger at wrist and hand level

S66.113- Strain of flexor muscle, fascia and tendon of left middle finger at wrist and hand level

S66.114- Strain of flexor muscle, fascia and tendon of right ring finger at wrist and hand level

S66.115- Strain of flexor muscle, fascia and tendon of left ring finger at wrist and hand level

S66.116- Strain of flexor muscle, fascia and tendon of right little finger at wrist and hand level

S66.117- Strain of flexor muscle, fascia and tendon of left little finger at wrist and hand level

S66.118- Strain of flexor muscle, fascia and tendon of other finger at wrist and hand level
Strain of flexor muscle, fascia and tendon of specified finger with unspecified laterality at wrist and hand level

S
6
5
-
S
6
6

S66.119- Strain of flexor muscle, fascia and tendon of <u>unspecified</u> finger at wrist and hand level

S66.12- <u>Laceration</u> of <u>flexor</u> muscle, fascia and tendon of <u>other and unspecified</u> <u>finger</u> at <u>wrist and hand level</u>

CC-A **S66.120-** Laceration of flexor muscle, fascia and tendon of <u>right</u> <u>index</u> finger at wrist and hand level

CC-A **S66.121-** Laceration of flexor muscle, fascia and tendon of <u>left</u> <u>index</u> finger at wrist and hand level

CC-A **S66.122-** Laceration of flexor muscle, fascia and tendon of <u>right</u> <u>middle</u> finger at wrist and hand level

CC-A **S66.123-** Laceration of flexor muscle, fascia and tendon of <u>left</u> <u>middle</u> finger at wrist and hand level

CC-A **S66.124-** Laceration of flexor muscle, fascia and tendon of <u>right</u> <u>ring</u> finger at wrist and hand level

CC-A **S66.125-** Laceration of flexor muscle, fascia and tendon of <u>left</u> <u>ring</u> finger at wrist and hand level

CC-A **S66.126-** Laceration of flexor muscle, fascia and tendon of <u>right</u> <u>little</u> finger at wrist and hand level

CC-A **S66.127-** Laceration of flexor muscle, fascia and tendon of <u>left</u> <u>little</u> finger at wrist and hand level

CC-A **S66.128-** Laceration of flexor muscle, fascia and tendon of <u>other</u> finger at wrist and hand level
      Laceration of flexor muscle, fascia and tendon of specified finger with unspecified laterality at wrist and hand level

CC-A **S66.129-** Laceration of flexor muscle, fascia and tendon of <u>unspecified</u> finger at wrist and hand level

S66.19- <u>Other injury</u> of <u>flexor</u> muscle, fascia and tendon of <u>other and unspecified</u> <u>finger</u> at <u>wrist and hand level</u>

S66.190- Other injury of flexor muscle, fascia and tendon of <u>right</u> <u>index</u> finger at wrist and hand level

S66.191- Other injury of flexor muscle, fascia and tendon of <u>left</u> <u>index</u> finger at wrist and hand level

S66.192- Other injury of flexor muscle, fascia and tendon of <u>right</u> <u>middle</u> finger at wrist and hand level

S66.193- Other injury of flexor muscle, fascia and tendon of <u>left</u> <u>middle</u> finger at wrist and hand level

S66.194- Other injury of flexor muscle, fascia and tendon of <u>right</u> <u>ring</u> finger at wrist and hand level

S66.195- Other injury of flexor muscle, fascia and tendon of <u>left</u> <u>ring</u> finger at wrist and hand level

S66.196- Other injury of flexor muscle, fascia and tendon of <u>right</u> <u>little</u> finger at wrist and hand level

S66.197- Other injury of flexor muscle, fascia and tendon of <u>left</u> <u>little</u> finger at wrist and hand level

S66.198- Other injury of flexor muscle, fascia and tendon of <u>other</u> finger at wrist and hand level
      Other injury of flexor muscle, fascia and tendon of specified finger with unspecified laterality at wrist and hand level

S66.199- Other injury of flexor muscle, fascia and tendon of <u>unspecified</u> finger at wrist and hand level

S66.2- <u>Injury</u> of <u>extensor</u> muscle, fascia and tendon of <u>thumb</u> at <u>wrist and hand level</u>

S66.20- <u>Unspecified</u> injury of <u>extensor</u> muscle, fascia and tendon of <u>thumb</u> at <u>wrist and hand level</u>

S66.201- Unspecified injury of extensor muscle, fascia and tendon of <u>right</u> thumb at wrist and hand level

S66.202- Unspecified injury of extensor muscle, fascia and tendon of <u>left</u> thumb at wrist and hand level

S66.209- Unspecified injury of extensor muscle, fascia and tendon of <u>unspecified</u> thumb at wrist and hand level

S66.21- Strain of <u>extensor</u> muscle, fascia and tendon of <u>thumb</u> at <u>wrist and hand level</u>

S66.211- Strain of extensor muscle, fascia and tendon of <u>right</u> thumb at wrist and hand level

S66.212- Strain of extensor muscle, fascia and tendon of <u>left</u> thumb at wrist and hand level

S66.219- Strain of extensor muscle, fascia and tendon of <u>unspecified</u> thumb at wrist and hand level

S66.22- <u>Laceration</u> of <u>extensor</u> muscle, fascia and tendon of <u>thumb</u> at <u>wrist and hand level</u>

CC-A **S66.221-** Laceration of extensor muscle, fascia and tendon of <u>right</u> thumb at wrist and hand level

CC-A **S66.222-** Laceration of extensor muscle, fascia and tendon of <u>left</u> thumb at wrist and hand level

CC-A **S66.229-** Laceration of extensor muscle, fascia and tendon of <u>unspecified</u> thumb at wrist and hand level

S66.29- <u>Other specified injury</u> of <u>extensor</u> muscle, fascia and tendon of <u>thumb</u> at <u>wrist and hand level</u>

S66.291- Other specified injury of extensor muscle, fascia and tendon of <u>right</u> thumb at wrist and hand level

S66.292- Other specified injury of extensor muscle, fascia and tendon of <u>left</u> thumb at wrist and hand level

S66.299- Other specified injury of extensor muscle, fascia and tendon of <u>unspecified</u> thumb at wrist and hand level

S66.3- <u>Injury</u> of <u>extensor</u> muscle, fascia and tendon of <u>other and unspecified</u> <u>finger</u> at <u>wrist and hand level</u>
    Excludes ❷: *Injury of extensor muscle, fascia and tendon of thumb at wrist and hand level (S66.2-)*

S66.30- <u>Unspecified</u> injury of <u>extensor</u> muscle, fascia and tendon of <u>other and unspecified</u> <u>finger</u> at <u>wrist and hand level</u>

S66.300- Unspecified injury of extensor muscle, fascia and tendon of <u>right</u> <u>index</u> finger at wrist and hand level

S66.301- Unspecified injury of extensor muscle, fascia and tendon of <u>left</u> <u>index</u> finger at wrist and hand level

S66.302- Unspecified injury of extensor muscle, fascia and tendon of <u>right</u> <u>middle</u> finger at wrist and hand level

S66.303- Unspecified injury of extensor muscle, fascia and tendon of <u>left</u> <u>middle</u> finger at wrist and hand level

S66.304- Unspecified injury of extensor muscle, fascia and tendon of <u>right</u> <u>ring</u> finger at wrist and hand level

S66.305- Unspecified injury of extensor muscle, fascia and tendon of <u>left</u> <u>ring</u> finger at wrist and hand level

S66.306- Unspecified injury of extensor muscle, fascia and tendon of <u>right</u> <u>little</u> finger at wrist and hand level

S66.307- Unspecified injury of extensor muscle, fascia and tendon of <u>left</u> <u>little</u> finger at wrist and hand level

S66.308- Unspecified injury of extensor muscle, fascia and tendon of <u>other</u> finger at wrist and hand level
      Unspecified injury of extensor muscle, fascia and tendon of specified finger with unspecified laterality at wrist and hand level

S66.309- Unspecified injury of extensor muscle, fascia and tendon of <u>unspecified</u> finger at wrist and hand level

S66.31- <u>Strain</u> of <u>extensor</u> muscle, fascia and tendon of <u>other and unspecified</u> <u>finger</u> at <u>wrist and hand level</u>

S66.310- Strain of extensor muscle, fascia and tendon of <u>right</u> <u>index</u> finger at wrist and hand level

S66.311- Strain of extensor muscle, fascia and tendon of <u>left</u> <u>index</u> finger at wrist and hand level

S66.312- Strain of extensor muscle, fascia and tendon of <u>right</u> <u>middle</u> finger at wrist and hand level

S66.313- Strain of extensor muscle, fascia and tendon of <u>left</u> <u>middle</u> finger at wrist and hand level

S66.314- Strain of extensor muscle, fascia and tendon of <u>right</u> <u>ring</u> finger at wrist and hand level

S66.315- Strain of extensor muscle, fascia and tendon of <u>left</u> <u>ring</u> finger at wrist and hand level

S66.316- Strain of extensor muscle, fascia and tendon of <u>right</u> <u>little</u> finger at wrist and hand level

S66.317- Strain of extensor muscle, fascia and tendon of <u>left</u> <u>little</u> finger at wrist and hand level

S66.318- Strain of extensor muscle, fascia and tendon of <u>other</u> finger at wrist and hand level
Strain of extensor muscle, fascia and tendon of specified finger with unspecified laterality at wrist and hand level

S66.319- Strain of extensor muscle, fascia and tendon of <u>unspecified</u> finger at wrist and hand level

S66.32- <u>Laceration</u> of <u>extensor</u> muscle, fascia and tendon of <u>other and unspecified finger</u> at <u>wrist and hand level</u>

CC-A **S66.320-** Laceration of extensor muscle, fascia and tendon of <u>right index</u> finger at wrist and hand level

CC-A **S66.321-** Laceration of extensor muscle, fascia and tendon of <u>left index</u> finger at wrist and hand level

CC-A **S66.322-** Laceration of extensor muscle, fascia and tendon of <u>right</u> middle finger at wrist and hand level

CC-A **S66.323-** Laceration of extensor muscle, fascia and tendon of <u>left middle</u> finger at wrist and hand level

CC-A **S66.324-** Laceration of extensor muscle, fascia and tendon of <u>right ring</u> finger at wrist and hand level

CC-A **S66.325-** Laceration of extensor muscle, fascia and tendon of <u>left ring</u> finger at wrist and hand level

CC-A **S66.326-** Laceration of extensor muscle, fascia and tendon of <u>right little</u> finger at wrist and hand level

CC-A **S66.327-** Laceration of extensor muscle, fascia and tendon of <u>left little</u> finger at wrist and hand level

CC-A **S66.328-** Laceration of extensor muscle, fascia and tendon of <u>other</u> finger at wrist and hand level
Laceration of extensor muscle, fascia and tendon of specified finger with unspecified laterality at wrist and hand level

CC-A **S66.329-** Laceration of extensor muscle, fascia and tendon of <u>unspecified</u> finger at wrist and hand level

S66.39- <u>Other injury</u> of <u>extensor</u> muscle, fascia and tendon of <u>other and unspecified finger</u> at <u>wrist and hand level</u>

S66.390- Other injury of extensor muscle, fascia and tendon of <u>right index</u> finger at wrist and hand level

S66.391- Other injury of extensor muscle, fascia and tendon of <u>left index</u> finger at wrist and hand level

S66.392- Other injury of extensor muscle, fascia and tendon of <u>right middle</u> finger at wrist and hand level

S66.393- Other injury of extensor muscle, fascia and tendon of <u>left middle</u> finger at wrist and hand level

S66.394- Other injury of extensor muscle, fascia and tendon of <u>right ring</u> finger at wrist and hand level

S66.395- Other injury of extensor muscle, fascia and tendon of <u>left ring</u> finger at wrist and hand level

S66.396- Other injury of extensor muscle, fascia and tendon of <u>right little</u> finger at wrist and hand level

S66.397- Other injury of extensor muscle, fascia and tendon of <u>left little</u> finger at wrist and hand level

S66.398- Other injury of extensor muscle, fascia and tendon of <u>other</u> finger at wrist and hand level
Other injury of extensor muscle, fascia and tendon of specified finger with unspecified laterality at wrist and hand level

S66.399- Other injury of extensor muscle, fascia and tendon of <u>unspecified</u> finger at wrist and hand level

S66.4- <u>Injury</u> of <u>intrinsic</u> muscle, fascia and tendon of <u>thumb</u> at wrist and hand level

S66.40- <u>Unspecified</u> injury of <u>intrinsic</u> muscle, fascia and tendon of <u>thumb</u> at <u>wrist and hand level</u>

S66.401- Unspecified injury of intrinsic muscle, fascia and tendon of <u>right</u> thumb at wrist and hand level

S66.402- Unspecified injury of intrinsic muscle, fascia and tendon of <u>left</u> thumb at wrist and hand level

S66.409- Unspecified injury of intrinsic muscle, fascia and tendon of <u>unspecified</u> thumb at wrist and hand level

S66.41- <u>Strain</u> of <u>intrinsic</u> muscle, fascia and tendon of <u>thumb</u> at <u>wrist and hand level</u>

S66.411- Strain of intrinsic muscle, fascia and tendon of <u>right</u> thumb at wrist and hand level

S66.412- Strain of intrinsic muscle, fascia and tendon of <u>left</u> thumb at wrist and hand level

S66.419- Strain of intrinsic muscle, fascia and tendon of <u>unspecified</u> thumb at wrist and hand level

S66.42- <u>Laceration</u> of <u>intrinsic</u> muscle, fascia and tendon of <u>thumb</u> at <u>wrist and hand level</u>

CC-A **S66.421-** Laceration of intrinsic muscle, fascia and tendon of <u>right</u> thumb at wrist and hand level

CC-A **S66.422-** Laceration of intrinsic muscle, fascia and tendon of <u>left</u> thumb at wrist and hand level

CC-A **S66.429-** Laceration of intrinsic muscle, fascia and tendon of <u>unspecified</u> thumb at wrist and hand level

S66.49- <u>Other specified injury</u> of <u>intrinsic</u> muscle, fascia and tendon of <u>thumb</u> at <u>wrist and hand level</u>

S66.491- Other specified injury of intrinsic muscle, and tendon of <u>right</u> thumb at wrist and hand level

S66.492- Other specified injury of intrinsic muscle, and tendon of <u>left</u> thumb at wrist and hand level

S66.499- Other specified injury of intrinsic muscle, and tendon of <u>unspecified</u> thumb at wrist and hand level

S66.5- <u>Injury</u> of <u>intrinsic</u> muscle, fascia and tendon of <u>other and unspecified finger</u> at <u>wrist and hand level</u>
Excludes ❷: injury of intrinsic muscle, fascia and tendon of thumb at wrist and hand level (S66.4-)

S66.50- <u>Unspecified</u> injury of <u>intrinsic</u> muscle, fascia and tendon of <u>other and unspecified finger</u> at <u>wrist and hand level</u>

S66.500- Unspecified injury of intrinsic muscle, fascia and tendon of <u>right index</u> finger at wrist and hand level

S66.501- Unspecified injury of intrinsic muscle, fascia and tendon of <u>left index</u> finger at wrist and hand level

S66.502- Unspecified injury of intrinsic muscle, fascia and tendon of <u>right middle</u> finger at wrist and hand level

S66.503- Unspecified injury of intrinsic muscle, fascia and tendon of <u>left middle</u> finger at wrist and hand level

S66.504- Unspecified injury of intrinsic muscle, fascia and tendon of <u>right ring</u> finger at wrist and hand level

S66.505- Unspecified injury of intrinsic muscle, fascia and tendon of <u>left ring</u> finger at wrist and hand level

S66.506- Unspecified injury of intrinsic muscle, fascia and tendon of <u>right little</u> finger at wrist and hand level

S66.507- Unspecified injury of intrinsic muscle, fascia and tendon of <u>left little</u> finger at wrist and hand level

S66.508- Unspecified injury of intrinsic muscle, fascia and tendon of <u>other</u> finger at wrist and hand level
Unspecified injury of intrinsic muscle, fascia and tendon of specified finger with unspecified laterality at wrist and hand level

S66.509- Unspecified injury of intrinsic muscle, fascia and tendon of <u>unspecified</u> finger at wrist and hand level

S66.51- <u>Strain</u> of <u>intrinsic</u> muscle, fascia and tendon of <u>other and unspecified finger</u> at <u>wrist and hand level</u>

S66.510- Strain of intrinsic muscle, fascia and tendon of <u>right index</u> finger at wrist and hand level

S66.511- Strain of intrinsic muscle, fascia and tendon of <u>left index</u> finger at wrist and hand level

S66.512- Strain of intrinsic muscle, fascia and tendon of <u>right middle</u> finger at wrist and hand level

S66.513- Strain of intrinsic muscle, fascia and tendon of <u>left middle</u> finger at wrist and hand level

S66.514- Strain of intrinsic muscle, fascia and tendon of <u>right ring</u> finger at wrist and hand level

S66.515- Strain of intrinsic muscle, fascia and tendon of <u>left ring</u> finger at wrist and hand level

S66 – S66

S66.516- Strain of intrinsic muscle, fascia and tendon of <u>right</u> <u>little</u> finger at wrist and hand level

S66.517- Strain of intrinsic muscle, fascia and tendon of <u>left</u> <u>little</u> finger at wrist and hand level

S66.518- Strain of intrinsic muscle, fascia and tendon of <u>other</u> finger at wrist and hand level
> Strain of intrinsic muscle, fascia and tendon of specified finger with unspecified laterality at wrist and hand level

S66.519- Strain of intrinsic muscle, fascia and tendon of <u>unspecified</u> finger at wrist and hand level

S66.52- <u>Laceration</u> of <u>intrinsic</u> muscle, fascia and tendon of <u>other and unspecified finger</u> at <u>wrist and hand level</u>

CC-A **S66.520-** Laceration of intrinsic muscle, fascia and tendon of <u>right</u> <u>index</u> finger at wrist and hand level

CC-A **S66.521-** Laceration of intrinsic muscle, fascia and tendon of <u>left</u> <u>index</u> finger at wrist and hand level

CC-A **S66.522-** Laceration of intrinsic muscle, fascia and tendon of <u>right</u> middle finger at wrist and hand level

CC-A **S66.523-** Laceration of intrinsic muscle, fascia and tendon of <u>left</u> <u>middle</u> finger at wrist and hand level

CC-A **S66.524-** Laceration of intrinsic muscle, fascia and tendon of <u>right</u> <u>ring</u> finger at wrist and hand level

CC-A **S66.525-** Laceration of intrinsic muscle, fascia and tendon of <u>left</u> <u>ring</u> finger at wrist and hand level

CC-A **S66.526-** Laceration of intrinsic muscle, fascia and tendon of <u>right</u> <u>little</u> finger at wrist and hand level

CC-A **S66.527-** Laceration of intrinsic muscle, fascia and tendon of <u>left</u> little finger at wrist and hand level

CC-A **S66.528-** Laceration of intrinsic muscle, fascia and tendon of <u>other</u> finger at wrist and hand level
> Laceration of intrinsic muscle, fascia and tendon of specified finger with unspecified laterality at wrist and hand level

CC-A **S66.529-** Laceration of intrinsic muscle, fascia and tendon of <u>unspecified</u> finger at wrist and hand level

S66.59- <u>Other injury</u> of <u>intrinsic</u> muscle, fascia and tendon of <u>other and unspecified finger</u> at <u>wrist and hand level</u>

S66.590- Other injury of intrinsic muscle, fascia and tendon of <u>right</u> <u>index</u> finger at wrist andhand level

S66.591- Other injury of intrinsic muscle, fascia and tendon of <u>left</u> <u>index</u> finger at wrist and hand level

S66.592- Other injury of intrinsic muscle, fascia and tendon of <u>right</u> <u>middle</u> finger at wrist and hand level

S66.593- Other injury of intrinsic muscle, fascia and tendon of <u>left</u> <u>middle</u> finger at wrist and hand level

S66.594- Other injury of intrinsic muscle, fascia and tendon of <u>right</u> <u>ring</u> finger at wrist and hand level

S66.595- Other injury of intrinsic muscle, fascia and tendon of <u>left</u> <u>ring</u> finger at wrist and hand level

S66.596- Other injury of intrinsic muscle, fascia and tendon of <u>right</u> <u>little</u> finger at wrist and hand level

S66.597- Other injury of intrinsic muscle, fascia and tendon of <u>left</u> <u>little</u> finger at wrist and hand level

S66.598- Other injury of intrinsic muscle, fascia and tendon of <u>other</u> finger at wrist and hand level
> Other injury of intrinsic muscle, fascia and tendon of specified finger with unspecified laterality at wrist and hand level

S66.599- Other injury of intrinsic muscle, fascia and tendon of <u>unspecified</u> finger at wrist and hand level

S66.8- <u>Injury</u> of <u>other specified</u> <u>muscles, fascia and tendons</u> at <u>wrist and hand level</u>

S66.80- <u>Unspecified</u> injury of <u>other specified</u> muscles, fascia and tendons at <u>wrist and hand level</u>

S66.801- Unspecified injury of other specified muscles, fascia and tendons at wrist and hand level, <u>right</u> hand

S66.802- Unspecified injury of other specified muscles, fascia and tendons at wrist and hand level, <u>left</u> hand

S66.809- Unspecified injury of other specified muscles, fascia and tendons at wrist and hand level, <u>unspecified</u> hand

S66.81- <u>Strain</u> of <u>other specified</u> muscles, fascia and tendons at <u>wrist and hand level</u>

S66.811- Strain of other specified muscles, fascia and tendons at wrist and hand level, <u>right</u> hand

S66.812- Strain of other specified muscles, fascia and tendons at wrist and hand level, <u>left</u> hand

S66.819- Strain of other specified muscles, fascia and tendons at wrist and hand level, <u>unspecified</u> hand

S66.82- <u>Laceration</u> of <u>other specified</u> muscles, fascia and tendons at <u>wrist and hand level</u>

CC-A **S66.821-** Laceration of other specified muscles, fascia and tendons at wrist and hand level, <u>right</u> hand

CC-A **S66.822-** Laceration of other specified muscles, fascia and tendons at wrist and hand level, <u>left</u> hand

CC-A **S66.829-** Laceration of other specified muscles, fascia and tendons at wrist and hand level, <u>unspecified</u> hand

S66.89- <u>Other injury</u> of <u>other specified</u> muscles, fascia and tendons at <u>wrist and hand level</u>

S66.891- Other injury of other specified muscles, fascia and tendons at wrist and hand level, <u>right</u> hand

S66.892- Other injury of other specified muscles, fascia and tendons at wrist and hand level, <u>left</u> hand

S66.899- Other injury of other specified muscles, fascia and tendons at wrist and hand level, <u>unspecified</u> hand

S66.9- Injury of <u>unspecified</u> muscle, fascia and tendon at <u>wrist and hand level</u>

S66.90- <u>Unspecified</u> injury of <u>unspecified</u> muscle, fascia and tendon at <u>wrist and hand level</u>

S66.901- Unspecified injury of unspecified muscle, fascia and tendon at wrist and hand level, <u>right</u> hand

S66.902- Unspecified injury of unspecified muscle, fascia and tendon at wrist and hand level, <u>left</u> hand

S66.909- Unspecified injury of unspecified muscle, fascia and tendon at wrist and hand level, <u>unspecified</u> hand

S66.91- <u>Strain</u> of <u>unspecified</u> muscle, fascia and tendon at <u>wrist and hand level</u>

S66.911- Strain of unspecified muscle, fascia and tendon at wrist and hand level, <u>right</u> hand

S66.912- Strain of unspecified muscle, fascia and tendon at wrist and hand level, <u>left</u> hand

S66.919- Strain of unspecified muscle, fascia and tendon at wrist and hand level, <u>unspecified</u> hand

S66.92- <u>Laceration</u> of <u>unspecified</u> muscle, fascia and tendon at <u>wrist and hand level</u>

CC-A **S66.921-** Laceration of unspecified muscle, fascia and tendon at wrist and hand level, <u>right</u> hand

CC-A **S66.922-** Laceration of unspecified muscle, fascia and tendon at wrist and hand level, <u>left</u> hand

CC-A **S66.929-** Laceration of unspecified muscle, fascia and tendon at wrist and hand level, <u>unspecified</u> hand

S66.99- <u>Other injury</u> of <u>unspecified</u> muscle, fascia and tendon at <u>wrist and hand level</u>

S66.991- Other injury of unspecified muscle, fascia and tendon at wrist and hand level, <u>right</u> hand

S66.992- Other injury of unspecified muscle, fascia and tendon at wrist and hand level, <u>left</u> hand

S66.999- Other injury of unspecified muscle, fascia and tendon at wrist and hand level, <u>unspecified</u> hand

S66 | S66

S67- Crushing injury of wrist, hand and fingers
Use additional code for all associated injuries, such as:
Fracture of wrist and hand (S62.-)
Open wound of wrist and hand (S61.-)
The appropriate 7th character is to be added to each code from category S67:
  A   Initial encounter
  D   Subsequent encounter
  S   Sequela

S67.0- Crushing injury of thumb
  S67.00x- Crushing injury of unspecified thumb
  S67.01x- Crushing injury of right thumb
  S67.02x- Crushing injury of left thumb

S67.1- Crushing injury of other and unspecified finger(s)
  Excludes ❷: crushing injury of thumb (S67.0-)
  S67.10x- Crushing injury of unspecified finger(s)
  S67.19- Crushing injury of other finger(s)
    S67.190- Crushing injury of right index finger
    S67.191- Crushing injury of left index finger
    S67.192- Crushing injury of right middle finger
    S67.193- Crushing injury of left middle finger
    S67.194- Crushing injury of right ring finger
    S67.195- Crushing injury of left ring finger
    S67.196- Crushing injury of right little finger
    S67.197- Crushing injury of left little finger
    S67.198- Crushing injury of other finger
      Crushing injury of specified finger with unspecified laterality

S67.2- Crushing injury of hand
  Excludes ❷: crushing injury of fingers (S67.1-)
          crushing injury of thumb (S67.0-)
  S67.20x- Crushing injury of unspecified hand
  S67.21x- Crushing injury of right hand
  S67.22x- Crushing injury of left hand

S67.3- Crushing injury of wrist
  S67.30x- Crushing injury of unspecified wrist
  S67.31x- Crushing injury of right wrist
  S67.32x- Crushing injury of left wrist

S67.4- Crushing injury of wrist and hand
  Excludes 1: crushing injury of hand alone (S67.2-)
          crushing injury of wrist alone (S67.3-)
  Excludes ❷: crushing injury of fingers (S67.1-)
          crushing injury of thumb (S67.0-)
  S67.40x- Crushing injury of unspecified wrist and hand
  S67.41x- Crushing injury of right wrist and hand
  S67.42x- Crushing injury of left wrist and hand

S67.9- Crushing injury of unspecified part(s) of wrist, hand and fingers
  S67.90x- Crushing injury of unspecified part(s) of unspecified wrist, hand and fingers
  S67.91x- Crushing injury of unspecified part(s) of right wrist, hand and fingers
  S67.92x- Crushing injury of unspecified part(s) of left wrist, hand and fingers

S68- Traumatic amputation of wrist, hand and fingers
Note: An amputation not identified as partial or complete should be coded to complete
The appropriate 7th character is to be added to each code from category S68:
  A   Initial encounter
  D   Subsequent encounter
  S   Sequela

S68.0- Traumatic metacarpophalangeal amputation of thumb
  Traumatic amputation of thumb NOS
  S68.01- Complete traumatic metacarpophalangeal amputation of thumb
    S68.011- Complete traumatic metacarpophalangeal amputation of right thumb

S68.012- Complete traumatic metacarpophalangeal amputation of left thumb
S68.019- Complete traumatic metacarpophalangeal amputation of unspecified thumb

S68.02- Partial traumatic metacarpophalangeal amputation of thumb
  S68.021- Partial traumatic metacarpophalangeal amputation of right thumb
  S68.022- Partial traumatic metacarpophalangeal amputation of left thumb
  S68.029- Partial traumatic metacarpophalangeal amputation of unspecified thumb

S68.1- Traumatic metacarpophalangeal amputation of other and unspecified finger
  Traumatic amputation of finger NOS
  Excludes ❷: traumatic metacarpophalangeal amputation of thumb (S68.0-)

S68.11- Complete traumatic metacarpophalangeal amputation of other and unspecified finger
  S68.110- Complete traumatic metacarpophalangeal amputation of right index finger
  S68.111- Complete traumatic metacarpophalangeal amputation of left index finger
  S68.112- Complete traumatic metacarpophalangeal amputation of right middle finger
  S68.113- Complete traumatic metacarpophalangeal amputation of left middle finger
  S68.114- Complete traumatic metacarpophalangeal amputation of right ring finger
  S68.115- Complete traumatic metacarpophalangeal amputation of left ring finger
  S68.116- Complete traumatic metacarpophalangeal amputation of right little finger
  S68.117- Complete traumatic metacarpophalangeal amputation of left little finger
  S68.118- Complete traumatic metacarpophalangeal amputation of other finger
    Complete traumatic metacarpophalangeal amputation of specified finger with unspecified laterality
  S68.119- Complete traumatic metacarpophalangeal amputation of unspecified finger

S68.12- Partial traumatic metacarpophalangeal amputation of other and unspecified finger
  S68.120- Partial traumatic metacarpophalangeal amputation of right index finger
  S68.121- Partial traumatic metacarpophalangeal amputation of left index finger
  S68.122- Partial traumatic metacarpophalangeal amputation of right middle finger
  S68.123- Partial traumatic metacarpophalangeal amputation of left middle finger
  S68.124- Partial traumatic metacarpophalangeal amputation of right ring finger
  S68.125- Partial traumatic metacarpophalangeal amputation of left ring finger
  S68.126- Partial traumatic metacarpophalangeal amputation of right little finger
  S68.127- Partial traumatic metacarpophalangeal amputation of left little finger
  S68.128- Partial traumatic metacarpophalangeal amputation of other finger
    Partial traumatic metacarpophalangeal amputation of specified finger with unspecified laterality
  S68.129- Partial traumatic metacarpophalangeal amputation of unspecified finger

S67 - S68

S68.4- Traumatic <u>amputation</u> of <u>hand</u> at <u>wrist level</u>
  Traumatic amputation of hand NOS
  Traumatic amputation of wrist

  S68.41- <u>Complete</u> traumatic <u>amputation</u> of <u>hand</u> at <u>wrist level</u>

  CC-A **S68.411-** Complete traumatic amputation of <u>right</u> hand at wrist level

  CC-A **S68.412-** Complete traumatic amputation of <u>left</u> hand at wrist level

  CC-A **S68.419-** Complete traumatic amputation of <u>unspecified</u> hand at wrist level

  S68.42- <u>Partial</u> traumatic <u>amputation</u> of <u>hand</u> at <u>wrist level</u>

  CC-A **S68.421-** Partial traumatic amputation of <u>right</u> hand at wrist level

  CC-A **S68.422-** Partial traumatic amputation of <u>left</u> hand at wrist level

  CC-A **S68.429-** Partial traumatic amputation of <u>unspecified</u> hand at wrist level

S68.5- Traumatic <u>transphalangeal</u> <u>amputation</u> of <u>thumb</u>
  Traumatic interphalangeal joint amputation of thumb

  S68.51- <u>Complete</u> traumatic <u>transphalangeal</u> <u>amputation</u> of <u>thumb</u>

  S68.511- Complete traumatic transphalangeal amputation of <u>right</u> thumb

  S68.512- Complete traumatic transphalangeal amputation of <u>left</u> thumb

  S68.519- Complete traumatic transphalangeal amputation of <u>unspecified</u> thumb

  S68.52- <u>Partial</u> traumatic <u>transphalangeal</u> <u>amputation</u> of <u>thumb</u>

  S68.521- Partial traumatic transphalangeal amputation of <u>right</u> thumb

  S68.522- Partial traumatic transphalangeal amputation of <u>left</u> thumb

  S68.529- Partial traumatic transphalangeal amputation of <u>unspecified</u> thumb

S68.6- Traumatic <u>transphalangeal</u> <u>amputation</u> of <u>other and unspecified</u> <u>finger</u>

  S68.61- <u>Complete</u> traumatic <u>transphalangeal</u> <u>amputation</u> of <u>other and unspecified</u> <u>finger(s)</u>

  S68.610- Complete traumatic transphalangeal amputation of <u>right</u> <u>index</u> finger

  S68.611- Complete traumatic transphalangeal amputation of <u>left</u> <u>index</u> finger

  S68.612- Complete traumatic transphalangeal amputation of <u>right</u> <u>middle</u> finger

  S68.613- Complete traumatic transphalangeal amputation of <u>left</u> <u>middle</u> finger

  S68.614- Complete traumatic transphalangeal amputation of <u>right</u> <u>ring</u> finger

  S68.615- Complete traumatic transphalangeal amputation of <u>left</u> <u>ring</u> finger

  S68.616- Complete traumatic transphalangeal amputation of <u>right</u> <u>little</u> finger

  S68.617- Complete traumatic transphalangeal amputation of <u>left</u> <u>little</u> finger

  S68.618- Complete traumatic transphalangeal amputation of <u>other</u> finger
  Complete traumatic transphalangeal amputation of specified finger with unspecified laterality

  S68.619- Complete traumatic transphalangeal amputation of <u>unspecified</u> finger

  S68.62- <u>Partial</u> traumatic <u>transphalangeal</u> <u>amputation</u> of <u>other and unspecified</u> <u>finger</u>

  S68.620- Partial traumatic transphalangeal amputation of <u>right</u> <u>index</u> finger

  S68.621- Partial traumatic transphalangeal amputation of <u>left</u> <u>index</u> finger

  S68.622- Partial traumatic transphalangeal amputation of <u>right</u> <u>middle</u> finger

  S68.623- Partial traumatic transphalangeal amputation of <u>left</u> <u>middle</u> finger

  S68.624- Partial traumatic transphalangeal amputation of <u>right</u> <u>ring</u> finger

  S68.625- Partial traumatic transphalangeal amputation of <u>left</u> <u>ring</u> finger

  S68.626- Partial traumatic transphalangeal amputation of <u>right</u> <u>little</u> finger

  S68.627- Partial traumatic transphalangeal amputation of <u>left</u> <u>little</u> finger

  S68.628- Partial traumatic transphalangeal amputation of <u>other</u> finger
  Partial traumatic transphalangeal amputation of specified finger with unspecified laterality

  S68.629- Partial traumatic transphalangeal amputation of <u>unspecified</u> finger

S68.7- Traumatic <u>transmetacarpal</u> <u>amputation</u> of <u>hand</u>

  S68.71- <u>Complete</u> traumatic <u>transmetacarpal</u> <u>amputation</u> of <u>hand</u>

  CC-A **S68.711-** Complete traumatic transmetacarpal amputation of <u>right</u> hand

  CC-A **S68.712-** Complete traumatic transmetacarpal amputation of <u>left</u> hand

  CC-A **S68.719-** Complete traumatic transmetacarpal amputation of <u>unspecified</u> hand

  S68.72- <u>Partial</u> traumatic <u>transmetacarpal</u> <u>amputation</u> of <u>hand</u>

  CC-A **S68.721-** Partial traumatic transmetacarpal amputation of <u>right</u> hand

  CC-A **S68.722-** Partial traumatic transmetacarpal amputation of <u>left</u> hand

  CC-A **S68.729-** Partial traumatic transmetacarpal amputation of <u>unspecified</u> hand

S69- Other and unspecified injuries of <u>wrist, hand and finger(s)</u>
  The appropriate 7th character is to be added to each code from category S69:
  A   <u>Initial</u> encounter
  D   <u>Subsequent</u> encounter
  S   <u>Sequela</u>

S69.8- <u>Other specified injuries</u> of <u>wrist, hand and finger(s)</u>

  S69.80x- Other specified injuries of <u>unspecified</u> wrist, hand and finger(s)

  S69.81x- Other specified injuries of <u>right</u> wrist, hand and finger(s)

  S69.82x- Other specified injuries of <u>left</u> wrist, hand and finger(s)

S69.9- <u>Unspecified injury</u> of <u>wrist, hand and finger(s)</u>

  S69.90x- Unspecified injury of <u>unspecified</u> wrist, hand and finger(s)

  S69.91x- Unspecified injury of <u>right</u> wrist, hand and finger(s)

  S69.92x- Unspecified injury of <u>left</u> wrist, hand and finger(s)

Injuries to the hip and thigh (S70-S79)

Excludes ❷: *burns and corrosions (T20-T32)*
  frostbite (T33-T34)
  snake bite (T63.0-)
  venomous insect bite or sting (T63.4-)

S70- <u>Superficial injury</u> of <u>hip and thigh</u>
  The appropriate 7th character is to be added to each code from category S70:
  A   <u>Initial</u> encounter
  D   <u>Subsequent</u> encounter
  S   <u>Sequela</u>

S70.0- <u>Contusion</u> of <u>hip</u>

  S70.00x- Contusion of <u>unspecified</u> hip

  S70.01x- Contusion of <u>right</u> hip

  S70.02x- Contusion of <u>left</u> hip

S70.1- <u>Contusion</u> of <u>thigh</u>

  S70.10x- Contusion of <u>unspecified</u> thigh

  S70.11x- Contusion of <u>right</u> thigh

  S70.12x- Contusion of <u>left</u> thigh

S 6 8 I S 7 0

Excludes 1: = NOT CODED HERE! (Do not code both)   *Excludes ❷:* = Not Included Here

S70.2- Other superficial injuries of hip
    S70.21- Abrasion of hip
        S70.211- Abrasion, right hip
        S70.212- Abrasion, left hip
        S70.219- Abrasion, unspecified hip
    S70.22- Blister (nonthermal) of hip
        S70.221- Blister (nonthermal), right hip
        S70.222- Blister (nonthermal), left hip
        S70.229- Blister (nonthermal), unspecified hip
    S70.24- External constriction of hip
        S70.241- External constriction, right hip
        S70.242- External constriction, left hip
        S70.249- External constriction, unspecified hip
    S70.25- Superficial foreign body of hip
        Splinter in the hip
        S70.251- Superficial foreign body, right hip
        S70.252- Superficial foreign body, left hip
        S70.259- Superficial foreign body, unspecified hip
    S70.26- Insect bite (nonvenomous) of hip
        S70.261- Insect bite (nonvenomous), right hip
        S70.262- Insect bite (nonvenomous), left hip
        S70.269- Insect bite (nonvenomous), unspecified hip
    S70.27- Other superficial bite of hip
        Excludes 1:   open bite of hip (S71.05-)
        S70.271- Other superficial bite of hip, right hip
        S70.272- Other superficial bite of hip, left hip
        S70.279- Other superficial bite of hip, unspecified hip
S70.3- Other superficial injuries of thigh
    S70.31- Abrasion of thigh
        S70.311- Abrasion, right thigh
        S70.312- Abrasion, left thigh
        S70.319- Abrasion, unspecified thigh
    S70.32- Blister (nonthermal) of thigh
        S70.321- Blister (nonthermal), right thigh
        S70.322- Blister (nonthermal), left thigh
        S70.329- Blister (nonthermal), unspecified thigh
    S70.34- External constriction of thigh
        S70.341- External constriction, right thigh
        S70.342- External constriction, left thigh
        S70.349- External constriction, unspecified thigh
    S70.35- Superficial foreign body of thigh
        Splinter in the thigh
        S70.351- Superficial foreign body, right thigh
        S70.352- Superficial foreign body, left thigh
        S70.359- Superficial foreign body, unspecified thigh
    S70.36- Insect bite (nonvenomous) of thigh
        S70.361- Insect bite (nonvenomous), right thigh
        S70.362- Insect bite (nonvenomous), left thigh
        S70.369- Insect bite (nonvenomous), unspecified thigh
    S70.37- Other superficial bite of thigh
        Excludes 1:   open bite of thigh (S71.15)
        S70.371- Other superficial bite of right thigh
        S70.372- Other superficial bite of left thigh
        S70.379- Other superficial bite of unspecified thigh
S70.9- Unspecified superficial injury of hip and thigh
    S70.91- Unspecified superficial injury of hip
        S70.911- Unspecified superficial injury of right hip
        S70.912- Unspecified superficial injury of left hip
        S70.919- Unspecified superficial injury of unspecified hip
    S70.92- Unspecified superficial injury of thigh
        S70.921- Unspecified superficial injury of right thigh
        S70.922- Unspecified superficial injury of left thigh
        S70.929- Unspecified superficial injury of unspecified thigh

S71- Open wound of hip and thigh
    Code also any associated wound infection
    Excludes 1:   open fracture of hip and thigh (S72.-)
                traumatic amputation of hip and thigh (S78.-)
    Excludes 2:   bite of venomous animal (T63.-)
                open wound of ankle, foot and toes (S91.-)
                open wound of knee and lower leg (S81.-)

> The appropriate 7th character is to be added to each code from category S71:
> **A**   **Initial** encounter
> **D**   **Subsequent** encounter
> **S**   **Sequela**

S71.0- Open wound of hip
    S71.00- Unspecified open wound of hip
        S71.001- Unspecified open wound, right hip
        S71.002- Unspecified open wound, left hip
        S71.009- Unspecified open wound, unspecified hip
    S71.01- Laceration without foreign body of hip
        S71.011- Laceration without foreign body, right hip
        S71.012- Laceration without foreign body, left hip
        S71.019- Laceration without foreign body, unspecified hip
    S71.02- Laceration with foreign body of hip
        S71.021- Laceration with foreign body, right hip
        S71.022- Laceration with foreign body, left hip
        S71.029- Laceration with foreign body, unspecified hip
    S71.03- Puncture wound without foreign body of hip
        S71.031- Puncture wound without foreign body, right hip
        S71.032- Puncture wound without foreign body, left hip
        S71.039- Puncture wound without foreign body, unspecified hip
    S71.04- Puncture wound with foreign body of hip
        S71.041- Puncture wound with foreign body, right hip
        S71.042- Puncture wound with foreign body, left hip
        S71.049- Puncture wound with foreign body, unspecified hip
    S71.05- Open bite of hip
        Bite of hip NOS
        Excludes 1:   superficial bite of hip (S70.26, S70.27)
        S71.051- Open bite, right hip
        S71.052- Open bite, left hip
        S71.059- Open bite, unspecified hip
S71.1- Open wound of thigh
    S71.10- Unspecified open wound of thigh
        S71.101- Unspecified open wound, right thigh
        S71.102- Unspecified open wound, left thigh
        S71.109- Unspecified open wound, unspecified thigh
    S71.11- Laceration without foreign body of thigh
        S71.111- Laceration without foreign body, right thigh
        S71.112- Laceration without foreign body, left thigh
        S71.119- Laceration without foreign body, unspecified thigh
    S71.12- Laceration with foreign body of thigh
        S71.121- Laceration with foreign body, right thigh
        S71.122- Laceration with foreign body, left thigh
        S71.129- Laceration with foreign body, unspecified thigh
    S71.13- Puncture wound without foreign body of thigh
        S71.131- Puncture wound without foreign body, right thigh
        S71.132- Puncture wound without foreign body, left thigh
        S71.139- Puncture wound without foreign body, unspecified thigh
    S71.14- Puncture wound with foreign body of thigh
        S71.141- Puncture wound with foreign body, right thigh
        S71.142- Puncture wound with foreign body, left thigh
        S71.149- Puncture wound with foreign body, unspecified thigh
    S71.15- Open bite of thigh
        Bite of thigh NOS
        Excludes 1:   superficial bite of thigh (S70.37-)
        S71.151- Open bite, right thigh

S70 - S71

S71.152- Open bite, <u>left</u> thigh

S71.159- Open bite, <u>unspecified</u> thigh

S72- <u>Fracture</u> of <u>femur</u>
> Note: A fracture not indicated as displaced or nondisplaced should be coded to displaced
> Note: A fracture not indicated as open or closed should be coded to closed
> Note: The open fracture designations are based on the Gustilo open fracture classification
> *Excludes 1:* *traumatic amputation of hip and thigh (S78.-)*
> *Excludes ❷:* *fracture of lower leg and ankle (S82.-)*
> *fracture of foot (S92.-)*
> *periprosthetic fracture of prosthetic implant of hip (T84.040, T84.041)*

The appropriate 7th character is to be added to all codes from category S72:

A <u>Initial</u> encounter for <u>closed</u> fracture

B <u>Initial</u> encounter for <u>open</u> fracture <u>type I or II</u>
<u>Initial</u> encounter for open fracture NOS

C <u>Initial</u> encounter for <u>open</u> fracture <u>type IIIA, IIIB, or IIIC</u>

D <u>Subsequent</u> encounter for <u>closed</u> fracture <u>with routine healing</u>

E <u>Subsequent</u> encounter for <u>open</u> fracture <u>type I or II</u> <u>with routine healing</u>

F <u>Subsequent</u> encounter for <u>open</u> fracture <u>type IIIA, IIIB, or IIIC with routine healing</u>

G <u>Subsequent</u> encounter for <u>closed</u> fracture <u>with delayed healing</u>

H <u>Subsequent</u> encounter for <u>open</u> fracture <u>type I or II</u> <u>with delayed healing</u>

J <u>Subsequent</u> encounter for <u>open</u> fracture <u>type IIIA, IIIB, or IIIC with delayed healing</u>

K <u>Subsequent</u> encounter for <u>closed</u> fracture <u>with nonunion</u>

M <u>Subsequent</u> encounter for <u>open</u> fracture <u>type I or II</u> <u>with nonunion</u>

N <u>Subsequent</u> encounter for <u>open</u> fracture <u>type IIIA, IIIB, or IIIC with nonunion</u>

P <u>Subsequent</u> encounter for <u>closed</u> fracture <u>with malunion</u>

Q <u>Subsequent</u> encounter for <u>open</u> fracture <u>type I or II</u> <u>with malunion</u>

R <u>Subsequent</u> encounter for <u>open</u> fracture <u>type IIIA, IIIB, or IIIC with malunion</u>

S <u>Sequela</u>

S72.0- <u>Fracture</u> of <u>head</u> and <u>neck</u> of <u>femur</u>
> *Excludes ❷: physeal fracture of upper end of femur (S79.0-)*

S72.00- Fracture of <u>unspecified part</u> of <u>neck</u> of femur
Fracture of hip NOS
Fracture of neck of femur NOS

S72.001- Fracture of unspecified part of neck of <u>right</u> femur
CC-K,M,N,P,Q,R MCC-A,B,C

S72.002- Fracture of unspecified part of neck of <u>left</u> femur
CC-K,M,N,P,Q,R MCC-A,B,C

S72.009- Fracture of unspecified part of neck of <u>unspecified</u> femur
CC-K,M,N,P,Q,R MCC-A,B,C

S72.01- <u>Unspecified</u> <u>intracapsular</u> fracture of femur
Subcapital fracture of femur

S72.011- Unspecified intracapsular fracture of <u>right</u> femur
CC-K,M,N,P,Q,R MCC-A,B,C

S72.012- Unspecified intracapsular fracture of <u>left</u> femur
CC-K,M,N,P,Q,R MCC-A,B,C

S72.019- Unspecified intracapsular fracture of <u>unspecified</u> femur
CC-K,M,N,P,Q,R MCC-A,B,C

S72.02- Fracture of <u>epiphysis</u> (separation) (upper) of femur
Transepiphyseal fracture of femur
> *Excludes 1:   capital femoral epiphyseal fracture (pediatric) of femur (S79.01-)*
> *Salter-Harris Type I physeal fracture of upper end of femur (S79.01-)*

S72.021- <u>Displaced</u> fracture of epiphysis (separation) (upper) of <u>right</u> femur
CC-K,M,N,P,Q,R MCC-A,B,C

S72.022- <u>Displaced</u> fracture of epiphysis (separation) (upper) of <u>left</u> femur
CC-K,M,N,P,Q,R MCC-A,B,C

S72.023- <u>Displaced</u> fracture of epiphysis (separation) (upper) of <u>unspecified</u> femur
CC-K,M,N,P,Q,R MCC-A,B,C

S72.024- <u>Nondisplaced</u> fracture of epiphysis (separation) (upper) of <u>right</u> femur
CC-K,M,N,P,Q,R MCC-A,B,C

S72.025- <u>Nondisplaced</u> fracture of epiphysis (separation) (upper) of <u>left</u> femur
CC-K,M,N,P,Q,R MCC-A,B,C

S72.026- <u>Nondisplaced</u> fracture of epiphysis (separation) (upper) of <u>unspecified</u> femur
CC-K,M,N,P,Q,R MCC-A,B,C

S72.03- <u>Midcervical</u> fracture of femur
Transcervical fracture of femur NOS

S72.031- <u>Displaced</u> midcervical fracture of <u>right</u> femur
CC-K,M,N,P,Q,R MCC-A,B,C

S72.032- <u>Displaced</u> midcervical fracture of <u>left</u> femur
CC-K,M,N,P,Q,R MCC-A,B,C

S72.033- <u>Displaced</u> midcervical fracture of <u>unspecified</u> femur
CC-K,M,N,P,Q,R MCC-A,B,C

S72.034- <u>Nondisplaced</u> midcervical fracture of <u>right</u> femur
CC-K,M,N,P,Q,R MCC-A,B,C

S72.035- <u>Nondisplaced</u> midcervical fracture of <u>left</u> femur
CC-K,M,N,P,Q,R MCC-A,B,C

S72.036- <u>Nondisplaced</u> midcervical fracture of <u>unspecified</u> femur
CC-K,M,N,P,Q,R MCC-A,B,C

S72.04- Fracture of <u>base of neck</u> of femur
Cervicotrochanteric fracture of femur

S72.041- <u>Displaced</u> fracture of base of neck of <u>right</u> femur
CC-K,M,N,P,Q,R MCC-A,B,C

S72.042- <u>Displaced</u> fracture of base of neck of <u>left</u> femur
CC-K,M,N,P,Q,R MCC-A,B,C

S72.043- <u>Displaced</u> fracture of base of neck of <u>unspecified</u> femur
CC-K,M,N,P,Q,R MCC-A,B,C

S72.044- <u>Nondisplaced</u> fracture of base of neck of <u>right</u> femur
CC-K,M,N,P,Q,R MCC-A,B,C

S72.045- <u>Nondisplaced</u> fracture of base of neck of <u>left</u> femur
CC-K,M,N,P,Q,R MCC-A,B,C

S72.046- <u>Nondisplaced</u> fracture of base of neck of <u>unspecified</u> femur
CC-K,M,N,P,Q,R MCC-A,B,C

S72.05- <u>Unspecified</u> fracture of <u>head</u> of femur
Fracture of head of femur NOS

S72.051- Unspecified fracture of head of <u>right</u> femur
CC-K,M,N,P,Q,R MCC-A,B,C

S72.052- Unspecified fracture of head of <u>left</u> femur
CC-K,M,N,P,Q,R MCC-A,B,C

S72.059- Unspecified fracture of head of <u>unspecified</u> femur
CC-K,M,N,P,Q,R MCC-A,B,C

S72.06- <u>Articular</u> fracture of <u>head</u> of femur

S72.061- <u>Displaced</u> articular fracture of head of <u>right</u> femur
CC-K,M,N,P,Q,R MCC-A,B,C

S72.062- <u>Displaced</u> articular fracture of head of <u>left</u> femur
CC-K,M,N,P,Q,R MCC-A,B,C

S72.063- <u>Displaced</u> articular fracture of head of <u>unspecified</u> femur
CC-K,M,N,P,Q,R MCC-A,B,C

S72.064- <u>Nondisplaced</u> articular fracture of head of <u>right</u> femur
CC-K,M,N,P,Q,R MCC-A,B,C

S72.065- <u>Nondisplaced</u> articular fracture of head of <u>left</u> femur
CC-K,M,N,P,Q,R MCC-A,B,C

S72.066- <u>Nondisplaced</u> articular fracture of head of <u>unspecified</u> femur
CC-K,M,N,P,Q,R MCC-A,B,C

S72.09- <u>Other fracture</u> of <u>head and neck</u> of femur

S72.091- Other fracture of head and neck of <u>right</u> femur
CC-K,M,N,P,Q,R MCC-A,B,C

S72.092- Other fracture of head and neck of <u>left</u> femur
CC-K,M,N,P,Q,R MCC-A,B,C

S71-S72

S72.099- Other fracture of head and neck of <u>unspecified</u> femur
CC-K,M,N,P,Q,R MCC-A,B,C

S72.1- <u>Pertrochanteric</u> fracture

S72.10- <u>Unspecified</u> trochanteric fracture of femur
Fracture of trochanter NOS

S72.101- Unspecified trochanteric fracture of <u>right</u> femur
CC-K,M,N,P,Q,R MCC-A,B,C

S72.102- Unspecified trochanteric fracture of <u>left</u> femur
CC-K,M,N,P,Q,R MCC-A,B,C

S72.109- Unspecified trochanteric fracture of <u>unspecified</u> femur
CC-K,M,N,P,Q,R MCC-A,B,C

S72.11- Fracture of <u>greater trochanter</u> of femur

S72.111- <u>Displaced</u> fracture of greater trochanter of <u>right</u> femur
CC-K,M,N,P,Q,R MCC-A,B,C

S72.112- <u>Displaced</u> fracture of greater trochanter of <u>left</u> femur
CC-K,M,N,P,Q,R MCC-A,B,C

S72.113- <u>Displaced</u> fracture of greater trochanter of <u>unspecified</u> femur
CC-K,M,N,P,Q,R MCC-A,B,C

S72.114- <u>Nondisplaced</u> fracture of greater trochanter of <u>right</u> femur
CC-K,M,N,P,Q,R MCC-A,B,C

S72.115- <u>Nondisplaced</u> fracture of greater trochanter of <u>left</u> femur
CC-K,M,N,P,Q,R MCC-A,B,C

S72.116- <u>Nondisplaced</u> fracture of greater trochanter of <u>unspecified</u> femur
CC-K,M,N,P,Q,R MCC-A,B,C

S72.12- Fracture of <u>lesser trochanter</u> of femur

S72.121- <u>Displaced</u> fracture of lesser trochanter of <u>right</u> femur
CC-K,M,N,P,Q,R MCC-A,B,C

S72.122- <u>Displaced</u> fracture of lesser trochanter of <u>left</u> femur
CC-K,M,N,P,Q,R MCC-A,B,C

S72.123- <u>Displaced</u> fracture of lesser trochanter of <u>unspecified</u> femur
CC-K,M,N,P,Q,R MCC-A,B,C

S72.124- <u>Nondisplaced</u> fracture of lesser trochanter of <u>right</u> femur
CC-K,M,N,P,Q,R MCC-A,B,C

S72.125- <u>Nondisplaced</u> fracture of lesser trochanter of <u>left</u> femur
CC-K,M,N,P,Q,R MCC-A,B,C

S72.126- <u>Nondisplaced</u> fracture of lesser trochanter of <u>unspecified</u> femur
CC-K,M,N,P,Q,R MCC-A,B,C

S72.13- <u>Apophyseal</u> fracture of femur
Excludes 1:   chronic (nontraumatic) slipped upper femoral epiphysis (M93.0-)

S72.131- <u>Displaced</u> apophyseal fracture of <u>right</u> femur
CC-K,M,N,P,Q,R MCC-A,B,C

S72.132- <u>Displaced</u> apophyseal fracture of <u>left</u> femur
CC-K,M,N,P,Q,R MCC-A,B,C

S72.133- <u>Displaced</u> apophyseal fracture of <u>unspecified</u> femur
CC-K,M,N,P,Q,R MCC-A,B,C

S72.134- <u>Nondisplaced</u> apophyseal fracture of <u>right</u> femur
CC-K,M,N,P,Q,R MCC-A,B,C

S72.135- <u>Nondisplaced</u> apophyseal fracture of <u>left</u> femur
CC-K,M,N,P,Q,R MCC-A,B,C

S72.136- <u>Nondisplaced</u> apophyseal fracture of <u>unspecified</u> femur
CC-K,M,N,P,Q,R MCC-A,B,C

S72.14- <u>Intertrochanteric</u> fracture of femur

S72.141- <u>Displaced</u> intertrochanteric fracture of <u>right</u> femur
CC-K,M,N,P,Q,R MCC-A,B,C

S72.142- <u>Displaced</u> intertrochanteric fracture of <u>left</u> femur
CC-K,M,N,P,Q,R MCC-A,B,C

S72.143- <u>Displaced</u> intertrochanteric fracture of <u>unspecified</u> femur
CC-K,M,N,P,Q,R MCC-A,B,C

S72.144- <u>Nondisplaced</u> intertrochanteric fracture of <u>right</u> femur
CC-K,M,N,P,Q,R MCC-A,B,C

S72.145- <u>Nondisplaced</u> intertrochanteric fracture of <u>left</u> femur
CC-K,M,N,P,Q,R MCC-A,B,C

S72.146- <u>Nondisplaced</u> intertrochanteric fracture of <u>unspecified</u> femur
CC-K,M,N,P,Q,R MCC-A,B,C

S72.2- <u>Subtrochanteric</u> fracture of femur

S72.21x- <u>Displaced</u> subtrochanteric fracture of <u>right</u> femur
CC-K,M,N,P,Q,R MCC-A,B,C

S72.22x- <u>Displaced</u> subtrochanteric fracture of <u>left</u> femur
CC-K,M,N,P,Q,R MCC-A,B,C

S72.23x- <u>Displaced</u> subtrochanteric fracture of <u>unspecified</u> femur
CC-K,M,N,P,Q,R MCC-A,B,C

S72.24x- <u>Nondisplaced</u> subtrochanteric fracture of <u>right</u> femur
CC-K,M,N,P,Q,R MCC-A,B,C

S72.25x- <u>Nondisplaced</u> subtrochanteric fracture of <u>left</u> femur
CC-K,M,N,P,Q,R MCC-A,B,C

S72.26x- <u>Nondisplaced</u> subtrochanteric fracture of <u>unspecified</u> femur
CC-K,M,N,P,Q,R MCC-A,B,C

S72.3- Fracture of <u>shaft</u> of femur

S72.30- <u>Unspecified</u> fracture of <u>shaft</u> of femur

S72.301- Unspecified fracture of shaft of <u>right</u> femur
CC-K,M,N,P,Q,R MCC-A,B,C

S72.302- Unspecified fracture of shaft of <u>left</u> femur
CC-K,M,N,P,Q,R MCC-A,B,C

S72.309- Unspecified fracture of shaft of <u>unspecified</u> femur
CC-K,M,N,P,Q,R MCC-A,B,C

S72.32- <u>Transverse</u> fracture of <u>shaft</u> of femur

S72.321- <u>Displaced</u> transverse fracture of shaft of <u>right</u> femur
CC-K,M,N,P,Q,R MCC-A,B,C

S72.322- <u>Displaced</u> transverse fracture of shaft of <u>left</u> femur
CC-K,M,N,P,Q,R MCC-A,B,C

S72.323- <u>Displaced</u> transverse fracture of shaft of <u>unspecified</u> femur
CC-K,M,N,P,Q,R MCC-A,B,C

S72.324- <u>Nondisplaced</u> transverse fracture of shaft of <u>right</u> femur
CC-K,M,N,P,Q,R MCC-A,B,C

S72.325- <u>Nondisplaced</u> transverse fracture of shaft of <u>left</u> femur
CC-K,M,N,P,Q,R MCC-A,B,C

S72.326- <u>Nondisplaced</u> transverse fracture of shaft of <u>unspecified</u> femur
CC-K,M,N,P,Q,R MCC-A,B,C

S72.33- <u>Oblique</u> fracture of <u>shaft</u> of femur

S72.331- <u>Displaced</u> oblique fracture of shaft of <u>right</u> femur
CC-K,M,N,P,Q,R MCC-A,B,C

S72.332- <u>Displaced</u> oblique fracture of shaft of <u>left</u> femur
CC-K,M,N,P,Q,R MCC-A,B,C

S72.333- <u>Displaced</u> oblique fracture of shaft of <u>unspecified</u> femur
CC-K,M,N,P,Q,R MCC-A,B,C

S72.334- <u>Nondisplaced</u> oblique fracture of shaft of <u>right</u> femur
CC-K,M,N,P,Q,R MCC-A,B,C

S72.335- <u>Nondisplaced</u> oblique fracture of shaft of <u>left</u> femur
CC-K,M,N,P,Q,R MCC-A,B,C

S72.336- <u>Nondisplaced</u> oblique fracture of shaft of <u>unspecified</u> femur
CC-K,M,N,P,Q,R MCC-A,B,C

S72.34- <u>Spiral</u> fracture of <u>shaft</u> of femur

S72.341- <u>Displaced</u> spiral fracture of shaft of <u>right</u> femur
CC-K,M,N,P,Q,R MCC-A,B,C

S72.342- <u>Displaced</u> spiral fracture of shaft of <u>left</u> femur
CC-K,M,N,P,Q,R MCC-A,B,C

S72.343- <u>Displaced</u> spiral fracture of shaft of <u>unspecified</u> femur
CC-K,M,N,P,Q,R MCC-A,B,C

S72.344- <u>Nondisplaced</u> spiral fracture of shaft of <u>right</u> femur
CC-K,M,N,P,Q,R MCC-A,B,C

S72.345- <u>Nondisplaced</u> spiral fracture of shaft of <u>left</u> femur
CC-K,M,N,P,Q,R MCC-A,B,C

S 7 2 - S 7 2

S72.346- <u>Nondisplaced</u> spiral fracture of shaft of <u>unspecified</u> femur
CC-K,M,N,P,Q,R MCC-A,B,C

S72.35- <u>Comminuted</u> fracture of <u>shaft</u> of femur

S72.351- <u>Displaced</u> comminuted fracture of shaft of <u>right</u> femur
CC-K,M,N,P,Q,R MCC-A,B,C

S72.352- <u>Displaced</u> comminuted fracture of shaft of <u>left</u> femur
CC-K,M,N,P,Q,R MCC-A,B,C

S72.353- <u>Displaced</u> comminuted fracture of shaft of <u>unspecified</u> femur
CC-K,M,N,P,Q,R MCC-A,B,C

S72.354- <u>Nondisplaced</u> comminuted fracture of shaft of <u>right</u> femur
CC-K,M,N,P,Q,R MCC-A,B,C

S72.355- <u>Nondisplaced</u> comminuted fracture of shaft of <u>left</u> femur
CC-K,M,N,P,Q,R MCC-A,B,C

S72.356- <u>Nondisplaced</u> comminuted fracture of shaft of <u>unspecified</u> femur
CC-K,M,N,P,Q,R MCC-A,B,C

S72.36- <u>Segmental</u> fracture of <u>shaft</u> of femur

S72.361- <u>Displaced</u> segmental fracture of shaft of <u>right</u> femur
CC-K,M,N,P,Q,R MCC-A,B,C

S72.362- <u>Displaced</u> segmental fracture of shaft of <u>left</u> femur
CC-K,M,N,P,Q,R MCC-A,B,C

S72.363- <u>Displaced</u> segmental fracture of shaft of <u>unspecified</u> femur
CC-K,M,N,P,Q,R MCC-A,B,C

S72.364- <u>Nondisplaced</u> segmental fracture of shaft of <u>right</u> femur
CC-K,M,N,P,Q,R MCC-A,B,C

S72.365- <u>Nondisplaced</u> segmental fracture of shaft of <u>left</u> femur
CC-K,M,N,P,Q,R MCC-A,B,C

S72.366- <u>Nondisplaced</u> segmental fracture of shaft of <u>unspecified</u> femur
CC-K,M,N,P,Q,R MCC-A,B,C

S72.39- <u>Other fracture</u> of <u>shaft</u> of femur

S72.391- Other fracture of shaft of <u>right</u> femur
CC-K,M,N,P,Q,R MCC-A,B,C

S72.392- Other fracture of shaft of <u>left</u> femur
CC-K,M,N,P,Q,R MCC-A,B,C

S72.399- Other fracture of shaft of <u>unspecified</u> femur
CC-K,M,N,P,Q,R MCC-A,B,C

S72.4- Fracture of <u>lower end</u> of femur
Fracture of distal end of femur
Excludes ❷: fracture of shaft of femur (S72.3-)
                physeal fracture of lower end of femur (S79.1-)

S72.40- <u>Unspecified</u> fracture of <u>lower end</u> of femur

S72.401- Unspecified fracture of lower end of <u>right</u> femur
CC-A,K,M,N,P,Q,R MCC-B,C

S72.402- Unspecified fracture of lower end of <u>left</u> femur
CC-A,K,M,N,P,Q,R MCC-B,C

S72.409- Unspecified fracture of lower end of <u>unspecified</u> femur
CC-A,K,M,N,P,Q,R MCC-B,C

S72.41- <u>Unspecified</u> <u>condyle</u> fracture of <u>lower end</u> of femur
Condyle fracture of femur NOS

S72.411- <u>Displaced</u> unspecified condyle fracture of lower end of <u>right</u> femur
CC-A,K,M,N,P,Q,R MCC-B,C

S72.412- <u>Displaced</u> unspecified condyle fracture of lower end of <u>left</u> femur
CC-A,K,M,N,P,Q,R MCC-B,C

S72.413- <u>Displaced</u> unspecified condyle fracture of lower end of <u>unspecified</u> femur
CC-A,K,M,N,P,Q,R MCC-B,C

S72.414- <u>Nondisplaced</u> unspecified condyle fracture of lower end of <u>right</u> femur
CC-A,K,M,N,P,Q,R MCC-B,C

S72.415- <u>Nondisplaced</u> unspecified condyle fracture of lower end of <u>left</u> femur
CC-A,K,M,N,P,Q,R MCC-B,C

S72.416- <u>Nondisplaced</u> unspecified condyle fracture of lower end of <u>unspecified</u> femur
CC-A,K,M,N,P,Q,R MCC-B,C

S72.42- Fracture of <u>lateral condyle</u> of femur

S72.421- <u>Displaced</u> fracture of lateral condyle of <u>right</u> femur
CC-A,K,M,N,P,Q,R MCC-B,C

S72.422- <u>Displaced</u> fracture of lateral condyle of <u>left</u> femur
CC-A,K,M,N,P,Q,R MCC-B,C

S72.423- <u>Displaced</u> fracture of lateral condyle of <u>unspecified</u> femur
CC-A,K,M,N,P,Q,R MCC-B,C

S72.424- <u>Nondisplaced</u> fracture of lateral condyle of <u>right</u> femur
CC-A,K,M,N,P,Q,R MCC-B,C

S72.425- <u>Nondisplaced</u> fracture of lateral condyle of <u>left</u> femur
CC-A,K,M,N,P,Q,R MCC-B,C

S72.426- <u>Nondisplaced</u> fracture of lateral condyle of <u>unspecified</u> femur
CC-A,K,M,N,P,Q,R MCC-B,C

S72.43- Fracture of <u>medial condyle</u> of femur

S72.431- <u>Displaced</u> fracture of medial condyle of <u>right</u> femur
CC-A,K,M,N,P,Q,R MCC-B,C

S72.432- <u>Displaced</u> fracture of medial condyle of <u>left</u> femur
CC-A,K,M,N,P,Q,R MCC-B,C

S72.433- <u>Displaced</u> fracture of medial condyle of <u>unspecified</u> femur
CC-A,K,M,N,P,Q,R MCC-B,C

S72.434- <u>Nondisplaced</u> fracture of medial condyle of <u>right</u> femur
CC-A,K,M,N,P,Q,R MCC-B,C

S72.435- <u>Nondisplaced</u> fracture of medial condyle of <u>left</u> femur
CC-A,K,M,N,P,Q,R MCC-B,C

S72.436- <u>Nondisplaced</u> fracture of medial condyle of <u>unspecified</u> femur
CC-A,K,M,N,P,Q,R MCC-B,C

S72.44- Fracture of <u>lower epiphysis</u> (separation) of femur
Excludes 1:   Salter-Harris Type I physeal fracture of lower end
                of femur (S79.11-)

S72.441- <u>Displaced</u> fracture of lower epiphysis (separation) of <u>right</u> femur
CC-A,K,M,N,P,Q,R MCC-B,C

S72.442- <u>Displaced</u> fracture of lower epiphysis (separation) of <u>left</u> femur
CC-A,K,M,N,P,Q,R MCC-B,C

S72.443- <u>Displaced</u> fracture of lower epiphysis (separation) of <u>unspecified</u> femur
CC-A,K,M,N,P,Q,R MCC-B,C

S72.444- <u>Nondisplaced</u> fracture of lower epiphysis (separation) of <u>right</u> femur
CC-A,K,M,N,P,Q,R MCC-B,C

S72.445- <u>Nondisplaced</u> fracture of lower epiphysis (separation) of <u>left</u> femur
CC-A,K,M,N,P,Q,R MCC-B,C

S72.446- <u>Nondisplaced</u> fracture of lower epiphysis (separation) of <u>unspecified</u> femur
CC-A,K,M,N,P,Q,R MCC-B,C

S72.45- <u>Supracondylar</u> fracture <u>without</u> intracondylar extension of lower end of femur
Supracondylar fracture of lower end of femur NOS
Excludes 1:   supracondylar fracture with intracondylar
                extension of lower end of femur (S72.46-)

S72.451- <u>Displaced</u> supracondylar fracture <u>without</u> intracondylar extension of lower end of <u>right</u> femur
CC-A,K,M,N,P,Q,R MCC-B,C

S72.452- <u>Displaced</u> supracondylar fracture <u>without</u> intracondylar extension of lower end of <u>left</u> femur
CC-A,K,M,N,P,Q,R MCC-B,C

S72.453- <u>Displaced</u> supracondylar fracture <u>without</u> intracondylar extension of lower end of <u>unspecified</u> femur
CC-A,K,M,N,P,Q,R MCC-B,C

S72.454- <u>Nondisplaced</u> supracondylar fracture <u>without</u> intracondylar extension of lower end of <u>right</u> femur
CC-A,K,M,N,P,Q,R MCC-B,C

S72 - S72

S72.455- Nondisplaced supracondylar fracture without intracondylar extension of lower end of left femur
CC-A,K,M,N,P,Q,R MCC-B,C

S72.456- Nondisplaced supracondylar fracture without intracondylar extension of lower end of unspecified femur
CC-A,K,M,N,P,Q,R MCC-B,C

S72.46- Supracondylar fracture with intracondylar extension of lower end of femur
  Excludes 1: supracondylar fracture without intracondylar extension of lower end of femur (S72.45-)

S72.461- Displaced supracondylar fracture with intracondylar extension of lower end of right femur
CC-A,K,M,N,P,Q,R MCC-B,C

S72.462- Displaced supracondylar fracture with intracondylar extension of lower end of left femur
CC-A,K,M,N,P,Q,R MCC-B,C

S72.463- Displaced supracondylar fracture with intracondylar extension of lower end of unspecified femur
CC-A,K,M,N,P,Q,R MCC-B,C

S72.464- Nondisplaced supracondylar fracture with intracondylar extension of lower end of right femur
CC-A,K,M,N,P,Q,R MCC-B,C

S72.465- Nondisplaced supracondylar fracture with intracondylar extension of lower end of left femur
CC-A,K,M,N,P,Q,R MCC-B,C

S72.466- Nondisplaced supracondylar fracture with intracondylar extension of lower end of unspecified femur
CC-A,K,M,N,P,Q,R MCC-B,C

S72.47- Torus fracture of lower end of femur

The appropriate 7th character is to be added to all codes in subcategory S72.47:
  A Initial encounter for closed fracture
  D Subsequent encounter for fracture with routine healing
  G Subsequent encounter for fracture with delayed healing
  K Subsequent encounter for fracture with nonunion
  P Subsequent encounter for fracture with malunion
  S Sequela

CC-A,K,P **S72.471-** Torus fracture of lower end of right femur
CC-A,K,P **S72.472-** Torus fracture of lower end of left femur
CC-A,K,P **S72.479-** Torus fracture of lower end of unspecified femur

S72.49- Other fracture of lower end of femur

S72.491- Other fracture of lower end of right femur
CC-A,K,M,N,P,Q,R MCC-B,C

S72.492- Other fracture of lower end of left femur
CC-A,K,M,N,P,Q,R MCC-B,C

S72.499- Other fracture of lower end of unspecified femur
CC-A,K,M,N,P,Q,R MCC-B,C

S72.8- Other fracture of femur

S72.8x- Other fracture of femur

S72.8x1- Other fracture of right femur
CC-K,M,N,P,Q,R MCC-A,B,C

S72.8x2- Other fracture of left femur
CC-K,M,N,P,Q,R MCC-A,B,C

S72.8x9- Other fracture of unspecified femur
CC-K,M,N,P,Q,R MCC-A,B,C

S72.9- Unspecified fracture of femur
  Fracture of thigh NOS
  Fracture of upper leg NOS
  Excludes 1: fracture of hip NOS (S72.00-, S72.01-)

S72.90x- Unspecified fracture of unspecified femur
CC-K,M,N,P,Q,R MCC-A,B,C

S72.91x- Unspecified fracture of right femur
CC-K,M,N,P,Q,R MCC-A,B,C

S72.92x- Unspecified fracture of left femur
CC-K,M,N,P,Q,R MCC-A,B,C

S73- Dislocation and sprain of joint and ligaments of hip
  Includes: Avulsion of joint or ligament of hip
       Laceration of cartilage, joint or ligament of hip
       Sprain of cartilage, joint or ligament of hip
       Traumatic hemarthrosis of joint or ligament of hip
       Traumatic rupture of joint or ligament of hip
       Traumatic subluxation of joint or ligament of hip
       Traumatic tear of joint or ligament of hip
  Code also any associated open wound
  Excludes ❷: strain of muscle, fascia and tendon of hip and thigh (S76.-)

The appropriate 7th character is to be added to each code from category S73:
  A Initial encounter
  D Subsequent encounter
  S Sequela

S73.0- Subluxation and dislocation of hip
  Excludes ❷: dislocation and subluxation of hip prosthesis (T84.020, T84.021)

S73.00- Unspecified subluxation and dislocation of hip
  Dislocation of hip NOS
  Subluxation of hip NOS

CC-A **S73.001-** Unspecified subluxation of right hip
CC-A **S73.002-** Unspecified subluxation of left hip
CC-A **S73.003-** Unspecified subluxation of unspecified hip
CC-A **S73.004-** Unspecified dislocation of right hip
CC-A **S73.005-** Unspecified dislocation of left hip
CC-A **S73.006-** Unspecified dislocation of unspecified hip

S73.01- Posterior subluxation and dislocation of hip
CC-A **S73.011-** Posterior subluxation of right hip
CC-A **S73.012-** Posterior subluxation of left hip
CC-A **S73.013-** Posterior subluxation of unspecified hip
CC-A **S73.014-** Posterior dislocation of right hip
CC-A **S73.015-** Posterior dislocation of left hip
CC-A **S73.016-** Posterior dislocation of unspecified hip

S73.02- Obturator subluxation and dislocation of hip
CC-A **S73.021-** Obturator subluxation of right hip
CC-A **S73.022-** Obturator subluxation of left hip
CC-A **S73.023-** Obturator subluxation of unspecified hip
CC-A **S73.024-** Obturator dislocation of right hip
CC-A **S73.025-** Obturator dislocation of left hip
CC-A **S73.026-** Obturator dislocation of unspecified hip

S73.03- Other anterior dislocation of hip
CC-A **S73.031-** Other anterior subluxation of right hip
CC-A **S73.032-** Other anterior subluxation of left hip
CC-A **S73.033-** Other anterior subluxation of unspecified hip
CC-A **S73.034-** Other anterior dislocation of right hip
CC-A **S73.035-** Other anterior dislocation of left hip
CC-A **S73.036-** Other anterior dislocation of unspecified hip

S73.04- Central dislocation of hip
CC-A **S73.041-** Central subluxation of right hip
CC-A **S73.042-** Central subluxation of left hip
CC-A **S73.043-** Central subluxation of unspecified hip
CC-A **S73.044-** Central dislocation of right hip
CC-A **S73.045-** Central dislocation of left hip
CC-A **S73.046-** Central dislocation of unspecified hip

S73.1- Sprain of hip
  AHA 14:4Q:p25 – Left hip labral tear (sprain)

S73.10- Unspecified sprain of hip
S73.101- Unspecified sprain of right hip
S73.102- Unspecified sprain of left hip
S73.109- Unspecified sprain of unspecified hip

S73.11- Iliofemoral ligament sprain of hip
S73.111- Iliofemoral ligament sprain of right hip
S73.112- Iliofemoral ligament sprain of left hip
S73.119- Iliofemoral ligament sprain of unspecified hip

S73.12- Ischiocapsular (ligament) sprain of hip
S73.121- Ischiocapsular ligament sprain of right hip
S73.122- Ischiocapsular ligament sprain of left hip

S 72 - S 73

S73.129- Ischiocapsular ligament sprain of <u>unspecified</u> hip
S73.19- <u>Other sprain</u> of hip
S73.191- Other sprain of <u>right</u> hip
S73.192- Other sprain of <u>left</u> hip
S73.199- Other sprain of <u>unspecified</u> hip

S74- <u>Injury of nerves</u> at <u>hip and thigh level</u>
Code also any associated open wound (S71.-)
Excludes ❷: injury of nerves at ankle and foot level (S94.-)
injury of nerves at lower leg level (S84.-)

The appropriate 7th character is to be added to each code from
category S74:
A <u>Initial</u> encounter
D <u>Subsequent</u> encounter
S <u>Sequela</u>

S74.0- Injury of <u>sciatic</u> nerve at <u>hip and thigh level</u>
S74.00x- Injury of sciatic nerve at hip and thigh level, <u>unspecified</u> leg
S74.01x- Injury of sciatic nerve at hip and thigh level, <u>right</u> leg
S74.02x- Injury of sciatic nerve at hip and thigh level, <u>left</u> leg

S74.1- Injury of <u>femoral</u> nerve at <u>hip and thigh level</u>
S74.10x- Injury of femoral nerve at hip and thigh level, <u>unspecified</u> leg
S74.11x- Injury of femoral nerve at hip and thigh level, <u>right</u> leg
S74.12x- Injury of femoral nerve at hip and thigh level, <u>left</u> leg

S74.2- Injury of <u>cutaneous sensory</u> nerve at <u>hip and thigh level</u>
S74.20x- Injury of cutaneous sensory nerve at hip and thigh level, <u>unspecified</u> leg
S74.21x- Injury of cutaneous sensory nerve at hip and high level, <u>right</u> leg
S74.22x- Injury of cutaneous sensory nerve at hip and thigh level, <u>left</u> leg

S74.8- Injury of <u>other nerves</u> at <u>hip and thigh level</u>
S74.8x- Injury of <u>other nerves</u> at <u>hip and thigh level</u>
S74.8x1- Injury of other nerves at hip and thigh level, <u>right</u> leg
S74.8x2- Injury of other nerves at hip and thigh level, <u>left</u> leg
S74.8x9- Injury of other nerves at hip and thigh level, <u>unspecified</u> leg

S74.9- Injury of <u>unspecified</u> nerve at <u>hip and thigh level</u>
S74.90x- Injury of unspecified nerve at hip and thigh level, <u>unspecified</u> leg
S74.91x- Injury of unspecified nerve at hip and thigh level, <u>right</u> leg
S74.92x- Injury of unspecified nerve at hip and thigh level, <u>left</u> leg

S75- <u>Injury of blood vessels</u> at <u>hip and thigh level</u>
Code also any associated open wound (S71.-)
Excludes ❷: injury of blood vessels at lower leg level (S85.-)
injury of popliteal artery (S85.0)

The appropriate 7th character is to be added to each code from
category S75:
A <u>Initial</u> encounter
D <u>Subsequent</u> encounter
S <u>Sequela</u>

S75.0- Injury of <u>femoral artery</u>
S75.00- <u>Unspecified</u> injury of <u>femoral artery</u>
MCC-A S75.001- Unspecified injury of femoral artery, <u>right</u> leg
MCC-A S75.002- Unspecified injury of femoral artery, <u>left</u> leg
MCC-A S75.009- Unspecified injury of femoral artery, <u>unspecified</u> leg
S75.01- <u>Minor laceration</u> of <u>femoral artery</u>
Incomplete transection of femoral artery
Laceration of femoral artery NOS
Superficial laceration of femoral artery
MCC-A S75.011- Minor laceration of femoral artery, <u>right</u> leg
MCC-A S75.012- Minor laceration of femoral artery, <u>left</u> leg
MCC-A S75.019- Minor laceration of femoral artery, <u>unspecified</u> leg

S75.02- <u>Major laceration</u> of <u>femoral artery</u>
Complete transection of femoral artery
Traumatic rupture of femoral artery
MCC-A S75.021- Major laceration of femoral artery, <u>right</u> leg
MCC-A S75.022- Major laceration of femoral artery, <u>left</u> leg
MCC-A S75.029- Major laceration of femoral artery, <u>unspecified</u> leg
S75.09- <u>Other specified injury</u> of <u>femoral artery</u>
MCC-A S75.091- Other specified injury of femoral artery, <u>right</u> leg
MCC-A S75.092- Other specified injury of femoral artery, <u>left</u> leg
MCC-A S75.099- Other specified injury of femoral artery, <u>unspecified</u> leg

S75.1- Injury of <u>femoral vein</u> at <u>hip and thigh level</u>
S75.10- <u>Unspecified</u> injury of <u>femoral vein</u> at <u>hip and thigh level</u>
MCC-A S75.101- Unspecified injury of femoral vein at hip and thigh level, <u>right</u> leg
MCC-A S75.102- Unspecified injury of femoral vein at hip and thigh level, <u>left</u> leg
MCC-A S75.109- Unspecified injury of femoral vein at hip and thigh level, <u>unspecified</u> leg
S75.11- <u>Minor laceration</u> of <u>femoral vein</u> at <u>hip and thigh level</u>
Incomplete transection of femoral vein at hip and thigh level
Laceration of femoral vein at hip and thigh level NOS
Superficial laceration of femoral vein at hip and thigh level
MCC-A S75.111- Minor laceration of femoral vein at hip and thigh level, <u>right</u> leg
MCC-A S75.112- Minor laceration of femoral vein at hip and thigh level, <u>left</u> leg
MCC-A S75.119- Minor laceration of femoral vein at hip and thigh level, <u>unspecified</u> leg
S75.12- <u>Major laceration</u> of <u>femoral vein</u> at <u>hip and thigh level</u>
Complete transection of femoral vein at hip and thigh level
Traumatic rupture of femoral vein at hip and thigh level
MCC-A S75.121- Major laceration of femoral vein at hip and thigh level, <u>right</u> leg
MCC-A S75.122- Major laceration of femoral vein at hip and thigh level, <u>left</u> leg
MCC-A S75.129- Major laceration of femoral vein at hip and thigh level, <u>unspecified</u> leg
S75.19- <u>Other specified injury</u> of <u>femoral vein</u> at <u>hip and thigh level</u>
MCC-A S75.191- Other specified injury of femoral vein at hip and thigh level, <u>right</u> leg
MCC-A S75.192- Other specified injury of femoral vein at hip and thigh level, <u>left</u> leg
MCC-A S75.199- Other specified injury of femoral vein at hip and thigh level, <u>unspecified</u> leg

S75.2- Injury of <u>greater saphenous vein</u> at <u>hip and thigh level</u>
Excludes 1: greater saphenous vein NOS (S85.3)
S75.20- <u>Unspecified</u> injury of <u>greater saphenous vein</u> at <u>hip and thigh level</u>
CC-A S75.201- Unspecified injury of greater saphenous vein at hip and thigh level, <u>right</u> leg
CC-A S75.202- Unspecified injury of greater saphenous vein at hip and thigh level, <u>left</u> leg
CC-A S75.209- Unspecified injury of greater saphenous vein at hip and thigh level, <u>unspecified</u> leg
S75.21- <u>Minor laceration</u> of <u>greater saphenous vein</u> at <u>hip and thigh level</u>
Incomplete transection of greater saphenous vein at hip and thigh level
Laceration of greater saphenous vein at hip and thigh level NOS
Superficial laceration of greater saphenous vein at hip and thigh level
CC-A S75.211- Minor laceration of greater saphenous vein at hip and thigh level, <u>right</u> leg
CC-A S75.212- Minor laceration of greater saphenous vein at hip and thigh level, <u>left</u> leg
CC-A S75.219- Minor laceration of greater saphenous vein at hip and thigh level, <u>unspecified</u> leg

S73 – S75

S75.22- Major laceration of greater saphenous vein at hip and thigh level
　　　　Complete transection of greater saphenous vein at hip and thigh level
　　　　Traumatic rupture of greater saphenous vein at hip and thigh level

CC-A **S75.221-** Major laceration of greater saphenous vein at hip and thigh level, right leg

CC-A **S75.222-** Major laceration of greater saphenous vein at hip and thigh level, left leg

CC-A **S75.229-** Major laceration of greater saphenous vein at hip and thigh level, unspecified leg

S75.29- Other specified injury of greater saphenous vein at hip and thigh level

CC-A **S75.291-** Other specified injury of greater saphenous vein at hip and thigh level, right leg

CC-A **S75.292-** Other specified injury of greater saphenous vein at hip and thigh level, left leg

CC-A **S75.299-** Other specified injury of greater saphenous vein at hip and thigh level, unspecified leg

S75.8- Injury of other blood vessels at hip and thigh level

S75.80- Unspecified injury of other blood vessels at hip and thigh level

CC-A **S75.801-** Unspecified injury of other blood vessels at hip and thigh level, right leg

CC-A **S75.802-** Unspecified injury of other blood vessels at hip and thigh level, left leg

CC-A **S75.809-** Unspecified injury of other blood vessels at hip and thigh level, unspecified leg

S75.81- Laceration of other blood vessels at hip and thigh level

CC-A **S75.811-** Laceration of other blood vessels at hip and thigh level, right leg

CC-A **S75.812-** Laceration of other blood vessels at hip and thigh level, left leg

CC-A **S75.819-** Laceration of other blood vessels at hip and thigh level, unspecified leg

S75.89- Other specified injury of other blood vessels at hip and thigh level

CC-A **S75.891-** Other specified injury of other blood vessels at hip and thigh level, right leg

CC-A **S75.892-** Other specified injury of other blood vessels at hip and thigh level, left leg

CC-A **S75.899-** Other specified injury of other blood vessels at hip and thigh level, unspecified leg

S75.9- Injury of unspecified blood vessel at hip and thigh level

S75.90- Unspecified injury of unspecified blood vessel at hip and thigh level

CC-A **S75.901-** Unspecified injury of unspecified blood vessel at hip and thigh level, right leg

CC-A **S75.902-** Unspecified injury of unspecified blood vessel at hip and thigh level, left leg

CC-A **S75.909-** Unspecified injury of unspecified blood vessel at hip and thigh level, unspecified leg

S75.91- Laceration of unspecified blood vessel at hip and thigh level

CC-A **S75.911-** Laceration of unspecified blood vessel at hip and thigh level, right leg

CC-A **S75.912-** Laceration of unspecified blood vessel at hip and thigh level, left leg

CC-A **S75.919-** Laceration of unspecified blood vessel at hip and thigh level, unspecified leg

S75.99- Other specified injury of unspecified blood vessel at hip and thigh level

CC-A **S75.991-** Other specified injury of unspecified blood vessel at hip and thigh level, right leg

CC-A **S75.992-** Other specified injury of unspecified blood vessel at hip and thigh level, left leg

CC-A **S75.999-** Other specified injury of unspecified blood vessel at hip and thigh level, unspecified leg

S76- Injury of muscle, fascia and tendon at hip and thigh level
　　Code also any associated open wound (S71.-)
　　Excludes ❷: injury of muscle, fascia and tendon at lower leg level (S86)
　　　　　　sprain of joint and ligament of hip (S73.1)

The appropriate 7th character is to be added to each code from category S76:
A　Initial encounter
D　Subsequent encounter
S　Sequela

S76.0- Injury of muscle, fascia and tendon of hip

S76.00- Unspecified injury of muscle, fascia and tendon of hip

S76.001- Unspecified injury of muscle, fascia and tendon of right hip

S76.002- Unspecified injury of muscle, fascia and tendon of left hip

S76.009- Unspecified injury of muscle, fascia and tendon of unspecified hip

S76.01- Strain of muscle, fascia and tendon of hip

S76.011- Strain of muscle, fascia and tendon of right hip

S76.012- Strain of muscle, fascia and tendon of left hip

S76.019- Strain of muscle, fascia and tendon of unspecified hip

S76.02- Laceration of muscle, fascia and tendon of hip

CC-A **S76.021-** Laceration of muscle, fascia and tendon of right hip

CC-A **S76.022-** Laceration of muscle, fascia and tendon of left hip

CC-A **S76.029-** Laceration of muscle, fascia and tendon of unspecified hip

S76.09- Other specified injury of muscle, fascia and tendon of hip

S76.091- Other specified injury of muscle, fascia and tendon of right hip

S76.092- Other specified injury of muscle, fascia and tendon of left hip

S76.099- Other specified injury of muscle, fascia and tendon of unspecified hip

S76.1- Injury of quadriceps muscle, fascia and tendon
　　Injury of patellar ligament (tendon)

S76.10- Unspecified injury of quadriceps muscle, fascia and tendon

S76.101- Unspecified injury of right quadriceps muscle, fascia and tendon

S76.102- Unspecified injury of left quadriceps muscle, fascia and tendon

S76.109- Unspecified injury of unspecified quadriceps muscle, fascia and tendon

S76.11- Strain of quadriceps muscle, fascia and tendon

S76.111- Strain of right quadriceps muscle, fascia and tendon

S76.112- Strain of left quadriceps muscle, fascia and tendon

S76.119- Strain of unspecified quadriceps muscle, fascia and tendon

S76.12- Laceration of quadriceps muscle, fascia and tendon

CC-A **S76.121-** Laceration of right quadriceps muscle, fascia and tendon

CC-A **S76.122-** Laceration of left quadriceps muscle, fascia and tendon

CC-A **S76.129-** Laceration of unspecified quadriceps muscle, fascia and tendon

S76.19- Other specified injury of quadriceps muscle, fascia and tendon

S76.191- Other specified injury of right quadriceps muscle, fascia and tendon

S76.192- Other specified injury of left quadriceps muscle, fascia and tendon

S76.199- Other specified injury of unspecified quadriceps muscle, fascia and tendon

S75 – S76

S76.2- Injry of <u>adductor muscle, fascia and tendon</u> of <u>thigh</u>

  S76.20- <u>Unspecified</u> injury of <u>adductor</u> muscle, fascia and tendon of <u>thigh</u>

    S76.201- Unspecified injury of adductor muscle, fascia and tendon of <u>right</u> thigh

    S76.202- Unspecified injury of adductor muscle, fascia and tendon of <u>left</u> thigh

    S76.209- Unspecified injury of adductor muscle, fascia and tendon of <u>unspecified</u> thigh

  S76.21- <u>Strain</u> of <u>adductor</u> muscle, fascia and tendon of <u>thigh</u>

    S76.211- Strain of adductor muscle, fascia and tendon of <u>right</u> thigh

    S76.212- Strain of adductor muscle, fascia and tendon of <u>left</u> thigh

    S76.219- Strain of adductor muscle, fascia and tendon of <u>unspecified</u> thigh

  S76.22- <u>Laceration</u> of <u>adductor</u> muscle, fascia and tendon of <u>thigh</u>

  CC-A **S76.221-** Laceration of adductor muscle, fascia and tendon of <u>right</u> thigh

  CC-A **S76.222-** Laceration of adductor muscle, fascia and tendon of <u>left</u> thigh

  CC-A **S76.229-** Laceration of adductor muscle, fascia and tendon of <u>unspecified</u> thigh

  S76.29- <u>Other injury</u> of <u>adductor</u> muscle, fascia and tendon of <u>thigh</u>

    S76.291- Other injury of adductor muscle, fascia and tendon of <u>right</u> thigh

    S76.292- Other injury of adductor muscle, fascia and tendon of <u>left</u> thigh

    S76.299- Other injury of adductor muscle, fascia and tendon of <u>unspecified</u> thigh

S76.3- Injury of <u>muscle, fascia and tendon</u> of the <u>posterior muscle group</u> at <u>thigh</u> level

  S76.30- <u>Unspecified</u> injury of muscle, fascia and tendon of the <u>posterior muscle group</u> at <u>thigh</u> level

    S76.301- Unspecified injury of muscle, fascia and tendon of the posterior muscle group at thigh level, <u>right</u> thigh

    S76.302- Unspecified injury of muscle, fascia and tendon of the posterior muscle group at thigh level, <u>left</u> thigh

    S76.309- Unspecified injury of muscle, fascia and tendon of the posterior muscle group at thigh level, <u>unspecified</u> thigh

  S76.31- <u>Strain</u> of muscle, fascia and tendon of the <u>posterior muscle group</u> at <u>thigh</u> level

    S76.311- Strain of muscle, fascia and tendon of the posterior muscle group at thigh level, <u>right</u> thigh

    S76.312- Strain of muscle, fascia and tendon of the posterior muscle group at thigh level, <u>left</u> thigh

    S76.319- Strain of muscle, fascia and tendon of the posterior muscle group at thigh level, <u>unspecified</u> thigh

  S76.32- <u>Laceration</u> of muscle, fascia and tendon of the <u>posterior muscle group</u> at <u>thigh</u> level

  CC-A **S76.321-** Laceration of muscle, fascia and tendon of the posterior muscle group at thigh level, <u>right</u> thigh

  CC-A **S76.322-** Laceration of muscle, fascia and tendon of the posterior muscle group at thigh level, <u>left</u> thigh

  CC-A **S76.329-** Laceration of muscle, fascia and tendon of the posterior muscle group at thigh level, <u>unspecified</u> thigh

  S76.39- <u>Other specified injury</u> of muscle, fascia and tendon of the <u>posterior muscle group</u> at <u>thigh</u> level

    S76.391- Other specified injury of muscle, fascia and tendon of the posterior muscle group at thigh level, <u>right</u> thigh

    S76.392- Other specified injury of muscle, fascia and tendon of the posterior muscle group at thigh level, <u>left</u> thigh

    S76.399- Other specified injury of muscle, fascia and tendon of the posterior muscle group at thigh level, <u>unspecified</u> thigh

S76.8- Injury of <u>other specified muscles, fascia and tendons</u> at <u>thigh</u> level

  S76.80- <u>Unspecified</u> injury of <u>other specified muscles, fascia and tendons</u> at <u>thigh</u> level

    S76.801- Unspecified injury of other specified muscles, fascia and tendons at thigh level, <u>right</u> thigh

    S76.802- Unspecified injury of other specified muscles, fascia and tendons at thigh level, <u>left</u> thigh

    S76.809- Unspecified injury of other specified muscles, fascia and tendons at thigh level, <u>unspecified</u> thigh

  S76.81- <u>Strain</u> of <u>other specified muscles, fascia and tendons</u> at <u>thigh</u> level

    S76.811- Strain of other specified muscles, fascia and tendons at thigh level, <u>right</u> thigh

    S76.812- Strain of other specified muscles, fascia and tendons at thigh level, <u>left</u> thigh

    S76.819- Strain of other specified muscles, fascia and tendons at thigh level, <u>unspecified</u> thigh

  S76.82- <u>Laceration</u> of <u>other specified muscles, fascia and tendons</u> at <u>thigh</u> level

  CC-A **S76.821-** Laceration of other specified muscles, fascia and tendons at thigh level, <u>right</u> thigh

  CC-A **S76.822-** Laceration of other specified muscles, fascia and tendons at thigh level, <u>left</u> thigh

  CC-A **S76.829-** Laceration of other specified muscles, fascia and tendons at thigh level, <u>unspecified</u> thigh

  S76.89- Other injury of <u>other specified muscles, fascia and tendons</u> at <u>thigh</u> level

    S76.891- Other injury of other specified muscles, fascia and tendons at thigh level, <u>right</u> thigh

    S76.892- Other injury of other specified muscles, fascia and tendons at thigh level, <u>left</u> thigh

    S76.899- Other injury of other specified muscles, fascia and tendons at thigh level, <u>unspecified</u> thigh

S76.9- Injury of <u>unspecified muscles, fascia and tendons</u> at <u>thigh</u> level

  S76.90- Unspecified injury of <u>unspecified muscles, fascia and tendons</u> at <u>thigh</u> level

    S76.901- Unspecified injury of unspecified muscles, fascia and tendons at thigh level, <u>right</u> thigh

    S76.902- Unspecified injury of unspecified muscles, fascia and tendons at thigh level, <u>left</u> thigh

    S76.909- Unspecified injury of unspecified muscles, fascia and tendons at thigh level, <u>unspecified</u> thigh

  S76.91- <u>Strain</u> of <u>unspecified muscles, fascia and tendons</u> at <u>thigh</u> level

    S76.911- Strain of unspecified muscles, fascia and tendons at thigh level, <u>right</u> thigh

    S76.912- Strain of unspecified muscles, fascia and tendons at thigh level, <u>left</u> thigh

    S76.919- Strain of unspecified muscles, fascia and tendons at thigh level, <u>unspecified</u> thigh

  S76.92- <u>Laceration</u> of <u>unspecified muscles, fascia and tendons</u> at <u>thigh</u> level

  CC-A **S76.921-** Laceration of unspecified muscles, fascia and tendons at thigh level, <u>right</u> thigh

  CC-A **S76.922-** Laceration of unspecified muscles, fascia and tendons at thigh level, <u>left</u> thigh

  CC-A **S76.929-** Laceration of unspecified muscles, fascia and tendons at thigh level, <u>unspecified</u> thigh

  S76.99- <u>Other specified injury</u> of <u>unspecified muscles, fascia and tendons</u> at <u>thigh</u> level

    S76.991- Other specified injury of unspecified muscles, fascia and tendons at thigh level, <u>right</u> thigh

    S76.992- Other specified injury of unspecified muscles, fascia and tendons at thigh level, <u>left</u> thigh

S76 – S76

S76.999- Other specified injury of unspecified muscles, fascia and tendons at thigh level, <u>unspecified</u> thigh

S77- <u>Crushing injury</u> of <u>hip</u> and <u>thigh</u>
Use additional code(s) for all associated injuries
Excludes ❷: crushing injury of ankle and foot (S97.-)
crushing injury of lower leg (S87.-)

The appropriate 7th character is to be added to each code from category S77:
A <u>Initial</u> encounter
D <u>Subsequent</u> encounter
S <u>Sequela</u>

S77.0- <u>Crushing</u> injury of <u>hip</u>
CC-A S77.00x- Crushing injury of <u>unspecified</u> hip
CC-A S77.01x- Crushing injury of <u>right</u> hip
CC-A S77.02x- Crushing injury of <u>left</u> hip

S77.1- <u>Crushing</u> injury of <u>thigh</u>
CC-A S77.10x- Crushing injury of <u>unspecified</u> thigh
CC-A S77.11x- Crushing injury of <u>right</u> thigh
CC-A S77.12x- Crushing injury of <u>left</u> thigh

S77.2- <u>Crushing</u> injury of <u>hip with thigh</u>
S77.20x- Crushing injury of <u>unspecified</u> hip with thigh
S77.21x- Crushing injury of <u>right</u> hip with thigh
S77.22x- Crushing injury of <u>left</u> hip with thigh

S78- <u>Traumatic amputation</u> of <u>hip</u> and <u>thigh</u>
Note: An amputation not identified as partial or complete should be coded to complete
Excludes 1: traumatic amputation of knee (S88.0-)

The appropriate 7th character is to be added to each code from category S78:
A <u>Initial</u> encounter
D <u>Subsequent</u> encounter
S <u>Sequela</u>

S78.0- Traumatic <u>amputation</u> at <u>hip joint</u>
S78.01- <u>Complete</u> traumatic <u>amputation</u> at <u>hip joint</u>
CC-A S78.011- Complete traumatic amputation at <u>right</u> hip joint
CC-A S78.012- Complete traumatic amputation at <u>left</u> hip joint
CC-A S78.019- Complete traumatic amputation at <u>unspecified</u> hip joint

S78.02- <u>Partial</u> traumatic <u>amputation</u> at <u>hip joint</u>
CC-A S78.021- Partial traumatic amputation at <u>right</u> hip joint
CC-A S78.022- Partial traumatic amputation at <u>left</u> hip joint
CC-A S78.029- Partial traumatic amputation at <u>unspecified</u> hip joint

S78.1- Traumatic <u>amputation</u> at <u>level between hip and knee</u>
Excludes 1: traumatic amputation of knee (S88.0-)
S78.11- <u>Complete</u> traumatic amputation at <u>level between hip and knee</u>
CC-A S78.111- Complete traumatic amputation at level between <u>right</u> hip and knee
CC-A S78.112- Complete traumatic amputation at level between <u>left</u> hip and knee
CC-A S78.119- Complete traumatic amputation at level between <u>unspecified</u> hip and knee
S78.12- <u>Partial</u> traumatic amputation at <u>level between hip and knee</u>
CC-A S78.121- Partial traumatic amputation at level between <u>right</u> hip and knee
CC-A S78.122- Partial traumatic amputation at level between <u>left</u> hip and knee
CC-A S78.129- Partial traumatic amputation at level between <u>unspecified</u> hip and knee

S78.9- Traumatic <u>amputation</u> of <u>hip and thigh</u>, <u>level unspecified</u>
S78.91- <u>Complete</u> traumatic <u>amputation</u> of <u>hip and thigh</u>, <u>level unspecified</u>
CC-A S78.911- Complete traumatic amputation of <u>right</u> hip and thigh, level unspecified
CC-A S78.912- Complete traumatic amputation of <u>left</u> hip and thigh, level unspecified

CC-A S78.919- Complete traumatic amputation of <u>unspecified</u> hip and thigh, level unspecified

S78.92- <u>Partial</u> traumatic <u>amputation</u> of <u>hip and thigh</u>, <u>level unspecified</u>
CC-A S78.921- Partial traumatic amputation of <u>right</u> hip and thigh, level unspecified
CC-A S78.922- Partial traumatic amputation of <u>left</u> hip and thigh, level unspecified
CC-A S78.929- Partial traumatic amputation of <u>unspecified</u> hip and thigh, level unspecified

S79- <u>Other and unspecified injuries</u> of <u>hip</u> and <u>thigh</u>
Note: A fracture not indicated as open or closed should be coded to closed

The appropriate 7th character is to be added to each code from subcategories S79.0 and S79.1:
A <u>Initial</u> encounter for closed fracture
D <u>Subsequent</u> encounter for fracture with routine healing
G <u>Subsequent</u> encounter for fracture with delayed healing
K <u>Subsequent</u> encounter for fracture with nonunion
P <u>Subsequent</u> encounter for fracture with malunion
S <u>Sequela</u>

S79.0- <u>Physeal fracture</u> of <u>upper end</u> of <u>femur</u>
Excludes 1: apophyseal fracture of upper end of femur (S72.13-)
nontraumatic slipped upper femoral epiphysis (M93.0-)

S79.00- <u>Unspecified physeal</u> fracture of <u>upper end</u> of <u>femur</u>
CC-K,P MCC-A S79.001- Unspecified physeal fracture of upper end of <u>right</u> femur
CC-K,P MCC-A S79.002- Unspecified physeal fracture of upper end of <u>left</u> femur
CC-K,P MCC-A S79.009- Unspecified physeal fracture of upper end of <u>unspecified</u> femur

S79.01- <u>Salter-Harris Type I</u> physeal fracture of <u>upper end</u> of <u>femur</u>
Acute on chronic slipped capital femoral epiphysis (traumatic)
Acute slipped capital femoral epiphysis (traumatic)
Capital femoral epiphyseal fracture
Excludes 1: chronic slipped upper femoral epiphysis (nontraumatic) (M93.02-)
CC-K,P MCC-A S79.011- Salter-Harris Type I physeal fracture of upper end of <u>right</u> femur
CC-K,P MCC-A S79.012- Salter-Harris Type I physeal fracture of upper end of <u>left</u> femur
CC-K,P MCC-A S79.019- Salter-Harris Type I physeal fracture of upper end of <u>unspecified</u> femur

S79.09- <u>Other physeal</u> fracture of <u>upper end</u> of <u>femur</u>
CC-K,P MCC-A S79.091- Other physeal fracture of upper end of <u>right</u> femur
CC-K,P MCC-A S79.092- Other physeal fracture of upper end of <u>left</u> femur
CC-K,P MCC-A S79.099- Other physeal fracture of upper end of <u>unspecified</u> femur

S79.1- <u>Physeal fracture</u> of <u>lower end</u> of <u>femur</u>
S79.10- <u>Unspecified physeal</u> fracture of <u>lower end</u> of <u>femur</u>
CC-A,K,P S79.101- Unspecified physeal fracture of lower end of <u>right</u> femur
CC-A,K,P S79.102- Unspecified physeal fracture of lower end of <u>left</u> femur
CC-A,K,P S79.109- Unspecified physeal fracture of lower end of <u>unspecified</u> femur

S79.11- <u>Salter-Harris Type I</u> physeal fracture of <u>lower end</u> of <u>femur</u>
CC-A,K,P S79.111- Salter-Harris Type I physeal fracture of lower end of <u>right</u> femur
CC-A,K,P S79.112- Salter-Harris Type I physeal fracture of lower end of <u>left</u> femur
CC-A,K,P S79.119- Salter-Harris Type I physeal fracture of lower end of <u>unspecified</u> femur

S79.12- <u>Salter-Harris Type II</u> physeal fracture of <u>lower end</u> of <u>femur</u>
CC-A,K,P S79.121- Salter-Harris Type II physeal fracture of lower end of <u>right</u> femur
CC-A,K,P S79.122- Salter-Harris Type II physeal fracture of lower end of <u>left</u> femur

CC-A,K,P **S79.129-** Salter-Harris Type II physeal fracture of lower end of <u>unspecified</u> femur

S79.13- <u>Salter-Harris Type III</u> physeal fracture of <u>lower end</u> of <u>femur</u>

CC-A,K,P **S79.131-** Salter-Harris Type III physeal fracture of lower end of <u>right</u> femur

CC-A,K,P **S79.132-** Salter-Harris Type III physeal fracture of lower end of <u>left</u> femur

CC-A,K,P **S79.139-** Salter-Harris Type III physeal fracture of lower end of <u>unspecified</u> femur

S79.14- <u>Salter-Harris Type IV</u> physeal fracture of <u>lower end</u> of <u>femur</u>

CC-A,K,P **S79.141-** Salter-Harris Type IV physeal fracture of lower end of <u>right</u> femur

CC-A,K,P **S79.142-** Salter-Harris Type IV physeal fracture of lower end of <u>left</u> femur

CC-A,K,P **S79.149-** Salter-Harris Type IV physeal fracture of lower end of <u>unspecified</u> femur

S79.19- <u>Other physeal</u> fracture of <u>lower end</u> of <u>femur</u>

CC-A,K,P **S79.191-** Other physeal fracture of lower end of <u>right</u> femur

CC-A,K,P **S79.192-** Other physeal fracture of lower end of <u>left</u> femur

CC-A,K,P **S79.199-** Other physeal fracture of lower end of <u>unspecified</u> femur

S79.8- <u>Other specified injuries</u> of <u>hip</u> and <u>thigh</u>
The appropriate 7th character is to be added to each code in subcategory S79.8:
A <u>Initial</u> encounter
D <u>Subsequent</u> encounter
S <u>Sequela</u>

S79.81- <u>Other specified injuries</u> of <u>hip</u>

S79.811- Other specified injuries of <u>right</u> hip

S79.812- Other specified injuries of <u>left</u> hip

S79.819- Other specified injuries of <u>unspecified</u> hip

S79.82- <u>Other specified injuries</u> of <u>thigh</u>

S79.821- Other specified injuries of <u>right</u> thigh

S79.822- Other specified injuries of <u>left</u> thigh

S79.829- Other specified injuries of <u>unspecified</u> thigh

S79.9- <u>Unspecified injury</u> of <u>hip</u> and <u>thigh</u>
The appropriate 7th character is to be added to each code in subcategory S79.9:
A <u>Initial</u> encounter
D <u>Subsequent</u> encounter
S <u>Sequela</u>

S79.91- <u>Unspecified</u> injury of <u>hip</u>

S79.911- Unspecified injury of <u>right</u> hip

S79.912- Unspecified injury of <u>left</u> hip

S79.919- Unspecified injury of <u>unspecified</u> hip

S79.92- <u>Unspecified</u> injury of <u>thigh</u>

S79.921- Unspecified injury of <u>right</u> thigh

S79.922- Unspecified injury of <u>left</u> thigh

S79.929- Unspecified injury of <u>unspecified</u> thigh

Injuries to the knee and lower leg (S80-S89)

Excludes ❷: *burns and corrosions (T20-T32)*
frostbite (T33-T34)
injuries of ankle and foot, except fracture of ankle and malleolus (S90-S99)
insect bite or sting, venomous (T63.4)

S80- <u>Superficial injury</u> of <u>knee</u> and <u>lower leg</u>
Excludes ❷: *superficial injury of ankle and foot (S90.-)*
The appropriate 7th character is to be added to each code from category S80:
A <u>Initial</u> encounter
D <u>Subsequent</u> encounter
S <u>Sequela</u>

S80.0- <u>Contusion</u> of <u>knee</u>

S80.00x- Contusion of <u>unspecified</u> knee

S80.01x- Contusion of <u>right</u> knee

S80.02x- Contusion of <u>left</u> knee

S80.1- <u>Contusion</u> of <u>lower leg</u>

S80.10x- Contusion of <u>unspecified</u> lower leg

S80.11x- Contusion of <u>right</u> lower leg

S80.12x- Contusion of <u>left</u> lower leg

S80.2- <u>Other superficial injuries</u> of <u>knee</u>

S80.21- <u>Abrasion</u> of knee

S80.211- Abrasion, <u>right</u> knee

S80.212- Abrasion, <u>left</u> knee

S80.219- Abrasion, <u>unspecified</u> knee

S80.22- <u>Blister</u> (nonthermal) of knee

S80.221- Blister (nonthermal), <u>right</u> knee

S80.222- Blister (nonthermal), <u>left</u> knee

S80.229- Blister (nonthermal), <u>unspecified</u> knee

S80.24- <u>External constriction</u> of knee

S80.241- External constriction, <u>right</u> knee

S80.242- External constriction, <u>left</u> knee

S80.249- External constriction, <u>unspecified</u> knee

S80.25- <u>Superficial foreign body</u> of knee
Splinter in the knee

S80.251- Superficial foreign body, <u>right</u> knee

S80.252- Superficial foreign body, <u>left</u> knee

S80.259- Superficial foreign body, <u>unspecified</u> knee

S80.26- <u>Insect bite (nonvenomous)</u> of knee

S80.261- Insect bite (nonvenomous), <u>right</u> knee

S80.262- Insect bite (nonvenomous), <u>left</u> knee

S80.269- Insect bite (nonvenomous), <u>unspecified</u> knee

S80.27- <u>Other superficial bite</u> of knee
Excludes 1: *open bite of knee (S81.05-)*

S80.271- Other superficial bite of <u>right</u> knee

S80.272- Other superficial bite of <u>left</u> knee

S80.279- Other superficial bite of <u>unspecified</u> knee

S80.8- <u>Other superficial injuries</u> of <u>lower leg</u>

S80.81- <u>Abrasion</u> of lower leg

S80.811- Abrasion, <u>right</u> lower leg

S80.812- Abrasion, <u>left</u> lower leg

S80.819- Abrasion, <u>unspecified</u> lower leg

S80.82- <u>Blister</u> (nonthermal) of lower leg

S80.821- Blister (nonthermal), <u>right</u> lower leg

S80.822- Blister (nonthermal), <u>left</u> lower leg

S80.829- Blister (nonthermal), <u>unspecified</u> lower leg

S80.84- <u>External constriction</u> of lower leg

S80.841- External constriction, <u>right</u> lower leg

S80.842- External constriction, <u>left</u> lower leg

S80.849- External constriction, <u>unspecified</u> lower leg

S80.85- <u>Superficial foreign body</u> of lower leg
Splinter in the lower leg

S80.851- Superficial foreign body, <u>right</u> lower leg

S80.852- Superficial foreign body, <u>left</u> lower leg

S80.859- Superficial foreign body, <u>unspecified</u> lower leg

S80.86- <u>Insect bite (nonvenomous)</u> of lower leg

S80.861- Insect bite (nonvenomous), <u>right</u> lower leg

S80.862- Insect bite (nonvenomous), <u>left</u> lower leg

S80.869- Insect bite (nonvenomous), <u>unspecified</u> lower leg

S80.87- <u>Other superficial bite</u> of lower leg
Excludes 1: *open bite of lower leg (S81.85-)*

S80.871- Other superficial bite, <u>right</u> lower leg

S80.872- Other superficial bite, <u>left</u> lower leg

S80.879- Other superficial bite, <u>unspecified</u> lower leg

S80.9- <u>Unspecified superficial injury</u> of <u>knee</u> and <u>lower leg</u>

S80.91- <u>Unspecified superficial injury</u> of <u>knee</u>

S80.911- Unspecified superficial injury of <u>right</u> knee

S80.912- Unspecified superficial injury of <u>left</u> knee

S80.919- Unspecified superficial injury of <u>unspecified</u> knee

S 7 9 - S 80

S80.92- Unspecified superficial injury of lower leg

    S80.921- Unspecified superficial injury of right lower leg

    S80.922- Unspecified superficial injury of left lower leg

    S80.929- Unspecified superficial injury of unspecified lower leg

S81- Open wound of knee and lower leg

  Code also any associated wound infection

  Excludes 1:   *open fracture of knee and lower leg (S82.-)*

               traumatic amputation of lower leg (S88.-)

  Excludes ❷: *open wound of ankle and foot (S91.-)*

  The appropriate 7th character is to be added to each code from category S81:

    A   Initial encounter

    D   Subsequent encounter

    S   Sequela

S81.0- Open wound of knee

  S81.00- Unspecified open wound of knee

    S81.001- Unspecified open wound, right knee

    S81.002- Unspecified open wound, left knee

    S81.009- Unspecified open wound, unspecified knee

  S81.01- Laceration without foreign body of knee

    S81.011- Laceration without foreign body, right knee

    S81.012- Laceration without foreign body, left knee

    S81.019- Laceration without foreign body, unspecified knee

  S81.02- Laceration with foreign body of knee

    S81.021- Laceration with foreign body, right knee

    S81.022- Laceration with foreign body, left knee

    S81.029- Laceration with foreign body, unspecified knee

  S81.03- Puncture wound without foreign body of knee

    S81.031- Puncture wound without foreign body, right knee

    S81.032- Puncture wound without foreign body, left knee

    S81.039- Puncture wound without foreign body, unspecified knee

  S81.04- Puncture wound with foreign body of knee

    S81.041- Puncture wound with foreign body, right knee

    S81.042- Puncture wound with foreign body, left knee

    S81.049- Puncture wound with foreign body, unspecified knee

  S81.05- Open bite of knee

    Bite of knee NOS

    Excludes 1:   *superficial bite of knee (S80.27-)*

    S81.051- Open bite, right knee

    S81.052- Open bite, left knee

    S81.059- Open bite, unspecified knee

S81.8- Open wound of lower leg

  S81.80- Unspecified open wound of lower leg

    S81.801- Unspecified open wound, right lower leg

    S81.802- Unspecified open wound, left lower leg

    S81.809- Unspecified open wound, unspecified lower leg

  S81.81- Laceration without foreign body of lower leg

    S81.811- Laceration without foreign body, right lower leg

    S81.812- Laceration without foreign body, left lower leg

    S81.819- Laceration without foreign body, unspecified lower leg

  S81.82- Laceration with foreign body of lower leg

    S81.821- Laceration with foreign body, right lower leg

    S81.822- Laceration with foreign body, left lower leg

    S81.829- Laceration with foreign body, unspecified lower leg

  S81.83- Puncture wound without foreign body of lower leg

    S81.831- Puncture wound without foreign body, right lower leg

    S81.832- Puncture wound without foreign body, left lower leg

    S81.839- Puncture wound without foreign body, unspecified lower leg

S81.84- Puncture wound with foreign body of lower leg

    S81.841- Puncture wound with foreign body, right lower leg

    S81.842- Puncture wound with foreign body, left lower leg

    S81.849- Puncture wound with foreign body, unspecified lower leg

S81.85- Open bite of lower leg

    Bite of lower leg NOS

    Excludes 1:   *superficial bite of lower leg (S80.86-, S80.87-)*

    S81.851- Open bite, right lower leg

    S81.852- Open bite, left lower leg

    S81.859- Open bite, unspecified lower leg

S82- Fracture of lower leg, including ankle

  AHA 15:1Q:p25 — Comminuted fracture of left distal tibia and fibula

  Note: A fracture not indicated as displaced or nondisplaced should be coded to displaced

  Note: A fracture not indicated as open or closed should be coded to closed

  Note: The open fracture designations are based on the Gustilo open fracture classification

  Includes: Fracture of malleolus

  Excludes 1:   *traumatic amputation of lower leg (S88.-)*

  Excludes ❷: *fracture of foot, except ankle (S92.-)*

               periprosthetic fracture of prosthetic implant of knee (T84.042, T84.043)

  The appropriate 7th character is to be added to all codes from category S82:

    A   Initial encounter for closed fracture

    B   Initial encounter for open fracture type I or II

        Initial encounter for open fracture NOS

    C   Initial encounter for open fracture type IIIA, IIIB, or IIIC

    D   Subsequent encounter for closed fracture with routine healing

    E   Subsequent encounter for open fracture type I or II with routine healing

    F   Subsequent encounter for open fracture type IIIA, IIIB, or IIIC with routine healing

    G   Subsequent encounter for closed fracture with delayed healing

    H   Subsequent encounter for open fracture type I or II with delayed healing

    J   Subsequent encounter for open fracture type IIIA, IIIB, or IIIC with delayed healing

    K   Subsequent encounter for closed fracture with nonunion

    M   Subsequent encounter for open fracture type I or II with nonunion

    N   Subsequent encounter for open fracture type IIIA, IIIB, or IIIC with nonunion

    P   Subsequent encounter for closed fracture with malunion

    Q   Subsequent encounter for open fracture type I or II with malunion

    R   Subsequent encounter for open fracture type IIIA, IIIB, or IIIC with malunion

    S   Sequela

S82.0- Fracture of patella

    Knee cap

  S82.00- Unspecified fracture of patella

    S82.001- Unspecified fracture of right patella

    CC-A,B,C,K,M,N,P,Q,R

    S82.002- Unspecified fracture of left patella

    CC-A,B,C,K,M,N,P,Q,R

    S82.009- Unspecified fracture of unspecified patella

    CC-A,B,C,K,M,N,P,Q,R

  S82.01- Osteochondral fracture of patella

    S82.011- Displaced osteochondral fracture of right patella

    CC-A,B,C,K,M,N,P,Q,R

    S82.012- Displaced osteochondral fracture of left patella

    CC-A,B,C,K,M,N,P,Q,R

    S82.013- Displaced osteochondral fracture of unspecified patella

    CC-A,B,C,K,M,N,P,Q,R

    S82.014- Nondisplaced osteochondral fracture of right patella

    CC-A,B,C,K,M,N,P,Q,R

    S82.015- Nondisplaced osteochondral fracture of left patella

    CC-A,B,C,K,M,N,P,Q,R

Excludes 1: = NOT CODED HERE! (Do not code both)

Excludes ❷: = Not Included Here

S82.016- <u>Nondisplaced</u> osteochondral fracture of <u>unspecified</u> patella
CC-A,B,C,K,M,N,P,Q,R

S82.02- <u>Longitudinal</u> fracture of <u>patella</u>

S82.021- <u>Displaced</u> longitudinal fracture of <u>right</u> patella
CC-A,B,C,K,M,N,P,Q,R

S82.022- <u>Displaced</u> longitudinal fracture of <u>left</u> patella
CC-A,B,C,K,M,N,P,Q,R

S82.023- <u>Displaced</u> longitudinal fracture of <u>unspecified</u> patella
CC-A,B,C,K,M,N,P,Q,R

S82.024- <u>Nondisplaced</u> longitudinal fracture of <u>right</u> patella
CC-A,B,C,K,M,N,P,Q,R

S82.025- <u>Nondisplaced</u> longitudinal fracture of <u>left</u> patella
CC-A,B,C,K,M,N,P,Q,R

S82.026- <u>Nondisplaced</u> longitudinal fracture of <u>unspecified</u> patella
CC-A,B,C,K,M,N,P,Q,R

S82.03- <u>Transverse</u> fracture of <u>patella</u>

S82.031- <u>Displaced</u> transverse fracture of <u>right</u> patella
CC-A,B,C,K,M,N,P,Q,R

S82.032- <u>Displaced</u> transverse fracture of <u>left</u> patella
CC-A,B,C,K,M,N,P,Q,R

S82.033- <u>Displaced</u> transverse fracture of <u>unspecified</u> patella
CC-A,B,C,K,M,N,P,Q,R

S82.034- <u>Nondisplaced</u> transverse fracture of <u>right</u> patella
CC-A,B,C,K,M,N,P,Q,R

S82.035- <u>Nondisplaced</u> transverse fracture of <u>left</u> patella
CC-A,B,C,K,M,N,P,Q,R

S82.036- <u>Nondisplaced</u> transverse fracture of <u>unspecified</u> patella
CC-A,B,C,K,M,N,P,Q,R

S82.04- <u>Comminuted</u> fracture of <u>patella</u>

S82.041- <u>Displaced</u> comminuted fracture of <u>right</u> patella
CC-A,B,C,K,M,N,P,Q,R

S82.042- <u>Displaced</u> comminuted fracture of <u>left</u> patella
CC-A,B,C,K,M,N,P,Q,R

S82.043- <u>Displaced</u> comminuted fracture of <u>unspecified</u> patella
CC-A,B,C,K,M,N,P,Q,R

S82.044- <u>Nondisplaced</u> comminuted fracture of <u>right</u> patella
CC-A,B,C,K,M,N,P,Q,R

S82.045- <u>Nondisplaced</u> comminuted fracture of <u>left</u> patella
CC-A,B,C,K,M,N,P,Q,R

S82.046- <u>Nondisplaced</u> comminuted fracture of <u>unspecified</u> patella
CC-A,B,C,K,M,N,P,Q,R

S82.09- <u>Other fracture</u> of <u>patella</u>

S82.091- Other fracture of <u>right</u> patella
CC-A,B,C,K,M,N,P,Q,R

S82.092- Other fracture of <u>left</u> patella
CC-A,B,C,K,M,N,P,Q,R

S82.099- Other fracture of <u>unspecified</u> patella
CC-A,B,C,K,M,N,P,Q,R

S82.1- <u>Fracture</u> of <u>upper end</u> of <u>tibia</u>
Fracture of proximal end of tibia
Excludes ❷: *fracture of shaft of tibia (S82.2-)*
physeal fracture of upper end of tibia (S89.0-)

S82.10- <u>Unspecified</u> fracture of <u>upper end</u> of <u>tibia</u>

S82.101- <u>Unspecified</u> fracture of upper end of <u>right</u> tibia
CC-A,K,M,N,P,Q,R MCC-B,C

S82.102- <u>Unspecified</u> fracture of upper end of <u>left</u> tibia
CC-A,K,M,N,P,Q,R MCC-B,C

S82.109- <u>Unspecified</u> fracture of upper end of <u>unspecified</u> tibia
CC-A,K,M,N,P,Q,R MCC-B,C

S82.11- <u>Fracture</u> of <u>tibial spine</u>

S82.111- <u>Displaced</u> fracture of <u>right</u> tibial spine
CC-A,K,M,N,P,Q,R MCC-B,C

S82.112- <u>Displaced</u> fracture of <u>left</u> tibial spine
CC-A,K,M,N,P,Q,R MCC-B,C

S82.113- <u>Displaced</u> fracture of <u>unspecified</u> tibial spine
CC-A,K,M,N,P,Q,R MCC-B,C

S82.114- <u>Nondisplaced</u> fracture of <u>right</u> tibial spine
CC-A,K,M,N,P,Q,R MCC-B,C

S82.115- <u>Nondisplaced</u> fracture of <u>left</u> tibial spine
CC-A,K,M,N,P,Q,R MCC-B,C

S82.116- <u>Nondisplaced</u> fracture of <u>unspecified</u> tibial spine
CC-A,K,M,N,P,Q,R MCC-B,C

S82.12- Fracture of <u>lateral condyle</u> of <u>tibia</u>

S82.121- <u>Displaced</u> fracture of lateral condyle of <u>right</u> tibia
CC-A,K,M,N,P,Q,R MCC-B,C

S82.122- <u>Displaced</u> fracture of lateral condyle of <u>left</u> tibia
CC-A,K,M,N,P,Q,R MCC-B,C

S82.123- <u>Displaced</u> fracture of lateral condyle of <u>unspecified</u> tibia
CC-A,K,M,N,P,Q,R MCC-B,C

S82.124- <u>Nondisplaced</u> fracture of lateral condyle of <u>right</u> tibia
CC-A,K,M,N,P,Q,R MCC-B,C

S82.125- <u>Nondisplaced</u> fracture of lateral condyle of <u>left</u> tibia
CC-A,K,M,N,P,Q,R MCC-B,C

S82.126- <u>Nondisplaced</u> fracture of lateral condyle of <u>unspecified</u> tibia
CC-A,K,M,N,P,Q,R MCC-B,C

S82.13- Fracture of <u>medial condyle</u> of <u>tibia</u>

S82.131- <u>Displaced</u> fracture of medial condyle of <u>right</u> tibia
CC-A,K,M,N,P,Q,R MCC-B,C

S82.132- <u>Displaced</u> fracture of medial condyle of <u>left</u> tibia
CC-A,K,M,N,P,Q,R MCC-B,C

S82.133- <u>Displaced</u> fracture of medial condyle of <u>unspecified</u> tibia
CC-A,K,M,N,P,Q,R MCC-B,C

S82.134- <u>Nondisplaced</u> fracture of medial condyle of <u>right</u> tibia
CC-A,K,M,N,P,Q,R MCC-B,C

S82.135- <u>Nondisplaced</u> fracture of medial condyle of <u>left</u> tibia
CC-A,K,M,N,P,Q,R MCC-B,C

S82.136- <u>Nondisplaced</u> fracture of medial condyle of <u>unspecified</u> tibia
CC-A,K,M,N,P,Q,R MCC-B,C

S82.14- <u>Bicondylar</u> fracture of <u>tibia</u>
Fracture of tibial plateau NOS

S82.141- <u>Displaced</u> bicondylar fracture of <u>right</u> tibia
CC-A,K,M,N,P,Q,R MCC-B,C

S82.142- <u>Displaced</u> bicondylar fracture of <u>left</u> tibia
CC-A,K,M,N,P,Q,R MCC-B,C

S82.143- <u>Displaced</u> bicondylar fracture of <u>unspecified</u> tibia
CC-A,K,M,N,P,Q,R MCC-B,C

S82.144- <u>Nondisplaced</u> bicondylar fracture of <u>right</u> tibia
CC-A,K,M,N,P,Q,R MCC-B,C

S82.145- <u>Nondisplaced</u> bicondylar fracture of <u>left</u> tibia
CC-A,K,M,N,P,Q,R MCC-B,C

S82.146- <u>Nondisplaced</u> bicondylar fracture of <u>unspecified</u> tibia
CC-A,K,M,N,P,Q,R MCC-B,C

S82.15- Fracture of <u>tibial tuberosity</u>

S82.151- <u>Displaced</u> fracture of <u>right</u> tibial tuberosity
CC-A,K,M,N,P,Q,R MCC-B,C

S82.152- <u>Displaced</u> fracture of <u>left</u> tibial tuberosity
CC-A,K,M,N,P,Q,R MCC-B,C

S82.153- <u>Displaced</u> fracture of <u>unspecified</u> tibial tuberosity
CC-A,K,M,N,P,Q,R MCC-B,C

S82.154- <u>Nondisplaced</u> fracture of <u>right</u> tibial tuberosity
CC-A,K,M,N,P,Q,R MCC-B,C

S82.155- <u>Nondisplaced</u> fracture of <u>left</u> tibial tuberosity
CC-A,K,M,N,P,Q,R MCC-B,C

S82.156- <u>Nondisplaced</u> fracture of <u>unspecified</u> tibial tuberosity
CC-A,K,M,N,P,Q,R MCC-B,C

S82
I
S82

S82.16-　Torus fracture of upper end of tibia
　　　The appropriate 7th character is to be added to all codes
　　　　in subcategory S82.16:
　　A　Initial encounter for closed fracture
　　D　Subsequent encounter for fracture with routine healing
　　G　Subsequent encounter for fracture with delayed healing
　　K　Subsequent encounter for fracture with nonunion
　　P　Subsequent encounter for fracture with malunion
　　S　Sequela

CC-A,K,P S82.161-　Torus fracture of upper end of right tibia
CC-A,K,P S82.162-　Torus fracture of upper end of left tibia
CC-A,K,P S82.169-　Torus fracture of upper end of unspecified tibia

S82.19-　Other fracture of upper end of tibia
　　S82.191-　Other fracture of upper end of right tibia
　　　CC-A,K,M,N,P,Q,R MCC-B,C
　　S82.192-　Other fracture of upper end of left tibia
　　　CC-A,K,M,N,P,Q,R MCC-B,C
　　S82.199-　Other fracture of upper end of unspecified tibia
　　　CC-A,K,M,N,P,Q,R MCC-B,C

S82.2-　Fracture of shaft of tibia
　S82.20-　Unspecified fracture of shaft of tibia
　　　Fracture of tibia NOS
　　S82.201-　Unspecified fracture of shaft of right tibia
　　　CC-A,K,M,N,P,Q,R MCC-B,C
　　S82.202-　Unspecified fracture of shaft of left tibia
　　　CC-A,K,M,N,P,Q,R MCC-B,C
　　S82.209-　Unspecified fracture of shaft of unspecified tibia
　　　CC-A,K,M,N,P,Q,R MCC-B,C

　S82.22-　Transverse fracture of shaft of tibia
　　S82.221-　Displaced transverse fracture of shaft of right tibia
　　　CC-A,K,M,N,P,Q,R MCC-B,C
　　S82.222-　Displaced transverse fracture of shaft of left tibia
　　　CC-A,K,M,N,P,Q,R MCC-B,C
　　S82.223-　Displaced transverse fracture of shaft of unspecified tibia
　　　CC-A,K,M,N,P,Q,R MCC-B,C
　　S82.224-　Nondisplaced transverse fracture of shaft of right tibia
　　　CC-A,K,M,N,P,Q,R MCC-B,C
　　S82.225-　Nondisplaced transverse fracture of shaft of left tibia
　　　CC-A,K,M,N,P,Q,R MCC-B,C
　　S82.226-　Nondisplaced transverse fracture of shaft of unspecified tibia
　　　CC-A,K,M,N,P,Q,R MCC-B,C

　S82.23-　Oblique fracture of shaft of tibia
　　　AHA 15:1Q:p8 – Nondisplaced oblique fracture of right tibia
　　S82.231-　Displaced oblique fracture of shaft of right tibia
　　　CC-A,K,M,N,P,Q,R MCC-B,C
　　S82.232-　Displaced oblique fracture of shaft of left tibia
　　　CC-A,K,M,N,P,Q,R MCC-B,C
　　S82.233-　Displaced oblique fracture of shaft of unspecified tibia
　　　CC-A,K,M,N,P,Q,R MCC-B,C
　　S82.234-　Nondisplaced oblique fracture of shaft of right tibia
　　　CC-A,K,M,N,P,Q,R MCC-B,C
　　S82.235-　Nondisplaced oblique fracture of shaft of left tibia
　　　CC-A,K,M,N,P,Q,R MCC-B,C
　　S82.236-　Nondisplaced oblique fracture of shaft of unspecified tibia
　　　CC-A,K,M,N,P,Q,R MCC-B,C

　S82.24-　Spiral fracture of shaft of tibia
　　　Toddler fracture
　　S82.241-　Displaced spiral fracture of shaft of right tibia
　　　CC-A,K,M,N,P,Q,R MCC-B,C
　　S82.242-　Displaced spiral fracture of shaft of left tibia
　　　CC-A,K,M,N,P,Q,R MCC-B,C
　　S82.243-　Displaced spiral fracture of shaft of unspecified tibia
　　　CC-A,K,M,N,P,Q,R MCC-B,C
　　S82.244-　Nondisplaced spiral fracture of shaft of right tibia
　　　CC-A,K,M,N,P,Q,R MCC-B,C

S82.245-　Nondisplaced spiral fracture of shaft of left tibia
　　CC-A,K,M,N,P,Q,R MCC-B,C
S82.246-　Nondisplaced spiral fracture of shaft of unspecified tibia
　　CC-A,K,M,N,P,Q,R MCC-B,C

S82.25-　Comminuted fracture of shaft of tibia
　　S82.251-　Displaced comminuted fracture of shaft of right tibia
　　　CC-A,K,M,N,P,Q,R MCC-B,C
　　S82.252-　Displaced comminuted fracture of shaft of left tibia
　　　CC-A,K,M,N,P,Q,R MCC-B,C
　　S82.253-　Displaced comminuted fracture of shaft of unspecified tibia
　　　CC-A,K,M,N,P,Q,R MCC-B,C
　　S82.254-　Nondisplaced comminuted fracture of shaft of right tibia
　　　CC-A,K,M,N,P,Q,R MCC-B,C
　　S82.255-　Nondisplaced comminuted fracture of shaft of left tibia
　　　CC-A,K,M,N,P,Q,R MCC-B,C
　　S82.256-　Nondisplaced comminuted fracture of shaft of unspecified tibia
　　　CC-A,K,M,N,P,Q,R MCC-B,C

S82.26-　Segmental fracture of shaft of tibia
　　S82.261-　Displaced segmental fracture of shaft of right tibia
　　　CC-A,K,M,N,P,Q,R MCC-B,C
　　S82.262-　Displaced segmental fracture of shaft of left tibia
　　　CC-A,K,M,N,P,Q,R MCC-B,C
　　S82.263-　Displaced segmental fracture of shaft of unspecified tibia
　　　CC-A,K,M,N,P,Q,R MCC-B,C
　　S82.264-　Nondisplaced segmental fracture of shaft of right tibia
　　　CC-A,K,M,N,P,Q,R MCC-B,C
　　S82.265-　Nondisplaced segmental fracture of shaft of left tibia
　　　CC-A,K,M,N,P,Q,R MCC-B,C
　　S82.266-　Nondisplaced segmental fracture of shaft of unspecified tibia
　　　CC-A,K,M,N,P,Q,R MCC-B,C

S82.29-　Other fracture of shaft of tibia
　　S82.291-　Other fracture of shaft of right tibia
　　　CC-A,K,M,N,P,Q,R MCC-B,C
　　S82.292-　Other fracture of shaft of left tibia
　　　CC-A,K,M,N,P,Q,R MCC-B,C
　　S82.299-　Other fracture of shaft of unspecified tibia
　　　CC-A,K,M,N,P,Q,R MCC-B,C

S82.3-　Fracture of lower end of tibia
　　Excludes 1:　bimalleolar fracture of lower leg (S82.84-)
　　　　　　　fracture of medial malleolus alone (S82.5-)
　　　　　　　Maisonneuve's fracture (S82.86-)
　　　　　　　pilon fracture of distal tibia (S82.87-)
　　　　　　　trimalleolar fractures of lower leg (S82.85-)

　S82.30-　Unspecified fracture of lower end of tibia
　　S82.301-　Unspecified fracture of lower end of right tibia
　　　CC-B,C,K,M,N,P,Q,R
　　S82.302-　Unspecified fracture of lower end of left tibia
　　　CC-B,C,K,M,N,P,Q,R
　　S82.309-　Unspecified fracture of lower end of unspecified tibia
　　　CC-B,C,K,M,N,P,Q,R

　S82.31-　Torus fracture of lower end of tibia
　　　The appropriate 7th character is to be added to all codes
　　　　in subcategory S82.31:
　　A　Initial encounter for closed fracture
　　D　Subsequent encounter for fracture with routine healing
　　G　Subsequent encounter for fracture with delayed healing
　　K　Subsequent encounter for fracture with nonunion
　　P　Subsequent encounter for fracture with malunion
　　S　Sequela

CC-A,K,P S82.311-　Torus fracture of lower end of right tibia
CC-A,K,P S82.312-　Torus fracture of lower end of left tibia
CC-A,K,P S82.319-　Torus fracture of lower end of unspecified tibia

S82 - S82

S82.39- Other fracture of lower end of tibia

S82.391- Other fracture of lower end of right tibia
CC-B,C,K,M,N,P,Q,R

S82.392- Other fracture of lower end of left tibia
CC-B,C,K,M,N,P,Q,R

S82.399- Other fracture of lower end of unspecified tibia
CC-B,C,K,M,N,P,Q,R

S82.4- Fracture of shaft of fibula
Excludes ❷:　fracture of lateral malleolus alone (S82.6-)

S82.40- Unspecified fracture of shaft of fibula

S82.401- Unspecified fracture of shaft of right fibula
CC-K,M,N,P,Q,R MCC-B,C

S82.402- Unspecified fracture of shaft of left fibula
CC-K,M,N,P,Q,R MCC-B,C

S82.409- Unspecified fracture of shaft of unspecified fibula
CC-K,M,N,P,Q,R MCC-B,C

S82.42- Transverse fracture of shaft of fibula

S82.421- Displaced transverse fracture of shaft of right fibula
CC-K,M,N,P,Q,R MCC-B,C

S82.422- Displaced transverse fracture of shaft of left fibula
CC-K,M,N,P,Q,R MCC-B,C

S82.423- Displaced transverse fracture of shaft of unspecified fibula
CC-K,M,N,P,Q,R MCC-B,C

S82.424- Nondisplaced transverse fracture of shaft of right fibula
CC-K,M,N,P,Q,R MCC-B,C

S82.425- Nondisplaced transverse fracture of shaft of left fibula
CC-K,M,N,P,Q,R MCC-B,C

S82.426- Nondisplaced transverse fracture of shaft of unspecified fibula
CC-K,M,N,P,Q,R MCC-B,C

S82.43- Oblique fracture of shaft of fibula

S82.431- Displaced oblique fracture of shaft of right fibula
CC-K,M,N,P,Q,R MCC-B,C

S82.432- Displaced oblique fracture of shaft of left fibula
CC-K,M,N,P,Q,R MCC-B,C

S82.433- Displaced oblique fracture of shaft of unspecified fibula
CC-K,M,N,P,Q,R MCC-B,C

S82.434- Nondisplaced oblique fracture of shaft of right fibula
CC-K,M,N,P,Q,R MCC-B,C

S82.435- Nondisplaced oblique fracture of shaft of left fibula
CC-K,M,N,P,Q,R MCC-B,C

S82.436- Nondisplaced oblique fracture of shaft of unspecified fibula
CC-K,M,N,P,Q,R MCC-B,C

S82.44- Spiral fracture of shaft of fibula

S82.441- Displaced spiral fracture of shaft of right fibula
CC-K,M,N,P,Q,R MCC-B,C

S82.442- Displaced spiral fracture of shaft of left fibula
CC-K,M,N,P,Q,R MCC-B,C

S82.443- Displaced spiral fracture of shaft of unspecified fibula
CC-K,M,N,P,Q,R MCC-B,C

S82.444- Nondisplaced spiral fracture of shaft of right fibula
CC-K,M,N,P,Q,R MCC-B,C

S82.445- Nondisplaced spiral fracture of shaft of left fibula
CC-K,M,N,P,Q,R MCC-B,C

S82.446- Nondisplaced spiral fracture of shaft of unspecified fibula
CC-K,M,N,P,Q,R MCC-B,C

S82.45- Comminuted fracture of shaft of fibula

S82.451- Displaced comminuted fracture of shaft of right fibula
CC-K,M,N,P,Q,R MCC-B,C

S82.452- Displaced comminuted fracture of shaft of left fibula
CC-K,M,N,P,Q,R MCC-B,C

S82.453- Displaced comminuted fracture of shaft of unspecified fibula
CC-K,M,N,P,Q,R MCC-B,C

S82.454- Nondisplaced comminuted fracture of shaft of right fibula
CC-K,M,N,P,Q,R MCC-B,C

S82.455- Nondisplaced comminuted fracture of shaft of left fibula
CC-K,M,N,P,Q,R MCC-B,C

S82.456- Nondisplaced comminuted fracture of shaft of unspecified fibula
CC-K,M,N,P,Q,R MCC-B,C

S82.46- Segmental fracture of shaft of fibula

S82.461- Displaced segmental fracture of shaft of right fibula
CC-K,M,N,P,Q,R MCC-B,C

S82.462- Displaced segmental fracture of shaft of left fibula
CC-K,M,N,P,Q,R MCC-B,C

S82.463- Displaced segmental fracture of shaft of unspecified fibula
CC-K,M,N,P,Q,R MCC-B,C

S82.464- Nondisplaced segmental fracture of shaft of right fibula
CC-K,M,N,P,Q,R MCC-B,C

S82.465- Nondisplaced segmental fracture of shaft of left fibula
CC-K,M,N,P,Q,R MCC-B,C

S82.466- Nondisplaced segmental fracture of shaft of unspecified fibula
CC-K,M,N,P,Q,R MCC-B,C

S82.49- Other fracture of shaft of fibula

S82.491- Other fracture of shaft of right fibula
CC-K,M,N,P,Q,R MCC-B,C

S82.492- Other fracture of shaft of left fibula
CC-K,M,N,P,Q,R MCC-B,C

S82.499- Other fracture of shaft of unspecified fibula
CC-K,M,N,P,Q,R MCC-B,C

S82.5- Fracture of medial malleolus
Excludes 1:　pilon fracture of distal tibia (S82.87-)
Salter-Harris type III of lower end of tibia (S89.13-)
Salter-Harris type IV of lower end of tibia (S89.14-)

S82.51x- Displaced fracture of medial malleolus of right tibia
CC-B,C,K,M,N,P,Q,R

S82.52x- Displaced fracture of medial malleolus of left tibia
CC-B,C,K,M,N,P,Q,R

S82.53x- Displaced fracture of medial malleolus of unspecified tibia
CC-B,C,K,M,N,P,Q,R

S82.54x- Nondisplaced fracture of medial malleolus of right tibia
CC-B,C,K,M,N,P,Q,R

S82.55x- Nondisplaced fracture of medial malleolus of left tibia
CC-B,C,K,M,N,P,Q,R

S82.56x- Nondisplaced fracture of medial malleolus of unspecified tibia
CC-B,C,K,M,N,P,Q,R

S82.6- Fracture of lateral malleolus
Excludes 1:　pilon fracture of distal tibia (S82.87-)

S82.61x- Displaced fracture of lateral malleolus of right fibula
CC-B,C,K,M,N,P,Q,R

S82.62x- Displaced fracture of lateral malleolus of left fibula
CC-B,C,K,M,N,P,Q,R

S82.63x- Displaced fracture of lateral malleolus of unspecified fibula
CC-B,C,K,M,N,P,Q,R

S82.64x- Nondisplaced fracture of lateral malleolus of right fibula
CC-B,C,K,M,N,P,Q,R

S82.65x- Nondisplaced fracture of lateral malleolus of left fibula
CC-B,C,K,M,N,P,Q,R

S82.66x- Nondisplaced fracture of lateral malleolus of unspecified fibula
CC-B,C,K,M,N,P,Q,R

S82 - S82 - S82

Excludes 1: = NOT CODED HERE! (Do not code both)　　　**1115**　　　*Excludes ❷: = Not Included Here*

S82.8- Other fractures of lower leg

S82.81- Torus fracture of upper end of fibula

The appropriate 7th character is to be added to all codes in subcategory S82.81:

- **A** Initial encounter for closed fracture
- **D** Subsequent encounter for fracture with routine healing
- **G** Subsequent encounter for fracture with delayed healing
- **K** Subsequent encounter for fracture with nonunion
- **P** Subsequent encounter for fracture with malunion
- **S** Sequela

CC-K,P **S82.811-** Torus fracture of upper end of right fibula

CC-K,P **S82.812-** Torus fracture of upper end of left fibula

CC-K,P **S82.819-** Torus fracture of upper end of unspecified fibula

S82.82- Torus fracture of lower end of fibula

The appropriate 7th character is to be added to all codes in subcategory S82.82:

- **A** Initial encounter for closed fracture
- **D** Subsequent encounter for fracture with routine healing
- **G** Subsequent encounter for fracture with delayed healing
- **K** Subsequent encounter for fracture with nonunion
- **P** Subsequent encounter for fracture with malunion
- **S** Sequela

CC-K,P **S82.821-** Torus fracture of lower end of right fibula

CC-K,P **S82.822-** Torus fracture of lower end of left fibula

CC-K,P **S82.829-** Torus fracture of lower end of unspecified fibula

S82.83- Other fracture of upper and lower end of fibula

S82.831- Other fracture of upper and lower end of right fibula
CC-K,M,N,P,Q,R MCC-B,C

S82.832- Other fracture of upper and lower end of left fibula
CC-K,M,N,P,Q,R MCC-B,C

S82.839- Other fracture of upper and lower end of unspecified fibula
CC-K,M,N,P,Q,R MCC-B,C

S82.84- Bimalleolar fracture of lower leg

S82.841- Displaced bimalleolar fracture of right lower leg
CC-B,C,K,M,N,P,Q,R

S82.842- Displaced bimalleolar fracture of left lower leg
CC-B,C,K,M,N,P,Q,R

S82.843- Displaced bimalleolar fracture of unspecified lower leg
CC-B,C,K,M,N,P,Q,R

S82.844- Nondisplaced bimalleolar fracture of right lower leg
CC-B,C,K,M,N,P,Q,R

S82.845- Nondisplaced bimalleolar fracture of left lower leg
CC-B,C,K,M,N,P,Q,R

S82.846- Nondisplaced bimalleolar fracture of unspecified lower leg
CC-B,C,K,M,N,P,Q,R

S82.85- Trimalleolar fracture of lower leg

S82.851- Displaced trimalleolar fracture of right lower leg
CC-B,C,K,M,N,P,Q,R

S82.852- Displaced trimalleolar fracture of left lower leg
CC-B,C,K,M,N,P,Q,R

S82.853- Displaced trimalleolar fracture of unspecified lower leg
CC-B,C,K,M,N,P,Q,R

S82.854- Nondisplaced trimalleolar fracture of right lower leg
CC-B,C,K,M,N,P,Q,R

S82.855- Nondisplaced trimalleolar fracture of left lower leg
CC-B,C,K,M,N,P,Q,R

S82.856- Nondisplaced trimalleolar fracture of unspecified lower leg
CC-B,C,K,M,N,P,Q,R

S82.86- Maisonneuve's fracture

S82.861- Displaced Maisonneuve's fracture of right leg
CC-K,M,N,P,Q,R MCC-B,C

S82.862- Displaced Maisonneuve's fracture of left leg
CC-K,M,N,P,Q,R MCC-B,C

S82.863- Displaced Maisonneuve's fracture of unspecified leg
CC-K,M,N,P,Q,R MCC-B,C

S82.864- Nondisplaced Maisonneuve's fracture of right leg
CC-K,M,N,P,Q,R MCC-B,C

S82.865- Nondisplaced Maisonneuve's fracture of left leg
CC-K,M,N,P,Q,R MCC-B,C

S82.866- Nondisplaced Maisonneuve's fracture of unspecified leg
CC-K,M,N,P,Q,R MCC-B,C

S82.87- Pilon fracture of tibia

S82.871- Displaced pilon fracture of right tibia
CC-B,C,K,M,N,P,Q,R

S82.872- Displaced pilon fracture of left tibia
CC-B,C,K,M,N,P,Q,R

S82.873- Displaced pilon fracture of unspecified tibia
CC-B,C,K,M,N,P,Q,R

S82.874- Nondisplaced pilon fracture of right tibia
CC-B,C,K,M,N,P,Q,R

S82.875- Nondisplaced pilon fracture of left tibia
CC-B,C,K,M,N,P,Q,R

S82.876- Nondisplaced pilon fracture of unspecified tibia
CC-B,C,K,M,N,P,Q,R

S82.89- Other fractures of lower leg

Fracture of ankle NOS

S82.891- Other fracture of right lower leg
CC-B,C,K,M,N,P,Q,R

S82.892- Other fracture of left lower leg
CC-B,C,K,M,N,P,Q,R

S82.899- Other fracture of unspecified lower leg
CC-B,C,K,M,N,P,Q,R

S82.9- Unspecified fracture of lower leg

S82.90x- Unspecified fracture of unspecified lower leg
CC-B,C,K,M,N,P,Q,R

S82.91x- Unspecified fracture of right lower leg
CC-B,C,K,M,N,P,Q,R

S82.92x- Unspecified fracture of left lower leg
CC-B,C,K,M,N,P,Q,R

S83- Dislocation and sprain of joints and ligaments of knee

Includes: Avulsion of joint or ligament of knee
Laceration of cartilage, joint or ligament of knee
Sprain of cartilage, joint or ligament of knee
Traumatic hemarthrosis of joint or ligament of knee
Traumatic rupture of joint or ligament of knee
Traumatic subluxation of joint or ligament of knee
Traumatic tear of joint or ligament of knee

Code also any associated open wound

Excludes 1: derangement of patella (M22.0-M22.3)
injury of patellar ligament (tendon) (S76.1-)
internal derangement of knee (M23.-)
old dislocation of knee (M24.36)
pathological dislocation of knee (M24.36)
recurrent dislocation of knee (M22.0)

Excludes ❷: strain of muscle, fascia and tendon of lower leg (S86.-)

The appropriate 7th character is to be added to each code from category S83:

- **A** Initial encounter
- **D** Subsequent encounter
- **S** Sequela

S83.0- Subluxation and dislocation of patella

S83.00- Unspecified subluxation and dislocation of patella

S83.001- Unspecified subluxation of right patella

S83.002- Unspecified subluxation of left patella

S83.003- Unspecified subluxation of unspecified patella

S83.004- Unspecified dislocation of right patella

S83.005- Unspecified dislocation of left patella

S83.006- Unspecified dislocation of unspecified patella

S83.01- Lateral subluxation and dislocation of patella

S83.011- Lateral subluxation of right patella

S83.012- Lateral subluxation of left patella

S83.013- Lateral subluxation of unspecified patella

S83.014- Lateral dislocation of right patella

S83.015- Lateral dislocation of left patella

S83.016- Lateral dislocation of unspecified patella
S83.09- Other subluxation and dislocation of patella
    S83.091- Other subluxation of right patella
    S83.092- Other subluxation of left patella
    S83.093- Other subluxation of unspecified patella
    S83.094- Other dislocation of right patella
    S83.095- Other dislocation of left patella
    S83.096- Other dislocation of unspecified patella
S83.1- Subluxation and dislocation of knee
    Excludes ❷: instability of knee prosthesis (T84.022, T84.023)
    S83.10- Unspecified subluxation and dislocation of knee
    S83.101- Unspecified subluxation of right knee
    S83.102- Unspecified subluxation of left knee
    S83.103- Unspecified subluxation of unspecified knee
    S83.104- Unspecified dislocation of right knee
    S83.105- Unspecified dislocation of left knee
    S83.106- Unspecified dislocation of unspecified knee
    S83.11- Anterior subluxation and dislocation of proximal end of tibia
        Posterior subluxation and dislocation of distal end of femur
    S83.111- Anterior subluxation of proximal end of tibia, right knee
    S83.112- Anterior subluxation of proximal end of tibia, left knee
    S83.113- Anterior subluxation of proximal end of tibia, unspecified knee
    S83.114- Anterior dislocation of proximal end of tibia, right knee
    S83.115- Anterior dislocation of proximal end of tibia, left knee
    S83.116- Anterior dislocation of proximal end of tibia, unspecified knee
    S83.12- Posterior subluxation and dislocation of proximal end of tibia
        Anterior dislocation of distal end of femur
    S83.121- Posterior subluxation of proximal end of tibia, right knee
    S83.122- Posterior subluxation of proximal end of tibia, left knee
    S83.123- Posterior subluxation of proximal end of tibia, unspecified knee
    S83.124- Posterior dislocation of proximal end of tibia, right knee
    S83.125- Posterior dislocation of proximal end of tibia, left knee
    S83.126- Posterior dislocation of proximal end of tibia, unspecified knee
    S83.13- Medial subluxation and dislocation of proximal end of tibia
    S83.131- Medial subluxation of proximal end of tibia, right knee
    S83.132- Medial subluxation of proximal end of tibia, left knee
    S83.133- Medial subluxation of proximal end of tibia, unspecified knee
    S83.134- Medial dislocation of proximal end of tibia, right knee
    S83.135- Medial dislocation of proximal end of tibia, left knee
    S83.136- Medial dislocation of proximal end of tibia, unspecified knee
    S83.14- Lateral subluxation and dislocation of proximal end of tibia
    S83.141- Lateral subluxation of proximal end of tibia, right knee
    S83.142- Lateral subluxation of proximal end of tibia, left knee

S83.143- Lateral subluxation of proximal end of tibia, unspecified knee
S83.144- Lateral dislocation of proximal end of tibia, right knee
S83.145- Lateral dislocation of proximal end of tibia, left knee
S83.146- Lateral dislocation of proximal end of tibia, unspecified knee
S83.19- Other subluxation and dislocation of knee
    S83.191- Other subluxation of right knee
    S83.192- Other subluxation of left knee
    S83.193- Other subluxation of unspecified knee
    S83.194- Other dislocation of right knee
    S83.195- Other dislocation of left knee
    S83.196- Other dislocation of unspecified knee
S83.2- Tear of meniscus, current injury
    Excludes 1: old bucket-handle tear (M23.2)
    S83.20- Tear of unspecified meniscus, current injury
        Tear of meniscus of knee NOS
    S83.200- Bucket-handle tear of unspecified meniscus, current injury, right knee
    S83.201- Bucket-handle tear of unspecified meniscus, current injury, left knee
    S83.202- Bucket-handle tear of unspecified meniscus, current injury, unspecified knee
    S83.203- Other tear of unspecified meniscus, current injury, right knee
    S83.204- Other tear of unspecified meniscus, current injury, left knee
    S83.205- Other tear of unspecified meniscus, current injury, unspecified knee
    S83.206- Unspecified tear of unspecified meniscus, current injury, right knee
    S83.207- Unspecified tear of unspecified meniscus, current injury, left knee
    S83.209- Unspecified tear of unspecified meniscus, current injury, unspecified knee
    S83.21- Bucket-handle tear of medial meniscus, current injury
    S83.211- Bucket-handle tear of medial meniscus, current injury, right knee
    S83.212- Bucket-handle tear of medial meniscus, current injury, left knee
    S83.219- Bucket-handle tear of medial meniscus, current injury, unspecified knee
    S83.22- Peripheral tear of medial meniscus, current injury
    S83.221- Peripheral tear of medial meniscus, current injury, right knee
    S83.222- Peripheral tear of medial meniscus, current injury, left knee
    S83.229- Peripheral tear of medial meniscus, current injury, unspecified knee
    S83.23- Complex tear of medial meniscus, current injury
    S83.231- Complex tear of medial meniscus, current injury, right knee
    S83.232- Complex tear of medial meniscus, current injury, left knee
    S83.239- Complex tear of medial meniscus, current injury, unspecified knee
    S83.24- Other tear of medial meniscus, current injury
    S83.241- Other tear of medial meniscus, current injury, right knee
    S83.242- Other tear of medial meniscus, current injury, left knee
    S83.249- Other tear of medial meniscus, current injury, unspecified knee
    S83.25- Bucket-handle tear of lateral meniscus, current injury
    S83.251- Bucket-handle tear of lateral meniscus, current injury, right knee

S 8 3 I S 8 3

S83.252- Bucket-handle tear of lateral meniscus, current injury, <u>left</u> knee

S83.259- Bucket-handle tear of lateral meniscus, current injury, <u>unspecified</u> knee

S83.26- <u>Peripheral tear</u> of <u>lateral meniscus, current injury</u>

S83.261- Peripheral tear of lateral meniscus, current injury, <u>right</u> knee

S83.262- Peripheral tear of lateral meniscus, current injury, <u>left</u> knee

S83.269- Peripheral tear of lateral meniscus, current injury, <u>unspecified</u> knee

S83.27- <u>Complex tear</u> of <u>lateral meniscus, current injury</u>

S83.271- Complex tear of lateral meniscus, current injury, <u>right</u> knee

S83.272- Complex tear of lateral meniscus, current injury, <u>left</u> knee

S83.279- Complex tear of lateral meniscus, current injury, <u>unspecified</u> knee

S83.28- <u>Other tear</u> of <u>lateral meniscus, current injury</u>

S83.281- Other tear of lateral meniscus, current injury, <u>right</u> knee

S83.282- Other tear of lateral meniscus, current injury, <u>left</u> knee

S83.289- Other tear of lateral meniscus, current injury, <u>unspecified</u> knee

S83.3- <u>Tear of articular cartilage</u> of <u>knee, current</u>

S83.30x- Tear of articular cartilage of <u>unspecified</u> knee, current

S83.31x- Tear of articular cartilage of <u>right</u> knee, current

S83.32x- Tear of articular cartilage of <u>left</u> knee, current

S83.4- <u>Sprain</u> of <u>collateral</u> ligament of <u>knee</u>

S83.40- Sprain of <u>unspecified collateral</u> ligament of <u>knee</u>

S83.401- Sprain of unspecified collateral ligament of <u>right</u> knee

S83.402- Sprain of unspecified collateral ligament of <u>left</u> knee

S83.409- Sprain of unspecified collateral ligament of <u>unspecified</u> knee

S83.41- <u>Sprain</u> of <u>medial collateral</u> ligament of <u>knee</u>
Sprain of tibial collateral ligament

S83.411- Sprain of medial collateral ligament of <u>right</u> knee

S83.412- Sprain of medial collateral ligament of <u>left</u> knee

S83.419- Sprain of medial collateral ligament of <u>unspecified</u> knee

S83.42- <u>Sprain</u> of <u>lateral collateral</u> ligament of <u>knee</u>
Sprain of fibular collateral ligament

S83.421- Sprain of lateral collateral ligament of <u>right</u> knee

S83.422- Sprain of lateral collateral ligament of <u>left</u> knee

S83.429- Sprain of lateral collateral ligament of <u>unspecified</u> knee

S83.5- <u>Sprain</u> of <u>cruciate</u> ligament of <u>knee</u>

S83.50- <u>Sprain</u> of <u>unspecified cruciate</u> ligament of <u>knee</u>

S83.501- Sprain of unspecified cruciate ligament of <u>right</u> knee

S83.502- Sprain of unspecified cruciate ligament of <u>left</u> knee

S83.509- Sprain of unspecified cruciate ligament of <u>unspecified</u> knee

S83.51- <u>Sprain</u> of <u>anterior cruciate</u> ligament of <u>knee</u>

S83.511- Sprain of anterior cruciate ligament of <u>right</u> knee

S83.512- Sprain of anterior cruciate ligament of <u>left</u> knee

S83.519- Sprain of anterior cruciate ligament of <u>unspecified</u> knee

S83.52- <u>Sprain</u> of <u>posterior cruciate</u> ligament of <u>knee</u>

S83.521- Sprain of posterior cruciate ligament of <u>right</u> knee

S83.522- Sprain of posterior cruciate ligament of <u>left</u> knee

S83.529- Sprain of posterior cruciate ligament of <u>unspecified</u> knee

S83.6- <u>Sprain</u> of the <u>superior tibiofibular joint and ligament</u>

S83.60x- Sprain of the superior tibiofibular joint and ligament, <u>unspecified</u> knee

S83.61x- Sprain of the superior tibiofibular joint and ligament, <u>right</u> knee

S83.62x- Sprain of the superior tibiofibular joint and ligament, <u>left</u> knee

S83.8- <u>Sprain</u> of <u>other specified parts</u> of <u>knee</u>

S83.8x- Sprain of <u>other specified parts</u> of <u>knee</u>

S83.8x1- Sprain of other specified parts of <u>right</u> knee

S83.8x2- Sprain of other specified parts of <u>left</u> knee

S83.8x9- Sprain of other specified parts of <u>unspecified</u> knee

S83.9- <u>Sprain</u> of <u>unspecified site</u> of <u>knee</u>

S83.90x- Sprain of unspecified site of <u>unspecified</u> knee

S83.91x- Sprain of unspecified site of <u>right</u> knee

S83.92x- Sprain of unspecified site of <u>left</u> knee

S84- <u>Injury of nerves</u> at <u>lower leg</u> level
Code also any associated open wound (S81-)
Excludes ❷: injury of nerves at ankle and foot level (S94-)

The appropriate 7th character is to be added to each code from category S84:
A   <u>Initial</u> encounter
D   <u>Subsequent</u> encounter
S   <u>Sequela</u>

S84.0- Injury of <u>tibial</u> nerve at <u>lower leg</u> level

S84.00x- Injury of tibial nerve at lower leg level, <u>unspecified</u> leg

S84.01x- Injury of tibial nerve at lower leg level, <u>right</u> leg

S84.02x- Injury of tibial nerve at lower leg level, <u>left</u> leg

S84.1- Injury of <u>peroneal</u> nerve at <u>lower leg</u> level

S84.10x- Injury of peroneal nerve at lower leg level, <u>unspecified</u> leg

S84.11x- Injury of peroneal nerve at lower leg level, <u>right</u> leg

S84.12x- Injury of peroneal nerve at lower leg level, <u>left</u> leg

S84.2- Injury of <u>cutaneous sensory</u> nerve at <u>lower leg</u> level

S84.20x- Injury of cutaneous sensory nerve at lower leg level, <u>unspecified</u> leg

S84.21x- Injury of cutaneous sensory nerve at lower leg level, <u>right</u> leg

S84.22x- Injury of cutaneous sensory nerve at lower leg level, <u>left</u> leg

S84.8- Injury of other nerves at lower leg level

S84.80- Injury of <u>other nerves</u> at <u>lower leg</u> level

S84.801- Injury of other nerves at lower leg level, <u>right</u> leg

S84.802- Injury of other nerves at lower leg level, <u>left</u> leg

S84.809- Injury of other nerves at lower leg level, <u>unspecified</u> leg

S84.9- Injury of <u>unspecified nerve</u> at <u>lower leg</u> level

S84.90x- Injury of unspecified nerve at lower leg level, <u>unspecified</u> leg

S84.91x- Injury of unspecified nerve at lower leg level, <u>right</u> leg

S84.92x- Injury of unspecified nerve at lower leg level, <u>left</u> leg

S85- <u>Injury of blood vessels</u> at <u>lower leg</u> level
Code also any associated open wound (S81.-)
Excludes ❷: injury of blood vessels at ankle and foot level (S95.-)

The appropriate 7th character is to be added to each code from category S85:
A   <u>Initial</u> encounter
D   <u>Subsequent</u> encounter
S   <u>Sequela</u>

S85.0- Injury of <u>popliteal artery</u>

S85.00- <u>Unspecified</u> injury of <u>popliteal artery</u>

MCC-A **S85.001-** Unspecified injury of popliteal artery, <u>right</u> leg

MCC-A **S85.002-** Unspecified injury of popliteal artery, <u>left</u> leg

MCC-A **S85.009-** Unspecified injury of popliteal artery, <u>unspecified</u> leg

S85.01- <u>Laceration</u> of <u>popliteal artery</u>

MCC-A **S85.011-** Laceration of popliteal artery, <u>right</u> leg

S83 - S85

© 2016 Channel Publishing Ltd

MCC-A **S85.012-**   Laceration of popliteal artery, <u>left</u> leg
MCC-A **S85.019-**   Laceration of popliteal artery, <u>unspecified</u> leg
S85.09-   <u>Other specified injury</u> of <u>popliteal artery</u>
MCC-A **S85.091-**   Other specified injury of popliteal artery, <u>right</u> leg
MCC-A **S85.092-**   Other specified injury of popliteal artery, <u>left</u> leg
MCC-A **S85.099-**   Other specified injury of popliteal artery, <u>unspecified</u> leg

S85.1-   Injury of <u>tibial artery</u>
    S85.10-   <u>Unspecified</u> injury of <u>unspecified tibial artery</u>
       Injury of tibial artery NOS
    CC-A **S85.101-**   Unspecified injury of unspecified tibial artery, <u>right</u> leg
    CC-A **S85.102-**   Unspecified injury of unspecified tibial artery, <u>left</u> leg
    CC-A **S85.109-**   Unspecified injury of unspecified tibial artery, <u>unspecified</u> leg
    S85.11-   <u>Laceration</u> of <u>unspecified tibial artery</u>
    CC-A **S85.111-**   Laceration of unspecified tibial artery, <u>right</u> leg
    CC-A **S85.112-**   Laceration of unspecified tibial artery, <u>left</u> leg
    CC-A **S85.119-**   Laceration of unspecified tibial artery, <u>unspecified</u> leg
    S85.12-   <u>Other specified injury</u> of <u>unspecified tibial artery</u>
    CC-A **S85.121-**   Other specified injury of unspecified tibial artery, <u>right</u> leg
    CC-A **S85.122-**   Other specified injury of unspecified tibial artery, <u>left</u> leg
    CC-A **S85.129-**   Other specified injury of unspecified tibial artery, <u>unspecified</u> leg
    S85.13-   <u>Unspecified</u> injury of <u>anterior tibial artery</u>
    CC-A **S85.131-**   Unspecified injury of anterior tibial artery, <u>right</u> leg
    CC-A **S85.132-**   Unspecified injury of anterior tibial artery, <u>left</u> leg
    CC-A **S85.139-**   Unspecified injury of anterior tibial artery, <u>unspecified</u> leg
    S85.14-   <u>Laceration</u> of <u>anterior tibial artery</u>
    CC-A **S85.141-**   Laceration of anterior tibial artery, <u>right</u> leg
    CC-A **S85.142-**   Laceration of anterior tibial artery, <u>left</u> leg
    CC-A **S85.149-**   Laceration of anterior tibial artery, <u>unspecified</u> leg
    S85.15-   <u>Other specified injury</u> of <u>anterior tibial artery</u>
    CC-A **S85.151-**   Other specified injury of anterior tibial artery, <u>right</u> leg
    CC-A **S85.152-**   Other specified injury of anterior tibial artery, <u>left</u> leg
    CC-A **S85.159-**   Other specified injury of anterior tibial artery, <u>unspecified</u> leg
    S85.16-   <u>Unspecified</u> injury of <u>posterior tibial artery</u>
    CC-A **S85.161-**   Unspecified injury of posterior tibial artery, <u>right</u> leg
    CC-A **S85.162-**   Unspecified injury of posterior tibial artery, <u>left</u> leg
    CC-A **S85.169-**   Unspecified injury of posterior tibial artery, <u>unspecified</u> leg
    S85.17-   <u>Laceration</u> of <u>posterior tibial artery</u>
    CC-A **S85.171-**   Laceration of posterior tibial artery, <u>right</u> leg
    CC-A **S85.172-**   Laceration of posterior tibial artery, <u>left</u> leg
    CC-A **S85.179**   Laceration of posterior tibial artery, <u>unspecified</u> leg
    S85.18-   <u>Other specified injury</u> of <u>posterior tibial artery</u>
    CC-A **S85.181-**   Other specified injury of posterior tibial artery, <u>right</u> leg
    CC-A **S85.182-**   Other specified injury of posterior tibial artery, <u>left</u> leg
    CC-A **S85.189**   Other specified injury of posterior tibial artery, <u>unspecified</u> leg

S85.2-   Injury of <u>peroneal artery</u>
    S85.20-   <u>Unspecified</u> injury of <u>peroneal artery</u>
    CC-A **S85.201-**   Unspecified injury of peroneal artery, <u>right</u> leg
    CC-A **S85.202-**   Unspecified injury of peroneal artery, <u>left</u> leg

CC-A **S85.209**   Unspecified injury of peroneal artery, <u>unspecified</u> leg
    S85.21-   <u>Laceration</u> of <u>peroneal artery</u>
    CC-A **S85.211-**   Laceration of peroneal artery, <u>right</u> leg
    CC-A **S85.212-**   Laceration of peroneal artery, <u>left</u> leg
    CC-A **S85.219-**   Laceration of peroneal artery, <u>unspecified</u> leg
    S85.29-   <u>Other specified injury</u> of <u>peroneal artery</u>
    CC-A **S85.291-**   Other specified injury of peroneal artery, <u>right</u> leg
    CC-A **S85.292-**   Other specified injury of peroneal artery, <u>left</u> leg
    CC-A **S85.299-**   Other specified injury of peroneal artery, <u>unspecified</u> leg

S85.3-   Injury of <u>greater saphenous vein</u> at <u>lower leg</u> level
       Injury of greater saphenous vein NOS
       Injury of saphenous vein NOS
    S85.30-   <u>Unspecified</u> injury of <u>greater saphenous vein</u> at <u>lower leg</u> level
    CC-A **S85.301-**   Unspecified injury of greater saphenous vein at lower leg level, <u>right</u> leg
    CC-A **S85.302-**   Unspecified injury of greater saphenous vein at lower leg level, <u>left</u> leg
    CC-A **S85.309-**   Unspecified injury of greater saphenous vein at lower leg level, <u>unspecified</u> leg
    S85.31-   <u>Laceration</u> of <u>greater saphenous vein</u> at <u>lower leg</u> level
    CC-A **S85.311-**   Laceration of greater saphenous vein at lower leg level, <u>right</u> leg
    CC-A **S85.312-**   Laceration of greater saphenous vein at lower leg level, <u>left</u> leg
    CC-A **S85.319-**   Laceration of greater saphenous vein at lower leg level, <u>unspecified</u> leg
    S85.39-   <u>Other specified injury</u> of <u>greater saphenous vein</u> at <u>lower leg</u> level
    CC-A **S85.391-**   Other specified injury of greater saphenous vein at lower leg level, <u>right</u> leg
    CC-A **S85.392-**   Other specified injury of greater saphenous vein at lower leg level, <u>left</u> leg
    CC-A **S85.399-**   Other specified injury of greater saphenous vein at lower leg level, <u>unspecified</u> leg

S85.4-   Injury of <u>lesser saphenous vein</u> at <u>lower leg</u> level
    S85.40-   <u>Unspecified</u> injury of <u>lesser saphenous vein</u> at <u>lower leg</u> level
    CC-A **S85.401-**   Unspecified injury of lesser saphenous vein at lower leg level, <u>right</u> leg
    CC-A **S85.402-**   Unspecified injury of lesser saphenous vein at lower leg level, <u>left</u> leg
    CC-A **S85.409-**   Unspecified injury of lesser saphenous vein at lower leg level, <u>unspecified</u> leg
    S85.41-   <u>Laceration</u> of <u>lesser saphenous vein</u> at <u>lower leg</u> level
    CC-A **S85.411-**   Laceration of lesser saphenous vein at lower leg level, <u>right</u> leg
    CC-A **S85.412-**   Laceration of lesser saphenous vein at lower leg level, <u>left</u> leg
    CC-A **S85.419-**   Laceration of lesser saphenous vein at lower leg level, <u>unspecified</u> leg
    S85.49-   <u>Other specified injury</u> of <u>lesser saphenous vein</u> at <u>lower leg</u> level
    CC-A **S85.491-**   Other specified injury of lesser saphenous vein at lower leg level, <u>right</u> leg
    CC-A **S85.492-**   Other specified injury of lesser saphenous vein at lower leg level, <u>left</u> leg
    CC-A **S85.499-**   Other specified injury of lesser saphenous vein at lower leg level, <u>unspecified</u> leg

S85.5-   Injury of <u>popliteal vein</u>
    S85.50-   <u>Unspecified</u> injury of <u>popliteal vein</u>
    MCC-A **S85.501-**   Unspecified injury of popliteal vein, <u>right</u> leg
    MCC-A **S85.502-**   Unspecified injury of popliteal vein, <u>left</u> leg
    MCC-A **S85.509-**   Unspecified injury of popliteal vein, <u>unspecified</u> leg
    S85.51-   <u>Laceration</u> of <u>popliteal vein</u>

Excludes 1: = NOT CODED HERE! (Do not code both)   **1119**   *Excludes ❷:* = Not Included Here

MCC-A **S85.511-** Laceration of popliteal vein, <u>right</u> leg

MCC-A **S85.512-** Laceration of popliteal vein, <u>left</u> leg

MCC-A **S85.519-** Laceration of popliteal vein, <u>unspecified</u> leg

S85.59- <u>Other specified injury</u> of <u>popliteal</u> <u>vein</u>

MCC-A **S85.591-** Other specified injury of popliteal vein, <u>right</u> leg

MCC-A **S85.592-** Other specified injury of popliteal vein, <u>left</u> leg

MCC-A **S85.599-** Other specified injury of popliteal vein, <u>unspecified</u> leg

S85.8- <u>Injury</u> of <u>other blood vessels</u> at <u>lower leg</u> level

S85.80- <u>Unspecified</u> injury of other blood vessels at <u>lower leg</u> level

CC-A **S85.801-** Unspecified injury of other blood vessels at lower leg level, <u>right</u> leg

CC-A **S85.802-** Unspecified injury of other blood vessels at lower leg level, <u>left</u> leg

CC-A **S85.809-** Unspecified injury of other blood vessels at lower leg level, <u>unspecified</u> leg

S85.81- <u>Laceration</u> of other blood vessels at <u>lower leg</u> level

CC-A **S85.811-** Laceration of other blood vessels at lower leg level, <u>right</u> leg

CC-A **S85.812-** Laceration of other blood vessels at lower leg level, <u>left</u> leg

CC-A **S85.819-** Laceration of other blood vessels at lower leg level, <u>unspecified</u> leg

S85.89- <u>Other specified injury</u> of <u>other blood vessels</u> at <u>lower leg</u> level

CC-A **S85.891-** Other specified injury of other blood vessels at lower leg level, <u>right</u> leg

CC-A **S85.892-** Other specified injury of other blood vessels at lower leg level, <u>left</u> leg

CC-A **S85.899-** Other specified injury of other blood vessels at lower leg level, <u>unspecified</u> leg

S85.9- <u>Injury</u> of <u>unspecified blood vessel</u> at <u>lower leg</u> level

S85.90- <u>Unspecified</u> injury of <u>unspecified blood vessel</u> at <u>lower leg</u> level

CC-A **S85.901-** Unspecified injury of unspecified blood vessel at lower leg level, <u>right</u> leg

CC-A **S85.902-** Unspecified injury of unspecified blood vessel at lower leg level, <u>left</u> leg

CC-A **S85.909-** Unspecified injury of unspecified blood vessel at lower leg level, <u>unspecified</u> leg

S85.91- <u>Laceration</u> of <u>unspecified blood vessel</u> at <u>lower leg</u> level

CC-A **S85.911-** Laceration of unspecified blood vessel at lower leg level, <u>right</u> leg

CC-A **S85.912-** Laceration of unspecified blood vessel at lower leg level, <u>left</u> leg

CC-A **S85.919-** Laceration of unspecified blood vessel at lower leg level, <u>unspecified</u> leg

S85.99- <u>Other specified injury</u> of <u>unspecified blood vessel</u> at <u>lower leg</u> level

CC-A **S85.991-** Other specified injury of unspecified blood vessel at lower leg level, <u>right</u> leg

CC-A **S85.992-** Other specified injury of unspecified blood vessel at lower leg level, <u>left</u> leg

CC-A **S85.999-** Other specified injury of unspecified blood vessel at lower leg level, <u>unspecified</u> leg

S86- <u>Injury</u> of <u>muscle, fascia and tendon</u> at <u>lower leg</u> level

Code also any associated open wound (S81.-)

Excludes ❷: *injury of muscle, fascia and tendon at ankle (S96.-)*
injury of patellar ligament (tendon) (S76.1-)
sprain of joints and ligaments of knee (S83.-)

The appropriate 7th character is to be added to each code from category S86:

A <u>Initial</u> encounter

D <u>Subsequent</u> encounter

S <u>Sequela</u>

S86.0- <u>Injury</u> of <u>Achilles</u> tendon

S86.00- <u>Unspecified</u> injury of <u>Achilles</u> tendon

S86.001- Unspecified injury of <u>right</u> Achilles tendon

S86.002- Unspecified injury of <u>left</u> Achilles tendon

S86.009- Unspecified injury of <u>unspecified</u> Achilles tendon

S86.01- <u>Strain</u> of <u>Achilles</u> tendon

S86.011- Strain of <u>right</u> Achilles tendon

S86.012- Strain of <u>left</u> Achilles tendon

S86.019- Strain of <u>unspecified</u> Achilles tendon

S86.02- <u>Laceration</u> of <u>Achilles</u> tendon

CC-A **S86.021-** Laceration of <u>right</u> Achilles tendon

CC-A **S86.022-** Laceration of <u>left</u> Achilles tendon

CC-A **S86.029-** Laceration of <u>unspecified</u> Achilles tendon

S86.09- <u>Other specified injury</u> of <u>Achilles</u> tendon

S86.091- Other specified injury of <u>right</u> Achilles tendon

S86.092- Other specified injury of <u>left</u> Achilles tendon

S86.099- Other specified injury of <u>unspecified</u> Achilles tendon

S86.1- <u>Injury</u> of <u>other muscle(s) and tendon(s)</u> of <u>posterior muscle group</u> at <u>lower leg</u> level

S86.10- <u>Unspecified</u> injury of other muscle(s) and tendon(s) of <u>posterior</u> muscle group at <u>lower leg</u> level

S86.101- Unspecified injury of other muscle(s) and tendon(s) of posterior muscle group at lower leg level, <u>right</u> leg

S86.102- Unspecified injury of other muscle(s) and tendon(s) of posterior muscle group at lower leg level, <u>left</u> leg

S86.109- Unspecified injury of other muscle(s) and tendon(s) of posterior muscle group at lower leg level, <u>unspecified</u> leg

S86.11- <u>Strain</u> of other muscle(s) and tendon(s) of <u>posterior</u> muscle group at <u>lower leg</u> level

S86.111- Strain of other muscle(s) and tendon(s) of posterior muscle group at lower leg level, <u>right</u> leg

S86.112- Strain of other muscle(s) and tendon(s) of posterior muscle group at lower leg level, <u>left</u> leg

S86.119- Strain of other muscle(s) and tendon(s) of posterior muscle group at lower leg level, <u>unspecified</u> leg

S86.12- <u>Laceration</u> of other muscle(s) and tendon(s) of <u>posterior</u> muscle group at <u>lower leg</u> level

CC-A **S86.121-** Laceration of other muscle(s) and tendon(s) of posterior muscle group at lower leg level, <u>right</u> leg

CC-A **S86.122-** Laceration of other muscle(s) and tendon(s) of posterior muscle group at lower leg level, <u>left</u> leg

CC-A **S86.129-** Laceration of other muscle(s) and tendon(s) of posterior muscle group at lower leg level, <u>unspecified</u> leg

S86.19- <u>Other injury</u> of other muscle(s) and tendon(s) of <u>posterior</u> muscle group at <u>lower leg</u> level

S86.191- Other injury of other muscle(s) and tendon(s) of posterior muscle group at lower leg level, <u>right</u> leg

S86.192- Other injury of other muscle(s) and tendon(s) of posterior muscle group at lower leg level, <u>left</u> leg

S86.199- Other injury of other muscle(s) and tendon(s) of posterior muscle group at lower leg level, <u>unspecified</u> leg

S85
–
S86

S86.2- Injury of muscle(s) and tendon(s) of anterior muscle group at lower leg level

S86.20- Unspecified injury of muscle(s) and tendon(s) of anterior muscle group at lower leg level

S86.201- Unspecified injury of muscle(s) and tendon(s) of anterior muscle group at lower leg level, right leg

S86.202- Unspecified injury of muscle(s) and tendon(s) of anterior muscle group at lower leg level, left leg

S86.209- Unspecified injury of muscle(s) and tendon(s) of anterior muscle group at lower leg level, unspecified leg

S86.21- Strain of muscle(s) and tendon(s) of anterior muscle group at lower leg level

S86.211- Strain of muscle(s) and tendon(s) of anterior muscle group at lower leg level, right leg

S86.212- Strain of muscle(s) and tendon(s) of anterior muscle group at lower leg level, left leg

S86.219- Strain of muscle(s) and tendon(s) of anterior muscle group at lower leg level, unspecified leg

S86.22- Laceration of muscle(s) and tendon(s) of anterior muscle group at lower leg level

CC-A **S86.221-** Laceration of muscle(s) and tendon(s) of anterior muscle group at lower leg level, right leg

CC-A **S86.222-** Laceration of muscle(s) and tendon(s) of anterior muscle group at lower leg level, left leg

CC-A **S86.229-** Laceration of muscle(s) and tendon(s) of anterior muscle group at lower leg level, unspecified leg

S86.29- Other injury of muscle(s) and tendon(s) of anterior muscle group at lower leg level

S86.291- Other injury of muscle(s) and tendon(s) of anterior muscle group at lower leg level, right leg

S86.292- Other injury of muscle(s) and tendon(s) of anterior muscle group at lower leg level, left leg

S86.299- Other injury of muscle(s) and tendon(s) of anterior muscle group at lower leg level, unspecified leg

S86.3- Injury of muscle(s) and tendon(s) of peroneal muscle group at lower leg level

S86.30- Unspecified injury of muscle(s) and tendon(s) of peroneal muscle group at lower leg level

S86.301- Unspecified injury of muscle(s) and tendon(s) of peroneal muscle group at lower leg level, right leg

S86.302- Unspecified injury of muscle(s) and tendon(s) of peroneal muscle group at lower leg level, left leg

S86.309- Unspecified injury of muscle(s) and tendon(s) of peroneal muscle group at lower leg level, unspecified leg

S86.31- Strain of muscle(s) and tendon(s) of peroneal muscle group at lower leg level

S86.311- Strain of muscle(s) and tendon(s) of peroneal muscle group at lower leg level, right leg

S86.312- Strain of muscle(s) and tendon(s) of peroneal muscle group at lower leg level, left leg

S86.319- Strain of muscle(s) and tendon(s) of peroneal muscle group at lower leg level, unspecified leg

S86.32- Laceration of muscle(s) and tendon(s) of peroneal muscle group at lower leg level

CC-A **S86.321-** Laceration of muscle(s) and tendon(s) of peroneal muscle group at lower leg level, right leg

CC-A **S86.322-** Laceration of muscle(s) and tendon(s) of peroneal muscle group at lower leg level, left leg

CC-A **S86.329-** Laceration of muscle(s) and tendon(s) of peroneal muscle group at lower leg level, unspecified leg

S86.39- Other injury of muscle(s) and tendon(s) of peroneal muscle group at lower leg level

S86.391- Other injury of muscle(s) and tendon(s) of peroneal muscle group at lower leg level, right leg

S86.392- Other injury of muscle(s) and tendon(s) of peroneal muscle group at lower leg level, left leg

S86.399- Other injury of muscle(s) and tendon(s) of peroneal muscle group at lower leg level, unspecified leg

S86.8- Injury of other muscles and tendons at lower leg level

S86.80- Unspecified injury of other muscles and tendons at lower leg level

S86.801- Unspecified injury of other muscle(s) and tendon(s) at lower leg level, right leg

S86.802- Unspecified injury of other muscle(s) and tendon(s) at lower leg level, left leg

S86.809- Unspecified injury of other muscle(s) and tendon(s) at lower leg level, unspecified leg

S86.81- Strain of other muscles and tendons at lower leg level

S86.811- Strain of other muscle(s) and tendon(s) at lower leg level, right leg

S86.812- Strain of other muscle(s) and tendon(s) at lower leg level, left leg

S86.819- Strain of other muscle(s) and tendon(s) at lower leg level, unspecified leg

S86.82- Laceration of other muscles and tendons at lower leg level

CC-A **S86.821-** Laceration of other muscle(s) and tendon(s) at lower leg level, right leg

CC-A **S86.822-** Laceration of other muscle(s) and tendon(s) at lower leg level, left leg

CC-A **S86.829-** Laceration of other muscle(s) and tendon(s) at lower leg level, unspecified leg

S86.89- Other injury of other muscles and tendons at lower leg level

S86.891- Other injury of other muscle(s) and tendon(s) at lower leg level, right leg

S86.892- Other injury of other muscle(s) and tendon(s) at lower leg level, left leg

S86.899- Other injury of other muscle(s) and tendon(s) at lower leg level, unspecified leg

S86.9- Injury of unspecified muscle and tendon at lower leg level

S86.90- Unspecified injury of unspecified muscle and tendon at lower leg level

S86.901- Unspecified injury of unspecified muscle(s) and tendon(s) at lower leg level, right leg

S86.902- Unspecified injury of unspecified muscle(s) and tendon(s) at lower leg level, left leg

S86.909- Unspecified injury of unspecified muscle(s) and tendon(s) at lower leg level, unspecified leg

S86.91- Strain of unspecified muscle and tendon at lower leg level

S86.911- Strain of unspecified muscle(s) and tendon(s) at lower leg level, right leg

S86.912- Strain of unspecified muscle(s) and tendon(s) at lower leg level, left leg

S86.919- Strain of unspecified muscle(s) and tendon(s) at lower leg level, unspecified leg

S86.92- Laceration of unspecified muscle and tendon at lower leg level

CC-A **S86.921-** Laceration of unspecified muscle(s) and tendon(s) at lower leg level, right leg

CC-A **S86.922-** Laceration of unspecified muscle(s) and tendon(s) at lower leg level, left leg

CC-A **S86.929-** Laceration of unspecified muscle(s) and tendon(s) at lower leg level, unspecified leg

S86.99- Other injury of unspecified muscle and tendon at lower leg level

S86.991- Other injury of unspecified muscle(s) and tendon(s) at lower leg level, right leg

S86.992- Other injury of unspecified muscle(s) and tendon(s) at lower leg level, left leg

S86.999- Other injury of unspecified muscle(s) and tendon(s) at lower leg level, unspecified leg

S86 – S86

S87- **Crushing injury** of **lower leg**
Use additional code(s) for all associated injuries
Excludes 2: *crushing injury of ankle and foot (S97.-)*

The appropriate 7th character is to be added to each code from category S87:
A   **Initial** encounter
D   **Subsequent** encounter
S   **Sequela**

S87.0- **Crushing** injury of **knee**
S87.00x- Crushing injury of **unspecified** knee
S87.01x- Crushing injury of **right** knee
S87.02x- Crushing injury of **left** knee

S87.8- **Crushing** injury of **lower leg**
S87.80x- Crushing injury of **unspecified** lower leg
S87.81x- Crushing injury of **right** lower leg
S87.82x- Crushing injury of **left** lower leg

S88- **Traumatic amputation** of **lower leg**
Note: An amputation not identified as partial or complete should be coded to complete
Excludes 1: *traumatic amputation of ankle and foot (S98.-)*

The appropriate 7th character is to be added to each code from category S88:
A   **Initial** encounter
D   **Subsequent** encounter
S   **Sequela**

S88.0- **Traumatic amputation** at **knee level**
S88.01- **Complete** traumatic amputation at knee level
CC-A **S88.011-** Complete traumatic amputation at knee level, **right** lower leg
CC-A **S88.012-** Complete traumatic amputation at knee level, **left** lower leg
CC-A **S88.019-** Complete traumatic amputation at knee level, **unspecified** lower leg
S88.02- **Partial** traumatic amputation at knee level
CC-A **S88.021-** Partial traumatic amputation at knee level, **right** lower leg
CC-A **S88.022-** Partial traumatic amputation at knee level, **left** lower leg
CC-A **S88.029-** Partial traumatic amputation at knee level, **unspecified** lower leg

S88.1- **Traumatic amputation** at level **between knee and ankle**
S88.11- **Complete** traumatic amputation at level between knee and ankle
CC-A **S88.111-** Complete traumatic amputation at level between knee and ankle, **right** lower leg
CC-A **S88.112-** Complete traumatic amputation at level between knee and ankle, **left** lower leg
CC-A **S88.119-** Complete traumatic amputation at level between knee and ankle, **unspecified** lower leg
S88.12- **Partial** traumatic amputation at level between knee and ankle
CC-A **S88.121-** Partial traumatic amputation at level between knee and ankle, **right** lower leg
CC-A **S88.122-** Partial traumatic amputation at level between knee and ankle, **left** lower leg
CC-A **S88.129-** Partial traumatic amputation at level between knee and ankle, **unspecified** lower leg

S88.9- **Traumatic amputation** of **lower leg, level unspecified**
S88.91- **Complete** traumatic amputation of lower leg, level unspecified
CC-A **S88.911-** Complete traumatic amputation of **right** lower leg, level unspecified
CC-A **S88.912-** Complete traumatic amputation of **left** lower leg, level unspecified
CC-A **S88.919-** Complete traumatic amputation of **unspecified** lower leg, level unspecified
S88.92- **Partial** traumatic amputation of lower leg, level unspecified

CC-A **S88.921-** Partial traumatic amputation of **right** lower leg, level unspecified
CC-A **S88.922-** Partial traumatic amputation of **left** lower leg, level unspecified
CC-A **S88.929-** Partial traumatic amputation of **unspecified** lower leg, level unspecified

S89- **Other and unspecified injuries** of **lower leg**
Note: A fracture not indicated as open or closed should be coded to closed
Excludes 2: *other and unspecified injuries of ankle and foot (S99.-)*

The appropriate 7th character is to be added to each code from subcategories S89.0, S89.1, S89.2, and S89.3:
A   **Initial** encounter for **closed** fracture
D   **Subsequent** encounter for fracture **with routine healing**
G   **Subsequent** encounter for fracture **with delayed healing**
K   **Subsequent** encounter for fracture **with nonunion**
P   **Subsequent** encounter for fracture **with malunion**
S   **Sequela**

S89.0- **Physeal** **fracture** of **upper end** of **tibia**
S89.00- **Unspecified** **physeal** fracture of **upper end** of **tibia**
CC-A,K,P **S89.001-** Unspecified physeal fracture of upper end of **right** tibia
CC-A,K,P **S89.002-** Unspecified physeal fracture of upper end of **left** tibia
CC-A,K,P **S89.009-** Unspecified physeal fracture of upper end of **unspecified** tibia
S89.01- **Salter-Harris Type I** physeal fracture of **upper end** of **tibia**
CC-A,K,P **S89.011-** Salter-Harris Type I physeal fracture of upper end of **right** tibia
CC-A,K,P **S89.012-** Salter-Harris Type I physeal fracture of upper end of **left** tibia
CC-A,K,P **S89.019-** Salter-Harris Type I physeal fracture of upper end of **unspecified** tibia
S89.02- **Salter-Harris Type II** physeal fracture of **upper end** of **tibia**
CC-A,K,P **S89.021-** Salter-Harris Type II physeal fracture of upper end of **right** tibia
CC-A,K,P **S89.022-** Salter-Harris Type II physeal fracture of upper end of **left** tibia
CC-A,K,P **S89.029-** Salter-Harris Type II physeal fracture of upper end of **unspecified** tibia
S89.03- **Salter-Harris Type III** physeal fracture of **upper end** of **tibia**
CC-A,K,P **S89.031-** Salter-Harris Type III physeal fracture of upper end of **right** tibia
CC-A,K,P **S89.032-** Salter-Harris Type III physeal fracture of upper end of **left** tibia
CC-A,K,P **S89.039-** Salter-Harris Type III physeal fracture of upper end of **unspecified** tibia
S89.04- **Salter-Harris Type IV** physeal fracture of **upper end** of **tibia**
CC-A,K,P **S89.041-** Salter-Harris Type IV physeal fracture of upper end of **right** tibia
CC-A,K,P **S89.042-** Salter-Harris Type IV physeal fracture of upper end of **left** tibia
CC-A,K,P **S89.049-** Salter-Harris Type IV physeal fracture of upper end of **unspecified** tibia
S89.09- **Other physeal** fracture of **upper end** of **tibia**
CC-A,K,P **S89.091-** Other physeal fracture of upper end of **right** tibia
CC-A,K,P **S89.092-** Other physeal fracture of upper end of **left** tibia
CC-A,K,P **S89.099-** Other physeal fracture of upper end of **unspecified** tibia

S89.1- **Physeal** fracture of **lower end** of **tibia**
S89.10- **Unspecified** **physeal** fracture of **lower end** of **tibia**
CC-K,P **S89.101-** Unspecified physeal fracture of lower end of **right** tibia
CC-K,P **S89.102-** Unspecified physeal fracture of lower end of **left** tibia
CC-K,P **S89.109-** Unspecified physeal fracture of lower end of **unspecified** tibia

S89.11- <u>Salter-Harris Type I</u> physeal fracture of <u>lower end</u> of <u>tibia</u>
CC-K,P S89.111- Salter-Harris Type I physeal fracture of lower end of <u>right</u> tibia
CC-K,P S89.112- Salter-Harris Type I physeal fracture of lower end of <u>left</u> tibia
CC-K,P S89.119- Salter-Harris Type I physeal fracture of lower end of <u>unspecified</u> tibia

S89.12- <u>Salter-Harris Type II</u> physeal fracture of <u>lower end</u> of <u>tibia</u>
CC-K,P S89.121- Salter-Harris Type II physeal fracture of lower end of <u>right</u> tibia
CC-K,P S89.122- Salter-Harris Type II physeal fracture of lower end of <u>left</u> tibia
CC-K,P S89.129- Salter-Harris Type II physeal fracture of lower end of <u>unspecified</u> tibia

S89.13- <u>Salter-Harris Type III</u> physeal fracture of <u>lower end</u> of <u>tibia</u>
    Excludes 1:   *fracture of medial malleolus (adult) (S82.5-)*
CC-K,P S89.131- Salter-Harris Type III physeal fracture of lower end of <u>right</u> tibia
CC-K,P S89.132- Salter-Harris Type III physeal fracture of lower end of <u>left</u> tibia
CC-K,P S89.139- Salter-Harris Type III physeal fracture of lower end of <u>unspecified</u> tibia

S89.14- <u>Salter-Harris Type IV</u> physeal fracture of <u>lower end</u> of <u>tibia</u>
    Excludes 1:   *fracture of medial malleolus (adult) (S82.5-)*
CC-K,P S89.141- Salter-Harris Type IV physeal fracture of lower end of <u>right</u> tibia
CC-K,P S89.142- Salter-Harris Type IV physeal fracture of lower end of <u>left</u> tibia
CC-K,P S89.149- Salter-Harris Type IV physeal fracture of lower end of <u>unspecified</u> tibia

S89.19- <u>Other physeal</u> fracture of <u>lower end</u> of <u>tibia</u>
CC-K,P S89.191- Other physeal fracture of lower end of <u>right</u> tibia
CC-K,P S89.192- Other physeal fracture of lower end of <u>left</u> tibia
CC-K,P S89.199- Other physeal fracture of lower end of <u>unspecified</u> tibia

S89.2- <u>Physeal fracture</u> of <u>upper end</u> of <u>fibula</u>
S89.20- <u>Unspecified physeal</u> fracture of <u>upper end</u> of <u>fibula</u>
CC-K,P S89.201- Unspecified physeal fracture of upper end of <u>right</u> fibula
CC-K,P S89.202- Unspecified physeal fracture of upper end of <u>left</u> fibula
CC-K,P S89.209- Unspecified physeal fracture of upper end of <u>unspecified</u> fibula

S89.21- <u>Salter-Harris Type I</u> physeal fracture of <u>upper end</u> of <u>fibula</u>
CC-K,P S89.211- Salter-Harris Type I physeal fracture of upper end of <u>right</u> fibula
CC-K,P S89.212- Salter-Harris Type I physeal fracture of upper end of <u>left</u> fibula
CC-K,P S89.219- Salter-Harris Type I physeal fracture of upper end of <u>unspecified</u> fibula

S89.22- <u>Salter-Harris Type II</u> physeal fracture of <u>upper end</u> of <u>fibula</u>
CC-K,P S89.221- Salter-Harris Type II physeal fracture of upper end of <u>right</u> fibula
CC-K,P S89.222- Salter-Harris Type II physeal fracture of upper end of <u>left</u> fibula
CC-K,P S89.229- Salter-Harris Type II physeal fracture of upper end of <u>unspecified</u> fibula

S89.29- <u>Other physeal</u> fracture of <u>upper end</u> of <u>fibula</u>
CC-K,P S89.291- Other physeal fracture of upper end of <u>right</u> fibula
CC-K,P S89.292- Other physeal fracture of upper end of <u>left</u> fibula
CC-K,P S89.299- Other physeal fracture of upper end of <u>unspecified</u> fibula

S89.3- <u>Physeal</u> fracture of <u>lower end</u> of <u>fibula</u>
S89.30- Unspecified physeal fracture of lower end of fibula
CC-K,P S89.301- Unspecified physeal fracture of lower end of <u>right</u> fibula
CC-K,P S89.302- Unspecified physeal fracture of lower end of <u>left</u> fibula
CC-K,P S89.309- Unspecified physeal fracture of lower end of <u>unspecified</u> fibula

S89.31- <u>Salter-Harris Type I</u> physeal fracture of <u>lower end</u> of <u>fibula</u>
CC-K,P S89.311- Salter-Harris Type I physeal fracture of lower end of <u>right</u> fibula
CC-K,P S89.312- Salter-Harris Type I physeal fracture of lower end of <u>left</u> fibula
CC-K,P S89.319- Salter-Harris Type I physeal fracture of lower end of <u>unspecified</u> fibula

S89.32- <u>Salter-Harris Type II</u> physeal fracture of <u>lower end</u> of <u>fibula</u>
CC-K,P S89.321- Salter-Harris Type II physeal fracture of lower end of <u>right</u> fibula
CC-K,P S89.322- Salter-Harris Type II physeal fracture of lower end of <u>left</u> fibula
CC-K,P S89.329- Salter-Harris Type II physeal fracture of lower end of <u>unspecified</u> fibula

S89.39- <u>Other physeal</u> fracture of <u>lower end</u> of <u>fibula</u>
CC-K,P S89.391- Other physeal fracture of lower end of <u>right</u> fibula
CC-K,P S89.392- Other physeal fracture of lower end of <u>left</u> fibula
CC-K,P S89.399- Other physeal fracture of lower end of <u>unspecified</u> fibula

S89.8- <u>Other specified injuries</u> of <u>lower leg</u>
The appropriate 7th character is to be added to each code in subcategory S89.8:
    A   <u>Initial</u> encounter
    D   <u>Subsequent</u> encounter
    S   <u>Sequela</u>
S89.80x- Other specified injuries of <u>unspecified</u> lower leg
S89.81x- Other specified injuries of <u>right</u> lower leg
S89.82x- Other specified injuries of <u>left</u> lower leg

S89.9- <u>Unspecified injury</u> of <u>lower leg</u>
The appropriate 7th character is to be added to each code in subcategory S89.9:
    A   <u>Initial</u> encounter
    D   <u>Subsequent</u> encounter
    S   <u>Sequela</u>
S89.90x- Unspecified injury of <u>unspecified</u> lower leg
S89.91x- Unspecified injury of <u>right</u> lower leg
S89.92x- Unspecified injury of <u>left</u> lower leg

Injuries to the ankle and foot (S90-S99)

Excludes ❷: *burns and corrosions (T20-T32)*
            fracture of ankle and malleolus (S82.-)
            frostbite (T33-T34)
            insect bite or sting, venomous (T63.4)

S90- <u>Superficial injury</u> of <u>ankle, foot and toes</u>
The appropriate 7th character is to be added to each code from category S90:
    A   <u>Initial</u> encounter
    D   <u>Subsequent</u> encounter
    S   <u>Sequela</u>

S90.0- <u>Contusion</u> of <u>ankle</u>
S90.00x- Contusion of <u>unspecified</u> ankle
S90.01x- Contusion of <u>right</u> ankle
S90.02x- Contusion of <u>left</u> ankle

S90.1- <u>Contusion</u> of <u>toe without</u> damage to nail
S90.11- <u>Contusion</u> of <u>great toe without</u> damage to nail
S90.111- Contusion of <u>right</u> great toe <u>without</u> damage to nail
S90.112- Contusion of <u>left</u> great toe <u>without</u> damage to nail

S89 - S90

Excludes 1: = NOT CODED HERE! (Do not code both)   **1123**   *Excludes ❷:* = Not Included Here

S90.119-   Contusion of <u>unspecified</u> great toe <u>without</u> damage to nail

S90.12-   <u>Contusion</u> of <u>lesser toe without</u> damage to nail

S90.121-   Contusion of <u>right</u> lesser toe(s) <u>without</u> damage to nail

S90.122-   Contusion of <u>left</u> lesser toe(s) <u>without</u> damage to nail

S90.129-   Contusion of <u>unspecified</u> lesser toe(s) <u>without</u> damage to nail
  Contusion of toe NOS

S90.2-   <u>Contusion</u> of <u>toe with damage to nail</u>

S90.21-   Contusion of <u>great toe with damage to nail</u>

S90.211-   Contusion of <u>right</u> great toe with damage to nail

S90.212-   Contusion of <u>left</u> great toe with damage to nail

S90.219-   Contusion of <u>unspecified</u> great toe with damage to nail

S90.22-   <u>Contusion</u> of <u>lesser toe with damage to nail</u>

S90.221-   Contusion of <u>right</u> lesser toe(s) with damage to nail

S90.222-   Contusion of <u>left</u> lesser toe(s) with damage to nail

S90.229-   Contusion of <u>unspecified</u> lesser toe(s) with damage to nail

S90.3-   <u>Contusion</u> of <u>foot</u>
  Excludes ❷: contusion of toes (S90.1-, S90.2-)

S90.30x-   Contusion of <u>unspecified</u> foot
  Contusion of foot NOS

S90.31x-   Contusion of <u>right</u> foot

S90.32x-   Contusion of <u>left</u> foot

S90.4-   <u>Other superficial injuries</u> of <u>toe</u>

S90.41-   <u>Abrasion</u> of <u>toe</u>

S90.411-   Abrasion, <u>right great</u> toe

S90.412-   Abrasion, <u>left great</u> toe

S90.413-   Abrasion, <u>unspecified great</u> toe

S90.414-   Abrasion, <u>right lesser</u> toe(s)

S90.415-   Abrasion, <u>left lesser</u> toe(s)

S90.416-   Abrasion, <u>unspecified lesser</u> toe(s)

S90.42-   <u>Blister</u> (nonthermal) of <u>toe</u>

S90.421-   Blister (nonthermal), <u>right great</u> toe

S90.422-   Blister (nonthermal), <u>left great</u> toe

S90.423-   Blister (nonthermal), <u>unspecified great</u> toe

S90.424-   Blister (nonthermal), <u>right lesser</u> toe(s)

S90.425-   Blister (nonthermal), <u>left lesser</u> toe(s)

S90.426-   Blister (nonthermal), <u>unspecified lesser</u> toe(s)

S90.44-   <u>External constriction</u> of <u>toe</u>
  Hair tourniquet syndrome of toe

S90.441-   External constriction, <u>right great</u> toe

S90.442-   External constriction, <u>left great</u> toe

S90.443-   External constriction, <u>unspecified great</u> toe

S90.444-   External constriction, <u>right lesser</u> toe(s)

S90.445-   External constriction, <u>left lesser</u> toe(s)

S90.446-   External constriction, <u>unspecified lesser</u> toe(s)

S90.45-   <u>Superficial foreign body</u> of <u>toe</u>
  Splinter in the toe

S90.451-   Superficial foreign body, <u>right great</u> toe

S90.452-   Superficial foreign body, <u>left great</u> toe

S90.453-   Superficial foreign body, <u>unspecified great</u> toe

S90.454-   Superficial foreign body, <u>right lesser</u> toe(s)

S90.455-   Superficial foreign body, <u>left lesser</u> toe(s)

S90.456-   Superficial foreign body, <u>unspecified lesser</u> toe(s)

S90.46-   <u>Insect bite (nonvenomous)</u> of toe

S90.461-   Insect bite (nonvenomous), <u>right great</u> toe

S90.462-   Insect bite (nonvenomous), <u>left great</u> toe

S90.463-   Insect bite (nonvenomous), <u>unspecified great</u> toe

S90.464-   Insect bite (nonvenomous), <u>right lesser</u> toe(s)

S90.465-   Insect bite (nonvenomous), <u>left lesser</u> toe(s)

S90.466-   Insect bite (nonvenomous), <u>unspecified lesser</u> toe(s)

S90.47-   <u>Other superficial bite</u> of toe
  Excludes 1:   open bite of toe (S91.15-, S91.25-)

S90.471-   Other superficial bite of <u>right great</u> toe

S90.472-   Other superficial bite of <u>left great</u> toe

S90.473-   Other superficial bite of <u>unspecified great</u> toe

S90.474-   Other superficial bite of <u>right lesser</u> toe(s)

S90.475-   Other superficial bite of <u>left lesser</u> toe(s)

S90.476-   Other superficial bite of <u>unspecified lesser</u> toe(s)

S90.5-   <u>Other superficial injuries</u> of <u>ankle</u>

S90.51-   <u>Abrasion</u> of <u>ankle</u>

S90.511-   Abrasion, <u>right</u> ankle

S90.512-   Abrasion, <u>left</u> ankle

S90.519-   Abrasion, <u>unspecified</u> ankle

S90.52-   <u>Blister</u> (nonthermal) of <u>ankle</u>

S90.521-   Blister (nonthermal), <u>right</u> ankle

S90.522-   Blister (nonthermal), <u>left</u> ankle

S90.529-   Blister (nonthermal), <u>unspecified</u> ankle

S90.54-   <u>External constriction</u> of <u>ankle</u>

S90.541-   External constriction, <u>right</u> ankle

S90.542-   External constriction, <u>left</u> ankle

S90.549-   External constriction, <u>unspecified</u> ankle

S90.55-   <u>Superficial foreign body</u> of <u>ankle</u>
  Splinter in the ankle

S90.551-   Superficial foreign body, <u>right</u> ankle

S90.552-   Superficial foreign body, <u>left</u> ankle

S90.559-   Superficial foreign body, <u>unspecified</u> ankle

S90.56-   <u>Insect bite (nonvenomous)</u> of <u>ankle</u>

S90.561-   Insect bite (nonvenomous), <u>right</u> ankle

S90.562-   Insect bite (nonvenomous), <u>left</u> ankle

S90.569-   Insect bite (nonvenomous), <u>unspecified</u> ankle

S90.57-   <u>Other superficial bite</u> of <u>ankle</u>
  Excludes 1:   open bite of ankle (S91.05-)

S90.571-   Other superficial bite of ankle, <u>right</u> ankle

S90.572-   Other superficial bite of ankle, <u>left</u> ankle

S90.579-   Other superficial bite of ankle, <u>unspecified</u> ankle

S90.8-   <u>Other superficial injuries</u> of <u>foot</u>

S90.81-   <u>Abrasion</u> of <u>foot</u>

S90.811-   Abrasion, <u>right</u> foot

S90.812-   Abrasion, <u>left</u> foot

S90.819-   Abrasion, <u>unspecified</u> foot

S90.82-   <u>Blister</u> (nonthermal) of <u>foot</u>

S90.821-   Blister (nonthermal), <u>right</u> foot

S90.822-   Blister (nonthermal), <u>left</u> foot

S90.829-   Blister (nonthermal), <u>unspecified</u> foot

S90.84-   <u>External constriction</u> of <u>foot</u>

S90.841-   External constriction, <u>right</u> foot

S90.842-   External constriction, <u>left</u> foot

S90.849-   External constriction, <u>unspecified</u> foot

S90.85-   <u>Superficial foreign body</u> of <u>foot</u>
  Splinter in the foot

S90.851-   Superficial foreign body, <u>right</u> foot

S90.852-   Superficial foreign body, <u>left</u> foot

S90.859-   Superficial foreign body, <u>unspecified</u> foot

S90.86-   <u>Insect bite (nonvenomous)</u> of <u>foot</u>

S90.861-   Insect bite (nonvenomous), <u>right</u> foot

S90.862-   Insect bite (nonvenomous), <u>left</u> foot

S90.869-   Insect bite (nonvenomous), <u>unspecified</u> foot

S90.87-   <u>Other superficial bite</u> of <u>foot</u>
  Excludes 1:   open bite of foot (S91.35-)

S90.871-   Other superficial bite of <u>right</u> foot

S90.872-   Other superficial bite of <u>left</u> foot

S90.879-   Other superficial bite of <u>unspecified</u> foot

Excludes 1: = NOT CODED HERE! (Do not code both)   *Excludes ❷:* = Not Included Here

S90.9- Unspecified superficial injury of ankle, foot and toe

  S90.91- Unspecified superficial injury of ankle

    S90.911- Unspecified superficial injury of right ankle

    S90.912- Unspecified superficial injury of left ankle

    S90.919- Unspecified superficial injury of unspecified ankle

  S90.92- Unspecified superficial injury of foot

    S90.921- Unspecified superficial injury of right foot

    S90.922- Unspecified superficial injury of left foot

    S90.929- Unspecified superficial injury of unspecified foot

  S90.93- Unspecified superficial injury of toes

    S90.931- Unspecified superficial injury of right great toe

    S90.932- Unspecified superficial injury of left great toe

    S90.933- Unspecified superficial injury of unspecified great toe

    S90.934- Unspecified superficial injury of right lesser toe(s)

    S90.935- Unspecified superficial injury of left lesser toe(s)

    S90.936- Unspecified superficial injury of unspecified lesser toe(s)

S91- Open wound of ankle, foot and toes
Code also any associated wound infection
Excludes 1: open fracture of ankle, foot and toes (S92.-with 7th character B)
          traumatic amputation of ankle and foot (S98.-)

> **The appropriate 7th character is to be added to each code from category S91:**
> **A** Initial encounter
> **D** Subsequent encounter
> **S** Sequela

  S91.0- Open wound of ankle

    S91.00- Unspecified open wound of ankle

      S91.001- Unspecified open wound, right ankle

      S91.002- Unspecified open wound, left ankle

      S91.009- Unspecified open wound, unspecified ankle

    S91.01- Laceration without foreign body of ankle

      S91.011- Laceration without foreign body, right ankle

      S91.012- Laceration without foreign body, left ankle

      S91.019- Laceration without foreign body, unspecified ankle

    S91.02- Laceration with foreign body of ankle

      S91.021- Laceration with foreign body, right ankle

      S91.022- Laceration with foreign body, left ankle

      S91.029- Laceration with foreign body, unspecified ankle

    S91.03- Puncture wound without foreign body of ankle

      S91.031- Puncture wound without foreign body, right ankle

      S91.032- Puncture wound without foreign body, left ankle

      S91.039- Puncture wound without foreign body, unspecified ankle

    S91.04- Puncture wound with foreign body of ankle

      S91.041- Puncture wound with foreign body, right ankle

      S91.042- Puncture wound with foreign body, left ankle

      S91.049- Puncture wound with foreign body, unspecified ankle

    S91.05- Open bite of ankle
      Excludes 1: superficial bite of ankle (S90.56-, S90.57-)

      S91.051- Open bite, right ankle

      S91.052- Open bite, left ankle

      S91.059- Open bite, unspecified ankle

  S91.1- Open wound of toe without damage to nail

    S91.10- Unspecified open wound of toe without damage to nail

      S91.101- Unspecified open wound of right great toe without damage to nail

      S91.102- Unspecified open wound of left great toe without damage to nail

      S91.103- Unspecified open wound of unspecified great toe without damage to nail

      S91.104- Unspecified open wound of right lesser toe(s) without damage to nail

      S91.105- Unspecified open wound of left lesser toe(s) without damage to nail

      S91.106- Unspecified open wound of unspecified lesser toe(s) without damage to nail

      S91.109- Unspecified open wound of unspecified toe(s) without damage to nail

    S91.11- Laceration without foreign body of toe without damage to nail

      S91.111- Laceration without foreign body of right great toe without damage to nail

      S91.112- Laceration without foreign body of left great toe without damage to nail

      S91.113- Laceration without foreign body of unspecified great toe without damage to nail

      S91.114- Laceration without foreign body of right lesser toe(s) without damage to nail

      S91.115- Laceration without foreign body of left lesser toe(s) without damage to nail

      S91.116- Laceration without foreign body of unspecified lesser toe(s) without damage to nail

      S91.119- Laceration without foreign body of unspecified toe without damage to nail

    S91.12- Laceration with foreign body of toe without damage to nail

      S91.121- Laceration with foreign body of right great toe without damage to nail

      S91.122- Laceration with foreign body of left great toe without damage to nail

      S91.123- Laceration with foreign body of unspecified great toe without damage to nail

      S91.124- Laceration with foreign body of right lesser toe(s) without damage to nail

      S91.125- Laceration with foreign body of left lesser toe(s) without damage to nail

      S91.126- Laceration with foreign body of unspecified lesser toe(s) without damage to nail

      S91.129- Laceration with foreign body of unspecified toe(s) without damage to nail

    S91.13- Puncture wound without foreign body of toe without damage to nail

      S91.131- Puncture wound without foreign body of right great toe without damage to nail

      S91.132- Puncture wound without foreign body of left great toe without damage to nail

      S91.133- Puncture wound without foreign body of unspecified great toe without damage to nail

      S91.134- Puncture wound without foreign body of right lesser toe(s) without damage to nail

      S91.135- Puncture wound without foreign body of left lesser toe(s) without damage to nail

      S91.136- Puncture wound without foreign body of unspecified lesser toe(s) without damage to nail

      S91.139- Puncture wound without foreign body of unspecified toe(s) without damage to nail

    S91.14- Puncture wound with foreign body of toe without damage to nail

      S91.141- Puncture wound with foreign body of right great toe without damage to nail

      S91.142- Puncture wound with foreign body of left great toe without damage to nail

      S91.143- Puncture wound with foreign body of unspecified great toe without damage to nail

      S91.144- Puncture wound with foreign body of right lesser toe(s) without damage to nail

      S91.145- Puncture wound with foreign body of left lesser toe(s) without damage to nail

      S91.146- Puncture wound with foreign body of unspecified lesser toe(s) without damage to nail

S90-S91

S91.149- Puncture wound <u>with foreign body</u> of <u>unspecified</u> toe(s) <u>without</u> damage to nail

S91.15- <u>Open bite</u> of <u>toe</u> <u>without</u> damage to nail
Bite of toe NOS
Excludes 1:   superficial bite of toe (S90.46-, S90.47-)

S91.151- Open bite of <u>right great</u> toe <u>without</u> damage to nail

S91.152- Open bite of <u>left great</u> toe <u>without</u> damage to nail

S91.153- Open bite of <u>unspecified great</u> toe <u>without</u> damage to nail

S91.154- Open bite of <u>right lesser</u> toe(s) <u>without</u> damage to nail

S91.155- Open bite of <u>left lesser</u> toe(s) <u>without</u> damage to nail

S91.156- Open bite of <u>unspecified lesser</u> toe(s) <u>without</u> damage to nail

S91.159- Open bite of <u>unspecified</u> toe(s) <u>without</u> damage to nail

S91.2- <u>Open wound</u> of <u>toe with damage to nail</u>

S91.20- <u>Unspecified open wound</u> of <u>toe with damage to nail</u>

S91.201- Unspecified open wound of <u>right great</u> toe <u>with damage to nail</u>

S91.202- Unspecified open wound of <u>left great</u> toe <u>with damage to nail</u>

S91.203- Unspecified open wound of <u>unspecified great</u> toe <u>with damage to nail</u>

S91.204- Unspecified open wound of <u>right lesser</u> toe(s) <u>with damage to nail</u>

S91.205- Unspecified open wound of <u>left lesser</u> toe(s) <u>with damage to nail</u>

S91.206- Unspecified open wound of <u>unspecified lesser</u> toe(s) <u>with damage to nail</u>

S91.209- Unspecified open wound of <u>unspecified</u> toe(s) <u>with damage to nail</u>

S91.21- <u>Laceration without</u> foreign body of toe <u>with damage to nail</u>

S91.211- Laceration <u>without</u> foreign body of <u>right great</u> toe <u>with damage to nail</u>

S91.212- Laceration <u>without</u> foreign body of <u>left great</u> toe <u>with damage to nail</u>

S91.213- Laceration <u>without</u> foreign body of <u>unspecified great</u> toe <u>with damage to nail</u>

S91.214- Laceration <u>without</u> foreign body of <u>right lesser</u> toe(s) <u>with damage to nail</u>

S91.215- Laceration <u>without</u> foreign body of <u>left lesser</u> toe(s) <u>with damage to nail</u>

S91.216- Laceration <u>without</u> foreign body of <u>unspecified lesser</u> toe(s) <u>with damage to nail</u>

S91.219- Laceration <u>without</u> foreign body of <u>unspecified</u> toe(s) <u>with damage to nail</u>

S91.22- <u>Laceration with foreign body</u> of <u>toe with damage to nail</u>

S91.221- Laceration <u>with foreign body</u> of <u>right great</u> toe <u>with damage to nail</u>

S91.222- Laceration <u>with foreign body</u> of <u>left great</u> toe <u>with damage to nail</u>

S91.223- Laceration <u>with foreign body</u> of <u>unspecified great</u> toe <u>with damage to nail</u>

S91.224- Laceration <u>with foreign body</u> of <u>right lesser</u> toe(s) <u>with damage to nail</u>

S91.225- Laceration <u>with foreign body</u> of <u>left lesser</u> toe(s) <u>with damage to nail</u>

S91.226- Laceration <u>with foreign body</u> of <u>unspecified lesser</u> toe(s) <u>with damage to nail</u>

S91.229- Laceration <u>with foreign body</u> of <u>unspecified</u> toe(s) <u>with damage to nail</u>

S91.23- <u>Puncture</u> wound <u>without</u> foreign body of <u>toe with damage to nail</u>

S91.231- Puncture wound <u>without</u> foreign body of <u>right great</u> toe <u>with damage to nail</u>

S91.232- Puncture wound <u>without</u> foreign body of <u>left great</u> toe <u>with damage to nail</u>

S91.233- Puncture wound <u>without</u> foreign body of <u>unspecified great</u> toe <u>with damage to nail</u>

S91.234- Puncture wound <u>without</u> foreign body of <u>right lesser</u> toe(s) <u>with damage to nail</u>

S91.235- Puncture wound <u>without</u> foreign body of <u>left lesser</u> toe(s) <u>with damage to nail</u>

S91.236- Puncture wound <u>without</u> foreign body of <u>unspecified lesser</u> toe(s) <u>with damage to nail</u>

S91.239- Puncture wound <u>without</u> foreign body of <u>unspecified</u> toe(s) <u>with damage to nail</u>

S91.24- <u>Puncture</u> wound <u>with foreign body</u> of <u>toe with damage to nail</u>

S91.241- Puncture wound <u>with foreign body</u> of <u>right great</u> toe <u>with damage to nail</u>

S91.242- Puncture wound <u>with foreign body</u> of <u>left great</u> toe <u>with damage to nail</u>

S91.243- Puncture wound <u>with foreign body</u> of <u>unspecified great</u> toe <u>with damage to nail</u>

S91.244- Puncture wound <u>with foreign body</u> of <u>right lesser</u> toe(s) <u>with damage to nail</u>

S91.245- Puncture wound <u>with foreign body</u> of <u>left lesser</u> toe(s) <u>with damage to nail</u>

S91.246- Puncture wound <u>with foreign body</u> of <u>unspecified lesser</u> toe(s) <u>with damage to nail</u>

S91.249- Puncture wound <u>with foreign body</u> of <u>unspecified</u> toe(s) <u>with damage to nail</u>

S91.25- <u>Open bite</u> of <u>toe with damage to nail</u>
Bite of toe with damage to nail NOS
Excludes 1:   superficial bite of toe (S90.46-, S90.47-)

S91.251- Open bite of <u>right great</u> toe <u>with damage to nail</u>

S91.252- Open bite of <u>left great</u> toe <u>with damage to nail</u>

S91.253- Open bite of <u>unspecified great</u> toe <u>with damage to nail</u>

S91.254- Open bite of <u>right lesser</u> toe(s) <u>with damage to nail</u>

S91.255- Open bite of <u>left lesser</u> toe(s) <u>with damage to nail</u>

S91.256- Open bite of <u>unspecified lesser</u> toe(s) <u>with damage to nail</u>

S91.259- Open bite of <u>unspecified</u> toe(s) <u>with damage to nail</u>

S91.3- <u>Open wound</u> of <u>foot</u>

S91.30- <u>Unspecified</u> open wound of <u>foot</u>

S91.301- Unspecified open wound, <u>right</u> foot

S91.302- Unspecified open wound, <u>left</u> foot

S91.309- Unspecified open wound, <u>unspecified</u> foot

S91.31- <u>Laceration without</u> foreign body of <u>foot</u>

S91.311- Laceration <u>without</u> foreign body, <u>right</u> foot

S91.312- Laceration <u>without</u> foreign body, <u>left</u> foot

S91.319- Laceration <u>without</u> foreign body, <u>unspecified</u> foot

S91.32- <u>Laceration with foreign body</u> of <u>foot</u>

S91.321- Laceration <u>with foreign body</u>, <u>right</u> foot

S91.322- Laceration <u>with foreign body</u>, <u>left</u> foot

S91.329- Laceration <u>with foreign body</u>, <u>unspecified</u> foot

S91.33- <u>Puncture</u> wound <u>without</u> foreign body of <u>foot</u>

S91.331- Puncture wound <u>without</u> foreign body, <u>right</u> foot

S91.332- Puncture wound <u>without</u> foreign body, <u>left</u> foot

S91.339- Puncture wound <u>without</u> foreign body, <u>unspecified</u> foot

S91.34- <u>Puncture</u> wound <u>with foreign body</u> of <u>foot</u>

S91.341- Puncture wound <u>with foreign body</u>, <u>right</u> foot

S91.342- Puncture wound <u>with foreign body</u>, <u>left</u> foot

S91 – S91

S91.349- Puncture wound <u>with foreign body</u>, <u>unspecified</u> foot

S91.35- <u>Open bite</u> of <u>foot</u>
   Excludes 1:   superficial bite of foot (S90.86-, S90.87-)

S91.351- Open bite, <u>right</u> foot
S91.352- Open bite, <u>left</u> foot
S91.359- Open bite, <u>unspecified</u> foot

S92- <u>Fracture</u> of <u>foot and toe</u>, <u>except ankle</u>
   Note: A fracture not indicated as displaced or nondisplaced should be coded to displaced
   Note: A fracture not indicated as open or closed should be coded to closed
   Excludes 1:   traumatic amputation of ankle and foot (S98.-)
   Excludes ❷: fracture of ankle (S82.-)
   *   fracture of malleolus (S82.-)*

> **The appropriate 7th character is to be added to each code from category S92:**
> **A** <u>Initial</u> encounter for <u>closed</u> fracture
> **B** <u>Initial</u> encounter for <u>open</u> fracture
> **D** <u>Subsequent</u> encounter for fracture <u>with routine healing</u>
> **G** <u>Subsequent</u> encounter for fracture <u>with delayed healing</u>
> **K** <u>Subsequent</u> encounter for fracture <u>with nonunion</u>
> **P** <u>Subsequent</u> encounter for fracture <u>with malunion</u>
> **S** <u>Sequela</u>

S92.0- <u>Fracture</u> of <u>calcaneus</u>
   Heel bone
   Os calcis
   Excludes ❷: physeal fracture of calcaneus (S99.0-)

S92.00- <u>Unspecified</u> fracture of <u>calcaneus</u>
CC-B,K,P S92.001- Unspecified fracture of <u>right</u> calcaneus
CC-B,K,P S92.002- Unspecified fracture of <u>left</u> calcaneus
CC-B,K,P S92.009- Unspecified fracture of <u>unspecified</u> calcaneus

S92.01- Fracture of <u>body</u> of <u>calcaneus</u>
CC-B,K,P S92.011- <u>Displaced</u> fracture of body of <u>right</u> calcaneus
CC-B,K,P S92.012- <u>Displaced</u> fracture of body of <u>left</u> calcaneus
CC-B,K,P S92.013- <u>Displaced</u> fracture of body of <u>unspecified</u> calcaneus
CC-B,K,P S92.014- <u>Nondisplaced</u> fracture of body of <u>right</u> calcaneus
CC-B,K,P S92.015- <u>Nondisplaced</u> fracture of body of <u>left</u> calcaneus
CC-B,K,P S92.016- <u>Nondisplaced</u> fracture of body of <u>unspecified</u> calcaneus

S92.02- Fracture of <u>anterior process</u> of <u>calcaneus</u>
CC-B,K,P S92.021- <u>Displaced</u> fracture of anterior process of <u>right</u> calcaneus
CC-B,K,P S92.022- <u>Displaced</u> fracture of anterior process of <u>left</u> calcaneus
CC-B,K,P S92.023- <u>Displaced</u> fracture of anterior process of <u>unspecified</u> calcaneus
CC-B,K,P S92.024- <u>Nondisplaced</u> fracture of anterior process of <u>right</u> calcaneus
CC-B,K,P S92.025- <u>Nondisplaced</u> fracture of anterior process of <u>left</u> calcaneus
CC-B,K,P S92.026- <u>Nondisplaced</u> fracture of anterior process of <u>unspecified</u> calcaneus

S92.03- <u>Avulsion</u> fracture of <u>tuberosity</u> of <u>calcaneus</u>
CC-B,K,P S92.031- <u>Displaced</u> avulsion fracture of tuberosity of <u>right</u> calcaneus
CC-B,K,P S92.032- <u>Displaced</u> avulsion fracture of tuberosity of <u>left</u> calcaneus
CC-B,K,P S92.033- <u>Displaced</u> avulsion fracture of tuberosity of <u>unspecified</u> calcaneus
CC-B,K,P S92.034- <u>Nondisplaced</u> avulsion fracture of tuberosity of <u>right</u> calcaneus
CC-B,K,P S92.035- <u>Nondisplaced</u> avulsion fracture of tuberosity of <u>left</u> calcaneus
CC-B,K,P S92.036- <u>Nondisplaced</u> avulsion fracture of tuberosity of <u>unspecified</u> calcaneus

S92.04- <u>Other fracture</u> of <u>tuberosity</u> of <u>calcaneus</u>
CC-B,K,P S92.041- <u>Displaced</u> other fracture of tuberosity of <u>right</u> calcaneus
CC-B,K,P S92.042- <u>Displaced</u> other fracture of tuberosity of <u>left</u> calcaneus

CC-B,K,P S92.043- <u>Displaced</u> other fracture of tuberosity of <u>unspecified</u> calcaneus
CC-B,K,P S92.044- <u>Nondisplaced</u> other fracture of tuberosity of <u>right</u> calcaneus
CC-B,K,P S92.045- <u>Nondisplaced</u> other fracture of tuberosity of <u>left</u> calcaneus
CC-B,K,P S92.046- <u>Nondisplaced</u> other fracture of tuberosity of <u>unspecified</u> calcaneus

S92.05- <u>Other extraarticular</u> fracture of <u>calcaneus</u>
CC-B,K,P S92.051- <u>Displaced</u> other extraarticular fracture of <u>right</u> calcaneus
CC-B,K,P S92.052- <u>Displaced</u> other extraarticular fracture of <u>left</u> calcaneus
CC-B,K,P S92.053- <u>Displaced</u> other extraarticular fracture of <u>unspecified</u> calcaneus
CC-B,K,P S92.054- <u>Nondisplaced</u> other extraarticular fracture of <u>right</u> calcaneus
CC-B,K,P S92.055- <u>Nondisplaced</u> other extraarticular fracture of <u>left</u> calcaneus
CC-B,K,P S92.056- <u>Nondisplaced</u> other extraarticular fracture of <u>unspecified</u> calcaneus

S92.06- <u>Intraarticular</u> fracture of <u>calcaneus</u>
CC-B,K,P S92.061- <u>Displaced</u> intraarticular fracture of <u>right</u> calcaneus
CC-B,K,P S92.062- <u>Displaced</u> intraarticular fracture of <u>left</u> calcaneus
CC-B,K,P S92.063- <u>Displaced</u> intraarticular fracture of <u>unspecified</u> calcaneus
CC-B,K,P S92.064- <u>Nondisplaced</u> intraarticular fracture of <u>right</u> calcaneus
CC-B,K,P S92.065- <u>Nondisplaced</u> intraarticular fracture of <u>left</u> calcaneus
CC-B,K,P S92.066- <u>Nondisplaced</u> intraarticular fracture of <u>unspecified</u> calcaneus

S92.1- <u>Fracture</u> of <u>talus</u>
   Astragalus

S92.10- <u>Unspecified</u> fracture of <u>talus</u>
CC-B,K,P S92.101- Unspecified fracture of <u>right</u> talus
CC-B,K,P S92.102- Unspecified fracture of <u>left</u> talus
CC-B,K,P S92.109- Unspecified fracture of <u>unspecified</u> talus

S92.11- Fracture of <u>neck</u> of <u>talus</u>
CC-B,K,P S92.111- <u>Displaced</u> fracture of neck of <u>right</u> talus
CC-B,K,P S92.112- <u>Displaced</u> fracture of neck of <u>left</u> talus
CC-B,K,P S92.113- <u>Displaced</u> fracture of neck of <u>unspecified</u> talus
CC-B,K,P S92.114- <u>Nondisplaced</u> fracture of neck of <u>right</u> talus
CC-B,K,P S92.115- <u>Nondisplaced</u> fracture of neck of <u>left</u> talus
CC-B,K,P S92.116- <u>Nondisplaced</u> fracture of neck of <u>unspecified</u> talus

S92.12- Fracture of <u>body</u> of <u>talus</u>
CC-B,K,P S92.121- <u>Displaced</u> fracture of body of <u>right</u> talus
CC-B,K,P S92.122- <u>Displaced</u> fracture of body of <u>left</u> talus
CC-B,K,P S92.123- <u>Displaced</u> fracture of body of <u>unspecified</u> talus
CC-B,K,P S92.124- <u>Nondisplaced</u> fracture of body of <u>right</u> talus
CC-B,K,P S92.125- <u>Nondisplaced</u> fracture of body of <u>left</u> talus
CC-B,K,P S92.126- <u>Nondisplaced</u> fracture of body of <u>unspecified</u> talus

S92.13- Fracture of <u>posterior process</u> of <u>talus</u>
CC-B,K,P S92.131- <u>Displaced</u> fracture of posterior process of <u>right</u> talus
CC-B,K,P S92.132- <u>Displaced</u> fracture of posterior process of <u>left</u> talus
CC-B,K,P S92.133- <u>Displaced</u> fracture of posterior process of <u>unspecified</u> talus
CC-B,K,P S92.134- <u>Nondisplaced</u> fracture of posterior process of <u>right</u> talus
CC-B,K,P S92.135- <u>Nondisplaced</u> fracture of posterior process of <u>left</u> talus
CC-B,K,P S92.136- <u>Nondisplaced</u> fracture of posterior process of <u>unspecified</u> talus

S92.14- <u>Dome</u> fracture of <u>talus</u>
   Excludes 1:   osteochondritis dissecans (M93.2)

S91-S92

CC-B,K,P S92.141- **Displaced** dome fracture of **right** talus

CC-B,K,P S92.142- **Displaced** dome fracture of **left** talus

CC-B,K,P S92.143- **Displaced** dome fracture of **unspecified** talus

CC-B,K,P S92.144- **Nondisplaced** dome fracture of **right** talus

CC-B,K,P S92.145- **Nondisplaced** dome fracture of **left** talus

CC-B,K,P S92.146- **Nondisplaced** dome fracture of **unspecified** talus

S92.15- **Avulsion** fracture (chip fracture) of **talus**

CC-B,K,P S92.151- **Displaced** avulsion fracture (chip fracture) of **right** talus

CC-B,K,P S92.152- **Displaced** avulsion fracture (chip fracture) of **left** talus

CC-B,K,P S92.153- **Displaced** avulsion fracture (chip fracture) of **unspecified** talus

CC-B,K,P S92.154- **Nondisplaced** avulsion fracture (chip fracture) of **right** talus

CC-B,K,P S92.155- **Nondisplaced** avulsion fracture (chip fracture) of **left** talus

CC-B,K,P S92.156- **Nondisplaced** avulsion fracture (chip fracture) of **unspecified** talus

S92.19- **Other fracture** of **talus**

CC-B,K,P S92.191- Other fracture of **right** talus

CC-B,K,P S92.192- Other fracture of **left** talus

CC-B,K,P S92.199- Other fracture of **unspecified** talus

S92.2- Fracture of **other and unspecified tarsal** bone(s)

S92.20- Fracture of **unspecified** tarsal bone(s)

CC-B,K,P S92.201- Fracture of **unspecified** tarsal bone(s) of **right** foot

CC-B,K,P S92.202- Fracture of **unspecified** tarsal bone(s) of **left** foot

CC-B,K,P S92.209- Fracture of **unspecified** tarsal bone(s) of **unspecified** foot

S92.21- Fracture of **cuboid** bone

CC-B,K,P S92.211- **Displaced** fracture of cuboid bone of **right** foot

CC-B,K,P S92.212- **Displaced** fracture of cuboid bone of **left** foot

CC-B,K,P S92.213- **Displaced** fracture of cuboid bone of **unspecified** foot

CC-B,K,P S92.214- **Nondisplaced** fracture of cuboid bone of **right** foot

CC-B,K,P S92.215- **Nondisplaced** fracture of cuboid bone of **left** foot

CC-B,K,P S92.216- **Nondisplaced** fracture of cuboid bone of **unspecified** foot

S92.22- Fracture of **lateral cuneiform**

CC-B,K,P S92.221- **Displaced** fracture of lateral cuneiform of **right** foot

CC-B,K,P S92.222- **Displaced** fracture of lateral cuneiform of **left** foot

CC-B,K,P S92.223- **Displaced** fracture of lateral cuneiform of **unspecified** foot

CC-B,K,P S92.224- **Nondisplaced** fracture of lateral cuneiform of **right** foot

CC-B,K,P S92.225- **Nondisplaced** fracture of lateral cuneiform of **left** foot

CC-B,K,P S92.226- **Nondisplaced** fracture of lateral cuneiform of **unspecified** foot

S92.23- Fracture of **intermediate cuneiform**

CC-B,K,P S92.231- **Displaced** fracture of intermediate cuneiform of **right** foot

CC-B,K,P S92.232- **Displaced** fracture of intermediate cuneiform of **left** foot

CC-B,K,P S92.233- **Displaced** fracture of intermediate cuneiform of **unspecified** foot

CC-B,K,P S92.234- **Nondisplaced** fracture of intermediate cuneiform of **right** foot

CC-B,K,P S92.235- **Nondisplaced** fracture of intermediate cuneiform of **left** foot

CC-B,K,P S92.236- **Nondisplaced** fracture of intermediate cuneiform of **unspecified** foot

S92.24- Fracture of **medial cuneiform**

CC-B,K,P S92.241- **Displaced** fracture of medial cuneiform of **right** foot

CC-B,K,P S92.242- **Displaced** fracture of medial cuneiform of **left** foot

CC-B,K,P S92.243- **Displaced** fracture of medial cuneiform of **unspecified** foot

CC-B,K,P S92.244- **Nondisplaced** fracture of medial cuneiform of **right** foot

CC-B,K,P S92.245- **Nondisplaced** fracture of medial cuneiform of **left** foot

CC-B,K,P S92.246- **Nondisplaced** fracture of medial cuneiform of **unspecified** foot

S92.25- Fracture of **navicular [scaphoid]** of **foot**

CC-B,K,P S92.251- **Displaced** fracture of navicular [scaphoid] of **right** foot

CC-B,K,P S92.252- **Displaced** fracture of navicular [scaphoid] of **left** foot

CC-B,K,P S92.253- **Displaced** fracture of navicular [scaphoid] of **unspecified** foot

CC-B,K,P S92.254- **Nondisplaced** fracture of navicular [scaphoid] of **right** foot

CC-B,K,P S92.255- **Nondisplaced** fracture of navicular [scaphoid] of **left** foot

CC-B,K,P S92.256- **Nondisplaced** fracture of navicular [scaphoid] of **unspecified** foot

S92.3- **Fracture** of **metatarsal** bone(s)

Excludes ❷: *physeal fracture of metatarsal (S99.1-)*

S92.30- Fracture of **unspecified metatarsal** bone(s)

CC-B,K,P S92.301- Fracture of **unspecified** metatarsal bone(s), **right** foot

CC-B,K,P S92.302- Fracture of **unspecified** metatarsal bone(s), **left** foot

CC-B,K,P S92.309- Fracture of **unspecified** metatarsal bone(s), **unspecified** foot

S92.31- Fracture of first metatarsal bone

CC-B,K,P S92.311- **Displaced** fracture of first metatarsal bone, **right** foot

CC-B,K,P S92.312- **Displaced** fracture of first metatarsal bone, **left** foot

CC-B,K,P S92.313- **Displaced** fracture of first metatarsal bone, **unspecified** foot

CC-B,K,P S92.314- **Nondisplaced** fracture of first metatarsal bone, **right** foot

CC-B,K,P S92.315- **Nondisplaced** fracture of first metatarsal bone, **left** foot

CC-B,K,P S92.316- **Nondisplaced** fracture of first metatarsal bone, **unspecified** foot

S92.32- Fracture of **second** metatarsal bone

CC-B,K,P S92.321- **Displaced** fracture of second metatarsal bone, **right** foot

CC-B,K,P S92.322- **Displaced** fracture of second metatarsal bone, **left** foot

CC-B,K,P S92.323- **Displaced** fracture of second metatarsal bone, **unspecified** foot

CC-B,K,P S92.324- **Nondisplaced** fracture of second metatarsal bone, **right** foot

CC-B,K,P S92.325- **Nondisplaced** fracture of second metatarsal bone, **left** foot

CC-B,K,P S92.326- **Nondisplaced** fracture of second metatarsal bone, **unspecified** foot

S92.33- Fracture of **third** metatarsal bone

CC-B,K,P S92.331- **Displaced** fracture of third metatarsal bone, **right** foot

CC-B,K,P S92.332- **Displaced** fracture of third metatarsal bone, **left** foot

CC-B,K,P S92.333- **Displaced** fracture of third metatarsal bone, **unspecified** foot

CC-B,K,P S92.334- **Nondisplaced** fracture of third metatarsal bone, **right** foot

CC-B,K,P S92.335- **Nondisplaced** fracture of third metatarsal bone, **left** foot

S92 – S92

CC-B,K,P **S92.336-** **Nondisplaced** fracture of third metatarsal bone, **unspecified** foot

S92.34- Fracture of **fourth** metatarsal bone

CC-B,K,P **S92.341-** **Displaced** fracture of fourth metatarsal bone, **right** foot

CC-B,K,P **S92.342-** **Displaced** fracture of fourth metatarsal bone, **left** foot

CC-B,K,P **S92.343-** **Displaced** fracture of fourth metatarsal bone, **unspecified** foot

CC-B,K,P **S92.344-** **Nondisplaced** fracture of fourth metatarsal bone, **right** foot

CC-B,K,P **S92.345-** **Nondisplaced** fracture of fourth metatarsal bone, **left** foot

CC-B,K,P **S92.346-** **Nondisplaced** fracture of fourth metatarsal bone, **unspecified** foot

S92.35- Fracture of **fifth** metatarsal bone

CC-B,K,P **S92.351-** **Displaced** fracture of fifth metatarsal bone, **right** foot

CC-B,K,P **S92.352-** **Displaced** fracture of fifth metatarsal bone, **left** foot

CC-B,K,P **S92.353-** **Displaced** fracture of fifth metatarsal bone, **unspecified** foot

CC-B,K,P **S92.354-** **Nondisplaced** fracture of fifth metatarsal bone, **right** foot

CC-B,K,P **S92.355-** **Nondisplaced** fracture of fifth metatarsal bone, **left** foot

CC-B,K,P **S92.356-** **Nondisplaced** fracture of fifth metatarsal bone, **unspecified** foot

S92.4- **Fracture** of **great toe**
  Excludes ❷: *physeal fracture of phalanx of toe (S99.2-)*

S92.40- **Unspecified** fracture of **great toe**

CC-K,P **S92.401-** **Displaced** unspecified fracture of **right** great toe

CC-K,P **S92.402-** **Displaced** unspecified fracture of **left** great toe

CC-K,P **S92.403-** **Displaced** unspecified fracture of **unspecified** great toe

CC-K,P **S92.404-** **Nondisplaced** unspecified fracture of **right** great toe

CC-K,P **S92.405-** **Nondisplaced** unspecified fracture of **left** great toe

CC-K,P **S92.406-** **Nondisplaced** unspecified fracture of **unspecified** great toe

S92.41- Fracture of **proximal phalanx** of **great toe**

CC-K,P **S92.411-** **Displaced** fracture of proximal phalanx of **right** great toe

CC-K,P **S92.412-** **Displaced** fracture of proximal phalanx of **left** great toe

CC-K,P **S92.413-** **Displaced** fracture of proximal phalanx of **unspecified** great toe

CC-K,P **S92.414-** **Nondisplaced** fracture of proximal phalanx of **right** great toe

CC-K,P **S92.415-** **Nondisplaced** fracture of proximal phalanx of **left** great toe

CC-K,P **S92.416-** **Nondisplaced** fracture of proximal phalanx of **unspecified** great toe

S92.42- Fracture of **distal phalanx** of **great toe**

CC-K,P **S92.421-** **Displaced** fracture of distal phalanx of **right** great toe

CC-K,P **S92.422-** **Displaced** fracture of distal phalanx of **left** great toe

CC-K,P **S92.423-** **Displaced** fracture of distal phalanx of **unspecified** great toe

CC-K,P **S92.424-** **Nondisplaced** fracture of distal phalanx of **right** great toe

CC-K,P **S92.425-** **Nondisplaced** fracture of distal phalanx of **left** great toe

CC-K,P **S92.426-** **Nondisplaced** fracture of distal phalanx of **unspecified** great toe

S92.49- **Other fracture** of **great toe**

CC-K,P **S92.491-** Other fracture of **right** great toe

CC-K,P **S92.492-** Other fracture of **left** great toe

CC-K,P **S92.499-** Other fracture of **unspecified** great toe

S92.5- **Fracture** of **lesser toe(s)**
  Excludes ❷: *physeal fracture of phalanx of toe (S99.2-)*

S92.50- **Unspecified** fracture of **lesser toe(s)**

CC-K,P **S92.501-** **Displaced** unspecified fracture of **right** lesser toe(s)

CC-K,P **S92.502-** **Displaced** unspecified fracture of **left** lesser toe(s)

CC-K,P **S92.503-** **Displaced** unspecified fracture of **unspecified** lesser toe(s)

CC-K,P **S92.504-** **Nondisplaced** unspecified fracture of **right** lesser toe(s)

CC-K,P **S92.505-** **Nondisplaced** unspecified fracture of **left** lesser toe(s)

CC-K,P **S92.506-** **Nondisplaced** unspecified fracture of **unspecified** lesser toe(s)

S92.51- Fracture of **proximal phalanx** of **lesser toe(s)**

CC-K,P **S92.511-** **Displaced** fracture of proximal phalanx of **right** lesser toe(s)

CC-K,P **S92.512-** **Displaced** fracture of proximal phalanx of **left** lesser toe(s)

CC-K,P **S92.513-** **Displaced** fracture of proximal phalanx of **unspecified** lesser toe(s)

CC-K,P **S92.514-** **Nondisplaced** fracture of proximal phalanx of **right** lesser toe(s)

CC-K,P **S92.515-** **Nondisplaced** fracture of proximal phalanx of **left** lesser toe(s)

CC-K,P **S92.516-** **Nondisplaced** fracture of proximal phalanx of **unspecified** lesser toe(s)

S92.52- Fracture of **medial phalanx** of **lesser toe(s)**

CC-K,P **S92.521-** **Displaced** fracture of medial phalanx of **right** lesser toe(s)

CC-K,P **S92.522-** **Displaced** fracture of medial phalanx of **left** lesser toe(s)

CC-K,P **S92.523-** **Displaced** fracture of medial phalanx of **unspecified** lesser toe(s)

CC-K,P **S92.524-** **Nondisplaced** fracture of medial phalanx of **right** lesser toe(s)

CC-K,P **S92.525-** **Nondisplaced** fracture of medial phalanx of **left** lesser toe(s)

CC-K,P **S92.526-** **Nondisplaced** fracture of medial phalanx of **unspecified** lesser toe(s)

S92.53- Fracture of **distal phalanx** of **lesser toe(s)**

CC-K,P **S92.531-** **Displaced** fracture of distal phalanx of **right** lesser toe(s)

CC-K,P **S92.532-** **Displaced** fracture of distal phalanx of **left** lesser toe(s)

CC-K,P **S92.533-** **Displaced** fracture of distal phalanx of **unspecified** lesser toe(s)

CC-K,P **S92.534-** **Nondisplaced** fracture of distal phalanx of **right** lesser toe(s)

CC-K,P **S92.535-** **Nondisplaced** fracture of distal phalanx of **left** lesser toe(s)

CC-K,P **S92.536-** **Nondisplaced** fracture of distal phalanx of **unspecified** lesser toe(s)

S92.59- **Other fracture** of **lesser toe(s)**

CC-K,P **S92.591-** Other fracture of **right** lesser toe(s)

CC-K,P **S92.592-** Other fracture of **left** lesser toe(s)

CC-K,P **S92.599-** Other fracture of **unspecified** lesser toe(s)

S92.8- **Other fracture** of **foot**, except ankle

S92.81- **Other** fracture of **foot**
  Sesamoid fracture of foot

CC-B,K,P **S92.811-** Other fracture of **right** foot

CC-B,K,P **S92.812-** Other fracture of **left** foot

CC-B,K,P **S92.819-** Other fracture of **unspecified** foot

S92.9- **Unspecified** fracture of foot and toe

S92.90- **Unspecified** fracture of **foot**

CC-B,K,P **S92.901-** Unspecified fracture of **right** foot

S 9 2 - S 9 2

CC-B,K,P **S92.902-** Unspecified fracture of <u>left</u> foot

CC-B,K,P **S92.909-** Unspecified fracture of <u>unspecified</u> foot

S92.91- <u>Unspecified</u> fracture of <u>toe</u>

CC-K,P **S92.911-** Unspecified fracture of <u>right</u> toe(s)

CC-K,P **S92.912-** Unspecified fracture of <u>left</u> toe(s)

CC-K,P **S92.919-** Unspecified fracture of <u>unspecified</u> toe(s)

S93- <u>Dislocation and sprain</u> of joints and ligaments at <u>ankle, foot and toe level</u>

Includes:
Avulsion of joint or ligament of ankle, foot and toe
Laceration of cartilage, joint or ligament of ankle, foot and toe
Sprain of cartilage, joint or ligament of ankle, foot and toe
Traumatic hemarthrosis of joint or ligament of ankle, foot and toe
Traumatic rupture of joint or ligament of ankle, foot and toe
Traumatic subluxation of joint or ligament of ankle, foot and toe
Traumatic tear of joint or ligament of ankle, foot and toe

Code also any associated open wound

Excludes ❷: *strain of muscle and tendon of ankle and foot (S96.-)*

The appropriate 7th character is to be added to each code from category S93:
A   <u>Initial</u> encounter
D   <u>Subsequent</u> encounter
S   <u>Sequela</u>

S93.0- Subluxation and dislocation of <u>ankle joint</u>
Subluxation and dislocation of astragalus
Subluxation and dislocation of fibula, lower end
Subluxation and dislocation of talus
Subluxation and dislocation of tibia, lower end

S93.01x- <u>Subluxation</u> of <u>right</u> ankle joint

S93.02x- <u>Subluxation</u> of <u>left</u> ankle joint

S93.03x- <u>Subluxation</u> of <u>unspecified</u> ankle joint

S93.04x- <u>Dislocation</u> of <u>right</u> ankle joint

S93.05x- <u>Dislocation</u> of <u>left</u> ankle joint

S93.06x- <u>Dislocation</u> of <u>unspecified</u> ankle joint

S93.1- Subluxation and dislocation of toe

S93.10- <u>Unspecified</u> subluxation and dislocation of <u>toe</u>
Dislocation of toe NOS
Subluxation of toe NOS

S93.101- Unspecified <u>subluxation</u> of <u>right</u> toe(s)

S93.102- Unspecified <u>subluxation</u> of <u>left</u> toe(s)

S93.103- Unspecified <u>subluxation</u> of <u>unspecified</u> toe(s)

S93.104- Unspecified <u>dislocation</u> of <u>right</u> toe(s)

S93.105- Unspecified <u>dislocation</u> of <u>left</u> toe(s)

S93.106- Unspecified <u>dislocation</u> of <u>unspecified</u> toe(s)

S93.11- <u>Dislocation</u> of <u>interphalangeal joint</u>

S93.111- Dislocation of interphalangeal joint of <u>right</u> <u>great</u> toe

S93.112- Dislocation of interphalangeal joint of <u>left</u> <u>great</u> toe

S93.113- Dislocation of interphalangeal joint of <u>unspecified</u> <u>great</u> toe

S93.114- Dislocation of interphalangeal joint of <u>right</u> <u>lesser</u> toe(s)

S93.115- Dislocation of interphalangeal joint of <u>left</u> <u>lesser</u> toe(s)

S93.116- Dislocation of interphalangeal joint of <u>unspecified</u> <u>lesser</u> toe(s)

S93.119- Dislocation of interphalangeal joint of <u>unspecified</u> toe(s)

S93.12- <u>Dislocation</u> of <u>metatarsophalangeal joint</u>

S93.121- Dislocation of metatarsophalangeal joint of <u>right</u> <u>great</u> toe

S93.122- Dislocation of metatarsophalangeal joint of <u>left</u> <u>great</u> toe

S93.123- Dislocation of metatarsophalangeal joint of <u>unspecified</u> <u>great</u> toe

S93.124- Dislocation of metatarsophalangeal joint of <u>right</u> <u>lesser</u> toe(s)

S93.125- Dislocation of metatarsophalangeal joint of <u>left</u> <u>lesser</u> toe(s)

S93.126- Dislocation of metatarsophalangeal joint of <u>unspecified</u> lesser toe(s)

S93.129- Dislocation of metatarsophalangeal joint of <u>unspecified</u> toe(s)

S93.13- <u>Subluxation</u> of <u>interphalangeal joint</u>

S93.131- Subluxation of interphalangeal joint of <u>right</u> <u>great</u> toe

S93.132- Subluxation of interphalangeal joint of <u>left</u> <u>great</u> toe

S93.133- Subluxation of interphalangeal joint of <u>unspecified</u> <u>great</u> toe

S93.134- Subluxation of interphalangeal joint of <u>right</u> <u>lesser</u> toe(s)

S93.135- Subluxation of interphalangeal joint of <u>left</u> <u>lesser</u> toe(s)

S93.136- Subluxation of interphalangeal joint of <u>unspecified</u> <u>lesser</u> toe(s)

S93.139- Subluxation of interphalangeal joint of <u>unspecified</u> toe(s)

S93.14- <u>Subluxation</u> of <u>metatarsophalangeal joint</u>

S93.141- Subluxation of metatarsophalangeal joint of <u>right</u> <u>great</u> toe

S93.142- Subluxation of metatarsophalangeal joint of <u>left</u> <u>great</u> toe

S93.143- Subluxation of metatarsophalangeal joint of <u>unspecified</u> <u>great</u> toe

S93.144- Subluxation of metatarsophalangeal joint of <u>right</u> <u>lesser</u> toe(s)

S93.145- Subluxation of metatarsophalangeal joint of <u>left</u> <u>lesser</u> toe(s)

S93.146- Subluxation of metatarsophalangeal joint of <u>unspecified</u> <u>lesser</u> toe(s)

S93.149- Subluxation of metatarsophalangeal joint of <u>unspecified</u> toe(s)

S93.3- Subluxation and dislocation of <u>foot</u>

Excludes ❷: *dislocation of toe (S93.1-)*

S93.30- <u>Unspecified</u> subluxation and dislocation of <u>foot</u>
Dislocation of foot NOS
Subluxation of foot NOS

S93.301- Unspecified <u>subluxation</u> of <u>right</u> foot

S93.302- Unspecified <u>subluxation</u> of <u>left</u> foot

S93.303- Unspecified <u>subluxation</u> of <u>unspecified</u> foot

S93.304- Unspecified <u>dislocation</u> of <u>right</u> foot

S93.305- Unspecified <u>dislocation</u> of <u>left</u> foot

S93.306- Unspecified <u>dislocation</u> of <u>unspecified</u> foot

S93.31- Subluxation and dislocation of <u>tarsal joint</u>

S93.311- <u>Subluxation</u> of tarsal joint of <u>right</u> foot

S93.312- <u>Subluxation</u> of tarsal joint of <u>left</u> foot

S93.313- <u>Subluxation</u> of tarsal joint of <u>unspecified</u> foot

S93.314- <u>Dislocation</u> of tarsal joint of <u>right</u> foot

S93.315- <u>Dislocation</u> of tarsal joint of <u>left</u> foot

S93.316- <u>Dislocation</u> of tarsal joint of <u>unspecified</u> foot

S93.32- Subluxation and dislocation of <u>tarsometatarsal joint</u>

S93.321- <u>Subluxation</u> of tarsometatarsal joint of <u>right</u> foot

S93.322- <u>Subluxation</u> of tarsometatarsal joint of <u>left</u> foot

S93.323- <u>Subluxation</u> of tarsometatarsal joint of <u>unspecified</u> foot

S93.324- <u>Dislocation</u> of tarsometatarsal joint of <u>right</u> foot

S93.325- <u>Dislocation</u> of tarsometatarsal joint of <u>left</u> foot

S93.326- <u>Dislocation</u> of tarsometatarsal joint of <u>unspecified</u> foot

S93.33- <u>Other</u> subluxation and dislocation of <u>foot</u>

S93.331- Other <u>subluxation</u> of <u>right</u> foot

S93.332- Other <u>subluxation</u> of <u>left</u> foot

S93.333- Other <u>subluxation</u> of <u>unspecified</u> foot

S93.334- Other <u>dislocation</u> of <u>right</u> foot

S93.335- Other <u>dislocation</u> of <u>left</u> foot

Excludes 1: = NOT CODED HERE! (Do not code both)

Excludes ❷: = Not Included Here

S93.336-   Other <u>dislocation</u> of <u>unspecified</u> foot

S93.4-   <u>Sprain</u> of <u>ankle</u>
Excludes ❷: injury of Achilles tendon (S86.0-)

S93.40-   <u>Sprain</u> of <u>unspecified ligament</u> of <u>ankle</u>
Sprain of ankle NOS
Sprained ankle NOS

S93.401-   Sprain of unspecified ligament of <u>right</u> ankle

S93.402-   Sprain of unspecified ligament of <u>left</u> ankle

S93.409-   Sprain of unspecified ligament of <u>unspecified</u> ankle

S93.41-   <u>Sprain</u> of <u>calcaneofibular</u> ligament

S93.411-   Sprain of calcaneofibular ligament of <u>right</u> ankle

S93.412-   Sprain of calcaneofibular ligament of <u>left</u> ankle

S93.419-   Sprain of calcaneofibular ligament of <u>unspecified</u> ankle

S93.42-   <u>Sprain</u> of <u>deltoid</u> ligament

S93.421-   Sprain of deltoid ligament of <u>right</u> ankle

S93.422-   Sprain of deltoid ligament of <u>left</u> ankle

S93.429-   Sprain of deltoid ligament of <u>unspecified</u> ankle

S93.43-   <u>Sprain</u> of <u>tibiofibular</u> ligament

S93.431-   Sprain of tibiofibular ligament of <u>right</u> ankle

S93.432-   Sprain of tibiofibular ligament of <u>left</u> ankle

S93.439-   Sprain of tibiofibular ligament of <u>unspecified</u> ankle

S93.49-   <u>Sprain</u> of <u>other ligament</u> of <u>ankle</u>
Sprain of internal collateral ligament
Sprain of talofibular ligament

S93.491-   Sprain of other ligament of <u>right</u> ankle

S93.492-   Sprain of other ligament of <u>left</u> ankle

S93.499-   Sprain of other ligament of <u>unspecified</u> ankle

S93.5-   <u>Sprain</u> of <u>toe</u>

S93.50-   <u>Unspecified sprain</u> of <u>toe</u>

S93.501-   Unspecified sprain of <u>right great</u> toe

S93.502-   Unspecified sprain of <u>left great</u> toe

S93.503-   Unspecified sprain of <u>unspecified great</u> toe

S93.504-   Unspecified sprain of <u>right lesser</u> toe(s)

S93.505-   Unspecified sprain of <u>left lesser</u> toe(s)

S93.506-   Unspecified sprain of <u>unspecified lesser</u> toe(s)

S93.509-   Unspecified sprain of <u>unspecified</u> toe(s)

S93.51-   <u>Sprain</u> of <u>interphalangeal joint</u> of <u>toe</u>

S93.511-   Sprain of interphalangeal joint of <u>right great</u> toe

S93.512-   Sprain of interphalangeal joint of <u>left great</u> toe

S93.513-   Sprain of interphalangeal joint of <u>unspecified great</u> toe

S93.514-   Sprain of interphalangeal joint of <u>right lesser</u> toe(s)

S93.515-   Sprain of interphalangeal joint of <u>left lesser</u> toe(s)

S93.516-   Sprain of interphalangeal joint of <u>unspecified lesser</u> toe(s)

S93.519-   Sprain of interphalangeal joint of <u>unspecified</u> toe(s)

S93.52-   <u>Sprain</u> of <u>metatarsophalangeal joint</u> of <u>toe</u>

S93.521-   Sprain of metatarsophalangeal joint of <u>right great</u> toe

S93.522-   Sprain of metatarsophalangeal joint of <u>left great</u> toe

S93.523-   Sprain of metatarsophalangeal joint of <u>unspecified great</u> toe

S93.524-   Sprain of metatarsophalangeal joint of <u>right lesser</u> toe(s)

S93.525-   Sprain of metatarsophalangeal joint of <u>left lesser</u> toe(s)

S93.526-   Sprain of metatarsophalangeal joint of <u>unspecified lesser</u> toe(s)

S93.529-   Sprain of metatarsophalangeal joint of <u>unspecified</u> toe(s)

S93.6-   <u>Sprain</u> of <u>foot</u>
*Excludes ❷: sprain of metatarsophalangeal joint of toe (S93.52-)
sprain of toe (S93.5-)*

S93.60-   <u>Unspecified sprain</u> of <u>foot</u>

S93.601-   Unspecified sprain of <u>right</u> foot

S93.602-   Unspecified sprain of <u>left</u> foot

S93.609-   Unspecified sprain of <u>unspecified</u> foot

S93.61-   <u>Sprain</u> of <u>tarsal ligament</u> of <u>foot</u>

S93.611-   Sprain of tarsal ligament of <u>right</u> foot

S93.612-   Sprain of tarsal ligament of <u>left</u> foot

S93.619-   Sprain of tarsal ligament of <u>unspecified</u> foot

S93.62-   <u>Sprain</u> of <u>tarsometatarsal ligament</u> of <u>foot</u>

S93.621-   Sprain of tarsometatarsal ligament of <u>right</u> foot

S93.622-   Sprain of tarsometatarsal ligament of <u>left</u> foot

S93.629-   Sprain of tarsometatarsal ligament of <u>unspecified</u> foot

S93.69-   <u>Other sprain</u> of <u>foot</u>

S93.691-   Other sprain of <u>right</u> foot

S93.692-   Other sprain of <u>left</u> foot

S93.699-   Other sprain of <u>unspecified</u> foot

S94-   <u>Injury of nerves</u> at <u>ankle and foot level</u>
Code also any associated open wound (S91.-)
The appropriate 7th character is to be added to each code from category S94:
A   <u>Initial</u> encounter
D   <u>Subsequent</u> encounter
S   <u>Sequela</u>

S94.0-   Injury of <u>lateral plantar nerve</u>

S94.00x-   Injury of lateral plantar nerve, <u>unspecified</u> leg

S94.01x-   Injury of lateral plantar nerve, <u>right</u> leg

S94.02x-   Injury of lateral plantar nerve, <u>left</u> leg

S94.1-   Injury of <u>medial plantar nerve</u>

S94.10x-   Injury of medial plantar nerve, <u>unspecified</u> leg

S94.11x-   Injury of medial plantar nerve, <u>right</u> leg

S94.12x-   Injury of medial plantar nerve, <u>left</u> leg

S94.2-   Injury of <u>deep peroneal nerve</u> at <u>ankle and foot level</u>
Injury of terminal, lateral branch of deep peroneal nerve

S94.20x-   Injury of deep peroneal nerve at ankle and foot level, <u>unspecified</u> leg

S94.21x-   Injury of deep peroneal nerve at ankle and foot level, <u>right</u> leg

S94.22x-   Injury of deep peroneal nerve at ankle and foot level, <u>left</u> leg

S94.3-   Injury of <u>cutaneous sensory nerve</u> at <u>ankle and foot level</u>

S94.30x-   Injury of cutaneous sensory nerve at ankle and foot level, <u>unspecified</u> leg

S94.31x-   Injury of cutaneous sensory nerve at ankle and foot level, <u>right</u> leg

S94.32x-   Injury of cutaneous sensory nerve at ankle and foot level, <u>left</u> leg

S94.8-   Injury of other nerves at ankle and foot level

S94.8x-   Injury of <u>other nerves</u> at <u>ankle and foot level</u>

S94.8x1-   Injury of other nerves at ankle and foot level, <u>right</u> leg

S94.8x2-   Injury of other nerves at ankle and foot level, <u>left</u> leg

S94.8x9-   Injury of other nerves at ankle and foot level, <u>unspecified</u> leg

S94.9-   Injury of <u>unspecified nerve</u> at <u>ankle and foot level</u>

S94.90x-   Injury of unspecified nerve at ankle and foot level, <u>unspecified</u> leg

S94.91x-   Injury of unspecified nerve at ankle and foot level, <u>right</u> leg

S94.92x-   Injury of unspecified nerve at ankle and foot level, <u>left</u> leg

S 9 3 - S 9 4

Excludes 1: = NOT CODED HERE! (Do not code both)   *Excludes ❷:* = Not Included Here

S95- Injury of blood vessels at ankle and foot level
Code also any associated open wound (S91.-)
Excludes ❷: injury of posterior tibial artery and vein (S85.1-, S85.8-)

The appropriate 7th character is to be added to each code from category S95:
A Initial encounter
D Subsequent encounter
S Sequela

S95.0- Injury of dorsal artery of foot

S95.00- Unspecified injury of dorsal artery of foot

CC-A **S95.001-** Unspecified injury of dorsal artery of right foot

CC-A **S95.002-** Unspecified injury of dorsal artery of left foot

CC-A **S95.009-** Unspecified injury of dorsal artery of unspecified foot

S95.01- Laceration of dorsal artery of foot

CC-A **S95.011-** Laceration of dorsal artery of right foot

CC-A **S95.012-** Laceration of dorsal artery of left foot

CC-A **S95.019-** Laceration of dorsal artery of unspecified foot

S95.09- Other specified injury of dorsal artery of foot

CC-A **S95.091-** Other specified injury of dorsal artery of right foot

CC-A **S95.092-** Other specified injury of dorsal artery of left foot

CC-A **S95.099-** Other specified injury of dorsal artery of unspecified foot

S95.1- Injury of plantar artery of foot

S95.10- Unspecified injury of plantar artery of foot

CC-A **S95.101-** Unspecified injury of plantar artery of right foot

CC-A **S95.102-** Unspecified injury of plantar artery of left foot

CC-A **S95.109-** Unspecified injury of plantar artery of unspecified foot

S95.11- Laceration of plantar artery of foot

CC-A **S95.111-** Laceration of plantar artery of right foot

CC-A **S95.112-** Laceration of plantar artery of left foot

CC-A **S95.119-** Laceration of plantar artery of unspecified foot

S95.19- Other specified injury of plantar artery of foot

CC-A **S95.191-** Other specified injury of plantar artery of right foot

CC-A **S95.192-** Other specified injury of plantar artery of left foot

CC-A **S95.199-** Other specified injury of plantar artery of unspecified foot

S95.2- Injury of dorsal vein of foot

S95.20- Unspecified injury of dorsal vein of foot

CC-A **S95.201-** Unspecified injury of dorsal vein of right foot

CC-A **S95.202-** Unspecified injury of dorsal vein of left foot

CC-A **S95.209-** Unspecified injury of dorsal vein of unspecified foot

S95.21- Laceration of dorsal vein of foot

CC-A **S95.211-** Laceration of dorsal vein of right foot

CC-A **S95.212-** Laceration of dorsal vein of left foot

CC-A **S95.219-** Laceration of dorsal vein of unspecified foot

S95.29- Other specified injury of dorsal vein of foot

CC-A **S95.291-** Other specified injury of dorsal vein of right foot

CC-A **S95.292-** Other specified injury of dorsal vein of left foot

CC-A **S95.299-** Other specified injury of dorsal vein of unspecified foot

S95.8- Injury of other blood vessels at ankle and foot level

S95.80- Unspecified injury of other blood vessels at ankle and foot level

CC-A **S95.801-** Unspecified injury of other blood vessels at ankle and foot level, right leg

CC-A **S95.802-** Unspecified injury of other blood vessels at ankle and foot level, left leg

CC-A **S95.809-** Unspecified injury of other blood vessels at ankle and foot level, unspecified leg

S95.81- Laceration of other blood vessels at ankle and foot level

CC-A **S95.811-** Laceration of other blood vessels at ankle and foot level, right leg

CC-A **S95.812-** Laceration of other blood vessels at ankle and foot level, left leg

CC-A **S95.819-** Laceration of other blood vessels at ankle and foot level, unspecified leg

S95.89- Other specified injury of other blood vessels at ankle and foot level

CC-A **S95.891-** Other specified injury of other blood vessels at ankle and foot level, right leg

CC-A **S95.892-** Other specified injury of other blood vessels at ankle and foot level, left leg

CC-A **S95.899-** Other specified injury of other blood vessels at ankle and foot level, unspecified leg

S95.9- Injury of unspecified blood vessel at ankle and foot level

S95.90- Unspecified injury of unspecified blood vessel at ankle and foot level

CC-A **S95.901-** Unspecified injury of unspecified blood vessel at ankle and foot level, right leg

CC-A **S95.902-** Unspecified injury of unspecified blood vessel at ankle and foot level, left leg

CC-A **S95.909-** Unspecified injury of unspecified blood vessel at ankle and foot level, unspecified leg

S95.91- Laceration of unspecified blood vessel at ankle and foot level

CC-A **S95.911-** Laceration of unspecified blood vessel at ankle and foot level, right leg

CC-A **S95.912-** Laceration of unspecified blood vessel at ankle and foot level, left leg

CC-A **S95.919-** Laceration of unspecified blood vessel at ankle and foot level, unspecified leg

S95.99- Other specified injury of unspecified blood vessel at ankle and foot level

CC-A **S95.991-** Other specified injury of unspecified blood vessel at ankle and foot level, right leg

CC-A **S95.992-** Other specified injury of unspecified blood vessel at ankle and foot level, left leg

CC-A **S95.999-** Other specified injury of unspecified blood vessel at ankle and foot level, unspecified leg

S96- Injury of muscle and tendon at ankle and foot level
Code also any associated open wound (S91.-)
Excludes ❷: injury of Achilles tendon (S86.0-)
sprain of joints and ligaments of ankle and foot (S93.-)

The appropriate 7th character is to be added to each code from category S96:
A Initial encounter
D Subsequent encounter
S Sequela

S96.0- Injury of muscle and tendon of long flexor muscle of toe at ankle and foot level

S96.00- Unspecified injury of muscle and tendon of long flexor muscle of toe at ankle and foot level

S96.001- Unspecified injury of muscle and tendon of long flexor muscle of toe at ankle and foot level, right foot

S96.002- Unspecified injury of muscle and tendon of long flexor muscle of toe at ankle and foot level, left foot

S96.009- Unspecified injury of muscle and tendon of long flexor muscle of toe at ankle and foot level, unspecified foot

S96.01- Strain of muscle and tendon of long flexor muscle of toe at ankle and foot level

S96.011- Strain of muscle and tendon of long flexor muscle of toe at ankle and foot level, right foot

S96.012- Strain of muscle and tendon of long flexor muscle of toe at ankle and foot level, left foot

S96.019- Strain of muscle and tendon of long flexor muscle of toe at ankle and foot level, unspecified foot

S96.02- Laceration of muscle and tendon of long flexor muscle of toe at ankle and foot level

CC-A **S96.021-** Laceration of muscle and tendon of long flexor muscle of toe at ankle and foot level, right foot

CC-A **S96.022-** Laceration of muscle and tendon of long flexor muscle of toe at ankle and foot level, <u>left</u> foot

CC-A **S96.029-** Laceration of muscle and tendon of long flexor muscle of toe at ankle and foot level, <u>unspecified</u> foot

S96.09- <u>Other injury</u> of muscle and tendon of <u>long flexor muscle</u> of <u>toe</u> at <u>ankle and foot level</u>

S96.091- Other injury of muscle and tendon of long flexor muscle of toe at ankle and foot level, <u>right</u> foot

S96.092- Other injury of muscle and tendon of long flexor muscle of toe at ankle and foot level, <u>left</u> foot

S96.099- Other injury of muscle and tendon of long flexor muscle of toe at ankle and foot level, <u>unspecified</u> foot

S96.1- <u>Injury</u> of muscle and tendon of <u>long extensor muscle</u> of <u>toe</u> at <u>ankle and foot level</u>

S96.10- <u>Unspecified</u> injury of muscle and tendon of <u>long extensor muscle</u> of <u>toe</u> at <u>ankle and foot level</u>

S96.101- Unspecified injury of muscle and tendon of long extensor muscle of toe at ankle and foot level, <u>right</u> foot

S96.102- Unspecified injury of muscle and tendon of long extensor muscle of toe at ankle and foot level, <u>left</u> foot

S96.109- Unspecified injury of muscle and tendon of long extensor muscle of toe at ankle and foot level, <u>unspecified</u> foot

S96.11- <u>Strain</u> of muscle and tendon of <u>long extensor muscle</u> of <u>toe</u> at <u>ankle and foot level</u>

S96.111- Strain of muscle and tendon of long extensor muscle of toe at ankle and foot level, <u>right</u> foot

S96.112- Strain of muscle and tendon of long extensor muscle of toe at ankle and foot level, <u>left</u> foot

S96.119- Strain of muscle and tendon of long extensor muscle of toe at ankle and foot level, <u>unspecified</u> foot

S96.12- <u>Laceration</u> of muscle and tendon of <u>long extensor muscle</u> of <u>toe</u> at <u>ankle and foot level</u>

CC-A **S96.121-** Laceration of muscle and tendon of long extensor muscle of toe at ankle and foot level, <u>right</u> foot

CC-A **S96.122-** Laceration of muscle and tendon of long extensor muscle of toe at ankle and foot level, <u>left</u> foot

CC-A **S96.129-** Laceration of muscle and tendon of long extensor muscle of toe at ankle and foot level, <u>unspecified</u> foot

S96.19- <u>Other specified injury</u> of muscle and tendon of <u>long extensor muscle</u> of <u>toe</u> at <u>ankle and foot level</u>

S96.191- Other specified injury of muscle and tendon of long extensor muscle of toe at ankle and foot level, <u>right</u> foot

S96.192- Other specified injury of muscle and tendon of long extensor muscle of toe at ankle and foot level, <u>left</u> foot

S96.199- Other specified injury of muscle and tendon of long extensor muscle of toe at ankle and foot level, <u>unspecified</u> foot

S96.2- <u>Injury</u> of <u>intrinsic muscle and tendon</u> at <u>ankle and foot level</u>

S96.20- <u>Unspecified</u> injury of <u>intrinsic muscle and tendon</u> at <u>ankle and foot level</u>

S96.201- Unspecified injury of intrinsic muscle and tendon at ankle and foot level, <u>right</u> foot

S96.202- Unspecified injury of intrinsic muscle and tendon at ankle and foot level, <u>left</u> foot

S96.209- Unspecified injury of intrinsic muscle and tendon at ankle and foot level, <u>unspecified</u> foot

S96.21- <u>Strain</u> of <u>intrinsic muscle and tendon</u> at <u>ankle and foot level</u>

S96.211- Strain of intrinsic muscle and tendon at ankle and foot level, <u>right</u> foot

S96.212- Strain of intrinsic muscle and tendon at ankle and foot level, <u>left</u> foot

S96.219- Strain of intrinsic muscle and tendon at ankle and foot level, <u>unspecified</u> foot

S96.22- <u>Laceration</u> of <u>intrinsic muscle and tendon</u> at <u>ankle and foot level</u>

CC-A **S96.221-** Laceration of intrinsic muscle and tendon at ankle and foot level, <u>right</u> foot

CC-A **S96.222-** Laceration of intrinsic muscle and tendon at ankle and foot level, <u>left</u> foot

CC-A **S96.229-** Laceration of intrinsic muscle and tendon at ankle and foot level, <u>unspecified</u> foot

S96.29- <u>Other specified injury</u> of <u>intrinsic muscle and tendon</u> at <u>ankle and foot level</u>

S96.291- Other specified injury of intrinsic muscle and tendon at ankle and foot level, <u>right</u> foot

S96.292- Other specified injury of intrinsic muscle and tendon at ankle and foot level, <u>left</u> foot

S96.299- Other specified injury of intrinsic muscle and tendon at ankle and foot level, <u>unspecified</u> foot

S96.8- <u>Injury</u> of <u>other specified muscles and tendons</u> at <u>ankle and foot level</u>

S96.80- <u>Unspecified</u> injury of <u>other specified muscles and tendons</u> at <u>ankle and foot level</u>

S96.801- Unspecified injury of other specified muscles and tendons at ankle and foot level, <u>right</u> foot

S96.802- Unspecified injury of other specified muscles and tendons at ankle and foot level, <u>left</u> foot

S96.809- Unspecified injury of other specified muscles and tendons at ankle and foot level, <u>unspecified</u> foot

S96.81- <u>Strain</u> of <u>other specified muscles and tendons</u> at <u>ankle and foot level</u>

S96.811- Strain of other specified muscles and tendons at ankle and foot level, <u>right</u> foot

S96.812- Strain of other specified muscles and tendons at ankle and foot level, <u>left</u> foot

S96.819- Strain of other specified muscles and tendons at ankle and foot level, <u>unspecified</u> foot

S96.82- <u>Laceration</u> of <u>other specified muscles and tendons</u> at <u>ankle and foot level</u>

CC-A **S96.821-** Laceration of other specified muscles and tendons at ankle and foot level, <u>right</u> foot

CC-A **S96.822-** Laceration of other specified muscles and tendons at ankle and foot level, <u>left</u> foot

CC-A **S96.829-** Laceration of other specified muscles and tendons at ankle and foot level, <u>unspecified</u> foot

S96.89- <u>Other specified injury</u> of <u>other specified muscles and tendons</u> at <u>ankle and foot level</u>

S96.891- Other specified injury of other specified muscles and tendons at ankle and foot level, <u>right</u> foot

S96.892- Other specified injury of other specified muscles and tendons at ankle and foot level, <u>left</u> foot

S96.899- Other specified injury of other specified muscles and tendons at ankle and foot level, <u>unspecified</u> foot

S96.9- <u>Injury</u> of <u>unspecified muscle and tendon</u> at <u>ankle and foot level</u>

S96.90- <u>Unspecified</u> injury of <u>unspecified muscle and tendon</u> at <u>ankle and foot level</u>

S96.901- Unspecified injury of unspecified muscle and tendon at ankle and foot level, <u>right</u> foot

S96.902- Unspecified injury of unspecified muscle and tendon at ankle and foot level, <u>left</u> foot

S96.909- Unspecified injury of unspecified muscle and tendon at ankle and foot level, <u>unspecified</u> foot

S96.91- <u>Strain</u> of <u>unspecified muscle and tendon</u> at <u>ankle and foot level</u>

S96.911- Strain of unspecified muscle and tendon at ankle and foot level, <u>right</u> foot

S 9 6 I S 9 6

Excludes 1: = NOT CODED HERE! (Do not code both)   **1133**   *Excludes ❷:* = Not Included Here

S96.912- Strain of unspecified muscle and tendon at ankle and foot level, <u>left</u> foot

S96.919- Strain of unspecified muscle and tendon at ankle and foot level, <u>unspecified</u> foot

S96.92- <u>Laceration</u> of <u>unspecified muscle and tendon</u> at <u>ankle and foot level</u>

CC-A S96.921- Laceration of unspecified muscle and tendon at ankle and foot level, <u>right</u> foot

CC-A S96.922- Laceration of unspecified muscle and tendon at ankle and foot level, <u>left</u> foot

CC-A S96.929- Laceration of unspecified muscle and tendon at ankle and foot level, <u>unspecified</u> foot

S96.99- <u>Other specified injury</u> of <u>unspecified muscle and tendon</u> at <u>ankle and foot level</u>

S96.991- Other specified injury of unspecified muscle and tendon at ankle and foot level, <u>right</u> foot

S96.992- Other specified injury of unspecified muscle and tendon at ankle and foot level, <u>left</u> foot

S96.999- Other specified injury of unspecified muscle and tendon at ankle and foot level, <u>unspecified</u> foot

S97- <u>Crushing injury</u> of <u>ankle and foot</u>
Use additional code(s) for all associated injuries

The appropriate 7th character is to be added to each code from category S97:
A <u>Initial</u> encounter
D <u>Subsequent</u> encounter
S <u>Sequela</u>

S97.0- <u>Crushing</u> injury of <u>ankle</u>
S97.00x- Crushing injury of <u>unspecified</u> ankle
S97.01x- Crushing injury of <u>right</u> ankle
S97.02x- Crushing injury of <u>left</u> ankle

S97.1- <u>Crushing</u> injury of <u>toe</u>
S97.10- <u>Crushing</u> injury of <u>unspecified toe(s)</u>
S97.101- Crushing injury of unspecified <u>right</u> toe(s)
S97.102- Crushing injury of unspecified <u>left</u> toe(s)
S97.109- Crushing injury of unspecified toe(s)
Crushing injury of toe NOS
S97.11- <u>Crushing</u> injury of <u>great toe</u>
S97.111- Crushing injury of <u>right</u> great toe
S97.112- Crushing injury of <u>left</u> great toe
S97.119- Crushing injury of <u>unspecified</u> great toe
S97.12- <u>Crushing</u> injury of <u>lesser toe(s)</u>
S97.121- Crushing injury of <u>right</u> lesser toe(s)
S97.122- Crushing injury of <u>left</u> lesser toe(s)
S97.129- Crushing injury of <u>unspecified</u> lesser toe(s)

S97.8- <u>Crushing</u> injury of <u>foot</u>
S97.80x- Crushing injury of <u>unspecified</u> foot
Crushing injury of foot NOS
S97.81x- Crushing injury of <u>right</u> foot
S97.82x- Crushing injury of <u>left</u> foot

S98- <u>Traumatic amputation</u> of <u>ankle and foot</u>
Note: An amputation not identified as partial or complete should be coded to complete

The appropriate 7th character is to be added to each code from category S98:
A <u>Initial</u> encounter
D <u>Subsequent</u> encounter
S <u>Sequela</u>

S98.0- <u>Traumatic amputation</u> of <u>foot</u> at <u>ankle level</u>
S98.01- <u>Complete</u> traumatic amputation of foot at ankle level
CC-A S98.011- Complete traumatic amputation of <u>right</u> foot at ankle level
CC-A S98.012- Complete traumatic amputation of <u>left</u> foot at ankle level
CC-A S98.019- Complete traumatic amputation of <u>unspecified</u> foot at ankle level

S98.02- <u>Partial</u> traumatic amputation of foot at ankle level
CC-A S98.021- Partial traumatic amputation of <u>right</u> foot at ankle level
CC-A S98.022- Partial traumatic amputation of <u>left</u> foot at ankle level
CC-A S98.029- Partial traumatic amputation of <u>unspecified</u> foot at ankle level

S98.1- <u>Traumatic amputation</u> of <u>one toe</u>
S98.11- <u>Complete</u> traumatic amputation of <u>great</u> toe
S98.111- Complete traumatic amputation of <u>right</u> great toe
S98.112- Complete traumatic amputation of <u>left</u> great toe
S98.119- Complete traumatic amputation of <u>unspecified</u> great toe
S98.12- <u>Partial</u> traumatic amputation of <u>great</u> toe
S98.121- Partial traumatic amputation of <u>right</u> great toe
S98.122- Partial traumatic amputation of <u>left</u> great toe
S98.129- Partial traumatic amputation of <u>unspecified</u> great toe
S98.13- <u>Complete</u> traumatic amputation of <u>one lesser toe</u>
Traumatic amputation of toe NOS
S98.131- Complete traumatic amputation of one <u>right</u> lesser toe
S98.132- Complete traumatic amputation of one <u>left</u> lesser toe
S98.139- Complete traumatic amputation of one <u>unspecified</u> lesser toe
S98.14- <u>Partial</u> traumatic amputation of <u>one lesser toe</u>
S98.141- Partial traumatic amputation of one <u>right</u> lesser toe
S98.142- Partial traumatic amputation of one <u>left</u> lesser toe
S98.149- Partial traumatic amputation of one <u>unspecified</u> lesser toe

S98.2- <u>Traumatic amputation</u> of <u>two or more lesser toes</u>
S98.21- <u>Complete</u> traumatic amputation of two or more lesser toes
S98.211- Complete traumatic amputation of two or more <u>right</u> lesser toes
S98.212- Complete traumatic amputation of two or more <u>left</u> lesser toes
S98.219- Complete traumatic amputation of two or more <u>unspecified</u> lesser toes
S98.22- <u>Partial</u> traumatic amputation of two or more lesser toes
S98.221- Partial traumatic amputation of two or more <u>right</u> lesser toes
S98.222- Partial traumatic amputation of two or more <u>left</u> lesser toes
S98.229- Partial traumatic amputation of two or more <u>unspecified</u> lesser toes

S98.3- <u>Traumatic amputation</u> of <u>midfoot</u>
S98.31- <u>Complete</u> traumatic amputation of midfoot
CC-A S98.311- Complete traumatic amputation of <u>right</u> midfoot
CC-A S98.312- Complete traumatic amputation of <u>left</u> midfoot
CC-A S98.319- Complete traumatic amputation of <u>unspecified</u> midfoot
S98.32- <u>Partial</u> traumatic amputation of midfoot
CC-A S98.321- Partial traumatic amputation of <u>right</u> midfoot
CC-A S98.322- Partial traumatic amputation of <u>left</u> midfoot
CC-A S98.329- Partial traumatic amputation of <u>unspecified</u> midfoot

S98.9- <u>Traumatic amputation</u> of <u>foot, level unspecified</u>
S98.91- <u>Complete</u> traumatic amputation of foot, <u>level unspecified</u>
CC-A S98.911- Complete traumatic amputation of <u>right</u> foot, level unspecified
CC-A S98.912- Complete traumatic amputation of <u>left</u> foot, level unspecified
CC-A S98.919- Complete traumatic amputation of <u>unspecified</u> foot, level unspecified

S98.92- Partial traumatic amputation of foot, level unspecified
CC-A **S98.921-** Partial traumatic amputation of right foot, level unspecified
CC-A **S98.922-** Partial traumatic amputation of left foot, level unspecified
CC-A **S98.929-** Partial traumatic amputation of unspecified foot, level unspecified

S99- Other and unspecified injuries of ankle and foot

S99.0- Physeal fracture of calcaneus
The appropriate 7th character is to be added to each code from subcategory S99.0:
A Initial encounter for closed fracture
B Initial encounter for open fracture
D Subsequent encounter for fracture with routine healing
G Subsequent encounter for fracture with delayed healing
K Subsequent encounter for fracture with nonunion
P Subsequent encounter for fracture with malunion
S Sequela

S99.00- Unspecified physeal fracture of calcaneus
S99.001- Unspecified physeal fracture of right calcaneus
S99.002- Unspecified physeal fracture of left calcaneus
S99.009- Unspecified physeal fracture of unspecified calcaneus

S99.01- Salter-Harris Type I physeal fracture of calcaneus
S99.011- Salter-Harris Type I physeal fracture of right calcaneus
S99.012- Salter-Harris Type I physeal fracture of left calcaneus
S99.019- Salter-Harris Type I physeal fracture of unspecified calcaneus

S99.02- Salter-Harris Type II physeal fracture of calcaneus
S99.021- Salter-Harris Type II physeal fracture of right calcaneus
S99.022- Salter-Harris Type II physeal fracture of left calcaneus
S99.029- Salter-Harris Type II physeal fracture of unspecified calcaneus

S99.03- Salter-Harris Type III physeal fracture of calcaneus
S99.031- Salter-Harris Type III physeal fracture of right calcaneus
S99.032- Salter-Harris Type III physeal fracture of left calcaneus
S99.039- Salter-Harris Type III physeal fracture of unspecified calcaneus

S99.04- Salter-Harris Type IV physeal fracture of calcaneus
S99.041- Salter-Harris Type IV physeal fracture of right calcaneus
S99.042- Salter-Harris Type IV physeal fracture of left calcaneus
S99.049- Salter-Harris Type IV physeal fracture of unspecified calcaneus

S99.09- Other physeal fracture of calcaneus
S99.091- Other physeal fracture of right calcaneus
S99.092- Other physeal fracture of left calcaneus
S99.099- Other physeal fracture of unspecified calcaneus

S99.1- Physeal fracture of metatarsal
The appropriate 7th character is to be added to each code from subcategory S99.1:
A Initial encounter for closed fracture
B Initial encounter for open fracture
D Subsequent encounter for fracture with routine healing
G Subsequent encounter for fracture with delayed healing
K Subsequent encounter for fracture with nonunion
P Subsequent encounter for fracture with malunion
S Sequela

S99.10- Unspecified physeal fracture of metatarsal
S99.101- Unspecified physeal fracture of right metatarsal
S99.102- Unspecified physeal fracture of left metatarsal
S99.109- Unspecified physeal fracture of unspecified metatarsal

S99.11- Salter-Harris Type I physeal fracture of metatarsal
S99.111- Salter-Harris Type I physeal fracture of right metatarsal
S99.112- Salter-Harris Type I physeal fracture of left metatarsal
S99.119- Salter-Harris Type I physeal fracture of unspecified metatarsal

S99.12- Salter-Harris Type II physeal fracture of metatarsal
S99.121- Salter-Harris Type II physeal fracture of right metatarsal
S99.122- Salter-Harris Type II physeal fracture of left metatarsal
S99.129- Salter-Harris Type II physeal fracture of unspecified metatarsal

S99.13- Salter-Harris Type III physeal fracture of metatarsal
S99.131- Salter-Harris Type III physeal fracture of right metatarsal
S99.132- Salter-Harris Type III physeal fracture of left metatarsal
S99.139- Salter-Harris Type III physeal fracture of unspecified metatarsal

S99.14- Salter-Harris Type IV physeal fracture of metatarsal
S99.141- Salter-Harris Type IV physeal fracture of right metatarsal
S99.142- Salter-Harris Type IV physeal fracture of left metatarsal
S99.149- Salter-Harris Type IV physeal fracture of unspecified metatarsal

S99.19- Other physeal fracture of metatarsal
S99.191- Other physeal fracture of right metatarsal
S99.192- Other physeal fracture of left metatarsal
S99.199- Other physeal fracture of unspecified metatarsal

S99.2- Physeal fracture of phalanx of toe
The appropriate 7th character is to be added to each code from subcategory S99.2:
A Initial encounter for closed fracture
B Initial encounter for open fracture
D Subsequent encounter for fracture with routine healing
G Subsequent encounter for fracture with delayed healing
K Subsequent encounter for fracture with nonunion
P Subsequent encounter for fracture with malunion
S Sequela

S99.20- Unspecified physeal fracture of phalanx of toe
S99.201- Unspecified physeal fracture of phalanx of right toe
S99.202- Unspecified physeal fracture of phalanx of left toe
S99.209- Unspecified physeal fracture of phalanx of unspecified toe

S99.21- Salter-Harris Type I physeal fracture of phalanx of toe
S99.211- Salter-Harris Type I physeal fracture of phalanx of right toe
S99.212- Salter-Harris Type I physeal fracture of phalanx of left toe

S98 - S99

S99.219- Salter-Harris <u>Type I</u> physeal fracture of phalanx of <u>unspecified</u> toe

S99.22- <u>Salter-Harris Type II</u> physeal fracture of phalanx of toe

S99.221- Salter-Harris <u>Type II</u> physeal fracture of phalanx of <u>right</u> toe

S99.222- Salter-Harris <u>Type II</u> physeal fracture of phalanx of <u>left</u> toe

S99.229- Salter-Harris <u>Type II</u> physeal fracture of phalanx of <u>unspecified</u> toe

S99.23- <u>Salter-Harris Type III</u> physeal fracture of phalanx of toe

S99.231- Salter-Harris <u>Type III</u> physeal fracture of phalanx of <u>right</u> toe

S99.232- Salter-Harris <u>Type III</u> physeal fracture of phalanx of <u>left</u> toe

S99.239- Salter-Harris <u>Type III</u> physeal fracture of phalanx of <u>unspecified</u> toe

S99.24- <u>Salter-Harris Type IV</u> physeal fracture of phalanx of toe

S99.241- Salter-Harris <u>Type IV</u> physeal fracture of phalanx of <u>right</u> toe

S99.242- Salter-Harris <u>Type IV</u> physeal fracture of phalanx of <u>left</u> toe

S99.249- Salter-Harris <u>Type IV</u> physeal fracture of phalanx of <u>unspecified</u> toe

S99.29- <u>Other</u> physeal fracture of phalanx of toe

S99.291- Other physeal fracture of phalanx of <u>right</u> toe

S99.292- Other physeal fracture of phalanx of <u>left</u> toe

S99.299- Other physeal fracture of phalanx of <u>unspecified</u> toe

S99.8- <u>Other specified injuries</u> of <u>ankle and foot</u>

The appropriate 7th character is to be added to each code from subcategory S99.8:
A <u>Initial</u> encounter
D <u>Subsequent</u> encounter
S <u>Sequela</u>

S99.81- <u>Other specified injuries</u> of <u>ankle</u>

S99.811- Other specified injuries of <u>right</u> ankle

S99.812- Other specified injuries of <u>left</u> ankle

S99.819- Other specified injuries of <u>unspecified</u> ankle

S99.82- <u>Other specified injuries</u> of <u>foot</u>

S99.821- Other specified injuries of <u>right</u> foot

S99.822- Other specified injuries of <u>left</u> foot

S99.829- Other specified injuries of <u>unspecified</u> foot

S99.9- <u>Unspecified injury</u> of <u>ankle and foot</u>

The appropriate 7th character is to be added to each code from subcategory S99.9:
A <u>Initial</u> encounter
D <u>Subsequent</u> encounter
S <u>Sequela</u>

S99.91- <u>Unspecified</u> injury of <u>ankle</u>

S99.911- Unspecified injury of <u>right</u> ankle

S99.912- Unspecified injury of <u>left</u> ankle

S99.919- Unspecified injury of <u>unspecified</u> ankle

S99.92- <u>Unspecified</u> injury of <u>foot</u>

S99.921- Unspecified injury of <u>right</u> foot

S99.922- Unspecified injury of <u>left</u> foot

S99.929- Unspecified injury of <u>unspecified</u> foot

Injury, poisoning and certain other consequences of external causes (T07-T88)

Injuries involving multiple body regions (T07)

Excludes 1: burns and corrosions (T20-T32)
frostbite (T33-T34)
insect bite or sting, venomous (T63.4)
sunburn (L55-)

T07   Unspecified multiple injuries
Excludes 1: injury NOS (T14-)

Injury of unspecified body region (T14)

T14-   Injury of unspecified body region
Excludes 1: multiple unspecified injuries (T07)

T14.8   Other injury of unspecified body region
Abrasion NOS
Contusion NOS
Crush injury NOS
Fracture NOS
Skin injury NOS
Vascular injury NOS

T14.9-   Unspecified injury

T14.90   Injury, unspecified
Injury NOS

T14.91   Suicide attempt
Attempted suicide NOS

Effects of foreign body entering through natural orifice (T15-T19)

Excludes ❷: foreign body accidentally left in operation wound (T81.5-)
foreign body in penetrating wound — see open wound by body region
residual foreign body in soft tissue (M79.5)
splinter, without open wound — see superficial injury by body region

T15-   Foreign body on external eye
Excludes ❷: foreign body in penetrating wound of orbit and eye ball (S05.4-, S05.5-)
open wound of eyelid and periocular area (S01.1-)
retained foreign body in eyelid (H02.8-)
retained (old) foreign body in penetrating wound of orbit and eye ball (H05.5-, H44.6-, H44.7-)
superficial foreign body of eyelid and periocular area (S00.25-)

The appropriate 7th character is to be added to each code from category T15:
A   Initial encounter
D   Subsequent encounter
S   Sequela

T15.0-   Foreign body in cornea
T15.00x-   Foreign body in cornea, unspecified eye
T15.01x-   Foreign body in cornea, right eye
T15.02x-   Foreign body in cornea, left eye

T15.1-   Foreign body in conjunctival sac
T15.10x-   Foreign body in conjunctival sac, unspecified eye
T15.11x-   Foreign body in conjunctival sac, right eye
T15.12x-   Foreign body in conjunctival sac, left eye

T15.8-   Foreign body in other and multiple parts of external eye
Foreign body in lacrimal punctum
T15.80x-   Foreign body in other and multiple parts of external eye, unspecified eye
T15.81x-   Foreign body in other and multiple parts of external eye, right eye
T15.82x-   Foreign body in other and multiple parts of external eye, left eye

T15.9-   Foreign body on external eye, part unspecified
T15.90x-   Foreign body on external eye, part unspecified, unspecified eye
T15.91x-   Foreign body on external eye, part unspecified, right eye
T15.92x-   Foreign body on external eye, part unspecified, left eye

T16-   Foreign body in ear
Includes: Foreign body in auditory canal
The appropriate 7th character is to be added to each code from category T16:
A   Initial encounter
D   Subsequent encounter
S   Sequela

T16.1xx-   Foreign body in right ear
T16.2xx-   Foreign body in left ear
T16.9xx-   Foreign body in ear, unspecified ear

T17-   Foreign body in respiratory tract
The appropriate 7th character is to be added to each code from category T17:
A   Initial encounter
D   Subsequent encounter
S   Sequela

T17.0xx-   Foreign body in nasal sinus
T17.1xx-   Foreign body in nostril
Foreign body in nose NOS
T17.2-   Foreign body in pharynx
Foreign body in nasopharynx
Foreign body in throat NOS
T17.20-   Unspecified foreign body in pharynx
T17.200-   Unspecified foreign body in pharynx causing asphyxiation
T17.208-   Unspecified foreign body in pharynx causing other injury
T17.21-   Gastric contents in pharynx
Aspiration of gastric contents into pharynx
Vomitus in pharynx
T17.210-   Gastric contents in pharynx causing asphyxiation
T17.218-   Gastric contents in pharynx causing other injury
T17.22-   Food in pharynx
Bones in pharynx
Seeds in pharynx
T17.220-   Food in pharynx causing asphyxiation
T17.228-   Food in pharynx causing other injury
T17.29-   Other foreign object in pharynx
T17.290-   Other foreign object in pharynx causing asphyxiation
T17.298-   Other foreign object in pharynx causing other injury
T17.3-   Foreign body in larynx
T17.30-   Unspecified foreign body in larynx
T17.300-   Unspecified foreign body in larynx causing asphyxiation
T17.308-   Unspecified foreign body in larynx causing other injury
T17.31-   Gastric contents in larynx
Aspiration of gastric contents into larynx
Vomitus in larynx
T17.310-   Gastric contents in larynx causing asphyxiation
T17.318-   Gastric contents in larynx causing other injury
T17.32-   Food in larynx
Bones in larynx
Seeds in larynx
T17.320-   Food in larynx causing asphyxiation
T17.328-   Food in larynx causing other injury
T17.39-   Other foreign object in larynx
T17.390-   Other foreign object in larynx causing asphyxiation
T17.398-   Other foreign object in larynx causing other injury

T17.4- Foreign body in <u>trachea</u>

   T17.40- <u>Unspecified</u> foreign body in trachea

CC-A **T17.400-** Unspecified foreign body in trachea <u>causing asphyxiation</u>

CC-A **T17.408-** Unspecified foreign body in trachea <u>causing other injury</u>

   T17.41- Gastric contents in <u>trachea</u>
        Aspiration of gastric contents into trachea
        Vomitus in trachea

CC-A **T17.410-** Gastric contents in trachea <u>causing asphyxiation</u>

CC-A **T17.418-** Gastric contents in trachea <u>causing other injury</u>

   T17.42- Food in <u>trachea</u>
        Bones in trachea
        Seeds in trachea

CC-A **T17.420-** Food in trachea <u>causing asphyxiation</u>

CC-A **T17.428-** Food in trachea <u>causing other injury</u>

   T17.49- <u>Other foreign object</u> in <u>trachea</u>

CC-A **T17.490-** Other foreign object in trachea <u>causing asphyxiation</u>

CC-A **T17.498-** Other foreign object in trachea <u>causing other injury</u>

T17.5- Foreign body in <u>bronchus</u>

   T17.50- <u>Unspecified</u> foreign body in <u>bronchus</u>

CC-A **T17.500-** Unspecified foreign body in bronchus <u>causing asphyxiation</u>

CC-A **T17.508-** Unspecified foreign body in bronchus <u>causing other injury</u>

   T17.51- <u>Gastric contents</u> in <u>bronchus</u>
        Aspiration of gastric contents into bronchus
        Vomitus in bronchus

CC-A **T17.510-** Gastric contents in bronchus <u>causing asphyxiation</u>

CC-A **T17.518-** Gastric contents in bronchus <u>causing other injury</u>

   T17.52- <u>Food in bronchus</u>
        Bones in bronchus
        Seeds in bronchus

CC-A **T17.520-** Food in bronchus <u>causing asphyxiation</u>

CC-A **T17.528-** Food in bronchus <u>causing other injury</u>

   T17.59- <u>Other foreign object</u> in <u>bronchus</u>

CC-A **T17.590-** Other foreign object in bronchus <u>causing asphyxiation</u>

CC-A **T17.598-** Other foreign object in bronchus <u>causing other injury</u>

T17.8- Foreign body <u>in other parts of respiratory tract</u>
     Foreign body in bronchioles
     Foreign body in lung

   T17.80- <u>Unspecified</u> foreign body <u>in other parts of respiratory tract</u>

CC-A **T17.800-** Unspecified foreign body in other parts of respiratory tract <u>causing asphyxiation</u>

CC-A **T17.808-** Unspecified foreign body in other parts of respiratory tract <u>causing other injury</u>

   T17.81- <u>Gastric contents</u> in other parts of <u>respiratory tract</u>
        Aspiration of gastric contents into other parts of respiratory tract
        Vomitus in other parts of respiratory tract

CC-A **T17.810-** Gastric contents in other parts of respiratory tract <u>causing asphyxiation</u>

CC-A **T17.818-** Gastric contents in other parts of respiratory tract <u>causing other injury</u>

   T17.82- <u>Food in other parts of respiratory tract</u>
        Bones in other parts of respiratory tract
        Seeds in other parts of respiratory tract

CC-A **T17.820-** Food in other parts of respiratory tract <u>causing asphyxiation</u>

CC-A **T17.828-** Food in other parts of respiratory tract <u>causing other injury</u>

   T17.89- <u>Other foreign object</u> <u>in other parts of respiratory tract</u>

CC-A **T17.890-** Other foreign object in other parts of respiratory tract <u>causing asphyxiation</u>

CC-A **T17.898-** Other foreign object in other parts of respiratory tract <u>causing other injury</u>

T17.9- Foreign body <u>in respiratory tract</u>, <u>part unspecified</u>

   T17.90- <u>Unspecified</u> foreign body in respiratory tract, part unspecified

     T17.900- Unspecified foreign body in respiratory tract, part unspecified <u>causing asphyxiation</u>

     T17.908- Unspecified foreign body in respiratory tract, part unspecified <u>causing other injury</u>

   T17.91- <u>Gastric contents in respiratory tract</u>, <u>part unspecified</u>
        Aspiration of gastric contents into respiratory tract, part unspecified
        Vomitus in trachea respiratory tract, part unspecified

     T17.910- Gastric contents in respiratory tract, part unspecified <u>causing asphyxiation</u>

     T17.918- Gastric contents in respiratory tract, part unspecified <u>causing other injury</u>

   T17.92- <u>Food in respiratory tract</u>, <u>part unspecified</u>
        Bones in respiratory tract, part unspecified
        Seeds in respiratory tract, part unspecified

     T17.920- Food in respiratory tract, part unspecified <u>causing asphyxiation</u>

     T17.928- Food in respiratory tract, part unspecified <u>causing other injury</u>

   T17.99- <u>Other foreign object</u> <u>in respiratory tract</u>, <u>part unspecified</u>

     T17.990- Other foreign object in respiratory tract, part unspecified in <u>causing asphyxiation</u>

     T17.998- Other foreign object in respiratory tract, part unspecified <u>causing other injury</u>

T18- <u>Foreign body</u> <u>in alimentary tract</u>
   Excludes ❷: foreign body in pharynx (T17.2-)

> The appropriate 7th character is to be added to each code from category T18:
> **A**   <u>Initial</u> encounter
> **D**   <u>Subsequent</u> encounter
> **S**   <u>Sequela</u>

T18.0xx- Foreign body in <u>mouth</u>

T18.1- Foreign body in <u>esophagus</u>
   Excludes ❷: foreign body in respiratory tract (T17.-)

   T18.10- <u>Unspecified</u> foreign body in <u>esophagus</u>

     T18.100- Unspecified foreign body in esophagus <u>causing compression of trachea</u>
        Unspecified foreign body in esophagus causing obstruction of respiration

     T18.108- Unspecified foreign body in esophagus <u>causing other injury</u>

   T18.11- <u>Gastric contents</u> in <u>esophagus</u>
        Vomitus in esophagus

     T18.110- Gastric contents in esophagus <u>causing compression of trachea</u>
        Gastric contents in esophagus causing obstruction of respiration

     T18.118- Gastric contents in esophagus <u>causing other injury</u>

   T18.12- <u>Food in esophagus</u>
        Bones in esophagus
        Seeds in esophagus

     T18.120- Food in esophagus <u>causing compression of trachea</u>
        Food in esophagus causing obstruction of respiration

     T18.128- Food in esophagus <u>causing other injury</u>

   T18.19- <u>Other foreign object</u> in <u>esophagus</u>

     T18.190- Other foreign object in esophagus <u>causing compression of trachea</u>
        Other foreign body in esophagus causing obstruction of respiration

     T18.198- Other foreign object in esophagus <u>causing other injury</u>

T18.2xx- Foreign body in <u>stomach</u>

T18.3xx- Foreign body in <u>small intestine</u>

T18.4xx- Foreign body in <u>colon</u>

T18.5xx- Foreign body in <u>anus and rectum</u>
     Foreign body in rectosigmoid (junction)

T18.8xx- Foreign body in <u>other parts of alimentary tract</u>

T18.9xx-   Foreign body of alimentary tract, part unspecified
     Foreign body in digestive system NOS
     Swallowed foreign body NOS

T19-   <u>Foreign body</u> in <u>genitourinary tract</u>
   Excludes ❷: *complications due to implanted mesh (T83.7-)*
        mechanical complications of contraceptive device (intrauterine)
        (vaginal) (T83.3-)
        presence of contraceptive device (intrauterine) (vaginal)
        (Z97.5)

   The appropriate 7th character is to be added to each code from
   category T19:
   A   <u>Initial</u> encounter
   D   <u>Subsequent</u> encounter
   S   <u>Sequela</u>

T19.0xx-   Foreign body in urethra
T19.1xx-   Foreign body in bladder
T19.2xx-   Foreign body in vulva and vagina — [♀]
T19.3xx-   Foreign body in uterus — [♀]
T19.4xx-   Foreign body in penis — [♂]
T19.8xx-   Foreign body in other parts of genitourinary tract
T19.9xx-   Foreign body in genitourinary tract, part unspecified

Burns and corrosions (T20-T32)

Includes: Burns (thermal) from electrical heating appliances
      Burns (thermal) from electricity
      Burns (thermal) from flame
      Burns (thermal) from friction
      Burns (thermal) from hot air and hot gases
      Burns (thermal) from hot objects
      Burns (thermal) from lightning
      Burns (thermal) from radiation
      Chemical burn [corrosion] (external) (internal)
      Scalds
Excludes ❷: *erythema [dermatitis] ab igne (L59.0)*
      radiation-related disorders of the skin and subcutaneous tissue
      (L55-L59)
      sunburn (L55.-)

Burns and corrosions of external body surface, specified by site (T20-T25)

Includes: Burns and corrosions of first degree [erythema]
      Burns and corrosions of second degree [blisters][epidermal loss]
      Burns and corrosions of third degree [deep necrosis of
         underlying tissue] [full- thickness skin loss]
Use additional code from category T31 or T32 to identify extent of body
surface involved

T20-   <u>Burn and corrosion</u> of <u>head, face, and neck</u>
   Excludes ❷: *burn and corrosion of ear drum (T28.41, T28.91)*
         burn and corrosion of eye and adnexa (T26.-)
         burn and corrosion of mouth and pharynx (T28.0)

   The appropriate 7th character is to be added to each code from
   category T20:
   A   <u>Initial</u> encounter
   D   <u>Subsequent</u> encounter
   S   <u>Sequela</u>

T20.0-   Burn of <u>unspecified degree</u> of head, face, and neck
     Use additional external cause code to identify the source, place and
     intent of the burn (X00-X19, X75-X77, X96-X98, Y92)

T20.00x-   Burn of <u>unspecified degree</u> of <u>head, face, and neck,</u>
     <u>unspecified</u> site

T20.01-   Burn of <u>unspecified degree</u> of <u>ear</u> [any part, except ear
     drum]
     Excludes ❷: *burn of ear drum (T28.41-)*

   T20.011-   Burn of <u>unspecified degree</u> of <u>right</u> ear [any part,
        except ear drum]
   T20.012-   Burn of <u>unspecified degree</u> of <u>left</u> ear [any part,
        except ear drum]
   T20.019-   Burn of <u>unspecified degree</u> of <u>unspecified</u> ear [any
        part, except ear drum]
T20.02x-   Burn of <u>unspecified degree</u> of lip(s)
T20.03x-   Burn of <u>unspecified degree</u> of chin
T20.04x-   Burn of <u>unspecified degree</u> of nose (septum)
T20.05x-   Burn of <u>unspecified degree</u> of scalp [any part]

T20.06x-   Burn of <u>unspecified degree</u> of forehead and cheek
T20.07x-   Burn of <u>unspecified degree</u> of neck
T20.09x-   Burn of <u>unspecified degree</u> of multiple sites of head,
     face, and neck

T20.1-   Burn of <u>first</u> degree of <u>head, face, and neck</u>
     Use additional external cause code to identify the source, place and
     intent of the burn (X00-X19, X75-X77, X96-X98, Y92)

T20.10x-   Burn of <u>first</u> degree of head, face, and neck,
     <u>unspecified</u> site

T20.11-   Burn of <u>first</u> degree of <u>ear</u> [any part, except ear drum]
     Excludes ❷: *burn of ear drum (T28.41-)*

   T20.111-   Burn of <u>first</u> degree of <u>right</u> ear [any part, except
        ear drum]
   T20.112-   Burn of <u>first</u> degree of <u>left</u> ear [any part, except ear
        drum]
   T20.119-   Burn of <u>first</u> degree of <u>unspecified</u> ear [any part,
        except ear drum]
T20.12x-   Burn of <u>first</u> degree of lip(s)
T20.13x-   Burn of <u>first</u> degree of chin
T20.14x-   Burn of <u>first</u> degree of nose (septum)
T20.15x-   Burn of <u>first</u> degree of scalp [any part]
T20.16x-   Burn of <u>first</u> degree of forehead and cheek
T20.17x-   Burn of <u>first</u> degree of neck
T20.19x-   Burn of <u>first</u> degree of multiple sites of head, face, and
     neck

T20.2-   Burn of <u>second</u> degree of head, face, and neck
     Use additional external cause code to identify the source, place and
     intent of the burn (X00-X19, X75-X77, X96-X98, Y92)

T20.20x-   Burn of <u>second</u> degree of head, face, and neck,
     <u>unspecified</u> site

T20.21-   Burn of <u>second</u> degree of <u>ear</u> [any part, except ear
     drum]
     Excludes ❷: *burn of ear drum (T28.41-)*

   T20.211-   Burn of <u>second</u> degree of <u>right</u> ear [any part,
        except ear drum]
   T20.212-   Burn of <u>second</u> degree of <u>left</u> ear [any part,
        except ear drum]
   T20.219-   Burn of <u>second</u> degree of <u>unspecified</u> ear [any part,
        except ear drum]
T20.22x-   Burn of <u>second</u> degree of lip(s)
T20.23x-   Burn of <u>second</u> degree of chin
T20.24x-   Burn of <u>second</u> degree of nose (septum)
T20.25x-   Burn of <u>second</u> degree of scalp [any part]
T20.26x-   Burn of <u>second</u> degree of forehead and cheek
T20.27x-   Burn of <u>second</u> degree of neck
T20.29x-   Burn of <u>second</u> degree of multiple sites of head, face,
     and neck

T20.3-   Burn of <u>third</u> degree of <u>head, face, and neck</u>
     Use additional external cause code to identify the source, place and
     intent of the burn (X00-X19, X75-X77, X96-X98, Y92)

CC-A **T20.30x-**   Burn of <u>third</u> degree of <u>head, face, and neck,</u>
     <u>unspecified</u> site

T20.31-   Burn of <u>third</u> degree of <u>ear</u> [any part, except ear drum]
     AHA 15:1Q:p18 – Status post third degree burn of left external
     ear
     Excludes ❷: *burn of ear drum (T28.41-)*

CC-A **T20.311-**   Burn of <u>third</u> degree of <u>right</u> ear [any part, except
        ear drum]
CC-A **T20.312-**   Burn of <u>third</u> degree of <u>left</u> ear [any part, except
        ear drum]
CC-A **T20.319-**   Burn of <u>third</u> degree of <u>unspecified</u> ear [any part,
        except ear drum]
CC-A **T20.32x-**   Burn of <u>third</u> degree of lip(s)
CC-A **T20.33x-**   Burn of <u>third</u> degree of chin
CC-A **T20.34x-**   Burn of <u>third</u> degree of nose (septum)
CC-A **T20.35x-**   Burn of <u>third</u> degree of scalp [any part]
CC-A **T20.36x-**   Burn of <u>third</u> degree of forehead and cheek
CC-A **T20.37x-**   Burn of <u>third</u> degree of neck

T18 - T20

CC-A **T20.39x-** Burn of third degree of multiple sites of head, face, and neck

T20.4- Corrosion of unspecified degree of head, face, and neck
Code first (T51-T65) to identify chemical and intent
Use additional external cause code to identify place (Y92)

T20.40x- Corrosion of unspecified degree of head, face, and neck, unspecified site

T20.41- Corrosion of unspecified degree of ear [any part, except ear drum]
Excludes ❷: corrosion of ear drum (T28.91-)

T20.411- Corrosion of unspecified degree of right ear [any part, except ear drum]

T20.412- Corrosion of unspecified degree of left ear [any part, except ear drum]

T20.419- Corrosion of unspecified degree of unspecified ear [any part, except ear drum]

T20.42x- Corrosion of unspecified degree of lip(s)

T20.43x- Corrosion of unspecified degree of chin

T20.44x- Corrosion of unspecified degree of nose (septum)

T20.45x- Corrosion of unspecified degree of scalp [any part]

T20.46x- Corrosion of unspecified degree of forehead and cheek

T20.47x- Corrosion of unspecified degree of neck

T20.49x- Corrosion of unspecified degree of multiple sites of head, face, and neck

T20.5- Corrosion of first degree of head, face, and neck
Code first (T51-T65) to identify chemical and intent
Use additional external cause code to identify place (Y92)

T20.50x- Corrosion of first degree of head, face, and neck, unspecified site

T20.51- Corrosion of first degree of ear [any part, except ear drum]
Excludes ❷: corrosion of ear drum (T28.91-)

T20.511- Corrosion of first degree of right ear [any part, except ear drum]

T20.512- Corrosion of first degree of left ear [any part, except ear drum]

T20.519- Corrosion of first degree of unspecified ear [any part, except ear drum]

T20.52x- Corrosion of first degree of lip(s)

T20.53x- Corrosion of first degree of chin

T20.54x- Corrosion of first degree of nose (septum)

T20.55x- Corrosion of first degree of scalp [any part]

T20.56x- Corrosion of first degree of forehead and cheek

T20.57x- Corrosion of first degree of neck

T20.59x- Corrosion of first degree of multiple sites of head, face, and neck

T20.6- Corrosion of second degree of head, face, and neck
Code first (T51-T65) to identify chemical and intent
Use additional external cause code to identify place (Y92)

T20.60x- Corrosion of second degree of head, face, and neck, unspecified site

T20.61- Corrosion of second degree of ear [any part, except ear drum]
Excludes ❷: corrosion of ear drum (T28.91-)

T20.611- Corrosion of second degree of right ear [any part, except ear drum]

T20.612- Corrosion of second degree of left ear [any part, except ear drum]

T20.619- Corrosion of second degree of unspecified ear [any part, except ear drum]

T20.62x- Corrosion of second degree of lip(s)

T20.63x- Corrosion of second degree of chin

T20.64x- Corrosion of second degree of nose (septum)

T20.65x- Corrosion of second degree of scalp [any part]

T20.66x- Corrosion of second degree of forehead and cheek

T20.67x- Corrosion of second degree of neck

T20.69x- Corrosion of second degree of multiple sites of head, face, and neck

T20.7- Corrosion of third degree of head, face, and neck
Code first (T51-T65) to identify chemical and intent
Use additional external cause code to identify place (Y92)

CC-A **T20.70x-** Corrosion of third degree of head, face, and neck, unspecified site

T20.71- Corrosion of third degree of ear [any part, except ear drum]
Excludes ❷: corrosion of ear drum (T28.91-)

CC-A **T20.711-** Corrosion of third degree of right ear [any part, except ear drum]

CC-A **T20.712-** Corrosion of third degree of left ear [any part, except ear drum]

CC-A **T20.719-** Corrosion of third degree of unspecified ear [any part, except ear drum]

CC-A **T20.72x-** Corrosion of third degree of lip(s)

CC-A **T20.73x-** Corrosion of third degree of chin

CC-A **T20.74x-** Corrosion of third degree of nose (septum)

CC-A **T20.75x-** Corrosion of third degree of scalp [any part]

CC-A **T20.76x-** Corrosion of third degree of forehead and cheek

CC-A **T20.77x-** Corrosion of third degree of neck

CC-A **T20.79x-** Corrosion of third degree of multiple sites of head, face, and neck

T21- Burn and corrosion of trunk
Includes: Burns and corrosion of hip region
Excludes ❷: burns and corrosion of axilla (T22.- with fifth character 4)
burns and corrosion of scapular region (T22.- with fifth character 6)
burns and corrosion of shoulder (T22. with fifth character 5)

The appropriate 7th character is to be added to each code from category T21:
A **Initial** encounter
D **Subsequent** encounter
S **Sequela**

T21.0- Burn of unspecified degree of trunk
Use additional external cause code to identify the source, place and intent of the burn (X00-X19, X75-X77, X96-X98, Y92)

T21.00x- Burn of unspecified degree of trunk, unspecified site

T21.01x- Burn of unspecified degree of chest wall
Burn of of unspecified degree of breast

T21.02x- Burn of unspecified degree of abdominal wall
Burn of unspecified degree of flank
Burn of unspecified degree of groin

T21.03x- Burn of unspecified degree of upper back
Burn of unspecified degree of interscapular region

T21.04x- Burn of unspecified degree of lower back

T21.05x- Burn of unspecified degree of buttock
Burn of unspecified degree of anus

T21.06x- Burn of unspecified degree of male genital region — [♂]
Burn of unspecified degree of penis
Burn of unspecified degree of scrotum
Burn of unspecified degree of testis

T21.07x- Burn of unspecified degree of female genital region — [♀]
Burn of unspecified degree of labium (majus) (minus)
Burn of unspecified degree of perineum
Burn of unspecified degree of vulva
Excludes ❷: burn of vagina (T28.3)

T21.09x- Burn of unspecified degree of other site of trunk

T21.1- Burn of first degree of trunk
Use additional external cause code to identify the source, place and intent of the burn (X00-X19, X75-X77, X96-X98, Y92)

T21.10x- Burn of first degree of trunk, unspecified site

T21.11x- Burn of first degree of chest wall
Burn of first degree of breast

T21.12x- Burn of first degree of abdominal wall
Burn of first degree of flank
Burn of first degree of groin

T21.13x- Burn of first degree of upper back
Burn of first degree of interscapular region

T21.14x- Burn of first degree of lower back

T20 - T21 *(side tab)*

T21.15x-   Burn of <u>first</u> degree of <u>buttock</u>
    Burn of first degree of anus

T21.16x-   Burn of <u>first</u> degree of <u>male genital region</u> — [♂]
    Burn of first degree of penis
    Burn of first degree of scrotum
    Burn of first degree of testis

T21.17x-   Burn of <u>first</u> degree of <u>female genital region</u> — [♀]
    Burn of first degree of labium (majus) (minus)
    Burn of first degree of perineum
    Burn of first degree of vulva
    Excludes ❷: burn of vagina (T28.3)

T21.19x-   Burn of <u>first</u> degree of <u>other</u> site of trunk

T21.2-   Burn of <u>second</u> degree of <u>trunk</u>
    Use additional external cause code to identify the source, place and
    intent of the burn (X00-X19, X75-X77, X96-X98, Y92)

T21.20x-   Burn of <u>second</u> degree of trunk, <u>unspecified</u> site

T21.21x-   Burn of <u>second</u> degree of <u>chest wall</u>
    Burn of second degree of breast

T21.22x-   Burn of <u>second</u> degree of <u>abdominal wall</u>
    Burn of second degree of flank
    Burn of second degree of groin

T21.23x-   Burn of <u>second</u> degree of <u>upper back</u>
    Burn of second degree of interscapular region

T21.24x-   Burn of <u>second</u> degree of <u>lower back</u>

T21.25x-   Burn of <u>second</u> degree of <u>buttock</u>
    Burn of second degree of anus

T21.26x-   Burn of <u>second</u> degree of <u>male genital region</u> — [♂]
    Burn of second degree of penis
    Burn of second degree of scrotum
    Burn of second degree of testis

T21.27x-   Burn of <u>second</u> degree of <u>female genital region</u> — [♀]
    Burn of second degree of labium (majus) (minus)
    Burn of second degree of perineum
    Burn of second degree of vulva
    Excludes ❷: burn of vagina (T28.3)

T21.29x-   Burn of <u>second</u> degree of <u>other</u> site of trunk

T21.3-   Burn of <u>third</u> degree of <u>trunk</u>
    Use additional external cause code to identify the source, place and
    intent of the burn (X00-X19, X75-X77, X96-X98, Y92)

CC-A T21.30x-   Burn of <u>third</u> degree of trunk, <u>unspecified</u> site

CC-A T21.31x-   Burn of <u>third</u> degree of <u>chest wall</u>
    Burn of third degree of breast

CC-A T21.32x-   Burn of <u>third</u> degree of <u>abdominal wall</u>
    Burn of third degree of flank
    Burn of third degree of groin

CC-A T21.33x-   Burn of <u>third</u> degree of <u>upper back</u>
    Burn of third degree of interscapular region

CC-A T21.34x-   Burn of <u>third</u> degree of <u>lower back</u>

CC-A T21.35x-   Burn of <u>third</u> degree of <u>buttock</u>
    Burn of third degree of anus

CC-A T21.36x-   Burn of <u>third</u> degree of <u>male genital region</u> — [♂]
    Burn of third degree of penis
    Burn of third degree of scrotum
    Burn of third degree of testis

CC-A T21.37x-   Burn of <u>third</u> degree of <u>female genital region</u> — [♀]
    Burn of third degree of labium (majus) (minus)
    Burn of third degree of perineum
    Burn of third degree of vulva
    Excludes ❷: burn of vagina (T28.3)

CC-A T21.39x-   Burn of <u>third</u> degree of <u>other</u> site of trunk

T21.4-   <u>Corrosion</u> of <u>unspecified degree</u> of <u>trunk</u>
    Code first (T51-T65) to identify chemical and intent
    Use additional external cause code to identify place (Y92)

T21.40x-   <u>Corrosion</u> of <u>unspecified degree</u> of <u>trunk</u>, <u>unspecified</u>
    site

T21.41x-   <u>Corrosion</u> of <u>unspecified degree</u> of <u>chest wall</u>
    Corrosion of unspecified degree of breast

T21.42x-   <u>Corrosion</u> of <u>unspecified degree</u> of <u>abdominal wall</u>
    Corrosion of unspecified degree of flank
    Corrosion of unspecified degree of groin

T21.43x-   <u>Corrosion</u> of <u>unspecified degree</u> of <u>upper back</u>
    Corrosion of unspecified degree of interscapular region

T21.44x-   <u>Corrosion</u> of <u>unspecified degree</u> of <u>lower back</u>

T21.45x-   <u>Corrosion</u> of <u>unspecified degree</u> of <u>buttock</u>
    Corrosion of unspecified degree of anus

T21.46x-   <u>Corrosion</u> of <u>unspecified degree</u> of <u>male genital</u>
    <u>region</u> — [♂]
    Corrosion of unspecified degree of penis
    Corrosion of unspecified degree of scrotum
    Corrosion of unspecified degree of testis

T21.47x-   <u>Corrosion</u> of <u>unspecified degree</u> of <u>female genital</u>
    <u>region</u> — [♀]
    Corrosion of unspecified degree of labium (majus) (minus)
    Corrosion of unspecified degree of perineum
    Corrosion of unspecified degree of vulva
    Excludes ❷: corrosion of vagina (T28.8)

T21.49x-   <u>Corrosion</u> of <u>unspecified degree</u> of <u>other</u> site of trunk

T21.5-   <u>Corrosion</u> of <u>first degree</u> of <u>trunk</u>
    Code first (T51-T65) to identify chemical and intent
    Use additional external cause code to identify place (Y92)

T21.50x-   <u>Corrosion</u> of <u>first</u> degree of <u>trunk</u>, <u>unspecified</u> site

T21.51x-   <u>Corrosion</u> of <u>first</u> degree of <u>chest wall</u>
    Corrosion of first degree of breast

T21.52x-   <u>Corrosion</u> of <u>first</u> degree of <u>abdominal wall</u>
    Corrosion of first degree of flank
    Corrosion of first degree of groin

T21.53x-   <u>Corrosion</u> of <u>first</u> degree of <u>upper back</u>
    Corrosion of first degree of interscapular region

T21.54x-   <u>Corrosion</u> of <u>first</u> degree of <u>lower back</u>

T21.55x-   <u>Corrosion</u> of <u>first</u> degree of <u>buttock</u>
    Corrosion of first degree of anus

T21.56x-   <u>Corrosion</u> of <u>first</u> degree of <u>male genital region</u> — [♂]
    Corrosion of first degree of penis
    Corrosion of first degree of scrotum
    Corrosion of first degree of testis

T21.57x-   <u>Corrosion</u> of <u>first</u> degree of <u>female genital region</u> —
    [♀]
    Corrosion of first degree of labium (majus) (minus)
    Corrosion of first degree of perineum
    Corrosion of first degree of vulva
    Excludes ❷: corrosion of vagina (T28.8)

T21.59x-   <u>Corrosion</u> of <u>first</u> degree of <u>other</u> site of trunk

T21.6-   <u>Corrosion</u> of <u>second</u> degree of <u>trunk</u>
    Code first (T51-T65) to identify chemical and Intent
    Use additional external cause code to identify place (Y92)

T21.60x-   <u>Corrosion</u> of <u>second</u> degree of <u>trunk</u>, <u>unspecified</u> site

T21.61x-   <u>Corrosion</u> of <u>second</u> degree of <u>chest wall</u>
    Corrosion of second degree of breast

T21.62x-   <u>Corrosion</u> of <u>second</u> degree of <u>abdominal wall</u>
    Corrosion of second degree of flank
    Corrosion of second degree of groin

T21.63x-   <u>Corrosion</u> of <u>second</u> degree of <u>upper back</u>
    Corrosion of second degree of interscapular region

T21.64x-   <u>Corrosion</u> of <u>second</u> degree of <u>lower back</u>

T21.65x-   <u>Corrosion</u> of <u>second</u> degree of <u>buttock</u>
    Corrosion of second degree of anus

T21.66x-   <u>Corrosion</u> of <u>second</u> degree of <u>male genital region</u> —
    [♂]
    Corrosion of second degree of penis
    Corrosion of second degree of scrotum
    Corrosion of second degree of testis

T21.67x-   <u>Corrosion</u> of <u>second</u> degree of <u>female genital region</u> —
    [♀]
    Corrosion of second degree of labium (majus) (minus)
    Corrosion of second degree of perineum
    Corrosion of second degree of vulva
    Excludes ❷: corrosion of vagina (T28.8)

T21.69x-   <u>Corrosion</u> of <u>second</u> degree of <u>other</u> site of trunk

T21.7-   <u>Corrosion</u> of <u>third</u> degree of <u>trunk</u>
    Code first (T51-T65) to identify chemical and intent
    Use additional external cause code to identify place (Y92)

CC-A T21.70x-   <u>Corrosion</u> of <u>third</u> degree of <u>trunk</u>, <u>unspecified</u> site

CC-A T21.71x-   <u>Corrosion</u> of <u>third</u> degree of <u>chest wall</u>
    Corrosion of third degree of breast

CC-A T21.72x-   <u>Corrosion</u> of <u>third</u> degree of <u>abdominal wall</u>
    Corrosion of third degree of flank
    Corrosion of third degree of groin

T21 - T21 - T21

CC-A **T21.73x-** <u>Corrosion</u> of <u>third</u> degree of <u>upper back</u>
Corrosion of third degree of interscapular region

CC-A **T21.74x-** <u>Corrosion</u> of <u>third</u> degree of <u>lower back</u>

CC-A **T21.75x-** <u>Corrosion</u> of <u>third</u> degree of <u>buttock</u>
Corrosion of third degree of anus

CC-A **T21.76x-** <u>Corrosion</u> of <u>third</u> degree of <u>male genital region</u> —[♂]
Corrosion of third degree of penis
Corrosion of third degree of scrotum
Corrosion of third degree of testis

CC-A **T21.77x-** <u>Corrosion</u> of <u>third</u> degree of <u>female genital region</u> —[♀]
Corrosion of third degree of labium (majus) (minus)
Corrosion of third degree of perineum
Corrosion of third degree of vulva
Excludes ❷: *corrosion of vagina (T28.8)*

CC-A **T21.79x-** <u>Corrosion</u> of <u>third</u> degree of <u>other</u> site of trunk

T22- <u>Burn and corrosion</u> of <u>shoulder and upper limb</u>, <u>except wrist and hand</u>
Excludes ❷: *burn and corrosion of interscapular region (T21.-)*
burn and corrosion of wrist and hand (T23.-)

The appropriate 7th character is to be added to each code from category T22:
A   <u>Initial</u> encounter
D   <u>Subsequent</u> encounter
S   <u>Sequela</u>

T22.0- Burn of <u>unspecified degree</u> of <u>shoulder and upper limb</u>, <u>except wrist and hand</u>
Use additional external cause code to identify the source, place and intent of the burn (X00-X19, X75-X77, X96-X98, Y92)

T22.00x- Burn of <u>unspecified degree</u> of <u>shoulder and upper limb</u>, except wrist and hand, <u>unspecified</u> site

T22.01- Burn of <u>unspecified degree</u> of <u>forearm</u>
T22.011- Burn of unspecified degree of <u>right</u> forearm
T22.012- Burn of unspecified degree of <u>left</u> forearm
T22.019- Burn of unspecified degree of <u>unspecified</u> forearm

T22.02- Burn of <u>unspecified degree</u> of <u>elbow</u>
T22.021- Burn of unspecified degree of <u>right</u> elbow
T22.022- Burn of unspecified degree of <u>left</u> elbow
T22.029- Burn of unspecified degree of <u>unspecified</u> elbow

T22.03- Burn of <u>unspecified degree</u> of <u>upper arm</u>
T22.031- Burn of unspecified degree of <u>right</u> upper arm
T22.032- Burn of unspecified degree of <u>left</u> upper arm
T22.039- Burn of unspecified degree of <u>unspecified</u> upper arm

T22.04- Burn of <u>unspecified degree</u> of <u>axilla</u>
T22.041- Burn of unspecified degree of <u>right</u> axilla
T22.042- Burn of unspecified degree of <u>left</u> axilla
T22.049- Burn of unspecified degree of <u>unspecified</u> axilla

T22.05- Burn of <u>unspecified degree</u> of <u>shoulder</u>
T22.051- Burn of unspecified degree of <u>right</u> shoulder
T22.052- Burn of unspecified degree of <u>left</u> shoulder
T22.059- Burn of unspecified degree of <u>unspecified</u> shoulder

T22.06- Burn of <u>unspecified degree</u> of <u>scapular region</u>
T22.061- Burn of unspecified degree of <u>right</u> scapular region
T22.062- Burn of unspecified degree of <u>left</u> scapular region
T22.069- Burn of unspecified degree of <u>unspecified</u> scapular region

T22.09- Burn of <u>unspecified degree</u> of <u>multiple</u> sites of shoulder and upper limb, except wrist and hand
T22.091- Burn of unspecified degree of multiple sites of <u>right</u> shoulder and upper limb, except wrist and hand
T22.092- Burn of unspecified degree of multiple sites of <u>left</u> shoulder and upper limb, except wrist and hand
T22.099- Burn of unspecified degree of multiple sites of <u>unspecified</u> shoulder and upper limb, except wrist and hand

T22.1- Burn of <u>first</u> degree of <u>shoulder and upper limb</u>, <u>except wrist and hand</u>
Use additional external cause code to identify the source, place and intent of the burn (X00-X19, X75-X77, X96-X98, Y92)

T22.10x- Burn of <u>first</u> degree of <u>shoulder and upper limb</u>, except wrist and hand, <u>unspecified</u> site

T22.11- Burn of <u>first</u> degree of <u>forearm</u>
T22.111- Burn of first degree of <u>right</u> forearm
T22.112- Burn of first degree of <u>left</u> forearm
T22.119- Burn of first degree of <u>unspecified</u> forearm

T22.12- Burn of <u>first</u> degree of <u>elbow</u>
T22.121- Burn of first degree of <u>right</u> elbow
T22.122- Burn of first degree of <u>left</u> elbow
T22.129- Burn of first degree of <u>unspecified</u> elbow

T22.13- Burn of <u>first</u> degree of <u>upper arm</u>
T22.131- Burn of first degree of <u>right</u> upper arm
T22.132- Burn of first degree of <u>left</u> upper arm
T22.139- Burn of first degree of <u>unspecified</u> upper arm

T22.14- Burn of <u>first</u> degree of <u>axilla</u>
T22.141- Burn of first degree of <u>right</u> axilla
T22.142- Burn of first degree of <u>left</u> axilla
T22.149- Burn of first degree of <u>unspecified</u> axilla

T22.15- Burn of <u>first</u> degree of <u>shoulder</u>
T22.151- Burn of first degree of <u>right</u> shoulder
T22.152- Burn of first degree of <u>left</u> shoulder
T22.159- Burn of first degree of <u>unspecified</u> shoulder

T22.16- Burn of <u>first</u> degree of <u>scapular region</u>
T22.161- Burn of first degree of <u>right</u> scapular region
T22.162- Burn of first degree of <u>left</u> scapular region
T22.169- Burn of first degree of <u>unspecified</u> scapular region

T22.19- Burn of <u>first</u> degree of <u>multiple</u> sites of shoulder and upper limb, except wrist and hand
T22.191- Burn of first degree of multiple sites of <u>right</u> shoulder and upper limb, except wrist and hand
T22.192- Burn of first degree of multiple sites of <u>left</u> shoulder and upper limb, except wrist and hand
T22.199- Burn of first degree of multiple sites of <u>unspecified</u> shoulder and upper limb, except wrist and hand

T22.2- Burn of <u>second</u> degree of <u>shoulder and upper limb</u>, <u>except wrist and hand</u>
Use additional external cause code to identify the source, place and intent of the burn (X00-X19, X75-X77, X96-X98, Y92)

T22.20x- Burn of <u>second</u> degree of <u>shoulder and upper limb</u>, except wrist and hand, <u>unspecified</u> site

T22.21- Burn of <u>second</u> degree of <u>forearm</u>
T22.211- Burn of second degree of <u>right</u> forearm
T22.212- Burn of second degree of <u>left</u> forearm
T22.219- Burn of second degree of <u>unspecified</u> forearm

T22.22- Burn of <u>second</u> degree of <u>elbow</u>
T22.221- Burn of second degree of <u>right</u> elbow
T22.222- Burn of second degree of <u>left</u> elbow
T22.229- Burn of second degree of <u>unspecified</u> elbow

T22.23- Burn of <u>second</u> degree of <u>upper arm</u>
T22.231- Burn of second degree of <u>right</u> upper arm
T22.232- Burn of second degree of <u>left</u> upper arm
T22.239- Burn of second degree of <u>unspecified</u> upper arm

T22.24- Burn of <u>second</u> degree of <u>axilla</u>
T22.241- Burn of second degree of <u>right</u> axilla
T22.242- Burn of second degree of <u>left</u> axilla
T22.249- Burn of second degree of <u>unspecified</u> axilla

T22.25- Burn of <u>second</u> degree of <u>shoulder</u>
T22.251- Burn of second degree of <u>right</u> shoulder
T22.252- Burn of second degree of <u>left</u> shoulder
T22.259- Burn of second degree of <u>unspecified</u> shoulder

T22.26- Burn of <u>second</u> degree of <u>scapular region</u>
T22.261- Burn of second degree of <u>right</u> scapular region

T22.262- Burn of second degree of <u>left</u> scapular region
T22.269- Burn of second degree of <u>unspecified</u> scapular region

T22.29- Burn of <u>second</u> degree of <u>multiple</u> sites of shoulder and upper limb, except wrist and hand
    T22.291- Burn of second degree of multiple sites of <u>right</u> shoulder and upper limb, except wrist and hand
    T22.292- Burn of second degree of multiple sites of <u>left</u> shoulder and upper limb, except wrist and hand
    T22.299- Burn of second degree of multiple sites of <u>unspecified</u> shoulder and upper limb, except wrist and hand

T22.3- Burn of <u>third</u> degree of <u>shoulder and upper limb</u>, <u>except wrist and hand</u>
    Use additional external cause code to identify the source, place and intent of the burn (X00-X19, X75-X77, X96-X98, Y92)

CC-A T22.30x- Burn of <u>third</u> degree of shoulder and upper limb, except wrist and hand, <u>unspecified</u> site

T22.31- Burn of <u>third</u> degree of <u>forearm</u>
CC-A T22.311- Burn of third degree of <u>right</u> forearm
CC-A T22.312- Burn of third degree of <u>left</u> forearm
CC-A T22.319- Burn of third degree of <u>unspecified</u> forearm

T22.32- Burn of <u>third</u> degree of <u>elbow</u>
CC-A T22.321- Burn of third degree of <u>right</u> elbow
CC-A T22.322- Burn of third degree of <u>left</u> elbow
CC-A T22.329- Burn of third degree of <u>unspecified</u> elbow

T22.33- Burn of <u>third</u> degree of <u>upper arm</u>
CC-A T22.331- Burn of third degree of <u>right</u> upper arm
CC-A T22.332- Burn of third degree of <u>left</u> upper arm
CC-A T22.339- Burn of third degree of <u>unspecified</u> upper arm

T22.34- Burn of <u>third</u> degree of <u>axilla</u>
CC-A T22.341- Burn of third degree of <u>right</u> axilla
CC-A T22.342- Burn of third degree of <u>left</u> axilla
CC-A T22.349- Burn of third degree of <u>unspecified</u> axilla

T22.35- Burn of <u>third</u> degree of <u>shoulder</u>
CC-A T22.351- Burn of third degree of <u>right</u> shoulder
CC-A T22.352- Burn of third degree of <u>left</u> shoulder
CC-A T22.359- Burn of third degree of <u>unspecified</u> shoulder

T22.36- Burn of <u>third</u> degree of <u>scapular region</u>
CC-A T22.361- Burn of third degree of <u>right</u> scapular region
CC-A T22.362- Burn of third degree of <u>left</u> scapular region
CC-A T22.369- Burn of third degree of <u>unspecified</u> scapular region

T22.39 Burn of <u>third</u> degree of <u>multiple</u> sites of shoulder and upper limb, except wrist and hand
CC-A T22.391- Burn of third degree of multiple sites of <u>right</u> shoulder and upper limb, except wrist and hand
CC-A T22.392- Burn of third degree of multiple sites of <u>left</u> shoulder and upper limb, except wrist and hand
CC-A T22.399- Burn of third degree of multiple sites of <u>unspecified</u> shoulder and upper limb, except wrist and hand

T22.4- <u>Corrosion</u> of <u>unspecified degree</u> of <u>shoulder and upper limb</u>, <u>except wrist and hand</u>
    Code first (T51-T65) to identify chemical and intent
    Use additional external cause code to identify place (Y92)

T22.40x- <u>Corrosion</u> of <u>unspecified degree</u> of <u>shoulder and upper limb</u>, <u>except wrist and hand</u>, <u>unspecified</u> site

T22.41- <u>Corrosion</u> of <u>unspecified degree</u> of <u>forearm</u>
    T22.411- Corrosion of unspecified degree of <u>right</u> forearm
    T22.412- Corrosion of unspecified degree of <u>left</u> forearm
    T22.419- Corrosion of unspecified degree of <u>unspecified</u> forearm

T22.42- <u>Corrosion</u> of <u>unspecified degree</u> of <u>elbow</u>
    T22.421- Corrosion of unspecified degree of <u>right</u> elbow
    T22.422- Corrosion of unspecified degree of <u>left</u> elbow
    T22.429- Corrosion of unspecified degree of <u>unspecified</u> elbow

T22.43- <u>Corrosion</u> of <u>unspecified degree</u> of <u>upper arm</u>
    T22.431- Corrosion of unspecified degree of <u>right</u> upper arm
    T22.432- Corrosion of unspecified degree of <u>left</u> upper arm
    T22.439- Corrosion of unspecified degree of <u>unspecified</u> upper arm

T22.44- <u>Corrosion</u> of <u>unspecified degree</u> of <u>axilla</u>
    T22.441- Corrosion of unspecified degree of <u>right</u> axilla
    T22.442- Corrosion of unspecified degree of <u>left</u> axilla
    T22.449- Corrosion of unspecified degree of <u>unspecified</u> axilla

T22.45- <u>Corrosion</u> of <u>unspecified degree</u> of <u>shoulder</u>
    T22.451- Corrosion of unspecified degree of <u>right</u> shoulder
    T22.452- Corrosion of unspecified degree of <u>left</u> shoulder
    T22.459- Corrosion of unspecified degree of <u>unspecified</u> shoulder

T22.46- <u>Corrosion</u> of <u>unspecified degree</u> of <u>scapular region</u>
    T22.461- Corrosion of unspecified degree of <u>right</u> scapular region
    T22.462- Corrosion of unspecified degree of <u>left</u> scapular region
    T22.469- Corrosion of unspecified degree of <u>unspecified</u> scapular region

T22.49- <u>Corrosion</u> of <u>unspecified degree</u> of <u>multiple</u> sites of shoulder and upper limb, except wrist and hand
    T22.491- Corrosion of unspecified degree of multiple sites of <u>right</u> shoulder and upper limb, except wrist and hand
    T22.492- Corrosion of unspecified degree of multiple sites of <u>left</u> shoulder and upper limb, except wrist and hand
    T22.499- Corrosion of unspecified degree of multiple sites of <u>unspecified</u> shoulder and upper limb, except wrist and hand

T22.5- <u>Corrosion</u> of <u>first</u> degree of <u>shoulder and upper limb</u>, <u>except wrist and hand</u>
    Code first (T51-T65) to identify chemical and intent
    Use additional external cause code to identify place (Y92)

T22.50x- <u>Corrosion</u> of <u>first</u> degree of <u>shoulder and upper limb</u>, except wrist and hand <u>unspecified</u> site

T22.51- <u>Corrosion</u> of <u>first</u> degree of <u>forearm</u>
    T22.511- Corrosion of first degree of <u>right</u> forearm
    T22.512- Corrosion of first degree of <u>left</u> forearm
    T22.519- Corrosion of first degree of <u>unspecified</u> forearm

T22.52- <u>Corrosion</u> of <u>first</u> degree of <u>elbow</u>
    T22.521- Corrosion of first degree of <u>right</u> elbow
    T22.522- Corrosion of first degree of <u>left</u> elbow
    T22.529- Corrosion of first degree of <u>unspecified</u> elbow

T22.53- <u>Corrosion</u> of <u>first</u> degree of <u>upper arm</u>
    T22.531- Corrosion of first degree of <u>right</u> upper arm
    T22.532- Corrosion of first degree of <u>left</u> upper arm
    T22.539- Corrosion of first degree of <u>unspecified</u> upper arm

T22.54- <u>Corrosion</u> of <u>first</u> degree of <u>axilla</u>
    T22.541- Corrosion of first degree of <u>right</u> axilla
    T22.542- Corrosion of first degree of <u>left</u> axilla
    T22.549- Corrosion of first degree of <u>unspecified</u> axilla

T22.55- <u>Corrosion</u> of <u>first</u> degree of <u>shoulder</u>
    T22.551- Corrosion of first degree of <u>right</u> shoulder
    T22.552- Corrosion of first degree of <u>left</u> shoulder
    T22.559- Corrosion of first degree of <u>unspecified</u> shoulder

T22.56- <u>Corrosion</u> of <u>first</u> degree of <u>scapular region</u>
    T22.561- Corrosion of first degree of <u>right</u> scapular region
    T22.562- Corrosion of first degree of <u>left</u> scapular region
    T22.569- Corrosion of first degree of <u>unspecified</u> scapular region

T22 - T22

T22.59- Corrosion of first degree of multiple sites of shoulder and upper limb, except wrist and hand

T22.591- Corrosion of first degree of multiple sites of right shoulder and upper limb, except wrist and hand

T22.592- Corrosion of first degree of multiple sites of left shoulder and upper limb, except wrist and hand

T22.599- Corrosion of first degree of multiple sites of unspecified shoulder and upper limb, except wrist and hand

T22.6- Corrosion of second degree of shoulder and upper limb, except wrist and hand
Code first (T51-T65) to identify chemical and intent
Use additional external cause code to identify place (Y92)

T22.60x- Corrosion of second degree of shoulder and upper limb, except wrist and hand, unspecified site

T22.61- Corrosion of second degree of forearm

T22.611- Corrosion of second degree of right forearm

T22.612- Corrosion of second degree of left forearm

T22.619- Corrosion of second degree of unspecified forearm

T22.62- Corrosion of second degree of elbow

T22.621- Corrosion of second degree of right elbow

T22.622- Corrosion of second degree of left elbow

T22.629- Corrosion of second degree of unspecified elbow

T22.63- Corrosion of second degree of upper arm

T22.631- Corrosion of second degree of right upper arm

T22.632- Corrosion of second degree of left upper arm

T22.639- Corrosion of second degree of unspecified upper arm

T22.64- Corrosion of second degree of axilla

T22.641- Corrosion of second degree of right axilla

T22.642- Corrosion of second degree of left axilla

T22.649- Corrosion of second degree of unspecified axilla

T22.65- Corrosion of second degree of shoulder

T22.651- Corrosion of second degree of right shoulder

T22.652- Corrosion of second degree of left shoulder

T22.659- Corrosion of second degree of unspecified shoulder

T22.66- Corrosion of second degree of scapular region

T22.661- Corrosion of second degree of right scapular region

T22.662- Corrosion of second degree of left scapular region

T22.669- Corrosion of second degree of unspecified scapular region

T22.69- Corrosion of second degree of multiple sites of shoulder and upper limb, except wrist and hand

T22.691- Corrosion of second degree of multiple sites of right shoulder and upper limb, except wrist and hand

T22.692- Corrosion of second degree of multiple sites of left shoulder and upper limb, except wrist and hand

T22.699- Corrosion of second degree of multiple sites of unspecified shoulder and upper limb, except wrist and hand

T22.7- Corrosion of third degree of shoulder and upper limb, except wrist and hand
Code first (T51-T65) to identify chemical and intent
Use additional external cause code to identify place (Y92)

CC-A T22.70x- Corrosion of third degree of shoulder and upper limb, except wrist and hand, unspecified site

T22.71- Corrosion of third degree of forearm

CC-A T22.711- Corrosion of third degree of right forearm

CC-A T22.712- Corrosion of third degree of left forearm

CC-A T22.719- Corrosion of third degree of unspecified forearm

T22.72- Corrosion of third degree of elbow

CC-A T22.721- Corrosion of third degree of right elbow

CC-A T22.722- Corrosion of third degree of left elbow

CC-A T22.729- Corrosion of third degree of unspecified elbow

T22.73- Corrosion of third degree of upper arm

CC-A T22.731- Corrosion of third degree of right upper arm

CC-A T22.732- Corrosion of third degree of left upper arm

CC-A T22.739- Corrosion of third degree of unspecified upper arm

T22.74- Corrosion of third degree of axilla

CC-A T22.741- Corrosion of third degree of right axilla

CC-A T22.742- Corrosion of third degree of left axilla

CC-A T22.749- Corrosion of third degree of unspecified axilla

T22.75- Corrosion of third degree of shoulder

CC-A T22.751- Corrosion of third degree of right shoulder

CC-A T22.752- Corrosion of third degree of left shoulder

CC-A T22.759- Corrosion of third degree of unspecified shoulder

T22.76- Corrosion of third degree of scapular region

CC-A T22.761- Corrosion of third degree of right scapular region

CC-A T22.762- Corrosion of third degree of left scapular region

CC-A T22.769- Corrosion of third degree of unspecified scapular region

T22.79- Corrosion of third degree of multiple sites of shoulder and upper limb, except wrist and hand

CC-A T22.791- Corrosion of third degree of multiple sites of right shoulder and upper limb, except wrist and hand

CC-A T22.792- Corrosion of third degree of multiple sites of left shoulder and upper limb, except wrist and hand

CC-A T22.799- Corrosion of third degree of multiple sites of unspecified shoulder and upper limb, except wrist and hand

T23- **Burn and corrosion of wrist and hand**
The appropriate 7th character is to be added to each code from category T23:
A Initial encounter
D Subsequent encounter
S Sequela

T23.0- Burn of unspecified degree of wrist and hand
Use additional external cause code to identify the source, place and intent of the burn (X00-X19, X75-X77, X96-X98, Y92)

T23.00- Burn of unspecified degree of hand, unspecified site

T23.001- Burn of unspecified degree of right hand, unspecified site

T23.002- Burn of unspecified degree of left hand, unspecified site

T23.009- Burn of unspecified degree of unspecified hand, unspecified site

T23.01- Burn of unspecified degree of thumb (nail)

T23.011- Burn of unspecified degree of right thumb (nail)

T23.012- Burn of unspecified degree of left thumb (nail)

T23.019- Burn of unspecified degree of unspecified thumb (nail)

T23.02- Burn of unspecified degree of single finger (nail) except thumb

T23.021- Burn of unspecified degree of single right finger (nail) except thumb

T23.022- Burn of unspecified degree of single left finger (nail) except thumb

T23.029- Burn of unspecified degree of unspecified single finger (nail) except thumb

T23.03- Burn of unspecified degree of multiple fingers (nail), not including thumb

T23.031- Burn of unspecified degree of multiple right fingers (nail), not including thumb

T23.032- Burn of unspecified degree of multiple left fingers (nail), not including thumb

T23.039- Burn of unspecified degree of unspecified multiple fingers (nail), not including thumb

T23.04- Burn of unspecified degree of multiple fingers (nail), including thumb

T23.041- Burn of unspecified degree of multiple right fingers (nail), including thumb

T23.042- Burn of unspecified degree of multiple left fingers (nail), including thumb

T22-T23

T23.049- Burn of unspecified degree of <u>unspecified</u> multiple fingers (nail), including thumb

T23.05- Burn of <u>unspecified degree</u> of <u>palm</u>
- **T23.051-** Burn of unspecified degree of <u>right</u> palm
- **T23.052-** Burn of unspecified degree of <u>left</u> palm
- **T23.059-** Burn of unspecified degree of <u>unspecified</u> palm

T23.06- Burn of <u>unspecified degree</u> of <u>back of hand</u>
- **T23.061-** Burn of unspecified degree of back of <u>right</u> hand
- **T23.062-** Burn of unspecified degree of back of <u>left</u> hand
- **T23.069-** Burn of unspecified degree of back of <u>unspecified</u> hand

T23.07- Burn of <u>unspecified degree</u> of <u>wrist</u>
- **T23.071-** Burn of unspecified degree of <u>right</u> wrist
- **T23.072-** Burn of unspecified degree of <u>left</u> wrist
- **T23.079-** Burn of unspecified degree of <u>unspecified</u> wrist

T23.09- Burn of <u>unspecified degree</u> of <u>multiple</u> sites of <u>wrist and hand</u>
- **T23.091-** Burn of unspecified degree of multiple sites of <u>right</u> wrist and hand
- **T23.092-** Burn of unspecified degree of multiple sites of <u>left</u> wrist and hand
- **T23.099-** Burn of unspecified degree of multiple sites of <u>unspecified</u> wrist and hand

T23.1- Burn of <u>first</u> degree of <u>wrist and hand</u>
Use additional external cause code to identify the source, place and intent of the burn (X00-X19, X75-X77, X96-X98, Y92)

T23.10- Burn of <u>first</u> degree of hand, <u>unspecified</u> site
- **T23.101-** Burn of first degree of <u>right</u> hand, unspecified site
- **T23.102-** Burn of first degree of <u>left</u> hand, unspecified site
- **T23.109-** Burn of first degree of <u>unspecified</u> hand, unspecified site

T23.11- Burn of <u>first</u> degree of <u>thumb</u> (nail)
- **T23.111-** Burn of first degree of <u>right</u> thumb (nail)
- **T23.112-** Burn of first degree of <u>left</u> thumb (nail)
- **T23.119-** Burn of first degree of <u>unspecified</u> thumb (nail)

T23.12- Burn of <u>first</u> degree of <u>single finger</u> (nail) <u>except thumb</u>
- **T23.121-** Burn of first degree of single <u>right</u> finger (nail) except thumb
- **T23.122-** Burn of first degree of single <u>left</u> finger (nail) except thumb
- **T23.129-** Burn of first degree of <u>unspecified</u> single finger (nail) except thumb

T23.13- Burn of <u>first</u> degree of <u>multiple fingers</u> (nail), <u>not including thumb</u>
- **T23.131-** Burn of first degree of multiple <u>right</u> fingers (nail), not including thumb
- **T23.132-** Burn of first degree of multiple <u>left</u> fingers (nail), not including thumb
- **T23.139-** Burn of first degree of <u>unspecified</u> multiple fingers (nail), not including thumb

T23.14- Burn of <u>first</u> degree of <u>multiple fingers</u> (nail), <u>including thumb</u>
- **T23.141-** Burn of first degree of multiple <u>right</u> fingers (nail), including thumb
- **T23.142-** Burn of first degree of multiple <u>left</u> fingers (nail), including thumb
- **T23.149-** Burn of first degree of <u>unspecified</u> multiple fingers (nail), including thumb

T23.15- Burn of <u>first</u> degree of <u>palm</u>
- **T23.151-** Burn of first degree of <u>right</u> palm
- **T23.152-** Burn of first degree of <u>left</u> palm
- **T23.159-** Burn of first degree of <u>unspecified</u> palm

T23.16- Burn of <u>first</u> degree of <u>back of hand</u>
- **T23.161-** Burn of first degree of back of <u>right</u> hand
- **T23.162-** Burn of first degree of back of <u>left</u> hand
- **T23.169-** Burn of first degree of back of <u>unspecified</u> hand

T23.17- Burn of <u>first</u> degree of <u>wrist</u>
- **T23.171-** Burn of first degree of <u>right</u> wrist
- **T23.172-** Burn of first degree of <u>left</u> wrist
- **T23.179-** Burn of first degree of <u>unspecified</u> wrist

T23.19- Burn of <u>first</u> degree of <u>multiple</u> sites of <u>wrist and hand</u>
- **T23.191-** Burn of first degree of multiple sites of <u>right</u> wrist and hand
- **T23.192-** Burn of first degree of multiple sites of <u>left</u> wrist and hand
- **T23.199-** Burn of first degree of multiple sites of <u>unspecified</u> wrist and hand

T23.2- Burn of <u>second</u> degree of <u>wrist and hand</u>
Use additional external cause code to identify the source, place and intent of the burn (X00-X19, X75-X77, X96-X98, Y92)

T23.20- Burn of <u>second</u> degree of hand, <u>unspecified</u> site
- **T23.201-** Burn of second degree of <u>right</u> hand, unspecified site
- **T23.202-** Burn of second degree of <u>left</u> hand, unspecified site
- **T23.209-** Burn of second degree of unspecified hand, <u>unspecified</u> site

T23.21- Burn of <u>second</u> degree of <u>thumb</u> (nail)
- **T23.211-** Burn of second degree of <u>right</u> thumb (nail)
- **T23.212-** Burn of second degree of <u>left</u> thumb (nail)
- **T23.219-** Burn of second degree of <u>unspecified</u> thumb (nail)

T23.22- Burn of <u>second</u> degree of <u>single finger</u> (nail) <u>except thumb</u>
- **T23.221-** Burn of second degree of single <u>right</u> finger (nail) except thumb
- **T23.222-** Burn of second degree of single <u>left</u> finger (nail) except thumb
- **T23.229-** Burn of second degree of <u>unspecified</u> single finger (nail) except thumb

T23.23- Burn of <u>second</u> degree of <u>multiple fingers</u> (nail), <u>not including thumb</u>
- **T23.231-** Burn of second degree of multiple <u>right</u> fingers (nail), not including thumb
- **T23.232-** Burn of second degree of multiple <u>left</u> fingers (nail), not including thumb
- **T23.239-** Burn of second degree of <u>unspecified</u> multiple fingers (nail), not including thumb

T23.24- Burn of <u>second</u> degree of <u>multiple fingers</u> (nail), <u>including thumb</u>
- **T23.241-** Burn of second degree of multiple <u>right</u> fingers (nail), including thumb
- **T23.242-** Burn of second degree of multiple <u>left</u> fingers (nail), including thumb
- **T23.249-** Burn of second degree of <u>unspecified</u> multiple fingers (nail), including thumb

T23.25- Burn of <u>second</u> degree of <u>palm</u>
- **T23.251-** Burn of second degree of <u>right</u> palm
- **T23.252-** Burn of second degree of <u>left</u> palm
- **T23.259-** Burn of second degree of <u>unspecified</u> palm

T23.26- Burn of <u>second</u> degree of <u>back of hand</u>
- **T23.261-** Burn of second degree of back of <u>right</u> hand
- **T23.262-** Burn of second degree of back of <u>left</u> hand
- **T23.269-** Burn of second degree of back of <u>unspecified</u> hand

T23.27- Burn of <u>second</u> degree of <u>wrist</u>
- **T23.271-** Burn of second degree of <u>right</u> wrist
- **T23.272-** Burn of second degree of <u>left</u> wrist
- **T23.279-** Burn of second degree of <u>unspecified</u> wrist

T23.29- Burn of <u>second</u> degree of <u>multiple</u> sites of <u>wrist and hand</u>
- **T23.291-** Burn of second degree of multiple sites of <u>right</u> wrist and hand
- **T23.292-** Burn of second degree of multiple sites of <u>left</u> wrist and hand

T 2 3 - T 2 3

T23.299- Burn of second degree of multiple sites of <u>unspecified</u> wrist and hand

T23.3- Burn of <u>third</u> degree of <u>wrist and hand</u>
Use additional external cause code to identify the source, place and intent of the burn (X00-X19, X75-X77, X96-X98, Y92)

T23.30- Burn of <u>third</u> degree of hand, <u>unspecified</u> site

CC-A T23.301- Burn of third degree of <u>right</u> hand, unspecified site

CC-A T23.302- Burn of third degree of <u>left</u> hand, unspecified site

CC-A T23.309- Burn of third degree of <u>unspecified</u> hand, unspecified site

T23.31- Burn of <u>third</u> degree of <u>thumb</u> (nail)

CC-A T23.311- Burn of third degree of <u>right</u> thumb (nail)

CC-A T23.312- Burn of third degree of <u>left</u> thumb (nail)

CC-A T23.319- Burn of third degree of <u>unspecified</u> thumb (nail)

T23.32- Burn of <u>third</u> degree of <u>single finger</u> (nail) except thumb

CC-A T23.321- Burn of third degree of single <u>right</u> finger (nail) except thumb

CC-A T23.322- Burn of third degree of single <u>left</u> finger (nail) except thumb

CC-A T23.329- Burn of third degree of <u>unspecified</u> single finger (nail) except thumb

T23.33- Burn of <u>third</u> degree of <u>multiple</u> fingers (nail), <u>not including thumb</u>

CC-A T23.331- Burn of third degree of multiple <u>right</u> fingers (nail), not including thumb

CC-A T23.332- Burn of third degree of multiple <u>left</u> fingers (nail), not including thumb

CC-A T23.339- Burn of third degree of <u>unspecified</u> multiple fingers (nail), not including thumb

T23.34- Burn of <u>third</u> degree of <u>multiple</u> fingers (nail), <u>including thumb</u>

CC-A T23.341- Burn of third degree of multiple <u>right</u> fingers (nail), including thumb

CC-A T23.342- Burn of third degree of multiple <u>left</u> fingers (nail), including thumb

CC-A T23.349- Burn of third degree of <u>unspecified</u> multiple fingers (nail), including thumb

T23.35- Burn of <u>third</u> degree of <u>palm</u>

CC-A T23.351- Burn of third degree of <u>right</u> palm

CC-A T23.352- Burn of third degree of <u>left</u> palm

CC-A T23.359- Burn of third degree of <u>unspecified</u> palm

T23.36- Burn of <u>third</u> degree of <u>back of hand</u>

CC-A T23.361- Burn of third degree of back of <u>right</u> hand

CC-A T23.362- Burn of third degree of back of <u>left</u> hand

CC-A T23.369- Burn of third degree of back of <u>unspecified</u> hand

T23.37- Burn of <u>third</u> degree of <u>wrist</u>

CC-A T23.371- Burn of third degree of <u>right</u> wrist

CC-A T23.372- Burn of third degree of <u>left</u> wrist

CC-A T23.379- Burn of third degree of <u>unspecified</u> wrist

T23.39- Burn of <u>third</u> degree of <u>multiple</u> sites of <u>wrist and hand</u>

CC-A T23.391- Burn of third degree of multiple sites of <u>right</u> wrist and hand

CC-A T23.392- Burn of third degree of multiple sites of <u>left</u> wrist and hand

CC-A T23.399- Burn of third degree of multiple sites of <u>unspecified</u> wrist and hand

T23.4- <u>Corrosion</u> of <u>unspecified degree</u> of <u>wrist and hand</u>
Code first (T51-T65) to identify chemical and intent
Use additional external cause code to identify place (Y92)

T23.40- <u>Corrosion</u> of <u>unspecified degree</u> of hand, <u>unspecified</u> site

T23.401- Corrosion of unspecified degree of <u>right</u> hand, unspecified site

T23.402- Corrosion of unspecified degree of <u>left</u> hand, unspecified site

T23.409- Corrosion of unspecified degree of <u>unspecified</u> hand, unspecified site

T23.41- <u>Corrosion</u> of <u>unspecified degree</u> of <u>thumb</u> (nail)

T23.411- Corrosion of unspecified degree of <u>right</u> thumb (nail)

T23.412- Corrosion of unspecified degree of <u>left</u> thumb (nail)

T23.419- Corrosion of unspecified degree of <u>unspecified</u> thumb (nail)

T23.42- <u>Corrosion</u> of <u>unspecified degree</u> of <u>single finger</u> (nail) <u>except thumb</u>

T23.421- Corrosion of unspecified degree of single <u>right</u> finger (nail) except thumb

T23.422- Corrosion of unspecified degree of single <u>left</u> finger (nail) except thumb

T23.429- Corrosion of unspecified degree of <u>unspecified</u> single finger (nail) except thumb

T23.43- <u>Corrosion</u> of <u>unspecified degree</u> of <u>multiple</u> fingers (nail), <u>not including thumb</u>

T23.431- Corrosion of unspecified degree of multiple <u>right</u> fingers (nail), not including thumb

T23.432- Corrosion of unspecified degree of multiple <u>left</u> fingers (nail), not including thumb

T23.439- Corrosion of unspecified degree of <u>unspecified</u> multiple fingers (nail), not including thumb

T23.44- <u>Corrosion</u> of <u>unspecified degree</u> of <u>multiple</u> fingers (nail), <u>including thumb</u>

T23.441- Corrosion of unspecified degree of multiple <u>right</u> fingers (nail), including thumb

T23.442- Corrosion of unspecified degree of multiple <u>left</u> fingers (nail), including thumb

T23.449- Corrosion of unspecified degree of <u>unspecified</u> multiple fingers (nail), including thumb

T23.45- <u>Corrosion</u> of <u>unspecified degree</u> of <u>palm</u>

T23.451- Corrosion of unspecified degree of <u>right</u> palm

T23.452- Corrosion of unspecified degree of <u>left</u> palm

T23.459- Corrosion of unspecified degree of <u>unspecified</u> palm

T23.46- <u>Corrosion</u> of <u>unspecified degree</u> of <u>back of hand</u>

T23.461- Corrosion of unspecified degree of back of <u>right</u> hand

T23.462- Corrosion of unspecified degree of back of <u>left</u> hand

T23.469- Corrosion of unspecified degree of back of <u>unspecified</u> hand

T23.47- <u>Corrosion</u> of <u>unspecified degree</u> of <u>wrist</u>

T23.471- Corrosion of unspecified degree of <u>right</u> wrist

T23.472- Corrosion of unspecified degree of <u>left</u> wrist

T23.479- Corrosion of unspecified degree of <u>unspecified</u> wrist

T23.49- <u>Corrosion</u> of <u>unspecified degree</u> of <u>multiple</u> sites of <u>wrist and hand</u>

T23.491- Corrosion of unspecified degree of multiple sites of <u>right</u> wrist and hand

T23.492- Corrosion of unspecified degree of multiple sites of <u>left</u> wrist and hand

T23.499- Corrosion of unspecified degree of multiple sites of <u>unspecified</u> wrist and hand

T23.5- <u>Corrosion</u> of <u>first</u> degree of <u>wrist and hand</u>
Code first (T51-T65) to identify chemical and intent
Use additional external cause code to identify place (Y92)

T23.50- <u>Corrosion</u> of <u>first</u> degree of hand, <u>unspecified</u> site

T23.501- Corrosion of first degree of <u>right</u> hand, unspecified site

T23.502- Corrosion of first degree of <u>left</u> hand, unspecified site

T23.509- Corrosion of first degree of <u>unspecified</u> hand, unspecified site

T23.51- <u>Corrosion</u> of <u>first</u> degree of <u>thumb</u> (nail)

T23.511- Corrosion of first degree of <u>right</u> thumb (nail)

T23 - T23

T23.512-   Corrosion of first degree of <u>left</u> thumb (nail)
T23.519-   Corrosion of first degree of <u>unspecified</u> thumb (nail)
T23.52-   <u>Corrosion</u> of <u>first</u> degree of <u>single finger</u> (nail) <u>except thumb</u>
T23.521-   Corrosion of first degree of single <u>right</u> finger (nail) except thumb
T23.522-   Corrosion of first degree of single <u>left</u> finger (nail) except thumb
T23.529-   Corrosion of first degree of <u>unspecified</u> single finger (nail) except thumb
T23.53-   <u>Corrosion</u> of <u>first</u> degree of <u>multiple fingers</u> (nail), <u>not including thumb</u>
T23.531-   Corrosion of first degree of multiple <u>right</u> fingers (nail), not including thumb
T23.532-   Corrosion of first degree of multiple <u>left</u> fingers (nail), not including thumb
T23.539-   Corrosion of first degree of <u>unspecified</u> multiple fingers (nail), not including thumb
T23.54-   <u>Corrosion</u> of <u>first</u> degree of <u>multiple fingers</u> (nail), <u>including thumb</u>
T23.541-   Corrosion of first degree of multiple <u>right</u> fingers (nail), including thumb
T23.542-   Corrosion of first degree of multiple <u>left</u> fingers (nail), including thumb
T23.549-   Corrosion of first degree of <u>unspecified</u> multiple fingers (nail), including thumb
T23.55-   <u>Corrosion</u> of <u>first</u> degree of <u>palm</u>
T23.551-   Corrosion of first degree of <u>right</u> palm
T23.552-   Corrosion of first degree of <u>left</u> palm
T23.559-   Corrosion of first degree of <u>unspecified</u> palm
T23.56-   <u>Corrosion</u> of <u>first</u> degree of <u>back of hand</u>
T23.561-   Corrosion of first degree of back of <u>right</u> hand
T23.562-   Corrosion of first degree of back of <u>left</u> hand
T23.569-   Corrosion of first degree of back of <u>unspecified</u> hand
T23.57-   <u>Corrosion</u> of <u>first</u> degree of <u>wrist</u>
T23.571-   Corrosion of first degree of <u>right</u> wrist
T23.572-   Corrosion of first degree of <u>left</u> wrist
T23.579-   Corrosion of first degree of <u>unspecified</u> wrist
T23.59-   <u>Corrosion</u> of <u>first</u> degree of <u>multiple</u> sites of <u>wrist and hand</u>
T23.591-   Corrosion of first degree of multiple sites of <u>right</u> wrist and hand
T23.592-   Corrosion of first degree of multiple sites of <u>left</u> wrist and hand
T23.599-   Corrosion of first degree of multiple sites of <u>unspecified</u> wrist and hand
T23.6-   <u>Corrosion</u> of <u>second</u> degree of <u>wrist and hand</u>
Code first (T51-T65) to identify chemical and intent
Use additional external cause code to identify place (Y92)
T23.60-   <u>Corrosion</u> of <u>second</u> degree of hand, <u>unspecified</u> site
T23.601-   Corrosion of second degree of <u>right</u> hand, unspecified site
T23.602-   Corrosion of second degree of <u>left</u> hand, unspecified site
T23.609-   Corrosion of second degree of <u>unspecified</u> hand, unspecified site
T23.61-   <u>Corrosion</u> of <u>second</u> degree of <u>thumb</u> (nail)
T23.611-   Corrosion of second degree of <u>right</u> thumb (nail)
T23.612-   Corrosion of second degree of <u>left</u> thumb (nail)
T23.619-   Corrosion of second degree of <u>unspecified</u> thumb (nail)
T23.62-   <u>Corrosion</u> of <u>second</u> degree of <u>single finger</u> (nail) <u>except thumb</u>
T23.621-   Corrosion of second degree of single <u>right</u> finger (nail) except thumb

T23.622-   Corrosion of second degree of single <u>left</u> finger (nail) except thumb
T23.629-   Corrosion of second degree of <u>unspecified</u> single finger (nail) except thumb
T23.63-   <u>Corrosion</u> of <u>second</u> degree of <u>multiple fingers</u> (nail), <u>not including thumb</u>
T23.631-   Corrosion of second degree of multiple <u>right</u> fingers (nail), not including thumb
T23.632-   Corrosion of second degree of multiple <u>left</u> fingers (nail), not including thumb
T23.639-   Corrosion of second degree of <u>unspecified</u> multiple fingers (nail), not including thumb
T23.64-   <u>Corrosion</u> of <u>second</u> degree of <u>multiple fingers</u> (nail), <u>including thumb</u>
T23.641-   Corrosion of second degree of multiple <u>right</u> fingers (nail), including thumb
T23.642-   Corrosion of second degree of multiple <u>left</u> fingers (nail), including thumb
T23.649-   Corrosion of second degree of <u>unspecified</u> multiple fingers (nail), including thumb
T23.65-   <u>Corrosion</u> of <u>second</u> degree of <u>palm</u>
T23.651-   Corrosion of second degree of <u>right</u> palm
T23.652-   Corrosion of second degree of <u>left</u> palm
T23.659-   Corrosion of second degree of <u>unspecified</u> palm
T23.66-   <u>Corrosion</u> of <u>second</u> degree of <u>back of hand</u>
T23.661-   Corrosion of second degree back of <u>right</u> hand
T23.662-   Corrosion of second degree back of <u>left</u> hand
T23.669-   Corrosion of second degree back of <u>unspecified</u> hand
T23.67-   <u>Corrosion</u> of <u>second</u> degree of <u>wrist</u>
T23.671-   Corrosion of second degree of <u>right</u> wrist
T23.672-   Corrosion of second degree of <u>left</u> wrist
T23.679-   Corrosion of second degree of <u>unspecified</u> wrist
T23.69-   <u>Corrosion</u> of <u>second</u> degree of <u>multiple</u> sites of <u>wrist and hand</u>
T23.691-   Corrosion of second degree of multiple sites of <u>right</u> wrist and hand
T23.692-   Corrosion of second degree of multiple sites of <u>left</u> wrist and hand
T23.699-   Corrosion of second degree of multiple sites of <u>unspecified</u> wrist and hand
T23.7-   <u>Corrosion</u> of <u>third</u> degree of <u>wrist and hand</u>
Code first (T51-T65) to identify chemical and intent
Use additional external cause code to identify place (Y92)
T23.70-   <u>Corrosion</u> of <u>third</u> degree of hand, <u>unspecified</u> site
CC-A T23.701-   Corrosion of third degree of <u>right</u> hand, unspecified site
CC-A T23.702-   Corrosion of third degree of <u>left</u> hand, unspecified site
CC-A T23.709-   Corrosion of third degree of <u>unspecified</u> hand, unspecified site
T23.71-   <u>Corrosion</u> of <u>third</u> degree of <u>thumb</u> (nail)
CC-A T23.711-   Corrosion of third degree of <u>right</u> thumb (nail)
CC-A T23.712-   Corrosion of third degree of <u>left</u> thumb (nail)
CC-A T23.719-   Corrosion of third degree of <u>unspecified</u> thumb (nail)
T23.72-   <u>Corrosion</u> of <u>third</u> degree of <u>single finger</u> (nail) <u>except thumb</u>
CC-A T23.721-   Corrosion of third degree of single <u>right</u> finger (nail) except thumb
CC-A T23.722-   Corrosion of third degree of single <u>left</u> finger (nail) except thumb
CC-A T23.729-   Corrosion of third degree of <u>unspecified</u> single finger (nail) except thumb
T23.73-   <u>Corrosion</u> of <u>third</u> degree of <u>multiple fingers</u> (nail), <u>not including thumb</u>
CC-A T23.731-   Corrosion of third degree of multiple <u>right</u> fingers (nail), not including thumb

T23 - T23

CC-A **T23.732-** Corrosion of third degree of multiple <u>left</u> fingers (nail), not including thumb

CC-A **T23.739-** Corrosion of third degree of <u>unspecified</u> multiple fingers (nail), not including thumb

T23.74- <u>Corrosion</u> of <u>third</u> degree of <u>multiple fingers</u> (nail), <u>including thumb</u>

CC-A **T23.741-** Corrosion of third degree of multiple <u>right</u> fingers (nail), including thumb

CC-A **T23.742-** Corrosion of third degree of multiple <u>left</u> fingers (nail), including thumb

CC-A **T23.749-** Corrosion of third degree of <u>unspecified</u> multiple fingers (nail), including thumb

T23.75- <u>Corrosion</u> of <u>third</u> degree of <u>palm</u>

CC-A **T23.751-** Corrosion of third degree of <u>right</u> palm

CC-A **T23.752-** Corrosion of third degree of <u>left</u> palm

CC-A **T23.759-** Corrosion of third degree of <u>unspecified</u> palm

T23.76- <u>Corrosion</u> of <u>third</u> degree of <u>back of hand</u>

CC-A **T23.761-** Corrosion of third degree of back of <u>right</u> hand

CC-A **T23.762-** Corrosion of third degree of back of <u>left</u> hand

CC-A **T23.769-** Corrosion of third degree back of <u>unspecified</u> hand

T23.77- <u>Corrosion</u> of <u>third</u> degree of <u>wrist</u>

CC-A **T23.771-** Corrosion of third degree of <u>right</u> wrist

CC-A **T23.772-** Corrosion of third degree of <u>left</u> wrist

CC-A **T23.779-** Corrosion of third degree of <u>unspecified</u> wrist

T23.79- <u>Corrosion</u> of <u>third</u> degree of <u>multiple</u> sites of <u>wrist and hand</u>

CC-A **T23.791-** Corrosion of third degree of multiple sites of <u>right</u> wrist and hand

CC-A **T23.792-** Corrosion of third degree of multiple sites of <u>left</u> wrist and hand

CC-A **T23.799-** Corrosion of third degree of multiple sites of <u>unspecified</u> wrist and hand

T24- <u>Burn and corrosion</u> of <u>lower limb, except ankle and foot</u>

Excludes ❷: *burn and corrosion of ankle and foot (T25.-)*
            burn and corrosion of hip region (T21.-)

The appropriate 7th character is to be added to each code from category T24:
A   <u>Initial</u> encounter
D   <u>Subsequent</u> encounter
S   <u>Sequela</u>

T24.0- Burn of <u>unspecified degree</u> of <u>lower limb, except ankle and foot</u>
Use additional external cause code to identify the source, place and intent of the burn (X00-X19, X75-X77, X96-X98, Y92)

T24.00- Burn of <u>unspecified degree</u> of <u>unspecified</u> site of <u>lower limb, except ankle and foot</u>

T24.001- Burn of unspecified degree of unspecified site of <u>right</u> lower limb, except ankle and foot

T24.002- Burn of unspecified degree of unspecified site of <u>left</u> lower limb, except ankle and foot

T24.009- Burn of unspecified degree of unspecified site of <u>unspecified</u> lower limb, except ankle and foot

T24.01- Burn of <u>unspecified degree</u> of <u>thigh</u>

T24.011- Burn of unspecified degree of <u>right</u> thigh

T24.012- Burn of unspecified degree of <u>left</u> thigh

T24.019- Burn of unspecified degree of <u>unspecified</u> thigh

T24.02- Burn of <u>unspecified degree</u> of <u>knee</u>

T24.021- Burn of unspecified degree of <u>right</u> knee

T24.022- Burn of unspecified degree of <u>left</u> knee

T24.029- Burn of unspecified degree of <u>unspecified</u> knee

T24.03- Burn of <u>unspecified degree</u> of <u>lower leg</u>

T24.031- Burn of unspecified degree of <u>right</u> lower leg

T24.032- Burn of unspecified degree of <u>left</u> lower leg

T24.039- Burn of unspecified degree of <u>unspecified</u> lower leg

T24.09- Burn of <u>unspecified degree</u> of <u>multiple</u> sites of <u>lower limb, except ankle and foot</u>

T24.091- Burn of unspecified degree of multiple sites of <u>right</u> lower limb, except ankle and foot

T24.092- Burn of unspecified degree of multiple sites of <u>left</u> lower limb, except ankle and foot

T24.099- Burn of unspecified degree of multiple sites of <u>unspecified</u> lower limb, except ankle and foot

T24.1- Burn of <u>first</u> degree of <u>lower limb, except ankle and foot</u>
Use additional external cause code to identify the source, place and intent of the burn (X00-X19, X75-X77, X96-X98, Y92)

T24.10- Burn of <u>first</u> degree of <u>unspecified</u> site of <u>lower limb, except ankle and foot</u>

T24.101- Burn of first degree of unspecified site of <u>right</u> lower limb, except ankle and foot

T24.102- Burn of first degree of unspecified site of <u>left</u> lower limb, except ankle and foot

T24.109- Burn of first degree of unspecified site of <u>unspecified</u> lower limb, except ankle and foot

T24.11- Burn of <u>first</u> degree of <u>thigh</u>

T24.111- Burn of first degree of <u>right</u> thigh

T24.112- Burn of first degree of <u>left</u> thigh

T24.119- Burn of first degree of <u>unspecified</u> thigh

T24.12- Burn of <u>first</u> degree of <u>knee</u>

T24.121- Burn of first degree of <u>right</u> knee

T24.122- Burn of first degree of <u>left</u> knee

T24.129- Burn of first degree of <u>unspecified</u> knee

T24.13- Burn of <u>first</u> degree of <u>lower leg</u>

T24.131- Burn of first degree of <u>right</u> lower leg

T24.132- Burn of first degree of <u>left</u> lower leg

T24.139- Burn of first degree of <u>unspecified</u> lower leg

T24.19- Burn of <u>first</u> degree of <u>multiple</u> sites of <u>lower limb, except ankle and foot</u>

T24.191- Burn of first degree of multiple sites of <u>right</u> lower limb, except ankle and foot

T24.192- Burn of first degree of multiple sites of <u>left</u> lower limb, except ankle and foot

T24.199- Burn of first degree of multiple sites of <u>unspecified</u> lower limb, except ankle and foot

T24.2- Burn of <u>second</u> degree of <u>lower limb, except ankle and foot</u>
Use additional external cause code to identify the source, place and intent of the burn (X00-X19, X75-X77, X96-X98, Y92)

T24.20- Burn of <u>second</u> degree of <u>unspecified</u> site of <u>lower limb, except ankle and foot</u>

T24.201- Burn of second degree of unspecified site of <u>right</u> lower limb, except ankle and foot

T24.202- Burn of second degree of unspecified site of <u>left</u> lower limb, except ankle and foot

T24.209- Burn of second degree of unspecified site of <u>unspecified</u> lower limb, except ankle and foot

T24.21- Burn of <u>second</u> degree of <u>thigh</u>

T24.211- Burn of second degree of <u>right</u> thigh

T24.212- Burn of second degree of <u>left</u> thigh

T24.219- Burn of second degree of <u>unspecified</u> thigh

T24.22- Burn of <u>second</u> degree of <u>knee</u>

T24.221- Burn of second degree of <u>right</u> knee

T24.222- Burn of second degree of <u>left</u> knee

T24.229- Burn of second degree of <u>unspecified</u> knee

T24.23- Burn of <u>second</u> degree of <u>lower leg</u>

T24.231- Burn of second degree of <u>right</u> lower leg

T24.232- Burn of second degree of <u>left</u> lower leg

T24.239- Burn of second degree of <u>unspecified</u> lower leg

T24.29- Burn of <u>second</u> degree of <u>multiple</u> sites of <u>lower limb, except ankle and foot</u>

T24.291- Burn of second degree of multiple sites of <u>right</u> lower limb, except ankle and foot

T24.292- Burn of second degree of multiple sites of <u>left</u> lower limb, except ankle and foot

T24.299- Burn of second degree of multiple sites of <u>unspecified</u> lower limb, except ankle and foot

T24.3- Burn of <u>third</u> degree of <u>lower limb, except ankle and foot</u>
Use additional external cause code to identify the source, place and intent of the burn (X00-X19, X75-X77, X96-X98, Y92)

T24.30- Burn of <u>third</u> degree of <u>unspecified</u> site of <u>lower limb, except ankle and foot</u>

CC-A **T24.301-** Burn of third degree of <u>unspecified</u> site of <u>right</u> lower limb, except ankle and foot

CC-A **T24.302-** Burn of third degree of <u>unspecified</u> site of <u>left</u> lower limb, except ankle and foot

CC-A **T24.309-** Burn of third degree of <u>unspecified</u> site of <u>unspecified</u> lower limb, except ankle and foot

T24.31- Burn of <u>third</u> degree of <u>thigh</u>

CC-A **T24.311-** Burn of third degree of <u>right</u> thigh

CC-A **T24.312-** Burn of third degree of <u>left</u> thigh

CC-A **T24.319-** Burn of third degree of <u>unspecified</u> thigh

T24.32- Burn of <u>third</u> degree of <u>knee</u>

CC-A **T24.321-** Burn of third degree of <u>right</u> knee

CC-A **T24.322-** Burn of third degree of <u>left</u> knee

CC-A **T24.329-** Burn of third degree of <u>unspecified</u> knee

T24.33- Burn of <u>third</u> degree of <u>lower leg</u>

CC-A **T24.331-** Burn of third degree of <u>right</u> lower leg

CC-A **T24.332-** Burn of third degree of <u>left</u> lower leg

CC-A **T24.339-** Burn of third degree of <u>unspecified</u> lower leg

T24.39- Burn of <u>third</u> degree of <u>multiple</u> sites of <u>lower limb, except ankle and foot</u>

CC-A **T24.391-** Burn of third degree of multiple sites of <u>right</u> lower limb, except ankle and foot

CC-A **T24.392-** Burn of third degree of multiple sites of <u>left</u> lower limb, except ankle and foot

CC-A **T24.399-** Burn of third degree of multiple sites of <u>unspecified</u> lower limb, except ankle and foot

T24.4- <u>Corrosion</u> of <u>unspecified degree</u> of <u>lower limb, except ankle and foot</u>
Code first (T51-T65) to identify chemical and intent
Use additional external cause code to identify place (Y92)

T24.40- <u>Corrosion</u> of <u>unspecified degree</u> of <u>unspecified</u> site of <u>lower limb, except ankle and foot</u>

T24.401- Corrosion of unspecified degree of <u>unspecified</u> site of <u>right</u> lower limb, except ankle and foot

T24.402- Corrosion of unspecified degree of <u>unspecified</u> site of <u>left</u> lower limb, except ankle and foot

T24.409- Corrosion of unspecified degree of <u>unspecified</u> site of <u>unspecified</u> lower limb, except ankle and foot

T24.41- <u>Corrosion</u> of <u>unspecified degree</u> of <u>thigh</u>

T24.411- Corrosion of unspecified degree of <u>right</u> thigh

T24.412- Corrosion of unspecified degree of <u>left</u> thigh

T24.419- Corrosion of unspecified degree of <u>unspecified</u> thigh

T24.42- <u>Corrosion</u> of <u>unspecified degree</u> of <u>knee</u>

T24.421- Corrosion of unspecified degree of <u>right</u> knee

T24.422- Corrosion of unspecified degree of <u>left</u> knee

T24.429- Corrosion of unspecified degree of <u>unspecified</u> knee

T24.43- <u>Corrosion</u> of <u>unspecified degree</u> of <u>lower leg</u>

T24.431- Corrosion of unspecified degree of <u>right</u> lower leg

T24.432- Corrosion of unspecified degree of <u>left</u> lower leg

T24.439- Corrosion of unspecified degree of <u>unspecified</u> lower leg

T24.49- <u>Corrosion</u> of <u>unspecified degree</u> of <u>multiple</u> sites of <u>lower limb, except ankle and foot</u>

T24.491- Corrosion of unspecified degree of multiple sites of <u>right</u> lower limb, except ankle and foot

T24.492- Corrosion of unspecified degree of multiple sites of <u>left</u> lower limb, except ankle and foot

T24.499- Corrosion of unspecified degree of multiple sites of <u>unspecified</u> lower limb, except ankle and foot

T24.5- <u>Corrosion</u> of <u>first</u> degree of <u>lower limb, except ankle and foot</u>
Code first (T51-T65) to identify chemical and intent
Use additional external cause code to identify place (Y92)

T24.50- <u>Corrosion</u> of <u>first</u> degree of <u>unspecified</u> site of <u>lower limb, except ankle and foot</u>

T24.501- Corrosion of first degree of unspecified site of <u>right</u> lower limb, except ankle and foot

T24.502- Corrosion of first degree of unspecified site of <u>left</u> lower limb, except ankle and foot

T24.509- Corrosion of first degree of unspecified site of <u>unspecified</u> lower limb, except ankle and foot

T24.51- <u>Corrosion</u> of <u>first</u> degree of <u>thigh</u>

T24.511- Corrosion of first degree of <u>right</u> thigh

T24.512- Corrosion of first degree of <u>left</u> thigh

T24.519- Corrosion of first degree of <u>unspecified</u> thigh

T24.52- <u>Corrosion</u> of <u>first</u> degree of <u>knee</u>

T24.521- Corrosion of first degree of <u>right</u> knee

T24.522- Corrosion of first degree of <u>left</u> knee

T24.529- Corrosion of first degree of <u>unspecified</u> knee

T24.53- <u>Corrosion</u> of <u>first</u> degree of <u>lower leg</u>

T24.531- Corrosion of first degree of <u>right</u> lower leg

T24.532- Corrosion of first degree of <u>left</u> lower leg

T24.539- Corrosion of first degree of <u>unspecified</u> lower leg

T24.59- <u>Corrosion</u> of <u>first</u> degree of <u>multiple</u> sites of <u>lower limb, except ankle and foot</u>

T24.591- Corrosion of first degree of multiple sites of <u>right</u> lower limb, except ankle and foot

T24.592- Corrosion of first degree of multiple sites of <u>left</u> lower limb, except ankle and foot

T24.599- Corrosion of first degree of multiple sites of <u>unspecified</u> lower limb, except ankle and foot

T24.6- <u>Corrosion</u> of <u>second</u> degree of <u>lower limb, except ankle and foot</u>
Code first (T51-T65) to identify chemical and intent
Use additional external cause code to identify place (Y92)

T24.60- <u>Corrosion</u> of <u>second</u> degree of <u>unspecified</u> site of <u>lower limb, except ankle and foot</u>

T24.601- Corrosion of second degree of unspecified site of <u>right</u> lower limb, except ankle and foot

T24.602- Corrosion of second degree of unspecified site of <u>left</u> lower limb, except ankle and foot

T24.609- Corrosion of second degree of unspecified site of <u>unspecified</u> lower limb, except ankle and foot

T24.61- <u>Corrosion</u> of <u>second</u> degree of <u>thigh</u>

T24.611- Corrosion of second degree of <u>right</u> thigh

T24.612- Corrosion of second degree of <u>left</u> thigh

T24.619- Corrosion of second degree of <u>unspecified</u> thigh

T24.62- <u>Corrosion</u> of <u>second</u> degree of <u>knee</u>

T24.621- Corrosion of second degree of <u>right</u> knee

T24.622- Corrosion of second degree of <u>left</u> knee

T24.629- Corrosion of second degree of <u>unspecified</u> knee

T24.63- <u>Corrosion</u> of <u>second</u> degree of <u>lower leg</u>

T24.631- Corrosion of second degree of <u>right</u> lower leg

T24.632- Corrosion of second degree of <u>left</u> lower leg

T24.639- Corrosion of second degree of <u>unspecified</u> lower leg

T24.69- <u>Corrosion</u> of <u>second</u> degree of <u>multiple</u> sites of <u>lower limb, except ankle and foot</u>

T24.691- Corrosion of second degree of multiple sites of <u>right</u> lower limb, except ankle and foot

T24.692- Corrosion of second degree of multiple sites of <u>left</u> lower limb, except ankle and foot

T24.699- Corrosion of second degree of multiple sites of <u>unspecified</u> lower limb, except ankle and foot

T24 - T24

Excludes 1: = NOT CODED HERE! (Do not code both)   **1149**   *Excludes ❷:* = Not Included Here

T24.7- Corrosion of third degree of lower limb, except ankle and foot
Code first (T51-T65) to identify chemical and intent
Use additional external cause code to identify place (Y92)

T24.70- Corrosion of third degree of unspecified site of lower limb, except ankle and foot

CC-A **T24.701-** Corrosion of third degree of unspecified site of right lower limb, except ankle and foot

CC-A **T24.702-** Corrosion of third degree of unspecified site of left lower limb, except ankle and foot

CC-A **T24.709-** Corrosion of third degree of unspecified site of unspecified lower limb, except ankle and foot

T24.71- Corrosion of third degree of thigh

CC-A **T24.711-** Corrosion of third degree of right thigh

CC-A **T24.712-** Corrosion of third degree of left thigh

CC-A **T24.719-** Corrosion of third degree of unspecified thigh

T24.72- Corrosion of third degree of knee

CC-A **T24.721-** Corrosion of third degree of right knee

CC-A **T24.722-** Corrosion of third degree of left knee

CC-A **T24.729-** Corrosion of third degree of unspecified knee

T24.73- Corrosion of third degree of lower leg

CC-A **T24.731-** Corrosion of third degree of right lower leg

CC-A **T24.732-** Corrosion of third degree of left lower leg

CC-A **T24.739-** Corrosion of third degree of unspecified lower leg

T24.79- Corrosion of third degree of multiple sites of lower limb, except ankle and foot

CC-A **T24.791-** Corrosion of third degree of multiple sites of right lower limb, except ankle and foot

CC-A **T24.792-** Corrosion of third degree of multiple sites of left lower limb, except ankle and foot

CC-A **T24.799-** Corrosion of third degree of multiple sites of unspecified lower limb, except ankle and foot

T25- Burn and corrosion of ankle and foot

The appropriate 7th character is to be added to each code from category T25:

A Initial encounter
D Subsequent encounter
S Sequela

T25.0- Burn of unspecified degree of ankle and foot
Use additional external cause code to identify the source, place and intent of the burn (X00-X19, X75-X77, X96-X98, Y92)

T25.01- Burn of unspecified degree of ankle

T25.011- Burn of unspecified degree of right ankle

T25.012- Burn of unspecified degree of left ankle

T25.019- Burn of unspecified degree of unspecified ankle

T25.02- Burn of unspecified degree of foot
Excludes ❷: burn of unspecified degree of toe(s) (nail) (T25.03-)

T25.021- Burn of unspecified degree of right foot

T25.022- Burn of unspecified degree of left foot

T25.029- Burn of unspecified degree of unspecified foot

T25.03- Burn of unspecified degree of toe(s) (nail)

T25.031- Burn of unspecified degree of right toe(s) (nail)

T25.032- Burn of unspecified degree of left toe(s) (nail)

T25.039- Burn of unspecified degree of unspecified toe(s) (nail)

T25.09- Burn of unspecified degree of multiple sites of ankle and foot

T25.091- Burn of unspecified degree of multiple sites of right ankle and foot

T25.092- Burn of unspecified degree of multiple sites of left ankle and foot

T25.099- Burn of unspecified degree of multiple sites of unspecified ankle and foot

T25.1- Burn of first degree of ankle and foot
Use additional external cause code to identify the source, place and intent of the burn (X00-X19, X75-X77, X96-X98, Y92)

T25.11- Burn of first degree of ankle

T25.111- Burn of first degree of right ankle

T25.112- Burn of first degree of left ankle

T25.119- Burn of first degree of unspecified ankle

T25.12- Burn of first degree of foot
Excludes ❷: burn of first degree of toe(s) (nail) (T25.13-)

T25.121- Burn of first degree of right foot

T25.122- Burn of first degree of left foot

T25.129- Burn of first degree of unspecified foot

T25.13- Burn of first degree of toe(s) (nail)

T25.131- Burn of first degree of right toe(s) (nail)

T25.132- Burn of first degree of left toe(s) (nail)

T25.139- Burn of first degree of unspecified toe(s) (nail)

T25.19- Burn of first degree of multiple sites of ankle and foot

T25.191- Burn of first degree of multiple sites of right ankle and foot

T25.192- Burn of first degree of multiple sites of left ankle and foot

T25.199- Burn of first degree of multiple sites of unspecified ankle and foot

T25.2- Burn of second degree of ankle and foot
Use additional external cause code to identify the source, place and intent of the burn (X00-X19, X75-X77, X96-X98, Y92)

T25.21- Burn of second degree of ankle

T25.211- Burn of second degree of right ankle

T25.212- Burn of second degree of left ankle

T25.219- Burn of second degree of unspecified ankle

T25.22- Burn of second degree of foot
Excludes ❷: burn of second degree of toe(s) (nail) (T25.23-)

T25.221- Burn of second degree of right foot

T25.222- Burn of second degree of left foot

T25.229- Burn of second degree of unspecified foot

T25.23- Burn of second degree of toe(s) (nail)

T25.231- Burn of second degree of right toe(s) (nail)

T25.232- Burn of second degree of left toe(s) (nail)

T25.239- Burn of second degree of unspecified toe(s) (nail)

T25.29- Burn of second degree of multiple sites of ankle and foot

T25.291- Burn of second degree of multiple sites of right ankle and foot

T25.292- Burn of second degree of multiple sites of left ankle and foot

T25.299- Burn of second degree of multiple sites of unspecified ankle and foot

T25.3- Burn of third degree of ankle and foot
Use additional external cause code to identify the source, place and intent of the burn (X00-X19, X75-X77, X96-X98, Y92)

T25.31- Burn of third degree of ankle

CC-A **T25.311-** Burn of third degree of right ankle

CC-A **T25.312-** Burn of third degree of left ankle

CC-A **T25.319-** Burn of third degree of unspecified ankle

T25.32- Burn of third degree of foot
Excludes ❷: burn of third degree of toe(s) (nail) (T25.33-)

CC-A **T25.321-** Burn of third degree of right foot

CC-A **T25.322-** Burn of third degree of left foot

CC-A **T25.329-** Burn of third degree of unspecified foot

T25.33- Burn of third degree of toe(s) (nail)

CC-A **T25.331-** Burn of third degree of right toe(s) (nail)

CC-A **T25.332-** Burn of third degree of left toe(s) (nail)

CC-A **T25.339-** Burn of third degree of unspecified toe(s) (nail)

T25.39- Burn of third degree of multiple sites of ankle and foot

CC-A **T25.391-** Burn of third degree of multiple sites of right ankle and foot

CC-A **T25.392-** Burn of third degree of multiple sites of left ankle and foot

CC-A **T25.399-** Burn of third degree of multiple sites of unspecified ankle and foot

T24 - T25

T25.4-   Corrosion of unspecified degree of ankle and foot
          Code first (T51-T65) to identify chemical and intent
          Use additional external cause code to identify place (Y92)

    T25.41- Corrosion of unspecified degree of ankle

        T25.411- Corrosion of unspecified degree of right ankle

        T25.412- Corrosion of unspecified degree of left ankle

        T25.419- Corrosion of unspecified degree of unspecified ankle

    T25.42- Corrosion of unspecified degree of foot
             Excludes ❷: corrosion of unspecified degree of toe(s) (nail)
                           (T25.43-)

        T25.421- Corrosion of unspecified degree of right foot

        T25.422- Corrosion of unspecified degree of left foot

        T25.429- Corrosion of unspecified degree of unspecified foot

    T25.43- Corrosion of unspecified degree of toe(s) (nail)

        T25.431- Corrosion of unspecified degree of right toe(s) (nail)

        T25.432- Corrosion of unspecified degree of left toe(s) (nail)

        T25.439- Corrosion of unspecified degree of unspecified toe(s) (nail)

    T25.49- Corrosion of unspecified degree of multiple sites of ankle and foot

        T25.491- Corrosion of unspecified degree of multiple sites of right ankle and foot

        T25.492- Corrosion of unspecified degree of multiple sites of left ankle and foot

        T25.499- Corrosion of unspecified degree of multiple sites of unspecified ankle and foot

T25.5-   Corrosion of first degree of ankle and foot
          Code first (T51-T65) to identify chemical and intent
          Use additional external cause code to identify place (Y92)

    T25.51- Corrosion of first degree of ankle

        T25.511- Corrosion of first degree of right ankle

        T25.512- Corrosion of first degree of left ankle

        T25.519- Corrosion of first degree of unspecified ankle

    T25.52- Corrosion of first degree of foot
             Excludes ❷: corrosion of first degree of toe(s) (nail) (T25.53-)

        T25.521- Corrosion of first degree of right foot

        T25.522- Corrosion of first degree of left foot

        T25.529- Corrosion of first degree of unspecified foot

    T25.53- Corrosion of first degree of toe(s) (nail)

        T25.531- Corrosion of first degree of right toe(s) (nail)

        T25.532- Corrosion of first degree of left toe(s) (nail)

        T25.539- Corrosion of first degree of unspecified toe(s) (nail)

    T25.59- Corrosion of first degree of multiple sites of ankle and foot

        T25.591- Corrosion of first degree of multiple sites of right ankle and foot

        T25.592- Corrosion of first degree of multiple sites of left ankle and foot

        T25.599- Corrosion of first degree of multiple sites of unspecified ankle and foot

T25.6-   Corrosion of second degree of ankle and foot
          Code first (T51-T65) to identify chemical and intent
          Use additional external cause code to identify place (Y92)

    T25.61- Corrosion of second degree of ankle

        T25.611- Corrosion of second degree of right ankle

        T25.612- Corrosion of second degree of left ankle

        T25.619- Corrosion of second degree of unspecified ankle

    T25.62- Corrosion of second degree of foot
             Excludes ❷: corrosion of second degree of toe(s) (nail)
                           (T25.63-)

        T25.621- Corrosion of second degree of right foot

        T25.622- Corrosion of second degree of left foot

        T25.629- Corrosion of second degree of unspecified foot

    T25.63- Corrosion of second degree of toe(s) (nail)

        T25.631- Corrosion of second degree of right toe(s) (nail)

        T25.632- Corrosion of second degree of left toe(s) (nail)

        T25.639- Corrosion of second degree of unspecified toe(s) (nail)

    T25.69   Corrosion of second degree of multiple sites of ankle and foot

        T25.691- Corrosion of second degree of right ankle and foot

        T25.692- Corrosion of second degree of left ankle and foot

        T25.699- Corrosion of second degree of unspecified ankle and foot

T25.7-   Corrosion of third degree of ankle and foot
          Code first (T51-T65) to identify chemical and intent
          Use additional external cause code to identify place (Y92)

    T25.71- Corrosion of third degree of ankle

  CC-A T25.711- Corrosion of third degree of right ankle

  CC-A T25.712- Corrosion of third degree of left ankle

  CC-A T25.719- Corrosion of third degree of unspecified ankle

    T25.72- Corrosion of third degree of foot
             Excludes ❷: corrosion of third degree of toe(s) (nail) (T25.73-)

  CC-A T25.721- Corrosion of third degree of right foot

  CC-A T25.722- Corrosion of third degree of left foot

  CC-A T25.729- Corrosion of third degree of unspecified foot

    T25.73- Corrosion of third degree of toe(s) (nail)

  CC-A T25.731- Corrosion of third degree of right toe(s) (nail)

  CC-A T25.732- Corrosion of third degree of left toe(s) (nail)

  CC-A T25.739- Corrosion of third degree of unspecified toe(s) (nail)

    T25.79- Corrosion of third degree of multiple sites of ankle and foot

  CC-A T25.791- Corrosion of third degree of multiple sites of right ankle and foot

  CC-A T25.792- Corrosion of third degree of multiple sites of left ankle and foot

  CC-A T25.799- Corrosion of third degree of multiple sites of unspecified ankle and foot

Burns and corrosions confined to eye and internal organs (T26-T28)

T26-   Burn and corrosion confined to eye and adnexa
        The appropriate 7th character is to be added to each code from category T26:
        A   Initial encounter
        D   Subsequent encounter
        S   Sequela

    T26.0- Burn of eyelid and periocular area
            Use additional external cause code to identify the source, place and intent of the burn (X00-X19, X75-X77, X96-X98, Y92)

        T26.00x- Burn of unspecified eyelid and periocular area

        T26.01x- Burn of right eyelid and periocular area

        T26.02x- Burn of left eyelid and periocular area

    T26.1- Burn of cornea and conjunctival sac
            Use additional external cause code to identify the source, place and intent of the burn (X00-X19, X75-X77, X96-X98, Y92)

        T26.10x- Burn of cornea and conjunctival sac, unspecified eye

        T26.11x- Burn of cornea and conjunctival sac, right eye

        T26.12x- Burn of cornea and conjunctival sac, left eye

    T26.2- Burn with resulting rupture and destruction of eyeball
            Use additional external cause code to identify the source, place and intent of the burn (X00-X19, X75-X77, X96-X98, Y92)

  CC-A T26.20x- Burn with resulting rupture and destruction of unspecified eyeball

  CC-A T26.21x- Burn with resulting rupture and destruction of right eyeball

  CC-A T26.22x- Burn with resulting rupture and destruction of left eyeball

    T26.3- Burns of other specified parts of eye and adnexa
            Use additional external cause code to identify the source, place and intent of the burn (X00-X19, X75-X77, X96-X98, Y92)

        T26.30x- Burns of other specified parts of unspecified eye and adnexa

T26.31x- Burns of other specified parts of <u>right</u> eye and adnexa

T26.32x- Burns of other specified parts of <u>left</u> eye and adnexa

T26.4- Burn of eye and adnexa, part <u>unspecified</u>
Use additional external cause code to identify the source, place and intent of the burn (X00-X19, X75-X77, X96-X98, Y92)

T26.40x- Burn of <u>unspecified</u> eye and adnexa, part <u>unspecified</u>

T26.41x- Burn of <u>right</u> eye and adnexa, part <u>unspecified</u>

T26.42x- Burn of <u>left</u> eye and adnexa, part <u>unspecified</u>

T26.5- <u>Corrosion</u> of <u>eyelid and periocular area</u>
Code first (T51-T65) to identify chemical and intent
Use additional external cause code to identify place (Y92)

T26.50x- Corrosion of <u>unspecified</u> eyelid and periocular area

T26.51x- Corrosion of <u>right</u> eyelid and periocular area

T26.52x- Corrosion of <u>left</u> eyelid and periocular area

T26.6- <u>Corrosion</u> of <u>cornea and conjunctival sac</u>
Code first (T51-T65) to identify chemical and intent
Use additional external cause code to identify place (Y92)

T26.60x- Corrosion of cornea and conjunctival sac, <u>unspecified</u> eye

T26.61x- Corrosion of cornea and conjunctival sac, <u>right</u> eye

T26.62x- Corrosion of cornea and conjunctival sac, <u>left</u> eye

T26.7- <u>Corrosion with resulting rupture and destruction of eyeball</u>
Code first (T51-T65) to identify chemical and intent
Use additional external cause code to identify place (Y92)

CC-A T26.70x- Corrosion with resulting rupture and destruction of <u>unspecified</u> eyeball

CC-A T26.71x- Corrosion with resulting rupture and destruction of <u>right</u> eyeball

CC-A T26.72x- Corrosion with resulting rupture and destruction of <u>left</u> eyeball

T26.8- <u>Corrosions</u> of <u>other specified parts</u> of <u>eye and adnexa</u>
Code first (T51-T65) to identify chemical and intent
Use additional external cause code to identify place (Y92)

T26.80x- Corrosions of other specified parts of <u>unspecified</u> eye and adnexa

T26.81x- Corrosions of other specified parts of <u>right</u> eye and adnexa

T26.82x- Corrosions of other specified parts of <u>left</u> eye and adnexa

T26.9- <u>Corrosion</u> of eye and adnexa, part <u>unspecified</u>
Code first (T51-T65) to identify chemical and intent
Use additional external cause code to identify place (Y92)

T26.90x- Corrosion of <u>unspecified</u> eye and adnexa, part <u>unspecified</u>

T26.91x- Corrosion of <u>right</u> eye and adnexa, part <u>unspecified</u>

T26.92x- Corrosion of <u>left</u> eye and adnexa, part <u>unspecified</u>

T27- <u>Burn and corrosion</u> of <u>respiratory tract</u>
Use additional external cause code to identify the source and intent of the burn (X00-X19, X75-X77, X96-X98)
Use additional external cause code to identify place (Y92)

The appropriate 7th character is to be added to each code from category T27:
A <u>Initial</u> encounter
D <u>Subsequent</u> encounter
S <u>Sequela</u>

T27.0xx- Burn of larynx and trachea
CC-A

T27.1xx- Burn involving larynx and trachea with lung
CC-A

T27.2xx- Burn of other parts of respiratory tract
CC-A Burn of thoracic cavity

T27.3xx- Burn of respiratory tract, part <u>unspecified</u>
CC-A Code first (T51-T65) to identify chemical and intent for codes T27.4-T27.7

T27.4xx- <u>Corrosion</u> of larynx and trachea
CC-A

T27.5xx- <u>Corrosion</u> involving larynx and trachea with lung
CC-A

T27.6xx- <u>Corrosion</u> of other parts of respiratory tract
CC-A

T27.7xx- <u>Corrosion</u> of respiratory tract, part <u>unspecified</u>
CC-A

T28- <u>Burn and corrosion</u> of <u>other internal organs</u>
Use additional external cause code to identify the source and intent of the burn (X00-X19, X75-X77, X96-X98)
Use additional external cause code to identify place (Y92)

The appropriate 7th character is to be added to each code from category T28:
A <u>Initial</u> encounter
D <u>Subsequent</u> encounter
S <u>Sequela</u>

T28.0xx- Burn of mouth and pharynx

T28.1xx- Burn of esophagus
CC-A

T28.2xx- Burn of other parts of alimentary tract
CC-A

T28.3xx- Burn of internal genitourinary organs

T28.4xx- Burns of other and unspecified internal organs

T28.40x- Burn of <u>unspecified</u> internal organ

T28.41- Burn of <u>ear drum</u>

T28.411- Burn of <u>right</u> ear drum

T28.412- Burn of <u>left</u> ear drum

T28.419- Burn of <u>unspecified</u> ear drum

T28.49x- Burn of <u>other</u> internal organ
Code first (T51-T65) to identify chemical and intent for T28.5-T28.9-

T28.5xx- <u>Corrosion</u> of mouth and pharynx

T28.6xx- <u>Corrosion</u> of esophagus
CC-A

T28.7xx- <u>Corrosion</u> of other parts of alimentary tract
CC-A

T28.8xx- <u>Corrosion</u> of internal genitourinary organs

T28.9xx- <u>Corrosions</u> of other and unspecified internal organs

T28.90x- Corrosions of <u>unspecified</u> internal organs

T28.91- Corrosions of <u>ear drum</u>

T28.911- Corrosions of <u>right</u> ear drum

T28.912- Corrosions of <u>left</u> ear drum

T28.919- Corrosions of <u>unspecified</u> ear drum

T28.99x- Corrosions of <u>other</u> internal organs

T
2
6
I
T
2
8

Burns and corrosions of multiple and unspecified body regions (T30-T32)

T30- <u>Burn and corrosion</u>, <u>body region unspecified</u>

    T30.0 Burn of <u>unspecified</u> body region, <u>unspecified degree</u>
        Note: This code is not for inpatient use. Code to specified site and degree of burns
          Burn NOS
          Multiple burns NOS

    T30.4 <u>Corrosion</u> of <u>unspecified</u> body region, <u>unspecified degree</u>
        Note: This code is not for inpatient use. Code to specified site and degree of corrosion
          Corrosion NOS
          Multiple corrosion NOS

T31- <u>Burns</u> <u>classified according to extent of body surface involved</u>
    Note: This category is to be used as the primary code only when the site of the burn is unspecified. It should be used as a supplementary code with categories T20-T25 when the site is specified.

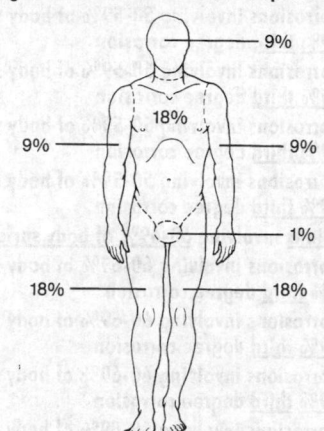

BODY SURFACE RULE OF NINES

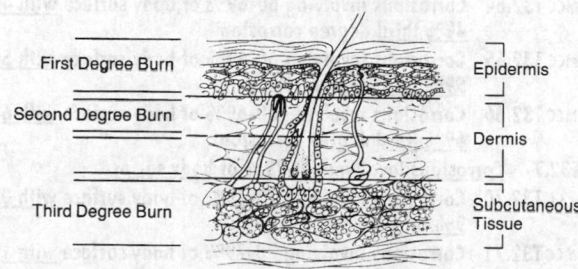

First Degree Burn — Epidermis
Second Degree Burn — Dermis
Third Degree Burn — Subcutaneous Tissue

EXTENT OF SKIN BURN

T31.0 Burns involving <u>less than 10% of body surface</u>

T31.1- Burns involving <u>10-19% of body surface</u>
  CC **T31.10** Burns involving 10-19% of body surface <u>with 0% to 9%</u> <u>third</u> degree burns
        Burns involving 10-19% of body surface NOS
  CC **T31.11** Burns involving 10-19% of body surface <u>with 10-19%</u> <u>third</u> degree burns

T31.2- Burns involving <u>20-29% of body surface</u>
  CC **T31.20** Burns involving 20-29% of body surface <u>with 0% to 9%</u> <u>third</u> degree burns
        Burns involving 20-29% of body surface NOS
  MCC **T31.21** Burns involving 20-29% of body surface <u>with 10-19%</u> <u>third</u> degree burns
  MCC **T31.22** Burns involving 20-29% of body surface <u>with 20-29%</u> <u>third</u> degree burns

T31.3- Burns involving <u>30-39% of body surface</u>
  CC **T31.30** Burns involving 30-39% of body surface <u>with 0% to 9%</u> <u>third</u> degree burns
        Burns involving 30-39% of body surface NOS
  MCC **T31.31** Burns involving 30-39% of body surface <u>with 10-19%</u> <u>third</u> degree burns
  MCC **T31.32** Burns involving 30-39% of body surface <u>with 20-29%</u> <u>third</u> degree burns

MCC **T31.33** Burns involving 30-39% of body surface <u>with 30-39%</u> <u>third</u> degree burns

T31.4- Burns involving <u>40-49% of body surface</u>
  CC **T31.40** Burns involving 40-49% of body surface <u>with 0% to 9%</u> <u>third</u> degree burns
        Burns involving 40-49% of body surface NOS
  MCC **T31.41** Burns involving 40-49% of body surface <u>with 10-19%</u> <u>third</u> degree burns
  MCC **T31.42** Burns involving 40-49% of body surface <u>with 20-29%</u> <u>third</u> degree burns
  MCC **T31.43** Burns involving 40-49% of body surface <u>with 30-39%</u> <u>third</u> degree burns
  MCC **T31.44** Burns involving 40-49% of body surface <u>with 40-49%</u> <u>third</u> degree burns

T31.5- Burns involving <u>50-59% of body surface</u>
  CC **T31.50** Burns involving 50-59% of body surface <u>with 0% to 9%</u> <u>third</u> degree burns
        Burns involving 50-59% of body surface NOS
  MCC **T31.51** Burns involving 50-59% of body surface <u>with 10-19%</u> <u>third</u> degree burns
  MCC **T31.52** Burns involving 50-59% of body surface <u>with 20-29%</u> <u>third</u> degree burns
  MCC **T31.53** Burns involving 50-59% of body surface <u>with 30-39%</u> <u>third</u> degree burns
  MCC **T31.54** Burns involving 50-59% of body surface <u>with 40-49%</u> <u>third</u> degree burns
  MCC **T31.55** Burns involving 50-59% of body surface <u>with 50-59%</u> <u>third</u> degree burns

T31.6- Burns involving <u>60-69% of body surface</u>
  CC **T31.60** Burns involving 60-69% of body surface <u>with 0% to 9%</u> <u>third</u> degree burns
        Burns involving 60-69% of body surface NOS
  MCC **T31.61** Burns involving 60-69% of body surface <u>with 10-19%</u> <u>third</u> degree burns
  MCC **T31.62** Burns involving 60-69% of body surface <u>with 20-29%</u> <u>third</u> degree burns
  MCC **T31.63** Burns involving 60-69% of body surface <u>with 30-39%</u> <u>third</u> degree burns
  MCC **T31.64** Burns involving 60-69% of body surface <u>with 40-49%</u> <u>third</u> degree burns
  MCC **T31.65** Burns involving 60-69% of body surface <u>with 50-59%</u> <u>third</u> degree burns
  MCC **T31.66** Burns involving 60-69% of body surface <u>with 60-69%</u> <u>third</u> degree burns

T31.7- Burns involving <u>70-79% of body surface</u>
  CC **T31.70** Burns involving 70-79% of body surface <u>with 0% to 9%</u> <u>third</u> degree burns
        Burns involving 70-79% of body surface NOS
  MCC **T31.71** Burns involving 70-79% of body surface <u>with 10-19%</u> <u>third</u> degree burns
  MCC **T31.72** Burns involving 70-79% of body surface <u>with 20-29%</u> <u>third</u> degree burns
  MCC **T31.73** Burns involving 70-79% of body surface <u>with 30-39%</u> <u>third</u> degree burns
  MCC **T31.74** Burns involving 70-79% of body surface <u>with 40-49%</u> <u>third</u> degree burns
  MCC **T31.75** Burns involving 70-79% of body surface <u>with 50-59%</u> <u>third</u> degree burns
  MCC **T31.76** Burns involving 70-79% of body surface <u>with 60-69%</u> <u>third</u> degree burns
  MCC **T31.77** Burns involving 70-79% of body surface <u>with 70-79%</u> <u>third</u> degree burns

T30 - T31

T31.8- Burns involving <u>80-89% of body surface</u>

cc **T31.80** Burns involving 80-89% of body surface <u>with 0% to 9% third</u> degree burns
Burns involving 80-89% of body surface NOS

MCC **T31.81** Burns involving 80-89% of body surface <u>with 10-19% third</u> degree burns

MCC **T31.82** Burns involving 80-89% of body surface <u>with 20-29% third</u> degree burns

MCC **T31.83** Burns involving 80-89% of body surface <u>with 30-39% third</u> degree burns

MCC **T31.84** Burns involving 80-89% of body surface <u>with 40-49% third</u> degree burns

MCC **T31.85** Burns involving 80-89% of body surface <u>with 50-59% third</u> degree burns

MCC **T31.86** Burns involving 80-89% of body surface <u>with 60-69% third</u> degree burns

MCC **T31.87** Burns involving 80-89% of body surface <u>with 70-79% third</u> degree burns

MCC **T31.88** Burns involving 80-89% of body surface <u>with 80-89% third</u> degree burns

T31.9- Burns involving <u>90% or more of body surface</u>

cc **T31.90** Burns involving 90% or more of body surface <u>with 0% to 9% third</u> degree burns
Burns involving 90% or more of body surface NOS

MCC **T31.91** Burns involving 90% or more of body surface <u>with 10-19% third</u> degree burns

MCC **T31.92** Burns involving 90% or more of body surface <u>with 20-29% third</u> degree burns

MCC **T31.93** Burns involving 90% or more of body surface <u>with 30-39% third</u> degree burns

MCC **T31.94** Burns involving 90% or more of body surface <u>with 40-49% third</u> degree burns

MCC **T31.95** Burns involving 90% or more of body surface <u>with 50-59% third</u> degree burns

MCC **T31.96** Burns involving 90% or more of body surface <u>with 60-69% third</u> degree burns

MCC **T31.97** Burns involving 90% or more of body surface <u>with 70-79% third</u> degree burns

MCC **T31.98** Burns involving 90% or more of body surface <u>with 80-89% third</u> degree burns

MCC **T31.99** Burns involving 90% or more of body surface <u>with 90% or more third</u> degree burns

T32- Corrosions <u>classified according to extent of body surface involved</u>
Note: This category is to be used as the primary code only when the site of the corrosion is unspecified. It may be used as a supplementary code with categories T20-T25 when the site is specified.

T32.0 Corrosions involving <u>less than 10% of body surface</u>

T32.1- Corrosions involving <u>10-19% of body surface</u>

cc **T32.10** Corrosions involving 10-19% of body surface <u>with 0% to 9% third</u> degree corrosion
Corrosions involving 10-19% of body surface NOS

cc **T32.11** Corrosions involving 10-19% of body surface <u>with 10-19% third</u> degree corrosion

T32.2- Corrosions involving <u>20-29% of body surface</u>

cc **T32.20** Corrosions involving 20-29% of body surface <u>with 0% to 9% third</u> degree corrosion

MCC **T32.21** Corrosions involving 20-29% of body surface <u>with 10-19% third</u> degree corrosion

MCC **T32.22** Corrosions involving 20-29% of body surface <u>with 20-29% third</u> degree corrosion

T32.3- Corrosions involving <u>30-39% of body surface</u>

cc **T32.30** Corrosions involving 30-39% of body surface <u>with 0% to 9% third</u> degree corrosion

MCC **T32.31** Corrosions involving 30-39% of body surface <u>with 10-19% third</u> degree corrosion

MCC **T32.32** Corrosions involving 30-39% of body surface <u>with 20-29% third</u> degree corrosion

MCC **T32.33** Corrosions involving 30-39% of body surface <u>with 30-39% third</u> degree corrosion

T32.4- Corrosions involving <u>40-49% of body surface</u>

cc **T32.40** Corrosions involving 40-49% of body surface <u>with 0% to 9% third</u> degree corrosion

MCC **T32.41** Corrosions involving 40-49% of body surface <u>with 10-19% third</u> degree corrosion

MCC **T32.42** Corrosions involving 40-49% of body surface <u>with 20-29% third</u> degree corrosion

MCC **T32.43** Corrosions involving 40-49% of body surface <u>with 30-39% third</u> degree corrosion

MCC **T32.44** Corrosions involving 40-49% of body surface <u>with 40-49% third</u> degree corrosion

T32.5- Corrosions involving <u>50-59% of body surface</u>

cc **T32.50** Corrosions involving 50-59% of body surface <u>with 0% to 9% third</u> degree corrosion

MCC **T32.51** Corrosions involving 50-59% of body surface <u>with 10-19% third</u> degree corrosion

MCC **T32.52** Corrosions involving 50-59% of body surface <u>with 20-29% third</u> degree corrosion

MCC **T32.53** Corrosions involving 50-59% of body surface <u>with 30-39% third</u> degree corrosion

MCC **T32.54** Corrosions involving 50-59% of body surface <u>with 40-49% third</u> degree corrosion

MCC **T32.55** Corrosions involving 50-59% of body surface <u>with 50-59% third</u> degree corrosion

T32.6- Corrosions involving <u>60-69% of body surface</u>

cc **T32.60** Corrosions involving 60-69% of body surface <u>with 0% to 9% third</u> degree corrosion

MCC **T32.61** Corrosions involving 60-69% of body surface <u>with 10-19% third</u> degree corrosion

MCC **T32.62** Corrosions involving 60-69% of body surface <u>with 20-29% third</u> degree corrosion

MCC **T32.63** Corrosions involving 60-69% of body surface <u>with 30-39% third</u> degree corrosion

MCC **T32.64** Corrosions involving 60-69% of body surface <u>with 40-49% third</u> degree corrosion

MCC **T32.65** Corrosions involving 60-69% of body surface <u>with 50-59% third</u> degree corrosion

MCC **T32.66** Corrosions involving 60-69% of body surface <u>with 60-69% third</u> degree corrosion

T32.7- Corrosions involving <u>70-79% of body surface</u>

cc **T32.70** Corrosions involving 70-79% of body surface <u>with 0% to 9% third</u> degree corrosion

MCC **T32.71** Corrosions involving 70-79% of body surface <u>with 10-19% third</u> degree corrosion

MCC **T32.72** Corrosions involving 70-79% of body surface <u>with 20-29% third</u> degree corrosion

MCC **T32.73** Corrosions involving 70-79% of body surface <u>with 30-39% third</u> degree corrosion

MCC **T32.74** Corrosions involving 70-79% of body surface <u>with 40-49% third</u> degree corrosion

MCC **T32.75** Corrosions involving 70-79% of body surface <u>with 50-59% third</u> degree corrosion

MCC **T32.76** Corrosions involving 70-79% of body surface <u>with 60-69% third</u> degree corrosion

MCC **T32.77** Corrosions involving 70-79% of body surface <u>with 70-79% third</u> degree corrosion

T32.8- Corrosions involving <u>80-89% of body surface</u>

cc **T32.80** Corrosions involving 80-89% of body surface <u>with 0% to 9% third</u> degree corrosion

MCC **T32.81** Corrosions involving 80-89% of body surface <u>with 10-19% third</u> degree corrosion

MCC **T32.82** Corrosions involving 80-89% of body surface <u>with 20-29% third</u> degree corrosion

MCC **T32.83** Corrosions involving 80-89% of body surface <u>with 30-39% third</u> degree corrosion

MCC **T32.84** Corrosions involving 80-89% of body surface <u>with 40-49% third</u> degree corrosion

---

Excludes 1: = NOT CODED HERE! (Do not code both)   **1154**   *Excludes* ❷: = Not Included Here

MCC **T32.85** Corrosions involving 80-89% of body surface <u>with 50-59% third</u> degree corrosion

MCC **T32.86** Corrosions involving 80-89% of body surface <u>with 60-69% third</u> degree corrosion

MCC **T32.87** Corrosions involving 80-89% of body surface <u>with 70-79% third</u> degree corrosion

MCC **T32.88** Corrosions involving 80-89% of body surface <u>with 80-89% third</u> degree corrosion

T32.9- <u>Corrosions</u> involving <u>90% or more of body surface</u>

CC **T32.90** Corrosions involving 90% or more of body surface <u>with 0% to 9% third</u> degree corrosion

MCC **T32.91** Corrosions involving 90% or more of body surface <u>with 10-19% third</u> degree corrosion

MCC **T32.92** Corrosions involving 90% or more of body surface <u>with 20-29% third</u> degree corrosion

MCC **T32.93** Corrosions involving 90% or more of body surface <u>with 30-39% third</u> degree corrosion

MCC **T32.94** Corrosions involving 90% or more of body surface <u>with 40-49% third</u> degree corrosion

MCC **T32.95** Corrosions involving 90% or more of body surface <u>with 50-59% third</u> degree corrosion

MCC **T32.96** Corrosions involving 90% or more of body surface <u>with 60-69% third</u> degree corrosion

MCC **T32.97** Corrosions involving 90% or more of body surface <u>with 70-79% third</u> degree corrosion

MCC **T32.98** Corrosions involving 90% or more of body surface <u>with 80-89% third</u> degree corrosion

MCC **T32.99** Corrosions involving 90% or more of body surface <u>with 90% or more third</u> degree corrosion

Frostbite (T33-T34)

Excludes ❷: hypothermia and other effects of reduced temperature (T68, T69.-)

T33- <u>Superficial</u> frostbite
Includes: Frostbite with partial thickness skin loss
The appropriate 7th character is to be added to each code from category T33:
A <u>Initial</u> encounter
D <u>Subsequent</u> encounter
S <u>Sequela</u>

T33.0- Superficial frostbite of head
  T33.01- Superficial frostbite of <u>ear</u>
  CC-A **T33.011-** Superficial frostbite of <u>right</u> ear
  CC-A **T33.012-** Superficial frostbite of <u>left</u> ear
  CC-A **T33.019-** Superficial frostbite of <u>unspecified</u> ear
CC-A **T33.02x-** Superficial frostbite of nose
CC-A **T33.09x-** Superficial frostbite of other part of head
T33.1xx- Superficial frostbite of neck
CC-A
T33.2xx- Superficial frostbite of thorax
CC-A
T33.3xx- Superficial frostbite of abdominal wall, lower back and pelvis
CC-A
T33.4- Superficial frostbite of <u>arm</u>
  Excludes ❷: superficial frostbite of wrist and hand (T33.5-)
CC-A **T33.40x-** Superficial frostbite of <u>unspecified</u> arm
CC-A **T33.41x-** Superficial frostbite of <u>right</u> arm
CC-A **T33.42x-** Superficial frostbite of <u>left</u> arm
T33.5- Superficial frostbite of wrist, hand, and fingers
  T33.51- Superficial frostbite of <u>wrist</u>
  CC-A **T33.511-** Superficial frostbite of <u>right</u> wrist
  CC-A **T33.512-** Superficial frostbite of <u>left</u> wrist
  CC-A **T33.519-** Superficial frostbite of <u>unspecified</u> wrist
  T33.52- Superficial frostbite of <u>hand</u>
    Excludes ❷: superficial frostbite of fingers (T33.53-)
  CC-A **T33.521-** Superficial frostbite of <u>right</u> hand
  CC-A **T33.522-** Superficial frostbite of <u>left</u> hand
  CC-A **T33.529-** Superficial frostbite of <u>unspecified</u> hand

  T33.53- Superficial frostbite of <u>finger(s)</u>
  CC-A **T33.531-** Superficial frostbite of <u>right</u> finger(s)
  CC-A **T33.532-** Superficial frostbite of <u>left</u> finger(s)
  CC-A **T33.539-** Superficial frostbite of <u>unspecified</u> finger(s)
T33.6- Superficial frostbite of <u>hip and thigh</u>
CC-A **T33.60x-** Superficial frostbite of <u>unspecified</u> hip and thigh
CC-A **T33.61x-** Superficial frostbite of <u>right</u> hip and thigh
CC-A **T33.62x-** Superficial frostbite of <u>left</u> hip and thigh
T33.7- Superficial frostbite of <u>knee and lower leg</u>
  Excludes ❷: superficial frostbite of ankle and foot (T33.8-)
CC-A **T33.70x-** Superficial frostbite of <u>unspecified</u> knee and lower leg
CC-A **T33.71x-** Superficial frostbite of <u>right</u> knee and lower leg
CC-A **T33.72x-** Superficial frostbite of <u>left</u> knee and lower leg
T33.8- Superficial frostbite of ankle, foot, and toe(s)
  T33.81- Superficial frostbite of <u>ankle</u>
  CC-A **T33.811-** Superficial frostbite of <u>right</u> ankle
  CC-A **T33.812-** Superficial frostbite of <u>left</u> ankle
  CC-A **T33.819-** Superficial frostbite of <u>unspecified</u> ankle
  T33.82- Superficial frostbite of <u>foot</u>
  CC-A **T33.821-** Superficial frostbite of <u>right</u> foot
  CC-A **T33.822-** Superficial frostbite of <u>left</u> foot
  CC-A **T33.829-** Superficial frostbite of <u>unspecified</u> foot
  T33.83- Superficial frostbite of <u>toe(s)</u>
  CC-A **T33.831-** Superficial frostbite of <u>right</u> toe(s)
  CC-A **T33.832-** Superficial frostbite of <u>left</u> toe(s)
  CC-A **T33.839-** Superficial frostbite of <u>unspecified</u> toe(s)
T33.9- Superficial frostbite of other and unspecified sites
CC-A **T33.90x-** Superficial frostbite of <u>unspecified</u> sites
    Superficial frostbite NOS
CC-A **T33.99x-** Superficial frostbite of <u>other</u> sites
    Superficial frostbite of leg NOS
    Superficial frostbite of trunk NOS

T34- <u>Frostbite</u> <u>with tissue necrosis</u>
The appropriate 7th character is to be added to each code from category T34:
A <u>Initial</u> encounter
D <u>Subsequent</u> encounter
S <u>Sequela</u>

T34.0- Frostbite <u>with tissue necrosis</u> of head
  T34.01- Frostbite <u>with tissue necrosis</u> of <u>ear</u>
  CC-A **T34.011-** Frostbite with tissue necrosis of <u>right</u> ear
  CC-A **T34.012-** Frostbite with tissue necrosis of <u>left</u> ear
  CC-A **T34.019-** Frostbite with tissue necrosis of <u>unspecified</u> ear
CC-A **T34.02x-** Frostbite <u>with tissue necrosis</u> of nose
CC-A **T34.09x-** Frostbite <u>with tissue necrosis</u> of other part of head
T34.1xx- Frostbite <u>with tissue necrosis</u> of neck
CC-A
T34.2xx- Frostbite <u>with tissue necrosis</u> of thorax
CC-A
T34.3xx- Frostbite <u>with tissue necrosis</u> of abdominal wall, lower back and pelvis
CC-A
T34.4- Frostbite <u>with tissue necrosis</u> of <u>arm</u>
  Excludes ❷: frostbite with tissue necrosis of wrist and hand (T34.5-)
CC-A **T34.40x-** Frostbite with tissue necrosis of <u>unspecified</u> arm
CC-A **T34.41x-** Frostbite with tissue necrosis of <u>right</u> arm
CC-A **T34.42x-** Frostbite with tissue necrosis of <u>left</u> arm
T34.5- Frostbite <u>with tissue necrosis</u> of wrist, hand, and finger(s)
  T34.51- Frostbite <u>with tissue necrosis</u> of <u>wrist</u>
  CC-A **T34.511-** Frostbite with tissue necrosis of <u>right</u> wrist
  CC-A **T34.512-** Frostbite with tissue necrosis of <u>left</u> wrist
  CC-A **T34.519-** Frostbite with tissue necrosis of <u>unspecified</u> wrist
  T34.52- Frostbite <u>with tissue necrosis</u> of <u>hand</u>
    Excludes ❷: frostbite with tissue necrosis of finger(s) (T34.53-)
  CC-A **T34.521-** Frostbite with tissue necrosis of <u>right</u> hand
  CC-A **T34.522-** Frostbite with tissue necrosis of <u>left</u> hand
  CC-A **T34.529-** Frostbite with tissue necrosis of <u>unspecified</u> hand

T32 - T34

T34.53- Frostbite <u>with tissue necrosis</u> of <u>finger(s)</u>

CC-A T34.531- Frostbite with tissue necrosis of <u>right</u> finger(s)

CC-A T34.532- Frostbite with tissue necrosis of <u>left</u> finger(s)

CC-A T34.539- Frostbite with tissue necrosis of <u>unspecified</u> finger(s)

T34.6- Frostbite <u>with tissue necrosis</u> of <u>hip and thigh</u>

CC-A T34.60x- Frostbite with tissue necrosis of <u>unspecified</u> hip and thigh

CC-A T34.61x- Frostbite with tissue necrosis of <u>right</u> hip and thigh

CC-A T34.62x- Frostbite with tissue necrosis of <u>left</u> hip and thigh

T34.7- Frostbite <u>with tissue necrosis</u> of <u>knee and lower leg</u>

> Excludes ❷: *frostbite with tissue necrosis of ankle and foot (T34.8-)*

CC-A T34.70x- Frostbite with tissue necrosis of <u>unspecified</u> knee and lower leg

CC-A T34.71x- Frostbite with tissue necrosis of <u>right</u> knee and lower leg

CC-A T34.72x- Frostbite with tissue necrosis of <u>left</u> knee and lower leg

T34.8- Frostbite <u>with tissue necrosis</u> of ankle, foot, and toe(s)

T34.81- Frostbite <u>with tissue necrosis</u> of <u>ankle</u>

CC-A T34.811- Frostbite with tissue necrosis of <u>right</u> ankle

CC-A T34.812- Frostbite with tissue necrosis of <u>left</u> ankle

CC-A T34.819- Frostbite with tissue necrosis of <u>unspecified</u> ankle

T34.82- Frostbite <u>with tissue necrosis</u> of <u>foot</u>

CC-A T34.821- Frostbite with tissue necrosis of <u>right</u> foot

CC-A T34.822- Frostbite with tissue necrosis of <u>left</u> foot

CC-A T34.829- Frostbite with tissue necrosis of <u>unspecified</u> foot

T34.83- Frostbite <u>with tissue necrosis</u> of <u>toe(s)</u>

CC-A T34.831- Frostbite with tissue necrosis of <u>right</u> toe(s)

CC-A T34.832- Frostbite with tissue necrosis of <u>left</u> toe(s)

CC-A T34.839- Frostbite with tissue necrosis of <u>unspecified</u> toe(s)

T34.9- Frostbite <u>with tissue necrosis</u> of other and unspecified sites

CC-A T34.90x- Frostbite with tissue necrosis of <u>unspecified</u> sites
> Frostbite with tissue necrosis NOS

CC-A T34.99x- Frostbite with tissue necrosis of <u>other</u> sites
> Frostbite with tissue necrosis of leg NOS
> Frostbite with tissue necrosis of trunk NOS

Poisoning by, adverse effects of and underdosing of drugs, medicaments and biological substances (T36-T50)

Includes: Adverse effect of correct substance properly administered
Poisoning by overdose of substance
Poisoning by wrong substance given or taken in error
Underdosing by (inadvertantly) (deliberately) taking less substance than prescribed or instructed

Code first, for adverse effects, the nature of the adverse effect, such as:
Adverse effect NOS (T88.7)
Aspirin gastritis (K29-)
Blood disorders (D56-D76)
Contact dermatitis (L23-L25)
Dermatitis due to substances taken internally (L27-)
Nephropathy (N14.0-N14.2)

Note: The drug giving rise to the adverse effect should be identified by use of codes from categories T36-T50 with fifth or sixth character 5.

Use additional code(s) to specify:
Manifestations of poisoning
Underdosing of medication regime (Z91.12-, Z91.13-)
Underdosing or failure in dosage during medical and surgical care (Y63.6, Y63.8-Y63.9)

> Excludes 1: *toxic reaction to local anesthesia in pregnancy (O29.3-)*
> Excludes ❷: *abuse and dependence of psychoactive substances (F10-F19)*
> *abuse of non-dependence-producing substances (F55-)*
> *drug reaction and poisoning affecting newborn (P00-P96)*
> *pathological drug intoxication (inebriation) (F10-F19)*

* Indicates the complete list of specific drugs and chemicals included in each drug and chemical category for codes T36-T65, taken directly from the Official Table of Drugs & Chemicals.

T36- Poisoning by, adverse effect of and underdosing of <u>systemic antibiotics</u>

> Excludes 1: *antineoplastic antibiotics (T45.1-)*
> *locally applied antibiotic NEC (T49.0)*
> *topically used antibiotic for ear, nose and throat (T49.6)*
> *topically used antibiotic for eye (T49.5)*

The appropriate 7th character is to be added to each code from category T36:

A <u>Initial</u> encounter

D <u>Subsequent</u> encounter

S <u>Sequela</u>

T36.0- Poisoning by, adverse effect of and underdosing of <u>penicillins</u>

<u>T36.0 - DRUGS/CHEMS*</u>		
Adicillin	Ciclacillin	Penethamate
Amdinocilline	Clemizole penicillin	Penicillin (any)
Amoxicillin	Clometocillin	Phenbenicillin
Ampicillin	Cloxacillin	Pheneticillin
Ancillin	Cyclacillin	Phenoxymethyl penicillin
Apalcillin	Dicloxacillin	Phenthicillin
Aspoxicillin	Epicillin	Piperacillin
Azidocillin	Flucloxacillin	Pivampicillin
Azlocillin	Hetacillin	Pivmecillinam
Bacampicillin	Hydrabamine penicillin	Procaine, benzylpenicillin
Benethamine penicillin	Imipenem	Procaine, penicillin G
Benzathine benzylpenicillin	Isoxazolyl penicillin	Propicillin
Benzathine penicillin	Mecillinam	Sodium nafcillin
Benzyl penicillin	Metampicillin	Sulbactam
Benzylpenicillin	Methicillin	Sulbenicillin
Carbenicillin	Methoxybenzyl penicillin	Sultamicillin
Carfecillin	Meticillin	Talampicillin
Carindacillin	Mezlocillin	Temocillin
Cephalosporins, N	Nafcillin	Ticarcillin
(adicillin)	Oxacillin	Xantocillin
	Penamecillin	

T36.0x- Poisoning by, adverse effect of and underdosing of penicillins

T36.0x1- Poisoning by penicillins, <u>accidental</u> (unintentional)
> Poisoning by penicillins NOS

T36.0x2- Poisoning by penicillins, <u>intentional</u> self-harm

T36.0x3- Poisoning by penicillins, <u>assault</u>

T36.0x4- Poisoning by penicillins, <u>undetermined</u>

T36.0x5- <u>Adverse effect</u> of penicillins

T36.0x6- <u>Underdosing</u> of penicillins

T34 - T36

T36.1-   **Poisoning by, adverse effect of and underdosing of cephalosporins and other beta-lactam antibiotics**

T36.1 - DRUGS/CHEMS*	Cefbuperazone	Cefteram
Antibiotic, cephalosporin (group)	Cefetamet	Ceftezole
Antibiotic, b-lactam NEC	Cefixime	Ceftizoxime
Aztreonam	Cefmenoxime	Ceftriaxone
Cefacetrile	Cefmetazole	Cefuroxime
Cefaclor	Cefminox	Cefuzonam
Cefadroxil	Cefonicid	Cephalexin
Cefalexin	Cefoperazone	Cephaloglycin
Cefaloglycin	Ceforanide	Cephaloridine
Cefaloridine	Cefotaxime	Cephalosporins
Cefalosporins	Cefotetan	Cephalothin
Cefalotin	Cefotiam	Cephalotin
Cefamandole	Cefoxitin	Cephradine
Cefamycin antibiotic	Cefpimizole	Clavulanic acid
Cefapirin	Cefpiramide	Flomoxef
Cefatrizine	Cefradine	Latamoxef
Cefazedone	Cefroxadine	
Cefazolin	Cefsulodin	
	Ceftazidime	

T36.1x-   **Poisoning by, adverse effect of and underdosing of <u>cephalosporins and other beta-lactam antibiotics</u>**

     T36.1x1-   **Poisoning by cephalosporins and other beta-lactam antibiotics, <u>accidental</u> (unintentional)**
         Poisoning by cephalosporins and other beta-lactam antibiotics NOS

     T36.1x2-   **Poisoning by cephalosporins and other beta-lactam antibiotics, <u>intentional</u> self-harm**

     T36.1x3-   **Poisoning by cephalosporins and other beta-lactam antibiotics, <u>assault</u>**

     T36.1x4-   **Poisoning by cephalosporins and other beta-lactam antibiotics, <u>undetermined</u>**

     T36.1x5-   **<u>Adverse effect</u> of cephalosporins and other beta-lactam antibiotics**

     T36.1x6-   **<u>Underdosing</u> of cephalosporins and other beta-lactam antibiotics**

T36.2-   **Poisoning by, adverse effect of and underdosing of chloramphenicol group**

T36.2 - DRUGS/CHEMS*	Chloramphenicol	Cloramfenicol
Antibiotic, chloramphenicol (group)	Chloromycetin	Thiamphenicol
	Cloponone	

T36.2x-   **Poisoning by, adverse effect of and underdosing of <u>chloramphenicol group</u>**

     T36.2x1-   **Poisoning by chloramphenicol group, <u>accidental</u> (unintentional)**
         Poisoning by chloramphenicol group NOS

     T36.2x2-   **Poisoning by chloramphenicol group, <u>intentional</u> self-harm**

     T36.2x3-   **Poisoning by chloramphenicol group, <u>assault</u>**

     T36.2x4-   **Poisoning by chloramphenicol group, <u>undetermined</u>**

     T36.2x5-   **<u>Adverse effect</u> of chloramphenicol group**

     T36.2x6-   **<u>Underdosing</u> of chloramphenicol group**

T36.3-   **Poisoning by, adverse effect of and underdosing of macrolides**

T36.3 - DRUGS/CHEMS*	Kitasamycin	Rokitamycin
Antibiotic, macrolides	Macrolide, antibiotic	Roxithromycin
Azithromycin	Midecamycin	Spiramycin
Erythromycin (salts)	Miokamycin	TAO
Ilotycin	Oleandomycin	Triacetyloleandomycin
Josamycin	Pristinamycin	Troleandomycin

T36.3x-   **Poisoning by, adverse effect of and underdosing of <u>macrolides</u>**

     T36.3x1-   **Poisoning by macrolides, <u>accidental</u> (unintentional)**
         Poisoning by macrolides NOS

     T36.3x2-   **Poisoning by macrolides, <u>intentional</u> self-harm**

     T36.3x3-   **Poisoning by macrolides, <u>assault</u>**

     T36.3x4-   **Poisoning by macrolides, <u>undetermined</u>**

     T36.3x5-   **<u>Adverse effect</u> of macrolides**

     T36.3x6-   **<u>Underdosing</u> of macrolides**

T36.4-   **Poisoning by, adverse effect of and underdosing of tetracyclines**

T36.4 - DRUGS/CHEMS*	Demeclocycline	Methacycline
Achromycin	Demethylchlortetracycline	Minocycline
Antibiotic, tetracycline (group)	Demethyltetracycline	Oxytetracycline
Aureomycin	DMCT	Penimepicycline
Chlormethylenecycline	Doxycycline	Polycycline
Chlortetracycline	Guamecycline	Rolitetracycline
Clomocycline	Lymecycline	Terramycin
Declomycin	Meclocycline	Tetracycline
	Metacycline	

T36.4x-   **Poisoning by, adverse effect of and underdosing of <u>tetracyclines</u>**

     T36.4x1-   **Poisoning by tetracyclines, <u>accidental</u> (unintentional)**
         Poisoning by tetracyclines NOS

     T36.4x2-   **Poisoning by tetracyclines, <u>intentional</u> self-harm**

     T36.4x3-   **Poisoning by tetracyclines, <u>assault</u>**

     T36.4x4-   **Poisoning by tetracyclines, <u>undetermined</u>**

     T36.4x5-   **<u>Adverse effect</u> of tetracyclines**

     T36.4x6-   **<u>Underdosing</u> of tetracyclines**

T36.5-   **Poisoning by, adverse effect of and underdosing of aminoglycosides**
     Poisoning by, adverse effect of and underdosing of streptomycin

T36.5 - DRUGS/CHEMS*	Bekanamycin	Netilmicin
Amikacin	Dibekacin	Novobiocin
Antibiotic, aminoglycoside	Dihydrostreptomycin	Paromomycin
Antibiotic, antimycobacterial	Framycetin	Ribostamycin
Anti-infective, antimycobacterial, antibiotics	Garamycin	Sisomicin
	Gentamicin	Spectinomycin
	Isepamicin	Streptoduocin
Antimycobacterial drug, antibiotics	Kanamycin	Streptomycin (derivative)
	Kantrex	Streptonivicin
	Micronomicin	Streptovarycin
Antituberculars, antibiotics	Mycifradin	Tobramycin
Astromicin	Neomycin (derivatives)	

T36.5x-   **Poisoning by, adverse effect of and underdosing of <u>aminoglycosides</u>**

     T36.5x1-   **Poisoning by aminoglycosides, <u>accidental</u> (unintentional)**
         Poisoning by aminoglycosides NOS

     T36.5x2-   **Poisoning by aminoglycosides, <u>intentional</u> self-harm**

     T36.5x3-   **Poisoning by aminoglycosides, <u>assault</u>**

     T36.5x4-   **Poisoning by aminoglycosides, <u>undetermined</u>**

     T36.5x5-   **<u>Adverse effect</u> of aminoglycosides**

     T36.5x6-   **<u>Underdosing</u> of aminoglycosides**

T36.6-   **Poisoning by, adverse effect of and underdosing of rifampicins**

T36.6 - DRUGS/CHEMS*	Rifamide	Rifaximin
Ansamycin	Rifampicin	
Isoniazid with rifampicin	Rifampin	
Rifabutin	Rifamycin	

T36.6x-   **Poisoning by, adverse effect of and underdosing of <u>rifampicins</u>**

     T36.6x1-   **Poisoning by rifampicins, <u>accidental</u> (unintentional)**
         Poisoning by rifampicins NOS

     T36.6x2-   **Poisoning by rifampicins, <u>intentional</u> self-harm**

     T36.6x3-   **Poisoning by rifampicins, <u>assault</u>**

     T36.6x4-   **Poisoning by rifampicins, <u>undetermined</u>**

     T36.6x5-   **<u>Adverse effect</u> of rifampicins**

     T36.6x6-   **<u>Underdosing</u> of rifampicins**

T36 - T36

Excludes 1: = NOT CODED HERE! (Do not code both)   **1157**   *Excludes ❷:* = Not Included Here

T36.7- Poisoning by, adverse effect of and underdosing of antifungal antibiotics, systemically used

T36.7 - DRUGS/CHEMS*		
Amphotericin B	Fungizone	Nilstat
Antibiotic, antifungal	Grifulvin	Nystatin
Antifungal, antibiotic	Griseofulvin	Pimaricin
(systemic)	Hachimycin	Trichomycin
Fulvicin	Mepartricin	
	Mycostatin	

T36.7x- Poisoning by, adverse effect of and underdosing of <u>antifungal antibiotics, systemically used</u>

T36.7x1- Poisoning by antifungal antibiotics, systemically used, <u>accidental</u> (unintentional)
Poisoning by antifungal antibiotics, systemically used NOS

T36.7x2- Poisoning by antifungal antibiotics, systemically used, <u>intentional</u> self-harm

T36.7x3- Poisoning by antifungal antibiotics, systemically used, <u>assault</u>

T36.7x4- Poisoning by antifungal antibiotics, systemically used, <u>undetermined</u>

T36.7x5- <u>Adverse effect</u> of antifungal antibiotics, systemically used

T36.7x6- <u>Underdosing</u> of antifungal antibiotics, systemically used

T36.8- Poisoning by, adverse effect of and underdosing of other systemic antibiotics

T36.8 - DRUGS/CHEMS*	Colistimethate	Neosporin
Aerosporin	Colistin	Norfloxacin
Albamycin	Co-trimoxazole	Ofloxacin
Amfomycin	Enoxacin	Polymyxin
Amphomycin	Enviomycin	Polymyxin B
Antibiotic, intestinal	Fleroxacin	Ristocetin
Antibiotic, polypeptide	Fosfomycin	Sodium fusidate
Antibiotic, specified NEC	Fugillin	Sulfamethoxazole with
Anti-infective, antibiotics,	Fumadil	trimethoprim
specified NEC	Fumagillin	Sulfomyxin
Betamicin	Fusafungine	Teicoplanin
Capreomycin	Fusidate (ethanolamine)	Trimethoprim with
Carbomycin	(sodium)	sulfamethoxazole
Cathomycin	Fusidic acid	Vancomycin
Ciprofloxacin	Lincomycin	Viomycin
Clindamycin	Magnamycin	Virginiamycin
Colimycin	Mycitracin	

T36.8x- Poisoning by, adverse effect of and underdosing of <u>other systemic antibiotics</u>

T36.8x1- Poisoning by other systemic antibiotics, <u>accidental</u> (unintentional)
Poisoning by other systemic antibiotics NOS

T36.8x2- Poisoning by other systemic antibiotics, <u>intentional</u> self-harm

T36.8x3- Poisoning by other systemic antibiotics, <u>assault</u>

T36.8x4- Poisoning by other systemic antibiotics, <u>undetermined</u>

T36.8x5- <u>Adverse effect</u> of other systemic antibiotics

T36.8x6- <u>Underdosing</u> of other systemic antibiotics

T36.9- Poisoning by, adverse effect of and underdosing of <u>unspecified systemic antibiotic</u>

T36.9 - DRUGS/CHEMS*
Antibiotic NEC
Anti-infective, antibiotics

T36.91x- Poisoning by unspecified systemic antibiotic, <u>accidental</u> (unintentional)
Poisoning by systemic antibiotic NOS

T36.92x- Poisoning by unspecified systemic antibiotic, <u>intentional</u> self-harm

T36.93x- Poisoning by unspecified systemic antibiotic, <u>assault</u>

T36.94x- Poisoning by unspecified systemic antibiotic, <u>undetermined</u>

T36.95x- <u>Adverse effect</u> of unspecified systemic antibiotic

T36.96x- <u>Underdosing</u> of unspecified systemic antibiotic

T37- Poisoning by, adverse effect of and underdosing of <u>other systemic anti-infectives and antiparasitics</u>

Excludes 1:   anti-infectives topically used for ear, nose and throat (T49.6-)
    anti-infectives topically used for eye (T49.5-)
    locally applied anti-infectives NEC (T49.0-)

The appropriate 7th character is to be added to each code from category T37:
A   <u>Initial</u> encounter
D   <u>Subsequent</u> encounter
S   <u>Sequela</u>

T37.0- Poisoning by, adverse effect of and underdosing of sulfonamides

T37.0 - DRUGS/CHEMS*	Sulfaethidole	Sulfaproxyline
Acedapsone	Sulfafurazole	Sulfapyridine
Acesulfamethoxypyridazine	Sulfaguanidine	Sulfapyrimidine
Acetylsulfamethoxypyrida	Sulfalene	Sulfasalazine
zine	Sulfaloxate	Sulfasuxidine
Azosulfamide	Sulfaloxic acid	Sulfasymazine
Azulfidine	Sulfamerazine	Sulfathiazole
Diaphenylsulfone	Sulfameter	Sulfisomidine
Disulfanilamide	Sulfamethazine	Sulfisoxazole
Neoprontosil	Sulfamethizole	Sulfonamide NEC
Phthalylsulfathiazole	Sulfamethoxazole	Sulphadiazine
Prontosil	Sulfamethoxydiazine	Sulphadimethoxine
Salazosulfapyridine	Sulfamethoxypyridazine	Sulphadimidine
Salicylazosulfapyridine	Sulfamethylthiazole	Sulphafurazole
Succinylsulfathiazole	Sulfametoxydiazine	Sulphamethizole
Sulfachlorpyridazine	Sulfamonomethoxine	Sulphamethoxazole
Sulfacitine	Sulfamoxole	Sulphaphenazole
Sulfadiasulfone sodium	Sulfanilamide	Sulphapyridine
Sulfadiazine	Sulfanilylguanidine	Sulphasalazine
Sulfadimethoxine	Sulfaperin	Trisulfapyrimidines
Sulfadimidine	Sulfaphenazole	
Sulfadoxine	Sulfaphenylthiazole	

T37.0x- Poisoning by, adverse effect of and underdosing of <u>sulfonamides</u>

T37.0x1- Poisoning by sulfonamides, <u>accidental</u> (unintentional)
Poisoning by sulfonamides NOS

T37.0x2- Poisoning by sulfonamides, <u>intentional</u> self-harm

T37.0x3- Poisoning by sulfonamides, <u>assault</u>

T37.0x4- Poisoning by sulfonamides, <u>undetermined</u>

T37.0x5- <u>Adverse effect</u> of sulfonamides

T37.0x6- <u>Underdosing</u> of sulfonamides

T37.1- **Poisoning by, adverse effect of and underdosing of antimycobacterial drugs**
Excludes 1:   rifampicins (T36.6-)
                streptomycin (T36.5-)

T37.1 - DRUGS/CHEMS*	Diaminodiphenylsulfone	Potassium aminosalicylate
Acetosulfone (sodium)	Diasone (sodium)	Promacetin
Aldesulfone sodium	Etambutol	Promin
Aminosalicylic acid	Ethambutol	Prothionamide
Aminosalylum	Ethionamide	Protionamide
Anti-infective,	Ethionamide	Pyrazinamide
antimycobacterial NEC	Ethyl chaulmoograte	Pyrazinoic acid (amide)
Antimycobacterial drug	Fenamisal	Rifampicin with isoniazid
NEC	Glucosulfone sodium	Rimifon
Antimycobacterial drug,	Glyconiazide	Salinazid
combination	INH	Sodium acetosulfone
Antituberculars	Isoniazid	Sodium glucosulfone
Avlosulfon	Isoniazid with	Sodium sulfoxone
Benzamidosalicylate	thioacetazone	Solapsone
(calcium)	Isonicotinic acid hydrazide	Solasulfone
Benzoylpas calcium	Izoniazid	Sulfonazide
Bromosalicylhydroxamic	Izoniazid with	Sulfones
acid	thioacetazone	Sulfoxone
Calcium	Methaniazide	Sulphadione
benzamidosalicylate	Morinamide	Terizidone
Chaulmosulfone	Morphazinamide	Thiambutosine
Clofazimine	Nydrazid	Thioacetazone
Cyanacetyl hydrazide	Para-aminosalicylic acid	Thioacetazone, with
Cycloserine	PAS	isoniazid
DADPS	Pasiniazid	Thiocarlide
Dapsone	Pentylsalicylamide	Tiocarlide
DDS	Pirazinamide	Trecator

T37.1x- **Poisoning by, adverse effect of and underdosing of antimycobacterial drugs**

T37.1x1- **Poisoning by antimycobacterial drugs, accidental (unintentional)**
Poisoning by antimycobacterial drugs NOS

T37.1x2- **Poisoning by antimycobacterial drugs, intentional self-harm**

T37.1x3- **Poisoning by antimycobacterial drugs, assault**

T37.1x4- **Poisoning by antimycobacterial drugs, undetermined**

T37.1x5- **Adverse effect of antimycobacterial drugs**

T37.1x6- **Underdosing of antimycobacterial drugs**

T37.2- **Poisoning by, adverse effect of and underdosing of antimalarials and drugs acting on other blood protozoa**
Excludes 1:   hydroxyquinoline derivatives (T37.8-)

T37.2 - DRUGS/CHEMS*	Chloroguanide	Pentaquine
8-Aminoquinoline drugs	Chloroquine	Primaquine
Amodiaquine	Chlorproguanil	Proguanil
Amopyroquin(e)	Cinchona	Pyrimethamine
Anti-infective, antimalarial	Cinchonine alkaloids	Pyrimethamine with
Anti-infective,	Cycloguanil embonate	sulfadoxine
antiprotozoal, blood	Daraprim	Quinacrine
Antimalarial	Eflornithine	Quinine
Antimalarial, prophylactic	Guanatol	Quinocide
NEC	Halofantrine	Schizontozide (blood)
Antimalarial, pyrimidine	Isopentaquine	(tissue)
derivative	Mefloquine	Sulfadoxine with
Antiprotozoal drug, blood	Mepacrine	pyrimethamine
Aralen	Paludrine	
Camoquin	Pamaquine (naphthoute)	

T37.2x- **Poisoning by, adverse effect of and underdosing of antimalarials and drugs acting on other blood protozoa**

T37.2x1- **Poisoning by antimalarials and drugs acting on other blood protozoa, accidental (unintentional)**
Poisoning by antimalarials and drugs acting on other blood protozoa NOS

T37.2x2- **Poisoning by antimalarials and drugs acting on other blood protozoa, intentional self-harm**

T37.2x3- **Poisoning by antimalarials and drugs acting on other blood protozoa, assault**

T37.2x4- **Poisoning by antimalarials and drugs acting on other blood protozoa, undetermined**

T37.2x5- **Adverse effect of antimalarials and drugs acting on other blood protozoa**

T37.2x6- **Underdosing of antimalarials and drugs acting on other blood protozoa**

T37.3- **Poisoning by, adverse effect of and underdosing of other antiprotozoal drugs**

T37.3 - DRUGS/CHEMS*	Clefamide	Ornidazole
Acetarsol	Dehydroemetine	Oxophenarsine
Acterol	DHE	Pentamidine
Aminitrozole	Difetarsone	Phanquinone
Anti-infective,	Diloxanide	Phanquone
antiprotozoal NEC	Emetine	Secnidazole
Antimony,	Etofamide	Sodium antimony
dimercaptosuccinate	Flagyl	gluconate
Antimony, sodium	Glaucarubin	Sodium stibogluconate
dimercaptosuccinate	Glycobiarsol	Stibogluconate
Antiprotozoal drug NEC	Hydroxystilbamidine	Stilbamidine (isetionate)
Antitrichomonal drug	Melarsonyl potassium	Teclozan
Arsthinol	Melarsoprol	Tenonitrozole
Azanidazole	Misonidazole	Tinidazole
Benznidazole	Nifurtimox	Trichomonacides NEC
Bialamicol	Nimorazole	Tryparsamide
Carbarsone	Nitrimidazine	

T37.3x- **Poisoning by, adverse effect of and underdosing of other antiprotozoal drugs**

T37.3x1- **Poisoning by other antiprotozoal drugs, accidental (unintentional)**
Poisoning by other antiprotozoal drugs NOS

T37.3x2- **Poisoning by other antiprotozoal drugs, intentional self-harm**

T37.3x3- **Poisoning by other antiprotozoal drugs, assault**

T37.3x4- **Poisoning by other antiprotozoal drugs, undetermined**

T37.3x5- **Adverse effect of other antiprotozoal drugs**

T37.3x6- **Underdosing of other antiprotozoal drugs**

T3 7 - T37

89

T37.4- Poisoning by, adverse effect of and underdosing of anthelminthics

T37.4 - DRUGS/CHEMS*	Dichlorophen	Piperazine
Alantolactone	Diethyl carbamazine	Praziquantel
Albendazole	Diethylcarbamazine	Pumpkin seed extract
Amphotalide	Dithiazanine iodide	Pyrantel
Anthelmintic NEC	Fenbendazole	Pyrvinium chloride
Anthiolimine	Filix mas	Santonin
Antifilarial drug	Flubendazole	Spigelia (root)
Antihelmintics	Helenin	Stibophen
Antihookworm drug	Ivermectin	Suramin (sodium)
Anti-infective, anthelmintic	Levamisole	Teroxalene
Antinematode drug	Lucanthone	Tetrachloroethylene,
Antiplatyhelmintic drug	Male fern extract	medicinal
Antischistosomal drug	Mebendazole	Tetramisole
Antitapeworm drug	Niclosamide	Thiabendazole
Antiwhipworm drug	Niridazole	Tiabendazole
Ascaridole	Nitrothiazol	Urea stibamine
Aspidium (oleoresin)	Oxamniquine	Veroxil
Bephenium	Oxantel	Viprynium
hydroxynaphthoate	Pelletierine tannate	Wormseed, American
Bithionol, anthelminthic	Perchloroethylene,	
Bitoscanate	medicinal	
Chenopodium	Pinkroot	

T37.4x- Poisoning by, adverse effect of and underdosing of anthelminthics

T37.4x1- Poisoning by anthelminthics, accidental (unintentional)

Poisoning by anthelminthics NOS

T37.4x2- Poisoning by anthelminthics, intentional self-harm

T37.4x3- Poisoning by anthelminthics, assault

T37.4x4- Poisoning by anthelminthics, undetermined

T37.4x5- Adverse effect of anthelminthics

T37.4x6- Underdosing of anthelminthics

T37.5- Poisoning by, adverse effect of and underdosing of antiviral drugs

Excludes 1: amantadine (T42.8-)
cytarabine (T45.1-)

T37.5 - DRUGS/CHEMS*	Dideoxyinosine	Metisazone
ABOB	Flumidin	Moroxydine
Aciclovir	Foscarnet sodium	Ribavirin
Acyclovir	Fosfonet sodium	Rimantadine
Adenine, arabinoside	Ganciclovir (sodium)	Thymopentin
Anti-infective, antiviral	Ibacitabine	Trifluridine
Antiviral drug NEC	Inosine pranobex	Tromantadine
Ara-A	Interferon (alpha) (beta)	Vidarabine
Azidothymidine	(gamma)	Virugon
AZT	Methisazone	Zalcitabine
Dideoxycytidine	Methisoprinol	Zidovudine

T37.5x- Poisoning by, adverse effect of and underdosing of antiviral drugs

T37.5x1- Poisoning by antiviral drugs, accidental (unintentional)

Poisoning by antiviral drugs NOS

T37.5x2- Poisoning by antiviral drugs, intentional self-harm

T37.5x3- Poisoning by antiviral drugs, assault

T37.5x4- Poisoning by antiviral drugs, undetermined

T37.5x5- Adverse effect of antiviral drugs

T37.5x6- Underdosing of antiviral drugs

T37.8- Poisoning by, adverse effect of and underdosing of other specified systemic anti-infectives and antiparasitics

Poisoning by, adverse effect of and underdosing of hydroxyquinoline derivatives

Excludes 1: antimalarial drugs (T37.2-)

T37.8 - DRUGS/CHEMS*	Fluconazole	Nifurtoinol
Akritoin	Flucytosine	Nitrofurantoin
Anti-infective, arsenical	Flumequine	Nitroxoline
Anti-infective, heavy metals	Flunidazole	Oxolinic acid
NEC	Fluorocytosine	Oxyquinoline (derivatives)
Antimony, anti-infectives	Furazolidone	Pefloxacin
Antimony, potassium	Hexamine (mandelate)	Pipemidic acid
(sodium) tartrate	Hexetidine	Piromidic acid
Antimony, tartrated	Hydroxychloroquine	Potassium antimony
Antiparasitic drug, specified	Hydroxyquinoline	'tartrate'
NEC	(derivatives) NEC	Quiniobine
Arsenic anti-infectives	Iodobismitol	Quinoline (derivatives) NEC
Arsphenamine (silver)	Iodochlorhydroxyquin	Rosoxacin
Bismarsen	Iodochlorhydroxyquinoline	Salvarsan 606 (neosilver)
Bismuth salts, anti-	Iodoquinol	(silver)
infectives	Itraconazole	Silver arsphenamine
Bismuth salts, subsalicylate	Lead, anti-infectives	Silver salvarsan
Bismuth salts,	Mandelic acid	Sodium cacodylate, anti-
sulfarsphenamine	Mapharsen	infective
Bithionol	Meglumine antimoniate	Stovarsal
Broxyquinoline	Mercury, anti-infective,	Sulfarsphenamine
Chiniofon	systemic	Tartar emetic
Cinoxacin	Methenamine (mandelate)	Tartrated antimony (anti-
Clioquinol	Methyl glucamine	infective)
Croconazole	antimonate	Thiobismol
Dichlorhydroxyquinoline	Metronidazole	Thiocarbarsone
Diiodohydroxyquin	Nalidixic acid	Tin, anti-infectives
Diiodohydroxyquinoline	Neoarsphenamine	Trimethoprim
Diodoquin	Neosalvarsan	Urinary anti-infective
Disinfectant, intestinal	Neosilversalvarsan	Vioform
Floraquin	Nifuratel	Xibornol

T37.8x- Poisoning by, adverse effect of and underdosing of other specified systemic anti-infectives and antiparasitics

T37.8x1- Poisoning by other specified systemic anti-infectives and antiparasitics, accidental (unintentional)

Poisoning by other specified systemic anti-infectives and antiparasitics NOS

T37.8x2- Poisoning by other specified systemic anti-infectives and antiparasitics, intentional self-harm

T37.8x3- Poisoning by other specified systemic anti-infectives and antiparasitics, assault

T37.8x4- Poisoning by other specified systemic anti-infectives and antiparasitics, undetermined

T37.8x5- Adverse effect of other specified systemic anti-infectives and antiparasitics

T37.8x6- Underdosing of other specified systemic anti-infectives and antiparasitics

T37.9- Poisoning by, adverse effect of and underdosing of unspecified systemic anti-infective and antiparasitics

T37.9 - DRUGS/CHEMS*	Anti-infective NEC	Ethoxazene
Acriflavine	Anti-infective, mixed	Furadantin
Ammonium mandelate	Antiparasitic drug	Furoxone
Antifungal, anti-infective	(systemic)	Nifuraldezone
NEC	Calcium mandelate	Serenium (hydrochloride)

T37.91x- Poisoning by unspecified systemic anti-infective and antiparasitics, accidental (unintentional)

Poisoning by, adverse effect of and underdosing of systemic anti-infective and antiparasitics NOS

T37.92x- Poisoning by unspecified systemic anti-infective and antiparasitics, intentional self-harm

T37.93x- Poisoning by unspecified systemic anti-infective and antiparasitics, assault

T37.94x- Poisoning by unspecified systemic anti-infective and antiparasitics, undetermined

T37.95x- Adverse effect of unspecified systemic anti-infective and antiparasitic

T37.96x- Underdosing of unspecified systemic anti-infectives and antiparasitics

T38- Poisoning by, adverse effect of and underdosing of <u>hormones and their synthetic substitutes and antagonists</u>, <u>not elsewhere classified</u>

Excludes 1:   *mineralocorticoids and their antagonists (T50.0-)*
        oxytocic hormones (T48.0-)
        parathyroid hormones and derivatives (T50.9-)

The appropriate 7th character is to be added to each code from category T38:

A   <u>Initial</u> encounter
D   <u>Subsequent</u> encounter
S   <u>Sequela</u>

T38.0- Poisoning by, adverse effect of and underdosing of glucocorticoids and synthetic analogues

Excludes 1:   *glucocorticoids, topically used (T49.-)*

T38.0 - DRUGS/CHEMS*	Corticosteroid	Glucocorticoids
Adrenal (extract, cortex or medulla) (glucocorticoids) (hormones) (mineralocorticoids)	Cortisone (acetate)	Glucocorticosteroid
	Cortivazol	Hormone, adrenal cortical steroids
	Cortogen	
	Cortone	Hydeltra
Aristocort	Cortril	Hydrocortone
Celestone	Decadron	Kenacort
Clocortolone	Deflazacort	Meprednisone
Cloprednol	Deltasone	Methyl prednisolone
Compound E (cortisone)	Deltra	Paramethasone
Compound F (hydrocortisone)	Dexamethasone	Percorten
	DOCA	Prednisolone
Cortate	Florinef	Prednisone
Cort-Dome	Fluohydrocortisone	Prednylidene
Cortef	Fluorinated corticosteroids	Steroid
	Fluprednisolone	

T38.0x- Poisoning by, adverse effect of and underdosing of <u>glucocorticoids and synthetic analogues</u>

T38.0x1- Poisoning by glucocorticoids and synthetic analogues, <u>accidental</u> (unintentional)
    Poisoning by glucocorticoids and synthetic analogues NOS

T38.0x2- Poisoning by glucocorticoids and synthetic analogues, <u>intentional</u> self-harm

T38.0x3- Poisoning by glucocorticoids and synthetic analogues, <u>assault</u>

T38.0x4- Poisoning by glucocorticoids and synthetic analogues, <u>undetermined</u>

T38.0x5- <u>Adverse effect</u> of glucocorticoids and synthetic analogues

T38.0x6- <u>Underdosing</u> of glucocorticoids and synthetic analogues

T38.1- Poisoning by, adverse effect of and underdosing of thyroid hormones and substitutes

T38.1 - DRUGS/CHEMS*	Levoid	Synthroid
Cytomel	Levothyroxine	Thyroglobulin
Detrothyronine	Levothyroxine sodium	Thyroid (hormone)
Dextrothyroxin	Liothyronine	Thyrolar
Dextrothyroxine sodium	Liotrix	Thyroxine
Euthroid	Proloid	Tiratricol
Hormone, thyroid	Sodium l-triiodothyronine	Titroid
l-thyroxine sodium	Sodium (L)- triiodothyronine	Triiodothyronine
Letter		

T38.1x- Poisoning by, adverse effect of and underdosing of <u>thyroid hormones and substitutes</u>

T38.1x1- Poisoning by thyroid hormones and substitutes, <u>accidental</u> (unintentional)
    Poisoning by thyroid hormones and substitutes NOS

T38.1x2- Poisoning by thyroid hormones and substitutes, <u>intentional</u> self-harm

T38.1x3- Poisoning by thyroid hormones and substitutes, <u>assault</u>

T38.1x4- Poisoning by thyroid hormones and substitutes, <u>undetermined</u>

T38.1x5- <u>Adverse effect</u> of thyroid hormones and substitutes
T38.1x6- <u>Underdosing</u> of thyroid hormones and substitutes

T38.2- Poisoning by, adverse effect of and underdosing of antithyroid drugs

T38.2 - DRUGS/CHEMS*	Methimazole	Sodium iodide I-131, therapeutic
Antithyroid drug NEC	Methyl thiouracil	
Benzylthiouracil	Methylthiouracil	Tapazole
Carbimazole	Potassium perchlorate, antithyroid	Thiamazole
Diiodotyrosine		Thiocarbamide
Iodine 131, therapeutic	Potassium perchlorate, medicinal	Thiouracil (benzyl) (methyl) (propyl)
Iodine for thyroid conditions (antithyroid)		
	Propyl thiouracil	Thiourea
Iothiouracil	Propylthiouracil	
Methiacil		

T38.2x- Poisoning by, adverse effect of and underdosing of <u>antithyroid drugs</u>

T38.2x1- Poisoning by antithyroid drugs, <u>accidental</u> (unintentional)
    Poisoning by antithyroid drugs NOS

T38.2x2- Poisoning by antithyroid drugs, <u>intentional</u> self-harm

T38.2x3- Poisoning by antithyroid drugs, <u>assault</u>

T38.2x4- Poisoning by antithyroid drugs, <u>undetermined</u>

T38.2x5- <u>Adverse effect</u> of antithyroid drugs

T38.2x6- <u>Underdosing</u> of antithyroid drugs

T38.3- Poisoning by, adverse effect of and underdosing of insulin and oral hypoglycemic [antidiabetic] drugs

T38.3 - DRUGS/CHEMS*	Glisolamide	Insulin, slow acting
Acetohexamide	Glisoxepide	Insulin, zinc, protamine injection
Antidiabetic NEC	Globin zinc insulin	
Antidiabetic, biguanide	Glucagon	Insulin, zinc, suspension (amorphous) (crystalline)
Antidiabetic, biguanide and sulfonyl combined	Glyburide	
	Glyclopyramide	
Antidiabetic, combined	Glycyclamide	Isophane insulin
Antidiabetic, sulfonylurea	Glymidine sodium	Lente lietin (insulin)
Biguanide derivatives, oral	Hormone, antidiabetic agents	Metformin
Buformin		Neutral insulin injection
Carbutamide	Iletin	NPH Iletin (insulin)
Chlorpropamide	Insular tissue extract	Orinase
DBI	Insulin (amorphous) (globin) (isophane) (Lente) (NPH) (Semilente) (Ultralente) (zinc)	Phenformin
Diabinese		Phenylethylbiguanide
Dimethyl diguanide		Protamine sulfate, zinc insulin
Dymelor		
Extended insulin zinc suspension		PZI
	Insulin, defalan	Sodium tolbutamide
Glibenclamide	Insulin, human	Sulfonylurea derivatives, oral
Glibornuride	Insulin, injection, soluble	
Gliclazide	Insulin, injection, soluble, biphasic	Tolazamide
Glimidine		Tolbutamide (sodium)
Glipizide	Insulin, intermediate acting	
Gliquidone	Insulin, protamine zinc	

T38.3x- Poisoning by, adverse effect of and underdosing of <u>insulin and oral hypoglycemic [antidiabetic] drugs</u>

T38.3x1- Poisoning by insulin and oral hypoglycemic [antidiabetic] drugs, <u>accidental</u> (unintentional)
    Poisoning by insulin and oral hypoglycemic [antidiabetic] drugs NOS

T38.3x2- Poisoning by insulin and oral hypoglycemic [antidiabetic] drugs, <u>intentional</u> self-harm

T38.3x3- Poisoning by insulin and oral hypoglycemic [antidiabetic] drugs, <u>assault</u>

T38.3x4- Poisoning by insulin and oral hypoglycemic [antidiabetic] drugs, <u>undetermined</u>

T38.3x5- <u>Adverse effect</u> of insulin and oral hypoglycemic [antidiabetic] drugs

T38.3x6- <u>Underdosing</u> of insulin and oral hypoglycemic [antidiabetic] drugs

T38 - T38

T38.4-   Poisoning by, adverse effect of and underdosing of oral contraceptives
   Poisoning by, adverse effect of and underdosing of multiple- and single-ingredient oral contraceptive preparations

T38.4 - DRUGS/CHEMS*		
Antifertility pill	Ethynodiol with mestranol diacetate	Norlestrin
Contraceptive (oral)	Etinodiol	Norlutin
Demulen	Etynodiol	Oracon
Enovid	Levonorgestrel	Oral contraceptives
Ethinylestradiol, with levonorgestrel	Lynestrenol	Ortho-Novum
	Norethindrone	Ovral
Ethinylestradiol, with norethisterone	Norethisterone (acetate) (enantate)	Ovulen
		Progestin, oral contraceptive
Ethynodiol	Norgestrel	Quingestanol
	Norgestrienone	

T38.4x-   Poisoning by, adverse effect of and underdosing of <u>oral contraceptives</u>

   T38.4x1-   Poisoning by oral contraceptives, <u>accidental</u> (unintentional)
      Poisoning by oral contraceptives NOS

   T38.4x2-   Poisoning by oral contraceptives, <u>intentional</u> self-harm

   T38.4x3-   Poisoning by oral contraceptives, <u>assault</u>

   T38.4x4-   Poisoning by oral contraceptives, <u>undetermined</u>

   T38.4x5-   <u>Adverse effect</u> of oral contraceptives

   T38.4x6-   <u>Underdosing</u> of oral contraceptives

T38.5-   Poisoning by, adverse effect of and underdosing of other estrogens and progestogens
   Poisoning by, adverse effect of and underdosing of estrogens and progestogens mixtures and substitutes

T38.5 - DRUGS/CHEMS*		
Allylestrenol	Estrogen, conjugated	Norethisterone with ethinylestradiol
Anhydrohydroxy-progesterone	Estrone	
	Estropipate	Noretynodrel
Antineoplastic combination, estrogen	Ethinylestradiol, ethinyloestradiol	Normethandrone
		Oestradiol
Chlormadinone	Ethisterone	Oestriol
Chlorotrianisene	Fosfestrol	Oestrogen
Chlortrianisene	Gestonorone caproate	Oestrone
Clomifene	Gonadal tissue extract, female	Ovarian hormone
Clomiphene		Ovarian stimulant
Conjugated estrogenic substances	Hexestrol	Oxendolone
	Hexoestrol	Piperazine estrone sulfate
Delalutin	Hormone, ovarian	Polyestradiol phosphate
Demegestone	Hydroxyestrone	Polyoestradiol phosphate
Desogestrel	Hydroxyprogesterone	Pregnandiol
Diaethylstiloestrolum	Hydroxyprogesterone caproate	Pregneninolone
Dienestrol	Isopregnenone	Premarin
Dienoestrol	Levonorgestrel with ethinylestradiol	Progesterone
Diethyl stilbestrol		Progestin
Diethylstilbestrol	Lipo-Lutin	Progestogen NEC
Diethylstilboestrol	Lutocylol	Progestone
Dimestrol	Lutromone	Proluton
Dimethisterone	Medrogestone	Promegestone
Dydrogesterone	Medroxyprogesterone acetate (depot)	Provera
Epiestriol		Quinestradiol
Epimestrol	Megestrol	Quinestradol
Estradiol	Mestranol	Quinestrol
Estradiol benzoate	Methallenestril	Steroid, antineoplastic, hormone, estrogen
Estriol	Methallenoestril	
Estrogen	Methylestrenolone	Stilbestrol
Estrogen, with progesterone	Methylestrenolone	Stilboestrol
	Nomegestrol	Tace

T38.5x-   Poisoning by, adverse effect of and underdosing of <u>other estrogens and progestogens</u>

   T38.5x1-   Poisoning by other estrogens and progestogens, <u>accidental</u> (unintentional)
      Poisoning by other estrogens and progestogens NOS

   T38.5x2-   Poisoning by other estrogens and progestogens, <u>intentional</u> self-harm

   T38.5x3-   Poisoning by other estrogens and progestogens, <u>assault</u>

   T38.5x4-   Poisoning by other estrogens and progestogens, <u>undetermined</u>

T38.5x5-   <u>Adverse effect</u> of other estrogens and progestogens
T38.5x6-   <u>Underdosing</u> of other estrogens and progestogens

T38.6-   Poisoning by, adverse effect of and underdosing of antigonadotrophins, antiestrogens, antiandrogens, not elsewhere classified
   Poisoning by, adverse effect of and underdosing of tamoxifen

T38.6 - DRUGS/CHEMS*		
Antiandrogen NEC	Danazol	Ormeloxifene
Antiestrogen NEC	Flutamide	Taleranol
Antigonadotrophin NEC	Mifepristone	Tamoxifen
Cyproterone	Nafoxidine	Toremifene
	Nilutamide	

T38.6x-   Poisoning by, adverse effect of and underdosing of <u>antigonadotrophins, antiestrogens, antiandrogens</u>, <u>not elsewhere classified</u>

   T38.6x1-   Poisoning by antigonadotrophins, antiestrogens, antiandrogens, not elsewhere classified, <u>accidental</u> (unintentional)
      Poisoning by antigonadotrophins, antiestrogens, antiandrogens, not elsewhere classified NOS

   T38.6x2-   Poisoning by antigonadotrophins, antiestrogens, antiandrogens, not elsewhere classified, <u>intentional</u> self-harm

   T38.6x3-   Poisoning by antigonadotrophins, antiestrogens, antiandrogens, not elsewhere classified, <u>assault</u>

   T38.6x4-   Poisoning by antigonadotrophins, antiestrogens, antiandrogens, not elsewhere classified, <u>undetermined</u>

   T38.6x5-   <u>Adverse effect</u> of antigonadotrophins, antiestrogens, antiandrogens, not elsewhere classified

   T38.6x6-   <u>Underdosing</u> of antigonadotrophins, antiestrogens, antiandrogens, not elsewhere classified

T38.7-   Poisoning by, adverse effect of and underdosing of androgens and anabolic congeners

T38.7 - DRUGS/CHEMS*		
Anabolic steroid	Ethylestrenol	Nandrolone
Androgen	Fluoxymesterone	Norethandrolone
Androgen-estrogen mixture	Gonadal tissue extract, male	Nortestosterone (furanpropionate)
Androstalone		
Androstanolone	Hormone, androgenic	Oxandrolone
Androsterone	Macrolide, anabolic drug	Oxymesterone
Antineoplastic steroid	Mepitiostane	Oxymetholone
Calusterone	Mestanolone	Prasterone
Chlorodehydromethyl-testosterone	Mesterolone	Stanolone
	Metandienone	Stanozolol
Congener, anabolic	Metandrostenolone	Steroid, anabolic
Dromostanolone	Metenolone	Steroid, androgenic
Drostanolone	Methandienone	Steroid, antineoplastic, hormone
Durabolin	Methandriol	
Epitiostanol	Methandrostenolone	Testolactone
Estanozolol	Methenolone	Testosterone
Estradiol with testosterone	Methyl androstanolone	Zeranol
Ethyl estranol	Methyl testosterone	
	Methyltestosterone	

T38.7x-   Poisoning by, adverse effect of and underdosing of <u>androgens and anabolic congeners</u>

   T38.7x1-   Poisoning by androgens and anabolic congeners, <u>accidental</u> (unintentional)
      Poisoning by androgens and anabolic congeners NOS

   T38.7x2-   Poisoning by androgens and anabolic congeners, <u>intentional</u> self-harm

   T38.7x3-   Poisoning by androgens and anabolic congeners, <u>assault</u>

   T38.7x4-   Poisoning by androgens and anabolic congeners, <u>undetermined</u>

   T38.7x5-   <u>Adverse effect</u> of androgens and anabolic congeners

   T38.7x6-   <u>Underdosing</u> of androgens and anabolic congeners

T38.8-　Poisoning by, adverse effect of and underdosing of other and unspecified hormones and synthetic substitutes

T38.80-　Poisoning by, adverse effect of and underdosing of underdosing of <u>unspecified hormones and synthetic substitutes</u>

T38.80 - DRUGS/CHEMS*
Hormone

T38.801-　Poisoning by unspecified hormones and synthetic substitutes, <u>accidental</u> (unintentional)
　　　　Poisoning by unspecified hormones and synthetic substitutes NOS

T38.802-　Poisoning by unspecified hormones and synthetic substitutes, <u>intentional</u> self-harm

T38.803-　Poisoning by unspecified hormones and synthetic substitutes, <u>assault</u>

T38.804-　Poisoning by unspecified hormones and synthetic substitutes, <u>undetermined</u>

T38.805-　<u>Adverse effect</u> of unspecified hormones and synthetic substitutes

T38.806-　<u>Underdosing</u> of unspecified hormones and synthetic substitutes

T38.81-　Poisoning by, adverse effect of and underdosing of <u>anterior pituitary [adenohypophyseal] hormones</u>

T38.81 - DRUGS/CHEMS*		
ACTH	HGH (human growth hormone)	Menotropins
Adrenocorticotrophic hormone	Hormone, anterior pituitary NEC	Pergonal
Adrenocorticotrophin	Hormone, follicle stimulating	Pituitary extracts, anterior
Alsactide		Prolactin
Anterior pituitary hormone NEC	Hormone, gonadotropic, pituitary	Seractide
Corticotropin	Hormone, growth	Somatotropin
Cosyntropin	Hormone, luteinizing	Somatrem
Follicle-stimulating hormone, human	Hormone, pituitary, anterior	Somatropin
FSH	Human growth hormone (HGH)	Tetracosactide
Gonadotropin, pituitary		Tetracosactrin
Growth hormone	Luteinizing hormone	Thyreotrophic hormone
		Thyrotrophin
		Thyrotropic hormone
		TSH
		Urofollitropin

T38.811-　Poisoning by anterior pituitary [adenohypophyseal] hormones, <u>accidental</u> (unintentional)
　　　　Poisoning by anterior pituitary [adenohypophyseal] hormones NOS

T38.812-　Poisoning by anterior pituitary [adenohypophyseal] hormones, <u>intentional</u> self-harm

T38.813-　Poisoning by anterior pituitary [adenohypophyseal] hormones, <u>assault</u>

T38.814-　Poisoning by anterior pituitary [adenohypophyseal] hormones, <u>undetermined</u>

T38.815-　<u>Adverse effect</u> of anterior pituitary [adenohypophyseal] hormones

T38.816-　<u>Underdosing</u> of anterior pituitary [adenohypophyseal] hormones

T38.89-　Poisoning by, adverse effect of and underdosing of <u>other hormones and synthetic substitutes</u>

T38.89 - DRUGS/CHEMS*	Hormone, antidiuretic	Pituitrin
ADH	Hormone, gonadotropic	Placental hormone
Antidiuretic hormone	Hormone, pituitary (posterior) NEC	Posterior pituitary hormone NEC
Buserelin		
Chorionic gonadotropin	Hormone, specified, NEC	Protirelin
DDAVP	Hypophysis, posterior	Sermorelin
Deamino-D-arginine vasopressin	Leuprolide	Somatorelin
	Lypressin	Terlipressin
Desmopressin	Lysine vasopressin	Thymus extract
Enterogastrone	Melanocyte-stimulating hormone	Vasopressin
Felypressin		Vasopressor drugs
Gonadorelin	Pitressin (tannate)	
Gonadotropin	Pituitary extracts (posterior)	
Gonadotropin, chorionic		

T38.891-　Poisoning by other hormones and synthetic substitutes, <u>accidental</u> (unintentional)
　　　　Poisoning by other hormones and synthetic substitutes NOS

T38.892-　Poisoning by other hormones and synthetic substitutes, <u>intentional</u> self-harm

T38.893-　Poisoning by other hormones and synthetic substitutes, <u>assault</u>

T38.894-　Poisoning by other hormones and synthetic substitutes, <u>undetermined</u>

T38.895-　<u>Adverse effect</u> of other hormones and synthetic substitutes

T38.896-　<u>Underdosing</u> of other hormones and synthetic substitutes

T38.9-　Poisoning by, adverse effect of and underdosing of other and unspecified hormone antagonists

T38.90-　Poisoning by, adverse effect of and underdosing of <u>unspecified hormone antagonists</u>

T38.90 - DRUGS/CHEMS*
Gonadal tissue extract

T38.901-　Poisoning by unspecified hormone antagonists, <u>accidental</u> (unintentional)
　　　　Poisoning by unspecified hormone antagonists NOS

T38.902-　Poisoning by unspecified hormone antagonists, <u>intentional</u> self-harm

T38.903-　Poisoning by unspecified hormone antagonists, <u>assault</u>

T38.904-　Poisoning by unspecified hormone antagonists, <u>undetermined</u>

T38.905-　<u>Adverse effect</u> of unspecified hormone antagonists

T38.906-　<u>Underdosing</u> of unspecified hormone antagonists

T38.99-　Poisoning by, adverse effect of and underdosing of <u>other hormone antagonists</u>

T38.99 - DRUGS/CHEMS*	Somatostatin
Octreotide	Trilostane

T38.991-　Poisoning by other hormone antagonists, <u>accidental</u> (unintentional)
　　　　Poisoning by other hormone antagonists NOS

T38.992-　Poisoning by other hormone antagonists, <u>intentional</u> self-harm

T38.993-　Poisoning by other hormone antagonists, <u>assault</u>

T38.994-　Poisoning by other hormone antagonists, <u>undetermined</u>

T38.995-　<u>Adverse effect</u> of other hormone antagonists

T38.996-　<u>Underdosing</u> of other hormone antagonists

T38 - T38

Excludes 1: = NOT CODED HERE! (Do not code both)　　　**1163**　　　*Excludes ❷:* = Not Included Here

T39- Poisoning by, adverse effect of and underdosing of <u>nonopioid analgesics, antipyretics and antirheumatics</u>

The appropriate 7th character is to be added to each code from category T39:
- A   <u>Initial</u> encounter
- D   <u>Subsequent</u> encounter
- S   <u>Sequela</u>

T39.0-   Poisoning by, adverse effect of and underdosing of <u>salicylates</u>

T39.01- Poisoning by, adverse effect of and underdosing of <u>aspirin</u>
Poisoning by, adverse effect of and underdosing of acetylsalicylic acid

T39.01 - DRUGS/CHEMS*	Aluminium bis	Calcium actylsalicylate
Acetylsalicylic acid (enteric coated) (salts)	(acetylsalicylate)	Calcium carbaspirin
Alka-seltzer	Aspirin (aluminum) (soluble)	Carbaspirin
Aluminium aspirin	Bufferin	Fiorinal
		Rhodine

T39.011-   Poisoning by aspirin, <u>accidental</u> (unintentional)
T39.012-   Poisoning by aspirin, <u>intentional</u> self-harm
T39.013-   Poisoning by aspirin, <u>assault</u>
T39.014-   Poisoning by aspirin, <u>undetermined</u>
T39.015-   <u>Adverse effect</u> of aspirin
T39.016-   <u>Underdosing</u> of aspirin

T39.09- Poisoning by, adverse effect of and underdosing of <u>other salicylates</u>

T39.09 - DRUGS/CHEMS*	Diflunisal	Salicylic acid, derivative
Aluminium salicylate	Magnesium salicylate	Salicylic acid, salts
Calcium salicylate	Salicylamide	Salsalate
Carbethyl salicylate	Salicylate NEC	Sodium salicylate
Choline salicylate	Salicylic acid, congeners	Sodium thiosalicylate

T39.091-   Poisoning by salicylates, <u>accidental</u> (unintentional)
Poisoning by salicylates NOS
T39.092-   Poisoning by salicylates, <u>intentional</u> self-harm
T39.093-   Poisoning by salicylates, <u>assault</u>
T39.094-   Poisoning by salicylates, <u>undetermined</u>
T39.095-   <u>Adverse effect</u> of salicylates
T39.096-   <u>Underdosing</u> of salicylates

T39.1-   Poisoning by, adverse effect of and underdosing of <u>4-Aminophenol derivatives</u>

T39.1 - DRUGS/CHEMS*	Analgesic, aromatic NEC	Para-acetamidophenol
P-Acetamidophenol	Aniline analgesic	Para-aminophenol derivatives
Acetaminophen	Aniline derivatives, therapeutic NEC	Paracetamol
Acetaminosalol	Bromo-seltzer	Phenacetin
Acetanilide	Exalgin	
Acetophenetedin	Panadol	
4-Aminophenol derivatives		

T39.1x-   Poisoning by, adverse effect of and underdosing of 4-Aminophenol derivatives

T39.1x1-   Poisoning by 4-Aminophenol derivatives, <u>accidental</u> (unintentional)
Poisoning by 4-Aminophenol derivatives NOS
T39.1x2-   Poisoning by 4-Aminophenol derivatives, <u>intentional</u> self-harm
T39.1x3-   Poisoning by 4-Aminophenol derivatives, <u>assault</u>
T39.1x4-   Poisoning by 4-Aminophenol derivatives, <u>undetermined</u>
T39.1x5-   <u>Adverse effect</u> of 4-Aminophenol derivatives
T39.1x6-   <u>Underdosing</u> of 4-Aminophenol derivatives

T39.2-   Poisoning by, adverse effect of and underdosing of pyrazolone derivatives

T39.2 - DRUGS/CHEMS*	Feprazone	Phenazone
Amidopyrine	Hydroxyphenylbutazone	Phenyl butazone
Aminofenazone	Indocin	Phenylbutazone
Aminophenazone	Isopropylaminophenazone	Propyphenazone
Aminopyrine	Kebuzone	Pyramidon
Analgesic, pyrazole	Ketazon	Pyrazole (derivatives)
Analgin	Metamizole sodium	Pyrazolone analgesic NEC
Antipyrine	Methampyrone	Ramifenazone
Azapropazone	Mofebutazone	Sulfamazone
Butazolidin	Monophenylbutazone	Sulfamidopyrine
Clofezone	Myochrysin(e)	Sulpyrine
Coal tar, medicinal, analgesics NEC	Nifenazone	Suxibuzone
Diphenylbutazone	Noramidopyrine	Tandearil, tanderil
Dipyrone	Noramidopyrine methanesulfonate sodium	
Fenazone	Oxyphenbutazone	
Fenylbutazone		

T39.2x-   Poisoning by, adverse effect of and underdosing of <u>pyrazolone derivatives</u>

T39.2x1-   Poisoning by pyrazolone derivatives, <u>accidental</u> (unintentional)
Poisoning by pyrazolone derivatives NOS
T39.2x2-   Poisoning by pyrazolone derivatives, <u>intentional</u> self-harm
T39.2x3-   Poisoning by pyrazolone derivatives, <u>assault</u>
T39.2x4-   Poisoning by pyrazolone derivatives, <u>undetermined</u>
T39.2x5-   <u>Adverse effect</u> of pyrazolone derivatives
T39.2x6-   <u>Underdosing</u> of pyrazolone derivatives

T39.3-   Poisoning by, adverse effect of and underdosing of <u>other nonsteroidal anti-inflammatory drugs [NSAID]</u>

T39.31-   Poisoning by, adverse effect of and underdosing of <u>propionic acid derivatives</u>
Poisoning by, adverse effect of and underdosing of fenoprofen
Poisoning by, adverse effect of and underdosing of flurbiprofen
Poisoning by, adverse effect of and underdosing of ibuprofen
Poisoning by, adverse effect of and underdosing of ketoprofen
Poisoning by, adverse effect of and underdosing of naproxen
Poisoning by, adverse effect of and underdosing of oxaprozin

T39.31 - DRUGS/CHEMS*	Carprofen	Naproxen
Aleve	Esflurbiprofen	Oxaprozin
Analgesic, anti-inflammatory NEC, propionic acid derivative	Fenoprofen	Suprofen
	Flurbiprofen	Tiaprofenic acid
	Ibufenac	
Anti-inflammatory drug, nonsteroidal, propionic acid derivative	Ibuprofen	
	Ibuproxam	
	Ketoprofen	

T39.311-   Poisoning by propionic acid derivatives, <u>accidental</u> (unintentional)
T39.312-   Poisoning by propionic acid derivatives, <u>intentional</u> self-harm
T39.313-   Poisoning by propionic acid derivatives, <u>assault</u>
T39.314-   Poisoning by propionic acid derivatives, <u>undetermined</u>
T39.315-   <u>Adverse effect</u> of propionic acid derivatives
T39.316-   <u>Underdosing</u> of propionic acid derivatives

T39.39-   Poisoning by, adverse effect of and underdosing of <u>other nonsteroidal anti-inflammatory drugs [NSAID]</u>

T39.39 - DRUGS/CHEMS*	Fenflumizole	Nimesulide
Anti-inflammatory drug NEC	Flufenamic acid	Piroxicam
	Indometacin	Proquazone
Anti-inflammatory drug, nonsteroidal NEC	Indomethacin	Sulindac
	Isoxicam	Tenoxicam
Anti-inflammatory drug, specified NEC	Meclofenamate	Tolmetin
	Meclofenamic acid	Ufenamate
Diclofenac	Mefenamic acid	Zomepirac
Etodolac	Nabumetone	

T39.391-   Poisoning by other nonsteroidal anti-inflammatory drugs [NSAID], <u>accidental</u> (unintentional)
Poisoning by other nonsteroidal anti-inflammatory drugs NOS

Excludes 1: = NOT CODED HERE! (Do not code both)   **1164**   *Excludes* ❷: = Not Included Here

T39.392- Poisoning by other nonsteroidal anti-inflammatory drugs [NSAID], <u>intentional</u> self-harm

T39.393- Poisoning by other nonsteroidal anti-inflammatory drugs [NSAID], <u>assault</u>

T39.394- Poisoning by other nonsteroidal anti-inflammatory drugs [NSAID], <u>undetermined</u>

T39.395- <u>Adverse effect</u> of other nonsteroidal anti-inflammatory drugs [NSAID]

T39.396- <u>Underdosing</u> of other nonsteroidal anti-inflammatory drugs [NSAID]

T39.4- Poisoning by, adverse effect of and underdosing of antirheumatics, not elsewhere classified

Excludes 1:   *poisoning by, adverse effect of and underdosing of glucocorticoids (T38.0-)*
               poisoning by, adverse effect of and underdosing of salicylates (T39.0-)

<u>T39.4</u> - DRUGS/CHEMS*	Auranofin	Glucosamine sulfate
Analgesic, antirheumatic NEC	Aurothioglucose	Gold salts
Antiphlogistic NEC	Aurothioglycanide	Indomethacin farnesil
Antirheumatic NEC	Aurothiomalate sodium	Sodium aurothiomalate
	Aurotioprol	Sodium aurothiosulfate

T39.4x- Poisoning by, adverse effect of and underdosing of <u>antirheumatics</u>, <u>not elsewhere classified</u>

T39.4x1- Poisoning by antirheumatics, not elsewhere classified, <u>accidental</u> (unintentional)
     Poisoning by antirheumatics, not elsewhere classified NOS

T39.4x2- Poisoning by antirheumatics, not elsewhere classified, <u>intentional</u> self-harm

T39.4x3- Poisoning by antirheumatics, not elsewhere classified, <u>assault</u>

T39.4x4- Poisoning by antirheumatics, not elsewhere classified, <u>undetermined</u>

T39.4x5- <u>Adverse effect</u> of antirheumatics, not elsewhere classified

T39.4x6- <u>Underdosing</u> of antirheumatics, not elsewhere classified

T39.8- Poisoning by, adverse effect of and underdosing of other nonopioid analgesics and antipyretics, not elsewhere classified

<u>T39.8</u> - DRUGS/CHEMS*	Fluradoline	Phenyramidol,
Acetylphenylhydrazine	Glafenine	phenyramidon
Analgesic, specified NEC	Jamaica dogwood (bark)	Piroxicam, beta-
Antipyretic, specified NEC	Ketorolac	cyclodextrin complex
Carbiphene	Lefetamine	Piscidia (bark) (erythrina)
Clonixin	Meptazinol	Pyrabital
Cropropamide	Methopholine	Pyridium
Crotethamide	Metofoline	Rimazolium metilsulfate
Cryogenine	Nefopam	Sumatriptan
Cyclopyrabital	Oxetorone	Tiaramide
Darvon	Pentosan polysulfate	Tinoridine
Diclonixine	(sodium)	Versidyne
Doloxene	Perisoxal	Viminol
Emorfazone	Phenazopyridine	Zactane
Etomide	Phenicarbazide	
Floctafenine		

T39.8x- Poisoning by, adverse effect of and underdosing of <u>other nonopioid analgesics and antipyretics</u>, <u>not elsewhere classified</u>

T39.8x1- Poisoning by other nonopioid analgesics and antipyretics, not elsewhere classified, <u>accidental</u> (unintentional)
     Poisoning by other nonopioid analgesics and antipyretics, not elsewhere classified NOS

T39.8x2- Poisoning by other nonopioid analgesics and antipyretics, not elsewhere classified, <u>intentional</u> self-harm

T39.8x3- Poisoning by other nonopioid analgesics and antipyretics, not elsewhere classified, <u>assault</u>

T39.8x4- Poisoning by other nonopioid analgesics and antipyretics, not elsewhere classified, <u>undetermined</u>

T39.8x5- <u>Adverse effect</u> of other nonopioid analgesics and antipyretics, not elsewhere classified

T39.8x6- <u>Underdosing</u> of other nonopioid analgesics and antipyretics, not elsewhere classified

T39.9- Poisoning by, adverse effect of and underdosing of <u>unspecified</u> <u>nonopioid analgesic, antipyretic and antirheumatic</u>

<u>T39.9</u> - DRUGS/CHEMS*	Analgesic, non-narcotic	Antipyretic
Analgesic	NEC	
Analgesic, anti-	Analgesic, non-narcotic	
inflammatory NEC	NEC, combination	

T39.91x- Poisoning by unspecified nonopioid analgesic, antipyretic and antirheumatic, <u>accidental</u> (unintentional)
     Poisoning by nonopioid analgesic, antipyretic and antirheumatic NOS

T39.92x- Poisoning by unspecified nonopioid analgesic, antipyretic and antirheumatic, <u>intentional</u> self-harm

T39.93x- Poisoning by unspecified nonopioid analgesic, antipyretic and antirheumatic, <u>assault</u>

T39.94x- Poisoning by unspecified nonopioid analgesic, antipyretic and antirheumatic, <u>undetermined</u>

T39.95x- <u>Adverse effect</u> of unspecified nonopioid analgesic, antipyretic and antirheumatic

T39.96x- <u>Underdosing</u> of unspecified nonopioid analgesic, antipyretic and antirheumatic

T40- Poisoning by, adverse effect of and underdosing of <u>narcotics and psychodysleptics [hallucinogens]</u>

Excludes ❷: *drug dependence and related mental and behavioral disorders due to psychoactive substance use (F10.-F19.-)*

The appropriate 7th character is to be added to each code from category T40:
A   <u>Initial</u> encounter
D   <u>Subsequent</u> encounter
S   <u>Sequela</u>

T40.0- Poisoning by, adverse effect of and underdosing of opium

<u>T40.0</u> - DRUGS/CHEMS*	Opium alkaloids,	Pantopon
Laudanum	standardized powdered	Papaveretum
Opium alkaloids (total)	Opium alkaloids, tincture	Paregoric
	(camphorated)	

T40.0x- Poisoning by, adverse effect of and underdosing of <u>opium</u>

T40.0x1- Poisoning by opium, <u>accidental</u> (unintentional)
     Poisoning by opium NOS

T40.0x2- Poisoning by opium, <u>intentional</u> self-harm

T40.0x3- Poisoning by opium, <u>assault</u>

T40.0x4- Poisoning by opium, <u>undetermined</u>

T40.0x5- <u>Adverse effect</u> of opium

T40.0x6- <u>Underdosing</u> of opium

T40.1- Poisoning by and adverse effect of heroin

<u>T40.1</u> - DRUGS/CHEMS*	Diacetylmorphine	Heroin
Acetomorphine	Diamorphine	

T40.1x- Poisoning by and adverse effect of <u>heroin</u>

T40.1x1- Poisoning by heroin, <u>accidental</u> (unintentional)
     Poisoning by heroin NOS

T40.1x2- Poisoning by heroin, <u>intentional</u> self-harm

T40.1x3- Poisoning by heroin, <u>assault</u>

T40.1x4- Poisoning by heroin, <u>undetermined</u>

T
3
9
-
T
4
0

T40.2- Poisoning by, adverse effect of and underdosing of other opioids

T40.2 - DRUGS/CHEMS*	Dihydrohydroxy-	Metopon
14-hydroxydihydro morphinone	morphinone	Morfin
Acemorphan	Dihydroisocodeine	Morphine
Acetorphine	Dihydromorphine	Morpholinylethylmorphine
Acetyldihydrocodeine	Dihydromorphinone	Nicomorphine
Acetyldihydrocodeinone	Dihydroxycodeinone	Nisentil
Alvodine	Dilaudid	Normorphine
Antitussive, codeine mixture	Dimethyl meperidine	Numorphan
Antitussive, opiate	Dionin	Opioid NEC
Benzomorphan	Drocode	Oxycodone
Benzyl morphine	Dromoran	Oxymorphone
Blue velvet	Ethyl morphine	Palfium
Cliradon	Ethylmorphine	Paracodin
Codeine	Etorphine	Parzone
Cough mixture, containing opiates	Eucodal	Percodan
Demerol	Heptalgin	Peronine
Desocodeine	Hycodan	Phenadoxone
Desomorphine	Hydrocodone	Phenomorphan
Dextrorphan	Hydromorphinol	Piminodine
Difencloxazine	Hydromorphinone	Pipadone
Dihydrocodeine	Hydromorphone	Prinadol
Dihydrocodein-one	Hydroxydihydrocodeinone	Promedol
Dihydrohydroxycodein-one	Leritine	Racemoramide
	Levo-dromoran	Racemorphan
	Methyl dihydromorphinone	Thebaine
	Methyl morphine NEC	
	Methylmorphine	

T40.2x- Poisoning by, adverse effect of and underdosing of **other opioids**

T40.2x1- Poisoning by other opioids, **accidental** (unintentional)
Poisoning by other opioids NOS

T40.2x2- Poisoning by other opioids, **intentional** self-harm

T40.2x3- Poisoning by other opioids, **assault**

T40.2x4- Poisoning by other opioids, **undetermined**

T40.2x5- **Adverse effect** of other opioids

T40.2x6- **Underdosing** of other opioids

T40.3- Poisoning by, adverse effect of and underdosing of methadone

T40.3 - DRUGS/CHEMS*	Dolophine	Methadone
Amidone	Levo-iso-methadone	Physeptone

T40.3x- Poisoning by, adverse effect of and underdosing of **methadone**

T40.3x1- Poisoning by methadone, **accidental** (unintentional)
Poisoning by methadone NOS

T40.3x2- Poisoning by methadone, **intentional** self-harm

T40.3x3- Poisoning by methadone, **assault**

T40.3x4- Poisoning by methadone, **undetermined**

T40.3x5- **Adverse effect** of methadone

T40.3x6- **Underdosing** of methadone

T40.4- Poisoning by, adverse effect of and underdosing of other synthetic narcotics

T40.4 - DRUGS/CHEMS*	Eptazocine	Pentazocine
Alfentanil	Ethoheptazine	Pethidine
Alphaprodine	Fentanyl	Phenazocine
Anileridine	Isonipecaine	Phenoperidine
Bezitramide	Ketobemidone	Piritramide
Buprenorphine	Levopropoxyphene	Profadol
Butorphanol	Levorphanol	Propoxyphene
Dextromoramide	Meperidine	Sufentanil
Dextropropoxyphene	Nalbuphine	Tilidine
Dipipanone	Narcotic, synthetic	Tramadol

T40.4x- Poisoning by, adverse effect of and underdosing of **other synthetic narcotics**

T40.4x1- Poisoning by other synthetic narcotics, **accidental** (unintentional)
Poisoning by other synthetic narcotics NOS

T40.4x2- Poisoning by other synthetic narcotics, **intentional** self-harm

T40.4x3- Poisoning by other synthetic narcotics, **assault**

T40.4x4- Poisoning by other synthetic narcotics, **undetermined**

T40.4x5- **Adverse effect** of other synthetic narcotics

T40.4x6- **Underdosing** of other synthetic narcotics

T40.5- Poisoning by, adverse effect of and underdosing of cocaine

T40.5 - DRUGS/CHEMS*	Cocaine
Coca (leaf)	Crack

T40.5x- Poisoning by, adverse effect of and underdosing of **cocaine**
AHA 16:2Q:p8 – Overdose of crack cocaine, intent

T40.5x1- Poisoning by cocaine, **accidental** (unintentional)
Poisoning by cocaine NOS

T40.5x2- Poisoning by cocaine, **intentional** self-harm

T40.5x3- Poisoning by cocaine, **assault**

T40.5x4- Poisoning by cocaine, **undetermined**

T40.5x5- **Adverse effect** of cocaine

T40.5x6- **Underdosing** of cocaine

T40.6- Poisoning by, adverse effect of and underdosing of other and unspecified narcotics

T40.60- Poisoning by, adverse effect of and underdosing of **unspecified** narcotics

T40.60 - DRUGS/CHEMS*	Analgesic, narcotic NEC, obstetric	Opiate NEC
Analgesic, narcotic NEC		
Analgesic, narcotic NEC, combination	Narcotic (drug)	
	Narcotic analgesic NEC	

T40.601- Poisoning by unspecified narcotics, **accidental** (unintentional)
Poisoning by narcotics NOS

T40.602- Poisoning by unspecified narcotics, **intentional** self-harm

T40.603- Poisoning by unspecified narcotics, **assault**

T40.604- Poisoning by unspecified narcotics, **undetermined**

T40.605- **Adverse effect** of unspecified narcotics

T40.606- **Underdosing** of unspecified narcotics

T40.69- Poisoning by, adverse effect of and underdosing of **other narcotics**

T40.69 - DRUGS/CHEMS*
Narcotic, specified NEC

T40.691- Poisoning by other narcotics, **accidental** (unintentional)
Poisoning by other narcotics NOS

T40.692- Poisoning by other narcotics, **intentional** self-harm

T40.693- Poisoning by other narcotics, **assault**

T40.694- Poisoning by other narcotics, **undetermined**

T40.695- **Adverse effect** of other narcotics

T40.696- **Underdosing** of other narcotics

T40-T40

Excludes 1: = NOT CODED HERE! (Do not code both)   1166   *Excludes ❷:* = Not Included Here

T40.7-   Poisoning by, adverse effect of and underdosing of cannabis (derivatives)

T40.7 - DRUGS/CHEMS*	Central nervous system	Lebanese red
Afghanistan black	depressants, cannabis	Marihuana
Bhang	sativa	Marijuana
Cannabinol	Dronabinol	Nabilone
Cannabis (derivatives)	Ganja	Pot
	Hashish	Tetrahydrocannabinol
	Indian hemp	THC

T40.7x- Poisoning by, adverse effect of and underdosing of cannabis (derivatives)

T40.7x1- Poisoning by cannabis (derivatives), accidental (unintentional)
   Poisoning by cannabis NOS

T40.7x2- Poisoning by cannabis (derivatives), intentional self-harm

T40.7x3- Poisoning by cannabis (derivatives), assault

T40.7x4- Poisoning by cannabis (derivatives), undetermined

T40.7x5- Adverse effect of cannabis (derivatives)

T40.7x6- Underdosing of cannabis (derivatives)

T40.8-   Poisoning by and adverse effect of lysergide [LSD]

T40.8 - DRUGS/CHEMS*	LSD
D-lysergic acid	Lysergic acid diethylamide
diethylamide	Lysergide

T40.8x- Poisoning by and adverse effect of lysergide [LSD]

T40.8x1- Poisoning by lysergide [LSD], accidental (unintentional)
   Poisoning by lysergide [LSD] NOS

T40.8x2- Poisoning by lysergide [LSD], intentional self-harm

T40.8x3- Poisoning by lysergide [LSD], assault

T40.8x4- Poisoning by lysergide [LSD], undetermined

T40.9-   Poisoning by, adverse effect of and underdosing of other and unspecified psychodysleptics [hallucinogens]

T40.90- Poisoning by, adverse effect of and underdosing of unspecified psychodysleptics [hallucinogens]

T40.90 - DRUGS/CHEMS*	Hallucinogen NEC
Central nervous system	Megahallucinogen
depressants,	Psychodysleptic drug NEC
hallucinogenics	Psychotomimetic agents

T40.901- Poisoning by unspecified psychodysleptics [hallucinogens], accidental (unintentional)

T40.902- Poisoning by unspecified psychodysleptics [hallucinogens], intentional self-harm

T40.903- Poisoning by unspecified psychodysleptics [hallucinogens], assault

T40.904- Poisoning by unspecified psychodysleptics [hallucinogens], undetermined

T40.905- Adverse effect of unspecified psychodysleptics [hallucinogens]

T40.906- Underdosing of unspecified psychodysleptics

T40.99- Poisoning by, adverse effect of and underdosing of other psychodysleptics [hallucinogens]

T40.99 - DRUGS/CHEMS*	Magic mushroom	Peyote
Bufotenine	Mescal buttons	Phencyclidine
Diethyltryptamine (DET)	Mescaline	Psilocin
Dimethyl tryptamine	Morning glory seeds	Psilocybin
Hawaiian Woodrose seeds	PCP, meaning phencyclidine	Psilocybine
Heavenly Blue (morning	Pearly Gates (morning	Yohimbic acid
glory)	glory seeds)	

T40.991- Poisoning by other psychodysleptics [hallucinogens], accidental (unintentional)
   Poisoning by other psychodysleptics [hallucinogens] NOS

T40.992- Poisoning by other psychodysleptics [hallucinogens], intentional self-harm

T40.993- Poisoning by other psychodysleptics [hallucinogens], assault

T40.994- Poisoning by other psychodysleptics [hallucinogens], undetermined

T40.995- Adverse effect of other psychodysleptics [hallucinogens]

T40.996- Underdosing of other psychodysleptics

T41-   Poisoning by, adverse effect of and underdosing of anesthetics and therapeutic gases

Excludes 1:   *benzodiazepines (T42.4-)*
   cocaine (T40.5-)
   complications of anesthesia during pregnancy (O29.-)
   complications of anesthesia during labor and delivery (O74.-)
   complications of anesthesia during the puerperium (O89.-)
   opioids (T40.0-T40.2-)

The appropriate 7th character is to be added to each code from category T41:
A   Initial encounter
D   Subsequent encounter
S   Sequela

T41.0-   Poisoning by, adverse effect of and underdosing of inhaled anesthetics

Excludes 1:   *oxygen (T41.5-)*

T41.0 - DRUGS/CHEMS*	Diethyl ether (vapor) – see	Fluothane
Anesthesia, endotracheal	also Ether	Fluroxene
Anesthesia, inhalation	Divinyl ether	Gas, anesthetic
Anesthetic, gaseous NEC	Enflurane	Halothane
Anesthetic, halogenated	Ether (vapor)	Isoflurane
hydrocarbon derivatives	Ether, anesthetic	Laughing gas
NEC	Ether, divinyl	Methoxyflurane
Central nervous system	Ether, ethyl (medicinal)	Nitrous oxide
depressants, anesthetic,	Ethyl bromide (anesthetic)	Trichloroethylene,
gases NEC	Ethyl chloride (anesthetic)	anesthetic (gas)
Chloroform, anesthetic	Ethyl chloride, anesthetic,	Trifluoroethyl vinyl ether
Chloroform, water,	inhaled	Trilene
concentrated	Ethylene, anesthetic	Vinesthene, vinethene
	(general)	Vinyl ether

T41.0x- Poisoning by, adverse effect of and underdosing of inhaled anesthetics

T41.0x1- Poisoning by inhaled anesthetics, accidental (unintentional)
   Poisoning by inhaled anesthetics NOS

T41.0x2- Poisoning by inhaled anesthetics, intentional self-harm

T41.0x3- Poisoning by inhaled anesthetics, assault

T41.0x4- Poisoning by inhaled anesthetics, undetermined

T41.0x5- Adverse effect of inhaled anesthetics

T41.0x6- Underdosing of inhaled anesthetics

T41.1-   Poisoning by, adverse effect of and underdosing of intravenous anesthetics
   Poisoning by, adverse effect of and underdosing of thiobarbiturates

T41.1 - DRUGS/CHEMS*	Butyl thiobarbital sodium	Pentothal
Alfadolone	Central nervous system	Sernyl
Alfaxalone	depressants, anesthetic,	Sodium thiopental
Alphadolone	intravenous	Surital
Alphaxalone	Etomidate	Thialbarbital
Anesthetic, intravenous	Evipal sodium	Thiamylal
NEC	Evipan sodium	Thiamylal sodium
Anesthetic, thiobarbiturate	Hexobarbital, sodium	Thiobarbital sodium
Barbiturate anesthetic	Intranarcon	Thiobarbiturate anesthetic
(intravenous)	Kemithal	Thiobutabarbital sodium
Brevital (sodium)	Methohexital	Thiopental (sodium)
Buthalitone (sodium)	Methohexitone	Thiopentone (sodium)

T41.1x- Poisoning by, adverse effect of and underdosing of intravenous anesthetics

T41.1x1- Poisoning by intravenous anesthetics, accidental (unintentional)
   Poisoning by intravenous anesthetics NOS

T41.1x2- Poisoning by intravenous anesthetics, intentional self-harm

T41.1x3- Poisoning by intravenous anesthetics, assault

T41.1x4- Poisoning by intravenous anesthetics, undetermined

T41.1x5- Adverse effect of intravenous anesthetics

T41.1x6- Underdosing of intravenous anesthetics

T40 – T41

T41.2- Poisoning by, adverse effect of and underdosing of other and unspecified general anesthetics

T41.20- Poisoning by, adverse effect of and underdosing of <u>unspecified general anesthetics</u>

T41.20 - DRUGS/CHEMS*		
Anesthesia, potentiated	Anesthetic, with muscle relaxant, general	Central nervous system depressants, anesthetic (general) NEC
Anesthesia, rectal	Anesthetic, general NEC	
Anesthesia, rectal, general	Anesthetic, rectal	Depressant, central nervous system, general anesthetic
Anesthetic, with muscle relaxant	Anesthetic, rectal, general	
		Premedication anesthetic

    T41.201- Poisoning by unspecified general anesthetics, <u>accidental</u> (unintentional)
        Poisoning by general anesthetics NOS

    T41.202- Poisoning by unspecified general anesthetics, <u>intentional</u> self-harm

    T41.203- Poisoning by unspecified general anesthetics, <u>assault</u>

    T41.204- Poisoning by unspecified general anesthetics, <u>undetermined</u>

    T41.205- <u>Adverse effect</u> of unspecified general anesthetics

    T41.206- <u>Underdosing</u> of unspecified general anesthetics

T41.29- Poisoning by, adverse effect of and underdosing of <u>other general anesthetics</u>

T41.29 - DRUGS/CHEMS*	Ketamine	Propofol
Cyclopropane	Minaxolone	Sodium oxybate
Disoprofol	Oxybate sodium	Tiletamine
Hexobarbital, rectal	Propanidid	Tribromoethanol, rectal

    T41.291- Poisoning by other general anesthetics, <u>accidental</u> (unintentional)
        Poisoning by other general anesthetics NOS

    T41.292- Poisoning by other general anesthetics, <u>intentional</u> self-harm

    T41.293- Poisoning by other general anesthetics, <u>assault</u>

    T41.294- Poisoning by other general anesthetics, <u>undetermined</u>

    T41.295- <u>Adverse effect</u> of other general anesthetics

    T41.296- <u>Underdosing</u> of other general anesthetics

T41.3- Poisoning by, adverse effect of and underdosing of local anesthetics

    Cocaine (topical)

    Excludes ❷: poisoning by cocaine used as a central nervous system stimulant (T40.5x1-T40.5x4)

T41.3 - DRUGS/CHEMS*	Blockain, infiltration (subcutaneous)	Cinchocaine, topical (surface)
Amethocaine (regional) (spinal)	Blockain, nerve block (peripheral) (plexus)	Citanest
Amyleine, regional	Blockain, topical (surface)	Citanest, infiltration (subcutaneous)
Amylocaine (regional) (infiltration) (nerve block) (spinal) (topical)	Bupivacaine	Citanest, nerve block (peripheral) (plexus)
	Bupivacaine, infiltration (subcutaneous)	Cocaine, topical anesthetic
Anesthesia, caudal	Bupivacaine, nerve block (peripheral) (plexus)	Cyclaine
Anesthesia, epidural		Cyclomethycaine
Anesthesia, local	Bupivacaine, spinal	Dibucaine
Anesthesia, mucosal	Butacaine	Dibucaine, topical (surface)
Anesthesia, nerve blocking	Butamben	Dimethocaine
Anesthesia, plexus blocking	Butanilicaine	Diperodon
Anesthesia, rectal, local	Butyl aminobenzoate	Dorsacaine
Anesthesia, regional	Butyn	Dyclone
Anesthesia, surface	Carbocaine	Dyclonine
Anesthetic, with muscle relaxant, local	Carbocaine, infiltration (subcutaneous)	Endocaine
Anesthetic, infiltration NEC		EPAB
Anesthetic, local NEC	Carbocaine, nerve block (peripheral) (plexus)	Ethocaine (infiltration) (topical)
Anesthetic, rectal, local	Carbocaine, topical (surface)	Ethocaine, nerve block (peripheral) (plexus)
Anesthetic, regional NEC		
Anesthetic, spinal NEC	Chloroprocaine	Ethocaine, spinal
Anesthetic, topical	Chloroprocaine, infiltration (subcutaneous)	Ethyl aminobenzoate
Aptocaine		Ethyl chloride, anesthetic (local)
Articaine	Chloroprocaine, nerve block (peripheral) (plexus)	
Benoxinate		Etidocaine
Benzamine	Chloroprocaine, spinal	Etidocaine, infiltration (subcutaneous)
Benzocaine	Cinchocaine	
Betoxycaine		
Blockain		

Excludes 1: = NOT CODED HERE! (Do not code both)

T41.3 - DRUGS/CHEMS* – Continued	Novocain, spinal	Procaine, spinal
Etidocaine, nerve (peripheral) (plexus)	Nupercaine (spinal anesthetic)	Proparacaine
		Propitocaine
Eucaine	Nupercaine, topical (surface)	Propitocaine, infiltration (subcutaneous)
Hexylcaine	Ophthaine	
Leucinocaine	Ophthetic	Propitocaine, nerve block (peripheral) (plexus)
Lidocaine	Orthocaine	
Lidocaine, regional	Oxetacaine	Propoxycaine
Lidocaine, spinal	Oxethazine	Propoxycaine, infiltration (subcutaneous)
Lignocaine	Oxybuprocaine	
Lignocaine, regional	Percaine (spinal)	Propoxycaine, nerve block (peripheral) (plexus)
Lignocaine, spinal	Percaine, topical (surface)	
Marcaine	Phenacaine	Propoxycaine, topical (surface)
Marcaine, infiltration (subcutaneous)	Piperocaine	Proxymetacaine
	Piperocaine, infiltration (subcutaneous)	Quotane
Marcaine, nerve block (peripheral) (plexus)		Stovaine
	Piperocaine, nerve block (peripheral) (plexus)	Stovaine, infiltration (subcutaneous)
Mepivacaine		
Mepivacaine epidural	Piperocaine, topical (surface)	Stovaine, nerve block (peripheral) (plexus)
Meprylcaine		
Metabutethamine	Pitkin's solution	Stovaine, spinal
Metycaine	Pontocaine (hydrochloride) (infiltration) (topical)	Stovaine, topical (surface)
Metycaine, infiltration (subcutaneous)		Surfacaine
	Pontocaine, nerve block (peripheral) (plexus)	Tetracaine
Metycaine, nerve block (peripheral) (plexus)		Tetracaine, nerve block (peripheral) (plexus)
	Pontocaine, spinal	
Metycaine, topical (surface)	Prilocaine	Tetracaine, regional
Nesacaine	Prilocaine, infiltration (subcutaneous)	Tetracaine, spinal
Nesacaine, infiltration (subcutaneous)		Trimecaine
	Prilocaine, nerve block (peripheral) (plexus)	Tronothane
Nesacaine, nerve block (peripheral) (plexus)		Xylocaine (infiltration) (topical)
	Prilocaine, regional	
Novocain (infiltration) (topical)	Procaine	Xylocaine, nerve block (peripheral) (plexus)
	Procaine, nerve block (peripheral) (plexus)	
Novocain, nerve block (peripheral) (plexus)	Procaine, regional	Xylocaine, spinal

T41.3x- Poisoning by, adverse effect of and underdosing of <u>local anesthetics</u>

    T41.3x1- Poisoning by local anesthetics, <u>accidental</u> (unintentional)
        Poisoning by local anesthetics NOS

    T41.3x2- Poisoning by local anesthetics, <u>intentional</u> self-harm

    T41.3x3- Poisoning by local anesthetics, <u>assault</u>

    T41.3x4- Poisoning by local anesthetics, <u>undetermined</u>

    T41.3x5- <u>Adverse effect</u> of local anesthetics

    T41.3x6- <u>Underdosing</u> of local anesthetics

T41.4- Poisoning by, adverse effect of and underdosing of <u>unspecified anesthetic</u>

T41.4 - DRUGS/CHEMS*	
Anesthetic NEC – see also Anesthesia	

    T41.41x- Poisoning by unspecified anesthetic, <u>accidental</u> (unintentional)
        Poisoning by anesthetic NOS

    T41.42x- Poisoning by unspecified anesthetic, <u>intentional</u> self-harm

    T41.43x- Poisoning by unspecified anesthetic, <u>assault</u>

    T41.44x- Poisoning by unspecified anesthetic, <u>undetermined</u>

    T41.45x- <u>Adverse effect</u> of unspecified anesthetic

    T41.46x- <u>Underdosing</u> of unspecified anesthetics

T41.5- Poisoning by, adverse effect of and underdosing of therapeutic gases

T41.5 - DRUGS/CHEMS*	Gas, therapeutic
Carbon dioxide, medicinal	Oxygen

T41.5x- Poisoning by, adverse effect of and underdosing of <u>therapeutic gases</u>

    T41.5x1- Poisoning by therapeutic gases, <u>accidental</u> (unintentional)
        Poisoning by therapeutic gases NOS

Excludes ❷: = Not Included Here

T41-T41

T41.5x2- Poisoning by therapeutic gases, <u>intentional</u> self-harm

T41.5x3- Poisoning by therapeutic gases, <u>assault</u>

T41.5x4- Poisoning by therapeutic gases, <u>undetermined</u>

T41.5x5- <u>Adverse effect</u> of therapeutic gases

T41.5x6- <u>Underdosing</u> of therapeutic gases

T42- Poisoning by, adverse effect of and underdosing of <u>antiepileptic, sedative-hypnotic and antiparkinsonism drugs</u>

    Excludes ❷: drug dependence and related mental and behavioral disorders due to psychoactive substance use (F10.-F19.-)

The appropriate 7th character is to be added to each code from category T42:

  A <u>Initial</u> encounter

  D <u>Subsequent</u> encounter

  S <u>Sequela</u>

T42.0- Poisoning by, adverse effect of and underdosing of hydantoin derivatives

T42.0 - DRUGS/CHEMS*	Epanutin	Methetoin
Albutoin	Ethotoin	Methoin
Anticonvulsant, hydantoin	Hydantoin derivative NEC	Phenantoin
Dilantin	Mephenytoin	Phenytoin
Diphenylhydantoin	Metetoin	

T42.0x- Poisoning by, adverse effect of and underdosing of <u>hydantoin derivatives</u>

T42.0x1- Poisoning by hydantoin derivatives, <u>accidental</u> (unintentional)

      Poisoning by hydantoin derivatives NOS

T42.0x2- Poisoning by hydantoin derivatives, <u>intentional</u> self-harm

T42.0x3- Poisoning by hydantoin derivatives, <u>assault</u>

T42.0x4- Poisoning by hydantoin derivatives, <u>undetermined</u>

T42.0x5- <u>Adverse effect</u> of hydantoin derivatives

T42.0x6- <u>Underdosing</u> of hydantoin derivatives

T42.1- Poisoning by, adverse effect of and underdosing of iminostilbenes

    Poisoning by, adverse effect of and underdosing of carbamazepine

T42.1 - DRUGS/CHEMS*	Iminostilbene	Tegretol
Carbamazepine	Oxcarbazepine	

T42.1x- Poisoning by, adverse effect of and underdosing of <u>iminostilbenes</u>

T42.1x1- Poisoning by iminostilbenes, <u>accidental</u> (unintentional)

      Poisoning by iminostilbenes NOS

T42.1x2- Poisoning by iminostilbenes, <u>intentional</u> self-harm

T42.1x3- Poisoning by iminostilbenes, <u>assault</u>

T42.1x4- Poisoning by iminostilbenes, <u>undetermined</u>

T42.1x5- <u>Adverse effect</u> of iminostilbenes

T42.1x6- <u>Underdosing</u> of iminostilbenes

T42.2- Poisoning by, adverse effect of and underdosing of succinimides and oxazolidinediones

T42.2 - DRUGS/CHEMS*	Mesuximide	Phensuximide
Aloxidone	Methsuximide	Succinimide, antiepileptic
Anticonvulsant, oxazolidinedione	Morsuximide	or anticonvulsant
	Oxazolidine derivatives	Tridione
Anticonvulsant, succinimide	Oxazolidinedione	Trimethadione
Ethadione	(derivative)	Troxidone
Ethosuximide	Paradione	
Isoethadione	Paramethadione	

T42.2x- Poisoning by, adverse effect of and underdosing of <u>succinimides and oxazolidinediones</u>

T42.2x1- Poisoning by succinimides and oxazolidinediones, <u>accidental</u> (unintentional)

      Poisoning by succinimides and oxazolidinediones NOS

T42.2x2- Poisoning by succinimides and oxazolidinediones, <u>intentional</u> self-harm

T42.2x3- Poisoning by succinimides and oxazolidinediones, <u>assault</u>

T42.2x4- Poisoning by succinimides and oxazolidinediones, <u>undetermined</u>

T42.2x5- <u>Adverse effect</u> of succinimides and oxazolidinediones

T42.2x6- <u>Underdosing</u> of succinimides and oxazolidinediones

T42.3- Poisoning by, adverse effect of and underdosing of barbiturates

    Excludes 1:   poisoning by, adverse effect of and underdosing of thiobarbiturates (T41.1-)

T42.3 - DRUGS/CHEMS*	Dormiral	Noptil
Agrypnal	Enhexymal	Nunol
Allobarbital	Eskabarb	Ortal (sodium)
Allylisopropylmalonylurea	Ethobral	Pentobarbital
Allypropymal	Etilfen	Pentobarbital, sodium
Alurate	Etoval	Pentobarbitone
Amobarbital (sodium)	Euneryl	Pentymal
Amylobarbitone	Evipal	Pernocton
Amytal (sodium)	Evipan	Pernoston
Anticonvulsant, barbiturate	Febarbamate	Phanodorm, phanodorn
Anticonvulsant, combination (with barbiturate)	Fenobarbital	Phemitone
	Gardenal	Phenemal
	Gardepanyl	Phenobal
Aprobarbital	Gemonil	Phenobarbital
Barbenyl	Heptabarb	Phenobarbital with
Barbital	Heptabarbital	mephenytoin
Barbital, sodium	Heptabarbitone	Phenobarbital with
Barbitone	Hexemal	phenytoin
Barbiturate NEC	Hexethal (sodium)	Phenobarbital, sodium
Barbiturate with tranquilizer	Hexobarbital	Phenobarbitone
	Ipral	Phenonyl
Brallobarbital	Lotusate	Phenylmethylbarbitone
Butabarbital (sodium)	Luminal	Phenytoin with
Butabarbitone	Meballymal	phenobarbital
Butabarpal	Mebaral	Probarbital
Butalbital	Mebumal	Propallylonal
Butallylonal	Medinal	Proxibarbal
Butethal	Medomin	Quinalbarbital
Butisol (sodium)	Mephebarbital	Quinalbarbitone sodium
Butobarbital	Mephenytoin with	Secbutabarbital
Butobarbital sodium	phenobarbital	Secbutabarbitone
Butobarbitone	Mephobarbital	Secobarbital
Carbrital	Metharbital	Seconal
Central nervous system depressants, barbiturates	Methitural	Sodium amytal
	Methobarbital, methobarbitone	Sodium barbiturate
		Somonal
Cyclobarbital	Methylhexabital	Soneryl
Cyclobarbitone	Methylphenobarbital	Talbutal
Delvinal	Mysoline	Veramon
Dial, sedative	Nealbarbital	Veronal
Diallylbarbituric acid	Nembutal	Vinbarbital, vinbarbitone
Diallymal	Neonal	Vinyl bital
Diemal	Neraval	Vinylbital
Diethyl barbituric acid	Neravan	
Difebarbamate	Neurobarb	

T42.3x- Poisoning by, adverse effect of and underdosing of <u>barbiturates</u>

T42.3x1- Poisoning by barbiturates, <u>accidental</u> (unintentional)

      Poisoning by barbiturates NOS

T42.3x2- Poisoning by barbiturates, <u>intentional</u> self-harm

T42.3x3- Poisoning by barbiturates, <u>assault</u>

T42.3x4- Poisoning by barbiturates, <u>undetermined</u>

T42.3x5- <u>Adverse effect</u> of barbiturates

T42.3x6- <u>Underdosing</u> of barbiturates

T41-T42

T42.4- Poisoning by, adverse effect of and underdosing of benzodiazepines

T42.4 - DRUGS/CHEMS*	Delorazepam	Nimetazepam
Alprazolam	Diazepam	Nitrazepam
Bentazepam	Estazolam	Nordazepam
Benzodiapin	Ethyl loflazepate	Oxazepam
Benzodiazepine NEC	Etizolam	Oxazolam
Bromazepam	Fludiazepam	Perlapine
Brotizolam	Flunitrazepam	Pinazepam
Camazepam	Flurazepam	Prazepam
Carpipramine	Flutazolam	Quazepam
Central nervous system	Flutoprazepam	Rohypnol
depressants,	Halazepam	Serax
benzodiazepines	Haloxazolam	Temazepam
Chlordiazepoxide	Ketazolam	Tetrazepam
Clobazam	Librium	Tofisopam
Clonazepam	Loprazolam	Tranquilizer,
Clorazepate (dipotassium)	Lorazepam	benzodiazepine NEC
Clotiazepam	Lormetazepam	Tranxene
Cloxazolam	Medazepam	Triazolam
Clozapine	Mexazolam	Valium
Dalmane	Midazolam	

T42.4x- Poisoning by, adverse effect of and underdosing of <u>benzodiazepines</u>

T42.4x1- Poisoning by benzodiazepines, <u>accidental</u> (unintentional)
    Poisoning by benzodiazepines NOS

T42.4x2- Poisoning by benzodiazepines, <u>intentional</u> self-harm

T42.4x3- Poisoning by benzodiazepines, <u>assault</u>

T42.4x4- Poisoning by benzodiazepines, <u>undetermined</u>

T42.4x5- <u>Adverse effect</u> of benzodiazepines

T42.4x6- <u>Underdosing</u> of benzodiazepines

T42.5- Poisoning by, adverse effect of and underdosing of mixed antiepileptics

T42.5 - DRUGS/CHEMS*	Antiepilepsy agent, mixed
Antiepilepsy agent, combination	

T42.5x- Poisoning by, adverse effect of and underdosing of <u>antiepileptics</u>

T42.5x1- Poisoning by mixed antiepileptics, <u>accidental</u> (unintentional)
    Poisoning by mixed antiepileptics NOS

T42.5x2- Poisoning by mixed antiepileptics, <u>intentional</u> self-harm

T42.5x3- Poisoning by mixed antiepileptics, <u>assault</u>

T42.5x4- Poisoning by mixed antiepileptics, <u>undetermined</u>

T42.5x5- <u>Adverse effect</u> of mixed antiepileptics

T42.5x6- <u>Underdosing</u> of mixed antiepileptics

T42.6- Poisoning by, adverse effect of and underdosing of other antiepileptic and sedative-hypnotic drugs
    Poisoning by, adverse effect of and underdosing of methaqualone
    Poisoning by, adverse effect of and underdosing of valproic acid
Excludes 1:   *poisoning by, adverse effect of and underdosing of carbamazepine (T42.1-)*

T42.6 - DRUGS/CHEMS*	Central nervous system	Petrichloral
Acecarbromal	depressants, sedatives	Phenacemide
Acetylcarbromal	sedative-hypnotics,	Phenergan
Acetylpheneturide	specified NEC	Pheneturide
Allylisopropylacetylurea	Chloral	Phthalimidoglutarimide
Allyltribromide	Chloral derivative	Placidyl
Ammonium bromide	Chloralhydrate	Potassium bromide
Anticonvulsant, hypnotic	Chloralamide	Primidone
NEC	Chloralodol	Progabide
Anticonvulsant,	Chlorbutol	Propionaldehyde
pyrimidinedione	Chlorethiazol	(medicinal)
Anticonvulsant, specified	Chloretone	Pyrithyldione
NEC	Chlorhexadol	Quaalude
Antiepilepsy agent,	Chlormethiazole	Sedative, mixed NEC
specified, NEC	Chlormezanone	Sedormid
Apronalide	Clomethiazole	Serenesil
Avomine	Cloral betaine	Sodium bromide
Barbexaclone	Croton, chloral	Sodium valproate
Beclamide	Dichloralphenazone	Somnos
Beta-Chlor	Diethylsulfone-	Sopor
Bromal (hydrate)	diethylmethane	Soporific drug, specified
Bromide salts	Divalproex	type NEC
Bromine compounds	Doriden	Sulfonal
(medicinal)	Dormison	Sulfonethylmethane
Bromine sedative	Ectylurea	Sulfonmethane
Bromisoval	Ethchlorvynol	Sulthiame
Bromisovalum	Ethinamate	Sultiame
Bromoform	Etifoxine	Tetronal
Bromural	Glutethimide	Toloxatone
Bromvaletone	Hexapropymate	Tranquilizer with hypnotic
Butyl chloral (hydrate)	Hypnotic, specified NEC	or sedative
Butylchloral hydrate	Lactuca (virosa) (extract)	Tribromacetaldehyde
Calcium bromide	Lactucarium	Tribromomethane
Calcium bromolactobionate	Lettuce opium	Trichloroethanol
Carbamate (sedative)	Levanil	Trichloroethyl phosphate
Carbromal	Levoprome	Triclofos
Central nervous system	Meparfynol	Trional
depressants, bromides	Methaqualone (compound)	Triple bromides
Central nervous system	Methyl parafynol	Valerian root
depressants, chloral	Methyl sulfonal	Valerian tincture
hydrate	Methylparafynol	Valmid
Central nervous system	Methylpentynol,	Valnoctamide
depressants, hypnotics,	methylpenthynol	Valproate (sodium)
specified NEC	Methyprylon	Valproic acid
Central nervous system	Niaprazine	Valpromide
depressants,	Noctec	Vigabatrin
paraldehyde	Noludar	Welldorm
Central nervous system	Paracetaldehyde	Zolpidem
depressants, sedatives	Paraldehyde	Zopiclone
sedative-hypnotics,	Pentaerythritol, chloral	
mixed NEC	Periclor	

T42.6x- Poisoning by, adverse effect of and underdosing of <u>other antiepileptic and sedative-hypnotic drugs</u>

T42.6x1- Poisoning by other antiepileptic and sedative-hypnotic drugs, <u>accidental</u> (unintentional)
    Poisoning by other antiepileptic and sedative-hypnotic drugs NOS

T42.6x2- Poisoning by other antiepileptic and sedative-hypnotic drugs, <u>intentional</u> self-harm

T42.6x3- Poisoning by other antiepileptic and sedative-hypnotic drugs, <u>assault</u>

T42.6x4- Poisoning by other antiepileptic and sedative-hypnotic drugs, <u>undetermined</u>

T42.6x5- <u>Adverse effect</u> of other antiepileptic and sedative-hypnotic drugs

T42.6x6- <u>Underdosing</u> of other antiepileptic and sedative-hypnotic drugs

T42 - T42

T42.7-   Poisoning by, adverse effect of and underdosing of unspecified <u>antiepileptic and sedative-hypnotic drugs</u>

T42.7 - DRUGS/CHEMS*	Central nervous system depressants, sedatives	Hypnotic
Anticonvulsant	sedative-hypnotics	Hypnotic, anticonvulsant
Antiepilepsy agent	Depressant, central nervous	Sedative NEC
Central nervous system	system (anesthetic) —	Sleeping draught, pill
depressants	see also Central nervous	Soporific
Central nervous system	system, depressant	Soporific drug
depressants, hypnotics		

T42.71x-   Poisoning by unspecified antiepileptic and sedative-hypnotic drugs, <u>accidental</u> (unintentional)
Poisoning by antiepileptic and sedative-hypnotic drugs NOS

T42.72x-   Poisoning by unspecified antiepileptic and sedative-hypnotic drugs, <u>intentional</u> self-harm

T42.73x-   Poisoning by unspecified antiepileptic and sedative-hypnotic drugs, <u>assault</u>

T42.74x-   Poisoning by unspecified antiepileptic and sedative-hypnotic drugs, <u>undetermined</u>

T42.75x-   <u>Adverse effect</u> of unspecified antiepileptic and sedative-hypnotic drugs

T42.76x-   <u>Underdosing</u> of unspecified antiepileptic and sedative-hypnotic drugs

T42.8-   Poisoning by, adverse effect of and underdosing of antiparkinsonism drugs and other central muscle-tone depressants
Poisoning by, adverse effect of and underdosing of amantadine

T42.8 - DRUGS/CHEMS*	Deprenyl	Muscle affecting agents,
Afloqualone	Depressant, central nervous	relaxants, central
Amantadine	system, muscle tone	nervous system
Antiparkinsonism drug NEC	Depressant, muscle tone,	Muscle-tone depressant,
Antirigidity drug NEC	central	central NEC
Baclofen	Diethazine	Muscle-tone depressant,
Benserazide	Difluoromethyldopa	central, specified NEC
Benzatropine	Disipal	Orphenadrine
Benztropine, antiparkinson	Dopa	(hydrochloride)
Bromocriptine	Idrocilamide	Pergolide
Cabergoline	L-dopa	Phenprobamate
Carbidopa (with levodopa)	Levodopa	Piribedil
Carisoprodol	Levodopa with carbidopa	Rela
Central nervous system	Lisuride	Relaxant, muscle, central
depressants, muscle	Mephenamin(e)	nervous system
relaxants	Mephenesin	Selegiline
Central nervous system	Mephenoxalone	Soma
muscle-tone depressants	Mesulergine	Styramate
Chlorphenesin	Metaxalone	Tizanidine
Chlorzoxazone	Metergoline	Tolserol
Dantrolene	Methocarbamol	Zoxazolamine
Deprenalin		

T42.8x-   Poisoning by, adverse effect of and underdosing of <u>antiparkinsonism drugs and other central muscle-tone depressants</u>

T42.8x1-   Poisoning by antiparkinsonism drugs and other central muscle-tone depressants, <u>accidental</u> (unintentional)
Poisoning by antiparkinsonism drugs and other central muscle-tone depressants NOS

T42.8x2-   Poisoning by antiparkinsonism drugs and other central muscle-tone depressants, <u>intentional</u> self-harm

T42.8x3-   Poisoning by antiparkinsonism drugs and other central muscle-tone depressants, <u>assault</u>

T42.8x4-   Poisoning by antiparkinsonism drugs and other central muscle-tone depressants, <u>undetermined</u>

T42.8x5-   <u>Adverse effect</u> of antiparkinsonism drugs and other central muscle-tone depressants

T42.8x6-   <u>Underdosing</u> of antiparkinsonism drugs and other central muscle-tone depressants

T43-   Poisoning by, adverse effect of and underdosing of <u>psychotropic drugs</u>, not elsewhere classified
Excludes 1:   appetite depressants (T50.5-)
barbiturates (T42.3-)
benzodiazepines (T42.4-)
methaqualone (T42.6-)
psychodysleptics [hallucinogens] (T40.7-T40.9-)
Excludes ❷: drug dependence and related mental and behavioral disorders due to psychoactive substance use (F10.- -F19.-)

The appropriate 7th character is to be added to each code from category T43:
A   <u>Initial</u> encounter
D   <u>Subsequent</u> encounter
S   <u>Sequela</u>

T43.0-   Poisoning by, adverse effect of and underdosing of tricyclic and tetracyclic antidepressants

T43.01-   Poisoning by, adverse effect of and underdosing of <u>tricyclic antidepressants</u>

T43.01 - DRUGS/CHEMS*	Desmethylimipramine	Noxiptiline
Allegron	Dibenzepin	Opipramol
Amineptine	Dosulepin	Pertofrane
Amitriptyline	Dothiepin	Protriptyline
Amitriptylinoxide	Doxepin	Quinupramine
Amoxapine	Imipramine	Saroten
Antidepressant, tricyclic	Iprindole	Sinequan
Butriptyline	Laroxyl	Tofranil
Chlorimipramine	Lofepramine	Trimipramine
Cianopramine	Melitracen	Tryptizol
Clomipramine	Metapramine	
Desipramine	Nortriptyline	

T43.011-   Poisoning by tricyclic antidepressants, <u>accidental</u> (unintentional)
Poisoning by tricyclic antidepressants NOS

T43.012-   Poisoning by tricyclic antidepressants, <u>intentional</u> self-harm

T43.013-   Poisoning by tricyclic antidepressants, <u>assault</u>

T43.014-   Poisoning by tricyclic antidepressants, <u>undetermined</u>

T43.015-   <u>Adverse effect</u> of tricyclic antidepressants

T43.016-   <u>Underdosing</u> of tricyclic antidepressants

T43.02-   Poisoning by, adverse effect of and underdosing of <u>tetracyclic antidepressants</u>

T43.02 - DRUGS/CHEMS*	Maprotiline	Mirtazapine
Antidepressant, tetracyclic	Mianserin	Oxaprotiline

T43.021-   Poisoning by tetracyclic antidepressants, <u>accidental</u> (unintentional)
Poisoning by tetracyclic antidepressants NOS

T43.022-   Poisoning by tetracyclic antidepressants, <u>intentional</u> self-harm

T43.023-   Poisoning by tetracyclic antidepressants, <u>assault</u>

T43.024-   Poisoning by tetracyclic antidepressants, <u>undetermined</u>

T43.025-   <u>Adverse effect</u> of tetracyclic antidepressants

T43.026-   <u>Underdosing</u> of tetracyclic antidepressants

T43.1-   Poisoning by, adverse effect of and underdosing of monoamine-oxidase-inhibitor antidepressants

T43.1x-   Poisoning by, adverse effect of and underdosing of <u>monoamine-oxidase-inhibitor antidepressants</u>

T43.1 - DRUGS/CHEMS*	Inhibitor, monoamine	Monoamine oxidase
Amiflamine	oxidase, hydrazine	inhibitor NEC
Antidepressant,	Iproclozide	Monoamine oxidase
monoamine oxidase	Iproniazid	inhibitor, hydrazine
inhibitor	Isocarboxazid	Nardil
Clorgiline	MAO inhibitors	Nialamide
Hydrazine monoamine	Marplan	Parnate
oxidase inhibitors	Marsilid	Phenelzine
Inhibitor, monoamine	Mebanazine	Pheniprazine
oxidase NEC	Moclobemide	Safrazine
		Tranylcypromine

T42 • T43

T43.1x1- Poisoning by monoamine-oxidase-inhibitor antidepressants, <u>accidental</u> (unintentional)
Poisoning by monoamine-oxidase-inhibitor antidepressants NOS

T43.1x2- Poisoning by monoamine-oxidase-inhibitor antidepressants, <u>intentional</u> self-harm

T43.1x3- Poisoning by monoamine-oxidase-inhibitor antidepressants, <u>assault</u>

T43.1x4- Poisoning by monoamine-oxidase-inhibitor antidepressants, <u>undetermined</u>

T43.1x5- <u>Adverse effect</u> of monoamine-oxidase-inhibitor antidepressants

T43.1x6- <u>Underdosing</u> of monoamine-oxidase-inhibitor antidepressants

T43.2- Poisoning by, adverse effect of and underdosing of other and unspecified antidepressants

T43.20- Poisoning by, adverse effect of and underdosing of <u>unspecified antidepressants</u>

T43.20 - DRUGS/CHEMS*	
Antidepressant	Psychotherapeutic drug,
Central nervous system	antidepressants — see
stimulants,	also Antidepressant
antidepressants	

T43.201- Poisoning by unspecified antidepressants, <u>accidental</u> (unintentional)
Poisoning by antidepressants NOS

T43.202- Poisoning by unspecified antidepressants, <u>intentional</u> self-harm

T43.203- Poisoning by unspecified antidepressants, <u>assault</u>

T43.204- Poisoning by unspecified antidepressants, <u>undetermined</u>

T43.205- <u>Adverse effect</u> of unspecified antidepressants

T43.206- <u>Underdosing</u> of unspecified antidepressants

T43.21- Poisoning by, adverse effect of and underdosing of <u>selective serotonin and norepinephrinere uptake inhibitors</u>
Poisoning by, adverse effect of and underdosing of SSNRI antidepressants

T43.21 - DRUGS/CHEMS*	
Antidepressant, selective	Antidepressant,
serotonin	triazolopyridine
norepinephrine	Trazodone
reuptake inhibitor	Venlafaxine

T43.211- Poisoning by selective serotonin and norepinephrine reuptake inhibitors, <u>accidental</u> (unintentional)

T43.212- Poisoning by selective serotonin and norepinephrine reuptake inhibitors, <u>intentional</u> self-harm

T43.213- Poisoning by selective serotonin and norepinephrine reuptake inhibitors, <u>assault</u>

T43.214- Poisoning by selective serotonin and norepinephrine reuptake inhibitors, <u>undetermined</u>

T43.215- <u>Adverse effect</u> of selective serotonin and norepinephrine reuptake inhibitors

T43.216- <u>Underdosing</u> of selective serotonin and norepinephrine reuptake inhibitors

T43.22- Poisoning by, adverse effect of and underdosing of <u>selective serotonin reuptake inhibitors</u>
Poisoning by, adverse effect of and underdosing of SSRI antidepressants

T43.22 - DRUGS/CHEMS*		
Antidepressant, selective	Citalopram	Indalpine
serotonin reuptake	Femoxetine	Prozac
inhibitor	Fluoxetine	Zimeldine
	Fluvoxamine	

T43.221- Poisoning by selective serotonin reuptake inhibitors, <u>accidental</u> (unintentional)

T43.222- Poisoning by selective serotonin reuptake inhibitors, <u>intentional</u> self-harm

T43.223- Poisoning by selective serotonin reuptake inhibitors, <u>assault</u>

T43.224- Poisoning by selective serotonin reuptake inhibitors, <u>undetermined</u>

T43.225- <u>Adverse effect</u> of selective serotonin reuptake inhibitors

T43.226- <u>Underdosing</u> of selective serotonin reuptake inhibitors

T43.29- Poisoning by, adverse effect of and underdosing of <u>other antidepressants</u>

T43.29 - DRUGS/CHEMS*		
Amfebutamone	Bupropion	Prazitone
Antidepressant, specified	Diclofensine	Thiazesim
NEC	Minaprine	Tianeptine
Bifemelane	Nomifensine	Viloxazine
	Oxitriptan	

T43.291- Poisoning by other antidepressants, <u>accidental</u> (unIntentional)
Poisoning by other antidepressants NOS

T43.292- Poisoning by other antidepressants, <u>intentional</u> self-harm

T43.293- Poisoning by other antidepressants, <u>assault</u>

T43.294- Poisoning by other antidepressants, <u>undetermined</u>

T43.295- <u>Adverse effect</u> of other antidepressants

T43.296- <u>Underdosing</u> of other antidepressants

T43.3- Poisoning by, adverse effect of and underdosing of phenothiazine antipsychotics and neuroleptics

T43.3 - DRUGS/CHEMS*		
Acepromazine	Mequitazine	Stemetil
Acetophenazine	Mesoridazine	Sulforidazine
Alimemazine	Methdilazine	Thiazinamium metilsulfate
Butaperazine	Methopromazine	Thiethylperazine
Carfenazine	Methotrimeprazine	Thiopropazate
Carphenazine	Methoxypromazine	Thioproperazine
Chlorpromazine	Metofenazate	Thioridazine
Compazine	Oxomemazine	Thorazine
Cyamemazine	Pecazine	Tindal
Dimetotiazine	Perazine	Tranquilizer,
Dioxopromethazine	Periciazine	dimethylamine
Dixyrazine	Perphenazine	Tranquilizer, ethylamine
Ethyl aminophenothiazine	Phenothiazine	Tranquilizer, penothiazine
Fentazin	(psychotropic) NEC	NEC
Fluopromazine	Piperacetazine	Tranquilizer,
Fluphenazine	Pipotiazine	phenothiazine-based
Isopromethazine	Plegicil	Tranquilizer, piperazine
Largactil	Prochlorperazine	NEC
Levomepromazine	Promazine	Tranquilizer, piperidine
Levopromazine	Promethazine (teoclate)	Tranquilizer, propylamine
Mellaril	Propylaminophenothiazine	Trifluoperazine
Mepazine	Sparine	Triflupromazine
	Stelazine	

T43.3x- Poisoning by, adverse effect of and underdosing of <u>phenothiazine antipsychotics and neuroleptics</u>

T43.3x1- Poisoning by phenothiazine antipsychotics and neuroleptics, <u>accidental</u> (unintentional)
Poisoning by phenothiazine antipsychotics and neuroleptics NOS

T43.3x2- Poisoning by phenothiazine antipsychotics and neuroleptics, <u>intentional</u> self-harm

T43.3x3- Poisoning by phenothiazine antipsychotics and neuroleptics, <u>assault</u>

T43.3x4- Poisoning by phenothiazine antipsychotics and neuroleptics, <u>undetermined</u>

T43.3x5- <u>Adverse effect</u> of phenothiazine antipsychotics and neuroleptics

T43.3x6- <u>Underdosing</u> of phenothiazine antipsychotics and neuroleptics

T43 - T43

© 2016 Channel Publishing, Ltd.

T43.4- Poisoning by, adverse effect of and underdosing of butyrophenone and thiothixene neuroleptics

T43.4 - DRUGS/CHEMS*	Flupentixol	Thiothixene
Benperidol	Haloperidol	Timiperone
Bromperidol	Lenperone	Tiotixene
Butyrophenone (-based	Melperone	Tranquilizer,
tranquilizers)	Methyl peridol	butyrophenone NEC
Chlorprothixene	Moperone	Trifluperidol
Clopenthixol	Pipamperone	Triperidol
Fluanisone	Spiperone	Zuclopenthixol
Flupentixol	Spiroperidol	

T43.4x- Poisoning by, adverse effect of and underdosing of butyrophenone and thiothixene neuroleptics

T43.4x1- Poisoning by butyrophenone and thiothixene neuroleptics, accidental (unintentional)
Poisoning by butyrophenone and thiothixene neuroleptics NOS

T43.4x2- Poisoning by butyrophenone and thiothixene neuroleptics, intentional self-harm

T43.4x3- Poisoning by butyrophenone and thiothixene neuroleptics, assault

T43.4x4- Poisoning by butyrophenone and thiothixene neuroleptics, undetermined

T43.4x5- Adverse effect of butyrophenone and thiothixene neuroleptics

T43.4x6- Underdosing of butyrophenone and thiothixene neuroleptics

T43.5- Poisoning by, adverse effect of and underdosing of other and unspecified antipsychotics and neuroleptics
Excludes 1: *poisoning by, adverse effect of and underdosing of rauwolfia (T46.5-)*

T43.50- Poisoning by, adverse effect of and underdosing of unspecified antipsychotics and neuroleptics

T43.50 - DRUGS/CHEMS*	Depressant,	Tranquilizer NEC
Antianxiety drug NEC	psychotherapeutic	Tranquilizer, major NEC
Antihallucinogen	Neuroleptic drug NEC	
Antipsychotic drug	Psychotherapeutic drug,	
Ataractic drug NEC	tranquilizers NEC	

T43.501- Poisoning by unspecified antipsychotics and neuroleptics, accidental (unintentional)
Poisoning by antipsychotics and neuroleptics NOS

T43.502- Poisoning by unspecified antipsychotics and neuroleptics, intentional self-harm

T43.503- Poisoning by unspecified antipsychotics and neuroleptics, assault

T43.504- Poisoning by unspecified antipsychotics and neuroleptics, undetermined

T43.505- Adverse effect of unspecified antipsychotics and neuroleptics

T43.506- Underdosing of unspecified antipsychotics and neuroleptics

T43.59- Poisoning by, adverse effect of and underdosing of other antipsychotics and neuroleptics

T43.59 - DRUGS/CHEMS*	Hydroxyzine	Raclopride
Aminophenylpyridone	Lithium gluconate	Remoxipride
Amisulpride	Lithium salts (carbonate)	Setoperone
Amperozide	Loxapine	Spirilene
Amphenidone	Mebutamate	Sulpiride
Antipsychotic drug,	Meprobam	Sultopride
specified NEC	Meprobamate	Taractan
Azacyclonol	Miltown	Tetrabenazine
Benzperidin	Molindone	Tiapride
Benzperidol	Mosapramine	Tranquilizer, carbamate
Buspirone	Nemonapride	Tranquilizer, hydroxyzine
Captodiame, captodiamine	Olanzapine	Tranquilizer, specified NEC
Clotiapine	Oxanamide	Tranquilizer, thioxanthene
Droperidol	Oxypertine	NEC
Emylcamate	Penfluridol	Tybamate
Enpiprazole	Phenaglycodol	Zotepine
Equanil	Pimozide	Zyprexa
Fluspirilene	Procalmidol	
Hydroxyphenamate	Prothipendyl	

T43.591- Poisoning by other antipsychotics and neuroleptics, accidental (unintentional)
Poisoning by other antipsychotics and neuroleptics NOS

T43.592- Poisoning by other antipsychotics and neuroleptics, intentional self-harm

T43.593- Poisoning by other antipsychotics and neuroleptics, assault

T43.594- Poisoning by other antipsychotics and neuroleptics, undetermined

T43.595- Adverse effect of other antipsychotics and neuroleptics

T43.596- Underdosing of other antipsychotics and neuroleptics

T43.6- Poisoning by, adverse effect of and underdosing of psychostimulants
Excludes 1: *poisoning by, adverse effect of and underdosing of cocaine (T40.5-)*

T43.60- Poisoning by, adverse effect of and underdosing of unspecified psychostimulant

T43.60 - DRUGS/CHEMS*	Psychostimulant	Stimulant, central nervous
Central nervous system	Stimulant, central nervous	system,
stimulants	system — see also	psychotherapeutic NEC —
Cerebral stimulants	Psychostimulant	see also
Cerebral stimulants,		Psychotherapeutic drug
psychotherapeutic		

T43.601- Poisoning by unspecified psychostimulants, accidental (unintentional)
Poisoning by psychostimulants NOS

T43.602- Poisoning by unspecified psychostimulants, intentional self-harm

T43.603- Poisoning by unspecified psychostimulants, assault

T43.604- Poisoning by unspecified psychostimulants, undetermined

T43.605- Adverse effect of unspecified psychostimulants

T43.606- Underdosing of unspecified psychostimulants

T43.61- Poisoning by, adverse effect of and underdosing of caffeine

T43.61 - DRUGS/CHEMS*	Psychostimulant, caffeine
Caffeine	

T43.611- Poisoning by caffeine, accidental (unintentional)
Poisoning by caffeine NOS

T43.612- Poisoning by caffeine, intentional self-harm

T43.613- Poisoning by caffeine, assault

T43.614- Poisoning by caffeine, undetermined

T43.615- Adverse effect of caffeine

T43.616- Underdosing of caffeine

T43 - T43

T43.62- Poisoning by, adverse effect of and underdosing of <u>amphetamines</u>
Poisoning by, adverse effect of and underdosing of methamphetamines

T43.62 - DRUGS/CHEMS*	Dexamphetamine	Methylenedioxyamphetamine
Amfetamine	Dexedrine	
Amfetaminil	Dextroamphetamine	Methylenedioxymethamphetamine
Amphetamine NEC	Ecstasy	tamine
Benzedrine (amphetamine)	MDMA	Psychostimulant,
Central nervous system	Metamfetamine	amphetamine
stimulants,	Methamphetamine	Speed
amphetamines	Methedrine	Tenamfetamine
Desoxyephedrine	Methyl amphetamine	
Dexamfetamine	Methylamphetamine	

   T43.621- Poisoning by amphetamines, <u>accidental</u> (unintentional)
      Poisoning by amphetamines NOS

   T43.622- Poisoning by amphetamines, <u>intentional</u> self-harm

   T43.623- Poisoning by amphetamines, <u>assault</u>

   T43.624- Poisoning by amphetamines, <u>undetermined</u>

   T43.625- <u>Adverse effect</u> of amphetamines

   T43.626- <u>Underdosing</u> of amphetamines

T43.63- Poisoning by, adverse effect of and underdosing of <u>methylphenidate</u>

T43.63 - DRUGS/CHEMS*	Psychostimulant,
Methyl phenidate	methylphenidate
Methylphenidate	Ritalin

   T43.631- Poisoning by methylphenidate, <u>accidental</u> (unintentional)
      Poisoning by methylphenidate NOS

   T43.632- Poisoning by methylphenidate, <u>intentional</u> self-harm

   T43.633- Poisoning by methylphenidate, <u>assault</u>

   T43.634- Poisoning by methylphenidate, <u>undetermined</u>

   T43.635- <u>Adverse effect</u> of methylphenidate

   T43.636- <u>Underdosing</u> of methylphenidate

T43.69- Poisoning by, adverse effect of and underdosing of <u>other psychostimulants</u>

T43.69 - DRUGS/CHEMS*	Etryptamine	Preludin
Catha (edulis) (tea)	Fencamfamine	Prolintane
Central nervous system	Fenetylline	Psychostimulant, specified
stimulants, specified NEC	Khat	NEC
Cerebral stimulants,	Meclofenoxate	Stimulant, central nervous
specified NEC	Pipradrol	system, specified NEC

   T43.691- Poisoning by other psychostimulants, <u>accidental</u> (unintentional)
      Poisoning by other psychostimulants NOS

   T43.692- Poisoning by other psychostimulants, <u>intentional</u> self-harm

   T43.693- Poisoning by other psychostimulants, <u>assault</u>

   T43.694- Poisoning by other psychostimulants, <u>undetermined</u>

   T43.695- <u>Adverse effect</u> of other psychostimulants

   T43.696- <u>Underdosing</u> of other psychostimulants

T43.8- Poisoning by, adverse effect of and underdosing of other psychotropic drugs

T43.8 - DRUGS/CHEMS*	Inhibitor, postsynaptic	Nizofenone
4-Aminobutyric acid	Lithane	Psychotherapeutic drug,
Eskalith	Lithonate	specified NEC
GABA	Memantine	Psychotropic drug, specified
Gamma-aminobutyric acid	Namenda	NEC

  T43.8x- Poisoning by, adverse effect of and underdosing of <u>other psychotropic drugs</u>

   T43.8x1- Poisoning by other psychotropic drugs, <u>accidental</u> (unintentional)
      Poisoning by other psychotropic drugs NOS

   T43.8x2- Poisoning by other psychotropic drugs, <u>intentional</u> self-harm

   T43.8x3- Poisoning by other psychotropic drugs, <u>assault</u>

   T43.8x4- Poisoning by other psychotropic drugs, <u>undetermined</u>

   T43.8x5- <u>Adverse effect</u> of other psychotropic drugs

   T43.8x6- <u>Underdosing</u> of other psychotropic drugs

T43.9- Poisoning by, adverse effect of and underdosing of <u>unspecified psychotropic drug</u>

T43.9 - DRUGS/CHEMS*	Psychotherapeutic drug	Psychotropic drug NEC
	NEC	

  T43.91x- Poisoning by unspecified psychotropic drug, <u>accidental</u> (unintentional)
     Poisoning by psychotropic drug NOS

  T43.92x- Poisoning by unspecified psychotropic drug, <u>intentional</u> self-harm

  T43.93x- Poisoning by unspecified psychotropic drug, <u>assault</u>

  T43.94x- Poisoning by unspecified psychotropic drug, <u>undetermined</u>

  T43.95x- <u>Adverse effect</u> of unspecified psychotropic drug

  T43.96x- <u>Underdosing</u> of unspecified psychotropic drug

T44- Poisoning by, adverse effect of and underdosing of <u>drugs primarily affecting the autonomic nervous system</u>

The appropriate 7th character is to be added to each code from category T44:
  A   <u>Initial</u> encounter
  D   <u>Subsequent</u> encounter
  S   <u>Sequela</u>

T44.0- Poisoning by, adverse effect of and underdosing of anticholinesterase agents

T44.0 - DRUGS/CHEMS*	DFP	Galantamine
Ambenonium (chloride)	Diflos	Isoflurophate
Anticholinesterase	Difluorophate	Neomycin with neostigmine
Anticholinesterase,	Diisopropylfluorophos	Neostigmine bromide
organophosphorus	phonate	Prostigmin
Anticholinesterase,	Distigmine (bromide)	Pyridostigmine bromide
reversible	Dyflos	Tacrine
Cholinergic	Edrophonium	Tetrahydroaminoacridine
organophosphorus	Edrophonium chloride	

  T44.0x- Poisoning by, adverse effect of and underdosing of <u>anticholinesterase agents</u>

   T44.0x1- Poisoning by anticholinesterase agents, <u>accidental</u> (unintentional)
      Poisoning by anticholinesterase agents NOS

   T44.0x2- Poisoning by anticholinesterase agents, <u>intentional</u> self-harm

   T44.0x3- Poisoning by anticholinesterase agents, <u>assault</u>

   T44.0x4- Poisoning by anticholinesterase agents, <u>undetermined</u>

   T44.0x5- <u>Adverse effect</u> of anticholinesterase agents

   T44.0x6- <u>Underdosing</u> of anticholinesterase agents

T44.1- Poisoning by, adverse effect of and underdosing of other parasympathomimetics [cholinergics]

T44.1 - DRUGS/CHEMS*	Carbachol	Parasympathomimetic drug
Aceclidine	Carbamylcholine chloride	NEC
Acetylcholine (chloride)	Cholinergic (drug) NEC	Pilocarpine
(derivative)	Cholinergic muscle tone	Pilocarpus (jaborandi)
Arecoline	enhancer	extract
Benzpyrinium bromide	Cholinergic trimethyl	
Bethanechol	ammonium propanediol	
Bethanechol chloride	Methacholine	

  T44.1x- Poisoning by, adverse effect of and underdosing of <u>other parasympathomimetics [cholinergics]</u>

   T44.1x1- Poisoning by other parasympathomimetics [cholinergics], <u>accidental</u> (unintentional)
      Poisoning by other parasympathomimetics [cholinergics] NOS

   T44.1x2- Poisoning by other parasympathomimetics [cholinergics], <u>intentional</u> self-harm

---

Excludes 1: = NOT CODED HERE! (Do not code both)

Excludes ❷: = Not Included Here

T43 - T44

T44.1x3- Poisoning by other parasympathomimetics [cholinergics], <u>assault</u>

T44.1x4- Poisoning by other parasympathomimetics [cholinergics], <u>undetermined</u>

T44.1x5- <u>Adverse effect</u> of other parasympathomimetics [cholinergics]

T44.1x6- <u>Underdosing</u> of other parasympathomimetics

T44.2- Poisoning by, adverse effect of and underdosing of ganglionic blocking drugs

T44.2 - DRUGS/CHEMS*		
Ganglionic blocking drug NEC	Pempidine	Tetraethylammonium chloride
Ganglionic blocking drug, specified NEC	Pentamethonium bromide	Tetrylammonium chloride
	Pentapyrrolinium (bitartrate)	Trimetaphan camsilate
Hexamethonium bromide	Pentolonium tartrate	Trimethaphan
Mecamylamine	Quarternary ammonium, ganglion blocking	Trimethidinium

T44.2x- Poisoning by, adverse effect of and underdosing of <u>ganglionic blocking drugs</u>

T44.2x1- Poisoning by ganglionic blocking drugs, <u>accidental</u> (unintentional)
Poisoning by ganglionic blocking drugs NOS

T44.2x2- Poisoning by ganglionic blocking drugs, <u>intentional</u> self-harm

T44.2x3- Poisoning by ganglionic blocking drugs, <u>assault</u>

T44.2x4- Poisoning by ganglionic blocking drugs, <u>undetermined</u>

T44.2x5- <u>Adverse effect</u> of ganglionic blocking drugs

T44.2x6- <u>Underdosing</u> of ganglionic blocking drugs

T44.3- Poisoning by, adverse effect of and underdosing of other parasympatholytics [anticholinergics and antimuscarinics] and spasmolytics
Poisoning by, adverse effect of and underdosing of papaverine

T44.3 - DRUGS/CHEMS*		
Adiphenine	Dibutoline sulfate	Methantheline
Alverine	Dicyclomine	Methanthelinium bromide
Ambutonium bromide	Dicycloverine	Methixene
Aminopentamide	Diisopromine	Methscopolamine bromide
Amprotropine	Diphemanil	Methyl atropine
Aniscoropine	Diphemanil metilsulfate	Methylatropine nitrate
Anisotropine methylbromide	Drotaverine	Methylbenactyzium bromide
	Duboisine	
Antagonist, extrapyramidal NEC	Dyphylline	Metixene
	Emepronium (salts)	Milverine
Anticholinergic NEC	Emepronium bromide	Moxaverine
Antimuscarinic NEC	Ethaverine	Muscle affecting agents, relaxants, smooth
Artane	Ethopropazine	
Atropine	Etomidoline	Mydriacyl
Atropine derivative	Etybenzatropine	Octatropine methyl bromide
Atropine methonitrate	Euphthalmine	
Belladonna alkaloids	Extrapyramidal antagonist NEC	Otilonium bromide
Belladonna extract	Fenoverine	Oxapium iodide
Belladonna herb	Flavoxate	Oxybutynin
Benactyzine	Flopropione	Oxyphencyclimine
Benaprizine	Gefarnate	Oxyphenonium bromide
Benzhexol	Glycopyrrolate	Papaverine
Benzilonium bromide	Glycopyrronium	Parasympatholytic NEC
Benztropine, anticholinergic	Glycopyrronium bromide	Penthienate bromide
	Hexasonium iodide	Phenglutarimide
Bevonium metilsulfate	Hexocyclium	Pinaverium bromide
Biperiden	Hexocyclium metilsulfate	Pipenzolate bromide
Bornaprine	Homatropine	Piperidolate
Butethamate	Homatropine methylbromide	Pipethanate
Butropium bromide		Poldine metilsulfate
Butyl scopolamine bromide	Hyoscine	Pramiverine
Camylofin	Hyoscyamine	Pridinol
Caramiphen	Hyoscyamus	Prifinium bromide
Carpronium chloride	Hyoscyamus, dry extract	Pro-Banthine
Chlorbenzoxamine	Isometheptene	Procyclidine
Cimetropium bromide	Isopropamide	Profenamine
Clidinium bromide	Isopropamide iodide	Profenil
Clorotepine	Levsin	Propantheline
Cogentin	Mebeverine	Propantheline bromide
Cyclodrine	Meladrazine	Quarternary ammonium, parasympatholytic
Cyclopentolate	Mepenzolate	
Cycrimine	Mepenzolate bromide	Relaxant, muscle, smooth NEC
Dexetimide	Mepiperphenidol	Rociverine

T44.3 - DRUGS/CHEMS* — Continued		
	Tiemonium	Trimebutine
Scopolamine	Tiemonium, iodide	Trimeprazine (tartrate)
Scopolia extract	Tifenamil	Triperiden
Smooth muscle relaxant	Tigloidine	Trithiozine
Spacoline	Timepidium bromide	Tritiozine
Spasmolytic, anticholinergics	Tiquizium bromide	Tropacine
	Tolperisone	Tropatepine
Spasmolytic, autonomic	Toquizine	Tropicamide
Spasmolytic, quaternary ammonium	Trasentine	Trospium chloride
	Triampyzine	Valethamate bromide
Sulmetozine	Tricyclamol chloride	
Thiphenamil	Tridihexethyl iodide	
	Trihexyphenidyl	

T44.3x- Poisoning by, adverse effect of and underdosing of <u>other parasympatholytics [anticholinergics and antimuscarinics] and spasmolytics</u>

T44.3x1- Poisoning by other parasympatholytics [anticholinergics and antimuscarinics] and spasmolytics, <u>accidental</u> (unintentional)
Poisoning by other parasympatholytics [anticholinergics and antimuscarinics] and spasmolytics NOS

T44.3x2- Poisoning by other parasympatholytics [anticholinergics and antimuscarinics] and spasmolytics, <u>intentional</u> self-harm

T44.3x3- Poisoning by other parasympatholytics [anticholinergics and antimuscarinics] and spasmolytics, <u>assault</u>

T44.3x4- Poisoning by other parasympatholytics [anticholinergics and antimuscarinics] and spasmolytics, <u>undetermined</u>

T44.3x5- <u>Adverse effect</u> of other parasympatholytics [anticholinergics and antimuscarinics] and spasmolytics

T44.3x6- <u>Underdosing</u> of other parasympatholytics [anticholinergics and antimuscarinics] and spasmolytics

T44.4- Poisoning by, adverse effect of and underdosing of predominantly alpha-adrenoreceptor agonists
Poisoning by, adverse effect of and underdosing of metaraminol

T44.4 - DRUGS/CHEMS*		
Agonist, predominantly alpha-adrenoreceptor	Etilefrine	Norfenefrine
	Gepefrine	Oxedrine
Aplonidine	Levarterenol	Paredrine
Apraclonidine (hydrochloride)	Metaraminol	Phenylephrine
	Methoxamine	Privine
Cyclopentamine	Noradrenaline	Propyl hexadrine
	Norepinephrine	

T44.4x- Poisoning by, adverse effect of and underdosing of <u>predominantly alpha-adrenoreceptor agonists</u>

T44.4x1- Poisoning by predominantly alpha-adrenoreceptor agonists, <u>accidental</u> (unintentional)
Poisoning by predominantly alpha-adrenoreceptor agonists NOS

T44.4x2- Poisoning by predominantly alpha-adrenoreceptor agonists, <u>intentional</u> self-harm

T44.4x3- Poisoning by predominantly alpha-adrenoreceptor agonists, <u>assault</u>

T44.4x4- Poisoning by predominantly alpha-adrenoreceptor agonists, <u>undetermined</u>

T44.4x5- <u>Adverse effect</u> of predominantly alpha-adrenoreceptor agonists

T44.4x6- <u>Underdosing</u> of predominantly alpha-adrenoreceptor agonists

T44 - T44

Excludes 1: = NOT CODED HERE! (Do not code both)   **1175**   *Excludes ❷:* = Not Included Here

T44.5- **Poisoning by, adverse effect of and underdosing of predominantly beta-adrenoreceptor agonists**

> Excludes 1: *poisoning by, adverse effect of and underdosing of beta-adrenoreceptor agonists used in asthmatherapy (T48.6-)*

T44.5 - DRUGS/CHEMS*	Beclomethasone	Procaterol
Adrenalin	Budesonide	Racepinefrin
Adrenaline	Dobutamine	Ritodrine
Agonist, predominantly	Epinephrine	Xamoterol
beta-adrenoreceptor	Isoetharine	
Angiotensin	Prenalterol	

T44.5x- **Poisoning by, adverse effect of and underdosing of <u>predominantly beta-adrenoreceptor agonists</u>**

T44.5x1- **Poisoning by predominantly beta-adrenoreceptor agonists, <u>accidental</u> (unintentional)**
> Poisoning by predominantly beta-adrenoreceptor agonists NOS

T44.5x2- **Poisoning by predominantly beta-adrenoreceptor agonists, <u>intentional</u> self-harm**

T44.5x3- **Poisoning by predominantly beta-adrenoreceptor agonists, <u>assault</u>**

T44.5x4- **Poisoning by predominantly beta-adrenoreceptor agonists, <u>undetermined</u>**

T44.5x5- **<u>Adverse effect</u> of predominantly beta-adrenoreceptor agonists**

T44.5x6- **<u>Underdosing</u> of predominantly beta-adrenoreceptor agonists**

T44.6- **Poisoning by, adverse effect of and underdosing of alpha-adrenoreceptor antagonists**

> Excludes 1: *poisoning by, adverse effect of and underdosing of ergot alkaloids (T48.0)*

T44.6 - DRUGS/CHEMS*	Dibenamine	Prazosin
Alpha adrenergic blocking	Dibenzyline	Priscol, Priscoline
drug	Doxazosin	Tamsulosin
Antagonist, alpha-	Flomax	Terazosin
adrenoreceptor	Hydergine	
Bunazosin	Indoramin	

T44.6x- **Poisoning by, adverse effect of and underdosing of <u>alpha-adrenoreceptor antagonists</u>**

T44.6x1- **Poisoning by alpha-adrenoreceptor antagonists, <u>accidental</u> (unintentional)**
> Poisoning by alpha-adrenoreceptor antagonists NOS

T44.6x2- **Poisoning by alpha-adrenoreceptor antagonists, <u>intentional</u> self-harm**

T44.6x3- **Poisoning by alpha-adrenoreceptor antagonists, <u>assault</u>**

T44.6x4- **Poisoning by alpha-adrenoreceptor antagonists, <u>undetermined</u>**

T44.6x5- **<u>Adverse effect</u> of alpha-adrenoreceptor antagonists**

T44.6x6- **<u>Underdosing</u> of alpha-adrenoreceptor antagonists**

T44.7- **Poisoning by, adverse effect of and underdosing of beta-adrenoreceptor antagonists**

T44.7 - DRUGS/CHEMS*	Bisoprolol	Nadolol
Acebutolol	Bopindolol	Oxprenolol
Adrenergic, blocking agent	Bunitrolol	Penbutolol
NEC, beta, heart	Bupranolol	Pindolol
Alprenolol	Carazolol	Practolol
Antagonist, beta-	Carteolol	Pronetalol
adrenoreceptor	Celiprolol	Propranolol
Atenolol	Esmolol	Sotalol
Beta adrenergic blocking	Indenolol	Tertatolol
agent, heart	Inderal	Timolol
Betaxolol	Mepindolol	Tolamolol
Bevantolol	Metoprolol	

T44.7x- **Poisoning by, adverse effect of and underdosing of <u>beta-adrenoreceptor antagonists</u>**

T44.7x1- **Poisoning by beta-adrenoreceptor antagonists, <u>accidental</u> (unintentional)**
> Poisoning by beta-adrenoreceptor antagonists NOS

T44.7x2- **Poisoning by beta-adrenoreceptor antagonists, <u>intentional</u> self-harm**

T44.7x3- **Poisoning by beta-adrenoreceptor antagonists, <u>assault</u>**

T44.7x4- **Poisoning by beta-adrenoreceptor antagonists, <u>undetermined</u>**

T44.7x5- **<u>Adverse effect</u> of beta-adrenoreceptor antagonists**

T44.7x6- **<u>Underdosing</u> of beta-adrenoreceptor antagonists**

T44.8- **Poisoning by, adverse effect of and underdosing of centrally-acting and adrenergic-neuron-blocking agents**

> Excludes 1: *poisoning by, adverse effect of and underdosing of clonidine (T46.5)*
> *poisoning by, adverse effect of and underdosing of guanethidine (T46.5)*

T44.8 - DRUGS/CHEMS*	Antiadrenergic NEC	Sympatholytic,
Adrenergic, blocking agent	Labetalol	haloalkylamine
NEC	Medroxalol	
Alfuzosin (hydrochloride)	Sympatholytic NEC	

T44.8x- **Poisoning by, adverse effect of and underdosing of <u>centrally-acting and adrenergic-neuron-blocking agents</u>**

T44.8x1- **Poisoning by centrally-acting and adrenergic-neuron-blocking agents, <u>accidental</u> (unintentional)**
> Poisoning by centrally-acting and adrenergic-neuron-blocking agents NOS

T44.8x2- **Poisoning by centrally-acting and adrenergic-neuron-blocking agents, <u>intentional</u> self-harm**

T44.8x3- **Poisoning by centrally-acting and adrenergic-neuron-blocking agents, <u>assault</u>**

T44.8x4- **Poisoning by centrally-acting and adrenergic-neuron-blocking agents, <u>undetermined</u>**

T44.8x5- **<u>Adverse effect</u> of centrally-acting and adrenergic-neuron-blocking agents**

T44.8x6- **<u>Underdosing</u> of centrally-acting and adrenergic-neuron-blocking agents**

T44.9- **Poisoning by, adverse effect of and underdosing of other and unspecified drugs primarily affecting the autonomic nervous system**
> Poisoning by, adverse effect of and underdosing of drug stimulating both alpha and beta-adrenoreceptors

T44.90- **Poisoning by, adverse effect of and underdosing of <u>unspecified drugs primarily affecting the autonomic nervous system</u>**

T44.90 - DRUGS/CHEMS*	Autonomic nervous system	Sympathomimetic NEC
Adrenergic NEC	agent NEC	

T44.901- **Poisoning by unspecified drugs primarily affecting the autonomic nervous system, <u>accidental</u> (unintentional)**
> Poisoning by unspecified drugs primarily affecting the autonomic nervous system NOS

T44.902- **Poisoning by unspecified drugs primarily affecting the autonomic nervous system, <u>intentional</u> self-harm**

T44.903- **Poisoning by unspecified drugs primarily affecting the autonomic nervous system, <u>assault</u>**

T44.904- **Poisoning by unspecified drugs primarily affecting the autonomic nervous system, <u>undetermined</u>**

T44.905- **<u>Adverse effect</u> of unspecified drugs primarily affecting the autonomic nervous system**

T44.906- **<u>Underdosing</u> of unspecified drugs primarily affecting the autonomic nervous system**

T44.99- **Poisoning by, adverse effect of and underdosing of <u>other drugs primarily affecting the autonomic nervous system</u>**

T44.99 - DRUGS/CHEMS*	Dopamine	Mephentermine
Adrenergic, specified NEC	Ephedra	Phenylpropanolamine
Amezinium metilsulfate	Ephedrine	Pseudoephedrine
Angiotensinamide	Ibopamine	Sympathomimetic, specified
Benzedrex	Isoephedrine	NEC

T44.991- **Poisoning by other drug primarily affecting the autonomic nervous system, <u>accidental</u> (unintentional)**
> Poisoning by other drugs primarily affecting the autonomic nervous system NOS

T44 - T44

T44.992- Poisoning by other drug primarily affecting the autonomic nervous system, <u>intentional</u> self-harm

T44.993- Poisoning by other drug primarily affecting the autonomic nervous system, <u>assault</u>

T44.994- Poisoning by other drug primarily affecting the autonomic nervous system, <u>undetermined</u>

T44.995- <u>Adverse effect</u> of other drug primarily affecting the autonomic nervous system

T44.996- <u>Underdosing</u> of other drug primarily affecting the autonomic nervous system

T45- Poisoning by, adverse effect of and underdosing of <u>primarily systemic and hematological agents</u>, <u>not elsewhere classified</u>

The appropriate 7th character is to be added to each code from category T45:

A <u>Initial</u> encounter
D <u>Subsequent</u> encounter
S <u>Sequela</u>

T45.0- Poisoning by, adverse effect of and underdosing of antiallergic and antiemetic drugs

Excludes 1: poisoning by, adverse effect of and underdosing of phenothiazine-based neuroleptics (T43.3)

T45.0 - DRUGS/CHEMS*		
Acrivastine	Cinnarizine	Methaphenilene
Alizapride	Clemastine	Methapyrilene
Antazolin(e)	Clemizole	Metoclopramide
Antiallergic NEC	Clorfenamine	Moxastine
Antiemetic drug	Cyclizine	Nytol
Antihistamine	Cyproheptadine	Ondansetron
Antinausea drug	Deptropine	Oxatomide
Antistine	Dexbrompheniramine	Percogesic – see also
Antivertigo drug	Dexchlorpheniramine	Acetaminophen
Astemizole	Dibenzheptropine	Periactin
Azatadine	Difenidol	Phenindamine
Azelastine	Dimenhydrinate	Pheniramine
Bamipine	Dimetane	Phenyltoloxamine
Benadryl	Dimethindene	Pimethixene
Benzhydramine (chloride)	Dimetindene	Pipamazine
Benzquinamide	Diphenhydramine	Pipoxizine
Bisulepin (hydrochloride)	Diphenidol	Piprinhydrinate
Bonine	Diphenylpyraline	Propiomazine
Bromazlne	Domperidone	Pyrathiazine
Bromodiphenhydramine	Doxylamine	Pyribenzamine
Brompheniramine	Dramamine	Pyrilamine
Buclizine	Embramine	Pyrrobutamine
Carbinoxamine	Granisetron	Rotoxamine
Cerium oxalate	Homochlorcyclizine	Setastine
Cerous oxalate	Isothipendyl	Sleep-eze
Cetirizine	Ketotifen	Sominex
Cetoxime	Levocabastine	Terfenadine
Chlorcyclizine	(hydrochloride)	Thenyldiamine
Chloropyramine	Loratidine	Thonzylamine (systemic)
Chloropyrilene	Magnesium thiosulfate	Tigan
Chlorothen	Marezine	Tranilast
Chlorphenamine	Mebhydrolin	Trimethobenzamide
Chlorphenamine	Meclizine (hydrochloride)	Trimeton
Chlorpheniramine	Meclozine	Tripelennamine
Chlorphenoxamine	Mephenhydramine	Triprolidine
Chlor-Trimeton	Mepyramine	Tritoqualine

T45.0x- Poisoning by, adverse effect of and underdosing of <u>antiallergic and antiemetic drugs</u>

T45.0x1- Poisoning by antiallergic and antiemetic drugs, <u>accidental</u> (unintentional)
Poisoning by antiallergic and antiemetic drugs NOS

T45.0x2- Poisoning by antiallergic and antiemetic drugs, <u>intentional</u> self-harm

T45.0x3- Poisoning by antiallergic and antiemetic drugs, <u>assault</u>

T45.0x4- Poisoning by antiallergic and antiemetic drugs, <u>undetermined</u>

T45.0x5- <u>Adverse effect</u> of antiallergic and antiemetic drugs

T45.0x6- <u>Underdosing</u> of antiallergic and antiemetic drugs

T45.1- Poisoning by, adverse effect of and underdosing of antineoplastic and immunosuppressive drugs

Excludes 1: poisoning by, adverse effect of and underdosing of tamoxifen (T38.6)

T45.1 - DRUGS/CHEMS*		
Aclarubicin	2-Deoxy-5-fluorouridine	Myleran
Actinomycin C	5-Deoxy-5-fluorouridine	Nimustine
Actinomycin D	Dibromodulcitol	Nitrogen mustard
Adriamycin	Dibromomannitol	Olivomycin
Alkylating drug NEC	Doxifluridine	Oncovin
(antimyeloproliferative)	Doxorubicin	Paroxypropione
(lymphatic)	DTIC	Pentostatin
Altretamine	Elliptinium acetate	Peplomycin
Amethopterin	Enocitabine	Phenyl hydrazine,
Aminoglutethimide	Epirubicin	antineoplastic
Aminopterin sodium	Estramustine	Phenylalanine mustard
Amsacrine	Ethyl carbamate	Pipobroman
Antagonist, folic acid	Etoglucid	Pirarubicin
Antagonist, pyrimidine	Etoposide	Plicamycin
Anthramycin	FAC (fluorouracil +	Porfiromycin
Antibiotic, anticancer	doxorubicin	Prednimustine
Antibiotic, antineoplastic	+ cyclophosphamide)	Procarbazine
Anticancer agents NEC	Floxuridine	Pteroyltriglutamate
Antimetabolite	Fluorodeoxyuridine	Purine analogue
Antimitotic agent	Fluorouracil	(antineoplastic)
Antineoplastic NEC	Folic acid, antagonist	Purinethol
Antineoplastic antibiotics	Ftorafur	Pyrimidine antagonist
Antineoplastic alkaloidal	Gold, colloidal (I98Au)	Razoxane
Antineoplastic combination	Goserelin	Rubidomycin
Ara-C	Hexamethylmelamine	Rufocromomycin
Asparaginase	Hormone, cancer therapy	Sarcolysin
Azacitidine	Hydroxycarbamide	Sarkomycin
Azaribine	Hydroxyurea	Semustine
Azaserine	Idarubicin	Sodium aminopterin
Azatepa	Ifosfamide	Streptozocin
Azathioprine	Imidazole-4-carboxamide	Streptozotocin
BCNU	Immunosuppressive drug	Tauromustine
Benzcarbimine	Inproquone	Tegafur
Bleomycin	Iproplatin	TEM
Broxuridine	Isophosphamide	Teniposide
Busulfan, busulphan	Leukeran	TEPA
Cactinomycin	Lomustine	ThalidomIde
Cancer chemotherapy drug	Lonidamine	Thioguanine
regimen	M-AMSA	Thiotepa
Carboplatin	Mannomustine	Tioguanine
Carboquone	Matulane	Treosulfan
Carmofur	Mechlorethamine	Tretamine
Carmustine	Melphalan	Triaziquone
Chlorambucil	Mercaptopurine	Trichlormethine
Chlorhexamide	Methotrexate	Trichlorotriethylamine
Chlormethine	Methyl CCNU	Triethanomelamine
Chloropurine	Metoprine	Triethylenemelamine
Chromic phosphate 32P	Mithramycin	Triethylenephosphoramide
Chromomycin A3	Mitobronitol	Triethylenethio-
Ciclosporin	Mitoguazone	phosphoramide
Cisplatin	Mitolactol	Trimetrexate
Colaspase	Mitomycin	Trimustine
Corynebacterium parvum	Mitopodozide	Trofosfamide
Cycloleucin	Mitotane	Uracil mustard
Cyclophosphamide	Mitoxantrone	Uramustine
Cyclosporin	Mopidamol	Urethane
Cytarabine	MOPP (mechlorethamine	Vinblastine
Cytosine arabinoside	+ vincristine +	Vincamine
Cytoxan	prednisone +	Vincristine
Dacarbazine	procarbazine)	Vindesine
Dactinomycin	Muromonab-CD3	Vinorelbine tartrate
Daunomycin	Mustard, nitrogen	Zinostatin
Daunorubicin	Mustine	Zorubicin
Demecolcine	M-vac	
	Myelobromal	

T45.1x- Poisoning by, adverse effect of and underdosing of <u>antineoplastic and immunosuppressive drugs</u>

T45.1x1- Poisoning by antineoplastic and immunosuppressive drugs, <u>accidental</u> (unintentional)
Poisoning by antineoplastic and immunosuppressive drugs NOS

T45.1x2- Poisoning by antineoplastic and immunosuppressive drugs, <u>intentional</u> self-harm

T45.1x3- Poisoning by antineoplastic and immunosuppressive drugs, <u>assault</u>

T4 · T45

T45.1x4- Poisoning by antineoplastic and immunosuppressive drugs, <u>undetermined</u>

T45.1x5- <u>Adverse effect</u> of antineoplastic and immunosuppressive drugs
AHA 14:4Q:p22 – Adverse effect of antineoplastic drug

T45.1x6- <u>Underdosing</u> of antineoplastic and immunosuppressive drugs

T45.2- Poisoning by, adverse effect of and underdosing of vitamins
Excludes ❷: *poisoning by, adverse effect of and underdosing of nicotinic acid (derivatives) (T46.7)*
poisoning by, adverse effect of and underdosing of iron (T45.4)
poisoning by, adverse effect of and underdosing of vitamin K (T45.7)

T45.2 - DRUGS/CHEMS*		
Acetiamine	Dexpanthenol	Retinol
Adenine	Dextro calcium	Riboflavin
Alfacalcidol	pantothenate	Thiamine
Alpha tocoferol (acetate)	Dextro pantothenyl alcohol	Tocoferol
Aneurine	Dihydrotachysterol	Tocopherol
Ascorbic acid	Ergocalciferol	Tocopherol acetate
Axerophthol	Esculin	Viosterol
Benfotiamine	Esculoside	Vitamin NEC
Betacarotene	Flavine adenine	Vitamin A
Biotin	dinucleotide	Vitamin B NEC
Bisbentiamine	Folic acid with ferrous salt	Vitamin B1
Bisbutiamine	Fursultiamine	Vitamin B2
Calcifediol	Ilopan	Vitamin B6
Calciferol	Lactoflavin	Vitamin B12
Calcitriol	Niacinamide	Vitamin B15
Calcium pantothenate	Nicotinamide	Vitamin C
Carotene	Octotiamine	Vitamin D
Cetotiamine	Oleovitamin A	Vitamin D2
Cevitamic acid	Pangamic acid	Vitamin D3
Cholecalciferol	Panthenol	Vitamin E
Cobalamine	Pantothenic acid	Vitamin E acetate
Cod-liver oil	Provitamin A	Vitamin PP
Colecalciferol	Pyridoxal phosphate	Yeast
Cozyme	Pyridoxine	Yeast, dried

T45.2x- Poisoning by, adverse effect of and underdosing of <u>vitamins</u>

T45.2x1- Poisoning by vitamins, <u>accidental</u> (unintentional)
Poisoning by vitamins NOS

T45.2x2- Poisoning by vitamins, <u>intentional</u> self-harm

T45.2x3- Poisoning by vitamins, <u>assault</u>

T45.2x4- Poisoning by vitamins, <u>undetermined</u>

T45.2x5- <u>Adverse effect</u> of vitamins

T45.2x6- <u>Underdosing</u> of vitamins
Excludes 1: *vitamin deficiencies (E50-E56)*

T45.3- Poisoning by, adverse effect of and underdosing of enzymes

T45.3 - DRUGS/CHEMS*		
Alglucerase	Chymotrypsin	Hyaluronidase
Alidase	Cocarboxylase	Hyazyme
Alpha amylase	Deoxyribonuclease	Pancreatic dornase
Brinase	(pancreatic)	Penicillinase
Bromelains	Diffusin	Pronase
Catalase	Enzodase	Serrapeptase
Chymar	Enzyme NEC	Streptodornase
Chymopapain	Enzyme, fibrolytic	Sutilains
	Enzyme, thrombolytic	Trypsin

T45.3x- Poisoning by, adverse effect of and underdosing of <u>enzymes</u>

T45.3x1- Poisoning by enzymes, <u>accidental</u> (unintentional)
Poisoning by enzymes NOS

T45.3x2- Poisoning by enzymes, <u>intentional</u> self-harm

T45.3x3- Poisoning by enzymes, <u>assault</u>

T45.3x4- Poisoning by enzymes, <u>undetermined</u>

T45.3x5- <u>Adverse effect</u> of enzymes

T45.3x6- <u>Underdosing</u> of enzymes

T45.4- Poisoning by, adverse effect of and underdosing of iron and its compounds

T45.4 - DRUGS/CHEMS*		
Calcium ferrous citrate	Ferrodextrane	Iron, dextran injection
Dextriferron	Ferropolimaler	Iron, salts
Ferric chloride	Ferrous phosphate	Iron, sorbitex
Ferric citrate	Ferrous salt	Iron, sorbitol citric acid
Ferric hydroxide, colloidal	Ferrous salt with folic acid	complex
Ferric hydroxide,	Ferrous fumarate,	Isomaltose, ferric complex
polymaltose	gluconate, lactate, salt	Jectofer
Ferric pyrophosphate	NEC, sulfate (medicinal)	Polyferose
Ferritin	Iron (compounds)	Sodium iron edetate
Ferrocholinate	(medicinal) NEC	
	Iron, ammonium	

T45.4x- Poisoning by, adverse effect of and underdosing of <u>iron and its compounds</u>

T45.4x1- Poisoning by iron and its compounds, <u>accidental</u> (unintentional)
Poisoning by iron and its compounds NOS

T45.4x2- Poisoning by iron and its compounds, <u>intentional</u> self-harm

T45.4x3- Poisoning by iron and its compounds, <u>assault</u>

T45.4x4- Poisoning by iron and its compounds, <u>undetermined</u>

T45.4x5- <u>Adverse effect</u> of iron and its compounds

T45.4x6- <u>Underdosing</u> of iron and its compounds
Excludes 1: *iron deficiency (E61.1)*

T45.5- Poisoning by, adverse effect of and underdosing of anticoagulants and antithrombotic drugs

T45.51- Poisoning by, adverse effect of and underdosing of <u>anticoagulants</u>
AHA 16:1Q:p14 – Duodenal ulcer with hemorrhage due to Coumadin therapy

T45.51 - DRUGS/CHEMS*		
Acenocoumarin	Diphenadione	Nicoumalone
Acenocoumarol	Drotrecogin alfa	Panwarfin
Anisindione	Enoxaparin (sodium)	Phenindione
Anticoagulant NEC	Ethyl biscoumacetate	Phenprocoumon
Bishydroxycoumarin	Ethylidene dicoumarin	Prothrombin synthesis
Bromindione	Ethylidene dicoumarol	inhibitor
Coumadin	Fluindione	Sintrom
Coumarin	Heparin (sodium)	Tioclomarol
Coumetarol	Heparin-fraction	Warfarin
Cumetharol	Heparinoid (systemic)	Xigris
Danilone	Indandione (derivatives)	Zovant
Dicoumarol, dicoumarin,	Indendione (derivatives)	
dicumarol	Inhibitor, prothrombin	
	synthesis	

T45.511- Poisoning by anticoagulants, <u>accidental</u> (unintentional)
Poisoning by anticoagulants NOS

T45.512- Poisoning by anticoagulants, <u>intentional</u> self-harm

T45.513- Poisoning by anticoagulants, <u>assault</u>

T45.514- Poisoning by anticoagulants, <u>undetermined</u>

T45.515- <u>Adverse effect</u> of anticoagulants
AHA 13:2Q:p34 – Warfarin induced skin necrosis

T45.516- <u>Underdosing</u> of anticoagulants

T45.52- Poisoning by, adverse effect of and underdosing of <u>antithrombotic drugs</u>
AHA 16:1Q:p15 – Hemorrhage due to Prasugrel (Effient®)
Poisoning by, adverse effect of and underdosing of antiplatelet drugs
Excludes ❷: *poisoning by, adverse effect of and underdosing of aspirin (T39.01-)*
poisoning by, adverse effect of and underdosing of acetylsalicylic acid (T39.01-)

T45.52 - DRUGS/CHEMS*		
Epoprostenol	Prostacyclin	Triflusal
Indobufen	Prostaglandin (I2)	
	Ticlopidine	

T45.521- Poisoning by antithrombotic drugs, <u>accidental</u> (unintentional)
Poisoning by antithrombotic drug NOS

T45.522- Poisoning by antithrombotic drugs, <u>intentional</u> self-harm

T45.523-   Poisoning by antithrombotic drugs, <u>assault</u>

T45.524-   Poisoning by antithrombotic drugs, <u>undetermined</u>

T45.525-   <u>Adverse effect</u> of antithrombotic drugs

T45.526-   <u>Underdosing</u> of antithrombotic drugs

T45.6-   Poisoning by, adverse effect of and underdosing of fibrinolysis-affecting drugs

T45.60-   Poisoning by, adverse effect of and underdosing of <u>unspecified fibrinolysis-affecting drugs</u>

T45.60 - DRUGS/CHEMS*
Fibrinolysis, affecting drug

T45.601-   Poisoning by unspecified fibrinolysis-affecting drugs, <u>accidental</u> (unintentional)
      Poisoning by fibrinolysis-affecting drug NOS

T45.602-   Poisoning by unspecified fibrinolysis-affecting drugs, <u>intentional</u> self-harm

T45.603-   Poisoning by unspecified fibrinolysis-affecting drugs, <u>assault</u>

T45.604-   Poisoning by unspecified fibrinolysis-affecting drugs, <u>undetermined</u>

T45.605-   <u>Adverse effect</u> of unspecified fibrinolysis-affecting drugs

T45.606-   <u>Underdosing</u> of unspecified fibrinolysis-affecting drugs

T45.61-   Poisoning by, adverse effect of and underdosing of <u>thrombolytic drugs</u>

T45.61 - DRUGS/CHEMS*	Plasminogen (tissue)	Thrombolysin
Alteplase	activator	Urokinase
Anistreplase	Rt-PA	
Fibrinolytic drug	Streptokinase	

T45.611-   Poisoning by thrombolytic drug, <u>accidental</u> (unintentional)
      Poisoning by thrombolytic drug NOS

T45.612-   Poisoning by thrombolytic drug, <u>intentional</u> self-harm

T45.613-   Poisoning by thrombolytic drug, <u>assault</u>

T45.614-   Poisoning by thrombolytic drug, <u>undetermined</u>

T45.615-   <u>Adverse effect</u> of thrombolytic drugs

T45.616-   <u>Underdosing</u> of thrombolytic drugs

T45.62-   Poisoning by, adverse effect of and underdosing of <u>hemostatic drugs</u>

T45.62 - DRUGS/CHEMS*	Epsilon amino-caproic acid	Inhibitor, fibrinolysis
Aminocaproic acid	Fibrinolysis, inhibitor NEC	Tranexamic acid
Antifibrinolytic drug	Hemostatic	
Aprotinin	Hemostatic, drug, systemic	

T45.621-   Poisoning by hemostatic drug, <u>accidental</u> (unintentional)
      Poisoning by hemostatic drug NOS

T45.622-   Poisoning by hemostatic drug, <u>intentional</u> self-harm

T45.623-   Poisoning by hemostatic drug, <u>assault</u>

T45.624-   Poisoning by hemostatic drug, <u>undetermined</u>

T45.625-   <u>Adverse effect</u> of hemostatic drug

T45.626-   <u>Underdosing</u> of hemostatic drugs

T45.69-   Poisoning by, adverse effect of and underdosing of <u>other fibrinolysis-affecting drugs</u>

T45.69 - DRUGS/CHEMS*	Ancrod
Aminomethylbenzoic acid	Fibrinolysin (human)

T45.691-   Poisoning by other fibrinolysis-affecting drugs, <u>accidental</u> (unintentional)
      Poisoning by other fibrinolysis-affecting drug NOS

T45.692-   Poisoning by other fibrinolysis-affecting drugs, <u>intentional</u> self-harm

T45.693-   Poisoning by other fibrinolysis-affecting drugs, <u>assault</u>

T45.694-   Poisoning by other fibrinolysis-affecting drugs, <u>undetermined</u>

T45.695-   <u>Adverse effect</u> of other fibrinolysis-affecting drugs

T45.696-   <u>Underdosing</u> of other fibrinolysis-affecting drugs

T45.7-   Poisoning by, adverse effect of and underdosing of anticoagulant antagonists, vitamin K and other coagulants

T45.7 - DRUGS/CHEMS*	Factor IX complex	Phytomenadione
Acetomenaphthone	Gelatin, absorbable	Phytonadione
Antagonist, anticoagulant	(sponge)	Protamine sulfate
Anticoagulant, antagonist	Gelfoam	Prothrombin activator
Antihemophilic globulin	Heparin, action reverser	Russel's viper venin
concentrate	Hexadimethrine (bromide)	Snake venom or bite,
Antihemophilic plasma,	Menadiol	hemocoagulase
dried	Menadiol sodium sulfate	Sponge, absorbable
Antiheparin drug	Menadione	(gelatin)
Coagulant NEC	Menadione sodium bisulfite	Thrombin
Cotarnine	Menaphthone	Thromboplastin
Cytozyme	Menaquinone	Vitamin K NEC
Etamsylate	Menatetrenone	Vitamin K1
Ethamsylate	Phylloquinone	Vitamin K2

T45.7x-   Poisoning by, adverse effect of and underdosing of <u>anticoagulant antagonists, vitamin K and other coagulants</u>

T45.7x1-   Poisoning by anticoagulant antagonists, vitamin K and other coagulants, <u>accidental</u> (unintentional)
      Poisoning by anticoagulant antagonists, vitamin K and other coagulants NOS

T45.7x2-   Poisoning by anticoagulant antagonists, vitamin K and other coagulants, <u>intentional</u> self-harm

T45.7x3-   Poisoning by anticoagulant antagonists, vitamin K and other coagulants, <u>assault</u>

T45.7x4-   Poisoning by anticoagulant antagonists, vitamin K and other coagulants, <u>undetermined</u>

T45.7x5-   <u>Adverse effect</u> of anticoagulant antagonists, vitamin K and other coagulants

T45.7x6-   <u>Underdosing</u> of anticoagulant antagonist, vitamin K and other coagulants
      Excludes 1:   *vitamin K deficiency (E56.1)*

T45.8-   Poisoning by, adverse effect of and underdosing of other primarily systemic and hematological agents
      Poisoning by, adverse effect of and underdosing of liver preparations and other antianemic agents
      Poisoning by, adverse effect of and underdosing of natural blood and blood products
      Poisoning by, adverse effect of and underdosing of plasma substitute
      Excludes ❷: *poisoning by, adverse effect of and underdosing of immunoglobulin (T50.Z1)*
             poisoning by, adverse effect of and underdosing of iron (T45.4)
             transfusion reactions (T80-)

T45.8x-   Poisoning by, adverse effect of and underdosing of <u>other primarily systemic and hematological agents</u>

T45.8 - DRUGS/CHEMS*	Calcium EDTA	Fibrinogen (human)
Albumin (bovine) (human	Calcium folinate	Folacin
serum (salt-poor))	Calcium leucovorin	Folic acid
(normal human serum)	Citrovorum (factor)	Folinic acid
Aminoethylisothiourium	Cobalt, medicinal (trace)	Gelatin (intravenous)
Antagonist, heavy metal	(chloride)	Haptendextran
Anti-anemic (drug)	Copper, medicinal (trace)	Heavy metal antidote
(preparation)	Cyanocobalamin	Hematin
Antidote, heavy metal	Deferoxamine	Hematinic preparation
Antihemophilic factor	Desferrioxamine	Hematological agent,
Antihemophilic fraction	Dextran (40) (70) (150)	specified NEC
Antihemophilic human	Dimercaprol (British anti-	HES
plasma	lewisite)	Hetastarch
BAL	Dimercaptopropanol	Human albumin
Blood (derivatives)	Edathamil disodium	Hydroxocobalamin
(natural) (plasma)	Edetate, disodium	Hydroxyethyl starch
(whole)	(calcium)	Leucovorin (factor)
Blood, dried	EPO	Liver extract
Blood, expander NEC	Epoetin alpha	Liver extract for parenteral
Blood, fraction NEC	Erythropoietin	use
Blood, substitute	Erythropoietin, human	Liver fraction 1
(macromolecular)	Factor I (fibrinogen)	Liver hydrolysate
British antilewisite	Factor III (thromboplastin)	LMD
Calcium disodium	Factor VIII (antihemophilic	Mecobalamin
edathamil	Factor) (concentrate)	
Calcium disodium edetate	Factor IX complex, human	

T45 - T45

T45.8 - DRUGS/CHEMS*	Polyvinylpyrrolidone	Sodium edetate
– Continued	Potassium aminobenzoate	Sodium feredetate
Natural blood (product)	Povidone	Sodium glutamate
Normal serum albumin	Pteroylglutamic acid	Sodium lactate (compound
(human), salt-poor	PVP	solution)
Oxypolygelatin	Red blood cells, packed	Sodium phosphate,
Packed red cells	Saccharated iron oxide	cellulose
Plasma	Serum, complement	Systemic drug, specified
Plasma expander NEC	(inhibitor)	NEC
Plasma protein fraction	Serum, hemolytic	Trace element NEC
(human)	complement	Trientine
Plasmanate	Sodium calcium edetate	Vitamin hematopoietic
Polygeline	Sodium dehydrocholate	Whole blood (human)
Polyvidone	Sodium dipantoyl ferrate	

T45.8x1- **Poisoning by other primarily systemic and hematological agents, <u>accidental</u> (unintentional)**
      Poisoning by other primarily systemic and hematological agents NOS

T45.8x2- **Poisoning by other primarily systemic and hematological agents, <u>intentional</u> self-harm**

T45.8x3- **Poisoning by other primarily systemic and hematological agents, <u>assault</u>**

T45.8x4- **Poisoning by other primarily systemic and hematological agents, <u>undetermined</u>**

T45.8x5- **<u>Adverse effect</u> of other primarily systemic and hematological agents**

T45.8x6- **<u>Underdosing</u> of other primarily systemic and hematological agents**

T45.9- **Poisoning by, adverse effect of and underdosing of <u>unspecified</u> primarily systemic and hematological agent**

T45.9 - DRUGS/CHEMS*	Hematological agent
Blood, drug affecting NEC	Systemic drug

T45.91x- **Poisoning by unspecified primarily systemic and hematological agent, <u>accidental</u> (unintentional)**
      Poisoning by primarily systemic and hematological agent NOS

T45.92x- **Poisoning by unspecified primarily systemic and hematological agent, <u>intentional</u> self-harm**

T45.93x- **Poisoning by unspecified primarily systemic and hematological agent, <u>assault</u>**

T45.94x- **Poisoning by unspecified primarily systemic and hematological agent, <u>undetermined</u>**

T45.95x- **<u>Adverse effect</u> of unspecified primarily systemic and hematological agent**

T45.96x- **<u>Underdosing</u> of unspecified primarily systemic and hematological agent**

T46- **Poisoning by, adverse effect of and underdosing of agents <u>primarily affecting the cardiovascular system</u>**
  Excludes 1:   poisoning by, adverse effect of and underdosing of metaraminol (T44.4)

> The appropriate 7th character is to be added to each code from category T46:
> A <u>Initial</u> encounter
> D <u>Subsequent</u> encounter
> S <u>Sequela</u>

T46.0- **Poisoning by, adverse effect of and underdosing of cardiac-stimulant glycosides and drugs of similar action**

T46.0 - DRUGS/CHEMS*	Digitalis lanata	Metildigoxin
Acetyldigitoxin	Digitalis purpurea	Oleandrin
Acetyldigoxin	Digitoxin	Ouabain(e)
Alpha acetyldigoxin	Digitoxose	Pengitoxin
b-acetyldigoxin	Digoxin	Peruvoside
Cardiotonic (glycoside) NEC	Digoxine	Proscillaridin
Cerberin	Gitalin	Squill
Ch'an su	Gitalin, amorphous	Strofantina
Convallaria glycosides	Gitaloxin	Strophanthin (g) (k)
Crataegus extract	Gitoxin	Strophanthus
Cymarin	Glycoside, cardiac	Strophantin
Deslanoside	(stimulant)	Strophantin-g
Digitalin(e)	Lanatosides	
Digitalis (leaf) (glycoside)	Meproscillarin	

T46.0x- **Poisoning by, adverse effect of and underdosing of <u>cardiac-stimulant glycosides and drugs of similar action</u>**

T46.0x1- **Poisoning by cardiac-stimulant glycosides and drugs of similar action, <u>accidental</u> (unintentional)**
      Poisoning by cardiac-stimulant glycosides and drugs of similar action NOS

T46.0x2- **Poisoning by cardiac-stimulant glycosides and drugs of similar action, <u>intentional</u> self-harm**

T46.0x3- **Poisoning by cardiac-stimulant glycosides and drugs of similar action, <u>assault</u>**

T46.0x4- **Poisoning by cardiac-stimulant glycosides and drugs of similar action, <u>undetermined</u>**

T46.0x5- **<u>Adverse effect</u> of cardiac-stimulant glycosides and drugs of similar action**

T46.0x6- **<u>Underdosing</u> of cardiac-stimulant glycosides and drugs of similar action**

T46.1- **Poisoning by, adverse effect of and underdosing of calcium-channel blockers**

T46.1 - DRUGS/CHEMS*	Iproveratril	Nisoldipine
Bepridil	Isradipine	Nitrendipine
Blockers, calcium channel	Lidoflazine	Oxodipine
Diltiazem	Monoxidine hydrochloride	Tiapamil
Felodipine	Nicardipine	Verapamil
Fendiline	Nifedipine	
Gallopamil	Nimodipine	

T46.1x- **Poisoning by, adverse effect of and underdosing of <u>calcium-channel blockers</u>**

T46.1x1- **Poisoning by calcium-channel blockers, <u>accidental</u> (unintentional)**
      Poisoning by calcium-channel blockers NOS

T46.1x2- **Poisoning by calcium-channel blockers, <u>intentional</u> self-harm**

T46.1x3- **Poisoning by calcium-channel blockers, <u>assault</u>**

T46.1x4- **Poisoning by calcium-channel blockers, <u>undetermined</u>**

T46.1x5- **<u>Adverse effect</u> of calcium-channel blockers**

T46.1x6- **<u>Underdosing</u> of calcium-channel blockers**

T45 - T46

T46.2-   Poisoning by, adverse effect of and underdosing of other antidysrhythmic drugs, not elsewhere classified

Excludes 1:   poisoning by, adverse effect of and underdosing of beta-adrenoreceptor antagonists (T44.7-)

T46.2 - DRUGS/CHEMS*	Cardiac rhythm regulator, specified NEC	Mexiletine
Adenosine (phosphate)		Pilsicainide (hydrochloride)
Ajmaline	Chinidin(e)	Prajmalium bitartrate
Amiodarone	Cibenzoline	Procainamide
Antidysrhythmic NEC	Depressant, cardiac	Pronestyl (hydrochloride)
Aprindine	Encainide	Propafenone
Bretylium tosilate	Flecainide	Quinaglute
Bunaftine	Hydroquinidine	Quinidine
Cardiac depressants	Lorajmine	Tocainide
Cardiac rhythm regulator	Lorcainide	

T46.2x-   Poisoning by, adverse effect of and underdosing of other antidysrhythmic drugs

T46.2x1-   Poisoning by other antidysrhythmic drugs, accidental (unintentional)
Poisoning by other antidysrhythmic drugs NOS

T46.2x2-   Poisoning by other antidysrhythmic drugs, intentional self-harm

T46.2x3-   Poisoning by other antidysrhythmic drugs, assault

T46.2x4-   Poisoning by other antidysrhythmic drugs, undetermined

T46.2x5-   Adverse effect of other antidysrhythmic drugs

T46.2x6-   Underdosing of other antidysrhythmic drugs

T46.3-   Poisoning by, adverse effect of and underdosing of coronary vasodilators

Poisoning by, adverse effect of and underdosing of dipyridamole

Excludes 1:   poisoning by, adverse effect of and underdosing of calcium-channel blockers (T46.1)

T46.3 - DRUGS/CHEMS*	Heptaminol	Pentaerythritol, tetranitrate NEC
Amikhelline	Hexadiline	
Amyl nitrite	Hexadylamine	Pentaerythrityl tetranitrate
Bendazol	Hexobendine	Pentrinat
Benziodarone	Ipriflavone	Perhexilene
Carbocromen	Isoamyl nitrite	Perhexiline (maleate)
Chromonar	Isosorbide dinitrate	Peritrate
Coronary vasodilator NEC	Itramin tosilate	Piridoxilate
Cromonar	Khellin	Prenylamine
Diisopropylamine	Khelloside	Propatylnitrate
Dilazep	Mannitol hexanitrate	Sorbide nitrate
Dimoxyline	Molsidomine	Sweet niter spirit
Dioxyline	Nicorandil	Tenitramine
Dipyridamole	Nitrate, organic	Terodiline
Efloxate	Nitrite, amyl (medicinal) (vapor)	Trapidil
Eritrityl tetranitrate		Triethanolamine, trinitrate (biphosphate)
Erythrityl tetranitrate	Nitroglycerin, nitro-glycerol (medicinal)	
Erythrol tetranitrate		Trinitrine
Etafenone	Nitrous ether spirit	Trolnitrate (phosphate)
Fenalcomine	Octyl nitrite	Vasodilator, coronary NEC
Fluorosol	Organonitrate NEC	Visnadine
Glyceryl nitrate	Oxyfedrine	
Glyceryl trinitrate	Pentaerythritol	

T46.3x-   Poisoning by, adverse effect of and underdosing of coronary vasodilators

T46.3x1-   Poisoning by coronary vasodilators, accidental (unintentional)
Poisoning by coronary vasodilators NOS

T46.3x2-   Poisoning by coronary vasodilators, intentional self-harm

T46.3x3-   Poisoning by coronary vasodilators, assault

T46.3x4-   Poisoning by coronary vasodilators, undetermined

T46.3x5-   Adverse effect of coronary vasodilators

T46.3x6-   Underdosing of coronary vasodilators

T46.4-   Poisoning by, adverse effect of and underdosing of angiotensin-converting-enzyme inhibitors

T46.4 - DRUGS/CHEMS*	Enalaprilat	Perindopril
Alacepril	Fosinopril	Quinapril
Benazepril	Fosinopril, sodium	Ramipril
Captopril	Inhibitor, angiotensin- converting enzyme	Spirapril
Cilazapril		Zofenopril
Enalapril	Lisinopril	

T46.4x-   Poisoning by, adverse effect of and underdosing of angiotensin-converting-enzyme inhibitors

T46.4x1-   Poisoning by angiotensin-converting-enzyme inhibitors, accidental (unintentional)
Poisoning by angiotensin-converting-enzyme inhibitors NOS

T46.4x2-   Poisoning by angiotensin-converting-enzyme inhibitors, intentional self-harm

T46.4x3-   Poisoning by angiotensin-converting-enzyme inhibitors, assault

T46.4x4-   Poisoning by angiotensin-converting-enzyme inhibitors, undetermined

T46.4x5-   Adverse effect of angiotensin-converting-enzyme inhibitors

T46.4x6-   Underdosing of angiotensin-converting-enzyme inhibitors

T46.5-   Poisoning by, adverse effect of and underdosing of other antihypertensive drugs

Excludes ❷: poisoning by, adverse effect of and underdosing of beta-adrenoreceptor antagonists (T44.7)
poisoning by, adverse effect of and underdosing of calcium-channel blockers (T46.1)
poisoning by, adverse effect of and underdosing of diuretics (T50.0-T50.2)

T46.5 - DRUGS/CHEMS*	Guanabenz	Protoveratrine(s) (A) (B)
Aldomet	Guanacline	Raudixin
Alkavervir	Guanadrel	Rautensin
Alseroxylon	Guanethidine	Rautina
Amiquinsin	Guanfacine	Rautotal
Antagonist, serotonin	Guanochlor	Rauwiloid
Antihypertensive drug NEC	Guanoclor	Rauwoldin
Apresoline	Guanoctine	Rauwolfia (alkaloids)
Benzapril hydrochloride	Guanoxabenz	Rescinnamine
Betanidine	Guanoxan	Reserpin(e)
Bethanidine	Harmonyl	Sandril
Budralazine	Hydralazine	Saralasin
Cadralazine	Hypotensive NEC	Serpasil
Clonidine	Indapamide	Singoserp
Cryptenamine (tannates)	Lacidipine	Sodium nitroferricyanide
Debrisoquine	Methoserpidine	Sodium nitroprusside
Deserpidine	Methyldopa	Syrosingopine
DHE 45	Methyldopate	Teprotide
Diazoxide	Methysergide	Todralazine
Dihydralazine	Metirosine	Tolonidine
Dihydrazine	Moderil	Urapidil
Dihydroergotamine	Nitroprusside	Veratrine
Endralazine	Pargyline	Veratrum, alkaloids
Ergotamine	Pinacidil	

T46.5x-   Poisoning by, adverse effect of and underdosing of other antihypertensive drugs

T46.5x1-   Poisoning by other antihypertensive drugs, accidental (unintentional)
Poisoning by other antihypertensive drugs NOS

T46.5x2-   Poisoning by other antihypertensive drugs, intentional self-harm

T46.5x3-   Poisoning by other antihypertensive drugs, assault

T46.5x4-   Poisoning by other antihypertensive drugs, undetermined

T46.5x5-   Adverse effect of other antihypertensive drugs

T46.5x6-   Underdosing of other antihypertensive drugs

T46 - T46

T46.6- Poisoning by, adverse effect of and underdosing of antihyperlipidemic and antiarteriosclerotic drugs

T46.6 - DRUGS/CHEMS*	Clinofibrate	Linolenic acid
Acipimox	Clofibrate	Lovastatin
Allyl disulfide	Clofibride	Mesoglycan
Aluminium clofibrate	Clotibric acid	Oleic acid
Antiarteriosclerotic drug	Colestipol	Pirozadil
Anticholesterolemic drug NEC	Colestyramine	Polidexide (sulfate)
	Cyamopsis tetragono-loba	Pravastatin
Antihyperlipidemic drug	Detaxtran	Probucol
Antilipemic drug NEC	Ethylparachloro-	Ronifibrate
b-benzalbutyramide	phenoxyisobutyrate	Safflower oil
Benfluorex	Etiroxate	Simfibrate
Benzalbutyramide	Etofibrate	Simvastatin
Benzyl nicotinate	Etofylline clofibrate	Sitosterols
Bezafibrate	Fenofibrate	Soysterol
Binifibrate	Gemfibrozil	Sunflower seed oil
b-sitosterol(s)	Guar gum (medicinal)	Triparanol
Cholesterol-lowering	Halofenate	Unsaturated fatty acid
agents	Ion exchange resin,	
Cholestyramine (resin)	cholestyramine	
Ciprofibrate	Linoleic acid	

T46.6x- Poisoning by, adverse effect of and underdosing of antihyperlipidemic and antiarteriosclerotic drugs

T46.6x1- Poisoning by antihyperlipidemic and antiarteriosclerotic drugs, accidental (unintentional)
Poisoning by antihyperlipidemic and antiarteriosclerotic drugs NOS

T46.6x2- Poisoning by antihyperlipidemic and antiarteriosclerotic drugs, intentional self-harm

T46.6x3- Poisoning by antihyperlipidemic and antiarteriosclerotic drugs, assault

T46.6x4- Poisoning by antihyperlipidemic and antiarteriosclerotic drugs, undetermined

T46.6x5- Adverse effect of antihyperlipidemic and antiarteriosclerotic drugs

T46.6x6- Underdosing of antihyperlipidemic and antiarteriosclerotic drugs

T46.7- Poisoning by, adverse effect of and underdosing of peripheral vasodilators
Poisoning by, adverse effect of and underdosing of nicotinic acid (derivatives)
Excludes 1: *poisoning by, adverse effect of and underdosing of papaverine (T44.3)*

T46.7 - DRUGS/CHEMS*	Etofylline	Pentoxifylline
Alprostadil	Flunarizine	Phenoxybenzamine
Aluminium nicotinate	Hepronicate	Phentolamine
Azapetine	Hydromethylpyridine	Prostaglandin E1
Bamethan (sulfate)	Ifenprodil	Raubasine
Bencyclane	Iloprost	Sildenafil
Betahistine	Inositol nicotinate	Suloctidil
Brovincamine	Isoxsuprine	Tadalafil
Buflomedil	Kallidinogenase	Tetranicotinoyl fructose
Buphenine	Kallikrein	Thurfyl nicotinate
Butalamine	Lipo-alprostadil	Thymoxamine
Cetiedil	Minoxidil	Tolazoline
Ciclonicate	Moxisylyte	Trimetazidine
Cinepazide	Naftidrofuryl (oxalate)	Vardenafil
Cyclandelate	Niacin	Vasodilan
Dihydroergocornine	Nicametate	Vasodilator, peripheral NEC
Dihydroergocristine	Nicergoline	Vinburnine
(mesilate)	Nicofuranose	Vinpocetine
Dihydroergokryptine	Nicotinic acid	Viquidil
Dihydroergotoxine	Nicotinyl alcohol	Vitamin B, nicotinic acid
Dihydroergotoxine mesilate	Nylidrin	Xanthinol nicotinate
Ergoloid mesylates	Pentifylline	Xantinol nicotinate

T46.7x- Poisoning by, adverse effect of and underdosing of peripheral vasodilators

T46.7x1- Poisoning by peripheral vasodilators, accidental (unintentional)
Poisoning by peripheral vasodilators NOS

T46.7x2- Poisoning by peripheral vasodilators, intentional self-harm

T46.7x3- Poisoning by peripheral vasodilators, assault

T46.7x4- Poisoning by peripheral vasodilators, undetermined

T46.7x5- Adverse effect of peripheral vasodilators

T46.7x6- Underdosing of peripheral vasodilators

T46.8- Poisoning by, adverse effect of and underdosing of antivaricose drugs, including sclerosing agents

T46.8 - DRUGS/CHEMS*	Monoethanolamine oleate	Sodium tetradecyl sulfate
Antivaricose drug	Phenol, in oil injection	Sotradecol
Dextrose, concentrated	Polidocanol	Varicose reduction drug
solution, intravenous	Sclerosing agent	Venous sclerosing drug NEC
Ethanolamine oleate	Sodium morrhuate	Zinc, antivaricose
Monoethanolamine	Sodium psylliate	

T46.8x- Poisoning by, adverse effect of and underdosing of antivaricose drugs, including sclerosing agents

T46.8x1- Poisoning by antivaricose drugs, including sclerosing agents, accidental (unintentional)
Poisoning by antivaricose drugs, including sclerosing agents NOS

T46.8x2- Poisoning by antivaricose drugs, including sclerosing agents, intentional self-harm

T46.8x3- Poisoning by antivaricose drugs, including sclerosing agents, assault

T46.8x4- Poisoning by antivaricose drugs, including sclerosing agents, undetermined

T46.8x5- Adverse effect of antivaricose drugs, including sclerosing agents

T46.8x6- Underdosing of antivaricose drugs, including sclerosing agents

T46.9- Poisoning by, adverse effect of and underdosing of other and unspecified agents primarily affecting the cardiovascular system

T46.90- Poisoning by, adverse effect of and underdosing of unspecified agents primarily affecting the cardiovascular system

T46.90 - DRUGS/CHEMS*	Cardiovascular drug NEC
Capillary-active drug NEC	

T46.901- Poisoning by unspecified agents primarily affecting the cardiovascular system, accidental (unintentional)

T46.902- Poisoning by unspecified agents primarily affecting the cardiovascular system, intentional self-harm

T46.903- Poisoning by unspecified agents primarily affecting the cardiovascular system, assault

T46.904- Poisoning by unspecified agents primarily affecting the cardiovascular system, undetermined

T46.905- Adverse effect of unspecified agents primarily affecting the cardiovascular system

T46.906- Underdosing of unspecified agents primarily affecting the cardiovascular system

T46.99- Poisoning by, adverse effect of and underdosing of other agents primarily affecting the cardiovascular system

T46.99 - DRUGS/CHEMS*	Calcium dobesilate	Naftazone
Aconite (wild)	Chlorisondamine chloride	Phenopyrazone
Aconitine	Diosmin	Pholedrine
Aconitum ferox	Escin	Rutinum
Adrenochrome (derivative)	Ethoxazorutoside	Rutoside
((mono) semicarbazone)	Flavodic acid	Tribenoside
Aurantiin	Hesperidin	Troxerutin
Benzopyrone	Leucocianidol	
Bioflavonoid(s)	Metescufylline	

T46.991- Poisoning by other agents primarily affecting the cardiovascular system, accidental (unintentional)

T46.992- Poisoning by other agents primarily affecting the cardiovascular system, intentional self-harm

T46.993- Poisoning by other agents primarily affecting the cardiovascular system, assault

T46.994- Poisoning by other agents primarily affecting the cardiovascular system, undetermined

T46 - T46

T46.995- <u>Adverse effect</u> of other agents primarily affecting the cardiovascular system

T46.996- <u>Underdosing</u> of other agents primarily affecting the cardiovascular system

T47- Poisoning by, adverse effect of and underdosing of <u>agents primarily affecting the gastrointestinal system</u>

> The appropriate 7th character is to be added to each code from category T47:
> **A**   <u>Initial</u> encounter
> **D**   <u>Subsequent</u> encounter
> **S**   <u>Sequela</u>

T47.0- Poisoning by, adverse effect of and underdosing of histamine H2-receptor blockers

T47.0 - DRUGS/CHEMS*	Famotidine	Roxatidine
Antagonist, H2 receptor	Nizatidine	
Cimetidine	Ranitidine	

T47.0x- Poisoning by, adverse effect of and underdosing of <u>histamine H2-receptor blockers</u>

T47.0x1- Poisoning by histamine H2-receptor blockers, <u>accidental</u> (unintentional)
  Poisoning by histamine H2-receptor blockers NOS

T47.0x2- Poisoning by histamine H2-receptor blockers, <u>intentional</u> self-harm

T47.0x3- Poisoning by histamine H2-receptor blockers, <u>assault</u>

T47.0x4- Poisoning by histamine H2-receptor blockers, <u>undetermined</u>

T47.0x5- <u>Adverse effect</u> of histamine H2-receptor blockers

T47.0x6- <u>Underdosing</u> of histamine H2-receptor blockers

T47.1- Poisoning by, adverse effect of and underdosing of other antacids and anti-gastric-secretion drugs

T47.1 - DRUGS/CHEMS*	Bismuth salts, aluminate	Misoprostol
Alexitol sodium	Burimamide	Omeprazole
Algeldrate	Calcium carbonate	Ornoprostil
Almagate	Carbenoxolone	Pepstatin
Almasilate	Cetraxate	Pirenzepine
Aloglutamol	Chalk, precipitated	Potassium glucaldrate
Aluminium carbonate (gel, basic)	Dihydroxyaluminum aminoacetate	Proglumide
Aluminium chlorhydroxide-complex	Dihydroxyaluminum sodium carbonate	Rolaids
Aluminium glycinate	Dimethicone	Simaldrate
Aluminium hydroxide (gel)	Dimeticone	Simethicone
Aluminium hydroxide-magnesium carb. gel	Enprostil	Soda, bicarb
Aluminium magnesium silicate	Hydrotalcite	Sodium bicarbonate
Aluminium phosphate	Magaldrate	Sodium glucaldrate
Aluminium silicate	Magnesia magma	Sodium polyhydroxyaluminium monocarbonate
Aluminium sodium silicate	Magnesium carbonate	Sucralfate
Antacid NEC	Magnesium hydroxide	Sulglicotide
Anti-gastric-secretion drug NEC	Magnesium oxide	Triple carbonate
Benexate	Magnesium trisilicate	Vitamin ulceroprotectant
	Methylpolysiloxane	
	Metiamide	
	Milk of magnesia	

T47.1x- Poisoning by, adverse effect of and underdosing of <u>other antacids and anti-gastric-secretion drugs</u>

T47.1x1- Poisoning by other antacids and anti-gastric-secretion drugs, <u>accidental</u> (unintentional)
  Poisoning by other antacids and anti-gastric-secretion drugs NOS

T47.1x2- Poisoning by other antacids and anti-gastric-secretion drugs, <u>intentional</u> self-harm

T47.1x3- Poisoning by other antacids and anti-gastric-secretion drugs, <u>assault</u>

T47.1x4- Poisoning by other antacids and anti-gastric-secretion drugs, <u>undetermined</u>

T47.1x5- <u>Adverse effect</u> of other antacids and anti-gastric-secretion drugs

T47.1x6- <u>Underdosing</u> of other antacids and anti-gastric-secretion drugs

T47.2- Poisoning by, adverse effect of and underdosing of stimulant laxatives

T47.2 - DRUGS/CHEMS*	Danthron	Phenolphthalein
Aloes	Dantron	Picosulfate (sodium)
Aloin	Dianthone	Potassium sulfate
Bisacodyl	Dihydroxyanthraquinone	Rhubarb, dry extract
Bisoxatin	Dulcolax	Rhubarb, tincture, compound
Bryonia	Elaterium	Scammony
Carter's Little Pills	Ex-Lax (phenolphthalein)	Senna
Cascara (sagrada)	Frangula	Sennoside A + B
Castor oil	Frangula, extract	Sodium phosphate, dibasic
Cathartic, anthracene derivative	Gamboge	Sodium phosphate, monobasic
Cathartic, contact	Hinkle's pills	Sodium picosulfate
Cathartic, irritant NEC	Jalap	Squirting cucumber (cathartic)
Cathartic, vegetable	Laxative, stimulant	Sulisatin
Chrysazin	Mineral oil, emulsion	Yellow phenolphthalein
Colocynth	Oleum ricini	
Croton (oil)	Oxyphenisatine	
	Phenisatin	

T47.2x- Poisoning by, adverse effect of and underdosing of <u>stimulant laxatives</u>

T47.2x1- Poisoning by stimulant laxatives, <u>accidental</u> (unintentional)
  Poisoning by stimulant laxatives NOS

T47.2x2- Poisoning by stimulant laxatives, <u>intentional</u> self-harm

T47.2x3- Poisoning by stimulant laxatives, <u>assault</u>

T47.2x4- Poisoning by stimulant laxatives, <u>undetermined</u>

T47.2x5- <u>Adverse effect</u> of stimulant laxatives

T47.2x6- <u>Underdosing</u> of stimulant laxatives

T47.3- Poisoning by, adverse effect of and underdosing of saline and osmotic laxatives

T47.3 - DRUGS/CHEMS*	Lactulose	Potassium bisulfote
Carbamide	Laxative, osmotic	Urea
Cathartic, saline	Laxative, saline	
Epsom salt	Mannitol	

T47.3x- Poisoning by and adverse effect of <u>saline and osmotic laxatives</u>

T47.3x1- Poisoning by saline and osmotic laxatives, <u>accidental</u> (unintentional)
  Poisoning by saline and osmotic laxatives NOS

T47.3x2- Poisoning by saline and osmotic laxatives, <u>intentional</u> self-harm

T47.3x3- Poisoning by saline and osmotic laxatives, <u>assault</u>

T47.3x4- Poisoning by saline and osmotic laxatives, <u>undetermined</u>

T47.3x5- <u>Adverse effect</u> of saline and osmotic laxatives

T47.3x6- <u>Underdosing</u> of saline and osmotic laxatives

T46-T47

T47.4- Poisoning by, adverse effect of and underdosing of other laxatives

T47.4 - DRUGS/CHEMS*	Fiber, dietary	Paraffin(s), liquid (medicinal)
Agar	Glycerin	Peach kernel oil (emulsion)
Arachis oil, cathartic	Glycerol	Peanut oil (emulsion) NEC
Atonia drug, intestinal	Ispagula	Petrolatum, liquid
Bran (wheat)	Ispagula, husk	Phosphate, laxative
Bulk filler, cathartic	Karaya (gum)	Poloxalkol
Calcium dioctyl sulfosuccinate	Konsyl	Poloxamer
Carboxymethyl-cellulose	Laxative NEC	Polycarbophil
Carmellose	Linseed	Psyllium hydrophilic mucilloid
Cathartic NEC	Liquid paraffin	Purgative NEC — see also Cathartic
Cathartic, bulk	Liquid petrolatum	
Cathartic, emollient NEC	Magnesium citrate	Soap, enema
Cathartic, mucilage	Magnesium sulfate	Sodium basic phosphate
Cellulose, cathartic	Metamucil	Sodium dioctyl sulfosuccinate
Cellulose, hydroxyethyl	Methyl cellulose	
Colace	Methylcellulose	Sodium sulfate
Dioctyl sulfosuccinate (calcium) (sodium)	Methylcellulose, laxative	Sorbitol
Docusate sodium	Mineral oil (laxative) (medicinal)	Sterculia
Ethylhydroxycellulose	Mucilage, plant	Tartrate, laxative
Fecal softener	Olive oil (medicinal) NEC	

T47.4x- Poisoning by, adverse effect of and underdosing of <u>other laxatives</u>

  T47.4x1- Poisoning by other laxatives, <u>accidental</u> (unintentional)
    Poisoning by other laxatives NOS

  T47.4x2- Poisoning by other laxatives, <u>intentional</u> self-harm

  T47.4x3- Poisoning by other laxatives, <u>assault</u>

  T47.4x4- Poisoning by other laxatives, <u>undetermined</u>

  T47.4x5- <u>Adverse effect</u> of other laxatives

  T47.4x6- <u>Underdosing</u> of other laxatives

T47.5- Poisoning by, adverse effect of and underdosing of digestants

T47.5 - DRUGS/CHEMS*	Decholin	Hydrochloric acid, medicinal (digestant)
Amylase	Dehydrocholic acid	
Anise oil	Diastase	Lipancreatin
Antiflatulent	Digestant NEC	Ox bile extract
Betaine	Dill	Pancreatin
b-galactosidase	Elastase	Pancrelipase
Bile salts	Enzyme, gastric	Papain
Carminative	Enzyme, intestinal	Papain, digestant
Chenodeoxycholic acid	Florantyrone	Peppermint (oil)
Chenodiol	b-Galactosidase	Pepsin
Cholagogues	Gastric enzymes	Pepsin, digestant
Choleretic	Gentian	Phenylpropanol
Cholic acid	Ginger	Protease
Citric acid	Glutamic acid	Tilactase
Cytochrome C		

T47.5x- Poisoning by, adverse effect of and underdosing of <u>digestants</u>

  T47.5x1- Poisoning by digestants, <u>accidental</u> (unintentional)
    Poisoning by digestants NOS

  T47.5x2- Poisoning by digestants, <u>intentional</u> self-harm

  T47.5x3- Poisoning by digestants, <u>assault</u>

  T47.5x4- Poisoning by digestants, <u>undetermined</u>

  T47.5x5- <u>Adverse effect</u> of digestants

  T47.5x6- <u>Underdosing</u> of digestants

T47.6- Poisoning by, adverse effect of and underdosing of antidiarrheal drugs

  Excludes ❷: poisoning by, adverse effect of and underdosing of systemic antibiotics and other anti-infectives (T36-T37)

T47.6 - DRUGS/CHEMS*	Charcoal	Lactobacillus acidophilus
Activated charcoal — see also Charcoal, medicinal	Charcoal, activated — see also Charcoal, medicinal	Lactobacillus acidophilus, compound
Aluminium tannate	Charcoal, medicinal (activated)	Lactobacillus bifidus, lyophilized
Amylopectin		
Antidiarrheal drug NEC	Charcoal, medicinal, antidiarrheal	Lactobacillus bulgaricus
Antidiarrheal drug, absorbent	Difenoxin	Lactobacillus sporogenes
Attapulgite	Diphenoxylate	Lignin hemicellulose
Bacillus, subtilis	Fetoxilate	Lomotil
Bismuth salts	Intestinal motility control drug	Loperamide
Bismuth salts, subcarbonate		Miyari bacteria
	Kaolin	Pectin
Carbo medicinalis	Kaolin, light	Saccharomyces boulardii

T47.6x- Poisoning by, adverse effect of and underdosing of <u>antidiarrheal drugs</u>

  T47.6x1- Poisoning by antidiarrheal drugs, <u>accidental</u> (unintentional)
    Poisoning by antidiarrheal drugs NOS

  T47.6x2- Poisoning by antidiarrheal drugs, <u>intentional</u> self-harm

  T47.6x3- Poisoning by antidiarrheal drugs, <u>assault</u>

  T47.6x4- Poisoning by antidiarrheal drugs, <u>undetermined</u>

  T47.6x5- <u>Adverse effect</u> of antidiarrheal drugs

  T47.6x6- <u>Underdosing</u> of antidiarrheal drugs

T47.7- Poisoning by, adverse effect of and underdosing of emetics

T47.7 - DRUGS/CHEMS*	Copper sulfate, cupric, medicinal, emetic	Emetic NEC
Apomorphine		Ipecac
Copper, emetic	Copper sulfate, medicinal, emetic	Mustard (emetic)
		Mustard, black

T47.7x- Poisoning by, adverse effect of and underdosing of <u>emetics</u>

  T47.7x1- Poisoning by emetics, <u>accidental</u> (unintentional)
    Poisoning by emetics NOS

  T47.7x2- Poisoning by emetics, <u>intentional</u> self-harm

  T47.7x3- Poisoning by emetics, <u>assault</u>

  T47.7x4- Poisoning by emetics, <u>undetermined</u>

  T47.7x5- <u>Adverse effect</u> of emetics

  T47.7x6- <u>Underdosing</u> of emetics

T47.8- Poisoning by, adverse effect of and underdosing of other agents primarily affecting gastrointestinal system

T47.8 - DRUGS/CHEMS*	Clebopride	Ion exchange resin, intestinal
Algin	Dimethyl polysiloxane	
Ammonium sulfonate resin	Gastrointestinal drug, biological	Liquorice, extract
Bacillus, lactobacillus		Mesalazine
Bromopride	Gastrointestinal drug, specified NEC	Olsalazine
Carrageenan		Pancreatic digestive secretion stimulant
Charcoal, medicinal, poison control	Glucurolactone	
	Hepatic secretion stimulant	Polysilane
Charcoal, medicinal, specified use other than for diarrhea	Intestinal motility control drug, biological	Sodium alginate
		Sodium amylosulfate
	Ion exchange resin, anion	Sulfated amylopectin
Cisapride		

T47.8x- Poisoning by, adverse effect of and underdosing of <u>other agents primarily affecting gastrointestinal system</u>

  T47.8x1- Poisoning by other agents primarily affecting gastrointestinal system, <u>accidental</u> (unintentional)
    Poisoning by other agents primarily affecting gastrointestinal system NOS

  T47.8x2- Poisoning by other agents primarily affecting gastrointestinal system, <u>intentional</u> self-harm

  T47.8x3- Poisoning by other agents primarily affecting gastrointestinal system, <u>assault</u>

  T47.8x4- Poisoning by other agents primarily affecting gastrointestinal system, <u>undetermined</u>

Excludes 1: = NOT CODED HERE! (Do not code both)   *Excludes ❷:* = Not Included Here

T47-T47

T47.8x5- <u>Adverse effect</u> of other agents primarily affecting gastrointestinal system

T47.8x6- <u>Underdosing</u> of other agents primarily affecting gastrointestinal system

T47.9- Poisoning by, adverse effect of and underdosing of <u>unspecified agents primarily affecting the gastrointestinal system</u>

T47.9 - DRUGS/CHEMS*
Gastrointestinal drug

T47.91x- Poisoning by unspecified agents primarily affecting the gastrointestinal system, <u>accidental</u> (unintentional)
 Poisoning by agents primarily affecting the gastrointestinal system NOS

T47.92x- Poisoning by unspecified agents primarily affecting the gastrointestinal system, <u>intentional</u> self-harm

T47.93x- Poisoning by unspecified agents primarily affecting the gastrointestinal system, <u>assault</u>

T47.94x- Poisoning by unspecified agents primarily affecting the gastrointestinal system, <u>undetermined</u>

T47.95x- <u>Adverse effect</u> of unspecified agents primarily affecting the gastrointestinal system

T47.96x- <u>Underdosing</u> of unspecified agents primarily affecting the gastrointestinal system

T48- Poisoning by, adverse effect of and underdosing of <u>agents primarily acting on smooth and skeletal muscles and the respiratory system</u>
The appropriate 7th character is to be added to each code from category T48:
A <u>Initial</u> encounter
D <u>Subsequent</u> encounter
S <u>Sequela</u>

T48.0- Poisoning by, adverse effect of and underdosing of oxytocic drugs
 Excludes 1: poisoning by, adverse effect of and underdosing of estrogens, progestogens and antagonists (T38.4-T38.6)

T48.0 - DRUGS/CHEMS*	Ergotrate	Oxytocin (synthetic)
Carboprost	Gemeprost	Pitocin
Dinoprost	Hormone, oxytocic	Prostaglandin E2
Dinoprostone	Methergine	Prostaglandin F2 alpha
Ergobasine	Methyl ergometrine	Sparteine
Ergometrine	Methyl ergonovine	Sulprostone
Ergonovine	Methylergometrine	Syntocinon
Ergot, derivative	Methylergonovine	Tocosamine
Ergot, medicinal (alkaloids)	Muscle affecting agents,	Vetrabutine
Ergot, prepared	oxytocic	
Ergotocine	Oxytocic drug NEC	

T48.0x- Poisoning by, adverse effect of and underdosing of <u>oxytocic drugs</u>

T48.0x1- Poisoning by oxytocic drugs, <u>accidental</u> (unintentional)
 Poisoning by oxytocic drugs NOS

T48.0x2- Poisoning by oxytocic drugs, <u>intentional</u> self-harm

T48.0x3- Poisoning by oxytocic drugs, <u>assault</u>

T48.0x4- Poisoning by oxytocic drugs, <u>undetermined</u>

T48.0x5- <u>Adverse effect</u> of oxytocic drugs

T48.0x6- <u>Underdosing</u> of oxytocic drugs

T48.1- Poisoning by, adverse effect of and underdosing of skeletal muscle relaxants [neuromuscular blocking agents]

T48.1 - DRUGS/CHEMS*	Gallamine (triethiodide)	Relaxant, muscle,
Adlatonium napadisilate	Hexafluorenium bromide	anesthetic
Alcuronium (chloride)	Hexafluronium (bromide)	Relaxant, muscle, skeletal
Anesthesia, muscle	Hexanuorenium	NEC
relaxation	Hexcarbacholine bromide	Skeletal muscle relaxants
Atracurium besilate	Laudexium	Spasmolytic, skeletal
Carbolonium (bromide)	Methocarbamol, skeletal	muscle NEC
Curare, curarine	muscle relaxant	Succinylcholine
Cyclobenzaprine	Mivacurium chloride	Suxamethonium (chloride)
Decamethonium (bromide)	Muscle affecting agents,	Suxethonium (chloride)
Dimethyl tubocurarine	relaxants, skeletal	Tubocurare
Dimethyltubocurarinium	Myoneural blocking agents	Tubocurarine (chloride)
chloride	Neuromuscular blocking	Urari
Fazadinium bromide	drug	Vecuronium bromide
Flaxedil	Pancuronium (bromide)	Woorali

T48.1x- Poisoning by, adverse effect of and underdosing of <u>skeletal muscle relaxants [neuromuscular blocking agents]</u>

T48.1x1- Poisoning by skeletal muscle relaxants [neuromuscular blocking agents], <u>accidental</u> (unintentional)
 Poisoning by skeletal muscle relaxants [neuromuscular blocking agents] NOS

T48.1x2- Poisoning by skeletal muscle relaxants [neuromuscular blocking agents], <u>intentional</u> self-harm

T48.1x3- Poisoning by skeletal muscle relaxants [neuromuscular blocking agents], <u>assault</u>

T48.1x4- Poisoning by skeletal muscle relaxants [neuromuscular blocking agents], <u>undetermined</u>

T48.1x5- <u>Adverse effect</u> of skeletal muscle relaxants [neuromuscular blocking agents]

T48.1x6- <u>Underdosing</u> of skeletal muscle relaxants [neuromuscular blocking agents]

T48.2- Poisoning by, adverse effect of and underdosing of other and unspecified drugs acting on muscles

T48.20- Poisoning by, adverse effect of and underdosing of <u>unspecified drugs acting on muscles</u>

T48.20 - DRUGS/CHEMS*	Muscle affecting agents,	Muscle-action drug NEC
Muscle affecting agents NEC	relaxants	

T48.201- Poisoning by unspecified drugs acting on muscles, <u>accidental</u> (unintentional)
 Poisoning by unspecified drugs acting on muscles NOS

T48.202- Poisoning by unspecified drugs acting on muscles, <u>intentional</u> self-harm

T48.203- Poisoning by unspecified drugs acting on muscles, <u>assault</u>

T48.204- Poisoning by unspecified drugs acting on muscles, <u>undetermined</u>

T48.205- <u>Adverse effect</u> of unspecified drugs acting on muscles

T48.206- <u>Underdosing</u> of unspecified drugs acting on muscles

T48.29- Poisoning by, adverse effect of and underdosing of <u>other drugs acting on muscles</u>

T48.29 - DRUGS/CHEMS*	Dipropyline	Metaproterenol
Botox	Hydrastine	Orciprenaline
Bruceine	Lututrin	Strychnine, medicinal

T48.291- Poisoning by other drugs acting on muscles, <u>accidental</u> (unintentional)
 Poisoning by other drugs acting on muscles NOS

T48.292- Poisoning by other drugs acting on muscles, <u>intentional</u> self-harm

T48.293- Poisoning by other drugs acting on muscles, <u>assault</u>

T48.294- Poisoning by other drugs acting on muscles, <u>undetermined</u>

T48.295- <u>Adverse effect</u> of other drugs acting on muscles

T48.296- <u>Underdosing</u> of other drugs acting on muscles

Excludes 1: = NOT CODED HERE! (Do not code both)   **1185**   *Excludes* ❷: = Not Included Here

T47 - T48

T48.3- **Poisoning by, adverse effect of and underdosing of antitussives**

T48.3 - DRUGS/CHEMS*	Dibunate sodium	Oxeladin (citrate)
Antitussive NEC	Dimemorfan	Oxolamine
Benproperine	Dimethoxanate	Pentoxyverine
Benzonatate	Dropropizine	Pholcodine
Bibenzonium bromide	Ethyl dibunate	Picoperine
Butamirate	Fedrilate	Pipazetate
Carbetapentane	Fominoben	Piperidione
Chlophedianol	Isoaminile (citrate)	Prenoxdiazine
Clobutinol	Levdropropizine	Romilar
Clofedanol	Methorate	Tessalon
Cloperastine	Narcotine	Thebacon
Clophedianol	Nectadon	Tipepidine
Dextromethorphan	Noscapine	Zipeprol

T48.3x- **Poisoning by, adverse effect of and underdosing of antitussives**

T48.3x1- **Poisoning by antitussives, accidental (unintentional)**
Poisoning by antitussives NOS

T48.3x2- **Poisoning by antitussives, intentional self-harm**

T48.3x3- **Poisoning by antitussives, assault**

T48.3x4- **Poisoning by antitussives, undetermined**

T48.3x5- **Adverse effect of antitussives**

T48.3x6- **Underdosing of antitussives**

T48.4- **Poisoning by, adverse effect of and underdosing of expectorants**

T48.4 - DRUGS/CHEMS*	Expectorant NEC	Mucomyst
Acetylcysteine	Glycerol, iodinated	Organidin
Ambroxol	Glyceryl gualacolate	Potassium iodide
Ammonium chloride, expectorant	Glycyrrhiza extract	Quillaja extract
Bromhexine	Glycyrrhizic acid	Respaire
Calcium iodide	Glycyrrhizinate potassium	Respiratory drug, expectorant NEC
Carbocisteine	Guaiacol derivatives	Senega syrup
S-Carboxymethyl-cysteine	Guaifenesin	Sobrerol
Cough mixture (syrup)	Guaimesal	Sodium dibunate
Cough mixture, expectorants	Guaiphenesin	Sputum viscosity-lowering drug
Creosote, medicinal (expectorant)	Hydriodic acid	Stepronin
Creosote, syrup	Iodide, potassium (expectorant) NEC	Sulfogaiacol
Deglycyrrhizinized extract of licorice	Iodinated glycerol	Superinone
Domiodol	Ipecacuanha	Tenoglicin
Dornase	Letosteine	Terpin (cis) hydrate
Eprazinone	Liquorice	Tyloxapol
	Mecysteine	
	Mesna	
	Mucolytic drug	

T48.4x- **Poisoning by, adverse effect of and underdosing of expectorants**

T48.4x1- **Poisoning by expectorants, accidental (unintentional)**
Poisoning by expectorants NOS

T48.4x2- **Poisoning by expectorants, intentional self-harm**

T48.4x3- **Poisoning by expectorants, assault**

T48.4x4- **Poisoning by expectorants, undetermined**

T48.4x5- **Adverse effect of expectorants**

T48.4x6- **Underdosing of expectorants**

T48.5- **Poisoning by, adverse effect of and underdosing of other anti-common-cold drugs**
Poisoning by, adverse effect of and underdosing of decongestants
Excludes 2: *poisoning by, adverse effect of and underdosing of antipyretics, NEC (T39.9-)*
poisoning by, adverse effect of and underdosing of non-steroidal antiinflammatory drugs (T39.3-)
poisoning by, adverse effect of and underdosing of salicylates (T39.0-)

T48.5 - DRUGS/CHEMS*	Decongestant, nasal, combination	Sympathomimetic, anti-common-cold
Amidefrine mesilate	Fenoxazoline	Thonzylamine, mucosal decongestant
Anti-common-cold drug NEC	Indanazoline	Tramazoline
APC	Menthol	Tuaminoheptane
Benzoin (tincture)	Metizoline	Tymazoline
Cinnamedrine	Naphazoline	Xylometazoline
Contac	Oxymetazoline	
Decongestant, nasal (mucosa)	Propylhexedrine	
	Respiratory drug, anti-common-cold NEC	

T48.5x- **Poisoning by, adverse effect of and underdosing of other anti-common-cold drugs**

T48.5x1- **Poisoning by other anti-common-cold drugs, accidental (unintentional)**
Poisoning by other anti-common-cold drugs NOS

T48.5x2- **Poisoning by other anti-common-cold drugs, intentional self-harm**

T48.5x3- **Poisoning by other anti-common-cold drugs, assault**

T48.5x4- **Poisoning by other anti-common-cold drugs, undetermined**

T48.5x5- **Adverse effect of other anti-common-cold drugs**

T48.5x6- **Underdosing of other anti-common-cold drugs**

T48.6- **Poisoning by, adverse effect of and underdosing of antiasthmatics, not elsewhere classified**
Poisoning by, adverse effect of and underdosing of beta-adrenoreceptor agonists used in asthma therapy
Excludes 1: *poisoning by, adverse effect of and underdosing of beta-adrenoreceptor agonists not used in asthma therapy (T44.5)*
poisoning by, adverse effect of and underdosing of anterior pituitary [adenohypophyseal] hormones (T38.8)

T48.6 - DRUGS/CHEMS*	Ethyl noradrenaline	Respiratory drug, antiasthmatic NEC
Acefylline piperazine	Ethylenediamine theophylline	Rimiterol
Acepifylline	Ethylnorepinephrine	Salbutamol
Albuterol	Fenoterol	Salmeterol
Ambuphylline	Flunisolide	Sodium cromoglicate
Aminophylline	Flutropium bromide	Spasmolytic, bronchial NEC
Amlexanox	Folium stramoniae	Stramonium
Antiasthmatic drug NEC	Glyphylline	Sympathomimetic, bronchodilator
Bambuterol	Hexoprenaline	Terbutaline
Bamifylline	Ibuterol	Theobromine (calcium salicylate)
Bitolterol	Ipratropium (bromide)	Theobromine, sodium salicylate
Bronchodilator NEC	Isoetarine	Theophyllamine
Broxaterol	Isoprenaline	Theophylline
Bufrolin	Isoproterenol	Theophylline, aminobenzoic acid
Bufylline	Levalbuterol	Theophylline, ethylenediamine
Butetamate	Levoproxyphylline	Theophylline, piperazine p-amino-benzoate
Carbuterol	Methoxyphenamine	Tretoquinol
Choline	Nedocromil	Tulobuterol
Choline theophyllinate	Oxitropium bromide	
Clenbuterol	Oxtriphylline	
Clorprenaline	Pemirolast (potassium)	
Cromoglicic acid	Pirbuterol	
Cromolyn	Protokylol	
Doxantrazole	Proxyphylline	
Enprofylline	Reproterol	
Etafedrine		
Etamiphyllin		

T48.6x- **Poisoning by, adverse effect of and underdosing of antiasthmatics**

T48.6x1- **Poisoning by antiasthmatics, accidental (unintentional)**
Poisoning by antiasthmatics NOS

Excludes 1: = NOT CODED HERE! (Do not code both)   *Excludes 2:* = Not Included Here

T48.6x2-　Poisoning by antiasthmatics, <u>intentional</u> self-harm

T48.6x3-　Poisoning by antiasthmatics, <u>assault</u>

T48.6x4-　Poisoning by antiasthmatics, <u>undetermined</u>

T48.6x5-　<u>Adverse effect</u> of antiasthmatics

T48.6x6-　<u>Underdosing</u> of antiasthmatics

T48.9-　Poisoning by, adverse effect of and underdosing of other and unspecified agents primarily acting on the respiratory system

T48.90-　Poisoning by, adverse effect of and underdosing of <u>unspecified agents primarily acting on the respiratory system</u>

T48.90 - DRUGS/CHEMS*	Stimulant, respiratory
Respiratory drug NEC	
Respiratory drug, stimulant	

T48.901-　Poisoning by unspecified agents primarily acting on the respiratory system, <u>accidental</u> (unintentional)

T48.902-　Poisoning by unspecified agents primarily acting on the respiratory system, <u>intentional</u> self-harm

T48.903-　Poisoning by unspecified agents primarily acting on the respiratory system, <u>assault</u>

T48.904-　Poisoning by unspecified agents primarily acting on the respiratory system, <u>undetermined</u>

T48.905-　<u>Adverse effect</u> of unspecified agents primarily acting on the respiratory system

T48.906-　<u>Underdosing</u> of unspecified agents primarily acting on the respiratory system

T48.99-　Poisoning by, adverse effect of and underdosing of <u>other agents primarily acting on the respiratory system</u>

T48.99 - DRUGS/CHEMS*	Helium, medicinal
Ammonia, aromatic spirit	

T48.991-　Poisoning by other agents primarily acting on the respiratory system, <u>accidental</u> (unintentional)

T48.992-　Poisoning by other agents primarily acting on the respiratory system, <u>intentional</u> self-harm

T48.993-　Poisoning by other agents primarily acting on the respiratory system, <u>assault</u>

T48.994-　Poisoning by other agents primarily acting on the respiratory system, <u>undetermined</u>

T48.995-　<u>Adverse effect</u> of other agents primarily acting on the respiratory system

T48.996-　<u>Underdosing</u> of other agents primarily acting on the respiratory system

T49-　Poisoning by, adverse effect of and underdosing of <u>topical agents primarily affecting skin and mucous membrane and by ophthalmological, otorhinorlaryngological and dental drugs</u>

Includes:　Poisoning by, adverse effect of and underdosing of glucocorticoids, topically used

The appropriate 7th character is to be added to each code from category T49:

A　<u>Initial</u> encounter

D　<u>Subsequent</u> encounter

S　<u>Sequela</u>

T49.0-　Poisoning by, adverse effect of and underdosing of local antifungal, anti-infective and anti-inflammatory drugs

T49.0 - DRUGS/CHEMS*	Buclosamide	Desonide
Achromycin, topical NEC	Butoconazole (nitrate)	Desoximetasone
Acriflavinium chloride	Cadexomer iodine	Dettol (external
Acrinol	Calomel	medication)
Acrisorcin	Camomile	Dexamethasone, topical
Adrenal, topical NEC	Candeptin	NEC
Aerosporin, topical NEC	Candicidin	Diamthazole
Akrinol	Carbamide, peroxide	Dibromopropamidine
Alclometasone	Carbol fuchsin	isethionate
Alkonium (bromide)	Carfusin	Dibrompropamidine
Allethrin	Castellani's paint	Dicophane
Aluminium acetate solution	Ceepryn	Diethyltoluamide
Aluminium sulfate	Celestone, topical	Diflorasone
Amcinonide	Cetalkonium (chloride)	Diflucortolone
Aminacrine	Cethexonium chloride	Diiodohydroxyquin, topical
Aminoacridine	Cetrimide	Dimazole
Ammoniated mercury	Cetrimonium (bromide)	Dixanthogen
Amphotericin B, topical	Cetylpyridinium chloride	Dodicin
Antibiotic, fungicidal (local)	Chamomile	Dofamium chloride
Antibiotic, local	Chloramine T	Domiphen (bromide)
Antifungal, disinfectant,	Chloramine, topical	Dye, antiseptic
local	Chloramphenicol, topical	Econazole
Antifungal, topical	NEC	Erythromycin, topical NEC
Anti-infective, bismuth,	Chlordantoin	Ethacridine
local	Chlorhexidine	Ethylene oxide, medicinal
Anti-infective, local NEC	Chlorhydroxyquinolin	Eurax
Anti-infective, local,	Chlorinated lime, and boric	Exalamide
specified NEC	acid solution	Fenticlor
Anti-infective, topical NEC	Chlorinated soda solution	Florinef, topical NEC
Anti-inflammatory drug,	Chlorobutanol	Fluclorolone acetonide
local	Chlorocresol	Fludrocortisone, topical
Antiparasitic drug, local	Chloromycetin, topical NEC	NEC
Antiprotozoal drug, local	Chloroxylenol	Fludroxycortide
Antiseptics (external)	Chlorphenesin, topical	Flumethasone
(medicinal)	(antifungal)	Fluocinolone (acetonide)
Argyrol	Chlorquinaldol	Fluocinonide
Aristocort, topical NEC	Chlorquinol	Fluocortin (butyl)
Asiaticoside	Ciclopirox (olamine)	Fluocortolone
Aureomycin, topical NEC	Clobetasol	Fluohydrocortisone, topical
Azelaic acid	Clobetasone	NEC
Bacimycin	Clodantoin	Fluonid
Bacitracin zinc	Clofenotane	Fluormetholone
Bacitracin zinc with	Clotrimazole	Fluorometholone
neomycin	Cloxiquine	Fluprednidene
Bacitracin zinc, topical NEC	Copper gluconate	Flurandrenolide
Basic fuchsin	Copper oleate	Flurandrenolone
Benisone	Cordran	Flurobate
Benzalkonium (chloride)	Cort-Dome, topical NEC	Fungizone, topical
Benzethonium (chloride)	Cortef, topical NEC	Furacin
Benzoic acid	Corticosteroid, topical NEC	Furazolium chloride
Benzoic acid with salicylic	Cortisol	Gamma-benzene
acid	Cortisol, topical NEC	hexachloride
Benzoxonium chloride	Cortisone, topical NEC	(medicinal)
Benzoyl peroxide	Cortril, topical NEC	Gamma-BHC (medicinal) –
Benzydamine	Creosol (compound)	see also Gamma-
Benzyl alcohol	Creosote (coal tar)	benzene hexachloride
Benzyl benzoate	(beechwood)	Garamycin, topical NEC
Benzyl Benzoic acid	Cresol(s)	Gentamicin, topical NEC
Betamethasone	Cresol(s) and soap solution	Gentian, violet
Betamethasone, topical	Cresyl acetate	Gexane
BHC (medicinal)	Cresylic acid	Glutaral (medicinal)
Bismuth salts, formic iodide	Crotamiton	Glutaraldehyde, medicinal
Bismuth salts,	Crystal violet	Glyceryl triacetate (topical)
glycolylarsenate	Cupric gluconate	Gramicidin
Boracic acid	Cupric oleate	Halcinolone
Boric acid	Dakin's solution	Halcinonide
Bromochlorosalicylanilide	Decadron, topical NEC	Halethazole
Bromosalicylchloranitide	Dequalinium (chloride)	

T48 - T49

<u>T49.0</u> - DRUGS/CHEMS*	Methyl paraben	Pyrogallol
– Continued	Methyl prednisolone,	Quarternary ammonium,
Halometasone	topical NEC	anti-infective
Haloprogin	Methyl rosaniline NEC	Retinoic acid
Halotex	Methylbenzethonium	Salicylhydroxamic acid
Halquinols	chloride	Silvadene
HCH, medicinal	Methylrosaniline	Silver
Hedaquinium	Methylrosanilinium	Silver, anti-infectives
Hexachlorophene	chloride	Silver, colloidal
Hexamidine	Micatin	Silver nitrate
Hydrargaphen	Miconazole	Sodium hypochlorite,
Hydrargyri amino-	Mometasone	medicinal (anti-
chloridum	Monistat	infective) (external)
Hydrocortisone	Monosulfiram	Sodium hyposulfite
(derivatives)	Mupirocin	Sodium perborate,
Hydrocortisone, aceponate	Mycifradin, topical	medicinal
Hydrocortisone, topical NEC	Mycostatin, topical	Sodium propionate
Hydrocortone, topical NEC	Myralact	Sporostacin
Hydrogen peroxide	Naftifine	Staphisagria or stavesacre
Hydroxytoluene, medicinal	Natamycin	(pediculicide)
Hypochlorite	Neomycin with bacitracin	Steroid, topical NEC
Ichthammol	Neomycin, topical NEC	Sulbentine
Ilotycin, topical NEC	Neosporin, topical NEC	Sulfacetamide
Iodide NEC – see also	Nilstat, topical	Sulfadiazine, silver
Iodine	Nitrofural	(topical)
Iodide, mercury (ointment)	Nitrofurazone	Sulfamylon
Iodide, methylate	Nitromersol	Sulfiram
Iodine (antiseptic, external)	Nitrozone	Sulfur, ointment
(tincture) NEC	Noxytiolin	Synalar
Iodine solution	Nystatin, topical	Terconazole
Iodochlorhydroxyquin,	Orthoboric acid	Tetracycline, topical NEC
topical	Oxiconazole	Tetramethylthiuram,
Iodoform	Oxychlorosene	medicinal
Isoconazole	Oxylone	Thimerosal
Ketoconazole	Parachlorophenol	Thiomersal
Kwell, anti-infective	(camphorated)	Thymol
(topical)	Paramethasone acetate	Ticlatone
Laurolinium	Peruvian balsam	Tioconazole
Lidex	Phenoctide	Tolciclate
Lindane, medicinal	Phenol	Tolnaftate
Locorten	Phenothrin	Tretinoin
Lysozyme	Phenoxyethanol	Triacetin
Mafenide	Phenylmercuric acetate	Triamcinolone
Magnesium peroxide	Phenylmercuric borate	Triamcinolone,
Malathion (medicinal)	Phenylmercuric nitrate	hexacetonide
Maphenide	Piketoprofen	Triamcinolone, topical NEC
Medrysone	Polymyxin B, topical NEC	Triclobisonium chloride
Melaleuca alternifolia oil	Polynoxylin	Triclocarban
Merbromin	Polyoxymethyleneurea	Triclosan
Mercaptobenzothiazole	Potassium iodate	Tridesilon
salts	Potassium permanganate,	Undecenoic acid
Mercurochrome	medicinal	Undecoylium
Mercury, ammoniated	Povidone, iodine	Undecylenic acid
Mercury, anti-infective,	Prednicarbate	(derivatives)
local	Prednisolone, steaglate	Urea peroxide
Mercury, anti-infective,	Prednisolone, topical NEC	Valisone
topical	Proflavine	Vioform, topical
Mercury, chloride	Propamidine	Zephiran (topical)
(ammoniated)	Propiolactone	Zinc, anti-infectives
Mercury, oxide, yellow	Propion gel	Zinc bacitracin
Merthiolate	Propionate (calcium)	Zinc peroxide
Mesulfen	(sodium)	Zinc sulfate, topical NEC
Metactesylacetate	Pyrethrum extract	Zinc undecylenate
Metaphen	Pyrogallic acid	

T49.0x- **Poisoning by, adverse effect of and underdosing of** <u>local antifungal, anti-infective and anti-inflammatory drugs</u>

T49.0x1- **Poisoning by local antifungal, anti-infective and anti-inflammatory drugs,** <u>accidental</u> **(unintentional)**
   Poisoning by local antifungal, anti-infective and anti-inflammatory drugs NOS

T49.0x2- **Poisoning by local antifungal, anti-infective and anti-inflammatory drugs,** <u>intentional</u> **self-harm**

T49.0x3- **Poisoning by local antifungal, anti-infective and anti-inflammatory drugs,** <u>assault</u>

T49.0x4- **Poisoning by local antifungal, anti-infective and anti-inflammatory drugs,** <u>undetermined</u>

T49.0x5- <u>Adverse effect</u> **of local antifungal, anti-infective and anti-inflammatory drugs**

T49.0x6- <u>Underdosing</u> **of local antifungal, anti-infective and anti-inflammatory drugs**

T49.1- **Poisoning by, adverse effect of and underdosing of antipruritics**

<u>T49.1</u> - DRUGS/CHEMS*	ESDT (ether-soluble tar	Pramocaine
Antipruritic drug NEC	distillate)	Pramoxine
Benzamine, lactate	Fluticasone propionate	Quinisocaine
b-eucaine	Juniper tar	Tar, distillate
Coal tar	Phenol, medicinal	Tar, medicinal
Dimethisoquin	Phenolic preparation	Tar, ointment

T49.1x- **Poisoning by, adverse effect of and underdosing of** <u>antipruritics</u>

T49.1x1- **Poisoning by antipruritics,** <u>accidental</u> **(unintentional)**
   Poisoning by antipruritics NOS

T49.1x2- **Poisoning by antipruritics,** <u>intentional</u> **self-harm**

T49.1x3- **Poisoning by antipruritics,** <u>assault</u>

T49.1x4- **Poisoning by antipruritics,** <u>undetermined</u>

T49.1x5- <u>Adverse effect</u> **of antipruritics**

T49.1x6- <u>Underdosing</u> **of antipruritics**

T49.2- **Poisoning by, adverse effect of and underdosing of local astringents and local detergents**

<u>T49.2</u> - DRUGS/CHEMS*	Detergent, local	Septisol
Acetic acid medicinal	Detergent, medicinal	Soap, medicinal, soft
(lotion)	Dial (soap)	Soap, superfatted
Aluminium acetate	Duponol (C) (EP)	Sodium lauryl (sulfate)
Aluminium chloride	Green soap	Sulfatostearate
Aluminium diacetate	Hamamelis	Tannic acid
Aluminium subacetate	Hexa-germ	Tannic acid, medicinal
Antihemorrhoidal	Iproheptine	(astringent)
preparation	Lauryl sulfoacetate	Thiram, medicinal
Antiperspirant NEC	Lead acetate	Vegetable extract,
Astringent (local)	Lowila	astringent
Astringent, specified NEC	Methyl salicylate	Witch hazel
Detergent	pHisoHex	
Detergent, external	Polyethanolamine alkyl	
medication	sulfate	

T49.2x- **Poisoning by, adverse effect of and underdosing of** <u>local astringents and local detergents</u>

T49.2x1- **Poisoning by local astringents and local detergents,** <u>accidental</u> **(unintentional)**
   Poisoning by local astringents and local detergents NOS

T49.2x2- **Poisoning by local astringents and local detergents,** <u>intentional</u> **self-harm**

T49.2x3- **Poisoning by local astringents and local detergents,** <u>assault</u>

T49.2x4- **Poisoning by local astringents and local detergents,** <u>undetermined</u>

T49.2x5- <u>Adverse effect</u> **of local astringents and local detergents**

T49.2x6- <u>Underdosing</u> **of local astringents and local detergents**

T49 - T49

T49.3-   Poisoning by, adverse effect of and underdosing of emollients, demulcents and protectants

T49.3 - DRUGS/CHEMS*		
Acetic acid with sodium acetate (ointment)	Filtering cream	Plaster dressing
Acrylic resin	Flaxseed (medicinal)	Plastic dressing
Allylthiourea	Homosalate	Polyethylene adhesive
Aluminium ointment (surgical) (topical)	Hydrophilic lotion	Protectant, skin NEC
Aluminium topical NEC	Hydrous wool fat	Pyroxylin
Aminobenzoic acid (-p)	Lanolin	Rose water ointment
Arachis oil	Liquid petrolatum, topical	Salicylate, methyl
Barrier cream	Mecrilate	Salol
Bentonite	Meladinin	Silicone, medicinal
Benzophenones	Melanizing agents	Solar lotion
Betula oil	Meloxine	Sulisobenzone
Calamine (lotion)	Methoxa-Dome	Sweet oil (birch)
Carbowax	Mexenone	Talc powder
Cellulose, nitrates (topical)	Mineral oil, topical	Talcum
Chlordiethyl benzamide	Nutmeg oil (liniment)	Thiosinamine
Cold cream	Octafonium (chloride)	Titanium dioxide
Collodion	Oil, wintergreen (bitter) NEC	Titanium ointment
Colophony adhesive	Oily preparation (for skin)	Titanium oxide
Corn starch	Ointment NEC	Trimethylpsoralen
Cornhusker's lotion	Oxsoralen	Trisoralen
Cottonseed oil	PABA	Ultraviolet light protectant
Cyanoacrylate adhesive	Padimate	Unna's boot
Demulcent (external)	Para-aminobenzoic acid	Vaseline
Demulcent, specified NEC	Peanut oil, topical	Wintergreen (oil)
Diethyl toluamide, medicinal	Petrolatum	Wool fat (hydrous)
Dimethyl phthlate	Petrolatum, hydrophilic	Xanthotoxin
Emollient NEC	Petrolatum, liquid, topical	Zinc, gelatin
	Petrolatum, red veterinary	Zinc oxide
	Petrolatum, white	Zinc oxide, plaster
	Phenyl salicylate	Zinc stearate

T49.3x-   Poisoning by, adverse effect of and underdosing of <u>emollients, demulcents and protectants</u>

    T49.3x1-   Poisoning by emollients, demulcents and protectants, <u>accidental</u> (unintentional)
       Poisoning by emollients, demulcents and protectants NOS

    T49.3x2-   Poisoning by emollients, demulcents and protectants, <u>intentional</u> self-harm

    T49.3x3-   Poisoning by emollients, demulcents and protectants, <u>assault</u>

    T49.3x4-   Poisoning by emollients, demulcents and protectants, <u>undetermined</u>

    T49.3x5-   <u>Adverse effect</u> of emollients, demulcents and protectants

    T49.3x6-   <u>Underdosing</u> of emollients, demulcents and protectants

T49.4-   Poisoning by, adverse effect of and underdosing of keratolytics, keratoplastics, and other hair treatment drugs and preparations

T49.4 - DRUGS/CHEMS*		
Allantoin	Dimethylamine sulfate	Salicylic acid with benzoic acid
Alum (medicinal)	Dithranol	Savin (oil)
Ammonium ichthyosulronate	Enzyme, local action	Selenium disulfide or sulfide
Anthralin	Enzyme, proteolytic	Selenium sulfide
Antiseborrheics	Ethyl chloride, local	Selsun
Bleaching agent (medicinal)	Ethyl fumarate	Silver nitrate, toughened (keratolytic)
Butantrone	Euresol	Silver sulfadiazine
Cade oil	Flowers of sulfur	Sulfur, sulfurated, sulfuric, sulfurous, sulfuryl (compounds NEC) (medicinal)
Cadmium sulfide (medicinal) NEC	Fumaric acid	
Capsicum	Hair dye	
Carbazochrome (salicylate) (sodium sulfonate)	Hair preparation NEC	Sulfur, medicinal (keratolytic) (ointment) NEC
Carbon dioxide, snow	Hemostyptic	
Cellulose, oxidized	Ichthyol	Thioglycolate
Chlorothymol	Isopropyl alcohol, medicinal	Tioxolone
Chloroxine	Keratolytic drug NEC	Triacetoxyanthracene
Chrysarobin	Keratolytic drug, anthracene	Trichloroacetic acid, medicinal
Coal tar, medicinal (ointment)	Keratoplastic NEC	Trioxysalen
Collagenase	Lassar's paste	Vleminckx's solution
Corn cures	Methyl nicotinate	White lotion (keratolytic)
Depilatory	Monobenzone	Xenysalate
Desloughing agent	Podophyllum (resin)	Zinc pyrithionate
Diachylon plaster	Preparation, local	
Dimethyl sulfoxide, medicinal	Pyrithione zinc	
	Resorcin, resorcinol, medicinal	
	Rubefacient	
	Salicylic acid	

T49.4x-   Poisoning by, adverse effect of and underdosing of <u>keratolytics, keratoplastics, and other hair treatment drugs and preparations</u>

    T49.4x1-   Poisoning by keratolytics, keratoplastics, and other hair treatment drugs and preparations, <u>accidental</u> (unintentional)
       Poisoning by keratolytics, keratoplastics, and other hair treatment drugs and preparations NOS

    T49.4x2-   Poisoning by keratolytics, keratoplastics, and other hair treatment drugs and preparations, <u>intentional</u> self-harm

    T49.4x3-   Poisoning by keratolytics, keratoplastics, and other hair treatment drugs and preparations, <u>assault</u>

    T49.4x4-   Poisoning by keratolytics, keratoplastics, and other hair treatment drugs and preparations, <u>undetermined</u>

    T49.4x5-   <u>Adverse effect</u> of keratolytics, keratoplastics, and other hair treatment drugs and preparations

    T49.4x6-   <u>Underdosing</u> of keratolytics, keratoplastics, and other hair treatment drugs and preparations

T49.5-   Poisoning by, adverse effect of and underdosing of ophthalmological drugs and preparations

T49.5 - DRUGS/CHEMS*		
Achromycin, ophthalmic preparation	Bacimycin, ophthalmic preparation	Colistin sulfate (eye preparation)
Adrenal, ophthalmic preparation	Bacitracin zinc, ophthalmic preparation	Contact lens solution
Aerosporin, ophthalmic preparation	Befunolol	Copper sulfate, cupric, medicinal, eye
Ammonium acid tartrate	Benzalkonium, ophthalmic preparation	Copper sulfate, medicinal, eye
Antibiotic, eye	Bibrocathol	Cort-Dome, ophthalmic preparation
Anticholinesterase, reversible, ophthalmological	Boracic acid, ophthalmic preparation	Cortef, ophthalmic preparation
Anti-infective, eye NEC	Boric acid, ophthalmic preparation	Corticosteroid, ophthalmic
Anti-infective, ophthalmic preparation	Chloramphenicol, ophthalmic preparation	Cortisol, ophthalmic preparation
Antiviral drug, eye	Chloromycetin, ophthalmic preparation	Cortisone, ophthalmic preparation
Argyrol, ophthalmic preparation	Chloroptic	Cortogen, ophthalmic preparation
Aristocort, ophthalmic preparation	Chymar, ophthalmic preparation	Cortone, ophthalmic preparation
Aureomycin, ophthalmic preparation	Chymotrypsin, ophthalmic preparation	Cortril, ophthalmic preparation

T 4 9 - T 4 9

Excludes 1: = NOT CODED HERE! (Do not code both)   **1189**   *Excludes ❷:* = Not Included Here

T49.5 - DRUGS/CHEMS* – Continued		
Cycloplegic drug	Hydrocortisone, ophthalmic preparation	Prednisolone, ophthalmic preparation
Decadron, ophthalmic preparation	Hydrocortone, ophthalmic preparation	Propylparaben (ophthalmic)
Demecarium (bromide)	Hydroxyamphetamine	Silver nitrate, ophthalmic preparation
Dendrid	Hypromellose	Silver, protein
Dexamethasone, ophthalmic preparation	Ilotycin, ophthalmic preparation	Sodium borate, cleanser, eye
Dipivefrine	Irrigating fluid, eye	Steroid, ophthalmic preparation
Echothiophate, echothiophate, ecothiopate	Lachesine	Stoxil
Levobunolol	Sulfacetamide, ophthalmic preparation
Ecothiopate iodide	Lubricant, eye	Sulfisoxazole, ophthalmic preparation
Edoxudine	Merthiolate, ophthalmic preparation	
Erythromycin, ophthalmic preparation	Methyl prednisolone, ophthalmic preparation	Sulfonamide, eye
Eserine	Methylparaben (ophthalmic)	Tear solution
Eucatropine	Metipranolol	Tetracycline, ophthalmic preparation
External medications, ophthalmic preparation	Miotic drug	Tetrahydrozoline
Mycitracin, ophthalmic preparation	Tetryzoline
Eye agents (anti-infective)	Mydriatic drug	Thimerosal, ophthalmic preparation
Eye drug NEC	Neomycin, ophthalmic preparation	
Florinef, ophthalmic preparation	Topical action drug, eye
Fludrocortisone, ophthalmic preparation	Neosporin, ophthalmic preparation	Triamcinolone, ophthalmic preparation
Fluohydrocortisone, ophthalmic preparation	Orthoboric acid, ophthalmic preparation	Tyrothricin, ophthalmic preparation
Fluorometholone, ophthalmic preparation	Oxylone, ophthalmic preparation	Visine
Zephiran, ophthalmic preparation
Fluorphenylalanine	Phospholine	Zinc sulfate
Garamycin, ophthalmic preparation	Physostigmine	Zinc sulfate, ophthalmic solution
Polymyxin B, ophthalmic preparation
Gentamicin, ophthalmic preparation	Polymyxin E sulfate (eye preparation)	
Herplex		

T49.5x- Poisoning by, adverse effect of and underdosing of ophthalmological drugs and preparations

T49.5x1- Poisoning by ophthalmological drugs and preparations, <u>accidental</u> (unintentional)
   Poisoning by ophthalmological drugs and preparations NOS

T49.5x2- Poisoning by ophthalmological drugs and preparations, <u>intentional</u> self-harm

T49.5x3- Poisoning by ophthalmological drugs and preparations, <u>assault</u>

T49.5x4- Poisoning by ophthalmological drugs and preparations, <u>undetermined</u>

T49.5x5- <u>Adverse effect</u> of ophthalmological drugs and preparations

T49.5x6- <u>Underdosing</u> of ophthalmological drugs and preparations

T49.6- Poisoning by, adverse effect of and underdosing of otorhinolaryngological drugs and preparations

T49.6 - DRUGS/CHEMS*		
Adrenal, ENT agent	Cetylpyridinium chloride, lozenges	Ear drug NEC
Aerosporin, ENT agent	Chloramphenicol, ENT agent	Ear preparations
Alkaline antiseptic solution (aromatic)	ENT preparations (anti-infectives)
Chloromycetin, ENT agent
Ambazone	Chloromycetin, otic solution	External medications, ENT agent
Amylmetacresol	Copper sulfate, cupric, medicinal, ear	
Antibiotic, ENT	Florinef, ENT agent
Antibiotic, throat	Copper sulfate, medicinal, ear	Fludrocortisone, ENT agent
Anti-infective, ENT	Fluohydrocortisone, ENT agent
Argyrol, ENT agent	Corbadrine	
Aristocort, ENT agent	Cort-Dome, ENT agent	Glycerol, borax
Bacitracin zinc, ENT agent	Cortef, ENT agent	Hydrocortisone, ENT agent
Biclotymol	Corticosteroid, ENT agent	Hydrocortone, ENT agent
Bisdequalinium (salts) (diacetate)	Cortisol, ENT agent	Levonordefrin
Cortisone, ENT agent	Lozenges (throat)
Boracic acid, ENT agent	Cortogen, ENT agent	Methyl prednisolone, ENT agent
Boric acid, ENT agent	Cortone, ENT agent	
Ceepryn, ENT agent	Cortril, ENT agent	Mouthwash (antiseptic) (zinc chloride)
Ceepryn, lozenges	Decadron, ENT agent	
Cetylpyridinium chloride, ENT agent	Dexamethasone, ENT agent	Nasal drug NEC
Dichlorobenzyl alcohol	Neomycin, ENT agent

T49.6 - DRUGS/CHEMS* – Continued		
Neosporin, ENT agent	Polymyxin B, ENT agent	Triamcinolone, ENT agent
Nose preparations	Prednisolone, ENT agent	Tyrothricin
Orthoboric acid, ENT agent	Steroid, ENT agent	Tyrothricin, ENT agent
Otorhinolaryngological drug NEC	Thenoic acid	Zinc chloride (mouthwash)
Throat drug NEC	Zinc sulfate, ENT agent
Topical action drug, ear, nose or throat	

T49.6x- Poisoning by, adverse effect of and underdosing of <u>otorhinolaryngological drugs and preparations</u>

T49.6x1- Poisoning by otorhinolaryngological drugs and preparations, <u>accidental</u> (unintentional)
   Poisoning by otorhinolaryngological drugs and preparations NOS

T49.6x2- Poisoning by otorhinolaryngological drugs and preparations, <u>intentional</u> self-harm

T49.6x3- Poisoning by otorhinolaryngological drugs and preparations, <u>assault</u>

T49.6x4- Poisoning by otorhinolaryngological drugs and preparations, <u>undetermined</u>

T49.6x5- <u>Adverse effect</u> of otorhinolaryngological drugs and preparations

T49.6x6- <u>Underdosing</u> of otorhinolaryngological drugs and preparations

T49.7- Poisoning by, adverse effect of and underdosing of <u>dental drugs, topically applied</u>

T49.7 - DRUGS/CHEMS*		
Dental drug, topical application NEC	External medications, dental agent	Oil, cloves
Pulp, devitalizing paste
Dentifrice	Fluoride, medicinal, dental use	Pulp, dressing
Dressing, live pulp	Stannous fluoride
Eucalyptus oil	Fluoride, stannous	
Fluoristan	

T49.7x- Poisoning by, adverse effect of and underdosing of <u>dental drugs, topically applied</u>

T49.7x1- Poisoning by dental drugs, topically applied, <u>accidental</u> (unintentional)
   Poisoning by dental drugs, topically applied NOS

T49.7x2- Poisoning by dental drugs, topically applied, <u>intentional</u> self-harm

T49.7x3- Poisoning by dental drugs, topically applied, <u>assault</u>

T49.7x4- Poisoning by dental drugs, topically applied, <u>undetermined</u>

T49.7x5- <u>Adverse effect</u> of dental drugs, topically applied

T49.7x6- <u>Underdosing</u> of dental drugs, topically applied

T49.8- Poisoning by, adverse effect of and underdosing of other topical agents
   Poisoning by, adverse effect of and underdosing of spermicides

T49.8 - DRUGS/CHEMS*		
Benoquin	Dextromoramide, topical	Octoxinol (9)
Camphor, medicinal	Elase	Panthenol, topical
Cantharides, cantharidin, cantharis	Enzyme, depolymizing	Podophyllotoxin
External medications, specified NEC	Preparation H
Carbamide, topical	Gelfilm	Santyl
Cell stimulants and proliferants	Heet	Scarlet red
Irrigating fluid (vaginal)	Skin agents, specified NEC
Charcoal, medicinal, topical	Lactic acid	Sodium borate, therapeutic
Chloresium	Local action drug NEC	Spanish fly
Contraceptive, vaginal	Lytta (vitatta)	Spermicide
Cosmetic preparation	Mucous membrane agents, specified NEC	Topical action drug, specified NEC
Cosmetics	Tosylchloramide sodium
Demelanizing agents	Nonoxinol	Urea, topical
Deodorant spray (feminine hygiene)	Nonylphenoxy (polyethoxy-ethanol)	Vaginal contraceptives

T49.8x- Poisoning by, adverse effect of and underdosing of <u>other topical agents</u>

T49.8x1- Poisoning by other topical agents, <u>accidental</u> (unintentional)
   Poisoning by other topical agents NOS

T49.8x2- Poisoning by other topical agents, <u>intentional</u> self-harm

T49.8x3- Poisoning by other topical agents, <u>assault</u>

T49.8x4- Poisoning by other topical agents, <u>undetermined</u>

T49 - T49

T49.8x5-   <u>Adverse effect</u> of other topical agents

T49.8x6-   <u>Underdosing</u> of other topical agents

T49.9-   Poisoning by, adverse effect of and underdosing of <u>unspecified</u> <u>topical</u> agent

<u>T49.9</u> - DRUGS/CHEMS*	Lotions NEC	Topical action drug NEC
External medications (skin) (mucous membrane)	Mucous membrane agents (external)	Topical action drug, skin (external)
Liniments NEC	Skin agents (external)	

T49.91x-   Poisoning by unspecified topical agent, <u>accidental</u> (unintentional)

T49.92x-   Poisoning by unspecified topical agent, <u>intentional</u> self-harm

T49.93x-   Poisoning by unspecified topical agent, <u>assault</u>

T49.94x-   Poisoning by unspecified topical agent, <u>undetermined</u>

T49.95x-   <u>Adverse effect</u> of unspecified topical agent

T49.96x-   <u>Underdosing</u> of unspecified topical agent

T50-   Poisoning by, adverse effect of and underdosing of <u>diuretics and other and unspecified drugs, medicaments and biological substances</u>

The appropriate 7th character is to be added to each code from category T50:
A   <u>Initial</u> encounter
D   <u>Subsequent</u> encounter
S   <u>Sequela</u>

T50.0-   Poisoning by, adverse effect of and underdosing of mineralocorticoids and their antagonists

<u>T50.0</u> - DRUGS/CHEMS*	Corticosteroid, mineral	Mineralocorticosteroid
Aldactone	Deoxycortone	Potassium canrenoate
Aldosterone	Desoxycorticosteroid	Salt-retaining
Antagonist, aldosterone	Desoxycortone	mineralocorticoid
Canrenoic acid	Fludrocortisone	Spironolactone
Canrenone	Fluorhydrocortisone	

T50.0x-   Poisoning by, adverse effect of and underdosing of <u>mineralocorticoids and their antagonists</u>

T50.0x1-   Poisoning by mineralocorticoids and their antagonists, <u>accidental</u> (unintentional)
    Poisoning by mineralocorticoids and their antagonists NOS

T50.0x2-   Poisoning by mineralocorticoids and their antagonists, <u>intentional</u> self-harm

T50.0x3-   Poisoning by mineralocorticoids and their antagonists, <u>assault</u>

T50.0x4-   Poisoning by mineralocorticoids and their antagonists, <u>undetermined</u>

T50.0x5-   <u>Adverse effect</u> of mineralocorticoids and their antagonists

T50.0x6-   <u>Underdosing</u> of mineralocorticoids and their antagonists

T50.1-   Poisoning by, adverse effect of and underdosing of loop [high-ceiling] diuretics

<u>T50.1</u> - DRUGS/CHEMS*	Ethacrynic acid	Piretanide
Bumetanide	Etozolin	Sodium ethacrynate
Diuretic, loop (high-ceiling)	Frusemide	Ticrynafen
Edecrin	Furosemide	Tienilic acid
Etacrynate sodium	Lasix	
Etacrynic acid	Lyovac Sodium Edecrin	

T50.1x-   Poisoning by, adverse effect of and underdosing of <u>loop [high-ceiling] diuretics</u>

T50.1x1-   Poisoning by loop [high-ceiling] diuretics, <u>accidental</u> (unintentional)
    Poisoning by loop [high-ceiling] diuretics NOS

T50.1x2-   Poisoning by loop [high-ceiling] diuretics, <u>intentional</u> self-harm

T50.1x3-   Poisoning by loop [high-ceiling] diuretics, <u>assault</u>

T50.1x4-   Poisoning by loop [high-ceiling] diuretics, <u>undetermined</u>

T50.1x5-   <u>Adverse effect</u> of loop [high-ceiling] diuretics

T50.1x6-   <u>Underdosing</u> of loop [high-ceiling] diuretics

T50.2-   Poisoning by, adverse effect of and underdosing of carbonic-anhydrase inhibitors, benzothiadiazides and other diuretics
    Poisoning by, adverse effect of and underdosing of acetazolamide

<u>T50.2</u> - DRUGS/CHEMS*	Diucardin	Mercurophylline
Acetazolamide	Diupres	Mercury, diuretic NEC
Altizide	Diuretic NEC	Mersalyl
Amiloride	Diuretic, benzothiadiazine	Methazolamide
Aminometradine	Diuretic, carbonic acid	Methyclothiazide
Amisometradine	anhydrase inhibitors	Meticrane
Anhydron	Diuretic, furfuryl NEC	Metolazone
Bendrofluazide	Diuretic, mercurial NEC	Osmotic diuretics
Bendroflumethiazide	Diuretic, osmotic	Penflutizide
Benzothiadiazides	Diuretic, purine NEC	Polythiazide
Benzthiazide	Diuretic, saluretic NEC	Purine diuretics
Benzylhydrochlorthiazide	Diuretic, sulfonamide	Quinethazone
Butizide	Diuretic, thiazide NEC	Regroton
Carbonic acid gas,	Diuretic, xanthine	Renese
anhydrase inhibitor NEC	Diurgin	Salicylate, theobromine
Cardrase	Diuril	calcium
Chlorazanil	Epitizide	Saluretic NEC
Chlormerodrin	Equisetum, diuretic	Saluron
Chlorothiazide	Ethamide	Sodium mersalate
Chlortalidone	Ethiazide	Teclothiazide
Chlorthalidone	Ethoxzolamide	Tetrachlormethiazide
Clofenamide	Fenquizone	Thiazides (diuretics)
Clopamide	Flumethiazide	Thiomercaptomerin
Clorexolone	Hydrochlorothiazide	Thiomerin
Cyclopenthiazide	Hydroflumethiazide	Tiamizide
Cyclothiazide	Hydromox	Triamterene
Diamox	Inhibitor, carbonic	Trichlormethiazide
Dichlorphenamide	anhydrase	Tripamide
Diclofenamide	Mefruside	Trometamol
Dihydroxypropyl	Meralluride	Tromethamine
theophylline	Merbaphen	Xanthine diuretics
Diphylline	Mercaptomerin	Xipamide
Diprophylline	Mercumatilin	Zaroxolyn
Disulfamide	Mercuramide	

T50.2x-   Poisoning by, adverse effect of and underdosing of <u>carbonic-anhydrase inhibitors, benzothiadiazides and other diuretics</u>

T50.2x1-   Poisoning by carbonic-anhydrase inhibitors, benzothiadiazides and other diuretics, <u>accidental</u> (unintentional)
    Poisoning by carbonic-anhydrase inhibitors, benzothiadiazides and other diuretics NOS

T50.2x2-   Poisoning by carbonic-anhydrase inhibitors, benzothiadiazides and other diuretics, <u>intentional</u> self-harm

T50.2x3-   Poisoning by carbonic-anhydrase inhibitors, benzothiadiazides and other diuretics, <u>assault</u>

T50.2x4-   Poisoning by carbonic-anhydrase inhibitors, benzothiadiazides and other diuretics, <u>undetermined</u>

T50.2x5-   <u>Adverse effect</u> of carbonic-anhydrase inhibitors, benzothiadiazides and other diuretics

T50.2x6-   <u>Underdosing</u> of carbonic-anhydrase inhibitors, benzothiadiazides and other diuretics

T50.3-   Poisoning by, adverse effect of and underdosing of electrolytic, caloric and water-balance agents
    Poisoning by, adverse effect of and underdosing of oral rehydration salts

<u>T50.3</u> - DRUGS/CHEMS*	Caloric agent	Hartmann's solution
Acetic acid irrigating solution	Carbacrylamine (resin)	Invert sugar
Amino acids	Cation exchange resin	Ion exchange resin, cation
Aminoacetic acid (derivatives)	Dextrose	Lactated potassic saline
	Dialysis solution (intraperitoneal)	Levulose
Antikaluretic	Electrolyte balance drug	Magnesium silicofluoride
Calcium	Electrolytes NEC	Mineral salt NEC
Calcium glubionate	Electrolytic agent NEC	Oral rehydration salts
Calcium gluconate	Fructose	Peritoneal dialysis solution
Calcium gluconogalactogluc- onate	Galactose	Polyaminostyrene resins
	Glucose	Potassic saline injection (lactated)
Calcium lactate	Glucose with sodium chloride	Potassium (salts) NEC
Calcium phosphate	Glycerol, intravenous	Potassium chloride
Calcium salts	Glycine	Potassium-removing resin
		Potassium-retaining drug

T49 - T50

T50.3 - DRUGS/CHEMS* – Continued	Sodium chloride with glucose	Sodium removing resins
Rehydration salts (oral)	Sodium cyclamate	Sodium salt NEC
Replacement solution	Sodium, free salt	Sodium-removing resin
Ringer (lactate) solution	Sodium hydrogen	Sucrose
Sodium acid phosphate	carbonate	Travert
Sodium biphosphate	Sodium polystyrene	Water balance drug
Sodium chloride	sulfonate	Water, distilled
		Water, purified

T50.3x- Poisoning by, adverse effect of and underdosing of <u>electrolytic, caloric and water-balance agents</u>

T50.3x1- Poisoning by electrolytic, caloric and water-balance agents, <u>accidental</u> (unintentional)
Poisoning by electrolytic, caloric and water-balance agents NOS

T50.3x2- Poisoning by electrolytic, caloric and water-balance agents, <u>intentional</u> self-harm

T50.3x3- Poisoning by electrolytic, caloric and water-balance agents, <u>assault</u>

T50.3x4- Poisoning by electrolytic, caloric and water-balance agents, <u>undetermined</u>

T50.3x5- <u>Adverse effect</u> of electrolytic, caloric and water-balance agents

T50.3x6- <u>Underdosing</u> of electrolytic, caloric and water-balance agents

T50.4- Poisoning by, adverse effect of and underdosing of drugs affecting uric acid metabolism

T50.4 - DRUGS/CHEMS*	Etebenecid	Sulfinpyrazone
Allopurinol	Ethebenecid	Sulphinpyrazone
Atophan	Neocinchophen	Tisopurine
Benemid	Oxipurinol	Urate oxidase
Benzbromarone	Phenoquin	Uric acid metabolism drug
Cinchophen	Probenecid	NEC
Colchicine	Spindle inactivator	Uricosuric agent

T50.4x- Poisoning by, adverse effect of and underdosing of <u>drugs affecting uric acid metabolism</u>

T50.4x1- Poisoning by drugs affecting uric acid metabolism, <u>accidental</u> (unintentional)
Poisoning by drugs affecting uric acid metabolism NOS

T50.4x2- Poisoning by drugs affecting uric acid metabolism, <u>intentional</u> self-harm

T50.4x3- Poisoning by drugs affecting uric acid metabolism, <u>assault</u>

T50.4x4- Poisoning by drugs affecting uric acid metabolism, <u>undetermined</u>

T50.4x5- <u>Adverse effect</u> of drugs affecting uric acid metabolism

T50.4x6- <u>Underdosing</u> of drugs affecting uric acid metabolism

T50.5- Poisoning by, adverse effect of and underdosing of appetite depressants

T50.5 - DRUGS/CHEMS*	Chlorphentermine	Fenproporex
Amfepramone	Clobenzorex	Levopropylhexedrine
Aminorex	Cloforex	Mazindol
Anorexiant (central)	Clortermine	Mefenorex
Anorexic agents	Depressant, appetite	Norpseudoephedrine
Appetite depressants, central	Depressant, appetite, central	Oxazimedrine
Benzamphetamine	Dexfenfluramine	Phenbutrazate
Benzfetamine	Diethyl propion	Phendimetrazine
Benzphetamine	Diethylpropion	Phenmetrazine
Bulk filler	Fenbutrazate	Phentermine
Cathine	Fenfluramine	

T50.5x- Poisoning by, adverse effect of and underdosing of <u>appetite depressants</u>

T50.5x1- Poisoning by appetite depressants, <u>accidental</u> (unintentional)
Poisoning by appetite depressants NOS

T50.5x2- Poisoning by appetite depressants, <u>intentional</u> self-harm

T50.5x3- Poisoning by appetite depressants, <u>assault</u>

T50.5x4- Poisoning by appetite depressants, <u>undetermined</u>

T50.5x5- <u>Adverse effect</u> of appetite depressants

T50.5x6- <u>Underdosing</u> of appetite depressants

T50.6- Poisoning by, adverse effect of and underdosing of antidotes and chelating agents
Poisoning by, adverse effect of and underdosing of alcohol deterrents

T50.6 - DRUGS/CHEMS*	Ethylenedinitrilotetra-acetate	Pralidoxime, chloride
Alcohol, deterrent NEC		Protopam
Antabuse	Fytic acid, nonasodium	Prussian blue, therapeutic
Antidote NEC	Glutathione	Pyridine, aldoxime
Calcium carbimide	Methylene blue	methiodide
Chelating agent NEC	Methylthionine chloride	Pyridine, aldoxime methyl
Cholinesterase reactivator	Methylthioninium chloride	chloride
Cysteamine	Nitrefazole	Sodium nitrite
Deterrent, alcohol	Obidoxime chloride	Sodium phytate
Detoxifying agent	PAM (pralidoxime)	Sodium thiosulfate
Disodium edetate	Penicillamine	Sodium versenate
Disulfiram	Potassium ferric	Tetraethylthiuram disulfide
EDTA	hexacyanoferrate	Trisodium hydrogen
Ethylenediaminetetra-acetic acid	(medicinal)	edetate
	Pralidoxime (iodide)	Versenate

T50.6x- Poisoning by, adverse effect of and underdosing of <u>antidotes and chelating agents</u>

T50.6x1- Poisoning by antidotes and chelating agents, <u>accidental</u> (unintentional)
Poisoning by antidotes and chelating agents NOS

T50.6x2- Poisoning by antidotes and chelating agents, <u>intentional</u> self-harm

T50.6x3- Poisoning by antidotes and chelating agents, <u>assault</u>

T50.6x4- Poisoning by antidotes and chelating agents, <u>undetermined</u>

T50.6x5- <u>Adverse effect</u> of antidotes and chelating agents

T50.6x6- <u>Underdosing</u> of antidotes and chelating agents

T50.7- Poisoning by, adverse effect of and underdosing of analeptics and opioid receptor antagonists

T50.7 - DRUGS/CHEMS*	Crotethamide with cropropamide	Nikethamide
Almitrine		Opiate, antagonists
Amiphenazole	Cyclazocine	Pemoline
Analeptic NEC	Dimefline	Pentetrazole
Antagonist, narcotic analgesic	Dimorpholamine	Pentylenetetrazole
	Doxapram	Picrotoxin
Antagonist, opiate	Etamivan	Pimeclone
Bemegride	Ethamivan	Prethcamide
Bicuculline	Leptazol	Stimulant, central nervous
Central nervous system stimulants, analeptics	Levallorphan	system, analeptics
	Lobeline	Stimulant, central nervous
Central nervous system stimulants, opiate antagonists	Morphine, antagonist	system, opiate
	Nalorphine	antagonist
	Naloxone	
Cropropamide with crotethamide	Naltrexone	
	Narcotic antagonist	

T50.7x- Poisoning by, adverse effect of and underdosing of <u>analeptics and opioid receptor antagonists</u>

T50.7x1- Poisoning by analeptics and opioid receptor antagonists, <u>accidental</u> (unintentional)
Poisoning by analeptics and opioid receptor antagonists NOS

T50.7x2- Poisoning by analeptics and opioid receptor antagonists, <u>intentional</u> self-harm

T50.7x3- Poisoning by analeptics and opioid receptor antagonists, <u>assault</u>

T50.7x4- Poisoning by analeptics and opioid receptor antagonists, <u>undetermined</u>

T50.7x5- <u>Adverse effect</u> of analeptics and opioid receptor antagonists

T50.7x6- <u>Underdosing</u> of analeptics and opioid receptor antagonists

T50
-
T50

T50.8-   Poisoning by, adverse effect of and underdosing of diagnostic agents

T50.8 - DRUGS/CHEMS*		
Acetrizoate (sodium)	Iodinated human serum albumin (131I)	Pentagastrin
Acetrizoic acid	Iodine 125 — see also	Peptavlon
Adipiodone	Radiation sickness, and	Phenobutiodil
Alcohol, diagnostic (gastric function)	Exposure to radioactivce isotopes	Phenol, red
Ametazole	Iodine 131 — see also	Phenolsulfonphthalein
Amidotrizoate	Radiation sickness, and	Propyl iodone
Aminohippuric acid	Exposure to radioactivce isotopes	Propyliodone
Angio-Conray		PSP (phenolsulfon-phthalein)
Azuresin	Iodine, diagnostic	Radioactive drug NEC
Barium, diagnostic agent	Iodipamide	Radio-opaque (drugs) (materials)
Barium, sulfate (medicinal)	Iodized (poppy seed) oil	Renografin
Bentiromide	Iodocholesterol (131I)	Rose bengal sodium (131I)
Betazole	Iodohippuric acid	Rubidium chloride Rb82
Biligrafin	Iodopanoic acid	Secretin
Bilopaque	Iodophthalein (sodium)	Selenomethionine (75Se)
Bromsulfophthalein	Iodopyracet	Sincalide
Bunamiodyl	Iodoxamic acid	Skin test antigen
Calcium ipodate	Iofendylate	Sodium acetrizoate
Cardiografin	Ioglycamic acid	Sodium amidotrizoate
Cardio-green	Iohexol	Sodium cacodylate (nonmedicinal) NEC
Ceruletide	Iopamidol	Sodium diatrizoate
Cholebrine	Iopanoic acid	Sodium indigotin disulfonate
Cholecystokinin	Iophenoic acid	
Cholografin	Iopodate, sodium	Sodium iodide I-131
Chromium sesquioxide	Iopodic acid	Sodium iodohippurate (131I)
Coccidioidin	Iopromide	
Congo red	Iopydol	Sodium iopodate
Contrast medium, radiography	Iotalamic acid	Sodium iothalamate
	Iothalamate	Sodium metrizoate
Diagnostic agent NEC	Iotrol	Sodium para-aminohippurate
Diatrizoate	Iotrolan	
Diodone	Iotroxate	Sodium pertechnetate Tc99m
Dye, diagnostic agents	Iotroxic acid	
Ethiodized oil (131 I)	Ioversol	Sodium tyropanoate
Evans blue	Ioxaglate	Sulfan blue (diagnostic dye)
Fludeoxyglucose (18F)	Ioxaglic acid	
Fluorescein	Ioxitalamic acid	Sulfobromophthalein (sodium)
Frei antigen	Ipodate, calcium	
Gadopentetic acid	Iprofenin	Sulfobromphthalein
Gastrografin	Lidofenin	Sulfonphthal, sulfonphthol
Histalog	Lygranum (skin test)	Sulkowitch's reagent
Histamine (phosphate)	Lymphogranuloma venereum antigen	Sulphan blue
Histoplasmin		Telepaque
Hypaque	Meglumine diatrizoate	Thorium dioxide suspension
Indigo carmine	Meglumine iodipamide	
Indocyanine green	Meglumine iotroxate	Toxin, diphtheria (Schick Test)
Inulin	Methiodal sodium	
Iobenzamic acid	Metrizamide	Tuberculin, purified protein derivative (PPD)
Iocarmic acid	Metrizoic acid	
Iocetamic acid	Metyrapone	Tyropanoate
Iodamide	Mumps skin test antigen	Urokon
Iodinated contrast medium	Oragrafin	Xenon (127Xe) (133Xe)
	Penicilloyl polylysine	

T50.8x- Poisoning by, adverse effect of and underdosing of diagnostic agents

T50.8x1- Poisoning by diagnostic agents, accidental (unintentional)
   Poisoning by diagnostic agents NOS

T50.8x2- Poisoning by diagnostic agents, intentional self-harm

T50.8x3- Poisoning by diagnostic agents, assault

T50.8x4- Poisoning by diagnostic agents, undetermined

T50.8x5- Adverse effect of diagnostic agents

T50.8x6- Underdosing of diagnostic agents

T50.A-   Poisoning by, adverse effect of and underdosing of bacterial vaccines

T50.A1- Poisoning by, adverse effect of and underdosing of pertussis vaccine, including combinations with a pertussis component

T50.A1 - DRUGS/CHEMS*		
Diphtheria, toxoid, with tetanus toxoid, with pertussis component	Tetanus toxoid or vaccine, toxoid, with diphtheria toxoid, with pertussis	Vaccine, pertussis, with diphtheria
Diphtheria, vaccine, combination, including pertussis	Triple vaccine, DPT	Vaccine, pertussis, with diphtheria, and tetanus
	Triple vaccine, including pertussis	Vaccine, pertussis, with other component
Pertussis immune serum vaccine (with diphtheria toxoid) (with tetanus toxoid)	Vaccine, bacterial with, pertussis component	
	Vaccine, diphtheria, with tetanus, and pertussis	
	Vaccine, pertussis	

T50.A11- Poisoning by pertussis vaccine, including combinations with a pertussis component, accidental (unintentional)

T50.A12- Poisoning by pertussis vaccine, including combinations with a pertussis component, intentional self-harm

T50.A13- Poisoning by pertussis vaccine, including combinations with a pertussis component, assault

T50.A14- Poisoning by pertussis vaccine, including combinations with a pertussis component, undetermined

T50.A15- Adverse effect of pertussis vaccine, including combinations with a pertussis component

T50.A16- Underdosing of pertussis vaccine, including combinations with a pertussis component

T50.A2- Poisoning by, adverse effect of and underdosing of mixed bacterial vaccines without a pertussis component

T50.A2 - DRUGS/CHEMS*		
Diphtheria, toxoid, with tetanus toxoid	Toxoid, combined	Vaccine, diphtheria, with tetanus
Diphtheria, vaccine, combination, without pertussis	Vaccine, bacterial with, other bacterial component	Vaccine, rickettsial, with bacterial component
	Vaccine, bacterial with, viral-rickettsial component	
Tetanus toxoid or vaccine, toxoid with diphtheria toxoid	Vaccine, bacterial, mixed NEC	

T50.A21- Poisoning by mixed bacterial vaccines without a pertussis component, accidental (unintentional)

T50.A22- Poisoning by mixed bacterial vaccines without a pertussis component, intentional self-harm

T50.A23- Poisoning by mixed bacterial vaccines without a pertussis component, assault

T50.A24- Poisoning by mixed bacterial vaccines without a pertussis component, undetermined

T50.A25- Adverse effect of mixed bacterial vaccines without a pertussis component

T50.A26- Underdosing of mixed bacterial vaccines without a pertussis component

T50.A9- Poisoning by, adverse effect of and underdosing of other bacterial vaccines

T50.A9 - DRUGS/CHEMS*		
BCG (vaccine)	Tetanus toxoid or vaccine	Vaccine, meningococcal
Cholera vaccine	Tetanus toxoid or vaccine, toxoid	Vaccine, paratyphoid
Diphtheria, toxoid		Vaccine, plague
Diphtheria, vaccine	Toxoid, diphtheria	Vaccine, rickettsial NEC
Meningococcal vaccine	Toxoid, tetanus	Vaccine, Rocky Mountain spotted fever
Menningovax (-AC) (-C)	Typhoid-paratyphoid vaccine	
Paratyphoid vaccine	Typhus vaccine	Vaccine, TAB
Plague vaccine	Vaccine, bacterial NEC	Vaccine, tetanus
Rickettsial vaccine NEC	Vaccine, BCG	Vaccine, typhoid
Rocky Mountain spotted fever vaccine	Vaccine, cholera	Vaccine, typhus
	Vaccine, diphtheria	

T50.A91- Poisoning by other bacterial vaccines, accidental (unintentional)

T50.A92- Poisoning by other bacterial vaccines, intentional self-harm

T50 - T5A

T50.A93-   Poisoning by other bacterial vaccines, <u>assault</u>

T50.A94-   Poisoning by other bacterial vaccines, <u>undetermined</u>

T50.A95-   <u>Adverse effect</u> of other bacterial vaccines

T50.A96-   <u>Underdosing</u> of other bacterial vaccines

T50.B-   Poisoning by, adverse effect of and underdosing of viral vaccines

   T50.B1-   Poisoning by, adverse effect of and underdosing of <u>smallpox vaccines</u>

T50.B1 - DRUGS/CHEMS*	Vaccine, smallpox
Smallpox vaccine	

T50.B11-   Poisoning by smallpox vaccines, <u>accidental</u> (unintentional)

T50.B12-   Poisoning by smallpox vaccines, <u>intentional</u> self-harm

T50.B13-   Poisoning by smallpox vaccines, <u>assault</u>

T50.B14-   Poisoning by smallpox vaccines, <u>undetermined</u>

T50.B15-   <u>Adverse effect</u> of smallpox vaccines

T50.B16-   <u>Underdosing</u> of smallpox vaccines

   T50.B9-   Poisoning by, adverse effect of and underdosing of <u>other viral vaccines</u>

T50.B9 - DRUGS/CHEMS*	Rabies vaccine	Vaccine, poliovirus
Diplovax	Rubella vaccine	Vaccine, rabies
Hepatitis B vaccine	Rubeola vaccine	Vaccine, respiratory
Influenza vaccine	Synagis	syncytial virus
Measles virus vaccine	Triple vaccine, MMR	Vaccine, rubella
(attenuated)	Vaccine, influenza	Vaccine, sabin oral
Meruvax	Vaccine, measles	Vaccine, viral NEC
Mumps vaccine	Vaccine, measles, with	Vaccine, yellow fever
Mumpsvax	mumps and rubella	Viral vaccine NEC
Orimune	Vaccine, mumps	Yellow fever vaccine
Poliomyelitis vaccine	Vaccine, poliomyelitis	

T50.B91-   Poisoning by other viral vaccines, <u>accidental</u> (unintentional)

T50.B92-   Poisoning by other viral vaccines, <u>intentional</u> self-harm

T50.B93-   Poisoning by other viral vaccines, <u>assault</u>

T50.B94-   Poisoning by other viral vaccines, <u>undetermined</u>

T50.B95-   <u>Adverse effect</u> of other viral vaccines

T50.B96-   <u>Underdosing</u> of other viral vaccines

T50.Z-   Poisoning by, adverse effect of and underdosing of other vaccines and biological substances

   T50.Z1-   Poisoning by, adverse effect of and underdosing of <u>immunoglobulin</u>

T50.Z1 - DRUGS/CHEMS*	Gamma globulin	Rabies immune globulin
AHLG	Gamulin	(human)
Anti-D immunoglobulin	Globulin, antilymphocytic	Rh (D) immune globulin
(human)	Globulin, antirhesus	(human)
Antidiphtheria serum	Globulin, antivenin	RhoGAM
Anti-human lymphocytic	Globulin, antiviral	Serum, antibotulinus
globulin	Hepatitis B immune	Serum, anticytotoxic
Antirabies hyperimmune	globulin	Serum, antidiphtheria
serum	Homo-tet	Serum, antimeningococcus
Antiscorpion sera	Horse anti-human	Serum, anti-Rh
Antitetanus	lymphocytic serum	Serum, anti-snake-bite
immunoglobulin	Human immune serum	Serum, antitetanic
Antitoxin	Hypertussis	Serum, antitoxic
Antitoxin, diphtheria	Immu-G	Serum, convalescent
Antitoxin, gas gangrene	Immuglobin	Serum, immune (human)
Antitoxin, tetanus	Immune globulin	Serum, protective NEC
Antivenin, antivenom	Immune serum globulin	Spider, antivenin
(sera)	Immunoglobin human	Tetanus toxoid or vaccine,
Antivenin, crotaline	(intravenous) (normal)	antitoxin
Antivenin, spider bite	Immunoglobin human,	Tetanus toxoid or vaccine,
Black widow spider	unmodified	immune globulin
antivenin	Immu-tetanus	(human)
Botulinus anti-toxin (type	Mumps immune globulin	Vaccinia immune globulin
A, B)	(human)	
Diphtheria, antitoxin	Pertussis immune serum	
Gamimune	(human)	

T50.Z11-   Poisoning by immunoglobulin, <u>accidental</u> (unintentional)

T50.Z12-   Poisoning by immunoglobulin, <u>intentional</u> self-harm

T50.Z13-   Poisoning by immunoglobulin, <u>assault</u>

T50.Z14-   Poisoning by immunoglobulin, <u>undetermined</u>

T50.Z15-   <u>Adverse effect</u> of immunoglobulin

T50.Z16-   <u>Underdosing</u> of immunoglobulin

   T50.Z9-   Poisoning by, adverse effect of and underdosing of <u>other vaccines and biological substances</u>

T50.Z9 - DRUGS/CHEMS*	Pegademase, bovine
Glandular extract	Vaccine NEC
(medicinal) NEC	Vaccine, antineoplastic

T50.Z91-   Poisoning by other vaccines and biological substances, <u>accidental</u> (unintentional)

T50.Z92-   Poisoning by other vaccines and biological substances, <u>intentional</u> self-harm

T50.Z93-   Poisoning by other vaccines and biological substances, <u>assault</u>

T50.Z94-   Poisoning by other vaccines and biological substances, <u>undetermined</u>

T50.Z95-   <u>Adverse effect</u> of other vaccines and biological substances

T50.Z96-   <u>Underdosing</u> of other vaccines and biological substances

T50.9-   Poisoning by, adverse effect of and underdosing of other and unspecified drugs, medicaments and biological substances

   T50.90-   Poisoning by, adverse effect of and underdosing of <u>unspecified drugs, medicaments and biological substances</u>

T50.90 - DRUGS/CHEMS*	Lactose (as excipient)	Salt-replacing drug
Acidifying agent NEC	Lipotropic drug NEC	Sodium-free salt
Adjunct, pharmaceutical	Medicament NEC	Soothing syrup
Alkalinizing agents	Nutritional supplement	Spray, medicinal NEC
(medicinal)	Pharmaceutical, adjunct	Starch
Alkalizing agent NEC	NEC	Stone-dissolving drug
Biological substance NEC	Pharmaceutical, excipient	Sweetener
Dietetic drug NEC	NEC	Tablets — see also specified
Drug NEC	Pharmaceutical, sweetener	substance
Dye, pharmaceutical NEC	Pharmaceutical, viscous	Tonic NEC
Elemental diet	agent	Viscous agent
Excipients, pharmaceutical	Preservative, medicinal	
Headache cures, drugs,	Saccharin	
powders NEC	Salt substitute	

T50.901-   Poisoning by unspecified drugs, medicaments and biological substances, <u>accidental</u> (unintentional)

T50.902-   Poisoning by unspecified drugs, medicaments and biological substances, <u>intentional</u> self-harm

T50.903-   Poisoning by unspecified drugs, medicaments and biological substances, <u>assault</u>

T50.904-   Poisoning by unspecified drugs, medicaments and biological substances, <u>undetermined</u>

T50.905-   <u>Adverse effect</u> of unspecified drugs, medicaments and biological substances

T50.906-   <u>Underdosing</u> of unspecified drugs, medicaments and biological substances

T50.99- Poisoning by, adverse effect of and underdosing of <u>other drugs, medicaments and biological substances</u>

T50.99 - DRUGS/CHEMS*	Diacetyl monoxime	Methylethyl cellulose
Acetohydroxamic acid	Drug, specified NEC	Monooctanoin
Acitretin	Elcatonin	Octanoin
Ammonium chloride	Epomediol	Orazamide
Arginine	Etidronate	Ornithine aspartate
Arginine glutamate	Etidronic acid (disodium	Oxalic acid, ammonium salt
Baking soda	salt)	Palm kernel oil
Bergapten	Etretinate	Parathormone
BHA	Fat suspension, intravenous	Parathyroid extract
Borate(s) buffer	Fluoride, medicinal NEC	Phenaphthazine reagent
Bromophenol blue reagent	Gallium citrate	Potassium citrate
Butylated hydroxy-anisole	Gelsemine	Protein hydrolysate
Calcitonin	Gluconic acid	Psoralens (medicinal)
Calcium chloride	Glycerophosphate	Serotonin
Calcium chloride,	Guaiac reagent	Silibinin
anhydrous	Hormone, parathyroid	Silymarin
Calculus-dissolving drug	(derivatives)	Sodium citrate
Canthaxanthin	Inositol	Sodium iodide
Cetomacrogol	Intravenous, amino acids	Sodium magnesium citrate
Chlorophyll	Intravenous, fat suspension	Sodium propyl
Choline chloride	Iodine 125, therapeutic	hydroxybenzoate
Choline dihydrogen citrate	Isotretinoin	Teriparatide (acetate)
Cianidanol	Levocarnitine	Thioctamide
Clodronic acid	Levoglutamide	Thioctic acid
Cochineal, medicinal	Macrogol	Tidiacic
products	Manganese, medicinal	Tiopronin
Coenzyme A	Methionine	Tragacanth
Cogalactoiso-merase	Methoxsalen	Ursodeoxycholic acid
Collagen	5-Methoxypsoralen (5-	Ursodiol
Colorant – see also Dye	MOP)	Vienna red, pharmaceutical
Cyclamate	8-Methoxypsoralen (8-	dye
Deanol (aceglumate)	MOP)	

T50.991- Poisoning by other drugs, medicaments and biological substances, <u>accidental</u> (unintentional)

T50.992- Poisoning by other drugs, medicaments and biological substances, <u>intentional</u> self-harm

T50.993- Poisoning by other drugs, medicaments and biological substances, <u>assault</u>

T50.994- Poisoning by other drugs, medicaments and biological substances, <u>undetermined</u>

T50.995- <u>Adverse effect</u> of other drugs, medicaments and biological substances

T50.996- <u>Underdosing</u> of other drugs, medicaments and biological substances

Toxic effects of substances chiefly nonmedicinal as to source (T51-T65)

Note: When no intent is indicated code to accidental. Undetermined intent is only for use when there is specific documentation in the record that the intent of the toxic effect cannot be determined.
Use additional code(s):
    For all associated manifestations of toxic effect, such as: respiratory conditions due to external agents (J60-J70)
    Personal history of foreign body fully removed (Z87.821)
    To identify any retained foreign body, if applicable (Z18.-)
Excludes 1:   contact with and (suspected) exposure to toxic substances (Z77.-)

T51- Toxic effect of <u>alcohol</u>

The appropriate 7th character is to be added to each code from category T51:
A   <u>Initial</u> encounter
D   <u>Subsequent</u> encounter
S   <u>Sequela</u>

T51.0- Toxic effect of ethanol
Toxic effect of ethyl alcohol
Excludes ❷: acute alcohol intoxication or "hangover" effects (F10.129, F10.229, F10.929)
        drunkenness (F10.129, F10.229, F10.929)
        pathological alcohol intoxication (F10.129, F10.229, F10.929)

T51.0 - DRUGS/CHEMS*	Alcohol, industrial	Ethyl alcohol, beverage
Absinthe (beverage)	Alcohol, preparation for	Grain alcohol
Alcohol, absolute	consumption	Industrial alcohol
(beverage)	Alcohol, surgical	Neutral spirits
Alcohol, beverage	Central nervous system	Neutral spirits, beverage
Alcohol, dehydrated	depressants, ethanol	Spirit(s) (neutral) NEC
(beverage)	Denatured alcohol	Spirit(s), beverage
Alcohol, denatured	Ethanol	Spirit(s), industrial
Alcohol, ethyl (beverage)	Ethanol, beverage	Spirit(s), surgical
Alcohol, grain (beverage)	Ethyl alcohol	

T51.0x- Toxic effect of <u>ethanol</u>
T51.0x1- Toxic effect of ethanol, <u>accidental</u> (unintentional)
    Toxic effect of ethanol NOS
T51.0x2- Toxic effect of ethanol, <u>intentional</u> self-harm
T51.0x3- Toxic effect of ethanol, <u>assault</u>
T51.0x4- Toxic effect of ethanol, <u>undetermined</u>

T51.1- Toxic effect of methanol
Toxic effect of methyl alcohol

T51.1 - DRUGS/CHEMS*	Antifreeze, alcohol	Methyl carbinol
Alcohol, antifreeze	Canned heat	Methylated spirit
Alcohol, methyl	Carbinol	Radiator alcohol
Alcohol, radiator	Methanol (vapor)	Wood alcohol or spirit
Alcohol, wood	Methyl alcohol	Zerone

T51.1x- Toxic effect of <u>methanol</u>
T51.1x1- Toxic effect of methanol, <u>accidental</u> (unintentional)
    Toxic effect of methanol NOS
T51.1x2- Toxic effect of methanol, <u>intentional</u> self-harm
T51.1x3- Toxic effect of methanol, <u>assault</u>
T51.1x4- Toxic effect of methanol, <u>undetermined</u>

T51.2- Toxic effect of 2-Propanol
Toxic effect of isopropyl alcohol

T51.2 - DRUGS/CHEMS*	Alcohol, rubbing	2-Propanol
2-propanol	Dimethyl carbinol	Rubbing alcohol
Alcohol, isopropyl	Isopropanol	
Alcohol, propyl, secondary	Isopropyl alcohol	

T51.2x- Toxic effect of <u>2-Propanol</u>
T51.2x1- Toxic effect of 2-Propanol, <u>accidental</u> (unintentional)
    Toxic effect of 2-Propanol NOS
T51.2x2- Toxic effect of 2-Propanol, <u>intentional</u> self-harm
T51.2x3- Toxic effect of 2-Propanol, <u>assault</u>
T51.2x4- Toxic effect of 2-Propanol, <u>undetermined</u>

T50 - T51

T51.3-   Toxic effect of fusel oil
Toxic effect of amyl alcohol
Toxic effect of butyl [1-butanol] alcohol
Toxic effect of propyl [1-propanol] alcohol

T51.3 - DRUGS/CHEMS*	Butanol	Methyl butanol
1-propanol	Butyl alcohol	Methyl propylcarbinol
Alcohol, amyl	Butyl carbinol	Pentanol
Alcohol, butyl	Diethyl carbinol	1-Propanol
Alcohol, propyl	Ethyl carbinol	Propyl alcohol
Amyl alcohol	Fusel oil (any) (amyl)	Propyl carbinol
Amylene hydrate	(butyl) (propyl), vapor	Trimethylcarbinol

T51.3x- Toxic effect of fusel oil

T51.3x1-   Toxic effect of fusel oil, accidental (unintentional)
Toxic effect of fusel oil NOS

T51.3x2-   Toxic effect of fusel oil, intentional self-harm

T51.3x3-   Toxic effect of fusel oil, assault

T51.3x4-   Toxic effect of fusel oil, undetermined

T51.8-   Toxic effect of other alcohols

T51.8 - DRUGS/CHEMS*	Antifreeze, ethylene glycol	Hexahydrocresol(s)
Alcohol, allyl	Bay rum	Hexahydrophenol
Alcohol, specified type NEC	Cyclohexanol	Hexalen
Allyl alcohol	Ethyl methylcarbinol	Methyl cyclohexanol

T51.8x- Toxic effect of other alcohols

T51.8x1-   Toxic effect of other alcohols, accidental (unintentional)
Toxic effect of other alcohols NOS

T51.8x2-   Toxic effect of other alcohols, intentional self-harm

T51.8x3-   Toxic effect of other alcohols, assault

T51.8x4-   Toxic effect of other alcohols, undetermined

T51.9-   Toxic effect of unspecified alcohol

T51.9 - DRUGS/CHEMS*
Alcohol

T51.91x-   Toxic effect of unspecified alcohol, accidental (unintentional)

T51.92x-   Toxic effect of unspecified alcohol, intentional self-harm

T51.93x-   Toxic effect of unspecified alcohol, assault

T51.94x-   Toxic effect of unspecified alcohol, undetermined

T52- Toxic effect of organic solvents
Excludes 1:   halogen derivatives of aliphatic and aromatic hydrocarbons (T53.-)

The appropriate 7th character is to be added to each code from category T52:
A   Initial encounter
D   Subsequent encounter
S   Sequela

T52.0-   Toxic effects of petroleum products
Toxic effects of gasoline [petrol]
Toxic effects of kerosene [paraffin oil]
Toxic effects of paraffin wax
Toxic effects of ether petroleum
Toxic effects of naphtha petroleum
Toxic effects of spirit petroleum

T52.0 - DRUGS/CHEMS*	Kerosene, kerosine,	Petrol
Automobile fuel	insecticide	Petrol, vapor
Benzol vapor	Kerosene, kerosine, vapor	Petrolatum, nonmedicinal
Brasso	Lighter fluid	Petroleum (products) NEC
Cigarette lighter fluid	Ligroin(e) (solvent)	Petroleum, solids
Coal tar, naphtha (solvent)	Lubricating oil NEC	Petroleum, solvents
Crude oil	Mineral oil, nonmedicinal	Petroleum, vapor
Ethyl formate NEC (solvent)	Mineral spirits	Solvent, industrial,
Ethylidene diethyl ether	Naphtha (painters')	naphtha
Fuel, automobile	(petroleum)	Solvent, industrial,
Fuel, automobile, vapor	Naphtha, solvent	petroleum
NEC	Naphtha, vapor	Spirit(s), mineral
Gas, oil	Oil, lubricating	Tar NEC
Gasoline	Paraffin(s) (wax)	Tractor fuel NEC
Gasoline, vapor	Paraffin(s), liquid,	Wax (paraffin) (petroleum)
Kerosene, kerosine (fuel)	nonmedicinal	Wax, floor
(solvent) NEC	Pesticide, kerosene	White spirit

T52.0x- Toxic effects of petroleum products

T52.0x1-   Toxic effect of petroleum products, accidental (unintentional)
Toxic effects of petroleum products NOS

T52.0x2-   Toxic effect of petroleum products, intentional self-harm

T52.0x3-   Toxic effect of petroleum products, assault

T52.0x4-   Toxic effect of petroleum products, undetermined

T52.1-   Toxic effects of benzene
Excludes 1:   homologues of benzene (T52.2)
nitroderivatives and aminoderivatives of benzene and its homologues (T65.3)

T52.1 - DRUGS/CHEMS*	Diphenylmethane dye)
Benzene	
Benzol (benzene)	

T52.1x- Toxic effects of benzene

T52.1x1-   Toxic effect of benzene, accidental (unintentional)
Toxic effects of benzene NOS

T52.1x2-   Toxic effect of benzene, intentional self-harm

T52.1x3-   Toxic effect of benzene, assault

T52.1x4-   Toxic effect of benzene, undetermined

T52.2-   Toxic effects of homologues of benzene
Toxic effects of toluene [methylbenzene]
Toxic effects of xylene [dimethylbenzene]

T52.2 - DRUGS/CHEMS*	Hexylresorcinol	Toluol (liquid)
Benzene, homologues	Hydroquinone	Toluol, vapor
(acetyl) (dimethyl)	Methyl benzene	Xylene (vapor)
(methyl) (solvent)	Methyl benzol	Xylol (vapor
Butyltoluene	Toluene (liquid)	

T52.2x- Toxic effects of homologues of benzene

T52.2x1-   Toxic effect of homologues of benzene, accidental (unintentional)
Toxic effects of homologues of benzene NOS

T52.2x2-   Toxic effect of homologues of benzene, intentional self-harm

T52.2x3-   Toxic effect of homologues of benzene, assault

T52.2x4-   Toxic effect of homologues of benzene, undetermined

T52.3-   Toxic effects of glycols

T52.3 - DRUGS/CHEMS*	Diethylene glycol	Ethylene glycol(s), dinitrate
Butyl carbitol	(monoacetate)	Ethylene glycol(s),
Butyl cellosolve	(monobutyl ether)	monobutyl ether
Carbitol	(monoethyl ether)	Glycols (ether)
	2-Ethoxyethanol	2-Methoxyethanol
	Ethylene dinitrate	Nitroglycol

T52.3x- Toxic effects of glycols

T52.3x1-   Toxic effect of glycols, accidental (unintentional)
Toxic effects of glycols NOS

T52.3x2-   Toxic effect of glycols, intentional self-harm

T52.3x3-   Toxic effect of glycols, assault

T52.3x4-   Toxic effect of glycols, undetermined

T52.4-   Toxic effects of ketones

T52.4 - DRUGS/CHEMS*	Dimethyl ketone	MEK (methyl ethyl ketone)
Acetone (chlorinated) (oils)	Dimethyl ketone, vapor	Methyl acetate
(vapor)	Hexanone, 2-hexanone	Methyl acetone
Acetophenone	Hexone	Methyl ethyl ketone
Butanone, 2-butanone	Hydroxymethylpenta-none	Methyl isobutyl ketone
Cyclohexanone	Ketols	
Diacetone alcohol	Ketone oils	

T52.4x- Toxic effects of ketones

T52.4x1-   Toxic effect of ketones, accidental (unintentional)
Toxic effects of ketones NOS

T52.4x2-   Toxic effect of ketones, intentional self-harm

T52.4x3-   Toxic effect of ketones, assault

T52.4x4-   Toxic effect of ketones, undetermined

T51-T52

T52.8-   Toxic effects of other organic solvents

T52.8 - DRUGS/CHEMS*	Diethylene dioxide	Hexahydrobenzol
Acetal	Dimethyl carbonate	Hexamethylene
Acetaldehyde (vapor)	Dimethyl sulfoxide	Isobutyl acetate
Acetic acid ester (solvent)	(nonmedicinal)	Isopropyl acetate
(vapor)	Dimethylformamide	Isopropyl ether
Acetic ether (vapor)	Dioxane	Limonene
Acetonitrile	Dipentene	Methyl benzoate
Amyl acetate	Epichlorhydrin,	Methyl carbonate
Amyl formate	epichlorohydrin	Methyl cyclohexane
Benzyl acetate	Ether, ethyl, nonmedicinal	Methyl cyclohexanone
Butyl acetate (secondary)	Ether, solvent	Methyl cyclohexyl acetate
Butyl butyrate	Ethyl acetate	Methyl sulfate, liquid
Butyl formate	Ethyl aldehyde, liquid	Nitropropane
Butyl lactate	Ethyl benzoate	Oil, Niobe
Butyl propionate	Ethyl carbonate	Paint solvent NEC
Cyclohexane	ether — see also Ether	Paint stripper
Cyclohexyl acetate	Ethyl hydroxyisobutyrate	Pimelic ketone
Decahydronaphthalene	NEC (solvent)	Pyridine
Decalin	Ethyl lactate NEC (solvent)	Solvent, industrial,
Dekalin	Ethyl oxybutyrate NEC	specified NEC
Dichlorhydrin	(solvent)	Stripper (paint) (solvent)
Dichloroethane	Ethylene chlorohydrin	Tetrahydrofuran
Dichlorohydrin, alpha-	Ethylene dichloride	Tetrahydronaphthalene
dichlorohydrin	Ethylene glycol(s)	Tetralin
Diethyl carbonate	Furfural	Turpentine (spirits of)
Diethyl oxide	Glue NEC	Turpentine, vapor

T52.8x- Toxic effects of other organic solvents

T52.8x1-   Toxic effect of other organic solvents, **accidental (unintentional)**
Toxic effects of other organic solvents NOS

T52.8x2-   Toxic effect of other organic solvents, **intentional self-harm**

T52.8x3-   Toxic effect of other organic solvents, **assault**

T52.8x4-   Toxic effect of other organic solvents, **undetermined**

T52.9-   Toxic effects of unspecified organic solvent

T52.9 - DRUGS/CHEMS*	Methyl cellosolve	Tricresyl phosphate, solvent
Cellosolve	Nail polish remover	Varnish, cleaner
Cleaner, of paint or varnish	Paint cleaner	
Dialkyl carbonate	Phosphate, solvent	
Industrial solvents (fumes)	Polyester resin hardener	
(vapors)	Solvent, industrial NEC	

T52.91x- Toxic effect of unspecified organic solvent, **accidental (unintentional)**

T52.92x- Toxic effect of unspecified organic solvent, **intentional self-harm**

T52.93x- Toxic effect of unspecified organic solvent, **assault**

T52.94x- Toxic effect of unspecified organic solvent, **undetermined**

T53-   Toxic effect of halogen derivatives of aliphatic and aromatic hydrocarbons

The appropriate 7th character is to be added to each code from category T53:
A   Initial encounter
D   Subsequent encounter
S   Sequela

T53.0-   Toxic effects of carbon tetrachloride
Toxic effects of tetrachloromethane

T53.0 - DRUGS/CHEMS*	Carbon tetrachloride, liquid	Carbon tetrachloride,
Carbon tetrachloride	(cleansing agent) NEC	solvent
(vapor) NEC		

T53.0x- Toxic effects of carbon tetrachloride

T53.0x1-   Toxic effect of carbon tetrachloride, **accidental (unintentional)**
Toxic effects of carbon tetrachloride NOS

T53.0x2-   Toxic effect of carbon tetrachloride, **intentional self-harm**

T53.0x3-   Toxic effect of carbon tetrachloride, **assault**

T53.0x4-   Toxic effect of carbon tetrachloride, **undetermined**

T53.1-   Toxic effects of chloroform
Toxic effects of trichloromethane

T53.1 - DRUGS/CHEMS*	Chloroform, solvent
Chloroform (fumes)	
(vapor)	

T53.1x- Toxic effects of chloroform

T53.1x1-   Toxic effect of chloroform, **accidental (unintentional)**
Toxic effects of chloroform NOS

T53.1x2-   Toxic effect of chloroform, **intentional** self-harm

T53.1x3-   Toxic effect of chloroform, **assault**

T53.1x4-   Toxic effect of chloroform, **undetermined**

T53.2-   Toxic effects of trichloroethylene
Toxic effects of trichloroethene

T53.2 - DRUGS/CHEMS*	Trichloroethylene (liquid)
Trichlorethane	(vapor)
Trichlorethylene	Trichloroethylene, vapor
Trichloroethane	NEC

T53.2x- Toxic effects of trichloroethylene

T53.2x1-   Toxic effect of trichloroethylene, **accidental (unintentional)**
Toxic effects of trichloroethylene NOS

T53.2x2-   Toxic effect of trichloroethylene, **intentional** self-harm

T53.2x3-   Toxic effect of trichloroethylene, **assault**

T53.2x4-   Toxic effect of trichloroethylene, **undetermined**

T53.3-   Toxic effects of tetrachloroethylene
Toxic effects of perchloroethylene
Toxic effect of tetrachloroethene

T53.3 - DRUGS/CHEMS*	Tetrachloroethylene
Perchloroethylene	(liquid)
Perchloroethylene, vapor	Tetrachloroethylene, vapor

T53.3x- Toxic effects of tetrachloroethylene

T53.3x1-   Toxic effect of tetrachloroethylene, **accidental (unintentional)**
Toxic effects of tetrachloroethylene NOS

T53.3x2-   Toxic effect of tetrachloroethylene, **intentional** self-harm

T53.3x3-   Toxic effect of tetrachloroethylene, **assault**

T53.3x4-   Toxic effect of tetrachloroethylene, **undetermined**

T53.4-   Toxic effects of dichloromethane
Toxic effects of methylene chloride

T53.4 - DRUGS/CHEMS*	Dichloromethane, vapor	Methylene chloride or
Dichloromethane (solvent)		dichloride (solvent) NEC

T53.4x- Toxic effects of dichloromethane

T53.4x1-   Toxic effect of dichloromethane, **accidental (unintentional)**
Toxic effects of dichloromethane NOS

T53.4x2-   Toxic effect of dichloromethane, **intentional** self-harm

T53.4x3-   Toxic effect of dichloromethane, **assault**

T53.4x4-   Toxic effect of dichloromethane, **undetermined**

T53.5-   Toxic effects of chlorofluorocarbons

T53.5 - DRUGS/CHEMS*	Fumes, freons	Refrigerant gas
Chlorofluorocarbons	Gas, refrigerant	(chlorofluoro-carbon)
Dichlorodifluoromethane	(chlorofluorocarbon)	Trichlorofluoromethane
Freon		NEC

T53.5x- Toxic effects of chlorofluorocarbons

T53.5x1-   Toxic effect of chlorofluorocarbons, **accidental (unintentional)**
Toxic effects of chlorofluorocarbons NOS

T53.5x2-   Toxic effect of chlorofluorocarbons, **intentional** self-harm

T53.5x3-   Toxic effect of chlorofluorocarbons, **assault**

T53.5x4-   Toxic effect of chlorofluorocarbons, **undetermined**

T52 - T53

T53.6- Toxic effects of other halogen derivatives of aliphatic hydrocarbons

T53.6 - DRUGS/CHEMS*	Chloropicrin (fumes)	HCH
Acetyl (bromide) (chloride)	Dibromoethane	Hexachlorocyclohexane
Acetylene dichloride	Sym-Dichloroethyl ether	Lindane (insecticide)
Acetylene tetrachloride (vapor)	Dichloroethylene	(nonmedicinal) (vapor)
Amyl chloride	Ethyl chloride, solvent	Pentachloroethane
Amylene dichloride	Ethylene chlorohydrin, vapor	Pentalin
BHC, nonmedicinal (vapor)	Ethylene dichloride, vapor	Sym-dichloroethyl ether
Chlorex	Ethylidene chloride NEC	Tetrachloroethane
Chlorinated camphene	Fluorocarbon monomer	Tetrachloroethane, vapor
Chlorobromomethane (fire extinguisher)	Gamma-benzene hexachloride,	Tetrachloroethane, vapor, paint or varnish
Chloroethylene	nonmedicinal, vapor	Trichloropropane

T53.6x- Toxic effects of <u>other halogen derivatives of aliphatic hydrocarbons</u>

T53.6x1- Toxic effect of other halogen derivatives of aliphatic hydrocarbons, <u>accidental</u> (unintentional)
Toxic effects of other halogen derivatives of aliphatic hydrocarbons NOS

T53.6x2- Toxic effect of other halogen derivatives of aliphatic hydrocarbons, <u>intentional</u> self-harm

T53.6x3- Toxic effect of other halogen derivatives of aliphatic hydrocarbons, <u>assault</u>

T53.6x4- Toxic effect of other halogen derivatives of aliphatic hydrocarbons, <u>undetermined</u>

T53.7- Toxic effects of other halogen derivatives of aromatic hydrocarbons

T53.7 - DRUGS/CHEMS*	Chlorodinitrobenzene	Dioxin
Chlorbenzene, chlorbenzol	Chlorodinitrobenzene, dust or vapor	Methoxychlor
Chlorinated diphenyl	Chlorodiphenyl	Methoxy-DDT
Chlorinated naphthalene, industrial (non-pesticide)	Chloronitrobenzene	Monochlorobenzene
	Chloronitrobenzene, dust or vapor	Orthodichlorobenzene
Chloroaniline		Pentachloronaphthalene
Chlorobenzene, chlorobenzol	Chlorophenol	TCDD
	Dichlorobenzene	2,3,7,8-Tetrachlorodibenzo-p-dioxin

T53.7x- Toxic effects of <u>other halogen derivatives of aromatic hydrocarbons</u>

T53.7x1- Toxic effect of other halogen derivatives of aromatic hydrocarbons, <u>accidental</u> (unintentional)
Toxic effects of other halogen derivatives of aromatic hydrocarbons NOS

T53.7x2- Toxic effect of other halogen derivatives of aromatic hydrocarbons, <u>intentional</u> self-harm

T53.7x3- Toxic effect of other halogen derivatives of aromatic hydrocarbons, <u>assault</u>

T53.7x4- Toxic effect of other halogen derivatives of aromatic hydrocarbons, <u>undetermined</u>

T53.9- Toxic effects of <u>unspecified halogen derivatives of aliphatic and aromatic hydrocarbons</u>

T53.9 - DRUGS/CHEMS*	Chlorinated hydrocarbons,
Chlorinated hydrocarbons NEC	solvents

T53.91x- Toxic effect of unspecified halogen derivatives of aliphatic and aromatic hydrocarbons, <u>accidental</u> (unintentional)

T53.92x- Toxic effect of unspecified halogen derivatives of aliphatic and aromatic hydrocarbons, <u>intentional</u> self-harm

T53.93x- Toxic effect of unspecified halogen derivatives of aliphatic and aromatic hydrocarbons, <u>assault</u>

T53.94x- Toxic effect of unspecified halogen derivatives of aliphatic and aromatic hydrocarbons, <u>undetermined</u>

T54- Toxic effect of <u>corrosive substances</u>
The appropriate 7th character is to be added to each code from category T54:
A <u>Initial</u> encounter
D <u>Subsequent</u> encounter
S <u>Sequela</u>

T54.0- Toxic effects of phenol and phenol homologues

T54.0 - DRUGS/CHEMS*	Hydroxytoluene	Phenol, nonmedicinal NEC
Aminophenol	(nonmedicinal)	
Carbolic acid — see also	Nitrophenol	
Phenol	Phenol, disinfectant	

T54.0x- Toxic effects of <u>phenol and phenol homologues</u>

T54.0x1- Toxic effect of phenol and phenol homologues, <u>accidental</u> (unintentional)
Toxic effects of phenol and phenol homologues NOS

T54.0x2- Toxic effect of phenol and phenol homologues, <u>intentional</u> self-harm

T54.0x3- Toxic effect of phenol and phenol homologues, <u>assault</u>

T54.0x4- Toxic effect of phenol and phenol homologues, <u>undetermined</u>

T54.1- Toxic effects of other corrosive organic compounds

T54.1 - DRUGS/CHEMS*	Aziridine (chelating)	Creolin, disinfectant
Acrolein, liquid	Corrosive aromatics	Disinfectant, aromatic
Aromatics, corrosive	Corrosive aromatics, disinfectant	Ethylene imine
Aromatics, corrosive, disinfectants	Creolin	Hydrazine
		Lysol

T54.1x- Toxic effects of <u>other corrosive organic compounds</u>

T54.1x1- Toxic effect of other corrosive organic compounds, <u>accidental</u> (unintentional)
Toxic effects of other corrosive organic compounds NOS

T54.1x2- Toxic effect of other corrosive organic compounds, <u>intentional</u> self-harm

T54.1x3- Toxic effect of other corrosive organic compounds, <u>assault</u>

T54.1x4- Toxic effect of other corrosive organic compounds, <u>undetermined</u>

T54.2- Toxic effects of corrosive acids and acid-like substances
Toxic effects of hydrochloric acid
Toxic effects of sulfuric acid

T54.2 - DRUGS/CHEMS*	Mineral acids	Phosphoric acid
Acetic acid	Nitric acid (liquid)	Picric (acid)
Acid (corrosive) NEC	Nitrohydrochloric acid	Saniflush (cleaner)
Aqua fortis	Nitrous acid (liquid)	Storage battery (cells) (acid)
Battery acid or fluid	Oil, vitriol (liquid)	
Corrosive acid NEC	Oil, vitriol, fumes	Sulfur, acid
Formic acid	Orthotolidine (reagent)	Sulfuric acid
Hydrazoic acid, azides	Osmic acid (liquid)	Trichloroacetic acid, trichloracetic acid
Hydrochloric acid (liquid)	Osmic acid, fumes	
Hydrofluoric acid (liquid)	Oxalic acid	

T54.2x- Toxic effects of <u>corrosive acids and acid-like substances</u>

T54.2x1- Toxic effect of corrosive acids and acid-like substances, <u>accidental</u> (unintentional)
Toxic effects of corrosive acids and acid-like substances NOS

T54.2x2- Toxic effect of corrosive acids and acid-like substances, <u>intentional</u> self-harm

T54.2x3- Toxic effect of corrosive acids and acid-like substances, <u>assault</u>

T54.2x4- Toxic effect of corrosive acids and acid-like substances, <u>undetermined</u>

T
5
3
-
T
5
4

T54.3- Toxic effects of corrosive alkalis and alkali-like substances
Toxic effects of potassium hydroxide
Toxic effects of sodium hydroxide

T54.3 - DRUGS/CHEMS*	Caustic(s) hydroxide	Potassium hydroxide
Alkali (caustic)	Caustic(s) potash	Quicklime
Ammonia, liquid	Caustic(s) soda	Soda (caustic)
(household)	Chloride of lime (bleach)	Sodium carbonate NEC
Ammonium carbonate	Chlorinated lime (bleach)	Sodium hydroxide
Ammonium compounds	Chlorine bleach	Sodium hypochlorite
(household) NEC	Disinfectant, alkaline	(bleach) NEC
Ammonium compounds,	Drano (drain cleaner)	Sodium hypochlorite,
industrial	Hydroxide, caustic	disinfectant
Calcium hydrate, hydroxide	Lime (chloride)	Sodium hypochlorite, vapor
Calcium hypochlorite	Lye (concentrated)	Triethanolamine NEC
Calcium oxide	Potash (caustic)	Triethanolamine, detergent
Caustic(s) alkali	Potassium carbonate	

T54.3x- Toxic effects of <u>corrosive alkalis and alkali-like</u> <u>substances</u>

T54.3x1- Toxic effect of corrosive alkalis and alkali-like substances, <u>accidental</u> (unintentional)
Toxic effects of corrosive alkalis and alkali-like substances NOS

T54.3x2- Toxic effect of corrosive alkalis and alkali-like substances, <u>intentional</u> self-harm

T54.3x3- Toxic effect of corrosive alkalis and alkali-like substances, <u>assault</u>

T54.3x4- Toxic effect of corrosive alkalis and alkali-like substances, <u>undetermined</u>

T54.9- Toxic effects of <u>unspecified corrosive substance</u>

T54.9 - DRUGS/CHEMS*	Clorox (bleach)	Oxidizing agent NEC
Bleach	Corrosive NEC	Purex (bleach)
Borate(s) cleanser	Corrosive fumes NEC	Sodium chlorate, herbicide
Borax (cleanser)	Corrosive, specified NEC	
Caustic(s) NEC	Fluoride, not pesticide NEC	
Caustic(s) specified NEC	Fumes, corrosive NEC	

T54.91x- Toxic effect of unspecified corrosive substance, <u>accidental</u> (unintentional)

T54.92x- Toxic effect of unspecified corrosive substance, <u>intentional</u> self-harm

T54.93x- Toxic effect of unspecified corrosive substance, <u>assault</u>

T54.94x- Toxic effect of unspecified corrosive substance, <u>undetermined</u>

T55- Toxic effect of <u>soaps and detergents</u>
The appropriate 7th character is to be added to each code from category T55:
A <u>Initial</u> encounter
D <u>Subsequent</u> encounter
S <u>Sequela</u>

T55.0- Toxic effect of soaps

T55.0 - DRUGS/CHEMS*	Soap (powder) (product)	Soft soap
Shampoo	Sodium perborate, soap	

T55.0x- Toxic effect of <u>soaps</u>

T55.0x1- Toxic effect of soaps, <u>accidental</u> (unintentional)
Toxic effect of soaps NOS

T55.0x2- Toxic effect of soaps, <u>intentional</u> self-harm

T55.0x3- Toxic effect of soaps, <u>assault</u>

T55.0x4- Toxic effect of soaps, <u>undetermined</u>

T55.1- Toxic effect of detergents

T55.1 - DRUGS/CHEMS*	Detergent, specified NEC
Detergent, nonmedicinal	

T55.1x- Toxic effect of <u>detergents</u>

T55.1x1- Toxic effect of detergents, <u>accidental</u> (unintentional)
Toxic effect of detergents NOS

T55.1x2- Toxic effect of detergents, <u>intentional</u> self-harm

T55.1x3- Toxic effect of detergents, <u>assault</u>

T55.1x4- Toxic effect of detergents, <u>undetermined</u>

T56- Toxic effect of <u>metals</u>
Includes: Toxic effects of fumes and vapors of metals
Toxic effects of metals from all sources, except medicinal substances
Use additional code to identify any retained metal foreign body, if applicable (Z18.0-, T18.1-)
Excludes 1: arsenic and its compounds (T57.0)
manganese and its compounds (T57.2)

The appropriate 7th character is to be added to each code from category T56:
A <u>Initial</u> encounter
D <u>Subsequent</u> encounter
S <u>Sequela</u>

T56.0- Toxic effects of lead and its compounds

T56.0 - DRUGS/CHEMS*	Lead carbonate, paint	Lead oxide
Antiknock (tetraethyl lead)	Lead chromate	Lead oxide, paint
Chromate, lead — see also	Lead chromate, paint	Lead paint
Lead	Lead dioxide	Lead salts
Chromate, lead paint	Lead, inorganic	Lead, specified compound
Lead (dust) (fumes)	Lead iodide	NEC
(vapor) NEC	Lead iodide, pigment	Lead, tetra-ethyl
Lead alkyl (fuel additive)	(paint)	Paint, lead (fumes)
Lead, antiknock compound	Lead monoxide (dust)	Tetraethyl, lead
(tetraethyl)	Lead monoxide, paint	
Lead carbonate	Lead, organic	

T56.0x- Toxic effects of <u>lead and its compounds</u>

T56.0x1- Toxic effect of lead and its compounds, <u>accidental</u> (unintentional)
Toxic effects of lead and its compounds NOS

T56.0x2- Toxic effect of lead and its compounds, <u>intentional</u> self-harm

T56.0x3- Toxic effect of lead and its compounds, <u>assault</u>

T56.0x4- Toxic effect of lead and its compounds, <u>undetermined</u>

T56.1- Toxic effects of mercury and its compounds

T56.1 - DRUGS/CHEMS*	Mercury, mercurial,	Mercury, chloride, fungicide
Corrosive sublimate	mercuric, mercurous	Mercury, fungicide
Ethyl mercuric chloride	(compounds) (cyanide)	Mercury, organic
Fulminate of mercury	(fumes) (nonmedicinal)	(fungicide)
	(vapor) NEC	

T56.1x- Toxic effects of <u>mercury and its compounds</u>

T56.1x1- Toxic effect of mercury and its compounds, <u>accidental</u> (unintentional)
Toxic effects of mercury and its compounds NOS

T56.1x2- Toxic effect of mercury and its compounds, <u>intentional</u> self-harm

T56.1x3- Toxic effect of mercury and its compounds, <u>assault</u>

T56.1x4- Toxic effect of mercury and its compounds, <u>undetermined</u>

T56.2- Toxic effects of chromium and its compounds

T56.2 - DRUGS/CHEMS*	Chromate, dust or mist	Chromium
Bichromates, fumes	Chromic acid	Chromyl chloride
Chromate	Chromic acid, dust or mist	Potassium bichromate

T56.2x- Toxic effects of <u>chromium and its compounds</u>

T56.2x1- Toxic effect of chromium and its compounds, <u>accidental</u> (unintentional)
Toxic effects of chromium and its compounds NOS

T56.2x2- Toxic effect of chromium and its compounds, <u>intentional</u> self-harm

T56.2x3- Toxic effect of chromium and its compounds, <u>assault</u>

T56.2x4- Toxic effect of chromium and its compounds, <u>undetermined</u>

T54 – T56

T56.3- Toxic effects of cadmium and its compounds

T56.3 - DRUGS/CHEMS*	
Cadmium (chloride) (fumes) (oxide)	

T56.3x- Toxic effects of cadmium and its compounds

T56.3x1- Toxic effect of cadmium and its compounds, accidental (unintentional)
　　　　Toxic effects of cadmium and its compounds NOS

T56.3x2- Toxic effect of cadmium and its compounds, intentional self-harm

T56.3x3- Toxic effect of cadmium and its compounds, assault

T56.3x4- Toxic effect of cadmium and its compounds, undetermined

T56.4- Toxic effects of copper and its compounds

T56.4 - DRUGS/CHEMS*		
Copper (dust) (fumes) (nonmedicinal) NEC	Copper sulfate, cupric	Cuprous sulfate — see also
Copper sulfate	Copper sulfate, cuprous	Copper sulfate
	Cupric sulfate	

T56.4x- Toxic effects of copper and its compounds

T56.4x1- Toxic effect of copper and its compounds, accidental (unintentional)
　　　　Toxic effects of copper and its compounds NOS

T56.4x2- Toxic effect of copper and its compounds, intentional self-harm

T56.4x3- Toxic effect of copper and its compounds, assault

T56.4x4- Toxic effect of copper and its compounds, undetermined

T56.5- Toxic effects of zinc and its compounds

T56.5 - DRUGS/CHEMS*	
Zinc (compounds) (fumes) (vapor) NEC	Zinc chromate
	Zinc, pesticides

T56.5x- Toxic effects of zinc and its compounds

T56.5x1- Toxic effect of zinc and its compounds, accidental (unintentional)
　　　　Toxic effects of zinc and its compounds NOS

T56.5x2- Toxic effect of zinc and its compounds, intentional self-harm

T56.5x3- Toxic effect of zinc and its compounds, assault

T56.5x4- Toxic effect of zinc and its compounds, undetermined

T56.6- Toxic effects of tin and its compounds

T56.6 - DRUGS/CHEMS*	
Tin (chloride) (dust) (oxide) NEC	

T56.6x- Toxic effects of tin and its compounds

T56.6x1- Toxic effect of tin and its compounds, accidental (unintentional)
　　　　Toxic effects of tin and its compounds NOS

T56.6x2- Toxic effect of tin and its compounds, intentional self-harm

T56.6x3- Toxic effect of tin and its compounds, assault

T56.6x4- Toxic effect of tin and its compounds, undetermined

T56.7- Toxic effects of beryllium and its compounds

T56.7 - DRUGS/CHEMS*	
Beryllium (compounds)	

T56.7x- Toxic effects of beryllium and its compounds

T56.7x1- Toxic effect of beryllium and its compounds, accidental (unintentional)
　　　　Toxic effects of beryllium and its compounds NOS

T56.7x2- Toxic effect of beryllium and its compounds, intentional self-harm

T56.7x3- Toxic effect of beryllium and its compounds, assault

T56.7x4- Toxic effect of beryllium and its compounds, undetermined

T56.8- Toxic effects of other metals

T56.81- Toxic effect of thallium

T56.81 - DRUGS/CHEMS*	
Metals, thallium	Thallium (compounds) (dust) NEC

T56.811- Toxic effect of thallium, accidental (unintentional)
　　　　Toxic effect of thallium NOS

T56.812- Toxic effect of thallium, intentional self-harm

T56.813- Toxic effect of thallium, assault

T56.814- Toxic effect of thallium, undetermined

T56.89- Toxic effects of other metals

T56.89 - DRUGS/CHEMS*		
Alum, nonmedicinal (ammonium) (potassium)	Golden sulfide of antimony	Silver, nonmedicinal (dust)
	Iron, nonmedicinal	Stibine
Antimony (compounds) (vapor) NEC	Lithium	Tellurium
	Magnesium NEC	Tellurium, fumes
Antimony, hydride	Metals, specified NEC	Titanium (compounds) (vapor)
Brass (fumes)	Nickel (carbonyl) (tetra-carbonyl) (fumes) (vapor)	Titanium tetrachloride
Cobalt (nonmedicinal) (fumes) (industrial)	Nickelocene	Titanocene
	Selenium NEC	Vanadium

T56.891- Toxic effect of other metals, accidental (unintentional)
　　　　Toxic effects of other metals NOS

T56.892- Toxic effect of other metals, intentional self-harm

T56.893- Toxic effect of other metals, assault

T56.894- Toxic effect of other metals, undetermined

T56.9- Toxic effects of unspecified metal

T56.9 - DRUGS/CHEMS*		
Metals (heavy) (nonmedicinal)	Metals, dust, fumes, or vapor NEC	Metals, light, dust, fumes, or vapor NEC
	Metals, light NEC	Smelter fumes NEC

T56.91x- Toxic effect of unspecified metal, accidental (unintentional)

T56.92x- Toxic effect of unspecified metal, intentional self-harm

T56.93x- Toxic effect of unspecified metal, assault

T56.94x- Toxic effect of unspecified metal, undetermined

T57- Toxic effect of other inorganic substances

The appropriate 7th character is to be added to each code from category T57:
A **Initial** encounter
D **Subsequent** encounter
S **Sequela**

T57.0- Toxic effect of arsenic and its compounds

T57.0 - DRUGS/CHEMS*		
Arsenate of lead	Diphenylchloroarsine, not in war	Lewisite (gas), not in war
Arsenate of lead, herbicide	Ethyl dichloroarsine (vapor)	Paris green
Arsenic, arsenicals (compounds) (dust) (vapor) NEC		Paris green, insecticide
	Fowler's solution	Pesticide, arsenic
Arsenic pesticide (dust) (fumes)	Hexahydrocresol(s) arsenide	Potassium arsenite (solution)
Arsine (gas)	Hexahydrocresol(s) arseniurated	Realgar
Cacodyl, cacodylic acid	Hexahydrocresol(s) sulfide, arseniurated	Scheele's green
Chlorovinyldichloro-arsine, not in war		Scheele's green, insecticide
	Hydrogen arsenide	Schweinfurth green
Copper arsenate, arsenite	Hydrogen, arseniureted	Schweinfurth green, insecticide
Cupric acetoarsenite	Hydrogen sulfide, arseniureted	Sodium arsenate
Cupric arsenate		Trioxide of arsenic
Dimethyl arsine, arsinic acid	Lead arsenate, arsenite (dust) (herbicide) (insecticide) (vapor)	Vienna green
		Vienna red
		White arsenic

T57.0x- Toxic effect of arsenic and its compounds

T57.0x1- Toxic effect of arsenic and its compounds, accidental (unintentional)
　　　　Toxic effect of arsenic and its compounds NOS

T57.0x2- Toxic effect of arsenic and its compounds, intentional self-harm

T57.0x3- Toxic effect of arsenic and its compounds, assault

T57.0x4- Toxic effect of arsenic and its compounds, undetermined

Excludes 1: = NOT CODED HERE! (Do not code both)　　　**1200**　　　Excludes ❷: = Not Included Here

T56 - T57

T57.1- Toxic effect of phosphorus and its compounds
Excludes 1:   *organophosphate insecticides (T60.0)*

T57.1 - DRUGS/CHEMS*	Phosphine, fumigant
Hydrogen phosphureted	Phosphorus (compound)
Phosphine	NEC

T57.1x- Toxic effect of <u>phosphorus and its compounds</u>

T57.1x1- Toxic effect of phosphorus and its compounds, <u>accidental</u> (unintentional)
Toxic effect of phosphorus and its compounds NOS

T57.1x2- Toxic effect of phosphorus and its compounds, <u>intentional</u> self-harm

T57.1x3- Toxic effect of phosphorus and its compounds, <u>assault</u>

T57.1x4- Toxic effect of phosphorus and its compounds, <u>undetermined</u>

T57.2- Toxic effect of manganese and its compounds

T57.2 - DRUGS/CHEMS*
Manganese (dioxide)
(salts)

T57.2x- Toxic effect of <u>manganese and its compounds</u>

T57.2x1- Toxic effect of manganese and its compounds, <u>accidental</u> (unintentional)
Toxic effect of manganese and its compounds NOS

T57.2x2- Toxic effect of manganese and its compounds, <u>intentional</u> self-harm

T57.2x3- Toxic effect of manganese and its compounds, <u>assault</u>

T57.2x4- Toxic effect of manganese and its compounds, <u>undetermined</u>

T57.3- Toxic effect of hydrogen cyanide

T57.3 - DRUGS/CHEMS*	Gas, cyanide	Hydrogen cyanide (salts)
Cyanide(s), dust or gas	HCN	Hydrogen cyanide, gas
(inhalation) NEC	Hexahydrocresol(s) cyanide	Prussic acid, vapor
Cyanide(s), hydrogen	Hydrocyanic acid (liquid)	

T57.3x- Toxic effect of <u>hydrogen cyanide</u>

T57.3x1- Toxic effect of hydrogen cyanide, <u>accidental</u> (unintentional)
Toxic effect of hydrogen cyanide NOS

T57.3x2- Toxic effect of hydrogen cyanide, <u>intentional</u> self-harm

T57.3x3- Toxic effect of hydrogen cyanide, <u>assault</u>

T57.3x4- Toxic effect of hydrogen cyanide, <u>undetermined</u>

T57.8- Toxic effect of other specified inorganic substances

T57.8 - DRUGS/CHEMS*	Boron	Hexahydrocresol(s)
Asbestos	Boron hydride NEC	sulfurated
Barium (carbonate)	Boron hydride, fumes or	Hydrogen chloride
(chloride) (sulfite)	gas	Potassium fluoride
Bichromates (calcium)	Calcium cyanide	Potassium nitrate
(potassium) (sodium)	Chloramine	Sodium bichromate
(crystals)	Decaborane	Sodium borate, cleanser
Borane complex	Hexahydrocresol(s)	
Borate(s)	Fluoride (liquid)	
Borate(s) sodium	Hexahydrocresol(s) sulfate	

T57.8x- Toxic effect of <u>other specified inorganic substances</u>

T57.8x1- Toxic effect of other specified inorganic substances, <u>accidental</u> (unintentional)
Toxic effect of other specified inorganic substances NOS

T57.8x2- Toxic effect of other specified inorganic substances, <u>intentional</u> self-harm

T57.8x3- Toxic effect of other specified inorganic substances, <u>assault</u>

T57.8x4- Toxic effect of other specified inorganic substances, <u>undetermined</u>

T57.9- Toxic effect of <u>unspecified inorganic substance</u>

T57.9 - DRUGS/CHEMS*
Inorganic substance

T57.91x- Toxic effect of unspecified inorganic substance, <u>accidental</u> (unintentional)

T57.92x- Toxic effect of unspecified inorganic substance, <u>intentional</u> self-harm

T57.93x- Toxic effect of unspecified inorganic substance, <u>assault</u>

T57.94x- Toxic effect of unspecified inorganic substance, <u>undetermined</u>

T58- Toxic effect of <u>carbon monoxide</u>
Includes: Asphyxiation from carbon monoxide
Toxic effect of carbon monoxide from all sources

The appropriate 7th character is to be added to each code from category T58:
A   <u>Initial</u> encounter
D   <u>Subsequent</u> encounter
S   <u>Sequela</u>

T58.0- Toxic effect of <u>carbon monoxide from motor vehicle exhaust</u>
Toxic effect of exhaust gas from gas engine
Toxic effect of exhaust gas from motor pump

T58.0 - DRUGS/CHEMS*	Carbon monoxide, exhaust	Exhaust gas (engine)
Carbon monoxide, exhaust	gas, gas engine	(motor vehicle)
gas (motor) not in	Carbon monoxide, exhaust	Fuel, automobile, exhaust
transit	gas, motor pump	gas, not in transit
Carbon monoxide, exhaust	Carbon monoxide, exhaust	Gas, exhaust
gas, combustion engine,	gas, motor vehicle, not	Gas, garage
any not in watercraft	in transit	Gas, motor exhaust, not in
Carbon monoxide, exhaust	Carbon monoxide, motor	transit
gas, farm tractor, not in	exhaust gas, not in	Motor exhaust gas
transit	transit	

T58.01x- Toxic effect of carbon monoxide from motor vehicle exhaust, <u>accidental</u> (unintentional)

T58.02x- Toxic effect of carbon monoxide from motor vehicle exhaust, <u>intentional</u> self-harm

T58.03x- Toxic effect of carbon monoxide from motor vehicle exhaust, <u>assault</u>

T58.04x- Toxic effect of carbon monoxide from motor vehicle exhaust, <u>undetermined</u>

T58.1- Toxic effect of <u>carbon monoxide from utility gas</u>
Toxic effect of acetylene
Toxic effect of gas NOS used for lighting, heating, cooking
Toxic effect of water gas

T58.1 - DRUGS/CHEMS*	Carbon monoxide, fuel,	Carbon monoxide, utility
Acetylene, incomplete	utility, in mobile	gas
combustion of	container	Carbon monoxide, utility
Butane, incomplete	Carbon monoxide, fuel,	gas, piped
combustion	piped (natural)	Carbon monoxide, water
Carbon monoxide, butane	Carbon monoxide,	gas
(distributed in mobile	illuminating gas	Gas, acetylene, incomplete
container)	Carbon monoxide, piped	combustion of
Carbon monoxide, butane,	gas (manufactured)	Gas, illuminating (after
distributed through	(natural)	combustion)
pipes	Carbon monoxide, propane	Gas, stove (after
Carbon monoxide, coal, gas	(distributed in mobile	combustion)
(piped)	container)	Gas, water
Carbon monoxide, fuel, gas	Carbon monoxide,	Illuminating gas (after
(piped)	propane, distributed	combustion)
Carbon monoxide, fuel,	through pipes	Natural gas, incomplete
gas, in mobile container	Carbon monoxide, stove	combustion
Carbon monoxide, fuel,	gas	Propane, incomplete
utility	Carbon monoxide, stove	combustion
	gas, piped	

T58.11x- Toxic effect of carbon monoxide from utility gas, <u>accidental</u> (unintentional)

T58.12x- Toxic effect of carbon monoxide from utility gas, <u>intentional</u> self-harm

T58.13x- Toxic effect of carbon monoxide from utility gas, <u>assault</u>

T58.14x- Toxic effect of carbon monoxide from utility gas, <u>undetermined</u>

T57 - T58

T58.2- Toxic effect of carbon monoxide from incomplete combustion of other domestic fuels
Toxic effect of carbon monoxide from incomplete combustion of coal, coke, kerosene, wood

T58.2 - DRUGS/CHEMS*		
Carbon monoxide, charcoal fumes	Carbon monoxide, kerosene (in domestic stoves, fireplaces)	Coke fumes or gas (carbon monoxide)
Carbon monoxide, coal	Carbon monoxide, wood (in domestic stoves, fireplaces)	Furnace (coal burning) (domestic), gas from
Carbon monoxide, coal, solid (in domestic stoves, fireplaces)		Gas, coal
	Charcoal, fumes (carbon monoxide)	Gas, from wood- or coal-burning stove or fireplace
Carbon monoxide, coke (in domestic stoves, fireplaces)	Coal (carbon monoxide from) — see also Carbon, monoxide, coal	
Carbon monoxide, fuel (in domestic use)		

T58.2x- Toxic effect of <u>carbon monoxide from incomplete combustion of other domestic fuels</u>

    T58.2x1- Toxic effect of carbon monoxide from incomplete combustion of other domestic fuels, <u>accidental</u> (unintentional)

    T58.2x2- Toxic effect of carbon monoxide from incomplete combustion of other domestic fuels, <u>intentional self-harm</u>

    T58.2x3- Toxic effect of carbon monoxide from incomplete combustion of other domestic fuels, <u>assault</u>

    T58.2x4- Toxic effect of carbon monoxide from incomplete combustion of other domestic fuels, <u>undetermined</u>

T58.8- Toxic effect of carbon monoxide from other source
Toxic effect of carbon monoxide from blast furnace gas
Toxic effect of carbon monoxide from fuels in industrial use
Toxic effect of carbon monoxide from kiln vapor

T58.8 - DRUGS/CHEMS*		
Blast furnace gas (carbon monoxide from)	Carbon monoxide, producer gas	Gas, blast furnace
Carbon monoxide, blast furnace gas	Carbon monoxide, specified source NEC	Gas, fuel, industrial use
		Gas, kiln
Carbon monoxide, industrial fuels or gases, any	Charcoal, fumes, industrial	Gas, producer
	Coke fumes or gas, industrial use	Kiln gas or vapor (carbon monoxide)
Carbon monoxide, kiln gas or vapor	Fuel, industrial, incomplete combustion	Producer gas
	Furnace, gas from, industrial	Vapor, kiln (carbon monoxide)

T58.8x- Toxic effect of <u>carbon monoxide from other source</u>

    T58.8x1- Toxic effect of carbon monoxide from other source, <u>accidental</u> (unintentional)

    T58.8x2- Toxic effect of carbon monoxide from other source, <u>intentional self-harm</u>

    T58.8x3- Toxic effect of carbon monoxide from other source, <u>assault</u>

    T58.8x4- Toxic effect of carbon monoxide from other source, <u>undetermined</u>

T58.9- Toxic effect of <u>carbon monoxide from unspecified source</u>

T58.9 - DRUGS/CHEMS*
Carbon monoxide (from incomplete combustion)

T58.91x- Toxic effect of carbon monoxide from unspecified source, <u>accidental</u> (unintentional)

T58.92x- Toxic effect of carbon monoxide from unspecified source, <u>intentional self-harm</u>

T58.93x- Toxic effect of carbon monoxide from unspecified source, <u>assault</u>

T58.94x- Toxic effect of carbon monoxide from unspecified source, <u>undetermined</u>

T59- Toxic effect of <u>other gases, fumes and vapors</u>
Includes: Aerosol propellants
Excludes 1: *chlorofluorocarbons (T53.5)*

The appropriate 7th character is to be added to each code from category T59:
A   <u>Initial</u> encounter
D   <u>Subsequent</u> encounter
S   <u>Sequela</u>

T59.0- Toxic effect of nitrogen oxides

T59.0 - DRUGS/CHEMS*	Nitric oxide (gas)
Fumes, nitrogen dioxide	Nitrogen

T59.0x- Toxic effect of <u>nitrogen oxides</u>

    T59.0x1- Toxic effect of nitrogen oxides, <u>accidental</u> (unintentional)
        Toxic effect of nitrogen oxides NOS

    T59.0x2- Toxic effect of nitrogen oxides, <u>intentional</u> self-harm

    T59.0x3- Toxic effect of nitrogen oxides, <u>assault</u>

    T59.0x4- Toxic effect of nitrogen oxides, <u>undetermined</u>

T59.1- Toxic effect of sulfur dioxide

T59.1 - DRUGS/CHEMS*	Smog
Fumes, sulfur dioxide	Sulfur, dioxide (gas)

T59.1x- Toxic effect of <u>sulfur dioxide</u>

    T59.1x1- Toxic effect of sulfur dioxide, <u>accidental</u> (unintentional)
        Toxic effect of sulfur dioxide NOS

    T59.1x2- Toxic effect of sulfur dioxide, <u>intentional</u> self-harm

    T59.1x3- Toxic effect of sulfur dioxide, <u>assault</u>

    T59.1x4- Toxic effect of sulfur dioxide, <u>undetermined</u>

T59.2- Toxic effect of formaldehyde

T59.2 - DRUGS/CHEMS*	Formalin
Formaldehyde (solution), gas or vapor	Formalin, vapor

T59.2x- Toxic effect of <u>formaldehyde</u>

    T59.2x1- Toxic effect of formaldehyde, <u>accidental</u> (unintentional)
        Toxic effect of formaldehyde NOS

    T59.2x2- Toxic effect of formaldehyde, <u>intentional</u> self-harm

    T59.2x3- Toxic effect of formaldehyde, <u>assault</u>

    T59.2x4- Toxic effect of formaldehyde, <u>undetermined</u>

T59.3- Toxic effect of lacrimogenic gas
Toxic effect of tear gas

T59.3 - DRUGS/CHEMS*	Chloroacetophenone	Lacrimogenic gas
Brombenzylcyanide	Ethyl iodoacetate	Mace
Bromobenzylcyanide	Gas, lacrimogenic	Methyl chloroformate
Chloroacetone	Gas, tear	Tear gas

T59.3x- Toxic effect of <u>lacrimogenic gas</u>

    T59.3x1- Toxic effect of lacrimogenic gas, <u>accidental</u> (unintentional)
        Toxic effect of lacrimogenic gas NOS

    T59.3x2- Toxic effect of lacrimogenic gas, <u>intentional</u> self-harm

    T59.3x3- Toxic effect of lacrimogenic gas, <u>assault</u>

    T59.3x4- Toxic effect of lacrimogenic gas, <u>undetermined</u>

T59.4- Toxic effect of chlorine gas

T59.4 - DRUGS/CHEMS*	Chlorine disinfectant
Chlorine (fumes) (gas)	Chlorine releasing agents
Chlorine compound gas NEC	NEC
	Gas, chlorine

T59.4x- Toxic effect of <u>chlorine gas</u>

    T59.4x1- Toxic effect of chlorine gas, <u>accidental</u> (unintentional)
        Toxic effect of chlorine gas NOS

    T59.4x2- Toxic effect of chlorine gas, <u>intentional</u> self-harm

    T59.4x3- Toxic effect of chlorine gas, <u>assault</u>

    T59.4x4- Toxic effect of chlorine gas, <u>undetermined</u>

T59.5-   Toxic effect of fluorine gas and hydrogen fluoride

T59.5 - DRUGS/CHEMS*	
Fluorine (gas)	Hydrogen fluoride
	Hydrogen fluoride, vapor

T59.5x-   Toxic effect of <u>fluorine gas and hydrogen fluoride</u>

   T59.5x1-   Toxic effect of fluorine gas and hydrogen fluoride, <u>accidental</u> (unintentional)
       Toxic effect of fluorine gas and hydrogen fluoride NOS

   T59.5x2-   Toxic effect of fluorine gas and hydrogen fluoride, <u>intentional</u> self-harm

   T59.5x3-   Toxic effect of fluorine gas and hydrogen fluoride, <u>assault</u>

   T59.5x4-   Toxic effect of fluorine gas and hydrogen fluoride, <u>undetermined</u>

T59.6-   Toxic effect of hydrogen sulfide

T59.6 - DRUGS/CHEMS*		
Hexahydrocresol(s) sulfide (gas)	Hydrogen sulfide	Sulfur, hydrogen
	Hydrogen, sulfureted	
	Hydrosulfuric acid (gas)	

T59.6x-   Toxic effect of <u>hydrogen sulfide</u>

   T59.6x1-   Toxic effect of hydrogen sulfide, <u>accidental</u> (unintentional)
       Toxic effect of hydrogen sulfide NOS

   T59.6x2-   Toxic effect of hydrogen sulfide, <u>intentional</u> self-harm

   T59.6x3-   Toxic effect of hydrogen sulfide, <u>assault</u>

   T59.6x4-   Toxic effect of hydrogen sulfide, <u>undetermined</u>

T59.7-   Toxic effect of carbon dioxide

T59.7 - DRUGS/CHEMS*		
Carbon dioxide (gas)	Carbon dioxide, nonmedicinal	Choke damp
	Carbonic acid gas	

T59.7x-   Toxic effect of <u>carbon dioxide</u>

   T59.7x1-   Toxic effect of carbon dioxide, <u>accidental</u> (unintentional)
       Toxic effect of carbon dioxide NOS

   T59.7x2-   Toxic effect of carbon dioxide, <u>intentional</u> self-harm

   T59.7x3-   Toxic effect of carbon dioxide, <u>assault</u>

   T59.7x4-   Toxic effect of carbon dioxide, <u>undetermined</u>

T59.8-   Toxic effect of other specified gases, fumes and vapors

  T59.81- Toxic effect of <u>smoke</u>
     AHA 13:4Q:p121 – Acute respiratory failure due to smoke inhalation
      Smoke inhalation
     Excludes ❷: toxic effect of cigarette (tobacco) smoke (T65.22-)

T59.81 - DRUGS/CHEMS*
Smoke NEC

   T59.811- Toxic effect of smoke, <u>accidental</u> (unintentional)
       Toxic effect of smoke NOS

   T59.812- Toxic effect of smoke, <u>intentional</u> self-harm

   T59.813- Toxic effect of smoke, <u>assault</u>

   T59.814- Toxic effect of smoke, <u>undetermined</u>

  T59.89- Toxic effect of <u>other specified gases, fumes and vapors</u>

T59.89 - DRUGS/CHEMS*		
Acetylene (gas)	Butane (distributed in mobile container)	Dichloroformoxine, not in war
Acetylene, industrial	Butane, distributed through pipes	Dimethyl sulfate (fumes)
Acridine, vapor		Dinitrobenzene, vapor
Acrolein (gas)	Cholinergic	Dinitrobenzol, vapor
Alcohol, vapor (from any type of alcohol)	organophosphorus, nerve gas	Domestic gas, prior to combustion
Ammonia (fumes) (gas) (vapor)	Coal tar, fumes	Dynamite, fumes
Ammonium compounds, fumes (any usage)	Combustion gas, prior to combustion	Ethidium chloride (vapor)
Amyl acetate, vapor	Cordite vapor	Ethyl aldehyde (vapor)
Anticholinesterase, organophosphorus, nerve gas	Cyanic acid (gas)	Ethylene (gas)
	Cyanogen (chloride) (gas) NEC	Ethylene oxide (fumigant) (nonmedicinal)
Boron trifluoride	Decaborane, fumes	Ferrovanadium (fumes)
Brake fluid vapor	Diazomethane (gas)	Firedamp
Bromine vapor	Diborane (gas)	Formic acid, vapor
	Dichloroethyl sulfide, not in war	

T59.89 - DRUGS/CHEMS* — Continued		
Fuel, gas (domestic use) — see also Carbon, monoxide, fuel, utility	Gas, illuminating, prior to combustion	Ligroin(e), vapor
Fuel, gas, utility	Gas, marsh	Liquefied petroleum gases
Fuel, gas, utility, in mobile container	Gas, mustard, not in war	Liquefied petroleum gases, piped (pure or mixed with air)
Fuel, gas, utility, piped (natural)	Gas, natural	Marsh gas
Fumes, hydrocarbons	Gas, petroleum (liquefied) (distributed in mobile containers)	Methane
Fumes, hydrocarbons, petroleum (liquefied)	Gas, petroleum, piped (pure or mixed with air)	Methanethiol
Fumes, hydrocarbons, petroleum, distributed through pipes (pure or mixed with air)	Gas, piped (manufactured) (natural) NEC	Methyl bromide (gas)
	Gas, refrigerant, not chlorofluoro-carbon	Methyl chloride (gas)
Fumes, petroleum (liquefied)	Gas, stove, prior to combustion	Methyl mercaptan
Fumes, petroleum, distributed through pipes (pure or mixed with air)	Gas, utility (for cooking, heating, or lighting) (piped) NEC	Methyl sulfate (fumes)
	Gas, utility, in mobile container	Natural gas (piped)
Fumes, polyester	Gas, utility, piped (natural)	Nitric acid, vapor
Fumes, specified source NEC — see also substance, specified	Helium (nonmedicinal) NEC	Nitroaniline, vapor
	Hexahydrocresol(s) cyanide, gas	Nitrous acid, fumes
Gas, acetylene	Hexahydrocresol(s) Fluoride, vapor	Oil, fumes
Gas, from utility, prior to combustion	Hydrocarbon gas	Ozone
Gas, fuel, prior to combustion	Hydrocarbon gas, liquefied (mobile container)	Paint fumes NEC
	Hydrocarbon gas, liquefied, piped (natural)	Phosgene (gas)
Gas, fuel, utility	Hydrochloric acid, vapor	Polyester fumes
Gas, fuel, utility, in mobile container	Hydrofluoric acid, vapor	Polyester resin hardener, fumes
Gas, fuel, utility, piped (natural)	Hydrogen	Polytetrafluoroethylene (inhaled)
	Hydroquinone, vapor	Propane (distributed in mobile container)
Gas, hydrocarbon NEC	Illuminating gas, prior to combustion	Propane, distributed through pipes
Gas, hydrocarbon, liquefied, piped	Industrial fumes	Propylene
	Iodine vapor	Pyridine, vapor
		Refrigerant gas, not chlorofluoro-carbon
		Selenium, fumes
		Sternutator gas
		Sulfur, vapor NEC
		Tar, fumes
		Toluidine, vapor
		Vapor, specified source NEC
		Vinyl chloride

   T59.891- Toxic effect of other specified gases, fumes and vapors, <u>accidental</u> (unintentional)

   T59.892- Toxic effect of other specified gases, fumes and vapors, <u>intentional</u> self-harm

   T59.893- Toxic effect of other specified gases, fumes and vapors, <u>assault</u>

   T59.894- Toxic effect of other specified gases, fumes and vapors, <u>undetermined</u>

T59.9-   Toxic effect of <u>unspecified gases, fumes and vapors</u>

T59.9 - DRUGS/CHEMS*		
Fumes (from)	Gas, nerve, not in war	Sewer gas
Gas	Gas, sewer	Vapor — see also Gas
Gas, air contaminants, source or type not specified	Gas, specified source NEC	
	Lung irritant (gas) NEC	
	Mustard gas, not in war	
	Nerve gas, not in war	

  T59.91x- Toxic effect of unspecified gases, fumes and vapors, <u>accidental</u> (unintentional)

  T59.92x- Toxic effect of unspecified gases, fumes and vapors, <u>intentional</u> self-harm

  T59.93x- Toxic effect of unspecified gases, fumes and vapors, <u>assault</u>

  T59.94x- Toxic effect of unspecified gases, fumes and vapors, <u>undetermined</u>

T59 - T59

T60-   **Toxic effect of <u>pesticides</u>**
    Includes: Toxic effect of wood preservatives

The appropriate 7th character is to be added to each code from category T60:
- A   <u>Initial</u> encounter
- D   <u>Subsequent</u> encounter
- S   <u>Sequela</u>

T60.0-   **Toxic effect of organophosphate and carbamate insecticides**

T60.0 - DRUGS/CHEMS*		
Aldicarb	Demephion -O and -S	Mevinphos
Anticholinesterase,	Demeton -O and -S	Mipafox
organophosphorus,	Diazinon	Naled
insecticide	Dicapthon	Octamethyl
Azinphos (ethyl) (methyl)	Dichlorvos	pyrophosphoramide
Benomyl	Dicrotophos	OMPA
Carbamate (insecticide)	Dimefox	Organophosphates
Carbamate, herbicide	Dimethoate	Paraoxon
Carbamate, insecticide	Dimethyl parathion	Parathion
Carbaril	Dimetilan	Phenylsulfthion
Carbaryl	Dioxathion	Phorate
Carbophenothion	Disulfoton	Phosdrin
Chlorfenvinphos	Dithiocarbamate	Phosfolan
Chlormephos	EPN	Phosphamidon
Chloropyrifos	Ethion	Phosphate, organic
Chlorthion	Fenthion	Phosphorus, pesticide
Chlorthiophos	Fluorophosphate insecticide	Propoxur
Cholinergic	HETP	Prothoate
organophosphorus,	Hexaethyl tetraphos-phate	Quinalphos
insecticide	Hexahydrocresol(s)	Schradan
Compound 3422	phophorated	TEPP
(parathion)	Insecticide, carbamate	Terbufos
Compound 3911 (phorate)	Insecticide,	Tetraethyl pyrophosphate
Compound 4049	corganophosphorus	Thiocarbamate (insecticide)
(malathion)	Leptophos	Thiofos
Compound 4069	Malathion, insecticide	Thionazin
(malathion)	Mephosfolan	Trichlorfon
Compound 4124	Metaphos	Trichloronate
(dicapthon)	Methyl demeton	Zineb
Coumaphos	Methyl parathion	
	Metrifonate	

T60.0x-   **Toxic effect of <u>organophosphate and carbamate insecticides</u>**

   T60.0x1-   **Toxic effect of organophosphate and carbamate insecticides, <u>accidental</u> (unintentional)**
      Toxic effect of organophosphate and carbamate insecticides NOS

   T60.0x2-   **Toxic effect of organophosphate and carbamate insecticides, <u>intentional</u> self-harm**

   T60.0x3-   **Toxic effect of organophosphate and carbamate insecticides, <u>assault</u>**

   T60.0x4-   **Toxic effect of organophosphate and carbamate insecticides, <u>undetermined</u>**

T60.1-   **Toxic effect of halogenated insecticides**
    Excludes 1:   chlorinated hydrocarbon (T53.-)

T60.1 - DRUGS/CHEMS*		
2,4,5-T (trichloropheno	Diflubenzuron	PCP, meaning
xyacetic acid)	Endrin	pentachlorophenol
Aldrin (dust)	Heptachlor	PCP, meaning
Chlordan(e) (dust)	Insecticide, cchlorinated	pentachlorophenol,
Chlorex, insecticide	Insecticide, corganochlorine	insecticide
Chlorinated naphthalene	Isobenzan	Pentachlorophenol
(insecticide)	Kelevan	(pesticide)
Chlorophenothane	Kwell (insecticide)	Pentachlorophenol,
Compound 269 (endrin)	Mirex	insecticide
Compound 497 (dieldrin)	Moth balls,	Permethrin
Compound 3956 (toxaphene)	paradichlorobenzene	Pesticide, chlorinated
Cryolite (vapor)	Naphthalene, chlorinated	Pesticide, organochlorine
Cryolite, insecticide	Naphthalene, chlorinated,	(compounds)
Cyhalothrin	vapor	Sodium monofluoroacetate
Cypermethrin	Naphthalene, insecticide or	(pesticide)
DDT (dust)	moth repellent,	Strobane
Deltamethrin	chlorinated	Tar, camphor
Dieldrin (vapor)	Naphthalene, vapor,	Toxaphene (dust) (spray)
	chlorinated	

T60.1x-   **Toxic effect of <u>halogenated insecticides</u>**

   T60.1x1-   **Toxic effect of halogenated insecticides, <u>accidental</u> (unintentional)**
      Toxic effect of halogenated insecticides NOS

   T60.1x2-   **Toxic effect of halogenated insecticides, <u>intentional</u> self-harm**

   T60.1x3-   **Toxic effect of halogenated insecticides, <u>assault</u>**

   T60.1x4-   **Toxic effect of halogenated insecticides, <u>undetermined</u>**

T60.2-   **Toxic effect of other insecticides**

T60.2 - DRUGS/CHEMS*		
Azadirachta	Endosulfan	Pesticide, naphthalene
Camphor, insecticide	Moth balls — see also	Phenothiazine, insecticide
Copper arsenate, arsenite,	Pesticides	Pyrethrin, pyrethrum
insecticide	Moth balls, naphthalene	(nonmedicinal)
Copper, insecticide	Naphthalene (non-	Rotenone
Cyphenothrin	chlorinated)	Sabadilla, pesticide
D-Con, insecticide	Naphthalene, insecticide or	Sodium selenate
DDE (bis(chlorophenyl)-	moth repellent	Tetramethrin
dichloroethylene)	Naphthalene, vapor	Vienna green, insecticide
Derris root	Nicotine (insecticide)	
	(spray) (sulfate) NEC	

T60.2x-   **Toxic effect of <u>other insecticides</u>**

   T60.2x1-   **Toxic effect of other insecticides, <u>accidental</u> (unintentional)**
      Toxic effect of other insecticides NOS

   T60.2x2-   **Toxic effect of other insecticides, <u>intentional</u> self-harm**

   T60.2x3-   **Toxic effect of other insecticides, <u>assault</u>**

   T60.2x4-   **Toxic effect of other insecticides, <u>undetermined</u>**

T60.3-   **Toxic effect of herbicides and fungicides**

T60.3 - DRUGS/CHEMS*		
2,4-D	Dichloronaphthoquinone	Paraquat
(dichlorophenoxyacetic	2,4-Dichlorophenoxyacetic	PCP, meaning
acid)	acid	pentachlorophenol,
Ammonium sulfamate	Dichloropropene	fungicide
Antifungal, nonmedicinal	Dichloropropionic acid	PCP, meaning
(spray)	Dinoseb	pentachlorophenol,
Auramine fungicide	Diquat (dibromide)	herbicide
Benzimidazole	Diuron	Pentachlorophenol,
Bordeaux mixture	DNBP	fungicide
Bromoxynil	Endothall	Pentachlorophenol,
Captafol	Ethylidene diacetate	herbicide
Captan	Fertilizers with herbicide	Plant food or fertilizer,
Chlorate (potassium)	mixture	containing herbicide
(sodium) NEC	Folpet	Propachlor
Chlorate, herbicide	Formaldehyde, fungicide	Propanil
Chloroacetic acid	Formalin, fungicide	Simazine
Chloropicrin, fungicide	Fungicide NEC	Sodium cacodylate,
Chlorothalonil	(nonmedicinal)	herbicide
Copper, fungicide	Glyphosate	2,4,5-T
Copper sulfate, cupric,	HCB	Tetramethylthiuram
fungicide	Herbicide NEC	(disulfide) NEC
Copper sulfate, fungicide	Hexachlorobenzene (vapor)	Thiram
Cupric acetate	MCPA	TMTD
Cycloheximide	Mecoprop	Triazine (herbicide)
2,4-D	Methyl isothiocyanate	Triazole (herbicide)
Dalapon (sodium)	Methylchlorophenoxy-acetic	2,4,5-
Dicamba	acid	Trichlorophenoxyacetic
Dichlobenil	Monochloroacetic acid	acid
Dichlone	Monuron	Verdigris
	Paraformaldehyde	Weed killers NEC

T60.3x-   **Toxic effect of <u>herbicides and fungicides</u>**

   T60.3x1-   **Toxic effect of herbicides and fungicides, <u>accidental</u> (unintentional)**
      Toxic effect of herbicides and fungicides NOS

   T60.3x2-   **Toxic effect of herbicides and fungicides, <u>intentional</u> self-harm**

   T60.3x3-   **Toxic effect of herbicides and fungicides, <u>assault</u>**

   T60.3x4-   **Toxic effect of herbicides and fungicides, <u>undetermined</u>**

T60 - T60

T60.4-   **Toxic effect of rodenticides**
    Excludes 1:   strychnine and its salts (T65.1)
                  thallium (T56.81-)

T60.4 - DRUGS/CHEMS*	Crimidine	Rough-on-rats
ANTU (alpha	D-Con, rodenticide	Scilla, rat poison
naphthylthiourea)	Diphacinone	Scillaren
Barium, pesticide	Diphenadione, rodenticide	Sodium fluoroacetate
Barium, rodenticide	Naphthylthiourea (ANTU)	(dust) (pesticide)
Brodifacoum	Norbormide	Squill, rat poison
Bromethalin	Pesticide, thallium	Thallium, pesticide
Chloralose	Pindone	Warfarin, rodenticide
Chlorophacinone	Pyriminil	Warfarin, sodium
Compound 1080 (sodium	Rat poison NEC	Zinc phosphide
fluoroacetate)	Red squill (scilliroside)	
Coumadin, rodenticide	Rodenticide NEC	

T60.4x- **Toxic effect of rodenticides**
    T60.4x1- **Toxic effect of rodenticides, accidental (unintentional)**
              Toxic effect of rodenticides NOS
    T60.4x2- **Toxic effect of rodenticides, intentional self-harm**
    T60.4x3- **Toxic effect of rodenticides, assault**
    T60.4x4- **Toxic effect of rodenticides, undetermined**

T60.8-   **Toxic effect of other pesticides**

T60.8 - DRUGS/CHEMS*	Fluoroacetate	Petroleum, pesticide
Acaricide	Fluoride (nonmedicinal)	Phenol, pesticide
Antimony, pesticide (vapor)	(pesticide) (sodium) NEC	Piperonyl butoxide
Azobenzene smoke,	Fluoroacetate	Seed disinfectant or
acaricide	Metaldehyde (snail killer)	dressing
Chlorinated pesticide NEC	NEC	Snail killer NEC
Chloropicrin, fumigant	Methyl bromide, fumigant	Tetradifon
Chloropicrin, pesticide	Pesticide, petroleum	
Deet	(distillate) (products)	
Dibromochloropropane	NEC	
Diethyl toluamide	Pesticide, specified	
(nonmedicinal)	ingredient NEC	

T60.8x- **Toxic effect of other pesticides**
    T60.8x1- **Toxic effect of other pesticides, accidental (unintentional)**
              Toxic effect of other pesticides NOS
    T60.8x2- **Toxic effect of other pesticides, intentional self-harm**
    T60.8x3- **Toxic effect of other pesticides, assault**
    T60.8x4- **Toxic effect of other pesticides, undetermined**

T60.9-   **Toxic effect of unspecified pesticide**

T60.9 - DRUGS/CHEMS*	Black leaf (40)	Pesticide, mixture (of
Pesticide (dust) (fumes)	D-Con	compounds)
(vapor) NEC	Fumigant NEC	Preservative, wood
Antrol – see also by specific	Horticulture agent with	Sulfur, pesticide (vapor)
chemical substance	pesticide	
Antrol, fungicide	Insecticide NEC	
Black flag	Insecticide, cmixed	

T60.91x- **Toxic effect of unspecified pesticide, accidental (unintentional)**
T60.92x- **Toxic effect of unspecified pesticide, intentional self-harm**
T60.93x- **Toxic effect of unspecified pesticide, assault**
T60.94x- **Toxic effect of unspecified pesticide, undetermined**

T61-   **Toxic effect of noxious substances eaten as seafood**
    Excludes 1:   allergic reaction to food, such as:
              anaphylactic reaction or shock due to adverse food reaction (T78.0-)
              bacterial foodborne intoxications (A05.-)
              dermatitis (L23.6, L25.4, L27.2)
              food protein-induced enterocolitis syndrome (K52.21)
              food protein-induced enteropathy (K52.22)
              gastroenteritis (noninfective) (K52.29)
         toxic effect of aflatoxin and other mycotoxins (T64)
         toxic effect of cyanides (T65.0-)
         toxic effect of harmful algae bloom (T65.82-)
         toxic effect of hydrogen cyanide (T57.3-)
         toxic effect of mercury (T56.1-)
         toxic effect of red tide (T65.82-)

The appropriate 7th character is to be added to each code from category T61:
   A   Initial encounter
   D   Subsequent encounter
   S   Sequela

T61.0-   **Ciguatera fish poisoning**

T61.0 - DRUGS/CHEMS*	Fish, ciguatera
Ciguatoxin	

T61.01x- **Ciguatera fish poisoning, accidental (unintentional)**
T61.02x- **Ciguatera fish poisoning, intentional self-harm**
T61.03x- **Ciguatera fish poisoning, assault**
T61.04x- **Ciguatera fish poisoning, undetermined**

T61.1-   **Scombroid fish poisoning**
         Histamine-like syndrome

T61.1 - DRUGS/CHEMS*	Scombrotoxin
Fish, scombroid	

T61.11x- **Scombroid fish poisoning, accidental (unintentional)**
T61.12x- **Scombroid fish poisoning, intentional self-harm**
T61.13x- **Scombroid fish poisoning, assault**
T61.14x- **Scombroid fish poisoning, undetermined**

T61.7-   **Other fish and shellfish poisoning**
    T61.77- **Other fish poisoning**

T61.77 - DRUGS/CHEMS*	Tetradotoxin
Fish, specified NEC	

        T61.771- **Other fish poisoning, accidental (unintentional)**
        T61.772- **Other fish poisoning, intentional self-harm**
        T61.773- **Other fish poisoning, assault**
        T61.774- **Other fish poisoning, undetermined**
    T61.78- **Other shellfish poisoning**

T61.78 - DRUGS/CHEMS*	Food, shellfish	Shellfish, noxious,
Fish, shell	Mussel, noxious	nonbacterial

        T61.781- **Other shellfish poisoning, accidental (unintentional)**
        T61.782- **Other shellfish poisoning, intentional self-harm**
        T61.783- **Other shellfish poisoning, assault**
        T61.784- **Other shellfish poisoning, undetermined**

T61.8-   **Toxic effect of other seafood**

T61.8 - DRUGS/CHEMS*	Food, seafood, specified	Seafood, specified NEC
	NEC	

T61.8x- **Toxic effect of other seafood**
    T61.8x1- **Toxic effect of other seafood, accidental (unintentional)**
    T61.8x2- **Toxic effect of other seafood, intentional self-harm**
    T61.8x3- **Toxic effect of other seafood, assault**
    T61.8x4- **Toxic effect of other seafood, undetermined**

T61.9-   **Toxic effect of unspecified seafood**

T61.9 - DRUGS/CHEMS*	Food, fish – see also Fish	Seafood
Fish, noxious, nonbacterial	Food, seafood	

T61.91x- **Toxic effect of unspecified seafood, accidental (unintentional)**
T61.92x- **Toxic effect of unspecified seafood, intentional self-harm**
T61.93x- **Toxic effect of unspecified seafood, assault**
T61.94x- **Toxic effect of unspecified seafood, undetermined**

T60 - T61

T62- Toxic effect of <u>other noxious substances eaten as food</u>

Excludes 1: allergic reaction to food, such as:
anaphylactic shock (reaction) due to adverse food reaction (T78.0-)
bacterial food borne intoxications (A05.-)
dermatitis (L23.6, L25.4, L27.2)
food protein-induced enterocolitis syndrome (K52.21)
food protein-induced enteropathy (K52.22)
gastroenteritis (noninfective) (K52.29)
toxic effect of aflatoxin and other mycotoxins (T64)
toxic effect of cyanides (T65.0-)
toxic effect of hydrogen cyanide (T57.3-)
toxic effect of mercury (T56.1-)

The appropriate 7th character is to be added to each code from category T62:
A   <u>Initial</u> encounter
D   <u>Subsequent</u> encounter
S   <u>Sequela</u>

T62.0- Toxic effect of ingested mushrooms

T62.0 - DRUGS/CHEMS*	Food, mushrooms	Mushroom, noxious
Amanita phalloides	Fungi, noxious, used as	Toadstool
Amanitine	food	

T62.0x- Toxic effect of <u>ingested mushrooms</u>

T62.0x1- Toxic effect of ingested mushrooms, <u>accidental</u> (unintentional)
Toxic effect of ingested mushrooms NOS

T62.0x2- Toxic effect of ingested mushrooms, <u>intentional</u> self-harm

T62.0x3- Toxic effect of ingested mushrooms, <u>assault</u>

T62.0x4- Toxic effect of ingested mushrooms, <u>undetermined</u>

T62.1- Toxic effect of ingested berries

T62.1 - DRUGS/CHEMS*	Deadly nightshade, berry	Plant, noxious, used as
Actaea spicata, berry	Elder berry, (unripe)	food, berries
Akee	Food, berries	Poisonous berries
Anamirta cocculus	Mezereon berries	Privet berries
Berries, poisonous	Nightshade, deadly, berry	Sambucus canadensis berry
Cocculus indicus	Phytolacca decandra	Solanine berries
Convallaria majalis, berry	berries	Solanum dulcamara berries
Daphne, berry		

T62.1x- Toxic effect of <u>ingested berries</u>

T62.1x1- Toxic effect of ingested berries, <u>accidental</u> (unintentional)
Toxic effect of ingested berries NOS

T62.1x2- Toxic effect of ingested berries, <u>intentional</u> self-harm

T62.1x3- Toxic effect of ingested berries, <u>assault</u>

T62.1x4- Toxic effect of ingested berries, <u>undetermined</u>

T62.2- Toxic effect of other ingested (parts of) plant(s)

T62.2 - DRUGS/CHEMS*	Cuckoopint	Jamaica ginger, root
Abrine	Cyclamen europaeum	Jatropha
Abrus (seed)	Cytisus laburnum	Jatropha curcas
Actaea spicata	Cytisus scoparius	Jequirity (bean)
Aethusa cynapium	Daphne (gnidium)	Jimson weed (stramonium)
African boxwood	(mezereum)	Jimson weed, seeds
Amygdaline	Darnel	Kosam seed
Anemone pulsatilla	Deadly nightshade — see	Laburnum (seeds)
Bearsfoot	also Belladonna	Laburnum, leaves
Bittersweet	Delphinium	Larkspur
Black henbane	Elder	Lathyrus (seed)
Brucia	Equisetum	Laurel, black or cherry
Buttercups	Food, plants	Ligustrum vulgare
Calabar bean	Food, seeds	Lily of the valley
Caladium seguinum	Fool's parsley	Lobelia
Cassava	Foxglove	Lolium temulentum
Castor bean	Gaultheria procumbens	Meadow saffron
Cerbera (odallam)	Gelsemium (sempervirens)	Melia azedarach
Chelidonium majus	Goldylocks	Mezereon
Cherry laurel	Gratiola officinalis	Monkshood
Cicuta maculata or virosa	Green hellebore	Myristica fragrans
Cicutoxin	Hedge hyssop	Nerium oleander
Claviceps purpurea	Hellebore (black) (green)	Nicotiana (plant)
Clematis vitalba	(white)	Nightshade, deadly
Colchicum	Hemlock	(solanum) — see also
Coniine	Henbane	Belladonna
Conium (maculatum)	Holly berries	Oleander
Convallaria majalis	Ilex	
Cowbane	Indian tobacco	

T62.2 - DRUGS/CHEMS* – Contiued	Prunus virginiana	Tansy
Physostigma venenosum	Pulsatilla	Thornapple
Phytolacca decandra	Ranunculus	Tobacco, Indian
Piper cubeba	Ricin	Urtica
Plant, noxious, used as food	Ricinus communis	Veratrum, album
	Rue	Veratrum, viride
Plant, noxious, used as food, seeds	Ruta (graveolens)	Water, hemlock
	Sabadilla (plant)	White hellebore
Plant, noxious, used as food, specified type NEC	Sambucus canadensis	Wild black cherry
	Sanguinaria canadensis	Wild poisonous plants NEC
Pokeweed (any part)	Seeds (poisonous)	Wisterine
Pride of China	Solanine	Yellow jasmine
Primula (veris)	Solanum dulcamara	Yew
Privet	Spurge flax	Zygadenus (venenosus)
Prunus laurocerasus	Spurges	
	Stramonium, natural state	

T62.2x- Toxic effect of <u>other ingested (parts of) plant(s)</u>

T62.2x1- Toxic effect of other ingested (parts of) plant(s), <u>accidental</u> (unintentional)
Toxic effect of other ingested (parts of) plant(s) NOS

T62.2x2- Toxic effect of other ingested (parts of) plant(s), <u>intentional</u> self-harm

T62.2x3- Toxic effect of other ingested (parts of) plant(s), <u>assault</u>

T62.2x4- Toxic effect of other ingested (parts of) plant(s), <u>undetermined</u>

T62.8- Toxic effect of other specified noxious substances eaten as food

T62.8 - DRUGS/CHEMS*	Food, specified NEC	Oil, bitter almond
Bitter almond oil	Meat, noxious	Pyrrolizidine alkaloids
Bone meal	Noxious foodstuff, specified	
Coffee	NEC	

T62.8x- Toxic effect of <u>other specified noxious substances eaten as food</u>

T62.8x1- Toxic effect of other specified noxious substances eaten as food, <u>accidental</u> (unintentional)
Toxic effect of other specified noxious substances eaten as food NOS

T62.8x2- Toxic effect of other specified noxious substances eaten as food, <u>intentional</u> self-harm

T62.8x3- Toxic effect of other specified noxious substances eaten as food, <u>assault</u>

T62.8x4- Toxic effect of other specified noxious substances eaten as food, <u>undetermined</u>

T62.9- Toxic effect of <u>unspecified noxious substance eaten as food</u>

T62.9 - DRUGS/CHEMS*	Food, foodstuffs, noxious, nonbacterial, NEC	Noxious foodstuff

T62.91x- Toxic effect of unspecified noxious substance eaten as food, <u>accidental</u> (unintentional)
Toxic effect of unspecified noxious substance eaten as food NOS

T62.92x- Toxic effect of unspecified noxious substance eaten as food, <u>intentional</u> self-harm

T62.93x- Toxic effect of unspecified noxious substance eaten as food, <u>assault</u>

T62.94x- Toxic effect of unspecified noxious substance eaten as food, <u>undetermined</u>

T62 - T62

T63- Toxic effect of <u>contact with venomous animals and plants</u>
Includes: Bite or touch of venomous animal
             Pricked or stuck by thorn or leaf
Excludes ❷: ingestion of toxic animal or plant (T61.-, T62.-)
The appropriate 7th character is to be added to each code from category T63:
  A   <u>Initial</u> encounter
  D   <u>Subsequent</u> encounter
  S   <u>Sequela</u>

T63.0-   Toxic effect of snake venom
  T63.00-   Toxic effect of <u>unspecified snake venom</u>

> **T63.00** - DRUGS/CHEMS*   Venom, snake
> Snake venom or bite

    T63.001-   Toxic effect of unspecified snake venom, <u>accidental</u> (unintentional)
        Toxic effect of unspecified snake venom NOS
    T63.002-   Toxic effect of unspecified snake venom, <u>intentional</u> self-harm
    T63.003-   Toxic effect of unspecified snake venom, <u>assault</u>
    T63.004-   Toxic effect of unspecified snake venom, <u>undetermined</u>

  T63.01-   Toxic effect of <u>rattlesnake venom</u>

> **T63.01** - DRUGS/CHEMS*   Venom, snake, rattlesnake
> Rattlesnake (venom)

    T63.011-   Toxic effect of rattlesnake venom, <u>accidental</u> (unintentional)
        Toxic effect of rattlesnake venom NOS
    T63.012-   Toxic effect of rattlesnake venom, <u>intentional</u> self-harm
    T63.013-   Toxic effect of rattlesnake venom, <u>assault</u>
    T63.014-   Toxic effect of rattlesnake venom, <u>undetermined</u>

  T63.02-   Toxic effect of <u>coral snake venom</u>

> **T63.02** - DRUGS/CHEMS*   Venom, snake, coral snake
> Coral snake (bite) (venom)

    T63.021-   Toxic effect of coral snake venom, <u>accidental</u> (unintentional)
        Toxic effect of coral snake venom NOS
    T63.022-   Toxic effect of coral snake venom, <u>Intentional</u> self-harm
    T63.023-   Toxic effect of coral snake venom, <u>assault</u>
    T63.024-   Toxic effect of coral snake venom, <u>undetermined</u>

  T63.03-   Toxic effect of <u>taipan venom</u>

> **T63.03** - DRUGS/CHEMS*
> Venom, snake, taipan

    T63.031-   Toxic effect of taipan venom, <u>accidental</u> (unintentional)
        Toxic effect of taipan venom NOS
    T63.032-   Toxic effect of taipan venom, <u>intentional</u> self-harm
    T63.033-   Toxic effect of taipan venom, <u>assault</u>
    T63.034-   Toxic effect of taipan venom, <u>undetermined</u>

  T63.04-   Toxic effect of <u>cobra venom</u>

> **T63.04** - DRUGS/CHEMS*   Venom, snake, cobra
> Cobra (venom)

    T63.041-   Toxic effect of cobra venom, <u>accidental</u> (unintentional)
        Toxic effect of cobra venom NOS
    T63.042-   Toxic effect of cobra venom, <u>intentional</u> self-harm
    T63.043-   Toxic effect of cobra venom, <u>assault</u>
    T63.044-   Toxic effect of cobra venom, <u>undetermined</u>

  T63.06-   Toxic effect of venom of <u>other North and South American snake</u>

> **T63.06** - DRUGS/CHEMS*   Fer de lance (bite) (venom) Water moccasin (venom)
> Copperhead snake (bite)   Venom, snake, American
>   (venom)   (North) (South) NEC

    T63.061-   Toxic effect of venom of other North and South American snake, <u>accidental</u> (unintentional)
        Toxic effect of venom of other North and South American snake NOS

    T63.062-   Toxic effect of venom of other North and South American snake, <u>intentional</u> self-harm
    T63.063-   Toxic effect of venom of other North and South American snake, <u>assault</u>
    T63.064-   Toxic effect of venom of other North and South American snake, <u>undetermined</u>

  T63.07-   Toxic effect of venom of <u>other Australian snake</u>

> **T63.07** - DRUGS/CHEMS*
> Venom, snake, Australian

    T63.071-   Toxic effect of venom of other Australian snake, <u>accidental</u> (unintentional)
        Toxic effect of venom of other Australian snake NOS
    T63.072-   Toxic effect of venom of other Australian snake, <u>intentional</u> self-harm
    T63.073-   Toxic effect of venom of other Australian snake, <u>assault</u>
    T63.074-   Toxic effect of venom of other Australian snake, <u>undetermined</u>

  T63.08-   Toxic effect of venom of <u>other African and Asian snake</u>

> **T63.08** - DRUGS/CHEMS*   Venom, snake, Asian
> Venom, snake, African NEC

    T63.081-   Toxic effect of venom of other African and Asian snake, <u>accidental</u> (unintentional)
        Toxic effect of venom of other African and Asian snake NOS
    T63.082-   Toxic effect of venom of other African and Asian snake, <u>intentional</u> self-harm
    T63.083-   Toxic effect of venom of other African and Asian snake, <u>assault</u>
    T63.084-   Toxic effect of venom of other African and Asian snake, <u>undetermined</u>

  T63.09-   Toxic effect of <u>venom of other snake</u>

> **T63.09** - DRUGS/CHEMS*   Venom, snake, specified
> Krait (venom)   NEC
> Sea snake (bite) (venom)   Viper (venom)

    T63.091-   Toxic effect of venom of other snake, <u>accidental</u> (unintentional)
        Toxic effect of venom of other snake NOS
    T63.092-   Toxic effect of venom of other snake, <u>intentional</u> self-harm
    T63.093-   Toxic effect of venom of other snake, <u>assault</u>
    T63.094-   Toxic effect of venom of other snake, <u>undetermined</u>

T63.1-   Toxic effect of <u>venom of other reptiles</u>
  T63.11-   Toxic effect of <u>venom of gila monster</u>

> **T63.11** - DRUGS/CHEMS*   Venom, reptile, gila
> Gila monster (venom)   monster

    T63.111-   Toxic effect of venom of gila monster, <u>accidental</u> (unintentional)
        Toxic effect of venom of gila monster NOS
    T63.112-   Toxic effect of venom of gila monster, <u>intentional</u> self-harm
    T63.113-   Toxic effect of venom of gila monster, <u>assault</u>
    T63.114-   Toxic effect of venom of gila monster, <u>undetermined</u>

  T63.12-   Toxic effect of <u>venom of other venomous lizard</u>

> **T63.12** - DRUGS/CHEMS*   Venom, lizard
> Lizard (bite) (venom)   Venom, reptile, lizard NEC

    T63.121-   Toxic effect of venom of other venomous lizard, <u>accidental</u> (unintentional)
        Toxic effect of venom of other venomous lizard NOS
    T63.122-   Toxic effect of venom of other venomous lizard, <u>intentional</u> self-harm
    T63.123-   Toxic effect of venom of other venomous lizard, <u>assault</u>
    T63.124-   Toxic effect of venom of other venomous lizard, <u>undetermined</u>

T63 - T63

T63.19- Toxic effect of <u>venom of other reptiles</u>

> **T63.19** - DRUGS/CHEMS*
> Venom, reptile

T63.191- Toxic effect of venom of other reptiles, <u>accidental</u> (unintentional)
Toxic effect of venom of other reptiles NOS

T63.192- Toxic effect of venom of other reptiles, <u>intentional</u> self-harm

T63.193- Toxic effect of venom of other reptiles, <u>assault</u>

T63.194- Toxic effect of venom of other reptiles, <u>undetermined</u>

T63.2- Toxic effect of venom of scorpion

> **T63.2** - DRUGS/CHEMS*
> Venom, scorpion

T63.2x- Toxic effect of <u>venom of scorpion</u>

T63.2x1- Toxic effect of venom of scorpion, <u>accidental</u> (unintentional)
Toxic effect of venom of scorpion NOS

T63.2x2- Toxic effect of venom of scorpion, <u>intentional</u> self-harm

T63.2x3- Toxic effect of venom of scorpion, <u>assault</u>

T63.2x4- Toxic effect of venom of scorpion, <u>undetermined</u>

T63.3- Toxic effect of venom of spider

T63.30- Toxic effect of <u>unspecified spider venom</u>

> **T63.30** - DRUGS/CHEMS*
> Venom, spider

T63.301- Toxic effect of unspecified spider venom, <u>accidental</u> (unintentional)

T63.302- Toxic effect of unspecified spider venom, <u>intentional</u> self-harm

T63.303- Toxic effect of unspecified spider venom, <u>assault</u>

T63.304- Toxic effect of unspecified spider venom, <u>undetermined</u>

T63.31- Toxic effect of <u>venom of black widow spider</u>

> **T63.31** - DRUGS/CHEMS*   Venom, spider, black widow
> Black widow spider (bite)

T63.311- Toxic effect of venom of black widow spider, <u>accidental</u> (unintentional)

T63.312- Toxic effect of venom of black widow spider, <u>intentional</u> self-harm

T63.313- Toxic effect of venom of black widow spider, <u>assault</u>

T63.314- Toxic effect of venom of black widow spider, <u>undetermined</u>

T63.32- Toxic effect of <u>venom of tarantula</u>

> **T63.32** - DRUGS/CHEMS*   Venom, spider, tarantula
> Tarantula (venomous)

T63.321- Toxic effect of venom of tarantula, <u>accidental</u> (unintentional)

T63.322- Toxic effect of venom of tarantula, <u>intentional</u> self-harm

T63.323- Toxic effect of venom of tarantula, <u>assault</u>

T63.324- Toxic effect of venom of tarantula, <u>undetermined</u>

T63.33- Toxic effect of <u>venom of brown recluse spider</u>

> **T63.33** - DRUGS/CHEMS*   Venom, spider, brown
> Brown recluse spider (bite)   recluse
> (venom)

T63.331- Toxic effect of venom of brown recluse spider, <u>accidental</u> (unintentional)

T63.332- Toxic effect of venom of brown recluse spider, <u>intentional</u> self-harm

T63.333- Toxic effect of venom of brown recluse spider, <u>assault</u>

T63.334- Toxic effect of venom of brown recluse spider, <u>undetermined</u>

T63.39- Toxic effect of <u>venom of other spider</u>

> **T63.39** - DRUGS/CHEMS*   Spider (bite) (venom)
> Brown spider (bite)   Venom, spider, specified
> (venom)   NEC

T63.391- Toxic effect of venom of other spider, <u>accidental</u> (unintentional)

T63.392- Toxic effect of venom of other spider, <u>intentional</u> self-harm

T63.393- Toxic effect of venom of other spider, <u>assault</u>

T63.394- Toxic effect of venom of other spider, <u>undetermined</u>

T63.4- Toxic effect of venom of other arthropods

T63.41- Toxic effect of <u>venom of centipedes and venomous millipedes</u>

> **T63.41** - DRUGS/CHEMS*   Millipede (tropical)   Venom, millipede (tropical)
> Centipede (bite)   (venomous)
> Venom, centipede

T63.411- Toxic effect of venom of centipedes and venomous millipedes, <u>accidental</u> (unintentional)

T63.412- Toxic effect of venom of centipedes and venomous millipedes, <u>intentional</u> self-harm

T63.413- Toxic effect of venom of centipedes and venomous millipedes, <u>assault</u>

T63.414- Toxic effect of venom of centipedes and venomous millipedes, <u>undetermined</u>

T63.42- Toxic effect of <u>venom of ants</u>

> **T63.42** - DRUGS/CHEMS*   Insect (sting), venomous,   Venom, ant
> Ant (bite) (sting)   ant

T63.421- Toxic effect of venom of ants, <u>accidental</u> (unintentional)

T63.422- Toxic effect of venom of ants, <u>intentional</u> self-harm

T63.423- Toxic effect of venom of ants, <u>assault</u>

T63.424- Toxic effect of venom of ants, <u>undetermined</u>

T63.43- Toxic effect of <u>venom of caterpillars</u>

> **T63.43** - DRUGS/CHEMS*   Insect (sting), venomous,
> Caterpillar (sting)   caterpillar

T63.431- Toxic effect of venom of caterpillars, <u>accidental</u> (unintentional)

T63.432- Toxic effect of venom of caterpillars, <u>intentional</u> self-harm

T63.433- Toxic effect of venom of caterpillars, <u>assault</u>

T63.434- Toxic effect of venom of caterpillars, <u>undetermined</u>

T63.44- Toxic effect of <u>venom of bees</u>

> **T63.44** - DRUGS/CHEMS*   Insect (sting), venomous,   Venom, bee
> Bee (sting) (venom)   bee

T63.441- Toxic effect of venom of bees, <u>accidental</u> (unintentional)

T63.442- Toxic effect of venom of bees, <u>intentional</u> self-harm

T63.443- Toxic effect of venom of bees, <u>assault</u>

T63.444- Toxic effect of venom of bees, <u>undetermined</u>

T63.45- Toxic effect of <u>venom of hornets</u>

> **T63.45** - DRUGS/CHEMS*   Insect (sting), venomous,   Venom, hornet
> Hornet (sting)   hornet

T63.451- Toxic effect of venom of hornets, <u>accidental</u> (unintentional)

T63.452- Toxic effect of venom of hornets, <u>intentional</u> self-harm

T63.453- Toxic effect of venom of hornets, <u>assault</u>

T63.454- Toxic effect of venom of hornets, <u>undetermined</u>

T63.46- Toxic effect of <u>venom of wasps</u>
Toxic effect of yellow jacket

> **T63.46** - DRUGS/CHEMS*   Venom, wasp
> Insect (sting), venomous,   Wasp (sting)
> wasp

T63.461- Toxic effect of venom of wasps, <u>accidental</u> (unintentional)

T63
I
T63

T63.462- Toxic effect of venom of wasps, <u>intentional</u> self-harm

T63.463- Toxic effect of venom of wasps, <u>assault</u>

T63.464- Toxic effect of venom of wasps, <u>undetermined</u>

T63.48- Toxic effect of <u>venom of other arthropod</u>

T63.48 - DRUGS/CHEMS*	Insect (sting), venomous	Venom, insect NEC
Arthropod (venomous) NEC	Venom, arthropod NEC	

T63.481- Toxic effect of venom of other arthropod, <u>accidental</u> (unintentional)

T63.482- Toxic effect of venom of other arthropod, <u>intentional</u> self-harm

T63.483- Toxic effect of venom of other arthropod, <u>assault</u>

T63.484- Toxic effect of venom of other arthropod, <u>undetermined</u>

T63.5- Toxic effect of <u>contact with venomous fish</u>
　　Excludes ❷: poisoning by ingestion of fish (T61.-)

T63.51- Toxic effect of <u>contact with stingray</u>

T63.51 - DRUGS/CHEMS*	Venom, sting ray
Venom, marine, sting ray	

T63.511- Toxic effect of contact with stingray, <u>accidental</u> (unintentional)

T63.512- Toxic effect of contact with stingray, <u>intentional</u> self-harm

T63.513- Toxic effect of contact with stingray, <u>assault</u>

T63.514- Toxic effect of contact with stingray, <u>undetermined</u>

T63.59- Toxic effect of <u>contact with other venomous fish</u>

T63.59 - DRUGS/CHEMS*	Venom, marine, fish
Venom, fish	

T63.591- Toxic effect of contact with other venomous fish, <u>accidental</u> (unintentional)

T63.592- Toxic effect of contact with other venomous fish, <u>intentional</u> self-harm

T63.593- Toxic effect of contact with other venomous fish, <u>assault</u>

T63.594- Toxic effect of contact with other venomous fish, <u>undetermlned</u>

T63.6- Toxic effect of <u>contact with other venomous marine animals</u>
　　Excludes 1: sea-snake venom (T63.09)
　　Excludes ❷: poisoning by ingestion of shellfish (T61.78-)

T63.61- Toxic effect of <u>contact with Portugese Man-o-war</u>
　　Toxic effect of contact with bluebottle

T63.61 - DRUGS/CHEMS*	Venom, marine, animals,
Venom, marine, animals,	Portugese Man-o-war
bluebottle	

T63.611- Toxic effect of contact with Portugese Man-o-war, <u>accidental</u> (unintentional)

T63.612- Toxic effect of contact with Portugese Man-o-war, <u>intentional</u> self-harm

T63.613- Toxic effect of contact with Portugese Man-o-war, <u>assault</u>

T63.614- Toxic effect of contact with Portugese Man-o-war, <u>undetermined</u>

T63.62- Toxic effect of <u>contact with other jellyfish</u>

T63.62 - DRUGS/CHEMS*	Venom, marine, animals,
Jellyfish (sting)	jellyfish NEC

T63.621- Toxic effect of contact with other jellyfish, <u>accidental</u> (unintentional)

T63.622- Toxic effect of contact with other jellyfish, <u>intentional</u> self-harm

T63.623- Toxic effect of contact with other jellyfish, <u>assault</u>

T63.624- Toxic effect of contact with other jellyfish, <u>undetermined</u>

T63.63- Toxic effect of <u>contact with sea anemone</u>

T63.63 - DRUGS/CHEMS*	Venom, marine, animals,
Sea anemone (sting)	sea anemone

T63.631- Toxic effect of contact with sea anemone, <u>accidental</u> (unintentional)

T63.632- Toxic effect of contact with sea anemone, <u>intentional</u> self-harm

T63.633- Toxic effect of contact with sea anemone, <u>assault</u>

T63.634- Toxic effect of contact with sea anemone, <u>undetermined</u>

T63.69- Toxic effect of <u>contact with other venomous marine animals</u>

T63.69 - DRUGS/CHEMS*	Nematocyst (sting)	Venom, marine, animals,
Coral (sting)	Sea cucumber (sting)	specified NEC
Marine (sting)	Sea urchin spine (puncture)	
Marine, animals (sting)	Venom, marine, animals	

T63.691- Toxic effect of contact with other venomous marine animals, <u>accidental</u> (unintentional)

T63.692- Toxic effect of contact with other venomous marine animals, <u>intentional</u> self-harm

T63.693- Toxic effect of contact with other venomous marine animals, <u>assault</u>

T63.694- Toxic effect of contact with other venomous marine animals, <u>undetermined</u>

T63.7- Toxic effect of contact with venomous plant

T63.71- Toxic effect of <u>contact with venomous marine plant</u>

T63.71 - DRUGS/CHEMS*	Venom, marine, plants
Marine, plants (sting)	Venom, plant, marine

T63.711- Toxic effect of contact with venomous marine plant, <u>accidental</u> (unintentional)

T63.712- Toxic effect of contact with venomous marine plant, <u>intentional</u> self-harm

T63.713- Toxic effect of contact with venomous marine plant, <u>assault</u>

T63.714- Toxic effect of contact with venomous marine plant, <u>undetermined</u>

T63.79- Toxic effect of <u>contact with other venomous plant</u>

T63.79 - DRUGS/CHEMS*
Venom, plant NEC

T63.791- Toxic effect of contact with other venomous plant, <u>accidental</u> (unintentional)

T63.792- Toxic effect of contact with other venomous plant, <u>intentional</u> self-harm

T63.793- Toxic effect of contact with other venomous plant, <u>assault</u>

T63.794- Toxic effect of contact with other venomous plant, <u>undetermined</u>

T63.8- Toxic effect of contact with other venomous animals

T63.81- Toxic effect of <u>contact with venomous frog</u>
　　Excludes 1: contact with nonvenomous frog (W62.0)

T63.81 - DRUGS/CHEMS*
Venom, frog

T63.811- Toxic effect of contact with venomous frog, <u>accidental</u> (unintentional)

T63.812- Toxic effect of contact with venomous frog, <u>intentional</u> self-harm

T63.813- Toxic effect of contact with venomous frog, <u>assault</u>

T63.814- Toxic effect of contact with venomous frog, <u>undetermined</u>

T63.82- Toxic effect of contact <u>with venomous toad</u>
　　Excludes 1: contact with nonvenomous toad (W62.1)

T63.82 - DRUGS/CHEMS*
Venom, toad

T63.821- Toxic effect of contact with venomous toad, <u>accidental</u> (unintentional)

T63.822- Toxic effect of contact with venomous toad, <u>intentional</u> self-harm

T63.823- Toxic effect of contact with venomous toad, <u>assault</u>

T63.824- Toxic effect of contact with venomous toad, <u>undetermined</u>

T63 - T63

Excludes 1: = NOT CODED HERE! (Do not code both)　　　**1209**　　　*Excludes ❷:* = Not Included Here

T63.83- Toxic effect of contact with other venomous amphibian
Excludes 1: contact with nonvenomous amphibian (W62.9)

> **T63.83 - DRUGS/CHEMS***
> Venom, amphibian NEC

T63.831- Toxic effect of contact with other venomous amphibian, accidental (unintentional)

T63.832- Toxic effect of contact with other venomous amphibian, intentional self-harm

T63.833- Toxic effect of contact with other venomous amphibian, assault

T63.834- Toxic effect of contact with other venomous amphibian, undetermined

T63.89- Toxic effect of contact with other venomous animals

> **T63.89 - DRUGS/CHEMS***
> Venom, animal NEC

T63.891- Toxic effect of contact with other venomous animals, accidental (unintentional)

T63.892- Toxic effect of contact with other venomous animals, intentional self-harm

T63.893- Toxic effect of contact with other venomous animals, assault

T63.894- Toxic effect of contact with other venomous animals, undetermined

T63.9- Toxic effect of contact with unspecified venomous animal

> **T63.9 - DRUGS/CHEMS***
> Venom, venomous (bite) (sting)

T63.91x- Toxic effect of contact with unspecified venomous animal, accidental (unintentional)

T63.92x- Toxic effect of contact with unspecified venomous animal, intentional self-harm

T63.93x- Toxic effect of contact with unspecified venomous animal, assault

T63.94x- Toxic effect of contact with unspecified venomous animal, undetermined

T64- Toxic effect of aflatoxin and other mycotoxin food contaminants
The appropriate 7th character is to be added to each code from category T64:
A   Initial encounter
D   Subsequent encounter
S   Sequela

T64.0- Toxic effect of aflatoxin

> **T64.0 - DRUGS/CHEMS***   Mycotoxins, aflatoxin
> Aflatoxin

T64.01x- Toxic effect of aflatoxin, accidental (unintentional)

T64.02x- Toxic effect of aflatoxin, intentional self-harm

T64.03x- Toxic effect of aflatoxin, assault

T64.04x- Toxic effect of aflatoxin, undetermined

T64.8- Toxic effect of other mycotoxin food contaminants

> **T64.8 - DRUGS/CHEMS***   Mycotoxins
> Ergot NEC   Mycotoxins, specified NEC

T64.81x- Toxic effect of other mycotoxin food contaminants, accidental (unintentional)

T64.82x- Toxic effect of other mycotoxin food contaminants, intentional self-harm

T64.83x- Toxic effect of other mycotoxin food contaminants, assault

T64.84x- Toxic effect of other mycotoxin food contaminants, undetermined

T65- Toxic effect of other and unspecified substances
The appropriate 7th character is to be added to each code from category T65:
A   Initial encounter
D   Subsequent encounter
S   Sequela

T65.0- Toxic effect of cyanides
Excludes 1: hydrogen cyanide (T57.3-)

> **T65.0 - DRUGS/CHEMS***   Cyanide(s), pesticide (dust)   Potassium cyanide
> 2,4-toluene diisocyanate   (fumes)   Prussic acid
> Aliphatic thiocyanates   Dicyanogen (gas)   Sodium cyanide
> Alkylisocyanate   Gas, dicyanogen   TDI (vapor)
> Cyanide(s) (compounds)   Gas, hydrocyanic acid   Toluene diisocyanate
>   (potassium) (sodium)   Hydrocyanic acid, gas   Tolylene-2,4-diisocyanate
>   NEC   Isocyanate
> Cyanide(s), fumigant   Pesticide, cyanide

T65.0x- Toxic effect of cyanides

T65.0x1- Toxic effect of cyanides, accidental (unintentional)
Toxic effect of cyanides NOS

T65.0x2- Toxic effect of cyanides, intentional self-harm

T65.0x3- Toxic effect of cyanides, assault

T65.0x4- Toxic effect of cyanides, undetermined

T65.1- Toxic effect of strychnine and its salts

> **T65.1 - DRUGS/CHEMS***   Nux vomica   Strychnine (nonmedicinal)
> Brucine   Pesticide, strychnine   (pesticide) (salts)

T65.1x- Toxic effect of strychnine and its salts

T65.1x1- Toxic effect of strychnine and its salts, accidental (unintentional)
Toxic effect of strychnine and its salts NOS

T65.1x2- Toxic effect of strychnine and its salts, intentional self-harm

T65.1x3- Toxic effect of strychnine and its salts, assault

T65.1x4- Toxic effect of strychnine and its salts, undetermined

T65.2- Toxic effect of tobacco and nicotine
Excludes ❷: nicotine dependence (F17.-)

T65.21- Toxic effect of chewing tobacco

> **T65.21 - DRUGS/CHEMS***
> Snuff

T65.211- Toxic effect of chewing tobacco, accidental (unintentional)
Toxic effect of chewing tobacco NOS

T65.212- Toxic effect of chewing tobacco, intentional self-harm

T65.213- Toxic effect of chewing tobacco, assault

T65.214- Toxic effect of chewing tobacco, undetermined

T65.22- Toxic effect of tobacco cigarettes
Toxic effect of tobacco smoke
Use additional code for exposure to second hand tobacco smoke (Z57.31, Z77.22)

> **T65.22 - DRUGS/CHEMS***   Nicotine from tobacco,   Tobacco smoke, second-
> Cigarettes (tobacco)   cigarettes   hand
>   Tobacco, cigarettes

T65.221- Toxic effect of tobacco cigarettes, accidental (unintentional)
Toxic effect of tobacco cigarettes NOS

T65.222- Toxic effect of tobacco cigarettes, intentional self-harm

T65.223- Toxic effect of tobacco cigarettes, assault

T65.224- Toxic effect of tobacco cigarettes, undetermined

T65.29- Toxic effect of other tobacco and nicotine

> **T65.29 - DRUGS/CHEMS***   Nicotine, not insecticide
> Nicotine from tobacco   Tobacco NEC

T65.291- Toxic effect of other tobacco and nicotine, accidental (unintentional)
Toxic effect of other tobacco and nicotine NOS

T65.292- Toxic effect of other tobacco and nicotine, intentional self-harm

T63 - T65

T65.293-   Toxic effect of other tobacco and nicotine, <u>assault</u>

T65.294-   Toxic effect of other tobacco and nicotine, <u>undetermined</u>

T65.3-   Toxic effect of nitroderivatives and aminoderivatives of benzene and its homologues
      Toxic effect of anilin [benzenamine]
      Toxic effect of nitrobenzene
      Toxic effect of trinitrotoluene

T65.3 - DRUGS/CHEMS*	Dinitrophenol	Phenyl enediamine
Aniline (dye) (liquid)	Diphenylamine	Phenyl hydrazine
Aniline vapor	DNOC	Phenylenediamine
Anisidine	Dynamite	Tetryl
Azobenzene smoke	Methoxyaniline	TNT (fumes)
Benzenamine	Methyl aminophenol	Toluylenediamine
Binitrobenzol	Nitramine	Trinitrobenzol
Dichlorbenzidine	Nitroaniline	Trinitrophenol
Dinitro (-ortho-)cresol	Nitrobenzene, nitrobenzol	Trinitrotoluene (fumes)
(pesticide) (spray)	Nitrobenzene, vapor	
Dinitrobenzene	Nitrodiphenyl	
Dinitrobenzol	Nitrosodimethylamine	
Dinitrobutylphenol	Nitrotoluene, nitrotoluol	
Dinitrocyclohexylphenol	Nitrotoluene, vapor	

T65.3x-   Toxic effect of <u>nitroderivatives and aminoderivatives of benzene and its homologues</u>

    T65.3x1-   Toxic effect of nitroderivatives and aminoderivatives of benzene and its homologues, <u>accidental</u> (unintentional)
        Toxic effect of nitroderivatives and aminoderivatives of benzene and its homologues NOS

    T65.3x2-   Toxic effect of nitroderivatives and aminoderivatives of benzene and its homologues, <u>intentional</u> self-harm

    T65.3x3-   Toxic effect of nitroderivatives and aminoderivatives of benzene and its homologues, <u>assault</u>

    T65.3x4-   Toxic effect of nitroderivatives and aminoderivatives of benzene and its homologues, <u>undetermined</u>

T65.4-   Toxic effect of carbon disulfide

T65.4 - DRUGS/CHEMS*	Carbon bisulfide vapor	Carbon disulfide, vapor
Carbon bisulfide (liquid)	Carbon disulfide (liquid)	Varnish

T65.4x-   Toxic effect of <u>carbon disulfide</u>

    T65.4x1-   Toxic effect of carbon disulfide, <u>accidental</u> (unintentional)
        Toxic effect of carbon disulfide NOS

    T65.4x2-   Toxic effect of carbon disulfide, <u>intentional</u> self-harm

    T65.4x3-   Toxic effect of carbon disulfide, <u>assault</u>

    T65.4x4-   Toxic effect of carbon disulfide, <u>undetermined</u>

T65.5-   Toxic effect of nitroglycerin and other nitric acids and esters
      Toxic effect of 1,2,3-Propanetriol trinitrate

T65.5 - DRUGS/CHEMS*	Nitroglycerin,
Nitroglycerin, nonmedicinal	nonmedicinal, fumes

T65.5x-   Toxic effect of <u>nitroglycerin and other nitric acids and esters</u>

    T65.5x1-   Toxic effect of nitroglycerin and other nitric acids and esters, <u>accidental</u> (unintentional)
        Toxic effect of nitroglycerin and other nitric acids and esters NOS

    T65.5x2-   Toxic effect of nitroglycerin and other nitric acids and esters, <u>intentional</u> self-harm

    T65.5x3-   Toxic effect of nitroglycerin and other nitric acids and esters, <u>assault</u>

    T65.5x4-   Toxic effect of nitroglycerin and other nitric acids and esters, <u>undetermined</u>

T65.6-   Toxic effect of paints and dyes, not elsewhere classified

T65.6 - DRUGS/CHEMS*	Cochineal	Oil, colors
Acridine	Dye NEC	Paint NEC
Auramine dye	Lacquer	Stains

T65.6x-   Toxic effect of <u>paints and dyes</u>, <u>not elsewhere classified</u>

    T65.6x1-   Toxic effect of paints and dyes, not elsewhere classified, <u>accidental</u> (unintentional)
        Toxic effect of paints and dyes NOS

    T65.6x2-   Toxic effect of paints and dyes, not elsewhere classified, <u>intentional</u> self-harm

    T65.6x3-   Toxic effect of paints and dyes, not elsewhere classified, <u>assault</u>

    T65.6x4-   Toxic effect of paints and dyes, not elsewhere classified, <u>undetermined</u>

T65.8-   Toxic effect of other specified substances

T65.81-   Toxic effect of <u>latex</u>

T65.81 - DRUGS/CHEMS*
Latex

    T65.811-   Toxic effect of latex, <u>accidental</u> (unintentional)
        Toxic effect of latex NOS

    T65.812-   Toxic effect of latex, <u>intentional</u> self-harm

    T65.813-   Toxic effect of latex, <u>assault</u>

    T65.814-   Toxic effect of latex, <u>undetermined</u>

T65.82-   Toxic effect of <u>harmful algae and algae toxins</u>
      Toxic effect of (harmful) algae bloom NOS
      Toxic effect of blue-green algae bloom
      Toxic effect of brown tide
      Toxic effect of cyanobacteria bloom
      Toxic effect of Florida red tide
      Toxic effect of pfiesteria piscicida
      Toxic effect of red tide

T65.82 - DRUGS/CHEMS*
Algae (harmful) (toxin)

    T65.821-   Toxic effect of harmful algae and algae toxins, <u>accidental</u> (unintentional)
        Toxic effect of harmful algae and algae toxins NOS

    T65.822-   Toxic effect of harmful algae and algae toxins, <u>Intentional</u> self-harm

    T65.823-   Toxic effect of harmful algae and algae toxins, <u>assault</u>

    T65.824-   Toxic effect of harmful algae and algae toxins, <u>undetermined</u>

T65.83-   Toxic effect of <u>fiberglass</u>

T65.83 - DRUGS/CHEMS*
Fiberglass

    T65.831-   Toxic effect of fiberglass, <u>accidental</u> (unintentional)
        Toxic effect of fiberglass NOS

    T65.832-   Toxic effect of fiberglass, <u>intentional</u> self-harm

    T65.833-   Toxic effect of fiberglass, <u>assault</u>

    T65.834-   Toxic effect of fiberglass, <u>undetermined</u>

T65 - T65

T65.89- Toxic effect of <u>other specified substances</u>

T65.89 - DRUGS/CHEMS*		
Acetaldehyde liquid	Naphthol	Reducing agent, industrial NEC
Acetic anhydride	Naphthylamine	Resorcin, resorcinol
Acrylamide	Nitrocellulose	(nonmedicinal)
Acrylonitrile	Nitrocellulose, lacquer	Scouring powder
Adhesive NEC	Nitronaphthalene	Silicone NEC
Amyl propionate	Oil (of)	Sodium bisulfate
Antiaris toxicaria	PBB (polybrominated	Sodium chlorate NEC
Auramine	biphenyls)	Sodium chromate
Benzidine	PCB	Sodium metasilicate
Bergamot oil	Permanganate	Sodium nitrate (oxidizing
Cleaner, cleansing agent,	Phosphate	agent)
type not specified	Phosphate, tricresyl	Sodium oxalate
Cleaner, specified type NEC	Phthalates	Sodium oxide/peroxide
Cordite	Phthalic anhydride	Sodium perborate
Diethylhexylphthalate	Pine oil (disinfectant)	(nonmedicinal) NEC
Dimethyl sulfate, liquid	Pitch	Soldering fluid
Disinfectant	Plant food or fertilizer NEC	Solid substance, specified
Epoxy resin	Polish (car) (floor)	NEC
Fertilizers NEC	(furniture) (metal)	Spray, cosmetic
Furniture polish	(porcelain) (silver)	Styrene
Glutaral, nonmedicinal	Polish, abrasive	Tartaric acid
Glutaraldehyde	Polish, porcelain	Thioglycolic acid
(nonmedicinal)	Polychlorinated biphenyl	Toilet deodorizer
Grease	Potassium chlorate NEC	Toluidine
Guano	Potassium ferric	Tricresyl phosphate
Ink	hexacyanoferrate,	Triorthocresyl phosphate
Isophorone	nonmedicinal	Triphenylphosphate
Jamaica ginger	Potassium oxalate	Vinyl acetate
Liquid, specified NEC	Potassium perchlorate	Vinyl bromide
Liquor creosolis compositus	(nonmedicinal) NEC	Vinylidene chloride
Methyl acrylate	Potassium permanganate	Wax, automobile
Methyl hydrazine	(nonmedicinal)	Whitewash
Methyl iodide	Preservative	Window cleaning fluid
Monosodium glutamate	(nonmedicinal)	
Myristicin	Prussian blue, commercial	
	Psoralene (nonmedicinal)	

T65.891- Toxic effect of other specified substances, <u>accidental</u> (unintentional)
    Toxic effect of other specified substances NOS

T65.892- Toxic effect of other specified substances, <u>intentional</u> self-harm

T65.893- Toxic effect of other specified substances, <u>assault</u>

T65.894- Toxic effect of other specified substances, <u>undetermined</u>

T65.9- Toxic effect of <u>unspecified substance</u>

T65.9 - DRUGS/CHEMS*		
Agricultural agent NEC	Bismuth salts,	Liquid substance
Aerosol spray NEC	nonmedicinal	Poison NEC
Air contaminant (s),	(compounds) NEC	Solid substance
source/type NOS	Chemical substance NEC	Spray (aerosol)
Antifreeze	Horticulture agent NEC	
	Ingested substance NEC	

T65.91x- Toxic effect of unspecified substance, <u>accidental</u> (unintentional)
    Poisoning NOS

T65.92x- Toxic effect of unspecified substance, <u>intentional</u> self-harm

T65.93x- Toxic effect of unspecified substance, <u>assault</u>

T65.94x- Toxic effect of unspecified substance, <u>undetermined</u>

Other and unspecified effects of external causes (T66-T78)

T66.xxx- Radiation sickness, <u>unspecified</u>
    Excludes 1:   radiation gastroenteritis and colitis (K52.0)
                   radiation pneumonitis (J70.0)
                   radiation related disorders of the skin and
                       subcutaneous tissue (L55-L59)
                   specified adverse effects of radiation, such as:
                       burns (T20-T31)
                       leukemia (C91-C95)
                       sunburn (L55.-)

> **The appropriate 7th character is to be added to code T66:**
> **A** **<u>Initial</u> encounter**
> **D** **<u>Subsequent</u> encounter**
> **S** **<u>Sequela</u>**

T67- Effects of heat and light
    Excludes 1:   erythema [dermatitis] ab igne (L59.0)
                   malignant hyperpyrexia due to anesthesia (T88.3)
                   radiation-related disorders of the skin and subcutaneous tissue
                       (L55-L59)
    Excludes ❷: burns (T20-T31)
                   sunburn (L55.-)
                   sweat disorder due to heat (L74-L75)

> **The appropriate 7th character is to be added to each code from category T67:**
> **A** **<u>Initial</u> encounter**
> **D** **<u>Subsequent</u> encounter**
> **S** **<u>Sequela</u>**

T67.0xx- Heatstroke and sunstroke
CC-A   Heat apoplexy
            Heat pyrexia
            Siriasis
            Thermoplegia
            Use additional code(s) to identify any associated complications of
                heatstroke, such as:
            Coma and stupor (R40.-)
            Systemic inflammatory response syndrome (R65.1-)

T67.1xx- Heat syncope
            Heat collapse

T67.2xx- Heat cramp

T67.3xx- Heat exhaustion, anhydrotic
            Heat prostration due to water depletion
            Excludes 1:   heat exhaustion due to salt depletion (T67.4)

T67.4xx- Heat exhaustion due to salt depletion
            Heat prostration due to salt (and water) depletion

T67.5xx- Heat exhaustion, <u>unspecified</u>
            Heat prostration NOS

T67.6xx- Heat fatigue, transient

T67.7xx- Heat edema

T67.8xx- Other effects of heat and light

T67.9xx- Effect of heat and light, <u>unspecified</u>

T68xxx- Hypothermia
            Accidental hypothermia
            Hypothermia NOS
            Use additional code to identify source of exposure:
            Exposure to excessive cold of man-made origin (W93)
            Exposure to excessive cold of natural origin (X31)
            Excludes 1:   hypothermia following anesthesia (T88.51)
                           hypothermia not associated with low environmental
                               temperature (R68.0)
                           hypothermia of newborn (P80.-)
            Excludes ❷: frostbite (T33-T34)

> **The appropriate 7th character is to be added to code T68:**
> **A** **<u>Initial</u> encounter**
> **D** **<u>Subsequent</u> encounter**
> **S** **<u>Sequela</u>**

T65-T68

T69-   <u>Other effects of reduced temperature</u>
Use additional code to identify source of exposure:
    Exposure to excessive cold of man-made origin (W93)
    Exposure to excessive cold of natural origin (X31)
    Excludes ❷: frostbite (T33-T34)
    The appropriate 7th character is to be added to each code from category T69:
      A   <u>Initial</u> encounter
      D   <u>Subsequent</u> encounter
      S   <u>Sequela</u>

   T69.0-   <u>Immersion</u> hand and foot
     T69.01-   Immersion <u>hand</u>
       T69.011-   Immersion hand, <u>right</u> hand
       T69.012-   Immersion hand, <u>left</u> hand
       T69.019-   Immersion hand, <u>unspecified</u> hand
     T69.02-   Immersion <u>foot</u>
        Trench foot
    CC-A **T69.021-**   Immersion foot, <u>right</u> foot
    CC-A **T69.022-**   Immersion foot, <u>left</u> foot
    CC-A **T69.029-**   Immersion foot, <u>unspecified</u> foot

   T69.1xx-   Chilblains
   T69.8xx-   Other specified effects of reduced temperature
   T69.9xx-   Effect of reduced temperature, unspecified

T70-   Effects of air pressure and water pressure
    The appropriate 7th character is to be added to each code from category T70:
      A   <u>Initial</u> encounter
      D   <u>Subsequent</u> encounter
      S   <u>Sequela</u>

   T70.0xx-   Otitic barotrauma
       Aero-otitis media
       Effects of change in ambient atmospheric pressure or water pressure on ears
   T70.1xx-   Sinus barotrauma
       Aerosinusitis
       Effects of change in ambient atmospheric pressure on sinuses
   T70.2-   Other and <u>unspecified</u> effects of high altitude
      Excludes ❷: polycythemia due to high altitude (D75.1)
     T70.20x-   Unspecified effects of high altitude
     T70.29x-   Other effects of high altitude
       Alpine sickness
       Anoxia due to high altitude
       Barotrauma NOS
       Hypobaropathy
       Mountain sickness
   T70.3xx-   Caisson disease [decompression sickness]
   CC-A   Compressed-air disease
       Diver's palsy or paralysis
   T70.4xx-   Effects of high-pressure fluids
       Hydraulic jet injection (industrial)
       Pneumatic jet injection (industrial)
       Traumatic jet injection (industrial)
   T70.8xx-   Other effects of air pressure and water pressure
   T70.9xx-   Effect of air pressure and water pressure, unspecified

T71-   <u>Asphyxiation</u>
    Mechanical suffocation
    Traumatic suffocation
    Excludes 1:   acute respiratory distress (syndrome) (J80)
         anoxia due to high altitude (T70.2)
         asphyxia NOS (R09.01)
         asphyxia from carbon monoxide (T58-)
         asphyxia from inhalation of food or foreign body (T17-)
         asphyxia from other gases, fumes and vapors (T59-)
         respiratory distress (syndrome) in newborn (P22-)
    The appropriate 7th character is to be added to each code from category T71:
      A   <u>Initial</u> encounter
      D   <u>Subsequent</u> encounter
      S   <u>Sequela</u>

   T71.1-   Asphyxiation due to <u>mechanical threat to breathing</u>
       Suffocation due to mechanical threat to breathing
     T71.11-   Asphyxiation due to <u>smothering under pillow</u>
    CC-A **T71.111-**   Asphyxiation due to smothering under pillow, <u>accidental</u>
        Asphyxiation due to smothering under pillow NOS
    CC-A **T71.112-**   Asphyxiation due to smothering under pillow, <u>intentional</u> self-harm
    CC-A **T71.113-**   Asphyxiation due to smothering under pillow, <u>assault</u>
    CC-A **T71.114-**   Asphyxiation due to smothering under pillow, <u>undetermined</u>
     T71.12-   Asphyxiation due to <u>plastic bag</u>
    CC-A **T71.121-**   Asphyxiation due to plastic bag, <u>accidental</u>
        Asphyxiation due to plastic bag NOS
    CC-A **T71.122-**   Asphyxiation due to plastic bag, <u>intentional</u> self-harm
    CC-A **T71.123-**   Asphyxiation due to plastic bag, <u>assault</u>
    CC-A **T71.124-**   Asphyxiation due to plastic bag, <u>undetermined</u>
     T71.13-   Asphyxiation due to <u>being trapped in bed linens</u>
    CC-A **T71.131-**   Asphyxiation due to being trapped in bed linens, <u>accidental</u>
        Asphyxiation due to being trapped in bed linens NOS
    CC-A **T71.132-**   Asphyxiation due to being trapped in bed linens, <u>intentional</u> self-harm
    CC-A **T71.133-**   Asphyxiation due to being trapped in bed linens, <u>assault</u>
    CC-A **T71.134-**   Asphyxiation due to being trapped in bed linens, <u>undetermined</u>
     T71.14-   Asphyxiation due to <u>smothering under another person's body (in bed)</u>
    CC-A **T71.141-**   Asphyxiation due to smothering under another person's body (in bed), <u>accidental</u>
        Asphyxiation due to smothering under another person's body (in bed) NOS
    CC-A **T71.143-**   Asphyxiation due to smothering under another person's body (in bed), <u>assault</u>
    CC-A **T71.144-**   Asphyxiation due to smothering under another person's body (in bed), <u>undetermined</u>
     T71.15-   Asphyxiation due to <u>smothering in furniture</u>
    CC-A **T71.151-**   Asphyxiation due to smothering in furniture, <u>accidental</u>
        Asphyxiation due to smothering in furniture NOS
    CC-A **T71.152-**   Asphyxiation due to smothering in furniture, <u>intentional</u> self-harm
    CC-A **T71.153-**   Asphyxiation due to smothering in furniture, <u>assault</u>
    CC-A **T71.154-**   Asphyxiation due to smothering in furniture, <u>undetermined</u>

T 6 9 - T 7 1

T71.16- Asphyxiation due to <u>hanging</u>
　　　Hanging by window shade cord
　　　Use additional code for any associated injuries, such as:
　　　　Crushing injury of neck (S17.-)
　　　　Fracture of cervical vertebrae (S12.0-S12.2-)
　　　　Open wound of neck (S11.-)

CC-A **T71.161-** Asphyxiation due to hanging, <u>accidental</u>
　　　　Asphyxiation due to hanging NOS
　　　　Hanging NOS

CC-A **T71.162-** Asphyxiation due to hanging, <u>intentional</u> self-harm

CC-A **T71.163-** Asphyxiation due to hanging, <u>assault</u>

CC-A **T71.164-** Asphyxiation due to hanging, <u>undetermined</u>

T71.19- Asphyxiation due to <u>mechanical threat to breathing due to other causes</u>

CC-A **T71.191-** Asphyxiation due to mechanical threat to breathing due to other causes, <u>accidental</u>
　　　　Asphyxiation due to other causes NOS

CC-A **T71.192-** Asphyxiation due to mechanical threat to breathing due to other causes, <u>intentional</u> self-harm

CC-A **T71.193-** Asphyxiation due to mechanical threat to breathing due to other causes, <u>assault</u>

CC-A **T71.194-** Asphyxiation due to mechanical threat to breathing due to other causes, <u>undetermined</u>

T71.2- Asphyxiation due to <u>systemic oxygen deficiency due to low oxygen content in ambient air</u>
　　　Suffocation due to systemic oxygen deficiency due to low oxygen content in ambient air

CC-A **T71.20x-** Asphyxiation due to systemic oxygen deficiency due to low oxygen content in ambient air due to <u>unspecified cause</u>

CC-A **T71.21x-** Asphyxiation due to <u>cave-in or falling earth</u>
　　　　Use additional code for any associated cataclysm (X34-X38)

T71.22- Asphyxiation due to <u>being trapped in a car trunk</u>

CC-A **T71.221-** Asphyxiation due to being trapped in a car trunk, <u>accidental</u>

CC-A **T71.222-** Asphyxiation due to being trapped in a car trunk, <u>intentional</u> self-harm

CC-A **T71.223-** Asphyxiation due to being trapped in a car trunk, <u>assault</u>

CC-A **T71.224-** Asphyxiation due to being trapped in a car trunk, <u>undetermined</u>

T71.23- Asphyxiation due to <u>being trapped in a (discarded) refrigerator</u>

CC-A **T71.231-** Asphyxiation due to being trapped in a (discarded) refrigerator, <u>accidental</u>

CC-A **T71.232-** Asphyxiation due to being trapped in a (discarded) refrigerator, <u>intentional</u> self-harm

CC-A **T71.233-** Asphyxiation due to being trapped in a (discarded) refrigerator, <u>assault</u>

CC-A **T71.234-** Asphyxiation due to being trapped in a (discarded) refrigerator, <u>undetermined</u>

CC-A **T71.29x-** Asphyxiation due to <u>being trapped in other low oxygen environment</u>

T71.9xx- Asphyxiation due to <u>unspecified cause</u>
CC-A　　Suffocation (by strangulation) due to unspecified cause
　　　Suffocation NOS
　　　Systemic oxygen deficiency due to low oxygen content in ambient air due to unspecified cause
　　　Systemic oxygen deficiency due to mechanical threat to breathing due to unspecified cause
　　　Traumatic asphyxia NOS

T73- Effects of other deprivation
　　The appropriate 7th character is to be added to each code from category T73:
　　A <u>Initial</u> encounter
　　D <u>Subsequent</u> encounter
　　S <u>Sequela</u>

T73.0xx- Starvation
　　　Deprivation of food

T73.1xx- Deprivation of water

T73.2xx- Exhaustion due to exposure

T73.3xx- Exhaustion due to excessive exertion
　　　Exhaustion due to overexertion

T73.8xx- Other effects of deprivation

T73.9xx- Effect of deprivation, unspecified

T74- Adult and child abuse, neglect and other maltreatment, <u>confirmed</u>
　　Use additional code, if applicable, to identify any associated current injury
　　Use additional external cause code to identify perpetrator, if known (Y07-)
　　Excludes 1:　abuse and maltreatment in pregnancy (O9A.3-, O9A.4-, O9A.5-)
　　　　　adult and child maltreatment, suspected (T76-)
　　The appropriate 7th character is to be added to each code from category T74:
　　A <u>Initial</u> encounter
　　D <u>Subsequent</u> encounter
　　S <u>Sequela</u>

T74.0- <u>Neglect or abandonment</u>, <u>confirmed</u>

CC-A **T74.01x-** <u>Adult</u> neglect or abandonment, <u>confirmed</u> — [Age/15-124]

CC-A **T74.02x-** <u>Child</u> neglect or abandonment, <u>confirmed</u> — [Age/0-17]

T74.1- <u>Physical abuse</u>, <u>confirmed</u>
　　　Excludes ❷:　sexual abuse (T74.2-)

CC-A **T74.11x-** <u>Adult</u> physical abuse, <u>confirmed</u> — [Age/15-124]

CC-A **T74.12x-** <u>Child</u> physical abuse, <u>confirmed</u> — [Age/0-17]
　　　Excludes ❷:　shaken infant syndrome (T74.4)

T74.2- <u>Sexual abuse</u>, <u>confirmed</u>
　　　Rape, confirmed
　　　Sexual assault, confirmed

CC-A **T74.21x-** <u>Adult</u> sexual abuse, <u>confirmed</u> — [Age/15-124]

CC-A **T74.22x-** <u>Child</u> sexual abuse, <u>confirmed</u> — [Age/0-17]

T74.3- <u>Psychological abuse</u>, <u>confirmed</u>

T74.31x- <u>Adult</u> psychological abuse, <u>confirmed</u> — [Age/15-124]

CC-A **T74.32x-** <u>Child</u> psychological abuse, <u>confirmed</u> — [Age/0-17]

T74.4xx- Shaken infant syndrome — [Age/0-17]
CC-A

T74.9- <u>Unspecified maltreatment</u>, <u>confirmed</u>

CC-A **T74.91x-** Unspecified <u>adult</u> maltreatment, <u>confirmed</u> — [Age/15-124]

CC-A **T74.92x-** Unspecified <u>child</u> maltreatment, <u>confirmed</u> — [Age/0-17]

T75- Other and unspecified effects of other external causes
　　Excludes 1:　adverse effects NEC (T78.-)
　　Excludes ❷:　burns (electric) (T20-T31)
　　The appropriate 7th character is to be added to each code from category T75:
　　A <u>Initial</u> encounter
　　D <u>Subsequent</u> encounter
　　S <u>Sequela</u>

T75.0- Effects of lightning
　　　Struck by lightning

T75.00x- Unspecified effects of lightning
　　　Struck by lightning NOS

T75.01x- Shock due to being struck by lightning

T75.09x- Other effects of lightning
　　　Use additional code for other effects of lightning

T75.1xx- Unspecified effects of drowning and nonfatal submersion
CC-A　　Immersion
　　　Excludes 1:　specified effects of drowning — code to effects

T71-T75

T75.2- Effects of vibration

    T75.20x- Unspecified effects of vibration

    T75.21x- Pneumatic hammer syndrome

    T75.22x- Traumatic vasospastic syndrome

    T75.23x- Vertigo from infrasound
        Excludes 1:   *vertigo NOS (R42)*

    T75.29- Other effects of vibration

T75.3xx- Motion sickness
    Airsickness
    Seasickness
    Travel sickness
    Use additional external cause code to identify vehicle or type of
       motion (Y92.81-, Y93.5-)

T75.4xx- Electrocution
    Shock from electric current
    Shock from electroshock gun (taser)

T75.8- Other specified effects of external causes

    T75.81x- Effects of abnormal gravitation [G] forces

    T75.82x- Effects of weightlessness

    T75.89x- Other specified effects of external causes

T76- Adult and child abuse, neglect and other maltreatment, <u>suspected</u>
    Use additional code, if applicable, to identify any associated current injury
    Excludes 1: *adult and child maltreatment, confirmed (T74.-)*
             suspected abuse and maltreatment in pregnancy (O9A.3-,
                O9A.4-, O9A.5-)
             suspected adult physical abuse, ruled out (Z04.71)
             suspected adult sexual abuse, ruled out (Z04.41)
             suspected child physical abuse, ruled out (Z04.72)
             suspected child sexual abuse, ruled out (Z04.42)

**The appropriate 7th character is to be added to each code from
    category T76:**
    A <u>Initial</u> encounter
    D <u>Subsequent</u> encounter
    S <u>Sequela</u>

T76.0- <u>Neglect or abandonment</u>, suspected

CC-A **T76.01x-** <u>Adult</u> neglect or abandonment, suspected — [Age/15-124]

CC-A **T76.02x-** <u>Child</u> neglect or abandonment, suspected — [Age/0-17]

T76.1- <u>Physical abuse</u>, suspected

CC-A **T76.11x-** <u>Adult</u> physical abuse, suspected — [Age/15-124]

CC-A **T76.12x-** <u>Child</u> physical abuse, suspected — [Age/0-17]

T76.2- <u>Sexual abuse</u>, suspected
    Rape, suspected
    Sexual abuse, suspected
    Excludes 1: *alleged abuse, ruled out (Z04.7)*

CC-A **T76.21x-** <u>Adult</u> sexual abuse, suspected — [Age/15-124]

CC-A **T76.22x-** <u>Child</u> sexual abuse, suspected — [Age/0-17]

T76.3- <u>Psychological abuse</u>, suspected

    T76.31x- <u>Adult</u> psychological abuse, suspected — [Age/15-124]

CC-A **T76.32x-** <u>Child</u> psychological abuse, suspected — [Age/0-17]

T76.9- <u>Unspecified maltreatment</u>, suspected

CC-A **T76.91x-** Unspecified <u>adult</u> maltreatment, suspected —
        [Age/15-124]

CC-A **T76.92x-** Unspecified <u>child</u> maltreatment, suspected — [Age/0-17]

T78- Adverse effects, <u>not elsewhere classified</u>
    Excludes ❷: *complications of surgical and medical care NEC (T80-T88)*
**The appropriate 7th character is to be added to each code from
    category T78:**
    A <u>Initial</u> encounter
    D <u>Subsequent</u> encounter
    S <u>Sequela</u>

T78.0- <u>Anaphylactic reaction due to food</u>
    Anaphylactic reaction due to adverse food reaction
    Anaphylactic shock or reaction due to nonpoisonous foods
    Anaphylactoid reaction due to food

CC-A **T78.00x-** Anaphylactic reaction due to unspecified food

CC-A **T78.01x-** Anaphylactic reaction due to peanuts

CC-A **T78.02x-** Anaphylactic reaction due to shellfish (crustaceans)

CC-A **T78.03x-** Anaphylactic reaction due to other fish

CC-A **T78.04x-** Anaphylactic reaction due to fruits and vegetables

CC-A **T78.05x-** Anaphylactic reaction due to tree nuts and seeds
        Excludes ❷: *anaphylactic reaction due to peanuts (T78.01)*

CC-A **T78.06x-** Anaphylactic reaction due to food additives

CC-A **T78.07x-** Anaphylactic reaction due to milk and dairy products

CC-A **T78.08x-** Anaphylactic reaction due to eggs

CC-A **T78.09x-** Anaphylactic reaction due to other food products

T78.1xx- Other adverse food reactions, <u>not elsewhere classified</u>
    Use additional code to identify the type of reaction, if applicable
    Excludes 1: *anaphylactic reaction or shock due to adverse food*
               reaction (T78.0-)
             anaphylactic reaction due to food (T78.0-)
             bacterial food borne intoxications (A05-)
    Excludes ❷: *allergic and dietetic gastroenteritis and colitis*
               (K52.29)
             allergic rhinitis due to food (J30.5)
             dermatitis due to food in contact with skin (L23.6,
               L24.6, L25.4)
             dermatitis due to ingested food (L27.2)
             food protein-induced enterocolitis syndrome (K52.21)
             food protein-induced enteropathy (K52.22)

T78.2xx- Anaphylactic shock, <u>unspecified</u>
CC-A   Allergic shock
    Anaphylactic reaction
    Anaphylaxis
    Excludes 1: *anaphylactic reaction or shock due to adverse effect*
               of correct medicinal substance properly
               administered (T88.6)
             anaphylactic reaction or shock due to adverse food
               reaction (T78.0-)
             anaphylactic reaction or shock due to serum (T80.5)

T78.3xx- Angioneurotic edema
    Allergic angioedema
    Giant urticaria
    Quincke's edema
    Excludes 1: *serum urticaria (T80.6-)*
             urticaria (L50-)

T78.4- Other and unspecified allergy
    Excludes 1: *specified types of allergic reaction such as:*
               allergic diarrhea (K52.29)
               allergic gastroenteritis and colitis (K52.29)
               dermatitis (L23-L25, L27.-)
               food protein-induced enterocolitis syndrome (K52.21)
               food protein-induced enteropathy (K52.22)
               hay fever (J30.1)

    T78.40x- Allergy, unspecified
        Allergic reaction NOS
        Hypersensitivity NOS

    T78.41x- Arthus phenomenon
        Arthus reaction

    T78.49x- Other allergy

T78.8xx- Other adverse effects, not elsewhere classified

Certain early complications of trauma (T79)

T79- Certain early complications of trauma, <u>not elsewhere classified</u>

　Excludes ❷:　acute respiratory distress syndrome (J80)
　　complications occurring during or following medical procedures (T80-T88)
　　complications of surgical and medical care NEC (T80-T88)
　　newborn respiratory distress syndrome (P22.0)

> The appropriate 7th character is to be added to each code from category T79:
> A　<u>Initial</u> encounter
> D　<u>Subsequent</u> encounter
> S　<u>Sequela</u>

T79.0xx- **Air embolism (traumatic)**
MCC-A
　Excludes 1:　air embolism complicating abortion or ectopic or molar pregnancy (O00-O07, O08.2)
　　air embolism complicating pregnancy, childbirth and the puerperium (O88.0)
　　air embolism following infusion, transfusion, and therapeutic injection (T80.0)
　　air embolism following procedure NEC (T81.7-)

T79.1xx- **Fat embolism (traumatic)**
MCC-A
　Excludes 1:　fat embolism complicating:
　　abortion or ectopic or molar pregnancy (O00-O07, O08.2)
　　pregnancy, childbirth and the puerperium (O88.8)

T79.2xx- **Traumatic secondary and recurrent hemorrhage and seroma**
CC-A

T79.4xx- **Traumatic shock**
MCC-A
　Shock (immediate) (delayed) following injury
　Excludes 1:　anaphylactic shock due to adverse food reaction (T78.0-)
　　anaphylactic shock due to correct medicinal substance properly administered (T88.6)
　　anaphylactic shock due to serum (T80.5-)
　　anaphylactic shock NOS (T78.2)
　　anesthetic shock (T88.2)
　　electric shock (T75.4)
　　nontraumatic shock NEC (R57-)
　　obstetric shock (O75.1)
　　postprocedural shock (T81.1-)
　　septic shock (R65.21)
　　shock complicating abortion or ectopic or molar pregnancy (O00-O07, O08.3)
　　shock due to lightning (T75.01)
　　shock NOS (R57.9)

T79.5xx- **Traumatic anuria**
MCC-A
　Crush syndrome
　Renal failure following crushing

T79.6xx- **Traumatic ischemia of muscle**
　Traumatic rhabdomyolysis
　Volkmann's ischemic contracture
　Excludes ❷:　anterior tibial syndrome (M76.8)
　　compartment syndrome (traumatic) (T79.A-)
　　nontraumatic ischemia of muscle (M62.2-)

T79.7xx- **Traumatic subcutaneous emphysema**
CC-A
　Excludes 1:　emphysema NOS (J43)
　　emphysema (subcutaneous) resulting from a procedure (T81.82)

T79.A- **Traumatic compartment syndrome**
　Excludes 1:　fibromyalgia (M79.7)
　　nontraumatic compartment syndrome (M79.A-)
　　traumatic ischemic infarction of muscle (T79.6)

CC-A **T79.A0x-** **Compartment syndrome, <u>unspecified</u>**
　Compartment syndrome NOS

T79.A1- **Traumatic compartment syndrome of <u>upper extremity</u>**
　Traumatic compartment syndrome of shoulder, arm, forearm, wrist, hand, and fingers

CC-A **T79.A11-** **Traumatic compartment syndrome of <u>right</u> upper extremity**

CC-A **T79.A12-** **Traumatic compartment syndrome of <u>left</u> upper extremity**

CC-A **T79.A19-** **Traumatic compartment syndrome of <u>unspecified</u> upper extremity**

T79.A2- **Traumatic compartment syndrome of <u>lower extremity</u>**
　Traumatic compartment syndrome of hip, buttock, thigh, leg, foot, and toes

CC-A **T79.A21-** **Traumatic compartment syndrome of <u>right</u> lower extremity**

CC-A **T79.A22-** **Traumatic compartment syndrome of <u>left</u> lower extremity**

CC-A **T79.A29-** **Traumatic compartment syndrome of <u>unspecified</u> lower extremity**

CC-A **T79.A3x-** **Traumatic compartment syndrome of <u>abdomen</u>**

CC-A **T79.A9x-** **Traumatic compartment syndrome of <u>other</u> sites**

T79.8xx- **Other early complications of trauma**

T79.9xx- **Unspecified early complication of trauma**

Complications of surgical and medical care, not elsewhere classified (T80-T88)

Use additional code for adverse effect, if applicable, to identify drug (T36-T50 with fifth or sixth character 5)
Use additional code(s) to identify the specified condition resulting from the complication
Use additional code to identify devices involved and details of circumstances (Y62-Y82)
　Excludes ❷:　any encounters with medical care for postprocedural conditions in which no complications are present, such as:
　　artificial opening status (Z93-)
　　closure of external stoma (Z43-)
　　fitting and adjustment of external prosthetic device (Z44-)
　　burns and corrosions from local applications and irradiation (T20-T32)
　　complications of surgical procedures during pregnancy, childbirth and the puerperium (O00-O9A)
　　mechanical complication of respirator [ventilator] (J95.850)
　　poisoning and toxic effects of drugs and chemicals (T36-T65 with fifth or sixth characters 1-4 or 6)
　　postprocedural fever (R50.82)
　　specified complications classified elsewhere, such as:
　　cerebrospinal fluid leak from spinal puncture (G97.0)
　　colostomy malfunction (K94.0-)
　　disorders of fluid and electrolyte imbalance (E86-E87)
　　functional disturbances following cardiac surgery (I97.0-I97.1)
　　intraoperative and postprocedural complications of specified body systems (D78-, E36-, E89-, G97.3-, G97.4, H59.3-, H59-, H95.2-, H95.3, I97.4-, I97.5, J95.6-, J95.7, K91.6-, L76-, M96-, N99-)
　　ostomy complications (J95.0-, K94.-, N99.5-)
　　postgastric surgery syndromes (K91.1)
　　postlaminectomy syndrome NEC (M96.1)
　　postmastectomy lymphedema syndrome (I97.2)
　　postsurgical blind-loop syndrome (K91.2)
　　ventilator associated pneumonia (J95.851)

T80- **Complications following <u>infusion, transfusion and therapeutic injection</u>**
　Includes:　Complications following perfusion
　Excludes ❷:　bone marrow transplant rejection (T86.01)
　　febrile nonhemolytic transfusion reaction (R50.84)
　　fluid overload due to transfusion (E87.71)
　　posttransfusion purpura (D69.51)
　　transfusion associated circulatory overload (TACO) (E87.71)
　　transfusion (red blood cell) associated hemochromatosis (E83.111)
　　transfusion related acute lung injury (TRALI) (J95.84)

> The appropriate 7th character is to be added to each code from category T80:
> A　<u>Initial</u> encounter
> D　<u>Subsequent</u> encounter
> S　<u>Sequela</u>

T80.0xx- <u>**Air embolism**</u> **following infusion, transfusion and**
MCC-A **therapeutic injection**

T80.1xx- <u>**Vascular**</u> **complications following infusion, transfusion and**
CC-A **therapeutic injection**
　Use additional code to identify the vascular complication
　Excludes ❷:　extravasation of vesicant agent (T80.81-)
　　infiltration of vesicant agent (T80.81-)
　　postprocedural vascular complications (T81.7-)
　　vascular complications specified as due to prosthetic devices, implants and grafts (T82.8-, T83.8-, T84.8-, T85.8-)

T 7 9 - T 8 0

T80.2-   **Infections** following infusion, transfusion and therapeutic injection
    Use additional code to identify the specific infection, such as:
        Sepsis (A41.9)
    Use additional code (R65.2-) to identify severe sepsis, if applicable
    *Excludes ❷: infections specified as due to prosthetic devices, implants and grafts (T82.6-T82.7, T83.5-T83.6, T84.5-T84.7, T85.7)
        postprocedural infections (T81.4-)*

T80.21-   Infection <u>due to central venous catheter</u>
        Infection due to pulmonary artery catheter (Swan-Ganz catheter)

CC-A **T80.211-**   <u>Bloodstream</u> infection due to central venous catheter
        Bloodstream infection due to Hickman catheter
        Bloodstream infection due to peripherally inserted central catheter (PICC)
        Bloodstream infection due to portacath (port-a-cath)
        Bloodstream infection due to pulmonary artery catheter
        Bloodstream infection due to triple lumen catheter
        Bloodstream infection due to umbilical venous catheter
        Catheter-related bloodstream infection (CRBSI) NOS
        Central line-associated bloodstream infection (CLABSI)

CC-A **T80.212-**   <u>Local</u> infection due to central venous catheter
        Exit or insertion site infection
        Local infection due to Hickman catheter
        Local infection due to peripherally inserted central catheter (PICC)
        Local infection due to portacath (port-a-cath)
        Local infection due to pulmonary artery catheter
        Local infection due to triple lumen catheter
        Local infection due to umbilical venous catheter
        Port or reservoir infection
        Tunnel infection

CC-A **T80.218-**   <u>Other</u> infection due to central venous catheter
        Other central line-associated infection
        Other infection due to Hickman catheter
        Other infection due to peripherally inserted central catheter (PICC)
        Other infection due to portacath (port-a-cath)
        Other infection due to pulmonary artery catheter
        Other infection due to triple lumen catheter
        Other infection due to umbilical venous catheter

CC-A **T80.219-**   <u>Unspecified</u> infection due to central venous catheter
        Central line-associated infection NOS
        Unspecified infection due to Hickman catheter
        Unspecified infection due to peripherally inserted central catheter (PICC)
        Unspecified infection due to portacath (port-a-cath)
        Unspecified infection due to pulmonary artery catheter
        Unspecified infection due to triple lumen catheter
        Unspecified infection due to umbilical venous catheter

CC-A **T80.22x-**   <u>Acute infection</u> following transfusion, infusion, or injection of <u>blood and blood products</u>

CC-A **T80.29x-**   Infection following <u>other infusion, transfusion and therapeutic injection</u>

T80.3-   <u>ABO incompatibility reaction</u> due to transfusion of blood or blood products
    Excludes 1:   minor blood group antigens reactions (Duffy) (E) (K(ell)) (Kidd) (Lewis) (M) (N) (P) (S) (T80.A)

CC-A **T80.30x-**   ABO incompatibility reaction due to transfusion of blood or blood products, <u>unspecified</u>
        ABO incompatibility blood transfusion NOS
        Reaction to ABO incompatibility from transfusion NOS

T80.31- ABO incompatibility <u>with hemolytic transfusion reaction</u>

CC-A **T80.310-**   ABO incompatibility with <u>acute</u> hemolytic transfusion reaction
        ABO incompatibility with hemolytic transfusion reaction less than 24 hours after transfusion
        Acute hemolytic transfusion reaction (AHTR) due to ABO incompatibility

CC-A **T80.311-**   ABO incompatibility with <u>delayed</u> hemolytic transfusion reaction
        ABO incompatibility with hemolytic transfusion reaction 24 hours or more after transfusion
        Delayed hemolytic transfusion reaction (DHTR) due to ABO incompatibility

CC-A **T80.319-**   ABO incompatibility with hemolytic transfusion reaction, <u>unspecified</u>
        ABO incompatibility with hemolytic transfusion reaction at unspecified time after transfusion
        Hemolytic transfusion reaction (HTR) due to ABO incompatibility NOS

CC-A **T80.39x-**   <u>Other</u> ABO incompatibility reaction due to transfusion of blood or blood products
        Delayed serologic transfusion reaction (DSTR) from ABO incompatibility
        Other ABO incompatible blood transfusion
        Other reaction to ABO incompatible blood transfusion

T80.4-   <u>Rh incompatibility reaction</u> due to transfusion of blood or blood products
        Reaction due to incompatibility of Rh antigens (C) (c) (D) (E) (e)

CC-A **T80.40x-**   Rh incompatibility reaction due to transfusion of blood or blood products, <u>unspecified</u>
        Reaction due to Rh factor in transfusion NOS
        Rh incompatible blood transfusion NOS

T80.41- Rh incompatibility <u>with hemolytic transfusion reaction</u>

CC-A **T80.410-**   Rh incompatibility with <u>acute</u> hemolytic transfusion reaction
        Acute hemolytic transfusion reaction (AHTR) due to Rh incompatibility
        Rh incompatibility with hemolytic transfusion reaction less than 24 hours after transfusion

CC-A **T80.411-**   Rh incompatibility with <u>delayed</u> hemolytic transfusion reaction
        Delayed hemolytic transfusion reaction (DHTR) due to Rh incompatibility
        Rh incompatibility with hemolytic transfusion reaction 24 hours or more after transfusion

CC-A **T80.419-**   Rh incompatibility with hemolytic transfusion reaction, <u>unspecified</u>
        Rh incompatibility with hemolytic transfusion reaction at unspecified time after transfusion
        Hemolytic transfusion reaction (HTR) due to Rh incompatibility NOS

CC-A **T80.49x-**   <u>Other</u> Rh incompatibility reaction due to transfusion of blood or blood products
        Delayed serologic transfusion reaction (DSTR) from Rh incompatibility
        Other reaction to Rh incompatible blood transfusion

T80.A-   <u>Non-ABO incompatibility reaction</u> due to transfusion of blood or blood products
        Reaction due to incompatibility of minor antigens (Duffy) (Kell) (Kidd) (Lewis) (M) (N) (P) (S)

CC-A **T80.A0x-**   Non-ABO incompatibility reaction due to transfusion of blood or blood products, <u>unspecified</u>
        Non-ABO antigen incompatibility reaction from transfusion NOS

T80.A1- Non-ABO incompatibility <u>with hemolytic transfusion reaction</u>

CC-A **T80.A10-**   Non-ABO incompatibility with <u>acute</u> hemolytic transfusion reaction
        Acute hemolytic transfusion reaction (AHTR) due to non-ABO incompatibility
        Non-ABO incompatibility with hemolytic transfusion reaction less than 24 hours after transfusion

CC-A **T80.A11-**   Non-ABO incompatibility with <u>delayed</u> hemolytic transfusion reaction
        Delayed hemolytic transfusion reaction (DHTR) due to non-ABO incompatibility
        Non-ABO incompatibility with hemolytic transfusion reaction 24 or more hours after transfusion

CC-A **T80.A19-**   Non-ABO incompatibility with hemolytic transfusion reaction, <u>unspecified</u>
        Hemolytic transfusion reaction (HTR) due to non-ABO incompatibility NOS
        Non-ABO incompatibility with hemolytic transfusion reaction at unspecified time after transfusion

CC-A **T80.A9x-**   <u>Other</u> non-ABO incompatibility reaction due to transfusion of blood or blood products
        Delayed serologic transfusion reaction (DSTR) from non-ABO incompatibility
        Other reaction to non-ABO incompatible blood transfusion

T80 - T80

T80.5- **Anaphylactic reaction due to serum**
    Allergic shock due to serum
    Anaphylactic shock due to serum
    Anaphylactoid reaction due to serum
    Anaphylaxis due to serum
    Excludes 1:   *ABO incompatibility reaction due to transfusion of*
         blood or blood products (T80.3-)
         allergic reaction or shock NOS (T78.2)
         anaphylactic reaction or shock NOS (T78.2)
         anaphylactic reaction or shock due to adverse effect of
          correct medicinal substance properly administered
          (T88.6)
         other serum reaction (T80.6-)

CC-A **T80.51x-** **Anaphylactic reaction due to administration of blood and blood products**

CC-A **T80.52x-** **Anaphylactic reaction due to vaccination**

CC-A **T80.59x-** **Anaphylactic reaction due to other serum**

T80.6- **Other serum reactions**
    Intoxication by serum
    Protein sickness
    Serum rash
    Serum sickness
    Serum urticaria
    Excludes ❷: *serum hepatitis (B16-B19)*

CC-A **T80.61x-** **Other serum reaction due to administration of blood and blood products**

CC-A **T80.62x-** **Other serum reaction due to vaccination**

CC-A **T80.69x-** **Other serum reaction due to other serum**

T80.8- **Other complications following infusion, transfusion and therapeutic injection**

    T80.81- **Extravasation of vesicant agent**
        Infiltration of vesicant agent

    CC-A **T80.810-** **Extravasation of vesicant antineoplastic chemotherapy**
        Infiltration of vesicant antineoplastic chemotherapy

    CC-A **T80.818-** **Extravasation of other vesicant agent**
        Infiltration of other vesicant agent

    T80.89x- **Other complications following infusion, transfusion and therapeutic injection**
        Delayed serologic transfusion reaction (DSTR), unspecified incompatibility
        Use additional code to identify graft-versus-host reaction, if applicable, (D89.81-)

T80.9- **Unspecified complication following infusion, transfusion and therapeutic injection**

    T80.90x- **Unspecified complication following infusion and therapeutic injection**

    T80.91- **Hemolytic transfusion reaction, unspecified incompatibility**
        Excludes 1:   *ABO incompatibility with hemolytic transfusion*
          reaction (T80.31-)
         Non-ABO incompatibility with hemolytic
          transfusion reaction (T80.A1-)
         Rh incompatibility with hemolytic transfusion
          reaction (T80.41-)

    CC-A **T80.910-** **Acute hemolytic transfusion reaction, unspecified incompatibility**

    CC-A **T80.911-** **Delayed hemolytic transfusion reaction, unspecified incompatibility**

    CC-A **T80.919-** **Hemolytic transfusion reaction, unspecified incompatibility, unspecified as acute ordelayed**
        Hemolytic transfusion reaction NOS

    T80.92x- **Unspecified transfusion reaction**
        Transfusion reaction NOS

T81- **Complications of procedures, <u>not elsewhere classified</u>**
    Use additional code for adverse effect, if applicable, to identify drug (T36-T50 with fifth or sixth character 5)
    Excludes ❷: *complications following immunization (T88.0-T88.1)*
         complications following infusion, transfusion and therapeutic
          injection (T80-)
         complications of transplanted organs and tissue (T86-)
         specified complications classified elsewhere, such as:
          complication of prosthetic devices, implants and grafts
           (T82-T85)
          dermatitis due to drugs and medicaments (L23.3, L24.4,
           L25.1, L27.0-L27.1)
          endosseous dental implant failure (M27.6-)
          floppy iris syndrome (IFIS) (intraoperative) H21.81
         intraoperative and postprocedural complications of specific
           body system (D78.-, E36.-, E89.-, G97.3-, G97.4,
           H59.3-, H59.-, H95.2-, H95.3, I97.4-, I97.5, J95,
           K91.-, L76.-, M96.-, N99.-)
          ostomy complications (J95.0-, K94.-, N99.5-)
          plateau iris syndrome (post-iridectomy) (postprocedural)
           H21.82
         poisoning and toxic effects of drugs and chemicals (T36-T65
           with fifth or sixth character 1-4 or 6)

The appropriate 7th character is to be added to each code from category T81:
  A   <u>Initial</u> encounter
  D   <u>Subsequent</u> encounter
  S   <u>Sequela</u>

T81.1- **Postprocedural shock**
    AHA 15:1Q:p23 – Penny lodged in proximal esophagus
    Shock during or resulting from a procedure, not elsewhere classified
    Excludes 1:   *anaphylactic shock NOS (T78.2)*
         anaphylactic shock due to correct substance properly
          administered (T88.6)
         anaphylactic shock due to serum (T80.5-)
         anesthetic shock (T88.2)
         electric shock (T75.4)
         obstetric shock (O75.1)
         septic shock (R65.21)
         shock following abortion or ectopic or molar pregnancy
          (O00-O07, O08.3)
         traumatic shock (T79.4)

CC-A **T81.10x-** **Postprocedural shock, unspecified**
    Collapse NOS during or resulting from a procedure, not elsewhere classified
    Postprocedural failure of peripheral circulation
    Postprocedural shock NOS

MCC-A **T81.11x-** **Postprocedural cardiogenic shock**

MCC-A **T81.12x-** **Postprocedural septic shock** — [Unacceptable PDX]
    Postprocedural endotoxic shock resulting from a procedure, not elsewhere classified
    Postprocedural gram-negative shock resulting from a procedure, not elsewhere classified
    Code first underlying infection
    Use additional code, to identify any associated acute organ dysfunction, if applicable

MCC-A **T81.19x-** **Other postprocedural shock**
    Postprocedural hypovolemic shock

T80 - T81

T81.3- <u>Disruption of wound</u>, not elsewhere classified

AHA 14:1Q:p23 – Nonhealing surgical wound

Disruption of any suture materials or other closure methods

Excludes 1: breakdown (mechanical) of permanent sutures (T85.612)

displacement of permanent sutures (T85.622)

disruption of cesarean delivery wound (O90.0)

disruption of perineal obstetric wound (O90.1)

mechanical complication of permanent sutures NEC (T85.692)

CC-A **T81.30x-** Disruption of wound, <u>unspecified</u>

Disruption of wound NOS

CC-A **T81.31x-** Disruption of <u>external</u> operation (surgical) wound, not elsewhere classified

Dehiscence of operation wound NOS

Disruption of operation wound NOS

Disruption or dehiscence of closure of cornea

Disruption or dehiscence of closure of mucosa

Disruption or dehiscence of closure of skin and subcutaneous tissue

Full-thickness skin disruption or dehiscence

Superficial disruption or dehiscence of operation wound

Excludes 1: dehiscence of amputation stump (T87.81)

CC-A **T81.32x-** Disruption of <u>internal</u> operation (surgical) wound, not elsewhere classified

Deep disruption or dehiscence of operation wound NOS

Disruption or dehiscence of closure of internal organ or other internal tissue

Disruption or dehiscence of closure of muscle or muscle flap

Disruption or dehiscence of closure of ribs or rib cage

Disruption or dehiscence of closure of skull or craniotomy

Disruption or dehiscence of closure of sternum or sternotomy

Disruption or dehiscence of closure of tendon or ligament

Disruption or dehiscence of closure of superficial or muscular fascia

CC-A **T81.33x-** Disruption of <u>traumatic</u> injury wound repair

Disruption or dehiscence of closure of traumatic laceration (external) (internal)

T81.4xx- Infection following a procedure

CC-A

AHA 14:1Q:p23 – Nonhealing surgical wound

Intra-abdominal abscess following a procedure

Postprocedural infection, not elsewhere classified

Sepsis following a procedure

Stitch abscess following a procedure

Subphrenic abscess following a procedure

Wound abscess following a procedure

Use additional code to identify infection

Use additional code (R65.2-) to identify severe sepsis, if applicable

Excludes 1: obstetric surgical wound infection (O86.0)

postprocedural fever NOS (R50.82)

postprocedural retroperitoneal abscess (K68.11)

Excludes ❷: bleb associated endophthalmitis (H59.4-)

infection due to infusion, transfusion and therapeutic injection (T80.2-)

infection due to prosthetic devices, implants and grafts (T82.6-T82.7, T83.5-T83.6, T84.5-T84.7, T85.7)

T81.5- Complications of foreign body accidentally left in body following procedure

AHA 14:4Q:p24 – Loose cement fragment in hip joint

T81.50- <u>Unspecified complication</u> of <u>foreign body accidentally left in body following procedure</u>

CC-A **T81.500-** Unspecified complication of foreign body accidentally left in body following <u>surgical operation</u>

CC-A **T81.501-** Unspecified complication of foreign body accidentally left in body following <u>infusion or transfusion</u>

CC-A **T81.502-** Unspecified complication of foreign body accidentally left in body following <u>kidney dialysis</u>

CC-A **T81.503-** Unspecified complication of foreign body accidentally left in body following <u>injection or immunization</u>

CC-A **T81.504-** Unspecified complication of foreign body accidentally left in body following <u>endoscopic examination</u>

CC-A **T81.505-** Unspecified complication of foreign body accidentally left in body following <u>heart catheterization</u>

CC-A **T81.506-** Unspecified complication of foreign body accidentally left in body following <u>aspiration, puncture or other catheterization</u>

CC-A **T81.507-** Unspecified complication of foreign body accidentally left in body following <u>removal of catheter or packing</u>

CC-A **T81.508-** Unspecified complication of foreign body accidentally left in body following <u>other procedure</u>

CC-A **T81.509-** Unspecified complication of foreign body accidentally left in body following <u>unspecified procedure</u>

T81.51- <u>Adhesions</u> due to <u>foreign body accidentally left in body following procedure</u>

CC-A **T81.510-** Adhesions due to foreign body accidentally left in body following <u>surgical operation</u>

CC-A **T81.511-** Adhesions due to foreign body accidentally left in body following <u>infusion or transfusion</u>

CC-A **T81.512-** Adhesions due to foreign body accidentally left in body following <u>kidney dialysis</u>

CC-A **T81.513-** Adhesions due to foreign body accidentally left in body following <u>injection or immunization</u>

CC-A **T81.514-** Adhesions due to foreign body accidentally left in body following <u>endoscopic examination</u>

CC-A **T81.515-** Adhesions due to foreign body accidentally left in body following <u>heart catheterization</u>

CC-A **T81.516-** Adhesions due to foreign body accidentally left in body following <u>aspiration, puncture or other catheterization</u>

CC-A **T81.517-** Adhesions due to foreign body accidentally left in body following <u>removal of catheter or packing</u>

CC-A **T81.518-** Adhesions due to foreign body accidentally left in body following <u>other procedure</u>

CC-A **T81.519-** Adhesions due to foreign body accidentally left in body following <u>unspecified procedure</u>

T81.52- <u>Obstruction</u> due to <u>foreign body accidentally left in body following procedure</u>

CC-A **T81.520-** Obstruction due to foreign body accidentally left in body following <u>surgical operation</u>

CC-A **T81.521-** Obstruction due to foreign body accidentally left in body following <u>infusion or transfusion</u>

CC-A **T81.522-** Obstruction due to foreign body accidentally left in body following <u>kidney dialysis</u>

CC-A **T81.523-** Obstruction due to foreign body accidentally left in body following <u>injection or immunization</u>

CC-A **T81.524-** Obstruction due to foreign body accidentally left in body following <u>endoscopic examination</u>

CC-A **T81.525-** Obstruction due to foreign body accidentally left in body following <u>heart catheterization</u>

CC-A **T81.526-** Obstruction due to foreign body accidentally left in body following <u>aspiration, puncture or other catheterization</u>

CC-A **T81.527-** Obstruction due to foreign body accidentally left in body following <u>removal of catheter or packing</u>

CC-A **T81.528-** Obstruction due to foreign body accidentally left in body following <u>other procedure</u>

CC-A **T81.529-** Obstruction due to foreign body accidentally left in body following <u>unspecified procedure</u>

T81.53- <u>Perforation</u> due to <u>foreign body accidentally left in body following procedure</u>

CC-A **T81.530-** Perforation due to foreign body accidentally left in body following <u>surgical operation</u>

CC-A **T81.531-** Perforation due to foreign body accidentally left in body following <u>infusion or transfusion</u>

CC-A **T81.532-** Perforation due to foreign body accidentally left in body following <u>kidney dialysis</u>

T81-T81

CC-A **T81.533-** Perforation due to foreign body accidentally left in body following <u>injection or immunization</u>

CC-A **T81.534-** Perforation due to foreign body accidentally <u>left</u> in body following <u>endoscopic examination</u>

CC-A **T81.535-** Perforation due to foreign body accidentally left in body following <u>heart catheterization</u>

CC-A **T81.536-** Perforation due to foreign body accidentally <u>left</u> in body following <u>aspiration, puncture or other catheterization</u>

CC-A **T81.537-** Perforation due to foreign body accidentally left in body following <u>removal of catheter or packing</u>

CC-A **T81.538-** Perforation due to foreign body accidentally <u>left</u> in body following <u>other procedure</u>

CC-A **T81.539-** Perforation due to foreign body accidentally left in body following <u>unspecified procedure</u>

T81.59- <u>Other complications</u> of <u>foreign body accidentally left in body following procedure</u>
    Excludes ❷: obstruction or perforation due to prosthetic devices and implants intentionally left in body (T82.0-T82.5, T83.0-T83.4, T83.7, T84.0-T84.4, T85.0-T85.6)

CC-A **T81.590-** Other complications of foreign body accidentally left in body following <u>surgical operation</u>

CC-A **T81.591-** Other complications of foreign body accidentally left in body following <u>infusion or transfusion</u>

CC-A **T81.592-** Other complications of foreign body accidentally left in body following <u>kidneydialysis</u>

CC-A **T81.593-** Other complications of foreign body accidentally left in body following <u>injection or immunization</u>

CC-A **T81.594-** Other complications of foreign body accidentally left in body following <u>endoscopic examination</u>

CC-A **T81.595-** Other complications of foreign body accidentally left in body following <u>heart catheterization</u>

CC-A **T81.596-** Other complications of foreign body accidentally left in body following <u>aspiration, puncture or other catheterization</u>

CC-A **T81.597-** Other complications of foreign body accidentally left in body following <u>removal of catheter or packing</u>

CC-A **T81.598-** Other complications of foreign body accidentally left in body following <u>other procedure</u>

CC-A **T81.599-** Other complications of foreign body accidentally left in body following <u>unspecified procedure</u>

T81.6- <u>Acute reaction</u> to <u>foreign substance accidentally left during a procedure</u>
    Excludes ❷: complications of foreign body accidentally left in body cavity or operation wound following procedure (T81.5-)

CC-A **T81.60x-** <u>Unspecified</u> acute reaction to foreign substance accidentally left during a procedure

CC-A **T81.61x-** <u>Aseptic peritonitis</u> due to foreign substance accidentally left during a procedure
    Chemical peritonitis

CC-A **T81.69x-** <u>Other acute reaction</u> to foreign substance accidentally left during a procedure

T81.7- <u>Vascular complications following a procedure</u>, <u>not elsewhere classified</u>
    Air embolism following procedure NEC
    Phlebitis or thrombophlebitis resulting from a procedure
    Excludes 1: embolism complicating abortion or ectopic or molar pregnancy (O00-O07, O08.2)
    embolism complicating pregnancy, childbirth and the puerperium (O88.-)
    traumatic embolism (T79.0)
    Excludes ❷: embolism due to prosthetic devices, implants and grafts (T82.8-, T83.81, T84.8-, T85.81-)
    embolism following infusion, transfusion and therapeutic injection (T80.0)

T81.71- Complication of <u>artery</u> following a procedure, not elsewhere classified

CC-A **T81.710-** Complication of <u>mesenteric</u> artery following a procedure, not elsewhere classified

CC-A **T81.711-** Complication of <u>renal</u> artery following a procedure, not elsewhere classified

CC-A **T81.718-** Complication of <u>other artery</u> following a procedure, not elsewhere classified

CC-A **T81.719-** Complication of <u>unspecified artery</u> following a procedure, not elsewhere classified

CC-A **T81.72x-** Complication of <u>vein</u> following a procedure, not elsewhere classified

T81.8- Other complications of procedures, <u>not elsewhere classified</u>
    Excludes ❷: hypothermia following anesthesia (T88.51)
    malignant hyperpyrexia due to anesthesia (T88.3)

T81.81x- Complication of inhalation therapy

T81.82x- Emphysema (subcutaneous) resulting from a procedure

CC-A **T81.83x-** Persistent postprocedural fistula

T81.89x- Other complications of procedures, not elsewhere classified
    AHA 14:1Q:p23 – Nonhealing surgical wound
    Use additional code to specify complication, such as:
    Postprocedural delirium (F05)

T81.9xx- Unspecified complication of procedure

T82- <u>Complications of cardiac and vascular prosthetic devices, implants and grafts</u>
    Excludes ❷: failure and rejection of transplanted organs and tissue (T86.-)

The appropriate 7th character is to be added to each code from category T82:
A <u>Initial</u> encounter
D <u>Subsequent</u> encounter
S <u>Sequela</u>

T82.0- <u>Mechanical</u> complication of <u>heart valve prosthesis</u>
    Mechanical complication of artificial heart valve
    Excludes 1: mechanical complication of biological heart valve graft (T82.22-)

CC-A **T82.01x-** Breakdown (mechanical) of heart valve prosthesis

CC-A **T82.02x-** Displacement of heart valve prosthesis
    Malposition of heart valve prosthesis

CC-A **T82.03x-** Leakage of heart valve prosthesis

CC-A **T82.09x-** Other mechanical complication of heart valve prosthesis
    Obstruction (mechanical) of heart valve prosthesis
    Perforation of heart valve prosthesis
    Protrusion of heart valve prosthesis

T82.1- <u>Mechanical</u> complication of <u>cardiac electronic device</u>
T82.11- Breakdown (mechanical) of cardiac electronic device

CC-A **T82.110-** Breakdown (mechanical) of cardiac electrode

CC-A **T82.111-** Breakdown (mechanical) of cardiac pulse generator (battery)

CC-A **T82.118-** Breakdown (mechanical) of other cardiac electronic device

CC-A **T82.119-** Breakdown (mechanical) of unspecified cardiac electronic device

T82.12- <u>Displacement</u> of <u>cardiac electronic device</u>
    Malposition of cardiac electronic device

CC-A **T82.120-** Displacement of cardiac electrode

CC-A **T82.121-** Displacement of cardiac pulse generator (battery)

CC-A **T82.128-** Displacement of other cardiac electronic device

CC-A **T82.129-** Displacement of unspecified cardiac electronic device

T82.19- <u>Other mechanical</u> complication of <u>cardiac electronic device</u>
    Leakage of cardiac electronic device
    Obstruction of cardiac electronic device
    Perforation of cardiac electronic device
    Protrusion of cardiac electronic device

CC-A **T82.190-** Other mechanical complication of cardiac electrode

CC-A **T82.191-** Other mechanical complication of cardiac pulse generator (battery)

CC-A **T82.198-** Other mechanical complication of other cardiac electronic device

CC-A **T82.199-** Other mechanical complication of unspecified cardiac device

T82.2- Mechanical complication of coronary artery bypass graft and biological heart valve graft
    Excludes 1:   *mechanical complication of artificial heart valve prosthesis (T82.0-)*

T82.21- Mechanical complication of coronary artery bypass graft

CC-A **T82.211-** Breakdown (mechanical) of coronary artery bypass graft

CC-A **T82.212-** Displacement of coronary artery bypass graft
    Malposition of coronary artery bypass graft

CC-A **T82.213-** Leakage of coronary artery bypass graft

CC-A **T82.218-** Other mechanical complication of coronary artery bypass graft
    Obstruction, mechanical of coronary artery bypass graft
    Perforation of coronary artery bypass graft
    Protrusion of coronary artery bypass graft

T82.22- Mechanical complication of biological heart valve graft

CC-A **T82.221-** Breakdown (mechanical) of biological heart valve graft

CC-A **T82.222-** Displacement of biological heart valve graft
    Malposition of biological heart valve graft

CC-A **T82.223-** Leakage of biological heart valve graft

CC-A **T82.228-** Other mechanical complication of biological heart valve graft
    Obstruction of biological heart valve graft
    Perforation of biological heart valve graft
    Protrusion of biological heart valve graft

T82.3- Mechanical complication of other vascular grafts

T82.31- Breakdown (mechanical) of other vascular grafts

CC-A **T82.310-** Breakdown (mechanical) of aortic (bifurcation) graft (replacement)

CC-A **T82.311-** Breakdown (mechanical) of carotid arterial graft (bypass)

CC-A **T82.312-** Breakdown (mechanical) of femoral arterial graft (bypass)

CC-A **T82.318-** Breakdown (mechanical) of other vascular grafts

CC-A **T82.319-** Breakdown (mechanical) of unspecified vascular grafts

T82.32- Displacement of other vascular grafts
    Malposition of other vascular grafts

CC-A **T82.320-** Displacement of aortic (bifurcation) graft (replacement)

CC-A **T82.321-** Displacement of carotid arterial graft (bypass)

CC-A **T82.322-** Displacement of femoral arterial graft (bypass)

CC-A **T82.328-** Displacement of other vascular grafts

CC-A **T82.329-** Displacement of unspecified vascular grafts

T82.33- Leakage of other vascular grafts

CC-A **T82.330-** Leakage of aortic (bifurcation) graft (replacement)

CC-A **T82.331-** Leakage of carotid arterial graft (bypass)

CC-A **T82.332-** Leakage of femoral arterial graft (bypass)

CC-A **T82.338-** Leakage of other vascular grafts

CC-A **T82.339-** Leakage of unspecified vascular graft

T82.39- Other mechanical complication of other vascular grafts
    Obstruction (mechanical) of other vascular grafts
    Perforation of other vascular grafts
    Protrusion of other vascular grafts

CC-A **T82.390-** Other mechanical complication of aortic (bifurcation) graft (replacement)

CC-A **T82.391-** Other mechanical complication of carotid arterial graft (bypass)

CC-A **T82.392-** Other mechanical complication of femoral arterial graft (bypass)

CC-A **T82.398-** Other mechanical complication of other vascular grafts

CC-A **T82.399-** Other mechanical complication of unspecified vascular grafts

T82.4- Mechanical complication of vascular dialysis catheter
    Mechanical complication of hemodialysis catheter
    Excludes 1:   *mechanical complication of intraperitoneal dialysis catheter (T85.62)*

CC-A **T82.41x-** Breakdown (mechanical) of vascular dialysis catheter

CC-A **T82.42x-** Displacement of vascular dialysis catheter
    Malposition of vascular dialysis catheter

CC-A **T82.43x-** Leakage of vascular dialysis catheter

CC-A **T82.49x-** Other complication of vascular dialysis catheter
    Obstruction (mechanical) of vascular dialysis catheter
    Perforation of vascular dialysis catheter
    Protrusion of vascular dialysis catheter

T82.5- Mechanical complication of other cardiac and vascular devices and implants
    Excludes ❷: *mechanical complication of epidural and subdural infusion catheter (T85.61)*

T82.51- Breakdown (mechanical) of other cardiac and vascular devices and implants

CC-A **T82.510-** Breakdown (mechanical) of surgically created arteriovenous fistula

CC-A **T82.511-** Breakdown (mechanical) of surgically created arteriovenous shunt

CC-A **T82.512-** Breakdown (mechanical) of artificial heart

CC-A **T82.513-** Breakdown (mechanical) of balloon (counterpulsation) device

CC-A **T82.514-** Breakdown (mechanical) of infusion catheter

CC-A **T82.515-** Breakdown (mechanical) of umbrella device

CC-A **T82.518-** Breakdown (mechanical) of other cardiac and vascular devices and implants

CC-A **T82.519-** Breakdown (mechanical) of unspecified cardiac and vascular devices and implants

T82.52- Displacement of other cardiac and vascular devices and implants
    Malposition of other cardiac and vascular devices and implants

CC-A **T82.520-** Displacement of surgically created arteriovenous fistula

CC-A **T82.521-** Displacement of surgically created arteriovenous shunt

CC-A **T82.522-** Displacement of artificial heart

CC-A **T82.523-** Displacement of balloon (counterpulsation) device

CC-A **T82.524-** Displacement of infusion catheter

CC-A **T82.525-** Displacement of umbrella device

CC-A **T82.528-** Displacement of other cardiac and vascular devices and implants

CC-A **T82.529-** Displacement of unspecified cardiac and vascular devices and implants

T82.53- Leakage of other cardiac and vascular devices and implants

CC-A **T82.530-** Leakage of surgically created arteriovenous fistula

CC-A **T82.531-** Leakage of surgically created arteriovenous shunt

CC-A **T82.532-** Leakage of artificial heart

CC-A **T82.533-** Leakage of balloon (counterpulsation) device

CC-A **T82.534-** Leakage of infusion catheter

CC-A **T82.535-** Leakage of umbrella device

CC-A **T82.538-** Leakage of other cardiac and vascular devices and implants

CC-A **T82.539-** Leakage of unspecified cardiac and vascular devices and implants

T82.59- Other mechanical complication of other cardiac and vascular devices and implants
    Obstruction (mechanical) of other cardiac and vascular devices and implants
    Perforation of other cardiac and vascular devices and implants
    Protrusion of other cardiac and vascular devices and implants

CC-A **T82.590-** Other mechanical complication of surgically created arteriovenous fistula

CC-A **T82.591-** Other mechanical complication of surgically created arteriovenous shunt

T82 - T82

CC-A **T82.592-** Other mechanical complication of artificial heart

CC-A **T82.593-** Other mechanical complication of balloon (counterpulsation) device

CC-A **T82.594-** Other mechanical complication of infusion catheter

CC-A **T82.595-** Other mechanical complication of umbrella device

CC-A **T82.598-** Other mechanical complication of other cardiac and vascular devices and implants

CC-A **T82.599-** Other mechanical complication of unspecified cardiac and vascular devices and implants

T82.6xx- <u>Infection and inflammatory reaction</u> due to <u>cardiac valve prosthesis</u>
CC-A
Use additional code to identify infection

T82.7xx- <u>Infection and inflammatory reaction</u> due to <u>other cardiac and vascular devices, implants and grafts</u>
CC-A
Use additional code to identify infection

T82.8- <u>Other specified complications</u> of <u>cardiac and vascular prosthetic devices, implants and grafts</u>

T82.81- <u>Embolism</u> due to cardiac and vascular prosthetic devices, implants and grafts

CC-A **T82.817-** Embolism due to cardiac prosthetic devices, implants and grafts

CC-A **T82.818-** Embolism due to vascular prosthetic devices, implants and grafts

T82.82- <u>Fibrosis</u> due to cardiac and vascular prosthetic devices, implants and grafts

CC-A **T82.827-** Fibrosis due to cardiac prosthetic devices, implants and grafts

CC-A **T82.828-** Fibrosis due to vascular prosthetic devices, implants and grafts

T82.83- <u>Hemorrhage</u> due to cardiac and vascular prosthetic devices, implants and grafts

CC-A **T82.837-** Hemorrhage due to cardiac prosthetic devices, implants and grafts

CC-A **T82.838-** Hemorrhage due to vascular prosthetic devices, implants and grafts

T82.84- <u>Pain</u> due to cardiac and vascular prosthetic devices, implants and grafts

CC-A **T82.847-** Pain due to cardiac prosthetic devices, implants and grafts

CC-A **T82.848-** Pain due to vascular prosthetic devices, implants and grafts

T82.85- <u>Stenosis</u> due to cardiac and vascular prosthetic devices, implants and grafts

CC-A **T82.855-** Stenosis of coronary artery stent
In-stent stenosis (restenosis) of coronary artery stent
Restenosis of coronary artery stent

CC-A **T82.856-** Stenosis of peripheral vascular stent
In-stent stenosis (restenosis) of peripheral vascular stent
Restenosis of peripheral vascular stent

CC-A **T82.857-** Stenosis of other cardiac prosthetic devices, implants and grafts

CC-A **T82.858-** Stenosis of other vascular prosthetic devices, implants and grafts

T82.86- <u>Thrombosis</u> of cardiac and vascular prosthetic devices, implants and grafts

CC-A **T82.867-** Thrombosis due to cardiac prosthetic devices, implants and grafts

CC-A **T82.868-** Thrombosis due to vascular prosthetic devices, implants and grafts

T82.89- <u>Other specified complication</u> of cardiac and vascular prosthetic devices, implants and grafts

CC-A **T82.897-** Other specified complication of cardiac prosthetic devices, implants and grafts

CC-A **T82.898-** Other specified complication of vascular prosthetic devices, implants and grafts

T82.9xx- <u>Unspecified</u> complication of cardiac and vascular prosthetic
CC-A
device, implant and graft

T83- <u>Complications of genitourinary prosthetic devices, implants and grafts</u>
Excludes ❷: failure and rejection of transplanted organs and tissue (T86.-)

The appropriate 7th character is to be added to each code from category T83:
A <u>Initial</u> encounter
D <u>Subsequent</u> encounter
S <u>Sequela</u>

T83.0- <u>Mechanical</u> complication of <u>urinary catheter</u>
Excludes ❷: complications of stoma of urinary tract (N99.5-)

T83.01- <u>Breakdown</u> (mechanical) of urinary catheter

CC-A **T83.010-** Breakdown (mechanical) of <u>cystostomy</u> catheter

T83.011- Breakdown (mechanical) of <u>indwelling urethral</u> catheter

T83.012- Breakdown (mechanical) of <u>nephrostomy</u> catheter

T83.018- Breakdown (mechanical) of <u>other</u> urinary catheter
Breakdown (mechanical) of Hopkins catheter
Breakdown (mechanical) of ileostomy catheter
Breakdown (mechanical) of urostomy catheter

T83.02- <u>Displacement</u> of urinary catheter
Malposition of urinary catheter

CC-A **T83.020-** Displacement of <u>cystostomy</u> catheter

T83.021- Displacement of <u>indwelling urethral</u> catheter

T83.022- Displacement of <u>nephrostomy</u> catheter

T83.028- Displacement of <u>other</u> urinary catheter
Displacement of Hopkins catheter
Displacement of ileostomy catheter
Displacement of urostomy catheter

T83.03- <u>Leakage</u> of urinary catheter

CC-A **T83.030-** Leakage of <u>cystostomy</u> catheter

T83.031- Leakage of <u>indwelling urethral</u> catheter

T83.032- Leakage of <u>nephrostomy</u> catheter

T83.038- Leakage of <u>other</u> urinary catheter
Leakage of Hopkins catheter
Leakage of ileostomy catheter
Leakage of urostomy catheter

T83.09- <u>Other mechanical</u> complication of urinary catheter
Obstruction (mechanical) of urinary catheter
Perforation of urinary catheter
Protrusion of urinary catheter

CC-A **T83.090-** Other mechanical complication of <u>cystostomy</u> catheter

T83.091- Other mechanical complication of <u>indwelling urethral</u> catheter

T83.092- Other mechanical complication of <u>nephrostomy</u> catheter

T83.098- Other mechanical complication of <u>other</u> urinary catheter
Other mechanical complication of Hopkins catheter
Other mechanical complication of ileostomy catheter
Other mechanical complication of urostomy catheter

T83.1- <u>Mechanical</u> complication of <u>other urinary devices and implants</u>

T83.11- <u>Breakdown</u> (mechanical) of other urinary devices and implants

CC-A **T83.110-** Breakdown (mechanical) of <u>urinary electronic stimulator device</u>
*Excludes ❷: breakdown (mechanical) of electrode (lead) for sacral nerve neurostimulator (T85.111)
breakdown (mechanical) of implanted electronic sacral neurostimulator, pulse generator or receiver (T85.113)*

CC-A **T83.111-** Breakdown (mechanical) of <u>implanted urinary sphincter</u>

CC-A **T83.112-** Breakdown (mechanical) of <u>indwelling ureteral stent</u>

CC-A **T83.113-** Breakdown (mechanical) of <u>other</u> urinary <u>stents</u>
Breakdown (mechanical) of ileal conduit stent
Breakdown (mechanical) of nephroureteral stent

CC-A **T83.118-** Breakdown (mechanical) of <u>other</u> urinary <u>devices</u> and implants

T82
-
T83

T83.12- **Displacement** of other urinary devices and implants
  Malposition of other urinary devices and implants

CC-A T83.120- Displacement of <u>urinary electronic stimulator device</u>
  Excludes ❷: *displacement of electrode (lead) for sacral nerve neurostimulator (T85.121)*
   displacement of implanted electronic sacral neurostimulator, pulse generator or receiver (T85.123)

CC-A T83.121- Displacement of <u>implanted urinary sphincter</u>

CC-A T83.122- Displacement of <u>indwelling ureteral stent</u>

CC-A T83.123- Displacement of <u>other</u> urinary <u>stents</u>
  Displacement of ileal conduit stent
  Displacement of nephroureteral stent

CC-A T83.128- Displacement of <u>other</u> urinary <u>devices</u> and implants

T83.19- <u>Other mechanical complication</u> of other urinary devices and implants
  Leakage of other urinary devices and implants
  Obstruction (mechanical) of other urinary devices and implants
  Perforation of other urinary devices and implants
  Protrusion of other urinary devices and implants

CC-A T83.190- Other mechanical complication of <u>urinary electronic stimulator device</u>
  Excludes ❷: *other mechanical complication of electrode (lead) for sacral nerve neurostimulator (T85.191)*
   other mechanical complication of implanted electronic sacral neurostimulator, pulse generator or receiver (T85.193)

CC-A T83.191- Other mechanical complication of <u>implanted urinary sphincter</u>

CC-A T83.192- Other mechanical complication of <u>indwelling ureteral stent</u>

CC-A T83.193- Other mechanical complication of <u>other</u> urinary <u>stent</u>
  Other mechanical complication of ileal conduit stent
  Other mechanical complication of nephroureteral stent

CC-A T83.198- Other mechanical complication of <u>other</u> urinary <u>devices</u> and implants

T83.2- <u>Mechanical</u> complication of <u>graft of urinary organ</u>

CC-A T83.21x- <u>Breakdown</u> (mechanical) of graft of urinary organ

CC-A T83.22x- <u>Displacement</u> of graft of urinary organ
  Malposition of graft of urinary organ

CC-A T83.23x- <u>Leakage</u> of graft of urinary organ

CC-A T83.24x- <u>Erosion</u> of graft of urinary organ

CC-A T83.25x- <u>Exposure</u> of graft of urinary organ

CC-A T83.29x- <u>Other</u> mechanical complication of graft of urinary organ
  Obstruction (mechanical) of graft of urinary organ
  Perforation of graft of urinary organ
  Protrusion of graft of urinary organ

T83.3- <u>Mechanical</u> complication of <u>intrauterine contraceptive device</u>

T83.31x- <u>Breakdown</u> (mechanical) of intrauterine contraceptive device — [♀]

T83.32x- <u>Displacement</u> of intrauterine contraceptive device — [♀]
  Malposition of intrauterine contraceptive device
  Missing string of intrauterine contraceptive device

T83.39x- <u>Other</u> mechanical complication of intrauterine contraceptive device — [♀]
  Leakage of intrauterine contraceptive device
  Obstruction (mechanical) of intrauterine contraceptive device
  Perforation of intrauterine contraceptive device
  Protrusion of intrauterine contraceptive device

T83.4- <u>Mechanical</u> complication of <u>other prosthetic devices, implants and grafts of genital tract</u>

T83.41- <u>Breakdown</u> (mechanical) of other prosthetic devices, implants and grafts of genital tract

CC-A T83.410- Breakdown (mechanical) of <u>implanted penile prosthesis</u> — [♂]
  Breakdown (mechanical) of penile prosthesis cylinder
  Breakdown (mechanical) of penile prosthesis pump
  Breakdown (mechanical) of penile prosthesis reservoir

CC-A T83.411- Breakdown (mechanical) of <u>implanted testicular prosthesis</u> — [♂]

CC-A T83.418- Breakdown (mechanical) of <u>other</u> prosthetic devices, implants and grafts of genital tract

T83.42- <u>Displacement</u> of other prosthetic devices, implants and grafts of genital tract
  Malposition of other prosthetic devices, implants and grafts of genital tract

CC-A T83.420- Displacement of <u>implanted penile prosthesis</u> — [♂]
  Displacement of penile prosthesis cylinder
  Displacement of penile prosthesis pump
  Displacement of penile prosthesis reservoir

CC-A T83.421- Displacement of <u>implanted testicular prosthesis</u> — [♂]

CC-A T83.428- Displacement of <u>other</u> prosthetic devices, implants and grafts of genital tract

T83.49- <u>Other mechanical complication</u> of other prosthetic devices, implants and grafts of genital tract
  Leakage of other prosthetic devices, implants and grafts of genital tract
  Obstruction, mechanical of other prosthetic devices, implants and grafts of genital tract
  Perforation of other prosthetic devices, implants and grafts of genital tract
  Protrusion of other prosthetic devices, implants and grafts of genital tract

CC-A T83.490- Other mechanical complication of <u>implanted penile prosthesis</u> — [♂]
  Other mechanical complication of penile prosthesis cylinder
  Other mechanical complication of penile prosthesis pump
  Other mechanical complication of penile prosthesis reservoir

CC-A T83.491- Other mechanical complication of <u>implanted testicular prosthesis</u> — [♂]

CC-A T83.498- Other mechanical complication of <u>other</u> prosthetic devices, implants and grafts of genital tract

T83.5- <u>Infection and inflammatory reaction</u> due to <u>prosthetic device, implant and graft in urinary system</u>
  Use additional code to identify infection

T83.51- Infection and inflammatory reaction due to urinary catheter
  Excludes ❷: *complications of stoma of urinary tract (N99.5-)*

CC-A T83.510- Infection and inflammatory reaction due to <u>cystostomy</u> catheter

CC-A T83.511- Infection and inflammatory reaction due to <u>indwelling urethral</u> catheter

CC-A T83.512- Infection and inflammatory reaction due to <u>nephrostomy</u> catheter

CC-A T83.518- Infection and inflammatory reaction due to <u>other</u> urinary catheter
  Infection and inflammatory reaction due to Hopkins catheter
  Infection and inflammatory reaction due to ileostomy catheter
  Infection and inflammatory reaction due to urostomy catheter

T83 - T83

T83.59- Infection and inflammatory reaction due to prosthetic device, implant and graft in urinary system

CC-A **T83.590-** Infection and inflammatory reaction due to implanted urinary neurostimulation device
Excludes ❷: *infection and inflammatory reaction due to electrode lead of sacral nerve neurostimulator (T85.732)*
infection and inflammatory reaction due to pulse generator or receiver of sacral nerve neurostimulator (T85.734)

CC-A **T83.591-** Infection and inflammatory reaction due to implanted urinary sphincter

CC-A **T83.592-** Infection and inflammatory reaction due to indwelling ureteral stent

CC-A **T83.593-** Infection and inflammatory reaction due to other urinary stents
Infection and inflammatory reaction due to ileal conduit stents
Infection and inflammatory reaction due to nephroureteral stent

CC-A **T83.598-** Infection and inflammatory reaction due to other prosthetic device, implant and graft in urinary system

T83.6- Infection and inflammatory reaction due to prosthetic device, implant and graft in genital tract
Use additional code to identify infection

CC-A **T83.61x-** Infection and inflammatory reaction due to implanted penile prosthesis
Infection and inflammatory reaction due to penile prosthesis cylinder
Infection and inflammatory reaction due to penile prosthesis pump
Infection and inflammatory reaction due to penile prosthesis reservoir

CC-A **T83.62x-** Infection and inflammatory reaction due to implanted testicular prosthesis

CC-A **T83.69x-** Infection and inflammatory reaction due to other prosthetic device, implant and graft in genital tract

T83.7- Complications due to implanted mesh and other prosthetic materials

T83.71- Erosion of implanted mesh and other prosthetic materials to surrounding organ or tissue

T83.711- Erosion of implanted vaginal mesh to surrounding organ or tissue — [♀]
Erosion of implanted vaginal mesh into pelvic floor muscles

CC-A **T83.712-** Erosion of implanted urethral mesh to surrounding organ or tissue
Erosion of implanted female urethral sling
Erosion of implanted male urethral sling
Erosion of implanted urethral mesh into pelvic floor muscles

CC-A **T83.713-** Erosion of implanted urethral bulking agent to surrounding organ or tissue

CC-A **T83.714-** Erosion of implanted ureteral bulking agent to surrounding organ or tissue

CC-A **T83.718-** Erosion of other implanted mesh to organ or tissue

CC-A **T83.719-** Erosion of other prosthetic materials to surrounding organ or tissue

T83.72- Exposure of implanted mesh and other prosthetic materials into surrounding organ or tissue
Extrusion of implanted mesh

T83.721- Exposure of implanted vaginal mesh into vagina — [♀]
Exposure of implanted vaginal mesh through vaginal wall

CC-A **T83.722-** Exposure of implanted urethral mesh into urethra
Exposure of implanted female urethral sling
Exposure of implanted male urethral sling
Exposure of implanted urethral mesh through urethral wall

CC-A **T83.723-** Exposure of implanted urethral bulking agent into urethra

CC-A **T83.724-** Exposure of implanted ureteral bulking agent into ureter

CC-A **T83.728-** Exposure of other implanted mesh into organ or tissue

CC-A **T83.729-** Exposure of other prosthetic materials into organ or tissue

CC-A **T83.79x-** Other specified complications due to other genitourinary prosthetic materials

T83.8- Other specified complications of genitourinary prosthetic devices, implants and grafts

CC-A **T83.81x-** Embolism due to genitourinary prosthetic devices, implants and grafts

CC-A **T83.82x-** Fibrosis due to genitourinary prosthetic devices, implants and grafts

CC-A **T83.83x-** Hemorrhage due to genitourinary prosthetic devices, implants and grafts

CC-A **T83.84x-** Pain due to genitourinary prosthetic devices, implants and grafts

CC-A **T83.85x-** Stenosis due to genitourinary prosthetic devices, implants and grafts

CC-A **T83.86x-** Thrombosis due to genitourinary prosthetic devices, implants and grafts

CC-A **T83.89x-** Other specified complication of genitourinary prosthetic devices, implants and grafts

T83.9xx- Unspecified complication of genitourinary prosthetic device, implant and graft
CC-A

T84- Complications of internal orthopedic prosthetic devices, implants and grafts
Excludes ❷: *failure and rejection of transplanted organs and tissues (T86.-)*
fracture of bone following insertion of orthopedic implant, joint prosthesis or bone plate (M96.6)

The appropriate 7th character is to be added to each code from category T84:
A Initial encounter
D Subsequent encounter
S Sequela

T84.0- Mechanical complication of internal joint prosthesis

T84.01- Broken internal joint prosthesis
Breakage (fracture) of prosthetic joint
Broken prosthetic joint implant
Excludes 1: *periprosthetic joint implant fracture (T84.04)*

CC-A **T84.010-** Broken internal right hip prosthesis

CC-A **T84.011-** Broken internal left hip prosthesis

CC-A **T84.012-** Broken internal right knee prosthesis

CC-A **T84.013-** Broken internal left knee prosthesis

CC-A **T84.018-** Broken internal joint prosthesis, other site
Use additional code to identify the joint (Z96.6-)

CC-A **T84.019-** Broken internal joint prosthesis, unspecified site

T84.02- Dislocation of internal joint prosthesis
Instability of internal joint prosthesis
Subluxation of internal joint prosthesis

CC-A **T84.020-** Dislocation of internal right hip prosthesis

CC-A **T84.021-** Dislocation of internal left hip prosthesis

CC-A **T84.022-** Instability of internal right knee prosthesis

CC-A **T84.023-** Instability of internal left knee prosthesis

CC-A **T84.028-** Dislocation of other internal joint prosthesis
Use additional code to identify the joint (Z96.6-)

CC-A **T84.029-** Dislocation of unspecified internal joint prosthesis

T84.03- Mechanical loosening of internal prosthetic joint
Aseptic loosening of prosthetic joint

CC-A **T84.030-** Mechanical loosening of internal right hip prosthetic joint

CC-A **T84.031-** Mechanical loosening of internal left hip prosthetic joint

CC-A **T84.032-** Mechanical loosening of internal right knee prosthetic joint

CC-A **T84.033-** Mechanical loosening of internal left knee prosthetic joint

T83-T84

© 2016 Channel Publishing, Ltd

CC-A **T84.038-** Mechanical loosening of <u>other</u> internal prosthetic joint
Use additional code to identify the joint (Z96.6-)

CC-A **T84.039-** Mechanical loosening of <u>unspecified</u> internal prosthetic joint

T84.05- <u>Periprosthetic osteolysis</u> of internal prosthetic joint
Use additional code to identify major osseous defect, if applicable (M89.7-)

CC-A **T84.050-** Periprosthetic osteolysis of internal prosthetic <u>right hip</u> joint

CC-A **T84.051-** Periprosthetic osteolysis of internal prosthetic <u>left hip</u> joint

CC-A **T84.052-** Periprosthetic osteolysis of internal prosthetic <u>right knee</u> joint

CC-A **T84.053-** Periprosthetic osteolysis of internal prosthetic <u>left knee</u> joint

CC-A **T84.058-** Periprosthetic osteolysis of <u>other</u> internal prosthetic joint
Use additional code to identify the joint (Z96.6-)

CC-A **T84.059-** Periprosthetic osteolysis of <u>unspecified</u> internal prosthetic joint

T84.06- <u>Wear of articular bearing surface</u> of internal prosthetic joint

CC-A **T84.060-** Wear of articular bearing surface of internal prosthetic <u>right hip</u> joint

CC-A **T84.061-** Wear of articular bearing surface of internal prosthetic <u>left hip</u> joint

CC-A **T84.062-** Wear of articular bearing surface of internal prosthetic <u>right knee</u> joint

CC-A **T84.063-** Wear of articular bearing surface of internal prosthetic <u>left knee</u> joint

CC-A **T84.068-** Wear of articular bearing surface of <u>other</u> internal prosthetic joint
Use additional code to identify the joint (Z96.6-)

CC-A **T84.069-** Wear of articular bearing surface of <u>unspecified</u> internal prosthetic joint

T84.09- <u>Other mechanical complication</u> of internal joint prosthesis
Prosthetic joint implant failure NOS

CC-A **T84.090-** Other mechanical complication of internal <u>right hip</u> prosthesis

CC-A **T84.091-** Other mechanical complication of internal <u>left hip</u> prosthesis

CC-A **T84.092-** Other mechanical complication of internal <u>right knee</u> prosthesis

CC-A **T84.093-** Other mechanical complication of internal <u>left knee</u> prosthesis

CC-A **T84.098-** Other mechanical complication of <u>other</u> internal joint prosthesis
Use additional code to identify the joint (Z96.6-)

CC-A **T84.099-** Other mechanical complication of <u>unspecified</u> internal joint prosthesis

T84.1- <u>Mechanical complication of internal fixation device of bones of limb</u>
Excludes ❷: *mechanical complication of internal fixation device of bones of feet (T84.2-)*
mechanical complication of internal fixation device of bones of fingers (T84.2-)
mechanical complication of internal fixation device of bones of hands (T84.2-)
mechanical complication of internal fixation device of bones of toes (T84.2-)

T84.11- <u>Breakdown</u> (mechanical) of internal fixation device of bones of limb

CC-A **T84.110-** Breakdown (mechanical) of internal fixation device of <u>right humerus</u>

CC-A **T84.111-** Breakdown (mechanical) of internal fixation device of <u>left humerus</u>

CC-A **T84.112-** Breakdown (mechanical) of internal fixation device of bone of <u>right forearm</u>

CC-A **T84.113-** Breakdown (mechanical) of internal fixation device of bone of <u>left forearm</u>

CC-A **T84.114-** Breakdown (mechanical) of internal fixation device of <u>right femur</u>

CC-A **T84.115-** Breakdown (mechanical) of internal fixation device of <u>left femur</u>

CC-A **T84.116-** Breakdown (mechanical) of internal fixation device of bone of <u>right lower leg</u>

CC-A **T84.117-** Breakdown (mechanical) of internal fixation device of bone of <u>left lower leg</u>

CC-A **T84.119-** Breakdown (mechanical) of internal fixation device of <u>unspecified</u> bone of limb

T84.12- <u>Displacement</u> of internal fixation device of bones of limb
Malposition of internal fixation device of bones of limb

CC-A **T84.120-** Displacement of internal fixation device of <u>right humerus</u>

CC-A **T84.121-** Displacement of internal fixation device of <u>left humerus</u>

CC-A **T84.122-** Displacement of internal fixation device of bone of <u>right forearm</u>

CC-A **T84.123-** Displacement of internal fixation device of bone of <u>left forearm</u>

CC-A **T84.124-** Displacement of internal fixation device of <u>right femur</u>

CC-A **T84.125-** Displacement of internal fixation device of <u>left femur</u>

CC-A **T84.126-** Displacement of internal fixation device of bone of <u>right lower leg</u>

CC-A **T84.127-** Displacement of internal fixation device of bone of <u>left lower leg</u>

CC-A **T84.129-** Displacement of internal fixation device of <u>unspecified</u> bone of limb

T84.19- <u>Other mechanical complication</u> of internal fixation device of bones of limb
Obstruction (mechanical) of internal fixation device of bones of limb
Perforation of internal fixation device of bones of limb
Protrusion of internal fixation device of bones of limb

CC-A **T84.190-** Other mechanical complication of internal fixation device of <u>right humerus</u>

CC-A **T84.191-** Other mechanical complication of internal fixation device of <u>left humerus</u>

CC-A **T84.192-** Other mechanical complication of internal fixation device of bone of <u>right forearm</u>

CC-A **T84.193-** Other mechanical complication of internal fixation device of bone of <u>left forearm</u>

CC-A **T84.194-** Other mechanical complication of internal fixation device of <u>right femur</u>

CC-A **T84.195-** Other mechanical complication of internal fixation device of <u>left femur</u>

CC-A **T84.196-** Other mechanical complication of internal fixation device of bone of <u>right lower leg</u>

CC-A **T84.197-** Other mechanical complication of internal fixation device of bone of <u>left lower leg</u>

CC-A **T84.199-** Other mechanical complication of internal fixation device of <u>unspecified</u> bone of limb

T84.2- <u>Mechanical complication of internal fixation device of other bones</u>

T84.21- <u>Breakdown</u> (mechanical) of internal fixation device of other bones

CC-A **T84.210-** Breakdown (mechanical) of internal fixation device of bones of <u>hand and fingers</u>

CC-A **T84.213-** Breakdown (mechanical) of internal fixation device of bones of <u>foot and toes</u>

CC-A **T84.216-** Breakdown (mechanical) of internal fixation device of <u>vertebrae</u>

CC-A **T84.218-** Breakdown (mechanical) of internal fixation device of <u>other bones</u>

Excludes 1: = NOT CODED HERE! (Do not code both)   **1225**   *Excludes ❷:* = Not Included Here

T84 - T84

T84.22- <u>Displacement</u> of internal fixation device of other bones
Malposition of internal fixation device of other bones

CC-A **T84.220-** Displacement of internal fixation device of bones of <u>hand and fingers</u>

CC-A **T84.223-** Displacement of internal fixation device of bones of <u>foot and toes</u>

CC-A **T84.226-** Displacement of internal fixation device of <u>vertebrae</u>

CC-A **T84.228-** Displacement of internal fixation device of <u>other bones</u>

T84.29- <u>Other mechanical complication</u> of internal fixation device of other bones
Obstruction (mechanical) of internal fixation device of other bones
Perforation of internal fixation device of other bones
Protrusion of internal fixation device of other bones

CC-A **T84.290-** Other mechanical complication of internal fixation device of bones of <u>hand and fingers</u>

CC-A **T84.293-** Other mechanical complication of internal fixation device of bones of <u>foot and toes</u>

CC-A **T84.296-** Other mechanical complication of internal fixation device of <u>vertebrae</u>

CC-A **T84.298-** Other mechanical complication of internal fixation device of <u>other bones</u>

T84.3- <u>Mechanical complication</u> of <u>other bone devices, implants and grafts</u>
Excludes ❷: other complications of bone graft (T86.83-)

T84.31- <u>Breakdown</u> (mechanical) of other bone devices, implants and grafts

CC-A **T84.310-** Breakdown (mechanical) of electronic bone stimulator

CC-A **T84.318-** Breakdown (mechanical) of other bone devices, implants and grafts

T84.32- <u>Displacement</u> of other bone devices, implants and grafts
Malposition of other bone devices, implants and grafts

CC-A **T84.320-** Displacement of electronic bone stimulator

CC-A **T84.328-** Displacement of other bone devices, implants and grafts
AHA 14:4Q:p28 – Dislodged proximal hooks and growing rods

T84.39- <u>Other mechanical complication</u> of other bone devices, implants and grafts
Obstruction (mechanical) of other bone devices, implants and grafts
Perforation of other bone devices, implants and grafts
Protrusion of other bone devices, implants and grafts

CC-A **T84.390-** Other mechanical complication of electronic bone stimulator

CC-A **T84.398-** Other mechanical complication of other bone devices, implants and grafts

T84.4- <u>Mechanical</u> complication of <u>other internal orthopedic devices, implants and grafts</u>

T84.41- <u>Breakdown</u> (mechanical) of other internal orthopedic devices, implants and grafts

CC-A **T84.410-** Breakdown (mechanical) of muscle and tendon graft

CC-A **T84.418-** Breakdown (mechanical) of other internal orthopedic devices, implants and grafts

T84.42- <u>Displacement</u> of other internal orthopedic devices, implants and grafts
Malposition of other internal orthopedic devices, implants and grafts

CC-A **T84.420-** Displacement of muscle and tendon graft

CC-A **T84.428-** Displacement of other internal orthopedic devices, implants and grafts

T84.49- <u>Other mechanical complication</u> of other internal orthopedic devices, implants and grafts
Mechanical complication of other internal orthopedic devices, implants and grafts NOS
Obstruction (mechanical) of other internal orthopedic devices, implants and grafts
Perforation of other internal orthopedic devices, implants and grafts
Protrusion of other internal orthopedic devices, implants and grafts

CC-A **T84.490-** Other mechanical complication of muscle and tendon graft

CC-A **T84.498-** Other mechanical complication of other internal orthopedic devices, implants and grafts

T84.5- <u>Infection and inflammatory reaction</u> due to <u>internal joint prosthesis</u>
AHA 15:1Q:p16 – Infection after a primary left total hip replacement
Use additional code to identify infection

CC-A **T84.50x-** Infection and inflammatory reaction due to <u>unspecified</u> internal joint prosthesis

CC-A **T84.51x-** Infection and inflammatory reaction due to internal <u>right hip</u> prosthesis

CC-A **T84.52x-** Infection and inflammatory reaction due to internal <u>left hip</u> prosthesis

CC-A **T84.53x-** Infection and inflammatory reaction due to internal <u>right knee</u> prosthesis

CC-A **T84.54x-** Infection and inflammatory reaction due to internal <u>left knee</u> prosthesis

CC-A **T84.59x-** Infection and inflammatory reaction due to <u>other</u> internal joint prosthesis

T84.6- <u>Infection and inflammatory reaction</u> due to <u>internal fixation device</u>
Use additional code to identify infection

CC-A **T84.60x-** Infection and inflammatory reaction due to internal fixation device of <u>unspecified</u> site

T84.61- Infection and inflammatory reaction due to internal fixation device of <u>arm</u>

CC-A **T84.610-** Infection and inflammatory reaction due to internal fixation device of <u>right humerus</u>

CC-A **T84.611-** Infection and inflammatory reaction due to internal fixation device of <u>left humerus</u>

CC-A **T84.612-** Infection and inflammatory reaction due to internal fixation device of <u>right radius</u>

CC-A **T84.613-** Infection and inflammatory reaction due to internal fixation device of <u>left radius</u>

CC-A **T84.614-** Infection and inflammatory reaction due to internal fixation device of <u>right ulna</u>

CC-A **T84.615-** Infection and inflammatory reaction due to internal fixation device of <u>left ulna</u>

CC-A **T84.619-** Infection and inflammatory reaction due to internal fixation device of <u>unspecified</u> bone of arm

T84.62- Infection and inflammatory reaction due to internal fixation device of <u>leg</u>

CC-A **T84.620-** Infection and inflammatory reaction due to internal fixation device of <u>right femur</u>

CC-A **T84.621-** Infection and inflammatory reaction due to internal fixation device of <u>left femur</u>

CC-A **T84.622-** Infection and inflammatory reaction due to internal fixation device of <u>right tibia</u>

CC-A **T84.623-** Infection and inflammatory reaction due to internal fixation device of <u>left tibia</u>

CC-A **T84.624-** Infection and inflammatory reaction due to internal fixation device of <u>right fibula</u>

CC-A **T84.625-** Infection and inflammatory reaction due to internal fixation device of <u>left fibula</u>

CC-A **T84.629-** Infection and inflammatory reaction due to internal fixation device of <u>unspecified</u> bone of leg

CC-A **T84.63x-** Infection and inflammatory reaction due to internal fixation device of <u>spine</u>

CC-A **T84.69x-** Infection and inflammatory reaction due to internal fixation device of <u>other site</u>

T84.7xx-   **Infection and inflammatory reaction** due to **other internal**
CC-A   **orthopedic prosthetic devices, implants and grafts**
    Use additional code to identify infection

T84.8-   **Other specified complications** of **internal orthopedic prosthetic devices, implants and grafts**

CC-A **T84.81x-**   **Embolism** due to internal orthopedic prosthetic devices, implants and grafts

CC-A **T84.82x-**   **Fibrosis** due to internal orthopedic prosthetic devices, implants and grafts

CC-A **T84.83x-**   **Hemorrhage** due to internal orthopedic prosthetic devices, implants and grafts

CC-A **T84.84x-**   **Pain** due to internal orthopedic prosthetic devices, implants and grafts

CC-A **T84.85x-**   **Stenosis** due to internal orthopedic prosthetic devices, implants and grafts

CC-A **T84.86x-**   **Thrombosis** due to internal orthopedic prosthetic devices, implants and grafts

CC-A **T84.89x-**   **Other specified complication** of internal orthopedic prosthetic devices, implants and grafts

T84.9xx-   **Unspecified** complication of internal orthopedic prosthetic
CC-A   device, implant and graft

T85-   **Complications of other internal prosthetic devices, implants and grafts**
    AHA 15:1Q:p15 – Graft prolapse
    Excludes ❷: failure and rejection of transplanted organs and tissue (T86-)

The appropriate 7th character is to be added to each code from
    category T85:
    A   **Initial** encounter
    D   **Subsequent** encounter
    S   **Sequela**

T85.0-   **Mechanical** complication of **ventricular intracranial (communicating) shunt**

CC-A **T85.01x-**   **Breakdown** (mechanical) of ventricular intracranial (communicating) shunt

CC-A **T85.02x-**   **Displacement** of ventricular intracranial (communicating) shunt
    Malposition of ventricular intracranial (communicating) shunt

CC-A **T85.03x-**   **Leakage** of ventricular intracranial (communicating) shunt

CC-A **T85.09x-**   **Other mechanical** complication of ventricular intracranial (communicating) shunt
    Obstruction (mechanical) of ventricular intracranial (communicating) shunt
    Perforation of ventricular intracranial (communicating) shunt
    Protrusion of ventricular intracranial (communicating) shunt

T85.1-   **Mechanical** complication of **implanted electronic stimulator of nervous system**

T85.11-   **Breakdown** (mechanical) of implanted electronic stimulator of nervous system

CC-A **T85.110-**   Breakdown (mechanical) of implanted electronic neurostimulator of **brain electrode (lead)**

CC-A **T85.111-**   Breakdown (mechanical) of implanted electronic neurostimulator of **peripheral nerve electrode (lead)**
    Breakdown of electrode (lead) for cranial nerve neurostimulators
    Breakdown of electrode (lead) for gastric neurostimulator
    Breakdown of electrode (lead) for sacral nerve neurostimulator
    Breakdown of electrode (lead) for vagal nerve neurostimulators

CC-A **T85.112-**   Breakdown (mechanical) of implanted electronic neurostimulator of **spinal cord electrode (lead)**

CC-A **T85.113-**   Breakdown (mechanical) of implanted electronic neurostimulator, **generator**
    Breakdown (mechanical) of implanted electronic neurostimulator generator, brain, peripheral, gastric, spinal
    Breakdown (mechanical) of implanted electronic sacral neurostimulator, pulse generator or receiver

CC-A **T85.118-**   Breakdown (mechanical) of **other** implanted electronic stimulator of nervous system

T85.12-   **Displacement** of implanted electronic stimulator of nervous system
    Malposition of implanted electronic stimulator of nervous system

CC-A **T85.120-**   Displacement of implanted electronic neurostimulator of **brain** electrode (lead)

CC-A **T85.121-**   Displacement of implanted electronic neurostimulator of **peripheral nerve** electrode (lead)
    Displacement of electrode (lead) for cranial nerve neurostimulators
    Displacement of electrode (lead) for gastric neurostimulator
    Displacement of electrode (lead) for sacral nerve neurostimulator
    Displacement of electrode (lead) for vagal nerve neurostimulators

CC-A **T85.122-**   Displacement of implanted electronic neurostimulator of **spinal cord** electrode (lead)

CC-A **T85.123-**   Displacement of implanted electronic neurostimulator, **generator**
    Displacement of implanted electronic neurostimulator generator, brain, peripheral, gastric, spinal
    Displacement of implanted electronic sacral neurostimulator, pulse generator or receiver

CC-A **T85.128-**   Displacement of **other** implanted electronic stimulator of nervous system

T85.19-   **Other mechanical** complication of implanted electronic stimulator of nervous system
    Leakage of implanted electronic stimulator of nervous system
    Obstruction (mechanical) of implanted electronic stimulator of nervous system
    Perforation of implanted electronic stimulator of nervous system
    Protrusion of implanted electronic stimulator of nervous system

CC-A **T85.190-**   Other mechanical complication of implanted electronic neurostimulator of **brain** electrode (lead)

CC-A **T85.191-**   Other mechanical complication of implanted electronic neurostimulator of **peripheral nerve** electrode (lead)
    Other mechanical complication of electrode (lead) for cranial nerve neurostimulators
    Other mechanical complication of electrode (lead) for gastric neurostimulator
    Other mechanical complication of electrode (lead) for sacral nerve neurostimulator
    Other mechanical complication of electrode (lead) for vagal nerve neurostimulators

CC-A **T85.192-**   Other mechanical complication of implanted electronic neurostimulator of **spinal cord** electrode (lead)

CC-A **T85.193-**   Other mechanical complication of implanted electronic neurostimulator, **generator**
    Other mechanical complication of implanted electronic neurostimulator generator, brain, peripheral, gastric, spinal
    Other mechanical complication of implanted electronic sacral neurostimulator, pulse generator or receiver

CC-A **T85.199-**   Other mechanical complication of **other** implanted electronic stimulator of nervous system

T85.2-   **Mechanical** complication of **intraocular lens**

CC-A **T85.21x-**   **Breakdown** (mechanical) of intraocular lens

CC-A **T85.22x-**   **Displacement** of intraocular lens
    Malposition of intraocular lens

CC-A **T85.29x-**   **Other mechanical** complication of intraocular lens
    Obstruction (mechanical) of intraocular lens
    Perforation of intraocular lens
    Protrusion of intraocular lens

T84 - T85

Excludes 1: = NOT CODED HERE! (Do not code both)   **1227**   *Excludes ❷: = Not Included Here*

T85.3- Mechanical complication of other ocular prosthetic devices, implants and grafts

> Excludes ❷: other complications of corneal graft (T86.84-)

T85.31- Breakdown (mechanical) of other ocular prosthetic devices, implants and grafts

CC-A **T85.310-** Breakdown (mechanical) of prosthetic orbit of right eye

CC-A **T85.311-** Breakdown (mechanical) of prosthetic orbit of left eye

T85.318- Breakdown (mechanical) of other ocular prosthetic devices, implants and grafts

T85.32- Displacement of other ocular prosthetic devices, implants and grafts

> Malposition of other ocular prosthetic devices, implants and grafts

CC-A **T85.320-** Displacement of prosthetic orbit of right eye

CC-A **T85.321-** Displacement of prosthetic orbit of left eye

T85.328- Displacement of other ocular prosthetic devices, implants and grafts

T85.39- Other mechanical complication of other ocular prosthetic devices, implants and grafts

> Obstruction (mechanical) of other ocular prosthetic devices, implants and grafts
>
> Perforation of other ocular prosthetic devices, implants and grafts
>
> Protrusion of other ocular prosthetic devices, implants and grafts

CC-A **T85.390-** Other mechanical complication of prosthetic orbit of right eye

CC-A **T85.391-** Other mechanical complication of prosthetic orbit of left eye

T85.398- Other mechanical complication of other ocular prosthetic devices, implants and grafts

T85.4- Mechanical complication of breast prosthesis and implant

CC-A **T85.41x-** Breakdown (mechanical) of breast prosthesis and implant

CC-A **T85.42x-** Displacement of breast prosthesis and implant

> Malposition of breast prosthesis and implant

CC-A **T85.43x-** Leakage of breast prosthesis and implant

CC-A **T85.44x-** Capsular contracture of breast implant

CC-A **T85.49x-** Other mechanicalm complication of breast prosthesis and implant

> Obstruction (mechanical) of breast prosthesis and implant
>
> Perforation of breast prosthesis and implant
>
> Protrusion of breast prosthesis and implant

T85.5- Mechanical complication of gastrointestinal prosthetic devices, implants and grafts

T85.51- Breakdown (mechanical) of gastrointestinal prosthetic devices, implants and grafts

CC-A **T85.510-** Breakdown (mechanical) of bile duct prosthesis

CC-A **T85.511-** Breakdown (mechanical) of esophageal anti-reflux device

CC-A **T85.518-** Breakdown (mechanical) of other gastrointestinal prosthetic devices, implants and grafts

T85.52- Displacement of gastrointestinal prosthetic devices, implants and grafts

> Malposition of gastrointestinal prosthetic devices, implants and grafts

CC-A **T85.520-** Displacement of bile duct prosthesis

CC-A **T85.521-** Displacement of esophageal anti-reflux device

CC-A **T85.528-** Displacement of other gastrointestinal prosthetic devices, implants and grafts

T85.59- Other mechanical complication of gastrointestinal prosthetic devices, implants and

> Obstruction, mechanical of gastrointestinal prosthetic devices, implants and grafts
>
> Perforation of gastrointestinal prosthetic devices, implants and grafts
>
> Protrusion of gastrointestinal prosthetic devices, implants and grafts

CC-A **T85.590-** Other mechanical complication of bile duct prosthesis

CC-A **T85.591-** Other mechanical complication of esophageal anti-reflux device

CC-A **T85.598-** Other mechanical complication of other gastrointestinal prosthetic devices, implants and grafts

T85.6- Mechanical complication of other specified internal and external prosthetic devices, implants and grafts

T85.61- Breakdown (mechanical) of other specified internal prosthetic devices, implants and grafts

CC-A **T85.610-** Breakdown (mechanical) of cranial or spinal infusion catheter

> Breakdown (mechanical) of epidural infusion catheter
>
> Breakdown (mechanical) of intrathecal infusion catheter
>
> Breakdown (mechanical) of subarachnoid infusion catheter
>
> Breakdown (mechanical) of subdural infusion catheter

CC-A **T85.611-** Breakdown (mechanical) of intraperitoneal dialysis catheter

> Excludes 1: mechanical complication of vascular dialysis catheter (T82.4-)

CC-A **T85.612-** Breakdown (mechanical) of permanent sutures

> Excludes 1: mechanical complication of permanent (wire) suture used in bone repair (T84.1-T84.2)

CC-A **T85.613-** Breakdown (mechanical) of artificial skin graft and decellularized allodermis

> Failure of artificial skin graft and decellularized allodermis
>
> Non-adherence of artificial skin graft and decellularized allodermis
>
> Poor incorporation of artificial skin graft and decellularized allodermis
>
> Shearing of artificial skin graft and decellularized allodermis

CC-A **T85.614-** Breakdown (mechanical) of insulin pump

CC-A **T85.615-** Breakdown (mechanical) of other nervous system device, implant or graft

> Breakdown (mechanical) of intrathecal infusion pump

CC-A **T85.618-** Breakdown (mechanical) of other specified internal prosthetic devices, implants and grafts

T85.62- Displacement of other specified internal prosthetic devices, implants and grafts

> Malposition of other specified internal prosthetic devices, implants and grafts

CC-A **T85.620-** Displacement of cranial or spinal infusion catheter

> Displacement of epidural infusion catheter
>
> Displacement of intrathecal infusion catheter
>
> Displacement of subarachnoid infusion catheter
>
> Displacement of subdural infusion catheter

CC-A **T85.621-** Displacement of intraperitoneal dialysis catheter

> Excludes 1: mechanical complication of vascular dialysis catheter (T82.4-)

CC-A **T85.622-** Displacement of permanent sutures

> Excludes 1: mechanical complication of permanent (wire) suture used in bone repair (T84.1-T84.2)

CC-A **T85.623-** Displacement of artificial skin graft and decellularized allodermis

> Dislodgement of artificial skin graft and decellularized allodermis
>
> Displacement of artificial skin graft and decellularized allodermis

CC-A **T85.624-** Displacement of insulin pump

CC-A **T85.625-** Displacement of other nervous system device, implant or graft

> Displacement of intrathecal infusion pump

CC-A **T85.628-** Displacement of other specified internal prosthetic devices, implants and grafts

T85.63- Leakage of other specified internal prosthetic devices, implants and grafts

CC-A **T85.630-** Leakage of cranial or spinal infusion catheter

> Leakage of epidural infusion catheter
>
> Leakage of intrathecal infusion catheter
>
> Leakage of subarachnoid infusion catheter
>
> Leakage of subdural infusion catheter

Excludes 1: = NOT CODED HERE! (Do not code both)

Excludes ❷: = Not Included Here

T85 - T85

CC-A **T85.631-** Leakage of <u>intraperitoneal dialysis catheter</u>
  Excludes 1:   *mechanical complication of vascular dialysis catheter (T82.4)*

CC-A **T85.633-** Leakage of <u>insulin pump</u>

CC-A **T85.635-** Leakage of other nervous system device, implant or graft
  Leakage of intrathecal infusion pump

CC-A **T85.638-** Leakage of <u>other</u> specified internal prosthetic devices, implants and grafts

T85.69- <u>Other mechanical</u> complication of other specified internal prosthetic devices, implants and grafts
  Obstruction, mechanical of other specified internal prosthetic devices, implants and grafts
  Perforation of other specified internal prosthetic devices, implants and grafts
  Protrusion of other specified internal prosthetic devices, implants and grafts

CC-A **T85.690-** Other mechanical complication of <u>cranial or spinal infusion catheter</u>
  Other mechanical complication of epidural infusion catheter
  Other mechanical complication of intrathecal infusion catheter
  Other mechanical complication of subarachnoid infusion catheter
  Other mechanical complication of subdural infusion catheter

CC-A **T85.691-** Other mechanical complication of <u>intraperitoneal dialysis catheter</u>
  Excludes 1:   *mechanical complication of vascular dialysis catheter (T82.4)*

CC-A **T85.692-** Other mechanical complication of <u>permanent sutures</u>
  Excludes 1:   *mechanical complication of permanent (wire) suture used in bone repair (T84.1-T84.2)*

CC-A **T85.693-** Other mechanical complication of <u>artificial skin graft and decellularized allodermis</u>

CC-A **T85.694-** Other mechanical complication of <u>insulin pump</u>

CC-A **T85.695-** Other mechanical complication of other nervous system device, implant or graft
  Other mechanical complication of intrathecal infusion pump

CC-A **T85.698-** Other mechanical complication of <u>other</u> specified internal prosthetic devices, implants and grafts
  Mechanical complication of nonabsorbable surgical material NOS

T85.7- <u>Infection and inflammatory reaction</u> due to <u>other internal prosthetic devices, implants and grafts</u>
  Use additional code to identify infection

CC-A **T85.71x-** Infection and inflammatory reaction due to <u>peritoneal dialysis catheter</u>

CC-A **T85.72x-** Infection and inflammatory reaction due to <u>insulin pump</u>

T85.73- <u>Infection and inflammatory reaction</u> due to <u>nervous system devices, implants and graft</u>

CC-A **T85.730-** Infection and inflammatory reaction due to <u>ventricular intracranial (communicating) shunt</u>

CC-A **T85.731-** Infection and inflammatory reaction due to implanted electronic <u>neurostimulator of brain</u>, electrode (lead)

CC-A **T85.732-** Infection and inflammatory reaction due to implanted electronic <u>neurostimulator of peripheral nerve</u>, electrode (lead)
  Infection and inflammatory reaction due to electrode (lead) for cranial nerve neurostimulators
  Infection and inflammatory reaction due to electrode (lead) for gastric neurostimulator
  Infection and inflammatory reaction due to electrode (lead) for sacral nerve neurostimulator
  Infection and inflammatory reaction due to electrode (lead) for vagal nerve neurostimulators

CC-A **T85.733-** Infection and inflammatory reaction due to implanted electronic <u>neurostimulator of spinal cord</u>, electrode (lead)

CC-A **T85.734-** Infection and inflammatory reaction due to implanted electronic <u>neurostimulator, generator</u>
  Generator pocket infection

CC-A **T85.735-** Infection and inflammatory reaction due to cranial or spinal <u>infusion catheter</u>
  Infection and inflammatory reaction due to epidural catheter
  Infection and inflammatory reaction due to intrathecal infusion catheter
  Infection and inflammatory reaction due to subarachnoid catheter
  Infection and inflammatory reaction due to subdural catheter

CC-A **T85.738-** Infection and inflammatory reaction due to <u>other</u> nervous system device, implant or graft
  Infection and inflammatory reaction due to intrathecal infusion pump

CC-A **T85.79x-** Infection and inflammatory reaction due to <u>other</u> internal prosthetic devices, implants and grafts

T85.8- <u>Other specified complications</u> of internal prosthetic devices, implants and grafts, not elsewhere classified

T85.81- <u>Embolism</u> due to internal prosthetic devices, implants and grafts, not elsewhere classified

CC-A,D **T85.810-** Embolism due to <u>nervous system</u> prosthetic devices, implants and grafts

T85.818- Embolism due to <u>other</u> internal prosthetic devices, implants and grafts

T85.82- <u>Fibrosis</u> due to internal prosthetic devices, implants and grafts, not elsewhere classified

CC-A,D **T85.820-** Fibrosis due to <u>nervous system</u> prosthetic devices, implants and grafts

T85.828- Fibrosis due to <u>other</u> internal prosthetic devices, implants and grafts

T85.83- <u>Hemorrhage</u> due to internal prosthetic devices, implants and grafts, not elsewhere classified

CC-A,D **T85.830-** Hemorrhage due to <u>nervous system</u> prosthetic devices, implants and grafts

T85.838- Hemorrhage due to <u>other</u> internal prosthetic devices, implants and grafts

T85.84- <u>Pain</u> due to internal prosthetic devices, implants and grafts, not elsewhere classified

CC-A,D **T85.840-** Pain due to <u>nervous system</u> prosthetic devices, implants and grafts

T85.848- Pain due to <u>other</u> internal prosthetic devices, implants and grafts

T85.85- <u>Stenosis</u> due to internal prosthetic devices, implants and grafts, not elsewhere classified

CC-A,D **T85.850-** Stenosis due to <u>nervous system</u> prosthetic devices, implants and grafts

T85.858- Stenosis due to <u>other</u> internal prosthetic devices, implants and grafts

T85.86- <u>Thrombosis</u> due to internal prosthetic devices, implants and grafts, not elsewhere classified

CC-A,D **T85.860-** Thrombosis due to <u>nervous system</u> prosthetic devices, implants and grafts

T85.868- Thrombosis due to <u>other</u> internal prosthetic devices, implants and grafts

T85.89- <u>Other specified complication</u> of internal prosthetic devices, implants and grafts, not elsewhere classified
  Erosion or breakdown of subcutaneous device pocket

CC-A,D **T85.890-** Other specified complication of nervous system prosthetic devices, implants and grafts

T85.898- Other specified complication of other internal prosthetic devices, implants and grafts

T85.9xx- <u>Unspecified</u> complication of internal prosthetic device, implant and graft
  Complication of internal prosthetic device, implant and graft NOS

T85-T85

T86- <u>Complications of transplanted organs and tissue</u>
Use additional code to identify other transplant complications, such as:
Graft-versus-host disease (D89.81-)
Malignancy associated with organ transplant (C80.2)
Post-transplant lymphoproliferative disorders (PTLD) (D47.Z1)

T86.0- Complications of <u>bone marrow transplant</u>

CC **T86.00** <u>Unspecified</u> complication of bone marrow transplant

CC **T86.01** Bone marrow transplant <u>rejection</u>

CC **T86.02** Bone marrow transplant <u>failure</u>

CC **T86.03** Bone marrow transplant <u>infection</u>

CC **T86.09** <u>Other</u> complications of bone marrow transplant

T86.1- Complications of <u>kidney transplant</u>

CC **T86.10** <u>Unspecified</u> complication of kidney transplant

CC **T86.11** Kidney transplant <u>rejection</u>

CC **T86.12** Kidney transplant <u>failure</u>
AHA 13:1Q:p24 – Kidney transplant failure with stage IV chronic kidney disease

CC **T86.13** Kidney transplant <u>infection</u>
Use additional code to specify infection

CC **T86.19** <u>Other</u> complication of kidney transplant

T86.2- Complications of <u>heart transplant</u>
Excludes 1: complication of:
artificial heart device (T82.5)
heart-lung transplant (T86.3)

CC **T86.20** <u>Unspecified</u> complication of heart transplant

CC **T86.21** Heart transplant <u>rejection</u>

CC **T86.22** Heart transplant <u>failure</u>

CC **T86.23** Heart transplant <u>infection</u>
Use additional code to specify infection

T86.29- <u>Other</u> complications of heart transplant

CC **T86.290** <u>Cardiac allograft vasculopathy</u>
Excludes 1: atherosclerosis of coronary arteries
(I25.75-, I25.76-, I25.81-)

CC **T86.298** <u>Other</u> complications of heart transplant

T86.3- Complications of <u>heart-lung transplant</u>

CC **T86.30** <u>Unspecified</u> complication of heart-lung transplant

CC **T86.31** Heart-lung transplant <u>rejection</u>

CC **T86.32** Heart-lung transplant <u>failure</u>

CC **T86.33** Heart-lung transplant <u>infection</u>
Use additional code to specify infection

CC **T86.39** <u>Other</u> complications of heart-lung transplant

T86.4- Complications of <u>liver transplant</u>

CC **T86.40** <u>Unspecified</u> complication of liver transplant

CC **T86.41** Liver transplant <u>rejection</u>

CC **T86.42** Liver transplant <u>failure</u>

CC **T86.43** Liver transplant <u>infection</u>
Use additional code to identify infection, such as:
Cytomegalovirus (CMV) infection (B25.-)

CC **T86.49** <u>Other</u> complications of liver transplant

CC **T86.5** Complications of <u>stem cell transplant</u>
Complications from stem cells from peripheral blood
Complications from stem cells from umbilical cord

T86.8- Complications of other transplanted organs and tissues

T86.81- Complications of <u>lung transplant</u>
Excludes 1: complication of heart-lung transplant (T86.3-)

CC **T86.810** Lung transplant <u>rejection</u>

CC **T86.811** Lung transplant <u>failure</u>

CC **T86.812** Lung transplant <u>infection</u>
Use additional code to specify infection

CC **T86.818** <u>Other</u> complications of lung transplant

CC **T86.819** <u>Unspecified</u> complication of lung transplant

T86.82- Complications of <u>skin graft (allograft) (autograft)</u>
Excludes ❷: complication of artificial skin graft (T85.693)

CC **T86.820** Skin graft (allograft) <u>rejection</u>

CC **T86.821** Skin graft (allograft) (autograft) <u>failure</u>

CC **T86.822** Skin graft (allograft) (autograft) <u>infection</u>
Use additional code to specify infection

CC **T86.828** <u>Other</u> complications of skin graft (allograft) (autograft)

CC **T86.829** <u>Unspecified</u> complication of skin graft (allograft) (autograft)

T86.83- Complications of <u>bone graft</u>
Excludes ❷: mechanical complications of bone graft (T84.3-)

CC **T86.830** Bone graft <u>rejection</u>

CC **T86.831** Bone graft <u>failure</u>

CC **T86.832** Bone graft <u>infection</u>
Use additional code to specify infection

CC **T86.838** <u>Other</u> complications of bone graft

CC **T86.839** <u>Unspecified</u> complication of bone graft

T86.84- Complications of <u>corneal transplant</u>
Excludes ❷: mechanical complications of corneal graft (T85.3-)

CC **T86.840** Corneal transplant <u>rejection</u>

CC **T86.841** Corneal transplant <u>failure</u>

CC **T86.842** Corneal transplant <u>infection</u>
Use additional code to specify infection

CC **T86.848** <u>Other</u> complications of corneal transplant

CC **T86.849** <u>Unspecified</u> complication of corneal transplant

T86.85- Complication of <u>intestine transplant</u>

CC **T86.850** Intestine transplant <u>rejection</u>

CC **T86.851** Intestine transplant <u>failure</u>

CC **T86.852** Intestine transplant <u>infection</u>
Use additional code to specify infection

CC **T86.858** <u>Other</u> complications of intestine transplant

CC **T86.859** <u>Unspecified</u> complication of intestine transplant

T86.89- Complications of <u>other transplanted tissue</u>
Transplant failure or rejection of pancreas

CC **T86.890** Other transplanted tissue <u>rejection</u>

CC **T86.891** Other transplanted tissue <u>failure</u>

CC **T86.892** Other transplanted tissue <u>infection</u>
Use additional code to specify infection

CC **T86.898** <u>Other</u> complications of other transplanted tissue

CC **T86.899** <u>Unspecified</u> complication of other transplanted tissue

T86.9- Complication of <u>unspecified transplanted organ and tissue</u>

CC **T86.90** <u>Unspecified</u> complication of unspecified transplanted organ and tissue

CC **T86.91** Unspecified transplanted organ and tissue <u>rejection</u>

CC **T86.92** Unspecified transplanted organ and tissue <u>failure</u>

CC **T86.93** Unspecified transplanted organ and tissue <u>infection</u>
Use additional code to specify infection

CC **T86.99** <u>Other</u> complications of unspecified transplanted organ and tissue

T86 – T86

T87- Complications peculiar to reattachment and amputation

T87.0- Complications of reattached (part of) upper extremity

    T87.0x- Complications of reattached (part of) upper extremity

      CC **T87.0x1** Complications of reattached (part of) right upper extremity

      CC **T87.0x2** Complications of reattached (part of) left upper extremity

      CC **T87.0x9** Complications of reattached (part of) unspecified upper extremity

T87.1- Complications of reattached (part of) lower extremity

    T87.1x- Complications of reattached (part of) lower extremity

      CC **T87.1x1** Complications of reattached (part of) right lower extremity

      CC **T87.1x2** Complications of reattached (part of) left lower extremity

      CC **T87.1x9** Complications of reattached (part of) unspecified lower extremity

CC **T87.2** Complications of other reattached body part

T87.3- Neuroma of amputation stump

    T87.30 Neuroma of amputation stump, unspecified extremity

    T87.31 Neuroma of amputation stump, right upper extremity

    T87.32 Neuroma of amputation stump, left upper extremity

    T87.33 Neuroma of amputation stump, right lower extremity

    T87.34 Neuroma of amputation stump, left lower extremity

T87.4- Infection of amputation stump

    CC **T87.40** Infection of amputation stump, unspecified extremity

    CC **T87.41** Infection of amputation stump, right upper extremity

    CC **T87.42** Infection of amputation stump, left upper extremity

    CC **T87.43** Infection of amputation stump, right lower extremity

    CC **T87.44** Infection of amputation stump, left lower extremity

T87.5- Necrosis of amputation stump

    T87.50 Necrosis of amputation stump, unspecified extremity

    T87.51 Necrosis of amputation stump, right upper extremity

    T87.52 Necrosis of amputation stump, left upper extremity

    T87.53 Necrosis of amputation stump, right lower extremity

    T87.54 Necrosis of amputation stump, left lower extremity

T87.8- Other complications of amputation stump

    T87.81 Dehiscence of amputation stump

    T87.89 Other complications of amputation stump

      Amputation stump contracture
      Amputation stump contracture of next proximal joint
      Amputation stump edema
      Amputation stump flexion
      Amputation stump hematoma

      Excludes ❷: *phantom limb syndrome (G54.6-G54.7)*

T87.9 Unspecified complications of amputation stump

T88- Other complications of surgical and medical care, not elsewhere classified

  Excludes ❷: *complication following infusion, transfusion and therapeutic injection (T80.-)*
    complication following procedure NEC (T81.-)
    complications of anesthesia in labor and delivery (O74.-)
    complications of anesthesia in pregnancy (O29.-)
    complications of anesthesia in puerperium (O89.-)
    complications of devices, implants and grafts (T82-T85)
    complications of obstetric surgery and procedure (O75.4)
    dermatitis due to drugs and medicaments (L23.3, L24.4, L25.1, L27.0-L27.1)
    poisoning and toxic effects of drugs and chemicals (T36-T65 with fifth or sixth character 1-4 or 6)
    specified complications classified elsewhere

The appropriate 7th character is to be added to each code from category T88:
  A Initial encounter
  D Subsequent encounter
  S Sequela

T88.0xx- Infection following immunization

CC-A Sepsis following immunization

T88.1xx- Other complications following immunization, not elsewhere classified

CC-A Generalized vaccinia
    Rash following immunization

    Excludes 1: *vaccinia not from vaccine (B08.011)*
    Excludes ❷: *anaphylactic shock due to serum (T80.5-)*
      other serum reactions (T80.6-)
      postimmunization arthropathy (M02.2)
      postimmunization encephalitis (G04.02)
      postimmunization fever (R50.83)

T88.2xx- Shock due to anesthesia

CC-A Use additional code for adverse effect, if applicable, to identify drug (T41- with fifth or sixth character 5)

    Excludes 1: *complications of anesthesia (in):*
      labor and delivery (O74-)
      pregnancy (O29-)
      puerperium (O89-)
      postprocedural shock NOS (T81.1-)

T88.3xx- Malignant hyperthermia due to anesthesia

CC-A Use additional code for adverse effect, if applicable, to identify drug (T41- with fifth or sixth character 5)

T88.4xx- Failed or difficult intubation

T88.5- Other complications of anesthesia

  Use additional code for adverse effect, if applicable, to identify drug (T41- with fifth or sixth character 5)

    T88.51x- Hypothermia following anesthesia

    T88.52x- Failed moderate sedation during procedure

      Failed conscious sedation during procedure

      Excludes ❷: *personal history of failed moderate sedation (Z92.83)*

    T88.53x- Unintended awareness under general anesthesia during procedure

      Excludes ❷: *personal history of unintended awareness under general anesthesia (Z92.84)*

    T88.59x- Other complications of anesthesia

T88.6xx- Anaphylactic reaction due to adverse effect of correct drug or medicament properly administered

CC-A Anaphylactic shock due to adverse effect of correct drug or medicament properly administered
    Anaphylactoid reaction NOS
  Use additional code for adverse effect, if applicable, to identify drug (T36-T50 with fifth or sixth character 5)

    Excludes 1: *anaphylactic reaction due to serum (T80.5)*

T88.7xx- Unspecified adverse effect of drug or medicament

    Drug hypersensitivity NOS
    Drug reaction NOS
  Use additional code for adverse effect, if applicable, to identify drug (T36-T50 with fifth or sixth character 5)

    Excludes 1: *specified adverse effects of drugs and medicaments (A00-R94 and T80-T88.6, T88.8)*

T88.8xx- Other specified complications of surgical and medical care, not elsewhere classified

  Use additional code to identify the complication

T88.9xx- Complication of surgical and medical care, unspecified

T87 - T88

T88 – T88

Chapter 20 – External causes of morbidity (V00-Y99)

Note: This chapter permits the classification of environmental events and circumstances as the cause of injury, and other adverse effects. Where a code from this section is applicable, it is intended that it shall be used secondary to a code from another chapter of the Classification indicating the nature of the condition. Most often, the condition will be classifiable to Chapter 19, Injury, poisoning and certain other consequences of external causes (S00-T88). Other conditions that may be stated to be due to external causes are classified in Chapters I to XVIII. For these conditions, codes from Chapter 20 should be used to provide additional information as to the cause of the condition.

This chapter contains the following blocks:

V00-X58	Accidents
V00-V99	Transport accidents
V00-V09	Pedestrian injured in transport accident
V10-V19	Pedal cycle rider injured in transport accident
V20-V29	Motorcycle rider injured in transport accident
V30-V39	Occupant of three-wheeled motor vehicle injured in transport accident
V40-V49	Car occupant injured in transport accident
V50-V59	Occupant of pick-up truck or van injured in transport accident
V60-V69	Occupant of heavy transport vehicle injured in transport accident
V70-V79	Bus occupant injured in transport accident
V80-V89	Other land transport accidents
V90-V94	Water transport accidents
V95-V97	Air and space transport accidents
V98-V99	Other and unspecified transport accidents
W00-W19	Slipping, tripping, stumbling and falls
W20-W49	Exposure to inanimate mechanical forces
W50-W64	Exposure to animate mechanical forces
W65-W74	Accidental non-transport drowning and submersion
W85-W99	Exposure to electric current, radiation and extreme ambient air temperature and pressure
X00-X08	Exposure to smoke, fire and flames
X10-X19	Contact with heat and hot substances
X30-X39	Exposure to forces of nature
X50	Overexertion and strenuous or repetitive movements
X52-X58	Accidental exposure to other specified factors
X71-X83	Intentional self-harm
X92-Y09	Assault
Y21-Y33	Event of undetermined intent
Y35-Y38	Legal intervention, operations of war, military operations, and terrorism
Y62-Y69	Misadventures to patients during surgical and medical care
Y70-Y82	Medical devices associated with adverse incidents in diagnostic and therapeutic use
Y83-Y84	Surgical and other medical procedures as the cause of abnormal reaction of the patient, or of later complication, without mention of misadventure at the time of the procedure
Y90-Y99	Supplementary factors related to causes of morbidity classified elsewhere

Accidents (V00-X58)

Transport accidents (V00-V99)

Note: This section is structured in 12 groups. Those relating to land transport accidents (V00-V89) reflect the victim's mode of transport and are subdivided to identify the victim's "counterpart" or the type of event. The vehicle of which the injured person is an occupant is identified in the first two characters since it is seen as the most important factor to identify for prevention purposes. A transport accident is one in which the vehicle involved must be moving or running or in use for transport purposes at the time of the accident.

Use additional code to identify:
Airbag injury (W22.1)
Type of street or road (Y92.4-)
Use of cellular telephone and other electronic equipment at the time of the transport accident (Y93.C-)

Excludes 1:   *agricultural vehicles in stationary use or maintenance (W31-)*
   assault by crashing of motor vehicle (Y03-)
   automobile or motor cycle in stationary use or maintenance — code to type of accident
   crashing of motor vehicle, undetermined intent (Y32)
   intentional self-harm by crashing of motor vehicle (X82)
Excludes ❷: *transport accidents due to cataclysm (X34-X38)*

Definitions related to transport accidents:
(a)   **A transport accident (V00-V99)** is any accident involving a device designed primarily for, or used at the time primarily for, conveying persons or goods from one place to another.

(b)   **A public highway [trafficway] or street** is the entire width between property lines (or other boundary lines) of land open to the public as a matter of right or custom for purposes of moving persons or property from one place to another. A roadway is that part of the public highway designed, improved and customarily used for vehicular traffic.

(c)   **A traffic accident** is any vehicle accident occurring on the public highway [i.e. originating on, terminating on, or involving a vehicle partially on the highway]. A vehicle accident is assumed to have occurred on the public highway unless another place is specified, except in the case of accidents involving only off-road motor vehicles, which are classified as nontraffic accidents unless the contrary is stated.

(d)   **A nontraffic accident** is any vehicle accident that occurs entirely in any place other than a public highway.

(e)   **A pedestrian** is any person involved in an accident who was not at the time of the accident riding in or on a motor vehicle, railway train, streetcar or animal-drawn or other vehicle, or on a pedal cycle or animal. This includes, a person changing a tire, working on a parked car, or a person on foot. It also includes the user of a pedestrian conveyance such as a babystroller, ice-skates, skis, sled, roller skates, a skateboard, nonmotorized or motorized wheelchair, motorized mobility scooter, or nonmotorized scooter.

(f)   **A driver** is an occupant of a transport vehicle who is operating or intending to operate it.

(g)   **A passenger** is any occupant of a transport vehicle other than the driver, except a person traveling on the outside of the vehicle.

(h)   **A person on the outside of a vehicle** is any person being transported by a vehicle but not occupying the space normally reserved for the driver or passengers, or the space intended for the transport of property. This includes a person traveling on the bodywork, bumper, fender, roof, running board or step of a vehicle, as well as, hanging on the outside of the vehicle.

(i)   **A pedal cycle** is any land transport vehicle operated solely by nonmotorized pedals including a bicycle or tricycle.

(j)   **A pedal cyclist** is any person riding a pedal cycle or in a sidecar or trailer attached to a pedal cycle.

(k)   **A motorcycle** is a two-wheeled motor vehicle with one or two riding saddles and sometimes with a third wheel for the support of a sidecar. The sidecar is considered part of the motorcycle. This includes a moped, motor scooter, or motorized bicycle.

(l)   **A motorcycle rider** is any person riding a motorcycle or in a sidecar or trailer attached to the motorcycle.

(m)   **A three-wheeled motor vehicle** is a motorized tricycle designed primarily for on-road use. This includes a motor-driven tricycle, a motorized rickshaw, or a three-wheeled motor car.

(n)   **A car [automobile]** is a four-wheeled motor vehicle designed primarily for carrying up to 7 persons. A trailer being towed by the car is considered part of the car. It does not include a van or minivan — see definition (o).

(o)   **A pick-up truck or van** is a four or six-wheeled motor vehicle designed for carrying passengers as well as property or cargo weighing less than the local limit for classification as a heavy goods vehicle, and not requiring a special driver's license. This includes a minivan and a sport-utility vehicle (SUV).

(p)   **A heavy transport vehicle** is a motor vehicle designed primarily for carrying property, meeting local criteria for classification as a heavy goods vehicle in terms of weight and requiring a special driver's license.

(q)   **A bus (coach)** is a motor vehicle designed or adapted primarily for carrying more than 10 passengers, and requiring a special driver's license.

(r)   **A railway train or railway vehicle** is any device, with or without freight or passenger cars coupled to it, designed for traffic on a railway track. This includes subterranean (subways) or elevated trains.

(s)   **A streetcar** is a device designed and used primarily for transporting passengers within a municipality, running on rails, usually subject to normal traffic control signals, and operated principally on a right-of-way that forms part of the roadway. This includes a tram or trolley that runs on rails. A trailer being towed by a streetcar is considered part of the streetcar.

(t)   **A special vehicle mainly used on industrial premises** is a motor vehicle designed primarily for use within the buildings and premises of industrial or commercial establishments. This includes battery-powered airport passenger vehicles or baggage/mail trucks, forklifts, coal-cars in a coal mine, logging cars and trucks used in mines or quarries.

(u)   **A special vehicle mainly used in agriculture** is a motor vehicle designed specifically for use in farming and agriculture (horticulture), to work the land, tend and harvest crops and transport materials on the farm. This includes harvesters, farm machinery and tractor and trailers.

(v)   **A special construction vehicle** is a motor vehicle designed specifically for use on construction and demolition sites. This includes bulldozers, diggers, earth levellers, dump trucks, backhoes, front-end loaders, pavers, and mechanical shovels.

V00 | V00

(w) **A special all-terrain vehicle** is a motor vehicle of special design to enable it to negotiate over rough or soft terrain, snow or sand. Examples of special design are high construction, special wheels and tires, tracks, and support on a cushion of air. This includes snow mobiles, all-terrain vehicles (ATV), and dune buggies. It does not include passenger vehicle designated as Sport Utility Vehicles (SUV).

(x) **A watercraft** is any device designed for transporting passengers or goods on water. This includes motor or sail boats, ships, and hovercraft.

(y) **An aircraft** is any device for transporting passengers or goods in the air. This includes hot-air balloons, gliders, helicopters and airplanes.

(z) **A military vehicle** is any motorized vehicle operating on a public roadway owned by the military and being operated by a member of the military.

Chapter-Specific Coding Guidelines

C. **Chapter-Specific Coding Guidelines**
In addition to general coding guidelines, there are guidelines for specific diagnoses and/or conditions in the classification. Unless otherwise indicated, these guidelines apply to all health care settings. Please refer to Section II for guidelines on the selection of principal diagnosis.

20. Chapter 20: External Causes of Morbidity (V00-Y99)

The external causes of morbidity codes should never be sequenced as the first-listed or principal diagnosis.

External cause codes are intended to provide data for injury research and evaluation of injury prevention strategies. These codes capture how the injury or health condition happened (cause), the intent (unintentional or accidental; or intentional, such as suicide or assault), the place where the event occurred the activity of the patient at the time of the event, and the person's status (e.g., civilian, military).

There is no national requirement for mandatory ICD-10-CM external cause code reporting. Unless a provider is subject to a state-based external cause code reporting mandate or these codes are required by a particular payer, reporting of ICD-10-CM codes in Chapter 20, External Causes of Morbidity, is not required. In the absence of a mandatory reporting requirement, providers are encouraged to voluntarily report external cause codes, as they provide valuable data for injury research and evaluation of injury prevention strategies.

a. **General External Cause Coding Guidelines**

1) **Used with any code in the range of A00.0-T88.9, Z00-Z99**
An external cause code may be used with any code in the range of A00.0-Z00-Z99, classification that is a health condition due to an external cause. Though they are most applicable to injuries, they are also valid for use with such things as infections or diseases due to an external source, and other health conditions, such as a heart attack that occurs during strenuous physical activity.

2) **External cause code used for length of treatment**
Assign the external cause code, with the appropriate 7th character (initial encounter, subsequent encounter or sequela) for each encounter for which the injury or condition is being treated.
Most categories in chapter 20 have a 7th character requirement for each applicable code. Most categories in this chapter have three 7th character values: A, initial encounter, D, subsequent encounter and S, sequela. While the patient may be seen by a new or different provider over the course of treatment for an injury or condition, assignment of the 7th character for external cause should match the 7th character of the code assigned for the associated injury or condition for the encounter.

3) **Use the full range of external cause codes**
Use the full range of external cause codes to completely describe the cause, the intent, the place of occurrence, and if applicable, the activity of the patient at the time of the event, and the patient's status, for all injuries, and other health conditions due to an external cause.

4) **Assign as many external cause codes as necessary**
Assign as many external cause codes as necessary to fully explain each cause. If only one external code can be recorded, assign the code most related to the principal diagnosis.

5) **The selection of the appropriate external cause code**
The selection of the appropriate external cause code is guided by the Alphabetic Index of External Causes and by Inclusion and Exclusion notes in the Tabular List.

6) **External cause code can never be a principal diagnosis**
An external cause code can never be a principal (first-listed) diagnosis.

7) **Combination external cause codes**
Certain of the external cause codes are combination codes that identify sequential events that result in an injury, such as a fall which results in striking against an object. The injury may be due to either event or both. The combination external cause code used should correspond to the sequence of events regardless of which caused the most serious injury.

8) **No external cause code needed in certain circumstances**
No external cause code from Chapter 20 is needed if the external cause and intent are included in a code from another chapter (e.g. T36.0x1- Poisoning by penicillins, accidental (unintentional)).

b. **Place of Occurrence Guideline**
Codes from category Y92, Place of occurrence of the external cause, are secondary codes for use after other external cause codes to identify the location of the patient at the time of injury or other condition.

Generally, a place of occurrence code is assigned only once, at the initial encounter for treatment. However, in the rare instance that a new injury occurs during hospitalization, an additional place of occurrence code may be assigned. No 7th characters are used for Y92.

Do not use place of occurrence code Y92.9 if the place is not stated or is not applicable.

c. **Activity Code**
Assign a code from category Y93, Activity code, to describe the activity of the patient at the time the injury or other health condition occurred.

An activity code is used only once, at the initial encounter for treatment. Only one code from Y93 should be recorded on a medical record.

The activity codes are not applicable to poisonings, adverse effects, misadventures or sequela.

Do not assign Y93.9, Unspecified activity, if the activity is not stated.

A code from category Y93 is appropriate for use with external cause and intent codes if identifying the activity provides additional information about the event.

d. **Place of Occurrence, Activity, and Status Codes Used with other External Cause Code**
When applicable, place of occurrence, activity, and external cause status codes are sequenced after the main external cause code(s). Regardless of the number of external cause codes assigned, there should be only one place of occurrence code, one activity code, and one external cause status code assigned to an encounter.

e. **If the Reporting Format Limits the Number of External Cause Codes**
If the reporting format limits the number of external cause codes that can be used in reporting clinical data, report the code for the cause/intent most related to the principal diagnosis. If the format permits capture of additional external cause codes, the cause/intent, including medical misadventures, of the additional events should be reported rather than the codes for place, activity, or external status.

f. **Multiple External Cause Coding Guidelines**
More than one external cause code is required to fully describe the external cause of an illness or injury. The assignment of external cause codes should be sequenced in the following priority:
If two or more events cause separate injuries, an external cause code should be assigned for each cause. The first-listed external cause code will be selected in the following order:

External codes for child and adult abuse take priority over all other external cause codes.
See Section I.C.19. Child and Adult abuse guidelines.

External cause codes for terrorism events take priority over all other external cause codes except child and adult abuse.

External cause codes for cataclysmic events take priority over all other external cause codes except child and adult abuse and terrorism.

External cause codes for transport accidents take priority over all other external cause codes except cataclysmic events, child and adult abuse and terrorism.

Activity and external cause status codes are assigned following all causal (intent) external cause codes.

The first-listed external cause code should correspond to the cause of the most serious diagnosis due to an assault, accident, or self-harm, following the order of hierarchy listed above.

V 0 0 – V 0 0

g.   Child and Adult Abuse Guideline
Adult and child abuse, neglect and maltreatment are classified as assault. Any of the assault codes may be used to indicate the external cause of any injury resulting from the confirmed abuse.

For confirmed cases of abuse, neglect and maltreatment, when the perpetrator is known, a code from Y07, Perpetrator of maltreatment and neglect, should accompany any other assault codes.

See Section I.C.19. Adult and child abuse, neglect and other maltreatment.

h.   Unknown or Undetermined Intent Guideline
If the intent (accident, self-harm, assault) of the cause of an injury or other condition is unknown or unspecified, code the intent as accidental intent. All transport accident categories assume accidental intent.

1)   Use of undetermined intent
External cause codes for events of undetermined intent are only for use if the documentation in the record specifies that the intent cannot be determined.

i.   Sequelae (Late Effects) of External Cause Guidelines

1)   Sequelae external cause codes
Sequela are reported using the external cause code with the 7th character "S" for sequela. These codes should be used with any report of a late effect or sequela resulting from a previous injury.

See Section I.B.10 Sequela (Late Effects).

2)   Sequela external cause code with a related current injury
A sequela external cause code should never be used with a related current nature of injury code.

3)   Use of sequela external cause codes for subsequent visits
Use a late effect external cause code for subsequent visits when a late effect of the initial injury is being treated. Do not use a late effect external cause code for subsequent visits for follow-up care (e.g., to assess healing, to receive rehabilitative therapy) of the injury when no late effect of the injury has been documented.

j.   Terrorism Guidelines

1)   Cause of injury identified by the Federal Government (FBI) as terrorism
When the cause of an injury is identified by the Federal Government (FBI) as terrorism, the first-listed external cause code should be a code from category Y38, Terrorism. The definition of terrorism employed by the FBI is found at the inclusion note at the beginning of category Y38. Use additional code for place of occurrence (Y92.-). More than one Y38 code may be assigned if the injury is the result of more than one mechanism of terrorism.

2)   Cause of an injury is suspected to be the result of terrorism
When the cause of an injury is suspected to be the result of terrorism a code from category Y38 should not be assigned. Suspected cases should be classified as assault.

3)   Code Y38.9, Terrorism, secondary effects
Assign code Y38.9, Terrorism, secondary effects, for conditions occurring subsequent to the terrorist event. This code should not be assigned for conditions that are due to the initial terrorist act.

It is acceptable to assign code Y38.9 with another code from Y38 if there is an injury due to the initial terrorist event and an injury that is a subsequent result of the terrorist event.

k.   External cause status
A code from category Y99, External cause status, should be assigned whenever any other external cause code is assigned for an encounter, including an Activity code, except for the events noted below. Assign a code from category Y99, External cause status, to indicate the work status of the person at the time the event occurred. The status code indicates whether the event occurred during military activity, whether a non-military person was at work, whether an individual including a student or volunteer was involved in a non-work activity at the time of the causal event.

A code from Y99, External cause status, should be assigned, when applicable, with other external cause codes, such as transport accidents and falls. The external cause status codes are not applicable to poisonings, adverse effects, misadventures or late effects.

Do not assign a code from category Y99 if no other external cause codes (cause, activity) are applicable for the encounter.

An external cause status code is used only once, at the initial encounter for treatment. Only one code from Y99 should be recorded on a medical record.

Do not assign code Y99.9, Unspecified external cause status, if the status is not stated.

Pedestrian injured in transport accident (V00-V09)

Includes:	**Person changing tire on transport vehicle** **Person examining engine of vehicle broken down in (on side of) road**
Excludes 1:	*fall due to non-transport collision with other person (W03)* *pedestrian on foot falling (slipping) on ice and snow (W00-)* *struck or bumped by another person (W51)*

V00-   Pedestrian conveyance accident
Use additional place of occurrence and activity external cause codes, if known (Y92-, Y93-)

Excludes 1:	*collision with another person without fall (W51)* *fall due to person on foot colliding with another person on foot (W03)* *fall from non-moving wheelchair, nonmotorized scooter and motorized mobility scooter without collision (W05-)* *pedestrian (conveyance) collision with other land transport vehicle (V01-V09)* *pedestrian on foot falling (slipping) on ice and snow (W00-)*

The appropriate 7th character is to be added to each code from category V00:

A	Initial encounter
D	**Subsequent encounter**
S	**Sequela**

V00.0-   Pedestrian on foot injured in collision with pedestrian conveyance

V00.01x-   Pedestrian on foot injured in collision with roller-skater

V00.02x-   Pedestrian on foot injured in collision with skateboarder

V00.09x-   Pedestrian on foot injured in collision with other pedestrian conveyance

V00.1-   Rolling-type pedestrian conveyance accident
> *Excludes 1:   accident with babystroller (V00.82-)*
> *accident with wheelchair (powered) (V00.81-)*
> *accident with motorized mobility scooter (V00.83-)*

V00.11-   In-line roller-skate accident

V00.111-   Fall from in-line roller-skates

V00.112-   In-line roller-skater colliding with stationary object

V00.118-   Other in-line roller-skate accident
> *Excludes 1:   roller-skater collision with other land transport vehicle (V01-V09 with 5th character 1)*

V00.12-   Non-in- line roller-skate accident

V00.121-   Fall from non-in-line roller-skates

V00.122-   Non-in-line roller-skater colliding with stationary object

V00.128-   Other non-in-line roller-skating accident
> *Excludes 1:   roller-skater collision with other land transport vehicle (V01-V09 with 5th character 1)*

V00.13-   Skateboard accident

V00.131-   Fall from skateboard

V00.132-   Skateboarder colliding with stationary object

V00.138-   Other skateboard accident
> *Excludes 1:   skateboarder collision with other land transport vehicle (V01-V09 with 5th character 2)*

V00.14-   Scooter (nonmotorized) accident
> *Excludes 1:   motorscooter accident (V20-V29)*

V00.141-   Fall from scooter (nonmotorized)

V00.142-   Scooter (nonmotorized) colliding with stationary object

V00.148-   Other scooter (nonmotorized) accident
> *Excludes 1:   scooter (nonmotorized) collision with other land transport vehicle (V01-V09 with fifth character 9)*

V00.15-   Heelies accident
> Rolling shoe
> Wheeled shoe
> Wheelies accident

V00.151-   Fall from heelies

V00.152-   Heelies colliding with stationary object

V00 - V00

V00.158-   Other heelies accident

V00.18- Accident on other rolling-type pedestrian conveyance

    V00.181-   Fall from other rolling-type pedestrian conveyance

    V00.182-   Pedestrian on other rolling-type pedestrian conveyance colliding with stationary object

    V00.188-   Other accident on other rolling-type pedestrian conveyance

V00.2-   <u>Gliding-type pedestrian</u> conveyance accident

   V00.21- Ice-skates accident

    V00.211-   Fall from ice-skates

    V00.212-   Ice-skater colliding with stationary object

    V00.218-   Other ice-skates accident
      Excludes 1:   *ice-skater collision with other land transport vehicle (V01-V09 with 5th digit 9)*

   V00.22- Sled accident

    V00.221-   Fall from sled

    V00.222-   Sledder colliding with stationary object

    V00.228-   Other sled accident
      Excludes 1:   *sled collision with other land transport vehicle (V01-V09 with 5th digit 9)*

  V00.28- Other gliding-type pedestrian conveyance accident

    V00.281-   Fall from other gliding-type pedestrian conveyance

    V00.282-   Pedestrian on other gliding-type pedestrian conveyance colliding with stationary object

    V00.288-   Other accident on other gliding-type pedestrian conveyance
      Excludes 1:   *gliding-type pedestrian conveyance collision with other land transport vehicle (V01-V09 with 5th digit 9)*

V00.3-   Flat-bottomed pedestrian conveyance accident

   V00.31- <u>Snowboard accident</u>

    V00.311-   Fall from snowboard

    V00.312-   Snowboarder colliding with stationary object

    V00.318-   Other snowboard accident
      Excludes 1:   *snowboarder collision with other land transport vehicle (V01-V09 with 5th digit 9)*

   V00.32- <u>Snow-ski accident</u>

    V00.321-   Fall from snow-skis
      AHA 15:1Q:p12 – Fell down while cross country skiing

    V00.322-   Snow-skier colliding with stationary object

    V00.328-   Other snow-ski accident
      Excludes 1:   *snow-skier collision with other land transport vehicle (V01-V09 with 5th digit 9)*

  V00.38- Other flat-bottomed pedestrian conveyance accident

    V00.381-   Fall from other flat-bottomed pedestrian conveyance

    V00.382-   Pedestrian on other flat-bottomed pedestrian conveyance colliding with stationary object

    V00.388-   Other accident on other flat-bottomed pedestrian conveyance

V00.8-   Accident on other pedestrian conveyance

   V00.81- Accident with <u>wheelchair</u> (powered)

    V00.811-   Fall from moving wheelchair (powered)
      Excludes 1:   *fall from non-moving wheelchair (W05.0)*

    V00.812-   Wheelchair (powered) colliding with stationary object

    V00.818-   Other accident with wheelchair (powered)

   V00.82- Accident with <u>babystroller</u>

    V00.821-   Fall from babystroller

    V00.822-   Babystroller colliding with stationary object

    V00.828-   Other accident with babystroller

   V00.83- Accident with <u>motorized mobility scooter</u>

    V00.831-   Fall from motorized mobility scooter
      Excludes 1:   *fall from non-moving motorized mobility scooter (W05.2)*

    V00.832-   Motorized mobility scooter colliding with stationary object

    V00.838-   Other accident with motorized mobility scooter

  V00.89- Accident on other pedestrian conveyance

    V00.891-   Fall from other pedestrian conveyance

    V00.892-   Pedestrian on other pedestrian conveyance colliding with stationary object

    V00.898-   Other accident on other pedestrian conveyance
      Excludes 1:   *other pedestrian (conveyance) collision with other land transport vehicle (V01-V09 with 5th digit 9)*

V01-   <u>Pedestrian injured in collision</u> with <u>pedal cycle</u>

The appropriate 7th character is to be added to each code from category V01:

A   <u>Initial</u> encounter
D   <u>Subsequent</u> encounter
S   <u>Sequela</u>

  V01.0-   <u>Pedestrian injured in collision</u> with <u>pedal cycle</u> in <u>nontraffic</u> accident

    V01.00x-   Pedestrian on foot injured in collision with pedal cycle in nontraffic accident
      Pedestrian NOS injured in collision with pedal cycle in nontraffic accident

    V01.01x-   Pedestrian on roller-skates injured in collision with pedal cycle in nontraffic accident

    V01.02x-   Pedestrian on skateboard injured in collision with pedal cycle in nontraffic accident

    V01.09x-   Pedestrian with other conveyance injured in collision with pedal cycle in nontraffic accident
      Pedestrian with babystroller injured in collision with pedal cycle in nontraffic accident
      Pedestrian on ice-skates injured in collision with pedal cycle in nontraffic accident
      Pedestrian on nonmotorized scooter injured in collision with pedal cycle in nontraffic accident
      Pedestrian on sled injured in collision with pedal cycle in nontraffic accident
      Pedestrian on snowboard injured in collision with pedal cycle in nontraffic accident
      Pedestrian on snow-skis injured in collision with pedal cycle in nontraffic accident
      Pedestrian in wheelchair (powered) injured in collision with pedal cycle in nontraffic accident
      Pedestrian in motorized mobility scooter injured in collision with pedal cycle in nontraffic accident

  V01.1-   <u>Pedestrian injured in collision</u> with <u>pedal cycle</u> in <u>traffic</u> accident

    V01.10x-   Pedestrian on foot injured in collision with pedal cycle in traffic accident
      Pedestrian NOS injured in collision with pedal cycle in traffic accident

    V01.11x-   Pedestrian on roller-skates injured in collision with pedal cycle in traffic accident

    V01.12x-   Pedestrian on skateboard injured in collision with pedal cycle in traffic accident

    V01.19x-   Pedestrian with other conveyance injured in collision with pedal cycle in traffic accident
      Pedestrian with babystroller injured in collision with pedal cycle in traffic accident
      Pedestrian on ice-skates injured in collision with pedal cycle in traffic accident
      Pedestrian on nonmotorized scooter injured in collision with pedal cycle in traffic accident
      Pedestrian on sled injured in collision with pedal cycle in traffic accident
      Pedestrian on snowboard injured in collision with pedal cycle in traffic accident
      Pedestrian on snow-skis injured in collision with pedal cycle in traffic accident
      Pedestrian in wheelchair (powered) injured in collision with pedal cycle in traffic accident
      Pedestrian in motorized mobility scooter injured in collision with pedal cycle in traffic accident

V01.9- **Pedestrian injured in collision** with **pedal cycle**, **unspecified** whether traffic or nontraffic accident

V01.90x- Pedestrian on foot injured in collision with pedal cycle, unspecified whether traffic or nontraffic accident
    Pedestrian NOS injured in collision with pedal cycle, unspecified whether traffic or nontraffic accident

V01.91x- Pedestrian on roller-skates injured in collision with pedal cycle, unspecified whether traffic or nontraffic accident

V01.92x- Pedestrian on skateboard injured in collision with pedal cycle, unspecified whether traffic or nontraffic accident

V01.99x- Pedestrian with other conveyance injured in collision with pedal cycle, unspecified whether traffic or nontraffic accident
    Pedestrian with babystroller injured in collision with pedal cycle, unspecified whether traffic or nontraffic accident
    Pedestrian on ice-skates injured in collision with pedal cycle unspecified, whether traffic or nontraffic accident
    Pedestrian on nonmotorized scooter injured in collision with pedal cycle, unspecified whether traffic or nontraffic accident
    Pedestrian on sled injured in collision with pedal cycle unspecified, whether traffic or nontraffic accident
    Pedestrian on snowboard injured in collision with pedal cycle, unspecified whether traffic or nontraffic accident
    Pedestrian on snow-skis injured in collision with pedal cycle, unspecified whether traffic or nontraffic accident
    Pedestrian in wheelchair (powered) injured in collision with pedal cycle, unspecified whether traffic or nontraffic accident
    Pedestrian in motorized mobility scooter injured in collision with pedal cycle, unspecified whether traffic or nontraffic accident

V02- **Pedestrian injured in collision** with **two- or three-wheeled motor vehicle**

The appropriate 7th character is to be added to each code from category V02:
A **Initial** encounter
D **Subsequent** encounter
S **Sequela**

V02.0- **Pedestrian Injured In collision** with **two- or three-wheeled motor vehicle** in **nontraffic** accident

V02.00x- Pedestrian on foot injured in collision with two- or three-wheeled motor vehicle in nontraffic accident
    Pedestrian NOS injured in collision with two- or three-wheeled motor vehicle in nontraffic accident

V02.01x- Pedestrian on roller-skates injured in collision with two- or three-wheeled motor vehicle in nontraffic accident

V02.02x- Pedestrian on skateboard injured in collision with two- or three-wheeled motor vehicle in nontraffic accident

V02.09x- Pedestrian with other conveyance injured in collision with two- or three-wheeled motorvehicle in nontraffic accident
    Pedestrian with babystroller injured in collision with two- or three-wheeled motor vehicle in nontraffic accident
    Pedestrian on ice-skates injured in collision with two- or three-wheeled motor vehicle in nontraffic accident
    Pedestrian on nonmotorized scooter injured in collision with two- or three-wheeled motor vehicle in nontraffic accident
    Pedestrian on sled injured in collision with two- or three-wheeled motor vehicle in nontraffic accident
    Pedestrian on snowboard injured in collision with two- or three-wheeled motor vehicle in nontraffic accident
    Pedestrian on snow-skis injured in collision with two- or three-wheeled motor vehicle in nontraffic accident
    Pedestrian in wheelchair (powered) injured in collision with two- or three-wheeled motor vehicle in nontraffic accident
    Pedestrian in motorized mobility scooter injured in collision with two- or three-wheeled motor vehicle in nontraffic accident

V02.1- **Pedestrian injured in collision** with **two- or three-wheeled motor vehicle** in **traffic** accident

V02.10x- Pedestrian on foot injured in collision with two- or three-wheeled motor vehicle in traffic accident
    Pedestrian NOS injured in collision with two- or three-wheeled motor vehicle in traffic accident

V02.11x- Pedestrian on roller-skates injured in collision with two- or three-wheeled motor vehicle intraffic accident

V02.12x- Pedestrian on skateboard injured in collision with two- or three-wheeled motor vehicle intraffic accident

V02.19x- Pedestrian with other conveyance injured in collision with two- or three-wheeled motorvehicle in traffic accident
    Pedestrian with babystroller injured in collision with two- or three-wheeled motor vehicle in traffic accident
    Pedestrian on ice-skates injured in collision with two- or three-wheeled motor vehicle in traffic accident
    Pedestrian on nonmotorized scooter injured in collision with two- or three-wheeled motor vehicle in traffic accident
    Pedestrian on sled injured in collision with two- or three-wheeled motor vehicle in traffic accident
    Pedestrian on snowboard injured in collision with two- or three-wheeled motor vehicle in traffic accident
    Pedestrian on snow-skis injured in collision with two- or three-wheeled motor vehicle in traffic accident
    Pedestrian in wheelchair (powered) injured in collision with two- or three-wheeled motor vehicle in traffic accident
    Pedestrian in motorized mobility scooter injured in collision with two- or three-wheeled motor vehicle in traffic accident

V02.9- **Pedestrian injured in collision** with **two- or three-wheeled motor vehicle**, **unspecified** whether traffic or nontraffic accident

V02.90x- Pedestrian on foot injured in collision with two- or three-wheeled motor vehicle, unspecified whether traffic or nontraffic accident
    Pedestrian NOS injured in collision with two- or three-wheeled motor vehicle, unspecified whether traffic or nontraffic accident

V02.91x- Pedestrian on roller-skates injured in collision with two- or three-wheeled motor vehicle, unspecified whether traffic or nontraffic accident

V02.92x- Pedestrian on skateboard injured in collision with two- or three-wheeled motor vehicle, unspecified whether traffic or nontraffic accident

V02.99x- Pedestrian with other conveyance injured in collision with two- or three-wheeled motor vehicle, unspecified whether traffic or nontraffic accident
    Pedestrian with babystroller injured in collision with two- or three-wheeled motor vehicle, unspecified whether traffic or nontraffic accident
    Pedestrian on ice-skates injured in collision with two- or three-wheeled motor vehicle, unspecified whether traffic or nontraffic accident
    Pedestrian on nonmotorized scooter injured in collision with two- or three-wheeled motor vehicle, unspecified whether traffic or nontraffic accident
    Pedestrian on sled injured in collision with two- or three-wheeled motor vehicle, unspecified whether traffic or nontraffic accident
    Pedestrian on snowboard injured in collision with two- or three-wheeled motor vehicle, unspecified whether traffic or nontraffic accident
    Pedestrian on snow-skis injured in collision with two- or three-wheeled motor vehicle, unspecified whether traffic or nontraffic accident
    Pedestrian in wheelchair (powered) injured in collision with two- or three-wheeled motor vehicle, unspecified whether traffic or nontraffic accident
    Pedestrian in motorized mobility scooter injured in collision with two- or three-wheeled motor vehicle, unspecified whether traffic or nontraffic accident

V01 - V02

V03- Pedestrian injured in collision with car, pick-up truck or van

The appropriate 7th character is to be added to each code from category V03:

A Initial encounter
D Subsequent encounter
S Sequela

V03.0- Pedestrian injured in collision with car, pick-up truck or van in nontraffic accident

V03.00x- Pedestrian on foot injured in collision with car, pick-up truck or van in nontraffic accident
Pedestrian NOS injured in collision with car, pick-up truck or van in nontraffic accident

V03.01x- Pedestrian on roller-skates injured in collision with car, pick-up truck or van in nontraffic accident

V03.02x- Pedestrian on skateboard injured in collision with car, pick-up truck or van in nontraffic accident

V03.09x- Pedestrian with other conveyance injured in collision with car, pick-up truck or van in nontraffic accident
Pedestrian with babystroller injured in collision with car, pick-up truck or van in nontraffic accident
Pedestrian on ice-skates injured in collision with car, pick-up truck or van in nontraffic accident
Pedestrian on nonmotorized scooter injured in collision with car, pick-up truck or van in nontraffic accident
Pedestrian on sled injured in collision with car, pick-up truck or van in nontraffic accident
Pedestrian on snowboard injured in collision with car, pick-up truck or van in nontraffic accident
Pedestrian on snow-skis injured in collision with car, pick-up truck or van in nontraffic accident
Pedestrian in wheelchair (powered) injured in collision with car, pick-up truck or van in nontraffic accident
Pedestrian in motorized mobility scooter injured in collision with car, pick-up truck or van in nontraffic accident

V03.1- Pedestrian injured in collision with car, pick-up truck or van in traffic accident

V03.10x- Pedestrian on foot injured in collision with car, pick-up truck or van in traffic accident
Pedestrian NOS injured in collision with car, pick-up truck or van in traffic accident

V03.11x- Pedestrian on roller-skates injured in collision with car, pick-up truck or van in traffic accident

V03.12x- Pedestrian on skateboard injured in collision with car, pick-up truck or van in traffic accident

V03.19x- Pedestrian with other conveyance injured in collision with car, pick-up truck or van in traffic accident
Pedestrian with babystroller injured in collision with car, pick-up truck or van in traffic accident
Pedestrian on ice-skates injured in collision with car, pick-up truck or van in traffic accident
Pedestrian on nonmotorized scooter injured in collision with car, pick-up truck or van in traffic accident
Pedestrian on sled injured in collision with car, pick-up truck or van in traffic accident
Pedestrian on snowboard injured in collision with car, pick-up truck or van in traffic accident
Pedestrian on snow-skis injured in collision with car, pick-up truck or van in traffic accident
Pedestrian in wheelchair (powered) injured in collision with car, pick-up truck or van in traffic accident
Pedestrian in motorized mobility scooter injured in collision with car, pick-up truck or van in traffic accident

V03.9- Pedestrian injured in collision with car, pick-up truck or van, unspecified whether traffic or nontraffic accident

V03.90x- Pedestrian on foot injured in collision with car, pick-up truck or van, unspecified whether traffic or nontraffic accident
Pedestrian NOS injured in collision with car, pick-up truck or van, unspecified whether traffic or nontraffic accident

V03.91x- Pedestrian on roller-skates injured in collision with car, pick-up truck or van, unspecified whether traffic or nontraffic accident

V03.92x- Pedestrian on skateboard injured in collision with car, pick-up truck or van, unspecified whether traffic or nontraffic accident

V03.99x- Pedestrian with other conveyance injured in collision with car, pick-up truck or van, unspecified whether traffic or nontraffic accident
Pedestrian with babystroller injured in collision with car, pick-up truck or van, unspecified whether traffic or nontraffic accident
Pedestrian on ice-skates injured in collision with car, pick-up truck or van, unspecified whether traffic or nontraffic accident
Pedestrian on nonmotorized scooter injured in collision with car, pick-up truck or van, unspecified whether traffic or nontraffic accident
Pedestrian on sled injured in collision with car, pick-up truck or van in nontraffic accident
Pedestrian on snowboard injured in collision with car, pick-up truck or van, unspecified whether traffic or nontraffic accident
Pedestrian on snow-skis injured in collision with car, pick-up truck or van, unspecified whether traffic or nontraffic accident
Pedestrian in wheelchair (powered) injured in collision with car, pick-up truck or van, unspecified whether traffic or nontraffic accident
Pedestrian in motorized mobility scooter injured in collision with car, pick-up truck or van, unspecified whether traffic or nontraffic accident

V04- Pedestrian injured in collision with heavy transport vehicle or bus
Excludes 1: pedestrian injured in collision with military vehicle (V09.01, V09.21)

The appropriate 7th character is to be added to each code from category V04:

A Initial encounter
D Subsequent encounter
S Sequela

V04.0- Pedestrian injured in collision with heavy transport vehicle or bus in nontraffic accident

V04.00x- Pedestrian on foot injured in collision with heavy transport vehicle or bus in nontraffic accident
Pedestrian NOS injured in collision with heavy transport vehicle or bus in nontraffic accident

V04.01x- Pedestrian on roller-skates injured in collision with heavy transport vehicle or bus in nontraffic accident

V04.02x- Pedestrian on skateboard injured in collision with heavy transport vehicle or bus in nontraffic accident

V04.09x- Pedestrian with other conveyance injured in collision with heavy transport vehicle or bus in nontraffic accident
Pedestrian with babystroller injured in collision with heavy transport vehicle or bus in nontraffic accident
Pedestrian on ice-skates injured in collision with heavy transport vehicle or bus in nontraffic accident
Pedestrian on nonmotorized scooter injured in collision with heavy transport vehicle or bus in nontraffic accident
Pedestrian on sled injured in collision with heavy transport vehicle or bus in nontraffic accident
Pedestrian on snowboard injured in collision with heavy transport vehicle or bus in nontraffic accident
Pedestrian on snow-skis injured in collision with heavy transport vehicle or bus in nontraffic accident
Pedestrian in wheelchair (powered) injured in collision with heavy transport vehicle or bus in nontraffic accident
Pedestrian in motorized mobility scooter injured in collision with heavy transport vehicle or bus in nontraffic accident

V04.1- Pedestrian injured in collision with heavy transport vehicle or bus in traffic accident

V04.10x- Pedestrian on foot injured in collision with heavy transport vehicle or bus in traffic accident
Pedestrian NOS injured in collision with heavy transport vehicle or bus in traffic accident

V04.11x- Pedestrian on roller-skates injured in collision with heavy transport vehicle or bus in traffic accident

V04.12x- Pedestrian on skateboard injured in collision with heavy transport vehicle or bus in traffic accident

V03-V04

V04.19x- Pedestrian with other conveyance injured in collision with heavy transport vehicle or bus in traffic accident
Pedestrian with babystroller injured in collision with heavy transport vehicle or bus in traffic accident
Pedestrian on ice-skates injured in collision with heavy transport vehicle or bus in traffic accident
Pedestrian on nonmotorized scooter injured in collision with heavy transport vehicle or bus in traffic accident
Pedestrian on sled injured in collision with heavy transport vehicle or bus in traffic accident
Pedestrian on snowboard injured in collision with heavy transport vehicle or bus in traffic accident
Pedestrian on snow-skis injured in collision with heavy transport vehicle or bus in traffic accident
Pedestrian in wheelchair (powered) injured in collision with heavy transport vehicle or bus in traffic accident
Pedestrian in motorized mobility scooter injured in collision with heavy transport vehicle or bus in traffic accident

V04.9- Pedestrian injured in collision with heavy transport vehicle or bus, unspecified whether traffic or nontraffic accident

V04.90x- Pedestrian on foot injured in collision with heavy transport vehicle or bus, unspecified whether traffic or nontraffic accident
Pedestrian NOS injured in collision with heavy transport vehicle or bus, unspecified whether traffic or nontraffic accident

V04.91x- Pedestrian on roller-skates injured in collision with heavy transport vehicle or bus, unspecified whether traffic or nontraffic accident

V04.92x- Pedestrian on skateboard injured in collision with heavy transport vehicle or bus, unspecified whether traffic or nontraffic accident

V04.99x- Pedestrian with other conveyance injured in collision with heavy transport vehicle or bus, unspecified whether traffic or nontraffic accident
Pedestrian with babystroller injured in collision with heavy transport vehicle or bus, unspecified whether traffic or nontraffic accident
Pedestrian on ice-skates injured in collision with heavy transport vehicle or bus, unspecified whether traffic or nontraffic accident
Pedestrian on nonmotorized scooter injured in collision with heavy transport vehicle or bus, unspecified whether traffic or nontraffic accident
Pedestrian on sled injured in collision with heavy transport vehicle or bus, unspecified whether traffic or nontraffic accident
Pedestrian on snowboard injured in collision with heavy transport vehicle or bus, unspecified whether traffic or nontraffic accident
Pedestrian on snow-skis injured in collision with heavy transport vehicle or bus, unspecified whether traffic or nontraffic accident
Pedestrian in wheelchair (powered) injured in collision with heavy transport vehicle or bus, unspecified whether traffic or nontraffic accident
Pedestrian in motorized mobility scooter injured in collision with heavy transport vehicle or bus, unspecified whether traffic or nontraffic accident

V05- Pedestrian injured in collision with railway train or railway vehicle
The appropriate 7th character is to be added to each code from category V05:
A   Initial encounter
D   Subsequent encounter
S   Sequela

V05.0- Pedestrian injured in collision with railway train or railway vehicle in nontraffic accident

V05.00x- Pedestrian on foot injured in collision with railway train or railway vehicle in nontraffic accident
Pedestrian NOS injured in collision with railway train or railway vehicle in nontraffic accident

V05.01x- Pedestrian on roller-skates injured in collision with railway train or railway vehicle in nontraffic accident

V05.02x- Pedestrian on skateboard injured in collision with railway train or railway vehicle in nontraffic accident

V05.09x- Pedestrian with other conveyance injured in collision with railway train or railway vehicle in nontraffic accident
Pedestrian with babystroller injured in collision with railway train or railway vehicle in nontraffic accident
Pedestrian on ice-skates injured in collision with railway train or railway vehicle in nontraffic accident
Pedestrian on nonmotorized scooter injured in collision with railway train or railway vehicle in nontraffic accident
Pedestrian on sled injured in collision with railway train or railway vehicle in nontraffic accident
Pedestrian on snowboard injured in collision with railway train or railway vehicle in nontraffic accident
Pedestrian on snow-skis injured in collision with railway train or railway vehicle in nontraffic accident
Pedestrian in wheelchair (powered) injured in collision with railway train or railway vehicle in nontraffic accident
Pedestrian in motorized mobility scooter injured in collision with railway train or railway vehicle in nontraffic accident

V05.1- Pedestrian injured in collision with railway train or railway vehicle in traffic accident

V05.10x- Pedestrian on foot injured in collision with railway train or railway vehicle in traffic accident
Pedestrian NOS injured in collision with railway train or railway vehicle in traffic accident

V05.11x- Pedestrian on roller-skates injured in collision with railway train or railway vehicle in traffic accident

V05.12x- Pedestrian on skateboard injured in collision with railway train or railway vehicle in traffic accident

V05.19x- Pedestrian with other conveyance injured in collision with railway train or railway vehicle in traffic accident
Pedestrian with babystroller injured in collision with railway train or railway vehicle in traffic accident
Pedestrian on ice-skates injured in collision with railway train or railway vehicle in traffic accident
Pedestrian on nonmotorized scooter injured in collision with railway train or railway vehicle in traffic accident
Pedestrian on sled injured in collision with railway train or railway vehicle in traffic accident
Pedestrian on snowboard injured in collision with railway train or railway vehicle in traffic accident
Pedestrian on snow-skis injured in collision with railway train or railway vehicle in traffic accident
Pedestrian in wheelchair (powered) injured in collision with railway train or railway vehicle in traffic accident
Pedestrian in motorized mobility scooter injured in collision with railway train or railway vehicle in traffic accident

V05.9- Pedestrian injured in collision with railway train or railway vehicle, unspecified whether traffic or nontraffic accident

V05.90x- Pedestrian on foot injured in collision with railway train or railway vehicle, unspecified whether traffic or nontraffic accident
Pedestrian NOS injured in collision with railway train or railway vehicle, unspecified whether traffic or nontraffic accident

V05.91x- Pedestrian on roller-skates injured in collision with railway train or railway vehicle, unspecified whether traffic or nontraffic accident

V05.92x- Pedestrian on skateboard injured in collision with railway train or railway vehicle, unspecified whether traffic or nontraffic accident

V 0 4 - V 0 5

V05.99x- Pedestrian with other conveyance injured in collision with railway train or railway vehicle, unspecified whether traffic or nontraffic accident
> Pedestrian with babystroller injured in collision with railway train or railway vehicle, unspecified whether traffic or nontraffic
> Pedestrian on ice-skates injured in collision with railway train or railway vehicle, unspecified whether traffic or nontraffic
> Pedestrian on nonmotorized scooter injured in collision with railway train or railway vehicle, unspecified whether traffic or nontraffic
> Pedestrian on sled injured in collision with railway train or railway vehicle, unspecified whether traffic or nontraffic
> Pedestrian on snowboard injured in collision with railway train or railway vehicle, unspecified whether traffic or nontraffic
> Pedestrian on snow-skis injured in collision with railway train or railway vehicle, unspecified whether traffic or nontraffic
> Pedestrian in wheelchair (powered) injured in collision with railway train or railway vehicle, unspecified whether traffic or nontraffic
> Pedestrian in motorized mobility scooter injured in collision with railway train or railway vehicle, unspecified whether traffic or nontraffic

V06- Pedestrian injured in collision with other nonmotor vehicle
- Includes: Collision with animal-drawn vehicle, animal being ridden, nonpowered streetcar
- Excludes 1: *pedestrian injured in collision with pedestrian conveyance (V00.0-)*

The appropriate 7th character is to be added to each code from category V06:
- A   Initial encounter
- D   Subsequent encounter
- S   Sequela

V06.0- Pedestrian injured in collision with other nonmotor vehicle in nontraffic accident

V06.00x- Pedestrian on foot injured in collision with other nonmotor vehicle in nontraffic accident
> Pedestrian NOS injured in collision with other nonmotor vehicle in nontraffic accident

V06.01x- Pedestrian on roller-skates injured in collision with other nonmotor vehicle in nontraffic accident

V06.02x- Pedestrian on skateboard injured in collision with other nonmotor vehicle in nontraffic accident

V06.09x- Pedestrian with other conveyance injured in collision with other nonmotor vehicle in nontraffic accident
> Pedestrian with babystroller injured in collision with other nonmotor vehicle in nontraffic accident
> Pedestrian on ice-skates injured in collision with other nonmotor vehicle in nontraffic accident
> Pedestrian on nonmotorized scooter injured in collision with other nonmotor vehicle in nontraffic accident
> Pedestrian on sled injured in collision with other nonmotor vehicle in nontraffic accident
> Pedestrian on snowboard injured in collision with other nonmotor vehicle in nontraffic accident
> Pedestrian on snow-skis injured in collision with other nonmotor vehicle in nontraffic accident
> Pedestrian in wheelchair (powered) injured in collision with other nonmotor vehicle in nontraffic accident
> Pedestrian in motorized mobility scooter injured in collision with other nonmotor vehicle in nontraffic accident

V06.1- Pedestrian injured in collision with other nonmotor vehicle in traffic accident

V06.10x- Pedestrian on foot injured in collision with other nonmotor vehicle in traffic accident
> Pedestrian NOS injured in collision with other nonmotor vehicle in traffic accident

V06.11x- Pedestrian on roller-skates injured in collision with other nonmotor vehicle in traffic accident

V06.12x- Pedestrian on skateboard injured in collision with other nonmotor vehicle in traffic accident

V06.19x- Pedestrian with other conveyance injured in collision with other nonmotor vehicle in traffic accident
> Pedestrian with babystroller injured in collision with other nonmotor vehicle in nontraffic accident
> Pedestrian on ice-skates injured in collision with other nonmotor vehicle in traffic accident
> Pedestrian on nonmotorized scooter injured in collision with other nonmotor vehicle in traffic accident
> Pedestrian on sled injured in collision with other nonmotor vehicle in traffic accident
> Pedestrian on snowboard injured in collision with other nonmotor vehicle in traffic accident
> Pedestrian on snow-skis injured in collision with other nonmotor vehicle in traffic accident
> Pedestrian in wheelchair (powered) injured in collision with other nonmotor vehicle in traffic accident
> Pedestrian in motorized mobility scooter injured in collision with other nonmotor vehicle in traffic accident

V06.9- Pedestrian injured in collision with other nonmotor vehicle, unspecified whether traffic or nontraffic accident

V06.90x- Pedestrian on foot injured in collision with other nonmotor vehicle, unspecified whether traffic or nontraffic accident
> Pedestrian NOS injured in collision with other nonmotor vehicle, unspecified whether traffic or nontraffic accident

V06.91x- Pedestrian on roller-skates injured in collision with other nonmotor vehicle, unspecified whether traffic or nontraffic accident

V06.92x- Pedestrian on skateboard injured in collision with other nonmotor vehicle, unspecified whether traffic or nontraffic accident

V06.99x- Pedestrian with other conveyance injured in collision with other nonmotor vehicle, unspecified whether traffic or nontraffic accident
> Pedestrian with babystroller injured in collision with other nonmotor vehicle, unspecified whether traffic or nontraffic accident
> Pedestrian on ice-skates injured in collision with other nonmotor vehicle, unspecified whether traffic or nontraffic accident
> Pedestrian on nonmotorized scooter injured in collision with other nonmotor vehicle, unspecified whether traffic or nontraffic accident
> Pedestrian on sled injured in collision with other nonmotor vehicle, unspecified whether traffic or nontraffic accident
> Pedestrian on snowboard injured in collision with other nonmotor vehicle, unspecified whether traffic or nontraffic accident
> Pedestrian on snow-skis injured in collision with other nonmotor vehicle, unspecified whether traffic or nontraffic accident
> Pedestrian in wheelchair (powered) injured in collision with other nonmotor vehicle, unspecified whether traffic or nontraffic accident
> Pedestrian in motorized mobility scooter injured in collision with other nonmotor vehicle, unspecified whether traffic or nontraffic accident

V09- Pedestrian injured in other and unspecified transport accidents

The appropriate 7th character is to be added to each code from category V09:
- A   Initial encounter
- D   Subsequent encounter
- S   Sequela

V09.0- Pedestrian injured in nontraffic accident involving other and unspecified motor vehicles

V09.00x- Pedestrian injured in nontraffic accident involving unspecified motor vehicles

V09.01x- Pedestrian injured in nontraffic accident involving military vehicle

V09.09x- Pedestrian injured in nontraffic accident involving other motor vehicles
> Pedestrian injured in nontraffic accident by special vehicle

V09.1xx- Pedestrian injured in unspecified nontraffic accident

V05 - V09

V09.2-   Pedestrian injured in traffic accident involving other and unspecified motor vehicles

    V09.20x-   Pedestrian injured in traffic accident involving unspecified motor vehicles

    V09.21x-   Pedestrian injured in traffic accident involving military vehicle

    V09.29x-   Pedestrian injured in traffic accident involving other motor vehicles

V09.3xx-   Pedestrian injured in unspecified traffic accident

V09.9xx-   Pedestrian injured in unspecified transport accident

Pedal cycle rider injured in transport accident (V10-V19)

Includes: Any non-motorized vehicle, excluding an animal-drawn vehicle, or a sidecar or trailer attached to the pedal cycle

Excludes ❷: rupture of pedal cycle tire (W37.0)

V10-   Pedal cycle rider injured in collision with pedestrian or animal
    Excludes 1:   pedal cycle rider collision with animal-drawn vehicle or animal being ridden (V16.-)

The appropriate 7th character is to be added to each code from category V10:
- **A**   **Initial** encounter
- **D**   **Subsequent** encounter
- **S**   **Sequela**

V10.0xx-   Pedal cycle driver injured in collision with pedestrian or animal in nontraffic accident

V10.1xx-   Pedal cycle passenger injured in collision with pedestrian or animal in nontraffic accident

V10.2xx-   Unspecified pedal cyclist injured in collision with pedestrian or animal in nontraffic accident

V10.3xx-   Person boarding or alighting a pedal cycle injured in collision with pedestrian or animal

V10.4xx-   Pedal cycle driver injured in collision with pedestrian or animal in traffic accident

V10.5xx-   Pedal cycle passenger injured in collision with pedestrian or animal in traffic accident

V10.9xx-   Unspecified pedal cyclist injured in collision with pedestrian or animal in traffic accident

V11-   Pedal cycle rider injured in collision with other pedal cycle

The appropriate 7th character is to be added to each code from category V11:
- **A**   **Initial** encounter
- **D**   **Subsequent** encounter
- **S**   **Sequela**

V11.0xx-   Pedal cycle driver injured in collision with other pedal cycle in nontraffic accident

V11.1xx-   Pedal cycle passenger injured in collision with other pedal cycle in nontraffic accident

V11.2xx-   Unspecified pedal cyclist injured in collision with other pedal cycle in nontraffic accident

V11.3xx-   Person boarding or alighting a pedal cycle injured in collision with other pedal cycle

V11.4xx-   Pedal cycle driver injured in collision with other pedal cycle in traffic accident

V11.5xx-   Pedal cycle passenger injured in collision with other pedal cycle in traffic accident

V11.9xx-   Unspecified pedal cyclist injured in collision with other pedal cycle in traffic accident

V12-   Pedal cycle rider injured in collision with two- or three-wheeled motor vehicle

The appropriate 7th character is to be added to each code from category V12:
- **A**   **Initial** encounter
- **D**   **Subsequent** encounter
- **S**   **Sequela**

V12.0xx-   Pedal cycle driver injured in collision with two- or three-wheeled motor vehicle in nontraffic accident

V12.1xx-   Pedal cycle passenger injured in collision with two- or three-wheeled motor vehicle in nontraffic accident

V12.2xx-   Unspecified pedal cyclist injured in collision with two- or three-wheeled motor vehicle in nontraffic accident

V12.3xx-   Person boarding or alighting a pedal cycle injured in collision with two- or three-wheeled motor vehicle

V12.4xx-   Pedal cycle driver injured in collision with two- or three-wheeled motor vehicle in traffic accident

V12.5xx-   Pedal cycle passenger injured in collision with two- or three-wheeled motor vehicle in traffic accident

V12.9xx-   Unspecified pedal cyclist injured in collision with two- or three-wheeled motor vehicle in traffic accident

V13-   Pedal cycle rider injured in collision with car, pick-up truck or van

The appropriate 7th character is to be added to each code from category V13:
- **A**   **Initial** encounter
- **D**   **Subsequent** encounter
- **S**   **Sequela**

V13.0xx-   Pedal cycle driver injured in collision with car, pick-up truck or van in nontraffic accident

V13.1xx-   Pedal cycle passenger injured in collision with car, pick-up truck or van in nontraffic accident

V13.2xx-   Unspecified pedal cyclist injured in collision with car, pick-up truck or van in nontraffic accident

V13.3xx-   Person boarding or alighting a pedal cycle injured in collision with car, pick-up truck or van

V13.4xx-   Pedal cycle driver injured in collision with car, pick-up truck or van in traffic accident

V13.5xx-   Pedal cycle passenger injured in collision with car, pick-up truck or van in traffic accident

V13.9xx-   Unspecified pedal cyclist injured in collision with car, pick-up truck or van in traffic accident

V14-   Pedal cycle rider injured in collision with heavy transport vehicle or bus
    Excludes 1:   pedal cycle rider injured in collision with military vehicle (V19.81)

The appropriate 7th character is to be added to each code from category V14:
- **A**   **Initial** encounter
- **D**   **Subsequent** encounter
- **S**   **Sequela**

V14.0xx-   Pedal cycle driver injured in collision with heavy transport vehicle or bus in nontraffic accident

V14.1xx-   Pedal cycle passenger injured in collision with heavy transport vehicle or bus in nontraffic accident

V14.2xx-   Unspecified pedal cyclist injured in collision with heavy transport vehicle or bus in nontraffic accident

V14.3xx-   Person boarding or alighting a pedal cycle injured in collision with heavy transport vehicle or bus

V14.4xx-   Pedal cycle driver injured in collision with heavy transport vehicle or bus in traffic accident

V14.5xx-   Pedal cycle passenger injured in collision with heavy transport vehicle or bus in traffic accident

V14.9xx-   Unspecified pedal cyclist injured in collision with heavy transport vehicle or bus in traffic accident

V15-   Pedal cycle rider injured in collision with railway train or railway vehicle

The appropriate 7th character is to be added to each code from category V15:
- **A**   **Initial** encounter
- **D**   **Subsequent** encounter
- **S**   **Sequela**

V15.0xx-   Pedal cycle driver injured in collision with railway train or railway vehicle in nontraffic accident

V15.1xx-   Pedal cycle passenger injured in collision with railway train or railway vehicle in nontraffic accident

V15.2xx-   Unspecified pedal cyclist injured in collision with railway train or railway vehicle in nontraffic accident

V15.3xx-   Person boarding or alighting a pedal cycle injured in collision with railway train or railway vehicle

V15.4xx-   Pedal cycle driver injured in collision with railway train or railway vehicle in traffic accident

V15.5xx-   Pedal cycle passenger injured in collision with railway train or railway vehicle in traffic accident

V09 - V15

V15.9xx- Unspecified pedal cyclist injured in collision with railway train or railway vehicle in traffic accident

V16- Pedal cycle rider injured in collision with other nonmotor vehicle
Includes: Collision with animal-drawn vehicle, animal being ridden, streetcar

The appropriate 7th character is to be added to each code from category V16:
 A Initial encounter
 D Subsequent encounter
 S Sequela

V16.0xx- Pedal cycle driver injured in collision with other nonmotor vehicle in nontraffic accident
V16.1xx- Pedal cycle passenger injured in collision with other nonmotor vehicle in nontraffic accident
V16.2xx- Unspecified pedal cyclist injured in collision with other nonmotor vehicle in nontraffic accident
V16.3xx- Person boarding or alighting a pedal cycle injured in collision with other nonmotor vehicle in nontraffic accident
V16.4xx- Pedal cycle driver injured in collision with other nonmotor vehicle in traffic accident
V16.5xx- Pedal cycle passenger injured in collision with other nonmotor vehicle in traffic accident
V16.9xx- Unspecified pedal cyclist injured in collision with other nonmotor vehicle in traffic accident

V17- Pedal cycle rider injured in collision with fixed or stationary object

The appropriate 7th character is to be added to each code from category V17:
 A Initial encounter
 D Subsequent encounter
 S Sequela

V17.0xx- Pedal cycle driver injured in collision with fixed or stationary object in nontraffic accident
V17.1xx- Pedal cycle passenger injured in collision with fixed or stationary object in nontraffic accident
V17.2xx- Unspecified pedal cyclist injured in collision with fixed or stationary object in nontraffic accident
V17.3xx- Person boarding or alighting a pedal cycle injured in collision with fixed or stationary object
V17.4xx- Pedal cycle driver injured in collision with fixed or stationary object in traffic accident
V17.5xx- Pedal cycle passenger injured in collision with fixed or stationary object in traffic accident
V17.9xx- Unspecified pedal cyclist injured in collision with fixed or stationary object in traffic accident

V18- Pedal cycle rider injured in noncollision transport accident
Includes: Fall or thrown from pedal cycle (without antecedent collision)
Overturning pedal cycle NOS
Overturning pedal cycle without collision

The appropriate 7th character is to be added to each code from category V18:
 A Initial encounter
 D Subsequent encounter
 S Sequela

V18.0xx- Pedal cycle driver injured in noncollision transport accident in nontraffic accident
V18.1xx- Pedal cycle passenger injured in noncollision transport accident in nontraffic accident
V18.2xx- Unspecified pedal cyclist injured in noncollision transport accident in nontraffic accident
V18.3xx- Person boarding or alighting a pedal cycle injured in noncollision transport accident
V18.4xx- Pedal cycle driver injured in noncollision transport accident in traffic accident
V18.5xx- Pedal cycle passenger injured in noncollision transport accident in traffic accident
V18.9xx- Unspecified pedal cyclist injured in noncollision transport accident in traffic accident

V19- Pedal cycle rider injured in other and unspecified transport accidents

The appropriate 7th character is to be added to each code from category V19:
 A Initial encounter
 D Subsequent encounter
 S Sequela

V19.0- Pedal cycle driver injured in collision with other and unspecified motor vehicles in nontraffic accident
  V19.00x- Pedal cycle driver injured in collision with unspecified motor vehicles in nontraffic accident
  V19.09x- Pedal cycle driver injured in collision with other motor vehicles in nontraffic accident
V19.1- Pedal cycle passenger injured in collision with other and unspecified motor vehicles in nontraffic accident
  V19.10x- Pedal cycle passenger injured in collision with unspecified motor vehicles in nontraffic accident
  V19.19x- Pedal cycle passenger injured in collision with other motor vehicles in nontraffic accident
V19.2- Unspecified pedal cyclist injured in collision with other and unspecified motor vehicles in nontraffic accident
  V19.20x- Unspecified pedal cyclist injured in collision with unspecified motor vehicles in nontraffic accident
   Pedal cycle collision NOS, nontraffic
  V19.29x- Unspecified pedal cyclist injured in collision with other motor vehicles in nontraffic accident
V19.3xx- Pedal cyclist (driver) (passenger) injured in unspecified nontraffic accident
   Pedal cycle accident NOS, nontraffic
   Pedal cyclist injured in nontraffic accident NOS
V19.4- Pedal cycle driver injured in collision with other and unspecified motor vehicles in traffic accident
  V19.40x- Pedal cycle driver injured in collision with unspecified motor vehicles in traffic accident
  V19.49x- Pedal cycle driver injured in collision with other motor vehicles in traffic accident
V19.5- Pedal cycle passenger injured in collision with other and unspecified motor vehicles in traffic accident
  V19.50x- Pedal cycle passenger injured in collision with unspecified motor vehicles in traffic accident
  V19.59x- Pedal cycle passenger injured in collision with other motor vehicles in traffic accident
V19.6- Unspecified pedal cyclist injured in collision with other and unspecified motor vehicles in traffic accident
  V19.60x- Unspecified pedal cyclist injured in collision with unspecified motor vehicles in traffic accident
   Pedal cycle collision NOS (traffic)
  V19.69x- Unspecified pedal cyclist injured in collision with other motor vehicles in traffic accident
V19.8- Pedal cyclist (driver) (passenger) injured in other specified transport accidents
  V19.81x- Pedal cyclist (driver) (passenger) injured in transport accident with military vehicle
  V19.88x- Pedal cyclist (driver) (passenger) injured in other specified transport accidents
V19.9xx- Pedal cyclist (driver) (passenger) injured in unspecified traffic accident
   Pedal cycle accident NOS

V15 - V19

Motorcycle rider injured in transport accident (V20-V29)

Includes: Moped
               Motorcycle with sidecar
               Motorized bicycle
               Motor scooter

Excludes 1:   *three-wheeled motor vehicle (V30-V39)*

V20-   **Motorcycle rider injured in collision** with **pedestrian or animal**

Excludes 1:   *motorcycle rider collision with animal-drawn vehicle or animal being ridden (V26.-)*

The appropriate 7th character is to be added to each code from category V20:

   A   **Initial** encounter
   D   **Subsequent** encounter
   S   **Sequela**

V20.0xx-   Motorcycle driver injured in collision with pedestrian or animal in nontraffic accident

V20.1xx-   Motorcycle passenger injured in collision with pedestrian or animal in nontraffic accident

V20.2xx-   Unspecified motorcycle rider injured in collision with pedestrian or animal in nontraffic accident

V20.3xx-   Person boarding or alighting a motorcycle injured in collision with pedestrian or animal

V20.4xx-   Motorcycle driver injured in collision with pedestrian or animal in traffic accident

V20.5xx-   Motorcycle passenger injured in collision with pedestrian or animal in traffic accident

V20.9xx-   Unspecified motorcycle rider injured in collision with pedestrian or animal in traffic accident

V21-   **Motorcycle rider injured in collision** with **pedal cycle**

The appropriate 7th character is to be added to each code from category V21:

   A   **Initial** encounter
   D   **Subsequent** encounter
   S   **Sequela**

V21.0xx-   Motorcycle driver injured in collision with pedal cycle in nontraffic accident

V21.1xx-   Motorcycle passenger injured in collision with pedal cycle in nontraffic accident

V21.2xx-   Unspecified motorcycle rider injured in collision with pedal cycle in nontraffic accident

V21.3xx-   Person boarding or alighting a motorcycle injured in collision with pedal cycle

V21.4xx-   Motorcycle driver injured in collision with pedal cycle in traffic accident

V21.5xx-   Motorcycle passenger injured in collision with pedal cycle in traffic accident

V21.9xx-   Unspecified motorcycle rider injured in collision with pedal cycle in traffic accident

V22-   **Motorcycle rider injured in collision** with **two- or three-wheeled motor vehicle**

The appropriate 7th character is to be added to each code from category V22:

   A   **Initial** encounter
   D   **Subsequent** encounter
   S   **Sequela**

V22.0xx-   Motorcycle driver injured in collision with two- or three-wheeled motor vehicle in nontraffic accident

V22.1xx-   Motorcycle passenger injured in collision with two- or three-wheeled motor vehicle in nontraffic accident

V22.2xx-   Unspecified motorcycle rider injured in collision with two- or three-wheeled motor vehicle in nontraffic accident

V22.3xx-   Person boarding or alighting a motorcycle injured in collision with two- or three-wheeled motor vehicle

V22.4xx-   Motorcycle driver injured in collision with two- or three-wheeled motor vehicle in traffic accident

V22.5xx-   Motorcycle passenger injured in collision with two- or three-wheeled motor vehicle in traffic accident

V22.9xx-   Unspecified motorcycle rider injured in collision with two- or three-wheeled motor vehicle in traffic accident

V23-   **Motorcycle rider injured in collision** with **car, pick-up truck or van**

The appropriate 7th character is to be added to each code from category V23:

   A   **Initial** encounter
   D   **Subsequent** encounter
   S   **Sequela**

V23.0xx-   Motorcycle driver injured in collision with car, pick-up truck or van in nontraffic accident

V23.1xx-   Motorcycle passenger injured in collision with car, pick-up truck or van in nontraffic accident

V23.2xx-   Unspecified motorcycle rider injured in collision with car, pick-up truck or van in nontraffic accident

V23.3xx-   Person boarding or alighting a motorcycle injured in collision with car, pick-up truck or van

V23.4xx-   Motorcycle driver injured in collision with car, pick-up truck or van in traffic accident

V23.5xx-   Motorcycle passenger injured in collision with car, pick-up truck or van in traffic accident

V23.9xx-   Unspecified motorcycle rider injured in collision with car, pick-up truck or van in traffic accident

V24-   **Motorcycle rider injured in collision** with **heavy transport vehicle or bus**

Excludes 1:   *motorcycle rider injured in collision with military vehicle (V29.81)*

The appropriate 7th character is to be added to each code from category V24:

   A   **Initial** encounter
   D   **Subsequent** encounter
   S   **Sequela**

V24.0xx-   Motorcycle driver injured in collision with heavy transport vehicle or bus in nontraffic accident

V24.1xx-   Motorcycle passenger injured in collision with heavy transport vehicle or bus in nontraffic accident

V24.2xx-   Unspecified motorcycle rider injured in collision with heavy transport vehicle or bus in nontraffic accident

V24.3xx-   Person boarding or alighting a motorcycle injured in collision with heavy transport vehicle or bus

V24.4xx-   Motorcycle driver injured in collision with heavy transport vehicle or bus in traffic accident

V24.5xx-   Motorcycle passenger injured in collision with heavy transport vehicle or bus in traffic accident

V24.9xx-   Unspecified motorcycle rider injured in collision with heavy transport vehicle or bus in traffic accident

V25-   **Motorcycle rider injured in collision** with **railway train or railway vehicle**

The appropriate 7th character is to be added to each code from category V25:

   A   **Initial** encounter
   D   **Subsequent** encounter
   S   **Sequela**

V25.0xx-   Motorcycle driver injured in collision with railway train or railway vehicle in nontraffic accident

V25.1xx-   Motorcycle passenger injured in collision with railway train or railway vehicle in nontraffic accident

V25.2xx-   Unspecified motorcycle rider injured in collision with railway train or railway vehicle in nontraffic accident

V25.3xx-   Person boarding or alighting a motorcycle injured in collision with railway train or railway vehicle

V25.4xx-   Motorcycle driver injured in collision with railway train or railway vehicle in traffic accident

V25.5xx-   Motorcycle passenger injured in collision with railway train or railway vehicle in traffic accident

V25.9xx-   Unspecified motorcycle rider injured in collision with railway train or railway vehicle in traffic accident

Excludes 1: = NOT CODED HERE! (Do not code both)   **1243**   *Excludes ❷:* = Not Included Here

V20 - V25

V26- Motorcycle rider injured in collision with other nonmotor vehicle
Includes: Collision with animal-drawn vehicle, animal being ridden, streetcar

The appropriate 7th character is to be added to each code from category V26:
A **Initial** encounter
D **Subsequent** encounter
S **Sequela**

V26.0xx- Motorcycle driver injured in collision with other nonmotor vehicle in nontraffic accident

V26.1xx- Motorcycle passenger injured in collision with other nonmotor vehicle in nontraffic accident

V26.2xx- Unspecified motorcycle rider injured in collision with other nonmotor vehicle in nontraffic accident

V26.3xx- Person boarding or alighting a motorcycle injured in collision with other nonmotor vehicle

V26.4xx- Motorcycle driver injured in collision with other nonmotor vehicle in traffic accident

V26.5xx- Motorcycle passenger injured in collision with other nonmotor vehicle in traffic accident

V26.9xx- Unspecified motorcycle rider injured in collision with other nonmotor vehicle in traffic accident

V27- Motorcycle rider injured in collision with fixed or stationary object

The appropriate 7th character is to be added to each code from category V27:
A **Initial** encounter
D **Subsequent** encounter
S **Sequela**

V27.0xx- Motorcycle driver injured in collision with fixed or stationary object in nontraffic accident

V27.1xx- Motorcycle passenger injured in collision with fixed or stationary object in nontraffic accident

V27.2xx- Unspecified motorcycle rider injured in collision with fixed or stationary object in nontraffic accident

V27.3xx- Person boarding or alighting a motorcycle injured in collision with fixed or stationary object

V27.4xx- Motorcycle driver injured in collision with fixed or stationary object in traffic accident

V27.5xx- Motorcycle passenger injured in collision with fixed or stationary object in traffic accident

V27.9xx- Unspecified motorcycle rider injured in collision with fixed or stationary object in traffic accident

V28- Motorcycle rider injured in noncollision transport accident
Includes: Fall or thrown from motorcycle (without antecedent collision)
Overturning motorcycle NOS
Overturning motorcycle without collision

The appropriate 7th character is to be added to each code from category V28:
A **Initial** encounter
D **Subsequent** encounter
S **Sequela**

V28.0xx- Motorcycle driver injured in noncollision transport accident in nontraffic accident

V28.1xx- Motorcycle passenger injured in noncollision transport accident in nontraffic accident

V28.2xx- Unspecified motorcycle rider injured in noncollision transport accident in nontraffic accident

V28.3xx- Person boarding or alighting a motorcycle injured in noncollision transport accident

V28.4xx- Motorcycle driver injured in noncollision transport accident in traffic accident

V28.5xx- Motorcycle passenger injured in noncollision transport accident in traffic accident

V28.9xx- Unspecified motorcycle rider injured in noncollision transport accident in traffic accident

V29- Motorcycle rider injured in other and unspecified transport accidents

The appropriate 7th character is to be added to each code from category V29:
A **Initial** encounter
D **Subsequent** encounter
S **Sequela**

V29.0- Motorcycle driver injured in collision with other and unspecified motor vehicles in nontraffic accident

V29.00x- Motorcycle driver injured in collision with unspecified motor vehicles in nontraffic accident

V29.09x- Motorcycle driver injured in collision with other motor vehicles in nontraffic accident

V29.1- Motorcycle passenger injured in collision with other and unspecified motor vehicles in nontraffic accident

V29.10x- Motorcycle passenger injured in collision with unspecified motor vehicles in nontraffic accident

V29.19x- Motorcycle passenger injured in collision with other motor vehicles in nontraffic accident

V29.2- Unspecified motorcycle rider injured in collision with other and unspecified motor vehicles in nontraffic accident

V29.20x- Unspecified motorcycle rider injured in collision with unspecified motor vehicles in nontraffic accident
Motorcycle collision NOS, nontraffic

V29.29x- Unspecified motorcycle rider injured in collision with other motor vehicles in nontraffic accident

V29.3xx- Motorcycle rider (driver) (passenger) injured in unspecified nontraffic accident
Motorcycle accident NOS, nontraffic
Motorcycle rider injured in nontraffic accident NOS

V29.4- Motorcycle driver injured in collision with other and unspecified motor vehicles in traffic accident

V29.40x- Motorcycle driver injured in collision with unspecified motor vehicles in traffic accident

V29.49x- Motorcycle driver injured in collision with other motor vehicles in traffic accident

V29.5- Motorcycle passenger injured in collision with other and unspecified motor vehicles in traffic accident

V29.50x- Motorcycle passenger injured in collision with unspecified motor vehicles in traffic accident

V29.59x- Motorcycle passenger injured in collision with other motor vehicles in traffic accident

V29.6- Unspecified motorcycle rider injured in collision with other and unspecified motor vehicles in traffic accident

V29.60x- Unspecified motorcycle rider injured in collision with unspecified motor vehicles in traffic accident
Motorcycle collision NOS (traffic)

V29.69x- Unspecified motorcycle rider injured in collision with other motor vehicles in traffic accident

V29.8- Motorcycle rider (driver) (passenger) injured in other specified transport accidents

V29.81x- Motorcycle rider (driver) (passenger) injured in transport accident with military vehicle

V29.88x- Motorcycle rider (driver) (passenger) injured in other specified transport accidents

V29.9xx- Motorcycle rider (driver) (passenger) injured in unspecified traffic accident
Motorcycle accident NOS

V
2
6
–
V
2
9

Occupant of three-wheeled motor vehicle injured in transport accident (V30-V39)

Includes: Motorized tricycle
              Motorized rickshaw
              Three-wheeled motor car
Excludes 1:   all-terrain vehicles (V86.-)
              motorcycle with sidecar (V20-V29)
              vehicle designed primarily for off-road use (V86.-)

V30- Occupant of three-wheeled motor vehicle injured in collision with pedestrian or animal
Excludes 1:   three-wheeled motor vehicle collision with animal-drawn vehicle or animal being ridden (V36.-)

The appropriate 7th character is to be added to each code from category V30:
- A   Initial encounter
- D   Subsequent encounter
- S   Sequela

V30.0xx- Driver of three-wheeled motor vehicle injured in collision with pedestrian or animal in nontraffic accident

V30.1xx- Passenger in three-wheeled motor vehicle injured in collision with pedestrian or animal in nontraffic accident

V30.2xx- Person on outside of three-wheeled motor vehicle injured in collision with pedestrian or animal in nontraffic accident

V30.3xx- Unspecified occupant of three-wheeled motor vehicle injured in collision with pedestrian or animal in nontraffic accident

V30.4xx- Person boarding or alighting a three-wheeled motor vehicle injured in collision with pedestrian or animal

V30.5xx- Driver of three-wheeled motor vehicle injured in collision with pedestrian or animal in traffic accident

V30.6xx- Passenger in three-wheeled motor vehicle injured in collision with pedestrian or animal in traffic accident

V30.7xx- Person on outside of three-wheeled motor vehicle injured in collision with pedestrian or animal in traffic accident

V30.9xx- Unspecified occupant of three-wheeled motor vehicle injured in collision with pedestrian or animal in traffic accident

V31- Occupant of three-wheeled motor vehicle injured in collision with pedal cycle

The appropriate 7th character is to be added to each code from category V31:
- A   Initial encounter
- D   Subsequent encounter
- S   Sequela

V31.0xx- Driver of three-wheeled motor vehicle injured in collision with pedal cycle in nontraffic accident

V31.1xx- Passenger in three-wheeled motor vehicle injured in collision with pedal cycle in nontraffic accident

V31.2xx- Person on outside of three-wheeled motor vehicle injured in collision with pedal cycle in nontraffic accident

V31.3xx- Unspecified occupant of three-wheeled motor vehicle injured in collision with pedal cycle in nontraffic accident

V31.4xx- Person boarding or alighting a three-wheeled motor vehicle injured in collision with pedal cycle

V31.5xx- Driver of three-wheeled motor vehicle injured in collision with pedal cycle in traffic accident

V31.6xx- Passenger in three-wheeled motor vehicle injured in collision with pedal cycle in traffic accident

V31.7xx- Person on outside of three-wheeled motor vehicle injured in collision with pedal cycle in traffic accident

V31.9xx- Unspecified occupant of three-wheeled motor vehicle injured in collision with pedal cycle in traffic accident

V32- Occupant of three-wheeled motor vehicle injured in collision with two- or three-wheeled motor vehicle

The appropriate 7th character is to be added to each code from category V32:
- A   Initial encounter
- D   Subsequent encounter
- S   Sequela

V32.0xx- Driver of three-wheeled motor vehicle injured in collision with two- or three-wheeled motor vehicle in nontraffic accident

V32.1xx- Passenger in three-wheeled motor vehicle injured in collision with two- or three-wheeled motor vehicle in nontraffic accident

V32.2xx- Person on outside of three-wheeled motor vehicle injured in collision with two- or three-wheeled motor vehicle in nontraffic accident

V32.3xx- Unspecified occupant of three-wheeled motor vehicle injured in collision with two- or three-wheeled motor vehicle in nontraffic accident

V32.4xx- Person boarding or alighting a three-wheeled motor vehicle injured in collision with two- or three-wheeled motor vehicle

V32.5xx- Driver of three-wheeled motor vehicle injured in collision with two- or three-wheeled motor vehicle in traffic accident

V32.6xx- Passenger in three-wheeled motor vehicle injured in collision with two- or three-wheeled motor vehicle in traffic accident

V32.7xx- Person on outside of three-wheeled motor vehicle injured in collision with two- or three-wheeled motor vehicle in traffic accident

V32.9xx- Unspecified occupant of three-wheeled motor vehicle injured in collision with two- or three-wheeled motor vehicle in traffic accident

V33- Occupant of three-wheeled motor vehicle injured in collision with car, pick-up truck or van

The appropriate 7th character is to be added to each code from category V33:
- A   Initial encounter
- D   Subsequent encounter
- S   Sequela

V33.0xx- Driver of three-wheeled motor vehicle injured in collision with car, pick-up truck or van in nontraffic accident

V33.1xx- Passenger in three-wheeled motor vehicle injured in collision with car, pick-up truck or van in nontraffic accident

V33.2xx- Person on outside of three-wheeled motor vehicle injured in collision with car, pick-up truck or van in nontraffic accident

V33.3xx- Unspecified occupant of three-wheeled motor vehicle injured in collision with car, pick-up truck or van in nontraffic accident

V33.4xx- Person boarding or alighting a three-wheeled motor vehicle injured in collision with car, pick-up truck or van

V33.5xx- Driver of three-wheeled motor vehicle injured in collision with car, pick-up truck or van in traffic accident

V33.6xx- Passenger in three-wheeled motor vehicle injured in collision with car, pick-up truck or van in traffic accident

V33.7xx- Person on outside of three-wheeled motor vehicle injured in collision with car, pick-up truck or van in traffic accident

V33.9xx- Unspecified occupant of three-wheeled motor vehicle injured in collision with car, pick-up truck or van in traffic accident

V30 - V33

V34- Occupant of three-wheeled motor vehicle injured in collision with heavy transport vehicle or bus

Excludes 1: occupant of three-wheeled motor vehicle injured in collision with military vehicle (V39.81)

The appropriate 7th character is to be added to each code from category V34:
- A Initial encounter
- D Subsequent encounter
- S Sequela

V34.0xx- Driver of three-wheeled motor vehicle injured in collision with heavy transport vehicle or bus in nontraffic accident

V34.1xx- Passenger in three-wheeled motor vehicle injured in collision with heavy transport vehicle or bus in nontraffic accident

V34.2xx- Person on outside of three-wheeled motor vehicle injured in collision with heavy transport vehicle or bus in nontraffic accident

V34.3xx- Unspecified occupant of three-wheeled motor vehicle injured in collision with heavy transport vehicle or bus in nontraffic accident

V34.4xx- Person boarding or alighting a three-wheeled motor vehicle injured in collision with heavy transport vehicle or bus

V34.5xx- Driver of three-wheeled motor vehicle injured in collision with heavy transport vehicle or bus in traffic accident

V34.6xx- Passenger in three-wheeled motor vehicle injured in collision with heavy transport vehicle or bus in traffic accident

V34.7xx- Person on outside of three-wheeled motor vehicle injured in collision with heavy transport vehicle or bus in traffic accident

V34.9xx- Unspecified occupant of three-wheeled motor vehicle injured in collision with heavy transport vehicle or bus in traffic accident

V35- Occupant of three-wheeled motor vehicle injured in collision with railway train or railway vehicle

The appropriate 7th character is to be added to each code from category V35:
- A Initial encounter
- D Subsequent encounter
- S Sequela

V35.0xx- Driver of three-wheeled motor vehicle injured in collision with railway train or railway vehicle in nontraffic accident

V35.1xx- Passenger in three-wheeled motor vehicle injured in collision with railway train or railway vehicle in nontraffic accident

V35.2xx- Person on outside of three-wheeled motor vehicle injured in collision with railway train or railway vehicle in nontraffic accident

V35.3xx- Unspecified occupant of three-wheeled motor vehicle injured in collision with railway train or railway vehicle in nontraffic accident

V35.4xx- Person boarding or alighting a three-wheeled motor vehicle injured in collision with railway train or railway vehicle

V35.5xx- Driver of three-wheeled motor vehicle injured in collision with railway train or railway vehicle in traffic accident

V35.6xx- Passenger in three-wheeled motor vehicle injured in collision with railway train or railway vehicle in traffic accident

V35.7xx- Person on outside of three-wheeled motor vehicle injured in collision with railway train or railway vehicle in traffic accident

V35.9xx- Unspecified occupant of three-wheeled motor vehicle injured in collision with railway train or railway vehicle in traffic accident

V36- Occupant of three-wheeled motor vehicle injured in collision with other nonmotor vehicle

Includes: Collision with animal-drawn vehicle, animal being ridden, streetcar

The appropriate 7th character is to be added to each code from category V36:
- A Initial encounter
- D Subsequent encounter
- S Sequela

V36.0xx- Driver of three-wheeled motor vehicle injured in collision with other nonmotor vehicle in nontraffic accident

V36.1xx- Passenger in three-wheeled motor vehicle injured in collision with other nonmotor vehicle in nontraffic accident

V36.2xx- Person on outside of three-wheeled motor vehicle injured in collision with other nonmotor vehicle in nontraffic accident

V36.3xx- Unspecified occupant of three-wheeled motor vehicle injured in collision with other nonmotor vehicle in nontraffic accident

V36.4xx- Person boarding or alighting a three-wheeled motor vehicle injured in collision with other nonmotor vehicle

V36.5xx- Driver of three-wheeled motor vehicle injured in collision with other nonmotor vehicle in traffic accident

V36.6xx- Passenger in three-wheeled motor vehicle injured in collision with other nonmotor vehicle in traffic accident

V36.7xx- Person on outside of three-wheeled motor vehicle injured in collision with other nonmotor vehicle in traffic accident

V36.9xx- Unspecified occupant of three-wheeled motor vehicle injured in collision with other nonmotor vehicle in traffic accident

V37- Occupant of three-wheeled motor vehicle injured in collision with fixed or stationary object

The appropriate 7th character is to be added to each code from category V37:
- A Initial encounter
- D Subsequent encounter
- S Sequela

V37.0xx- Driver of three-wheeled motor vehicle injured in collision with fixed or stationary object in nontraffic accident

V37.1xx- Passenger in three-wheeled motor vehicle injured in collision with fixed or stationary object in nontraffic accident

V37.2xx- Person on outside of three-wheeled motor vehicle injured in collision with fixed or stationary object in nontraffic accident

V37.3xx- Unspecified occupant of three-wheeled motor vehicle injured in collision with fixed or stationary object in nontraffic accident

V37.4xx- Person boarding or alighting a three-wheeled motor vehicle injured in collision with fixed or stationary object

V37.5xx- Driver of three-wheeled motor vehicle injured in collision with fixed or stationary object in traffic accident

V37.6xx- Passenger in three-wheeled motor vehicle injured in collision with fixed or stationary object in traffic accident

V37.7xx- Person on outside of three-wheeled motor vehicle injured in collision with fixed or stationary object in traffic accident

V37.9xx- Unspecified occupant of three-wheeled motor vehicle injured in collision with fixed or stationary object in traffic accident

V34-V37

Excludes 1: = NOT CODED HERE! (Do not code both)

Excludes ❷: = Not Included Here

V38- **Occupant of three-wheeled motor vehicle injured** in **noncollision transport accident**
  Includes: Fall or thrown from three-wheeled motor vehicle
              Overturning of three-wheeled motor vehicle NOS
              Overturning of three-wheeled motor vehicle without collision

The appropriate 7th character is to be added to each code from category V38:
  A   **Initial** encounter
  D   **Subsequent** encounter
  S   **Sequela**

V38.0xx- Driver of three-wheeled motor vehicle injured in noncollision transport accident in nontraffic accident

V38.1xx- Passenger in three-wheeled motor vehicle injured in noncollision transport accident in nontraffic accident

V38.2xx- Person on outside of three-wheeled motor vehicle injured in noncollision transport accident in nontraffic accident

V38.3xx- Unspecified occupant of three-wheeled motor vehicle injured in noncollision transport accident in nontraffic accident

V38.4xx- Person boarding or alighting a three-wheeled motor vehicle injured in noncollision transport accident

V38.5xx- Driver of three-wheeled motor vehicle injured in noncollision transport accident in traffic accident

V38.6xx- Passenger in three-wheeled motor vehicle injured in noncollision transport accident in traffic accident

V38.7xx- Person on outside of three-wheeled motor vehicle injured in noncollision transport accident in traffic accident

V38.9xx- Unspecified occupant of three-wheeled motor vehicle injured in noncollision transport accident in traffic accident

V39- **Occupant of three-wheeled motor vehicle injured** in **other and unspecified transport accidents**

The appropriate 7th character is to be added to each code from category V39:
  A   **Initial** encounter
  D   **Subsequent** encounter
  S   **Sequela**

V39.0- Driver of three-wheeled motor vehicle injured in collision with other and unspecified motor vehicles in nontraffic accident

V39.00x- Driver of three-wheeled motor vehicle injured in collision with unspecified motor vehicles in nontraffic accident

V39.09x- Driver of three-wheeled motor vehicle injured in collision with other motor vehicles in nontraffic accident

V39.1- Passenger in three-wheeled motor vehicle injured in collision with other and unspecified motor vehicles in nontraffic accident

V39.10x- Passenger in three-wheeled motor vehicle injured in collision with unspecified motor vehicles in nontraffic accident

V39.19x- Passenger in three-wheeled motor vehicle injured in collision with other motor vehicles in nontraffic accident

V39.2- Unspecified occupant of three-wheeled motor vehicle injured in collision with other and unspecified motor vehicles in nontraffic accident

V39.20x- Unspecified occupant of three-wheeled motor vehicle injured in collision with unspecified motor vehicles in nontraffic accident
              Collision NOS involving three-wheeled motor vehicle, nontraffic

V39.29x- Unspecified occupant of three-wheeled motor vehicle injured in collision with other motor vehicles in nontraffic accident

V39.3xx- Occupant (driver) (passenger) of three-wheeled motor vehicle injured in unspecified nontraffic accident
              Accident NOS involving three-wheeled motor vehicle, nontraffic
              Occupant of three-wheeled motor vehicle injured in nontraffic accident NOS

V39.4- Driver of three-wheeled motor vehicle injured in collision with other and unspecified motor vehicles in traffic accident

V39.40x- Driver of three-wheeled motor vehicle injured in collision with unspecified motor vehicles in traffic accident

V39.49x- Driver of three-wheeled motor vehicle injured in collision with other motor vehicles in traffic accident

V39.5- Passenger in three-wheeled motor vehicle injured in collision with other and unspecified motor vehicles in traffic accident

V39.50x- Passenger in three-wheeled motor vehicle injured in collision with unspecified motor vehicles in traffic accident

V39.59x- Passenger in three-wheeled motor vehicle injured in collision with other motor vehicles in traffic accident

V39.6- Unspecified occupant of three-wheeled motor vehicle injured in collision with other and unspecified motor vehicles in traffic accident

V39.60x- Unspecified occupant of three-wheeled motor vehicle injured in collision with unspecified motor vehicles in traffic accident
              Collision NOS involving three-wheeled motor vehicle (traffic)

V39.69x- Unspecified occupant of three-wheeled motor vehicle injured in collision with other motor vehicles in traffic accident

V39.8- Occupant (driver) (passenger) of three-wheeled motor vehicle injured in other specified transport accidents

V39.81x- Occupant (driver) (passenger) of three-wheeled motor vehicle injured in transport accident with military vehicle

V39.89x- Occupant (driver) (passenger) of three-wheeled motor vehicle injured in other specified transport accidents

V39.9xx- Occupant (driver) (passenger) of three-wheeled motor vehicle injured in unspecified traffic accident
              Accident NOS involving three-wheeled motor vehicle

Car occupant injured in transport accident (V40-V49)

  Includes: A four-wheeled motor vehicle designed primarily for carrying passengers
              Automobile (pulling a trailer or camper)
  Excludes 1: bus (V50-V59)
              minibus (V50-V59)
              minivan (V50-V59)
              motorcoach (V70-V79)
              pick-up truck (V50-V59)
              sport utility vehicle (SUV) (V50-V59)

V40- **Car occupant injured in collision** with **pedestrian or animal**
  Excludes 1:   car collision with animal-drawn vehicle or animal being ridden (V46.-)

The appropriate 7th character is to be added to each code from category V40:
  A   **Initial** encounter
  D   **Subsequent** encounter
  S   **Sequela**

V40.0xx- Car driver injured in collision with pedestrian or animal in nontraffic accident

V40.1xx- Car passenger injured in collision with pedestrian or animal in nontraffic accident

V40.2xx- Person on outside of car injured in collision with pedestrian or animal in nontraffic accident

V40.3xx- Unspecified car occupant injured in collision with pedestrian or animal in nontraffic accident

V40.4xx- Person boarding or alighting a car injured in collision with pedestrian or animal

V40.5xx- Car driver injured in collision with pedestrian or animal in traffic accident

V40.6xx- Car passenger injured in collision with pedestrian or animal in traffic accident

V40.7xx- Person on outside of car injured in collision with pedestrian or animal in traffic accident

V
3
8
–
V
4
0

V40.9xx- Unspecified car occupant injured in collision with pedestrian or animal in traffic accident

V41- <u>Car occupant injured in collision</u> with <u>pedal cycle</u>

The appropriate 7th character is to be added to each code from category V41:
A <u>Initial</u> encounter
D <u>Subsequent</u> encounter
S <u>Sequela</u>

V41.0xx- Car driver injured in collision with pedal cycle in nontraffic accident

V41.1xx- Car passenger injured in collision with pedal cycle in nontraffic accident

V41.2xx- Person on outside of car injured in collision with pedal cycle in nontraffic accident

V41.3xx- Unspecified car occupant injured in collision with pedal cycle in nontraffic accident

V41.4xx- Person boarding or alighting a car injured in collision with pedal cycle

V41.5xx- Car driver injured in collision with pedal cycle in traffic accident

V41.6xx- Car passenger injured in collision with pedal cycle in traffic accident

V41.7xx- Person on outside of car injured in collision with pedal cycle in traffic accident

V41.9xx- Unspecified car occupant injured in collision with pedal cycle in traffic accident

V42- <u>Car occupant injured in collision</u> with <u>two- or three-wheeled motor vehicle</u>

The appropriate 7th character is to be added to each code from category V42:
A <u>Initial</u> encounter
D <u>Subsequent</u> encounter
S <u>Sequela</u>

V42.0xx- Car driver injured in collision with two- or three-wheeled motor vehicle in nontraffic accident

V42.1xx- Car passenger injured in collision with two- or three-wheeled motor vehicle in nontraffic accident

V42.2xx- Person on outside of car injured in collision with two- or three-wheeled motor vehicle in nontraffic accident

V42.3xx- Unspecified car occupant injured in collision with two- or three-wheeled motor vehicle in nontraffic accident

V42.4xx- Person boarding or alighting a car injured in collision with two- or three-wheeled motor vehicle

V42.5xx- Car driver injured in collision with two- or three-wheeled motor vehicle in traffic accident

V42.6xx- Car passenger injured in collision with two- or three-wheeled motor vehicle in traffic accident

V42.7xx- Person on outside of car injured in collision with two- or three-wheeled motor vehicle in traffic accident

V42.9xx- Unspecified car occupant injured in collision with two- or three-wheeled motor vehicle in traffic accident

V43- <u>Car occupant injured in collision</u> with <u>car, pick-up truck or van</u>

The appropriate 7th character is to be added to each code from category V43:
A <u>Initial</u> encounter
D <u>Subsequent</u> encounter
S <u>Sequela</u>

V43.0- Car driver injured in collision with car, pick-up truck or van in nontraffic accident

V43.01x- Car driver injured in collision with sport utility vehicle in nontraffic accident

V43.02x- Car driver injured in collision with other type car in nontraffic accident

V43.03x- Car driver injured in collision with pick-up truck in nontraffic accident

V43.04x- Car driver injured in collision with van in nontraffic accident

V43.1- Car passenger injured in collision with car, pick-up truck or van in nontraffic accident

V43.11x- Car passenger injured in collision with sport utility vehicle in nontraffic accident

V43.12x- Car passenger injured in collision with other type car in nontraffic accident

V43.13x- Car passenger injured in collision with pick-up in nontraffic accident

V43.14x- Car passenger injured in collision with van in nontraffic accident

V43.2- Person on outside of car injured in collision with car, pick-up truck or van in nontraffic accident

V43.21x- Person on outside of car injured in collision with sport utility vehicle in nontraffic accident

V43.22x- Person on outside of car injured in collision with other type car in nontraffic accident

V43.23x- Person on outside of car injured in collision with pick-up truck in nontraffic accident

V43.24x- Person on outside of car injured in collision with van in nontraffic accident

V43.3- Unspecified car occupant injured in collision with car, pick-up truck or van in nontraffic accident

V43.31x- Unspecified car occupant injured in collision with sport utility vehicle in nontraffic accident

V43.32x- Unspecified car occupant injured in collision with other type car in nontraffic accident

V43.33x- Unspecified car occupant injured in collision with pick-up truck in nontraffic accident

V43.34x- Unspecified car occupant injured in collision with van in nontraffic accident

V43.4- Person boarding or alighting a car injured in collision with car, pick-up truck or van

V43.41x- Person boarding or alighting a car injured in collision with sport utility vehicle

V43.42x- Person boarding or alighting a car injured in collision with other type car

V43.43x- Person boarding or alighting a car injured in collision with pick-up truck

V43.44x- Person boarding or alighting a car injured in collision with van

V43.5- Car driver injured in collision with car, pick-up truck or van in traffic accident

V43.51x- Car driver injured in collision with sport utility vehicle in traffic accident

V43.52x- Car driver injured in collision with other type car in traffic accident

V43.53x- Car driver injured in collision with pick-up truck in traffic accident

V43.54x- Car driver injured in collision with van in traffic accident

V43.6- Car passenger injured in collision with car, pick-up truck or van in traffic accident

V43.61x- Car passenger injured in collision with sport utility vehicle in traffic accident

AHA 15:1Q:p5 – Car passenger injured in collision with sport utility vehicle in traffic accident

V43.62x- Car passenger injured in collision with other type car in traffic accident

V43.63x- Car passenger injured in collision with pick-up truck in traffic accident

V43.64x- Car passenger injured in collision with van in traffic accident

V43.7- Person on outside of car injured in collision with car, pick-up truck or van in traffic accident

V43.71x- Person on outside of car injured in collision with sport utility vehicle in traffic accident

V43.72x- Person on outside of car injured in collision with other type car in traffic accident

V40 - V43

Excludes 1: = NOT CODED HERE! (Do not code both)   *Excludes ❷:* = Not Included Here

V43.73x- Person on outside of car injured in collision with pick-up truck in traffic accident

V43.74x- Person on outside of car injured in collision with van in traffic accident

V43.9- Unspecified car occupant injured in collision with car, pick-up truck or van in traffic accident

V43.91x- Unspecified car occupant injured in collision with sport utility vehicle in traffic accident

V43.92x- Unspecified car occupant injured in collision with other type car in traffic accident

V43.93x- Unspecified car occupant injured in collision with pick-up truck in traffic accident

V43.94x- Unspecified car occupant injured in collision with van in traffic accident

V44- <u>Car occupant injured in collision</u> with <u>heavy transport vehicle or bus</u>

> *Excludes 1:* *car occupant injured in collision with military vehicle (V49.81)*

> The appropriate 7th character is to be added to each code from category V44:
> **A** <u>Initial</u> encounter
> **D** <u>Subsequent</u> encounter
> **S** <u>Sequela</u>

V44.0xx- Car driver injured in collision with heavy transport vehicle or bus in nontraffic accident

V44.1xx- Car passenger injured in collision with heavy transport vehicle or bus in nontraffic accident

V44.2xx- Person on outside of car injured in collision with heavy transport vehicle or bus in nontraffic accident

V44.3xx- Unspecified car occupant injured in collision with heavy transport vehicle or bus in nontraffic accident

V44.4xx- Person boarding or alighting a car injured in collision with heavy transport vehicle or bus

V44.5xx- Car driver injured in collision with heavy transport vehicle or bus in traffic accident

V44.6xx- Car passenger injured in collision with heavy transport vehicle or bus in traffic accident

V44.7xx- Person on outside of car injured in collision with heavy transport vehicle or bus in traffic accident

V44.9xx- Unspecified car occupant injured in collision with heavy transport vehicle or bus in traffic accident

V45- <u>Car occupant injured in collision</u> with <u>railway train or railway vehicle</u>

> The appropriate 7th character is to be added to each code from category V45:
> **A** <u>Initial</u> encounter
> **D** <u>Subsequent</u> encounter
> **S** <u>Sequela</u>

V45.0xx- Car driver injured in collision with railway train or railway vehicle in nontraffic accident

V45.1xx- Car passenger injured in collision with railway train or railway vehicle in nontraffic accident

V45.2xx- Person on outside of car injured in collision with railway train or railway vehicle in nontraffic accident

V45.3xx- Unspecified car occupant injured in collision with railway train or railway vehicle in nontraffic accident

V45.4xx- Person boarding or alighting a car injured in collision with railway train or railway vehicle

V45.5xx- Car driver injured in collision with railway train or railway vehicle in traffic accident

V45.6xx- Car passenger injured in collision with railway train or railway vehicle in traffic accident

V45.7xx- Person on outside of car injured in collision with railway train or railway vehicle in traffic accident

V45.9xx- Unspecified car occupant injured in collision with railway train or railway vehicle in traffic accident

V46- <u>Car occupant injured in collision</u> with <u>other nonmotor vehicle</u>

> Includes: Collision with animal-drawn vehicle, animal being ridden, streetcar

> The appropriate 7th character is to be added to each code from category V46:
> **A** <u>Initial</u> encounter
> **D** <u>Subsequent</u> encounter
> **S** <u>Sequela</u>

V46.0xx- Car driver injured in collision with other nonmotor vehicle in nontraffic accident

V46.1xx- Car passenger injured in collision with other nonmotor vehicle in nontraffic accident

V46.2xx- Person on outside of car injured in collision with other nonmotor vehicle in nontraffic accident

V46.3xx- Unspecified car occupant injured in collision with other nonmotor vehicle in nontraffic accident

V46.4xx- Person boarding or alighting a car injured in collision with other nonmotor vehicle

V46.5xx- Car driver injured in collision with other nonmotor vehicle in traffic accident

V46.6xx- Car passenger injured in collision with other nonmotor vehicle in traffic accident

V46.7xx- Person on outside of car injured in collision with other nonmotor vehicle in traffic accident

V46.9xx- Unspecified car occupant injured in collision with other nonmotor vehicle in traffic accident

V47- <u>Car occupant injured in collision</u> with <u>fixed or stationary object</u>

> The appropriate 7th character is to be added to each code from category V47:
> **A** <u>Initial</u> encounter
> **D** <u>Subsequent</u> encounter
> **S** <u>Sequela</u>

V47.0xx- Car driver injured in collision with fixed or stationary object in nontraffic accident

V47.1xx- Car passenger injured in collision with fixed or stationary object in nontraffic accident

V47.2xx- Person on outside of car injured in collision with fixed or stationary object in nontraffic accident

V47.3xx- Unspecified car occupant injured in collision with fixed or stationary object in nontraffic accident

V47.4xx- Person boarding or alighting a car injured in collision with fixed or stationary object

V47.5xx- Car driver injured in collision with fixed or stationary object in traffic accident

V47.6xx- Car passenger injured in collision with fixed or stationary object in traffic accident

V47.7xx- Person on outside of car injured in collision with fixed or stationary object in traffic accident

V47.9xx- Unspecified car occupant injured in collision with fixed or stationary object in traffic accident

V48- <u>Car occupant injured in noncollision transport accident</u>

> Includes: Overturning car NOS
>   Overturning car without collision

> The appropriate 7th character is to be added to each code from category V48:
> **A** <u>Initial</u> encounter
> **D** <u>Subsequent</u> encounter
> **S** <u>Sequela</u>

V48.0xx- Car driver injured in noncollision transport accident in nontraffic accident

V48.1xx- Car passenger injured in noncollision transport accident in nontraffic accident

V48.2xx- Person on outside of car injured in noncollision transport accident in nontraffic accident

V48.3xx- Unspecified car occupant injured in noncollision transport accident in nontraffic accident

V48.4xx- Person boarding or alighting a car injured in noncollision transport accident

V48.5xx- Car driver injured in noncollision transport accident in traffic accident

---

Excludes 1: = NOT CODED HERE! (Do not code both)   **1249**   *Excludes ❷:* = Not Included Here

V48.6xx- Car passenger injured in noncollision transport accident in traffic accident

V48.7xx- Person on outside of car injured in noncollision transport accident in traffic accident

V48.9xx- Unspecified car occupant injured in noncollision transport accident in traffic accident

V49- Car occupant injured in other and unspecified transport accidents

The appropriate 7th character is to be added to each code from category V49:
A   Initial encounter
D   Subsequent encounter
S   Sequela

V49.0- Driver injured in collision with other and unspecified motor vehicles in nontraffic accident

  V49.00x- Driver injured in collision with unspecified motor vehicles in nontraffic accident

  V49.09x- Driver injured in collision with other motor vehicles in nontraffic accident

V49.1- Passenger injured in collision with other and unspecified motor vehicles in nontraffic accident

  V49.10x- Passenger injured in collision with unspecified motor vehicles in nontraffic accident

  V49.19x- Passenger injured in collision with other motor vehicles in nontraffic accident

V49.2- Unspecified car occupant injured in collision with other and unspecified motor vehicles in nontraffic accident

  V49.20x- Unspecified car occupant injured in collision with unspecified motor vehicles in nontraffic accident
      Car collision NOS, nontraffic

  V49.29x- Unspecified car occupant injured in collision with other motor vehicles in nontraffic accident

V49.3xx- Car occupant (driver) (passenger) injured in unspecified nontraffic accident
      Car accident NOS, nontraffic
      Car occupant injured in nontraffic accident NOS

V49.4- Driver injured in collision with other and unspecified motor vehicles in traffic accident

  V49.40x- Driver injured in collision with unspecified motor vehicles in traffic accident

  V49.49x- Driver injured in collision with other motor vehicles in traffic accident

V49.5- Passenger injured in collision with other and unspecified motor vehicles in traffic accident

  V49.50x- Passenger injured in collision with unspecified motor vehicles in traffic accident

  V49.59x- Passenger injured in collision with other motor vehicles in traffic accident

V49.6- Unspecified car occupant injured in collision with other and unspecified motor vehicles in traffic accident

  V49.60x- Unspecified car occupant injured in collision with unspecified motor vehicles in traffic accident
      Car collision NOS (traffic)

  V49.69x- Unspecified car occupant injured in collision with other motor vehicles in traffic accident

V49.8- Car occupant (driver) (passenger) injured in other specified transport accidents

  V49.81x- Car occupant (driver) (passenger) injured in transport accident with military vehicle

  V49.88x- Car occupant (driver) (passenger) injured in other specified transport accidents

V49.9xx- Car occupant (driver) (passenger) injured in unspecified traffic accident
      Car accident NOS

Occupant of pick-up truck or van injured in transport accident (V50-V59)

Includes: A four or six wheel motor vehicle designed primarily for carrying passengers and property but weighing less than the local limit for classification as a heavy goods vehicle
        Minibus
        Minivan
        Sport utility vehicle (SUV)
        Truck
        Van

Excludes 1:   heavy transport vehicle (V60-V69)

V50- Occupant of pick-up truck or van injured in collision with pedestrian or animal

Excludes 1:   pick-up truck or van collision with animal-drawn vehicle or animal being ridden (V56.-)

The appropriate 7th character is to be added to each code from category V50:
A   Initial encounter
D   Subsequent encounter
S   Sequela

  V50.0xx- Driver of pick-up truck or van injured in collision with pedestrian or animal in nontraffic accident

  V50.1xx- Passenger in pick-up truck or van injured in collision with pedestrian or animal in nontraffic accident

  V50.2xx- Person on outside of pick-up truck or van injured in collision with pedestrian or animal in nontraffic accident

  V50.3xx- Unspecified occupant of pick-up truck or van injured in collision with pedestrian or animal in nontraffic accident

  V50.4xx- Person boarding or alighting a pick-up truck or van injured in collision with pedestrian or animal

  V50.5xx- Driver of pick-up truck or van injured in collision with pedestrian or animal in traffic accident

  V50.6xx- Passenger in pick-up truck or van injured in collision with pedestrian or animal in traffic accident

  V50.7xx- Person on outside of pick-up truck or van injured in collision with pedestrian or animal in traffic accident

  V50.9xx- Unspecified occupant of pick-up truck or van injured in collision with pedestrian or animal in traffic accident

V51- Occupant of pick-up truck or van injured in collision with pedal cycle

The appropriate 7th character is to be added to each code from category V51:
A   Initial encounter
D   Subsequent encounter
S   Sequela

  V51.0xx- Driver of pick-up truck or van injured in collision with pedal cycle in nontraffic accident

  V51.1xx- Passenger in pick-up truck or van injured in collision with pedal cycle in nontraffic accident

  V51.2xx- Person on outside of pick-up truck or van injured in collision with pedal cycle in nontraffic accident

  V51.3xx- Unspecified occupant of pick-up truck or van injured in collision with pedal cycle in nontraffic accident

  V51.4xx- Person boarding or alighting a pick-up truck or van injured in collision with pedal cycle

  V51.5xx- Driver of pick-up truck or van injured in collision with pedal cycle in traffic accident

  V51.6xx- Passenger in pick-up truck or van injured in collision with pedal cycle in traffic accident

  V51.7xx- Person on outside of pick-up truck or van injured in collision with pedal cycle in traffic accident

  V51.9xx- Unspecified occupant of pick-up truck or van injured in collision with pedal cycle in traffic accident

V48
–
V51

V52- **Occupant of pick-up truck or van injured in collision** with **two- or three-wheeled motor vehicle**

The appropriate 7th character is to be added to each code from category V52:
- **A** **Initial** encounter
- **D** **Subsequent** encounter
- **S** **Sequela**

V52.0xx- Driver of pick-up truck or van injured in collision with two- or three-wheeled motor vehicle in nontraffic accident

V52.1xx- Passenger in pick-up truck or van injured in collision with two- or three-wheeled motor vehicle in nontraffic accident

V52.2xx- Person on outside of pick-up truck or van injured in collision with two- or three-wheeled motor vehicle in nontraffic accident

V52.3xx- Unspecified occupant of pick-up truck or van injured in collision with two- or three-wheeled motor vehicle in nontraffic accident

V52.4xx- Person boarding or alighting a pick-up truck or van injured in collision with two- or three-wheeled motor vehicle

V52.5xx- Driver of pick-up truck or van injured in collision with two- or three-wheeled motor vehicle in traffic accident

V52.6xx- Passenger in pick-up truck or van injured in collision with two- or three-wheeled motor vehicle in traffic accident

V52.7xx- Person on outside of pick-up truck or van injured in collision with two- or three-wheeled motor vehicle in traffic accident

V52.9xx- Unspecified occupant of pick-up truck or van injured in collision with two- or three-wheeled motor vehicle in traffic accident

V53- **Occupant of pick-up truck or van injured in collision** with **car, pick-up truck or van**

The appropriate 7th character is to be added to each code from category V53:
- **A** **Initial** encounter
- **D** **Subsequent** encounter
- **S** **Sequela**

V53.0xx- Driver of pick-up truck or van injured in collision with car, pick-up truck or van in nontraffic accident

V53.1xx- Passenger in pick-up truck or van injured in collision with car, pick-up truck or van in nontraffic accident

V53.2xx- Person on outside of pick-up truck or van injured in collision with car, pick-up truck or van in nontraffic accident

V53.3xx- Unspecified occupant of pick-up truck or van injured in collision with car, pick-up truck or van in nontraffic accident

V53.4xx- Person boarding or alighting a pick-up truck or van injured in collision with car, pick-up truck or van

V53.5xx- Driver of pick-up truck or van injured in collision with car, pick-up truck or van in traffic accident

V53.6xx- Passenger in pick-up truck or van injured in collision with car, pick-up truck or van in traffic accident

V53.7xx- Person on outside of pick-up truck or van injured in collision with car, pick-up truck or van in traffic accident

V53.9xx- Unspecified occupant of pick-up truck or van injured in collision with car, pick-up truck or van in traffic accident

V54- **Occupant of pick-up truck or van injured in collision** with **heavy transport vehicle or bus**

Excludes 1:   *occupant of pick-up truck or van injured in collision with military vehicle (V59.81)*

The appropriate 7th character is to be added to each code from category V54:
- **A** **Initial** encounter
- **D** **Subsequent** encounter
- **S** **Sequela**

V54.0xx- Driver of pick-up truck or van injured in collision with heavy transport vehicle or bus in nontraffic accident

V54.1xx- Passenger in pick-up truck or van injured in collision with heavy transport vehicle or bus in nontraffic accident

V54.2xx- Person on outside of pick-up truck or van injured in collision with heavy transport vehicle or bus in nontraffic accident

V54.3xx- Unspecified occupant of pick-up truck or van injured in collision with heavy transport vehicle or bus in nontraffic accident

V54.4xx- Person boarding or alighting a pick-up truck or van injured in collision with heavy transport vehicle or bus

V54.5xx- Driver of pick-up truck or van injured in collision with heavy transport vehicle or bus in traffic accident

V54.6xx- Passenger in pick-up truck or van injured in collision with heavy transport vehicle or bus in traffic accident

V54.7xx- Person on outside of pick-up truck or van injured in collision with heavy transport vehicle or bus in traffic accident

V54.9xx- Unspecified occupant of pick-up truck or van injured in collision with heavy transport vehicle or bus in traffic accident

V55- **Occupant of pick-up truck or van injured in collision** with **railway train or railway vehicle**

The appropriate 7th character is to be added to each code from category V55:
- **A** **Initial** encounter
- **D** **Subsequent** encounter
- **S** **Sequela**

V55.0xx- Driver of pick-up truck or van injured in collision with railway train or railway vehicle in nontraffic accident

V55.1xx- Passenger in pick-up truck or van injured in collision with railway train or railway vehicle in nontraffic accident

V55.2xx- Person on outside of pick-up truck or van injured in collision with railway train or railway vehicle in nontraffic accident

V55.3xx- Unspecified occupant of pick-up truck or van injured in collision with railway train or railway vehicle in nontraffic accident

V55.4xx- Person boarding or alighting a pick-up truck or van injured in collision with railway train or railway vehicle

V55.5xx- Driver of pick-up truck or van injured in collision with railway train or railway vehicle in traffic accident

V55.6xx- Passenger in pick-up truck or van injured in collision with railway train or railway vehicle in traffic accident

V55.7xx- Person on outside of pick-up truck or van injured in collision with railway train or railway vehicle in traffic accident

V55.9xx- Unspecified occupant of pick-up truck or van injured in collision with railway train or railway vehicle in traffic accident

V56- **Occupant of pick-up truck or van injured in collision** with **other nonmotor vehicle**

Includes: Collision with animal-drawn vehicle, animal being ridden, streetcar

The appropriate 7th character is to be added to each code from category V56:
- **A** **Initial** encounter
- **D** **Subsequent** encounter
- **S** **Sequela**

V56.0xx- Driver of pick-up truck or van injured in collision with other nonmotor vehicle in nontraffic accident

V56.1xx- Passenger in pick-up truck or van injured in collision with other nonmotor vehicle in nontraffic accident

V56.2xx- Person on outside of pick-up truck or van injured in collision with other nonmotor vehicle in nontraffic accident

V56.3xx- Unspecified occupant of pick-up truck or van injured in collision with other nonmotor vehicle in nontraffic accident

V56.4xx- Person boarding or alighting a pick-up truck or van injured in collision with other nonmotor vehicle

V56.5xx- Driver of pick-up truck or van injured in collision with other nonmotor vehicle in traffic accident

V56.6xx- Passenger in pick-up truck or van injured in collision with other nonmotor vehicle in traffic accident

V56.7xx- Person on outside of pick-up truck or van injured in collision with other nonmotor vehicle in traffic accident

V52 - V56

V56.9xx- Unspecified occupant of pick-up truck or van injured in collision with other nonmotor vehicle in traffic accident

V57- Occupant of pick-up truck or van injured in collision with fixed or stationary object

The appropriate 7th character is to be added to each code from category V57:
- **A** Initial encounter
- **D** Subsequent encounter
- **S** Sequela

V57.0xx- Driver of pick-up truck or van injured in collision with fixed or stationary object in nontraffic accident

V57.1xx- Passenger in pick-up truck or van injured in collision with fixed or stationary object in nontraffic accident

V57.2xx- Person on outside of pick-up truck or van injured in collision with fixed or stationary object in nontraffic accident

V57.3xx- Unspecified occupant of pick-up truck or van injured in collision with fixed or stationary object in nontraffic accident

V57.4xx- Person boarding or alighting a pick-up truck or van injured in collision with fixed or stationary object

V57.5xx- Driver of pick-up truck or van injured in collision with fixed or stationary object in traffic accident

V57.6xx- Passenger in pick-up truck or van injured in collision with fixed or stationary object in traffic accident

V57.7xx- Person on outside of pick-up truck or van injured in collision with fixed or stationary object in traffic accident

V57.9xx- Unspecified occupant of pick-up truck or van injured in collision with fixed or stationary object in traffic accident

V58- Occupant of pick-up truck or van injured in noncollision transport accident

Includes: Overturning pick-up truck or van NOS
Overturning pick-up truck or van without collision

The appropriate 7th character is to be added to each code from category V58:
- **A** Initial encounter
- **D** Subsequent encounter
- **S** Sequela

V58.0xx- Driver of pick-up truck or van injured in noncollision transport accident in nontraffic accident

V58.1xx- Passenger in pick-up truck or van injured in noncollision transport accident in nontraffic accident

V58.2xx- Person on outside of pick-up truck or van injured in noncollision transport accident in nontraffic accident

V58.3xx- Unspecified occupant of pick-up truck or van injured in noncollision transport accident in nontraffic accident

V58.4xx- Person boarding or alighting a pick-up truck or van injured in noncollision transport accident

V58.5xx- Driver of pick-up truck or van injured in noncollision transport accident in traffic accident

V58.6xx- Passenger in pick-up truck or van injured in noncollision transport accident in traffic accident

V58.7xx- Person on outside of pick-up truck or van injured in noncollision transport accident in traffic accident

V58.9xx- Unspecified occupant of pick-up truck or van injured in noncollision transport accident in traffic accident

V59- Occupant of pick-up truck or van injured in other and unspecified transport accidents

The appropriate 7th character is to be added to each code from category V59:
- **A** Initial encounter
- **D** Subsequent encounter
- **S** Sequela

V59.0- Driver of pick-up truck or van injured in collision with other and unspecified motor vehicles in nontraffic accident

V59.00x- Driver of pick-up truck or van injured in collision with unspecified motor vehicles in nontraffic accident

V59.09x- Driver of pick-up truck or van injured in collision with other motor vehicles in nontraffic accident

V59.1- Passenger in pick-up truck or van injured in collision with other and unspecified motor vehicles in nontraffic accident

V59.10x- Passenger in pick-up truck or van injured in collision with unspecified motor vehicles in nontraffic accident

V59.19x- Passenger in pick-up truck or van injured in collision with other motor vehicles in nontraffic accident

V59.2- Unspecified occupant of pick-up truck or van injured in collision with other and unspecified motor vehicles in nontraffic accident

V59.20x- Unspecified occupant of pick-up truck or van injured in collision with unspecified motor vehicles in nontraffic accident

Collision NOS involving pick-up truck or van, nontraffic

V59.29x- Unspecified occupant of pick-up truck or van injured in collision with other motor vehicles in nontraffic accident

V59.3xx- Occupant (driver) (passenger) of pick-up truck or van injured in unspecified nontraffic accident

Accident NOS involving pick-up truck or van, nontraffic
Occupant of pick-up truck or van injured in nontraffic accident NOS

V59.4- Driver of pick-up truck or van injured in collision with other and unspecified motor vehicles in traffic accident

V59.40x- Driver of pick-up truck or van injured in collision with unspecified motor vehicles in traffic accident

V59.49x- Driver of pick-up truck or van injured in collision with other motor vehicles in traffic accident

V59.5- Passenger in pick-up truck or van injured in collision with other and unspecified motor vehicles in traffic accident

V59.50x- Passenger in pick-up truck or van injured in collision with unspecified motor vehicles in traffic accident

V59.59x- Passenger in pick-up truck or van injured in collision with other motor vehicles in traffic accident

V59.6- Unspecified occupant of pick-up truck or van injured in collision with other and unspecified motor vehicles in traffic accident

V59.60x- Unspecified occupant of pick-up truck or van injured in collision with unspecified motor vehicles in traffic accident

Collision NOS involving pick-up truck or van (traffic)

V59.69x- Unspecified occupant of pick-up truck or van injured in collision with other motor vehicles in traffic accident

V59.8- Occupant (driver) (passenger) of pick-up truck or van injured in other specified transport accidents

V59.81x- Occupant (driver) (passenger) of pick-up truck or van injured in transport accident with military vehicle

V59.88x- Occupant (driver) (passenger) of pick-up truck or van injured in other specified transport accidents

V59.9xx- Occupant (driver) (passenger) of pick-up truck or van injured in unspecified traffic accident

Accident NOS involving pick-up truck or van

V56 - V59

Occupant of heavy transport vehicle injured in transport accident (V60-V69)

Includes: 18 wheeler
Armored car
Panel truck
Excludes 1: bus
motorcoach

V60- Occupant of heavy transport vehicle injured in collision with pedestrian or animal
Excludes 1: *heavy transport vehicle collision with animal-drawn vehicle or animal being ridden (V66.-)*

The appropriate 7th character is to be added to each code from category V60:
A Initial encounter
D Subsequent encounter
S Sequela

V60.0xx- Driver of heavy transport vehicle injured in collision with pedestrian or animal in nontraffic accident

V60.1xx- Passenger in heavy transport vehicle injured in collision with pedestrian or animal in nontraffic accident

V60.2xx- Person on outside of heavy transport vehicle injured in collision with pedestrian or animal in nontraffic accident

V60.3xx- Unspecified occupant of heavy transport vehicle injured in collision with pedestrian or animal in nontraffic accident

V60.4xx- Person boarding or alighting a heavy transport vehicle injured in collision with pedestrian or animal

V60.5xx- Driver of heavy transport vehicle injured in collision with pedestrian or animal in traffic accident

V60.6xx- Passenger in heavy transport vehicle injured in collision with pedestrian or animal in traffic accident

V60.7xx- Person on outside of heavy transport vehicle injured in collision with pedestrian or animal in traffic accident

V60.9xx- Unspecified occupant of heavy transport vehicle injured in collision with pedestrian or animal in traffic accident

V61- Occupant of heavy transport vehicle injured in collision with pedal cycle

The appropriate 7th character is to be added to each code from category V61:
A Initial encounter
D Subsequent encounter
S Sequela

V61.0xx- Driver of heavy transport vehicle injured in collision with pedal cycle in nontraffic accident

V61.1xx- Passenger in heavy transport vehicle injured in collision with pedal cycle in nontraffic accident

V61.2xx- Person on outside of heavy transport vehicle injured in collision with pedal cycle in nontraffic accident

V61.3xx- Unspecified occupant of heavy transport vehicle injured in collision with pedal cycle in nontraffic accident

V61.4xx- Person boarding or alighting a heavy transport vehicle injured in collision with pedal cycle while boarding or alighting

V61.5xx- Driver of heavy transport vehicle injured in collision with pedal cycle in traffic accident

V61.6xx- Passenger in heavy transport vehicle injured in collision with pedal cycle in traffic accident

V61.7xx- Person on outside of heavy transport vehicle injured in collision with pedal cycle in traffic accident

V61.9xx- Unspecified occupant of heavy transport vehicle injured in collision with pedal cycle in traffic accident

V62- Occupant of heavy transport vehicle injured in collision with two- or three-wheeled motor vehicle

The appropriate 7th character is to be added to each code from category V62:
A Initial encounter
D Subsequent encounter
S Sequela

V62.0xx- Driver of heavy transport vehicle injured in collision with two- or three-wheeled motor vehicle in nontraffic accident

V62.1xx- Passenger in heavy transport vehicle injured in collision with two- or three-wheeled motor vehicle in nontraffic accident

V62.2xx- Person on outside of heavy transport vehicle injured in collision with two- or three-wheeled motor vehicle in nontraffic accident

V62.3xx- Unspecified occupant of heavy transport vehicle injured in collision with two- or three-wheeled motor vehicle in nontraffic accident

V62.4xx- Person boarding or alighting a heavy transport vehicle injured in collision with two- or three-wheeled motor vehicle

V62.5xx- Driver of heavy transport vehicle injured in collision with two- or three-wheeled motor vehicle in traffic accident

V62.6xx- Passenger in heavy transport vehicle injured in collision with two- or three-wheeled motor vehicle in traffic accident

V62.7xx- Person on outside of heavy transport vehicle injured in collision with two- or three-wheeled motor vehicle in traffic accident

V62.9xx- Unspecified occupant of heavy transport vehicle injured in collision with two- or three-wheeled motor vehicle in traffic accident

V63- Occupant of heavy transport vehicle injured in collision with car, pick-up truck or van

The appropriate 7th character is to be added to each code from category V63:
A Initial encounter
D Subsequent encounter
S Sequela

V63.0xx- Driver of heavy transport vehicle injured in collision with car, pick-up truck or van in nontraffic accident

V63.1xx- Passenger in heavy transport vehicle injured in collision with car, pick-up truck or van in nontraffic accident

V63.2xx- Person on outside of heavy transport vehicle injured in collision with car, pick-up truck or van in nontraffic accident

V63.3xx- Unspecified occupant of heavy transport vehicle injured In collision with car, pick-up truck or van in nontraffic accident

V63.4xx- Person boarding or alighting a heavy transport vehicle injured in collision with car, pick-up truck or van

V63.5xx- Driver of heavy transport vehicle injured in collision with car, pick-up truck or van in traffic accident

V63.6xx- Passenger in heavy transport vehicle injured in collision with car, pick-up truck or van In traffic accident

V63.7xx- Person on outside of heavy transport vehicle injured in collision with car, pick-up truck or van in traffic accident

V63.9xx- Unspecified occupant of heavy transport vehicle injured in collision with car, pick-up truck or van in traffic accident

V64- Occupant of heavy transport vehicle injured in collision with heavy transport vehicle or bus
Excludes 1: *occupant of heavy transport vehicle injured in collision with military vehicle (V69.81)*

The appropriate 7th character is to be added to each code from category V64:
A Initial encounter
D Subsequent encounter
S Sequela

V64.0xx- Driver of heavy transport vehicle injured in collision with heavy transport vehicle or bus in nontraffic accident

V64.1xx- Passenger in heavy transport vehicle injured in collision with heavy transport vehicle or bus in nontraffic accident

V64.2xx- Person on outside of heavy transport vehicle injured in collision with heavy transport vehicle or bus in nontraffic accident

V64.3xx- Unspecified occupant of heavy transport vehicle injured in collision with heavy transport vehicle or bus in nontraffic accident

V64.4xx- Person boarding or alighting a heavy transport vehicle injured in collision with heavy transport vehicle or bus while boarding or alighting

V60 - V64

V64.5xx- Driver of heavy transport vehicle injured in collision with heavy transport vehicle or bus in traffic accident

V64.6xx- Passenger in heavy transport vehicle injured in collision with heavy transport vehicle or bus in traffic accident

V64.7xx- Person on outside of heavy transport vehicle injured in collision with heavy transport vehicle or bus in traffic accident

V64.9xx- Unspecified occupant of heavy transport vehicle injured in collision with heavy transport vehicle or bus in traffic accident

V65- Occupant of heavy transport vehicle injured in collision with railway train or railway vehicle

> The appropriate 7th character is to be added to each code from category V65:
> **A** Initial encounter
> **D** Subsequent encounter
> **S** Sequela

V65.0xx- Driver of heavy transport vehicle injured in collision with railway train or railway vehicle in nontraffic accident

V65.1xx- Passenger in heavy transport vehicle injured in collision with railway train or railway vehicle in nontraffic accident

V65.2xx- Person on outside of heavy transport vehicle injured in collision with railway train or railway vehicle in nontraffic accident

V65.3xx- Unspecified occupant of heavy transport vehicle injured in collision with railway train or railway vehicle in nontraffic accident

V65.4xx- Person boarding or alighting a heavy transport vehicle injured in collision with railway train or railway vehicle

V65.5xx- Driver of heavy transport vehicle injured in collision with railway train or railway vehicle in traffic accident

V65.6xx- Passenger in heavy transport vehicle injured in collision with railway train or railway vehicle in traffic accident

V65.7xx- Person on outside of heavy transport vehicle injured in collision with railway train or railway vehicle in traffic accident

V65.9xx- Unspecified occupant of heavy transport vehicle injured in collision with railway train or railway vehicle in traffic accident

V66- Occupant of heavy transport vehicle injured in collision with other nonmotor vehicle

> Includes: Collision with animal-drawn vehicle, animal being ridden, streetcar

> The appropriate 7th character is to be added to each code from category V66:
> **A** Initial encounter
> **D** Subsequent encounter
> **S** Sequela

V66.0xx- Driver of heavy transport vehicle injured in collision with other nonmotor vehicle in nontraffic accident

V66.1xx- Passenger in heavy transport vehicle injured in collision with other nonmotor vehicle in nontraffic accident

V66.2xx- Person on outside of heavy transport vehicle injured in collision with other nonmotor vehicle in nontraffic accident

V66.3xx- Unspecified occupant of heavy transport vehicle injured in collision with other nonmotor vehicle in nontraffic accident

V66.4xx- Person boarding or alighting a heavy transport vehicle injured in collision with other nonmotor vehicle

V66.5xx- Driver of heavy transport vehicle injured in collision with other nonmotor vehicle in traffic accident

V66.6xx- Passenger in heavy transport vehicle injured in collision with other nonmotor vehicle in traffic accident

V66.7xx- Person on outside of heavy transport vehicle injured in collision with other nonmotor vehicle in traffic accident

V66.9xx- Unspecified occupant of heavy transport vehicle injured in collision with other nonmotor vehicle in traffic accident

V67- Occupant of heavy transport vehicle injured in collision with fixed or stationary object

> The appropriate 7th character is to be added to each code from category V67:
> **A** Initial encounter
> **D** Subsequent encounter
> **S** Sequela

V67.0xx- Driver of heavy transport vehicle injured in collision with fixed or stationary object in nontraffic accident

V67.1xx- Passenger in heavy transport vehicle injured in collision with fixed or stationary object in nontraffic accident

V67.2xx- Person on outside of heavy transport vehicle injured in collision with fixed or stationary object in nontraffic accident

V67.3xx- Unspecified occupant of heavy transport vehicle injured in collision with fixed or stationary object in nontraffic accident

V67.4xx- Person boarding or alighting a heavy transport vehicle injured in collision with fixed or stationary object

V67.5xx- Driver of heavy transport vehicle injured in collision with fixed or stationary object in traffic accident

V67.6xx- Passenger in heavy transport vehicle injured in collision with fixed or stationary object in traffic accident

V67.7xx- Person on outside of heavy transport vehicle injured in collision with fixed or stationary object in traffic accident

V67.9xx- Unspecified occupant of heavy transport vehicle injured in collision with fixed or stationary object in traffic accident

V68- Occupant of heavy transport vehicle injured in noncollision transport accident

> Includes: Overturning heavy transport vehicle NOS
> Overturning heavy transport vehicle without collision

> The appropriate 7th character is to be added to each code from category V68:
> **A** Initial encounter
> **D** Subsequent encounter
> **S** Sequela

V68.0xx- Driver of heavy transport vehicle injured in noncollision transport accident in nontraffic accident

V68.1xx- Passenger in heavy transport vehicle injured in noncollision transport accident in nontraffic accident

V68.2xx- Person on outside of heavy transport vehicle injured in noncollision transport accident in nontraffic accident

V68.3xx- Unspecified occupant of heavy transport vehicle injured in noncollision transport accident in nontraffic accident

V68.4xx- Person boarding or alighting a heavy transport vehicle injured in noncollision transport accident

V68.5xx- Driver of heavy transport vehicle injured in noncollision transport accident in traffic accident

V68.6xx- Passenger in heavy transport vehicle injured in noncollision transport accident in traffic accident

V68.7xx- Person on outside of heavy transport vehicle injured in noncollision transport accident in traffic accident

V68.9xx- Unspecified occupant of heavy transport vehicle injured in noncollision transport accident in traffic accident

V69- Occupant of heavy transport vehicle injured in other and unspecified transport accidents

> The appropriate 7th character is to be added to each code from category V69:
> **A** Initial encounter
> **D** Subsequent encounter
> **S** Sequela

V69.0- Driver of heavy transport vehicle injured in collision with other and unspecified motor vehicles in nontraffic accident

V69.00x- Driver of heavy transport vehicle injured in collision with unspecified motor vehicles in nontraffic accident

V69.09x- Driver of heavy transport vehicle injured in collision with other motor vehicles in nontraffic accident

V 6 4 - V 6 9

V69.1-   Passenger in heavy transport vehicle injured in collision with other and unspecified motor vehicles in nontraffic accident

V69.10x-   Passenger in heavy transport vehicle injured in collision with unspecified motor vehicles in nontraffic accident

V69.19x-   Passenger in heavy transport vehicle injured in collision with other motor vehicles in nontraffic accident

V69.2-   Unspecified occupant of heavy transport vehicle injured in collision with other and unspecified motor vehicles in nontraffic accident

V69.20x-   Unspecified occupant of heavy transport vehicle injured in collision with unspecified motor vehicles in nontraffic accident
   Collision NOS involving heavy transport vehicle, nontraffic

V69.29x-   Unspecified occupant of heavy transport vehicle injured in collision with other motor vehicles in nontraffic accident

V69.3xx-   Occupant (driver) (passenger) of heavy transport vehicle injured in unspecified nontraffic accident
   Accident NOS involving heavy transport vehicle, nontraffic
   Occupant of heavy transport vehicle injured in nontraffic accident NOS

V69.4-   Driver of heavy transport vehicle injured in collision with other and unspecified motor vehicles intraffic accident

V69.40x-   Driver of heavy transport vehicle injured in collision with unspecified motor vehicles in traffic accident

V69.49x-   Driver of heavy transport vehicle injured in collision with other motor vehicles in traffic accident

V69.5-   Passenger in heavy transport vehicle injured in collision with other and unspecified motor vehicles in traffic accident

V69.50x-   Passenger in heavy transport vehicle injured in collision with unspecified motor vehicles in traffic accident

V69.59x-   Passenger in heavy transport vehicle injured in collision with other motor vehicles in traffic accident

V69.6-   Unspecified occupant of heavy transport vehicle injured in collision with other and unspecified motor vehicles in traffic accident

V69.60x-   Unspecified occupant of heavy transport vehicle injured in collision with unspecified motor vehicles in traffic accident
   Collision NOS involving heavy transport vehicle (traffic)

V69.69x-   Unspecified occupant of heavy transport vehicle injured in collision with other motor vehicles in traffic accident

V69.8-   Occupant (driver) (passenger) of heavy transport vehicle injured in other specified transport accidents

V69.81x-   Occupant (driver) (passenger) of heavy transport vehicle injured in transport accidents with military vehicle

V69.88x-   Occupant (driver) (passenger) of heavy transport vehicle injured in other specified transport accidents

V69.9xx-   Occupant (driver) (passenger) of heavy transport vehicle injured in unspecified traffic accident
   Accident NOS involving heavy transport vehicle

Bus occupant injured in transport accident (V70-V79)

Includes: Motorcoach
Excludes 1:   *minibus (V50-V59)*

V70-   Bus occupant injured in collision with pedestrian or animal
   Excludes 1:   bus collision with animal-drawn vehicle or animal being ridden (V76.-)

The appropriate 7th character is to be added to each code from category V70:
A   Initial encounter
D   Subsequent encounter
S   Sequela

V70.0xx-   Driver of bus injured in collision with pedestrian or animal in nontraffic accident

V70.1xx-   Passenger on bus injured in collision with pedestrian or animal in nontraffic accident

V70.2xx-   Person on outside of bus injured in collision with pedestrian or animal in nontraffic accident

V70.3xx-   Unspecified occupant of bus injured in collision with pedestrian or animal in nontraffic accident

V70.4xx-   Person boarding or alighting from bus injured in collision with pedestrian or animal

V70.5xx-   Driver of bus injured in collision with pedestrian or animal in traffic accident

V70.6xx-   Passenger on bus injured in collision with pedestrian or animal in traffic accident

V70.7xx-   Person on outside of bus injured in collision with pedestrian or animal in traffic accident

V70.9xx-   Unspecified occupant of bus injured in collision with pedestrian or animal in traffic accident

V71-   Bus occupant injured in collision with pedal cycle

The appropriate 7th character is to be added to each code from category V71:
A   Initial encounter
D   Subsequent encounter
S   Sequela

V71.0xx-   Driver of bus injured in collision with pedal cycle in nontraffic accident

V71.1xx-   Passenger on bus injured in collision with pedal cycle in nontraffic accident

V71.2xx-   Person on outside of bus injured in collision with pedal cycle in nontraffic accident

V71.3xx-   Unspecified occupant of bus injured in collision with pedal cycle in nontraffic accident

V71.4xx-   Person boarding or alighting from bus injured in collision with pedal cycle

V71.5xx-   Driver of bus injured in collision with pedal cycle in traffic accident

V71.6xx-   Passenger on bus injured in collision with pedal cycle in traffic accident

V71.7xx-   Person on outside of bus injured in collision with pedal cycle in traffic accident

V71.9xx-   Unspecified occupant of bus injured in collision with pedal cycle in traffic accident

V72-   Bus occupant injured in collision with two- or three-wheeled motor vehicle

The appropriate 7th character is to be added to each code from category V72:
A   Initial encounter
D   Subsequent encounter
S   Sequela

V72.0xx-   Driver of bus injured in collision with two- or three-wheeled motor vehicle in nontraffic accident

V72.1xx-   Passenger on bus injured in collision with two- or three-wheeled motor vehicle in nontraffic accident

V72.2xx-   Person on outside of bus injured in collision with two- or three-wheeled motor vehicle in nontraffic accident

V72.3xx-   Unspecified occupant of bus injured in collision with two- or three-wheeled motor vehicle in nontraffic accident

V
6
9
ı
V
7
2

V72.4xx- Person boarding or alighting from bus injured in collision with two- or three-wheeled motor vehicle

V72.5xx- Driver of bus injured in collision with two- or three-wheeled motor vehicle in traffic accident

V72.6xx- Passenger on bus injured in collision with two- or three-wheeled motor vehicle in traffic accident

V72.7xx- Person on outside of bus injured in collision with two- or three-wheeled motor vehicle in traffic accident

V72.9xx- Unspecified occupant of bus injured in collision with two- or three-wheeled motor vehicle in traffic accident

V73- Bus occupant injured in collision with car, pick-up truck or van

The appropriate 7th character is to be added to each code from category V73:
- **A** Initial encounter
- **D** Subsequent encounter
- **S** Sequela

V73.0xx- Driver of bus injured in collision with car, pick-up truck or van in nontraffic accident

V73.1xx- Passenger on bus injured in collision with car, pick-up truck or van in nontraffic accident

V73.2xx- Person on outside of bus injured in collision with car, pick-up truck or van in nontraffic accident

V73.3xx- Unspecified occupant of bus injured in collision with car, pick-up truck or van in nontraffic accident

V73.4xx- Person boarding or alighting from bus injured in collision with car, pick-up truck or van

V73.5xx- Driver of bus injured in collision with car, pick-up truck or van in traffic accident

V73.6xx- Passenger on bus injured in collision with car, pick-up truck or van in traffic accident

V73.7xx- Person on outside of bus injured in collision with car, pick-up truck or van in traffic accident

V73.9xx- Unspecified occupant of bus injured in collision with car, pick-up truck or van in traffic accident

V74- Bus occupant injured in collision with heavy transport vehicle or bus

Excludes 1: bus occupant injured in collision with military vehicle (V79.81)

The appropriate 7th character is to be added to each code from category V74:
- **A** Initial encounter
- **D** Subsequent encounter
- **S** Sequela

V74.0xx- Driver of bus injured in collision with heavy transport vehicle or bus in nontraffic accident

V74.1xx- Passenger on bus injured in collision with heavy transport vehicle or bus in nontraffic accident

V74.2xx- Person on outside of bus injured in collision with heavy transport vehicle or bus in nontraffic accident

V74.3xx- Unspecified occupant of bus injured in collision with heavy transport vehicle or bus in nontraffic accident

V74.4xx- Person boarding or alighting from bus injured in collision with heavy transport vehicle or bus

V74.5xx- Driver of bus injured in collision with heavy transport vehicle or bus in traffic accident

V74.6xx- Passenger on bus injured in collision with heavy transport vehicle or bus in traffic accident

V74.7xx- Person on outside of bus injured in collision with heavy transport vehicle or bus in traffic accident

V74.9xx- Unspecified occupant of bus injured in collision with heavy transport vehicle or bus in traffic accident

V75- Bus occupant injured in collision with railway train or railway vehicle

The appropriate 7th character is to be added to each code from category V75:
- **A** Initial encounter
- **D** Subsequent encounter
- **S** Sequela

V75.0xx- Driver of bus injured in collision with railway train or railway vehicle in nontraffic accident

V75.1xx- Passenger on bus injured in collision with railway train or railway vehicle in nontraffic accident

V75.2xx- Person on outside of bus injured in collision with railway train or railway vehicle in nontraffic accident

V75.3xx- Unspecified occupant of bus injured in collision with railway train or railway vehicle in nontraffic accident

V75.4xx- Person boarding or alighting from bus injured in collision with railway train or railway vehicle

V75.5xx- Driver of bus injured in collision with railway train or railway vehicle in traffic accident

V75.6xx- Passenger on bus injured in collision with railway train or railway vehicle in traffic accident

V75.7xx- Person on outside of bus injured in collision with railway train or railway vehicle in traffic accident

V75.9xx- Unspecified occupant of bus injured in collision with railway train or railway vehicle in traffic accident

V76- Bus occupant injured in collision with other nonmotor vehicle

Includes: Collision with animal-drawn vehicle, animal being ridden, streetcar

The appropriate 7th character is to be added to each code from category V76:
- **A** Initial encounter
- **D** Subsequent encounter
- **S** Sequela

V76.0xx- Driver of bus injured in collision with other nonmotor vehicle in nontraffic accident

V76.1xx- Passenger on bus injured in collision with other nonmotor vehicle in nontraffic accident

V76.2xx- Person on outside of bus injured in collision with other nonmotor vehicle in nontraffic accident

V76.3xx- Unspecified occupant of bus injured in collision with other nonmotor vehicle in nontraffic accident

V76.4xx- Person boarding or alighting from bus injured in collision with other nonmotor vehicle

V76.5xx- Driver of bus injured in collision with other nonmotor vehicle in traffic accident

V76.6xx- Passenger on bus injured in collision with other nonmotor vehicle in traffic accident

V76.7xx- Person on outside of bus injured in collision with other nonmotor vehicle in traffic accident

V76.9xx- Unspecified occupant of bus injured in collision with other nonmotor vehicle in traffic accident

V77- Bus occupant injured in collision with fixed or stationary object

The appropriate 7th character is to be added to each code from category V77:
- **A** Initial encounter
- **D** Subsequent encounter
- **S** Sequela

V77.0xx- Driver of bus injured in collision with fixed or stationary object in nontraffic accident

V77.1xx- Passenger on bus injured in collision with fixed or stationary object in nontraffic accident

V77.2xx- Person on outside of bus injured in collision with fixed or stationary object in nontraffic accident

V77.3xx- Unspecified occupant of bus injured in collision with fixed or stationary object in nontraffic accident

V77.4xx- Person boarding or alighting from bus injured in collision with fixed or stationary object

V77.5xx- Driver of bus injured in collision with fixed or stationary object in traffic accident

V77.6xx- Passenger on bus injured in collision with fixed or stationary object in traffic accident

V77.7xx- Person on outside of bus injured in collision with fixed or stationary object in traffic accident

V77.9xx- Unspecified occupant of bus injured in collision with fixed or stationary object in traffic accident

V72-V77

V78- **Bus occupant injured** in **noncollision** **transport accident**
Includes: Overturning bus NOS
            Overturning bus without collision

The appropriate 7th character is to be added to each code from category
V78:
A   Initial encounter
D   Subsequent encounter
S   Sequela

V78.0xx- Driver of bus injured in noncollision transport accident in nontraffic accident

V78.1xx- Passenger on bus injured in noncollision transport accident in nontraffic accident

V78.2xx- Person on outside of bus injured in noncollision transport accident in nontraffic accident

V78.3xx- Unspecified occupant of bus injured in noncollision transport accident in nontraffic accident

V78.4xx- Person boarding or alighting from bus injured in noncollision transport accident

V78.5xx- Driver of bus injured in noncollision transport accident in traffic accident

V78.6xx- Passenger on bus injured in noncollision transport accident in traffic accident

V78.7xx- Person on outside of bus injured in noncollision transport accident in traffic accident

V78.9xx- Unspecified occupant of bus injured in noncollision transport accident in traffic accident

V79- **Bus occupant injured** in **other and unspecified transport accidents**

The appropriate 7th character is to be added to each code from category
V79:
A   Initial encounter
D   Subsequent encounter
S   Sequela

V79.0- Driver of bus injured in collision with other and unspecified motor vehicles in nontraffic accident

V79.00x- Driver of bus injured in collision with unspecified motor vehicles in nontraffic accident

V79.09x- Driver of bus injured in collision with other motor vehicles in nontraffic accident

V79.1- Passenger on bus injured in collision with other and unspecified motor vehicles in nontraffic accident

V79.10x- Passenger on bus injured in collision with unspecified motor vehicles in nontraffic accident

V79.19x- Passenger on bus injured in collision with other motor vehicles in nontraffic accident

V79.2- Unspecified bus occupant injured in collision with other and unspecified motor vehicles in nontraffic accident

V79.20x- Unspecified bus occupant injured in collision with unspecified motor vehicles in nontraffic accident
Bus collision NOS, nontraffic

V79.29x- Unspecified bus occupant injured in collision with other motor vehicles in nontraffic accident

V79.3xx- Bus occupant (driver) (passenger) injured in unspecified nontraffic accident
Bus accident NOS, nontraffic
Bus occupant injured in nontraffic accident NOS

V79.4- Driver of bus injured in collision with other and unspecified motor vehicles in traffic accident

V79.40x- Driver of bus injured in collision with unspecified motor vehicles in traffic accident

V79.49x- Driver of bus injured in collision with other motor vehicles in traffic accident

V79.5- Passenger on bus injured in collision with other and unspecified motor vehicles in traffic accident

V79.50x- Passenger on bus injured in collision with unspecified motor vehicles in traffic accident

V79.59x- Passenger on bus injured in collision with other motor vehicles in traffic accident

V79.6- Unspecified bus occupant injured in collision with other and unspecified motor vehicles in traffic accident

V79.60x- Unspecified bus occupant injured in collision with unspecified motor vehicles in traffic accident
Bus collision NOS (traffic)

V79.69x- Unspecified bus occupant injured in collision with other motor vehicles in traffic accident

V79.8- Bus occupant (driver) (passenger) injured in other specified transport accidents

V79.81x- Bus occupant (driver) (passenger) injured in transport accidents with military vehicle

V79.88x- Bus occupant (driver) (passenger) injured in other specified transport accidents

V79.9xx- Bus occupant (driver) (passenger) injured in unspecified traffic accident
Bus accident NOS

Other land transport accidents (V80-V89)

V80- **Animal-rider or occupant of animal-drawn vehicle injured in transport accident**

The appropriate 7th character is to be added to each code from category
V80:
A   Initial encounter
D   Subsequent encounter
S   Sequela

V80.0- Animal-rider or occupant of animal drawn vehicle injured **by fall from or being thrown from animal or animal-drawn vehicle in noncollision accident**

V80.01- Animal-rider injured by fall from or being thrown from animal in noncollision accident

V80.010- Animal-rider injured by fall from or being thrown from horse in noncollision accident

V80.018- Animal-rider injured by fall from or being thrown from other animal in noncollision accident

V80.02x- Occupant of animal-drawn vehicle injured by fall from or being thrown from animal-drawn vehicle in noncollision accident
Overturning animal-drawn vehicle NOS
Overturning animal-drawn vehicle without collision

V80.1- Animal-rider or occupant of animal-drawn vehicle injured in **collision with pedestrian or animal**
Excludes 1:   *animal-rider or animal-drawn vehicle collision with animal-drawn vehicle or animal being ridden (V80.7)*

V80.11x- Animal-rider injured in collision with pedestrian or animal

V80.12x- Occupant of animal-drawn vehicle injured in collision with pedestrian or animal

V80.2- Animal-rider or occupant of animal-drawn vehicle injured in **collision with pedal cycle**

V80.21x- Animal-rider injured in collision with pedal cycle

V80.22x- Occupant of animal-drawn vehicle injured in collision with pedal cycle

V80.3- Animal-rider or occupant of animal-drawn vehicle injured in **collision with two- or three-wheeled motor vehicle**

V80.31x- Animal-rider injured in collision with two- or three-wheeled motor vehicle

V80.32x- Occupant of animal-drawn vehicle injured in collision with two- or three-wheeled motor vehicle

V80.4- Animal-rider or occupant of animal-drawn vehicle injured in **collision with car, pick-up truck, van, heavy transport vehicle or bus**
Excludes 1:   *animal-rider injured in collision with military vehicle (V80.910)*
                occupant of animal-drawn vehicle injured in collision with military vehicle (V80.920)

V80.41x- Animal-rider injured in collision with car, pick-up truck, van, heavy transport vehicle or bus

V78 - V80

V80.42x- Occupant of animal-drawn vehicle injured in collision with car, pick-up truck, van, heavy transport vehicle or bus

V80.5- Animal-rider or occupant of animal-drawn vehicle injured in collision with other specified motor vehicle

V80.51x- Animal-rider injured in collision with other specified motor vehicle

V80.52x- Occupant of animal-drawn vehicle injured in collision with other specified motor vehicle

V80.6- Animal-rider or occupant of animal-drawn vehicle injured in collision with railway train or railway vehicle

V80.61x- Animal-rider injured in collision with railway train or railway vehicle

V80.62x- Occupant of animal-drawn vehicle injured in collision with railway train or railway vehicle

V80.7- Animal-rider or occupant of animal-drawn vehicle injured in collision with other nonmotor vehicles

V80.71- Animal-rider or occupant of animal-drawn vehicle injured in collision with animal being ridden

V80.710- Animal-rider injured in collision with other animal being ridden

V80.711- Occupant of animal-drawn vehicle injured in collision with animal being ridden

V80.72- Animal-rider or occupant of animal-drawn vehicle injured in collision with other animal-drawn vehicle

V80.720- Animal-rider injured in collision with animal-drawn vehicle

V80.721- Occupant of animal-drawn vehicle injured in collision with other animal-drawn vehicle

V80.73- Animal-rider or occupant of animal-drawn vehicle injured in collision with streetcar

V80.730- Animal-rider injured in collision with streetcar

V80.731- Occupant of animal-drawn vehicle injured in collision with streetcar

V80.79- Animal-rider or occupant of animal-drawn vehicle injured in collision with other nonmotor vehicles

V80.790- Animal-rider injured in collision with other nonmotor vehicles

V80.791- Occupant of animal-drawn vehicle injured in collision with other nonmotor vehicles

V80.8- Animal-rider or occupant of animal-drawn vehicle injured in collision with fixed or stationary object

V80.81x- Animal-rider injured in collision with fixed or stationary object

V80.82x- Occupant of animal-drawn vehicle injured in collision with fixed or stationary object

V80.9- Animal-rider or occupant of animal-drawn vehicle injured in other and unspecified transport accidents

V80.91- Animal-rider injured in other and unspecified transport accidents

V80.910- Animal-rider injured in transport accident with military vehicle

V80.918- Animal-rider injured in other transport accident

V80.919- Animal-rider injured in unspecified transport accident

Animal rider accident NOS

V80.92- Occupant of animal-drawn vehicle injured in other and unspecified transport accidents

V80.920- Occupant of animal-drawn vehicle injured in transport accident with military vehicle

V80.928- Occupant of animal-drawn vehicle injured in other transport accident

V80.929- Occupant of animal-drawn vehicle injured in unspecified transport accident

Animal-drawn vehicle accident NOS

V81- Occupant of railway train or railway vehicle injured in transport accident

Includes: Derailment of railway train or railway vehicle
Person on outside of train

Excludes 1: *streetcar (V82.-)*

The appropriate 7th character is to be added to each code from category V81:

A Initial encounter
D Subsequent encounter
S Sequela

V81.0xx- Occupant of railway train or railway vehicle injured in collision with motor vehicle in nontraffic accident

Excludes 1: *occupant of railway train or railway vehicle injured due to collision with military vehicle (V81.83)*

V81.1xx- Occupant of railway train or railway vehicle injured in collision with motor vehicle in traffic accident

Excludes 1: *occupant of railway train or railway vehicle injured due to collision with military vehicle (V81.83)*

V81.2xx- Occupant of railway train or railway vehicle injured in collision with or hit by rolling stock

V81.3xx- Occupant of railway train or railway vehicle injured in collision with other object

Railway collision NOS

V81.4xx- Person injured while boarding or alighting from railway train or railway vehicle

V81.5xx- Occupant of railway train or railway vehicle injured by fall in railway train or railway vehicle

V81.6xx- Occupant of railway train or railway vehicle injured by fall from railway train or railway vehicle

V81.7xx- Occupant of railway train or railway vehicle injured in derailment without antecedent collision

V81.8- Occupant of railway train or railway vehicle injured in other specified railway accidents

V81.81x- Occupant of railway train or railway vehicle injured due to explosion or fire on train

V81.82x- Occupant of railway train or railway vehicle injured due to object falling onto train

Occupant of railway train or railway vehicle injured due to falling earth onto train
Occupant of railway train or railway vehicle injured due to falling rocks onto train
Occupant of railway train or railway vehicle injured due to falling snow onto train
Occupant of railway train or railway vehicle injured due to falling trees onto train

V81.83x- Occupant of railway train or railway vehicle injured due to collision with military vehicle

V81.89x- Occupant of railway train or railway vehicle injured due to other specified railway accident

V81.9xx- Occupant of railway train or railway vehicle injured in unspecified railway accident

Railway accident NOS

V82- Occupant of powered streetcar injured in transport accident

Includes: Interurban electric car
Person on outside of streetcar
Tram (car)
Trolley (car)

Excludes 1: *bus (V70-V79)*
motorcoach (V70-V79)
nonpowered streetcar (V76.-)
train (V81.-)

The appropriate 7th character is to be added to each code from category V82:

A Initial encounter
D Subsequent encounter
S Sequela

V82.0xx- Occupant of streetcar injured in collision with motor vehicle in nontraffic accident

V82.1xx- Occupant of streetcar injured in collision with motor vehicle in traffic accident

V82.2xx- Occupant of streetcar injured in collision with or hit by rolling stock

V80 - V82

© 2016 Channel Publishing, Ltd.

V82.3xx- Occupant of streetcar injured in collision with other object
>Excludes 1: collision with animal-drawn vehicle or animal being ridden (V82.8)

V82.4xx- Person injured while boarding or alighting from streetcar

V82.5xx- Occupant of streetcar injured by fall in streetcar
>Excludes 1: fall in streetcar:
>while boarding or alighting (V82.4)
>with antecedent collision (V82.0-V82.3)

V82.6xx- Occupant of streetcar injured by fall from streetcar
>Excludes 1: fall from streetcar:
>while boarding or alighting (V82.4)
>with antecedent collision (V82.0-V82.3)

V82.7xx- Occupant of streetcar injured in derailment without antecedent collision
>Excludes 1: occupant of streetcar injured in derailment with antecedent collision (V82.0-V82.3)

V82.8xx- Occupant of streetcar injured in other specified transport accidents
>Streetcar collision with military vehicle
>Streetcar collision with train or nonmotor vehicles

V82.9xx- Occupant of streetcar injured in unspecified traffic accident
>Streetcar accident NOS

V83- Occupant of special vehicle mainly used on industrial premises injured in transport accident
>Includes: Battery-powered airport passenger vehicle
>Battery-powered truck (baggage) (mail)
>Voal-car in mine
>Forklift (truck)
>Logging car
>Self-propelled industrial truck
>Station baggage truck (powered)
>Tram, truck, or tub (powered) in mine or quarry
>Excludes 1: special construction vehicles (V85.-)
>special industrial vehicle in stationary use or maintenance (W31.-)

The appropriate 7th character is to be added to each code from category V83:
A   Initial encounter
D   Subsequent encounter
S   Sequela

V83.0xx- Driver of special industrial vehicle injured in traffic accident

V83.1xx- Passenger of special industrial vehicle injured in traffic accident

V83.2xx- Person on outside of special industrial vehicle injured in traffic accident

V83.3xx- Unspecified occupant of special industrial vehicle injured in traffic accident

V83.4xx- Person injured while boarding or alighting from special industrial vehicle

V83.5xx- Driver of special industrial vehicle injured in nontraffic accident

V83.6xx- Passenger of special industrial vehicle injured in nontraffic accident

V83.7xx- Person on outside of special industrial vehicle injured in nontraffic accident

V83.9xx- Unspecified occupant of special industrial vehicle injured in nontraffic accident
>Special-industrial-vehicle accident NOS

V84- Occupant of special vehicle mainly used in agriculture injured in transport accident
>Includes: Self-propelled farm machinery
>Tractor (and trailer)
>Excludes 1: animal-powered farm machinery accident (W30.8-)
>contact with combine harvester (W30.0)
>special agricultural vehicle in stationary use or maintenance (W30.-)

The appropriate 7th character is to be added to each code from category V84:
A   Initial encounter
D   Subsequent encounter
S   Sequela

V84.0xx- Driver of special agricultural vehicle injured in traffic accident

V84.1xx- Passenger of special agricultural vehicle injured in traffic accident

V84.2xx- Person on outside of special agricultural vehicle injured in traffic accident

V84.3xx- Unspecified occupant of special agricultural vehicle injured in traffic accident

V84.4xx- Person injured while boarding or alighting from special agricultural vehicle

V84.5xx- Driver of special agricultural vehicle injured in nontraffic accident

V84.6xx- Passenger of special agricultural vehicle injured in nontraffic accident

V84.7xx- Person on outside of special agricultural vehicle injured in nontraffic accident

V84.9xx- Unspecified occupant of special agricultural vehicle injured in nontraffic accident
>Special-agricultural vehicle accident NOS

V85- Occupant of special construction vehicle injured in transport accident
>Includes: Bulldozer
>Digger
>Dump truck
>Earth-leveller
>Mechanical shovel
>Road-roller
>Excludes 1: special industrial vehicle (V83.-)
>special construction vehicle in stationary use or maintenance (W31.-)

The appropriate 7th character is to be added to each code from category V85:
A   Initial encounter
D   Subsequent encounter
S   Sequela

V85.0xx- Driver of special construction vehicle injured in traffic accident

V85.1xx- Passenger of special construction vehicle injured in traffic accident

V85.2xx- Person on outside of special construction vehicle injured in traffic accident

V85.3xx- Unspecified occupant of special construction vehicle injured in traffic accident

V85.4xx- Person injured while boarding or alighting from special construction vehicle

V85.5xx- Driver of special construction vehicle injured in nontraffic accident

V85.6xx- Passenger of special construction vehicle injured in nontraffic accident

V85.7xx- Person on outside of special construction vehicle injured in nontraffic accident

V85.9xx- Unspecified occupant of special construction vehicle injured in nontraffic accident
>Special-construction-vehicle accident NOS

V86- Occupant of special all-terrain or other off-road motor vehicle, injured in transport accident
>Excludes 1: special all-terrain vehicle in stationary use or maintenance (W31.-)
>sport-utility vehicle (V50-V59)
>three-wheeled motor vehicle designed for on-road use (V30-V39)

The appropriate 7th character is to be added to each code from category V86:
A   Initial encounter
D   Subsequent encounter
S   Sequela

V86.0- Driver of special all-terrain or other off-road motor vehicle injured in traffic accident

V86.01x- Driver of ambulance or fire engine injured in traffic accident

V86.02x- Driver of snowmobile injured in traffic accident

V86.03x- Driver of dune buggy injured in traffic accident

V86.04x- Driver of military vehicle injured in traffic accident

V82 – V86

V86.09x- **Driver of other special all-terrain or other off-road motor vehicle injured in traffic accident**
Driver of dirt bike injured in traffic accident
Driver of go cart injured in traffic accident
Driver of golf cart injured in traffic accident

V86.1- **Passenger of special all-terrain or other off-road motor vehicle injured in traffic accident**

V86.11x- **Passenger of ambulance or fire engine injured in traffic accident**

V86.12x- **Passenger of snowmobile injured in traffic accident**

V86.13x- **Passenger of dune buggy injured in traffic accident**

V86.14x- **Passenger of military vehicle injured in traffic accident**

V86.19x- **Passenger of other special all-terrain or other off-road motor vehicle injured in traffic accident**
Passenger of dirt bike injured in traffic accident
Passenger of go cart injured in traffic accident
Passenger of golf cart injured in traffic accident

V86.2- **Person on outside of special all-terrain or other off-road motor vehicle injured in traffic accident**

V86.21x- **Person on outside of ambulance or fire engine injured in traffic accident**

V86.22x- **Person on outside of snowmobile injured in traffic accident**

V86.23x- **Person on outside of dune buggy injured in traffic accident**

V86.24x- **Person on outside of military vehicle injured in traffic accident**

V86.29x- **Person on outside of other special all-terrain or other off-road motor vehicle injured in traffic accident**
Person on outside of dirt bike injured in traffic accident
Person on outside of go cart in traffic accident
Person on outside of golf cart injured in traffic accident

V86.3- **Unspecified occupant of special all-terrain or other off-road motor vehicle injured in traffic accident**

V86.31x- **Unspecified occupant of ambulance or fire engine injured in traffic accident**

V86.32x- **Unspecified occupant of snowmobile injured in traffic accident**

V86.33x- **Unspecified occupant of dune buggy injured in traffic accident**

V86.34x- **Unspecified occupant of military vehicle injured in traffic accident**

V86.39x- **Unspecified occupant of other special all-terrain or other off-road motor vehicle injured in traffic accident**
Unspecified occupant of dirt bike injured in traffic accident
Unspecified occupant of go cart injured in traffic accident
Unspecified occupant of golf cart injured in traffic accident

V86.4- **Person injured while boarding or alighting from special all-terrain or other off-road motor vehicle**

V86.41x- **Person injured while boarding or alighting from ambulance or fire engine**

V86.42x- **Person injured while boarding or alighting from snowmobile**

V86.43x- **Person injured while boarding or alighting from dune buggy**

V86.44x- **Person injured while boarding or alighting from military vehicle**

V86.49x- **Person injured while boarding or alighting from other special all-terrain or other off-road motor vehicle**
Person injured while boarding or alighting from dirt bike
Person injured while boarding or alighting from go cart
Person injured while boarding or alighting from golf cart

V86.5- **Driver of special all-terrain or other off-road motor vehicle injured in nontraffic accident**

V86.51x- **Driver of ambulance or fire engine injured in nontraffic accident**

V86.52x- **Driver of snowmobile injured in nontraffic accident**

V86.53x- **Driver of dune buggy injured in nontraffic accident**

V86.54x- **Driver of military vehicle injured in nontraffic accident**

V86.59x- **Driver of other special all-terrain or other off-road motor vehicle injured in nontraffic accident**
Driver of dirt bike injured in nontraffic accident
Driver of go cart injured in nontraffic accident
Driver of golf cart injured in nontraffic accident

V86.6- **Passenger of special all-terrain or other off-road motor vehicle injured in nontraffic accident**

V86.61x- **Passenger of ambulance or fire engine injured in nontraffic accident**

V86.62x- **Passenger of snowmobile injured in nontraffic accident**

V86.63x- **Passenger of dune buggy injured in nontraffic accident**

V86.64x- **Passenger of military vehicle injured in nontraffic accident**

V86.69x- **Passenger of other special all-terrain or other off-road motor vehicle injured in nontraffic accident**
Passenger of dirt bike injured in nontraffic accident
Passenger of go cart injured in nontraffic accident
Passenger of golf cart injured in nontraffic accident

V86.7- **Person on outside of special all-terrain or other off-road motor vehicle injured in nontraffic accident**

V86.71x- **Person on outside of ambulance or fire engine injured in nontraffic accident**

V86.72x- **Person on outside of snowmobile injured in nontraffic accident**

V86.73x- **Person on outside of dune buggy injured in nontraffic accident**

V86.74x- **Person on outside of military vehicle injured in nontraffic accident**

V86.79x- **Person on outside of other special all-terrain or other off-road motor vehicles injured in nontraffic accident**
Person on outside of dirt bike injured in nontraffic accident
Person on outside of go cart injured in nontraffic accident
Person on outside of golf cart injured in nontraffic accident

V86.9- **Unspecified occupant of special all-terrain or other off-road motor vehicle injured in nontraffic accident**

V86.91x- **Unspecified occupant of ambulance or fire engine injured in nontraffic accident**

V86.92x- **Unspecified occupant of snowmobile injured in nontraffic accident**

V86.93x- **Unspecified occupant of dune buggy injured in nontraffic accident**

V86.94x- **Unspecified occupant of military vehicle injured in nontraffic accident**

V86.99x- **Unspecified occupant of other special all-terrain or other off-road motor vehicle injured in nontraffic accident**
All-terrain motor-vehicle accident NOS
Off-road motor-vehicle accident NOS
Other motor-vehicle accident NOS
Unspecified occupant of dirt bike injured in nontraffic accident
Unspecified occupant of go cart injured in nontraffic accident
Unspecified occupant of golf cart injured in nontraffic accident

V87- <u>**Traffic accident of specified type but victim's mode of transport unknown**</u>
Excludes 1:   *collision involving:*
            pedal cycle (V10-V19)
            pedestrian (V01-V09)

The appropriate 7th character is to be added to each code from category V87:
    A   <u>**Initial**</u> encounter
    D   <u>**Subsequent**</u> encounter
    S   <u>**Sequela**</u>

V87.0xx- **Person injured in collision between car and two- or three-wheeled powered vehicle (traffic)**

V87.1xx- **Person injured in collision between other motor vehicle and two- or three-wheeled motor vehicle (traffic)**

V87.2xx- **Person injured in collision between car and pick-up truck or van (traffic)**

V87.3xx- **Person injured in collision between car and bus (traffic)**

V 8 6 - V 8 7

V87.4xx- Person injured in collision between car and heavy transport vehicle (traffic)

V87.5xx- Person injured in collision between heavy transport vehicle and bus (traffic)

V87.6xx- Person injured in collision between railway train or railway vehicle and car (traffic)

V87.7xx- Person injured in collision between other specified motor vehicles (traffic)

V87.8xx- Person injured in other specified noncollision transport accidents involving motor vehicle (traffic)

V87.9xx- Person injured in other specified (collision) (noncollision) transport accidents involving nonmotor vehicle (traffic)

V88- Nontraffic accident of specified type but victim's mode of transport unknown

Excludes 1: collision involving:
  pedal cycle (V10-V19)
  pedestrian (V01-V09)

The appropriate 7th character is to be added to each code from category V88:
  A **Initial** encounter
  D **Subsequent** encounter
  S **Sequela**

V88.0xx- Person injured in collision between car and two- or three-wheeled motor vehicle, nontraffic

V88.1xx- Person injured in collision between other motor vehicle and two- or three-wheeled motor vehicle, nontraffic

V88.2xx- Person injured in collision between car and pick-up truck or van, nontraffic

V88.3xx- Person injured in collision between car and bus, nontraffic

V88.4xx- Person injured in collision between car and heavy transport vehicle, nontraffic

V88.5xx- Person injured in collision between heavy transport vehicle and bus, nontraffic

V88.6xx- Person injured in collision between railway train or railway vehicle and car, nontraffic

V88.7xx- Person injured in collision between other specified motor vehicle, nontraffic

V88.8xx- Person Injured In other specified noncollision transport accidents involving motor vehicle, nontraffic

V88.9xx- Person injured in other specified (collision)(noncollision) transport accidents involving nonmotor vehicle, nontraffic

V89- Motor- or nonmotor-vehicle accident, type of vehicle unspecified

The appropriate 7th character is to be added to each code from category V89:
  A **Initial** encounter
  D **Subsequent** encounter
  S **Sequela**

V89.0xx- Person injured in unspecified motor-vehicle accident, nontraffic
  Motor-vehicle accident NOS, nontraffic

V89.1xx- Person injured in unspecified nonmotor-vehicle accident, nontraffic
  Nonmotor-vehicle accident NOS (nontraffic)

V89.2xx- Person injured in unspecified motor-vehicle accident, traffic
  Motor-vehicle accident [MVA] NOS
  Road (traffic) accident [RTA] NOS

V89.3xx- Person injured in unspecified nonmotor-vehicle accident, traffic
  Nonmotor-vehicle traffic accident NOS

V89.9xx- Person injured in unspecified vehicle accident
  Collision NOS

Water transport accidents (V90-V94)

V90- Drowning and submersion due to accident to watercraft
  Excludes 1: civilian water transport accident involving military watercraft (V94.81-)
    fall into water not from watercraft (W16.-)
    military watercraft accident in military or war operations (Y36.0-, Y37.0-)
    water-transport-related drowning or submersion without accident to watercraft (V92.-)

The appropriate 7th character is to be added to each code from category V90:
  A **Initial** encounter
  D **Subsequent** encounter
  S **Sequela**

V90.0- Drowning and submersion due to watercraft overturning

V90.00x- Drowning and submersion due to merchant ship overturning

V90.01x- Drowning and submersion due to passenger ship overturning
  Drowning and submersion due to Ferry-boat overturning
  Drowning and submersion due to Liner overturning

V90.02x- Drowning and submersion due to fishing boat overturning

V90.03x- Drowning and submersion due to other powered watercraft overturning
  Drowning and submersion due to Hovercraft (on open water) overturning
  Drowning and submersion due to Jet ski overturning

V90.04x- Drowning and submersion due to sailboat overturning

V90.05x- Drowning and submersion due to canoe or kayak overturning

V90.06x- Drowning and submersion due to (nonpowered) inflatable craft overturning

V90.08x- Drowning and submersion due to other unpowered watercraft overturning
  Drowning and submersion due to windsurfer overturning

V90.09x- Drowning and submersion due to unspecified watercraft overturning
  Drowning and submersion due to boat NOS overturning
  Drowning and submersion due to ship NOS overturning
  Drowning and submersion due to watercraft NOS overturning

V90.1- Drowning and submersion due to watercraft sinking

V90.10x- Drowning and submersion due to merchant ship sinking

V90.11x- Drowning and submersion due to passenger ship sinking
  Drowning and submersion due to Ferry-boat sinking
  Drowning and submersion due to Liner sinking

V90.12x- Drowning and submersion due to fishing boat sinking

V90.13x- Drowning and submersion due to other powered watercraft sinking
  Drowning and submersion due to Hovercraft (on open water) sinking
  Drowning and submersion due to Jet ski sinking

V90.14x- Drowning and submersion due to sailboat sinking

V90.15x- Drowning and submersion due to canoe or kayak sinking

V90.16x- Drowning and submersion due to (nonpowered) inflatable craft sinking

V90.18x- Drowning and submersion due to other unpowered watercraft sinking

V90.19x- Drowning and submersion due to unspecified watercraft sinking
  Drowning and submersion due to boat NOS sinking
  Drowning and submersion due to ship NOS sinking
  Drowning and submersion due to watercraft NOS sinking

V90.2- Drowning and submersion due to falling or jumping from burning watercraft

V90.20x- Drowning and submersion due to falling or jumping from burning merchant ship

V
8
7
I
V
9
0

V90.21x- Drowning and submersion due to falling or jumping from burning passenger ship
> Drowning and submersion due to falling or jumping from burning Ferry-boat
> Drowning and submersion due to falling or jumping from burning Liner

V90.22x- Drowning and submersion due to falling or jumping from burning fishing boat

V90.23x- Drowning and submersion due to falling or jumping from other burning powered watercraft
> Drowning and submersion due to falling and jumping from burning Hovercraft (on open water)
> Drowning and submersion due to falling and jumping from burning Jet ski

V90.24x- Drowning and submersion due to falling or jumping from burning sailboat

V90.25x- Drowning and submersion due to falling or jumping from burning canoe or kayak

V90.26x- Drowning and submersion due to falling or jumping from burning (nonpowered) inflatable craft

V90.27x- Drowning and submersion due to falling or jumping from burning water-skis

V90.28x- Drowning and submersion due to falling or jumping from other burning unpowered watercraft
> Drowning and submersion due to falling and jumping from burning surf-board
> Drowning and submersion due to falling and jumping from burning windsurfer

V90.29x- Drowning and submersion due to falling or jumping from unspecified burning watercraft
> Drowning and submersion due to falling or jumping from burning boat NOS
> Drowning and submersion due to falling or jumping from burning ship NOS
> Drowning and submersion due to falling or jumping from burning watercraft NOS

V90.3- Drowning and submersion <u>due to falling or jumping from crushed watercraft</u>

V90.30x- Drowning and submersion due to falling or jumping from crushed merchant ship

V90.31x- Drowning and submersion due to falling or jumping from crushed passenger ship
> Drowning and submersion due to falling and jumping from crushed Ferry boat
> Drowning and submersion due to falling and jumping from crushed Liner

V90.32x- Drowning and submersion due to falling or jumping from crushed fishing boat

V90.33x- Drowning and submersion due to falling or jumping from other crushed powered watercraft
> Drowning and submersion due to falling and jumping from crushed Hovercraft
> Drowning and submersion due to falling and jumping from crushed Jet ski

V90.34x- Drowning and submersion due to falling or jumping from crushed sailboat

V90.35x- Drowning and submersion due to falling or jumping from crushed canoe or kayak

V90.36x- Drowning and submersion due to falling or jumping from crushed (nonpowered) inflatable craft

V90.37x- Drowning and submersion due to falling or jumping from crushed water-skis

V90.38x- Drowning and submersion due to falling or jumping from other crushed unpowered watercraft
> Drowning and submersion due to falling and jumping from crushed surf-board
> Drowning and submersion due to falling and jumping from crushed windsurfer

V90.39x- Drowning and submersion due to falling or jumping from crushed unspecified watercraft
> Drowning and submersion due to falling and jumping from crushed boat NOS
> Drowning and submersion due to falling and jumping from crushed ship NOS
> Drowning and submersion due to falling and jumping from crushed watercraft NOS

V90.8- Drowning and submersion <u>due to other accident to watercraft</u>

V90.80x- Drowning and submersion due to other accident to merchant ship

V90.81x- Drowning and submersion due to other accident to passenger ship
> Drowning and submersion due to other accident to Ferry-boat
> Drowning and submersion due to other accident to Liner

V90.82x- Drowning and submersion due to other accident to fishing boat

V90.83x- Drowning and submersion due to other accident to other powered watercraft
> Drowning and submersion due to other accident to Hovercraft (on open water)
> Drowning and submersion due to other accident to Jet ski

V90.84x- Drowning and submersion due to other accident to sailboat

V90.85x- Drowning and submersion due to other accident to canoe or kayak

V90.86x- Drowning and submersion due to other accident to (nonpowered) inflatable craft

V90.87x- Drowning and submersion due to other accident to water-skis

V90.88x- Drowning and submersion due to other accident to other unpowered watercraft
> Drowning and submersion due to other accident to surf-board
> Drowning and submersion due to other accident to windsurfer

V90.89x- Drowning and submersion due to other accident to unspecified watercraft
> Drowning and submersion due to other accident to boat NOS
> Drowning and submersion due to other accident to ship NOS
> Drowning and submersion due to other accident to watercraft NOS

V91- <u>Other injury due to accident to watercraft</u>
Includes: Any injury except drowning and submersion as a result of an accident to watercraft
Excludes 1: *civilian water transport accident involving military watercraft (V94.81-)*
military watercraft accident in military or war operations (Y36, Y37.-)
Excludes ❷: *drowning and submersion due to accident to watercraft (V90.-)*

The appropriate 7th character is to be added to each code from category V91:
A <u>Initial</u> encounter
D <u>Subsequent</u> encounter
S <u>Sequela</u>

V91.0- <u>Burn</u> due to watercraft on fire
Excludes 1: *burn from localized fire or explosion on board ship without accident to watercraft (V93.-)*

V91.00x- Burn due to merchant ship on fire

V91.01x- Burn due to passenger ship on fire
> Burn due to Ferry-boat on fire
> Burn due to Liner on fire

V91.02x- Burn due to fishing boat on fire

V91.03x- Burn due to other powered watercraft on fire
> Burn due to Hovercraft (on open water) on fire
> Burn due to Jet ski on fire

V91.04x- Burn due to sailboat on fire

V91.05x- Burn due to canoe or kayak on fire

V91.06x- Burn due to (nonpowered) inflatable craft on fire

V91.07x- Burn due to water-skis on fire

V91.08x- Burn due to other unpowered watercraft on fire

V91.09x- Burn due to unspecified watercraft on fire
> Burn due to boat NOS on fire
> Burn due to ship NOS on fire
> Burn due to watercraft NOS on fire

V90-V91

V91.1- <u>Crushed</u> between watercraft and other watercraft or other object due to collision
    Crushed by lifeboat after abandoning ship in a collision
    NOTE: Select the specified type of watercraft that the victim was on at the time of the collision

V91.10x- Crushed between merchant ship and other watercraft or other object due to collision

V91.11x- Crushed between passenger ship and other watercraft or other object due to collision
    Crushed between Ferry-boat and other watercraft or other object due to collision
    Crushed between Liner and other watercraft or other object due to collision

V91.12x- Crushed between fishing boat and other watercraft or other object due to collision

V91.13x- Crushed between other powered watercraft and other watercraft or other object due to collision
    Crushed between Hovercraft (on open water) and other watercraft or other object due to collision
    Crushed between Jet ski and other watercraft or other object due to collision

V91.14x- Crushed between sailboat and other watercraft or other object due to collision

V91.15x- Crushed between canoe or kayak and other watercraft or other object due to collision

V91.16x- Crushed between (nonpowered) inflatable craft and other watercraft or other object due to collision

V91.18x- Crushed between other unpowered watercraft and other watercraft or other object due to collision
    Crushed between surfboard and other watercraft or other object due to collision
    Crushed between windsurfer and other watercraft or other object due to collision

V91.19x- Crushed between unspecified watercraft and other watercraft or other object due to collision
    Crushed between boat NOS and other watercraft or other object due to collision
    Crushed between ship NOS and other watercraft or other object due to collision
    Crushed between watercraft NOS and other watercraft or other object due to collision

V91.2- <u>Fall</u> due to collision between watercraft and other watercraft or other object
    Fall while remaining on watercraft after collision
    Note: Select the specified type of watercraft that the victim was on at the time of the collision
    Excludes 1:   *crushed between watercraft and other watercraft and other object due to collision (V91.1-)*
        drowning and submersion due to falling from crushed watercraft (V90.3-)

V91.20x- Fall due to collision between merchant ship and other watercraft or other object

V91.21x- Fall due to collision between passenger ship and other watercraft or other object
    Fall due to collision between Ferry-boat and other watercraft or other object
    Fall due to collision between Liner and other watercraft or other object

V91.22x- Fall due to collision between fishing boat and other watercraft or other object

V91.23x- Fall due to collision between other powered watercraft and other watercraft or other object
    Fall due to collision between Hovercraft (on open water) and other watercraft or other object
    Fall due to collision between Jet ski and other watercraft or other object

V91.24x- Fall due to collision between sailboat and other watercraft or other object

V91.25x- Fall due to collision between canoe or kayak and other watercraft or other object

V91.26x- Fall due to collision between (nonpowered) inflatable craft and other watercraft or other object

V91.29x- Fall due to collision between unspecified watercraft and other watercraft or other object
    Fall due to collision between boat NOS and other watercraft or other object
    Fall due to collision between ship NOS and other watercraft or other object
    Fall due to collision between watercraft NOS and other watercraft or other object

V91.3- <u>Hit or struck by falling object</u> due to accident to watercraft
    Hit or struck by falling object (part of damaged watercraft or other object) after falling or jumping from damaged watercraft
    Excludes ❷: *drowning or submersion due to fall or jumping from damaged watercraft (V90.2-, V90.3-)*

V91.30x- Hit or struck by falling object due to accident to merchant ship

V91.31x- Hit or struck by falling object due to accident to passenger ship
    Hit or struck by falling object due to accident to Ferry-boat
    Hit or struck by falling object due to accident to Liner

V91.32x- Hit or struck by falling object due to accident to fishing boat

V91.33x- Hit or struck by falling object due to accident to other powered watercraft
    Hit or struck by falling object due to accident to Hovercraft (on open water)
    Hit or struck by falling object due to accident to Jet ski

V91.34x- Hit or struck by falling object due to accident to sailboat

V91.35x- Hit or struck by falling object due to accident to canoe or kayak

V91.36x- Hit or struck by falling object due to accident to (nonpowered) inflatable craft

V91.37x- Hit or struck by falling object due to accident to water-skis
    Hit by water-skis after jumping off of waterskis

V91.38x- Hit or struck by falling object due to accident to other unpowered watercraft
    Hit or struck by surf-board after falling off damaged surf-board
    Hit or struck by object after falling off damaged windsurfer

V91.39x- Hit or struck by falling object due to accident to unspecified watercraft
    Hit or struck by falling object due to accident to boat NOS
    Hit or struck by falling object due to accident to ship NOS
    Hit or struck by falling object due to accident to watercraft NOS

V91.8- <u>Other injury</u> due to other accident to watercraft

V91.80x- Other injury due to other accident to merchant ship

V91.81x- Other injury due to other accident to passenger ship
    Other injury due to other accident to Ferry-boat
    Other injury due to other accident to Liner

V91.82x- Other injury due to other accident to fishing boat

V91.83x- Other injury due to other accident to other powered watercraft
    Other injury due to other accident to Hovercraft (on open water)
    Other injury due to other accident to Jet ski

V91.84x- Other injury due to other accident to sailboat

V91.85x- Other injury due to other accident to canoe or kayak

V91.86x- Other injury due to other accident to (nonpowered) inflatable craft

V91.87x- Other injury due to other accident to water-skis

V91.88x- Other injury due to other accident to other unpowered watercraft
    Other injury due to other accident to surf-board
    Other injury due to other accident to windsurfer

V91.89x- Other injury due to other accident to unspecified watercraft
    Other injury due to other accident to boat NOS
    Other injury due to other accident to ship NOS
    Other injury due to other accident to watercraft NOS

V 9 1 - V 9 1

V92- <u>Drowning and submersion</u> <u>due to accident on board watercraft,</u> <u>without accident to watercraft</u>

 Excludes 1: *civilian water transport accident involving military watercraft (V94.81-)*
     drowning or submersion due to accident to watercraft (V90-V91)
     drowning or submersion of diver who voluntarily jumps from boat not involved in an accident (W16.711, W16.721)
     fall into water without watercraft (W16.-)
     military watercraft accident in military or war operations (Y36, Y37)

The appropriate 7th character is to be added to each code from category V92:
A   <u>Initial</u> encounter
D   <u>Subsequent</u> encounter
S   <u>Sequela</u>

V92.0-   Drowning and submersion <u>due to fall off watercraft</u>
    Drowning and submersion due to fall from gangplank of watercraft
    Drowning and submersion due to fall overboard watercraft
   Excludes ❷: *hitting head on object or bottom of body of water due to fall from watercraft (V94.0-)*

  V92.00x-   Drowning and submersion due to fall off merchant ship
  V92.01x-   Drowning and submersion due to fall off passenger ship
     Drowning and submersion due to fall off Ferry-boat
     Drowning and submersion due to fall off Liner
  V92.02x-   Drowning and submersion due to fall off fishing boat
  V92.03x-   Drowning and submersion due to fall off other powered watercraft
     Drowning and submersion due to fall off Hovercraft (on open water)
     Drowning and submersion due to fall off Jet ski
  V92.04x-   Drowning and submersion due to fall off sailboat
  V92.05x-   Drowning and submersion due to fall off canoe or kayak
  V92.06x-   Drowning and submersion due to fall off (nonpowered) inflatable craft
  V92.07x-   Drowning and submersion due to fall off water-skis
   Excludes 1: *drowning and submersion due to falling off burning water-skis (V90.27)*
      drowning and submersion due to falling off crushed water-skis (V90.37)
      hit by boat while water-skiing NOS (V94.-)
  V92.08x-   Drowning and submersion due to fall off other unpowered watercraft
     Drowning and submersion due to fall off surf-board
     Drowning and submersion due to fall off windsurfer
   Excludes 1: *drowning and submersion due to fall off burning unpowered watercraft (V90.28)*
      drowning and submersion due to fall off crushed unpowered watercraft (V90.38)
      drowning and submersion due to fall off damaged unpowered watercraft (V90.88)
      drowning and submersion due to rider of nonpowered watercraft being hit by other watercraft (V94.-)
      other injury due to rider of nonpowered watercraft being hit by other watercraft (V94.-)
  V92.09x-   Drowning and submersion due to fall off unspecified watercraft
     Drowning and submersion due to fall off boat NOS
     Drowning and submersion due to fall off ship
     Drowning and submersion due to fall off watercraft NOS

V92.1-   Drowning and submersion <u>due to being thrown overboard by motion of watercraft</u>
   Excludes 1: *drowning and submersion due to fall off surf-board (V92.08)*
      drowning and submersion due to fall off water-skis (V92.07)
      drowning and submersion due to fall off windsurfer (V92.08)

  V92.10x-   Drowning and submersion due to being thrown overboard by motion of merchant ship

  V92.11x-   Drowning and submersion due to being thrown overboard by motion of passenger ship
     Drowning and submersion due to being thrown overboard by motion of Ferry-boat
     Drowning and submersion due to being thrown overboard by motion of Liner
  V92.12x-   Drowning and submersion due to being thrown overboard by motion of fishing boat
  V92.13x-   Drowning and submersion due to being thrown overboard by motion of other powered watercraft
     Drowning and submersion due to being thrown overboard by motion of Hovercraft
  V92.14x-   Drowning and submersion due to being thrown overboard by motion of sailboat
  V92.15x-   Drowning and submersion due to being thrown overboard by motion of canoe or kayak
  V92.16x-   Drowning and submersion due to being thrown overboard by motion of (nonpowered) inflatable craft
  V92.19x-   Drowning and submersion due to being thrown overboard by motion of unspecified watercraft
     Drowning and submersion due to being thrown overboard by motion of boat NOS
     Drowning and submersion due to being thrown overboard by motion of ship NOS
     Drowning and submersion due to being thrown overboard by motion of watercraft NOS

V92.2-   Drowning and submersion <u>due to being washed overboard from watercraft</u>
   Code first any associated cataclysm (X37.0-)

  V92.20x-   Drowning and submersion due to being washed overboard from merchant ship
  V92.21x-   Drowning and submersion due to being washed overboard from passenger ship
     Drowning and submersion due to being washed overboard from Ferry-boat
     Drowning and submersion due to being washed overboard from Liner
  V92.22x-   Drowning and submersion due to being washed overboard from fishing boat
  V92.23x-   Drowning and submersion due to being washed overboard from other powered watercraft
     Drowning and submersion due to being washed overboard from Hovercraft (on open water)
     Drowning and submersion due to being washed overboard from Jet ski
  V92.24x-   Drowning and submersion due to being washed overboard from sailboat
  V92.25x-   Drowning and submersion due to being washed overboard from canoe or kayak
  V92.26x-   Drowning and submersion due to being washed overboard from (nonpowered) inflatable craft
  V92.27x-   Drowning and submersion due to being washed overboard from water-skis
   Excludes 1: *drowning and submersion due to fall off water-skis (V92.07)*
  V92.28x-   Drowning and submersion due to being washed overboard from other unpowered watercraft
     Drowning and submersion due to being washed overboard from surf-board
     Drowning and submersion due to being washed overboard from windsurfer
  V92.29x-   Drowning and submersion due to being washed overboard from unspecified watercraft
     Drowning and submersion due to being washed overboard from boat NOS
     Drowning and submersion due to being washed overboard from ship NOS
     Drowning and submersion due to being washed overboard from watercraft NOS

V92 - V92

V93- <u>Other injury due to accident on board watercraft</u>, <u>without accident to</u> <u>watercraft</u>

> *Excludes 1:*   *civilian water transport accident involving military watercraft*
> *(V94.81-)*
> *other injury due to accident to watercraft (V91.-)*
> *military watercraft accident in military or war operations*
> *(Y36, Y37.-)*
>
> *Excludes ❷:*   *drowning and submersion due to accident on board watercraft,*
> *without accident to watercraft (V92.-)*

> The appropriate 7th character is to be added to each code from category
> V93:
> **A**   <u>Initial</u> encounter
> **D**   <u>Subsequent</u> encounter
> **S**   <u>Sequela</u>

V93.0- <u>Burn</u> due to localized fire on board watercraft
> *Excludes 1:   burn due to watercraft on fire (V91.0-)*

V93.00x- Burn due to localized fire on board merchant vessel

V93.01x- Burn due to localized fire on board passenger vessel
> Burn due to localized fire on board Ferry-boat
> Burn due to localized fire on board Liner

V93.02x- Burn due to localized fire on board fishing boat

V93.03x- Burn due to localized fire on board other powered
watercraft
> Burn due to localized fire on board Hovercraft
> Burn due to localized fire on board Jet ski

V93.04x- Burn due to localized fire on board sailboat

V93.09x- Burn due to localized fire on board unspecified
watercraft
> Burn due to localized fire on board boat NOS
> Burn due to localized fire on board ship NOS
> Burn due to localized fire on board watercraft NOS

V93.1- <u>Other burn</u> on board watercraft
> Burn due to source other than fire on board watercraft
> *Excludes 1:   burn due to watercraft on fire (V91.0-)*

V93.10x- Other burn on board merchant vessel

V93.11x- Other burn on board passenger vessel
> Other burn on board Ferry-boat
> Other burn on board Liner

V93.12x- Other burn on board fishing boat

V93.13x- Other burn on board other powered watercraft
> Other burn on board Hovercraft
> Other burn on board Jet ski

V93.14x- Other burn on board sailboat

V93.19x- Other burn on board unspecified watercraft
> Other burn on board boat NOS
> Other burn on board ship NOS
> Other burn on board watercraft NOS

V93.2- <u>Heat exposure</u> on board watercraft
> *Excludes 1:   exposure to man-made heat not aboard watercraft*
> *(W92)*
> *exposure to natural heat while on board watercraft*
> *(X30)*
> *exposure to sunlight while on board watercraft (X32)*
> *Excludes ❷: burn due to fire on board watercraft (V93.0-)*

V93.20x- Heat exposure on board merchant ship

V93.21x- Heat exposure on board passenger ship
> Heat exposure on board Ferry-boat
> Heat exposure on board Liner

V93.22x- Heat exposure on board fishing boat

V93.23x- Heat exposure on board other powered watercraft
> Heat exposure on board hovercraft

V93.24x- Heat exposure on board sailboat

V93.29x- Heat exposure on board unspecified watercraft
> Heat exposure on board boat NOS
> Heat exposure on board ship NOS
> Heat exposure on board watercraft NOS

V93.3- <u>Fall</u> on board watercraft
> *Excludes 1:   fall due to collision of watercraft (V91.2-)*

V93.30x- Fall on board merchant ship

V93.31x- Fall on board passenger ship
> Fall on board Ferry-boat
> Fall on board Liner

V93.32x- Fall on board fishing boat

V93.33x- Fall on board other powered watercraft
> Fall on board Hovercraft (on open water)
> Fall on board Jet ski

V93.34x- Fall on board sailboat

V93.35x- Fall on board canoe or kayak

V93.36x- Fall on board (nonpowered) inflatable craft

V93.38x- Fall on board other unpowered watercraft

V93.39x- Fall on board unspecified watercraft
> Fall on board boat NOS
> Fall on board ship NOS
> Fall on board watercraft NOS

V93.4- <u>Struck by falling object</u> on board watercraft
> Hit by falling object on board watercraft
> *Excludes 1:   struck by falling object due to accident to watercraft*
> *(V91.3)*

V93.40x- Struck by falling object on merchant ship

V93.41x- Struck by falling object on passenger ship
> Struck by falling object on Ferry-boat
> Struck by falling object on Liner

V93.42x- Struck by falling object on fishing boat

V93.43x- Struck by falling object on other powered watercraft
> Struck by falling object on Hovercraft

V93.44x- Struck by falling object on sailboat

V93.48x- Struck by falling object on other unpowered watercraft

V93.49x- Struck by falling object on unspecified watercraft

V93.5- <u>Explosion</u> on board watercraft
> Boiler explosion on steamship
> *Excludes ❷: fire on board watercraft (V93.0-)*

V93.50x- Explosion on board merchant ship

V93.51x- Explosion on board passenger ship
> Explosion on board Ferry-boat
> Explosion on board Liner

V93.52x- Explosion on board fishing boat

V93.53x- Explosion on board other powered watercraft
> Explosion on board Hovercraft
> Explosion on board Jet ski

V93.54x- Explosion on board sailboat

V93.59x- Explosion on board unspecified watercraft
> Explosion on board boat NOS
> Explosion on board ship NOS
> Explosion on board watercraft NOS

V93.6- <u>Machinery accident</u> on board watercraft
> *Excludes 1:   machinery explosion on board watercraft (V93.4-)*
> *machinery fire on board watercraft (V93.0-)*

V93.60x- Machinery accident on board merchant ship

V93.61x- Machinery accident on board passenger ship
> Machinery accident on board Ferry-boat
> Machinery accident on board Liner

V93.62x- Machinery accident on board fishing boat

V93.63x- Machinery accident on board other powered watercraft
> Machinery accident on board Hovercraft

V93.64x- Machinery accident on board sailboat

V93.69x- Machinery accident on board unspecified watercraft
> Machinery accident on board boat NOS
> Machinery accident on board ship NOS
> Machinery accident on board watercraft NOS

V93.8- <u>Other injury</u> due to other accident on board watercraft
> Accidental poisoning by gases or fumes on watercraft

V93.80x- Other injury due to other accident on board merchant
ship

V93.81x- Other injury due to other accident on board passenger
ship
> Other injury due to other accident on board Ferry-boat
> Other injury due to other accident on board Liner

V93.82x- Other injury due to other accident on board fishing
boat

V93.83x- Other injury due to other accident on board other
powered watercraft
> Other injury due to other accident on board Hovercraft
> Other injury due to other accident on board Jet ski

V93.84x- Other injury due to other accident on board sailboat

V93.85x- Other injury due to other accident on board canoe or
kayak

Excludes 1: = NOT CODED HERE! (Do not code both)   1265   *Excludes ❷:* = Not Included Here

V
9
3
|
V
9
3

V93.86x- Other injury due to other accident on board (nonpowered) inflatable craft

V93.87x- Other injury due to other accident on board water-skis
Hit or struck by object while waterskiing

V93.88x- Other injury due to other accident on board other unpowered watercraft
Hit or struck by object while surfing
Hit or struck by object while on board windsurfer

V93.89x- Other injury due to other accident on board unspecified watercraft
Other injury due to other accident on board boat NOS
Other injury due to other accident on board ship NOS
Other injury due to other accident on board watercraft NOS

V94- **Other and unspecified water transport accidents**
Excludes 1: military watercraft accidents in military or war operations (Y36, Y37)

The appropriate 7th character is to be added to each code from category V94:
A **Initial** encounter
D **Subsequent** encounter
S **Sequela**

V94.0xx- Hitting object or bottom of body of water due to fall from watercraft
Excludes ❷: drowning and submersion due to fall from watercraft (V92.0-)

V94.1- Bather struck by watercraft
Swimmer hit by watercraft

V94.11x- Bather struck by powered watercraft

V94.12x- Bather struck by nonpowered watercraft

V94.2- Rider of nonpowered watercraft struck by other watercraft

V94.21x- Rider of nonpowered watercraft struck by other nonpowered watercraft
Canoer hit by other nonpowered watercraft
Surfer hit by other nonpowered watercraft
Windsurfer hit by other nonpowered watercraft

V94.22x- Rider of nonpowered watercraft struck by powered watercraft
Canoer hit by motorboat
Surfer hit by motorboat
Windsurfer hit by motorboat

V94.3- Injury to rider of (inflatable) watercraft being pulled behind other watercraft

V94.31x- Injury to rider of (inflatable) recreational watercraft being pulled behind other watercraft
Injury to rider of inner-tube pulled behind motor boat

V94.32x- Injury to rider of non-recreational watercraft being pulled behind other watercraft
Injury to occupant of dingy being pulled behind boat or ship
Injury to occupant of life-raft being pulled behind boat or ship

V94.4xx- Injury to barefoot water-skier
Injury to person being pulled behind boat or ship

V94.8- Other water transport accident

V94.81- Water transport accident involving military watercraft

V94.810- Civilian watercraft involved in water transport accident with military watercraft
Passenger on civilian watercraft injured due to accident with military watercraft

V94.811- Civilian in water injured by military watercraft

V94.818- Other water transport accident involving military watercraft

V94.89x- Other water transport accident

V94.9xx- Unspecified water transport accident
Water transport accident NOS

Air and space transport accidents (V95-V97)

Excludes 1: military aircraft accidents in military or war operations (Y36, Y37)

V95- **Accident to powered aircraft causing injury to occupant**
The appropriate 7th character is to be added to each code from category V95:
A **Initial** encounter
D **Subsequent** encounter
S **Sequela**

V95.0- **Helicopter** accident injuring occupant

V95.00x- Unspecified helicopter accident injuring occupant

V95.01x- Helicopter crash injuring occupant

V95.02x- Forced landing of helicopter injuring occupant

V95.03x- Helicopter collision injuring occupant
Helicopter collision with any object, fixed, movable or moving

V95.04x- Helicopter fire injuring occupant

V95.05x- Helicopter explosion injuring occupant

V95.09x- Other helicopter accident injuring occupant

V95.1- **Ultralight, microlight or powered-glider** accident injuring occupant

V95.10x- Unspecified ultralight, microlight or powered-glider accident injuring occupant

V95.11x- Ultralight, microlight or powered-glider crash injuring occupant

V95.12x- Forced landing of ultralight, microlight or powered-glider injuring occupant

V95.13x- Ultralight, microlight or powered-glider collision injuring occupant
Ultralight, microlight or powered-glider collision with any object, fixed, movable or moving

V95.14x- Ultralight, microlight or powered-glider fire injuring occupant

V95.15x- Ultralight, microlight or powered-glider explosion injuring occupant

V95.19x- Other ultralight, microlight or powered-glider accident injuring occupant

V95.2- **Other private fixed-wing aircraft** accident injuring occupant

V95.20x- Unspecified accident to other private fixed-wing aircraft, injuring occupant

V95.21x- Other private fixed-wing aircraft crash injuring occupant

V95.22x- Forced landing of other private fixed-wing aircraft injuring occupant

V95.23x- Other private fixed-wing aircraft collision injuring occupant
Other private fixed-wing aircraft collision with any object, fixed, movable or moving

V95.24x- Other private fixed-wing aircraft fire injuring occupant

V95.25x- Other private fixed-wing aircraft explosion injuring occupant

V95.29x- Other accident to other private fixed-wing aircraft injuring occupant

V95.3- **Commercial fixed-wing aircraft accident** injuring occupant

V95.30x- Unspecified accident to commercial fixed-wing aircraft injuring occupant

V95.31x- Commercial fixed-wing aircraft crash injuring occupant

V95.32x- Forced landing of commercial fixed-wing aircraft injuring occupant

V95.33x- Commercial fixed-wing aircraft collision injuring occupant
Commercial fixed-wing aircraft collision with any object, fixed, movable or moving

V95.34x- Commercial fixed-wing aircraft fire injuring occupant

V95.35x- Commercial fixed-wing aircraft explosion injuring occupant

V95.39x- Other accident to commercial fixed-wing aircraft injuring occupant

V95.4-   Spacecraft accident injuring occupant
    V95.40x-   Unspecified spacecraft accident injuring occupant
    V95.41x-   Spacecraft crash injuring occupant
    V95.42x-   Forced landing of spacecraft injuring occupant
    V95.43x-   Spacecraft collision injuring occupant
         Spacecraft collision with any object, fixed, moveable or moving
    V95.44x-   Spacecraft fire injuring occupant
    V95.45x-   Spacecraft explosion injuring occupant
    V95.49x-   Other spacecraft accident injuring occupant
V95.8xx-   Other powered aircraft accidents injuring occupant
V95.9xx-   Unspecified aircraft accident injuring occupant
    Aircraft accident NOS
    Air transport accident NOS

V96-   Accident to nonpowered aircraft causing injury to occupant
    The appropriate 7th character is to be added to each code from category V96:
    A   Initial encounter
    D   Subsequent encounter
    S   Sequela
V96.0-   Balloon accident injuring occupant
    V96.00x-   Unspecified balloon accident injuring occupant
    V96.01x-   Balloon crash injuring occupant
    V96.02x-   Forced landing of balloon injuring occupant
    V96.03x-   Balloon collision injuring occupant
         Balloon collision with any object, fixed, moveable or moving
    V96.04x-   Balloon fire injuring occupant
    V96.05x-   Balloon explosion injuring occupant
    V96.09x-   Other balloon accident injuring occupant
V96.1-   Hang-glider accident injuring occupant
    V96.10x-   Unspecified hang-glider accident injuring occupant
    V96.11x-   Hang-glider crash injuring occupant
    V96.12x-   Forced landing of hang-glider injuring occupant
    V96.13x-   Hang-glider collision injuring occupant
         Hang-glider collision with any object, fixed, moveable or moving
    V96.14x-   Hang-glider fire injuring occupant
    V96.15x-   Hang-glider explosion injuring occupant
    V96.19x-   Other hang-glider accident injuring occupant
V96.2-   Glider (nonpowered) accident injuring occupant
    V96.20x-   Unspecified glider (nonpowered) accident injuring occupant
    V96.21x-   Glider (nonpowered) crash injuring occupant
    V96.22x-   Forced landing of glider (nonpowered) injuring occupant
    V96.23x-   Glider (nonpowered) collision injuring occupant
         Glider (nonpowered) collision with any object, fixed, moveable or moving
    V96.24x-   Glider (nonpowered) fire injuring occupant
    V96.25x-   Glider (nonpowered) explosion injuring occupant
    V96.29x-   Other glider (nonpowered) accident injuring occupant
V96.8xx-   Other nonpowered-aircraft accidents injuring occupant
    Kite carrying a person accident injuring occupant
V96.9xx-   Unspecified nonpowered-aircraft accident injuring occupant
    Nonpowered-aircraft accident NOS

V97-   Other specified air transport accidents
    The appropriate 7th character is to be added to each code from category V97:
    A   Initial encounter
    D   Subsequent encounter
    S   Sequela
V97.0xx-   Occupant of aircraft injured in other specified air transport accidents
    Fall in, on or from aircraft in air transport accident
    Excludes 1:   accident while boarding or alighting aircraft (V97.1)
V97.1xx-   Person injured while boarding or alighting from aircraft

V97.2-   Parachutist accident
    V97.21x-   Parachutist entangled in object
         Parachutist landing in tree
    V97.22x-   Parachutist injured on landing
    V97.29x-   Other parachutist accident
V97.3-   Person on ground injured in air transport accident
    V97.31x-   Hit by object falling from aircraft
         Hit by crashing aircraft
         Injured by aircraft hitting house
         Injured by aircraft hitting car
    V97.32x-   Injured by rotating propeller
    V97.33x-   Sucked into jet engine
    V97.39x-   Other injury to person on ground due to air transport accident
V97.8-   Other air transport accidents, not elsewhere classified
    Excludes 1:   aircraft accident NOS (V95.9)
    exposure to changes in air pressure during ascent or descent (W94.-)
    V97.81-   Air transport accident involving military aircraft
        V97.810-   Civilian aircraft involved in air transport accident with military aircraft
            Passenger in civilian aircraft injured due to accident with military aircraft
        V97.811-   Civilian injured by military aircraft
        V97.818-   Other air transport accident involving military aircraft
    V97.89x-   Other air transport accidents, not elsewhere classified
        Injury from machinery on aircraft

Other and unspecified transport accidents (V98-V99)

Excludes 1:   vehicle accident, type of vehicle unspecified (V89.-)

V98-   Other specified transport accidents
    The appropriate 7th character is to be added to each code from category V98:
    A   Initial encounter
    D   Subsequent encounter
    S   Sequela
V98.0xx-   Accident to, on or involving cable-car, not on rails
    Caught or dragged by cable-car, not on rails
    Fall or jump from cable-car, not on rails
    Object thrown from or in cable-car, not on rails
V98.1xx-   Accident to, on or involving land-yacht
V98.2xx-   Accident to, on or involving ice yacht
V98.3xx-   Accident to, on or involving ski lift
    Accident to, on or involving ski chair-lift
    Accident to, on or involving ski-lift with gondola
V98.8xx-   Other specified transport accidents

V99.xxx-   Unspecified transport accident
    The appropriate 7th character is to be added to code V99
    A   Initial encounter
    D   Subsequent encounter
    S   Sequela

V95 – V99

Other external causes of accidental injury (W00-X58)

Slipping, tripping, stumbling and falls (W00-W19)

Excludes 1:   *assault involving a fall (Y01-Y02)*
               fall from animal (V80.-)
               fall (in) (from) machinery (in operation) (W28-W31)
               fall (in) (from) transport vehicle (V01-V99)
               intentional self-harm involving a fall (X80-X81)
Excludes ❷: *at risk for fall (history of fall) Z91.81*
               fall (in) (from) burning building (X00.-)
               fall into fire (X00-X04, X08-X09)

W00- __Fall__ due to __ice and snow__
    Includes: Pedestrian on foot falling (slipping) on ice and snow
    Excludes 1:   *fall on (from) ice and snow involving pedestrian conveyance (V00.-)*
               fall from stairs and steps not due to ice and snow (W10.-)

The appropriate 7th character is to be added to each code from category W00:
    A   __Initial__ encounter
    D   __Subsequent__ encounter
    S   __Sequela__

W00.0xx-   Fall on same level due to ice and snow
W00.1xx-   Fall from stairs and steps due to ice and snow
W00.2xx-   Other fall from one level to another due to ice and snow
W00.9xx-   Unspecified fall due to ice and snow

W01- __Fall on same level from slipping, tripping and stumbling__
    Includes: Fall on moving sidewalk
    Excludes 1:   *fall due to bumping (striking) against object (W18.0-)*
               fall in shower or bathtub (W18.2-)
               fall on same level NOS (W18.30)
               fall on same level from slipping, tripping and stumbling due to ice or snow (W00.0)
               fall off or from toilet (W18.1-)
               slipping, tripping and stumbling NOS (W18.40)
               slipping, tripping and stumbling without falling (W18.4-)

The appropriate 7th character is to be added to each code from category W01:
    A   __Initial__ encounter
    D   __Subsequent__ encounter
    S   __Sequela__

W01.0xx-   Fall on same level from slipping, tripping and stumbling __without__ subsequent striking against object
        Falling over animal

W01.1-   Fall on same level from slipping, tripping and stumbling __with__ __subsequent striking against object__

    W01.10x-   Fall on same level from slipping, tripping and stumbling with subsequent striking against unspecified object

    W01.11-   Fall on same level from slipping, tripping and stumbling with subsequent striking against __sharp__ object

        W01.110-   Fall on same level from slipping, tripping and stumbling with subsequent striking against sharp __glass__

        W01.111-   Fall on same level from slipping, tripping and stumbling with subsequent striking against __power tool or machine__

        W01.118-   Fall on same level from slipping, tripping and stumbling with subsequent striking against __other__ sharp object

        W01.119-   Fall on same level from slipping, tripping and stumbling with subsequent striking against __unspecified__ sharp object

    W01.19-   Fall on same level from slipping, tripping and stumbling __with subsequent striking against other object__

        W01.190-   Fall on same level from slipping, tripping and stumbling with subsequent striking against __furniture__

        W01.198-   Fall on same level from slipping, tripping and stumbling with subsequent striking against __other__ object

W03.xxx-   Other __fall__ on __same level__ due to __collision with another person__
    AHA 15:1Q:p8 – Tripped over another player
        Fall due to non-transport collision with other person
    Excludes 1:   *collision with another person without fall (W51)*
               crushed or pushed by a crowd or human stampede (W52)
               fall involving pedestrian conveyance (V00-V09)
               fall due to ice or snow (W00)
               fall on same level NOS (W18.30)

The appropriate 7th character is to be added to code W03:
    A   __Initial__ encounter
    D   __Subsequent__ encounter
    S   __Sequela__

W04.xxx-   __Fall while being carried or supported by other persons__
        Accidentally dropped while being carried

The appropriate 7th character is to be added to code W04:
    A   __Initial__ encounter
    D   __Subsequent__ encounter
    S   __Sequela__

W05- __Fall__ from __non-moving__ wheelchair, nonmotorized scooter and motorized mobility scooter
    Excludes 1:   *fall from moving wheelchair (powered) (V00.811)*
               fall from moving motorized mobility scooter (V00.831)
               fall from nonmotorized scooter (V00.141)

The appropriate 7th character is to be added to each code from category W05:
    A   __Initial__ encounter
    D   __Subsequent__ encounter
    S   __Sequela__

W05.0xx-   Fall from non-moving __wheelchair__
W05.1xx-   Fall from non-moving __nonmotorized scooter__
W05.2xx-   Fall from non-moving __motorized mobility scooter__

W06.xxx-   __Fall from bed__
The appropriate 7th character is to be added to code W06:
    A   __Initial__ encounter
    D   __Subsequent__ encounter
    S   __Sequela__

W07.xxx-   __Fall from chair__
The appropriate 7th character is to be added to code W07:
    A   __Initial__ encounter
    D   __Subsequent__ encounter
    S   __Sequela__

W08.xxx-   __Fall from other furniture__
The appropriate 7th character is to be added to code W08:
    A   __Initial__ encounter
    D   __Subsequent__ encounter
    S   __Sequela__

W09- __Fall__ on and from __playground equipment__
    Excludes 1:   *fall involving recreational machinery (W31)*

The appropriate 7th character is to be added to each code from category W09:
    A   __Initial__ encounter
    D   __Subsequent__ encounter
    S   __Sequela__

W09.0xx-   Fall on or from playground slide
W09.1xx-   Fall from playground swing
W09.2xx-   Fall on or from jungle gym
W09.8xx-   Fall on or from other playground equipment

W10- __Fall__ on and from __stairs and steps__
    Excludes 1:   *Fall from stairs and steps due to ice and snow (W00.1)*

The appropriate 7th character is to be added to each code from category W10:
    A   __Initial__ encounter
    D   __Subsequent__ encounter
    S   __Sequela__

W10.0xx-   Fall (on) (from) escalator
W10.1xx-   Fall (on) (from) sidewalk curb
W10.2xx-   Fall (on) (from) incline
        Fall (on) (from) ramp
W10.8xx-   Fall (on) (from) other stairs and steps
W10.9xx-   Fall (on) (from) unspecified stairs and steps

W00-W10

W11.xxx- <u>Fall</u> on and from <u>ladder</u>
The appropriate 7th character is to be added to code W11:
A **Initial** encounter
D **Subsequent** encounter
S **Sequela**

W12.xxx- <u>Fall</u> on and from <u>scaffolding</u>
The appropriate 7th character is to be added to code W12:
A **Initial** encounter
D **Subsequent** encounter
S **Sequela**

W13- <u>Fall</u> from, out of or through <u>building or structure</u>
The appropriate 7th character is to be added to each code from category W13:
A **Initial** encounter
D **Subsequent** encounter
S **Sequela**

W13.0xx- Fall from, out of or through balcony
Fall from, out of or through railing

W13.1xx- Fall from, out of or through bridge

W13.2xx- Fall from, out of or through roof

W13.3xx- Fall through floor

W13.4xx- Fall from, out of or through window
Excludes ❷: fall with subsequent striking against sharp glass (W01.110)

W13.8xx- Fall from, out of or through other building or structure
Fall from, out of or through viaduct
Fall from, out of or through wall
Fall from, out of or through flag-pole

W13.9xx- Fall from, out of or through building, not otherwise specified
Excludes 1: collapse of a building or structure (W20.-)
fall or jump from burning building or structure (X00.-)

W14.xxx- <u>Fall</u> from <u>tree</u>
The appropriate 7th character is to be added to code W14:
A **Initial** encounter
D **Subsequent** encounter
S **Sequela**

W15.xxx- <u>Fall</u> from <u>cliff</u>
The appropriate 7th character is to be added to code W15:
A **Initial** encounter
D **Subsequent** encounter
S **Sequela**

W16- <u>Fall</u>, jump or diving <u>into water</u>
Excludes 1: accidental non-watercraft drowning and submersion not involving fall (W65-W74)
effects of air pressure from diving (W94.-)
fall into water from watercraft (V90-V94)
hitting an object or against bottom when falling from watercraft (V94.0)
Excludes ❷: striking or hitting diving board (W21.4)
The appropriate 7th character is to be added to each code from category W16:
A **Initial** encounter
D **Subsequent** encounter
S **Sequela**

W16.0- <u>Fall</u> into <u>swimming pool</u>
Fall into swimming pool NOS
Excludes 1: fall into empty swimming pool (W17.3)

W16.01-Fall into swimming pool <u>striking water surface</u>
W16.011- Fall into swimming pool striking water surface <u>causing drowning and submersion</u>
Excludes 1: drowning and submersion while in swimming pool without fall (W67)
W16.012- Fall into swimming pool striking water surface <u>causing other injury</u>

W16.02-Fall into swimming pool <u>striking bottom</u>
W16.021- Fall into swimming pool striking bottom <u>causing drowning and submersion</u>
Excludes 1: drowning and submersion while in swimming pool without fall (W67)

W16.022- Fall into swimming pool striking bottom <u>causing other injury</u>

W16.03-Fall into swimming pool <u>striking wall</u>
W16.031- Fall into swimming pool striking wall <u>causing drowning and submersion</u>
Excludes 1: drowning and submersion while in swimming pool without fall (W67)
W16.032- Fall into swimming pool striking wall causing other injury

W16.1- <u>Fall</u> into <u>natural body of water</u>
Fall into lake
Fall into open sea
Fall into river
Fall into stream

W16.11-Fall into natural body of water <u>striking water surface</u>
W16.111- Fall into natural body of water striking water surface <u>causing drowning and submersion</u>
Excludes 1: drowning and submersion while in natural body of water without fall (W69)
W16.112- Fall into natural body of water striking water surface <u>causing other injury</u>

W16.12-Fall into natural body of <u>water striking bottom</u>
W16.121- Fall into natural body of water striking bottom <u>causing drowning and submersion</u>
Excludes 1: drowning and submersion while in natural body of water without fall (W69)
W16.122- Fall into natural body of water striking bottom <u>causing other injury</u>

W16.13-Fall into natural body of <u>water striking side</u>
W16.131- Fall into natural body of water striking side <u>causing drowning and submersion</u>
Excludes 1: drowning and submersion while in natural body of water without fall (W69)
W16.132- Fall into natural body of water striking side <u>causing other injury</u>

W16.2- <u>Fall</u> in (into) <u>filled bathtub or bucket of water</u>
W16.21-Fall in (into) filled <u>bathtub</u>
Excludes 1: fall into empty bathtub (W18.2)
W16.211- Fall in (into) filled bathtub <u>causing drowning and submersion</u>
Excludes 1: drowning and submersion while in filled bathtub without fall (W65)
W16.212- Fall in (into) filled bathtub <u>causing other injury</u>

W16.22-Fall in (into) <u>bucket of water</u>
W16.221- Fall in (into) bucket of water <u>causing drowning and submersion</u>
W16.222- Fall in (into) bucket of water <u>causing other injury</u>

W16.3- <u>Fall</u> into <u>other water</u>
Fall into fountain
Fall into reservoir

W16.31-Fall into other water <u>striking water surface</u>
W16.311- Fall into other water striking water surface <u>causing drowning and submersion</u>
Excludes 1: drowning and submersion while in other water without fall (W73)
W16.312- Fall into other water striking water surface <u>causing other injury</u>

W16.32-Fall into other water <u>striking bottom</u>
W16.321- Fall into other water striking bottom <u>causing drowning and submersion</u>
Excludes 1: drowning and submersion while in other water without fall (W73)
W16.322- Fall into other water striking bottom <u>causing other injury</u>

W16.33-Fall into other water <u>striking wall</u>
W16.331- Fall into other water striking wall <u>causing drowning and submersion</u>
Excludes 1: drowning and submersion while in other water without fall (W73)
W16.332 Fall into other water striking wall <u>causing other injury</u>

Excludes 1: = NOT CODED HERE! (Do not code both) **1269** *Excludes ❷:* = Not Included Here

W11 - W16

W16.4- Fall into unspecified water
    W16.41x- Fall into unspecified water <u>causing drowning and submersion</u>
    W16.42x- Fall into unspecified water <u>causing other injury</u>

W16.5- <u>Jumping or diving</u> into <u>swimming pool</u>
    W16.51-Jumping or diving into swimming pool <u>striking water surface</u>
        W16.511- Jumping or diving into swimming pool striking water surface causing drowning and submersion
        Excludes 1: drowning and submersion while in swimming pool without jumping or diving (W67)
        W16.512- Jumping or diving into swimming pool striking water surface <u>causing other injury</u>
    W16.52-Jumping or diving into swimming pool <u>striking bottom</u>
        W16.521- Jumping or diving into swimming pool striking bottom <u>causing drowning and submersion</u>
        Excludes 1: drowning and submersion while in swimming pool without jumping or diving (W67)
        W16.522- Jumping or diving into swimming pool striking bottom <u>causing other injury</u>
    W16.53-Jumping or diving into swimming pool <u>striking wall</u>
        W16.531- Jumping or diving into swimming pool striking wall <u>causing drowning and submersion</u>
        Excludes 1: drowning and submersion while in swimming pool without jumping or diving (W67)
        W16.532- Jumping or diving into swimming pool striking wall <u>causing other injury</u>

W16.6- <u>Jumping or diving</u> into <u>natural body of water</u>
    Jumping or diving into lake
    Jumping or diving into open sea
    Jumping or diving into river
    Jumping or diving into stream
    W16.61-Jumping or diving into natural body of water <u>striking water surface</u>
        W16.611- Jumping or diving into natural body of water striking water surface <u>causing drowning and submersion</u>
        Excludes 1: drowning and submersion while in natural body of water without jumping or diving (W69)
        W16.612- Jumping or diving into natural body of water striking water surface <u>causing other injury</u>
    W16.62-Jumping or diving into natural body of water <u>striking bottom</u>
        W16.621- Jumping or diving into natural body of water striking bottom <u>causing drowning and submersion</u>
        Excludes 1: drowning and submersion while in natural body of water without jumping ordiving (W69)
        W16.622- Jumping or diving into natural body of water striking bottom <u>causing other injury</u>

W16.7- Jumping or diving from <u>boat</u>
    Excludes 1: fall from boat into water — see watercraft accident (V90-V94)
    W16.71-Jumping or diving from boat <u>striking water surface</u>
        W16.711- Jumping or diving from boat striking water surface <u>causing drowning and submersion</u>
        W16.712- Jumping or diving from boat striking water surface <u>causing other injury</u>
    W16.72-Jumping or diving from boat <u>striking bottom</u>
        W16.721- Jumping or diving from boat striking bottom <u>causing drowning and submersion</u>
        W16.722- Jumping or diving from boat striking bottom <u>causing other injury</u>

W16.8- Jumping or diving into <u>other water</u>
    Jumping or diving into fountain
    Jumping or diving into reservoir
    W16.81-Jumping or diving into other water <u>striking water surface</u>
        W16.811- Jumping or diving into other water striking water surface <u>causing drowning and submersion</u>
        Excludes 1: drowning and submersion while in other water without jumping or diving (W73)
        W16.812- Jumping or diving into other water striking water surface <u>causing other injury</u>
    W16.82-Jumping or diving into other water <u>striking bottom</u>
        W16.821- Jumping or diving into other water striking bottom <u>causing drowning and submersion</u>
        Excludes 1: drowning and submersion while in other water without jumping or diving (W73)
        W16.822- Jumping or diving into other water striking bottom <u>causing other injury</u>
    W16.83-Jumping or diving into other water <u>striking wall</u>
        W16.831- Jumping or diving into other water striking wall <u>causing drowning and submersion</u>
        Excludes 1: drowning and submersion while in other water without jumping or diving (W73)
        W16.832- Jumping or diving into other water striking wall <u>causing other injury</u>

W16.9- Jumping or diving into <u>unspecified water</u>
    W16.91x- Jumping or diving into unspecified water <u>causing drowning and submersion</u>
    W16.92x- Jumping or diving into unspecified water <u>causing other injury</u>

W17- <u>Other fall from one level to another</u>
    The appropriate 7th character is to be added to each code from category W17:
    A   <u>Initial</u> encounter
    D   <u>Subsequent</u> encounter
    S   <u>Sequela</u>

W17.0xx- Fall into well
W17.1xx- Fall into storm drain or manhole
W17.2xx- Fall into hole
    Fall into pit
W17.3xx- Fall into empty swimming pool
    Excludes 1: fall into filled swimming pool (W16.0-)
W17.4xx- Fall from dock
W17.8- Other fall from one level to another
    W17.81x- Fall down embankment (hill)
    W17.82x- Fall from (out of) grocery cart
        Fall due to grocery cart tipping over
    W17.89x- Other fall from one level to another
        Fall from cherry picker
        Fall from lifting device
        Fall from mobile elevated work platform [MEWP]
        Fall from sky lift

W18- <u>Other slipping, tripping and stumbling and falls</u>
    The appropriate 7th character is to be added to each code from category W18:
    A   <u>Initial</u> encounter
    D   <u>Subsequent</u> encounter
    S   <u>Sequela</u>

W18.0- Fall due to <u>bumping against object</u>
    Striking against object with subsequent fall
    Excludes 1: fall on same level due to slipping, tripping, or stumbling with subsequent striking against object (W01.1-)
    W18.00x- Striking against unspecified object with subsequent fall
    W18.01x- Striking against sports equipment with subsequent fall
    W18.02x- Striking against glass with subsequent fall
    W18.09x- Striking against other object with subsequent fall
W18.1- Fall from or off <u>toilet</u>
    W18.11x- Fall from or off toilet without subsequent striking against object
        Fall from (off) toilet NOS

W16 – W18

© 2016 Channel Publishing, Ltd.

W18.12x- Fall from or off toilet with subsequent striking against object

W18.2xx- Fall in (into) <u>shower or empty bathtub</u>
Excludes 1: fall in full bathtub causing drowning or submersion (W16.21-)

W18.3- Other and unspecified fall on same level
W18.30x- Fall on same level, unspecified
W18.31x- Fall on same level due to stepping on an object
Fall on same level due to stepping on an animal
Excludes 1: slipping, tripping and stumbling without fall due to stepping on animal (W18.41)
W18.39x- Other fall on same level

W18.4- Slipping, tripping and stumbling <u>without falling</u>
Excludes 1: collision with another person without fall (W51)
W18.40x- Slipping, tripping and stumbling without falling, unspecified
W18.41x- Slipping, tripping and stumbling without falling due to stepping on object
Slipping, tripping and stumbling without falling due to stepping on animal
Excludes 1: slipping, tripping and stumbling with fall due to stepping on animal (W18.31)
W18.42x- Slipping, tripping and stumbling without falling due to stepping into hole or opening
W18.43x- Slipping, tripping and stumbling without falling due to stepping from one level to another
W18.49x- Other slipping, tripping and stumbling without falling

W19.xxx- <u>Unspecified fall</u>
Accidental fall NOS
The appropriate 7th character is to be added to code W19:
A <u>Initial</u> encounter
D <u>Subsequent</u> encounter
S <u>Sequela</u>

Exposure to inanimate mechanical forces (W20-W49)

Excludes 1: assault (X92-Y09)
contact or collision with animals or persons (W50-W64)
exposure to inanimate mechanical forces involving military or war operations (Y36-, Y37-)
intentional self-harm (X71-X83)

W20- <u>Struck by</u> <u>thrown, projected or falling object</u>
Code first any associated:
Cataclysm (X34-X39)
Lightning strike (T75.00)
Excludes 1: falling object in machinery accident (W24, W28-W31)
falling object in transport accident (V01-V99)
object set in motion by explosion (W35-W40)
object set in motion by firearm (W32-W34)
struck by thrown sports equipment (W21.-)
The appropriate 7th character is to be added to each code from category W20:
A <u>Initial</u> encounter
D <u>Subsequent</u> encounter
S <u>Sequela</u>

W20.0xx- Struck by falling object in cave-in
Excludes ❷: asphyxiation due to cave-in (T71.21)
W20.1xx- Struck by object due to collapse of building
Excludes 1: struck by object due to collapse of burning building (X00.2, X02.2)
W20.8xx- Other cause of strike by thrown, projected or falling object
Excludes 1: struck by thrown sports equipment (W21.-)

W21- <u>Striking against or struck</u> by <u>sports equipment</u>
Excludes 1: assault with sports equipment (Y08.0-)
striking against or struck by sports equipment with subsequent fall (W18.01)
The appropriate 7th character is to be added to each code from category W21:
A <u>Initial</u> encounter
D <u>Subsequent</u> encounter
S <u>Sequela</u>

W21.0- Struck by <u>hit or thrown ball</u>
W21.00x- Struck by hit or thrown ball, unspecified type
W21.01x- Struck by football

W21.02x- Struck by soccer ball
W21.03x- Struck by baseball
W21.04x- Struck by golf ball
W21.05x- Struck by basketball
W21.06x- Struck by volleyball
W21.07x- Struck by softball
W21.09x- Struck by other hit or thrown ball

W21.1- Struck by <u>bat, racquet or club</u>
W21.11x- Struck by baseball bat
W21.12x- Struck by tennis racquet
W21.13x- Struck by golf club
W21.19x- Struck by other bat, racquet or club

W21.2- Struck by <u>hockey stick or puck</u>
W21.21-Struck by hockey <u>stick</u>
W21.210- Struck by ice hockey stick
W21.211- Struck by field hockey stick
W21.22-Struck by hockey <u>puck</u>
W21.220- Struck by ice hockey puck
W21.221- Struck by field hockey puck

W21.3- Struck by <u>sports foot wear</u>
W21.31x- Struck by shoe cleats
Stepped on by shoe cleats
W21.32x- Struck by skate blades
Skated over by skate blades
W21.39x- Struck by other sports foot wear

W21.4xx- Striking against <u>diving board</u>
Use additional code for subsequent falling into water, if applicable (W16.-)

W21.8- Striking against or struck by <u>other</u> sports equipment
W21.81x- Striking against or struck by football helmet
W21.89x- Striking against or struck by other sports equipment

W21.9xx- Striking against or struck by <u>unspecified</u> sports equipment

W22- <u>Striking</u> against or struck by <u>other objects</u>
Excludes 1: striking against or struck by object with subsequent fall (W18.09)
The appropriate 7th character is to be added to each code from category W22:
A <u>Initial</u> encounter
D <u>Subsequent</u> encounter
S <u>Sequela</u>

W22.0- Striking against <u>stationary object</u>
Excludes 1: striking against stationary sports equipment (W21.8)
W22.01x- Walked into wall
W22.02x- Walked into lamppost
W22.03x- Walked into furniture
W22.04-Striking against wall of swimming pool
W22.041- Striking against wall of swimming pool causing drowning and submersion
Excludes 1: drowning and submersion while swimming without striking against wall (W67)
W22.042- Striking against wall of swimming pool causing other injury
W22.09x- Striking against other stationary object

W22.1- Striking against or struck by <u>automobile airbag</u>
W22.10x- Striking against or struck by unspecified automobile airbag
W22.11x- Striking against or struck by driver side automobile airbag
W22.12x- Striking against or struck by front passenger side automobile airbag
W22.19x- Striking against or struck by other automobile airbag

W22.8xx- Striking against or struck by other objects
Striking against or struck by object NOS
Excludes 1: struck by thrown, projected or falling object (W20.-)

W18 - W22

W23- <u>Caught, crushed, jammed or pinched</u> <u>in or between objects</u>

Excludes 1:   *injury caused by cutting or piercing instruments (W25-W27)*
        injury caused by firearms malfunction (W32.1, W33.1-, W34.1-)
        injury caused by lifting and transmission devices (W24.-)
        injury caused by machinery (W28-W31)
        injury caused by nonpowered hand tools (W27.-)
        injury caused by transport vehicle being used as a means of transportation (V01-V99)
        injury caused by struck by thrown, projected or falling object (W20.-)

The appropriate 7th character is to be added to each code from category W23:
- **A** <u>Initial</u> encounter
- **D** <u>Subsequent</u> encounter
- **S** <u>Sequela</u>

W23.0xx- Caught, crushed, jammed, or pinched between moving objects

W23.1xx- Caught, crushed, jammed, or pinched between stationary objects

W24- Contact with lifting and transmission devices, not elsewhere classified

Excludes 1:   *transport accidents (V01-V99)*

The appropriate 7th character is to be added to each code from category W24:
- **A** <u>Initial</u> encounter
- **D** <u>Subsequent</u> encounter
- **S** <u>Sequela</u>

W24.0xx- Contact with lifting devices, not elsewhere classified
    Contact with chain hoist
    Contact with drive belt
    Contact with pulley (block)

W24.1xx- Contact with transmission devices, not elsewhere classified
    Contact with transmission belt or cable

W25.xxx- <u>Contact with sharp glass</u>
    Code first any associated:
    Injury due to flying glass from explosion or firearm discharge (W32-W40)
    Transport accident (V00-V99)

Excludes 1:   *fall on same level due to slipping, tripping and stumbling with subsequent striking against sharp glass (W01.10)*
        striking against sharp glass with subsequent fall (W18.02)

Excludes ❷: *glass embedded in skin (W45.-)*

The appropriate 7th character is to be added to code W25:
- **A** <u>Initial</u> encounter
- **D** <u>Subsequent</u> encounter
- **S** <u>Sequela</u>

W26- Contact with <u>other sharp objects</u>

Excludes ❷: *sharp object(s) embedded in skin (W45.-)*

The appropriate 7th character is to be added to each code from category W26:
- **A** <u>Initial</u> encounter
- **D** <u>Subsequent</u> encounter
- **S** <u>Sequela</u>

W26.0xx- Contact with knife
    Excludes 1:   *contact with electric knife (W29.1)*

W26.1xx- Contact with sword or dagger

W26.2xx- Contact with edge of stiff paper
    Paper cut

W26.8xx- Contact with other sharp object(s), not elsewhere classified
    Contact with tin can lid

W26.9xx- Contact with unspecified sharp object(s)

W27- Contact with <u>nonpowered hand tool</u>

The appropriate 7th character is to be added to each code from category W27:
- **A** <u>Initial</u> encounter
- **D** <u>Subsequent</u> encounter
- **S** <u>Sequela</u>

W27.0xx- Contact with <u>workbench tool</u>
    Contact with auger
    Contact with axe
    Contact with chisel
    Contact with handsaw
    Contact with screwdriver

W27.1xx- Contact with <u>garden tool</u>
    Contact with hoe
    Contact with nonpowered lawn mower
    Contact with pitchfork
    Contact with rake

W27.2xx- Contact with <u>scissors</u>

W27.3xx- Contact with <u>needle (sewing)</u>
    Excludes 1:   *contact with hypodermic needle (W46.-)*

W27.4xx- Contact with <u>kitchen utensil</u>
    Contact with fork
    Contact with ice-pick
    Contact with can-opener NOS

W27.5xx- Contact with <u>paper-cutter</u>

W27.8xx- Contact with <u>other nonpowered hand tool</u>
    Contact with nonpowered sewing machine
    Contact with shovel

W28.xxx- Contact with <u>powered lawn mower</u>
    Powered lawn mower (commercial) (residential)
    Excludes 1:   *contact with nonpowered lawn mower (W27.1)*
    Excludes ❷: *exposure to electric current (W86-)*

The appropriate 7th character is to be added to code W28:
- **A** <u>Initial</u> encounter
- **D** <u>Subsequent</u> encounter
- **S** <u>Sequela</u>

W29- Contact with <u>other powered hand tools and household machinery</u>

Excludes 1:   *contact with commercial machinery (W31.82)*
        contact with hot household appliance (X15)
        contact with nonpowered hand tool (W27.-)
        exposure to electric current (W86)

The appropriate 7th character is to be added to each code from category W29:
- **A** <u>Initial</u> encounter
- **D** <u>Subsequent</u> encounter
- **S** <u>Sequela</u>

W29.0xx- Contact with powered <u>kitchen</u> appliance
    Contact with blender
    Contact with can-opener
    Contact with garbage disposal
    Contact with mixer

W29.1xx- Contact with electric knife

W29.2xx- Contact with other powered <u>household</u> machinery
    Contact with electric fan
    Contact with powered dryer (clothes) (powered) (spin)
    Contact with washing-machine
    Contact with sewing machine

W29.3xx- Contact with powered <u>garden</u> and <u>outdoor</u> hand tools and machinery
    Contact with chainsaw
    Contact with edger
    Contact with garden cultivator (tiller)
    Contact with hedge trimmer
    Contact with other powered garden tool
    Excludes 1:   *contact with powered lawn mower (W28)*

W29.4xx- Contact with <u>nail gun</u>

W29.8xx- Contact with <u>other</u> powered powered hand tools and household machinery
    Contact with do-it-yourself tool NOS

W30- Contact with <u>agricultural</u> machinery
    Includes: Animal-powered farm machine
    Excludes 1:   *agricultural transport vehicle accident (V01-V99)*
        explosion of grain store (W40.8)
        exposure to electric current (W86.-)

The appropriate 7th character is to be added to each code from category W30:
- **A** <u>Initial</u> encounter
- **D** <u>Subsequent</u> encounter
- **S** <u>Sequela</u>

W30.0xx- Contact with combine harvester
    Contact with reaper
    Contact with thresher

W30.1xx- Contact with power take-off devices (PTO)

W30.2xx- Contact with hay derrick

W30.3xx- Contact with grain storage elevator
    Excludes 1:   *explosion of grain store (W40.8)*

**W
2
3
-
W
3
0**

W30.8- Contact with other specified agricultural machinery

W30.81x- Contact with agricultural transport vehicle in stationary use
    Contact with agricultural transport vehicle under repair, not on public roadway
    Excludes 1:   *agricultural transport vehicle accident (V01-V99)*

W30.89x- Contact with other specified agricultural machinery

W30.9xx- Contact with unspecified agricultural machinery
    Contact with farm machinery NOS

W31- Contact with other and unspecified machinery
    Excludes 1:   *contact with agricultural machinery (W30.-)*
                contact with machinery in transport under own power or being towed by a vehicle (V01-V99)
                exposure to electric current (W86)

> The appropriate 7th character is to be added to each code from category W31:
> **A**   Initial encounter
> **D**   Subsequent encounter
> **S**   Sequela

W31.0xx- Contact with mining and earth-drilling machinery
    Contact with bore or drill (land) (seabed)
    Contact with shaft hoist
    Contact with shaft lift
    Contact with undercutter

W31.1xx- Contact with metalworking machines
    Contact with abrasive wheel
    Contact with forging machine
    Contact with lathe
    Contact with mechanical shears
    Contact with metal drilling machine
    Contact with milling machine
    Contact with power press
    Contact with rolling-mill
    Contact with metal sawing machine

W31.2xx- Contact with powered woodworking and forming machines
    Contact with band saw
    Contact with bench saw
    Contact with circular saw
    Contact with molding machine
    Contact with overhead plane
    Contact with powered saw
    Contact with radial saw
    Contact with sander
    Excludes 1:   *nonpowered woodworking tools (W27.0)*

W31.3xx- Contact with prime movers
    Contact with gas turbine
    Contact with internal combustion engine
    Contact with steam engine
    Contact with water driven turbine

W31.8- Contact with other specified machinery

W31.81x- Contact with recreational machinery
    Contact with roller coaster

W31.82x- Contact with other commercial machinery
    Contact with commercial electric fan
    Contact with commercial kitchen appliances
    Contact with commercial powered dryer (clothes) (powered) (spin)
    Contact with commercial washing-machine
    Contact with commercial sewing machine
    Excludes 1:   *contact with household machinery (W29.-)*
                contact with powered lawn mower (W28)

W31.83x- Contact with special construction vehicle in stationary use
    Contact with special construction vehicle under repair, not on public roadway
    Excludes 1:   *special construction vehicle accident (V01-V99)*

W31.89x- Contact with other specified machinery

W31.9xx- Contact with unspecified machinery
    Contact with machinery NOS

W32- Accidental handgun discharge and malfunction
    Includes: Accidental discharge and malfunction of gun for single hand use
               Accidental discharge and malfunction of pistol
               Accidental discharge and malfunction of revolver
    Handgun discharge and malfunction NOS
    Excludes 1:   *accidental airgun discharge and malfunction (W34.010, W34.110)*
                accidental BB gun discharge and malfunction (W34.010, W34.110)
                accidental pellet gun discharge and malfunction (W34.010, W34.110)
                accidental shotgun discharge and malfunction (W33.01, W33.11)
                assault by handgun discharge (X93)
                handgun discharge involving legal intervention (Y35.0-)
                handgun discharge involving military or war operations (Y36.4-)
                intentional self-harm by handgun discharge (X72)
                Very pistol discharge and malfunction (W34.09, W34.19)

> The appropriate 7th character is to be added to each code from category W32:
> **A**   Initial encounter
> **D**   Subsequent encounter
> **S**   Sequela

W32.0xx- Accidental handgun discharge

W32.1xx- Accidental handgun malfunction
    Injury due to explosion of handgun (parts)
    Injury due to malfunction of mechanism or component of handgun
    Injury due to recoil of handgun
    Powder burn from handgun

W33- Accidental rifle, shotgun and larger firearm discharge and malfunction
    Includes: Rifle, shotgun and larger firearm discharge and malfunction NOS
    Excludes 1:   *accidental airgun discharge and malfunction (W34.010, W34.110)*
                accidental BB gun discharge and malfunction (W34.010, W34.110)
                accidental handgun discharge and malfunction (W32.-)
                accidental pellet gun discharge and malfunction (W34.010, W34.110)
                assault by rifle, shotgun and larger firearm discharge (X94)
                firearm discharge involving legal intervention (Y35.0-)
                firearm discharge involving military or war operations (Y36.4-)
                intentional self-harm by rifle, shotgun and larger firearm discharge (X73)

> The appropriate 7th character is to be added to each code from category W33:
> **A**   Initial encounter
> **D**   Subsequent encounter
> **S**   Sequela

W33.0- Accidental rifle, shotgun and larger firearm discharge

W33.00x- Accidental discharge of unspecified larger firearm
    Discharge of unspecified larger firearm NOS

W33.01x- Accidental discharge of shotgun
    Discharge of shotgun NOS

W33.02x- Accidental discharge of hunting rifle
    Discharge of hunting rifle NOS

W33.03x- Accidental discharge of machine gun
    Discharge of machine gun NOS

W33.09x- Accidental discharge of other larger firearm
    Discharge of other larger firearm NOS

W33.1- Accidental rifle, shotgun and larger firearm malfunction
    Injury due to explosion of rifle, shotgun and larger firearm (parts)
    Injury due to malfunction of mechanism or component of rifle, shotgun and larger firearm
    Injury due to piercing, cutting, crushing or pinching due to (by) slide trigger mechanism, scope or other gunpart
    Injury due to recoil of rifle, shotgun and larger firearm
    Powder burn from rifle, shotgun and larger firearm

W33.10x- Accidental malfunction of unspecified larger firearm
    Malfunction of unspecified larger firearm NOS

W33.11x- Accidental malfunction of shotgun
    Malfunction of shotgun NOS

© 2016 Channel Publishing, Ltd.

W30 – W33

W33.12x- Accidental malfunction of hunting rifle
Malfunction of hunting rifle NOS

W33.13x- Accidental malfunction of machine gun
Malfunction of machine gun NOS

W33.19x- Accidental malfunction of other larger firearm
Malfunction of other larger firearm NOS

W34- Accidental discharge and malfunction from other and unspecified firearms and guns

The appropriate 7th character is to be added to each code from category W34:
A   Initial encounter
D   Subsequent encounter
S   Sequela

W34.0- Accidental discharge from other and unspecified firearms and guns
AHA 15:1Q:p17 – Accidental gunshot wound

W34.00x- Accidental discharge from unspecified firearms or gun
Discharge from firearm NOS
Gunshot wound NOS
Shot NOS

W34.01- Accidental discharge of gas, air or spring-operated guns

W34.010- Accidental discharge of airgun
Accidental discharge of BB gun
Accidental discharge of pellet gun

W34.011- Accidental discharge of paintball gun
Accidental injury due to paintball discharge

W34.018- Accidental discharge of other gas, air or spring-operated gun

W34.09x- Accidental discharge from other specified firearms
Accidental discharge from Very pistol [flare]

W34.1- Accidental malfunction from other and unspecified firearms and guns

W34.10x- Accidental malfunction from unspecified firearms or gun
Firearm malfunction NOS

W34.11- Accidental malfunction of gas, air or spring-operated guns

W34.110- Accidental malfunction of airgun
Accidental malfunction of BB gun
Accidental malfunction of pellet gun

W34.111- Accidental malfunction of paintball gun
Accidental injury due to paintball gun malfunction

W34.118- Accidental malfunction of other gas, air or spring-operated gun

W34.19x- Accidental malfunction from other specified firearms
Accidental malfunction from Very pistol [flare]

W35.xxx- Explosion and rupture of boiler
Excludes 1:   explosion and rupture of boiler on watercraft (V93.4)

The appropriate 7th character is to be added to code W35:
A   Initial encounter
D   Subsequent encounter
S   Sequela

W36- Explosion and rupture of gas cylinder
The appropriate 7th character is to be added to each code from category W36:
A   Initial encounter
D   Subsequent encounter
S   Sequela

W36.1xx- Explosion and rupture of aerosol can
W36.2xx- Explosion and rupture of air tank
W36.3xx- Explosion and rupture of pressurized-gas tank
W36.8xx- Explosion and rupture of other gas cylinder
W36.9xx- Explosion and rupture of unspecified gas cylinder

W37- Explosion and rupture of pressurized tire, pipe or hose
The appropriate 7th character is to be added to each code from category W37:
A   Initial encounter
D   Subsequent encounter
S   Sequela

W37.0xx- Explosion of bicycle tire
W37.8xx- Explosion and rupture of other pressurized tire, pipe or hose

W38.xxx- Explosion and rupture of other specified pressurized devices
The appropriate 7th character is to be added to code W38
A   Initial encounter
D   Subsequent encounter
S   Sequela

W39.xxx- Discharge of firework
The appropriate 7th character is to be added to code W39
A   Initial encounter
D   Subsequent encounter
S   Sequela

W40- Explosion of other materials
Excludes 1:   assault by explosive material (X96)
explosion involving legal intervention (Y35.1-)
explosion involving military or war operations (Y36.0-, Y36.2-)
intentional self-harm by explosive material (X75)

The appropriate 7th character is to be added to each code from category W40:
A   Initial encounter
D   Subsequent encounter
S   Sequela

W40.0xx- Explosion of blasting material
Explosion of blasting cap
Explosion of detonator
Explosion of dynamite
Explosion of explosive (any) used in blasting operations

W40.1xx- Explosion of explosive gases
Explosion of acetylene
Explosion of butane
Explosion of coal gas
Explosion in mine NOS
Explosion of explosive gas
Explosion of fire damp
Explosion of gasoline fumes
Explosion of methane
Explosion of propane

W40.8xx- Explosion of other specified explosive materials
Explosion in dump NOS
Explosion in factory NOS
Explosion in grain store
Explosion in munitions
Excludes 1:   explosion involving legal intervention (Y35.1-)
explosion involving military or war operations (Y36.0-, Y36.2-)

W40.9xx- Explosion of unspecified explosive materials
Explosion NOS

W42- Exposure to noise
The appropriate 7th character is to be added to each code from category W42:
A   Initial encounter
D   Subsequent encounter
S   Sequela

W42.0xx- Exposure to supersonic waves
W42.9xx- Exposure to other noise
Exposure to sound waves NOS

W33 – W42

W45- <u>Foreign body or object</u> <u>entering through skin</u>
Includes: Foreign body or object embedded in skin
              Nail embedded in skin
Excludes ❷: *contact with hand tools (nonpowered) (powered) (W27-W29)*
              contact with other sharp object(s) (W26.-)
              contact with sharp glass (W25.-)
              struck by objects (W20-W22)

The appropriate 7th character is to be added to each code from category
     W45:
  A   <u>Initial</u> encounter
  D   <u>Subsequent</u> encounter
  S   <u>Sequela</u>

W45.0xx- Nail entering through skin

W45.8xx- Other foreign body or object entering through skin
              Splinter in skin NOS

W46- Contact <u>with</u> <u>hypodermic needle</u>
The appropriate 7th character is to be added to each code from category
     W46:
  A   <u>Initial</u> encounter
  D   <u>Subsequent</u> encounter
  S   <u>Sequela</u>

W46.0xx- Contact with hypodermic needle
              Hypodermic needle stick NOS

W46.1xx- Contact with contaminated hypodermic needle

W49- Exposure to other inanimate mechanical forces
Includes: Exposure to abnormal gravitational [G] forces
              Exposure to inanimate mechanical forces NEC
Excludes 1: *exposure to inanimate mechanical forces involving military or*
              war operations (Y36.-, Y37.-)

The appropriate 7th character is to be added to each code from category
     W49:
  A   <u>Initial</u> encounter
  D   <u>Subsequent</u> encounter
  S   <u>Sequela</u>

W49.0- Item causing external constriction
  W49.01x- Hair causing external constriction
  W49.02x- String or thread causing external constriction
  W49.03x- Rubber band causing external constriction
  W49.04x- Ring or other jewelry causing external constriction
  W49.09x- Other specified item causing external constriction

W49.9xx- Exposure to other inanimate mechanical forces

Exposure to animate mechanical forces (W50-W64)

Excludes 1: *toxic effect of contact with venomous animals and plants*
              (T63.-)

W50- <u>Accidental</u> hit, strike, kick, twist, bite or scratch by <u>another person</u>
Includes: Hit, strike, kick, twist, bite, or scratch by another person NOS
Excludes 1: *assault by bodily force (Y04)*
              struck by objects (W20-W22)

The appropriate 7th character is to be added to each code from category
     W50:
  A   <u>Initial</u> encounter
  D   <u>Subsequent</u> encounter
  S   <u>Sequela</u>

W50.0xx- Accidental hit or strike by another person
              Hit or strike by another person NOS

W50.1xx- Accidental kick by another person
              Kick by another person NOS

W50.2xx- Accidental twist by another person
              AHA 15:1Q:p7 – Brother twisted his right elbow
              Twist by another person NOS

W50.3xx- Accidental bite by another person
              Human bite
              Bite by another person NOS

W50.4xx- Accidental scratch by another person
              Scratch by another person NOS

W51.xxx- <u>Accidental</u> striking against or bumped into by <u>another person</u>
Excludes 1: *assault by striking against or bumping into by another*
              person (Y04.2)
              fall due to collision with another person (W03)
The appropriate 7th character is to be added to code W51:
  A   <u>Initial</u> encounter
  D   <u>Subsequent</u> encounter
  S   <u>Sequela</u>

W52.xxx- <u>Crushed</u>, pushed or stepped on <u>by crowd or human stampede</u>
              Crushed, pushed or stepped on by crowd or human stampede with
              or without fall
The appropriate 7th character is to be added to code W52:
  A   <u>Initial</u> encounter
  D   <u>Subsequent</u> encounter
  S   <u>Sequela</u>

W53- Contact <u>with</u> <u>rodent</u>
Includes: Contact with saliva, feces or urine of rodent
The appropriate 7th character is to be added to each code from category
     W53:
  A   <u>Initial</u> encounter
  D   <u>Subsequent</u> encounter
  S   <u>Sequela</u>

W53.0- Contact with <u>mouse</u>
  W53.01x- Bitten by mouse
  W53.09x- Other contact with mouse

W53.1- Contact with <u>rat</u>
  W53.11x- Bitten by rat
  W53.19x- Other contact with rat

W53.2- Contact with <u>squirrel</u>
  W53.21x- Bitten by squirrel
  W53.29x- Other contact with squirrel

W53.8- Contact with <u>other</u> rodent
  W53.81x- Bitten by other rodent
  W53.89x- Other contact with other rodent

W54- Contact <u>with</u> <u>dog</u>
Includes: Contact with saliva, feces or urine of dog
The appropriate 7th character is to be added to each code from category
     W54:
  A   <u>Initial</u> encounter
  D   <u>Subsequent</u> encounter
  S   <u>Sequela</u>

W54.0xx- Bitten by dog

W54.1xx- Struck by dog
              Knocked over by dog

W54.8xx- Other contact with dog

W55- Contact <u>with</u> <u>other mammals</u>
Includes: Contact with saliva, feces or urine of mammal
Excludes 1: *animal being ridden- see transport accidents*
              bitten or struck by dog (W54)
              bitten or struck by rodent (W53.-)
              contact with marine mammals (W56.-)

The appropriate 7th character is to be added to each code from category
     W55:
  A   <u>Initial</u> encounter
  D   <u>Subsequent</u> encounter
  S   <u>Sequela</u>

W55.0- Contact with <u>cat</u>
  W55.01x- Bitten by cat
  W55.03x- Scratched by cat
  W55.09x- Other contact with cat

W55.1- Contact with <u>horse</u>
  W55.11x- Bitten by horse
  W55.12x- Struck by horse
  W55.19x- Other contact with horse

W55.2- Contact with <u>cow</u>
              Contact with bull
  W55.21x- Bitten by cow
  W55.22x- Struck by cow
              Gored by bull
  W55.29x- Other contact with cow

W45 | W55

Excludes 1: = NOT CODED HERE! (Do not code both)   **1275**   *Excludes ❷:* = Not Included Here

W55.3- Contact with <u>other hoof stock</u>
 Contact with goats
 Contact with sheep
  W55.31x- Bitten by other hoof stock
  W55.32x- Struck by other hoof stock
 Gored by goat
 Gored by ram
  W55.39x- Other contact with other hoof stock

W55.4- Contact with <u>pig</u>
  W55.41x- Bitten by pig
  W55.42x- Struck by pig
  W55.49x- Other contact with pig

W55.5- Contact with <u>raccoon</u>
  W55.51x- Bitten by raccoon
  W55.52x- Struck by raccoon
  W55.59x- Other contact with raccoon

W55.8- Contact with <u>other mammals</u>
  W55.81x- Bitten by other mammals
  W55.82x- Struck by other mammals
  W55.89x- Other contact with other mammals

W56- Contact with <u>nonvenomous marine animal</u>
  Excludes 1:   *contact with venomous marine animal (T63.-)*
  The appropriate 7th character is to be added to each code from category
 W56:
  A <u>Initial</u> encounter
  D <u>Subsequent</u> encounter
  S <u>Sequela</u>

W56.0- Contact with <u>dolphin</u>
  W56.01x- Bitten by dolphin
  W56.02x- Struck by dolphin
  W56.09x- Other contact with dolphin

W56.1- Contact with <u>sea lion</u>
  W56.11x- Bitten by sea lion
  W56.12x- Struck by sea lion
  W56.19x- Other contact with sea lion

W56.2- Contact with <u>orca</u>
 Contact with killer whale
  W56.21x- Bitten by orca
  W56.22x- Struck by orca
  W56.29x- Other contact with orca

W56.3- Contact with <u>other marine mammals</u>
  W56.31x- Bitten by other marine mammals
  W56.32x- Struck by other marine mammals
  W56.39x- Other contact with other marine mammals

W56.4- Contact with <u>shark</u>
  W56.41x- Bitten by shark
  W56.42x- Struck by shark
  W56.49x- Other contact with shark

W56.5- Contact with <u>other fish</u>
  W56.51x- Bitten by other fish
  W56.52x- Struck by other fish
  W56.59x- Other contact with other fish

W56.8- Contact with <u>other nonvenomous marine animals</u>
  W56.81x- Bitten by other nonvenomous marine animals
  W56.82x- Struck by other nonvenomous marine animals
  W56.89x- Other contact with other nonvenomous marine animals

W57.xxx- <u>Bitten or stung</u> by <u>nonvenomous insect and other</u>
 <u>nonvenomous arthropods</u>
  Excludes 1:   *contact with venomous insects and arthropods (T63.2-,*
 T63.3-, T63.4-)
  The appropriate 7th character is to be added to code W57:
  A <u>Initial</u> encounter
  D <u>Subsequent</u> encounter
  S <u>Sequela</u>

W58- <u>Contact with</u> <u>crocodile or alligator</u>
  The appropriate 7th character is to be added to each code from category
 W58:
  A <u>Initial</u> encounter
  D <u>Subsequent</u> encounter
  S <u>Sequela</u>

W58.0- Contact with <u>alligator</u>
  W58.01x- Bitten by alligator
  W58.02x- Struck by alligator
  W58.03x- Crushed by alligator
  W58.09x- Other contact with alligator

W58.1- Contact with <u>crocodile</u>
  W58.11x- Bitten by crocodile
  W58.12x- Struck by crocodile
  W58.13x- Crushed by crocodile
  W58.19x- Other contact with crocodile

W59- Contact with <u>other nonvenomous reptiles</u>
  Excludes 1:   *contact with venomous reptile (T63.0-, T63.1-)*
  The appropriate 7th character is to be added to each code from category
 W59:
  A <u>Initial</u> encounter
  D <u>Subsequent</u> encounter
  S <u>Sequela</u>

W59.0- Contact with <u>nonvenomous lizards</u>
  W59.01x- Bitten by nonvenomous lizards
  W59.02x- Struck by nonvenomous lizards
  W59.09x- Other contact with nonvenomous lizards
 Exposure to nonvenomous lizards

W59.1- Contact with <u>nonvenomous snakes</u>
  W59.11x- Bitten by nonvenomous snake
  W59.12x- Struck by nonvenomous snake
  W59.13x- Crushed by nonvenomous snake
  W59.19x- Other contact with nonvenomous snake

W59.2- Contact with <u>turtles</u>
  Excludes 1:   *contact with tortoises (W59.8-)*
  W59.21x- Bitten by turtle
  W59.22x- Struck by turtle
  W59.29x- Other contact with turtle
 Exposure to turtles

W59.8- Contact with <u>other nonvenomous reptiles</u>
  W59.81x- Bitten by other nonvenomous reptiles
  W59.82x- Struck by other nonvenomous reptiles
  W59.83x- Crushed by other nonvenomous reptiles
  W59.89x- Other contact with other nonvenomous reptiles

W60.xxx- Contact with <u>nonvenomous plant thorns and spines and sharp</u>
 <u>leaves</u>
  Excludes 1:   *contact with venomous plants (T63.7-)*
  The appropriate 7th character is to be added to code W60
  A <u>Initial</u> encounter
  D <u>Subsequent</u> encounter
  S <u>Sequela</u>

W61- Contact with <u>birds (domestic) (wild)</u>
  Includes: Contact with excreta of birds
  The appropriate 7th character is to be added to each code from category
 W61:
  A <u>Initial</u> encounter
  D <u>Subsequent</u> encounter
  S <u>Sequela</u>

W61.0- Contact with <u>parrot</u>
  W61.01x- Bitten by parrot
  W61.02x- Struck by parrot
  W61.09x- Other contact with parrot
 Exposure to parrots

W 5 5 - W 6 1

W61.1- Contact with <u>macaw</u>
  W61.11x- Bitten by macaw
  W61.12x- Struck by macaw
  W61.19x- Other contact with macaw
    Exposure to macaws
W61.2- Contact with <u>other psittacines</u>
  W61.21x- Bitten by other psittacines
  W61.22x- Struck by other psittacines
  W61.29x- Other contact with other psittacines
    Exposure to other psittacines
W61.3- Contact with <u>chicken</u>
  W61.32x- Struck by chicken
  W61.33x- Pecked by chicken
  W61.39x- Other contact with chicken
    Exposure to chickens
W61.4- Contact with <u>turkey</u>
  W61.42x- Struck by turkey
  W61.43x- Pecked by turkey
  W61.49x- Other contact with turkey
W61.5- Contact with <u>goose</u>
  W61.51x- Bitten by goose
  W61.52x- Struck by goose
  W61.59x- Other contact with goose
W61.6- Contact with <u>duck</u>
  W61.61x- Bitten by duck
  W61.62x- Struck by duck
  W61.69x- Other contact with duck
W61.9- Contact with <u>other birds</u>
  W61.91x- Bitten by other birds
  W61.92x- Struck by other birds
  W61.99x- Other contact with other birds
    Contact with bird NOS

W62- Contact with <u>nonvenomous amphibians</u>
  Excludes 1:   contact with venomous amphibians (T63.81-R63.83)
  The appropriate 7th character is to be added to each code from category
    W62:
    A <u>Initial</u> encounter
    D <u>Subsequent</u> encounter
    S <u>Sequela</u>
W62.0xx- Contact with nonvenomous frogs
W62.1xx- Contact with nonvenomous toads
W62.9xx- Contact with other nonvenomous amphibians

W64.xxx- <u>Exposure to other animate mechanical forces</u>
  Includes: Exposure to nonvenomous animal NOS
  Excludes 1:   contact with venomous animal (T63.-)
  The appropriate 7th character is to be added to code W64:
    A <u>Initial</u> encounter
    D <u>Subsequent</u> encounter
    S <u>Sequela</u>

Accidental non-transport drowning and submersion (W65-W74)

Excludes 1:   accidental drowning and submersion due to fall into water (W16.-)
    accidental drowning and submersion due to water transport accident (V90.-, V92.-)
Excludes ❷: accidental drowning and submersion due to cataclysm (X34-X39)

W65.xxx- <u>Accidental drowning and submersion while in bath-tub</u>
  Excludes 1:   accidental drowning and submersion due to fall in (into) bathtub (W16.211)
  The appropriate 7th character is to be added to code W65:
    A <u>Initial</u> encounter
    D <u>Subsequent</u> encounter
    S <u>Sequela</u>

W67.xxx- <u>Accidental drowning and submersion while in swimming-pool</u>
  Excludes 1:   accidental drowning and submersion due to fall into swimming pool (W16.011, W16.021, W16.031)
    accidental drowning and submersion due to striking into wall of swimming pool (W22.041)
  The appropriate 7th character is to be added to code W67:
    A <u>Initial</u> encounter
    D <u>Subsequent</u> encounter
    S <u>Sequela</u>

W69.xxx- <u>Accidental drowning and submersion while in natural water</u>
  Accidental drowning and submersion while in lake
  Accidental drowning and submersion while in open sea
  Accidental drowning and submersion while in river
  Accidental drowning and submersion while in stream
  Excludes 1:   accidental drowning and submersion due to fall into natural body of water (W16.111, W16.121, W16.131)
  The appropriate 7th character is to be added to code W69:
    A <u>Initial</u> encounter
    D <u>Subsequent</u> encounter
    S <u>Sequela</u>

W73.xxx- <u>Other specified cause of accidental non-transport drowning and submersion</u>
  Accidental drowning and submersion while in quenching tank
  Accidental drowning and submersion while in reservoir
  Excludes 1:   accidental drowning and submersion due to fall into other water (W16.311, W16.321, W16.331)
  The appropriate 7th character is to be added to code W73:
    A <u>Initial</u> encounter
    D <u>Subsequent</u> encounter
    S <u>Sequela</u>

W74.xxx- <u>Unspecified cause of accidental drowning and submersion</u>
  Drowning NOS
  The appropriate 7th character is to be added to code W74:
    A <u>Initial</u> encounter
    D <u>Subsequent</u> encounter
    S <u>Sequela</u>

Exposure to electric current, radiation and extreme ambient air temperature and pressure (W85-W99)

Excludes 1:   exposure to:
      lightning (T75.0-)
      natural cold (X31)
      natural heat (X30)
      natural radiation NOS (X39)
      radiological procedure and radiotherapy (Y84.2)
      sunlight (X32)
      failure in dosage of radiation or temperature during surgical and medical care (Y63.2-Y63.5)

W85.xxx- <u>Exposure to electric transmission lines</u>
  Broken power line
  The appropriate 7th character is to be added to code W85:
    A <u>Initial</u> encounter
    D <u>Subsequent</u> encounter
    S <u>Sequela</u>

W61
I
W85

W86- Exposure to other specified electric current
The appropriate 7th character is to be added to each code from category W86:
- A   Initial encounter
- D   Subsequent encounter
- S   Sequela

W86.0xx- Exposure to domestic wiring and appliances

W86.1xx- Exposure to industrial wiring, appliances and electrical machinery
Exposure to conductors
Exposure to control apparatus
Exposure to electrical equipment and machinery
Exposure to transformers

W86.8xx- Exposure to other electric current
Exposure to wiring and appliances in or on farm (not farmhouse)
Exposure to wiring and appliances outdoors
Exposure to wiring and appliances in or on public building
Exposure to wiring and appliances in or on residential institutions
Exposure to wiring and appliances in or on schools

W88- Exposure to ionizing radiation
Excludes 1:   exposure to sunlight (X32)
The appropriate 7th character is to be added to each code from category W88:
- A   Initial encounter
- D   Subsequent encounter
- S   Sequela

W88.0xx- Exposure to X-rays

W88.1xx- Exposure to radioactive isotopes

W88.8xx- Exposure to other ionizing radiation

W89- Exposure to man-made visible and ultraviolet light
Includes: Exposure to welding light (arc)
Excludes 1:   exposure to sunlight (X32)
The appropriate 7th character is to be added to each code from category W89:
- A   Initial encounter
- D   Subsequent encounter
- S   Sequela

W89.0xx- Exposure to welding light (arc)

W89.1xx- Exposure to tanning bed

W89.8xx- Exposure to other man-made visible and ultraviolet light

W89.9xx- Exposure to unspecified man-made visible and ultraviolet light

W90- Exposure to other nonionizing radiation
Excludes 1:   exposure to sunlight (X32)
The appropriate 7th character is to be added to each code from category W90:
- A   Initial encounter
- D   Subsequent encounter
- S   Sequela

W90.0xx- Exposure to radiofrequency

W90.1xx- Exposure to infrared radiation

W90.2xx- Exposure to laser radiation

W90.8xx- Exposure to other nonionizing radiation

W92.xxx- Exposure to excessive heat of man-made origin
The appropriate 7th character is to be added to code W92:
- A   Initial encounter
- D   Subsequent encounter
- S   Sequela

W93- Exposure to excessive cold of man-made origin
The appropriate 7th character is to be added to each code from category W93:
- A   Initial encounter
- D   Subsequent encounter
- S   Sequela

W93.0- Contact with or inhalation of dry ice

W93.01x- Contact with dry ice

W93.02x- Inhalation of dry ice

W93.1- Contact with or inhalation of liquid air

W93.11x- Contact with liquid air
Contact with liquid hydrogen
Contact with liquid nitrogen

W93.12x- Inhalation of liquid air
Inhalation of liquid hydrogen
Inhalation of liquid nitrogen

W93.2xx- Prolonged exposure in deep freeze unit or refrigerator

W93.8xx- Exposure to other excessive cold of man-made origin

W94- Exposure to high and low air pressure and changes in air pressure
The appropriate 7th character is to be added to each code from category W94:
- A   Initial encounter
- D   Subsequent encounter
- S   Sequela

W94.0xx- Exposure to prolonged high air pressure

W94.1- Exposure to prolonged low air pressure

W94.11x- Exposure to residence or prolonged visit at high altitude

W94.12x- Exposure to other prolonged low air pressure

W94.2- Exposure to rapid changes in air pressure during ascent

W94.21x- Exposure to reduction in atmospheric pressure while surfacing from deep-water diving

W94.22x- Exposure to reduction in atmospheric pressure while surfacing from underground

W94.23x- Exposure to sudden change in air pressure in aircraft during ascent

W94.29x- Exposure to other rapid changes in air pressure during ascent

W94.3- Exposure to rapid changes in air pressure during descent

W94.31x- Exposure to sudden change in air pressure in aircraft during descent

W94.32x- Exposure to high air pressure from rapid descent in water

W94.39x- Exposure to other rapid changes in air pressure during descent

W99.xxx- Exposure to other man-made environmental factors
The appropriate 7th character is to be added to code W99:
- A   Initial encounter
- D   Subsequent encounter
- S   Sequela

Exposure to smoke, fire and flames (X00-X08)

Excludes 1:   arson (X97)
Excludes ❷: explosions (W35-W40)
lightning (T75.0-)
transport accident (V01-V99)

X00- Exposure to uncontrolled fire in building or structure
Includes: Conflagration in building or structure
Code first any associated cataclysm
Excludes ❷: exposure to ignition or melting of nightwear (X05)
exposure to ignition or melting of other clothing and apparel (X06.-)
exposure to other specified smoke, fire and flames (X08.-)
The appropriate 7th character is to be added to each code from category X00:
- A   Initial encounter
- D   Subsequent encounter
- S   Sequela

X00.0xx- Exposure to flames in uncontrolled fire in building or structure

X00.1xx- Exposure to smoke in uncontrolled fire in building or structure

X00.2xx- Injury due to collapse of burning building or structure in uncontrolled fire
Excludes 1:   injury due to collapse of building not on fire (W20.1)

X00.3xx- Fall from burning building or structure in uncontrolled fire

X00.4xx- Hit by object from burning building or structure in uncontrolled fire

X00.5xx- Jump from burning building or structure in uncontrolled fire

X00.8xx- Other exposure to uncontrolled fire in building or structure

W86
I
X00

© 2016 Channel Publishing, Ltd.

X01- Exposure to <u>uncontrolled fire</u>, <u>not in</u> building or structure
Includes: Exposure to forest fire

The appropriate 7th character is to be added to each code from category X01:
   A   <u>Initial</u> encounter
   D   <u>Subsequent</u> encounter
   S   <u>Sequela</u>

X01.0xx-   Exposure to <u>flames</u> in uncontrolled fire, not in building or structure
X01.1xx-   Exposure to <u>smoke</u> in uncontrolled fire, not in building or structure
X01.3xx-   <u>Fall</u> due to uncontrolled fire, not in building or structure
X01.4xx-   <u>Hit</u> by object due to uncontrolled fire, not in building or structure
X01.8xx-   <u>Other</u> exposure to uncontrolled fire, not in building or structure

X02- Exposure to <u>controlled fire</u> in <u>building or structure</u>
Includes: Exposure to fire in fireplace
            Exposure to fire in stove

The appropriate 7th character is to be added to each code from category X02:
   A   <u>Initial</u> encounter
   D   <u>Subsequent</u> encounter
   S   <u>Sequela</u>

X02.0xx-   Exposure to <u>flames</u> in controlled fire in building or structure
X02.1xx-   Exposure to <u>smoke</u> in controlled fire in building or structure
X02.2xx-   Injury due to <u>collapse</u> of burning building or structure in controlled fire
   Excludes 1:   injury due to collapse of building not on fire (W20.1)
X02.3xx-   <u>Fall</u> from burning building or structure in controlled fire
X02.4xx-   <u>Hit by object</u> from burning building or structure in controlled fire
X02.5xx-   <u>Jump</u> from burning building or structure in controlled fire
X02.8xx-   <u>Other</u> exposure to controlled fire in building or structure

X03- Exposure to <u>controlled fire</u>, <u>not in</u> building or structure
Includes: Exposure to bon fire
            Exposure to camp-fire
            Exposure to trash fire

The appropriate 7th character is to be added to each code from category X03:
   A   <u>Initial</u> encounter
   D   <u>Subsequent</u> encounter
   S   <u>Sequela</u>

X03.0xx-   Exposure to <u>flames</u> in controlled fire, not in building or structure
X03.1xx-   Exposure to <u>smoke</u> in controlled fire, not in building or structure
X03.3xx-   <u>Fall</u> due to controlled fire, not in building or structure
X03.4xx-   <u>Hit by object</u> due to controlled fire, not in building or structure
X03.8xx-   <u>Other</u> exposure to controlled fire, not in building or structure

X04.xxx- Exposure to ignition of highly flammable material
Includes: Exposure to ignition of gasoline
            Exposure to ignition of kerosene
            Exposure to ignition of petrol
Excludes ❷: exposure to ignition or melting of nightwear (X05)
             exposure to ignition or melting of other clothing and apparel (X06)

The appropriate 7th character is to be added to code X04:
   A   <u>Initial</u> encounter
   D   <u>Subsequent</u> encounter
   S   <u>Sequela</u>

X05.xxx- Exposure to <u>ignition or melting of nightwear</u>
Excludes ❷: exposure to uncontrolled fire in building or structure (X00.-)
             exposure to uncontrolled fire, not in building or structure (X01.-)
             exposure to controlled fire in building or structure (X02.-)
             exposure to controlled fire, not in building or structure (X03.-)
             exposure to ignition of highly flammable materials (X04.-)

The appropriate 7th character is to be added to code X05:
   A   <u>Initial</u> encounter
   D   <u>Subsequent</u> encounter
   S   <u>Sequela</u>

X06- Exposure to <u>ignition or melting of other clothing and apparel</u>
Excludes ❷: exposure to uncontrolled fire in building or structure (X00.-)
             exposure to uncontrolled fire, not in building or structure (X01.-)
             exposure to controlled fire in building or structure (X02.-)
             exposure to controlled fire, not in building or structure (X03.-)
             exposure to ignition of highly flammable materials (X04.-)

The appropriate 7th character is to be added to each code from category X06:
   A   <u>Initial</u> encounter
   D   <u>Subsequent</u> encounter
   S   <u>Sequela</u>

X06.0xx-   Exposure to ignition of plastic jewelry
X06.1xx-   Exposure to melting of plastic jewelry
X06.2xx-   Exposure to ignition of other clothing and apparel
X06.3xx-   Exposure to melting of other clothing and apparel

X08- Exposure to <u>other specified smoke, fire and flames</u>
The appropriate 7th character is to be added to each code from category X08:
   A   <u>Initial</u> encounter
   D   <u>Subsequent</u> encounter
   S   <u>Sequela</u>

X08.0-   Exposure to <u>bed fire</u>
            Exposure to mattress fire
X08.00x-   Exposure to bed fire due to unspecified burning material
X08.01x-   Exposure to bed fire due to burning cigarette
X08.09x-   Exposure to bed fire due to other burning material
X08.1-   Exposure to <u>sofa fire</u>
X08.10x-   Exposure to sofa fire due to unspecified burning material
X08.11x-   Exposure to sofa fire due to burning cigarette
X08.19x-   Exposure to sofa fire due to other burning material
X08.2-   Exposure to <u>other furniture fire</u>
X08.20x-   Exposure to other furniture fire due to unspecified burning material
X08.21x-   Exposure to other furniture fire due to burning cigarette
X08.29x-   Exposure to other furniture fire due to other burning material
X08.8xx-   Exposure to <u>other specified smoke, fire and flames</u>

Contact with heat and hot substances (X10-X19)

Excludes 1:   exposure to excessive natural heat (X30)
             exposure to fire and flames (X00-X09)

X10- Contact with <u>hot drinks, food, fats and cooking oils</u>
The appropriate 7th character is to be added to each code from category X10:
   A   <u>Initial</u> encounter
   D   <u>Subsequent</u> encounter
   S   <u>Sequela</u>

X10.0xx-   Contact with hot drinks
X10.1xx-   Contact with hot food
X10.2xx-   Contact with fats and cooking oils

X01 - X10

X11-   Contact with hot tap-water
  Includes: Contact with boiling tap-water
                   Contact with boiling water NOS
  Excludes 1:   contact with water heated on stove (X12)

  The appropriate 7th character is to be added to each code from category
         X11:
         A   Initial encounter
         D   Subsequent encounter
         S   Sequela

X11.0xx-   Contact with hot water in bath or tub
         Excludes 1:   contact with running hot water in bath or tub (X11.1)

X11.1xx-   Contact with running hot water
                   Contact with hot water running out of hose
                   Contact with hot water running out of tap

X11.8xx-   Contact with other hot tap-water
                   Contact with hot water in bucket
                   Contact with hot tap-water NOS

X12.xxx-   Contact with other hot fluids
                   Contact with water heated on stove
         Excludes 1:   hot (liquid) metals (X18)

  The appropriate 7th character is to be added to code X12:
         A   Initial encounter
         D   Subsequent encounter
         S   Sequela

X13-   Contact with steam and other hot vapors
  The appropriate 7th character is to be added to each code from category
         X13:
         A   Initial encounter
         D   Subsequent encounter
         S   Sequela

X13.0xx-   Inhalation of steam and other hot vapors

X13.1xx-   Other contact with steam and other hot vapors

X14-   Contact with hot air and other hot gases
  The appropriate 7th character is to be added to each code from category
         X14:
         A   Initial encounter
         D   Subsequent encounter
         S   Sequela

X14.0xx-   Inhalation of hot air and gases

X14.1xx-   Other contact with hot air and other hot gases

X15-   Contact with hot household appliances
  Excludes 1:   contact with heating appliances (X16)
                   contact with powered household appliances (W29.-)
                   exposure to controlled fire in building or structure due to
                      household appliance (X02.8)
                   exposure to household appliances electrical current (W86.0)

  The appropriate 7th character is to be added to each code from category
         X15:
         A   Initial encounter
         D   Subsequent encounter
         S   Sequela

X15.0xx-   Contact with hot stove (kitchen)

X15.1xx-   Contact with hot toaster

X15.2xx-   Contact with hotplate

X15.3xx-   Contact with hot saucepan or skillet

X15.8xx-   Contact with other hot household appliances
                   Contact with cooker
                   Contact with kettle
                   Contact with light bulbs

X16.xxx-   Contact with hot heating appliances, radiators and pipes
         Excludes 1:   contact with powered appliances (W29.-)
                   exposure to controlled fire in building or structure due
                      to appliance (X02.8)
                   exposure to industrial appliances electrical current
                      (W86.1)

  The appropriate 7th character is to be added to code X16:
         A   Initial encounter
         D   Subsequent encounter
         S   Sequela

X17.xxx-   Contact with hot engines, machinery and tools
         Excludes 1:   contact with hot heating appliances, radiators and pipes
                      (X16)
                   contact with hot household appliances (X15)

  The appropriate 7th character is to be added to code X17:
         A   Initial encounter
         D   Subsequent encounter
         S   Sequela

X18.xxx-   Contact with other hot metals
                   Contact with liquid metal

  The appropriate 7th character is to be added to code X18:
         A   Initial encounter
         D   Subsequent encounter
         S   Sequela

X19.xxx-   Contact with other heat and hot substances
         Excludes 1:   objects that are not normally hot, e.g., an object made
                      hot by a house fire (X00-X09)

  The appropriate 7th character is to be added to code X19:
         A   Initial encounter
         D   Subsequent encounter
         S   Sequela

Exposure to forces of nature (X30-X39)

X30.xxx-   Exposure to excessive natural heat
                   Exposure to excessive heat as the cause of sunstroke
                   Exposure to heat NOS
         Excludes 1:   excessive heat of man-made origin (W92)
                   exposure to man-made radiation (W89)
                   exposure to sunlight (X32)
                   exposure to tanning bed (W89)

  The appropriate 7th character is to be added to code X30:
         A   Initial encounter
         D   Subsequent encounter
         S   Sequela

X31.xxx-   Exposure to excessive natural cold
                   Excessive cold as the cause of chilblains NOS
                   Excessive cold as the cause of immersion foot or hand
                   Exposure to cold NOS
                   Exposure to weather conditions
         Excludes 1:   cold of man-made origin (W93.-)
                   contact with or inhalation of dry ice (W93.-)
                   contact with or inhalation of liquefied gas (W93.-)

  The appropriate 7th character is to be added to code X31:
         A   Initial encounter
         D   Subsequent encounter
         S   Sequela

X32.xxx-   Exposure to sunlight
         Excludes 1:   man-made radiation (tanning bed) (W89)

  The appropriate 7th character is to be added to code X32:
         A   Initial encounter
         D   Subsequent encounter
         S   Sequela

X34.xxx-   Earthquake
         Excludes ❷: tidal wave (tsunami) due to earthquake (X37.41)

  The appropriate 7th character is to be added to code X34:
         A   Initial encounter
         D   Subsequent encounter
         S   Sequela

X35.xxx-   Volcanic eruption
         Excludes ❷: tidal wave (tsunami) due to volcanic eruption (X37.41)

  The appropriate 7th character is to be added to code X35:
         A   Initial encounter
         D   Subsequent encounter
         S   Sequela

X11-X35

X36- Avalanche, landslide and other earth movements
Includes: Victim of mudslide of cataclysmic nature
Excludes 1: *earthquake (X34)*
Excludes ❷: *transport accident involving collision with avalanche or landslide not in motion (V01-V99)*

The appropriate 7th character is to be added to each code from category X36:
A **Initial** encounter
D **Subsequent** encounter
S **Sequela**

X36.0xx- Collapse of dam or man-made structure causing earth movement
X36.1xx- Avalanche, landslide, or mudslide

X37- Cataclysmic storm
The appropriate 7th character is to be added to each code from category X37:
A **Initial** encounter
D **Subsequent** encounter
S **Sequela**

X37.0xx- Hurricane
Storm surge
Typhoon
X37.1xx- Tornado
Cyclone
Twister
X37.2xx- Blizzard (snow) (ice)
X37.3xx- Dust storm
X37.4- Tidalwave
X37.41x- Tidal wave due to earthquake or volcanic eruption
Tidal wave NOS
Tsunami
X37.42x- Tidal wave due to storm
X37.43x- Tidal wave due to landslide
X37.8xx- Other cataclysmic storms
Cloudburst
Torrential rain
Excludes ❷: *flood (X38)*
X37.9xx- Unspecified cataclysmic storm
Storm NOS
Excludes 1: *collapse of dam or man-made structure causing earth movement (X39.0)*

X38.xxx- Flood
Flood arising from remote storm
Flood of cataclysmic nature arising from melting snow
Flood resulting directly from storm
Excludes 1: *collapse of dam or man-made structure causing earth movement (X39.0)*
tidal wave NOS (X37.41)
tidal wave caused by storm (X37.2)

The appropriate 7th character is to be added to code X38:
A **Initial** encounter
D **Subsequent** encounter
S **Sequela**

X39- Exposure to other forces of nature
The appropriate 7th character is to be added to each code from category X39:
A **Initial** encounter
D **Subsequent** encounter
S **Sequela**

X39.0- Exposure to natural radiation
Excludes 1: *contact with and (suspected) exposure to radon and other naturally occuring radiation (Z77.123)*
exposure to man-made radiation (W88-W90)
exposure to sunlight (X32)
X39.01x- Exposure to radon
X39.08x- Exposure to other natural radiation
X39.8xx- Other exposure to forces of nature

Overexertion and strenuous or repetitive movements (X50)

X50- Overexertion and strenuous or repetitive movement or load
The appropriate 7th character is to be added to each code from category X50:
A **Initial** encounter
D **Subsequent** encounter
S **Sequela**

X50.0xx- Overexertion from strenuous movements
Lifting heavy objects
Lifting weights
X50.1xx- Overexertion from prolonged static or awkward postures
Prolonged bending
Prolonged kneeling
Prolonged reaching
Prolonged sitting
Prolonged standing
Prolonged twisting
Static bending
Static kneeling
Static reaching
Static sitting
Static standing
Static twisting
X50.3xx- Overexertion from repetitive movements
Use of hand as hammer
Excludes ❷: *overuse from prolonged static or awkward postures (X50.1)*
X50.9xx- Other and unspecified overexertion or strenuous movements or postures
Contact pressure
Contact stress

Accidental exposure to other specified factors (X52-X58)

X52.xxx- Prolonged stay in weightless environment
Weightlessness in spacecraft (simulator)
The appropriate 7th character is to be added to code X52:
A **Initial** encounter
D **Subsequent** encounter
S **Sequela**

X58.xxx- Exposure to other specified factors
Accident NOS
Exposure NOS
The appropriate 7th character is to be added to code X58:
A **Initial** encounter
D **Subsequent** encounter
S **Sequela**

Intentional self-harm (X71-X83)

Purposely self-inflicted injury
Suicide (attempted)

X71- Intentional self-harm by drowning and submersion
The appropriate 7th character is to be added to each code from category X71:
A **Initial** encounter
D **Subsequent** encounter
S **Sequela**

X71.0xx- Intentional self-harm by drowning and submersion while in bathtub
X71.1xx- Intentional self-harm by drowning and submersion while in swimming pool
X71.2xx- Intentional self-harm by drowning and submersion after jump into swimming pool
X71.3xx- Intentional self-harm by drowning and submersion in natural water
X71.8xx- Other intentional self-harm by drowning and submersion
X71.9xx- Intentional self-harm by drowning and submersion, unspecified

X
3
6
|
X
7
1

X72.xxx- Intentional self-harm by handgun discharge
Intentional self-harm by gun for single hand use
Intentional self-harm by pistol
Intentional self-harm by revolver
Excludes 1:   Very pistol (X74.8)
The appropriate 7th character is to be added to code X72:
- A   **Initial** encounter
- D   **Subsequent** encounter
- S   **Sequela**

X73- Intentional self-harm by rifle, shotgun and larger firearm discharge
Excludes 1:   airgun (X74.01)
The appropriate 7th character is to be added to each code from category X73:
- A   **Initial** encounter
- D   **Subsequent** encounter
- S   **Sequela**

X73.0xx- Intentional self-harm by shotgun discharge

X73.1xx- Intentional self-harm by hunting rifle discharge

X73.2xx- Intentional self-harm by machine gun discharge

X73.8xx- Intentional self-harm by other larger firearm discharge

X73.9xx- Intentional self-harm by unspecified larger firearm discharge

X74- Intentional self-harm by other and unspecified firearm and gun discharge
The appropriate 7th character is to be added to each code from category X74:
- A   **Initial** encounter
- D   **Subsequent** encounter
- S   **Sequela**

X74.0- Intentional self-harm by gas, air or spring-operated guns

X74.01x- Intentional self-harm by airgun
Intentional self-harm by BB gun discharge
Intentional self-harm by pellet gun discharge

X74.02x- Intentional self-harm by paintball gun

X74.09x- Intentional self-harm by other gas, air or spring-operated gun

X74.8xx- Intentional self-harm by other firearm discharge
Intentional self-harm by Very pistol [flare] discharge

X74.9xx- Intentional self-harm by unspecified firearm discharge

X75.xxx- Intentional self-harm by explosive material
The appropriate 7th character is to be added to code X75:
- A   **Initial** encounter
- D   **Subsequent** encounter
- S   **Sequela**

X76.xxx- Intentional self-harm by smoke, fire and flames
The appropriate 7th character is to be added to code X76:
- A   **Initial** encounter
- D   **Subsequent** encounter
- S   **Sequela**

X77- Intentional self-harm by steam, hot vapors and hot objects
The appropriate 7th character is to be added to each code from category X77:
- A   **Initial** encounter
- D   **Subsequent** encounter
- S   **Sequela**

X77.0xx- Intentional self-harm by steam or hot vapors

X77.1xx- Intentional self-harm by hot tap water

X77.2xx- Intentional self-harm by other hot fluids

X77.3xx- Intentional self-harm by hot household appliances

X77.8xx- Intentional self-harm by other hot objects

X77.9xx- Intentional self-harm by unspecified hot objects

X78- Intentional self-harm by sharp object
The appropriate 7th character is to be added to each code from category X78:
- A   **Initial** encounter
- D   **Subsequent** encounter
- S   **Sequela**

X78.0xx- Intentional self-harm by sharp glass

X78.1xx- Intentional self-harm by knife

X78.2xx- Intentional self-harm by sword or dagger

X78.8xx- Intentional self-harm by other sharp object

X78.9xx- Intentional self-harm by unspecified sharp object

X79.xxx- Intentional self-harm by blunt object
The appropriate 7th character is to be added to code X79:
- A   **Initial** encounter
- D   **Subsequent** encounter
- S   **Sequela**

X80.xxx- Intentional self-harm by jumping from a high place
Intentional fall from one level to another
The appropriate 7th character is to be added to code X80:
- A   **Initial** encounter
- D   **Subsequent** encounter
- S   **Sequela**

X81- Intentional self-harm by jumping or lying in front of moving object
The appropriate 7th character is to be added to each code from category X81:
- A   **Initial** encounter
- D   **Subsequent** encounter
- S   **Sequela**

X81.0xx- Intentional self-harm by jumping or lying in front of motor vehicle

X81.1xx- Intentional self-harm by jumping or lying in front of (subway) train

X81.8xx- Intentional self-harm by jumping or lying in front of other moving object

X82- Intentional self-harm by crashing of motor vehicle
The appropriate 7th character is to be added to each code from category X82:
- A   **Initial** encounter
- D   **Subsequent** encounter
- S   **Sequela**

X82.0xx- Intentional collision of motor vehicle with other motor vehicle

X82.1xx- Intentional collision of motor vehicle with train

X82.2xx- Intentional collision of motor vehicle with tree

X82.8xx- Other intentional self-harm by crashing of motor vehicle

X83- Intentional self-harm by other specified means
Excludes 1:   intentional self-harm by poisoning or contact with toxic substance — see Table of Drugs and Chemicals
The appropriate 7th character is to be added to each code from category X83:
- A   **Initial** encounter
- D   **Subsequent** encounter
- S   **Sequela**

X83.0xx- Intentional self-harm by crashing of aircraft

X83.1xx- Intentional self-harm by electrocution

X83.2xx- Intentional self-harm by exposure to extremes of cold

X83.8xx- Intentional self-harm by other specified means

Assault (X92-Y09)

Includes: Homicide
Injuries inflicted by another person with intent to injure or kill, by any means
Excludes 1:   injuries due to legal intervention (Y35.-)
injuries due to operations of war (Y36.-)
injuries due to terrorism (Y38.-)

X92- Assault by drowning and submersion
The appropriate 7th character is to be added to each code from category X92:
- A   **Initial** encounter
- D   **Subsequent** encounter
- S   **Sequela**

X92.0xx- Assault by drowning and submersion while in bathtub

X92.1xx- Assault by drowning and submersion while in swimming pool

X92.2xx- Assault by drowning and submersion after push into swimming pool

X92.3xx- Assault by drowning and submersion in natural water

X92.8xx- Other assault by drowning and submersion

X92.9xx- Assault by drowning and submersion, unspecified

X72-X92

X93.xxx-   Assault by **handgun discharge**
       Assault by discharge of gun for single hand use
       Assault by discharge of pistol
       Assault by discharge of revolver
       Excludes 1:   *Very pistol (X95.8)*
       The appropriate 7th character is to be added to code X93:
          A   Initial encounter
          D   Subsequent encounter
          S   Sequela

X94-   Assault by **rifle, shotgun and larger firearm discharge**
       Excludes 1:   *airgun (X95.01)*
       The appropriate 7th character is to be added to each code from category X94:
          A   Initial encounter
          D   Subsequent encounter
          S   Sequela

X94.0xx-   Assault by shotgun
X94.1xx-   Assault by hunting rifle
X94.2xx-   Assault by machine gun
X94.8xx-   Assault by other larger firearm discharge
X94.9xx-   Assault by unspecified larger firearm discharge

X95-   Assault by **other and unspecified firearm and gun discharge**
       The appropriate 7th character is to be added to each code from category X95:
          A   Initial encounter
          D   Subsequent encounter
          S   Sequela

X95.0-   Assault by gas, air or spring-operated guns
   X95.01x-   Assault by airgun discharge
          Assault by BB gun discharge
          Assault by pellet gun discharge
   X95.02x-   Assault by paintball gun discharge
   X95.09x-   Assault by other gas, air or spring-operated gun
X95.8xx-   Assault by other firearm discharge
          Assault by Very pistol [flare] discharge
X95.9xx-   Assault by unspecified firearm discharge

X96-   Assault by **explosive material**
       Excludes 1:   *incendiary device (X97)*
                   terrorism involving explosive material (Y38.2-)
       The appropriate 7th character is to be added to each code from category X96:
          A   Initial encounter
          D   Subsequent encounter
          S   Sequela

X96.0xx-   Assault by antipersonnel bomb
       Excludes 1:   *antipersonnel bomb use in military or war (Y36.2-)*
X96.1xx-   Assault by gasoline bomb
X96.2xx-   Assault by letter bomb
X96.3xx-   Assault by fertilizer bomb
X96.4xx-   Assault by pipe bomb
X96.8xx-   Assault by other specified explosive
X96.9xx-   Assault by unspecified explosive

X97.xxx-   Assault by **smoke, fire and flames**
       Assault by arson
       Assault by cigarettes
       Assault by incendiary device
       The appropriate 7th character is to be added to code X97:
          A   Initial encounter
          D   Subsequent encounter
          S   Sequela

X98-   Assault by **steam, hot vapors and hot objects**
       The appropriate 7th character is to be added to each code from category X98:
          A   Initial encounter
          D   Subsequent encounter
          S   Sequela

X98.0xx-   Assault by steam or hot vapors
X98.1xx-   Assault by hot tap water
X98.2xx-   Assault by hot fluids
X98.3xx-   Assault by hot household appliances

X98.8xx-   Assault by other hot objects
X98.9xx-   Assault by unspecified hot objects

X99-   Assault by **sharp object**
       Excludes 1:   *assault by strike by sports equipment (Y08.0-)*
       The appropriate 7th character is to be added to each code from category X99:
          A   Initial encounter
          D   Subsequent encounter
          S   Sequela

X99.0xx-   Assault by sharp glass
X99.1xx-   Assault by knife
X99.2xx-   Assault by sword or dagger
X99.8xx-   Assault by other sharp object
X99.9xx-   Assault by unspecified sharp object
       Assault by stabbing NOS

Y00.xxx-   Assault by **blunt object**
       Excludes 1:   *assault by strike by sports equipment (Y08.0-)*
       The appropriate 7th character is to be added to code Y00:
          A   Initial encounter
          D   Subsequent encounter
          S   Sequela

Y01.xxx-   Assault by **pushing from high place**
       The appropriate 7th character is to be added to code Y01:
          A   Initial encounter
          D   Subsequent encounter
          S   Sequela

Y02-   Assault by **pushing or placing victim in front of moving object**
       The appropriate 7th character is to be added to each code from category Y02:
          A   Initial encounter
          D   Subsequent encounter
          S   Sequela

Y02.0xx-   Assault by pushing or placing victim in front of motor vehicle
Y02.1xx-   Assault by pushing or placing victim in front of (subway) train
Y02.8xx-   Assault by pushing or placing victim in front of other moving object

Y03-   Assault by **crashing of motor vehicle**
       The appropriate 7th character is to be added to each code from category Y03:
          A   Initial encounter
          D   Subsequent encounter
          S   Sequela

Y03.0xx-   Assault by being hit or run over by motor vehicle
Y03.8xx-   Other assault by crashing of motor vehicle

Y04-   Assault by **bodily force**
       Excludes 1:   *assault by:*
                 submersion (X92.-)
                 use of weapon (X93-X95, X99, Y00)
       The appropriate 7th character is to be added to each code from category Y04:
          A   Initial encounter
          D   Subsequent encounter
          S   Sequela

Y04.0xx-   Assault by unarmed brawl or fight
Y04.1xx-   Assault by human bite
Y04.2xx-   Assault by strike against or bumped into by another person
Y04.8xx-   Assault by other bodily force
       Assault by bodily force NOS

X93 | Y04

Y07- **Perpetrator** of <u>assault, maltreatment and neglect</u>
Note: Codes from this category are for use only in cases of confirmed abuse (T74-)
Note: Selection of the correct perpetrator code is based on the relationship between the perpetrator and the victim
Includes: Perpetrator of abandonment
Perpetrator of emotional neglect
Perpetrator of mental cruelty
Perpetrator of physical abuse
Perpetrator of physical neglect
Perpetrator of sexual abuse
Perpetrator of torture

Y07.0- <u>Spouse or partner</u>, perpetrator of maltreatment and neglect
Spouse or partner, perpetrator of maltreatment and neglect against spouse or partner

Y07.01 Husband, perpetrator of maltreatment and neglect

Y07.02 Wife, perpetrator of maltreatment and neglect

Y07.03 Male partner, perpetrator of maltreatment and neglect

Y07.04 Female partner, perpetrator of maltreatment and neglect

Y07.1- <u>Parent</u> (adoptive) (biological), perpetrator of maltreatment and neglect

Y07.11 Biological father, perpetrator of maltreatment and neglect

Y07.12 Biological mother, perpetrator of maltreatment and neglect

Y07.13 Adoptive father, perpetrator of maltreatment and neglect

Y07.14 Adoptive mother, perpetrator of maltreatment and neglect

Y07.4- <u>Other family member</u>, perpetrator of maltreatment and neglect

Y07.41- <u>Sibling</u>, perpetrator of maltreatment and neglect
Excludes 1:   stepsibling, perpetrator of maltreatment and neglect (Y07.435, Y07.436)

Y07.410 Brother, perpetrator of maltreatment and neglect

Y07.411 Sister, perpetrator of maltreatment and neglect

Y07.42- Foster parent, perpetrator of maltreatment and neglect

Y07.420 Foster father, perpetrator of maltreatment and neglect

Y07.421 Foster mother, perpetrator of maltreatment and neglect

Y07.43- <u>Stepparent or stepsibling</u>, perpetrator of maltreatment and neglect

Y07.430 Stepfather, perpetrator of maltreatment and neglect

Y07.432 Male friend of parent (co-residing in household), perpetrator of maltreatment and neglect

Y07.433 Stepmother, perpetrator of maltreatment and neglect

Y07.434 Female friend of parent (co-residing in household), perpetrator of maltreatment and neglect

Y07.435 Stepbrother, perpetrator or maltreatment and neglect

Y07.436 Stepsister, perpetrator of maltreatment and neglect

Y07.49- <u>Other family member</u>, perpetrator of maltreatment and neglect

Y07.490 Male cousin, perpetrator of maltreatment and neglect

Y07.491 Female cousin, perpetrator of maltreatment and neglect

Y07.499 Other family member, perpetrator of maltreatment and neglect

Y07.5- <u>Non-family member</u>, perpetrator of maltreatment and neglect

Y07.50 <u>Unspecified</u> non-family member, perpetrator of maltreatment and neglect

Y07.51- <u>Daycare provider</u>, perpetrator of maltreatment and neglect

Y07.510 At-home childcare provider, perpetrator of maltreatment and neglect

Y07.511 Daycare center childcare provider, perpetrator of maltreatment and neglect

Y07.512 At-home adultcare provider, perpetrator of maltreatment and neglect

Y07.513 Adultcare center provider, perpetrator of maltreatment and neglect

Y07.519 Unspecified daycare provider, perpetrator of maltreatment and neglect

Y07.52- <u>Healthcare provider</u>, perpetrator of maltreatment and neglect

Y07.521 Mental health provider, perpetrator of maltreatment and neglect

Y07.528 Other therapist or healthcare provider, perpetrator of maltreatment and neglect
Nurse perpetrator of maltreatment and neglect
Occupational therapist perpetrator of maltreatment and neglect
Physical therapist perpetrator of maltreatment and neglect
Speech therapist perpetrator of maltreatment and neglect

Y07.529 Unspecified healthcare provider, perpetrator of maltreatment and neglect

Y07.53 <u>Teacher or instructor</u>, perpetrator of maltreatment and neglect
Coach, perpetrator of maltreatment and neglect

Y07.59 <u>Other non-family</u> member, perpetrator of maltreatment and neglect

Y07.9 Unspecified perpetrator of maltreatment and neglect

Y08- <u>Assault</u> by <u>other specified means</u>
The appropriate 7th character is to be added to each code from category Y08:
A   <u>Initial</u> encounter
D   <u>Subsequent</u> encounter
S   <u>Sequela</u>

Y08.0- Assault by strike by sport equipment

Y08.01x- Assault by strike by hockey stick

Y08.02x- Assault by strike by baseball bat

Y08.09x- Assault by strike by other specified type of sport equipment

Y08.8- Assault by other specified means

Y08.81x- Assault by crashing of aircraft

Y08.89x- Assault by other specified means

Y09 Assault by unspecified means
Assassination (attempted) NOS
Homicide (attempted) NOS
Manslaughter (attempted) NOS
Murder (attempted) NOS

Event of undetermined intent (Y21-Y33)

Note: Undetermined intent is only for use when there is specific documentation in the record that the intent of the injury cannot be determined. If no such documentation is present, code to accidental (unintentional).

Y21- Drowning and submersion, <u>undetermined intent</u>
The appropriate 7th character is to be added to each code from category Y21:
A   <u>Initial</u> encounter
D   <u>Subsequent</u> encounter
S   <u>Sequela</u>

Y21.0xx- Drowning and submersion while in bathtub, undetermined intent

Y21.1xx- Drowning and submersion after fall into bathtub, undetermined intent

Y21.2xx- Drowning and submersion while in swimming pool, undetermined intent

Y21.3xx- Drowning and submersion after fall into swimming pool, undetermined intent

Y21.4xx- Drowning and submersion in natural water, undetermined intent

Y21.8xx- Other drowning and submersion, undetermined intent

Y21.9xx- Unspecified drowning and submersion, undetermined intent

Y07 - Y21

Y22.xxx-   Handgun discharge, <u>undetermined intent</u>
- Discharge of gun for single hand use, undetermined intent
- Discharge of pistol, undetermined intent
- Discharge of revolver, undetermined intent

Excludes ➋: Very pistol (Y24.8)

The appropriate 7th character is to be added to code Y22:
- **A**   <u>Initial</u> encounter
- **D**   <u>Subsequent</u> encounter
- **S**   <u>Sequela</u>

Y23-   Rifle, shotgun and larger firearm discharge, <u>undetermined intent</u>

Excludes ➋: airgun (Y24.0)

The appropriate 7th character is to be added to each code from category Y23:
- **A**   <u>Initial</u> encounter
- **D**   <u>Subsequent</u> encounter
- **S**   <u>Sequela</u>

Y23.0xx-   Shotgun discharge, undetermined intent

Y23.1xx-   Hunting rifle discharge, undetermined intent

Y23.2xx-   Military firearm discharge, undetermined intent

Y23.3xx-   Machine gun discharge, undetermined intent

Y23.8xx-   Other larger firearm discharge, undetermined intent

Y23.9xx-   Unspecified larger firearm discharge, undetermined intent

Y24-   Other and unspecified firearm discharge, <u>undetermined intent</u>

The appropriate 7th character is to be added to each code from category Y24:
- **A**   <u>Initial</u> encounter
- **D**   <u>Subsequent</u> encounter
- **S**   <u>Sequela</u>

Y24.0xx-   Airgun discharge, undetermined intent
- BB gun discharge, undetermined intent
- Pellet gun discharge, undetermined intent

Y24.8xx-   Other firearm discharge, undetermined intent
- Paintball gun discharge, undetermined intent
- Very pistol [flare] discharge, undetermined intent

Y24.9xx-   Unspecified firearm discharge, undetermined intent

Y25.xxx-   Contact with explosive material, <u>undetermined intent</u>

The appropriate 7th character is to be added to code Y25:
- **A**   <u>Initial</u> encounter
- **D**   <u>Subsequent</u> encounter
- **S**   <u>Sequela</u>

Y26.xxx-   Exposure to smoke, fire and flames, <u>undetermined intent</u>

The appropriate 7th character is to be added to code Y26:
- **A**   <u>Initial</u> encounter
- **D**   <u>Subsequent</u> encounter
- **S**   <u>Sequela</u>

Y27-   Contact with steam, hot vapors and hot objects, <u>undetermined intent</u>

The appropriate 7th character is to be added to each code from category Y27:
- **A**   <u>Initial</u> encounter
- **D**   <u>Subsequent</u> encounter
- **S**   <u>Sequela</u>

Y27.0xx-   Contact with steam and hot vapors, undetermined intent

Y27.1xx-   Contact with hot tap water, undetermined intent

Y27.2xx-   Contact with hot fluids, undetermined intent

Y27.3xx-   Contact with hot household appliance, undetermined intent

Y27.8xx-   Contact with other hot objects, undetermined intent

Y27.9xx-   Contact with unspecified hot objects, undetermined intent

Y28-   Contact with sharp object, <u>undetermined intent</u>

The appropriate 7th character is to be added to each code from category Y28:
- **A**   <u>Initial</u> encounter
- **D**   <u>Subsequent</u> encounter
- **S**   <u>Sequela</u>

Y28.0xx-   Contact with sharp glass, undetermined intent

Y28.1xx-   Contact with knife, undetermined intent

Y28.2xx-   Contact with sword or dagger, undetermined intent

Y28.8xx-   Contact with other sharp object, undetermined intent

Y28.9xx-   Contact with unspecified sharp object, undetermined intent

---

Y29.xxx-   Contact with blunt object, <u>undetermined intent</u>

The appropriate 7th character is to be added to code Y29:
- **A**   <u>Initial</u> encounter
- **D**   <u>Subsequent</u> encounter
- **S**   <u>Sequela</u>

Y30.xxx-   Falling, jumping or pushed from a high place, <u>undetermined intent</u>
- Victim falling from one level to another, undetermined intent

The appropriate 7th character is to be added to code Y30:
- **A**   <u>Initial</u> encounter
- **D**   <u>Subsequent</u> encounter
- **S**   <u>Sequela</u>

Y31.xxx-   Falling, lying or running before or into moving object, <u>undetermined intent</u>

The appropriate 7th character is to be added to code Y31:
- **A**   <u>Initial</u> encounter
- **D**   <u>Subsequent</u> encounter
- **S**   <u>Sequela</u>

Y32.xxx-   Crashing of motor vehicle, <u>undetermined intent</u>

The appropriate 7th character is to be added to code Y32:
- **A**   <u>Initial</u> encounter
- **D**   <u>Subsequent</u> encounter
- **S**   <u>Sequela</u>

Y33.xxx-   Other specified events, <u>undetermined intent</u>

The appropriate 7th character is to be added to code Y33:
- **A**   <u>Initial</u> encounter
- **D**   <u>Subsequent</u> encounter
- **S**   <u>Sequela</u>

Legal intervention, operations of war, military operations, and terrorism (Y35-Y38)

Y35-   <u>Legal intervention</u>

Includes: Any injury sustained as a result of an encounter with any law enforcement official, serving in any capacity at the time of the encounter, whether on-duty or off-duty. Includes: injury to law enforcement official, suspect and bystander

The appropriate 7th character is to be added to code Y35:
- **A**   <u>Initial</u> encounter
- **D**   <u>Subsequent</u> encounter
- **S**   <u>Sequela</u>

Y35.0-   Legal intervention involving <u>firearm discharge</u>

Y35.00-   Legal intervention involving unspecified firearm discharge
- Legal intervention involving gunshot wound
- Legal intervention involving shot NOS

Y35.001-   Legal intervention involving <u>unspecified firearm</u> discharge, <u>law enforcement official injured</u>

Y35.002-   Legal intervention involving unspecified firearm discharge, <u>bystander</u> injured

Y35.003-   Legal intervention involving unspecified firearm discharge, <u>suspect</u> injured

Y35.01-   Legal intervention involving injury by <u>machine gun</u>

Y35.011-   Legal intervention involving injury by machine gun, <u>law enforcement official injured</u>

Y35.012-   Legal intervention involving injury by machine gun, <u>bystander</u> injured

Y35.013-   Legal intervention involving injury by machine gun, <u>suspect</u> injured

Y35.02-   Legal intervention involving injury by <u>handgun</u>

Y35.021-   Legal intervention involving injury by handgun, <u>law enforcement official injured</u>

Y35.022-   Legal intervention involving injury by handgun, <u>bystander</u> injured

Y35.023-   Legal intervention involving injury by handgun, <u>suspect</u> injured

Y35.03-   Legal intervention involving injury by <u>rifle pellet</u>

Y35.031-   Legal intervention involving injury by rifle pellet, <u>law enforcement official injured</u>

Y35.032-   Legal intervention involving injury by rifle pellet, <u>bystander</u> injured

Y22-Y35

Y35.033- Legal intervention involving injury by rifle pellet, <u>suspect</u> injured

Y35.04- Legal intervention involving injury by <u>rubber bullet</u>

Y35.041- Legal intervention involving injury by rubber bullet, <u>law enforcement official injured</u>

Y35.042- Legal intervention involving injury by rubber bullet, <u>bystander</u> injured

Y35.043- Legal intervention involving injury by rubber bullet, <u>suspect</u> injured

Y35.09- Legal intervention involving <u>other firearm discharge</u>

Y35.091- Legal intervention involving other firearm discharge, <u>law enforcement official injured</u>

Y35.092- Legal intervention involving other firearm discharge, <u>bystander</u> injured

Y35.093- Legal intervention involving other firearm discharge, <u>suspect</u> injured

Y35.1- Legal intervention involving <u>explosives</u>

Y35.10- Legal intervention involving unspecified explosives

Y35.101- Legal intervention involving unspecified explosives, <u>law enforcement official injured</u>

Y35.102- Legal intervention involving unspecified explosives, <u>bystander</u> injured

Y35.103- Legal intervention involving unspecified explosives, <u>suspect</u> injured

Y35.11- Legal intervention involving injury by <u>dynamite</u>

Y35.111- Legal intervention involving injury by dynamite, law <u>enforcement official injured</u>

Y35.112- Legal intervention involving injury by dynamite, <u>bystander</u> injured

Y35.113- Legal intervention involving injury by dynamite, <u>suspect</u> injured

Y35.12- Legal intervention involving injury by <u>explosive shell</u>

Y35.121- Legal intervention involving injury by explosive shell, <u>law enforcement official injured</u>

Y35.122- Legal intervention involving injury by explosive shell, <u>bystander</u> injured

Y35.123- Legal intervention involving injury by explosive shell, <u>suspect</u> injured

Y35.19- Legal intervention involving <u>other explosives</u>
Legal intervention involving injury by grenade
Legal intervention involving injury by mortar bomb

Y35.191- Legal intervention involving other explosives, <u>law enforcement official injured</u>

Y35.192- Legal intervention involving other explosives, <u>bystander</u> injured

Y35.193- Legal intervention involving other explosives, <u>suspect</u> injured

Y35.2- Legal intervention involving <u>gas</u>
Legal intervention involving asphyxiation by gas
Legal intervention involving poisoning by gas

Y35.20- Legal intervention involving <u>unspecified</u> gas

Y35.201- Legal intervention involving unspecified gas, <u>law enforcement official injured</u>

Y35.202- Legal intervention involving unspecified gas, <u>bystander</u> injured

Y35.203- Legal intervention involving unspecified gas, <u>suspect</u> injured

Y35.21- Legal intervention involving injury by <u>tear gas</u>

Y35.211- Legal intervention involving injury by tear gas, <u>law enforcement official injured</u>

Y35.212- Legal intervention involving injury by tear gas, <u>bystander</u> injured

Y35.213- Legal intervention involving injury by tear gas, <u>suspect</u> injured

Y35.29- Legal intervention involving <u>other gas</u>

Y35.291- Legal intervention involving other gas, <u>law enforcement official injured</u>

Y35.292- Legal intervention involving other gas, <u>bystander</u> injured

Y35.293- Legal intervention involving other gas, <u>suspect</u> injured

Y35.3- Legal intervention involving <u>blunt objects</u>
Legal intervention involving being hit or struck by blunt object

Y35.30- Legal intervention involving <u>unspecified</u> blunt objects

Y35.301- Legal intervention involving unspecified blunt objects, <u>law enforcement official injured</u>

Y35.302- Legal intervention involving unspecified blunt objects, <u>bystander</u> injured

Y35.303- Legal intervention involving unspecified blunt objects, <u>suspect</u> injured

Y35.31- Legal intervention involving <u>baton</u>

Y35.311- Legal intervention involving baton, <u>law enforcement official injured</u>

Y35.312- Legal intervention involving baton, <u>bystander</u> injured

Y35.313- Legal intervention involving baton, <u>suspect</u> injured

Y35.39- Legal intervention involving <u>other blunt objects</u>

Y35.391- Legal intervention involving other blunt objects, <u>law enforcement official injured</u>

Y35.392- Legal intervention involving other blunt objects, <u>bystander</u> injured

Y35.393- Legal intervention involving other blunt objects, <u>suspect</u> injured

Y35.4- Legal intervention involving <u>sharp objects</u>
Legal intervention involving being cut by sharp objects
Legal intervention involving being stabbed by sharp objects

Y35.40- Legal intervention involving <u>unspecified</u> sharp objects

Y35.401- Legal intervention involving unspecified sharp objects, <u>law enforcement official injured</u>

Y35.402- Legal intervention involving unspecified sharp objects, <u>bystander</u> injured

Y35.403- Legal intervention involving unspecified sharp objects, <u>suspect</u> injured

Y35.41- Legal intervention involving <u>bayonet</u>

Y35.411- Legal intervention involving bayonet, <u>law enforcement official injured</u>

Y35.412- Legal intervention involving bayonet, <u>bystander</u> injured

Y35.413- Legal intervention involving bayonet, <u>suspect</u> injured

Y35.49- Legal intervention involving <u>other sharp objects</u>

Y35.491- Legal intervention involving other sharp objects, <u>law enforcement official injured</u>

Y35.492- Legal intervention involving other sharp objects, <u>bystander</u> injured

Y35.493- Legal intervention involving other sharp objects, <u>suspect</u> injured

Y35.8- Legal intervention involving <u>other specified means</u>

Y35.81- Legal intervention involving <u>manhandling</u>

Y35.811- Legal intervention involving manhandling, <u>law enforcement official injured</u>

Y35.812- Legal intervention involving manhandling, <u>bystander</u> injured

Y35.813- Legal intervention involving manhandling, <u>suspect</u> injured

Y35.89- Legal intervention involving <u>other specified means</u>

Y35.891- Legal intervention involving other specified means, <u>law enforcement official injured</u>

Y35.892- Legal intervention involving other specified means, <u>bystander</u> injured

Y35.893- Legal intervention involving other specified means, <u>suspect</u> injured

Y35.9- Legal intervention, <u>means unspecified</u>

Y35.91- Legal intervention, means unspecified, <u>law enforcement official injured</u>

Y35.92- Legal intervention, means unspecified, <u>bystander</u> injured

Y35.93- Legal intervention, means unspecified, <u>suspect</u> injured

Y35 - Y35

Excludes 1: = NOT CODED HERE! (Do not code both)   **1286**   *Excludes ❷:* = Not Included Here

Y36- Operations of war
  AHA 14:3Q:p4 – Encounters for treatment of conditions due to war
  Includes: Injuries to military personnel and civilians caused by war, civil
       insurrection, and peacekeeping missions
  *Excludes 1: injury to military personnel occurring during peacetime military
       operations (Y37.-)
       military vehicles involved in transport accidents with non-
       military vehicle during peacetime (V09.01, V09.21,
       V19.81, V29.81, V39.81, V49.81, V59.81, V69.81, V79.81)*

The appropriate 7th character is to be added to each code from category
    Y36:
  A **Initial** encounter
  D **Subsequent** encounter
  S **Sequela**

Y36.0- War operations involving **explosion of marine weapons**
  Y36.00- War operations involving explosion of **unspecified** marine
      weapon
      War operations involving underwater blast NOS
    Y36.000- War operations involving explosion of unspecified
        marine weapon, **military** personnel
    Y36.001- War operations involving explosion of unspecified
        marine weapon, **civilian**
  Y36.01- War operations involving explosion of **depth-charge**
    Y36.010- War operations involving explosion of depth-
        charge, **military** personnel
    Y36.011- War operations involving explosion of depth-
        charge, **civilian**
  Y36.02- War operations involving explosion of **marine mine**
      War operations involving explosion of marine mine, at sea or
      in harbor
    Y36.020- War operations involving explosion of marine
        mine, **military** personnel
    Y36.021- War operations involving explosion of marine
        mine, **civilian**
  Y36.03- War operations involving explosion of **sea-based artillery
      shell**
    Y36.030- War operations involving explosion of sea-based
        artillery shell, **military** personnel
    Y36.031- War operations involving explosion of sea-based
        artillery shell, **civilian**
  Y36.04- War operations involving explosion of **torpedo**
    Y36.040- War operations involving explosion of torpedo,
        military personnel
    Y36.041- War operations involving explosion of torpedo,
        civilian
  Y36.05- War operations involving **accidental detonation of
      onboard marine weapons**
    Y36.050- War operations involving accidental detonation of
        onboard marine weapons, **military** personnel
    Y36.051- War operations involving accidental detonation of
        onboard marine weapons, **civilian**
  Y36.09- War operations involving explosion of **other marine
      weapons**
    Y36.090- War operations involving explosion of other
        marine weapons, **military** personnel
    Y36.091- War operations involving explosion of other
        marine weapons, **civilian**
Y36.1- War operations involving **destruction of aircraft**
  Y36.10- War operations involving **unspecified** destruction of
      aircraft
    Y36.100- War operations involving unspecified destruction
        of aircraft, **military** personnel
    Y36.101- War operations involving unspecified destruction
        of aircraft, **civilian**

Y36.11- War operations involving destruction of aircraft **due to
    enemy fire or explosives**
      War operations involving destruction of aircraft due to air to
      air missile
      War operations involving destruction of aircraft due to
      explosive placed on aircraft
      War operations involving destruction of aircraft due to rocket
      propelled grenade [RPG]
      War operations involving destruction of aircraft due to small
      arms fire
      War operations involving destruction of aircraft due to surface
      to air missile
  Y36.110- War operations involving destruction of aircraft
      due to enemy fire or explosives, **military** personnel
  Y36.111- War operations involving destruction of aircraft
      due to enemy fire or explosives, **civilian**
Y36.12- War operations involving destruction of aircraft **due to
    collision with other aircraft**
  Y36.120- War operations involving destruction of aircraft
      due to collision with other aircraft, **military**
      personnel
  Y36.121- War operations involving destruction of aircraft
      due to collision with other aircraft, **civilian**
Y36.13- War operations involving destruction of aircraft **due to
    onboard fire**
  Y36.130- War operations involving destruction of aircraft
      due to onboard fire, **military** personnel
  Y36.131- War operations involving destruction of aircraft
      due to onboard fire, **civilian**
Y36.14- War operations involving destruction of aircraft due to
    **accidental detonation of onboard munitions and
    explosives**
  Y36.140- War operations involving destruction of aircraft
      due to accidental detonation of onboard munitions
      and explosives, **military** personnel
  Y36.141- War operations involving destruction of aircraft
      due to accidental detonation of onboard munitions
      and explosives, **civilian**
Y36.19- War operations involving **other destruction of aircraft**
  Y36.190- War operations involving other destruction of
      aircraft, **military** personnel
  Y36.191- War operations involving other destruction of
      aircraft, **civilian**
Y36.2- War operations involving **other explosions and fragments**
  *Excludes 1: war operations involving explosion of aircraft (Y36.1-)
      war operations involving explosion of marine weapons
      (Y36.0-)
      war operations involving explosion of nuclear weapons
      (Y36.5-)
      war operations involving explosion occurring after
      cessation of hostilities (Y36.8-)*
  Y36.20- War operations involving **unspecified** explosion and
      fragments
      War operations involving air blast NOS
      War operations involving blast NOS
      War operations involving blast fragments NOS
      War operations involving blast wave NOS
      War operations involving blast wind NOS
      War operations involving explosion NOS
      War operations involving explosion of bomb NOS
    Y36.200- War operations involving unspecified explosion
        and fragments, **military** personnel
    Y36.201- War operations involving unspecified explosion
        and fragments, **civilian**
  Y36.21- War operations involving explosion of **aerial bomb**
    Y36.210- War operations involving explosion of aerial bomb,
        military personnel
    Y36.211- War operations involving explosion of aerial bomb,
        civilian
  Y36.22- War operations involving explosion of **guided missile**
    Y36.220- War operations involving explosion of guided
        missile, **military** personnel
    Y36.221- War operations involving explosion of guided
        missile, **civilian**

Y36 – Y36

Y36.23- <u>War</u> operations involving explosion of <u>improvised explosive device [IED]</u>
    War operations involving explosion of person-borne improvised explosive device [IED]
    War operations involving explosion of vehicle-borne improvised explosive device [IED]
    War operations involving explosion of roadside improvised explosive device [IED]

    Y36.230- <u>War</u> operations involving explosion of improvised explosive device [IED], <u>military</u> personnel

    Y36.231- <u>War</u> operations involving explosion of improvised explosive device [IED], <u>civilian</u>

Y36.24- <u>War</u> operations involving explosion due to <u>accidental detonation and discharge of own munitions or munitions launch device</u>

    Y36.240- <u>War</u> operations involving explosion due to accidental detonation and discharge of own munitions or munitions launch-device, <u>military</u> personnel

    Y36.241- <u>War</u> operations involving explosion due to accidental detonation and discharge of own munitions or munitions launch device, <u>civilian</u>

Y36.25- <u>War</u> operations involving <u>fragments from munitions</u>

    Y36.250- <u>War</u> operations involving fragments from munitions, <u>military</u> personnel

    Y36.251- <u>War</u> operations involving fragments from munitions, <u>civilian</u>

Y36.26 <u>War</u> operations involving fragments of <u>improvised explosive device [IED]</u>
    War operations involving fragments of person-borne improvised explosive device [IED]
    War operations involving fragments of vehicle-borne improvised explosive device [IED]
    War operations involving fragments of roadside improvised explosive device [IED]

    Y36.260- <u>War</u> operations involving fragments of improvised explosive device [IED], <u>military</u> personnel

    Y36.261- <u>War</u> operations involving fragments of improvised explosive device [IED], <u>civilian</u>

Y36.27- <u>War</u> operations involving <u>fragments from weapons</u>

    Y36.270- <u>War</u> operations involving fragments from weapons, <u>military</u> personnel

    Y36.271- <u>War</u> operations involving fragments from weapons, <u>civilian</u>

Y36.29- <u>War</u> operations involving <u>other explosions and fragments</u>
    War operations involving explosion of grenade
    War operations involving explosions of land mine
    War operations involving shrapnel NOS

    Y36.290- <u>War</u> operations involving other explosions and fragments, <u>military</u> personnel

    Y36.291- <u>War</u> operations involving other explosions and fragments, <u>civilian</u>

Y36.3- <u>War</u> operations involving <u>fires, conflagrations and hot substances</u>
    War operations involving smoke, fumes, and heat from fires, conflagrations and hot substances
    Excludes 1: *war operations involving fires and conflagrations aboard military aircraft (Y36.1-)*
           war operations involving fires and conflagrations aboard military watercraft (Y36.0-)
           war operations involving fires and conflagrations caused indirectly by conventional weapons (Y36.2-)
           war operations involving fires and thermal effects of nuclear weapons (Y36.53-)

    Y36.30- <u>War</u> operations involving <u>unspecified</u> fire, conflagration and hot substance

    Y36.300- <u>War</u> operations involving unspecified fire, conflagration and hot substance, <u>military</u> personnel

    Y36.301- <u>War</u> operations involving unspecified fire, conflagration and hot substance, <u>civilian</u>

Y36.31- <u>War</u> operations involving <u>gasoline bomb</u>
    War operations involving incendiary bomb
    War operations involving petrol bomb

    Y36.310- <u>War</u> operations involving gasoline bomb, <u>military</u> personnel

    Y36.311- <u>War</u> operations involving gasoline bomb, <u>civilian</u>

Y36.32- <u>War</u> operations involving <u>incendiary bullet</u>

    Y36.320- <u>War</u> operations involving incendiary bullet, <u>military</u> personnel

    Y36.321- <u>War</u> operations involving incendiary bullet, <u>civilian</u>

Y36.33- <u>War</u> operations involving <u>flamethrower</u>

    Y36.330- <u>War</u> operations involving flamethrower, <u>military</u> personnel

    Y36.331- <u>War</u> operations involving flamethrower, <u>civilian</u>

Y36.39- <u>War</u> operations involving <u>other</u> fires, conflagrations and hot substances

    Y36.390- <u>War</u> operations involving other fires, conflagrations and hot substances, <u>military</u> personnel

    Y36.391- <u>War</u> operations involving other fires, conflagrations and hot substances, <u>civilian</u>

Y36.4- <u>War operations involving firearm discharge and other forms of conventional warfare</u>

    Y36.41- <u>War</u> operations involving <u>rubber bullets</u>

    Y36.410- <u>War</u> operations involving rubber bullets, <u>military</u> personnel

    Y36.411- <u>War</u> operations involving rubber bullets, <u>civilian</u>

    Y36.42- <u>War</u> operations involving <u>firearms pellets</u>

    Y36.420- <u>War</u> operations involving firearms pellets, <u>military</u> personnel

    Y36.421- <u>War</u> operations involving firearms pellets, <u>civilian</u>

    Y36.43- <u>War</u> operations involving <u>other</u> firearms discharge
    War operations involving bullets NOS
    Excludes 1: *war operations involving munitions fragments (Y36.25-)*
           war operations involving incendiary bullets (Y36.32-)

    Y36.430- <u>War</u> operations involving other firearms discharge, <u>military</u> personnel

    Y36.431- <u>War</u> operations involving other firearms discharge, <u>civilian</u>

    Y36.44- <u>War</u> operations involving <u>unarmed hand to hand combat</u>
    Excludes 1: *war operations involving combat using blunt or piercing object (Y36.45-)*
           war operations involving intentional restriction of air and airway (Y36.46-)
           war operations involving unintentional restriction of air and airway (Y36.47-)

    Y36.440- <u>War</u> operations involving unarmed hand to hand combat, <u>military</u> personnel

    Y36.441- <u>War</u> operations involving unarmed hand to hand combat, <u>civilian</u>

    Y36.45- <u>War</u> operations involving combat <u>using blunt or piercing object</u>

    Y36.450- <u>War</u> operations involving combat using blunt or piercing object, <u>military</u> personnel

    Y36.451- <u>War</u> operations involving combat using blunt or piercing object, <u>civilian</u>

    Y36.46- <u>War</u> operations involving <u>intentional restriction of air and airway</u>

    Y36.460- <u>War</u> operations involving intentional restriction of air and airway, <u>military</u> personnel

    Y36.461- <u>War</u> operations involving intentional restriction of air and airway, <u>civilian</u>

    Y36.47- <u>War</u> operations involving <u>unintentional restriction of air and airway</u>

    Y36.470- <u>War</u> operations involving unintentional restriction of air and airway, <u>military</u> personnel

    Y36.471- <u>War</u> operations involving unintentional restriction of air and airway, <u>civilian</u>

Y36 I Y36

Y36.49- **War** operations involving <u>other</u> forms of conventional warfare

     Y36.490- **War** operations involving other forms of conventional warfare, <u>military</u> personnel

     Y36.491- **War** operations involving other forms of conventional warfare, <u>civilian</u>

Y36.5- **War** operations involving <u>nuclear weapons</u>
     War operations involving dirty bomb NOS

Y36.50- **War** operations involving <u>unspecified</u> effect of nuclear weapon

     Y36.500- **War** operations involving unspecified effect of nuclear weapon, <u>military</u> personnel

     Y36.501- **War** operations involving unspecified effect of nuclear weapon, <u>civilian</u>

Y36.51- **War** operations involving <u>direct blast effect</u> of nuclear weapon
     War operations involving blast pressure of nuclear weapon

     Y36.510- **War** operations involving direct blast effect of nuclear weapon, <u>military</u> personnel

     Y36.511- **War** operations involving direct blast effect of nuclear weapon, <u>civilian</u>

Y36.52- **War** operations involving <u>indirect blast effect</u> of nuclear weapon
     War operations involving being thrown by blast of nuclear weapon
     War operations involving being struck or crushed by blast debris of nuclear weapon

     Y36.520- **War** operations involving indirect blast effect of nuclear weapon, <u>military</u> personnel

     Y36.521- **War** operations involving indirect blast effect of nuclear weapon, <u>civilian</u>

Y36.53- **War** operations involving <u>thermal radiation effect</u> of nuclear weapon
     War operations involving direct heat from nuclear weapon
     War operation involving fireball effects from nuclear weapon

     Y36.530- **War** operations involving thermal radiation effect of nuclear weapon, <u>military</u> personnel

     Y36.531- **War** operations involving thermal radiation effect of nuclear weapon, <u>civilian</u>

Y36.54- **War** operation involving <u>nuclear radiation effects</u> of nuclear weapon
     War operation involving acute radiation exposure from nuclear weapon
     War operation involving exposure to immediate ionizing radiation from nuclear weapon
     War operation involving fallout exposure from nuclear weapon
     War operation involving secondary effects of nuclear weapons

     Y36.540- **War** operation involving nuclear radiation effects of nuclear weapon, <u>military</u> personnel

     Y36.541- **War** operation involving nuclear radiation effects of nuclear weapon, <u>civilian</u>

Y36.59- **War** operation involving <u>other</u> effects of nuclear weapons

     Y36.590- **War** operation involving other effects of nuclear weapons, <u>military</u> personnel

     Y36.591- **War** operation involving other effects of nuclear weapons, <u>civilian</u>

Y36.6- **War** operations involving <u>biological weapons</u>

Y36.6x- **War** operations involving biological weapons

     Y36.6x0- **War** operations involving biological weapons, <u>military</u> personnel

     Y36.6x1- **War** operations involving biological weapons, <u>civilian</u>

Y36.7- **War** operations involving <u>chemical weapons and other forms of unconventional warfare</u>
     Excludes 1:   *war operations involving incendiary devices (Y36.3-, Y36.5-)*

Y36.7x- **War** operations involving <u>chemical weapons and other forms of unconventional warfare</u>

     Y36.7x0- **War** operations involving chemical weapons and other forms of unconventional warfare, <u>military</u> personnel

Y36.7x1- **War** operations involving chemical weapons and other forms of unconventional warfare, <u>civilian</u>

Y36.8- **War** operations occurring <u>after cessation of hostilities</u>
     War operations classifiable to categories Y36.0-Y36.8 but occurring after cessation of hostilities

Y36.81- Explosion of <u>mine</u> placed during <u>war</u> operations but <u>exploding after</u> cessation of hostilities

     Y36.810- Explosion of mine placed during <u>war</u> operations but exploding after cessation of hostilities, <u>military</u> personnel

     Y36.811- Explosion of mine placed during <u>war</u> operations but exploding after cessation of hostilities, <u>civilian</u>

Y36.82- Explosion of <u>bomb</u> placed during <u>war</u> operations but <u>exploding after</u> cessation of hostilities

     Y36.820- Explosion of bomb placed during <u>war</u> operations but exploding after cessation of hostilities, <u>military</u> personnel

     Y36.821- Explosion of bomb placed during <u>war</u> operations but exploding after cessation of hostilities, <u>civilian</u>

Y36.88- <u>Other</u> <u>war</u> operations <u>occurring after</u> cessation of hostilities

     Y36.880- Other <u>war</u> operations occurring after cessation of hostilities, <u>military</u> personnel

     Y36.881- Other <u>war</u> operations occurring after cessation of hostilities, <u>civilian</u>

Y36.89- <u>Unspecified</u> <u>war</u> operations <u>occurring after</u> cessation of hostilities

     Y36.890- Unspecified <u>war</u> operations occurring after cessation of hostilities, <u>military</u> personnel

     Y36.891- Unspecified <u>war</u> operations occurring after cessation of hostilities, <u>civilian</u>

Y36.9- Other and unspecified <u>war</u> operations

Y36.90- **War** operations, <u>unspecified</u>

Y36.91- **War** operations involving <u>unspecified weapon of mass destruction [WMD]</u>

Y36.92- **War** operations involving <u>friendly fire</u>

Y37- **Military operations**
   Includes: Injuries to military personnel and civilians <u>occurring during peacetime</u> on military property and <u>during routine military exercises and operations</u>
   Excludes 1:   *military aircraft involved in aircraft accident with civilian aircraft (V97.81-)*
     military vehicles involved in transport accident with civilian vehicle (V09.01, V09.21, V19.81, V29.81, V39.81, V49.81, V59.81, V69.81, V79.81)
     military watercraft involved in water transport accident with civilian watercraft (V94.81-)
     war operations (Y36.-)

The appropriate 7th character is to be added to each code from category Y37:
A   <u>Initial</u> encounter
D   <u>Subsequent</u> encounter
S   <u>Sequela</u>

Y37.0- **Military** operations involving <u>explosion of marine weapons</u>

Y37.00- **Military** operations involving explosion of <u>unspecified</u> marine weapon
     Military operations involving underwater blast NOS

     Y37.000- **Military** operations involving explosion of unspecified marine weapon, <u>military</u> personnel

     Y37.001- **Military** operations involving explosion of unspecified marine weapon, <u>civilian</u>

Y37.01- **Military** operations involving explosion of <u>depth-charge</u>

     Y37.010- **Military** operations involving explosion of depth-charge, <u>military</u> personnel

     Y37.011- **Military** operations involving explosion of depth-charge, <u>civilian</u>

Y37.02- **Military** operations involving explosion of <u>marine mine</u>
     Military operations involving explosion of marine mine, at sea or in harbor

     Y37.020- **Military** operations involving explosion of marine mine, <u>military</u> personnel

Y36 – Y37

Y37.021- Military operations involving explosion of marine mine, <u>civilian</u>

Y37.03- Military operations involving explosion of <u>sea-based artillery shell</u>

Y37.030- Military operations involving explosion of sea-based artillery shell, <u>military</u> personnel

Y37.031- Military operations involving explosion of sea-based artillery shell, <u>civilian</u>

Y37.04- Military operations involving explosion of <u>torpedo</u>

Y37.040- Military operations involving explosion of torpedo, <u>military</u> personnel

Y37.041- Military operations involving explosion of torpedo, <u>civilian</u>

Y37.05- Military operations involving <u>accidental detonation of onboard marine weapons</u>

Y37.050- Military operations involving accidental detonation of onboard marine weapons, <u>military</u> personnel

Y37.051- Military operations involving accidental detonation of onboard marine weapons, <u>civilian</u>

Y37.09- Military operations involving explosion of <u>other marine weapons</u>

Y37.090- Military operations involving explosion of other marine weapons, <u>military</u> personnel

Y37.091- Military operations involving explosion of other marine weapons, <u>civilian</u>

Y37.1- Military operations involving <u>destruction of aircraft</u>

Y37.10- Military operations involving <u>unspecified</u> destruction of aircraft

Y37.100- Military operations involving unspecified destruction of aircraft, <u>military</u> personnel

Y37.101- Military operations involving unspecified destruction of aircraft, <u>civilian</u>

Y37.11- Military operations involving destruction of aircraft <u>due to enemy fire or explosives</u>

Military operations involving destruction of aircraft due to air to air missile

Military operations involving destruction of aircraft due to explosive placed on aircraft

Military operations involving destruction of aircraft due to rocket propelled grenade [RPG]

Military operations involving destruction of aircraft due to small arms fire

Military operations involving destruction of aircraft due to surface to air missile

Y37.110- Military operations involving destruction of aircraft due to enemy fire or explosives, <u>military</u> personnel

Y37.111- Military operations involving destruction of aircraft due to enemy fire or explosives, <u>civilian</u>

Y37.12- Military operations involving destruction of aircraft <u>due to collision with other aircraft</u>

Y37.120- Military operations involving destruction of aircraft due to collision with other aircraft, <u>military</u> personnel

Y37.121- Military operations involving destruction of aircraft due to collision with other aircraft, <u>civilian</u>

Y37.13- Military operations involving destruction of aircraft <u>due to onboard fire</u>

Y37.130- Military operations involving destruction of aircraft due to onboard fire, <u>military</u> personnel

Y37.131- Military operations involving destruction of aircraft due to onboard fire, <u>civilian</u>

Y37.14- Military operations involving destruction of aircraft <u>due to accidental detonation of onboard munitions and explosives</u>

Y37.140- Military operations involving destruction of aircraft due to accidental detonation of onboard munitions and explosives, <u>military</u> personnel

Y37.141- Military operations involving destruction of aircraft due to accidental detonation of onboard munitions and explosives, <u>civilian</u>

Y37.19- Military operations involving <u>other destruction of aircraft</u>

Y37.190- Military operations involving other destruction of aircraft, <u>military</u> personnel

Y37.191- Military operations involving other destruction of aircraft, <u>civilian</u>

Y37.2- Military operations involving <u>other explosions and fragments</u>

Excludes 1: *military operations involving explosion of aircraft (Y37.1-)*
military operations involving explosion of marine weapons (Y37.0-)
military operations involving explosion of nuclear weapons (Y37.5-)

Y37.20- Military operations involving <u>unspecified</u> explosion and fragments

Military operations involving air blast NOS
Military operations involving blast NOS
Military operations involving blast fragments NOS
Military operations involving blast wave NOS
Military operations involving blast wind NOS
Military operations involving explosion NOS
Military operations involving explosion of bomb NOS

Y37.200- Military operations involving unspecified explosion and fragments, <u>military</u> personnel

Y37.201- Military operations involving unspecified explosion and fragments, <u>civilian</u>

Y37.21- Military operations involving explosion of <u>aerial bomb</u>

Y37.210- Military operations involving explosion of aerial bomb, <u>military</u> personnel

Y37.211- Military operations involving explosion of aerial bomb, <u>civilian</u>

Y37.22- Military operations involving explosion of <u>guided missile</u>

Y37.220- Military operations involving explosion of guided missile, <u>military</u> personnel

Y37.221- Military operations involving explosion of guided missile, <u>civilian</u>

Y37.23- Military operations involving explosion of <u>improvised explosive device [IED]</u>

Military operations involving explosion of person-borne improvised explosive device [IED]
Military operations involving explosion of vehicle-borne improvised explosive device [IED]
Military operations involving explosion of roadside improvised explosive device [IED]

Y37.230- Military operations involving explosion of improvised explosive device [IED], <u>military</u> personnel

Y37.231- Military operations involving explosion of improvised explosive device [IED], <u>civilian</u>

Y37.24- Military operations involving explosion due to <u>accidental detonation and discharge of own munitions or munitions launch device</u>

Y37.240- Military operations involving explosion due to accidental detonation and discharge of own munitions or munitions launch device, <u>military</u> personnel

Y37.241- Military operations involving explosion due to accidental detonation and discharge of own munitions or munitions launch device, <u>civilian</u>

Y37.25- Military operations involving <u>fragments from munitions</u>

Y37.250- Military operations involving fragments from munitions, <u>military</u> personnel

Y37.251- Military operations involving fragments from munitions, <u>civilian</u>

Y37.26- Military operations involving <u>fragments of improvised explosive device [IED]</u>

Military operations involving fragments of person-borne improvised explosive device [IED]
Military operations involving fragments of vehicle-borne improvised explosive device [IED]
Military operations involving fragments of roadside improvised explosive device [IED]

Y37.260- Military operations involving fragments of improvised explosive device [IED], <u>military</u> personnel

Y37 - Y37

Y37.261-   Military operations involving fragments of improvised explosive device [IED], <u>civilian</u>

Y37.27-   Military operations involving <u>fragments from weapons</u>

     Y37.270-   Military operations involving fragments from weapons, <u>military</u> personnel

     Y37.271-   Military operations involving fragments from weapons, <u>civilian</u>

Y37.29-   Military operations involving <u>other explosions and fragments</u>
     Military operations involving explosion of grenade
     Military operations involving explosions of land mine
     Military operations involving shrapnel NOS

     Y37.290-   Military operations involving other explosions and fragments, <u>military</u> personnel

     Y37.291-   Military operations involving other explosions and fragments, <u>civilian</u>

Y37.3-   Military operations involving <u>fires, conflagrations and hot substances</u>
     Military operations involving smoke, fumes, and heat from fires, conflagrations and hot substances
     Excludes 1:   *military operations involving fires and conflagrations aboard military aircraft (Y37.1-)*
         military operations involving fires and conflagrations aboard military watercraft (Y37.0-)
         military operations involving fires and conflagrations caused indirectly by conventional weapons (Y37.2-)
         military operations involving fires and thermal effects of nuclear weapons (Y36.53-)

     Y37.30-   Military operations involving <u>unspecified</u> fire, conflagration and hot substance

         Y37.300-   Military operations involving unspecified fire, conflagration and hot substance, <u>military</u> personnel

         Y37.301-   Military operations involving unspecified fire, conflagration and hot substance, <u>civilian</u>

     Y37.31-   Military operations involving <u>gasoline bomb</u>
         Military operations involving incendiary bomb
         Military operations involving petrol bomb

         Y37.310-   Military operations involving gasoline bomb, <u>military</u> personnel

         Y37.311-   Military operations involving gasoline bomb, <u>civilian</u>

     Y37.32-   Military operations involving <u>incendiary bullet</u>

         Y37.320-   Military operations involving incendiary bullet, <u>military</u> personnel

         Y37.321-   Military operations involving incendiary bullet, <u>civilian</u>

     Y37.33-   Military operations involving <u>flamethrower</u>

         Y37.330-   Military operations involving flamethrower, <u>military</u> personnel

         Y37.331-   Military operations involving flamethrower, <u>civilian</u>

     Y37.39-   Military operations involving <u>other</u> fires, conflagrations and hot substances

         Y37.390-   Military operations involving other fires, conflagrations and hot substances, <u>military</u> personnel

         Y37.391-   Military operations involving other fires, conflagrations and hot substances, <u>civilian</u>

Y37.4-   Military operations involving <u>firearm discharge and other forms of conventional warfare</u>

     Y37.41-   Military operations involving <u>rubber bullets</u>

         Y37.410-   Military operations involving rubber bullets, <u>military</u> personnel

         Y37.411-   Military operations involving rubber bullets, <u>civilian</u>

     Y37.42-   Military operations involving <u>firearms pellets</u>

         Y37.420-   Military operations involving firearms pellets, <u>military</u> personnel

         Y37.421-   Military operations involving firearms pellets, <u>civilian</u>

Y37.43-   Military operations involving <u>other</u> firearms discharge
     Military operations involving bullets NOS
     Excludes 1:   *military operations involving munitions fragments (Y37.25-)*
         military operations involving incendiary bullets (Y37.32-)

     Y37.430-   Military operations involving other firearms discharge, <u>military</u> personnel

     Y37.431-   Military operations involving other firearms discharge, <u>civilian</u>

Y37.44-   Military operations <u>involving unarmed hand to hand combat</u>
     Excludes 1:   *military operations involving combat using blunt or piercing object (Y37.45-)*
         military operations involving intentional restriction of air and airway (Y37.46-)
         military operations involving unintentional restriction of air and airway (Y37.47-)

     Y37.440-   Military operations involving unarmed hand to hand combat, <u>military</u> personnel

     Y37.441-   Military operations involving unarmed hand to hand combat, <u>civilian</u>

Y37.45-   Military operations involving <u>combat using blunt or piercing object</u>

     Y37.450-   Military operations involving combat using blunt or piercing object, <u>military</u> personnel

     Y37.451-   Military operations involving combat using blunt or piercing object, <u>civilian</u>

Y37.46-   Military operations involving <u>intentional restriction of air and airway</u>

     Y37.460-   Military operations involving intentional restriction of air and airway, <u>military</u> personnel

     Y37.461-   Military operations involving intentional restriction of air and airway, <u>civilian</u>

Y37.47-   Military operations involving <u>unintentional restriction of air and airway</u>

     Y37.470-   Military operations involving unintentional restriction of air and airway, <u>military</u> personnel

     Y37.471-   Military operations involving unintentional restriction of air and airway, <u>civilian</u>

Y37.49-   Military operations involving <u>other</u> forms of conventional warfare

     Y37.490-   Military operations involving other forms of conventional warfare, <u>military</u> personnel

     Y37.491-   Military operations involving other forms of conventional warfare, <u>civilian</u>

Y37.5-   Military operations involving <u>nuclear weapons</u>
     Military operation involving dirty bomb NOS

     Y37.50-   Military operations involving <u>unspecified</u> effect of nuclear weapon

         Y37.500-   Military operations involving unspecified effect of nuclear weapon, <u>military</u> personnel

         Y37.501-   Military operations involving unspecified effect of nuclear weapon, <u>civilian</u>

     Y37.51-   Military operations involving <u>direct blast effect</u> of nuclear weapon
         Military operations involving blast pressure of nuclear weapon

         Y37.510-   Military operations involving direct blast effect of nuclear weapon, <u>military</u> personnel

         Y37.511-   Military operations involving direct blast effect of nuclear weapon, <u>civilian</u>

     Y37.52-   Military operations involving <u>indirect blast effect</u> of nuclear weapon
         Military operations involving being thrown by blast of nuclear weapon
         Military operations involving being struck or crushed by blast debris of nuclear weapon

         Y37.520-   Military operations involving indirect blast effect of nuclear weapon, <u>military</u> personnel

         Y37.521-   Military operations involving indirect blast effect of nuclear weapon, <u>civilian</u>

Excludes 1: = NOT CODED HERE! (Do not code both)   *Excludes ❷:* = Not Included Here

Y37 - Y37   Y37.Y37

Y37.53- Military operations involving <u>thermal radiation effect</u> of nuclear weapon
> Military operations involving direct heat from nuclear weapon
> Military operation involving fireball effects from nuclear weapon

Y37.530- Military operations involving thermal radiation effect of nuclear weapon, <u>military</u> personnel

Y37.531- Military operations involving thermal radiation effect of nuclear weapon, <u>civilian</u>

Y37.54- Military operation involving <u>nuclear radiation effects</u> of nuclear weapon
> Military operation involving acute radiation exposure from nuclear weapon
> Military operation involving exposure to immediate ionizing radiation from nuclear weapon
> Military operation involving fallout exposure from nuclear weapon
> Military operation involving secondary effects of nuclear weapons

Y37.540- Military operation involving nuclear radiation effects of nuclear weapon, <u>military</u> personnel

Y37.541- Military operation involving nuclear radiation effects of nuclear weapon, <u>civilian</u>

Y37.59- Military operation involving <u>other</u> effects of nuclear weapons

Y37.590- Military operation involving other effects of nuclear weapons, <u>military</u> personnel

Y37.591- Military operation involving other effects of nuclear weapons, <u>civilian</u>

Y37.6- Military operations involving <u>biological weapons</u>

Y37.6x- Military operations involving biological weapons

Y37.6x0- Military operations involving biological weapons, <u>military</u> personnel

Y37.6x1- Military operations involving biological weapons, <u>civilian</u>

Y37.7- Military operations involving <u>chemical weapons and other forms of unconventional warfare</u>
> *Excludes 1:*   *military operations involving incendiary devices (Y36.3-, Y36.5-)*

Y37.7x- Military operations involving <u>chemical weapons</u> and other forms of unconventional warfare

Y37.7x0- Military operations involving chemical weapons and other forms of unconventional warfare, <u>military</u> personnel

Y37.7x1- Military operations involving chemical weapons and other forms of unconventional warfare, <u>civilian</u>

Y37.9- Other and unspecified military operations

Y37.90x- Military operations, <u>unspecified</u>

Y37.91x- Military operations involving <u>unspecified weapon of mass destruction [WMD]</u>

Y37.92x- Military operations involving <u>friendly fire</u>

Y38- <u>Terrorism</u>
Note: These codes are for use to identify injuries resulting from the unlawful use of force or violence against persons or property to intimidate or coerce a Government, the civilian population, or any segment thereof, in furtherance of political or social objective
Use additional code for place of occurrence (Y92.-)
The appropriate 7th character is to be added to each code from category Y38:
> A <u>Initial</u> encounter
> D <u>Subsequent</u> encounter
> S <u>Sequela</u>

Y38.0- Terrorism involving <u>explosion of marine weapons</u>
> Terrorism involving depth-charge
> Terrorism involving marine mine
> Terrorism involving mine NOS, at sea or in harbor
> Terrorism involving sea-based artillery shell
> Terrorism involving torpedo
> Terrorism involving underwater blast

Y38.0x- Terrorism involving explosion of <u>marine weapons</u>

Y38.0x1- Terrorism involving explosion of marine weapons, <u>public safety official</u> injured

Y38.0x2- Terrorism involving explosion of marine weapons, <u>civilian</u> injured

Y38.0x3- Terrorism involving explosion of marine weapons, <u>terrorist</u> injured

Y38.1- Terrorism involving <u>destruction of aircraft</u>
> Terrorism involving aircraft burned
> Terrorism involving aircraft exploded
> Terrorism involving aircraft being shot down
> Terrorism involving aircraft used as a weapon

Y38.1x- Terrorism involving destruction of aircraft

Y38.1x1- Terrorism involving destruction of aircraft, <u>public safety official</u> injured

Y38.1x2- Terrorism involving destruction of aircraft, <u>civilian</u> injured

Y38.1x3- Terrorism involving destruction of aircraft, <u>terrorist</u> injured

Y38.2- Terrorism involving <u>other explosions and fragments</u>
> Terrorism involving antipersonnel (fragments) bomb
> Terrorism involving blast NOS
> Terrorism involving explosion NOS
> Terrorism involving explosion of breech block
> Terrorism involving explosion of cannon block
> Terrorism involving explosion (fragments) of artillery shell
> Terrorism involving explosion (fragments) of bomb
> Terrorism involving explosion (fragments) of grenade
> Terrorism involving explosion (fragments) of guided missile
> Terrorism involving explosion (fragments) of land mine
> Terrorism involving explosion of mortar bomb
> Terrorism involving explosion of munitions
> Terrorism involving explosion (fragments) of rocket
> Terrorism involving explosion (fragments) of shell
> Terrorism involving shrapnel
> Terrorism involving mine NOS, on land
> *Excludes 1:*   *terrorism involving explosion of nuclear weapon (Y38.5)*
> *terrorism involving suicide bomber (Y38.81)*

Y38.2x- Terrorism involving other explosions and fragments

Y38.2x1- Terrorism involving other explosions and fragments, <u>public safety official</u> injured

Y38.2x2- Terrorism involving other explosions and fragments, <u>civilian</u> injured

Y38.2x3- Terrorism involving other explosions and fragments, <u>terrorist</u> injured

Y38.3- Terrorism involving <u>fires, conflagration and hot substances</u>
> Terrorism involving conflagration NOS
> Terrorism involving fire NOS
> Terrorism involving petrol bomb
> *Excludes 1:*   *terrorism involving fire or heat of nuclear weapon (Y38.5)*

Y38.3x- Terrorism involving fires, conflagration and hot substances

Y38.3x1- Terrorism involving fires, conflagration and hot substances, <u>public safety official</u> injured

Y38.3x2- Terrorism involving fires, conflagration and hot substances, <u>civilian</u> injured

Y38.3x3- Terrorism involving fires, conflagration and hot substances, <u>terrorist</u> injured

Y38.4- Terrorism involving <u>firearms</u>
> Terrorism involving carbine bullet
> Terrorism involving machine gun bullet
> Terrorism involving pellets (shotgun)
> Terrorism involving pistol bullet
> Terrorism involving rifle bullet
> Terrorism involving rubber (rifle) bullet

Y38.4x- Terrorism involving firearms

Y38.4x1- Terrorism involving firearms, <u>public safety official</u> injured

Y38.4x2- Terrorism involving firearms, <u>civilian</u> injured

Y38.4x3- Terrorism involving firearms, <u>terrorist</u> injured

Y38.5- Terrorism involving <u>nuclear weapons</u>
> Terrorism involving blast effects of nuclear weapon
> Terrorism involving exposure to ionizing radiation from nuclear weapon
> Terrorism involving fireball effect of nuclear weapon
> Terrorism involving heat from nuclear weapon

Y38.5x- Terrorism involving nuclear weapons

Y38.5x1- Terrorism involving nuclear weapons, <u>public safety official</u> injured

Y37-Y38

Y38.5x2- Terrorism involving nuclear weapons, <u>civilian</u> injured

Y38.5x3- Terrorism involving nuclear weapons, <u>terrorist</u> injured

Y38.6- Terrorism involving <u>biological weapons</u>
Terrorism involving anthrax
Terrorism involving cholera
Terrorism involving smallpox

Y38.6x- Terrorism involving biological weapons

Y38.6x1- Terrorism involving biological weapons, <u>public safety official</u> injured

Y38.6x2- Terrorism involving biological weapons, <u>civilian</u> injured

Y38.6x3- Terrorism involving biological weapons, <u>terrorist</u> injured

Y38.7- Terrorism involving <u>chemical weapons</u>
Terrorism involving gases, fumes, chemicals
Terrorism involving hydrogen cyanide
Terrorism involving phosgene
Terrorism involving sarin

Y38.7x- Terrorism involving chemical weapons

Y38.7x1- Terrorism involving chemical weapons, <u>public safety official</u> injured

Y38.7x2- Terrorism involving chemical weapons, <u>civilian</u> injured

Y38.7x3- Terrorism involving chemical weapons, <u>terrorist</u> injured

Y38.8- Terrorism involving <u>other and unspecified means</u>

Y38.80x- Terrorism involving <u>unspecified</u> means
Terrorism NOS

Y38.81- Terrorism involving <u>suicide bomber</u>

Y38.811- Terrorism involving suicide bomber, <u>public safety official</u> injured

Y38.812- Terrorism involving suicide bomber, <u>civilian</u> injured

Y38.89- Terrorism involving <u>other means</u>
Terrorism involving drowning and submersion
Terrorism involving lasers
Terrorism involving piercing or stabbing instruments

Y38.891- Terrorism involving other means, <u>public safety official</u> injured

Y38.892- Terrorism involving other means, <u>civilian</u> injured

Y38.893- Terrorism involving other means, <u>terrorist</u> injured

Y38.9- Terrorism, <u>secondary effects</u>
Note: This code is for use to identify conditions occurring subsequent to a terrorist attack not those that are due to the initial terrorist attack.

Y38.9x- Terrorism, secondary effects

Y38.9x1- Terrorism, secondary effects, <u>public safety official</u> injured

Y38.9x2- Terrorism, secondary effects, <u>civilian</u> injured

Complications of medical and surgical care (Y62-Y84)

Includes: Complications of medical devices
Surgical and medical procedures as the cause of abnormal reaction of the patient, or of later complication, without mention of misadventure at the time of the procedure

Misadventures to patients during surgical and medical care (Y62-Y69)

Excludes 1: *surgical and medical procedures as the cause of abnormal reaction of the patient, without mention of misadventure at the time of the procedure (Y83-Y84)*

Excludes ❷: *breakdown or malfunctioning of medical device (during procedure) (after implantation) (ongoing use) (Y70-Y82)*

Y62- <u>Failure of sterile precautions</u> during surgical and medical care

Y62.0 Failure of sterile precautions during <u>surgical operation</u>

Y62.1 Failure of sterile precautions during <u>infusion or transfusion</u>

Y62.2 Failure of sterile precautions during <u>kidney dialysis and other perfusion</u>

Y62.3 Failure of sterile precautions during <u>injection or immunization</u>

Y62.4 Failure of sterile precautions during <u>endoscopic examination</u>

Y62.5 Failure of sterile precautions during <u>heart catheterization</u>

Y62.6 Failure of sterile precautions during <u>aspiration, puncture and other catheterization</u>

Y62.8 Failure of sterile precautions during <u>other</u> surgical and medical care

Y62.9 Failure of sterile precautions during <u>unspecified</u> surgical and medical care

Y63- <u>Failure in dosage</u> during surgical and medical care
Excludes ❷: accidental overdose of drug or wrong drug given in error (T36-T50)

Y63.0 <u>Excessive amount</u> of blood or other fluid given during transfusion or infusion

Y63.1 <u>Incorrect dilution</u> of fluid used during infusion

Y63.2 <u>Overdose of radiation</u> given during therapy

Y63.3 <u>Inadvertent exposure</u> of patient to radiation during medical care

Y63.4 Failure in dosage in <u>electroshock or insulin-shock therapy</u>

Y63.5 <u>Inappropriate temperature</u> in local application and packing

Y63.6 <u>Underdosing</u> and <u>nonadministration</u> of necessary drug, medicament or biological substance

Y63.8 Failure in dosage during <u>other</u> surgical and medical care

Y63.9 Failure in dosage during <u>unspecified</u> surgical and medical care

Y64- <u>Contaminated</u> medical or biological substances

Y64.0 Contaminated medical or biological substance, <u>transfused or infused</u>

Y64.1 Contaminated medical or biological substance, <u>injected or used for immunization</u>

Y64.8 Contaminated medical or biological substance <u>administered by other means</u>

Y64.9 Contaminated medical or biological substance administered by <u>unspecified</u> means
Administered contaminated medical or biological substance NOS

Y65- <u>Other misadventures</u> during surgical and medical care

Y65.0 <u>Mismatched</u> blood in transfusion

Y65.1 <u>Wrong fluid used in infusion</u> — [Wrong Procedure Performed]

Y65.2 <u>Failure in suture or ligature</u> during surgical operation — [Wrong Procedure Performed]

Y65.3 <u>Endotracheal tube wrongly placed</u> during anesthetic procedure — [Wrong Procedure Performed]

Y65.4 <u>Failure to introduce or to remove</u> other tube or instrument

Y65.5- Performance of <u>wrong procedure</u> (operation)

Y65.51 Performance of wrong procedure (operation) on correct patient
Wrong device implanted into correct surgical site
Excludes 1: performance of correct procedure (operation) on wrong side or body part (Y65.53)

Excludes 1: = NOT CODED HERE! (Do not code both)

Excludes ❷: = Not Included Here

Y38 - Y65

Y65.52 Performance of procedure (operation) on patient not scheduled for surgery

Performance of procedure (operation) intended for another patient

Performance of procedure (operation) on wrong patient

Y65.53 Performance of correct procedure (operation) on <u>wrong side or body part</u>

Performance of correct procedure (operation) on wrong side

Performance of correct procedure (operation) on wrong site

Y65.8 <u>Other</u> specified misadventures during surgical and medical care

Y66 <u>Nonadministration</u> of <u>surgical and medical care</u>

Premature cessation of surgical and medical care

Excludes 1:   *DNR status (Z66)*

palliative care (Z51.5)

Y69 <u>Unspecified</u> misadventure during surgical and medical care

Medical devices associated with adverse incidents in diagnostic and therapeutic use (Y70-Y82)

Includes: Breakdown or malfunction of medical devices (during use) (after implantation) (ongoing use)

Excludes ❷: *breakdown or malfunctioning of medical device (after implantation) (during procedure) (ongoing use) (Y70-Y82)*

later complications following use of medical devices without breakdown or malfunctioning of device (Y83-Y84)

misadventure to patients during surgical and medical care, classifiable to (Y62-Y69)

surgical and other medical procedures as the cause of abnormal reaction of the patient, or of later complication, without mention of misadventure at the time of the procedure (Y83-Y84)

Y70- <u>Anesthesiology devices</u> <u>associated with adverse incidents</u>

Y70.0 Diagnostic and monitoring anesthesiology devices associated with adverse incidents

Y70.1 Therapeutic (nonsurgical) and rehabilitative anesthesiology devices associated with adverse incidents

Y70.2 Prosthetic and other implants, materials and accessory anesthesiology devices associated with adverse incidents

Y70.3 Surgical instruments, materials and anesthesiology devices (including sutures) associated with adverse incidents

Y70.8 Miscellaneous anesthesiology devices associated with adverse incidents, not elsewhere classified

Y71- <u>Cardiovascular devices</u> <u>associated with adverse incidents</u>

Y71.0 Diagnostic and monitoring cardiovascular devices associated with adverse incidents

Y71.1 Therapeutic (nonsurgical) and rehabilitative cardiovascular devices associated with adverse incidents

Y71.2 Prosthetic and other implants, materials and accessory cardiovascular devices associated with adverse incidents

Y71.3 Surgical instruments, materials and cardiovascular devices (including sutures) associated with adverse incidents

Y71.8 Miscellaneous cardiovascular devices associated with adverse incidents, not elsewhere classified

Y72- <u>Otorhinolaryngological devices</u> <u>associated with adverse incidents</u>

Y72.0 Diagnostic and monitoring otorhinolaryngological devices associated with adverse incidents

Y72.1 Therapeutic (nonsurgical) and rehabilitative otorhinolaryngological devices associated with adverse incidents

Y72.2 Prosthetic and other implants, materials and accessory otorhinolaryngological devices associated with adverse incidents

Y72.3 Surgical instruments, materials and otorhinolaryngological devices (including sutures) associated with adverse incidents

Y72.8 Miscellaneous otorhinolaryngological devices associated with adverse incidents, not elsewhere classified

Y73- <u>Gastroenterology and urology devices</u> <u>associated with adverse incidents</u>

Y73.0 Diagnostic and monitoring gastroenterology and urology devices associated with adverse incidents

Y73.1 Therapeutic (nonsurgical) and rehabilitative gastroenterology and urology devices associated with adverse incidents

Y73.2 Prosthetic and other implants, materials and accessory gastroenterology and urology devices associated with adverse incidents

Y73.3 Surgical instruments, materials and gastroenterology and urology devices (including sutures) associated with adverse incidents

Y73.8 Miscellaneous gastroenterology and urology devices associated with adverse incidents, not elsewhere classified

Y74- <u>General hospital and personal-use devices</u> <u>associated with adverse incidents</u>

Y74.0 <u>Diagnostic</u> and monitoring general hospital and personal-use devices associated with adverse incidents

Y74.1 <u>Therapeutic</u> (nonsurgical) and rehabilitative general hospital and personal-use devices associated with adverse incidents

Y74.2 <u>Prosthetic</u> and other implants, materials and accessory general hospital and personal-use devices associated with adverse incidents

Y74.3 <u>Surgical</u> instruments, materials and general hospital and personal-use devices (including sutures) associated with adverse incidents

Y74.8 <u>Miscellaneous</u> general hospital and personal-use devices associated with adverse incidents, not elsewhere classified

Y75- <u>Neurological devices</u> <u>associated with adverse incidents</u>

Y75.0 <u>Diagnostic</u> and monitoring neurological devices associated with adverse incidents

Y75.1 <u>Therapeutic</u> (nonsurgical) and rehabilitative neurological devices associated with adverse incidents

Y75.2 <u>Prosthetic</u> and other implants, materials and neurological devices associated with adverse incidents

Y75.3 <u>Surgical</u> instruments, materials and neurological devices (including sutures) associated with adverse incidents

Y75.8 <u>Miscellaneous</u> neurological devices associated with adverse incidents, not elsewhere classified

Y76- <u>Obstetric and gynecological devices</u> <u>associated with adverse incidents</u>

Y76.0 <u>Diagnostic</u> and monitoring obstetric and gynecological devices associated with adverse incidents — [♀]

Y76.1 <u>Therapeutic</u> (nonsurgical) and rehabilitative obstetric and gynecological devices associated with adverse incidents — [♀]

Y76.2 <u>Prosthetic</u> and other implants, materials and accessory obstetric and gynecological devices associated with adverse incidents — [♀]

Y76.3 <u>Surgical</u> instruments, materials and obstetric and gynecological devices (including sutures) associated with adverse incidents — [♀]

Y76.8 <u>Miscellaneous</u> obstetric and gynecological devices associated with adverse incidents, not elsewhere classified — [♀]

Y77- <u>Ophthalmic devices</u> <u>associated with adverse incidents</u>

Y77.0 <u>Diagnostic</u> and monitoring ophthalmic devices associated with adverse incidents

Y77.1 <u>Therapeutic</u> (nonsurgical) and rehabilitative ophthalmic devices associated with adverse incidents

Y77.2 <u>Prosthetic</u> and other implants, materials and accessory ophthalmic devices associated with adverse incidents

Y77.3 <u>Surgical</u> instruments, materials and ophthalmic devices (including sutures) associated with adverse incidents

Y77.8 <u>Miscellaneous</u> ophthalmic devices associated with adverse incidents, not elsewhere classified

Y65 - Y77

Y78-　Radiological devices associated with adverse incidents

Y78.0　**Diagnostic** and monitoring radiological devices associated with adverse incidents

Y78.1　**Therapeutic** (nonsurgical) and rehabilitative radiological devices associated with adverse incidents

Y78.2　**Prosthetic** and other implants, materials and accessory radiological devices associated with adverse incidents

Y78.3　**Surgical** instruments, materials and radiological devices (including sutures) associated with adverse incidents

Y78.8　**Miscellaneous** radiological devices associated with adverse incidents, not elsewhere classified

Y79-　Orthopedic devices associated with adverse incidents

Y79.0　**Diagnostic** and monitoring orthopedic devices associated with adverse incidents

Y79.1　**Therapeutic** (nonsurgical) and rehabilitative orthopedic devices associated with adverse incidents

Y79.2　**Prosthetic** and other implants, materials and accessory orthopedic devices associated with adverse incidents

Y79.3　**Surgical** instruments, materials and orthopedic devices (including sutures) associated with adverse incidents

Y79.8　**Miscellaneous** orthopedic devices associated with adverse incidents, not elsewhere classified

Y80-　Physical medicine devices associated with adverse incidents

Y80.0　**Diagnostic** and monitoring physical medicine devices associated with adverse incidents

Y80.1　**Therapeutic** (nonsurgical) and rehabilitative physical medicine devices associated with adverse incidents

Y80.2　**Prosthetic** and other implants, materials and accessory physical medicine devices associated with adverse incidents

Y80.3　**Surgical** instruments, materials and physical medicine devices (including sutures) associated with adverse incidents

Y80.8　**Miscellaneous** physical medicine devices associated with adverse incidents, not elsewhere classified

Y81-　General- and plastic-surgery devices associated with adverse incidents

Y81.0　**Diagnostic** and monitoring general- and plastic-surgery devices associated with adverse incidents

Y81.1　**Therapeutic** (nonsurgical) and rehabilitative general- and plastic-surgery devices associated with adverse incidents

Y81.2　**Prosthetic** and other implants, materials and accessory general- and plastic-surgery devices associated with adverse incidents

Y81.3　**Surgical** instruments, materials and general- and plastic-surgery devices (including sutures) associated with adverse incidents

Y81.8　**Miscellaneous** general- and plastic-surgery devices associated with adverse incidents, not elsewhere classified

Y82-　Other and unspecified medical devices associated with adverse incidents

Y82.8　**Other** medical devices associated with adverse incidents

Y82.9　**Unspecified** medical devices associated with adverse incidents

Surgical and other medical procedures as the cause of abnormal reaction of the patient, or of later complication, without mention of misadventure at the time of the procedure (Y83-Y84)

Excludes 1:　*misadventures to patients during surgical and medical care, classifiable to (Y62-Y69)*

Excludes ❷:　*breakdown or malfunctioning of medical device (after implantation) (during procedure) (ongoing use) (Y70-Y82)*

Y83-　Surgical operation and other surgical procedures as the cause of abnormal reaction of the patient, or of later complication, without mention of misadventure at the time of the procedure

Y83.0　Surgical operation with **transplant** of whole organ as the cause of abnormal reaction of the patient, or of later complication, without mention of misadventure at the time of the procedure

Y83.1　Surgical operation with **implant** of artificial internal device as the cause of abnormal reaction of the patient, or of later complication, without mention of misadventure at the time of the procedure

Y83.2　Surgical operation with **anastomosis**, bypass or graft as the cause of abnormal reaction of the patient, or of later complication, without mention of misadventure at the time of the procedure

Y83.3　Surgical operation with **formation** of external stoma as the cause of abnormal reaction of the patient, or of later complication, without mention of misadventure at the time of the procedure

Y83.4　**Other** reconstructive surgery as the cause of abnormal reaction of the patient, or of later complication, without mention of misadventure at the time of the procedure

Y83.5　**Amputation** of limb(s) as the cause of abnormal reaction of the patient, or of later complication, without mention of misadventure at the time of the procedure

Y83.6　Removal of other **organ** (partial) (total) as the cause of abnormal reaction of the patient, or of later complication, without mention of misadventure at the time of the procedure

Y83.8　**Other** surgical procedures as the cause of abnormal reaction of the patient, or of later complication, without mention of misadventure at the time of the procedure

Y83.9　Surgical procedure, **unspecified** as the cause of abnormal reaction of the patient, or of later complication, without mention of misadventure at the time of the procedure

Y84-　Other medical procedures as the cause of abnormal reaction of the patient, or of later complication, without mention of misadventure at the time of the procedure

Y84.0　**Cardiac catheterization** as the cause of abnormal reaction of the patient, or of later complication, without mention of misadventure at the time of the procedure

Y84.1　**Kidney dialysis** as the cause of abnormal reaction of the patient, or of later complication, without mention of misadventure at the time of the procedure

Y84.2　**Radiological procedure and radiotherapy** as the cause of abnormal reaction of the patient, or of later complication, without mention of misadventure at the time of the procedure

Y84.3　**Shock therapy** as the cause of abnormal reaction of the patient, or of later complication, without mention of misadventure at the time of the procedure

Y84.4　**Aspiration of fluid** as the cause of abnormal reaction of the patient, or of later complication, without mention of misadventure at the time of the procedure

Y84.5　**Insertion of gastric or duodenal sound** as the cause of abnormal reaction of the patient, or of later complication, without mention of misadventure at the time of the procedure

Y84.6　**Urinary catheterization** as the cause of abnormal reaction of the patient, or of later complication, without mention of misadventure at the time of the procedure

Y78 | Y84

Y84.7 <u>Blood-sampling</u> as the cause of abnormal reaction of the patient, or of later complication, without mention of misadventure at the time of the procedure

Y84.8 <u>Other</u> medical procedures as the cause of abnormal reaction of the patient, or of later complication, without mention of misadventure at the time of the procedure
AHA 14:4Q:p24 – Durotomy secondary to previous epidural injections

Y84.9 Medical procedure, <u>unspecified</u> as the cause of abnormal reaction of the patient, or of later complication, without mention of misadventure at the time of the procedure

Supplementary factors related to causes of morbidity classified elsewhere (Y90-Y99)

Note: These categories may be used to provide supplementary information concerning causes of morbidity. They are not to be used for single-condition coding.

Y90- <u>Evidence of alcohol involvement determined by blood alcohol level</u>
Code first any associated alcohol related disorders (F10)

Y90.0 Blood alcohol level of less than 20 mg/100 ml

Y90.1 Blood alcohol level of 20-39 mg/100 ml

Y90.2 Blood alcohol level of 40-59 mg/100 ml

Y90.3 Blood alcohol level of 60-79 mg/100 ml

Y90.4 Blood alcohol level of 80-99 mg/100 ml

Y90.5 Blood alcohol level of 100-119 mg/100 ml

Y90.6 Blood alcohol level of 120-199 mg/100 ml

Y90.7 Blood alcohol level of 200-239 mg/100 ml

Y90.8 Blood alcohol level of 240 mg/100 ml or more

Y90.9 Presence of alcohol in blood, level not specified

Y92- <u>Place of occurrence</u> of the <u>external cause</u>
Note: The following category is for use, when relevant, to identify the place of occurrence of the external cause. Use in conjunction with an activity code.
Note: Place of occurrence should be recorded only at the initial encounter for treatment.

Y92.0- <u>Non-institutional (private) residence</u> as the place of occurrence of the external cause
Excludes 1: *abandoned or derelict house (Y92.89)*
home under construction but not yet occupied (Y92.6-)
institutional place of residence (Y92.1-)

Y92.00- <u>Unspecified</u> non-institutional (private) residence as the place of occurrence of the external cause

Y92.000 <u>Kitchen</u> of unspecified non-institutional (private) residence as the place of occurrence of the external cause

Y92.001 <u>Dining room</u> of unspecified non-institutional (private) residence as the place of occurrence of the external cause

Y92.002 <u>Bathroom</u> of unspecified non-institutional (private) residence single-family (private) house as the place of occurrence of the external cause

Y92.003 <u>Bedroom</u> of unspecified non-institutional (private) residence as the place of occurrence of the external cause

Y92.007 <u>Garden or yard</u> in unspecified non-institutional (private) residence as the place of occurrence of the external cause

Y92.008 <u>Other</u> place in unspecified non-institutional (private) residence as the place of occurrence of the external cause

Y92.009 <u>Unspecified</u> place in unspecified non-institutional (private) residence as the place of occurrence of the external cause
Home (NOS) as the place of occurrence of the external cause

Y92.01- <u>Single-family</u> non-institutional (private) house as the place of occurrence of the external cause
Farmhouse as the place of occurrence of the external cause
Excludes 1: *barn (Y92.71)*
chicken coop or hen house (Y92.72)
farm field (Y92.73)
orchard (Y92.74)
single family mobile home or trailer (Y92.02-)
slaughter house (Y92.86)

Y92.010 <u>Kitchen</u> of single-family (private) house as the place of occurrence of the external cause

Y92.011 <u>Dining room</u> of single-family (private) house as the place of occurrence of the external cause

Y92.012 <u>Bathroom</u> of single-family (private) house as the place of occurrence of the external cause

Y92.013 <u>Bedroom</u> of single-family (private) house as the place of occurrence of the external cause

Y92.014 <u>Private driveway</u> to single-family (private) house as the place of occurrence of the external cause

Y92.015 <u>Private garage</u> of single-family (private) house as the place of occurrence of the external cause

Y92.016 <u>Swimming-pool</u> in single-family (private) house or garden as the place of occurrence of the external cause

Y92.017 <u>Garden or yard</u> in single-family (private) house as the place of occurrence of the external cause

Y92.018 <u>Other</u> place in single-family (private) house as the place of occurrence of the external cause

Y92.019 <u>Unspecified</u> place in single-family (private) house as the place of occurrence of the external cause

Y92.02- <u>Mobile home</u> as the place of occurrence of the external cause

Y92.020 <u>Kitchen</u> in mobile home as the place of occurrence of the external cause

Y92.021 <u>Dining room</u> in mobile home as the place of occurrence of the external cause

Y92.022 <u>Bathroom</u> in mobile home as the place of occurrence of the external cause

Y92.023 <u>Bedroom</u> in mobile home as the place of occurrence of the external cause

Y92.024 <u>Driveway</u> of mobile home as the place of occurrence of the external cause

Y92.025 <u>Garage</u> of mobile home as the place of occurrence of the external cause

Y92.026 <u>Swimming-pool</u> of mobile home as the place of occurrence of the external cause

Y92.027 <u>Garden or yard</u> of mobile home as the place of occurrence of the external cause

Y92.028 <u>Other</u> place in mobile home as the place of occurrence of the external cause

Y92.029 <u>Unspecified</u> place in mobile home as the place of occurrence of the external cause

Y92.03- <u>Apartment</u> as the place of occurrence of the external cause
Condominium as the place of occurrence of the external cause
Co-op apartment as the place of occurrence of the external cause

Y92.030 <u>Kitchen</u> in apartment as the place of occurrence of the external cause

Y92.031 <u>Bathroom</u> in apartment as the place of occurrence of the external cause

Y92.032 <u>Bedroom</u> in apartment as the place of occurrence of the external cause

Y92.038 <u>Other</u> place in apartment as the place of occurrence of the external cause

Y92.039 <u>Unspecified</u> place in apartment as the place of occurrence of the external cause

Y84 - Y92

Y92.04- Boarding-house as the place of occurrence of the external cause

    Y92.040 Kitchen in boarding-house as the place of occurrence of the external cause

    Y92.041 Bathroom in boarding-house as the place of occurrence of the external cause

    Y92.042 Bedroom in boarding-house as the place of occurrence of the external cause

    Y92.043 Driveway of boarding-house as the place of occurrence of the external cause

    Y92.044 Garage of boarding-house as the place of occurrence of the external cause

    Y92.045 Swimming-pool of boarding-house as the place of occurrence of the external cause

    Y92.046 Garden or yard of boarding-house as the place of occurrence of the external cause

    Y92.048 Other place in boarding-house as the place of occurrence of the external cause

    Y92.049 Unspecified place in boarding-house as the place of occurrence of the external cause

Y92.09- Other non-institutional residence as the place of occurrence of the external cause

    Y92.090 Kitchen in other non-institutional residence as the place of occurrence of the external cause

    Y92.091 Bathroom in other non-institutional residence as the place of occurrence of the external cause

    Y92.092 Bedroom in other non-institutional residence as the place of occurrence of the external cause

    Y92.093 Driveway of other non-institutional residence as the place of occurrence of the external cause

    Y92.094 Garage of other non-institutional residence as the place of occurrence of the external cause

    Y92.095 Swimming-pool of other non-institutional residence as the place of occurrence of the external cause

    Y92.096 Garden or yard of other non-institutional residence as the place of occurrence of the external cause

    Y92.098 Other place in other non-institutional residence as the place of occurrence of the external cause

    Y92.099 Unspecified place in other non-institutional residence as the place of occurrence of the external cause

Y92.1- Institutional (nonprivate) residence as the place of occurrence of the external cause

    Y92.10 Unspecified residential institution as the place of occurrence of the external cause

Y92.11- Children's home and orphanage as the place of occurrence of the external cause

    Y92.110 Kitchen in children's home and orphanage as the place of occurrence of the external cause

    Y92.111 Bathroom in children's home and orphanage as the place of occurrence of the external cause

    Y92.112 Bedroom in children's home and orphanage as the place of occurrence of the external cause

    Y92.113 Driveway of children's home and orphanage as the place of occurrence of the external cause

    Y92.114 Garage of children's home and orphanage as the place of occurrence of the external cause

    Y92.115 Swimming-pool of children's home and orphanage as the place of occurrence of the external cause

    Y92.116 Garden or yard of children's home and orphanage as the place of occurrence of the external cause

    Y92.118 Other place in children's home and orphanage as the place of occurrence of the external cause

    Y92.119 Unspecified place in children's home and orphanage as the place of occurrence of the external cause

Y92.12- Nursing home as the place of occurrence of the external cause

    Home for the sick as the place of occurrence of the external cause

    Hospice as the place of occurrence of the external cause

    Y92.120 Kitchen in nursing home as the place of occurrence of the external cause

    Y92.121 Bathroom in nursing home as the place of occurrence of the external cause

    Y92.122 Bedroom in nursing home as the place of occurrence of the external cause

    Y92.123 Driveway of nursing home as the place of occurrence of the external cause

    Y92.124 Garage of nursing home as the place of occurrence of the external cause

    Y92.125 Swimming-pool of nursing home as the place of occurrence of the external cause

    Y92.126 Garden or yard of nursing home as the place of occurrence of the external cause

    Y92.128 Other place in nursing home as the place of occurrence of the external cause

    Y92.129 Unspecified place in nursing home as the place of occurrence of the external cause

Y92.13- Military base as the place of occurrence of the external cause

    Excludes 1:   *military training grounds (Y92.83)*

    Y92.130 Kitchen on military base as the place of occurrence of the external cause

    Y92.131 Mess hall on military base as the place of occurrence of the external cause

    Y92.133 Barracks on military base as the place of occurrence of the external cause

    Y92.135 Garage on military base as the place of occurrence of the external cause

    Y92.136 Swimming-pool on military base as the place of occurrence of the external cause

    Y92.137 Garden or yard on military base as the place of occurrence of the external cause

    Y92.138 Other place on military base as the place of occurrence of the external cause

    Y92.139 Unspecified place military base as the place of occurrence of the external cause

Y92.14- Prison as the place of occurrence of the external cause

    Y92.140 Kitchen in prison as the place of occurrence of the external cause

    Y92.141 Dining room in prison as the place of occurrence of the external cause

    Y92.142 Bathroom in prison as the place of occurrence of the external cause

    Y92.143 Cell of prison as the place of occurrence of the external cause

    Y92.146 Swimming-pool of prison as the place of occurrence of the external cause

    Y92.147 Courtyard of prison as the place of occurrence of the external cause

    Y92.148 Other place in prison as the place of occurrence of the external cause

    Y92.149 Unspecified place in prison as the place of occurrence of the external cause

Y92.15- Reform school as the place of occurrence of the external cause

    Y92.150 Kitchen in reform school as the place of occurrence of the external cause

    Y92.151 Dining room in reform school as the place of occurrence of the external cause

    Y92.152 Bathroom in reform school as the place of occurrence of the external cause

    Y92.153 Bedroom in reform school as the place of occurrence of the external cause

Y92 - Y92

Y92.154 <u>Driveway</u> of reform school as the place of occurrence of the external cause

Y92.155 <u>Garage</u> of reform school as the place of occurrence of the external cause

Y92.156 <u>Swimming-pool</u> of reform school as the place of occurrence of the external cause

Y92.157 <u>Garden or yard</u> of reform school as the place of occurrence of the external cause

Y92.158 <u>Other</u> place in reform school as the place of occurrence of the external cause

Y92.159 <u>Unspecified</u> place in reform school as the place of occurrence of the external cause

Y92.16- <u>School dormitory</u> as the place of occurrence of the external cause

> Excludes 1:   reform school as the place of occurrence of the external cause (Y92.15-)
> school buildings and grounds as the place of occurrence of the external cause (Y92.2-)
> school sports and athletic areas as the place of occurrence of the external cause (Y92.3-)

Y92.160 <u>Kitchen</u> in school dormitory as the place of occurrence of the external cause

Y92.161 <u>Dining room</u> in school dormitory as the place of occurrence of the external cause

Y92.162 <u>Bathroom</u> in school dormitory as the place of occurrence of the external cause

Y92.163 <u>Bedroom</u> in school dormitory as the place of occurrence of the external cause

Y92.168 <u>Other</u> place in school dormitory as the place of occurrence of the external cause

Y92.169 <u>Unspecified</u> place in school dormitory as the place of occurrence of the external cause

Y92.19- <u>Other specified residential institution</u> as the place of occurrence of the external cause

Y92.190 <u>Kitchen</u> in other specified residential institution as the place of occurrence of the external cause

Y92.191 <u>Dining room</u> in other specified residential institution as the place of occurrence of the external cause

Y92.192 <u>Bathroom</u> in other specified residential institution as the place of occurrence of the external cause

Y92.193 <u>Bedroom</u> in other specified residential institution as the place of occurrence of the external cause

Y92.194 <u>Driveway</u> of other specified residential institution as the place of occurrence of the external cause

Y92.195 <u>Garage</u> of other specified residential institution as the place of occurrence of the external cause

Y92.196 <u>Pool</u> of other specified residential institution as the place of occurrence of the external cause

Y92.197 <u>Garden or yard</u> of other specified residential institution as the place of occurrence of the external cause

Y92.198 <u>Other</u> place in other specified residential institution as the place of occurrence of the external cause

Y92.199 <u>Unspecified</u> place in other specified residential institution as the place of occurrence of the external cause

Y92.2- <u>School, other institution and public administrative area</u> as the place of occurrence of the external cause

> Building and adjacent grounds used by the general public or by a particular group of the public
> Excludes 1:   building under construction as the place of occurrence of the external cause (Y92.6)
> residential institution as the place of occurrence of the external cause (Y92.1)
> school dormitory as the place of occurrence of the external cause (Y92.16-)
> sports and athletics area of schools as the place of occurrence of the external cause (Y92.3-)

Y92.21- <u>School (private) (public) (state)</u> as the place of occurrence of the external cause

Y92.210 <u>Daycare center</u> as the place of occurrence of the external cause

Y92.211 <u>Elementary school</u> as the place of occurrence of the external cause

> Kindergarten as the place of occurrence of the external cause

Y92.212 <u>Middle school</u> as the place of occurrence of the external cause

Y92.213 <u>High school</u> as the place of occurrence of the external cause

Y92.214 <u>College</u> as the place of occurrence of the external cause

> University as the place of occurrence of the external cause

Y92.215 <u>Trade school</u> as the place of occurrence of the external cause

Y92.218 <u>Other</u> school as the place of occurrence of the external cause

Y92.219 <u>Unspecified</u> school as the place of occurrence of the external cause

Y92.22 <u>Religious institution</u> as the place of occurrence of the external cause

> Church as the place of occurrence of the external cause
> Mosque as the place of occurrence of the external cause
> Synagogue as the place of occurrence of the external cause

Y92.23- <u>Hospital</u> as the place of occurrence of the external cause

> Excludes 1:   ambulatory (outpatient) health services establishments (Y92.53-)
> home for the sick as the place of occurrence of the external cause (Y92.12-)
> hospice as the place of occurrence of the external cause (Y92.12-)
> nursing home as the place of occurrence of the external cause (Y92.12-)

Y92.230 <u>Patient room</u> in hospital as the place of occurrence of the external cause

Y92.231 <u>Patient bathroom</u> in hospital as the place of occurrence of the external cause

Y92.232 <u>Corridor</u> of hospital as the place of occurrence of the external cause

Y92.233 <u>Cafeteria</u> of hospital as the place of occurrence of the external cause

Y92.234 <u>Operating room</u> of hospital as the place of occurrence of the external cause

Y92.238 <u>Other</u> place in hospital as the place of occurrence of the external cause

Y92.239 <u>Unspecified</u> place in hospital as the place of occurrence of the external cause

Y92.24- <u>Public administrative building</u> as the place of occurrence of the external cause

Y92.240 <u>Courthouse</u> as the place of occurrence of the external cause

Y92.241 <u>Library</u> as the place of occurrence of the external cause

Y92.242 <u>Post office</u> as the place of occurrence of the external cause

Y92.243 <u>City hall</u> as the place of occurrence of the external cause

Y92 – Y92

Y92.248   **Other** public administrative building as the place of occurrence of the external cause

Y92.25-   **Cultural building** as the place of occurrence of the external cause

Y92.250   **Art Gallery** as the place of occurrence of the external cause

Y92.251   **Museum** as the place of occurrence of the external cause

Y92.252   **Music hall** as the place of occurrence of the external cause

Y92.253   **Opera house** as the place of occurrence of the external cause

Y92.254   **Theater (live)** as the place of occurrence of the external cause

Y92.258   **Other** cultural public building as the place of occurrence of the external cause

Y92.26   **Movie house or cinema** as the place of occurrence of the external cause

Y92.29   **Other** specified public building as the place of occurrence of the external cause
Assembly hall as the place of occurrence of the external cause
Clubhouse as the place of occurrence of the external cause

Y92.3-   **Sports and athletics area** as the place of occurrence of the external cause

Y92.31-   **Athletic court** as the place of occurrence of the external cause
Excludes 1:   *tennis court in private home or garden (Y92.09)*

Y92.310   **Basketball** court as the place of occurrence of the external cause

Y92.311   **Squash** court as the place of occurrence of the external cause

Y92.312   **Tennis** court as the place of occurrence of the external cause

Y92.318   **Other** athletic court as the place of occurrence of the external cause

Y92.32-   **Athletic field** as the place of occurrence of the external cause

Y92.320   **Baseball** field as the place of occurrence of the external cause

Y92.321   **Football** field as the place of occurrence of the external cause

Y92.322   **Soccer** field as the place of occurrence of the external cause

Y92.328   **Other** athletic field as the place of occurrence of the external cause
Cricket field as the place of occurrence of the external cause
Hockey field as the place of occurrence of the external cause

Y92.33-   **Skating rink** as the place of occurrence of the external cause

Y92.330   **Ice skating** rink (indoor) (outdoor) as the place of occurrence of the external cause

Y92.331   **Roller skating** rink as the place of occurrence of the external cause

Y92.34   **Swimming pool (public)** as the place of occurrence of the external cause
Excludes 1:   *swimming pool in private home or garden (Y92.016)*

Y92.39   **Other** specified sports and athletic area as the place of occurrence of the external cause
Golf-course as the place of occurrence of the external cause
Gymnasium as the place of occurrence of the external cause
Riding-school as the place of occurrence of the external cause
Stadium as the place of occurrence of the external cause

Y92.4-   **Street, highway and other paved roadways** as the place of occurrence of the external cause
Excludes 1:   *private driveway of residence (Y92.014, Y92.024, Y92.043, Y92.093, Y92.113, Y92.123, Y92.154, Y92.194)*

Y92.41-   **Street and highway** as the place of occurrence of the external cause

Y92.410   **Unspecified** street and highway as the place of occurrence of the external cause
Road NOS as the place of occurrence of the external cause

Y92.411   **Interstate highway** as the place of occurrence of the external cause
Freeway as the place of occurrence of the external cause
Motorway as the place of occurrence of the external cause

Y92.412   **Parkway** as the place of occurrence of the external cause

Y92.413   **State road** as the place of occurrence of the external cause

Y92.414   **Local residential or business street** as the place of occurrence of the external cause

Y92.415   **Exit ramp or entrance ramp** of street or highway as the place of occurrence of the external cause

Y92.48-   **Other paved roadways** as the place of occurrence of the external cause

Y92.480   **Sidewalk** as the place of occurrence of the external cause

Y92.481   **Parking lot** as the place of occurrence of the external cause

Y92.482   **Bike path** as the place of occurrence of the external cause

Y92.488   **Other** paved roadways as the place of occurrence of the external cause

Y92.5-   **Trade and service area** as the place of occurrence of the external cause
Excludes 1:   *garage in private home (Y92.015)*
schools and other public administration buildings (Y92.2-)

Y92.51-   **Private commercial establishments** as the place of occurrence of the external cause

Y92.510   **Bank** as the place of occurrence of the external cause

Y92.511   **Restaurant or café** as the place of occurrence of the external cause

Y92.512   **Supermarket,** store or market as the place of occurrence of the external cause

Y92.513   **Shop (commercial)** as the place of occurrence of the external cause

Y92.52-   **Service areas** as the place of occurrence of the external cause

Y92.520   **Airport** as the place of occurrence of the external cause

Y92.521   **Bus station** as the place of occurrence of the external cause

Y92.522   **Railway station** as the place of occurrence of the external cause

Y92.523   **Highway rest stop** as the place of occurrence of the external cause

Y92.524   **Gas station** as the place of occurrence of the external cause
Petroleum station as the place of occurrence of the external cause
Service station as the place of occurrence of the external cause

Y92 - Y92

Y92.53- <u>Ambulatory health services establishments</u> as the place of occurrence of the external cause

Y92.530 Ambulatory <u>surgery center</u> as the place of occurrence of the external cause
> Outpatient surgery center, including that connected with a hospital as the place of occurrence of the external cause
> Same day surgery center, including that connected with a hospital as the place of occurrence of the external cause

Y92.531 Health care <u>provider office</u> as the place of occurrence of the external cause
> Physician office as the place of occurrence of the external cause

Y92.532 <u>Urgent care center</u> as the place of occurrence of the external cause

Y92.538 <u>Other</u> ambulatory health services establishments as the place of occurrence of the external cause

Y92.59 <u>Other</u> trade areas as the place of occurrence of the external cause
> Office building as the place of occurrence of the external cause
> Casino as the place of occurrence of the external cause
> Garage (commercial) as the place of occurrence of the external cause
> Hotel as the place of occurrence of the external cause
> Radio or television station as the place of occurrence of the external cause
> Shopping mall as the place of occurrence of the external cause
> Warehouse as the place of occurrence of the external cause

Y92.6- <u>Industrial and construction area</u> as the place of occurrence of the external cause

Y92.61 <u>Building [any] under construction</u> as the place of occurrence of the external cause

Y92.62 <u>Dock or shipyard</u> as the place of occurrence of the external cause
> Dockyard as the place of occurrence of the external cause
> Dry dock as the place of occurrence of the external cause
> Shipyard as the place of occurrence of the external cause

Y92.63 <u>Factory</u> as the place of occurrence of the external cause
> Factory building as the place of occurrence of the external cause
> Factory premises as the place of occurrence of the external cause
> Industrial yard as the place of occurrence of the external cause

Y92.64 <u>Mine or pit</u> as the place of occurrence of the external cause
> Mine as the place of occurrence of the external cause

Y92.65 <u>Oil rig</u> as the place of occurrence of the external cause
> Pit (coal) (gravel) (sand) as the place of occurrence of the external cause

Y92.69 <u>Other</u> specified industrial and construction area as the place of occurrence of the external cause
> Gasworks as the place of occurrence of the external cause
> Power-station (coal) (nuclear) (oil) as the place of occurrence of the external cause
> Tunnel under construction as the place of occurrence of the external cause
> Workshop as the place of occurrence of the external cause

Y92.7- <u>Farm</u> as the place of occurrence of the external cause
> Ranch as the place of occurrence of the external cause

Excludes 1: *farmhouse and home premises of farm (Y92.01-)*

Y92.71 <u>Barn</u> as the place of occurrence of the external cause

Y92.72 <u>Chicken coop</u> as the place of occurrence of the external cause
> Hen house as the place of occurrence of the external cause

Y92.73 <u>Farm field</u> as the place of occurrence of the external cause

Y92.74 <u>Orchard</u> as the place of occurrence of the external cause

Y92.79 <u>Other</u> farm location as the place of occurrence of the external cause

Y92.8- <u>Other</u> places as the place of occurrence of the external cause

Y92.81- <u>Transport vehicle</u> as the place of occurrence of the external cause

Excludes 1: *transport accidents (V00-V99)*

Y92.810 <u>Car</u> as the place of occurrence of the external cause

Y92.811 <u>Bus</u> as the place of occurrence of the external cause

Y92.812 <u>Truck</u> as the place of occurrence of the external cause

Y92.813 <u>Airplane</u> as the place of occurrence of the external cause

Y92.814 <u>Boat</u> as the place of occurrence of the external cause

Y92.815 <u>Train</u> as the place of occurrence of the external cause

Y92.816 <u>Subway</u> car as the place of occurrence of the external cause

Y92.818 <u>Other</u> transport vehicle as the place of occurrence of the external cause

Y92.82- <u>Wilderness area</u>

Y92.820 <u>Desert</u> as the place of occurrence of the external cause

Y92.821 <u>Forest</u> as the place of occurrence of the external cause

Y92.828 <u>Other</u> wilderness area as the place of occurrence of the external cause
> Swamp as the place of occurrence of the external cause
> Mountain as the place of occurrence of the external cause
> Marsh as the place of occurrence of the external cause
> Prairie as the place of occurrence of the external cause

Y92.83- <u>Recreation area</u> as the place of occurrence of the external cause

Y92.830 <u>Public park</u> as the place of occurrence of the external cause

Y92.831 <u>Amusement park</u> as the place of occurrence of the external cause

Y92.832 <u>Beach</u> as the place of occurrence of the external cause
> Seashore as the place of occurrence of the external cause

Y92.833 <u>Campsite</u> as the place of occurrence of the external cause

Y92.834 <u>Zoological garden (Zoo)</u> as the place of occurrence of the external cause

Y92.838 <u>Other</u> recreation area as the place of occurrence of the external cause

Y92.84 <u>Military training ground</u> as the place of occurrence of the external cause

Y92.85 <u>Railroad track</u> as the place of occurrence of the external cause

Y92.86 <u>Slaughter house</u> as the place of occurrence of the external cause

Y92.89 <u>Other</u> specified places as the place of occurrence of the external cause
> Derelict house as the place of occurrence of the external cause

Y92.9 <u>Unspecified</u> place or not applicable

Y92 - Y92

Y93- **Activity codes**

Note: Category Y93 is provided for use to indicate the activity of the person seeking healthcare for an injury or health condition, such as a heart attack while shoveling snow, which resulted from, or was contributed to, by the activity. These codes are appropriate for use for both acute injuries, such as those from chapter 19, and conditions that are due to the long-term, cumulative effects of an activity, such as those from chapter 13. They are also appropriate for use with external cause codes for cause and intent if identifying the activity providesadditional information on the event. These codes should be used in conjunction with codes for external cause status (Y99) and place of occurrence (Y92).

This section contains the following broad activity categories:

Y93.0   Activities involving walking and running
Y93.1   Activities involving water and water craft
Y93.2   Activities involving ice and snow
Y93.3   Activities involving climbing, rappelling, and jumping off
Y93.4   Activities involving dancing and other rhythmic movement
Y93.5   Activities involving other sports and athletics played individually
Y93.6   Activities involving other sports and athletics played as a team or group
Y93.7   Activities involving other specified sports and athletics
Y93.A   Activities involving other cardiorespiratory exercise
Y93.B   Activities involving other muscle strengthening exercises
Y93.C   Activities involving computer technology and electronic devices
Y93.D   Activities involving arts and handcrafts
Y93.E   Activities involving personal hygiene and interior property and clothing maintenance
Y93.F   Activities involving caregiving
Y93.G   Activities involving food preparation, cooking and grilling
Y93.H   Activities involving exterior property and land maintenance, building and construction
Y93.I   Activities involving roller coasters and other types of external motion
Y93.J   Activities involving playing musical Instrument
Y93.K   Activities involving animal care
Y93.8   Activities, other specified
Y93.9   Activity, unspecified

Y93.0- **Activities involving walking and running**
Excludes 1:   activity, walking an animal (Y93.K1)
                     activity, walking or running on a treadmill (Y93.A1)

Y93.01   **Activity, walking, marching and hiking**
Activity, walking, marching and hiking on level or elevated terrain
Excludes 1:   activity, mountain climbing (Y93.31)

Y93.02   **Activity, running**

Y93.1- **Activities involving water and water craft**
Excludes 1:   activities involving ice (Y93.2-)

Y93.11   **Activity, swimming**
Y93.12   **Activity, springboard and platform diving**
Y93.13   **Activity, water polo**
Y93.14   **Activity, water aerobics and water exercise**
Y93.15   **Activity, underwater diving and snorkeling**
Activity, SCUBA diving
Y93.16   **Activity, rowing, canoeing, kayaking, rafting and tubing**
Activity, canoeing, kayaking, rafting and tubing in calm and turbulent water
Y93.17   **Activity, water skiing and wake boarding**
Y93.18   **Activity, surfing, windsurfing and boogie boarding**
Activity, water sliding
Y93.19   **Activity, other involving water and watercraft**
Activity involving water NOS
Activity, parasailing
Activity, water survival training and testing

Y93.2- **Activities involving ice and snow**
Excludes 1:   activity, shoveling ice and snow (Y93.H1)

Y93.21   **Activity, ice skating**
Activity, figure skating (singles) (pairs)
Activity, ice dancing
Excludes 1:   activity, ice hockey (Y93.22)
Y93.22   **Activity, ice hockey**
Y93.23   **Activity, snow (alpine) (downhill) skiing, snow boarding, sledding, tobogganing and snowtubing**
Excludes 1:   activity, cross country skiing (Y93.24)
Y93.24   **Activity, cross country skiing**
Activity, nordic skiing
Y93.29   **Activity, other involving ice and snow**
Activity involving ice and snow NOS

Y93.3- **Activities involving climbing, rappelling and jumping off**
Excludes 1:   activity, hiking on level or elevated terrain (Y93.01)
                     activity, jumping rope (Y93.56)
                     activity, trampoline jumping (Y93.44)

Y93.31   **Activity, mountain climbing, rock climbing and wall climbing**
Y93.32   **Activity, rappelling**
Y93.33   **Activity, BASE jumping**
Activity, Building, Antenna, Span, Earth jumping
Y93.34   **Activity, bungee jumping**
Y93.35   **Activity, hang gliding**
Y93.39   **Activity, other involving climbing, rappelling and jumping off**

Y93.4- **Activities involving dancing and other rhythmic movement**
Excludes 1:   activity, martial arts (Y93.75)

Y93.41   **Activity, dancing**
Y93.42   **Activity, yoga**
Y93.43   **Activity, gymnastics**
Activity, rhythmic gymnastics
Excludes 1:   activity, trampolining (Y93.44)
Y93.44   **Activity, trampolining**
Y93.45   **Activity, cheerleading**
Y93.49   **Activity, other involving dancing and other rhythmic movements**

Y93.5- **Activities involving other sports and athletics played individually**
Excludes 1:   activity, dancing (Y93.41)
                     activity, gymnastic (Y93.43)
                     activity, trampolining (Y93.44)
                     activity, yoga (Y93.42)

Y93.51   **Activity, roller skating (inline) and skateboarding**
Y93.52   **Activity, horseback riding**
Y93.53   **Activity, golf**
Y93.54   **Activity, bowling**
Y93.55   **Activity, bike riding**
Y93.56   **Activity, jumping rope**
Y93.57   **Activity, non-running track and field events**
Excludes 1:   activity, running (any form) (Y93.02)
Y93.59   **Activity, other involving other sports and athletics played individually**
Excludes 1:   activities involving climbing, rappelling, and jumping (Y93.3-)
                     activities involving ice and snow (Y93.2-)
                     activities involving walking and running (Y93.0-)
                     activities involving water and watercraft (Y93.1-)

Y93.6- **Activities involving other sports and athletics played as a team or group**
Excludes 1:   activity, ice hockey (Y93.22)
                     activity, water polo (Y93.13)

Y93.61   **Activity, american tackle football**
Activity, football NOS
Y93.62   **Activity, american flag or touch football**
Y93.63   **Activity, rugby**
Y93.64   **Activity, baseball**
Activity, softball

© 2016 Channel Publishing, Ltd.

Y93 I Y93

Y93.65 Activity, lacrosse and field hockey
AHA 15:1Q:p8 – Playing lacrosse

Y93.66 Activity, soccer

Y93.67 Activity, basketball

Y93.68 Activity, volleyball (beach) (court)

Y93.6A Activity, physical games generally associated with school recess, summer camp and children
Activity, capture the flag
Activity, dodge ball
Activity, four square
Activity, kickball

Y93.69 Activity, other involving other sports and athletics played as a team or group
Activity, cricket

Y93.7- Activities involving other specified sports and athletics

Y93.71 Activity, boxing

Y93.72 Activity, wrestling

Y93.73 Activity, racquet and hand sports
Activity, handball
Activity, racquetball
Activity, squash
Activity, tennis

Y93.74 Activity, frisbee
Activity, ultimate frisbee

Y93.75 Activity, martial arts
Activity, combatives

Y93.79 Activity, other specified sports and athletics
Excludes 1:   sports and athletics activities specified in categories Y93.0-Y93.6

Y93.A- Activities involving other cardiorespiratory exercise
Activities involving physical training

Y93.A1 Activity, exercise machines primarily for cardiorespiratory conditioning
Activity, elliptical and stepper machines
Activity, stationary bike
Activity, treadmill

Y93.A2 Activity, calisthenics
Activity, jumping jacks
Activity, warm up and cool down

Y93.A3 Activity, aerobic and step exercise

Y93.A4 Activity, circuit training

Y93.A5 Activity, obstacle course
Activity, challenge course
Activity, confidence course

Y93.A6 Activity, grass drills
Activity, guerilla drills

Y93.A9 Activity, other involving cardiorespiratory exercise
Excludes 1:   activities involving cardiorespiratory exercise specified in categories Y93.0-Y93.7

Y93.B- Activities involving other muscle strengthening exercises

Y93.B1 Activity, exercise machines primarily for muscle strengthening

Y93.B2 Activity, push-ups, pull-ups, sit-ups

Y93.B3 Activity, free weights
Activity, barbells
Activity, dumbbells

Y93.B4 Activity, pilates

Y93.B9 Activity, other involving muscle strengthening exercises
Excludes 1:   activities involving muscle strengthening specified in categories Y93.0-Y93.A

Y93.C- Activities involving computer technology and electronic devices
Excludes 1:   activity, electronic musical keyboard or instruments (Y93.J-)

Y93.C1 Activity, computer keyboarding
Activity, electronic game playing using keyboard or other stationary device

Y93.C2 Activity, hand held interactive electronic device
Activity, cellular telephone and communication device
Activity, electronic game playing using interactive device
Excludes 1:   activity, electronic game playing using keyboard or other stationary device (Y93.C1)

Y93.C9 Activity, other involving computer technology and electronic devices

Y93.D- Activities involving arts and handcrafts
Excludes 1:   activities involving playing musical instrument (Y93.J-)

Y93.D1 Activity, knitting and crocheting

Y93.D2 Activity, sewing

Y93.D3 Activity, furniture building and finishing
Activity, furniture repair

Y93.D9 Activity, other involving arts and handcrafts

Y93.E- Activities involving personal hygiene and interior property and clothing maintenance
Excludes 1:   activities involving cooking and grilling (Y93.G-)
activities involving exterior property and land maintenance, building and construction (Y93.H-)
activities involving caregiving (Y93.F-)
activity, dishwashing (Y93.G1)
activity, food preparation (Y93.G1)
activity, gardening (Y93.H2)

Y93.E1 Activity, personal bathing and showering

Y93.E2 Activity, laundry

Y93.E3 Activity, vacuuming

Y93.E4 Activity, ironing

Y93.E5 Activity, floor mopping and cleaning

Y93.E6 Activity, residential relocation
Activity, packing up and unpacking involved in moving to a new residence

Y93.E8 Activity, other personal hygiene

Y93.E9 Activity, other interior property and clothing maintenance

Y93.F- Activities involving caregiving
Activity involving the provider of caregiving

Y93.F1 Activity, caregiving, bathing

Y93.F2 Activity, caregiving, lifting

Y93.F9 Activity, other caregiving

Y93.G- Activities involving food preparation, cooking and grilling

Y93.G1 Activity, food preparation and clean up
Activity, dishwashing

Y93.G2 Activity, grilling and smoking food

Y93.G3 Activity, cooking and baking
Activity, use of stove, oven and microwave oven

Y93.G9 Activity, other involving cooking and grilling

Y93.H- Activities involving exterior property and land maintenance, building and construction

Y93.H1 Activity, digging, shoveling and raking
Activity, dirt digging
Activity, raking leaves
Activity, snow shoveling

Y93.H2 Activity, gardening and landscaping
Activity, pruning, trimming shrubs, weeding

Y93.H3 Activity, building and construction

Y93.H9 Activity, other involving exterior property and land maintenance, building and construction

Y93.I- Activities involving roller coasters and other types of external motion

Y93.I1 Activity, roller coaster riding

Y93.I9 Activity, other involving external motion

Y93.J- Activities involving playing musical instrument
Activity involving playing electric musical instrument

Y93.J1 Activity, piano playing
Activity, musical keyboard (electronic) playing

Y93.J2 Activity, drum and other percussion instrument playing

Y93.J3 Activity, string instrument playing

Y93.J4 Activity, winds and brass instrument playing

Y93.K- Activities involving animal care
Excludes 1:   activity, horseback riding (Y93.52)

Y93.K1 Activity, walking an animal

Y93.K2 Activity, milking an animal

Y93.K3 Activity, grooming and shearing an animal

Y93.K9 Activity, other involving animal care

Excludes 1: = NOT CODED HERE! (Do not code both)

Excludes ❷: = Not Included Here

Y93 - Y93

Y93.8- **Activities, <u>other specified</u>**

    Y93.81 **Activity, refereeing a sports activity**

    Y93.82 **Activity, spectator at an event**

    Y93.83 **Activity, rough housing and horseplay**
        AHA 15:1Q:p7 – Rough housing

    Y93.84 **Activity, sleeping**

    Y93.85 **Activity, choking game**
        Activity, blackout game
        Activity, fainting game
        Activity, pass out game

    Y93.89 **Activity, other specified**

Y93.9 **Activity, <u>unspecified</u>**

Y95 **Nosocomial condition**
    AHA 13:4Q:p119 – Healthcare associated pneumonia

Y99- **<u>External cause status</u>**
    Note: A single code from category Y99 should be used in conjunction with
        the external cause code(s) assigned to a record to indicate the status
        of the person at the time the event occurred.

Y99.0 **Civilian activity done for income or pay**
    Civilian activity done for financial or other compensation
    Excludes 1:   *military activity (Y99.1)*
                       volunteer activity (Y99.2)

Y99.1 **Military activity**
    Excludes 1:   *activity of off duty military personnel (Y99.8)*

Y99.2 **Volunteer activity**
    Excludes 1:   *activity of child or other family member assisting in*
                       compensated work of other family member (Y99.8)

Y99.8 **Other external cause status**
    Activity NEC
    Activity of child or other family member assisting in compensated
        work of other family member
    Hobby not done for income
    Leisure activity
    Off-duty activity of military personnel
    Recreation or sport not for income or while a student
    Student activity
    Excludes 1:   *civilian activity done for income or compensation*
                     (Y99.0)
                     military activity (Y99.1)

Y99.9 **Unspecified external cause status**

Y93 – Y99

Excludes 1: = NOT CODED HERE! (Do not code both) *Excludes ❷:* = Not Included Here

Chapter 21 – Factors influencing health status and contact with health services (Z00-Z99)

Note: Z codes represent reasons for encounters. A corresponding procedure code must accompany a Z code if a procedure is performed. Categories Z00-Z99 are provided for occasions when circumstances other than a disease, injury or external cause classifiable to categories A00-Y89 are recorded as "diagnoses" or "problems". This can arise in two main ways:

(a) When a person who may or may not be sick encounters the health services for some specific purpose, such as to receive limited care or service for a current condition, to donate an organ or tissue, to receive prophylactic vaccination (immunization), or to discuss a problem which is in itself not a disease or injury.

(b) When some circumstance or problem is present which influences the person's health status but is not in itself a current illness or injury.

This chapter contains the following blocks:

Z00-Z13	Persons encountering health services for examinations
Z14-Z15	Genetic carrier and genetic susceptibility to disease
Z16	Resistance to antimicrobial drugs
Z17	Estrogen receptor status
Z18	Retained foreign body fragments
Z19	Hormone sensitivity malignancy status
Z20-Z29	Persons with potential health hazards related to communicable diseases
Z30-Z39	Persons encountering health services in circumstances related to reproduction
Z40-Z53	Encounters for other specific health care
Z55-Z65	Persons with potential health hazards related to socioeconomic and psychosocial circumstances
Z66	Do not resuscitate status
Z67	Blood type
Z68	Body mass index (BMI)
Z69-Z76	Persons encountering health services in other circumstances
Z77-Z99	Persons with potential health hazards related to family and personal history and certain conditions influencing health status

Chapter-Specific Coding Guidelines

C. Chapter-Specific Coding Guidelines

In addition to general coding guidelines, there are guidelines for specific diagnoses and/or conditions in the classification. Unless otherwise indicated, these guidelines apply to all health care settings. Please refer to Section II for guidelines on the selection of principal diagnosis.

21. Chapter 21: Factors Influencing Health Status and Contact with Health Services (Z00-Z99)

Note: The chapter specific guidelines provide additional information about the use of Z codes for specified encounters.

a. Use of Z codes in any healthcare setting

Z codes are for use in any healthcare setting. Z codes may be used as either a first-listed (principal diagnosis code in the inpatient setting) or secondary code, depending on the circumstances of the encounter.

Certain Z codes may only be used as first-listed or principal diagnosis.

b. Z Codes indicate a reason for an encounter

Z codes are not procedure codes. A corresponding procedure code must accompany a Z code to describe any procedure performed.

c. Categories of Z Codes

1) Contact/Exposure

Category Z20 indicates contact with, and suspected exposure to, communicable diseases. These codes are for patients who do not show any sign or symptom of a disease but are suspected to have been exposed to it by close personal contact with an infected individual or are in an area where a disease is epidemic.

Category Z77, Other contact with and (suspected) exposures hazardous to health, indicates contact with and suspected exposures hazardous to health.

Contact/exposure codes may be used as a first-listed code to explain an encounter for testing, or, more commonly, as a secondary code to identify a potential risk.

2) Inoculations and vaccinations

Code Z23 is for encounters for inoculations and vaccinations. It indicates that a patient is being seen to receive a prophylactic inoculation against a disease. Procedure codes are required to identify the actual administration of the injection and the type(s) of immunizations given. Code Z23 may be used as a secondary code if the inoculation is given as a routine part of preventive health care, such as a well-baby visit.

3) Status

Status codes indicate that a patient is either a carrier of a disease or has the sequelae or residual of a past disease or condition. This includes such things as the presence of prosthetic or mechanical devices resulting from past treatment. A status code is informative, because the status may affect the course of treatment and its outcome. A status code is distinct from a history code. The history code indicates that the patient no longer has the condition.

A status code should not be used with a diagnosis code from one of the body system chapters, if the diagnosis code includes the information provided by the status code. For example, code Z94.1, Heart transplant status, should not be used with a code from subcategory T86.2, Complications of heart transplant. The status code does not provide additional information. The complication code indicates that the patient is a heart transplant patient.

For encounters for weaning from a mechanical ventilator, assign a code from subcategory J96.1, Chronic respiratory failure, followed by code Z99.11, Dependence on respirator [ventilator] status.

The status Z codes/categories are:

Z14	Genetic carrier

Genetic carrier status indicates that a person carries a gene, associated with a particular disease, which may be passed to offspring who may develop that disease. The person does not have the disease and is not at risk of developing the disease.

Z15	Genetic susceptibility to disease

Genetic susceptibility indicates that a person has a gene that increases the risk of that person developing the disease.

Codes from category Z15 should not be used as principal or first-listed codes. If the patient has the condition to which he/she is susceptible, and that condition is the reason for the encounter, the code for the current condition should be sequenced first. If the patient is being seen for follow-up after completed treatment for this condition, and the condition no longer exists, a follow-up code should be sequenced first, followed by the appropriate personal history and genetic susceptibility codes. If the purpose of the encounter is genetic counseling associated with procreative management, code Z31.5, Encounter for genetic counseling, should be assigned as the first-listed code, followed by a code from category Z15. Additional codes should be assigned for any applicable family or personal history.

Z16	Resistance to antimicrobial drugs

This code indicates that a patient has a condition that is resistant to antimicrobial drug treatment. Sequence the infection code first.

Z17	Estrogen receptor status
Z18	Retained foreign body fragments
Z19	Hormone sensitivity malignancy status
Z21	Asymptomatic HIV infection status

This code indicates that a patient has tested positive for HIV but has manifested no signs or symptoms of the disease.

Z22	Carrier of infectious disease

Carrier status indicates that a person harbors the specific organisms of a disease without manifest symptoms and is capable of transmitting the infection.

Z28.3	Underimmunization status
Z33.1	Pregnant state, incidental

This code is a secondary code only for use when the pregnancy is in no way complicating the reason for visit. Otherwise, a code from the obstetric chapter is required.

Z66	Do not resuscitate

This code may be used when it is documented by the provider that a patient is on do not resuscitate status at any time during the stay.

Z67	Blood type
Z68	Body mass index (BMI)

As with all other secondary diagnosis codes, the BMI codes should only be assigned when they meet the definition of a reportable diagnosis (see Section III, Reporting Additional Diagnoses).

Z74.01	Bed confinement status
Z76.82	Awaiting organ transplant status
Z78	Other specified health status

Code Z78.1, Physical restraint status, may be used when it is documented by the provider that a patient has been put in restraints during the current encounter. Please note that this code should not be reported when it is documented by the provider that a patient is temporarily restrained during a procedure.

Z00 - Z00

Z79 Long-term (current) drug therapy
Codes from this category indicate a patient's continuous use of a prescribed drug (including such things as aspirin therapy) for the long-term treatment of a condition or for prophylactic use. It is not for use for patients who have addictions to drugs. This subcategory is not for use of medications for detoxification or maintenance programs to prevent withdrawal symptoms in patients with drug dependence (e.g., methadone maintenance for opiate dependence). Assign the appropriate code for the drug dependence instead.

Assign a code from Z79 if the patient is receiving a medication for an extended period as a prophylactic measure (such as for the prevention of deep vein thrombosis) or as treatment of a chronic condition (such as arthritis) or a disease requiring a lengthy course of treatment (such as cancer). Do not assign a code from category Z79 for medication being administered for a brief period of time to treat an acute illness or injury (such as a course of antibiotics to treat acute bronchitis).

Z88 Allergy status to drugs, medicaments and biological substances
Except: Z88.9, Allergy status to unspecified drugs, medicaments and biological substances status

Z89 Acquired absence of limb

Z90 Acquired absence of organs, not elsewhere classified

Z91.0- Allergy status, other than to drugs and biological substances

Z92.82 Status post administration of tPA (rtPA) in a different facility within the last 24 hours prior to admission to a current facility.
Assign code Z92.82, Status post administration of tPA (rtPA) in a different facility within the last 24 hours prior to admission to current facility, as a secondary diagnosis when a patient is received by transfer into a facility and documentation indicates they were administered tissue plasminogen activator (tPA) within the last 24 hours prior to admission to the current facility.

This guideline applies even if the patient is still receiving the tPA at the time they are received into the current facility.

The appropriate code for the condition for which the tPA was administered (such as cerebrovascular disease or myocardial infarction) should be assigned first.

Code Z92.82 is only applicable to the receiving facility record and not to the transferring facility record.

Z93 Artificial opening status

Z94 Transplanted organ and tissue status

Z95 Presence of cardiac and vascular implants and grafts

Z96 Presence of other functional implants

Z97 Presence of other devices

Z98 Other postprocedural states
Assign code Z98.85, Transplanted organ removal status, to indicate that a transplanted organ has been previously removed. This code should not be assigned for the encounter in which the transplanted organ is removed. The complication necessitating removal of the transplant organ should be assigned for that encounter.

See section I.C19. for information on the coding of organ transplant complications.

Z99 Dependence on enabling machines and devices, not elsewhere classified
Note: Categories Z89-Z90 and Z93-Z99 are for use only if there are no complications or malfunctions of the organ or tissue replaced, the amputation site or the equipment on which the patient is dependent.

4) History (of)
There are two types of history Z codes, personal and family. Personal history codes explain a patient's past medical condition that no longer exists and is not receiving any treatment, but that has the potential for recurrence, and therefore may require continued monitoring.

Family history codes are for use when a patient has a family member(s) who has had a particular disease that causes the patient to be at higher risk of also contracting the disease.

Personal history codes may be used in conjunction with follow-up codes and family history codes may be used in conjunction with screening codes to explain the need for a test or procedure. History codes are also acceptable on any medical record regardless of the reason for visit. A history of an illness, even if no longer present, is important information that may alter the type of treatment ordered.

The history Z code categories are:
Z80 Family history of primary malignant neoplasm
Z81 Family history of mental and behavioral disorders
Z82 Family history of certain disabilities and chronic diseases (leading to disablement)
Z83 Family history of other specific disorders
Z84 Family history of other conditions

Z85 Personal history of malignant neoplasm
Z86 Personal history of certain other diseases
Z87 Personal history of other diseases and conditions
Z91.4- Personal history of psychological trauma, not elsewhere classified
Z91.5 Personal history of self-harm
Z91.8- Other specified personal risk factors, not elsewhere classified
Exception: Z91.83, Wandering in diseases classified elsewhere
Z92 Personal history of medical treatment
Except: Z92.0, Personal history of contraception
Except: Z92.82, Status post administration of tPA (rtPA) in a different facility within the last 24 hours prior to admission to a current facility

5) Screening
Screening is the testing for disease or disease precursors in seemingly well individuals so that early detection and treatment can be provided for those who test positive for the disease (e.g., screening mammogram).

The testing of a person to rule out or confirm a suspected diagnosis because the patient has some sign or symptom is a diagnostic examination, not a screening. In these cases, the sign or symptom is used to explain the reason for the test.

A screening code may be a first-listed code if the reason for the visit is specifically the screening exam. It may also be used as an additional code if the screening is done during an office visit for other health problems. A screening code is not necessary if the screening is inherent to a routine examination, such as a pap smear done during a routine pelvic examination.

Should a condition be discovered during the screening then the code for the condition may be assigned as an additional diagnosis.

The Z code indicates that a screening exam is planned. A procedure code is required to confirm that the screening was performed.

The screening Z codes/categories:
Z11 Encounter for screening for infectious and parasitic diseases
Z12 Encounter for screening for malignant neoplasms
Z13 Encounter for screening for other diseases and disorders
Except: Z13.9, Encounter for screening, unspecified
Z36 Encounter for antenatal screening for mother

6) Observation
There are ~~two~~ three observation Z code categories. They are for use in very limited circumstances when a person is being observed for a suspected condition that is ruled out. The observation codes are not for use if an injury or illness or any signs or symptoms related to the suspected condition are present. In such cases the diagnosis/symptom code is used with the corresponding external cause code.

The observation codes are to be used as principal diagnosis only. The only exception to this is when the principal diagnosis is required to be a code from category Z38, Liveborn infants according to place of birth and type of delivery. Then a code from category Z05, Encounter for observation and evaluation of newborn for suspected diseases and conditions ruled out, is sequenced after the Z38 code. Additional codes may be used in addition to the observation code but only if they are unrelated to the suspected condition being observed.

Codes from subcategory Z03.7, Encounter for suspected maternal and fetal conditions ruled out, may either be used as a first-listed or as an additional code assignment depending on the case. They are for use in very limited circumstances on a maternal record when an encounter is for a suspected maternal or fetal condition that is ruled out during that encounter (for example, a maternal or fetal condition may be suspected due to an abnormal test result). These codes should not be used when the condition is confirmed. In those cases, the confirmed condition should be coded. In addition, these codes are not for use if an illness or any signs or symptoms related to the suspected condition or problem are present. In such cases the diagnosis/symptom code is used.

Additional codes may be used in addition to the code from subcategory Z03.7, but only if they are unrelated to the suspected condition being evaluated.

Codes from subcategory Z03.7 may not be used for encounters for antenatal screening of mother. *See Section I.C.21. Screening.*

For encounters for suspected fetal condition that are inconclusive following testing and evaluation, assign the appropriate code from category O35, O36, O40 or O41.

The observation Z code categories:
Z03 Encounter for medical observation for suspected diseases and conditions ruled out
Z04 Encounter for examination and observation for other reasons
Except: Z04.9, Encounter for examination and observation for unspecified reason
Z05 Encounter for observation and evaluation of newborn for suspected diseases and conditions ruled out

Z00-Z00

7) Aftercare

Aftercare visit codes cover situations when the initial treatment of a disease has been performed and the patient requires continued care during the healing or recovery phase, or for the long-term consequences of the disease. The aftercare Z code should not be used if treatment is directed at a current, acute disease. The diagnosis code is to be used in these cases. Exceptions to this rule are codes Z51.0, Encounter for antineoplastic radiation therapy, and codes from subcategory Z51.1, Encounter for antineoplastic chemotherapy and immunotherapy. These codes are to be first-listed, followed by the diagnosis code when a patient's encounter is solely to receive radiation therapy, chemotherapy, or immunotherapy for the treatment of a neoplasm. If the reason for the encounter is more than one type of antineoplastic therapy, code Z51.0 and a code from subcategory Z51.1 may be assigned together, in which case one of these codes would be reported as a secondary diagnosis.

The aftercare Z codes should also not be used for aftercare for injuries. For aftercare of an injury, assign the acute injury code with the appropriate 7th character (for subsequent encounter).

The aftercare codes are generally first-listed to explain the specific reason for the encounter. An aftercare code may be used as an additional code when some type of aftercare is provided in addition to the reason for admission and no diagnosis code is applicable. An example of this would be the closure of a colostomy during an encounter for treatment of another condition.

Aftercare codes should be used in conjunction with other aftercare codes or diagnosis codes to provide better detail on the specifics of an aftercare encounter visit, unless otherwise directed by the classification. Should a patient receive multiple types of antineoplastic therapy during the same encounter, code Z51.0, Encounter for antineoplastic radiation therapy, and codes from subcategory Z51.1, Encounter for antineoplastic chemotherapy and immunotherapy, may be used together on a record. The sequencing of multiple aftercare codes depends on the circumstances of the encounter.

Certain aftercare Z code categories need a secondary diagnosis code to describe the resolving condition or sequelae. For others, the condition is included in the code title.

Additional Z code aftercare category terms include fitting and adjustment, and attention to artificial openings.

Status Z codes may be used with aftercare Z codes to indicate the nature of the aftercare. For example code Z95.1, Presence of aortocoronary bypass graft, may be used with code Z48.812, Encounter for surgical aftercare following surgery on the circulatory system, to indicate the surgery for which the aftercare is being performed. A status code should not be used when the aftercare code indicates the type of status, such as using Z43.0, Encounter for attention to tracheostomy, with Z93.0, Tracheostomy status.

The aftercare Z category/codes:

Z42	Encounter for plastic and reconstructive surgery following medical procedure or healed injury
Z43	Encounter for attention to artificial openings
Z44	Encounter for fitting and adjustment of external prosthetic device
Z45	Encounter for adjustment and management of implanted device
Z46	Encounter for fitting and adjustment of other devices
Z47	Orthopedic aftercare
Z48	Encounter for other postprocedural aftercare
Z49	Encounter for care involving renal dialysis
Z51	Encounter for other aftercare and medical care

8) Follow-up

The follow-up codes are used to explain continuing surveillance following completed treatment of a disease, condition, or injury. They imply that the condition has been fully treated and no longer exists. They should not be confused with aftercare codes, or injury codes with a 7th character for subsequent encounter, that explain ongoing care of a healing condition or its sequelae. Follow-up codes may be used in conjunction with history codes to provide the full picture of the healed condition and its treatment. The follow-up code is sequenced first, followed by the history code.

A follow-up code may be used to explain multiple visits. Should a condition be found to have recurred on the follow-up visit, then the diagnosis code for the condition should be assigned in place of the follow-up code.

The follow-up Z code categories:

Z08	Encounter for follow-up examination after completed treatment for malignant neoplasm
Z09	Encounter for follow-up examination after completed treatment for conditions other than malignant neoplasm
Z39	Encounter for maternal postpartum care and examination

9) Donor

Codes in category Z52, Donors of organs and tissues, are used for living individuals who are donating blood or other body tissue. These codes are only for individuals donating for others, not for self-donations. They are not used to identify cadaveric donations.

10) Counseling

Counseling Z codes are used when a patient or family member receives assistance in the aftermath of an illness or injury, or when support is required in coping with family or social problems. They are not used in conjunction with a diagnosis code when the counseling component of care is considered integral to standard treatment. The counseling Z codes/categories:

Z30.0-	Encounter for general counseling and advice on contraception
Z31.5	Encounter for genetic counseling
Z31.6-	Encounter for general counseling and advice on procreation
Z32.2	Encounter for childbirth instruction
Z32.3	Encounter for childcare instruction
Z69	Encounter for mental health services for victim and perpetrator of abuse
Z70	Counseling related to sexual attitude, behavior and orientation
Z71	Persons encountering health services for other counseling and medical advice, not elsewhere classified
Z76.81	Expectant mother prebirth pediatrician visit

11) Encounters for Obstetrical and Reproductive Services

See Section I.C.15. Pregnancy, Childbirth, and the Puerperium, for further instruction on the use of these codes.

Z codes for pregnancy are for use in those circumstances when none of the problems or complications included in the codes from the Obstetrics chapter exist (a routine prenatal visit or postpartum care). Codes in category Z34, Encounter for supervision of normal pregnancy, are always first-listed and are not to be used with any other code from the OB chapter.

Codes in category Z3A, Weeks of gestation, may be assigned to provide additional information about the pregnancy. Category Z3A codes should not be assigned for pregnancies with abortive outcomes (categories O00-O08), elective termination of pregnancy (code Z33.32), nor for postpartum conditions, as category Z3A is not applicable to these conditions. The date of the admission should be used to determine weeks of gestation for inpatient admissions that encompass more than one gestational week.

The outcome of delivery, category Z37, should be included on all maternal delivery records. It is always a secondary code. Codes in category Z37 should not be used on the newborn record.

Z codes for family planning (contraceptive) or procreative management and counseling should be included on an obstetric record either during the pregnancy or the postpartum stage, if applicable.

Z codes/categories for obstetrical and reproductive services:

Z30	Encounter for contraceptive management
Z31	Encounter for procreative management
Z32.2	Encounter for childbirth instruction
Z32.3	Encounter for childcare instruction
Z33	Pregnant state
Z34	Encounter for supervision of normal pregnancy
Z36	Encounter for antenatal screening of mother
Z3A	Weeks of gestation
Z37	Outcome of delivery
Z39	Encounter for maternal postpartum care and examination
Z76.81	Expectant mother prebirth pediatrician visit

12) Newborns and Infants

See Section I.C.16. Newborn (Perinatal) Guidelines, for further instruction on the use of these codes.

Newborn Z codes/categories:

Z76.1	Encounter for health supervision and care of foundling
Z00.1-	Encounter for routine child health examination
Z38	Liveborn infants according to place of birth and type of delivery

13) Routine and administrative examinations

The Z codes allow for the description of encounters for routine examinations, such as, a general check-up, or, examinations for administrative purposes, such as, a pre-employment physical. The codes are not to be used if the examination is for diagnosis of a suspected condition or for treatment purposes. In such cases the diagnosis code is used. During a routine exam, should a diagnosis or condition be discovered, it should be coded as an additional code. Pre-existing and chronic conditions and history codes may also be included as additional codes as long as the examination is for administrative purposes and not focused on any particular condition.

Z00 - Z00

Some of the codes for routine health examinations distinguish between "with" and "without" abnormal findings. Code assignment depends on the information that is known at the time the encounter is being coded. For example, if no abnormal findings were found during the examination, but the encounter is being coded before test results are back, it is acceptable to assign the code for "without abnormal findings." When assigning a code for "with abnormal findings," additional code(s) should be assigned to identify the specific abnormal finding(s).

Pre-operative examination and pre-procedural laboratory examination Z codes are for use only in those situations when a patient is being cleared for a procedure or surgery and no treatment is given.

The Z codes/categories for routine and administrative examinations:

Z00   Encounter for general examination without complaint, suspected or reported diagnosis
Z01   Encounter for other special examination without complaint, suspected or reported diagnosis
Z02   Encounter for administrative examination
     Except: Z02.9, Encounter for administrative examinations, unspecified
Z32.0-   Encounter for pregnancy test

14) Miscellaneous Z codes

The miscellaneous Z codes capture a number of other health care encounters that do not fall into one of the other categories. Certain of these codes identify the reason for the encounter; others are for use as additional codes that provide useful information on circumstances that may affect a patient's care and treatment.

Prophylactic Organ Removal

For encounters specifically for prophylactic removal of an organ (such as prophylactic removal of breasts due to a genetic susceptibility to cancer or a family history of cancer), the principal or first-listed code should be a code from category Z40, Encounter for prophylactic surgery, followed by the appropriate codes to identify the associated risk factor (such as genetic susceptibility or family history).

If the patient has a malignancy of one site and is having prophylactic removal at another site to prevent either a new primary malignancy or metastatic disease, a code for the malignancy should also be assigned in addition to a code from subcategory Z40.0, Encounter for prophylactic surgery for risk factors related to malignant neoplasms. A Z40.0 code should not be assigned if the patient is having organ removal for treatment of a malignancy, such as the removal of the testes for the treatment of prostate cancer.

Miscellaneous Z codes/categories:

Z28   Immunization not carried out
     Except: Z28.3, Underimmunization status
Z29   Encounter for other prophylactic measures
Z40   Encounter for prophylactic surgery
Z41   Encounter for procedures for purposes other than remedying health state
     Except: Z41.9, Encounter for procedure for purposes other than remedying health state, unspecified
Z53   Persons encountering health services for specific procedures and treatment, not carried out
Z55   Problems related to education and literacy
Z56   Problems related to employment and unemployment
Z57   Occupational exposure to risk factors
Z58   Problems related to physical environment
Z59   Problems related to housing and economic circumstances
Z60   Problems related to social environment
Z62   Problems related to upbringing
Z63   Other problems related to primary support group, including family circumstances
Z64   Problems related to certain psychosocial circumstances
Z65   Problems related to other psychosocial circumstances
Z72   Problems related to lifestyle
     Note: These codes should be assigned only when the documentation specifies that the patient has an associated problem
Z73   Problems related to life management difficulty
Z74   Problems related to care provider dependency
     Except: Z74.01, Bed confinement status
Z75   Problems related to medical facilities and other health care
Z76.0   Encounter for issue of repeat prescription
Z76.3   Healthy person accompanying sick person
Z76.4   Other boarder to healthcare facility
Z76.5   Malingerer [conscious simulation]
Z91.1-   Patient's noncompliance with medical treatment and regimen
Z91.83   Wandering in diseases classified elsewhere
Z91.89   Other specified personal risk factors, not elsewhere classified

15) Nonspecific Z codes

Certain Z codes are so non-specific, or potentially redundant with other codes in the classification, that there can be little justification for their use in the inpatient setting. Their use in the outpatient setting should be limited to those instances when there is no further documentation to permit more precise coding. Otherwise, any sign or symptom or any other reason for visit that is captured in another code should be used.

Nonspecific Z codes/categories:

Z02.9   Encounter for administrative examinations, unspecified
Z04.9   Encounter for examination and observation for unspecified reason
Z13.9   Encounter for screening, unspecified
Z41.9   Encounter for procedure for purposes other than remedying health state, unspecified
Z52.9   Donor of unspecified organ or tissue
Z86.59   Personal history of other mental and behavioral disorders
Z88.9   Allergy status to unspecified drugs, medicaments and biological substances status
Z92.0   Personal history of contraception

16) Z Codes That May Only be Principal/First-Listed Diagnosis

The following Z codes/categories may only be reported as the principal/first-listed diagnosis, except when there are multiple encounters on the same day and the medical records for the encounters are combined:

Z00   Encounter for general examination without complaint, suspected or reported diagnosis Except: Z00.6
Z01   Encounter for other special examination without complaint, suspected or reported diagnosis
Z02   Encounter for administrative examination
Z03   Encounter for medical observation for suspected diseases and conditions ruled out
Z04   Encounter for examination and observation for other reasons
Z31.81   Encounter for male factor infertility in female patient
~~Z31.82   Encounter for Rh incompatibility status~~
Z31.83   Encounter for assisted reproductive fertility procedure cycle
Z31.84   Encounter for fertility preservation procedure
Z34   Encounter for supervision of normal pregnancy
Z39   Encounter for maternal postpartum care and examination
Z38   Liveborn infants according to place of birth and type of delivery
Z42   Encounter for plastic and reconstructive surgery following medical procedure or healed injury
Z51.0   Encounter for antineoplastic radiation therapy
Z51.1-   Encounter for antineoplastic chemotherapy and immunotherapy
Z52   Donors of organs and tissues
     Except: Z52.9, Donor of unspecified organ or tissue
Z76.1   Encounter for health supervision and care of foundling
Z76.2   Encounter for health supervision and care of other healthy infant and child
Z99.12   Encounter for respirator [ventilator] dependence during power failure

Z00 - Z99

Persons encountering health services for examinations (Z00-Z13)

Note: Nonspecific abnormal findings disclosed at the time of these examinations are classified to categories R70-R94.
Excludes 1: *examinations related to pregnancy and reproduction (Z30-Z36, Z39.-)*

Z00- Encounter for <u>general examination</u> <u>without</u> complaint, suspected or reported diagnosis
   Excludes 1: *encounter for examination for administrative purposes (Z02.-)*
   Excludes ❷: *encounter for pre-procedural examinations (Z01.81-)*
      special screening examinations (Z11-Z13)

Z00.0- Encounter for general adult medical examination
   Encounter for adult periodic examination (annual) (physical) and any associated laboratory and radiologic examinations
   Excludes 1: *encounter for examination of sign or symptom- code to sign or symptom*
      general health check-up of infant or child (Z00.12.-)

   Z00.00 Encounter for general adult medical examination <u>without abnormal findings</u> — [Age/15-124] [Unacceptable PDX]
      AHA 16:1Q:p36 – Adult exam with history of COPD and smoking
      Encounter for adult health check-up NOS

   Z00.01 Encounter for general adult medical examination <u>with abnormal findings</u> — [Age/15-124] [Unacceptable PDX]
      AHA 16:1Q:p36 – Adult exam with acute exacerbation of COPD
      AHA 16:1Q:p35 – Adult exam with elevated blood pressure
      Use additional code to identify abnormal findings

Z00.1- Encounter for newborn, infant and child health examinations

   Z00.11- <u>Newborn health examination</u>
      Health check for child under 29 days old
      Use additional code to identify any abnormal findings
      Excludes 1: *health check for child over 28 days old (Z00.12-)*

      Z00.110 Health examination for newborn <u>under 8 days old</u> — [Age/0] [Unacceptable PDX]
         Health check for newborn under 8 days old

      Z00.111 Health examination for newborn <u>8 to 28 days old</u> — [Age/0] [Unacceptable PDX]
         Health check for newborn 8 to 28 days old
         Newborn weight check

   Z00.12- Encounter for <u>routine child health examination</u>
      Encounter for development testing of infant or child
      Health check (routine) for child over 28 days old
      Excludes 1: *health check for child under 29 days old (Z00.11-)*
      health supervision of foundling or other healthy infant or child (Z76.1-Z76.2)
      newborn health examination (Z00.11-)

      Z00.121 Encounter for routine child health examination <u>with abnormal findings</u> — [Age/0-17] [Unacceptable PDX]
         AHA 16:1Q:p35 – Well-child exam with acute exacerbation of mild persistent asthma
         AHA 16:1Q:p34 – Well-infant exam with findings of otitis media
         Use additional code to identify abnormal findings

      Z00.129 Encounter for routine child health examination <u>without</u> abnormal findings — [Age/0-17] [Unacceptable PDX]
         AHA 16:1Q:p34 – Well-child exam with previous diagnosis of viral bronchitis
         Encounter for routine child health examination NOS

Z00.2 Encounter for examination for period of rapid growth in childhood — [Age/0-17] [Unacceptable PDX]

Z00.3 Encounter for examination for adolescent development state — [Age/0-17] [Unacceptable PDX]
   Encounter for puberty development state

Z00.5 Encounter for examination of potential donor of organ and tissue — [Unacceptable PDX]

Z00.6 Encounter for examination for normal comparison and control in clinical research program
   Examination of participant or control in clinical research program

Z00.7- Encounter for <u>examination for period of delayed growth in childhood</u>

   Z00.70 Encounter for examination for period of delayed growth in childhood <u>without</u> abnormal findings — [Age/0-17] [Unacceptable PDX]

   Z00.71 Encounter for examination for period of delayed growth in childhood <u>with abnormal findings</u> — [Age/0-17] [Unacceptable PDX]
      Use additional code to identify abnormal findings

Z00.8 Encounter for other general examination — [Unacceptable PDX]
   Encounter for health examination in population surveys

Z01- Encounter for <u>other special examination</u> <u>without</u> complaint, suspected or reported diagnosis
   Includes: Routine examination of specific system
   Note: Codes from category Z01 represent the reason for the encounter. A separate procedure code is required to identify any examinations or procedures performed.
   Excludes 1: *encounter for examination for administrative purposes (Z02.-)*
      encounter for examination for suspected conditions, proven not to exist (Z03.-)
      encounter for laboratory and radiologic examinations as a component of general medical examinations (Z00.0-)
      encounter for laboratory, radiologic and imaging examinations for sign(s) and symptom(s) — code to the sign(s) or symptom(s)
   Excludes ❷: *screening examinations (Z11-Z13)*

Z01.0- Encounter for <u>examination of eyes and vision</u>
   Excludes 1: *examination for driving license (Z02.4)*

   Z01.00 Encounter for examination of eyes and vision <u>without</u> abnormal findings
      Encounter for examination of eyes and vision NOS

   Z01.01 Encounter for examination of eyes and vision <u>with abnormal findings</u>
      Use additional code to identify abnormal findings

Z01.1- Encounter for <u>examination of ears and hearing</u>

   Z01.10 Encounter for examination of ears and hearing <u>without</u> abnormal findings — [Unacceptable PDX]
      Encounter for examination of ears and hearing NOS

   Z01.11- Encounter for examination of ears and hearing <u>with abnormal findings</u>

      Z01.110 Encounter for hearing examination following failed hearing screening — [Unacceptable PDX]

      Z01.118 Encounter for examination of ears and hearing with other abnormal findings — [Unacceptable PDX]
         Use additional code to identify abnormal findings

   Z01.12 Encounter for hearing conservation and treatment — [Unacceptable PDX]

Z01.2- Encounter for <u>dental examination and cleaning</u>

   Z01.20 Encounter for dental examination and cleaning <u>without</u> abnormal findings — [Unacceptable PDX]
      Encounter for dental examination and cleaning NOS

   Z01.21 Encounter for dental examination and cleaning <u>with abnormal findings</u> — [Unacceptable PDX]
      Use additional code to identify abnormal findings

Z01.3- Encounter for <u>examination of blood pressure</u>

   Z01.30 Encounter for examination of blood pressure <u>without</u> abnormal findings — [Unacceptable PDX]
      Encounter for examination of blood pressure NOS

   Z01.31 Encounter for examination of blood pressure <u>with abnormal findings</u> — [Unacceptable PDX]
      Use additional code to identify abnormal findings

Z00-Z01

Excludes 1: = NOT CODED HERE! (Do not code both)   **1309**   *Excludes ❷:* = Not Included Here

Z01.4- Encounter for <u>gynecological examination</u>
 Excludes ❷: *pregnancy examination or test (Z32.0-)*
    routine examination for contraceptive maintenance
    (Z30.4-)

 Z01.41- Encounter for <u>routine</u> gynecological examination
  Encounter for general gynecological examination with or
   without cervical smear
  Encounter for gynecological examination (general) (routine)
   NOS
  Encounter for pelvic examination (annual) (periodic)
  Use additional code:
  For screening for human papillomavirus, if applicable,
   (Z11.51)
  For screening vaginal pap smear, if applicable (Z12.72)
  To identify acquired absence of uterus, if applicable (Z90.71-)
  Excludes 1: *gynecologic examination status-post hysterectomy*
    for malignant condition (Z08)
    screening cervical pap smear not a part of a
    routine gynecological examination (Z12.4)

  Z01.411 Encounter for gynecological examination (general)
   (routine) <u>with abnormal findings</u> — [♀]
   Use additional code to identify abnormal findings

  Z01.419 Encounter for gynecological examination (general)
   (routine) <u>without</u> abnormal findings — [♀]

 Z01.42 Encounter for cervical smear to confirm findings of recent
  normal smear following initial abnormal smear — [♀]

Z01.8- Encounter for other specified special examinations

 Z01.81- Encounter for <u>preprocedural examinations</u>
  Encounter for preoperative examinations
  Encounter for radiological and imaging examinations as part
   of preprocedural examination

  Z01.810 Encounter for preprocedural <u>cardiovascular</u>
   examination

  Z01.811 Encounter for preprocedural <u>respiratory</u>
   examination

  Z01.812 Encounter for preprocedural <u>laboratory</u>
   examination — [Unacceptable PDX]
   Blood and urine tests prior to treatment or procedure

  Z01.818 Encounter for <u>other</u> preprocedural examination —
   [Unacceptable PDX]
   Encounter for preprocedural examination NOS
   Encounter for examinations prior to antineoplastic
   chemotherapy

 Z01.82 Encounter for allergy testing — [Unacceptable PDX]
  Excludes 1: *encounter for antibody response examination*
    (Z01.84)

 Z01.83 Encounter for blood typing — [Unacceptable PDX]
  Encounter for Rh typing

 Z01.84 Encounter for antibody response examination —
  [Unacceptable PDX]
  Encounter for immunity status testing
  Excludes 1: *encounter for allergy testing (Z01.82)*

 Z01.89 Encounter for other specified special examinations —
  [Unacceptable PDX]

Z02- Encounter for <u>administrative examination</u>

 Z02.0 Encounter for examination for admission to educational
  institution — [Unacceptable PDX]
  Encounter for examination for admission to preschool (education)
  Encounter for examination for re-admission to school following
   illness or medical treatment

 Z02.1 Encounter for pre-employment examination

 Z02.2 Encounter for examination for admission to residential
  institution — [Unacceptable PDX]
  Excludes 1: *examination for admission to prison (Z02.89)*

 Z02.3 Encounter for examination for recruitment to armed forces

 Z02.4 Encounter for examination for driving license —
  [Unacceptable PDX]

 Z02.5 Encounter for examination for participation in sport —
  [Unacceptable PDX]
  Excludes 1: *blood-alcohol and blood-drug test (Z02.83)*

 Z02.6 Encounter for examination for insurance purposes —
  [Unacceptable PDX]

 Z02.7- Encounter for issue of medical certificate
  Excludes 1: *encounter for general medical examination (Z00-Z01,*
    Z02.0-Z02.6, Z02.8-Z02.9)

  Z02.71 Encounter for disability determination — [Unacceptable PDX]
   Encounter for issue of medical certificate of incapacity
   Encounter for issue of medical certificate of invalidity

  Z02.79 Encounter for issue of other medical certificate —
   [Unacceptable PDX]

 Z02.8- Encounter for other administrative examinations

  Z02.81 Encounter for paternity testing

  Z02.82 Encounter for adoption services — [Unacceptable PDX]

  Z02.83 Encounter for blood-alcohol and blood-drug test
   Use additional code for findings of alcohol or drugs in blood
   (R78.-)

  Z02.89 Encounter for other administrative examinations —
   [Unacceptable PDX]
   Encounter for examination for admission to prison
   Encounter for examination for admission to summer camp
   Encounter for immigration examination
   Encounter for naturalization examination
   Encounter for premarital examination
   Excludes 1: *health supervision of foundling or other healthy*
     infant or child (Z76.1-Z76.2)

 Z02.9 Encounter for administrative examinations, unspecified —
  [Unacceptable PDX]

Z03- Encounter for <u>medical observation for suspected diseases and
conditions</u> <u>ruled out</u>
 Note: This category is to be used when a person without a diagnosis is
  suspected of having an abnormal condition, without signs or
  symptoms, which requires study, but after examination and
  observation, is ruled out. This category is also for use for
  administrative and legal observation status.
 Excludes 1: *contact with and (suspected) exposures hazardous to health*
    (Z77.-)
    newborn observation for suspected condition, ruled out (P00-
    P04)
    person with feared complaint in whom no diagnosis is made
    (Z71.1)
    signs or symptoms under study — code to signs or symptoms

 Z03.6 Encounter for observation for suspected toxic effect from
  ingested substance ruled out
  Encounter for observation for suspected adverse effect from drug
  Encounter for observation for suspected poisoning

 Z03.7- Encounter for <u>suspected maternal and fetal conditions</u> ruled
  out
  Encounter for suspected maternal and fetal conditions not found
  Excludes 1: *known or suspected fetal anomalies affecting*
    management of mother, not ruled out (O26.-,
    O35.-, O36.-, O40.-, O41.-)

  Z03.71 Encounter for suspected problem <u>with amniotic cavity and
   membrane</u> ruled out — [♀, Age/12-55] [Unacceptable PDX]
   Encounter for suspected oligohydramnios ruled out
   Encounter for suspected polyhydramnios ruled out

  Z03.72 Encounter for suspected <u>placental problem</u> ruled out —
   [♀, Age/12-55] [Unacceptable PDX]

  Z03.73 Encounter for suspected <u>fetal anomaly</u> ruled out —
   [♀, Age/12-55] [Unacceptable PDX]

  Z03.74 Encounter for suspected <u>problem with fetal growth</u> ruled
   out — [♀, Age/12-55] [Unacceptable PDX]

  Z03.75 Encounter for suspected <u>cervical shortening</u> ruled out —
   [♀, Age/12-55] [Unacceptable PDX]

  Z03.79 Encounter for <u>other</u> suspected maternal and fetal
   conditions <u>ruled out</u> — [♀, Age/12-55] [Unacceptable PDX]

 Z03.8- Encounter for observation for other suspected diseases and
  conditions ruled out

  Z03.81- Encounter for observation for suspected exposure to
   biological agents ruled out

   Z03.810 Encounter for observation for suspected exposure
    to anthrax ruled out

   Z03.818 Encounter for observation for suspected exposure
    to other biological agents ruled out

  Z03.89 Encounter for observation for other suspected diseases
   and conditions ruled out

Excludes 1: = NOT CODED HERE! (Do not code both)   **1310**   *Excludes ❷:* = Not Included Here

Z04- **Encounter for examination and observation for other reasons**
Includes: Encounter for examination for medicolegal reasons
Note: This category is to be used when a person without a diagnosis is suspected of having an abnormal condition, without signs or symptoms, which requires study, but after examination and observation, is ruled out. This category is also for use for administrative and legal observation status.

Z04.1 **Encounter for examination and observation following transport accident**
Excludes 1:   encounter for examination and observation following work accident (Z04.2)

Z04.2 **Encounter for examination and observation following work accident**

Z04.3 **Encounter for examination and observation following other accident**

Z04.4- **Encounter for examination and observation following <u>alleged rape</u>**
Encounter for examination and observation of victim following alleged rape
Encounter for examination and observation of victim following alleged sexual abuse

    Z04.41 **Encounter for examination and observation following alleged <u>adult</u> rape** — [Age/15-124]
Suspected adult rape, ruled out
Suspected adult sexual abuse, ruled out

    Z04.42 **Encounter for examination and observation following alleged <u>child</u> rape** — [Age/0-17]
Suspected child rape, ruled out
Suspected child sexual abuse, ruled out

Z04.6 **Encounter for general psychiatric examination, requested by authority**

Z04.7- **Encounter for examination and observation following <u>alleged physical abuse</u>**

    Z04.71 **Encounter for examination and observation following alleged <u>adult</u> physical abuse** — [Age/15-124]
Suspected adult physical abuse, ruled out
Excludes 1:   confirmed case of adult physical abuse (T74.-)
encounter for examination and observation following alleged adult sexual abuse (Z04.41)
suspected case of adult physical abuse, not ruled out (T76.-)

    Z04.72 **Encounter for examination and observation following alleged <u>child</u> physical abuse** — [Age/0-17]
Suspected child physical abuse, ruled out
Excludes 1:   confirmed case of child physical abuse (T74.-)
encounter for examination and observation following alleged child sexual abuse (Z04.42)
suspected case of child physical abuse, not ruled out (T76.-)

Z04.8 **Encounter for examination and observation for other specified reasons** — [Unacceptable PDX]
Encounter for examination and observation for request for expert evidence

Z04.9 **Encounter for examination and observation for unspecified reason** — [Unacceptable PDX]
Encounter for observation NOS

Z05- **Encounter for observation and examination of <u>newborn</u> for suspected diseases and <u>conditions ruled out</u>**
This category is to be used for newborns, within the neonatal period (the first 28 days of life), who are suspected of having an abnormal condition unrelated to exposure from the mother or the birth process, but without signs or symptoms, and which, after examination and observation, is ruled out.
Excludes ❷: newborn observation for suspected condition, related to exposure from the mother or birth process (P00-P04)

Z05.0 **Observation and evaluation of newborn for suspected <u>cardiac</u> condition ruled out** — [Age/0] [Unacceptable PDX]

Z05.1 **Observation and evaluation of newborn for suspected <u>infectious</u> condition ruled out** — [Age/0] [Unacceptable PDX]

Z05.2 **Observation and evaluation of newborn for suspected <u>neurological</u> condition ruled out** — [Age/0] [Unacceptable PDX]

Z05.3 **Observation and evaluation of newborn for suspected <u>respiratory</u> condition ruled out** — [Age/0] [Unacceptable PDX]

Z05.4- **Observation and evaluation of newborn for suspected <u>genetic, metabolic or immunologic</u> condition ruled out**

    Z05.41 **Observation and evaluation of newborn for suspected <u>genetic</u> condition ruled out** — [Age/0] [Unacceptable PDX]

    Z05.42 **Observation and evaluation of newborn for suspected <u>metabolic</u> condition ruled out** — [Age/0] [Unacceptable PDX]

    Z05.43 **Observation and evaluation of newborn for suspected <u>immunologic</u> condition ruled out** — [Age/0] [Unacceptable PDX]

Z05.5 **Observation and evaluation of newborn for suspected <u>gastrointestinal</u> condition ruled out** — [Age/0] [Unacceptable PDX]

Z05.6 **Observation and evaluation of newborn for suspected <u>genitourinary</u> condition ruled out** — [Age/0] [Unacceptable PDX]

Z05.7- **Observation and evaluation of newborn for suspected <u>skin, subcutaneous, musculoskeletal and connective tissue</u> condition ruled out**

    Z05.71 **Observation and evaluation of newborn for suspected <u>skin and subcutaneous tissue</u> condition ruled out** — [Age/0] [Unacceptable PDX]

    Z05.72 **Observation and evaluation of newborn for suspected <u>musculoskeletal</u> condition ruled out** — [Age/0] [Unacceptable PDX]

    Z05.73 **Observation and evaluation of newborn for suspected <u>connective tissue</u> condition ruled out** — [Age/0] [Unacceptable PDX]

Z05.8 **Observation and evaluation of newborn for <u>other specified</u> suspected condition ruled out** — [Age/0] [Unacceptable PDX]

Z05.9 **Observation and evaluation of newborn for <u>unspecified</u> suspected condition ruled out** — [Age/0] [Unacceptable PDX]

Z08 **Encounter for follow-up examination after completed treatment for malignant neoplasm** — [Unacceptable PDX]
Medical surveillance following completed treatment
Use additional code to identify any acquired absence of organs (Z90.-)
Use additional code to identify the personal history of malignant neoplasm (Z85.-)
Excludes 1:   aftercare following medical care (Z43-Z49, Z51)

Z09 **Encounter for follow-up examination after completed treatment for conditions other than malignant neoplasm** — [Unacceptable PDX]
Medical surveillance following completed treatment
Use additional code to identify any applicable history of disease code (Z86.- Z87.-)
Excludes 1:   aftercare following medical care (Z43-Z49, Z51)
surveillance of contraception (Z30.4-)
surveillance of prosthetic and other medical devices (Z44-Z46)

Z11- **Encounter for screening for infectious and parasitic diseases**
Note: Screening is the testing for disease or disease precursors in asymptomatic individuals so that early detection and treatment can be provided for those who test positive for the disease.
Excludes 1:   encounter for diagnostic examination — code to sign or symptom

Z11.0 **Encounter for screening for intestinal infectious diseases** — [Unacceptable PDX]

Z11.1 **Encounter for screening for respiratory tuberculosis** — [Unacceptable PDX]

Z11.2 **Encounter for screening for other bacterial diseases** — [Unacceptable PDX]

Z11.3 **Encounter for screening for infections with a predominantly sexual mode of transmission** — [Unacceptable PDX]
Excludes ❷: encounter for screening for human immunodeficiency virus [HIV] (Z11.4)
encounter for screening for human papillomavirus (Z11.51)

Z11.4 **Encounter for screening for human immunodeficiency virus [HIV]** — [Unacceptable PDX]

Z04 - Z11

Z11.5- **Encounter for screening for other viral diseases**
Excludes ❷: *encounter for screening for viral intestinal disease (Z11.0)*

Z11.51 **Encounter for screening for human papillomavirus (HPV)** — [Unacceptable PDX]

Z11.59 **Encounter for screening for other viral diseases** — [Unacceptable PDX]

Z11.6 **Encounter for screening for other protozoal diseases and helminthiases** — [Unacceptable PDX]
Excludes ❷: *encounter for screening for protozoal intestinal disease (Z11.0)*

Z11.8 **Encounter for screening for other infectious and parasitic diseases** — [Unacceptable PDX]
Encounter for screening for chlamydia
Encounter for screening for rickettsial
Encounter for screening for spirochetal
Encounter for screening for mycoses

Z11.9 **Encounter for screening for infectious and parasitic diseases, unspecified** — [Unacceptable PDX]

Z12- **Encounter for screening for malignant neoplasms**
AHA 15:1Q:p24 – Screening mammogram
Note: Screening is the testing for disease or disease precursors in asymptomatic individuals so that early detection and treatment can be provided for those who test positive for the disease.
Use additional code to identify any family history of malignant neoplasm (Z80.-)
Excludes 1: *encounter for diagnostic examination — code to sign or symptom*

Z12.0 **Encounter for screening for malignant neoplasm of stomach** — [Unacceptable PDX]

Z12.1- **Encounter for screening for malignant neoplasm of intestinal tract**

Z12.10 **Encounter for screening for malignant neoplasm of intestinal tract, unspecified** — [Unacceptable PDX]

Z12.11 **Encounter for screening for malignant neoplasm of colon** — [Unacceptable PDX]
Encounter for screening colonoscopy NOS

Z12.12 **Encounter for screening for malignant neoplasm of rectum** — [Unacceptable PDX]

Z12.13 **Encounter for screening for malignant neoplasm of small intestine** — [Unacceptable PDX]

Z12.2 **Encounter for screening for malignant neoplasm of respiratory organs** — [Unacceptable PDX]

Z12.3- **Encounter for screening for malignant neoplasm of breast**

Z12.31 **Encounter for screening mammogram for malignant neoplasm of breast** — [Unacceptable PDX]
Excludes 1: *inconclusive mammogram (R92.2)*

Z12.39 **Encounter for other screening for malignant neoplasm of breast** — [Unacceptable PDX]

Z12.4 **Encounter for screening for malignant neoplasm of cervix** — [♀] [Unacceptable PDX]
Encounter for screening pap smear for malignant neoplasm of cervix
Excludes 1: *when screening is part of general gynecological examination (Z01.4-)*
Excludes ❷: *encounter for screening for human papillomavirus (Z11.51)*

Z12.5 **Encounter for screening for malignant neoplasm of prostate** — [♂]

Z12.6 **Encounter for screening for malignant neoplasm of bladder** — [Unacceptable PDX]

Z12.7- **Encounter for screening for malignant neoplasm of other genitourinary organs**

Z12.71 **Encounter for screening for malignant neoplasm of testis** — [♂] [Unacceptable PDX]

Z12.72 **Encounter for screening for malignant neoplasm of vagina** — [♀] [Unacceptable PDX]
Vaginal pap smear status-post hysterectomy for non-malignant condition
Use additional code to identify acquired absence of uterus (Z90.71-)
Excludes 1: *vaginal pap smear status-post hysterectomy for malignant conditions (Z08)*

Z12.73 **Encounter for screening for malignant neoplasm of ovary** — [♀] [Unacceptable PDX]

Z12.79 **Encounter for screening for malignant neoplasm of other genitourinary organs** — [Unacceptable PDX]

Z12.8- **Encounter for screening for malignant neoplasm of other sites**

Z12.81 **Encounter for screening for malignant neoplasm of oral cavity** — [Unacceptable PDX]

Z12.82 **Encounter for screening for malignant neoplasm of nervous system** — [Unacceptable PDX]

Z12.83 **Encounter for screening for malignant neoplasm of skin** — [Unacceptable PDX]

Z12.89 **Encounter for screening for malignant neoplasm of other sites** — [Unacceptable PDX]

Z12.9 **Encounter for screening for malignant neoplasm, site unspecified** — [Unacceptable PDX]

Z13- **Encounter for screening for other diseases and disorders**
Note: Screening is the testing for disease or disease precursors in asymptomatic individuals so that early detection and treatment can be provided for those who test positive for the disease.
Excludes 1: *encounter for diagnostic examination — code to sign or symptom*

Z13.0 **Encounter for screening for diseases of the blood and blood-forming organs and certain disorders involving the immune mechanism** — [Unacceptable PDX]

Z13.1 **Encounter for screening for diabetes mellitus** — [Unacceptable PDX]

Z13.2- **Encounter for screening for nutritional, metabolic and other endocrine disorders**

Z13.21 **Encounter for screening for nutritional disorder** — [Unacceptable PDX]

Z13.22- **Encounter for screening for metabolic disorder**

Z13.220 **Encounter for screening for lipoid disorders** — [Unacceptable PDX]
Encounter for screening for cholesterol level
Encounter for screening for hypercholesterolemia
Encounter for screening for hyperlipidemia

Z13.228 **Encounter for screening for other metabolic disorders** — [Unacceptable PDX]

Z13.29 **Encounter for screening for other suspected endocrine disorder** — [Unacceptable PDX]
Excludes 1: *encounter for screening for diabetes mellitus (Z13.1)*

Z13.4 **Encounter for screening for certain developmental disorders in childhood** — [Age/0-17] [Unacceptable PDX]
Encounter for screening for developmental handicaps in early childhood
Excludes 1: *routine development testing of infant or child (Z00.1-)*

Z13.5 **Encounter for screening for eye and ear disorders** — [Unacceptable PDX]
Excludes ❷: *encounter for general hearing examination (Z01.1-)*
encounter for general vision examination (Z01.0-)

Z13.6 **Encounter for screening for cardiovascular disorders** — [Unacceptable PDX]

Z13.7- **Encounter for screening for genetic and chromosomal anomalies**
Excludes 1: *genetic testing for procreative management (Z31.4-)*

Z13.71 **Encounter for nonprocreative screening for genetic disease carrier status** — [Unacceptable PDX]

Z13.79 **Encounter for other screening for genetic and chromosomal anomalies** — [Unacceptable PDX]

Z13.8- **Encounter for screening for other specified diseases and disorders**
Excludes ❷: *screening for malignant neoplasms (Z12.-)*

Z13.81- **Encounter for screening for digestive system disorders**

Z13.810 **Encounter for screening for upper gastrointestinal disorder** — [Unacceptable PDX]

Z13.811 **Encounter for screening for lower gastrointestinal disorder** — [Unacceptable PDX]
Excludes 1: *encounter for screening for intestinal infectious disease (Z11.0)*

Z13.818 **Encounter for screening for other digestive system disorders** — [Unacceptable PDX]

Excludes 1: = NOT CODED HERE! (Do not code both)

Excludes ❷: = Not Included Here

Z11 - Z13

Z13.82- Encounter for screening for musculoskeletal disorder

Z13.820 Encounter for screening for osteoporosis — [Unacceptable PDX]

Z13.828 Encounter for screening for other musculoskeletal disorder — [Unacceptable PDX]

Z13.83 Encounter for screening for respiratory disorder NEC — [Unacceptable PDX]
> Excludes 1: encounter for screening for respiratory tuberculosis (Z11.1)

Z13.84 Encounter for screening for dental disorders — [Unacceptable PDX]

Z13.85- Encounter for screening for nervous system disorders

Z13.850 Encounter for screening for traumatic brain injury — [Unacceptable PDX]

Z13.858 Encounter for screening for other nervous system disorders — [Unacceptable PDX]

Z13.88 Encounter for screening for disorder due to exposure to contaminants — [Unacceptable PDX]
> Excludes 1: those exposed to contaminants without suspected disorders (Z57.-, Z77.-)

Z13.89 Encounter for screening for other disorder — [Unacceptable PDX]
> Encounter for screening for genitourinary disorders

Z13.9 Encounter for screening, unspecified — [Unacceptable PDX]

Genetic carrier and genetic susceptibility to disease (Z14-Z15)

Z14- Genetic carrier

Z14.0- Hemophilia A carrier

Z14.01 Asymptomatic hemophilia A carrier — [Unacceptable PDX]

Z14.02 Symptomatic hemophilia A carrier — [Unacceptable PDX]

Z14.1 Cystic fibrosis carrier — [Unacceptable PDX]

Z14.8 Genetic carrier of other disease — [Unacceptable PDX]

Z15- Genetic susceptibility to disease
> Includes: Confirmed abnormal gene
> Use additional code, if applicable, for any associated family history of the disease (Z80-Z84)
> Excludes 1: chromosomal anomalies (Q90-Q99)

Z15.0- Genetic susceptibility to malignant neoplasm
> Code first, if applicable, any current malignant neoplasm (C00-C75, C81-C96)
> Use additional code, if applicable, for any personal history of malignant neoplasm (Z85-)

Z15.01 Genetic susceptibility to malignant neoplasm of breast — [Unacceptable PDX]

Z15.02 Genetic susceptibility to malignant neoplasm of ovary — [♀] [Unacceptable PDX]

Z15.03 Genetic susceptibility to malignant neoplasm of prostate — [♂] [Unacceptable PDX]

Z15.04 Genetic susceptibility to malignant neoplasm of endometrium — [♀] [Unacceptable PDX]

Z15.09 Genetic susceptibility to other malignant neoplasm — [Unacceptable PDX]

Z15.8- Genetic susceptibility to other disease

Z15.81 Genetic susceptibility to multiple endocrine neoplasia [MEN] — [Unacceptable PDX]
> Excludes 1: multiple endocrine neoplasia [MEN] syndromes (E31.2-)

Z15.89 Genetic susceptibility to other disease — [Unacceptable PDX]

Resistance to antimicrobial drugs (Z16)

Z16- Resistance to antimicrobial drugs
> Note: The codes in this category are provided for use as additional codes to identify the resistance and nonresponsiveness of a condition to antimicrobial drugs.
> Code first the infection
> Excludes 1: methicillin resistant Staphylococcus aureus infection (A49.02)
> methicillin resistant Staphylococcus aureus infection in diseases classified elsewhere (B95.62)
> methicillin resistant Staphylococcus aureus pneumonia (J15.212)
> sepsis due to methicillin resistant Staphylococcus aureus (A41.02)

Z16.1- Resistance to beta lactam antibiotics

Z16.10 Resistance to unspecified beta lactam antibiotics — [Unacceptable PDX]

Z16.11 Resistance to penicillins — [Unacceptable PDX]
> Resistance to amoxicillin
> Resistance to ampicillin

Z16.12 Extended spectrum beta lactamase (ESBL) resistance — [Unacceptable PDX]

Z16.19 Resistance to other specified beta lactam antibiotics — [Unacceptable PDX]
> Resistance to cephalosporins

Z16.2- Resistance to other antibiotics

Z16.20 Resistance to unspecified antibiotic — [Unacceptable PDX]
> Resistance to antibiotics NOS

Z16.21 Resistance to vancomycin — [Unacceptable PDX]

Z16.22 Resistance to vancomycin related antibiotics — [Unacceptable PDX]

Z16.23 Resistance to quinolones and fluoroquinolones — [Unacceptable PDX]

Z16.24 Resistance to multiple antibiotics — [Unacceptable PDX]

Z16.29 Resistance to other single specified antibiotic — [Unacceptable PDX]
> Resistance to aminoglycosides
> Resistance to macrolides
> Resistance to sulfonamides
> Resistance to tetracyclines

Z16.3- Resistance to other antimicrobial drugs
> Excludes 1: resistance to antibiotics (Z16.1-, Z16.2-)

Z16.30 Resistance to unspecified antimicrobial drugs — [Unacceptable PDX]
> Drug resistance NOS

Z16.31 Resistance to antiparasitic drug(s) — [Unacceptable PDX]
> Resistance to quinine and related compounds

Z16.32 Resistance to antifungal drug(s) — [Unacceptable PDX]

Z16.33 Resistance to antiviral drug(s) — [Unacceptable PDX]

Z16.34- Resistance to antimycobacterial drug(s)
> Resistance to tuberculostatics

Z16.341 Resistance to single antimycobacterial drug — [Unacceptable PDX]
> Resistance to antimycobacterial drug NOS

Z16.342 Resistance to multiple antimycobacterial drugs — [Unacceptable PDX]

Z16.35 Resistance to multiple antimicrobial drugs — [Unacceptable PDX]
> Excludes 1: resistance to multiple antibiotics only (Z16.24)

Z16.39 Resistance to other specified antimicrobial drug — [Unacceptable PDX]

Estrogen receptor status (Z17)

Z17- Estrogen receptor status
> Code first malignant neoplasm of breast (C50-)

Z17.0 Estrogen receptor positive status [ER+] — [Unacceptable PDX]

Z17.1 Estrogen receptor negative status [ER-] — [Unacceptable PDX]

Z13 - Z17

Retained foreign body fragments (Z18)

Z18- Retained foreign body fragments
Includes: Embedded fragment (status)
            Embedded splinter (status)
            Retained foreign body status
Excludes 1:   artificial joint prosthesis status (Z96.6-)
              foreign body accidentally left during a procedure (T81.5-)
              foreign body entering through orifice (T15-T19)
              in situ cardiac device (Z95.-)
              organ or tissue replaced by means other than transplant (Z96.-, Z97.-)
              organ or tissue replaced by transplant (Z94.-)
              personal history of retained foreign body fully removed Z87.821
              superficial foreign body (non-embedded splinter) — code to superficial foreign body, by site

Z18.0- Retained radioactive fragments
  Z18.01 Retained depleted uranium fragments — [Unacceptable PDX]
  Z18.09 Other retained radioactive fragments — [Unacceptable PDX]
          Other retained depleted isotope fragments
          Retained nontherapeutic radioactive fragments

Z18.1- Retained metal fragments
  Excludes 1:   retained radioactive metal fragments (Z18.01-Z18.09)
  Z18.10 Retained metal fragments, unspecified — [Unacceptable PDX]
          Retained metal fragment NOS
  Z18.11 Retained magnetic metal fragments — [Unacceptable PDX]
  Z18.12 Retained nonmagnetic metal fragments — [Unacceptable PDX]

Z18.2   Retained plastic fragments — [Unacceptable PDX]
        Acrylics fragments
        Diethylhexylphthalates fragments
        Isocyanate fragments

Z18.3- Retained organic fragments
  Z18.31 Retained animal quills or spines — [Unacceptable PDX]
  Z18.32 Retained tooth — [Unacceptable PDX]
  Z18.33 Retained wood fragments — [Unacceptable PDX]
  Z18.39 Other retained organic fragments — [Unacceptable PDX]

Z18.8- Other specified retained foreign body
  Z18.81 Retained glass fragments — [Unacceptable PDX]
  Z18.83 Retained stone or crystalline fragments — [Unacceptable PDX]
          Retained concrete or cement fragments
  Z18.89 Other specified retained foreign body fragments — [Unacceptable PDX]

Z18.9   Retained foreign body fragments, unspecified material — [Unacceptable PDX]

Hormone sensitivity malignancy status (Z19)

Z19- Hormone sensitivity malignancy status
      Code first malignant neoplasm – see Table of Neoplasms, by site, malignant
Z19.1   Hormone sensitive malignancy status — [Unacceptable PDX]
Z19.2   Hormone resistant malignancy status — [Unacceptable PDX]
        Castrate resistant prostate malignancy status

Persons with potential health hazards related to communicable diseases (Z20-Z29)

Z20- Contact with and (suspected) exposure to communicable diseases
      Excludes 1:   carrier of infectious disease (Z22.-)
                    diagnosed current infectious or parasitic disease — see Alphabetic Index
      Excludes ❷: personal history of infectious and parasitic diseases (Z86.1-)
Z20.0- Contact with and (suspected) exposure to intestinal infectious diseases
  Z20.01 Contact with and (suspected) exposure to intestinal infectious diseases due to Escherichia coli (E. coli)
  Z20.09 Contact with and (suspected) exposure to other intestinal infectious diseases — [Unacceptable PDX]
Z20.1   Contact with and (suspected) exposure to tuberculosis — [Unacceptable PDX]
Z20.2   Contact with and (suspected) exposure to infections with a predominantly sexual mode of transmission — [Unacceptable PDX]

Z20.3   Contact with and (suspected) exposure to rabies — [Unacceptable PDX]
Z20.4   Contact with and (suspected) exposure to rubella — [Unacceptable PDX]
Z20.5   Contact with and (suspected) exposure to viral hepatitis
Z20.6   Contact with and (suspected) exposure to human immunodeficiency virus [HIV]
      Excludes 1:   asymptomatic human immunodeficiency virus [HIV] HIV infection status (Z21)
Z20.7   Contact with and (suspected) exposure to pediculosis, acariasis and other infestations — [Unacceptable PDX]
Z20.8- Contact with and (suspected) exposure to other communicable diseases
  Z20.81- Contact with and (suspected) exposure to other bacterial communicable diseases
    Z20.810 Contact with and (suspected) exposure to anthrax — [Unacceptable PDX]
    Z20.811 Contact with and (suspected) exposure to meningococcus
    Z20.818 Contact with and (suspected) exposure to other bacterial communicable diseases — [Unacceptable PDX]
  Z20.82- Contact with and (suspected) exposure to other viral communicable diseases
    Z20.820 Contact with and (suspected) exposure to varicella
    Z20.828 Contact with and (suspected) exposure to other viral communicable diseases
  Z20.89 Contact with and (suspected) exposure to other communicable diseases — [Unacceptable PDX]
Z20.9   Contact with and (suspected) exposure to unspecified communicable disease — [Unacceptable PDX]

Z21 Asymptomatic human immunodeficiency virus [HIV] infection status — [Questionable Admission]
      HIV positive NOS
      Code first human immunodeficiency virus [HIV] disease complicating pregnancy, childbirth and the puerperium, if applicable (O98.7-)
      Excludes 1:   acquired immunodeficiency syndrome (B20)
                    contact with human immunodeficiency virus [HIV] (Z20.6)
                    exposure to human immunodeficiency virus [HIV] (Z20.6)
                    human immunodeficiency virus [HIV] disease (B20)
                    inconclusive laboratory evidence of human immunodeficiency virus [HIV] (R75)

Z22- Carrier of infectious disease
      Includes: Colonization status
                  Suspected carrier
      Excludes ❷: carrier of viral hepatitis (B18.-)
Z22.0   Carrier of typhoid — [Unacceptable PDX]
Z22.1   Carrier of other intestinal infectious diseases — [Unacceptable PDX]
Z22.2   Carrier of diphtheria — [Unacceptable PDX]
Z22.3- Carrier of other specified bacterial diseases
  Z22.31 Carrier of bacterial disease due to meningococci — [Unacceptable PDX]
  Z22.32- Carrier of bacterial disease due to staphylococci
    Z22.321 Carrier or suspected carrier of methicillin susceptible Staphylococcus aureus — [Unacceptable PDX]
            MSSA colonization
    Z22.322 Carrier or suspected carrier of methicillin resistant Staphylococcus aureus — [Unacceptable PDX]
            MRSA colonization
  Z22.33- Carrier of bacterial disease due to streptococci
    Z22.330 Carrier of Group B streptococcus — [Unacceptable PDX]
            Excludes 1:   carrier of streptococcus group B (GBS) complicating pregnancy, childbirth and the puerperium (O99.-)
    Z22.338 Carrier of other streptococcus — [Unacceptable PDX]
  Z22.39 Carrier of other specified bacterial diseases — [Unacceptable PDX]
Z22.4   Carrier of infections with a predominantly sexual mode of transmission — [Unacceptable PDX]

Z22.6   **Carrier of human T-lymphotropic virus type-1 [HTLV-1] infection** — [Unacceptable PDX]

Z22.8   **Carrier of other infectious diseases** — [Unacceptable PDX]

Z22.9   **Carrier of infectious disease, unspecified** — [Unacceptable PDX]

Z23   **Encounter for immunization** — [Unacceptable PDX]
Code first any routine childhood examination
Note: Procedure codes are required to identify the types of immunizations given.

Z28-   **Immunization <u>not carried out and underimmunization status</u>**
Includes: Vaccination not carried out

Z28.0-   **Immunization <u>not carried out because of contraindication</u>**

Z28.01   **Immunization not carried out because of <u>acute illness</u> of patient** — [Unacceptable PDX]

Z28.02   **Immunization not carried out because of <u>chronic illness</u> or condition of patient** — [Unacceptable PDX]

Z28.03   **Immunization not carried out because of <u>immune compromised state</u> of patient** — [Unacceptable PDX]

Z28.04   **Immunization not carried out because of <u>patient allergy</u> to vaccine or component** — [Unacceptable PDX]

Z28.09   **Immunization not carried out because of <u>other</u> contraindication** — [Unacceptable PDX]

Z28.1   **Immunization <u>not carried out because of patient decision for reasons of belief or group pressure</u>** — [Unacceptable PDX]
Immunization not carried out because of religious belief

Z28.2-   **Immunization <u>not carried out because of patient decision for other and unspecified reason</u>**

Z28.20   **Immunization not carried out because of patient decision for unspecified reason** — [Unacceptable PDX]

Z28.21   **Immunization not carried out because of patient refusal** — [Unacceptable PDX]

Z28.29   **Immunization not carried out because of patient decision for other reason** — [Unacceptable PDX]

Z28.3   **<u>Underimmunization status</u>** — [Unacceptable PDX]
Delinquent immunization status
Lapsed immunization schedule status

Z28.8-   **Immunization <u>not carried out for other reason</u>**

Z28.81   **Immunization not carried out <u>due to patient having had the disease</u>** — [Unacceptable PDX]

Z28.82   **Immunization not carried out <u>because of caregiver refusal</u>** — [Unacceptable PDX]
Immunization not carried out because of guardian refusal
Immunization not carried out because of parent refusal
Excludes 1:   *immunization not carried out because of caregiver refusal because of religious belief (Z28.1)*

Z28.89   **Immunization not carried out for <u>other</u> reason** — [Unacceptable PDX]

Z28.9   **Immunization not carried out for unspecified reason** — [Unacceptable PDX]

Z29-   **Encounter for <u>other prophylactic</u> measures**
Excludes 1:   *desensitization to allergens (Z51.6)*
prophylactic surgery (Z40.-)

Z29.1-   **Encounter for prophylactic <u>immunotherapy</u>**
Encounter for administration of immunoglobulin

Z29.11   **Encounter for prophylactic immunotherapy for <u>respiratory syncytial virus</u> (RSV)** — [Unacceptable PDX]

Z29.12   **Encounter for prophylactic <u>antivenin</u>** — [Unacceptable PDX]

Z29.13   **Encounter for prophylactic <u>Rho(D)</u> immune globulin** — [Unacceptable PDX]

Z29.14   **Encounter for prophylactic <u>rabies</u> immune globin** — [Unacceptable PDX]

Z29.3   **Encounter for prophylactic <u>fluoride</u> administration** — [Unacceptable PDX]

Z29.8   **Encounter for <u>other</u> specified prophylactic measures** — [Unacceptable PDX]

Z29.9   **Encounter for prophylactic measures, <u>unspecified</u>** — [Unacceptable PDX]

Persons encountering health services in circumstances related to reproduction (Z30-Z39)

Z30-   **<u>Encounter for contraceptive management</u>**

Z30.0-   **Encounter for general counseling and advice on contraception**

Z30.01-   **Encounter for <u>initial prescription of contraceptives</u>**
Excludes 1:   *encounter for surveillance of contraceptives (Z30.4-)*

Z30.011   **Encounter for initial prescription of contraceptive pills** — [♀] [Unacceptable PDX]

Z30.012   **Encounter for prescription of emergency contraception** — [♀] [Unacceptable PDX]
Encounter for postcoital contraception

Z30.013   **Encounter for initial prescription of injectable contraceptive** — [♀] [Unacceptable PDX]

Z30.014   **Encounter for initial prescription of intrauterine contraceptive device** — [♀] [Unacceptable PDX]
Excludes 1:   *encounter for insertion of intrauterine contraceptive device (Z30.430, Z30.432)*

Z30.015   **Encounter for initial prescription of vaginal ring hormonal contraceptive** — [♀] [Unacceptable PDX]

Z30.016   **Encounter for initial prescription of transdermal patch hormonal contraceptive device** — [♀] [Unacceptable PDX]

Z30.017   **Encounter for initial prescription of implantable subdermal contraceptive** — [♀] [Unacceptable PDX]

Z30.018   **Encounter for initial prescription of other contraceptives** — [♀] [Unacceptable PDX]
Encounter for initial prescription of barrier contraception
Encounter for initial prescription of diaphragm

Z30.019   **Encounter for initial prescription of contraceptives, unspecified** — [♀] [Unacceptable PDX]

Z30.02   **Counseling and instruction in natural family planning to avoid pregnancy** — [Unacceptable PDX]

Z30.09   **Encounter for other general counseling and advice on contraception** — [Unacceptable PDX]
Encounter for family planning advice NOS

Z30.2   **Encounter for sterilization**

Z30.4-   **Encounter for <u>surveillance of contraceptives</u>**

Z30.40   **Encounter for surveillance of contraceptives, unspecified** — [Unacceptable PDX]

Z30.41   **Encounter for surveillance of <u>contraceptive pills</u>** — [♀] [Unacceptable PDX]
Encounter for repeat prescription for contraceptive pill

Z30.42   **Encounter for surveillance of <u>injectable contraceptive</u>** — [♀] [Unacceptable PDX]

Z30.43-   **Encounter for surveillance of <u>intrauterine contraceptive device</u>**

Z30.430   **Encounter for <u>insertion</u> of intrauterine contraceptive device** — [♀] [Unacceptable PDX]

Z30.431   **Encounter for <u>routine checking</u> of intrauterine contraceptive device** — [♀] [Unacceptable PDX]

Z30.432   **Encounter for <u>removal</u> of intrauterine contraceptive device** — [♀] [Unacceptable PDX]

Z30.433   **Encounter for <u>removal and reinsertion</u> of intrauterine contraceptive device** — [♀] [Unacceptable PDX]
Encounter for replacement of intrauterine contraceptive device

Z30.44   **Encounter for surveillance of vaginal ring hormonal contraceptive device** — [♀] [Unacceptable PDX]

Z30.45   **Encounter for surveillance of transdermal patch hormonal contraceptive device** — [♀] [Unacceptable PDX]

Z30.46   **Encounter for surveillance of implantable subdermal contraceptive** — [♀] [Unacceptable PDX]
Encounter for checking, reinsertion or removal of implantable subdermal contraceptive

Z22 - Z30

Z30.49 Encounter for surveillance of other contraceptives — [♀]
[Unacceptable PDX]
Encounter for surveillance of barrier contraception
Encounter for surveillance of diaphragm

Z30.8 Encounter for other contraceptive management —
[Unacceptable PDX]
Encounter for postvasectomy sperm count
Encounter for routine examination for contraceptive maintenance
Excludes 1: *sperm count following sterilization reversal (Z31.42)*
sperm count for fertility testing (Z31.41)

Z30.9 Encounter for contraceptive management, unspecified —
[Unacceptable PDX]

Z31- Encounter for procreative management
Excludes 1: *complications associated with artificial fertilization (N98.-)*
female infertility (N97.-)
male infertility (N46.-)

Z31.0 Encounter for reversal of previous sterilization

Z31.4- Encounter for procreative investigation and testing
Excludes 1: *postvasectomy sperm count (Z30.8)*

Z31.41 Encounter for fertility testing — [Unacceptable PDX]
Encounter for fallopian tube patency testing
Encounter for sperm count for fertility testing

Z31.42 Aftercare following sterilization reversal —
[Unacceptable PDX]
Sperm count following sterilization reversal

Z31.43- Encounter for genetic testing of female for procreative management
Use additional code for recurrent pregnancy loss, if applicable (N96, O26.2-)
Excludes 1: *nonprocreative genetic testing (Z13.7-)*

Z31.430 Encounter of female for testing for genetic disease carrier status for procreative management — [♀]
[Unacceptable PDX]

Z31.438 Encounter for other genetic testing of female for procreative management — [♀] [Unacceptable PDX]

Z31.44- Encounter for genetic testing of male for procreative management
Excludes 1: *nonprocreative genetic testing (Z13.7-)*

Z31.440 Encounter of male for testing for genetic disease carrier status for procreative management — [♂]
[Unacceptable PDX]

Z31.441 Encounter for testing of male partner of patient with recurrent pregnancy loss — [♂, Age/15-124]
[Unacceptable PDX]

Z31.448 Encounter for other genetic testing of male for procreative management — [♂, Age/15-124]
[Unacceptable PDX]

Z31.49 Encounter for other procreative investigation and testing — [Unacceptable PDX]

Z31.5 Encounter for genetic counseling — [Unacceptable PDX]

Z31.6- Encounter for general counseling and advice on procreation

Z31.61 Procreative counseling and advice using natural family planning — [Unacceptable PDX]

Z31.62 Encounter for fertility preservation counseling —
[Unacceptable PDX]
Encounter for fertility preservation counseling prior to cancer therapy
Encounter for fertility preservation counseling prior to surgical removal of gonads

Z31.69 Encounter for other general counseling and advice on procreation — [Unacceptable PDX]

Z31.7 Encounter for procreative management and counseling for gestational carrier — [Unacceptable PDX]
Excludes 1: *pregnant state, gestational carrier (Z33.3)*

Z31.8- Encounter for other procreative management

Z31.81 Encounter for male factor infertility in female patient — [♀] [Unacceptable PDX]

Z31.82 Encounter for Rh incompatibility status — [♀]
[Unacceptable PDX]
AHA 14:4Q:p17 – Prophylactic injection of anti-D antibodies during prenatal visit

Z31.83 Encounter for assisted reproductive fertility procedure cycle — [♀] [Unacceptable PDX]
Patient undergoing in vitro fertilization cycle
Use additional code to identify the type of infertility
Excludes 1: *pre-cycle diagnosis and testing — code to reason for encounter*

Z31.84 Encounter for fertility preservation procedure —
[Unacceptable PDX]
Encounter for fertility preservation procedure prior to cancer therapy
Encounter for fertility preservation procedure prior to surgical removal of gonads

Z31.89 Encounter for other procreative management —
[Unacceptable PDX]

Z31.9 Encounter for procreative management, unspecified —
[Unacceptable PDX]

Z32- Encounter for pregnancy test and childbirth and childcare instruction

Z32.0- Encounter for pregnancy test

Z32.00 Encounter for pregnancy test, result unknown — [♀]
Encounter for pregnancy test NOS

Z32.01 Encounter for pregnancy test, result positive —
[♀, Age/12-55]

Z32.02 Encounter for pregnancy test, result negative — [♀]

Z32.2 Encounter for childbirth instruction — [Unacceptable PDX]

Z32.3 Encounter for childcare instruction — [Unacceptable PDX]
Encounter for prenatal or postpartum childcare instruction

Z33- Pregnant state

Z33.1 Pregnant state, incidental — [♀, Age/12-55] [Unacceptable PDX]
Pregnant state NOS
Excludes 1: *complications of pregnancy (O00-O9A)*
pregnant state, gestational carrier (Z33.3)

Z33.2 Encounter for elective termination of pregnancy —
[♀, Age/12-55]
Excludes 1: *early fetal death with retention of dead fetus (O02.1)*
late fetal death (O36.4)
spontaneous abortion (O03)

Z33.3 Pregnant state, gestational carrier — [♀, Age/12-55]
[Unacceptable PDX]
Excludes 1: *encounter for procreative management and counseling for gestational carrier (Z31.7)*

Z34- Encounter for supervision of normal pregnancy
Excludes 1: *any complication of pregnancy (O00-O9A)*
encounter for pregnancy test (Z32.0-)
encounter for supervision of high risk pregnancy (O09-)

Z34.0- Encounter for supervision of normal first pregnancy

Z34.00 Encounter for supervision of normal first pregnancy, unspecified trimester — [♀, Age/12-55] [Unacceptable PDX]

Z34.01 Encounter for supervision of normal first pregnancy, first trimester — [♀, Age/12-55] [Unacceptable PDX]

Z34.02 Encounter for supervision of normal first pregnancy, second trimester — [♀, Age/12-55] [Unacceptable PDX]

Z34.03 Encounter for supervision of normal first pregnancy, third trimester — [♀, Age/12-55] [Unacceptable PDX]

Z34.8- Encounter for supervision of other normal pregnancy
AHA 14:4Q:p17 – Prophylactic injection of anti-D antibodies during prenatal visit

Z34.80 Encounter for supervision of other normal pregnancy, unspecified trimester — [♀, Age/12-55] [Unacceptable PDX]

Z34.81 Encounter for supervision of other normal pregnancy, first trimester — [♀, Age/12-55] [Unacceptable PDX]

Z34.82 Encounter for supervision of other normal pregnancy, second trimester — [♀, Age/12-55] [Unacceptable PDX]

Z34.83 Encounter for supervision of other normal pregnancy, third trimester — [♀, Age/12-55] [Unacceptable PDX]

Z34.9- Encounter for supervision of normal pregnancy, unspecified

Z34.90 Encounter for supervision of normal pregnancy, unspecified, unspecified trimester — [♀, Age/12-55]
[Unacceptable PDX]

Z34.91 Encounter for supervision of normal pregnancy, unspecified, first trimester — [♀, Age/12-55] [Unacceptable PDX]

Z30 – Z34

Z34.92 Encounter for supervision of normal pregnancy, unspecified, <u>second trimester</u> — [♀, Age/12-55]
[Unacceptable PDX]

Z34.93 Encounter for supervision of normal pregnancy, unspecified, <u>third trimester</u> — [♀, Age/12-55] [Unacceptable PDX]

Z36 Encounter for antenatal screening of mother — [♀, Age/12-55]
[Unacceptable PDX]

Excludes 1: *abnormal findings on antenatal screening of mother (O28.-)*
diagnostic examination- code to sign or symptom
encounter for suspected maternal and fetal conditions ruled out (Z03.7-)
suspected fetal condition affecting management of pregnancy — code to condition in Chapter 15

Excludes ❷: *genetic counseling and testing (Z31.43-, Z31.5)*
routine prenatal care (Z34)

Z3A- <u>Weeks of gestation</u>

AHA 13:2Q:p33 – Use date of admission for weeks of gestation
AHA 14:1Q:p14 – Discrepancies in documentation of gestational age
AHA 14:3Q:p17 – Weeks of gestation not applicable in ectopic pregnancies
Note: Codes from category Z3A are for use, only on the maternal record, to indicate the weeks of gestation of the pregnancy, if known.
Code first complications of pregnancy, childbirth and the puerperium (O00-O9A)

Z3A.0- Weeks of gestation of pregnancy, unspecified or less than 10 weeks

Z3A.00 Weeks of gestation of pregnancy not specified — [♀, Age/12-55] [Unacceptable PDX]

Z3A.01 Less than 8 weeks of gestation of pregnancy — [♀, Age/12-55] [Unacceptable PDX]

Z3A.08 8 weeks of gestation of pregnancy — [♀, Age/12-55] [Unacceptable PDX]

Z3A.09 9 weeks of gestation of pregnancy — [♀, Age/12-55] [Unacceptable PDX]

Z3A.1- Weeks of gestation of pregnancy, weeks 10-19

Z3A.10 10 weeks of gestation of pregnancy — [♀, Age/12-55] [Unacceptable PDX]

Z3A.11 11 weeks of gestation of pregnancy — [♀, Age/12-55] [Unacceptable PDX]

Z3A.12 12 weeks of gestation of pregnancy — [♀, Age/12-55] [Unacceptable PDX]

Z3A.13 13 weeks of gestation of pregnancy — [♀, Age/12-55] [Unacceptable PDX]

Z3A.14 14 weeks of gestation of pregnancy — [♀, Age/12-55] [Unacceptable PDX]

Z3A.15 15 weeks of gestation of pregnancy — [♀, Age/12-55] [Unacceptable PDX]

Z3A.16 16 weeks of gestation of pregnancy — [♀, Age/12-55] [Unacceptable PDX]

Z3A.17 17 weeks of gestation of pregnancy — [♀, Age/12-55] [Unacceptable PDX]

Z3A.18 18 weeks of gestation of pregnancy — [♀, Age/12-55] [Unacceptable PDX]

Z3A.19 19 weeks of gestation of pregnancy — [♀, Age/12-55] [Unacceptable PDX]

Z3A.2- Weeks of gestation of pregnancy, weeks 20-29

Z3A.20 20 weeks of gestation of pregnancy — [♀, Age/12-55] [Unacceptable PDX]

Z3A.21 21 weeks of gestation of pregnancy — [♀, Age/12-55] [Unacceptable PDX]

Z3A.22 22 weeks of gestation of pregnancy — [♀, Age/12-55] [Unacceptable PDX]

Z3A.23 23 weeks of gestation of pregnancy — [♀, Age/12-55] [Unacceptable PDX]

Z3A.24 24 weeks of gestation of pregnancy — [♀, Age/12-55] [Unacceptable PDX]

Z3A.25 25 weeks of gestation of pregnancy — [♀, Age/12-55] [Unacceptable PDX]

Z3A.26 26 weeks of gestation of pregnancy — [♀, Age/12-55] [Unacceptable PDX]

Z3A.27 27 weeks of gestation of pregnancy — [♀, Age/12-55] [Unacceptable PDX]

Z3A.28 28 weeks of gestation of pregnancy — [♀, Age/12-55] [Unacceptable PDX]

Z3A.29 29 weeks of gestation of pregnancy — [♀, Age/12-55] [Unacceptable PDX]

Z3A.3- Weeks of gestation of pregnancy, weeks 30-39

Z3A.30 30 weeks of gestation of pregnancy — [♀, Age/12-55] [Unacceptable PDX]

Z3A.31 31 weeks of gestation of pregnancy — [♀, Age/12-55] [Unacceptable PDX]

Z3A.32 32 weeks of gestation of pregnancy — [♀, Age/12-55] [Unacceptable PDX]

Z3A.33 33 weeks of gestation of pregnancy — [♀, Age/12-55] [Unacceptable PDX]

Z3A.34 34 weeks of gestation of pregnancy — [♀, Age/12-55] [Unacceptable PDX]

Z3A.35 35 weeks of gestation of pregnancy — [♀, Age/12-55] [Unacceptable PDX]

Z3A.36 36 weeks of gestation of pregnancy — [♀, Age/12-55] [Unacceptable PDX]

Z3A.37 37 weeks of gestation of pregnancy — [♀, Age/12-55] [Unacceptable PDX]

Z3A.38 38 weeks of gestation of pregnancy — [♀, Age/12-55] [Unacceptable PDX]

Z3A.39 39 weeks of gestation of pregnancy — [♀, Age/12-55] [Unacceptable PDX]

Z3A.4- Weeks of gestation of pregnancy, weeks 40 or greater

Z3A.40 40 weeks of gestation of pregnancy — [♀, Age/12-55] [Unacceptable PDX]

Z3A.41 41 weeks of gestation of pregnancy — [♀, Age/12-55] [Unacceptable PDX]

Z3A.42 42 weeks of gestation of pregnancy — [♀, Age/12-55] [Unacceptable PDX]

Z3A.49 Greater than 42 weeks of gestation of pregnancy — [♀, Age/12-55] [Unacceptable PDX]

AHA 14:4Q:p23 – 42 weeks of gestation or more

Z37- <u>Outcome of delivery</u>
Note: This category is intended for use as an additional code to identify the outcome of delivery on the mother's record. It is not for use on the newborn record.
Excludes 1: *stillbirth (P95)*

Z37.0 Single live birth — [♀, Age/12-55] [Unacceptable PDX]

Z37.1 Single stillbirth — [♀, Age/12-55] [Unacceptable PDX]

Z37.2 Twins, both liveborn — [♀, Age/12-55] [Unacceptable PDX]

Z37.3 Twins, one liveborn and one stillborn — [♀, Age/12-55] [Unacceptable PDX]

Z37.4 Twins, both stillborn — [♀, Age/12-55] [Unacceptable PDX]

Z37.5- Other multiple births, all liveborn

Z37.50 Multiple births, unspecified, all liveborn — [♀, Age/12-55] [Unacceptable PDX]

Z37.51 Triplets, all liveborn — [♀, Age/12-55] [Unacceptable PDX]

Z37.52 Quadruplets, all liveborn — [♀, Age/12-55] [Unacceptable PDX]

Z37.53 Quintuplets, all liveborn — [♀, Age/12-55] [Unacceptable PDX]

Z37.54 Sextuplets, all liveborn — [♀, Age/12-55] [Unacceptable PDX]

Z37.59 Other multiple births, all liveborn — [♀, Age/12-55] [Unacceptable PDX]

Z37.6- Other multiple births, some liveborn

Z37.60 Multiple births, unspecified, some liveborn — [♀, Age/12-55] [Unacceptable PDX]

Z37.61 Triplets, some liveborn — [♀, Age/12-55] [Unacceptable PDX]

Z37.62 Quadruplets, some liveborn — [♀, Age/12-55] [Unacceptable PDX]

Z37.63 Quintuplets, some liveborn — [♀, Age/12-55] [Unacceptable PDX]

Z37.64 Sextuplets, some liveborn — [♀, Age/12-55] [Unacceptable PDX]

Z37.69 Other multiple births, some liveborn — [♀, Age/12-55] [Unacceptable PDX]

Z37.7 Other multiple births, all stillborn — [♀, Age/12-55] [Unacceptable PDX]

Z34 - Z37

Excludes 1: = NOT CODED HERE! (Do not code both)

Excludes ❷: = Not Included Here

Z37.9   **Outcome of delivery, unspecified** — [♀, Age/12-55]
[Unacceptable PDX]
   Multiple birth NOS
   Single birth NOS

Z38-   **Liveborn infants according to place of birth and type of delivery**
Note: This category is for use as the principal code on the initial record of a newborn baby. It is to be used for the initial birth record only. It is not to be used on the mother's record.

AHA 15:2Q:p15 – Physician reporting of Z38 category codes

Z38.0-   **Single liveborn infant, born in hospital**
   Single liveborn infant, born in birthing center or other health care facility

Z38.00   **Single liveborn infant, delivered vaginally** — [Age/0]

Z38.01   **Single liveborn infant, delivered by cesarean** — [Age/0]

Z38.1   **Single liveborn infant, born outside hospital** — [Age/0]

Z38.2   **Single liveborn infant, unspecified as to place of birth** — [Age/0]
   Single liveborn infant NOS

Z38.3-   **Twin liveborn infant, born in hospital**

Z38.30   **Twin liveborn infant, delivered vaginally** — [Age/0]

Z38.31   **Twin liveborn infant, delivered by cesarean** — [Age/0]

Z38.4   **Twin liveborn infant, born outside hospital** — [Age/0]

Z38.5   **Twin liveborn infant, unspecified as to place of birth** — [Age/0]

Z38.6-   **Other multiple liveborn infant, born in hospital**

Z38.61   **Triplet liveborn infant, delivered vaginally** — [Age/0]

Z38.62   **Triplet liveborn infant, delivered by cesarean** — [Age/0]

Z38.63   **Quadruplet liveborn infant, delivered vaginally** — [Age/0]

Z38.64   **Quadruplet liveborn Infant, delivered by cesarean** — [Age/0]

Z38.65   **Quintuplet liveborn infant, delivered vaginally** — [Age/0]

Z38.66   **Quintuplet liveborn infant, delivered by cesarean** — [Age/0]

Z38.68   **Other multiple liveborn infant, delivered vaginally** — [Age/0]

Z38.69   **Other multiple liveborn infant, delivered by cesarean** — [Age/0]

Z38.7   **Other multiple liveborn infant, born outside hospital** — [Age/0]

Z38.8   **Other multiple liveborn infant, unspecified as to place of birth** — [Age/0]

Z39-   **Encounter for maternal postpartum care and examination**

Z39.0   **Encounter for care and examination of mother immediately after delivery** — [♀, Age/12-55]
   Care and observation in uncomplicated cases when the delivery occurs outside a healthcare facility
   Excludes 1:   care for postpartum complication — see Alphabetic index

Z39.1   **Encounter for care and examination of lactating mother** — [♀, Age/12-55] [Unacceptable PDX]
   Encounter for supervision of lactation
   Excludes 1:   disorders of lactation (O92.-)

Z39.2   **Encounter for routine postpartum follow-up** — [♀, Age/12-55]
[Unacceptable PDX]

Encounters for other specific health care (Z40-Z53)

NOTE: Categories Z40-Z53 are intended for use to indicate a reason for care. They may be used for patients who have already been treated for a disease or injury, but who are receiving aftercare or prophylactic care, or care to consolidate the treatment, or to deal with a residual state.
Excludes ❷: follow-up examination for medical surveillance after treatment (Z08-Z09)

Z40-   **Encounter for prophylactic surgery**
Excludes 1:   organ donations (Z52.-)
   therapeutic organ removal — code to condition

Z40.0-   **Encounter for prophylactic surgery for risk factors related to malignant neoplasms**
   Admission for prophylactic organ removal
   Use additional code to identify risk factor

Z40.00   **Encounter for prophylactic removal of unspecified organ**

Z40.01   **Encounter for prophylactic removal of breast**

Z40.02   **Encounter for prophylactic removal of ovary** — [♀]

Z40.09   **Encounter for prophylactic removal of other organ**

Z40.8   **Encounter for other prophylactic surgery** — [Unacceptable PDX]

Z40.9   **Encounter for prophylactic surgery, unspecified** —
[Unacceptable PDX]

Z41-   **Encounter for procedures for purposes other than remedying health state**

Z41.1   **Encounter for cosmetic surgery**
   Encounter for cosmetic breast implant
   Encounter for cosmetic procedure
   Excludes 1:   encounter for plastic and reconstructive surgery following medical procedure or healed injury (Z42-)
   encounter for post-mastectomy breast implantation (Z42.1)

Z41.2   **Encounter for routine and ritual male circumcision** — [♂]

Z41.3   **Encounter for ear piercing** — [Unacceptable PDX]

Z41.8   **Encounter for other procedures for purposes other than remedying health state**

Z41.9   **Encounter for procedure for purposes other than remedying health state, unspecified** — [Unacceptable PDX]

Z42-   **Encounter for plastic and reconstructive surgery following medical procedure or healed injury**
Excludes 1:   encounter for cosmetic plastic surgery (Z41.1)
   encounter for plastic surgery for treatment of current injury — code to relevent injury

Z42.1   **Encounter for breast reconstruction following mastectomy** — [Age/15-124]
   Excludes 1:   deformity and disproportion of reconstructed breast (N65.1-)

Z42.8   **Encounter for other plastic and reconstructive surgery following medical procedure or healed injury**

Z43-   **Encounter for attention to artificial openings**
Includes: Closure of artificial openings
   Passage of sounds or bougies through artificial openings
   Reforming artificial openings
   Removal of catheter from artificial openings
   Toilet or cleansing of artificial openings
Excludes 1:   artificial opening status only, without need for care (Z93.-)
   complications of external stoma (J95.0-, K94.-, N99.5-)
Excludes ❷: fitting and adjustment of prosthetic and other devices (Z44-Z46)

Z43.0   **Encounter for attention to tracheostomy**

CC **Z43.1**   **Encounter for attention to gastrostomy**

Z43.2   **Encounter for attention to ileostomy**

Z43.3   **Encounter for attention to colostomy**

Z43.4   **Encounter for attention to other artificial openings of digestive tract**

Z43.5   **Encounter for attention to cystostomy**

Z43.6   **Encounter for attention to other artificial openings of urinary tract**
   Encounter for attention to nephrostomy
   Encounter for attention to ureterostomy
   Encounter for attention to urethrostomy

Z43.7   **Encounter for attention to artificial vagina**

Z43.8   **Encounter for attention to other artificial openings**

Excludes 1: = NOT CODED HERE! (Do not code both)   **1318**   Excludes ❷: = Not Included Here

Z43.9   Encounter for attention to unspecified artificial opening —
[Unacceptable PDX]

Z44-   Encounter for <u>fitting and adjustment of external prosthetic device</u>
   Includes: Removal or replacement of external prosthetic device
   Excludes 1:   malfunction or other complications of device — see
                     Alphabetical Index
                 presence of prosthetic device (Z97.-)

Z44.0-   Encounter for fitting and adjustment of <u>artificial arm</u>

   Z44.00- Encounter for fitting and adjustment of <u>unspecified</u>
   artificial arm

      Z44.001   Encounter for fitting and adjustment of unspecified
      <u>right</u> artificial arm

      Z44.002   Encounter for fitting and adjustment of unspecified
      <u>left</u> artificial arm

      Z44.009   Encounter for fitting and adjustment of unspecified
      artificial arm, <u>unspecified</u> arm

   Z44.01- Encounter for fitting and adjustment of <u>complete</u> artificial
   arm

      Z44.011   Encounter for fitting and adjustment of complete
      <u>right</u> artificial arm

      Z44.012   Encounter for fitting and adjustment of complete
      <u>left</u> artificial arm

      Z44.019   Encounter for fitting and adjustment of complete
      artificial arm, <u>unspecified</u> arm

   Z44.02- Encounter for fitting and adjustment of <u>partial</u> artificial
   arm

      Z44.021   Encounter for fitting and adjustment of partial
      artificial <u>right</u> arm

      Z44.022   Encounter for fitting and adjustment of partial
      artificial <u>left</u> arm

      Z44.029   Encounter for fitting and adjustment of partial
      artificial arm, <u>unspecified</u> arm

Z44.1-   Encounter for <u>fitting and adjustment of artificial leg</u>

   Z44.10- Encounter for fitting and adjustment of unspecified
   artificial leg

      Z44.101   Encounter for fitting and adjustment of unspecified
      <u>right</u> artificial leg

      Z44.102   Encounter for fitting and adjustment of unspecified
      <u>left</u> artificial leg

      Z44.109   Encounter for fitting and adjustment of unspecified
      artificial leg, <u>unspecified</u> leg

   Z44.11- Encounter for fitting and adjustment of <u>complete</u> artificial
   leg

      Z44.111   Encounter for fitting and adjustment of complete
      <u>right</u> artificial leg

      Z44.112   Encounter for fitting and adjustment of complete
      <u>left</u> artificial leg

      Z44.119   Encounter for fitting and adjustment of complete
      artificial leg, <u>unspecified</u> leg

   Z44.12- Encounter for fitting and adjustment of <u>partial</u> artificial
   leg

      Z44.121   Encounter for fitting and adjustment of partial
      artificial <u>right</u> leg

      Z44.122   Encounter for fitting and adjustment of partial
      artificial <u>left</u> leg

      Z44.129   Encounter for fitting and adjustment of partial
      artificial leg, unspecified leg

Z44.2-   Encounter for <u>fitting and adjustment of artificial eye</u>
   Excludes 1:   mechanical complication of ocular prosthesis (T85.3)

   Z44.20   Encounter for fitting and adjustment of artificial eye,
   <u>unspecified</u>

   Z44.21   Encounter for fitting and adjustment of artificial <u>right</u> eye

   Z44.22   Encounter for fitting and adjustment of artificial <u>left</u> eye

Z44.3-   Encounter for <u>fitting and adjustment of external breast
prosthesis</u>
   Excludes 1:   complications of breast implant (T85.4-)
                 encounter for adjustment or removal of breast implant
                     (Z45.81-)
                 encounter for initial breast implant insertion for
                     cosmetic breast augmentation (Z41.1)
                 encounter for breast reconstruction following
                     mastectomy (Z42.1)

   Z44.30   Encounter for fitting and adjustment of external breast
   prosthesis, <u>unspecified</u> breast

   Z44.31   Encounter for fitting and adjustment of external <u>right</u>
   breast prosthesis

   Z44.32   Encounter for fitting and adjustment of external <u>left</u>
   breast prosthesis

Z44.8   Encounter for fitting and adjustment of other external
prosthetic devices

Z44.9   Encounter for fitting and adjustment of unspecified external
prosthetic device — [Unacceptable PDX]

Z45-   Encounter for <u>adjustment and management of implanted device</u>
   Includes: Removal or replacement of implanted device
   Excludes 1:   malfunction or other complications of device — see
                     Alphabetical Index
                 presence of prosthetic and other devices (Z95-Z97)
   Excludes ❷: encounter for fitting and adjustment of non-implanted device
                     (Z46-)

Z45.0-   Encounter for adjustment and management of <u>cardiac device</u>

   Z45.01- Encounter for adjustment and management of cardiac
   <u>pacemaker</u>
      Encounter for adjustment and management of cardiac
      resynchronization therapy pacemaker (CRT-P)
   Excludes 1:   encounter for adjustment and management of
                     automatic implantable cardiac defibrillator
                     with synchronous cardiac pacemaker (Z45.02)

      Z45.010   Encounter for checking and testing of cardiac
      pacemaker <u>pulse generator [battery]</u> —
      [Questionable Admission]
         Encounter for replacing cardiac pacemaker pulse
         generator [battery]

      Z45.018   Encounter for adjustment and management of
      <u>other part of cardiac pacemaker</u> —
      [Questionable Admission]

   Z45.02   Encounter for adjustment and management of automatic
   implantable <u>cardiac defibrillator</u> — [Questionable Admission]
      Encounter for adjustment and management of automatic
      implantable cardiac defibrillator with synchronous
      cardiac pacemaker
      Encounter for adjustment and management of cardiac
      resynchronization therapy defibrillator (CRT-D)

   Z45.09   Encounter for adjustment and management of other
   cardiac device — [Questionable Admission]

Z45.1   Encounter for adjustment and management of <u>infusion pump</u>

Z45.2   Encounter for adjustment and management of <u>vascular access
device</u>
      Encounter for adjustment and management of vascular catheters
   Excludes 1:   encounter for adjustment and management of renal
                     dialysis catheter (Z49.01)

Z45.3-   Encounter for <u>adjustment and management of implanted
devices of the special senses</u>

   Z45.31   Encounter for adjustment and management of implanted
   visual substitution device

   Z45.32- Encounter for adjustment and management of <u>implanted
   hearing device</u>
   Excludes 1:   Encounter for fitting and adjustment of hearing
                     aide (Z46.1)

      Z45.320   Encounter for adjustment and management of <u>bone
      conduction device</u>

      Z45.321   Encounter for adjustment and management of
      <u>cochlear device</u>

      Z45.328   Encounter for adjustment and management of
      <u>other</u> implanted hearing device

Excludes 1: = NOT CODED HERE! (Do not code both)   1319   Excludes ❷ = Not Included Here

Z43 - Z45

Z45.4- Encounter for <u>adjustment and management of implanted nervous system device</u>
AHA 14:3Q:p19 – Replacement of Baclofen pump and catheter

Z45.41 Encounter for adjustment and management of <u>cerebrospinal fluid drainage device</u>
Encounter for adjustment and management of cerebral ventricular (communicating) shunt

Z45.42 Encounter for adjustment and management of <u>neuropacemaker</u> (brain) (peripheral nerve) (spinal cord)

Z45.49 Encounter for adjustment and management of <u>other</u> implanted nervous system device
AHA 14:4Q:p26 – Encounter for adjustment of vertical expandable prosthetic titanium rib (VEPTR)
AHA 14:4Q:p27 – Encounter for open lengthening of growing rods

Z45.8- Encounter for adjustment and management of <u>other implanted devices</u>

Z45.81- Encounter for <u>adjustment or removal of breast implant</u>
Encounter for elective implant exchange (different material) (different size)
Encounter removal of tissue expander without synchronous insertion of permanent implant
Excludes 1: complications of breast implant (T85.4-)
encounter for initial breast implant insertion for cosmetic breast augmentation (Z41.1)
encounter for breast reconstruction following mastectomy (Z42.1)

Z45.811 Encounter for adjustment or removal of <u>right</u> breast implant

Z45.812 Encounter for adjustment or removal of <u>left</u> breast implant

Z45.819 Encounter for adjustment or removal of <u>unspecified</u> breast implant

Z45.82 Encounter for adjustment or removal of myringotomy device (stent) (tube) — [Unacceptable PDX]

Z45.89 Encounter for adjustment and management of other implanted devices — [Unacceptable PDX]

Z45.9 Encounter for adjustment and management of unspecified implanted device — [Unacceptable PDX]

Z46- Encounter for <u>fitting and adjustment of other devices</u>
Includes: Removal or replacement of other device
Excludes 1: malfunction or other complications of device — see Alphabetical Index
Excludes ❷: encounter for fitting and management of implanted devices (Z45-)
issue of repeat prescription only (Z76.0)
presence of prosthetic and other devices (Z95-Z97)

Z46.0 Encounter for fitting and adjustment of <u>spectacles and contact lenses</u> — [Unacceptable PDX]

Z46.1 Encounter for fitting and adjustment of <u>hearing aid</u> — [Unacceptable PDX]
Excludes 1: encounter for adjustment and management of implanted hearing device (Z45.32-)

Z46.2 Encounter for fitting and adjustment of other devices related to nervous system and special senses
Excludes ❷: encounter for adjustment and management of implanted nervous system device (Z45.4-)
encounter for adjustment and management of implanted visual substitution device (Z45.31)

Z46.3 Encounter for fitting and adjustment of <u>dental prosthetic device</u>
Encounter for fitting and adjustment of dentures

Z46.4 Encounter for fitting and adjustment of <u>orthodontic</u> device — [Unacceptable PDX]

Z46.5- Encounter for fitting and adjustment of <u>other gastrointestinal appliance and device</u>
Excludes 1: encounter for attention to artificial openings of digestive tract (Z43.1-Z43.4)

Z46.51 Encounter for fitting and adjustment of <u>gastric lap band</u> — [Unacceptable PDX]

Z46.59 Encounter for fitting and adjustment of <u>other</u> gastrointestinal appliance and device — [Unacceptable PDX]

Z46.6 Encounter for fitting and adjustment of <u>urinary device</u> — [Unacceptable PDX]
Excludes ❷: attention to artificial openings of urinary tract (Z43.5, Z43.6)

Z46.8- Encounter for fitting and adjustment of other specified devices

Z46.81 Encounter for fitting and adjustment of <u>insulin pump</u> — [Unacceptable PDX]
Encounter for insulin pump titration
Encounter for insulin pump instruction and training

Z46.82 Encounter for fitting and adjustment of <u>non-vascular catheter</u>

Z46.89 Encounter for fitting and adjustment of <u>other</u> specified devices — [Unacceptable PDX]
Encounter for fitting and adjustment of wheelchair

Z46.9 Encounter for fitting and adjustment of unspecified device — [Unacceptable PDX]

Z47- <u>Orthopedic aftercare</u>
Excludes 1: aftercare for healing fracture — code to fracture with 7th character D

Z47.1 Aftercare following <u>joint replacement</u> surgery
Use additional code to identify the joint (Z96.6-)

Z47.2 Encounter for <u>removal of internal fixation device</u>
Excludes 1: encounter for adjustment of internal fixation device for fracture treatment — code to fracture with appropriate 7th character
encounter for removal of external fixation device — code to fracture with 7th character D
infection or inflammatory reaction to internal fixation device (T84.6-)
mechanical complication of internal fixation device (T84.1-)

Z47.3- Aftercare following <u>explanation of joint prosthesis</u>
AHA 15:1Q:p16 – Insertion of new hip prosthesis after removal of previous
Aftercare following explanation of joint prosthesis, staged procedure
Encounter for joint prosthesis insertion following prior explanation of joint prosthesis

Z47.31 Aftercare following explanation of <u>shoulder</u> joint prosthesis
Excludes 1: acquired absence of shoulder joint following prior explanation of shoulder joint prosthesis (Z89.23-)
shoulder joint prosthesis explanation status (Z89.23-)

Z47.32 Aftercare following explanation of <u>hip</u> joint prosthesis
Excludes 1: acquired absence of hip joint following prior explanation of hip joint prosthesis (Z89.62-)
hip joint prosthesis explanation status (Z89.62-)

Z47.33 Aftercare following explanation of <u>knee</u> joint prosthesis
Excludes 1: acquired absence of knee joint following prior explanation of knee joint prosthesis (Z89.52-)
knee joint prosthesis explanation status (Z89.52-)

Z47.8- Encounter for <u>other orthopedic aftercare</u>

Z47.81 Encounter for orthopedic aftercare <u>following surgical amputation</u>
Use additional code to identify the limb amputated (Z89.-)

Z47.82 Encounter for orthopedic aftercare <u>following scoliosis surgery</u>

Z47.89 Encounter for <u>other</u> orthopedic aftercare

Z48- Encounter for <u>other postprocedural aftercare</u>
Excludes 1: encounter for follow-up examination after completed treatment (Z08-Z09)
Excludes ❷: encounter for attention to artificial openings (Z43.-)
encounter for fitting and adjustment of prosthetic and other devices (Z44-Z46)

Z48.0- Encounter for attention to dressings, sutures and drains
Excludes 1: encounter for planned postprocedural wound closure (Z48.1)

Z48.00 Encounter for change or removal of nonsurgical wound dressing — [Unacceptable PDX]
Encounter for change or removal of wound dressing NOS

Z
4
5
-
Z
4
8

Z48.01 Encounter for change or removal of surgical wound dressing — [Unacceptable PDX]

Z48.02 Encounter for removal of sutures — [Unacceptable PDX]
Encounter for removal of staples

Z48.03 Encounter for change or removal of drains

Z48.1 Encounter for planned postprocedural wound closure
Excludes 1:   encounter for attention to dressings and sutures (Z48.0-)

Z48.2- Encounter for <u>aftercare following organ transplant</u>

cc **Z48.21** Encounter for aftercare following <u>heart</u> transplant

cc **Z48.22** Encounter for aftercare following <u>kidney</u> transplant

cc **Z48.23** Encounter for aftercare following <u>liver</u> transplant

cc **Z48.24** Encounter for aftercare following <u>lung</u> transplant

Z48.28- Encounter for aftercare following <u>multiple</u> organ transplant

   cc **Z48.280** Encounter for aftercare following <u>heart-lung transplant</u>

    Z48.288 Encounter for aftercare following <u>multiple organ transplant</u>

Z48.29- Encounter for aftercare following <u>other</u> organ transplant

   cc **Z48.290** Encounter for aftercare following <u>bone marrow</u> transplant

    Z48.298 Encounter for aftercare following <u>other</u> organ transplant

Z48.3 Aftercare following <u>surgery for neoplasm</u>
Use additional code to identify the neoplasm

Z48.8- Encounter for other specified postprocedural aftercare

Z48.81- Encounter for surgical aftercare following surgery on specified body systems
Note: These codes identify the body system requiring aftercare. They are for use in conjunction with other aftercare codes to fully explain the aftercare encounter. The condition treated should also be coded if still present.
*Excludes 1:   aftercare for injury — code the injury with 7th character D
aftercare following surgery for neoplasm (Z48.3)*
*Excludes ❷: aftercare following organ transplant (Z48.2-)
orthopedic aftercare (Z47.-)*

Z48.810 Encounter for surgical aftercare following surgery on the sense organs

Z48.811 Encounter for surgical aftercare following surgery on the nervous system
Excludes ❷: encounter for surgical aftercare following surgery on the sense organs (Z48.810)

Z48.812 Encounter for surgical aftercare following surgery on the circulatory system

Z48.813 Encounter for surgical aftercare following surgery on the respiratory system

Z48.814 Encounter for surgical aftercare following surgery on the teeth or oral cavity

Z48.815 Encounter for surgical aftercare following surgery on the digestive system

Z48.816 Encounter for surgical aftercare following surgery on the genitourinary system
Excludes 1:   encounter for aftercare following sterilization reversal (Z31.42)

Z48.817 Encounter for surgical aftercare following surgery on the skin and subcutaneous tissue

Z48.89 Encounter for other specified surgical aftercare

Z49- Encounter for care involving renal dialysis
Code also associated end stage renal disease (N18.6)

Z49.0- Preparatory care for renal dialysis
Encounter for dialysis instruction and training

Z49.01 Encounter for fitting and adjustment of <u>extracorporeal dialysis catheter</u>
Removal or replacement of renal dialysis catheter
Toilet or cleansing of renal dialysis catheter

Z49.02 Encounter for fitting and adjustment of <u>peritoneal dialysis catheter</u> — [Unacceptable PDX]

Z49.3- Encounter for adequacy testing for <u>dialysis</u>

Z49.31 Encounter for adequacy testing for <u>hemodialysis</u> — [Unacceptable PDX]

Z49.32 Encounter for adequacy testing for <u>peritoneal dialysis</u> — [Unacceptable PDX]
Encounter for peritoneal equilibration test

Z51- Encounter for other aftercare and medical care
Code also condition requiring care
Excludes 1:   follow-up examination after treatment (Z08-Z09)

Z51.0 Encounter for <u>antineoplastic radiation therapy</u>

Z51.1- Encounter for antineoplastic chemotherapy and immunotherapy
Excludes ❷: encounter for chemotherapy and immunotherapy for nonneoplastic condition — code to condition

Z51.11 Encounter for <u>antineoplastic chemotherapy</u>
AHA 15:3Q:p19 – Admitted for chemotherapy

Z51.12 Encounter for <u>antineoplastic immunotherapy</u>

Z51.5 Encounter for <u>palliative care</u> — [Unacceptable PDX]

Z51.6 Encounter for <u>desensitization to allergens</u> — [Unacceptable PDX]

Z51.8- Encounter for other specified aftercare
Excludes 1:   holiday relief care (Z75.5)

Z51.81 Encounter for therapeutic drug level monitoring
Code also any long-term (current) drug therapy (Z79.-)
Excludes 1:   encounter for blood-drug test for administrative or medicolegal reasons (Z02.83)

Z51.89 Encounter for other specified aftercare — [Unacceptable PDX, Requires Secondary DX]

Z52- <u>Donors of organs and tissues</u>
AHA 12:4Q:p99 – Domino liver transplant
Includes: Autologous and other living donors
*Excludes 1:   cadaveric donor — omit code
examination of potential donor (Z00.5)*

Z52.0- <u>Blood donor</u>

Z52.00- <u>Unspecified</u> blood donor

Z52.000 Unspecified donor, whole blood — [Unacceptable PDX]

Z52.001 Unspecified donor, stem cells — [Unacceptable PDX]

Z52.008 Unspecified donor, other blood — [Unacceptable PDX]

Z52.01- <u>Autologous</u> blood donor

Z52.010 Autologous donor, whole blood — [Unacceptable PDX]

Z52.011 Autologous donor, stem cells — [Unacceptable PDX]

Z52.018 Autologous donor, other blood — [Unacceptable PDX]

Z52.09- <u>Other blood</u> donor
Volunteer donor

Z52.090 Other blood donor, whole blood — [Unacceptable PDX]

Z52.091 Other blood donor, stem cells — [Unacceptable PDX]

Z52.098 Other blood donor, other blood — [Unacceptable PDX]

Z52.1- <u>Skin</u> donor

Z52.10 Skin donor, unspecified

Z52.11 Skin donor, autologous

Z52.19 Skin donor, other

Z52.2- <u>Bone</u> donor

Z52.20 Bone donor, unspecified

Z52.21 Bone donor, autologous

Z52.29 Bone donor, other

Z52.3 Bone marrow donor

Z52.4 Kidney donor

Z52.5 Cornea donor

Z52.6 Liver donor

Z52.8- Donor of other specified organs or tissues

Z52.81- <u>Egg (Oocyte) donor</u>

Z52.810 Egg (Oocyte) donor <u>under age 35, anonymous recipient</u> — [♀] [Unacceptable PDX]
Egg donor under age 35 NOS

Z52.811 Egg (Oocyte) donor <u>under age 35, designated</u> recipient — [♀] [Unacceptable PDX]

Z52.812 Egg (Oocyte) donor <u>age 35 and over, anonymous recipient</u> — [♀] [Unacceptable PDX]
Egg donor age 35 and over NOS

Z 4 8 I Z 5 2

Excludes 1: = NOT CODED HERE! (Do not code both)   1321   *Excludes ❷: = Not Included Here*

Z52.813 Egg (Oocyte) donor _age 35 and over_, _designated recipient_ — [♀] [Unacceptable PDX]

Z52.819 Egg (Oocyte) donor, _unspecified_ — [♀] [Unacceptable PDX]

Z52.89 Donor of other specified organs or tissues

Z52.9 Donor of unspecified organ or tissue
Donor NOS

Z53- Persons encountering health services for _specific procedures and treatment, not carried out_

Z53.0- Procedure and treatment not carried out because of _contraindication_

Z53.01 Procedure and treatment not carried out _due to patient smoking_ — [Unacceptable PDX]

Z53.09 Procedure and treatment not carried out _because of other contraindication_ — [Unacceptable PDX]

Z53.1 Procedure and treatment not carried out _because of patient's decision for reasons of belief and group pressure_ — [Unacceptable PDX]

Z53.2- Procedure and treatment not carried out _because of patient's decision for other and unspecified reasons_

Z53.20 Procedure and treatment not carried out because of patient's decision for unspecified reasons — [Unacceptable PDX]

Z53.21 Procedure and treatment not carried out due to patient leaving prior to being seen by healthcare provider — [Unacceptable PDX]

Z53.29 Procedure and treatment not carried out because of patient's decision for other reasons — [Unacceptable PDX]

Z53.3- _Procedure converted to open procedure_

Z53.31 _Laparoscopic_ surgical procedure converted to open procedure — [Unacceptable PDX]

Z53.32 _Thoracoscopic_ surgical procedure converted to open procedure — [Unacceptable PDX]

Z53.33 _Arthroscopic_ surgical procedure converted to open procedure — [Unacceptable PDX]

Z53.39 _Other specified_ procedure converted to open procedure — [Unacceptable PDX]

Z53.8 Procedure and treatment _not carried out for other reasons_ — [Unacceptable PDX]

Z53.9 Procedure and treatment _not carried out, unspecified reason_ — [Unacceptable PDX]

Persons with potential health hazards related to socioeconomic and psychosocial circumstances (Z55-Z65)

Z55- Problems related to education and literacy
Excludes 1: _disorders of psychological development (F80-F89)_

Z55.0 Illiteracy and low-level literacy — [Unacceptable PDX]

Z55.1 Schooling unavailable and unattainable — [Unacceptable PDX]

Z55.2 Failed school examinations — [Unacceptable PDX]

Z55.3 Underachievement in school — [Unacceptable PDX]

Z55.4 Educational maladjustment and discord with teachers and classmates — [Unacceptable PDX]

Z55.8 Other problems related to education and literacy — [Unacceptable PDX]
Problems related to inadequate teaching

Z55.9 Problems related to education and literacy, unspecified — [Unacceptable PDX]
Academic problems NOS

Z56- Problems related to employment and unemployment
Excludes ❷: _occupational exposure to risk factors (Z57.-)_
problems related to housing and economic circumstances (Z59.-)

Z56.0 Unemployment, unspecified — [Unacceptable PDX]

Z56.1 Change of job — [Age/15-124] [Unacceptable PDX]

Z56.2 Threat of job loss — [Unacceptable PDX]

Z56.3 Stressful work schedule — [Unacceptable PDX]

Z56.4 Discord with boss and workmates — [Unacceptable PDX]

Z56.5 Uncongenial work environment — [Unacceptable PDX]
Difficult conditions at work

Z56.6 Other physical and mental strain related to work — [Unacceptable PDX]

Z56.8- Other problems related to employment

Z56.81 Sexual harassment on the job — [Unacceptable PDX]

Z56.82 Military deployment status — [Unacceptable PDX]
Individual (civilian or military) currently deployed in theater or in support of military war, peacekeeping and humanitarian operations

Z56.89 Other problems related to employment — [Unacceptable PDX]

Z56.9 Unspecified problems related to employment — [Unacceptable PDX]
Occupational problems NOS

Z57- Occupational exposure to risk factors

Z57.0 Occupational exposure to noise — [Unacceptable PDX]

Z57.1 Occupational exposure to radiation — [Unacceptable PDX]

Z57.2 Occupational exposure to dust — [Unacceptable PDX]

Z57.3- Occupational exposure to other air contaminants

Z57.31 Occupational exposure to environmental tobacco smoke — [Unacceptable PDX]
Excludes ❷: _exposure to environmental tobacco smoke (Z77.22)_

Z57.39 Occupational exposure to other air contaminants — [Unacceptable PDX]

Z57.4 Occupational exposure to toxic agents in agriculture — [Unacceptable PDX]
Occupational exposure to solids, liquids, gases or vapors in agriculture

Z57.5 Occupational exposure to toxic agents in other industries — [Unacceptable PDX]
Occupational exposure to solids, liquids, gases or vapors in other industries

Z57.6 Occupational exposure to extreme temperature — [Unacceptable PDX]

Z57.7 Occupational exposure to vibration — [Unacceptable PDX]

Z57.8 Occupational exposure to other risk factors — [Unacceptable PDX]

Z57.9 Occupational exposure to unspecified risk factor — [Unacceptable PDX]

Z59- Problems related to housing and economic circumstances
Excludes ❷: _problems related to upbringing (Z62.-)_

Z59.0 Homelessness — [Unacceptable PDX]

Z59.1 Inadequate housing — [Unacceptable PDX]
Lack of heating
Restriction of space
Technical defects in home preventing adequate care
Unsatisfactory surroundings
Excludes 1: _problems related to the natural and physical environment (Z77.1-)_

Z59.2 Discord with neighbors, lodgers and landlord — [Unacceptable PDX]

Z59.3 Problems related to living in residential institution — [Unacceptable PDX]
Boarding-school resident
Excludes 1: _institutional upbringing (Z62.2)_

Z59.4 Lack of adequate food and safe drinking water — [Unacceptable PDX]
Inadequate drinking water supply
Excludes 1: _effects of hunger (T73.0)_
inappropriate diet or eating habits (Z72.4)
malnutrition (E40-E46)

Z59.5 Extreme poverty — [Unacceptable PDX]

Z59.6 Low income — [Unacceptable PDX]

Z59.7 Insufficient social insurance and welfare support — [Unacceptable PDX]

Z59.8 Other problems related to housing and economic circumstances — [Unacceptable PDX]
Foreclosure on loan
Isolated dwelling
Problems with creditors

Z59.9 Problem related to housing and economic circumstances, unspecified — [Unacceptable PDX]

Z52-Z59

Z60-   Problems related to social environment

Z60.0   Problems of adjustment to life-cycle transitions —
[Unacceptable PDX]
        Empty nest syndrome
        Phase of life problem
        Problem with adjustment to retirement [pension]

Z60.2   Problems related to living alone — [Unacceptable PDX]

Z60.3   Acculturation difficulty — [Unacceptable PDX]
        Problem with migration
        Problem with social transplantation

Z60.4   Social exclusion and rejection — [Unacceptable PDX]
        Exclusion and rejection on the basis of personal characteristics,
            such as unusual physical appearance, illness or behavior.
        *Excludes 1:   target of adverse discrimination such as for racial or
                religious reasons (Z60.5)*

**Z60.5   Target of (perceived) adverse discrimination and
        persecution —** [Unacceptable PDX]
        Excludes 1:   social exclusion and rejection (Z60.4)

Z60.8   Other problems related to social environment —
[Unacceptable PDX]

Z60.9   Problem related to social environment, unspecified —
[Unacceptable PDX]

Z62-   Problems related to upbringing
    Includes: Current and past negative life events in childhood
                Current and past problems of a child related to upbringing
    *Excludes ❷: maltreatment syndrome (T74.-)
                problems related to housing and economic circumstances
                    (Z59.-)*

Z62.0   Inadequate parental supervision and control —
[Unacceptable PDX]

Z62.1   Parental overprotection — [Unacceptable PDX]

Z62.2-   Upbringing away from parents
        Excludes 1:   problems with boarding school (Z59.3)

    Z62.21   Child in welfare custody — [Age/0-17] [Unacceptable PDX]
            Child in care of non-parental family member
            Child in foster care
            *Excludes ❷: problem for parent due to child in welfare custody
                    (Z63.5)*

    Z62.22   Institutional upbringing — [Unacceptable PDX]
            Child living in orphanage or group home

    Z62.29   Other upbringing away from parents — [Unacceptable PDX]

Z62.3   Hostility towards and scapegoating of child — [Age/0-17]
[Unacceptable PDX]

Z62.6   Inappropriate (excessive) parental pressure — [Unacceptable PDX]

Z62.8-   Other specified problems related to upbringing

    Z62.81- Personal history of abuse in childhood

        **Z62.810   Personal history of physical and sexual abuse in
                childhood —** [Unacceptable PDX]
                *Excludes 1:   current child physical abuse (T74.12-,
                        T76.12-)
                        current child sexual abuse (T74.22-,
                        T76.22-)*

        **Z62.811   Personal history of psychological abuse in
                childhood —** [Unacceptable PDX]
                *Excludes 1:   current child psychological abuse (T74.32-,
                        T76.32-)*

        Z62.812   Personal history of neglect in childhood —
                [Unacceptable PDX]
                Excludes 1:   current child neglect (T74.02, T76.02-)

        **Z62.819   Personal history of unspecified abuse in
                childhood —** [Unacceptable PDX]
                Excludes 1:   current child abuse NOS (T74.92, T76.92-)

    Z62.82- Parent-child conflict

        Z62.820   Parent-biological child conflict — [Unacceptable PDX]
                Parent-child problem NOS

        Z62.821   Parent-adopted child conflict — [Unacceptable PDX]

        Z62.822   Parent-foster child conflict — [Unacceptable PDX]

    Z62.89- Other specified problems related to upbringing

        Z62.890   Parent-child estrangement NEC — [Unacceptable PDX]

        Z62.891   Sibling rivalry — [Unacceptable PDX]

        Z62.898   Other specified problems related to upbringing —
                [Unacceptable PDX]

Z62.9   Problem related to upbringing, unspecified — [Unacceptable PDX]

**Z63-   Other problems related to primary support group, including family
        circumstances**
    *Excludes ❷: maltreatment syndrome (T74.-, T76)
                parent-child problems (Z62.-)
                problems related to negative life events in childhood (Z62.-)
                problems related to upbringing (Z62.-)*

Z63.0   Problems in relationship with spouse or partner —
[Unacceptable PDX]
        *Excludes 1:   counseling for spousal or partner abuse problems
                (Z69.1)
                counseling related to sexual attitude, behavior, and
                orientation (Z70.-)*

Z63.1   Problems in relationship with in-laws — [Unacceptable PDX]

Z63.3-   Absence of family member
        *Excludes 1:   absence of family member due to disappearance and
                death (Z63.4)
                absence of family member due to separation and
                divorce (Z63.5)*

    Z63.31   Absence of family member due to military deployment —
            [Unacceptable PDX]
            Individual or family affected by other family member being on
                military deployment
            *Excludes 1:   family disruption due to return of family member
                    from military deployment (Z63.71)*

    Z63.32   Other absence of family member — [Unacceptable PDX]

Z63.4   Disappearance and death of family member — [Unacceptable PDX]
        AHA 14:1Q:p25 – Bereavement
        Assumed death of family member
        Bereavement

Z63.5   Disruption of family by separation and divorce —
[Unacceptable PDX]
        Marital estrangement

Z63.6   Dependent relative needing care at home — [Unacceptable PDX]

Z63.7-   Other stressful life events affecting family and household

    **Z63.71   Stress on family due to return of family member from
            military deployment —** [Unacceptable PDX]
            Individual or family affected by family member having
                returned from military deployment (current or past
                conflict)

    Z63.72   Alcoholism and drug addiction in family — [Unacceptable PDX]

    **Z63.79   Other stressful life events affecting family and
            household —** [Unacceptable PDX]
            Anxiety (normal) about sick person in family
            Health problems within family
            Ill or disturbed family member
            Isolated family

Z63.8   Other specified problems related to primary support group —
[Unacceptable PDX]
        Family discord NOS
        Family estrangement NOS
        High expressed emotional level within family
        Inadequate family support NOS
        Inadequate or distorted communication within family

Z63.9   Problem related to primary support group, unspecified —
[Unacceptable PDX]
        Relationship disorder NOS

Z64-   Problems related to certain psychosocial circumstances

Z64.0   Problems related to unwanted pregnancy — [♀]
[Unacceptable PDX]

Z64.1   Problems related to multiparity — [♀] [Unacceptable PDX]

Z64.4   Discord with counselors — [Unacceptable PDX]
        Discord with probation officer
        Discord with social worker

Z65-   Problems related to other psychosocial circumstances

**Z65.0   Conviction in civil and criminal proceedings without
        imprisonment —** [Unacceptable PDX]

Z65.1   Imprisonment and other incarceration — [Unacceptable PDX]

Z65.2   Problems related to release from prison — [Unacceptable PDX]

Z65.3   Problems related to other legal circumstances —
[Unacceptable PDX]
        Arrest
        Child custody or support proceedings
        Litigation
        Prosecution

Z60 - Z65

Excludes 1: = NOT CODED HERE! (Do not code both)   **1323**   *Excludes ❷:* = Not Included Here

Z65.4 Victim of crime and terrorism — [Unacceptable PDX]
Victim of torture

Z65.5 Exposure to disaster, war and other hostilities — [Unacceptable PDX]
Excludes 1: target of perceived discrimination or persecution (Z60.5)

Z65.8 Other specified problems related to psychosocial circumstances — [Unacceptable PDX]

Z65.9 Problem related to unspecified psychosocial circumstances — [Unacceptable PDX]

Do not resuscitate status (Z66)

Z66 Do not resuscitate — [Unacceptable PDX]
DNR status

Blood type (Z67)

Z67- Blood type

Z67.1- Type A blood

    Z67.10 Type A blood, Rh positive — [Unacceptable PDX]

    Z67.11 Type A blood, Rh negative — [Unacceptable PDX]

Z67.2- Type B blood

    Z67.20 Type B blood, Rh positive — [Unacceptable PDX]

    Z67.21 Type B blood, Rh negative — [Unacceptable PDX]

Z67.3- Type AB blood

    Z67.30 Type AB blood, Rh positive — [Unacceptable PDX]

    Z67.31 Type AB blood, Rh negative — [Unacceptable PDX]

Z67.4- Type O blood

    Z67.40 Type O blood, Rh positive — [Unacceptable PDX]

    Z67.41 Type O blood, Rh negative — [Unacceptable PDX]

Z67.9- Unspecified blood type

    Z67.90 Unspecified blood type, Rh positive — [Unacceptable PDX]

    Z67.91 Unspecified blood type, Rh negative — [Unacceptable PDX]

Body mass index [BMI] (Z68)

Z68- Body mass index [BMI]
Kilograms per meters squared
Note: BMI adult codes are for use for persons 21 years of age or older.
Note: BMI pediatric codes are for use for persons 2-20 years of age. These percentiles are based on the growth charts published by the Centers for Disease Control and Prevention (CDC).

CC **Z68.1** Body mass index (BMI) 19 or less, adult — [Age/15-124] [Unacceptable PDX]

Z68.2- Body mass index (BMI) 20-29, adult

    Z68.20 Body mass index (BMI) 20.0-20.9, adult — [Age/15-124] [Unacceptable PDX]

    Z68.21 Body mass index (BMI) 21.0-21.9, adult — [Age/15-124] [Unacceptable PDX]

    Z68.22 Body mass index (BMI) 22.0-22.9, adult — [Age/15-124] [Unacceptable PDX]

    Z68.23 Body mass index (BMI) 23.0-23.9, adult — [Age/15-124] [Unacceptable PDX]

    Z68.24 Body mass index (BMI) 24.0-24.9, adult — [Age/15-124] [Unacceptable PDX]

    Z68.25 Body mass index (BMI) 25.0-25.9, adult — [Age/15-124] [Unacceptable PDX]

    Z68.26 Body mass index (BMI) 26.0-26.9, adult — [Age/15-124] [Unacceptable PDX]

    Z68.27 Body mass index (BMI) 27.0-27.9, adult — [Age/15-124] [Unacceptable PDX]

    Z68.28 Body mass index (BMI) 28.0-28.9, adult — [Age/15-124] [Unacceptable PDX]

    Z68.29 Body mass index (BMI) 29.0-29.9, adult — [Age/15-124] [Unacceptable PDX]

Z68.3- Body mass index (BMI) 30-39, adult

    Z68.30 Body mass index (BMI) 30.0-30.9, adult — [Age/15-124] [Unacceptable PDX]

    Z68.31 Body mass index (BMI) 31.0-31.9, adult — [Age/15-124] [Unacceptable PDX]

    Z68.32 Body mass index (BMI) 32.0-32.9, adult — [Age/15-124] [Unacceptable PDX]

    Z68.33 Body mass index (BMI) 33.0-33.9, adult — [Age/15-124] [Unacceptable PDX]

    Z68.34 Body mass index (BMI) 34.0-34.9, adult — [Age/15-124] [Unacceptable PDX]

    Z68.35 Body mass index (BMI) 35.0-35.9, adult — [Age/15-124] [Unacceptable PDX]

    Z68.36 Body mass index (BMI) 36.0-36.9, adult — [Age/15-124] [Unacceptable PDX]

    Z68.37 Body mass index (BMI) 37.0-37.9, adult — [Age/15-124] [Unacceptable PDX]

    Z68.38 Body mass index (BMI) 38.0-38.9, adult — [Age/15-124] [Unacceptable PDX]

    Z68.39 Body mass index (BMI) 39.0-39.9, adult — [Age/15-124] [Unacceptable PDX]

Z68.4- Body mass index (BMI) 40 or greater, adult

CC **Z68.41** Body mass index (BMI) 40.0-44.9, adult — [Age/15-124] [Unacceptable PDX]

CC **Z68.42** Body mass index (BMI) 45.0-49.9, adult — [Age/15-124] [Unacceptable PDX]

CC **Z68.43** Body mass index (BMI) 50.0-59.9, adult — [Age/15-124] [Unacceptable PDX]

CC **Z68.44** Body mass index (BMI) 60.0-69.9, adult — [Age/15-124] [Unacceptable PDX]

CC **Z68.45** Body mass index (BMI) 70 or greater, adult — [Age/15-124] [Unacceptable PDX]

Z68.5- Body mass index (BMI) pediatric

    Z68.51 Body mass index (BMI) pediatric, less than 5th percentile for age — [Unacceptable PDX]

    Z68.52 Body mass index (BMI) pediatric, 5th percentile to less than 85th percentile for age — [Unacceptable PDX]

    Z68.53 Body mass index (BMI) pediatric, 85th percentile to less than 95th percentile for age — [Unacceptable PDX]

    Z68.54 Body mass index (BMI) pediatric, greater than or equal to 95th percentile for age — [Unacceptable PDX]

Persons encountering health services in other circumstances (Z69-Z76)

Z69- Encounter for mental health services for victim and perpetrator of abuse
Includes: Counseling for victims and perpetrators of abuse

Z69.0- Encounter for mental health services for child abuse problems

    Z69.01- Encounter for mental health services for parental child abuse

        Z69.010 Encounter for mental health services for victim of parental child abuse — [Age/0-17]

        Z69.011 Encounter for mental health services for perpetrator of parental child abuse — [Unacceptable PDX]
        Excludes 1: encounter for mental health services for non-parental child abuse (Z69.02-)

    Z69.02- Encounter for mental health services for non-parental child abuse

        Z69.020 Encounter for mental health services for victim of non-parental child abuse — [Age/0-17]

        Z69.021 Encounter for mental health services for perpetrator of non-parental child abuse — [Unacceptable PDX]

Z69.1- Encounter for mental health services for spousal or partner abuse problems

    Z69.11 Encounter for mental health services for victim of spousal or partner abuse — [Unacceptable PDX]

Z 65 - Z 69

Z69.12 Encounter for mental health services for <u>perpetrator</u> of spousal or partner abuse — [Unacceptable PDX]

Z69.8- Encounter for mental health services for victim or perpetrator of <u>other</u> abuse

   Z69.81 Encounter for mental health services for <u>victim</u> of other abuse — [Unacceptable PDX]
      Encounter for rape victim counseling

   Z69.82 Encounter for mental health services for <u>perpetrator</u> of other abuse — [Unacceptable PDX]

Z70- Counseling related to sexual attitude, behavior and orientation
  Includes: Encounter for mental health services for sexual attitude, behavior and orientation
  Excludes ❷: contraceptive or procreative counseling (Z30-Z31)

  Z70.0 Counseling related to sexual attitude — [Unacceptable PDX]

  Z70.1 Counseling related to patient's sexual behavior and orientation — [Unacceptable PDX]
    Patient concerned regarding impotence
    Patient concerned regarding non-responsiveness
    Patient concerned regarding promiscuity
    Patient concerned regarding sexual orientation

  Z70.2 Counseling related to sexual behavior and orientation of third party — [Unacceptable PDX]
    Advice sought regarding sexual behavior and orientation of child
    Advice sought regarding sexual behavior and orientation of partner
    Advice sought regarding sexual behavior and orientation of spouse

  Z70.3 Counseling related to combined concerns regarding sexual attitude, behavior and orientation — [Unacceptable PDX]

  Z70.8 Other sex counseling — [Unacceptable PDX]
    Encounter for sex education

  Z70.9 Sex counseling, unspecified — [Unacceptable PDX]

Z71- Persons encountering health services for other counseling and medical advice, not elsewhere classified
  Excludes ❷: contraceptive or procreation counseling (Z30-Z31)
    sex counseling (Z70.-)

  Z71.0 Person encountering health services to consult on behalf of another person — [Unacceptable PDX]
    Person encountering health services to seek advice or treatment for non-attending third party
    Excludes ❷: anxiety (normal) about sick person in family (Z63.7)
      expectant (adoptive) parent(s) pre-birth pediatrician visit (Z76.81)

  Z71.1 Person with feared health complaint in whom no diagnosis is made — [Unacceptable PDX]
    Person encountering health services with feared condition which was not demonstrated
    Person encountering health services in which problem was normal state
    "Worried well"
    Excludes 1: medical observation for suspected diseases and conditions proven not to exist (Z03.-)

  Z71.2 Person consulting for explanation of examination or test findings — [Unacceptable PDX]

  Z71.3 Dietary counseling and surveillance — [Unacceptable PDX]
    Use additional code for any associated underlying medical condition
    Use additional code to identify body mass index (BMI), if known (Z68.-)

  Z71.4- <u>Alcohol abuse counseling and surveillance</u>
    Use additional code for alcohol abuse or dependence (F10.-)
   Z71.41 Alcohol abuse counseling and surveillance of <u>alcoholic</u> — [Unacceptable PDX]
   Z71.42 Counseling for <u>family member of alcoholic</u> — [Unacceptable PDX]
    Counseling for significant other, partner, or friend of alcoholic

  Z71.5- Drug abuse counseling and surveillance
    Use additional code for drug abuse or dependence (F11-F16, F18-F19)
   Z71.51 Drug abuse counseling and surveillance of drug abuser — [Unacceptable PDX]
   Z71.52 Counseling for <u>family member of drug abuser</u> — [Unacceptable PDX]
    Counseling for significant other, partner, or friend of drug abuser

  Z71.6 Tobacco abuse counseling — [Unacceptable PDX]
    Use additional code for nicotine dependence (F17.-)

Z71.7 Human immunodeficiency virus [HIV] counseling — [Unacceptable PDX]

Z71.8- Other specified counseling
  Excludes ❷: counseling for contraception (Z30.0-)
    counseling for genetics (Z31.5)
    counseling for procreative management (Z31.6-)
  Z71.81 Spiritual or religious counseling — [Unacceptable PDX]
  Z71.89 Other specified counseling — [Unacceptable PDX]

Z71.9 Counseling, unspecified — [Unacceptable PDX]
  Encounter for medical advice NOS

Z72- Problems related to lifestyle
  Excludes ❷: problems related to life-management difficulty (Z73.-)
    problems related to socioeconomic and psychosocial circumstances (Z55-Z65)

  Z72.0 Tobacco use — [Unacceptable PDX]
    Tobacco use NOS
    Excludes 1: history of tobacco dependence (Z87.891)
      nicotine dependence (F17.2-)
      tobacco dependence (F17.2-)
      tobacco use during pregnancy (O99.33-)

  Z72.3 Lack of physical exercise — [Unacceptable PDX]

  Z72.4 Inappropriate diet and eating habits — [Unacceptable PDX]
    Excludes 1: behavioral eating disorders of infancy or childhood (F98.2.-F98.3)
      eating disorders (F50.-)
      lack of adequate food (Z59.4)
      malnutrition and other nutritional deficiencies (E40-E64)

  Z72.5- High risk sexual behavior
    Promiscuity
    Excludes 1: paraphilias (F65)
   Z72.51 High risk heterosexual behavior — [Unacceptable PDX]
   Z72.52 High risk homosexual behavior — [Unacceptable PDX]
   Z72.53 High risk bisexual behavior — [Unacceptable PDX]

  Z72.6 Gambling and betting — [Unacceptable PDX]
    Excludes 1: compulsive or pathological gambling (F63.0)

  Z72.8- Other problems related to lifestyle
   Z72.81- Antisocial behavior
    Excludes 1: conduct disorders (F91.-)
    Z72.810 Child and adolescent antisocial behavior — [Age/0-17]
      Antisocial behavior (child) (adolescent) without manifest psychiatric disorder
      Delinquency NOS
      Group delinquency
      Offenses in the context of gang membership
      Stealing in company with others
      Truancy from school
    Z72.811 Adult antisocial behavior — [Age/15-124]
      Adult antisocial behavior without manifest psychiatric disorder

   Z72.82- Problems related to sleep
    Z72.820 Sleep deprivation
      Lack of adequate sleep
      Excludes 1: insomnia (G47.0-)
    Z72.821 Inadequate sleep hygiene — [Unacceptable PDX]
      Bad sleep habits
      Irregular sleep habits
      Unhealthy sleep wake schedule
      Excludes 1: insomnia (F51.0-, G47.0-)

   Z72.89 Other problems related to lifestyle — [Unacceptable PDX]
    Self-damaging behavior

  Z72.9 Problem related to lifestyle, unspecified — [Unacceptable PDX]

Z73- Problems related to life management difficulty
  Excludes ❷: problems related to socioeconomic and psychosocial circumstances (Z55-Z65)

  Z73.0 Burn-out — [Unacceptable PDX]
  Z73.1 Type A behavior pattern — [Unacceptable PDX]
  Z73.2 Lack of relaxation and leisure — [Unacceptable PDX]
  Z73.3 Stress, not elsewhere classified — [Unacceptable PDX]
    Physical and mental strain NOS
    Excludes 1: stress related to employment or unemployment (Z56.-)

Z69 - Z73

Z73.4 Inadequate social skills, not elsewhere classified — [Unacceptable PDX]

Z73.5 Social role conflict, not elsewhere classified — [Unacceptable PDX]

Z73.6 Limitation of activities due to disability — [Unacceptable PDX]
> Excludes 1: care-provider dependency (Z74.-)

Z73.8- Other problems related to life management difficulty

Z73.81- Behavioral insomnia of childhood

Z73.810 Behavioral insomnia of childhood, sleep-onset association type — [Age/0-17] [Unacceptable PDX]

Z73.811 Behavioral insomnia of childhood, limit setting type — [Age/0-17] [Unacceptable PDX]

Z73.812 Behavioral insomnia of childhood, combined type — [Age/0-17] [Unacceptable PDX]

Z73.819 Behavioral insomnia of childhood, unspecified type — [Age/0-17] [Unacceptable PDX]

Z73.82 Dual sensory impairment — [Unacceptable PDX]

Z73.89 Other problems related to life management difficulty — [Unacceptable PDX]

Z73.9 Problem related to life management difficulty, unspecified — [Unacceptable PDX]

Z74- Problems related to care provider dependency
> Excludes ❷: dependence on enabling machines or devices NEC (Z99.-)

Z74.0- Reduced mobility

Z74.01 Bed confinement status — [Unacceptable PDX]
> Bedridden

Z74.09 Other reduced mobility — [Unacceptable PDX]
> Chairridden
> Reduced mobility NOS
> Excludes ❷: wheelchair dependence (Z99.3)

Z74.1 Need for assistance with personal care — [Unacceptable PDX]

Z74.2 Need for assistance at home and no other household member able to render care — [Unacceptable PDX]

Z74.3 Need for continuous supervision — [Unacceptable PDX]

Z74.8 Other problems related to care provider dependency — [Unacceptable PDX]

Z74.9 Problem related to care provider dependency, unspecified — [Unacceptable PDX]

Z75- Problems related to medical facilities and other health care

Z75.0 Medical services not available in home — [Unacceptable PDX]
> Excludes 1: no other household member able to render care (Z74.2)

Z75.1 Person awaiting admission to adequate facility elsewhere — [Unacceptable PDX]

Z75.2 Other waiting period for investigation and treatment — [Unacceptable PDX]

Z75.3 Unavailability and inaccessibility of health-care facilities — [Unacceptable PDX]
> Excludes 1: bed unavailable (Z75.1)

Z75.4 Unavailability and inaccessibility of other helping agencies — [Unacceptable PDX]

Z75.5 Holiday relief care — [Unacceptable PDX]

Z75.8 Other problems related to medical facilities and other health care — [Unacceptable PDX]

Z75.9 Unspecified problem related to medical facilities and other health care — [Unacceptable PDX]

Z76- Persons encountering health services in other circumstances
> AHA 14:2Q:p10 – Encounter for Neulasta to prevent infection

Z76.0 Encounter for issue of repeat prescription — [Unacceptable PDX]
> Encounter for issue of repeat prescription for appliance
> Encounter for issue of repeat prescription for medicaments
> Encounter for issue of repeat prescription for spectacles
> Excludes ❷: issue of medical certificate (Z02.7)
> repeat prescription for contraceptive (Z30.4-)

Z76.1 Encounter for health supervision and care of foundling

Z76.2 Encounter for health supervision and care of other healthy infant and child — [Age/0-17] [Unacceptable PDX]
> Encounter for medical or nursing care or supervision of healthy infant under circumstances such as adverse socioeconomic conditions at home
> Encounter for medical or nursing care or supervision of healthy infant under circumstances such as awaiting foster or adoptive placement
> Encounter for medical or nursing care or supervision of healthy infant under circumstances such as maternal illness
> Encounter for medical or nursing care or supervision of healthy infant under circumstances such as number of children at home preventing or interfering with normal care

Z76.3 Healthy person accompanying sick person

Z76.4 Other boarder to healthcare facility
> Excludes 1: homelessness (Z59.0)

Z76.5 Malingerer [conscious simulation]
> Person feigning illness (with obvious motivation)
> Excludes 1: factitious disorder (F68.1-)
> peregrinating patient (F68.1-)

Z76.8- Persons encountering health services in other specified circumstances

Z76.81 Expectant parent(s) prebirth pediatrician visit — [Unacceptable PDX]
> Pre-adoption pediatrician visit for adoptive parent(s)

Z76.82 Awaiting organ transplant status — [Unacceptable PDX]
> Patient waiting for organ availability

Z76.89 Persons encountering health services in other specified circumstances — [Unacceptable PDX]
> Persons encountering health services NOS

Persons with potential health hazards related to family and personal history and certain conditions influencing health status (Z77-Z99)

> Code also any follow-up examination (Z08-Z09)

Z77- Other contact with and (suspected) exposures hazardous to health
> Includes: Contact with and (suspected) exposures to potential hazards to health
> Excludes ❷: contact with and (suspected) exposure to communicable diseases (Z20.-)
> exposure to (parental) (environmental) tobacco smoke in the perinatal period (P96.81)
> newborn affected by noxious substances transmitted via placenta or breast milk (P04.-)
> occupational exposure to risk factors (Z57.-)
> retained foreign body (Z18.-)
> retained foreign body fully removed (Z87.821)
> toxic effects of substances chiefly nonmedicinal as to source (T51-T65)

Z77.0- Contact with and (suspected) exposure to hazardous, chiefly nonmedicinal, chemicals

Z77.01- Contact with and (suspected) exposure to hazardous metals

Z77.010 Contact with and (suspected) exposure to arsenic — [Unacceptable PDX]

Z77.011 Contact with and (suspected) exposure to lead — [Unacceptable PDX]

Z77.012 Contact with and (suspected) exposure to uranium — [Unacceptable PDX]
> Excludes 1: retained depleted uranium fragments (Z18.01)

Z77.018 Contact with and (suspected) exposure to other hazardous metals — [Unacceptable PDX]
> Contact with and (suspected) exposure to chromium compounds
> Contact with and (suspected) exposure to nickel dust

Z77.02- Contact with and (suspected) exposure to hazardous aromatic compounds

Z77.020 Contact with and (suspected) exposure to aromatic amines — [Unacceptable PDX]

Z77.021 Contact with and (suspected) exposure to benzene — [Unacceptable PDX]

Z77.028   **Contact with and (suspected) exposure to other hazardous aromatic compounds** — [Unacceptable PDX]
Aromatic dyes NOS
Polycyclic aromatic hydrocarbons

Z77.09-   **Contact with and (suspected) exposure to other hazardous, chiefly nonmedicinal, chemicals**

Z77.090   **Contact with and (suspected) exposure to asbestos** — [Unacceptable PDX]

Z77.098   **Contact with and (suspected) exposure to other hazardous, chiefly nonmedicinal, chemicals** — [Unacceptable PDX]
Dyes NOS

Z77.1-   **Contact with and (suspected) exposure to environmental pollution and hazards in the physical environment**

Z77.11-   **Contact with and (suspected) exposure to environmental pollution**

Z77.110   **Contact with and (suspected) exposure to air pollution** — [Unacceptable PDX]

Z77.111   **Contact with and (suspected) exposure to water pollution** — [Unacceptable PDX]

Z77.112   **Contact with and (suspected) exposure to soil pollution** — [Unacceptable PDX]

Z77.118   **Contact with and (suspected) exposure to other environmental pollution** — [Unacceptable PDX]

Z77.12-   **Contact with and (suspected) exposure to hazards in the physical environment**

Z77.120   **Contact with and (suspected) exposure to mold (toxic)** — [Unacceptable PDX]

Z77.121   **Contact with and (suspected) exposure to harmful algae and algae toxins** — [Unacceptable PDX]
Contact with and (suspected) exposure to (harmful) algae bloom NOS
Contact with and (suspected) exposure to blue-green algae bloom
Contact with and (suspected) exposure to brown tide
Contact with and (suspected) exposure to cyanobacteria bloom
Contact with and (suspected) exposure to Florida red tide
Contact with and (suspected) exposure to pfiesteria piscicida
Contact with and (suspected) exposure to red tide

Z77.122   **Contact with and (suspected) exposure to noise** — [Unacceptable PDX]

Z77.123   **Contact with and (suspected) exposure to radon and other naturally occuring radiation** — [Unacceptable PDX]
*Excludes ❷: radiation exposure as the cause of a confirmed condition (W88-W90, X39.0-)
radiation sickness NOS (T66)*

Z77.128   **Contact with and (suspected) exposure to other hazards in the physical environment** — [Unacceptable PDX]

Z77.2-   **Contact with and (suspected) exposure to other hazardous substances**

Z77.21   **Contact with and (suspected) exposure to potentially hazardous body fluids** — [Unacceptable PDX]

Z77.22   **Contact with and (suspected) exposure to environmental tobacco smoke (acute) (chronic)** — [Unacceptable PDX]
Exposure to second hand tobacco smoke (acute) (chronic)
Passive smoking (acute) (chronic)
*Excludes 1:   nicotine dependence (F17.-)
tobacco use (Z72.0)*
Excludes ❷: occupational exposure to environmental tobacco smoke (Z57.31)

Z77.29   **Contact with and (suspected) exposure to other hazardous substances** — [Unacceptable PDX]
AHA 16:2Q:p33 – Wheezing due to exposure to electronic cigarette vapors

Z77.9   **Other contact with and (suspected) exposures hazardous to health** — [Unacceptable PDX]

Z78-   **Other specified health status**
*Excludes ❷: asymptomatic human immunodeficiency virus [HIV] infection status (Z21)
postprocedural status (Z93-Z99)
sex reassignment status (Z87.890)*

Z78.0   **Asymptomatic menopausal state** — [♀, Age/15-124] [Unacceptable PDX]
Menopausal state NOS
Postmenopausal status NOS
Excludes ❷: symptomatic menopausal state (N95.1)

Z78.1   **Physical restraint status** — [Unacceptable PDX]
Excludes 1:   physical restraint due to a procedure — omit code

Z78.9   **Other specified health status** — [Unacceptable PDX]

Z79-   **Long term (current) drug therapy**
Includes: Long term (current) drug use for prophylactic purposes
Code also any therapeutic drug level monitoring (Z51.81)
*Excludes ❷: drug abuse and dependence (F11-F19)
drug use complicating pregnancy, childbirth, and the puerperium (O99.32-)
long term (current) use of oral antidiabetic drugs (Z79.84)
long term (current) use of oral hypoglycemic drugs (Z79.84)*

Z79.0-   **Long term (current) use of anticoagulants and antithrombotics/antiplatelets**
Excludes ❷: long term (current) use of aspirin (Z79.82)

Z79.01   **Long term (current) use of anticoagulants**

Z79.02   **Long term (current) use of antithrombotics/antiplatelets** — [Unacceptable PDX]

Z79.1   **Long term (current) use of non-steroidal anti-inflammatories (NSAID)** — [Unacceptable PDX]
Excludes ❷: long term (current) use of aspirin (Z79.82)

Z79.2   **Long term (current) use of antibiotics** — [Unacceptable PDX]

Z79.3   **Long term (current) use of hormonal contraceptives**
Long term (current) use of birth control pill or patch

Z79.4   **Long term (current) use of insulin**

Z79.5-   **Long term (current) use of steroids**

Z79.51   **Long term (current) use of inhaled steroids** — [Unacceptable PDX]

Z79.52   **Long term (current) use of systemic steroids** — [Unacceptable PDX]

Z79.8-   **Other long term (current) drug therapy**

Z79.81-   **Long term (current) use of agents affecting estrogen receptors and estrogen levels**
Code first, if applicable:
Malignant neoplasm of breast (C50.-)
Malignant neoplasm of prostate (C61)
Use additional code, if applicable, to identify:
Estrogen receptor positive status (Z17.0)
Family history of breast cancer (Z80.3)
Genetic susceptibility to malignant neoplasm (cancer) (Z15.0-)
Personal history of breast cancer (Z85.3)
Personal history of prostate cancer (Z85.46)
Postmenopausal status (Z78.0)
Excludes 1:   hormone replacement therapy (postmenopausal) (Z79.890)

Z79.810   **Long term (current) use of selective estrogen receptor modulators (SERMs)** — [Unacceptable PDX]
Long term (current) use of raloxifene (Evista)
Long term (current) use of tamoxifen (Nolvadex)
Long term (current) use of toremifene (Fareston)

Z79.811   **Long term (current) use of aromatase inhibitors** — [Unacceptable PDX]
Long term (current) use of anastrozole (Arimidex)
Long term (current) use of exemestane (Aromasin)
Long term (current) use of letrozole (Femara)

Z79.818   **Long term (current) use of other agents affecting estrogen receptors and estrogen levels** — [Unacceptable PDX]
Long term (current) use of estrogen receptor downregulators
Long term (current) use of fulvestrant (Faslodex)
Long term (current) use of gonadotropin-releasing hormone (GnRH) agonist
Long term (current) use of goserelin acetate (Zoladex)
Long term (current) use of leuprolide acetate (leuprorelin) (Lupron)
Long term (current) use of megestrol acetate (Megace)

Z77 – Z79

Excludes 1: = NOT CODED HERE! (Do not code both)   *Excludes ❷: = Not Included Here*

Z79.82 Long term (current) use of aspirin

Z79.83 Long term (current) use of bisphosphonates —
[Unacceptable PDX]

Z79.84 Long term (current) use of oral hypoglycemic drugs —
[Unacceptable PDX]
Long term (current) use of oral antidiabetic drugs
Excludes ❷: long term (current) use of insulin (Z79.4)

Z79.89- Other long term (current) drug therapy

Z79.890 Hormone replacement therapy
(postmenopausal) — [Unacceptable PDX]

Z79.891 Long term (current) use of opiate analgesic
Long term (current) use of methadone for pain management
Excludes 1: methadone use NOS (F11.9-)
use of methadone for treatment of heroin addiction (F11.2-)

Z79.899 Other long term (current) drug therapy
AHA 15:3Q:p21 — Immunocompromised state due to immunosuppresant medication

Z80- Family history of primary malignant neoplasm

Z80.0 Family history of malignant neoplasm of digestive organs —
[Unacceptable PDX]
Conditions classifiable to C15-C26

Z80.1 Family history of malignant neoplasm of trachea, bronchus and lung — [Unacceptable PDX]
Conditions classifiable to C33-C34

Z80.2 Family history of malignant neoplasm of other respiratory and intrathoracic organs — [Unacceptable PDX]
Conditions classifiable to C30-C32, C37-C39

Z80.3 Family history of malignant neoplasm of breast —
[Unacceptable PDX]
Conditions classifiable to C50.-

Z80.4- Family history of malignant neoplasm of genital organs
Conditions classifiable to C51-C63

Z80.41 Family history of malignant neoplasm of ovary —
[Unacceptable PDX]

Z80.42 Family history of malignant neoplasm of prostate —
[Unacceptable PDX]

Z80.43 Family history of malignant neoplasm of testis —
[Unacceptable PDX]

Z80.49 Family history of malignant neoplasm of other genital organs — [Unacceptable PDX]

Z80.5- Family history of malignant neoplasm of urinary tract
Conditions classifiable to C64-C68

Z80.51 Family history of malignant neoplasm of kidney —
[Unacceptable PDX]

Z80.52 Family history of malignant neoplasm of bladder —
[Unacceptable PDX]

Z80.59 Family history of malignant neoplasm of other urinary tract organ — [Unacceptable PDX]

Z80.6 Family history of leukemia — [Unacceptable PDX]
Conditions classifiable to C91-C95

Z80.7 Family history of other malignant neoplasms of lymphoid, hematopoietic and related tissues — [Unacceptable PDX]
Conditions classifiable to C81-C90, C96.-

Z80.8 Family history of malignant neoplasm of other organs or systems — [Unacceptable PDX]
Conditions classifiable to C00-C14, C40-C49, C69-C79

Z80.9 Family history of malignant neoplasm, unspecified —
[Unacceptable PDX]
Conditions classifiable to C80.1

Z81- Family history of mental and behavioral disorders

Z81.0 Family history of intellectual disabilities — [Unacceptable PDX]
Conditions classifiable to F70-F79

Z81.1 Family history of alcohol abuse and dependence —
[Unacceptable PDX]
Conditions classifiable to F10.-

Z81.2 Family history of tobacco abuse and dependence —
[Unacceptable PDX]
Conditions classifiable to F17.-

Z81.3 Family history of other psychoactive substance abuse and dependence — [Unacceptable PDX]
Conditions classifiable to F11-F16, F18-F19

Z81.4 Family history of other substance abuse and dependence —
[Unacceptable PDX]
Conditions classifiable to F55

Z81.8 Family history of other mental and behavioral disorders —
[Unacceptable PDX]
Conditions classifiable elsewhere in F01-F99

Z82- Family history of certain disabilities and chronic diseases (leading to disablement)

Z82.0 Family history of epilepsy and other diseases of the nervous system — [Unacceptable PDX]
Conditions classifiable to G00-G99

Z82.1 Family history of blindness and visual loss — [Unacceptable PDX]
Conditions classifiable to H54.-

Z82.2 Family history of deafness and hearing loss — [Unacceptable PDX]
Conditions classifiable to H90-H91

Z82.3 Family history of stroke — [Unacceptable PDX]
Conditions classifiable to I60-I64

Z82.4- Family history of ischemic heart disease and other diseases of the circulatory system
Conditions classifiable to I00-I52, I65-I99

Z82.41 Family history of sudden cardiac death — [Unacceptable PDX]

Z82.49 Family history of ischemic heart disease and other diseases of the circulatory system — [Unacceptable PDX]

Z82.5 Family history of asthma and other chronic lower respiratory diseases — [Unacceptable PDX]
Conditions classifiable to J40-J47
Excludes ❷: family history of other diseases of the respiratory system (Z83.6)

Z82.6- Family history of arthritis and other diseases of the musculoskeletal system and connective tissue
Conditions classifiable to M00-M99

Z82.61 Family history of arthritis — [Unacceptable PDX]

Z82.62 Family history of osteoporosis — [Unacceptable PDX]

Z82.69 Family history of other diseases of the musculoskeletal system and connective tissue — [Unacceptable PDX]

Z82.7- Family history of congenital malformations, deformations and chromosomal abnormalities
Conditions classifiable to Q00-Q99

Z82.71 Family history of polycystic kidney — [Unacceptable PDX]

Z82.79 Family history of other congenital malformations, deformations and chromosomal abnormalities —
[Unacceptable PDX]

Z82.8 Family history of other disabilities and chronic diseases leading to disablement, not elsewhere classified —
[Unacceptable PDX]

Z83- Family history of other specific disorders
Excludes ❷: contact with and (suspected) exposure to communicable disease in the family (Z20.-)

Z83.0 Family history of human immunodeficiency virus [HIV] disease — [Unacceptable PDX]
Conditions classifiable to B20

Z83.1 Family history of other infectious and parasitic diseases —
[Unacceptable PDX]
Conditions classifiable to A00-B19, B25-B94, B99

Z83.2 Family history of diseases of the blood and blood-forming organs and certain disorders involving the immune mechanism — [Unacceptable PDX]
Conditions classifiable to D50-D89

Z83.3 Family history of diabetes mellitus — [Unacceptable PDX]
Conditions classifiable to E08-E13

Z83.4- Family history of other endocrine, nutritional and metabolic diseases
Conditions classifiable to E00-E07, E15-E88

Z83.41 Family history of multiple endocrine neoplasia [MEN] syndrome — [Unacceptable PDX]

Z83.42 Family history of familial hypercholesterolemia —
[Unacceptable PDX]

Z79 - Z83

Z83.49 Family history of other endocrine, nutritional and metabolic diseases — [Unacceptable PDX]

Z83.5- Family history of eye and ear disorders

Z83.51- Family history of eye disorders
Conditions classifiable to H00-H53, H55-H59
Excludes ❷: family history of blindness and visual loss (Z82.1)

Z83.511 Family history of glaucoma — [Unacceptable PDX]

Z83.518 Family history of other specified eye disorder — [Unacceptable PDX]

Z83.52 Family history of ear disorders — [Unacceptable PDX]
Conditions classifiable to H60-H83, H92-H95
Excludes ❷: family history of deafness and hearing loss (Z82.2)

Z83.6 Family history of other diseases of the respiratory system — [Unacceptable PDX]
Conditions classifiable to J00-J39, J60-J99
Excludes ❷: family history of asthma and other chronic lower respiratory diseases (Z82.5)

Z83.7- Family history of diseases of the digestive system
Conditions classifiable to K00-K93

Z83.71 Family history of colonic polyps — [Unacceptable PDX]
Excludes 1:   family history of malignant neoplasm of digestive organs (Z80.0)

Z83.79 Family history of other diseases of the digestive system — [Unacceptable PDX]

Z84- Family history of other conditions

Z84.0 Family history of diseases of the skin and subcutaneous tissue — [Unacceptable PDX]
Conditions classifiable to L00-L99

Z84.1 Family history of disorders of kidney and ureter — [Unacceptable PDX]
Conditions classifiable to N00-N29

Z84.2 Family history of other diseases of the genitourinary system — [Unacceptable PDX]
Conditions classifiable to N30-N99

Z84.3 Family history of consanguinity — [Unacceptable PDX]

Z84.8- Family history of other specified conditions

Z84.81 Family history of carrier of genetic disease — [Unacceptable PDX]

Z84.82 Family history of sudden infant death syndrome — [Unacceptable PDX]
Family history of SIDS

Z84.89 Family history of other specified conditions — [Unacceptable PDX]

Z85- Personal history of malignant neoplasm
Code first any follow-up examination after treatment of malignant neoplasm (Z08)
Use additional code to identify:
Alcohol use and dependence (F10.-)
Exposure to environmental tobacco smoke (Z77.22)
History of tobacco dependence (Z87.891)
Occupational exposure to environmental tobacco smoke (Z57.31)
Tobacco dependence (F17.-)
Tobacco use (Z72.0)
*Excludes ❷: personal history of benign neoplasm (Z86.01-)
    personal history of carcinoma-in-situ (Z86.00-)*

Z85.0- Personal history of malignant neoplasm of digestive organs

Z85.00 Personal history of malignant neoplasm of unspecified digestive organ — [Unacceptable PDX]

Z85.01 Personal history of malignant neoplasm of esophagus — [Unacceptable PDX]
Conditions classifiable to C15

Z85.02- Personal history of malignant neoplasm of stomach

Z85.020 Personal history of malignant carcinoid tumor of stomach — [Unacceptable PDX]
Conditions classifiable to C7A.092

Z85.028 Personal history of other malignant neoplasm of stomach — [Unacceptable PDX]
Conditions classifiable to C16

Z85.03- Personal history of malignant neoplasm of large intestine

Z85.030 Personal history of malignant carcinoid tumor of large intestine — [Unacceptable PDX]
Conditions classifiable to C7A.022-C7A.025, C7A.029

Z85.038 Personal history of other malignant neoplasm of large intestine — [Unacceptable PDX]
Conditions classifiable to C18

Z85.04- Personal history of malignant neoplasm of rectum, rectosigmoid junction, and anus

Z85.040 Personal history of malignant carcinoid tumor of rectum — [Unacceptable PDX]
Conditions classifiable to C7A.026

Z85.048 Personal history of other malignant neoplasm of rectum, rectosigmoid junction, and anus — [Unacceptable PDX]
Conditions classifiable to C19-C21

Z85.05 Personal history of malignant neoplasm of liver — [Unacceptable PDX]
Conditions classifiable to C22

Z85.06- Personal history of malignant neoplasm of small intestine

Z85.060 Personal history of malignant carcinoid tumor of small intestine — [Unacceptable PDX]
Conditions classifiable to C7A.01-

Z85.068 Personal history of other malignant neoplasm of small intestine — [Unacceptable PDX]
Conditions classifiable to C17

Z85.07 Personal history of malignant neoplasm of pancreas — [Unacceptable PDX]
Conditions classifiable to C25

Z85.09 Personal history of malignant neoplasm of other digestive organs — [Unacceptable PDX]

Z85.1- Personal history of malignant neoplasm of trachea, bronchus and lung

Z85.11- Personal history of malignant neoplasm of bronchus and lung

Z85.110 Personal history of malignant carcinoid tumor of bronchus and lung — [Unacceptable PDX]
Conditions classifiable to C7A.090

Z85.118 Personal history of other malignant neoplasm of bronchus and lung — [Unacceptable PDX]
Conditions classifiable to C34

Z85.12 Personal history of malignant neoplasm of trachea — [Unacceptable PDX]
Conditions classifiable to C33

Z85.2- Personal history of malignant neoplasm of other respiratory and intrathoracic organs

Z85.20 Personal history of malignant neoplasm of unspecified respiratory organ — [Unacceptable PDX]

Z85.21 Personal history of malignant neoplasm of larynx — [Unacceptable PDX]
Conditions classifiable to C32

Z85.22 Personal history of malignant neoplasm of nasal cavities, middle ear, and accessory sinuses — [Unacceptable PDX]
Conditions classifiable to C30-C31

Z85.23- Personal history of malignant neoplasm of thymus

Z85.230 Personal history of malignant carcinoid tumor of thymus — [Unacceptable PDX]
Conditions classifiable to C7A.091

Z85.238 Personal history of other malignant neoplasm of thymus — [Unacceptable PDX]
Conditions classifiable to C37

Z85.29 Personal history of malignant neoplasm of other respiratory and intrathoracic organs — [Unacceptable PDX]

Z85.3 Personal history of malignant neoplasm of breast — [Unacceptable PDX]
Conditions classifiable to C50.-

Z83 - Z85

Z85.4- <u>Personal history</u> of <u>malignant neoplasm</u> of <u>genital organs</u>
Conditions classifiable to C51-C63

Z85.40 Personal history of malignant neoplasm of unspecified female genital organ — [♀] [Unacceptable PDX]

Z85.41 Personal history of malignant neoplasm of cervix uteri — [♀] [Unacceptable PDX]

Z85.42 Personal history of malignant neoplasm of other parts of uterus — [♀] [Unacceptable PDX]

Z85.43 Personal history of malignant neoplasm of ovary — [♀] [Unacceptable PDX]

Z85.44 Personal history of malignant neoplasm of other female genital organs — [♀] [Unacceptable PDX]

Z85.45 Personal history of malignant neoplasm of unspecified male genital organ — [♂] [Unacceptable PDX]

Z85.46 Personal history of malignant neoplasm of prostate — [♂] [Unacceptable PDX]

Z85.47 Personal history of malignant neoplasm of testis — [♂] [Unacceptable PDX]

Z85.48 Personal history of malignant neoplasm of epididymis — [♂] [Unacceptable PDX]

Z85.49 Personal history of malignant neoplasm of other male genital organs — [♂] [Unacceptable PDX]

Z85.5- <u>Personal history</u> of <u>malignant neoplasm</u> of <u>urinary tract</u>
Conditions classifiable to C64-C68

Z85.50 Personal history of malignant neoplasm of unspecified urinary tract organ — [Unacceptable PDX]

Z85.51 Personal history of malignant neoplasm of bladder — [Unacceptable PDX]

Z85.52- Personal history of malignant neoplasm of kidney
Excludes 1: *personal history of malignant neoplasm of renal pelvis (Z85.53)*

Z85.520 Personal history of malignant carcinoid tumor of kidney — [Unacceptable PDX]
Conditions classifiable to C7A.093

Z85.528 Personal history of other malignant neoplasm of kidney — [Unacceptable PDX]
Conditions classifiable to C64

Z85.53 Personal history of malignant neoplasm of renal pelvis — [Unacceptable PDX]

Z85.54 Personal history of malignant neoplasm of ureter — [Unacceptable PDX]

Z85.59 Personal history of malignant neoplasm of other urinary tract organ — [Unacceptable PDX]

Z85.6 <u>Personal history</u> of <u>leukemia</u> — [Unacceptable PDX]
Conditions classifiable to C91-C95
Excludes 1: *leukemia in remission C91.0-C95.9 with 5th character 1*

Z85.7- <u>Personal history</u> of other <u>malignant neoplasms</u> of <u>lymphoid, hematopoietic and related tissues</u>

Z85.71 Personal history of Hodgkin lymphoma — [Unacceptable PDX]
Conditions classifiable to C81

Z85.72 Personal history of non-Hodgkin lymphomas — [Unacceptable PDX]
Conditions classifiable to C82-C85

Z85.79 Personal history of other malignant neoplasms of lymphoid, hematopoietic and related tissues — [Unacceptable PDX]
Conditions classifiable to C88-C90, C96
Excludes 1: *multiple myeloma in remission (C90.01)*
plasma cell leukemia in remission (C90.11)
plasmacytoma in remission (C90.21)

Z85.8- <u>Personal history</u> of <u>malignant neoplasms</u> of <u>other organs and systems</u>
Conditions classifiable to C00-C14, C40-C49, C69-C79, C7A.098, C76-C79

Z85.81- Personal history of malignant neoplasm of lip, oral cavity, and pharynx

Z85.810 Personal history of malignant neoplasm of tongue — [Unacceptable PDX]

Z85.818 Personal history of malignant neoplasm of other sites of lip, oral cavity, and pharynx — [Unacceptable PDX]

Z85.819 Personal history of malignant neoplasm of unspecified site of lip, oral cavity, and pharynx — [Unacceptable PDX]

Z85.82- <u>Personal history</u> of <u>malignant neoplasm</u> of <u>skin</u>

Z85.820 Personal history of malignant melanoma of skin — [Unacceptable PDX]
Conditions classifiable to C43

Z85.821 Personal history of Merkel cell carcinoma — [Unacceptable PDX]
Conditions classifiable to C4A

Z85.828 Personal history of other malignant neoplasm of skin — [Unacceptable PDX]
Conditions classifiable to C44

Z85.83- <u>Personal history</u> of <u>malignant neoplasm</u> of <u>bone and soft tissue</u>

Z85.830 Personal history of malignant neoplasm of bone — [Unacceptable PDX]

Z85.831 Personal history of malignant neoplasm of soft tissue — [Unacceptable PDX]
Excludes ❷: *personal history of malignant neoplasm of skin (Z85.82-)*

Z85.84- <u>Personal history</u> of <u>malignant neoplasm</u> of <u>eye and nervous tissue</u>

Z85.840 Personal history of malignant neoplasm of eye — [Unacceptable PDX]

Z85.841 Personal history of malignant neoplasm of brain — [Unacceptable PDX]

Z85.848 Personal history of malignant neoplasm of other parts of nervous tissue — [Unacceptable PDX]

Z85.85- <u>Personal history</u> of <u>malignant neoplasm</u> of <u>endocrine glands</u>

Z85.850 Personal history of malignant neoplasm of thyroid — [Unacceptable PDX]

Z85.858 Personal history of malignant neoplasm of other endocrine glands — [Unacceptable PDX]

Z85.89 <u>Personal history</u> of <u>malignant neoplasm</u> of <u>other</u> organs and systems — [Unacceptable PDX]

Z85.9 <u>Personal history</u> of <u>malignant neoplasm, unspecified</u> — [Unacceptable PDX]
Conditions classifiable to C7A.00, C80.1

Z86- <u>Personal history</u> of <u>certain other diseases</u>
Code first any follow-up examination after treatment (Z09)

Z86.0- <u>Personal history</u> of <u>in situ and benign neoplasms</u> and <u>neoplasms of uncertain behavior</u>
Excludes ❷: *personal history of malignant neoplasms (Z85.-)*

Z86.00- Personal history of <u>in situ neoplasm</u>
Conditions classifiable to D00-D09

Z86.000 Personal history of in situ neoplasm of breast — [Unacceptable PDX]

Z86.001 Personal history of in situ neoplasm of cervix uteri — [♀] [Unacceptable PDX]
Personal history of cervical intraepithelial neoplasia III [CIN III]

Z86.008 Personal history of in situ neoplasm of other site — [Unacceptable PDX]
Personal history of vaginal intraepithelial neoplasia III [VAIN III]
Personal history of vulvar intraepithelial neoplasia III [VIN III]

Z86.01- Personal history of <u>benign neoplasm</u>

Z86.010 Personal history of colonic polyps — [Unacceptable PDX]

Z86.011 Personal history of benign neoplasm of the brain — [Unacceptable PDX]

Z86.012 Personal history of benign carcinoid tumor — [Unacceptable PDX]

Z86.018 Personal history of other benign neoplasm — [Unacceptable PDX]

Z85-Z86

Excludes 1: = NOT CODED HERE! (Do not code both)

Excludes ❷: = Not Included Here

Z86.03 Personal history of neoplasm of uncertain behavior — [Unacceptable PDX]

Z86.1- Personal history of infectious and parasitic diseases
  Conditions classifiable to A00-B89, B99
  Excludes 1:   personal history of infectious diseases specific to a body system
                sequelae of infectious and parasitic diseases (B90-B94)

Z86.11 Personal history of tuberculosis — [Unacceptable PDX]

Z86.12 Personal history of poliomyelitis — [Unacceptable PDX]

Z86.13 Personal history of malaria — [Unacceptable PDX]

Z86.14 Personal history of methicillin resistant Staphylococcus aureus infection — [Unacceptable PDX]
  Personal history of MRSA infection

Z86.19 Personal history of other infectious and parasitic diseases — [Unacceptable PDX]

Z86.2 Personal history of diseases of the blood and blood-forming organs and certain disorders involving the immune mechanism — [Unacceptable PDX]
  Conditions classifiable to D50-D89

Z86.3- Personal history of endocrine, nutritional and metabolic diseases
  Conditions classifiable to E00-E88

Z86.31 Personal history of diabetic foot ulcer — [Unacceptable PDX]
  Excludes ❷: current diabetic foot ulcer (E08.621, E09.621, E10.621, E11.621, E13.621)

Z86.32 Personal history of gestational diabetes — [♀] [Unacceptable PDX]
  Pesonal history of conditions classifiable to O24.4-
  Excludes 1:   gestational diabetes mellitus in current pregnancy (O24.4-)

Z86.39 Personal history of other endocrine, nutritional and metabolic disease — [Unacceptable PDX]

Z86.5- Personal history of mental and behavioral disorders
  Conditions classifiable to F40-F59

Z86.51 Personal history of combat and operational stress reaction — [Age/15-124] [Unacceptable PDX]

Z86.59 Personal history of other mental and behavioral disorders — [Unacceptable PDX]

Z86.6- Personal history of diseases of the nervous system and sense organs
  Conditions classifiable to G00-G99, H00-H95

Z86.61 Personal history of infections of the central nervous system — [Unacceptable PDX]
  Personal history of encephalitis
  Personal history of meningitis

Z86.69 Personal history of other diseases of the nervous system and sense organs — [Unacceptable PDX]

Z86.7- Personal history of diseases of the circulatory system
  Conditions classifiable to I00-I99
  Excludes ❷: old myocardial infarction (I25.2)
                personal history of anaphylactic shock (Z87.892)
                postmyocardial infarction syndrome (I24.1)

Z86.71- Personal history of venous thrombosis and embolism

Z86.711 Personal history of pulmonary embolism — [Unacceptable PDX]

Z86.718 Personal history of other venous thrombosis and embolism — [Unacceptable PDX]

Z86.72 Personal history of thrombophlebitis — [Unacceptable PDX]

Z86.73 Personal history of transient ischemic attack (TIA), and cerebral infarction without residual deficits — [Unacceptable PDX]
  Personal history of prolonged reversible ischemic neurological deficit (PRIND)
  Personal history of stroke NOS without residual deficits
  Excludes 1:   personal history of traumatic brain injury (Z87.820)
                sequelae of cerebrovascular disease (I69.-)

Z86.74 Personal history of sudden cardiac arrest — [Unacceptable PDX]
  Personal history of sudden cardiac death successfully resuscitated

Z86.79 Personal history of other diseases of the circulatory system — [Unacceptable PDX]

Z87- Personal history of other diseases and conditions
  Code first any follow-up examination after treatment (Z09)

Z87.0- Personal history of diseases of the respiratory system
  Conditions classifiable to J00-J99

Z87.01 Personal history of pneumonia (recurrent) — [Unacceptable PDX]

Z87.09 Personal history of other diseases of the respiratory system — [Unacceptable PDX]

Z87.1- Personal history of diseases of the digestive system
  Conditions classifiable to K00-K93

Z87.11 Personal history of peptic ulcer disease — [Unacceptable PDX]

Z87.19 Personal history of other diseases of the digestive system — [Unacceptable PDX]

Z87.2 Personal history of diseases of the skin and subcutaneous tissue — [Unacceptable PDX]
  Conditions classifiable to L00-L99
  Excludes ❷: personal history of diabetic foot ulcer (Z86.31)

Z87.3- Personal history of diseases of the musculoskeletal system and connective tissue
  Conditions classifiable to M00-M99
  Excludes ❷: personal history of (healed) traumatic fracture (Z87.81)

Z87.31- Personal history of (healed) nontraumatic fracture

Z87.310 Personal history of (healed) osteoporosis fracture — [Unacceptable PDX]
  Personal history of (healed) fragility fracture
  Personal history of (healed) collapsed vertebra due to osteoporosis

Z87.311 Personal history of (healed) other pathological fracture — [Unacceptable PDX]
  Personal history of (healed) collapsed vertebra NOS
  Excludes ❷: personal history of osteoporosis fracture (Z87.310)

Z87.312 Personal history of (healed) stress fracture — [Unacceptable PDX]
  Personal history of (healed) fatigue fracture

Z87.39 Personal history of other diseases of the musculoskeletal system and connective tissue — [Unacceptable PDX]

Z87.4- Personal history of diseases of genitourinary system
  Conditions classifiable to N00-N99

Z87.41- Personal history of dysplasia of the female genital tract
  Excludes 1:   personal history of intraepithelial neoplasia III of female genital tract (Z87.001, Z87.008)
                personal history of malignant neoplasm of female genital tract (Z85.40-Z85.44)

Z87.410 Personal history of cervical dysplasia — [♀] [Unacceptable PDX]

Z87.411 Personal history of vaginal dysplasia — [♀] [Unacceptable PDX]

Z87.412 Personal history of vulvar dysplasia — [♀] [Unacceptable PDX]

Z87.42 Personal history of other diseases of the female genital tract — [♀] [Unacceptable PDX]

Z87.43- Personal history of diseases of male genital organs

Z87.430 Personal history of prostatic dysplasia — [♂] [Unacceptable PDX]
  Excludes 1:   personal history of malignant neoplasm of prostate (Z85.46)

Z87.438 Personal history of other diseases of male genital organs — [♂] [Unacceptable PDX]

Z87.44- Personal history of diseases of urinary system
  Excludes 1:   personal history of malignant neoplasm of cervix uteri (Z85.41)

Z87.440 Personal history of urinary (tract) infections — [Unacceptable PDX]

Z87.441 Personal history of nephrotic syndrome — [Unacceptable PDX]

Z87.442 Personal history of urinary calculi — [Unacceptable PDX]
  Personal history of kidney stones

Z87.448 Personal history of other diseases of urinary system — [Unacceptable PDX]

Excludes 1: = NOT CODED HERE! (Do not code both)   **1331**   Excludes ❷: = Not Included Here

Z 8 6 - Z 8 7

Z87.5- <u>Personal history</u> of <u>complications of pregnancy, childbirth and the puerperium</u>
Conditions classifiable to O00-O9A
Excludes ②: *recurrent pregnancy loss (N96)*

Z87.51 Personal history of pre-term labor — [♀] [Unacceptable PDX]
Excludes 1: *current pregnancy with history of pre-term labor (O09.21-)*

Z87.59 Personal history of other complications of pregnancy, childbirth and the puerperium — [♀] [Unacceptable PDX]
Personal history of trophoblastic disease

Z87.7- <u>Personal history</u> of (corrected) <u>congenital malformations</u>
Conditions classifiable to Q00-Q89 that have been repaired or corrected
Excludes 1: *congenital malformations that have been partially corrected or repair but which still require medical treatment — code to condition*
Excludes ②: *other postprocedural states (Z98.-)*
personal history of medical treatment (Z92.-)
presence of cardiac and vascular implants and grafts (Z95.-)
presence of other devices (Z97.-)
presence of other functional implants (Z96.-)
transplanted organ and tissue status (Z94.-)

Z87.71- Personal history of (corrected) <u>congenital malformations of genitourinary system</u>

Z87.710 Personal history of (corrected) hypospadias — [♂] [Unacceptable PDX]

Z87.718 Personal history of other specified (corrected) congenital malformations of genitourinary system — [Unacceptable PDX]

Z87.72- Personal history of (corrected) <u>congenital malformations of nervous system and senseorgans</u>

Z87.720 Personal history of (corrected) congenital malformations of eye — [Unacceptable PDX]

Z87.721 Personal history of (corrected) congenital malformations of ear — [Unacceptable PDX]

Z87.728 Personal history of other specified (corrected) congenital malformations of nervous system and sense organs — [Unacceptable PDX]

Z87.73- Personal history of (corrected) <u>congenital malformations of digestive system</u>

Z87.730 Personal history of (corrected) cleft lip and palate — [Unacceptable PDX]

Z87.738 Personal history of other specified (corrected) congenital malformations of digestive system — [Unacceptable PDX]

Z87.74 Personal history of (corrected) <u>congenital malformations of heart and circulatory system</u> — [Unacceptable PDX]

Z87.75 Personal history of (corrected) <u>congenital malformations of respiratory system</u> — [Unacceptable PDX]

Z87.76 Personal history of (corrected) <u>congenital malformations of integument, limbs and musculoskeletal system</u> — [Unacceptable PDX]

Z87.79- Personal history of <u>other</u> (corrected) congenital malformations

Z87.790 Personal history of (corrected) congenital malformations of face and neck — [Unacceptable PDX]

Z87.798 Personal history of other (corrected) congenital malformations — [Unacceptable PDX]

Z87.8- <u>Personal history</u> of <u>other</u> specified conditions
Excludes ②: *personal history of self harm (Z91.5)*

Z87.81 Personal history of (healed) traumatic fracture — [Unacceptable PDX]
Excludes ②: *personal history of (healed) nontraumatic fracture (Z87.31-)*

Z87.82- Personal history of <u>other (healed) physical injury and trauma</u>
Conditions classifiable to S00-T88, except traumatic fractures

Z87.820 Personal history of traumatic brain injury — [Unacceptable PDX]
Excludes 1: *personal history of transient ischemic attack (TIA), and cerebral infarction without residual deficits (Z86.73)*

Z87.821 Personal history of retained foreign body fully removed — [Unacceptable PDX]

Z87.828 Personal history of other (healed) physical injury and trauma — [Unacceptable PDX]

Z87.89- Personal history of <u>other</u> specified conditions

Z87.890 Personal history of sex reassignment

Z87.891 Personal history of nicotine dependence — [Unacceptable PDX]
Excludes 1: *current nicotine dependence (F17.2-)*

Z87.892 Personal history of anaphylaxis — [Unacceptable PDX]
Code also allergy status, such as:
Allergy status to drugs, medicaments and biological substances (Z88-)
Allergy status, other than to drugs and biological substances (Z91.0-)

Z87.898 Personal history of other specified conditions — [Unacceptable PDX]
AHA 13:1Q:p21 – Methamphetamine abuse in prolonged remission

Z88- <u>Allergy status to drugs, medicaments and biological substances</u>
Excludes ②: *allergy status, other than to drugs and biological substances (Z91.0-)*

Z88.0 Allergy status to penicillin — [Unacceptable PDX]

Z88.1 Allergy status to other antibiotic agents status — [Unacceptable PDX]

Z88.2 Allergy status to sulfonamides status — [Unacceptable PDX]

Z88.3 Allergy status to other anti-infective agents status — [Unacceptable PDX]

Z88.4 Allergy status to anesthetic agent status — [Unacceptable PDX]

Z88.5 Allergy status to narcotic agent status — [Unacceptable PDX]

Z88.6 Allergy status to analgesic agent status — [Unacceptable PDX]

Z88.7 Allergy status to serum and vaccine status — [Unacceptable PDX]

Z88.8 Allergy status to other drugs, medicaments and biological substances status — [Unacceptable PDX]

Z88.9 Allergy status to unspecified drugs, medicaments and biological substances status — [Unacceptable PDX]

Z89- <u>Acquired absence of limb</u>
Includes: Amputation status
Postprocedural loss of limb
Post-traumatic loss of limb
Excludes 1: *acquired deformities of limbs (M20-M21)*
congenital absence of limbs (Q71-Q73)

Z89.0- Acquired absence of thumb and other finger(s)

Z89.01- Acquired absence of <u>thumb</u>

Z89.011 Acquired absence of <u>right</u> thumb — [Unacceptable PDX]

Z89.012 Acquired absence of <u>left</u> thumb — [Unacceptable PDX]

Z89.019 Acquired absence of <u>unspecified</u> thumb — [Unacceptable PDX]

Z89.02- Acquired absence of <u>other finger(s)</u>
Excludes ②: *acquired absence of thumb (Z89.01-)*

Z89.021 Acquired absence of <u>right</u> finger(s) — [Unacceptable PDX]

Z89.022 Acquired absence of <u>left</u> finger(s) — [Unacceptable PDX]

Z89.029 Acquired absence of <u>unspecified</u> finger(s) — [Unacceptable PDX]

Z89.1- Acquired absence of hand and wrist

Z89.11- Acquired absence of <u>hand</u>

Z89.111 Acquired absence of <u>right</u> hand — [Unacceptable PDX]

Z89.112 Acquired absence of <u>left</u> hand — [Unacceptable PDX]

Z89.119 Acquired absence of <u>unspecified</u> hand — [Unacceptable PDX]

Z
8
7
–
Z
8
9

Z89.12- Acquired absence of <u>wrist</u>
  Disarticulation at wrist
  Z89.121 Acquired absence of <u>right</u> wrist — [Unacceptable PDX]
  Z89.122 Acquired absence of <u>left</u> wrist — [Unacceptable PDX]
  Z89.129 Acquired absence of <u>unspecified</u> wrist — [Unacceptable PDX]

Z89.2- Acquired absence of upper limb above wrist
  Z89.20- Acquired absence of <u>upper limb, unspecified level</u>
    Z89.201 Acquired absence of <u>right</u> upper limb, unspecified level — [Unacceptable PDX]
    Z89.202 Acquired absence of <u>left</u> upper limb, unspecified level — [Unacceptable PDX]
    Z89.209 Acquired absence of <u>unspecified</u> upper limb, unspecified level — [Unacceptable PDX]
      Acquired absence of arm NOS
  Z89.21- Acquired absence of <u>upper limb below elbow</u>
    Z89.211 Acquired absence of <u>right</u> upper limb below elbow — [Unacceptable PDX]
    Z89.212 Acquired absence of <u>left</u> upper limb below elbow — [Unacceptable PDX]
    Z89.219 Acquired absence of <u>unspecified</u> upper limb below elbow — [Unacceptable PDX]
  Z89.22- Acquired absence of <u>upper limb above elbow</u>
    Disarticulation at elbow
    Z89.221 Acquired absence of <u>right</u> upper limb above elbow — [Unacceptable PDX]
    Z89.222 Acquired absence of <u>left</u> upper limb above elbow — [Unacceptable PDX]
    Z89.229 Acquired absence of <u>unspecified</u> upper limb above elbow — [Unacceptable PDX]
  Z89.23- Acquired absence of <u>shoulder</u>
    Acquired absence of shoulder joint following explantation of shoulder joint prosthesis, with or without presence of antibiotic-impregnated cement spacer
    Z89.231 Acquired absence of <u>right</u> shoulder — [Unacceptable PDX]
    Z89.232 Acquired absence of <u>left</u> shoulder — [Unacceptable PDX]
    Z89.239 Acquired absence of <u>unspecified</u> shoulder — [Unacceptable PDX]

Z89.4- Acquired absence of toe(s), foot, and ankle
  Z89.41- Acquired absence of <u>great toe</u>
    Z89.411 Acquired absence of <u>right</u> great toe — [Unacceptable PDX]
    Z89.412 Acquired absence of <u>left</u> great toe — [Unacceptable PDX]
    Z89.419 Acquired absence of <u>unspecified</u> great toe — [Unacceptable PDX]
  Z89.42- Acquired absence of <u>other toe(s)</u>
    Excludes ❷: acquired absence of great toe (Z89.41-)
    Z89.421 Acquired absence of other <u>right</u> toe(s) — [Unacceptable PDX]
    Z89.422 Acquired absence of other <u>left</u> toe(s) — [Unacceptable PDX]
    Z89.429 Acquired absence of other toe(s), <u>unspecified</u> side — [Unacceptable PDX]
  Z89.43- Acquired absence of <u>foot</u>
    Z89.431 Acquired absence of <u>right</u> foot — [Unacceptable PDX]
    Z89.432 Acquired absence of <u>left</u> foot — [Unacceptable PDX]
    Z89.439 Acquired absence of <u>unspecified</u> foot — [Unacceptable PDX]
  Z89.44- Acquired absence of <u>ankle</u>
    Disarticulation of ankle
    Z89.441 Acquired absence of <u>right</u> ankle — [Unacceptable PDX]
    Z89.442 Acquired absence of <u>left</u> ankle — [Unacceptable PDX]
    Z89.449 Acquired absence of <u>unspecified</u> ankle — [Unacceptable PDX]

Z89.5- Acquired absence of <u>leg below knee</u>
  Z89.51- Acquired absence of leg below knee
    Z89.511 Acquired absence of <u>right</u> leg below knee — [Unacceptable PDX]
    Z89.512 Acquired absence of <u>left</u> leg below knee — [Unacceptable PDX]
    Z89.519 Acquired absence of <u>unspecified</u> leg below knee — [Unacceptable PDX]
  Z89.52- Acquired absence of knee
    Acquired absence of knee joint following explantation of knee joint prosthesis, with or without presence of antibiotic-impregnated cement spacer
    Z89.521 Acquired absence of <u>right</u> knee — [Unacceptable PDX]
    Z89.522 Acquired absence of <u>left</u> knee — [Unacceptable PDX]
    Z89.529 Acquired absence of <u>unspecified</u> knee — [Unacceptable PDX]

Z89.6- Acquired absence of leg above knee
  Z89.61- Acquired absence of <u>leg above knee</u>
    Acquired absence of leg NOS
    Disarticulation at knee
    Z89.611 Acquired absence of <u>right</u> leg above knee — [Unacceptable PDX]
    Z89.612 Acquired absence of <u>left</u> leg above knee — [Unacceptable PDX]
    Z89.619 Acquired absence of <u>unspecified</u> leg above knee — [Unacceptable PDX]
  Z89.62- Acquired absence of <u>hip</u>
    Acquired absence of hip joint following explantation of hip joint prosthesis, with or without presence of antibiotic-impregnated cement spacer
    Disarticulation at hip
    Z89.621 Acquired absence of <u>right</u> hip joint — [Unacceptable PDX]
    Z89.622 Acquired absence of <u>left</u> hip joint — [Unacceptable PDX]
    Z89.629 Acquired absence of <u>unspecified</u> hip joint — [Unacceptable PDX]

Z89.9 Acquired absence of limb, unspecified — [Unacceptable PDX]

Z90- <u>Acquired absence</u> of organs, <u>not elsewhere classified</u>
  Includes: Postprocedural or post-traumatic loss of body part NEC
  Excludes 1:   congenital absence — see Alphabetical Index
  Excludes ❷: postprocedural absence of endocrine glands (E89.-)
  Z90.0- Acquired absence of part of head and neck
    Z90.01 Acquired absence of eye — [Unacceptable PDX]
    Z90.02 Acquired absence of larynx — [Unacceptable PDX]
    Z90.09 Acquired absence of other part of head and neck — [Unacceptable PDX]
      Acquired absence of nose
      Excludes ❷: teeth (K08.1)
  Z90.1- Acquired absence of <u>breast and nipple</u>
    Z90.10 Acquired absence of <u>unspecified</u> breast and nipple
    Z90.11 Acquired absence of <u>right</u> breast and nipple
    Z90.12 Acquired absence of <u>left</u> breast and nipple
    Z90.13 Acquired absence of <u>bilateral</u> breasts and nipples
  Z90.2 Acquired absence of lung [part of] — [Unacceptable PDX]
  Z90.3 Acquired absence of stomach [part of] — [Unacceptable PDX]
  Z90.4- Acquired absence of other specified parts of digestive tract
    Z90.41 Acquired absence of pancreas
      Code also exocrine pancreatic insufficiency (K86.81)
      Use additional code to identify any associated:
        Insulin use (Z79.4)
        Diabetes mellitus, postpancreatectomy (E13.-)
      Z90.410 Acquired total absence of pancreas — [Unacceptable PDX]
        Acquired absence of pancreas NOS
      Z90.411 Acquired partial absence of pancreas — [Unacceptable PDX]
    Z90.49 Acquired absence of other specified parts of digestive tract — [Unacceptable PDX]
  Z90.5 Acquired absence of kidney — [Unacceptable PDX]

Z90.6 **Acquired absence of other parts of urinary tract —**
[Unacceptable PDX]
Acquired absence of bladder

Z90.7- **Acquired absence of genital organ(s)**
Excludes 1:   *personal history of sex reassignment (Z87.890)*
Excludes ❷: *female genital mutilation status (N90.81-)*

Z90.71- **Acquired absence of cervix and uterus**

Z90.710 **Acquired absence of <u>both cervix and uterus</u> — [♀]**
[Unacceptable PDX]
Acquired absence of uterus NOS
Status post total hysterectomy

Z90.711 **Acquired absence of <u>uterus with remaining cervical</u>
<u>stump</u> — [♀]** [Unacceptable PDX]
Status post partial hysterectomy with remaining
cervical stump

Z90.712 **Acquired absence of <u>cervix with remaining</u>
<u>uterus</u> — [♀]** [Unacceptable PDX]

Z90.72- **Acquired absence of <u>ovaries</u>**

Z90.721 **Acquired absence of ovaries, <u>unilateral</u> — [♀]**
[Unacceptable PDX]

Z90.722 **Acquired absence of ovaries, <u>bilateral</u> — [♀]**
[Unacceptable PDX]

Z90.79 **Acquired absence of other genital organ(s) —**
[Unacceptable PDX]

Z90.8- **Acquired absence of other organs**

Z90.81 **Acquired absence of spleen — [Unacceptable PDX]**

Z90.89 **Acquired absence of other organs — [Unacceptable PDX]**

Z91- **Personal risk factors, not elsewhere classified**
Excludes ❷: *contact with and (suspected) exposures hazardous to health*
(Z77-)
exposure to pollution and other problems related to physical
environment (Z77.1-)
occupational exposure to risk factors (Z57-)
personal history of physical injury and trauma (Z87.81,
Z87.82-)

Z91.0- **<u>Allergy status</u>, other than to drugs and biological substances**
Excludes ❷: *allergy status to drugs, medicaments, and biological*
substances (Z88-)

Z91.01- **<u>Food</u> allergy status**
Excludes ❷: *food additives allergy status (Z91.02)*

Z91.010 **Allergy to peanuts — [Unacceptable PDX]**

Z91.011 **Allergy to milk products — [Unacceptable PDX]**
Excludes 1:   *lactose intolerance (E73-)*

Z91.012 **Allergy to eggs — [Unacceptable PDX]**

Z91.013 **Allergy to seafood — [Unacceptable PDX]**
Allergy to shellfish
Allergy to octopus or squid ink

Z91.018 **Allergy to other foods — [Unacceptable PDX]**
Allergy to nuts other than peanuts

Z91.02 **<u>Food additives</u> allergy status — [Unacceptable PDX]**

Z91.03- **<u>Insect</u> allergy status**

Z91.030 **Bee allergy status — [Unacceptable PDX]**

Z91.038 **Other insect allergy status — [Unacceptable PDX]**

Z91.04- **<u>Nonmedicinal substance</u> allergy status**

Z91.040 **Latex allergy status — [Unacceptable PDX]**
Latex sensitivity status

Z91.041 **Radiographic dye allergy status — [Unacceptable PDX]**
Allergy status to contrast media used for diagnostic
X-ray procedure

Z91.048 **Other nonmedicinal substance allergy status —**
[Unacceptable PDX]

Z91.09 **<u>Other</u> allergy status, other than to drugs and biological
substances — [Unacceptable PDX]**

Z91.1- <u>Patient's noncompliance with medical treatment and regimen</u>

Z91.11 **Patient's noncompliance with <u>dietary regimen</u> —**
[Unacceptable PDX]

Z91.12- **Patient's <u>intentional underdosing</u> of medication regimen**
Code first underdosing of medication (T36-T50) with fifth or sixth
character 6
Excludes 1:   *adverse effect of prescribed drug taken as*
directed — code to adverse effect
poisoning (overdose) — code to poisoning

Z91.120 **Patient's intentional underdosing of medication
regimen <u>due to financial hardship</u> —**
[Unacceptable PDX]

Z91.128 **Patient's intentional underdosing of medication
regimen <u>for other reason</u> — [Unacceptable PDX]**

Z91.13- **Patient's <u>unintentional underdosing</u> of medication
regimen**
Code first underdosing of medication (T36-T50) with fifth or
sixth character 6
Excludes 1:   *adverse effect of prescribed drug taken as*
directed — code to adverse effect
poisoning (overdose) — code to poisoning

Z91.130 **Patient's unintentional underdosing of medication
regimen <u>due to age-related debility</u> —**
[Unacceptable PDX]

Z91.138 **Patient's unintentional underdosing of medication
regimen <u>for other reason</u> — [Unacceptable PDX]**

Z91.14 **Patient's <u>other noncompliance</u> <u>with medication</u>
<u>regimen</u> — [Unacceptable PDX]**
Patient's underdosing of medication NOS

Z91.15 **Patient's <u>noncompliance</u> <u>with renal dialysis</u> —**
[Unacceptable PDX]

Z91.19 **Patient's <u>noncompliance</u> <u>with other</u> medical treatment
and regimen — [Unacceptable PDX]**

Z91.4- **Personal history of psychological trauma, not elsewhere
classified**

Z91.41- **Personal history of adult abuse**
Excludes ❷: *personal history of abuse in childhood (Z62.81-)*

Z91.410 **Personal history of adult physical and sexual
abuse — [Age/15-124] [Unacceptable PDX]**
Excludes 1:   *current adult physical abuse (T74.11,*
T76.11)
current adult sexual abuse (T74.21, T76.11)

Z91.411 **Personal history of adult psychological abuse —**
[Age/15-124] [Unacceptable PDX]

Z91.412 **Personal history of adult neglect — [Age/15-124]**
[Unacceptable PDX]
Excludes 1:   *current adult neglect (T74.01, T76.01)*

Z91.419 **Personal history of unspecified adult abuse —**
[Age/15-124] [Unacceptable PDX]

Z91.49 **Other personal history of psychological trauma, not
elsewhere classified — [Unacceptable PDX]**

Z91.5 **Personal history of self-harm — [Unacceptable PDX]**
Personal history of parasuicide
Personal history of self-poisoning
Personal history of suicide attempt

Z91.8- **Other specified personal risk factors, not elsewhere classified**

Z91.81 **<u>History of falling</u> — [Unacceptable PDX]**
At risk for falling

Z91.82 **Personal history of military deployment — [Age/15-124]**
[Unacceptable PDX]
Individual (civilian or military) with past history of military
war, peacekeeping and humanitarian deployment
(current or past conflict)
Returned from military deployment

Z91.83 **Wandering in diseases classified elsewhere —**
[Not Allowed as PDX]
Code first underlying disorder, such as:
Alzheimer's disease (G30.-)
Autism or pervasive developmental disorder (F84.-)
Intellectual disabilities (F70-F79)
Unspecified dementia with behavioral disturbance (F03.9-)

Z91.89 **Other specified personal risk factors, not elsewhere
classified — [Unacceptable PDX]**

Z90-Z91

Z92-   <u>Personal history</u> of medical treatment

Excludes ❷: *postprocedural states (Z98-)*

Z92.0   Personal history of <u>contraception</u> — [Unacceptable PDX]

Excludes 1:   *counseling or management of current contraceptive practices (Z30-)*
long term (current) use of contraception (Z79.3)
presence of (intrauterine) contraceptive device (Z97.5)

Z92.2-   Personal history of <u>drug therapy</u>

Excludes ❷: *long term (current) drug therapy (Z79-)*

Z92.21   Personal history of antineoplastic chemotherapy — [Unacceptable PDX]

Z92.22   Personal history of monoclonal drug therapy — [Unacceptable PDX]

Z92.23   Personal history of estrogen therapy — [Unacceptable PDX]

Z92.24-   Personal history of steroid therapy

Z92.240   Personal history of inhaled steroid therapy — [Unacceptable PDX]

Z92.241   Personal history of systemic steroid therapy — [Unacceptable PDX]

Personal history of steroid therapy NOS

Z92.25   Personal history of <u>immunosupression therapy</u> — [Unacceptable PDX]

Excludes ❷: *personal history of steroid therapy (Z92.24)*

Z92.29   Personal history of other drug therapy — [Unacceptable PDX]

Z92.3   Personal history of <u>irradiation</u> — [Unacceptable PDX]

Personal history of exposure to therapeutic radiation

Excludes 1:   *exposure to radiation in the physical environment (Z77.12)*
occupational exposure to radiation (Z57.1)

Z92.8-   Personal history of <u>other</u> medical treatment

Z92.81   Personal history of extracorporeal membrane oxygenation (ECMO) — [Unacceptable PDX]

Z92.82   Status post administration of tPA (rtPA) in a different facility within the last 24 hours prior to admission to current facility — [Unacceptable PDX]

AHA 13:4Q:p124 – tPA (rtPA) in a different facility within the last 24 hours

Code first condition requiring tPA administration, such as:
Acute cerebral infarction (I63-)
Acute myocardial infarction (I21-, I22-)

Z92.83   Personal history of failed moderate sedation — [Unacceptable PDX]

Personal history of failed conscious sedation

Excludes ❷: *failed moderate sedation during procedure (T88.52)*

Z92.84   Personal history of unintended awareness under general anesthesia — [Unacceptable PDX]

Excludes ❷: *unintended awareness under general anesthesia during procedure (T88.53)*

Z92.89   Personal history of other medical treatment — [Unacceptable PDX]

Z93-   <u>Artificial opening status</u>

Excludes 1:   *artificial openings requiring attention or management (Z43.-)*
complications of external stoma (J95.0-, K94.-, N99.5-)

Z93.0   Tracheostomy status — [Unacceptable PDX]

Z93.1   Gastrostomy status — [Unacceptable PDX]

Z93.2   Ileostomy status — [Unacceptable PDX]

Z93.3   Colostomy status — [Unacceptable PDX]

Z93.4   Other artificial openings of gastrointestinal tract status — [Unacceptable PDX]

Z93.5-   Cystostomy status

Z93.50   Unspecified cystostomy status — [Unacceptable PDX]

Z93.51   Cutaneous-vesicostomy status — [Unacceptable PDX]

Z93.52   Appendico-vesicostomy status — [Unacceptable PDX]

Z93.59   Other cystostomy status — [Unacceptable PDX]

Z93.6   Other artificial openings of urinary tract status — [Unacceptable PDX]

Nephrostomy status
Ureterostomy status
Urethrostomy status

Z93.8   Other artificial opening status — [Unacceptable PDX]

Z93.9   Artificial opening status, unspecified — [Unacceptable PDX]

Z94-   <u>Transplanted organ and tissue status</u>

Includes: Organ or tissue replaced by heterogenous or homogenous transplant

Excludes 1:   *complications of transplanted organ or tissue — see Alphabetical Index*

Excludes ❷: *presence of vascular grafts (Z95.-)*

cc **Z94.0**   Kidney transplant status — [Unacceptable PDX]

cc **Z94.1**   Heart transplant status — [Unacceptable PDX]

Excludes 1:   *artificial heart status (Z95.812)*
heart-valve replacement status (Z95.2-Z95.4)

cc **Z94.2**   Lung transplant status — [Unacceptable PDX]

cc **Z94.3**   Heart and lungs transplant status — [Unacceptable PDX]

cc **Z94.4**   Liver transplant status — [Unacceptable PDX]

Z94.5   Skin transplant status — [Unacceptable PDX]

Autogenous skin transplant status

Z94.6   Bone transplant status — [Unacceptable PDX]

Z94.7   Corneal transplant status — [Unacceptable PDX]

Z94.8-   Other transplanted organ and tissue status

cc **Z94.81**   Bone marrow transplant status — [Unacceptable PDX]

cc **Z94.82**   Intestine transplant status — [Unacceptable PDX]

cc **Z94.83**   Pancreas transplant status — [Unacceptable PDX]

cc **Z94.84**   Stem cells transplant status — [Unacceptable PDX]

Z94.89   Other transplanted organ and tissue status — [Unacceptable PDX]

Z94.9   Transplanted organ and tissue status, unspecified — [Unacceptable PDX]

Z95-   <u>Presence of cardiac and vascular implants and grafts</u>

Excludes 1:   *complications of cardiac and vascular devices, implants and grafts (T82.-)*

Z95.0   Presence of cardiac pacemaker — [Unacceptable PDX]

Presence of cardiac resynchronization therapy (CRT-P) pacemaker

Excludes 1:   *adjustment or management of cardiac device (Z45.0-)*
adjustment or management of cardiac pacemaker (Z45.0)
presence of automatic (implantable) cardiac defibrillator with synchronous cardiac pacemaker (Z95.810)

Z95.1   Presence of aortocoronary bypass graft — [Unacceptable PDX]

Presence of coronary artery bypass graft

Z95.2   Presence of prosthetic heart valve — [Unacceptable PDX]

Presence of heart valve NOS

Z95.3   Presence of xenogenic heart valve — [Unacceptable PDX]

Z95.4   Presence of other heart-valve replacement — [Unacceptable PDX]

Z95.5   Presence of coronary angioplasty implant and graft — [Unacceptable PDX]

Excludes 1:   *coronary angioplasty status without implant and graft (Z98.61)*

Z95.8-   Presence of other cardiac and vascular implants and grafts

Z95.81-   Presence of other cardiac implants and grafts

Z95.810   Presence of automatic (implantable) cardiac defibrillator — [Unacceptable PDX]

Presence of automatic (implantable) cardiac defibrillator with synchronous cardiac pacemaker
Presence of cardiac resynchronization therapy defibrillator (CRT-D)
Presence of cardioverter-defibrillator (ICD)

cc **Z95.811**   Presence of heart assist device — [Unacceptable PDX]

cc **Z95.812**   Presence of fully implantable artificial heart — [Unacceptable PDX]

Z95.818   Presence of other cardiac implants and grafts — [Unacceptable PDX]

Z95.82-   Presence of other vascular implants and grafts

Z95.820   Peripheral vascular angioplasty status with implants and grafts — [Unacceptable PDX]

Excludes 1:   *peripheral vascular angioplasty without implant and graft (Z98.62)*

Z95.828   Presence of other vascular implants and grafts — [Unacceptable PDX]

Presence of intravascular prosthesis NEC

Excludes 1: = NOT CODED HERE! (Do not code both)   **1335**   *Excludes ❷:* = Not Included Here

Z 9 2 - Z 9 5

Z95.9 Presence of cardiac and vascular implant and graft, unspecified — [Unacceptable PDX]

Z96- Presence of other functional implants

> *Excludes ❷:* *complications of internal prosthetic devices, implants and grafts (T82-T85)*
> *fitting and adjustment of prosthetic and other devices (Z44-Z46)*

Z96.0 Presence of urogenital implants — [Unacceptable PDX]

Z96.1 Presence of intraocular lens — [Unacceptable PDX]
> Presence of pseudophakia

Z96.2- Presence of otological and audiological implants

  Z96.20 Presence of otological and audiological implant, unspecified — [Unacceptable PDX]

  Z96.21 Cochlear implant status — [Unacceptable PDX]

  Z96.22 Myringotomy tube(s) status — [Unacceptable PDX]

  Z96.29 Presence of other otological and audiological implants — [Unacceptable PDX]
> Presence of bone-conduction hearing device
> Presence of eustachian tube stent
> Stapes replacement

Z96.3 Presence of artificial larynx — [Unacceptable PDX]

Z96.4- Presence of endocrine implants

  Z96.41 Presence of insulin pump (external) (internal) — [Unacceptable PDX]

  Z96.49 Presence of other endocrine implants — [Unacceptable PDX]

Z96.5 Presence of tooth-root and mandibular implants — [Unacceptable PDX]

Z96.6- Presence of orthopedic joint implants
> AHA 15:1Q:p16 – Presence of left artificial hip joint

  Z96.60 Presence of unspecified orthopedic joint implant — [Unacceptable PDX]

  Z96.61- Presence of artificial <u>shoulder</u> joint

    Z96.611 Presence of <u>right</u> artificial shoulder joint — [Unacceptable PDX]

    Z96.612 Presence of <u>left</u> artificial shoulder joint — [Unacceptable PDX]

    Z96.619 Presence of <u>unspecified</u> artificial shoulder joint — [Unacceptable PDX]

  Z96.62- Presence of artificial <u>elbow</u> joint

    Z96.621 Presence of <u>right</u> artificial elbow joint — [Unacceptable PDX]

    Z96.622 Presence of <u>left</u> artificial elbow joint — [Unacceptable PDX]

    Z96.629 Presence of <u>unspecified</u> artificial elbow joint — [Unacceptable PDX]

  Z96.63- Presence of artificial <u>wrist</u> joint

    Z96.631 Presence of <u>right</u> artificial wrist joint — [Unacceptable PDX]

    Z96.632 Presence of <u>left</u> artificial wrist joint — [Unacceptable PDX]

    Z96.639 Presence of <u>unspecified</u> artificial wrist joint — [Unacceptable PDX]

  Z96.64- Presence of artificial <u>hip</u> joint
> Hip-joint replacement (partial) (total)

    Z96.641 Presence of <u>right</u> artificial hip joint — [Unacceptable PDX]

    Z96.642 Presence of <u>left</u> artificial hip joint — [Unacceptable PDX]

    Z96.643 Presence of artificial hip joint, <u>bilateral</u> — [Unacceptable PDX]

    Z96.649 Presence of <u>unspecified</u> artificial hip joint — [Unacceptable PDX]

Z96.65- Presence of artificial <u>knee</u> joint

  Z96.651 Presence of <u>right</u> artificial knee joint — [Unacceptable PDX]

  Z96.652 Presence of <u>left</u> artificial knee joint — [Unacceptable PDX]

  Z96.653 Presence of artificial knee joint, <u>bilateral</u> — [Unacceptable PDX]

  Z96.659 Presence of <u>unspecified</u> artificial knee joint — [Unacceptable PDX]

Z96.66- Presence of artificial <u>ankle</u> joint

  Z96.661 Presence of <u>right</u> artificial ankle joint — [Unacceptable PDX]

  Z96.662 Presence of <u>left</u> artificial ankle joint — [Unacceptable PDX]

  Z96.669 Presence of <u>unspecified</u> artificial ankle joint — [Unacceptable PDX]

Z96.69- Presence of <u>other</u> orthopedic joint implants

  Z96.691 Finger-joint replacement of <u>right</u> hand — [Unacceptable PDX]

  Z96.692 Finger-joint replacement of <u>left</u> hand — [Unacceptable PDX]

  Z96.693 Finger-joint replacement, <u>bilateral</u> — [Unacceptable PDX]

  Z96.698 Presence of other orthopedic joint implants — [Unacceptable PDX]

Z96.7 Presence of other bone and tendon implants — [Unacceptable PDX]
> Presence of skull plate

Z96.8- Presence of other specified functional implants

  Z96.81 Presence of artificial skin — [Unacceptable PDX]

  Z96.89 Presence of other specified functional implants — [Unacceptable PDX]

Z96.9 Presence of functional implant, unspecified — [Unacceptable PDX]

Z97- Presence of other devices

> *Excludes 1:* *complications of internal prosthetic devices, implants and grafts (T82-T85)*
> *fitting and adjustment of prosthetic and other devices (Z44-Z46)*
> *Excludes ❷:* *presence of cerebrospinal fluid drainage device (Z98.2)*

Z97.0 Presence of artificial eye — [Unacceptable PDX]

Z97.1- Presence of artificial limb (complete) (partial)

  Z97.10 Presence of artificial limb (complete) (partial), <u>unspecified</u> — [Unacceptable PDX]

  Z97.11 Presence of artificial <u>right arm</u> (complete) (partial) — [Unacceptable PDX]

  Z97.12 Presence of artificial <u>left arm</u> (complete) (partial) — [Unacceptable PDX]

  Z97.13 Presence of artificial <u>right leg</u> (complete) (partial) — [Unacceptable PDX]

  Z97.14 Presence of artificial <u>left leg</u> (complete) (partial) — [Unacceptable PDX]

  Z97.15 Presence of artificial <u>arms</u>, <u>bilateral</u> (complete) (partial) — [Unacceptable PDX]

  Z97.16 Presence of artificial <u>legs</u>, <u>bilateral</u> (complete) (partial) — [Unacceptable PDX]

Z97.2 Presence of dental prosthetic device (complete) (partial) — [Unacceptable PDX]
> Presence of dentures (complete) (partial)

Z97.3 Presence of spectacles and contact lenses — [Unacceptable PDX]

Z97.4 Presence of external hearing-aid — [Unacceptable PDX]

Z97.5 Presence of (intrauterine) contraceptive device — [♀] [Unacceptable PDX]
> *Excludes 1:* *checking, reinsertion or removal of implantable subdermal contraceptive (Z30.46)*
> *checking, reinsertion or removal of intrauterine contraceptive device (Z30.43-)*

Z97.8 Presence of other specified devices — [Unacceptable PDX]

Z98- <u>Other postprocedural states</u>
Excludes ❷: *aftercare (Z43-Z49, Z51)*
follow-up medical care (Z08-Z09)
postprocedural complication — see Alphabetical Index

Z98.0 **Intestinal bypass and anastomosis status** — [Unacceptable PDX]
Excludes ❷: *bariatric surgery status (Z98.84)*
gastric bypass status (Z98.84)
obesity surgery status (Z98.84)

Z98.1 **Arthrodesis status** — [Unacceptable PDX]

Z98.2 **Presence of cerebrospinal fluid drainage device** —
[Unacceptable PDX]
Presence of CSF shunt

Z98.3 **Post therapeutic collapse of lung status** — [Unacceptable PDX]
Code first underlying disease

Z98.4- **Cataract extraction status**
Use additional code to identify intraocular lens implant status (Z96.1)
Excludes 1: *aphakia (H27.0)*

    Z98.41 **Cataract extraction status, <u>right</u> eye** — [Unacceptable PDX]

    Z98.42 **Cataract extraction status, <u>left</u> eye** — [Unacceptable PDX]

    Z98.49 **Cataract extraction status, <u>unspecified</u> eye** —
[Unacceptable PDX]

Z98.5- **Sterilization status**
Excludes 1: *female infertility (N97.-)*
male infertility (N46.-)

    Z98.51 **Tubal ligation status** — [♀] [Unacceptable PDX]

    Z98.52 **Vasectomy status** — [♂, Age/15-124] [Unacceptable PDX]

Z98.6- <u>Angioplasty status</u>

    Z98.61 **<u>Coronary</u> angioplasty status** — [Unacceptable PDX]
Excludes 1: *coronary angioplasty status with implant and graft (Z95.5)*

    Z98.62 **<u>Peripheral vascular</u> angioplasty status** — [Unacceptable PDX]
Excludes 1: *peripheral vascular angioplasty status with implant and graft (Z95.820)*

Z98.8- **Other specified postprocedural states**

    Z98.81- **Dental procedure status**

        Z98.810 **Dental sealant status** — [Unacceptable PDX]

        Z98.811 **Dental restoration status** — [Unacceptable PDX]
Dental crown status
Dental fillings status

        Z98.818 **Other dental procedure status** — [Unacceptable PDX]

    Z98.82 **Breast implant status** — [Unacceptable PDX]
Excludes 1: *breast implant removal status (Z98.86)*

    Z98.83 **Filtering (vitreous) bleb after glaucoma surgery status** —
[Unacceptable PDX]
Excludes 1: *Inflammation (infection) of postprocedural bleb (H59.4-)*

    Z98.84 **<u>Bariatric surgery status</u>** — [Unacceptable PDX]
Gastric banding status
Gastric bypass status for obesity
Obesity surgery status
Excludes 1: *bariatric surgery status complicating pregnancy, childbirth, or the puerperium (O99.84)*
Excludes ❷: *intestinal bypass and anastomosis status (Z98.0)*

    Z98.85 **Transplanted organ removal status** — [Unacceptable PDX]
Transplanted organ previously removed due to complication, failure, rejection or infection
Excludes 1: *encounter for removal of transplanted organ — code to complication of transplanted organ (T86.-)*

    Z98.86 **Personal history of breast implant removal** —
[Unacceptable PDX]

    Z98.87- **Personal history of in utero procedure**

        Z98.870 **Personal history of in utero procedure during pregnancy** — [♀] [Unacceptable PDX]
Excludes ❷: *complications from in utero procedure for current pregnancy (O35.7)*
supervision of current pregnancy with history of in utero procedure during previous pregnancy (O09.82-)

        Z98.871 **Personal history of in utero procedure while a fetus** — [Unacceptable PDX]

    Z98.89- **Other specified postprocedural states**

        Z98.890 **Other specified postprocedural states** —
[Unacceptable PDX]
Personal history of surgery, not elsewhere classified

        Z98.891 **History of uterine scar from previous surgery** —
[Unacceptable PDX]
Excludes 1: *maternal care due to uterine scar from previous surgery (O34.2-)*

Z99- <u>Dependence on enabling machines and devices, not elsewhere classified</u>
Excludes 1: *cardiac pacemaker status (Z95.0)*

Z99.0 **Dependence on aspirator** — [Unacceptable PDX]

Z99.1- **Dependence on respirator**
Dependence on ventilator

  CC **Z99.11** **Dependence on <u>respirator [ventilator] status</u>**

  CC **Z99.12** **Encounter for <u>respirator [ventilator] dependence during power failure</u>**
Excludes 1: *mechanical complication of respirator [ventilator] (J95.850)*

Z99.2 **Dependence on <u>renal dialysis</u>** — [Unacceptable PDX]
Hemodialysis status
Peritoneal dialysis status
Presence of arteriovenous shunt for dialysis
Renal dialysis status NOS
Excludes 1: *encounter for fitting and adjustment of dialysis catheter (Z49.0-)*
Excludes ❷: *noncompliance with renal dialysis (Z91.15)*

Z99.3 **Dependence on wheelchair** — [Unacceptable PDX]
Wheelchair confinement status
Code first cause of dependence, such as:
Muscular dystrophy (G71.0)
Obesity (E66.-)

Z99.8- **Dependence on other enabling machines and devices**

    Z99.81 **Dependence on <u>supplemental oxygen</u>** — [Unacceptable PDX]
Dependence on long-term oxygen

    Z99.89 **Dependence on other enabling machines and devices** —
[Unacceptable PDX]
Dependence on machine or device NOS

Z98-Z99

Z99-Z99